DecisionHealth | home care matters
a Simplify *Compliance* brand

Your Complete ICD-10 Coding Solution

Enhance your coding knowledge and improve your accuracy with these ICD-10 resources from DecisionHealth:

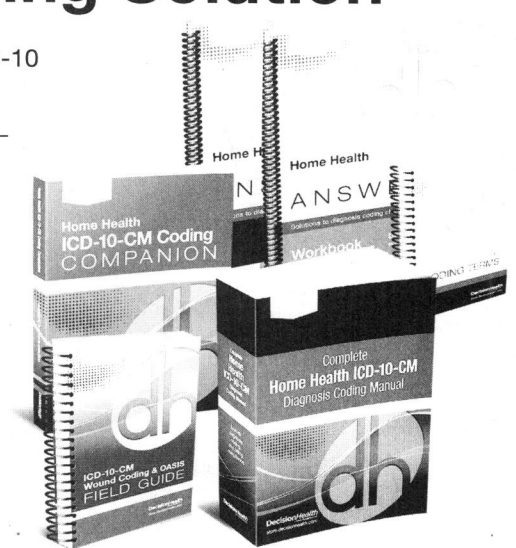

▸ **Complete Home Health ICD-10-CM Diagnosis Coding Manual, 2020** – Code accurately in ICD-10 with 71,000 codes to choose from, along with brand new conventions and guidelines.

▸ **Home Health ICD-10-CM Coding Companion, 2020** – The perfect go-to guide for every home health coder to use in conjunction with the ICD-10 manual to help you code faster and more accurately.

▸ **Home Health ICD-10-CM Coding Answers, 2020** – Practice coding 200 home health scenarios, and get a bonus plain English guide of common coding terms.

▸ **ICD-10-CM Wound Coding & OASIS Field Guide, 2020** – Use this on-the-go reference to choose the right ICD-10 codes and complete the OASIS for the most common home health wounds.

Use the convenient form below to place your order today!

☑ **YES!** I want new 2020 ICD-10-CM coding resources from DecisionHealth. Please complete this form and return with your payment in the enclosed reply envelope.

Product Description	Code	Price	Qty*	Subtotal
Complete Home Health ICD-10-CM Diagnosis Coding Manual, 2020	DHPABHHICD20	$219	___	$_____
Home Health ICD-10 Manual and Companion, 2020	DHPAPIXCOM20	$319	___	$_____
Home Health ICD-10 Companion and Answers, 2020	DHPAPIXCMA20	$298	___	$_____
ICD-10-CM Wound Coding & OASIS Field Guide, 2020	DHPABI10WD20	$199	___	$_____
Home Health ICD-10 Manual, Companion and Answers, 2020	DHPAPIXAMC20	$429	___	$_____
Home Health ICD-10 Manual and Answers, 2020	DHPAPIXMAN20	$299	___	$_____

*For orders of 5 or more, please call Peggy Hall at 1-855-225-5341 x.6041.

**$14.95 for one item and $6 for each additional item.

***Residents of CA, CO, CT, FL, GA, ID, IL, KS, MD, MA, ME, MI, MN, NJ, NM, NY, NC, NV, OH, PA, RI, SC, TN, TX, UT, VA, WI, and WA add applicable sales tax.

S & H**	
Subtotal	
Sales Tax***	$_____
TOTAL	$_____

For faster service, call toll-free **1-855-CALL-DH1**, or visit *store.decisionhealth.com.*

CONTACT INFORMATION:

Name:_____

Title:_____

Organization:_____

Street:_____

City/State/Zip:_____

Phone:_____ Fax:_____

Email_____

PAYMENT OPTIONS:

☐ **CHECK ENCLOSED** f̶ ̶ ̶ ̶ ̶ ̶ ̶ ̶made payable to DecisionHealth (Fed̶

☐ **Charge my credit**

☐ Visa ☐ Ma̶

Name:_____

Card #:_____ Exp._____

Signature:_____

Home Health Events

Ultimate Coding & OASIS Training Series

Don't risk your agency's revenue and productivity—Join us in a city near you!

Prepare to tackle code changes, and work through the new coding guidelines and ever-changing OASIS guidance. Get in-depth, hands-on ICD-10 and OASIS training from the top home health experts in the nation.

Learn more and register at:
decisionhealth.com/ultimatetraining

DATES AND LOCATIONS:
OCTOBER 21–24, 2019 | FRANKLIN, TN
NOVEMBER 4–7, 2019 | KING OF PRUSSIA, PA
2020 dates and locations coming soon!

Home Health Administrator's Summit

MAY 13–15, 2020
HILTON LAKE BUENA VISTA – DISNEY SPRINGS | ORLANDO, FL

Get strategies for growth & operational efficiencies, achieve regulatory compliance, position your business for growth. Join hundreds of home health financial and clinical veterans alike and gain key regulatory insights and tools to set you up for success in the coming year.

Learn more and register at:
hhadminsummit.com

Annual Home Health Coding Summit

Your one-stop shop for beginner, intermediate and advanced code training! Join the nation's top home health coding experts for an agenda packed with ICD-10 guidance, tools and best practices to sharpen your coding skills, protect your agency against audits and navigate regulations that could endanger your reimbursement.

Look for 2020 dates and location at:
homehealthcodingsummit.com

Home Health Payment Summit

Get the guidance you need to protect your reimbursement and prime your agency to succeed under the Patient-Driven Groupings Model (PDGM).

Look for 2020 dates and location at:
hhpaymentsummit.com

AHCC's Home Health Compliance Conference

SEPTEMBER 23–26, 2019
THE WESTIN PEACHTREE PLAZA | ATLANTA, GA

Set your agency up for success and join us for in-depth sessions on compliance, the new CoPs with a focus on QAPI, OASIS changes, documentation, outcomes improvement and care-transition programs.

Learn more and register at:
hhcomplianceconference.com

Home of **BMSC** & Caring Professionals

Raise the bar for organizational excellence!

BMSC credentials represent achievement of a gold standard of knowledge for the operation of a home care or hospice organization. Position your agency as an industry leader with a reputation for excellence.

Benefits of BMSC Credentials for your agency!

- 🎁 Demonstrates your agency's good-faith effort to comply with coding, OASIS or regulatory guidance; can be a deciding factor in appeals

- 🎁 Shows your agency reinforces a professional commitment to excellence

- 🎁 Increases agency's productivity and profitability through efficient coders

 ## BMSC Credentials:

Home Care Coding Specialist – Diagnosis (HCS-D)
Possessed by professionals skilled in classifying medical data from home health patient records

Home Care Coding Specialist – Hospice (HCS-H)
Earned by professionals skilled in classifying medical data from hospice patient records

Home Care Clinical Specialist – OASIS (HCS-O)
Held by clinicians who demonstrate clinical skills and judgment necessary to assess a patient's condition correctly

Home Care Specialist - Compliance (HCS-C)
Gained by professionals skilled in establishing, implementing, and monitoring an agency's compliance program

To learn more about AHCC and BMSC credentials, visit:
ahcc.decisionhealth.com/credentials

Home health agencies hire the industry's
BEST!

Identify your agency as an industry leader with Board of Medical Specialty Coding & Compliance (BMSC) credentialed coder and clinician personnel.

84% OF **EMPLOYERS**

consider BMSC credentials **important when hiring**

64% OF **EMPLOYERS**

require a BMSC credential

Complete Home Health

ICD-10-CM

Diagnosis Coding Manual

Ensure diagnosis coding and billing compliance

International Classification of Diseases,
10th Revision, Clinical Modification (ICD-10-CM)

2020 EDITION

Published by:

All the codes, indexes and other material in the International Classification of Diseases, 10th Revision, Clinical Modification (ICD-10-CM) are taken from official ICD-10-CM data tables and instructions from the National Center for Health Statistics (NCHS) and authorized for use by Medicare providers by the Centers for Medicare and Medicaid Services (CMS). NCHS serves as the World Health Organization (WHO) Collaborating Center for the Family of International Classifications for North America, and in this capacity is responsible for coordination of all official disease classification activities in the United States relating to the ICD and its use, interpretation, and periodic revision.

The tips and related content found in this coding manual are derived from CMS guidance, the official coding guidelines and Coding Clinic guidance. Additional proprietary information contained herein is compiled from DecisionHealth products *Home Health Line*, *Home Health Coding Center* and *Diagnosis Coding Pro for Home Health*.

Every reasonable effort has been made to ensure the accuracy of the information contained herein. However, the ultimate responsibility for correct coding lies with the provider of services. DecisionHealth, its employees, agents and staff make no representation, warranty or guarantee that use of the content herein ensures payment or will prevent disputes with Medicare or other third-party payers, and will not bear responsibility or liability for the results or consequences resulting from the use of this book.

COPYRIGHT © 2019

Product Code: DHPABHHICD20
ISBN: 978-1-68308-945-2

DecisionHealth
a Simplify *Compliance* brand

Subject Matter Expert Contributors

Lisa Selman-Holman, JD, BSN, RN, HCS-D, HCS-O, COS-C, is a 30-year veteran of home care as a registered nurse and attorney. She is the founder of Selman-Holman & Associates, a home care management and consulting company based in Denton, Texas, and the coding service CoDR – Coding Done Right. She is the Chair of the Board of Medical Specialty Coding and Compliance (BMSC) and one of the developers of the HCS-D examinations. Lisa is an AHIMA Approved ICD-10-CM/PCS Trainer.

Megan Batty, HCS-D, HCS-H, is a coding consultant and an independent coding expert in the world of home health. She previously worked for *DecisionHealth* for 10 years as a graduate fellow, editor and junior product manager. She has covered multiple aspects of home health for *Home Health Line* and *OASIS & Outcomes Solutions*, but spent the majority of her time writing about home health diagnosis coding as the executive editor of *Diagnosis Coding Pro for Home Health*. She's worked on many of *DecisionHealth's* industry-leading coding products, including the *Complete Home Health ICD-10-CM Diagnosis Coding Manual, ICD-10-CM Coding & OASIS Field Guide, Home Health Coding Companion and Documentation Trainer*, and she was the developer of the *Wound Coding & OASIS Field Guide*.

Also contributing subject matter expertise to the Coding Manual:
J'non Griffin, RN, MHA, WCC, HCS-D, HCS-H, COS-C, AHIMA-Approved ICD-10-CM Trainer/Ambassador, is the president of Home Health Solutions, LLC. Griffin offers home health consulting on many topics including quality assurance and performance improvement, program development, coding and OASIS review, staff education and plan of care compilation. Griffin has experience as a field nurse, director and executive with home health and hospice agencies.

DecisionHealth's 2020 Complete Home Health ICD-10-CM Diagnosis Coding Manual Team

Maria Tsigas, Product Director, Information, Print Subscription Products and Services

Susana Lambert, Production Editor & Coordinator

Dmitriy Bonin, Database Developer

Diana Chi, .NET Web Developer

Orit Keselman, QA Tester

Luba Tsaturova, Business Analyst

AnnMarie Lemoine, Team Lead, Creative Layout

Nicole Grande, Senior Layout Artist

DecisionHealth
100 Winners Circle, Suite 300
Brentwood, TN 37027
store.decisionhealth.com

Table of Contents

Understanding this Manual

Before you can code a patient's diagnosis, it's important to understand how to use the ICD-10-CM manual. ICD-10-CM code(s) establish medical necessity for services rendered, and can impact the episodic payment a home health agency (HHA) receives under the Medicare Prospective Payment System (PPS) and in the new Patient Driven Groupings Model (PDGM) payment system set to take effect 1/1/20.

DecisionHealth's *Complete Home Health ICD-10-CM Diagnosis Coding Manual* contains many icons and highlights that call attention to key indicators and serve as triggers to alert you to instances when you may need additional information to accurately assign a specific code. **IMPORTANT:** We have updated this 2020 Home Health Coding Manual with the new PDGM payment icons, but remember the PPS system, including PPS case-mix and supply values are in effect until 12/31/19.

Here are the icons used in this Manual, and what they are calling attention to:

- **SP** This icon indicates the code is an acceptable primary diagnosis in PDGM and depending on its clinical group, will generate case-mix points and determine payment amount. **IMPORTANT:** This list is current as of the 1/1/20 PPS proposed rule. To view a list of all PDGM acceptable primary diagnoses along with their assigned clinical group, visit **decisionhealth.com/pdf/pdgm.zip.** If CMS updates the list after the Manual has published, we will upload the new list to this folder.

- **IQ** This icon indicates "questionable encounter" and appears on those codes that are NOT acceptable as primary diagnoses in PDGM. Under PDGM, failure to use a primary diagnosis code that fits into one of the clinical groups could result in claims getting kicked back to providers. **IMPORTANT:** This list is current as of the 1/1/20 PPS proposed rule. To view a list of all questionable encounter codes, visit **decisionhealth.com/pdf/pdgm.zip.** If CMS updates the list after the Manual has published, we will upload the new list to this folder.

- **SH** **SL** These icons are placed on those codes that can generate either a High or Low comorbidity adjustment in PDGM. In addition to assigning one principal diagnosis, you can assign up to 24 secondary diagnoses, and receive a comorbidity adjustment. **Only one adjustment is applied per episode.** Comorbidity adjustments fall into one of three categories: no, low or high. The adjustments are designed to account for the additional resource use required for patients with complex needs. To qualify for a **low** comorbidity adjustment, the claim must include **one secondary diagnosis** found within one of 12 comorbidity subgroups associated with higher resource use. To qualify for a **high** comorbidity adjustment, the claim must include **two or more secondary diagnoses** that fall within 34 comorbidity subgroup interactions that account for 18 distinct comorbidity subgroups. **IMPORTANT:** This list is current as of the 1/1/20 PPS proposed rule. To view a list of of those codes eligible for the low and high adjustment along with their subgroups, visit **decisionhealth.com/pdf/pdgm.zip.** If CMS updates the list after the Manual has published, we will upload the new list to this folder.

- **SP** **IQ** When both these icons appear on a code, it indicates that one or more of the 7th character codes are acceptable primary diagnoses and one or more are not acceptable. Note, you will find most of these instances in Chapter 19. To view a list of all PDGM acceptable primary diagnoses, visit **decisionhealth.com/pdf/pdgm.zip**.

- **4 5 6 7** These icons indicate that an additional character is required to make the code valid. When a 7th character is required, there is a box indicating what the 7th character means. Also, all codes requiring a 7th character will have a dash at the end of them indicating they are not valid until a 7th character is added. The 7th character is used in certain chapters to provide information about the characteristic of the encounter. For example in Chapter 19 (Injury, poisoning and certain other consequences of external causes), the 7th character indicates one of the following:

  - A = Initial encounter
  - D = Subsequent encounter
  - S = Sequela

  Additional examples of 7th character use can be found in Chapters 13 (musculoskeletal), 15 – 16 (obstetrics) and 20 (external causes).

- **X7** This icon appears on codes that require a 7th character but are less than six characters. ICD-10-CM utilizes a placeholder character "X" for these codes. The placeholder "X" should be assigned for all characters less than six, and the 7th character must always be the 7th character of the code. Where a placeholder exists, the X must be used in order for the code to be considered a valid code. For these codes, we've already placed the X placeholders in the code for you; however, you will still need to choose the appropriate 7th character. An example of the **X7** is at category T36 (Poisoning by, adverse effect of and underdosing of systemic antibiotics).

- Unspecified This indicator appears on codes that are described as 'unspecified'. Codes titled "unspecified" are for use when the information in the medical record is insufficient to assign a more specific code. For those categories for which an unspecified code is not provided, the "other specified" code may represent both other and unspecified. Diagnoses codes that are too vague — meaning the code does not provide adequate information to support the need for home health services — won't fit into any of the groupings under PDGM; therefore it is imperative for home health coders to be as specific as possible when coding a condition.

- ✚ This indicator appears on codes with the instruction to "use additional code when documentation is present." Also, when a code contains instructions to "use additional code," "code first," and/or "code also," these instructions are highlighted in red to alert you that an additional code is required when assigning that particular code.

- Ⓜ This icon indicates a manifestation code. Be alerted to these codes because they can never be coded alone and are never allowed to be listed as the primary diagnosis. Icons and educational notes help coders spot manifestation codes and sequence them properly – the etiology, or underlying condition, is sequenced first followed by the manifestation. In addition to the icon, these codes are highlighted in yellow with italic font in the Tabular to emphasize their importance. For example, see category F02 (Dementia in other diseases classified elsewhere) in the Tabular. In the Alphabetic Index, the etiology and manifestation conditions are listed together with the etiology code listed first followed by the manifestation code in brackets. For example, when you look up "dementia, with Parkinsonism" in the Index, code G31.83 (Parkinsonism) is listed first, followed by the manifestation code *[F02.80]*.

- ▤ Be alerted to codes that require you to identify the specific side of the body, or both sides. Note, for bilateral sites, the final character of the codes indicates laterality. Example: L89.012 (Pressure ulcer of **right** elbow, stage 2).

- **Px** Z codes (found in Chapter 21) may be used as either a first-listed or secondary code, depending on the circumstances of the encounter. Certain Z codes may only be used as first-listed or principal diagnosis – these are indicated with a **Px** icon in the Tabular. The Z codes that may only be reported as the principal/first-listed diagnosis also are listed in the ICD-10 guidelines.

- ⊞ Look for this icon in the Tabular List to help identify acceptable hospice non-cancer diagnoses. *Note:* This is not an exhaustive list; it is just a starting point. Because of the expansion in coding diagnoses that contribute to the prognosis of 6 months or less, there are hundreds of codes that can be coded by hospice. The ones marked in the Manual with the hospice icon are those listed in the PGBA hospice LCD as well as those categories that are common hospice non-cancer diagnoses, such as I69 and I50. For more information on coding hospice diagnoses, see the Hospice section in the back of the Manual.

- ▲★ These icons in the Tabular alert you to codes that were newly added ★ or revised ▲ for the upcoming code year.

Tips, guidelines, alerts and definitions

This Manual provides our exclusive *DecisionHealth* content in the form of tips, guidelines, alerts and definitions in the Tabular that guide you on how to use a specific code to avoid common mistakes. Keep an eye out for the following indicators in the Tabular:

- **CODING TIPS ✓** Tips specific to home health ICD-10 coding that guide you, raise red flags and will help you code correctly.

- **GUIDELINES** ICD-10 guidelines embedded in the Tabular at the code level to alert you to the specific home health rules you need to be aware of to code accurately.

- **ALERTS** Specific "Alerts" on codes that are being denied with information on how to properly assign them to avoid having the claim denied.

- **DEFINITION** Definitions appear throughout to help you identify diseases and conditions to enhance coding and critical thinking skills.

Additional features

Other features of the Manual that help coders make the right choices and improve coding skills include:

- Home health **scenarios:** More than 100 home health scenarios and code assignment answers can be used to teach and learn proper coding. Look for these at the back of each Tabular chapter. Note that some disease chapters that are uncommon in home health, do not have scenarios. **Important:** Chapter 18 contains examples of scenarios in which it would be common to assign a symptom code in the primary position. However, these scenarios have been updated to demonstrate the importance of securing a more definitive diagnosis. Remember, most symptom codes do not fit into any of the groupings under PDGM, and assigning one in the primary position could result in a claim denial.

- Narrative **chapter introductions** quickly give a sense of the codes you'll find in that specific disease chapter. The introductory comments before each chapter highlight the basics of what is covered in the section, including sequencing issues and guidance for assigning the top home care diagnoses. All introductions are written in plain English to help home health staff understand what is in the chapter.

- **Hospice coding primer:** In the back of the book you'll find hospice coding guidance based on the Hospice Wage Index rule and expert analysis to ensure accurate coding of hospice claims.

- **Official coding guidelines:** The FY2020 official coding guidelines are in a separate packet, delivered with your Coding Manual.

Defining ICD-10-CM & its conventions

Background on ICD-10

The National Center for Health Statistics (NCHS), the federal agency responsible for use of the International Statistical Classification of Diseases and Related Health Problems, 10th revision (ICD-10) in the United States, has developed a clinical modification for morbidity purposes. The ICD-10 was initially used to code and classify mortality data from death certificates, having replaced ICD-9 for this purpose as of Jan. 1, 1999. ICD-10-CM then replaced ICD-9-CM, volumes 1 and 2 as of Oct. 1, 2015.

The World Health Organization (WHO) owns and publishes the ICD-10 classification, and authorized the development of an adaptation of ICD-10 for use in the United States.

ICD-10-CM was developed following a thorough evaluation by a technical advisory panel and additional consultation with physician groups, clinical coders, and others to assure clinical accuracy and utility.

The American Hospital Association (AHA) and the American Health Information Management Association (AHIMA) conducted a field test for ICD-10-CM in summer 2003.

The clinical modification represents a significant improvement over ICD-9-CM. Specific improvements include: the addition of information relevant to ambulatory and managed care encounters; expanded injury codes; the creation of combination diagnosis/symptom codes to reduce the number of codes needed to fully describe a condition; the addition of sixth and seventh characters; laterality; and greater specificity in code assignment. The new structure allows further expansion than was possible with ICD-9-CM.

On Jan. 16, 2009, the Department of Health and Human Services (HHS) published a final rule adopting ICD-10-CM (and ICD-10-PCS) to replace ICD-9-CM in HIPAA-covered transactions, effective Oct. 1, 2013. However, that effective date was postponed twice and the implementation finally occurred on Oct. 1, 2015. *[www.cdc.gov/nchs/icd/icd10cm.htm#10update.]*

What is ICD-10-CM?

ICD-10-CM, or the International Classification of Diseases, 10th Edition, Clinical Modification, applies to all covered entities. A number of other countries have also moved to ICD-10, including:

- United Kingdom (1995);
- France (1997);
- Australia (1998);
- Germany (2000); and
- Canada (2001).

The ICD-10-CM system is an improvement in that it provides a higher level of detail and the ability to expand to capture new technologies and advancements in clinical medicine. ICD-10-CM will lead to more accurate payment for services rendered, and facilitate evaluation of medical processes and outcomes, according to CMS.

ICD-10-CM/PCS consists of two parts:

- **ICD-10-CM for diagnosis coding:** This is the diagnosis classification system developed by the Centers for Disease Control and Prevention for use in all U.S. health care treatment settings. It consists of the Alphabetic Index an the Tabular List, and uses 3–7 alpha and numeric digits and full code titles;

- **ICD-10-PCS for inpatient procedure coding:** This is the procedure classification system developed by the Centers for Medicare & Medicaid Services (CMS) for use in the U.S. for inpatient hospital settings **ONLY. Home health does *not* use ICD-10 procedure codes.**

Breakdown of ICD-10-CM

To select a code that corresponds to a diagnosis or reason for the visit documented in the medical record, first locate the term in the Alphabetic Index, and then verify the code in the Tabular List. Make sure to read and adhere to all instructional notations that appear in both the Alphabetic Index and the Tabular List.

You must use both the Alphabetic Index and Tabular List when locating and assigning a code. The Alphabetic Index does not always provide the full code. Selection of the full code, including laterality and any applicable 7th character, can only be done in the Tabular List. A dash (-) at the end of an Alphabetic Index entry or Tabular code indicates that additional characters are required. Even when a dash is not included at the Alphabetic Index, you must refer to the Tabular List to verify that no 7th character is required.

Tabular List

The Tabular List is a numerical listing of the ICD-10 codes and their descriptors classified to etiology of conditions or to conditions that affect a specific body system. The Tabular List explains the details of how coding a particular condition must be done. Includes and Excludes 1 and 2 notes give more guidance, and can help validate code selection or steer you to another area.

ICD-10-CM diagnosis codes are composed of codes with 3, 4, 5, 6 or 7 characters. Codes with three characters are included as the heading of a category that may be further subdivided by the use of fourth and/or fifth characters and/or sixth characters, which provide greater detail.

A three-character code is to be used only if it is not further subdivided. A code is invalid if it has not been coded to the full number of characters required for that code, including the 7th character, if applicable.

The tabular code list contains categories, subcategories and codes. Characters for categories, subcategories and codes may be either a letter or a number. All categories are three characters. Subcategories are either 4 or 5 characters. Codes may be 3, 4, 5, 6 or 7 characters.

Here's an example:

M1a: Chronic Gout

> **M1a.3**: Chronic gout due to renal impairment

>> **M1a.33**: Chronic gout due to renal impairment, wrist

>>> **M1a.332**: Chronic gout due to renal impairment, left wrist

The appropriate code or codes from A00.0 through T88.9-, Z00.- – Z99.89 must be used to identify diagnoses, symptoms, conditions, problems, complaints or other reason(s) for the encounter/visit.

Codes that describe symptoms and signs, as opposed to diagnoses, are acceptable for reporting purposes when a related definitive diagnosis has not been established (confirmed) by the provider. ICD-10 Chapter 18, Symptoms, Signs, and Abnormal Clinical and Laboratory Findings, Not Elsewhere Classified (codes R00.0 - R99), contains many, but not all codes for symptoms.

Alphabetic Index

You should not code directly from the Alphabetic Index. First, review the medical record to extract the pertinent written descriptions of the disease or symptoms. Then, look up the condition, injury, or sign/symptom in the Index, and then verify the code(s) in the Tabular Listing.

The Alphabetic Index is an index of diseases, injuries, symptoms and other reasons for a patient encounter. The main terms are in boldface type and should never be referenced by anatomical site. When using the Index, you would reference the "condition," or other key words to locate potential diagnosis assignment.

When consulting the Alphabetic Index, several codes listed may seem applicable at first. To determine which one is correct, consult the Tabular List. In reviewing the Tabular List, pay attention to the chapter and subsection in which the code appears. This can help in the selection of the correct code when several alternatives may appear suitable. Follow all instructional notes at the category and specific code areas.

Subterms are indented under the main term and indicate the site, type, or etiology for conditions or injuries. More specificity in the condition will be further indented to the right, as needed. Connecting words such as "with," "due to," "in," or "associated with" indicate a relationship between the main term and the subterm.

The word "with" or "in" should be interpreted to mean "associated with" or "due to" when it appears in a code title, the Alphabetic Index, or an instructional note in the Tabular List. The classification presumes a causal relationship between the two conditions linked by these terms. These conditions should be coded as related even in the absence of provider documentation explicitly linking them, unless the documentation clearly states the conditions are unrelated or when another guideline exists that specifically requires a documented linkage between two conditions (e.g., sepsis guideline for "acute organ dysfunction that is not clearly associated with the sepsis"), according to the official coding guidelines conventions.

Another important coding convention is the etiology/manifestation convention. When two codes are required to indicate etiology and manifestation, the manifestation code will appear italicized and in [brackets] following the etiology code. The conditions are to be assigned as listed: the etiology code precedes the *[manifestation code]* in sequencing.

Neoplasm Table

In the Alphabetic Index also contains the Neoplasm Table. The Neoplasm Table appears at the end of the Alphabetic Index.

In the Neoplasm Table, codes listed with a dash (–) following the code have a required 5th character for laterality. The tabular list must be reviewed for the complete code.

Table of Drugs and Chemicals

After the Neoplasm Table is the Table of Drugs and Chemicals. This table contains a classification of drugs and other chemical substances associated with poisonings and external causes of adverse effects. The table's rows identify the substance and the columns define the intent: poisoning, accidental (unintentional); poisoning, intentional self-harm; poisoning, assault; poisoning, undetermined; adverse effect; and underdosing.

There often is confusion as to when coding a poisoning is appropriate versus when coding an adverse effect is appropriate. In ICD-10, when the drug was correctly prescribed and properly administered and the patient experienced a problem, it is an adverse effect. Assign the code for the nature of the adverse effect followed by the code for the adverse effect of the drug (T36-T50).

Unlike an adverse effect, a poisoning involves a scenario in which the drug was *not* taken correctly. Poisoning codes have an associated intent: accidental, intentional self-harm, assault and undetermined. List the poisoning code first, followed by the symptoms (effects).

Index to External Cause of Injuries

The final section of the Alphabetic Index is the Index to External Cause of Injuries. This section classifies environmental events, circumstances, and conditions as the *cause of* injury, poisoning and other adverse effects. The Index to External Cause of Injuries is organized by main terms that describe the accident, circumstance, event, or specific agent causing the injury or other adverse effect.

ICD-10-CM Guidelines

All necessary coding guidance can be found in the ICD-10-CM Coding Guidelines and the instructional notes embedded within the Tabular.

ICD-10-CM Conventions

The conventions for ICD-10-CM are the general rules for use independent of the guidelines. These conventions are incorporated within the Alphabetic Index and Tabular List as instructional notes. You should take note of the following key conventions:

Abbreviations

- NEC – Not elsewhere classifiable: This abbreviation represents "other specified." When a specific code is not available for a condition, the Alphabetic Index directs the coder to the "other specified" code in the Tabular List.

- NOS – Not otherwise specified: This abbreviation is the equivalent of unspecified.

Punctuation

- [ ] Brackets are used in the Tabular List to enclose synonyms, alternative wording or explanatory phrases. Brackets are used in the Alphabetic Index to identify manifestation codes.

- ( ) Parentheses are used in both the Alphabetic Index and Tabular List to enclose supplementary words that may be present or absent in the statement of a disease or procedure without affecting the code number to which it is assigned. The terms within the parentheses are referred to as nonessential modifiers.

The nonessential modifiers in the Alphabetic Index to Diseases apply to subterms following a main term except when a nonessential modifier and a subentry are mutually exclusive, the subentry takes precedence. For example, in the ICD-10-CM Alphabetic Index under the main term Enteritis, "acute" is a nonessential modifier and "chronic" is a subentry. In this case, the nonessential modifier "acute" does not apply to the subentry "chronic."

- : Colons are used in the Tabular List after an incomplete term, which needs one or more of the modifiers following the colon to make it assignable to a given category.

Instructional Notations

- INCLUDES This note appears immediately under a three character code title to further define, or give examples of, the content of the category.

- **Excludes Notes:** ICD-10 has two types of excludes notes. Each type of note has a different definition.

  - EXCLUDES 1 Excludes 1 means "not coded here." An Excludes 1 note indicates that the code excluded should ***never*** be used at the same time as the code above the Excludes 1 note. An Excludes 1 is used when two conditions cannot occur together, such as a congenital form versus an acquired form of the same condition. ***Note:*** You may code two conditions together, even if one or both of them is listed in an Excludes 1 note, as long as they are ***not related***.

  - EXCLUDES 2 Excludes 2 means "not included here." An Excludes 2 note indicates that the condition excluded is not part of the condition represented by the code, but a patient may have both conditions at the same time. When an Excludes 2 note appears under a code, it is acceptable to use both the code and the excluded code together, when appropriate.

Laterality

Some ICD-10-CM codes indicate laterality, specifying whether the condition occurs on the left, right or is bilateral. If no bilateral code is provided and the condition is bilateral, assign separate codes for both the left and right side. If the side is not identified in the medical record, assign the code for the unspecified side.

Deep dive into ICD-10 conventions & guidelines

The coding conventions always take precedence over the coding guidelines.

A keen understanding of how coding conventions and guidelines interact will help you navigate through thorny scenarios where guidance sometimes is contradictory, and where getting it wrong can lead to claim rejections and cash-flow interruptions.

Section I of the *Official Coding Guidelines* encases the coding conventions, general coding guidelines and chapter-specific coding guidelines. While conventions always supersede both sets of guidelines, general and chapter-specific guidelines carry the same weight.

Build your foundation with ICD-10 conventions

The following are a few of the ***ICD-10 coding conventions***, along with specific examples that will apply to home health. Master these before moving on to studying ICD-10 coding guidelines, as these instructions will always take precedence:

Etiology-manifestation sequencing *[I.A.13]*: A manifestation code must be sequenced directly after its etiology, and it can never be coded primary. As a convention, this sequencing instruction will trump other instructions in the guidelines, such as the rule to sequence a residual code before its related sequela code *[I.B.10]*.

The 7th character *[I.A.5]*: Certain ICD-10 codes require the use of a 7th character, such as fracture codes, which are coded on home health claims instead of an aftercare code. The code will be considered invalid if the 7th character is not included, or isn't assigned in the 7th position. ***Example:*** Consider the code for a fracture of the shaft of the right fibula in ICD-10, S82.401. By itself, S82.401 is invalid; it needs a 7th character, such as "D" for subsequent encounter for closed fracture with routine healing. "D" will be the 7th character most commonly used for the care of fractures in home health.

The placeholder character *[I.A.4]*: A placeholder character "x" is used to fill in unused spaces with certain ICD-10 codes that require a 7th character designation, but the most subdivided form of the code doesn't contain at least six characters. ***Example:*** Home health will often use these placeholder characters with external cause codes found in Chapter 20. Many of these codes are made up of only four characters, but require a 7th character to describe the type of encounter, whether initial (A), subsequent (D) or sequela (S). Consider X10.2 for Contact with fats and cooking oils, which is only four digits, but needs the 7th character to be valid. This code requires two placeholder x's to result in X10.2xxD (Contact with fat and cooking oils, subsequent encounter). Note that when placeholders are required, the x's must be used in order for the code to be valid. ***Note:*** Invalid codes due to missing 7th characters or placeholder x's were among the top reasons for claims being returned for provider (RTP'd) in the first several months following the ICD-10 implementation.

Excludes 1 and Excludes 2 notes *[I.A.12.a/b]*: ICD-10 employs two types of Excludes notes.

An **Excludes 1** note means that two conditions can ***never*** be coded together. ***Example***: An Excludes 1 note at the E10.- category level (Type 1 diabetes mellitus) lists E11.- which is the category that contains codes for Type 2 diabetes mellitus. This means you can never assign a code from the E10.- category along with a code from the E11.- category. ***Note:*** You may code two conditions together, even if one or both of them is listed in an Excludes 1 note, as long as they are ***not related***.

An **Excludes 2** note implies that two conditions ***could be coded*** on the same claim if appropriate. ***Example***: A home health patient could have both an acute bronchitis infection on top of chronic obstructive bronchitis, a form of COPD. The ICD-10 code for acute obstructive bronchitis is J20.9, and it carries an Excludes 2 note that lists codes from the J44.- category (Other chronic obstructive pulmonary disease). The Excludes 2 note communicates that the acute bronchitis is not the same as chronic obstructive bronchitis, but they can be assigned together if both are diagnosed.

The word "with" or "in" should be interpreted to mean "associated with" or "due to" when it appears in a code title, the Alphabetic Index, or an instructional note in the Tabular List. The classification presumes a causal relationship between the two conditions linked by these terms. These conditions should be coded as related even in the absence of provider documentation explicitly linking them, unless the documentation clearly states the conditions are unrelated or when another guideline exists that specifically requires a documented linkage between two conditions (e.g., sepsis guideline for "acute organ dysfunction that is not clearly associated with the sepsis").

Take note of key ICD-10 guidelines

Further your grasp of ICD-10 by developing a thorough understanding of *ICD-10 coding guidelines*, once you'd laid a firm foundation on the coding conventions. These ICD-10 guidelines will have a direct impact on home health coding:

Laterality *[I.B.13]*: The ICD-10 code set provides a way to capture laterality — that is, a right or left side, or bilateral, designation. *Example*: Consider the M17.- category for Osteoarthritis of knee. A fourth character of "0" indicates that the condition is primary and bilateral (on both sides). If that patient's osteoarthritis is primary and confined to his right knee, for example, the correct code would be M17.11 (Unilateral primary osteoarthritis, right knee).

Coders can assign a unilateral code in the case of a patient who had a condition on both sides of the body, but for whom treatment resolved the condition on one side and it still exists on the other. An example of this would be a patient whose cataract in one eye is resolved through surgery but who still has a cataract in the other eye. However, if the treatment on the first side didn't resolve the condition completely, the bilateral code should still be used, according to coding guidelines.

Sequelae *[I.B.10]*: What were known as late effects in ICD-9 are *sequela* in ICD-10, and are governed by the rules in this guideline. The condition currently at hand, that resulted from the past illness or injury, i.e. the residual, is to be coded *before* the sequela form of the code for the now-resolved illness or injury. *Example:* Consider a woman being treated in home health for a contracture of her right hand that resulted from a third-degree burn suffered several years ago. The contracture is the residual and is coded with M24.541 (Contracture, right hand). It is immediately followed by the sequela form of the code for the injury that caused it, the burn, T23.301S (Burn of third degree of right hand, unspecified site, sequela). Notice the 7th character "S" on the code, which designates it as a sequela, as opposed to an active condition.

Signs, Symptoms and Unspecified Codes. *[I.B.18]*: This guideline expounds upon existing conventions and guidelines to explain the appropriate use of unspecified codes when there isn't sufficient documentation available to code a more definitive diagnosis, and of signs and symptoms codes in the absence of a confirmed diagnosis. *Unspecified code example:* Assign J44.9 (Chronic obstructive pulmonary disease, unspecified) if you don't have further information regarding a patient's COPD diagnosis. *Symptom code example:* Assign R06.00 (Dyspnea, unspecified) for a patient receiving therapy to address problems with ADLs as a result of severe shortness of breath, but for whom no underlying diagnosis, such as congestive heart failure, has been confirmed.

Steps to Accurate Coding

Recording diagnoses is the responsibility of the attending physician. As of Jan. 1, 1998, physicians are required by law to provide the diagnosis information for Medicare and Medicaid patients (*Balanced Budget Act, HR 2015 Sec 4317*). Failure to do so can result in prosecution. The physician must supply the diagnosis code for all services and testing performed or ordered, including home health care. Although the law provides for the physician to provide the diagnosis codes, home health providers do not always find this to be true. OASIS assessment strategies allow diagnosis information to be obtained through assessment with verification from the physician. The plan of care lists the conditions that require or may impact home health care; these conditions are listed in following forms: plan of care, OASIS and the claim form (UB-04).

Warning: The hospital discharge diagnosis is not always the reason home care is provided. There should be close scrutiny of the primary diagnosis assigned. The home health PPS rule states that the only clinicians who can determine the primary and secondary or other diagnoses are the assessing clinicians, including the registered nurse, and physical, occupational, or speech therapists. The assigned codes on the OASIS comprehensive assessment must match the home health plan of care, as well as those on the home health claim submitted.

Basic Coding Steps

Review the plan of care and assessment to find the reason(s) for home health services. The need for medically necessary skilled services is used in judging the relevancy of a diagnosis to the plan of care (POC) and to the OASIS. A review of qualifications for various skilled services under the home health benefit can be found in Chapter 7 of the Medicare Benefit Policy Manual.

To select a code in the classification that corresponds to a diagnosis or reason for visit documented in a medical record, first locate the term in the Alphabetic Index, and then verify the code in the Tabular List. You should read and be guided by instructional notations that appear in both the Alphabetic Index and Tabular list. It is essential to use both the Alphabetic Index and Tabular List when locating and assigning a code. The format of the Alphabetic Index and the Tabular list are dictionary style: Main terms in the Alphabetic Index are set flush with the left- hand margin and printed in bold type.

The Alphabetic Index does not always provide the full code. Selection of the full code, including laterality and 7th character, can only be completed in the Tabular. A dash (-) at the end of a code at the Alphabetic Index will indicate that additional characters are required. Even if a dash is not included at the Alphabetic Index

entry, it is necessary to refer to the Tabular List to verify that no 7th character is required.

Follow any instructions that direct you to "see" another code. This is a crucial step that must be completed.

Identify any manifestation code (these codes will have two selections with a code in brackets following the main code). This pair is to be assigned with the etiology preceding the manifestation. For example: Dementia with Lewy Bodies: G31.83 first listed, *[F02.80]* follows etiology.

General Coding Guidelines

The ICD-10-CM coding guidelines are revised and approved by the American Hospital Association, the American Health Information Management Association, the Centers for Medicare and Medicaid Services and the National Center for Health Statistics. They state:

1. The appropriate code or codes from A00.0 through T88.9, Z00.0-Z99.8 are used to identify diagnoses, symptoms, conditions, problems, complaints, or other reason(s) for encounter/visit.

2. For accurate reporting of ICD-10-CM diagnosis codes, the documentation should describe the patient's condition using terminology that includes specific diagnoses as well as symptoms, problems, or reasons for the encounter. There are ICD-10-CM codes to describe all of these.

3. Codes that describe symptoms and signs, as opposed to diagnoses, are acceptable for reporting purposes when a diagnosis has not been established (confirmed) by the physician. Chapter 18, Symptoms, Signs and Abnormal Clinical and Laboratory Findings, Note Elsewhere Classified (codes R00.0-R99), contains many, but not all, codes for symptoms.

4. ICD-10-CM is composed of codes with three, four, five, six or seven characters. Codes with three characters are included in ICD-10-CM as the headings for categories of codes that may be further subdivided by the use of fourth and/ or fifth characters and/or sixth characters, which provide greater specificity.

A three-character code is to be used only if it is not further subdivided. A code is invalid if it has not been coded to the full number of characters required for that code, including the seventh character, if applicable.

Rules for selecting the primary and secondary diagnoses codes come from OASIS requirements and ICD-10-CM guidelines. OASIS instructions state to follow the official guidelines for coding.

In the Alphabetic Index, reference the entire "indented" series of codes following a main term. These indented terms underneath the main bold term are called "sub entries." Their purpose is to add specificity to the code.

These "sub entries" change the code term and increase the specificity of a code. The first code at the main bold term is usually an unspecified code, also known as 'not otherwise specified' (NOS). Only use NOS codes if you do not have access to more specific information.

The word "with" in the Alphabetic Index is sequenced immediately following the main term, not in alphabetical order.

The word "with" or "in" should be interpreted to mean "associated with" or "due to" when it appears in a code title, the Alphabetic Index, or an instructional note in the Tabular List. The classification presumes a causal relationship between the two conditions linked by these terms in the Alphabetic Index or Tabular List, according to the official coding guidelines.

These conditions should be coded as related even in the absence of provider documentation explicitly linking them, unless the documentation clearly states the conditions are unrelated. For conditions not specifically linked by these relational terms in the classification, provider documentation must link the conditions in order to code them as related.

An example is diabetes and the manifestations listed underneath the word 'with' in the alphabetical index, but the convention also applies to other instances where the word 'with' is a sub entry under a main term in the alpha listing. However, if there is ever uncertainty as to the relationship between two conditions, query the physician.

Write down the code possibilities and verify in the Tabular List the accurate code assignment. Be sure to read the notes at the Tabular List for the accurate code assignment and sequencing. The patient's primary focus of care for the home health episode will be the principal code choice, unless official coding guidelines otherwise apply.

Assign the code(s) selected in proper sequence. List first the ICD-10-CM code for the diagnosis, condition, problem, or other reason for the home health visit documented in the medical record as chiefly responsible for the services provided. List additional codes that describe any coexisting conditions managed during the episode of care.

If more than one diagnosis is treated concurrently, the diagnosis that represents the most acute condition and requires the most intensive services should be entered first. The primary diagnosis is the diagnosis most related to the POC; most acute diagnosis; and the chief reason for providing home care. The secondary or other diagnoses must be relevant to the care rendered. Include conditions actively addressed and any comorbid conditions

affecting the patient's responsiveness to treatment and rehabilitative prognosis, even if the condition is not the focus of any home health treatment itself. A diagnosis, once listed, must be supported by documentation in the comprehensive assessment (OASIS) and in the plan of care.

Do not assign a diagnosis documented as "probable," "suspected," "questionable," "rule-out," or "working." Rather, code the condition(s) to the highest degree of certainty for the visit, such as symptoms, signs, or other reasons.

Chronic conditions treated on an ongoing basis may be coded and reported as many times as the patient receives treatment and care for the condition. A chronic condition, even if not the focus of care, will always impact the care and should be coded as a pertinent diagnosis. These diagnoses also should be addressed in the plan of care. Do not code conditions that are resolved, i.e. no longer exist, or do not impact the home health plan of care.

As a home care provider, you should try to select an ICD-10 code from Chapters 1 – 19 that best describes the patient's current, active condition under treatment. However, be aware that there also are additional codes (supplemental classification) that are important to coding. Z codes identify conditions other than illness that result in the use of health care services. For example, Z47.1 describes aftercare following joint replacement surgery. In addition, V, W, X, and Y codes classify external causes of morbidity, such as X11.0- (Contact with hot water in a bath or tub), and include codes for adverse effects and poisonings.

Code to the highest level of specificity

The diagnosis codes are made up of three, four, five, six, or seven characters. When coding the patient's condition, the ICD-10-CM code must be taken to the highest level of specificity.

If a three-character category further subdivides into 4th, 5th, 6th, or 7th characters, the completed code must include the appropriate 4th, 5th, 6th, and 7th characters, as indicated. A three-character code category is to be used only if it is not further subdivided into 4th, 5th, 6th, or 7th character requirements. For example, Unspecified viral encephalitis (A86), Unspecified mood disorder (F39), Microencephalopathy (Q02), Unspecified urinary incontinence (R32), Nondiabetic hypoglycemic coma (E15), are all examples where three characters represent the highest specificity.

Where 4th, 5th, 6th and/or 7th character subclassifications are provided, they must be assigned or the result will be an invalid Medicare claim. Assigning the highest degree of specificity will enable Medicare to properly classify the severity of the patient's condition. Additionally, you will avoid having your Medicare claim rejected.

Using combination codes

ICD-10-CM includes a number of codes referred to as "combination codes." A combination code is a single code used to classify two diagnoses, or a diagnosis with an associated secondary process (manifestation), or a diagnosis with an associated complication. Not all conditions may be captured by the use of combination codes, but some may, and in those cases, the combination code should be assigned. Assign only the combination code when that code fully identifies the diagnostic conditions involved or when the Alphabetic Index so directs. Multiple coding should not be used when the classification provides a combination code that clearly identifies all of the elements documented in the diagnosis.

For example, many diabetes codes in the ICD-10-CM code set utilize combination codes to capture both the diabetes and a manifestation of the diabetes within one ICD-10 code. Type 2 diabetes mellitus with unspecified diabetic retinopathy with macular edema is coded to E11.311. This is an example of using a combination code that classifies a diagnosis with an associated secondary process (manifestation) within the combination code. No second code is assigned for the retinopathy or macular edema, as the single combination code includes these conditions.

Only when the combination code lacks specificity in describing the manifestation or complication, an additional code should be used. In such a case, sequencing guidelines for the specific combination code will indicate to "use an additional code." For example, when assigning the combination code E11.22, Type 2 diabetes with diabetic chronic kidney disease, an additional code is required to identify the stage of chronic kidney disease. Instructions at the code level will indicate to use an additional code to identify the stage of chronic kidney disease (N18.1 – N18.6), which should be sequenced following the E11.22 code.

Manifestation coding steps

In certain cases, ICD-10-CM requires that more than one code be assigned to report a condition. This requirement, termed "etiology/manifestation coding" often involves both a disease (etiology) and one of its manifestations. The ICD-10-CM manual clearly shows the instances where manifestation coding is required. You'll notice that these codes are listed in the Alphabetic Index with the etiology code listed first, followed by the manifestation code italicized in brackets. The code appearing in brackets is always to be sequenced second. Additionally, these codes appear in the Tabular List with a "code first" note at the manifestation code and a "use additional code" note at the etiology code. Coding conventions require that these sequencing guidelines be followed and failure to follow

correct sequencing for a manifestation/etiology code pair may result in return of the claim to the provider.

To help you identify them, manifestation codes in the Tabular List are italicized and highlighted in yellow with an 'M' to the left of the code. Manifestation codes may never appear in the principal diagnosis field, and must be preceded by the code for the underlying condition (etiology). Every manifestation code in the Tabular List is accompanied by instructions to report the etiology first.

The sequencing instructions in the ICD-10-CM Coding Guidelines for manifestation coding for a single condition are only intended to apply to diagnoses that are required to be sequenced a certain way by the coding guidelines, e.g., manifestations, sequelae, complications.

Therefore, unless an agency encounters such a situation when consulting the Alphabetic Index or Tabular List, it should continue to list the primary reason for home care in the principal diagnosis field as it has always done. ICD-10-CM guidelines, except in the case of manifestation coding and other specific sequencing guidelines, do not direct users to report the root cause of a patient's health problems when a more proximate diagnosis is available. For example, consider neurogenic bladder in a stable MS patient or radiculitis in a stable MS patient. In these cases, when the proximate diagnosis (neurogenic bladder or radiculitis) is the main reason for home care, it is reported as the primary diagnosis, and the underlying condition (MS) is a secondary diagnosis. Always consult the Official Coding Guidelines and instructions for guidance on sequencing.

Sequela coding steps

A "sequela" is the residual effect (condition produced) after the acute phase of an injury or illness has terminated. The residual effect may be apparent early, such as after an acute phase of illness (e.g., CVA), or it may occur much later, a year or more, as with a previous injury. Examples of sequelae include: scar formation due to a healed burn, deviated septum due to a nasal fracture, and infertility due to tubal occlusion from old tuberculosis. Coding of sequelae generally requires two codes sequenced in the following order: the condition or nature of the sequela is sequenced first. The sequela code is sequenced second.

An exception to this general sequencing guideline includes instances where the code for the sequela is followed by a manifestation code identified in the Tabular List, or the sequela code has been expanded (at the 4th, 5th or 6th character levels) to include the manifestation(s) (for example, I69.391, Dysphagia following cerebral infarction, should be sequenced prior to the code for the type of dysphagia).

To identify the sequela code, reference the word "sequela" in the Alphabetic Index.

Coding from the Table of Drugs and Chemicals

Knowing when to use a code to indicate a poisoning or an adverse event can be tricky. Consider the following ICD-10-CM rules when coding poisonings and adverse events.

A substance used incorrectly is poisoning in ICD-10 terms. However, it's also considered a poisoning if the patient's condition is caused by the interaction between a therapeutic drug used correctly and a nonprescription drug or alcohol. For example, a patient may present with acute liver failure because he correctly took Valium, but he also consumed ethyl alcohol. This would be considered a poisoning.

When a patient presents with a poisoning, list the combination code for the drug or substance causing the poisoning code first (and the circumstance), then follow with a code for the effect of the poisoning.

In the Valium and alcohol example above, you would first code T51.0X1D (accidental poisoning by alcohol, subsequent encounter), followed by T42.4X1D (accidental poisoning due to Valium, subsequent episode) followed by K72.00 (Acute hepatic failure without coma).

Check the documentation for the following clues that the condition is considered a poisoning: wrong medication given or taken, wrong dosage given or taken, medication given to or taken by the wrong person, intoxication (other than cumulative, see "adverse effect"), or the term "overdose."

ICD-10-CM also includes codes for underdosing of a medication. Underdosing refers to taking less than is prescribed by a provider or manufacturer's instruction. Do not assign codes for underdosing as a primary diagnosis under any condition. Rather, the medical condition for which the underdosed medication was prescribed should be assigned, if this condition relapsed or exacerbated. A code for non-compliance (Z91.12-, Z91.13-) should be assigned with a code for underdosing when appropriate.

A substance used correctly, but with an unintended reaction, is considered an adverse effect for ICD-10 purposes. This includes a bad interaction between two or more therapeutic drugs that have been used correctly.

When coding an adverse effect, sequence the nature of the adverse effect first, then follow with the appropriate combination code from T36 – T50 for the adverse effect of the drug.

Terms you might see in your physician's documentation that signal an adverse effect include: "allergic reaction," "cumulative effect" of a drug (toxicity), "hypersensitivity" to a drug, "idiosyncratic reaction," "paradoxical reaction," or "synergistic reaction."

Remember to always check the Tabular List when coding from the Table of Drugs and Chemicals.

What happens if you choose the wrong code?

If a diagnosis is listed on the billing form and no supporting documentation is found in the medical record, there may be financial consequences for the home health entity, and the discrepancy is an audit liability.

Conditions for which there is no supporting documentation should not be reported. Query the physician if there are questions on documentation.

CMS has software programs that scan forms (OASIS, UB-04) for discrepancies (i.e., final diagnosis code submitted not matching the codes on the UB-04, OASIS, etc.). This could suspend payment and require additional document review by the MAC and other government contractors.

Prospective audits should be conducted by the home health agency to ensure accurate capture of the appropriate ICD-10-CM codes as well as consistency across forms (plan of care, OASIS and UB-04). Careful attention must be paid to the differences in the coding rules between home health agencies and hospitals/physicians.

Also consider that correct coding is a requirement of HIPAA compliance.

Get the details on how PDGM works

As the 2020 Home Health Coding Manual went to press, the new home health payment system, the Patient-Driven Groupings Model (PDGM), was set to take effect Jan. 1, 2020. The details of the PDGM system contained in this article are based on the 1/1/20 PPS proposed rule. If CMS updates PDGM after the Manual has published, we will upload those details to decisionhealth.com/pdf/pdgm.zip.

The new payment model utilizes 30-day payment periods and stops using the number of therapy visits to determine payment. LUPA thresholds under PDGM will range from two to six visits, depending on the specific HHRG.

CMS will use specific, individual patient characteristics to determine payments in PDGM.

The primary diagnosis code on the claim will determine which clinical group the episode falls into.

Once a primary diagnosis grouping is assigned, the classification is further refined by determining the level of care and assistance required by the patient and assigning a functional status of high, medium or low.

The terminology used here has been among the most confusing aspects of the new model, and it is important to note that a functional status of high or low doesn't refer to the patient's functional abilities but instead indicates the patient's level of functional impairment.

It reflects the level of assistance and resource use required for that patient. A high rating means the patient has a high impairment, requires the highest level of care and assistance and is expected to require high use of agency resources.

Additional factors impacting the payment formula include whether the patient is new to home health or has previously received services, and whether the patient was admitted to home health from the community or an institutional setting.

Coding impacts clinical values

The **primary diagnosis** code on the claim will determine which of the **clinical groups** below the episode falls into:

- Musculoskeletal rehabilitation
- Neuro/ stroke rehabilitation
- Wounds – post-op wound aftercare and skin/non-surgical wound care
- Behavioral health
- Complex nursing interventions
- Medication Management, teaching and assessment (MMTA), which is further subdivided into 7 subgroups:
  - MMTA – Surgical aftercare
  - MMTA – Cardiac/circulatory
  - MMTA – Endocrine
  - MMTA – GI/GU
  - MMTA – Infectious disease/ neoplasms/ blood-forming diseases
  - MMTA – Respiratory
  - MMTA – Other

List all diagnoses relevant to the plan of care — not just the six allowed on the OASIS — on the home health claim. In addition to assigning one principal diagnosis, you can assign up to **24 secondary diagnoses**, and receive a **comorbidity adjustment**. A certain combination of secondary diagnoses within designated categories will lead to a comorbidity adjustment. **Only one adjustment is applied per episode.** Comorbidity adjustments fall into one of three categories: none, low or high. The adjustments are designed to account for the additional resource use required for patients with complex needs.

To qualify for a **low comorbidity adjustment**, the claim must include **one secondary diagnosis** found within one of 12 comorbidity subgroups associated with higher resource use. To qualify for a **high comorbidity adjustment**, the claim must include **two or more secondary diagnoses** that fall within 34 comorbidity subgroup interactions that account for 18 distinct comorbidity subgroups. [*See comorbidity subgroups for low and high in tables below.*]

Patients with heart failure and patients with Parkinson's disease are two examples of subgroups that will be eligible for an adjustment.

Primary Diagnosis Clinical Groups

Clinical groups	The primary reason for the home health encounter is to provide the following
Musculoskeletal Rehabilitation	Therapy (physical, occupational or speech) for a musculoskeletal condition.
Neuro/Stroke Rehabilitation	Therapy (physical, occupational or speech) for a neurological condition or stroke.
Wounds — Post-Op Wound Aftercare and Skin/Non-Surgical Wound Care.	Assessment, treatment & evaluation of a surgical wound(s); assessment, treatment and evaluation of non-surgical wounds, ulcers, burns and other lesions.
Behavioral Health Care	Assessment, treatment and evaluation of psychiatric conditions, including substance use disorders.
Complex Nursing Interventions	Assessment, treatment and evaluation of complex medical and surgical conditions including IV, total parenteral nutrition (TPN), enteral nutrition, ventilator and ostomies
Medication Management, Teaching and Assessment (MMTA) — Surgical aftercare	Assessment, evaluation, teaching and medication management for surgical aftercare
MMTA — Cardiac/circulatory	Assessment, evaluation, teaching and medication management for cardiac or other circulatory related conditions
MMTA — Endocrine	Assessment, evaluation, teaching and medication management for endocrine related conditions
MMTA — GI/GU	Assessment, evaluation, teaching and medication management for gastrointestinal or genitourinary related conditions
MMTA — Infectious disease/ neoplasms/ blood-forming diseases	Assessment, evaluation, teaching and medication management for conditions related to infectious diseases, neoplasms and blood-forming diseases
MMTA — Respiratory	Assessment, evaluation, teaching and medication management for respiratory related conditions
MMTA — Other	Assessment, evaluation, teaching and medication management for a variety of medical and surgical conditions not classified in one of the previously listed groups

Source: CMS

Average resource use by clinical group under PDGM

Among the six clinical groups under the Patient-Driven Groupings Model, Medication management, teaching and assessment (MMTA) has by far the greatest percent of periods. That's according to an CMS analysis of 2017 Medicare claims data.

Clinical group	Percent of periods
MMTA	55.2%
MS rehab	18.4%
Neuro	10.4%
Wound	9.0%
Complex	3.5%
Behavioral health	3.3%

Source: CMS analysis of 2017 Medicare claims data

LOW comorbidity adjustment interaction subgroups

The chart below lists the 12 subgroups that lead to low comorbidity adjustments under PDGM. Claims with a secondary diagnosis in one of these subgroups will qualify for a low comorbidity adjustment.

Comorbidity subgroup	Description
Cerebral 4	Includes sequelae of cerebrovascular diseases
Circulatory 10	Includes varicose veins with ulceration
Circulatory 9	Includes acute and chronic embolisms and thrombosis
Heart 10	Includes cardiac dysrhythmias
Heart 11	Includes heart failure
Neoplasms 1	Includes oral cancers
Neuro 10	Includes peripheral and polyneuropathies
Neuro 5	Includes Parkinson's disease
Neuro 7	Includes hemiplegia, paraplegia and quadriplegia
Skin 1	Includes cutaneous abscess, cellulitis and lymphangitis
Skin 3	Include diseases of arteries, arterioles and capillaries with ulceration and non-pressure chronic ulcers
Skin 4	Includes Stage 2, 3, 4 and unstageable pressure ulcers by site

Source: 2020 PPS proposed rule

HIGH comorbidity adjustment interaction subgroups

The chart below lists the subgroups that lead to high comorbidity adjustments under PDGM. Claims with secondary diagnoses within interacting categories will qualify for a high comorbidity adjustment.

Comorbidity subgroup interaction	Comorbidity subgroup	Description	Comorbidity subgroup	Description
1	Behavioral 2	Includes depression and bipolar disorder	Skin 3	Includes diseases of arteries, arterioles and capillaries with ulceration and non-pressure, chronic ulcers
2	Cerebral 4	Includes sequelae of cerebral vascular diseases	Circulatory 4	Includes hypertensive chronic kidney disease
3	Cerebral 4	Includes sequelae of cerebral vascular diseases	Heart 11	Includes heart failure
4	Cerebral 4	Includes sequelae of cerebral vascular diseases	Neuro 10	Includes peripheral and polyneuropathies
5	Circulatory 4	Includes hypertensive chronic kidney disease	Skin 1	Includes cutaneous abscess, cellulitis, lymphangitis
6	Circulatory 4	Includes hypertensive chronic kidney disease	Skin 3	Includes diseases of arteries, arterioles and capillaries with ulceration and non-pressure, chronic ulcers
7	Circulatory 4	Includes hypertensive chronic kidney disease	Skin 4	Includes Stage 2, 3, 4 and unstageable pressure ulcers by site
8	Circulatory 7	Includes atherosclerosis	Skin 3	Includes diseases of arteries, arterioles and capillaries with ulceration and non-pressure, chronic ulcers
9	Endocrine 3	Includes diabetes with complications	Neuro 5	Includes Parkinson's disease
10	Endocrine 3	Includes diabetes with complications	Neuro 7	Includes hemiplegia, paraplegia and quadriplegia
11	Endocrine 3	Includes diabetes with complications	Skin 1	Includes cutaneous abscess, cellulitis, lymphangitis
12	Endocrine 3	Includes diabetes with complications	Skin 3	Includes diseases of arteries, arterioles and capillaries with ulceration and non-pressure, chronic ulcers
13	Heart 10	Includes cardiac dysrhythmias	Skin 3	Includes diseases of arteries, arterioles and capillaries with ulceration and non-pressure, chronic ulcers
14	Heart 10	Includes cardiac dysrhythmias	Skin 4	Includes Stage 2, 3, 4 and unstageable pressure ulcers by site
15	Heart 11	Includes heart failure	Neuro 10	Includes peripheral and polyneuropathies
16	Heart 11	Includes heart failure	Neuro 5	Includes Parkinson's disease
17	Heart 11	Includes heart failure	Skin 1	Includes cutaneous abscess, cellulitis, lymphangitis
18	Heart 11	Includes heart failure	Skin 3	Includes diseases of arteries, arterioles and capillaries with ulceration and non-pressure, chronic ulcers
19	Heart 11	Includes heart failure	Skin 4	Includes Stage 2, 3, 4 and unstageable pressure ulcers by site
20	Heart 12	Includes other heart diseases	Skin 3	Includes diseases of arteries, arterioles and capillaries with ulceration and non-pressure, chronic ulcers
21	Heart 12	Includes other heart diseases	Skin 4	Includes Stage 2, 3, 4 and unstageable pressure ulcers by site
22	Neuro 10	Includes peripheral and polyneuropathies	Neuro 5	Includes Parkinson's disease
23	Neuro 10	Includes peripheral and polyneuropathies	Skin 3	Includes diseases of arteries, arterioles and capillaries with ulceration and non-pressure, chronic ulcers
24	Neuro 3	Includes dementias	Skin 3	Includes diseases of arteries, arterioles and capillaries with ulceration and non-pressure, chronic ulcers

HIGH comorbidity adjustment interaction subgroups (cont.)

Comorbidity subgroup interaction	Comorbidity subgroup	Description	Comorbidity subgroup	Description
25	Neuro 3	Includes dementias	Skin 4	Includes Stage 2, 3, 4 and unstageable pressure ulcers by site
26	Neuro 5	Includes Parkinson's disease	Renal 3	Includes nephrogenic diabetes insipidus
27	Neuro 7	Includes hemiplegia, paraplegia and quadriplegia	Renal 3	Includes nephrogenic diabetes insipidus
28	Renal 1	Includes Chronic kidney disease and ESRD	Skin 3	Includes diseases of arteries, arterioles and capillaries with ulceration and non-pressure, chronic ulcers
29	Renal 1	Includes Chronic kidney disease and ESRD	Skin 4	Includes Stage 2, 3, 4 and unstageable pressure ulcers by site
30	Renal 3	Includes nephrogenic diabetes insipidus	Skin 4	Includes Stage 2, 3, 4 and unstageable pressure ulcers by site
31	Resp 5	Includes COPD and asthma	Skin 3	Includes diseases of arteries, arterioles and capillaries with ulceration and non-pressure, chronic ulcers
32	Resp 5	Includes COPD and asthma	Skin 4	Includes Stage 2, 3, 4 and unstageable pressure ulcers by site
33	Skin 1	Includes cutaneous abscess, cellulitis, lymphangitis	Skin 3	Includes diseases of arteries, arterioles and capillaries with ulceration and non-pressure, chronic ulcers
34	Skin 3	Includes diseases of arteries, arterioles and capillaries with ulceration and non-pressure, chronic ulcers	Skin 4	Includes Stage 2, 3, 4 and unstageable pressure ulcers by site

Source: CMS

Avoid listing questionable codes

Under PDGM, failure to use a primary diagnosis code that fits into one of the clinical groups, means you're using a **questionable encounter** code, which could result in claims getting kicked back to providers, payment delays and potential red flags for auditors.

The red flags would come because if claims are sent back to the agency and then resubmitted with a new primary diagnosis code, it may appear to auditors that the agency isn't confirming the diagnoses with the physician but recoding to resubmit quickly.

Common home health diagnosis codes M62.81 (Muscle weakness (generalized)), R26.89 (Other abnormalities of gait and mobility), M19.91 (Primary osteoarthritis, unspecified site) and R13.10 (Primary osteoarthritis, unspecified site) are among the 20 most common questionable encounter codes under PDGM, according to an analysis from Strategic Healthcare Programs (SHP) in Santa Barbara, Calif.

To avoid these issues, take steps to identify which questionable encounter codes your agency uses and work to gather more detailed information that will lead to more specific, acceptable codes instead.

CMS states that "the majority of the R codes (codes that describe signs and symptoms, as opposed to diagnoses) are not appropriate as principal diagnosis codes for grouping home health periods into clinical groups."

Top 10 questionable encounter codes in PDGM

Muscle weakness (generalized) was by far the most commonly-used primary diagnosis that would be deemed questionable under the Patient-Driven Groupings Model, according to 2017 data from Santa Barbara, Calif.-based Strategic Healthcare Programs.

Diagnosis code	Description	Primary diagnosis category	Questionable encounters	Percentage of starts of care (SOC) with a questionable encounter
M62.81	Muscle weakness (generalized)	Musculoskeletal/connective tissue	115,322	25.9%
R26.89	Other abnormalities of gait and mobility	Symptoms/signs/ill-defined	27,994	6.3%
R26.81	Unsteadiness on feet	Symptoms/signs/ill-defined	17,513	3.9%
R29.6	Repeated falls	Symptoms/signs/ill-defined	16,226	3.6%
R53.1	Weakness	Symptoms/signs/ill-defined	16,146	3.6%
R26.9	Unspecified abnormalities of gait and mobility	Symptoms/signs/ill-defined	14,210	3.2%
R26.2	Difficulty in walking not elsewhere classified	Symptoms/signs/ill-defined	9,796	2.2%
M19.91	Primary osteoarthritis, unspecified site	Musculoskeletal/connective tissue	7,216	1.6%
M19.90	Unspecified osteoarthritis, unspecified site	Musculoskeletal/connective tissue	6,968	1.6%
M06.9	Rheumatoid arthritis, unspecified	Musculoskeletal/connective tissue	6,526	1.5%

Source: Strategic Healthcare Programs (SHP), Santa Barbara, Calif.

Tips to ensure coding accuracy in PDGM

Coding accuracy, specificity and detail will drive the PDGM. Here are a few areas to focus on:

• **Get specific.** Diagnoses codes that are too vague — meaning the code does not provide adequate information to support the need for home health services — won't fit into any of the groupings under PDGM. Neither will manifestation codes that are subject to a manifestation/etiology convention and require the etiology code to be reported as the principal diagnosis.

One example of a code that's too vague: H57.9 (Unspecified disorder of eye and adnexa).

You'll also need to watch out for code-first sequencing conventions such as G99.2 (Myelopathy in diseases classified elsewhere), and codes that are unlikely to be used in home care or restricted to acute care settings.

Note: If you needed another reason to avoid simply copying codes previously used by the hospital or clinic where the patient had an inpatient stay, this is one.

However, CMS makes an exception for non-specific coding involving urinary tract infections. Realizing that home health clinicians can't really determine the exact site of a urinary tract infection without physician confirmation, N39.0 (Urinary tract infection, site not specified) will be grouped under the MMTA GI/GU grouping.

• **Understand what to do if the primary diagnosis changes.** Two 30-day payment periods are allowed to have two different case-mix groups to reflect changes in patient condition, CMS says. However, similar to PPS, the case mix group cannot be adjusted within each 30-day period.

If the primary diagnosis changes between the first and second 30-day period, only the claim for the second 30-day period should reflect the new diagnosis. If, for example, the patient suffers a fall before the start of a second, contiguous 30-day period, agencies shouldn't change the claim for the first 30-day period.

CMS explains that the revised Home Health Conditions of Participation (CoPs) already require agencies update the comprehensive assessment if a patient experiences a significant change in condition [§484.55(d)(1)(ii); G546]. In this scenario, a follow-up assessment should be submitted at the start of the second 30-day payment period to reflect the change in functional level. The second 30-day claim would then be grouped into the appropriate case-mix group.

- **Take heed of the process for returning claims.** CMS clearly outlines the expectation for what will happen when a claim is returned to the provider because it doesn't have a primary diagnosis that fits into one of the available clinical groups.

CMS notes that updating the primary diagnosis with a more specific or appropriate code would not be considered "up-coding," as long as there is documentation clearly supporting the need for services and that the physician signs and dates any changes in the plan of care.

When a claim is returned for more specific coding, CMS expects the diagnosis on the plan of care to be corrected, too.

- **Know when wound care grouping is appropriate.** CMS states that for a payment period to be grouped into the wound category, the diagnosis on the claim must reflect a break in skin integrity "for which clinical practice guidelines involve wound care necessitating skilled nursing services."

A diagnosis simply indicating infection may or may not demand wound care.

Resources

- The CY 2020 PDGM Grouper Tool is available at https://go.cms.gov/2znxqAa.
- Find comorbidity groups within the PDGM grouper tool at https://go.cms.gov/1RoGVoi.
- LUPA thresholds under PDGM will range from two to six visits, depending on the specific HHRG. View those thresholds in an updated file called "PDGM Case Mix Weights and LUPA Thresholds" at https://go.cms.gov/1RoGVoi.
- CMS has released an updated file called "PDGM agency level impacts." It's also available at https://go.cms.gov/1RoGVoi. The file lists agencies by CMS certification number and explains the total money they're estimated to make under the current system and how much money they would be estimated to make if PDGM was in effect.

FY2020 Code Change Summary

Starting Oct. 1, 2019, coders will have 25 new codes to specifically capture deep tissue injuries (DTIs).

For the home health industry, these additions are the most significant updates among the FY2020 ICD-10 code changes.

Overall, the list of changes includes 273 new codes, 30 revised codes, an additional 98 revisions to Tabular instructions, and 21 codes set to be rendered invalid.

Prior to Oct. 1, 2019, deep tissue injuries were coded as unstageable pressure ulcers. That's incorrect by definition, according to an initial proposal for the codes discussed at the ICD-10 Coordination & Maintenance Committee meeting in September 2018.

Among the new codes are **L89.026** (Pressure-induced deep tissue damage of left elbow) and **L89.156** (Pressure-induced deep tissue damage of sacral region).

Also of note is a revision to the description of code **J44.0** (Chronic obstructive pulmonary disease with (acute) lower respiratory infection). The word "acute" is placed in parenthesis, making it a non-essential modifier, which means you can use J44.0 regardless of whether "acute" has been documented by the physician.

Notable Tabular revisions

- The "code also" note at **I21.A** (Myocardial infarction type 2) is now a **"code first"** note.

- The Excludes 1 note at **I25.81** (Atherosclerosis of other coronary vessels without angina pectoris) is now an **Excludes 2** note (excluding atherosclerotic heart disease of native coronary artery without angina pectoris (I25.10)). An Excludes 2 note indicates that the condition excluded is not part of the condition represented by the code, but a patient may have both conditions at the same time, and therefore it is acceptable to use both the code and the excluded code together, when appropriate.

- The note on code **Z68** (Body mass index [BMI]) has been revised to state "BMI adult codes are for use for persons **20 years** of age or older," and "BMI pediatric codes are for use for persons 2-**19 years** of age." Previously the adult age limit started at 21 years, and the pediatric limit maxed at 20 years of age.

New codes for atrial fibrillation

You now have four new codes in the I48.- category to capture different forms of persistent and chronic atrial fibrillation.

Note that with the new, more specific codes, however, agencies would have to get more detailed information from physicians to code the atrial fibrillation accurately.

The new codes include: **I48.11** (Longstanding persistent atrial fibrillation); **I48.19** (Other persistent atrial fibrillation); **I48.20** (Chronic atrial fibrillation, unspecified) and **I48.21** (Permanent atrial fibrillation).

The Mayo Clinic provides the following definitions:

- **Persistent** — Heart rhythm doesn't go back to normal on its own. If you have persistent atrial fibrillation, you'll need treatment such as an electrical shock or medications in order to restore your heart rhythm.

- **Longstanding persistent** — The issue is continuous and lasts longer than 12 months.

- **Permanent** — Abnormal heart rhythm can't be restored. You'll have atrial fibrillation permanently, and you'll often require medications to control your heart rate.

Remember, it's the physician who has to determine if it's chronic or permanent.

Other notable highlights

- **8** new codes would allow reporting of **chronic embolism** and **thrombosis** of the peroneal vein and calf muscular vein (**I82.551-I82.559** and **I82.561-I82.569**). In addition, **8** codes would allow for reporting of **acute embolism** and **thrombosis** of those veins (**I82.451 – I82.459** and **I82.461-I82.469**).

- **8** new codes for **phlebitis** and **thrombophlebitis** (**I80.241-I80.249** and **I80.251-I80.259**) would allow more specific coding for laterality and location.

- **18** new T codes are for **poisoning, adverse effects** or **underdosing** of multiple unspecified drugs, medicaments and biological substances (**T50.91-**). You'll use the appropriate seventh character to describe the encounter: initial, subsequent or sequela. The new poisoning codes are divided into four causes: accidental, intentional, assault and undetermined. For example, T50.913S. (Poisoning by multiple unspecified drugs, medicaments and biological substances, assault, sequela).

- **T40.906-** (Underdosing of unspecified psychodysleptics) and **T40.996-** (Underdosing of other psychodysleptics) were revised to include the term "[hallucinogens]" in the title. **T44.1x6-** (Underdosing of other parasympathomimetics) is revised to include the term "cholinergics" in the title.

- **M77.51** (Other enthesopathy of right foot) and **M77.52** (Other enthesopathy of left foot) are revised to include "and ankle" in the title.

Quick Reference Guide to Alphabetic Index Search Terms

Use this tool to help you more efficiently locate correct codes in the alphabetic index

Diagnosis	Term to search for in the index
Pressure ulcer	Search "ulcer, pressure" and then to body site affected
Pseudogout	Search under "chondrocalcinosis"
Chronic nephritis due to systemic lupus erythematosus	Search under "lupus, nephritis"
Hip fracture	Search under "fracture, femur, upper end, neck"
Alzheimer's disease	Search under "disease, Alzheimer's"
Crohn's disease	Search under "Enteritis, regional"
Status of replaced joint	Ankle: Search under "presence, ankle joint implant"
	Elbow: Search under "presence, elbow joint implant"
	Finger: Search under "presence, finger joint implant"
	Hip: Search under "presence, hip joint implant"
	Knee: Search under "presence, knee joint implant"
	Shoulder: Search under "presence, shoulder joint implant"
	Wrist: Search under "presence, wrist joint implant"
	Specified NEC: Search under "presence, joint implant, specified joint NEC"
Heart failure	Search under "failure, heart"
COPD (Chronic obstructive pulmonary disease)	Search under "disease, pulmonary, chronic obstructive"
PVD (peripheral vascular disease)	Search under "disease, vascular, peripheral"
Diabetic ulcer	Search under "diabetes, with, foot ulcer"
	OR
	Search under "diabetes, with, skin ulcer NEC"
Amputation stump infection	Search under "complication, amputation stump NEC, infection or inflammation"
Coronary artery disease	Search under "disease, heart, ischemic, atherosclerotic"
Coronary artery disease with angina	Of native vessel: Search under "arteriosclerosis, coronary, native vessel, with angina pectoris"
	Of bypass graft: Search under "arteriosclerosis, coronary, bypass graft, with angina pectoris"
Toe ulcer	Search under "ulcer, lower limb, toe"
Gastric ulcer	Search under "ulcer, stomach"
Lower limb amputation status	Above knee: Search under "absence, extremity, lower"
	Below knee: Search under "absence, extremity, below knee"
Upper limb amputation status	Above elbow: Search under "absence, arm, above elbow"
	Below elbow: Search under "absence, arm, below elbow"
Osteomyelitis in the foot	Acute: Search under "osteomyelitis, acute, metatarsus"
	Chronic: Search under "osteomyelitis, chronic, metatarsus"
Parkinson's disease	Search under "Parkinsonism"
Major recurrent depression	Search under "disorder, depressive, recurrent"

Quick Reference Guide to Alphabetic Index Search Terms (cont.)

Diagnosis	Term to search for in the index
Surgical wound infection	Search under "Complication, surgical procedure, wound infection"
Cerebral autosomal dominant, with subcortical infarcts and leukoencephalopathy (CADASIL)	Search under "Arteriopathy, cerebral autosomal dominant, with subcortical infarcts and leukoencephalopathy (CADASIL)" or "CADASIL (cerebral autosomal dominant arteriopathy with subcortical infarcts andleukoencephalopathy)"
Elevated blood pressure reading, no diagnosis of hypertension	Search under "Hypertension, transient"
Lacunar infarction or stroke	Search under "Infarct, lacunar"
Paraplegia due to current injury	Code to injury with seventh character A
Paraplegia as sequela of previous injury	Code to injury with seventh character S
Postprocedural sepsis	Search under "Sepsis, postprocedural"

Source: Megan Batty, HCS-D and Vonnie Blevins, HCS-D, 2018

ICD-10-CM Official Guidelines
for Coding and Reporting FY2020
(October 1, 2019 – September 30, 2020)

The FY2020 Coding Guidelines are included in a separate packet that was delivered with your 2020 Coding Manual.

A

Aarskog's syndrome Q87.19
Abandonment — *see* Maltreatment
Abasia (-astasia) (hysterical) F44.4
Abderhalden-Kaufmann-Lignac syndrome (cystinosis) E72.04
Abdomen, abdominal — *see also* condition
  acute R10.0
  angina K55.1
  muscle deficiency syndrome Q79.4
Abdominalgia — *see* Pain, abdominal
Abduction contracture, hip or other joint — *see* Contraction, joint
Aberrant (congenital) — *see also* Malposition, congenital
  adrenal gland Q89.1
  artery (peripheral) Q27.8
    basilar NEC Q28.1
    cerebral Q28.3
    coronary Q24.5
    digestive system Q27.8
    eye Q15.8
    lower limb Q27.8
    precerebral Q28.1
    pulmonary Q25.79
    renal Q27.2
    retina Q14.1
    specified site NEC Q27.8
    subclavian Q27.8
    upper limb Q27.8
    vertebral Q28.1
  breast Q83.8
  endocrine gland NEC Q89.2
  hepatic duct Q44.5
  pancreas Q45.3
  parathyroid gland Q89.2
  pituitary gland Q89.2
  sebaceous glands, mucous membrane, mouth, congenital Q38.6
  spleen Q89.09
  subclavian artery Q27.8
  thymus (gland) Q89.2
  thyroid gland Q89.2
  vein (peripheral) NEC Q27.8
    cerebral Q28.3
    digestive system Q27.8
    lower limb Q27.8
    precerebral Q28.1
    specified site NEC Q27.8
    upper limb Q27.8
Aberration
  distintal — *see* Disturbance, visual
  mental F99
Abetalipoproteinemia E78.6
Abiotrophy R68.89
Ablatio, ablation
  retinae — *see* Detachment, retina
Ablepharia, ablepharon Q10.3
Abnormal, abnormality, abnormalities — *see also* Anomaly
  acid-base balance (mixed) E87.4
  albumin R77.0
  alphafetoprotein R77.2
  alveolar ridge K08.9
  anatomical relationship Q89.9
  apertures, congenital, diaphragm Q79.1
  auditory perception H93.29-
    diplacusis — *see* Diplacusis
    hyperacusis — *see* Hyperacusis
    recruitment — *see* Recruitment, auditory
    threshold shift — *see* Shift, auditory threshold
  autosomes Q99.9
    fragile site Q95.5
  basal metabolic rate R94.8
  biosynthesis, testicular androgen E29.1
  bleeding time R79.1
  blood-gas level R79.81
  blood level (of)
    cobalt R79.0
    copper R79.0
    iron R79.0
    lithium R78.89
    magnesium R79.0
    mineral NEC R79.0

Abnormal, abnormality, abnormalities - *continued*
  blood level (of) - *continued*
    zinc R79.0
  blood pressure
    elevated R03.0
    low reading (nonspecific) R03.1
  blood sugar R73.09
  bowel sounds R19.15
    absent R19.11
    hyperactive R19.12
  brain scan R94.02
  breathing R06.9
  caloric test R94.138
  cerebrospinal fluid R83.9
    cytology R83.6
    drug level R83.2
    enzyme level R83.0
    hormones R83.1
    immunology R83.4
    microbiology R83.5
    nonmedicinal level R83.3
    specified type NEC R83.8
  chemistry, blood R79.9
    C-reactive protein R79.82
    drugs — *see* Findings, abnormal, in blood
    gas level R79.81
    minerals R79.0
    pancytopenia D61.818
    PTT R79.1
    specified NEC R79.89
    toxins — *see* Findings, abnormal, in blood
  chest sounds (friction) (rales) R09.89
  chromosome, chromosomal Q99.9
    with more than three X chromosomes, female Q97.1
    analysis result R89.8
      bronchial washings R84.8
      cerebrospinal fluid R83.8
      cervix uteri NEC R87.89
      nasal secretions R84.8
      nipple discharge R89.8
      peritoneal fluid R85.89
      pleural fluid R84.8
      prostatic secretions R86.8
      saliva R85.89
      seminal fluid R86.8
      sputum R84.8
      synovial fluid R89.8
      throat scrapings R84.8
      vagina R87.89
      vulva R87.89
      wound secretions R89.8
    dicentric replacement Q93.2
    ring replacement Q93.2
    sex Q99.8
      female phenotype Q97.9
        specified NEC Q97.8
      male phenotype Q98.9
        specified NEC Q98.8
      structural male Q98.6
    specified NEC Q99.8
  clinical findings NEC R68.89
  coagulation D68.9
    newborn, transient P61.6
    profile R79.1
    time R79.1
  communication — *see* Fistula
  conjunctiva, vascular H11.41-
  coronary artery Q24.5
  cortisol-binding globulin E27.8
  course, eustachian tube Q17.8
  creatinine clearance R94.4
  cytology
    anus R85.619
      atypical squamous cells cannot exclude high grade squamous intraepithelial lesion (ASC-H) R85.611
      atypical squamous cells of undetermined significance (ASC-US) R85.610
      cytologic evidence of malignancy R85.614
      high grade squamous intraepithelial lesion (HGSIL) R85.613
      human papillomavirus (HPV) DNA test

Abnormal, abnormality, abnormalities - *continued*
  cytology - *continued*
    anus - *continued*
      human papillomavirus (HPV) DNA test - *continued*
        high risk positive R85.81
        low risk postive R85.82
      inadequate smear R85.615
      low grade squamous intraepithelial lesion (LGSIL) R85.612
      satisfactory anal smear but lacking transformation zone R85.616
      specified NEC R85.618
      unsatisfactory smear R85.615
    female genital organs — *see* Abnormal, Papanicolaou (smear)
  dark adaptation curve H53.61
  dentofacial NEC — *see* Anomaly, dentofacial
  development, developmental Q89.9
    central nervous system Q07.9
  diagnostic imaging
    abdomen, abdominal region NEC R93.5
    biliary tract R93.2
    bladder R93.41
    breast R92.8
    central nervous system NEC R90.89
    cerebrovascular NEC R90.89
    coronary circulation R93.1
    digestive tract NEC R93.3
    gastrointestinal (tract) R93.3
    genitourinary organs R93.89
    head R93.0
    heart R93.1
    intrathoracic organ NEC R93.89
    kidney R93.42-
    limbs R93.6
    liver R93.2
    lung (field) R91.8
    musculoskeletal system NEC R93.7
    renal pelvis R93.41
    retroperitoneum R93.5
    site specified NEC R93.89
    skin and subcutaneous tissue R93.89
    skull R93.09
    testis R93.81-
    urinary organs specified NEC R93.49
    ureter R93.41
  direction, teeth, fully erupted M26.30
  ear ossicles, acquired NEC H74.39-
    ankylosis — *see* Ankylosis, ear ossicles
    discontinuity — *see* Discontinuity, ossicles, ear
    partial loss — *see* Loss, ossicles, ear (partial)
  Ebstein Q22.5
  echocardiogram R93.1
  echoencephalogram R90.81
  echogram — *see* Abnormal, diagnostic imaging
  electrocardiogram [ECG] [EKG] R94.31
  electroencephalogram [EEG] R94.01
  electrolyte — *see* Imbalance, electrolyte
  electromyogram [EMG] R94.131
  electro-oculogram [EOG] R94.110
  electrophysiological intracardiac studies R94.39
  electroretinogram [ERG] R94.111
  erythrocytes
    congenital, with perinatal jaundice D58.9
  feces (color) (contents) (mucus) R19.5
  finding — *see* Findings, abnormal, without diagnosis
  fluid
    amniotic — *see* Abnormal, specimen, specified
    cerebrospinal — *see* Abnormal, cerebrospinal fluid
    peritoneal — *see* Abnormal, specimen, digestive organs
    pleural — *see* Abnormal, specimen, respiratory organs
    synovial — *see* Abnormal, specimen, specified

normality, abnormalities -

continued

x (bronchial washings) (pleural
fluid) — *see* Abnormal, specimen,
respiratory organs
vaginal — *see* Abnormal, specimen,
female genital organs
form
teeth K00.2
uterus — *see* Anomaly, uterus
function studies
auditory R94.120
bladder R94.8
brain R94.09
cardiovascular R94.30
ear R94.128
endocrine NEC R94.7
eye NEC R94.118
kidney R94.4
liver R94.5
nervous system
central NEC R94.09
peripheral NEC R94.138
pancreas R94.8
placenta R94.8
pulmonary R94.2
special senses NEC R94.128
spleen R94.8
thyroid R94.6
vestibular R94.121
gait — *see* Gait
hysterical F44.4
gastrin secretion E16.4
globulin R77.1
cortisol-binding E27.8
thyroid-binding E07.89
glomerular, minor — *see also* N00-N07 with
fourth character .0 N05.0
glucagon secretion E16.3
glucose tolerance (test) (non-fasting) R73.09
gravitational (G) forces or states (effect
of) T75.81
hair (color) (shaft) L67.9
specified NEC L67.8
hard tissue formation in pulp (dental) K04.3
head movement R25.0
heart
rate R00.9
specified NEC R00.8
shadow R93.1
sounds NEC R01.2
hemoglobin (disease) — *see also* Disease,
hemoglobin D58.2
trait — *see* Trait, hemoglobin, abnormal
histology NEC R89.7
immunological findings R89.4
in serum R76.9
specified NEC R76.8
increase in appetite R63.2
involuntary movement — *see* Abnormal,
movement, involuntary
jaw closure M26.51
karyotype R89.8
kidney function test R94.4
knee jerk R29.2
leukocyte (cell) (differential) NEC D72.9
liver function test R94.5
loss of
height R29.890
weight R63.4
mammogram NEC R92.8
calcification (calculus) R92.1
microcalcification R92.0
Mantoux test R76.11
movement (disorder) — *see also* Disorder,
movement
head R25.0
involuntary R25.9
fasciculation R25.3
of head R25.0
spasm R25.2
specified type NEC R25.8
tremor R25.1
myoglobin (Aberdeen) (Annapolis) R89.7

Abnormal, abnormality, abnormalities -
continued

neonatal screening P09
oculomotor study R94.113
palmar creases Q82.8
Papanicolaou (smear)
anus R85.619
atypical squamous cells cannot exclude
high grade squamous intraepithelial
lesion (ASC-H) R85.611
atypical squamous cells of undetermined
significance (ASC-US) R85.610
cytologic evidence of
malignancy R85.614
high grade squamous intraepithelial
lesion (HGSIL) R85.613
human papillomavirus (HPV) DNA test
high risk positive R85.81
low risk postive R85.82
inadequate smear R85.615
low grade squamous intraepithelial
lesion (LGSIL) R85.612
satisfactory anal smear but lacking
transformation zone R85.616
specified NEC R85.618
unsatisfactory smear R85.615
bronchial washings R84.6
cerebrospinal fluid R83.6
cervix R87.619
atypical squamous cells cannot exclude
high grade squamous intraepithelial
lesion (ASC-H) R87.611
atypical squamous cells of undetermined
significance (ASC-US) R87.610
cytologic evidence of
malignancy R87.614
high grade squamous intraepithelial
lesion (HGSIL) R87.613
inadequate smear R87.615
low grade squamous intraepithelial
lesion (LGSIL) R87.612
non-atypical endometrial cells R87.618
satisfactory cervical smear but lacking
transformation zone R87.616
specified NEC R87.618
thin preparaton R87.619
unsatisfactory smear R87.615
nasal secretions R84.6
nipple discharge R89.6
peritoneal fluid R85.69
pleural fluid R84.6
prostatic secretions R86.6
saliva R85.69
seminal fluid R86.6
sites NEC R89.6
sputum R84.6
synovial fluid R89.6
throat scrapings R84.6
vagina R87.629
atypical squamous cells cannot exclude
high grade squamous intraepithelial
lesion (ASC-H) R87.621
atypical squamous cells of undetermined
significance (ASC-US) R87.620
cytologic evidence of
malignancy R87.624
high grade squamous intraepithelial
lesion (HGSIL) R87.623
inadequate smear R87.625
low grade squamous intraepithelial
lesion (LGSIL) R87.622
specified NEC R87.628
thin preparation R87.629
unsatisfactory smear R87.625
vulva R87.69
wound secretions R89.6
partial thromboplastin time (PTT) R79.1
pelvis (bony) — *see* Deformity, pelvis
percussion, chest (tympany) R09.89
periods (grossly) — *see* Menstruation
phonocardiogram R94.39
plantar reflex R29.2
plasma
protein R77.9
specified NEC R77.8

Abnormal, abnormality, abnormalities -
continued

plasma - *continued*
viscosity R70.1
pleural (folds) Q34.0
posture R29.3
product of conception O02.9
specified type NEC O02.89
prothrombin time (PT) R79.1
pulmonary
artery, congenital Q25.79
function, newborn P28.89
test results R94.2
pulsations in neck R00.2
pupillary H21.56-
function (reaction) (reflex) — *see*
Anomaly, pupil, function
radiological examination — *see* Abnormal,
diagnostic imaging
red blood cell (s) (morphology)
(volume) R71.8
reflex — *see* Reflex
renal function test R94.4
response to nerve stimulation R94.130
retinal correspondence H53.31
retinal function study R94.111
rhythm, heart — *see also* Arrhythmia
saliva — *see* Abnormal, specimen, digestive
organs
scan
kidney R94.4
liver R93.2
thyroid R94.6
secretion
gastrin E16.4
glucagon E16.3
semen, seminal fluid — *see* Abnormal,
specimen, male genital organs
serum level (of)
acid phosphatase R74.8
alkaline phosphatase R74.8
amylase R74.8
enzymes R74.9
specified NEC R74.8
lipase R74.8
triacylglycerol lipase R74.8
shape
gravid uterus — *see* Anomaly, uterus
sinus venosus Q21.1
size, tooth, teeth K00.2
spacing, tooth, teeth, fully erupted M26.30
specimen
digestive organs (peritoneal fluid)
(saliva) R85.9
cytology R85.69
drug level R85.2
enzyme level R85.0
histology R85.7
hormones R85.1
immunology R85.4
microbiology R85.5
nonmedicinal level R85.3
specified type NEC R85.89
female genital organs (secretions)
(smears) R87.9
cytology R87.69
cervix R87.619
human papillomavirus (HPV) DNA
test
high risk positive R87.810
low risk positive R87.820
inadequate (unsatisfactory)
smear R87.615
non-atypical endometrial
cells R87.618
specified NEC R87.618
vagina R87.629
human papillomavirus (HPV) DNA
test
high risk positive R87.811
low risk positive R87.821
inadequate (unsatisfactory)
smear R87.625
vulva R87.69
drug level R87.2

Abnormal, abnormality, abnormalities - *continued*

specimen - *continued*

female genital organs (secretions) (smears) - *continued*

enzyme level R87.0
histological R87.7
hormones R87.1
immunology R87.4
microbiology R87.5
nonmedicinal level R87.3
specified type NEC R87.89
male genital organs (prostatic secretions) (semen) R86.9
cytology R86.6
drug level R86.2
enzyme level R86.0
histological R86.7
hormones R86.1
immunology R86.4
microbiology R86.5
nonmedicinal level R86.3
specified type NEC R86.8
nipple discharge — *see* Abnormal, specimen, specified
respiratory organs (bronchial washings) (nasal secretions) (pleural fluid) (sputum) R84.9
cytology R84.6
drug level R84.2
enzyme level R84.0
histology R84.7
hormones R84.1
immunology R84.4
microbiology R84.5
nonmedicinal level R84.3
specified type NEC R84.8
specified organ, system and tissue NOS R89.9
cytology R89.6
drug level R89.2
enzyme level R89.0
histology R89.7
hormones R89.1
immunology R89.4
microbiology R89.5
nonmedicinal level R89.3
specified type NEC R89.8
synovial fluid — *see* Abnormal, specimen, specified
thorax (bronchial washings) (pleural fluids) — *see* Abnormal, specimen, respiratory organs
vagina (secretion) (smear) R87.629
vulva (secretion) (smear) R87.69
wound secretion — *see* Abnormal, specimen, specified
spermatozoa — *see* Abnormal, specimen, male genital organs
sputum (amount) (color) (odor) R09.3
stool (color) (contents) (mucus) R19.5
bloody K92.1
guaiac positive R19.5
synchondrosis Q78.8
thermography — *see also* Abnormal, diagnostic imaging R93.89
thyroid-binding globulin E07.89
tooth, teeth (form) (size) K00.2
toxicology (findings) R78.9
transport protein E88.09
tumor marker NEC R97.8
ultrasound results — *see* Abnormal, diagnostic imaging
umbilical cord complicating delivery O69.9
urination NEC R39.198
urine (constituents) R82.90
bile R82.2
cytological examination R82.89
drugs R82.5
fat R82.0
glucose R81
heavy metals R82.6
hemoglobin R82.3
histological examination R82.89
ketones R82.4

Abnormal, abnormality, abnormalities - *continued*

urine (constituents) - *continued*

microbiological examination (culture) R82.79
myoglobin R82.1
positive culture R82.79
protein — *see* Proteinuria
specified substance NEC R82.998
chromoabnormality NEC R82.91
substances nonmedical R82.6
uterine hemorrhage — *see* Hemorrhage, uterus
vectorcardiogram R94.39
visually evoked potential (VEP) R94.112
white blood cells D72.9
specified NEC D72.89
X-ray examination — *see* Abnormal, diagnostic imaging
Abnormity (any organ or part) — *see* Anomaly
Abocclusion M26.29
hemolytic disease (newborn) P55.1
incompatibility reaction ABO — *see* Complication(s), transfusion, incompatibility reaction, ABO
Abolition, language R48.8
Aborter, habitual or recurrent — *see* Loss (of), pregnancy, recurrent
Abortion (complete) (spontaneous) O03.9
with
retained products of conception — *see* Abortion, incomplete
attempted (elective) (failed) O07.4
complicated by O07.30
afibrinogenemia O07.1
cardiac arrest O07.36
chemical damage of pelvic organ (s) O07.34
circulatory collapse O07.31
cystitis O07.38
defibrination syndrome O07.1
electrolyte imbalance O07.33
embolism (air) (amniotic fluid) (blood clot) (fat) (pulmonary) (septic) (soap) O07.2
endometritis O07.0
genital tract and pelvic infection O07.0
hemolysis O07.1
hemorrhage (delayed) (excessive) O07.1
infection
genital tract or pelvic O07.0
urinary tract tract O07.38
intravascular coagulation O07.1
laceration of pelvic organ (s) O07.34
metabolic disorder O07.33
oliguria O07.32
oophoritis O07.0
parametritis O07.0
pelvic peritonitis O07.0
perforation of pelvic organ (s) O07.34
renal failure or shutdown O07.32
salpingitis or salpingo-oophoritis O07.0
sepsis O07.37
shock O07.31
specified condition NEC O07.39
tubular necrosis (renal) O07.32
uremia O07.32
urinary tract infection O07.38
venous complication NEC O07.35
embolism (air) (amniotic fluid) (blood clot) (fat) (pulmonary) (septic) (soap) O07.2
complicated (by) (following) O03.80
afibrinogenemia O03.6
cardiac arrest O03.86
chemical damage of pelvic organ (s) O03.84
circulatory collapse O03.81
cystitis O03.88
defibrination syndrome O03.6
electrolyte imbalance O03.83
embolism (air) (amniotic fluid) (blood clot) (fat) (pulmonary) (septic) (soap) O03.7

Abortion (complete) (spontaneous) - *continued*

complicated (by) (following) - *continued*

endometritis O03.5
genital tract and pelvic infection O03.5
hemolysis O03.6
hemorrhage (delayed) (excessive) O03.6
infection
genital tract or pelvic O03.5
urinary tract O03.88
intravascular coagulation O03.6
laceration of pelvic organ (s) O03.84
metabolic disorder O03.83
oliguria O03.82
oophoritis O03.5
parametritis O03.5
pelvic peritonitis O03.5
perforation of pelvic organ (s) O03.84
renal failure or shutdown O03.82
salpingitis or salpingo-oophoritis O03.5
sepsis O03.87
shock O03.81
specified condition NEC O03.89
tubular necrosis (renal) O03.82
uremia O03.82
urinary tract infection O03.88
venous complication NEC O03.85
embolism (air) (amniotic fluid) (blood clot) (fat) (pulmonary) (septic) (soap) O03.7
failed — *see* Abortion, attempted
habitual or recurrent N96
with current abortion — *see* categories O03-O04
without current pregnancy N96
care in current pregnancy O26.2-
incomplete (spontaneous) O03.4
complicated (by) (following) O03.30
afibrinogenemia O03.1
cardiac arrest O03.36
chemical damage of pelvic organ (s) O03.34
circulatory collapse O03.31
cystitis O03.38
defibrination syndrome O03.1
electrolyte imbalance O03.33
embolism (air) (amniotic fluid) (blood clot) (fat) (pulmonary) (septic) (soap) O03.2
endometritis O03.0
genital tract and pelvic infection O03.0
hemolysis O03.1
hemorrhage (delayed) (excessive) O03.1
infection
genital tract or pelvic O03.0
urinary tract O03.38
intravascular coagulation O03.1
laceration of pelvic organ (s) O03.34
metabolic disorder O03.33
oliguria O03.32
oophoritis O03.0
parametritis O03.0
pelvic peritonitis O03.0
perforation of pelvic organ (s) O03.34
renal failure or shutdown O03.32
salpingitis or salpingo-oophoritis O03.0
sepsis O03.37
shock O03.31
specified condition NEC O03.39
tubular necrosis (renal) O03.32
uremia O03.32
urinary infection O03.38
venous complication NEC O03.35
embolism (air) (amniotic fluid) (blood clot) (fat) (pulmonary) (septic) (soap) O03.2
induced (encounter for) Z33.2
complicated by O04.80
afibrinogenemia O04.6
cardiac arrest O04.86
chemical damage of pelvic organ (s) O04.84
circulatory collapse O04.81
cystitis O04.88
defibrination syndrome O04.6

Abortion (complete) (spontaneous) - *continued*

  induced (encounter for) - *continued*

    complicated by - *continued*

      electrolyte imbalance O04.83

      embolism (air) (amniotic fluid) (blood clot) (fat) (pulmonary) (septic) (soap) O04.7

      endometritis O04.5

      genital tract and pelvic infection O04.5

      hemolysis O04.6

      hemorrhage (delayed) (excessive) O04.6

      infection

        genital tract or pelvic O04.5

        urinary tract O04.88

      intravascular coagulation O04.6

      laceration of pelvic organ (s) O04.84

      metabolic disorder O04.83

      oliguria O04.82

      oophoritis O04.5

      parametritis O04.5

      pelvic peritonitis O04.5

      perforation of pelvic organ (s) O04.84

      renal failure or shutdown O04.82

      salpingitis or salpingo-oophoritis O04.5

      sepsis O04.87

      shock O04.81

      specified condition NEC O04.89

      tubular necrosis (renal) O04.82

      uremia O04.82

      urinary tract infection O04.88

      venous complication NEC O04.85

        embolism (air) (amniotic fluid) (blood clot) (fat) (pulmonary) (septic) (soap) O04.7

  missed O02.1

  spontaneous — *see* Abortion (complete) (spontaneous)

    threatened O20.0

  threatened (spontaneous) O20.0

  tubal O00.10-

    with intrauterine pregnancy O00.11-

Abortus fever A23.1

Aboulomania F60.7

Abrami's disease D59.8

Abramov-Fiedler myocarditis (acute isolated myocarditis) I40.1

Abrasion T14.8

  abdomen, abdominal (wall) S30.811

  alveolar process S00.512

  ankle S90.51-

  antecubital space — *see* Abrasion, elbow

  anus S30.817

  arm (upper) S40.81-

  auditory canal — *see* Abrasion, ear

  auricle — *see* Abrasion, ear

  axilla — *see* Abrasion, arm

  back, lower S30.810

  breast S20.11-

  brow S00.81

  buttock S30.810

  calf — *see* Abrasion, leg

  canthus — *see* Abrasion, eyelid

  cheek S00.81

    internal S00.512

  chest wall — *see* Abrasion, thorax

  chin S00.81

  clitoris S30.814

  cornea S05.0-

  costal region — *see* Abrasion, thorax

  dental K03.1

  digit (s)

    foot — *see* Abrasion, toe

    hand — *see* Abrasion, finger

  ear S00.41-

  elbow S50.31-

  epididymis S30.813

  epigastric region S30.811

  epiglottis S10.11

  esophagus (thoracic) S27.818

    cervical S10.11

  eyebrow — *see* Abrasion, eyelid

  eyelid S00.21-

  face S00.81

  finger (s) S60.41-

Abrasion - *continued*

  finger (s) - *continued*

    index S60.41-

    little S60.41-

    middle S60.41-

    ring S60.41-

  flank S30.811

  foot (except toe (s) alone) S90.81-

    toe — *see* Abrasion, toe

  forearm S50.81-

    elbow only — *see* Abrasion, elbow

  forehead S00.81

  genital organs, external

    female S30.816

    male S30.815

  groin S30.811

  gum S00.512

  hand S60.51-

  head S00.91

    ear — *see* Abrasion, ear

    eyelid — *see* Abrasion, eyelid

    lip S00.511

    nose S00.31

    oral cavity S00.512

    scalp S00.01

    specified site NEC S00.81

  heel — *see* Abrasion, foot

  hip S70.21-

  inguinal region S30.811

  interscapular region S20.419

  jaw S00.81

  knee S80.21-

  labium (majus) (minus) S30.814

  larynx S10.11

  leg (lower) S80.81-

    knee — *see* Abrasion, knee

    upper — *see* Abrasion, thigh

  lip S00.511

  lower back S30.810

  lumbar region S30.810

  malar region S00.81

  mammary — *see* Abrasion, breast

  mastoid region S00.81

  mouth S00.512

  nail

    finger — *see* Abrasion, finger

    toe — *see* Abrasion, toe

  nape S10.91

  nasal S00.31

  neck S10.91

    specified site NEC S10.81

    throat S10.11

  nose S00.31

  occipital region S00.01

  oral cavity S00.512

  orbital region — *see* Abrasion, eyelid

  palate S00.512

  palm — *see* Abrasion, hand

  parietal region S00.01

  pelvis S30.810

  penis S30.812

  perineum

    female S30.814

    male S30.810

  periocular area — *see* Abrasion, eyelid

  phalanges

    finger — *see* Abrasion, finger

    toe — *see* Abrasion, toe

  pharynx S10.11

  pinna — *see* Abrasion, ear

  popliteal space — *see* Abrasion, knee

  prepuce S30.812

  pubic region S30.810

  pudendum

    female S30.816

    male S30.815

  sacral region S30.810

  scalp S00.01

  scapular region — *see* Abrasion, shoulder

  scrotum S30.813

  shin — *see* Abrasion, leg

  shoulder S40.21-

  skin NEC T14.8

  sternal region S20.319

  submaxillary region S00.81

Abrasion - *continued*

  submental region S00.81

  subungual

    finger (s) — *see* Abrasion, finger

    toe (s) — *see* Abrasion, toe

  supraclavicular fossa S10.81

  supraorbital S00.81

  temple S00.81

  temporal region S00.81

  testis S30.813

  thigh S70.31-

  thorax, thoracic (wall) S20.91

    back S20.41-

    front S20.31-

  throat S10.11

  thumb S60.31-

  toe (s) (lesser) S90.416

    great S90.41-

  tongue S00.512

  tooth, teeth (dentifrice) (habitual) (hard tissues) (occupational) (ritual) (traditional) K03.1

  trachea S10.11

  tunica vaginalis S30.813

  tympanum, tympanic membrane — *see* Abrasion, ear

  uvula S00.512

  vagina S30.814

  vocal cords S10.11

  vulva S30.814

  wrist S60.81-

Abrism — *see* Poisoning, food, noxious, plant

Abruptio placentae O45.9-

  with

    afibrinogenemia O45.01-

    coagulation defect O45.00-

      specified NEC O45.09-

    disseminated intravascular coagulation O45.01-

    hypofibrinogenemia O45.01-

  specified NEC O45.8-

Abruption, placenta — *see* Abruptio placentae

Abscess (connective tissue) (embolic) (fistulous) (infective) (metastatic) (multiple) (pernicious) (pyogenic) (septic) L02.91

  with

    diverticular disease (intestine) K57.80

      with bleeding K57.81

      large intestine K57.20

        with

          bleeding K57.21

          small intestine K57.40

            with bleeding K57.41

      small intestine K57.00

        with

          bleeding K57.01

          large intestine K57.40

            with bleeding K57.41

    lymphangitis - code by site under Abscess

  abdomen, abdominal

    cavity K65.1

    wall L02.211

  abdominopelvic K65.1

  accessory sinus — *see* Sinusitis

  adrenal (capsule) (gland) E27.8

  alveolar K04.7

    with sinus K04.6

  amebic A06.4

    brain (and liver or lung abscess) A06.6

    genitourinary tract A06.82

    liver (without mention of brain or lung abscess) A06.4

    lung (and liver) (without mention of brain abscess) A06.5

    specified site NEC A06.89

    spleen A06.89

  anerobic A48.0

  ankle — *see* Abscess, lower limb

  anorectal K61.2

  antecubital space — *see* Abscess, upper limb

  antrum (chronic) (Highmore) — *see* Sinusitis, maxillary

  anus K61.0

Abscess (connective tissue) (embolic) (fistulous) (infective) (metastatic) (multiple) (pernicious) (pyogenic) (septic) - *continued*
  apical (tooth) K04.7
    with sinus (alveolar) K04.6
  appendix K35.33
  areola (acute) (chronic) (nonpuerperal) N61.1
    puerperal, postpartum or gestational — *see* Infection, nipple
  arm (any part) — *see* Abscess, upper limb
  artery (wall) I77.89
  atheromatous I77.2
  auricle, ear — *see* Abscess, ear, external
  axilla (region) L02.41-
    lymph gland or node L04.2
  back (any part, except buttock) L02.212
  Bartholin's gland N75.1
    with
      abortion — *see* Abortion, by type
      complicated by, sepsis
      ectopic or molar pregnancy O08.0
      following ectopic or molar pregnancy O08.0
  Bezold's — *see* Mastoiditis, acute
  bilharziasis B65.1
  bladder (wall) — *see* Cystitis, specified type NEC
  bone (subperiosteal) — *see also* Osteomyelitis, specified type NEC
    accessory sinus (chronic) — *see* Sinusitis
    chronic or old — *see* Osteomyelitis, chronic
    jaw (lower) (upper) M27.2
    mastoid — *see* Mastoiditis, acute, subperiosteal
    petrous — *see* Petrositis
    spinal (tuberculous) A18.01
      nontuberculous — *see* Osteomyelitis, vertebra
  bowel K63.0
  brain (any part) (cystic) (otogenic) G06.0
    amebic (with abscess of any other site) A06.6
    gonococcal A54.82
    pheomycotic (chromomycotic) B43.1
    tuberculous A17.81
  breast (acute) (chronic) (nonpuerperal) N61.1
    newborn P39.0
    puerperal, postpartum, gestational — *see* Mastitis, obstetric, purulent
  broad ligament N73.2
    acute N73.0
    chronic N73.1
  Brodie's (localized) (chronic) M86.8X-
  bronchi J98.09
  buccal cavity K12.2
  bulbourethral gland N34.0
  bursa M71.00
    ankle M71.07-
    elbow M71.02-
    foot M71.07-
    hand M71.04-
    hip M71.05-
    knee M71.06-
    multiple sites M71.09
    pharyngeal J39.1
    shoulder M71.01-
    specified site NEC M71.08
    wrist M71.03-
  buttock L02.31
  canthus — *see* Blepharoconjunctivitis
  cartilage — *see* Disorder, cartilage, specified type NEC
  cecum K35.33
  cerebellum, cerebellar G06.0
    sequelae G09
  cerebral (embolic) G06.0
    sequelae G09
  cervical (meaning neck) L02.11
    lymph gland or node L04.0
  cervix (stump) (uteri) — *see* Cervicitis
  cheek (external) L02.01
    inner K12.2
  chest J86.9

Abscess (connective tissue) (embolic) (fistulous) (infective) (metastatic) (multiple) (pernicious) (pyogenic) (septic) - *continued*
  chest - *continued*
    with fistula J86.0
    wall L02.213
  chin L02.01
  choroid — *see* Inflammation, chorioretinal
  circumtonsillar J36
  cold (lung) (tuberculous) — *see also* Tuberculosis, abscess, lung
    articular — *see* Tuberculosis, joint
  colon (wall) K63.0
  colostomy K94.02
  conjunctiva — *see* Conjunctivitis, acute
  cornea H16.31-
  corpus
    cavernosum N48.21
    luteum — *see* Oophoritis
  Cowper's gland N34.0
  cranium G06.0
  cul-de-sac (Douglas') (posterior) — *see* Peritonitis, pelvic, female
  cutaneous — *see* Abscess, by site
  dental K04.7
    with sinus (alveolar) K04.6
  dentoalveolar K04.7
    with sinus K04.6
  diaphragm, diaphragmatic K65.1
  Douglas' cul-de-sac or pouch — *see* Peritonitis, pelvic, female
  Dubois A50.59
  ear (middle) — *see also* Otitis, media, suppurative
    acute — *see* Otitis, media, suppurative, acute
    external H60.0-
  entamebic — *see* Abscess, amebic
  enterostomy K94.12
  epididymis N45.4
  epidural G06.2
    brain G06.0
    spinal cord G06.1
  epiglottis J38.7
  epiploon, epiploic K65.1
  erysipelatous — *see* Erysipelas
  esophagus K20.8
  ethmoid (bone) (chronic) (sinus) J32.2
  external auditory canal — *see* Abscess, ear, external
  extradural G06.2
    brain G06.0
      sequelae G09
    spinal cord G06.1
  extraperitoneal K68.19
  eye — *see* Endophthalmitis, purulent
  eyelid H00.03-
  face (any part, except ear, eye and nose) L02.01
  fallopian tube — *see* Salpingitis
  fascia M72.8
  fauces J39.1
  fecal K63.0
  femoral (region) — *see* Abscess, lower limb
  filaria, filarial — *see* Infestation, filarial
  finger (any) — *see also* Abscess, hand
    nail — *see* Cellulitis, finger
  foot L02.61-
  forehead L02.01
  frontal sinus (chronic) J32.1
  gallbladder K81.0
  genital organ or tract
    female (external) N76.4
    male N49.9
      multiple sites N49.8
      specified NEC N49.8
  gestational mammary O91.11-
  gestational subareolar O91.11-
  gingival — *see* Periodontitis, localized
  gland, glandular (lymph) (acute) — *see* Lymphadenitis, acute
  gluteal (region) L02.31
  gonorrheal — *see* Gonococcus
  groin L02.214
  gum — *see* Periodontitis, localized

Abscess (connective tissue) (embolic) (fistulous) (infective) (metastatic) (multiple) (pernicious) (pyogenic) (septic) - *continued*
  hand L02.51-
  head NEC L02.811
    face (any part, except ear, eye and nose) L02.01
  heart — *see* Carditis
  heel — *see* Abscess, foot
  helminthic — *see* Infestation, helminth
  hepatic (cholangitic) (hematogenic) (lymphogenic) (pylephlebitic) K75.0
    amebic A06.4
  hip (region) — *see* Abscess, lower limb
  horseshoe K61.31
  ileocecal K35.33
  ileostomy (bud) K94.12
  iliac (region) L02.214
    fossa K35.33
  infraclavicular (fossa) — *see* Abscess, upper limb
  inguinal (region) L02.214
    lymph gland or node L04.1
  intersphincteric K61.4
  intestine, intestinal NEC K63.0
    rectal K61.1
  intra-abdominal — *see also* Abscess, peritoneum K65.1
    following procedure T81.43
      obstetrical O86.03
    postprocedural T81.49
      retroperitoneal K68.11
  intracranial G06.0
  intramammary — *see* Abscess, breast
  intramuscular, following procedure T81.42
    obstetrical O86.02
  intraorbital — *see* Abscess, orbit
  intraperitoneal K65.1
  intrasphincteric (anus) K61.4
  intraspinal G06.1
  intratonsillar J36
  ischiorectal (fossa) (specified NEC) K61.39
  jaw (bone) (lower) (upper) M27.2
  joint — *see* Arthritis, pyogenic or pyemic
    spine (tuberculous) A18.01
      nontuberculous — *see* Spondylopathy, infective
  kidney N15.1
    with calculus N20.0
      with hydronephrosis N13.6
    puerperal (postpartum) O86.21
  knee — *see also* Abscess, lower limb
    joint M00.9
  labium (majus) (minus) N76.4
  lacrimal
    caruncle — *see* Inflammation, lacrimal, passages, acute
    gland — *see* Dacryoadenitis
    passages (duct) (sac) — *see* Inflammation, lacrimal, passages, acute
  lacunar N34.0
  larynx J38.7
  lateral (alveolar) K04.7
    with sinus K04.6
  leg (any part) — *see* Abscess, lower limb
  lens H27.8
  lingual K14.0
    tonsil J36
  lip K13.0
  Littre's gland N34.0
  liver (cholangitic) (hematogenic) (lymphogenic) (pylephlebitic) (pyogenic) K75.0
    amebic (due to Entamoeba histolytica) (dysenteric) (tropical) A06.4
      with
        brain abscess (and liver or lung abscess) A06.6
        lung abscess A06.5
  loin (region) L02.211
  lower limb L02.41-
  lumbar (tuberculous) A18.01
    nontuberculous L02.212
  lung (miliary) (putrid) J85.2
    with pneumonia J85.1

Abscess (connective tissue) (embolic) (fistulous) (infective) (metastatic) (multiple) (pernicious) (pyogenic) (septic) - *continued*
  lung (miliary) (putrid) - *continued*
    with pneumonia - *continued*
      due to specified organism (see
        Pneumonia, in (due to))
    amebic (with liver abscess) A06.5
      with
        brain abscess A06.6
        pneumonia A06.5
  lymph, lymphatic, gland or node (acute) —
    see also Lymphadenitis, acute
    mesentery I88.0
  malar M27.2
  mammary gland — *see* Abscess, breast
  marginal, anus K61.0
  mastoid — *see* Mastoiditis, acute
  maxilla, maxillary M27.2
    molar (tooth) K04.7
      with sinus K04.6
    premolar K04.7
    sinus (chronic) J32.0
  mediastinum J85.3
  meibomian gland — *see* Hordeolum
  meninges G06.2
  mesentery, mesenteric K65.1
  mesosalpinx — *see* Salpingitis
  mons pubis L02.215
  mouth (floor) K12.2
  muscle — *see* Myositis, infective
  myocardium I40.0
  nabothian (follicle) — *see* Cervicitis
  nasal J32.9
  nasopharyngeal J39.1
  navel L02.216
    newborn P38.9
      with mild hemorrhage P38.1
      without hemorrhage P38.9
  neck (region) L02.11
    lymph gland or node L04.0
  nephritic — *see* Abscess, kidney
  nipple N61.1
    associated with
      lactation — *see* Pregnancy, complicated
        by
      pregnancy — *see* Pregnancy,
        complicated by
  nose (external) (fossa) (septum) J34.0
    sinus (chronic) — *see* Sinusitis
  omentum K65.1
  operative wound T81.49
  orbit, orbital — *see* Cellulitis, orbit
  otogenic G06.0
  ovary, ovarian (corpus luteum) — *see*
    Oophoritis
  oviduct — *see* Oophoritis
  palate (soft) K12.2
    hard M27.2
  palmar (space) — *see* Abscess, hand
  pancreas (duct) — *see* Pancreatitis, acute
  parafrenal N48.21
  parametric, parametrium N73.2
    acute N73.0
    chronic N73.1
  paranephric N15.1
  parapancreatic — *see* Pancreatitis, acute
  parapharyngeal J39.0
  pararectal K61.1
  parasinus — *see* Sinusitis
  parauterine — *see also* Disease, pelvis,
    inflammatory N73.2
  paravaginal — *see* Vaginitis
  parietal region (scalp) L02.811
  parodontal — *see* Periodontitis, aggressive,
    localized
  parotid (duct) (gland) K11.3
    region K12.2
  pectoral (region) L02.213
  pelvis, pelvic
    female — *see* Disease, pelvis,
      inflammatory
    male, peritoneal K65.1
  penis N48.21

Abscess (connective tissue) (embolic) (fistulous) (infective) (metastatic) (multiple) (pernicious) (pyogenic) (septic) - *continued*
  penis - *continued*
    gonococcal (accessory gland)
      (periurethral) A54.1
  perianal K61.0
  periapical K04.7
    with sinus (alveolar) K04.6
  periappendicular K35.33
  pericardial I30.1
  pericecal K35.33
  pericemental — *see* Periodontitis, aggressive,
    localized
  pericholecystic — *see* Cholecystitis, acute
  pericoronal — *see* Periodontitis, aggressive,
    localized
  peridental — *see* Periodontitis, aggressive,
    localized
  perimetric — *see also* Disease, pelvis,
    inflammatory N73.2
  perinephric, perinephritic — *see* Abscess,
    kidney
  perineum, perineal (superficial) L02.215
    urethra N34.0
  periodontal (parietal) — *see* Periodontitis,
    aggressive, localized
    apical K04.7
  periosteum, periosteal — *see also*
    Osteomyelitis, specified type NEC
    with osteomyelitis — *see also*
      Osteomyelitis, specified type NEC
    acute — *see* Osteomyelitis, acute
    chronic — *see* Osteomyelitis, chronic
  peripharyngeal J39.0
  peripleuritic J86.9
    with fistula J86.0
  periprostatic N41.2
  perirectal K61.1
  perirenal (tissue) — *see* Abscess, kidney
  perisinuous (nose) — *see* Sinusitis
  peritoneum, peritoneal (perforated)
    (ruptured) K65.1
    with appendicitis — *see also*
      Appendicitis K35.33
    pelvic
      female — *see* Peritonitis, pelvic, female
      male K65.1
    postoperative T81.49
    puerperal, postpartum, childbirth O85
    tuberculous A18.31
  peritonsillar J36
  perityphlic K35.33
  periureteral N28.89
  periurethral N34.0
    gonococcal (accessory gland)
      (periurethral) A54.1
  periuterine — *see also* Disease, pelvis,
    inflammatory N73.2
  perivesical — *see* Cystitis, specified type
    NEC
  petrous bone — *see* Petrositis
  phagedenic NOS L02.91
    chancroid A57
  pharynx, pharyngeal (lateral) J39.1
  pilonidal L05.01
  pituitary (gland) E23.6
  pleura J86.9
    with fistula J86.0
  popliteal — *see* Abscess, lower limb
  postcecal K35.33
  postlaryngeal J38.7
  postnasal J34.0
  postoperative (any site) — *see also* Infection,
    postoperative wound T81.49
    retroperitoneal K68.11
  postpharyngeal J39.0
  posttonsillar J36
  post-typhoid A01.09
  pouch of Douglas — *see* Peritonitis, pelvic,
    female
  premammary — *see* Abscess, breast
  prepatellar — *see* Abscess, lower limb
  prostate N41.2
    gonococcal (acute) (chronic) A54.22

Abscess (connective tissue) (embolic) (fistulous) (infective) (metastatic) (multiple) (pernicious) (pyogenic) (septic) - *continued*
  psoas muscle K68.12
  puerperal - code by site under Puerperal,
    abscess
  pulmonary — *see* Abscess, lung
  pulp, pulpal (dental) K04.01
    irreversible K04.02
    reversible K04.01
  rectovaginal septum K63.0
  rectovesical — *see* Cystitis, specified type
    NEC
  rectum K61.1
  renal — *see* Abscess, kidney
  retina — *see* Inflammation, chorioretinal
  retrobulbar — *see* Abscess, orbit
  retrocecal K65.1
  retrolaryngeal J38.7
  retromammary — *see* Abscess, breast
  retroperitoneal NEC K68.19
    postprocedural K68.11
  retropharyngeal J39.0
  retrouterine — *see* Peritonitis, pelvic, female
  retrovesical — *see* Cystitis, specified type
    NEC
  root, tooth K04.7
    with sinus (alveolar) K04.6
  round ligament — *see also* Disease, pelvis,
    inflammatory N73.2
  rupture (spontaneous) NOS L02.91
  sacrum (tuberculous) A18.01
    nontuberculous M46.28
  salivary (duct) (gland) K11.3
  scalp (any part) L02.811
  scapular — *see* Osteomyelitis, specified type
    NEC
  sclera — *see* Scleritis
  scrofulous (tuberculous) A18.2
  scrotum N49.2
  seminal vesicle N49.0
  septal, dental K04.7
    with sinus (alveolar) K04.6
  serous — *see* Periostitis
  shoulder (region) — *see* Abscess, upper limb
  sigmoid K63.0
  sinus (accessory) (chronic) (nasal) — *see*
    also Sinusitis
    intracranial venous (any) G06.0
  Skene's duct or gland N34.0
  skin — *see* Abscess, by site
  specified site NEC L02.818
  spermatic cord N49.1
  sphenoidal (sinus) (chronic) J32.3
  spinal cord (any part) (staphylococcal) G06.1
    tuberculous A17.81
  spine (column) (tuberculous) A18.01
    epidural G06.1
    nontuberculous — *see* Osteomyelitis,
      vertebra
  spleen D73.3
    amebic A06.89
  stitch T81.41
    following an obstetrical procedure O86.01
  subarachnoid G06.2
    brain G06.0
    spinal cord G06.1
  subareolar — *see* Abscess, breast
  subcecal K35.33
  subcutaneous — *see also* Abscess, by site
    following procedure T81.41
      obstetrical O86.01
    pheomycotic (chromomycotic) B43.2
  subdiaphragmatic K65.1
  subdural G06.2
    brain G06.0
      sequelae G09
    spinal cord G06.1
  sub-fascial, following an obstetrical
    procedure O86.02
  subgaleal L02.811
  subhepatic K65.1
  sublingual K12.2
    gland K11.3
  submammary — *see* Abscess, breast

Abscess (connective tissue) (embolic) (fistulous) (infective) (metastatic) (multiple) (pernicious) (pyogenic) (septic) - *continued*
submandibular (region) (space) (triangle) K12.2
  gland K11.3
submaxillary (region) L02.01
  gland K11.3
submental L02.01
  gland K11.3
subperiosteal — *see* Osteomyelitis, specified type NEC
subphrenic K65.1
  following an obstetrical procedure O86.03
  postoperative T81.43
suburethral N34.0
sudoriparous L75.8
supraclavicular (fossa) — *see* Abscess, upper limb
supralevator K61.5
suprapelvic, acute N73.0
suprarenal (capsule) (gland) E27.8
sweat gland L74.8
tear duct — *see* Inflammation, lacrimal, passages, acute
temple L02.01
temporal region L02.01
temporosphenoidal G06.0
tendon (sheath) M65.00
  ankle M65.07-
  foot M65.07-
  forearm M65.03-
  hand M65.04-
  lower leg M65.06-
  pelvic region M65.05-
  shoulder region M65.01-
  specified site NEC M65.08
  thigh M65.05-
  upper arm M65.02-
testis N45.4
thigh — *see* Abscess, lower limb
thorax J86.9
  with fistula J86.0
throat J39.1
thumb — *see also* Abscess, hand
  nail — *see* Cellulitis, finger
thymus (gland) E32.1
thyroid (gland) E06.0
toe (any) — *see also* Abscess, foot
  nail — *see* Cellulitis, toe
tongue (staphylococcal) K14.0
tonsil (s) (lingual) J36
tonsillopharyngeal J36
tooth, teeth (root) K04.7
  with sinus (alveolar) K04.6
  supporting structures NEC — *see* Periodontitis, aggressive, localized
trachea J39.8
trunk L02.219
  abdominal wall L02.211
  back L02.212
  chest wall L02.213
  groin L02.214
  perineum L02.215
  umbilicus L02.216
tubal — *see* Salpingitis
tuberculous — *see* Tuberculosis, abscess
tubo-ovarian — *see* Salpingo-oophoritis
tunica vaginalis N49.1
umbilicus L02.216
upper
  limb L02.41-
  respiratory J39.8
urethral (gland) N34.0
urinary N34.0
uterus, uterine (wall) — *see also* Endometritis
  ligament — *see also* Disease, pelvis, inflammatory N73.2
  neck — *see* Cervicitis
uvula K12.2
vagina (wall) — *see* Vaginitis
vaginorectal — *see* Vaginitis
vas deferens N49.1
vermiform appendix K35.33

Abscess (connective tissue) (embolic) (fistulous) (infective) (metastatic) (multiple) (pernicious) (pyogenic) (septic) - *continued*
vertebra (column) (tuberculous) A18.01
  nontuberculous — *see* Osteomyelitis, vertebra
vesical — *see* Cystitis, specified type NEC
vesico-uterine pouch — *see* Peritonitis, pelvic, female
vitreous (humor) — *see* Endophthalmitis, purulent
vocal cord J38.3
von Bezold's — *see* Mastoiditis, acute
vulva N76.4
vulvovaginal gland N75.1
web space — *see* Abscess, hand
wound T81.49
wrist — *see* Abscess, upper limb

Absence (of) (organ or part) (complete or partial)
adrenal (gland) (congenital) Q89.1
  acquired E89.6
albumin in blood E88.09
alimentary tract (congenital) Q45.8
  upper Q40.8
alveolar process (acquired) — *see* Anomaly, alveolar
ankle (acquired) Z89.44-
anus (congenital) Q42.3
  with fistula Q42.2
aorta (congenital) Q25.41
appendix, congenital Q42.8
arm (acquired) Z89.20-
  above elbow Z89.22-
    congenital (with hand present) — *see* Agenesis, arm, with hand present
    and hand — *see* Agenesis, forearm, and hand
  below elbow Z89.21-
    congenital (with hand present) — *see* Agenesis, arm, with hand present
    and hand — *see* Agenesis, forearm, and hand
  congenital — *see* Defect, reduction, upper limb
  shoulder (following explanation of shoulder joint prosthesis) (joint) (with or without presence of antibiotic-impregnated cement spacer) Z89.23-
    congenital (with hand present) — *see* Agenesis, arm, with hand present
artery (congenital) (peripheral) Q27.8
  brain Q28.3
  coronary Q24.5
  pulmonary Q25.79
  specified NEC Q27.8
  umbilical Q27.0
atrial septum (congenital) Q21.1
auditory canal (congenital) (external) Q16.1
auricle (ear) , congenital Q16.0
bile, biliary duct, congenital Q44.5
bladder (acquired) Z90.6
  congenital Q64.5
bowel sounds R19.11
brain Q00.0
  part of Q04.3
breast (s) (and nipple (s)) (acquired) Z90.1-
  congenital Q83.8
broad ligament Q50.6
bronchus (congenital) Q32.4
canaliculus lacrimalis, congenital Q10.4
cerebellum (vermis) Q04.3
cervix (acquired) (with uterus) Z90.710
  with remaining uterus Z90.712
  congenital Q51.5
chin, congenital Q18.8
cilia (congenital) Q10.3
  acquired — *see* Madarosis
clitoris (congenital) Q52.6
coccyx, congenital Q76.49
cold sense R20.8
congenital
  lumen — *see* Atresia
  organ or site NEC — *see* Agenesis
  septum — *see* Imperfect, closure

Absence (of) (organ or part) (complete or partial) - *continued*
corpus callosum Q04.0
cricoid cartilage, congenital Q31.8
diaphragm (with hernia) , congenital Q79.1
digestive organ (s) or tract, congenital Q45.8
  acquired NEC Z90.49
  upper Q40.8
ductus arteriosus Q28.8
duodenum (acquired) Z90.49
  congenital Q41.0
ear, congenital Q16.9
  acquired H93.8-
  auricle Q16.0
  external Q16.0
  inner Q16.5
  lobe, lobule Q17.8
  middle, except ossicles Q16.4
    ossicles Q16.3
  ossicles Q16.3
ejaculatory duct (congenital) Q55.4
endocrine gland (congenital) NEC Q89.2
  acquired E89.89
epididymis (congenital) Q55.4
  acquired Z90.79
epiglottis, congenital Q31.8
esophagus (congenital) Q39.8
  acquired (partial) Z90.49
eustachian tube (congenital) Q16.2
extremity (acquired) Z89.9
  congenital Q73.0
  knee (following explanation of knee joint prosthesis) (joint) (with or without presence of antibiotic-impregnated cement spacer) Z89.52-
  lower (above knee) Z89.619
    below knee Z89.51-
  upper — *see* Absence, arm
eye (acquired) Z90.01
  congenital Q11.1
  muscle (congenital) Q10.3
eyeball (acquired) Z90.01
eyelid (fold) (congenital) Q10.3
  acquired Z90.01
face, specified part NEC Q18.8
fallopian tube (s) (acquired) Z90.79
  congenital Q50.6
family member (causing problem in home) NEC — *see also* Disruption, family Z63.32
femur, congenital — *see* Defect, reduction, lower limb, longitudinal, femur
fibrinogen (congenital) D68.2
  acquired D65
finger (s) (acquired) Z89.02-
  congenital — *see* Agenesis, hand
foot (acquired) Z89.43-
  congenital — *see* Agenesis, foot
forearm (acquired) — *see* Absence, arm, below elbow
gallbladder (acquired) Z90.49
  congenital Q44.0
gamma globulin in blood D80.1
  hereditary D80.0
genital organs
  acquired (female) (male) Z90.79
  female, congenital Q52.8
    external Q52.71
    internal NEC Q52.8
  male, congenital Q55.8
genitourinary organs, congenital NEC
  female Q52.8
  male Q55.8
globe (acquired) Z90.01
  congenital Q11.1
glottis, congenital Q31.8
hand and wrist (acquired) Z89.11-
  congenital — *see* Agenesis, hand
head, part (acquired) NEC Z90.09
heat sense R20.8
hip (following explanation of hip joint prosthesis) (joint) (with or without presence of antibiotic-impregnated cement spacer) Z89.62-
hymen (congenital) Q52.4

Absence (of) (organ or part) (complete or partial) - *continued*
ileum (acquired) Z90.49
  congenital Q41.2
immunoglobulin, isolated NEC D80.3
  IgA D80.2
  IgG D80.3
  IgM D80.4
incus (acquired) — *see* Loss, ossicles, ear
  congenital Q16.3
inner ear, congenital Q16.5
intestine (acquired) (small) Z90.49
  congenital Q41.9
    specified NEC Q41.8
  large Z90.49
    congenital Q42.9
      specified NEC Q42.8
iris, congenital Q13.1
jejunum (acquired) Z90.49
  congenital Q41.1
joint
  acquired
    hip (following explantation of hip joint prosthesis) (with or without presence of antibiotic-impregnated cement spacer) Z89.62-
    knee (following explantation of knee joint prosthesis) (with or without presence of antibiotic-impregnated cement spacer) Z89.52-
    shoulder (following explantation of shoulder joint prosthesis) (with or without presence of antibiotic-impregnated cement spacer) Z89.23-
  congenital NEC Q74.8
kidney (s) (acquired) Z90.5
  congenital Q60.2
    bilateral Q60.1
    unilateral Q60.0
knee (following explantation of knee joint prosthesis) (joint) (with or without presence of antibiotic-impregnated cement spacer) Z89.52-
labyrinth, membranous Q16.5
larynx (congenital) Q31.8
  acquired Z90.02
leg (acquired) (above knee) Z89.61-
  below knee (acquired) Z89.51-
  congenital — *see* Defect, reduction, lower limb
lens (acquired) — *see also* Aphakia
  congenital Q12.3
  post cataract extraction Z98.4-
limb (acquired) — *see* Absence, extremity
lip Q38.6
liver (congenital) Q44.7
lung (fissure) (lobe) (bilateral) (unilateral) (congenital) Q33.3
  acquired (any part) Z90.2
menstruation — *see* Amenorrhea
muscle (congenital) (pectoral) Q79.8
  ocular Q10.3
neck, part Q18.8
neutrophil — *see* Agranulocytosis
nipple (s) (with breast (s)) (acquired) Z90.1-
  congenital Q83.2
nose (congenital) Q30.1
  acquired Z90.09
organ
  of Corti, congenital Q16.5
  or site, congenital NEC Q89.8
    acquired NEC Z90.89
osseous meatus (ear) Q16.4
ovary (acquired)
  bilateral Z90.722
  congenital
    bilateral Q50.02
    unilateral Q50.01
  unilateral Z90.721
oviduct (acquired)
  bilateral Z90.722
  congenital Q50.6
  unilateral Z90.721
pancreas (congenital) Q45.0

Absence (of) (organ or part) (complete or partial) - *continued*
pancreas (congenital) - *continued*
  acquired Z90.410
    complete Z90.410
    partial Z90.411
    total Z90.410
parathyroid gland (acquired) E89.2
  congenital Q89.2
patella, congenital Q74.1
penis (congenital) Q55.5
  acquired Z90.79
pericardium (congenital) Q24.8
pituitary gland (congenital) Q89.2
  acquired E89.3
prostate (acquired) Z90.79
  congenital Q55.4
pulmonary valve Q22.0
punctum lacrimale (congenital) Q10.4
radius, congenital — *see* Defect, reduction, upper limb, longitudinal, radius
rectum (congenital) Q42.1
  with fistula Q42.0
  acquired Z90.49
respiratory organ NOS Q34.9
rib (acquired) Z90.89
  congenital Q76.6
sacrum, congenital Q76.49
salivary gland (s) , congenital Q38.4
scrotum, congenital Q55.29
seminal vesicles (congenital) Q55.4
  acquired Z90.79
septum
  atrial (congenital) Q21.1
  between aorta and pulmonary artery Q21.4
  ventricular (congenital) Q20.4
sex chromosome
  female phenotype Q97.8
  male phenotype Q98.8
skull bone (congenital) Q75.8
  with
    anencephaly Q00.0
    encephalocele — *see* Encephalocele
    hydrocephalus Q03.9
      with spina bifida — *see* Spina bifida, by site, with hydrocephalus
    microcephaly Q02
spermatic cord, congenital Q55.4
spine, congenital Q76.49
spleen (congenital) Q89.01
  acquired Z90.81
sternum, congenital Q76.7
stomach (acquired) (partial) Z90.3
  congenital Q40.2
superior vena cava, congenital Q26.8
teeth, tooth (congenital) K00.0
  acquired (complete) K08.109
    class I K08.101
    class II K08.102
    class III K08.103
    class IV K08.104
    due to
      caries K08.139
        class I K08.131
        class II K08.132
        class III K08.133
        class IV K08.134
      periodontal disease K08.129
        class I K08.121
        class II K08.122
        class III K08.123
        class IV K08.124
      specified NEC K08.199
        class I K08.191
        class II K08.192
        class III K08.193
        class IV K08.194
      trauma K08.119
        class I K08.111
        class II K08.112
        class III K08.113
        class IV K08.114
    partial K08.409
      class I K08.401
      class II K08.402

Absence (of) (organ or part) (complete or partial) - *continued*
teeth, tooth (congenital) - *continued*
  acquired (complete) - *continued*
    partial - *continued*
      class III K08.403
      class IV K08.404
      due to
        caries K08.439
          class I K08.431
          class II K08.432
          class III K08.433
          class IV K08.434
        periodontal disease K08.429
          class I K08.421
          class II K08.422
          class III K08.423
          class IV K08.424
        specified NEC K08.499
          class I K08.491
          class II K08.492
          class III K08.493
          class IV K08.494
        trauma K08.419
          class I K08.411
          class II K08.412
          class III K08.413
          class IV K08.414
tendon (congenital) Q79.8
testis (congenital) Q55.0
  acquired Z90.79
thumb (acquired) Z89.01-
  congenital — *see* Agenesis, hand
thymus gland Q89.2
thyroid (gland) (acquired) E89.0
  cartilage, congenital Q31.8
  congenital E03.1
toe (s) (acquired) Z89.42-
  with foot — *see* Absence, foot and ankle
  congenital — *see* Agenesis, foot
  great Z89.41-
tongue, congenital Q38.3
trachea (cartilage) , congenital Q32.1
transverse aortic arch, congenital Q25.49
tricuspid valve Q22.4
umbilical artery, congenital Q27.0
upper arm and forearm with hand present, congenital — *see* Agenesis, arm, with hand present
ureter (congenital) Q62.4
  acquired Z90.6
urethra, congenital Q64.5
uterus (acquired) Z90.710
  with cervix Z90.710
  with remaining cervical stump Z90.711
  congenital Q51.0
uvula, congenital Q38.5
vagina, congenital Q52.0
vas deferens (congenital) Q55.4
  acquired Z90.79
vein (peripheral) congenital NEC Q27.8
  cerebral Q28.3
  digestive system Q27.8
  great Q26.8
  lower limb Q27.8
  portal Q26.5
  precerebral Q28.1
  specified site NEC Q27.8
  upper limb Q27.8
vena cava (inferior) (superior) , congenital Q26.8
ventricular septum Q20.4
vertebra, congenital Q76.49
vulva, congenital Q52.71
wrist (acquired) Z89.12-
Absorbent system disease I87.8
Absorption
carbohydrate, disturbance K90.49
chemical — *see* Table of Drugs and Chemicals
  through placenta (newborn) P04.9
    environmental substance P04.6
    nutritional substance P04.5
    obstetric anesthetic or analgesic drug P04.0

Absorption - *continued*
  drug NEC — *see* Table of Drugs and
      Chemicals
    addictive
      through placenta (newborn) — *see also*
          Newborn, affected by, maternal,
          use of P04.40
        cocaine P04.41
        hallucinogens P04.42
        specified drug NEC P04.49
    medicinal
      through placenta (newborn) P04.19
    through placenta (newborn) P04.19
      obstetric anesthetic or analgesic
          drug P04.0
  fat, disturbance K90.49
    pancreatic K90.3
  noxious substance — *see* Table of Drugs and
      Chemicals
  protein, disturbance K90.49
  starch, disturbance K90.49
  toxic substance — *see* Table of Drugs and
      Chemicals
  uremic — *see* Uremia
Abstinence symptoms, syndrome
  alcohol F10.239
    with delirium F10.231
  cocaine F14.23
  neonatal P96.1
  nicotine — *see* Dependence, drug, nicotine,
      with, withdrawal
  opioid F11.93
    with dependence F11.23
  psychoactive NEC F19.939
    with
      delirium F19.931
      dependence F19.239
        with
          delirium F19.231
          perceptual disturbance F19.232
        uncomplicated F19.230
      perceptual disturbance F19.932
    uncomplicated F19.930
  sedative F13.939
    with
      delirium F13.931
      dependence F13.239
        with
          delirium F13.231
          perceptual disturbance F13.232
        uncomplicated F13.230
      perceptual disturbance F13.932
    uncomplicated F13.930
  stimulant NEC F15.93
    with dependence F15.23
Abulia R68.89
Abulomania F60.7
Abuse
  adult — *see* Maltreatment, adult
    as reason for
      couple seeking advice (including
          offender) Z63.0
  alcohol (non-dependent) F10.10
    with
      anxiety disorder F10.180
      intoxication F10.129
        with delirium F10.121
        uncomplicated F10.120
      mood disorder F10.14
      other specified disorder F10.188
      psychosis F10.159
        delusions F10.150
        hallucinations F10.151
      sexual dysfunction F10.181
      sleep disorder F10.182
      unspecified disorder F10.19
    counseling and surveillance Z71.41
    in remission (early) (sustained) F10.11
  amphetamine (or related substance) — *see
      also* Abuse, drug, stimulant NEC
    stimulant NEC F15.10
      with
        anxiety disorder F15.180
        intoxication F15.129
          with

Abuse - *continued*
  amphetamine (or related substance) -
      continued
    stimulant NEC - *continued*
      with - *continued*
        intoxication - *continued*
          with - *continued*
            delirium F15.121
            perceptual disturbance F15.122
  analgesics (non-prescribed) (over the
      counter) F55.8
  antacids F55.0
  antidepressants — *see* Abuse, drug,
      psychoactive NEC
  anxiolytic — *see* Abuse, drug, sedative
  barbiturates — *see* Abuse, drug, sedative
  caffeine — *see* Abuse, drug, stimulant NEC
  cannabis, cannabinoids — *see* Abuse, drug,
      cannabis
  child — *see* Maltreatment, child
  cocaine — *see* Abuse, drug, cocaine
  drug NEC (non-dependent) F19.10
    with sleep disorder F19.182
    amphetamine type — *see* Abuse, drug,
        stimulant NEC
    analgesics (non-prescribed) (over the
        counter) F55.8
    antacids F55.0
    antidepressants — *see* Abuse, drug,
        psychoactive NEC
    anxiolytics — *see* Abuse, drug, sedative
    barbiturates — *see* Abuse, drug, sedative
    caffeine — *see* Abuse, drug, stimulant
        NEC
    cannabis F12.10
      with
        anxiety disorder F12.180
        intoxication F12.129
          with
            delirium F12.121
            perceptual disturbance F12.122
          uncomplicated F12.120
        other specified disorder F12.188
        psychosis F12.159
          delusions F12.150
          hallucinations F12.151
        unspecified disorder F12.19
      in remission (early) (sustained) F12.11
    cocaine F14.10
      with
        anxiety disorder F14.180
        intoxication F14.129
          with
            delirium F14.121
            perceptual disturbance F14.122
          uncomplicated F14.120
        mood disorder F14.14
        other specified disorder F14.188
        psychosis F14.159
          delusions F14.150
          hallucinations F14.151
        sexual dysfunction F14.181
        sleep disorder F14.182
        unspecified disorder F14.19
      in remission (early) (sustained) F14.11
    counseling and surveillance Z71.51
    hallucinogen F16.10
      with
        anxiety disorder F16.180
        flashbacks F16.183
        intoxication F16.129
          with
            delirium F16.121
            perceptual disturbance F16.122
          uncomplicated F16.120
        mood disorder F16.14
        other specified disorder F16.188
        perception disorder,
            persisting F16.183
        psychosis F16.159
          delusions F16.150
          hallucinations F16.151
        unspecified disorder F16.19
      in remission (early) (sustained) F16.11
    hashish — *see* Abuse, drug, cannabis

Abuse - *continued*
  drug NEC (non-dependent) - *continued*
    herbal or folk remedies F55.1
    hormones F55.3
    hypnotics — *see* Abuse, drug, sedative
    inhalant F18.10
      with
        anxiety disorder F18.180
        dementia, persisting F18.17
        intoxication F18.129
          with delirium F18.121
          uncomplicated F18.120
        mood disorder F18.14
        other specified disorder F18.188
        psychosis F18.159
          delusions F18.150
          hallucinations F18.151
        unspecified disorder F18.19
      in remission (early) (sustained) F18.11
    in remission (early) (sustained) F19.11
    laxatives F55.2
    LSD — *see* Abuse, drug, hallucinogen
    marihuana — *see* Abuse, drug, cannabis
    morphine type (opioids) — *see* Abuse,
        drug, opioid
    opioid F11.10
      with
        intoxication F11.129
          with
            delirium F11.121
            perceptual disturbance F11.122
          uncomplicated F11.120
        mood disorder F11.14
        other specified disorder F11.188
        psychosis F11.159
          delusions F11.150
          hallucinations F11.151
        sexual dysfunction F11.181
        sleep disorder F11.182
        unspecified disorder F11.19
      in remission (early) (sustained) F11.11
    PCP (phencyclidine) (or related
        substance) — *see* Abuse, drug,
        hallucinogen
    psychoactive NEC F19.10
      with
        amnestic disorder F19.16
        anxiety disorder F19.180
        dementia F19.17
        intoxication F19.129
          with
            delirium F19.121
            perceptual disturbance F19.122
          uncomplicated F19.120
        mood disorder F19.14
        other specified disorder F19.188
        psychosis F19.159
          delusions F19.150
          hallucinations F19.151
        sexual dysfunction F19.181
        sleep disorder F19.182
        unspecified disorder F19.19
    sedative, hypnotic or anxiolytic F13.10
      with
        anxiety disorder F13.180
        intoxication F13.129
          with delirium F13.121
          uncomplicated F13.120
        mood disorder F13.14
        other specified disorder F13.188
        psychosis F13.159
          delusions F13.150
          hallucinations F13.151
        sexual dysfunction F13.181
        sleep disorder F13.182
        unspecified disorder F13.19
      in remission (early) (sustained) F13.11
    solvent — *see* Abuse, drug, inhalant
    steroids F55.3
    stimulant NEC F15.10
      with
        anxiety disorder F15.180
        intoxication F15.129
          with
            delirium F15.121

Abuse - *continued*
  drug NEC (non-dependent) - *continued*
    stimulant NEC - *continued*
      with - *continued*
        intoxication - *continued*
          with - *continued*
            perceptual disturbance F15.122
            uncomplicated F15.120
          mood disorder F15.14
          other specified disorder F15.188
          psychosis F15.159
            delusions F15.150
            hallucinations F15.151
          sexual dysfunction F15.181
          sleep disorder F15.182
          unspecified disorder F15.19
        in remission (early) (sustained) F15.11
      tranquilizers — *see* Abuse, drug, sedative
      vitamins F55.4
    hallucinogens — *see* Abuse, drug, hallucinogen
    hashish — *see* Abuse, drug, cannabis
    herbal or folk remedies F55.1
    hormones F55.3
    hypnotic — *see* Abuse, drug, sedative
    inhalant — *see* Abuse, drug, inhalant
    laxatives F55.2
    LSD — *see* Abuse, drug, hallucinogen
    marihuana — *see* Abuse, drug, cannabis
    morphine type (opioids) — *see* Abuse, drug, opioid
    non-psychoactive substance NEC F55.8
      antacids F55.0
      folk remedies F55.1
      herbal remedies F55.1
      hormones F55.3
      laxatives F55.2
      steroids F55.3
      vitamins F55.4
    opioids — *see* Abuse, drug, opioid
    PCP (phencyclidine) (or related substance) — *see* Abuse, drug, hallucinogen
    physical (adult) (child) — *see* Maltreatment
    psychoactive substance — *see* Abuse, drug, psychoactive NEC
    psychological (adult) (child) — *see* Maltreatment
    sedative — *see* Abuse, drug, sedative
    sexual — *see* Maltreatment
    solvent — *see* Abuse, drug, inhalant
    steroids F55.3
    vitamins F55.4
Acalculia R48.8
  developmental F81.2
Acanthamebiasis (with) B60.10
  conjunctiva B60.12
  keratoconjunctivitis B60.13
  meningoencephalitis B60.11
  other specified B60.19
Acanthocephaliasis B83.8
Acanthocheilonemiasis B74.4
Acanthocytosis E78.6
Acantholysis L11.9
Acanthosis (acquired) (nigricans) L83
  benign Q82.8
  congenital Q82.8
  seborrheic L82.1
    inflamed L82.0
  tongue K14.3
Acapnia E87.3
Acarbia E87.2
Acardia, acardius Q89.8
Acardiacus amorphus Q89.8
Acardiotrophia I51.4
Acariasis B88.0
  scabies B86
Acarodermatitis (urticarioides) B88.0
Acarophobia F40.218
Acatalasemia, acatalasia E80.3
Acathisia (drug induced) G25.71
Accelerated atrioventricular conduction I45.6
Accentuation of personality traits (type A) Z73.1

Accessory (congenital)
  adrenal gland Q89.1
  anus Q43.4
  appendix Q43.4
  atrioventricular conduction I45.6
  auditory ossicles Q16.3
  auricle (ear) Q17.0
  biliary duct or passage Q44.5
  bladder Q64.79
  blood vessels NEC Q27.9
    coronary Q24.5
  bone NEC Q79.8
  breast tissue, axilla Q83.1
  carpal bones Q74.0
  cecum Q43.4
  chromosome (s) NEC (nonsex) Q92.9
    with complex rearrangements NEC Q92.5
      seen only at prometaphase Q92.8
    partial Q92.9
    sex
      female phenotype Q97.8
    13 — *see* Trisomy, 13
    18 — *see* Trisomy, 18
    21 — *see* Trisomy, 21
  coronary artery Q24.5
  cusp (s) , heart valve NEC Q24.8
    pulmonary Q22.3
  cystic duct Q44.5
  digit (s) Q69.9
  ear (auricle) (lobe) Q17.0
  endocrine gland NEC Q89.2
  eye muscle Q10.3
  eyelid Q10.3
  face bone (s) Q75.8
  fallopian tube (fimbria) (ostium) Q50.6
  finger (s) Q69.0
  foreskin N47.8
  frontonasal process Q75.8
  gallbladder Q44.1
  genital organ (s)
    female Q52.8
      external Q52.79
      internal NEC Q52.8
    male Q55.8
  genitourinary organs NEC Q89.8
    female Q52.8
    male Q55.8
  hallux Q69.2
  heart Q24.8
    valve NEC Q24.8
      pulmonary Q22.3
  hepatic ducts Q44.5
  hymen Q52.4
  intestine (large) (small) Q43.4
  kidney Q63.0
  lacrimal canal Q10.6
  leaflet, heart valve NEC Q24.8
  ligament, broad Q50.6
  liver Q44.7
    duct Q44.5
  lobule (ear) Q17.0
  lung (lobe) Q33.1
  muscle Q79.8
  navicular of carpus Q74.0
  nervous system, part NEC Q07.8
  nipple Q83.3
  nose Q30.8
  organ or site not listed — *see* Anomaly, by site
  ovary Q50.31
  oviduct Q50.6
  pancreas Q45.3
  parathyroid gland Q89.2
  parotid gland (and duct) Q38.4
  pituitary gland Q89.2
  preauricular appendage Q17.0
  prepuce N47.8
  renal arteries (multiple) Q27.2
  rib Q76.6
    cervical Q76.5
  roots (teeth) K00.2
  salivary gland Q38.4
  sesamoid bones Q74.8
    foot Q74.2
    hand Q74.0

Accessory (congenital) - *continued*
  skin tags Q82.8
  spleen Q89.09
  sternum Q76.7
  submaxillary gland Q38.4
  tarsal bones Q74.2
  teeth, tooth K00.1
  tendon Q79.8
  thumb Q69.1
  thymus gland Q89.2
  thyroid gland Q89.2
  toes Q69.2
  tongue Q38.3
  tooth, teeth K00.1
  tragus Q17.0
  ureter Q62.5
  urethra Q64.79
  urinary organ or tract NEC Q64.8
  uterus Q51.28
  vagina Q52.10
  valve, heart NEC Q24.8
    pulmonary Q22.3
  vertebra Q76.49
  vocal cords Q31.8
  vulva Q52.79
Accident
  birth — *see* Birth, injury
  cardiac — *see* Infarct, myocardium
  cerebral I63.9
  cerebrovascular (embolic) (ischemic) (thrombotic) I63.9
    aborted I63.9
    hemorrhagic — *see* Hemorrhage, intracranial, intracerebral
    old (without sequelae) Z86.73
      with sequelae (of) — *see* Sequelae, infarction, cerebral
  coronary — *see* Infarct, myocardium
  craniovascular I63.9
  vascular, brain I63.9
Accidental — *see* condition
Accommodation (disorder) — *see also* condition
  hysterical paralysis of F44.89
  insufficiency of H52.4
  paresis — *see* Paresis, of accommodation
  spasm — *see* Spasm, of accommodation
Accouchement — *see* Delivery
Accreta placenta O43.21-
Accretio cordis (nonrheumatic) I31.0
Accretions, tooth, teeth K03.6
Acculturation difficulty Z60.3
Accumulation secretion, prostate N42.89
Acephalia, acephalism, acephalus, acephaly Q00.0
Acephalobrachia monster Q89.8
Acephalochirus monster Q89.8
Acephalogaster Q89.8
Acephalostomus monster Q89.8
Acephalothorax Q89.8
Acerophobia F40.298
Acetonemia R79.89
  in Type 1 diabetes E10.10
    with coma E10.11
Acetonuria R82.4
Achalasia (cardia) (esophagus) K22.0
  congenital Q39.5
  pylorus Q40.0
  sphincteral NEC K59.8
Ache (s) — *see* Pain
Acheilia Q38.6
Achillobursitis — *see* Tendinitis, Achilles
Achillodynia — *see* Tendinitis, Achilles
Achlorhydria, achlorhydric (neurogenic) K31.83
  anemia D50.8
  diarrhea K31.83
  psychogenic F45.8
  secondary to vagotomy K91.1
Achluophobia F40.228
Acholia K82.8
Acholuric jaundice (familial) (splenomegalic) — *see also* Spherocytosis
  acquired D59.8

Achondrogenesis Q77.0
Achondroplasia (osteosclerosis congenita) Q77.4
Achroma, cutis L80
Achromat (ism) , achromatopsia (acquired) (congenital) H53.51
Achromia parasitica B36.0
Achromia, congenital — *see* Albinism
Achylia gastrica K31.89
  psychogenic F45.8
Acid
  burn — *see* Corrosion
  deficiency
    amide nicotinic E52
    ascorbic E54
    folic E53.8
    nicotinic E52
    pantothenic E53.8
  intoxication E87.2
  peptic disease K30
  phosphatase deficiency E83.39
  stomach K30
    psychogenic F45.8
Acidemia E87.2
  argininosuccinic E72.22
  isovaleric E71.110
  metabolic (newborn) P19.9
    first noted before onset of labor P19.0
    first noted during labor P19.1
    noted at birth P19.2
  methylmalonic E71.120
  pipecolic E72.3
  propionic E71.121
Acidity, gastric (high) K30
  psychogenic F45.8
Acidocytopenia — *see* Agranulocytosis
Acidocytosis D72.1
Acidopenia — *see* Agranulocytosis
Acidosis (lactic) (respiratory) E87.2
  in Type 1 diabetes E10.10
    with coma E10.11
  kidney, tubular N25.89
  lactic E87.2
  metabolic NEC E87.2
    with respiratory acidosis E87.4
    hyperchloremic, of newborn P74.421
    late, of newborn P74.0
  mixed metabolic and respiratory, newborn P84
  newborn P84
  renal (hyperchloremic) (tubular) N25.89
  respiratory E87.2
    complicated by
      metabolic
        acidosis E87.4
        alkalosis E87.4
Aciduria
  4-hydroxybutyric E72.81
  argininosuccinic E72.22
  gamma-hydroxybutyric E72.81
  glutaric (type I) E72.3
    type II E71.313
    type III E71.5-
  orotic (congenital) (hereditary) (pyrimidine deficiency) E79.8
    anemia D53.0
Acladiosis (skin) B36.0
Aclasis, diaphyseal Q78.6
Acleistocardia Q21.1
Aclusion — *see* Anomaly, dentofacial, malocclusion
Acne L70.9
  artificialis L70.8
  atrophica L70.2
  cachecticorum (Hebra) L70.8
  conglobata L70.1
  cystic L70.0
  decalvans L66.2
  excoriée (des jeunes filles) L70.5
  frontalis L70.2
  indurata L70.0
  infantile L70.4
  keloid L73.0
  lupoid L70.2
  necrotic, necrotica (miliaris) L70.2

Acne - *continued*
  neonatal L70.4
  nodular L70.0
  occupational L70.8
  picker's L70.5
  pustular L70.0
  rodens L70.2
  rosacea L71.9
  specified NEC L70.8
  tropica L70.3
  varioliformis L70.2
  vulgaris L70.0
Acnitis (primary) A18.4
Acosta's disease T70.29
Acoustic — *see* condition
Acousticophobia F40.298
Acquired — *see also* condition
  immunodeficiency syndrome (AIDS) B20
Acrania Q00.0
Acroangiodermatitis I78.9
Acroasphyxia, chronic I73.89
Acrobystitis N47.7
Acrocephalopolysyndactyly Q87.0
Acrocephalosyndactyly Q87.0
Acrocephaly Q75.0
Acrochondrohyperplasia — *see* Syndrome, Marfan's
Acrocyanosis I73.89
  newborn P28.2
    meaning transient blue hands and feet - omit code
Acrodermatitis L30.8
  atrophicans (chronica) L90.4
  continua (Hallopeau) L40.2
  enteropathica (hereditary) E83.2
  Hallopeau's L40.2
  infantile papular L44.4
  perstans L40.2
  pustulosa continua L40.2
  recalcitrant pustular L40.2
Acrodynia — *see* Poisoning, mercury
Acromegaly, acromegalia E22.0
Acromelalgia I73.81
Acromicria, acromikria Q79.8
Acronyx L60.0
Acropachy, thyroid — *see* Thyrotoxicosis
Acroparesthesia (simple) (vasomotor) I73.89
Acropathy, thyroid — *see* Thyrotoxicosis
Acrophobia F40.241
Acroposthitis N47.7
Acroscleriasis, acroscleroderma, acrosclerosis — *see* Sclerosis, systemic
Acrosphacelus I96
Acrospiroma, eccrine — *see* Neoplasm, skin, benign
Acrostealgia — *see* Osteochondropathy
Acrotrophodynia — *see* Immersion
ACTH ectopic syndrome E24.3
Actinic — *see* condition
Actinobacillosis, actinobacillus A28.8
  mallei A24.0
  muris A25.1
Actinomyces israelii (infection) — *see* Actinomycosis
Actinomycetoma (foot) B47.1
Actinomycosis, actinomycotic A42.9
  with pneumonia A42.0
  abdominal A42.1
  cervicofacial A42.2
  cutaneous A42.89
  gastrointestinal A42.1
  pulmonary A42.0
  sepsis A42.7
  specified site NEC A42.89
Actinoneuritis G62.82
Action, heart
  disorder I49.9
  irregular I49.9
    psychogenic F45.8
Activated protein C resistance D68.51
Activation
  mast cell (disorder) (syndrome) D89.40
    idiopathic D89.42
    monoclonal D89.41
    secondary D89.43

Activation - *continued*
  mast cell (disorder) (syndrome) - *continued*
    specified type NEC D89.49
Active — *see* condition
Acute — *see also* condition
  abdomen R10.0
  gallbladder — *see* Cholecystitis, acute
Acyanotic heart disease (congenital) Q24.9
Acystia Q64.5
Adair-Dighton syndrome (brittle bones and blue sclera, deafness) Q78.0
Adamantinoblastoma — *see* Ameloblastoma
Adamantinoma — *see also* Cyst, calcifying odontogenic
  long bones C40.90
    lower limb C40.2-
    upper limb C40.0-
  malignant C41.1
    jaw (bone) (lower) C41.1
      upper C41.0
  tibial C40.2-
Adamantoblastoma — *see* Ameloblastoma
Adams-Stokes (-Morgagni) disease or syndrome I45.9
Adaption reaction — *see* Disorder, adjustment
Addiction — *see also* Dependence F19.20
  alcohol, alcoholic (ethyl) (methyl) (wood) (without remission) F10.20
    with remission F10.21
  drug — *see* Dependence, drug
  ethyl alcohol (without remission) F10.20
    with remission F10.21
  heroin — *see* Dependence, drug, opioid
  methyl alcohol (without remission) F10.20
    with remission F10.21
  methylated spirit (without remission) F10.20
    with remission F10.21
  morphine (-like substances) — *see* Dependence, drug, opioid
  nicotine — *see* Dependence, drug, nicotine
  opium and opioids — *see* Dependence, drug, opioid
  tobacco — *see* Dependence, drug, nicotine
Addison-Biermer anemia (pernicious) D51.0
Addisonian crisis E27.2
Addison's
  anemia (pernicious) D51.0
  disease (bronze) or syndrome E27.1
    tuberculous A18.7
  keloid L94.0
Addison-Schilder complex E71.528
Additional — *see also* Accessory
  chromosome (s) Q99.8
    sex — *see* Abnormal, chromosome, sex
    21 — *see* Trisomy, 21
Adduction contracture, hip or other joint — *see* Contraction, joint
Adenitis — *see also* Lymphadenitis
  acute, unspecified site L04.9
  axillary I88.9
    acute L04.2
    chronic or subacute I88.1
  Bartholin's gland N75.8
  bulbourethral gland — *see* Urethritis
  cervical I88.9
    acute L04.0
    chronic or subacute I88.1
  chancroid (Hemophilus ducreyi) A57
  chronic, unspecified site I88.1
  Cowper's gland — *see* Urethritis
  due to Pasteurella multocida (P. septica) A28.0
  epidemic, acute B27.09
  gangrenous L04.9
  gonorrheal NEC A54.89
  groin I88.9
    acute L04.1
    chronic or subacute I88.1
  infectious (acute) (epidemic) B27.09
  inguinal I88.9
    acute L04.1
    chronic or subacute I88.1
  lymph gland or node, except mesenteric I88.9
    acute — *see* Lymphadenitis, acute

Adenitis - *continued*
  lymph gland or node, except mesenteric -
    continued
      chronic or subacute I88.1
  mesenteric (acute) (chronic) (nonspecific)
    (subacute) I88.0
  parotid gland (suppurative) — *see*
    Sialoadenitis
  salivary gland (any) (suppurative) — *see*
    Sialoadenitis
  scrofulous (tuberculous) A18.2
  Skene's duct or gland — *see* Urethritis
  strumous, tuberculous A18.2
  subacute, unspecified site I88.1
  sublingual gland (suppurative) — *see*
    Sialoadenitis
  submandibular gland (suppurative) — *see*
    Sialoadenitis
  submaxillary gland (suppurative) — *see*
    Sialoadenitis
  tuberculous — *see* Tuberculosis, lymph
    gland
  urethral gland — *see* Urethritis
  Wharton's duct (suppurative) — *see*
    Sialoadenitis
Adenoacanthoma — *see* Neoplasm,
  malignant, by site
Adenoameloblastoma — *see* Cyst, calcifying
  odontogenic
Adenocarcinoid (tumor) — *see* Neoplasm,
  malignant, by site
Adenocarcinoma — *see also* Neoplasm,
  malignant, by site
  acidophil
    specified site — *see* Neoplasm, malignant,
      by site
    unspecified site C75.1
  adrenal cortical C74.0-
  alveolar — *see* Neoplasm, lung, malignant
  apocrine
    breast — *see* Neoplasm, breast, malignant
    in situ
      breast D05.8-
      specified site NEC — *see* Neoplasm,
        skin, in situ
      unspecified site D04.9
    specified site NEC — *see* Neoplasm, skin,
      malignant
    unspecified site C44.99
  basal cell
    specified site — *see* Neoplasm, skin,
      malignant
    unspecified site C08.9
  basophil
    specified site — *see* Neoplasm, malignant,
      by site
    unspecified site C75.1
  bile duct type C22.1
    liver C22.1
    specified site NEC — *see* Neoplasm,
      malignant, by site
    unspecified site C22.1
  bronchiolar — *see* Neoplasm, lung,
    malignant
  bronchioloalveolar — *see* Neoplasm, lung,
    malignant
  ceruminous C44.29-
  cervix, in situ — *see also* Carcinoma, cervix
    uteri, in situ D06.9
  chromophobe
    specified site — *see* Neoplasm, malignant,
      by site
    unspecified site C75.1
  diffuse type
    specified site — *see* Neoplasm, malignant,
      by site
    unspecified site C16.9
  duct
    infiltrating
      with Paget's disease — *see* Neoplasm,
        breast, malignant
      specified site — *see* Neoplasm,
        malignant, by site
      unspecified site (female) C50.91-
        male C50.92-

Adenocarcinoma - *continued*
  duct - *continued*
    specified site — *see* Neoplasm, malignant,
      by site
    unspecified site
      female C56.9
      male C61
  eosinophil
    specified site — *see* Neoplasm, malignant,
      by site
    unspecified site C75.1
  follicular
    with papillary C73
    moderately differentiated C73
    specified site — *see* Neoplasm, malignant,
      by site
    trabecular C73
    unspecified site C73
    well differentiated C73
  Hurthle cell C73
  in
    adenomatous
      polyposis coli C18.9
  infiltrating duct
    with Paget's disease — *see* Neoplasm,
      breast, malignant
    specified site — *see* Neoplasm, by site,
      malignant
    unspecified site (female) C50.91-
      male C50.92-
  inflammatory
    specified site — *see* Neoplasm, by site,
      malignant
    unspecified site (female) C50.91-
      male C50.92-
  intestinal type
    specified site — *see* Neoplasm, by site,
      malignant
    unspecified site C16.9
  intracystic papillary
  intraductal
    breast D05.1-
    noninfiltrating
      breast D05.1-
      papillary
        with invasion
          specified site — *see* Neoplasm, by
            site, malignant
          unspecified site (female) C50.91-
            male C50.92-
          breast D05.1-
          specified site NEC — *see* Neoplasm,
            in situ, by site
          unspecified site D05.1-
      specified site NEC — *see* Neoplasm, in
        situ, by site
      unspecified site D05.1-
    papillary
      with invasion
        specified site — *see* Neoplasm,
          malignant, by site
        unspecified site (female) C50.91-
          male C50.92-
      breast D05.1-
      specified site — *see* Neoplasm, in situ,
        by site
      unspecified site D05.1-
    specified site NEC — *see* Neoplasm, in
      situ, by site
    unspecified site D05.1-
  islet cell
    with exocrine, mixed
      specified site — *see* Neoplasm,
        malignant, by site
      unspecified site C25.9
    pancreas C25.4
    specified site NEC — *see* Neoplasm,
      malignant, by site
    unspecified site C25.4
  lobular
    in situ
      breast D05.0-
      specified site NEC — *see* Neoplasm, in
        situ, by site
      unspecified site D05.0-

Adenocarcinoma - *continued*
  lobular - *continued*
    specified site — *see* Neoplasm, malignant,
      by site
    unspecified site (female) C50.91-
      male C50.92-
  mucoid — *see also* Neoplasm, malignant, by
    site
    cell
      specified site — *see* Neoplasm,
        malignant, by site
      unspecified site C75.1
  nonencapsulated sclerosing C73
  papillary
    with follicular C73
    follicular variant C73
    intraductal (noninfiltrating)
      with invasion
        specified site — *see* Neoplasm,
          malignant, by site
        unspecified site (female) C50.91-
          male C50.92-
      breast D05.1-
      specified site NEC — *see* Neoplasm, in
        situ, by site
      unspecified site D05.1-
    serous
      specified site — *see* Neoplasm,
        malignant, by site
      unspecified site C56.9
  papillocystic
    specified site — *see* Neoplasm, malignant,
      by site
    unspecified site C56.9
  pseudomucinous
    specified site — *see* Neoplasm, malignant,
      by site
    unspecified site C56.9
  renal cell C64-
  sebaceous — *see* Neoplasm, skin, malignant
  serous — *see also* Neoplasm, malignant, by
    site
    papillary
      specified site — *see* Neoplasm,
        malignant, by site
      unspecified site C56.9
  sweat gland — *see* Neoplasm, skin,
    malignant
  water-clear cell C75.0
Adenocarcinoma-in-situ — *see also*
  Neoplasm, in situ, by site
  breast D05.9-
Adenofibroma
  clear cell — *see* Neoplasm, benign, by site
  endometrioid D27.9
    borderline malignancy D39.10
    malignant C56-
  mucinous
    specified site — *see* Neoplasm, benign, by
      site
    unspecified site D27.9
  papillary
    specified site — *see* Neoplasm, benign, by
      site
    unspecified site D27.9
  prostate — *see* Enlargement, enlarged,
    prostate
  serous
    specified site — *see* Neoplasm, benign, by
      site
    unspecified site D27.9
  specified site — *see* Neoplasm, benign, by
    site
  unspecified site D27.9
Adenofibrosis
  breast — *see* Fibroadenosis, breast
  endometrioid N80.0
Adenoiditis (chronic) J35.02
  with tonsillitis J35.03
  acute J03.90
    recurrent J03.91
    specified organism NEC J03.80
      recurrent J03.81
    staphylococcal J03.80
      recurrent J03.81

Adenoiditis (chronic) - *continued*
  acute - *continued*
    streptococcal J03.00
    recurrent J03.01
Adenoids — *see* condition
Adenolipoma — *see* Neoplasm, benign, by site
Adenolipomatosis, Launois-Bensaude E88.89
Adenolymphoma
  specified site — *see* Neoplasm, benign, by site
  unspecified site D11.9
Adenoma — *see also* Neoplasm, benign, by site
  acidophil
    specified site — *see* Neoplasm, benign, by site
    unspecified site D35.2
  acidophil-basophil, mixed
    specified site — *see* Neoplasm, benign, by site
    unspecified site D35.2
  adrenal (cortical) D35.00
    clear cell D35.00
    compact cell D35.00
    glomerulosa cell D35.00
    heavily pigmented variant D35.00
    mixed cell D35.00
  alpha-cell
    pancreas D13.7
    specified site NEC — *see* Neoplasm, benign, by site
    unspecified site D13.7
  alveolar D14.30
  apocrine
    breast D24-
    specified site NEC — *see* Neoplasm, skin, benign, by site
    unspecified site D23.9
  basal cell D11.9
  basophil
    specified site — *see* Neoplasm, benign, by site
    unspecified site D35.2
  basophil-acidophil, mixed
    specified site — *see* Neoplasm, benign, by site
    unspecified site D35.2
  beta-cell
    pancreas D13.7
    specified site NEC — *see* Neoplasm, benign, by site
    unspecified site D13.7
  bile duct D13.4
    common D13.5
    extrahepatic D13.5
    intrahepatic D13.4
    specified site NEC — *see* Neoplasm, benign, by site
    unspecified site D13.4
  black D35.00
  bronchial D38.1
    cylindroid type — *see* Neoplasm, lung, malignant
  ceruminous D23.2-
  chief cell D35.1
  chromophobe
    specified site — *see* Neoplasm, benign, by site
    unspecified site D35.2
  colloid
    specified site — *see* Neoplasm, benign, by site
    unspecified site D34
  duct
  eccrine, papillary — *see* Neoplasm, skin, benign
  endocrine, multiple
    single specified site — *see* Neoplasm, uncertain behavior, by site
    two or more specified sites D44-
    unspecified site D44.9
  endometrioid — *see also* Neoplasm, benign
    borderline malignancy — *see* Neoplasm, uncertain behavior, by site
  eosinophil

Adenoma - *continued*
  eosinophil - *continued*
    specified site — *see* Neoplasm, benign, by site
    unspecified site D35.2
  fetal
    specified site — *see* Neoplasm, benign, by site
    unspecified site D34
  follicular
    specified site — *see* Neoplasm, benign, by site
    unspecified site D34
  hepatocellular D13.4
  Hurthle cell D34
  islet cell
    pancreas D13.7
    specified site NEC — *see* Neoplasm, benign, by site
    unspecified site D13.7
  liver cell D13.4
  macrofollicular
    specified site — *see* Neoplasm, benign, by site
    unspecified site D34
  malignant, malignum — *see* Neoplasm, malignant, by site
  microcystic
    pancreas D13.6
    specified site NEC — *see* Neoplasm, benign, by site
    unspecified site D13.6
  microfollicular
    specified site — *see* Neoplasm, benign, by site
    unspecified site D34
  mucoid cell
    specified site — *see* Neoplasm, benign, by site
    unspecified site D35.2
  multiple endocrine
    single specified site — *see* Neoplasm, uncertain behavior, by site
    two or more specified sites D44-
    unspecified site D44.9
  nipple D24-
  papillary — *see also* Neoplasm, benign, by site
    eccrine — *see* Neoplasm, skin, benign, by site
  Pick's tubular
    specified site — *see* Neoplasm, benign, by site
    unspecified site
      female D27.9
      male D29.20
  pleomorphic
    carcinoma in — *see* Neoplasm, salivary gland, malignant
    specified site — *see* Neoplasm, malignant, by site
    unspecified site C08.9
  polypoid — *see also* Neoplasm, benign
    adenocarcinoma in — *see* Neoplasm, malignant, by site
    adenocarcinoma in situ — *see* Neoplasm, in situ, by site
  prostate — *see* Neoplasm, benign, prostate
  rete cell D29.20
  sebaceous — *see* Neoplasm, skin, benign
  Sertoli cell
    specified site — *see* Neoplasm, benign, by site
    unspecified site
      female D27.9
      male D29.20
  skin appendage — *see* Neoplasm, skin, benign
  sudoriferous gland — *see* Neoplasm, skin, benign
  sweat gland — *see* Neoplasm, skin, benign
  testicular
    specified site — *see* Neoplasm, benign, by site
    unspecified site

Adenoma - *continued*
  testicular - *continued*
    unspecified site - *continued*
      female D27.9
      male D29.20
  tubular — *see also* Neoplasm, benign, by site
    adenocarcinoma in — *see* Neoplasm, malignant, by site
    adenocarcinoma in situ — *see* Neoplasm, in situ, by site
    Pick's
      specified site — *see* Neoplasm, benign, by site
      unspecified site
        female D27.9
        male D29.20
  tubulovillous — *see also* Neoplasm, benign, by site
    adenocarcinoma in — *see* Neoplasm, malignant, by site
    adenocarcinoma in situ — *see* Neoplasm, in situ, by site
  villous — *see* Neoplasm, uncertain behavior, by site
    adenocarcinoma in — *see* Neoplasm, malignant, by site
    adenocarcinoma in situ — *see* Neoplasm, in situ, by site
  water-clear cell D35.1
Adenomatosis
  endocrine (multiple) E31.20
    single specified site — *see* Neoplasm, uncertain behavior, by site
  erosive of nipple D24-
  pluriendocrine — *see* Adenomatosis, endocrine
  pulmonary D38.1
    malignant — *see* Neoplasm, lung, malignant
  specified site — *see* Neoplasm, benign, by site
  unspecified site D12.6
Adenomatous
  goiter (nontoxic) E04.9
    with hyperthyroidism — *see* Hyperthyroidism, with, goiter, nodular
    toxic — *see* Hyperthyroidism, with, goiter, nodular
Adenomyoma — *see also* Neoplasm, benign, by site
  prostate — *see* Enlarged, prostate
Adenomyometritis N80.0
Adenomyosis N80.0
Adenopathy (lymph gland) R59.9
  generalized R59.1
  inguinal R59.0
  localized R59.0
  mediastinal R59.0
  mesentery R59.0
  syphilitic (secondary) A51.49
  tracheobronchial R59.0
    tuberculous A15.4
      primary (progressive) A15.7
  tuberculous — *see also* Tuberculosis, lymph gland
    tracheobronchial A15.4
      primary (progressive) A15.7
Adenosalpingitis — *see* Salpingitis
Adenosarcoma — *see* Neoplasm, malignant, by site
Adenosclerosis I88.8
Adenosis (sclerosing) breast — *see* Fibroadenosis, breast
Adenovirus, as cause of disease classified elsewhere B97.0
Adentia (complete) (partial) — *see* Absence, teeth
Adherent — *see also* Adhesions
  labia (minora) N90.89
  pericardium (nonrheumatic) I31.0
    rheumatic I09.2
  placenta (with hemorrhage) O72.0
    without hemorrhage O73.0
  prepuce, newborn N47.0

Adherent - *continued*
scar (skin) L90.5
tendon in scar L90.5
Adhesions, adhesive (postinfective) K66.0
with intestinal obstruction K56.50
complete K56.52
incomplete K56.51
partial K56.51
abdominal (wall) — *see* Adhesions,
peritoneum
appendix K38.8
bile duct (common) (hepatic) K83.8
bladder (sphincter) N32.89
bowel — *see* Adhesions, peritoneum
cardiac I31.0
rheumatic I09.2
cecum — *see* Adhesions, peritoneum
cervicovaginal N88.1
congenital Q52.8
postpartal O90.89
old N88.1
cervix N88.1
ciliary body NEC — *see* Adhesions, iris
clitoris N90.89
colon — *see* Adhesions, peritoneum
common duct K83.8
congenital — *see also* Anomaly, by site
fingers — *see* Syndactylism, complex,
fingers
omental, anomalous Q43.3
peritoneal Q43.3
tongue (to gum or roof of mouth) Q38.3
conjunctiva (acquired) H11.21-
congenital Q15.8
cystic duct K82.8
diaphragm — *see* Adhesions, peritoneum
due to foreign body — *see* Foreign body
duodenum — *see* Adhesions, peritoneum
ear
middle H74.1-
epididymis N50.89
epidural — *see* Adhesions, meninges
epiglottis J38.7
eyelid H02.59
female pelvis N73.6
gallbladder K82.8
globe H44.89
heart I31.0
rheumatic I09.2
ileocecal (coil) — *see* Adhesions, peritoneum
ileum — *see* Adhesions, peritoneum
intestine — *see also* Adhesions, peritoneum
with obstruction K56.50
complete K56.52
incomplete K56.51
partial K56.51
intra-abdominal — *see* Adhesions,
peritoneum
iris H21.50-
anterior H21.51-
goniosynechiae H21.52-
posterior H21.54-
to corneal graft T85.898
joint — *see* Ankylosis
knee M23.8X
temporomandibular M26.61-
labium (majus) (minus) , congenital Q52.5
liver — *see* Adhesions, peritoneum
lung J98.4
mediastinum J98.59
meninges (cerebral) (spinal) G96.12
congenital Q07.8
tuberculous (cerebral) (spinal) A17.0
mesenteric — *see* Adhesions, peritoneum
nasal (septum) (to turbinates) J34.89
ocular muscle — *see* Strabismus, mechanical
omentum — *see* Adhesions, peritoneum
ovary N73.6
congenital (to cecum, kidney or
omentum) Q50.39
paraovarian N73.6
pelvic (peritoneal)
female N73.6
postprocedural N99.4
male — *see* Adhesions, peritoneum

Adhesions, adhesive (postinfective) -
continued
pelvic (peritoneal) - *continued*
postpartal (old) N73.6
tuberculous A18.17
penis to scrotum (congenital) Q55.8
periappendiceal — *see also* Adhesions,
peritoneum
pericardium (nonrheumatic) I31.0
focal I31.8
rheumatic I09.2
tuberculous A18.84
pericholecystic K82.8
perigastric — *see* Adhesions, peritoneum
periovarian N73.6
periprostatic N42.89
perirectal — *see* Adhesions, peritoneum
perirenal N28.89
peritoneum, peritoneal (postinfective) K66.0
with obstruction (intestinal) K56.50
complete K56.52
incomplete K56.51
partial K56.51
congenital Q43.3
pelvic, female N73.6
postprocedural N99.4
postpartal, pelvic N73.6
postprocedural K66.0
to uterus N73.6
peritubal N73.6
periureteral N28.89
periuterine N73.6
perivesical N32.89
perivesicular (seminal vesicle) N50.89
pleura, pleuritic J94.8
tuberculous NEC A15.6
pleuropericardial J94.8
postoperative (gastrointestinal tract) K66.0
with obstruction — *see also* Obstruction,
intestine, postoperative K91.30
due to foreign body accidentally left in
wound — *see* Foreign body,
accidentally left during a procedure
pelvic peritoneal N99.4
urethra — *see* Stricture, urethra,
postprocedural
vagina N99.2
postpartal, old (vulva or perineum) N90.89
preputial, prepuce N47.5
pulmonary J98.4
pylorus — *see* Adhesions, peritoneum
sciatic nerve — *see* Lesion, nerve, sciatic
seminal vesicle N50.89
shoulder (joint) — *see* Capsulitis, adhesive
sigmoid flexure — *see* Adhesions,
peritoneum
spermatic cord (acquired) N50.89
congenital Q55.4
spinal canal G96.12
stomach — *see* Adhesions, peritoneum
subscapular — *see* Capsulitis, adhesive
temporomandibular M26.61-
tendinitis — *see also* Tenosynovitis,
specified type NEC
shoulder — *see* Capsulitis, adhesive
testis N44.8
tongue, congenital (to gum or roof of
mouth) Q38.3
acquired K14.8
trachea J39.8
tubo-ovarian N73.6
tunica vaginalis N44.8
uterus N73.6
internal N85.6
to abdominal wall N73.6
vagina (chronic) N89.5
postoperative N99.2
vitreomacular H43.82-
vitreous H43.89
vulva N90.89
Adiaspiromycosis B48.8
Adie (-Holmes) pupil or syndrome — *see*
Anomaly, pupil, function, tonic pupil
Adiponecrosis neonatorum P83.88

Adiposis — *see also* Obesity
cerebralis E23.6
dolorosa E88.2
Adiposity — *see also* Obesity
heart — *see* Degeneration, myocardial
localized E65
Adiposogenital dystrophy E23.6
Adjustment
disorder — *see* Disorder, adjustment
implanted device — *see* Encounter (for),
adjustment (of)
prosthesis, external — *see* Fitting
reaction — *see* Disorder, adjustment
**Administration of tPA (rtPA) in a different
facility within the last 24 hours prior to
admission to current facility** Z92.82
Admission (for) — *see also* Encounter (for)
adjustment (of)
artificial
arm Z44.00-
complete Z44.01-
partial Z44.02-
eye Z44.2
leg Z44.10-
complete Z44.11-
partial Z44.12-
brain neuropacemaker Z46.2
implanted Z45.42
breast
implant Z45.81
prosthesis (external) Z44.3
colostomy belt Z46.89
contact lenses Z46.0
cystostomy device Z46.6
dental prosthesis Z46.3
device NEC
abdominal Z46.89
implanted Z45.89
cardiac Z45.09
defibrillator (with synchronous
cardiac pacemaker) Z45.02
pacemaker (cardiac
resynchronization therapy
(CRT-P)) Z45.018
pulse generator Z45.010
resynchronization therapy
defibrillator (CRT-D) Z45.02
hearing device Z45.328
bone conduction Z45.320
cochlear Z45.321
infusion pump Z45.1
nervous system Z45.49
CSF drainage Z45.41
hearing device — *see* Admission,
adjustment, device, implanted,
hearing device
neuropacemaker Z45.42
visual substitution Z45.31
specified NEC Z45.89
vascular access Z45.2
visual substitution Z45.31
nervous system Z46.2
implanted — *see* Admission,
adjustment, device, implanted,
nervous system
orthodontic Z46.4
prosthetic Z44.9
arm — *see* Admission, adjustment,
artificial, arm
breast Z44.3
dental Z46.3
eye Z44.2
leg — *see* Admission, adjustment,
artificial, leg
specified type NEC Z44.8
substitution
auditory Z46.2
implanted — *see* Admission,
adjustment, device, implanted,
hearing device
nervous system Z46.2
implanted — *see* Admission,
adjustment, device, implanted,
nervous system
visual Z46.2

Admission (for) - *continued*
adjustment (of) - *continued*
device NEC - *continued*
substitution - *continued*
visual - *continued*
implanted Z45.31
urinary Z46.6
hearing aid Z46.1
implanted — *see* Admission,
adjustment, device, implanted,
hearing device
ileostomy device Z46.89
intestinal appliance or device NEC Z46.89
neuropacemaker (brain) (peripheral nerve)
(spinal cord) Z46.2
implanted Z45.42
orthodontic device Z46.4
orthopedic (brace) (cast) (device)
(shoes) Z46.89
pacemaker (cardiac resynchronization
therapy (CRT-P))
cardiac Z45.018
pulse generator Z45.010
nervous system Z46.2
implanted Z45.42
portacath (port-a-cath) Z45.2
prosthesis Z44.9
arm — *see* Admission, adjustment,
artificial, arm
breast Z44.3
dental Z46.3
eye Z44.2
leg — *see* Admission, adjustment,
artificial, leg
specified NEC Z44.8
spectacles Z46.0
aftercare — *see also* Aftercare Z51.89
postpartum
immediately after delivery Z39.0
routine follow-up Z39.2
radiation therapy (antineoplastic) Z51.0
attention to artificial opening (of) Z43.9
artificial vagina Z43.7
colostomy Z43.3
cystostomy Z43.5
enterostomy Z43.4
gastrostomy Z43.1
ileostomy Z43.2
jejunostomy Z43.4
nephrostomy Z43.6
specified site NEC Z43.8
intestinal tract Z43.4
urinary tract Z43.6
tracheostomy Z43.0
ureterostomy Z43.6
urethrostomy Z43.6
breast augmentation or reduction Z41.1
breast reconstruction following
mastectomy Z42.1
change of
dressing (nonsurgical) Z48.00
neuropacemaker device (brain) (peripheral
nerve) (spinal cord) Z46.2
implanted Z45.42
surgical dressing Z48.01
circumcision, ritual or routine (in absence of
diagnosis) Z41.2
clinical research investigation (control)
(normal comparison) (participant) Z00.6
contraceptive management Z30.9
cosmetic surgery NEC Z41.1
counseling — *see also* Counseling
dietary Z71.3
gestational carrier Z31.7
HIV Z71.7
human immunodeficiency virus Z71.7
nonattending third party Z71.0
procreative management NEC Z31.69
delivery, full-term, uncomplicated O80
cesarean, without indication O82
desensitization to allergens Z51.6
dietary surveillance and counseling Z71.3
ear piercing Z41.3
examination at health care facility (adult) —
see also Examination Z00.00

Admission (for) - *continued*
examination at health care facility (adult) -
continued
with abnormal findings Z00.01
clinical research investigation (control)
(normal comparison)
(participant) Z00.6
dental Z01.20
with abnormal findings Z01.21
donor (potential) Z00.5
ear Z01.10
with abnormal findings NEC Z01.118
eye Z01.00
with abnormal findings Z01.01
following failed vision
screening Z01.020
with abnormal findings Z01.021
general, specified reason NEC Z00.8
hearing Z01.10
with abnormal findings NEC Z01.118
infant or child (over 28 days
old) Z00.129
with abnormal findings Z00.121
postpartum checkup Z39.2
psychiatric (general) Z00.8
requested by authority Z04.6
vision Z01.00
with abnormal findings Z01.01
following failed vision
screening Z01.020
with abnormal findings Z01.021
infant or child (over 28 days
old) Z00.129
with abnormal findings Z00.121
fitting (of)
artificial
arm — *see* Admission, adjustment,
artificial, arm
eye Z44.2
leg — *see* Admission, adjustment,
artificial, leg
brain neuropacemaker Z46.2
implanted Z45.42
breast prosthesis (external) Z44.3
colostomy belt Z46.89
contact lenses Z46.0
cystostomy device Z46.6
dental prosthesis Z46.3
dentures Z46.3
device NEC
abdominal Z46.89
nervous system Z46.2
implanted — *see* Admission,
adjustment, device, implanted,
nervous system
orthodontic Z46.4
prosthetic Z44.9
breast Z44.3
dental Z46.3
eye Z44.2
substitution
auditory Z46.2
implanted — *see* Admission,
adjustment, device, implanted,
hearing device
nervous system Z46.2
implanted — *see* Admission,
adjustment, device, implanted,
nervous system
visual Z46.2
implanted Z45.31
hearing aid Z46.1
ileostomy device Z46.89
intestinal appliance or device NEC Z46.89
neuropacemaker (brain) (peripheral nerve)
(spinal cord) Z46.2
implanted Z45.42
orthodontic device Z46.4
orthopedic device (brace) (cast)
(shoes) Z46.89
prosthesis Z44.9
arm — *see* Admission, adjustment,
artificial, arm
breast Z44.3
dental Z46.3

Admission (for) - *continued*
fitting (of) - *continued*
prosthesis - *continued*
eye Z44.2
leg — *see* Admission, adjustment,
artificial, leg
specified type NEC Z44.8
spectacles Z46.0
follow-up examination Z09
intrauterine device management Z30.431
initial prescription Z30.014
mental health evaluation Z00.8
requested by authority Z04.6
observation — *see* Observation
Papanicolaou smear, cervix Z12.4
for suspected malignant neoplasm Z12.4
plastic and reconstructive surgery following
medical procedure or healed injury
NEC Z42.8
plastic surgery, cosmetic NEC Z41.1
postpartum observation
immediately after delivery Z39.0
routine follow-up Z39.2
poststerilization (for restoration) Z31.0
aftercare Z31.42
procreative management Z31.9
prophylactic (measure) — *see also*
Encounter, prophylactic measures
organ removal Z40.00
breast Z40.01
fallopian tube (s) Z40.03
with ovary (s) Z40.02
ovary (s) Z40.02
specified organ NEC Z40.09
testes Z40.09
vaccination Z23
psychiatric examination (general) Z00.8
requested by authority Z04.6
radiation therapy (antineoplastic) Z51.0
reconstructive surgery following medical
procedure or healed injury NEC Z42.8
removal of
cystostomy catheter Z43.5
drains Z48.03
dressing (nonsurgical) Z48.00
implantable subdermal
contraceptive Z30.46
intrauterine contraceptive device Z30.432
neuropacemaker (brain) (peripheral nerve)
(spinal cord) Z46.2
implanted Z45.42
staples Z48.02
surgical dressing Z48.01
sutures Z48.02
ureteral stent Z46.6
respirator [ventilator] use during power
failure Z99.12
restoration of organ continuity
(poststerilization) Z31.0
aftercare Z31.42
sensitivity test — *see also* Test, skin
allergy NEC Z01.82
Mantoux Z11.1
tuboplasty following previous
sterilization Z31.0
aftercare Z31.42
vasoplasty following previous
sterilization Z31.0
aftercare Z31.42
vision examination Z01.00
with abnormal findings Z01.01
following failed vision screening Z01.020
with abnormal findings Z01.021
infant or child (over 28 days old) Z00.129
with abnormal findings Z00.121
waiting period for admission to other
facility Z75.1
Adnexitis (suppurative) — *see* Salpingo-
oophoritis
Adolescent X-linked
adrenoleukodystrophy E71.521
Adrenal (gland) — *see* condition
Adrenalism, tuberculous A18.7
Adrenalitis, adrenitis E27.8
autoimmune E27.1

Adrenalitis, adrenitis - *continued*
  meningococcal, hemorrhagic A39.1
Adrenarche, premature E27.0
Adrenocortical syndrome — *see* Cushing's, syndrome
Adrenogenital syndrome E25.9
  acquired E25.8
  congenital E25.0
  salt loss E25.0
Adrenogenitalism, congenital E25.0
Adrenoleukodystrophy E71.529
  neonatal E71.511
  X-linked E71.529
    Addison only phenotype E71.528
    Addison-Schilder E71.528
    adolescent E71.521
    adrenomyeloneuropathy E71.522
    childhood cerebral E71.520
    other specified E71.528
Adrenomyeloneuropathy E71.522
Adventitious bursa — *see* Bursopathy, specified type NEC
Adverse effect — *see* Table of Drugs and Chemicals, categories T36-T50, with 6th character 5
Advice — *see* Counseling
Adynamia (episodica) (hereditary) (periodic) G72.3
Aeration lung imperfect, newborn — *see* Atelectasis
Aerobullosis T70.3
Aerocele — *see* Embolism, air
Aerodermectasia
  subcutaneous (traumatic) T79.7
Aerodontalgia T70.29
Aeroembolism T70.3
Aerogenes capsulatus infection A48.0
Aero-otitis media T70.0
Aerophagy, aerophagia (psychogenic) F45.8
Aerophobia F40.228
Aerosinusitis T70.1
Aerotitis T70.0
Affection — *see* Disease
Afibrinogenemia — *see also* Defect, coagulation D68.8
  acquired D65
  congenital D68.2
  following ectopic or molar pregnancy O08.1
  in abortion — *see* Abortion, by type, complicated by, afibrinogenemia
  puerperal O72.3
African
  sleeping sickness B56.9
  tick fever A68.1
  trypanosomiasis B56.9
    gambian B56.0
    rhodesian B56.1
Aftercare — *see also* Care Z51.89
  following surgery (for) (on)
    amputation Z47.81
    attention to
      drains Z48.03
      dressings (nonsurgical) Z48.00
        surgical Z48.01
      sutures Z48.02
    circulatory system Z48.812
    delayed (planned) wound closure Z48.1
    digestive system Z48.815
    explantation of joint prosthesis (staged procedure)
      hip Z47.32
      knee Z47.33
      shoulder Z47.31
    genitourinary system Z48.816
    joint replacement Z47.1
    neoplasm Z48.3
    nervous system Z48.811
    oral cavity Z48.814
    organ transplant
      bone marrow Z48.290
      heart Z48.21
      heart-lung Z48.280
      kidney Z48.22
      liver Z48.23
      lung Z48.24

Aftercare - *continued*
  following surgery (for) (on) - *continued*
    organ transplant - *continued*
      multiple organs NEC Z48.288
      specified NEC Z48.298
    orthopedic NEC Z47.89
    planned wound closure Z48.1
    removal of internal fixation device Z47.2
    respiratory system Z48.813
    scoliosis Z47.82
    sense organs Z48.810
    skin and subcutaneous tissue Z48.817
    specified body system
      circulatory Z48.812
      digestive Z48.815
      genitourinary Z48.816
      nervous Z48.811
      oral cavity Z48.814
      respiratory Z48.813
      sense organs Z48.810
      skin and subcutaneous tissue Z48.817
      teeth Z48.814
    specified NEC Z48.89
    spinal Z47.89
    teeth Z48.814
  fracture - code to fracture with seventh character D
  involving
    removal of
      drains Z48.03
      dressings (nonsurgical) Z48.00
      staples Z48.02
      surgical dressings Z48.01
      sutures Z48.02
  neuropacemaker (brain) (peripheral nerve) (spinal cord) Z46.2
    implanted Z45.42
  orthopedic NEC Z47.89
  postprocedural — *see* Aftercare, following surgery
After-cataract — *see* Cataract, secondary
Agalactia (primary) O92.3
  elective, secondary or therapeutic O92.5
Agammaglobulinemia (acquired (secondary)) (nonfamilial) D80.1
  with
    immunoglobulin-bearing B-lymphocytes D80.1
    lymphopenia D81.9
  autosomal recessive (Swiss type) D80.0
  Bruton's X-linked D80.0
  common variable (CVAgamma) D80.1
  congenital sex-linked D80.0
  hereditary D80.0
  lymphopenic D81.9
  Swiss type (autosomal recessive) D80.0
  X-linked (with growth hormone deficiency) (Bruton) D80.0
Aganglionosis (bowel) (colon) Q43.1
Age (old) — *see* Senility
Agenesis
  adrenal (gland) Q89.1
  alimentary tract (complete) (partial) NEC Q45.8
    upper Q40.8
  anus, anal (canal) Q42.3
    with fistula Q42.2
  aorta Q25.41
  appendix Q42.8
  arm (complete) Q71.0-
    with hand present Q71.1-
  artery (peripheral) Q27.9
    brain Q28.3
    coronary Q24.5
    pulmonary Q25.79
    specified NEC Q27.8
    umbilical Q27.0
  auditory (canal) (external) Q16.1
  auricle (ear) Q16.0
  bile duct or passage Q44.5
  bladder Q64.5
  bone Q79.9
  brain Q00.0
    part of Q04.3
  breast (with nipple present) Q83.8

Agenesis - *continued*
  breast (with nipple present) - *continued*
    with absent nipple Q83.0
  bronchus Q32.4
  canaliculus lacrimalis Q10.4
  carpus — *see* Agenesis, hand
  cartilage Q79.9
  cecum Q42.8
  cerebellum Q04.3
  cervix Q51.5
  chin Q18.8
  cilia Q10.3
  circulatory system, part NOS Q28.9
  clavicle Q74.0
  clitoris Q52.6
  coccyx Q76.49
  colon Q42.9
    specified NEC Q42.8
  corpus callosum Q04.0
  cricoid cartilage Q31.8
  diaphragm (with hernia) Q79.1
  digestive organ (s) or tract (complete) (partial) NEC Q45.8
    upper Q40.8
  ductus arteriosus Q28.8
  duodenum Q41.0
  ear Q16.9
    auricle Q16.0
    lobe Q17.8
  ejaculatory duct Q55.4
  endocrine (gland) NEC Q89.2
  epiglottis Q31.8
  esophagus Q39.8
  eustachian tube Q16.2
  eye Q11.1
    adnexa Q15.8
  eyelid (fold) Q10.3
  face
    bones NEC Q75.8
    specified part NEC Q18.8
  fallopian tube Q50.6
  femur — *see* Defect, reduction, lower limb, longitudinal, femur
  fibula — *see* Defect, reduction, lower limb, longitudinal, fibula
  finger (complete) (partial) — *see* Agenesis, hand
  foot (and toes) (complete) (partial) Q72.3-
  forearm (with hand present) — *see* Agenesis, arm, with hand present
    and hand Q71.2-
  gallbladder Q44.0
  gastric Q40.2
  genitalia, genital (organ (s))
    female Q52.8
      external Q52.71
      internal NEC Q52.8
    male Q55.8
  glottis Q31.8
  hair Q84.0
  hand (and fingers) (complete) (partial) Q71.3-
  heart Q24.8
    valve NEC Q24.8
      pulmonary Q22.0
  hepatic Q44.7
  humerus — *see* Defect, reduction, upper limb
  hymen Q52.4
  ileum Q41.2
  incus Q16.3
  intestine (small) Q41.9
    large Q42.9
      specified NEC Q42.8
  iris (dilator fibers) Q13.1
  jaw M26.09
  jejunum Q41.1
  kidney (s) (partial) Q60.2
    bilateral Q60.1
    unilateral Q60.0
  labium (majus) (minus) Q52.71
  labyrinth, membranous Q16.5
  lacrimal apparatus Q10.4
  larynx Q31.8
  leg (complete) Q72.0-
    with foot present Q72.1-

Agenesis - *continued*
leg (complete) - *continued*
lower leg (with foot present) — *see* Agenesis, leg, with foot present and foot Q72.2-
lens Q12.3
limb (complete) Q73.0
lower — *see* Agenesis, leg
upper — *see* Agenesis, arm
lip Q38.0
liver Q44.7
lung (fissure) (lobe) (bilateral) (unilateral) Q33.3
mandible, maxilla M26.09
metacarpus — *see* Agenesis, hand
metatarsus — *see* Agenesis, foot
muscle Q79.8
eyelid Q10.3
ocular Q15.8
musculoskeletal system NEC Q79.8
nail (s) Q84.3
neck, part Q18.8
nerve Q07.8
nervous system, part NEC Q07.8
nipple Q83.2
nose Q30.1
nuclear Q07.8
organ
of Corti Q16.5
or site not listed — *see* Anomaly, by site
osseous meatus (ear) Q16.1
ovary
bilateral Q50.02
unilateral Q50.01
oviduct Q50.6
pancreas Q45.0
parathyroid (gland) Q89.2
parotid gland (s) Q38.4
patella Q74.1
pelvic girdle (complete) (partial) Q74.2
penis Q55.5
pericardium Q24.8
pituitary (gland) Q89.2
prostate Q55.4
punctum lacrimale Q10.4
radioulnar — *see* Defect, reduction, upper limb
radius — *see* Defect, reduction, upper limb, longitudinal, radius
rectum Q42.1
with fistula Q42.0
renal Q60.2
bilateral Q60.1
unilateral Q60.0
respiratory organ NEC Q34.8
rib Q76.6
roof of orbit Q75.8
round ligament Q52.8
sacrum Q76.49
salivary gland Q38.4
scapula Q74.0
scrotum Q55.29
seminal vesicles Q55.4
septum
atrial Q21.1
between aorta and pulmonary artery Q21.4
ventricular Q20.4
shoulder girdle (complete) (partial) Q74.0
skull (bone) Q75.8
with
anencephaly Q00.0
encephalocele — *see* Encephalocele
hydrocephalus Q03.9
with spina bifida — *see* Spina bifida, by site, with hydrocephalus
microcephaly Q02
spermatic cord Q55.4
spinal cord Q06.0
spine Q76.49
spleen Q89.01
sternum Q76.7
stomach Q40.2
submaxillary gland (s) (congenital) Q38.4
tarsus — *see* Agenesis, foot
tendon Q79.8

Agenesis - *continued*
testicle Q55.0
thymus (gland) Q89.2
thyroid (gland) E03.1
cartilage Q31.8
tibia — *see* Defect, reduction, lower limb, longitudinal, tibia
tibiofibular — *see* Defect, reduction, lower limb, specified type NEC
toe (and foot) (complete) (partial) — *see* Agenesis, foot
tongue Q38.3
trachea (cartilage) Q32.1
ulna — *see* Defect, reduction, upper limb, longitudinal, ulna
upper limb — *see* Agenesis, arm
ureter Q62.4
urethra Q64.5
urinary tract NEC Q64.8
uterus Q51.0
uvula Q38.5
vagina Q52.0
vas deferens Q55.4
vein (s) (peripheral) Q27.9
brain Q28.3
great NEC Q26.8
portal Q26.5
vena cava (inferior) (superior) Q26.8
vermis of cerebellum Q04.3
vertebra Q76.49
vulva Q52.71
Ageusia R43.2
Agitated — *see* condition
Agitation R45.1
Aglossia (congenital) Q38.3
Aglossia-adactylia syndrome Q87.0
Aglycogenosis E74.00
Agnosia (body image) (other senses) (tactile) R48.1
developmental F88
verbal R48.1
auditory R48.1
developmental F80.2
developmental F80.2
visual (object) R48.3
Agoraphobia F40.00
with panic disorder F40.01
without panic disorder F40.02
Agrammatism R48.8
Agranulocytopenia — *see* Agranulocytosis
Agranulocytosis (chronic) (cyclical) (genetic) (infantile) (periodic) (pernicious) — *see also* Neutropenia D70.9
congenital D70.0
cytoreductive cancer chemotherapy sequela D70.1
drug-induced D70.2
due to cytoreductive cancer chemotherapy D70.1
due to infection D70.3
secondary D70.4
drug-induced D70.2
due to cytoreductive cancer chemotherapy D70.1
Agraphia (absolute) R48.8
with alexia R48.0
developmental F81.81
Ague (dumb) — *see* Malaria
Agyria Q04.3
Ahumada-del Castillo syndrome E23.0
Aichomophobia F40.298
AIDS (related complex) B20
Ailment heart — *see* Disease, heart
Ailurophobia F40.218
AIN — *see* Neoplasia, intraepithelial, anal
Ainhum (disease) L94.6
AIPHI (acute idiopathic pulmonary hemorrhage in infants (over 28 days old)) R04.81
Air
anterior mediastinum J98.2
compressed, disease T70.3
conditioner lung or pneumonitis J67.7
embolism (artery) (cerebral) (any site) T79.0
with ectopic or molar pregnancy O08.2

Air - *continued*
embolism (artery) (cerebral) (any site) - *continued*
due to implanted device NEC — *see* Complications, by site and type, specified NEC
following
abortion — *see* Abortion by type, complicated by, embolism
ectopic or molar pregnancy O08.2
infusion, therapeutic injection or transfusion T80.0
in pregnancy, childbirth or puerperium — *see* Embolism, obstetric
traumatic T79.0
hunger, psychogenic F45.8
rarefied, effects of — *see* Effect, adverse, high altitude
sickness T75.3
Airplane sickness T75.3
Akathisia (drug-induced) (treatment-induced) G25.71
neuroleptic induced (acute) G25.71
tardive G25.71
Akinesia R29.898
Akinetic mutism R41.89
Akureyri's disease G93.3
Alactasia, congenital E73.0
Alagille's syndrome Q44.7
Alastrim B03
Albers-Schönberg syndrome Q78.2
Albert's syndrome — *see* Tendinitis, Achilles
Albinism, albino E70.30
with hematologic abnormality E70.339
Chédiak-Higashi syndrome E70.330
Hermansky-Pudlak syndrome E70.331
other specified E70.338
I E70.320
II E70.321
ocular E70.319
autosomal recessive E70.311
other specified E70.318
X-linked E70.310
oculocutaneous E70.329
other specified E70.328
tyrosinase (ty) negative E70.320
tyrosinase (ty) positive E70.321
other specified E70.39
Albinismus E70.30
Albright (-McCune) (-Sternberg) syndrome Q78.1
Albuminous — *see* condition
Albuminuria, albuminuric (acute) (chronic) (subacute) — *see also* Proteinuria R80.9
complicating pregnancy — *see* Proteinuria, gestational
with
gestational hypertension — *see* Pre-eclampsia
pre-existing hypertension — *see* Hypertension, complicating pregnancy, pre-existing, with, pre-eclampsia
gestational — *see* Proteinuria, gestational
with
gestational hypertension — *see* Pre-eclampsia
pre-existing hypertension — *see* Hypertension, complicating pregnancy, pre-existing, with, pre-eclampsia
orthostatic R80.2
postural R80.2
pre-eclamptic — *see* Pre-eclampsia
scarlatinal A38.8
Albuminurophobia F40.298
Alcaptonuria E70.29
Alcohol, alcoholic, alcohol-induced
addiction (without remission) F10.20
with remission F10.21
amnestic disorder, persisting F10.96
with dependence F10.26
anxiety disorder F10.980
bipolar and related disorder F10.94
depressive disorder F10.94

Alcohol, alcoholic, alcohol-induced - *continued*
  major neurocognitive disorder, amnestic-confabulatory type F10.96
  major neurocognitive disorder, nonamnestic-confabulatory type F10.97
  mild neurocognitive disorder F10.988
  psychotic disorder F10.959
  sexual dysfunction F10.981
  sleep disorder F10.982
  brain syndrome, chronic F10.97
    with dependence F10.27
  cardiopathy I42.6
  counseling and surveillance Z71.41
    family member Z71.42
  delirium (acute) (tremens)
    (withdrawal) F10.231
    with intoxication F10.921
    in
      abuse F10.121
      dependence F10.221
  dementia F10.97
    with dependence F10.27
  deterioration F10.97
    with dependence F10.27
  hallucinosis (acute) F10.951
    in
      abuse F10.151
      dependence F10.251
  insanity F10.959
  intoxication (acute) (without dependence) F10.129
    with
      delirium F10.121
      dependence F10.229
        with delirium F10.221
        uncomplicated F10.220
      uncomplicated F10.120
  jealousy F10.988
  Korsakoff's, Korsakov's, Korsakow's F10.26
  liver K70.9
    acute — *see* Disease, liver, alcoholic, hepatitis
  mania (acute) (chronic) F10.959
  paranoia, paranoid (type) psychosis F10.950
  pellagra E52
  poisoning, accidental (acute) NEC — *see* Table of Drugs and Chemicals, alcohol, poisoning
  psychosis — *see* Psychosis, alcoholic
  withdrawal (without convulsions) F10.239
    with delirium F10.231
Alcoholism (chronic) (without remission) F10.20
  with
    psychosis — *see* Psychosis, alcoholic
  remission F10.21
  Korsakov's F10.96
    with dependence F10.26
Alder (-Reilly) anomaly or syndrome (leukocyte granulation) D72.0
Aldosteronism E26.9
  familial (type I) E26.02
  glucocorticoid-remediable E26.02
  primary (due to (bilateral) adrenal hyperplasia) E26.09
  primary NEC E26.09
  secondary E26.1
  specified NEC E26.89
Aldosteronoma D44.10
Aldrich (-Wiskott) syndrome (eczema-thrombocytopenia) D82.0
Alektorophobia F40.218
Aleppo boil B55.1
Aleukemic — *see* condition
Aleukia
  congenital D70.0
  hemorrhagica D61.9
    congenital D61.09
  splenica D73.1
Alexia R48.0
  developmental F81.0
  secondary to organic lesion R48.0
Algoneurodystrophy M89.00
  ankle M89.07-

Algoneurodystrophy - *continued*
  foot M89.07-
  forearm M89.03-
  hand M89.04-
  lower leg M89.06-
  multiple sites M89.0-
  shoulder M89.01-
  specified site NEC M89.08
  thigh M89.05-
  upper arm M89.02-
Algophobia F40.298
Alienation, mental — *see* Psychosis
Alkalemia E87.3
Alkalosis E87.3
  metabolic E87.3
    with respiratory acidosis E87.4
    of newborn P74.41
  respiratory E87.3
Alkaptonuria E70.29
Allen-Masters syndrome N83.8
Allergy, allergic (reaction) (to) T78.40
  air-borne substance NEC (rhinitis) J30.89
  alveolitis (extrinsic) J67.9
    due to
      Aspergillus clavatus J67.4
      Cryptostroma corticale J67.6
      organisms (fungal, thermophilic actinomycete) growing in ventilation (air conditioning) systems J67.7
    specified type NEC J67.8
  anaphylactic reaction or shock T78.2
  angioneurotic edema T78.3
  animal (dander) (epidermal) (hair) (rhinitis) J30.81
  bee sting (anaphylactic shock) — *see* Toxicity, venom, arthropod, bee
  biological — *see* Allergy, drug
  colitis — *see also* Colitis, allergic K52.29
  dander (animal) (rhinitis) J30.81
  dandruff (rhinitis) J30.81
  dental restorative material (existing) K08.55
  dermatitis — *see* Dermatitis, contact, allergic
  diathesis — *see* History, allergy
  drug, medicament & biological (any) (external) (internal) T78.40
    correct substance properly administered — *see* Table of Drugs and Chemicals, by drug, adverse effect
    wrong substance given or taken NEC (by accident) — *see* Table of Drugs and Chemicals, by drug, poisoning
  due to pollen J30.1
  dust (house) (stock) (rhinitis) J30.89
    with asthma — *see* Asthma, allergic extrinsic
  eczema — *see* Dermatitis, contact, allergic
  epidermal (animal) (rhinitis) J30.81
  feathers (rhinitis) J30.89
  food (any) (ingested) NEC T78.1
    anaphylactic shock — *see* Shock, anaphylactic, due to food
    dermatitis — *see* Dermatitis, due to, food
    dietary counseling and surveillance Z71.3
    in contact with skin L23.6
    rhinitis J30.5
    status (without reaction) Z91.018
      eggs Z91.012
      milk products Z91.011
      peanuts Z91.010
      seafood Z91.013
      specified NEC Z91.018
    gastrointestinal — *see also* specific type of allergic reaction
      meaning colitis — *see also* Colitis, allergic K52.29
      meaning gastroenteritis — *see also* Gastroenteritis, allergic K52.29
      meaning other adverse food reaction not elsewhere classified T78.1
  grain J30.1
  grass (hay fever) (pollen) J30.1
    asthma — *see* Asthma, allergic extrinsic
  hair (animal) (rhinitis) J30.81

Allergy, allergic (reaction) (to) - *continued*
  history (of) — *see* History, allergy
  horse serum — *see* Allergy, serum
  inhalant (rhinitis) J30.89
    pollen J30.1
  kapok (rhinitis) J30.89
  medicine — *see* Allergy, drug
  milk protein — *see also* Allergy, food Z91.011
    anaphylactic reaction T78.07
    dermatitis L27.2
    enterocolitis syndrome K52.21
    enteropathy K52.22
    gastroenteritis K52.29
    gastroesophageal reflux — *see also* Reaction, adverse, food K21.9
      with esophagitis K21.0
    proctocolitis K52.82
  nasal, seasonal due to pollen J30.1
  pneumonia J82
  pollen (any) (hay fever) J30.1
    asthma — *see* Asthma, allergic extrinsic
  primrose J30.1
  primula J30.1
  proctocolitis K52.82
  purpura D69.0
  ragweed (hay fever) (pollen) J30.1
    asthma — *see* Asthma, allergic extrinsic
  rose (pollen) J30.1
  seasonal NEC J30.2
  Senecio jacobae (pollen) J30.1
  serum — *see also* Reaction, serum T80.69
    anaphylactic shock T80.59
  shock (anaphylactic) T78.2
    due to
      administration of blood and blood products T80.51
      adverse effect of correct medicinal substance properly administered T88.6
      immunization T80.52
      serum NEC T80.59
      vaccination T80.52
  specific NEC T78.49
  tree (any) (hay fever) (pollen) J30.1
    asthma — *see* Asthma, allergic extrinsic
  upper respiratory J30.9
  urticaria L50.0
  vaccine — *see* Allergy, serum
  wheat — *see* Allergy, food
Allescheriasis B48.2
Alligator skin disease Q80.9
Allocheiria, allochiria R20.8
Almeida's disease — *see* Paracoccidioidomycosis
Alopecia (hereditaria) (seborrheica) L65.9
  androgenic L64.9
    drug-induced L64.0
    specified NEC L64.8
  areata L63.9
    ophiasis L63.2
    specified NEC L63.8
    totalis L63.0
    universalis L63.1
  cicatricial L66.9
    specified NEC L66.8
  circumscripta L63.9
  congenital, congenitalis Q84.0
  due to cytotoxic drugs NEC L65.8
  mucinosa L65.2
  postinfective NEC L65.8
  postpartum L65.0
  premature L64.8
  specific (syphilitic) A51.32
  specified NEC L65.8
  syphilitic (secondary) A51.32
  totalis (capitis) L63.0
  universalis (entire body) L63.1
  X-ray L58.1
Alpers' disease G31.81
Alpine sickness T70.29
Alport syndrome Q87.81
ALTE (apparent life threatening event) in newborn and infant R68.13

Alteration (of) , Altered
  awareness
    transient R40.4
    unintended under general anesthesia,
      during procedureT88.53
  mental status R41.82
  pattern of family relationships affecting
    child Z62.898
  sensation
    following
      cerebrovascular disease I69.998
        cerebral infarction I69.398
        intracerebral hemorrhage I69.198
        nontraumatic intracranial hemorrhage
          NEC I69.298
        specified disease NEC I69.898
        subarachnoid hemorrhage I69.098
Alternating — *see* condition
Altitude, high (effects) — *see* Effect, adverse,
    high altitude
Aluminosis (of lung) J63.0
Alveolitis
  allergic (extrinsic) — *see* Pneumonitis,
    hypersensitivity
  due to
    Aspergillus clavatus J67.4
    Cryptostroma corticale J67.6
  fibrosing (cryptogenic) (idiopathic) J84.112
  jaw M27.3
  sicca dolorosa M27.3
Alveolus, alveolar — *see* condition
Alymphocytosis D72.810
  thymic (with immunodeficiency) D82.1
Alymphoplasia, thymic D82.1
Alzheimer's disease or sclerosis — *see*
    Disease, Alzheimer's
Amastia (with nipple present) Q83.8
  with absent nipple Q83.0
Amathophobia F40.228
Amaurosis (acquired) (congenital) — *see*
    also Blindness
  fugax G45.3
  hysterical F44.6
  Leber's congenital H35.50
  uremic — *see* Uremia
Amaurotic idiocy (infantile) (juvenile)
    (late) E75.4
Amaxophobia F40.248
Ambiguous genitalia Q56.4
Amblyopia (congenital) (ex anopsia)
    (partial) (suppression) H53.00-
  anisometropic — *see* Amblyopia, refractive
  deprivation H53.01-
  hysterical F44.6
  nocturnal — *see also* Blindness, night
    vitamin A deficiency E50.5
  refractive H53.02-
  strabismic H53.03-
  suspect H53.04-
  tobacco H53.8
  toxic NEC H53.8
  uremic — *see* Uremia
Ameba, amebic (histolytica) — *see also*
    Amebiasis
  abscess (liver) A06.4
Amebiasis A06.9
  with abscess — *see* Abscess, amebic
  acute A06.0
  chronic (intestine) A06.1
    with abscess — *see* Abscess, amebic
  cutaneous A06.7
  cutis A06.7
  cystitis A06.81
  genitourinary tract NEC A06.82
  hepatic — *see* Abscess, liver, amebic
  intestine A06.0
  nondysenteric colitis A06.2
  skin A06.7
  specified site NEC A06.89
Ameboma (of intestine) A06.3
Amelia Q73.0
  lower limb — *see* Agenesis, leg
  upper limb — *see* Agenesis, arm

Ameloblastoma — *see also* Cyst, calcifying
    odontogenic
  long bones C40.9-
    lower limb C40.2-
    upper limb C40.0-
  malignant C41.1
    jaw (bone) (lower) C41.1
    upper C41.0
  tibial C40.2-
Amelogenesis imperfecta K00.5
  nonhereditaria (segmentalis) K00.4
Amenorrhea N91.2
  hyperhormonal E28.8
  primary N91.0
  secondary N91.1
Amentia — *see* Disability, intellectual
  Meynert's (nonalcoholic) F04
American
  leishmaniasis B55.2
  mountain tick fever A93.2
Ametropia — *see* Disorder, refraction
AMH (asymptomatic microscopic
    hematuria) R31.21
Amianthosis J61
Amimia R48.8
Amino-acid disorder E72.9
  anemia D53.0
Aminoacidopathy E72.9
Aminoaciduria E72.9
Amnes (t) ic syndrome (post-traumatic) F04
  induced by
    alcohol F10.96
      with dependence F10.26
    psychoactive NEC F19.96
      with
        abuse F19.16
        dependence F19.26
    sedative F13.96
      with dependence F13.26
Amnesia R41.3
  anterograde R41.1
  auditory R48.8
  dissociative F44.0
    with dissociative fugue F44.1
  hysterical F44.0
  postictal in epilepsy — *see* Epilepsy
  psychogenic F44.0
  retrograde R41.2
  transient global G45.4
Amnion, amniotic — *see* condition
Amnionitis — *see* Pregnancy, complicated by
Amok F68.8
Amoral traits F60.89
Amphetamine (or other stimulant) -induced
  anxiety disorder F15.980
  bipolar and related disorder F15.94
  delirium F15.921
  depressive disorder F15.94
  obsessive-compulsive and related
    disorder F15.988
  psychotic disorder F15.959
  sexual dysfunction F15.981
  sleep disorder F15.982
  stimulant withdrawal F15.23
Ampulla
  lower esophagus K22.8
  phrenic K22.8
Amputation — *see also* Absence, by site,
    acquired
  neuroma (postoperative) (traumatic) — *see*
    Complications, amputation stump,
    neuroma
  stump (surgical)
    abnormal, painful, or with complication
      (late) — *see* Complications,
      amputation stump
    healed or old NOS Z89.9
  traumatic (complete) (partial)
    arm (upper) (complete) S48.91-
      at
        elbow S58.01-
          partial S58.02-
        shoulder joint (complete) S48.01-
          partial S48.02-
        between

Amputation - *continued*
  traumatic (complete) (partial) - *continued*
    arm (upper) (complete) - *continued*
      between - *continued*
        elbow and wrist (complete) S58.11-
          partial S58.12-
        shoulder and elbow
          (complete) S48.11-
          partial S48.12-
        partial S48.92-
    breast (complete) S28.21-
      partial S28.22-
    clitoris (complete) S38.211
      partial S38.212
    ear (complete) S08.11-
      partial S08.12-
    finger (complete)
        (metacarpophalangeal) S68.11-
      index S68.11-
      little S68.11-
      middle S68.11-
      partial S68.12-
        index S68.12-
        little S68.12-
        middle S68.12-
        ring S68.12-
      ring S68.11-
      thumb — *see* Amputation, traumatic,
        thumb
      transphalangeal (complete) S68.61-
        index S68.61-
        little S68.61-
        middle S68.61-
        partial S68.62-
          index S68.62-
          little S68.62-
          middle S68.62-
          ring S68.62-
        ring S68.61-
    foot (complete) S98.91-
      at ankle level S98.01-
        partial S98.02-
      midfoot S98.31-
        partial S98.32-
      partial S98.92-
    forearm (complete) S58.91-
      at elbow level (complete) S58.01-
        partial S58.02-
      between elbow and wrist
        (complete) S58.11-
        partial S58.12-
      partial S58.92-
    genital organ (s) (external)
      female (complete) S38.211
        partial S38.212
      male
        penis (complete) S38.221
          partial S38.222
        scrotum (complete) S38.231
          partial S38.232
        testes (complete) S38.231
          partial S38.232
    hand (complete) (wrist level) S68.41-
      finger (s) alone — *see* Amputation,
        traumatic, finger
      partial S68.42-
      thumb alone — *see* Amputation,
        traumatic, thumb
      transmetacarpal (complete) S68.71-
        partial S68.72-
    head
      ear — *see* Amputation, traumatic, ear
      nose (partial) S08.812
        complete S08.811
      part S08.89
        scalp S08.0
    hip (and thigh) (complete) S78.91-
      at hip joint (complete) S78.01-
        partial S78.02-
      between hip and knee
        (complete) S78.11-
        partial S78.12-
      partial S78.92-
    labium (majus) (minus)
        (complete) S38.21-

Amputation - *continued*
  traumatic (complete) (partial) - *continued*
    labium (majus) (minus) (complete) - *continued*
      partial S38.21-
      leg (lower) S88.91-
        at knee level S88.01-
          partial S88.02-
        between knee and ankle S88.11-
          partial S88.12-
        partial S88.92-
      nose (partial) S08.812
        complete S08.811
      penis (complete) S38.221
        partial S38.222
      scrotum (complete) S38.231
        partial S38.232
      shoulder — *see* Amputation, traumatic, arm
        at shoulder joint — *see* Amputation, traumatic, arm, at shoulder joint
      testes (complete) S38.231
        partial S38.232
      thigh — *see* Amputation, traumatic, hip
      thorax, part of S28.1
        breast — *see* Amputation, traumatic, breast
      thumb (complete) (metacarpophalangeal) S68.01-
        partial S68.02-
      transphalangeal (complete) S68.51-
        partial S68.52-
      toe (lesser) S98.13-
        great S98.11-
          partial S98.12-
        more than one S98.21-
          partial S98.22-
        partial S98.14-
      vulva (complete) S38.211
        partial S38.212
Amputee (bilateral) (old) Z89.9
Amsterdam dwarfism Q87.19
Amusia R48.8
  developmental F80.89
Amyelencephalus, amyelencephaly Q00.0
Amyelia Q06.0
Amygdalitis — *see* Tonsillitis
Amygdalolith J35.8
Amyloid heart (disease) E85.4 *[I43]*
Amyloidosis (generalized) (primary) E85.9
  with lung involvement E85.4 *[J99]*
  familial E85.2
  genetic E85.2
  heart E85.4 *[I43]*
  hemodialysis-associated E85.3
  light chain (AL) E85.81
  liver E85.4 *[K77]*
  localized E85.4
  neuropathic heredofamilial E85.1
  non-neuropathic heredofamilial E85.0
  organ limited E85.4
  Portuguese E85.1
  pulmonary E85.4 *[J99]*
  secondary systemic E85.3
  senile systemic (SSA) E85.82
  skin (lichen) (macular) E85.4 *[L99]*
  specified NEC E85.89
  subglottic E85.4 *[J99]*
  wild-type transthyretin-related (ATTR) E85.82
Amylopectinosis (brancher enzyme deficiency) E74.03
Amylophagia — *see* Pica
Amyoplasia congenita Q79.8
Amyotonia M62.89
  congenita G70.2
Amyotrophia, amyotrophy, amyotrophic G71.8
  congenita Q79.8
  diabetic — *see* Diabetes, amyotrophy
  lateral sclerosis G12.21
  neuralgic G54.5
  spinal progressive G12.25
Anacidity, gastric K31.83
  psychogenic F45.8

Anaerosis of newborn P28.89
Analbuminemia E88.09
Analgesia — *see* Anesthesia
Analphalipoproteinemia E78.6
Anaphylactic
  purpura D69.0
  shock or reaction — *see* Shock, anaphylactic
Anaphylactoid shock or reaction — *see* Shock, anaphylactic
Anaphylactoid syndrome of pregnancy O88.01-
Anaphylaxis — *see* Shock, anaphylactic
Anaplasia cervix — *see also* Dysplasia, cervix N87.9
Anaplasmosis, human A77.49
Anarthria R47.1
Anasarca R60.1
  cardiac — *see* Failure, heart, congestive
  lung J18.2
  newborn P83.2
  nutritional E43
  pulmonary J18.2
  renal N04.9
Anastomosis
  aneurysmal — *see* Aneurysm
  arteriovenous ruptured brain I60.8
    intracerebral I61.8
    intraparenchymal I61.8
    intraventricular I61.5
    subarachnoid I60.8
  intestinal K63.89
    complicated NEC K91.89
      involving urinary tract N99.89
  retinal and choroidal vessels (congenital) Q14.8
Anatomical narrow angle H40.03-
Ancylostoma, ancylostomiasis (braziliense) (caninum) (ceylanicum) (duodenale) B76.0
  Necator americanus B76.1
Andersen's disease (glycogen storage) E74.09
Anderson-Fabry disease E75.21
Andes disease T70.29
Andrews' disease (bacterid) L08.89
Androblastoma
  benign
    specified site — *see* Neoplasm, benign, by site
    unspecified site
      female D27.9
      male D29.20
  malignant
    specified site — *see* Neoplasm, malignant, by site
    unspecified site
      female C56.9
      male C62.90
  specified site — *see* Neoplasm, uncertain behavior, by site
  tubular
    with lipid storage
      specified site — *see* Neoplasm, benign, by site
      unspecified site
        female D27.9
        male D29.20
    specified site — *see* Neoplasm, benign, by site
    unspecified site
      female D27.9
      male D29.20
  unspecified site
    female D39.10
    male D40.10
Androgen insensitivity syndrome — *see also* Syndrome, androgen insensitivity E34.50
Androgen resistance syndrome — *see also* Syndrome, androgen insensitivity E34.50
Android pelvis Q74.2
  with disproportion (fetopelvic) O33.3
    causing obstructed labor O65.3
Androphobia F40.290

Anectasis, pulmonary (newborn) — *see* Atelectasis
Anemia (essential) (general) (hemoglobin deficiency) (infantile) (primary) (profound) D64.9
  with (due to) (in)
    disorder of
      anaerobic glycolysis D55.2
      pentose phosphate pathway D55.1
    koilonychia D50.9
  achlorhydric D50.8
  achrestic D53.1
  Addison (-Biermer) (pernicious) D51.0
  agranulocytic — *see* Agranulocytosis
  amino-acid-deficiency D53.0
  aplastic D61.9
    congenital D61.09
    drug-induced D61.1
    due to
      drugs D61.1
      external agents NEC D61.2
      infection D61.2
      radiation D61.2
    idiopathic D61.3
    red cell (pure) D60.9
      chronic D60.0
      congenital D61.01
      specified type NEC D60.8
      transient D60.1
    specified type NEC D61.89
    toxic D61.2
  aregenerative
    congenital D61.09
  asiderotic D50.9
  atypical (primary) D64.9
  Baghdad spring D55.0
  Balantidium coli A07.0
  Biermer's (pernicious) D51.0
  blood loss (chronic) D50.0
    acute D62
  bothriocephalus B70.0 *[D63.8]*
  brickmaker's B76.9 *[D63.8]*
  cerebral I67.89
  childhood D58.9
  chlorotic D50.8
  chronic
    blood loss D50.0
    hemolytic D58.9
      idiopathic D59.9
    simple D53.9
  chronica congenita aregenerativa D61.09
  combined system disease NEC D51.0 *[G32.0]*
    due to dietary vitamin B12 deficiency D51.3 *[G32.0]*
  complicating pregnancy, childbirth or puerperium — *see* Pregnancy, complicated by (management affected by), anemia
  congenital P61.4
    aplastic D61.09
    due to isoimmunization NOS P55.9
    dyserythropoietic, dyshematopoietic D64.4
    following fetal blood loss P61.3
    Heinz body D58.2
    hereditary hemolytic NOS D58.9
    pernicious D51.0
    spherocytic D58.0
  Cooley's (erythroblastic) D56.1
  cytogenic D51.0
  deficiency D53.9
    2, 3 diphosphoglycurate mutase D55.2
    2, 3 PG D55.2
    6 phosphogluconate dehydrogenase D55.1
    6-PGD D55.1
    amino-acid D53.0
    combined B12 and folate D53.1
    enzyme D55.9
      drug-induced (hemolytic) D59.2
      glucose-6-phosphate dehydrogenase (G6PD) D55.0
      glycolytic D55.2
      nucleotide metabolism D55.3
      related to hexose monophosphate (HMP) shunt pathway NEC D55.1

Anemia (essential) (general) (hemoglobin deficiency) (infantile) (primary) (profound) - *continued*
  deficiency - *continued*
    enzyme - *continued*
      specified type NEC D55.8
    erythrocytic glutathione D55.1
    folate D52.9
      dietary D52.0
      drug-induced D52.1
    folic acid D52.9
      dietary D52.0
      drug-induced D52.1
    G SH D55.1
    GGS-R D55.1
    glucose-6-phosphate dehydrogenase D55.0
    glutathione reductase D55.1
    glyceraldehyde phosphate
        dehydrogenase D55.2
    G6PD D55.0
    hexokinase D55.2
    iron D50.9
      secondary to blood loss (chronic) D50.0
    nutritional D53.9
      with
        poor iron absorption D50.8
        specified deficiency NEC D53.8
    phosphofructo-aldolase D55.2
    phosphoglycerate kinase D55.2
    PK D55.2
    protein D53.0
    pyruvate kinase D55.2
    transcobalamin II D51.2
    triose-phosphate isomerase D55.2
    vitamin B12 NOS D51.9
      dietary D51.3
      due to
        intrinsic factor deficiency D51.0
        selective vitamin B12 malabsorption
            with proteinuria D51.1
      pernicious D51.0
      specified type NEC D51.8
  Diamond-Blackfan (congenital
      hypoplastic) D61.01
  dibothriocephalus B70.0 *[D63.8]*
  dimorphic D53.1
  diphasic D53.1
  Diphyllobothrium
      (Dibothriocephalus) B70.0 *[D63.8]*
  due to (in) (with)
    antineoplastic chemotherapy D64.81
    blood loss (chronic) D50.0
      acute D62
    chemotherapy, antineoplastic D64.81
    chronic disease classified elsewhere
        NEC D63.8
    chronic kidney disease D63.1
    deficiency
      amino-acid D53.0
      copper D53.8
      folate (folic acid) D52.9
        dietary D52.0
        drug-induced D52.1
      molybdenum D53.8
      protein D53.0
      zinc D53.8
    dietary vitamin B12 deficiency D51.3
    disorder of
      glutathione metabolism D55.1
      nucleotide metabolism D55.3
    drug — *see* Anemia, by type — *see also*
        Table of Drugs and Chemicals
    end stage renal disease D63.1
    enzyme disorder D55.9
    fetal blood loss P61.3
    fish tapeworm (D.latum) infestation B70.0
        [D63.8]
    hemorrhage (chronic) D50.0
      acute D62
    impaired absorption D50.9
    loss of blood (chronic) D50.0
      acute D62
    myxedema E03.9 *[D63.8]*
    Necator americanus B76.1 *[D63.8]*
    prematurity P61.2

Anemia (essential) (general) (hemoglobin deficiency) (infantile) (primary) (profound) - *continued*
  due to (in) (with) - *continued*
    selective vitamin B12 malabsorption with
        proteinuria D51.1
    transcobalamin II deficiency D51.2
  Dyke-Young type (secondary)
      (symptomatic) D59.1
  dyserythropoietic (congenital) D64.4
  dyshematopoietic (congenital) D64.4
  Egyptian B76.9 *[D63.8]*
  elliptocytosis — *see* Elliptocytosis
  enzyme-deficiency, drug-induced D59.2
  epidemic — *see also* Ancylostomiasis B76.9
      [D63.8]
  erythroblastic
    familial D56.1
    newborn — *see also* Disease,
        hemolytic P55.9
    of childhood D56.1
  erythrocytic glutathione deficiency D55.1
  erythropoietin-resistant anemia (EPO
      resistant anemia) D63.1
  Faber's (achlorhydric anemia) D50.9
  factitious (self-induced blood letting) D50.0
  familial erythroblastic D56.1
  Fanconi's (congenital pancytopenia) D61.09
  favism D55.0
  fish tapeworm (D. latum) infestation B70.0
      [D63.8]
  folate (folic acid) deficiency D52.9
  glucose-6-phosphate dehydrogenase (G6PD)
      deficiency D55.0
  glutathione-reductase deficiency D55.1
  goat's milk D52.0
  granulocytic — *see* Agranulocytosis
  Heinz body, congenital D58.2
  hemolytic D58.9
    acquired D59.9
      with hemoglobinuria NEC D59.6
      autoimmune NEC D59.1
      infectious D59.4
      specified type NEC D59.8
      toxic D59.4
    acute D59.9
      due to enzyme deficiency specified type
          NEC D55.8
      Lederer's D59.1
    autoimmune D59.1
      drug-induced D59.0
    chronic D58.9
      idiopathic D59.9
    cold type (secondary)
        (symptomatic) D59.1
    congenital (spherocytic) — *see*
        Spherocytosis
    due to
      cardiac conditions D59.4
      drugs (nonautoimmune) D59.2
        autoimmune D59.0
      enzyme disorder D55.9
        drug-induced D59.2
      presence of shunt or other internal
          prosthetic device D59.4
    familial D58.9
    hereditary D58.9
      due to enzyme disorder D55.9
        specified type NEC D55.8
      specified type NEC D58.8
    idiopathic (chronic) D59.9
    mechanical D59.4
    microangiopathic D59.4
    nonautoimmune D59.4
      drug-induced D59.2
    nonspherocytic
      congenital or hereditary NEC D55.8
        glucose-6-phosphate dehydrogenase
            deficiency D55.0
        pyruvate kinase deficiency D55.2
        type
          I D55.1
          II D55.2
      type
        I D55.1

Anemia (essential) (general) (hemoglobin deficiency) (infantile) (primary) (profound) - *continued*
  hemolytic - *continued*
    nonspherocytic - *continued*
      type - *continued*
        II D55.2
    secondary D59.4
      autoimmune D59.1
    specified (hereditary) type NEC D58.8
    Stransky-Regala type — *see also*
        Hemoglobinopathy D58.8
    symptomatic D59.4
      autoimmune D59.1
    toxic D59.4
    warm type (secondary)
        (symptomatic) D59.1
  hemorrhagic (chronic) D50.0
    acute D62
  Herrick's D57.1
  hexokinase deficiency D55.2
  hookworm B76.9 *[D63.8]*
  hypochromic (idiopathic) (microcytic)
      (normoblastic) D50.9
    due to blood loss (chronic) D50.0
      acute D62
    familial sex-linked D64.0
    pyridoxine-responsive D64.3
    sideroblastic, sex-linked D64.0
  hypoplasia, red blood cells D61.9
    congenital or familial D61.01
  hypoplastic (idiopathic) D61.9
    congenital or familial (of
        childhood) D61.01
  hypoproliferative (refractive) D61.9
  idiopathic D64.9
    aplastic D61.3
    hemolytic, chronic D59.9
  in (due to) (with)
    chronic kidney disease D63.1
    end stage renal disease D63.1
    failure, kidney (renal) D63.1
    neoplastic disease — *see also*
        Neoplasm D63.0
  intertropical — *see also*
      Ancylostomiasis D63.8
  iron deficiency D50.9
    secondary to blood loss (chronic) D50.0
      acute D62
    specified type NEC D50.8
  Joseph-Diamond-Blackfan (congenital
      hypoplastic) D61.01
  Lederer's (hemolytic) D59.1
  leukoerythroblastic D61.82
  macrocytic D53.9
    nutritional D52.0
    tropical D52.8
  malarial — *see also* Malaria B54 *[D63.8]*
  malignant (progressive) D51.0
  malnutrition D53.9
  marsh — *see also* Malaria B54 *[D63.8]*
  Mediterranean (with other
      hemoglobinopathy) D56.9
  megaloblastic D53.1
    combined B12 and folate deficiency D53.1
    hereditary D51.1
    nutritional D52.0
    orotic aciduria D53.0
    refractory D53.1
    specified type NEC D53.1
  megalocytic D53.1
  microcytic (hypochromic) D50.9
    due to blood loss (chronic) D50.0
      acute D62
    familial D56.8
  microdrepanocytosis D57.40
  microelliptopoikilocytic (Rietti-Greppi-
      Micheli) D56.9
  miner's B76.9 *[D63.8]*
  myelodysplastic D46.9
  myelofibrosis D75.81
  myelogenous D64.89
  myelopathic D64.89
  myelophthisic D61.82
  myeloproliferative D47.Z9

Anemia (essential) (general) (hemoglobin deficiency) (infantile) (primary) (profound) - *continued*
  newborn P61.4
    due to
      ABO (antibodies, isoimmunization, maternal/fetal incompatibility) P55.1
      Rh (antibodies, isoimmunization, maternal/fetal incompatibility) P55.0
    following fetal blood loss P61.3
    posthemorrhagic (fetal) P61.3
  nonspherocytic hemolytic — see Anemia, hemolytic, nonspherocytic
  normocytic (infectional) D64.9
    due to blood loss (chronic) D50.0
      acute D62
    myelophthisic D61.82
  nutritional (deficiency) D53.9
    with
      poor iron absorption D50.8
      specified deficiency NEC D53.8
    megaloblastic D52.0
  of prematurity P61.2
  orotaciduric (congenital) (hereditary) D53.0
  osteosclerotic D64.89
  ovalocytosis (hereditary) — see Elliptocytosis
  paludal — see also Malaria B54 *[D63.8]*
  pernicious (congenital) (malignant) (progressive) D51.0
  pleochromic D64.89
    of sprue D52.8
  posthemorrhagic (chronic) D50.0
    acute D62
    newborn P61.3
  postoperative (postprocedural)
    due to (acute) blood loss D62
      chronic blood loss D50.0
    specified NEC D64.9
  postpartum O90.81
  pressure D64.89
  progressive D64.9
    malignant D51.0
    pernicious D51.0
  protein-deficiency D53.0
  pseudoleukemica infantum D64.89
  pure red cell D60.9
    congenital D61.01
  pyridoxine-responsive D64.3
  pyruvate kinase deficiency D55.2
  refractory D46.4
    with
      excess of blasts D46.20
        1 (RAEB 1) D46.21
        2 (RAEB 2) D46.22
        in transformation (RAEB T) — see Leukemia, acute myeloblastic
      hemochromatosis D46.1
      sideroblasts (ring) (RARS) D46.1
    megaloblastic D53.1
    sideroblastic D46.1
    sideropenic D50.9
    without ring sideroblasts, so stated D46.0
    without sideroblasts without excess of blasts D46.0
  Rietti-Greppi-Micheli D56.9
  scorbutic D53.2
  secondary to
    blood loss (chronic) D50.0
      acute D62
    hemorrhage (chronic) D50.0
      acute D62
  semiplastic D61.89
  sickle-cell — see Disease, sickle-cell
  sideroblastic D64.3
    hereditary D64.0
    hypochromic, sex-linked D64.0
    pyridoxine-responsive NEC D64.3
    refractory D46.1
    secondary (due to)
      disease D64.1
      drugs and toxins D64.2
    specified type NEC D64.3

Anemia (essential) (general) (hemoglobin deficiency) (infantile) (primary) (profound) - *continued*
  sideropenic (refractory) D50.9
    due to blood loss (chronic) D50.0
      acute D62
  simple chronic D53.9
  specified type NEC D64.89
  spherocytic (hereditary) — see Spherocytosis
  splenic D64.89
  splenomegalic D64.89
  stomatocytosis D58.8
  syphilitic (acquired) (late) A52.79 *[D63.8]*
  target cell D64.89
  thalassemia D56.9
  thrombocytopenic — see Thrombocytopenia
  toxic D61.2
  tropical B76.9 *[D63.8]*
    macrocytic D52.8
  tuberculous A18.89 *[D63.8]*
  vegan D51.3
  vitamin
    B6-responsive D64.3
    B12 deficiency (dietary) pernicious D51.0
  von Jaksch's D64.89
  Witts' (achlorhydric anemia) D50.8
Anemophobia F40.228
Anencephalus, anencephaly Q00.0
Anergasia — see Psychosis, organic
Anesthesia, anesthetic R20.0
  complication or reaction NEC — see also Complications, anesthesia T88.59
  due to
    correct substance properly administered — see Table of Drugs and Chemicals, by drug, adverse effect
    overdose or wrong substance given — see Table of Drugs and Chemicals, by drug, poisoning
  unintended awareness under general anesthesia during procedure T88.53
    personal history of Z92.84
  cornea H18.81-
  dissociative F44.6
  functional (hysterical) F44.6
  hyperesthetic, thalamic G89.0
  hysterical F44.6
  local skin lesion R20.0
  sexual (psychogenic) F52.1
  shock (due to) T88.2
  skin R20.0
  testicular N50.9
Anetoderma (maculosum) (of) L90.8
  Jadassohn-Pellizzari L90.2
  Schweniger-Buzzi L90.1
Aneurin deficiency E51.9
Aneurysm (anastomotic) (artery) (cirsoid) (diffuse) (false) (fusiform) (multiple) (saccular) I72.9
  abdominal (aorta) I71.4
    ruptured I71.3
    syphilitic A52.01
  aorta, aortic (nonsyphilitic) I71.9
    abdominal I71.4
      ruptured I71.3
    arch I71.2
      ruptured I71.1
    arteriosclerotic I71.9
      ruptured I71.8
    ascending I71.2
      ruptured I71.1
    congenital Q25.43
    descending I71.9
      abdominal I71.4
        ruptured I71.3
      ruptured I71.8
      thoracic I71.2
        ruptured I71.1
    root Q25.43
      ruptured I71.8
    sinus, congenital Q25.43
    syphilitic A52.01
    thoracic I71.2
      ruptured I71.1

Aneurysm (anastomotic) (artery) (cirsoid) (diffuse) (false) (fusiform) (multiple) (saccular) - *continued*
  aorta, aortic (nonsyphilitic) - *continued*
    thoracoabdominal I71.6
      ruptured I71.5
    thorax, thoracic (arch) I71.2
      ruptured I71.1
    transverse I71.2
      ruptured I71.1
    valve (heart) — see also Endocarditis, aortic I35.8
  arteriosclerotic I72.9
    cerebral I67.1
      ruptured — see Hemorrhage, intracranial, subarachnoid
  arteriovenous (congenital) — see also Malformation, arteriovenous
    acquired I77.0
      brain I67.1
        ruptured — see Aneurysm, arteriovenous, brain, ruptured
      coronary I25.41
      pulmonary I28.0
    brain Q28.2
      ruptured I60.8
        intracerebral I61.8
        intraparenchymal I61.8
        intraventricular I61.5
        subarachnoid I60.8
    peripheral — see Malformation, arteriovenous, peripheral
    precerebral vessels Q28.0
    specified site NEC — see also Malformation, arteriovenous
      acquired I77.0
  basal — see Aneurysm, brain
  basilar (trunk) I72.5
  berry (congenital) (nonruptured) I67.1
    ruptured I60.7
  brain I67.1
    arteriosclerotic I67.1
      ruptured — see Hemorrhage, intracranial, subarachnoid
    arteriovenous (congenital) (nonruptured) Q28.2
      acquired I67.1
        ruptured — see Aneurysm, arteriovenous, brain, ruptured I60.8
      ruptured — see Aneurysm, arteriovenous, brain, ruptured I60.8
    berry (congenital) (nonruptured) I67.1
      ruptured — see also Hemorrhage, intracranial, subarachnoid I60.7
    congenital Q28.3
      ruptured I60.7
    meninges I67.1
      ruptured I60.8
    miliary (congenital) (nonruptured) I67.1
      ruptured — see also Hemorrhage, intracranial, subarachnoid I60.7
    mycotic I33.0
      ruptured — see Hemorrhage, intracranial, subarachnoid
    syphilitic (hemorrhage) A52.05
  cardiac (false) — see also Aneurysm, heart I25.3
  carotid artery (common) (external) I72.0
    internal (intracranial) I67.1
      extracranial portion I72.0
      ruptured into brain I60.0-
    syphilitic A52.09
      intracranial A52.05
  cavernous sinus I67.1
    arteriovenous (congenital) (nonruptured) Q28.3
      ruptured I60.8
  celiac I72.8
  central nervous system, syphilitic A52.05
  cerebral — see Aneurysm, brain
  chest — see Aneurysm, thorax
  circle of Willis I67.1
    congenital Q28.3
      ruptured I60.6

Aneurysm (anastomotic) (artery) (cirsoid) (diffuse) (false) (fusiform) (multiple) (saccular) - *continued*
  circle of Willis - *continued*
    ruptured I60.6
  common iliac artery I72.3
  congenital (peripheral) Q27.8
    aorta (root) (sinus) Q25.43
    brain Q28.3
      ruptured I60.7
    coronary Q24.5
    digestive system Q27.8
    lower limb Q27.8
    pulmonary Q25.79
    retina Q14.1
    specified site NEC Q27.8
    upper limb Q27.8
  conjunctiva — *see* Abnormality, conjunctiva, vascular
  conus arteriosus — *see* Aneurysm, heart
  coronary (arteriosclerotic) (artery) I25.41
    arteriovenous, congenital Q24.5
    congenital Q24.5
    ruptured — *see* Infarct, myocardium
    · syphilitic A52.06
    vein I25.89
  cylindroid (aorta) I71.9
    ruptured I71.8
    syphilitic A52.01
  ductus arteriosus Q25.0
  endocardial, infective (any valve) I33.0
  femoral (artery) (ruptured) I72.4
  gastroduodenal I72.8
  gastroepiploic I72.8
  heart (wall) (chronic or with a stated duration of over 4 weeks) I25.3
    valve — *see* Endocarditis
  hepatic I72.8
  iliac (common) (artery) (ruptured) I72.3
  infective I72.9
    endocardial (any valve) I33.0
  innominate (nonsyphilitic) I72.8
    syphilitic A52.09
  interauricular septum — *see* Aneurysm, heart
  interventricular septum — *see* Aneurysm, heart
  intrathoracic (nonsyphilitic) I71.2
    ruptured I71.1
    syphilitic A52.01
  lower limb I72.4
  lung (pulmonary artery) I28.1
  mediastinal (nonsyphilitic) I72.8
    syphilitic A52.09
  miliary (congenital) I67.1
    ruptured — *see* Hemorrhage, intracerebral, subarachnoid, intracranial
  mitral (heart) (valve) I34.8
  mural — *see* Aneurysm, heart
  mycotic I72.9
    endocardial (any valve) I33.0
    ruptured, brain — *see* Hemorrhage, intracerebral, subarachnoid
  myocardium — *see* Aneurysm, heart
  neck I72.0
  pancreaticoduodenal I72.8
  patent ductus arteriosus Q25.0
  peripheral NEC I72.8
    congenital Q27.8
      digestive system Q27.8
      lower limb Q27.8
      specified site NEC Q27.8
      upper limb Q27.8
  popliteal (artery) (ruptured) I72.4
  precerebral
    congenital (nonruptured) Q28.1
    specified site, NEC I72.5
  pulmonary I28.1
    arteriovenous Q25.72
      acquired I28.0
    syphilitic A52.09
    valve (heart) — *see* Endocarditis, pulmonary
  racemose (peripheral) I72.9
    congenital — *see* Aneurysm, congenital
  radial I72.1

Aneurysm (anastomotic) (artery) (cirsoid) (diffuse) (false) (fusiform) (multiple) (saccular) - *continued*
  Rasmussen NEC A15.0
  renal (artery) I72.2
  retina — *see also* Disorder, retina, microaneurysms
    congenital Q14.1
    diabetic — *see* E08-E13 with .3-
  sinus of Valsalva Q25.49
  specified NEC I72.8
  spinal (cord) I72.8
    syphilitic (hemorrhage) A52.09
  splenic I72.8
  subclavian (artery) (ruptured) I72.8
    syphilitic A52.09
  superior mesenteric I72.8
  syphilitic (aorta) A52.01
    central nervous system A52.05
    congenital (late) A50.54 *[I79.0]*
    spine, spinal A52.09
  thoracoabdominal (aorta) I71.6
    ruptured I71.5
    syphilitic A52.01
  thorax, thoracic (aorta) (arch) (nonsyphilitic) I71.2
    ruptured I71.1
    syphilitic A52.01
  traumatic (complication) (early) , specified site — *see* Injury, blood vessel
  tricuspid (heart) (valve) I07.8
  ulnar I72.1
  upper limb (ruptured) I72.1
  valve, valvular — *see* Endocarditis
  venous — *see also* Varix I86.8
    congenital Q27.8
      digestive system Q27.8
      lower limb Q27.8
      specified site NEC Q27.8
      upper limb Q27.8
  ventricle — *see* Aneurysm, heart
  vertebral artery I72.6
  visceral NEC I72.8
Angelman syndrome Q93.51
Anger R45.4
Angiectasis, angiectopia I99.8
Angiitis I77.6
  allergic granulomatous M30.1
  hypersensitivity M31.0
  necrotizing M31.9
    specified NEC M31.8
  nervous system, granulomatous I67.7
Angina (attack) (cardiac) (chest) (heart) (pectoris) (syndrome) (vasomotor) I20.9
  with
    atherosclerotic heart disease — *see* Arteriosclerosis, coronary (artery), documented spasm I20.1
  abdominal K55.1
  accelerated — *see* Angina, unstable
  agranulocytic — *see* Agranulocytosis
  angiospastic — *see* Angina, with documented spasm
  aphthous B08.5
  crescendo — *see* Angina, unstable
  croupous J05.0
  cruris I73.9
  de novo effort — *see* Angina, unstable
  diphtheritic, membranous A36.0
  equivalent I20.8
  exudative, chronic J37.0
  following acute myocardial infarction I23.7
  gangrenous diphtheritic A36.0
  intestinal K55.1
  Ludovici K12.2
  Ludwig's K12.2
  malignant diphtheritic A36.0
  membranous J05.0
    diphtheritic A36.0
    Vincent's A69.1
  mesenteric K55.1
  monocytic — *see* Mononucleosis, infectious
  of effort — *see* Angina, specified NEC
  phlegmonous J36
    diphtheritic A36.0

Angina (attack) (cardiac) (chest) (heart) (pectoris) (syndrome) (vasomotor) - *continued*
  post-infarctional I23.7
  pre-infarctional — *see* Angina, unstable
  Prinzmetal — *see* Angina, with documented spasm
  progressive — *see* Angina, unstable
  pseudomembranous A69.1
  pultaceous, diphtheritic A36.0
  spasm-induced — *see* Angina, with documented spasm
  specified NEC I20.8
  stable I20.8
  stenocardia — *see* Angina, specified NEC
  stridulous, diphtheritic A36.2
  tonsil J36
  trachealis J05.0
  unstable I20.0
  variant — *see* Angina, with documented spasm
  Vincent's A69.1
  worsening effort — *see* Angina, unstable
Angioblastoma — *see* Neoplasm, connective tissue, uncertain behavior
Angiocholecystitis — *see* Cholecystitis, acute
Angiocholitis — *see also* Cholecystitis, acute K83.09
Angiodysgenesis spinalis G95.19
Angiodysplasia (cecum) (colon) K55.20
  with bleeding K55.21
  duodenum (and stomach) K31.819
    with bleeding K31.811
  stomach (and duodenum) K31.819
    with bleeding K31.811
Angioedema (allergic) (any site) (with urticaria) T78.3
  hereditary D84.1
Angioendothelioma — *see* Neoplasm, uncertain behavior, by site
  benign D18.00
    intra-abdominal D18.03
    intracranial D18.02
    skin D18.01
    specified site NEC D18.09
  bone — *see* Neoplasm, bone, malignant
  Ewing's — *see* Neoplasm, bone, malignant
Angioendotheliomatosis C85.8-
Angiofibroma — *see also* Neoplasm, benign, by site
  juvenile
    specified site — *see* Neoplasm, benign, by site
    unspecified site D10.6
Angiohemophilia (A) (B) D68.0
Angioid streaks (choroid) (macula) (retina) H35.33
Angiokeratoma — *see* Neoplasm, skin, benign
  corporis diffusum E75.21
Angioleiomyoma — *see* Neoplasm, connective tissue, benign
Angiolipoma — *see also* Lipoma
  infiltrating — *see* Lipoma
Angioma — *see also* Hemangioma, by site
  capillary I78.1
  hemorrhagicum hereditaria I78.0
  intra-abdominal D18.03
  intracranial D18.02
  malignant — *see* Neoplasm, connective tissue, malignant
  plexiform D18.00
    intra-abdominal D18.03
    intracranial D18.02
    skin D18.01
    specified site NEC D18.09
  senile I78.1
  serpiginosum L81.7
  skin D18.01
  specified site NEC D18.09
  spider I78.1
  stellate I78.1
  venous Q28.3
Angiomatosis Q82.8
  bacillary A79.89
  encephalotrigeminal Q85.8

Angiomatosis - *continued*
  hemorrhagic familial I78.0
  hereditary familial I78.0
  liver K76.4
Angiomyolipoma — *see* Lipoma
Angiomyoliposarcoma — *see* Neoplasm,
  connective tissue, malignant
Angiomyoma — *see* Neoplasm, connective
  tissue, benign
Angiomyosarcoma — *see* Neoplasm,
  connective tissue, malignant
Angiomyxoma — *see* Neoplasm, connective
  tissue, uncertain behavior
Angioneurosis F45.8
Angioneurotic edema (allergic) (any site)
  (with urticaria) T78.3
  hereditary D84.1
Angiopathia, angiopathy I99.9
  cerebral I67.9
    amyloid E85.4 *[I68.0]*
  diabetic (peripheral) — *see* Diabetes,
    angiopathy
  peripheral I73.9
    diabetic — *see* Diabetes, angiopathy
    specified type NEC I73.89
  retinae syphilitica A52.05
  retinalis (juvenilis)
    diabetic — *see* Diabetes, retinopathy
    proliferative — *see* Retinopathy,
      proliferative
Angiosarcoma — *see also* Neoplasm,
  connective tissue, malignant
  liver C22.3
Angiosclerosis — *see* Arteriosclerosis
Angiospasm (peripheral) (traumatic) (vessel)
  I73.9
  brachial plexus G54.0
  cerebral G45.9
  cervical plexus G54.2
  nerve
    arm — *see* Mononeuropathy, upper limb
      axillary G54.0
      median — *see* Lesion, nerve, median
      ulnar — *see* Lesion, nerve, ulnar
    axillary G54.0
    leg — *see* Mononeuropathy, lower limb
    median — *see* Lesion, nerve, median
    plantar — *see* Lesion, nerve, plantar
    ulnar — *see* Lesion, nerve, ulnar
Angiospastic disease or edema I73.9
Angiostrongyliasis
  due to
    Parastrongylus
      cantonensis B83.2
      costaricensis B81.3
    intestinal B81.3
Anguillulosis — *see* Strongyloidiasis
Angulation
  cecum — *see* Obstruction, intestine
  coccyx (acquired) (*see also* subcategory
    M43.8)
    congenital NEC Q76.49
  femur (acquired) — *see also* Deformity,
    limb, specified type NEC, thigh
    congenital Q74.2
  intestine (large) (small) — *see* Obstruction,
    intestine
  sacrum (acquired) (*see also* subcategory
    M43.8)
    congenital NEC Q76.49
  sigmoid (flexure) — *see* Obstruction,
    intestine
  spine — *see* Dorsopathy, deforming,
    specified NEC
  tibia (acquired) — *see also* Deformity, limb,
    specified type NEC, lower leg
    congenital Q74.2
  ureter N13.5
    with infection N13.6
  wrist (acquired) — *see also* Deformity, limb,
    specified type NEC, forearm
    congenital Q74.0
Angulus infectiosus (lips) K13.0
Anhedonia R45.84
  sexual F52.0

Anhidrosis L74.4
Anhydration E86.0
Anhydremia E86.0
Anidrosis L74.4
Aniridia (congenital) Q13.1
Anisakiasis (infection) (infestation) B81.0
Anisakis larvae infestation B81.0
Aniseikonia H52.32
Anisocoria (pupil) H57.02
  congenital Q13.2
Anisocytosis R71.8
Anisometropia (congenital) H52.31
Ankle — *see* condition
Ankyloblepharon (eyelid) (acquired) — *see*
  also Blepharophimosis
  filiforme (adnatum) (congenital) Q10.3
  total Q10.3
Ankyloglossia Q38.1
Ankylosis (fibrous) (osseous) (joint) M24.60
  ankle M24.67-
  arthrodesis status Z98.1
  cricoarytenoid (cartilage) (joint)
    (larynx) J38.7
  dental K03.5
  ear ossicles H74.31-
  elbow M24.62-
  foot M24.67-
  hand M24.64-
  hip M24.65-
  incostapedial joint (infectional) — *see*
    Ankylosis, ear ossicles
  jaw (temporomandibular) M26.61-
  knee M24.66-
  lumbosacral (joint) M43.27
  postoperative (status) Z98.1
  produced by surgical fusion, status Z98.1
  sacro-iliac (joint) M43.28
  shoulder M24.61-
  spine (joint) — *see also* Fusion, spine
    spondylitic — *see* Spondylitis, ankylosing
  surgical Z98.1
  temporomandibular M26.61-
  tooth, teeth (hard tissues) K03.5
  wrist M24.63-
Ankylostoma — *see* Ancylostoma
Ankylostomiasis — *see* Ancylostomiasis
Ankylurethria — *see* Stricture, urethra
Annular — *see also* condition
  detachment, cervix N88.8
  organ or site, congenital NEC — *see*
    Distortion
  pancreas (congenital) Q45.1
Anodontia (complete) (partial) (vera) K00.0
  acquired K08.10
Anomaly, anomalous (congenital)
  (unspecified type) Q89.9
  abdominal wall NEC Q79.59
  acoustic nerve Q07.8
  adrenal (gland) Q89.1
  Alder (-Reilly) (leukocyte
    granulation) D72.0
  alimentary tract Q45.9
    upper Q40.9
  alveolar M26.70
    hyperplasia M26.79
      mandibular M26.72
      maxillary M26.71
    hypoplasia M26.79
      mandibular M26.74
      maxillary M26.73
    ridge (process) M26.79
    specified NEC M26.79
  ankle (joint) Q74.2
  anus Q43.9
  aorta (arch) NEC Q25.40
    coarctation (preductal) (postductal) Q25.1
  aortic cusp or valve Q23.9
  appendix Q43.8
  apple peel syndrome Q41.1
  aqueduct of Sylvius Q03.0
    with spina bifida — *see* Spina bifida, with
      hydrocephalus
  arm Q74.0
  arteriovenous NEC
    coronary Q24.5

Anomaly, anomalous (congenital)
(unspecified type) - *continued*
  arteriovenous NEC - *continued*
    gastrointestinal Q27.33
      acquired — *see* Angiodysplasia
  artery (peripheral) Q27.9
    basilar NEC Q28.1
    cerebral Q28.3
    coronary Q24.5
    digestive system Q27.8
    eye Q15.8
    great Q25.9
      specified NEC Q25.8
    lower limb Q27.8
    peripheral Q27.9
      specified NEC Q27.8
    pulmonary NEC Q25.79
    renal Q27.2
    retina Q14.1
    specified site NEC Q27.8
    subclavian Q27.8
      origin Q25.48
    umbilical Q27.0
    upper limb Q27.8
    vertebral NEC Q28.1
  aryteno-epiglottic folds Q31.8
  atrial
    bands or folds Q20.8
    septa Q21.1
  atrioventricular
    excitation I45.6
    septum Q21.0
  auditory canal Q17.8
  auricle
    ear Q17.8
      causing impairment of hearing Q16.9
    heart Q20.8
  Axenfeld's Q15.0
  back Q89.9
  band
    atrial Q20.8
    heart Q24.8
    ventricular Q24.8
  Bartholin's duct Q38.4
  biliary duct or passage Q44.5
  bladder Q64.70
    absence Q64.5
    diverticulum Q64.6
    exstrophy Q64.10
      cloacal Q64.12
      extroversion Q64.19
      specified type NEC Q64.19
      supravesical fissure Q64.11
    neck obstruction Q64.31
    specified type NEC Q64.79
  bone Q79.9
    arm Q74.0
    face Q75.9
    leg Q74.2
    pelvic girdle Q74.2
    shoulder girdle Q74.0
    skull Q75.9
      with
        anencephaly Q00.0
        encephalocele — *see* Encephalocele
        hydrocephalus Q03.9
          with spina bifida — *see* Spina
            bifida, by site, with
            hydrocephalus
        microcephaly Q02
  brain (multiple) Q04.9
    vessel Q28.3
  breast Q83.9
  broad ligament Q50.6
  bronchus Q32.4
  bulbus cordis Q21.9
  bursa Q79.9
  canal of Nuck Q52.4
  canthus Q10.3
  capillary Q27.9
  cardiac Q24.9
    chambers Q20.9
      specified NEC Q20.8
    septal closure Q21.9
      specified NEC Q21.8

Anomaly, anomalous (congenital)
(unspecified type) - *continued*
  cardiac - *continued*
    valve NEC Q24.8
      pulmonary Q22.3
  cardiovascular system Q28.8
  carpus Q74.0
  caruncle, lacrimal Q10.6
  cascade stomach Q40.2
  cauda equina Q06.3
  cecum Q43.9
  cerebral Q04.9
    vessels Q28.3
  cervix Q51.9
  Chédiak-Higashi (-Steinbrinck) (congenital
      gigantism of peroxidase
      granules) E70.330
  cheek Q18.9
  chest wall Q67.8
    bones Q76.9
  chin Q18.9
  chordae tendineae Q24.8
  choroid Q14.3
    plexus Q07.8
  chromosomes, chromosomal Q99.9
    D (1) — *see* condition, chromosome 13
    E (3) — *see* condition, chromosome 18
    G — *see* condition, chromosome 21
    sex
      female phenotype Q97.8
      gonadal dysgenesis (pure) Q99.1
      Klinefelter's Q98.4
      male phenotype Q98.9
      Turner's Q96.9
    specified NEC Q99.8
  cilia Q10.3
  circulatory system Q28.9
  clavicle Q74.0
  clitoris Q52.6
  coccyx Q76.49
  colon Q43.9
  common duct Q44.5
  communication
    coronary artery Q24.5
    left ventricle with right atrium Q21.0
  concha (ear) Q17.3
  connection
    portal vein Q26.5
    pulmonary venous Q26.4
      partial Q26.3
      total Q26.2
    renal artery with kidney Q27.2
  cornea (shape) Q13.4
  coronary artery or vein Q24.5
  cranium — *see* Anomaly, skull
  cricoid cartilage Q31.8
  cystic duct Q44.5
  dental
    alveolar — *see* Anomaly, alveolar
    arch relationship M26.20
      specified NEC M26.29
  dentofacial M26.9
    alveolar — *see* Anomaly, alveolar
    dental arch relationship M26.20
      specified NEC M26.29
    functional M26.50
      specified NEC M26.59
    jaw-cranial base relationship M26.10
      asymmetry M26.12
        maxillary M26.11
      specified type NEC M26.19
    jaw size M26.00
      macrogenia M26.05
      mandibular
        hyperplasia M26.03
        hypoplasia M26.04
      maxillary
        hyperplasia M26.01
        hypoplasia M26.02
      microgenia M26.06
      specified type NEC M26.09
    malocclusion M26.4
      dental arch relationship NEC M26.29

Anomaly, anomalous (congenital)
(unspecified type) - *continued*
  dentofacial - *continued*
    malocclusion - *continued*
      jaw-cranial base relationship — *see*Ano
          maly, dentofacial, jaw-cranial base
          relationship
      jaw size — *see* Anomaly, dentofacial,
          jaw size
    specified type NEC M26.89
    temporomandibular joint M26.60-
      adhesions M26.61-
      ankylosis M26.61-
      arthralgia M26.62-
      articular disc M26.63-
      specified type NEC M26.69
    tooth position, fully erupted M26.30
      specified NEC M26.39
  dermatoglyphic Q82.8
  diaphragm (apertures) NEC Q79.1
  digestive organ (s) or tract Q45.9
    lower Q43.9
    upper Q40.9
  distance, interarch (excessive)
      (inadequate) M26.25
  distribution, coronary artery Q24.5
  ductus
    arteriosus Q25.0
    botalli Q25.0
  duodenum Q43.9
  dura (brain) Q04.9
    spinal cord Q06.9
  ear (external) Q17.9
    causing impairment of hearing Q16.9
    inner Q16.5
    middle (causing impairment of
        hearing) Q16.4
      ossicles Q16.3
  Ebstein's (heart) (tricuspid valve) Q22.5
  ectodermal Q82.9
  Eisenmenger's (ventricular septal
      defect) Q21.8
  ejaculatory duct Q55.4
  elbow Q74.0
  endocrine gland NEC Q89.2
  epididymis Q55.4
  epiglottis Q31.8
  esophagus Q39.9
  eustachian tube Q17.8
  eye Q15.9
    anterior segment Q13.9
      specified NEC Q13.89
    posterior segment Q14.9
      specified NEC Q14.8
    ptosis (eyelid) Q10.0
    specified NEC Q15.8
  eyebrow Q18.8
  eyelid Q10.3
    ptosis Q10.0
  face Q18.9
    bone (s) Q75.9
  fallopian tube Q50.6
  fascia Q79.9
  femur NEC Q74.2
  fibula NEC Q74.2
  finger Q74.0
  fixation, intestine Q43.3
  flexion (joint) NOS Q74.9
    hip or thigh Q65.89
  foot NEC Q74.2
    varus (congenital) Q66.3-
  foramen
    Botalli Q21.1
    ovale Q21.1
  forearm Q74.0
  forehead Q75.8
  form, teeth K00.2
  fovea centralis Q14.1
  frontal bone — *see* Anomaly, skull
  gallbladder (position) (shape) (size) Q44.1
  Gartner's duct Q52.4
  gastrointestinal tract Q45.9
  genitalia, genital organ (s) or system
    female Q52.9
      external Q52.70

Anomaly, anomalous (congenital)
(unspecified type) - *continued*
  genitalia, genital organ (s) or system -
      continued
    female - *continued*
      internal NOS Q52.9
    male Q55.9
      hydrocele P83.5
      specified NEC Q55.8
  genitourinary NEC
    female Q52.9
    male Q55.9
  Gerbode Q21.0
  glottis Q31.8
  granulation or granulocyte, genetic
      (constitutional) (leukocyte) D72.0
  gum Q38.6
  gyri Q07.9
  hair Q84.2
  hand Q74.0
  hard tissue formation in pulp K04.3
  head — *see* Anomaly, skull
  heart Q24.9
    auricle Q20.8
    bands or folds Q24.8
    fibroelastosis cordis I42.4
    obstructive NEC Q22.6
    patent ductus arteriosus (Botalli) Q25.0
    septum Q21.9
      auricular Q21.1
      interatrial Q21.1
      interventricular Q21.0
        with pulmonary stenosis or atresia,
            dextraposition of aorta and
            hypertrophy of right
            ventricle Q21.3
      specified NEC Q21.8
      ventricular Q21.0
        with pulmonary stenosis or atresia,
            dextraposition of aorta and
            hypertrophy of right
            ventricle Q21.3
    tetralogy of Fallot Q21.3
    valve NEC Q24.8
      aortic
        bicuspid valve Q23.1
        insufficiency Q23.1
        stenosis Q23.0
          subaortic Q24.4
      mitral
        insufficiency Q23.3
        stenosis Q23.2
      pulmonary Q22.3
        atresia Q22.0
        insufficiency Q22.2
        stenosis Q22.1
          infundibular Q24.3
          subvalvular Q24.3
      tricuspid
        atresia Q22.4
        stenosis Q22.4
    ventricle Q20.8
  heel NEC Q74.2
  Hegglin's D72.0
  hemianencephaly Q00.0
  hemicephaly Q00.0
  hemicrania Q00.0
  hepatic duct Q44.5
  hip NEC Q74.2
  hourglass stomach Q40.2
  humerus Q74.0
  hydatid of Morgagni
    female Q50.5
    male (epididymal) Q55.4
      testicular Q55.29
  hymen Q52.4
  hypersegmentation of neutrophils,
      hereditary D72.0
  hypophyseal Q89.2
  ileocecal (coil) (valve) Q43.9
  ileum Q43.9
  ilium NEC Q74.2
  integument Q84.9
    specified NEC Q84.8

Anomaly, anomalous (congenital)
(unspecified type) - *continued*
    interarch distance (excessive)
        (inadequate) M26.25
    intervertebral cartilage or disc Q76.49
    intestine (large) (small) Q43.9
        with anomalous adhesions, fixation or
            malrotation Q43.3
    iris Q13.2
    ischium NEC Q74.2
    jaw — *see* Anomaly, dentofacial
        alveolar — *see* Anomaly, alveolar
    jaw-cranial base relationship — *see*
        Anomaly, dentofacial, jaw-cranial base
        relationship
    jejunum Q43.8
    joint Q74.9
        specified NEC Q74.8
    Jordan's D72.0
    kidney (s) (calyx) (pelvis) Q63.9
        artery Q27.2
        specified NEC Q63.8
    Klippel-Feil (brevicollis) Q76.1
    knee Q74.1
    labium (majus) (minus) Q52.70
    labyrinth, membranous Q16.5
    lacrimal apparatus or duct Q10.6
    larynx, laryngeal (muscle) Q31.9
        web (bed) Q31.0
    lens Q12.9
    leukocytes, genetic D72.0
        granulation (constitutional) D72.0
    lid (fold) Q10.3
    ligament Q79.9
        broad Q50.6
        round Q52.8
    limb Q74.9
        lower NEC Q74.2
            reduction deformity — *see* Defect,
                reduction, lower limb
        upper Q74.0
    lip Q38.0
    liver Q44.7
        duct Q44.5
    lower limb NEC Q74.2
    lumbosacral (joint) (region) Q76.49
        kyphosis — *see* Kyphosis, congenital
        lordosis — *see* Lordosis, congenital
    lung (fissure) (lobe) Q33.9
    mandible — *see* Anomaly, dentofacial
    maxilla — *see* Anomaly, dentofacial
    May (-Hegglin) D72.0
    meatus urinarius NEC Q64.79
    meningeal bands or folds Q07.9
        constriction of Q07.8
        spinal Q06.9
    meninges Q07.9
        cerebral Q04.8
        spinal Q06.9
    meningocele Q05.9
    mesentery Q45.9
    metacarpus Q74.0
    metatarsus NEC Q74.2
    middle ear Q16.4
        ossicles Q16.3
    mitral (leaflets) (valve) Q23.9
        insufficiency Q23.3
        specified NEC Q23.8
        stenosis Q23.2
    mouth Q38.6
    Müllerian — *see also* Anomaly, by site
        uterus NEC Q51.818
    multiple NEC Q89.7
    muscle Q79.9
        eyelid Q10.3
    musculoskeletal system, except limbs Q79.9
    myocardium Q24.8
    nail Q84.6
    narrowness, eyelid Q10.3
    nasal sinus (wall) Q30.8
    neck (any part) Q18.9
    nerve Q07.9
        acoustic Q07.8
        optic Q07.8
    nervous system (central) Q07.9

Anomaly, anomalous (congenital)
(unspecified type) - *continued*
    nipple Q83.9
    nose, nasal (bones) (cartilage) (septum)
        (sinus) Q30.9
        specified NEC Q30.8
    ocular muscle Q15.8
    omphalomesenteric duct Q43.0
    opening, pulmonary veins Q26.4
    optic
        disc Q14.2
        nerve Q07.8
    opticociliary vessels Q13.2
    orbit (eye) Q10.7
    organ Q89.9
        of Corti Q16.5
    origin
        artery
            innominate Q25.8
            pulmonary Q25.79
            renal Q27.2
            subclavian Q25.48
    osseous meatus (ear) Q16.1
    ovary Q50.39
    oviduct Q50.6
    palate (hard) (soft) NEC Q38.5
    pancreas or pancreatic duct Q45.3
    papillary muscles Q24.8
    parathyroid gland Q89.2
    paraurethral ducts Q64.79
    parotid (gland) Q38.4
    patella Q74.1
    Pelger-Huët (hereditary
        hyposegmentation) D72.0
    pelvic girdle NEC Q74.2
    pelvis (bony) NEC Q74.2
        rachitic E64.3
    penis (glans) Q55.69
    pericardium Q24.8
    peripheral vascular system Q27.9
    Peter's Q13.4
    pharynx Q38.8
    pigmentation L81.9
        congenital Q82.8
    pituitary (gland) Q89.2
    pleural (folds) Q34.0
    portal vein Q26.5
        connection Q26.5
    position, tooth, teeth, fully erupted M26.30
        specified NEC M26.39
    precerebral vessel Q28.1
    prepuce Q55.69
    prostate Q55.4
    pulmonary Q33.9
        artery NEC Q25.79
        valve Q22.3
            atresia Q22.0
            insufficiency Q22.2
            specified type NEC Q22.3
            stenosis Q22.1
                infundibular Q24.3
                subvalvular Q24.3
        venous connection Q26.4
            partial Q26.3
            total Q26.2
    pupil Q13.2
        function H57.00
            anisocoria H57.02
            Argyll Robertson pupil H57.01
            miosis H57.03
            mydriasis H57.04
            specified type NEC H57.09
            tonic pupil H57.05-
    pylorus Q40.3
    radius Q74.0
    rectum Q43.9
    reduction (extremity) (limb)
        femur (longitudinal) — *see* Defect,
            reduction, lower limb, longitudinal,
            femur
        fibula (longitudinal) — *see* Defect,
            reduction, lower limb, longitudinal,
            fibula
        lower limb — *see* Defect, reduction, lower
            limb

Anomaly, anomalous (congenital)
(unspecified type) - *continued*
    reduction (extremity) (limb) - *continued*
        radius (longitudinal) — *see* Defect,
            reduction, upper limb, longitudinal,
            radius
        tibia (longitudinal) — *see* Defect,
            reduction, lower limb, longitudinal,
            tibia
        ulna (longitudinal) — *see* Defect,
            reduction, upper limb, longitudinal,
            ulna
        upper limb — *see* Defect, reduction, upper
            limb
    refraction — *see* Disorder, refraction
    renal Q63.9
        artery Q27.2
        pelvis Q63.9
            specified NEC Q63.8
    respiratory system Q34.9
        specified NEC Q34.8
    retina Q14.1
    rib Q76.6
        cervical Q76.5
    Rieger's Q13.81
    rotation — *see* Malrotation
        hip or thigh Q65.89
    round ligament Q52.8
    sacroiliac (joint) NEC Q74.2
    sacrum NEC Q76.49
        kyphosis — *see* Kyphosis, congenital
        lordosis — *see* Lordosis, congenital
    saddle nose, syphilitic A50.57
    salivary duct or gland Q38.4
    scapula Q74.0
    scrotum — *see* Malformation, testis and
        scrotum
    sebaceous gland Q82.9
    seminal vesicles Q55.4
    sense organs NEC Q07.8
    sex chromosomes NEC — *see also* Anomaly,
        chromosomes
        female phenotype Q97.8
        male phenotype Q98.9
    shoulder (girdle) (joint) Q74.0
    sigmoid (flexure) Q43.9
    simian crease Q82.8
    sinus of Valsalva Q25.49
    skeleton generalized Q78.9
    skin (appendage) Q82.9
    skull Q75.9
        with
            anencephaly Q00.0
            encephalocele — *see* Encephalocele
            hydrocephalus Q03.9
                with spina bifida — *see* Spina bifida,
                    by site, with hydrocephalus
            microcephaly Q02
    specified organ or site NEC Q89.8
    spermatic cord Q55.4
    spine, spinal NEC Q76.49
        column NEC Q76.49
            kyphosis — *see* Kyphosis, congenital
            lordosis — *see* Lordosis, congenital
        cord Q06.9
        nerve root Q07.8
    spleen Q89.09
        agenesis Q89.01
    stenonian duct Q38.4
    sternum NEC Q76.7
    stomach Q40.3
    submaxillary gland Q38.4
    tarsus NEC Q74.2
    tendon Q79.9
    testis — *see* Malformation, testis and
        scrotum
    thigh NEC Q74.2
    thorax (wall) Q67.8
        bony Q76.9
    throat Q38.8
    thumb Q74.0
    thymus gland Q89.2
    thyroid (gland) Q89.2
        cartilage Q31.8
    tibia NEC Q74.2

DecisionHealth's FY 2020 Complete Home Health ICD-10-CM Diagnosis Coding Manual

Anomaly, anomalous (congenital) (unspecified type) - *continued*
    tibia NEC - *continued*
        saber A50.56
    toe Q74.2
    tongue Q38.3
    tooth, teeth K00.9
        eruption K00.6
        position, fully erupted M26.30
        spacing, fully erupted M26.30
    trachea (cartilage) Q32.1
    tragus Q17.9
    tricuspid (leaflet) (valve) Q22.9
        atresia or stenosis Q22.4
        Ebstein's Q22.5
    Uhl's (hypoplasia of myocardium, right
            ventricle) Q24.8
    ulna Q74.0
    umbilical artery Q27.0
    urachus Q64.4
    ureter Q62.8
        obstructive NEC Q62.39
            cecoureterocele Q62.32
            orthotopic ureterocele Q62.31
    urethra Q64.70
        absence Q64.5
        double Q64.74
        fistula to rectum Q64.73
        obstructive Q64.39
            stricture Q64.32
        prolapse Q64.71
        specified type NEC Q64.79
    urinary tract Q64.9
    uterus Q51.9
        with only one functioning horn Q51.4
    uvula Q38.5
    vagina Q52.4
    valleculae Q31.8
    valve (heart) NEC Q24.8
        coronary sinus Q24.5
        inferior vena cava Q24.8
        pulmonary Q22.3
        sinus coronario Q24.5
        venae cavae inferioris Q24.8
    vas deferens Q55.4
    vascular Q27.9
        brain Q28.3
        ring Q25.45
    vein (s) (peripheral) Q27.9
        brain Q28.3
        cerebral Q28.3
        coronary Q24.5
        developmental Q28.3
        great Q26.9
            specified NEC Q26.8
    vena cava (inferior) (superior) Q26.9
    venous — *see* Anomaly, vein(s)
    venous return Q26.8
    ventricular
        bands or folds Q24.8
        septa Q21.0
    vertebra Q76.49
        kyphosis — *see* Kyphosis, congenital
        lordosis — *see* Lordosis, congenital
    vesicourethral orifice Q64.79
    vessel (s) Q27.9
        optic papilla Q14.2
        precerebral Q28.1
    vitelline duct Q43.0
    vitreous body or humor Q14.0
    vulva Q52.70
    wrist (joint) Q74.0
Anomia R48.8
Anonychia (congenital) Q84.3
    acquired L60.8
**Anophthalmos, anophthalmus (congenital)
    (globe)** Q11.1
    acquired Z90.01

Anopia, anopsia H53.46-
    quadrant H53.46-
Anorchia, anorchism, anorchidism Q55.0
Anorexia R63.0
    hysterical F44.89
    nervosa F50.00
        atypical F50.9
        binge-eating type F50.2
            with purging F50.02
        restricting type F50.01
Anorgasmy, psychogenic (female) F52.31
    male F52.32
Anosmia R43.0
    hysterical F44.6
    postinfectional J39.8
Anosognosia R41.89
Anosteoplasia Q78.9
Anovulatory cycle N97.0
Anoxemia R09.02
    newborn P84
Anoxia (pathological) R09.02
    altitude T70.29
    cerebral G93.1
        complicating
            anesthesia (general) (local) or other
                sedation T88.59
            in labor and delivery O74.3
            in pregnancy O29.21-
            postpartum, puerperal O89.2
        delivery (cesarean) (instrumental) O75.4
        during a procedure G97.81
        newborn P84
        resulting from a procedure G97.82
    due to
        drowning T75.1
        high altitude T70.29
    heart — *see* Insufficiency, coronary
    intrauterine P84
    myocardial — *see* Insufficiency, coronary
    newborn P84
    spinal cord G95.11
    systemic (by suffocation) (low content in
        atmosphere) — *see* Asphyxia, traumatic
Anteflexion — *see* Anteversion
Antenatal
    care (normal pregnancy) Z34.90
    screening (encounter for) of mother — *see
        also* Encounter, antenatal
        screening Z36.9
Antepartum — *see* condition
Anterior — *see* condition
Antero-occlusion M26.220
Anteversion
    cervix — *see* Anteversion, uterus
    femur (neck) , congenital Q65.89
    uterus, uterine (cervix) (postinfectional)
        (postpartal, old) N85.4
        congenital Q51.818
        in pregnancy or childbirth — *see*
            Pregnancy, complicated by
Anthophobia F40.228
Anthracosilicosis J60
Anthracosis (lung) (occupational) J60
    lingua K14.3
Anthrax A22.9
    with pneumonia A22.1
    cerebral A22.8
    colitis A22.2
    cutaneous A22.0
    gastrointestinal A22.2
    inhalation A22.1
    intestinal A22.2
    meningitis A22.8
    pulmonary A22.1
    respiratory A22.1
    sepsis A22.7
    specified manifestation NEC A22.8
Anthropoid pelvis Q74.2
    with disproportion (fetopelvic) O33.0
Anthropophobia F40.10
    generalized F40.11

Antibodies, maternal (blood group) — *see*
    Isoimmunization, affecting management
    of pregnancy
    anti-D — *see* Isoimmunization, affecting
        management of pregnancy, Rh
    newborn P55.0
Antibody
    anticardiolipin R76.0
        with
            hemorrhagic disorder D68.312
            hypercoagulable state D68.61
    antiphosphatidylglycerol R76.0
        with
            hemorrhagic disorder D68.312
            hypercoagulable state D68.61
    antiphosphatidylinositol R76.0
        with
            hemorrhagic disorder D68.312
            hypercoagulable state D68.61
    antiphosphatidylserine R76.0
        with
            hemorrhagic disorder D68.312
            hypercoagulable state D68.61
    antiphospholipid R76.0
        with
            hemorrhagic disorder D68.312
            hypercoagulable state D68.61
Anticardiolipin syndrome D68.61
Anticoagulant, circulating (intrinsic) — *see
    also* - Disorder, hemorrhagic D68.318
    drug-induced (extrinsic) — *see also* -
        Disorder, hemorrhagic D68.32
    iatrogenic D68.32
Antidiuretic hormone syndrome E22.2
Antimonial cholera — *see* Poisoning,
    antimony
Antiphospholipid
    antibody
        with hemorrhagic disorder D68.312
    syndrome D68.61
Antisocial personality F60.2
Antithrombinemia — *see* Circulating
    anticoagulants
Antithromboplastinemia D68.318
Antithromboplastinogenemia D68.318
Antitoxin complication or reaction — *see*
    Complications, vaccination
Antlophobia F40.228
Antritis J32.0
    maxilla J32.0
        acute J01.00
            recurrent J01.01
    stomach K29.60
        with bleeding K29.61
Antrum, antral — *see* condition
Anuria R34
    calculous (impacted) (recurrent) — *see also*
        Calculus, urinary N20.9
    following
        abortion — *see* Abortion by type
            complicated by, renal failure
        ectopic or molar pregnancy O08.4
    newborn P96.0
    postprocedural N99.0
    postrenal N13.8
    traumatic (following crushing) T79.5
Anus, anal — *see* condition
Anusitis K62.89
Anxiety F41.9
    depression F41.8
    episodic paroxysmal F41.0
    generalized F41.1
    hysteria F41.8
    neurosis F41.1
    panic type F41.0
    reaction F41.1
    separation, abnormal (of childhood) F93.0
    specified NEC F41.8
    state F41.1
Aorta, aortic — *see* condition
Aortectasia — *see* Ectasia, aorta
    with aneurysm — *see* Aneurysm, aorta
Aortitis (nonsyphilitic) (calcific) I77.6
    arteriosclerotic I70.0
    Doehle-Heller A52.02

Aortitis (nonsyphilitic) (calcific) - *continued*
luetic A52.02
rheumatic — *see* Endocarditis, acute,
rheumatic
specific (syphilitic) A52.02
syphilitic A52.02
congenital A50.54 *[I79.1]*
Apathetic thyroid storm — *see*
Thyrotoxicosis
Apathy R45.3
Apeirophobia F40.228
Apepsia K30
psychogenic F45.8
Aperistalsis, esophagus K22.0
Apertognathia M26.29
Apert's syndrome Q87.0
Aphagia R13.0
psychogenic F50.9
Aphakia (acquired) (postoperative) H27.0-
congenital Q12.3
**Aphasia (amnestic) (global) (nominal)
(semantic) (syntactic)** R47.01
acquired, with epilepsy (Landau-Kleffner
syndrome) — *see* Epilepsy, specified
NEC
auditory (developmental) F80.2
developmental (receptive type) F80.2
expressive type F80.1
Wernicke's F80.2
following
cerebrovascular disease I69.920
cerebral infarction I69.320
intracerebral hemorrhage I69.120
nontraumatic intracranial hemorrhage
NEC I69.220
specified disease NEC I69.820
subarachnoid hemorrhage I69.020
primary progressive G31.01 *[F02.80]*
with behavioral disturbance G31.01
[F02.81]
progressive isolated G31.01 *[F02.80]*
with behavioral disturbance G31.01
[F02.81]
sensory F80.2
syphilis, tertiary A52.19
Wernicke's (developmental) F80.2
Aphonia (organic) R49.1
hysterical F44.4
psychogenic F44.4
Aphthae, aphthous — *see also* condition
Bednar's K12.0
cachectic K14.0
epizootic B08.8
fever B08.8
oral (recurrent) K12.0
stomatitis (major) (minor) K12.0
thrush B37.0
ulcer (oral) (recurrent) K12.0
genital organ (s) NEC
female N76.6
male N50.89
larynx J38.7
Apical — *see* condition
Apiphobia F40.218
Aplasia — *see also* Agenesis
abdominal muscle syndrome Q79.4
alveolar process (acquired) — *see* Anomaly,
alveolar
congenital Q38.6
aorta (congenital) Q25.41
axialis extracorticalis (congenita) E75.29
bone marrow (myeloid) D61.9
congenital D61.01
brain Q00.0
part of Q04.3
bronchus Q32.4
cementum K00.4
cerebellum Q04.3
cervix (congenital) Q51.5
congenital pure red cell D61.01
corpus callosum Q04.0
cutis congenita Q84.8
erythrocyte congenital D61.01
extracortical axial E75.29
eye Q11.1

Aplasia - *continued*
fovea centralis (congenital) Q14.1
gallbladder, congenital Q44.0
iris Q13.1
labyrinth, membranous Q16.5
limb (congenital) Q73.8
lower — *see* Defect, reduction, lower limb
upper — *see* Agenesis, arm
lung, congenital (bilateral) (unilateral) Q33.3
pancreas Q45.0
parathyroid-thymic D82.1
Pelizaeus-Merzbacher E75.29
penis Q55.5
prostate Q55.4
red cell (with thymoma) D60.9
acquired D60.9
due to drugs D60.9
adult D60.9
chronic D60.0
congenital D61.01
constitutional D61.01
due to drugs D60.9
hereditary D61.01
of infants D61.01
primary D61.01
pure D61.01
due to drugs D60.9
specified type NEC D60.8
transient D60.1
round ligament Q52.8
skin Q84.8
spermatic cord Q55.4
spleen Q89.01
testicle Q55.0
thymic, with immunodeficiency D82.1
thyroid (congenital) (with myxedema) E03.1
uterus Q51.0
ventral horn cell Q06.1
Apnea, apneic (of) (spells) R06.81
newborn NEC P28.4
obstructive P28.4
sleep (central) (obstructive)
(primary) P28.3
prematurity P28.4
sleep G47.30
central (primary) G47.31
idiopathic G47.31
in conditions classified
elsewhere G47.37
obstructive (adult) (pediatric) G47.33
hypopnea G47.33
primary central G47.31
specified NEC G47.39
Apneumatosis, newborn P28.0
Apocrine metaplasia (breast) — *see*
Dysplasia, mammary, specified type NEC
Apophysitis (bone) — *see also*
Osteochondropathy
calcaneus M92.8
juvenile M92.8
**Apoplectiform convulsions (cerebral
ischemia)** I67.82
Apoplexia, apoplexy, apoplectic
adrenal A39.1
heart (auricle) (ventricle) — *see* Infarct,
myocardium
heat T67.01
hemorrhagic (stroke) — *see* Hemorrhage,
intracranial
meninges, hemorrhagic — *see* Hemorrhage,
intracranial, subarachnoid
uremic N18.9 *[I68.8]*
Appearance
bizarre R46.1
specified NEC R46.89
very low level of personal hygiene R46.0
Appendage
epididymal (organ of Morgagni) Q55.4
intestine (epiploic) Q43.8
preauricular Q17.0
testicular (organ of Morgagni) Q55.29
Appendicitis (pneumococcal) (retrocecal)
K37
with
gangrene K35.891

Appendicitis (pneumococcal) (retrocecal) -
continued
with - *continued*
perforation NOS K35.32
peritoneal abscess K35.33
peritonitis NEC K35.33
generalized (with perforation or
rupture) K35.20
with abscess K35.21
localized K35.30
with
gangrene K35.31
perforation K35.32
and abscess K35.33
rupture (with localized
peritonitis) K35.32
acute (catarrhal) (fulminating) (gangrenous)
(obstructive) (retrocecal)
(suppurative) K35.80
with
gangrene K35.891
peritoneal abscess K35.33
peritonitis NEC K35.33
generalized (with perforation or
rupture) K35.20
with abscess K35.21
localized K35.30
with
gangrene K35.31
perforation K35.32
and abscess K35.33
specified NEC K35.890
with gangrene K35.891
amebic A06.89
chronic (recurrent) K36
exacerbation — *see* Appendicitis, acute
gangrenous — *see* Appendicitis, acute
healed (obliterative) K36
interval K36
neurogenic K36
obstructive K36
recurrent K36
relapsing K36
ruptured NOS (with localized
peritonitis) K35.32
subacute (adhesive) K36
subsiding K36
suppurative — *see* Appendicitis, acute
tuberculous A18.32
Appendicopathia oxyurica B80
Appendix, appendicular — *see also* condition
epididymis Q55.4
Morgagni
female Q50.5
male (epididymal) Q55.4
testicular Q55.29
testis Q55.29
Appetite
depraved — *see* Pica
excessive R63.2
lack or loss — *see also* Anorexia R63.0
nonorganic origin F50.89
psychogenic F50.89
perverted (hysterical) — *see* Pica
Apple peel syndrome Q41.1
Apprehension state F41.1
Apprehensiveness, abnormal F41.9
Approximal wear K03.0
**Apraxia (classic) (ideational) (ideokinetic)
(ideomotor) (motor) (verbal)** R48.2
following
cerebrovascular disease I69.990
cerebral infarction I69.390
intracerebral hemorrhage I69.190
nontraumatic intracranial hemorrhage
NEC I69.290
specified disease NEC I69.890
subarachnoid hemorrhage I69.090
oculomotor, congenital H51.8
Aptyalism K11.7
Apudoma — *see* Neoplasm, uncertain
behavior, by site
Aqueous misdirection H40.83-
Arabicum elephantiasis — *see* Infestation,
filarial

Arachnitis — *see* Meningitis
Arachnodactyly — *see* Syndrome, Marfan's
Arachnoiditis (acute) (adhesive) (basal)
  (brain) (cerebrospinal) — *see* Meningitis
Arachnophobia F40.210
Arboencephalitis, Australian A83.4
Arborization block (heart) I45.5
ARC (AIDS-related complex) B20
Arch
  aortic Q25.49
  bovine Q25.49
Arches — *see* condition
Arcuate uterus Q51.810
Arcuatus uterus Q51.810
Arcus (cornea) senilis — *see* Degeneration,
  cornea, senile
Arc-welder's lung J63.4
Areflexia R29.2
Areola — *see* condition
Argentaffinoma — *see also* Neoplasm,
  uncertain behavior, by site
  malignant — *see* Neoplasm, malignant, by
    site
  syndrome E34.0
Argininemia E72.21
Arginosuccinic aciduria E72.22
Argyll Robertson phenomenon, pupil or
  syndrome (syphilitic) A52.19
  atypical H57.09
  nonsyphilitic H57.09
Argyria, argyriasis
  conjunctival H11.13-
  from drug or medicament — *see* Table of
    Drugs and Chemicals, by substance
Argyrosis, conjunctival H11.13-
Arhinencephaly Q04.1
Ariboflavinosis E53.0
Arm — *see* condition
Arnold-Chiari disease, obstruction or
  syndrome (type II) Q07.00
  with
    hydrocephalus Q07.02
      with spina bifida Q07.03
    spina bifida Q07.01
      with hydrocephalus Q07.03
  type III — *see* Encephalocele
  type IV Q04.8
Aromatic amino-acid metabolism disorder
  E70.9
  specified NEC E70.8
Arousals, confusional G47.51
Arrest, arrested
  cardiac I46.9
    complicating
      abortion — *see* Abortion, by type,
        complicated by, cardiac arrest
      anesthesia (general) (local) or other
        sedation — *see* Table of Drugs and
        Chemicals, by drug,
      in labor and delivery O74.2
      in pregnancy O29.11-
      postpartum, puerperal O89.1
    delivery (cesarean) (instrumental) O75.4
    due to
      cardiac condition I46.2
      specified condition NEC I46.8
    intraoperative I97.71-
    newborn P29.81
    personal history, successfully
      resuscitated Z86.74
    postprocedural I97.12-
    obstetric procedure O75.4
  cardiorespiratory — *see* Arrest, cardiac
  circulatory — *see* Arrest, cardiac
  deep transverse O64.0
  development or growth
    bone — *see* Disorder, bone, development
      or growth
    child R62.50
    tracheal rings Q32.1
  epiphyseal
    complete
      femur M89.15-
      humerus M89.12-
      tibia M89.16-

Arrest, arrested - *continued*
  epiphyseal - *continued*
    complete - *continued*
      ulna M89.13-
      forearm M89.13-
        specified NEC M89.13-
        ulna — *see* Arrest, epiphyseal, by type,
          ulna
      lower leg M89.16-
        specified NEC M89.168
        tibia — *see* Arrest, epiphyseal, by type,
          tibia
    partial
      femur M89.15-
      humerus M89.12-
      tibia M89.16-
      ulna M89.13-
    specified NEC M89.18
  granulopoiesis — *see* Agranulocytosis
  growth plate — *see* Arrest, epiphyseal
  heart — *see* Arrest, cardiac
  legal, anxiety concerning Z65.3
  physeal — *see* Arrest, epiphyseal
  respiratory R09.2
    newborn P28.81
  sinus I45.5
  spermatogenesis (complete) — *see*
    Azoospermia
  incomplete — *see* Oligospermia
  transverse (deep) O64.0
Arrhenoblastoma
  benign
    specified site — *see* Neoplasm, benign, by
      site
    unspecified site
      female D27.9
      male D29.20
  malignant
    specified site — *see* Neoplasm, malignant,
      by site
    unspecified site
      female C56.9
      male C62.90
  specified site — *see* Neoplasm, uncertain
    behavior, by site
  unspecified site
    female D39.10
    male D40.10
Arrhythmia (auricle) (cardiac) (juvenile)
  (nodal) (reflex) (sinus)
  (supraventricular) (transitory)
  (ventricle) (ventricle) I49.9
  block I45.9
  extrasystolic I49.49
  newborn
    bradycardia P29.12
    occurring before birth P03.819
      before onset of labor P03.810
      during labor P03.811
    tachycardia P29.11
  psychogenic F45.8
  specified NEC I49.8
  vagal R55
  ventricular re-entry I47.0
Arrillaga-Ayerza syndrome (pulmonary
  sclerosis with pulmonary
  hypertension) I27.0
Arsenical pigmentation L81.8
  from drug or medicament — *see* Table of
    Drugs and Chemicals
Arsenism — *see* Poisoning, arsenic
Arterial — *see* condition
Arteriofibrosis — *see* Arteriosclerosis
Arteriolar sclerosis — *see* Arteriosclerosis
Arteriolith — *see* Arteriosclerosis
Arteriolitis I77.6
  necrotizing, kidney I77.5
  renal — *see* Hypertension, kidney
Arteriolosclerosis — *see* Arteriosclerosis
Arterionephrosclerosis — *see* Hypertension,
  kidney

Arteriopathy I77.9
  cerebral autosomal dominant, with
    subcortical infarcts and
    leukoencephalopathy
    (CADASIL) I67.850
Arteriosclerosis, arteriosclerotic (diffuse)
  (obliterans) (of) (senile) (with
  calcification) I70.90
  aorta I70.0
  arteries of extremities — *see*
    Arteriosclerosis, extremities
  brain I67.2
  bypass graft
    coronary — *see* Arteriosclerosis, coronary,
      bypass graft
    extremities — *see* Arteriosclerosis,
      extremities, bypass graft
  cardiac — *see* Disease, heart, ischemic,
    atherosclerotic
  cardiopathy — *see* Disease, heart, ischemic,
    atherosclerotic
  cardiorenal — *see* Hypertension, cardiorenal
  cardiovascular — *see* Disease, heart,
    ischemic, atherosclerotic
  carotid — *see also* Occlusion, artery,
    carotid I65.2-
  central nervous system I67.2
  cerebral I67.2
  cerebrovascular I67.2
  coronary (artery) I25.10
    due to
      calcified coronary lesion
        (severely) I25.84
      lipid rich plaque I25.83
    bypass graft I25.810
      with
        angina pectoris I25.709
          with documented spasm I25.701
          specified type NEC I25.708
          unstable I25.700
        ischemic chest pain I25.709
      autologous artery I25.810
        with
          angina pectoris I25.729
            with documented spasm I25.721
            specified type I25.728
            unstable I25.720
          ischemic chest pain I25.729
      autologous vein I25.810
        with
          angina pectoris I25.719
            with documented spasm I25.711
            specified type I25.718
            unstable I25.710
          ischemic chest pain I25.719
      nonautologous biological I25.810
        with
          angina pectoris I25.739
            with documented spasm I25.731
            specified type I25.738
            unstable I25.730
          ischemic chest pain I25.739
      specified type NEC I25.810
        with
          angina pectoris I25.799
            with documented spasm I25.791
            specified type I25.798
            unstable I25.790
          ischemic chest pain I25.799
    native vessel
      with
        angina pectoris I25.119
          with documented spasm I25.111
          specified type NEC I25.118
          unstable I25.110
        ischemic chest pain I25.119
    transplanted heart I25.811
      bypass graft I25.812
        with
          angina pectoris I25.769
            with documented spasm I25.761
            specified type I25.768
            unstable I25.760
          ischemic chest pain I25.769
      native coronary artery I25.811

Arteriosclerosis, arteriosclerotic (diffuse) (obliterans) (of) (senile) (with calcification) - *continued*
  coronary (artery) - *continued*
    transplanted heart - *continued*
      native coronary artery - *continued*
        with
          angina pectoris I25.759
            with documented spasm I25.751
            specified type I25.758
            unstable I25.750
          ischemic chest pain I25.759
  extremities (native arteries) I70.209
    bypass graft I70.309
      autologous vein graft I70.409
        leg I70.409
          with
            gangrene (and intermittent claudication, rest pain and ulcer) I70.469
            intermittent claudication I70.419
            rest pain (and intermittent claudication) I70.429
          bilateral I70.403
            with
              gangrene (and intermittent claudication, rest pain and ulcer) I70.463
              intermittent claudication I70.413
              rest pain (and intermittent claudication) I70.423
            specified type NEC I70.493
          left I70.402
            with
              gangrene (and intermittent claudication, rest pain and ulcer) I70.462
              intermittent claudication I70.412
              rest pain (and intermittent claudication) I70.422
              ulceration (and intermittent claudication and rest pain) I70.449
                ankle I70.443
                calf I70.442
                foot site NEC I70.445
                heel I70.444
                lower leg NEC I70.448
                midfoot I70.444
                thigh I70.441
            specified type NEC I70.492
          right I70.401
            with
              gangrene (and intermittent claudication, rest pain and ulcer) I70.461
              intermittent claudication I70.411
              rest pain (and intermittent claudication) I70.421
              ulceration (and intermittent claudication and rest pain) I70.439
                ankle I70.433
                calf I70.432
                foot site NEC I70.435
                heel I70.434
                lower leg NEC I70.438
                midfoot I70.434
                thigh I70.431
            specified type NEC I70.491
          specified type NEC I70.499
      specified NEC I70.408
        with
          gangrene (and intermittent claudication, rest pain and ulcer) I70.468
          intermittent claudication I70.418
          rest pain (and intermittent claudication) I70.428
          ulceration (and intermittent claudication and rest pain) I70.45

Arteriosclerosis, arteriosclerotic (diffuse) (obliterans) (of) (senile) (with calcification) - *continued*
  extremities (native arteries) - *continued*
    bypass graft - *continued*
      autologous vein graft - *continued*
        specified NEC - *continued*
          specified type NEC I70.498
        leg I70.309
          with
            gangrene (and intermittent claudication, rest pain and ulcer) I70.369
            intermittent claudication I70.319
            rest pain (and intermittent claudication) I70.329
          bilateral I70.303
            with
              gangrene (and intermittent claudication, rest pain and ulcer) I70.363
              intermittent claudication I70.313
              rest pain (and intermittent claudication) I70.323
            specified type NEC I70.393
          left I70.302
            with
              gangrene (and intermittent claudication, rest pain and ulcer) I70.362
              intermittent claudication I70.312
              rest pain (and intermittent claudication) I70.322
              ulceration (and intermittent claudication and rest pain) I70.349
                ankle I70.343
                calf I70.342
                foot site NEC I70.345
                heel I70.344
                lower leg NEC I70.348
                midfoot I70.344
                thigh I70.341
            specified type NEC I70.392
          right I70.301
            with
              gangrene (and intermittent claudication, rest pain and ulcer) I70.361
              intermittent claudication I70.311
              rest pain (and intermittent claudication) I70.321
              ulceration (and intermittent claudication and rest pain) I70.339
                ankle I70.333
                calf I70.332
                foot site NEC I70.335
                heel I70.334
                lower leg NEC I70.338
                midfoot I70.334
                thigh I70.331
            specified type NEC I70.391
          specified type NEC I70.399
      nonautologous biological graft I70.509
        leg I70.509
          with
            gangrene (and intermittent claudication, rest pain and ulcer) I70.569
            intermittent claudication I70.519
            rest pain (and intermittent claudication) I70.529
          bilateral I70.503
            with
              gangrene (and intermittent claudication, rest pain and ulcer) I70.563
              intermittent claudication I70.513
              rest pain (and intermittent claudication) I70.523
            specified type NEC I70.593
          left I70.502
            with

Arteriosclerosis, arteriosclerotic (diffuse) (obliterans) (of) (senile) (with calcification) - *continued*
  extremities (native arteries) - *continued*
    bypass graft - *continued*
      nonautologous biological graft - *continued*
        leg - *continued*
          left - *continued*
            with - *continued*
              gangrene (and intermittent claudication, rest pain and ulcer) I70.562
              intermittent claudication I70.512
              rest pain (and intermittent claudication) I70.522
              ulceration (and intermittent claudication and rest pain) I70.549
                ankle I70.543
                calf I70.542
                foot site NEC I70.545
                heel I70.544
                lower leg NEC I70.548
                midfoot I70.544
                thigh I70.541
            specified type NEC I70.592
          right I70.501
            with
              gangrene (and intermittent claudication, rest pain and ulcer) I70.561
              intermittent claudication I70.511
              rest pain (and intermittent claudication) I70.521
              ulceration (and intermittent claudication and rest pain) I70.539
                ankle I70.533
                calf I70.532
                foot site NEC I70.535
                heel I70.534
                lower leg NEC I70.538
                midfoot I70.534
                thigh I70.531
            specified type NEC I70.591
          specified type NEC I70.599
        specified NEC I70.508
          with
            gangrene (and intermittent claudication, rest pain and ulcer) I70.568
            intermittent claudication I70.518
            rest pain (and intermittent claudication) I70.528
            ulceration (and intermittent claudication and rest pain) I70.55
            specified type NEC I70.598
      nonbiological graft I70.609
        leg I70.609
          with
            gangrene (and intermittent claudication, rest pain and ulcer) I70.669
            intermittent claudication I70.619
            rest pain (and intermittent claudication) I70.629
          bilateral I70.603
            with
              gangrene (and intermittent claudication, rest pain and ulcer) I70.663
              intermittent claudication I70.613
              rest pain (and intermittent claudication) I70.623
            specified type NEC I70.693
          left I70.602
            with
              gangrene (and intermittent claudication, rest pain and ulcer) I70.662

Arteriosclerosis, arteriosclerotic (diffuse) (obliterans) (of) (senile) (with calcification) - *continued*
  extremities (native arteries) - *continued*
    bypass graft - *continued*
      nonbiological graft - *continued*
        leg - *continued*
          left - *continued*
            with - *continued*
              intermittent
                claudication I70.612
              rest pain (and intermittent
                claudication) I70.622
              ulceration (and intermittent
                claudication and rest
                pain) I70.649
              ankle I70.643
              calf I70.642
              foot site NEC I70.645
              heel I70.644
              lower leg NEC I70.648
              midfoot I70.644
              thigh I70.641
            specified type NEC I70.692
          right I70.601
            with
              gangrene (and intermittent
                claudication, rest pain and
                ulcer) I70.661
              intermittent
                claudication I70.611
              rest pain (and intermittent
                claudication) I70.621
              ulceration (and intermittent
                claudication and rest
                pain) I70.639
              ankle I70.633
              calf I70.632
              foot site NEC I70.635
              heel I70.634
              lower leg NEC I70.638
              midfoot I70.634
              thigh I70.631
            specified type NEC I70.691
          specified type NEC I70.699
        specified NEC I70.608
          with
            gangrene (and intermittent
              claudication, rest pain and
              ulcer) I70.668
            intermittent claudication I70.618
            rest pain (and intermittent
              claudication) I70.628
            ulceration (and intermittent
              claudication and rest
              pain) I70.65
          specified type NEC I70.698
      specified graft NEC I70.709
        leg I70.709
          with
            gangrene (and intermittent
              claudication, rest pain and
              ulcer) I70.769
            intermittent claudication I70.719
            rest pain (and intermittent
              claudication) I70.729
          bilateral I70.703
            with
              gangrene (and intermittent
                claudication, rest pain and
                ulcer) I70.763
              intermittent
                claudication I70.713
              rest pain (and intermittent
                claudication) I70.723
            specified type NEC I70.793
          left I70.702
            with
              gangrene (and intermittent
                claudication, rest pain and
                ulcer) I70.762
              intermittent
                claudication I70.712
              rest pain (and intermittent
                claudication) I70.722

Arteriosclerosis, arteriosclerotic (diffuse) (obliterans) (of) (senile) (with calcification) - *continued*
  extremities (native arteries) - *continued*
    bypass graft - *continued*
      specified graft NEC - *continued*
        leg - *continued*
          left - *continued*
            with - *continued*
              ulceration (and intermittent
                claudication and rest
                pain) I70.749
              ankle I70.743
              calf I70.742
              foot site NEC I70.745
              heel I70.744
              lower leg NEC I70.748
              midfoot I70.744
              thigh I70.741
            specified type NEC I70.792
          right I70.701
            with
              gangrene (and intermittent
                claudication, rest pain and
                ulcer) I70.761
              intermittent
                claudication I70.711
              rest pain (and intermittent
                claudication) I70.721
              ulceration (and intermittent
                claudication and rest
                pain) I70.739
              ankle I70.733
              calf I70.732
              foot site NEC I70.735
              heel I70.734
              lower leg NEC I70.738
              midfoot I70.734
              thigh I70.731
            specified type NEC I70.791
          specified type NEC I70.799
        specified NEC I70.708
          with
            gangrene (and intermittent
              claudication, rest pain and
              ulcer) I70.768
            intermittent claudication I70.718
            rest pain (and intermittent
              claudication) I70.728
            ulceration (and intermittent
              claudication and rest
              pain) I70.75
          specified type NEC I70.798
      specified NEC I70.308
        with
          gangrene (and intermittent
            claudication, rest pain and
            ulcer) I70.368
          intermittent claudication I70.318
          rest pain (and intermittent
            claudication) I70.328
          ulceration (and intermittent
            claudication and rest
            pain) I70.35
        specified type NEC I70.398
      leg I70.209
        with
          gangrene (and intermittent
            claudication, rest pain and
            ulcer) I70.269
          intermittent claudication I70.219
          rest pain (and intermittent
            claudication) I70.229
        bilateral I70.203
          with
            gangrene (and intermittent
              claudication, rest pain and
              ulcer) I70.263
            intermittent claudication I70.213
            rest pain (and intermittent
              claudication) I70.223
          specified type NEC I70.293
        left I70.202
          with

Arteriosclerosis, arteriosclerotic (diffuse) (obliterans) (of) (senile) (with calcification) - *continued*
  extremities (native arteries) - *continued*
    leg - *continued*
      left - *continued*
        with - *continued*
          gangrene (and intermittent
            claudication, rest pain and
            ulcer) I70.262
          intermittent claudication I70.212
          rest pain (and intermittent
            claudication) I70.222
          ulceration (and intermittent
            claudication and rest
            pain) I70.249
          ankle I70.243
          calf I70.242
          foot site NEC I70.245
          heel I70.244
          lower leg NEC I70.248
          midfoot I70.244
          thigh I70.241
        specified type NEC I70.292
      right I70.201
        with
          gangrene (and intermittent
            claudication, rest pain and
            ulcer) I70.261
          intermittent claudication I70.211
          rest pain (and intermittent
            claudication) I70.221
          ulceration (and intermittent
            claudication and rest
            pain) I70.239
          ankle I70.233
          calf I70.232
          foot site NEC I70.235
          · heel I70.234
          lower leg NEC I70.238
          midfoot I70.234
          thigh I70.231
        specified type NEC I70.291
      specified type NEC I70.299
    specified site NEC I70.208
      with
        gangrene (and intermittent
          claudication, rest pain and
          ulcer) I70.268
        intermittent claudication I70.218
        rest pain (and intermittent
          claudication) I70.228
        ulceration (and intermittent
          claudication and rest pain) I70.25
      specified type NEC I70.298
  generalized I70.91
  heart (disease) — *see* Arteriosclerosis,
    coronary (artery),
  kidney — *see* Hypertension, kidney
  medial — *see* Arteriosclerosis, extremities
  mesenteric (artery) K55.1
  Mönckeberg's — *see* Arteriosclerosis,
    extremities
  myocarditis I51.4
  peripheral (of extremities) — *see*
    Arteriosclerosis, extremities
  pulmonary (idiopathic) I27.0
  renal (arterioles) — *see also* Hypertension,
    kidney
    artery I70.1
  retina (vascular) I70.8 *[H35.0-]*
  specified artery NEC I70.8
  spinal (cord) G95.19
  vertebral (artery) I67.2
Arteriospasm I73.9
Arteriovenous — *see* condition
Arteritis I77.6
  allergic M31.0
  aorta (nonsyphilitic) I77.6
    syphilitic A52.02
  aortic arch M31.4
  brachiocephalic M31.4
  brain I67.7
    syphilitic A52.04
  cerebral I67.7

Arteritis - *continued*
  cerebral - *continued*
    in
      diseases classified elsewhere I68.2
      systemic lupus erythematosus M32.19
    listerial A32.89
    syphilitic A52.04
    tuberculous A18.89
  coronary (artery) I25.89
    rheumatic I01.8
      chronic I09.89
    syphilitic A52.06
  cranial (left) (right) , giant cell M31.6
  deformans — *see* Arteriosclerosis
  giant cell NEC M31.6
    with polymyalgia rheumatica M31.5
  necrosing or necrotizing M31.9
    specified NEC M31.8
  nodosa M30.0
  obliterans — *see* Arteriosclerosis
  pulmonary I28.8
  rheumatic — *see* Fever, rheumatic
  senile — *see* Arteriosclerosis
  suppurative I77.2
  syphilitic (general) A52.09
    brain A52.04
    coronary A52.06
    spinal A52.09
  temporal, giant cell M31.6
  young female aortic arch syndrome M31.4
Artery, arterial — *see also* condition
  abscess I77.89
  single umbilical Q27.0
Arthralgia (allergic) — *see also* Pain, joint
  in caisson disease T70.3
  temporomandibular M26.62-
Arthritis, arthritic (acute) (chronic)
  (nonpyogenic) (subacute) M19.90
  allergic — *see* Arthritis, specified form NEC
  ankylosing (crippling) (spine) — *see also*
    Spondylitis, ankylosing
    sites other than spine — *see* Arthritis,
      specified form NEC
  atrophic — *see* Osteoarthritis
    spine — *see* Spondylitis, ankylosing
  back — *see* Spondylopathy, inflammatory
  blennorrhagic (gonococcal) A54.42
  Charcot's — *see* Arthropathy, neuropathic
    diabetic — *see* Diabetes, arthropathy,
      neuropathic
    syringomyelic G95.0
  chylous (filarial) (*see also* category M01)
    B74.9
  climacteric (any site) NEC — *see* Arthritis,
    specified form NEC
  crystal (-induced) — *see* Arthritis, in,
    crystals
  deformans — *see* Osteoarthritis
  degenerative — *see* Osteoarthritis
  due to or associated with
    acromegaly E22.0
    brucellosis — *see* Brucellosis
    caisson disease T70.3
    diabetes — *see* Diabetes, arthropathy
    dracontiasis (*see also* category M01) B72
    enteritis NEC
      regional — *see* Enteritis, regional
    erysipelas (*see also* category M01) A46
    erythema
      epidemic A25.1
      nodosum L52
    filariasis NOS B74.9
    glanders A24.0
    helminthiasis (*see also* category M01)
      B83.9
    hemophilia D66 *[M36.2]*
    Henoch- (Schönlein) purpura D69.0
      [M36.4]
    human parvovirus (*see also* category M01)
      B97.6
    infectious disease NEC — *see* category
      M01
    leprosy (*see also* category M01) — *see*
      also Leprosy A30.9
    Lyme disease A69.23

Arthritis, arthritic (acute) (chronic)
(nonpyogenic) (subacute) - *continued*
  due to or associated with - *continued*
    mycobacteria (*see also* category M01)
      A31.8
    parasitic disease NEC (*see also* category
      M01) B89
    paratyphoid fever (see also category
      M01) — *see also* Fever,
      paratyphoid A01.4
    rat bite fever (*see also* category M01)
      A25.1
    regional enteritis — *see* Enteritis, regional
    respiratory disorder NOS J98.9
    serum sickness — *see also* Reaction,
      serum T80.69
    syringomyelia G95.0
    typhoid fever A01.04
  epidemic erythema A25.1
  febrile — *see* Fever, rheumatic
  gonococcal A54.42
  gouty (acute) — *see* Gout
  in (due to)
    acromegaly (*see also* subcategory M14.8-)
      E22.0
    amyloidosis (*see also* subcategory M14.8-)
      E85.4
    bacterial disease (*see also* subcategory
      M01) A49.9
    Behçet's syndrome M35.2
    caisson disease (*see also* subcategory
      M14.8-) T70.3
    coliform bacilli (Escherichia coli) — *see*
      Arthritis, in, pyogenic organism NEC
    crystals M11.9
      dicalcium phosphate — *see* Arthritis, in,
        crystals, specified type NEC
      hydroxyapatite M11.0-
      pyrophosphate — *see* Arthritis, in,
        crystals, specified type NEC
      specified type NEC M11.80
        ankle M11.87-
        elbow M11.82-
        foot joint M11.87-
        hand joint M11.84-
        hip M11.85-
        knee M11.86-
        multiple sites M11.8-
        shoulder M11.81-
        vertebrae M11.88
        wrist M11.83-
    dermatoarthritis, lipoid E78.81
    dracontiasis (dracunculiasis) (*see also*
      category M01) B72
    endocrine disorder NEC (*see also*
      subcategory M14.8-) E34.9
    enteritis, infectious NEC (*see also* category
      M01) A09
      specified organism NEC (*see also*
        category M01) A08.8
    erythema
      multiforme (*see also* subcategory
        M14.8-) L51.9
      nodosum (*see also* subcategory M14.8-)
        L52
    gout — *see* Gout
    helminthiasis NEC (*see also* category M01)
      B83.9
    hemochromatosis (*see also* subcategory
      M14.8-) E83.118
    hemoglobinopathy NEC D58.2 *[M36.3]*
    hemophilia NEC D66 *[M36.2]*
    Hemophilus influenzae M00.8- *[B96.3]*
    Henoch (-Schönlein) purpura D69.0
      [M36.4]
    hyperparathyroidism NEC (*see also*
      subcategory M14.8-) E21.3
    hypersensitivity reaction NEC T78.49
      [M36.4]
    hypogammaglobulinemia (*see also*
      subcategory M14.8-) D80.1
    hypothyroidism NEC (*see also*
      subcategory M14.8-) E03.9
    infection — *see* Arthritis, pyogenic or
      pyemic

Arthritis, arthritic (acute) (chronic)
(nonpyogenic) (subacute) - *continued*
  in (due to) - *continued*
    infection - *continued*
      spine — *see* Spondylopathy, infective
    infectious disease NEC — *see* category
      M01
    leprosy (*see also* category M01) A30.9
    leukemia NEC C95.9- *[M36.1]*
    lipoid dermatoarthritis E78.81
    Lyme disease A69.23
    Mediterranean fever, familial (*see also*
      subcategory M14.8-) M04.1
    Meningococcus A39.83
    metabolic disorder NEC (*see also*
      subcategory M14.8-) E88.9
    multiple myelomatosis C90.0- *[M36.1]*
    mumps B26.85
    mycosis NEC (*see also* category M01) B49
    myelomatosis (multiple) C90.0- *[M36.1]*
    neurological disorder NEC G98.0
    ochronosis (*see also* subcategory M14.8-)
      E70.29
    O'nyong-nyong (*see also* category M01)
      A92.1
    parasitic disease NEC (*see also* category
      M01) B89
    paratyphoid fever (*see also* category M01)
      A01.4
    Pseudomonas — *see* Arthritis, pyogenic,
      bacterial NEC
    psoriasis L40.50
    pyogenic organism NEC — *see* Arthritis,
      pyogenic, bacterial NEC
    Reiter's disease — *see* Reiter's disease
    respiratory disorder NEC (*see also*
      subcategory M14.8-) J98.9
    reticulosis, malignant (*see also*
      subcategory M14.8-) C86.0
    rubella B06.82
    Salmonella (arizonae) (cholerae-suis)
      (enteritidis) (typhimurium) A02.23
    sarcoidosis D86.86
    specified bacteria NEC — *see* Arthritis,
      pyogenic, bacterial NEC
    sporotrichosis B42.82
    syringomyelia G95.0
    thalassemia NEC D56.9 *[M36.3]*
    tuberculosis — *see* Tuberculosis, arthritis
    typhoid fever A01.04
    urethritis, Reiter's — *see* Reiter's disease
    viral disease NEC (*see also* category M01)
      B34.9
  infectious or infective — *see also* Arthritis,
    pyogenic or pyemic
    spine — *see* Spondylopathy, infective
  juvenile M08.90
    with systemic onset — *see* Still's disease
    ankle M08.97-
    elbow M08.92-
    foot joint M08.97-
    hand joint M08.94-
    hip M08.95-
    knee M08.96-
    multiple site M08.99
    pauciarticular M08.40
      ankle M08.47-
      elbow M08.42-
      foot joint M08.47-
      hand joint M08.44-
      hip M08.45-
      knee M08.46-
      shoulder M08.41-
      vertebrae M08.48
      wrist M08.43-
    psoriatic L40.54
    rheumatoid — *see* Arthritis, rheumatoid,
      juvenile
    shoulder M08.91-
    vertebra M08.98
    specified type NEC M08.80
      ankle M08.87-
      elbow M08.82-
      foot joint M08.87-
      hand joint M08.84-

Arthritis, arthritic (acute) (chronic) (nonpyogenic) (subacute) - *continued*
- juvenile - *continued*
  - specified type NEC - *continued*
    - hip M08.85-
    - knee M08.86-
    - multiple site M08.89
    - shoulder M08.81-
    - specified joint NEC M08.88
    - vertebrae M08.88
    - wrist M08.83-
    - wrist M08.93-
  - meaning osteoarthritis — *see* Osteoarthritis
- meningococcal A39.83
- menopausal (any site) NEC — *see* Arthritis, specified form NEC
- mutilans (psoriatic) L40.52
- mycotic NEC (*see also* category M01) B49
- neuropathic (Charcot) — *see* Arthropathy, neuropathic
  - diabetic — *see* Diabetes, arthropathy, neuropathic
  - nonsyphilitic NEC G98.0
  - syringomyelic G95.0
- ochronotic (*see also* subcategory M14.8-) E70.29
- palindromic (any site) — *see* Rheumatism, palindromic
- pneumococcal M00.10
  - ankle M00.17-
  - elbow M00.12-
  - foot joint — *see* Arthritis, pneumococcal, ankle
  - hand joint M00.14-
  - hip M00.15-
  - knee M00.16-
  - multiple site M00.19
  - shoulder M00.11-
  - vertebra M00.18
  - wrist M00.13-
- postdysenteric — *see* Arthropathy, postdysenteric
- postmeningococcal A39.84
- postrheumatic, chronic — *see* Arthropathy, postrheumatic, chronic
- primary progressive — *see also* Arthritis, specified form NEC
  - spine — *see* Spondylitis, ankylosing
- psoriatic L40.50
- purulent (any site except spine) — *see* Arthritis, pyogenic or pyemic
  - spine — *see* Spondylopathy, infective
- pyogenic or pyemic (any site except spine) M00.9
  - bacterial NEC M00.80
    - ankle M00.87-
    - elbow M00.82-
    - foot joint — *see* Arthritis, pyogenic, bacterial NEC, ankle
    - hand joint M00.84-
    - hip M00.85-
    - knee M00.86-
    - multiple site M00.89
    - shoulder M00.81-
    - vertebra M00.88
    - wrist M00.83-
  - pneumococcal — *see* Arthritis, pneumococcal
  - spine — *see* Spondylopathy, infective
  - staphylococcal — *see* Arthritis, staphylococcal
  - streptococcal — *see* Arthritis, streptococcal NEC
  - pneumococcal — *see* Arthritis, pneumococcal
- reactive — *see* Reiter's disease
- rheumatic — *see also* Arthritis, rheumatoid
  - acute or subacute — *see* Fever, rheumatic
- rheumatoid M06.9
  - with
    - carditis — *see* Rheumatoid, carditis
    - endocarditis — *see* Rheumatoid, carditis
    - heart involvement NEC — *see* Rheumatoid, carditis

Arthritis, arthritic (acute) (chronic) (nonpyogenic) (subacute) - *continued*
- rheumatoid - *continued*
  - with - *continued*
    - lung involvement — *see* Rheumatoid, lung
    - myocarditis — *see* Rheumatoid, carditis
    - myopathy — *see* Rheumatoid, myopathy
    - pericarditis — *see* Rheumatoid, carditis
    - polyneuropathy — *see* Rheumatoid, polyneuropathy
    - rheumatoid factor — *see* Arthritis, rheumatoid, seropositive
    - splenoadenomegaly and leukopenia — *see* Felty's syndrome
    - vasculitis — *see* Rheumatoid, vasculitis
    - visceral involvement NEC — *see* Rheumatoid, arthritis, with involvement of organs NEC
  - juvenile (with or without rheumatoid factor) M08.00
    - ankle M08.07-
    - elbow M08.02-
    - foot joint M08.07-
    - hand joint M08.04-
    - hip M08.05-
    - knee M08.06-
    - multiple site M08.09
    - shoulder M08.01-
    - vertebra M08.08
    - wrist M08.03-
  - seronegative M06.00
    - ankle M06.07-
    - elbow M06.02-
    - foot joint M06.07-
    - hand joint M06.04-
    - hip M06.05-
    - knee M06.06-
    - multiple site M06.09
    - shoulder M06.01-
    - vertebra M06.08
    - wrist M06.03-
  - seropositive M05.9
    - specified NEC M05.80
      - ankle M05.87-
      - elbow M05.82-
      - foot joint M05.87-
      - hand joint M05.84-
      - hip M05.85-
      - knee M05.86-
      - multiple sites M05.89
      - shoulder M05.81-
      - vertebra — *see* Spondylitis, ankylosing
      - wrist M05.83-
    - without organ involvement M05.70
      - ankle M05.77-
      - elbow M05.72-
      - foot joint M05.77-
      - hand joint M05.74-
      - hip M05.75-
      - knee M05.76-
      - multiple sites M05.79
      - shoulder M05.71-
      - vertebra — *see* Spondylitis, ankylosing
      - wrist M05.73-
    - specified type NEC M06.80
      - ankle M06.87-
      - elbow M06.82-
      - foot joint M06.87-
      - hand joint M06.84-
      - hip M06.85-
      - knee M06.86-
      - multiple site M06.89
      - shoulder M06.81-
      - vertebra M06.88
      - wrist M06.83-
  - spine — *see* Spondylitis, ankylosing
- rubella B06.82
- scorbutic (*see also* subcategory M14.8-) E54
- senile or senescent — *see* Osteoarthritis
- septic (any site except spine) — *see* Arthritis, pyogenic or pyemic
  - spine — *see* Spondylopathy, infective

Arthritis, arthritic (acute) (chronic) (nonpyogenic) (subacute) - *continued*
- serum (nontherapeutic) (therapeutic) — *see* Arthropathy, postimmunization
- specified form NEC M13.80
  - ankle M13.87-
  - elbow M13.82-
  - foot joint M13.87-
  - hand joint M13.84-
  - hip M13.85-
  - knee M13.86-
  - multiple site M13.89
  - shoulder M13.81-
  - specified joint NEC M13.88
  - wrist M13.83-
- spine — *see also* Spondylopathy, inflammatory
  - infectious or infective NEC — *see* Spondylopathy, infective
  - Marie-Strümpell — *see* Spondylitis, ankylosing
  - pyogenic — *see* Spondylopathy, infective
  - rheumatoid — *see* Spondylitis, ankylosing
  - traumatic (old) — *see* Spondylopathy, traumatic
  - tuberculous A18.01
- staphylococcal M00.00
  - ankle M00.07-
  - elbow M00.02-
  - foot joint — *see* Arthritis, staphylococcal, ankle
  - hand joint M00.04-
  - hip M00.05-
  - knee M00.06-
  - multiple site M00.09
  - shoulder M00.01-
  - vertebra M00.08
  - wrist M00.03-
- streptococcal NEC M00.20
  - ankle M00.27-
  - elbow M00.22-
  - foot joint — *see* Arthritis, streptococcal, ankle
  - hand joint M00.24-
  - hip M00.25-
  - knee M00.26-
  - multiple site M00.29
  - shoulder M00.21-
  - vertebra M00.28
  - wrist M00.23-
- suppurative — *see* Arthritis, pyogenic or pyemic
- syphilitic (late) A52.16
  - congenital A50.55 *[M12.80]*
- syphilitica deformans (Charcot) A52.16
- temporomandibular M26.69
- toxic of menopause (any site) — *see* Arthritis, specified form NEC
- transient — *see* Arthropathy, specified form NEC
- traumatic (chronic) — *see* Arthropathy, traumatic
- tuberculous A18.02
  - spine A18.01
- uratic — *see* Gout
- urethritica (Reiter's) — *see* Reiter's disease
- vertebral — *see* Spondylopathy, inflammatory
- villous (any site) — *see* Arthropathy, specified form NEC

Arthrocele — *see* Effusion, joint
Arthrodesis status Z98.1
Arthrodynia — *see also* Pain, joint
Arthrodysplasia Q74.9
Arthrofibrosis, joint — *see* Ankylosis
Arthrogryposis (congenital) Q68.8
- multiplex congenita Q74.3
Arthrokatadysis M24.7
Arthropathy — *see also* Arthritis M12.9
- Charcot's — *see* Arthropathy, neuropathic
  - diabetic — *see* Diabetes, arthropathy, neuropathic
  - syringomyelic G95.0
- cricoarytenoid J38.7

Arthropathy - *continued*
crystal (-induced) — *see* Arthritis, in,
   crystals
diabetic NEC — *see* Diabetes, arthropathy
distal interphalangeal, psoriatic L40.51
enteropathic M07.60
   ankle M07.67-
   elbow M07.62-
   foot joint M07.67-
   hand joint M07.64-
   hip M07.65-
   knee M07.66-
   multiple site M07.69
   shoulder M07.61-
   vertebra M07.68
   wrist M07.63-
following intestinal bypass M02.00
   ankle M02.07-
   elbow M02.02-
   foot joint M02.07-
   hand joint M02.04-
   hip M02.05-
   knee M02.06-
   multiple site M02.09
   shoulder M02.01-
   vertebra M02.08
   wrist M02.03-
gouty — *see also* Gout
   in (due to)
      Lesch-Nyhan syndrome E79.1 *[M14.8-]*
      sickle-cell disorders D57- *[M14.8-]*
hemophilic NEC D66 *[M36.2]*
   in (due to)
      hyperparathyroidism NEC E21.3
         [M14.8-]
      metabolic disease NOS E88.9 *[M14.8-]*
in (due to)
   acromegaly E22.0 *[M14.8-]*
   amyloidosis E85.4 *[M14.8-]*
   blood disorder NOS D75.9 *[M36.3]*
   diabetes — *see* Diabetes, arthropathy
   endocrine disease NOS E34.9 *[M14.8-]*
   erythema
      multiforme L51.9 *[M14.8-]*
      nodosum L52 *[M14.8-]*
   hemochromatosis E83.118 *[M14.8-]*
   hemoglobinopathy NEC D58.2 *[M36.3]*
   hemophilia NEC D66 *[M36.2]*
   Henoch-Schönlein purpura D69.0 *[M36.4]*
   hyperthyroidism E05.90 *[M14.8-]*
   hypothyroidism E03.9 *[M14.8-]*
   infective endocarditis I33.0 *[M12.80]*
   leukemia NEC C95.9- *[M36.1]*
   malignant histiocytosis C96.A *[M36.1]*
   metabolic disease NOS E88.9 *[M14.8-]*
   multiple myeloma C90.0- *[M36.1]*
   neoplastic disease NOS (see also
      Neoplasm) D49.9 *[M36.1]*
   nutritional deficiency (*see also*
      subcategory M14.8-) E63.9
   psoriasis NOS L40.50
   sarcoidosis D86.86
   syphilis (late) A52.77
      congenital A50.55 *[M12.80]*
   thyrotoxicosis (*see also* subcategory
      M14.8-) E05.90
   ulcerative colitis K51.90 *[M07.60]*
   viral hepatitis (postinfectious) NEC B19.9
      [M12.80]
   Whipple's disease (*see also* subcategory
      M14.8-) K90.81
Jaccoud — *see* Arthropathy, postrheumatic,
   chronic
juvenile — *see* Arthritis, juvenile
   psoriatic L40.54
mutilans (psoriatic) L40.52
neuropathic (Charcot) M14.60
   ankle M14.67-
   diabetic — *see* Diabetes, arthropathy,
      neuropathic
   elbow M14.62-
   foot joint M14.67-
   hand joint M14.64-
   hip M14.65-
   knee M14.66-

Arthropathy - *continued*
neuropathic (Charcot) - *continued*
   multiple site M14.69
   nonsyphilitic NEC G98.0
   shoulder M14.61-
   syringomyelic G95.0
   vertebra M14.68
   wrist M14.63-
osteopulmonary — *see* Osteoarthropathy,
   hypertrophic, specified NEC
postdysenteric M02.10
   ankle M02.17-
   elbow M02.12-
   foot joint M02.17-
   hand joint M02.14-
   hip M02.15-
   knee M02.16-
   multiple site M02.19
   shoulder M02.11-
   vertebra M02.18
   wrist M02.13-
postimmunization M02.20
   ankle M02.27-
   elbow M02.22-
   foot joint M02.27-
   hand joint M02.24-
   hip M02.25-
   knee M02.26-
   multiple site M02.29
   shoulder M02.21-
   vertebra M02.28
   wrist M02.23-
postinfectious NEC B99 *[M12.80]*
   in (due to)
      enteritis due to Yersinia
         enterocolitica A04.6 *[M12.80]*
      syphilis A52.77
      viral hepatitis NEC B19.9 *[M12.80]*
postrheumatic, chronic (Jaccoud) M12.00
   ankle M12.07-
   elbow M12.02-
   foot joint M12.07-
   hand joint M12.04-
   hip M12.05-
   knee M12.06-
   multiple site M12.09
   shoulder M12.01-
   specified joint NEC M12.08
   vertebrae M12.08
   wrist M12.03-
psoriatic NEC L40.59
   interphalangeal, distal L40.51
reactive M02.9
   in (due to)
      infective endocarditis I33.0 *[M02.9]*
   specified type NEC M02.80
      ankle M02.87-
      elbow M02.82-
      foot joint M02.87-
      hand joint M02.84-
      hip M02.85-
      knee M02.86-
      multiple site M02.89
      shoulder M02.81-
      vertebra M02.88
      wrist M02.83-
specified form NEC M12.80
   ankle M12.87-
   elbow M12.82-
   foot joint M12.87-
   hand joint M12.84-
   hip M12.85-
   knee M12.86-
   multiple site M12.89
   shoulder M12.81-
   specified joint NEC M12.88
   vertebrae M12.88
   wrist M12.83-
syringomyelic G95.0
tabes dorsalis A52.16
tabetic A52.16
transient — *see* Arthropathy, specified form
   NEC
traumatic M12.50
   ankle M12.57-

Arthropathy - *continued*
traumatic - *continued*
   elbow M12.52-
   foot joint M12.57-
   hand joint M12.54-
   hip M12.55-
   knee M12.56-
   multiple site M12.59
   shoulder M12.51-
   specified joint NEC M12.58
   vertebrae M12.58
   wrist M12.53-
Arthropyosis — *see* Arthritis, pyogenic or
   pyemic
Arthrosis (deformans) (degenerative)
   (localized) — *see also*
   Osteoarthritis M19.90
spine — *see* Spondylosis
Arthus' phenomenon or reaction T78.41
   due to
      drug — *see* Table of Drugs and Chemicals,
         by drug
Articular — *see* condition
Articulation, reverse (teeth) M26.24
Artificial
   insemination complication — *see*
      Complications, artificial, fertilization
   opening status (functioning) (without
      complication) Z93.9
      anus (colostomy) Z93.3
      colostomy Z93.3
      cystostomy Z93.50
         appendico-vesicostomy Z93.52
         cutaneous Z93.51
         specified NEC Z93.59
      enterostomy Z93.4
      gastrostomy Z93.1
      ileostomy Z93.2
      intestinal tract NEC Z93.4
      jejunostomy Z93.4
      nephrostomy Z93.6
      specified site NEC Z93.8
      tracheostomy Z93.0
      ureterostomy Z93.6
      urethrostomy Z93.6
      urinary tract NEC Z93.6
      vagina Z93.8
      vagina status Z93.8
Arytenoid — *see* condition
Asbestosis (occupational) J61
Ascariasis B77.9
   with
      complications NEC B77.89
      intestinal complications B77.0
      pneumonia, pneumonitis B77.81
Ascaridosis, ascaridiasis — *see* Ascariasis
Ascaris (infection) (infestation)
   (lumbricoides) — *see* Ascariasis
Ascending — *see* condition
ASC-H (atypical squamous cells cannot
   exclude high grade squamous
   intraepithelial lesion on cytologic
   smear)
   anus R85.611
   cervix R87.611
   vagina R87.621
Aschoff's bodies — *see* Myocarditis,
   rheumatic
Ascites (abdominal) R18.8
   cardiac — *see also* Failure, heart,
      right I50.810
   chylous (nonfilarial) I89.8
      filarial — *see* Infestation, filarial
   due to
      cirrhosis, alcoholic K70.31
      hepatitis
         alcoholic K70.11
         chronic active K71.51
      S. japonicum B65.2
   heart — *see also* Failure, heart, right I50.810
   malignant R18.0
   pseudochylous R18.8
   syphilitic A52.74
   tuberculous A18.31

ASC-US (atypical squamous cells of undetermined significance on cytologic smear)
  anus R85.610
  cervix R87.610
  vagina R87.620
Aseptic — *see* condition
Asherman's syndrome N85.6
Asialia K11.7
Asiatic cholera — *see* Cholera
Asimultagnosia (simultanagnosia) R48.3
Askin's tumor — *see* Neoplasm, connective tissue, malignant
Asocial personality F60.2
Asomatognosia R41.4
Aspartylglucosaminuria E77.1
Asperger's disease or syndrome F84.5
Aspergilloma — *see* Aspergillosis
Aspergillosis (with pneumonia) B44.9
  bronchopulmonary, allergic B44.81
  disseminated B44.7
  generalized B44.7
  pulmonary NEC B44.1
    allergic B44.81
    invasive B44.0
  specified NEC B44.89
  tonsillar B44.2
Aspergillus (flavus) (fumigatus) (infection) (terreus) — *see* Aspergillosis
Aspermatogenesis — *see* Azoospermia
Aspermia (testis) — *see* Azoospermia
Asphyxia, asphyxiation (by) R09.01
  antenatal P84
  birth P84
  bunny bag — *see* Asphyxia, due to, mechanical threat to breathing, trapped in bed clothes
  crushing S28.0
  drowning T75.1
  gas, fumes, or vapor — *see* Table of Drugs and Chemicals
  inhalation — *see* Inhalation
  intrauterine P84
  local I73.00
    with gangrene I73.01
  mucus — *see also* Foreign body, respiratory tract, causing asphyxia
  newborn P84
  pathological R09.01
  postnatal P84
    mechanical — *see* Asphyxia, due to, mechanical threat to breathing
  prenatal P84
  reticularis R23.1
  strangulation — *see* Asphyxia, due to, mechanical threat to breathing
  submersion T75.1
  traumatic T71.9
    due to
      crushed chest S28.0
      foreign body (in) — *see* Foreign body, respiratory tract, causing asphyxia
      low oxygen content of ambient air T71.20
        due to
          being trapped in low oxygen environment T71.29
            in car trunk T71.221
              circumstances
                undetermined T71.224
              done with intent to harm by another person T71.223
              self T71.222
            in refrigerator T71.231
              circumstances
                undetermined T71.234
              done with intent to harm by another person T71.233
              self T71.232
          cave-in T71.21
      mechanical threat to breathing (accidental) T71.191
        circumstances undetermined T71.194
        done with intent to harm by another person T71.193

Asphyxia, asphyxiation (by) - *continued*
  traumatic - *continued*
    due to - *continued*
      mechanical threat to breathing (accidental) - *continued*
        done with intent to harm by - *continued*
          self T71.192
        hanging T71.161
          circumstances
            undetermined T71.164
          done with intent to harm by another person T71.163
            self T71.162
        plastic bag T71.121
          circumstances
            undetermined T71.124
          done with intent to harm by another person T71.123
            self T71.122
        smothering
          in furniture T71.151
            circumstances
              undetermined T71.154
            done with intent to harm by another person T71.153
              self T71.152
        under
          another person's body T71.141
            circumstances
              undetermined T71.144
            done with intent to harm T71.143
          pillow T71.111
            circumstances
              undetermined T71.114
            done with intent to harm by another person T71.113
              self T71.112
        trapped in bed clothes T71.131
          circumstances
            undetermined T71.134
          done with intent to harm by another person T71.133
            self T71.132
  vomiting, vomitus — *see* Foreign body, respiratory tract, causing asphyxia
Aspiration
  amniotic (clear) fluid (newborn) P24.10
    with
      pneumonia (pneumonitis) P24.11
      respiratory symptoms P24.11
  blood
    newborn (without respiratory symptoms) P24.20
      with
        pneumonia (pneumonitis) P24.21
        respiratory symptoms P24.21
      specified age NEC — *see* Foreign body, respiratory tract
  bronchitis J69.0
  food or foreign body (with asphyxiation) — *see* Asphyxia, food
  liquor (amnii) (newborn) P24.10
    with
      pneumonia (pneumonitis) P24.11
      respiratory symptoms P24.11
  meconium (newborn) (without respiratory symptoms) P24.00
    with
      pneumonitis (pneumonitis) P24.01
      respiratory symptoms P24.01
  milk (newborn) (without respiratory symptoms) P24.30
    with
      pneumonia (pneumonitis) P24.31
      respiratory symptoms P24.31
    specified age NEC — *see* Foreign body, respiratory tract
  mucus — *see also* Foreign body, by site, causing asphyxia
    newborn P24.10
      with
        pneumonia (pneumonitis) P24.11
        respiratory symptoms P24.11

Aspiration - *continued*
  neonatal P24.9
    specific NEC (without respiratory symptoms) P24.80
      with
        pneumonia (pneumonitis) P24.81
        respiratory symptoms P24.81
  newborn P24.9
    specific NEC (without respiratory symptoms) P24.80
      with
        pneumonia (pneumonitis) P24.81
        respiratory symptoms P24.81
  pneumonia J69.0
  pneumonitis J69.0
  syndrome of newborn — *see* Aspiration, by substance, with pneumonia
  vernix caseosa (newborn) P24.80
    with
      pneumonia (pneumonitis) P24.81
      respiratory symptoms P24.81
  vomitus — *see also* Foreign body, respiratory tract
    newborn (without respiratory symptoms) P24.30
      with
        pneumonia (pneumonitis) P24.31
        respiratory symptoms P24.31
Asplenia (congenital) Q89.01
  postsurgical Z90.81
Assam fever B55.0
Assault, sexual — *see* Maltreatment
Assmann's focus NEC A15.0
Astasia (-abasia) (hysterical) F44.4
Asteatosis cutis L85.3
Astereognosia, astereognosis R48.1
Asterixis R27.8
  in liver disease K71.3
Asteroid hyalitis — *see* Deposit, crystalline
Asthenia, asthenic R53.1
  cardiac — *see also* Failure, heart I50.9
    psychogenic F45.8
  cardiovascular — *see also* Failure, heart I50.9
    psychogenic F45.8
  heart — *see also* Failure, heart I50.9
    psychogenic F45.8
  hysterical F44.4
  myocardial — *see also* Failure, heart I50.9
    psychogenic F45.8
  nervous F48.8
  neurocirculatory F45.8
  neurotic F48.8
  psychogenic F48.8
  psychoneurotic F48.8
  psychophysiologic F48.8
  reaction (psychophysiologic) F48.8
  senile R54
Asthenopia — *see also* Discomfort, visual
  hysterical F44.6
  psychogenic F44.6
Asthenospermia — *see* Abnormal, specimen, male genital organs
Asthma, asthmatic (bronchial) (catarrh) (spasmodic) J45.909
  with
    chronic obstructive bronchitis J44.9
      with
        acute lower respiratory infection J44.0
        exacerbation (acute) J44.1
    chronic obstructive pulmonary disease J44.9
      with
        acute lower respiratory infection J44.0
        exacerbation (acute) J44.1
    exacerbation (acute) J45.901
    hay fever — *see* Asthma, allergic extrinsic
    rhinitis, allergic — *see* Asthma, allergic extrinsic
    status asthmaticus J45.902
  allergic extrinsic J45.909
    with
      exacerbation (acute) J45.901
      status asthmaticus J45.902
  atopic — *see* Asthma, allergic extrinsic

Asthma, asthmatic (bronchial) (catarrh) (spasmodic) - *continued*
  cardiac — *see* Failure, ventricular, left
  cardiobronchial I50.1
  childhood J45.909
    with
      exacerbation (acute) J45.901
      status asthmaticus J45.902
  chronic obstructive J44.9
    with
      acute lower respiratory infection J44.0
      exacerbation (acute) J44.1
  collier's J60
  cough variant J45.991
  detergent J69.8
  due to
    detergent J69.8
    inhalation of fumes J68.3
  eosinophilic J82
  extrinsic, allergic — *see* Asthma, allergic extrinsic
  grinder's J62.8
  hay — *see* Asthma, allergic extrinsic
  heart I50.1
  idiosyncratic — *see* Asthma, nonallergic
  intermittent (mild) J45.20
    with
      exacerbation (acute) J45.21
      status asthmaticus J45.22
  intrinsic, nonallergic — *see* Asthma, nonallergic
  Kopp's E32.8
  late-onset J45.909
    with
      exacerbation (acute) J45.901
      status asthmaticus J45.902
  mild intermittent J45.20
    with
      exacerbation (acute) J45.21
      status asthmaticus J45.22
  mild persistent J45.30
    with
      exacerbation (acute) J45.31
      status asthmaticus J45.32
  Millar's (laryngismus stridulus) J38.5
  miner's J60
  mixed J45.909
    with
      exacerbation (acute) J45.901
      status asthmaticus J45.902
  moderate persistent J45.40
    with
      exacerbation (acute) J45.41
      status asthmaticus J45.42
  nervous — *see* Asthma, nonallergic
  nonallergic (intrinsic) J45.909
    with
      exacerbation (acute) J45.901
      status asthmaticus J45.902
  persistent
    mild J45.30
      with
        exacerbation (acute) J45.31
        status asthmaticus J45.32
    moderate J45.40
      with
        exacerbation (acute) J45.41
        status asthmaticus J45.42
    severe J45.50
      with
        exacerbation (acute) J45.51
        status asthmaticus J45.52
  platinum J45.998
  pneumoconiotic NEC J64
  potter's J62.8
  predominantly allergic J45.909
  psychogenic F54
  pulmonary eosinophilic J82
  red cedar J67.8
  Rostan's I50.1
  sandblaster's J62.8
  sequoiosis J67.8
  severe persistent J45.50
    with
      exacerbation (acute) J45.51

Asthma, asthmatic (bronchial) (catarrh) (spasmodic) - *continued*
  severe persistent - *continued*
    with - *continued*
      status asthmaticus J45.52
  specified NEC J45.998
  stonemason's J62.8
  thymic E32.8
  tuberculous — *see* Tuberculosis, pulmonary
  Wichmann's (laryngismus stridulus) J38.5
  wood J67.8
Astigmatism (compound) (congenital) H52.20-
  irregular H52.21-
  regular H52.22-
Astraphobia F40.220
Astroblastoma
  specified site — *see* Neoplasm, malignant, by site
  unspecified site C71.9
Astrocytoma (cystic)
  anaplastic
    specified site — *see* Neoplasm, malignant, by site
    unspecified site C71.9
  fibrillary
    specified site — *see* Neoplasm, malignant, by site
    unspecified site C71.9
  fibrous
    specified site — *see* Neoplasm, malignant, by site
    unspecified site C71.9
  gemistocytic
    specified site — *see* Neoplasm, malignant, by site
    unspecified site C71.9
  juvenile
    specified site — *see* Neoplasm, malignant, by site
    unspecified site C71.9
  pilocytic
    specified site — *see* Neoplasm, malignant, by site
    unspecified site C71.9
  piloid
    specified site — *see* Neoplasm, malignant, by site
    unspecified site C71.9
  protoplasmic
    specified site — *see* Neoplasm, malignant, by site
    unspecified site C71.9
  specified site NEC — *see* Neoplasm, malignant, by site
  subependymal D43.2
    giant cell
      specified site — *see* Neoplasm, uncertain behavior, by site
      unspecified site D43.2
    specified site — *see* Neoplasm, uncertain behavior, by site
    unspecified site D43.2
  unspecified site C71.9
Astroglioma
  specified site — *see* Neoplasm, malignant, by site
  unspecified site C71.9
Asymbolia R48.8
Asymmetry — *see also* Distortion
  between native and reconstructed breast N65.1
  face Q67.0
  jaw (lower) — *see* Anomaly, dentofacial, jaw-cranial base relationship, asymmetry
Asynergia, asynergy R27.8
  ventricular I51.89
Asystole (heart) — *see* Arrest, cardiac
At risk
  for
    dental caries Z91.849
      high Z91.843
      low Z91.841
      moderate Z91.842

At risk - *continued*
  for - *continued*
    falling Z91.81
Ataxia, ataxy, ataxic R27.0
  acute R27.8
  brain (hereditary) G11.9
  cerebellar (hereditary) G11.9
    with defective DNA repair G11.3
    alcoholic G31.2
    early-onset G11.1
    in
      alcoholism G31.2
      myxedema E03.9 *[G13.2]*
      neoplastic disease — *see also* Neoplasm D49.9 *[G32.81]*
      specified disease NEC G32.81
    late-onset (Marie's) G11.2
  cerebral (hereditary) G11.9
  congenital nonprogressive G11.0
  family, familial — *see* Ataxia, hereditary
  following
    cerebrovascular disease I69.993
      cerebral infarction I69.393
      intracerebral hemorrhage I69.193
      nontraumatic intracranial hemorrhage NEC I69.293
      specified disease NEC I69.893
      subarachnoid hemorrhage I69.093
  Friedreich's (heredofamilial) (cerebellar) (spinal) G11.1
  gait R26.0
    hysterical F44.4
  general R27.8
  gluten M35.9 *[G32.81]*
    with celiac disease K90.0 *[G32.81]*
  hereditary G11.9
    with neuropathy G60.2
    cerebellar — *see* Ataxia, cerebellar
    spastic G11.4
    specified NEC G11.8
    spinal (Friedreich's) G11.1
  heredofamilial — *see* Ataxia, hereditary
  Hunt's G11.1
  hysterical F44.4
  locomotor (progressive) (syphilitic) (partial) (spastic) A52.11
    diabetic — *see* Diabetes, ataxia
  Marie's (cerebellar) (heredofamilial) (late-onset) G11.2
  nonorganic origin F44.4
  nonprogressive, congenital G11.0
  psychogenic F44.4
  Roussy-Lévy G60.0
  Sanger-Brown's (hereditary) G11.2
  spastic hereditary G11.4
  spinal
    hereditary (Friedreich's) G11.1
    progressive (syphilitic) A52.11
  spinocerebellar, X-linked recessive G11.1
  telangiectasia (Louis-Bar) G11.3
Ataxia-telangiectasia (Louis-Bar) G11.3
Atelectasis (massive) (partial) (pressure) (pulmonary) J98.11
  newborn P28.10
    due to resorption P28.11
    partial P28.19
    primary P28.0
    secondary P28.19
  primary (newborn) P28.0
  tuberculous — *see* Tuberculosis, pulmonary
Atelocardia Q24.9
Atelomyelia Q06.1
Atheroembolism
  of
    extremities
      lower I75.02-
      upper I75.01-
    kidney I75.81
    specified NEC I75.89
Atheroma, atheromatous — *see also* Arteriosclerosis I70.90
  aorta, aortic I70.0
    valve — *see also* Endocarditis, aortic I35.8
  aorto-iliac I70.0
  artery — *see* Arteriosclerosis

Atheroma, atheromatous - *continued*
  basilar (artery) I67.2
  carotid (artery) (common) (internal) I67.2
  cerebral (arteries) I67.2
  coronary (artery) I25.10
    with angina pectoris — *see*
      Arteriosclerosis, coronary (artery),
    degeneration — *see* Arteriosclerosis
  heart, cardiac — *see* Disease, heart,
    ischemic, atherosclerotic
  mitral (valve) I34.8
  myocardium, myocardial — *see* Disease,
    heart, ischemic, atherosclerotic
  pulmonary valve (heart) — *see also*
    Endocarditis, pulmonary I37.8
  tricuspid (heart) (valve) I36.8
  valve, valvular — *see* Endocarditis
  vertebral (artery) I67.2
Atheromatosis — *see* Arteriosclerosis
Atherosclerosis — *see also* Arteriosclerosis
  coronary
    artery I25.10
      with angina pectoris — *see*
        Arteriosclerosis, coronary (artery),
      due to
        calcified coronary lesion
          (severely) I25.84
        lipid rich plaque I25.83
    transplanted heart I25.811
      bypass graft I25.812
        with angina pectoris — *see*
          Arteriosclerosis, coronary (artery),
      native coronary artery I25.811
        with angina pectoris — *see*
          Arteriosclerosis, coronary (artery),
Athetosis (acquired) R25.8
  bilateral (congenital) G80.3
  congenital (bilateral) (double) G80.3
  double (congenital) G80.3
  unilateral R25.8
Athlete's
  foot B35.3
  heart I51.7
Athrepsia E41
Athyrea (acquired) — *see also*
    Hypothyroidism
  congenital E03.1
Atonia, atony, atonic
  bladder (sphincter) (neurogenic) N31.2
  capillary I78.8
  cecum K59.8
    psychogenic F45.8
  colon — *see* Atony, intestine
  congenital P94.2
  esophagus K22.8
  intestine K59.8
    psychogenic F45.8
  stomach K31.89
    neurotic or psychogenic F45.8
  uterus (during labor) O62.2
    with hemorrhage (postpartum) O72.1
    postpartum (with hemorrhage) O72.1
      without hemorrhage O75.89
Atopy — *see* History, allergy
Atransferrinemia, congenital E88.09
Atresia, atretic
  alimentary organ or tract NEC Q45.8
    upper Q40.8
  ani, anus, anal (canal) Q42.3
    with fistula Q42.2
  aorta (ring) Q25.29
  aortic (orifice) (valve) Q23.0
    arch Q25.21
    congenital with hypoplasia of ascending
      aorta and defective development of
      left ventricle (with mitral
      stenosis) Q23.4
    in hypoplastic left heart syndrome Q23.4
  aqueduct of Sylvius Q03.0
    with spina bifida — *see* Spina bifida, with
      hydrocephalus
  artery NEC Q27.8
    cerebral Q28.3
    coronary Q24.5
    digestive system Q27.8

Atresia, atretic - *continued*
  artery NEC - *continued*
    eye Q15.8
    lower limb Q27.8
    pulmonary Q25.5
    specified site NEC Q27.8
    umbilical Q27.0
    upper limb Q27.8
  auditory canal (external) Q16.1
  bile duct (common) (congenital)
    (hepatic) Q44.2
    acquired — *see* Obstruction, bile duct
  bladder (neck) Q64.39
    obstruction Q64.31
  bronchus Q32.4
  cecum Q42.8
  cervix (acquired) N88.2
    congenital Q51.828
    in pregnancy or childbirth — *see* Anomaly,
      cervix, in pregnancy or childbirth
    causing obstructed labor O65.5
  choana Q30.0
  colon Q42.9
    specified NEC Q42.8
  common duct Q44.2
  cricoid cartilage Q31.8
  cystic duct Q44.2
    acquired K82.8
      with obstruction K82.0
  digestive organs NEC Q45.8
  duodenum Q41.0
  ear canal Q16.1
  ejaculatory duct Q55.4
  epiglottis Q31.8
  esophagus Q39.0
    with tracheoesophageal fistula Q39.1
  eustachian tube Q17.8
  fallopian tube (congenital) Q50.6
    acquired N97.1
  follicular cyst N83.0-
  foramen of
    Luschka Q03.1
      with spina bifida — *see* Spina bifida,
        with hydrocephalus
    Magendie Q03.1
      with spina bifida — *see* Spina bifida,
        with hydrocephalus
  gallbladder Q44.1
  genital organ
    external
      female Q52.79
      male Q55.8
    internal
      female Q52.8
      male Q55.8
  glottis Q31.8
  gullet Q39.0
    with tracheoesophageal fistula Q39.1
  heart valve NEC Q24.8
    pulmonary Q22.0
    tricuspid Q22.4
  hymen Q52.3
    acquired (postinfective) N89.6
  ileum Q41.2
  intestine (small) Q41.9
    large Q42.9
      specified NEC Q42.8
  iris, filtration angle Q15.0
  jejunum Q41.1
  lacrimal apparatus Q10.4
  larynx Q31.8
  meatus urinarius Q64.33
  mitral valve Q23.2
    in hypoplastic left heart syndrome Q23.4
  nares (anterior) (posterior) Q30.0
  nasopharynx Q34.8
  nose, nostril Q30.0
    acquired J34.89
  organ or site NEC Q89.8
  osseous meatus (ear) Q16.1
  oviduct (congenital) Q50.6
    acquired N97.1
  parotid duct Q38.4
    acquired K11.8
  pulmonary (artery) Q25.5

Atresia, atretic - *continued*
  pulmonary (artery) - *continued*
    valve Q22.0
    pulmonic Q22.0
    pupil Q13.2
    rectum Q42.1
      with fistula Q42.0
    salivary duct Q38.4
      acquired K11.8
    sublingual duct Q38.4
      acquired K11.8
    submandibular duct Q38.4
      acquired K11.8
    submaxillary duct Q38.4
      acquired K11.8
    thyroid cartilage Q31.8
    trachea Q32.1
    tricuspid valve Q22.4
    ureter Q62.10
      pelvic junction Q62.11
      vesical orifice Q62.12
    ureteropelvic junction Q62.11
    ureterovesical orifice Q62.12
    urethra (valvular) Q64.39
      stricture Q64.32
    urinary tract NEC Q64.8
    uterus Q51.818
      acquired N85.8
    vagina (congenital) Q52.4
      acquired (postinfectional) (senile) N89.5
    vas deferens Q55.3
    vascular NEC Q27.8
      cerebral Q28.3
      digestive system Q27.8
      lower limb Q27.8
      specified site NEC Q27.8
      upper limb Q27.8
    vein NEC Q27.8
      digestive system Q27.8
      great Q26.8
      lower limb Q27.8
      portal Q26.5
      pulmonary Q26.4
        partial Q26.3
        total Q26.2
      specified site NEC Q27.8
      upper limb Q27.8
    vena cava (inferior) (superior) Q26.8
    vesicourethral orifice Q64.31
    vulva Q52.79
      acquired N90.5
Atrichia, atrichosis — *see* Alopecia
Atrophia — *see also* Atrophy
  cutis senilis L90.8
    due to radiation L57.8
  gyrata of choroid and retina H31.23
  senilis R54
    dermatological L90.8
      due to radiation (nonionizing)
        (solar) L57.8
  unguium L60.3
    congenita Q84.6
Atrophie blanche (en plaque) (de
  Milian) L95.0
Atrophoderma, atrophodermia (of) L90.9
  diffusum (idiopathic) L90.4
  maculatum L90.8
    et striatum L90.8
      due to syphilis A52.79
    syphilitic A51.39
  neuriticum L90.8
  Pasini and Pierini L90.3
  pigmentosum Q82.1
  reticulatum symmetricum faciei L66.4
  senile L90.8
    due to radiation (nonionizing)
      (solar) L57.8
  vermiculata (cheeks) L66.4
Atrophy, atrophic (of)
  adrenal (capsule) (gland) E27.49
    primary (autoimmune) E27.1
  alveolar process or ridge
    (edentulous) K08.20
  anal sphincter (disuse) N81.84
  appendix K38.8

Atrophy, atrophic (of) - *continued*
arteriosclerotic — *see* Arteriosclerosis
bile duct (common) (hepatic) K83.8
bladder N32.89
　neurogenic N31.8
blanche (en plaque) (of Milian) L95.0
bone (senile) NEC — *see also* Disorder,
　　bone, specified type NEC
　due to
　　tabes dorsalis (neurogenic) A52.11
brain (cortex) (progressive) G31.9
　frontotemporal circumscribed G31.01
　　[F02.80]
　　with behavioral disturbance G31.01
　　　[F02.81]
　senile NEC G31.1
breast N64.2
　obstetric — *see* Disorder, breast, specified
　　type NEC
buccal cavity K13.79
cardiac — *see* Degeneration, myocardial
cartilage (infectional) (joint) — *see* Disorder,
　　cartilage, specified NEC
cerebellar — *see* Atrophy, brain
cerebral — *see* Atrophy, brain
cervix (mucosa) (senile) (uteri) N88.8
　menopausal N95.8
Charcot-Marie-Tooth G60.0
choroid (central) (macular) (myopic)
　　(retina) H31.10-
　diffuse secondary H31.12-
　gyrate H31.23
　senile H31.11-
ciliary body — *see* Atrophy, iris
conjunctiva (senile) H11.89
corpus cavernosum N48.89
cortical — *see* Atrophy, brain
cystic duct K82.8
Déjérine-Thomas G23.8
disuse NEC — *see* Atrophy, muscle
Duchenne-Aran G12.21
ear H93.8-
edentulous alveolar ridge K08.20
endometrium (senile) N85.8
　cervix N88.8
enteric K63.89
epididymis N50.89
eyeball — *see* Disorder, globe, degenerated
　　condition, atrophy
eyelid (senile) — *see* Disorder, eyelid,
　　degenerative
facial (skin) L90.9
fallopian tube (senile) N83.32-
　with ovary N83.33-
fascioscapulohumeral (Landouzy-
　　Déjérine) G71.02
fatty, thymus (gland) E32.8
gallbladder K82.8
gastric K29.40
　with bleeding K29.41
gastrointestinal K63.89
glandular I89.8
globe H44.52-
gum — *see* Recession, gingival
hair L67.8
heart (brown) — *see* Degeneration,
　　myocardial
hemifacial Q67.4
　Romberg G51.8
infantile E41
　paralysis, acute — *see* Poliomyelitis,
　　paralytic
intestine K63.89
iris (essential) (progressive) H21.26-
　specified NEC H21.29
kidney (senile) (terminal) — *see also*
　　Sclerosis, renal N26.1
　congenital or infantile Q60.5
　　bilateral Q60.4
　　unilateral Q60.3
　hydronephrotic — *see* Hydronephrosis
lacrimal gland (primary) H04.14-
　secondary H04.15-
Landouzy-Déjérine G71.02
laryngitis, infective J37.0

Atrophy, atrophic (of) - *continued*
larynx J38.7
Leber's optic (hereditary) H47.22
lip K13.0
liver (yellow) K72.90
　with coma K72.91
　acute, subacute K72.00
　　with coma K72.01
　chronic K72.10
　　with coma K72.11
lung (senile) J98.4
macular (dermatological) L90.8
　syphilitic, skin A51.39
　　striated A52.79
mandible (edentulous) K08.20
　minimal K08.21
　moderate K08.22
　severe K08.23
maxilla K08.20
　minimal K08.24
　moderate K08.25
　severe K08.26
muscle, muscular (diffuse) (general)
　　(idiopathic) (primary) M62.50
　ankle M62.57-
　Duchenne-Aran G12.21
　foot M62.57-
　forearm M62.53-
　hand M62.54-
　infantile spinal G12.0
　lower leg M62.56-
　multiple sites M62.59
　myelopathic — *see* Atrophy, muscle,
　　spinal
　myotonic G71.11
　neuritic G58.9
　neuropathic (peroneal) (progressive) G60.0
　pelvic (disuse) N81.84
　peroneal G60.0
　progressive (bulbar) G12.21
　　adult G12.1
　　infantile (spinal) G12.0
　　spinal G12.25
　　　adult G12.1
　　　infantile G12.0
　pseudohypertrophic G71.02
　shoulder region M62.51-
　specified site NEC M62.58
　spinal G12.9
　　adult form G12.1
　　Aran-Duchenne G12.21
　　childhood form, type II G12.1
　　distal G12.1
　　hereditary NEC G12.1
　　infantile, type I (Werdnig-
　　　Hoffmann) G12.0
　　juvenile form, type III (Kugelberg-
　　　Welander) G12.1
　　progressive G12.25
　　scapuloperoneal form G12.1
　　specified NEC G12.8
　　syphilitic A52.78
　thigh M62.55-
　upper arm M62.52-
myocardium — *see* Degeneration,
　　myocardial
myometrium (senile) N85.8
　cervix N88.8
myopathic NEC — *see* Atrophy, muscle
myotonia G71.11
nail L60.3
nasopharynx J31.1
nerve — *see also* Disorder, nerve
　abducens — *see* Strabismus, paralytic,
　　sixth nerve
　accessory G52.8
　acoustic or auditory — *see* subcategory
　　H93.3
　cranial G52.9
　　eighth (auditory) — *see* subcategory
　　　H93.3
　　eleventh (accessory) G52.8
　　fifth (trigeminal) G50.8
　　first (olfactory) G52.0

Atrophy, atrophic (of) - *continued*
nerve - *continued*
　cranial - *continued*
　　fourth (trochlear) — *see* Strabismus,
　　　paralytic, fourth nerve
　　second (optic) H47.20
　　sixth (abducens) — *see* Strabismus,
　　　paralytic, sixth nerve
　　tenth (pneumogastric) (vagus) G52.2
　　third (oculomotor) — *see* Strabismus,
　　　paralytic, third nerve
　　twelfth (hypoglossal) G52.3
　hypoglossal G52.3
　oculomotor — *see* Strabismus, paralytic,
　　third nerve
　olfactory G52.0
　optic (papillomacular bundle)
　　syphilitic (late) A52.15
　　congenital A50.44
　pneumogastric G52.2
　trigeminal G50.8
　trochlear — *see* Strabismus, paralytic,
　　fourth nerve
　vagus (pneumogastric) G52.2
neurogenic, bone, tabetic A52.11
nutritional E41
old age R54
olivopontocerebellar G23.8
optic (nerve) H47.20
　glaucomatous H47.23-
　hereditary H47.22
　primary H47.21-
　specified type NEC H47.29-
　syphilitic (late) A52.15
　congenital A50.44
orbit H05.31-
ovary (senile) N83.31-
　with fallopian tube N83.33-
oviduct (senile) — *see* Atrophy, fallopian
　　tube
palsy, diffuse (progressive) G12.22
pancreas (duct) (senile) K86.89
parotid gland K11.0
pelvic muscle N81.84
penis N48.89
pharynx J39.2
pluriglandular E31.8
　autoimmune E31.0
polyarthritis M15.9
prostate N42.89
pseudohypertrophic (muscle) G71.02
renal — *see also* Sclerosis, renal N26.1
retina, retinal (postinfectional) H35.89
rhinitis J31.0
salivary gland K11.0
scar L90.5
sclerosis, lobar (of brain) G31.09 *[F02.80]*
　with behavioral disturbance G31.09
　　[F02.81]
scrotum N50.89
seminal vesicle N50.89
senile R54
　due to radiation (nonionizing)
　　(solar) L57.8
skin (patches) (spots) L90.9
　degenerative (senile) L90.8
　due to radiation (nonionizing)
　　(solar) L57.8
　senile L90.8
spermatic cord N50.89
spinal (acute) (cord) G95.89
　muscular — *see* Atrophy, muscle, spinal
　paralysis G12.20
　　acute — *see* Poliomyelitis, paralytic
　　meaning progressive muscular
　　　atrophy G12.25
spine (column) — *see* Spondylopathy,
　　specified NEC
spleen (senile) D73.0
stomach K29.40
　with bleeding K29.41
striate (skin) L90.6
　syphilitic A52.79
subcutaneous L90.9
sublingual gland K11.0

Atrophy, atrophic (of) - *continued*
submandibular gland K11.0
submaxillary gland K11.0
Sudeck's — *see* Algoneurodystrophy
suprarenal (capsule) (gland) E27.49
  primary E27.1
systemic affecting central nervous system
    in
      myxedema E03.9 *[G13.2]*
      neoplastic disease — *see also*
        Neoplasm D49.9 *[G13.1]*
      specified disease NEC G13.8
tarso-orbital fascia, congenital Q10.3
testis N50.0
thenar, partial — *see* Syndrome, carpal
    tunnel
thymus (fatty) E32.8
thyroid (gland) (acquired) E03.4
  with cretinism E03.1
  congenital (with myxedema) E03.1
tongue (senile) K14.8
  papillae K14.4
trachea J39.8
tunica vaginalis N50.89
turbinate J34.89
tympanic membrane (nonflaccid) H73.82-
    flaccid H73.81-
upper respiratory tract J39.8
uterus, uterine (senile) N85.8
  cervix N88.8
  due to radiation (intended effect) N85.8
    adverse effect or misadventure N99.89
vagina (senile) N95.2
vas deferens N50.89
vascular I99.8
vertebra (senile) — *see* Spondylopathy,
    specified NEC
vulva (senile) N90.5
Werdnig-Hoffmann G12.0
yellow — *see* Failure, hepatic
Attack, attacks
with alteration of consciousness (with
    automatisms) — *see* Epilepsy,
    localization-related, symptomatic, with
    complex partial seizures
Adams-Stokes I45.9
akinetic — *see* Epilepsy, generalized,
    specified NEC
angina — *see* Angina
atonic — *see* Epilepsy, generalized, specified
    NEC
benign shuddering G25.83
cataleptic — *see* Catalepsy
coronary — *see* Infarct, myocardium
cyanotic, newborn P28.2
drop NEC R55
epileptic — *see* Epilepsy
heart — *see* infarct, myocardium
hysterical F44.9
jacksonian — *see* Epilepsy, localization-
    related, symptomatic, with simple
    partial seizures
myocardium, myocardial — *see* Infarct,
    myocardium
myoclonic — *see* Epilepsy, generalized,
    specified NEC
panic F41.0
psychomotor — *see* Epilepsy, localization-
    related, symptomatic, with complex
    partial seizures
salaam — *see* Epilepsy, spasms
schizophreniform, brief F23
shuddering, benign G25.83
Stokes-Adams I45.9
syncope R55
transient ischemic (TIA) G45.9
  specified NEC G45.8
unconsciousness R55
  hysterical F44.89
vasomotor R55
vasovagal (paroxysmal) (idiopathic) R55
without alteration of consciousness — *see*
    Epilepsy, localization-related,
    symptomatic, with simple partial
    seizures

Attention (to)
artificial
  opening (of) Z43.9
    digestive tract NEC Z43.4
      colon Z43.3
      ilium Z43.2
      stomach Z43.1
    specified NEC Z43.8
    trachea Z43.0
    urinary tract NEC Z43.6
      cystostomy Z43.5
      nephrostomy Z43.6
      ureterostomy Z43.6
      urethrostomy Z43.6
    vagina Z43.7
  colostomy Z43.3
  cystostomy Z43.5
  deficit disorder or syndrome F98.8
    with hyperactivity — *see* Disorder,
        attention-deficit hyperactivity
  gastrostomy Z43.1
  ileostomy Z43.2
  jejunostomy Z43.4
  nephrostomy Z43.6
  surgical dressings Z48.01
  sutures Z48.02
  tracheostomy Z43.0
  ureterostomy Z43.6
  urethrostomy Z43.6
Attrition
gum — *see* Recession, gingival
tooth, teeth (excessive) (hard tissues) K03.0
Atypical, atypism — *see also* condition
cells (on cytolgocial smear) (endocervical)
    (endometrial) (glandular)
  cervix R87.619
  vagina R87.629
cervical N87.9
endometrium N85.9
  hyperplasia N85.00
parenting situation Z62.9
Auditory — *see* condition
Aujeszky's disease B33.8
Aurantiasis, cutis E67.1
Auricle, auricular — *see also* condition
cervical Q18.2
Auriculotemporal syndrome G50.8
**Austin Flint murmur (aortic
    insufficiency)** I35.1
Australian
Q fever A78
X disease A83.4
Autism, autistic (childhood) (infantile) F84.0
atypical F84.9
spectrum disorder F84.0
Autodigestion R68.89
**Autoerythrocyte sensitization
    (syndrome)** D69.2
Autographism L50.3
Autoimmune
disease (systemic) M35.9
inhibitors to clotting factors D68.311
lymphoproliferative syndrome
    [ALPS] D89.82
thyroiditis E06.3
Autointoxication R68.89
Automatism G93.89
with temporal sclerosis G93.81
epileptic — *see* Epilepsy, localization-
    related, symptomatic, with complex
    partial seizures
paroxysmal, idiopathic — *see* Epilepsy,
    localization-related, symptomatic, with
    complex partial seizures
Autonomic, autonomous
bladder (neurogenic) N31.2
hysteria seizure F44.5
Autosensitivity, erythrocyte D69.2
Autosensitization, cutaneous L30.2
Autosome — *see* condition by chromosome
    involved
Autotopagnosia R48.1
Autotoxemia R68.89
Autumn — *see* condition
Avellis' syndrome G46.8

Aversion
oral R63.3
  newborn P92.-
  nonorganic origin F98.2
sexual F52.1
Aviator's
disease or sickness — *see* Effect, adverse,
    high altitude
ear T70.0
Avitaminosis (multiple) — *see also*
    Deficiency, vitamin E56.9
B E53.9
  with
    beriberi E51.11
    pellagra E52
B2 E53.0
B6 E53.1
B12 E53.8
D E55.9
  with rickets E55.0
G E53.0
K E56.1
nicotinic acid E52
**AVNRT (atrioventricular nodal re-entrant
    tachycardia)** I47.1
**AVRT (atrioventricular nodal re-entrant
    tachycardia)** I47.1
Avulsion (traumatic)
blood vessel — *see* Injury, blood vessel
bone — *see* Fracture, by site
cartilage — *see also* Dislocation, by site
  symphyseal (inner) , complicating
      delivery O71.6
external site other than limb — *see* Wound,
    open, by site
eye S05.7-
head (intracranial)
  external site NEC S08.89
  scalp S08.0
internal organ or site — *see* Injury, by site
joint — *see also* Dislocation, by site
  capsule — *see* Sprain, by site
kidney S37.06-
ligament — *see* Sprain, by site
limb — *see also* Amputation, traumatic, by
    site
  skin and subcutaneous tissue — *see*
      Wound, open, by site
muscle — *see* Injury, muscle
nerve (root) — *see* Injury, nerve
scalp S08.0
skin and subcutaneous tissue — *see* Wound,
    open, by site
spleen S36.032
symphyseal cartilage (inner) , complicating
    delivery O71.6
tendon — *see* Injury, muscle
tooth S03.2
Awareness of heart beat R00.2
Axenfeld's
anomaly or syndrome Q15.0
degeneration (calcareous) Q13.4
Axilla, axillary — *see also* condition
breast Q83.1
Axonotmesis — *see* Injury, nerve
**Ayerza's disease or syndrome (pulmonary
    artery sclerosis with pulmonary
    hypertension)** I27.0
Azoospermia (organic) N46.01
due to
  drug therapy N46.021
  efferent duct obstruction N46.023
  infection N46.022
  radiation N46.024
  specified cause NEC N46.029
  systemic disease N46.025
Azotemia R79.89
meaning uremia N19
Aztec ear Q17.3
Azygos
continuation inferior vena cava Q26.8
lobe (lung) Q33.1

B

Baastrup's disease — *see* Kissing spine
Babesiosis B60.0

Babington's disease (familial hemorrhagic telangiectasia) I78.0
Babinski's syndrome A52.79
Baby
crying constantly R68.11
floppy (syndrome) P94.2
Bacillary — *see* condition
Bacilluria R82.71
Bacillus — *see also* Infection, bacillus
abortus infection A23.1
anthracis infection A22.9
coli infection — *see also* Escherichia coli B96.20
Flexner's A03.1
mallei infection A24.0
Shiga's A03.0
suipestifer infection — *see* Infection, salmonella
Back — *see* condition
Backache (postural) M54.9
sacroiliac M53.3
specified NEC M54.89
Backflow — *see* Reflux
Backward reading (dyslexia) F81.0
Bacteremia R78.81
with sepsis — *see* Sepsis
Bactericholia — *see* Cholecystitis, acute
Bacterid, bacteride (pustular) L40.3
Bacterium, bacteria, bacterial
agent NEC, as cause of disease classified elsewhere B96.89
in blood — *see* Bacteremia
in urine — *see* Bacteriuria
Bacteriuria, bacteruria R82.71
asymptomatic R82.71
Bacteroides
fragilis, as cause of disease classified elsewhere B96.6
Bad
heart — *see* Disease, heart
trip
due to drug abuse — *see* Abuse, drug, hallucinogen
due to drug dependence — *see* Dependence, drug, hallucinogen
Baelz's disease (cheilitis glandularis apostematosa) K13.0
Baerensprung's disease (eczema marginatum) B35.6
Bagasse disease or pneumonitis J67.1
Bagassosis J67.1
Baker's cyst — *see* Cyst, Baker's
Bakwin-Krida syndrome (metaphyseal dysplasia) Q78.5
Balancing side interference M26.56
Balanitis (circinata) (erosiva) (gangrenosa) (phagedenic) (vulgaris) N48.1
amebic A06.82
candidal B37.42
due to Haemophilus ducreyi A57
gonococcal (acute) (chronic) A54.23
xerotica obliterans N48.0
Balanoposthitis N47.6
gonococcal (acute) (chronic) A54.23
ulcerative (specific) A63.8
Balanorrhagia — *see* Balanitis
Balantidiasis, balantidiosis A07.0
Bald tongue K14.4
Baldness — *see also* Alopecia
male-pattern — *see* Alopecia, androgenic
Balkan grippe A78
Balloon disease — *see* Effect, adverse, high altitude
Balo's disease (concentric sclerosis) G37.5
Bamberger-Marie disease — *see* Osteoarthropathy, hypertrophic, specified type NEC
Bancroft's filariasis B74.0
Band (s)
adhesive — *see* Adhesions, peritoneum
anomalous or congenital — *see also* Anomaly, by site
heart (atrial) (ventricular) Q24.8
intestine Q43.3
omentum Q43.3

Band (s) - *continued*
cervix N88.1
constricting, congenital Q79.8
gallbladder (congenital) Q44.1
intestinal (adhesive) — *see* Adhesions, peritoneum
obstructive
intestine K56.50
complete K56.52
incomplete K56.51
partial K56.51
peritoneum K56.50
complete K56.52
incomplete K56.51
partial K56.51
periappendiceal, congenital Q43.3
peritoneal (adhesive) — *see* Adhesions, peritoneum
uterus N73.6
internal N85.6
vagina N89.5
Bandemia D72.825
Bandl's ring (contraction) , complicating delivery O62.4
Bangkok hemorrhagic fever A91
Bang's disease (brucella abortus) A23.1
Bankruptcy, anxiety concerning Z59.8
Bannister's disease T78.3
hereditary D84.1
Banti's disease or syndrome (with cirrhosis) (with portal hypertension) K76.6
Bar, median, prostate — *see* Enlargement, enlarged, prostate
Barcoo disease or rot — *see* Ulcer, skin
Barlow's disease E54
Barodontalgia T70.29
Baron Münchausen syndrome — *see* Disorder, factitious
Barosinusitis T70.1
Barotitis T70.0
Barotrauma T70.29
odontalgia T70.29
otitic T70.0
sinus T70.1
Barraquer (-Simons) disease or syndrome (progressive lipodystrophy) E88.1
Barré-Guillain disease or syndrome G61.0
Barrel chest M95.4
Barré-Liéou syndrome (posterior cervical sympathetic) M53.0
Barrett's
disease — *see* Barrett's, esophagus
esophagus K22.70
with dysplasia K22.719
high grade K22.711
low grade K22.710
without dysplasia K22.70
syndrome — *see* Barrett's, esophagus
ulcer K22.10
with bleeding K22.11
without bleeding K22.10
Bársony (-Polgár) (-Teschendorf) syndrome (corkscrew esophagus) K22.4
Barth syndrome E78.71
Bartholinitis (suppurating) N75.8
gonococcal (acute) (chronic) (with abscess) A54.1
Bartonellosis A44.9
cutaneous A44.1
mucocutaneous A44.1
specified NEC A44.8
systemic A44.0
Barton's fracture S52.56-
Bartter's syndrome E26.81
Basal — *see* condition
Basan's (hidrotic) ectodermal dysplasia Q82.4
Baseball finger — *see* Dislocation, finger
Basedow's disease (exophthalmic goiter) — *see* Hyperthyroidism, with, goiter
Basic — *see* condition
Basilar — *see* condition
Bason's (hidrotic) ectodermal dysplasia Q82.4

Basopenia — *see* Agranulocytosis
Basophilia D72.824
Basophilism (cortico-adrenal) (Cushing's) (pituitary) E24.0
Bassen-Kornzweig disease or syndrome E78.6
Bat ear Q17.5
Bateman's
disease B08.1
purpura (senile) D69.2
Bathing cramp T75.1
Bathophobia F40.248
Batten (-Mayou) disease E75.4
retina E75.4 *[H36]*
Batten-Steinert syndrome G71.11
Battered — *see* Maltreatment
Battey Mycobacterium infection A31.0
Battle exhaustion F43.0
Battledore placenta O43.19-
Baumgarten-Cruveilhier cirrhosis, disease or syndrome K74.69
Bauxite fibrosis (of lung) J63.1
Bayle's disease (general paresis) A52.17
Bazin's disease (primary) (tuberculous) A18.4
Beach ear — *see* Swimmer's, ear
Beaded hair (congenital) Q84.1
Béal conjunctivitis or syndrome B30.2
Beard's disease (neurasthenia) F48.8
Beat (s)
atrial, premature I49.1
ectopic I49.49
elbow — *see* Bursitis, elbow
escaped, heart I49.49
hand — *see* Bursitis, hand
knee — *see* Bursitis, knee
premature I49.40
atrial I49.1
auricular I49.1
supraventricular I49.1
Beau's
disease or syndrome — *see* Degeneration, myocardial
lines (transverse furrows on fingernails) L60.4
Bechterev's syndrome — *see* Spondylitis, ankylosing
Becker's
cardiomyopathy I42.8
disease
idiopathic mural endomyocardial disease I42.3
myotonia congenita, recessive form G71.12
dystrophy G71.01
pigmented hairy nevus D22.5
Beck's syndrome (anterior spinal artery occlusion) I65.8
Beckwith-Wiedemann syndrome Q87.3
Bed confinement status Z74.01
Bed sore — *see* Ulcer, pressure, by site
Bedbug bite (s) — *see* Bite(s), by site, superficial, insect
Bedclothes, asphyxiation or suffocation by — *see* Asphyxia, traumatic, due to, mechanical, trapped
Bednar's
aphthae K12.0
tumor — *see* Neoplasm, malignant, by site
Bedridden Z74.01
Bedsore — *see* Ulcer, pressure, by site
Bedwetting — *see* Enuresis
Bee sting (with allergic or anaphylactic shock) — *see* Toxicity, venom, arthropod, bee
Beer drinker's heart (disease) I42.6
Begbie's disease (exophthalmic goiter) — *see* Hyperthyroidism, with, goiter
Behavior
antisocial
adult Z72.811
child or adolescent Z72.810
disorder, disturbance — *see* Disorder, conduct
disruptive — *see* Disorder, conduct

Behavior - *continued*
  drug seeking Z76.5
  inexplicable R46.2
  marked evasiveness R46.5
  obsessive-compulsive R46.81
  overactivity R46.3
  poor responsiveness R46.4
  self-damaging (life-style) Z72.89
  sleep-incompatible Z72.821
  slowness R46.4
  specified NEC R46.89
  strange (and inexplicable) R46.2
  suspiciousness R46.5
  type A pattern Z73.1
  undue concern or preoccupation with
    stressful events R46.6
  verbosity and circumstantial detail obscuring
    reason for contact R46.7
Behçet's disease or syndrome M35.2
Behr's disease — *see* Degeneration, macula
**Beigel's disease or morbus (white
  piedra)** B36.2
Bejel A65
Bekhterev's syndrome — *see* Spondylitis,
  ankylosing
Belching — *see* Eructation
Bell's
  mania F30.8
  palsy, paralysis G51.0
    infant or newborn P11.3
  spasm G51.3-
**Bence Jones albuminuria or proteinuria
  NEC** R80.3
Bends T70.3
Benedikt's paralysis or syndrome G46.3
Benign — *see also* condition
  prostatic hyperplasia — *see* Hyperplasia,
    prostate
Bennett's fracture (displaced) S62.21-
Benson's disease — *see* Deposit, crystalline
Bent
  back (hysterical) F44.4
  nose M95.0
    congenital Q67.4
Bereavement (uncomplicated) Z63.4
Bergeron's disease (hysterical chorea) F44.4
Berger's disease — *see* Nephropathy, IgA
Beriberi (dry) E51.11
  heart (disease) E51.12
  polyneuropathy E51.11
  wet E51.12
    involving circulatory system E51.11
**Berlin's disease or edema
  (traumatic)** S05.8X-
Berlock (berloque) dermatitis L56.2
Bernard-Horner syndrome G90.2
**Bernard-Soulier disease or
  thrombopathia** D69.1
Bernhardt (-Roth) disease — *see*
  Mononeuropathy, lower limb, meralgia
  paresthetica
Bernheim's syndrome — *see* Failure, heart,
  right
Bertielliasis B71.8
Berylliosis (lung) J63.2
Besnier-Boeck (-Schaumann) disease — *see*
  Sarcoidosis
Besnier's
  lupus pernio D86.3
  prurigo L20.0
Bestiality F65.89
Best's disease H35.50
Betalipoproteinemia, broad or floating E78.2
**Beta-mercaptolactate-cysteine
  disulfiduria** E72.09
Betting and gambling Z72.6
  pathological (compulsive) F63.0
Bezoar T18.9
  intestine T18.3
  stomach T18.2
Bezold's abscess — *see* Mastoiditis, acute
Bianchi's syndrome R48.8
Bicornate or bicornis uterus Q51.3
  in pregnancy or childbirth O34.00
    causing obstructed labor O65.5

Bicuspid aortic valve Q23.1
Biedl-Bardet syndrome Q87.89
Bielschowsky (-Jansky) disease E75.4
**Biermer's (pernicious) anemia or
  disease** D51.0
Biett's disease L93.0
Bifid (congenital)
  apex, heart Q24.8
  clitoris Q52.6
  kidney Q63.8
  nose Q30.2
  patella Q74.1
  scrotum Q55.29
  toe NEC Q74.2
  tongue Q38.3
  ureter Q62.8
  uterus Q51.3
  uvula Q35.7
Biforis uterus (suprasimplex) Q51.3
Bifurcation (congenital)
  gallbladder Q44.1
  kidney pelvis Q63.8
  renal pelvis Q63.8
  rib Q76.6
  tongue, congenital Q38.3
  trachea Q32.1
  ureter Q62.8
  urethra Q64.74
  vertebra Q76.49
Big spleen syndrome D73.1
Bigeminal pulse R00.8
Bilateral — *see* condition
Bile
  duct — *see* condition
  pigments in urine R82.2
Bilharziasis — *see also* Schistosomiasis
  chyluria B65.0
  cutaneous B65.3
  galacturia B65.0
  hematochyluria B65.0
  intestinal B65.1
  lipemia B65.9
  lipuria B65.0
  oriental B65.2
  piarhemia B65.9
  pulmonary NOS B65.9 *[J99]*
    pneumonia B65.9 *[J17]*
  tropical hematuria B65.0
  vesical B65.0
Biliary — *see* condition
Bilirubin metabolism disorder E80.7
  specified NEC E80.6
Bilirubinemia, familial nonhemolytic E80.4
Bilirubinuria R82.2
Biliuria R82.2
Bilocular stomach K31.2
Binswanger's disease I67.3
Biparta, bipartite
  carpal scaphoid Q74.0
  patella Q74.1
  vagina Q52.10
Bird
  face Q75.8
  fancier's disease or lung J67.2
Birth
  complications in mother — *see* Delivery,
    complicated
  compression during NOS P15.9
  defect — *see* Anomaly
  immature (less than 37 completed weeks) —
    see Preterm, newborn
    extremely (less than 28 completed
      weeks) — *see* Immaturity, extreme
  inattention, at or after — *see* Maltreatment,
    child, neglect
  injury NOS P15.9
    basal ganglia P11.1
    brachial plexus NEC P14.3
    brain (compression) (pressure) P11.2
    central nervous system NOS P11.9
    cerebellum P11.1
    cerebral hemorrhage P10.1
    external genitalia P15.5
    eye P15.3
    face P15.4

Birth - *continued*
  injury NOS - *continued*
    fracture
      bone P13.9
        specified NEC P13.8
      clavicle P13.4
      femur P13.2
      humerus P13.3
      long bone, except femur P13.3
      radius and ulna P13.3
      skull P13.0
      spine P11.5
      tibia and fibula P13.3
    intracranial P11.2
    laceration or hemorrhage P10.9
      specified NEC P10.8
    intraventricular hemorrhage P10.2
    laceration
      brain P10.1
      by scalpel P15.8
      peripheral nerve P14.9
    liver P15.0
    meninges
      brain P11.1
      spinal cord P11.5
    nerve
      brachial plexus P14.3
      cranial NEC (except facial) P11.4
      facial P11.3
      peripheral P14.9
      phrenic (paralysis) P14.2
    paralysis
      facial nerve P11.3
      spinal P11.5
    penis P15.5
    rupture
      spinal cord P11.5
    scalp P12.9
    scalpel wound P15.8
    scrotum P15.5
    skull NEC P13.1
      fracture P13.0
    specified type NEC P15.8
    spinal cord P11.5
    spine P11.5
    spleen P15.1
    sternomastoid (hematoma) P15.2
    subarachnoid hemorrhage P10.3
    subcutaneous fat necrosis P15.6
    subdural hemorrhage P10.0
    tentorial tear P10.4
    testes P15.5
    vulva P15.5
  lack of care, at or after — *see* Maltreatment,
    child, neglect
  neglect, at or after — *see* Maltreatment,
    child, neglect
  palsy or paralysis, newborn, NOS (birth
    injury) P14.9
  premature (infant) — *see* Preterm, newborn
  shock, newborn P96.89
  trauma — *see* Birth, injury
  weight
    low (2499 grams or less) — *see* Low,
      birthweight
    extremely (999 grams or less) — *see*
      Low, birthweight, extreme
    4000 grams to 4499 grams P08.1
    4500 grams or more P08.0
Birthmark Q82.5
Birt-Hogg-Dube syndrome Q87.89
Bisalbuminemia E88.09
Biskra's button B55.1
Bite (s) (animal) (human)
  abdomen, abdominal
    wall S31.159
      with penetration into peritoneal
        cavity S31.659
      epigastric region S31.152
        with penetration into peritoneal
          cavity S31.652
      left
        lower quadrant S31.154
          with penetration into peritoneal
            cavity S31.654

Bite (s) (animal) (human) - *continued*
abdomen, abdominal - *continued*
  wall - *continued*
    left - *continued*
      upper quadrant S31.151
        with penetration into peritoneal
          cavity S31.651
      periumbilic region S31.155
        with penetration into peritoneal
          cavity S31.655
    right
      lower quadrant S31.153
        with penetration into peritoneal
          cavity S31.653
      upper quadrant S31.150
        with penetration into peritoneal
          cavity S31.650
    superficial NEC S30.871
      insect S30.861
alveolar (process) — *see* Bite, oral cavity
amphibian (venomous) — *see* Venom, bite, amphibian
animal — *see also* Bite, by site
  venomous — *see* Venom
ankle S91.05-
  superficial NEC S90.57-
    insect S90.56-
antecubital space — *see* Bite, elbow
anus S31.835
  superficial NEC S30.877
    insect S30.867
arm (upper) S41.15-
  lower — *see* Bite, forearm
  superficial NEC S40.87-
    insect S40.86-
arthropod NEC — *see* Venom, bite, arthropod
auditory canal (external) (meatus) — *see* Bite, ear
auricle, ear — *see* Bite, ear
axilla — *see* Bite, arm
back — *see also* Bite, thorax, back
  lower S31.050
    with penetration into retroperitoneal
      space S31.051
    superficial NEC S30.870
      insect S30.860
bedbug — *see* Bite(s), by site, superficial, insect
breast S21.05-
  superficial NEC S20.17-
    insect S20.16-
brow — *see* Bite, head, specified site NEC
buttock S31.805
  left S31.825
  right S31.815
  superficial NEC S30.870
    insect S30.860
calf — *see* Bite, leg
canaliculus lacrimalis — *see* Bite, eyelid
canthus, eye — *see* Bite, eyelid
centipede — *see* Toxicity, venom, arthropod, centipede
cheek (external) S01.45-
  superficial NEC S00.87
    insect S00.86
  internal — *see* Bite, oral cavity
chest wall — *see* Bite, thorax
chigger B88.0
chin — *see* Bite, head, specified site NEC
clitoris — *see* Bite, vulva
costal region — *see* Bite, thorax
digit (s)
  hand — *see* Bite, finger
  toe — *see* Bite, toe
ear (canal) (external) S01.35-
  superficial NEC S00.47-
    insect S00.46-
elbow S51.05-
  superficial NEC S50.37-
    insect S50.36-
epididymis — *see* Bite, testis
epigastric region — *see* Bite, abdomen
epiglottis — *see* Bite, neck, specified site NEC

Bite (s) (animal) (human) - *continued*
esophagus, cervical S11.25
  superficial NEC S10.17
    insect S10.16
eyebrow — *see* Bite, eyelid
eyelid S01.15-
  superficial NEC S00.27-
    insect S00.26-
face NEC — *see* Bite, head, specified site NEC
finger (s) S61.259
  with
    damage to nail S61.359
  index S61.258
    with
      damage to nail S61.358
    left S61.251
      with
        damage to nail S61.351
    right S61.250
      with
        damage to nail S61.350
    superficial NEC S60.478
      insect S60.46-
  little S61.25-
    with
      damage to nail S61.35-
    superficial NEC S60.47-
      insect S60.46-
  middle S61.25-
    with
      damage to nail S61.35-
    superficial NEC S60.47-
      insect S60.46-
  ring S61.25-
    with
      damage to nail S61.35-
    superficial NEC S60.47-
      insect S60.46-
  superficial NEC S60.479
    insect S60.469
  thumb — *see* Bite, thumb
flank — *see* Bite, abdomen, wall
flea — *see* Bite, by site, superficial, insect
foot (except toe (s) alone) S91.35-
  superficial NEC S90.87-
    insect S90.86-
  toe — *see* Bite, toe
forearm S51.85-
  elbow only — *see* Bite, elbow
  superficial NEC S50.87-
    insect S50.86-
forehead — *see* Bite, head, specified site NEC
genital organs, external
  female S31.552
    superficial NEC S30.876
      insect S30.866
    vagina and vulva — *see* Bite, vulva
  male S31.551
    penis — *see* Bite, penis
    scrotum — *see* Bite, scrotum
    superficial NEC S30.875
      insect S30.865
    testes — *see* Bite, testis
groin — *see* Bite, abdomen, wall
gum — *see* Bite, oral cavity
hand S61.45-
  finger — *see* Bite, finger
  superficial NEC S60.57-
    insect S60.56-
  thumb — *see* Bite, thumb
head S01.95
  cheek — *see* Bite, cheek
  ear — *see* Bite, ear
  eyelid — *see* Bite, eyelid
  lip — *see* Bite, lip
  nose — *see* Bite, nose
  oral cavity — *see* Bite, oral cavity
  scalp — *see* Bite, scalp
  specified site NEC S01.85
    superficial NEC S00.87
      insect S00.86
  superficial NEC S00.97
    insect S00.96

Bite (s) (animal) (human) - *continued*
head - *continued*
  temporomandibular area — *see* Bite, cheek
heel — *see* Bite, foot
hip S71.05-
  superficial NEC S70.27-
    insect S70.26-
hymen S31.45
hypochondrium — *see* Bite, abdomen, wall
hypogastric region — *see* Bite, abdomen, wall
inguinal region — *see* Bite, abdomen, wall
insect — *see* Bite, by site, superficial, insect
instep — *see* Bite, foot
interscapular region — *see* Bite, thorax, back
jaw — *see* Bite, head, specified site NEC
knee S81.05-
  superficial NEC S80.27-
    insect S80.26-
labium (majus) (minus) — *see* Bite, vulva
lacrimal duct — *see* Bite, eyelid
larynx S11.015
  superficial NEC S10.17
    insect S10.16
leg (lower) S81.85-
  ankle — *see* Bite, ankle
  foot — *see* Bite, foot
  knee — *see* Bite, knee
  superficial NEC S80.87-
    insect S80.86-
  toe — *see* Bite, toe
  upper — *see* Bite, thigh
lip S01.551
  superficial NEC S00.571
    insect S00.561
lizard (venomous) — *see* Venom, bite, reptile
loin — *see* Bite, abdomen, wall
lower back — *see* Bite, back, lower
lumbar region — *see* Bite, back, lower
malar region — *see* Bite, head, specified site NEC
mammary — *see* Bite, breast
marine animals (venomous) — *see* Toxicity, venom, marine animal
mastoid region — *see* Bite, head, specified site NEC
mouth — *see* Bite, oral cavity
nail
  finger — *see* Bite, finger
  toe — *see* Bite, toe
nape — *see* Bite, neck, specified site NEC
nasal (septum) (sinus) — *see* Bite, nose
nasopharynx — *see* Bite, head, specified site NEC
neck S11.95
  involving
    cervical esophagus — *see* Bite, esophagus, cervical
    larynx — *see* Bite, larynx
    pharynx — *see* Bite, pharynx
    thyroid gland S11.15
    trachea — *see* Bite, trachea
  specified site NEC S11.85
    superficial NEC S10.87
      insect S10.86
  superficial NEC S10.97
    insect S10.96
  throat S11.85
    superficial NEC S10.17
      insect S10.16
nose (septum) (sinus) S01.25
  superficial NEC S00.37
    insect S00.36
occipital region — *see* Bite, scalp
oral cavity S01.552
  superficial NEC S00.572
    insect S00.562
orbital region — *see* Bite, eyelid
palate — *see* Bite, oral cavity
palm — *see* Bite, hand
parietal region — *see* Bite, scalp
pelvis S31.050
  with penetration into retroperitoneal
    space S31.051
  superficial NEC S30.870

Bite (s) (animal) (human) - *continued*
  pelvis - *continued*
    superficial NEC - *continued*
      insect S30.860
    penis S31.25
      superficial NEC S30.872
        insect S30.862
    perineum
      female — *see* Bite, vulva
      male — *see* Bite, pelvis
    periocular area (with or without lacrimal
      passages) — *see* Bite, eyelid
    phalanges
      finger — *see* Bite, finger
      toe — *see* Bite, toe
    pharynx S11.25
      superficial NEC S10.17
        insect S10.16
    pinna — *see* Bite, ear
    poisonous — *see* Venom
    popliteal space — *see* Bite, knee
    prepuce — *see* Bite, penis
    pubic region — *see* Bite, abdomen, wall
    rectovaginal septum — *see* Bite, vulva
    red bug B88.0
    reptile NEC — *see also* Venom, bite, reptile
      nonvenomous — *see* Bite, by site
      snake — *see* Venom, bite, snake
    sacral region — *see* Bite, back, lower
    sacroiliac region — *see* Bite, back, lower
    salivary gland — *see* Bite, oral cavity
    scalp S01.05
      superficial NEC S00.07
        insect S00.06
    scapular region — *see* Bite, shoulder
    scrotum S31.35
      superficial NEC S30.873
        insect S30.863
    sea-snake (venomous) — *see* Toxicity,
      venom, snake, sea snake
    shin — *see* Bite, leg
    shoulder S41.05-
      superficial NEC S40.27-
        insect S40.26-
    snake — *see also* Venom, bite, snake
      nonvenomous — *see* Bite, by site
    spermatic cord — *see* Bite, testis
    spider (venomous) — *see* Toxicity, venom,
      spider
      nonvenomous — *see* Bite, by site,
        superficial, insect
    sternal region — *see* Bite, thorax, front
    submaxillary region — *see* Bite, head,
      specified site NEC
    submental region — *see* Bite, head, specified
      site NEC
    subungual
      finger (s) — *see* Bite, finger
      toe — *see* Bite, toe
    superficial — *see* Bite, by site, superficial
    supraclavicular fossa S11.85
    supraorbital — *see* Bite, head, specified site
      NEC
    temple, temporal region — *see* Bite, head,
      specified site NEC
    temporomandibular area — *see* Bite, cheek
    testis S31.35
      superficial NEC S30.873
        insect S30.863
    thigh S71.15-
      superficial NEC S70.37-
        insect S70.36-
    thorax, thoracic (wall) S21.95
      back S21.25-
        with penetration into thoracic
          cavity S21.45-
      breast — *see* Bite, breast
      front S21.15-
        with penetration into thoracic
          cavity S21.35-
      superficial NEC S20.97
        back S20.47-
        front S20.37-
        insect S20.96
          back S20.46-

Bite (s) (animal) (human) - *continued*
  thorax, thoracic (wall) - *continued*
    superficial NEC - *continued*
      insect - *continued*
        front S20.36-
    throat — *see* Bite, neck, throat
    thumb S61.05-
      with
        damage to nail S61.15-
      superficial NEC S60.37-
        insect S60.36-
    thyroid S11.15
      superficial NEC S10.87
        insect S10.86
    toe (s) S91.15-
      with
        damage to nail S91.25-
      great S91.15-
        with
          damage to nail S91.25-
      lesser S91.15-
        with
          damage to nail S91.25-
      superficial NEC S90.47-
        great S90.47-
        insect S90.46-
          great S90.46-
    tongue S01.552
    trachea S11.025
      superficial NEC S10.17
        insect S10.16
    tunica vaginalis — *see* Bite, testis
    tympanum, tympanic membrane — *see* Bite,
      ear
    umbilical region S31.155
    uvula — *see* Bite, oral cavity
    vagina — *see* Bite, vulva
    venomous — *see* Venom
    vocal cords S11.035
      superficial NEC S10.17
        insect S10.16
    vulva S31.45
      superficial NEC S30.874
        insect S30.864
    wrist S61.55-
      superficial NEC S60.87-
        insect S60.86-
Biting, cheek or lip K13.1
Biventricular failure (heart) I50.82
Björck (-Thorson) syndrome (malignant
    carcinoid) E34.0
Black
  death A20.9
  eye S00.1-
  hairy tongue K14.3
  heel (foot) S90.3-
  lung (disease) J60
  palm (hand) S60.22-
Blackfan-Diamond anemia or syndrome
    (congenital hypoplastic anemia) D61.01
Blackhead L70.0
Blackout R55
Bladder — *see* condition
Blast (air) (hydraulic) (immersion)
    (underwater)
  blindness S05.8X-
  injury
    abdomen or thorax — *see* Injury, by site
    ear (acoustic nerve trauma) — *see* Injury,
      nerve, acoustic, specified type NEC
    syndrome NEC T70.8
Blastoma — *see* Neoplasm, malignant, by site
  pulmonary — *see* Neoplasm, lung, malignant
Blastomycosis, blastomycotic B40.9
  Brazilian — *see* Paracoccidioidomycosis
  cutaneous B40.3
  disseminated B40.7
  European — *see* Cryptococcosis
  generalized B40.7
  keloidal B48.0
  North American B40.9
  primary pulmonary B40.0
  pulmonary B40.2
    acute B40.0
    chronic B40.1

Blastomycosis, blastomycotic - *continued*
  skin B40.3
  South American — *see*
    Paracoccidioidomycosis
  specified NEC B40.89
Bleb (s) R23.8
  emphysematous (lung) (solitary) J43.9
  endophthalmitis H59.43
  filtering (vitreous) , after glaucoma
    surgery Z98.83
  inflammed (infected) ,
    postprocedural H59.40
    stage 1 H59.41
    stage 2 H59.42
    stage 3 H59.43
  lung (ruptured) J43.9
    congenital — *see* Atelectasis
    newborn P25.8
  subpleural (emphysematous) J43.9
Blebitis, postprocedural H59.40
  stage 1 H59.41
  stage 2 H59.42
  stage 3 H59.43
Bleeder (familial) (hereditary) — *see*
    Hemophilia
Bleeding — *see also* Hemorrhage
  anal K62.5
  anovulatory N97.0
  atonic, following delivery O72.1
  capillary I78.8
    puerperal O72.2
  contact (postcoital) N93.0
  due to uterine subinvolution N85.3
  ear — *see* Otorrhagia
  excessive, associated with menopausal
    onset N92.4
  familial — *see* Defect, coagulation
  following intercourse N93.0
  gastrointestinal K92.2
  hemorrhoids — *see* Hemorrhoids
  intermenstrual (regular) N92.3
    irregular N92.1
  intraoperative — *see* Complication,
    intraoperative, hemorrhage
  irregular N92.6
  menopausal N92.4
  newborn, intraventricular — *see* Newborn,
    affected by, hemorrhage,
    intraventricular
  nipple N64.59
  nose R04.0
  ovulation N92.3
  perimenopausal N92.4
  postclimacteric N95.0
  postcoital N93.0
  postmenopausal N95.0
  postoperative — *see* Complication,
    postprocedural, hemorrhage
  preclimacteric N92.4
  pre-pubertal vaginal N93.1
  puberty (excessive, with onset of menstrual
    periods) N92.2
  rectum, rectal K62.5
    newborn P54.3
  tendencies — *see* Defect, coagulation
  throat R04.1
  tooth socket (post-extraction) K91.840
  umbilical stump P51.9
  uterus, uterine NEC N93.9
    climacteric N92.4
    dysfunctional or functional N93.8
    menopausal N92.4
    preclimacteric or premenopausal N92.4
    unrelated to menstrual cycle N93.9
  vagina, vaginal (abnormal) N93.9
    dysfunctional or functional N93.8
    newborn P54.6
    pre-pubertal N93.1
  vicarious N94.89
Blennorrhagia, blennorrhagic — *see*
    Gonorrhea
Blennorrhea (acute) (chronic) — *see also*
    Gonorrhea
  inclusion (neonatal) (newborn) P39.1

Blennorrhea (acute) (chronic) - *continued*
lower genitourinary tract
(gonococcal) A54.00
neonatorum (gonococcal ophthalmia) A54.31
Blepharelosis — *see* Entropion
Blepharitis (angularis) (ciliaris) (eyelid)
(marginal) (nonulcerative) H01.009
herpes zoster B02.39
left H01.006
lower H01.005
upper H01.004
upper and lower H01.00B
right H01.003
lower H01.002
upper H01.001
upper and lower H01.00A
squamous H01.029
left H01.026
lower H01.025
upper H01.024
upper and lower H01.02B
right H01.023
lower H01.022
upper H01.021
upper and lower H01.02A
ulcerative H01.019
left H01.016
lower H01.015
upper H01.014
upper and lower H01.01B
right H01.013
lower H01.012
upper H01.011
upper and lower H01.01A
Blepharochalasis H02.30
congenital Q10.0
left H02.36
lower H02.35
upper H02.34
right H02.33
lower H02.32
upper H02.31
Blepharoclonus H02.59
Blepharoconjunctivitis H10.50-
angular H10.52-
contact H10.53-
ligneous H10.51-
Blepharophimosis (eyelid) H02.529
congenital Q10.3
left H02.526
lower H02.525
upper H02.524
right H02.523
lower H02.522
upper H02.521
Blepharoptosis H02.40-
congenital Q10.0
mechanical H02.41-
myogenic H02.42-
neurogenic H02.43-
paralytic H02.43-
Blepharopyorrhea, gonococcal A54.39
Blepharospasm G24.5
drug induced G24.01
Blighted ovum O02.0
Blind — *see also* Blindness
bronchus (congenital) Q32.4
loop syndrome K90.2
congenital Q43.8
sac, fallopian tube (congenital) Q50.6
spot, enlarged — *see* Defect, visual field,
localized, scotoma, blind spot area
tract or tube, congenital NEC — *see* Atresia,
by site
Blindness (acquired) (congenital) (both eyes)
H54.0X-
blast S05.8X-
color — *see* Deficiency, color vision
concussion S05.8X-
cortical H47.619
left brain H47.612
right brain H47.611
day H53.11
due to injury (current episode) S05.9-

Blindness (acquired) (congenital) (both eyes)
- *continued*
due to injury (current episode) - *continued*
sequelae -- code to injury with seventh
character S
eclipse (total) — *see* Retinopathy, solar
emotional (hysterical) F44.6
face H53.16
hysterical F44.6
legal (both eyes) (USA definition) H54.8
mind R48.8
night H53.60
abnormal dark adaptation curve H53.61
acquired H53.62
congenital H53.63
specified type NEC H53.69
vitamin A deficiency E50.5
one eye (other eye normal) H54.40
left (normal vision on right) H54.42-
low vision on right H54.12-
low vision, other eye H54.10
right (normal vision on left) H54.41-
low vision on left H54.11-
psychic R48.8
river B73.01
snow — *see* Photokeratitis
sun, solar — *see* Retinopathy, solar
transient — *see* Disturbance, vision,
subjective, loss, transient
traumatic (current episode) S05.9-
word (developmental) F81.0
acquired R48.0
secondary to organic lesion R48.0
Blister (nonthermal)
abdominal wall S30.821
alveolar process S00.522
ankle S90.52-
antecubital space — *see* Blister, elbow
anus S30.827
arm (upper) S40.82-
auditory canal — *see* Blister, ear
auricle — *see* Blister, ear
axilla — *see* Blister, arm
back, lower S30.820
beetle dermatitis L24.89
breast S20.12-
brow S00.82
calf — *see* Blister, leg
canthus — *see* Blister, eyelid
cheek S00.82
internal S00.522
chest wall — *see* Blister, thorax
chin S00.82
costal region — *see* Blister, thorax
digit (s)
foot — *see* Blister, toe
hand — *see* Blister, finger
due to burn — *see* Burn, by site, second
degree
ear S00.42-
elbow S50.32-
epiglottis S10.12
esophagus, cervical S10.12
eyebrow — *see* Blister, eyelid
eyelid S00.22-
face S00.82
fever B00.1
finger (s) S60.429
index S60.42-
little S60.42-
middle S60.42-
ring S60.42-
foot (except toe (s) alone) S90.82-
toe — *see* Blister, toe
forearm S50.82-
elbow only — *see* Blister, elbow
forehead S00.82
fracture - omit code
genital organ
female S30.826
male S30.825
gum S00.522
hand S60.52-
head S00.92
ear — *see* Blister, ear

Blister (nonthermal) - *continued*
head - *continued*
eyelid — *see* Blister, eyelid
lip S00.521
nose S00.32
oral cavity S00.522
scalp S00.02
specified site NEC S00.82
heel — *see* Blister, foot
hip S70.22-
interscapular region S20.429
jaw S00.82
knee S80.22-
larynx S10.12
leg (lower) S80.82-
knee — *see* Blister, knee
upper — *see* Blister, thigh
lip S00.521
malar region S00.82
mammary — *see* Blister, breast
mastoid region S00.82
mouth S00.522
multiple, skin, nontraumatic R23.8
nail
finger — *see* Blister, finger
toe — *see* Blister, toe
nasal S00.32
neck S10.92
specified site NEC S10.82
throat S10.12
nose S00.32
occipital region S00.02
oral cavity S00.522
orbital region — *see* Blister, eyelid
palate S00.522
palm — *see* Blister, hand
parietal region S00.02
pelvis S30.820
penis S30.822
periocular area — *see* Blister, eyelid
phalanges
finger — *see* Blister, finger
toe — *see* Blister, toe
pharynx S10.12
pinna — *see* Blister, ear
popliteal space — *see* Blister, knee
scalp S00.02
scapular region — *see* Blister, shoulder
scrotum S30.823
shin — *see* Blister, leg
shoulder S40.22-
sternal region S20.329
submaxillary region S00.82
submental region S00.82
subungual
finger (s) — *see* Blister, finger
toe (s) — *see* Blister, toe
supraclavicular fossa S10.82
supraorbital S00.82
temple S00.82
temporal region S00.82
testis S30.823
thermal — *see* Burn, second degree, by site
thigh S70.32-
thorax, thoracic (wall) S20.92
back S20.42-
front S20.32-
throat S10.12
thumb S60.32-
toe (s) S90.42-
great S90.42-
tongue S00.522
trachea S10.12
tympanum, tympanic membrane — *see*
Blister, ear
upper arm — *see* Blister, arm (upper)
uvula S00.522
vagina S30.824
vocal cords S10.12
vulva S30.824
wrist S60.82-
Bloating R14.0
Bloch-Sulzberger disease or syndrome Q82.3
Block, blocked
alveolocapillary J84.10

Block, blocked - *continued*
  arborization (heart) I45.5
  arrhythmic I45.9
  atrioventricular (incomplete) (partial) I44.30
    with atrioventricular dissociation I44.2
    complete I44.2
      congenital Q24.6
    congenital Q24.6
    first degree I44.0
    second degree (types I and II) I44.1
    specified NEC I44.39
    third degree I44.2
    types I and II I44.1
  auriculoventricular — *see* Block,
      atrioventricular
  bifascicular (cardiac) I45.2
  bundle-branch (complete) (false)
      (incomplete) I45.4
    bilateral I45.2
    left I44.7
      with right bundle branch block I45.2
      hemiblock I44.60
        anterior I44.4
        posterior I44.5
      incomplete I44.7
        with right bundle branch block I45.2
    right I45.10
      with
        left bundle branch block I45.2
        left fascicular block I45.2
      specified NEC I45.19
      Wilson's type I45.19
  cardiac I45.9
  conduction I45.9
    complete I44.2
  fascicular (left) I44.60
    anterior I44.4
    posterior I44.5
    right I45.0
    specified NEC I44.69
  foramen Magendie (acquired) G91.1
    congenital Q03.1
      with spina bifida — *see* Spina bifida, by
        site, with hydrocephalus
  heart I45.9
    bundle branch I45.4
      bilateral I45.2
    complete (atrioventricular) I44.2
    congenital Q24.6
    first degree (atrioventricular) I44.0
    second degree (atrioventricular) I44.1
    specified type NEC I45.5
    third degree (atrioventricular) I44.2
  hepatic vein I82.0
  intraventricular (nonspecific) I45.4
    bundle branch
      bilateral I45.2
  kidney N28.9
    postcystoscopic or postprocedural N99.0
  Mobitz (types I and II) I44.1
  myocardial — *see* Block, heart
  nodal I45.5
  organ or site, congenital NEC — *see* Atresia,
      by site
  portal (vein) I81
  second degree (types I and II) I44.1
  sinoatrial I45.5
  sinoauricular I45.5
  third degree I44.2
  trifascicular I45.3
  tubal N97.1
  vein NOS I82.90
  Wenckebach (types I and II) I44.1
Blockage — *see* Obstruction
Blocq's disease F44.4
Blood
  constituents, abnormal R78.9
  disease D75.9
  donor — *see* Donor, blood
  dyscrasia D75.9
    with
      abortion — *see* Abortion, by type,
        complicated by, hemorrhage
      ectopic pregnancy O08.1
      molar pregnancy O08.1

Blood - *continued*
  dyscrasia - *continued*
    following ectopic or molar
        pregnancy O08.1
    newborn P61.9
    puerperal, postpartum O72.3
  flukes NEC — *see* Schistosomiasis
  in
    feces K92.1
      occult R19.5
    urine — *see* Hematuria
  mole O02.0
  occult in feces R19.5
  pressure
    decreased, due to shock following
        injury T79.4
    examination only Z01.30
    fluctuating I99.8
    high — *see* Hypertension
      borderline R03.0
      incidental reading, without diagnosis of
          hypertension R03.0
    low — *see also* Hypotension
      incidental reading, without diagnosis of
          hypotension R03.1
  spitting — *see* Hemoptysis
  staining cornea — *see* Pigmentation, cornea,
      stromal
  transfusion
    reaction or complication — *see*
        Complications, transfusion
  type
    A (Rh positive) Z67.10
      Rh negative Z67.11
    AB (Rh positive) Z67.30
      Rh negative Z67.31
    B (Rh positive) Z67.20
      Rh negative Z67.21
    O (Rh positive) Z67.40
      Rh negative Z67.41
    Rh (positive) Z67.90
      negative Z67.91
  vessel rupture — *see* Hemorrhage
  vomiting — *see* Hematemesis
Blood-forming organs, disease D75.9
Bloodgood's disease — *see* Mastopathy, cystic
**Bloom (-Machacek) (-Torre)
  syndrome** Q82.8
Blount's disease or osteochondrosis — *see*
  Osteochondrosis, juvenile, tibia
Blue
  baby Q24.9
  diaper syndrome E72.09
  dome cyst (breast) — *see* Cyst, breast
  dot cataract Q12.0
  nevus D22.9
  sclera Q13.5
    with fragility of bone and deafness Q78.0
  toe syndrome I75.02-
Blueness — *see* Cyanosis
Blues, postpartal O90.6
  baby O90.6
Blurring, visual H53.8
Blushing (abnormal) (excessive) R23.2
BMI — *see* Body, mass index
Boarder, hospital NEC Z76.4
  accompanying sick person Z76.3
  healthy infant or child Z76.2
    foundling Z76.1
Bockhart's impetigo L01.02
**Bodechtel-Guttman disease (subacute
  sclerosing panencephalitis)** A81.1
**Boder-Sedgwick syndrome (ataxia-
  telangiectasia)** G11.3
Body, bodies
  Aschoff's — *see* Myocarditis, rheumatic
  asteroid, vitreous — *see* Deposit, crystalline
  cytoid (retina) — *see* Occlusion, artery,
      retina
  drusen (degenerative) (macula) (retinal) —
      see also Degeneration, macula, drusen
  optic disc — *see* Drusen, optic disc
  foreign — *see* Foreign body
  loose
    joint, except knee — *see* Loose, body, joint

Body, bodies - *continued*
  loose - *continued*
    joint, except knee - *continued*
      knee M23.4-
    sheath, tendon — *see* Disorder, tendon,
        specified type NEC
  mass index (BMI)
    adult
      19.9 or less Z68.1
      20.0-20.9 Z68.20
      21.0-21.9 Z68.21
      22.0-22.9 Z68.22
      23.0-23.9 Z68.23
      24.0-24.9 Z68.24
      25.0-25.9 Z68.25
      26.0-26.9 Z68.26
      27.0-27.9 Z68.27
      28.0-28.9 Z68.28
      29.0-29.9 Z68.29
      30.0-30.9 Z68.30
      31.0-31.9 Z68.31
      32.0-32.9 Z68.32
      33.0-33.9 Z68.33
      34.0-34.9 Z68.34
      35.0-35.9 Z68.35
      36.0-36.9 Z68.36
      37.0-37.9 Z68.37
      38.0-38.9 Z68.38
      39.0-39.9 Z68.39
      40.0-44.9 Z68.41
      45.0-49.9 Z68.42
      50.0-59.9 Z68.43
      60.0-69.9 Z68.44
      70 and over Z68.45
    pediatric
      5th percentile to less than 85th percentile
          for age Z68.52
      85th percentile to less than 95th
          percentile for age Z68.53
      greater than or equal to ninety-fifth
          percentile for age Z68.54
      less than fifth percentile for age Z68.51
  Mooser's A75.2
  rice — *see also* Loose, body, joint
    knee M23.4-
  rocking F98.4
Boeck's
  disease or sarcoid — *see* Sarcoidosis
  lupoid (miliary) D86.3
**Boerhaave's syndrome (spontaneous
  esophageal rupture)** K22.3
Boggy
  cervix N88.8
  uterus N85.8
Boil — *see also* Furuncle, by site
  Aleppo B55.1
  Baghdad B55.1
  Delhi B55.1
  lacrimal
    gland — *see* Dacryoadenitis
    passages (duct) (sac) — *see* Inflammation,
        lacrimal, passages, acute
  Natal B55.1
  orbit, orbital — *see* Abscess, orbit
  tropical B55.1
Bold hives — *see* Urticaria
Bombé, iris — *see* Membrane, pupillary
Bone — *see* condition
Bonnevie-Ullrich syndrome — *see
  also* Turner's syndrome Q87.19
Bonnier's syndrome — *see* subcategory H81.8
Bonvale dam fever T73.3
Bony block of joint — *see* Ankylosis
**BOOP (bronchiolitis obliterans organized
  pneumonia)** J84.89
Borderline
  diabetes mellitus R73.03
  hypertension R03.0
  osteopenia M85.8-
  pelvis, with obstruction during labor O65.1
  personality F60.3
Borna disease A83.9
Bornholm disease B33.0
Boston exanthem A88.0
Botalli, ductus (patent) (persistent) Q25.0

Bothriocephalus latus infestation B70.0
Botulism (foodborne intoxication) A05.1
  infant A48.51
  non-foodborne A48.52
  wound A48.52
Bouba — *see* Yaws
Bouchard's nodes (with arthropathy) M15.2
Bouffée délirante F23
Bouillaud's disease or syndrome (rheumatic heart disease) I01.9
Bourneville's disease Q85.1
Boutonniere deformity (finger) — *see* Deformity, finger, boutonniere
Bouveret (-Hoffmann) syndrome (paroxysmal tachycardia) I47.9
Bovine heart — *see* Hypertrophy, cardiac
Bowel — *see* condition
Bowen's
  dermatosis (precancerous) — *see* Neoplasm, skin, in situ
  disease — *see* Neoplasm, skin, in situ
  epithelioma — *see* Neoplasm, skin, in situ
  type
    epidermoid carcinoma-in-situ — *see* Neoplasm, skin, in situ
    intraepidermal squamous cell carcinoma — *see* Neoplasm, skin, in situ
Bowing
  femur — *see also* Deformity, limb, specified type NEC, thigh
    congenital Q68.3
  fibula — *see also* Deformity, limb, specified type NEC, lower leg
    congenital Q68.4
  forearm — *see* Deformity, limb, specified type NEC, forearm
  leg (s) , long bones, congenital Q68.5
  radius — *see* Deformity, limb, specified type NEC, forearm
  tibia — *see also* Deformity, limb, specified type NEC, lower leg
    congenital Q68.4
Bowleg (s) (acquired) M21.16-
  congenital Q68.5
  rachitic E64.3
Boyd's dysentery A03.2
Brachial — *see* condition
Brachycardia R00.1
Brachycephaly Q75.0
Bradley's disease A08.19
Bradyarrhythmia, cardiac I49.8
Bradycardia (sinoatrial) (sinus) (vagal) R00.1
  neonatal P29.12
  reflex G90.09
  tachycardia syndrome I49.5
Bradykinesia R25.8
Bradypnea R06.89
Bradytachycardia I49.5
Brailsford's disease or osteochondrosis — *see* Osteochondrosis, juvenile, radius
Brain — *see also* condition
  death G93.82
  syndrome — *see* Syndrome, brain
Branched-chain amino-acid disorder E71.2
Branchial — *see* condition
  cartilage, congenital Q18.2
Branchiogenic remnant (in neck) Q18.0
Brandt's syndrome (acrodermatitis enteropathica) E83.2
Brash (water) R12
Bravais-jacksonian epilepsy — *see* Epilepsy, localization-related, symptomatic, with simple partial seizures
Braxton Hicks contractions — *see* False, labor
Brazilian leishmaniasis B55.2
BRBPR K62.5
Break, retina (without detachment) H33.30-
  with retinal detachment — *see* Detachment, retina
  horseshoe tear H33.31-
  multiple H33.33-

Break, retina (without detachment) - *continued*
  round hole H33.32-
Breakdown
  device, graft or implant — *see also* Complications, by site and type, mechanical T85.618
    arterial graft NEC — *see* Complication, cardiovascular device, mechanical, vascular
    breast (implant) T85.41
    catheter NEC T85.618
      cystostomy T83.010
      Hopkins T83.018
      ileostomy T83.018
      dialysis (renal) T82.41
        intraperitoneal T85.611
      infusion NEC T82.514
        cranial T85.610
        epidural T85.610
        intrathecal T85.610
        spinal T85.610
        subarachnoid T85.610
        subdural T85.610
      nephrostomy T83.012
      urethral indwelling T83.011
      urinary NEC T83.018
      urostomy T83.018
    electronic (electrode) (pulse generator) (stimulator)
      bone T84.310
      cardiac T82.119
        electrode T82.110
        pulse generator T82.111
        specified type NEC T82.118
      nervous system — *see* Complication, prosthetic device, mechanical, electronic nervous system stimulator
      urinary — *see* Complication, genitourinary, device, urinary, mechanical
    fixation, internal (orthopedic) NEC — *see* Complication, fixation device, mechanical
    gastrointestinal — *see* Complications, prosthetic device, mechanical, gastrointestinal device
    genital NEC T83.418
      intrauterine contraceptive device T83.31
      penile prosthesis (cylinder) (implanted) (pump) (resevoir) T83.410
      testicular prosthesis T83.411
    heart NEC — *see* Complication, cardiovascular device, mechanical
    intrathecal infusion pump T85.615
    joint prosthesis — *see* Complications..., joint prosthesis, internal, mechanical, by site
    nervous system, specified device NEC T85.615
    ocular NEC — *see* Complications, prosthetic device, mechanical, ocular device
    orthopedic NEC — *see* Complication, orthopedic, device, mechanical
    specified NEC T85.618
    subcutaneous device pocket
      nervous system prosthetic device, implant, or graft T85.890
      other internal prosthetic device, implant, or graft T85.898
    sutures, permanent T85.612
      used in bone repair — *see* Complications, fixation device, internal (orthopedic), mechanical
    urinary NEC T83.118
      graft T83.21
      sphincter, implanted T83.111
      stent (ileal conduit) (nephroureteral) T83.113
      ureteral indwelling T83.112
    vascular NEC — *see* Complication, cardiovascular device, mechanical
    ventricular intracranial shunt T85.01

Breakdown - *continued*
  nervous F48.8
  perineum O90.1
  respirator J95.850
    specified NEC J95.859
  ventilator J95.850
    specified NEC J95.859
Breast — *see also* condition
  buds E30.1
    in newborn P96.89
  dense R92.2
  nodule — *see also* Lump, breast N63.0
Breath
  foul R19.6
  holder, child R06.89
  holding spell R06.89
  shortness R06.02
Breathing
  labored — *see* Hyperventilation
  mouth R06.5
    causing malocclusion M26.5
  periodic R06.3
    high altitude G47.32
Breathlessness R06.81
Breda's disease — *see* Yaws
Breech presentation (mother) O32.1
  causing obstructed labor O64.1
  footling O32.8
    causing obstructed labor O64.8
  incomplete O32.8
    causing obstructed labor O64.8
Breisky's disease N90.4
Brennemann's syndrome I88.0
Brenner
  tumor (benign) D27.9
    borderline malignancy D39.1-
    malignant C56
    proliferating D39.1-
Bretonneau's disease or angina A36.0
Breus' mole O02.0
Brevicollis Q76.49
Brickmakers' anemia B76.9 *[D63.8]*
Bridge, myocardial Q24.5
Bright red blood per rectum (BRBPR) K62.5
Bright's disease — *see also* Nephritis
  arteriosclerotic — *see* Hypertension, kidney
Brill (-Zinsser) disease (recrudescent typhus) A75.1
Brill-Symmers' disease C82.90
Brion-Kayser disease — *see* Fever, parathyroid
Briquet's disorder or syndrome F45.0
Brissaud's
  infantilism or dwarfism E23.0
  motor-verbal tic F95.2
Brittle
  bones disease Q78.0
  nails L60.3
    congenital Q84.6
Broad — *see also* condition
  beta disease E78.2
  ligament laceration syndrome N83.8
Broad- or floating -betalipoproteinemia E78.2
Brock's syndrome (atelectasis due to enlarged lymph nodes) J98.19
Brocq-Duhring disease (dermatitis herpetiformis) L13.0
Brodie's abscess or disease M86.8X-
Broken
  arches — *see also* Deformity, limb, flat foot
  arm (meaning upper limb) — *see* Fracture, arm
  back — *see* Fracture, vertebra
  bone — *see* Fracture
  implant or internal device — *see* Complications, by site and type, mechanical
  leg (meaning lower limb) — *see* Fracture, leg
  nose S02.2
  tooth, teeth — *see* Fracture, tooth
Bromhidrosis, bromidrosis L75.0
Bromidism, bromism G92
  due to

Bromidism, bromism - *continued*
  due to - *continued*
    correct substance properly
      administered — *see* Table of Drugs
      and Chemicals, by drug, adverse
      effect
    overdose or wrong substance given or
      taken — *see* Table of Drugs and
      Chemicals, by drug, poisoning
  chronic (dependence) F13.20
Bromidrosiphobia F40.298
Bronchi, bronchial — *see* condition
Bronchiectasis (cylindrical) (diffuse)
  (fusiform) (localized) (saccular) J47.9
  with
    acute
      bronchitis J47.0
      lower respiratory infection J47.0
    exacerbation (acute) J47.1
  congenital Q33.4
  tuberculous NEC — *see* Tuberculosis,
    pulmonary
Bronchiolectasis — *see* Bronchiectasis
Bronchiolitis (acute) (infective) (subacute)
  J21.9
  with
    bronchospasm or obstruction J21.9
    influenza, flu or grippe — *see* Influenza,
      with, respiratory manifestations NEC
  chemical (chronic) J68.4
    acute J68.0
  chronic (fibrosing) (obliterative) J44.9
  due to
    external agent — *see* Bronchitis, acute, due
      to
    human metapneumovirus J21.1
    respiratory syncytial virus (RSV) J21.0
    specified organism NEC J21.8
  fibrosa obliterans J44.9
  influenzal — *see* Influenza, with, respiratory
    manifestations NEC
  obliterans J42
    with organizing pneumonia
      (BOOP) J84.89
  obliterative (chronic) (subacute) J44.9
    due to fumes or vapors J68.4
    due to chemicals, gases, fumes or vapors
      (inhalation) J68.4
  respiratory, interstitial lung disease J84.115
Bronchitis (diffuse) (fibrinous) (hypostatic)
  (infective) (membranous) J40
  with
    influenza, flu or grippe — *see* Influenza,
      with, respiratory manifestations NEC
    obstruction (airway) (lung) J44.9
    tracheitis (15 years of age and above) J40
      acute or subacute J20.9
      chronic J42
      under 15 years of age J20.9
  acute or subacute (with bronchospasm or
    obstruction) J20.9
    with
      bronchiectasis J47.0
      chronic obstructive pulmonary
        disease J44.0
    chemical (due to gases, fumes or
      vapors) J68.0
    due to
      fumes or vapors J68.0
      Haemophilus influenzae J20.1
      Mycoplasma pneumoniae J20.0
      radiation J70.0
      specified organism NEC J20.8
      Streptococcus J20.2
      virus
        coxsackie J20.3
        echovirus J20.7
        parainfluenzae J20.4
        respiratory syncytial (RSV) J20.5
        rhinovirus J20.6
    viral NEC J20.8
  allergic (acute) J45.909
    with
      exacerbation (acute) J45.901
      status asthmaticus J45.902

Bronchitis (diffuse) (fibrinous) (hypostatic)
  (infective) (membranous) - *continued*
  arachidic T17.528
  aspiration (due to fumes or vapors) J68.0
  asthmatic J45.9
    chronic J44.9
      with
        acute lower respiratory infection J44.0
        exacerbation (acute) J44.1
  capillary — *see* Pneumonia, broncho
  caseous (tuberculous) A15.5
  Castellani's A69.8
  catarrhal (15 years of age and above) J40
    acute — *see* Bronchitis, acute
    chronic J41.0
    under 15 years of age J20.9
  chemical (acute) (subacute) J68.0
    chronic J68.4
    due to fumes or vapors J68.0
      chronic J68.4
  chronic J42
    with
      airways obstruction J44.9
      tracheitis (chronic) J42
    asthmatic (obstructive) J44.9
    catarrhal J41.0
    chemical (due to fumes or vapors) J68.4
    due to
      chemicals, gases, fumes or vapors
        (inhalation) J68.4
      radiation J70.1
      tobacco smoking J41.0
    emphysematous J44.9
    mucopurulent J41.1
    non-obstructive J41.0
    obliterans J44.9
    obstructive J44.9
    purulent J41.1
    simple J41.0
  croupous — *see* Bronchitis, acute
  due to gases, fumes or vapors
    (chemical) J68.0
  emphysematous (obstructive) J44.9
  exudative — *see* Bronchitis, acute
  fetid J41.1
  grippal — *see* Influenza, with, respiratory
    manifestations NEC
  in those under 15 years age — *see* Bronchitis,
    acute
    chronic — *see* Bronchitis, chronic
  influenzal — *see* Influenza, with, respiratory
    manifestations NEC
  mixed simple and mucopurulent J41.8
  moulder's J62.8
  mucopurulent (chronic) (recurrent) J41.1
    acute or subacute J20.9
    simple (mixed) J41.8
  obliterans (chronic) J44.9
  obstructive (chronic) (diffuse) J44.9
  pituitous J41.1
  pneumococcal, acute or subacute J20.2
  pseudomembranous, acute or subacute — *see*
    Bronchitis, acute
  purulent (chronic) (recurrent) J41.1
    acute or subacute — *see* Bronchitis, acute
  putrid J41.1
  senile (chronic) J42
  simple and mucopurulent (mixed) J41.8
  smokers' J41.0
  spirochetal NEC A69.8
  subacute — *see* Bronchitis, acute
  suppurative (chronic) J41.1
    acute or subacute — *see* Bronchitis, acute
  tuberculous A15.5
  under 15 years of age — *see* Bronchitis, acute
    chronic — *see* Bronchitis, chronic
  viral NEC, acute or subacute — *see also*
    Bronchitis, acute J20.8
Bronchoalveolitis J18.0
Bronchoaspergillosis B44.1
Bronchocele meaning goiter E04.0
Broncholithiasis J98.09
  tuberculous NEC A15.5
Bronchomalacia J98.09
  congenital Q32.2

Bronchomycosis NOS B49 *[J99]*
  candidal B37.1
Bronchopleuropneumonia — *see* Pneumonia,
  broncho
Bronchopneumonia — *see* Pneumonia,
  broncho
Bronchopneumonitis — *see* Pneumonia,
  broncho
Bronchopulmonary — *see* condition
Bronchopulmonitis — *see* Pneumonia,
  broncho
Bronchorrhagia (see Hemoptysis)
Bronchorrhea J98.09
  acute J20.9
  chronic (infective) (purulent) J42
Bronchospasm (acute) J98.01
  with
    bronchiolitis, acute J21.9
    bronchitis, acute (conditions in J20) — *see*
      Bronchitis, acute
  due to external agent — *see* condition,
    respiratory, acute, due to
  exercise induced J45.990
Bronchospirochetosis A69.8
  Castellani A69.8
Bronchostenosis J98.09
Bronchus — *see* condition
Brontophobia F40.220
Bronze baby syndrome P83.88
Brooke's tumor — *see* Neoplasm, skin, benign
Brown enamel of teeth (hereditary) K00.5
Brown's sheath syndrome H50.61-
Brown-Séquard disease, paralysis or
  syndrome G83.81
Bruce sepsis A23.0
Brucellosis (infection) A23.9
  abortus A23.1
  canis A23.3
  dermatitis A23.9
  melitensis A23.0
  mixed A23.8
  sepsis A23.9
    melitensis A23.0
    specified NEC A23.8
  suis A23.2
Bruck-de Lange disease Q87.19
Bruck's disease — *see* Deformity, limb
BRUE (brief resolved unexplained
  event) R68.13
Brugsch's syndrome Q82.8
Bruise (skin surface intact) — *see also*
  Contusion
  with
    open wound — *see* Wound, open
  internal organ — *see* Injury, by site
  newborn P54.5
  scalp, due to birth injury, newborn P12.3
  umbilical cord O69.5
Bruit (arterial) R09.89
  cardiac R01.1
Brush burn — *see* Abrasion, by site
Bruton's X-linked
  agammaglobulinemia D80.0
Bruxism
  psychogenic F45.8
  sleep related G47.63
Bubbly lung syndrome P27.0
Bubo I88.8
  blennorrhagic (gonococcal) A54.89
  chancroidal A57
  climatic A55
  due to Haemophilus ducreyi A57
  gonococcal A54.89
  indolent (nonspecific) I88.8
  inguinal (nonspecific) I88.8
    chancroidal A57
    climatic A55
    due to H. ducreyi A57
    infective I88.8
  scrofulous (tuberculous) A18.2
  soft chancre A57
  suppurating — *see* Lymphadenitis, acute
  syphilitic (primary) A51.0
    congenital A50.07
  tropical A55

Bubo - *continued*
virulent (chancroidal) A57
Bubonic plague A20.0
Bubonocele — *see* Hernia, inguinal
Buccal — *see* condition
Buchanan's disease or
osteochondrosis M91.0
Buchem's syndrome (hyperostosis
corticalis) M85.2
Bucket-handle fracture or tear (semilunar
cartilage) — *see* Tear, meniscus
Budd-Chiari syndrome (hepatic vein
thrombosis) I82.0
Budgerigar fancier's disease or lung J67.2
Buds
breast E30.1
in newborn P96.89
Buerger's disease (thromboangiitis
obliterans) I73.1
Bulbar — *see* condition
Bulbus cordis (left ventricle)
(persistent) Q21.8
Bulimia (nervosa) F50.2
atypical F50.9
normal weight F50.9
Bulky
stools R19.5
uterus N85.2
Bulla (e) R23.8
lung (emphysematous) (solitary) J43.9
newborn P25.8
Bullet wound — *see also* Wound, open
fracture - code as Fracture, by site
internal organ — *see* Injury, by site
Bundle
branch block (complete) (false)
(incomplete) — *see* Block, bundle-
branch
of His — *see* condition
Bunion M21.61-
tailor's M21.62-
Bunionette M21.62-
Buphthalmia, buphthalmos
(congenital) Q15.0
Burdwan fever B55.0
Bürger-Grütz disease or syndrome E78.3
Buried
penis (congenital) Q55.64
acquired N48.83
roots K08.3
Burke's syndrome K86.89
Burkitt
cell leukemia C91.0-
lymphoma (malignant) C83.7-
small noncleaved, diffuse C83.7-
spleen C83.77
undifferentiated C83.7-
tumor C83.7-
type
acute lymphoblastic leukemia C91.0-
undifferentiated C83.7-
Burn (electricity) (flame) (hot gas, liquid or
hot object) (radiation) (steam) (thermal)
T30.0
abdomen, abdominal (muscle) (wall) T21.02
first degree T21.12
second degree T21.22
third degree T21.32
above elbow T22.039
first degree T22.139
left T22.032
first degree T22.132
second degree T22.232
third degree T22.332
right T22.031
first degree T22.131
second degree T22.231
third degree T22.331
second degree T22.239
third degree T22.339
acid (caustic) (external) (internal) — *see*
Corrosion, by site
alimentary tract NEC T28.2
esophagus T28.1
mouth T28.0

Burn (electricity) (flame) (hot gas, liquid or
hot object) (radiation) (steam) (thermal) -
continued
alimentary tract NEC - *continued*
pharynx T28.0
alkaline (caustic) (external) (internal) — *see*
Corrosion, by site
ankle T25.019
first degree T25.119
left T25.012
first degree T25.112
second degree T25.212
third degree T25.312
multiple with foot — *see* Burn, lower,
limb, multiple, ankle and foot
right T25.011
first degree T25.111
second degree T25.211
third degree T25.311
second degree T25.219
third degree T25.319
anus — *see* Burn, buttock
arm (lower) (upper) — *see* Burn, upper, limb
axilla T22.049
first degree T22.149
left T22.042
first degree T22.142
second degree T22.242
third degree T22.342
right T22.041
first degree T22.141
second degree T22.241
third degree T22.341
second degree T22.249
third degree T22.349
back (lower) T21.04
first degree T21.14
second degree T21.24
third degree T21.34
upper T21.03
first degree T21.13
second degree T21.23
third degree T21.33
blisters - code as Burn, second degree, by site
breast (s) — *see* Burn, chest wall
buttock (s) T21.05
first degree T21.15
second degree T21.25
third degree T21.35
calf T24.039
first degree T24.139
left T24.032
first degree T24.132
second degree T24.232
third degree T24.332
right T24.031
first degree T24.131
second degree T24.231
third degree T24.331
second degree T24.239
third degree T24.339
canthus (eye) — *see* Burn, eyelid
caustic acid or alkaline — *see* Corrosion, by
site
cervix T28.3
cheek T20.06
first degree T20.16
second degree T20.26
third degree T20.36
chemical (acids) (alkalines) (caustics)
(external) (internal) — *see* Corrosion,
by site
chest wall T21.01
first degree T21.11
second degree T21.21
third degree T21.31
chin T20.03
first degree T20.13
second degree T20.23
third degree T20.33
colon T28.2
conjunctiva (and cornea) — *see* Burn, cornea
cornea (and conjunctiva) T26.1-
chemical — *see* Corrosion, cornea

Burn (electricity) (flame) (hot gas, liquid or
hot object) (radiation) (steam) (thermal) -
continued
corrosion (external) (internal) — *see*
Corrosion, by site
deep necrosis of underlying tissue - code as
Burn, third degree, by site
dorsum of hand T23.069
first degree T23.169
left T23.062
first degree T23.162
second degree T23.262
third degree T23.362
right T23.061
first degree T23.161
second degree T23.261
third degree T23.361
second degree T23.269
third degree T23.369
due to ingested chemical agent — *see*
Corrosion, by site
ear (auricle) (external) (canal) T20.01
first degree T20.11
second degree T20.21
third degree T20.31
elbow T22.029
first degree T22.129
left T22.022
first degree T22.122
second degree T22.222
third degree T22.322
right T22.021
first degree T22.121
second degree T22.221
third degree T22.321
second degree T22.229
third degree T22.329
epidermal loss - code as Burn, second
degree, by site
erythema, erythematous - code as Burn, first
degree, by site
esophagus T28.1
extent (percentage of body surface)
less than 10 percent T31.0
10-19 percent T31.10
with 0-9 percent third degree
burns T31.10
with 10-19 percent third degree
burns T31.11
20-29 percent T31.20
with 0-9 percent third degree
burns T31.20
with 10-19 percent third degree
burns T31.21
with 20-29 percent third degree
burns T31.22
30-39 percent T31.30
with 0-9 percent third degree
burns T31.30
with 10-19 percent third degree
burns T31.31
with 20-29 percent third degree
burns T31.32
with 30-39 percent third degree
burns T31.33
40-49 percent T31.40
with 0-9 percent third degree
burns T31.40
with 10-19 percent third degree
burns T31.41
with 20-29 percent third degree
burns T31.42
with 30-39 percent third degree
burns T31.43
with 40-49 percent third degree
burns T31.44
50-59 percent T31.50
with 0-9 percent third degree
burns T31.50
with 10-19 percent third degree
burns T31.51
with 20-29 percent third degree
burns T31.52
with 30-39 percent third degree
burns T31.53

Burn (electricity) (flame) (hot gas, liquid or hot object) (radiation) (steam) (thermal) - *continued*
- extent (percentage of body surface) - *continued*
  - 50-59 percent - *continued*
    - with 40-49 percent third degree burns T31.54
    - with 50-59 percent third degree burns T31.55
  - 60-69 percent T31.60
    - with 0-9 percent third degree burns T31.60
    - with 10-19 percent third degree burns T31.61
    - with 20-29 percent third degree burns T31.62
    - with 30-39 percent third degree burns T31.63
    - with 40-49 percent third degree burns T31.64
    - with 50-59 percent third degree burns T31.65
    - with 60-69 percent third degree burns T31.66
  - 70-79 percent T31.70
    - with 0-9 percent third degree burns T31.70
    - with 10-19 percent third degree burns T31.71
    - with 20-29 percent third degree burns T31.72
    - with 30-39 percent third degree burns T31.73
    - with 40-49 percent third degree burns T31.74
    - with 50-59 percent third degree burns T31.75
    - with 60-69 percent third degree burns T31.76
    - with 70-79 percent third degree burns T31.77
  - 80-89 percent T31.80
    - with 0-9 percent third degree burns T31.80
    - with 10-19 percent third degree burns T31.81
    - with 20-29 percent third degree burns T31.82
    - with 30-39 percent third degree burns T31.83
    - with 40-49 percent third degree burns T31.84
    - with 50-59 percent third degree burns T31.85
    - with 60-69 percent third degree burns T31.86
    - with 70-79 percent third degree burns T31.87
    - with 80-89 percent third degree burns T31.88
  - 90 percent or more T31.90
    - with 0-9 percent third degree burns T31.90
    - with 10-19 percent third degree burns T31.91
    - with 20-29 percent third degree burns T31.92
    - with 30-39 percent third degree burns T31.93
    - with 40-49 percent third degree burns T31.94
    - with 50-59 percent third degree burns T31.95
    - with 60-69 percent third degree burns T31.96
    - with 70-79 percent third degree burns T31.97
    - with 80-89 percent third degree burns T31.98
    - with 90 percent or more third degree burns T31.99
- extremity — *see* Burn, limb
- eye (s) and adnexa T26.4-

Burn (electricity) (flame) (hot gas, liquid or hot object) (radiation) (steam) (thermal) - *continued*
- eye (s) and adnexa - *continued*
  - with resulting rupture and destruction of eyeball T26.2-
  - conjunctival sac — *see* Burn, cornea
  - cornea — *see* Burn, cornea
  - lid — *see* Burn, eyelid
  - periocular area — *see* Burn, eyelid
  - specified site NEC T26.3-
- eyeball — *see* Burn, eye
- eyelid (s) T26.0-
  - chemical — *see* Corrosion, eyelid
- face — *see* Burn, head
- finger T23.029
  - first degree T23.129
  - left T23.022
    - first degree T23.122
    - second degree T23.222
    - third degree T23.322
  - multiple sites (without thumb) T23.039
    - with thumb T23.049
      - first degree T23.149
      - left T23.042
        - first degree T23.142
        - second degree T23.242
        - third degree T23.342
      - right T23.041
        - first degree T23.141
        - second degree T23.241
        - third degree T23.341
      - second degree T23.249
      - third degree T23.349
    - first degree T23.139
    - left T23.032
      - first degree T23.132
      - second degree T23.232
      - third degree T23.332
    - right T23.031
      - first degree T23.131
      - second degree T23.231
      - third degree T23.331
    - second degree T23.239
    - third degree T23.339
  - right T23.021
    - first degree T23.121
    - second degree T23.221
    - third degree T23.321
  - second degree T23.229
  - third degree T23.329
- flank — *see* Burn, abdominal wall
- foot T25.029
  - first degree T25.129
  - left T25.022
    - first degree T25.122
    - second degree T25.222
    - third degree T25.322
  - multiple with ankle — *see* Burn, lower, limb, multiple, ankle and foot
  - right T25.021
    - first degree T25.121
    - second degree T25.221
    - third degree T25.321
  - second degree T25.229
  - third degree T25.329
- forearm T22.019
  - first degree T22.119
  - left T22.012
    - first degree T22.112
    - second degree T22.212
    - third degree T22.312
  - right T22.011
    - first degree T22.111
    - second degree T22.211
    - third degree T22.311
  - second degree T22.219
  - third degree T22.319
- forehead T20.06
  - first degree T20.16
  - second degree T20.26
  - third degree T20.36
- fourth degree - code as Burn, third degree, by site
- friction — *see* Burn, by site

Burn (electricity) (flame) (hot gas, liquid or hot object) (radiation) (steam) (thermal) - *continued*
- from swallowing caustic or corrosive substance NEC — *see* Corrosion, by site
- full thickness skin loss - code as Burn, third degree, by site
- gastrointestinal tract NEC T28.2
  - from swallowing caustic or corrosive substance T28.7
- genital organs
  - external
    - female T21.07
      - first degree T21.17
      - second degree T21.27
      - third degree T21.37
    - male T21.06
      - first degree T21.16
      - second degree T21.26
      - third degree T21.36
  - internal T28.3
    - from caustic or corrosive substance T28.8
- groin — *see* Burn, abdominal wall
- hand (s) T23.009
  - back — *see* Burn, dorsum of hand
  - finger — *see* Burn, finger
  - first degree T23.109
  - left T23.002
    - first degree T23.102
    - second degree T23.202
    - third degree T23.302
  - multiple sites with wrist T23.099
    - first degree T23.199
    - left T23.092
      - first degree T23.192
      - second degree T23.292
      - third degree T23.392
    - right T23.091
      - first degree T23.191
      - second degree T23.291
      - third degree T23.391
    - second degree T23.299
    - third degree T23.399
  - palm — *see* Burn, palm
  - right T23.001
    - first degree T23.101
    - second degree T23.201
    - third degree T23.301
  - second degree T23.209
  - third degree T23.309
  - thumb — *see* Burn, thumb
- head (and face) (and neck) T20.00
  - cheek — *see* Burn, cheek
  - chin — *see* Burn, chin
  - ear — *see* Burn, ear
  - eye (s) only — *see* Burn, eye
  - first degree T20.10
  - forehead — *see* Burn, forehead
  - lip — *see* Burn, lip
  - multiple sites T20.09
    - first degree T20.19
    - second degree T20.29
    - third degree T20.39
  - neck — *see* Burn, neck
  - nose — *see* Burn, nose
  - scalp — *see* Burn, scalp
  - second degree T20.20
  - third degree T20.30
- hip (s) — *see* Burn, thigh
- inhalation — *see* Burn, respiratory tract
  - caustic or corrosive substance (fumes) — *see* Corrosion, respiratory tract
- internal organ (s) T28.40
  - alimentary tract T28.2
    - esophagus T28.1
  - eardrum T28.41
  - esophagus T28.1
  - from caustic or corrosive substance (swallowing) NEC — *see* Corrosion, by site
  - genitourinary T28.3
  - mouth T28.0
  - pharynx T28.0

Burn (electricity) (flame) (hot gas, liquid or hot object) (radiation) (steam) (thermal) - *continued*

    internal organ (s) - *continued*
        respiratory tract — *see* Burn, respiratory tract
        specified organ NEC T28.49
    interscapular region — *see* Burn, back, upper
    intestine (large) (small) T28.2
    knee T24.029
        first degree T24.129
        left T24.022
            first degree T24.122
            second degree T24.222
            third degree T24.322
        right T24.021
            first degree T24.121
            second degree T24.221
            third degree T24.321
        second degree T24.229
        third degree T24.329
    labium (majus) (minus) — *see* Burn, genital organs, external, female
    lacrimal apparatus, duct, gland or sac — *see* Burn, eye, specified site NEC
    larynx T27.0
        with lung T27.1
    leg (s) (lower) (upper) — *see* Burn, lower, limb
    lightning — *see* Burn, by site
    limb (s)
        lower (except ankle or foot alone) — *see* Burn, lower, limb
        upper — *see* Burn, upper limb
    lip (s) T20.02
        first degree T20.12
        second degree T20.22
        third degree T20.32
    lower
        back — *see* Burn, back
        limb T24.009
            ankle — *see* Burn, ankle
            calf — *see* Burn, calf
            first degree T24.109
            foot — *see* Burn, foot
            hip — *see* Burn, thigh
            knee — *see* Burn, knee
            left T24.002
                first degree T24.102
                second degree T24.202
                third degree T24.302
                multiple sites, except ankle and foot T24.099
                ankle and foot T25.099
                    first degree T25.199
                    left T25.092
                        first degree T25.192
                        second degree T25.292
                        third degree T25.392
                    right T25.091
                        first degree T25.191
                        second degree T25.291
                        third degree T25.391
                    second degree T25.299
                    third degree T25.399
                first degree T24.199
                left T24.092
                    first degree T24.192
                    second degree T24.292
                    third degree T24.392
                right T24.091
                    first degree T24.191
                    second degree T24.291
                    third degree T24.391
                second degree T24.299
                third degree T24.399
            right T24.001
                first degree T24.101
                second degree T24.201
                third degree T24.301
            second degree T24.209
            thigh — *see* Burn, thigh
            third degree T24.309
            toe — *see* Burn, toe
    lung (with larynx and trachea) T27.1

Burn (electricity) (flame) (hot gas, liquid or hot object) (radiation) (steam) (thermal) - *continued*

    mouth T28.0
    neck T20.07
        first degree T20.17
        second degree T20.27
        third degree T20.37
    nose (septum) T20.04
        first degree T20.14
        second degree T20.24
        third degree T20.34
    ocular adnexa — *see* Burn, eye
    orbit region — *see* Burn, eyelid
    palm T23.059
        first degree T23.159
        left T23.052
            first degree T23.152
            second degree T23.252
            third degree T23.352
        right T23.051
            first degree T23.151
            second degree T23.251
            third degree T23.351
        second degree T23.259
        third degree T23.359
    partial thickness - code as Burn, degree, by site
    pelvis — *see* Burn, trunk
    penis — *see* Burn, genital organs, external, male
    perineum
        female — *see* Burn, genital organs, external, female
        male — *see* Burn, genital organs, external, male
    periocular area — *see* Burn, eyelid
    pharynx T28.0
    rectum T28.2
    respiratory tract T27.3
        larynx — *see* Burn, larynx
        specified part NEC T27.2
        trachea — *see* Burn, trachea
    sac, lacrimal — *see* Burn, eye, specified site NEC
    scalp T20.05
        first degree T20.15
        second degree T20.25
        third degree T20.35
    scapular region T22.069
        first degree T22.169
        left T22.062
            first degree T22.162
            second degree T22.262
            third degree T22.362
        right T22.061
            first degree T22.161
            second degree T22.261
            third degree T22.361
        second degree T22.269
        third degree T22.369
    sclera — *see* Burn, eye, specified site NEC
    scrotum — *see* Burn, genital organs, external, male
    shoulder T22.059
        first degree T22.159
        left T22.052
            first degree T22.152
            second degree T22.252
            third degree T22.352
        right T22.051
            first degree T22.151
            second degree T22.251
            third degree T22.351
        second degree T22.259
        third degree T22.359
    stomach T28.2
    temple — *see* Burn, head
    testis — *see* Burn, genital organs, external, male
    thigh T24.019
        first degree T24.119
        left T24.012
            first degree T24.112
            second degree T24.212

Burn (electricity) (flame) (hot gas, liquid or hot object) (radiation) (steam) (thermal) - *continued*

    thigh - *continued*
        left - *continued*
            third degree T24.312
        right T24.011
            first degree T24.111
            second degree T24.211
            third degree T24.311
        second degree T24.219
        third degree T24.319
    thorax (external) — *see* Burn, trunk
    throat (meaning pharynx) T28.0
    thumb (s) T23.019
        first degree T23.119
        left T23.012
            first degree T23.112
            second degree T23.212
            third degree T23.312
        multiple sites with fingers T23.049
            first degree T23.149
            left T23.042
                first degree T23.142
                second degree T23.242
                third degree T23.342
            right T23.041
                first degree T23.141
                second degree T23.241
                third degree T23.341
            second degree T23.249
            third degree T23.349
        right T23.011
            first degree T23.111
            second degree T23.211
            third degree T23.311
        second degree T23.219
        third degree T23.319
    toe T25.039
        first degree T25.139
        left T25.032
            first degree T25.132
            second degree T25.232
            third degree T25.332
        right T25.031
            first degree T25.131
            second degree T25.231
            third degree T25.331
        second degree T25.239
        third degree T25.339
    tongue T28.0
    tonsil (s) T28.0
    trachea T27.0
        with lung T27.1
    trunk T21.00
        abdominal wall — *see* Burn, abdominal wall
        anus — *see* Burn, buttock
        axilla — *see* Burn, upper limb
        back — *see* Burn, back
        breast — *see* Burn, chest wall
        buttock — *see* Burn, buttock
        chest wall — *see* Burn, chest wall
        first degree T21.10
        flank — *see* Burn, abdominal wall
        genital
            female — *see* Burn, genital organs, external, female
            male — *see* Burn, genital organs, external, male
        groin — *see* Burn, abdominal wall
        interscapular region — *see* Burn, back, upper
        labia — *see* Burn, genital organs, external, female
        lower back — *see* Burn, back
        penis — *see* Burn, genital organs, external, male
        perineum
            female — *see* Burn, genital organs, external, female
            male — *see* Burn, genital organs, external, male
        scapula region — *see* Burn, scapular region

Burn (electricity) (flame) (hot gas, liquid or hot object) (radiation) (steam) (thermal) - *continued*
  trunk - *continued*
    scrotum — *see* Burn, genital organs, external, male
    second degree T21.20
    specified site NEC T21.09
      first degree T21.19
      second degree T21.29
      third degree T21.39
    testes — *see* Burn, genital organs, external, male
    third degree T21.30
    upper back — *see* Burn, back, upper
    vulva — *see* Burn, genital organs, external, female
  unspecified site with extent of body surface involved specified
    less than 10 percent T31.0
    10-19 percent (0-9 percent third degree) T31.10
      with 10-19 percent third degree T31.11
    20-29 percent (0-9 percent third degree) T31.20
      with
        10-19 percent third degree T31.21
        20-29 percent third degree T31.22
    30-39 percent (0-9 percent third degree) T31.30
      with
        10-19 percent third degree T31.31
        20-29 percent third degree T31.32
        30-39 percent third degree T31.33
    40-49 percent (0-9 percent third degree) T31.40
      with
        10-19 percent third degree T31.41
        20-29 percent third degree T31.42
        30-39 percent third degree T31.43
        40-49 percent third degree T31.44
    50-59 percent (0-9 percent third degree) T31.50
      with
        10-19 percent third degree T31.51
        20-29 percent third degree T31.52
        30-39 percent third degree T31.53
        40-49 percent third degree T31.54
        50-59 percent third degree T31.55
    60-69 percent (0-9 percent third degree) T31.60
      with
        10-19 percent third degree T31.61
        20-29 percent third degree T31.62
        30-39 percent third degree T31.63
        40-49 percent third degree T31.64
        50-59 percent third degree T31.65
        60-69 percent third degree T31.66
    70-79 percent (0-9 percent third degree) T31.70
      with
        10-19 percent third degree T31.71
        20-29 percent third degree T31.72
        30-39 percent third degree T31.73
        40-49 percent third degree T31.74
        50-59 percent third degree T31.75
        60-69 percent third degree T31.76
        70-79 percent third degree T31.77
    80-89 percent (0-9 percent third degree) T31.80
      with
        10-19 percent third degree T31.81
        20-29 percent third degree T31.82
        30-39 percent third degree T31.83
        40-49 percent third degree T31.84
        50-59 percent third degree T31.85
        60-69 percent third degree T31.86
        70-79 percent third degree T31.87
        80-89 percent third degree T31.88
    90 percent or more (0-9 percent third degree) T31.90
      with
        10-19 percent third degree T31.91
        20-29 percent third degree T31.92
        30-39 percent third degree T31.93

Burn (electricity) (flame) (hot gas, liquid or hot object) (radiation) (steam) (thermal) - *continued*
  unspecified site with extent of body surface involved specified - *continued*
    90 percent or more (0-9 percent third degree) - *continued*
      with - *continued*
        40-49 percent third degree T31.94
        50-59 percent third degree T31.95
        60-69 percent third degree T31.96
        70-79 percent third degree T31.97
        80-89 percent third degree T31.98
        90-99 percent third degree T31.99
  upper limb T22.00
    above elbow — *see* Burn, above elbow
    axilla — *see* Burn, axilla
    elbow — *see* Burn, elbow
    first degree T22.10
    forearm — *see* Burn, forearm
    hand — *see* Burn, hand
    interscapular region — *see* Burn, back, upper
    multiple sites T22.099
      first degree T22.199
      left T22.092
        first degree T22.192
        second degree T22.292
        third degree T22.392
      right T22.091
        first degree T22.191
        second degree T22.291
        third degree T22.391
      second degree T22.299
      third degree T22.399
    scapular region — *see* Burn, scapular region
    second degree T22.20
    shoulder — *see* Burn, shoulder
    third degree T22.30
    wrist — *see* Burn, wrist
  uterus T28.3
  vagina T28.3
  vulva — *see* Burn, genital organs, external, female
  wrist T23.079
    first degree T23.179
    left T23.072
      first degree T23.172
      second degree T23.272
      third degree T23.372
    multiple sites with hand T23.099
      first degree T23.199
      left T23.092
        first degree T23.192
        second degree T23.292
        third degree T23.392
      right T23.091
        first degree T23.191
        second degree T23.291
        third degree T23.391
      second degree T23.299
      third degree T23.399
    right T23.071
      first degree T23.171
      second degree T23.271
      third degree T23.371
    second degree T23.279
    third degree T23.379

Burnett's syndrome E83.52
Burning
  feet syndrome E53.9
  sensation R20.8
  tongue K14.6
Burn-out (state) Z73.0
Burns' disease or osteochondrosis — *see* Osteochondrosis, juvenile, ulna
Bursa — *see* condition
Bursitis M71.9
  Achilles — *see* Tendinitis, Achilles
  adhesive — *see* Bursitis, specified NEC
  ankle — *see* Enthesopathy, lower limb, ankle, specified type NEC
  calcaneal — *see* Enthesopathy, foot, specified type NEC

Bursitis - *continued*
  collateral ligament, tibial — *see* Bursitis, tibial collateral
  due to use, overuse, pressure — *see also* Disorder, soft tissue, due to use, specified type NEC
    specified NEC — *see* Disorder, soft tissue, due to use, specified NEC
  Duplay's M75.0
  elbow NEC M70.3-
    olecranon M70.2-
  finger — *see* Disorder, soft tissue, due to use, specified type NEC, hand
  foot — *see* Enthesopathy, foot, specified type NEC
  gonococcal A54.49
  gouty — *see* Gout
  hand M70.1-
  hip NEC M70.7-
    trochanteric M70.6-
  infective NEC M71.10
    abscess — *see* Abscess, bursa
    ankle M71.17-
    elbow M71.12-
    foot M71.17-
    hand M71.14-
    hip M71.15-
    knee M71.16-
    multiple sites M71.19
    shoulder M71.11-
    specified site NEC M71.18
    wrist M71.13-
  ischial — *see* Bursitis, hip
  knee NEC M70.5-
    prepatellar M70.4-
  occupational NEC — *see also* Disorder, soft tissue, due to, use
  olecranon — *see* Bursitis, elbow, olecranon
  pharyngeal J39.1
  popliteal — *see* Bursitis, knee
  prepatellar M70.4-
  radiohumeral M77.8
  rheumatoid M06.20
    ankle M06.27-
    elbow M06.22-
    foot joint M06.27-
    hand joint M06.24-
    hip M06.25-
    knee M06.26-
    multiple site M06.29
    shoulder M06.21-
    vertebra M06.28
    wrist M06.23-
  scapulohumeral — *see* Bursitis, shoulder
  semimembranous muscle (knee) — *see* Bursitis, knee
  shoulder M75.5-
    adhesive — *see* Capsulitis, adhesive
  specified NEC M71.50
    ankle M71.57-
    due to use, overuse or pressure — *see* Disorder, soft tissue, due to, use
    elbow M71.52-
    foot M71.57-
    hand M71.54-
    hip M71.55-
    knee M71.56-
    shoulder — *see* Bursitis, shoulder
    specified site NEC M71.58
    tibial collateral M76.4-
    wrist M71.53-
  subacromial — *see* Bursitis, shoulder
  subcoracoid — *see* Bursitis, shoulder
  subdeltoid — *see* Bursitis, shoulder
  syphilitic A52.78
  Thornwaldt, Tornwaldt J39.2
  tibial collateral M76.4-
  toe — *see* Enthesopathy, foot, specified type NEC
  trochanteric (area) — *see* Bursitis, hip, trochanteric
  wrist — *see* Bursitis, hand
Bursopathy M71.9
  specified type NEC M71.80
    ankle M71.87-

Bursopathy - *continued*
  specified type NEC - *continued*
    elbow M71.82-
    foot M71.87-
    hand M71.84-
    hip M71.85-
    knee M71.86-
    multiple sites M71.89
    shoulder M71.81-
    specified site NEC M71.88
    wrist M71.83-
Burst stitches or sutures (complication of surgery) T81.31
    external operation wound T81.31
    internal operation wound T81.32
Buruli ulcer A31.1
Bury's disease L95.1
Buschke's
    disease B45.3
    scleredema — *see* Sclerosis, systemic
Busse-Buschke disease B45.3
Buttock — *see* condition
Button
    Biskra B55.1
    Delhi B55.1
    oriental B55.1
Buttonhole deformity (finger) — *see* Deformity, finger, boutonniere
Bwamba fever A92.8
Byssinosis J66.0
Bywaters' syndrome T79.5

C

Cachexia R64
    cancerous R64
    cardiac — *see* Disease, heart
    dehydration E86.0
    due to malnutrition R64
    exophthalmic — *see* Hyperthyroidism
    heart — *see* Disease, heart
    hypophyseal E23.0
    hypopituitary E23.0
    lead — *see* Poisoning, lead
    malignant R64
    marsh — *see* Malaria
    nervous F48.8
    old age R54
    paludal — *see* Malaria
    pituitary E23.0
    renal N28.9
    saturnine — *see* Poisoning, lead
    senile R54
    Simmonds' E23.0
    splenica D73.0
    strumipriva E03.4
    tuberculous NEC — *see* Tuberculosis
CADASIL (cerebral autosomal dominant arteriopathy with subcortical infarcts and leukoencephalopathy) I67.850
Café, au lait spots L81.3
Caffeine-induced
    anxiety disorder F15.980
    sleep disorder F15.982
Caffey's syndrome Q78.8
Caisson disease T70.3
Cake kidney Q63.1
Caked breast (puerperal, postpartum) O92.79
Calabar swelling B74.3
Calcaneal spur — *see* Spur, bone, calcaneal
Calcaneo-apophysitis M92.8
Calcareous — *see* condition
Calcicosis J62.8
Calciferol (vitamin D) deficiency E55.9
    with rickets E55.0
Calcification
    adrenal (capsule) (gland) E27.49
      tuberculous E35 *[B90.8]*
    aorta I70.0
    artery (annular) — *see* Arteriosclerosis
    auricle (ear) — *see* Disorder, pinna, specified type NEC
    basal ganglia G23.8
    bladder N32.89
      due to Schistosoma hematobium B65.0
    brain (cortex) — *see* Calcification, cerebral

Calcification - *continued*
    bronchus J98.09
    bursa M71.40
      ankle M71.47-
      elbow M71.42-
      foot M71.47-
      hand M71.44-
      hip M71.45-
      knee M71.46-
      multiple sites M71.49
      shoulder M75.3-
      specified site NEC M71.48
      wrist M71.43-
    cardiac — *see* Degeneration, myocardial
    cerebral (cortex) G93.89
      artery I67.2
    cervix (uteri) N88.8
    choroid plexus G93.89
    conjunctiva — *see* Concretion, conjunctiva
    corpora cavernosa (penis) N48.89
    cortex (brain) — *see* Calcification, cerebral
    dental pulp (nodular) K04.2
    dentinal papilla K00.4
    fallopian tube N83.8
    falx cerebri G96.19
    gallbladder K82.8
    general E83.59
    heart — *see also* Degeneration, myocardial
      valve — *see* Endocarditis
    idiopathic infantile arterial (IIAC) Q28.8
    intervertebral cartilage or disc (postinfective) — *see* Disorder, disc, specified NEC
    intracranial — *see* Calcification, cerebral
    joint — *see* Disorder, joint, specified type NEC
    kidney N28.89
      tuberculous N29 *[B90.1]*
    larynx (senile) J38.7
    lens — *see* Cataract, specified NEC
    lung (active) (postinfectional) J98.4
      tuberculous B90.9
    lymph gland or node (postinfectional) I89.8
      tuberculous — *see also* Tuberculosis, lymph gland B90.8
    mammographic R92.1
    massive (paraplegic) — *see* Myositis, ossificans, in, quadriplegia
    medial — *see* Arteriosclerosis, extremities
    meninges (cerebral) (spinal) G96.19
    metastatic E83.59
    Mönckeberg's — *see* Arteriosclerosis, extremities
    muscle M61.9
      due to burns — *see* Myositis, ossificans, in, burns
      paralytic — *see* Myositis, ossificans, in, quadriplegia
      specified type NEC M61.40
        ankle M61.47-
        foot M61.47-
        forearm M61.43-
        hand M61.44-
        lower leg M61.46-
        multiple sites M61.49
        pelvic region M61.45-
        shoulder region M61.41-
        specified site NEC M61.48
        thigh M61.45-
        upper arm M61.42-
    myocardium, myocardial — *see* Degeneration, myocardial
    ovary N83.8
    pancreas K86.89
    penis N48.89
    periarticular — *see* Disorder, joint, specified type NEC
    pericardium — *see also* Pericarditis I31.1
    pineal gland E34.8
    pleura J94.8
      postinfectional J94.8
      tuberculous NEC B90.9
    pulpal (dental) (nodular) K04.2
    sclera H15.89
    spleen D73.89

Calcification - *continued*
    subcutaneous L94.2
    suprarenal (capsule) (gland) E27.49
    tendon (sheath) — *see also* Tenosynovitis, specified type NEC
      with bursitis, synovitis or tenosynovitis — *see* Tendinitis, calcific
    trachea J39.8
    ureter N28.89
    uterus N85.8
    vitreous — *see* Deposit, crystalline
Calcified — *see* Calcification
Calcinosis (interstitial) (tumoral) (universalis) E83.59
    with Raynaud's phenomenon, esophageal dysfunction, sclerodactyly, telangiectasia (CREST syndrome) M34.1
    circumscripta (skin) L94.2
    cutis L94.2
Calciphylaxis — *see also* Calcification, by site E83.59
Calcium
    deposits — *see* Calcification, by site
    metabolism disorder E83.50
    salts or soaps in vitreous — *see* Deposit, crystalline
Calciuria R82.994
Calculi — *see* Calculus
Calculosis, intrahepatic — *see* Calculus, bile duct
Calculus, calculi, calculous
    ampulla of Vater — *see* Calculus, bile duct
    anuria (impacted) (recurrent) — *see also* Calculus, urinary N20.9
    appendix K38.1
    bile duct (common) (hepatic) K80.50
      with
        calculus of gallbladder — *see* Calculus, gallbladder and bile duct
        cholangitis K80.30
          with
            cholecystitis — *see* Calculus, bile duct, with cholecystitis
            obstruction K80.31
          acute K80.32
            with
              chronic cholangitis K80.36
                with obstruction K80.37
              obstruction K80.33
          chronic K80.34
            with
              acute cholangitis K80.36
                with obstruction K80.37
              obstruction K80.35
        cholecystitis (with cholangitis) K80.40
          with obstruction K80.41
          acute K80.42
            with
              chronic cholecystitis K80.46
                with obstruction K80.47
              obstruction K80.43
          chronic K80.44
            with
              acute cholecystitis K80.46
                with obstruction K80.47
              obstruction K80.45
        obstruction K80.51
    biliary — *see also* Calculus, gallbladder
      specified NEC K80.80
        with obstruction K80.81
    bilirubin, multiple — *see* Calculus, gallbladder
    bladder (encysted) (impacted) (urinary) (diverticulum) N21.0
    bronchus J98.09
    calyx (kidney) (renal) — *see* Calculus, kidney
    cholesterol (pure) (solitary) — *see* Calculus, gallbladder
    common duct (bile) — *see* Calculus, bile duct
    conjunctiva — *see* Concretion, conjunctiva
    cystic N21.0
    duct — *see* Calculus, gallbladder

Calculus, calculi, calculous - *continued*
  dental (subgingival) (supragingival) K03.6
  diverticulum
    bladder N21.0
    kidney N20.0
  epididymis N50.89
  gallbladder K80.20
    with
      bile duct calculus — *see* Calculus,
        gallbladder and bile duct
      cholecystitis K80.10
        with obstruction K80.11
        acute K80.00
          with
            chronic cholecystitis K80.12
              with obstruction K80.13
            obstruction K80.01
        chronic K80.10
          with
            acute cholecystitis K80.12
              with obstruction K80.13
            obstruction K80.11
        specified NEC K80.18
          with obstruction K80.19
        obstruction K80.21
  gallbladder and bile duct K80.70
    with
      cholecystitis K80.60
        with obstruction K80.61
        acute K80.62
          with
            chronic cholecystitis K80.66
              with obstruction K80.67
            obstruction K80.63
        chronic K80.64
          with
            acute cholecystitis K80.66
              with obstruction K80.67
            obstruction K80.65
        obstruction K80.71
  hepatic (duct) — *see* Calculus, bile duct
  hepatobiliary K80.80
    with obstruction K80.81
  ileal conduit N21.8
  intestinal (impaction) (obstruction) K56.49
  kidney (impacted) (multiple) (pelvis)
    (recurrent) (staghorn) N20.0
    with calculus, ureter N20.2
    congenital Q63.8
  lacrimal passages — *see* Dacryolith
  liver (impacted) — *see* Calculus, bile duct
  lung J98.4
  mammographic R92.1
  nephritic (impacted) (recurrent) — *see*
    Calculus, kidney
  nose J34.89
  pancreas (duct) K86.89
  parotid duct or gland K11.5
  pelvis, encysted — *see* Calculus, kidney
  prostate N42.0
  pulmonary J98.4
  pyelitis (impacted) (recurrent) N20.0
    with hydronephrosis N13.6
  pyelonephritis (impacted) (recurrent) — *see*
    category N20
    with hydronephrosis N13.6
  renal (impacted) (recurrent) — *see* Calculus,
    kidney
  salivary (duct) (gland) K11.5
  seminal vesicle N50.89
  staghorn — *see* Calculus, kidney
  Stensen's duct K11.5
  stomach K31.89
  sublingual duct or gland K11.5
    congenital Q38.4
  submandibular duct, gland or region K11.5
  submaxillary duct, gland or region K11.5
  suburethral N21.8
  tonsil J35.8
  tooth, teeth (subgingival)
    (supragingival) K03.6
  tunica vaginalis N50.89
  ureter (impacted) (recurrent) N20.1
    with calculus, kidney N20.2
      with hydronephrosis N13.2

Calculus, calculi, calculous - *continued*
  ureter (impacted) (recurrent) - *continued*
    with calculus, kidney - *continued*
      with hydronephrosis - *continued*
        with infection N13.6
  urethra (impacted) N21.1
  urinary (duct) (impacted) (passage)
    (tract) N20.9
    with hydronephrosis N13.2
      with infection N13.6
    in (due to)
      lower N21.9
        specified NEC N21.8
  vagina N89.8
  vesical (impacted) N21.0
  Wharton's duct K11.5
  xanthine E79.8 *[N22]*
Calicectasis N28.89
Caliectasis N28.89
California
  disease B38.9
  encephalitis A83.5
Caligo cornea — *see* Opacity, cornea, central
Callositas, callosity (infected) L84
Callus (infected) L84
  bone — *see* Osteophyte
  excessive, following fracture - code as
    Sequelae of fracture
CALME (childhood asymmetric labium
  majus enlargement) N90.61
Calorie deficiency or malnutrition — *see*
  also Malnutrition E46
Calvé-Perthes disease — *see* Legg-Calvé-
  Perthes disease
Calvé's disease — *see* Osteochondrosis,
  juvenile, spine
Calvities — *see* Alopecia, androgenic
Cameroon fever — *see* Malaria
Camptocormia (hysterical) F44.4
Camurati-Engelmann syndrome Q78.3
Canal — *see also* condition
  atrioventricular common Q21.2
Canaliculitis (lacrimal) (acute) (subacute)
  H04.33-
  Actinomyces A42.89
  chronic H04.42-
Canavan's disease E75.29
Canceled procedure (surgical) Z53.9
  because of
    contraindication Z53.09
      smoking Z53.01
    left against medical advice (AMA) Z53.29
    patient's decision Z53.20
      for reasons of belief or group
        pressure Z53.1
      specified reason NEC Z53.29
    specified reason NEC Z53.8
Cancer — *see also* Neoplasm, by site,
  malignant
  bile duct type liver C22.1
  blood — *see* Leukemia
  breast — *see also* Neoplasm, breast,
    malignant C50.91-
  hepatocellular C22.0
  lung — *see also* Neoplasm, lung,
    malignant C34.90-
  ovarian — *see also* Neoplasm ovary,
    malignant C56.9-
  unspecified site (primary) C80.1
Cancerous — *see* Neoplasm, malignant, by
  site
Cancer (o) phobia F45.29
Cancrum oris A69.0
Candidiasis, candidal B37.9
  balanitis B37.42
  bronchitis B37.1
  cheilitis B37.83
  congenital P37.5
  cystitis B37.41
  disseminated B37.7
  endocarditis B37.6
  enteritis B37.82
  esophagitis B37.81
  intertrigo B37.2
  lung B37.1

Candidiasis, candidal - *continued*
  meningitis B37.5
  mouth B37.0
  nails B37.2
  neonatal P37.5
  onychia B37.2
  oral B37.0
  osteomyelitis B37.89
  otitis externa B37.84
  paronychia B37.2
  perionyxis B37.2
  pneumonia B37.1
  proctitis B37.82
  pulmonary B37.1
  pyelonephritis B37.49
  sepsis B37.7
  skin B37.2
  specified site NEC B37.89
  stomatitis B37.0
  systemic B37.7
  urethritis B37.41
  urogenital site NEC B37.49
  vagina B37.3
  vulva B37.3
  vulvovaginitis B37.3
Candidid L30.2
Candidosis — *see* Candidiasis
Candiru infection or infestation B88.8
Canities (premature) L67.1
  congenital Q84.2
Canker (mouth) (sore) K12.0
  rash A38.9
Cannabinosis J66.2
Cannabis induced
  anxiety disorder F12.980
  psychotic disorder F12.959
  sleep disorder F12.988
Canton fever A75.9
Cantrell's syndrome Q87.89
Capillariasis (intestinal) B81.1
  hepatic B83.8
Capillary — *see* condition
Caplan's syndrome — *see* Rheumatoid, lung
Capsule — *see* condition
Capsulitis (joint) — *see also* Enthesopathy
  adhesive (shoulder) M75.0-
  hepatic K65.8
  labyrinthine — *see* Otosclerosis, specified
    NEC
  thyroid E06.9
Caput
  crepitus Q75.8
  medusae I86.8
  succedaneum P12.81
Car sickness T75.3
Carapata (disease) A68.0
Carate — *see* Pinta
Carbon lung J60
Carbuncle L02.93
  abdominal wall L02.231
  anus K61.0
  auditory canal, external — *see* Abscess, ear,
    external
  auricle ear — *see* Abscess, ear, external
  axilla L02.43-
  back (any part) L02.232
  breast N61.1
  buttock L02.33
  cheek (external) L02.03
  chest wall L02.233
  chin L02.03
  corpus cavernosum N48.21
  ear (any part) (external) (middle) — *see*
    Abscess, ear, external
  external auditory canal — *see* Abscess, ear,
    external
  eyelid — *see* Abscess, eyelid
  face NEC L02.03
  femoral (region) — *see* Carbuncle, lower
    limb
  finger — *see* Carbuncle, hand
  flank L02.231
  foot L02.63-
  forehead L02.03
  genital — *see* Abscess, genital

Carbuncle - *continued*
  gluteal (region) L02.33
  groin L02.234
  hand L02.53-
  head NEC L02.831
  heel — *see* Carbuncle, foot
  hip — *see* Carbuncle, lower limb
  kidney — *see* Abscess, kidney
  knee — *see* Carbuncle, lower limb
  labium (majus) (minus) N76.4
  lacrimal
    gland — *see* Dacryoadenitis
    passages (duct) (sac) — *see* Inflammation,
      lacrimal, passages, acute
  leg — *see* Carbuncle, lower limb
  lower limb L02.43-
  malignant A22.0
  navel L02.236
  neck L02.13
  nose (external) (septum) J34.0
  orbit, orbital — *see* Abscess, orbit
  palmar (space) — *see* Carbuncle, hand
  partes posteriores L02.33
  pectoral region L02.233
  penis N48.21
  perineum L02.235
  pinna — *see* Abscess, ear, external
  popliteal — *see* Carbuncle, lower limb
  scalp L02.831
  seminal vesicle N49.0
  shoulder — *see* Carbuncle, upper limb
  specified site NEC L02.838
  temple (region) L02.03
  thumb — *see* Carbuncle, hand
  toe — *see* Carbuncle, foot
  trunk L02.239
    abdominal wall L02.231
    back L02.232
    chest wall L02.233
    groin L02.234
    perineum L02.235
    umbilicus L02.236
  umbilicus L02.236
  upper limb L02.43-
  urethra N34.0
  vulva N76.4
Carbunculus — *see* Carbuncle
Carcinoid (tumor) — *see* Tumor, carcinoid
Carcinoidosis E34.0
Carcinoma (malignant) — *see also*
    Neoplasm, by site, malignant
  acidophil
    specified site — *see* Neoplasm, malignant,
      by site
    unspecified site C75.1
  acidophil-basophil, mixed
    specified site — *see* Neoplasm, malignant,
      by site
    unspecified site C75.1
  adnexal (skin) — *see* Neoplasm, skin,
    malignant
  adrenal cortical C74.0-
  alveolar — *see* Neoplasm, lung, malignant
    cell — *see* Neoplasm, lung, malignant
  ameloblastic C41.1
    upper jaw (bone) C41.0
  apocrine
    breast — *see* Neoplasm, breast, malignant
    specified site NEC — *see* Neoplasm, skin,
      malignant
    unspecified site C44.99
  basal cell (pigmented) (see also Neoplasm,
    skin, malignant) C44.91
    fibro-epithelial — *see* Neoplasm, skin,
      malignant
    morphea — *see* Neoplasm, skin, malignant
    multicentric — *see* Neoplasm, skin,
      malignant
  basaloid
  basal-squamous cell, mixed — *see*
    Neoplasm, skin, malignant
  basophil
    specified site — *see* Neoplasm, malignant,
      by site
    unspecified site C75.1

Carcinoma (malignant) - *continued*
  basophil-acidophil, mixed
    specified site — *see* Neoplasm, malignant,
      by site
    unspecified site C75.1
  basosquamous — *see* Neoplasm, skin,
    malignant
  bile duct
    with hepatocellular, mixed C22.0
    liver C22.1
    specified site NEC — *see* Neoplasm,
      malignant, by site
    unspecified site C22.1
  branchial or branchiogenic C10.4
  bronchial or bronchogenic — *see* Neoplasm,
    lung, malignant
  bronchiolar — *see* Neoplasm, lung,
    malignant
  bronchioloalveolar — *see* Neoplasm, lung,
    malignant
  C cell
    specified site — *see* Neoplasm, malignant,
      by site
    unspecified site C73
  ceruminous C44.29-
  cervix uteri
    in situ D06.9
      endocervix D06.0
      exocervix D06.1
      specified site NEC D06.7
  chorionic
    specified site — *see* Neoplasm, malignant,
      by site
    unspecified site
      female C58
      male C62.90
  chromophobe
    specified site — *see* Neoplasm, malignant,
      by site
    unspecified site C75.1
  cloacogenic
    specified site — *see* Neoplasm, malignant,
      by site
    unspecified site C21.2
  diffuse type
    specified site — *see* Neoplasm, malignant,
      by site
    unspecified site C16.9
  duct (cell)
    with Paget's disease — *see* Neoplasm,
      breast, malignant
    infiltrating
      with lobular carcinoma (in situ)
        specified site — *see* Neoplasm,
          malignant, by site
        unspecified site (female) C50.91-
          male C50.92-
      specified site — *see* Neoplasm,
        malignant, by site
      unspecified site (female) C50.91-
        male C50.92-
  ductal
    with lobular
      specified site — *see* Neoplasm,
        malignant, by site
      unspecified site (female) C50.91-
        male C50.92-
  ductular, infiltrating
    specified site — *see* Neoplasm, malignant,
      by site
    unspecified site (female) C50.91-
      male C50.92-
  embryonal
    liver C22.7
  endometrioid
    specified site — *see* Neoplasm, malignant,
      by site
    unspecified site
      female C56.9
      male C61
  eosinophil
    specified site — *see* Neoplasm, malignant,
      by site
    unspecified site C75.1

Carcinoma (malignant) - *continued*
  epidermoid — *see also* Neoplasm, skin
      malignant
    in situ, Bowen's type — *see* Neoplasm,
      skin, in situ
  fibroepithelial, basal cell — *see* Neoplasm,
    skin, malignant
  follicular
    with papillary (mixed) C73
    moderately differentiated C73
    pure follicle C73
    specified site — *see* Neoplasm, malignant,
      by site
    trabecular C73
    unspecified site C73
    well differentiated C73
  generalized, with unspecified primary
    site C80.0
  glycogen-rich — *see* Neoplasm, breast,
    malignant
  granulosa cell C56-
  hepatic cell C22.0
  hepatocellular C22.0
    with bile duct, mixed C22.0
    fibrolamellar C22.0
  hepatocholangiolitic C22.0
  Hurthle cell C73
  in
    adenomatous
      polyposis coli C18.9
    pleomorphic adenoma — *see* Neoplasm,
      salivary glands, malignant
    situ — *see* Carcinoma-in-situ
  infiltrating
    duct
      with lobular
        specified site — *see* Neoplasm,
          malignant, by site
        unspecified site (female) C50.91-
          male C50.92-
      with Paget's disease — *see* Neoplasm,
        breast, malignant
      specified site — *see* Neoplasm,
        malignant
      unspecified site (female) C50.91-
        male C50.92-
    ductular
      specified site — *see* Neoplasm,
        malignant
      unspecified site (female) C50.91-
        male C50.92-
    lobular
      specified site — *see* Neoplasm,
        malignant
      unspecified site (female) C50.91-
        male C50.92-
  inflammatory
    specified site — *see* Neoplasm, malignant
    unspecified site (female) C50.91-
      male C50.92-
  intestinal type
    specified site — *see* Neoplasm, malignant,
      by site
    unspecified site C16.9
  intracystic
    noninfiltrating — *see* Neoplasm, in situ, by
      site
  intraductal (noninfiltrating)
    with Paget's disease — *see* Neoplasm,
      breast, malignant
    breast D05.1-
    papillary
      with invasion
        specified site — *see* Neoplasm,
          malignant, by site
        unspecified site (female) C50.91-
          male C50.92-
      breast D05.1-
      specified site NEC — *see* Neoplasm, in
        situ, by site
      unspecified site (female) D05.1-
    specified site NEC — *see* Neoplasm, in
      situ, by site
    unspecified site (female) D05.1-
  intraepidermal — *see* Neoplasm, in situ

Carcinoma (malignant) - *continued*
  intraepidermal - *continued*
    squamous cell, Bowen's type — *see*
      Neoplasm, skin, in situ
    intraepithelial — *see* Neoplasm, in situ, by
      site
      squamous cell — *see* Neoplasm, in situ, by
        site
    intraosseous C41.1
      upper jaw (bone) C41.0
    islet cell
      with exocrine, mixed
        specified site — *see* Neoplasm,
          malignant, by site
        unspecified site C25.9
      pancreas C25.4
      specified site NEC — *see* Neoplasm,
        malignant, by site
      unspecified site C25.4
    juvenile, breast — *see* Neoplasm, breast,
      malignant
    large cell
      small cell
        specified site — *see* Neoplasm,
          malignant, by site
        unspecified site C34.90
    Leydig cell (testis)
      specified site — *see* Neoplasm, malignant,
        by site
      unspecified site
        female C56.9
        male C62.90
    lipid-rich (female) C50.91-
      male C50.92-
    liver cell C22.0
    liver NEC C22.7
    lobular (infiltrating)
      with intraductal
        specified site — *see* Neoplasm,
          malignant, by site
        unspecified site (female) C50.91-
          male C50.92-
      noninfiltrating
        breast D05.0-
        specified site NEC — *see* Neoplasm, in
          situ, by site
        unspecified site D05.0-
      specified site — *see* Neoplasm, malignant,
        by site
      unspecified site (female) C50.91-
        male C50.92-
    medullary
      with
        amyloid stroma
          specified site — *see* Neoplasm,
            malignant, by site
          unspecified site C73
        lymphoid stroma
          specified site — *see* Neoplasm,
            malignant, by site
          unspecified site (female) C50.91-
            male C50.92-
    Merkel cell C4A.9
      anal margin C4A.51
      anal skin C4A.51
      canthus C4A.1-
      ear and external auricular canal C4A.2-
      external auricular canal C4A.2-
      eyelid, including canthus C4A.1-
      face C4A.30
        specified NEC C4A.39
      hip C4A.7-
      lip C4A.0
      lower limb, including hip C4A.7-
      neck C4A.4
      nodal presentation C7B.1
      nose C4A.31
      overlapping sites C4A.8
      perianal skin C4A.51
      scalp C4A.4
      secondary C7B.1
      shoulder C4A.6-
      skin of breast C4A.52
      trunk NEC C4A.59
      upper limb, including shoulder C4A.6-

Carcinoma (malignant) - *continued*
  Merkel cell - *continued*
    visceral metastatic C7B.1
    metastatic — *see* Neoplasm, secondary, by
      site
    metatypical — *see* Neoplasm, skin,
      malignant
    morphea, basal cell — *see* Neoplasm, skin,
      malignant
    mucoid
      cell
        specified site — *see* Neoplasm,
          malignant, by site
        unspecified site C75.1
    neuroendocrine — *see also* Tumor,
      neuroendocrine
      high grade, any site C7A.1
      poorly differentiated, any site C7A.1
    nonencapsulated sclerosing C73
    noninfiltrating
      intracystic — *see* Neoplasm, in situ, by site
      intraductal
        breast D05.1-
        papillary
          breast D05.1-
          specified site NEC — *see* Neoplasm,
            in situ, by site
          unspecified site D05.1-
        specified site — *see* Neoplasm, in situ,
          by site
        unspecified site D05.1-
      lobular
        breast D05.0-
        specified site NEC — *see* Neoplasm, in
          situ, by site
        unspecified site (female) D05.0-
    oat cell
      specified site — *see* Neoplasm, malignant,
        by site
      unspecified site C34.90
    odontogenic C41.1
      upper jaw (bone) C41.0
    papillary
      with follicular (mixed) C73
      follicular variant C73
      intraductal (noninfiltrating)
        with invasion
          specified site — *see* Neoplasm,
            malignant, by site
          unspecified site (female) C50.91-
            male C50.92-
        breast D05.1-
        specified site NEC — *see* Neoplasm, in
          situ, by site
        unspecified site D05.1-
      serous
        specified site — *see* Neoplasm,
          malignant, by site
        surface
          specified site — *see* Neoplasm,
            malignant, by site
          unspecified site C56.9
        unspecified site C56.9
    papillocystic
      specified site — *see* Neoplasm, malignant,
        by site
      unspecified site C56.9
    parafollicular cell
      specified site — *see* Neoplasm, malignant,
        by site
      unspecified site C73
    pilomatrix — *see* Neoplasm, skin, malignant
    pseudomucinous
      specified site — *see* Neoplasm, malignant,
        by site
      unspecified site C56.9
    renal cell C64-
    Schmincke — *see* Neoplasm, nasopharynx,
      malignant
    Schneiderian
      specified site — *see* Neoplasm, malignant,
        by site
      unspecified site C30.0
    sebaceous — *see* Neoplasm, skin, malignant

Carcinoma (malignant) - *continued*
  secondary — *see also* Neoplasm, secondary,
    by site
    Merkel cell C7B.1
  secretory, breast — *see* Neoplasm, breast,
    malignant
  serous
    papillary
      specified site — *see* Neoplasm,
        malignant, by site
      unspecified site C56.9
    surface, papillary
      specified site — *see* Neoplasm,
        malignant, by site
      unspecified site C56.9
  Sertoli cell
    specified site — *see* Neoplasm, malignant,
      by site
    unspecified site C62.90
      female C56.9
      male C62.90
  skin appendage — *see* Neoplasm, skin,
    malignant
  small cell
    fusiform cell
      specified site — *see* Neoplasm,
        malignant, by site
      unspecified site C34.90
    intermediate cell
      specified site — *see* Neoplasm,
        malignant, by site
      unspecified site C34.90
    large cell
      specified site — *see* Neoplasm,
        malignant, by site
      unspecified site C34.90
  solid
    with amyloid stroma
      specified site — *see* Neoplasm,
        malignant, by site
      unspecified site C73
    microinvasive
      specified site — *see* Neoplasm,
        malignant, by site
      unspecified site C53.9
  sweat gland — *see* Neoplasm, skin,
    malignant
  theca cell C56.-
  thymic C37
  unspecified site (primary) C80.1
  water-clear cell C75.0
Carcinoma-in-situ — *see also* Neoplasm, in
  situ, by site
  breast NOS D05.9-
    specified type NEC D05.8-
  epidermoid — *see also* Neoplasm, in situ, by
    site
    with questionable stromal invasion
      cervix D06.9
      specified site NEC — *see* Neoplasm, in
        situ, by site
      unspecified site D06.9
    Bowen's type — *see* Neoplasm, skin, in
      situ
  intraductal
    breast D05.1-
    specified site NEC — *see* Neoplasm, in
      situ, by site
    unspecified site D05.1-
  lobular
    with
      infiltrating duct
        breast (female) C50.91-
          male C50.92-
        specified site NEC — *see* Neoplasm,
          malignant
        unspecified site (female) C50.91-
          male C50.92-
      intraductal
        breast D05.8-
        specified site NEC — *see* Neoplasm,
          in situ, by site
        unspecified site (female) D05.8-
    breast D05.0-

Carcinoma-in-situ - *continued*
  lobular - *continued*
    specified site NEC — *see* Neoplasm, in situ, by site
    unspecified site D05.0-
  squamous cell — *see also* Neoplasm, in situ, by site
    with questionable stromal invasion
      cervix D06.9
      specified site NEC — *see* Neoplasm, in situ, by site
      unspecified site D06.9
Carcinomaphobia F45.29
Carcinomatosis C80.0
  peritonei C78.6
  unspecified site (primary) (secondary) C80.0
Carcinosarcoma — *see* Neoplasm, malignant, by site
  embryonal — *see* Neoplasm, malignant, by site
Cardia, cardial — *see* condition
Cardiac — *see also* condition
  death, sudden — *see* Arrest, cardiac
  pacemaker
    in situ Z95.0
    management or adjustment Z45.018
  tamponade I31.4
Cardialgia — *see* Pain, precordial
Cardiectasis — *see* Hypertrophy, cardiac
Cardiochalasia K21.9
Cardiomalacia I51.5
Cardiomegalia glycogenica diffusa E74.02 *[143]*
Cardiomegaly — *see also* Hypertrophy, cardiac
  congenital Q24.8
  glycogen E74.02 *[143]*
  idiopathic I51.7
Cardiomyoliposis I51.5
Cardiomyopathy (familial) (idiopathic) I42.9
  alcoholic I42.6
  amyloid E85.4 *[143]*
    transthyretin-related (ATTR) familial E85.4 *[143]*
  arteriosclerotic — *see* Disease, heart, ischemic, atherosclerotic
  beriberi E51.12
  cobalt-beer I42.6
  congenital I42.4
  congestive I42.0
  constrictive NOS I42.5
  dilated I42.0
  due to
    alcohol I42.6
    beriberi E51.12
    cardiac glycogenosis E74.02 *[143]*
    drugs I42.7
    external agents NEC I42.7
    Friedreich's ataxia G11.1
    myotonia atrophica G71.11 *[143]*
    progressive muscular dystrophy G71.09 *[143]*
  glycogen storage E74.02 *[143]*
  hypertensive — *see* Hypertension, heart
  hypertrophic (nonobstructive) I42.2
    obstructive I42.1
      congenital Q24.8
  in
    Chagas' disease (chronic) B57.2
      acute B57.0
    sarcoidosis D86.85
  ischemic I25.5
  metabolic E88.9 *[143]*
    thyrotoxic E05.90 *[143]*
      with thyroid storm E05.91 *[143]*
  newborn I42.8
    congenital I42.4
  non-ischemic — *see also* by cause I42.8
  nutritional E63.9 *[143]*
    beriberi E51.12
  obscure of Africa I42.8
  peripartum O90.3
  postpartum O90.3
  restrictive NEC I42.5
  rheumatic I09.0

Cardiomyopathy (familial) (idiopathic) - *continued*
  secondary I42.9
  specified NEC I42.8
  stress induced I51.81
  takotsubo I51.81
  thyrotoxic E05.90 *[143]*
    with thyroid storm E05.91 *[143]*
  toxic NEC I42.7
  transthyretin-related (ATTR) familial amyloid E85.4
  tuberculous A18.84
  viral B33.24
Cardionephritis — *see* Hypertension, cardiorenal
Cardionephropathy — *see* Hypertension, cardiorenal
Cardionephrosis — *see* Hypertension, cardiorenal
Cardiopathia nigra I27.0
Cardiopathy — *see also* Disease, heart I51.9
  idiopathic I42.9
  mucopolysaccharidosis E76.3 *[152]*
Cardiopericarditis — *see* Pericarditis
Cardiophobia F45.29
Cardiorenal — *see* condition
Cardiorrhexis — *see* Infarct, myocardium
Cardiosclerosis — *see* Disease, heart, ischemic, atherosclerotic
Cardiosis — *see* Disease, heart
Cardiospasm (esophagus) (reflex) (stomach) K22.0
  congenital Q39.5
    with megaesophagus Q39.5
Cardiostenosis — *see* Disease, heart
Cardiosymphysis I31.0
Cardiovascular — *see* condition
Carditis (acute) (bacterial) (chronic) (subacute) I51.89
  meningococcal A39.50
  rheumatic — *see* Disease, heart, rheumatic
  rheumatoid — *see* Rheumatoid, carditis
  viral B33.20
Care (of) (for) (following)
  child (routine) Z76.2
  family member (handicapped) (sick)
    creating problem for family Z63.6
    provided away from home for holiday relief Z75.5
    unavailable, due to
      absence (person rendering care) (sufferer) Z74.2
      inability (any reason) of person rendering care Z74.2
  foundling Z76.1
  holiday relief Z75.5
  improper — *see* Maltreatment
  lack of (at or after birth) (infant) — *see* Maltreatment, child, neglect
  lactating mother Z39.1
  palliative Z51.5
  postpartum
    immediately after delivery Z39.0
    routine follow-up Z39.2
  respite Z75.5
  unavailable, due to
    absence of person rendering care Z74.2
    inability (any reason) of person rendering care Z74.2
  well-baby Z76.2
Caries
  bone NEC A18.03
  dental (dentino enamel junction) (early childhood) (of dentine) (pre-eruptive) (recurrent) (to the pulp) K02.9
    arrested (coronal) (root) K02.3
    chewing surface
      limited to enamel K02.51
      penetrating into dentin K02.52
      penetrating into pulp K02.53
    coronal surface
      chewing surface
        limited to enamel K02.51
        penetrating into dentin K02.52
        penetrating into pulp K02.53

Caries - *continued*
  dental (dentino enamel junction) (early childhood) (of dentine) (pre-eruptive) (recurrent) (to the pulp) - *continued*
    coronal surface - *continued*
      pit and fissure surface
        limited to enamel K02.51
        penetrating into dentin K02.52
        penetrating into pulp K02.53
      smooth surface
        limited to enamel K02.61
        penetrating into dentin K02.62
        penetrating into pulp K02.63
    pit and fissure surface
      limited to enamel K02.51
      penetrating into dentin K02.52
      penetrating into pulp K02.53
    primary, cervical origin K02.52
    root K02.7
    smooth surface
      limited to enamel K02.61
      penetrating into dentin K02.62
      penetrating into pulp K02.63
  external meatus — *see* Disorder, ear, external, specified type NEC
  hip (tuberculous) A18.02
  initial (tooth)
    chewing surface K02.51
    pit and fissure surface K02.51
    smooth surface K02.61
  knee (tuberculous) A18.02
  labyrinth — *see* subcategory H83.8
  limb NEC (tuberculous) A18.03
  mastoid process (chronic) — *see* Mastoiditis, chronic
    tuberculous A18.03
  middle ear — *see* subcategory H74.8
  nose (tuberculous) A18.03
  orbit (tuberculous) A18.03
  ossicles, ear — *see* Abnormal, ear ossicles
  petrous bone — *see* Petrositis
  root (dental) (tooth) K02.7
  sacrum (tuberculous) A18.01
  spine, spinal (column) (tuberculous) A18.01
  syphilitic A52.77
    congenital (early) A50.02 *[M90.80]*
  tooth, teeth — *see* Caries, dental
  tuberculous A18.03
  vertebra (column) (tuberculous) A18.01
Carious teeth — *see* Caries, dental
Carneous mole O02.0
Carnitine insufficiency E71.40
Carotenemia (dietary) E67.1
Carotenosis (cutis) (skin) E67.1
Carotid body or sinus syndrome G90.01
Carotidynia G90.01
Carpal tunnel syndrome — *see* Syndrome, carpal tunnel
Carpenter's syndrome Q87.0
Carpopedal spasm — *see* Tetany
Carr-Barr-Plunkett syndrome Q97.1
Carrier (suspected) of
  amebiasis Z22.1
  bacterial disease NEC Z22.39
    diphtheria Z22.2
    intestinal infectious NEC Z22.1
    typhoid Z22.0
    meningococcal Z22.31
    sexually transmitted Z22.4
    specified NEC Z22.39
    staphylococcal (Methicillin susceptible) Z22.321
      Methicillin resistant Z22.322
    streptococcal Z22.338
      group B Z22.330
        complicating pregnancy or delivery O99.82-
    typhoid Z22.0
  cholera Z22.1
  diphtheria Z22.2
  gastrointestinal pathogens NEC Z22.1
  genetic Z14.8
    cystic fibrosis Z14.1
    hemophilia A (asymptomatic) Z14.01
      symptomatic Z14.02

Carrier (suspected) of - *continued*
gestational, pregnant Z33.1
gonorrhea Z22.4
HAA (hepatitis Australian-antigen) B18.8
HB (c) (s) -AG B18.1
hepatitis (viral) B18.9
Australia-antigen (HAA) B18.8
B surface antigen (HBsAg) B18.1
with acute delta- (super) infection B17.0
C B18.2
specified NEC B18.8
human T-cell lymphotropic virus type-1
(HTLV-1) infection Z22.6
infectious organism Z22.9
specified NEC Z22.8
meningococci Z22.31
Salmonella typhosa Z22.0
serum hepatitis — *see* Carrier, hepatitis
staphylococci (Methicillin
susceptible) Z22.321
Methicillin resistant Z22.322
streptococci Z22.338
group B Z22.330
complicating pregnancy or
delivery O99.82-
syphilis Z22.4
typhoid Z22.0
venereal disease NEC Z22.4
Carrion's disease A44.0
Carter's relapsing fever (Asiatic) A68.1
Cartilage — *see* condition
Caruncle (inflamed)
conjunctiva (acute) — *see* Conjunctivitis,
acute
labium (majus) (minus) N90.89
lacrimal — *see* Inflammation, lacrimal,
passages
myrtiform N89.8
urethral (benign) N36.2
Cascade stomach K31.2
**Caseation lymphatic gland
(tuberculous)** A18.2
**Cassidy (-Scholte) syndrome (malignant
carcinoid)** E34.0
Castellani's disease A69.8
Castration, traumatic, male S38.231
Casts in urine R82.998
Cat
cry syndrome Q93.4
ear Q17.3
eye syndrome Q92.8
Catabolism, senile R54
Catalepsy (hysterical) F44.2
schizophrenic F20.2
Cataplexy (idiopathic) — *see* - Narcolepsy
Cataract (cortical) (immature) (incipient)
H26.9
with
neovascularization — *see* Cataract,
complicated
age-related — *see* Cataract, senile
anterior
and posterior axial embryonal Q12.0
pyramidal Q12.0
associated with
galactosemia E74.21 *[H28]*
myotonic disorders G71.19 *[H28]*
blue Q12.0
central Q12.0
cerulean Q12.0
complicated H26.20
with
neovascularization H26.21-
ocular disorder H26.22-
glaucomatous flecks H26.23-
congenital Q12.0
coraliform Q12.0
coronary Q12.0
crystalline Q12.0
diabetic — *see* Diabetes, cataract
drug-induced H26.3-
due to
ocular disorder — *see* Cataract,
complicated
radiation H26.8

Cataract (cortical) (immature) (incipient) -
continued
electric H26.8
extraction status Z98.4-
glass-blower's H26.8
heat ray H26.8
heterochromic — *see* Cataract, complicated
hypermature — *see* Cataract, senile,
morgagnian type
in (due to)
chronic iridocyclitis — *see* Cataract,
complicated
diabetes — *see* Diabetes, cataract
endocrine disease E34.9 *[H28]*
eye disease — *see* Cataract, complicated
hypoparathyroidism E20.9 *[H28]*
malnutrition-dehydration E46 *[H28]*
metabolic disease E88.9 *[H28]*
myotonic disorders G71.19 *[H28]*
nutritional disease E63.9 *[H28]*
infantile — *see* Cataract, presenile
irradiational — *see* Cataract, specified NEC
juvenile — *see* Cataract, presenile
malnutrition-dehydration E46 *[H28]*
morgagnian — *see* Cataract, senile,
morgagnian type
myotonic G71.19 *[H28]*
myxedema E03.9 *[H28]*
nuclear
embryonal Q12.0
sclerosis — *see* Cataract, senile, nuclear
presenile H26.00-
combined forms H26.06-
cortical H26.01-
lamellar — *see* Cataract, presenile, cortical
nuclear H26.03-
specified NEC H26.09
subcapsular polar (anterior) H26.04-
posterior H26.05-
zonular — *see* Cataract, presenile, cortical
secondary H26.40
Soemmering's ring H26.41-
specified NEC H26.49-
to eye disease — *see* Cataract, complicated
senile H25.9
brunescens — *see* Cataract, senile, nuclear
combined forms H25.81-
coronary — *see* Cataract, senile, incipient
cortical H25.01-
hypermature — *see* Cataract, senile,
morgagnian type
incipient (mature) (total) H25.09-
cortical — *see* Cataract, senile, cortical
subcapsular — *see* Cataract, senile,
subcapsular
morgagnian type (hypermature) H25.2-
nuclear (sclerosis) H25.1-
polar subcapsular (anterior) (posterior) —
see Cataract, senile, incipient
punctate — *see* Cataract, senile, incipient
specified NEC H25.89
subcapsular polar (anterior) H25.03-
posterior H25.04-
snowflake — *see* Diabetes, cataract
specified NEC H26.8
toxic — *see* Cataract, drug-induced
traumatic H26.10-
localized H26.11-
partially resolved H26.12-
total H26.13-
zonular (perinuclear) Q12.0
Cataracta — *see also* Cataract
brunescens — *see* Cataract, senile, nuclear
centralis pulverulenta Q12.0
cerulea Q12.0
complicata — *see* Cataract, complicated
congenita Q12.0
coralliformis Q12.0
coronaria Q12.0
diabetic — *see* Diabetes, cataract
membranacea
accreta — *see* Cataract, secondary
congenita Q12.0
nigra — *see* Cataract, senile, nuclear
sunflower — *see* Cataract, complicated

**Catarrh, catarrhal (acute) (febrile)
(infectious) (inflammation)** — *see also*
condition J00
bronchial — *see* Bronchitis
chest — *see* Bronchitis
chronic J31.0
due to congenital syphilis A50.03
enteric — *see* Enteritis
eustachian H68.009
fauces — *see* Pharyngitis
gastrointestinal — *see* Enteritis
gingivitis K05.00
nonplaque induced K05.01
plaque induced K05.00
hay — *see* Fever, hay
intestinal — *see* Enteritis
larynx, chronic J37.0
liver B15.9
with hepatic coma B15.0
lung — *see* Bronchitis
middle ear, chronic — *see* Otitis, media,
nonsuppurative, chronic, serous
mouth K12.1
nasal (chronic) — *see* Rhinitis
nasobronchial J31.1
nasopharyngeal (chronic) J31.1
acute J00
pulmonary — *see* Bronchitis
spring (eye) (vernal) — *see* Conjunctivitis,
acute, atopic
summer (hay) — *see* Fever, hay
throat J31.2
tubotympanal — *see also* Otitis, media,
nonsuppurative
chronic — *see* Otitis, media,
nonsuppurative, chronic, serous
Catatonia (schizophrenic) F20.2
Catatonic
disorder due to known physiologic
condition F06.1
schizophrenia F20.2
stupor R40.1
Cat-scratch — *see also* Abrasion
disease or fever A28.1
Cauda equina — *see* condition
Cauliflower ear M95.1-
Causalgia (upper limb) G56.4-
lower limb G57.7-
Cause
external, general effects T75.89
Caustic burn — *see* Corrosion, by site
**Cavare's disease (familial periodic
paralysis)** G72.3
Cave-in, injury
crushing (severe) — *see* Crush
suffocation — *see* Asphyxia, traumatic, due
to low oxygen, due to cave-in
Cavernitis (penis) N48.29
Cavernositis N48.29
Cavernous — *see* condition
Cavitation of lung — *see also* Tuberculosis,
pulmonary
nontuberculous J98.4
Cavities, dental — *see* Caries, dental
Cavity
lung — *see* Cavitation of lung
optic papilla Q14.2
pulmonary — *see* Cavitation of lung
Cavovarus foot, congenital Q66.1-
Cavus foot (congenital) Q66.7-
acquired — *see* Deformity, limb, foot,
specified NEC
Cazenave's disease L10.2
Cecitis K52.9
with perforation, peritonitis, or rupture K65.8
Cecoureterocele Q62.32
Cecum — *see* condition
Celiac
artery compression syndrome I77.4
disease (with steatorrhea) K90.0
infantilism K90.0
Cell (s) , cellular — *see also* condition
in urine R82.998

Cellulitis (diffuse) (phlegmonous) (septic) (suppurative) L03.90
abdominal wall L03.311
anaerobic A48.0
ankle — *see* Cellulitis, lower limb
anus K61.0
arm — *see* Cellulitis, upper limb
auricle (ear) — *see* Cellulitis, ear
axilla L03.11-
back (any part) L03.312
breast (acute) (nonpuerperal)
   (subacute) N61.0
   nipple N61.0
broad ligament
   acute N73.0
buttock L03.317
cervical (meaning neck) L03.221
cervix (uteri) — *see* Cervicitis
cheek (external) L03.211
   internal K12.2
chest wall L03.313
chronic L03.90
clostridial A48.0
corpus cavernosum N48.22
digit
   finger — *see* Cellulitis, finger
   toe — *see* Cellulitis, toe
Douglas' cul-de-sac or pouch
   acute N73.0
drainage site (following operation) T81.49
ear (external) H60.1-
eosinophilic (granulomatous) L98.3
erysipelatous — *see* Erysipelas
external auditory canal — *see* Cellulitis, ear
eyelid — *see* Abscess, eyelid
face NEC L03.211
finger (intrathecal) (periosteal)
   (subcutaneous) (subcuticular) L03.01-
foot — *see* Cellulitis, lower limb
gangrenous — *see* Gangrene
genital organ NEC
   female (external) N76.4
   male N49.9
      multiple sites N49.8
      specified NEC N49.8
gluteal (region) L03.317
gonococcal A54.89
groin L03.314
hand — *see* Cellulitis, upper limb
head NEC L03.811
   face (any part, except ear, eye and
      nose) L03.211
heel — *see* Cellulitis, lower limb
hip — *see* Cellulitis, lower limb
jaw (region) L03.211
knee — *see* Cellulitis, lower limb
labium (majus) (minus) — *see* Vulvitis
lacrimal passages — *see* Inflammation,
   lacrimal, passages
larynx J38.7
leg — *see* Cellulitis, lower limb
lip K13.0
lower limb L03.11-
   toe — *see* Cellulitis, toe
mouth (floor) K12.2
multiple sites, so stated L03.90
nasopharynx J39.1
navel L03.316
   newborn P38.9
      with mild hemorrhage P38.1
      without hemorrhage P38.9
neck (region) L03.221
nipple (acute) (nonpuerperal)
   (subacute) N61.0
nose (septum) (external) J34.0
orbit, orbital H05.01-
palate (soft) K12.2
pectoral (region) L03.313
pelvis, pelvic (chronic)
   female — *see also* Disease, pelvis,
      inflammatory N73.2
      acute N73.0
   following ectopic or molar
      pregnancy O08.0
   male K65.0

Cellulitis (diffuse) (phlegmonous) (septic) (suppurative) - continued
penis N48.22
perineal, perineum L03.315
periorbital L03.213
perirectal K61.1
peritonsillar J36
periurethral N34.0
periuterine — *see also* Disease, pelvis,
   inflammatory N73.2
   acute N73.0
pharynx J39.1
preseptal L03.213
rectum K61.1
retroperitoneal K68.9
round ligament
   acute N73.0
scalp (any part) L03.811
scrotum N49.2
seminal vesicle N49.0
shoulder — *see* Cellulitis, upper limb
specified site NEC L03.818
submandibular (region) (space)
   (triangle) K12.2
   gland K11.3
submaxillary (region) K12.2
   gland K11.3
thigh — *see* Cellulitis, lower limb
thumb (intrathecal) (periosteal)
   (subcutaneous) (subcuticular) — *see*
      Cellulitis, finger
toe (intrathecal) (periosteal) (subcutaneous)
   (subcuticular) L03.03-
tonsil J36
trunk L03.319
   abdominal wall L03.311
   back (any part) L03.312
   buttock L03.317
   chest wall L03.313
   groin L03.314
   perineal, perineum L03.315
   umbilicus L03.316
tuberculous (primary) A18.4
umbilicus L03.316
upper limb L03.11-
   axilla — *see* Cellulitis, axilla
   finger — *see* Cellulitis, finger
   thumb — *see* Cellulitis, finger
vaccinal T88.0
vocal cord J38.3
vulva — *see* Vulvitis
wrist — *see* Cellulitis, upper limb
Cementoblastoma, benign — *see* Cyst,
   calcifying odontogenic
Cementoma — *see* Cyst, calcifying
   odontogenic
Cementoperiostitis — *see* Periodontitis
Cementosis K03.4
Central auditory processing disorder H93.25
Central pain syndrome G89.0
Cephalematocele, cephal (o) hematocele
   newborn P52.8
      birth injury P10.8
   traumatic — *see* Hematoma, brain
Cephalematoma, cephalhematoma
   (calcified)
   newborn (birth injury) P12.0
   traumatic — *see* Hematoma, brain
Cephalgia, cephalalgia — *see also* Headache
   histamine G44.009
      intractable G44.001
      not intractable G44.009
   trigeminal autonomic (TAC) NEC G44.099
      intractable G44.091
      not intractable G44.099
Cephalic — *see* condition
Cephalitis — *see* Encephalitis
Cephalocele — *see* Encephalocele
Cephalomenia N94.89
Cephalopelvic — *see* condition
Cerclage (with cervical incompetence) in
   pregnancy — *see* Incompetence, cervix,
   in pregnancy
Cerebellitis — *see* Encephalitis
Cerebellum, cerebellar — *see* condition

Cerebral — *see* condition
Cerebritis — *see* Encephalitis
Cerebro-hepato-renal syndrome Q87.89
Cerebromalacia — *see* Softening, brain
   sequelae of cerebrovascular disease I69.398
Cerebroside lipidosis E75.22
Cerebrospasticity (congenital) G80.1
Cerebrospinal — *see* condition
Cerebrum — *see* condition
Ceroid-lipofuscinosis, neuronal E75.4
Cerumen (accumulation) (impacted) H61.2-
Cervical — *see also* condition
   auricle Q18.2
   dysplasia in pregnancy — *see* Abnormal,
      cervix, in pregnancy or childbirth
   erosion in pregnancy — *see* Abnormal,
      cervix, in pregnancy or childbirth
   fibrosis in pregnancy — *see* Abnormal,
      cervix, in pregnancy or childbirth
   fusion syndrome Q76.1
   rib Q76.5
   shortening (complicating
      pregnancy) O26.87-
Cervicalgia M54.2
Cervicitis (acute) (chronic) (nonvenereal)
   (senile (atrophic)) (subacute) (with
   ulceration) N72
   with
      abortion — *see* Abortion, by type
      complicated by genital tract and
         pelvic infection
      ectopic pregnancy O08.0
      molar pregnancy O08.0
   chlamydial A56.09
   gonococcal A54.03
   herpesviral A60.03
   puerperal (postpartum) O86.11
   syphilitic A52.76
   trichomonal A59.09
   tuberculous A18.16
Cervicocolpitis (emphysematosa) (see also
   Cervicitis) N72
Cervix — *see* condition
Cesarean delivery, previous, affecting
   management of pregnancy O34.219
   classical (vertical) scar O34.212
   low transverse scar O34.211
Céstan (-Chenais) paralysis or
   syndrome G46.3
Céstan-Raymond syndrome I65.8
Cestode infestation B71.9
   specified type NEC B71.8
Cestodiasis B71.9
Chabert's disease A22.9
Chacaleh E53.8
Chafing L30.4
Chagas' (-Mazza) disease (chronic) B57.2
   with
      cardiovascular involvement NEC B57.2
      digestive system involvement B57.30
         megacolon B57.32
         megaesophagus B57.31
         other specified B57.39
      megacolon B57.32
      megaesophagus B57.31
      myocarditis B57.2
      nervous system involvement B57.40
         meningitis B57.41
         meningoencephalitis B57.42
         other specified B57.49
      specified organ involvement NEC B57.5
   acute (with) B57.1
      cardiovascular NEC B57.0
      myocarditis B57.0
Chagres fever B50.9
Chairridden Z74.09
Chalasia (cardiac sphincter) K21.9
Chalazion H00.19
   left H00.16
      lower H00.15
      upper H00.14
   right H00.13
      lower H00.12
      upper H00.11

Chalcosis — *see also* Disorder, globe, degenerative, chalcosis
  cornea — *see* Deposit, cornea
  crystalline lens — *see* Cataract, complicated
  retina H35.89
Chalicosis (pulmonum) J62.8
Chancre (any genital site) (hard) (hunterian) (mixed) (primary) (seronegative) (seropositive) (syphilitic) A51.0
  congenital A50.07
  conjunctiva NEC A51.2
  Ducrey's A57
  extragenital A51.2
  eyelid A51.2
  lip A51.2
  nipple A51.2
  Nisbet's A57
  of
    carate A67.0
    pinta A67.0
    yaws A66.0
  palate, soft A51.2
  phagedenic A57
  simple A57
  soft A57
    bubo A57
    palate A51.2
  urethra A51.0
  yaws A66.0
Chancroid (anus) (genital) (penis) (perineum) (rectum) (urethra) (vulva) A57
Chandler's disease (osteochondritis dissecans, hip) — *see* Osteochondritis, dissecans, hip
Change (s) (in) (of) — *see also* Removal
  arteriosclerotic — *see* Arteriosclerosis
  bone — *see also* Disorder, bone
    diabetic — *see* Diabetes, bone change
  bowel habit R19.4
  cardiorenal (vascular) — *see* Hypertension, cardiorenal
  cardiovascular — *see* Disease, cardiovascular
  circulatory I99.9
  cognitive (mild) (organic) R41.89
  color, tooth, teeth
    during formation K00.8
    posteruptive K03.7
  contraceptive device Z30.433
  corneal membrane H18.30
    Bowman's membrane fold or rupture H18.31-
    Descemet's membrane fold H18.32-
      rupture H18.33-
  coronary — *see* Disease, heart, ischemic
  degenerative, spine or vertebra — *see* Spondylosis
  dental pulp, regressive K04.2
  dressing (nonsurgical) Z48.00
    surgical Z48.01
  heart — *see* Disease, heart
  hip joint — *see* Derangement, joint, hip
  hyperplastic larynx J38.7
  hypertrophic
    nasal sinus J34.89
    turbinate, nasal J34.3
    upper respiratory tract J39.8
  indwelling catheter Z46.6
  inflammatory — *see also* Inflammation
    sacroiliac M46.1
  job, anxiety concerning Z56.1
  joint — *see* Derangement, joint
  life — *see* Menopause
  mental status R41.82
  minimal (glomerular) — *see also* N00-N07
    with fourth character .0 N05.0
  myocardium, myocardial — *see* Degeneration, myocardial
  of life — *see* Menopause
  pacemaker Z45.018
    pulse generator Z45.010
  personality (enduring) F68.8
    due to (secondary to)

Change (s) (in) (of) - *continued*
  personality (enduring) - *continued*
    due to (secondary to) - *continued*
      general medical condition F07.0
    secondary (nonspecific) F60.89
  regressive, dental pulp K04.2
  renal — *see* Disease, renal
  retina H35.9
    myopic — *see also* Myopia, degenerative H44.2-
  sacroiliac joint M53.3
  senile — *see also* condition R54
  sensory R20.8
  skin R23.9
    acute, due to ultraviolet radiation L56.9
      specified NEC L56.8
    chronic, due to nonionizing radiation L57.9
      specified NEC L57.8
    cyanosis R23.0
    flushing R23.2
    pallor R23.1
    petechiae R23.3
    specified change NEC R23.8
    swelling — *see* Mass, localized
    texture R23.4
  trophic
    arm — *see* Mononeuropathy, upper limb
    leg — *see* Mononeuropathy, lower limb
  vascular I99.9
  vasomotor I73.9
  voice R49.9
    psychogenic F44.4
    specified NEC R49.8
Changing sleep-work schedule, affecting sleep G47.26
Changuinola fever A93.1
Chapping skin T69.8
Charcot-Marie-Tooth disease, paralysis or syndrome G60.0
Charcot's
  arthropathy — *see* Arthropathy, neuropathic
  cirrhosis K74.3
  disease (tabetic arthropathy) A52.16
  joint (disease) (tabetic) A52.16
    diabetic — *see* Diabetes, with, arthropathy
    syringomyelic G95.0
  syndrome (intermittent claudication) I73.9
CHARGE association Q89.8
Charley-horse (quadriceps) M62.831
  traumatic (quadriceps) S76.11-
Charlouis' disease — *see* Yaws
Cheadle's disease E54
Checking (of)
  cardiac pacemaker (battery) (electrode (s)) Z45.018
    pulse generator Z45.010
  implantable subdermal contraceptive Z30.46
  intrauterine contraceptive device Z30.431
  wound Z48.0-
    due to injury - code to Injury, by site, using appropriate seventh character for subsequent encounter
Check-up — *see* Examination
Chédiak-Higashi (-Steinbrinck) syndrome (congenital gigantism of peroxidase granules) E70.330
Cheek — *see* condition
Cheese itch B88.0
Cheese-washer's lung J67.8
Cheese-worker's lung J67.8
Cheilitis (acute) (angular) (catarrhal) (chronic) (exfoliative) (gangrenous) (glandular) (infectional) (suppurative) (ulcerative) (vesicular) K13.0
  actinic (due to sun) L56.8
    other than from sun L59.8
  candidal B37.83
Cheilodynia K13.0
Cheiloschisis — *see* Cleft, lip
Cheilosis (angular) K13.0
  with pellagra E52
  due to
    vitamin B2 (riboflavin) deficiency E53.0
Cheiromegaly M79.89

Cheiropompholyx L30.1
Cheloid — *see* Keloid
Chemical burn — *see* Corrosion, by site
Chemodectoma — *see* Paraganglioma, nonchromaffin
Chemosis, conjunctiva — *see* Edema, conjunctiva
Chemotherapy (session) (for)
  cancer Z51.11
  neoplasm Z51.11
Cherubism M27.8
Chest — *see* condition
Cheyne-Stokes breathing (respiration) R06.3
Chiari's
  disease or syndrome (hepatic vein thrombosis) I82.0
  malformation
    type I G93.5
    type II — *see* Spina bifida
  net Q24.8
Chicago disease B40.9
Chickenpox — *see* Varicella
Chiclero ulcer or sore B55.1
Chigger (infestation) B88.0
Chignon (disease) B36.8
  newborn (from vacuum extraction) (birth injury) P12.1
Chilaiditi's syndrome (subphrenic displacement, colon) Q43.3
Chilblain (s) (lupus) T69.1
Child
  custody dispute Z65.3
Childbirth — *see* Delivery
Childhood
  cerebral X-linked adrenoleukodystrophy E71.520
  period of rapid growth Z00.2
Chill (s) R68.83
  with fever R50.9
  congestive in malarial regions B54
  without fever R68.83
Chilomastigiasis A07.8
Chimera 46,XX/46,XY Q99.0
Chin — *see* condition
Chinese dysentery A03.9
Chionophobia F40.228
Chitral fever A93.1
Chlamydia, chlamydial A74.9
  cervicitis A56.09
  conjunctivitis A74.0
  cystitis A56.01
  endometritis A56.11
  epididymitis A56.19
  female
    pelvic inflammatory disease A56.11
    pelviperitonitis A56.11
  orchitis A56.19
  peritonitis A74.81
  pharyngitis A56.4
  proctitis A56.3
  psittaci (infection) A70
  salpingitis A56.11
  sexually-transmitted infection NEC A56.8
  specified NEC A74.89
  urethritis A56.01
  vulvovaginitis A56.02
Chlamydiosis — *see* Chlamydia
Chloasma (skin) (idiopathic) (symptomatic) L81.1
  eyelid H02.719
    hyperthyroid E05.90 *[H02.719]*
      with thyroid storm E05.91 *[H02.719]*
    left H02.716
      lower H02.715
      upper H02.714
    right H02.713
      lower H02.712
      upper H02.711
Chloroma C92.3-
Chlorosis D50.9
  Egyptian B76.9 *[D63.8]*
  miner's B76.9 *[D63.8]*
Chlorotic anemia D50.8
Chocolate cyst (ovary) N80.1

Choked
 disc or disk — *see* Papilledema
 on food, phlegm, or vomitus NOS — *see* Foreign body, by site
 while vomiting NOS — *see* Foreign body, by site
Chokes (resulting from bends) T70.3
Choking sensation R09.89
Cholangiectasis K83.8
Cholangiocarcinoma
 with hepatocellular carcinoma, combined C22.0
 liver C22.1
 specified site NEC — *see* Neoplasm, malignant, by site
 unspecified site C22.1
Cholangiohepatitis K83.8
 due to fluke infestation B66.1
Cholangiohepatoma C22.0
Cholangiolitis (acute) (chronic) (extrahepatic) (gangrenous) (intrahepatic) K83.09
 paratyphoidal — *see* Fever, paratyphoid
 typhoidal A01.09
Cholangioma D13.4
 malignant — *see* Cholangiocarcinoma
Cholangitis (ascending) (recurrent) (secondary) (stenosing) (suppurative) K83.09
 with calculus, bile duct — *see* Calculus, bile duct, with cholangitis
 chronic nonsuppurative destructive K74.3
 primary K83.09
  sclerosing K83.01
 sclerosing K83.09
Cholecystectasia K82.8
Cholecystitis K81.9
 with
  calculus, stones in
   bile duct (common) (hepatic) — *see* Calculus, bile duct, with cholecystitis
   cystic duct — *see* Calculus, gallbladder, with cholecystitis
   gallbladder — *see* Calculus, gallbladder, with cholecystitis
  choledocholithiasis — *see* Calculus, bile duct, with cholecystitis
  cholelithiasis — *see* Calculus, gallbladder, with cholecystitis
 gangrene of gallbladder K82.A1
 perforation of gallbladder K82.A2
 acute (emphysematous) (gangrenous) (suppurative) K81.0
  with
   calculus, stones in
    cystic duct — *see* Calculus, gallbladder, with cholecystitis, acute
    gallbladder — *see* Calculus, gallbladder, with cholecystitis, acute
   choledocholithiasis — *see* Calculus, bile duct, with cholecystitis, acute
   cholelithiasis — *see* Calculus, gallbladder, with cholecystitis, acute
  chronic cholecystitis K81.2
   with gallbladder calculus K80.12
    with obstruction K80.13
 chronic K81.1
  with acute cholecystitis K81.2
   with gallbladder calculus K80.12
    with obstruction K80.13
 emphysematous (acute) — *see* Cholecystitis, acute
 gangrenous — *see* Cholecystitis, acute
 paratyphoidal, current A01.4
 suppurative — *see* Cholecystitis, acute
 typhoidal A01.09
Cholecystolithiasis — *see* Calculus, gallbladder
Choledochitis (suppurative) K83.09
Choledocholith — *see* Calculus, bile duct

Choledocholithiasis (common duct) (hepatic duct) — *see* Calculus, bile duct
 cystic — *see* Calculus, gallbladder
 typhoidal A01.09
Cholelithiasis (cystic duct) (gallbladder) (impacted) (multiple) — *see* Calculus, gallbladder
 bile duct (common) (hepatic) — *see* Calculus, bile duct
 hepatic duct — *see* Calculus, bile duct
 specified NEC K80.80
  with obstruction K80.81
Cholemia — *see also* Jaundice
 familial (simple) (congenital) E80.4
 Gilbert's E80.4
Choleperitoneum, choleperitonitis K65.3
Cholera (Asiatic) (epidemic) (malignant) A00.9
 antimonial — *see* Poisoning, antimony
 classical A00.0
 due to Vibrio cholerae 01 A00.9
  biovar cholerae A00.0
  biovar eltor A00.1
  el tor A00.1
 el tor A00.1
Cholerine — *see* Cholera
Cholestasis NEC K83.1
 with hepatocyte injury K71.0
 due to total parenteral nutrition (TPN) K76.89
 pure K71.0
Cholesteatoma (ear) (middle) (with reaction) H71.9-
 attic H71.0-
 external ear (canal) H60.4-
 mastoid H71.2-
 postmastoidectomy cavity (recurrent) — *see* Complications, postmastoidectomy, recurrent cholesteatoma
 recurrent (postmastoidectomy) — *see* Complications, postmastoidectomy, recurrent cholesteatoma
 tympanum H71.1-
Cholesteatosis, diffuse H71.3-
Cholesteremia E78.00
Cholesterin in vitreous — *see* Deposit, crystalline
Cholesterol
 deposit
  retina H35.89
  vitreous — *see* Deposit, crystalline
 elevated (high) E78.00
  with elevated (high) triglycerides E78.2
  screening for Z13.220
 imbibition of gallbladder K82.4
Cholesterolemia (essential) (pure) E78.00
 familial E78.01
 hereditary E78.01
Cholesterolosis, cholesterosis (gallbladder) K82.4
 cerebrotendinous E75.5
Cholocolic fistula K82.3
Choluria R82.2
Chondritis M94.8X9
 auricle H61.03-
 costal (Tietze's) M94.0
 external ear H61.03-
 patella, posttraumatic — *see* Chondromalacia, patella
 pinna H61.03-
 purulent M94.8X-
 tuberculous NEC A18.02
  intervertebral A18.01
Chondroblastoma — *see also* Neoplasm, bone, benign
 malignant — *see* Neoplasm, bone, malignant
Chondrocalcinosis M11.20
 ankle M11.27-
 elbow M11.22-
 familial M11.10
  ankle M11.17-
  elbow M11.12-
  foot joint M11.17-
  hand joint M11.14-
  hip M11.15-

Chondrocalcinosis - *continued*
 familial - *continued*
  knee M11.16-
  multiple site M11.19
  shoulder M11.11-
  vertebrae M11.18
  wrist M11.13-
 foot joint M11.27-
 hand joint M11.24-
 hip M11.25-
 knee M11.26-
 multiple site M11.29
 shoulder M11.21-
 vertebrae M11.28
 specified type NEC M11.20
  ankle M11.27-
  elbow M11.22-
  foot joint M11.27-
  hand joint M11.24-
  hip M11.25-
  knee M11.26-
  multiple site M11.29
  shoulder M11.21-
  vertebrae M11.28
  wrist M11.23-
 wrist M11.23-
Chondrodermatitis nodularis helicis or anthelicis — *see* Perichondritis, ear
Chondrodysplasia Q78.9
 with hemangioma Q78.4
 calcificans congenita Q77.3
 fetalis Q77.4
 metaphyseal (Jansen's) (McKusick's) (Schmid's) Q78.8
 punctata Q77.3
Chondrodystrophy, chondrodystrophia (familial) (fetalis) (hypoplastic) Q78.9
 calcificans congenita Q77.3
 myotonic (congenital) G71.13
 punctata Q77.3
Chondroectodermal dysplasia Q77.6
Chondrogenesis imperfecta Q77.4
Chondrolysis M94.35-
Chondroma — *see also* Neoplasm, cartilage, benign
 juxtacortical — *see* Neoplasm, bone, benign
 periosteal — *see* Neoplasm, bone, benign
Chondromalacia (systemic) M94.20
 acromioclavicular joint M94.21-
 ankle M94.27-
 elbow M94.22-
 foot joint M94.27-
 glenohumeral joint M94.21-
 hand joint M94.24-
 hip M94.25-
 knee M94.26-
  patella M22.4-
 multiple sites M94.29
 patella M22.4-
 rib M94.28
 sacroiliac joint M94.259
 shoulder M94.21-
 sternoclavicular joint M94.21-
 vertebral joint M94.28
 wrist M94.23-
Chondromatosis — *see also* Neoplasm, cartilage, uncertain behavior
 internal Q78.4
Chondromyxosarcoma — *see* Neoplasm, cartilage, malignant
Chondro-osteodysplasia (Morquio-Brailsford type) E76.219
Chondro-osteodystrophy E76.29
Chondro-osteoma — *see* Neoplasm, bone, benign
Chondropathia tuberosa M94.0
Chondrosarcoma — *see* Neoplasm, cartilage, malignant
 juxtacortical — *see* Neoplasm, bone, malignant
 mesenchymal — *see* Neoplasm, connective tissue, malignant
 myxoid — *see* Neoplasm, cartilage, malignant

Chordee (nonvenereal) N48.89
  congenital Q54.4
  gonococcal A54.09
Chorditis (fibrinous) (nodosa) (tuberosa) J38.2
Chordoma — *see* Neoplasm, vertebral (column), malignant
Chorea (chronic) (gravis) (posthemiplegic) (senile) (spasmodic) G25.5
  with
    heart involvement I02.0
      active or acute (conditions in I01-) I02.0
        rheumatic I02.9
          with valvular disorder I02.0
      rheumatic heart disease (chronic) (inactive) (quiescent) - code to rheumatic heart condition involved
  drug-induced G25.4
  habit F95.8
  hereditary G10
  Huntington's G10
  hysterical F44.4
  minor I02.9
    with heart involvement I02.0
  progressive G25.5
    hereditary G10
  rheumatic (chronic) I02.9
    with heart involvement I02.0
  Sydenham's I02.9
    with heart involvement — *see* Chorea, with rheumatic heart disease
  nonrheumatic G25.5
Choreoathetosis (paroxysmal) G25.5
Chorioadenoma (destruens) D39.2
Chorioamnionitis O41.12-
Chorioangioma D26.7
Choriocarcinoma — *see* Neoplasm, malignant, by site
  combined with
    embryonal carcinoma — *see* Neoplasm, malignant, by site
    other germ cell elements — *see* Neoplasm, malignant, by site
    teratoma — *see* Neoplasm, malignant, by site
  specified site — *see* Neoplasm, malignant, by site
  unspecified site
    female C58
    male C62.90
Chorioencephalitis (acute) (lymphocytic) (serous) A87.2
Chorioepithelioma — *see* Choriocarcinoma
Choriomeningitis (acute) (lymphocytic) (serous) A87.2
Chorionepithelioma — *see* Choriocarcinoma
Chorioretinitis — *see also* Inflammation, chorioretinal
  disseminated — *see also* Inflammation, chorioretinal, disseminated
    in neurosyphilis A52.19
  Egyptian B76.9 *[D63.8]*
  focal — *see also* Inflammation, chorioretinal, focal
  histoplasmic B39.9 *[H32]*
  in (due to)
    histoplasmosis B39.9 *[H32]*
    syphilis (secondary) A51.43
      late A52.71
    toxoplasmosis (acquired) B58.01
      congenital (active) P37.1 *[H32]*
    tuberculosis A18.53
  juxtapapillary, juxtapapillaris — *see* Inflammation, chorioretinal, focal, juxtapapillary
  leprous A30.9 *[H32]*
  miner's B76.9 *[D63.8]*
  progressive myopia (degeneration) — *see also* Myopia, degenerative H44.2-
  syphilitic (secondary) A51.43
    congenital (early) A50.01 *[H32]*
      late A50.32
    late A52.71
  tuberculous A18.53
Chorioretinopathy, central serous H35.71-

Choroid — *see* condition
Choroideremia H31.21
Choroiditis — *see* Chorioretinitis
Choroidopathy — *see* Disorder, choroid
Choroidoretinitis — *see* Chorioretinitis
Choroidoretinopathy, central serous — *see* Chorioretinopathy, central serous
Christian-Weber disease M35.6
Christmas disease D67
Chromaffinoma — *see also* Neoplasm, benign, by site
  malignant — *see* Neoplasm, malignant, by site
Chromatopsia — *see* Deficiency, color vision
Chromhidrosis, chromidrosis L75.1
Chromoblastomycosis — *see* Chromomycosis
Chromoconversion R82.91
Chromomycosis B43.9
  brain abscess B43.1
  cerebral B43.1
  cutaneous B43.0
  skin B43.0
  specified NEC B43.8
  subcutaneous abscess or cyst B43.2
Chromophytosis B36.0
Chromosome — *see* condition by chromosome involved
  D (1) — *see* condition, chromosome 13
  E (3) — *see* condition, chromosome 18
  G — *see* condition, chromosome 21
Chromotrichomycosis B36.8
Chronic — *see* condition
  fracture — *see* Fracture, pathological
Churg-Strauss syndrome M30.1
Chyle cyst, mesentery I89.8
Chylocele (nonfilarial) I89.8
  filarial — *see also* Infestation, filarial B74.9 *[N51]*
  tunica vaginalis N50.89
    filarial — *see also* Infestation, filarial B74.9 *[N51]*
Chylomicronemia (fasting) (with hyperprebetalipoproteinemia) E78.3
Chylopericardium I31.3
  acute I30.9
Chylothorax (nonfilarial) I89.8
  filarial — *see also* Infestation, filarial B74.9 *[J91.8]*
Chylous — *see* condition
Chyluria (nonfilarial) R82.0
  due to
    bilharziasis B65.0
    Brugia (malayi) B74.1
      timori B74.2
    schistosomiasis (bilharziasis) B65.0
    Wuchereria (bancrofti) B74.0
  filarial — *see* Infestation, filarial
Cicatricial (deformity) — *see* Cicatrix
Cicatrix (adherent) (contracted) (painful) (vicious) — *see also* Scar L90.5
  adenoid (and tonsil) J35.8
  alveolar process M26.79
  anus K62.89
  auricle — *see* Disorder, pinna, specified type NEC
  bile duct (common) (hepatic) K83.8
  bladder N32.89
  bone — *see* Disorder, bone, specified type NEC
  brain G93.89
  cervix (postoperative) (postpartal) N88.1
  common duct K83.8
  cornea H17.9
    tuberculous A18.59
  duodenum (bulb) , obstructive K31.5
  esophagus K22.2
  eyelid — *see* Disorder, eyelid function
  hypopharynx J39.2
  lacrimal passages — *see* Obstruction, lacrimal
  larynx J38.7
  lung J98.4
  middle ear — *see* subcategory H74.8
  mouth K13.79
  muscle M62.89

Cicatrix (adherent) (contracted) (painful) (vicious) - *continued*
  muscle - *continued*
    with contracture — *see* Contraction, muscle NEC
  nasopharynx J39.2
  palate (soft) K13.79
  penis N48.89
  pharynx J39.2
  prostate N42.89
  rectum K62.89
  retina — *see* Scar, chorioretinal
  semilunar cartilage — *see* Derangement, meniscus
  seminal vesicle N50.89
  skin L90.5
    infected L08.89
    postinfective L90.5
    tuberculous B90.8
  specified site NEC L90.5
  throat J39.2
  tongue K14.8
  tonsil (and adenoid) J35.8
  trachea J39.8
  tuberculous NEC B90.9
  urethra N36.8
  uterus N85.8
  vagina N89.8
    postoperative N99.2
  vocal cord J38.3
  wrist, constricting (annular) L90.5
CIDP (chronic inflammatory demyelinating polyneuropathy) G61.81
CIN — *see* Neoplasia, intraepithelial, cervix
CINCA (chronic infantile neurological, cutaneous and articular syndrome) M04.2
Cinchonism — *see* Deafness, ototoxic
  correct substance properly administered — *see* Table of Drugs and Chemicals, by drug, adverse effect
  overdose or wrong substance given or taken — *see* Table of Drugs and Chemicals, by drug, poisoning
Circle of Willis — *see* condition
Circular — *see* condition
Circulating anticoagulants — *see also* - Disorder, hemorrhagic D68.318
  due to drugs — *see also* - Disorder, hemorrhagic D68.32
  following childbirth O72.3
Circulation
  collateral, any site I99.8
  defective (lower extremity) I99.9
    congenital Q28.9
  embryonic Q28.9
  failure (peripheral) R57.9
    newborn P29.89
  fetal, persistent P29.38
  heart, incomplete Q28.9
Circulatory system — *see* condition
Circulus senilis (cornea) — *see* Degeneration, cornea, senile
Circumcision (in absence of medical indication) (ritual) (routine) Z41.2
Circumscribed — *see* condition
Circumvallate placenta O43.11-
Cirrhosis, cirrhotic (hepatic) (liver) K74.60
  alcoholic K70.30
    with ascites K70.31
  atrophic — *see* Cirrhosis, liver
  Baumgarten-Cruveilhier K74.69
  biliary (cholangiolitic) (cholangitic) (hypertrophic) (obstructive) (pericholangiolitic) K74.5
    due to
      Clonorchiasis B66.1
      flukes B66.3
    primary K74.3
    secondary K74.4
  cardiac (of liver) K76.1
  Charcot's K74.3
  cholangiolitic, cholangitic, cholostatic (primary) K74.3
  congestive K76.1

Cirrhosis, cirrhotic (hepatic) (liver) - *continued*
 Cruveilhier-Baumgarten K74.69
 cryptogenic (liver) K74.69
 due to
  hepatolenticular degeneration E83.01
  Wilson's disease E83.01
  xanthomatosis E78.2
 fatty K76.0
  alcoholic K70.0
 Hanot's (hypertrophic) K74.3
 hepatic — *see* Cirrhosis, liver
 hypertrophic K74.3
 Indian childhood K74.69
 kidney — *see* Sclerosis, renal
 Laennec's K70.30
  with ascites K70.31
  alcoholic K70.30
   with ascites K70.31
  nonalcoholic K74.69
 liver K74.60
  alcoholic K70.30
   with ascites K70.31
  fatty K70.0
  congenital P78.81
  syphilitic A52.74
 lung (chronic) J84.10
 macronodular K74.69
  alcoholic K70.30
   with ascites K70.31
 micronodular K74.69
  alcoholic K70.30
   with ascites K70.31
 mixed type K74.69
 monolobular K74.3
 nephritis — *see* Sclerosis, renal
 nutritional K74.69
  alcoholic K70.30
   with ascites K70.31
 obstructive — *see* Cirrhosis, biliary
 ovarian N83.8
 pancreas (duct) K86.89
 pigmentary E83.110
 portal K74.69
  alcoholic K70.30
   with ascites K70.31
 postnecrotic K74.69
  alcoholic K70.30
   with ascites K70.31
 pulmonary J84.10
 renal — *see* Sclerosis, renal
 spleen D73.2
 stasis K76.1
 Todd's K74.3
 unilobar K74.3
 xanthomatous (biliary) K74.5
  due to xanthomatosis (familial) (metabolic) (primary) E78.2
Cistern, subarachnoid R93.0
Citrullinemia E72.23
Citrullinuria E72.23
Civatte's disease or poikiloderma L57.3
Clam digger's itch B65.3
Clammy skin R23.1
Clap — *see* Gonorrhea
Clarke-Hadfield syndrome (pancreatic infantilism) K86.89
Clark's paralysis G80.9
Clastothrix L67.8
Claude Bernard-Horner syndrome G90.2
 traumatic — *see* Injury, nerve, cervical sympathetic
Claude's disease or syndrome G46.3
Claudicatio venosa intermittens I87.8
Claudication (intermittent) I73.9
 cerebral (artery) G45.9
 spinal cord (arteriosclerotic) G95.19
  syphilitic A52.09
 venous (axillary) I87.8
Claustrophobia F40.240
Clavus (infected) L84
Clawfoot (congenital) Q66.89
 acquired — *see* Deformity, limb, clawfoot

Clawhand (acquired) — *see also* Deformity, limb, clawhand
 congenital Q68.1
Clawtoe (congenital) Q66.89
 acquired — *see* Deformity, toe, specified NEC
Clay eating — *see* Pica
Cleansing of artificial opening — *see* Attention to, artificial, opening
Cleft (congenital) — *see also* Imperfect, closure
 alveolar process M26.79
 branchial (persistent) Q18.2
  cyst Q18.0
  fistula Q18.0
  sinus Q18.0
 cricoid cartilage, posterior Q31.8
 foot Q72.7
 hand Q71.6
 lip (unilateral) Q36.9
  with cleft palate Q37.9
   hard Q37.1
    with soft Q37.5
   soft Q37.3
    with hard Q37.5
  bilateral Q36.0
   with cleft palate Q37.8
    hard Q37.0
     with soft Q37.4
    soft Q37.2
     with hard Q37.4
  median Q36.1
 nose Q30.2
 palate Q35.9
  with cleft lip (unilateral) Q37.9
   bilateral Q37.8
  hard Q35.1
   with
    cleft lip (unilateral) Q37.1
     bilateral Q37.0
    soft Q35.5
     with cleft lip (unilateral) Q37.5
      bilateral Q37.4
  medial Q35.5
  soft Q35.3
   with
    cleft lip (unilateral) Q37.3
     bilateral Q37.2
    hard Q35.5
     with cleft lip (unilateral) Q37.5
      bilateral Q37.4
 penis Q55.69
 scrotum Q55.29
 thyroid cartilage Q31.8
 uvula Q35.7
Cleidocranial dysostosis Q74.0
Cleptomania F63.2
Clicking hip (newborn) R29.4
Climacteric (female) — *see also* Menopause
 arthritis (any site) NEC — *see* Arthritis, specified form NEC
 depression (single episode) F32.89
  recurrent episode F33.8
 melancholia (single episode) F32.89
  recurrent episode F33.8
 male (symptoms) (syndrome) NEC N50.89
 paranoid state F22
 polyarthritis NEC — *see* Arthritis, specified form NEC
 symptoms (female) N95.1
Clinical research investigation (clinical trial) (control subject) (normal comparison) (participant) Z00.6
Clitoris — *see* condition
Cloaca (persistent) Q43.7
Clonorchiasis, clonorchis infection (liver) B66.1
Clonus R25.8
Closed bite M26.29
Clostridium (C.) perfringens, as cause of disease classified elsewhere B96.7
Closure
 congenital, nose Q30.0
 cranial sutures, premature Q75.0

Closure - *continued*
 defective or imperfect NEC — *see* Imperfect, closure
 fistula, delayed — *see* Fistula
 foramen ovale, imperfect Q21.1
 hymen N89.6
 interauricular septum, defective Q21.1
 interventricular septum, defective Q21.0
 lacrimal duct — *see also* Stenosis, lacrimal, duct
  congenital Q10.5
 nose (congenital) Q30.0
  acquired M95.0
 of artificial opening — *see* Attention to, artificial, opening
 primary angle, without glaucoma damage H40.06-
 vagina N89.5
 valve — *see* Endocarditis
 vulva N90.5
Clot (blood) — *see also* Embolism
 artery (obstruction) (occlusion) — *see* Embolism
 bladder N32.89
 brain (intradural or extradural) — *see* Occlusion, artery, cerebral
 circulation I74.9
 heart — *see also* Infarct, myocardium
  not resulting in infarction I51.3
 vein — *see* Thrombosis
Clouded state R40.1
 epileptic — *see* Epilepsy, specified NEC
 paroxysmal — *see* Epilepsy, specified NEC
Cloudy antrum, antra J32.0
Clouston's (hidrotic) ectodermal dysplasia Q82.4
Clubbed nail
 pachydermoperiostosis M89.40 *[L62]*
Clubbing of finger (s) (nails) R68.3
Clubfinger R68.3
 congenital Q68.1
Clubfoot (congenital) Q66.89
 acquired — *see* Deformity, limb, clubfoot
 equinovarus Q66.0-
 paralytic — *see* Deformity, limb, clubfoot
Clubhand (congenital) (radial) Q71.4-
 acquired — *see* Deformity, limb, clubhand
Clubnail R68.3
 congenital Q84.6
Clump, kidney Q63.1
Clumsiness, clumsy child syndrome F82
Cluttering F80.81
Clutton's joints A50.51 *[M12.80]*
Coagulation, intravascular (diffuse) (disseminated) — *see also* Defibrination syndrome
 complicating abortion — *see* Abortion, by type, complicated by, intravascular coagulation
 following ectopic or molar pregnancy O08.1
Coagulopathy — *see also* Defect, coagulation
 consumption D65
 intravascular D65
 newborn P60
Coalition
 calcaneo-scaphoid Q66.89
 tarsal Q66.89
Coalminer's
 elbow — *see* Bursitis, elbow, olecranon
 lung or pneumoconiosis J60
Coalworker's lung or pneumoconiosis J60
Coarctation
 aorta (preductal) (postductal) Q25.1
 pulmonary artery Q25.71
Coated tongue K14.3
Coats' disease (exudative retinopathy) — *see* Retinopathy, exudative
Cocaine-induced
 anxiety disorder F14.980
 bipolar and related disorder F14.94
 depressive disorder F14.94
 obsessive-compulsive and related disorder F14.988
 psychotic disorder F14.959
 sleep disorder F14.982

Cocaine-induced - *continued*
  sexual dysfunction F14.981
Cocainism — *see* Disorder, cocaine use
Coccidioidomycosis B38.9
  cutaneous B38.3
  disseminated B38.7
  generalized B38.7
  meninges B38.4
  prostate B38.81
  pulmonary B38.2
    acute B38.0
    chronic B38.1
  skin B38.3
  specified NEC B38.89
Coccidioidosis — *see* Coccidioidomycosis
Coccidiosis (intestinal) A07.3
Coccydynia, coccygodynia M53.3
Coccyx — *see* condition
Cochin-China diarrhea K90.1
Cockayne's syndrome Q87.19
Cocked up toe — *see* Deformity, toe, specified
  NEC
Cock's peculiar tumor L72.3
Codman's tumor — *see* Neoplasm, bone,
  benign
Coenurosis B71.8
Coffee-worker's lung J67.8
Cogan's syndrome H16.32-
  oculomotor apraxia H51.8
Coitus, painful (female) N94.10
  male N53.12
  psychogenic F52.6
Cold J00
  with influenza, flu, or grippe — *see*
    Influenza, with, respiratory
    manifestations NEC
  agglutinin disease or hemoglobinuria
    (chronic) D59.1
  bronchial — *see* Bronchitis
  chest — *see* Bronchitis
  common (head) J00
  effects of T69.9
    specified effect NEC T69.8
  excessive, effects of T69.9
    specified effect NEC T69.8
  exhaustion from T69.8
  exposure to T69.9
    specified effect NEC T69.8
  head J00
  injury syndrome (newborn) P80.0
  on lung — *see* Bronchitis
  rose J30.1
  sensitivity, auto-immune D59.1
  symptoms J00
  virus J00
Coldsore B00.1
Colibacillosis A49.8
  as the cause of other disease — *see also*
    Escherichia coli B96.20
  generalized A41.50
Colic (bilious) (infantile) (intestinal)
  (recurrent) (spasmodic) R10.83
  abdomen R10.83
    psychogenic F45.8
  appendix, appendicular K38.8
  bile duct — *see* Calculus, bile duct
  biliary — *see* Calculus, bile duct
  common duct — *see* Calculus, bile duct
  cystic duct — *see* Calculus, gallbladder
  Devonshire NEC — *see* Poisoning, lead
  gallbladder — *see* Calculus, gallbladder
  gallstone — *see* Calculus, gallbladder
    gallbladder or cystic duct — *see* Calculus,
      gallbladder
  hepatic (duct) — *see* Calculus, bile duct
  hysterical F45.8
  kidney N23
  lead NEC — *see* Poisoning, lead
  mucous K58.9
    with diarrhea K58.0
    psychogenic F54
  nephritic N23
  painter's NEC — *see* Poisoning, lead
  pancreas K86.89
  psychogenic F45.8

Colic (bilious) (infantile) (intestinal)
(recurrent) (spasmodic) - *continued*
  renal N23
  saturnine NEC — *see* Poisoning, lead
  ureter N23
  urethral N36.8
    due to calculus N21.1
  uterus NEC N94.89
    menstrual — *see* Dysmenorrhea
  worm NOS B83.9
Colicystitis — *see* Cystitis
Colitis (acute) (catarrhal) (chronic)
  (noninfective) (hemorrhagic) — *see also*
    Enteritis K52.9
  allergic K52.29
    with
      food protein-induced enterocolitis
        syndrome K52.21
      proctocolitis K52.82
  amebic (acute) — *see also* Amebiasis A06.0
    nondysenteric A06.2
  anthrax A22.2
  bacillary — *see* Infection, Shigella
  balantidial A07.0
  Clostridium difficile
    not specified as recurrent A04.72
    recurrent A04.71
  coccidial A07.3
  collagenous K52.831
  cystica superficialis K52.89
  dietary counseling and surveillance
    (for) Z71.3
  dietetic — *see also* Colitis, allergic K52.29
  drug-induced K52.1
  due to radiation K52.0
  eosinophilic K52.82
  food hypersensitivity — *see also* Colitis,
    allergic K52.29
  giardial A07.1
  granulomatous — *see* Enteritis, regional,
    large intestine
  indeterminate, so stated K52.3
  infectious — *see* Enteritis, infectious
  ischemic K55.9
    acute (subacute) — *see also* Ischemia,
      intestine, acute K55.039
    chronic K55.1
    due to mesenteric artery
      insufficiency K55.1
    fulminant (acute) — *see also* Ischemia,
      intestine, acute K55.039
  left sided K51.50
    with
      abscess K51.514
      complication K51.519
        specified NEC K51.518
      fistula K51.513
      obstruction K51.512
      rectal bleeding K51.511
  lymphocytic K52.832
  membranous
    psychogenic F54
  microscopic K52.839
    specified NEC K52.838
  mucous — *see* Syndrome, irritable, bowel
    psychogenic F54
  noninfective K52.9
    specified NEC K52.89
  polyposa — *see* Polyp, colon, inflammatory
  protozoal A07.9
  pseudomembranous
    not specified as recurrent A04.72
    recurrent A04.71
  pseudomucinous — *see* Syndrome, irritable,
    bowel
  regional — *see* Enteritis, regional, large
    intestine
    infectious A09
  segmental — *see* Enteritis, regional, large
    intestine
  septic — *see* Enteritis, infectious
  spastic K58.9
    with diarrhea K58.0
    psychogenic F54
  staphylococcal A04.8

Colitis (acute) (catarrhal) (chronic)
  (noninfective) (hemorrhagic) - *continued*
  staphylococcal - *continued*
    foodborne A05.0
  subacute ischemic — *see also* Ischemia,
    intestine, acute K55.039
  thromboulcerative — *see also* Ischemia,
    intestine, acute K55.039
  toxic NEC K52.1
    due to Clostridium difficile
      not specified as recurrent A04.72
      recurrent A04.71
  transmural — *see* Enteritis, regional, large
    intestine
  trichomonal A07.8
  tuberculous (ulcerative) A18.32
  ulcerative (chronic) K51.90
    with
      complication K51.919
        abscess K51.914
        fistula K51.913
        obstruction K51.912
        rectal bleeding K51.911
        specified complication NEC K51.918
    enterocolitis — *see* Enterocolitis,
      ulcerative
    ileocolitis — *see* Ileocolitis, ulcerative
    mucosal proctocolitis — *see* Proctocolitis,
      mucosal
    proctitis — *see* Proctitis, ulcerative
    pseudopolyposis — *see* Polyp, colon,
      inflammatory
    psychogenic F54
    rectosigmoiditis — *see* Rectosigmoiditis,
      ulcerative
    specified type NEC K51.80
      with
        complication K51.819
          abscess K51.814
          fistula K51.813
          obstruction K51.812
          rectal bleeding K51.811
          specified complication
            NEC K51.818
Collagenosis, collagen disease (nonvascular)
  (vascular) M35.9
  cardiovascular I42.8
  reactive perforating L87.1
  specified NEC M35.8
Collapse R55
  adrenal E27.2
  cardiorespiratory R57.0
  cardiovascular R57.0
    newborn P29.89
  circulatory (peripheral) R57.9
    during or after labor and delivery O75.1
    following ectopic or molar
      pregnancy O08.3
    newborn P29.89
  during or
    after labor and delivery O75.1
    resulting from a procedure, not elsewhere
      classified T81.10
  external ear canal — *see* Stenosis, external
    ear canal
  general R55
  heart — *see* Disease, heart
  heat T67.1
  hysterical F44.89
  labyrinth, membranous (congenital) Q16.5
  lung (massive) — *see also* Atelectasis J98.19
    pressure due to anesthesia (general) (local)
      or other sedation T88.2
      during labor and delivery O74.1
      in pregnancy O29.02-
      postpartum, puerperal O89.09
  myocardial — *see* Disease, heart
  nervous F48.8
  neurocirculatory F45.8
  nose M95.0
  postoperative T81.10
  pulmonary — *see also* Atelectasis J98.19
    newborn — *see* Atelectasis
  trachea J39.8
  tracheobronchial J98.09

Collapse - *continued*
valvular — *see* Endocarditis
vascular (peripheral) R57.9
during or after labor and delivery O75.1
following ectopic or molar
pregnancy O08.3
newborn P29.89
vertebra M48.50-
cervical region M48.52-
cervicothoracic region M48.53-
in (due to)
metastasis — *see* Collapse, vertebra, in,
specified disease NEC
osteoporosis — *see also*
Osteoporosis M80.88
cervical region M80.88
cervicothoracic region M80.88
lumbar region M80.88
lumbosacral region M80.88
multiple sites M80.88
occipito-atlanto-axial region M80.88
sacrococcygeal region M80.88
thoracic region M80.88
thoracolumbar region M80.88
specified disease NEC M48.50-
cervical region M48.52-
cervicothoracic region M48.53-
lumbar region M48.56-
lumbosacral region M48.57-
occipito-atlanto-axial region M48.51-
sacrococcygeal region M48.58-
thoracic region M48.54-
thoracolumbar region M48.55-
lumbar region M48.56-
lumbosacral region M48.57-
occipito-atlanto-axial region M48.51-
sacrococcygeal region M48.58-
thoracic region M48.54-
thoracolumbar region M48.55-
Collateral — *see also* condition
circulation (venous) I87.8
dilation, veins I87.8
Colles' fracture S52.53-
Collet (-Sicard) syndrome G52.7
Collier's asthma or lung J60
Collodion baby Q80.2
Colloid nodule (of thyroid) (cystic) E04.1
Coloboma (iris) Q13.0
eyelid Q10.3
fundus Q14.8
lens Q12.2
optic disc (congenital) Q14.2
acquired H47.31-
Coloenteritis — *see* Enteritis
Colon — *see* condition
Colonization
MRSA (Methicillin resistant Staphylococcus aureus) Z22.322
MSSA (Methicillin susceptible Staphylococcus aureus) Z22.321
status — *see* Carrier (suspected) of
Coloptosis K63.4
Color blindness — *see* Deficiency, color vision
Colostomy
attention to Z43.3
fitting or adjustment Z46.89
malfunctioning K94.03
status Z93.3
Colpitis (acute) — *see* Vaginitis
Colpocele N81.5
Colpocystitis — *see* Vaginitis
Colpospasm N94.2
Column, spinal, vertebral — *see* condition
Coma R40.20
with
motor response (none) R40.231
abnormal R40.233
abnormal extensor posturing to pain or noxious stimuli (< 2 years of age) R40.232
abnormal flexure posturing to pain or noxious stimuli (0-5 years of age) R40.233
extension R40.232

Coma - *continued*
with - *continued*
motor response (none) - *continued*
extensor posturing to pain or noxious stimuli (2-5 years of age) R40.232
flexion/decorticate posturing (< 2 years of age) R40.233
flexion withdrawal R40.234
localizes pain (2-5 years of age) R40.235
normal or spontaneous movement (< 2 years of age) R40.236
obeys commands (2-5 years of age) R40.236
score of
1 R40.231
2 R40.232
3 R40.233
4 R40.234
5 R40.235
6 R40.236
withdraws from pain or noxious stimuli (0-5 years of age) R40.234
withdraws to touch (< 2 years of age) R40.235
opening of eyes (never) R40.211
in response to
pain R40.212
sound R40.213
score of
1 R40.211
2 R40.212
3 R40.213
4 R40.214
spontaneous R40.214
verbal response (none) R40.221
confused conversation R40.224
cooing or babbling or crying appropriately (< 2 years of age) R40.225
inappropriate crying or screaming (< 2 years of age) R40.223
inappropriate words R40.223
inappropriate words (2-5 years of age) R40.224
incomprehensible sounds (2-5 years of age) R40.222
incomprehensible words R40.222
irritable cries (< 2 years of age) R40.224
moans/grunts to pain; restless (< 2 years old) R40.222
oriented R40.225
score of
1 R40.221
2 R40.222
3 R40.223
4 R40.224
5 R40.225
screaming (2-5 years of age) R40.223
uses appropriate words (2- 5 years of age) R40.225
eclamptic — *see* Eclampsia
epileptic — *see* Epilepsy
Glasgow, scale score — *see* Glasgow coma scale
hepatic — *see* Failure, hepatic, by type, with coma
hyperglycemic (diabetic) — *see* Diabetes, by type, with hyperosmolarity, with coma
hyperosmolar (diabetic) — *see* Diabetes, by type, with hyperosmolarity, with coma
hypoglycemic (diabetic) — *see* Diabetes, by type, with hypoglycemia, with coma
nondiabetic E15
in diabetes — *see* Diabetes, coma
insulin-induced — *see* Coma, hypoglycemic
ketoacidotic (diabetic) — *see* Diabetes, by type, with ketoacidosis, with coma
myxedematous E03.5
newborn P91.5
persistent vegetative state R40.3
specified NEC, without documented Glasgow coma scale score, or with partial Glasgow coma scale score reported R40.244
Comatose — *see* Coma

Combat fatigue F43.0
Combined — *see* condition
Comedo, comedones (giant) L70.0
Comedocarcinoma — *see also* Neoplasm, breast, malignant
noninfiltrating
breast D05.8-
specified site — *see* Neoplasm, in situ, by site
unspecified site D05.8-
Comedomastitis — *see* Ectasia, mammary duct
Comminuted fracture - code as Fracture, closed
Common
arterial trunk Q20.0
atrioventricular canal Q21.2
atrium Q21.1
cold (head) J00
truncus (arteriosus) Q20.0
variable immunodeficiency — *see* Immunodeficiency, common variable
ventricle Q20.4
Commotio, commotion (current)
brain — *see* Injury, intracranial, concussion
cerebri — *see* Injury, intracranial, concussion
retinae S05.8X-
spinal cord — *see* Injury, spinal cord, by region
spinalis — *see* Injury, spinal cord, by region
Communication
between
base of aorta and pulmonary artery Q21.4
left ventricle and right atrium Q20.5
pericardial sac and pleural sac Q34.8
pulmonary artery and pulmonary vein, congenital Q25.72
congenital between uterus and digestive or urinary tract Q51.7
Compartment syndrome (deep) (posterior) (traumatic) T79.A0
abdomen T79.A3
lower extremity (hip, buttock, thigh, leg, foot, toes) T79.A2
nontraumatic
abdomen M79.A3
lower extremity (hip, buttock, thigh, leg, foot, toes) M79.A2-
specified site NEC M79.A9
upper extremity (shoulder, arm, forearm, wrist, hand, fingers) M79.A1-
specified site NEC T79.A9
upper extremity (shoulder, arm, forearm, wrist, hand, fingers) T79.A1
Compensation
failure — *see* Disease, heart
neurosis, psychoneurosis — *see* Disorder, factitious
Complaint — *see also* Disease
bowel, functional K59.9
psychogenic F45.8
intestine, functional K59.9
psychogenic F45.8
kidney — *see* Disease, renal
miners' J60
Complete — *see* condition
Complex
Addison-Schilder E71.528
cardiorenal — *see* Hypertension, cardiorenal
Costen's M26.69
disseminated mycobacterium avium-intracellulare (DMAC) A31.2
Eisenmenger's (ventricular septal defect) I27.83
hypersexual F52.8
jumped process, spine — *see* Dislocation, vertebra
primary, tuberculous A15.7
Schilder-Addison E71.528
subluxation (vertebral) M99.19
abdomen M99.19
acromioclavicular M99.17
cervical region M99.11
cervicothoracic M99.11
costochondral M99.18

Complex - *continued*
  subluxation (vertebral) - *continued*
    costovertebral M99.18
    head region M99.10
    hip M99.15
    lower extremity M99.16
    lumbar region M99.13
    lumbosacral M99.13
    occipitocervical M99.10
    pelvic region M99.15
    pubic M99.15
    rib cage M99.18
    sacral region M99.14
    sacrococcygeal M99.14
    sacroiliac M99.14
    specified NEC M99.19
    sternochondral M99.18
    sternoclavicular M99.17
    thoracic region M99.12
    thoracolumbar M99.12
    upper extremity M99.17
  Taussig-Bing (transposition, aorta and overriding pulmonary artery) Q20.1

Complication (s) (from) (of)
  accidental puncture or laceration during a procedure (of) — *see* Complications, intraoperative (intraprocedural), puncture or laceration
  amputation stump (surgical) (late) NEC T87.9
    dehiscence T87.81
    infection or inflammation T87.40
      lower limb T87.4-
      upper limb T87.4-
    necrosis T87.50
      lower limb T87.5-
      upper limb T87.5-
    neuroma T87.30
      lower limb T87.3-
      upper limb T87.3-
    specified type NEC T87.89
  anastomosis (and bypass) — *see also* Complications, prosthetic device or implant
    intestinal (internal) NEC K91.89
      involving urinary tract N99.89
    urinary tract (involving intestinal tract) N99.89
    vascular — *see* Complications, cardiovascular device or implant
  anesthesia, anesthetic — *see also* Anesthesia, complication T88.59
    brain, postpartum, puerperal O89.2
    cardiac
      in
        labor and delivery O74.2
        pregnancy O29.19-
      postpartum, puerperal O89.1
    central nervous system
      in
        labor and delivery O74.3
        pregnancy O29.29-
      postpartum, puerperal O89.2
    difficult or failed intubation T88.4
      in pregnancy O29.6-
    failed sedation (conscious) (moderate) during procedure T88.52
    general, unintended awareness during procedure T88.53
    hyperthermia, malignant T88.3
    hypothermia T88.51
    intubation failure T88.4
    malignant hyperthermia T88.3
    pulmonary
      in
        labor and delivery O74.1
        pregnancy NEC O29.09-
      postpartum, puerperal O89.09
    shock T88.2
    spinal and epidural
      in
        labor and delivery NEC O74.6
          headache O74.5
        pregnancy NEC O29.5X-
      postpartum, puerperal NEC O89.5

Complication (s) (from) (of) - *continued*
  anesthesia, anesthetic - *continued*
    spinal and epidural - *continued*
      postpartum, puerperal NEC - *continued*
        headache O89.4
    unintended awareness under general anesthesia during procedure T88.53
  anti-reflux device — *see* Complications, esophageal anti-reflux device
  aortic (bifurcation) graft — *see* Complications, graft, vascular
  aortocoronary (bypass) graft — *see* Complications, coronary artery (bypass) graft
  aortofemoral (bypass) graft — *see* Complications, extremity artery (bypass) graft
  arteriovenous
    fistula, surgically created T82.9
      embolism T82.818
      fibrosis T82.828
      hemorrhage T82.838
      infection or inflammation T82.7
      mechanical
        breakdown T82.510
        displacement T82.520
        leakage T82.530
        malposition T82.520
        obstruction T82.590
        perforation T82.590
        protrusion T82.590
      pain T82.848
      specified type NEC T82.898
      stenosis T82.858
      thrombosis T82.868
    shunt, surgically created T82.9
      embolism T82.818
      fibrosis T82.828
      hemorrhage T82.838
      infection or inflammation T82.7
      mechanical
        breakdown T82.511
        displacement T82.521
        leakage T82.531
        malposition T82.521
        obstruction T82.591
        perforation T82.591
        protrusion T82.591
      pain T82.848
      specified type NEC T82.898
      stenosis T82.858
      thrombosis T82.868
  arthroplasty — *see* Complications, joint prosthesis
  artificial
    fertilization or insemination N98.9
      attempted introduction (of)
        embryo in embryo transfer N98.3
        ovum following in vitro fertilization N98.2
      hyperstimulation of ovaries N98.1
      infection N98.0
      specified NEC N98.8
    heart T82.9
      embolism T82.817
      fibrosis T82.827
      hemorrhage T82.837
      infection or inflammation T82.7
      mechanical
        breakdown T82.512
        displacement T82.522
        leakage T82.532
        malposition T82.522
        obstruction T82.592
        perforation T82.592
        protrusion T82.592
      pain T82.847
      specified type NEC T82.897
      stenosis T82.857
      thrombosis T82.867
    opening
      cecostomy — *see* Complications, colostomy
      colostomy — *see* Complications, colostomy

Complication (s) (from) (of) - *continued*
  artificial - *continued*
    opening - *continued*
      cystostomy — *see* Complications, cystostomy
      enterostomy — *see* Complications, enterostomy
      gastrostomy — *see* Complications, gastrostomy
      ileostomy — *see* Complications, enterostomy
      jejunostomy — *see* Complications, enterostomy
      nephrostomy — *see* Complications, stoma, urinary tract
      tracheostomy — *see* Complications, tracheostomy
      ureterostomy — *see* Complications, stoma, urinary tract
      urethrostomy — *see* Complications, stoma, urinary tract
  balloon implant or device
    gastrointestinal T85.9
      embolism T85.818
      fibrosis T85.828
      hemorrhage T85.838
      infection and inflammation T85.79
      pain T85.848
      specified type NEC T85.898
      stenosis T85.858
      thrombosis T85.868
    vascular (counterpulsation) T82.9
      embolism T82.818
      fibrosis T82.828
      hemorrhage T82.838
      infection or inflammation T82.7
      mechanical
        breakdown T82.513
        displacement T82.523
        leakage T82.533
        malposition T82.523
        obstruction T82.593
        perforation T82.593
        protrusion T82.593
      pain T82.848
      specified type NEC T82.898
      stenosis T82.858
      thrombosis T82.868
  bariatric procedure
    gastric band procedure K95.09
      infection K95.01
    specified procedure NEC K95.89
      infection K95.81
  bile duct implant (prosthetic) T85.9
    embolism T85.818
    fibrosis T85.828
    hemorrhage T85.838
    infection and inflammation T85.79
    mechanical
      breakdown T85.510
      displacement T85.520
      malfunction T85.510
      malposition T85.520
      obstruction T85.590
      perforation T85.590
      protrusion T85.590
      specified NEC T85.590
    pain T85.848
    specified type NEC T85.898
    stenosis T85.858
    thrombosis T85.868
  bladder device (auxiliary) — *see* Complications, genitourinary, device or implant, urinary system
  bleeding (postoperative) — *see* Complication, postoperative, hemorrhage
    intraoperative — *see* Complication, intraoperative, hemorrhage
  blood vessel graft — *see* Complications, graft, vascular
  bone
    device NEC T84.9
      embolism T84.81
      fibrosis T84.82

Complication (s) (from) (of) - *continued*
   bone - *continued*
     device NEC - *continued*
      hemorrhage T84.83
      infection or inflammation T84.7
      mechanical
       breakdown T84.318
       displacement T84.328
       malposition T84.328
       obstruction T84.398
       perforation T84.398
       protrusion T84.398
      pain T84.84
      specified type NEC T84.89
      stenosis T84.85
      thrombosis T84.86
     graft — *see* Complications, graft, bone
     growth stimulator (electrode) — *see*
       Complications, electronic stimulator
       device, bone
     marrow transplant — *see* Complications,
       transplant, bone, marrow
   brain neurostimulator (electrode) — *see*
     Complications, electronic stimulator
     device, brain
   breast implant (prosthetic) T85.9
     capsular contracture T85.44
     embolism T85.818
     fibrosis T85.828
     hemorrhage T85.838
     infection and inflammation T85.79
     mechanical
      breakdown T85.41
      displacement T85.42
      leakage T85.43
      malposition T85.42
      obstruction T85.49
      perforation T85.49
      protrusion T85.49
      specified NEC T85.49
     pain T85.848
     specified type NEC T85.898
     stenosis T85.858
     thrombosis T85.868
   bypass — *see also* Complications, prosthetic
     device or implant
     aortocoronary — *see* Complications,
      coronary artery (bypass) graft
     arterial — *see also* Complications, graft,
      vascular
      extremity — *see* Complications,
       extremity artery (bypass) graft
   cardiac — *see also* Disease, heart
     device, implant or graft T82.9
      embolism T82.817
      fibrosis T82.827
      hemorrhage T82.837
      infection or inflammation T82.7
       valve prosthesis T82.6
      mechanical
       breakdown T82.519
        specified device NEC T82.518
       displacement T82.529
        specified device NEC T82.528
       leakage T82.539
        specified device NEC T82.538
       malposition T82.529
        specified device NEC T82.528
       obstruction T82.599
        specified device NEC T82.598
       perforation T82.599
        specified device NEC T82.598
       protrusion T82.599
        specified device NEC T82.598
      pain T82.847
      specified type NEC T82.897
      stenosis T82.857
      thrombosis T82.867
   cardiovascular device, graft or implant T82.9
     aortic graft — *see* Complications, graft,
      vascular
     arteriovenous
      fistula, artificial — *see* Complication,
       arteriovenous, fistula, surgically
       created

Complication (s) (from) (of) - *continued*
   cardiovascular device, graft or implant -
    continued
    arteriovenous - *continued*
     shunt — *see* Complication,
      arteriovenous, shunt, surgically
      created
    artificial heart — *see* Complication,
     artificial, heart
    balloon (counterpulsation) device — *see*
     Complication, balloon implant,
     vascular
    carotid artery graft — *see* Complications,
     graft, vascular
    coronary bypass graft — *see* Complication,
     coronary artery (bypass) graft
    dialysis catheter (vascular) — *see*
     Complication, catheter, dialysis
    electronic T82.9
     electrode T82.9
      embolism T82.817
      fibrosis T82.827
      hemorrhage T82.837
      infection T82.7
      mechanical
       breakdown T82.110
       displacement T82.120
       leakage T82.190
       obstruction T82.190
       perforation T82.190
       protrusion T82.190
       specified type NEC T82.190
      pain T82.847
      specified NEC T82.897
      stenosis T82.857
      thrombosis T82.867
     embolism T82.817
     fibrosis T82.827
     hemorrhage T82.837
     infection T82.7
     mechanical
      breakdown T82.119
      displacement T82.129
      leakage T82.199
      obstruction T82.199
      perforation T82.199
      protrusion T82.199
      specified type NEC T82.199
     pain T82.847
     pulse generator T82.9
      embolism T82.817
      fibrosis T82.827
      hemorrhage T82.837
      infection T82.7
      mechanical
       breakdown T82.111
       displacement T82.121
       leakage T82.191
       obstruction T82.191
       perforation T82.191
       protrusion T82.191
       specified type NEC T82.191
      pain T82.847
      specified NEC T82.897
      stenosis T82.857
      thrombosis T82.867
     specified condition NEC T82.897
     specified device NEC T82.9
      embolism T82.817
      fibrosis T82.827
      hemorrhage T82.837
      infection T82.7
      mechanical
       breakdown T82.118
       displacement T82.128
       leakage T82.198
       obstruction T82.198
       perforation T82.198
       protrusion T82.198
       specified type NEC T82.198
      pain T82.847
      specified NEC T82.897
      stenosis T82.857
      thrombosis T82.867
     stenosis T82.857

Complication (s) (from) (of) - *continued*
   cardiovascular device, graft or implant -
    continued
    electronic - *continued*
     thrombosis T82.867
    extremity artery graft — *see* Complication,
     extremity artery (bypass) graft
    femoral artery graft — *see* Complication,
     extremity artery (bypass) graft
    heart-lung transplant — *see* Complication,
     transplant, heart, with lung
    heart
     transplant — *see* Complication,
      transplant, heart
     valve — *see* Complication, prosthetic
      device, heart valve
      graft — *see* Complication, heart,
       valve, graft
    infection or inflammation T82.7
    umbrella device — *see* Complication,
     umbrella device, vascular
    vascular graft (or anastomosis) — *see*
     Complication, graft, vascular
   carotid artery (bypass) graft — *see*
     Complications, graft, vascular
   catheter (device) NEC — *see also*
     Complications, prosthetic device or
     implant
    cranial infusion
     infection and inflammation T85.735
     mechanical
      breakdown T85.610
      displacement T85.620
      leakage T85.630
      malfunction T85.690
      malposition T85.620
      obstruction T85.690
      perforation T85.690
      protrusion T85.690
      specified NEC T85.690
    cystostomy T83.9
     embolism T83.81
     fibrosis T83.82
     hemorrhage T83.83
     infection and inflammation T83.510
     mechanical
      breakdown T83.010
      displacement T83.020
      leakage T83.030
      malposition T83.020
      obstruction T83.090
      perforation T83.090
      protrusion T83.090
      specified NEC T83.090
     pain T83.84
     specified type NEC T83.89
     stenosis T83.85
     thrombosis T83.86
    dialysis (vascular) T82.9
     embolism T82.818
     fibrosis T82.828
     hemorrhage T82.838
     infection and inflammation T82.7
     intraperitoneal — *see* Complications,
      catheter, intraperitoneal
     mechanical
      breakdown T82.41
      displacement T82.42
      leakage T82.43
      malposition T82.42
      obstruction T82.49
      perforation T82.49
      protrusion T82.49
     pain T82.848
     specified type NEC T82.898
     stenosis T82.858
     thrombosis T82.868
    epidural infusion T85.9
     embolism T85.810
     fibrosis T85.820
     hemorrhage T85.830
     infection and inflammation T85.735
     mechanical
      breakdown T85.610
      displacement T85.620

Complication (s) (from) (of) - *continued*
catheter (device) NEC - *continued*
epidural infusion - *continued*
mechanical - *continued*
leakage T85.630
malfunction T85.610
malposition T85.620
obstruction T85.690
perforation T85.690
protrusion T85.690
specified NEC T85.690
pain T85.840
specified type NEC T85.890
stenosis T85.850
thrombosis T85.860
intraperitoneal dialysis T85.9
embolism T85.818
fibrosis T85.828
hemorrhage T85.838
infection and inflammation T85.71
mechanical
breakdown T85.611
displacement T85.621
leakage T85.631
malfunction T85.611
malposition T85.621
obstruction T85.691
perforation T85.691
protrusion T85.691
specified NEC T85.691
pain T85.848
specified type NEC T85.898
stenosis T85.858
thrombosis T85.868
intrathecal infusion
infection and inflammation T85.735
mechanical
breakdown T85.610
displacement T85.620
leakage T85.630
malfunction T85.690
malposition T85.620
obstruction T85.690
perforation T85.690
protrusion T85.690
specified NEC T85.690
intravenous infusion T82.9
embolism T82.818
fibrosis T82.828
hemorrhage T82.838
infection or inflammation T82.7
mechanical
breakdown T82.514
displacement T82.524
leakage T82.534
malposition T82.524
obstruction T82.594
perforation T82.594
protrusion T82.594
pain T82.848
specified type NEC T82.898
stenosis T82.858
thrombosis T82.868
spinal infusion
infection and inflammation T85.735
mechanical
breakdown T85.610
displacement T85.620
leakage T85.630
malfunction T85.690
malposition T85.620
obstruction T85.690
perforation T85.690
protrusion T85.690
specified NEC T85.690
subarachnoid infusion
infection and inflammation T85.735
mechanical
breakdown T85.610
displacement T85.620
leakage T85.630
malfunction T85.690
malposition T85.620
obstruction T85.690
perforation T85.690

Complication (s) (from) (of) - *continued*
catheter (device) NEC - *continued*
subarachnoid infusion - *continued*
mechanical - *continued*
protrusion T85.690
specified NEC T85.690
subdural infusion T85.9
embolism T85.810
fibrosis T85.820
hemorrhage T85.830
infection and inflammation T85.735
mechanical
breakdown T85.610
displacement T85.620
leakage T85.630
malfunction T85.610
malposition T85.620
obstruction T85.690
perforation T85.690
protrusion T85.690
specified NEC T85.690
pain T85.840
specified type NEC T85.890
stenosis T85.850
thrombosis T85.860
urethral T83.9
displacement T83.028
embolism T83.81
fibrosis T83.82
hemorrhage T83.83
indwelling
breakdown T83.011
displacement T83.021
infection and inflammation T83.511
leakage T83.031
specified complication NEC T83.091
infection and inflammation T83.511
leakage T83.038
malposition T83.028
mechanical
breakdown T83.011
obstruction (mechanical) T83.091
pain T83.84
perforation T83.091
protrusion T83.091
specified type NEC T83.091
stenosis T83.85
thrombosis T83.86
urinary NEC
breakdown T83.018
displacement T83.028
infection and inflammation T83.518
leakage T83.038
specified complication NEC T83.098
cecostomy (stoma) — *see* Complications, colostomy
cesarean delivery wound NEC O90.89
disruption O90.0
hematoma O90.2
infection (following delivery) O86.00
chemotherapy (antineoplastic) NEC T88.7
chin implant (prosthetic) — *see* Complication, prosthetic device or implant, specified NEC
circulatory system I99.8
intraoperative I97.88
postprocedural I97.89
following cardiac surgery — *see also* Infarct, myocardium, associated with revascularization procedure I97.19-
postcardiotomy syndrome I97.0
hypertension I97.3
lymphedema after mastectomy I97.2
postcardiotomy syndrome I97.0
specified NEC I97.89
colostomy (stoma) K94.00
hemorrhage K94.01
infection K94.02
malfunction K94.03
mechanical K94.03
specified complication NEC K94.09
contraceptive device, intrauterine — *see* Complications, intrauterine, contraceptive device

Complication (s) (from) (of) - *continued*
cord (umbilical) — *see* Complications, umbilical cord
corneal graft — *see* Complications, graft, cornea
coronary artery (bypass) graft T82.9
atherosclerosis — *see* Arteriosclerosis, coronary (artery),
embolism T82.818
fibrosis T82.828
hemorrhage T82.838
infection and inflammation T82.7
mechanical
breakdown T82.211
displacement T82.212
leakage T82.213
malposition T82.212
obstruction T82.218
perforation T82.218
protrusion T82.218
specified NEC T82.218
pain T82.848
specified type NEC T82.898
stenosis T82.858
thrombosis T82.868
counterpulsation device (balloon) , intra-aortic — *see* Complications, balloon implant, vascular
cystostomy (stoma) N99.518
catheter — *see* Complications, catheter, cystostomy
hemorrhage N99.510
infection N99.511
malfunction N99.512
specified type NEC N99.518
delivery — *see also* Complications, obstetric O75.9
procedure (instrumental) (manual) (surgical) O75.4
specified NEC O75.89
dialysis (peritoneal) (renal) — *see also* Complications, infusion
catheter (vascular) — *see* Complication, catheter, dialysis
peritoneal, intraperitoneal — *see* Complications, catheter, intraperitoneal
dorsal column (spinal) neurostimulator — *see* Complications, electronic stimulator device, spinal cord
drug NEC T88.7
ear procedure — *see also* Disorder, ear
intraoperative H95.88
hematoma — *see* Complications, intraoperative, hemorrhage (hematoma) (of), ear
hemorrhage — *see* Complications, intraoperative, hemorrhage (hematoma) (of), ear
laceration — *see* Complications, intraoperative, puncture or laceration..., ear
specified NEC H95.88
postoperative H95.89
external ear canal stenosis H95.81-
hematoma — *see* Complications, postprocedural, hematoma (of), ear
hemorrhage — *see* Complications, postprocedural, hemorrhage (of), ear
postmastoidectomy — *see* Complications, postmastoidectomy
seroma — *see* Complications, postprocedural, seroma (of), mastoid process
specified NEC H95.89
ectopic pregnancy O08.9
damage to pelvic organs O08.6
embolism O08.2
genital infection O08.0
hemorrhage (delayed) (excessive) O08.1
metabolic disorder O08.5
renal failure O08.4
shock O08.3
specified type NEC O08.0

Complication (s) (from) (of) - *continued*
  ectopic pregnancy - *continued*
    venous complication NEC O08.7
  electronic stimulator device
    bladder (urinary) — *see* Complications,
      electronic stimulator device, urinary
    bone T84.9
      breakdown T84.310
      displacement T84.320
      embolism T84.81
      fibrosis T84.82
      hemorrhage T84.83
      infection or inflammation T84.7
      malfunction T84.310
      malposition T84.320
      mechanical NEC T84.390
      obstruction T84.390
      pain T84.84
      perforation T84.390
      protrusion T84.390
      specified type NEC T84.89
      stenosis T84.85
      thrombosis T84.86
    brain T85.9
      embolism T85.810
      fibrosis T85.820
      hemorrhage T85.830
      infection and inflammation T85.731
      mechanical
        breakdown T85.110
        displacement T85.120
        leakage T85.190
        malposition T85.120
        obstruction T85.190
        perforation T85.190
        protrusion T85.190
        specified NEC T85.190
      pain T85.840
      specified type NEC T85.890
      stenosis T85.850
      thrombosis T85.860
    cardiac (defibrillator) (pacemaker) — *see*
      Complications, cardiovascular device
      or implant, electronic
    generator (brain) (gastric) (peripheral)
      (sacral) (spinal)
      breakdown T85.113
      displacement T85.123
      leakage T85.193
      malposition T85.123
      obstruction T85.193
      perforation T85.193
      protrusion T85.193
      specified type NEC T85.193
    muscle T84.9
      breakdown T84.418
      displacement T84.428
      embolism T84.81
      fibrosis T84.82
      hemorrhage T84.83
      infection or inflammation T84.7
      mechanical NEC T84.498
      pain T84.84
      specified type NEC T84.89
      stenosis T84.85
      thrombosis T84.86
    nervous system T85.9
      brain — *see* Complications, electronic
        stimulator device, brain
      cranial nerve — *see* Complications,
        electronic stimulator device,
        peripheral nerve
      embolism T85.810
      fibrosis T85.820
      gastric nerve — *see* Complications,
        electronic stimulator device,
        peripheral nerve
      hemorrhage T85.830
      infection and inflammation T85.738
      mechanical
        breakdown T85.118
        displacement T85.128
        leakage T85.199
        malposition T85.128
        obstruction T85.199

Complication (s) (from) (of) - *continued*
  electronic stimulator device - *continued*
    nervous system - *continued*
      mechanical - *continued*
        perforation T85.199
        protrusion T85.199
        specified NEC T85.199
      pain T85.840
      peripheral nerve — *see* Complications,
        electronic stimulator device,
        peripheral nerve
      sacral nerve — *see* Complications,
        electronic stimulator device,
        peripheral nerve
      specified type NEC T85.890
      spinal cord — *see* Complications,
        electronic stimulator device, spinal
        cord
      stenosis T85.850
      thrombosis T85.860
      vagal nerve — *see* Complications,
        electronic stimulator device,
        peripheral nerve
    peripheral nerve T85.9
      embolism T85.810
      fibrosis T85.820
      hemorrhage T85.830
      infection and inflammation T85.732
      mechanical
        breakdown T85.111
        displacement T85.121
        leakage T85.191
        malposition T85.121
        obstruction T85.191
        perforation T85.191
        protrusion T85.191
        specified NEC T85.191
      pain T85.840
      specified type NEC T85.890
      stenosis T85.850
      thrombosis T85.860
    spinal cord T85.9
      embolism T85.810
      fibrosis T85.820
      hemorrhage T85.830
      infection and inflammation T85.733
      mechanical
        breakdown T85.112
        displacement T85.122
        leakage T85.192
        malposition T85.122
        obstruction T85.192
        perforation T85.192
        protrusion T85.192
        specified NEC T85.192
      pain T85.840
      specified type NEC T85.890
      stenosis T85.850
      thrombosis T85.860
    urinary T83.9
      embolism T83.81
      fibrosis T83.82
      hemorrhage T83.83
      infection and inflammation T83.598
      mechanical
        breakdown T83.110
        displacement T83.120
        malposition T83.120
        perforation T83.190
        protrusion T83.190
        specified NEC T83.190
      pain T83.84
      specified type NEC T83.89
      stenosis T83.85
      thrombosis T83.86
  electroshock therapy T88.9
    specified NEC T88.8
  endocrine E34.9
    postprocedural
      adrenal hypofunction E89.6
      hypoinsulinemia E89.1
      hypoparathyroidism E89.2
      hypopituitarism E89.3
      hypothyroidism E89.0
      ovarian failure E89.40

Complication (s) (from) (of) - *continued*
  endocrine - *continued*
    postprocedural - *continued*
      ovarian failure - *continued*
        asymptomatic E89.40
        symptomatic E89.41
        specified NEC E89.89
        testicular hypofunction E89.5
  endodontic treatment NEC M27.59
  enterostomy (stoma) K94.10
    hemorrhage K94.11
    infection K94.12
    malfunction K94.13
    mechanical K94.13
    specified complication NEC K94.19
  episiotomy, disruption O90.1
  esophageal anti-reflux device T85.9
    embolism T85.818
    fibrosis T85.828
    hemorrhage T85.838
    infection and inflammation T85.79
    mechanical
      breakdown T85.511
      displacement T85.521
      malfunction T85.511
      malposition T85.521
      obstruction T85.591
      perforation T85.591
      protrusion T85.591
      specified NEC T85.591
    pain T85.848
    specified type NEC T85.898
    stenosis T85.858
    thrombosis T85.868
  esophagostomy K94.30
    hemorrhage K94.31
    infection K94.32
    malfunction K94.33
    mechanical K94.33
    specified complication NEC K94.39
  extracorporeal circulation T80.90
  extremity artery (bypass) graft T82.9
    arteriosclerosis — *see* Arteriosclerosis,
      extremities, bypass graft
    embolism T82.818
    fibrosis T82.828
    hemorrhage T82.838
    infection and inflammation T82.7
    mechanical
      breakdown T82.318
        femoral artery T82.312
      displacement T82.328
        femoral artery T82.322
      leakage T82.338
        femoral artery T82.332
      malposition T82.328
        femoral artery T82.322
      obstruction T82.398
        femoral artery T82.392
      perforation T82.398
        femoral artery T82.392
      protrusion T82.398
        femoral artery T82.392
    pain T82.848
    specified type NEC T82.898
    stenosis T82.858
    thrombosis T82.868
  eye H57.9
    corneal graft — *see* Complications, graft,
      cornea
    implant (prosthetic) T85.9
      embolism T85.818
      fibrosis T85.828
      hemorrhage T85.838
      infection and inflammation T85.79
      mechanical
        breakdown T85.318
        displacement T85.328
        leakage T85.398
        malposition T85.328
        obstruction T85.398
        perforation T85.398
        protrusion T85.398
        specified NEC T85.398
      pain T85.848

Complication (s) (from) (of) - *continued*
eye - *continued*
  implant (prosthetic) - *continued*
    specified type NEC T85.898
    stenosis T85.858
    thrombosis T85.868
  intraocular lens — *see* Complications,
    intraocular lens
  orbital prosthesis — *see* Complications,
    orbital prosthesis
female genital N94.9
  device, implant or graft NEC — *see*
    Complications, genitourinary, device
    or implant, genital tract
femoral artery (bypass) graft — *see*
  Complication, extremity artery (bypass)
  graft
fixation device, internal (orthopedic) T84.9
  infection and inflammation T84.60
    arm T84.61-
      humerus T84.61-
      radius T84.61-
      ulna T84.61-
    leg T84.629
      femur T84.62-
      fibula T84.62-
      tibia T84.62-
    specified site NEC T84.69
    spine T84.63
  mechanical
    breakdown
      limb T84.119
        carpal T84.210
        femur T84.11-
        fibula T84.11-
        humerus T84.11-
        metacarpal T84.210
        metatarsal T84.213
        phalanx
          foot T84.213
          hand T84.210
        radius T84.11-
        tarsal T84.213
        tibia T84.11-
        ulna T84.11-
      specified bone NEC T84.218
      spine T84.216
    displacement
      limb T84.129
        carpal T84.220
        femur T84.12-
        fibula T84.12-
        humerus T84.12-
        metacarpal T84.220
        metatarsal T84.223
        phalanx
          foot T84.223
          hand T84.220
        radius T84.12-
        tarsal T84.223
        tibia T84.12-
        ulna T84.12-
      specified bone NEC T84.228
      spine T84.226
    malposition — *see* Complications,
      fixation device, internal,
      mechanical, displacement
    obstruction — *see* Complications,
      fixation device, internal,
      mechanical, specified type NEC
    perforation — *see* Complications,
      fixation device, internal,
      mechanical, specified type NEC
    protrusion — *see* Complications,
      fixation device, internal,
      mechanical, specified type NEC
    specified type NEC
      limb T84.199
        carpal T84.290
        femur T84.19-
        fibula T84.19-
        humerus T84.19-
        metacarpal T84.290
        metatarsal T84.293
        phalanx

Complication (s) (from) (of) - *continued*
fixation device, internal (orthopedic) -
continued
  mechanical - *continued*
    specified type NEC - *continued*
      limb - *continued*
        phalanx - *continued*
          foot T84.293
          hand T84.290
        radius T84.19-
        tarsal T84.293
        tibia T84.19-
        ulna T84.19-
      specified bone NEC T84.298
      vertebra T84.296
    specified type NEC T84.89
      embolism T84.81
      fibrosis T84.82
      hemorrhage T84.83
      pain T84.84
      specified complication NEC T84.89
      stenosis T84.85
      thrombosis T84.86
following
  acute myocardial infarction NEC I23.8
    aneurysm (false) (of cardiac wall) (of
      heart wall) (ruptured) I23.3
    angina I23.7
    atrial
      septal defect I23.1
      thrombosis I23.6
    cardiac wall rupture I23.3
    chordae tendinae rupture I23.4
    defect
      septal
        atrial (heart) I23.1
        ventricular (heart) I23.2
    hemopericardium I23.0
    papillary muscle rupture I23.5
    rupture
      cardiac wall I23.3
        with hemopericardium I23.0
      chordae tendineae I23.4
      papillary muscle I23.5
    specified NEC I23.8
    thrombosis
      atrium I23.6
      auricular appendage I23.6
      ventricle (heart) I23.6
    ventricular
      septal defect I23.2
      thrombosis I23.6
  ectopic or molar pregnancy O08.9
    cardiac arrest O08.81
    sepsis O08.82
    specified type NEC O08.89
    urinary tract infection O08.83
  termination of pregnancy — *see* Abortion
gastrointestinal K92.9
  bile duct prosthesis — *see* Complications,
    bile duct implant
  esophageal anti-reflux device — *see*
    Complications, esophageal anti-reflux
    device
  postoperative
    colostomy — *see* Complications,
      colostomy
    dumping syndrome K91.1
    enterostomy — *see* Complications,
      enterostomy
    gastrostomy — *see* Complications,
      gastrostomy
    malabsorption NEC K91.2
    obstruction — *see also* Obstruction,
      intestine, postoperative K91.30
    postcholecystectomy syndrome K91.5
    specified NEC K91.89
    vomiting after GI surgery K91.0
  prosthetic device or implant
    bile duct prosthesis — *see*
      Complications, bile duct implant
    esophageal anti-reflux device — *see*
      Complications, esophageal anti-
      reflux device
    specified type NEC

Complication (s) (from) (of) - *continued*
gastrointestinal - *continued*
  prosthetic device or implant - *continued*
    specified type NEC - *continued*
      embolism T85.818
      fibrosis T85.828
      hemorrhage T85.838
      mechanical
        breakdown T85.518
        displacement T85.528
        malfunction T85.518
        malposition T85.528
        obstruction T85.598
        perforation T85.598
        protrusion T85.598
        specified NEC T85.598
      pain T85.848
      specified complication NEC T85.898
      stenosis T85.858
      thrombosis T85.868
gastrostomy (stoma) K94.20
  hemorrhage K94.21
  infection K94.22
  malfunction K94.23
  mechanical K94.23
  specified complication NEC K94.29
genitourinary
  device or implant T83.9
    genital tract T83.9
      infection or inflammation T83.69
      intrauterine contraceptive device —
        see Complications, intrauterine,
        contraceptive device
      mechanical — *see* Complications, by
        device, mechanical
      mesh — *see* Complications, prosthetic
        device or implant, mesh
      penile prosthesis — *see*
        Complications, prosthetic device,
        penile
      specified type NEC T83.89
        embolism T83.81
        fibrosis T83.82
        hemorrhage T83.83
        pain T83.84
        specified complication NEC T83.89
        stenosis T83.85
        thrombosis T83.86
      vaginal mesh — *see* Complications,
        prosthetic device or implant,
        mesh
  urinary system T83.9
    cystostomy catheter — *see*
      Complication, catheter,
      cystostomy
    electronic stimulator — *see*
      Complications, electronic
      stimulator device, urinary
    indwelling urethral catheter — *see*
      Complications, catheter, urethral,
      indwelling
    infection or inflammation T83.598
      indwelling urethral catheter T83.511
    kidney transplant — *see*
      Complication, transplant, kidney
    organ graft — *see* Complication, graft,
      urinary organ
    specified type NEC T83.89
      embolism T83.81
      fibrosis T83.82
      hemorrhage T83.83
      mechanical T83.198
        breakdown T83.118
        displacement T83.128
        malfunction T83.118
        malposition T83.128
        obstruction T83.198
        perforation T83.198
        protrusion T83.198
        specified NEC T83.198
      sphincter, implanted T83.191
      stent (ileal conduit)
        (nephroureteral) T83.193
      ureteral indwelling T83.192
      pain T83.84

Complication (s) (from) (of) - *continued*
genitourinary - *continued*
  device or implant - *continued*
    urinary system - *continued*
      stent (ileal conduit) (nephroureteral) -
        continued
        specified complication NEC T83.89
        stenosis T83.85
        thrombosis T83.86
      sphincter implant — *see*
        Complications, implant, urinary
        sphincter
  postprocedural
    pelvic peritoneal adhesions N99.4
    renal failure N99.0
    specified NEC N99.89
    stoma — *see* Complications, stoma,
      urinary tract
    urethral stricture — *see* Stricture,
      urethra, postprocedural
  vaginal
    adhesions N99.2
    vault prolapse N99.3
graft (bypass) (patch) — *see also*
    Complications, prosthetic device or
    implant
  aorta — *see* Complications, graft, vascular
  arterial — *see* Complication, graft,
    vascular
  bone T86.839
    failure T86.831
    infection T86.832
    mechanical T84.318
      breakdown T84.318
      displacement T84.328
      protrusion T84.398
      specified type NEC T84.398
    rejection T86.830
    specified type NEC T86.838
  carotid artery — *see* Complications, graft,
    vascular
  cornea T86.849
    failure T86.841
    infection T86.842
    mechanical T85.398
      breakdown T85.318
      displacement T85.328
      protrusion T85.398
      specified type NEC T85.398
    rejection T86.840
    retroprosthetic membrane T85.398
    specified type NEC T86.848
  femoral artery (bypass) — *see*
    Complication, extremity artery
    (bypass) graft
  genital organ or tract — *see*
    Complications, genitourinary, device
    or implant, genital tract
  muscle T84.9
    breakdown T84.410
    displacement T84.420
    embolism T84.81
    fibrosis T84.82
    hemorrhage T84.83
    infection and inflammation T84.7
    mechanical NEC T84.490
    pain T84.84
    specified type NEC T84.89
    stenosis T84.85
    thrombosis T84.86
  nerve — *see* Complication, prosthetic
    device or implant, specified NEC
  skin — *see* Complications, prosthetic
    device or implant, skin graft
  tendon T84.9
    breakdown T84.410
    displacement T84.420
    embolism T84.81
    fibrosis T84.82
    hemorrhage T84.83
    infection and inflammation T84.7
    mechanical NEC T84.490
    pain T84.84
    specified type NEC T84.89
    stenosis T84.85

Complication (s) (from) (of) - *continued*
graft (bypass) (patch) - *continued*
  tendon - *continued*
    thrombosis T84.86
  urinary organ T83.9
    embolism T83.81
    fibrosis T83.82
    hemorrhage T83.83
    infection and inflammation T83.598
      indwelling urethral catheter T83.511
    mechanical
      breakdown T83.21
      displacement T83.22
      erosion T83.24
      exposure T83.25
      leakage T83.23
      malposition T83.22
      obstruction T83.29
      perforation T83.29
      protrusion T83.29
      specified NEC T83.29
    pain T83.84
    specified type NEC T83.89
    stenosis T83.85
    thrombosis T83.86
  vascular T82.9
    embolism T82.818
    femoral artery — *see* Complication,
      extremity artery (bypass) graft
    fibrosis T82.828
    hemorrhage T82.838
    mechanical
      breakdown T82.319
        aorta (bifurcation) T82.310
        carotid artery T82.311
        specified vessel NEC T82.318
      displacement T82.329
        aorta (bifurcation) T82.320
        carotid artery T82.321
        specified vessel NEC T82.328
      leakage T82.339
        aorta (bifurcation) T82.330
        carotid artery T82.331
        specified vessel NEC T82.338
      malposition T82.329
        aorta (bifurcation) T82.320
        carotid artery T82.321
        specified vessel NEC T82.328
      obstruction T82.399
        aorta (bifurcation) T82.390
        carotid artery T82.391
        specified vessel NEC T82.398
      perforation T82.399
        aorta (bifurcation) T82.390
        carotid artery T82.391
        specified vessel NEC T82.398
      protrusion T82.399
        aorta (bifurcation) T82.390
        carotid artery T82.391
        specified vessel NEC T82.398
    pain T82.848
    specified complication NEC T82.898
    stenosis T82.858
    thrombosis T82.868
heart I51.9
  assist device
    infection and inflammation T82.7
    following acute myocardial infarction —
      see Complications, following, acute
      myocardial infarction
    postoperative — *see* Complications,
      circulatory system
    transplant — *see* Complication, transplant,
      heart
      and lung (s) — *see* Complications,
        transplant, heart, with lung
  valve
    graft (biological) T82.9
      embolism T82.817
      fibrosis T82.827
      hemorrhage T82.837
      infection and inflammation T82.7
      mechanical T82.228
        breakdown T82.221
        displacement T82.222

Complication (s) (from) (of) - *continued*
heart - *continued*
  valve - *continued*
    graft (biological) - *continued*
      mechanical - *continued*
        leakage T82.223
        malposition T82.222
        obstruction T82.228
        perforation T82.228
        protrusion T82.228
      pain T82.847
      specified type NEC T82.897
      stenosis T82.857
      thrombosis T82.867
    prosthesis T82.9
      embolism T82.817
      fibrosis T82.827
      hemorrhage T82.837
      infection or inflammation T82.6
      mechanical T82.09
        breakdown T82.01
        displacement T82.02
        leakage T82.03
        malposition T82.02
        obstruction T82.09
        perforation T82.09
        protrusion T82.09
      pain T82.847
      specified type NEC T82.897
        mechanical T82.09
      stenosis T82.857
      thrombosis T82.867
hematoma
  intraoperative — *see* Complication,
    intraoperative, hemorrhage
  postprocedural — *see* Complication,
    postprocedural, hematoma
hemodialysis — *see* Complications, dialysis
hemorrhage
  intraoperative — *see* Complication,
    intraoperative, hemorrhage
  postprocedural — *see* Complication,
    postprocedural, hemorrhage
ileostomy (stoma) — *see* Complications,
  enterostomy
immunization (procedure) — *see*
  Complications, vaccination
implant — *see also* Complications, by site
  and type
  urinary sphincter T83.9
    embolism T83.81
    fibrosis T83.82
    hemorrhage T83.83
    infection and inflammation T83.591
    mechanical
      breakdown T83.111
      displacement T83.121
      leakage T83.191
      malposition T83.121
      obstruction T83.191
      perforation T83.191
      protrusion T83.191
      specified NEC T83.191
    pain T83.84
    specified type NEC T83.89
    stenosis T83.85
    thrombosis T83.86
infusion (procedure) T80.90
  air embolism T80.0
  blood — *see* Complications, transfusion
  catheter — *see* Complications, catheter
  infection T80.29
  pump — *see* Complications,
    cardiovascular, device or implant
  sepsis T80.29
  serum reaction — *see also* Reaction,
    serum T80.69
    anaphylactic shock — *see also* Shock,
      anaphylactic T80.59
  specified type NEC T80.89
inhalation therapy NEC T81.81
injection (procedure) T80.90
  drug reaction — *see* Reaction, drug
  infection T80.29
  sepsis T80.29

Complication (s) (from) (of) - *continued*
 injection (procedure) - *continued*
  serum (prophylactic) (therapeutic) — *see* Complications, vaccination
  specified type NEC T80.89
  vaccine (any) — *see* Complications, vaccination
 inoculation (any) — *see* Complications, vaccination
 insulin pump
  infection and inflammation T85.72
  mechanical
   breakdown T85.614
   displacement T85.624
   leakage T85.633
   malposition T85.624
   obstruction T85.694
   perforation T85.694
   protrusion T85.694
   specified NEC T85.694
 intestinal pouch NEC K91.858
 intraocular lens (prosthetic) T85.9
  embolism T85.818
  fibrosis T85.828
  hemorrhage T85.838
  infection and inflammation T85.79
  mechanical
   breakdown T85.21
   displacement T85.22
   malposition T85.22
   obstruction T85.29
   perforation T85.29
   protrusion T85.29
   specified NEC T85.29
  pain T85.848
  specified type NEC T85.898
  stenosis T85.858
  thrombosis T85.868
 intraoperative (intraprocedural)
  cardiac arrest — *see also* Infarct, myocardium, associated with revascularization procedure
   during cardiac surgery I97.710
   during other surgery I97.711
  cardiac functional disturbance NEC — *see also* Infarct, myocardium, associated with revascularization procedure
   during cardiac surgery I97.790
   during other surgery I97.791
  hemorrhage (hematoma) (of)
   circulatory system organ or structure
    during cardiac bypass I97.411
    during cardiac catheterization I97.410
    during other circulatory system procedure I97.418
    during other procedure I97.42
   digestive system organ
    during procedure on digestive system K91.61
    during procedure on other organ K91.62
   ear
    during procedure on ear and mastoid process H95.21
    during procedure on other organ H95.22
   endocrine system organ or structure
    during procedure on endocrine system organ or structure E36.01
    during procedure on other organ E36.02
   eye and adnexa
    during ophthalmic procedure H59.11-
    during other procedure H59.12-
   genitourinary organ or structure
    during procedure on genitourinary organ or structure N99.61
    during procedure on other organ N99.62
   mastoid process
    during procedure on ear and mastoid process H95.21
    during procedure on other organ H95.22
   musculoskeletal structure

Complication (s) (from) (of) - *continued*
 intraoperative (intraprocedural) - *continued*
  hemorrhage (hematoma) (of) - *continued*
   musculoskeletal structure - *continued*
    during musculoskeletal surgery M96.810
    during non-orthopedic surgery M96.811
    during orthopedic surgery M96.810
   nervous system
    during a nervous system procedure G97.31
    during other procedure G97.32
   respiratory system
    during other procedure J95.62
    during procedure on respiratory system organ or structure J95.61
   skin and subcutaneous tissue
    during a dermatologic procedure L76.01
    during a procedure on other organ L76.02
   spleen
    during a procedure on other organ D78.02
    during a procedure on the spleen D78.01
  puncture or laceration (accidental) (unintentional) (of)
   brain
    during a nervous system procedure G97.48
    during other procedure G97.49
   circulatory system organ or structure
    during circulatory system procedure I97.51
    during other procedure I97.52
   digestive system
    during procedure on digestive system K91.71
    during procedure on other organ K91.72
   ear
    during procedure on ear and mastoid process H95.31
    during procedure on other organ H95.32
   endocrine system organ or structure
    during procedure on endocrine system organ or structure E36.11
    during procedure on other organ E36.12
   eye and adnexa
    during ophthalmic procedure H59.21-
    during other procedure H59.22-
   genitourinary organ or structure
    during procedure on genitourinary organ or structure N99.71
    during procedure on other organ N99.72
   mastoid process
    during procedure on ear and mastoid process H95.31
    during procedure on other organ H95.32
   musculoskeletal structure
    during musculoskeletal surgery M96.820
    during non-orthopedic surgery M96.821
    during orthopedic surgery M96.820
   nervous system
    during a nervous system procedure G97.48
    during other procedure G97.49
   respiratory system
    during other procedure J95.72
    during procedure on respiratory system organ or structure J95.71
   skin and subcutaneous tissue
    during a dermatologic procedure L76.11
    during a procedure on other organ L76.12
   spleen

Complication (s) (from) (of) - *continued*
 intraoperative (intraprocedural) - *continued*
  puncture or laceration (accidental) (unintentional) (of) - *continued*
   spleen - *continued*
    during a procedure on other organ D78.12
    during a procedure on the spleen D78.11
   specified NEC
    circulatory system I97.88
    digestive system K91.81
    ear H95.88
    endocrine system E36.8
    eye and adnexa H59.88
    genitourinary system N99.81
    mastoid process H95.88
    musculoskeletal structure M96.89
    nervous system G97.81
    respiratory system J95.88
    skin and subcutaneous tissue L76.81
    spleen D78.81
 intraperitoneal catheter (dialysis) (infusion) — *see* Complications, catheter, intraperitoneal
 intrathecal infusion pump
  infection and inflammation T85.738
  mechanical
   breakdown T85.615
   displacement T85.625
   leakage T85.635
   malfunction T85.695
   malposition T85.625
   obstruction T85.695
   perforation T85.695
   protrusion T85.695
   specified NEC T85.695
 intrauterine
  contraceptive device
   embolism T83.81
   fibrosis T83.82
   hemorrhage T83.83
   infection and inflammation T83.69
   mechanical
    breakdown T83.31
    displacement T83.32
    malposition T83.32
    obstruction T83.39
    perforation T83.39
    protrusion T83.39
    specified NEC T83.39
   pain T83.84
   specified type NEC T83.89
   stenosis T83.85
   thrombosis T83.86
  procedure (fetal) , to newborn P96.5
 jejunostomy (stoma) — *see* Complications, enterostomy
 joint prosthesis, internal T84.9
  breakage (fracture) T84.01-
  dislocation T84.02-
  fracture T84.01-
  infection or inflammation T84.50
   hip T84.5-
   knee T84.5-
   specified joint NEC T84.59
  instability T84.02-
  malposition — *see* Complications, joint prosthesis, mechanical, displacement
  mechanical
   breakage, broken T84.01-
   dislocation T84.02-
   fracture T84.01-
   instability T84.02-
   leakage — *see* Complications, joint prosthesis, mechanical, specified NEC
   loosening T84.039
    hip T84.03-
    knee T84.03-
    specified joint NEC T84.038
   obstruction — *see* Complications, joint prosthesis, mechanical, specified NEC

Complication (s) (from) (of) - *continued*
 joint prosthesis, internal - *continued*
  mechanical - *continued*
   perforation — *see* Complications, joint
     prosthesis, mechanical, specified
     NEC
    osteolysis T84.059
     hip T84.05-
     knee T84.05-
     other specified joint T84.058
    periprosthetic T84.059
    protrusion — *see* Complications, joint
     prosthesis, mechanical, specified
     NEC
    specified complication NEC T84.099
     hip T84.09-
     knee T84.09-
     other specified joint T84.098
    subluxation T84.02-
    wear of articular bearing
      surface T84.069
     hip T84.06-
     knee T84.06-
     other specified joint T84.068
   specified joint NEC T84.89
    embolism T84.81
    fibrosis T84.82
    hemorrhage T84.83
    pain T84.84
    specified complication NEC T84.89
    stenosis T84.85
    thrombosis T84.86
   subluxation T84.02-
 kidney transplant — *see* Complications,
   transplant, kidney
 labor O75.9
  specified NEC O75.89
 liver transplant (immune or nonimmune) —
   see Complications, transplant, liver
 lumbar puncture G97.1
  cerebrospinal fluid leak G97.0
  headache or reaction G97.1
 lung transplant — *see* Complications,
   transplant, lung
  and heart — *see* Complications, transplant,
   lung, with heart
 male genital N50.9
  device, implant or graft — *see*
    Complications, genitourinary, device
    or implant, genital tract
  postprocedural or postoperative — *see*
    Complications, genitourinary,
    postprocedural
  specified NEC N99.89
 mastoid (process) procedure
  intraoperative H95.88
   hematoma — *see* Complications,
     intraoperative, hemorrhage
     (hematoma) (of), mastoid process
   hemorrhage — *see* Complications,
     intraoperative, hemorrhage
     (hematoma) (of), mastoid process
   laceration — *see* Complications,
     intraoperative, puncture or
     laceration..., mastoid process
   specified NEC H95.88
  postmastoidectomy — *see* Complications,
    postmastoidectomy
  postoperative H95.89
   external ear canal stenosis H95.81-
   hematoma — *see* Complications...,
     postprocedural, hematoma (of),
     mastoid process
   hemorrhage — *see* Complications...,
     postprocedural, hemorrhage (of),
     mastoid process
   postmastoidectomy — *see*
     Complications, postmastoidectomy
   seroma — *see* Complications,
     postprocedural, seroma (of),
     mastoid process
   specified NEC H95.89
  mastoidectomy cavity — *see* Complications,
    postmastoidectomy

Complication (s) (from) (of) - *continued*
 mechanical — *see* Complications, by site and
   type, mechanical
 medical procedures — *see also*
   Complication(s), intraoperative T88.9
 metabolic E88.9
  postoperative E89.89
   specified NEC E89.89
 molar pregnancy NOS O08.9
  damage to pelvic organs O08.6
  embolism O08.2
  genital infection O08.0
  hemorrhage (delayed) (excessive) O08.1
  metabolic disorder O08.5
  renal failure O08.4
  shock O08.3
  specified type NEC O08.0
  venous complication NEC O08.7
 musculoskeletal system — *see also*
   Complication, intraoperative
   (intraprocedural), by site
  device, implant or graft NEC — *see*
    Complications, orthopedic, device or
    implant
  internal fixation (nail) (plate) (rod) — *see*
    Complications, fixation device,
    internal
  joint prosthesis — *see* Complications, joint
    prosthesis
  postoperative (postprocedural) M96.89
   with osteoporosis — *see* Osteoporosis
   fracture following insertion of device —
     see Fracture, following insertion of
     orthopedic implant, joint prosthesis
     or bone plate
   joint instability after prosthesis
     removal M96.89
   lordosis M96.4
   postlaminectomy syndrome NEC M96.1
    kyphosis M96.3
   pseudarthrosis M96.0
   specified complication NEC M96.89
  post radiation M96.89
   kyphosis M96.2
   scoliosis M96.5
   specified complication NEC M96.89
 nephrostomy (stoma) — *see* Complications,
   stoma, urinary tract, external NEC
 nervous system G98.8
  central G96.9
   device, implant or graft — *see also*
     Complication, prosthetic device or
     implant, specified NEC
    electronic stimulator (electrode (s)) —
      see Complications, electronic
      stimulator device
    specified NEC
     infection and inflammation T85.738
     mechanical T85.695
      breakdown T85.615
      displacement T85.625
      leakage T85.635
      malfunction T85.695
      malposition T85.625
      obstruction T85.695
      perforation T85.695
      protrusion T85.695
      specified NEC T85.695
    ventricular shunt — *see* Complications,
      ventricular shunt
   electronic stimulator (electrode (s)) — *see*
     Complications, electronic stimulator
     device
   postprocedural G97.82
    intracranial hypotension G97.2
    specified NEC G97.82
    spinal fluid leak G97.0
  newborn, due to intrauterine (fetal)
    procedure P96.5
 nonabsorbable (permanent) sutures — *see*
   Complication, sutures, permanent
 obstetric O75.9
  procedure (instrumental) (manual)
    (surgical) specified NEC O75.4
  specified NEC O75.89

Complication (s) (from) (of) - *continued*
 obstetric - *continued*
  surgical wound NEC O90.89
   hematoma O90.2
   infection O86.00
 ocular lens implant — *see* Complications,
   intraocular lens
 ophthalmologic
  postprocedural bleb — *see* Blebitis
 orbital prosthesis T85.9
  embolism T85.818
  fibrosis T85.828
  hemorrhage T85.838
  infection and inflammation T85.79
  mechanical
   breakdown T85.31-
   displacement T85.32-
   malposition T85.32-
   obstruction T85.39-
   perforation T85.39-
   protrusion T85.39-
   specified NEC T85.39-
  pain T85.848
  specified type NEC T85.898
  stenosis T85.858
  thrombosis T85.868
 organ or tissue transplant (partial) (total) —
   see Complications, transplant
 orthopedic — *see also* Disorder, soft tissue
  device or implant T84.9
   bone
    device or implant — *see*
      Complication, bone, device NEC
    graft — *see* Complication, graft, bone
   breakdown T84.418
   displacement T84.428
   electronic bone stimulator — *see*
     Complications, electronic
     stimulator device, bone
   embolism T84.81
   fibrosis T84.82
   fixation device — *see* Complication,
     fixation device, internal
   hemorrhage T84.83
   infection or inflammation T84.7
   joint prosthesis — *see* Complication,
     joint prosthesis, internal
   malfunction T84.418
   malposition T84.428
   mechanical NEC T84.498
   muscle graft — *see* Complications, graft,
     muscle
   obstruction T84.498
   pain T84.84
   perforation T84.498
   protrusion T84.498
   specified complication NEC T84.89
   stenosis T84.85
   tendon graft — *see* Complications, graft,
     tendon
   thrombosis T84.86
  fracture (following insertion of device) —
    see Fracture, following insertion of
    orthopedic implant, joint prosthesis or
    bone plate
  postprocedural M96.89
   fracture — *see* Fracture, following
     insertion of orthopedic implant,
     joint prosthesis or bone plate
   postlaminectomy syndrome NEC M96.1
    kyphosis M96.3
    lordosis M96.4
   postradiation
    kyphosis M96.2
    scoliosis M96.5
   pseudarthrosis post-fusion M96.0
   specified type NEC M96.89
 pacemaker (cardiac) — *see* Complications,
   cardiovascular device or implant,
   electronic
 pancreas transplant — *see* Complications,
   transplant, pancreas
 penile prosthesis (implant) — *see*
   Complications, prosthetic device, penile
 perfusion NEC T80.90

Complication (s) (from) (of) - *continued*
perineal repair (obstetrical) NEC O90.89
  disruption O90.1
  hematoma O90.2
  infection (following delivery) O86.09
phototherapy T88.9
  specified NEC T88.8
postmastoidectomy NEC H95.19-
  cyst, mucosal H95.13-
  granulation H95.12-
  inflammation, chronic H95.11-
  recurrent cholesteatoma H95.0-
postoperative — *see* Complications,
  postprocedural
circulatory — *see* Complications,
  circulatory system
ear — *see* Complications, ear
endocrine — *see* Complications, endocrine
eye — *see* Complications, eye
lumbar puncture G97.1
  cerebrospinal fluid leak G97.0
nervous system (central) (peripheral) —
  see Complications, nervous system
respiratory system — *see* Complications,
  respiratory system
postprocedural — *see also* Complications,
  surgical procedure
cardiac arrest — *see also* Infarct,
  myocardium, associated with
  revascularization procedure
  following cardiac surgery I97.120
  following other surgery I97.121
cardiac functional disturbance NEC — *see*
  also Infarct, myocardium, associated
  with revascularization procedure
  following cardiac surgery I97.190
  following other surgery I97.191
cardiac insufficiency
  following cardiac surgery I97.110
  following other surgery I97.111
chorioretinal scars following retinal
  surgery H59.81-
following cataract surgery
  cataract (lens) fragments H59.02-
  cystoid macular edema H59.03-
  specified NEC H59.09-
  vitreous (touch) syndrome H59.01-
heart failure
  following cardiac surgery I97.130
  following other surgery I97.131
hematoma (of)
  circulatory system organ or structure
    following cardiac bypass I97.631
    following cardiac
      catheterization I97.630
    following other circulatory system
      procedure I97.638
    following other procedure I97.621
  digestive system
    following procedure on digestive
      system K91.870
    following procedure on other
      organ K91.871
  ear
    following other procedure H95.52
    following procedure on ear and
      mastoid process H95.51
  endocrine system
    following endocrine system
      procedure E89.820
    following other procedure E89.821
  eye and adnexa
    following ophthalmic
      procedure H59.33-
    following other procedure H59.34-
  genitourinary organ or structure
    following procedure on genitourinary
      organ or structure N99.840
    following procedure on other
      organ N99.841
  mastoid process
    following other procedure H95.52
    following procedure on ear and
      mastoid process H95.51
  musculoskeletal structure

Complication (s) (from) (of) - *continued*
postprocedural - *continued*
  hematoma (of) - *continued*
    musculoskeletal structure - *continued*
      following musculoskeletal
        surgery M96.840
      following non-orthopedic
        surgery M96.841
      following orthopedic surgery M96.840
    nervous system
      following nervous system
        procedure G97.61
      following other procedure G97.62
    respiratory system
      following other procedure J95.861
      following procedure on respiratory
        system organ or structure J95.860
    skin and subcutaneous tissue
      following dermatologic
        procedure L76.31
      following procedure on other
        organ L76.32
    spleen
      following procedure on other
        organ D78.32
      following procedure on the
        spleen D78.31
  hemorrhage (of)
    circulatory system organ or structure
      following cardiac bypass I97.611
      following cardiac
        catheterization I97.610
      following other circulatory system
        procedure I97.618
      following other procedure I97.620
    digestive system
      following procedure on digestive
        system K91.840
      following procedure on other
        organ K91.841
    ear
      following other procedure H95.42
      following procedure on ear and
        mastoid process H95.41
    endocrine system
      following endocrine system
        procedure E89.810
      following other procedure E89.811
    eye and adnexa
      following ophthalmic
        procedure H59.31-
      following other procedure H59.32-
    genitourinary organ or structure
      following procedure on genitourinary
        organ or structure N99.820
      following procedure on other
        organ N99.821
    mastoid process
      following other procedure H95.42
      following procedure on ear and
        mastoid process H95.41
    musculoskeletal structure
      following musculoskeletal
        surgery M96.830
      following non-orthopedic
        surgery M96.831
      following orthopedic surgery M96.830
    nervous system
      following nervous system
        procedure G97.51
      following other procedure G97.52
    respiratory system
      following other procedure J95.831
      following procedure on respiratory
        system organ or structure J95.830
    skin and subcutaneous tissue
      following dermatologic
        procedure L76.21
      following a procedure on other
        organ L76.22
    spleen
      following procedure on other
        organ D78.22
      following procedure on the
        spleen D78.21

Complication (s) (from) (of) - *continued*
postprocedural - *continued*
  seroma (of)
    circulatory system organ or structure
      following cardiac bypass I97.641
      following cardiac
        catheterization I97.640
      following other circulatory system
        procedure I97.648
      following other procedure I97.622
    digestive system
      following procedure on digestive
        system K91.872
      following procedure on other
        organ K91.873
    ear
      following other procedure H95.54
      following procedure on ear and
        mastoid process H95.53
    endocrine system
      following endocrine system
        procedure E89.822
      following other procedure E89.823
    eye and adnexa
      following ophthalmic
        procedure H59.35-
      following other procedure H59.36-
    genitourinary organ or structure
      following procedure on genitourinary
        organ or structure N99.842
      following procedure on other
        organ N99.843
    mastoid process
      following other procedure H95.54
      following procedure on ear and
        mastoid process H95.53
    musculoskeletal structure
      following musculoskeletal
        surgery M96.842
      following non-orthopedic
        surgery M96.843
      following orthopedic surgery M96.842
    nervous system
      following nervous system
        procedure G97.63
      following other procedure G97.64
    respiratory system
      following other procedure J95.863
      following procedure on respiratory
        system organ or structure J95.862
    skin and subcutaneous tissue
      following dermatologic
        procedure L76.33
      following procedure on other
        organ L76.34
    spleen
      following procedure on other
        organ D78.34
      following procedure on the
        spleen D78.33
  specified NEC
    circulatory system I97.89
    digestive K91.89
    ear H95.89
    endocrine E89.89
    eye and adnexa H59.89
    genitourinary N99.89
    mastoid process H95.89
    metabolic E89.89
    musculoskeletal structure M96.89
    nervous system G97.82
    respiratory system J95.89
    skin and subcutaneous tissue L76.82
    spleen D78.89
pregnancy NEC — *see* Pregnancy,
  complicated by
prosthetic device or implant T85.9
  bile duct — *see* Complications, bile duct
    implant
  breast — *see* Complications, breast
    implant
  bulking agent
    ureteral
      erosion T83.714
      exposure T83.724

Complication (s) (from) (of) - *continued*
  prosthetic device or implant - *continued*
    bulking agent - *continued*
      urethral
        erosion T83.713
        exposure T83.723
    cardiac and vascular NEC — *see*
      Complications, cardiovascular device
      or implant
    corneal transplant — *see* Complications,
      graft, cornea
    electronic nervous system stimulator —
      see Complications, electronic
      stimulator device
    epidural infusion catheter — *see*
      Complications, catheter, epidural
    esophageal anti-reflux device — *see*
      Complications, esophageal anti-reflux
      device
    genital organ or tract — *see*
      Complications, genitourinary, device
      or implant, genital tract
      specified NEC T83.79
    heart valve — *see* Complications, heart,
      valve, prosthesis
    infection or inflammation T85.79
      intestine transplant T86.892
      liver transplant T86.43
      lung transplant T86.812
      pancreas transplant T86.892
      skin graft T86.822
    intraocular lens — *see* Complications,
      intraocular lens
    intraperitoneal (dialysis) catheter — *see*
      Complications, catheter,
      intraperitoneal
    joint — *see* Complications, joint
      prosthesis, internal
    mechanical NEC T85.698
      dialysis catheter (vascular) — *see also*
        Complication, catheter, dialysis,
        mechanical
      peritoneal — *see* Complication,
        catheter, intraperitoneal,
        mechanical
    gastrointestinal device T85.598
    ocular device T85.398
    subdural (infusion) catheter T85.690
    suture, permanent T85.692
      that for bone repair — *see*
        Complications, fixation device,
        internal (orthopedic), mechanical
    ventricular shunt
      breakdown T85.01
      displacement T85.02
      leakage T85.03
      malposition T85.02
      obstruction T85.09
      perforation T85.09
      protrusion T85.09
      specified NEC T85.09
  mesh
    erosion (to surrounding organ or
      tissue) T83.718
      urethral (into pelvic floor
        muscles) T83.712
      vaginal (into pelvic floor
        muscles) T83.711
    exposure (into surrounding organ or
      tissue) T83.728
      urethral (through urethral
        wall) T83.722
      vaginal (into vagina) (through vaginal
        wall) T83.721
  orbital — *see* Complications, orbital
    prosthesis
  penile T83.9
    embolism T83.81
    fibrosis T83.82
    hemorrhage T83.83
    infection and inflammation T83.61
    mechanical
      breakdown T83.410
      displacement T83.420
      leakage T83.490

Complication (s) (from) (of) - *continued*
  prosthetic device or implant - *continued*
    penile - *continued*
      mechanical - *continued*
        malposition T83.420
        obstruction T83.490
        perforation T83.490
        protrusion T83.490
        specified NEC T83.490
      pain T83.84
      specified type NEC T83.89
      stenosis T83.85
      thrombosis T83.86
    prosthetic materials NEC
      erosion (to surrounding organ or
        tissue) T83.718
      exposure (into surrounding organ or
        tissue) T83.728
    skin graft T86.829
      artificial skin or decellularized
        allodermis
        embolism T85.818
        fibrosis T85.828
        hemorrhage T85.838
        infection and inflammation T85.79
        mechanical
          breakdown T85.613
          displacement T85.623
          malfunction T85.613
          malposition T85.623
          obstruction T85.693
          perforation T85.693
          protrusion T85.693
          specified NEC T85.693
        pain T85.848
        specified type NEC T85.898
        stenosis T85.858
        thrombosis T85.868
      failure T86.821
      infection T86.822
      rejection T86.820
      specified NEC T86.828
    sling
      urethral (female) (male)
        erosion T83.712
        exposure T83.722
    specified NEC T85.9
      embolism T85.818
      fibrosis T85.828
      hemorrhage T85.838
      infection and inflammation T85.79
      mechanical
        breakdown T85.618
        displacement T85.628
        leakage T85.638
        malfunction T85.618
        malposition T85.628
        obstruction T85.698
        perforation T85.698
        protrusion T85.698
        specified NEC T85.698
      pain T85.848
      specified type NEC T85.898
      stenosis T85.858
      thrombosis T85.868
    subdural infusion catheter — *see*
      Complications, catheter, subdural
    sutures — *see* Complications, sutures
    urinary organ or tract NEC — *see*
      Complications, genitourinary, device
      or implant, urinary system
    vascular — *see* Complications,
      cardiovascular device or implant
    ventricular shunt — *see* Complications,
      ventricular shunt (device)
  puerperium — *see* Puerperal
  puncture, spinal G97.1
    cerebrospinal fluid leak G97.0
    headache or reaction G97.1
  pyelogram N99.89
  radiation
    kyphosis M96.2
    scoliosis M96.5
  reattached
    extremity (infection) (rejection)

Complication (s) (from) (of) - *continued*
  reattached - *continued*
    extremity (infection) (rejection) -
      continued
      lower T87.1X-
      upper T87.0X-
    specified body part NEC T87.2
  reconstructed breast
    asymmetry between native and
      reconstructed breast N65.1
    deformity N65.0
    disproportion between native and
      reconstructed breast N65.1
    excess tissue N65.0
    misshappen N65.0
  reimplant NEC — *see also* Complications,
    prosthetic device or implant
    limb (infection) (rejection) — *see*
      Complications, reattached, extremity
    organ (partial) (total) — *see*
      Complications, transplant
    prosthetic device NEC — *see*
      Complications, prosthetic device
  renal N28.9
    allograft — *see* Complications, transplant,
      kidney
    dialysis — *see* Complications, dialysis
  respirator
    mechancial J95.850
      specified NEC J95.859
  respiratory system J98.9
    device, implant or graft — *see*
      Complication, prosthetic device or
      implant, specified NEC
    lung transplant — *see* Complications,
      prosthetic device or implant, lung
      transplant
    postoperative J95.89
      air leak J95.812
      Mendelson's syndrome (chemical
        pneumonitis) J95.4
      pneumothorax J95.811
      pulmonary insufficiency (acute) (after
        nonthoracic surgery) J95.2
        chronic J95.3
        following thoracic surgery J95.1
      respiratory failure (acute) J95.821
        acute and chronic J95.822
      specified NEC J95.89
      subglottic stenosis J95.5
    tracheostomy complication — *see*
      Complications, tracheostomy
    therapy T81.89
  sedation during labor and delivery O74.9
    cardiac O74.2
    central nervous system O74.3
    pulmonary NEC O74.1
  shunt — *see also* Complications, prosthetic
    device or implant
    arteriovenous — *see* Complications,
      arteriovenous, shunt
    ventricular (communicating) — *see*
      Complications, ventricular shunt
  skin
    graft T86.829
      failure T86.821
      infection T86.822
      rejection T86.820
      specified type NEC T86.828
  spinal
    anesthesia — *see* Complications,
      anesthesia, spinal
    catheter (epidural) (subdural) — *see*
      Complications, catheter
    puncture or tap G97.1
      cerebrospinal fluid leak G97.0
      headache or reaction G97.1
  stent
    bile duct — *see* Complications, bile duct
      prosthesis
    ureteral indwelling
      breakdown T83.112
      displacement T83.122
      leakage T83.192
      malposition T83.122

Complication (s) (from) (of) - *continued*
stent - *continued*
  ureteral indwelling - *continued*
    obstruction T83.192
    perforation T83.192
    protrusion T83.192
    specified NEC T83.192
    urinary NEC (ileal conduit)
      (nephroureteral) T83.193
      embolism T83.81
      fibrosis T83.82
      hemorrhage T83.83
      infection and inflammation T83.593
      mechanical
        breakdown T83.113
        displacement T83.123
        leakage T83.193
        malposition T83.123
        obstruction T83.193
        perforation T83.193
        protrusion T83.193
        specified NEC T83.193
      pain T83.84
      specified type NEC T83.89
      stenosis T83.85
      thrombosis T83.86
  vascular
    end stent stenosis — *see* Restenosis,
      stent
    in stent stenosis — *see* Restenosis, stent
stoma
  digestive tract
    colostomy — *see* Complications,
      colostomy
    enterostomy — *see* Complications,
      enterostomy
    esophagostomy — *see* Complications,
      esophagostomy
    gastrostomy — *see* Complications,
      gastrostomy
  urinary tract N99.528
    continent N99.538
      hemorrhage N99.530
      herniation N99.533
      infection N99.531
      malfunction N99.532
      specified type NEC N99.538
      stenosis N99.534
    cystostomy — *see* Complications,
      cystostomy
    external NOS N99.528
    hemorrhage N99.520
    herniation N99.523
    incontinent N99.528
      hemorrhage N99.520
      herniation N99.523
      infection N99.521
      malfunction N99.522
      specified type NEC N99.528
      stenosis N99.524
    infection N99.521
    malfunction N99.522
    specified type NEC N99.528
    stenosis N99.524
stomach banding — *see* Complication(s),
  bariatric procedure
stomach stapling — *see* Complication(s),
  bariatric procedure
surgical material, nonabsorbable — *see*
  Complication, suture, permanent
surgical procedure (on) T81.9
  amputation stump (late) — *see*
    Complications, amputation stump
  cardiac — *see* Complications, circulatory
    system
  cholesteatoma, recurrent — *see*
    Complications, postmastoidectomy,
    recurrent cholesteatoma
  circulatory (early) — *see* Complications,
    circulatory system
  digestive system — *see* Complications,
    gastrointestinal
  dumping syndrome
    (postgastrectomy) K91.1
  ear — *see* Complications, ear

Complication (s) (from) (of) - *continued*
surgical procedure (on) - *continued*
  elephantiasis or lymphedema I97.89
    postmastectomy I97.2
  emphysema (surgical) T81.82
  endocrine — *see* Complications, endocrine
  eye — *see* Complications, eye
  fistula (persistent postoperative) T81.83
  foreign body inadvertently left in wound
    (sponge) (suture) (swab) — *see*
    Foreign body, accidentally left during
    a procedure
  gastrointestinal — *see* Complications,
    gastrointestinal
  genitourinary NEC N99.89
  hematoma
    intraoperative — *see* Complication,
      intraoperative, hemorrhage
    postprocedural — *see* Complication,
      postprocedural, hematoma
  hemorrhage
    intraoperative — *see* Complication,
      intraoperative, hemorrhage
    postprocedural — *see* Complication,
      postprocedural, hemorrhage
  hepatic failure K91.82
  hyperglycemia
    (postpancreatectomy) E89.1
  hypoinsulinemia
    (postpancreatectomy) E89.1
  hypoparathyroidism
    (postparathyroidectomy) E89.2
  hypopituitarism
    (posthypophysectomy) E89.3
  hypothyroidism (post-
    thyroidectomy) E89.0
  intestinal obstruction — *see also*
    Obstruction, intestine,
    postoperative K91.30
  intracranial hypotension following
    ventricular shunting
    (ventriculostomy) G97.2
  lymphedema I97.89
    postmastectomy I97.2
  malabsorption (postsurgical) NEC K91.2
    osteoporosis — *see* Osteoporosis,
      postsurgical malabsorption
  mastoidectomy cavity NEC — *see*
    Complications, postmastoidectomy
  metabolic E89.89
    specified NEC E89.89
  musculoskeletal — *see* Complications,
    musculoskeletal system
  nervous system (central) (peripheral) —
    see Complications, nervous system
  ovarian failure E89.40
    asymptomatic E89.40
    symptomatic E89.41
  peripheral vascular — *see* Complications,
    surgical procedure, vascular
  postcardiotomy syndrome I97.0
  postcholecystectomy syndrome K91.5
  postcommissurotomy syndrome I97.0
  postgastrectomy dumping syndrome K91.1
  postlaminectomy syndrome NEC M96.1
    kyphosis M96.3
  postmastectomy lymphedema
    syndrome I97.2
  postmastoidectomy cholesteatoma — *see*
    Complications, postmastoidectomy,
    recurrent cholesteatoma
  postvagotomy syndrome K91.1
  postvalvulotomy syndrome I97.0
  pulmonary insufficiency (acute) J95.2
    chronic J95.3
    following thoracic surgery J95.1
  reattached body part — *see* Complications,
    reattached
  respiratory — *see* Complications,
    respiratory system
  shock (hypovolemic) T81.19
  spleen (postoperative) D78.89
    intraoperative D78.81
  stitch abscess T81.41
  subglottic stenosis (postsurgical) J95.5

Complication (s) (from) (of) - *continued*
surgical procedure (on) - *continued*
  testicular hypofunction E89.5
  transplant — *see* Complications, organ or
    tissue transplant
  urinary NEC N99.89
  vaginal vault prolapse
    (posthysterectomy) N99.3
  vascular (peripheral)
    artery T81.719
      mesenteric T81.710
      renal T81.711
      specified NEC T81.718
    vein T81.72
  wound infection T81.49
suture, permanent (wire) NEC T85.9
  with repair of bone — *see* Complications,
    fixation device, internal
  embolism T85.818
  fibrosis T85.828
  hemorrhage T85.838
  infection and inflammation T85.79
  mechanical
    breakdown T85.612
    displacement T85.622
    malfunction T85.612
    malposition T85.622
    obstruction T85.692
    perforation T85.692
    protrusion T85.692
    specified NEC T85.692
  pain T85.848
  specified type NEC T85.898
  stenosis T85.858
  thrombosis T85.868
tracheostomy J95.00
  granuloma J95.09
  hemorrhage J95.01
  infection J95.02
  malfunction J95.03
  mechanical J95.03
  obstruction J95.03
  specified type NEC J95.09
  tracheo-esophageal fistula J95.04
transfusion (blood) (lymphocytes)
  (plasma) T80.92
  air emblism T80.0
  circulatory overload E87.71
  febrile nonhemolytic transfusion
    reaction R50.84
  hemolysis T80.89
  hemochromatosis E83.111
  hemolytic reaction (antigen
    unspecified) T80.919
  incompatibility reaction (antigen
    unspecified) T80.919
    ABO T80.30
      delayed serologic (DSTR) T80.39
      hemolytic transfusion reaction (HTR)
        (unspecified time after
        transfusion) T80.319
        acute (AHTR) (less than 24 hours
          after transfusion) T80.310
        delayed (DHTR) (24 hours or more
          after transfusion) T80.311
        specified NEC T80.39
    acute (antigen unspecified) T80.910
    delayed (antigen unspecified) T80.911
    delayed serologic (DSTR) T80.89
    Non-ABO (minor antigens (Duffy) (K)
      (Kell) (Kidd) (Lewis) (M) (N) (P)
      (S)) T80.A0
      delayed serologic (DSTR) T80.A9
      hemolytic transfusion reaction (HTR)
        (unspecified time after
        transfusion) T80.A19
        acute (AHTR) (less than 24 hours
          after transfusion) T80.A10
        delayed (DHTR) (24 hours or more
          after transfusion) T80.A11
      specified NEC T80.A9
    Rh (antigens (C) (c) (D) (E) (e))
      (factor) T80.40
      delayed serologic (DSTR) T80.49

Complication (s) (from) (of) - *continued*
transfusion (blood) (lymphocytes) (plasma) - *continued*
  incompatibility reaction (antigen unspecified) - *continued*
    Rh (antigens (C) (c) (D) (E) (e)) (factor) - *continued*
      hemolytic transfusion reaction (HTR) (unspecified time after transfusion) T80.419
        acute (AHTR) (less than 24 hours after transfusion) T80.410
        delayed (DHTR) (24 hours or more after transfusion) T80.411
        specified NEC T80.49
  infection T80.29
    acute T80.22
  reaction NEC T80.89
  sepsis T80.29
  shock T80.89
transplant T86.90
  bone T86.839
    failure T86.831
    infection T86.832
    rejection T86.830
    specified type NEC T86.838
  bone marrow T86.00
    failure T86.02
    infection T86.03
    rejection T86.01
    specified type NEC T86.09
  cornea T86.849
    failure T86.841
    infection T86.842
    rejection T86.840
    specified type NEC T86.848
  failure T86.92
  heart T86.20
    with lung T86.30
    cardiac allograft vasculopathy T86.290
      failure T86.32
      infection T86.33
      rejection T86.31
      specified type NEC T86.39
    failure T86.22
    infection T86.23
    rejection T86.21
    specified type NEC T86.298
  infection T86.93
  intestine T86.859
    failure T86.851
    infection T86.852
    rejection T86.850
    specified type NEC T86.858
  kidney T86.10
    failure T86.12
    infection T86.13
    rejection T86.11
    specified type NEC T86.19
  liver T86.40
    failure T86.42
    infection T86.43
    rejection T86.41
    specified type NEC T86.49
  lung T86.819
    with heart T86.30
      failure T86.32
      infection T86.33
      rejection T86.31
      specified type NEC T86.39
    failure T86.811
    infection T86.812
    rejection T86.810
    specified type NEC T86.818
  malignant neoplasm C80.2
  pancreas T86.899
    failure T86.891
    infection T86.892
    rejection T86.890
    specified type NEC T86.898
  peripheral blood stem cells T86.5
  post-transplant lymphoproliferative disorder (PTLD) D47.Z1
  rejection T86.91
  skin T86.829

Complication (s) (from) (of) - *continued*
transplant - *continued*
  skin - *continued*
    failure T86.821
    infection T86.822
    rejection T86.820
    specified type NEC T86.828
  specified
    tissue T86.899
      failure T86.891
      infection T86.892
      rejection T86.890
      specified type NEC T86.898
    type NEC T86.99
  stem cell (from peripheral blood) (from umbilical cord) T86.5
  umbilical cord stem cells T86.5
trauma (early) T79.9
  specified NEC T79.8
ultrasound therapy NEC T88.9
umbilical cord NEC
  complicating delivery O69.9
    specified NEC O69.89
umbrella device, vascular T82.9
  embolism T82.818
  fibrosis T82.828
  hemorrhage T82.838
  infection or inflammation T82.7
  mechanical
    breakdown T82.515
    displacement T82.525
    leakage T82.535
    malposition T82.525
    obstruction T82.595
    perforation T82.595
    protrusion T82.595
  pain T82.848
  specified type NEC T82.898
  stenosis T82.858
  thrombosis T82.868
urethral catheter — *see* Complications, catheter, urethral, indwelling
vaccination T88.1
  anaphylaxis NEC T80.52
  arthropathy — *see* Arthropathy, postimmunization
  cellulitis T88.0
  encephalitis or encephalomyelitis G04.02
  infection (general) (local) NEC T88.0
  meningitis G03.8
  myelitis G04.02
  protein sickness T80.62
  rash T88.1
  reaction (allergic) T88.1
    serum T80.62
  sepsis T88.0
  serum intoxication, sickness, rash, or other serum reaction NEC T80.62
    anaphylactic shock T80.52
  shock (allergic) (anaphylactic) T80.52
  vaccinia (generalized) (localized) T88.1
vas deferens device or implant — *see* Complications, genitourinary, device or implant, genital tract
vascular I99.9
  device or implant T82.9
    embolism T82.818
    fibrosis T82.828
    hemorrhage T82.838
    infection or inflammation T82.7
    mechanical
      breakdown T82.519
        specified device NEC T82.518
      displacement T82.529
        specified device NEC T82.528
      leakage T82.539
        specified device NEC T82.538
      malposition T82.529
        specified device NEC T82.528
      obstruction T82.599
        specified device NEC T82.598
      perforation T82.599
        specified device NEC T82.598
      protrusion T82.599
        specified device NEC T82.598

Complication (s) (from) (of) - *continued*
vascular - *continued*
  device or implant - *continued*
    pain T82.848
    specified type NEC T82.898
    stenosis T82.858
    thrombosis T82.868
  dialysis catheter — *see* Complication, catheter, dialysis
  following infusion, therapeutic injection or transfusion T80.1
  graft T82.9
    embolism T82.818
    fibrosis T82.828
    hemorrhage T82.838
    mechanical
      breakdown T82.319
        aorta (bifurcation) T82.310
        carotid artery T82.311
        specified vessel NEC T82.318
      displacement T82.329
        aorta (bifurcation) T82.320
        carotid artery T82.321
        specified vessel NEC T82.328
      leakage T82.339
        aorta (bifurcation) T82.330
        carotid artery T82.331
        specified vessel NEC T82.338
      malposition T82.329
        aorta (bifurcation) T82.320
        carotid artery T82.321
        specified vessel NEC T82.328
      obstruction T82.399
        aorta (bifurcation) T82.390
        carotid artery T82.391
        specified vessel NEC T82.398
      perforation T82.399
        aorta (bifurcation) T82.390
        carotid artery T82.391
        specified vessel NEC T82.398
      protrusion T82.399
        aorta (bifurcation) T82.390
        carotid artery T82.391
        specified vessel NEC T82.398
    pain T82.848
    specified complication NEC T82.898
    stenosis T82.858
    thrombosis T82.868
  postoperative — *see* Complications, postoperative, circulatory
  vena cava device (filter) (sieve) (umbrella) — *see* Complications, umbrella device, vascular
ventilation therapy NEC T81.81
ventilator
  mechanical J95.850
    specified NEC J95.859
ventricular (communicating) shunt (device) T85.9
  embolism T85.810
  fibrosis T85.820
  hemorrhage T85.830
  infection and inflammation T85.730
  mechanical
    breakdown T85.01
    displacement T85.02
    leakage T85.03
    malposition T85.02
    obstruction T85.09
    perforation T85.09
    protrusion T85.09
    specified NEC T85.09
  pain T85.840
  specified type NEC T85.890
  stenosis T85.850
  thrombosis T85.860
wire suture, permanent (implanted) — *see* Complications, suture, permanent
Compressed air disease T70.3
Compression
  with injury - code by Nature of injury
  artery I77.1
    celiac, syndrome I77.4
  brachial plexus G54.0
  brain (stem) G93.5

Compression - *continued*
  brain (stem) - *continued*
    due to
      contusion (diffuse) — *see* Injury,
        intracranial, diffuse
        focal — *see* Injury, intracranial, focal
      injury NEC — *see* Injury, intracranial,
        diffuse
      traumatic — *see* Injury, intracranial,
        diffuse
  bronchus J98.09
  cauda equina G83.4
  celiac (artery) (axis) I77.4
  cerebral — *see* Compression, brain
  cervical plexus G54.2
  cord
    spinal — *see* Compression, spinal
    umbilical — *see* Compression, umbilical
      cord
  cranial nerve G52.9
    eighth — *see* subcategory H93.3
    eleventh G52.8
    fifth G50.8
    first G52.0
    fourth — *see* Strabismus, paralytic, fourth
      nerve
    ninth G52.1
    second — *see* Disorder, nerve, optic
    seventh G51.8
    sixth — *see* Strabismus, paralytic, sixth
      nerve
    tenth G52.2
    third — *see* Strabismus, paralytic, third
      nerve
    twelfth G52.3
  diver's squeeze T70.3
  during birth (newborn) P15.9
  esophagus K22.2
  eustachian tube — *see* Obstruction,
    eustachian tube, cartilaginous
  facies Q67.1
  fracture
    nontraumatic NOS — *see* Collapse,
      vertebra
    pathological — *see* Fracture, pathological
    traumatic — *see* Fracture, traumatic
  heart — *see* Disease, heart
  intestine — *see* Obstruction, intestine
  laryngeal nerve, recurrent G52.2
    with paralysis of vocal cords and
      larynx J38.00
      bilateral J38.02
      unilateral J38.01
  lumbosacral plexus G54.1
  lung J98.4
  lymphatic vessel I89.0
  medulla — *see* Compression, brain
  nerve — *see also* Disorder, nerve G58.9
    arm NEC — *see* Mononeuropathy, upper
      limb
    axillary G54.0
    cranial — *see* Compression, cranial nerve
    leg NEC — *see* Mononeuropathy, lower
      limb
    median (in carpal tunnel) — *see*
      Syndrome, carpal tunnel
    optic — *see* Disorder, nerve, optic
    plantar — *see* Lesion, nerve, plantar
    posterior tibial (in tarsal tunnel) — *see*
      Syndrome, tarsal tunnel
    root or plexus NOS (in) G54.9
      intervertebral disc disorder NEC — *see*
        Disorder, disc, with, radiculopathy
        with myelopathy — *see* Disorder,
          disc, with, myelopathy
      neoplastic disease — *see also*
        Neoplasm D49.9 *[G55]*
      spondylosis — *see* Spondylosis, with
        radiculopathy
    sciatic (acute) — *see* Lesion, nerve, sciatic
    sympathetic G90.8
    traumatic — *see* Injury, nerve
    ulnar — *see* Lesion, nerve, ulnar
    upper extremity NEC — *see*
      Mononeuropathy, upper limb

Compression - *continued*
  spinal (cord) G95.20
    by displacement of intervertebral disc
      NEC — *see also* Disorder, disc, with,
      myelopathy
    nerve root NOS G54.9
      due to displacement of intervertebral
        disc NEC — *see* Disorder, disc,
        with, radiculopathy
        with myelopathy — *see* Disorder,
          disc, with, myelopathy
      specified NEC G95.29
    spondylogenic (cervical) (lumbar,
      lumbosacral) (thoracic) — *see*
      Spondylosis, with myelopathy NEC
    anterior — *see* Syndrome, anterior,
      spinal artery, compression
    traumatic — *see* Injury, spinal cord, by
      region
  subcostal nerve (syndrome) — *see*
    Mononeuropathy, upper limb, specified
    NEC
  sympathetic nerve NEC G90.8
  syndrome T79.5
  trachea J39.8
  ulnar nerve (by scar tissue) — *see* Lesion,
    nerve, ulnar
  umbilical cord
    complicating delivery O69.2
      cord around neck O69.1
      prolapse O69.0
      specified NEC O69.2
  ureter N13.5
  vein I87.1
  vena cava (inferior) (superior) I87.1
Compulsion, compulsive
  gambling F63.0
  neurosis F42.8
  personality F60.5
  states F42.8
  swearing F42.8
    in Gilles de la Tourette's syndrome F95.2
  tics and spasms F95.9
Concato's disease (pericardial polyserositis)
  A19.9
  nontubercular I31.1
  pleural — *see* Pleurisy, with effusion
Concavity chest wall M95.4
Concealed penis Q55.64
Concern (normal) about sick person in
  family Z63.6
Concrescence (teeth) K00.2
Concretio cordis I31.1
  rheumatic I09.2
Concretion — *see also* Calculus
  appendicular K38.1
  canaliculus — *see* Dacryolith
  clitoris N90.89
  conjunctiva H11.12-
  eyelid — *see* Disorder, eyelid, specified type
    NEC
  lacrimal passages — *see* Dacryolith
  prepuce (male) N47.8
  salivary gland (any) K11.5
  seminal vesicle N50.89
  tonsil J35.8
Concussion (brain) (cerebral) (current)
  S06.0X9
  with
    loss of consciousness of 30 minutes or
      less S06.0X1
    loss of consciousness of unspecified
      duration S06.0X9
  blast (air) (hydraulic) (immersion)
    (underwater)
    abdomen or thorax — *see* Injury, blast, by
      site
    ear with acoustic nerve injury — *see*
      Injury, nerve, acoustic, specified type
      NEC
  cauda equina S34.3
  conus medullaris S34.02
  ocular S05.8X-
  spinal (cord)
    cervical S14.0

Concussion (brain) (cerebral) (current) -
continued
  spinal (cord) - *continued*
    lumbar S34.01
    sacral S34.02
    thoracic S24.0
  syndrome F07.81
  without loss of consciousness S06.0X0
Condition — *see* Disease
Conditions arising in the perinatal
  period — *see* Newborn, affected by
Conduct disorder — *see* Disorder, conduct
Condyloma A63.0
  acuminatum A63.0
  gonorrheal A54.09
  latum A51.31
  syphilitic A51.31
    congenital A50.07
  venereal, syphilitic A51.31
Conflagration — *see also* Burn
  asphyxia (by inhalation of gases, fumes or
    vapors) — *see also* Table of Drugs and
    Chemicals T59.9-
Conflict (with) — *see also* Discord
  family Z73.9
  marital Z63.0
    involving divorce or estrangement Z63.5
  parent-child Z62.820
    parent-adopted child Z62.821
    parent-biological child Z62.820
    parent-foster child Z62.822
  social role NEC Z73.5
Confluent — *see* condition
Confusion, confused R41.0
  epileptic F05
  mental state (psychogenic) F44.89
  psychogenic F44.89
  reactive (from emotional stress,
    psychological trauma) F44.89
Confusional arousals G47.51
Congelation T69.9
Congenital — *see also* condition
  aortic septum Q25.49
  intrinsic factor deficiency D51.0
  malformation — *see* Anomaly
Congestion, congestive
  bladder N32.89
  bowel K63.89
  brain G93.89
  breast N64.59
  bronchial J98.09
  catarrhal J31.0
  chest R09.89
  chill, malarial — *see* Malaria
  circulatory NEC I99.8
  duodenum K31.89
  eye — *see* Hyperemia, conjunctiva
  facial, due to birth injury P15.4
  general R68.89
  glottis J37.0
  heart — *see* Failure, heart, congestive
  hepatic K76.1
  hypostatic (lung) — *see* Edema, lung
  intestine K63.89
  kidney N28.89
  labyrinth — *see* subcategory H83.8
  larynx J37.0
  liver K76.1
  lung R09.89
    active or acute — *see* Pneumonia
  malaria, malarial — *see* Malaria
  nasal R09.81
  nose R09.81
  orbit, orbital — *see also* Exophthalmos
    inflammatory (chronic) — *see*
      Inflammation, orbit
  ovary N83.8
  pancreas K86.89
  pelvic, female N94.89
  pleural J94.8
  prostate (active) N42.1
  pulmonary — *see* Congestion, lung
  renal N28.89
  retina H35.81
  seminal vesicle N50.1

Congestion, congestive - *continued*
  spinal cord G95.19
  spleen (chronic) D73.2
  stomach K31.89
  trachea — *see* Tracheitis
  urethra N36.8
  uterus N85.8
    with subinvolution N85.3
  venous (passive) I87.8
  viscera R68.89
Congestive — *see* Congestion
Conical
  cervix (hypertrophic elongation) N88.4
  cornea — *see* Keratoconus
  teeth K00.2
Conjoined twins Q89.4
Conjugal maladjustment Z63.0
  involving divorce or estrangement Z63.5
Conjunctiva — *see* condition
Conjunctivitis (staphylococcal)
    (streptococcal) NOS H10.9
  Acanthamoeba B60.12
  acute H10.3-
    atopic H10.1-
    mucopurulent H10.02-
      follicular H10.01-
    chemical — *see also* Corrosion,
        cornea H10.21-
    pseudomembranous H10.22-
    serous except viral H10.23-
      viral — *see* Conjunctivitis, viral
    toxic H10.21-
  adenoviral (acute) (follicular) B30.1
  allergic (acute) — *see* Conjunctivitis, acute,
      atopic
    chronic H10.45
      vernal H10.44
  anaphylactic — *see* Conjunctivitis, acute,
      atopic
  Apollo B30.3
  atopic (acute) — *see* Conjunctivitis, acute,
      atopic
  Béal's B30.2
  blennorrhagic (gonococcal)
      (neonatorum) A54.31
  chemical (acute) — *see also* Corrosion,
      cornea H10.21-
  chlamydial A74.0
    due to trachoma A71.1
    neonatal P39.1
  chronic (nodosa) (petrificans)
      (phlyctenular) H10.40-
    allergic H10.45
      vernal H10.44
    follicular H10.43-
    giant papillary H10.41-
    simple H10.42-
    vernal H10.44
  coxsackievirus 24 B30.3
  diphtheritic A36.86
  due to
    dust — *see* Conjunctivitis, acute, atopic
    filariasis B74.9
    mucocutaneous leishmaniasis B55.2
  enterovirus type 70 (hemorrhagic) B30.3
  epidemic (viral) B30.9
    hemorrhagic B30.3
  gonococcal (neonatorum) A54.31
  granular (trachomatous) A71.1
    sequelae (late effect) B94.0
  hemorrhagic (acute) (epidemic) B30.3
  herpes zoster B02.31
  in (due to)
    Acanthamoeba B60.12
    adenovirus (acute) (follicular) B30.1
    Chlamydia A74.0
    coxsackievirus 24 B30.3
    diphtheria A36.86
    enterovirus type 70 (hemorrhagic) B30.3
    filariasis B74.9
    gonococci A54.31
    herpes (simplex) virus B00.53
      zoster B02.31
    infectious disease NEC B99
    meningococci A39.89

Conjunctivitis (staphylococcal)
    (streptococcal) NOS - *continued*
  in (due to) - *continued*
    mucocutaneous leishmaniasis B55.2
    rosacea H10.82-
    syphilis (late) A52.71
    zoster B02.31
  inclusion A74.0
  infantile P39.1
    gonococcal A54.31
  Koch-Weeks' — *see* Conjunctivitis, acute,
      mucopurulent
  light — *see* Conjunctivitis, acute, atopic
  ligneous — *see* Blepharoconjunctivitis,
      ligneous
  meningococcal A39.89
  mucopurulent — *see* Conjunctivitis, acute,
      mucopurulent
  neonatal P39.1
    gonococcal A54.31
  Newcastle B30.8
  of Béal B30.2
  parasitic
    filariasis B74.9
    mucocutaneous leishmaniasis B55.2
  Parinaud's H10.89
  petrificans H10.89
  rosacea H10.82-
  specified NEC H10.89
  swimming-pool B30.1
  trachomatous A71.1
    acute A71.0
    sequelae (late effect) B94.0
  traumatic NEC H10.89
  tuberculous A18.59
  tularemic A21.1
  tularensis A21.1
  viral B30.9
    due to
      adenovirus B30.1
      enterovirus B30.3
    specified NEC B30.8
Conjunctivochalasis H11.82-
Connective tissue — *see* condition
Conn's syndrome E26.01
Conradi (-Hunermann) disease Q77.3
Consanguinity Z84.3
  counseling Z71.89
Conscious simulation (of illness) Z76.5
Consecutive — *see* condition
Consolidation lung (base) — *see* Pneumonia,
    lobar
Constipation (atonic) (neurogenic) (simple)
    (spastic) K59.00
  chronic K59.09
    idiopathic K59.04
  drug-induced K59.03
  functional K59.04
  outlet dysfunction K59.02
  psychogenic F45.8
  slow transit K59.01
  specified NEC K59.09
Constitutional — *see also* condition
  substandard F60.7
Constitutionally substandard F60.7
Constriction — *see also* Stricture
  auditory canal — *see* Stenosis, external ear
      canal
  bronchial J98.09
  duodenum K31.5
  esophagus K22.2
  external
    abdomen, abdominal (wall) S30.841
    alveolar process S00.542
    ankle S90.54-
    antecubital space — *see* Constriction,
        external, forearm
    arm (upper) S40.84-
    auricle — *see* Constriction, external, ear
    axilla — *see* Constriction, external, arm
    back, lower S30.840
    breast S20.14-
    brow S00.84
    buttock S30.840
    calf — *see* Constriction, external, leg

Constriction - *continued*
  external - *continued*
    canthus — *see* Constriction, external,
        eyelid
    cheek S00.84
      internal S00.542
    chest wall — *see* Constriction, external,
        thorax
    chin S00.84
    clitoris S30.844
    costal region — *see* Constriction, external,
        thorax
    digit (s)
      foot — *see* Constriction, external, toe
      hand — *see* Constriction, external,
          finger
    ear S00.44-
    elbow S50.34-
    epididymis S30.843
    epigastric region S30.841
    esophagus, cervical S10.14
    eyebrow — *see* Constriction, external,
        eyelid
    eyelid S00.24-
    face S00.84
    finger (s) S60.44-
      index S60.44-
      little S60.44-
      middle S60.44-
      ring S60.44-
    flank S30.841
    foot (except toe (s) alone) S90.84-
      toe — *see* Constriction, external, toe
    forearm S50.84-
      elbow only — *see* Constriction, external,
          elbow
    forehead S00.84
    genital organs, external
      female S30.846
      male S30.845
    groin S30.841
    gum S00.542
    hand S60.54-
    head S00.94
      ear — *see* Constriction, external, ear
      eyelid — *see* Constriction, external,
          eyelid
      lip S00.541
      nose S00.34
      oral cavity S00.542
      scalp S00.04
      specified site NEC S00.84
    heel — *see* Constriction, external, foot
    hip S70.24-
    inguinal region S30.841
    interscapular region S20.449
    jaw S00.84
    knee S80.24-
    labium (majus) (minus) S30.844
    larynx S10.14
    leg (lower) S80.84-
      knee — *see* Constriction, external, knee
      upper — *see* Constriction, external,
          thigh
    lip S00.541
    lower back S30.840
    lumbar region S30.840
    malar region S00.84
    mammary — *see* Constriction, external,
        breast
    mastoid region S00.84
    mouth S00.542
    nail
      finger — *see* Constriction, external,
          finger
      toe — *see* Constriction, external, toe
    nasal S00.34
    neck S10.94
      specified site NEC S10.84
      throat S10.14
    nose S00.34
    occipital region S00.04
    oral cavity S00.542
    orbital region — *see* Constriction, external,
        eyelid

Constriction - *continued*
external - *continued*
palate S00.542
palm — *see* Constriction, external, hand
parietal region S00.04
pelvis S30.840
penis S30.842
perineum
female S30.844
male S30.840
periocular area — *see* Constriction, external, eyelid
phalanges
finger — *see* Constriction, external, finger
toe — *see* Constriction, external, toe
pharynx S10.14
pinna — *see* Constriction, external, ear
popliteal space — *see* Constriction, external, knee
prepuce S30.842
pubic region S30.840
pudendum
female S30.846
male S30.845
sacral region S30.840
scalp S00.04
scapular region — *see* Constriction, external, shoulder
scrotum S30.843
shin — *see* Constriction, external, leg
shoulder S40.24-
sternal region S20.349
submaxillary region S00.84
submental region S00.84
subungual
finger (s) — *see* Constriction, external, finger
toe (s) — *see* Constriction, external, toe
supraclavicular fossa S10.84
supraorbital S00.84
temple S00.84
temporal region S00.84
testis S30.843
thigh S70.34-
thorax, thoracic (wall) S20.94
back S20.44-
front S20.34-
throat S10.14
thumb S60.34-
toe (s) (lesser) S90.44-
great S90.44-
tongue S00.542
trachea S10.14
tunica vaginalis S30.843
uvula S00.542
vagina S30.844
vulva S30.844
wrist S60.84-
gallbladder — *see* Obstruction, gallbladder
intestine — *see* Obstruction, intestine
larynx J38.6
congenital Q31.8
specified NEC Q31.8
subglottic Q31.1
organ or site, congenital NEC — *see* Atresia, by site
prepuce (acquired) (congenital) N47.1
pylorus (adult hypertrophic) K31.1
congenital or infantile Q40.0
newborn Q40.0
ring dystocia (uterus) O62.4
spastic — *see also* Spasm
ureter N13.5
ureter N13.5
with infection N13.6
urethra — *see* Stricture, urethra
visual field (peripheral) (functional) — *see* Defect, visual field
Constrictive — *see* condition
Consultation
medical — *see* Counseling, medical
religious Z71.81
specified reason NEC Z71.89
spiritual Z71.81

Consultation - *continued*
without complaint or sickness Z71.9
feared complaint unfounded Z71.1
specified reason NEC Z71.89
Consumption — *see* Tuberculosis
Contact (with) — *see also* Exposure (to)
acariasis Z20.7
AIDS virus Z20.6
air pollution Z77.110
algae and algae toxins Z77.121
algae bloom Z77.121
anthrax Z20.810
aromatic amines Z77.020
aromatic (hazardous) compounds NEC Z77.028
aromatic dyes NOS Z77.028
arsenic Z77.010
asbestos Z77.090
bacterial disease NEC Z20.818
benzene Z77.021
blue-green algae bloom Z77.121
body fluids (potentially hazardous) Z77.21
brown tide Z77.121
chemicals (chiefly nonmedicinal) (hazardous) NEC Z77.098
cholera Z20.09
chromium compounds Z77.018
communicable disease Z20.9
bacterial NEC Z20.818
specified NEC Z20.89
viral NEC Z20.828
Zika virus Z20.821
cyanobacteria bloom Z77.121
dyes Z77.098
Escherichia coli (E. coli) Z20.01
fiberglass — *see* Table of Drugs and Chemicals, fiberglass
German measles Z20.4
gonorrhea Z20.2
hazardous metals NEC Z77.018
hazardous substances NEC Z77.29
hazards in the physical environment NEC Z77.128
hazards to health NEC Z77.9
HIV Z20.6
HTLV-III/LAV Z20.6
human immunodeficiency virus (HIV) Z20.6
infection Z20.9
specified NEC Z20.89
infestation (parasitic) NEC Z20.7
intestinal infectious disease NEC Z20.09
Escherichia coli (E. coli) Z20.01
lead Z77.011
meningococcus Z20.811
mold (toxic) Z77.120
nickel dust Z77.018
noise Z77.122
parasitic disease Z20.7
pediculosis Z20.7
pfiesteria piscicida Z77.121
poliomyelitis Z20.89
pollution
air Z77.110
environmental NEC Z77.118
soil Z77.112
water Z77.111
polycyclic aromatic hydrocarbons Z77.028
rabies Z20.3
radiation, naturally occurring NEC Z77.123
radon Z77.123
red tide (Florida) Z77.121
rubella Z20.4
sexually-transmitted disease Z20.2
smallpox (laboratory) Z20.89
syphilis Z20.2
tuberculosis Z20.1
uranium Z77.012
varicella Z20.820
venereal disease Z20.2
viral disease NEC Z20.828
viral hepatitis Z20.5
water pollution Z77.111
Zika virus Z20.821
Contamination, food — *see* Intoxication, foodborne

Contraception, contraceptive
advice Z30.09
counseling Z30.09
device (intrauterine) (in situ) Z97.5
causing menorrhagia T83.83
checking Z30.431
complications — *see* Complications, intrauterine, contraceptive device
in place Z97.5
initial prescription Z30.014
reinsertion Z30.433
removal Z30.432
replacement Z30.433
emergency (postcoital) Z30.012
initial prescription Z30.019
barrier Z30.018
diaphragm Z30.018
injectable Z30.013
intrauterine device Z30.014
pills Z30.011
postcoital (emergency) Z30.012
specified type NEC Z30.018
subdermal implantable Z30.017
transdermal patch hormonal Z30.016
vaginal ring hormonal Z30.015
maintenance Z30.40
barrier Z30.49
diaphragm Z30.49
examination Z30.8
injectable Z30.42
intrauterine device Z30.431
pills Z30.41
specified type NEC Z30.49
subdermal implantable Z30.46
transdermal patch hormonal Z30.45
vaginal ring hormonal Z30.44
management Z30.9
specified NEC Z30.8
postcoital (emergency) Z30.012
prescription Z30.019
repeat Z30.40
sterilization Z30.2
surveillance (drug) — *see* Contraception, maintenance
Contraction (s) , contracture, contracted
Achilles tendon — *see also* Short, tendon, Achilles
congenital Q66.89
amputation stump (surgical) (flexion) (late) (next proximal joint) T87.89
anus K59.8
bile duct (common) (hepatic) K83.8
bladder N32.89
neck or sphincter N32.0
bowel, cecum, colon or intestine, any part — *see* Obstruction, intestine
Braxton Hicks — *see* False, labor
breast implant, capsular T85.44
bronchial J98.09
burn (old) — *see* Cicatrix
cervix — *see* Stricture, cervix
cicatricial — *see* Cicatrix
conjunctiva, trachomatous, active A71.1
sequelae (late effect) B94.0
Dupuytren's M72.0
eyelid — *see* Disorder, eyelid function
fascia (lata) (postural) M72.8
Dupuytren's M72.0
palmar M72.0
plantar M72.2
finger NEC — *see also* Deformity, finger
congenital Q68.1
joint — *see* Contraction, joint, hand
flaccid — *see* Contraction, paralytic
gallbladder K82.0
heart valve — *see* Endocarditis
hip — *see* Contraction, joint, hip
hourglass
bladder N32.89
congenital Q64.79
gallbladder K82.0
congenital Q44.1
stomach K31.89
congenital Q40.2
psychogenic F45.8

Contraction (s) , contracture, contracted - *continued*
hourglass - *continued*
  uterus (complicating delivery) O62.4
hysterical F44.4
internal os — *see* Stricture, cervix
joint (abduction) (acquired) (adduction)
  (flexion) (rotation) M24.50
  ankle M24.57-
  congenital NEC Q68.8
    hip Q65.89
  elbow M24.52-
  foot joint M24.57-
  hand joint M24.54-
  hip M24.55-
    congenital Q65.89
  hysterical F44.4
  knee M24.56-
  shoulder M24.51-
  wrist M24.53-
kidney (granular) (secondary) N26.9
  congenital Q63.8
  hydronephritic — *see* Hydronephrosis
    Page N26.2
  pyelonephritic — *see* Pyelitis, chronic
  tuberculous A18.11
ligament — *see also* Disorder, ligament
  congenital Q79.8
muscle (postinfective) (postural)
  NEC M62.40
  with contracture of joint — *see*
    Contraction, joint
  ankle M62.47-
  congenital Q79.8
    sternocleidomastoid Q68.0
  extraocular — *see* Strabismus
  eye (extrinsic) — *see* Strabismus
  foot M62.47-
  forearm M62.43-
  hand M62.44-
  hysterical F44.4
  ischemic (Volkmann's) T79.6
  lower leg M62.46-
  multiple sites M62.49
  pelvic region M62.45-
  posttraumatic — *see* Strabismus, paralytic
  psychogenic F45.8
    conversion reaction F44.4
  shoulder region M62.41-
  specified site NEC M62.48
  thigh M62.45-
  upper arm M62.42-
neck — *see* Torticollis
ocular muscle — *see* Strabismus
organ or site, congenital NEC — *see* Atresia,
  by site
outlet (pelvis) — *see* Contraction, pelvis
palmar fascia M72.0
paralytic
  joint — *see* Contraction, joint
  muscle — *see also* Contraction, muscle
    NEC
    ocular — *see* Strabismus, paralytic
pelvis (acquired) (general) M95.5
  with disproportion (fetopelvic) O33.1
    causing obstructed labor O65.1
  inlet O33.2
  mid-cavity O33.3
  outlet O33.3
plantar fascia M72.2
premature
  atrium I49.1
  auriculoventricular I49.49
  heart I49.49
  junctional I49.2
  supraventricular I49.1
  ventricular I49.3
prostate N42.89
pylorus NEC — *see also* Pylorospasm
  psychogenic F45.8
rectum, rectal (sphincter) K59.8
ring (Bandl's) (complicating delivery) O62.4
scar — *see* Cicatrix
spine — *see* Dorsopathy, deforming

Contraction (s) , contracture, contracted - *continued*
sternocleidomastoid (muscle) ,
  congenital Q68.0
stomach K31.89
  hourglass K31.89
    congenital Q40.2
    psychogenic F45.8
  psychogenic F45.8
tendon (sheath) M62.40
  with contracture of joint — *see*
    Contraction, joint
  Achilles — *see* Short, tendon, Achilles
  ankle M62.47-
    Achilles — *see* Short, tendon, Achilles
  foot M62.47-
  forearm M62.43-
  hand M62.44-
  lower leg M62.46-
  multiple sites M62.49
  neck M62.48
  pelvic region M62.45-
  shoulder region M62.41-
  specified site NEC M62.48
  thigh M62.45-
  thorax M62.48
  trunk M62.48
  upper arm M62.42-
toe — *see* Deformity, toe, specified NEC
ureterovesical orifice (postinfectional) N13.5
  with infection N13.6
urethra — *see also* Stricture, urethra
  orifice N32.0
uterus N85.8
  abnormal NEC O62.9
  clonic (complicating delivery) O62.4
  dyscoordinate (complicating
    delivery) O62.4
  hourglass (complicating delivery) O62.4
  hypertonic O62.4
  hypotonic NEC O62.2
  inadequate
    primary O62.0
    secondary O62.1
  incoordinate (complicating delivery) O62.4
  poor O62.2
  tetanic (complicating delivery) O62.4
vagina (outlet) N89.5
vesical N32.89
  neck or urethral orifice N32.0
visual field — *see* Defect, visual field,
  generalized
Volkmann's (ischemic) T79.6
Contusion (skin surface intact) T14.8
abdomen, abdominal (muscle) (wall) S30.1
adnexa, eye NEC S05.8X-
adrenal gland S37.812
alveolar process S00.532
ankle S90.0-
antecubital space — *see* Contusion, forearm
anus S30.3
arm (upper) S40.02-
  lower (with elbow) — *see* Contusion,
    forearm
auditory canal — *see* Contusion, ear
auricle — *see* Contusion, ear
axilla — *see* Contusion, arm, upper
back — *see also* Contusion, thorax, back
  lower S30.0
bile duct S36.13
bladder S37.22
bone NEC T14.8
brain (diffuse) — *see* Injury, intracranial,
  diffuse
  focal — *see* Injury, intracranial, focal
brainstem S06.38-
breast S20.0-
broad ligament S37.892
brow S00.83
buttock S30.0
canthus, eye S00.1-
cauda equina S34.3
cerebellar, traumatic S06.37-
cerebral S06.33-
  left side S06.32-

Contusion (skin surface intact) - *continued*
cerebral - *continued*
  right side S06.31-
cheek S00.83
  internal S00.532
chest (wall) — *see* Contusion, thorax
chin S00.83
clitoris S30.23
colon — *see* Injury, intestine, large,
  contusion
common bile duct S36.13
conjunctiva S05.1-
  with foreign body (in conjunctival sac) —
    see Foreign body, conjunctival sac
conus medullaris (spine) S34.139
cornea — *see* Contusion, eyeball
  with foreign body — *see* Foreign body,
    cornea
corpus cavernosum S30.21
cortex (brain) (cerebral) — *see* Injury,
  intracranial, diffuse
  focal — *see* Injury, intracranial, focal
costal region — *see* Contusion, thorax
cystic duct S36.13
diaphragm S27.802
duodenum S36.420
ear S00.43-
elbow S50.0-
  with forearm — *see* Contusion, forearm
epididymis S30.22
epigastric region S30.1
epiglottis S10.0
esophagus (thoracic) S27.812
  cervical S10.0
eyeball S05.1-
eyebrow S00.1-
eyelid (and periocular area) S00.1-
face NEC S00.83
fallopian tube S37.529
  bilateral S37.522
  unilateral S37.521
femoral triangle S30.1
finger (s) S60.00
  with damage to nail (matrix) S60.10
  index S60.02-
    with damage to nail S60.12-
  little S60.05-
    with damage to nail S60.15-
  middle S60.03-
    with damage to nail S60.13-
  ring S60.04-
    with damage to nail S60.14-
  thumb — *see* Contusion, thumb
flank S30.1
foot (except toe (s) alone) S90.3-
  toe — *see* Contusion, toe
forearm S50.1-
  elbow only — *see* Contusion, elbow
forehead S00.83
gallbladder S36.122
genital organs, external
  female S30.202
  male S30.201
globe (eye) — *see* Contusion, eyeball
groin S30.1
gum S00.532
hand S60.22-
  finger (s) — *see* Contusion, finger
  wrist — *see* Contusion, wrist
head S00.93
  ear — *see* Contusion, ear
  eyelid — *see* Contusion, eyelid
  lip S00.531
  nose S00.33
  oral cavity S00.532
  scalp S00.03
  specified part NEC S00.83
heart — *see also* Injury, heart S26.91
heel — *see* Contusion, foot
hepatic duct S36.13
hip S70.0-
ileum S36.428
iliac region S30.1
inguinal region S30.1
interscapular region S20.229

Contusion (skin surface intact) - *continued*
intra-abdominal organ S36.92
  colon — *see* Injury, intestine, large, contusion
  liver S36.112
  pancreas — *see* Contusion, pancreas
  rectum S36.62
  small intestine — *see* Injury, intestine, small, contusion
  specified organ NEC S36.892
  spleen — *see* Contusion, spleen
  stomach S36.32
iris (eye) — *see* Contusion, eyeball
jaw S00.83
jejunum S36.428
kidney S37.01-
  major (greater than 2 cm) S37.02-
  minor (less than 2 cm) S37.01-
knee S80.0-
labium (majus) (minus) S30.23
lacrimal apparatus, gland or sac S05.8X-
larynx S10.0
leg (lower) S80.1-
  knee — *see* Contusion, knee
lens — *see* Contusion, eyeball
lip S00.531
liver S36.112
lower back S30.0
lumbar region S30.0
lung S27.329
  bilateral S27.322
  unilateral S27.321
malar region S00.83
mastoid region S00.83
membrane, brain — *see* Injury, intracranial, diffuse
  focal — *see* Injury, intracranial, focal
mesentery S36.892
mesosalpinx S37.892
mouth S00.532
muscle — *see* Contusion, by site
nail
  finger — *see* Contusion, finger, with damage to nail
  toe — *see* Contusion, toe, with damage to nail
nasal S00.33
neck S10.93
  specified site NEC S10.83
  throat S10.0
nerve — *see* Injury, nerve
newborn P54.5
nose S00.33
occipital
  lobe (brain) — *see* Injury, intracranial, diffuse
  focal — *see* Injury, intracranial, focal
  region (scalp) S00.03
orbit (region) (tissues) S05.1-
ovary S37.429
  bilateral S37.422
  unilateral S37.421
palate S00.532
pancreas S36.229
  body S36.221
  head S36.220
  tail S36.222
parietal
  lobe (brain) — *see* Injury, intracranial, diffuse
  focal — *see* Injury, intracranial, focal
  region (scalp) S00.03
pelvic organ S37.92
  adrenal gland S37.812
  bladder S37.22
  fallopian tube — *see* Contusion, fallopian tube
  kidney — *see* Contusion, kidney
  ovary — *see* Contusion, ovary
  prostate S37.822
  specified organ NEC S37.892
  ureter S37.12
  urethra S37.32
  uterus S37.62
pelvis S30.0

Contusion (skin surface intact) - *continued*
penis S30.21
perineum
  female S30.23
  male S30.0
periocular area S00.1-
peritoneum S36.81
periurethral tissue — *see* Contusion, urethra
pharynx S10.0
pinna — *see* Contusion, ear
popliteal space — *see* Contusion, knee
prepuce S30.21
prostate S37.822
pubic region S30.1
pudendum
  female S30.202
  male S30.201
quadriceps femoris — *see* Contusion, thigh
rectum S36.62
retroperitoneum S36.892
round ligament S37.892
sacral region S30.0
scalp S00.03
  due to birth injury P12.3
scapular region — *see* Contusion, shoulder
sclera — *see* Contusion, eyeball
scrotum S30.22
seminal vesicle S37.892
shoulder S40.01-
skin NEC T14.8
small intestine — *see* Injury, intestine, small, contusion
spermatic cord S30.22
spinal cord — *see* Injury, spinal cord, by region
  cauda equina S34.3
  conus medullaris S34.139
spleen S36.029
  major S36.021
  minor S36.020
sternal region S20.219
stomach S36.32
subconjunctival S05.1-
subcutaneous NEC T14.8
submaxillary region S00.83
submental region S00.83
subperiosteal NEC T14.8
subungual
  finger — *see* Contusion, finger, with damage to nail
  toe — *see* Contusion, toe, with damage to nail
supraclavicular fossa S10.83
supraorbital S00.83
suprarenal gland S37.812
temple (region) S00.83
temporal
  lobe (brain) — *see* Injury, intracranial, diffuse
  focal — *see* Injury, intracranial, focal
  region S00.83
testis S30.22
thigh S70.1-
thorax (wall) S20.20
  back S20.22-
  front S20.21-
throat S10.0
thumb S60.01-
  with damage to nail S60.11-
toe (s) (lesser) S90.12-
  with damage to nail S90.22-
  great S90.11-
    with damage to nail S90.21-
tongue S00.532
trachea (cervical) S10.0
  thoracic S27.52
tunica vaginalis S30.22
tympanum, tympanic membrane — *see* Contusion, ear
ureter S37.12
urethra S37.32
urinary organ NEC S37.892
uterus S37.62
uvula S00.532
vagina S30.23

Contusion (skin surface intact) - *continued*
vas deferens S37.892
vesical S37.22
vocal cord (s) S10.0
vulva S30.23
wrist S60.21-
Conus (congenital) (any type) Q14.8
cornea — *see* Keratoconus
medullaris syndrome G95.81
Conversion hysteria, neurosis or reaction F44.9
Converter, tuberculosis (test reaction) R76.11
Conviction (legal) , anxiety concerning Z65.0
with imprisonment Z65.1
Convulsions (idiopathic) — *see also* Seizure(s) R56.9
apoplectiform (cerebral ischemia) I67.82
dissociative F44.5
epileptic — *see* Epilepsy
epileptiform, epileptoid — *see* Seizure, epileptiform
ether (anesthetic) — *see* Table of Drugs and Chemicals, by drug
febrile R56.00
  with status epilepticus G40.901
  complex R56.01
    with status epilepticus G40.901
  simple R56.00
hysterical F44.5
infantile P90
  epilepsy — *see* Epilepsy
jacksonian — *see* Epilepsy, localization-related, symptomatic, with simple partial seizures
myoclonic G25.3
newborn P90
obstetrical (nephritic) (uremic) — *see* Eclampsia
paretic A52.17
post traumatic R56.1
psychomotor — *see* Epilepsy, localization-related, symptomatic, with complex partial seizures
recurrent R56.9
reflex R25.8
scarlatinal A38.8
tetanus, tetanic — *see* Tetanus
thymic E32.8
Convulsive — *see also* Convulsions
Cooley's anemia D56.1
Coolie itch B76.9
Cooper's
disease — *see* Mastopathy, cystic
hernia — *see* Hernia, abdomen, specified site NEC
Copra itch B88.0
Coprophagy F50.89
Coprophobia F40.298
Coproporphyria, hereditary E80.29
Cor
biloculare Q20.8
bovis, bovinum — *see* Hypertrophy, cardiac
pulmonale (chronic) I27.81
  acute I26.09
triatriatum, triatrium Q24.2
triloculare Q20.8
  biatrium Q20.4
  biventriculare Q21.1
Corbus' disease (gangrenous balanitis) N48.1
Cord — *see also* condition
around neck
  complicating delivery O69.81
    with compression O69.1
  bladder G95.89
  tabetic A52.19
Cordis ectopia Q24.8
Corditis (spermatic) N49.1
Corectopia Q13.2
Cori's disease (glycogen storage) E74.03
Corkhandler's disease or lung J67.3
Corkscrew esophagus K22.4
Corkworker's disease or lung J67.3
Corn (infected) L84

Cornea — *see also* condition
  donor Z52.5
  plana Q13.4
Cornelia de Lange syndrome Q87.19
Cornu cutaneum L85.8
Cornual gestation or pregnancy O00.80
  with intrauterine pregnancy O00.81
Coronary (artery) — *see* condition
Coronavirus, as cause of disease classified
  elsewhere B97.29
  SARS-associated B97.21
Corpora — *see also* condition
  amylacea, prostate N42.89
  cavernosa — *see* condition
Corpulence — *see* Obesity
Corpus — *see* condition
Corrected transposition Q20.5
Corrosion (injury) (acid) (caustic) (chemical)
  (lime) (external) (internal) T30.4
  abdomen, abdominal (muscle) (wall) T21.42
    first degree T21.52
    second degree T21.62
    third degree T21.72
  above elbow T22.439
    first degree T22.539
    left T22.432
      first degree T22.532
      second degree T22.632
      third degree T22.732
    right T22.431
      first degree T22.531
      second degree T22.631
      third degree T22.731
    second degree T22.639
    third degree T22.739
  alimentary tract NEC T28.7
  ankle T25.419
    first degree T25.519
    left T25.412
      first degree T25.512
      second degree T25.612
      third degree T25.712
    multiple with foot — *see* Corrosion, lower,
      limb, multiple, ankle and foot
    right T25.411
      first degree T25.511
      second degree T25.611
      third degree T25.711
    second degree T25.619
    third degree T25.719
  anus — *see* Corrosion, buttock
  arm (s) (meaning upper limb (s)) — *see*
    Corrosion, upper limb
  axilla T22.449
    first degree T22.549
    left T22.442
      first degree T22.542
      second degree T22.642
      third degree T22.742
    right T22.441
      first degree T22.541
      second degree T22.641
      third degree T22.741
    second degree T22.649
    third degree T22.749
  back (lower) T21.44
    first degree T21.54
    second degree T21.64
    third degree T21.74
    upper T21.43
      first degree T21.53
      second degree T21.63
      third degree T21.73
  blisters - code as Corrosion, second degree,
    by site
  breast (s) — *see* Corrosion, chest wall
  buttock (s) T21.45
    first degree T21.55
    second degree T21.65
    third degree T21.75
  calf T24.439
    first degree T24.539
    left T24.432
      first degree T24.532
      second degree T24.632

Corrosion (injury) (acid) (caustic) (chemical)
(lime) (external) (internal) - *continued*
  calf - *continued*
    left - *continued*
      third degree T24.732
    right T24.431
      first degree T24.531
      second degree T24.631
      third degree T24.731
    second degree T24.639
    third degree T24.739
  canthus (eye) — *see* Corrosion, eyelid
  cervix T28.8
  cheek T20.46
    first degree T20.56
    second degree T20.66
    third degree T20.76
  chest wall T21.41
    first degree T21.51
    second degree T21.61
    third degree T21.71
  chin T20.43
    first degree T20.53
    second degree T20.63
    third degree T20.73
  colon T28.7
  conjunctiva (and cornea) — *see* Corrosion,
    cornea
  cornea (and conjunctiva) T26.6-
  deep necrosis of underlying tissue - code as
    Corrosion, third degree, by site
  dorsum of hand T23.469
    first degree T23.569
    left T23.462
      first degree T23.562
      second degree T23.662
      third degree T23.762
    right T23.461
      first degree T23.561
      second degree T23.661
      third degree T23.761
    second degree T23.669
    third degree T23.769
  ear (auricle) (external) (canal) T20.41
    drum T28.91
    first degree T20.51
    second degree T20.61
    third degree T20.71
  elbow T22.429
    first degree T22.529
    left T22.422
      first degree T22.522
      second degree T22.622
      third degree T22.722
    right T22.421
      first degree T22.521
      second degree T22.621
      third degree T22.721
    second degree T22.629
    third degree T22.729
  entire body — *see* Corrosion, multiple body
    regions
  epidermal loss - code as Corrosion, second
    degree, by site
  epiglottis T27.4
  erythema, erythematous - code as Corrosion,
    first degree, by site
  esophagus T28.6
  extent (percentage of body surface)
    less than 10 percent T32.0
    10-19 percent (0-9 percent third
      degree) T32.10
      with 10-19 percent third degree T32.11
    20-29 percent (0-9 percent third
      degree) T32.20
      with
        10-19 percent third degree T32.21
        20-29 percent third degree T32.22
    30-39 percent (0-9 percent third
      degree) T32.30
      with
        10-19 percent third degree T32.31
        20-29 percent third degree T32.32
        30-39 percent third degree T32.33

Corrosion (injury) (acid) (caustic) (chemical)
(lime) (external) (internal) - *continued*
  extent (percentage of body surface) -
    continued
    40-49 percent (0-9 percent third
      degree) T32.40
      with
        10-19 percent third degree T32.41
        20-29 percent third degree T32.42
        30-39 percent third degree T32.43
        40-49 percent third degree T32.44
    50-59 percent (0-9 percent third
      degree) T32.50
      with
        10-19 percent third degree T32.51
        20-29 percent third degree T32.52
        30-39 percent third degree T32.53
        40-49 percent third degree T32.54
        50-59 percent third degree T32.55
    60-69 percent (0-9 percent third
      degree) T32.60
      with
        10-19 percent third degree T32.61
        20-29 percent third degree T32.62
        30-39 percent third degree T32.63
        40-49 percent third degree T32.64
        50-59 percent third degree T32.65
        60-69 percent third degree T32.66
    70-79 percent (0-9 percent third
      degree) T32.70
      with
        10-19 percent third degree T32.71
        20-29 percent third degree T32.72
        30-39 percent third degree T32.73
        40-49 percent third degree T32.74
        50-59 percent third degree T32.75
        60-69 percent third degree T32.76
        70-79 percent third degree T32.77
    80-89 percent (0-9 percent third
      degree) T32.80
      with
        10-19 percent third degree T32.81
        20-29 percent third degree T32.82
        30-39 percent third degree T32.83
        40-49 percent third degree T32.84
        50-59 percent third degree T32.85
        60-69 percent third degree T32.86
        70-79 percent third degree T32.87
        80-89 percent third degree T32.88
    90 percent or more (0-9 percent third
      degree) T32.90
      with
        10-19 percent third degree T32.91
        20-29 percent third degree T32.92
        30-39 percent third degree T32.93
        40-49 percent third degree T32.94
        50-59 percent third degree T32.95
        60-69 percent third degree T32.96
        70-79 percent third degree T32.97
        80-89 percent third degree T32.98
        90-99 percent third degree T32.99
  extremity — *see* Corrosion, limb
  eye (s) and adnexa T26.9-
    with resulting rupture and destruction of
      eyeball T26.7-
    conjunctival sac — *see* Corrosion, cornea
    cornea — *see* Corrosion, cornea
    lid — *see* Corrosion, eyelid
    periocular area — *see* Corrosion eyelid
    specified site NEC T26.8-
  eyeball — *see* Corrosion, eye
  eyelid (s) T26.5-
  face — *see* Corrosion, head
  finger T23.429
    first degree T23.529
    left T23.422
      first degree T23.522
      second degree T23.622
      third degree T23.722
    multiple sites (without thumb) T23.439
      with thumb T23.449
        first degree T23.549
        left T23.442
          first degree T23.542
          second degree T23.642

Corrosion (injury) (acid) (caustic) (chemical) (lime) (external) (internal) - *continued*
  finger - *continued*
    multiple sites (without thumb) - *continued*
      with thumb - *continued*
        left - *continued*
          third degree T23.742
        right T23.441
          first degree T23.541
          second degree T23.641
          third degree T23.741
        second degree T23.649
        third degree T23.749
      first degree T23.539
      left T23.432
        first degree T23.532
        second degree T23.632
        third degree T23.732
      right T23.431
        first degree T23.531
        second degree T23.631
        third degree T23.731
      second degree T23.639
      third degree T23.739
    right T23.421
      first degree T23.521
      second degree T23.621
      third degree T23.721
    second degree T23.629
    third degree T23.729
  flank — *see* Corrosion, abdomen
  foot T25.429
    first degree T25.529
    left T25.422
      first degree T25.522
      second degree T25.622
      third degree T25.722
    multiple with ankle — *see* Corrosion, lower, limb, multiple, ankle and foot
    right T25.421
      first degree T25.521
      second degree T25.621
      third degree T25.721
    second degree T25.629
    third degree T25.729
  forearm T22.419
    first degree T22.519
    left T22.412
      first degree T22.512
      second degree T22.612
      third degree T22.712
    right T22.411
      first degree T22.511
      second degree T22.611
      third degree T22.711
    second degree T22.619
    third degree T22.719
  forehead T20.46
    first degree T20.56
    second degree T20.66
    third degree T20.76
  fourth degree - code as Corrosion, third degree, by site
  full thickness skin loss - code as Corrosion, third degree, by site
  gastrointestinal tract NEC T28.7
  genital organs
    external
      female T21.47
        first degree T21.57
        second degree T21.67
        third degree T21.77
      male T21.46
        first degree T21.56
        second degree T21.66
        third degree T21.76
    internal T28.8
  groin — *see* Corrosion, abdominal wall
  hand (s) T23.409
    back — *see* Corrosion, dorsum of hand
    finger — *see* Corrosion, finger
    first degree T23.509
    left T23.402
      first degree T23.502
      second degree T23.602

Corrosion (injury) (acid) (caustic) (chemical) (lime) (external) (internal) - *continued*
  hand (s) - *continued*
    left - *continued*
      third degree T23.702
    multiple sites with wrist T23.499
      first degree T23.599
      left T23.492
        first degree T23.592
        second degree T23.692
        third degree T23.792
      right T23.491
        first degree T23.591
        second degree T23.691
        third degree T23.791
      second degree T23.699
      third degree T23.799
    palm — *see* Corrosion, palm
    right T23.401
      first degree T23.501
      second degree T23.601
      third degree T23.701
    second degree T23.609
    third degree T23.709
    thumb — *see* Corrosion, thumb
  head (and face) (and neck) T20.40
    cheek — *see* Corrosion, cheek
    chin — *see* Corrosion, chin
    ear — *see* Corrosion, ear
    eye (s) only — *see* Corrosion, eye
    first degree T20.50
    forehead — *see* Corrosion, forehead
    lip — *see* Corrosion, lip
    multiple sites T20.49
      first degree T20.59
      second degree T20.69
      third degree T20.79
    neck — *see* Corrosion, neck
    nose — *see* Corrosion, nose
    scalp — *see* Corrosion, scalp
    second degree T20.60
    third degree T20.70
  hip (s) — *see* Corrosion, lower, limb
  inhalation — *see* Corrosion, respiratory tract
  internal organ (s) — *see also* Corrosion, by site T28.90
    alimentary tract T28.7
      esophagus T28.6
    esophagus T28.6
    genitourinary T28.8
    mouth T28.5
    pharynx T28.5
    specified organ NEC T28.99
  interscapular region — *see* Corrosion, back, upper
  intestine (large) (small) T28.7
  knee T24.429
    first degree T24.529
    left T24.422
      first degree T24.522
      second degree T24.622
      third degree T24.722
    right T24.421
      first degree T24.521
      second degree T24.621
      third degree T24.721
    second degree T24.629
    third degree T24.729
  labium (majus) (minus) — *see* Corrosion, genital organs, external, female
  lacrimal apparatus, duct, gland or sac — *see* Corrosion, eye, specified site NEC
  larynx T27.4
    with lung T27.5
  leg (s) (meaning lower limb (s)) — *see* Corrosion, lower limb
  limb (s)
    lower — *see* Corrosion, lower, limb
    upper — *see* Corrosion, upper limb
  lip (s) T20.42
    first degree T20.52
    second degree T20.62
    third degree T20.72
  lower
    back — *see* Corrosion, back

Corrosion (injury) (acid) (caustic) (chemical) (lime) (external) (internal) - *continued*
  lower - *continued*
    limb T24.409
      ankle — *see* Corrosion, ankle
      calf — *see* Corrosion, calf
      first degree T24.509
      foot — *see* Corrosion, foot
      knee — *see* Corrosion, knee
      left T24.402
        first degree T24.502
        second degree T24.602
        third degree T24.702
      multiple sites, except ankle and foot T24.499
        ankle and foot T25.499
          first degree T25.599
          left T25.492
            first degree T25.592
            second degree T25.692
            third degree T25.792
          right T25.491
            first degree T25.591
            second degree T25.691
            third degree T25.791
          second degree T25.699
          third degree T25.799
        first degree T24.599
        left T24.492
          first degree T24.592
          second degree T24.692
          third degree T24.792
        right T24.491
          first degree T24.591
          second degree T24.691
          third degree T24.791
        second degree T24.699
        third degree T24.799
      right T24.401
        first degree T24.501
        second degree T24.601
        third degree T24.701
      second degree T24.609
      hip — *see* Corrosion, thigh
      thigh — *see* Corrosion, thigh
      third degree T24.709
  lung (with larynx and trachea) T27.5
  mouth T28.5
  neck T20.47
    first degree T20.57
    second degree T20.67
    third degree T20.77
  nose (septum) T20.44
    first degree T20.54
    second degree T20.64
    third degree T20.74
  ocular adnexa — *see* Corrosion, eye
  orbit region — *see* Corrosion, eyelid
  palm T23.459
    first degree T23.559
    left T23.452
      first degree T23.552
      second degree T23.652
      third degree T23.752
    right T23.451
      first degree T23.551
      second degree T23.651
      third degree T23.751
    second degree T23.659
    third degree T23.759
  partial thickness - code as Corrosion, unspecified degree, by site
  pelvis — *see* Corrosion, trunk
  penis — *see* Corrosion, genital organs, external, male
  perineum
    female — *see* Corrosion, genital organs, external, female
    male — *see* Corrosion, genital organs, external, male
  periocular area — *see* Corrosion, eyelid
  pharynx T28.5
  rectum T28.7
  respiratory tract T27.7
    larynx — *see* Corrosion, larynx

Corrosion (injury) (acid) (caustic) (chemical) (lime) (external) (internal) - *continued*
 respiratory tract - *continued*
  specified part NEC T27.6
  trachea — *see* Corrosion, larynx
 sac, lacrimal — *see* Corrosion, eye, specified site NEC
 scalp T20.45
  first degree T20.55
  second degree T20.65
  third degree T20.75
 scapular region T22.469
  first degree T22.569
  left T22.462
   first degree T22.562
   second degree T22.662
   third degree T22.762
  right T22.461
   first degree T22.561
   second degree T22.661
   third degree T22.761
  second degree T22.669
  third degree T22.769
 sclera — *see* Corrosion, eye, specified site NEC
 scrotum — *see* Corrosion, genital organs, external, male
 shoulder T22.459
  first degree T22.559
  left T22.452
   first degree T22.552
   second degree T22.652
   third degree T22.752
  right T22.451
   first degree T22.551
   second degree T22.651
   third degree T22.751
  second degree T22.659
  third degree T22.759
 stomach T28.7
 temple — *see* Corrosion, head
 testis — *see* Corrosion, genital organs, external, male
 thigh T24.419
  first degree T24.519
  left T24.412
   first degree T24.512
   second degree T24.612
   third degree T24.712
  right T24.411
   first degree T24.511
   second degree T24.611
   third degree T24.711
  second degree T24.619
  third degree T24.719
 thorax (external) — *see* Corrosion, trunk
 throat (meaning pharynx) T28.5
 thumb (s) T23.419
  first degree T23.519
  left T23.412
   first degree T23.512
   second degree T23.612
   third degree T23.712
  multiple sites with fingers T23.449
   first degree T23.549
   left T23.442
    first degree T23.542
    second degree T23.642
    third degree T23.742
   right T23.441
    first degree T23.541
    second degree T23.641
    third degree T23.741
   second degree T23.649
   third degree T23.749
  right T23.411
   first degree T23.511
   second degree T23.611
   third degree T23.711
  second degree T23.619
  third degree T23.719
 toe T25.439
  first degree T25.539
  left T25.432
   first degree T25.532

Corrosion (injury) (acid) (caustic) (chemical) (lime) (external) (internal) - *continued*
 toe - *continued*
  left - *continued*
   second degree T25.632
   third degree T25.732
  right T25.431
   first degree T25.531
   second degree T25.631
   third degree T25.731
  second degree T25.639
  third degree T25.739
 tongue T28.5
 tonsil (s) T28.5
 total body — *see* Corrosion, multiple body regions
 trachea T27.4
  with lung T27.5
 trunk T21.40
  abdominal wall — *see* Corrosion, abdominal wall
  anus — *see* Corrosion, buttock
  axilla — *see* Corrosion, upper limb
  back — *see* Corrosion, back
  breast — *see* Corrosion, chest wall
  buttock — *see* Corrosion, buttock
  chest wall — *see* Corrosion, chest wall
  first degree T21.50
  flank — *see* Corrosion, abdominal wall
  genital
   female — *see* Corrosion, genital organs, external, female
   male — *see* Corrosion, genital organs, external, male
  groin — *see* Corrosion, abdominal wall
  interscapular region — *see* Corrosion, back, upper
  labia — *see* Corrosion, genital organs, external, female
  lower back — *see* Corrosion, back
  penis — *see* Corrosion, genital organs, external, male
  perineum
   female — *see* Corrosion, genital organs, external, female
   male — *see* Corrosion, genital organs, external, male
  scapular region — *see* Corrosion, upper limb
  scrotum — *see* Corrosion, genital organs, external, male
  second degree T21.60
  shoulder — *see* Corrosion, upper limb
  specified site NEC T21.49
   first degree T21.59
   second degree T21.69
   third degree T21.79
  testes — *see* Corrosion, genital organs, external, male
  third degree T21.70
  upper back — *see* Corrosion, back, upper
  vagina T28.8
  vulva — *see* Corrosion, genital organs, external, female
 unspecified site with extent of body surface involved specified
  less than 10 percent T32.0
  10-19 percent (0-9 percent third degree) T32.10
   with 10-19 percent third degree T32.11
  20-29 percent (0-9 percent third degree) T32.20
   with
    10-19 percent third degree T32.21
    20-29 percent third degree T32.22
  30-39 percent (0-9 percent third degree) T32.30
   with
    10-19 percent third degree T32.31
    20-29 percent third degree T32.32
    30-39 percent third degree T32.33
  40-49 percent (0-9 percent third degree) T32.40
   with
    10-19 percent third degree T32.41

Corrosion (injury) (acid) (caustic) (chemical) (lime) (external) (internal) - *continued*
 unspecified site with extent of body surface involved specified - *continued*
  40-49 percent (0-9 percent third degree) - *continued*
   with - *continued*
    20-29 percent third degree T32.42
    30-39 percent third degree T32.43
    40-49 percent third degree T32.44
  50-59 percent (0-9 percent third degree) T32.50
   with
    10-19 percent third degree T32.51
    20-29 percent third degree T32.52
    30-39 percent third degree T32.53
    40-49 percent third degree T32.54
    50-59 percent third degree T32.55
  60-69 percent (0-9 percent third degree) T32.60
   with
    10-19 percent third degree T32.61
    20-29 percent third degree T32.62
    30-39 percent third degree T32.63
    40-49 percent third degree T32.64
    50-59 percent third degree T32.65
    60-69 percent third degree T32.66
  70-79 percent (0-9 percent third degree) T32.70
   with
    10-19 percent third degree T32.71
    20-29 percent third degree T32.72
    30-39 percent third degree T32.73
    40-49 percent third degree T32.74
    50-59 percent third degree T32.75
    60-69 percent third degree T32.76
    70-79 percent third degree T32.77
  80-89 percent (0-9 percent third degree) T32.80
   with
    10-19 percent third degree T32.81
    20-29 percent third degree T32.82
    30-39 percent third degree T32.83
    40-49 percent third degree T32.84
    50-59 percent third degree T32.85
    60-69 percent third degree T32.86
    70-79 percent third degree T32.87
    80-89 percent third degree T32.88
  90 percent or more (0-9 percent third degree) T32.90
   with
    10-19 percent third degree T32.91
    20-29 percent third degree T32.92
    30-39 percent third degree T32.93
    40-49 percent third degree T32.94
    50-59 percent third degree T32.95
    60-69 percent third degree T32.96
    70-79 percent third degree T32.97
    80-89 percent third degree T32.98
    90-99 percent third degree T32.99
 upper limb (axilla) (scapular region) T22.40
  above elbow — *see* Corrosion, above elbow
  axilla — *see* Corrosion, axilla
  elbow — *see* Corrosion, elbow
  first degree T22.50
  forearm — *see* Corrosion, forearm
  hand — *see* Corrosion, hand
  interscapular region — *see* Corrosion, back, upper
  multiple sites T22.499
   first degree T22.599
   left T22.492
    first degree T22.592
    second degree T22.692
    third degree T22.792
   right T22.491
    first degree T22.591
    second degree T22.691
    third degree T22.791
   second degree T22.699
   third degree T22.799
  scapular region — *see* Corrosion, scapular region
  second degree T22.60

Corrosion (injury) (acid) (caustic) (chemical) (lime) (external) (internal) - *continued*
  upper limb (axilla) (scapular region) - *continued*
    shoulder — *see* Corrosion, shoulder
    third degree T22.70
    wrist — *see* Corrosion, hand
  uterus T28.8
  vagina T28.8
  vulva — *see* Corrosion, genital organs, external, female
  wrist T23.479
    first degree T23.579
    left T23.472
      first degree T23.572
      second degree T23.672
      third degree T23.772
    multiple sites with hand T23.499
      first degree T23.599
      left T23.492
        first degree T23.592
        second degree T23.692
        third degree T23.792
      right T23.491
        first degree T23.591
        second degree T23.691
        third degree T23.791
      second degree T23.699
      third degree T23.799
    right T23.471
      first degree T23.571
      second degree T23.671
      third degree T23.771
    second degree T23.679
    third degree T23.779
Corrosive burn — *see* Corrosion
Corsican fever — *see* Malaria
Cortical — *see* condition
Cortico-adrenal — *see* condition
Coryza (acute) J00
  with grippe or influenza — *see* Influenza, with, respiratory manifestations NEC
  syphilitic
    congenital (chronic) A50.05
Costen's syndrome or complex M26.69
Costiveness — *see* Constipation
Costochondritis M94.0
Cot death R99
Cotard's syndrome F22
Cotia virus B08.8
Cotton wool spots (retinal) H35.81
Cotungo's disease — *see* Sciatica
Cough (affected) (chronic) (epidemic) (nervous) R05
  with hemorrhage — *see* Hemoptysis
  bronchial R05
    with grippe or influenza — *see* Influenza, with, respiratory manifestations NEC
  functional F45.8
  hysterical F45.8
  laryngeal, spasmodic R05
  psychogenic F45.8
  smokers' J41.0
  tea taster's B49
Counseling (for) Z71.9
  abuse NEC
    perpetrator Z69.82
    victim Z69.81
  alcohol abuser Z71.41
    family Z71.42
  child abuse
    nonparental
      perpetrator Z69.021
      victim Z69.020
    parental
      perpetrator Z69.011
      victim Z69.010
  consanguinity Z71.89
  contraceptive Z30.09
  dietary Z71.3
  drug abuser Z71.51
    family member Z71.52
  exercise Z71.82
  family Z71.89

Counseling (for) - *continued*
  fertility preservation (prior to cancer therapy) (prior to removal of gonads) Z31.62
  for non-attending third party Z71.0
    related to sexual behavior or orientation Z70.2
  genetic
    nonprocreative Z71.83
    procreative NEC Z31.5
  gestational carrier Z31.7
  health (advice) (education) (instruction) — *see* Counseling, medical
    risk for travel (international) Z71.84
  human immunodeficiency virus (HIV) Z71.7
  impotence Z70.1
  insulin pump use Z46.81
  medical (for) Z71.9
    boarding school resident Z59.3
    consanguinity Z71.89
    feared complaint and no disease found Z71.1
    human immunodeficiency virus (HIV) Z71.7
    institutional resident Z59.3
    on behalf of another Z71.0
      related to sexual behavior or orientation Z70.2
    person living alone Z60.2
    specified reason NEC Z71.89
  natural family planning
    procreative Z31.61
    to avoid pregnancy Z30.02
  perpetrator (of)
    abuse NEC Z69.82
    child abuse
      non-parental Z69.021
      parental Z69.011
    rape NEC Z69.82
    spousal abuse Z69.12
  procreative NEC Z31.69
    fertility preservation (prior to cancer therapy) (prior to removal of gonads) Z31.62
    using natural family planning Z31.61
  promiscuity Z70.1
  rape victim Z69.81
  religious Z71.81
  safety for travel (international) Z71.84
  sex, sexual (related to) Z70.9
    attitude (s) Z70.0
    behavior or orientation Z70.1
    combined concerns Z70.3
    non-responsiveness Z70.1
    on behalf of third party Z70.2
    specified reason NEC Z70.8
  specified reason NEC Z71.89
  spiritual Z71.81
  spousal abuse (perpetrator) Z69.12
    victim Z69.11
  substance abuse Z71.89
    alcohol Z71.41
    drug Z71.51
    tobacco Z71.6
  tobacco use Z71.6
  travel (international) Z71.84
  use (of)
    insulin pump Z46.81
  victim (of)
    abuse Z69.81
    child abuse
      by parent Z69.010
      non-parental Z69.020
    rape NEC Z69.81
Coupled rhythm R00.8
Couvelaire syndrome or uterus (complicating delivery) O45.8X-
Cowperitis — *see* Urethritis
Cowper's gland — *see* condition
Cowpox B08.010
  due to vaccination T88.1
Coxa
  magna M91.4-
  plana M91.2-
  valga (acquired) — *see also* Deformity, limb, specified type NEC, thigh

Coxa - *continued*
  valga (acquired) - *continued*
    congenital Q65.81
    sequelae (late effect) of rickets E64.3
  vara (acquired) — *see also* Deformity, limb, specified type NEC, thigh
    congenital Q65.82
    sequelae (late effect) of rickets E64.3
Coxalgia, coxalgic (nontuberculous) — *see also* Pain, joint, hip
  tuberculous A18.02
Coxitis — *see* Monoarthritis, hip
Coxsackie (virus) (infection) B34.1
  as cause of disease classified elsewhere B97.11
  carditis B33.20
  central nervous system NEC A88.8
  endocarditis B33.21
  enteritis A08.39
  meningitis (aseptic) A87.0
  myocarditis B33.22
  pericarditis B33.23
  pharyngitis B08.5
  pleurodynia B33.0
  specific disease NEC B33.8
Crabs, meaning pubic lice B85.3
Crack baby P04.41
Cracked nipple N64.0
  associated with
    lactation O92.13
    pregnancy O92.11-
    puerperium O92.12
Cracked tooth K03.81
Cradle cap L21.0
Craft neurosis F48.8
Cramp (s) R25.2
  abdominal — *see* Pain, abdominal
  bathing T75.1
  colic R10.83
    psychogenic F45.8
  due to immersion T75.1
  fireman T67.2
  heat T67.2
  immersion T75.1
  intestinal — *see* Pain, abdominal
    psychogenic F45.8
  leg, sleep related G47.62
  limb (lower) (upper) NEC R25.2
    sleep related G47.62
  linotypist's F48.8
    organic G25.89
  muscle (limb) (general) R25.2
    due to immersion T75.1
    psychogenic F45.8
  occupational (hand) F48.8
    organic G25.89
  salt-depletion E87.1
  sleep related, leg G47.62
  stoker's T67.2
  swimmer's T75.1
  telegrapher's F48.8
    organic G25.89
  typist's F48.8
    organic G25.89
  uterus N94.89
    menstrual — *see* Dysmenorrhea
  writer's F48.8
    organic G25.89
Cranial — *see* condition
Craniocleidodysostosis Q74.0
Craniofenestria (skull) Q75.8
Craniolacunia (skull) Q75.8
Craniopagus Q89.4
Craniopathy, metabolic M85.2
Craniopharyngeal — *see* condition
Craniopharyngioma D44.4
Craniorachischisis (totalis) Q00.1
Cranioschisis Q75.8
Craniostenosis Q75.0
Craniosynostosis Q75.0
Craniotabes (cause unknown) M83.8
  neonatal P96.3
  rachitic E64.3
  syphilitic A50.56
Cranium — *see* condition

Craw-craw — *see* Onchocerciasis
Creaking joint — *see* Derangement, joint, specified type NEC
Creeping
  eruption B76.9
  palsy or paralysis G12.22
Crenated tongue K14.8
Creotoxism A05.9
Crepitus
  caput Q75.8
  joint — *see* Derangement, joint, specified type NEC
Crescent or conus choroid, congenital Q14.3
CREST syndrome M34.1
Cretin, cretinism (congenital) (endemic) (nongoitrous) (sporadic) E00.9
  pelvis
    with disproportion (fetopelvic) O33.0
      causing obstructed labor O65.0
  type
    hypothyroid E00.1
    mixed E00.2
    myxedematous E00.1
    neurological E00.0
Creutzfeldt-Jakob disease or syndrome (with dementia) A81.00
  familial A81.09
  iatrogenic A81.09
  specified NEC A81.09
  sporadic A81.09
  variant (vCJD) A81.01
Crib death R99
Cribriform hymen Q52.3
Cri-du-chat syndrome Q93.4
Crigler-Najjar disease or syndrome E80.5
Crime, victim of Z65.4
Crimean hemorrhagic fever A98.0
Criminalism F60.2
Crisis
  abdomen R10.0
  acute reaction F43.0
  addisonian E27.2
  adrenal (cortical) E27.2
  celiac K90.0
  Dietl's N13.8
  emotional — *see also* Disorder, adjustment
    acute reaction to stress F43.0
    specific to childhood and adolescence F93.8
  glaucomatocyclitic — *see* Glaucoma, secondary, inflammation
  heart — *see* Failure, heart
  nitritoid I95.2
    correct substance properly administered — *see* Table of Drugs and Chemicals, by drug, adverse effect
    overdose or wrong substance given or taken — *see* Table of Drugs and Chemicals, by drug, poisoning
  oculogyric H51.8
    psychogenic F45.8
  Pel's (tabetic) A52.11
  psychosexual identity F64.2
  renal N28.0
  sickle-cell D57.00
    with
      acute chest syndrome D57.01
      splenic sequestration D57.02
  state (acute reaction) F43.0
  tabetic A52.11
  thyroid — *see* Thyrotoxicosis with thyroid storm
  thyrotoxic — *see* Thyrotoxicosis with thyroid storm
Crocq's disease (acrocyanosis) I73.89
Crohn's disease — *see* Enteritis, regional
Crooked septum, nasal J34.2
Cross syndrome E70.328
Crossbite (anterior) (posterior) M26.24
Cross-eye — *see* Strabismus, convergent concomitant
Croup, croupous (catarrhal) (infectious) (inflammatory) (nondiphtheritic) J05.0
  bronchial J20.9

Croup, croupous (catarrhal) (infectious) (inflammatory) (nondiphtheritic) - *continued*
  diphtheritic A36.2
  false J38.5
  spasmodic J38.5
    diphtheritic A36.2
  stridulous J38.5
    diphtheritic A36.2
Crouzon's disease Q75.1
Crowding, tooth, teeth, fully erupted M26.31
CRST syndrome M34.1
Cruchet's disease A85.8
Cruelty in children — *see also* Disorder, conduct
Crural ulcer — *see* Ulcer, lower limb
Crush, crushed, crushing T14.8
  abdomen S38.1
  ankle S97.0-
  arm (upper) (and shoulder) S47.-
  axilla — *see* Crush, arm
  back, lower S38.1
  buttock S38.1
  cheek S07.0
  chest S28.0
  cranium S07.1
  ear S07.0
  elbow S57.0-
  extremity
    lower
      ankle — *see* Crush, ankle
      below knee — *see* Crush, leg
      foot — *see* Crush, foot
      hip — *see* Crush, hip
      knee — *see* Crush, knee
      thigh — *see* Crush, thigh
      toe — *see* Crush, toe
    upper
      below elbow S67.9-
      elbow — *see* Crush, elbow
      finger — *see* Crush, finger
      forearm — *see* Crush, forearm
      hand — *see* Crush, hand
      thumb — *see* Crush, thumb
      upper arm — *see* Crush, arm
      wrist — *see* Crush, wrist
  face S07.0
  finger (s) S67.1-
    with hand (and wrist) — *see* Crush, hand, specified site NEC
    index S67.19-
    little S67.19-
    middle S67.19-
    ring S67.19-
    thumb — *see* Crush, thumb
  foot S97.8-
    toe — *see* Crush, toe
  forearm S57.8-
  genitalia, external
    female S38.002
      vagina S38.03
      vulva S38.03
    male S38.001
      penis S38.01
      scrotum S38.02
      testis S38.02
  hand (except fingers alone) S67.2-
    with wrist S67.4-
  head S07.9
    specified NEC S07.8
  heel — *see* Crush, foot
  hip S77.0-
    with thigh S77.2-
  internal organ (abdomen, chest, or pelvis) NEC T14.8
  knee S87.0-
  labium (majus) (minus) S38.03
  larynx S17.0
  leg (lower) S87.8-
    knee — *see* Crush, knee
  lip S07.0
  lower
    back S38.1
    leg — *see* Crush, leg
  neck S17.9
  nerve — *see* Injury, nerve

Crush, crushed, crushing - *continued*
  nose S07.0
  pelvis S38.1
  penis S38.01
  scalp S07.8
  scapular region — *see* Crush, arm
  scrotum S38.02
  severe, unspecified site T14.8
  shoulder (and upper arm) — *see* Crush, arm
  skull S07.1
  syndrome (complication of trauma) T79.5
  testis S38.02
  thigh S77.1-
    with hip S77.2-
  throat S17.8
  thumb S67.0-
    with hand (and wrist) — *see* Crush, hand, specified site NEC
  toe (s) S97.10-
    great S97.11-
    lesser S97.12-
  trachea S17.0
  vagina S38.03
  vulva S38.03
  wrist S67.3-
    with hand S67.4-
Crusta lactea L21.0
Crusts R23.4
Crutch paralysis — *see* Injury, brachial plexus
Cruveilhier-Baumgarten cirrhosis, disease or syndrome K74.69
Cruveilhier's atrophy or disease G12.8
Crying (constant) (continuous) (excessive)
  child, adolescent, or adult R45.83
  infant (baby) (newborn) R68.11
Cryofibrinogenemia D89.2
Cryoglobulinemia (essential) (idiopathic) (mixed) (primary) (purpura) (secondary) (vasculitis) D89.1
  with lung involvement D89.1 *[J99]*
Cryptitis (anal) (rectal) K62.89
Cryptococcosis, cryptococcus (infection) (neoformans) B45.9
  bone B45.3
  cerebral B45.1
  cutaneous B45.2
  disseminated B45.7
  generalized B45.7
  meningitis B45.1
  meningocerebralis B45.1
  osseous B45.3
  pulmonary B45.0
  skin B45.2
  specified NEC B45.8
Cryptopapillitis (anus) K62.89
Cryptophthalmos Q11.2
  syndrome Q87.0
Cryptorchid, cryptorchism, cryptorchidism Q53.9
  bilateral Q53.20
    abdominal Q53.211
    perineal Q53.22
  unilateral Q53.10
    abdominal Q53.111
    perineal Q53.12
Cryptosporidiosis A07.2
  hepatobiliary B88.8
  respiratory B88.8
Cryptostromosis J67.6
Crystalluria R82.998
Cubitus
  congenital Q68.8
  valgus (acquired) M21.0-
    congenital Q68.8
    sequelae (late effect) of rickets E64.3
  varus (acquired) M21.1-
    congenital Q68.8
    sequelae (late effect) of rickets E64.3
Cultural deprivation or shock Z60.3
Curling esophagus K22.4
Curling's ulcer — *see* Ulcer, peptic, acute
Curschmann (-Batten) (-Steinert) disease or syndrome G71.11
Curse, Ondine's — *see* Apnea, sleep

Curvature
  organ or site, congenital NEC — *see*
    Distortion
  penis (lateral) Q55.61
  Pott's (spinal) A18.01
  radius, idiopathic, progressive
    (congenital) Q74.0
  spine (acquired) (angular) (idiopathic)
    (incorrect) (postural) — *see* Dorsopathy,
    deforming
    congenital Q67.5
    due to or associated with
      Charcot-Marie-Tooth disease (*see also*
        subcategory M49.8) G60.0
      osteitis
        deformans M88.88
        fibrosa cystica (*see also* subcategory
          M49.8) E21.0
      tuberculosis (Pott's curvature) A18.01
    sequelae (late effect) of rickets E64.3
    tuberculous A18.01
Cushingoid due to steroid therapy E24.2
  correct substance properly administered —
    see Table of Drugs and Chemicals, by
    drug, adverse effect
  overdose or wrong substance given or
    taken — *see* Table of Drugs and
    Chemicals, by drug, poisoning
Cushing's
  syndrome or disease E24.9
    drug-induced E24.2
    iatrogenic E24.2
    pituitary-dependent E24.0
    specified NEC E24.8
  ulcer — *see* Ulcer, peptic, acute
Cusp, Carabelli - omit code
Cut (external) — *see also* Laceration
  muscle — *see* Injury, muscle
Cutaneous — *see also* condition
  hemorrhage R23.3
  larva migrans B76.9
Cutis — *see also* condition
  hyperelastica Q82.8
    acquired L57.4
  laxa (hyperelastica) — *see* Dermatolysis
  marmorata R23.8
  osteosis L94.2
  pendula — *see* Dermatolysis
  rhomboidalis nuchae L57.2
  verticis gyrata Q82.8
    acquired L91.8
Cyanosis R23.0
  due to
    patent foramen botalli Q21.1
    persistent foramen ovale Q21.1
  enterogenous D74.8
  paroxysmal digital — *see* Raynaud's disease
    with gangrene I73.01
  retina, retinal H35.89
Cyanotic heart disease I24.9
  congenital Q24.9
Cycle
  anovulatory N97.0
  menstrual, irregular N92.6
Cyclencephaly Q04.9
Cyclical vomiting, in migraine, — *see also*
  Vomiting, cyclical G43.A0
  psychogenic F50.89
Cyclitis — *see also* Iridocyclitis H20.9
  chronic — *see* Iridocyclitis, chronic
  Fuchs' heterochromic H20.81-
  granulomatous — *see* Iridocyclitis, chronic
  lens-induced — *see* Iridocyclitis, lens-
    induced
  posterior H30.2-
Cycloid personality F34.0
Cyclophoria H50.54
Cyclopia, cyclops Q87.0
Cyclopism Q87.0
Cyclosporiasis A07.4
Cyclothymia F34.0
Cyclothymic personality F34.0
Cyclotropia H50.41-

Cylindroma — *see also* Neoplasm, malignant,
  by site
  eccrine dermal — *see* Neoplasm, skin,
    benign
  skin — *see* Neoplasm, skin, benign
Cylindruria R82.998
Cynanche
  diphtheritic A36.2
  tonsillaris J36
Cynophobia F40.218
Cynorexia R63.2
Cyphosis — *see* Kyphosis
Cyprus fever — *see* Brucellosis
Cyst (colloid) (mucous) (simple) (retention)
  adenoid (infected) J35.8
  adrenal gland E27.8
    congenital Q89.1
  air, lung J98.4
  allantoic Q64.4
  alveolar process (jaw bone) M27.40
  amnion, amniotic O41.8X-
  aneurysmal M27.49
  anterior
    chamber (eye) — *see* Cyst, iris
    nasopalatine K09.1
  antrum J34.1
  anus K62.89
  apical (tooth) (periodontal) K04.8
  appendix K38.8
  arachnoid, brain (acquired) G93.0
    congenital Q04.6
  arytenoid J38.7
  Baker's M71.2-
    ruptured M66.0
    tuberculous A18.02
  Bartholin's gland N75.0
  bile duct (common) (hepatic) K83.5
  bladder (multiple) (trigone) N32.89
  blue dome (breast) — *see* Cyst, breast
  bone (local) NEC M85.60
    aneurysmal M85.50
      ankle M85.57-
      foot M85.57-
      forearm M85.53-
      hand M85.54-
      jaw M27.49
      lower leg M85.56-
      multiple site M85.59
      neck M85.58
      rib M85.58
      shoulder M85.51-
      skull M85.58
      specified site NEC M85.58
      thigh M85.55-
      toe M85.57-
      upper arm M85.52-
      vertebra M85.58
    solitary M85.40
      ankle M85.47-
      fibula M85.46-
      foot M85.47-
      hand M85.44-
      humerus M85.42-
      jaw M27.49
      neck M85.48
      pelvis M85.45-
      radius M85.43-
      rib M85.48
      shoulder M85.41-
      skull M85.48
      specified site NEC M85.48
      tibia M85.46-
      toe M85.47-
      ulna M85.43-
      vertebra M85.48
    specified type NEC M85.60
      ankle M85.67-
      foot M85.67-
      forearm M85.63-
      hand M85.64-
      jaw M27.40
        developmental
          (nonodontogenic) K09.1
        odontogenic K09.0
        latent M27.0

Cyst (colloid) (mucous) (simple) (retention) -
continued
  bone (local) NEC - *continued*
    specified type NEC - *continued*
      lower leg M85.66-
      multiple site M85.69
      neck M85.68
      rib M85.68
      shoulder M85.61-
      skull M85.68
      specified site NEC M85.68
      thigh M85.65-
      toe M85.67-
      upper arm M85.62-
      vertebra M85.68
  brain (acquired) G93.0
    congenital Q04.6
    hydatid B67.99 *[G94]*
    third ventricle (colloid) , congenital Q04.6
  branchial (cleft) Q18.0
  branchiogenic Q18.0
  breast (benign) (blue dome) (pedunculated)
    (solitary) N60.0-
    involution — *see* Dysplasia, mammary,
      specified type NEC
    sebaceous — *see* Dysplasia, mammary,
      specified type NEC
  broad ligament (benign) N83.8
  bronchogenic (mediastinal)
    (sequestration) J98.4
    congenital Q33.0
  buccal K09.8
  bulbourethral gland N36.8
  bursa, bursal NEC M71.30
    with rupture — *see* Rupture, synovium
    ankle M71.37-
    elbow M71.32-
    foot M71.37-
    hand M71.34-
    hip M71.35-
    multiple sites M71.39
    pharyngeal J39.2
    popliteal space — *see* Cyst, Baker's
    shoulder M71.31-
    specified site NEC M71.38
    wrist M71.33-
  calcifying odontogenic D16.5
    upper jaw (bone) (maxilla) D16.4
  canal of Nuck (female) N94.89
    congenital Q52.4
  canthus — *see* Cyst, conjunctiva
  carcinomatous — *see* Neoplasm, malignant,
    by site
  cauda equina G95.89
  cavum septi pellucidi — *see* Cyst, brain
  celomic (pericardium) Q24.8
  cerebellopontine (angle) — *see* Cyst, brain
  cerebellum — *see* Cyst, brain
  cerebral — *see* Cyst, brain
  cervical lateral Q18.0
  cervix NEC N88.8
    embryonic Q51.6
    nabothian N88.8
  chiasmal optic NEC — *see* Disorder, optic,
    chiasm
  chocolate (ovary) N80.1
  choledochus, congenital Q44.4
  chorion O41.8X-
  choroid plexus G93.0
    congenital Q04.6
  ciliary body — *see* Cyst, iris
  clitoris N90.7
  colon K63.89
  common (bile) duct K83.5
  congenital NEC Q89.8
    adrenal gland Q89.1
    epiglottis Q31.8
    esophagus Q39.8
    fallopian tube Q50.4
    kidney Q61.00
      more than one (multiple) Q61.02
        specified as polycystic Q61.3
          adult type Q61.2
          infantile type NEC Q61.19
            collecting duct dilation Q61.11

Cyst (colloid) (mucous) (simple) (retention) - *continued*

congenital NEC - *continued*

kidney - *continued*

solitary Q61.01

larynx Q31.8

liver Q44.6

lung Q33.0

mediastinum Q34.1

ovary Q50.1

oviduct Q50.4

periurethral (tissue) Q64.79

prepuce Q55.69

salivary gland (any) Q38.4

sublingual Q38.6

submaxillary gland Q38.6

thymus (gland) Q89.2

tongue Q38.3

ureterovesical orifice Q62.8

vulva Q52.79

conjunctiva H11.44-

cornea H18.89-

corpora quadrigemina G93.0

corpus

albicans N83.29-

luteum (hemorrhagic) (ruptured) N83.1-

Cowper's gland (benign) (infected) N36.8

cranial meninges G93.0

craniobuccal pouch E23.6

craniopharyngeal pouch E23.6

cystic duct K82.8

Cysticercus — *see* Cysticercosis

Dandy-Walker Q03.1

with spina bifida — *see* Spina bifida

dental (root) K04.8

developmental K09.0

eruption K09.0

primordial K09.0

dentigerous (mandible) (maxilla) K09.0

dermoid — *see* Neoplasm, benign, by site

with malignant transformation C56.-

implantation

external area or site (skin) NEC L72.0

iris — *see* Cyst, iris, implantation

vagina N89.8

vulva N90.7

mouth K09.8

oral soft tissue K09.8

sacrococcygeal — *see* Cyst, pilonidal

developmental K09.1

odontogenic K09.0

oral region (nonodontogenic) K09.1

ovary, ovarian Q50.1

dura (cerebral) G93.0

spinal G96.19

ear (external) Q18.1

echinococcal — *see* Echinococcus

embryonic

cervix uteri Q51.6

fallopian tube Q50.4

vagina Q52.4

endometrium, endometrial (uterus) N85.8

ectopic — *see* Endometriosis

enterogenous Q43.8

epidermal, epidermoid (inclusion) (see also Cyst, skin) L72.0

mouth K09.8

oral soft tissue K09.8

epididymis N50.3

epiglottis J38.7

epiphysis cerebri E34.8

epithelial (inclusion) L72.0

epoophoron Q50.5

eruption K09.0

esophagus K22.8

ethmoid sinus J34.1

external female genital organs NEC N90.7

eye NEC H57.89

congenital Q15.8

eyelid (sebaceous) H02.829

infected — *see* Hordeolum

left H02.826

lower H02.825

upper H02.824

right H02.823

Cyst (colloid) (mucous) (simple) (retention) - *continued*

eyelid (sebaceous) - *continued*

right - *continued*

lower H02.822

upper H02.821

fallopian tube N83.8

congenital Q50.4

fimbrial (twisted) Q50.4

fissural (oral region) K09.1

follicle (graafian) (hemorrhagic) N83.0-

nabothian N88.8

follicular (atretic) (hemorrhagic) (ovarian) N83.0-

dentigerous K09.0

odontogenic K09.0

skin L72.9

specified NEC L72.8

frontal sinus J34.1

gallbladder K82.8

ganglion — *see* Ganglion

Gartner's duct Q52.4

gingiva K09.0

gland of Moll — *see* Cyst, eyelid

globulomaxillary K09.1

graafian follicle (hemorrhagic) N83.0-

granulosal lutein (hemorrhagic) N83.1-

hemangiomatous D18.00

intra-abdominal D18.03

intracranial D18.02

skin D18.01

specified site NEC D18.09

hemorrhagic M27.49

hydatid — *see also* Echinococcus B67.90

brain B67.99 *[G94]*

liver — *see also* Cyst, liver, hydatid B67.8

lung NEC B67.99 *[J99]*

Morgagni

female Q50.5

male (epididymal) Q55.4

testicular Q55.29

specified site NEC B67.99

hymen N89.8

embryonic Q52.4

hypopharynx J39.2

hypophysis, hypophyseal (duct) (recurrent) E23.6

cerebri E23.6

implantation (dermoid)

external area or site (skin) NEC L72.0

iris — *see* Cyst, iris, implantation

vagina N89.8

vulva N90.7

incisive canal K09.1

inclusion (epidermal) (epithelial) (epidermoid) (squamous) L72.0

not of skin - code under Cyst, by site

intestine (large) (small) K63.89

intracranial — *see* Cyst, brain

intraligamentous — *see also* Disorder, ligament

knee — *see* Derangement, knee

intrasellar E23.6

iris H21.309

exudative H21.31-

idiopathic H21.30-

implantation H21.32-

parasitic H21.33-

pars plana (primary) H21.34-

exudative H21.35-

jaw (bone) M27.40

aneurysmal M27.49

hemorrhagic M27.49

traumatic M27.49

developmental (odontogenic) K09.0

fissural K09.1

joint NEC — *see* Disorder, joint, specified type NEC

kidney (acquired) N28.1

calyceal — *see* Hydronephrosis

congenital Q61.00

more than one (multiple) Q61.02

specified as polycystic Q61.3

adult type (autosomal dominant) Q61.2

Cyst (colloid) (mucous) (simple) (retention) - *continued*

kidney (acquired) - *continued*

more than one (multiple) - *continued*

specified as polycystic - *continued*

infantile type (autosomal recessive) NEC Q61.19

collecting duct dilation Q61.11

pyelogenic — *see* Hydronephrosis

simple N28.1

solitary (single) Q61.01

acquired N28.1

labium (majus) (minus) N90.7

sebaceous N90.7

lacrimal — *see also* Disorder, lacrimal system, specified NEC

gland H04.13-

passages or sac — *see* Disorder, lacrimal system, specified NEC

larynx J38.7

lateral periodontal K09.0

lens H27.8

congenital Q12.8

lip (gland) K13.0

liver (idiopathic) (simple) K76.89

congenital Q44.6

hydatid B67.8

granulosus B67.0

multilocularis B67.5

lung J98.4

congenital Q33.0

giant bullous J43.9

lutein N83.1-

lymphangiomatous D18.1

lymphoepithelial, oral soft tissue K09.8

macula — *see* Degeneration, macula, hole

malignant — *see* Neoplasm, malignant, by site

mammary gland — *see* Cyst, breast

mandible M27.40

dentigerous K09.0

radicular K04.8

maxilla M27.40

dentigerous K09.0

radicular K04.8

medial, face and neck Q18.8

median

anterior maxillary K09.1

palatal K09.1

mediastinum, congenital Q34.1

meibomian (gland) — *see* Chalazion

infected — *see* Hordeolum

membrane, brain G93.0

meninges (cerebral) G93.0

spinal G96.19

meniscus, knee — *see* Derangement, knee, meniscus, cystic

mesentery, mesenteric K66.8

chyle I89.8

mesonephric duct

female Q50.5

male Q55.4

milk N64.89

Morgagni (hydatid)

female Q50.5

male (epididymal) Q55.4

testicular Q55.29

mouth K09.8

Müllerian duct Q50.4

appendix testis Q55.29

cervix Q51.6

fallopian tube Q50.4

female Q50.4

male Q55.29

prostatic utricle Q55.4

vagina (embryonal) Q52.4

multilocular (ovary) D39.10

benign — *see* Neoplasm, benign, by site

myometrium N85.8

nabothian (follicle) (ruptured) N88.8

nasoalveolar K09.1

nasolabial K09.1

nasopalatine (anterior) (duct) K09.1

nasopharynx J39.2

Cyst (colloid) (mucous) (simple) (retention) - *continued*

neoplastic — *see* Neoplasm, uncertain
behavior, by site
benign — *see* Neoplasm, benign, by site
nervous system NEC G96.8
neuroenteric (congenital) Q06.8
nipple — *see* Cyst, breast
nose (turbinates) J34.1
sinus J34.1
odontogenic, developmental K09.0
omentum (lesser) K66.8
congenital Q45.8
ora serrata — *see* Cyst, retina, ora serrata
oral
region K09.9
developmental (nonodontogenic) K09.1
specified NEC K09.8
soft tissue K09.9
specified NEC K09.8
orbit H05.81-
ovary, ovarian (twisted) N83.20-
adherent N83.20-
chocolate N80.1
corpus
albicans N83.29-
luteum (hemorrhagic) N83.1-
dermoid D27.9
developmental Q50.1
due to failure of involution NEC N83.20-
endometrial N80.1
follicular (graafian) (hemorrhagic) N83.0-
hemorrhagic N83.20-
in pregnancy or childbirth O34.8-
with obstructed labor O65.5
multilocular D39.10
pseudomucinous D27.9
retention N83.29-
serous N83.20-
specified NEC N83.29-
theca lutein (hemorrhagic) N83.1-
tuberculous A18.18
oviduct N83.8
palate (median) (fissural) K09.1
palatine papilla (jaw) K09.1
pancreas, pancreatic (hemorrhagic)
(true) K86.2
congenital Q45.2
false K86.3
paralabral
hip M24.85-
shoulder S43.43-
paramesonephric duct Q50.4
female Q50.4
male Q55.29
paranephric N28.1
paraphysis, cerebri, congenital Q04.6
parasitic B89
parathyroid (gland) E21.4
paratubal N83.8
paraurethral duct N36.8
paroophoron Q50.5
parotid gland K11.6
parovarian Q50.5
pelvis, female N94.89
in pregnancy or childbirth O34.8-
causing obstructed labor O65.5
penis (sebaceous) N48.89
periapical K04.8
pericardial (congenital) Q24.8
acquired (secondary) I31.8
pericoronal K09.0
periodontal K04.8
lateral K09.0
peripelvic (lymphatic) N28.1
peritoneum K66.8
chylous I89.8
periventricular, acquired, newborn P91.1
pharynx (wall) J39.2
pilar L72.11
pilonidal (infected) (rectum) L05.91
with abscess L05.01
malignant C44.59-
pituitary (duct) (gland) E23.6
placenta O43.19-

Cyst (colloid) (mucous) (simple) (retention) - *continued*

pleura J94.8
popliteal — *see* Cyst, Baker's
porencephalic Q04.6
acquired G93.0
postanal (infected) — *see* Cyst, pilonidal
postmastoidectomy cavity (mucosal) — *see*
Complications, postmastoidectomy, cyst
preauricular Q18.1
prepuce N47.4
congenital Q55.69
primordial (jaw) K09.0
prostate N42.83
pseudomucinous (ovary) D27.9
pupillary, miotic H21.27-
radicular (residual) K04.8
radiculodental K04.8
ranular K11.8
Rathke's pouch E23.6
rectum (epithelium) (mucous) K62.89
renal — *see* Cyst, kidney
residual (radicular) K04.8
retention (ovary) N83.29-
salivary gland K11.6
retina H33.19-
ora serrata H33.11-
parasitic H33.12-
retroperitoneal K68.9
sacrococcygeal (dermoid) — *see* Cyst,
pilonidal
salivary gland or duct (mucous extravasation
or retention) K11.6
Sampson's N80.1
sclera H15.89
scrotum L72.9
sebaceous L72.3
sebaceous (duct) (gland) L72.3
breast — *see* Dysplasia, mammary,
specified type NEC
eyelid — *see* Cyst, eyelid
genital organ NEC
female N94.89
male N50.89
scrotum L72.3
semilunar cartilage (knee) (multiple) — *see*
Derangement, knee, meniscus, cystic
seminal vesicle N50.89
serous (ovary) N83.20-
sinus (accessory) (nasal) J34.1
Skene's gland N36.8
skin L72.9
breast — *see* Dysplasia, mammary,
specified type NEC
epidermal, epidermoid L72.0
epithelial L72.0
eyelid — *see* Cyst, eyelid
genital organ NEC
female N90.7
male N50.89
inclusion L72.0
scrotum L72.9
sebaceous L72.3
sweat gland or duct L74.8
solitary
bone — *see* Cyst, bone, solitary
jaw M27.40
kidney N28.1
spermatic cord N50.89
sphenoid sinus J34.1
spinal meninges G96.19
spleen NEC D73.4
congenital Q89.09
hydatid — *see also* Echinococcus B67.99
[D77]
Stafne's M27.0
subarachnoid intrasellar R93.0
subcutaneous, pheomycotic
(chromomycotic) B43.2
subdural (cerebral) G93.0
spinal cord G96.19
sublingual gland K11.6
submandibular gland K11.6
submaxillary gland K11.6
suburethral N36.8

Cyst (colloid) (mucous) (simple) (retention) - *continued*

suprarenal gland E27.8
suprasellar — *see* Cyst, brain
sweat gland or duct L74.8
synovial — *see also* Cyst, bursa
ruptured — *see* Rupture, synovium
tarsal — *see* Chalazion
tendon (sheath) — *see* Disorder, tendon,
specified type NEC
testis N44.2
tunica albuginea N44.1
theca lutein (ovary) N83.1-
Thornwaldt's J39.2
thymus (gland) E32.8
thyroglossal duct (infected)
(persistent) Q89.2
thyrolingual duct (infected)
(persistent) Q89.2
thyroid (gland) E04.1
tongue K14.8
tonsil J35.8
tooth — *see* Cyst, dental
Tornwaldt's J39.2
trichilemmal (proliferating) L72.12
trichodermal L72.12
tubal (fallopian) N83.8
inflammatory — *see* Salpingitis, chronic
tubo-ovarian N83.8
inflammatory N70.13
tunica
albuginea testis N44.1
vaginalis N50.89
turbinate (nose) J34.1
Tyson's gland N48.89
urachus, congenital Q64.4
ureter N28.89
ureterovesical orifice N28.89
urethra, urethral (gland) N36.8
uterine ligament N83.8
uterus (body) (corpus) (recurrent) N85.8
embryonic Q51.818
cervix Q51.6
vagina, vaginal (implantation) (inclusion)
(squamous cell) (wall) N89.8
embryonic Q52.4
vallecula, vallecular (epiglottis) J38.7
vesical (orifice) N32.89
vitreous body H43.89
vulva (implantation) (inclusion) N90.7
congenital Q52.79
sebaceous gland N90.7
vulvovaginal gland N90.7
wolffian
female Q50.5
male Q55.4
Cystadenocarcinoma — *see* Neoplasm,
malignant, by site
bile duct C22.1
endometrioid — *see* Neoplasm, malignant,
by site
specified site — *see* Neoplasm, malignant,
by site
unspecified site
female C56.9
male C61
mucinous
papillary
specified site — *see* Neoplasm,
malignant, by site
unspecified site C56.9
specified site — *see* Neoplasm, malignant,
by site
unspecified site C56.9
papillary
mucinous
specified site — *see* Neoplasm,
malignant, by site
unspecified site C56.9
pseudomucinous
specified site — *see* Neoplasm,
malignant, by site
unspecified site C56.9
serous

Cystadenocarcinoma - *continued*
  papillary - *continued*
    serous - *continued*
      specified site — *see* Neoplasm,
        malignant, by site
      unspecified site C56.9
    specified site — *see* Neoplasm, malignant,
      by site
    unspecified site C56.9
  pseudomucinous
    papillary
      specified site — *see* Neoplasm,
        malignant, by site
      unspecified site C56.9
    specified site — *see* Neoplasm, malignant,
      by site
    unspecified site C56.9
  serous
    papillary
      specified site — *see* Neoplasm,
        malignant, by site
      unspecified site C56.9
    specified site — *see* Neoplasm, malignant,
      by site
    unspecified site C56.9
Cystadenofibroma
  clear cell — *see* Neoplasm, benign, by site
  endometrioid D27.9
    borderline malignancy D39.1-
    malignant C56.-
  mucinous
    specified site — *see* Neoplasm, benign, by
      site
    unspecified site D27.9
  serous
    specified site — *see* Neoplasm, benign, by
      site
    unspecified site D27.9
  specified site — *see* Neoplasm, benign, by
    site
  unspecified site D27.9
Cystadenoma — *see also* Neoplasm, benign,
    by site
  bile duct D13.4
  endometrioid — *see* Neoplasm, benign, by
      site
    borderline malignancy — *see* Neoplasm,
      uncertain behavior, by site
    malignant — *see* Neoplasm, malignant, by
      site
  mucinous
    borderline malignancy
      ovary C56.-
      specified site NEC — *see* Neoplasm,
        uncertain behavior, by site
      unspecified site C56.9
    papillary
      borderline malignancy
        ovary C56.-
        specified site NEC — *see* Neoplasm,
          uncertain behavior, by site
        unspecified site C56.9
      specified site — *see* Neoplasm, benign,
        by site
      unspecified site D27.9
    specified site — *see* Neoplasm, benign, by
      site
    unspecified site D27.9
  papillary
    borderline malignancy
      ovary C56.-
      specified site NEC — *see* Neoplasm,
        uncertain behavior, by site
      unspecified site C56.9
    lymphomatosum
      specified site — *see* Neoplasm, benign,
        by site
      unspecified site D11.9
    mucinous
      borderline malignancy
        ovary C56.-
        specified site NEC — *see* Neoplasm,
          uncertain behavior, by site
        unspecified site C56.9

Cystadenoma - *continued*
  papillary - *continued*
    mucinous - *continued*
      specified site — *see* Neoplasm, benign,
        by site
      unspecified site D27.9
    pseudomucinous
      borderline malignancy
        ovary C56.-
        specified site NEC — *see* Neoplasm,
          uncertain behavior, by site
        unspecified site C56.9
      specified site — *see* Neoplasm, benign,
        by site
      unspecified site D27.9
    serous
      borderline malignancy
        ovary C56.-
        specified site NEC — *see* Neoplasm,
          uncertain behavior, by site
        unspecified site C56.9
      specified site — *see* Neoplasm, benign,
        by site
      unspecified site D27.9
  pseudomucinous
    borderline malignancy
      ovary C56.-
      specified site NEC — *see* Neoplasm,
        uncertain behavior, by site
      unspecified site C56.9
    papillary
      borderline malignancy
        ovary C56.-
        specified site NEC — *see* Neoplasm,
          uncertain behavior, by site
        unspecified site C56.9
      specified site — *see* Neoplasm, benign,
        by site
      unspecified site D27.9
    specified site — *see* Neoplasm, benign, by
      site
    unspecified site D27.9
  serous
    borderline malignancy
      ovary C56.-
      specified site NEC — *see* Neoplasm,
        uncertain behavior, by site
      unspecified site C56.9
    papillary
      borderline malignancy
        ovary C56.-
        specified site NEC — *see* Neoplasm,
          uncertain behavior, by site
        unspecified site C56.9
      specified site — *see* Neoplasm, benign,
        by site
      unspecified site D27.9
    specified site — *see* Neoplasm, benign, by
      site
    unspecified site D27.9
Cystathionine synthase deficiency E72.11
Cystathioninemia E72.19
Cystathioninuria E72.19
Cystic — *see also* condition
  breast (chronic) — *see* Mastopathy, cystic
  corpora lutea (hemorrhagic) N83.1-
  duct — *see* condition
  eyeball (congenital) Q11.0
  fibrosis — *see* Fibrosis, cystic
  kidney (congenital) Q61.9
    adult type Q61.2
    infantile type NEC Q61.19
      collecting duct dilatation Q61.11
    medullary Q61.5
  liver, congenital Q44.6
  lung disease J98.4
    congenital Q33.0
  mastitis, chronic — *see* Mastopathy, cystic
  medullary, kidney Q61.5
  meniscus — *see* Derangement, knee,
    meniscus, cystic
  ovary N83.20-

Cysticercosis, cysticerciasis B69.9
  with
    epileptiform fits B69.0
    myositis B69.81
  brain B69.0
  central nervous system B69.0
  cerebral B69.0
  ocular B69.1
  specified NEC B69.89
Cysticercus cellulose infestation — *see*
    Cysticercosis
Cystinosis (malignant) E72.04
Cystinuria E72.01
Cystitis (exudative) (hemorrhagic) (septic)
    (suppurative) N30.90
  with
    fibrosis — *see* Cystitis, chronic, interstitial
    hematuria N30.91
    leukoplakia — *see* Cystitis, chronic,
      interstitial
    malakoplakia — *see* Cystitis, chronic,
      interstitial
    metaplasia — *see* Cystitis, chronic,
      interstitial
    prostatitis N41.3
  acute N30.00
    with hematuria N30.01
    of trigone N30.30
      with hematuria N30.31
  allergic — *see* Cystitis, specified type NEC
  amebic A06.81
  bilharzial B65.9 *[N33]*
  blennorrhagic (gonococcal) A54.01
  bullous — *see* Cystitis, specified type NEC
  calculous N21.0
  chlamydial A56.01
  chronic N30.20
    with hematuria N30.21
    interstitial N30.10
      with hematuria N30.11
    of trigone N30.30
      with hematuria N30.31
    specified NEC N30.20
      with hematuria N30.21
  cystic (a) — *see* Cystitis, specified type NEC
  diphtheritic A36.85
  echinococcal
    granulosus B67.39
    multilocularis B67.69
  emphysematous — *see* Cystitis, specified
    type NEC
  encysted — *see* Cystitis, specified type NEC
  eosinophilic — *see* Cystitis, specified type
    NEC
  follicular — *see* Cystitis, of trigone
  gangrenous — *see* Cystitis, specified type
    NEC
  glandularis — *see* Cystitis, specified type
    NEC
  gonococcal A54.01
  incrusted — *see* Cystitis, specified type NEC
  interstitial (chronic) — *see* Cystitis, chronic,
    interstitial
  irradiation N30.40
    with hematuria N30.41
  irritation — *see* Cystitis, specified type NEC
  malignant — *see* Cystitis, specified type
    NEC
  of trigone N30.30
    with hematuria N30.31
  panmural — *see* Cystitis, chronic, interstitial
  polyposa — *see* Cystitis, specified type NEC
  prostatic N41.3
  puerperal (postpartum) O86.22
  radiation — *see* Cystitis, irradiation
  specified type NEC N30.80
    with hematuria N30.81
  subacute — *see* Cystitis, chronic
  submucous — *see* Cystitis, chronic,
    interstitial
  syphilitic (late) A52.76
  trichomonal A59.03
  tuberculous A18.12
  ulcerative — *see* Cystitis, chronic, interstitial

Cystocele (-urethrocele)
female N81.10
with prolapse of uterus — see Prolapse,
uterus
lateral N81.12
midline N81.11
paravaginal N81.12
in pregnancy or childbirth O34.8-
causing obstructed labor O65.5
male N32.89
Cystolithiasis N21.0
Cystoma — see also Neoplasm, benign, by site
endometrial, ovary N80.1
mucinous
specified site — see Neoplasm, benign, by
site
unspecified site D27.9
serous
specified site — see Neoplasm, benign, by
site
unspecified site D27.9
simple (ovary) N83.29-
Cystoplegia N31.2
Cystoptosis N32.89
Cystopyelitis — see Pyelonephritis
Cystorrhagia N32.89
Cystosarcoma phyllodes D48.6-
benign D24-
malignant — see Neoplasm, breast,
malignant
Cystostomy
attention to Z43.5
complication — see Complications,
cystostomy
status Z93.50
appendico-vesicostomy Z93.52
cutaneous Z93.51
specified NEC Z93.59
Cystourethritis — see Urethritis
Cystourethrocele — see also Cystocele
female N81.10
with uterine prolapse — see Prolapse,
uterus
lateral N81.12
midline N81.11
paravaginal N81.12
male N32.89
Cytomegalic inclusion disease
congenital P35.1
Cytomegalovirus infection B25.9
Cytomycosis (reticuloendothelial) B39.4
Cytopenia D75.9
refractory
with multilineage dysplasia D46.A
and ring sideroblasts (RCMD
RS) D46.B
**Czerny's disease (periodic hydrarthrosis of
the knee)** — see Effusion, joint, knee

D

Da Costa's syndrome F45.8
**Daae (-Finsen) disease (epidemic
pleurodynia)** B33.0
Dabney's grip B33.0
Dacryoadenitis, dacryadenitis H04.00-
acute H04.01-
chronic H04.02-
Dacryocystitis H04.30-
acute H04.32-
chronic H04.41-
neonatal P39.1
phlegmonous H04.31-
syphilitic A52.71
congenital (early) A50.01
trachomatous, active A71.1
sequelae (late effect) B94.0
Dacryocystoblennorrhea — see Inflammation,
lacrimal, passages, chronic
Dacryocystocele — see Disorder, lacrimal
system, changes
Dacryolith, dacryolithiasis H04.51-
Dacryoma — see Disorder, lacrimal system,
changes
Dacryopericystitis — see Dacryocystitis
Dacryops H04.11-

Dacryostenosis — see also Stenosis, lacrimal
congenital Q10.5
Dactylitis
bone — see Osteomyelitis
sickle-cell D57.00
Hb C D57.219
Hb SS D57.00
specified NEC D57.819
skin L08.9
syphilitic A52.77
tuberculous A18.03
Dactylolysis spontanea (ainhum) L94.6
Dactylosymphysis Q70.9
fingers — see Syndactylism, complex,
fingers
toes — see Syndactylism, complex, toes
Damage
arteriosclerotic — see Arteriosclerosis
brain (nontraumatic) G93.9
anoxic, hypoxic G93.1
resulting from a procedure G97.82
child NEC G80.9
due to birth injury P11.2
cardiorenal (vascular) — see Hypertension,
cardiorenal
cerebral NEC — see Damage, brain
coccyx, complicating delivery O71.6
coronary — see Disease, heart, ischemic
deep tissue, pressure-induced — see also
L89 with final character .6
eye, birth injury P15.3
liver (nontraumatic) K76.9
alcoholic K70.9
due to drugs — see Disease, liver, toxic
toxic — see Disease, liver, toxic
medication T88.7
pelvic
joint or ligament, during delivery O71.6
organ NEC
during delivery O71.5
following ectopic or molar
pregnancy O08.6
renal — see Disease, renal
subendocardium, subendocardial — see
Degeneration, myocardial
vascular I99.9
**Dana-Putnam syndrome (subacute
combined sclerosis with pernicious
anemia)** — see Degeneration, combined
**Danbolt (-Cross) syndrome (acrodermatitis
enteropathica)** E83.2
Dandruff L21.0
Dandy-Walker syndrome Q03.1
with spina bifida — see Spina bifida
Danlos' syndrome — see also Syndrome,
Ehlers-Danlos Q79.60
Darier (-White) disease (congenital) Q82.8
meaning erythema annulare
centrifugum L53.1
Darier-Roussy sarcoid D86.3
Darling's disease or histoplasmosis B39.4
Darwin's tubercle Q17.8
Dawson's (inclusion body) encephalitis A81.1
De Beurmann (-Gougerot) disease B42.1
De la Tourette's syndrome F95.2
De Lange's syndrome Q87.19
De Morgan's spots (senile angiomas) I78.1
De Quervain's
disease (tendon sheath) M65.4
syndrome E34.51
thyroiditis (subacute granulomatous
thyroiditis) E06.1
De Toni-Fanconi (-Debré) syndrome E72.09
with cystinosis E72.04
Dead
fetus, retained (mother) O36.4
early pregnancy O02.1
labyrinth — see subcategory H83.2
ovum, retained O02.0
Deaf nonspeaking NEC H91.3
Deafmutism (acquired) (congenital) NEC
H91.3
hysterical F44.6
syphilitic, congenital (see also subcategory
H94.8) A50.09

**Deafness (acquired) (complete) (hereditary)
(partial)** H91.9-
with blue sclera and fragility of bone Q78.0
auditory fatigue — see Deafness, specified
type NEC
aviation T70.0
nerve injury — see Injury, nerve, acoustic,
specified type NEC
boilermaker's — see subcategory H83.3
central — see Deafness, sensorineural
conductive H90.2
and sensorineural
mixed H90.8
bilateral H90.6
bilateral H90.0
unilateral H90.1-
with restricted hearing on the
contralateral side H90.A-
congenital H90.5
with blue sclera and fragility of
bone Q78.0
due to toxic agents — see Deafness, ototoxic
emotional (hysterical) F44.6
functional (hysterical) F44.6
high frequency H91.9-
hysterical F44.6
low frequency H91.9-
mental R48.8
mixed conductive and sensorineural H90.8
bilateral H90.6
unilateral H90.7-
nerve — see Deafness, sensorineural
neural — see Deafness, sensorineural
noise-induced (see also subcategory H83.3)
nerve injury — see Injury, nerve, acoustic,
specified type NEC
nonspeaking H91.3
ototoxic — see subcategory H91.0
perceptive — see Deafness, sensorineural
psychogenic (hysterical) F44.6
sensorineural H90.5
and conductive
mixed H90.8
bilateral H90.6
bilateral H90.3
unilateral H90.4-
with restricted hearing on the
contralateral side H90.A-
sensory — see Deafness, sensorineural
specified type NEC — see subcategory
H91.8
sudden (idiopathic) H91.2-
syphilitic A52.15
transient ischemic H93.01-
traumatic — see Injury, nerve, acoustic,
specified type NEC
word (developmental) H93.25
**Death (cause unknown) (of) (unexplained)
(unspecified cause)** R99
brain G93.82
cardiac (sudden) (with successful
resuscitation) - code to underlying
disease
family history of Z82.41
personal history of Z86.74
family member (assumed) Z63.4
Debility (chronic) (general) (nervous) R53.81
congenital or neonatal NOS P96.9
nervous R53.81
old age R54
senile R54
Débove's disease (splenomegaly) R16.1
Decalcification
bone — see Osteoporosis
teeth K03.89
Decapsulation, kidney N28.89
Decay
dental — see Caries, dental
senile R54
tooth, teeth — see Caries, dental
Deciduitis (acute)
following ectopic or molar pregnancy O08.0
Decline (general) — see Debility
cognitive, age-associated R41.81

Decompensation
  cardiac (acute) (chronic) — *see* Disease,
      heart
  cardiovascular — *see* Disease,
      cardiovascular
  heart — *see* Disease, heart
  hepatic — *see* Failure, hepatic
  myocardial (acute) (chronic) — *see* Disease,
      heart
  respiratory J98.8
Decompression sickness T70.3
Decrease (d)
  absolute neutrophile count — *see*
      Neutropenia
  blood
    platelets — *see* Thrombocytopenia
    pressure R03.1
      due to shock following
        injury T79.4
        operation T81.19
  estrogen E28.39
    postablative E89.40
      asymptomatic E89.40
      symptomatic E89.41
  fragility of erythrocytes D58.8
  function
    lipase (pancreatic) K90.3
    ovary in hypopituitarism E23.0
    parenchyma of pancreas K86.89
    pituitary (gland) (anterior) (lobe) E23.0
      posterior (lobe) E23.0
  functional activity R68.89
  glucose R73.09
  hematocrit R71.0
  hemoglobin R71.0
  leukocytes D72.819
    specified NEC D72.818
  libido R68.82
  lymphocytes D72.810
  platelets D69.6
  respiration, due to shock following
      injury T79.4
  sexual desire R68.82
  tear secretion NEC — *see* Syndrome, dry eye
  tolerance
    fat K90.49
    glucose R73.09
    pancreatic K90.3
    salt and water E87.8
  vision NEC H54.7
  white blood cell count D72.819
    specified NEC D72.818
Decubitus (ulcer) — *see* Ulcer, pressure, by
    site
  cervix N86
Deepening acetabulum — *see* Derangement,
    joint, specified type NEC, hip
Defect, defective Q89.9
  3-beta-hydroxysteroid dehydrogenase E25.0
  11-hydroxylase E25.0
  21-hydroxylase E25.0
  abdominal wall, congenital Q79.59
  antibody immunodeficiency D80.9
  aorticopulmonary septum Q21.4
  atrial septal (ostium secundum type) Q21.1
    following acute myocardial infarction
        (current complication) I23.1
    ostium primum type Q21.2
  atrioventricular
    canal Q21.2
    septum Q21.2
  auricular septal Q21.1
  bilirubin excretion NEC E80.6
  biosynthesis, androgen (testicular) E29.1
  bulbar septum Q21.0
  catalase E80.3
  cell membrane receptor complex (CR3) D71
  circulation I99.9
    congenital Q28.9
    newborn Q28.9
  coagulation (factor) — *see also* Deficiency,
      factor D68.9
    with
      ectopic pregnancy O08.1
      molar pregnancy O08.1

Defect, defective - *continued*
  coagulation (factor) - *continued*
    acquired D68.4
    antepartum with hemorrhage — *see*
        Hemorrhage, antepartum, with
        coagulation defect
    due to
      liver disease D68.4
      vitamin K deficiency D68.4
    hereditary NEC D68.2
    intrapartum O67.0
    newborn, transient P61.6
    postpartum O99.13
      with hemorrhage O72.3
    specified type NEC D68.8
  complement system D84.1
  conduction (heart) I45.9
    bone — *see* Deafness, conductive
  congenital, organ or site not listed — *see*
      Anomaly, by site
  coronary sinus Q21.1
  cushion, endocardial Q21.2
  degradation, glycoprotein E77.1
  dental bridge, crown, fillings — *see* Defect,
      dental restoration
  dental restoration K08.50
    specified NEC K08.59
  dentin (hereditary) K00.5
  Descemet's membrane, congenital Q13.89
  developmental — *see also* Anomaly
    cauda equina Q06.3
  diaphragm
    with elevation, eventration or hernia — *see*
        Hernia, diaphragm
    congenital Q79.1
      with hernia Q79.0
      gross (with hernia) Q79.0
  ectodermal, congenital Q82.9
  Eisenmenger's Q21.8
  enzyme
    catalase E80.3
    peroxidase E80.3
  esophagus, congenital Q39.9
  extensor retinaculum M62.89
  fibrin polymerization D68.2
  filling
    bladder R93.41
    kidney R93.42-
    renal pelvis R93.41
    stomach R93.3
    ureter R93.41
    urinary organs, specified NEC R93.49
  GABA (gamma aminobutyric acid)
      metabolic E72.81
  Gerbode Q21.0
  glycoprotein degradation E77.1
  Hageman (factor) D68.2
  hearing — *see* Deafness
  high grade F70
  interatrial septal Q21.1
  interauricular septal Q21.1
  interventricular septal Q21.0
    with dextroposition of aorta, pulmonary
        stenosis and hypertrophy of right
        ventricle Q21.3
    in tetralogy of Fallot Q21.3
  learning (specific) — *see* Disorder, learning
  lymphocyte function antigen-1 (LFA-
      1) D84.0
  lysosomal enzyme, post-translational
      modification E77.0
  major osseous M89.70
    ankle M89.77-
    carpus M89.74-
    clavicle M89.71-
    femur M89.75-
    fibula M89.76-
    fingers M89.74-
    foot M89.77-
    forearm M89.73-
    hand M89.74-
    humerus M89.72-
    lower leg M89.76-
    metacarpus M89.74-
    metatarsus M89.77-

Defect, defective - *continued*
  major osseous - *continued*
    multiple sites M89.79
    pelvic region M89.75-
    pelvis M89.75-
    radius M89.73-
    scapula M89.71-
    shoulder region M89.71-
    specified NEC M89.78
    tarsus M89.77-
    thigh M89.75-
    tibia M89.76-
    toes M89.77-
    ulna M89.73-
  mental — *see* Disability, intellectual
  modification, lysosomal enzymes, post-
      translational E77.0
  obstructive, congenital
    renal pelvis Q62.39
    ureter Q62.39
      atresia — *see* Atresia, ureter
      cecoureterocele Q62.32
      megaureter Q62.2
      orthotopic ureterocele Q62.31
  osseous, major M89.70
    ankle M89.77-
    carpus M89.74-
    clavicle M89.71-
    femur M89.75-
    fibula M89.76-
    fingers M89.74-
    foot M89.77-
    forearm M89.73-
    hand M89.74-
    humerus M89.72-
    lower leg M89.76-
    metacarpus M89.74-
    metatarsus M89.77-
    multiple sites M89.9
    pelvic region M89.75-
    pelvis M89.75-
    radius M89.73-
    scapula M89.71-
    shoulder region M89.71-
    specified NEC M89.78
    tarsus M89.77-
    thigh M89.75-
    tibia M89.76-
    toes M89.77-
    ulna M89.73-
  osteochondral NEC — *see also*
      Deformity M95.8
  ostium
    primum Q21.2
    secundum Q21.1
  peroxidase E80.3
  placental blood supply — *see* Insufficiency,
      placental
  platelets, qualitative D69.1
    constitutional D68.0
  postural NEC, spine — *see* Dorsopathy,
      deforming
  reduction
    limb Q73.8
      lower Q72.9-
        absence — *see* Agenesis, leg
        foot — *see* Agenesis, foot
        longitudinal
          femur Q72.4-
          fibula Q72.6-
          tibia Q72.5-
        specified type NEC Q72.89-
        split foot Q72.7-
      specified type NEC Q73.8
      upper Q71.9-
        absence — *see* Agenesis, arm
        forearm — *see* Agenesis, forearm
        hand — *see* Agenesis, hand
        lobster-claw hand Q71.6-
        longitudinal
          radius Q71.4-
          ulna Q71.5-
        specified type NEC Q71.89-
  renal pelvis Q63.8
    obstructive Q62.39

Defect, defective - *continued*
  respiratory system, congenital Q34.9
  restoration, dental K08.50
    specified NEC K08.59
  retinal nerve bundle fibers H35.89
  septal (heart) NOS Q21.9
    acquired (atrial) (auricular) (ventricular)
      (old) I51.0
    atrial Q21.1
      concurrent with acute myocardial
        infarction — *see* Infarct,
        myocardium
      following acute myocardial infarction
        (current complication) I23.1
      ventricular — *see also* Defect, ventricular
        septal Q21.0
    sinus venosus Q21.1
  speech R47.9
    developmental F80.9
    specified NEC R47.89
  Taussig-Bing (aortic transposition and
    overriding pulmonary artery) Q20.1
  teeth, wedge K03.1
  vascular (local) I99.9
    congenital Q27.9
  ventricular septal Q21.0
    concurrent with acute myocardial
      infarction — *see* Infarct, myocardium
    following acute myocardial infarction
      (current complication) I23.2
    in tetralogy of Fallot Q21.3
  vision NEC H54.7
  visual field H53.40
    bilateral
      heteronymous H53.47
      homonymous H53.46-
    generalized contraction H53.48-
    localized
      arcuate H53.43-
      scotoma (central area) H53.41-
        blind spot area H53.42-
      sector H53.43-
      specified type NEC H53.45-
  voice R49.9
    specified NEC R49.8
  wedge, tooth, teeth (abrasion) K03.1
Deferentitis N49.1
  gonorrheal (acute) (chronic) A54.23
Defibrination (syndrome) D65
  antepartum — *see* Hemorrhage, antepartum,
    with coagulation defect, disseminated
    intravascular coagulation
  following ectopic or molar pregnancy O08.1
  intrapartum O67.0
  newborn P60
  postpartum O72.3
Deficiency, deficient
  3-beta hydroxysteroid dehydrogenase E25.0
  5-alpha reductase (with male
    pseudohermaphroditism) E29.1
  11-hydroxylase E25.0
  21-hydroxylase E25.0
  abdominal muscle syndrome Q79.4
  accelerator globulin (Ac G) (blood) D68.2
  AC globulin (congenital) (hereditary) D68.2
    acquired D68.4
  acid phosphatase E83.39
  activating factor (blood) D68.2
  ADA2 (adenosine deaminase 2) D81.32
  adenosine deaminase (ADA) D81.30
    with severe combined immunodeficiency
      (SCID) D81.31
    partial (type 1) D81.39
    specified NEC D81.39
    type 1 (without SCID) (without severe
      combined immunodeficiency) D81.39
    type 2 D81.32
  aldolase (hereditary) E74.19
  alpha-1-antitrypsin E88.01
  amino-acids E72.9
  anemia — *see* Anemia
  aneurin E51.9
  antibody with
    hyperimmunoglobulinemia D80.6
    near-normal immunoglobins D80.6

Deficiency, deficient - *continued*
  antidiuretic hormone E23.2
  anti-hemophilic
    factor (A) D66
      B D67
      C D68.1
    globulin (AHG) NEC D66
  antithrombin (antithrombin III) D68.59
  ascorbic acid E54
  attention (disorder) (syndrome) F98.8
    with hyperactivity — *see* Disorder,
      attention-deficit hyperactivity
  autoprothrombin
    I D68.2
    II D67
    C D68.2
  beta-glucuronidase E76.29
  biotin E53.8
  biotin-dependent carboxylase D81.819
  biotinidase D81.810
  brancher enzyme (amylopectinosis) E74.03
  calciferol E55.9
    with
      adult osteomalacia M83.8
      rickets — *see* Rickets
  calcium (dietary) E58
  calorie, severe E43
    with marasmus E41
    and kwashiorkor E42
  cardiac — *see* Insufficiency, myocardial
  carnitine E71.40
    due to
      hemodialysis E71.43
      inborn errors of metabolism E71.42
      Valproic acid therapy E71.43
    iatrogenic E71.43
    muscle palmityltransferase E71.314
    primary E71.41
    secondary E71.448
  carotene E50.9
  central nervous system G96.8
  ceruloplasmin (Wilson) E83.01
  choline E53.8
  Christmas factor D67
  chromium E61.4
  clotting (blood) — *see also* Deficiency,
    coagulation factor D68.9
  clotting factor NEC (hereditary) — *see also*
    Deficiency, factor D68.2
  coagulation NOS D68.9
    with
      ectopic pregnancy O08.1
      molar pregnancy O08.1
    acquired (any) D68.4
    antepartum hemorrhage — *see*
      Hemorrhage, antepartum, with
      coagulation defect
    clotting factor NEC — *see also*
      Deficiency, factor D68.2
    due to
      hyperprothrombinemia D68.4
      liver disease D68.4
      vitamin K deficiency D68.4
    newborn, transient P61.6
    postpartum O72.3
    specified NEC D68.8
  cognitive F09
  color vision H53.50
    achromatopsia H53.51
    acquired H53.52
    deuteranomaly H53.53
    protanomaly H53.54
    specified type NEC H53.59
    tritanomaly H53.55
  combined glucocorticoid and
    mineralocorticoid E27.49
  contact factor D68.2
  copper (nutritional) E61.0
  corticoadrenal E27.40
    primary E27.1
  craniofacial axis Q75.0
  cyanocobalamin E53.8
  C1 esterase inhibitor (C1-INH) D84.1
  debrancher enzyme (limit
    dextrinosis) E74.03

Deficiency, deficient - *continued*
  dehydrogenase
    long chain/very long chain acyl
      CoA E71.310
      medium chain acyl CoA E71.311
      short chain acyl CoA E71.312
  diet E63.9
  dihydropyrimidine dehydrogenase
    (DPD) E88.89
  disaccharidase E73.9
  edema — *see* Malnutrition, severe
  endocrine E34.9
  energy-supply — *see* Malnutrition
  enzymes, circulating NEC E88.09
  ergosterol E55.9
    with
      adult osteomalacia M83.8
      rickets — *see* Rickets
  essential fatty acid (EFA) E63.0
  factor — *see also* Deficiency, coagulation
    Hageman D68.2
    I (congenital) (hereditary) D68.2
    II (congenital) (hereditary) D68.2
    IX (congenital) (functional) (hereditary)
      (with functional defect) D67
    multiple (congenital) D68.8
      acquired D68.4
    V (congenital) (hereditary) D68.2
    VII (congenital) (hereditary) D68.2
    VIII (congenital) (functional) (hereditary)
      (with functional defect) D66
      with vascular defect D68.0
    X (congenital) (hereditary) D68.2
    XI (congenital) (hereditary) D68.1
    XII (congenital) (hereditary) D68.2
    XIII (congenital) (hereditary) D68.2
  femoral, proximal focal (congenital) — *see*
    Defect, reduction, lower limb,
    longitudinal, femur
  fibrin-stabilizing factor (congenital)
    (hereditary) D68.2
    acquired D68.4
  fibrinase D68.2
  fibrinogen (congenital) (hereditary) D68.2
    acquired D65
  folate E53.8
  folic acid E53.8
  foreskin N47.3
  fructokinase E74.11
  fructose 1,6-diphosphatase E74.19
  fructose-1-phosphate aldolase E74.19
  GABA (gamma aminobutyric acid)
    transaminase E72.81
  GABA-T (gamma aminobutyric acid
    transaminase) E72.81
  galactokinase E74.29
  galactose-1-phosphate uridyl
    transferase E74.29
  gammaglobulin in blood D80.1
    hereditary D80.0
  glass factor D68.2
  glucocorticoid E27.49
    mineralocorticoid E27.49
  glucose-6-phosphatase E74.01
  glucose-6-phosphate dehydrogenase
    anemia D55.0
    without anemia D75.A
  glucuronyl transferase E80.5
  glycogen synthetase E74.09
  gonadotropin (isolated) E23.0
  growth hormone (idiopathic) (isolated) E23.0
  Hageman factor D68.2
  hemoglobin D64.9
  hepatophosphorylase E74.09
  homogentisate 1,2-dioxygenase E70.29
  hormone
    anterior pituitary (partial) NEC E23.0
      growth E23.0
    growth (isolated) E23.0
    pituitary E23.0
    testicular E29.1
  hypoxanthine- (guanine)
    -phosphoribosyltransferase (HG- PRT)
    (total H-PRT) E79.1
  immunity D84.9

Deficiency, deficient - *continued*
immunity - *continued*
 cell-mediated D84.8
  with thrombocytopenia and
   eczema D82.0
 combined D81.9
 humoral D80.9
 IgA (secretory) D80.2
 IgG D80.3
 IgM D80.4
immuno — *see* Immunodeficiency
immunoglobulin, selective
 A (IgA) D80.2
 G (IgG) (subclasses) D80.3
 M (IgM) D80.4
inositol (B complex) E53.8
intrinsic
 factor (congenital) D51.0
 sphincter N36.42
  with urethral hypermobility N36.43
iodine E61.8
 congenital syndrome — *see* Syndrome,
  iodine-deficiency, congenital
iron E61.1
 anemia D50.9
kalium E87.6
kappa-light chain D80.8
labile factor (congenital) (hereditary) D68.2
 acquired D68.4
lacrimal fluid (acquired) — *see also*
 Syndrome, dry eye
 congenital Q10.6
lactase
 congenital E73.0
 secondary E73.1
Laki-Lorand factor D68.2
lecithin cholesterol acyltransferase E78.6
lipocaic K86.89
lipoprotein (familial) (high density) E78.6
liver phosphorylase E74.09
lysosomal alpha-1, 4 glucosidase E74.02
magnesium E61.2
major histocompatibility complex
 class I D81.6
 class II D81.7
manganese E61.3
menadione (vitamin K) E56.1
 newborn P53
mental (familial) (hereditary) — *see*
 Disability, intellectual
methylenetetrahydrofolate reductase
 (MTHFR) E72.12
mevalonate kinase M04.1
mineral NEC E61.8
mineralocorticoid E27.49
 with glucocorticoid E27.49
molybdenum (nutritional) E61.5
moral F60.2
multiple nutrient elements E61.7
multiple sulfatase (MSD) E75.26
muscle
 carnitine (palmityltransferase) E71.314
 phosphofructokinase E74.09
myoadenylate deaminase E79.2
myocardial — *see* Insufficiency, myocardial
myophosphorylase E74.04
NADH diaphorase or reductase
 (congenital) D74.0
NADH-methemoglobin reductase
 (congenital) D74.0
natrium E87.1
niacin (amide) (-tryptophan) E52
nicotinamide E52
nicotinic acid E52
number of teeth — *see* Anodontia
nutrient element E61.9
 multiple E61.7
 specified NEC E61.8
nutrition, nutritional E63.9
 sequelae — *see* Sequelae, nutritional
  deficiency
 specified NEC E63.8
of interleukin 1 receptor antagonist
 [DIRA] M04.8
ornithine transcarbamylase E72.4

Deficiency, deficient - *continued*
ovarian E28.39
oxygen — *see* Anoxia
pantothenic acid E53.8
parathyroid (gland) E20.9
perineum (female) N81.89
phenylalanine hydroxylase E70.1
phosphoenolpyruvate carboxykinase E74.4
phosphofructokinase E74.19
phosphomannomutuse E74.8
phosphomannose isomerase E74.8
phosphomannosyl mutase E74.8
phosphorylase kinase, liver E74.09
pituitary hormone (isolated) E23.0
plasma thromboplastin
 antecedent (PTA) D68.1
 component (PTC) D67
plasminogen (type 1) (type 2) E88.02
platelet NEC D69.1
 constitutional D68.0
polyglandular E31.8
 autoimmune E31.0
potassium (K) E87.6
prepuce N47.3
proaccelerin (congenital) (hereditary) D68.2
 acquired D68.4
proconvertin factor (congenital)
 (hereditary) D68.2
 acquired D68.4
protein — *see also* Malnutrition E46
 anemia D53.0
 C D68.59
 S D68.59
prothrombin (congenital) (heredItary) D68.2
 acquired D68.4
Prower factor D68.2
pseudocholinesterase E88.09
PTA (plasma thromboplastin
 antecedent) D68.1
PTC (plasma thromboplastin
 component) D67
purine nucleoside phosphorylase
 (PNP) D81.5
pyracin (alpha) (beta) E53.1
pyridoxal E53.1
pyridoxamine E53.1
pyridoxine (derivatives) E53.1
pyruvate
 carboxylase E74.4
 dehydrogenase E74.4
riboflavin (vitamin B2) E53.0
salt E87.1
secretion
 ovary E28.39
 salivary gland (any) K11.7
 urine R34
selenium (dietary) E59
serum antitrypsin, familial E88.01
short stature homeobox gene (SHOX)
 with
  dyschondrosteosis Q78.8
  short stature (idiopathic) E34.3
  Turner's syndrome Q96.9
sodium (Na) E87.1
SPCA (factor VII) D68.2
sphincter, intrinsic N36.42
 with urethral hypermobility N36.43
stable factor (congenital) (hereditary) D68.2
 acquired D68.4
Stuart-Prower (factor X) D68.2
succinic semialdehyde
 dehydrogenase E72.81
sucrase E74.39
sulfatase E75.26
sulfite oxidase E72.19
thiamin, thiaminic (chloride) E51.9
 beriberi (dry) E51.11
  wet E51.12
thrombokinase D68.2
 newborn P53
thyroid (gland) — *see* Hypothyroidism
tocopherol E56.0
tooth bud K00.0
transcobalamine II (anemia) D51.2
vanadium E61.6

Deficiency, deficient - *continued*
vascular I99.9
vasopressin E23.2
vertical ridge K06.8
viosterol — *see* Deficiency, calciferol
vitamin (multiple) NOS E56.9
 A E50.9
  with
   Bitot's spot (corneal) E50.1
   follicular keratosis E50.8
   keratomalacia E50.4
   manifestations NEC E50.8
   night blindness E50.5
   scar of cornea, xerophthalmic E50.6
   xeroderma E50.8
   xerophthalmia E50.7
   xerosis
    conjunctival E50.0
     and Bitot's spot E50.1
    cornea E50.2
     and ulceration E50.3
  sequelae E64.1
 B (complex) NOS E53.9
  with
   beriberi (dry) E51.11
    wet E51.12
   pellagra E52
 B1 NOS E51.9
  beriberi (dry) E51.11
   with circulatory system
    manifestations E51.11
   wet E51.12
 B12 E53.8
 B2 (riboflavin) E53.0
 B6 E53.1
 C E54
  sequelae E64.2
 D E55.9
  with
   adult osteomalacia M83.8
   rickets — *see* Rickets
  25-hydroxylase E83.32
 E E56.0
 folic acid E53.8
 G E53.0
 group B E53.9
  specified NEC E53.8
 H (biotin) E53.8
 K E56.1
  of newborn P53
 nicotinic E52
 P E56.8
 PP (pellagra-preventing) E52
 specified NEC E56.8
 thiamin E51.9
  beriberi — *see* Beriberi
 zinc, dietary E60
Deficit — *see also* Deficiency
attention and concentration R41.840
 following
  cerebral infarction I69.310
  cerebrovascular disease I69.910
   specified disease NEC I69.810
  nontraumatic
   intracerebral hemorrhage I69.110
   specified intracranial hemorrhage
    NEC I69.210
   subarachnoid hemorrhage I69.010
 disorder — *see* Attention, deficit
cognitive
 communication R41.841
 emotional
  following
   cerebral infarction I69.315
   cerebrovascular disease I69.915
    specified disease NEC I69.815
   nontraumatic
    intracerebral hemorrhage I69.115
    specified intracranial hemorrhage
     NEC I69.215
    subarachnoid hemorrhage I69.015
 following
  cerebral infarction I69.319
  cerebrovascular disease I69.919
   specified disease NEC I69.819

Deficit - *continued*
  cognitive - *continued*
    following - *continued*
      nontraumatic
        intracerebral hemorrhage I69.119
        specified intracranial hemorrhage
          NEC I69.219
        subarachnoid hemorrhage I69.019
    social
      following
        cerebral infarction I69.315
        cerebrovascular disease I69.915
          specified disease NEC I69.815
        nontraumatic
          intracerebral hemorrhage I69.115
          specified intracranial hemorrhage
            NEC I69.215
          subarachnoid hemorrhage I69.015
  cognitive NEC R41.89
    following
      cerebral infarction I69.318
      cerebrovascular disease I69.918
        specified disease NEC I69.818
      nontraumatic
        intracerebral hemorrhage I69.118
        specified intracranial hemorrhage
          NEC I69.218
        subarachnoid hemorrhage I69.018
  concentration R41.840
  executive function R41.844
    following
      cerebral infarction I69.314
      cerebrovascular disease I69.914
        specified disease NEC I69.814
      nontraumatic
        intracerebral hemorrhage I69.114
        specified intracranial hemorrhage
          NEC I69.214
        subarachnoid hemorrhage I69.014
  frontal lobe R41.844
    following
      cerebral infarction I69.314
      cerebrovascular disease I69.914
        specified disease NEC I69.814
      nontraumatic
        intracerebral hemorrhage I69.114
        specified intracranial hemorrhage
          NEC I69.214
        subarachnoid hemorrhage I69.014
  memory
    following
      cerebral infarction I69.311
      cerebrovascular disease I69.911
        specified disease NEC I69.811
      nontraumatic
        intracerebral hemorrhage I69.111
        specified intracranial hemorrhage
          NEC I69.211
        subarachnoid hemorrhage I69.011
  neurologic NEC R29.818
    ischemic
      reversible (RIND) I63.9
        prolonged (PRIND) I63.9
  oxygen R09.02
  prolonged reversible ischemic neurologic
    (PRIND) I63.9
  psychomotor R41.843
    following
      cerebral infarction I69.313
      cerebrovascular disease I69.913
        specified disease NEC I69.813
      nontraumatic
        intracerebral hemorrhage I69.113
        specified intracranial hemorrhage
          NEC I69.213
        subarachnoid hemorrhage I69.013
  visuospatial R41.842
    following
      cerebral infarction I69.312
      cerebrovascular disease I69.912
        specified disease NEC I69.812
      nontraumatic
        intracerebral hemorrhage I69.112
        specified intracranial hemorrhage
          NEC I69.212

Deficit - *continued*
  visuospatial - *continued*
    following - *continued*
      nontraumatic - *continued*
        subarachnoid hemorrhage I69.012
Deflection
  radius — *see* Deformity, limb, specified type
    NEC, forearm
  septum (acquired) (nasal) (nose) J34.2
  spine — *see* Curvature, spine
  turbinate (nose) J34.2
Defluvium
  capillorum — *see* Alopecia
  ciliorum — *see* Madarosis
  unguium L60.8
Deformity Q89.9
  abdomen, congenital Q89.9
  abdominal wall
    acquired M95.8
    congenital Q79.59
  acquired (unspecified site) M95.9
  adrenal gland Q89.1
  alimentary tract, congenital Q45.9
    upper Q40.9
  ankle (joint) (acquired) — *see also*
    Deformity, limb, lower leg
    abduction — *see* Contraction, joint, ankle
    congenital Q68.8
    contraction — *see* Contraction, joint, ankle
    specified type NEC — *see* Deformity,
      limb, foot, specified NEC
  anus (acquired) K62.89
    congenital Q43.9
  aorta (arch) (congenital) Q25.40
    acquired I77.89
  aortic
    arch, acquired I77.89
    cusp or valve (congenital) Q23.8
      acquired — *see also* Endocarditis,
        aortic I35.8
  arm (acquired) (upper) — *see also*
    Deformity, limb, upper arm
    congenital Q68.8
    forearm — *see* Deformity, limb, forearm
  artery (congenital) (peripheral) NOS Q27.9
    acquired I77.89
    coronary (acquired) I25.9
      congenital Q24.5
    umbilical Q27.0
  atrial septal Q21.1
  auditory canal (external) (congenital) — *see*
    also Malformation, ear, external
    acquired — *see* Disorder, ear, external,
      specified type NEC
  auricle
    ear (congenital) — *see also* Malformation,
      ear, external
      acquired — *see* Disorder, pinna,
        deformity
  back — *see* Dorsopathy, deforming
  bile duct (common) (congenital)
    (hepatic) Q44.5
    acquired K83.8
  biliary duct or passage (congenital) Q44.5
    acquired K83.8
  bladder (neck) (trigone) (sphincter)
    (acquired) N32.89
    congenital Q64.79
  bone (acquired) NOS M95.9
    congenital Q79.9
    turbinate M95.0
  brain (congenital) Q04.9
    acquired G93.89
    reduction Q04.3
  breast (acquired) N64.89
    congenital Q83.9
    reconstructed N65.0
  bronchus (congenital) Q32.4
    acquired NEC J98.09
  bursa, congenital Q79.9
  canaliculi (lacrimalis) (acquired) — *see also*
    Disorder, lacrimal system, changes
    congenital Q10.6
  canthus, acquired — *see* Disorder, eyelid,
    specified type NEC

Deformity - *continued*
  capillary (acquired) I78.8
  cardiovascular system, congenital Q28.9
  caruncle, lacrimal (acquired) — *see also*
    Disorder, lacrimal system, changes
    congenital Q10.6
  cascade, stomach K31.2
  cecum (congenital) Q43.9
    acquired K63.89
  cerebral, acquired G93.89
    congenital Q04.9
  cervix (uterus) (acquired) NEC N88.8
    congenital Q51.9
  cheek (acquired) M95.2
    congenital Q18.9
  chest (acquired) (wall) M95.4
    congenital Q67.8
    sequelae (late effect) of rickets E64.3
  chin (acquired) M95.2
    congenital Q18.9
  choroid (congenital) Q14.3
    acquired H31.8
    plexus Q07.8
      acquired G96.19
  cicatricial — *see* Cicatrix
  cilia, acquired — *see* Disorder, eyelid,
    specified type NEC
  clavicle (acquired) M95.8
    congenital Q68.8
  clitoris (congenital) Q52.6
    acquired N90.89
  clubfoot — *see* Clubfoot
  coccyx (acquired) — *see* subcategory M43.8
  colon (congenital) Q43.9
    acquired K63.89
  concha (ear) , congenital — *see also*
    Malformation, ear, external
    acquired — *see* Disorder, pinna, deformity
  cornea (acquired) H18.70
    congenital Q13.4
    descemetocele — *see* Descemetocele
    ectasia — *see* Ectasia, cornea
    specified NEC H18.79-
    staphyloma — *see* Staphyloma, cornea
  coronary artery (acquired) I25.9
    congenital Q24.5
  cranium (acquired) — *see* Deformity, skull
  cricoid cartilage (congenital) Q31.8
    acquired J38.7
  cystic duct (congenital) Q44.5
    acquired K82.8
  Dandy-Walker Q03.1
    with spina bifida — *see* Spina bifida
  diaphragm (congenital) Q79.1
    acquired J98.6
  digestive organ NOS Q45.9
  ductus arteriosus Q25.0
  duodenal bulb K31.89
  duodenum (congenital) Q43.9
    acquired K31.89
  dura — *see* Deformity, meninges
  ear (acquired) — *see also* Disorder, pinna,
    deformity
    congenital (external) Q17.9
      internal Q16.5
      middle Q16.4
        ossicles Q16.3
      ossicles Q16.3
  ectodermal (congenital) NEC Q84.9
  ejaculatory duct (congenital) Q55.4
    acquired N50.89
  elbow (joint) (acquired) — *see also*
    Deformity, limb, upper arm
    congenital Q68.8
    contraction — *see* Contraction, joint,
      elbow
  endocrine gland NEC Q89.2
  epididymis (congenital) Q55.4
    acquired N50.89
  epiglottis (congenital) Q31.8
    acquired J38.7
  esophagus (congenital) Q39.9
    acquired K22.8
  eustachian tube (congenital) NEC Q17.8
  eye, congenital Q15.9

Deformity - *continued*
  eyebrow (congenital) Q18.8
  eyelid (acquired) — *see also* Disorder,
      eyelid, specified type NEC
    congenital Q10.3
  face (acquired) M95.2
    congenital Q18.9
  fallopian tube, acquired N83.8
  femur (acquired) — *see* Deformity, limb,
      specified type NEC, thigh
  fetal
    with fetopelvic disproportion O33.7
    causing obstructed labor O66.3
  finger (acquired) M20.00-
    boutonniere M20.02-
    congenital Q68.1
    flexion contracture — *see* Contraction,
        joint, hand
    mallet finger M20.01-
    specified NEC M20.09-
    swan-neck M20.03-
  flexion (joint) (acquired) — *see also*
      Deformity, limb, flexion M21.20
    congenital NOS Q74.9
      hip Q65.89
  foot (acquired) — *see also* Deformity, limb,
      lower leg
    cavovarus (congenital) Q66.1-
    congenital NOS Q66.9-
      specified type NEC Q66.89
    specified type NEC — *see* Deformity,
        limb, foot, specified NEC
    valgus (congenital) Q66.6
      acquired — *see* Deformity, valgus, ankle
    varus (congenital) NEC Q66.3-
      acquired — *see* Deformity, varus, ankle
  forearm (acquired) — *see also* Deformity,
      limb, forearm
    congenital Q68.8
  forehead (acquired) M95.2
    congenital Q75.8
  frontal bone (acquired) M95.2
    congenital Q75.8
  gallbladder (congenital) Q44.1
    acquired K82.8
  gastrointestinal tract (congenital) NOS Q45.9
    acquired K63.89
  genitalia, genital organ (s) or system NEC
    female (congenital) Q52.9
      acquired N94.89
      external Q52.70
    male (congenital) Q55.9
      acquired N50.89
  globe (eye) (congenital) Q15.8
    acquired H44.89
  gum, acquired NEC K06.8
  hand (acquired) — *see* Deformity, limb, hand
    congenital Q68.1
  head (acquired) M95.2
    congenital Q75.8
  heart (congenital) Q24.9
    septum Q21.9
      auricular Q21.1
      ventricular Q21.0
    valve (congenital) NEC Q24.8
      acquired — *see* Endocarditis
  heel (acquired) — *see* Deformity, foot
  hepatic duct (congenital) Q44.5
    acquired K83.8
  hip (joint) (acquired) — *see also* Deformity,
      limb, thigh
    congenital Q65.9
    due to (previous) juvenile
        osteochondrosis — *see* Coxa, plana
    flexion — *see* Contraction, joint, hip
  hourglass — *see* Contraction, hourglass
  humerus (acquired) M21.82-
    congenital Q74.0
  hypophyseal (congenital) Q89.2
  ileocecal (coil) (valve) (acquired) K63.89
    congenital Q43.9
  ileum (congenital) Q43.9
    acquired K63.89
  ilium (acquired) M95.5
    congenital Q74.2

Deformity - *continued*
  integument (congenital) Q84.9
  intervertebral cartilage or disc (acquired) —
      see Disorder, disc, specified NEC
  intestine (large) (small) (congenital)
      NOS Q43.9
    acquired K63.89
  intrinsic minus or plus (hand) — *see*
      Deformity, limb, specified type NEC,
      forearm
  iris (acquired) H21.89
    congenital Q13.2
  ischium (acquired) M95.5
    congenital Q74.2
  jaw (acquired) (congenital) M26.9
  joint (acquired) NEC M21.90
    congenital Q68.8
    elbow M21.92-
    hand M21.94-
    hip M21.95-
    knee M21.96-
    shoulder M21.92-
    wrist M21.93-
  kidney (s) (calyx) (pelvis) (congenital) Q63.9
    acquired N28.89
    artery (congenital) Q27.2
      acquired I77.89
  Klippel-Feil (brevicollis) Q76.1
  knee (acquired) NEC — *see also* Deformity,
      limb, lower leg
    congenital Q68.2
  labium (majus) (minus) (congenital) Q52.79
    acquired N90.89
  lacrimal passages or duct (congenital)
      NEC Q10.6
    acquired — *see* Disorder, lacrimal system,
        changes
  larynx (muscle) (congenital) Q31.8
    acquired J38.7
    web (glottic) Q31.0
  leg (upper) (acquired) NEC — *see also*
      Deformity, limb, thigh
    congenital Q68.8
    lower leg — *see* Deformity, limb, lower
        leg
  lens (acquired) H27.8
    congenital Q12.9
  lid (fold) (acquired) — *see also* Disorder,
      eyelid, specified type NEC
    congenital Q10.3
  ligament (acquired) — *see* Disorder,
      ligament
    congenital Q79.9
  limb (acquired) M21.90
    clawfoot M21.53-
    clawhand M21.51-
    clubfoot M21.54-
    clubhand M21.52-
    congenital, except reduction
        deformity Q74.9
    flat foot M21.4-
    flexion M21.20
      ankle M21.27-
      elbow M21.22-
      finger M21.24-
      hip M21.25-
      knee M21.26-
      shoulder M21.21-
      toe M21.27-
      wrist M21.23-
    foot
      claw — *see* Deformity, limb, clawfoot
      club — *see* Deformity, limb, clubfoot
      drop M21.37-
      flat — *see* Deformity, limb, flat foot
      specified NEC M21.6X-
    forearm M21.93-
    hand M21.94-
    lower leg M21.96-
    specified type NEC M21.80
      forearm M21.83-
      lower leg M21.86-
      thigh M21.85-
      upper arm M21.82-
    thigh M21.95-

Deformity - *continued*
  limb (acquired) - *continued*
    unequal length M21.70
      short site is
        femur M21.75-
        fibula M21.76-
        humerus M21.72-
        radius M21.73-
        tibia M21.76-
        ulna M21.73-
      upper arm M21.92-
    valgus — *see* Deformity, valgus
    varus — *see* Deformity, varus
    wrist drop M21.33-
  lip (acquired) NEC K13.0
    congenital Q38.0
  liver (congenital) Q44.7
    acquired K76.89
  lumbosacral (congenital) (joint)
      (region) Q76.49
    acquired — *see* subcategory M43.8
    kyphosis — *see* Kyphosis, congenital
    lordosis — *see* Lordosis, congenital
  lung (congenital) Q33.9
    acquired J98.4
  lymphatic system, congenital Q89.9
  Madelung's (radius) Q74.0
  mandible (acquired) (congenital) M26.9
  maxilla (acquired) (congenital) M26.9
  meninges or membrane (congenital) Q07.9
    cerebral Q04.8
      acquired G96.19
    spinal cord (congenital) G96.19
      acquired G96.19
  metacarpus (acquired) — *see* Deformity,
      limb, forearm
    congenital Q74.0
  metatarsus (acquired) — *see* Deformity, foot
    congenital Q66.9-
  middle ear (congenital) Q16.4
    ossicles Q16.3
  mitral (leaflets) (valve) I05.8
    parachute Q23.2
    stenosis, congenital Q23.2
  mouth (acquired) K13.79
    congenital Q38.6
  multiple, congenital NEC Q89.7
  muscle (acquired) M62.89
    congenital Q79.9
      sternocleidomastoid Q68.0
  musculoskeletal system (acquired) M95.9
    congenital Q79.9
    specified NEC M95.8
  nail (acquired) L60.8
    congenital Q84.6
  nasal — *see* Deformity, nose
  neck (acquired) M95.3
    congenital Q18.9
      sternocleidomastoid Q68.0
  nervous system (congenital) Q07.9
  nipple (congenital) Q83.9
    acquired N64.89
  nose (acquired) (cartilage) M95.0
    bone (turbinate) M95.0
    congenital Q30.9
      bent or squashed Q67.4
    saddle M95.0
      syphilitic A50.57
    septum (acquired) J34.2
      congenital Q30.8
    sinus (wall) (congenital) Q30.8
      acquired M95.0
    syphilitic (congenital) A50.57
      late A52.73
  ocular muscle (congenital) Q10.3
    acquired — *see* Strabismus, mechanical
  opticociliary vessels (congenital) Q13.2
  orbit (eye) (acquired) H05.30
    atrophy — *see* Atrophy, orbit
    congenital Q10.7
    due to
      bone disease NEC H05.32-
      trauma or surgery H05.33-
    enlargement — *see* Enlargement, orbit
    exostosis — *see* Exostosis, orbit

Deformity - *continued*
  organ of Corti (congenital) Q16.5
  ovary (congenital) Q50.39
    acquired N83.8
  oviduct, acquired N83.8
  palate (congenital) Q38.5
    acquired M27.8
    cleft (congenital) — *see* Cleft, palate
  pancreas (congenital) Q45.3
    acquired K86.89
  parathyroid (gland) Q89.2
  parotid (gland) (congenital) Q38.4
    acquired K11.8
  patella (acquired) — *see* Disorder, patella,
    specified NEC
  pelvis, pelvic (acquired) (bony) M95.5
    with disproportion (fetopelvic) O33.0
      causing obstructed labor O65.0
    congenital Q74.2
    rachitic sequelae (late effect) E64.3
  penis (glans) (congenital) Q55.69
    acquired N48.89
  pericardium (congenital) Q24.8
    acquired — *see* Pericarditis
  pharynx (congenital) Q38.8
    acquired J39.2
  pinna, acquired — *see also* Disorder, pinna,
    deformity
    congenital Q17.9
  pituitary (congenital) Q89.2
  posture — *see* Dorsopathy, deforming
  prepuce (congenital) Q55.69
    acquired N47.8
  prostate (congenital) Q55.4
    acquired N42.89
  pupil (congenital) Q13.2
    acquired — *see* Abnormality, pupillary
  pylorus (congenital) Q40.3
    acquired K31.89
  rachitic (acquired) , old or healed E64.3
  radius (acquired) — *see also* Deformity,
    limb, forearm
    congenital Q68.8
  rectum (congenital) Q43.9
    acquired K62.89
  reduction (extremity) (limb) , congenital —
      see also condition and site Q73.8
    brain Q04.3
    lower — *see* Defect, reduction, lower limb
    upper — *see* Defect, reduction, upper limb
  renal — *see* Deformity, kidney
  respiratory system (congenital) Q34.9
  rib (acquired) M95.4
    congenital Q76.6
      cervical Q76.5
  rotation (joint) (acquired) — *see* Deformity,
      limb, specified site NEC
    congenital Q74.9
    hip — *see* Deformity, limb, specified type
      NEC, thigh
    congenital Q65.89
  sacroiliac joint (congenital) Q74.2
    acquired — *see* subcategory M43.8
  sacrum (acquired) — *see* subcategory M43.8
  saddle
    back — *see* Lordosis
    nose M95.0
      syphilitic A50.57
  salivary gland or duct (congenital) Q38.4
    acquired K11.8
  scapula (acquired) M95.8
    congenital Q68.8
  scrotum (congenital) — *see also*
      Malformation, testis and scrotum
    acquired N50.89
  seminal vesicles (congenital) Q55.4
    acquired N50.89
  septum, nasal (acquired) J34.2
  shoulder (joint) (acquired) — *see* Deformity,
      limb, upper arm
    congenital Q74.0
    contraction — *see* Contraction, joint,
      shoulder
  sigmoid (flexure) (congenital) Q43.9
    acquired K63.89

Deformity - *continued*
  skin (congenital) Q82.9
  skull (acquired) M95.2
    congenital Q75.8
      with
        anencephaly Q00.0
        encephalocele — *see* Encephalocele
        hydrocephalus Q03.9
          with spina bifida — *see* Spina
            bifida, by site, with
            hydrocephalus
        microcephaly Q02
  soft parts, organs or tissues (of pelvis)
    in pregnancy or childbirth NEC O34.8-
      causing obstructed labor O65.5
  spermatic cord (congenital) Q55.4
    acquired N50.89
    torsion — *see* Torsion, spermatic cord
  spinal — *see* Dorsopathy, deforming
    column (acquired) — *see* Dorsopathy,
      deforming
    congenital Q67.5
    cord (congenital) Q06.9
      acquired G95.89
    nerve root (congenital) Q07.9
  spine (acquired) — *see also* Dorsopathy,
      deforming
    congenital Q67.5
    rachitic E64.3
    specified NEC — *see* Dorsopathy,
      deforming, specified NEC
  spleen
    acquired D73.89
    congenital Q89.09
  Sprengel's (congenital) Q74.0
  sternocleidomastoid (muscle) ,
      congenital Q68.0
  sternum (acquired) M95.4
    congenital NEC Q76.7
  stomach (congenital) Q40.3
    acquired K31.89
  submandibular gland (congenital) Q38.4
  submaxillary gland (congenital) Q38.4
    acquired K11.8
  talipes — *see* Talipes
  testis (congenital) — *see also* Malformation,
      testis and scrotum
    acquired N44.8
    torsion — *see* Torsion, testis
  thigh (acquired) — *see also* Deformity, limb,
      thigh
    congenital NEC Q68.8
  thorax (acquired) (wall) M95.4
    congenital Q67.8
    sequelae of rickets E64.3
  thumb (acquired) — *see also* Deformity,
      finger
    congenital NEC Q68.1
  thymus (tissue) (congenital) Q89.2
  thyroid (gland) (congenital) Q89.2
    cartilage Q31.8
      acquired J38.7
  tibia (acquired) — *see also* Deformity, limb,
      specified type NEC, lower leg
    congenital NEC Q68.8
    saber (syphilitic) A50.56
  toe (acquired) M20.6-
    congenital Q66.9-
    hallux rigidus M20.2-
    hallux valgus M20.1-
    hallux varus M20.3-
    hammer toe M20.4-
    specified NEC M20.5X-
  tongue (congenital) Q38.3
    acquired K14.8
  tooth, teeth K00.2
  trachea (rings) (congenital) Q32.1
    acquired J39.8
  transverse aortic arch (congenital) Q25.49
  tricuspid (leaflets) (valve) I07.8
    atresia or stenosis Q22.4
    Ebstein's Q22.5
  trunk (acquired) M95.8
    congenital Q89.9

Deformity - *continued*
  ulna (acquired) — *see also* Deformity, limb,
      forearm
    congenital NEC Q68.8
  urachus, congenital Q64.4
  ureter (opening) (congenital) Q62.8
    acquired N28.89
  urethra (congenital) Q64.79
    acquired N36.8
  urinary tract (congenital) Q64.9
    urachus Q64.4
  uterus (congenital) Q51.9
    acquired N85.8
  uvula (congenital) Q38.5
  vagina (acquired) N89.8
    congenital Q52.4
  valgus NEC M21.00
    ankle M21.07-
    elbow M21.02-
    hip M21.05-
    knee M21.06-
  valve, valvular (congenital) (heart) Q24.8
    acquired — *see* Endocarditis
  varus NEC M21.10
    ankle M21.17-
    elbow M21.12-
    hip M21.15
    knee M21.16-
    tibia — *see* Osteochondrosis, juvenile,
      tibia
  vas deferens (congenital) Q55.4
    acquired N50.89
  vein (congenital) Q27.9
    great Q26.9
  vertebra — *see* Dorsopathy, deforming
  vertical talus (congenital) Q66.80
    left foot Q66.82
    right foot Q66.81
  vesicourethral orifice (acquired) N32.89
    congenital NEC Q64.79
  vessels of optic papilla (congenital) Q14.2
  visual field (contraction) — *see* Defect,
      visual field
  vitreous body, acquired H43.89
  vulva (congenital) Q52.79
    acquired N90.89
  wrist (joint) (acquired) — *see also*
      Deformity, limb, forearm
    congenital Q68.8
    contraction — *see* Contraction, joint, wrist
Degeneration, degenerative
  adrenal (capsule) (fatty) (gland) (hyaline)
      (infectional) E27.8
  amyloid — *see also* Amyloidosis E85.9
  anterior cornua, spinal cord G12.29
  anterior labral S43.49-
  aorta, aortic I70.0
    fatty I77.89
  aortic valve (heart) — *see* Endocarditis,
      aortic
  arteriovascular — *see* Arteriosclerosis
  artery, arterial (atheromatous)
      (calcareous) — *see also* Arteriosclerosis
    cerebral, amyloid E85.4 *[I68.0]*
    medial — *see* Arteriosclerosis, extremities
  articular cartilage NEC — *see* Derangement,
      joint, articular cartilage, by site
  atheromatous — *see* Arteriosclerosis
  basal nuclei or ganglia G23.9
    specified NEC G23.8
  bone NEC — *see* Disorder, bone, specified
      type NEC
  brachial plexus G54.0
  brain (cortical) (progressive) G31.9
    alcoholic G31.2
    arteriosclerotic I67.2
    childhood G31.9
      specified NEC G31.89
    cystic G31.89
      congenital Q04.6
    in
      alcoholism G31.2
      beriberi E51.2
      cerebrovascular disease I67.9
      congenital hydrocephalus Q03.9

Degeneration, degenerative - *continued*
  brain (cortical) (progressive) - *continued*
    in - *continued*
      congenital hydrocephalus - *continued*
        with spina bifida — *see also* Spina
            bifida
      Fabry-Anderson disease E75.21
      Gaucher's disease E75.22
      Hunter's syndrome E76.1
      lipidosis
        cerebral E75.4
        generalized E75.6
      mucopolysaccharidosis — *see*
          Mucopolysaccharidosis
      myxedema E03.9 *[G32.89]*
      neoplastic disease — *see also*
          Neoplasm D49.6 *[G32.89]*
      Niemann-Pick disease E75.249
          [G32.89]
      sphingolipidosis E75.3 *[G32.89]*
      vitamin B12 deficiency E53.8 *[G32.89]*
    senile NEC G31.1
  breast N64.89
  Bruch's membrane — *see* Degeneration,
      choroid
  capillaries (fatty) I78.8
    amyloid E85.89 *[I79.8]*
  cardiac — *see also* Degeneration, myocardial
    valve, valvular — *see* Endocarditis
  cardiorenal — *see* Hypertension, cardiorenal
  cardiovascular — *see also* Disease,
      cardiovascular
    renal — *see* Hypertension, cardiorenal
  cerebellar NOS G31.9
    alcoholic G31.2
    primary (hereditary) (sporadic) G11.9
  cerebral — *see* Degeneration, brain
  cerebrovascular I67.9
    due to hypertension I67.4
  cervical plexus G54.2
  cervix N88.8
    due to radiation (intended effect) N88.8
      adverse effect or misadventure N99.89
  chamber angle H21.21-
  changes, spine or vertebra — *see*
      Spondylosis
  chorioretinal — *see also* Degeneration,
      choroid
    hereditary H31.20
  choroid (colloid) (drusen) H31.10-
    atrophy — *see* Atrophy, choroidal
    hereditary — *see* Dystrophy, choroidal,
        hereditary
  ciliary body H21.22-
  cochlear — *see* subcategory H83.8
  combined (spinal cord) (subacute) E53.8
      [G32.0]
    with anemia (pernicious) D51.0 *[G32.0]*
      due to dietary vitamin B12
          deficiency D51.3 *[G32.0]*
    in (due to)
      vitamin B12 deficiency E53.8 *[G32.0]*
        anemia D51.9 *[G32.0]*
  conjunctiva H11.10
    concretions — *see* Concretion, conjunctiva
    deposits — *see* Deposit, conjunctiva
    pigmentations — *see* Pigmentation,
        conjunctiva
    pinguecula — *see* Pinguecula
    xerosis — *see* Xerosis, conjunctiva
  cornea H18.40
    calcerous H18.43
      band keratopathy H18.42-
    familial, hereditary — *see* Dystrophy,
        cornea
    hyaline (of old scars) H18.49
    keratomalacia — *see* Keratomalacia
    nodular H18.45-
    peripheral H18.46-
    senile H18.41-
    specified type NEC H18.49
  cortical (cerebellar)
      (parenchymatous) G31.89
    alcoholic G31.2
    diffuse, due to arteriopathy I67.2

Degeneration, degenerative - *continued*
  corticobasal G31.85
  cutis L98.8
    amyloid E85.4 *[L99]*
  dental pulp K04.2
  disc disease — *see* Degeneration,
      intervertebral disc NEC
  dorsolateral (spinal cord) — *see*
      Degeneration, combined
  extrapyramidal G25.9
  eye, macular — *see also* Degeneration,
      macula
    congenital or hereditary — *see* Dystrophy,
        retina
  facet joints — *see* Spondylosis
  fatty
    liver NEC K76.0
      alcoholic K70.0
  grey matter (brain) (Alpers') G31.81
  heart — *see also* Degeneration, myocardial
    amyloid E85.4 *[I43]*
    atheromatous — *see* Disease, heart,
        ischemic, atherosclerotic
    ischemic — *see* Disease, heart, ischemic
  hepatolenticular (Wilson's) E83.01
  hepatorenal K76.7
  hyaline (diffuse) (generalized)
    localized — *see* Degeneration, by site
  infrapatellar fat pad M79.4
  intervertebral disc NOS
    with
      myelopathy — *see* Disorder, disc, with,
          myelopathy
      radiculitis or radiculopathy — *see*
          Disorder, disc, with, radiculopathy
    cervical, cervicothoracic — *see* Disorder,
        disc, cervical, degeneration
      with
        myelopathy — *see* Disorder, disc,
            cervical, with myelopathy
        neuritis, radiculitis or
            radiculopathy — *see* Disorder,
            disc, cervical, with neuritis
    lumbar region M51.36
      with
        myelopathy M51.06
        neuritis, radiculitis, radiculopathy or
            sciatica M51.16
    lumbosacral region M51.37
      with
        neuritis, radiculitis, radiculopathy or
            sciatica M51.17
    sacrococcygeal region M53.3
    thoracic region M51.34
      with
        myelopathy M51.04
        neuritis, radiculitis,
            radiculopathy M51.14
    thoracolumbar region M51.35
      with
        myelopathy M51.05
        neuritis, radiculitis,
            radiculopathy M51.15
  intestine, amyloid E85.4
  iris (pigmentary) H21.23-
  ischemic — *see* Ischemia
  joint disease — *see* Osteoarthritis
  kidney N28.89
    amyloid E85.4 *[N29]*
    cystic, congenital Q61.9
    fatty N28.89
    polycystic Q61.3
      adult type (autosomal dominant) Q61.2
      infantile type (autosomal recessive)
          NEC Q61.19
        collecting duct dilatation Q61.11
  Kuhnt-Junius — *see also* Degeneration,
      macula H35.32-
  lens — *see* Cataract
  lenticular (familial) (progressive) (Wilson's)
      (with cirrhosis of liver) E83.01
  liver (diffuse) NEC K76.89
    amyloid E85.4 *[K77]*
    cystic K76.89
      congenital Q44.6

Degeneration, degenerative - *continued*
  liver (diffuse) NEC - *continued*
    fatty NEC K76.0
      alcoholic K70.0
    hypertrophic K76.89
    parenchymatous, acute or subacute K72.00
      with coma K72.01
    pigmentary K76.89
    toxic (acute) K71.9
  lung J98.4
  lymph gland I89.8
    hyaline I89.8
  macula, macular (acquired) (age-related)
      (senile) H35.30
    angioid streaks H35.33
    atrophic age-related H35.31-
    congenital or hereditary — *see* Dystrophy,
        retina
    cystoid H35.35-
    drusen H35.36-
    dry age-related H35.31-
    exudative H35.32-
    hole H35.34-
    nonexudative H35.31-
    puckering H35.37-
    toxic H35.38-
    wet age-related H35.32-
  membranous labyrinth, congenital (causing
      impairment of hearing) Q16.5
  meniscus — *see* Derangement, meniscus
  mitral — *see* Insufficiency, mitral
  Mönckeberg's — *see* Arteriosclerosis,
      extremities
  motor centers, senile G31.1
  multi-system G90.3
  mural — *see* Degeneration, myocardial
  muscle (fatty) (fibrous) (hyaline)
      (progressive) M62.89
    heart — *see* Degeneration, myocardial
  myelin, central nervous system G37.9
  myocardial, myocardium (fatty) (hyaline)
      (senile) I51.5
    with rheumatic fever (conditions in
        I00) I09.0
      active, acute or subacute I01.2
        with chorea I02.0
      inactive or quiescent (with chorea) I09.0
    hypertensive — *see* Hypertension, heart
    rheumatic — *see* Degeneration,
        myocardial, with rheumatic fever
    syphilitic A52.06
  nasal sinus (mucosa) J32.9
    frontal J32.1
    maxillary J32.0
  nerve — *see* Disorder, nerve
  nervous system G31.9
    alcoholic G31.2
    amyloid E85.4 *[G99.8]*
    autonomic G90.9
    fatty G31.89
    specified NEC G31.89
  nipple N64.89
  olivopontocerebellar (hereditary)
      (familial) G23.8
  osseous labyrinth — *see* subcategory H83.8
  ovary N83.8
    cystic N83.20-
    microcystic N83.20-
  pallidal pigmentary (progressive) G23.0
  pancreas K86.89
    tuberculous A18.83
  penis N48.89
  pigmentary (diffuse) (general)
    localized — *see* Degeneration, by site
    pallidal (progressive) G23.0
  pineal gland E34.8
  pituitary (gland) E23.6
  popliteal fat pad M79.4
  posterolateral (spinal cord) — *see*
      Degeneration, combined
  pulmonary valve (heart) I37.8
  pulp (tooth) K04.2
  pupillary margin H21.24-
  renal — *see* Degeneration, kidney
  retina H35.9

Degeneration, degenerative - *continued*
  retina - *continued*
    hereditary (cerebroretinal) (congenital)
      (juvenile) (macula) (peripheral)
      (pigmentary) — *see* Dystrophy, retina
    Kuhnt-Junius — *see also* Degeneration,
      macula H35.32-
    macula (cystic) (exudative) (hole)
      (nonexudative) (pseudohole) (senile)
      (toxic) — *see* Degeneration, macula
    peripheral H35.40
      lattice H35.41-
      microcystoid H35.42-
      paving stone H35.43-
      secondary
        pigmentary H35.45-
        vitreoretinal H35.46-
      senile reticular H35.44-
    pigmentary (primary) — *see also*
      Dystrophy, retina
      secondary — *see* Degeneration, retina,
        peripheral, secondary
    posterior pole — *see* Degeneration, macula
  saccule, congenital (causing impairment of
    hearing) Q16.5
  senile R54
    brain G31.1
    cardiac, heart or myocardium — *see*
      Degeneration, myocardial
    motor centers G31.1
    vascular — *see* Arteriosclerosis
  sinus (cystic) — *see also* Sinusitis
    polypoid J33.1
  skin L98.8
    amyloid E85.4 *[L99]*
    colloid L98.8
  spinal (cord) G31.89
    amyloid E85.4 *[G32.89]*
    combined (subacute) — *see* Degeneration,
      combined
    dorsolateral — *see* Degeneration,
      combined
    familial NEC G31.89
    fatty G31.89
    funicular — *see* Degeneration, combined
    posterolateral — *see* Degeneration,
      combined
    subacute combined — *see* Degeneration,
      combined
    tuberculous A17.81
  spleen D73.0
    amyloid E85.4 *[D77]*
  stomach K31.89
  striatonigral G23.2
  suprarenal (capsule) (gland) E27.8
  synovial membrane (pulpy) — *see* Disorder,
    synovium, specified type NEC
  tapetoretinal — *see* Dystrophy, retina
  thymus (gland) E32.8
    fatty E32.8
  thyroid (gland) E07.89
  tricuspid (heart) (valve) I07.9
  tuberculous NEC — *see* Tuberculosis
  turbinate J34.89
  uterus (cystic) N85.8
  vascular (senile) — *see* Arteriosclerosis
    hypertensive — *see* Hypertension
  vitreoretinal, secondary — *see* Degeneration,
    retina, peripheral, secondary,
    vitreoretinal
  vitreous (body) H43.81-
  Wallerian — *see* Disorder, nerve
  Wilson's hepatolenticular E83.01
Deglutition
  paralysis R13.0
    hysterical F44.4
  pneumonia J69.0
Degos' disease I77.89
Dehiscence (of)
  amputation stump T87.81
  cesarean wound O90.0
  closure of
    cornea T81.31
    craniotomy T81.32
    fascia (muscular) (superficial) T81.32

Dehiscence (of) - *continued*
  closure of - *continued*
    internal organ or tissue T81.32
    laceration (external) (internal) T81.33
    ligament T81.32
    mucosa T81.31
    muscle or muscle flap T81.32
    ribs or rib cage T81.32
    skin and subcutaneous tissue (full-
      thickness) (superficial) T81.31
    skull T81.32
    sternum (sternotomy) T81.32
    tendon T81.32
    traumatic laceration (external)
      (internal) T81.33
  episiotomy O90.1
  operation wound NEC T81.31
    external operation wound
      (superficial) T81.31
    internal operation wound (deep) T81.32
  perineal wound (postpartum) O90.1
  traumatic injury wound repair T81.33
  wound T81.30
    traumatic repair T81.33
Dehydration E86.0
  newborn P74.1
Déjérine-Roussy syndrome G89.0
Déjérine-Sottas disease or neuropathy
  (hypertrophic) G60.0
Déjérine-Thomas atrophy G23.8
Delay, delayed
  any plane in pelvis
    complicating delivery O66.9
  birth or delivery NOS O63.9
  closure, ductus arteriosus (Botalli) P29.38
  coagulation — *see* Defect, coagulation
  conduction (cardiac) (ventricular) I45.9
  delivery, second twin, triplet, etc O63.2
  development R62.50
    global F88
    intellectual (specific) F81.9
    language F80.9
      due to hearing loss F80.4
    learning F81.9
    pervasive F84.9
    physiological R62.50
      specified stage NEC R62.0
    reading F81.0
    sexual E30.0
    speech F80.9
      due to hearing loss F80.4
    spelling F81.81
  ejaculation F52.32
  gastric emptying K30
  menarche E30.0
  menstruation (cause unknown) N91.0
  milestone R62.0
  passage of meconium (newborn) P76.0
  primary respiration P28.9
  puberty (constitutional) E30.0
  separation of umbilical cord P96.82
  sexual maturation, female E30.0
  sleep phase syndrome G47.21
  union, fracture — *see* Fracture, by site
  vaccination Z28.9
Deletion (s)
  autosome Q93.9
    identified by fluorescence in situ
      hybridization (FISH) Q93.89
    identified by in situ hybridization
      (ISH) Q93.89
  chromosome
    with complex rearrangements NEC Q93.7
    part of NEC Q93.59
    seen only at prometaphase Q93.89
    short arm
      4 Q93.3
      5p Q93.4
      22q11.2 Q93.81
    specified NEC Q93.89
  long arm chromosome 18 or 21 Q93.89
    with complex rearrangements NEC Q93.7
  microdeletions NEC Q93.88
Delhi boil or button B55.1

Delinquency (juvenile) (neurotic) F91.8
  group Z72.810
Delinquent immunization status Z28.3
Delirium, delirious (acute or subacute) (not
  alcohol- or drug-induced) (with
  dementia) R41.0
  alcoholic (acute) (tremens)
    (withdrawal) F10.921
    with intoxication F10.921
      in
        abuse F10.121
        dependence F10.221
  due to (secondary to)
    alcohol
      intoxication F10.921
        in
          abuse F10.121
          dependence F10.221
      withdrawal F10.231
    amphetamine intoxication F15.921
      in
        abuse F15.121
        dependence F15.221
    anxiolytic
      intoxication F13.921
        in
          abuse F13.121
          dependence F13.221
      withdrawal F13.231
    cannabis intoxication (acute) F12.921
      in
        abuse F12.121
        dependence F12.221
    cocaine intoxication (acute) F14.921
      in
        abuse F14.121
        dependence F14.221
    general medical condition F05
    hallucinogen intoxication F16.921
      in
        abuse F16.121
        dependence F16.221
    hypnotic
      intoxication F13.921
        in
          abuse F13.121
          dependence F13.221
      withdrawal F13.231
    inhalant intoxication (acute) F18.921
      in
        abuse F18.121
        dependence F18.221
    multiple etiologies F05
    opioid intoxication (acute) F11.921
      in
        abuse F11.121
        dependence F11.221
    other (or unknown) substance F19.921
    phencyclidine intoxication (acute) F16.921
      in
        abuse F16.121
        dependence F16.221
    psychoactive substance NEC intoxication
      (acute) F19.921
      in
        abuse F19.121
        dependence F19.221
    sedative
      intoxication F13.921
        in
          abuse F13.121
          dependence F13.221
      withdrawal F13.231
    unknown etiology R41.0
  exhaustion F43.0
  hysterical F44.89
  postprocedural (postoperative) F05
  puerperal F05
  thyroid — *see* Thyrotoxicosis with thyroid
    storm
  traumatic — *see* Injury, intracranial
  tremens (alcohol-induced) F10.231
    sedative-induced F13.231
Delivery (childbirth) (labor)
  arrested active phase O62.1

Delivery (childbirth) (labor) - *continued*
  cesarean (for)
    abnormal
      pelvis (bony) (deformity) (major) NEC
        with disproportion
          (fetopelvic) O33.0
          with obstructed labor O65.0
      presentation or position O32.9
    abruptio placentae — *see also* Abruptio
      placentae O45.9-
    acromion presentation O32.2
    atony, uterus O62.2
    breech presentation O32.1
      incomplete O32.8
    brow presentation O32.3
    cephalopelvic disproportion O33.9
    cerclage O34.3-
    chin presentation O32.3
    cicatrix of cervix O34.4-
    contracted pelvis (general)
      inlet O33.2
      outlet O33.3
    cord presentation or prolapse O69.0
    cystocele O34.8-
    deformity (acquired) (congenital)
      pelvic organs or tissues NEC O34.8-
      pelvis (bony) NEC O33.0
    disproportion NOS O33.9
    eclampsia — *see* Eclampsia
    face presentation O32.3
    failed
      forceps O66.5
      induction of labor O61.9
        instrumental O61.1
        mechanical O61.1
        medical O61.0
        specified NEC O61.8
        surgical O61.1
      trial of labor NOS O66.40
        following previous cesarean
          delivery O66.41
      vacuum extraction O66.5
      ventouse O66.5
    fetal-maternal hemorrhage O43.01-
    hemorrhage (intrapartum) O67.9
      with coagulation defect O67.0
      specified cause NEC O67.8
    high head at term O32.4
    hydrocephalic fetus O33.6
    incarceration of uterus O34.51-
    incoordinate uterine action O62.4
    increased size, fetus O33.5
    inertia, uterus O62.2
      primary O62.0
      secondary O62.1
    lateroversion, uterus O34.59-
    mal lie O32.9
    malposition
      fetus O32.9
      pelvic organs or tissues NEC O34.8-
      uterus NEC O34.59-
    malpresentation NOS O32.9
    oblique presentation O32.2
    occurring after 37 completed weeks of
      gestation but before 39 completed
      weeks gestation due to (spontaneous)
      onset of labor O75.82
    oversize fetus O33.5
    pelvic tumor NEC O34.8-
    placenta previa O44.0-
      complete O44.0-
        with hemorrhage O44.1-
    placental insufficiency O36.51-
    planned, occurring after 37 completed
      weeks of gestation but before 39
      completed weeks gestation due to
      (spontaneous) onset of labor O75.82
    polyp, cervix O34.4-
      causing obstructed labor O65.5
    poor dilatation, cervix O62.0
    pre-eclampsia O14.94
      mild O14.04
      moderate O14.04
      severe O14.14

Delivery (childbirth) (labor) - *continued*
  cesarean (for) - *continued*
    pre-eclampsia - *continued*
      severe - *continued*
        with hemolysis, elevated liver
          enzymes and low platelet count
          (HELLP) O14.24
    previous
      cesarean delivery O34.219
        classical (vertical) scar O34.212
        low transverse scar O34.211
      surgery (to)
        cervix O34.4-
        gynecological NEC O34.8-
        rectum O34.7-
        uterus O34.29
        vagina O34.6-
    prolapse
      arm or hand O32.2
      uterus O34.52-
    prolonged labor NOS O63.9
    rectocele O34.8-
    retroversion
      uterus O34.53-
    rigid
      cervix O34.4-
      pelvic floor O34.8-
      perineum O34.7-
      vagina O34.6-
      vulva O34.7-
    sacculation, pregnant uterus O34.59-
    scar (s)
      cervix O34.4-
      cesarean delivery O34.219
        classical (vertical) O34.212
        low transverse O34.211
      transmural uterine O34.29
      uterus O34.29
    Shirodkar suture in situ O34.3-
    shoulder presentation O32.2
    stenosis or stricture, cervix O34.4-
    streptococcus group B (GBS) carrier
      state O99.824
    transmural uterine scar O34.29
    transverse presentation or lie O32.2
    tumor, pelvic organs or tissues
      NEC O34.8-
      cervix O34.4-
    umbilical cord presentation or
      prolapse O69.0
    without indication O82
  completely normal case O80
  complicated O75.9
    by
      abnormal, abnormality (of)
        forces of labor O62.9
          specified type NEC O62.8
        glucose O99.814
        uterine contractions NOS O62.9
      abruptio placentae — *see also* Abruptio
        placentae O45.9-
      abuse
        physical O9A.32
        psychological O9A.52
        sexual O9A.42
      adherent placenta O72.0
        without hemorrhage O73.0
      alcohol use O99.314
      anemia (pre-existing) O99.02
      anesthetic death O74.8
      annular detachment of cervix O71.3
      atony, uterus O62.2
      attempted vacuum extraction and
        forceps O66.5
      Bandl's ring O62.4
      bariatric surgery status O99.844
      biliary tract disorder O26.62
      bleeding — *see* Delivery, complicated
        by, hemorrhage
      blood disorder NEC O99.12
      cervical dystocia (hypotonic) O62.2
        primary O62.0
        secondary O62.1
      circulatory system disorder O99.42

Delivery (childbirth) (labor) - *continued*
  complicated - *continued*
    by - *continued*
      compression of cord (umbilical)
        NEC O69.2
      condition NEC O99.89
      contraction, contracted ring O62.4
      cord (umbilical)
        around neck
          with compression O69.1
          without compression O69.81
        bruising O69.5
        complication O69.9
          specified NEC O69.89
        compression NEC O69.2
        entanglement O69.2
          without compression O69.82
        hematoma O69.5
        presentation O69.0
        prolapse O69.0
        short O69.3
        thrombosis (vessels) O69.5
        vascular lesion O69.5
      Couvelaire uterus O45.8X-
      damage to (injury to) NEC
        perineum O71.82
        periurethral tissue O71.82
        vulva O71.82
      delay following rupture of membranes
        (spontaneous) — *see* Pregnancy,
        complicated by, premature rupture
        of membranes
      depressed fetal heart tones O76
      diabetes O24.92
        gestational O24.429
          diet controlled O24.420
          insulin controlled O24.424
          oral drug controlled (antidiabetic)
            (hypoglycemic) O24.425
        pre-existing O24.32
          specified NEC O24.82
          type 1 O24.02
          type 2 O24.12
      diastasis recti (abdominis) O71.89
      dilatation
        bladder O66.8
        cervix incomplete, poor or slow O62.0
      disease NEC O99.89
      disruptio uteri — *see* Delivery,
        complicated by, rupture, uterus
      drug use O99.324
      dysfunction, uterus NOS O62.9
        hypertonic O62.4
        hypotonic O62.2
          primary O62.0
          secondary O62.1
        incoordinate O62.4
      eclampsia O15.1
      embolism (pulmonary) — *see*
        Embolism, obstetric
      endocrine, nutritional or metabolic
        disease NEC O99.284
      failed
        attempted vaginal birth after previous
          cesarean delivery O66.41
        induction of labor O61.9
          instrumental O61.1
          mechanical O61.1
          medical O61.0
          specified NEC O61.8
          surgical O61.1
        trial of labor O66.40
      female genital mutilation O65.5
      fetal
        abnormal acid-base balance O68
        acidemia O68
        acidosis O68
        alkalosis O68
        death, early O02.1
        deformity O66.3
        heart rate or rhythm (abnormal) (non-
          reassuring) O76
        hypoxia O77.8
        stress O77.9
          due to drug administration O77.1

Delivery (childbirth) (labor) - *continued*
complicated - *continued*
  by - *continued*
    fetal - *continued*
      stress - *continued*
        electrocardiographic evidence of O77.8
        specified NEC O77.8
        ultrasound evidence of O77.8
    fever during labor O75.2
    gastric banding status O99.844
    gastric bypass status O99.844
    gastrointestinal disease NEC O99.62
    gestational
      diabetes O24.429
        diet controlled O24.420
        insulin (and diet) controlled O24.424
        oral drug controlled (antidiabetic) (hypoglycemic) O24.425
      edema O12.04
        with proteinuria O12.24
      proteinuria O12.14
    gonorrhea O98.22
    hematoma O71.7
      ischial spine O71.7
      pelvic O71.7
      vagina O71.7
      vulva or perineum O71.7
    hemorrhage (uterine) O67.9
      associated with
        afibrinogenemia O67.0
        coagulation defect O67.0
        hyperfibrinolysis O67.0
        hypofibrinogenemia O67.0
      due to
        low implantation of placenta O44.5-
        low lying placenta O44.5-
        placenta previa O44.1-
          marginal O44.3-
          partial O44.3-
        premature separation of placenta (normally implanted) — *see also* Abruptio placentae O45.9-
        retained placenta O72.0
        uterine leiomyoma O67.8
      placenta NEC O67.8
      postpartum NEC (atonic) (immediate) O72.1
        with retained or trapped placenta O72.0
        delayed O72.2
        secondary O72.2
        third stage O72.0
    hourglass contraction, uterus O62.4
    hypertension, hypertensive (pre-existing) — *see* Hypertension, complicated by, childbirth (labor)
    hypotension O26.5-
    incomplete dilatation (cervix) O62.0
    incoordinate uterus contractions O62.4
    inertia, uterus O62.2
      during latent phase of labor O62.0
      primary O62.0
      secondary O62.1
    infection (maternal) O98.92
      carrier state NEC O99.834
      gonorrhea O98.22
      human immunodeficiency virus (HIV) O98.72
      sexually transmitted NEC O98.32
      specified NEC O98.82
      syphilis O98.12
      tuberculosis O98.02
      viral hepatitis O98.42
      viral NEC O98.52
    injury (to mother) — *see also* Delivery, complicated, by, damage to O71.9
    intrauterine fetal death, early O02.1
    inversion, uterus O71.2
    laceration (perineal) O70.9
      anus (sphincter) O70.4

laceration (perineal) - *continued*
  anus (sphincter) - *continued*
    with third degree laceration — *see also* Delivery, complicated, by, laceration, perineum, third degree O70.20
      with mucosa O70.3
      without third degree laceration O70.4
  bladder (urinary) O71.5
  bowel O71.5
  cervix (uteri) O71.3
  fourchette O70.0
  hymen O70.0
  labia O70.0
  pelvic
    floor O70.1
    organ NEC O71.5
  perineum, perineal O70.9
    first degree O70.0
    fourth degree O70.3
    muscles O70.1
    second degree O70.1
    skin O70.0
    slight O70.0
    third degree O70.20
      with
        both external anal sphincter (EAS) and internal anal sphincter (IAS) torn (IIIc) O70.23
        less than 50% of external anal sphincter (EAS) thickness torn (IIIa) O70.21
        more than 50% external anal sphincter (EAS) thickness torn (IIIb) O70.22
      IIIa O70.21
      IIIb O70.22
      IIIc O70.23
  peritoneum (pelvic) O71.5
  rectovaginal (septum) (without perineal laceration) O71.4
    with perineum — *see also* Delivery, complicated, by, laceration, perineum, third degree O70.20
      with anal or rectal mucosa O70.3
    specified NEC O71.89
  sphincter ani — *see* Delivery, complicated, by, laceration, anus (sphincter)
  urethra O71.5
  uterus O71.81
    before labor O71.81
  vagina, vaginal (deep) (high) (without perineal laceration) O71.4
    with perineum O70.0
    muscles, with perineum O70.1
  vulva O70.0
liver disorder O26.62
malignancy O9A.12
malnutrition O25.2
malposition, malpresentation
  placenta O44.0-
    with hemorrhage O44.1-
  uterus or cervix O65.5
  without obstruction — *see also* Delivery, complicated by, obstruction O32.9
    breech O32.1
    compound O32.6
    face (brow) (chin) O32.3
    footling O32.8
    high head O32.4
    oblique O32.2
    specified NEC O32.8
    transverse O32.2
    unstable lie O32.0
meconium in amniotic fluid O77.0
mental disorder NEC O99.344
metrorrhexis — *see* Delivery, complicated by, rupture, uterus

nervous system disorder O99.354
obesity (pre-existing) O99.214
obesity surgery status O99.844
obstetric trauma O71.9
  specified NEC O71.89
obstructed labor
  due to
    breech (complete) (frank) presentation O64.1
      incomplete O64.8
    brow presentation O64.3
    buttock presentation O64.1
    chin presentation O64.2
    compound presentation O64.5
    contracted pelvis O65.1
    deep transverse arrest O64.0
    deformed pelvis O65.0
    dystocia (fetal) O66.9
      due to
        conjoined twins O66.3
        fetal
          abnormality NEC O66.3
          ascites O66.3
          hydrops O66.3
          meningomyelocele O66.3
          sacral teratoma O66.3
          tumor O66.3
        hydrocephalic fetus O66.3
        shoulder O66.0
    face presentation O64.2
    fetopelvic disproportion O65.4
    footling presentation O64.8
    impacted shoulders O66.0
    incomplete rotation of fetal head O64.0
    large fetus O66.2
    locked twins O66.1
    malposition O64.9
      specified NEC O64.8
    malpresentation O64.9
      specified NEC O64.8
    multiple fetuses NEC O66.6
    pelvic
      abnormality (maternal) O65.9
        organ O65.5
        specified NEC O65.8
      contraction
        inlet O65.2
        mid-cavity O65.3
        outlet O65.3
    persistent (position)
      occipitoiliac O64.0
      occipitoposterior O64.0
      occipitosacral O64.0
      occipitotransverse O64.0
    prolapsed arm O64.4
    shoulder presentation O64.4
    specified NEC O66.8
pathological retraction ring, uterus O62.4
penetration, pregnant uterus by instrument O71.1
perforation — *see* Delivery, complicated by, laceration
placenta, placental
  ablatio — *see also* Abruptio placentae O45.9-
  abnormality O43.9-
    specified NEC O43.89-
  abruptio — *see also* Abruptio placentae O45.9-
  accreta O43.21-
  adherent (with hemorrhage) O72.0
    without hemorrhage O73.0
  detachment (premature) — *see also* Abruptio placentae O45.9-
  disorder O43.9-
    specified NEC O43.89-
  hemorrhage NEC O67.8
  increta O43.22-
  low (implantation) (lying) O44.4-
    with hemorrhage O44.5-

Delivery (childbirth) (labor) - *continued*
complicated - *continued*
by - *continued*
placenta, placental - *continued*
malformation O43.10-
malposition O44.0-
without hemorrhage O44.1-
percreta O43.23-
previa (central) (complete) (lateral) (total) O44.0-
with hemorrhage O44.1-
marginal O44.2-
with hemorrhage O44.3-
partial O44.2-
with hemorrhage O44.3-
retained (with hemorrhage) O72.0
without hemorrhage O73.0
separation (premature) O45.9-
specified NEC O45.8X-
vicious insertion O44.1-
precipitate labor O62.3
premature rupture, membranes — *see also* Pregnancy, complicated by, premature rupture of membranes O42.90
prolapse
arm or hand O32.2
cord (umbilical) O69.0
foot or leg O32.8
uterus O34.52-
prolonged labor O63.9
first stage O63.0
second stage O63.1
protozoal disease (maternal) O98.62
respiratory disease NEC O99.52
retained membranes or portions of placenta O72.2
without hemorrhage O73.1
retarded birth O63.9
retention of secundines (with hemorrhage) O72.0
without hemorrhage O73.0
partial O72.2
without hemorrhage O73.1
rupture
bladder (urinary) O71.5
cervix O71.3
pelvic organ NEC O71.5
urethra O71.5
uterus (during or after labor) O71.1
before labor O71.0-
separation, pubic bone (symphysis pubis) O71.6
shock O75.1
shoulder presentation O64.4
skin disorder NEC O99.72
spasm, cervix O62.4
stenosis or stricture, cervix O65.5
streptococcus group B (GBS) carrier state O99.824
subluxation of symphysis (pubis) O26.72
syphilis (maternal) O98.12
tear — *see* Delivery, complicated by, laceration
tetanic uterus O62.4
trauma (obstetrical) — *see also* Delivery, complicated, by, damage to O71.9
non-obstetric O9A.22
periurethral O71.82
specified NEC O71.89
tuberculosis (maternal) O98.02
tumor, pelvic organs or tissues NEC O65.5
umbilical cord around neck
with compression O69.1
without compression O69.81
uterine inertia O62.2
during latent phase of labor O62.0
primary O62.0
secondary O62.1
vasa previa O69.4
velamentous insertion of cord O43.12-
specified complication NEC O75.89
delayed NOS O63.9

Delivery (childbirth) (labor) - *continued*
delayed NOS - *continued*
following rupture of membranes
artificial O75.5
second twin, triplet, etc. O63.2
forceps, low following failed vacuum extraction O66.5
missed (at or near term) O36.4
normal O80
obstructed — *see* Delivery, complicated by, obstructed labor
precipitate O62.3
preterm — *see also* Pregnancy, complicated by, preterm labor O60.10
spontaneous O80
term pregnancy NOS O80
uncomplicated O80
vaginal, following previous cesarean delivery O34.219
classical (vertical) scar O34.212
low transverse scar O34.211
Delusions (paranoid) — *see* Disorder, delusional
Dementia (degenerative (primary)) (old age) (persisting) F03.90
with
aggressive behavior F03.91
behavioral disturbance F03.91
combative behavior F03.91
Lewy bodies G31.83 *[F02.80]*
with behavioral disturbance G31.83 *[F02.81]*
Parkinsonism G31.83 *[F02.80]*
with behavioral disturbance G31.83 *[F02.81]*
Parkinson's disease G20 *[F02.80]*
with behavioral disturbance G20 *[F02.81]*
violent behavior F03.91
alcoholic F10.97
with dependence F10.27
Alzheimer's type — *see* Disease, Alzheimer's
arteriosclerotic — *see* Dementia, vascular
atypical, Alzheimer's type — *see* Disease, Alzheimer's, specified NEC
congenital — *see* Disability, intellectual
frontal (lobe) G31.09 *[F02.80]*
with behavioral disturbance G31.09 *[F02.81]*
frontotemporal G31.09 *[F02.80]*
with behavioral disturbance G31.09 *[F02.81]*
specified NEC G31.09 *[F02.80]*
with behavioral disturbance G31.09 *[F02.81]*
in (due to)
alcohol F10.97
with dependence F10.27
Alzheimer's disease — *see* Disease, Alzheimer's
arteriosclerotic brain disease — *see* Dementia, vascular
cerebral lipidoses E75.- *[F02.80]*
with behavioral disturbance E75.- *[F02.81]*
Creutzfeldt-Jakob disease — *see also* Creutzfeldt-Jakob disease or syndrome (with dementia) A81.00
epilepsy G40.- *[F02.80]*
with behavioral disturbance G40.- *[F02.81]*
hepatolenticular degeneration E83.01 *[F02.80]*
with behavioral disturbance E83.01 *[F02.81]*
human immunodeficiency virus (HIV) disease B20 *[F02.80]*
with behavioral disturbance B20 *[F02.81]*
Huntington's disease or chorea G10 *[F02.80]*
with behavioral disturbance G10 *[F02.81]*
hypercalcemia E83.52 *[F02.80]*

Dementia (degenerative (primary)) (old age) (persisting) - *continued*
in (due to) - *continued*
hypercalcemia - *continued*
with behavioral disturbance E83.52 *[F02.81]*
hypothyroidism, acquired E03.9 *[F02.80]*
with behavioral disturbance E03.9 *[F02.81]*
due to iodine deficiency E01.8 *[F02.80]*
with behavioral disturbance E01.8 *[F02.81]*
inhalants F18.97
with dependence F18.27
multiple
etiologies F03
sclerosis G35 *[F02.80]*
with behavioral disturbance G35 *[F02.81]*
neurosyphilis A52.17 *[F02.80]*
with behavioral disturbance A52.17 *[F02.81]*
juvenile A50.49 *[F02.80]*
with behavioral disturbance A50.49 *[F02.81]*
niacin deficiency E52 *[F02.80]*
with behavioral disturbance E52 *[F02.81]*
paralysis agitans G20 *[F02.80]*
with behavioral disturbance G20 *[F02.81]*
Parkinson's disease G20 *[F02.80]*
pellagra E52 *[F02.80]*
with behavioral disturbance E52 *[F02.81]*
Pick's G31.01 *[F02.80]*
with behavioral disturbance G31.01 *[F02.81]*
polyarteritis nodosa M30.0 *[F02.80]*
with behavioral disturbance M30.0 *[F02.81]*
psychoactive drug F19.97
with dependence F19.27
inhalants F18.97
with dependence F18.27
sedatives, hypnotics or anxiolytics F13.97
with dependence F13.27
sedatives, hypnotics or anxiolytics F13.97
with dependence F13.27
systemic lupus erythematosus M32.- *[F02.80]*
with behavioral disturbance M32.- *[F02.81]*
trypanosomiasis
African B56.9 *[F02.80]*
with behavioral disturbance B56.9 *[F02.81]*
unknown etiology F03
vitamin B12 deficiency E53.8 *[F02.80]*
with behavioral disturbance E53.8 *[F02.81]*
volatile solvents F18.97
with dependence F18.27
with behavioral disturbance G31.83 *[F02.81]*
infantile, infantilis F84.3
Lewy body G31.83 *[F02.80]*
with behavioral disturbance G31.83 *[F02.81]*
multi-infarct — *see* Dementia, vascular
paralytica, paralytic (syphilitic) A52.17 *[F02.80]*
with behavioral disturbance A52.17 *[F02.81]*
juvenilis A50.45
paretic A52.17
praecox — *see* Schizophrenia
presenile F03
Alzheimer's type — *see* Disease, Alzheimer's, early onset
primary degenerative F03
progressive, syphilitic A52.17
senile F03
with acute confusional state F05

Dementia (degenerative (primary)) (old age) (persisting) - *continued*
  senile - *continued*
    Alzheimer's type — *see* Disease, Alzheimer's, late onset
    depressed or paranoid type F03
    vascular (acute onset) (mixed) (multi-infarct) (subcortical) F01.50
      with behavioral disturbance F01.51
Demineralization, bone — *see* Osteoporosis
Demodex folliculorum (infestation) B88.0
Demophobia F40.248
Demoralization R45.3
Demyelination, demyelinization
  central nervous system G37.9
    specified NEC G37.8
  corpus callosum (central) G37.1
  disseminated, acute G36.9
    specified NEC G36.8
  global G35
  in optic neuritis G36.0
Dengue (classical) (fever) A90
  hemorrhagic A91
  sandfly A93.1
Dennie-Marfan syphilitic syndrome A50.45
Dens evaginatus, in dente or invaginatus K00.2
Dense breasts R92.2
Density
  increased, bone (disseminated) (generalized) (spotted) — *see* Disorder, bone, density and structure, specified type NEC
  lung (nodular) J98.4
Dental — *see also* condition
  examination Z01.20
    with abnormal findings Z01.21
  restoration
    aesthetically inadequate or displeasing K08.56
    defective K08.50
      specified NEC K08.59
    failure of marginal integrity K08.51
    failure of periodontal anatomical integrity K08.54
Dentia praecox K00.6
Denticles (pulp) K04.2
Dentigerous cyst K09.0
Dentin
  irregular (in pulp) K04.3
  opalescent K00.5
  secondary (in pulp) K04.3
  sensitive K03.89
Dentinogenesis imperfecta K00.5
Dentinoma — *see* Cyst, calcifying odontogenic
Dentition (syndrome) K00.7
  delayed K00.6
  difficult K00.7
  precocious K00.6
  premature K00.6
  retarded K00.6
Dependence (on) (syndrome) F19.20
  with remission F19.21
  alcohol (ethyl) (methyl) (without remission) F10.20
    with
      amnestic disorder, persisting F10.26
      anxiety disorder F10.280
      dementia, persisting F10.27
      intoxication F10.229
        with delirium F10.221
        uncomplicated F10.220
      mood disorder F10.24
      psychotic disorder F10.259
        with
          delusions F10.250
          hallucinations F10.251
      remission F10.21
      sexual dysfunction F10.281
      sleep disorder F10.282
      specified disorder NEC F10.288
      withdrawal F10.239
        with
          delirium F10.231
          perceptual disturbance F10.232

Dependence (on) (syndrome) - *continued*
  alcohol (ethyl) (methyl) (without remission) - *continued*
    with - *continued*
      withdrawal - *continued*
        uncomplicated F10.230
      counseling and surveillance Z71.41
  amobarbital — *see* Dependence, drug, sedative
  amphetamine (s) (type) — *see* Dependence, drug, stimulant NEC
  amytal (sodium) — *see* Dependence, drug, sedative
  analgesic NEC F55.8
  anesthetic (agent) (gas) (general) (local) NEC — *see* Dependence, drug, psychoactive NEC
  anxiolytic NEC — *see* Dependence, drug, sedative
  barbital (s) — *see* Dependence, drug, sedative
  barbiturate (s) (compounds) (drugs classifiable to T42) — *see* Dependence, drug, sedative
  benzedrine — *see* Dependence, drug, stimulant NEC
  bhang — *see* Dependence, drug, cannabis
  bromide (s) NEC — *see* Dependence, drug, sedative
  caffeine — *see* Dependence, drug, stimulant NEC
  cannabis (sativa) (indica) (resin) (derivatives) (type) — *see* Dependence, drug, cannabis
  chloral (betaine) (hydrate) — *see* Dependence, drug, sedative
  chlordiazepoxide — *see* Dependence, drug, sedative
  coca (leaf) (derivatives) — *see* Dependence, drug, cocaine
  cocaine — *see* Dependence, drug, cocaine
  codeine — *see* Dependence, drug, opioid
  combinations of drugs F19.20
  dagga — *see* Dependence, drug, cannabis
  demerol — *see* Dependence, drug, opioid
  dexamphetamine — *see* Dependence, drug, stimulant NEC
  dexedrine — *see* Dependence, drug, stimulant NEC
  dextromethorphan — *see* Dependence, drug, opioid
  dextromoramide — *see* Dependence, drug, opioid
  dextro-nor-pseudo-ephedrine — *see* Dependence, drug, stimulant NEC
  dextrorphan — *see* Dependence, drug, opioid
  diazepam — *see* Dependence, drug, sedative
  dilaudid — *see* Dependence, drug, opioid
  D-lysergic acid diethylamide — *see* Dependence, drug, hallucinogen
  drug NEC F19.20
    with sleep disorder F19.282
    cannabis F12.20
      with
        anxiety disorder F12.280
        intoxication F12.229
          with
            delirium F12.221
            perceptual disturbance F12.222
          uncomplicated F12.220
        other specified disorder F12.288
        psychosis F12.259
          delusions F12.250
          hallucinations F12.251
        unspecified disorder F12.29
        withdrawal F12.23
      in remission F12.21
    cocaine F14.20
      with
        anxiety disorder F14.280
        intoxication F14.229
          with
            delirium F14.221
            perceptual disturbance F14.222
          uncomplicated F14.220

Dependence (on) (syndrome) - *continued*
  drug NEC - *continued*
    cocaine - *continued*
      with - *continued*
        mood disorder F14.24
        other specified disorder F14.288
        psychosis F14.259
          delusions F14.250
          hallucinations F14.251
        sexual dysfunction F14.281
        sleep disorder F14.282
        unspecified disorder F14.29
        withdrawal F14.23
      in remission F14.21
      withdrawal symptoms in newborn P96.1
    counseling and surveillance Z71.51
    hallucinogen F16.20
      with
        anxiety disorder F16.280
        flashbacks F16.283
        intoxication F16.229
          with delirium F16.221
          uncomplicated F16.220
        mood disorder F16.24
        other specified disorder F16.288
        perception disorder, persisting F16.283
        psychosis F16.259
          delusions F16.250
          hallucinations F16.251
        unspecified disorder F16.29
      in remission F16.21
    in remission F19.21
    inhalant F18.20
      with
        anxiety disorder F18.280
        dementia, persisting F18.27
        intoxication F18.229
          with delirium F18.221
          uncomplicated F18.220
        mood disorder F18.24
        other specified disorder F18.288
        psychosis F18.259
          delusions F18.250
          hallucinations F18.251
        unspecified disorder F18.29
      in remission F18.21
    nicotine F17.200
      with disorder F17.209
      in remission F17.201
      specified disorder NEC F17.208
      withdrawal F17.203
      chewing tobacco F17.220
        with disorder F17.229
        in remission F17.221
        specified disorder NEC F17.228
        withdrawal F17.223
      cigarettes F17.210
        with disorder F17.219
        in remission F17.211
        specified disorder NEC F17.218
        withdrawal F17.213
      specified product NEC F17.290
        with disorder F17.299
        remission F17.291
        specified disorder NEC F17.298
        withdrawal F17.293
    opioid F11.20
      with
        intoxication F11.229
          with
            delirium F11.221
            perceptual disturbance F11.222
          uncomplicated F11.220
        mood disorder F11.24
        other specified disorder F11.288
        psychosis F11.259
          delusions F11.250
          hallucinations F11.251
        sexual dysfunction F11.281
        sleep disorder F11.282
        unspecified disorder F11.29
        withdrawal F11.23
      in remission F11.21
    psychoactive NEC F19.20

Dependence (on) (syndrome) - *continued*
drug NEC - *continued*
psychoactive NEC - *continued*
with
amnestic disorder F19.26
anxiety disorder F19.280
dementia F19.27
intoxication F19.229
with
delirium F19.221
perceptual disturbance F19.222
uncomplicated F19.220
mood disorder F19.24
other specified disorder F19.288
psychosis F19.259
delusions F19.250
hallucinations F19.251
sexual dysfunction F19.281
sleep disorder F19.282
unspecified disorder F19.29
withdrawal F19.239
with
delirium F19.231
perceptual disturbance F19.232
uncomplicated F19.230
sedative, hypnotic or anxiolytic F13.20
with
amnestic disorder F13.26
anxiety disorder F13.280
dementia, persisting F13.27
intoxication F13.229
with delirium F13.221
uncomplicated F13.220
mood disorder F13.24
other specified disorder F13.288
psychosis F13.259
delusions F13.250
hallucinations F13.251
sexual dysfunction F13.281
sleep disorder F13.282
unspecified disorder F13.29
withdrawal F13.239
with
delirium F13.231
perceptual disturbance F13.232
uncomplicated F13.230
in remission F13.21
stimulant NEC F15.20
with
anxiety disorder F15.280
intoxication F15.229
with
delirium F15.221
perceptual disturbance F15.222
uncomplicated F15.220
mood disorder F15.24
other specified disorder F15.288
psychosis F15.259
delusions F15.250
hallucinations F15.251
sexual dysfunction F15.281
sleep disorder F15.282
unspecified disorder F15.29
withdrawal F15.23
in remission F15.21
ethyl
alcohol (without remission) F10.20
with remission F10.21
bromide — *see* Dependence, drug,
sedative
carbamate F19.20
chloride F19.20
morphine — *see* Dependence, drug, opioid
ganja — *see* Dependence, drug, cannabis
glue (airplane) (sniffing) — *see* Dependence,
drug, inhalant
glutethimide — *see* Dependence, drug,
sedative
hallucinogenics — *see* Dependence, drug,
hallucinogen
hashish — *see* Dependence, drug, cannabis
hemp — *see* Dependence, drug, cannabis
heroin (salt) (any) — *see* Dependence, drug,
opioid

Dependence (on) (syndrome) - *continued*
hypnotic NEC — *see* Dependence, drug,
sedative
Indian hemp — *see* Dependence, drug,
cannabis
inhalants — *see* Dependence, drug, inhalant
khat — *see* Dependence, drug, stimulant
NEC
laudanum — *see* Dependence, drug, opioid
LSD (-25) (derivatives) — *see* Dependence,
drug, hallucinogen
luminal — *see* Dependence, drug, sedative
lysergic acid — *see* Dependence, drug,
hallucinogen
maconha — *see* Dependence, drug, cannabis
marihuana — *see* Dependence, drug,
cannabis
meprobamate — *see* Dependence, drug,
sedative
mescaline — *see* Dependence, drug,
hallucinogen
methadone — *see* Dependence, drug, opioid
methamphetamine (s) — *see* Dependence,
drug, stimulant NEC
methaqualone — *see* Dependence, drug,
sedative
methyl
alcohol (without remission) F10.20
with remission F10.21
bromide — *see* Dependence, drug,
sedative
morphine — *see* Dependence, drug, opioid
phenidate — *see* Dependence, drug,
stimulant NEC
sulfonal — *see* Dependence, drug, sedative
morphine (sulfate) (sulfite) (type) — *see*
Dependence, drug, opioid
narcotic (drug) NEC — *see* Dependence,
drug, opioid
nembutal — *see* Dependence, drug, sedative
neraval — *see* Dependence, drug, sedative
neravan — *see* Dependence, drug, sedative
neurobarb — *see* Dependence, drug, sedative
nicotine — *see* Dependence, drug, nicotine
nitrous oxide F19.20
nonbarbiturate sedatives and tranquilizers
with similar effect — *see* Dependence,
drug, sedative
on
artificial heart (fully implantable)
(mechanical) Z95.812
aspirator Z99.0
care provider (because of) Z74.9
impaired mobility Z74.09
need for
assistance with personal care Z74.1
continuous supervision Z74.3
no other household member able to
render care Z74.2
specified reason NEC Z74.8
machine Z99.89
enabling NEC Z99.89
specified type NEC Z99.89
renal dialysis (hemodialysis)
(peritoneal) Z99.2
respirator Z99.11
ventilator Z99.11
wheelchair Z99.3
opiate — *see* Dependence, drug, opioid
opioids — *see* Dependence, drug, opioid
opium (alkaloids) (derivatives) (tincture) —
see Dependence, drug, opioid
oxygen (long-term) (supplemental) Z99.81
paraldehyde — *see* Dependence, drug,
sedative
paregoric — *see* Dependence, drug, opioid
PCP (phencyclidine) (or related
substance) — *see* Dependence, drug,
hallucinogen
pentobarbital — *see* Dependence, drug,
sedative
pentobarbitone (sodium) — *see* Dependence,
drug, sedative
pentothal — *see* Dependence, drug, sedative

Dependence (on) (syndrome) - *continued*
peyote — *see* Dependence, drug,
hallucinogen
phencyclidine (PCP) (or related
substance) — *see* Dependence, drug,
hallucinogen
phenmetrazine — *see* Dependence, drug,
stimulant NEC
phenobarbital — *see* Dependence, drug,
sedative
polysubstance F19.20
psilocibin, psilocin, psilocyn, psilocyline —
see Dependence, drug, hallucinogen
psychostimulant NEC — *see* Dependence,
drug, stimulant NEC
secobarbital — *see* Dependence, drug,
sedative
seconal — *see* Dependence, drug, sedative
sedative NEC — *see* Dependence, drug,
sedative
specified drug NEC — *see* Dependence, drug
stimulant NEC — *see* Dependence, drug,
stimulant NEC
substance NEC — *see* Dependence, drug
supplemental oxygen Z99.81
tobacco — *see* Dependence, drug, nicotine
counseling and surveillance Z71.6
tranquilizer NEC — *see* Dependence, drug,
sedative
vitamin B6 E53.1
volatile solvents — *see* Dependence, drug,
inhalant
Dependency
care-provider Z74.9
passive F60.7
reactions (persistent) F60.7
Depersonalization (in neurotic state)
(neurotic) (syndrome) F48.1
Depletion
extracellular fluid E86.9
plasma E86.1
potassium E87.6
nephropathy N25.89
salt or sodium E87.1
causing heat exhaustion or
prostration T67.4
nephropathy N28.9
volume NOS E86.9
Deployment (current) (military) status
Z56.82
in theater or in support of military war,
peacekeeping and humanitarian
operations Z56.82
personal history of Z91.82
military war, peacekeeping and
humanitarian deployment (current or
past conflict) Z91.82
returned from Z91.82
Depolarization, premature I49.40
atrial I49.1
junctional I49.2
specified NEC I49.49
ventricular I49.3
Deposit
bone in Boeck's sarcoid D86.89
calcareous, calcium — *see* Calcification
cholesterol
retina H35.89
vitreous (body) (humor) — *see* Deposit,
crystalline
conjunctiva H11.11-
cornea H18.00-
argentous H18.02-
due to metabolic disorder H18.03-
Kayser-Fleischer ring H18.04-
pigmentation — *see* Pigmentation, cornea
crystalline, vitreous (body) (humor) H43.2-
hemosiderin in old scars of cornea — *see*
Pigmentation, cornea, stromal
metallic in lens — *see* Cataract, specified
NEC
skin R23.8
tooth, teeth (betel) (black) (green) (materia
alba) (orange) (tobacco) K03.6
urate, kidney — *see* Calculus, kidney

Depraved appetite — *see* Pica
Depressed
  HDL cholesterol E78.6
Depression (acute) (mental) F32.9
  agitated (single episode) F32.2
  anaclitic — *see* Disorder, adjustment
  anxiety F41.8
    persistent F34.1
  arches — *see also* Deformity, limb, flat foot
  atypical (single episode) F32.89
    recurrent episode F33.8
  basal metabolic rate R94.8
  bone marrow D75.89
  central nervous system R09.2
  cerebral R29.818
    newborn P91.4
  cerebrovascular I67.9
  chest wall M95.4
  climacteric (single episode) F32.89
    recurrent episode F33.8
  endogenous (without psychotic
      symptoms) F33.2
    with psychotic symptoms F33.3
  functional activity R68.89
  hysterical F44.89
  involutional (single episode) F32.89
    recurrent episode F33.8
  major F32.9
    with psychotic symptoms F32.3
    recurrent — *see* Disorder, depressive,
        recurrent
  manic-depressive — *see* Disorder,
      depressive, recurrent
  masked (single episode) F32.89
  medullary G93.89
  menopausal (single episode) F32.89
    recurrent episode F33.8
  metatarsus — *see* Depression, arches
  monopolar F33.9
  nervous F34.1
  neurotic F34.1
  nose M95.0
  postnatal (NOS) F53.0
  postpartum (NOS) F53.0
  post-psychotic of schizophrenia F32.89
  post-schizophrenic F32.89
  psychogenic (reactive) (single episode) F32.9
  psychoneurotic F34.1
  psychotic (single episode) F32.3
    recurrent F33.3
  reactive (psychogenic) (single episode) F32.9
    psychotic (single episode) F32.3
  recurrent — *see* Disorder, depressive,
      recurrent
  respiratory center G93.89
  seasonal — *see* Disorder, depressive,
      recurrent
  senile F03
  severe, single episode F32.2
  situational F43.21
  skull Q67.4
  specified NEC (single episode) F32.89
  sternum M95.4
  visual field — *see* Defect, visual field
  vital (recurrent) (without psychotic
      symptoms) F33.2
    with psychotic symptoms F33.3
    single episode F32.2
Deprivation
  cultural Z60.3
  effects NOS T73.9
    specified NEC T73.8
  emotional NEC Z65.8
    affecting infant or child — *see*
        Maltreatment, child, psychological
  food T73.0
  protein — *see* Malnutrition
  sleep Z72.820
  social Z60.4
    affecting infant or child — *see*
        Maltreatment, child, psychological
  specified NEC T73.8
  vitamins — *see* Deficiency, vitamin
  water T73.1

Derangement
  ankle (internal) — *see* Derangement, joint,
      ankle
  cartilage (articular) NEC — *see*
      Derangement, joint, articular cartilage,
      by site
    recurrent — *see* Dislocation, recurrent
  cruciate ligament, anterior, current injury —
      see Sprain, knee, cruciate, anterior
  elbow (internal) — *see* Derangement, joint,
      elbow
  hip (joint) (internal) (old) — *see*
      Derangement, joint, hip
  joint (internal) M24.9
    ankylosis — *see* Ankylosis
    articular cartilage M24.10
      ankle M24.17-
      elbow M24.12-
      foot M24.17-
      hand M24.14-
      hip M24.15-
      knee NEC M23.9-
      loose body — *see* Loose, body
      shoulder M24.11-
      wrist M24.13-
    contracture — *see* Contraction, joint
    current injury — *see also* Dislocation
      knee, meniscus or cartilage — *see* Tear,
          meniscus
    dislocation
      pathological — *see* Dislocation,
          pathological
      recurrent — *see* Dislocation, recurrent
    knee — *see* Derangement, knee
    ligament — *see* Disorder, ligament
    loose body — *see* Loose, body
    recurrent — *see* Dislocation, recurrent
    specified type NEC M24.80
      ankle M24.87-
      elbow M24.82-
      foot joint M24.87-
      hand joint M24.84-
      hip M24.85-
      shoulder M24.81-
      wrist M24.83-
    temporomandibular M26.69
  knee (recurrent) M23.9-
    ligament disruption, spontaneous M23.60-
      anterior cruciate M23.61-
      capsular M23.67-
      instability, chronic M23.5-
      lateral collateral M23.64-
      medial collateral M23.63-
      posterior cruciate M23.62-
    loose body M23.4-
    meniscus M23.30-
      cystic M23.00-
        lateral M23.002
          anterior horn M23.04-
          posterior horn M23.05-
          specified NEC M23.06-
        medial M23.005
          anterior horn M23.01-
          posterior horn M23.02-
          specified NEC M23.03-
      degenerate — *see* Derangement, knee,
          meniscus, specified NEC
      detached — *see* Derangement, knee,
          meniscus, specified NEC
      due to old tear or injury M23.20-
        lateral M23.20-
          anterior horn M23.24-
          posterior horn M23.25-
          specified NEC M23.26-
        medial M23.20-
          anterior horn M23.21-
          posterior horn M23.22-
          specified NEC M23.23-
      retained — *see* Derangement, knee,
          meniscus, specified NEC
      specified NEC M23.30-
        lateral M23.30-
          anterior horn M23.34-
          posterior horn M23.35-
          specified NEC M23.36-

Derangement - *continued*
  knee (recurrent) - *continued*
    meniscus - *continued*
      specified NEC - *continued*
        medial M23.30-
          anterior horn M23.31-
          posterior horn M23.32-
          specified NEC M23.33-
      old M23.8X-
    specified NEC — *see* subcategory M23.8
  low back NEC — *see* Dorsopathy, specified
      NEC
  meniscus — *see* Derangement, knee,
      meniscus
  mental — *see* Psychosis
  patella, specified NEC — *see* Disorder,
      patella, derangement NEC
  semilunar cartilage (knee) — *see*
      Derangement, knee, meniscus, specified
      NEC
  shoulder (internal) — *see* Derangement,
      joint, shoulder
Dercum's disease E88.2
Derealization (neurotic) F48.1
Dermal — *see* condition
Dermaphytid — *see* Dermatophytosis
Dermatitis (eczematous) L30.9
  ab igne L59.0
  acarine B88.0
  actinic (due to sun) L57.8
    other than from sun L59.8
  allergic — *see* Dermatitis, contact, allergic
  ambustionis, due to burn or scald — *see*
      Burn
  amebic A06.7
  ammonia L22
  arsenical (ingested) L27.8
  artefacta L98.1
    psychogenic F54
  atopic L20.9
    psychogenic F54
    specified NEC L20.89
  autoimmune progesterone L30.8
  berlock, berloque L56.2
  blastomycotic B40.3
  blister beetle L24.89
  bullous, bullosa L13.9
    mucosynechial, atrophic L12.1
    seasonal L30.8
    specified NEC L13.8
  calorica L59.0
    due to burn or scald — *see* Burn
  caterpillar L24.89
  cercarial B65.3
  combustionis L59.0
    due to burn or scald — *see* Burn
  congelationis T69.1
  contact (occupational) L25.9
    allergic L23.9
      due to
        adhesives L23.1
        cement L23.5
        chemical products NEC L23.5
        chromium L23.0
        cosmetics L23.2
        dander (cat) (dog) L23.81
        drugs in contact with skin L23.3
        dyes L23.4
        food in contact with skin L23.6
        hair (cat) (dog) L23.81
        insecticide L23.5
        metals L23.0
        nickel L23.0
        plants, non-food L23.7
        plastic L23.5
        rubber L23.5
        specified agent NEC L23.89
    due to
      cement L25.3
      chemical products NEC L25.3
      cosmetics L25.0
      dander (cat) (dog) L23.81
      drugs in contact with skin L25.1
      dyes L25.2
      food in contact with skin L25.4

Dermatitis (eczematous) - *continued*
contact (occupational) - *continued*
due to - *continued*
hair (cat) (dog) L23.81
plants, non-food L25.5
specified agent NEC L25.8
irritant L24.9
due to
cement L24.5
chemical products NEC L24.5
cosmetics L24.3
detergents L24.0
drugs in contact with skin L24.4
food in contact with skin L24.6
oils and greases L24.1
plants, non-food L24.7
solvents L24.2
specified agent NEC L24.89
contusiformis L52
diabetic — *see* E08-E13 with .620
diaper L22
diphtheritica A36.3
dry skin L85.3
due to
acetone (contact) (irritant) L24.2
acids (contact) (irritant) L24.5
adhesive (s) (allergic) (contact)
(plaster) L23.1
irritant L24.5
alcohol (irritant) (skin contact) (substances
in category T51) L24.2
taken internally L27.8
alkalis (contact) (irritant) L24.5
arsenic (ingested) L27.8
carbon disulfide (contact) (irritant) L24.2
caustics (contact) (irritant) L24.5
cement (contact) L25.3
cereal (ingested) L27.2
chemical (s) NEC L25.3
taken internally L27.8
chlorocompounds L24.2
chromium (contact) (irritant) L24.81
coffee (ingested) L27.2
cold weather L30.8
cosmetics (contact) L25.0
allergic L23.2
irritant L24.3
cyclohexanes L24.2
dander (cat) (dog) L23.81
Demodex species B88.0
Dermanyssus gallinae B88.0
detergents (contact) (irritant) L24.0
dichromate L24.81
drugs and medicaments (generalized)
(internal use) L27.0
external — *see* Dermatitis, due to, drugs,
in contact with skin
in contact with skin L25.1
allergic L23.3
irritant L24.4
localized skin eruption L27.1
specified substance — *see* Table of
Drugs and Chemicals
dyes (contact) L25.2
allergic L23.4
irritant L24.89
epidermophytosis — *see* Dermatophytosis
esters L24.2
external irritant NEC L24.9
fish (ingested) L27.2
flour (ingested) L27.2
food (ingested) L27.2
in contact with skin L25.4
fruit (ingested) L27.2
furs (allergic) (contact) L23.81
glues — *see* Dermatitis, due to, adhesives
glycols L24.2
greases NEC (contact) (irritant) L24.1
hair (cat) (dog) L23.81
hot
objects and materials — *see* Burn
weather or places L59.0
hydrocarbons L24.2
infrared rays L59.8
ingestion, ingested substance L27.9

Dermatitis (eczematous) - *continued*
due to - *continued*
ingestion, ingested substance - *continued*
chemical NEC L27.8
drugs and medicaments — *see*
Dermatitis, due to, drugs
food L27.2
specified NEC L27.8
insecticide in contact with skin L24.5
internal agent L27.9
drugs and medicaments (generalized) —
see Dermatitis, due to, drugs
food L27.2
irradiation — *see* Dermatitis, due to,
radioactive substance
ketones L24.2
lacquer tree (allergic) (contact) L23.7
light (sun) NEC L57.8
acute L56.8
other L59.8
Liponyssoides sanguineus B88.0
low temperature L30.8
meat (ingested) L27.2
metals, metal salts (contact)
(irritant) L24.81
milk (ingested) L27.2
nickel (contact) (irritant) L24.81
nylon (contact) (irritant) L24.5
oils NEC (contact) (irritant) L24.1
paint solvent (contact) (irritant) L24.2
petroleum products (contact) (irritant)
(substances in T52.0) L24.2
plants NEC (contact) L25.5
allergic L23.7
irritant L24.7
plasters (adhesive) (any) (allergic)
(contact) L23.1
irritant L24.5
plastic (contact) L25.3
preservatives (contact) — *see* Dermatitis,
due to, chemical, in contact with skin
primrose (allergic) (contact) L23.7
primula (allergic) (contact) L23.7
radiation L59.8
nonionizing (chronic exposure) L57.8
sun NEC L57.8
acute L56.8
radioactive substance L58.9
acute L58.0
chronic L58.1
radium L58.9
acute L58.0
chronic L58.1
ragweed (allergic) (contact) L23.7
Rhus (allergic) (contact) (diversiloba)
(radicans) (toxicodendron) (venenata)
(verniciflua) L23.7
rubber (contact) L24.5
Senecio jacobaea (allergic) (contact) L23.7
solvents (contact) (irritant) (substances in
categories T52) L24.2
specified agent NEC (contact) L25.8
allergic L23.89
irritant L24.89
sunshine NEC L57.8
acute L56.8
tetrachlorethylene (contact) (irritant) L24.2
toluene (contact) (irritant) L24.2
turpentine (contact) L24.2
ultraviolet rays (sun NEC) (chronic
exposure) L57.8
acute L56.8
vaccine or vaccination L27.0
specified substance — *see* Table of
Drugs and Chemicals
varicose veins — *see* Varix, leg, with,
inflammation
X-rays L58.9
acute L58.0
chronic L58.1
dyshydrotic L30.1
dysmenorrheica N94.6
escharotica — *see* Burn
exfoliative, exfoliativa (generalized) L26
neonatorum L00

Dermatitis (eczematous) - *continued*
eyelid — *see also* Dermatosis, eyelid
allergic H01.119
left H01.116
lower H01.115
upper H01.114
right H01.113
lower H01.112
upper H01.111
contact — *see* Dermatitis, eyelid, allergic
due to
Demodex species B88.0
herpes (zoster) B02.39
simplex B00.59
eczematous H01.139
left H01.136
lower H01.135
upper H01.134
right H01.133
lower H01.132
upper H01.131
facta, factitia, factitial L98.1
psychogenic F54
flexural NEC L20.82
friction L30.4
fungus B36.9
specified type NEC B36.8
gangrenosa, gangrenous infantum L08.0
harvest mite B88.0
heat L59.0
herpesviral, vesicular (ear) (lip) B00.1
herpetiformis (bullous) (erythematous)
(pustular) (vesicular) L13.0
juvenile L12.2
senile L12.0
hiemalis L30.8
hypostatic, hypostatica — *see* Varix, leg,
with, inflammation
infectious eczematoid L30.3
infective L30.3
irritant — *see* Dermatitis, contact, irritant
Jacquet's (diaper dermatitis) L22
Leptus B88.0
lichenified NEC L28.0
medicamentosa (generalized) (internal
use) — *see* Dermatitis, due to drugs
mite B88.0
multiformis L13.0
juvenile L12.2
napkin L22
neurotica L13.0
nummular L30.0
papillaris capillitii L73.0
pellagrous E52
perioral L71.0
photocontact L56.2
polymorpha dolorosa L13.0
pruriginosa L13.0
pruritic NEC L30.8
psychogenic F54
purulent L08.0
pustular
contagious B08.02
subcorneal L13.1
pyococcal L08.0
pyogenica L08.0
repens L40.2
Ritter's (exfoliativa) L00
Schamberg's L81.7
schistosome B65.3
seasonal bullous L30.8
seborrheic L21.9
infantile L21.1
specified NEC L21.8
sensitization NOS L23.9
septic L08.0
solare L57.8
specified NEC L30.8
stasis I87.2
with
varicose ulcer — *see* Varix, leg, with,
ulcer, with inflammation
varicose veins — *see* Varix, leg, with,
inflammation

Dermatitis (eczematous) - *continued*
stasis - *continued*
due to postthrombotic syndrome — *see* Syndrome, postthrombotic
suppurative L08.0
traumatic NEC L30.4
trophoneurotica L13.0
ultraviolet (sun) (chronic exposure) L57.8
acute L56.8
varicose — *see* Varix, leg, with, inflammation
vegetans L10.1
verrucosa B43.0
vesicular, herpesviral B00.1
Dermatoarthritis, lipoid E78.81
Dermatochalasis, eyelid H02.839
left H02.836
lower H02.835
upper H02.834
right H02.833
lower H02.832
upper H02.831
Dermatofibroma (lenticulare) — *see* Neoplasm, skin, benign
protuberans — *see* Neoplasm, skin, uncertain behavior
Dermatofibrosarcoma (pigmented) (protuberans) — *see* Neoplasm, skin, malignant
Dermatographia L50.3
Dermatolysis (exfoliativa) (congenital) Q82.8
acquired L57.4
eyelids — *see* Blepharochalasis
palpebrarum — *see* Blepharochalasis
senile L57.4
Dermatomegaly NEC Q82.8
Dermatomucosomyositis M33.10
with
myopathy M33.12
respiratory involvement M33.11
specified organ involvement NEC M33.19
Dermatomycosis B36.9
furfuracea B36.0
specified type NEC B36.8
Dermatomyositis (acute) (chronic) — *see also* Dermatopolymyositis
adult — *see also* Dermatomyositis, specified NEC M33.10
in (due to) neoplastic disease — *see also* Neoplasm D49.9 *[M36.0]*
juvenile M33.00
with
myopathy M33.02
respiratory involvement M33.01
specified organ involvement NEC M33.09
without myopathy M33.03
specified NEC M33.10
with
myopathy M33.12
respiratory involvement M33.11
specified organ involvement NEC M33.19
without myopathy M33.13
Dermatoneuritis of children — *see* Poisoning, mercury
Dermatophilosis A48.8
Dermatophytid L30.2
Dermatophytide — *see* Dermatophytosis
Dermatophytosis (epidermophyton) (infection) (Microsporum) (tinea) (Trichophyton) B35.9
beard B35.0
body B35.4
capitis B35.0
corporis B35.4
deep-seated B35.8
disseminated B35.8
foot B35.3
granulomatous B35.8
groin B35.6
hand B35.2
nail B35.1
perianal (area) B35.6
scalp B35.0

Dermatophytosis (epidermophyton) (infection) (Microsporum) (tinea) (Trichophyton) - *continued*
specified NEC B35.8
Dermatopolymyositis M33.90
with
myopathy M33.92
respiratory involvement M33.91
specified organ involvement NEC M33.99
in neoplastic disease — *see also* Neoplasm D49.9 *[M36.0]*
juvenile M33.00
with
myopathy M33.02
respiratory involvement M33.01
specified organ involvement NEC M33.09
specified NEC M33.10
myopathy M33.12
respiratory involvement M33.11
specified organ involvement NEC M33.19
without myopathy M33.93
Dermatopolyneuritis — *see* Poisoning, mercury
Dermatorrhexis — *see also* Syndrome, Ehlers-Danlos Q79.60
acquired L57.4
Dermatosclerosis — *see also* Scleroderma
localized L94.0
Dermatosis L98.9
Andrews' L08.89
Bowen's — *see* Neoplasm, skin, in situ
bullous L13.9
specified NEC L13.8
exfoliativa L26
eyelid (noninfectious)
dermatitis — *see* Dermatitis, eyelid
discoid lupus erythematosus — *see* Lupus, erythematosus, eyelid
xeroderma — *see* Xeroderma, acquired, eyelid
factitial L98.1
febrile neutrophilic L98.2
gonococcal A54.89
herpetiformis L13.0
juvenile L12.2
linear IgA L13.8
menstrual NEC L98.8
neutrophilic, febrile L98.2
occupational — *see* Dermatitis, contact
papulosa nigra L82.1
pigmentary L81.9
progressive L81.7
Schamberg's L81.7
psychogenic F54
purpuric, pigmented L81.7
pustular, subcorneal L13.1
transient acantholytic L11.1
Dermographia, dermographism L50.3
Dermoid (cyst) — *see also* Neoplasm, benign, by site
with malignant transformation C56-
due to radiation (nonionizing) L57.8
Dermopathy
infiltrative with thyrotoxicosis — *see* Thyrotoxicosis
nephrogenic fibrosing L90.8
Dermophytosis — *see* Dermatophytosis
Descemetocele H18.73-
Descemet's membrane — *see* condition
Descending — *see* condition
Descensus uteri — *see* Prolapse, uterus
Desert
rheumatism B38.0
sore — *see* Ulcer, skin
Desertion (newborn) — *see* Maltreatment
Desmoid (extra-abdominal) (tumor) — *see* Neoplasm, connective tissue, uncertain behavior
abdominal D48.1
Despondency F32.9
Desquamation, skin R23.4
Destruction, destructive — *see also* Damage
articular facet — *see also* Derangement, joint, specified type NEC

Destruction, destructive - *continued*
articular facet - *continued*
knee M23.8X-
vertebra — *see* Spondylosis
bone — *see also* Disorder, bone, specified type NEC
syphilitic A52.77
joint — *see also* Derangement, joint, specified type NEC
sacroiliac M53.3
rectal sphincter K62.89
septum (nasal) J34.89
tuberculous NEC — *see* Tuberculosis
tympanum, tympanic membrane (nontraumatic) — *see* Disorder, tympanic membrane, specified NEC
vertebral disc — *see* Degeneration, intervertebral disc
Destructiveness — *see also* Disorder, conduct
adjustment reaction — *see* Disorder, adjustment
Desultory labor O62.2
Detachment
cartilage — *see* Sprain
cervix, annular N88.8
complicating delivery O71.3
choroid (old) (postinfectional) (simple) (spontaneous) H31.40-
hemorrhagic H31.41-
serous H31.42-
ligament — *see* Sprain
meniscus (knee) — *see also* Derangement, knee, meniscus, specified NEC
current injury — *see* Tear, meniscus
due to old tear or injury — *see* Derangement, knee, meniscus, due to old tear
retina (without retinal break) (serous) H33.2-
with retinal:
break H33.00-
giant H33.03-
multiple H33.02-
single H33.01-
dialysis H33.04-
pigment epithelium — *see* Degeneration, retina, separation of layers, pigment epithelium detachment
rhegmatogenous — *see* Detachment, retina, with retinal, break
specified NEC H33.8
total H33.05-
traction H33.4-
vitreous (body) H43.81
Detergent asthma J69.8
Deterioration
epileptic F06.8
general physical R53.81
heart, cardiac — *see* Degeneration, myocardial
mental — *see* Psychosis
myocardial, myocardium — *see* Degeneration, myocardial
senile (simple) R54
Deuteranomaly (anomalous trichromat) H53.53
Deuteranopia (complete) (incomplete) H53.53
Development
abnormal, bone Q79.9
arrested R62.50
bone — *see* Arrest, development or growth, bone
child R62.50
due to malnutrition E45
defective, congenital — *see also* Anomaly, by site
cauda equina Q06.3
left ventricle Q24.8
in hypoplastic left heart syndrome Q23.4
valve Q24.8
pulmonary Q22.3
delayed — *see also* Delay, development R62.50
arithmetical skills F81.2
language (skills) (expressive) F80.1

Development - *continued*
  delayed - *continued*
    learning skill F81.9
    mixed skills F88
    motor coordination F82
    reading F81.0
    specified learning skill NEC F81.89
    speech F80.9
    spelling F81.81
    written expression F81.81
  imperfect, congenital — *see also* Anomaly, by site
    heart Q24.9
    lungs Q33.6
  incomplete
    bronchial tree Q32.4
    organ or site not listed — *see* Hypoplasia, by site
    respiratory system Q34.9
  sexual, precocious NEC E30.1
  tardy, mental — *see also* Disability, intellectual F79
Developmental — *see* condition
  testing, infant or child — *see* Examination, child
Devergie's disease (pityriasis rubra pilaris) L44.0
Deviation (in)
  conjugate palsy (eye) (spastic) H51.0
  esophagus (acquired) K22.8
  eye, skew H51.8
  midline (jaw) (teeth) (dental arch) M26.29
    specified site NEC — *see* Malposition
  nasal septum J34.2
    congenital Q67.4
  opening and closing of the mandible M26.53
  organ or site, congenital NEC — *see* Malposition, congenital
  septum (nasal) (acquired) J34.2
    congenital Q67.4
  sexual F65.9
    bestiality F65.89
    erotomania F52.8
    exhibitionism F65.2
    fetishism, fetishistic F65.0
      transvestism F65.1
    frotteurism F65.81
    masochism F65.51
    multiple F65.89
    necrophilia F65.89
    nymphomania F52.8
    pederosis F65.4
    pedophilia F65.4
    sadism, sadomasochism F65.52
    satyriasis F52.8
    specified type NEC F65.89
    transvestism F64.1
    voyeurism F65.3
  teeth, midline M26.29
  trachea J39.8
  ureter, congenital Q62.61
Device
  cerebral ventricle (communicating) in situ Z98.2
  contraceptive — *see* Contraceptive, device
  drainage, cerebrospinal fluid, in situ Z98.2
Devic's disease G36.0
Devil's
  grip B33.0
  pinches (purpura simplex) D69.2
Devitalized tooth K04.99
Devonshire colic — *see* Poisoning, lead
Dextraposition, aorta Q20.3
  in tetralogy of Fallot Q21.3
Dextrinosis, limit (debrancher enzyme deficiency) E74.03
Dextrocardia (true) Q24.0
  with
    complete transposition of viscera Q89.3
    situs inversus Q89.3
Dextrotransposition, aorta Q20.3
d-glycericacidemia E72.59
Dhat syndrome F48.8
Dhobi itch B35.6
Di George's syndrome D82.1

Di Guglielmo's disease C94.0-
Diabetes, diabetic (mellitus) (sugar) E11.9
  with
    amyotrophy E11.44
    arthropathy NEC E11.618
    autonomic (poly) neuropathy E11.43
    cataract E11.36
    Charcot's joints E11.610
    chronic kidney disease E11.22
    circulatory complication NEC E11.59
    complication E11.8
      specified NEC E11.69
    dermatitis E11.620
    foot ulcer E11.621
    gangrene E11.52
    gastroparalysis E11.43
    gastroparesis E11.43
    glomerulonephrosis, intracapillary E11.21
    glomerulosclerosis, intercapillary E11.21
    hyperglycemia E11.65
    hyperosmolarity E11.00
      with coma E11.01
    hypoglycemia E11.649
      with coma E11.641
    ketoacidosis E11.10
      with coma E11.11
    kidney complications NEC E11.29
    Kimmelstiel-Wilson disease E11.21
    loss of protective sensation (LOPS) — *see* Diabetes, by type, with neuropathy
    mononeuropathy E11.41
    myasthenia E11.44
    necrobiosis lipoidica E11.620
    nephropathy E11.21
    neuralgia E11.42
    neurologic complication NEC E11.49
    neuropathic arthropathy E11.610
    neuropathy E11.40
    ophthalmic complication NEC E11.39
    oral complication NEC E11.638
    osteomyelitis E11.69
    periodontal disease E11.630
    peripheral angiopathy E11.51
      with gangrene E11.52
    polyneuropathy E11.42
    renal complication NEC E11.29
    renal tubular degeneration E11.29
    retinopathy E11.319
      with macular edema E11.311
        resolved following treatment E11.37
      nonproliferative E11.329
        with macular edema E11.321
        mild E11.329
          with macular edema E11.321
        moderate E11.339
          with macular edema E11.331
        severe E11.349
          with macular edema E11.341
      proliferative E11.359
        with
          combined traction retinal detachment and rhegmatogenous retinal detachment E11.354
          macular edema E11.351
          stable proliferative diabetic retinopathy E11.355
          traction retinal detachment involving the macula E11.352
          traction retinal detachment not involving the macula E11.353
    skin complication NEC E11.628
    skin ulcer NEC E11.622
  brittle — *see* Diabetes, type 1
  bronzed E83.110
  complicating pregnancy — *see* Pregnancy, complicated by, diabetes
  dietary counseling and surveillance Z71.3
  due to
    autoimmune process — *see* Diabetes, type 1
    immune mediated pancreatic islet beta-cell destruction — *see* Diabetes, type 1
    due to drug or chemical E09.9
      with

Diabetes, diabetic (mellitus) (sugar) - *continued*
  due to drug or chemical - *continued*
    with - *continued*
      amyotrophy E09.44
      arthropathy NEC E09.618
      autonomic (poly) neuropathy E09.43
      cataract E09.36
      Charcot's joints E09.610
      chronic kidney disease E09.22
      circulatory complication NEC E09.59
      complication E09.8
        specified NEC E09.69
      dermatitis E09.620
      foot ulcer E09.621
      gangrene E09.52
      gastroparalysis E09.43
      gastroparesis E09.43
      glomerulonephrosis, intracapillary E09.21
      glomerulosclerosis, intercapillary E09.21
      hyperglycemia E09.65
      hyperosmolarity E09.00
        with coma E09.01
      hypoglycemia E09.649
        with coma E09.641
      ketoacidosis E09.10
        with coma E09.11
      kidney complications NEC E09.29
      Kimmelstiel-Wilson disease E09.21
      mononeuropathy E09.41
      myasthenia E09.44
      necrobiosis lipoidica E09.620
      nephropathy E09.21
      neuralgia E09.42
      neurologic complication NEC E09.49
      neuropathic arthropathy E09.610
      neuropathy E09.40
      ophthalmic complication NEC E09.39
      oral complication NEC E09.638
      periodontal disease E09.630
      peripheral angiopathy E09.51
        with gangrene E09.52
      polyneuropathy E09.42
      renal complication NEC E09.29
      renal tubular degeneration E09.29
      retinopathy E09.319
        with macular edema E09.311
        resolved following treatment E09.37
        nonproliferative E09.329
          with macular edema E09.321
          mild E09.329
            with macular edema E09.321
          moderate E09.339
            with macular edema E09.331
          severe E09.349
            with macular edema E09.341
        proliferative E09.359
          with
            combined traction retinal detachment and rhegmatogenous retinal detachment E09.354
            macular edema E09.351
            stable proliferative diabetic retinopathy E09.355
            traction retinal detachment involving the macula E09.352
            traction retinal detachment not involving the macula E09.353
      skin complication NEC E09.628
      skin ulcer NEC E09.622
  due to underlying condition E08.9
    with
      amyotrophy E08.44
      arthropathy NEC E08.618
      autonomic (poly) neuropathy E08.43
      cataract E08.36
      Charcot's joints E08.610
      chronic kidney disease E08.22
      circulatory complication NEC E08.59
      complication E08.8

Diabetes, diabetic (mellitus) (sugar) - *continued*
  due to underlying condition - *continued*
    with - *continued*
      complication - *continued*
        specified NEC E08.69
      dermatitis E08.620
      foot ulcer E08.621
      gangrene E08.52
      gastroparalysis E08.43
      gastroparesis E08.43
      glomerulonephrosis,
        intracapillary E08.21
      glomerulosclerosis,
        intercapillary E08.21
      hyperglycemia E08.65
      hyperosmolarity E08.00
        with coma E08.01
      hypoglycemia E08.649
        with coma E08.641
      ketoacidosis E08.10
        with coma E08.11
      kidney complications NEC E08.29
      Kimmelsteil-WIlson disease E08.21
      mononeuropathy E08.41
      myasthenia E08.44
      necrobiosis lipoidica E08.620
      nephropathy E08.21
      neuralgia E08.42
      neurologic complication NEC E08.49
      neuropathic arthropathy E08.610
      neuropathy E08.40
      ophthalmic complication NEC E08.39
      oral complication NEC E08.638
      periodontal disease E08.630
      peripheral angiopathy E08.51
        with gangrene E08.52
      polyneuropathy E08.42
      renal complication NEC E08.29
      renal tubular degeneration E08.29
      retinopathy E08.319
        with macular edema E08.311
        resolved following treatment E08.37
        nonproliferative E08.329
          with macular edema E08.321
          mild E08.329
            with macular edema E08.321
          moderate E08.339
            with macular edema E08.331
          severe E08,349
            with macular edema E08.341
        proliferative E08.359
          with
            combined traction retinal
              detachment and
              rhegmatogenous retinal
              detachment E08.354
            macular edema E08.351
            stable proliferative diabetic
              retinopathy E08.355
            traction retinal detachment
              involving the
              macula E08.352
            traction retinal detachment not
              involving the
              macula E08.353
      skin complication NEC E08.628
      skin ulcer NEC E08.622
  gestational (in pregnancy) O24.419
    affecting newborn P70.0
    diet controlled O24.410
    in childbirth O24.429
      diet controlled O24.420
      insulin (and diet) controlled O24.424
      oral drug controlled (antidiabetic)
        (hypoglycemic) O24.425
    insulin (and diet) controlled O24.414
    oral drug controlled (antidiabetic)
      (hypoglycemic) O24.415
    puerperal O24.439
      diet controlled O24.430
      insulin (and diet) controlled O24.434
      oral drug controlled (antidiabetic)
        (hypoglycemic) O24.435
  hepatogenous E13.9

Diabetes, diabetic (mellitus) (sugar) - *continued*
  idiopathic — *see* Diabetes, type 1
  inadequately controlled - code to Diabetes,
    by type, with hyperglycemia
  insipidus E23.2
    nephrogenic N25.1
    pituitary E23.2
    vasopressin resistant N25.1
  insulin dependent - code to type of diabetes
  juvenile-onset — *see* Diabetes, type 1
  ketosis-prone — *see* Diabetes, type 1
  latent R73.03
  neonatal (transient) P70.2
  non-insulin dependent - code to type of
    diabetes
  out of control - code to Diabetes, by type,
    with hyperglycemia
  phosphate E83.39
  poorly controlled - code to Diabetes, by type,
    with hyperglycemia
  postpancreatectomy — *see* Diabetes,
    specified type NEC
  postprocedural — *see* Diabetes, specified
    type NEC
  secondary diabetes mellitus NEC — *see*
    Diabetes, specified type NEC
  specified type NEC E13.9
    with
      amyotrophy E13.44
      arthropathy NEC E13.618
      autonomic (poly) neuropathy E13.43
      cataract E13.36
      Charcot's joints E13.610
      chronic kidney disease E13.22
      circulatory complication NEC E13.59
      complication E13.8
        specified NEC E13.69
      dermatitis E13.620
      foot ulcer E13.621
      gangrene E13.52
      gastroparalysis E13.43
      gastroparesis E13.43
      glomerulonephrosis,
        intracapillary E13.21
      glomerulosclerosis,
        intercapillary E13.21
      hyperglycemia E13.65
      hyperosmolarity E13.00
        with coma E13.01
      hypoglycemia E13.649
        with coma E13.641
      ketoacidosis E13.10
        with coma E13.11
      kidney complications NEC E13.29
      Kimmelsteil-Wilson disease E13.21
      mononeuropathy E13.41
      myasthenia E13.44
      necrobiosis lipoidica E13.620
      nephropathy E13.21
      neuralgia E13.42
      neurologic complication NEC E13.49
      neuropathic arthropathy E13.610
      neuropathy E13.40
      ophthalmic complication NEC E13.39
      oral complication NEC E13.638
      periodontal disease E13.630
      peripheral angiopathy E13.51
        with gangrene E13.52
      polyneuropathy E13.42
      renal complication NEC E13.29
      renal tubular degeneration E13.29
      retinopathy E13.319
        with macular edema E13.311
        resolved following treatment E13.37
        nonproliferative E13.329
          with macular edema E13.321
          mild E13.329
            with macular edema E13.321
          moderate E13.339
            with macular edema E13.331
          severe E13.349
            with macular edema E13.341
        proliferative E13.359
          with

Diabetes, diabetic (mellitus) (sugar) - *continued*
  specified type NEC - *continued*
    with - *continued*
      retinopathy - *continued*
        proliferative - *continued*
          with - *continued*
            combined traction retinal
              detachment and
              rhegmatogenous retinal
              detachment
              E13.354
            macular edema E13.351
            stable proliferative diabetic
              retinopathy E13.355
            traction retinal detachment
              involving the
              macula E13.352
            traction retinal detachment not
              involving the
              macula E13.353
      skin complication NEC E13.628
      skin ulcer NEC E13.622
  steroid-induced — *see* Diabetes, due to, drug
    or chemical
  type 1 E10.9
    with
      amyotrophy E10.44
      arthropathy NEC E10.618
      autonomic (poly) neuropathy E10.43
      cataract E10.36
      Charcot's joints E10.610
      chronic kidney disease E10.22
      circulatory complication NEC E10.59
      complication E10.8
        specified NEC E10.69
      dermatitis E10.620
      foot ulcer E10.621
      gangrene E10.52
      gastroparalysis E10.43
      gastroparesis E10.43
      glomerulonephrosis,
        intracapillary E10.21
      glomerulosclerosis,
        intercapillary E10.21
      hyperglycemia E10.65
      hypoglycemia E10.649
        with coma E10.641
      ketoacidosis E10.10
        with coma E10.11
      kidney complications NEC E10.29
      Kimmelsteil-Wilson disease E10.21
      mononeuropathy E10.41
      myasthenia E10.44
      necrobiosis lipoidica E10.620
      nephropathy E10.21
      neuralgia E10.42
      neurologic complication NEC E10.49
      neuropathic arthropathy E10.610
      neuropathy E10.40
      ophthalmic complication NEC E10.39
      oral complication NEC E10.638
      osteomyelitis E10.69
      periodontal disease E10.630
      peripheral angiopathy E10.51
        with gangrene E10.52
      polyneuropathy E10.42
      renal complication NEC E10.29
      renal tubular degeneration E10.29
      retinopathy E10.319
        with macular edema E10.311
        resolved following treatment E10.37
        nonproliferative E10.329
          with macular edema E10.321
          mild E10.329
            with macular edema E10.321
          moderate E10.339
            with macular edema E10.331
          severe E10.349
            with macular edema E10.341
        proliferative E10.359
          with
            combined traction retinal
              detachment and
              rhegmatogenous retinal
              detachment E10.354

Diabetes, diabetic (mellitus) (sugar) - *continued*
  type 1 - *continued*
    with - *continued*
      retinopathy - *continued*
        proliferative - *continued*
          with - *continued*
            macular edema E10.351
            stable proliferative diabetic
              retinopathy E10.355
            traction retinal detachment
              involving the
              macula E10.352
            traction retinal detachment not
              involving the
              macula E10.353
      skin complication NEC E10.628
      skin ulcer NEC E10.622
  type 2 E11.9
    with
      amyotrophy E11.44
      arthropathy NEC E11.618
      autonomic (poly) neuropathy E11.43
      cataract E11.36
      Charcot's joints E11.610
      chronic kidney disease E11.22
      circulatory complication NEC E11.59
      complication E11.8
        specified NEC E11.69
      dermatitis E11.620
      foot ulcer E11.621
      gangrene E11.52
      gastroparalysis E11.43
      gastroparesis E11.43
      glomerulonephrosis,
        intracapillary E11.21
      glomerulosclerosis, intercapillary E11.21
      hyperglycemia E11.65
      hyperosmolarity E11.00
        with coma E11.01
      hypoglycemia E11.649
        with coma E11.641
      ketoacidosis E11.10
        with coma E11.11
      kidney complications NEC E11.29
      Kimmelstiel-Wilson disease E11.21
      mononeuropathy E11.41
      myasthenia E11.44
      necrobiosis lipoidica E11.620
      nephropathy E11.21
      neuralgia E11.42
      neurologic complication NEC E11.49
      neuropathic arthropathy E11.610
      neuropathy E11.40
      ophthalmic complication NEC E11.39
      oral complication NEC E11.638
      osteomyelitis E11.69
      periodontal disease E11.630
      peripheral angiopathy E11.51
        with gangrene E11.52
      polyneuropathy E11.42
      renal complication NEC E11.29
      renal tubular degeneration E11.29
      retinopathy E11.319
        with macular edema E11.311
        resolved following treatment E11.37
        nonproliferative E11.329
          with macular edema E11.321
          mild E11.329
            with macular edema E11.321
          moderate E11.339
            with macular edema E11.331
          severe E11.349
            with macular edema E11.341
        proliferative E11.359
          with
            combined traction retinal
              detachment and
              rhegmatogenous retinal
              detachment E11.354
            macular edema E11.351
            stable proliferative diabetic
              retinopathy E11.355

Diabetes, diabetic (mellitus) (sugar) - *continued*
  type 2 - *continued*
    with - *continued*
      retinopathy - *continued*
        proliferative - *continued*
          with - *continued*
            traction retinal detachment
              involving the
              macula E11.352
            traction retinal detachment not
              involving the
              macula E11.353
      skin complication NEC E11.628
      skin ulcer NEC E11.622
    uncontrolled
      meaning
        hyperglycemia — *see* Diabetes, by type,
          with, hyperglycemia
        hypoglycemia — *see* Diabetes, by type,
          with, hypoglycemia
Diacyclothrombopathia D69.1
Diagnosis deferred R69
Dialysis (intermittent) (treatment)
  noncompliance (with) Z91.15
  renal (hemodialysis) (peritoneal) ,
    status Z99.2
  retina, retinal — *see* Detachment, retina, with
    retinal, dialysis
Diamond-Blackfan anemia (congenital
  hypoplastic) D61.01
Diamond-Gardener syndrome
  (autoerythrocyte sensitization) D69.2
Diaper rash L22
Diaphoresis (excessive) R61
Diaphragm — *see* condition
Diaphragmalgia R07.1
Diaphragmatitis, diaphragmitis J98.6
Diaphysial aclasis Q78.6
Diaphysitis — *see* Osteomyelitis, specified
  type NEC
Diarrhea, diarrheal (disease) (infantile)
  (inflammatory) R19.7
  achlorhydric K31.83
  allergic K52.29
    due to
      colitis — *see* Colitis, allergic
      enteritis — *see* Enteritis, allergic
  amebic — *see also* Amebiasis A06.0
    with abscess — *see* Abscess, amebic
    acute A06.0
    chronic A06.1
    nondysenteric A06.2
  bacillary — *see* Dysentery, bacillary
  balantidial A07.0
  cachectic NEC K52.89
  Chilomastix A07.8
  choleriformis A00.1
  chronic (noninfectious) K52.9
  coccidial A07.3
  Cochin-China K90.1
    strongyloidiasis B78.0
  Dientamoeba A07.8
  dietetic — *see also* Diarrhea, allergic K52.29
  drug-induced K52.1
  due to
    bacteria A04.9
      specified NEC A04.8
    Campylobacter A04.5
    Capillaria philippinensis B81.1
    Clostridium difficile
      not specified as recurrent A04.72
      recurrent A04.71
    Clostridium perfringens (C) (F) A04.8
    Cryptosporidium A07.2
    drugs K52.1
    Escherichia coli A04.4
      enteroaggregative A04.4
      enterohemorrhagic A04.3
      enteroinvasive A04.2
      enteropathogenic A04.0
      enterotoxigenic A04.1
      specified NEC A04.4
    food hypersensitivity — *see also* Diarrhea,
      allergic K52.29

Diarrhea, diarrheal (disease) (infantile)
(inflammatory) - *continued*
  due to - *continued*
    Necator americanus B76.1
    S. japonicum B65.2
    specified organism NEC A08.8
      bacterial A04.8
      viral A08.39
    Staphylococcus A04.8
    Trichuris trichiuria B79
    virus — *see* Enteritis, viral
    Yersinia enterocolitica A04.6
  dysenteric A09
  endemic A09
  epidemic A09
  flagellate A07.9
  Flexner's (ulcerative) A03.1
  functional K59.1
    following gastrointestinal surgery K91.89
    psychogenic F45.8
  Giardia lamblia A07.1
  giardial A07.1
  hill K90.1
  infectious A09
  malarial — *see* Malaria
  mite B88.0
  mycotic NEC B49
  neonatal (noninfectious) P78.3
  nervous F45.8
  neurogenic K59.1
  noninfectious K52.9
  postgastrectomy K91.1
  postvagotomy K91.1
  protozoal A07.9
    specified NEC A07.8
  psychogenic F45.8
  specified
    bacterium NEC A04.8
    virus NEC A08.39
  strongyloidiasis B78.0
  toxic K52.1
  trichomonal A07.8
  tropical K90.1
  tuberculous A18.32
  viral — *see* Enteritis, viral
Diastasis
  cranial bones M84.88
    congenital NEC Q75.8
  joint (traumatic) — *see* Dislocation
  muscle M62.00
    ankle M62.07-
    congenital Q79.8
    foot M62.07-
    forearm M62.03-
    hand M62.04-
    lower leg M62.06-
    pelvic region M62.05-
    shoulder region M62.01-
    specified site NEC M62.08
    thigh M62.05-
    upper arm M62.02-
  recti (abdomen)
    complicating delivery O71.89
    congenital Q79.59
Diastema, tooth, teeth, fully erupted M26.32
Diastematomyelia Q06.2
Diataxia, cerebral G80.4
Diathesis
  allergic — *see* History, allergy
  bleeding (familial) D69.9
  cystine (familial) E72.00
  gouty — *see* Gout
  hemorrhagic (familial) D69.9
    newborn NEC P53
  spasmophilic R29.0
Diaz's disease or osteochondrosis (juvenile)
  (talus) — *see* Osteochondrosis, juvenile,
  tarsus
Dibothriocephalus, dibothriocephaliasis
  (latus) (infection) (infestation) B70.0
  larval B70.1
Dicephalus, dicephaly Q89.4
Dichotomy, teeth K00.2

Dichromat, dichromatopsia (congenital) — *see* Deficiency, color vision
Dichuchwa A65
Dicroceliasis B66.2
Didelphia, didelphys — *see* Double uterus
Didymytis N45.1
  with orchitis N45.3
Dietary
  inadequacy or deficiency E63.9
  surveillance and counseling Z71.3
Dietl's crisis N13.8
Dieulafoy lesion (hemorrhagic)
  duodenum K31.82
  esophagus K22.8
  intestine (colon) K63.81
  stomach K31.82
Difficult, difficulty (in)
  acculturation Z60.3
  feeding R63.3
    newborn P92.9
      breast P92.5
      specified NEC P92.8
    nonorganic (infant or child) F98.29
  intubation, in anesthesia T88.4
  mechanical, gastroduodenal stoma K91.89
    causing obstruction — *see also*
      Obstruction, intestine,
      postoperative K91.30
  micturition
    need to immediately re-void R39.191
    position dependent R39.192
    specified NEC R39.198
  reading (developmental) F81.0
    secondary to emotional disorders F93.9
  spelling (specific) F81.81
    with reading disorder F81.89
    due to inadequate teaching Z55.8
  swallowing — *see* Dysphagia
  walking R26.2
  work
    conditions NEC Z56.5
    schedule Z56.3
Diffuse — *see* condition
DiGeorge's syndrome (thymic hypoplasia) D82.1
Digestive — *see* condition
Dihydropyrimidine dehydrogenase disease (DPD) E88.89
Diktyoma — *see* Neoplasm, malignant, by site
Dilaceration, tooth K00.4
Dilatation
  anus K59.8
    venule — *see* Hemorrhoids
  aorta (focal) (general) — *see* Ectasia, aorta
    with aneurysm — *see* Aneurysm, aorta
    congenital Q25.44
  artery — *see* Aneurysm
  bladder (sphincter) N32.89
    congenital Q64.79
  blood vessel I99.8
  bronchial J47.9
    with
      exacerbation (acute) J47.1
      lower respiratory infection J47.0
  calyx (due to obstruction) — *see* Hydronephrosis
  capillaries I78.8
  cardiac (acute) (chronic) — *see also* Hypertrophy, cardiac
    congenital Q24.8
      valve NEC Q24.8
        pulmonary Q22.3
    valve — *see* Endocarditis
  cavum septi pellucidi Q06.8
  cervix (uteri) — *see also* Incompetency, cervix
    incomplete, poor, slow complicating delivery O62.0
  colon K59.39
    congenital Q43.1
    psychogenic F45.8
    toxic K59.31
  common duct (acquired) K83.8
    congenital Q44.5

Dilatation - *continued*
  cystic duct (acquired) K82.8
    congenital Q44.5
  duct, mammary — *see* Ectasia, mammary duct
  duodenum K59.8
  esophagus K22.8
    congenital Q39.5
    due to achalasia K22.0
  eustachian tube, congenital Q17.8
  gallbladder K82.8
  gastric — *see* Dilatation, stomach
  heart (acute) (chronic) — *see also* Hypertrophy, cardiac
    congenital Q24.8
    valve — *see* Endocarditis
  ileum K59.8
    psychogenic F45.8
  jejunum K59.8
    psychogenic F45.8
  kidney (calyx) (collecting structures) (cystic) (parenchyma) (pelvis) (idiopathic) N28.89
  lacrimal passages or duct — *see* Disorder, lacrimal system, changes
  lymphatic vessel I89.0
  mammary duct — *see* Ectasia, mammary duct
  Meckel's diverticulum (congenital) Q43.0
    malignant — *see* Table of Neoplasms, small intestine, malignant
  myocardium (acute) (chronic) — *see* Hypertrophy, cardiac
  organ or site, congenital NEC — *see* Distortion
  pancreatic duct K86.89
  pericardium — *see* Pericarditis
  pharynx J39.2
  prostate N42.89
  pulmonary
    artery (idiopathic) I28.8
    valve, congenital Q22.3
  pupil H57.04
  rectum K59.39
  saccule, congenital Q16.5
  salivary gland (duct) K11.8
  sphincter ani K62.89
  stomach K31.89
    acute K31.0
    psychogenic F45.8
  submaxillary duct K11.8
  trachea, congenital Q32.1
  ureter (idiopathic) N28.82
    congenital Q62.2
    due to obstruction N13.4
  urethra (acquired) N36.8
  vasomotor I73.9
  vein I86.8
  ventricular, ventricle (acute) (chronic) — *see also* Hypertrophy, cardiac
    cerebral, congenital Q04.8
  venule NEC I86.8
  vesical orifice N32.89
Dilated, dilation — *see* Dilatation
Diminished, diminution
  hearing (acuity) — *see* Deafness
  sense or sensation (cold) (heat) (tactile) (vibratory) R20.8
  vision NEC H54.7
  vital capacity R94.2
Diminuta taenia B71.0
Dimitri-Sturge-Weber disease Q85.8
Dimple
  congenital sacral Q82.6
  parasacral Q82.6
  pilonidal or postanal — *see* Cyst, pilonidal
Dioctophyme renalis (infection) (infestation) B83.8
Dipetalonemiasis B74.4
Diphallus Q55.69
Diphtheria, diphtheritic (gangrenous) (hemorrhagic) A36.9
  carrier (suspected) Z22.2
  cutaneous A36.3
  faucial A36.0

Diphtheria, diphtheritic (gangrenous) (hemorrhagic) - *continued*
  infection of wound A36.3
  laryngeal A36.2
  myocarditis A36.81
  nasal, anterior A36.89
  nasopharyngeal A36.1
  neurological complication A36.89
  pharyngeal A36.0
  specified site NEC A36.89
  tonsillar A36.0
Diphyllobothriasis (intestine) B70.0
  larval B70.1
Diplacusis H93.22-
Diplegia (upper limbs) G83.0
  congenital (cerebral) G80.8
  facial G51.0
  lower limbs G82.20
  spastic G80.1
Diplococcus, diplococcal — *see* condition
Diplopia H53.2
Dipsomania F10.20
  with
    psychosis — *see* Psychosis, alcoholic
    remission F10.21
Dipylidiasis B71.1
DIRA (deficiency of interleukin 1 receptor antagonist) M04.8
Direction, teeth, abnormal, fully erupted M26.30
Dirofilariasis B74.8
Dirt-eating child F98.3
Disability, disabilities
  heart — *see* Disease, heart
  intellectual F79
    with
      autistic features F84.9
    mild (I.Q.50-69) F70
    moderate (I.Q.35-49) F71
    profound (I.Q. under 20) F73
    severe (I.Q.20-34) F72
    specified level NEC F78
  knowledge acquisition F81.9
  learning F81.9
  limiting activities Z73.6
  spelling, specific F81.81
Disappearance of family member Z63.4
Disarticulation — *see* Amputation
  meaning traumatic amputation — *see* Amputation, traumatic
Discharge (from)
  abnormal finding in — *see* Abnormal, specimen
  breast (female) (male) N64.52
  diencephalic autonomic idiopathic — *see* Epilepsy, specified NEC
  ear — *see also* Otorrhea
    blood — *see* Otorrhagia
  excessive urine R35.8
  nipple N64.52
  penile R36.9
  postnasal R09.82
  prison, anxiety concerning Z65.2
  urethral R36.9
    without blood R36.0
    hematospermia R36.1
  vaginal N89.8
Discitis, diskitis M46.40
  cervical region M46.42
  cervicothoracic region M46.43
  lumbar region M46.46
  lumbosacral region M46.47
  multiple sites M46.49
  occipito-atlanto-axial region M46.41
  pyogenic — *see* Infection, intervertebral disc, pyogenic
  sacrococcygeal region M46.48
  thoracic region M46.44
  thoracolumbar region M46.45
Discoid
  meniscus (congenital) Q68.6
  semilunar cartilage (congenital) — *see* Derangement, knee, meniscus, specified NEC

Discoloration
  nails L60.8
  teeth (posteruptive) K03.7
    during formation K00.8
Discomfort
  chest R07.89
  visual H53.14-
Discontinuity, ossicles, ear H74.2-
Discord (with)
  boss Z56.4
  classmates Z55.4
  counselor Z64.4
  employer Z56.4
  family Z63.8
  fellow employees Z56.4
  in-laws Z63.1
  landlord Z59.2
  lodgers Z59.2
  neighbors Z59.2
  probation officer Z64.4
  social worker Z64.4
  teachers Z55.4
  workmates Z56.4
Discordant connection
  atrioventricular (congenital) Q20.5
  ventriculoarterial Q20.3
Discrepancy
  centric occlusion maximum
    intercuspation M26.55
  leg length (acquired) — *see* Deformity, limb,
    unequal length
    congenital — *see* Defect, reduction, lower
      limb
  uterine size date O26.84-
Discrimination
  ethnic Z60.5
  political Z60.5
  racial Z60.5
  religious Z60.5
  sex Z60.5
Disease, diseased — *see also* Syndrome
  absorbent system I87.8
  acid-peptic K30
  Acosta's T70.29
  Adams-Stokes (-Morgagni) (syncope with
    heart block) I45.9
  Addison's anemia (pernicious) D51.0
  adenoids (and tonsils) J35.9
  adrenal (capsule) (cortex) (gland)
    (medullary) E27.9
    hyperfunction E27.0
    specified NEC E27.8
  ainhum L94.6
  airway
    obstructive, chronic J44.9
      due to
        cotton dust J66.0
        specific organic dusts NEC J66.8
    reactive — *see* Asthma
  akamushi (scrub typhus) A75.3
  Albers-Schönberg (marble bones) Q78.2
  Albert's — *see* Tendinitis, Achilles
  alimentary canal K63.9
  alligator-skin Q80.9
    acquired L85.0
  alpha heavy chain C88.3
  alpine T70.29
  altitude T70.20
  alveolar ridge
    edentulous K06.9
      specified NEC K06.8
  alveoli, teeth K08.9
  Alzheimer's G30.9 *[F02.80]*
    with behavioral disturbance G30.9
      [F02.81]
    early onset G30.0 *[F02.80]*
      with behavioral disturbance G30.0
        [F02.81]
    late onset G30.1 *[F02.80]*
      with behavioral disturbance G30.1
        [F02.81]
    specified NEC G30.8 *[F02.80]*
      with behavioral disturbance G30.8
        [F02.81]
  amyloid — *see* Amyloidosis

Disease, diseased - *continued*
  Andersen's (glycogenosis IV) E74.09
  Andes T70.29
  Andrews' (bacterid) L08.89
  angiospastic I73.9
    cerebral G45.9
    vein I87.8
  anterior
    chamber H21.9
    horn cell G12.29
  antiglomerular basement membrane (anti-
    GBM) antibody M31.0
    tubulo-interstitial nephritis N12
  antral — *see* Sinusitis, maxillary
  anus K62.9
    specified NEC K62.89
  aorta (nonsyphilitic) I77.9
    syphilitic NEC A52.02
  aortic (heart) (valve) I35.9
    rheumatic I06.9
  Apollo B30.3
  aponeuroses — *see* Enthesopathy
  appendix K38.9
    specified NEC K38.8
  aqueous (chamber) H21.9
  Arnold-Chiari — *see* Arnold-Chiari disease
  arterial I77.9
    occlusive — *see* Occlusion, by site
    due to stricture or stenosis I77.1
    peripheral I73.9
  arteriocardiorenal — *see* Hypertension,
    cardiorenal
  arteriolar (generalized) (obliterative) I77.9
  arteriorenal — *see* Hypertension, kidney
  arteriosclerotic — *see also* Arteriosclerosis
    cardiovascular — *see* Disease, heart,
      ischemic, atherosclerotic
    coronary (artery) — *see* Disease, heart,
      ischemic, atherosclerotic
    heart — *see* Disease, heart, ischemic,
      atherosclerotic
  artery I77.9
    cerebral I67.9
    coronary I25.10
      with angina pectoris — *see*
        Arteriosclerosis, coronary (artery)
    peripheral I73.9
  arthropod-borne NOS (viral) A94
    specified type NEC A93.8
  atticoantral, chronic H66.20
    left H66.22
      with right H66.23
    right H66.21
      with left H66.23
  auditory canal — *see* Disorder, ear, external
  auricle, ear NEC — *see* Disorder, pinna
  Australian X A83.4
  autoimmune (systemic) NOS M35.9
    hemolytic (cold type) (warm type) D59.1
      drug-induced D59.0
    thyroid E06.3
  autoinflammatory M04.9
    NOD2-associated M04.8
    specified type NEC M04.8
  aviator's — *see* Effect, adverse, high altitude
  Ayerza's (pulmonary artery sclerosis with
    pulmonary hypertension) I27.0
  Babington's (familial hemorrhagic
    telangiectasia) I78.0
  bacterial A49.9
    specified NEC A48.8
    zoonotic A28.9
      specified type NEC A28.8
  Baelz's (cheilitis glandularis
    apostematosa) K13.0
  bagasse J67.1
  balloon — *see* Effect, adverse, high altitude
  Bang's (brucella abortus) A23.1
  Bannister's T78.3
  barometer makers' — *see* Poisoning, mercury
  Barraquer (-Simons') (progressive
    lipodystrophy) E88.1
  Barrett's — *see* Barrett's, esophagus
  Bartholin's gland N75.9
  basal ganglia G25.9

Disease, diseased - *continued*
  basal ganglia - *continued*
    degenerative G23.9
      specified NEC G23.8
    specified NEC G25.89
  Basedow's (exophthalmic goiter) — *see*
    Hyperthyroidism, with, goiter (diffuse)
  Bateman's B08.1
  Batten-Steinert G71.11
  Battey A31.0
  Beard's (neurasthenia) F48.8
  Becker
    idiopathic mural endomyocardial I42.3
    myotonia congenita G71.12
  Begbie's (exophthalmic goiter) — *see*
    Hyperthyroidism, with, goiter (diffuse)
  behavioral, organic F07.9
  Beigel's (white piedra) B36.2
  Benson's — *see* Deposit, crystalline
  Bernard-Soulier (thrombopathy) D69.1
  Bernhardt (-Roth) — *see* Mononeuropathy,
    lower limb, meralgia paresthetica
  Biermer's (pernicious anemia) D51.0
  bile duct (common) (hepatic) K83.9
    with calculus, stones — *see* Calculus, bile
      duct
    specified NEC K83.8
  biliary (tract) K83.9
    specified NEC K83.8
  Billroth's — *see* Spina bifida
  bird fancier's J67.2
  black lung J60
  bladder N32.9
    in (due to)
      schistosomiasis (bilharziasis) B65.0
        [N33]
    specified NEC N32.89
  bleeder's D66
  blood D75.9
    forming organs D75.9
    vessel I99.9
  Bloodgood's — *see* Mastopathy, cystic
  Bodechtel-Guttmann (subacute sclerosing
    panencephalitis) A81.1
  bone — *see also* Disorder, bone
    aluminum M83.4
    fibrocystic NEC
      jaw M27.49
  bone-marrow D75.9
  Borna A83.9
  Bornholm (epidemic pleurodynia) B33.0
  Bouchard's (myopathic dilatation of the
    stomach) K31.0
  Bouillaud's (rheumatic heart disease) I01.9
  Bourneville (-Brissaud) (tuberous
    sclerosis) Q85.1
  Bouveret (-Hoffmann) (paroxysmal
    tachycardia) I47.9
  bowel K63.9
    functional K59.9
    psychogenic F45.8
  brain G93.9
    arterial, artery I67.9
    arteriosclerotic I67.2
    congenital Q04.9
    degenerative — *see* Degeneration, brain
    inflammatory — *see* Encephalitis
    organic G93.9
      arteriosclerotic I67.2
    parasitic NEC B71.9 *[G94]*
    senile NEC G31.1
    specified NEC G93.89
  breast — *see also* Disorder, breast N64.9
    cystic (chronic) — *see* Mastopathy, cystic
    fibrocystic — *see* Mastopathy, cystic
    Paget's
      female, unspecified side C50.91-
      male, unspecified side C50.92-
    specified NEC N64.89
  Breda's — *see* Yaws
  Bretonneau's (diphtheritic malignant
    angina) A36.0
  Bright's — *see* Nephritis
    arteriosclerotic — *see* Hypertension,
      kidney

Disease, diseased - *continued*
Brill's (recrudescent typhus) A75.1
Brill-Zinsser (recrudescent typhus) A75.1
Brion-Kayser — *see* Fever, paratyphoid
broad
  beta E78.2
  ligament (noninflammatory) N83.9
    inflammatory — *see* Disease, pelvis, inflammatory
    specified NEC N83.8
Brocq-Duhring (dermatitis herpetiformis) L13.0
Brocq's
  meaning
    dermatitis herpetiformis L13.0
    prurigo L28.2
bronchopulmonary J98.4
bronchus NEC J98.09
bronze Addison's E27.1
  tuberculous A18.7
budgerigar fancier's J67.2
bullous L13.9
  chronic of childhood L12.2
  specified NEC L13.8
Buerger's (thromboangiitis obliterans) I73.1
Bürger-Grütz (essential familial hyperlipemia) E78.3
bursa — *see* Bursopathy
caisson T70.3
California — *see* Coccidioidomycosis
capillaries I78.9
  specified NEC I78.8
Carapata A68.0
cardiac — *see* Disease, heart
cardiopulmonary, chronic I27.9
cardiorenal (hepatic) (hypertensive) (vascular) — *see* Hypertension, cardiorenal
cardiovascular (atherosclerotic) I25.10
  with angina pectoris — *see* Arteriosclerosis, coronary (artery),
  congenital Q28.9
  newborn P29.9
    specified NEC P29.89
  hypertensive — *see* Hypertension, heart
  renal (hypertensive) — *see* Hypertension, cardiorenal
  syphilitic (asymptomatic) A52.00
cartilage — *see* Disorder, cartilage
Castellani's A69.8
Castleman (unicentric) (multicentric) D47.Z2
  HHV-8-associated — *see also* Herpesvirus, human, 8 D47.Z2
cat-scratch A28.1
Cavare's (familial periodic paralysis) G72.3
cecum K63.9
celiac (adult) (infantile) (with steatorrhea) K90.0
cellular tissue L98.9
central core G71.2
cerebellar, cerebellum — *see* Disease, brain
cerebral — *see also* Disease, brain
  degenerative — *see* Degeneration, brain
cerebrospinal G96.9
cerebrovascular I67.9
  acute I67.89
    embolic I63.4-
    thrombotic I63.3-
  arteriosclerotic I67.2
  hereditary NEC I67.858
  specified NEC I67.89
cervix (uteri) (noninflammatory) N88.9
  inflammatory — *see* Cervicitis
  specified NEC N88.8
Chabert's A22.9
Chandler's (osteochondritis dissecans, hip) — *see* Osteochondritis, dissecans, hip
Charlouis — *see* Yaws
Chédiak-Steinbrinck (-Higashi) (congenital gigantism of peroxidase granules) E70.330
chest J98.9
Chiari's (hepatic vein thrombosis) I82.0
Chicago B40.9

Disease, diseased - *continued*
Chignon B36.8
chigo, chigoe B88.1
childhood granulomatous D71
Chinese liver fluke B66.1
chlamydial A74.9
  specified NEC A74.89
cholecystic K82.9
choroid H31.9
  specified NEC H31.8
Christmas D67
chronic bullous of childhood L12.2
chylomicron retention E78.3
ciliary body H21.9
  specified NEC H21.89
circulatory (system) NEC I99.8
  newborn P29.9
  syphilitic A52.00
    congenital A50.54
coagulation factor deficiency (congenital) — *see* Defect, coagulation
coccidioidal — *see* Coccidioidomycosis
cold
  agglutinin or hemoglobinuria D59.1
    paroxysmal D59.6
  hemagglutinin (chronic) D59.1
collagen NOS (nonvascular) (vascular) M35.9
  specified NEC M35.8
colon K63.9
  functional K59.9
    congenital Q43.2
  ischemic — *see also* Ischemia, intestine, acute K55.039
colonic inflammatory bowel, unclassified (IBDU) K52.3
combined system — *see* Degeneration, combined
compressed air T70.3
Concato's (pericardial polyserositis) A19.9
  nontubercular I31.1
  pleural — *see* Pleurisy, with effusion
conjunctiva H11.9
  chlamydial A74.0
  specified NEC H11.89
  viral B30.9
    specified NEC B30.8
connective tissue, systemic (diffuse) M35.9
  in (due to)
    hypogammaglobulinemia D80.1 [M36.8]
    ochronosis E70.29 [M36.8]
  specified NEC M35.8
Conor and Bruch's (boutonneuse fever) A77.1
Cooper's — *see* Mastopathy, cystic
Cori's (glycogenosis III) E74.03
corkhandler's or corkworker's J67.3
cornea H18.9
  specified NEC H18.89-
coronary (artery) — *see* Disease, heart, ischemic, atherosclerotic
  congenital Q24.5
  ostial, syphilitic (aortic) (mitral) (pulmonary) A52.03
corpus cavernosum N48.9
  specified NEC N48.89
Cotugno's — *see* Sciatica
coxsackie (virus) NEC B34.1
cranial nerve NOS G52.9
Creutzfeldt-Jakob — *see* Creutzfeldt-Jakob disease or syndrome
Crocq's (acrocyanosis) I73.89
Crohn's — *see* Enteritis, regional
Curschmann G71.11
cystic
  breast (chronic) — *see* Mastopathy, cystic
  kidney, congenital Q61.9
  liver, congenital Q44.6
  lung J98.4
    congenital Q33.0
cytomegalic inclusion (generalized) B25.9
  with pneumonia B25.0
  congenital P35.1
cytomegaloviral B25.9

Disease, diseased - *continued*
cytomegaloviral - *continued*
  specified NEC B25.8
Czerny's (periodic hydrarthrosis of the knee) — *see* Effusion, joint, knee
Daae (-Finsen) (epidemic pleurodynia) B33.0
Darling's — *see* Histoplasmosis capsulati
Débove's (splenomegaly) R16.1
deer fly — *see* Tularemia
Degos' I77.89
demyelinating, demyelinizating (nervous system) G37.9
  multiple sclerosis G35
  specified NEC G37.8
dense deposit — *see also* N00-N07 with fourth character .6 N05.6
deposition, hydroxyapatite — *see* Disease, hydroxyapatite deposition
de Quervain's (tendon sheath) M65.4
  thyroid (subacute granulomatous thyroiditis) E06.1
Devergie's (pityriasis rubra pilaris) L44.0
Devic's G36.0
diaphorase deficiency D74.0
diaphragm J98.6
diarrheal, infectious NEC A09
digestive system K92.9
  specified NEC K92.89
disc, degenerative — *see* Degeneration, intervertebral disc
discogenic — *see also* Displacement, intervertebral disc NEC
  with myelopathy — *see* Disorder, disc, with, myelopathy
diverticular — *see* Diverticula
Dubois (thymus) A50.59 *[E35]*
Duchenne-Griesinger G71.01
Duchenne's
  muscular dystrophy G71.01
  pseudohypertrophy, muscles G71.01
ductless glands E34.9
Duhring's (dermatitis herpetiformis) L13.0
duodenum K31.9
  specified NEC K31.89
Dupré's (meningism) R29.1
Dupuytren's (muscle contracture) M72.0
Durand-Nicholas-Favre (climatic bubo) A55
Duroziez's (congenital mitral stenosis) Q23.2
ear — *see* Disorder, ear
Eberth's — *see* Fever, typhoid
Ebola (virus) A98.4
Ebstein's heart Q22.5
Echinococcus — *see* Echinococcus
echovirus NEC B34.1
Eddowes' (brittle bones and blue sclera) Q78.0
edentulous (alveolar) ridge K06.9
  specified NEC K06.8
Edsall's T67.2
Eichstedt's (pityriasis versicolor) B36.0
Eisenmenger's (irreversible) I27.83
Ellis-van Creveld (chondroectodermal dysplasia) Q77.6
end stage renal (ESRD) N18.6
  due to hypertension I12.0
endocrine glands or system NEC E34.9
endomyocardial (eosinophilic) I42.3
English (rickets) E55.0
enteroviral, enterovirus NEC B34.1
  central nervous system NEC A88.8
epidemic B99.9
  specified NEC B99.8
epididymis N50.9
Erb (-Landouzy) G71.02
Erdheim-Chester (ECD) E88.89
esophagus K22.9
  functional K22.4
  psychogenic F45.8
  specified NEC K22.8
Eulenburg's (congenital paramyotonia) G71.19
eustachian tube — *see* Disorder, eustachian tube
external

Disease, diseased - *continued*
- external - *continued*
  - auditory canal — *see* Disorder, ear, external
  - ear — *see* Disorder, ear, external
- extrapyramidal G25.9
  - specified NEC G25.89
- eye H57.9
  - anterior chamber H21.9
  - inflammatory NEC H57.89
  - muscle (external) — *see* Strabismus
  - specified NEC H57.89
  - syphilitic — *see* Oculopathy, syphilitic
- eyeball H44.9
  - specified NEC H44.89
- eyelid — *see* Disorder, eyelid
  - specified NEC — *see* Disorder, eyelid, specified type NEC
- eyeworm of Africa B74.3
- facial nerve (seventh) G51.9
  - newborn (birth injury) P11.3
- Fahr (of brain) G23.8
- Fahr Volhard (of kidney) I12.-
- fallopian tube (noninflammatory) N83.9
  - inflammatory — *see* Salpingo-oophoritis
  - specified NEC N83.8
- familial periodic paralysis G72.3
- Fanconi's (congenital pancytopenia) D61.09
- fascia NEC — *see also* Disorder, muscle
  - inflammatory — *see* Myositis
  - specified NEC M62.89
- Fauchard's (periodontitis) — *see* Periodontitis
- Favre-Durand-Nicolas (climatic bubo) A55
- Fede's K14.0
- Feer's — *see* Poisoning, mercury
- female pelvic inflammatory — *see also* Disease, pelvis, inflammatory N73.9
  - syphilitic (secondary) A51.42
  - tuberculous A18.17
- Fernels' (aortic aneurysm) I71.9
- fibrocaseous of lung — *see* Tuberculosis, pulmonary
- fibrocystic — *see* Fibrocystic disease
- Fiedler's (leptospiral jaundice) A27.0
- fifth B08.3
- file-cutter's — *see* Poisoning, lead
- fish-skin Q80.9
  - acquired L85.0
- Flajani (-Basedow) (exophthalmic goiter) — *see* Hyperthyroidism, with, goiter (diffuse)
- flax-dresser's J66.1
- fluke — *see* Infestation, fluke
- foot and mouth B08.8
- foot process N04.9
- Forbes' (glycogenosis III) E74.03
- Fordyce-Fox (apocrine miliaria) L75.2
- Fordyce's (ectopic sebaceous glands) (mouth) Q38.6
- Forestier's (rhizomelic pseudopolyarthritis) M35.3
  - meaning ankylosing hyperostosis — *see* Hyperostosis, ankylosing
- Fothergill's
  - neuralgia — *see* Neuralgia, trigeminal
  - scarlatina anginosa A38.9
- Fournier (gangrene) N49.3
  - female N76.89
- fourth B08.8
- Fox (-Fordyce) (apocrine miliaria) L75.2
- Francis' — *see* Tularemia
- Franklin C88.2
- Frei's (climatic bubo) A55
- Friedreich's
  - combined systemic or ataxia G11.1
  - myoclonia G25.3
- frontal sinus — *see* Sinusitis, frontal
- fungus NEC B49
- Gaisböck's (polycythemia hypertonica) D75.1
- gallbladder K82.9
  - calculus — *see* Calculus, gallbladder
  - cholecystitis — *see* Cholecystitis
  - cholesterolosis K82.4

Disease, diseased - *continued*
- gallbladder - *continued*
  - fistula — *see* Fistula, gallbladder
  - hydrops K82.1
  - obstruction — *see* Obstruction, gallbladder
  - perforation K82.2
  - specified NEC K82.8
- gamma heavy chain C88.2
- Gamna's (siderotic splenomegaly) D73.2
- Gamstorp's (adynamia episodica hereditaria) G72.3
- Gandy-Nanta (siderotic splenomegaly) D73.2
- ganister J62.8
- gastric — *see* Disease, stomach
- gastroesophageal reflux (GERD) K21.9
  - with esophagitis K21.0
- gastrointestinal (tract) K92.9
  - amyloid E85.4
  - functional K59.9
    - psychogenic F45.8
  - specified NEC K92.89
- Gee (-Herter) (-Heubner) (-Thaysen) (nontropical sprue) K90.0
- genital organs
  - female N94.9
  - male N50.9
- Gerhardt's (erythromelalgia) I73.81
- Gibert's (pityriasis rosea) L42
- Gierke's (glycogenosis I) E74.01
- Gilles de la Tourette's (motor-verbal tic) F95.2
- gingiva K06.9
  - plaque induced K05.00
  - specified NEC K06.8
- gland (lymph) I89.9
- Glanzmann's (hereditary hemorrhagic thrombasthenia) D69.1
- glass-blower's (cataract) — *see* Cataract, specified NEC
  - salivary gland hypertrophy K11.1
- Glisson's — *see* Rickets
- globe H44.9
  - specified NEC H44.89
- glomerular — *see also* Glomerulonephritis
  - with edema — *see* Nephrosis
  - acute — *see* Nephritis, acute
  - chronic — *see* Nephritis, chronic
  - minimal change N05.0
  - rapidly progressive N01.9
- glycogen storage E74.00
  - Andersen's E74.09
  - Cori's E74.03
  - Forbes' E74.03
  - generalized E74.00
  - glucose-6-phosphatase deficiency E74.01
  - heart E74.02 *[I43]*
  - hepatorenal E74.09
  - Hers' E74.09
  - liver and kidney E74.09
  - McArdle's E74.04
  - muscle phosphofructokinase E74.09
  - myocardium E74.02 *[I43]*
  - Pompe's E74.02
  - Tauri's E74.09
  - type 0 E74.09
  - type I E74.01
  - type II E74.02
  - type III E74.03
  - type IV E74.09
  - type V E74.04
  - type VI-XI E74.09
  - Von Gierke's E74.01
- Goldstein's (familial hemorrhagic telangiectasia) I78.0
- gonococcal NOS A54.9
- graft-versus-host (GVH) D89.813
  - acute D89.810
  - acute on chronic D89.812
  - chronic D89.811
- grainhandler's J67.8
- granulomatous (childhood) (chronic) D71
- Graves' (exophthalmic goiter) — *see* Hyperthyroidism, with, goiter (diffuse)
- Griesinger's — *see* Ancylostomiasis
- Grisel's M43.6

Disease, diseased - *continued*
- Gruby's (tinea tonsurans) B35.0
- Guillain-Barré G61.0
- Guinon's (motor-verbal tic) F95.2
- gum K06.9
- gynecological N94.9
- H (Hartnup's) E72.02
- Haff — *see* Poisoning, mercury
- Hageman (congenital factor XII deficiency) D68.2
- hair (color) (shaft) L67.9
  - follicles L73.9
    - specified NEC L73.8
- Hamman's (spontaneous mediastinal emphysema) J98.2
- hand, foot and mouth B08.4
- Hansen's — *see* Leprosy
- Hantavirus, with pulmonary manifestations B33.4
  - with renal manifestations A98.5
- Harada's H30.81-
- Hartnup (pellagra-cerebellar ataxia-renal aminoaciduria) E72.02
- Hart's (pellagra-cerebellar ataxia-renal aminoaciduria) E72.02
- Hashimoto's (struma lymphomatosa) E06.3
- Hb — *see* Disease, hemoglobin
- heart (organic) I51.9
  - with
    - pulmonary edema (acute) — *see also* Failure, ventricular, left I50.1
    - rheumatic fever (conditions in I00)
      - active I01.9
        - with chorea I02.0
        - specified NEC I01.8
      - inactive or quiescent (with chorea) I09.9
        - specified NEC I09.89
  - amyloid E85.4 *[I43]*
  - aortic (valve) I35.9
  - arteriosclerotic or sclerotic (senile) — *see* Disease, heart, ischemic, atherosclerotic
  - artery, arterial — *see* Disease, heart, ischemic, atherosclerotic
  - beer drinkers' I42.6
  - beriberi (wet) E51.12
  - black I27.0
  - congenital Q24.9
    - cyanotic Q24.9
    - specified NEC Q24.8
  - coronary — *see* Disease, heart, ischemic
  - cryptogenic I51.9
  - fibroid — *see* Myocarditis
  - functional I51.89
    - psychogenic F45.8
  - glycogen storage E74.02 *[I43]*
  - gonococcal A54.83
  - hypertensive — *see* Hypertension, heart
  - hyperthyroid — *see also* Hyperthyroidism E05.90 *[I43]*
    - with thyroid storm E05.91 *[I43]*
  - ischemic (chronic or with a stated duration of over 4 weeks) I25.9
    - atherosclerotic (of) I25.10
      - with angina pectoris — *see* Arteriosclerosis, coronary (artery)
      - coronary artery bypass graft — *see* Arteriosclerosis, coronary (artery),
      - cardiomyopathy I25.5
    - diagnosed on ECG or other special investigation, but currently presenting no symptoms I25.6
    - silent I25.6
    - specified form NEC I25.89
  - kyphoscoliotic I27.1
  - meningococcal A39.50
    - endocarditis A39.51
    - myocarditis A39.52
    - pericarditis A39.53
  - mitral I05.9
    - specified NEC I05.8
  - muscular — *see* Degeneration, myocardial

Disease, diseased - *continued*
  heart (organic) - *continued*
    psychogenic (functional) F45.8
    pulmonary (chronic) I27.9
      in schistosomiasis B65.9 *[152]*
      specified NEC I27.89
    rheumatic (chronic) (inactive) (old)
        (quiescent) (with chorea) I09.9
      active or acute I01.9
        with chorea (acute) (rheumatic)
          (Sydenham's) I02.0
      specified NEC I09.89
    senile — *see* Myocarditis
    syphilitic A52.06
      aortic A52.03
        aneurysm A52.01
      congenital A50.54 *[152]*
    thyrotoxic — *see also*
        Thyrotoxicosis E05.90 *[143]*
      with thyroid storm E05.91 *[143]*
    valve, valvular (obstructive)
        (regurgitant) — *see also* Endocarditis
      congenital NEC Q24.8
        pulmonary Q22.3
    vascular — *see* Disease, cardiovascular
  heavy chain NEC C88.2
    alpha C88.3
    gamma C88.2
    mu C88.2
  Hebra's
    pityriasis
      maculata et circinata L42
      rubra pilaris L44.0
    prurigo L28.2
  hematopoietic organs D75.9
  hemoglobin or Hb
    abnormal (mixed) NEC D58.2
      with thalassemia D56.9
    AS genotype D57.3
    Bart's D56.0
    C (Hb-C) D58.2
      with other abnormal hemoglobin
        NEC D58.2
      elliptocytosis D58.1
      Hb-S D57.2-
      sickle-cell D57.2-
      thalassemia D56.8
    Constant Spring D58.2
    D (Hb-D) D58.2
    E (Hb-E) D58.2
    E-beta thalassemia D56.5
    elliptocytosis D58.1
    H (Hb-H) (thalassemia) D56.0
      with other abnormal hemoglobin
        NEC D56.9
      Constant Spring D56.0
    I thalassemia D56.9
    M D74.0
    S or SS D57.1
    SC D57.2-
    SD D57.8-
    SE D57.8-
    spherocytosis D58.0
    unstable, hemolytic D58.2
  hemolytic (newborn) P55.9
    autoimmune (cold type) (warm
        type) D59.1
    drug-induced D59.0
    due to or with
      incompatibility
        ABO (blood group) P55.1
        blood (group) (Duffy) (K) (Kell)
          (Kidd) (Lewis) (M) (S)
          NEC P55.8
        Rh (blood group) (factor) P55.0
      Rh negative mother P55.0
    specified type NEC P55.8
    unstable hemoglobin D58.2
  hemorrhagic D69.9
    newborn P53
  Henoch (-Schönlein) (purpura
      nervosa) D69.0
  hepatic — *see* Disease, liver
  hepatobiliary K83.9
    toxic K71.9

Disease, diseased - *continued*
  hepatolenticular E83.01
  heredodegenerative NEC
    spinal cord G95.89
  herpesviral, disseminated B00.7
  Hers' (glycogenosis VI) E74.09
  Herter (-Gee) (-Heubner) (nontropical
      sprue) K90.0
  Heubner-Herter (nontropical sprue) K90.0
  high fetal gene or hemoglobin
      thalassemia D56.9
  Hildenbrand's — *see* Typhus
  hip (joint) M25.9
    congenital Q65.89
    suppurative M00.9
    tuberculous A18.02
  His (-Werner) (trench fever) A79.0
  Hodgson's I71.2
    ruptured I71.1
  Holla — *see* Spherocytosis
  hookworm B76.9
    specified NEC B76.8
  host-versus-graft D89.813
    acute D89.810
    acute on chronic D89.812
    chronic D89.811
  human immunodeficiency virus (HIV) B20
  Huntington's G10
    with dementia G10 *[F02.80]*
  Hutchinson's (cheiropompholyx) — *see*
      Hutchinson's disease
  hyaline (diffuse) (generalized)
    membrane (lung) (newborn) P22.0
      adult J80
  hydatid — *see* Echinococcus
  hydroxyapatite deposition M11.00
    ankle M11.07-
    elbow M11.02-
    foot joint M11.07-
    hand joint M11.04-
    hip M11.05-
    knee M11.06-
    multiple site M11.09
    shoulder M11.01-
    vertebra M11.08
    wrist M11.03-
  hyperkinetic — *see* Hyperkinesia
  hypertensive — *see* Hypertension
  hypophysis E23.7
  Iceland G93.3
  I-cell E77.0
  immune D89.9
  immunoproliferative (malignant) C88.9
    small intestinal C88.3
    specified NEC C88.8
  inclusion B25.9
    salivary gland B25.9
  infectious, infective B99.9
    congenital P37.9
      specified NEC P37.8
      viral P35.9
        specified type NEC P35.8
    specified NEC B99.8
  inflammatory
    penis N48.29
      abscess N48.21
      cellulitis N48.22
    prepuce N47.7
      balanoposthitis N47.6
    tubo-ovarian — *see* Salpingo-oophoritis
  intervertebral disc — *see also* Disorder, disc
    with myelopathy — *see* Disorder, disc,
        with, myelopathy
    cervical, cervicothoracic — *see* Disorder,
        disc, cervical
      with
        myelopathy — *see* Disorder, disc,
          cervical, with myelopathy
        neuritis, radiculitis or
          radiculopathy — *see* Disorder,
          disc, cervical, with neuritis
      specified NEC — *see* Disorder, disc,
          cervical, specified type NEC
    lumbar (with)
      myelopathy M51.06

Disease, diseased - *continued*
  intervertebral disc - *continued*
    lumbar (with) - *continued*
      neuritis, radiculitis, radiculopathy or
          sciatica M51.16
      specified NEC M51.86
    lumbosacral (with)
      neuritis, radiculitis, radiculopathy or
          sciatica M51.17
      specified NEC M51.87
    specified NEC — *see* Disorder, disc,
        specified NEC
    thoracic (with)
      myelopathy M51.04
      neuritis, radiculitis or
          radiculopathy M51.14
      specified NEC M51.84
    thoracolumbar (with)
      myelopathy M51.05
      neuritis, radiculitis or
          radiculopathy M51.15
      specified NEC M51.85
  intestine K63.9
    functional K59.9
      psychogenic F45.8
      specified NEC K59.8
    organic K63.9
    protozoal A07.9
    specified NEC K63.89
  iris H21.9
    specified NEC H21.89
  iron metabolism or storage E83.10
  island (scrub typhus) A75.3
  itai-itai — *see* Poisoning, cadmium
  Jakob-Creutzfeldt — *see* Creutzfeldt-Jakob
      disease or syndrome
  jaw M27.9
    fibrocystic M27.49
    specified NEC M27.8
  jigger B88.1
  joint — *see also* Disorder, joint
    Charcot's — *see* Arthropathy, neuropathic
        (Charcot)
    degenerative — *see* Osteoarthritis
      multiple M15.9
      spine — *see* Spondylosis
    hypertrophic — *see* Osteoarthritis
    sacroiliac M53.3
    specified NEC — *see* Disorder, joint,
        specified type NEC
    spine NEC — *see* Dorsopathy
    suppurative — *see* Arthritis, pyogenic or
        pyemic
  Jourdain's (acute gingivitis) K05.00
    nonplaque induced K05.01
    plaque induced K05.00
  Kaschin-Beck (endemic
      polyarthritis) M12.10
    ankle M12.17-
    elbow M12.12-
    foot joint M12.17-
    hand joint M12.14-
    hip M12.15-
    knee M12.16-
    multiple site M12.19
    shoulder M12.11-
    vertebra M12.18
    wrist M12.13-
  Katayama B65.2
  Kedani (scrub typhus) A75.3
  Keshan E59
  kidney (functional) (pelvis) N28.9
    chronic N18.9
      hypertensive — *see* Hypertension,
          kidney
      stage 1 N18.1
      stage 2 (mild) N18.2
      stage 3 (moderate) N18.3
      stage 4 (severe) N18.4
      stage 5 N18.5
    complicating pregnancy — *see* Pregnancy,
        complicated by, renal disease
    cystic (congenital) Q61.9
    diabetic — *see* E08-E13 with .22
    fibrocystic (congenital) Q61.8

Disease, diseased - *continued*

  kidney (functional) (pelvis) - *continued*
    hypertensive — *see* Hypertension, kidney
    in (due to)
      schistosomiasis (bilharziasis) B65.9
        [N29]
    multicystic Q61.4
    polycystic Q61.3
      adult type Q61.2
      childhood type NEC Q61.19
        collecting duct dilatation Q61.11
  Kimmelstiel (-Wilson) (intercapillary
    polycystic (congenital)
    glomerulosclerosis) — *see* E08-E13
    with .21
  Kimura D21.9
    specified site (see Neoplasm, connective
      tissue benign)
  Kinnier Wilson's (hepatolenticular
    degeneration) E83.01
  kissing — *see* Mononucleosis, infectious
  Klebs' — *see also* Glomerulonephritis N05.-
  Klippel-Feil (brevicollis) Q76.1
  Köhler-Pellegrini-Stieda (calcification, knee
    joint) — *see* Bursitis, tibial collateral
  Kok Q89.8
  König's (osteochondritis dissecans) — *see*
    Osteochondritis, dissecans
  Korsakoff's (nonalcoholic) F04
    alcoholic F10.96
      with dependence F10.26
  Kostmann's (infantile genetic
    agranulocytosis) D70.0
  kuru A81.81
  Kyasanur Forest A98.2
  labyrinth, ear — *see* Disorder, ear, inner
  lacrimal system — *see* Disorder, lacrimal
    system
  Lafora's — *see* Epilepsy, generalized,
    idiopathic
  Lancereaux-Mathieu (leptospiral
    jaundice) A27.0
  Landry's G61.0
  Larrey-Weil (leptospiral jaundice) A27.0
  larynx J38.7
  legionnaires' A48.1
    nonpneumonic A48.2
  Lenegre's I44.2
  lens H27.9
    specified NEC H27.8
  Lev's (acquired complete heart block) I44.2
  Lewy body (dementia) G31.83 *[F02.80]*
    with behavioral disturbance G31.83
      [F02.81]
  Lichtheim's (subacute combined sclerosis
    with pernicious anemia) D51.0
  Lightwood's (renal tubular acidosis) N25.89
  Lignac's (cystinosis) E72.04
  lip K13.0
  lipid-storage E75.6
    specified NEC E75.5
  Lipschütz's N76.6
  liver (chronic) (organic) K76.9
    alcoholic (chronic) K70.9
      acute — *see* Disease, liver, alcoholic,
        hepatitis
      cirrhosis K70.30
        with ascites K70.31
      failure K70.40
        with coma K70.41
      fatty liver K70.0
      fibrosis K70.2
      hepatitis K70.10
        with ascites K70.11
      sclerosis K70.2
    cystic, congenital Q44.6
    drug-induced (idiosyncratic) (toxic)
      (predictable) (unpredictable) — *see*
      Disease, liver, toxic
    end stage K72.90
      due to hepatitis — *see* Hepatitis
    fatty, nonalcoholic (NAFLD) K76.0
      alcoholic K70.0
    fibrocystic (congenital) Q44.6
    fluke

Disease, diseased - *continued*

  liver (chronic) (organic) - *continued*
    fluke - *continued*
      Chinese B66.1
      oriental B66.1
      sheep B66.3
    gestational alloimmune (GALD) P78.84
    glycogen storage E74.09 *[K77]*
    in (due to)
      schistosomiasis (bilharziasis) B65.9
        [K77]
    inflammatory K75.9
      alcoholic K70.1
      specified NEC K75.89
    polycystic (congenital) Q44.6
    toxic K71.9
      with
        cholestasis K71.0
        cirrhosis (liver) K71.7
        fibrosis (liver) K71.7
        focal nodular hyperplasia K71.8
        hepatic granuloma K71.8
        hepatic necrosis K71.10
          with coma K71.11
        hepatitis NEC K71.6
          acute K71.2
          chronic
            active K71.50
              with ascites K71.51
            lobular K71.4
            persistent K71.3
        lupoid K71.50
          with ascites K71.51
        peliosis hepatis K71.8
        veno-occlusive disease (VOD) of
          liver K71.8
    veno-occlusive K76.5
  Lobo's (keloid blastomycosis) B48.0
  Lobstein's (brittle bones and blue
    sclera) Q78.0
  Ludwig's (submaxillary cellulitis) K12.2
  lumbosacral region M53.87
  lung J98.4
    black J60
    congenital Q33.9
    cystic J98.4
      congenital Q33.0
    fibroid (chronic) — *see* Fibrosis, lung
    fluke B66.4
      oriental B66.4
    in
      amyloidosis E85.4 *[J99]*
      sarcoidosis D86.0
      Sjögren's syndrome M35.02
      systemic
        lupus erythematosus M32.13
        sclerosis M34.81
    interstitial J84.9
      of childhood, specified NEC J84.848
      respiratory bronchiolitis J84.115
      specified NEC J84.89
    obstructive (chronic) J43.9
      with
        acute
          bronchitis J44.0
          exacerbation NEC J44.1
          lower respiratory infection J44.0
        alveolitis, allergic J67.9
        asthma J44.9
        bronchiectasis J47.9
          with
            exacerbation (acute) J47.1
            lower respiratory infection J47.0
        bronchitis J44.9
          with
            exacerbation (acute) J44.1
            lower respiratory infection J44.0
        emphysema J43.9
        hypersensitivity pneumonitis J67.9
      decompensated J44.1
        with
          exacerbation (acute) J44.1
    polycystic J98.4
      congenital Q33.0

Disease, diseased - *continued*

  lung - *continued*
    rheumatoid (diffuse) (interstitial) — *see*
      Rheumatoid, lung
  Lutembacher's (atrial septal defect with
    mitral stenosis) Q21.1
  Lyme A69.20
  lymphatic (gland) (system) (channel)
    (vessel) I89.9
  lymphoproliferative D47.9
    specified NEC D47.Z9
    T-gamma D47.Z9
    X-linked D82.3
  Magitot's M27.2
  malarial — *see* Malaria
  malignant — *see also* Neoplasm, malignant,
    by site
  Manson's B65.1
  maple bark J67.6
  maple-syrup-urine E71.0
  Marburg (virus) A98.3
  Marion's (bladder neck obstruction) N32.0
  Marsh's (exophthalmic goiter) — *see*
    Hyperthyroidism, with, goiter (diffuse)
  mastoid (process) — *see* Disorder, ear,
    middle
  Mathieu's (leptospiral jaundice) A27.0
  Maxcy's A75.2
  McArdle (-Schmid-Pearson) (glycogenosis
    V) E74.04
  mediastinum J98.59
  medullary center (idiopathic)
    (respiratory) G93.89
  Meige's (chronic hereditary edema) Q82.0
  meningococcal — *see* Infection,
    meningococcal
  mental F99
    organic F09
  mesenchymal M35.9
  mesenteric embolic — *see also* Ischemia,
    intestine, acute K55.039
  metabolic, metabolism E88.9
    bilirubin E80.7
  metal-polisher's J62.8
  metastatic — *see also* Neoplasm, secondary,
    by site C79.9
  microvascular - code to condition
  microvillus
    atrophy Q43.8
    inclusion (MVD) Q43.8
  middle ear — *see* Disorder, ear, middle
  Mikulicz' (dryness of mouth, absent or
    decreased lacrimation) K11.8
  Milroy's (chronic hereditary edema) Q82.0
  Minamata — *see* Poisoning, mercury
  minicore G71.2
  Minor's G95.19
  Minot's (hemorrhagic disease, newborn) P53
  Minot-von Willebrand-Jürgens
    (angiohemophilia) D68.0
  Mitchell's (erythromelalgia) I73.81
  mitral (valve) I05.9
    nonrheumatic I34.9
  mixed connective tissue M35.1
  moldy hay J67.0
  Monge's T70.29
  Morgagni-Adams-Stokes (syncope with heart
    block) I45.9
  Morgagni's (syndrome) (hyperostosis
    frontalis interna) M85.2
  Morton's (with metatarsalgia) — *see* Lesion,
    nerve, plantar
  Morvan's G60.8
  motor neuron (bulbar) (mixed type)
    (spinal) G12.20
    amyotrophic lateral sclerosis G12.21
    familial G12.24
    progressive bulbar palsy G12.22
    specified NEC G12.29
  moyamoya I67.5
  mu heavy chain disease C88.2
  multicore G71.2
  muscle — *see also* Disorder, muscle
    inflammatory — *see* Myositis
    ocular (external) — *see* Strabismus

Disease, diseased - *continued*
musculoskeletal system, soft tissue — *see also* Disorder, soft tissue
  specified NEC — *see* Disorder, soft tissue, specified type NEC
mushroom workers' J67.5
mycotic B49
myelodysplastic, not classified C94.6
myeloproliferative, not classified C94.6
  chronic D47.1
myocardium, myocardial — *see also* Degeneration, myocardial I51.5
  primary (idiopathic) I42.9
myoneural G70.9
Naegeli's D69.1
nails L60.9
  specified NEC L60.8
Nairobi (sheep virus) A93.8
nasal J34.9
nemaline body G71.2
nerve — *see* Disorder, nerve
nervous system G98.8
  autonomic G90.9
  central G96.9
    specified NEC G96.8
  congenital Q07.9
  parasympathetic G90.9
  specified NEC G98.8
  sympathetic G90.9
  vegetative G90.9
neuromuscular system G70.9
Newcastle B30.8
Nicolas (-Durand) -Favre (climatic bubo) A55
nipple N64.9
  Paget's C50.01-
    female C50.01-
    male C50.02-
Nishimoto (-Takeuchi) I67.5
nonarthropod-borne NOS (viral) B34.9
  enterovirus NEC B34.1
nonautoimmune hemolytic D59.4
  drug-induced D59.2
Nonne-Milroy-Meige (chronic hereditary edema) Q82.0
nose J34.9
nucleus pulposus — *see* Disorder, disc
nutritional E63.9
oast-house-urine E72.19
  ocular
    herpesviral B00.50
    zoster B02.30
obliterative vascular I77.1
Ohara's — *see* Tularemia
Opitz's (congestive splenomegaly) D73.2
Oppenheim-Urbach (necrobiosis lipoidica diabeticorum) — *see* E08-E13 with .620
optic nerve NEC — *see* Disorder, nerve, optic
orbit — *see* Disorder, orbit
Oriental liver fluke B66.1
Oriental lung fluke B66.4
Ormond's N13.5
Oropouche virus A93.0
Osler-Rendu (familial hemorrhagic telangiectasia) I78.0
osteofibrocystic E21.0
Otto's M24.7
outer ear — *see* Disorder, ear, external
ovary (noninflammatory) N83.9
  cystic N83.20-
  inflammatory — *see* Salpingo-oophoritis
  polycystic E28.2
  specified NEC N83.8
Owren's (congenital) — *see* Defect, coagulation
pancreas K86.9
  cystic K86.2
  fibrocystic E84.9
  specified NEC K86.89
panvalvular I08.9
  specified NEC I08.8
parametrium (noninflammatory) N83.9
parasitic B89
  cerebral NEC B71.9 *[G94]*

Disease, diseased - *continued*
parasitic - *continued*
  intestinal NOS B82.9
  mouth B37.0
  skin NOS B88.9
  specified type — *see* Infestation
  tongue B37.0
parathyroid (gland) E21.5
  specified NEC E21.4
Parkinson's G20
parodontal K05.6
Parrot's (syphilitic osteochondritis) A50.02
Parry's (exophthalmic goiter) — *see* Hyperthyroidism, with, goiter (diffuse)
Parson's (exophthalmic goiter) — *see* Hyperthyroidism, with, goiter (diffuse)
Paxton's (white piedra) B36.2
pearl-worker's — *see* Osteomyelitis, specified type NEC
Pellegrini-Stieda (calcification, knee joint) — *see* Bursitis, tibial collateral
pelvis, pelvic
  female NOS N94.9
    specified NEC N94.89
  gonococcal (acute) (chronic) A54.24
  inflammatory (female) N73.9
    acute N73.0
    chlamydial A56.11
    chronic N73.1
    specified NEC N73.8
    syphilitic (secondary) A51.42
      late A52.76
    tuberculous A18.17
  organ, female N94.9
  peritoneum, female NEC N94.89
penis N48.9
  inflammatory N48.29
    abscess N48.21
    cellulitis N48.22
  specified NEC N48.89
periapical tissues NOS K04.90
periodontal K05.6
  specified NEC K05.5
periosteum — *see* Disorder, bone, specified type NEC
peripheral
  arterial I73.9
  autonomic nervous system G90.9
  nerves — *see* Polyneuropathy
  vascular NOS I73.9
peritoneum K66.9
  pelvic, female NEC N94.89
  specified NEC K66.8
persistent mucosal (middle ear) H66.20
  left H66.22
    with right H66.23
  right H66.21
    with left H66.23
Petit's — *see* Hernia, abdomen, specified site NEC
pharynx J39.2
  specified NEC J39.2
Phocas' — *see* Mastopathy, cystic
photochromogenic (acid-fast bacilli) (pulmonary) A31.0
  nonpulmonary A31.9
Pick's G31.01 *[F02.80]*
  with behavioral disturbance G31.01 *[F02.81]*
  brain G31.01 *[F02.80]*
    with behavioral disturbance G31.01 *[F02.81]*
  of pericardium (pericardial pseudocirrhosis of liver) I31.1
pigeon fancier's J67.2
pineal gland E34.8
pink — *see* Poisoning, mercury
Pinkus' (lichen nitidus) L44.1
pinworm B80
Piry virus A93.8
pituitary (gland) E23.7
pituitary-snuff-taker's J67.8
pleura (cavity) J94.9
  specified NEC J94.8
pneumatic drill (hammer) T75.21

Disease, diseased - *continued*
Pollitzer's (hidradenitis suppurativa) L73.2
polycystic
  kidney or renal Q61.3
    adult type Q61.2
    childhood type NEC Q61.19
      collecting duct dilatation Q61.11
  liver or hepatic Q44.6
  lung or pulmonary J98.4
    congenital Q33.0
  ovary, ovaries E28.2
  spleen Q89.09
polyethylene T84.05-
Pompe's (glycogenosis II) E74.02
Posadas-Wernicke B38.9
Potain's (pulmonary edema) — *see* Edema, lung
prepuce N47.8
  inflammatory N47.7
    balanoposthitis N47.6
Pringle's (tuberous sclerosis) Q85.1
prion, central nervous system A81.9
  specified NEC A81.89
prostate N42.9
  specified NEC N42.89
protozoal B64
  acanthamebiasis — *see* Acanthamebiasis
  African trypanosomiasis — *see* African trypanosomiasis
  babesiosis B60.0
  Chagas disease — *see* Chagas disease
  intestine, intestinal A07.9
  leishmaniasis — *see* Leishmaniasis
  malaria — *see* Malaria
  naegleriasis B60.2
  pneumocystosis B59
  specified organism NEC B60.8
  toxoplasmosis — *see* Toxoplasmosis
pseudo-Hurler's E77.0
psychiatric F99
psychotic — *see* Psychosis
Puente's (simple glandular cheilitis) K13.0
puerperal — *see also* Puerperal O90.89
pulmonary — *see also* Disease, lung
  artery I28.9
  chronic obstructive J44.9
    with
      acute bronchitis J44.0
      exacerbation (acute) J44.1
      lower respiratory infection (acute) J44.0
    decompensated J44.1
      with
        exacerbation (acute) J44.1
  heart I27.9
    specified NEC I27.89
  hypertensive (vascular) — *see also* Hypertension, pulmonary I27.20
    primary (idiopathic) I27.0
  valve I37.9
    rheumatic I09.89
pulp (dental) NOS K04.90
pulseless M31.4
Putnam's (subacute combined sclerosis with pernicious anemia) D51.0
Pyle (-Cohn) (metaphyseal dysplasia) Q78.5
ragpicker's or ragsorter's A22.1
Raynaud's — *see* Raynaud's disease
reactive airway — *see* Asthma
Reclus' (cystic) — *see* Mastopathy, cystic
rectum K62.9
  specified NEC K62.89
Refsum's (heredopathia atactica polyneuritiformis) G60.1
renal (functional) (pelvis) — *see also* Disease, kidney N28.9
  with
    edema — *see* Nephrosis
    glomerular lesion — *see* Glomerulonephritis
      with edema — *see* Nephrosis
    interstitial nephritis N12
  acute N28.9
  chronic — *see also* Disease, kidney, chronic N18.9

Disease, diseased - *continued*
  renal (functional) (pelvis) - *continued*
    cystic, congenital Q61.9
    diabetic — *see* E08-E13 with .22
    end-stage (failure) N18.6
      due to hypertension I12.0
    fibrocystic (congenital) Q61.8
    hypertensive — *see* Hypertension, kidney
    lupus M32.14
    phosphate-losing (tubular) N25.0
    polycystic (congenital) Q61.3
      adult type Q61.2
      childhood type NEC Q61.19
        collecting duct dilatation Q61.11
    rapidly progressive N01.9
    subacute N01.9
  Rendu-Osler-Weber (familial hemorrhagic
    telangiectasia) I78.0
  renovascular (arteriosclerotic) — *see*
    Hypertension, kidney
  respiratory (tract) J98.9
    acute or subacute NOS J06.9
      due to
        chemicals, gases, fumes or vapors
          (inhalation) J68.3
        external agent J70.9
          specified NEC J70.8
        radiation J70.0
        smoke inhalation J70.5
      noninfectious J39.8
    chronic NOS J98.9
      due to
        chemicals, gases, fumes or
          vapors J68.4
        external agent J70.9
          specified NEC J70.8
        radiation J70.1
      newborn P27.9
        specified NEC P27.8
    due to
      chemicals, gases, fumes or vapors J68.9
        acute or subacute NEC J68.3
        chronic J68.4
      external agent J70.9
        specified NEC J70.8
    newborn P28.9
      specified type NEC P28.89
    upper J39.9
      acute or subacute J06.9
      noninfectious NEC J39.8
      specified NEC J39.8
      streptococcal J06.9
  retina, retinal H35.9
    Batten's or Batten-Mayou E75.4 *[H36]*
    specified NEC H35.89
  rheumatoid — *see* Arthritis, rheumatoid
  rickettsial NOS A79.9
    specified type NEC A79.89
  Riga (-Fede) (cachectic aphthae) K14.0
  Riggs' (compound periodontitis) — *see*
    Periodontitis
  Ritter's L00
  Rivalta's (cervicofacial actinomycosis) A42.2
  Robles' (onchocerciasis) B73.01
  Roger's (congenital interventricular septal
    defect) Q21.0
  Rosenthal's (factor XI deficiency) D68.1
  Rossbach's (hyperchlorhydria) K31.89
    psychogenic F45.8
  Ross River B33.1
  Rotes Quérol — *see* Hyperostosis,
    ankylosing
  Roth (-Bernhardt) — *see* Mononeuropathy,
    lower limb, meralgia paresthetica
  Runeberg's (progressive pernicious
    anemia) D51.0
  sacroiliac NEC M53.3
  salivary gland or duct K11.9
    inclusion B25.9
    specified NEC K11.8
    virus B25.9
  sandworm B76.9
  Schimmelbusch's — *see* Mastopathy, cystic
  Schmorl's — *see* Schmorl's disease or nodes

Disease, diseased - *continued*
  Schönlein (-Henoch) (purpura
    rheumatica) D69.0
  Schottmüller's — *see* Fever, paratyphoid
  Schultz's (agranulocytosis) — *see*
    Agranulocytosis
  Schwalbe-Ziehen-Oppenheim G24.1
  Schwartz-Jampel G71.13
  sclera H15.9
    specified NEC H15.89
  scrofulous (tuberculous) A18.2
  scrotum N50.9
  sebaceous glands L73.9
  semilunar cartilage, cystic — *see also*
    Derangement, knee, meniscus, cystic
  seminal vesicle N50.9
  serum NEC — *see also* Reaction,
    serum T80.69
  sexually transmitted A64
    anogenital
      herpesviral infection — *see* Herpes,
        anogenital
      warts A63.0
    chancroid A57
    chlamydial infection — *see* Chlamydia
    gonorrhea — *see* Gonorrhea
    granuloma inguinale A58
    specified organism NEC A63.8
    syphilis — *see* Syphilis
    trichomoniasis — *see* Trichomoniasis
  Sézary C84.1-
  shimamushi (scrub typhus) A75.3
  shipyard B30.0
  sickle-cell D57.1
    with crisis (vasoocclusive pain) D57.00
      with
        acute chest syndrome D57.01
        splenic sequestration D57.02
    elliptocytosis D57.8-
    Hb-C D57.20
      with crisis (vasoocclusive pain) D57.219
        with
          acute chest syndrome D57.211
          splenic sequestration D57.212
      without crisis D57.20
    Hb-SD D57.80
      with crisis D57.819
        with
          acute chest syndrome D57.811
          splenic sequestration D57.812
    Hb-SE D57.80
      with crisis D57.819
        with
          acute chest syndrome D57.811
          splenic sequestration D57.812
    specified NEC D57.80
      with crisis D57.819
        with
          acute chest syndrome D57.811
          splenic sequestration D57.812
    spherocytosis D57.80
      with crisis D57.819
        with
          acute chest syndrome D57.811
          splenic sequestration D57.812
    thalassemia D57.40
      with crisis (vasoocclusive pain) D57.419
        with
          acute chest syndrome D57.411
          splenic sequestration D57.412
      without crisis D57.40
  silo-filler's J68.8
    bronchitis J68.0
    pneumonitis J68.0
    pulmonary edema J68.1
  simian B00.4
  Simons' (progressive lipodystrophy) E88.1
  sin nombre virus B33.4
  sinus — *see* Sinusitis
  Sirkari's B55.0
  sixth B08.20
    due to human herpesvirus 6 B08.21
    due to human herpesvirus 7 B08.22
  skin L98.9

Disease, diseased - *continued*
  skin - *continued*
    due to metabolic disorder NEC E88.9
      [L99]
    specified NEC L98.8
  slim (HIV) B20
  small vessel I73.9
  Sneddon-Wilkinson (subcorneal pustular
    dermatosis) L13.1
  South African creeping B88.0
  spinal (cord) G95.9
    congenital Q06.9
    specified NEC G95.89
  spine — *see also* Spondylopathy
    joint — *see* Dorsopathy
    tuberculous A18.01
  spinocerebellar (hereditary) G11.9
    specified NEC G11.8
  spleen D73.9
    amyloid E85.4 *[D77]*
    organic D73.9
    polycystic Q89.09
    postinfectional D73.89
  sponge-diver's — *see* Toxicity, venom,
    marine animal, sea anemone
  Startle Q89.8
  Steinert's G71.11
  Sticker's (erythema infectiosum) B08.3
  Stieda's (calcification, knee joint) — *see*
    Bursitis, tibial collateral
  Stokes' (exophthalmic goiter) — *see*
    Hyperthyroidism, with, goiter (diffuse)
  Stokes-Adams (syncope with heart
    block) I45.9
  stomach K31.9
    functional, psychogenic F45.8
    specified NEC K31.89
  stonemason's J62.8
  storage
    glycogen — *see* Disease, glycogen storage
    mucopolysaccharide — *see*
      Mucopolysaccharidosis
  striatopallidal system NEC G25.89
  Stuart-Prower (congenital factor X
    deficiency) D68.2
  Stuart's (congenital factor X
    deficiency) D68.2
  subcutaneous tissue — *see* Disease, skin
  supporting structures of teeth K08.9
    specified NEC K08.89
  suprarenal (capsule) (gland) E27.9
    hyperfunction E27.0
    specified NEC E27.8
  sweat glands L74.9
    specified NEC L74.8
  Sweeley-Klionsky E75.21
  Swift (-Feer) — *see* Poisoning, mercury
  swimming-pool granuloma A31.1
  Sylvest's (epidemic pleurodynia) B33.0
  sympathetic nervous system G90.9
  synovium — *see* Disorder, synovium
  syphilitic — *see* Syphilis
  systemic tissue mast cell D47.02
  tanapox (virus) B08.71
  Tangier E78.6
  Tarral-Besnier (pityriasis rubra pilaris) L44.0
  Tauri's E74.09
  tear duct — *see* Disorder, lacrimal system
  tendon, tendinous — *see also* Disorder,
    tendon
    nodular — *see* Trigger finger
  terminal vessel I73.9
  testis N50.9
  thalassemia Hb-S — *see* Disease, sickle-cell,
    thalassemia
  Thaysen-Gee (nontropical sprue) K90.0
  Thomsen G71.12
  throat J39.2
    septic J02.0
  thromboembolic — *see* Embolism
  thymus (gland) E32.9
    specified NEC E32.8
  thyroid (gland) E07.9
    heart — *see also* Hyperthyroidism E05.90
      [I43]

Disease, diseased - *continued*
  thyroid (gland) - *continued*
    heart - *continued*
      with thyroid storm E05.91 *[I43]*
      specified NEC E07.89
  Tietze's M94.0
  tongue K14.9
    specified NEC K14.8
  tonsils, tonsillar (and adenoids) J35.9
  tooth, teeth K08.9
    hard tissues K03.9
      specified NEC K03.89
    pulp NEC K04.99
    specified NEC K08.89
  Tourette's F95.2
  trachea NEC J39.8
  tricuspid I07.9
    nonrheumatic I36.9
  triglyceride-storage E75.5
  trophoblastic — *see* Mole, hydatidiform
  tsutsugamushi A75.3
  tube (fallopian) (noninflammatory) N83.9
    inflammatory — *see* Salpingitis
    specified NEC N83.8
  tuberculous NEC — *see* Tuberculosis
  tubo-ovarian (noninflammatory) N83.9
    inflammatory — *see* Salpingo-oophoritis
    specified NEC N83.8
  tubotympanic, chronic — *see* Otitis, media,
    suppurative, chronic, tubotympanic
  tubulo-interstitial N15.9
    specified NEC N15.8
  tympanum — *see* Disorder, tympanic
    membrane
  Uhl's Q24.8
  Underwood's (sclerema neonatorum) P83.0
  Unverricht (-Lundborg) — *see* Epilepsy,
    generalized, idiopathic
  Urbach-Oppenheim (necrobiosis lipoidica
    diabeticorum) — *see* E08-E13 with .620
  ureter N28.9
    in (due to)
      schistosomiasis (bilharziasis) B65.0
        [N29]
  urethra N36.9
    specified NEC N36.8
  urinary (tract) N39.9
    bladder N32.9
      specified NEC N32.89
    specified NEC N39.8
  uterus (noninflammatory) N85.9
    infective — *see* Endometritis
    inflammatory — *see* Endometritis
    specified NEC N85.8
  uveal tract (anterior) H21.9
    posterior H31.9
  vagabond's B85.1
  vagina, vaginal (noninflammatory) N89.9
    inflammatory NEC N76.89
    specified NEC N89.8
  valve, valvular I38
    multiple I08.9
      specified NEC I08.8
  van Creveld-von Gierke (glycogenosis
    I) E74.01
  vas deferens N50.9
  vascular I99.9
    arteriosclerotic — *see* Arteriosclerosis
    ciliary body NEC — *see* Disorder, iris,
      vascular
    hypertensive — *see* Hypertension
    iris NEC — *see* Disorder, iris, vascular
    obliterative I77.1
      peripheral I73.9
    occlusive I99.8
    peripheral (occlusive) I73.9
      in diabetes mellitus — *see* E08-E13 with
        .51
  vasomotor I73.9
  vasospastic I73.9
  vein I87.9
  venereal — *see also* Disease, sexually
    transmitted A64
    chlamydial NEC A56.8
      anus A56.3

Disease, diseased - *continued*
  venereal - *continued*
    chlamydial NEC - *continued*
      genitourinary NOS A56.2
      pharynx A56.4
      rectum A56.3
    fifth A55
    sixth A55
    specified nature or type NEC A63.8
  vertebra, vertebral — *see also*
    Spondylopathy
    disc — *see* Disorder, disc
  vibration — *see* Vibration, adverse effects
  viral, virus — *see also* Disease, by type of
    virus B34.9
    arbovirus NOS A94
    arthropod-borne NOS A94
    congenital P35.9
      specified NEC P35.8
    Hanta (with renal manifestations)
      (Dobrava) (Puumala) (Seoul) A98.5
      with pulmonary manifestations (Andes)
        (Bayou) (Bermejo) (Black Creek
        Canal) (Choclo) (Juquitiba)
        (Laguna negra) (Lechiguanas)
        (New York) (Oran) (Sin
        nombre) B33.4
    Hantaan (Korean hemorrhagic
      fever) A98.5
    human immunodeficiency (HIV) B20
    Kunjin A83.4
    nonarthropod-borne NOS B34.9
    Powassan A84.8
    Rocio (encephalitis) A83.6
    Sin nombre (Hantavirus) (cardio)
      -pulmonary syndrome) B33.4
    Tahyna B33.8
    vesicular stomatitis A93.8
  vitreous H43.9
    specified NEC H43.89
  vocal cord J38.3
  Volkmann's, acquired T79.6
  von Eulenburg's (congenital
    paramyotonia) G71.19
  von Gierke's (glycogenosis I) E74.01
  von Graefe's — *see* Strabismus, paralytic,
    ophthalmoplegia, progressive
  von Willebrand (-Jürgens)
    (angiohemophilia) D68.0
  Vrolik's (osteogenesis imperfecta) Q78.0
  vulva (noninflammatory) N90.9
    inflammatory NEC N76.89
    specified NEC N90.89
  Wallgren's (obstruction of splenic vein with
    collateral circulation) I87.8
  Wassilieff's (leptospiral jaundice) A27.0
  wasting NEC R64
    due to malnutrition E41
  Waterhouse-Friderichsen A39.1
  Wegner's (syphilitic osteochondritis) A50.02
  Weil's (leptospiral jaundice of lung) A27.0
  Weir Mitchell's (erythromelalgia) I73.81
  Werdnig-Hoffmann G12.0
  Wermer's E31.21
  Werner-His (trench fever) A79.0
  Werner-Schultz (neutropenic
    splenomegaly) D73.81
  Wernicke-Posadas B38.9
  whipworm B79
  white blood cells D72.9
    specified NEC D72.89
  white matter R90.82
  white-spot, meaning lichen sclerosus et
    atrophicus L90.0
    penis N48.0
    vulva N90.4
  Wilkie's K55.1
  Wilkinson-Sneddon (subcorneal pustular
    dermatosis) L13.1
  Willis' — *see* Diabetes
  Wilson's (hepatolenticular
    degeneration) E83.01
  woolsorter's A22.1
  yaba monkey tumor B08.72
  yaba pox (virus) B08.72

Disease, diseased - *continued*
  Zika virus A92.5
    congenital P35.4
  zoonotic, bacterial A28.9
    specified type NEC A28.8
Disfigurement (due to scar) L90.5
Disgerminoma — *see* Dysgerminoma
**DISH (diffuse idiopathic skeletal
  hyperostosis)** — *see* Hyperostosis,
  ankylosing
Disinsertion, retina — *see* Detachment, retina
Dislocatable hip, congenital Q65.6
Dislocation (articular)
  with fracture — *see* Fracture
  acromioclavicular (joint) S43.10-
    with displacement
      100%-200% S43.12-
      more than 200% S43.13-
    inferior S43.14-
    posterior S43.15-
  ankle S93.0-
  astragalus — *see* Dislocation, ankle
  atlantoaxial S13.121
  atlantooccipital S13.111
  atloidooccipital S13.111
  breast bone S23.29
  capsule, joint - code by site under
    Dislocation
  carpal (bone) — *see* Dislocation, wrist
  carpometacarpal (joint) NEC S63.05-
    thumb S63.04-
  cartilage (joint) - code by site under
    Dislocation
  cervical spine (vertebra) — *see* Dislocation,
    vertebra, cervical
  chronic — *see* Dislocation, recurrent
  clavicle — *see* Dislocation,
    acromioclavicular joint
  coccyx S33.2
  congenital NEC Q68.8
  coracoid — *see* Dislocation, shoulder
  costal cartilage S23.29
  costochondral S23.29
  cricoarytenoid articulation S13.29
  cricothyroid articulation S13.29
  dorsal vertebra — *see* Dislocation, vertebra,
    thoracic
  ear ossicle — *see* Discontinuity, ossicles, ear
  elbow S53.10-
    congenital Q68.8
    pathological — *see* Dislocation,
      pathological NEC, elbow
    radial head alone — *see* Dislocation, radial
      head
    recurrent — *see* Dislocation, recurrent,
      elbow
    traumatic S53.10-
      anterior S53.11-
      lateral S53.14-
      medial S53.13-
      posterior S53.12-
      specified type NEC S53.19-
  eye, nontraumatic — *see* Luxation, globe
  eyeball, nontraumatic — *see* Luxation, globe
  femur
    distal end — *see* Dislocation, knee
    proximal end — *see* Dislocation, hip
  fibula
    distal end — *see* Dislocation, ankle
    proximal end — *see* Dislocation, knee
  finger S63.25-
    index S63.25-
    interphalangeal S63.27-
      distal S63.29-
        index S63.29-
        little S63.29-
        middle S63.29-
        ring S63.29-
      index S63.27-
      little S63.27-
      middle S63.27-
      proximal S63.28-
        index S63.28-
        little S63.28-
        middle S63.28-

Dislocation (articular) - *continued*
  finger - *continued*
    interphalangeal - *continued*
      proximal - *continued*
        ring S63.28-
        ring S63.27-
      little S63.25-
      metacarpophalangeal S63.26-
        index S63.26-
        little S63.26-
        middle S63.26-
        ring S63.26-
      middle S63.25-
      recurrent — *see* Dislocation, recurrent,
        finger
      ring S63.25-
      thumb — *see* Dislocation, thumb
  foot S93.30-
    recurrent — *see* Dislocation, recurrent,
      foot
    specified site NEC S93.33-
    tarsal joint S93.31-
    tarsometatarsal joint S93.32-
    toe — *see* Dislocation, toe
  fracture — *see* Fracture
  glenohumeral (joint) — *see* Dislocation,
    shoulder
  glenoid — *see* Dislocation, shoulder
  habitual — *see* Dislocation, recurrent
  hip S73.00-
    anterior S73.03-
      obturator S73.02-
    central S73.04-
    congenital (total) Q65.2
      bilateral Q65.1
      partial Q65.5
        bilateral Q65.4
        unilateral Q65.3-
      unilateral Q65.0-
    developmental M24.85-
    pathological — *see* Dislocation,
      pathological NEC, hip
    posterior S73.01-
    recurrent — *see* Dislocation, recurrent, hip
  humerus, proximal end — *see* Dislocation,
    shoulder
  incomplete — *see* Subluxation, by site
  incus — *see* Discontinuity, ossicles, ear
  infracoracoid — *see* Dislocation, shoulder
  innominate (pubic junction) (sacral
    junction) S33.39
    acetabulum — *see* Dislocation, hip
  interphalangeal (joint (s))
    finger S63.279
      distal S63.29-
        index S63.29-
        little S63.29-
        middle S63.29-
        ring S63.29-
      index S63.27-
      little S63.27-
      middle S63.27-
      proximal S63.28-
        index S63.28-
        little S63.28-
        middle S63.28-
        ring S63.28-
      ring S63.27-
    foot or toe — *see* Dislocation, toe
    thumb S63.12-
  jaw (cartilage) (meniscus) S03.0-
  joint prosthesis — *see* Complications, joint
    prosthesis, mechanical, displacement,
    by site
  knee S83.106
    cap — *see* Dislocation, patella
    congenital Q68.2
    old M23.8X-
    patella — *see* Dislocation, patella
    pathological — *see* Dislocation,
      pathological NEC, knee
    proximal tibia
      anteriorly S83.11-
      laterally S83.14-
      medially S83.13-

Dislocation (articular) - *continued*
  knee - *continued*
    proximal tibia - *continued*
      posteriorly S83.12-
    recurrent — *see also* Derangement, knee,
      specified NEC
    specified type NEC S83.19-
  lacrimal gland H04.16-
  lens (complete) H27.10
    anterior H27.12-
    congenital Q12.1
    ocular implant — *see* Complications,
      intraocular lens
    partial H27.11-
    posterior H27.13-
    traumatic S05.8X-
  ligament - code by site under Dislocation
  lumbar (vertebra) — *see* Dislocation,
    vertebra, lumbar
  lumbosacral (vertebra) — *see also*
    Dislocation, vertebra, lumbar
    congenital Q76.49
  mandible S03.0-
  meniscus (knee) — *see* Tear, meniscus
    other sites - code by site under Dislocation
  metacarpal (bone)
    distal end — *see* Dislocation, finger
    proximal end S63.06-
  metacarpophalangeal (joint)
    finger S63.26-
      index S63.26-
      little S63.26-
      middle S63.26-
      ring S63.26-
    thumb S63.11-
  metatarsal (bone) — *see* Dislocation, foot
  metatarsophalangeal (joint (s)) — *see*
    Dislocation, toe
  midcarpal (joint) S63.03-
  midtarsal (joint) — *see* Dislocation, foot
  neck S13.20
    specified site NEC S13.29
    vertebra — *see* Dislocation, vertebra,
      cervical
  nose (septal cartilage) S03.1
  occipitoatloid S13.111
  old — *see* Derangement, joint, specified type
    NEC
  ossicles, ear — *see* Discontinuity, ossicles,
    ear
  partial — *see* Subluxation, by site
  patella S83.006
    congenital Q74.1
    lateral S83.01-
    recurrent (nontraumatic) M22.0-
      incomplete M22.1-
    specified type NEC S83.09-
  pathological NEC M24.30
    ankle M24.37-
    elbow M24.32-
    foot joint M24.37-
    hand joint M24.34-
    hip M24.35-
    knee M24.36-
    lumbosacral joint — *see* subcategory
      M53.2
    pelvic region — *see* Dislocation,
      pathological, hip
    sacroiliac — *see* subcategory M53.2
    shoulder M24.31-
    wrist M24.33-
  pelvis NEC S33.30
    specified NEC S33.39
  phalanx
    finger or hand — *see* Dislocation, finger
    foot or toe — *see* Dislocation, toe
  prosthesis, internal — *see* Complications,
    prosthetic device, by site, mechanical
  radial head S53.006
    anterior S53.01-
    posterior S53.02-
    specified type NEC S53.09-
  radiocarpal (joint) S63.02-
  radiohumeral (joint) — *see* Dislocation,
    radial head

Dislocation (articular) - *continued*
  radioulnar (joint)
    distal S63.01-
    proximal — *see* Dislocation, elbow
  radius
    distal end — *see* Dislocation, wrist
    proximal end — *see* Dislocation, radial
      head
  recurrent M24.40
    ankle M24.47-
    elbow M24.42-
    finger M24.44-
    foot joint M24.47-
    hand joint M24.44-
    hip M24.45-
    knee M24.46-
      patella — *see* Dislocation, patella,
        recurrent
    patella — *see* Dislocation, patella,
      recurrent
    sacroiliac — *see* subcategory M53.2
    shoulder M24.41-
    toe M24.47-
    vertebra (*see also* subcategory M43.5)
      atlantoaxial M43.4
        with myelopathy M43.3
    wrist M24.43-
  rib (cartilage) S23.29
  sacrococcygeal S33.2
  sacroiliac (joint) (ligament) S33.2
    congenital Q74.2
    recurrent — *see* subcategory M53.2
  sacrum S33.2
  scaphoid (bone) (hand) (wrist) — *see*
    Dislocation, wrist
    foot — *see* Dislocation, foot
  scapula — *see* Dislocation, shoulder, girdle,
    scapula
  semilunar cartilage, knee — *see* Tear,
    meniscus
  septal cartilage (nose) S03.1
  septum (nasal) (old) J34.2
  sesamoid bone - code by site under
    Dislocation
  shoulder (blade) (ligament) (joint)
    (traumatic) S43.006
    acromioclavicular — *see* Dislocation,
      acromioclavicular
    chronic — *see* Dislocation, recurrent,
      shoulder
    congenital Q68.8
    girdle S43.30-
      scapula S43.31-
      specified site NEC S43.39-
    humerus S43.00-
      anterior S43.01-
      inferior S43.03-
      posterior S43.02-
    pathological — *see* Dislocation,
      pathological NEC, shoulder
    recurrent — *see* Dislocation, recurrent,
      shoulder
    specified type NEC S43.08-
  spine
    cervical — *see* Dislocation, vertebra,
      cervical
    congenital Q76.49
    due to birth trauma P11.5
    lumbar — *see* Dislocation, vertebra,
      lumbar
    thoracic — *see* Dislocation, vertebra,
      thoracic
  spontaneous — *see* Dislocation, pathological
  sternoclavicular (joint) S43.206
    anterior S43.21-
    posterior S43.22-
  sternum S23.29
  subglenoid — *see* Dislocation, shoulder
  symphysis pubis S33.4
  talus — *see* Dislocation, ankle
  tarsal (bone (s)) (joint (s)) — *see*
    Dislocation, foot
  tarsometatarsal (joint (s)) — *see* Dislocation,
    foot
  temporomandibular (joint) S03.0-

Dislocation (articular) - *continued*
thigh, proximal end — *see* Dislocation, hip
thorax S23.20
  specified site NEC S23.29
  vertebra — *see* Dislocation, vertebra
thumb S63.10-
  interphalangeal joint — *see* Dislocation,
    interphalangeal (joint), thumb
  metacarpophalangeal joint — *see*
    Dislocation, metacarpophalangeal
    (joint), thumb
thyroid cartilage S13.29
tibia
  distal end — *see* Dislocation, ankle
  proximal end — *see* Dislocation, knee
tibiofibular (joint)
  distal — *see* Dislocation, ankle
  superior — *see* Dislocation, knee
toe (s) S93.106
  great S93.10-
    interphalangeal joint S93.11-
    metatarsophalangeal joint S93.12-
  interphalangeal joint S93.119
  lesser S93.106
    interphalangeal joint S93.11-
    metatarsophalangeal joint S93.12-
  metatarsophalangeal joint S93.12-
tooth S03.2
trachea S23.29
ulna
  distal end S63.07-
  proximal end — *see* Dislocation, elbow
ulnohumeral (joint) — *see* Dislocation,
  elbow
vertebra (articular process) (body)
  (traumatic)
  cervical S13.101
    atlantoaxial joint S13.121
    atlantooccipital joint S13.111
    atloidooccipital joint S13.111
    joint between
      C0 and C1 S13.111
      C1 and C2 S13.121
      C2 and C3 S13.131
      C3 and C4 S13.141
      C4 and C5 S13.151
      C5and C6 S13.161
      C6and C7 S13.171
      C7and T1 S13.181
    occipitoatloid joint S13.111
  congenital Q76.49
  lumbar S33.101
    joint between
      L1and L2 S33.111
      L2and L3 S33.121
      L3 and L4 S33.131
      L4and L5 S33.141
  nontraumatic — *see* Displacement,
    intervertebral disc
  partial — *see* Subluxation, by site
  recurrent NEC — *see* subcategory M43.5
  thoracic S23.101
    joint between
      T1 and T2 S23.111
      T2 and T3 S23.121
      T3 and T4 S23.123
      T4 and T5 S23.131
      T5 and T6 S23.133
      T6 and T7 S23.141
      T7 and T8 S23.143
      T8 and T9 S23.151
      T9 and T10 S23.153
      T10 and T11 S23.161
      T11 and T12 S23.163
      T12 and L1 S23.171
wrist (carpal bone) S63.006
  carpometacarpal joint — *see* Dislocation,
    carpometacarpal (joint)
  distal radioulnar joint — *see* Dislocation,
    radioulnar (joint), distal
  metacarpal bone, proximal — *see*
    Dislocation, metacarpal (bone),
    proximal end
  midcarpal — *see* Dislocation, midcarpal
    (joint)

Dislocation (articular) - *continued*
wrist (carpal bone) - *continued*
  radiocarpal joint — *see* Dislocation,
    radiocarpal (joint)
  recurrent — *see* Dislocation, recurrent,
    wrist
  specified site NEC S63.09-
  ulna — *see* Dislocation, ulna, distal end
xiphoid cartilage S23.29
Disorder (of) — *see also* Disease
acantholytic L11.9
  specified NEC L11.8
acute
  psychotic — *see* Psychosis, acute
  stress F43.0
adjustment (grief) F43.20
  with
    anxiety F43.22
      with depressed mood F43.23
    conduct disturbance F43.24
      with emotional disturbance F43.25
    depressed mood F43.21
      with anxiety F43.23
    other specified symptom F43.29
adrenal (capsule) (gland) (medullary) E27.9
  specified NEC E27.8
adrenogenital E25.9
  drug-induced E25.8
  iatrogenic E25.8
  idiopathic E25.8
adult personality (and behavior) F69
  specified NEC F68.8
affective (mood) — *see* Disorder, mood
aggressive, unsocialized F91.1
alcohol-related F10.99
  with
    amnestic disorder, persisting F10.96
    anxiety disorder F10.980
    dementia, persisting F10.97
    intoxication F10.929
      with delirium F10.921
      uncomplicated F10.920
    mood disorder F10.94
    other specified F10.988
    psychotic disorder F10.959
      with
        delusions F10.950
        hallucinations F10.951
    sexual dysfunction F10.981
    sleep disorder F10.982
alcohol use
  mild F10.10
    with
      alcohol-induced
        anxiety disorder F10.180
        bipolar and related disorder F10.14
        depressive disorder F10.14
        psychotic disorder F10.159
        sexual dysfunction F10.181
        sleep disorder F10.182
      alcohol intoxication F10.129
        delirium F10.121
    in remission (early) (sustained) F10.11
  moderate or severe F10.20
    with
      alcohol-induced
        anxiety disorder F10.280
        bipolar and related disorder F10.24
        depressive disorder F10.24
        major neurocognitive disorder,
          amnestic-confabulatory
          type F10.26
        major neurocognitive disorder,
          nonamnestic-confabulatory
          type F10.27
        mild neurocognitive
          disorder F10.288
        psychotic disorder F10.259
        sexual dysfunction F10.281
        sleep disorder F10.282
      alcohol intoxication F10.229
        delirium F10.221
    in remission (early) (sustained) F10.21
allergic — *see* Allergy
alveolar NEC J84.09

Disorder (of) - *continued*
amino-acid
  cystathioninuria E72.19
  cystinosis E72.04
  cystinuria E72.01
  glycinuria E72.09
  homocystinuria E72.11
  metabolism — *see* Disturbance,
    metabolism, amino-acid
  specified NEC E72.89
  neonatal, transitory P74.8
  renal transport NEC E72.09
  transport NEC E72.09
amnesic, amnestic
  alcohol-induced F10.96
    with dependence F10.26
  due to (secondary to) general medical
    condition F04
  psychoactive NEC-induced F19.96
    with
      abuse F19.16
      dependence F19.26
  sedative, hypnotic or anxiolytic-
    induced F13.96
    with dependence F13.26
amphetamine-type substance use
  mild F15.10
    in remission (early) (sustained) F15.11
  moderate F15.20
    in remission (early) (sustained) F15.21
  severe F15.20
    in remission (early) (sustained) F15.21
amphetamine (or other stimulant) use
  mild
    with
      amphetamine (or other stimulant)
        -induced
        anxiety disorder F15.180
        bipolar and related disorder F15.14
        depressive disorder F15.14
        obsessive-compulsive and related
          disorder F15.188
        psychotic disorder F15.159
        sexual dysfunction F15.181
      amphetamine, cocaine, or other
        stimulant intoxication
        with perceptual
          disturbances F15.122
        without perceptual
          disturbances F15.129
      intoxication delirium F15.121
  moderate or severe
    with
      amphetamine (or other stimulant)
        -induced
        anxiety disorder F15.280
        obsessive-compulsive and related
          disorder F15.288
        sexual dysfunction F15.281
        bipolar and related disorder F15.24
        depressive disorder F15.24
        psychotic disorder F15.259
      amphetamine, cocaine, or other
        stimulant intoxication
        with perceptual
          disturbances F15.222
        without perceptual
          disturbances F15.229
      intoxication delirium F15.221
anaerobic glycolysis with anemia D55.2
anxiety F41.9
  due to (secondary to)
    alcohol F10.980
      in
        abuse F10.180
        dependence F10.280
    amphetamine F15.980
      in
        abuse F15.180
        dependence F15.280
    anxiolytic F13.980
      in
        abuse F13.180
        dependence F13.280
    caffeine F15.980

Disorder (of) - *continued*
　anxiety - *continued*
　　due to (secondary to) - *continued*
　　　caffeine - *continued*
　　　　in
　　　　　abuse F15.180
　　　　　dependence F15.280
　　　　cannabis F12.980
　　　　　in
　　　　　　abuse F12.180
　　　　　　dependence F12.280
　　　　cocaine F14.980
　　　　　in
　　　　　　abuse F14.180
　　　　　　dependence F14.180
　　　　general medical condition F06.4
　　　　hallucinogen F16.980
　　　　　in
　　　　　　abuse F16.180
　　　　　　dependence F16.280
　　　　hypnotic F13.980
　　　　　in
　　　　　　abuse F13.180
　　　　　　dependence F13.280
　　　　inhalant F18.980
　　　　　in
　　　　　　abuse F18.180
　　　　　　dependence F18.280
　　　　phencyclidine F16.980
　　　　　in
　　　　　　abuse F16.180
　　　　　　dependence F16.280
　　　　psychoactive substance NEC F19.980
　　　　　in
　　　　　　abuse F19.180
　　　　　　dependence F19.280
　　　　sedative F13.980
　　　　　in
　　　　　　abuse F13.180
　　　　　　dependence F13.280
　　　　volatile solvents F18.980
　　　　　in
　　　　　　abuse F18.180
　　　　　　dependence F18.280
　　generalized F41.1
　　illness F45.21
　　mixed
　　　with depression (mild) F41.8
　　　specified NEC F41.3
　　organic F06.4
　　phobic F40.9
　　　of childhood F40.8
　　specified NEC F41.8
　aortic valve — *see* Endocarditis, aortic
　aromatic amino-acid metabolism E70.9
　　specified NEC E70.8
　arteriole NEC I77.89
　artery NEC I77.89
　articulation — *see* Disorder, joint
　attachment (childhood)
　　disinhibited F94.2
　　reactive F94.1
　attention-deficit hyperactivity (adolescent)
　　(adult) (child) F90.9
　　combined
　　　presentation F90.2
　　　type F90.2
　　hyperactive
　　　impulsive presentation F90.1
　　　type F90.1
　　inattentive
　　　presentation F90.0
　　　type F90.0
　　specified type NEC F90.8
　attention-deficit without hyperactivity
　　(adolescent) (adult) (child) F98.8
　auditory processing (central) H93.25
　autistic F84.0
　autism spectrum F84.0
　autoimmune D89.89
　autonomic nervous system G90.9
　　specified NEC G90.8
　avoidant
　　child or adolescent F40.10
　　restrictive food intake F50.82

Disorder (of) - *continued*
　balance
　　acid-base E87.8
　　　mixed E87.4
　　electrolyte E87.8
　　fluid NEC E87.8
　behavioral (disruptive) — *see* Disorder,
　　conduct
　beta-amino-acid metabolism E72.89
　bile acid and cholesterol metabolism E78.70
　　Barth syndrome E78.71
　　other specified E78.79
　　Smith-Lemli-Opitz syndrome E78.72
　bilirubin excretion E80.6
　binge eating F50.81
　binocular
　　movement H51.9
　　　convergence
　　　　excess H51.12
　　　　insufficiency H51.11
　　　internuclear ophthalmoplegia — *see*
　　　　Ophthalmoplegia, internuclear
　　　palsy of conjugate gaze H51.0
　　　specified type NEC H51.8
　　vision NEC — *see* Disorder, vision,
　　　binocular
　bipolar (I) (type 1) F31.9
　　and related due to a known physiological
　　　condition
　　　with
　　　　manic features F06.33
　　　　manic- or hypomanic-like
　　　　　episodes F06.33
　　　　mixed features F06.34
　　current (or most recent) episode
　　　depressed F31.9
　　　　with psychotic features F31.5
　　　　without psychotic features F31.30
　　　　　mild F31.31
　　　　　moderate F31.32
　　　　　severe (without psychotic
　　　　　　features) F31.4
　　　　　　with psychotic features F31.5
　　　hypomanic F31.0
　　　manic F31.9
　　　　with psychotic features F31.2
　　　　without psychotic features F31.10
　　　　　mild F31.11
　　　　　moderate F31.12
　　　　　severe (without psychotic
　　　　　　features) F31.13
　　　　　　with psychotic features F31.2
　　　mixed F31.60
　　　　mild F31.61
　　　　moderate F31.62
　　　　severe (without psychotic
　　　　　features) F31.63
　　　　　with psychotic features F31.64
　　　severe depression (without psychotic
　　　　features) F31.4
　　　　with psychotic features F31.5
　　in remission (currently) F31.70
　　　in full remission
　　　　most recent episode
　　　　　depressed F31.76
　　　　　hypomanic F31.72
　　　　　manic F31.74
　　　　　mixed F31.78
　　　in partial remission
　　　　most recent episode
　　　　　depressed F31.75
　　　　　hypomanic F31.71
　　　　　manic F31.73
　　　　　mixed F31.77
　　specified NEC F31.89
　　II (type 2) F31.81
　　organic F06.30
　　single manic episode F30.9
　　　mild F30.11
　　　moderate F30.12
　　　severe (without psychotic
　　　　symptoms) F30.13
　　　　with psychotic symptoms F30.2
　bladder N32.9
　　functional NEC N31.9

Disorder (of) - *continued*
　bladder - *continued*
　　in schistosomiasis B65.0 *[N33]*
　　specified NEC N32.89
　bleeding D68.9
　blood D75.9
　　in congenital early syphilis A50.09 *[D77]*
　body dysmorphic F45.22
　bone M89.9
　　continuity M84.9
　　　specified type NEC M84.80
　　　　ankle M84.87-
　　　　fibula M84.86-
　　　　foot M84.87-
　　　　hand M84.84-
　　　　humerus M84.82-
　　　　neck M84.88
　　　　pelvis M84.859
　　　　radius M84.83-
　　　　rib M84.88
　　　　shoulder M84.81-
　　　　skull M84.88
　　　　thigh M84.85-
　　　　tibia M84.86-
　　　　ulna M84.83-
　　　　vertebra M84.88
　　density and structure M85.9
　　　cyst — *see also* Cyst, bone, specified
　　　　type NEC
　　　　aneurysmal — *see* Cyst, bone,
　　　　　aneurysmal
　　　　solitary — *see* Cyst, bone, solitary
　　　diffuse idiopathic skeletal
　　　　hyperostosis — *see* Hyperostosis,
　　　　　ankylosing
　　　fibrous dysplasia (monostotic) — *see*
　　　　Dysplasia, fibrous, bone
　　　fluorosis — *see* Fluorosis, skeletal
　　　hyperostosis of skull M85.2
　　　osteitis condensans — *see* Osteitis,
　　　　condensans
　　　specified type NEC M85.8-
　　　　ankle M85.87-
　　　　foot M85.87-
　　　　forearm M85.83-
　　　　hand M85.84-
　　　　lower leg M85.86-
　　　　multiple sites M85.89
　　　　neck M85.88
　　　　rib M85.88
　　　　shoulder M85.81-
　　　　skull M85.88
　　　　thigh M85.85-
　　　　upper arm M85.82-
　　　　vertebra M85.88
　　development and growth NEC M89.20
　　　carpus M89.24-
　　　clavicle M89.21-
　　　femur M89.25-
　　　fibula M89.26-
　　　finger M89.24-
　　　humerus M89.22-
　　　ilium M89.259
　　　ischium M89.259
　　　metacarpus M89.24-
　　　metatarsus M89.27-
　　　multiple sites M89.29
　　　neck M89.28
　　　radius M89.23-
　　　rib M89.28
　　　scapula M89.21-
　　　skull M89.28
　　　tarsus M89.27-
　　　tibia M89.26-
　　　toe M89.27-
　　　ulna M89.23-
　　　vertebra M89.28
　　　specified type NEC M89.8X-
　　brachial plexus G54.0
　　branched-chain amino-acid
　　　metabolism E71.2
　　　specified NEC E71.19
　　breast N64.9
　　　agalactia — *see* Agalactia
　　　associated with

Disorder (of) - *continued*
　breast - *continued*
　　associated with - *continued*
　　　lactation O92.70
　　　　specified NEC O92.79
　　　pregnancy O92.20
　　　　specified NEC O92.29
　　　puerperium O92.20
　　　　specified NEC O92.29
　　　cracked nipple — *see* Cracked nipple
　　　galactorrhea — *see* Galactorrhea
　　　hypogalactia O92.4
　　　lactation disorder NEC O92.79
　　　mastitis — *see* Mastitis
　　　nipple infection — *see* Infection, nipple
　　　retracted nipple — *see* Retraction, nipple
　　　specified type NEC N64.89
　Briquet's F45.0
　bullous, in diseases classified elsewhere L14
　caffeine use
　　mild
　　　with
　　　　caffeine-induced
　　　　　anxiety disorder F15.180
　　　　　sleep disorder F15.182
　　　moderate or severe
　　　　with
　　　　　caffeine-induced
　　　　　　anxiety disorder F15.280
　　　　　　sleep disorder F15.282
　cannabis use
　　mild F12.10
　　　with
　　　　cannabis-induced
　　　　　anxiety disorder F12.180
　　　　　psychotic disorder F12.159
　　　　　sleep disorder F12.188
　　　　cannabis intoxication
　　　　　delirium F12.121
　　　　　with perceptual
　　　　　　disturbances F12.122
　　　　　without perceptual
　　　　　　disturbances F12.129
　　　in remission (early) (sustained) F12.11
　　moderate or severe F12.20
　　　with
　　　　cannabis-induced
　　　　　anxiety disorder F12.280
　　　　　psychotic disorder F12.259
　　　　　sleep disorder F12.288
　　　　cannabis intoxication
　　　　　with perceptual
　　　　　　disturbances F12.222
　　　　　without perceptual
　　　　　　disturbances F12.229
　　　　　delirium F12.221
　　　in remission (early) (sustained) F12.21
　carbohydrate
　　absorption, intestinal NEC E74.39
　　metabolism (congenital) E74.9
　　　specified NEC E74.8
　cardiac, functional I51.89
　carnitine metabolism E71.40
　cartilage M94.9
　　articular NEC — *see* Derangement, joint,
　　　articular cartilage
　　chondrocalcinosis — *see*
　　　Chondrocalcinosis
　　specified type NEC M94.8X-
　　　articular — *see* Derangement, joint,
　　　　articular cartilage
　　　multiple sites M94.8X0
　catatonia (due to known physiological
　　condition) (with another mental
　　disorder) F06.1
　catatonic
　　due to (secondary to) known physiological
　　　condition F06.1
　　organic F06.1
　central auditory processing H93.25
　cervical
　　region NEC M53.82
　　root (nerve) NEC G54.2
　character NOS F60.9
　childhood disintegrative NEC F84.3

Disorder (of) - *continued*
　cholesterol and bile acid metabolism E78.70
　　Barth syndrome E78.71
　　other specified E78.79
　　Smith-Lemli-Opitz syndrome E78.72
　choroid H31.9
　　atrophy — *see* Atrophy, choroid
　　degeneration — *see* Degeneration, choroid
　　detachment — *see* Detachment, choroid
　　dystrophy — *see* Dystrophy, choroid
　　hemorrhage — *see* Hemorrhage, choroid
　　rupture — *see* Rupture, choroid
　　scar — *see* Scar, chorioretinal
　　solar retinopathy — *see* Retinopathy, solar
　　specified type NEC H31.8
　ciliary body — *see* Disorder, iris
　　degeneration — *see* Degeneration, ciliary
　　　body
　coagulation (factor) — *see also* Defect,
　　coagulation D68.9
　　newborn, transient P61.6
　cocaine use
　　mild F14.10
　　　with
　　　　amphetamine, cocaine, or other
　　　　　stimulant intoxication
　　　　　with perceptual
　　　　　　disturbances F14.122
　　　　　without perceptual
　　　　　　disturbances F14.129
　　　　cocaine-induced
　　　　　anxiety disorder F14.180
　　　　　bipolar and related disorder F14.14
　　　　　depressive disorder F14.14
　　　　　obsessive-compulsive and related
　　　　　　disorder F14.188
　　　　　psychotic disorder F14.159
　　　　　sexual dysfunction F14.181
　　　　　sleep disorder F14.182
　　　　cocaine intoxication delirium F14.121
　　　in remission (early) (sustained) F14.11
　　moderate or severe F14.20
　　　with
　　　　amphetamine, cocaine, or other
　　　　　stimulant intoxication
　　　　　with perceptual
　　　　　　disturbances F14.222
　　　　　without perceptual
　　　　　　disturbances F14.229
　　　　cocaine-induced
　　　　　anxiety disorder F14.280
　　　　　bipolar and related disorder F14.24
　　　　　depressive disorder F14.24
　　　　　obsessive-compulsive and related
　　　　　　disorder F14.288
　　　　　psychotic disorder F14.259
　　　　　sexual dysfunction F14.281
　　　　　sleep disorder F14.282
　　　　cocaine intoxication delirium F14.221
　　　in remission (early) (sustained) F14.21
　coccyx NEC M53.3
　cognitive F09
　　due to (secondary to) general medical
　　　condition F09
　　persisting R41.89
　　　due to
　　　　alcohol F10.97
　　　　　with dependence F10.27
　　　　anxiolytics F13.97
　　　　　with dependence F13.27
　　　　hypnotics F13.97
　　　　　with dependence F13.27
　　　　sedatives F13.97
　　　　　with dependence F13.27
　　　　specified substance NEC F19.97
　　　　　with
　　　　　　abuse F19.17
　　　　　　dependence F19.27
　communication F80.9
　　social pragmatic F80.82
　conduct (childhood) F91.9
　　adjustment reaction — *see* Disorder,
　　　adjustment
　　adolescent onset type F91.2
　　childhood onset type F91.1

Disorder (of) - *continued*
　conduct (childhood) - *continued*
　　compulsive F63.9
　　confined to family context F91.0
　　depressive F91.8
　　group type F91.2
　　hyperkinetic — *see* Disorder, attention-
　　　deficit hyperactivity
　　oppositional defiance F91.3
　　socialized F91.2
　　solitary aggressive type F91.1
　　specified NEC F91.8
　　unsocialized (aggressive) F91.1
　conduction, heart I45.9
　congenital glycosylation (CDG) E74.8
　conjunctiva H11.9
　　infection — *see* Conjunctivitis
　connective tissue, localized L94.9
　　specified NEC L94.8
　conversion (functional neurological symptom
　　disorder)
　　with
　　　abnormal movement F44.4
　　　anesthesia or sensory loss F44.6
　　　attacks or seizures F44.5
　　　mixed symptoms F44.7
　　　special sensory symptoms F44.6
　　　speech symptoms F44.4
　　　swallowing symptoms F44.4
　　　weakness or paralysis F44.4
　convulsive (secondary) — *see* Convulsions
　cornea H18.9
　　deformity — *see* Deformity, cornea
　　degeneration — *see* Degeneration, cornea
　　deposits — *see* Deposit, cornea
　　due to contact lens H18.82-
　　　specified as edema — *see* Edema,
　　　　cornea
　　edema — *see* Edema, cornea
　　keratitis — *see* Keratitis
　　keratoconjunctivitis — *see*
　　　Keratoconjunctivitis
　　membrane change — *see* Change, corneal
　　　membrane
　　neovascularization — *see*
　　　Neovascularization, cornea
　　scar — *see* Opacity, cornea
　　specified type NEC H18.89-
　　ulcer — *see* Ulcer, cornea
　corpus cavernosum N48.9
　cranial nerve — *see* Disorder, nerve, cranial
　cyclothymic F34.0
　defiant oppositional F91.3
　delusional (persistent) (systematized) F22
　　induced F24
　depersonalization F48.1
　depressive F32.9
　　due to known physiological condition
　　　with
　　　　depressive features F06.31
　　　　major depressive-like episode F06.32
　　　　mixed features F06.34
　　major F32.9
　　　with psychotic symptoms F32.3
　　　in remission (full) F32.5
　　　　partial F32.4
　　　recurrent F33.9
　　　　with psychotic features F33.3
　　　single episode F32.9
　　　　mild F32.0
　　　　moderate F32.1
　　　　severe (without psychotic
　　　　　symptoms) F32.2
　　　　　with psychotic symptoms F32.3
　　organic F06.31
　　persistent F34.1
　　recurrent F33.9
　　　current episode
　　　　mild F33.0
　　　　moderate F33.1
　　　　severe (without psychotic
　　　　　symptoms) F33.2
　　　　　with psychotic symptoms F33.3
　　　in remission F33.40
　　　　full F33.42

Disorder (of) - *continued*
  depressive - *continued*
    recurrent - *continued*
      in remission - *continued*
        partial F33.41
        specified NEC F33.8
      single episode — *see* Episode, depressive
      specified NEC F32.89
  developmental F89
    arithmetical skills F81.2
    coordination (motor) F82
    expressive writing F81.81
    language F80.9
      expressive F80.1
      mixed receptive and expressive F80.2
      receptive type F80.2
      specified NEC F80.89
    learning F81.9
      arithmetical F81.2
      reading F81.0
    mixed F88
    motor coordination or function F82
    pervasive F84.9
      specified NEC F84.8
    phonological F80.0
    reading F81.0
    scholastic skills — *see also* Disorder,
        learning
      mixed F81.89
    specified NEC F88
    speech F80.9
      articulation F80.0
      specified NEC F80.89
    written expression F81.81
  diaphragm J98.6
  digestive (system) K92.9
    newborn P78.9
      specified NEC P78.89
    postprocedural — *see* Complication,
        gastrointestinal
    psychogenic F45.8
  disc (intervertebral) M51.9
    with
      myelopathy
        cervical region M50.00
        cervicothoracic region M50.03
        high cervical region M50.01
        lumbar region M51.06
        mid-cervical region M50.020
        sacrococcygeal region M53.3
        thoracic region M51.04
        thoracolumbar region M51.05
      radiculopathy
        cervical region M50.10
        cervicothoracic region M50.13
        high cervical region M50.11
        lumbar region M51.16
        lumbosacral region M51.17
        mid-cervical region M50.120
        sacrococcygeal region M53.3
        thoracic region M51.14
        thoracolumbar region M51.15
    cervical M50.90
      with
        myelopathy M50.00
          C2-C3 M50.01
          C3-C4 M50.01
          C4-C5 M50.021
          C5-C6 M50.022
          C6-C7 M50.023
          C7-T1 M50.03
          cervicothoracic region M50.03
          high cervical region M50.01
          mid-cervical region M50.020
        neuritis, radiculitis or
            radiculopathy M50.10
          C2-C3 M50.11
          C3-C4 M50.11
          C4-C5 M50.121
          C5-C6 M50.122
          C6-C7 M50.123
          C7-T1 M50.13
          cervicothoracic region M50.13
          high cervical region M50.11
          mid-cervical region M50.120

Disorder (of) - *continued*
  disc (intervertebral) - *continued*
    cervical - *continued*
      C2-C3 M50.91
      C3-C4 M50.91
      C4-C5 M50.921
      C5-C6 M50.922
      C6-C7 M50.923
      C7-T1 M50.93
      cervicothoracic region M50.93
      degeneration M50.30
        C2-C3 M50.31
        C3-C4 M50.31
        C4-C5 M50.321
        C5-C6 M50.322
        C6-C7 M50.323
        C7-T1 M50.33
        cervicothoracic region M50.33
        high cervical region M50.31
        mid-cervical region M50.320
      displacement M50.20
        C2-C3 M50.21
        C3-C4 M50.21
        C4-C5 M50.221
        C5-C6 M50.222
        C6-C7 M50.223
        C7-T1 M50.23
        cervicothoracic region M50.23
        high cervical region M50.21
        mid-cervical region M50.220
      high cervical region M50.91
      mid-cervical region M50.920
      specified type NEC M50.80
        C2-C3 M50.81
        C3-C4 M50.81
        C4-C5 M50.821
        C5-C6 M50.822
        C6-C7 M50.823
        C7-T1 M50.83
        cervicothoracic region M50.83
        high cervical region M50.81
        mid-cervical region M50.820
    specified NEC
      lumbar region M51.86
      lumbosacral region M51.87
      sacrococcygeal region M53.3
      thoracic region M51.84
      thoracolumbar region M51.85
  disinhibited attachment (childhood) F94.2
  disintegrative, childhood NEC F84.3
  disruptive F91.9
    mood dysregulation F34.81
    specified NEC F91.8
  disruptive behavior — *see* Disorder, conduct
  dissocial personality F60.2
  dissociative F44.9
    affecting
      motor function F44.4
        and sensation F44.7
      sensation F44.6
        and motor function F44.7
    brief reactive F43.0
    due to (secondary to) general medical
        condition F06.8
    mixed F44.7
    organic F06.8
    other specified NEC F44.89
  double heterozygous sickling — *see* Disease,
      sickle-cell
  dream anxiety F51.5
  drug induced hemorrhagic D68.32
  drug related F19.99
    abuse — *see* Abuse, drug
    dependence — *see* Dependence, drug
  dysmorphic body F45.22
  dysthymic F34.1
  ear H93.9-
    bleeding — *see* Otorrhagia
    deafness — *see* Deafness
    degenerative H93.09-
    discharge — *see* Otorrhea
    external H61.9-
      auditory canal stenosis — *see* Stenosis,
          external ear canal

Disorder (of) - *continued*
  ear - *continued*
    external - *continued*
      exostosis — *see* Exostosis, external ear
          canal
      impacted cerumen — *see* Impaction,
          cerumen
      otitis — *see* Otitis, externa
      perichondritis — *see* Perichondritis, ear
      pinna — *see* Disorder, pinna
      specified type NEC H61.89-
        in diseases classified
            elsewhere H62.8X-
    inner H83.9-
      vestibular dysfunction — *see* Disorder,
          vestibular function
    middle H74.9-
      adhesive H74.1-
      ossicle — *see* Abnormal, ear ossicles
      polyp — *see* Polyp, ear (middle)
      specified NEC, in diseases classified
          elsewhere H75.8-
    postprocedural — *see* Complications, ear,
        procedure
    specified NEC, in diseases classified
        elsewhere H94.8-
  eating (adult) (psychogenic) F50.9
    anorexia — *see* Anorexia
    binge F50.81
    bulimia F50.2
    child F98.29
      pica F98.3
      rumination disorder F98.21
    pica F50.89
      childhood F98.3
  electrolyte (balance) NEC E87.8
    with
      abortion — *see* Abortion by type
          complicated by specified condition
          NEC
      ectopic pregnancy O08.5
      molar pregnancy O08.5
    acidosis (metabolic) (respiratory) E87.2
    alkalosis (metabolic) (respiratory) E87.3
  elimination, transepidermal L87.9
    specified NEC L87.8
  emotional (persistent) F34.9
    of childhood F93.9
      specified NEC F93.8
  endocrine E34.9
    postprocedural E89.89
    specified NEC E89.89
  erectile (male) (organic) — *see also*
      Dysfunction, sexual, male,
      erectile N52.9
    nonorganic F52.21
  erythematous — *see* Erythema
  esophagus K22.9
    functional K22.4
    psychogenic F45.8
  eustachian tube H69.9-
    infection — *see* Salpingitis, eustachian
    obstruction — *see* Obstruction, eustachian
        tube
    patulous — *see* Patulous, eustachian tube
    specified NEC H69.8-
  exhibitionistic F65.2
  extrapyramidal G25.9
    in diseases classified elsewhere — *see*
        category G26
    specified type NEC G25.89
  eye H57.9
    postprocedural — *see* Complication,
        postprocedural, eye
  eyelid H02.9
    cyst — *see* Cyst, eyelid
    degenerative H02.70
      chloasma — *see* Chloasma, eyelid
      madarosis — *see* Madarosis
      specified type NEC H02.79
      vitiligo — *see* Vitiligo, eyelid
      xanthelasma — *see* Xanthelasma
    dermatochalasis — *see* Dermatochalasis
    edema — *see* Edema, eyelid
    elephantiasis — *see* Elephantiasis, eyelid

Disorder (of) - *continued*
eyelid - *continued*
foreign body, retained — *see* Foreign body, retained, eyelid
function H02.59
abnormal innervation syndrome — *see* Syndrome, abnormal innervation
blepharochalasis — *see* Blepharochalasis
blepharoclonus — *see* Blepharoclonus
blepharophimosis — *see* Blepharophimosis
blepharoptosis — *see* Blepharoptosis
lagophthalmos — *see* Lagophthalmos
lid retraction — *see* Retraction, lid
hypertrichosis — *see* Hypertrichosis, eyelid
specified type NEC H02.89
vascular H02.879
left H02.876
lower H02.875
upper H02.874
right H02.873
lower H02.872
upper H02.871
factitious
by proxy F68.A
imposed on another F68.A
imposed on self F68.10
with predominantly
psychological symptoms F68.11
with physical symptoms F68.13
physical symptoms F68.12
with psychological symptoms F68.13
factor, coagulation — *see* Defect, coagulation
fatty acid
metabolism E71.30
specified NEC E71.39
oxidation
LCAD E71.310
MCAD E71.311
SCAD E71.312
specified deficiency NEC E71.318
feeding (infant or child) — *see also* Disorder, eating R63.3
or eating disorder F50.9
specified NEC F50.9
feigned (with obvious motivation) Z76.5
without obvious motivation — *see* Disorder, factitious
female
hypoactive sexual desire F52.0
orgasmic F52.31
sexual interest/arousal F52.22
fetishistic F65.0
fibroblastic M72.9
specified NEC M72.8
fluency
adult onset F98.5
childhood onset F80.81
following
cerebral infarction I69.323
cerebrovascular disease I69.923
specified disease NEC I69.823
intracerebral hemorrhage I69.123
nontraumatic intracranial hemorrhage NEC I69.223
subarachnoid hemorrhage I69.023
in conditions classified elsewhere R47.82
fluid balance E87.8
follicular (skin) L73.9
specified NEC L73.8
frotteuristic F65.81
fructose metabolism E74.10
essential fructosuria E74.11
fructokinase deficiency E74.11
fructose-1, 6-diphosphatase deficiency E74.19
hereditary fructose intolerance E74.12
other specified E74.19
functional polymorphonuclear neutrophils D71

Disorder (of) - *continued*
gallbladder, biliary tract and pancreas in diseases classified elsewhere K87
gambling F63.0
gamma aminobutyric acid (GABA) metabolism E72.81
gamma-glutamyl cycle E72.89
gastric (functional) K31.9
motility K30
psychogenic F45.8
secretion K30
gastrointestinal (functional) NOS K92.9
newborn P78.9
psychogenic F45.8
gender-identity or -role F64.9
childhood F64.2
effect on relationship F66
of adolescence or adulthood F64.0
nontranssexual F64.8
specified NEC F64.8
uncertainty F66
genito-pelvic pain penetration F52.6
genitourinary system
female N94.9
male N50.9
psychogenic F45.8
globe H44.9
degenerated condition H44.50
absolute glaucoma H44.51-
atrophy H44.52-
leucocoria H44.53-
degenerative H44.30
chalcosis H44.31-
myopia — *see also* Myopia, degenerative H44.2-
siderosis H44.32-
specified type NEC H44.39-
endophthalmitis — *see* Endophthalmitis
foreign body, retained — *see* Foreign body, intraocular, old, retained
hemophthalmos — *see* Hemophthalmos
hypotony H44.40
due to
ocular fistula H44.42-
specified disorder NEC H44.43-
flat anterior chamber H44.41-
primary H44.44-
luxation — *see* Luxation, globe
specified type NEC H44.89
glomerular (in) N05.9
amyloidosis E85.4 *[N08]*
cryoglobulinemia D89.1 *[N08]*
disseminated intravascular coagulation D65 *[N08]*
Fabry's disease E75.21 *[N08]*
familial lecithin cholesterol acyltransferase deficiency E78.6 *[N08]*
Goodpasture's syndrome M31.0
hemolytic-uremic syndrome D59.3
Henoch (-Schönlein) purpura D69.0 *[N08]*
malariae malaria B52.0
microscopic polyangiitis M31.7 *[N08]*
multiple myeloma C90.0- *[N08]*
mumps B26.83
schistosomiasis B65.9 *[N08]*
sepsis NEC A41.- *[N08]*
streptococcal A40.- *[N08]*
sickle-cell disorders D57.- *[N08]*
strongyloidiasis B78.9 *[N08]*
subacute bacterial endocarditis I33.0 *[N08]*
syphilis A52.75
systemic lupus erythematosus M32.14
thrombotic thrombocytopenic purpura M31.1 *[N08]*
Waldenström macroglobulinemia C88.0 *[N08]*
Wegener's granulomatosis M31.31
gluconeogenesis E74.4
glucosaminoglycan metabolism — *see* Disorder, metabolism, glucosaminoglycan
glycine metabolism E72.50
d-glycericacidemia E72.59
hyperhydroxyprolinemia E72.59
hyperoxaluria R82.992

Disorder (of) - *continued*
glycine metabolism - *continued*
hyperoxaluria - *continued*
primary E72.53
hyperprolinemia E72.59
non-ketotic hyperglycinemia E72.51
oxalosis E72.53
oxaluria E72.53
sarcosinemia E72.59
trimethylaminuria E72.52
glycoprotein metabolism E77.9
specified NEC E77.8
habit (and impulse) F63.9
involving sexual behavior NEC F65.9
specified NEC F63.89
hallucinogen use
mild F16.10
with
hallucinogen-induced
anxiety disorder F16.180
bipolar and related disorder F16.14
depressive disorder F16.14
psychotic disorder F16.159
hallucinogen intoxication delirium F16.121
other hallucinogen intoxication F16.129
in remission (early) (sustained) F16.11
moderate or severe F16.20
with
hallucinogen-induced
anxiety disorder F16.280
bipolar and related disorder F16.24
depressive disorder F16.24
psychotic disorder F16.259
hallucinogen intoxication delirium F16.221
other hallucinogen intoxication F16.229
in remission (early) (sustained) F16.21
heart action I49.9
hematological D75.9
newborn (transient) P61.9
specified NEC P61.8
hematopoietic organs D75.9
hemorrhagic NEC D69.9
drug-induced D68.32
due to
extrinsic circulating anticoagulants D68.32
increase in
anti-IIa D68.32
anti-Xa D68.32
intrinsic
circulating anticoagulants D68.318
increase in
antithrombin D68.318
anti-VIIIa D68.318
anti-IXa D68.318
anti-XIa D68.318
following childbirth O72.3
hemostasis — *see* Defect, coagulation
histidine metabolism E70.40
histidinemia E70.41
other specified E70.49
hoarding F42.3
hyperkinetic — *see* Disorder, attention-deficit hyperactivity
hyperleucine-isoleucinemia E71.19
hypervalinemia E71.19
hypoactive sexual desire F52.0
hypochondriacal F45.20
body dysmorphic F45.22
neurosis F45.21
other specified F45.29
identity
dissociative F44.81
of childhood F93.8
illness anxiety F45.21
immune mechanism (immunity) D89.9
specified type NEC D89.89
impaired renal tubular function N25.9
specified NEC N25.89
impulse (control) F63.9
inflammatory

Disorder (of) - *continued*
  inflammatory - *continued*
    pelvic, in diseases classified elsewhere —
      see category N74
    penis N48.29
      abscess N48.21
      cellulitis N48.22
  inhalant use
    mild F18.10
      with
        inhalant-induced
          anxiety disorder F18.180
          depressive disorder F18.14
          major neurocognitive
            disorder F18.17
          mild neurocognitive
            disorder F18.188
          psychotic disorder F18.159
        inhalant intoxication F18.129
        inhalant intoxication delirium F18.121
      in remission (early) (sustained) F18.11
    moderate or severe F18.20
      with
        inhalant-induced
          anxiety disorder F18.280
          depressive disorder F18.24
          major neurocognitive
            disorder F18.27
          mild neurocognitive
            disorder F18.288
          psychotic disorder F18.259
        inhalant intoxication F18.229
        inhalant intoxication delirium F18.221
      in remission (early) (sustained) F18.21
  integument, newborn P83.9
    specified NEC P83.88
  intermittent explosive F63.81
  internal secretion pancreas — *see* Increased,
      secretion, pancreas, endocrine
  intestine, intestinal
    carbohydrate absorption NEC E74.39
      postoperative K91.2
    functional NEC K59.9
      postoperative K91.89
    psychogenic F45.8
    vascular K55.9
      chronic K55.1
      specified NEC K55.8
  intraoperative (intraprocedural) — *see*
      Complications, intraoperative
  involuntary emotional expression
      (IEED) F48.2
  iris H21.9
    adhesions — *see* Adhesions, iris
    atrophy — *see* Atrophy, iris
    chamber angle recession — *see* Recession,
      chamber angle
    cyst — *see* Cyst, iris
    degeneration — *see* Degeneration, iris
    in diseases classified elsewhere H22
    iridodialysis — *see* Iridodialysis
    iridoschisis — *see* Iridoschisis
    miotic pupillary cyst — *see* Cyst, pupillary
    pupillary
      abnormality — *see* Abnormality,
        pupillary
      membrane — *see* Membrane, pupillary
    specified type NEC H21.89
    vascular NEC H21.1X-
  iron metabolism E83.10
    specified NEC E83.19
  isovaleric acidemia E71.110
  jaw, developmental M27.0
    temporomandibular — *see also* Anomaly,
      dentofacial, temporomandibular
      joint M26.60-
  joint M25.9
    derangement — *see* Derangement, joint
    effusion — *see* Effusion, joint
    fistula — *see* Fistula, joint
    hemarthrosis — *see* Hemarthrosis
    instability — *see* Instability, joint
    osteophyte — *see* Osteophyte
    pain — *see* Pain, joint
    psychogenic F45.8

Disorder (of) - *continued*
  joint - *continued*
    specified type NEC M25.80
      ankle M25.87-
      elbow M25.82-
      foot joint M25.87-
      hand joint M25.84-
      hip M25.85-
      knee M25.86-
      shoulder M25.81-
      wrist M25.83-
    stiffness — *see* Stiffness, joint
  ketone metabolism E71.32
  kidney N28.9
    functional (tubular) N25.9
    in
      schistosomiasis B65.9 *[N29]*
    tubular function N25.9
      specified NEC N25.89
  lacrimal system H04.9
    changes H04.69
      fistula — *see* Fistula, lacrimal
    gland H04.19
      atrophy — *see* Atrophy, lacrimal gland
      cyst — *see* Cyst, lacrimal, gland
      dacryops — *see* Dacryops
      dislocation — *see* Dislocation, lacrimal
        gland
      dry eye syndrome — *see* Syndrome, dry
        eye
      infection — *see* Dacryoadenitis
      granuloma — *see* Granuloma, lacrimal
      inflammation — *see* Inflammation,
        lacrimal
      obstruction — *see* Obstruction, lacrimal
    specified NEC H04.89
  lactation NEC O92.79
  language (developmental) F80.9
    expressive F80.1
    mixed receptive and expressive F80.2
    receptive F80.2
  late luteal phase dysphoric N94.89
  learning (specific) F81.9
    acalculia R48.8
    alexia R48.0
    mathematics F81.2
    reading F81.0
    specified
      with impairment in
        mathematics F81.2
        reading F81.0
        written expression F81.81
      specified NEC F81.89
    spelling F81.81
    written expression F81.81
  lens H27.9
    aphakia — *see* Aphakia
    cataract — *see* Cataract
    dislocation — *see* Dislocation, lens
    specified type NEC H27.8
  ligament M24.20
    ankle M24.27-
    attachment, spine — *see* Enthesopathy,
      spinal
    elbow M24.22-
    foot joint M24.27-
    hand joint M24.24-
    hip M24.25-
    knee — *see* Derangement, knee, specified
      NEC
    shoulder M24.21-
    vertebra M24.28
    wrist M24.23-
  ligamentous attachments — *see also*
      Enthesopathy
    spine — *see* Enthesopathy, spinal
  lipid
    metabolism, congenital E78.9
    storage E75.6
      specified NEC E75.5
  lipoprotein
    deficiency (familial) E78.6
    metabolism E78.9
      specified NEC E78.89
  liver K76.9

Disorder (of) - *continued*
  liver - *continued*
    malarial B54 *[K77]*
  low back — *see also* Dorsopathy, specified
      NEC
  lumbosacral
    plexus G54.1
    root (nerve) NEC G54.4
  lung, interstitial, drug-induced J70.4
    acute J70.2
    chronic J70.3
  lymphoproliferative, post-transplant
      (PTLD) D47.Z1
  lysine and hydroxylysine metabolism E72.3
  major neurocognitive — *see* Dementia, in
      (due to)
  male
    erectile (organic) — *see also* Dysfunction,
      sexual, male, erectile N52.9
      nonorganic F52.21
    hypoactive sexual desire F52.0
    orgasmic F52.32
  manic F30.9
    organic F06.33
  mast cell activation — *see* Activation, mast
      cell
  mastoid — *see also* Disorder, ear, middle
    postprocedural — *see* Complications, ear,
      procedure
  meniscus — *see* Derangement, knee,
      meniscus
  menopausal N95.9
    specified NEC N95.8
  menstrual N92.6
    psychogenic F45.8
    specified NEC N92.5
  mental (or behavioral) (nonpsychotic) F99
    due to (secondary to)
      amphetamine
        due to drug abuse — *see* Abuse, drug,
          stimulant
        due to drug dependence — *see*
          Dependence, drug, stimulant
      brain disease, damage and
        dysfunction F09
      caffeine use
        due to drug abuse — *see* Abuse, drug,
          stimulant
        due to drug dependence — *see*
          Dependence, drug, stimulant
      cannabis use
        due to drug abuse — *see* Abuse, drug,
          cannabis
        due to drug dependence — *see*
          Dependence, drug, cannabis
      general medical condition F09
      sedative or hypnotic use
        due to drug abuse — *see* Abuse, drug,
          sedative
        due to drug dependence — *see*
          Dependence, drug, sedative
      tobacco (nicotine) use — *see*
        Dependence, drug, nicotine
    following organic brain damage F07.9
      frontal lobe syndrome F07.0
      personality change F07.0
      postconcussional syndrome F07.81
      specified NEC F07.89
    infancy, childhood or adolescence F98.9
    neurotic — *see* Neurosis
    organic or symptomatic F09
    presenile, psychotic F03
    problem NEC
    psychoneurotic — *see* Neurosis
    psychotic — *see* Psychosis
    puerperal F53.0
    senile, psychotic NEC F03
  metabolic, amino acid, transitory,
      newborn P74.8
  metabolism NOS E88.9
    amino-acid E72.9
      aromatic E70.9
        albinism — *see* Albinism
        histidine E70.40
          histidinemia E70.41

Disorder (of) - *continued*
  metabolism NOS - *continued*
    amino-acid - *continued*
      aromatic - *continued*
        histidine - *continued*
          other specified E70.49
        hyperphenylalaninemia E70.1
          classical phenylketonuria E70.0
        other specified E70.8
        tryptophan E70.5
        tyrosine E70.20
          hypertyrosinemia E70.21
          other specified E70.29
      branched chain E71.2
        3-methylglutaconic aciduria E71.111
        hyperleucine-isoleucinemia E71.19
        hypervalinemia E71.19
        isovaleric acidemia E71.110
        maple syrup urine disease E71.0
        methylmalonic acidemia E71.120
        organic aciduria NEC E71.118
        other specified E71.19
        proprionate NEC E71.128
        proprionic acidemia E71.121
      glycine E72.50
        d-glycericacidemia E72.59
        hyperhydroxyprolinemia E72.59
        hyperoxaluria R82.992
          primary E72.53
        hyperprolinemia E72.59
        non-ketotic hyperglycinemia E72.51
        other specified E72.59
        sarcosinemia E72.59
        trimethylaminuria E72.52
      hydroxylysine E72.3
      lysine E72.3
      ornithine E72.4
      other specified E72.89
        beta-amino acid E72.89
        gamma-glutamyl cycle E72.89
        straight-chain E72.89
      sulfur-bearing E72.10
        homocystinuria E72.11
        methylenetetrahydrofolate reductase
          deficiency E72.12
        other specified E72.19
  bile acid and cholesterol
    metabolism E78.70
  bilirubin E80.7
    specified NEC E80.6
  calcium E83.50
    hypercalcemia E83.52
    hypocalcemia E83.51
    other specified E83.59
  carbohydrate E74.9
    specified NEC E74.8
  cholesterol and bile acid
    metabolism E78.70
  congenital E88.9
  copper E83.00
    Wilson's disease E83.01
    specified type NEC E83.09
  cystinuria E72.01
  fructose E74.10
  galactose E74.20
  glucosaminoglycan E76.9
    mucopolysaccharidosis — *see*
      Mucopolysaccharidosis
    specified NEC E76.8
  glutamine E72.89
  glycine E72.50
  glycogen storage (hepatorenal) E74.09
  glycoprotein E77.9
    specified NEC E77.8
  glycosaminoglycan E76.9
    specified NEC E76.8
  in labor and delivery O75.89
  iron E83.10
  isoleucine E71.19
  leucine E71.19
  lipoid E78.9
  lipoprotein E78.9
    specified NEC E78.89
  magnesium E83.40
    hypermagnesemia E83.41

Disorder (of) - *continued*
  metabolism NOS - *continued*
    magnesium - *continued*
      hypomagnesemia E83.42
      other specified E83.49
    mineral E83.9
      specified NEC E83.89
    mitochondrial E88.40
      MELAS syndrome E88.41
      MERRF syndrome (myoclonic epilepsy
        associated with ragged-red
        fibers) E88.42
      other specified E88.49
    ornithine E72.4
    phosphatases E83.30
    phosphorus E83.30
      acid phosphatase deficiency E83.39
      hypophosphatasia E83.39
      hypophosphatemia E83.39
        familial E83.31
      other specified E83.39
      pseudovitamin D deficiency E83.32
    plasma protein NEC E88.09
    porphyrin — *see* Porphyria
    postprocedural E89.89
      specified NEC E89.89
    purine E79.9
      specified NEC E79.8
    pyrimidine E79.9
      specified NEC E79.8
    pyruvate E74.4
    serine E72.89
    sodium E87.8
    specified NEC E88.89
    threonine E72.89
    valine E71.19
    zinc E83.2
  methylmalonic acidemia E71.120
  micturition NEC — *see also* Difficulty,
    micturition R39.198
    feeling of incomplete emptying R39.14
    hesitancy R39.11
    poor stream R39.12
    psychogenic F45.8
    split stream R39.13
    straining R39.16
    urgency R39.15
  mild neurocognitive G31.84
  mitochondrial metabolism E88.40
  mitral (valve) — *see* Endocarditis, mitral
  mixed
    anxiety and depressive F41.8
    of scholastic skills (developmental) F81.89
    receptive expressive language F80.2
  mood F39
    bipolar — *see* Disorder, bipolar
    depressive — *see* Disorder, depressive
    due to (secondary to)
      alcohol F10.94
      amphetamine F15.94
        in
          abuse F15.14
          dependence F15.24
      anxiolytic F13.94
        in
          abuse F13.14
          dependence F13.24
      cocaine F14.94
        in
          abuse F14.14
          dependence F14.24
      general medical condition F06.30
      hallucinogen F16.94
        in
          abuse F16.14
          dependence F16.24
      hypnotic F13.94
        in
          abuse F13.14
          dependence F13.24
      inhalant F18.94
        in
          abuse F18.14
          dependence F18.24
      opioid F11.94

Disorder (of) - *continued*
  mood - *continued*
    due to (secondary to) - *continued*
      opioid - *continued*
        in
          abuse F11.14
          dependence F11.24
      phencyclidine (PCP) F16.94
        in
          abuse F16.14
          dependence F16.24
      physiological condition F06.30
        with
          depressive features F06.31
          major depressive-like
            episode F06.32
          manic features F06.33
          mixed features F06.34
      psychoactive substance NEC F19.94
        in
          abuse F19.14
          dependence F19.24
      sedative F13.94
        in
          abuse F13.14
          dependence F13.24
      volatile solvents F18.94
        in
          abuse F18.14
          dependence F18.24
    manic episode F30.9
      with psychotic symptoms F30.2
      in remission (full) F30.4
        partial F30.3
      specified type NEC F30.8
      without psychotic symptoms F30.10
        mild F30.11
        moderate F30.12
        severe F30.13
    organic F06.30
      right hemisphere F07.89
    persistent F34.9
      cyclothymia F34.0
      dysthymia F34.1
      specified type NEC F34.89
    recurrent F39
    right hemisphere organic F07.89
  movement G25.9
    drug-induced G25.70
      akathisia G25.71
      specified NEC G25.79
    hysterical F44.4
    in diseases classified elsewhere — *see*
      category G26
    periodic limb G47.61
      sleep related G47.61
    specified NEC G25.89
    sleep related NEC G47.69
    stereotyped F98.4
    treatment-induced G25.9
  multiple personality F44.81
  muscle M62.9
    attachment, spine — *see* Enthesopathy,
      spinal
    in trichinellosis — *see* Trichinellosis, with
      muscle disorder
    psychogenic F45.8
    specified type NEC M62.89
    tone, newborn P94.9
      specified NEC P94.8
  muscular
    attachments — *see also* Enthesopathy
      spine — *see* Enthesopathy, spinal
    urethra N36.44
  musculoskeletal system, soft tissue — *see*
    Disorder, soft tissue
    postprocedural M96.89
    psychogenic F45.8
  myoneural G70.9
    due to lead G70.1
    specified NEC G70.89
    toxic G70.1
  myotonic NEC G71.19
  nail, in diseases classified elsewhere L62

Disorder (of) - *continued*

neck region NEC — *see* Dorsopathy, specified NEC

neonatal onset multisystemic inflammatory (NOMID) M04.2

nerve G58.9

  abducent NEC — *see* Strabismus, paralytic, sixth nerve

  accessory G52.8

  acoustic — *see* subcategory H93.3

  auditory — *see* subcategory H93.3

  auriculotemporal G50.8

  axillary G54.0

  cerebral — *see* Disorder, nerve, cranial

  cranial G52.9

    eighth — *see* subcategory H93.3

    eleventh G52.8

    fifth G50.9

    first G52.0

    fourth NEC — *see* Strabismus, paralytic, fourth nerve

    multiple G52.7

    ninth G52.1

    second NEC — *see* Disorder, nerve, optic

    seventh NEC G51.8

    sixth NEC — *see* Strabismus, paralytic, sixth nerve

    specified NEC G52.8

    tenth G52.2

    third NEC — *see* Strabismus, paralytic, third nerve

    twelfth G52.3

  entrapment — *see* Neuropathy, entrapment

  facial G51.9

    specified NEC G51.8

  femoral — *see* Lesion, nerve, femoral

  glossopharyngeal NEC G52.1

  hypoglossal G52.3

  intercostal G58.0

  lateral

    cutaneous of thigh — *see* Mononeuropathy, lower limb, meralgia paresthetica

    popliteal — *see* Lesion, nerve, popliteal

  lower limb — *see* Mononeuropathy, lower limb

  medial popliteal — *see* Lesion, nerve, popliteal, medial

  median NEC — *see* Lesion, nerve, median

  multiple G58.7

  oculomotor NEC — *see* Strabismus, paralytic, third nerve

  olfactory G52.0

  optic NEC H47.09-

    hemorrhage into sheath — *see* Hemorrhage, optic nerve

    ischemic H47.01-

  peroneal — *see* Lesion, nerve, popliteal

  phrenic G58.8

  plantar — *see* Lesion, nerve, plantar

  pneumogastric G52.2

  posterior tibial — *see* Syndrome, tarsal tunnel

  radial — *see* Lesion, nerve, radial

  recurrent laryngeal G52.2

  root G54.9

    cervical G54.2

    lumbosacral G54.1

    specified NEC G54.8

    thoracic G54.3

  sciatic NEC — *see* Lesion, nerve, sciatic

  specified NEC G58.8

    lower limb — *see* Mononeuropathy, lower limb, specified NEC

    upper limb — *see* Mononeuropathy, upper limb, specified NEC

  sympathetic G90.9

  tibial — *see* Lesion, nerve, popliteal, medial

  trigeminal G50.9

    specified NEC G50.8

  trochlear NEC — *see* Strabismus, paralytic, fourth nerve

  ulnar — *see* Lesion, nerve, ulnar

Disorder (of) - *continued*

nerve - *continued*

  upper limb — *see* Mononeuropathy, upper limb

  vagus G52.2

nervous system G98.8

  autonomic (peripheral) G90.9

    specified NEC G90.8

  central G96.9

    specified NEC G96.8

  parasympathetic G90.9

  specified NEC G98.8

  sympathetic G90.9

  vegetative G90.9

neurocognitive R41.9

  major

    with

      aggressive behavior F01.51

      combative behavior F01.51

      violent behavior F01.51

    due to vascular disease, with behavioral disturbance F01.51

    in (due to) (other diseases classified elsewhere) — *see also* Dementia, in (due to) F02.80

      with

        aggressive behavior F02.81

        combative behavior F02.81

        violent behavior F02.81

      without behavioral disturbance F01.50

  mild G31.84

neurodevelopmental F89

  specified NEC F88

neurohypophysis NEC E23.3

neurological NEC R29.818

neuromuscular G70.9

  hereditary NEC G71.9

  specified NEC G70.89

  toxic G70.1

neurotic F48.9

  specified NEC F48.8

neutrophil, polymorphonuclear D71

nicotine use — *see* Dependence, drug, nicotine

nightmare F51.5

non-rapid eye movement sleep arousal

  sleep terror type F51.4

  sleepwalking type F51.3

nose J34.9

  specified NEC J34.89

obsessive-compulsive F42.9

  and related disorder due to a known physiological condition F06.8

odontogenesis NOS K00.9

opioid use

  with

    opioid-induced psychotic disorder F11.959

      with

        delusions F11.950

        hallucinations F11.951

  due to drug abuse — *see* Abuse, drug, opioid

  due to drug dependence — *see* Dependence, drug, opioid

  mild F11.10

    with

      opioid-induced

        anxiety disorder F11.188

        depressive disorder F11.14

        sexual dysfunction F11.181

      opioid intoxication

        with perceptual disturbances F11.122

        delirium F11.121

        without perceptual disturbances F11.129

    in remission (early) (sustained) F11.11

  moderate or severe F11.20

    with

      opioid-induced

        anxiety disorder F11.288

        anxiety disorder F11.988

        depressive disorder F11.24

        depressive disorder F11.94

Disorder (of) - *continued*

opioid use - *continued*

  moderate or severe - *continued*

    with - *continued*

      opioid-induced - *continued*

        sexual dysfunction F11.281

        sexual dysfunction F11.981

      opioid intoxication

        with perceptual disturbances F11.222

        delirium F11.221

        without perceptual disturbances F11.229

    in remission (early) (sustained) F11.21

oppositional defiant F91.3

optic

  chiasm H47.49

    due to

      inflammatory disorder H47.41

      neoplasm H47.42

      vascular disorder H47.43

  disc H47.39-

    coloboma — *see* Coloboma, optic disc

    drusen — *see* Drusen, optic disc

    pseudopapilledema — *see* Pseudopapilledema

  radiations — *see* Disorder, visual, pathway

  tracts — *see* Disorder, visual, pathway

orbit H05.9

  cyst — *see* Cyst, orbit

  deformity — *see* Deformity, orbit

  edema — *see* Edema, orbit

  enophthalmos — *see* Enophthalmos

  exophthalmos — *see* Exophthalmos

  hemorrhage — *see* Hemorrhage, orbit

  inflammation — *see* Inflammation, orbit

  myopathy — *see* Myopathy, extraocular muscles

  retained foreign body — *see* Foreign body, orbit, old

  specified type NEC H05.89

organic

  anxiety F06.4

  catatonic F06.1

  delusional F06.2

  dissociative F06.8

  emotionally labile (asthenic) F06.8

  mood (affective) F06.30

  schizophrenia-like F06.2

orgasmic (female) F52.31

  male F52.32

ornithine metabolism E72.4

overanxious F41.1

  of childhood F93.8

pain

  with related psychological factors F45.42

  exclusively related to psychological factors F45.41

  genito-pelvic penetration disorder F52.6

pancreatic internal secretion E16.9

  specified NEC E16.8

panic F41.0

  with agoraphobia F40.01

papulosquamous L44.9

  in diseases classified elsewhere L45

  specified NEC L44.8

paranoid F22

  induced F24

  shared F24

paraphilic F65.9

  specified NEC F65.89

parathyroid (gland) E21.5

  specified NEC E21.4

parietoalveolar NEC J84.09

paroxysmal, mixed R56.9

patella M22.9-

  chondromalacia — *see* Chondromalacia, patella

  derangement NEC M22.3X-

  recurrent

    dislocation — *see* Dislocation, patella, recurrent

    subluxation — *see* Dislocation, patella, recurrent, incomplete

  specified NEC M22.8X-

Disorder (of) - *continued*
patellofemoral M22.2X-
pedophilic F65.4
pentose phosphate pathway with
 anemia D55.1
perception, due to hallucinogens F16.983
 in
 abuse F16.183
 dependence F16.283
peripheral nervous system NEC G64
peroxisomal E71.50
 biogenesis
 neonatal adrenoleukodystrophy E71.511
 specified disorder NEC E71.518
 Zellweger syndrome E71.510
 rhizomelic chondrodysplasia
 punctata E71.540
 specified form NEC E71.548
 group 1 E71.518
 group 2 E71.53
 group 3 E71.542
 X-linked adrenoleukodystrophy E71.529
 adolescent E71.521
 adrenomyeloneuropathy E71.522
 childhood E71.520
 specified form NEC E71.528
 Zellweger-like syndrome E71.541
persistent
 (somatoform) pain F45.41
 affective (mood) F34.9
personality — *see also* Personality F60.9
 affective F34.0
 aggressive F60.3
 amoral F60.2
 anankastic F60.5
 antisocial F60.2
 anxious F60.6
 asocial F60.2
 asthenic F60.7
 avoidant F60.6
 borderline F60.3
 change (secondary) due to general medical
 condition F07.0
 compulsive F60.5
 cyclothymic F34.0
 dependent (passive) F60.7
 depressive F34.1
 dissocial F60.2
 emotional instability F60.3
 expansive paranoid F60.0
 explosive F60.3
 following organic brain damage F07.9
 histrionic F60.4
 hyperthymic F34.0
 hypothymic F34.1
 hysterical F60.4
 immature F60.89
 inadequate F60.7
 labile F60.3
 mixed (nonspecific) F60.89
 moral deficiency F60.2
 narcissistic F60.81
 negativistic F60.89
 obsessional F60.5
 obsessive (-compulsive) F60.5
 organic F07.9
 overconscientious F60.5
 paranoid F60.0
 passive (-dependent) F60.7
 passive-aggressive F60.89
 pathological NEC F60.9
 pseudosocial F60.2
 psychopathic F60.2
 schizoid F60.1
 schizotypal F21
 self-defeating F60.7
 specified NEC F60.89
 type A F60.5
 unstable (emotional) F60.3
pervasive, developmental F84.9
phencyclidine use
 mild F16.10
 with
 phencyclidine-induced
 anxiety disorder F16.180

Disorder (of) - *continued*
phencyclidine use - *continued*
 mild - *continued*
 with - *continued*
 phencyclidine-induced - *continued*
 bipolar and related disorder F16.14
 depressive disorder F16.14
 psychotic disorder F16.159
 phencyclidine intoxication F16.129
 phencyclidine intoxication
 delirium F16.121
 in remission (early) (sustained) F16.11
 moderate or severe F16.20
 with
 phencyclidine-induced
 anxiety disorder F16.280
 bipolar and related disorder F16.24
 depressive disorder F16.24
 psychotic disorder F16.259
 phencyclidine intoxication F16.229
 phencyclidine intoxication
 delirium F16.221
 in remission (early) (sustained) F16.21
phobic anxiety, childhood F40.8
phosphate-losing tubular N25.0
pigmentation L81.9
 choroid, congenital Q14.3
 diminished melanin formation L81.6
 iron L81.8
 specified NEC L81.8
pinna (noninfective) H61.10-
 deformity, acquired H61.11-
 hematoma H61.12-
 perichondritis — *see* Perichondritis, ear
 specified type NEC H61.19-
pituitary gland E23.7
 iatrogenic (postprocedural) E89.3
 specified NEC E23.6
platelets D69.1
plexus G54.9
 specified NEC G54.8
polymorphonuclear neutrophils D71
porphyrin metabolism — *see* Porphyria
postconcussional F07.81
posthallucinogen perception F16.983
 in
 abuse F16.183
 dependence F16.283
postmenopausal N95.9
 specified NEC N95.8
postprocedural (postoperative) — *see*
 Complications, postprocedural
post-transplant lymphoproliferative D47.Z1
post-traumatic stress (PTSD) F43.10
 acute F43.11
 chronic F43.12
premenstrual dysphoric (PMDD) F32.81
prepuce N47.8
propionic acidemia E71.121
prostate N42.9
 specified NEC N42.89
psychogenic NOS — *see also*
 condition F45.9
 anxiety F41.8
 appetite F50.9
 asthenic F48.8
 cardiovascular (system) F45.8
 compulsive F42.8
 cutaneous F54
 depressive F32.9
 digestive (system) F45.8
 dysmenorrheic F45.8
 dyspneic F45.8
 endocrine (system) F54
 eye NEC F45.8
 feeding — *see* Disorder, eating
 functional NEC F45.8
 gastric F45.8
 gastrointestinal (system) F45.8
 genitourinary (system) F45.8
 heart (function) (rhythm) F45.8
 hyperventilatory F45.8
 hypochondriacal — *see* Disorder,
 hypochondriacal
 intestinal F45.8

Disorder (of) - *continued*
psychogenic NOS - *continued*
 joint F45.8
 learning F81.9
 limb F45.8
 lymphatic (system) F45.8
 menstrual F45.8
 micturition F45.8
 monoplegic NEC F44.4
 motor F44.4
 muscle F45.8
 musculoskeletal F45.8
 neurocirculatory F45.8
 obsessive F42.8
 occupational F48.8
 organ or part of body NEC F45.8
 paralytic NEC F44.4
 phobic F40.9
 physical NEC F45.8
 rectal F45.8
 respiratory (system) F45.8
 rheumatic F45.8
 sexual (function) F52.9
 skin (allergic) (eczematous) F54
 sleep F51.9
 specified part of body NEC F45.8
 stomach F45.8
psychological F99
 associated with
 disease classified elsewhere F54
 sexual
 development F66
 relationship F66
 uncertainty about gender identity F64.9
psychomotor NEC F44.4
 hysterical F44.4
psychoneurotic — *see also* Neurosis
 mixed NEC F48.8
psychophysiologic — *see* Disorder,
 somatoform
psychosexual F65.9
 development F66
 identity of childhood F64.2
psychosomatic NOS — *see* Disorder,
 somatoform
 multiple F45.0
 undifferentiated F45.1
psychotic — *see* Psychosis
 transient (acute) F23
puberty E30.9
 specified NEC E30.8
pulmonary (valve) — *see* Endocarditis,
 pulmonary
purine metabolism E79.9
pyrimidine metabolism E79.9
pyruvate metabolism E74.4
reactive attachment (childhood) F94.1
reading R48.0
 developmental (specific) F81.0
receptive language F80.2
receptor, hormonal, peripheral — *see also*
 Syndrome, androgen
 insensitivity E34.50
recurrent brief depressive F33.8
reflex R29.2
refraction H52.7
 aniseikonia H52.32
 anisometropia H52.31
 astigmatism — *see* Astigmatism
 hypermetropia — *see* Hypermetropia
 myopia — *see* Myopia
 presbyopia H52.4
 specified NEC H52.6
relationship F68.8
 due to sexual orientation F66
REM sleep behavior G47.52
renal function, impaired (tubular) N25.9
resonance R49.9
 specified NEC R49.8
respiratory function, impaired — *see also*
 Failure, respiration
 postprocedural — *see* Complication,
 postoperative, respiratory system
 psychogenic F45.8
retina H35.9

Disorder (of) - *continued*
retina - *continued*
angioid streaks H35.33
changes in vascular appearance H35.01-
degeneration — *see* Degeneration, retina
dystrophy (hereditary) — *see* Dystrophy, retina
edema H35.81
hemorrhage — *see* Hemorrhage, retina
ischemia H35.82
macular degeneration — *see* Degeneration, macula
microaneurysms H35.04-
microvascular abnormality NEC H35.09
neovascularization — *see* Neovascularization, retina
retinopathy — *see* Retinopathy
separation of layers H35.70
central serous chorioretinopathy H35.71-
pigment epithelium detachment (serous) H35.72-
hemorrhagic H35.73-
specified type NEC H35.89
telangiectasis — *see* Telangiectasis, retina
vasculitis — *see* Vasculitis, retina
retroperitoneal K68.9
right hemisphere organic affective F07.89
rumination (infant or child) F98.21
sacrum, sacrococcygeal NEC M53.3
schizoaffective F25.9
bipolar type F25.0
depressive type F25.1
manic type F25.0
mixed type F25.0
specified NEC F25.8
schizoid of childhood F84.5
schizophrenia spectrum and other psychotic disorder F29
specified NEC F28
schizophreniform F20.81
brief F23
schizotypal (personality) F21
secretion, thyrocalcitonin E07.0
sedative, hypnotic, or anxiolytic use
mild F13.10
with
sedative, hypnotic, or anxiolytic-induced
anxiety disorder F13.180
bipolar and related disorder F13.14
depressive disorder F13.14
psychotic disorder F13.159
sexual dysfunction F13.181
sedative, hypnotic, or anxiolytic intoxication F13.129
sedative, hypnotic, or anxiolytic intoxication delirium F13.121
in remission (early) (sustained) F13.11
moderate or severe F13.20
with
sedative, hypnotic, or anxiolytic-induced
anxiety disorder F13.280
bipolar and related disorder F13.24
depressive disorder F13.24
major neurocognitive disorder F13.27
mild neurocognitive disorder F13.288
psychotic disorder F13.259
sexual dysfunction F13.281
sedative, hypnotic, or anxiolytic intoxication F13.229
sedative, hypnotic, or anxiolytic intoxication delirium F13.221
in remission (early) (sustained) F13.21
seizure — *see also* Epilepsy G40.909
intractable G40.919
with status epilepticus G40.911
semantic pragmatic F80.89
with autism F84.0
sense of smell R43.1
psychogenic F45.8
separation anxiety, of childhood F93.0
sexual

Disorder (of) - *continued*
sexual - *continued*
arousal, female F52.22
aversion F52.1
function, psychogenic F52.9
interest/arousal, female F52.22
masochism F65.51
maturation F66
nonorganic F52.9
preference — *see also* Deviation, sexual F65.9
fetishistic transvestism F65.1
relationship F66
sadism F65.52
shyness, of childhood and adolescence F40.10
sibling rivalry F93.8
sickle-cell (sickling) (homozygous) — *see* Disease, sickle-cell
heterozygous D57.3
specified type NEC D57.8-
trait D57.3
sinus (nasal) J34.9
specified NEC J34.89
skin L98.9
atrophic L90.9
specified NEC L90.8
granulomatous L92.9
specified NEC L92.8
hypertrophic L91.9
specified NEC L91.8
infiltrative NEC L98.6
newborn P83.9
specified NEC P83.88
picking F42.4
psychogenic (allergic) (eczematous) F54
sleep G47.9
breathing-related — *see* Apnea, sleep
circadian rhythm G47.20
advance sleep phase type G47.22
delayed sleep phase type G47.21
due to
alcohol
abuse F10.182
dependence F10.282
use F10.982
amphetamines
abuse F15.182
dependence F15.282
use F15.982
caffeine
abuse F15.182
dependence F15.282
use F15.982
cocaine
abuse F14.182
dependence F14.282
use F14.982
drug NEC
abuse F19.182
dependence F19.282
use F19.982
opioid
abuse F11.182
dependence F11.282
use F11.982
psychoactive substance NEC
abuse F19.182
dependence F19.282
use F19.982
sedative, hypnotic, or anxiolytic
abuse F13.182
dependence F13.282
use F13.982
stimulant NEC
abuse F15.182
dependence F15.282
use F15.982
free running type G47.24
in conditions classified elsewhere G47.27
irregular sleep wake type G47.23
jet lag type G47.25
non-24-hour sleep-wake type G47.24
shift work type G47.26

Disorder (of) - *continued*
sleep - *continued*
circadian rhythm - *continued*
specified NEC G47.29
due to
alcohol
abuse F10.182
dependence F10.282
use F10.982
amphetamine
abuse F15.182
dependence F15.282
use F15.982
anxiolytic
abuse F13.182
dependence F13.282
use F13.982
caffeine
abuse F15.182
dependence F15.282
use F15.982
cocaine
abuse F14.182
dependence F14.282
use F14.982
drug NEC
abuse F19.182
dependence F19.282
use F19.982
hypnotic
abuse F13.182
dependence F13.282
use F13.982
opioid
abuse F11.182
dependence F11.282
use F11.982
psychoactive substance NEC
abuse F19.182
dependence F19.282
use F19.982
sedative
abuse F13.182
dependence F13.282
use F13.982
stimulant NEC
abuse F15.182
dependence F15.282
use F15.982
emotional F51.9
excessive somnolence — *see* Hypersomnia
hypersomnia type — *see* Hypersomnia
initiating or maintaining — *see* Insomnia
nightmares F51.5
nonorganic F51.9
specified NEC F51.8
parasomnia type G47.50
specified NEC G47.8
terrors F51.4
walking F51.3
sleep-wake pattern or schedule — *see also* Disorder, sleep, circadian rhythm G47.9
specified NEC G47.8
social
anxiety (of childhood) F40.10
generalized F40.11
functioning in childhood F94.9
specified NEC F94.8
pragmatic F80.82
soft tissue M79.9
ankle M79.9
due to use, overuse and pressure M70.90
ankle M70.97-
bursitis — *see* Bursitis
foot M70.97-
forearm M70.93-
hand M70.94-
lower leg M70.96-
multiple sites M70.99
pelvic region M70.95-
shoulder region M70.91-
specified site NEC M70.98
specified type NEC M70.80
ankle M70.87-

Disorder (of) - *continued*
soft tissue - *continued*
  due to use, overuse and pressure -
   continued
    specified type NEC - *continued*
     foot M70.87-
     forearm M70.83-
     hand M70.84-
     lower leg M70.86-
     multiple sites M70.89
     pelvic region M70.85-
     shoulder region M70.81-
     specified site NEC M70.88
     thigh M70.85-
     upper arm M70.82-
    thigh M70.95-
    upper arm M70.92-
  foot M79.9
  forearm M79.9
  hand M79.9
  lower leg M79.9
  multiple sites M79.9
  occupational — *see* Disorder, soft tissue,
    due to use, overuse and pressure
  pelvic region M79.9
  shoulder region M79.9
  specified type NEC M79.89
  thigh M79.9
  upper arm M79.9
somatic symptom F45.1
somatization F45.0
somatoform F45.9
  pain (persistent) F45.41
  somatization (multiple) (long-
    lasting) F45.0
  specified NEC F45.8
  undifferentiated F45.1
somnolence, excessive — *see* Hypersomnia
specific
  arithmetical F81.2
  developmental, of motor F82
  reading F81.0
  speech and language F80.9
  spelling F81.81
  written expression F81.81
speech R47.9
  articulation (functional) (specific) F80.0
  developmental F80.9
  specified NEC R47.89
speech-sound F80.0
spelling (specific) F81.81
spine — *see also* Dorsopathy
  ligamentous or muscular attachments,
    peripheral — *see* Enthesopathy, spinal
  specified NEC — *see* Dorsopathy,
    specified NEC
stereotyped, habit or movement F98.4
stimulant use (other) (unspecified)
  mild F15.10
    in remission (early) (sustained) F15.11
  moderate or severe F15.20
    in remission (early) (sustained) F15.21
stomach (functional) — *see* Disorder, gastric
stress F43.9
  acute F43.0
  post-traumatic F43.10
    acute F43.11
    chronic F43.12
substance use (other) (unknown)
  mild F19.10
    with substance-induced
     anxiety disorder F19.180
     bipolar and related disorder F19.14
     depressive disorder F19.14
     major neurocognitive disorder F19.17
     mild neurocognitive disorder F19.188
     obsessive-compulsive and related
      disorder F19.188
     sexual dysfunction F19.181
     substance intoxication F19.129
     substance intoxication delirium F19.121
  moderate or severe F19.20
    with substance-induced
     anxiety disorder F19.280
     bipolar and related disorder F19.24

Disorder (of) - *continued*
substance use (other) (unknown) - *continued*
  moderate or severe - *continued*
    with substance-induced - *continued*
     depressive disorder F19.24
     major neurocognitive disorder F19.27
     mild neurocognitive disorder F19.288
     obsessive-compulsive and related
      disorder F19.288
     sexual dysfunction F19.281
    in remission (early) (sustained) F19.21
    substance intoxication F19.229
    substance intoxication delirium F19.221
sulfur-bearing amino-acid
  metabolism E72.10
sweat gland (eccrine) L74.9
  apocrine L75.9
    specified NEC L75.8
  specified NEC L74.8
synovium M67.90
  acromioclavicular M67.91-
  ankle M67.97-
  elbow M67.92-
  foot M67.97-
  forearm M67.93-
  hand M67.94-
  hip M67.95-
  knee M67.96-
  multiple sites M67.99
  rupture — *see* Rupture, synovium
  shoulder M67.91-
  specified type NEC M67.80
    acromioclavicular M67.81-
    ankle M67.87-
    elbow M67.82-
    foot M67.87-
    hand M67.84-
    hip M67.85-
    knee M67.86-
    multiple sites M67.89
    wrist M67.83-
  synovitis — *see* Synovitis
  upper arm M67.92-
  wrist M67.93-
temperature regulation, newborn P81.9
  specified NEC P81.8
temporomandibular joint M26.60-
tendon M67.90
  acromioclavicular M67.91-
  ankle M67.97-
  contracture — *see* Contracture, tendon
  elbow M67.92-
  foot M67.97-
  forearm M67.93-
  hand M67.94-
  hip M67.95-
  knee M67.96-
  multiple sites M67.99
  rupture — *see* Rupture, tendon
  shoulder M67.91-
  specified type NEC M67.80
    acromioclavicular M67.81-
    ankle M67.87-
    elbow M67.82-
    foot M67.87-
    hand M67.84-
    hip M67.85-
    knee M67.86-
    multiple sites M67.89
    trunk M67.88
    wrist M67.83-
  synovitis — *see* Synovitis
  tendinitis — *see* Tendinitis
  tenosynovitis — *see* Tenosynovitis
  trunk M67.98
  upper arm M67.92-
  wrist M67.93-
thoracic root (nerve) NEC G54.3
thyrocalcitonin hypersecretion E07.0
thyroid (gland) E07.9
  function NEC, neonatal, transitory P72.2
  iodine-deficiency related E01.8
  specified NEC E07.89
tic — *see* Tic
tobacco use

Disorder (of) - *continued*
tobacco use - *continued*
  chewing tobacco (mild) (moderate)
    (severe)
    in remission (early) (sustained) F17.221
  cigarettes (mild) (moderate) (severe)
    in remission (early) (sustained) F17.211
  mild F17.200
    in remission (early) (sustained) F17.201
  moderate F17.200
    in remission (early) (sustained) F17.201
  severe F17.200
    in remission (early) (sustained) F17.201
  specified product NEC (mild) (moderate)
    (severe)
    in remission (early) (sustained) F17.291
tooth K08.9
  development K00.9
    specified NEC K00.8
  eruption K00.6
Tourette's F95.2
trance and possession F44.89
transvestic F65.1
trauma and stressor-related F43.9
  other specified F43.8
tricuspid (valve) — *see* Endocarditis,
  tricuspid
tryptophan metabolism E70.5
tubular, phosphate-losing N25.0
tubulo-interstitial (in)
  brucellosis A23.9 *[N16]*
  cystinosis E72.04
  diphtheria A36.84
  glycogen storage disease E74.00 *[N16]*
  leukemia NEC C95.9- *[N16]*
  lymphoma NEC C85.9- *[N16]*
  mixed cryoglobulinemia D89.1 *[N16]*
  multiple myeloma C90.0- *[N16]*
  Salmonella infection A02.25
  sarcoidosis D86.84
  sepsis A41.9 *[N16]*
    streptococcal A40.9 *[N16]*
  systemic lupus erythematosus M32.15
  toxoplasmosis B58.83
  transplant rejection T86.91 *[N16]*
  Wilson's disease E83.01 *[N16]*
tubulo-renal function, impaired N25.9
  specified NEC N25.89
tympanic membrane H73.9-
  atrophy — *see* Atrophy, tympanic
    membrane
  infection — *see* Myringitis
  perforation — *see* Perforation, tympanum
  specified NEC H73.89-
unsocialized aggressive F91.1
urea cycle metabolism E72.20
  argininemia E72.21
  arginosuccinic aciduria E72.22
  citrullinemia E72.23
  ornithine transcarbamylase
    deficiency E72.4
  other specified E72.29
ureter (in) N28.9
  schistosomiasis B65.0 *[N29]*
  tuberculosis A18.11
urethra N36.9
  specified NEC N36.8
urinary system N39.9
  specified NEC N39.8
valve, heart
  aortic — *see* Endocarditis, aortic
  mitral — *see* Endocarditis, mitral
  pulmonary — *see* Endocarditis, pulmonary
  rheumatic
    aortic — *see* Endocarditis, aortic,
     rheumatic
    mitral — *see* Endocarditis, mitral
    pulmonary — *see* Endocarditis,
     pulmonary, rheumatic
    tricuspid — *see* Endocarditis, tricuspid
  tricuspid — *see* Endocarditis, tricuspid
vestibular function H81.9-
  specified NEC — *see* subcategory H81.8
  in diseases classified elsewhere H82.-
vertigo — *see* Vertigo

Disorder (of) - *continued*
  vision, binocular H53.30
    abnormal retinal correspondence H53.31
    diplopia H53.2
    fusion with defective stereopsis H53.32
    simultaneous perception H53.33
    suppression H53.34
  visual
    cortex
      blindness H47.619
        left brain H47.612
        right brain H47.611
      due to
        inflammatory disorder H47.629
          left brain H47.622
          right brain H47.621
        neoplasm H47.639
          left brain H47.632
          right brain H47.631
        vascular disorder H47.649
          left brain H47.642
          right brain H47.641
    pathway H47.9
      due to
        inflammatory disorder H47.51-
        neoplasm H47.52-
        vascular disorder H47.53-
      optic chiasm — *see* Disorder, optic,
        chiasm
  vitreous body H43.9
    crystalline deposits — *see* Deposit,
      crystalline
    degeneration — *see* Degeneration, vitreous
    hemorrhage — *see* Hemorrhage, vitreous
    opacities — *see* Opacity, vitreous
    prolapse — *see* Prolapse, vitreous
    specified type NEC H43.89
  voice R49.9
    specified type NEC R49.8
  volatile solvent use
    due to drug abuse — *see* Abuse, drug,
      inhalant
    due to drug dependence — *see*
      Dependence, drug, inhalant
  voyeuristic F65.3
  white blood cells D72.9
    specified NEC D72.89
  withdrawing, child or adolescent F40.10
Disorientation R41.0
Displacement, displaced
  acquired traumatic of bone, cartilage, joint,
    tendon NEC — *see* Dislocation
  adrenal gland (congenital) Q89.1
  appendix, retrocecal (congenital) Q43.8
  auricle (congenital) Q17.4
  bladder (acquired) N32.89
    congenital Q64.19
  brachial plexus (congenital) Q07.8
  brain stem, caudal (congenital) Q04.8
  canaliculus (lacrimalis) , congenital Q10.6
  cardia through esophageal hiatus
    (congenital) Q40.1
  cerebellum, caudal (congenital) Q04.8
  cervix — *see* Malposition, uterus
  colon (congenital) Q43.3
  device, implant or graft — *see also*
    Complications, by site and type,
    mechanical T85.628
    arterial graft NEC — *see* Complication,
      cardiovascular device, mechanical,
      vascular
    breast (implant) T85.42
    catheter NEC T85.628
      dialysis (renal) T82.42
        intraperitoneal T85.621
      infusion NEC T82.524
        spinal (epidural) (subdural) T85.620
      urinary
        cystostomy T83.020
        Hopkins T83.028
        ileostomy T83.028
        indwelling T83.021
        nephrostomy T83.022
        specified NEC T83.028
        urostomy T83.028

Displacement, displaced - *continued*
  device, implant or graft - *continued*
    electronic (electrode) (pulse generator)
      (stimulator) — *see* Complication,
      electronic stimulator
    fixation, internal (orthopedic) NEC — *see*
      Complication, fixation device,
      mechanical
    gastrointestinal — *see* Complications,
      prosthetic device, mechanical,
      gastrointestinal device
    genital NEC T83.428
      intrauterine contraceptive device
        (string) T83.32
      penile prosthesis (cylinder) (implanted)
        (pump) (resevoir) T83.420
      testicular prosthesis T83.421
    heart NEC — *see* Complication,
      cardiovascular device, mechanical
    joint prosthesis — *see* Complications, joint
      prosthesis, mechanical
    ocular — *see* Complications, prosthetic
      device, mechanical, ocular device
    orthopedic NEC — *see* Complication,
      orthopedic, device or graft,
      mechanical
    specified NEC T85.628
    urinary NEC T83.128
      graft T83.22
      sphincter, implanted T83.121
      stent (ileal conduit)
        (nephroureteral) T83.123
      ureteral indwelling T83.122
    vascular NEC — *see* Complication,
      cardiovascular device, mechanical
    ventricular intracranial shunt T85.02
  electronic stimulator
    bone T84.320
    cardiac — *see* Complications, cardiac
      device, electronic
    nervous system — *see* Complication,
      prosthetic device, mechanical,
      electronic nervous system stimulator
    urinary — *see* Complications, electronic
      stimulator, urinary
  esophageal mucosa into cardia of stomach,
    congenital Q39.8
  esophagus (acquired) K22.8
    congenital Q39.8
  eyeball (acquired) (lateral) (old) — *see*
    Displacement, globe
    congenital Q15.8
    current — *see* Avulsion, eye
  fallopian tube (acquired) N83.4-
    congenital Q50.6
    opening (congenital) Q50.6
  gallbladder (congenital) Q44.1
  gastric mucosa (congenital) Q40.2
  globe (acquired) (old) (lateral) H05.21-
    current — *see* Avulsion, eye
  heart (congenital) Q24.8
    acquired I51.89
  hymen (upward) (congenital) Q52.4
  intervertebral disc NEC
    with myelopathy — *see* Disorder, disc,
      with, myelopathy
    cervical, cervicothoracic (with) M50.20
      myelopathy — *see* Disorder, disc,
        cervical, with myelopathy
      neuritis, radiculitis or radiculopathy —
        see Disorder, disc, cervical, with
        neuritis
    due to trauma — *see* Dislocation, vertebra
    lumbar region M51.26
      with
        myelopathy M51.06
        neuritis, radiculitis, radiculopathy or
          sciatica M51.16
    lumbosacral region M51.27
      with
        neuritis, radiculitis, radiculopathy or
          sciatica M51.17
    sacrococcygeal region M53.3
    thoracic region M51.24
      with

Displacement, displaced - *continued*
  intervertebral disc NEC - *continued*
    thoracic region - *continued*
      with - *continued*
        myelopathy M51.04
        neuritis, radiculitis,
          radiculopathy M51.14
      thoracolumbar region M51.25
        with
          myelopathy M51.05
          neuritis, radiculitis,
            radiculopathy M51.15
  intrauterine device (string) T83.32
  kidney (acquired) N28.83
    congenital Q63.2
  lachrymal, lacrimal apparatus or duct
    (congenital) Q10.6
  lens, congenital Q12.1
  macula (congenital) Q14.1
  Meckel's diverticulum Q43.0
    malignant — *see* Table of Neoplasms,
      small intestine, malignant
  nail (congenital) Q84.6
    acquired L60.8
  opening of Wharton's duct in mouth Q38.4
  organ or site, congenital NEC — *see*
    Malposition, congenital
  ovary (acquired) N83.4-
    congenital Q50.39
    free in peritoneal cavity
      (congenital) Q50.39
    into hernial sac N83.4-
  oviduct (acquired) N83.4-
    congenital Q50.6
  parathyroid (gland) E21.4
  parotid gland (congenital) Q38.4
  punctum lacrimale (congenital) Q10.6
  sacro-iliac (joint) (congenital) Q74.2
    current injury S33.2
    old — *see* subcategory M53.2
  salivary gland (any) (congenital) Q38.4
  spleen (congenital) Q89.09
  stomach, congenital Q40.2
  sublingual duct Q38.4
  tongue (downward) (congenital) Q38.3
  tooth, teeth, fully erupted M26.30
    horizontal M26.33
    vertical M26.34
  trachea (congenital) Q32.1
  ureter or ureteric opening or orifice
    (congenital) Q62.62
  uterine opening of oviducts or fallopian
    tubes Q50.6
  uterus, uterine — *see* Malposition, uterus
  ventricular septum Q21.0
    with rudimentary ventricle Q20.4
Disproportion
  between native and reconstructed
    breast N65.1
  fiber-type G71.2
Disruptio uteri — *see* Rupture, uterus
Disruption (of)
  ciliary body NEC H21.89
  closure of
    cornea T81.31
    craniotomy T81.32
    fascia (muscular) (superficial) T81.32
    internal organ or tissue T81.32
    laceration (external) (internal) T81.33
    ligament T81.32
    mucosa T81.31
    muscle or muscle flap T81.32
    ribs or rib cage T81.32
    skin and subcutaneous tissue (full-
      thickness) (superficial) T81.31
    skull T81.32
    sternum (sternotomy) T81.32
    tendon T81.32
    traumatic laceration (external)
      (internal) T81.33
  family Z63.8
    due to
      absence of family member due to
        military deployment Z63.31
      absence of family member NEC Z63.32

Disruption (of) - *continued*
  family - *continued*
    due to - *continued*
      alcoholism and drug addiction in
        family Z63.72
      bereavement Z63.4
      death (assumed) or disappearance of
        family member Z63.4
      divorce or separation Z63.5
      drug addiction in family Z63.72
      return of family member from military
        deployment (current or past
        conflict) Z63.71
      stressful life events NEC Z63.79
  iris NEC H21.89
  ligament (s) — *see also* Sprain
    knee
      current injury — *see* Dislocation, knee
      old (chronic) — *see* Derangement, knee,
        ligament, instability, chronic
      spontaneous NEC — *see* Derangement,
        knee, disruption ligament
  ossicular chain — *see* Discontinuity, ossicles,
    ear
  pelvic ring (stable) S32.810
    unstable S32.811
  wound T81.30
    episiotomy O90.1
    operation T81.31
      cesarean O90.0
      external operation wound
        (superficial) T81.31
      internal operation wound (deep) T81.32
    perineal (obstetric) O90.1
    traumatic injury repair T81.33
    traumatic injury wound repair T81.33
Dissatisfaction with
  employment Z56.9
  school environment Z55.4
Dissecting — *see* condition
Dissection
  aorta I71.00
    abdominal I71.02
    thoracic I71.01
    thoracoabdominal I71.03
  artery I77.70
    basilar (trunk) I77.75
    carotid I77.71
    cerebral (nonruptured) I67.0
      ruptured — *see* Hemorrhage,
        intracranial, subarachnoid
    coronary I25.42
    extremity
      lower I77.77
      upper I77.76
    iliac I77.72
    precerebral
      congenital (nonruptured) Q28.1
      specified site NEC I77.75
    renal I77.73
    specified NEC I77.79
    vertebral I77.74
  precerebral artery, congenital
    (nonruptured) Q28.1
  Heartland A93.8
  traumatic — *see* Wound, open, by site
  vascular I99.8
  wound — *see* Wound, open
Disseminated — *see* condition
Dissociation
  auriculoventricular or atrioventricular (AV)
    (any degree) (isorhythmic) I45.89
    with heart block I44.2
  interference I45.89
Dissociative reaction, state F44.9
Dissolution, vertebra — *see* Osteoporosis
Distension, distention
  abdomen R14.0
  bladder N32.89
  cecum K63.89
  colon K63.89
  gallbladder K82.8
  intestine K63.89
  kidney N28.89
  liver K76.89

Distension, distention - *continued*
  seminal vesicle N50.89
  stomach K31.89
    acute K31.0
    psychogenic F45.8
  ureter — *see* Dilatation, ureter
  uterus N85.8
Distoma hepaticum infestation B66.3
Distomiasis B66.9
  bile passages B66.3
  hemic B65.9
  hepatic B66.3
    due to Clonorchis sinensis B66.1
  intestinal B66.5
  liver B66.3
    due to Clonorchis sinensis B66.1
  lung B66.4
  pulmonary B66.4
Distomolar (fourth molar) K00.1
**Disto-occlusion (Division I) (Division
  II)** M26.212
Distortion (s) (congenital)
  adrenal (gland) Q89.1
  arm NEC Q68.8
  bile duct or passage Q44.5
  bladder Q64.79
  brain Q04.9
  cervix (uteri) Q51.9
  chest (wall) Q67.8
    bones Q76.8
  clavicle Q74.0
  clitoris Q52.6
  coccyx Q76.49
  common duct Q44.5
  coronary Q24.5
  cystic duct Q44.5
  ear (auricle) (external) Q17.3
    inner Q16.5
    middle Q16.4
      ossicles Q16.3
  endocrine NEC Q89.2
  eustachian tube Q17.8
  eye (adnexa) Q15.8
  face bone (s) NEC Q75.8
  fallopian tube Q50.6
  femur NEC Q68.8
  fibula NEC Q68.8
  finger (s) Q68.1
  foot Q66.9-
  genitalia, genital organ (s)
    female Q52.8
      external Q52.79
      internal NEC Q52.8
  gyri Q04.8
  hand bone (s) Q68.1
  heart (auricle) (ventricle) Q24.8
    valve (cusp) Q24.8
  hepatic duct Q44.5
  humerus NEC Q68.8
  hymen Q52.4
  intrafamilial communications Z63.8
  jaw NEC M26.89
  labium (majus) (minus) Q52.79
  leg NEC Q68.8
  lens Q12.8
  liver Q44.7
  lumbar spine Q76.49
    with disproportion O33.8
      causing obstructed labor O65.0
  lumbosacral (joint) (region) Q76.49
    kyphosis — *see* Kyphosis, congenital
    lordosis — *see* Lordosis, congenital
  nerve Q07.8
  nose Q30.8
  organ
    of Corti Q16.5
    or site not listed — *see* Anomaly, by site
  ossicles, ear Q16.3
  oviduct Q50.6
  pancreas Q45.3
  parathyroid (gland) Q89.2
  pituitary (gland) Q89.2
  radius NEC Q68.8
  sacroiliac joint Q74.2
  sacrum Q76.49

Distortion (s) (congenital) - *continued*
  scapula Q74.0
  shoulder girdle Q74.0
  skull bone (s) NEC Q75.8
    with
      anencephalus Q00.0
      encephalocele — *see* Encephalocele
      hydrocephalus Q03.9
        with spina bifida — *see* Spina bifida,
          with hydrocephalus
      microcephaly Q02
  spinal cord Q06.8
  spine Q76.49
    kyphosis — *see* Kyphosis, congenital
    lordosis — *see* Lordosis, congenital
  spleen Q89.09
  sternum NEC Q76.7
  thorax (wall) Q67.8
    bony Q76.8
  thymus (gland) Q89.2
  thyroid (gland) Q89.2
  tibia NEC Q68.8
  toe (s) Q66.9-
  tongue Q38.3
  trachea (cartilage) Q32.1
  ulna NEC Q68.8
  ureter Q62.8
  urethra Q64.79
    causing obstruction Q64.39
  uterus Q51.9
  vagina Q52.4
  vertebra Q76.49
    kyphosis — *see* Kyphosis, congenital
    lordosis — *see* Lordosis, congenital
  visual — *see also* Disturbance, vision
    shape and size H53.15
  vulva Q52.79
  wrist (bones) (joint) Q68.8
Distress
  abdomen — *see* Pain, abdominal
  acute respiratory R06.03
    syndrome (adult) (child) J80
  epigastric R10.13
  fetal P84
    complicating pregnancy — *see* Stress, fetal
  gastrointestinal (functional) K30
    psychogenic F45.8
  intestinal (functional) NOS K59.9
    psychogenic F45.8
  maternal, during labor and delivery O75.0
  relationship, with spouse or intimate
    partner Z63.0
  respiratory (adult) (child) R06.03
    newborn P22.9
      specified NEC P22.8
    orthopnea R06.01
    psychogenic F45.8
    shortness of breath R06.02
    specified type NEC R06.09
Distribution vessel, atypical Q27.9
  coronary artery Q24.5
  precerebral Q28.1
Districhiasis L68.8
Disturbance (s) — *see also* Disease
  absorption K90.9
    calcium E58
    carbohydrate K90.49
    fat K90.49
      pancreatic K90.3
    protein K90.49
    starch K90.49
    vitamin — *see* Deficiency, vitamin
  acid-base equilibrium E87.8
    mixed E87.4
  activity and attention (with hyperkinesis) —
    see Disorder, attention-deficit
    hyperactivity
  amino acid transport E72.00
  assimilation, food K90.9
  auditory nerve, except deafness — *see*
    subcategory H93.3
  behavior — *see* Disorder, conduct
  blood clotting (mechanism) — *see also*
    Defect, coagulation D68.9
  cerebral

Disturbance (s) - *continued*
cerebral - *continued*
  nerve — *see* Disorder, nerve, cranial
  status, newborn P91.9
    specified NEC P91.88
circulatory I99.9
conduct — *see also* Disorder, conduct F91.9
  adjustment reaction — *see* Disorder,
    adjustment
  compulsive F63.9
  disruptive F91.9
  hyperkinetic — *see* Disorder, attention-
    deficit hyperactivity
  socialized F91.2
  specified NEC F91.8
  unsocialized F91.1
coordination R27.8
cranial nerve — *see* Disorder, nerve, cranial
deep sensibility — *see* Disturbance,
  sensation
digestive K30
  psychogenic F45.8
electrolyte — *see also* Imbalance, electrolyte
  newborn, transitory P74.49
    hyperammonemia P74.6
    hyperchloremia P74.421
    hyperchloremic metabolic
      acidosis P74.421
    hypochloremia P74.422
    potassium balance
      hyperkalemia P74.31
      hypokalemia P74.32
    sodium balance
      hypernatremia P74.21
      hyponatremia P74.22
    specified type NEC P74.49
emotions specific to childhood and
  adolescence F93.9
  with
    anxiety and fearfulness NEC F93.8
    elective mutism F94.0
    oppositional disorder F91.3
    sensitivity (withdrawal) F40.10
    shyness F40.10
    social withdrawal F40.10
  involving relationship problems F93.8
  mixed F93.8
  specified NEC F93.8
endocrine (gland) E34.9
  neonatal, transitory P72.9
    specified NEC P72.8
equilibrium R42
fructose metabolism E74.10
gait — *see* Gait
  hysterical F44.4
  psychogenic F44.4
gastrointestinal (functional) K30
  psychogenic F45.8
habit, child F98.9
hearing, except deafness and tinnitus — *see*
  Abnormal, auditory perception
heart, functional (conditions in I44-I50)
  due to presence of (cardiac)
    prosthesis I97.19-
  postoperative I97.89
    cardiac surgery — *see also* Infarct,
      myocardium, associated with
      revascularization procedure I97.19-
hormones E34.9
innervation uterus (parasympathetic)
  (sympathetic) N85.8
keratinization NEC
  gingiva K05.10
    nonplaque induced K05.11
    plaque induced K05.10
  lip K13.0
  oral (mucosa) (soft tissue) K13.29
  tongue K13.29
learning (specific) — *see* Disorder, learning
memory — *see* Amnesia
  mild, following organic brain
    damage F06.8
mental F99
  associated with diseases classified
    elsewhere F54

Disturbance (s) - *continued*
metabolism E88.9
  with
    abortion — *see* Abortion, by type with
      other specified complication
    ectopic pregnancy O08.5
    molar pregnancy O08.5
  amino-acid E72.9
    aromatic E70.9
    branched-chain E71.2
    straight-chain E72.89
    sulfur-bearing E72.10
  ammonia E72.20
  arginine E72.21
  arginosuccinic acid E72.22
  carbohydrate E74.9
  cholesterol E78.9
  citrulline E72.23
  cystathionine E72.19
  general E88.9
  glutamine E72.89
  histidine E70.40
  homocystine E72.19
  hydroxylysine E72.3
  in labor or delivery O75.89
  iron E83.10
  lipoid E78.9
  lysine E72.3
  methionine E72.19
  neonatal, transitory P74.9
    calcium and magnesium P71.9
      specified type NEC P71.8
    carbohydrate metabolism P70.9
      specified type NEC P70.8
    specified NEC P74.8
  ornithine E72.4
  phosphate E83.39
  sodium NEC E87.8
  threonine E72.89
  tryptophan E70.5
  tyrosine E70.20
  urea cycle E72.20
motor R29.2
nervous, functional R45.0
neuromuscular mechanism (eye) , due to
  syphilis A52.15
nutritional E63.9
  nail L60.3
ocular motion H51.9
  psychogenic F45.8
oculogyric H51.8
  psychogenic F45.8
oculomotor H51.9
  psychogenic F45.8
olfactory nerve R43.1
optic nerve NEC — *see* Disorder, nerve,
  optic
oral epithelium, including tongue
  NEC K13.29
perceptual due to
  alcohol withdrawal F10.232
  amphetamine intoxication F15.922
    in
      abuse F15.122
      dependence F15.222
  anxiolytic withdrawal F13.232
  cannabis intoxication (acute) F12.922
    in
      abuse F12.122
      dependence F12.222
  cocaine intoxication (acute) F14.922
    in
      abuse F14.122
      dependence F14.222
  hypnotic withdrawal F13.232
  opioid intoxication (acute) F11.922
    in
      abuse F11.122
      dependence F11.222
  phencyclidine intoxication (acute) F16.122
  sedative withdrawal F13.232
personality (pattern) (trait) — *see also*
  Disorder, personality F60.9
  following organic brain damage F07.9
polyglandular E31.9

Disturbance (s) - *continued*
polyglandular - *continued*
  specified NEC E31.8
potassium balance, newborn
  hyperkalemia P74.31
  hypokalemia P74.32
psychogenic F45.9
psychomotor F44.4
psychophysical visual H53.16
pupillary — *see* Anomaly, pupil, function
reflex R29.2
rhythm, heart I49.9
salivary secretion K11.7
sensation (cold) (heat) (localization) (tactile
  discrimination) (texture) (vibratory)
  NEC R20.9
  hysterical F44.6
  skin R20.9
    anesthesia R20.0
    hyperesthesia R20.3
    hypoesthesia R20.1
    paresthesia R20.2
    specified type NEC R20.8
  smell R43.9
    and taste (mixed) R43.8
    anosmia R43.0
    parosmia R43.1
    specified NEC R43.8
  taste R43.9
    and smell (mixed) R43.8
    parageusia R43.2
    specified NEC R43.8
sensory — *see* Disturbance, sensation
situational (transient) — *see also* Disorder,
  adjustment
  acute F43.0
sleep G47.9
  nonorganic origin F51.9
smell — *see* Disturbance, sensation, smell
sociopathic F60.2
sodium balance, newborn
  hypernatremia P74.21
  hyponatremia P74.22
speech R47.9
  developmental F80.9
  specified NEC R47.89
stomach (functional) K31.9
sympathetic (nerve) G90.9
taste — *see* Disturbance, sensation, taste
temperature
  regulation, newborn P81.9
    specified NEC P81.8
  sense R20.8
    hysterical F44.6
tooth
  eruption K00.6
  formation K00.4
  structure, hereditary NEC K00.5
touch — *see* Disturbance, sensation
vascular I99.9
  arteriosclerotic — *see* Arteriosclerosis
vasomotor I73.9
vasospastic I73.9
vision, visual H53.9
  following
    cerebral infarction I69.398
    cerebrovascular disease I69.998
      specified NEC I69.898
    intracerebral hemorrhage I69.198
    nontraumatic intracranial hemorrhage
      NEC I69.298
    specified disease NEC I69.898
    subarachnoid hemorrhage I69.098
  psychophysical H53.16
  specified NEC H53.8
  subjective H53.10
    day blindness H53.11
    discomfort H53.14-
    distortions of shape and size H53.15
    loss
      sudden H53.13-
      transient H53.12-
    specified type NEC H53.19
voice R49.9
  psychogenic F44.4

Disturbance (s) - *continued*
  voice - *continued*
    specified NEC R49.8
Diuresis R35.8
Diver's palsy, paralysis or squeeze T70.3
Diverticulitis (acute) K57.92
  bladder — *see* Cystitis
  ileum — *see* Diverticulitis, intestine, small
  intestine K57.92
    with
      abscess, perforation or
        peritonitis K57.80
          with bleeding K57.81
      bleeding K57.93
    congenital Q43.8
    large K57.32
      with
        abscess, perforation or
          peritonitis K57.20
            with bleeding K57.21
        bleeding K57.33
        small intestine K57.52
          with
            abscess, perforation or
              peritonitis K57.40
                with bleeding K57.41
            bleeding K57.53
      small K57.12
        with
          abscess, perforation or
            peritonitis K57.00
              with bleeding K57.01ˑ
          bleeding K57.13
          large intestine K57.52
            with
              abscess, perforation or
                peritonitis K57.40
                  with bleeding K57.41
              bleeding K57.53
Diverticulosis K57.90
  with bleeding K57.91
  large intestine K57.30
    with
      bleeding K57.31
      small intestine K57.50
        with bleeding K57.51
  small intestine K57.10
    with
      bleeding K57.11
      large intestine K57.50
        with bleeding K57.51
Diverticulum, diverticula (multiple) K57.90
  appendix (noninflammatory) K38.2
  bladder (sphincter) N32.3
    congenital Q64.6
  bronchus (congenital) Q32.4
    acquired J98.09
  calyx, calyceal (kidney) N28.89
  cardia (stomach) K31.4
  cecum — *see* Diverticulosis, intestine, large
    congenital Q43.8
  colon — *see* Diverticulosis, intestine, large
    congenital Q43.8
  duodenum — *see* Diverticulosis, intestine,
    small
    congenital Q43.8
  epiphrenic (esophagus) K22.5
  esophagus (congenital) Q39.6
    acquired (epiphrenic) (pulsion)
      (traction) K22.5
  eustachian tube — *see* Disorder, eustachian
    tube, specified NEC
  fallopian tube N83.8
  gastric K31.4
  heart (congenital) Q24.8
  ileum — *see* Diverticulosis, intestine, small
  jejunum — *see* Diverticulosis, intestine,
    small
  kidney (pelvis) (calyces) N28.89
    with calculus — *see* Calculus, kidney
  Meckel's (displaced) (hypertrophic) Q43.0
    malignant — *see* Table of Neoplasms,
      small intestine, malignant
  midthoracic K22.5

Diverticulum, diverticula (multiple) -
  continued
  organ or site, congenital NEC — *see*
    Distortion
  pericardium (congenital) (cyst) Q24.8
    acquired I31.8
  pharyngoesophageal (congenital) Q39.6
    acquired K22.5
  pharynx (congenital) Q38.7
  rectosigmoid — *see* Diverticulosis, intestine,
    large
    congenital Q43.8
  rectum — *see* Diverticulosis, intestine, large
  Rokitansky's K22.5
  seminal vesicle N50.89
  sigmoid — *see* Diverticulosis, intestine, large
    congenital Q43.8
  stomach (acquired) K31.4
    congenital Q40.2
  trachea (acquired) J39.8
  ureter (acquired) N28.89
    congenital Q62.8
  ureterovesical orifice N28.89
  urethra (acquired) N36.1
    congenital Q64.79
  ventricle, left (congenital) Q24.8
  vesical N32.3
    congenital Q64.6
  Zenker's (esophagus) K22.5
Division
  cervix uteri (acquired) N88.8
  glans penis Q55.69
  labia minora (congenital) Q52.79
  ligament (partial or complete) (current) —
    see also Sprain
    with open wound — *see* Wound, open
  muscle (partial or complete) (current) — *see
    also* Injury, muscle
    with open wound — *see* Wound, open
  nerve (traumatic) — *see* Injury, nerve
  spinal cord — *see* Injury, spinal cord, by
    region
  vein I87.8
Divorce, causing family disruption Z63.5
Dix-Hallpike neurolabyrinthitis — *see*
  Neuronitis, vestibular
Dizziness R42
  hysterical F44.89
  psychogenic F45.8
**DMAC (disseminated mycobacterium
  avium- intracellulare complex)** A31.2
DNR (do not resuscitate) Z66
**Doan-Wiseman syndrome (primary splenic
  neutropenia)** — *see* Agranulocytosis
Doehle-Heller aortitis A52.02
Dog bite — *see* Bite
Dohle body panmyelopathic syndrome D72.0
Dolichocephaly Q67.2
Dolichocolon Q43.8
Dolichostenomelia — *see* Syndrome, Marfan's
Donohue's syndrome E34.8
Donor (organ or tissue) Z52.9
  blood (whole) Z52.000
    autologous Z52.010
    specified component (lymphocytes)
      (platelets) NEC Z52.008
      autologous Z52.018
      specified donor NEC Z52.098
    specified donor NEC Z52.090
    stem cells Z52.001
      autologous Z52.011
      specified donor NEC Z52.091
  bone Z52.20
    autologous Z52.21
    marrow Z52.3
    specified type NEC Z52.29
  cornea Z52.5
  egg (Oocyte) Z52.819
    age 35 and over Z52.812
      anonymous recipient Z52.812
      designated recipient Z52.813
    under age 35 Z52.810
      anonymous recipient Z52.810
      designated recipient Z52.811
  kidney Z52.4

Donor (organ or tissue) - *continued*
  liver Z52.6
  lung Z52.89
  lymphocyte — *see* Donor, blood, specified
    components NEC
  Oocyte — *see* Donor, egg
  platelets Z52.008
  potential, examination of Z00.5
  semen Z52.89
  skin Z52.10
    autologous Z52.11
    specified type NEC Z52.19
  specified organ or tissue NEC Z52.89
  sperm Z52.89
Donovanosis A58
Dorsalgia M54.9
  psychogenic F45.41
  specified NEC M54.89
Dorsopathy M53.9
  deforming M43.9
    specified NEC — *see* subcategory M43.8
  specified NEC M53.80
    cervical region M53.82
    cervicothoracic region M53.83
    lumbar region M53.86
    lumbosacral region M53.87
    occipito-atlanto-axial region M53.81
    sacrococcygeal region M53.88
    thoracic region M53.84
    thoracolumbar region M53.85
Double
  albumin E88.09
  aortic arch Q25.45
  auditory canal Q17.8
  auricle (heart) Q20.8
  bladder Q64.79
  cervix Q51.820
    with doubling of uterus (and
      vagina) Q51.10
      with obstruction Q51.11
  inlet ventricle Q20.4
  kidney with double pelvis (renal) Q63.0
  meatus urinarius Q64.75
  monster Q89.4
  outlet
    left ventricle Q20.2
    right ventricle Q20.1
  pelvis (renal) with double ureter Q62.5
  tongue Q38.3
  ureter (one or both sides) Q62.5
    with double pelvis (renal) Q62.5
  urethra Q64.74
  urinary meatus Q64.75
  uterus Q51.20
    with
      doubling of cervix (and vagina) Q51.10
        with obstruction Q51.11
      complete Q51.21
      in pregnancy or childbirth O34.0-
        causing obstructed labor O65.5
      partial Q51.22
      specified NEC Q51.28
  vagina Q52.10
    with doubling of uterus (and
      cervix) Q51.10
      with obstruction Q51.11
  vision H53.2
  vulva Q52.79
Douglas' pouch, cul-de-sac — *see* condition
Down syndrome Q90.9
  meiotic nondisjunction Q90.0
  mitotic nondisjunction Q90.1
  mosaicism Q90.1
  translocation Q90.2
**DPD (dihydropyrimidine dehydrogenase
  deficiency)** E88.89
Dracontiasis B72
Dracunculiasis, dracunculosis B72
Dream state, hysterical F44.89
Drepanocytic anemia — *see* Disease, sickle-
  cell
Dresbach's syndrome (elliptocytosis) D58.1
Dreschlera (hawaiiensis) (infection) B43.8
Dressler's syndrome I24.1

Drift, ulnar — *see* Deformity, limb, specified type NEC, forearm
Drinking (alcohol)
  excessive, to excess NEC (without dependence) F10.10
    habitual (continual) (without remission) F10.20
    with remission F10.21
Drip, postnasal (chronic) R09.82
  due to
    allergic rhinitis — *see* Rhinitis, allergic
    common cold J00
    gastroesophageal reflux — *see* Reflux, gastroesophageal
    nasopharyngitis — *see* Nasopharyngitis
    other know condition - code to condition
    sinusitis — *see* Sinusitis
Droop
  facial R29.810
    cerebrovascular disease I69.992
      cerebral infarction I69.392
      intracerebral hemorrhage I69.192
      nontraumatic intracranial hemorrhage NEC I69.292
      specified disease NEC I69.892
      subarachnoid hemorrhage I69.092
Drop (in)
  attack NEC R55
  finger — *see* Deformity, finger
  foot — *see* Deformity, limb, foot, drop
  hematocrit (precipitous) R71.0
  hemoglobin R71.0
  toe — *see* Deformity, toe, specified NEC
  wrist — *see* Deformity, limb, wrist drop
Dropped heart beats I45.9
Dropsy, dropsical — *see also* Hydrops
  abdomen R18.8
  brain — *see* Hydrocephalus
  cardiac, heart — *see* Failure, heart, congestive
  gangrenous — *see* Gangrene
  heart — *see* Failure, heart, congestive
  kidney — *see* Nephrosis
  lung — *see* Edema, lung
  newborn due to isoimmunization P56.0
  pericardium — *see* Pericarditis
Drowned, drowning (near) T75.1
Drowsiness R40.0
Drug
  abuse counseling and surveillance Z71.51
  addiction — *see* Dependence
  dependence — *see* Dependence
  habit — *see* Dependence
  harmful use — *see* Abuse, drug
  induced fever R50.2
  overdose — *see* Table of Drugs and Chemicals, by drug, poisoning
  poisoning — *see* Table of Drugs and Chemicals, by drug, poisoning
  resistant organism infection — *see also* Resistant, organism, to, drug Z16.30
  therapy
    long term (current) (prophylactic) — *see* Therapy, drug long-term (current) (prophylactic)
    short term - omit code
  wrong substance given or taken in error — *see* Table of Drugs and Chemicals, by drug, poisoning
Drunkenness (without dependence) F10.129
  acute in alcoholism F10.229
  chronic (without remission) F10.20
    with remission F10.21
  pathological (without dependence) F10.129
    with dependence F10.229
  sleep F51.9
Drusen
  macula (degenerative) (retina) — *see* Degeneration, macula, drusen
  optic disc H47.32-
Dry, dryness — *see also* condition
  larynx J38.7
  mouth R68.2
    due to dehydration E86.0
  nose J34.89

Dry, dryness - *continued*
  socket (teeth) M27.3
  throat J39.2
DSAP L56.5
Duane's syndrome H50.81-
Dubin-Johnson disease or syndrome E80.6
Dubois' disease (thymus gland) A50.59 *[E35]*
Dubowitz' syndrome Q87.19
Duchenne-Aran muscular atrophy G12.21
Duchenne-Griesinger disease G71.01
Duchenne's
  disease or syndrome
    motor neuron disease G12.22
    muscular dystrophy G71.01
    locomotor ataxia (syphilitic) A52.11
  paralysis
    birth injury P14.0
    due to or associated with
      motor neuron disease G12.22
      muscular dystrophy G71.01
Ducrey's chancre A57
Duct, ductus — *see* condition
Duhring's disease (dermatitis herpetiformis) L13.0
Dullness, cardiac (decreased) (increased) R01.2
Dumb ague — *see* Malaria
Dumbness — *see* Aphasia
Dumdum fever B55.0
Dumping syndrome (postgastrectomy) K91.1
Duodenitis (nonspecific) (peptic) K29.80
  with bleeding K29.81
Duodenocholangitis — *see* Cholangitis
Duodenum, duodenal — *see* condition
Duplay's bursitis or periarthritis — *see* Tendinitis, calcific, shoulder
Duplication, duplex — *see also* Accessory
  alimentary tract Q45.8
  anus Q43.4
  appendix (and cecum) Q43.4
  biliary duct (any) Q44.5
  bladder Q64.79
  cecum (and appendix) Q43.4
  cervix Q51.820
  chromosome NEC
    with complex rearrangements NEC Q92.5
    seen only at prometaphase Q92.8
  cystic duct Q44.5
  digestive organs Q45.8
  esophagus Q39.8
  frontonasal process Q75.8
  intestine (large) (small) Q43.4
  kidney Q63.0
  liver Q44.7
  pancreas Q45.3
  penis Q55.69
  respiratory organs NEC Q34.8
  salivary duct Q38.4
  spinal cord (incomplete) Q06.2
  stomach Q40.2
Dupré's disease (meningism) R29.1
Dupuytren's contraction or disease M72.0
Durand-Nicolas-Favre disease A55
Durotomy (inadvertent) (incidental) G97.41
Duroziez's disease (congenital mitral stenosis) Q23.2
Dutton's relapsing fever (West African) A68.1
Dwarfism E34.3
  achondroplastic Q77.4
  congenital E34.3
  constitutional E34.3
  hypochondroplastic Q77.4
  hypophyseal E23.0
  infantile E34.3
  Laron-type E34.3
  Lorain (-Levi) type E23.0
  metatropic Q77.8
  nephrotic-glycosuric (with hypophosphatemic rickets) E72.09
  nutritional E45
  pancreatic K86.89
  pituitary E23.0
  renal N25.0
  thanatophoric Q77.1

Dyke-Young anemia (secondary) (symptomatic) D59.1
Dysacusis — *see* Abnormal, auditory perception
Dysadrenocortism E27.9
  hyperfunction E27.0
Dysarthria R47.1
  following
    cerebral infarction I69.322
    cerebrovascular disease I69.922
      specified disease NEC I69.822
    intracerebral hemorrhage I69.122
    nontraumatic intracranial hemorrhage NEC I69.222
    subarachnoid hemorrhage I69.022
Dysautonomia (familial) G90.1
Dysbarism T70.3
Dysbasia R26.2
  angiosclerotica intermittens I73.9
  hysterical F44.4
  lordotica (progressiva) G24.1
  nonorganic origin F44.4
  psychogenic F44.4
Dysbetalipoproteinemia (familial) E78.2
Dyscalculia R48.8
  developmental F81.2
Dyschezia K59.00
Dyschondroplasia (with hemangiomata) Q78.4
Dyschromia (skin) L81.9
Dyscollagenosis M35.9
Dyscranio-pygo-phalangy Q87.0
Dyscrasia
  blood (with) D75.9
    antepartum hemorrhage — *see* Hemorrhage, antepartum, with coagulation defect
    newborn P61.9
      specified type NEC P61.8
    intrapartum hemorrhage O67.0
    puerperal, postpartum O72.3
  polyglandular, pluriglandular E31.9
Dysendocrinism E34.9
Dysentery, dysenteric (catarrhal) (diarrhea) (epidemic) (hemorrhagic) (infectious) (sporadic) (tropical) A09
  abscess, liver A06.4
  amebic — *see also* Amebiasis A06.0
    with abscess — *see* Abscess, amebic
    acute A06.0
    chronic A06.1
  arthritis (*see also* category M01) A09
    bacillary (*see also* category M01) A03.9
  bacillary A03.9
    arthritis (*see also* category M01) A03.9
    Boyd A03.2
    Flexner A03.1
    Schmitz (-Stutzer) A03.0
    Shiga (-Kruse) A03.0
    Shigella A03.9
      boydii A03.2
      dysenteriae A03.0
      flexneri A03.1
      group A A03.0
      group B A03.1
      group C A03.2
      group D A03.3
      sonnei A03.3
      specified type NEC A03.8
    Sonne A03.3
    specified type NEC A03.8
  balantidial A07.0
  Balantidium coli A07.0
  Boyd's A03.2
  candidal B37.82
  Chilomastix A07.8
  Chinese A03.9
  coccidial A07.3
  Dientamoeba (fragilis) A07.8
  Embadomonas A07.8
  Entamoeba, entamebic — *see* Dysentery, amebic
  Flexner-Boyd A03.2
  Flexner's A03.1
  Giardia lamblia A07.1

Dysentery, dysenteric (catarrhal) (diarrhea) (epidemic) (hemorrhagic) (infectious) (sporadic) (tropical) - *continued*
Hiss-Russell A03.1
Lamblia A07.1
leishmanial B55.0
malarial — *see* Malaria
metazoal B82.0
monilial B37.82
protozoal A07.9
Salmonella A02.0
schistosomal B65.1
Schmitz (-Stutzer) A03.0
Shiga (-Kruse) A03.0
Shigella NOS — *see* Dysentery, bacillary
Sonne A03.3
strongyloidiasis B78.0
trichomonal A07.8
viral — *see also* Enteritis, viral A08.4
Dysequilibrium R42
Dysesthesia R20.8
hysterical F44.6
Dysfibrinogenemia (congenital) D68.2
Dysfunction
adrenal E27.9
hyperfunction E27.0
autonomic
due to alcohol G31.2
somatoform F45.8
bladder N31.9
neurogenic NOS — *see* Dysfunction,
bladder, neuromuscular
neuromuscular NOS N31.9
atonic (motor) (sensory) N31.2
autonomous N31.2
flaccid N31.2
nonreflex N31.2
reflex N31.1
specified NEC N31.8
uninhibited N31.0
bleeding, uterus N93.8
cerebral G93.89
colon K59.9
psychogenic F45.8
colostomy K94.03
cystic duct K82.8
cystostomy (stoma) — *see* Complications,
cystostomy
ejaculatory N53.19
anejaculatory orgasm N53.13
painful N53.12
premature F52.4
retarded N53.11
endocrine NOS E34.9
endometrium N85.8
enterostomy K94.13
erectile — *see* Dysfunction, sexual, male,
erectile
gallbladder K82.8
gastrostomy (stoma) K94.23
gland, glandular NOS E34.9
meibomian, of eyelid — *see* Dysfunction,
meibomian gland
heart I51.89
hemoglobin D75.89
hepatic K76.89
hypophysis E23.7
hypothalamic NEC E23.3
ileostomy (stoma) K94.13
jejunostomy (stoma) K94.13
kidney — *see* Disease, renal
labyrinthine — *see* subcategory H83.2
left ventricular, following sudden emotional
stress I51.81
liver K76.89
male — *see* Dysfunction, sexual, male
meibomian gland, of eyelid H02.889
left H02.886
lower H02.885
upper H02.884
upper and lower eyelids H02.88B
right H02.883
lower H02.882
upper H02.881
upper and lower eyelids H02.88A

Dysfunction - *continued*
orgasmic (female) F52.31
male F52.32
ovary E28.9
specified NEC E28.8
papillary muscle I51.89
parathyroid E21.4
physiological NEC R68.89
psychogenic F59
pineal gland E34.8
pituitary (gland) E23.3
platelets D69.1
polyglandular E31.9
specified NEC E31.8
psychophysiologic F59
psychosexual F52.9
with
dyspareunia F52.6
premature ejaculation F52.4
vaginismus F52.5
pylorus K31.9
rectum K59.9
psychogenic F45.8
reflex (sympathetic) — *see* Syndrome, pain,
complex regional I
segmental — *see* Dysfunction, somatic
senile R54
sexual (due to) R37
alcohol F10.981
amphetamine F15.981
in
abuse F15.181
dependence F15.281
anxiolytic F13.981
in
abuse F13.181
dependence F13.281
cocaine F14.981
in
abuse F14.181
dependence F14.281
excessive sexual drive F52.8
failure of genital response (male) F52.21
female F52.22
female N94.9
aversion F52.1
dyspareunia N94.10
psychogenic F52.6
frigidity F52.22
nymphomania F52.8
orgasmic F52.31
psychogenic F52.9
aversion F52.1
dyspareunia F52.6
frigidity F52.22
nymphomania F52.8
orgasmic F52.31
vaginismus F52.5
vaginismus N94.2
psychogenic F52.5
hypnotic F13.981
in
abuse F13.181
dependence F13.281
inhibited orgasm (female) F52.31
male F52.32
lack
of sexual enjoyment F52.1
or loss of sexual desire F52.0
male N53.9
anejaculatory orgasm N53.13
ejaculatory N53.19
painful N53.12
premature F52.4
retarded N53.11
erectile N52.9
drug induced N52.2
due to
disease classified elsewhere N52.1
drug N52.2
postoperative (postprocedural) N52.39
following
cryotherapy N52.37
interstitial seed therapy N52.36
prostate ablative therapy N52.37

Dysfunction - *continued*
sexual (due to) - *continued*
male - *continued*
erectile - *continued*
postoperative (postprocedural) -
continued
following - *continued*
prostatectomy N52.34
radical N52.31
radiation therapy N52.35
radical cystectomy N52.32
ultrasound ablative
therapy N52.37
urethral surgery N52.33
psychogenic F52.21
specified cause NEC N52.8
vasculogenic
arterial insufficiency N52.01
with corporo-venous
occlusive N52.03
corporo-venous occlusive N52.02
with arterial insufficiency N52.03
impotence — *see* Dysfunction, sexual,
male, erectile
psychogenic F52.9
aversion F52.1
erectile F52.21
orgasmic F52.32
premature ejaculation F52.4
satyriasis F52.8
specified type NEC F52.8
specified type NEC N53.8
nonorganic F52.9
specified NEC F52.8
opioid F11.981
in
abuse F11.181
dependence F11.281
orgasmic dysfunction (female) F52.31
male F52.32
premature ejaculation F52.4
psychoactive substances NEC F19.981
in
abuse F19.181
dependence F19.281
psychogenic F52.9
sedative F13.981
in
abuse F13.181
dependence F13.281
sexual aversion F52.1
vaginismus (nonorganic)
(psychogenic) F52.5
sinoatrial node I49.5
somatic M99.09
abdomen M99.09
acromioclavicular M99.07
cervical region M99.01
cervicothoracic M99.01
costochondral M99.08
costovertebral M99.08
head region M99.00
hip M99.05
lower extremity M99.06
lumbar region M99.03
lumbosacral M99.03
occipitocervical M99.00
pelvic region M99.05
pubic M99.05
rib cage M99.08
sacral region M99.04
sacrococcygeal M99.04
sacroiliac M99.04
specified NEC M99.09
sternochondral M99.08
sternoclavicular M99.07
thoracic region M99.02
thoracolumbar M99.02
upper extremity M99.07
somatoform autonomic F45.8
stomach K31.89
psychogenic F45.8
suprarenal E27.9
hyperfunction E27.0
symbolic R48.9

Dysfunction - *continued*
  symbolic - *continued*
    specified type NEC R48.8
  temporomandibular (joint) M26.69
    joint-pain syndrome M26.62-
  testicular (endocrine) E29.9
    specified NEC E29.8
  thymus E32.9
  thyroid E07.9
  ureterostomy (stoma) — *see* Complications,
      stoma, urinary tract
  urethrostomy (stoma) — *see* Complications,
      stoma, urinary tract
  uterus, complicating delivery O62.9
    hypertonic O62.4
    hypotonic O62.2
      primary O62.0
      secondary O62.1
  ventricular I51.9
    with congestive heart failure — *see also*
        Failure, heart I50.9
    left, reversible, following sudden
        emotional stress I51.81
Dysgenesis
  gonadal (due to chromosomal
      anomaly) Q96.9
    pure Q99.1
  renal Q60.5
    bilateral Q60.4
    unilateral Q60.3
  reticular D72.0
  tidal platelet D69.3
Dysgerminoma
  specified site — *see* Neoplasm, malignant,
      by site
  unspecified site
    female C56.9
    male C62.90
Dysgeusia R43.2
Dysgraphia R27.8
Dyshidrosis, dysidrosis L30.1
Dyskaryotic cervical smear R87.619
Dyskeratosis L85.8
  cervix — *see* Dysplasia, cervix
  congenital Q82.8
  uterus NEC N85.8
Dyskinesia G24.9
  biliary (cystic duct or gallbladder) K82.8
  drug induced
    orofacial G24.01
  esophagus K22.4
  hysterical F44.4
  intestinal K59.8
  nonorganic origin F44.4
  orofacial (idiopathic) G24.4
    drug induced G24.01
  psychogenic F44.4
  subacute, drug induced G24.01
  tardive G24.01
    neuroleptic induced G24.01
  trachea J39.8
  tracheobronchial J98.09
Dyslalia (developmental) F80.0
Dyslexia R48.0
  developmental F81.0
Dyslipidemia E78.5
  depressed HDL cholesterol E78.6
  elevated fasting triglycerides E78.1
Dysmaturity — *see also* Light for dates
  pulmonary (newborn) (Wilson-Mikity) P27.0
Dysmenorrhea (essential) (exfoliative) N94.6
  congestive (syndrome) N94.6
  primary N94.4
  psychogenic F45.8
  secondary N94.5
Dysmetabolic syndrome X E88.81
Dysmetria R27.8
Dysmorphism (due to)
  alcohol Q86.0
  exogenous cause NEC Q86.8
  hydantoin Q86.1
  warfarin Q86.2
Dysmorphophobia (nondelusional) F45.22
  delusional F22
Dysnomia R47.01

Dysorexia R63.0
  psychogenic F50.89
Dysostosis
  cleidocranial, cleidocranialis Q74.0
  craniofacial Q75.1
  Fairbank's (idiopathic familial generalized
      osteophytosis) Q78.9
  mandibulofacial (incomplete) Q75.4
  multiplex E76.01
  oculomandibular Q75.5
Dyspareunia (female) N94.10
  deep N94.12
  male N53.12
  nonorganic F52.6
  psychogenic F52.6
  secondary N94.19
  specified NEC N94.19
  superficial (introital) N94.11
Dyspepsia R10.13
  atonic K30
  functional (allergic) (congenital)
      (gastrointestinal) (occupational)
      (reflex) K30
  intestinal K59.8
  nervous F45.8
  neurotic F45.8
  psychogenic F45.8
Dysphagia R13.10
  cervical R13.19
  following
    cerebral infarction I69.391
    cerebrovascular disease I69.991
      specified NEC I69.891
    intracerebral hemorrhage I69.191
    nontraumatic intracranial hemorrhage
        NEC I69.291
      specified disease NEC I69.891
    subarachnoid hemorrhage I69.091
  functional (hysterical) F45.8
  hysterical F45.8
  nervous (hysterical) F45.8
  neurogenic R13.19
  oral phase R13.11
  oropharyngeal phase R13.12
  pharyngeal phase R13.13
  pharyngoesophageal phase R13.14
  psychogenic F45.8
  sideropenic D50.1
  spastica K22.4
  specified NEC R13.19
Dysphagocytosis, congenital D71
Dysphasia R47.02
  developmental
    expressive type F80.1
    receptive type F80.2
  following
    cerebrovascular disease I69.921
      cerebral infarction I69.321
      intracerebral hemorrhage I69.121
      nontraumatic intracranial hemorrhage
          NEC I69.221
        specified disease NEC I69.821
      subarachnoid hemorrhage I69.021
Dysphonia R49.0
  functional F44.4
  hysterical F44.4
  psychogenic F44.4
  spastica J38.3
Dysphoria
  gender F64.9
    in
      adolescence and adulthood F64.0
      children F64.2
    specified NEC F64.8
  postpartal O90.6
Dyspituitarism E23.3
Dysplasia — *see also* Anomaly
  acetabular, congenital Q65.89
  alveolar capillary, with vein
      misalignment J84.843
  anus (histologically confirmed) (mild)
      (moderate) K62.82
    severe D01.3
  arrhythmogenic right ventricular I42.8
  arterial, fibromuscular I77.3

Dysplasia - *continued*
  asphyxiating thoracic (congenital) Q77.2
  brain Q07.9
  bronchopulmonary, perinatal P27.1
  cervix (uteri) N87.9
    mild N87.0
    moderate N87.1
    severe D06.9
  chondroectodermal Q77.6
  colon D12.6
  craniometaphyseal Q78.8
  dentinal K00.5
  diaphyseal, progressive Q78.3
  dystrophic Q77.5
  ectodermal (anhidrotic) (congenital)
      (hereditary) Q82.4
    hydrotic Q82.8
  epithelial, uterine cervix — *see* Dysplasia,
      cervix
  eye (congenital) Q11.2
  fibrous
    bone NEC (monostotic) M85.00
      ankle M85.07-
      foot M85.07-
      forearm M85.03-
      hand M85.04-
      lower leg M85.06-
      multiple site M85.09
      neck M85.08
      rib M85.08
      shoulder M85.01-
      skull M85.08
      specified site NEC M85.08
      thigh M85.05-
      toe M85.07-
      upper arm M85.02-
      vertebra M85.08
    diaphyseal, progressive Q78.3
    jaw M27.8
    polyostotic Q78.1
  florid osseous — *see also* Cyst, calcifying
      odontogenic
  high grade, focal D12.6
  hip, congenital Q65.89
  joint, congenital Q74.8
  kidney Q61.4
    multicystic Q61.4
  leg Q74.2
  lung, congenital (not associated with short
      gestation) Q33.6
  mammary (gland) (benign) N60.9-
    cyst (solitary) — *see* Cyst, breast
    cystic — *see* Mastopathy, cystic
    duct ectasia — *see* Ectasia, mammary duct
    fibroadenosis — *see* Fibroadenosis, breast
    fibrosclerosis — *see* Fibrosclerosis, breast
    specified type NEC N60.8-
  metaphyseal Q78.5
  muscle Q79.8
  oculodentodigital Q87.0
  periapical (cemental) (cemento-osseous) —
      see Cyst, calcifying odontogenic
  periosteum — *see* Disorder, bone, specified
      type NEC
  polyostotic fibrous Q78.1
  prostate — *see also* Neoplasia,
      intraepithelial, prostate N42.30
    severe D07.5
    specified NEC N42.39
  renal Q61.4
    multicystic Q61.4
  retinal, congenital Q14.1
  right ventricular, arrhythmogenic I42.8
  septo-optic Q04.4
  skin L98.8
  spinal cord Q06.1
  spondyloepiphyseal Q77.7
  thymic, with immunodeficiency D82.1
  vagina N89.3
    mild N89.0
    moderate N89.1
    severe NEC D07.2
  vulva N90.3
    mild N90.0
    moderate N90.1

Dysplasia - *continued*
  vulva - *continued*
    severe NEC D07.1
Dysplasminogenemia E88.02
Dyspnea (nocturnal) (paroxysmal) R06.00
  asthmatic (bronchial) J45.909
    with
      exacerbation (acute) J45.901
      bronchitis J45.909
        with
          exacerbation (acute) J45.901
          status asthmaticus J45.902
        chronic J44.9
        status asthmaticus J45.902
    cardiac — *see* Failure, ventricular, left
  cardiac — *see* Failure, ventricular, left
  functional F45.8
  hyperventilation R06.4
  hysterical F45.8
  newborn P28.89
  orthopnea R06.01
  psychogenic F45.8
  shortness of breath R06.02
  specified type NEC R06.09
Dyspraxia R27.8
  developmental (syndrome) F82
Dysproteinemia E88.09
Dysreflexia, autonomic G90.4
Dysrhythmia
  cardiac I49.9
    newborn
      bradycardia P29.12
        occurring before birth P03.819
          before onset of labor P03.810
          during labor P03.811
      tachycardia P29.11
    postoperative I97.89
  cerebral or cortical — *see* Epilepsy
Dyssomnia — *see* Disorder, sleep
Dyssynergia
  biliary K83.8
  bladder sphincter N36.44
  cerebellaris myoclonica (Hunt's ataxia) G11.1
Dysthymia F34.1
Dysthyroidism E07.9
Dystocia O66.9
  affecting newborn P03.1
  cervical (hypotonic) O62.2
    affecting newborn P03.6
    primary O62.0
    secondary O62.1
  contraction ring O62.4
  fetal O66.9
    abnormality NEC O66.3
    conjoined twins O66.3
    oversize O66.2
  maternal O66.9
  positional O64.9
  shoulder (girdle) O66.0
    causing obstructed labor O66.0
  uterine NEC O62.4
Dystonia G24.9
  cervical G24.3
  deformans progressiva G24.1
  drug induced NEC G24.09
    acute G24.02
    specified NEC G24.09
  familial G24.1
  idiopathic G24.1
    familial G24.1
    nonfamilial G24.2
    orofacial G24.4
  lenticularis G24.8
  musculorum deformans G24.1
  neuroleptic induced (acute) G24.02
  orofacial (idiopathic) G24.4
  oromandibular G24.4
    due to drug G24.01
  specified NEC G24.8
  torsion (familial) (idiopathic) G24.1
    acquired G24.8
    genetic G24.1
    symptomatic (nonfamilial) G24.2
Dystonic movements R25.8

Dystrophy, dystrophia
  adiposogenital E23.6
  autosomal recessive, childhood type, muscular dystrophy resembling Duchenne or Becker G71.01
  Becker's type G71.01
  cervical sympathetic G90.2
  choroid (hereditary) H31.20
    central areolar H31.22
    choroideremia H31.21
    gyrate atrophy H31.23
    specified type NEC H31.29
  cornea (hereditary) H18.50
    endothelial H18.51
    epithelial H18.52
    granular H18.53
    lattice H18.54
    macular H18.55
    specified type NEC H18.59
  Duchenne's type G71.01
  due to malnutrition E45
  Erb's G71.02
  Fuchs' H18.51
  Gower's muscular G71.01
  hair L67.8
  infantile neuraxonal G31.89
  Landouzy-Déjérine G71.02
  Leyden-Möbius G71.09
  muscular G71.00
    autosomal recessive, childhood type, muscular dystrophy resembling Duchenne or Becker G71.01
    benign (Becker type) G71.01
      scapuloperoneal with early contractures [Emery-Dreifuss] G71.09
    congenital (hereditary) (progressive) (with specific morphological abnormalities of the muscle fiber) G71.09
      myotonic G71.11
    distal G71.09
    Duchenne type G71.01
    Emery-Dreifuss G71.09
    Erb type G71.02
    facioscapulohumeral G71.02
    Gower's G71.01
    hereditary (progressive) G71.09
    Landouzy-Déjérine type G71.02
    limb-girdle G71.09
    myotonic G71.11
    progressive (hereditary) G71.09
      Charcot-Marie (-Tooth) type G60.0
    pseudohypertrophic (infantile) G71.01
    scapulohumeral G71.02
    scapuloperoneal G71.09
    severe (Duchenne type) G71.01
    specified type NEC G71.09
  myocardium, myocardial — *see* Degeneration, myocardial
  myotonic, myotonica G71.11
  nail L60.3
    congenital Q84.6
  nutritional E45
  ocular G71.09
  oculocerebrorenal E72.03
  oculopharyngeal G71.09
  ovarian N83.8
  polyglandular E31.8
  reflex (neuromuscular) (sympathetic) — *see* Syndrome, pain, complex regional I
  retinal (hereditary) H35.50
    in
      lipid storage disorders E75.6 *[H36]*
      systemic lipidoses E75.6 *[H36]*
    involving
      pigment epithelium H35.54
      sensory area H35.53
    pigmentary H35.52
    vitreoretinal H35.51
  Salzmann's nodular — *see* Degeneration, cornea, nodular
  scapuloperoneal G71.09
  skin NEC L98.8
  sympathetic (reflex) — *see* Syndrome, pain, complex regional I
    cervical G90.2

Dystrophy, dystrophia - *continued*
  tapetoretinal H35.54
  thoracic, asphyxiating Q77.2
  unguium L60.3
    congenital Q84.6
  vitreoretinal H35.51
  vulva N90.4
  yellow (liver) — *see* Failure, hepatic
Dysuria R30.0
  psychogenic F45.8

E

Eales' disease H35.06-
Ear — *see also* condition
  piercing Z41.3
  tropical NEC B36.9 *[H62.40]*
    in
      aspergillosis B44.89
      candidiasis B37.84
      moniliasis B37.84
  wax (impacted) H61.20
    left H61.22
      with right H61.23
    right H61.21
      with left H61.23
Earache — *see* subcategory H92.0
Early satiety R68.81
Eaton-Lambert syndrome — *see* Syndrome, Lambert-Eaton
Eberth's disease (typhoid fever) A01.00
Ebola virus disease A98.4
Ebstein's anomaly or syndrome (heart) Q22.5
Eccentro-osteochondrodysplasia E76.29
Ecchondroma — *see* Neoplasm, bone, benign
Ecchondrosis D48.0
Ecchymosis R58
  conjunctiva — *see* Hemorrhage, conjunctiva
  eye (traumatic) — *see* Contusion, eyeball
  eyelid (traumatic) — *see* Contusion, eyelid
  newborn P54.5
  spontaneous R23.3
  traumatic — *see* Contusion
Echinococciasis — *see* Echinococcus
Echinococcosis — *see* Echinococcus
Echinococcus (infection) B67.90
  granulosus B67.4
    bone B67.2
    liver B67.0
    lung B67.1
    multiple sites B67.32
    specified site NEC B67.39
    thyroid B67.31
  liver NOS B67.8
    granulosus B67.0
    multilocularis B67.5
  lung NEC B67.99
    granulosus B67.1
    multilocularis B67.69
  multilocularis B67.7
    liver B67.5
    multiple sites B67.61
    specified site NEC B67.69
  specified site NEC B67.99
    granulosus B67.39
    multilocularis B67.69
  thyroid NEC B67.99
    granulosus B67.31
    multilocularis B67.69 *[E35]*
Echinorhynchiasis B83.8
Echinostomiasis B66.8
Echolalia R48.8
Echovirus, as cause of disease classified elsewhere B97.12
Eclampsia, eclamptic (coma) (convulsions) (delirium) (with hypertension) NEC O15.9
  complicating
    labor and delivery O15.1
    postpartum O15.2
    pregnancy O15.0-
    puerperium O15.2
Economic circumstances affecting care Z59.9
Economo's disease A85.8
Ectasia, ectasis
  annuloaortic I35.8

Ectasia, ectasis - *continued*
  aorta I77.819
    with aneurysm — *see* Aneurysm, aorta
    abdominal I77.811
    thoracic I77.810
    thoracoabdominal I77.812
  breast — *see* Ectasia, mammary duct
  capillary I78.8
  cornea H18.71-
  gastric antral vascular (GAVE) K31.819
    with hemorrhage K31.811
    without hemorrhage K31.819
  mammary duct N60.4-
  salivary gland (duct) K11.8
  sclera — *see* Sclerectasia
Ecthyma L08.0
  contagiosum B08.02
  gangrenosum L08.0
  infectiosum B08.02
Ectocardia Q24.8
Ectodermal dysplasia (anhidrotic) Q82.4
Ectodermosis erosiva pluriorificialis L51.1
Ectopic, ectopia (congenital)
  abdominal viscera Q45.8
    due to defect in anterior abdominal
      wall Q79.59
  ACTH syndrome E24.3
  adrenal gland Q89.1
  anus Q43.5
  atrial beats I49.1
  beats I49.49
    atrial I49.1
    ventricular I49.3
  bladder Q64.10
  bone and cartilage in lung Q33.5
  brain Q04.8
  breast tissue Q83.8
  cardiac Q24.8
  cerebral Q04.8
  cordis Q24.8
  endometrium — *see* Endometriosis
  gastric mucosa Q40.2
  gestation — *see* Pregnancy, by site
  heart Q24.8
  hormone secretion NEC E34.2
  kidney (crossed) (pelvis) Q63.2
  lens, lentis Q12.1
  mole — *see* Pregnancy, by site
  organ or site NEC — *see* Malposition,
    congenital
  pancreas Q45.3
  pregnancy — *see* Pregnancy, ectopic
  pupil — *see* Abnormality, pupillary
  renal Q63.2
  sebaceous glands of mouth Q38.6
  spleen Q89.09
  testis Q53.00
    bilateral Q53.02
    unilateral Q53.01
  thyroid Q89.2
  tissue in lung Q33.5
  ureter Q62.63
  ventricular beats I49.3
  vesicae Q64.10
Ectromelia Q73.8
  lower limb — *see* Defect, reduction, limb,
    lower, specified type NEC
  upper limb — *see* Defect, reduction, limb,
    upper, specified type NEC
Ectropion H02.109
  cervix N86
    with cervicitis N72
  congenital Q10.1
  eyelid H02.109
    cicatricial H02.119
      left H02.116
        lower H02.115
        upper H02.114
      right H02.113
        lower H02.112
        upper H02.111
    congenital Q10.1
    left H02.106
      lower H02.105
      upper H02.104

Ectropion - *continued*
  eyelid - *continued*
    mechanical H02.129
      left H02.126
        lower H02.125
        upper H02.124
      right H02.123
        lower H02.122
        upper H02.121
    paralytic H02.159
      left H02.156
        lower H02.155
        upper H02.154
      right H02.153
        lower H02.152
        upper H02.151
    right H02.103
      lower H02.102
      upper H02.101
    senile H02.139
      left H02.136
        lower H02.135
        upper H02.134
      right H02.133
        lower H02.132
        upper H02.131
    spastic H02.149
      left H02.146
        lower H02.145
        upper H02.144
      right H02.143
        lower H02.142
        upper H02.141
  iris H21.89
  lip (acquired) K13.0
    congenital Q38.0
  urethra N36.8
  uvea H21.89
Eczema (acute) (chronic) (erythematous)
  (fissum) (rubrum) (squamous) — *see*
    also Dermatitis L30.9
  contact — *see* Dermatitis, contact
  dyshydrotic L30.1
  external ear — *see* Otitis, externa, acute,
    eczematoid
  flexural L20.82
  herpeticum B00.0
  hypertrophicum L28.0
  hypostatic — *see* Varix, leg, with,
    inflammation
  impetiginous L01.1
  infantile (due to any substance) L20.83
    intertriginous L21.1
    seborrheic L21.1
  intertriginous NEC L30.4
    infantile L21.1
  intrinsic (allergic) L20.84
  lichenified NEC L28.0
  marginatum (hebrae) B35.6
  pustular L30.3
  stasis I87.2
    with varicose veins — *see* Varix, leg, with,
      inflammation
  vaccination, vaccinatum T88.1
  varicose — *see* Varix, leg, with,
    inflammation
Eczematid L30.2
Eddowes (-Spurway) syndrome Q78.0
Edema, edematous (infectious) (pitting)
  (toxic) R60.9
  with nephritis — *see* Nephrosis
  allergic T78.3
  amputation stump (surgical) (sequelae (late
    effect)) T87.89
  angioneurotic (allergic) (any site) (with
    urticaria) T78.3
    hereditary D84.1
  angiospastic I73.9
  Berlin's (traumatic) S05.8X-
  brain (cytotoxic) (vasogenic) G93.6
    due to birth injury P11.0
    newborn (anoxia or hypoxia) P52.4
      birth injury P11.0
    traumatic — *see* Injury, intracranial,
      cerebral edema

Edema, edematous (infectious) (pitting)
(toxic) - *continued*
  cardiac — *see* Failure, heart, congestive
  cardiovascular — *see* Failure, heart,
    congestive
  cerebral — *see* Edema, brain
  cerebrospinal — *see* Edema, brain
  cervix (uteri) (acute) N88.8
    puerperal, postpartum O90.89
  chronic hereditary Q82.0
  circumscribed, acute T78.3
    hereditary D84.1
  conjunctiva H11.42-
  cornea H18.2-
    idiopathic H18.22-
    secondary H18.23-
      due to contact lens H18.21-
  due to
    lymphatic obstruction I89.0
    salt retention E87.0
  epiglottis — *see* Edema, glottis
  essential, acute T78.3
    hereditary D84.1
  extremities, lower — *see* Edema, legs
  eyelid NEC H02.849
    left H02.846
      lower H02.845
      upper H02.844
    right H02.843
      lower H02.842
      upper H02.841
  familial, hereditary Q82.0
  famine — *see* Malnutrition, severe
  generalized R60.1
  glottis, glottic, glottidis (obstructive)
    (passive) J38.4
    allergic T78.3
    hereditary D84.1
  heart — *see* Failure, heart, congestive
  heat T67.7
  hereditary Q82.0
  inanition — *see* Malnutrition, severe
  intracranial G93.6
  iris H21.89
  joint — *see* Effusion, joint
  larynx — *see* Edema, glottis
  legs R60.0
    due to venous obstruction I87.1
    hereditary Q82.0
  localized R60.0
    due to venous obstruction I87.1
  lower limbs — *see* Edema, legs
  lung J81.1
    with heart condition or failure — *see*
      Failure, ventricular, left
    acute J81.0
    chemical (acute) J68.1
      chronic J68.1
    chronic J81.1
    due to
      chemicals, gases, fumes or vapors
        (inhalation) J68.1
      external agent J70.9
        specified NEC J70.8
      radiation J70.1
    due to
      chemicals, fumes or vapors
        (inhalation) J68.1
      external agent J70.9
        specified NEC J70.8
      high altitude T70.29
      near drowning T75.1
      radiation J70.0
    meaning failure, left ventricle I50.1
  lymphatic I89.0
    due to mastectomy I97.2
  macula H35.81
    cystoid, following cataract surgery — *see*
      Complications, postprocedural,
      following cataract surgery
    diabetic — *see* Diabetes, by type, with,
      retinopathy, with macular edema
  malignant — *see* Gangrene, gas
  Milroy's Q82.0
  nasopharynx J39.2

Edema, edematous (infectious) (pitting) (toxic) - *continued*
  newborn P83.30
    hydrops fetalis — *see* Hydrops, fetalis
    specified NEC P83.39
  nutritional — *see also* Malnutrition, severe
    with dyspigmentation, skin and hair E40
  optic disc or nerve — *see* Papilledema
  orbit H05.22-
  pancreas K86.89
  papilla, optic — *see* Papilledema
  penis N48.89
  periodic T78.3
    hereditary D84.1
  pharynx J39.2
  pulmonary — *see* Edema, lung
  Quincke's T78.3
    hereditary D84.1
  renal — *see* Nephrosis
  retina H35.81
    diabetic — *see* Diabetes, by type, with, retinopathy, with macular edema
  salt E87.0
  scrotum N50.89
  seminal vesicle N50.89
  spermatic cord N50.89
  spinal (cord) (vascular) (nontraumatic) G95.19
  starvation — *see* Malnutrition, severe
  stasis — *see* Hypertension, venous, (chronic)
  subglottic — *see* Edema, glottis
  supraglottic — *see* Edema, glottis
  testis N44.8
  tunica vaginalis N50.89
  vas deferens N50.89
  vulva (acute) N90.89
Edentulism — *see* Absence, teeth, acquired
Edsall's disease T67.2
Educational handicap Z55.9
  specified NEC Z55.8
Edward's syndrome — *see* Trisomy, 18
Effect (s) (of) (from) — *see* Effect, adverse NEC
Effect, adverse
  abnormal gravitational (G) forces or states T75.81
  abuse — *see* Maltreatment
  air pressure T70.9
    specified NEC T70.8
  altitude (high) — *see* Effect, adverse, high altitude
  anesthesia — *see also* Anesthesia T88.59
    in labor and delivery O74.9
    local, toxic
      in labor and delivery O74.4
      in pregnancy NEC O29.3-
      postpartum, puerperal O89.3
    postpartum, puerperal O89.9
    specified NEC T88.59
      in labor and delivery O74.8
      postpartum, puerperal O89.8
    spinal and epidural T88.59
      headache T88.59
        in labor and delivery O74.5
        postpartum, puerperal O89.4
      specified NEC
        in labor and delivery O74.6
        postpartum, puerperal O89.5
  antitoxin — *see* Complications, vaccination
  atmospheric pressure T70.9
    due to explosion T70.8
    high T70.3
    low — *see* Effect, adverse, high altitude
    specified effect NEC T70.8
  biological, correct substance properly administered — *see* Effect, adverse, drug
  blood (derivatives) (serum) (transfusion) — *see* Complications, transfusion
  chemical substance — *see* Table of Drugs and Chemicals
  cold (temperature) (weather) T69.9
    chilblains T69.1
    frostbite — *see* Frostbite
    specified effect NEC T69.8

Effect, adverse - *continued*
  drugs and medicaments T88.7
    specified drug — *see* Table of Drugs and Chemicals, by drug, adverse effect
    specified effect - code to condition
  electric current, electricity (shock) T75.4
    burn — *see* Burn
  exertion (excessive) T73.3
  exposure — *see* Exposure
  external cause NEC T75.89
  foodstuffs T78.1
    allergic reaction — *see* Allergy, food
      causing anaphylaxis — *see* Shock, anaphylactic, due to food
    noxious — *see* Poisoning, food, noxious
  gases, fumes, or vapors T59.9-
    specified agent — *see* Table of Drugs and Chemicals
  glue (airplane) sniffing
    due to drug abuse — *see* Abuse, drug, inhalant
    due to drug dependence — *see* Dependence, drug, inhalant
  heat — *see* Heat
  high altitude NEC T70.29
    anoxia T70.29
    on
      ears T70.0
      sinuses T70.1
    polycythemia D75.1
  high pressure fluids T70.4
  hot weather — *see* Heat
  hunger T73.0
  immersion, foot — *see* Immersion
  immunization — *see* Complications, vaccination
  immunological agents — *see* Complications, vaccination
  infrared (radiation) (rays) NOS T66
    dermatitis or eczema L59.8
  infusion — *see* Complications, infusion
  lack of care of infants — *see* Maltreatment, child
  lightning — *see* Lightning
  medical care T88.9
    specified NEC T88.8
  medicinal substance, correct, properly administered — *see* Effect, adverse, drug
  motion T75.3
  noise, on inner ear — *see* subcategory H83.3
  overheated places — *see* Heat
  psychosocial, of work environment Z56.5
  radiation (diagnostic) (infrared) (natural source) (therapeutic) (ultraviolet) (X-ray) NOS T66
    dermatitis or eczema — *see* Dermatitis, due to, radiation
    fibrosis of lung J70.1
    pneumonitis J70.0
    pulmonary manifestations
      acute J70.0
      chronic J70.1
    skin L59.9
  radioactive substance NOS
    dermatitis or eczema — *see* Radiodermatitis
  reduced temperature T69.9
    immersion foot or hand — *see* Immersion
    specified effect NEC T69.8
  serum NEC — *see also* Reaction, serum T80.69
    specified NEC T78.8
    external cause NEC T75.89
  strangulation — *see* Asphyxia, traumatic
  submersion T75.1
  thirst T73.1
  toxic — *see* Toxicity
  transfusion — *see* Complications, transfusion
  ultraviolet (radiation) (rays) NOS T66
    burn — *see* Burn
    dermatitis or eczema — *see* Dermatitis, due to, ultraviolet rays
      acute L56.8

Effect, adverse - *continued*
  vaccine (any) — *see* Complications, vaccination
  vibration — *see* Vibration, adverse effects
  water pressure NEC T70.9
    specified NEC T70.8
  weightlessness T75.82
  whole blood — *see* Complications, transfusion
  work environment Z56.5
Effects, late — *see* Sequelae
Effluvium
  anagen L65.1
  telogen L65.0
Effort syndrome (psychogenic) F45.8
Effusion
  amniotic fluid — *see* Pregnancy, complicated by, prematue rupture of membranes
  brain (serous) G93.6
  bronchial — *see* Bronchitis
  cerebral G93.6
  cerebrospinal — *see also* Meningitis
    vessel G93.6
  chest — *see* Effusion, pleura
  chylous, chyliform (pleura) J94.0
  intracranial G93.6
  joint M25.40
    ankle M25.47-
    elbow M25.42-
    foot joint M25.47-
    hand joint M25.44-
    hip M25.45-
    knee M25.46-
    shoulder M25.41-
    specified joint NEC M25.48
    wrist M25.43-
  malignant pleural J91.0
  meninges — *see* Meningitis
  pericardium, pericardial (noninflammatory) I31.3
    acute — *see* Pericarditis, acute
  peritoneal (chronic) R18.8
  pleura, pleurisy, pleuritic, pleuropericardial J90
    chylous, chyliform J94.0
    due to systemic lupus erythematosis M32.13
    in conditions classified elsewhere J91.8
    influenzal — *see* Influenza, with, respiratory manifestations NEC
    malignant J91.0
    newborn P28.89
    tuberculous NEC A15.6
      primary (progressive) A15.7
  spinal — *see* Meningitis
  thorax, thoracic — *see* Effusion, pleura
Egg shell nails L60.3
  congenital Q84.6
Egyptian splenomegaly B65.1
Ehlers-Danlos syndrome — *see also* Syndrome, Ehlers-Danlos Q79.60
Ehrlichiosis A77.40
  due to
    E. chafeensis A77.41
    E. sennetsu A79.81
    specified organism NEC A77.49
Eichstedt's disease B36.0
Eisenmenger's
  complex or syndrome I27.83
  defect Q21.8
Ejaculation
  delayed F52.32
  painful N53.12
  premature F52.4
  retarded N53.11
  retrograde N53.14
  semen, painful N53.12
    psychogenic F52.6
Ekbom's syndrome (restless legs) G25.81
Ekman's syndrome (brittle bones and blue sclera) Q78.0
Elastic skin Q82.8
  acquired L57.4
Elastofibroma — *see* Neoplasm, connective tissue, benign

Elastoma (juvenile) Q82.8
  Miescher's L87.2
Elastomyofibrosis I42.4
Elastosis
  actinic, solar L57.8
  atrophicans (senile) L57.4
  perforans serpiginosa L87.2
  senilis L57.4
Elbow — *see* condition
Electric current, electricity, effects
    (concussion) (fatal) (nonfatal) (shock)
    T75.4
  burn — *see* Burn
Electric feet syndrome E53.8
Electrocution T75.4
  from electroshock gun (taser) T75.4
Electrolyte imbalance E87.8
  with
    abortion — *see* Abortion by type,
      complicated by, electrolyte imbalance
    ectopic pregnancy O08.5
    molar pregnancy O08.5
Elephantiasis (nonfilarial) I89.0
  arabicum — *see* Infestation, filarial
  bancroftian B74.0
  congenital (any site) (hereditary) Q82.0
  due to
    Brugia (malayi) B74.1
      timori B74.2
    mastectomy I97.2
    Wuchereria (bancrofti) B74.0
  eyelid H02.859
    left H02.856
      lower H02.855
      upper H02.854
    right H02.853
      lower H02.852
      upper H02.851
  filarial, filariensis — *see* Infestation, filarial
  glandular I89.0
  graecorum A30.9
  lymphangiectatic I89.0
  lymphatic vessel I89.0
    due to mastectomy I97.2
  scrotum (nonfilarial) I89.0
  streptococcal I89.0
  surgical I97.89
    postmastectomy I97.2
  telangiectodes I89.0
  vulva (nonfilarial) N90.89
Elevated, elevation
  antibody titer R76.0
  basal metabolic rate R94.8
  blood pressure — *see also* Hypertension
    reading (incidental) (isolated)
      (nonspecific) , no diagnosis of
      hypertension R03.0
  blood sugar R73.9
  body temperature (of unknown origin) R50.9
  C-reactive protein (CRP) R79.82
  cancer antigen 125 [CA 125] R97.1
  carcinoembryonic antigen [CEA] R97.0
  cholesterol E78.00
    with high triglycerides E78.2
  conjugate, eye H51.0
  diaphragm, congenital Q79.1
  erythrocyte sedimentation rate R70.0
  fasting glucose R73.01
  fasting triglycerides E78.1
  finding on laboratory examination — *see*
    Findings, abnormal, inconclusive,
    without diagnosis, by type of exam
  GFR (glomerular filtration rate) — *see*
    Findings, abnormal, inconclusive,
    without diagnosis, by type of exam
  glucose tolerance (oral) R73.02
  immunoglobulin level R76.8
  indoleacetic acid R82.5
  lactic acid dehydrogenase (LDH) level R74.0
  leukocytes D72.829
  lipoprotein a (Lp (a)) level E78.41
  liver function
    study R94.5
    test R79.89
      alkaline phosphatase R74.8

Elevated, elevation - *continued*
  liver function - *continued*
    test - *continued*
      aminotransferase R74.0
      bilirubin R17
      hepatic enzyme R74.8
      lactate dehydrogenase R74.0
  Lp (a) (lipoprotein (a)) E78.41
  lymphocytes D72.820
  prostate specific antigen [PSA] R97.20
  Rh titer — *see* Complication(s), transfusion,
    incompatibility reaction, Rh (factor)
  scapula, congenital Q74.0
  sedimentation rate R70.0
  SGOT R74.0
  SGPT R74.0
  transaminase level R74.0
  triglycerides E78.1
    with high cholesterol E78.2
  tumor associated antigens [TAA] NEC R97.8
  tumor specific antigens [TSA] NEC R97.8
  urine level of
    catecholamine R82.5
    indoleacetic acid R82.5
    17-ketosteroids R82.5
    steroids R82.5
    vanillylmandelic acid (VMA) R82.5
  venous pressure I87.8
  white blood cell count D72.829
    specified NEC D72.828
Elliptocytosis (congenital) (hereditary) D58.1
  Hb C (disease) D58.1
  hemoglobin disease D58.1
  sickle-cell (disease) D57.8-
    trait D57.3
Ellison-Zollinger syndrome E16.4
Ellis-van Creveld syndrome
    (chondroectodermal dysplasia) Q77.6
Elongated, elongation (congenital) — *see*
    also Distortion
  bone Q79.9
  cervix (uteri) Q51.828
    acquired N88.4
    hypertrophic N88.4
  colon Q43.8
  common bile duct Q44.5
  cystic duct Q44.5
  frenulum, penis Q55.69
  labia minora (acquired) N90.69
  ligamentum patellae Q74.1
  petiolus (epiglottidis) Q31.8
  tooth, teeth K00.2
  uvula Q38.6
Eltor cholera A00.1
Emaciation (due to malnutrition) E41
Embadomoniasis A07.8
Embedded tooth, teeth K01.0
  root only K08.3
Embolic — *see* condition
Embolism (multiple) (paradoxical) I74.9
  air (any site) (traumatic) T79.0
    following
      abortion — *see* Abortion by type
        complicated by embolism
      ectopic pregnancy O08.2
      infusion, therapeutic injection or
        transfusion T80.0
      molar pregnancy O08.2
      procedure NEC
        artery T81.719
          mesenteric T81.710
          renal T81.711
          specified NEC T81.718
        vein T81.72
    in pregnancy, childbirth or puerperium —
      see Embolism, obstetric
  amniotic fluid (pulmonary) — *see also*
    Embolism, obstetric
    following
      abortion — *see* Abortion by type
        complicated by embolism
      ectopic pregnancy O08.2
      molar pregnancy O08.2
  aorta, aortic I74.10
    abdominal I74.09

Embolism (multiple) (paradoxical) -
continued
  aorta, aortic - *continued*
    abdominal - *continued*
      saddle I74.01
    bifurcation I74.09
    saddle I74.01
    thoracic I74.11
  artery I74.9
    auditory, internal I65.8
    basilar — *see* Occlusion, artery, basilar
    carotid (common) (internal) — *see*
      Occlusion, artery, carotid
    cerebellar (anterior inferior) (posterior
      inferior) (superior) I66.3
    cerebral — *see* Occlusion, artery, cerebral
    choroidal (anterior) I65.8
    communicating posterior I65.8
    coronary — *see also* Infarct, myocardium
      not resulting in infarction I24.0
    extremity I74.4
      lower I74.3
      upper I74.2
    hypophyseal I65.8
    iliac I74.5
    limb I74.4
      lower I74.3
      upper I74.2
    mesenteric (with gangrene) — *see also*
      Ischemia, intestine, acute K55.059
    ophthalmic — *see* Occlusion, artery, retina
    peripheral I74.4
    pontine I65.8
    precerebral — *see* Occlusion, artery,
      precerebral
    pulmonary — *see* Embolism, pulmonary
    renal N28.0
    retinal — *see* Occlusion, artery, retina
    septic I76
    specified NEC I74.8
    vertebral — *see* Occlusion, artery,
      vertebral
  basilar (artery) I65.1
  blood clot
    following
      abortion — *see* Abortion by type
        complicated by embolism
      ectopic or molar pregnancy O08.2
    in pregnancy, childbirth or puerperium —
      see Embolism, obstetric
  brain — *see also* Occlusion, artery, cerebral
    following
      abortion — *see* Abortion by type
        complicated by embolism
      ectopic or molar pregnancy O08.2
    puerperal, postpartum, childbirth — *see*
      Embolism, obstetric
  capillary I78.8
  cardiac — *see also* Infarct, myocardium
    not resulting in infarction I51.3
  carotid (artery) (common) (internal) — *see*
    Occlusion, artery, carotid
  cavernous sinus (venous) — *see* Embolism,
    intracranial venous sinus
  cerebral — *see* Occlusion, artery, cerebral
  cholesterol — *see* Atheroembolism
  coronary (artery or vein) (systemic) — *see*
    Occlusion, coronary
  due to device, implant or graft — *see also*
    Complications, by site and type,
    specified NEC
    arterial graft NEC T82.818
    breast (implant) T85.818
    catheter NEC T85.818
      dialysis (renal) T82.818
        intraperitoneal T85.818
      infusion NEC T82.818
        spinal (epidural) (subdural) T85.810
      urinary (indwelling) T83.81
    electronic (electrode) (pulse generator)
      (stimulator)
      bone T84.81
      cardiac T82.817
      nervous system (brain) (peripheral
        nerve) (spinal) T85.810

Embolism (multiple) (paradoxical) - *continued*
  due to device, implant or graft - *continued*
    electronic (electrode) (pulse generator)
      (stimulator) - *continued*
        urinary T83.81
    fixation, internal (orthopedic) NEC T84.81
    gastrointestinal (bile duct)
      (esophagus) T85.818
    genital NEC T83.81
    heart (graft) (valve) T82.817
    joint prosthesis T84.81
    ocular (corneal graft) (orbital
      implant) T85.818
    orthopedic (bone graft) NEC T86.838
    specified NEC T85.818
    urinary (graft) NEC T83.81
    vascular NEC T82.818
    ventricular intracranial shunt T85.810
  extremities
    lower — *see* Embolism, vein, lower
      extremity
      arterial I74.3
    upper I74.2
  eye H34.9
  fat (cerebral) (pulmonary) (systemic) T79.1
    following
      abortion — *see* Abortion by type
        complicated by embolism
      ectopic or molar pregnancy O08.2
    complicating delivery — *see* Embolism,
      obstetric
  following
    abortion — *see* Abortion by type
      complicated by embolism
    ectopic or molar pregnancy O08.2
    infusion, therapeutic injection or
      transfusion
      air T80.0
  heart (fatty) — *see also* Infarct, myocardium
    not resulting in infarction I51.3
  hepatic (vein) I82.0
  in pregnancy, childbirth or puerperium — *see*
    Embolism, obstetric
  intestine (artery) (vein) (with gangrene) —
    see also Ischemia, intestine,
    acute K55.039
  intracranial — *see also* Occlusion, artery,
    cerebral
    venous sinus (any) G08
      nonpyogenic I67.6
  intraspinal venous sinuses or veins G08
    nonpyogenic G95.19
  kidney (artery) N28.0
  lateral sinus (venous) — *see* Embolism,
    intracranial, venous sinus
  leg — *see* Embolism, vein, lower extremity
    arterial I74.3
  longitudinal sinus (venous) — *see* Embolism,
    intracranial, venous sinus
  lung (massive) — *see* Embolism, pulmonary
  meninges I66.8
  mesenteric (artery) (vein) (with
    gangrene) — *see also* Ischemia,
    intestine, acute K55.059
  obstetric (in) (pulmonary)
    childbirth O88.22
      air O88.02
      amniotic fluid O88.12
      blood clot O88.22
      fat O88.82
      pyemic O88.32
      septic O88.32
      specified type NEC O88.82
    pregnancy O88.21-
      air O88.01-
      amniotic fluid O88.11-
      blood clot O88.21-
      fat O88.81-
      pyemic O88.31-
      septic O88.31-
      specified type NEC O88.81-
    puerperal O88.23
      air O88.03
      amniotic fluid O88.13

Embolism (multiple) (paradoxical) - *continued*
  obstetric (in) (pulmonary) - *continued*
    puerperal - *continued*
      blood clot O88.23
      fat O88.83
      pyemic O88.33
      septic O88.33
      specified type NEC O88.83
  ophthalmic — *see* Occlusion, artery, retina
  penis N48.81
  peripheral artery NOS I74.4
  pituitary E23.6
  popliteal (artery) I74.3
  portal (vein) I81
  postoperative, postrpocedural
    artery T81.719
      mesenteric T81.710
      renal T81.711
      specified NEC T81.718
    vein T81.72
  precerebral artery — *see* Occlusion, artery,
    precerebral
  puerperal — *see* Embolism, obstetric
  pulmonary (acute) (artery) (vein) I26.99
    with acute cor pulmonale I26.09
    chronic I27.82
    following
      abortion — *see* Abortion by type
        complicated by embolism
      ectopic or molar pregnancy O08.2
    healed or old Z86.711
    in pregnancy, childbirth or puerperium —
      see Embolism, obstetric
    multiple subsegmental without acute cor
      pulmonale I26.94
    personal history of Z86.711
    saddle I26.92
      with acute cor pulmonale I26.02
    septic I26.90
      with acute cor pulmonale I26.01
    single subsegmental without acute cor
      pulmonale I26.93
    subsegmental NOS I26.93
  pyemic (multiple) I76
    following
      abortion — *see* Abortion by type
        complicated by embolism
      ectopic or molar pregnancy O08.2
    Hemophilus influenzae A41.3
    pneumococcal A40.3
      with pneumonia J13
    puerperal, postpartum, childbirth (any
      organism) — *see* Embolism, obstetric
    specified organism NEC A41.89
    staphylococcal A41.2
    streptococcal A40.9
  renal (artery) N28.0
    vein I82.3
  retina, retinal — *see* Occlusion, artery, retina
  saddle
    abdominal aorta I74.01
    pulmonary artery I26.92
      with acute cor pulmonale I26.02
  septic (arterial) I76
    complicating abortion — *see* Abortion, by
      type, complicated by, embolism
  sinus — *see* Embolism, intracranial, venous
    sinus
  soap complicating abortion — *see* Abortion,
    by type, complicated by, embolism
  spinal cord G95.19
    pyogenic origin G06.1
  spleen, splenic (artery) I74.8
  upper extremity I74.2
  vein (acute) I82.90
    antecubital I82.61-
      chronic I82.71-
    axillary I82.A1-
      chronic I82.A2-
    basilic I82.61-
      chronic I82.71-
    brachial I82.62-
      chronic I82.72-
    brachiocephalic (innominate) I82.290

Embolism (multiple) (paradoxical) - *continued*
  vein (acute) - *continued*
    brachiocephalic (innominate) - *continued*
      chronic I82.291
    cephalic I82.61-
      chronic I82.71-
    chronic I82.91
    deep (DVT) I82.40-
      calf I82.4Z-
        chronic I82.5Z-
      lower leg I82.4Z-
        chronic I82.5Z-
      thigh I82.4Y-
        chronic I82.5Y-
      upper leg I82.4Y
        chronic I82.5y--
    femoral I82.41-
      chronic I82.51-
    iliac (iliofemoral) I82.42-
      chronic I82.52-
    innominate I82.290
      chronic I82.291
    internal jugular I82.C1-
      chronic I82.C2-
    lower extremity
      deep I82.40-
        chronic I82.50-
        specified NEC I82.49-
          chronic NEC I82.59-
      distal
        deep I82.4Z-
      proximal
        deep I82.4Y-
          chronic I82.5Y-
      superficial I82.81-
    popliteal I82.43-
      chronic I82.53-
    radial I82.62-
      chronic I82.72-
    renal I82.3
    saphenous (greater) (lesser) I82.81-
    specified NEC I82.890
      chronic NEC I82.891
    subclavian I82.B1-
      chronic I82.B2-
    thoracic NEC I82.290
      chronic I82.291
    tibial I82.44-
      chronic I82.54-
    ulnar I82.62-
      chronic I82.72-
    upper extremity I82.60-
      chronic I82.70-
      deep I82.62-
        chronic I82.72-
      superficial I82.61-
        chronic I82.71-
  vena cava
    inferior (acute) I82.220
      chronic I82.221
    superior (acute) I82.210
      chronic I82.211
  venous sinus G08
  vessels of brain — *see* Occlusion, artery,
    cerebral
Embolus — *see* Embolism
Embryoma — *see also* Neoplasm, uncertain
  behavior, by site
  benign — *see* Neoplasm, benign, by site
  kidney C64.-
  liver C22.0
  malignant — *see also* Neoplasm, malignant,
    by site
    kidney C64.-
    liver C22.0
    testis C62.9-
      descended (scrotal) C62.1-
      undescended C62.0-
  testis C62.9-
    descended (scrotal) C62.1-
    undescended C62.0-
Embryonic
  circulation Q28.9
  heart Q28.9

Embryonic - *continued*
vas deferens Q55.4
Embryopathia NOS Q89.9
Embryotoxon Q13.4
Emesis — *see* Vomiting
Emotional lability R45.86
Emotionality, pathological F60.3
Emotogenic disease — *see* Disorder,
  psychogenic
Emphysema (atrophic) (bullous) (chronic)
  (interlobular) (lung) (obstructive)
  (pulmonary) (senile) (vesicular) J43.9
  cellular tissue (traumatic) T79.7
    surgical T81.82
  centrilobular J43.2
  compensatory J98.3
  congenital (interstitial) P25.0
  conjunctiva H11.89
  connective tissue (traumatic) T79.7
    surgical T81.82
  due to chemicals, gases, fumes or
    vapors J68.4
  eyelid (s) — *see* Disorder, eyelid, specified
    type NEC
    surgical T81.82
    traumatic T79.7
  interstitial J98.2
    congenital P25.0
    perinatal period P25.0
  laminated tissue T79.7
    surgical T81.82
  mediastinal J98.2
    newborn P25.2
  orbit, orbital — *see* Disorder, orbit, specified
    type NEC
  panacinar J43.1
  panlobular J43.1
  specified NEC J43.8
  subcutaneous (traumatic) T79.7
    nontraumatic J98.2
    postprocedural T81.82
    surgical T81.82
  surgical T81.82
  thymus (gland) (congenital) E32.8
  traumatic (subcutaneous) T79.7
  unilateral J43.0
Empty nest syndrome Z60.0
Empyema (acute) (chest) (double) (pleura)
  (supradiaphragmatic) (thorax) J86.9
  with fistula J86.0
  accessory sinus (chronic) — *see* Sinusitis
  antrum (chronic) — *see* Sinusitis, maxillary
  brain (any part) — *see* Abscess, brain
  ethmoidal (chronic) (sinus) — *see* Sinusitis,
    ethmoidal
  extradural — *see* Abscess, extradural
  frontal (chronic) (sinus) — *see* Sinusitis,
    frontal
  gallbladder K81.0
  mastoid (process) (acute) — *see* Mastoiditis,
    acute
  maxilla, maxillary M27.2
    sinus (chronic) — *see* Sinusitis, maxillary
  nasal sinus (chronic) — *see* Sinusitis
  sinus (accessory) (chronic) (nasal) — *see*
    Sinusitis
  sphenoidal (sinus) (chronic) — *see* Sinusitis,
    sphenoidal
  subarachnoid — *see* Abscess, extradural
  subdural — *see* Abscess, subdural
  tuberculous A15.6
  ureter — *see* Ureteritis
  ventricular — *see* Abscess, brain
En coup de sabre lesion L94.1
Enamel pearls K00.2
Enameloma K00.2
Enanthema, viral B09
Encephalitis (chronic) (hemorrhagic)
  (idiopathic) (nonepidemic) (spurious)
  (subacute) G04.90
  acute — *see also* Encephalitis, viral A86
    disseminated G04.00
      infectious G04.01
      noninfectious G04.81

Encephalitis (chronic) (hemorrhagic)
(idiopathic) (nonepidemic) (spurious)
(subacute) - *continued*
  acute - *continued*
    disseminated - *continued*
      postimmunization
        (postvaccination) G04.02
      postinfectious G04.01
    inclusion body A85.8
    necrotizing hemorrhagic G04.30
      postimmunization G04.32
      postinfectious G04.31
      specified NEC G04.39
  arboviral, arbovirus NEC A85.2
  arthropod-borne NEC (viral) A85.2
  Australian A83.4
  California (virus) A83.5
  Central European (tick-borne) A84.1
  Czechoslovakian A84.1
  Dawson's (inclusion body) A81.1
  diffuse sclerosing A81.1
  disseminated, acute G04.00
  due to
    cat scratch disease A28.1
    human immunodeficiency virus (HIV)
      disease B20 *[G05.3]*
    malaria — *see* Malaria
    rickettsiosis — *see* Rickettsiosis
    smallpox inoculation G04.02
    typhus — *see* Typhus
  Eastern equine A83.2
  endemic (viral) A86
  epidemic NEC (viral) A86
  equine (acute) (infectious) (viral) A83.9
    Eastern A83.2
    Venezuelan A92.2
    Western A83.1
  Far Eastern (tick-borne) A84.0
  following vaccination or other immunization
    procedure G04.02
  herpes zoster B02.0
  herpesviral B00.4
    due to herpesvirus 6 B10.01
    due to herpesvirus 7 B10.09
    specified NEC B10.09
  Ilheus (virus) A83.8
  inclusion body A81.1
  in (due to)
    actinomycosis A42.82
    adenovirus A85.1
    African trypanosomiasis B56.9 *[G05.3]*
    Chagas' disease (chronic) B57.42
    cytomegalovirus B25.8
    enterovirus A85.0
    herpes (simplex) virus B00.4
      due to herpesvirus 6 B10.01
      due to herpesvirus 7 B10.09
      specified NEC B10.09
    infectious disease NEC B99 *[G05.3]*
    influenza — *see* Influenza, with,
      encephalopathy
    listeriosis A32.12
    measles B05.0
    mumps B26.2
    naegleriasis B60.2
    parasitic disease NEC B89 *[G05.3]*
    poliovirus A80.9 *[G05.3]*
    rubella B06.01
    syphilis
      congenital A50.42
      late A52.14
    systemic lupus erythematosus M32.19
    toxoplasmosis (acquired) B58.2
      congenital P37.1
    tuberculosis A17.82
    zoster B02.0
  infectious (acute) (virus) NEC A86
  Japanese (B type) A83.0
  La Crosse A83.5
  lead — *see* Poisoning, lead
  lethargica (acute) (infectious) A85.8
  louping ill A84.8
  lupus erythematosus, systemic M32.19
  lymphatica A87.2
  Mengo A85.8

Encephalitis (chronic) (hemorrhagic)
(idiopathic) (nonepidemic) (spurious)
(subacute) - *continued*
  meningococcal A39.81
  Murray Valley A83.4
  otitic NEC H66.40 *[G05.3]*
  parasitic NOS B71.9
  periaxial G37.0
  periaxialis (concentrica) (diffuse) G37.5
  postchickenpox B01.11
  postexanthematous NEC B09
  postimmunization G04.02
  postinfectious NEC G04.01
  postmeasles B05.0
  postvaccinal G04.02
  postvaricella B01.11
  postviral NEC A86
  Powassan A84.8
  Rasmussen G04.81
  Rio Bravo A85.8
  Russian
    autumnal A83.0
    spring-summer (taiga) A84.0
  saturnine — *see* Poisoning, lead
  specified NEC G04.81
  St. Louis A83.3
  subacute sclerosing A81.1
  summer A83.0
  suppurative G04.81
  tick-borne A84.9
  Torula, torular (cryptococcal) B45.1
  toxic NEC G92
  trichinosis B75 *[G05.3]*
  type
    B A83.0
    C A83.3
  van Bogaert's A81.1
  Venezuelan equine A92.2
  Vienna A85.8
  viral, virus A86
    arthropod-borne NEC A85.2
      mosquito-borne A83.9
        Australian X disease A83.4
        California virus A83.5
        Eastern equine A83.2
        Japanese (B type) A83.0
        Murray Valley A83.4
        specified NEC A83.8
        St. Louis A83.3
        type B A83.0
        type C A83.3
        Western equine A83.1
      tick-borne A84.9
        biundulant A84.1
        central European A84.1
        Czechoslovakian A84.1
        diphasic meningoencephalitis A84.1
        Far Eastern A84.0
        Russian spring-summer (taiga) A84.0
        specified NEC A84.8
      specified type NEC A85.8
    Western equine A83.1
Encephalocele Q01.9
  frontal Q01.0
  nasofrontal Q01.1
  occipital Q01.2
  specified NEC Q01.8
Encephalocystocele — *see* Encephalocele
Encephaloduroarteriomyosynangiosis
  (EDAMS) I67.5
Encephalomalacia (brain) (cerebellar)
  (cerebral) — *see* Softening, brain
Encephalomeningitis — *see*
  Meningoencephalitis
Encephalomeningocele — *see* Encephalocele
Encephalomeningomyelitis — *see*
  Meningoencephalitis
Encephalomyelitis — *see also*
  Encephalitis G04.90
  acute disseminated G04.00
    infectious G04.01
    noninfectious G04.81
    postimmunization G04.02
    postinfectious G04.01
  acute necrotizing hemorrhagic G04.30

Encephalomyelitis - *continued*
acute necrotizing hemorrhagic - *continued*
  postimmunization G04.32
  postinfectious G04.31
  specified NEC G04.39
benign myalgic G93.3
equine A83.9
  Eastern A83.2
  Venezuelan A92.2
  Western A83.1
in diseases classified elsewhere G05.3
myalgic, benign G93.3
postchickenpox B01.11
postinfectious NEC G04.01
postmeasles B05.0
postvaccinal G04.02
postvaricella B01.11
rubella B06.01
specified NEC G04.81
Venezuelan equine A92.2
Encephalomyelocele — *see* Encephalocele
Encephalomyelomeningitis — *see*
  Meningoencephalitis
Encephalomyelopathy G96.9
Encephalomyeloradiculitis (acute) G61.0
Encephalomyeloradiculoneuritis (acute)
  (Guillain-Barré) G61.0
Encephalomyeloradiculopathy G96.9
Encephalopathia hyperbilirubinemica,
  newborn P57.9
due to isoimmunization (conditions in
  P55) P57.0
Encephalopathy (acute) G93.40
acute necrotizing hemorrhagic G04.30
  postimmunization G04.32
  postinfectious G04.31
  specified NEC G04.39
alcoholic G31.2
anoxic — *see* Damage, brain, anoxic
arteriosclerotic I67.2
centrolobar progressive (Schilder) G37.0
congenital Q07.9
degenerative, in specified disease
  NEC G32.89
demyelinating callosal G37.1
due to
  drugs - — *see also* Table of Drugs and
    Chemicals G92
hepatic — *see* Failure, hepatic
hyperbilirubinemic, newborn P57.9
  due to isoimmunization (conditions in
    P55) P57.0
hypertensive I67.4
hypoglycemic E16.2
hypoxic — *see* Damage, brain, anoxic
hypoxic ischemic P91.60
  mild P91.61
  moderate P91.62
  severe P91.63
in (due to) (with)
  birth injury P11.1
  hyperinsulinism E16.1 *[G94]*
  influenza — *see* Influenza, with,
    encephalopathy
  lack of vitamin — *see also* Deficiency,
    vitamin E56.9 *[G32.89]*
  neoplastic disease (see also
    Neoplasm) D49.9 *[G13.1]*
  serum — *see also* Reaction, serum T80.69
  syphilis A52.17
  trauma (postconcussional) F07.81
    current injury — *see* Injury, intracranial
  vaccination G04.02
lead — *see* Poisoning, lead
metabolic G93.41
  drug induced G92
  toxic G92
myoclonic, early, symptomatic — *see*
  Epilepsy, generalized, specified NEC
necrotizing, subacute (Leigh) G31.82
neonatal P91.819
  in diseases classified elsewhere P91.811
pellagrous E52 *[G32.89]*
portosystemic — *see* Failure, hepatic
postcontusional F07.81

Encephalopathy (acute) - *continued*
postcontusional - *continued*
  current injury — *see* Injury, intracranial,
    diffuse
posthypoglycemic (coma) E16.1 *[G94]*
postradiation G93.89
saturnine — *see* Poisoning, lead
septic G93.41
specified NEC G93.49
spongiform, subacute (viral) A81.09
toxic G92
  metabolic G92
traumatic (postconcussional) F07.81
  current injury — *see* Injury, intracranial
vitamin B deficiency NEC E53.9 *[G32.89]*
  vitamin B1 E51.2
Wernicke's E51.2
Encephalorrhagia — *see* Hemorrhage,
  intracranial, intracerebral
Encephalosis, posttraumatic F07.81
Enchondroma — *see also* Neoplasm, bone,
  benign
Enchondromatosis (cartilaginous)
  (multiple) Q78.4
Encopresis R15.9
functional F98.1
nonorganic origin F98.1
psychogenic F98.1
Encounter (with health service) (for) Z76.89
adjustment and management (of)
  breast implant Z45.81
  implanted device NEC Z45.89
  myringotomy device (stent) (tube) Z45.82
  neurostimulator (brain) (gastric)
    (peripheral nerve) (sacral nerve)
    (spinal cord) (vagus nerve) Z45.42
administrative purpose only Z02.9
  examination for
    adoption Z02.82
    armed forces Z02.3
    disability determination Z02.71
    driving license Z02.4
    employment Z02.1
    insurance Z02.6
    medical certificate NEC Z02.79
    paternity testing Z02.81
    residential institution admission Z02.2
    school admission Z02.0
    sports Z02.5
  specified reason NEC Z02.89
aftercare — *see* Aftercare
antenatal screening Z36.9
  cervical length Z36.86
  chromosomal anomalies Z36.0
  congenital cardiac abnormalities Z36.83
  elevated maternal serum alphafetoprotein
    level Z36.1
  fetal growth retardation Z36.4
  fetal lung maturity Z36.84
  fetal macrosomia Z36.88
  hydrops fetalis Z36.81
  intrauterine growth restriction (IUGR)
    /small-for-dates Z36.4
  isoimmunization Z36.5
  large-for-dates Z36.88
  malformations Z36.3
  non-visualized anatomy on a previous
    scan Z36.2
  nuchal translucency Z36.82
  raised alphafetoprotein level Z36.1
  risk of pre-term labor Z36.86
  specified type NEC Z36.89
  specified follow-up NEC Z36.2
  specified genetic defects NEC Z36.8A
  Streptococcus B Z36.85
  suspected anomaly Z36.3
  uncertain dates Z36.87
assisted reproductive fertility procedure
  cycle Z31.83
blood typing Z01.83
  Rh typing Z01.83
breast augmentation or reduction Z41.1
breast implant exchange (different material)
  (different size) Z45.81

Encounter (with health service) (for) -
continued
breast reconstruction following
  mastectomy Z42.1
check-up — *see* Examination
chemotherapy for neoplasm Z51.11
colonoscopy, screening Z12.11
counseling — *see* Counseling
delivery, full-term, uncomplicated O80
  cesarean, without indication O82
desensitization to allergens Z51.6
ear piercing Z41.3
examination — *see* Examination
expectant parent (s) (adoptive) pre-birth
  pediatrician visit Z76.81
fertility preservation procedure (prior to
  cancer therapy) (prior to removal of
  gonads) Z31.84
fitting (of) — *see* Fitting (and adjustment)
  (of)
genetic
  counseling
    nonprocreative Z71.83
    procreative Z31.5
  testing — *see* Test, genetic
hearing conservation and treatment Z01.12
immunotherapy for neoplasm Z51.12
in vitro fertilization cycle Z31.83
instruction (in)
  childbirth Z32.2
  child care (postpartal) (prenatal) Z32.3
  natural family planning
    procreative Z31.61
    to avoid pregnancy Z30.02
insulin pump titration Z46.81
joint prosthesis insertion following prior
  explantation of joint prosthesis (staged
  procedure)
  hip Z47.32
  knee Z47.33
  shoulder Z47.31
laboratory (as part of a general medical
  examination) Z00.00
  with abnormal findings Z00.01
mental health services (for)
  abuse NEC
    perpetrator Z69.82
    victim Z69.81
  child abuse
    nonparental
      perpetrator Z69.021
      victim Z69.020
    parental
      perpetrator Z69.011
      victim Z69.010
  child neglect
    nonparental
      perpetrator Z69.021
      victim Z69.020
    parental
      perpetrator Z69.011
      victim Z69.010
  child psychological abuse
    nonparental
      perpetrator Z69.021
      victim Z69.020
    parental
      perpetrator Z69.011
      victim Z69.010
  child sexual abuse
    nonparental
      perpetrator Z69.021
      victim Z69.020
    parental
      perpetrator Z69.011
      victim Z69.010
  non-spousal adult abuse
    perpetrator Z69.82
    victim Z69.81
  spousal or partner
    abuse
      perpetrator Z69.12
      victim Z69.11
    neglect
      perpetrator Z69.12

Encounter (with health service) (for) - *continued*
  mental health services (for) - *continued*
    spousal or partner - *continued*
      neglect - *continued*
        victim Z69.11
      psychological abuse
        perpetrator Z69.12
        victim Z69.11
      violence
        perpetrator (physical) (sexual) Z69.12
        victim (physical) Z69.11
          sexual Z69.81
  observation (for) (ruled out)
    exposure to (suspected)
      anthrax Z03.810
      biological agent NEC Z03.818
  pediatrician visit, by expectant parent (s) (adoptive) Z76.81
  placental sample (taken vaginally) — *see also* Encounter, antenatal screening Z36.9
  plastic and reconstructive surgery following medical procedure or healed injury NEC Z42.8
  pregnancy
    supervision of — *see* Pregnancy, supervision of
    test Z32.00
      result negative Z32.02
      result positive Z32.01
  procreative management and counseling for gestational carrier Z31.7
  prophylactic measures Z29.9
    antivenin Z29.12
    fluoride administration Z29.3
    immunotherapy for respiratory syncytial virus (RSV) Z29.11
    rabies immune globin Z29.14
    Rho (D) immune globulin Z29.13
    specified NEC Z29.8
  radiation therapy (antineoplastic) Z51.0
  radiological (as part of a general medical examination) Z00.00
    with abnormal findings Z00.01
  reconstructive surgery following medical procedure or healed injury NEC Z42.8
  removal (of) — *see also* Removal
    artificial
      arm Z44.00-
        complete Z44.01-
        partial Z44.02-
      eye Z44.2-
      leg Z44.10-
        complete Z44.11-
        partial Z44.12-
    breast implant Z45.81
      tissue expander (with or without synchronous insertion of permanent implant) Z45.81
    device Z46.9
      specified NEC Z46.89
    external
      fixation device - code to fracture with seventh character D
      prosthesis, prosthetic device Z44.9
        breast Z44.3-
        specified NEC Z44.8
    implanted device NEC Z45.89
    insulin pump Z46.81
    internal fixation device Z47.2
    myringotomy device (stent) (tube) Z45.82
    nervous system device NEC Z46.2
      brain neuropacemaker Z46.2
      visual substitution device Z46.2
        implanted Z45.31
    non-vascular catheter Z46.82
    orthodontic device Z46.4
    stent
      ureteral Z46.6
    urinary device Z46.6
  repeat cervical smear to confirm findings of recent normal smear following initial abnormal smear Z01.42

Encounter (with health service) (for) - *continued*
  respirator [ventilator] use during power failure Z99.12
  Rh typing Z01.83
  screening — *see* Screening
  specified NEC Z76.89
  sterilization Z30.2
  suspected condition, ruled out
    amniotic cavity and membrane Z03.71
    cervical shortening Z03.75
    fetal anomaly Z03.73
    fetal growth Z03.74
    maternal and fetal conditions NEC Z03.79
    oligohydramnios Z03.71
    placental problem Z03.72
    polyhydramnios Z03.71
  suspected exposure (to) , ruled out
    anthrax Z03.810
    biological agents NEC Z03.818
  termination of pregnancy, elective Z33.2
  testing — *see* Test
  therapeutic drug level monitoring Z51.81
  titration, insulin pump Z46.81
  to determine fetal viability of pregnancy O36.80
  training
    insulin pump Z46.81
  X-ray of chest (as part of a general medical examination) Z00.00
    with abnormal findings Z00.01
Encystment — *see* Cyst
Endarteritis (bacterial, subacute) (infective) I77.6
  brain I67.7
  cerebral or cerebrospinal I67.7
  deformans — *see* Arteriosclerosis
  embolic — *see* Embolism
  obliterans — *see also* Arteriosclerosis
    pulmonary I28.8
  pulmonary I28.8
  retina — *see* Vasculitis, retina
  senile — *see* Arteriosclerosis
  syphilitic A52.09
    brain or cerebral A52.04
    congenital A50.54 *[I79.8]*
  tuberculous A18.89
Endemic — *see* condition
Endocarditis (chronic) (marantic) (nonbacterial) (thrombotic) (valvular) I38
  with rheumatic fever (conditions in I00)
    active — *see* Endocarditis, acute, rheumatic
    inactive or quiescent (with chorea) I09.1
  acute or subacute I33.9
    infective I33.0
    rheumatic (aortic) (mitral) (pulmonary) (tricuspid) I01.1
      with chorea (acute) (rheumatic) (Sydenham's) I02.0
  aortic (heart) (nonrheumatic) (valve) I35.8
    with
      mitral disease I08.0
        with tricuspid (valve) disease I08.3
        active or acute I01.1
          with chorea (acute) (rheumatic) (Sydenham's) I02.0
      rheumatic fever (conditions in I00)
        active — *see* Endocarditis, acute, rheumatic
        inactive or quiescent (with chorea) I06.9
      tricuspid (valve) disease I08.2
        with mitral (valve) disease I08.3
    acute or subacute I33.9
    arteriosclerotic I35.8
    rheumatic I06.9
      with mitral disease I08.0
        with tricuspid (valve) disease I08.3
        active or acute I01.1
          with chorea (acute) (rheumatic) (Sydenham's) I02.0
      active or acute I01.1

Endocarditis (chronic) (marantic) (nonbacterial) (thrombotic) (valvular) - *continued*
  aortic (heart) (nonrheumatic) (valve) - *continued*
    rheumatic - *continued*
      active or acute - *continued*
        with chorea (acute) (rheumatic) (Sydenham's) I02.0
      specified NEC I06.8
    specified cause NEC I35.8
    syphilitic A52.03
  arteriosclerotic I38
  atypical verrucous (Libman-Sacks) M32.11
  bacterial (acute) (any valve) (subacute) I33.0
  candidal B37.6
  congenital Q24.8
  constrictive I33.0
  Coxiella burnetii A78 *[I39]*
  Coxsackie B33.21
  due to
    prosthetic cardiac valve T82.6
    Q fever A78 *[I39]*
    Serratia marcescens I33.0
    typhoid (fever) A01.02
  gonococcal A54.83
  infectious or infective (acute) (any valve) (subacute) I33.0
  lenta (acute) (any valve) (subacute) I33.0
  Libman-Sacks M32.11
  listerial A32.82
  Löffler's I42.3
  malignant (acute) (any valve) (subacute) I33.0
  meningococcal A39.51
  mitral (chronic) (double) (fibroid) (heart) (inactive) (valve) (with chorea) I05.9
    with
      aortic (valve) disease I08.0
        with tricuspid (valve) disease I08.3
        active or acute I01.1
          with chorea (acute) (rheumatic) (Sydenham's) I02.0
      rheumatic fever (conditions in I00)
        active — *see* Endocarditis, acute, rheumatic
        inactive or quiescent (with chorea) I05.9
      tricuspid (valve) disease I08.1
        with aortic (valve) disease I08.3
    active or acute I01.1
      with chorea (acute) (rheumatic) (Sydenham's) I02.0
    bacterial I33.0
    arteriosclerotic I34.8
    nonrheumatic I34.8
      acute or subacute I33.9
    specified NEC I05.8
  monilial B37.6
  multiple valves I08.9
    specified disorders I08.8
  mycotic (acute) (any valve) (subacute) I33.0
  pneumococcal (acute) (any valve) (subacute) I33.0
  pulmonary (chronic) (heart) (valve) I37.8
    with rheumatic fever (conditions in I00)
      active — *see* Endocarditis, acute, rheumatic
      inactive or quiescent (with chorea) I09.89
        with aortic, mitral or tricuspid disease I08.8
    acute or subacute I33.9
      rheumatic I01.1
        with chorea (acute) (rheumatic) (Sydenham's) I02.0
    arteriosclerotic I37.8
    congenital Q22.2
    rheumatic (chronic) (inactive) (with chorea) I09.89
      active or acute I01.1
        with chorea (acute) (rheumatic) (Sydenham's) I02.0
    syphilitic A52.03
  purulent (acute) (any valve) (subacute) I33.0

Endocarditis (chronic) (marantic) (nonbacterial) (thrombotic) (valvular) - *continued*
    Q fever A78 [I39]
    rheumatic (chronic) (inactive) (with chorea) I09.1
        active or acute (aortic) (mitral) (pulmonary) (tricuspid) I01.1
           with chorea (acute) (rheumatic) (Sydenham's) I02.0
    rheumatoid — *see* Rheumatoid, carditis
    septic (acute) (any valve) (subacute) I33.0
    streptococcal (acute) (any valve) (subacute) I33.0
    subacute — *see* Endocarditis, acute
    suppurative (acute) (any valve) (subacute) I33.0
    syphilitic A52.03
    toxic I33.9
    tricuspid (chronic) (heart) (inactive) (rheumatic) (valve) (with chorea) I07.9
        with
           aortic (valve) disease I08.2
               mitral (valve) disease I08.3
           mitral (valve) disease I08.1
               aortic (valve) disease I08.3
           rheumatic fever (conditions in I00)
               active — *see* Endocarditis, acute, rheumatic
               inactive or quiescent (with chorea) I07.8
    active or acute I01.1
        with chorea (acute) (rheumatic) (Sydenham's) I02.0
    arteriosclerotic I36.8
    nonrheumatic I36.8
        acute or subacute I33.9
    specified cause, except rheumatic I36.8
    tuberculous — *see* Tuberculosis, endocarditis
    typhoid A01.02
    ulcerative (acute) (any valve) (subacute) I33.0
    vegetative (acute) (any valve) (subacute) I33.0
    verrucous (atypical) (nonbacterial) (nonrheumatic) M32.11
Endocardium, endocardial — *see also* condition
    cushion defect Q21.2
Endocervicitis — *see also* Cervicitis
    due to intrauterine (contraceptive) device T83.69
    hyperplastic N72
Endocrine — *see* condition
Endocrinopathy, pluriglandular E31.9
Endodontic
    overfill M27.52
    underfill M27.53
Endodontitis K04.01
    irreversible K04.02
    reversible K04.01
Endomastoiditis — *see* Mastoiditis
Endometrioma N80.9
Endometriosis N80.9
    appendix N80.5
    bladder N80.8
    bowel N80.5
    broad ligament N80.3
    cervix N80.0
    colon N80.5
    cul-de-sac (Douglas') N80.3
    exocervix N80.0
    fallopian tube N80.2
    female genital organ NEC N80.8
    gallbladder N80.8
    in scar of skin N80.6
    internal N80.0
    intestine N80.5
    lung N80.8
    myometrium N80.0
    ovary N80.1
    parametrium N80.3
    pelvic peritoneum N80.3
    peritoneal (pelvic) N80.3
    rectovaginal septum N80.4

Endometriosis - *continued*
    rectum N80.5
    round ligament N80.3
    skin (scar) N80.6
    specified site NEC N80.8
    stromal D39.0
    thorax N80.8
    umbilicus N80.8
    uterus (internal) N80.0
    vagina N80.4
    vulva N80.8
Endometritis (decidual) (nonspecific) (purulent) (senile) (atrophic) (suppurative) N71.9
    with ectopic pregnancy O08.0
    acute N71.0
    blenorrhagic (gonococcal) (acute) (chronic) A54.24
    cervix, cervical (with erosion or ectropion) — *see also* Cervicitis
        hyperplastic N72
    chlamydial A56.11
    chronic N71.1
    following
        abortion — *see* Abortion by type complicated by genital infection
        ectopic or molar pregnancy O08.0
    gonococcal, gonorrheal (acute) (chronic) A54.24
    hyperplastic — *see also* Hyperplasia, endometrial N85.00-
        cervix N72
    puerperal, postpartum, childbirth O86.12
    subacute N71.0
    tuberculous A18.17
Endometrium — *see* condition
Endomyocardiopathy, South African I42.3
Endomyocarditis — *see* Endocarditis
Endomyofibrosis I42.3
Endomyometritis — *see* Endometritis
Endopericarditis — *see* Endocarditis
Endoperineuritis — *see* Disorder, nerve
Endophlebitis — *see* Phlebitis
Endophthalmia — *see* Endophthalmitis, purulent
Endophthalmitis (acute) (infective) (metastatic) (subacute) H44.009
    bleb associated H59.4 — *see also* Bleb, inflamed (infected), postprocedural
    gonorrheal A54.39
    in (due to)
        cysticercosis B69.1
        onchocerciasis B73.01
        toxocariasis B83.0
    panuveitis — *see* Panuveitis
    parasitic H44.12-
    purulent H44.00-
        panophthalmitis — *see* Panophthalmitis
        vitreous abscess H44.02-
    specified NEC H44.19
    sympathetic — *see* Uveitis, sympathetic
Endosalpingioma D28.2
Endosalpingiosis N94.89
Endosteitis — *see* Osteomyelitis
Endothelioma, bone — *see* Neoplasm, bone, malignant
Endotheliosis (hemorrhagic infectional) D69.8
Endotoxemia - code to condition
Endotrachelitis — *see* Cervicitis
Engelmann (-Camurati) syndrome Q78.3
English disease — *see* Rickets
Engman's disease L30.3
Engorgement
    breast N64.59
        newborn P83.4
        puerperal, postpartum O92.79
    lung (passive) — *see* Edema, lung
    pulmonary (passive) — *see* Edema, lung
    stomach K31.89
    venous, retina — *see* Occlusion, retina, vein, engorgement
Enlargement, enlarged — *see also* Hypertrophy
    adenoids J35.2

Enlargement, enlarged - *continued*
    adenoids - *continued*
        with tonsils J35.3
    alveolar ridge K08.89
        congenital — *see* Anomaly, alveolar
    apertures of diaphragm (congenital) Q79.1
    gingival K06.1
    heart, cardiac — *see* Hypertrophy, cardiac
    labium majus, childhood asymmetric (CALME) N90.61
    lacrimal gland, chronic H04.03-
    liver — *see* Hypertrophy, liver
    lymph gland or node R59.9
        generalized R59.1
        localized R59.0
    orbit H05.34-
    organ or site, congenital NEC — *see* Anomaly, by site
    parathyroid (gland) E21.0
    pituitary fossa R93.0
    prostate N40.0
        with lower urinary tract symptoms (LUTS) N40.1
        without lower urinary tract symtpoms (LUTS) N40.0
    sella turcica R93.0
    spleen — *see* Splenomegaly
    thymus (gland) (congenital) E32.0
    thyroid (gland) — *see* Goiter
    tongue K14.8
    tonsils J35.1
        with adenoids J35.3
    uterus N85.2
    vestibular aqueduct Q16.5
Enophthalmos H05.40-
    due to
        orbital tissue atrophy H05.41-
        trauma or surgery H05.42-
Enostosis M27.8
Entamebic, entamebiasis — *see* Amebiasis
Entanglement
    umbilical cord (s) O69.82
        with compression O69.2
        around neck (with compression) O69.81
           with compression O69.1
           without compression O69.81
        of twins in monoamniotic sac O69.2
        without compression O69.82
Enteralgia — *see* Pain, abdominal
Enteric — *see* condition
Enteritis (acute) (diarrheal) (hemorrhagic) (noninfective) K52.9
    adenovirus A08.2
    aertrycke infection A02.0
    allergic K52.29
        with
           eosinophilic gastritis or gastroenteritis K52.81
           food protein-induced enterocolitis syndrome K52.21
           food protein-induced enteropathy K52.22
           FPIES K52.21
    amebic (acute) A06.0
        with abscess — *see* Abscess, amebic
        chronic A06.1
           with abscess — *see* Abscess, amebic
           nondysenteric A06.2
        nondysenteric A06.2
    astrovirus A08.32
    bacillary NOS A03.9
    bacterial A04.9
        specified NEC A04.8
    calicivirus A08.31
    candidal B37.82
    Chilomastix A07.8
    choleriformis A00.1
    chronic (noninfectious) K52.9
        ulcerative — *see* Colitis, ulcerative
    cicatrizing (chronic) — *see* Enteritis, regional, small intestine
    Clostridium
        botulinum (food poisoning) A05.1
        difficile
           not specified as recurrent A04.72

Enteritis (acute) (diarrheal) (hemorrhagic)
(noninfective) - *continued*
  Clostridium - *continued*
    difficile - *continued*
      recurrent A04.71
  coccidial A07.3
  coxsackie virus A08.39
  dietetic — *see also* Enteritis, allergic K52.29
  drug-induced K52.1
  due to
    astrovirus A08.32
    calicivirus A08.31
    coxsackie virus A08.39
    drugs K52.1
    echovirus A08.39
    enterovirus NEC A08.39
    food hypersensitivity — *see also* Enteritis,
      allergic K52.29
    infectious organism (bacterial) (viral) —
      see Enteritis, infectious
    torovirus A08.39
    Yersinia enterocolitica A04.6
  echovirus A08.39
  eltor A00.1
  enterovirus NEC A08.39
  eosinophilic K52.81
  epidemic (infectious) A09
  fulminant — *see also* Ischemia, intestine,
    acute K55.019
  gangrenous — *see* Enteritis, infectious
  giardial A07.1
  infectious NOS A09
  due to
    adenovirus A08.2
    Aerobacter aerogenes A04.8
    Arizona (bacillus) A02.0
    bacteria NOS A04.9
      specified NEC A04.8
    Campylobacter A04.5
    Clostridium difficile
      not specified as recurrent A04.72
      recurrent A04.71
    Clostridium perfringens A04.8
    Enterobacter aerogenes A04.8
    enterovirus A08.39
    Escherichia coli A04.4
      enteroaggregative A04.4
      enterohemorrhagic A04.3
      enteroinvasive A04.2
      enteropathogenic A04.0
      enterotoxigenic A04.1
      specified NEC A04.4
    specified
      bacteria NEC A04.8
      virus NEC A08.39
    Staphylococcus A04.8
    virus NEC A08.4
      specified type NEC A08.39
    Yersinia enterocolitica A04.6
    specified organism NEC A08.8
  influenzal — *see* Influenza, with, digestive
    manifestations
  ischemic K55.9
    acute — *see also* Ischemia, intestine,
      acute K55.019
    chronic K55.1
  microsporidial A07.8
  mucomembranous, myxomembranous — *see*
    Syndrome, irritable bowel
  mucous — *see* Syndrome, irritable bowel
  necroticans A05.2
  necrotizing of newborn — *see* Enterocolitis,
    necrotizing, in newborn
  neurogenic — *see* Syndrome, irritable bowel
  newborn necrotizing — *see* Enterocolitis,
    necrotizing, in newborn
  noninfectious K52.9
  norovirus A08.11
  parasitic NEC B82.9
  paratyphoid (fever) — *see* Fever, paratyphoid
  protozoal A07.9
    specified NEC A07.8
  radiation K52.0
  regional (of) K50.90
    with

Enteritis (acute) (diarrheal) (hemorrhagic)
(noninfective) - *continued*
  regional (of) - *continued*
    with - *continued*
      complication K50.919
        abscess K50.914
        fistula K50.913
        intestinal obstruction K50.912
        rectal bleeding K50.911
        specified complication NEC K50.918
    colon — *see* Enteritis, regional, large
      intestine
    duodenum — *see* Enteritis, regional, small
      intestine
    ileum — *see* Enteritis, regional, small
      intestine
    jejunum — *see* Enteritis, regional, small
      intestine
    large bowel — *see* Enteritis, regional, large
      intestine
    large intestine (colon) (rectum) K50.10
      with
        complication K50.119
          abscess K50.114
          fistula K50.113
          intestinal obstruction K50.112
          rectal bleeding K50.111
          small intestine (duodenum) (ileum)
            (jejunum) involvement K50.80
            with
              complication K50.819
                abscess K50.814
                fistula K50.813
                intestinal
                  obstruction K50.812
                rectal bleeding K50.811
                specified complication
                  NEC K50.818
          specified complication
            NEC K50.118
    rectum — *see* Enteritis, regional, large
      intestine
    small intestine (duodenum) (ileum)
      (jejunum) K50.00
      with
        complication K50.019
          abscess K50.014
          fistula K50.013
          intestinal obstruction K50.012
          large intestine (colon) (rectum)
            involvement K50.80
            with
              complication K50.819
                abscess K50.814
                fistula K50.813
                intestinal
                  obstruction K50.812
                rectal bleeding K50.811
                specified complication
                  NEC K50.818
        rectal bleeding K50.011
        specified complication
          NEC K50.018
  rotaviral A08.0
  Salmonella, salmonellosis (arizonae)
    (cholerae-suis) (enteritidis)
    (typhimurium) A02.0
  segmental — *see* Enteritis, regional
  septic A09
  Shigella — *see* Infection, Shigella
  small round structured NEC A08.19
  spasmodic, spastic — *see* Syndrome, irritable
    bowel
  staphylococcal A04.8
    due to food A05.0
  torovirus A08.39
  toxic NEC K52.1
    due to Clostridium difficile
      not specified as recurrent A04.72
      recurrent A04.71
  trichomonal A07.8
  tuberculous A18.32
  typhosa A01.00
  ulcerative (chronic) — *see* Colitis, ulcerative
  viral A08.4

Enteritis (acute) (diarrheal) (hemorrhagic)
(noninfective) - *continued*
  viral - *continued*
    adenovirus A08.2
    enterovirus A08.39
    Rotavirus A08.0
    small round structured NEC A08.19
    specified NEC A08.39
    virus specified NEC A08.39
Enterobiasis B80
Enterobius vermicularis (infection)
  (infestation) B80
Enterocele — *see also* Hernia, abdomen
  pelvic, pelvis (acquired) (congenital) N81.5
  vagina, vaginal (acquired) (congenital)
    NEC N81.5
Enterocolitis — *see also* Enteritis K52.9
  due to Clostridium difficile
    not specified as recurrent A04.72
    recurrent A04.71
  fulminant ischemic — *see also* Ischemia,
    intestine, acute K55.059
  granulomatous — *see* Enteritis, regional
  hemorrhagic (acute) — *see also* Ischemia,
    intestine, acute K55.059
  chronic K55.1
  infectious NEC A09
  ischemic K55.9
  necrotizing K55.30
    with
      perforation K55.33
      pneumatosis K55.32
        and perforation K55.33
    due to Clostridium difficile
      not specified as recurrent A04.72
      recurrent A04.71
    in non-newborn K55.30
      stage 1 (without pneumatosis, without
        perforation) K55.31
      stage 2 (with pneumatosis, without
        perforation) K55.32
      stage 3 (with pneumatosis, with
        perforation) K55.33
    in newborn P77.9
      stage 1 (without pneumatosis, without
        perforation) P77.1
      stage 2 (with pneumatosis, without
        perforation) P77.2
      stage 3 (with pneumatosis, with
        perforation) P77.3
    without pneumatosis or perforation K55.31
  noninfectious K52.9
  newborn — *see* Enterocolitis, necrotizing,
    in newborn
  pseudomembranous (newborn)
    not specified as recurrent A04.72
    recurrent A04.71
  radiation K52.0
    newborn — *see* Enterocolitis, necrotizing,
      in newborn
  ulcerative (chronic) — *see* Pancolitis,
    ulcerative (chronic)
Enterogastritis — *see* Enteritis
Enteropathy K63.9
  food protein-induced K52.22
  celiac-gluten-sensitive K90.0
    non-celiac K90.41
  hemorrhagic, terminal — *see also* Ischemia,
    intestine, acute K55.059
  protein-losing K90.49
Enteroperitonitis — *see* Peritonitis
Enteroptosis K63.4
Enterorrhagia K92.2
Enterospasm — *see also* Syndrome, irritable,
  bowel
  psychogenic F45.8
Enterostenosis — *see also* Obstruction,
  intestine, specified NEC K56.699
Enterostomy
  complication — *see* Complication,
    enterostomy
  status Z93.4
Enterovirus, as cause of disease classified
  elsewhere B97.10
  coxsackievirus B97.11

Enterovirus, as cause of disease classified elsewhere - *continued*
  echovirus B97.12
  other specified B97.19
Enthesopathy (peripheral) M77.9
  Achilles tendinitis — *see* Tendinitis, Achilles
  ankle and tarsus M77.5-
    specified type NEC — *see* Enthesopathy, foot, specified type NEC
  anterior tibial syndrome M76.81-
  calcaneal spur — *see* Spur, bone, calcaneal
  elbow region M77.8
    lateral epicondylitis — *see* Epicondylitis, lateral
    medial epicondylitis — *see* Epicondylitis, medial
  foot NEC M77.9
    metatarsalgia — *see* Metatarsalgia
    specified type NEC M77.5-
  forearm M77.9
  gluteal tendinitis — *see* Tendinitis, gluteal
  hand M77.9
  hip — *see* Enthesopathy, lower limb, specified type NEC
  iliac crest spur — *see* Spur, bone, iliac crest
  iliotibial band syndrome — *see* Syndrome, iliotibial band
  knee — *see* Enthesopathy, lower limb, lower leg, specified type NEC
  lateral epicondylitis — *see* Epicondylitis, lateral
  lower limb (excluding foot) M76.9
    Achilles tendinitis — *see* Tendinitis, Achilles
    ankle and tarsus M77.5-
      specified type NEC — *see* Enthesopathy, foot, specified type NEC
    anterior tibial syndrome M76.81-
    gluteal tendinitis — *see* Tendinitis, gluteal
    iliac crest spur — *see* Spur, bone, iliac crest
    iliotibial band syndrome — *see* Syndrome, iliotibial band
    patellar tendinitis — *see* Tendinitis, patellar
    pelvic region — *see* Enthesopathy, lower limb, specified type NEC
    peroneal tendinitis — *see* Tendinitis, peroneal
    posterior tibial syndrome M76.82-
    psoas tendinitis — *see* Tendinitis, psoas
    specified type NEC M76.89-
    tibial collateral bursitis — *see* Bursitis, tibial collateral
  medial epicondylitis — *see* Epicondylitis, medial
  metatarsalgia — *see* Metatarsalgia
  multiple sites M77.9
  patellar tendinitis — *see* Tendinitis, patellar
  pelvis M77.9
  periarthritis of wrist — *see* Periarthritis, wrist
  peroneal tendinitis — *see* Tendinitis, peroneal
  posterior tibial syndrome M76.82-
  psoas tendinitis — *see* Tendinitis, psoas
  shoulder M77.9
  shoulder region — *see* Lesion, shoulder
  specified site NEC M77.9
  specified type NEC M77.8
  spinal M46.00
    cervical region M46.02
    cervicothoracic region M46.03
    lumbar region M46.06
    lumbosacral region M46.07
    multiple sites M46.09
    occipito-atlanto-axial region M46.01
    sacrococcygeal region M46.08
    thoracic region M46.04
    thoracolumbar region M46.05
  tibial collateral bursitis — *see* Bursitis, tibial collateral
  upper arm M77.9
  wrist and carpus NEC M77.8
    calcaneal spur — *see* Spur, bone, calcaneal

Enthesopathy (peripheral) - *continued*
  wrist and carpus NEC - *continued*
    periarthritis of wrist — *see* Periarthritis, wrist
Entomophobia F40.218
Entomophthoromycosis B46.8
Entrance, air into vein — *see* Embolism, air
Entrapment, nerve — *see* Neuropathy, entrapment
Entropion (eyelid) (paralytic) H02.009
  cicatricial H02.019
    left H02.016
      lower H02.015
      upper H02.014
    right H02.013
      lower H02.012
      upper H02.011
  congenital Q10.2
  left H02.006
    lower H02.005
    upper H02.004
  mechanical H02.029
    left H02.026
      lower H02.025
      upper H02.024
    right H02.023
      lower H02.022
      upper H02.021
  right H02.003
    lower H02.002
    upper H02.001
  senile H02.039
    left H02.036
      lower H02.035
      upper H02.034
    right H02.033
      lower H02.032
      upper H02.031
  spastic H02.049
    left H02.046
      lower H02.045
      upper H02.044
    right H02.043
      lower H02.042
      upper H02.041
Enucleated eye (traumatic, current) S05.7-
Enuresis R32
  functional F98.0
  habit disturbance F98.0
  nocturnal N39.44
    psychogenic F98.0
  nonorganic origin F98.0
  psychogenic F98.0
Eosinopenia — *see* Agranulocytosis
Eosinophilia (allergic) (hereditary) (idiopathic) (secondary) D72.1
  with
    angiolymphoid hyperplasia (ALHE) D18.01
  infiltrative J82
  Löffler's J82
  peritoneal — *see* Peritonitis, eosinophilic
  pulmonary NEC J82
  tropical (pulmonary) J82
Eosinophilia-myalgia syndrome M35.8
Ependymitis (acute) (cerebral) (chronic) (granular) — *see* Encephalomyelitis
Ependymoblastoma
  specified site — *see* Neoplasm, malignant, by site
  unspecified site C71.9
Ependymoma (epithelial) (malignant)
  anaplastic
    specified site — *see* Neoplasm, malignant, by site
    unspecified site C71.9
  benign
    specified site — *see* Neoplasm, benign, by site
    unspecified site D33.2
  myxopapillary D43.2
    specified site — *see* Neoplasm, uncertain behavior, by site
    unspecified site D43.2
  papillary D43.2

Ependymoma (epithelial) (malignant) - *continued*
  papillary - *continued*
    specified site — *see* Neoplasm, uncertain behavior, by site
    unspecified site D43.2
  specified site — *see* Neoplasm, malignant, by site
  unspecified site C71.9
Ependymopathy G93.89
Ephelis, ephelides L81.2
Epiblepharon (congenital) Q10.3
Epicanthus, epicanthic fold (eyelid) (congenital) Q10.3
Epicondylitis (elbow)
  lateral M77.1-
  medial M77.0-
Epicystitis — *see* Cystitis
Epidemic — *see* condition
Epidermidalization, cervix — *see* Dysplasia, cervix
Epidermis, epidermal — *see* condition
Epidermodysplasia verruciformis B07.8
Epidermolysis
  bullosa (congenital) Q81.9
    acquired L12.30
      drug-induced L12.31
      specified cause NEC L12.35
    dystrophica Q81.2
    letalis Q81.1
    simplex Q81.0
    specified NEC Q81.8
  necroticans combustiformis L51.2
    due to drug — *see* Table of Drugs and Chemicals, by drug
Epidermophytid — *see* Dermatophytosis
Epidermophytosis (infected) — *see* Dermatophytosis
Epididymis — *see* condition
Epididymitis (acute) (nonvenereal) (recurrent) (residual) N45.1
  with orchitis N45.3
  blennorrhagic (gonococcal) A54.23
  caseous (tuberculous) A18.15
  chlamydial A56.19
  filarial — *see also* Infestation, filarial B74.9 *[N51]*
  gonococcal A54.23
  syphilitic A52.76
  tuberculous A18.15
Epididymo-orchitis — *see also* Epididymitis N45.3
Epidural — *see* condition
Epigastrium, epigastric — *see* condition
Epigastrocele — *see* Hernia, ventral
Epiglottis — *see* condition
Epiglottitis, epiglottiditis (acute) J05.10
  with obstruction J05.11
  chronic J37.0
Epignathus Q89.4
Epilepsia partialis continua — *see also* Kozhevnikof's epilepsy G40.1-
Epilepsy, epileptic, epilepsia (attack) (cerebral) (convulsion) (fit) (seizure) G40.909
  Note: the following terms are to be considered equivalent to intractable: pharmacoresistant (pharmacologically resistant) , treatment resistant, refractory (medically) and poorly controlled
  with
    complex partial seizures — *see* Epilepsy, localization-related, symptomatic, with complex partial seizures
    grand mal seizures on awakening — *see* Epilepsy, generalized, specified NEC
    myoclonic absences — *see* Epilepsy, generalized, specified NEC
    myoclonic-astatic seizures — *see* Epilepsy, generalized, specified NEC
    simple partial seizures — *see* Epilepsy, localization-related, symptomatic, with simple partial seizures
  akinetic — *see* Epilepsy, generalized, specified NEC

Epilepsy, epileptic, epilepsia (attack) (cerebral) (convulsion) (fit) (seizure) - *continued*
  benign childhood with centrotemporal EEG spikes — *see* Epilepsy, localization-related, idiopathic
  benign myoclonic in infancy G40.80-
  Bravais-jacksonian — *see* Epilepsy, localization-related, symptomatic, with simple partial seizures
  childhood
    with occipital EEG paroxysms — *see* Epilepsy, localization-related, idiopathic
    absence G40.A09
      intractable G40.A19
        with status epilepticus G40.A11
        without status epilepticus G40.A19
      not intractable G40.A09
        with status epilepticus G40.A01
        without status epilepticus G40.A09
  climacteric — *see* Epilepsy, specified NEC
  cysticercosis B69.0
  deterioration (mental) F06.8
  due to syphilis A52.19
  focal — *see* Epilepsy, localization-related, symptomatic, with simple partial seizures
  generalized
    idiopathic G40.309
      intractable G40.319
        with status epilepticus G40.311
        without status epilepticus G40.319
      not intractable G40.309
        with status epilepticus G40.301
        without status epilepticus G40.309
    specified NEC G40.409
      intractable G40.419
        with status epilepticus G40.411
        without status epilepticus G40.419
      not intractable G40.409
        with status epilepticus G40.401
        without status epilepticus G40.409
  impulsive petit mal — *see* Epilepsy, juvenile myoclonic
  intractable G40.919
    with status epilepticus G40.911
    without status epilepticus G40.919
  juvenile absence G40.A09
    intractable G40.A19
      with status epilepticus G40.A11
      without status epilepticus G40.A19
    not intractable G40.A09
      with status epilepticus G40.A01
      without status epilepticus G40.A09
  juvenile myoclonic G40.B09
    intractable G40.B19
      with status epilepticus G40.B11
      without status epilepticus G40.B19
    not intractable G40.B09
      with status epilepticus G40.B01
      without status epilepticus G40.B09
  localization-related (focal) (partial)
    idiopathic G40.009
      with seizures of localized onset G40.009
        intractable G40.019
          with status epilepticus G40.011
          without status epilepticus G40.019
        not intractable G40.009
          with status epilepticus G40.001
          without status epilepticus G40.009
    symptomatic
      with complex partial seizures G40.209
        intractable G40.219
          with status epilepticus G40.211
          without status epilepticus G40.219
        not intractable G40.209
          with status epilepticus G40.201
          without status epilepticus G40.209
      with simple partial seizures G40.109
        intractable G40.119
          with status epilepticus G40.111
          without status epilepticus G40.119
        not intractable G40.109
          with status epilepticus G40.101

Epilepsy, epileptic, epilepsia (attack) (cerebral) (convulsion) (fit) (seizure) - *continued*
  localization-related (focal) (partial) - *continued*
    symptomatic - *continued*
      with simple partial seizures - *continued*
        not intractable - *continued*
          without status epilepticus G40.109
  myoclonus, myoclonic — *see* Epilepsy, generalized, specified NEC
  progressive — *see* Epilepsy, generalized, idiopathic
  not intractable G40.909
    with status epilepticus G40.901
    without status epilepticus G40.909
  on awakening — *see* Epilepsy, generalized, specified NEC
  parasitic NOS B71.9 [G94]
  partialis continua — *see also* Kozhevnikof's epilepsy G40.1-
  peripheral — *see* Epilepsy, specified NEC
  procursiva — *see* Epilepsy, localization-related, symptomatic, with simple partial seizures
  progressive (familial) myoclonic — *see* Epilepsy, generalized, idiopathic
  reflex — *see* Epilepsy, specified NEC
  related to
    alcohol G40.509
      not intractable G40.509
        with status epilepticus G40.501
        without status epliepticus G40.509
    drugs G40.509
      not intractable G40.509
        with status epilepticus G40.501
        without status epliepticus G40.509
    external causes G40.509
      not intractable G40.509
        with status epilepticus G40.501
        without status epliepticus G40.509
    hormonal changes G40.509
      not intractable G40.509
        with status epilepticus G40.501
        without status epliepticus G40.509
    sleep deprivation G40.509
      not intractable G40.509
        with status epilepticus G40.501
        without status epliepticus G40.509
    stress G40.509
      not intractable G40.509
        with status epilepticus G40.501
        without status epliepticus G40.509
  somatomotor — *see* Epilepsy, localization-related, symptomatic, with simple partial seizures
  somatosensory — *see* Epilepsy, localization-related, symptomatic, with simple partial seizures
  spasms G40.822
    intractable G40.824
      with status epilepticus G40.823
      without status epilepticus G40.824
    not intractable G40.822
      with status epilepticus G40.821
      without status epilepticus G40.822
  specified NEC G40.802
    intractable G40.804
      with status epilepticus G40.803
      without status epilepticus G40.804
    not intractable G40.802
      with status epilepticus G40.801
      without status epilepticus G40.802
  syndromes
    generalized
      idiopathic G40.309
        intractable G40.319
          with status epilepticus G40.311
          without status epilepticus G40.319
        not intractable G40.309
          with status epilepticus G40.301
          without status epilepticus G40.309
      specified NEC G40.409
        intractable G40.419
          with status epilepticus G40.411

Epilepsy, epileptic, epilepsia (attack) (cerebral) (convulsion) (fit) (seizure) - *continued*
  syndromes - *continued*
    generalized - *continued*
      specified NEC - *continued*
        intractable - *continued*
          without status epilepticus G40.419
        not intractable G40.409
          with status epilepticus G40.401
          without status epilepticus G40.409
    localization-related (focal) (partial)
      idiopathic G40.009
        with seizures of localized onset G40.009
          intractable G40.019
            with status epilepticus G40.011
            without status epilepticus G40.019
          not intractable G40.009
            with status epilepticus G40.001
            without status epilepticus G40.009
      symptomatic
        with complex partial seizures G40.209
          intractable G40.219
            with status epilepticus G40.211
            without status epilepticus G40.219
          not intractable G40.209
            with status epilepticus G40.201
            without status epilepticus G40.209
        with simple partial seizures G40.109
          intractable G40.119
            with status epilepticus G40.111
            without status epilepticus G40.119
          not intractable G40.109
            with status epilepticus G40.101
            without status epilepticus G40.109
    specified NEC G40.802
      intractable G40.804
        with status epilepticus G40.803
        without status epilepticus G40.804
      not intractable G40.802
        with status epilepticus G40.801
        without status epilepticus G40.802
    tonic (-clonic) — *see* Epilepsy, generalized, specified NEC
    twilight F05
    uncinate (gyrus) — *see* Epilepsy, localization-related, symptomatic, with complex partial seizures
    Unverricht (-Lundborg) (familial myoclonic) — *see* Epilepsy, generalized, idiopathic
    visceral — *see* Epilepsy, specified NEC
    visual — *see* Epilepsy, specified NEC
Epiloia Q85.1
Epimenorrhea N92.0
Epipharyngitis — *see* Nasopharyngitis
Epiphora H04.20-
  due to
    excess lacrimation H04.21-
    insufficient drainage H04.22-
Epiphyseal arrest — *see* Arrest, epiphyseal
Epiphyseolysis, epiphysiolysis — *see* Osteochondropathy
Epiphysitis — *see also* Osteochondropathy
  juvenile M92.9
  syphilitic (congenital) A50.02
Epiplocele — *see* Hernia, abdomen
Epiploitis — *see* Peritonitis
Epiplosarcomphalocele — *see* Hernia, umbilicus
Episcleritis (suppurative) H15.10-
  in (due to)
    syphilis A52.71
    tuberculosis A18.51
  nodular H15.12-
  periodica fugax H15.11-
    angioneurotic — *see* Edema, angioneurotic
  syphilitic (late) A52.71

Episcleritis (suppurative) - *continued*
tuberculous A18.51
Episode
affective, mixed F39
depersonalization (in neurotic state) F48.1
depressive F32.9
major F32.9
mild F32.0
moderate F32.1
severe (without psychotic
symptoms) F32.2
with psychotic symptoms F32.3
recurrent F33.9
brief F33.8
specified NEC F32.89
hypomanic F30.8
manic F30.9
with
psychotic symptoms F30.2
remission (full) F30.4
partial F30.3
other specified F30.8
recurrent F31.89
without psychotic symptoms F30.10
mild F30.11
moderate F30.12
severe (without psychotic
symptoms) F30.13
with psychotic symptoms F30.2
psychotic F23
organic F06.8
schizophrenic (acute) NEC, brief F23
Epispadias (female) (male) Q64.0
Episplenitis D73.89
Epistaxis (multiple) R04.0
hereditary I78.0
vicarious menstruation N94.89
Epithelioma (malignant) — *see also*
Neoplasm, malignant, by site
adenoides cysticum — *see* Neoplasm, skin,
benign
basal cell — *see* Neoplasm, skin, malignant
benign — *see* Neoplasm, benign, by site
Bowen's — *see* Neoplasm, skin, in situ
calcifying, of Malherbe — *see* Neoplasm,
skin, benign
external site — *see* Neoplasm, skin,
malignant
intraepidermal, Jadassohn — *see* Neoplasm,
skin, benign
squamous cell — *see* Neoplasm, malignant,
by site
Epitheliomatosis pigmented Q82.1
**Epitheliopathy, multifocal placoid
pigment** H30.14-
Epithelium, epithelial — *see* condition
**Epituberculosis (with atelectasis)
(allergic)** A15.7
Eponychia Q84.6
Epstein's
nephrosis or syndrome — *see* Nephrosis
pearl K09.8
Epulis (gingiva) (fibrous) (giant cell) K06.8
Equinia A24.0
Equinovarus (congenital) (talipes) Q66.0-
acquired — *see* Deformity, limb, clubfoot
Equivalent
convulsive (abdominal) — *see* Epilepsy,
specified NEC
epileptic (psychic) — *see* Epilepsy,
localization-related, symptomatic, with
complex partial seizures
**Erb (-Duchenne) paralysis (birth injury)
(newborn)** P14.0
Erb-Goldflam disease or syndrome G70.00
with exacerbation (acute) G70.01
in crisis G70.01
Erb's
disease G71.02
palsy, paralysis (brachial) (birth)
(newborn) P14.0
spinal (spastic) syphilitic A52.17
pseudohypertrophic muscular
dystrophy G71.02

**Erdheim's syndrome (acromegalic
macrospondylitis)** E22.0
Erection, painful (persistent) — *see* Priapism
Ergosterol deficiency (vitamin D) E55.9
with
adult osteomalacia M83.8
rickets — *see* Rickets
Ergotism — *see also* Poisoning, food, noxious,
plant
from ergot used as drug (migraine
therapy) — *see* Table of Drugs and
Chemicals
Erosio interdigitalis blastomycetica B37.2
Erosion
artery I77.2
without rupture I77.89
bone — *see* Disorder, bone, density and
structure, specified NEC
bronchus J98.09
cartilage (joint) — *see* Disorder, cartilage,
specified type NEC
cervix (uteri) (acquired) (chronic)
(congenital) N86
with cervicitis N72
cornea (nontraumatic) — *see* Ulcer, cornea
recurrent H18.83-
traumatic — *see* Abrasion, cornea
dental (idiopathic) (occupational) (due to
diet, drugs or vomiting) K03.2
duodenum, postpyloric — *see* Ulcer,
duodenum
esophagus K22.10
with bleeding K22.11
gastric — *see* Ulcer, stomach
gastrojejunal — *see* Ulcer, gastrojejunal
implanted mesh — *see* Complications,
prosthetic devise or implant, mesh
intestine K63.3
lymphatic vessel I89.8
pylorus, pyloric (ulcer) — *see* Ulcer, stomach
spine, aneurysmal A52.09
stomach — *see* Ulcer, stomach
subcutaneous device pocket
nervous system prosthetic device, implant,
or graft T85.890
other internal prosthetic device, implant, or
graft T85.898
teeth (idiopathic) (occupational) (due to diet,
drugs or vomiting) K03.2
urethra N36.8
uterus N85.8
Erotomania F52.8
Error
metabolism, inborn -- se Disorder,
metabolism
refractive — *see* Disorder, refraction
Eructation R14.2
nervous or psychogenic F45.8
Eruption
creeping B76.9
drug (generalized) (taken internally) L27.0
fixed L27.1
in contact with skin — *see* Dermatitis, due
to drugs
localized L27.1
Hutchinson, summer L56.4
Kaposi's varicelliform B00.0
napkin L22
polymorphous light (sun) L56.4
recalcitrant pustular L13.8
ringed R23.8
skin (nonspecific) R21
creeping (meaning hookworm) B76.9
due to inoculation/vaccination
(generalized) — *see also* Dermatitis,
due to, vaccine L27.0
localized L27.1
erysipeloid A26.0
feigned L98.1
Kaposi's varicelliform B00.0
lichenoid L28.0
meaning dermatitis — *see* Dermatitis
toxic NEC L53.0
tooth, teeth, abnormal (incomplete) (late)
(premature) (sequence) K00.6

Eruption - *continued*
vesicular R23.8
**Erysipelas (gangrenous) (infantile)
(newborn) (phlegmonous) (suppurative)**
A46
external ear A46 *[H62.40]*
puerperal, postpartum O86.89
Erysipeloid A26.9
cutaneous (Rosenbach's) A26.0
disseminated A26.8
sepsis A26.7
specified NEC A26.8
**Erythema, erythematous (infectional)
(inflammation)** L53.9
ab igne L59.0
annulare (centrifugum) (rheumaticum) L53.1
arthriticum epidemicum A25.1
brucellum — *see* Brucellosis
chronic figurate NEC L53.3
chronicum migrans (Borrelia
burgdorferi) A69.20
diaper L22
due to
chemical NEC L53.0
in contact with skin L24.5
drug (internal use) — *see* Dermatitis, due
to, drugs
elevatum diutinum L95.1
endemic E52
epidemic, arthritic A25.1
figuratum perstans L53.3
gluteal L22
heat - code by site under Burn, first degree
ichthyosiforme congenitum bullous Q80.3
in diseases classified elsewhere L54
induratum (nontuberculous) L52
tuberculous A18.4
infectiosum B08.3
intertrigo L30.4
iris L51.9
marginatum L53.2
in (due to) acute rheumatic fever I00
medicamentosum — *see* Dermatitis, due to,
drugs
migrans A26.0
chronicum A69.20
tongue K14.1
multiforme (major) (minor) L51.9
bullous, bullosum L51.1
conjunctiva L51.1
nonbullous L51.0
pemphigoides L12.0
specified NEC L51.8
napkin L22
neonatorum P83.88
toxic P83.1
nodosum L52
tuberculous A18.4
palmar L53.8
pernio T69.1
rash, newborn P83.88
scarlatiniform (recurrent) (exfoliative) L53.8
solare L55.0
specified NEC L53.8
toxic, toxicum NEC L53.0
newborn P83.1
tuberculous (primary) A18.4
Erythematous, erythematosus — *see*
condition
Erythermalgia (primary) I73.81
Erythralgia I73.81
Erythrasma L08.1
Erythredema (polyneuropathy) — *see*
Poisoning, mercury
Erythremia (acute) C94.0-
chronic D45
secondary D75.1
Erythroblastopenia — *see also* Aplasia, red
cell D60.9
congenital D61.01
Erythroblastophthisis D61.09
Erythroblastosis (fetalis) (newborn) P55.9
due to
ABO (antibodies) (incompatibility)
(isoimmunization) P55.1

Erythroblastosis (fetalis) (newborn) - *continued*
  due to - *continued*
    Rh (antibodies) (incompatibility) (isoimmunization) P55.0
Erythrocyanosis (crurum) I73.89
Erythrocythemia — *see* Erythremia
Erythrocytosis (megalosplenic) (secondary) D75.1
  familial D75.0
  oval, hereditary — *see* Elliptocytosis
  secondary D75.1
  stress D75.1
Erythroderma (secondary) — *see also* Erythema L53.9
  bullous ichthyosiform, congenital Q80.3
  desquamativum L21.1
  ichthyosiform, congenital (bullous) Q80.3
  neonatorum P83.88
  psoriaticum L40.8
Erythrodysesthesia, palmar plantar (PPE) L27.1
Erythrogenesis imperfecta D61.09
Erythroleukemia C94.0-
Erythromelalgia I73.81
Erythrophagocytosis D75.89
Erythrophobia F40.298
Erythroplakia, oral epithelium, and tongue K13.29
Erythroplasia (Queyrat) D07.4
  specified site — *see* Neoplasm, skin, in situ
  unspecified site D07.4
Escherichia coli (E. coli) , as cause of disease classified elsewhere B96.20
  non-O157 Shiga toxin-producing (with known O group) B96.22
  non-Shiga toxin-producing B96.29
  O157 with confirmation of Shiga toxin when H antigen is unknown, or is not H7 B96.21
  O157:H- (nonmotile) with confirmation of Shiga toxin B96.21
  O157:H7 with or without confirmation of Shiga toxin-production B96.21
  Shiga toxin-producing (with unspecified O group) (STEC) B96.23
  O157 B96.21
  O157:H7 with or without confirmation of Shiga toxin-production B96.21
    specified NEC B96.22
  specified NEC B96.29
Esophagismus K22.4
Esophagitis (acute) (alkaline) (chemical) (chronic) (infectional) (necrotic) (peptic) (postoperative) K20.9
  candidal B37.81
  due to gastrointestinal reflux disease K21.0
  eosinophilic K20.0
  reflux K21.0
  specified NEC K20.8
  tuberculous A18.83
  ulcerative K22.10
    with bleeding K22.11
Esophagocele K22.5
Esophagomalacia K22.8
Esophagospasm K22.4
Esophagostenosis K22.2
Esophagostomiasis B81.8
Esophagotracheal — *see* condition
Esophagus — *see* condition
Esophoria H50.51
  convergence, excess H51.12
  divergence, insufficiency H51.8
Esotropia — *see* Strabismus, convergent concomitant
Espundia B55.2
Essential — *see* condition
Esthesioneuroblastoma C30.0
Esthesioneurocytoma C30.0
Esthesioneuroepithelioma C30.0
Esthiomene A55
Estivo-autumnal malaria (fever) B50.9
Estrangement (marital) Z63.5
  parent-child NEC Z62.890
Estriasis — *see* Myiasis

Ethanolism — *see* Alcoholism
Etherism — *see* Dependence, drug, inhalant
Ethmoid, ethmoidal — *see* condition
Ethmoiditis (chronic) (nonpurulent) (purulent) — *see also* Sinusitis, ethmoidal
  influenzal — *see* Influenza, with, respiratory manifestations NEC
  Woakes' J33.1
Ethylism — *see* Alcoholism
Eulenburg's disease (congenital paramyotonia) G71.19
Eumycetoma B47.0
Eunuchoidism E29.1
  hypogonadotropic E23.0
European blastomycosis — *see* Cryptococcosis
Eustachian — *see* condition
Evaluation (for) (of)
  development state
    adolescent Z00.3
    period of
      delayed growth in childhood Z00.70
        with abnormal findings Z00.71
      rapid growth in childhood Z00.2
      puberty Z00.3
  growth and developmental state (period of rapid growth) Z00.2
    delayed growth Z00.70
      with abnormal findings Z00.71
  mental health (status) Z00.8
    requested by authority Z04.6
  period of
    delayed growth in childhood Z00.70
      with abnormal findings Z00.71
    rapid growth in childhood Z00.2
  suspected condition — *see* Observation
Evans syndrome D69.41
Event
  apparent life threatening in newborn and infant (ALTE) R68.13
  brief resolved unexplained event (BRUE) R68.13
Eventration — *see also* Hernia, ventral
  colon into chest — *see* Hernia, diaphragm
  diaphragm (congenital) Q79.1
Eversion
  bladder N32.89
  cervix (uteri) N86
    with cervicitis N72
  foot NEC — *see also* Deformity, valgus, ankle
    congenital Q66.6
  punctum lacrimale (postinfectional) (senile) H04.52-
  ureter (meatus) N28.89
  urethra (meatus) N36.8
  uterus N81.4
Evidence
  cytologic
    of malignancy on anal smear R85.614
    of malignancy on cervical smear R87.614
    of malignancy on vaginal smear R87.624
Evisceration
  birth injury P15.8
  traumatic NEC
    eye — *see* Enucleated eye
Evulsion — *see* Avulsion
Ewing's sarcoma or tumor — *see* Neoplasm, bone, malignant
Examination (for) (following) (general) (of) (routine) Z00.00
  with abnormal findings Z00.01
  abuse, physical (alleged) , ruled out
    adult Z04.71
    child Z04.72
  adolescent (development state) Z00.3
  alleged rape or sexual assault (victim) , ruled out
    adult Z04.41
    child Z04.42
  allergy Z01.82
  annual (adult) (periodic) (physical) Z00.00
    with abnormal findings Z00.01
    gynecological Z01.419

Examination (for) (following) (general) (of) (routine) - *continued*
  annual (adult) (periodic) (physical) - *continued*
    gynecological - *continued*
      with abnormal findings Z01.411
  antibody response Z01.84
  blood — *see* Examination, laboratory
  blood pressure Z01.30
    with abnormal findings Z01.31
  cancer staging — *see* Neoplasm, malignant, by site
  cervical Papanicolaou smear Z12.4
    as part of routine gynecological examination Z01.419
    with abnormal findings Z01.411
  child (over 28 days old) Z00.129
    with abnormal findings Z00.121
    under 28 days old — *see* Newborn, examination
  clinical research control or normal comparison (control) (participant) Z00.6
  contraceptive (drug) maintenance (routine) Z30.8
    device (intrauterine) Z30.431
  dental Z01.20
    with abnormal findings Z01.21
  developmental — *see* Examination, child
  donor (potential) Z00.5
  ear Z01.10
    with abnormal findings NEC Z01.118
  eye Z01.00
    with abnormal findings Z01.01
    following failed vision screening Z01.020
      with abnormal findings Z01.021
  following
    accident NEC Z04.3
      transport Z04.1
      work Z04.2
    assault, alleged, ruled out
      adult Z04.71
      child Z04.72
    motor vehicle accident Z04.1
    treatment (for) Z09
      combined NEC Z09
        fracture Z09
        malignant neoplasm Z08
      malignant neoplasm Z08
      mental disorder Z09
      specified condition NEC Z09
  follow-up (routine) (following) Z09
    chemotherapy NEC Z09
      malignant neoplasm Z08
    fracture Z09
    malignant neoplasm Z08
    postpartum Z39.2
    psychotherapy Z09
    radiotherapy NEC Z09
      malignant neoplasm Z08
    surgery NEC Z09
      malignant neoplasm Z08
  forced sexual exploitation Z04.81
  forced labor exploitation Z04.82
  gynecological Z01.419
    with abnormal findings Z01.411
    for contraceptive maintenance Z30.8
  health — *see* Examination, medical
  hearing Z01.10
    with abnormal findings NEC Z01.118
    infant or child (over 28 days old) Z00.129
      with abnormal findings Z00.121
    following failed hearing screening Z01.110
  immunity status testing Z01.84
  laboratory (as part of a general medical examination) Z00.00
    with abnormal findings Z00.01
    preprocedural Z01.812
  lactating mother Z39.1
  medical (adult) (for) (of) Z00.00
    with abnormal findings Z00.01
    administrative purpose only Z02.9
      specified NEC Z02.89
    admission to
      armed forces Z02.3
      old age home Z02.2

Examination (for) (following) (general) (of) (routine) - *continued*
  medical (adult) (for) (of) - *continued*
    admission to - *continued*
      prison Z02.89
      residential institution Z02.2
      school Z02.0
        following illness or medical
          treatment Z02.0
      summer camp Z02.89
    adoption Z02.82
    blood alcohol or drug level Z02.83
    camp (summer) Z02.89
    clinical research, normal subject (control)
      (participant) Z00.6
    control subject in clinical research (normal
      comparison) (participant) Z00.6
    donor (potential) Z00.5
    driving license Z02.4
    general (adult) Z00.00
      with abnormal findings Z00.01
    immigration Z02.89
    insurance purposes Z02.6
    marriage Z02.89
    medicolegal reasons NEC Z04.89
    naturalization Z02.89
    participation in sport Z02.5
    paternity testing Z02.81
    population survey Z00.8
    pre-employment Z02.1
    pre-operative — *see* Examination, pre-
      procedural
    pre-procedural
      cardiovascular Z01.810
      respiratory Z01.811
      specified NEC Z01.818
    preschool children
      for admission to school Z02.0
    prisoners
      for entrance into prison Z02.89
    recruitment for armed forces Z02.3
    specified NEC Z00.8
    sport competition Z02.5
  medicolegal reason NEC Z04.89
    following
      forced sexual exploitation Z04.81
      forced labor exploitation Z04.82
  newborn — *see* Newborn, examination
  pelvic (annual) (periodic) Z01.419
    with abnormal findings Z01.411
  period of rapid growth in childhood Z00.2
  periodic (adult) (annual) (routine) Z00.00
    with abnormal findings Z00.01
  physical (adult) — *see also* Examination,
    medical Z00.00
    sports Z02.5
  postpartum
    immediately after delivery Z39.0
    routine follow-up Z39.2
  prenatal (normal pregnancy) — *see also*
    Pregnancy, normal Z34.9-
  pre-chemotherapy (antineoplastic) Z01.818
  pre-procedural (pre-operative)
    cardiovascular Z01.810
    laboratory Z01.812
    respiratory Z01.811
    specified NEC Z01.818
  prior to chemotherapy
    (antineoplastic) Z01.818
  psychiatric NEC Z00.8
    follow-up not needing further care Z09
    requested by authority Z04.6
  radiological (as part of a general medical
    examination) Z00.00
    with abnormal findings Z00.01
  repeat cervical smear to confirm findings of
    recent normal smear following initial
    abnormal smear Z01.42
  skin (hypersensitivity) Z01.82
  special — *see also* Examination, by
    type Z01.89
    specified type NEC Z01.89
  specified type or reason NEC Z04.89
  teeth Z01.20
    with abnormal findings Z01.21

Examination (for) (following) (general) (of) (routine) - *continued*
  urine — *see* Examination, laboratory
  vision Z01.00
    with abnormal findings Z01.01
    following failed vision screening Z01.020
      with abnormal findings Z01.021
    infant or child (over 28 days old) Z00.129
      with abnormal findings Z00.121
Exanthem, exanthema — *see also* Rash
  with enteroviral vesicular stomatitis B08.4
  Boston A88.0
  epidemic with meningitis A88.0 *[G02]*
  subitum B08.20
    due to human herpesvirus 6 B08.21
    due to human herpesvirus 7 B08.22
  viral, virus B09
    specified type NEC B08.8
Excess, excessive, excessively
  alcohol level in blood R78.0
  androgen (ovarian) E28.1
  attrition, tooth, teeth K03.0
  carotene, carotin (dietary) E67.1
  cold, effects of T69.9
    specified effect NEC T69.8
  convergence H51.12
  crying
    in child, adolescent, or adult R45.83
    in infant R68.11
  development, breast N62
  divergence H51.8
  drinking (alcohol) NEC (without
    dependence) F10.10
    habitual (continual) (without
      remission) F10.20
  eating R63.2
  estrogen E28.0
  fat — *see also* Obesity
    in heart — *see* Degeneration, myocardial
    localized E65
  foreskin N47.8
  gas R14.0
  glucagon E16.3
  heat — *see* Heat
  intermaxillary vertical dimension of fully
    erupted teeth M26.37
  interocclusal distance of fully erupted
    teeth M26.37
  kalium E87.5
  large
    colon K59.39
      congenital Q43.8
    infant P08.0
    organ or site, congenital NEC — *see*
      Anomaly, by site
  long
    organ or site, congenital NEC — *see*
      Anomaly, by site
  menstruation (with regular cycle) N92.0
    with irregular cycle N92.1
  napping Z72.821
  natrium E87.0
  number of teeth K00.1
  nutrient (dietary) NEC R63.2
  potassium (K) E87.5
  salivation K11.7
  secretion — *see also* Hypersecretion
    milk O92.6
    sputum R09.3
    sweat R61
  sexual drive F52.8
  short
    organ or site, congenital NEC — *see*
      Anomaly, by site
    umbilical cord in labor or delivery O69.3
  skin L98.7
    and subcutaneous tissue L98.7
    eyelid (acquired) — *see* Blepharochalasis
      congenital Q10.3
  sodium (Na) E87.0
  spacing of fully erupted teeth M26.32
  sputum R09.3
  sweating R61
  thirst R63.1
    due to deprivation of water T73.1

Excess, excessive, excessively - *continued*
  tuberosity of jaw M26.07
  vitamin
    A (dietary) E67.0
      administered as drug (prolonged
        intake) — *see* Table of Drugs and
        Chemicals, vitamins, adverse effect
      overdose or wrong substance given or
        taken — *see* Table of Drugs and
        Chemicals, vitamins, poisoning
    D (dietary) E67.3
      administered as drug (prolonged
        intake) — *see* Table of Drugs and
        Chemicals, vitamins, adverse effect
      overdose or wrong substance given or
        taken — *see* Table of Drugs and
        Chemicals, vitamins, poisoning
  weight
    gain R63.5
    loss R63.4
**Excitability, abnormal, under minor stress
  (personality disorder)** F60.3
Excitation
  anomalous atrioventricular I45.6
  psychogenic F30.8
  reactive (from emotional stress,
    psychological trauma) F30.8
Excitement
  hypomanic F30.8
  manic F30.9
  mental, reactive (from emotional stress,
    psychological trauma) F30.8
  state, reactive (from emotional stress,
    psychological trauma) F30.8
Excoriation (traumatic) — *see also* Abrasion
  neurotic L98.1
  skin picking disorder F42.4
Exfoliation
  due to erythematous conditions according to
    extent of body surface involved L49.0
    10-19 percent of body surface L49.1
    20-29 percent of body surface L49.2
    30-39 percent of body surface L49.3
    40-49 percent of body surface L49.4
    50-59 percent of body surface L49.5
    60-69 percent of body surface L49.6
    70-79 percent of body surface L49.7
    80-89 percent of body surface L49.8
    90-99 percent of body surface L49.9
    less than 10 percent of body surface L49.0
  teeth, due to systemic causes K08.0
Exfoliative — *see* condition
Exhaustion, exhaustive (physical NEC)
  R53.83
  battle F43.0
  cardiac — *see* Failure, heart
  delirium F43.0
  due to
    cold T69.8
    excessive exertion T73.3
    exposure T73.2
    neurasthenia F48.8
  heart — *see* Failure, heart
  heat — *see also* Heat, exhaustion T67.5
    due to
      salt depletion T67.4
      water depletion T67.3
  maternal, complicating delivery O75.81
  mental F48.8
  myocardium, myocardial — *see* Failure,
    heart
  nervous F48.8
  old age R54
  psychogenic F48.8
  psychosis F43.0
  senile R54
  vital NEC Z73.0
Exhibitionism F65.2
Exocervicitis — *see* Cervicitis
Exomphalos Q79.2
  meaning hernia — *see* Hernia, umbilicus
Exophoria H50.52
  convergence, insufficiency H51.11
  divergence, excess H51.8

Exophthalmos H05.2-
congenital Q15.8
constant NEC H05.24-
displacement, globe — *see* Displacement,
globe
due to thyrotoxicosis (hyperthyroidism) —
see Hyperthyroidism, with, goiter
(diffuse)
dysthyroid — *see* Hyperthyroidism, with,
goiter (diffuse)
goiter — *see* Hyperthyroidism, with, goiter
(diffuse)
intermittent NEC H05.25-
malignant — *see* Hyperthyroidism, with,
goiter (diffuse)
orbital
edema — *see* Edema, orbit
hemorrhage — *see* Hemorrhage, orbit
pulsating NEC H05.26-
thyrotoxic, thyrotropic — *see*
Hyperthyroidism, with, goiter (diffuse)
Exostosis — *see also* Disorder, bone
cartilaginous — *see* Neoplasm, bone, benign
congenital (multiple) Q78.6
external ear canal H61.81-
gonococcal A54.49
jaw (bone) M27.8
multiple, congenital Q78.6
orbit H05.35-
osteocartilaginous — *see* Neoplasm, bone,
benign
syphilitic A52.77
Exotropia — *see* Strabismus, divergent
concomitant
Explanation of
investigation finding Z71.2
medication Z71.89
Exposure (to) — *see also* Contact,
with T75.89
acariasis Z20.7
AIDS virus Z20.6
air pollution Z77.110
algae and algae toxins Z77.121
algae bloom Z77.121
anthrax Z20.810
aromatic amines Z77.020
aromatic (hazardous) compounds
NEC Z77.028
aromatic dyes NOS Z77.028
arsenic Z77.010
asbestos Z77.090
bacterial disease NEC Z20.818
benzene Z77.021
blue-green algae bloom Z77.121
body fluids (potentially hazardous) Z77.21
brown tide Z77.121
chemicals (chiefly nonmedicinal)
(hazardous) NEC Z77.098
cholera Z20.09
chromium compounds Z77.018
cold, effects of T69.9
specified effect NEC T69.8
communicable disease Z20.9
bacterial NEC Z20.818
specified NEC Z20.89
viral NEC Z20.828
Zika virus Z20.821
cyanobacteria bloom Z77.121
disaster Z65.5
discrimination Z60.5
dyes Z77.098
effects of T73.9
environmental tobacco smoke (acute)
(chronic) Z77.22
Escherichia coli (E. coli) Z20.01
exhaustion due to T73.2
fiberglass — *see* Table of Drugs and
Chemicals, fiberglass
German measles Z20.4
gonorrhea Z20.2
hazardous metals NEC Z77.018
hazardous substances NEC Z77.29
hazards in the physical environment
NEC Z77.128
hazards to health NEC Z77.9

Exposure (to) - *continued*
human immunodeficiency virus (HIV) Z20.6
human T-lymphotropic virus type-1 (HTLV-
1) Z20.89
implanted
mesh — *see* Complications, prosthetic
devise or implant, mesh
prosthetic materials NEC — *see*
Complications, prosthetic materials
NEC
infestation (parasitic) NEC Z20.7
intestinal infectious disease NEC Z20.09
Escherichia coli (E. coli) Z20.01
lead Z77.011
meningococcus Z20.811
mold (toxic) Z77.120
nickel dust Z77.018
noise Z77.122
occupational
air contaminants NEC Z57.39
dust Z57.2
environmental tobacco smoke Z57.31
extreme temperature Z57.6
noise Z57.0
radiation Z57.1
risk factors Z57.9
specified NEC Z57.8
toxic agents (gases) (liquids) (solids)
(vapors) in agriculture Z57.4
toxic agents (gases) (liquids) (solids)
(vapors) in industry NEC Z57.5
vibration Z57.7
parasitic disease NEC Z20.7
pediculosis Z20.7
persecution Z60.5
pfiesteria piscicida Z77.121
poliomyelitis Z20.89
polycyclic aromatic hydrocarbons Z77.028
pollution
air Z77.110
environmental NEC Z77.118
soil Z77.112
water Z77.111
prenatal (drugs) (toxic chemicals) — *see*
Newborn, affected by, noxious
substances transmitted via placenta or
breast milk
rabies Z20.3
radiation, naturally occurring NEC Z77.123
radon Z77.123
red tide (Florida) Z77.121
rubella Z20.4
second hand tobacco smoke (acute)
(chronic) Z77.22
in the perinatal period P96.81
sexually-transmitted disease Z20.2
smallpox (laboratory) Z20.89
syphilis Z20.2
terrorism Z65.4
torture Z65.4
tuberculosis Z20.1
uranium Z77.012
varicella Z20.820
venereal disease Z20.2
viral disease NEC Z20.828
war Z65.5
water pollution Z77.111
Zika virus Z20.821
Exsanguination — *see* Hemorrhage
Exstrophy
abdominal contents Q45.8
bladder Q64.10
cloacal Q64.12
specified type NEC Q64.19
supravesical fissure Q64.11
Extensive — *see* condition
Extra — *see also* Accessory
marker chromosomes (normal
individual) Q92.61
in abnormal individual Q92.62
rib Q76.6
cervical Q76.5
Extrasystoles (supraventricular) I49.49
atrial I49.1
auricular I49.1

Extrasystoles (supraventricular) - *continued*
junctional I49.2
ventricular I49.3
Extrauterine gestation or pregnancy — *see*
Pregnancy, by site
Extravasation
blood R58
chyle into mesentery I89.8
pelvicalyceal N13.8
pyelosinus N13.8
urine (from ureter) R39.0
vesicant agent
antineoplastic chemotherapy T80.810
other agent NEC T80.818
Extremity — *see* condition, limb
Extrophy — *see* Exstrophy
Extroversion
bladder Q64.19
uterus N81.4
complicating delivery O71.2
postpartal (old) N81.4
Extruded tooth (teeth) M26.34
Extrusion
breast implant (prosthetic) T85.42
eye implant (globe) (ball) T85.328
intervertebral disc — *see* Displacement,
intervertebral disc
ocular lens implant (prosthetic) — *see*
Complications, intraocular lens
vitreous — *see* Prolapse, vitreous
Exudate
pleural — *see* Effusion, pleura
retina H35.89
Exudative — *see* condition
Eye, eyeball, eyelid — *see* condition
Eyestrain — *see* Disturbance, vision,
subjective
Eyeworm disease of Africa B74.3

F

**Faber's syndrome (achlorhydric
anemia)** D50.9
Fabry (-Anderson) disease E75.21
Faciocephalalgia, autonomic — *see
also* Neuropathy, peripheral,
autonomic G90.09
Factor (s)
psychic, associated with diseases classified
elsewhere F54
psychological
affecting physical conditions F54
or behavioral
affecting general medical condition F54
associated with disorders or diseases
classified elsewhere F54
Fahr disease (of brain) G23.8
Fahr Volhard disease (of kidney) I12.-
Failure, failed
abortion — *see* Abortion, attempted
aortic (valve) I35.8
rheumatic I06.8
attempted abortion — *see* Abortion,
attempted
biventricular I50.82
due to left heart failure I50.814
bone marrow — *see* Anemia, aplastic
cardiac — *see* Failure, heart
cardiorenal (chronic) — *see also* Failure,
renal, and Failure, heart I50.9
hypertensive I13.2
cardiorespiratory — *see also* Failure,
heart R09.2
cardiovascular (chronic) — *see* Failure, heart
cerebrovascular I67.9
cervical dilatation in labor O62.0
circulation, circulatory (peripheral) R57.9
newborn P29.89
compensation — *see* Disease, heart
compliance with medical treatment or
regimen — *see* Noncompliance
congestive — *see* Failure, heart, congestive
dental implant (endosseous) M27.69
due to
failure of dental prosthesis M27.63
lack of attached gingiva M27.62

Failure, failed - *continued*
  dental implant (endosseous) - *continued*
    due to - *continued*
      occlusal trauma (poor prosthetic
        design) M27.62
      parafunctional habits M27.62
      periodontal infection (peri-
        implantitis) M27.62
      poor oral hygiene M27.62
    osseointegration M27.61
      due to
        complications of systemic
          disease M27.61
        poor bone quality M27.61
      iatrogenic M27.61
    post-osseointegration
      biological M27.62
        due to complications of systemic
          disease M27.62
        iatrogenic M27.62
      mechanical M27.63
    pre-integration M27.61
    pre-osseointegration M27.61
    specified NEC M27.69
  descent of head (at term) of pregnancy
    (mother) O32.4
  endosseous dental implant — *see* Failure,
    dental implant
  engagement of head (term of pregnancy)
    (mother) O32.4
  erection (penile) — *see also* Dysfunction,
    sexual, male, erectile N52.9
    nonorganic F52.21
  examination (s) , anxiety concerning Z55.2
  expansion terminal respiratory units
    (newborn) (primary) P28.0
  forceps NOS (with subsequent cesarean
    delivery) O66.5
  gain weight (child over 28 days old) R62.51
    adult R62.7
    newborn P92.6
  genital response (male) F52.21
    female F52.22
  heart (acute) (senile) (sudden) I50.9
    with
      acute pulmonary edema — *see* Failure,
        ventricular, left
      decompensation — *see also* Failure,
        heart, by type as diastolic or
        systolic, acute and chronic I50.9
      dilatation — *see* Disease, heart
      hypertension — *see* Hypertension, heart
      normal ejection fraction — *see* Failure,
        heart, diastolic
      preserved ejection fraction — *see*
        Failure, heart, diastolic
      reduced ejection fraction — *see* Failure,
        heart, systolic
    arteriosclerotic I70.90
    biventricular I50.82
      due to left heart failure I50.814
    combined left-right sided I50.82
      due to left heart failure I50.814
    compensated — *see also* Failure, heart, by
      type as diastolic or systolic,
      chronic I50.9
    complicating
      anesthesia (general) (local) or other
        sedation
        in labor and delivery O74.2
        in pregnancy O29.12-
        postpartum, puerperal O89.1
      delivery (cesarean) (instrumental) O75.4
    congestive I50.9
      with rheumatic fever (conditions in I00)
        active I01.8
        inactive or quiescent (with
          chorea) I09.81
      newborn P29.0
      rheumatic (chronic) (inactive) (with
        chorea) I09.81
        active or acute I01.8
          with chorea I02.0

Failure, failed - *continued*
  heart (acute) (senile) (sudden) - *continued*
    decompensated — *see also* Failure, heart,
      by type as diastolic or systolic, acute
      and chronic I50.9
    degenerative — *see* Degeneration,
      myocardial
    diastolic (congestive) (left
      ventricular) I50.30
      acute (congestive) I50.31
        and (on) chronic (congestive) I50.33
      chronic (congestive) I50.32
        and (on) acute (congestive) I50.33
      combined with systolic
        (congestive) I50.40
        acute (congestive) I50.41
          and (on) chronic (congestive) I50.43
        chronic (congestive) I50.42
          and (on) acute (congestive) I50.43
    due to presence of cardiac
      prosthesis I97.13-
    end stage — *see also* Failure, heart, by
      type as diastolic or systolic,
      chronic I50.84
    following cardiac surgery I97.13-
    high output NOS I50.83
    hypertensive — *see* Hypertension, heart
    left (ventricular) — *see also* Failure,
      ventricular, left
      combined diastolic and systolic — *see*
        Failure, heart, diastolic, combined
        with systolic
      diastolic — *see* Failure, heart, diastolic
      systolic — *see* Failure, heart, systolic
    low output (syndrome) NOS I50.9
    newborn P29.0
    organic — *see* Disease, heart
    peripartum O90.3
    postprocedural I97.13-
    rheumatic (chronic) (inactive) I09.9
    right (isolated) (ventricular) I50.810
      acute I50.811
        and (on) chronic I50.813
      chronic I50.812
        and acute I50.813
      secondary to left heart failure I50.814
    specified NEC I50.89
    Note: heart failure stages A, B, C, and D are
      based on the American College of
      Cardiology and American Heart
      Association stages of heart failure,
      which complement and should not be
      confused with the New York Heart
      Association Classification of Heart
      Failure, into Class I, Class II, Class III,
      and Class IV
    stage A Z91.89
    stage B — *see also* Failure, heart, by type
      as diastolic or systolic I50.9
    stage C — *see also* Failure, heart, by type
      as diastolic or systolic I50.9
    stage D — *see also* Failure, heart, by type
      as diastolic or systolic, chronic I50.84
    systolic (congestive) (left
      ventricular) I50.20
      acute (congestive) I50.21
        and (on) chronic (congestive) I50.23
      chronic (congestive) I50.22
        and (on) acute (congestive) I50.23
      combined with diastolic
        (congestive) I50.40
        acute (congestive) I50.41
          and (on) chronic (congestive) I50.43
        chronic (congestive) I50.42
          and (on) acute (congestive) I50.43
    thyrotoxic — *see also*
      Thyrotoxicosis E05.90 *[143]*
      with
        high output — *see also*
          Thyrotoxicosis I50.83
        thyroid storm E05.91 *[143]*
          high output — *see also*
            Thyrotoxicosis I50.83
    valvular — *see* Endocarditis
  hepatic K72.90

Failure, failed - *continued*
  hepatic - *continued*
    with coma K72.91
    acute or subacute K72.00
      with coma K72.01
      due to drugs K71.10
        with coma K71.11
    alcoholic (acute) (chronic)
      (subacute) K70.40
      with coma K70.41
    chronic K72.10
      with coma K72.11
      due to drugs (acute) (subacute)
        (chronic) K71.10
        with coma K71.11
    due to drugs (acute) (subacute)
      (chronic) K71.10
      with coma K71.11
    postprocedural K91.82
  hepatorenal K76.7
  induction (of labor) O61.9
    abortion — *see* Abortion, attempted
    by
      oxytocic drugs O61.0
      prostaglandins O61.0
    instrumental O61.1
    mechanical O61.1
    medical O61.0
    specified NEC O61.8
    surgical O61.1
  intubation during anesthesia T88.4
    in pregnancy O29.6-
    labor and delivery O74.7
    postpartum, puerperal O89.6
  involution, thymus (gland) E32.0
  kidney — *see also* Disease, kidney,
    chronic N19
    acute — *see also* Failure, renal,
      acute N17.9-
    diabetic — *see* E08-E13 with .22
  lactation (complete) O92.3
    partial O92.4
  Leydig's cell, adult E29.1
  liver — *see* Failure, hepatic
  menstruation at puberty N91.0
  mitral I05.8
  myocardial, myocardium — *see also* Failure,
    heart I50.9
    chronic — *see also* Failure, heart,
      congestive I50.9
    congestive — *see also* Failure, heart,
      congestive I50.9
  orgasm (female) (psychogenic) F52.31
    male F52.32
  ovarian (primary) E28.39
    iatrogenic E89.40
      asymptomatic E89.40
      symptomatic E89.41
    postprocedural (postablative)
      (postirradiation) (postsurgical) E89.40
      asymptomatic E89.40
      symptomatic E89.41
  ovulation causing infertility N97.0
  polyglandular, autoimmune E31.0
  prosthetic joint implant — *see*
    Complications, joint prosthesis,
    mechanical, breakdown, by site
  renal N19
    with
      tubular necrosis (acute) N17.0
    acute N17.9
      with
        cortical necrosis N17.1
        medullary necrosis N17.2
        tubular necrosis N17.0
      specified NEC N17.8
    chronic N18.9
      hypertensive — *see* Hypertension,
        kidney
    congenital P96.0
    end stage (chronic) N18.6
      due to hypertension I12.0
    following

Failure, failed - *continued*
  renal - *continued*
    following - *continued*
      abortion — *see* Abortion by type
        complicated by specified condition
        NEC
      crushing T79.5
      ectopic or molar pregnancy O08.4
      labor and delivery (acute) O90.4
      hypertensive — *see* Hypertension, kidney
      postprocedural N99.0
  respiration, respiratory J96.90
    with
      hypercapnia J96.92
      hypercarbia J96.92
      hypoxia J96.91
    acute J96.00
      with
        hypercapnia J96.02
        hypercarbia J96.02
        hypoxia J96.01
    center G93.89
    acute and (on) chronic J96.20
      with
        hypercapnia J96.22
        hypercarbia J96.22
        hypoxia J96.21
    chronic J96.10
      with
        hypercapnia J96.12
        hypercarbia J96.12
        hypoxia J96.11
    newborn P28.5
    postprocedural (acute) J95.821
      acute and chronic J95.822
  rotation
    cecum Q43.3
    colon Q43.3
    intestine Q43.3
    kidney Q63.2
  sedation (conscious) (moderate) during
    procedure T88.52
    history of Z92.83
  segmentation — *see also* Fusion
    fingers — *see* Syndactylism, complex,
      fingers
    vertebra Q76.49
      with scoliosis Q76.3
  seminiferous tubule, adult E29.1
  senile (general) R54
  sexual arousal (male) F52.21
    female F52.22
  testicular endocrine function E29.1
  to thrive (child over 28 days old) R62.51
    adult R62.7
    newborn P92.6
  transplant T86.92
    bone T86.831
      marrow T86.02
    cornea T86.841
    heart T86.22
      with lung (s) T86.32
    intestine T86.851
    kidney T86.12
    liver T86.42
    lung (s) T86.811
      with heart T86.32
    pancreas T86.891
    skin (allograft) (autograft) T86.821
    specified organ or tissue NEC T86.891
    stem cell (peripheral blood) (umbilical
      cord) T86.5
  trial of labor (with subsequent cesarean
    delivery) O66.40
    following previous cesarean
      delivery O66.41
  tubal ligation N99.89
  urinary — *see* Disease, kidney, chronic
  vacuum extraction NOS (with subsequent
    cesarean delivery) O66.5
  vasectomy N99.89
  ventouse NOS (with subsequent cesarean
    delivery) O66.5
  ventricular — *see also* Failure, heart I50.9
    left — *see also* Failure, heart, left I50.1

Failure, failed - *continued*
  ventricular - *continued*
    left - *continued*
      with rheumatic fever (conditions in I00)
        active I01.8
          with chorea I02.0
        inactive or quiescent (with
          chorea) I09.81
      rheumatic (chronic) (inactive) (with
        chorea) I09.81
        active or acute I01.8
          with chorea I02.0
    right — *see* Failure, heart, right
    vital centers, newborn P91.88
Fainting (fit) R55
Fallen arches — *see* Deformity, limb, flat foot
Falling, falls (repeated) R29.6
  any organ or part — *see* Prolapse
Fallopian
  insufflation Z31.41
  tube — *see* condition
Fallot's
  pentalogy Q21.8
  tetrad or tetralogy Q21.3
  triad or trilogy Q22.3
False — *see also* condition
  croup J38.5
  joint — *see* Nonunion, fracture
  labor (pains) O47.9
    at or after 37 completed weeks of
      gestation O47.1
    before 37 completed weeks of
      gestation O47.0-
  passage, urethra (prostatic) N36.5
  pregnancy F45.8
Family, familial — *see also* condition
  disruption Z63.8
    involving divorce or separation Z63.5
  Li-Fraumeni (syndrome) Z15.01
  planning advice Z30.09
  problem Z63.9
    specified NEC Z63.8
  retinoblastoma C69.2-
Famine (effects of) T73.0
  edema — *see* Malnutrition, severe
Fanconi (-de Toni) (-Debré) syndrome
  E72.09
  with cystinosis E72.04
Fanconi's anemia (congenital
  pancytopenia) D61.09
Farber's disease or syndrome E75.29
Farcy A24.0
Farmer's
  lung J67.0
  skin L57.8
Farsightedness — *see* Hypermetropia
Fascia — *see* condition
Fasciculation R25.3
Fasciitis M72.9
  diffuse (eosinophilic) M35.4
  infective M72.8
    necrotizing M72.6
  necrotizing M72.6
  nodular M72.4
  perirenal (with ureteral obstruction) N13.5
    with infection N13.6
  plantar M72.2
  specified NEC M72.8
  traumatic (old) M72.8
    current - code by site under Sprain
Fascioliasis B66.3
Fasciolopsis, fasciolopsiasis (intestinal) B66.5
Fascioscapulohumeral myopathy G71.02
Fast pulse R00.0
Fat
  embolism — *see* Embolism, fat
  excessive — *see also* Obesity
    in heart — *see* Degeneration, myocardial
  in stool R19.5
  localized (pad) E65
    heart — *see* Degeneration, myocardial
    knee M79.4
    retropatellar M79.4
  necrosis
    breast N64.1

Fat - *continued*
  necrosis - *continued*
    mesentery K65.4
    omentum K65.4
    pad E65
    knee M79.4
Fatigue R53.83
  auditory deafness — *see* Deafness
  chronic R53.82
  combat F43.0
  general R53.83
    psychogenic F48.8
  heat (transient) T67.6
  muscle M62.89
  myocardium — *see* Failure, heart
  neoplasm-related R53.0
  nervous, neurosis F48.8
  operational F48.8
  psychogenic (general) F48.8
  senile R54
  voice R49.8
Fatness — *see* Obesity
Fatty — *see also* condition
  apron E65
  degeneration — *see* Degeneration, fatty
  heart (enlarged) — *see* Degeneration,
    myocardial
  liver NEC K76.0
    alcoholic K70.0
    nonalcoholic K76.0
  necrosis — *see* Degeneration, fatty
Fauces — *see* condition
Fauchard's disease (periodontitis) — *see*
  Periodontitis
Faucitis J02.9
Favism (anemia) D55.0
Favus — *see* Dermatophytosis
Fazio-Londe disease or syndrome G12.1
Fear complex or reaction F40.9
Fear of — *see* Phobia
Feared complaint unfounded Z71.1
Febris, febrile — *see also* Fever
  flava — *see also* Fever, yellow A95.9
  melitensis A23.0
  pestis — *see* Plague
  recurrens — *see* Fever, relapsing
  rubra A38.9
Fecal
  incontinence R15.9
  smearing R15.1
  soiling R15.1
  urgency R15.2
Fecalith (impaction) K56.41
  appendix K38.1
  congenital P76.8
Fede's disease K14.0
Feeble rapid pulse due to shock following
  injury T79.4
Feeble-minded F70
Feeding
  difficulties R63.3
  problem R63.3
    newborn P92.9
      specified NEC P92.8
    nonorganic (adult) — *see* Disorder, eating
Feeling (of)
  foreign body in throat R09.89
Feer's disease — *see* Poisoning, mercury
Feet — *see* condition
Feigned illness Z76.5
Feil-Klippel syndrome (brevicollis) Q76.1
Feinmesser's (hidrotic) ectodermal
  dysplasia Q82.4
Felinophobia F40.218
Felon — *see also* Cellulitis, digit
  with lymphangitis — *see* Lymphangitis,
    acute, digit
Felty's syndrome M05.00
  ankle M05.07-
  elbow M05.02-
  foot joint M05.07-
  hand joint M05.04-
  hip M05.05-
  knee M05.06-
  multiple site M05.09

Felty's syndrome - *continued*
  shoulder M05.01-
  vertebra — *see* Spondylitis, ankylosing
  wrist M05.03-
Female genital cutting status — *see* Female
    genital mutilation status (FGM)
Female genital mutilation status (FGM)
    N90.810
  specified NEC N90.818
  type I (clitorectomy status) N90.811
  type II (clitorectomy with excision of labia
    minora status) N90.812
  type III (infibulation status) N90.813
  type IV N90.818
Femur, femoral — *see* condition
Fenestration, fenestrated — *see also*
    Imperfect, closure
  aortico-pulmonary Q21.4
  cusps, heart valve NEC Q24.8
    pulmonary Q22.3
  pulmonic cusps Q22.3
Fernell's disease (aortic aneurysm) I71.9
Fertile eunuch syndrome E23.0
Fetid
  breath R19.6
  sweat L75.0
Fetishism F65.0
  transvestic F65.1
Fetus, fetal — *see also* condition
  alcohol syndrome (dysmorphic) Q86.0
  compressus O31.0-
  hydantoin syndrome Q86.1
  lung tissue P28.0
  papyraceous O31.0-
Fever (inanition) (of unknown origin)
    (persistent) (with chills) (with rigor)
    R50.9
  abortus A23.1
  Aden (dengue) A90
  African tick-borne A68.1
  American
    mountain (tick) A93.2
      spotted A77.0
  aphthous B08.8
  arbovirus, arboviral A94
    hemorrhagic A94
    specified NEC A93.8
  Argentinian hemorrhagic A96.0
  Assam B55.0
  Australian Q A78
  Bangkok hemorrhagic A91
  Barmah forest A92.8
  Bartonella A44.0
  bilious, hemoglobinuric B50.8
  blackwater B50.8
  blister B00.1
  Bolivian hemorrhagic A96.1
  Bonvale dam T73.3
  boutonneuse A77.1
  brain — *see* Encephalitis
  Brazilian purpuric A48.4
  breakbone A90
  Bullis A77.0
  Bunyamwera A92.8
  Burdwan B55.0
  Bwamba A92.8
  Cameroon — *see* Malaria
  Canton A75.9
  catarrhal (acute) J00
    chronic J31.0
  cat-scratch A28.1
  Central Asian hemorrhagic A98.0
  cerebral — *see* Encephalitis
  cerebrospinal meningococcal A39.0
  Chagres B50.9
  Chandipura A92.8
  Changuinola A93.1
  Charcot's (biliary) (hepatic) (intermittent) —
    see Calculus, bile duct
  Chikungunya (viral) (hemorrhagic) A92.0
  Chitral A93.1
  Colombo — *see* Fever, paratyphoid
  Colorado tick (virus) A93.2
  congestive (remittent) — *see* Malaria
  Congo virus A98.0

**Fever (inanition) (of unknown origin)
  (persistent) (with chills) (with rigor)** -
  continued
  continued malarial B50.9
  Corsican — *see* Malaria
  Crimean-Congo hemorrhagic A98.0
  Cyprus — *see* Brucellosis
  dandy A90
  deer fly — *see* Tularemia
  dengue (virus) A90
    hemorrhagic A91
    sandfly A93.1
  desert B38.0
  drug induced R50.2
  due to
    conditions classified elsewhere R50.81
    heat T67.01
  enteric A01.00
  enteroviral exanthematous (Boston
    exanthem) A88.0
  ephemeral (of unknown origin) R50.9
  epidemic hemorrhagic A98.5
  erysipelatous — *see* Erysipelas
  estivo-autumnal (malarial) B50.9
  famine A75.0
  five day A79.0
  following delivery O86.4
  Fort Bragg A27.89
  gastroenteric A01.00
  gastromalarial — *see* Malaria
  Gibraltar — *see* Brucellosis
  glandular — *see* Mononucleosis, infectious
  Guama (viral) A92.8
  Haverhill A25.1
  hay (allergic) J30.1
    with asthma (bronchial) J45.909
      with
        exacerbation (acute) J45.901
        status asthmaticus J45.902
    due to
      allergen other than pollen J30.89
      pollen, any plant or tree J30.1
  heat (effects) T67.01
  hematuric, bilious B50.8
  hemoglobinuric (malarial) (bilious) B50.8
  hemorrhagic (arthropod-borne) NOS A94
    with renal syndrome A98.5
    arenaviral A96.9
      specified NEC A96.8
    Argentinian A96.0
    Bangkok A91
    Bolivian A96.1
    Central Asian A98.0
    Chikungunya A92.0
    Crimean-Congo A98.0
    dengue (virus) A91
    epidemic A98.5
    Junin (virus) A96.0
    Korean A98.5
    Kyasanur forest A98.2
    Machupo (virus) A96.1
    mite-borne A93.8
    mosquito-borne A92.8
    Omsk A98.1
    Philippine A91
    Russian A98.5
    Singapore A91
    Southeast Asia A91
    Thailand A91
    tick-borne NEC A93.8
    viral A99
      specified NEC A98.8
  hepatic — *see* Cholecystitis
  herpetic — *see* Herpes
  icterohemorrhagic A27.0
  Indiana A93.8
  infective B99.9
    specified NEC B99.8
  intermittent (bilious) — *see also* Malaria
    of unknown origin R50.9
    pernicious B50.9
  iodide R50.2
  Japanese river A75.3
  jungle — *see also* Malaria
    yellow A95.0

**Fever (inanition) (of unknown origin)
  (persistent) (with chills) (with rigor)** -
  continued
  Junin (virus) hemorrhagic A96.0
  Katayama B65.2
  kedani A75.3
  Kenya (tick) A77.1
  Kew Garden A79.1
  Korean hemorrhagic A98.5
  Lassa A96.2
  Lone Star A77.0
  Machupo (virus) hemorrhagic A96.1
  malaria, malarial — *see* Malaria
  Malta A23.9
  Marseilles A77.1
  marsh — *see* Malaria
  Mayaro (viral) A92.8
  Mediterranean — *see also* Brucellosis A23.9
    familial M04.1
    tick A77.1
  meningeal — *see* Meningitis
  Meuse A79.0
  Mexican A75.2
  mianeh A68.1
  miasmatic — *see* Malaria
  mosquito-borne (viral) A92.9
    hemorrhagic A92.8
  mountain — *see also* Brucellosis
    meaning Rocky Mountain spotted
      fever A77.0
    tick (American) (Colorado) (viral) A93.2
  Mucambo (viral) A92.8
  mud A27.9
  Neapolitan — *see* Brucellosis
  neutropenic D70.9
  newborn P81.9
    environmental P81.0
  Nine-Mile A78
  non-exanthematous tick A93.2
  North Asian tick-borne A77.2
  Omsk hemorrhagic A98.1
  O'nyong-nyong (viral) A92.1
  Oropouche (viral) A93.0
  Oroya A44.0
  paludal — *see* Malaria
  Panama (malarial) B50.9
  Pappataci A93.1
  paratyphoid A01.4
    A A01.1
    B A01.2
    C A01.3
  parrot A70
  periodic (Mediterranean) M04.1
  persistent (of unknown origin) R50.9
  petechial A39.0
  pharyngoconjunctival B30.2
  Philippine hemorrhagic A91
  phlebotomus A93.1
  Piry (virus) A93.8
  Pixuna (viral) A92.8
  Plasmodium ovale B53.0
  polioviral (nonparalytic) A80.4
  Pontiac A48.2
  postimmunization R50.83
  postoperative R50.82
    due to infection T81.40
  posttransfusion R50.84
  postvaccination R50.83
  presenting with conditions classified
    elsewhere R50.81
  pretibial A27.89
  puerperal O86.4
  Q A78
  quadrilateral A78
  quartan (malaria) B52.9
  Queensland (coastal) (tick) A77.3
  quintan A79.0
  rabbit — *see* Tularemia
  rat-bite A25.9
    due to
      Spirillum A25.0
      Streptobacillus moniliformis A25.1
  recurrent — *see* Fever, relapsing
  relapsing (Borrelia) A68.9
    Carter's (Asiatic) A68.1

Fever (inanition) (of unknown origin) (persistent) (with chills) (with rigor) - *continued*
   relapsing (Borrelia) - *continued*
     Dutton's (West African) A68.1
     Koch's A68.9
     louse-borne A68.0
     Novy's
       louse-borne A68.0
       tick-borne A68.1
     Obermeyer's (European) A68.0
     tick-borne A68.1
   remittent (bilious) (congestive) (gastric) — *see* Malaria
   rheumatic (active) (acute) (chronic) (subacute) I00
     with central nervous system involvement I02.9
     active with heart involvement — *see* category I01
     inactive or quiescent with
       cardiac hypertrophy I09.89
       carditis I09.9
       endocarditis I09.1
         aortic (valve) I06.9
           with mitral (valve) disease I08.0
         mitral (valve) I05.9
           with aortic (valve) disease I08.0
         pulmonary (valve) I09.89
         tricuspid (valve) I07.8
       heart disease NEC I09.89
       heart failure (congestive) (conditions in category I50.) I09.81
       left ventricular failure (conditions in I50.1- I50.4-) I09.81
       myocarditis, myocardial degeneration (conditions in I51.4) I09.0
       pancarditis I09.9
       pericarditis I09.2
   Rift Valley (viral) A92.4
   Rocky Mountain spotted A77.0
   rose J30.1
   Ross River B33.1
   Russian hemorrhagic A98.5
   San Joaquin (Valley) B38.0
   sandfly A93.1
   Sao Paulo A77.0
   scarlet A38.9
   seven day (leptospirosis) (autumnal) (Japanese) A27.89
   dengue A90
   shin-bone A79.0
   Singapore hemorrhagic A91
   solar A90
   Songo A98.5
   sore B00.1
   South African tick-bite A68.1
   Southeast Asia hemorrhagic A91
   spinal — *see* Meningitis
   spirillary A25.0
   splenic — *see* Anthrax
   spotted A77.9
     American A77.0
     Brazilian A77.0
     cerebrospinal meningitis A39.0
     Colombian A77.0
     due to Rickettsia
       australis A77.3
       conorii A77.1
       rickettsii A77.0
       sibirica A77.2
       specified type NEC A77.8
     Ehrlichiosis A77.40
       due to
         E. chafeensis A77.41
         specified organism NEC A77.49
     Rocky Mountain A77.0
   steroid R50.2
   streptobacillary A25.1
   subtertian B50.9
   Sumatran mite A75.3
   sun A90
   swamp A27.9
   swine A02.8
   sylvatic, yellow A95.0

Fever (inanition) (of unknown origin) (persistent) (with chills) (with rigor) - *continued*
   Tahyna B33.8
   tertian — *see* Malaria, tertian
   Thailand hemorrhagic A91
   thermic T67.01
   three-day A93.1
   tick
     American mountain A93.2
     Colorado A93.2
     Kemerovo A93.8
     Mediterranean A77.1
     mountain A93.2
     nonexanthematous A93.2
     Quaranfil A93.8
   tick-bite NEC A93.8
   tick-borne (hemorrhagic) NEC A93.8
   trench A79.0
   tsutsugamushi A75.3
   typhogastric A01.00
   typhoid (abortive) (hemorrhagic) (intermittent) (malignant) A01.00
     complicated by
       arthritis A01.04
       heart involvement A01.02
       meningitis A01.01
       osteomyelitis A01.05
       pneumonia A01.03
       specified NEC A01.09
   typhomalarial — *see* Malaria
   typhus — *see* Typhus (fever)
   undulant — *see* Brucellosis
   unknown origin R50.9
   uveoparotid D86.89
   valley B38.0
   Venezuelan equine A92.2
   vesicular stomatitis A93.8
   viral hemorrhagic — *see* Fever, hemorrhagic, by type of virus
   Volhynian A79.0
   Wesselsbron (viral) A92.8
   West
     African B50.8
     Nile (viral) A92.30
       with
         complications NEC A92.39
         cranial nerve disorders A92.32
         encephalitis A92.31
         encephalomyelitis A92.31
         neurologic manifestation NEC A92.32
         optic neuritis A92.32
         polyradiculitis A92.32
   Whitmore's — *see* Melioidosis
   Wolhynian A79.0
   worm B83.9
   yellow A95.9
     jungle A95.0
     sylvatic A95.0
     urban A95.1
   Zika virus A92.5
Fibrillation
   atrial or auricular (established) I48.91
     chronic I48.20
       persistent I48.19
     paroxysmal I48.0
     permanent I48.21
     persistent (chronic) (NOS) (other) I48.19
       longstanding I48.11
   cardiac I49.8
   heart I49.8
   muscular M62.89
   ventricular I49.01
Fibrin
   ball or bodies, pleural (sac) J94.1
   chamber, anterior (eye) (gelatinous exudate) — *see* Iridocyclitis, acute
Fibrinogenolysis — *see* Fibrinolysis
Fibrinogenopenia D68.8
   acquired D65
   congenital D68.2
Fibrinolysis (hemorrhagic) (acquired) D65
   antepartum hemorrhage — *see* Hemorrhage, antepartum, with coagulation defect
   following

Fibrinolysis (hemorrhagic) (acquired) - *continued*
   following - *continued*
     abortion — *see* Abortion by type
       complicated by hemorrhage
     ectopic or molar pregnancy O08.1
   intrapartum O67.0
   newborn, transient P60
   postpartum O72.3
Fibrinopenia (hereditary) D68.2
   acquired D68.4
Fibrinopurulent — *see* condition
Fibrinous — *see* condition
Fibroadenoma
   cellular intracanalicular D24-
   giant D24-
   intracanalicular
     cellular D24-
     giant D24-
     specified site — *see* Neoplasm, benign, by site
     unspecified site D24-
   juvenile D24-
   pericanalicular
     specified site — *see* Neoplasm, benign, by site
     unspecified site D24-
   phyllodes D24-
   prostate D29.1
   specified site NEC — *see* Neoplasm, benign, by site
   unspecified site D24-
Fibroadenosis, breast (chronic) (cystic) (diffuse) (periodic) (segmental) N60.2-
Fibroangioma — *see also* Neoplasm, benign, by site
   juvenile
     specified site — *see* Neoplasm, benign, by site
     unspecified site D10.6
Fibrochondrosarcoma — *see* Neoplasm, cartilage, malignant
Fibrocystic
   disease — *see also* Fibrosis, cystic
     breast — *see* Mastopathy, cystic
     jaw M27.49
     kidney (congenital) Q61.8
     liver Q44.6
     pancreas E84.9
   kidney (congenital) Q61.8
Fibrodysplasia ossificans progressiva — *see* Myositis, ossificans, progressiva
Fibroelastosis (cordis) (endocardial) (endomyocardial) I42.4
Fibroid (tumor) — *see also* Neoplasm, connective tissue, benign
   disease, lung (chronic) — *see* Fibrosis, lung
   heart (disease) — *see* Myocarditis
   in pregnancy or childbirth O34.1-
     causing obstructed labor O65.5
   induration, lung (chronic) — *see* Fibrosis, lung
   lung — *see* Fibrosis, lung
   pneumonia (chronic) — *see* Fibrosis, lung
   uterus — *see also* Leiomyoma, uterus D25.9
Fibrolipoma — *see* Lipoma
Fibroliposarcoma — *see* Neoplasm, connective tissue, malignant
Fibroma — *see also* Neoplasm, connective tissue, benign
   ameloblastic — *see* Cyst, calcifying odontogenic
   bone (nonossifying) — *see* Disorder, bone, specified type NEC
   ossifying — *see* Neoplasm, bone, benign
   cementifying — *see* Neoplasm, bone, benign
   chondromyxoid — *see* Neoplasm, bone, benign
   desmoplastic — *see* Neoplasm, connective tissue, uncertain behavior
   durum — *see* Neoplasm, connective tissue, benign
   fascial — *see* Neoplasm, connective tissue, benign

Fibroma - *continued*
  invasive — *see* Neoplasm, connective tissue, uncertain behavior
  molle — *see* Lipoma
  myxoid — *see* Neoplasm, connective tissue, benign
  nasopharynx, nasopharyngeal (juvenile) D10.6
  nonosteogenic (nonossifying) — *see* Dysplasia, fibrous
  odontogenic (central) — *see* Cyst, calcifying odontogenic
  ossifying — *see* Neoplasm, bone, benign
  periosteal — *see* Neoplasm, bone, benign
  soft — *see* Lipoma
Fibromatosis M72.9
  abdominal — *see* Neoplasm, connective tissue, uncertain behavior
  aggressive — *see* Neoplasm, connective tissue, uncertain behavior
  congenital generalized — *see* Neoplasm, connective tissue, uncertain behavior
  Dupuytren's M72.0
  gingival K06.1
  palmar (fascial) M72.0
  plantar (fascial) M72.2
  pseudosarcomatous (proliferative) (subcutaneous) M72.4
  retroperitoneal D48.3
  specified NEC M72.8
Fibromyalgia M79.7
Fibromyoma — *see also* Neoplasm, connective tissue, benign
  uterus (corpus) — *see also* Leiomyoma, uterus
    in pregnancy or childbirth — *see* Fibroid, in pregnancy or childbirth
      causing obstructed labor O65.5
Fibromyositis M79.7
Fibromyxolipoma D17.9
Fibromyxoma — *see* Neoplasm, connective tissue, benign
Fibromyxosarcoma — *see* Neoplasm, connective tissue, malignant
Fibro-odontoma, ameloblastic — *see* Cyst, calcifying odontogenic
Fibro-osteoma — *see* Neoplasm, bone, benign
Fibroplasia, retrolental H35.17-
Fibropurulent — *see* condition
Fibrosarcoma — *see also* Neoplasm, connective tissue, malignant
  ameloblastic C41.1
    upper jaw (bone) C41.0
  congenital — *see* Neoplasm, connective tissue, malignant
  fascial — *see* Neoplasm, connective tissue, malignant
  infantile — *see* Neoplasm, connective tissue, malignant
  odontogenic C41.1
    upper jaw (bone) C41.0
  periosteal — *see* Neoplasm, bone, malignant
Fibrosclerosis
  breast N60.3-
  multifocal M35.5
  penis (corpora cavernosa) N48.6
Fibrosis, fibrotic
  adrenal (gland) E27.8
  amnion O41.8X-
  anal papillae K62.89
  arteriocapillary — *see* Arteriosclerosis
  bladder N32.89
    interstitial — *see* Cystitis, chronic, interstitial
    localized submucosal — *see* Cystitis, chronic, interstitial
    panmural — *see* Cystitis, chronic, interstitial
  breast — *see* Fibrosclerosis, breast
  capillary — *see also* Arteriosclerosis I70.90
    lung (chronic) — *see* Fibrosis, lung
  cardiac — *see* Myocarditis
  cervix N88.8
  chorion O41.8X-
  corpus cavernosum (sclerosing) N48.6

Fibrosis, fibrotic - *continued*
  cystic (of pancreas) E84.9
    with
      distal intestinal obstruction syndrome E84.19
      fecal impaction E84.19
      intestinal manifestations NEC E84.19
      pulmonary manifestations E84.0
      specified manifestations NEC E84.8
  due to device, implant or graft — *see also* Complications, by site and type, specified NEC T85.828
    arterial graft NEC T82.828
    breast (implant) T85.828
    catheter NEC T85.828
      dialysis (renal) T82.828
        intraperitoneal T85.828
      infusion NEC T82.828
        spinal (epidural) (subdural) T85.820
      urinary (indwelling) T83.82
    electronic (electrode) (pulse generator) (stimulator)
      bone T84.82
      cardiac T82.827
      nervous system (brain) (peripheral nerve) (spinal) T85.820
      urinary T83.82
    fixation, internal (orthopedic) NEC T84.82
    gastrointestinal (bile duct) (esophagus) T85.828
    genital NEC T83.82
    heart NEC T82.827
    joint prosthesis T84.82
    ocular (corneal graft) (orbital implant) NEC T85.828
    orthopedic NEC T84.82
    specified NEC T85.828
    urinary NEC T83.82
    vascular NEC T82.828
    ventricular intracranial shunt T85.820
  ejaculatory duct N50.89
  endocardium — *see* Endocarditis
  endomyocardial (tropical) I42.3
  epididymis N50.89
  eye muscle — *see* Strabismus, mechanical
  heart — *see* Myocarditis
  hepatic — *see* Fibrosis, liver
  hepatolienal (portal hypertension) K76.6
  hepatosplenic (portal hypertension) K76.6
  infrapatellar fat pad M79.4
  intrascrotal N50.89
  kidney N26.9
  liver K74.0
    with sclerosis K74.2
    alcoholic K70.2
  lung (atrophic) (chronic) (confluent) (massive) (perialveolar) (peribronchial) J84.10
    with
      anthracosilicosis J60
      anthracosis J60
      asbestosis J61
      bagassosis J67.1
      bauxite J63.1
      berylliosis J63.2
      byssinosis J66.0
      calcicosis J62.8
      chalicosis J62.8
      dust reticulation J64
      farmer's lung J67.0
      ganister disease J62.8
      graphite J63.3
      pneumoconiosis NOS J64
      siderosis J63.4
      silicosis J62.8
    capillary J84.10
    congenital P27.8
    diffuse (idiopathic) J84.10
      chemicals, gases, fumes or vapors (inhalation) J68.4
      interstitial J84.10
        acute J84.114
      talc J62.0
    following radiation J70.1
    idiopathic J84.112

Fibrosis, fibrotic - *continued*
  lung (atrophic) (chronic) (confluent) (massive) (perialveolar) (peribronchial) - *continued*
    postinflammatory J84.10
    silicotic J62.8
    tuberculous — *see* Tuberculosis, pulmonary
  lymphatic gland I89.8
  median bar — *see* Hyperplasia, prostate
  mediastinum (idiopathic) J98.59
  meninges G96.19
  myocardium, myocardial — *see* Myocarditis
  ovary N83.8
  oviduct N83.8
  pancreas K86.89
  penis NEC N48.6
  pericardium I31.0
  perineum, in pregnancy or childbirth O34.7-
    causing obstructed labor O65.5
  pleura J94.1
  popliteal fat pad M79.4
  prostate (chronic) — *see* Hyperplasia, prostate
  pulmonary — *see also* Fibrosis, lung J84.10
    congenital P27.8
    idiopathic J84.112
  rectal sphincter K62.89
  retroperitoneal, idiopathic (with ureteral obstruction) N13.5
    with infection N13.6
  sclerosing mesenteric (idiopathic) K65.4
  scrotum N50.89
  seminal vesicle N50.89
  senile R54
  skin L90.5
  spermatic cord N50.89
  spleen D73.89
    in schistosomiasis (bilharziasis) B65.9 *[D77]*
  subepidermal nodular — *see* Neoplasm, skin, benign
  submucous (oral) (tongue) K13.5
  testis N44.8
    chronic, due to syphilis A52.76
  thymus (gland) E32.8
  tongue, submucous K13.5
  tunica vaginalis N50.89
  uterus (non-neoplastic) N85.8
  vagina N89.8
  valve, heart — *see* Endocarditis
  vas deferens N50.89
  vein I87.8
Fibrositis (periarticular) M79.7
  nodular, chronic (Jaccoud's) (rheumatoid) — *see* Arthropathy, postrheumatic, chronic
Fibrothorax J94.1
Fibrotic — *see* Fibrosis
Fibrous — *see* condition
Fibroxanthoma — *see also* Neoplasm, connective tissue, benign
  atypical — *see* Neoplasm, connective tissue, uncertain behavior
  malignant — *see* Neoplasm, connective tissue, malignant
Fibroxanthosarcoma — *see* Neoplasm, connective tissue, malignant
Fiedler's
  disease (icterohemorrhagic leptospirosis) A27.0
  myocarditis (acute) I40.1
Fifth disease B08.3
  venereal A55
Filaria, filarial, filariasis — *see* Infestation, filarial
Filatov's disease — *see* Mononucleosis, infectious
File-cutter's disease — *see* Poisoning, lead
Filling defect
  biliary tract R93.2
  bladder R93.41
  duodenum R93.3
  gallbladder R93.2
  gastrointestinal tract R93.3
  intestine R93.3

Filling defect - *continued*
  kidney R93.42-
  stomach R93.3
  ureter R93.41
  urinary organs, specified NEC R93.49
Fimbrial cyst Q50.4
Financial problem affecting care NOS Z59.9
  bankruptcy Z59.8
  foreclosure on loan Z59.8
Findings, abnormal, inconclusive, without diagnosis — *see also* Abnormal
  17-ketosteroids, elevated R82.5
  acetonuria R82.4
  alcohol in blood R78.0
  anisocytosis R71.8
  antenatal screening of mother O28.9
    biochemical O28.1
    chromosomal O28.5
    cytological O28.2
    genetic O28.5
    hematological O28.0
    radiological O28.4
    specified NEC O28.8
    ultrasonic O28.3
  antibody titer, elevated R76.0
  anticardiolipin antibody R76.0
  antiphosphatidylglycerol antibody R76.0
  antiphosphatidylinositol antibody R76.0
  antiphosphatidylserine antibody R76.0
  antiphospholipid antibody R76.0
  bacteriuria R82.71
  bicarbonate E87.8
  bile in urine R82.2
  blood sugar R73.09
    high R73.9
    low (transient) E16.2
  body fluid or substance, specified NEC R88.8
  casts, urine R82.998
  catecholamines R82.5
  cells, urine R82.998
  chloride E87.8
  cholesterol E78.9
    high E78.00
      with high triglycerides E78.2
  chyluria R82.0
  cloudy
    dialysis effluent R88.0
    urine R82.90
  creatinine clearance R94.4
  crystals, urine R82.998
  culture
    blood R78.81
    positive — *see* Positive, culture
  echocardiogram R93.1
  electrolyte level, urinary R82.998
  function study NEC R94.8
    bladder R94.8
    endocrine NEC R94.7
      thyroid R94.6
    kidney R94.4
    liver R94.5
    pancreas R94.8
    placenta R94.8
    pulmonary R94.2
    spleen R94.8
  gallbladder, nonvisualization R93.2
  glucose (tolerance test) (non-fasting) R73.09
  glycosuria R81
  heart
    shadow R93.1
    sounds R01.2
  hematinuria R82.3
  hematocrit drop (precipitous) R71.0
  hemoglobinuria R82.3
  human papillomavirus (HPV) DNA test positive
    cervix
      high risk R87.810
      low risk R87.820
    vagina
      high risk R87.811
      low risk R87.821
  in blood (of substance not normally found in blood) R78.9

Findings, abnormal, inconclusive, without diagnosis - *continued*
  in blood (of substance not normally found in blood) - *continued*
    addictive drug NEC R78.4
    alcohol (excessive level) R78.0
    cocaine R78.2
    hallucinogen R78.3
    heavy metals (abnormal level) R78.79
    lead R78.71
    lithium (abnormal level) R78.89
    opiate drug R78.1
    psychotropic drug R78.5
    specified substance NEC R78.89
    steroid agent R78.6
  indoleacetic acid, elevated R82.5
  ketonuria R82.4
  lactic acid dehydrogenase (LDH) R74.0
  liver function test R79.89
  mammogram NEC R92.8
    calcification (calculus) R92.1
    inconclusive result (due to dense breasts) R92.2
    microcalcification R92.0
  mediastinal shift R93.89
  melanin, urine R82.998
  myoglobinuria R82.1
  neonatal screening P09
  nonvisualization of gallbladder R93.2
  odor of urine NOS R82.90
  Papanicolaou cervix R87.619
    non-atypical endometrial cells R87.618
  pneumoencephalogram R93.0
  poikilocytosis R71.8
  potassium (deficiency) E87.6
    excess E87.5
  PPD R76.11
  radiologic (X-ray) R93.89
    abdomen R93.5
    biliary tract R93.2
    breast R92.8
    gastrointestinal tract R93.3
    genitourinary organs R93.89
    head R93.0
    inconclusive due to excess body fat of patient R93.9
    intrathoracic organs NEC R93.1
    musculoskeletal
      limbs R93.6
      other than limb R93.7
    placenta R93.89
    retroperitoneum R93.5
    skin R93.89
    skull R93.0
    subcutaneous tissue R93.89
    testis R93.81-
  red blood cell (count) (morphology) (sickling) (volume) R71.8
  scan NEC R94.8
    bladder R94.8
    bone R94.8
    kidney R94.4
    liver R93.2
    lung R94.2
    pancreas R94.8
    placental R94.8
    spleen R94.8
    thyroid R94.6
  sedimentation rate, elevated R70.0
  SGOT R74.0
  SGPT R74.0
  sodium (deficiency) E87.1
    excess E87.0
  specified body fluid NEC R88.8
  stress test R94.39
  thyroid (function) (metabolic rate) (scan) (uptake) R94.6
  transaminase (level) R74.0
  triglycerides E78.9
    high E78.1
      with high cholesterol E78.2
  tuberculin skin test (without active tuberculosis) R76.11
  urine R82.90
    acetone R82.4

Findings, abnormal, inconclusive, without diagnosis - *continued*
  urine - *continued*
    bacteria R82.71
    bile R82.2
    casts or cells R82.998
    chyle R82.0
    culture positive R82.79
    glucose R81
    hemoglobin R82.3
    ketone R82.4
    sugar R81
  vanillylmandelic acid (VMA) , elevated R82.5
  vectorcardiogram (VCG) R94.39
  ventriculogram R93.0
  white blood cell (count) (differential) (morphology) D72.9
  xerography R92.8
Finger — *see* condition
Fire, Saint Anthony's — *see* Erysipelas
Fire-setting
  pathological (compulsive) F63.1
Fish hook stomach K31.89
Fishmeal-worker's lung J67.8
Fissure, fissured
  anus, anal K60.2
    acute K60.0
    chronic K60.1
    congenital Q43.8
  ear, lobule, congenital Q17.8
  epiglottis (congenital) Q31.8
  larynx J38.7
    congenital Q31.8
  lip K13.0
    congenital — *see* Cleft, lip
  nipple N64.0
    associated with
      lactation O92.13
      pregnancy O92.11-
      puerperium O92.12
  nose Q30.2
  palate (congenital) — *see* Cleft, palate
  skin R23.4
  spine (congenital) — *see also* Spina bifida
    with hydrocephalus — *see* Spina bifida, by site, with hydrocephalus
  tongue (acquired) K14.5
    congenital Q38.3
Fistula (cutaneous) L98.8
  abdomen (wall) K63.2
    bladder N32.2
    intestine NEC K63.2
    ureter N28.89
    uterus N82.5
  abdominorectal K63.2
  abdominosigmoidal K63.2
  abdominothoracic J86.0
  abdominouterine N82.5
    congenital Q51.7
  abdominovesical N32.2
  accessory sinuses — *see* Sinusitis
  actinomycotic — *see* Actinomycosis
  alveolar antrum — *see* Sinusitis, maxillary
  alveolar process K04.6
  anorectal K60.5
  antrobuccal — *see* Sinusitis, maxillary
  antrum — *see* Sinusitis, maxillary
  anus, anal (recurrent) (infectional) K60.3
    congenital Q43.6
      with absence, atresia and stenosis Q42.2
    tuberculous A18.32
  aorta-duodenal I77.2
  appendix, appendicular K38.3
  arteriovenous (acquired) (nonruptured) I77.0
    brain I67.1
      congenital Q28.2
        ruptured — *see* Fistula, arteriovenous, brain, ruptured
      ruptured I60.8
        intracerebral I61.8
        intraparenchymal I61.8
        intraventricular I61.5
        subarachnoid I60.8

Fistula (cutaneous) - *continued*
arteriovenous (acquired) (nonruptured) -
continued
cerebral — *see* Fistula, arteriovenous,
brain
congenital (peripheral) — *see also*
Malformation, arteriovenous
brain Q28.2
ruptured — *see* Fistula, arteriovenous,
brain, ruptured
coronary Q24.5
pulmonary Q25.72
coronary I25.41
congenital Q24.5
pulmonary I28.0
congenital Q25.72
surgically created (for dialysis) Z99.2
complication — *see* Complication,
arteriovenous, fistula, surgically
created
traumatic — *see* Injury, blood vessel
artery I77.2
aural (mastoid) — *see* Mastoiditis, chronic
auricle — *see also* Disorder, pinna, specified
type NEC
congenital Q18.1
Bartholin's gland N82.8
bile duct (common) (hepatic) K83.3
with calculus, stones — *see* Calculus, bile
duct
biliary (tract) — *see* Fistula, bile duct
bladder (sphincter) NEC — *see also* Fistula,
vesico- N32.2
into seminal vesicle N32.2
bone — *see also* Disorder, bone, specified
type NEC
with osteomyelitis, chronic — *see*
Osteomyelitis, chronic, with draining
sinus
brain G93.89
arteriovenous (acquired) — *see also*
Fistula, arteriovenous, brain I67.1
congenital Q28.2
branchial (cleft) Q18.0
branchiogenous Q18.0
breast N61.0
puerperal, postpartum or gestational, due
to mastitis (purulent) — *see* Mastitis,
obstetric, purulent
bronchial J86.0
bronchocutaneous, bronchomediastinal,
bronchopleural,
bronchopleuromediastinal
(infective) J86.0
tuberculous NEC A15.5
bronchoesophageal J86.0
congenital Q39.2
with atresia of esophagus Q39.1
bronchovisceral J86.0
buccal cavity (infective) K12.2
cecosigmoidal K63.2
cecum K63.2
cerebrospinal (fluid) G96.0
cervical, lateral Q18.1
cervicoaural Q18.1
cervicosigmoidal N82.4
cervicovesical N82.1
cervix N82.8
chest (wall) J86.0
cholecystenteric — *see* Fistula, gallbladder
cholecystocolic — *see* Fistula, gallbladder
cholecystocolonic — *see* Fistula, gallbladder
cholecystoduodenal — *see* Fistula,
gallbladder
cholecystogastric — *see* Fistula, gallbladder
cholecystointestinal — *see* Fistula,
gallbladder
choledochoduodenal — *see* Fistula, bile duct
cholocolic K82.3
coccyx — *see* Sinus, pilonidal
colon K63.2
colostomy K94.09
colovesical N32.1
common duct — *see* Fistula, bile duct

Fistula (cutaneous) - *continued*
congenital, site not listed — *see* Anomaly, by
site
coronary, arteriovenous I25.41
congenital Q24.5
costal region J86.0
cul-de-sac, Douglas' N82.8
cystic duct — *see also* Fistula, gallbladder
congenital Q44.5
dental K04.6
diaphragm J86.0
duodenum K31.6
ear (external) (canal) — *see* Disorder, ear,
external, specified type NEC
enterocolic K63.2
enterocutaneous K63.2
enterouterine N82.4
congenital Q51.7
enterovaginal N82.4
congenital Q52.2
large intestine N82.3
small intestine N82.2
enterovesical N32.1
epididymis N50.89
tuberculous A18.15
esophagobronchial J86.0
congenital Q39.2
with atresia of esophagus Q39.1
esophagocutaneous K22.8
esophagopleural-cutaneous J86.0
esophagotracheal J86.0
congenital Q39.2
with atresia of esophagus Q39.1
esophagus K22.8
congenital Q39.2
with atresia of esophagus Q39.1
ethmoid — *see* Sinusitis, ethmoidal
eyeball (cornea) (sclera) — *see* Disorder,
globe, hypotony
eyelid H01.8
fallopian tube, external N82.5
fecal K63.2
congenital Q43.6
from periapical abscess K04.6
frontal sinus — *see* Sinusitis, frontal
gallbladder K82.3
with calculus, cholelithiasis, stones — *see*
Calculus, gallbladder
gastric K31.6
gastrocolic K31.6
congenital Q40.2
tuberculous A18.32
gastroenterocolic K31.6
gastroesophageal K31.6
gastrojejunal K31.6
gastrojejunocolic K31.6
genital tract (female) N82.9
specified NEC N82.8
to intestine NEC N82.4
to skin N82.5
hepatic artery-portal vein, congenital Q26.6
hepatopleural J86.0
hepatopulmonary J86.0
ileorectal or ileosigmoidal K63.2
ileovaginal N82.2
ileovesical N32.1
ileum K63.2
in ano K60.3
tuberculous A18.32
inner ear (labyrinth) — *see* subcategory
H83.1
intestine NEC K63.2
intestinocolonic (abdominal) K63.2
intestinoureteral N28.89
intestinouterine N82.4
intestinovaginal N82.4
large intestine N82.3
small intestine N82.2
intestinovesical N32.1
ischiorectal (fossa) K61.39
jejunum K63.2
joint M25.10
ankle M25.17-
elbow M25.12-
foot joint M25.17-

Fistula (cutaneous) - *continued*
joint - *continued*
hand joint M25.14-
hip M25.15-
knee M25.16-
shoulder M25.11-
specified joint NEC M25.18
tuberculous — *see* Tuberculosis, joint
vertebrae M25.18
wrist M25.13-
kidney N28.89
labium (majus) (minus) N82.8
labyrinth — *see* subcategory H83.1
lacrimal (gland) (sac) H04.61-
lacrimonasal duct — *see* Fistula, lacrimal
laryngotracheal, congenital Q34.8
larynx J38.7
lip K13.0
congenital Q38.0
lumbar, tuberculous A18.01
lung J86.0
lymphatic I89.8
mammary (gland) N61.0
mastoid (process) (region) — *see*
Mastoiditis, chronic
maxillary J32.0
medial, face and neck Q18.8
mediastinal J86.0
mediastinobronchial J86.0
mediastinocutaneous J86.0
middle ear — *see* subcategory H74.8
mouth K12.2
nasal J34.89
sinus — *see* Sinusitis
nasopharynx J39.2
nipple N64.0
nose J34.89
oral (cutaneous) K12.2
maxillary J32.0
nasal (with cleft palate) — *see* Cleft, palate
orbit, orbital — *see* Disorder, orbit, specified
type NEC
oroantral J32.0
oviduct, external N82.5
palate (hard) M27.8
pancreatic K86.89
pancreaticoduodenal K86.89
parotid (gland) K11.4
region K12.2
penis N48.89
perianal K60.3
pericardium (pleura) (sac) — *see* Pericarditis
pericecal K63.2
perineorectal K60.4
perineosigmoidal K63.2
perineum, perineal (with urethral
involvement) NEC N36.0
tuberculous A18.13
ureter N28.89
perirectal K60.4
tuberculous A18.32
peritoneum K65.9
pharyngoesophageal J39.2
pharynx J39.2
branchial cleft (congenital) Q18.0
pilonidal (infected) (rectum) — *see* Sinus,
pilonidal
pleura, pleural, pleurocutaneous,
pleuroperitoneal J86.0
tuberculous NEC A15.6
pleuropericardial I31.8
portal vein-hepatic artery, congenital Q26.6
postauricular H70.81-
postoperative, persistent T81.83
specified site — *see* Fistula, by site
preauricular (congenital) Q18.1
prostate N42.89
pulmonary J86.0
arteriovenous I28.0
congenital Q25.72
tuberculous — *see* Tuberculosis,
pulmonary
pulmonoperitoneal J86.0
rectolabial N82.4
rectosigmoid (intercommunicating) K63.2

Fistula (cutaneous) - *continued*
  rectoureteral N28.89
  rectourethral N36.0
    congenital Q64.73
  rectouterine N82.4
    congenital Q51.7
  rectovaginal N82.3
    congenital Q52.2
    tuberculous A18.18
  rectovesical N32.1
    congenital Q64.79
  rectovesicovaginal N82.3
  rectovulval N82.4
    congenital Q52.79
  rectum (to skin) K60.4
    congenital Q43.6
      with absence, atresia and stenosis Q42.0
    tuberculous A18.32
  renal N28.89
  retroauricular — *see* Fistula, postauricular
  salivary duct or gland (any) K11.4
    congenital Q38.4
  scrotum (urinary) N50.89
    tuberculous A18.15
  semicircular canals — *see* subcategory H83.1
  sigmoid K63.2
    to bladder N32.1
  sinus — *see* Sinusitis
  skin L98.8
    to genital tract (female) N82.5
  splenocolic D73.89
  stercoral K63.2
  stomach K31.6
  sublingual gland K11.4
  submandibular gland K11.4
  submaxillary (gland) K11.4
    region K12.2
  thoracic J86.0
    duct I89.8
  thoracoabdominal J86.0
  thoracogastric J86.0
  thoracointestinal J86.0
  thorax J86.0
  thyroglossal duct Q89.2
  thyroid E07.89
  trachea, congenital (external) (internal) Q32.1
  tracheoesophageal J86.0
    congenital Q39.2
      with atresia of esophagus Q39.1
    following tracheostomy J95.04
  traumatic arteriovenous — *see* Injury, blood vessel, by site
  tuberculous - code by site under Tuberculosis
  typhoid A01.09
  umbilicourinary Q64.8
  urachus, congenital Q64.4
  ureter (persistent) N28.89
  ureteroabdominal N28.89
  ureterorectal N28.89
  ureterosigmoido-abdominal N28.89
  ureterovaginal N82.1
  ureterovesical N32.2
  urethra N36.0
    congenital Q64.79
    tuberculous A18.13
  urethroperineal N36.0
  urethroperineovesical N32.2
  urethrorectal N36.0
    congenital Q64.73
  urethroscrotal N50.89
  urethrovaginal N82.1
  urethrovesical N32.2
  urinary (tract) (persistent) (recurrent) N36.0
  uteroabdominal N82.5
    congenital Q51.7
  uteroenteric, uterointestinal N82.4
    congenital Q51.7
  uterorectal N82.4
    congenital Q51.7
  uteroureteric N82.1
  uterourethral Q51.7
  uterovaginal N82.8
  uterovesical N82.1
    congenital Q51.7

Fistula (cutaneous) - *continued*
  uterus N82.8
  vagina (postpartal) (wall) N82.8
  vaginocutaneous (postpartal) N82.5
  vaginointestinal NEC N82.4
    large intestine N82.3
    small intestine N82.2
  vaginoperineal N82.5
  vasocutaneous, congenital Q55.7
  vesical NEC N32.2
  vesicoabdominal N32.2
  vesicocervicovaginal N82.1
  vesicocolic N32.1
  vesicocutaneous N32.2
  vesicoenteric N32.1
  vesicointestinal N32.1
  vesicometrorectal N82.4
  vesicoperineal N32.2
  vesicorectal N32.1
    congenital Q64.79
  vesicosigmoidal N32.1
  vesicosigmoidovaginal N82.3
  vesicoureteral N32.2
  vesicoureterovaginal N82.1
  vesicourethral N32.2
  vesicourethrorectal N32.1
  vesicouterine N82.1
    congenital Q51.7
  vesicovaginal N82.0
  vulvorectal N82.4
    congenital Q52.79
Fit R56.9
  epileptic — *see* Epilepsy
  fainting R55
  hysterical F44.5
  newborn P90
Fitting (and adjustment) (of)
  artificial
    arm — *see* Admission, adjustment, artificial, arm
    breast Z44.3
    eye Z44.2
    leg — *see* Admission, adjustment, artificial, leg
  automatic implantable cardiac defibrillator (with synchronous cardiac pacemaker) Z45.02
  brain neuropacemaker Z46.2
    implanted Z45.42
  cardiac defibrillator — *see* Fitting (and adjustment) (of), automatic implantable cardiac defibrillator
  catheter, non-vascular Z46.82
  colostomy belt Z46.89
  contact lenses Z46.0
  CRT-D (resynchronization therapy defibrillator) Z45.02
  CRT-P (cardiac resynchronization therapy pacemaker) Z45.018
    pulse generator Z45.010
  cystostomy device Z46.6
  defibrillator, cardiac — *see* Fitting (and adjustment) (of), automatic implantable cardiac defibrillator
  dentures Z46.3
  device NOS Z46.9
    abdominal Z46.89
    gastrointestinal NEC Z46.59
    implanted NEC Z45.89
    nervous system Z46.2
      implanted — *see* Admission, adjustment, device, implanted, nervous system
    orthodontic Z46.4
    orthoptic Z46.0
    orthotic Z46.89
    prosthetic (external) Z44.9
      breast Z44.3
      dental Z46.3
      eye Z44.2
      specified NEC Z44.8
    specified NEC Z46.89
    substitution
      auditory Z46.2

Fitting (and adjustment) (of) - *continued*
  device NOS - *continued*
    substitution - *continued*
      auditory - *continued*
        implanted — *see* Admission, adjustment, device, implanted, hearing device
        nervous system Z46.2
          implanted — *see* Admission, adjustment, device, implanted, nervous system
        visual Z46.2
          implanted Z45.31
        urinary Z46.6
  gastric lap band Z46.51
  gastrointestinal appliance NEC Z46.59
  glasses (reading) Z46.0
  hearing aid Z46.1
  ileostomy device Z46.89
  insulin pump Z46.81
  intestinal appliance NEC Z46.89
  myringotomy device (stent) (tube) Z45.82
  neuropacemaker Z46.2
    implanted Z45.42
  non-vascular catheter Z46.82
  orthodontic device Z46.4
  orthopedic device (brace) (cast) (corset) (shoes) Z46.89
  pacemaker (cardiac) (cardiac resynchronization therapy (CRT-P)) Z45.018
    nervous system (brain) (peripheral nerve) (spinal cord) Z46.2
      implanted Z45.42
    pulse generator Z45.010
  portacath (port-a-cath) Z45.2
  prosthesis (external) Z44.9
    arm — *see* Admission, adjustment, artificial, arm
    breast Z44.3
    dental Z46.3
    eye Z44.2
    leg — *see* Admission, adjustment, artificial, leg
    specified NEC Z44.8
  spectacles Z46.0
  wheelchair Z46.89
Fitzhugh-Curtis syndrome
  due to
    Chlamydia trachomatis A74.81
    Neisseria gonorrhorea (gonococcal peritonitis) A54.85
Fitz's syndrome (acute hemorrhagic pancreatitis) — *see also* Pancreatitis, acute K85.80
Fixation
  joint — *see* Ankylosis
  larynx J38.7
  stapes — *see* Ankylosis, ear ossicles
    deafness — *see* Deafness, conductive
  uterus (acquired) — *see* Malposition, uterus
  vocal cord J38.3
Flabby ridge K06.8
Flaccid — *see also* condition
  palate, congenital Q38.5
Flail
  chest S22.5
    newborn (birth injury) P13.8
  joint (paralytic) M25.20
    ankle M25.27-
    elbow M25.22-
    foot joint M25.27-
    hand joint M25.24-
    hip M25.25-
    knee M25.26-
    shoulder M25.21-
    specified joint NEC M25.28
    wrist M25.23-
Flajani's disease — *see* Hyperthyroidism, with, goiter (diffuse)
Flap, liver K71.3
Flashbacks (residual to hallucinogen use) F16.283

Flat
  chamber (eye) — *see* Disorder, globe, hypotony, flat anterior chamber
  chest, congenital Q67.8
  foot (acquired) (fixed type) (painful) (postural) — *see also* Deformity, limb, flat foot
    congenital (rigid) (spastic (everted)) Q66.5-
    rachitic sequelae (late effect) E64.3
  organ or site, congenital NEC — *see* Anomaly, by site
  pelvis M95.5
    with disproportion (fetopelvic) O33.0
      causing obstructed labor O65.0
    congenital Q74.2
Flatau-Schilder disease G37.0
Flatback syndrome M40.30
  lumbar region M40.36
  lumbosacral region M40.37
  thoracolumbar region M40.35
Flattening
  head, femur M89.8X5
  hip — *see* Coxa, plana
  lip (congenital) Q18.8
  nose (congenital) Q67.4
    acquired M95.0
Flatulence R14.3
  psychogenic F45.8
Flatus R14.3
  vaginalis N89.8
Flax-dresser's disease J66.1
Flea bite — *see* Injury, bite, by site, superficial, insect
Flecks, glaucomatous (subcapsular) — *see* Cataract, complicated
Fleischer (-Kayser) ring (cornea) H18.04-
Fleshy mole O02.0
Flexibilitas cerea — *see* Catalepsy
Flexion
  amputation stump (surgical) T87.89
  cervix — *see* Malposition, uterus
  contracture, joint — *see* Contraction, joint
  deformity, joint — *see also* Deformity, limb, flexion M21.20
    hip, congenital Q65.89
  uterus — *see also* Malposition, uterus
    lateral — *see* Lateroversion, uterus
Flexner-Boyd dysentery A03.2
Flexner's dysentery A03.1
Flexure — *see* Flexion
Flint murmur (aortic insufficiency) I35.1
Floater, vitreous — *see* Opacity, vitreous
Floating
  cartilage (joint) — *see also* Loose, body, joint
    knee — *see* Derangement, knee, loose body
  gallbladder, congenital Q44.1
  kidney N28.89
    congenital Q63.8
  spleen D73.89
Flooding N92.0
Floor — *see* condition
Floppy
  baby syndrome (nonspecific) P94.2
  iris syndrome (intraoperative) (IFIS) H21.81
  nonrheumatic mitral valve syndrome I34.1
Flu — *see also* Influenza
  avian — *see also* Influenza, due to, identified novel influenza A virus J09.X2
  bird — *see also* Influenza, due to, identified novel influenza A virus J09.X2
  intestinal NEC A08.4
  swine (viruses that normally cause infections in pigs) — *see also* Influenza, due to, identified novel influenza A virus J09.X2
Fluctuating blood pressure I99.8
Fluid
  abdomen R18.8
  chest J94.8
  heart — *see* Failure, heart, congestive
  joint — *see* Effusion, joint
  loss (acute) E86.9

Fluid - *continued*
  lung — *see* Edema, lung
  overload E87.70
    specified NEC E87.79
  peritoneal cavity R18.8
  pleural cavity J94.8
  retention R60.9
Flukes NEC — *see also* Infestation, fluke
  blood NEC — *see* Schistosomiasis
  liver B66.3
Fluor (vaginalis) N89.8
  trichomonal or due to Trichomonas (vaginalis) A59.00
Fluorosis
  dental K00.3
  skeletal M85.10
    ankle M85.17-
    foot M85.17-
    forearm M85.13-
    hand M85.14-
    lower leg M85.16-
    multiple site M85.19
    neck M85.18
    rib M85.18
    shoulder M85.11-
    skull M85.18
    specified site NEC M85.18
    thigh M85.15-
    toe M85.17-
    upper arm M85.12-
    vertebra M85.18
Flush syndrome E34.0
Flushing R23.2
  menopausal N95.1
Flutter
  atrial or auricular I48.92
    atypical I48.4
    type I I48.3
    type II I48.4
    typical I48.3
  heart I49.8
    atrial or auricular I48.92
      atypical I48.4
      type I I48.3
      type II I48.4
      typical I48.3
    ventricular I49.02
  ventricular I49.02
FNHTR (febrile nonhemolytic transfusion reaction) R50.84
Fochier's abscess - code by site under Abscess
Focus, Assmann's — *see* Tuberculosis, pulmonary
Fogo selvagem L10.3
Foix-Alajouanine syndrome G95.19
Fold, folds (anomalous) — *see also* Anomaly, by site
  Descemet's membrane — *see* Change, corneal membrane, Descemet's, fold
  epicanthic Q10.3
  heart Q24.8
Folie à deux F24
Follicle
  cervix (nabothian) (ruptured) N88.8
  graafian, ruptured, with hemorrhage N83.0-
  nabothian N88.8
Follicular — *see* condition
Folliculitis (superficial) L73.9
  abscedens et suffodiens L66.3
  cyst N83.0-
  decalvans L66.2
  deep — *see* Furuncle, by site
  gonococcal (acute) (chronic) A54.01
  keloid, keloidalis L73.0
  pustular L01.02
  ulerythematosa reticulata L66.4
Folliculome lipidique
  specified site — *see* Neoplasm, benign, by site
  unspecified site
    female D27.9
    male D29.20
Følling's disease E70.0
Follow-up — *see* Examination, follow-up

Fong's syndrome (hereditary osteo-onychodysplasia) Q87.2
Food
  allergy L27.2
  asphyxia (from aspiration or inhalation) — *see* Foreign body, by site
  choked on — *see* Foreign body, by site
  deprivation T73.0
    specified kind of food NEC E63.8
  intoxication — *see* Poisoning, food
  lack of T73.0
  poisoning — *see* Poisoning, food
  rejection NEC — *see* Disorder, eating
  strangulation or suffocation — *see* Foreign body, by site
  toxemia — *see* Poisoning, food
Foot — *see* condition
Foramen ovale (nonclosure) (patent) (persistent) Q21.1
Forbes' glycogen storage disease E74.03
Fordyce-Fox disease L75.2
Fordyce's disease (mouth) Q38.6
Forearm — *see* condition
Foreign body
  with
    laceration — *see* Laceration, by site, with foreign body
    puncture wound — *see* Puncture, by site, with foreign body
  accidentally left following a procedure T81.509
  aspiration T81.506
    resulting in
      adhesions T81.516
      obstruction T81.526
      perforation T81.536
      specified complication NEC T81.596
  cardiac catheterization T81.505
    resulting in
      acute reaction T81.60
        aseptic peritonitis T81.61
        specified NEC T81.69
      adhesions T81.515
      obstruction T81.525
      perforation T81.535
      specified complication NEC T81.595
  causing
    acute reaction T81.60
      aseptic peritonitis T81.61
      specified complication NEC T81.69
    adhesions T81.519
    aseptic peritonitis T81.61
    obstruction T81.529
    perforation T81.539
    specified complication NEC T81.599
  endoscopy T81.504
    resulting in
      adhesions T81.514
      obstruction T81.524
      perforation T81.534
      specified complication NEC T81.594
  immunization T81.503
    resulting in
      adhesions T81.513
      obstruction T81.523
      perforation T81.533
      specified complication NEC T81.593
  infusion T81.501
    resulting in
      adhesions T81.511
      obstruction T81.521
      perforation T81.531
      specified complication NEC T81.591
  injection T81.503
    resulting in
      adhesions T81.513
      obstruction T81.523
      perforation T81.533
      specified complication NEC T81.593
  kidney dialysis T81.502
    resulting in
      adhesions T81.512
      obstruction T81.522
      perforation T81.532
      specified complication NEC T81.592

Foreign body - *continued*
accidentally left following a procedure - *continued*
  packing removal T81.507
    resulting in
      acute reaction T81.60
        aseptic peritonitis T81.61
        specified NEC T81.69
      adhesions T81.517
      obstruction T81.527
      perforation T81.537
      specified complication NEC T81.597
  puncture T81.506
    resulting in
      adhesions T81.516
      obstruction T81.526
      perforation T81.536
      specified complication NEC T81.596
  specified procedure NEC T81.508
    resulting in
      acute reaction T81.60
        aseptic peritonitis T81.61
        specified NEC T81.69
      adhesions T81.518
      obstruction T81.528
      perforation T81.538
      specified complication NEC T81.598
  surgical operation T81.500
    resulting in
      acute reaction T81.60
        aseptic peritonitis T81.61
        specified NEC T81.69
      adhesions T81.510
      obstruction T81.520
      perforation T81.530
      specified complication NEC T81.590
  transfusion T81.501
    resulting in
      adhesions T81.511
      obstruction T81.521
      perforation T81.531
      specified complication NEC T81.591
alimentary tract T18.9
  anus T18.5
  colon T18.4
  esophagus — *see* Foreign body, esophagus
  mouth T18.0
  multiple sites T18.8
  rectosigmoid (junction) T18.5
  rectum T18.5
  small intestine T18.3
  specified site NEC T18.8
  stomach T18.2
anterior chamber (eye) S05.5-
auditory canal — *see* Foreign body, entering through orifice, ear
bronchus T17.508
  causing
    asphyxiation T17.500
      food (bone) (seed) T17.520
      gastric contents (vomitus) T17.510
      specified type NEC T17.590
    injury NEC T17.508
      food (bone) (seed) T17.528
      gastric contents (vomitus) T17.518
      specified type NEC T17.598
canthus — *see* Foreign body, conjunctival sac
ciliary body (eye) S05.5-
conjunctival sac T15.1-
cornea T15.0-
entering through orifice
  accessory sinus T17.0
  alimentary canal T18.9
    multiple parts T18.8
    specified part NEC T18.8
  alveolar process T18.0
  antrum (Highmore's) T17.0
  anus T18.5
  appendix T18.4
  auditory canal — *see* Foreign body, entering through orifice, ear
  auricle — *see* Foreign body, entering through orifice, ear
  bladder T19.1

Foreign body - *continued*
entering through orifice - *continued*
  bronchioles — *see* Foreign body, respiratory tract, specified site NEC
  bronchus (main) — *see* Foreign body, bronchus
  buccal cavity T18.0
  canthus (inner) — *see* Foreign body, conjunctival sac
  cecum T18.4
  cervix (canal) (uteri) T19.3
  colon T18.4
  conjunctival sac — *see* Foreign body, conjunctival sac
  cornea — *see* Foreign body, cornea
  digestive organ or tract NOS T18.9
    multiple parts T18.8
    specified part NEC T18.8
  duodenum T18.3
  ear (external) T16.-
  esophagus — *see* Foreign body, esophagus
  eye (external) NOS T15.9-
    conjunctival sac — *see* Foreign body, conjunctival sac
    cornea — *see* Foreign body, cornea
    specified part NEC T15.8-
    eyeball — *see also* Foreign body, entering through orifice, eye, specified part NEC
    with penetrating wound — *see* Puncture, eyeball
    eyelid — *see also* Foreign body, conjunctival sac
    with
      laceration — *see* Laceration, eyelid, with foreign body
      puncture — *see* Puncture, eyelid, with foreign body
      superficial injury — *see* Foreign body, superficial, eyelid
  gastrointestinal tract T18.9
    multiple parts T18.8
    specified part NEC T18.8
  genitourinary tract T19.9
    multiple parts T19.8
    specified part NEC T19.8
  globe — *see* Foreign body, entering through orifice, eyeball
  gum T18.0
  Highmore's antrum T17.0
  hypopharynx — *see* Foreign body, pharynx
  ileum T18.3
  intestine (small) T18.3
    large T18.4
  lacrimal apparatus (punctum) — *see* Foreign body, entering through orifice, eye, specified part NEC
  large intestine T18.4
  larynx — *see* Foreign body, larynx
  lung — *see* Foreign body, respiratory tract, specified site NEC
  maxillary sinus T17.0
  mouth T18.0
  nasal sinus T17.0
  nasopharynx — *see* Foreign body, pharynx
  nose (passage) T17.1
  nostril T17.1
  oral cavity T18.0
  palate T18.0
  penis T19.4
  pharynx — *see* Foreign body, pharynx
  piriform sinus — *see* Foreign body, pharynx
  rectosigmoid (junction) T18.5
  rectum T18.5
  respiratory tract — *see* Foreign body, respiratory tract
  sinus (accessory) (frontal) (maxillary) (nasal) T17.0
    piriform — *see* Foreign body, pharynx
  small intestine T18.3
  stomach T18.2
  suffocation by — *see* Foreign body, by site

Foreign body - *continued*
entering through orifice - *continued*
  tear ducts or glands — *see* Foreign body, entering through orifice, eye, specified part NEC
  throat — *see* Foreign body, pharynx
  tongue T18.0
  tonsil, tonsillar (fossa) — *see* Foreign body, pharynx
  trachea — *see* Foreign body, trachea
  ureter T19.8
  urethra T19.0
  uterus (any part) T19.3
  vagina T19.2
  vulva T19.2
esophagus T18.108
  causing
    injury NEC T18.108
      food (bone) (seed) T18.128
      gastric contents (vomitus) T18.118
      specified type NEC T18.198
    tracheal compression T18.100
      food (bone) (seed) T18.120
      gastric contents (vomitus) T18.110
      specified type NEC T18.190
feeling of, in throat R09.89
fragment — *see* Retained, foreign body fragments (type of)
genitourinary tract T19.9
  bladder T19.1
  multiple parts T19.8
  penis T19.4
  specified site NEC T19.8
  urethra T19.0
  uterus T19.3
    IUD Z97.5
  vagina T19.2
    contraceptive device Z97.5
  vulva T19.2
granuloma (old) (soft tissue) — *see also* Granuloma, foreign body
  skin L92.3
in
  laceration — *see* Laceration, by site, with foreign body
  puncture wound — *see* Puncture, by site, with foreign body
  soft tissue (residual) M79.5
inadvertently left in operation wound — *see* Foreign body, accidentally left during a procedure
ingestion, ingested NOS T18.9
inhalation or inspiration — *see* Foreign body, by site
internal organ, not entering through a natural orifice - code as specific injury with foreign body
intraocular S05.5-
  old, retained (nonmagnetic) H44.70-
    anterior chamber H44.71-
    ciliary body H44.72-
    iris H44.72-
    lens H44.73-
    magnetic H44.60-
      anterior chamber H44.61-
      ciliary body H44.62-
      iris H44.62-
      lens H44.63-
      posterior wall H44.64-
      specified site NEC H44.69-
      vitreous body H44.65-
    posterior wall H44.74-
    specified site NEC H44.79-
    vitreous body H44.75-
iris — *see* Foreign body, intraocular
lacrimal punctum — *see* Foreign body, entering through orifice, eye, specified part NEC
larynx T17.308
  causing
    asphyxiation T17.300
      food (bone) (seed) T17.320
      gastric contents (vomitus) T17.310
      specified type NEC T17.390
    injury NEC T17.308

Foreign body - *continued*
larynx - *continued*
  causing - *continued*
    injury NEC - *continued*
      food (bone) (seed) T17.328
      gastric contents (vomitus) T17.318
      specified type NEC T17.398
lens — *see* Foreign body, intraocular
ocular muscle S05.4-
  old, retained — *see* Foreign body, orbit, old
old or residual
  soft tissue (residual) M79.5
operation wound, left accidentally — *see* Foreign body, accidentally left during a procedure
orbit S05.4-
  old, retained H05.5-
pharynx T17.208
  causing
    asphyxiation T17.200
      food (bone) (seed) T17.220
      gastric contents (vomitus) T17.210
      specified type NEC T17.290
    injury NEC T17.208
      food (bone) (seed) T17.228
      gastric contents (vomitus) T17.218
      specified type NEC T17.298
respiratory tract T17.908
  bronchioles — *see* Foreign body, respiratory tract, specified site NEC
  bronchus — *see* Foreign body, bronchus
  causing
    asphyxiation T17.900
      food (bone) (seed) T17.920
      gastric contents (vomitus) T17.910
      specified type NEC T17.990
    injury NEC T17.908
      food (bone) (seed) T17.928
      gastric contents (vomitus) T17.918
      specified type NEC T17.998
  larynx — *see* Foreign body, larynx
  lung — *see* Foreign body, respiratory tract, specified site NEC
  multiple parts — *see* Foreign body, respiratory tract, specified site NEC
nasal sinus T17.0
nasopharynx — *see* Foreign body, pharynx
nose T17.1
nostril T17.1
pharynx — *see* Foreign body, pharynx
specified site NEC T17.808
  causing
    asphyxiation T17.800
      food (bone) (seed) T17.820
      gastric contents (vomitus) T17.810
      specified type NEC T17.890
    injury NEC T17.808
      food (bone) (seed) T17.828
      gastric contents (vomitus) T17.818
      specified type NEC T17.898
throat — *see* Foreign body, pharynx
trachea — *see* Foreign body, trachea
retained (old) (nonmagnetic) (in)
anterior chamber (eye) — *see* Foreign body, intraocular, old, retained, anterior chamber
  magnetic — *see* Foreign body, intraocular, old, retained, magnetic, anterior chamber
ciliary body — *see* Foreign body, intraocular, old, retained, ciliary body
  magnetic — *see* Foreign body, intraocular, old, retained, magnetic, ciliary body
eyelid H02.819
  left H02.816
    lower H02.815
    upper H02.814
  right H02.813
    lower H02.812
    upper H02.811
fragments — *see* Retained, foreign body fragments (type of)

Foreign body - *continued*
retained (old) (nonmagnetic) (in) - *continued*
  globe — *see* Foreign body, intraocular, old, retained
    magnetic — *see* Foreign body, intraocular, old, retained, magnetic
  intraocular — *see* Foreign body, intraocular, old, retained
    magnetic — *see* Foreign body, intraocular, old, retained, magnetic
  iris — *see* Foreign body, intraocular, old, retained, iris
    magnetic — *see* Foreign body, intraocular, old, retained, magnetic, iris
  lens — *see* Foreign body, intraocular, old, retained, lens
    magnetic — *see* Foreign body, intraocular, old, retained, magnetic, lens
  muscle — *see* Foreign body, retained, soft tissue
  orbit — *see* Foreign body, orbit, old
  posterior wall of globe — *see* Foreign body, intraocular, old, retained, posterior wall
    magnetic — *see* Foreign body, intraocular, old, retained, magnetic, posterior wall
  retrobulbar — *see* Foreign body, orbit, old, retrobulbar
  soft tissue M79.5
  vitreous — *see* Foreign body, intraocular, old, retained, vitreous body
    magnetic — *see* Foreign body, intraocular, old, retained, magnetic, vitreous body
retina S05.5-
superficial, without open wound
  abdomen, abdominal (wall) S30.851
  alveolar process S00.552
  ankle S90.55-
  antecubital space — *see* Foreign body, superficial, forearm
  anus S30.857
  arm (upper) S40.85-
  auditory canal — *see* Foreign body, superficial, ear
  auricle — *see* Foreign body, superficial, ear
  axilla — *see* Foreign body, superficial, arm
  back, lower S30.850
  breast S20.15-
  brow S00.85
  buttock S30.850
  calf — *see* Foreign body, superficial, leg
  canthus — *see* Foreign body, superficial, eyelid
  cheek S00.85
    internal S00.552
  chest wall — *see* Foreign body, superficial, thorax
  chin S00.85
  clitoris S30.854
  costal region — *see* Foreign body, superficial, thorax
  digit (s)
    hand — *see* Foreign body, superficial, finger
    foot — *see* Foreign body, superficial, toe
  ear S00.45-
  elbow S50.35-
  epididymis S30.853
  epigastric region S30.851
  epiglottis S10.15
  esophagus, cervical S10.15
  eyebrow — *see* Foreign body, superficial, eyelid
  eyelid S00.25-
  face S00.85
  finger (s) S60.459
    index S60.45-
    little S60.45-
    middle S60.45-
    ring S60.45-

Foreign body - *continued*
superficial, without open wound - *continued*
  flank S30.851
  foot (except toe (s) alone) S90.85-
    toe — *see* Foreign body, superficial, toe
  forearm S50.85-
    elbow only — *see* Foreign body, superficial, elbow
  forehead S00.85
  genital organs, external
    female S30.856
    male S30.855
  groin S30.851
  gum S00.552
  hand S60.55-
  head S00.95
    ear — *see* Foreign body, superficial, ear
    eyelid — *see* Foreign body, superficial, eyelid
    lip S00.551
    nose S00.35
    oral cavity S00.552
    scalp S00.05
    specified site NEC S00.85
  heel — *see* Foreign body, superficial, foot
  hip S70.25-
  inguinal region S30.851
  interscapular region S20.459
  jaw S00.85
  knee S80.25-
  labium (majus) (minus) S30.854
  larynx S10.15
  leg (lower) S80.85-
    knee — *see* Foreign body, superficial, knee
    upper — *see* Foreign body, superficial, thigh
  lip S00.551
  lower back S30.850
  lumbar region S30.850
  malar region S00.85
  mammary — *see* Foreign body, superficial, breast
  mastoid region S00.85
  mouth S00.552
  nail
    finger — *see* Foreign body, superficial, finger
    toe — *see* Foreign body, superficial, toe
  nape S10.85
  nasal S00.35
  neck S10.95
    specified site NEC S10.85
    throat S10.15
  nose S00.35
  occipital region S00.05
  oral cavity S00.552
  orbital region — *see* Foreign body, superficial, eyelid
  palate S00.552
  palm — *see* Foreign body, superficial, hand
  parietal region S00.05
  pelvis S30.850
  penis S30.852
  perineum
    female S30.854
    male S30.850
  periocular area — *see* Foreign body, superficial, eyelid
  phalanges
    finger — *see* Foreign body, superficial, finger
    toe — *see* Foreign body, superficial, toe
  pharynx S10.15
  pinna — *see* Foreign body, superficial, ear
  popliteal space — *see* Foreign body, superficial, knee
  prepuce S30.852
  pubic region S30.850
  pudendum
    female S30.856
    male S30.855
  sacral region S30.850
  scalp S00.05

Foreign body - *continued*
  superficial, without open wound - *continued*
    scapular region — *see* Foreign body,
      superficial, shoulder
    scrotum S30.853
    shin — *see* Foreign body, superficial, leg
    shoulder S40.25-
    sternal region S20.359
    submaxillary region S00.85
    submental region S00.85
    subungual
      finger (s) — *see* Foreign body,
        superficial, finger
      toe (s) — *see* Foreign body, superficial,
        toe
    supraclavicular fossa S10.85
    supraorbital S00.85
    temple S00.85
    temporal region S00.85
    testis S30.853
    thigh S70.35-
    thorax, thoracic (wall) S20.95
      back S20.45-
      front S20.35-
    throat S10.15
    thumb S60.35-
    toe (s) (lesser) S90.456
      great S90.45-
    tongue S00.552
    trachea S10.15
    tunica vaginalis S30.853
    tympanum, tympanic membrane — *see*
      Foreign body, superficial, ear
    uvula S00.552
    vagina S30.854
    vocal cords S10.15
    vulva S30.854
    wrist S60.85-
  swallowed T18.9
  trachea T17.408
    causing
      asphyxiation T17.400
        food (bone) (seed) T17.420
        gastric contents (vomitus) T17.410
        specified type NEC T17.490
      injury NEC T17.408
        food (bone) (seed) T17.428
        gastric contents (vomitus) T17.418
        specified type NEC T17.498
  type of fragment — *see* Retained, foreign
    body fragments (type of)
  vitreous (humor) S05.5-
Forestier's disease (rhizomelic
  pseudopolyarthritis) M35.3
  meaning ankylosing hyperostosis — *see*
    Hyperostosis, ankylosing
Formation
  hyalin in cornea — *see* Degeneration, cornea
  sequestrum in bone (due to infection) — *see*
    Osteomyelitis, chronic
  valve
    colon, congenital Q43.8
    ureter (congenital) Q62.39
Formication R20.2
Fort Bragg fever A27.89
Fossa — *see also* condition
  pyriform — *see* condition
Foster-Kennedy syndrome H47.14-
Fothergill's
  disease (trigeminal neuralgia) — *see also*
    Neuralgia, trigeminal
  scarlatina anginosa A38.9
Foul breath R19.6
Foundling Z76.1
Fournier disease or gangrene N49.3
  female N76.89
Fourth
  cranial nerve — *see* condition
  molar K00.1
Foville's (peduncular) disease or
  syndrome G46.3
Fox (-Fordyce) disease (apocrine
  miliaria) L75.2
FPIES (food protein-induced enterocolitis
  syndrome) K52.21

Fracture, burst — *see* Fracture, traumatic, by
  site
Fracture, chronic — *see* Fracture,
  pathological, by site
Fracture, insufficiency — *see* Fracture,
  pathological, by site
Fracture, nontraumatic, NEC
  atypical
    femur M84.750-
      complete
        oblique M84.759
          left side M84.758
          right side M84.757
        transverse M84.756
          left side M84.755
          right side M84.754
      incomplete M84.753
        left side M84.752
        right side M84.751
Fracture, pathological (pathologic) — *see*
  also Fracture, traumatic M84.40
  ankle M84.47-
  carpus M84.44-
  clavicle M84.41-
  compression (not due to trauma) — *see also*
    Collapse, vertebra M48.50-
  dental implant M27.63
  dental restorative material K08.539
    with loss of material K08.531
    without loss of material K08.530
  due to
    neoplastic disease NEC — *see also*
      Neoplasm M84.50
      ankle M84.57-
      carpus M84.54-
      clavicle M84.51-
      femur M84.55-
      fibula M84.56-
      finger M84.54-
      hip M84.559
      humerus M84.52-
      ilium M84.550
      ischium M84.550
      metacarpus M84.54-
      metatarsus M84.57-
      neck M84.58
      pelvis M84.550
      radius M84.53-
      rib M84.58
      scapula M84.51-
      skull M84.58
      specified site NEC M84.58
      tarsus M84.57-
      tibia M84.56-
      toe M84.57-
      ulna M84.53-
      vertebra M84.58
    osteoporosis M80.00
      disuse — *see* Osteoporosis, specified
        type NEC, with pathological
        fracture
      drug-induced — *see* Osteoporosis, drug
        induced, with pathological fracture
      idiopathic — *see* Osteoporosis, specified
        type NEC, with pathological
        fracture
      postmenopausal — *see* Osteoporosis,
        postmenopausal, with pathological
        fracture
      postoophorectomy — *see* Osteoporosis,
        postoophorectomy, with
        pathological fracture
      postsurgical malabsorption — *see*
        Osteoporosis, specified type NEC,
        with pathological fracture
      specified cause NEC — *see*
        Osteoporosis, specified type NEC,
        with pathological fracture
    specified disease NEC M84.60
      ankle M84.67-
      carpus M84.64-
      clavicle M84.61-
      femur M84.65-
      fibula M84.66-
      finger M84.64-

Fracture, pathological (pathologic) -
continued
  due to - *continued*
    specified disease NEC - *continued*
      hip M84.65-
      humerus M84.62-
      ilium M84.650
      ischium M84.650
      metacarpus M84.64-
      metatarsus M84.67-
      neck M84.68
      radius M84.63-
      rib M84.68
      scapula M84.61-
      skull M84.68
      tarsus M84.67-
      tibia M84.66-
      toe M84.67-
      ulna M84.63-
      vertebra M84.68
  femur M84.45-
  fibula M84.46-
  finger M84.44-
  hip M84.459
  humerus M84.42-
  ilium M84.454
  ischium M84.454
  joint prosthesis — *see* Complications, joint
    prosthesis, mechanical, breakdown, by
    site
    periprosthetic — *see* Fracture,
      pathological, periprosthetic
  metacarpus M84.44-
  metatarsus M84.47-
  neck M84.48
  pelvis M84.454
  periprosthetic M97.9
    ankle M97.2-
    elbow M97.4-
    finger M97.8
    hip M97.0-
    knee M97.1-
    other specified joint M97.8
    shoulder M97.3-
    spinal joint M97.8
    toe joint M97.8
    wrist joint M97.8
  radius M84.43-
  restorative material (dental) K08.539
    with loss of material K08.531
    without loss of material K08.530
  rib M84.48
  scapula M84.41-
  skull M84.48
  tarsus M84.47-
  tibia M84.46-
  toe M84.47-
  ulna M84.43-
  vertebra M84.48
Fracture, traumatic (abduction) (adduction)
  (separation) — *see also* Fracture,
    pathological T14.8
  acetabulum S32.40-
    column
      anterior (displaced) (iliopubic) S32.43-
        nondisplaced S32.436
      posterior (displaced)
        (ilioischial) S32.443
        nondisplaced S32.44-
    dome (displaced) S32.48-
      nondisplaced S32.48
    specified NEC S32.49-
    transverse (displaced) S32.45-
      with associated posterior wall fracture
        (displaced) S32.46-
        nondisplaced S32.46-
      nondisplaced S32.45-
    wall
      anterior (displaced) S32.41-
        nondisplaced S32.41-
      medial (displaced) S32.47-
        nondisplaced S32.47-
      posterior (displaced) S32.42-
        with associated transverse fracture
        (displaced) S32.46-

Fracture, traumatic (abduction) (adduction) (separation) - *continued*
  acetabulum - *continued*
    wall - *continued*
      posterior (displaced) - *continued*
        with associated transverse fracture (displaced) - *continued*
          nondisplaced S32.46-
      nondisplaced S32.42-
  acromion — *see* Fracture, scapula, acromial process
  ankle S82.899
    bimalleolar (displaced) S82.84-
      nondisplaced S82.84-
    lateral malleolus only (displaced) S82.6-
      nondisplaced S82.6-
    medial malleolus (displaced) S82.5-
      associated with Maisonneuve's fracture — *see* Fracture, Maisonneuve's
      nondisplaced S82.5-
    talus — *see* Fracture, tarsal, talus
    trimalleolar (displaced) S82.85-
      nondisplaced S82.85-
  arm (upper) — *see also* Fracture, humerus, shaft
    humerus — *see* Fracture, humerus
    radius — *see* Fracture, radius
    ulna — *see* Fracture, ulna
  astragalus — *see* Fracture, tarsal, talus
  atlas — *see* Fracture, neck, cervical vertebra, first
  axis — *see* Fracture, neck, cervical vertebra, second
  back — *see* Fracture, vertebra
  Barton's — *see* Barton's fracture
  base of skull — *see* Fracture, skull, base
  basicervical (basal) (femoral) S72.0
  Bennett's — *see* Bennett's fracture
  bimalleolar — *see* Fracture, ankle, bimalleolar
  blow-out S02.3-
  bone NEC T14.8
    birth injury P13.9
    following insertion of orthopedic implant, joint prosthesis or bone plate — *see* Fracture, following insertion of orthopedic implant, joint prosthesis or bone plate
    in (due to) neoplastic disease NEC — *see* Fracture, pathological, due to, neoplastic disease
    pathological (cause unknown) — *see* Fracture, pathological
  breast bone — *see* Fracture, sternum
  bucket handle (semilunar cartilage) — *see* Tear, meniscus
  burst — *see* Fracture, traumatic, by site
  calcaneus — *see* Fracture, tarsal, calcaneus
  carpal bone (s) S62.10-
    capitate (displaced) S62.13-
      nondisplaced S62.13-
    cuneiform — *see* Fracture, carpal bone, triquetrum
    hamate (body) (displaced) S62.143
      hook process (displaced) S62.15-
        nondisplaced S62.15-
      nondisplaced S62.14-
    larger multangular — *see* Fracture, carpal bones, trapezium
    lunate (displaced) S62.12-
      nondisplaced S62.12-
    navicular S62.00-
      distal pole (displaced) S62.01-
        nondisplaced S62.01-
      middle third (displaced) S62.02-
        nondisplaced S62.02-
      proximal third (displaced) S62.03-
        nondisplaced S62.03-
      volar tuberosity — *see* Fracture, carpal bones, navicular, distal pole
    os magnum — *see* Fracture, carpal bones, capitate
    pisiform (displaced) S62.16-
      nondisplaced S62.16-

Fracture, traumatic (abduction) (adduction) (separation) - *continued*
  carpal bone (s) - *continued*
    semilunar — *see* Fracture, carpal bones, lunate
    smaller multangular — *see* Fracture, carpal bones, trapezoid
    trapezium (displaced) S62.17-
      nondisplaced S62.17-
    trapezoid (displaced) S62.18-
      nondisplaced S62.18-
    triquetrum (displaced) S62.11-
      nondisplaced S62.11-
    unciform — *see* Fracture, carpal bones, hamate
  cervical — *see* Fracture, vertebra, cervical
  clavicle S42.00-
    acromial end (displaced) S42.03-
      nondisplaced S42.03-
    birth injury P13.4
    lateral end — *see* Fracture, clavicle, acromial end
    shaft (displaced) S42.02-
      nondisplaced S42.02-
    sternal end (anterior) (displaced) S42.01-
      nondisplaced S42.01-
      posterior S42.01-
  coccyx S32.2
  collapsed — *see* Collapse, vertebra
  collar bone — *see* Fracture, clavicle
  Colles' — *see* Colles' fracture
  coronoid process — *see* Fracture, ulna, upper end, coronoid process
  corpus cavernosum penis S39.840
  costochondral cartilage S23.41
  costochondral, costosternal junction — *see* Fracture, rib
  cranium — *see* Fracture, skull
  cricoid cartilage S12.8
  cuboid (ankle) — *see* Fracture, tarsal, cuboid
  cuneiform
    foot — *see* Fracture, tarsal, cuneiform
    wrist — *see* Fracture, carpal, triquetrum
  delayed union — *see* Delay, union, fracture
  dental restorative material K08.539
    with loss of material K08.531
    without loss of material K08.530
  due to
    birth injury — *see* Birth, injury, fracture
    osteoporosis — *see* Osteoporosis, with fracture
  Dupuytren's — *see* Fracture, ankle, lateral malleolus
  elbow S42.40-
  ethmoid (bone) (sinus) — *see* Fracture, skull, base
  face bone S02.92
  fatigue — *see also* Fracture, stress
    vertebra M48.40
      cervical region M48.42
      cervicothoracic region M48.43
      lumbar region M48.46
      lumbosacral region M48.47
      occipito-atlanto-axial region M48.41
      sacrococcygeal region M48.48
      thoracic region M48.44
      thoracolumbar region M48.45
  femur, femoral S72.9-
    basicervical (basal) S72.0
    birth injury P13.2
    capital epiphyseal S79.01-
    condyles, epicondyles — *see* Fracture, femur, lower end
    distal end — *see* Fracture, femur, lower end
    epiphysis
      head — *see* Fracture, femur, upper end, epiphysis
      lower — *see* Fracture, femur, lower end, epiphysis
      upper — *see* Fracture, femur, upper end, epiphysis
    following insertion of implant, prosthesis or plate M96.66-

Fracture, traumatic (abduction) (adduction) (separation) - *continued*
  femur, femoral - *continued*
    head — *see* Fracture, femur, upper end, head
    intertrochanteric — *see* Fracture, femur, trochanteric
    intratrochanteric — *see* Fracture, femur, trochanteric
    lower end S72.40-
      condyle (displaced) S72.41-
        lateral (displaced) S72.42-
          nondisplaced S72.42-
        medial (displaced) S72.43-
          nondisplaced S72.43-
        nondisplaced S72.41-
      epiphysis (displaced) S72.44-
        nondisplaced S72.44-
      physeal S79.10-
        Salter-Harris
          Type I S79.11-
          Type II S79.12-
          Type III S79.13-
          Type IV S79.14-
        specified NEC S79.19-
      specified NEC S72.49-
      supracondylar (displaced) S72.45-
        with intracondylar extension (displaced) S72.46-
          nondisplaced S72.46-
        nondisplaced S72.45-
      torus S72.47-
    neck — *see* Fracture, femur, upper end, neck
    pertrochanteric — *see* Fracture, femur, trochanteric
    shaft (lower third) (middle third) (upper third) S72.30-
      comminuted (displaced) S72.35-
        nondisplaced S72.35-
      oblique (displaced) S72.33-
        nondisplaced S72.33-
      segmental (displaced) S72.36-
        nondisplaced S72.36-
      specified NEC S72.39-
      spiral (displaced) S72.34-
        nondisplaced S72.34-
      transverse (displaced) S72.32-
        nondisplaced S72.32-
    specified site NEC — *see* subcategory S72.8
    subcapital (displaced) S72.01-
    subtrochanteric (region) (section) (displaced) S72.2-
      nondisplaced S72.2-
    transcervical — *see* Fracture, femur, midcervical
    transtrochanteric — *see* Fracture, femur, trochanteric
    trochanteric S72.10-
      apophyseal (displaced) S72.13-
        nondisplaced S72.13-
      greater trochanter (displaced) S72.11-
        nondisplaced S72.11-
      intertrochanteric (displaced) S72.14-
        nondisplaced S72.14-
      lesser trochanter (displaced) S72.12-
        nondisplaced S72.12-
    upper end S72.00-
      apophyseal (displaced) S72.13-
        nondisplaced S72.13-
      cervicotrochanteric — *see* Fracture, femur, upper end, neck, base
      epiphysis (displaced) S72.02-
        nondisplaced S72.02-
      head S72.05-
        articular (displaced) S72.06-
          nondisplaced S72.06-
        specified NEC S72.09-
      intertrochanteric (displaced) S72.14-
        nondisplaced S72.14-
      intracapsular S72.01-
      midcervical (displaced) S72.03-
        nondisplaced S72.03-
      neck S72.00-

Fracture, traumatic (abduction) (adduction) (separation) - *continued*
femur, femoral - *continued*
upper end - *continued*
neck - *continued*
base (displaced) S72.04-
nondisplaced S72.04-
specified NEC S72.09-
pertrochanteric — *see* Fracture, femur, upper end, trochanteric
physeal S79.00-
Salter-Harris type I S79.01-
specified NEC S79.09-
subcapital (displaced) S72.01-
subtrochanteric (displaced) S72.2-
nondisplaced S72.2-
transcervical — *see* Fracture, femur, upper end, midcervical
trochanteric S72.10-
greater (displaced) S72.11-
nondisplaced S72.11-
lesser (displaced) S72.12-
nondisplaced S72.12-
fibula (shaft) (styloid) S82.40-
comminuted (displaced) S82.45-
nondisplaced S82.45-
following insertion of implant, prosthesis or plate M96.67-
involving ankle or malleolus — *see* Fracture, fibula, lateral malleolus
lateral malleolus (displaced) S82.6-
nondisplaced S82.6-
lower end
physeal S89.30-
Salter-Harris
Type I S89.31-
Type II S89.32-
specified NEC S89.39-
specified NEC S82.83-
torus S82.82-
oblique (displaced) S82.43-
nondisplaced S82.43-
segmental (displaced) S82.46-
nondisplaced S82.46-
specified NEC S82.49-
spiral (displaced) S82.44-
nondisplaced S82.44-
transverse (displaced) S82.42-
nondisplaced S82.42-
upper end
physeal S89.20-
Salter-Harris
Type I S89.21-
Type II S89.22-
specified NEC S89.29-
specified NEC S82.83-
torus S82.81-
finger (except thumb) S62.60-
distal phalanx (displaced) S62.63-
nondisplaced S62.66-
index S62.60-
distal phalanx (displaced) S62.63-
nondisplaced S62.66-
middle phalanx (displaced) S62.62-
nondisplaced S62.65-
proximal phalanx (displaced) S62.61-
nondisplaced S62.64-
little S62.60-
distal phalanx (displaced) S62.63-
nondisplaced S62.66-
middle phalanx (displaced) S62.62-
nondisplaced S62.65-
proximal phalanx (displaced) S62.61-
nondisplaced S62.64-
middle phalanx (displaced) S62.62-
nondisplaced S62.65-
middle S62.60-
distal phalanx (displaced) S62.63-
nondisplaced S62.66-
middle phalanx (displaced) S62.62-
nondisplaced S62.65-
proximal phalanx (displaced) S62.61-
nondisplaced S62.64-
proximal phalanx (displaced) S62.61-
nondisplaced S62.64-

Fracture, traumatic (abduction) (adduction) (separation) - *continued*
finger (except thumb) - *continued*
ring S62.60-
distal phalanx (displaced) S62.63-
nondisplaced S62.66-
middle phalanx (displaced) S62.62-
nondisplaced S62.65-
proximal phalanx (displaced) S62.61-
nondisplaced S62.64-
thumb — *see* Fracture, thumb
following insertion (intraoperative) (postoperative) of orthopedic implant, joint prosthesis or bone plate M96.69
femur M96.66-
fibula M96.67-
humerus M96.62-
pelvis M96.65
radius M96.63-
specified bone NEC M96.69
tibia M96.67-
ulna M96.63-
foot S92.90-
astragalus — *see* Fracture, tarsal, talus
calcaneus — *see* Fracture, tarsal, calcaneus
cuboid — *see* Fracture, tarsal, cuboid
cuneiform — *see* Fracture, tarsal, cuneiform
metatarsal — *see* Fracture, metatarsal
navicular — *see* Fracture, tarsal, navicular
sesamoid S92.81-
specified NEC S92.81-
talus — *see* Fracture, tarsal, talus
tarsal — *see* Fracture, tarsal
toe — *see* Fracture, toe
forearm S52.9-
radius — *see* Fracture, radius
ulna — *see* Fracture, ulna
fossa (anterior) (middle) (posterior) S02.19
fragility — *see* Fracture, pathological, due to osteoporosis
frontal (bone) (skull) S02.0
sinus S02.19
glenoid (cavity) (scapula) — *see* Fracture, scapula, glenoid cavity
greenstick — *see* Fracture, by site
hallux — *see* Fracture, toe, great
hand S62.9-
carpal — *see* Fracture, carpal bone
finger (except thumb) — *see* Fracture, finger
metacarpal — *see* Fracture, metacarpal
navicular (scaphoid) (hand) — *see* Fracture, carpal bone, navicular
thumb — *see* Fracture, thumb
healed or old
with complications - code by Nature of the complication
heel bone — *see* Fracture, tarsal, calcaneus
Hill-Sachs S42.29-
hip — *see* Fracture, femur, neck
humerus S42.30-
anatomical neck — *see* Fracture, humerus, upper end
articular process — *see* Fracture, humerus, lower end
capitellum — *see* Fracture, humerus, lower end, condyle, lateral
distal end — *see* Fracture, humerus, lower end
epiphysis
lower — *see* Fracture, humerus, lower end, physeal
upper — *see* Fracture, humerus, upper end, physeal
external condyle — *see* Fracture, humerus, lower end, condyle, lateral
following insertion of implant, prosthesis or plate M96.62-
great tuberosity — *see* Fracture, humerus, upper end, greater tuberosity
intercondylar — *see* Fracture, humerus, lower end

Fracture, traumatic (abduction) (adduction) (separation) - *continued*
humerus - *continued*
internal epicondyle — *see* Fracture, humerus, lower end, epicondyle, medial
lesser tuberosity — *see* Fracture, humerus, upper end, lesser tuberosity
lower end S42.40-
condyle
lateral (displaced) S42.45-
nondisplaced S42.45-
medial (displaced) S42.46-
nondisplaced S42.46-
epicondyle
lateral (displaced) S42.43-
nondisplaced S42.43-
medial (displaced) S42.44-
incarcerated S42.44-
nondisplaced S42.44-
physeal S49.10-
Salter-Harris
Type I S49.11-
Type II S49.12-
Type III S49.13-
Type IV S49.14-
specified NEC S49.19-
specified NEC (displaced) S42.49-
nondisplaced S42.49-
supracondylar (simple) (displaced) S42.41-
with intercondylar fracture — *see* Fracture, humerus, lower end
comminuted (displaced) S42.42-
nondisplaced S42.42-
nondisplaced S42.41-
torus S42.48-
transcondylar (displaced) S42.47-
nondisplaced S42.47-
proximal end — *see* Fracture, humerus, upper end
shaft S42.30-
comminuted (displaced) S42.35-
nondisplaced S42.35-
greenstick S42.31-
oblique (displaced) S42.33-
nondisplaced S42.33-
segmental (displaced) S42.36-
nondisplaced S42.36-
specified NEC S42.39-
spiral (displaced) S42.34-
nondisplaced S42.34-
transverse (displaced) S42.32-
nondisplaced S42.32-
supracondylar — *see* Fracture, humerus, lower end
surgical neck — *see* Fracture, humerus, upper end, surgical neck
trochlea — *see* Fracture, humerus, lower end, condyle, medial
tuberosity — *see* Fracture, humerus, upper end
upper end S42.20-
anatomical neck — *see* Fracture, humerus, upper end, specified NEC
articular head — *see* Fracture, humerus, upper end, specified NEC
epiphysis — *see* Fracture, humerus, upper end, physeal
greater tuberosity (displaced) S42.25-
nondisplaced S42.25-
lesser tuberosity (displaced) S42.26-
nondisplaced S42.26-
physeal S49.00-
Salter-Harris
Type I S49.01-
Type II S49.02-
Type III S49.03-
Type IV S49.04-
specified NEC S49.09-
specified NEC (displaced) S42.29-
nondisplaced S42.29-
surgical neck (displaced) S42.21-
four-part S42.24-
nondisplaced S42.21-

Fracture, traumatic (abduction) (adduction) (separation) - *continued*
  humerus - *continued*
    upper end - *continued*
      surgical neck (displaced) - *continued*
        three-part S42.23-
        two-part (displaced) S42.22-
          nondisplaced S42.22-
      torus S42.27-
      transepiphyseal — *see* Fracture, humerus, upper end, physeal
  hyoid bone S12.8
  ilium S32.30-
    with disruption of pelvic ring — *see* Disruption, pelvic ring
    avulsion (displaced) S32.31-
      nondisplaced S32.31-
    specified NEC S32.39-
  impaction, impacted - code as Fracture, by site
  innominate bone — *see* Fracture, ilium
  instep — *see* Fracture, foot
  ischium S32.60-
    with disruption of pelvic ring — *see* Disruption, pelvic ring
    avulsion (displaced) S32.61-
      nondisplaced S32.61-
    specified NEC S32.69-
  jaw (bone) (lower) — *see* Fracture, mandible
    upper — *see* Fracture, maxilla
  joint prosthesis — *see* Complications, joint prosthesis, mechanical, breakdown, by site
    periprosthetic — *see* Fracture, traumatic, periprosthetic
  knee cap — *see* Fracture, patella
  larynx S12.8
  late effects — *see* Sequelae, fracture
  leg (lower) S82.9-
    ankle — *see* Fracture, ankle
    femur — *see* Fracture, femur
    fibula — *see* Fracture, fibula
    malleolus — *see* Fracture, ankle
    patella — *see* Fracture, patella
    specified site NEC S82.89-
    tibia — *see* Fracture, tibia
  lumbar spine — *see* Fracture, vertebra, lumbar
  lumbosacral spine S32.9
  Maisonneuve's (displaced) S82.86-
    nondisplaced S82.86-
  malar bone — *see also* Fracture, maxilla S02.400
    left side S02.40B
    right side S02.40A
  malleolus — *see* Fracture, ankle
  malunion — *see* Fracture, by site
  mandible (lower jaw (bone)) S02.609
    alveolus S02.67-
    angle (of jaw) S02.65-
    body, unspecified S02.600
      left side S02.602
      right side S02.601
    condylar process S02.61-
    coronoid process S02.63-
    ramus, unspecified S02.64-
    specified site NEC S02.69
    subcondylar process S02.62-
    symphysis S02.66
  manubrium (sterni) S22.21
    dissociation from sternum S22.23
  march — *see* Fracture, traumatic, stress, by site
  maxilla, maxillary (bone) (sinus) (superior) (upper jaw) S02.401
    alveolus S02.42
    inferior — *see* Fracture, mandible
    LeFort I S02.411
    LeFort II S02.412
    LeFort III S02.413
    left side S02.40D
    right side S02.40C
  metacarpal S62.309
    base (displaced) S62.319
      nondisplaced S62.349

Fracture, traumatic (abduction) (adduction) (separation) - *continued*
  metacarpal - *continued*
    fifth S62.30-
      base (displaced) S62.31-
        nondisplaced S62.34-
      neck (displaced) S62.33-
        nondisplaced S62.36-
      shaft (displaced) S62.32-
        nondisplaced S62.35-
      specified NEC S62.398
    first S62.20-
      base NEC (displaced) S62.23-
        nondisplaced S62.23-
      Bennett's — *see* Bennett's fracture
      neck (displaced) S62.25-
        nondisplaced S62.25-
      shaft (displaced) S62.24-
        nondisplaced S62.24-
      specified NEC S62.29-
    fourth S62.30-
      base (displaced) S62.31-
        nondisplaced S62.34-
      neck (displaced) S62.33-
        nondisplaced S62.36-
      shaft (displaced) S62.32-
        nondisplaced S62.35-
      specified NEC S62.39-
    neck (displaced) S62.33-
      nondisplaced S62.36-
    Rolando's — *see* Rolando's fracture
    second S62.30-
      base (displaced) S62.31-
        nondisplaced S62.34-
      neck (displaced) S62.33-
        nondisplaced S62.36-
      shaft (displaced) S62.32-
        nondisplaced S62.35-
      specified NEC S62.39-
    shaft (displaced) S62.32-
      nondisplaced S62.35-
    third S62.30-
      base (displaced) S62.31-
        nondisplaced S62.34-
      neck (displaced) S62.33-
        nondisplaced S62.36-
      shaft (displaced) S62.32-
        nondisplaced S62.35-
      specified NEC S62.39-
    specified NEC S62.399
  metastatic — *see* Fracture, pathological, due to, neoplastic disease — *see also* Neoplasm
  metatarsal bone S92.30-
    fifth (displaced) S92.35-
      nondisplaced S92.35-
    first (displaced) S92.31-
      nondisplaced S92.31-
    fourth (displaced) S92.34-
      nondisplaced S92.34-
    physeal S99.10-
      Salter-Harris
        Type I S99.11-
        Type II S99.12-
        Type III S99.13-
        Type IV S99.14-
      specified NEC S99.19-
    second (displaced) S92.32-
      nondisplaced S92.32-
    third (displaced) S92.33-
      nondisplaced S92.33-
  Monteggia's — *see* Monteggia's fracture
  multiple
    hand (and wrist) NEC — *see* Fracture, by site
    ribs — *see* Fracture, rib, multiple
  nasal (bone (s)) S02.2
  navicular (scaphoid) (foot) — *see also* Fracture, tarsal, navicular
    hand — *see* Fracture, carpal, navicular
  neck S12.9
    cervical vertebra S12.9
      fifth (displaced) S12.400
        nondisplaced S12.401

Fracture, traumatic (abduction) (adduction) (separation) - *continued*
  neck - *continued*
    cervical vertebra - *continued*
      fifth (displaced) - *continued*
        specified type NEC (displaced) S12.490
          nondisplaced S12.491
      first (displaced) S12.000
        burst (stable) S12.01
          unstable S12.02
        lateral mass (displaced) S12.040
          nondisplaced S12.041
        nondisplaced S12.001
        posterior arch (displaced) S12.030
          nondisplaced S12.031
        specified type NEC (displaced) S12.090
          nondisplaced S12.091
      fourth (displaced) S12.300
        nondisplaced S12.301
        specified type NEC (displaced) S12.390
          nondisplaced S12.391
      second (displaced) S12.100
        nondisplaced S12.101
        dens (anterior) (displaced) (type II) S12.110
          nondisplaced S12.112
          posterior S12.111
        specified type NEC (displaced) S12.120
          nondisplaced S12.121
        specified type NEC (displaced) S12.190
          nondisplaced S12.191
      seventh (displaced) S12.600
        nondisplaced S12.601
        specified type NEC (displaced) S12.690
          nondisplaced S12.691
      sixth (displaced) S12.500
        nondisplaced S12.501
        specified type NEC (displaced) S12.590
          nondisplaced S12.591
      third (displaced) S12.200
        nondisplaced S12.201
        specified type NEC (displaced) S12.290
          nondisplaced S12.291
    hyoid bone S12.8
    larynx S12.8
    specified site NEC S12.8
    thyroid cartilage S12.8
    trachea S12.8
  neoplastic NEC — *see* Fracture, pathological, due to, neoplastic disease
  neural arch — *see* Fracture, vertebra
  newborn — *see* Birth, injury, fracture
  nontraumatic — *see* Fracture, pathological
  nonunion — *see* Nonunion, fracture
  nose, nasal (bone) (septum) S02.2
  occiput — *see* Fracture, skull, base, occiput
  odontoid process — *see* Fracture, neck, cervical vertebra, second
  olecranon (process) (ulna) — *see* Fracture, ulna, upper end, olecranon process
  orbit, orbital (bone) (region) S02.85
    floor (blow-out) S02.3-
    roof S02.12-
    wall S02.85
      lateral S02.84-
      medial S02.83-
  os
    calcis — *see* Fracture, tarsal, calcaneus
    magnum — *see* Fracture, carpal, capitate
    pubis — *see* Fracture, pubis
  palate S02.8-
  parietal bone (skull) S02.0
  patella S82.00-
    comminuted (displaced) S82.04-
      nondisplaced S82.04-
    longitudinal (displaced) S82.02-
      nondisplaced S82.02-

Fracture, traumatic (abduction) (adduction) (separation) - continued

patella - *continued*
  osteochondral (displaced) S82.01-
    nondisplaced S82.01-
  specified NEC S82.09-
  transverse (displaced) S82.03-
    nondisplaced S82.03-
pedicle (of vertebral arch) — *see* Fracture, vertebra
pelvis, pelvic (bone) S32.9
  acetabulum — *see* Fracture, acetabulum
  circle — *see* Disruption, pelvic ring
  following insertion of implant, prosthesis or plate M96.65
  ilium — *see* Fracture, ilium
  ischium — *see* Fracture, ischium
  multiple
    with disruption of pelvic ring (circle) — *see* Disruption, pelvic ring
    without disruption of pelvic ring (circle) S32.82
  pubis — *see* Fracture, pubis
  specified site NEC S32.89
  sacrum — *see* Fracture, sacrum
periprosthetic, around internal prosthetic joint M97.9
  ankle M97.2-
  elbow M97.4-
  finger M97.8
  hip M97.0-
  knee M97.1--
  shoulder M97.3-
  specified joint NEC M97.8
  spine M97.8
  toe M97.8
  wrist M97.8
phalanx
  foot — *see* Fracture, toe
  hand — *see* Fracture, finger
pisiform — *see* Fracture, carpal, pisiform
pond — *see* Fracture, skull
prosthetic device, internal — *see* Complications, prosthetic device, by site, mechanical
pubis S32.50-
  with disruption of pelvic ring — *see* Disruption, pelvic ring
  specified site NEC S32.59-
  superior rim S32.51-
radius S52.9-
  distal end — *see* Fracture, radius, lower end
  following insertion of implant, prosthesis or plate M96.63-
  head — *see* Fracture, radius, upper end, head
  lower end S52.50-
    Barton's — *see* Barton's fracture
    Colles' — *see* Colles' fracture
    extraarticular NEC S52.55-
    intraarticular NEC S52.57-
    physeal S59.20-
      Salter-Harris
        Type I S59.21-
        Type II S59.22-
        Type III S59.23-
        Type IV S59.24-
      specified NEC S59.29-
    Smith's — *see* Smith's fracture
    specified NEC S52.59-
    styloid process (displaced) S52.51-
      nondisplaced S52.51-
    torus S52.52-
  neck — *see* Fracture, radius, upper end
  proximal end — *see* Fracture, radius, upper end
  shaft S52.30-
    bent bone S52.38-
    comminuted (displaced) S52.35-
      nondisplaced S52.35-
    Galeazzi's — *see* Galeazzi's fracture
    greenstick S52.31-
    oblique (displaced) S52.33-
      nondisplaced S52.33-

Fracture, traumatic (abduction) (adduction) (separation) - continued

radius - *continued*
  shaft - *continued*
    segmental (displaced) S52.36-
      nondisplaced S52.36-
    specified NEC S52.39-
    spiral (displaced) S52.34-
      nondisplaced S52.34-
    transverse (displaced) S52.32-
      nondisplaced S52.32-
  upper end S52.10-
    head (displaced) S52.12-
      nondisplaced S52.12-
    neck (displaced) S52.13-
      nondisplaced S52.13-
    specified NEC S52.18-
    physeal S59.10-
      Salter-Harris
        Type I S59.11-
        Type II S59.12-
        Type III S59.13-
        Type IV S59.14-
      specified NEC S59.19-
    torus S52.11-
  ramus
    inferior or superior, pubis — *see* Fracture, pubis
    mandible — *see* Fracture, mandible
restorative material (dental) K08.539
  with loss of material K08.531
  without loss of material K08.530
rib S22.3-
  with flail chest — *see* Flail, chest
  multiple S22.4-
    with flail chest — *see* Flail, chest
root, tooth — *see* Fracture, tooth
sacrum S32.10
  specified NEC S32.19
  Type
    1 S32.14
    2 S32.15
    3 S32.16
    4 S32.17
  Zone
    I S32.119
      displaced (minimally) S32.111
        severely S32.112
      nondisplaced S32.110
    II S32.129
      displaced (minimally) S32.121
        severely S32.122
      nondisplaced S32.120
    III S32.139
      displaced (minimally) S32.131
        severely S32.132
      nondisplaced S32.130
scaphoid (hand) — *see also* Fracture, carpal, navicular
  foot — *see* Fracture, tarsal, navicular
scapula S42.10-
  acromial process (displaced) S42.12-
    nondisplaced S42.12-
  body (displaced) S42.11-
    nondisplaced S42.11-
  coracoid process (displaced) S42.13-
    nondisplaced S42.13-
  glenoid cavity (displaced) S42.14-
    nondisplaced S42.14-
  neck (displaced) S42.15-
    nondisplaced S42.15-
  specified NEC S42.19-
semilunar bone, wrist — *see* Fracture, carpal, lunate
sequelae — *see* Sequelae, fracture
sesamoid bone
  foot S92.81-
  hand — *see* Fracture, carpal
  other — *see* Fracture, traumatic, by site
shepherd's — *see* Fracture, tarsal, talus
shoulder (girdle) S42.9-
  blade — *see* Fracture, scapula
sinus (ethmoid) (frontal) S02.19
skull S02.91
  base S02.10-

Fracture, traumatic (abduction) (adduction) (separation) - continued

skull - *continued*
  base - *continued*
    occiput S02.119
    condyle S02.113
      type I S02.110
        left side S02.11B
        right side S02.11A
      type II S02.111
        left side S02.11D
        right side S02.11C
      type III S02.112
        left side S02.11F
        right side S02.11E
      specified NEC S02.118
        left side S02.11H
        right side S02.11G
    specified NEC S02.19
  birth injury P13.0
  frontal bone S02.0
  parietal bone S02.0
  specified site NEC S02.8-
  temporal bone S02.19
  vault S02.0
Smith's — *see* Smith's fracture
sphenoid (bone) (sinus) S02.19
spine — *see* Fracture, vertebra
spinous process — *see* Fracture, vertebra
spontaneous (cause unknown) — *see* Fracture, pathological
stave (of thumb) — *see* Fracture, metacarpal, first
sternum S22.20
  with flail chest — *see* Flail, chest
  body S22.22
  manubrium S22.21
  xiphoid (process) S22.24
stress M84.30
  ankle M84.37-
  carpus M84.34-
  clavicle M84.31-
  femoral neck M84.359
  femur M84.35-
  fibula M84.36-
  finger M84.34-
  hip M84.359
  humerus M84.32-
  ilium M84.350
  ischium M84.350
  metacarpus M84.34-
  metatarsus M84.37-
  neck — *see* Fracture, fatigue, vertebra
  pelvis M84.350
  radius M84.33-
  rib M84.38
  scapula M84.31-
  skull M84.38
  tarsus M84.37-
  tibia M84.36-
  toe M84.37-
  ulna M84.33-
  vertebra — *see* Fracture, fatigue, vertebra
supracondylar, elbow — *see* Fracture, humerus, lower end, supracondylar
symphysis pubis — *see* Fracture, pubis
talus (ankle bone) — *see* Fracture, tarsal, talus
tarsal bone (s) S92.20-
  astragalus — *see* Fracture, tarsal, talus
  calcaneus S92.00-
    anterior process (displaced) S92.02-
      nondisplaced S92.02-
    body (displaced) S92.01-
      nondisplaced S92.01-
    extraarticular NEC (displaced) S92.05-
      nondisplaced S92.05-
    intraarticular (displaced) S92.06-
      nondisplaced S92.06-
    physeal S99.00-
      Salter-Harris
        Type I S99.01-
        Type II S99.02-
        Type III S99.03-
        Type IV S99.04-

Fracture, traumatic (abduction) (adduction) (separation) - *continued*
tarsal bone (s) - *continued*
calcaneus - *continued*
physeal - *continued*
specified NEC S99.09-
tuberosity (displaced) S92.04-
avulsion (displaced) S92.03-
nondisplaced S92.03-
nondisplaced S92.04-
cuboid (displaced) S92.21-
nondisplaced S92.21-
cuneiform
intermediate (displaced) S92.23-
nondisplaced S92.23-
lateral (displaced) S92.22-
nondisplaced S92.22-
medial (displaced) S92.24-
nondisplaced S92.24-
navicular (displaced) S92.25-
nondisplaced S92.25-
scaphoid — *see* Fracture, tarsal, navicular
talus S92.10-
avulsion (displaced) S92.15-
nondisplaced S92.15-
body (displaced) S92.12-
nondisplaced S92.12-
dome (displaced) S92.14-
nondisplaced S92.14-
head (displaced) S92.12-
nondisplaced S92.12-
lateral process (displaced) S92.14-
nondisplaced S92.14-
neck (displaced) S92.11-
nondisplaced S92.11-
posterior process (displaced) S92.13-
nondisplaced S92.13-
specified NEC S92.19-
temporal bone (styloid) S02.19
thorax (bony) S22.9
with flail chest — *see* Flail, chest
rib S22.3-
multiple S22.4-
with flail chest — *see* Flail, chest
sternum S22.20
body S22.22
manubrium S22.21
xiphoid process S22.24
vertebra (displaced) S22.009
burst (stable) S22.001
unstable S22.002
eighth S22.069
burst (stable) S22.061
unstable S22.062
specified type NEC S22.068
wedge compression S22.060
eleventh S22.089
burst (stable) S22.081
unstable S22.082
specified type NEC S22.088
wedge compression S22.080
fifth S22.059
burst (stable) S22.051
unstable S22.052
specified type NEC S22.058
wedge compression S22.050
first S22.019
burst (stable) S22.011
unstable S22.012
specified type NEC S22.018
wedge compression S22.010
fourth S22.049
burst (stable) S22.041
unstable S22.042
specified type NEC S22.048
wedge compression S22.040
ninth S22.079
burst (stable) S22.071
unstable S22.072
specified type NEC S22.078
wedge compression S22.070
nondisplaced S22.001
second S22.029
burst (stable) S22.021
unstable S22.022

Fracture, traumatic (abduction) (adduction) (separation) - *continued*
thorax (bony) - *continued*
vertebra (displaced) - *continued*
second - *continued*
specified type NEC S22.028
wedge compression S22.020
seventh S22.069
burst (stable) S22.061
unstable S22.062
specified type NEC S22.068
wedge compression S22.060
sixth S22.059
burst (stable) S22.051
unstable S22.052
specified type NEC S22.058
wedge compression S22.050
specified type NEC S22.008
tenth S22.079
burst (stable) S22.071
unstable S22.072
specified type NEC S22.078
wedge compression S22.070
third S22.039
burst (stable) S22.031
unstable S22.032
specified type NEC S22.038
wedge compression S22.030
twelfth S22.089
burst (stable) S22.081
unstable S22.082
specified type NEC S22.088
wedge compression S22.080
wedge compression S22.000
thumb S62.50-
distal phalanx (displaced) S62.52-
nondisplaced S62.52-
proximal phalanx (displaced) S62.51-
nondisplaced S62.51-
thyroid cartilage S12.8
tibia (shaft) S82.20-
comminuted (displaced) S82.25-
nondisplaced S82.25-
condyles — *see* Fracture, tibia, upper end
distal end — *see* Fracture, tibia, lower end
epiphysis
lower — *see* Fracture, tibia, lower end
upper — *see* Fracture, tibia, upper end
following insertion of implant, prosthesis
or plate M96.67-
head (involving knee joint) — *see*
Fracture, tibia, upper end
intercondyloid eminence — *see* Fracture,
tibia, upper end
involving ankle or malleolus — *see*
Fracture, ankle, medial malleolus
lower end S82.30-
physeal S89.10-
Salter-Harris
Type I S89.11-
Type II S89.12-
Type III S89.13-
Type IV S89.14-
specified NEC S89.19-
pilon (displaced) S82.87-
nondisplaced S82.87-
specified NEC S82.39-
torus S82.31-
malleolus — *see* Fracture, ankle, medial
malleolus
oblique (displaced) S82.23-
nondisplaced S82.23-
pilon — *see* Fracture, tibia, lower end,
pilon
proximal end — *see* Fracture, tibia, upper
end
segmental (displaced) S82.26-
nondisplaced S82.26-
specified NEC S82.29-
spine — *see* Fracture, tibia, upper end,
spine
spiral (displaced) S82.24-
nondisplaced S82.24-
transverse (displaced) S82.22-
nondisplaced S82.22-

Fracture, traumatic (abduction) (adduction) (separation) - *continued*
tibia (shaft) - *continued*
tuberosity — *see* Fracture, tibia, upper end,
tuberosity
upper end S82.10-
bicondylar (displaced) S82.14-
nondisplaced S82.14-
lateral condyle (displaced) S82.12-
nondisplaced S82.12-
medial condyle (displaced) S82.13-
nondisplaced S82.13-
physeal S89.00-
Salter-Harris
Type I S89.01-
Type II S89.02-
Type III S89.03-
Type IV S89.04-
specified NEC S89.09-
plateau — *see* Fracture, tibia, upper end,
bicondylar
spine (displaced) S82.11-
nondisplaced S82.11-
torus S82.16-
specified NEC S82.19-
tuberosity (displaced) S82.15-
nondisplaced S82.15-
toe S92.91-
great (displaced) S92.40-
distal phalanx (displaced) S92.42-
nondisplaced S92.42-
nondisplaced S92.40-
proximal phalanx (displaced) S92.41-
nondisplaced S92.41-
specified NEC S92.49-
lesser (displaced) S92.50-
distal phalanx (displaced) S92.53-
nondisplaced S92.53-
middle phalanx (displaced) S92.52-
nondisplaced S92.52-
nondisplaced S92.50-
proximal phalanx (displaced) S92.51-
nondisplaced S92.51-
specified NEC S92.59-
physeal
phalanx S99.20-
Salter-Harris
Type I S99.21-
Type II S99.22-
Type III S99.23-
Type IV S99.24-
specified NEC S99.29-
tooth (root) S02.5
trachea (cartilage) S12.8
transverse process — *see* Fracture, vertebra
trapezium or trapezoid bone — *see* Fracture,
carpal
trimalleolar — *see* Fracture, ankle,
trimalleolar
triquetrum (cuneiform of carpus) — *see*
Fracture, carpal, triquetrum
trochanter — *see* Fracture, femur,
trochanteric
tuberosity (external) — *see* Fracture,
traumatic, by site
ulna (shaft) S52.20-
bent bone S52.28-
coronoid process — *see* Fracture, ulna,
upper end, coronoid process
distal end — *see* Fracture, ulna, lower end
following insertion of implant, prosthesis
or plate M96.63-
head S52.60-
lower end S52.60-
physeal S59.00-
Salter-Harris
Type I S59.01-
Type II S59.02-
Type III S59.03-
Type IV S59.04-
specified NEC S59.09-
specified NEC S52.69-
styloid process (displaced) S52.61-
nondisplaced S52.61-
torus S52.62-

Fracture, traumatic (abduction) (adduction) (separation) - *continued*
ulna (shaft) - *continued*
proximal end — *see* Fracture, ulna, upper end
shaft S52.20-
comminuted (displaced) S52.25-
nondisplaced S52.25-
greenstick S52.21-
Monteggia's — *see* Monteggia's fracture
oblique (displaced) S52.23-
nondisplaced S52.23-
segmental (displaced) S52.26-
nondisplaced S52.26-
specified NEC S52.29-
spiral (displaced) S52.24-
nondisplaced S52.24-
transverse (displaced) S52.22-
nondisplaced S52.22-
upper end S52.00-
coronoid process (displaced) S52.04-
nondisplaced S52.04-
olecranon process (displaced) S52.02-
with intraarticular extension S52.03-
nondisplaced S52.02-
with intraarticular extension S52.03-
specified NEC S52.09-
torus S52.01-
unciform — *see* Fracture, carpal, hamate
vault of skull S02.0
vertebra, vertebral (arch) (body) (column)
(neural arch) (pedicle) (spinous process)
(transverse process)
atlas — *see* Fracture, neck, cervical
vertebra, first
axis — *see* Fracture, neck, cervical
vertebra, second
cervical (teardrop) S12.9
axis — *see* Fracture, neck, cervical
vertebra, second
first (atlas) — *see* Fracture, neck,
cervical vertebra, first
second (axis) — *see* Fracture, neck,
cervical vertebra, second
chronic M84.48
coccyx S32.2
dorsal — *see* Fracture, thorax, vertebra
lumbar S32.009
burst (stable) S32.001
unstable S32.002
fifth S32.059
burst (stable) S32.051
unstable S32.052
specified type NEC S32.058
wedge compression S32.050
first S32.019
burst (stable) S32.011
unstable S32.012
specified type NEC S32.018
wedge compression S32.010
fourth S32.049
burst (stable) S32.041
unstable S32.042
specified type NEC S32.048
wedge compression S32.040
second S32.029
burst (stable) S32.021
unstable S32.022
specified type NEC S32.028
wedge compression S32.020
specified type NEC S32.008
third S32.039
burst (stable) S32.031
unstable S32.032
specified type NEC S32.038
wedge compression S32.030
wedge compression S32.000
metastatic — *see* Collapse, vertebra, in,
specified disease NEC — *see also*
Neoplasm
newborn (birth injury) P11.5
sacrum S32.10
specified NEC S32.19
Type
1 S32.14

Fracture, traumatic (abduction) (adduction) (separation) - *continued*
vertebra, vertebral (arch) (body) (column)
(neural arch) (pedicle) (spinous process)
(transverse process) - *continued*
sacrum - *continued*
Type - *continued*
2 S32.15
3 S32.16
4 S32.17
Zone
I S32.119
displaced (minimally) S32.111
severely S32.112
nondisplaced S32.110
II S32.129
displaced (minimally) S32.121
severely S32.122
nondisplaced S32.120
III S32.139
displaced (minimally) S32.131
severely S32.132
nondisplaced S32.130
thoracic — *see* Fracture, thorax, vertebra
vertex S02.0
vomer (bone) S02.2
wrist S62.10-
carpal — *see* Fracture, carpal bone
navicular (scaphoid) (hand) — *see*
Fracture, carpal, navicular
xiphisternum, xiphoid (process) S22.24
zygoma S02.402
left side S02.40F
right side S02.40E
Fragile, fragility
autosomal site Q95.5
bone, congenital (with blue sclera) Q78.0
capillary (hereditary) D69.8
hair L67.8
nails L60.3
non-sex chromosome site Q95.5
X chromosome Q99.2
Fragilitas
crinium L67.8
ossium (with blue sclerae) (hereditary) Q78.0
unguium L60.3
congenital Q84.6
**Fragments, cataract (lens) , following
cataract surgery** H59.02-
retained foreign body — *see* Retained,
foreign body fragments (type of)
Frailty (frail) R54
mental R41.81
Frambesia, frambesial (tropica) — *see also*
Yaws
initial lesion or ulcer A66.0
primary A66.0
Frambeside
gummatous A66.4
of early yaws A66.2
Frambesioma A66.1
**Franceschetti-Klein (-Wildervanck) disease
or syndrome** Q75.4
Francis' disease — *see* Tularemia
Franklin disease C88.2
Frank's essential thrombocytopenia D69.3
Fraser's syndrome Q87.0
Freckle (s) L81.2
malignant melanoma in — *see* Melanoma
melanotic (Hutchinson's) — *see* Melanoma,
in situ
retinal D49.81
Frederickson's hyperlipoproteinemia, type
I and V E78.3
IIA E78.00
IIB and III E78.2
IV E78.1
Freeman Sheldon syndrome Q87.0
Freezing — *see also* Effect, adverse,
cold T69.9
**Freiberg's disease (infraction of metatarsal
head or osteochondrosis)** — *see*
Osteochondrosis, juvenile, metatarsus
Frei's disease A55
Fremitus, friction, cardiac R01.2

Frenum, frenulum
external os Q51.828
tongue (shortening) (congenital) Q38.1
Frequency micturition (nocturnal) R35.0
psychogenic F45.8
Frey's syndrome
auriculotemporal G50.8
hyperhidrosis L74.52
Friction
burn — *see* Burn, by site
fremitus, cardiac R01.2
precordial R01.2
sounds, chest R09.89
**Friderichsen-Waterhouse syndrome or
disease** A39.1
Friedländer's B (bacillus) NEC — *see
also* condition A49.8
Friedreich's
ataxia G11.1
combined systemic disease G11.1
facial hemihypertrophy Q67.4
sclerosis (cerebellum) (spinal cord) G11.1
Frigidity F52.22
Fröhlich's syndrome E23.6
Frontal — *see also* condition
lobe syndrome F07.0
Frostbite (superficial) T33.90
with
partial thickness skin loss — *see* Frostbite
(superficial), by site
tissue necrosis T34.90
abdominal wall T33.3
with tissue necrosis T34.3
ankle T33.81-
with tissue necrosis T34.81-
arm T33.4-
with tissue necrosis T34.4-
finger (s) — *see* Frostbite, finger
hand — *see* Frostbite, hand
wrist — *see* Frostbite, wrist
ear T33.01-
with tissue necrosis T34.01-
face T33.09
with tissue necrosis T34.09
finger T33.53-
with tissue necrosis T34.53-
foot T33.82-
with tissue necrosis T34.82-
hand T33.52-
with tissue necrosis T34.52-
head T33.09
with tissue necrosis T34.09
ear — *see* Frostbite, ear
nose — *see* Frostbite, nose
hip (and thigh) T33.6-
with tissue necrosis T34.6-
knee T33.7-
with tissue necrosis T34.7-
leg T33.9-
with tissue necrosis T34.9-
ankle — *see* Frostbite, ankle
foot — *see* Frostbite, foot
knee — *see* Frostbite, knee
lower T33.7-
with tissue necrosis T34.7-
thigh — *see* Frostbite, hip
toe — *see* Frostbite, toe
limb
lower T33.99
with tissue necrosis T34.99
upper — *see* Frostbite, arm
neck T33.1
with tissue necrosis T34.1
nose T33.02
with tissue necrosis T34.02
pelvis T33.3
with tissue necrosis T34.3
specified site NEC T33.99
with tissue necrosis T34.99
thigh — *see* Frostbite, hip
thorax T33.2
with tissue necrosis T34.2
toes T33.83-
with tissue necrosis T34.83-
trunk T33.99

Frostbite (superficial) - *continued*
  trunk - *continued*
    with tissue necrosis T34.99
    wrist T33.51-
      with tissue necrosis T34.51-
Frotteurism F65.81
Frozen — *see also* Effect, adverse, cold T69.9
  pelvis (female) N94.89
    male K66.8
  shoulder — *see* Capsulitis, adhesive
Fructokinase deficiency E74.11
Fructose 1,6 diphosphatase deficiency E74.19
Fructosemia (benign) (essential) E74.12
Fructosuria (benign) (essential) E74.11
Fuchs'
  black spot (myopic) — *see also* Myopia, degenerative H44.2-
  dystrophy (corneal endothelium) H18.51
  heterochromic cyclitis — *see* Cyclitis, Fuchs' heterochromic
Fucosidosis E77.1
Fugue R68.89
  dissociative F44.1
  hysterical (dissociative) F44.1
  postictal in epilepsy — *see* Epilepsy
  reaction to exceptional stress (transient) F43.0
Fulminant, fulminating — *see* condition
Functional — *see also* condition
  bleeding (uterus) N93.8
Functioning, intellectual, borderline R41.83
Fundus — *see* condition
Fungemia NOS B49
Fungus, fungous
  cerebral G93.89
  disease NOS B49
  infection — *see* Infection, fungus
Funiculitis (acute) (chronic) (endemic) N49.1
  gonococcal (acute) (chronic) A54.23
  tuberculous A18.15
Funnel
  breast (acquired) M95.4
    congenital Q67.6
    sequelae (late effect) of rickets E64.3
  chest (acquired) M95.4
    congenital Q67.6
    sequelae (late effect) of rickets E64.3
  pelvis (acquired) M95.5
    with disproportion (fetopelvic) O33.3
      causing obstructed labor O65.3
    congenital Q74.2
FUO (fever of unknown origin) R50.9
Furfur L21.0
  microsporon B36.0
Furrier's lung J67.8
Furrowed K14.5
  nail (s) (transverse) L60.4
    congenital Q84.6
  tongue K14.5
    congenital Q38.3
Furuncle L02.92
  abdominal wall L02.221
  ankle — *see* Furuncle, lower limb
  anus K61.0
  antecubital space — *see* Furuncle, upper limb
  arm — *see* Furuncle, upper limb
  auditory canal, external — *see* Abscess, ear, external
  auricle (ear) — *see* Abscess, ear, external
  axilla (region) L02.42-
  back (any part) L02.222
  breast N61.1
  buttock L02.32
  cheek (external) L02.02
  chest wall L02.223
  chin L02.02
  corpus cavernosum N48.21
  ear, external — *see* Abscess, ear, external
  external auditory canal — *see* Abscess, ear, external
  eyelid — *see* Abscess, eyelid
  face L02.02
  femoral (region) — *see* Furuncle, lower limb

Furuncle - *continued*
  finger — *see* Furuncle, hand
  flank L02.221
  foot L02.62-
  forehead L02.02
  gluteal (region) L02.32
  groin L02.224
  hand L02.52-
  head L02.821
    face L02.02
  hip — *see* Furuncle, lower limb
  kidney — *see* Abscess, kidney
  knee — *see* Furuncle, lower limb
  labium (majus) (minus) N76.4
  lacrimal
    gland — *see* Dacryoadenitis
    passages (duct) (sac) — *see* Inflammation, lacrimal, passages, acute
  leg (any part) — *see* Furuncle, lower limb
  lower limb L02.42-
  malignant A22.0
  mouth K12.2
  navel L02.226
  neck L02.12
  nose J34.0
  orbit, orbital — *see* Abscess, orbit
  palmar (space) — *see* Furuncle, hand
  partes posteriores L02.32
  pectoral region L02.223
  penis N48.21
  perineum L02.225
  pinna — *see* Abscess, ear, external
  popliteal — *see* Furuncle, lower limb
  prepatellar — *see* Furuncle, lower limb
  scalp L02.821
  seminal vesicle N49.0
  shoulder — *see* Furuncle, upper limb
  specified site NEC L02.828
  submandibular K12.2
  temple (region) L02.02
  thumb — *see* Furuncle, hand
  toe — *see* Furuncle, foot
  trunk L02.229
    abdominal wall L02.221
    back L02.222
    chest wall L02.223
    groin L02.224
    perineum L02.225
    umbilicus L02.226
  umbilicus L02.226
  upper limb L02.42-
  vulva N76.4
Furunculosis — *see* Furuncle
Fused — *see* Fusion, fused
Fusion, fused (congenital)
  astragaloscaphoid Q74.2
  atria Q21.1
  auditory canal Q16.1
  auricles, heart Q21.1
  binocular with defective stereopsis H53.32
  bone Q79.8
  cervical spine M43.22
  choanal Q30.0
  commissure, mitral valve Q23.2
  cusps, heart valve NEC Q24.8
    mitral Q23.2
    pulmonary Q22.1
    tricuspid Q22.4
  ear ossicles Q16.3
  fingers Q70.0-
  hymen Q52.3
  joint (acquired) — *see also* Ankylosis
    congenital Q74.8
  kidneys (incomplete) Q63.1
  labium (majus) (minus) Q52.5
  larynx and trachea Q34.8
  limb, congenital Q74.8
    lower Q74.2
    upper Q74.0
  lobes, lung Q33.8
  lumbosacral (acquired) M43.27
    arthrodesis status Z98.1
    congenital Q76.49
    postprocedural status Z98.1
  nares, nose, nasal, nostril (s) Q30.0

Fusion, fused (congenital) - *continued*
  organ or site not listed — *see* Anomaly, by site
  ossicles Q79.9
    auditory Q16.3
  pulmonic cusps Q22.1
  ribs Q76.6
  sacroiliac (joint) (acquired) M43.28
    arthrodesis status Z98.1
    congenital Q74.2
    postprocedural status Z98.1
  spine (acquired) NEC M43.20
    arthrodesis status Z98.1
    cervical region M43.22
    cervicothoracic region M43.23
    congenital Q76.49
    lumbar M43.26
    lumbosacral region M43.27
    occipito-atlanto-axial region M43.21
    postoperative status Z98.1
    sacrococcygeal region M43.28
    thoracic region M43.24
    thoracolumbar region M43.25
  sublingual duct with submaxillary duct at opening in mouth Q38.4
  testes Q55.1
  toes Q70.2-
  tooth, teeth K00.2
  trachea and esophagus Q39.8
  twins Q89.4
  vagina Q52.4
  ventricles, heart Q21.0
  vertebra (arch) — *see* Fusion, spine
  vulva Q52.5
Fusospirillosis (mouth) (tongue) (tonsil) A69.1
Fussy baby R68.12

G

Gain in weight (abnormal) (excessive) — *see also* Weight, gain
Gaisböck's disease (polycythemia hypertonica) D75.1
Gait abnormality R26.9
  ataxic R26.0
  falling R29.6
  hysterical (ataxic) (staggering) F44.4
  paralytic R26.1
  spastic R26.1
  specified type NEC R26.89
  staggering R26.0
  unsteadiness R26.81
  walking difficulty NEC R26.2
Galactocele (breast) N64.89
  puerperal, postpartum O92.79
Galactokinase deficiency E74.29
Galactophoritis N61.0
  gestational, puerperal, postpartum O91.2-
Galactorrhea O92.6
  not associated with childbirth N64.3
Galactosemia (classic) (congenital) E74.21
Galactosuria E74.29
Galacturia R82.0
  schistosomiasis (bilharziasis) B65.0
GALD (gestational alloimmune liver disease) P78.84
Galeazzi's fracture S52.37-
Galen's vein — *see* condition
Galeophobia F40.218
Gall duct — *see* condition
Gallbladder — *see also* condition
  acute K81.0
Gallop rhythm R00.8
Gallstone (colic) (cystic duct) (gallbladder) (impacted) (multiple) — *see also* Calculus, gallbladder
  with
    cholecystitis — *see* Calculus, gallbladder, with cholecystitis
  bile duct (common) (hepatic) — *see* Calculus, bile duct
  causing intestinal obstruction K56.3
  specified NEC K80.80
    with obstruction K80.81
Gambling Z72.6
  pathological (compulsive) F63.0

Gammopathy (of undetermined significance [MGUS]) D47.2
  associated with lymphoplasmacytic dyscrasia D47.2
  monoclonal D47.2
  polyclonal D89.0
Gamna's disease (siderotic splenomegaly) D73.1
Gamophobia F40.298
Gampsodactylia (congenital) Q66.7-
Gamstorp's disease (adynamia episodica hereditaria) G72.3
Gandy-Nanta disease (siderotic splenomegaly) D73.1
Gang
  membership offenses Z72.810
Gangliocytoma D36.10
Ganglioglioma — *see* Neoplasm, uncertain behavior, by site
Ganglion (compound) (diffuse) (joint) (tendon (sheath)) M67.40
  ankle M67.47-
  foot M67.47-
  forearm M67.43-
  hand M67.44-
  lower leg M67.46-
  multiple sites M67.49
  of yaws (early) (late) A66.6
  pelvic region M67.45-
  periosteal — *see* Periostitis
  shoulder region M67.41-
  specified site NEC M67.48
  thigh region M67.45-
  tuberculous A18.09
  upper arm M67.42-
  wrist M67.43-
Ganglioneuroblastoma — *see* Neoplasm, nerve, malignant
Ganglioneuroma D36.10
  malignant — *see* Neoplasm, nerve, malignant
Ganglioneuromatosis D36.10
Ganglionitis
  fifth nerve — *see* Neuralgia, trigeminal
  gasserian (postherpetic) (postzoster) B02.21
  geniculate G51.1
    newborn (birth injury) P11.3
    postherpetic, postzoster B02.21
  herpes zoster B02.21
  postherpetic geniculate B02.21
Gangliosidosis E75.10
  GM1 E75.19
  GM2 E75.00
    other specified E75.09
    Sandhoff disease E75.01
    Tay-Sachs disease E75.02
  GM3 E75.19
  mucolipidosis IV E75.11
Gangosa A66.5
Gangrene, gangrenous (connective tissue) (dropsical) (dry) (moist) (skin) (ulcer)
  — *see also* Necrosis I96
  with diabetes (mellitus) — *see* Diabetes, gangrene
  abdomen (wall) I96
  alveolar M27.3
  appendix K35.80
    with
      peritonitis, localized — *see also* Appendicitis K35.31
  arteriosclerotic (general) (senile) — *see* Arteriosclerosis, extremities, with, gangrene
  auricle I96
  Bacillus welchii A48.0
  bladder (infectious) — *see* Cystitis, specified type NEC
  bowel, cecum, or colon — *see* Gangrene, intestine
  Clostridium perfringens or welchii A48.0
  cornea H18.89-
  corpora cavernosa N48.29
    noninfective N48.89
  cutaneous, spreading I96
  decubital — *see* Ulcer, pressure, by site

Gangrene, gangrenous (connective tissue) (dropsical) (dry) (moist) (skin) (ulcer) - *continued*
  diabetic (any site) — *see* Diabetes, gangrene
  epidemic — *see* Poisoning, food, noxious, plant
  epididymis (infectional) N45.1
  erysipelas — *see* Erysipelas
  emphysematous — *see* Gangrene, gas
  extremity (lower) (upper) I96
  Fournier N49.3
    female N76.89
  fusospirochetal A69.0
  gallbladder — *see* Cholecystitis, acute
  gas (bacillus) A48.0
    following
      abortion — *see* Abortion by type complicated by infection
      ectopic or molar pregnancy O08.0
  glossitis K14.0
  hernia — *see* Hernia, by site, with gangrene
  intestine, intestinal (hemorrhagic) (massive) — *see also* Infarct, intestine K55.069
    with
      mesenteric embolism — *see also* Infarct, intestine K55.069
      obstruction — *see* Obstruction, intestine
  laryngitis J04.0
  limb (lower) (upper) I96
  lung J85.0
    spirochetal A69.8
  lymphangitis I89.1
  Meleney's (synergistic) — *see* Ulcer, skin
  mesentery — *see also* Infarct, intestine K55.069
    with
      embolism — *see also* Infarct, intestine K55.069
      intestinal obstruction — *see* Obstruction, intestine
  mouth A69.0
  ovary — *see* Oophoritis
  pancreas — *see* Pancreatitis, acute
  penis N48.29
    noninfective N48.89
  perineum I96
  pharynx — *see also* Pharyngitis
    Vincent's A69.1
  presenile I73.1
  progressive synergistic — *see* Ulcer, skin
  pulmonary J85.0
  pulpal (dental) K04.1
  quinsy J36
  Raynaud's (symmetric gangrene) I73.01
  retropharyngeal J39.2
  scrotum N49.3
    noninfective N50.89
  senile (atherosclerotic) — *see* Arteriosclerosis, extremities, with, gangrene
  spermatic cord N49.1
    noninfective N50.89
  spine I96
  spirochetal NEC A69.8
  spreading cutaneous I96
  stomatitis A69.0
  symmetrical I73.01
  testis (infectional) N45.2
    noninfective N44.8
  throat — *see also* Pharyngitis
    diphtheritic A36.0
    Vincent's A69.1
  thyroid (gland) E07.89
  tooth (pulp) K04.1
  tuberculous NEC — *see* Tuberculosis
  tunica vaginalis N49.1
    noninfective N50.89
  umbilicus I96
  uterus — *see* Endometritis
  uvulitis K12.2
  vas deferens N49.1
    noninfective N50.89
  vulva N76.89
Ganister disease J62.8

Ganser's syndrome (hysterical) F44.89
Gardner-Diamond syndrome (autoerythrocyte sensitization) D69.2
Gargoylism E76.01
Garré's disease, osteitis (sclerosing) , osteomyelitis — *see* Osteomyelitis, specified type NEC
Garrod's pad, knuckle M72.1
Gartner's duct
  cyst Q52.4
  persistent Q50.6
Gas R14.3
  asphyxiation, inhalation, poisoning, suffocation NEC — *see* Table of Drugs and Chemicals
  excessive R14.0
  gangrene A48.0
    following
      abortion — *see* Abortion by type complicated by infection
      ectopic or molar pregnancy O08.0
  on stomach R14.0
  pains R14.1
Gastralgia — *see also* Pain, abdominal
Gastrectasis K31.0
  psychogenic F45.8
Gastric — *see* condition
Gastrinoma
  malignant
    pancreas C25.4
    specified site NEC — *see* Neoplasm, malignant, by site
    unspecified site C25.4
  specified site — *see* Neoplasm, uncertain behavior
  unspecified site D37.9
Gastritis (simple) K29.70
  with bleeding K29.71
  acute (erosive) K29.00
    with bleeding K29.01
  alcoholic K29.20
    with bleeding K29.21
  allergic K29.60
    with bleeding K29.61
  atrophic (chronic) K29.40
    with bleeding K29.41
  chronic (antral) (fundal) K29.50
    with bleeding K29.51
    atrophic K29.40
      with bleeding K29.41
    superficial K29.30
      with bleeding K29.31
  dietary counseling and surveillance Z71.3
  due to diet deficiency E63.9
  eosinophilic K52.81
  giant hypertrophic K29.60
    with bleeding K29.61
  granulomatous K29.60
    with bleeding K29.61
  hypertrophic (mucosa) K29.60
    with bleeding K29.61
  nervous F54
  spastic K29.60
    with bleeding K29.61
  specified NEC K29.60
    with bleeding K29.61
  superficial chronic K29.30
    with bleeding K29.31
  tuberculous A18.83
  viral NEC A08.4
Gastrocarcinoma — *see* Neoplasm, malignant, stomach
Gastrocolic — *see* condition
Gastrodisciasis, gastrodiscoidiasis B66.8
Gastroduodenitis K29.90
  with bleeding K29.91
  virus, viral A08.4
    specified type NEC A08.39
Gastrodynia — *see* Pain, abdominal
Gastroenteritis (acute) (chronic) (noninfectious) — *see also* Enteritis K52.9
  allergic K52.29
    with

Gastroenteritis (acute) (chronic) (noninfectious) - *continued*
  allergic - *continued*
    with - *continued*
      eosinophilic gastritis or gastroenteritis K52.81
      food protein-induced enterocolitis syndrome K52.21
      food protein-induced enteropathy K52.22
    dietetic — *see also* Gastroenteritis, allergic K52.29
  drug-induced K52.1
  due to
    Cryptosporidium A07.2
    drugs K52.1
    food poisoning — *see* Intoxication, foodborne
    radiation K52.0
  eosinophilic K52.81
  epidemic (infectious) A09
  food hypersensitivity — *see also* Gastroenteritis, allergic K52.29
  infectious — *see* Enteritis, infectious
  influenzal — *see* Influenza, with gastroenteritis
  noninfectious K52.9
    specified NEC K52.89
  rotaviral A08.0
  Salmonella A02.0
  toxic K52.1
  viral NEC A08.4
    acute infectious A08.39
      type Norwalk A08.11
    infantile (acute) A08.39
    Norwalk agent A08.11
    rotaviral A08.0
    severe of infants A08.39
    specified type NEC A08.39
Gastroenteropathy — *see also* Gastroenteritis K52.9
  acute, due to Norwalk agent A08.11
  acute, due to Norovirus A08.11
  infectious A09
Gastroenteroptosis K63.4
Gastroesophageal laceration- hemorrhage syndrome K22.6
Gastrointestinal — *see* condition
Gastrojejunal — *see* condition
Gastrojejunitis — *see also* Enteritis K52.9
Gastrojejunocolic — *see* condition
Gastroliths K31.89
Gastromalacia K31.89
Gastroparalysis K31.84
  diabetic — *see* Diabetes, gastroparalysis
Gastroparesis K31.84
  diabetic — *see* Diabetes, by type, with gastroparesis
Gastropathy K31.9
  congestive portal K31.89
  erythematous K29.70
  exudative K90.89
  portal hypertensive K31.89
Gastroptosis K31.89
Gastrorrhagia K92.2
  psychogenic F45.8
Gastroschisis (congenital) Q79.3
Gastrospasm (neurogenic) (reflex) K31.89
  neurotic F45.8
  psychogenic F45.8
Gastrostaxis — *see* Gastritis, with bleeding
Gastrostenosis K31.89
Gastrostomy
  attention to Z43.1
  status Z93.1
Gastrosuccorrhea (continuous) (intermittent) K31.89
  neurotic F45.8
  psychogenic F45.8
Gatophobia F40.218
Gaucher's disease or splenomegaly (adult) (infantile) E75.22
Gee (-Herter) (-Thaysen) disease (nontropical sprue) K90.0

Gélineau's syndrome G47.419
  with cataplexy G47.411
Gemination, tooth, teeth K00.2
Gemistocytoma
  specified site — *see* Neoplasm, malignant, by site
  unspecified site C71.9
General, generalized — *see* condition
Genetic
  carrier (status)
    cystic fibrosis Z14.1
    hemophilia A (asymptomatic) Z14.01
      symptomatic Z14.02
    specified NEC Z14.8
  susceptibility to disease NEC Z15.89
    malignant neoplasm Z15.09
      breast Z15.01
      endometrium Z15.04
      ovary Z15.02
      prostate Z15.03
      specified NEC Z15.09
    multiple endocrine neoplasia Z15.81
Genital — *see* condition
Genito-anorectal syndrome A55
Genitourinary system — *see* condition
Genu
  congenital Q74.1
  extrorsum (acquired) — *see also* Deformity, varus, knee
    congenital Q74.1
    sequelae (late effect) of rickets E64.3
  introrsum (acquired) — *see also* Deformity, valgus, knee
    congenital Q74.1
    sequelae (late effect) of rickets E64.3
  rachitic (old) E64.3
  recurvatum (acquired) — *see also* Deformity, limb, specified type NEC, lower leg
    congenital Q68.2
    sequelae (late effect) of rickets E64.3
  valgum (acquired) (knock-knee) M21.06-
    congenital Q74.1
    sequelae (late effect) of rickets E64.3
  varum (acquired) (bowleg) M21.16-
    congenital Q74.1
    sequelae (late effect) of rickets E64.3
Geographic tongue K14.1
Geophagia — *see* Pica
Geotrichosis B48.3
  stomatitis B48.3
Gephyrophobia F40.242
Gerbode defect Q21.0
GERD (gastroesophageal reflux disease) K21.9
Gerhardt's
  disease (erythromelalgia) I73.81
  syndrome (vocal cord paralysis) J38.00
    bilateral J38.02
    unilateral J38.01
German measles — *see also* Rubella
  exposure to Z20.4
Germinoblastoma (diffuse) C85.9-
  follicular C82.9-
Germinoma — *see* Neoplasm, malignant, by site
Gerontoxon — *see* Degeneration, cornea, senile
Gerstmann's syndrome R48.8
  developmental F81.2
Gerstmann-Sträussler-Scheinker syndrome (GSS) A81.82
Gestation (period) — *see also* Pregnancy
  ectopic — *see* Pregnancy, by site
  multiple O30.9-
    greater than quadruplets — *see* Pregnancy, multiple (gestation), specified NEC
    specified NEC — *see* Pregnancy, multiple (gestation), specified NEC
Gestational
  mammary abscess O91.11-
  purulent mastitis O91.11-
  subareolar abscess O91.11-
Ghon tubercle, primary infection A15.7
Ghost
  teeth K00.4

Ghost - *continued*
  vessels (cornea) H16.41-
Ghoul hand A66.3
Gianotti-Crosti disease L44.4
Giant
  cell
    epulis K06.8
    peripheral granuloma K06.8
  esophagus, congenital Q39.5
  kidney, congenital Q63.3
  urticaria T78.3
    hereditary D84.1
Giardiasis A07.1
Gibert's disease or pityriasis L42
Giddiness R42
  hysterical F44.89
  psychogenic F45.8
Gierke's disease (glycogenosis I) E74.01
Gigantism (cerebral) (hypophyseal) (pituitary) E22.0
  constitutional E34.4
Gilbert's disease or syndrome E80.4
Gilchrist's disease B40.9
Gilford-Hutchinson disease E34.8
Gilles de la Tourette's disease or syndrome (motor-verbal tic) F95.2
Gingivitis K05.10
  acute (catarrhal) K05.00
    necrotizing A69.1
    nonplaque induced K05.01
    plaque induced K05.00
  chronic (desquamative) (hyperplastic) (simple marginal) (pregnancy associated) (ulcerative) K05.10
    nonplaque induced K05.11
    plaque induced K05.10
  expulsiva — *see* Periodontitis
  necrotizing ulcerative (acute) A69.1
  pellagrous E52
    acute necrotizing A69.1
  Vincent's A69.1
Gingivoglossitis K14.0
Gingivopericementitis — *see* Periodontitis
Gingivosis — *see* Gingivitis, chronic
Gingivostomatitis K05.10
  herpesviral B00.2
  necrotizing ulcerative (acute) A69.1
Gland, glandular — *see* condition
Glanders A24.0
Glanzmann (-Naegeli) disease or thrombasthenia D69.1
Glasgow coma scale
  total score
    3-8 R40.243
    9-12 R40.242
    13-15 R40.241
Glass-blower's disease (cataract) — *see* Cataract, specified NEC
Glaucoma H40.9
  with
    increased episcleral venous pressure H40.81-
    pseudoexfoliation of lens — *see* Glaucoma, open angle, primary, capsular
  absolute H44.51-
  angle-closure (primary) H40.20-
    acute (attack) (crisis) H40.21-
    chronic H40.22-
    intermittent H40.23-
    residual stage H40.24-
  borderline H40.00-
  capsular (with pseudoexfoliation of lens) — *see* Glaucoma, open angle, primary, capsular
  childhood Q15.0
  closed angle — *see* Glaucoma, angle-closure
  congenital Q15.0
  corticosteroid-induced — *see* Glaucoma, secondary, drugs
  hypersecretion H40.82-
  in (due to)
    amyloidosis E85.4 *[H42]*
    aniridia Q13.1 *[H42]*

Glaucoma - *continued*
  in (due to) - *continued*
    concussion of globe — *see* Glaucoma, secondary, trauma
    dislocation of lens — *see* Glaucoma, secondary
    disorder of lens NEC — *see* Glaucoma, secondary
    drugs — *see* Glaucoma, secondary, drugs
    endocrine disease NOS E34.9 *[H42]*
    eye
      inflammation — *see* Glaucoma, secondary, inflammation
      trauma — *see* Glaucoma, secondary, trauma
    hypermature cataract — *see* Glaucoma, secondary
    iridocyclitis — *see* Glaucoma, secondary, inflammation
    lens disorder — *see* Glaucoma, secondary, Lowe's syndrome E72.03 *[H42]*
    metabolic disease NOS E88.9 *[H42]*
    ocular disorders NEC — *see* Glaucoma, secondary
    onchocerciasis B73.02
    pupillary block — *see* Glaucoma, secondary
    retinal vein occlusion — *see* Glaucoma, secondary
    Rieger's anomaly Q13.81 *[H42]*
    rubeosis of iris — *see* Glaucoma, secondary
    tumor of globe — *see* Glaucoma, secondary
  infantile Q15.0
  low tension — *see* Glaucoma, open angle, primary, low-tension
  malignant H40.83-
  narrow angle — *see* Glaucoma, angle-closure
  newborn Q15.0
  noncongestive (chronic) — *see* Glaucoma, open angle
  nonobstructive — *see* Glaucoma, open angle
  obstructive — *see also* Glaucoma, angle-closure
    due to lens changes — *see* Glaucoma, secondary
  open angle H40.10-
    primary H40.11-
      capsular (with pseudoexfoliation of lens) H40.14-
      low-tension H40.12-
      pigmentary H40.13-
      residual stage H40.15-
  phacolytic — *see* Glaucoma, secondary
  pigmentary — *see* Glaucoma, open angle, primary, pigmentary
  postinfectious — *see* Glaucoma, secondary, inflammation
  secondary (to) H40.5-
    drugs H40.6-
    inflammation H40.4-
    trauma H40.3-
  simple (chronic) H40.11-
  simplex H40.11-
  specified type NEC H40.89
  suspect H40.00-
  syphilitic A52.71
  traumatic — *see also* Glaucoma, secondary, trauma
    newborn (birth injury) P15.3
  tuberculous A18.59
Glaucomatous flecks (subcapsular) — *see* Cataract, complicated
Glazed tongue K14.4
Gleet (gonococcal) A54.01
Glénard's disease K63.4
Glioblastoma (multiforme)
  with sarcomatous component
    specified site — *see* Neoplasm, malignant, by site
    unspecified site C71.9
  giant cell
    specified site — *see* Neoplasm, malignant, by site

Glioblastoma (multiforme) - *continued*
  giant cell - *continued*
    unspecified site C71.9
  specified site — *see* Neoplasm, malignant, by site
  unspecified site C71.9
Glioma (malignant)
  astrocytic
    specified site — *see* Neoplasm, malignant, by site
    unspecified site C71.9
  mixed
    specified site — *see* Neoplasm, malignant, by site
    unspecified site C71.9
  nose Q30.8
  specified site NEC — *see* Neoplasm, malignant, by site
  subependymal D43.2
    specified site — *see* Neoplasm, uncertain behavior, by site
    unspecified site D43.2
  unspecified site C71.9
Gliomatosis cerebri C71.0
Glioneuroma — *see* Neoplasm, uncertain behavior, by site
Gliosarcoma
  specified site — *see* Neoplasm, malignant, by site
  unspecified site C71.9
Gliosis (cerebral) G93.89
  spinal G95.89
Glisson's disease — *see* Rickets
Globinuria R82.3
Globus (hystericus) F45.8
Glomangioma D18.00
  intra-abdominal D18.03
  intracranial D18.02
  skin D18.01
  specified site NEC D18.09
Glomangiomyoma D18.00
  intra-abdominal D18.03
  intracranial D18.02
  skin D18.01
  specified site NEC D18.09
Glomangiosarcoma — *see* Neoplasm, connective tissue, malignant
Glomerular
  disease in syphilis A52.75
  nephritis — *see* Glomerulonephritis
Glomerulitis — *see* Glomerulonephritis
Glomerulonephritis — *see also* Nephritis N05.9
  with
    edema — *see* Nephrosis
    minimal change N05.0
    minor glomerular abnormality N05.0
  acute N00.9
  chronic N03.9
  crescentic (diffuse) NEC — *see also* N00-N07 with fourth character .7 N05.7
  dense deposit — *see also* N00-N07 with fourth character .6 N05.6
  diffuse
    crescentic — *see also* N00-N07 with fourth character .7 N05.7
    endocapillary proliferative — *see also* N00-N07 with fourth character .4 N05.4
    membranous — *see also* N00-N07 with fourth character .2 N05.2
    mesangial proliferative — *see also* N00-N07 with fourth character .3 N05.3
    mesangiocapillary — *see also* N00-N07 with fourth character .5 N05.5
    sclerosing N18.9
  endocapillary proliferative (diffuse) NEC — *see also* N00-N07 with fourth character .4 N05.4
  extracapillary NEC — *see also* N00-N07 with fourth character .7 N05.7
  focal (and segmental) — *see also* N00-N07 with fourth character .1 N05.1

Glomerulonephritis - *continued*
  hypocomplementemic — *see* Glomerulonephritis, membranoproliferative
  IgA — *see* Nephropathy, IgA
  immune complex (circulating) NEC N05.8
  in (due to)
    amyloidosis E85.4 *[N08]*
    bilharziasis B65.9 *[N08]*
    cryoglobulinemia D89.1 *[N08]*
    defibrination syndrome D65 *[N08]*
    diabetes mellitus — *see* Diabetes, glomerulosclerosis
    disseminated intravascular coagulation D65 *[N08]*
    Fabry (-Anderson) disease E75.21 *[N08]*
    Goodpasture's syndrome M31.0
    hemolytic-uremic syndrome D59.3
    Henoch (-Schönlein) purpura D69.0 *[N08]*
    lecithin cholesterol acyltransferase deficiency E78.6 *[N08]*
    microscopic polyangiitis M31.7 *[N08]*
    multiple myeloma C90.0- *[N08]*
    Plasmodium malariae B52.0
    schistosomiasis B65.9 *[N08]*
    sepsis A41.9 *[N08]*
    streptococcal A40- *[N08]*
    sickle-cell disorders D57.- *[N08]*
    strongyloidiasis B78.9 *[N08]*
    subacute bacterial endocarditis I33.0 *[N08]*
    syphilis (late) congenital A50.59 *[N08]*
    systemic lupus erythematosus M32.14
    thrombotic thrombocytopenic purpura M31.1 *[N08]*
    typhoid fever A01.09
    Waldenström macroglobulinemia C88.0 *[N08]*
    Wegener's granulomatosis M31.31
  latent or quiescent N03.9
  lobular, lobulonodular — *see* Glomerulonephritis, membranoproliferative
  membranoproliferative (diffuse) (type 1 or 3) — *see also* N00-N07 with fourth character .5 N05.5
    dense deposit (type 2) NEC — *see also* N00-N07 with fourth character .6 N05.6
  membranous (diffuse) NEC — *see also* N00-N07 with fourth character .2 N05.2
  mesangial
    IgA/IgG — *see* Nephropathy, IgA
    proliferative (diffuse) NEC — *see also* N00-N07 with fourth character .3 N05.3
  mesangiocapillary (diffuse) NEC — *see also* N00-N07 with fourth character .5 N05.5
  necrotic, necrotizing NEC — *see also* N00-N07 with fourth character .8 N05.8
  nodular — *see* Glomerulonephritis, membranoproliferative
  poststreptococcal NEC N05.9
    acute N00.9
    chronic N03.9
    rapidly progressive N01.9
  proliferative NEC — *see also* N00-N07 with fourth character .8 N05.8
    diffuse (lupus) M32.14
  rapidly progressive N01.9
  sclerosing, diffuse N18.9
  specified pathology NEC — *see also* N00-N07 with fourth character .8 N05.8
  subacute N01.9
Glomerulopathy — *see* Glomerulonephritis
Glomerulosclerosis — *see also* Sclerosis, renal
  intercapillary (nodular) (with diabetes) — *see* Diabetes, glomerulosclerosis
  intracapillary — *see* Diabetes, glomerulosclerosis
Glossagra K14.6
Glossalgia K14.6
Glossitis (chronic superficial) (gangrenous) (Moeller's) K14.0
  areata exfoliativa K14.1

Glossitis (chronic superficial) (gangrenous) (Moeller's) - *continued*
- atrophic K14.4
- benign migratory K14.1
- cortical superficial, sclerotic K14.0
- Hunter's D51.0
- interstitial, sclerous K14.0
- median rhomboid K14.2
- pellagrous E52
- superficial, chronic K14.0

Glossocele K14.8

Glossodynia K14.6
- exfoliativa K14.4

Glossoncus K14.8

Glossopathy K14.9

Glossophytia K14.3

Glossoplegia K14.8

Glossoptosis K14.8

Glossopyrosis K14.6

Glossotrichia K14.3

Glossy skin L90.8

Glottis — *see* condition

Glottitis — *see also* Laryngitis J04.0

Glucagonoma
- pancreas
  - benign D13.7
  - malignant C25.4
  - uncertain behavior D37.8
- specified site NEC
  - benign — *see* Neoplasm, benign, by site
  - malignant — *see* Neoplasm, malignant, by site
  - uncertain behavior — *see* Neoplasm, uncertain behavior, by site
- unspecified site
  - benign D13.7
  - malignant C25.4
  - uncertain behavior D37.8

Glucoglycinuria E72.51

Glucose-galactose malabsorption E74.39

Glue
- ear — *see* Otitis, media, nonsuppurative, chronic, mucoid
- sniffing (airplane) — *see* Abuse, drug, inhalant
  - dependence — *see* Dependence, drug, inhalant

Glutaric aciduria E72.3

Glycinemia E72.51

Glycinuria (renal) (with ketosis) E72.09

Glycogen
- infiltration — *see* Disease, glycogen storage
- storage disease — *see* Disease, glycogen storage

Glycogenosis (diffuse) (generalized) — *see also* Disease, glycogen storage
- cardiac E74.02 *[I43]*
- diabetic, secondary — *see* Diabetes, glycogenosis, secondary
- pulmonary interstitial J84.842

Glycopenia E16.2

Glycosuria R81
- renal E74.8

Gnathostoma spinigerum (infection) (infestation) , gnathostomiasis (wandering swelling) B83.1

Goiter (plunging) (substernal) E04.9
- with
  - hyperthyroidism (recurrent) — *see* Hyperthyroidism, with, goiter
  - thyrotoxicosis — *see* Hyperthyroidism, with, goiter
- adenomatous — *see* Goiter, nodular
- cancerous C73
- congenital (nontoxic) E03.0
  - diffuse E03.0
  - parenchymatous E03.0
  - transitory, with normal functioning P72.0
- cystic E04.2
  - due to iodine-deficiency E01.1
- due to
  - enzyme defect in synthesis of thyroid hormone E07.1
  - iodine-deficiency (endemic) E01.2
- dyshormonogenetic (familial) E07.1

Goiter (plunging) (substernal) - *continued*
- endemic (iodine-deficiency) E01.2
  - diffuse E01.0
  - multinodular E01.1
- exophthalmic — *see* Hyperthyroidism, with, goiter
- iodine-deficiency (endemic) E01.2
  - diffuse E01.0
  - multinodular E01.1
  - nodular E01.1
- lingual Q89.2
- lymphadenoid E06.3
- malignant C73
- multinodular (cystic) (nontoxic) E04.2
  - toxic or with hyperthyroidism E05.20
    - with thyroid storm E05.21
- neonatal NEC P72.0
- nodular (nontoxic) (due to) E04.9
  - with
    - hyperthyroidism E05.20
      - with thyroid storm E05.21
    - thyrotoxicosis E05.20
      - with thyroid storm E05.21
  - endemic E01.1
  - iodine-deficiency E01.1
  - sporadic E04.9
  - toxic E05.20
    - with thyroid storm E05.21
- nontoxic E04.9
  - diffuse (colloid) E04.0
  - multinodular E04.2
  - simple E04.0
  - specified NEC E04.8
  - uninodular E04.1
- simple E04.0
- toxic — *see* Hyperthyroidism, with, goiter
- uninodular (nontoxic) E04.1
  - toxic or with hyperthyroidism E05.10
    - with thyroid storm E05.11

Goiter-deafness syndrome E07.1

Goldberg syndrome Q89.8

Goldberg-Maxwell syndrome E34.51

Goldblatt's hypertension or kidney I70.1

Goldenhar (-Gorlin) syndrome Q87.0

Goldflam-Erb disease or syndrome G70.00
- with exacerbation (acute) G70.01
- in crisis G70.01

Goldscheider's disease Q81.8

Goldstein's disease (familial hemorrhagic telangiectasia) I78.0

Golfer's elbow — *see* Epicondylitis, medial

Gonadoblastoma
- specified site — *see* Neoplasm, uncertain behavior, by site
- unspecified site
  - female D39.10
  - male D40.10

Gonecystitis — *see* Vesiculitis

Gongylonemiasis B83.8

Goniosynechiae — *see* Adhesions, iris, goniosynechiae

Gonococcemia A54.86

Gonococcus, gonococcal (disease) (infection) — *see also* condition A54.9
- anus A54.6
- bursa, bursitis A54.49
- conjunctiva, conjunctivitis (neonatorum) A54.31
- endocardium A54.83
- eye A54.30
  - conjunctivitis A54.31
  - iridocyclitis A54.32
  - keratitis A54.33
  - newborn A54.31
  - other specified A54.39
- fallopian tubes (acute) (chronic) A54.24
- genitourinary (organ) (system) (tract) (acute)
  - lower A54.00
    - with abscess (accessory gland) (periurethral) A54.1
  - upper — *see also* condition A54.29
- heart A54.83
- iridocyclitis A54.32
- joint A54.42
- lymphatic (gland) (node) A54.89

Gonococcus, gonococcal (disease) (infection) - *continued*
- meninges, meningitis A54.81
- musculoskeletal A54.40
  - arthritis A54.42
  - osteomyelitis A54.43
  - other specified A54.49
  - spondylopathy A54.41
- pelviperitonitis A54.24
- pelvis (acute) (chronic) A54.24
- pharynx A54.5
- proctitis A54.6
- pyosalpinx (acute) (chronic) A54.24
- rectum A54.6
- skin A54.89
- specified site NEC A54.89
- tendon sheath A54.49
- throat A54.5
- urethra (acute) (chronic) A54.01
  - with abscess (accessory gland) (periurethral) A54.1
- vulva (acute) (chronic) A54.02

Gonocytoma
- specified site — *see* Neoplasm, uncertain behavior, by site
- unspecified site
  - female D39.10
  - male D40.10

Gonorrhea (acute) (chronic) A54.9
- Bartholin's gland (acute) (chronic) (purulent) A54.02
  - with abscess (accessory gland) (periurethral) A54.1
- bladder A54.01
- cervix A54.03
- conjunctiva, conjunctivitis (neonatorum) A54.31
- contact Z20.2
- Cowper's gland (with abscess) A54.1
- exposure to Z20.2
- fallopian tube (acute) (chronic) A54.24
- kidney (acute) (chronic) A54.21
- lower genitourinary tract A54.00
  - with abscess (accessory gland) (periurethral) A54.1
- ovary (acute) (chronic) A54.24
- pelvis (acute) (chronic) A54.24
  - female pelvic inflammatory disease A54.24
- penis A54.09
- prostate (acute) (chronic) A54.22
- seminal vesicle (acute) (chronic) A54.23
- specified site not listed — *see also* Gonococcus A54.89
- spermatic cord (acute) (chronic) A54.23
- urethra A54.01
  - with abscess (accessory gland) (periurethral) A54.1
- vagina A54.02
- vas deferens (acute) (chronic) A54.23
- vulva A54.02

Goodall's disease A08.19

Goodpasture's syndrome M31.0

Gopalan's syndrome (burning feet) E53.0

Gorlin-Chaudry-Moss syndrome Q87.0

Gottron's papules L94.4

Gougerot-Blum syndrome (pigmented purpuric lichenoid dermatitis) L81.7

Gougerot-Carteaud disease or syndrome (confluent reticulate papillomatosis) L83

Gougerot's syndrome (trisymptomatic) L81.7

Gouley's syndrome (constrictive pericarditis) I31.1

Goundou A66.6

Gout, chronic — *see also* Gout, gouty M1A.9
- drug-induced M1A.20
  - ankle M1A.27-
  - elbow M1A.22-
  - foot joint M1A.27-
  - hand joint M1A.24-
  - hip M1A.25-
  - knee M1A.26-
  - multiple site M1A.29-

Gout, chronic - *continued*
  drug-induced - *continued*
    shoulder M1A.21-
    vertebrae M1A.28
    wrist M1A.23-
  idiopathic M1A.00
    ankle M1A.07-
    elbow M1A.02-
    foot joint M1A.07-
    hand joint M1A.04-
    hip M1A.05-
    knee M1A.06-
    multiple site M1A.09
    shoulder M1A.01-
    vertebrae M1A.08
    wrist M1A.03-
  in (due to) renal impairment M1A.30
    ankle M1A.37-
    elbow M1A.32-
    foot joint M1A.37-
    hand joint M1A.34-
    hip M1A.35-
    knee M1A.36-
    multiple site M1A.39
    shoulder M1A.31-
    vertebrae M1A.38
    wrist M1A.33-
  lead-induced M1A.10
    ankle M1A.17-
    elbow M1A.12-
    foot joint M1A.17-
    hand joint M1A.14-
    hip M1A.15-
    knee M1A.16-
    multiple site M1A.19
    shoulder M1A.11-
    vertebrae M1A.18
    wrist M1A.13-
  primary — *see* Gout, chronic, idiopathic
  saturnine — *see* Gout, chronic, lead-induced
  secondary NEC M1A.40
    ankle M1A.47-
    elbow M1A.42-
    foot joint M1A.47-
    hand joint M1A.44-
    hip M1A.45-
    knee M1A.46-
    multiple site M1A.49
    shoulder M1A.41-
    vertebrae M1A.48
    wrist M1A.43-
  syphilitic (*see also* subcategory M14.8-)
    A52.77
  tophi M1A.9
Gout, gouty (acute) (attack) (flare) — *see also* Gout, chronic M10.9
  drug-induced M10.20
    ankle M10.27-
    elbow M10.22-
    foot joint M10.27-
    hand joint M10.24-
    hip M10.25-
    knee M10.26-
    multiple site M10.29
    shoulder M10.21-
    vertebrae M10.28
    wrist M10.23-
  idiopathic M10.00
    ankle M10.07-
    elbow M10.02-
    foot joint M10.07-
    hand joint M10.04-
    hip M10.05-
    knee M10.06-
    multiple site M10.09
    shoulder M10.01-
    vertebrae M10.08
    wrist M10.03-
  in (due to) renal impairment M10.30
    ankle M10.37-
    elbow M10.32-
    foot joint M10.37-
    hand joint M10.34-
    hip M10.35-
    knee M10.36-

Gout, gouty (acute) (attack) (flare) - *continued*
  in (due to) renal impairment - *continued*
    multiple site M10.39
    shoulder M10.31-
    vertebrae M10.38
    wrist M10.33-
  lead-induced M10.10
    ankle M10.17-
    elbow M10.12-
    foot joint M10.17-
    hand joint M10.14-
    hip M10.15-
    knee M10.16-
    multiple site M10.19
    shoulder M10.11-
    vertebrae M10.18
    wrist M10.13-
  primary — *see* Gout, idiopathic
  saturnine — *see* Gout, lead-induced
  secondary NEC M10.40
    ankle M10.47-
    elbow M10.42-
    foot joint M10.47-
    hand joint M10.44-
    hip M10.45-
    knee M10.46-
    multiple site M10.49
    shoulder M10.41-
    vertebrae M10.48
    wrist M10.43-
  syphilitic (*see also* subcategory M14.8-)
    A52.77
  tophi — *see* Gout, chronic
Gower's
  muscular dystrophy G71.01
  syndrome (vasovagal attack) R55
Gradenigo's syndrome — *see* Otitis, media, suppurative, acute
Graefe's disease — *see* Strabismus, paralytic, ophthalmoplegia, progressive
Graft-versus-host disease D89.813
  acute D89.810
  acute on chronic D89.812
  chronic D89.811
Grain mite (itch) B88.0
Grainhandler's disease or lung J67.8
Grand mal — *see* Epilepsy, generalized, specified NEC
Grand multipara status only (not pregnant) Z64.1
  pregnant — *see* Pregnancy, complicated by, grand multiparity
Granite worker's lung J62.8
Granular — *see also* condition
  inflammation, pharynx J31.2
  kidney (contracting) — *see* Sclerosis, renal
  liver K74.69
Granulation tissue (abnormal) (excessive) L92.9
  postmastoidectomy cavity — *see* Complications, postmastoidectomy, granulation
Granulocytopenia (primary) (malignant) — *see* Agranulocytosis
Granuloma L92.9
  abdomen K66.8
    from residual foreign body L92.3
    pyogenicum L98.0
  actinic L57.5
  annulare (perforating) L92.0
  apical K04.5
  aural — *see* Otitis, externa, specified NEC
  beryllium (skin) L92.3
  bone
    eosinophilic C96.6
    from residual foreign body — *see* Osteomyelitis, specified type NEC
    lung C96.6
  brain (any site) G06.0
    schistosomiasis B65.9 *[G07]*
  canaliculus lacrimalis — *see* Granuloma, lacrimal
  candidal (cutaneous) B37.2
  cerebral (any site) G06.0

Granuloma - *continued*
  coccidioidal (primary) (progressive) B38.7
    lung B38.1
    meninges B38.4
  colon K63.89
  conjunctiva H11.22-
  dental K04.5
  ear, middle — *see* Cholesteatoma
  eosinophilic C96.6
    bone C96.6
    lung C96.6
    oral mucosa K13.4
    skin L92.2
  eyelid H01.8
  facial (e) L92.2
  foreign body (in soft tissue) NEC M60.20
    ankle M60.27-
    foot M60.27-
    forearm M60.23-
    hand M60.24-
    in operation wound — *see* Foreign body, accidentally left during a procedure
    lower leg M60.26-
    pelvic region M60.25-
    shoulder region M60.21-
    skin L92.3
    specified site NEC M60.28
    subcutaneous tissue L92.3
    thigh M60.25-
    upper arm M60.22-
  gangraenescens M31.2
  genito-inguinale A58
  giant cell (central) (reparative) (jaw) M27.1
    gingiva (peripheral) K06.8
  gland (lymph) I88.8
  hepatic NEC K75.3
    in (due to)
      berylliosis J63.2 *[K77]*
      sarcoidosis D86.89
  Hodgkin C81.9
  ileum K63.89
  infectious B99.9
    specified NEC B99.8
  inguinale (Donovan) (venereal) A58
  intestine NEC K63.89
  intracranial (any site) G06.0
  intraspinal (any part) G06.1
  iridocyclitis — *see* Iridocyclitis, chronic
  jaw (bone) (central) M27.1
    reparative giant cell M27.1
  kidney — *see also* Infection, kidney N15.8
  lacrimal H04.81-
  larynx J38.7
  lethal midline (faciale) (e)) M31.2
  liver NEC — *see* Granuloma, hepatic
  lung (infectious) — *see also* Fibrosis, lung
    coccidioidal B38.1
    eosinophilic C96.6
  Majocchi's B35.8
  malignant (facial) (e)) M31.2
  mandible (central) M27.1
  midline (lethal) M31.2
  monilial (cutaneous) B37.2
  nasal sinus — *see* Sinusitis
  operation wound T81.89
    foreign body — *see* Foreign body, accidentally left during a procedure
    stitch T81.89
    talc — *see* Foreign body, accidentally left during a procedure
  oral mucosa K13.4
  orbit, orbital H05.11-
  paracoccidioidal B41.8
  penis, venereal A58
  periapical K04.5
  peritoneum K66.8
    due to ova of helminths NOS — *see also* Helminthiasis B83.9 *[K67]*
  postmastoidectomy cavity — *see* Complications, postmastoidectomy, recurrent cholesteatoma
  prostate N42.89
  pudendi (ulcerating) A58
  pulp, internal (tooth) K03.3
  pyogenic, pyogenicum (of) (skin) L98.0

Granuloma - *continued*
pyogenic, pyogenicum (of) (skin) - *continued*
gingiva K06.8
maxillary alveolar ridge K04.5
oral mucosa K13.4
rectum K62.89
reticulohistiocytic D76.3
rubrum nasi L74.8
Schistosoma — *see* Schistosomiasis
septic (skin) L98.0
silica (skin) L92.3
sinus (accessory) (infective) (nasal) — *see*
Sinusitis
skin L92.9
from residual foreign body L92.3
pyogenicum L98.0
spine
syphilitic (epidural) A52.19
tuberculous A18.01
stitch (postoperative) T81.89
suppurative (skin) L98.0
swimming pool A31.1
talc — *see also* Granuloma, foreign body
in operation wound — *see* Foreign body,
accidentally left during a procedure
telangiectaticum (skin) L98.0
tracheostomy J95.09
trichophyticum B35.8
tropicum A66.4
umbilical P83.81
umbilicus P83.81
urethra N36.8
uveitis — *see* Iridocyclitis, chronic
vagina A58
venereum A58
vocal cord J38.3
Granulomatosis L92.9
lymphoid C83.8-
miliary (listerial) A32.89
necrotizing, respiratory M31.30
progressive septic D71
specified NEC L92.8
Wegener's M31.30
with renal involvement M31.31
Granulomatous tissue (abnormal)
(excessive) L92.9
Granulosis rubra nasi L74.8
Graphite fibrosis (of lung) J63.3
Graphospasm F48.8
organic G25.89
Grating scapula M89.8X1
Gravel (urinary) — *see* Calculus, urinary
Graves' disease — *see* Hyperthyroidism, with,
goiter
Gravis — *see* condition
Grawitz tumor C64.-
Gray syndrome (newborn) P93.0
Grayness, hair (premature) L67.1
congenital Q84.2
Green sickness D50.8
Greenfield's disease
meaning
concentric sclerosis (encephalitis
periaxialis concentrica) G37.5
metachromatic leukodystrophy E75.25
Greenstick fracture - code as Fracture, by
site
Grey syndrome (newborn) P93.0
Grief F43.21
prolonged F43.29
reaction — *see also* Disorder,
adjustment F43.20
Griesinger's disease B76.0
Grinder's lung or pneumoconiosis J62.8
Grinding, teeth
psychogenic F45.8
sleep related G47.63
Grip
Dabney's B33.0
devil's B33.0
Grippe, grippal — *see also* Influenza
Balkan A78
summer, of Italy A93.1
Grisel's disease M43.6
Groin — *see* condition

Grooved tongue K14.5
Ground itch B76.9
Grover's disease or syndrome L11.1
Growing pains, children R29.898
Growth (fungoid) (neoplastic) (new) — *see*
also Neoplasm
adenoid (vegetative) J35.8
benign — *see* Neoplasm, benign, by site
malignant — *see* Neoplasm, malignant, by
site
rapid, childhood Z00.2
secondary — *see* Neoplasm, secondary, by
site
Gruby's disease B35.0
Gubler-Millard paralysis or syndrome G46.3
Guerin-Stern syndrome Q74.3
Guidance, insufficient anterior
(occlusal) M26.54
Guillain-Barré disease or syndrome G61.0
sequelae G65.0
Guinea worms (infection) (infestation) B72
Guinon's disease (motor-verbal tic) F95.2
Gull's disease E03.4
Gum — *see* condition
Gumboil K04.7
with sinus K04.6
Gumma (syphilitic) A52.79
artery A52.09
cerebral A52.04
bone A52.77
of yaws (late) A66.6
brain A52.19
cauda equina A52.19
central nervous system A52.3
ciliary body A52.71
congenital A50.59
eyelid A52.71
heart A52.06
intracranial A52.19
iris A52.71
kidney A52.75
larynx A52.73
leptomeninges A52.19
liver A52.74
meninges A52.19
myocardium A52.06
nasopharynx A52.73
neurosyphilitic A52.3
nose A52.73
orbit A52.71
palate (soft) A52.79
penis A52.76
pericardium A52.06
pharynx A52.73
pituitary A52.79
scrofulous (tuberculous) A18.4
skin A52.79
specified site NEC A52.79
spinal cord A52.19
tongue A52.79
tonsil A52.73
trachea A52.73
tuberculous A18.4
ulcerative due to yaws A66.4
ureter A52.75
yaws A66.4
bone A66.6
Gunn's syndrome Q07.8
Gunshot wound — *see also* Wound, open
fracture - code as Fracture, by site
internal organs — *see* Injury, by site
Gynandrism Q56.0
Gynandroblastoma
specified site — *see* Neoplasm, uncertain
behavior, by site
unspecified site
female D39.10
male D40.10
Gynecological examination (periodic)
(routine) Z01.419
with abnormal findings Z01.411
Gynecomastia N62
Gynephobia F40.291
Gyrate scalp Q82.8

H

H (Hartnup's) disease E72.02
Haas' disease or osteochondrosis (juvenile)
(head of humerus) — *see*
Osteochondrosis, juvenile, humerus
Habit, habituation
bad sleep Z72.821
chorea F95.8
disturbance, child F98.9
drug — *see* Dependence, drug
irregular sleep Z72.821
laxative F55.2
spasm — *see* Tic
tic — *see* Tic
Haemophilus (H.) influenzae, as cause of
disease classified elsewhere B96.3
Haff disease — *see* Poisoning, mercury
Hageman's factor defect, deficiency or
disease D68.2
Haglund's disease or osteochondrosis
(juvenile) (os tibiale externum) — *see*
Osteochondrosis, juvenile, tarsus
Hailey-Hailey disease Q82.8
Hair — *see also* condition
plucking F63.3
in stereotyped movement disorder F98.4
tourniquet syndrome — *see also*
Constriction, external, by site
finger S60.44-
penis S30.842
thumb S60.34-
toe S90.44-
Hairball in stomach T18.2
Hair-pulling, pathological
(compulsive) F63.3
Hairy black tongue K14.3
Half vertebra Q76.49
Halitosis R19.6
Hallerman-Streiff syndrome Q87.0
Hallervorden-Spatz disease G23.0
Hallopeau's acrodermatitis or disease L40.2
Hallucination R44.3
auditory R44.0
gustatory R44.2
olfactory R44.2
specified NEC R44.2
tactile R44.2
visual R44.1
Hallucinosis (chronic) F28
alcoholic (acute) F10.951
in
abuse F10.151
dependence F10.251
drug-induced F19.951
cannabis F12.951
cocaine F14.951
hallucinogen F16.151
in
abuse F19.151
cannabis F12.151
cocaine F14.151
hallucinogen F16.151
inhalant F18.151
opioid F11.151
sedative, anxiolytic or
hypnotic F13.151
stimulant NEC F15.151
dependence F19.251
cannabis F12.251
cocaine F14.251
hallucinogen F16.251
inhalant F18.251
opioid F11.251
sedative, anxiolytic or
hypnotic F13.251
stimulant NEC F15.251
inhalant F18.951
opioid F11.951
sedative, anxiolytic or hypnotic F13.951
stimulant NEC F15.951
organic F06.0
Hallux
deformity (acquired) NEC M20.5X-
limitus M20.5X-
malleus (acquired) NEC M20.3-

Hallux - *continued*
  rigidus (acquired) M20.2-
    congenital Q74.2
    sequelae (late effect) of rickets E64.3
  valgus (acquired) M20.1-
    congenital Q66.6
  varus (acquired) M20.3-
    congenital Q66.3-
Halo, visual H53.19
Hamartoma, hamartoblastoma Q85.9
  epithelial (gingival) , odontogenic, central or
    peripheral — *see* Cyst, calcifying
    odontogenic
Hamartosis Q85.9
Hamman-Rich syndrome J84.114
Hammer toe (acquired) NEC — *see also*
  Deformity, toe, hammer toe
  congenital Q66.89
  sequelae (late effect) of rickets E64.3
Hand — *see* condition
Hand-foot syndrome L27.1
Handicap, handicapped
  educational Z55.9
  specified NEC Z55.8
Hand-Schüller-Christian disease or
  syndrome C96.5
Hanging (asphyxia) (strangulation)
  (suffocation) — *see* Asphyxia, traumatic,
  due to mechanical threat
Hangnail — *see also* Cellulitis, digit
  with lymphangitis — *see* Lymphangitis,
    acute, digit
Hangover (alcohol) F10.129
Hanhart's syndrome Q87.0
Hanot-Chauffard (-Troisier)
  syndrome E83.19
Hanot's cirrhosis or disease K74.3
Hansen's disease — *see* Leprosy
Hantaan virus disease (Korean hemorrhagic
  fever) A98.5
Hantavirus disease (with renal
  manifestations) (Dobrava) (Puumala)
  (Seoul) A98.5
  with pulmonary manifestations (Andes)
    (Bayou) (Bermejo) (Black Creek Canal)
    (Choclo) (Juquitiba) (Laguna negra)
    (Lechiguanas) (New York) (Oran) (Sin
    nombre) B33.4
Happy puppet syndrome Q93.51
Harada's disease or syndrome H30.81-
Hardening
  artery — *see* Arteriosclerosis
  brain G93.89
Harelip (complete) (incomplete) — *see* Cleft,
  lip
Harlequin (newborn) Q80.4
Harley's disease D59.6
Harmful use (of)
  alcohol F10.10
  anxiolytics — *see* Abuse, drug, sedative
  cannabinoids — *see* Abuse, drug, cannabis
  cocaine — *see* Abuse, drug, cocaine
  drug — *see* Abuse, drug
  hallucinogens — *see* Abuse, drug,
    hallucinogen
  hypnotics — *see* Abuse, drug, sedative
  opioids — *see* Abuse, drug, opioid
  PCP (phencyclidine) — *see* Abuse, drug,
    hallucinogen
  sedatives — *see* Abuse, drug, sedative
  stimulants NEC — *see* Abuse, drug,
    stimulant
Harris' lines — *see* Arrest, epiphyseal
Hartnup's disease E72.02
Harvester's lung J67.0
Harvesting ovum for in vitro
  fertilization Z31.83
Hashimoto's disease or thyroiditis E06.3
Hashitoxicosis (transient) E06.3
Hassal-Henle bodies or warts
  (cornea) H18.49
Haut mal — *see* Epilepsy, generalized,
  specified NEC
Haverhill fever A25.1
Hay fever — *see also* Fever, hay J30.1

Hayem-Widal syndrome D59.8
Haygarth's nodes M15.8
Haymaker's lung J67.0
Hb (abnormal)
  Bart's disease D56.0
  disease — *see* Disease, hemoglobin
  trait — *see* Trait
Head — *see* condition
Headache R51
  allergic NEC G44.89
  associated with sexual activity G44.82
  chronic daily R51
  cluster G44.009
    chronic G44.029
      intractable G44.021
      not intractable G44.029
    episodic G44.019
      intractable G44.011
      not intractable G44.019
    intractable G44.001
    not intractable G44.009
  cough (primary) G44.83
  daily chronic R51
  drug-induced NEC G44.40
    intractable G44.41
    not intractable G44.40
  exertional (primary) G44.84
  histamine G44.009
    intractable G44.001
    not intractable G44.009
  hypnic G44.81
  lumbar puncture G97.1
  medication overuse G44.40
    intractable G44.41
    not intractable G44.40
  menstrual — *see* Migraine, menstrual
  migraine (type) — *see also*
    Migraine G43.909
  nasal septum R51
  neuralgiform, short lasting unilateral, with
    conjunctival injection and tearing
    (SUNCT) G44.059
    intractable G44.051
    not intractable G44.059
  new daily persistent (NDPH) G44.52
  orgasmic G44.82
  periodic syndromes in adults and
    children G43.C0
    with refractory migraine G43.C1
      intractable G43.C1
      not intractable G43.C0
    without refractory migraine G43.C0
  postspinal puncture G97.1
  post-traumatic G44.309
    acute G44.319
      intractable G44.311
      not intractable G44.319
    chronic G44.329
      intractable G44.321
      not intractable G44.329
    intractable G44.301
    not intractable G44.309
  pre-menstrual — *see* Migraine, menstrual
  preorgasmic G44.82
  primary
    cough G44.83
    exertional G44.84
    stabbing G44.85
    thunderclap G44.53
  rebound G44.40
    intractable G44.41
    not intractable G44.40
  short lasting unilateral neuralgiform, with
    conjunctival injection and tearing
    (SUNCT) G44.059
    intractable G44.051
    not intractable G44.059
  specified syndrome NEC G44.89
  spinal and epidural anesthesia -
    induced T88.59
    in labor and delivery O74.5
    in pregnancy O29.4-
    postpartum, puerperal O89.4
  spinal fluid loss (from puncture) G97.1
  stabbing (primary) G44.85

Headache - *continued*
  tension (-type) G44.209
    chronic G44.229
      intractable G44.221
      not intractable G44.229
    episodic G44.219
      intractable G44.211
      not intractable G44.219
    intractable G44.201
    not intractable G44.209
  thunderclap (primary) G44.53
  vascular NEC G44.1
Healthy
  infant
    accompanying sick mother Z76.3
    receiving care Z76.2
  person accompanying sick person Z76.3
Hearing examination Z01.10
  with abnormal findings NEC Z01.118
  infant or child (over 28 days old) Z00.129
    with abnormal findings Z00.121
  following failed hearing screening Z01.110
  for hearing conservation and
    treatment Z01.12
Heart — *see* condition
Heart beat
  abnormality R00.9
    specified NEC R00.8
  awareness R00.2
  rapid R00.0
  slow R00.1
Heartburn R12
  psychogenic F45.8
Heartland virus disease A93.8
Heat (effects) T67.9
  apoplexy T67.01
  burn — *see also* Burn L55.9
  collapse T67.1
  cramps T67.2
  dermatitis or eczema L59.0
  edema T67.7
  erythema - code by site under Burn, first
    degree
  excessive T67.9
    specified effect NEC T67.8
  exhaustion T67.5
    anhydrotic T67.3
    due to
      salt (and water) depletion T67.4
      water depletion T67.3
        with salt depletion T67.4
  fatigue (transient) T67.6
  fever T67.01
  hyperpyrexia T67.01
  prickly L74.0
  prostration — *see* Heat, exhaustion
  pyrexia T67.01
  rash L74.0
  specified effect NEC T67.8
  stroke T67.01
    exertional T67.02
    specified NEC T67.09
  sunburn — *see* Sunburn
  syncope T67.1
Heavy-for-dates NEC (infant) (4000g to
  4499g) P08.1
  exceptionally (4500g or more) P08.0
Hebephrenia, hebephrenic
  (schizophrenia) F20.1
Heberden's disease or nodes (with
  arthropathy) M15.1
Hebra's
  pityriasis L26
  prurigo L28.2
Heel — *see* condition
Heerfordt's disease D86.89
Hegglin's anomaly or syndrome D72.0
Heilmeyer-Schoner disease D45
Heine-Medin disease A80.9
Heinz body anemia, congenital D58.2
Heliophobia F40.228
Heller's disease or syndrome F84.3
HELLP syndrome (hemolysis, elevated liver
  enzymes and low platelet count) O14.2-
  complicating

HELLP syndrome (hemolysis, elevated liver enzymes and low platelet count) - *continued*
  complicating - *continued*
    childbirth O14.24
    puerperium O14.25
Helminthiasis — *see also* Infestation, helminth
  Ancylostoma B76.0
  intestinal B82.0
    mixed types (types classifiable to more than one of the titles B65.0-B81.3 and B81.8) B81.4
    specified type NEC B81.8
    mixed types (intestinal) (types classifiable to more than one of the titles B65.0-B81.3 and B81.8) B81.4
  Necator (americanus) B76.1
  specified type NEC B83.8
Heloma L84
Hemangioblastoma — *see* Neoplasm, connective tissue, uncertain behavior
  malignant — *see* Neoplasm, connective tissue, malignant
Hemangioendothelioma — *see also* Neoplasm, uncertain behavior, by site
  benign D18.00
    intra-abdominal D18.03
    intracranial D18.02
    skin D18.01
    specified site NEC D18.09
  bone (diffuse) — *see* Neoplasm, bone, malignant
  epithelioid — *see also* Neoplasm, uncertain behavior, by site
    malignant — *see* Neoplasm, malignant, by site
  malignant — *see* Neoplasm, connective tissue, malignant
Hemangiofibroma — *see* Neoplasm, benign, by site
Hemangiolipoma — *see* Lipoma
Hemangioma D18.00
  arteriovenous D18.00
    intra-abdominal D18.03
    intracranial D18.02
    skin D18.01
    specified site NEC D18.09
  capillary I78.1
    intra-abdominal D18.03
    intracranial D18.02
    skin D18.01
    specified site NEC D18.09
  cavernous D18.00
    intra-abdominal D18.03
    intracranial D18.02
    skin D18.01
    specified site NEC D18.09
  epithelioid D18.00
    intra-abdominal D18.03
    intracranial D18.02
    skin D18.01
    specified site NEC D18.09
  histiocytoid D18.00
    intra-abdominal D18.03
    intracranial D18.02
    skin D18.01
    specified site NEC D18.09
  infantile D18.00
    intra-abdominal D18.03
    intracranial D18.02
    skin D18.01
    specified site NEC D18.09
  intra-abdominal D18.03
  intracranial D18.02
  intramuscular D18.00
    intra-abdominal D18.03
    intracranial D18.02
    skin D18.01
    specified site NEC D18.09
  intrathoracic structures D18.09
  juvenile D18.00
  malignant — *see* Neoplasm,connective tissue, malignant
  plexiform D18.00
    intra-abdominal D18.03
    intracranial D18.02

Hemangioma - *continued*
  plexiform - *continued*
    skin D18.01
    specified site NEC D18.09
  racemose D18.00
    intra-abdominal D18.03
    intracranial D18.02
    skin D18.01
    specified site NEC D18.09
  sclerosing — *see* Neoplasm,skin, benign
  simplex D18.00
    intra-abdominal D18.03
    intracranial D18.02
    skin D18.01
    specified site NEC D18.09
  skin D18.01
  specified site NEC D18.09
  venous D18.00
    intra-abdominal D18.03
    intracranial D18.02
    skin D18.01
    specified site NEC D18.09
  verrucous keratotic D18.00
    intra-abdominal D18.03
    intracranial D18.02
    skin D18.01
    specified site NEC D18.09
Hemangiomatosis (systemic) I78.8
  involving single site — *see* Hemangioma
Hemangiopericytoma — *see also* Neoplasm, connective tissue, uncertain behavior
  benign — *see* Neoplasm, connective tissue, benign
  malignant — *see* Neoplasm, connective tissue, malignant
Hemangiosarcoma — *see* Neoplasm, connective tissue, malignant
Hemarthrosis (nontraumatic) M25.00
  ankle M25.07-
  elbow M25.02-
  foot joint M25.07-
  hand joint M25.04-
  hip M25.05-
  in hemophilic arthropathy — *see* Arthropathy, hemophilic
  knee M25.06-
  shoulder M25.01-
  specified joint NEC M25.08
  traumatic — *see* Sprain, by site
  vertebrae M25.08
  wrist M25.03-
Hematemesis K92.0
  with ulcer - code by site under Ulcer, with hemorrhage K27.4
  newborn, neonatal P54.0
    due to swallowed maternal blood P78.2
Hematidrosis L74.8
Hematinuria — *see also* Hemoglobinuria
  malarial B50.8
Hematobilia K83.8
Hematocele
  female NEC N94.89
    with ectopic pregnancy O00.90
      with intrauterine pregnancy O00.91
    ovary N83.8
  male N50.1
Hematochezia — *see also* Melena K92.1
Hematochyluria — *see also* Infestation, filarial
  schistosomiasis (bilharziasis) B65.0
Hematocolpos (with hematometra or hematosalpinx) N89.7
Hematocornea — *see* Pigmentation, cornea, stromal
Hematogenous — *see* condition
Hematoma (traumatic) (skin surface intact) — *see also* Contusion
  with
    injury of internal organs — *see* Injury, by site
    open wound — *see* Wound, open
  amputation stump (surgical) (late) T87.89
  aorta, dissecting I71.00
    abdominal I71.02
    thoracic I71.01

Hematoma (traumatic) (skin surface intact) - *continued*
  aorta, dissecting - *continued*
    thoracoabdominal I71.03
  aortic intramural — *see* Dissection, aorta
  arterial (complicating trauma) — *see* Injury, blood vessel, by site
  auricle — *see* Contusion, ear
    nontraumatic — *see* Disorder, pinna, hematoma
  birth injury NEC P15.8
  brain (traumatic)
    with
      cerebral laceration or contusion (diffuse) — *see* Injury, intracranial, diffuse
      focal — *see* Injury, intracranial, focal
    cerebellar, traumatic S06.37-
    newborn NEC P52.4
      birth injury P10.1
    intracerebral, traumatic — *see* Injury, intracranial, intracerebral hemorrhage
    nontraumatic — *see* Hemorrhage, intracranial
    subarachnoid, arachnoid, traumatic — *see* Injury, intracranial, subarachnoid hemorrhage
    subdural, traumatic — *see* Injury, intracranial, subdural hemorrhage
  breast (nontraumatic) N64.89
  broad ligament (nontraumatic) N83.7
    traumatic S37.892
  cerebellar, traumatic S06.37-
  cerebral — *see* Hematoma, brain
  cerebrum S06.36-
    left S06.35-
    right S06.34-
  cesarean delivery wound O90.2
  complicating delivery (perineal) (pelvic) (vagina) (vulva) O71.7
  corpus cavernosum (nontraumatic) N48.89
  epididymis (nontraumatic) N50.1
  epidural (traumatic) — *see* Injury, intracranial, epidural hemorrhage
    spinal — *see* Injury, spinal cord, by region
  episiotomy O90.2
  face, birth injury P15.4
  genital organ NEC (nontraumatic)
    female (nonobstetric) N94.89
      traumatic S30.202
    male N50.1
      traumatic S30.201
  internal organs — *see* Injury, by site
  intracerebral, traumatic — *see* Injury, intracranial, intracerebral hemorrhage
  intraoperative — *see* Complications, intraoperative, hemorrhage
  labia (nontraumatic) (nonobstetric) N90.89
  liver (subcapsular) (nontraumatic) K76.89
    birth injury P15.0
  mediastinum — *see* Injury, intrathoracic
  mesosalpinx (nontraumatic) N83.7
    traumatic S37.898
  muscle - code by site under Contusion
  nontraumatic
    muscle M79.81
    soft tissue M79.81
  obstetrical surgical wound O90.2
  orbit, orbital (nontraumatic) — *see also* Hemorrhage, orbit
    traumatic — *see* Contusion, orbit
  pelvis (female) (nontraumatic) (nonobstetric) N94.89
    obstetric O71.7
    traumatic — *see* Injury, by site
  penis (nontraumatic) N48.89
    birth injury P15.5
  perianal (nontraumatic) K64.5
  perineal S30.23
    complicating delivery O71.7
  perirenal — *see* Injury, kidney
  pinna — *see* Contusion, ear
    nontraumatic — *see* Disorder, pinna, hematoma
  placenta O43.89-

Hematoma (traumatic) (skin surface intact) -
continued
  postoperative (postprocedural) — *see*
    Complication, postprocedural,
    hematoma
  retroperitoneal (nontraumatic) K66.1
    traumatic S36.892
  scrotum, superficial S30.22
    birth injury P15.5
  seminal vesicle (nontraumatic) N50.1
    traumatic S37.892
  spermatic cord (traumatic) S37.892
    nontraumatic N50.1
  spinal (cord) (meninges) — *see also* Injury,
    spinal cord, by region
    newborn (birth injury) P11.5
  spleen D73.5
    intraoperative — *see* Complications,
      intraoperative, hemorrhage, spleen
    postprocedural (postoperative) — *see*
      Complications, postprocedural,
      hemorrhage, spleen
  sternocleidomastoid, birth injury P15.2
  sternomastoid, birth injury P15.2
  subarachnoid (traumatic) — *see* Injury,
    intracranial, subarachnoid hemorrhage
    newborn (nontraumatic) P52.5
      due to birth injury P10.3
    nontraumatic — *see* Hemorrhage,
      intracranial, subarachnoid
  subdural (traumatic) — *see* Injury,
    intracranial, subdural hemorrhage
    newborn (localized) P52.8
      birth injury P10.0
    nontraumatic — *see* Hemorrhage,
      intracranial, subdural
    superficial, newborn P54.5
  testis (nontraumatic) N50.1
    birth injury P15.5
  tunica vaginalis (nontraumatic) N50.1
  umbilical cord, complicating delivery O69.5
  uterine ligament (broad)
    (nontraumatic) N83.7
    traumatic S37.892
  vagina (ruptured) (nontraumatic) N89.8
    complicating delivery O71.7
  vas deferens (nontraumatic) N50.1
    traumatic S37.892
  vitreous — *see* Hemorrhage, vitreous
  vulva (nontraumatic) (nonobstetric) N90.89
    complicating delivery O71.7
    newborn (birth injury) P15.5
Hematometra N85.7
  with hematocolpos N89.7
Hematomyelia (central) G95.19
  newborn (birth injury) P11.5
  traumatic T14.8
Hematomyelitis G04.90
Hematoperitoneum — *see* Hemoperitoneum
Hematophobia F40.230
Hematopneumothorax (see Hemothorax)
Hematopoiesis, cyclic D70.4
Hematoporphyria — *see* Porphyria
Hematorachis, hematorrhachis G95.19
  newborn (birth injury) P11.5
Hematosalpinx N83.6
  with
    hematocolpos N89.7
    hematometra N85.7
      with hematocolpos N89.7
    infectional — *see* Salpingitis
Hematospermia R36.1
Hematothorax (see Hemothorax)
Hematuria R31.9
  due to sulphonamide, sulfonamide — *see*
    Table of Drugs and Chemicals, by drug
  benign (familial) (of childhood) — *see also*
    Hematuria, idiopathic
    essential microscopic R31.1
  endemic — *see also* Schistosomiasis B65.0
  gross R31.0
  idiopathic N02.9
    with glomerular lesion
      crescentic (diffuse)
        glomerulonephritis N02.7

Hematuria - *continued*
  idiopathic - *continued*
    with glomerular lesion - *continued*
      dense deposit disease N02.6
      endocapillary proliferative
        glomerulonephritis N02.4
      focal and segmental hyalinosis or
        sclerosis N02.1
      membranoproliferative (diffuse) N02.5
      membranous (diffuse) N02.2
      mesangial proliferative (diffuse) N02.3
      mesangiocapillary (diffuse) N02.5
      minor abnormality N02.0
      proliferative NEC N02.8
      specified pathology NEC N02.8
  intermittent — *see* Hematuria, idiopathic
  malarial B50.8
  microscopic NEC (with symptoms) R31.29
    asymptomatic R31.21
    benign essential R31.1
  paroxysmal — *see also* Hematuria,
    idiopathic
    nocturnal D59.5
  persistent — *see* Hematuria, idiopathic
  recurrent — *see* Hematuria, idiopathic
  tropical — *see also* Schistosomiasis B65.0
  tuberculous A18.13
Hemeralopia (day blindness) H53.11
  vitamin A deficiency E50.5
Hemi-akinesia R41.4
Hemianalgesia R20.0
Hemianencephaly Q00.0
Hemianesthesia R20.0
Hemianopia, hemianopsia (heteronymous)
  H53.47
  homonymous H53.46-
  syphilitic A52.71
Hemiathetosis R25.8
Hemiatrophy R68.89
  cerebellar G31.9
  face, facial, progressive (Romberg) G51.8
  tongue K14.8
Hemiballism (us) G25.5
Hemicardia Q24.8
Hemicephalus, hemicephaly Q00.0
Hemichorea G25.5
Hemicolitis, left — *see* Colitis, left sided
Hemicrania
  congenital malformation Q00.0
  continua G44.51
  meaning migraine — *see also*
    Migraine G43.909
  paroxysmal G44.039
    chronic G44.049
      intractable G44.041
      not intractable G44.049
    episodic G44.039
      intractable G44.031
      not intractable G44.039
    intractable G44.031
    not intractable G44.039
Hemidystrophy — *see* Hemiatrophy
Hemiectromelia Q73.8
Hemihypalgesia R20.8
Hemihypesthesia R20.1
Hemi-inattention R41.4
Hemimelia Q73.8
  lower limb — *see* Defect, reduction, lower
    limb, specified type NEC
  upper limb — *see* Defect, reduction, upper
    limb, specified type NEC
Hemiparalysis — *see* Hemiplegia
Hemiparesis — *see* Hemiplegia
Hemiparesthesia R20.2
Hemiparkinsonism G20
Hemiplegia G81.9-
  alternans facialis G83.89
  ascending NEC G81.90
    spinal G95.89
  congenital (cerebral) G80.8
    spastic G80.2
  embolic (current episode) I63.4-
  flaccid G81.0-
  following
    cerebrovascular disease I69.959

Hemiplegia - *continued*
  following - *continued*
    cerebrovascular disease - *continued*
      cerebral infarction I69.35-
      intracerebral hemorrhage I69.15-
      nontraumatic intracranial hemorrhage
        NEC I69.25-
      specified disease NEC I69.85-
      stroke NOS I69.35-
      subarachnoid hemorrhage I69.05-
  hysterical F44.4
  newborn NEC P91.88
    birth injury P11.9
  spastic G81.1-
    congenital G80.2
  thrombotic (current episode) I63.3-
Hemisection, spinal cord — *see* Injury, spinal
  cord, by region
Hemispasm (facial) R25.2
Hemisporosis B48.8
Hemitremor R25.1
Hemivertebra Q76.49
  failure of segmentation with scoliosis Q76.3
  fusion with scoliosis Q76.3
Hemochromatosis E83.119
  with refractory anemia D46.1
  due to repeated red blood cell
    transfusion E83.111
  hereditary (primary) E83.110
  neonatal P78.84
  primary E83.110
  specified NEC E83.118
Hemoglobin — *see also* condition
  abnormal (disease) — *see* Disease,
    hemoglobin
  AS genotype D57.3
  Constant Spring D58.2
  E-beta thalassemia D56.5
  fetal, hereditary persistence (HPFH) D56.4
  H Constant Spring D56.0
  low NOS D64.9
  S (Hb S) , heterozygous D57.3
Hemoglobinemia D59.9
  due to blood transfusion T80.89
  paroxysmal D59.6
    nocturnal D59.5
Hemoglobinopathy (mixed) D58.2
  with thalassemia D56.8
  sickle-cell D57.1
    with thalassemia D57.40
      with crisis (vasoocclusive pain) D57.419
      with
        acute chest syndrome D57.411
        splenic sequestration D57.412
      without crisis D57.40
Hemoglobinuria R82.3
  with anemia, hemolytic, acquired (chronic)
    NEC D59.6
  cold (agglutinin) (paroxysmal) (with
    Raynaud's syndrome) D59.6
  due to exertion or hemolysis NEC D59.6
  intermittent D59.6
  malarial B50.8
  march D59.6
  nocturnal (paroxysmal) D59.5
  paroxysmal (cold) D59.6
    nocturnal D59.5
Hemolymphangioma D18.1
Hemolysis
  intravascular
    with
      abortion — *see* Abortion, by type,
        complicated by, hemorrhage
      ectopic or molar pregnancy O08.1
      hemorrhage
        antepartum — *see* Hemorrhage,
          antepartum, with coagulation
          defect
        intrapartum — *see also* Hemorrhage,
          complicating, delivery O67.0
      postpartum O72.3
  neonatal (excessive) P58.9
    specified NEC P58.8
Hemolytic — *see* condition

Hemopericardium I31.2
following acute myocardial infarction
(current complication) I23.0
newborn P54.8
traumatic — see Injury, heart, with
hemopericardium
Hemoperitoneum K66.1
infectional K65.9
traumatic S36.899
with open wound — see Wound, open,
with penetration into peritoneal cavity
Hemophilia (classical) (familial) (hereditary)
D66
A D66
B D67
C D68.1
acquired D68.311
autoimmune D68.311
calcipriva — see also Defect,
coagulation D68.4
nonfamilial — see also Defect,
coagulation D68.4
secondary D68.311
vascular D68.0
Hemophthalmos H44.81-
Hemopneumothorax — see also Hemothorax
traumatic S27.2
Hemoptysis R04.2
newborn P26.9
tuberculous — see Tuberculosis, pulmonary
Hemorrhage, hemorrhagic (concealed) R58
abdomen R58
accidental antepartum — see Hemorrhage,
antepartum
acute idiopathic pulmonary, in
infants R04.81
adenoid J35.8
adrenal (capsule) (gland) E27.49
medulla E27.8
newborn P54.4
after delivery — see Hemorrhage,
postpartum
alveolar
lung, newborn P26.8
process K08.89
alveolus K08.89
amputation stump (surgical) T87.89
anemia (chronic) D50.0
acute D62
antepartum (with) O46.90
with coagulation defect O46.00-
afibrinogenemia O46.01-
disseminated intravascular
coagulation O46.02-
hypofibrinogenemia O46.01-
specified defect NEC O46.09-
before 20 weeks gestation O20.9
specified type NEC O20.8
threatened abortion O20.0
due to
abruptio placenta — see also Abruptio
placentae O45.9-
leiomyoma, uterus — see Hemorrhage,
antepartum, specified cause NEC
placenta previa O44.1-
specified cause NEC — see subcategory
O46.8X-
anus (sphincter) K62.5
apoplexy (stroke) — see Hemorrhage,
intracranial, intracerebral
arachnoid — see Hemorrhage, intracranial,
subarachnoid
artery R58
brain — see Hemorrhage, intracranial,
intracerebral
basilar (ganglion) I61.0
bladder N32.89
bowel K92.2
newborn P54.3
brain (miliary) (nontraumatic) — see
Hemorrhage, intracranial, intracerebral
due to
birth injury P10.1
syphilis A52.05

Hemorrhage, hemorrhagic (concealed) -
continued
brain (miliary) (nontraumatic) - continued
epidural or extradural (traumatic) — see
Injury, intracranial, epidural
hemorrhage
newborn P52.4
birth injury P10.1
subarachnoid — see Hemorrhage,
intracranial, subarachnoid
subdural — see Hemorrhage, intracranial,
subdural
brainstem (nontraumatic) I61.3
traumatic S06.38-
breast N64.59
bronchial tube — see Hemorrhage, lung
bronchopulmonary — see Hemorrhage, lung
bronchus — see Hemorrhage, lung
bulbar I61.5
capillary I78.8
primary D69.8
cecum K92.2
cerebellar, cerebellum (nontraumatic) I61.4
newborn P52.6
traumatic S06.37-
cerebral, cerebrum — see also Hemorrhage,
intracranial, intracerebral
newborn (anoxic) P52.4
birth injury P10.1
lobe I61.1
cerebromeningeal I61.8
cerebral, cerebrum — see Hemorrhage,
intracranial, intracerebral
cerebrospinal — see Hemorrhage,
intracranial, intracerebral
cervix (uteri) (stump) NEC N88.8
chamber, anterior (eye) — see Hyphema
childbirth — see Hemorrhage, complicating,
delivery
choroid H31.30-
expulsive H31.31-
ciliary body — see Hyphema
cochlea — see subcategory H83.8
colon K92.2
complicating
abortion — see Abortion, by type,
complicated by, hemorrhage
delivery O67.9
associated with coagulation defect
(afibrinogenemia) (DIC)
(hyperfibrinolysis) O67.0
specified cause NEC O67.8
surgical procedure — see Hemorrhage,
intraoperative
conjunctiva H11.3-
newborn P54.8
cord, newborn (stump) P51.9
corpus luteum (ruptured) cyst N83.1-
cortical (brain) I61.1
cranial — see Hemorrhage, intracranial
cutaneous R23.3
due to autosensitivity, erythrocyte D69.2
newborn P54.5
delayed
following ectopic or molar
pregnancy O08.1
postpartum O72.2
diathesis (familial) D69.9
disease D69.9
newborn P53
specified type NEC D69.8
due to or associated with
afibrinogenemia or other coagulation
defect (conditions in categories D65-
D69)
antepartum — see Hemorrhage,
antepartum, with coagulation defect
intrapartum O67.0
dental implant M27.61
device, implant or graft — see also
Complications, by site and type,
specified NEC T85.838
arterial graft NEC T82.838
breast T85.838
catheter NEC T85.838
dialysis (renal) T82.838
intraperitoneal T85.838

Hemorrhage, hemorrhagic (concealed) -
continued
due to or associated with - continued
device, implant or graft - continued
catheter NEC - continued
infusion NEC T82.838
spinal (epidural) (subdural) T85.830
urinary (indwelling) T83.83
electronic (electrode) (pulse generator)
(stimulator)
bone T84.83
cardiac T82.837
nervous system (brain) (peripheral
nerve) (spinal) T85.830
urinary T83.83
fixation, internal (orthopedic)
NEC T84.83
gastrointestinal (bile duct)
(esophagus) T85.838
genital NEC T83.83
heart NEC T82.837
joint prosthesis T84.83
ocular (corneal graft) (orbital implant)
NEC T85.838
orthopedic NEC T84.83
bone graft T86.838
specified NEC T85.838
urinary NEC T83.83
vascular NEC T82.838
ventricular intracranial shunt T85.830
duodenum, duodenal K92.2
ulcer — see Ulcer, duodenum, with
hemorrhage
dura mater — see Hemorrhage, intracranial,
subdural
endotracheal — see Hemorrhage, lung
epicranial subaponeurotic (massive) , birth
injury P12.2
epidural (traumatic) — see also Injury,
intracranial, epidural hemorrhage
nontraumatic I62.1
esophagus K22.8
varix I85.01
secondary I85.11
excessive, following ectopic gestation
(subsequent episode) O08.1
extradural (traumatic) — see Injury,
intracranial, epidural hemorrhage
birth injury P10.8
newborn (anoxic) (nontraumatic) P52.8
nontraumatic I62.1
eye NEC H57.89
fundus — see Hemorrhage, retina
lid — see Disorder, eyelid, specified type
NEC
fallopian tube N83.6
fibrinogenolysis — see Fibrinolysis
fibrinolytic (acquired) — see Fibrinolysis
from
ear (nontraumatic) — see Otorrhagia
tracheostomy stoma J95.01
fundus, eye — see Hemorrhage, retina
funis — see Hemorrhage, umbilicus, cord
gastric — see Hemorrhage, stomach
gastroenteric K92.2
newborn P54.3
gastrointestinal (tract) K92.2
newborn P54.3
genital organ, male N50.1
genitourinary (tract) NOS R31.9
gingiva K06.8
globe (eye) — see Hemophthalmos
graafian follicle cyst (ruptured) N83.0-
gum K06.8
heart I51.89
hypopharyngeal (throat) R04.1
intermenstrual (regular) N92.3
irregular N92.1
internal (organs) NEC R58
capsule I61.0
ear — see subcategory H83.8
newborn P54.8
intestine K92.2
newborn P54.3
intra-abdominal R58

Hemorrhage, hemorrhagic (concealed) - *continued*
- intra-alveolar (lung) , newborn P26.8
- intracerebral (nontraumatic) — *see* Hemorrhage, intracranial, intracerebral
- intracranial (nontraumatic) I62.9
  - birth injury P10.9
  - epidural, nontraumatic I62.1
  - extradural, nontraumatic I62.1
  - newborn P52.9
    - specified NEC P52.8
  - intracerebral (nontraumatic) (in) I61.9
    - brain stem I61.3
    - cerebellum I61.4
    - newborn P52.4
      - birth injury P10.1
    - hemisphere I61.2
      - cortical (superficial) I61.1
      - subcortical (deep) I61.0
    - intraoperative
      - during a nervous system procedure G97.31
      - during other procedure G97.32
    - intraventricular I61.5
    - multiple localized I61.6
    - postprocedural
      - following a nervous system procedure G97.51
      - following other procedure G97.52
    - specified NEC I61.8
    - superficial I61.1
    - traumatic (diffuse) — *see* Injury, intracranial, diffuse
      - focal — *see* Injury, intracranial, focal
  - subarachnoid (nontraumatic) (from) I60.9
    - newborn P52.5
      - birth injury P10.3
    - intracranial (cerebral) artery I60.7
      - anterior communicating I60.2
      - basilar I60.4
      - carotid siphon and bifurcation I60.0-
      - communicating I60.7
        - anterior I60.2
        - posterior I60.3-
      - middle cerebral I60.1-
      - posterior communicating I60.3-
      - specified artery NEC I60.6
      - vertebral I60.5-
    - specified NEC I60.8
    - traumatic S06.6X-
  - subdural (nontraumatic) I62.00
    - acute I62.01
    - birth injury P10.0
    - chronic I62.03
    - newborn (anoxic) (hypoxic) P52.8
      - birth injury P10.0
    - spinal G95.19
    - subacute I62.02
    - traumatic — *see* Injury, intracranial, subdural hemorrhage
  - traumatic — *see* Injury, intracranial, focal brain injury
- intramedullary NEC G95.19
- intraocular — *see* Hemophthalmos
- intraoperative, intraprocedural — *see* Complication, hemorrhage (hematoma), intraoperative (intraprocedural), by site
- intrapartum — *see* Hemorrhage, complicating, delivery
- intrapelvic
  - female N94.89
  - male K66.1
- intraperitoneal K66.1
- intrapontine I61.3
- intraprocedural — *see* Complication, hemorrhage (hematoma), intraoperative (intraprocedural), by site
- intrauterine N85.7
  - complicating delivery — *see also* Hemorrhage, complicating, delivery O67.9
  - postpartum — *see* Hemorrhage, postpartum
- intraventricular I61.5

Hemorrhage, hemorrhagic (concealed) - *continued*
- intraventricular - *continued*
  - newborn (nontraumatic) — *see also* Newborn, affected by, hemorrhage P52.3
    - due to birth injury P10.2
    - grade
      - 1 P52.0
      - 2 P52.1
      - 3 P52.21
      - 4 P52.22
- intravesical N32.89
- iris (postinfectional) (postinflammatory) (toxic) — *see* Hyphema
- joint (nontraumatic) — *see* Hemarthrosis
- kidney N28.89
- knee (joint) (nontraumatic) — *see* Hemarthrosis, knee
- labyrinth — *see* subcategory H83.8
- lenticular striate artery I61.0
- ligature, vessel — *see* Hemorrhage, postoperative
- liver K76.89
- lung R04.89
  - newborn P26.9
    - massive P26.1
    - specified NEC P26.8
  - tuberculous — *see* Tuberculosis, pulmonary
- massive umbilical, newborn P51.0
- mediastinum — *see* Hemorrhage, lung
- medulla I61.3
- membrane (brain) I60.8
  - spinal cord — *see* Hemorrhage, spinal cord
- meninges, meningeal (brain) (middle) I60.8
  - spinal cord — *see* Hemorrhage, spinal cord
- mesentery K66.1
- metritis — *see* Endometritis
- mouth K13.79
- mucous membrane NEC R58
  - newborn P54.8
- muscle M62.89
- nail (subungual) L60.8
- nasal turbinate R04.0
  - newborn P54.8
- navel, newborn P51.9
- newborn P54.9
  - specified NEC P54.8
- nipple N64.59
- nose R04.0
  - newborn P54.8
- omentum K66.1
- optic nerve (sheath) H47.02-
- orbit, orbital H05.23-
- ovary NEC N83.8
- oviduct N83.6
- pancreas K86.89
- parathyroid (gland) (spontaneous) E21.4
- parturition — *see* Hemorrhage, complicating, delivery
- penis N48.89
- pericardium, pericarditis I31.2
- peritoneum, peritoneal K66.1
- peritonsillar tissue J35.8
  - due to infection J36
- petechial R23.3
  - due to autosensitivity, erythrocyte D69.2
- pituitary (gland) E23.6
- pleura — *see* Hemorrhage, lung
- polioencephalitis, superior E51.2
- polymyositis — *see* Polymyositis
- pons, pontine I61.3
- posterior fossa (nontraumatic) I61.8
  - newborn P52.6
- postmenopausal N95.0
- postnasal R04.0
- postoperative — *see* Complications, postprocedural, hemorrhage, by site
- postpartum NEC (following delivery of placenta) O72.1
  - delayed or secondary O72.2
  - retained placenta O72.0
  - third stage O72.0
- pregnancy — *see* Hemorrhage, antepartum

Hemorrhage, hemorrhagic (concealed) - *continued*
- preretinal — *see* Hemorrhage, retina
- prostate N42.1
- puerperal — *see* Hemorrhage, postpartum
  - delayed or secondary O72.2
- pulmonary R04.89
  - newborn P26.9
    - massive P26.1
    - specified NEC P26.8
  - tuberculous — *see* Tuberculosis, pulmonary
- purpura (primary) D69.3
- rectum (sphincter) K62.5
  - newborn P54.2
- recurring, following initial hemorrhage at time of injury T79.2
- renal N28.89
- respiratory passage or tract R04.9
  - specified NEC R04.89
- retina, retinal (vessels) H35.6-
  - diabetic — *see* Diabetes, retinal, hemorrhage
- retroperitoneal R58
- scalp R58
- scrotum N50.1
- secondary (nontraumatic) R58
  - following initial hemorrhage at time of injury T79.2
- seminal vesicle N50.1
- skin R23.3
  - newborn P54.5
- slipped umbilical ligature P51.8
- spermatic cord N50.1
- spinal (cord) G95.19
  - newborn (birth injury) P11.5
- spleen D73.5
  - intraoperative — *see* Complications, intraoperative, hemorrhage, spleen
  - postprocedural — *see* Complications, postprocedural, hemorrhage, spleen
- stomach K92.2
  - newborn P54.3
  - ulcer — *see* Ulcer, stomach, with hemorrhage
- subarachnoid (nontraumatic) — *see* Hemorrhage, intracranial, subarachnoid
- subconjunctival — *see also* Hemorrhage, conjunctiva
  - birth injury P15.3
- subcortical (brain) I61.0
- subcutaneous R23.3
- subdiaphragmatic R58
- subdural (acute) (nontraumatic) — *see* Hemorrhage, intracranial, subdural
- subependymal
  - newborn P52.0
    - with intraventricular extension P52.1
    - and intracerebral extension P52.22
- subgaleal P12.2
- subhyaloid — *see* Hemorrhage, retina
- subperiosteal — *see* Disorder, bone, specified type NEC
- subretinal — *see* Hemorrhage, retina
- subtentorial — *see* Hemorrhage, intracranial, subdural
- subungual L60.8
- suprarenal (capsule) (gland) E27.49
  - newborn P54.4
- tentorium (traumatic) NEC — *see* Hemorrhage, brain
  - newborn (birth injury) P10.4
- testis N50.1
- third stage (postpartum) O72.0
- thorax — *see* Hemorrhage, lung
- throat R04.1
- thymus (gland) E32.8
- thyroid (cyst) (gland) E07.89
- tongue K14.8
- tonsil J35.8
- trachea — *see* Hemorrhage, lung
- tracheobronchial R04.89
  - newborn P26.0
- traumatic - code to specific injury
  - cerebellar — *see* Hemorrhage, brain

Hemorrhage, hemorrhagic (concealed) - *continued*
  traumatic - code to specific injury - *continued*
    intracranial — *see* Hemorrhage, brain
    recurring or secondary (following initial hemorrhage at time of injury) T79.2
  tuberculous NEC — *see also* Tuberculosis, pulmonary A15.0
  tunica vaginalis N50.1
  ulcer - code by site under Ulcer, with hemorrhage K27.4
  umbilicus, umbilical
    cord
      after birth, newborn P51.9
      complicating delivery O69.5
    newborn P51.9
      massive P51.0
      slipped ligature P51.8
    stump P51.9
  urethra (idiopathic) N36.8
  uterus, uterine (abnormal) N93.9
    climacteric N92.4
    complicating delivery — *see* Hemorrhage, complicating, delivery
    dysfunctional or functional N93.8
    intermenstrual (regular) N92.3
      irregular N92.1
    postmenopausal N95.0
    postpartum — *see* Hemorrhage, postpartum
    preclimacteric or premenopausal N92.4
    prepubertal N93.8
    pubertal N92.2
  vagina (abnormal) N93.9
    newborn P54.6
  vas deferens N50.1
  vasa previa O69.4
  ventricular I61.5
  vesical N32.89
  viscera NEC R58
    newborn P54.8
  vitreous (humor) (intraocular) H43.1-
  vulva N90.89
Hemorrhoids (bleeding) (without mention of degree) K64.9
  1st degree (grade/stage I) (without prolapse outside of anal canal) K64.0
  2nd degree (grade/stage II) (that prolapse with straining but retract spontaneously) K64.1
  3rd degree (grade/stage III) (that prolapse with straining and require manual replacement back inside anal canal) K64.2
  4th degree (grade/stage IV) (with prolapsed tissue that cannot be manually replaced) K64.3
  complicating
    pregnancy O22.4
    puerperium O87.2
  external K64.4
    with
      thrombosis K64.5
  internal (without mention of degree) K64.8
  prolapsed K64.8
  skin tags
    anus K64.4
    residual K64.4
  specified NEC K64.8
  strangulated — *see also* Hemorrhoids, by degree K64.8
  thrombosed — *see also* Hemorrhoids, by degree K64.5
  ulcerated — *see also* Hemorrhoids, by degree K64.8
Hemosalpinx N83.6
  with
    hematocolpos N89.7
    hematometra N85.7
      with hematocolpos N89.7
Hemosiderosis (dietary) E83.19
  pulmonary, idiopathic E83.1- *[J84.03]*
  transfusion T80.89

Hemothorax (bacterial) (nontuberculous) J94.2
  newborn P54.8
  traumatic S27.1
    with pneumothorax S27.2
  tuberculous NEC A15.6
Henoch (-Schönlein) disease or syndrome (purpura) D69.0
Henpue, henpuye A66.6
Hepar lobatum (syphilitic) A52.74
Hepatalgia K76.89
Hepatitis K75.9
  acute B17.9
    with coma K72.01
    with hepatic failure — *see* Failure, hepatic
    alcoholic — *see* Hepatitis, alcoholic
    infectious B17.9
    non-viral K72.0
    viral B17.9
  alcoholic (acute) (chronic) K70.10
    with ascites K70.11
  amebic — *see* Abscess, liver, amebic
  anicteric, (viral) — *see* Hepatitis, viral
  antigen-associated (HAA) — *see* Hepatitis, B
  Australia-antigen (positive) — *see* Hepatitis, B
  autoimmune K75.4
  B B19.10
    with hepatic coma B19.11
    acute B16.9
      with
        delta-agent (coinfection) (without hepatic coma) B16.1
          with hepatic coma B16.0
        hepatic coma (without delta-agent coinfection) B16.2
    chronic B18.1
      with delta-agent B18.0
  bacterial NEC K75.89
  C (viral) B19.20
    with hepatic coma B19.21
    acute B17.10
      with hepatic coma B17.11
    chronic B18.2
  catarrhal (acute) B15.9
    with hepatic coma B15.0
  cholangiolitic K75.89
  cholestatic K75.89
  chronic K73.9
    active NEC K73.2
    lobular NEC K73.1
    persistent NEC K73.0
    specified NEC K73.8
  cytomegaloviral B25.1
  due to ethanol (acute) (chronic) — *see* Hepatitis, alcoholic
  epidemic B15.9
    with hepatic coma B15.0
  fulminant NEC (viral) — *see* Hepatitis, viral
  neonatal giant cell P59.29
  granulomatous NEC K75.3
  herpesviral B00.81
  history of
    B Z86.19
    C Z86.19
  homologous serum — *see* Hepatitis, viral, type B
  in (due to)
    mumps B26.81
    toxoplasmosis (acquired) B58.1
      congenital (active) P37.1 *[K77]*
  infectious, infective B15.9
    acute (subacute) B17.9
    chronic B18.9
  inoculation — *see* Hepatitis, viral, type B
  interstitial (chronic) K74.69
  lupoid NEC K75.4
  malignant NEC (with hepatic failure) K72.90
    with coma K72.91
  neonatal (idiopathic) (toxic) P59.29
  newborn P59.29
  postimmunization — *see* Hepatitis, viral, type B
  post-transfusion — *see* Hepatitis, viral, type B

Hepatitis - *continued*
  reactive, nonspecific K75.2
  serum — *see* Hepatitis, viral, type B
  specified type NEC
    with hepatic failure — *see* Failure, hepatic
  syphilitic (late) A52.74
    congenital (early) A50.08 *[K77]*
      late A50.59 *[K77]*
    secondary A51.45
  toxic — *see also* Disease, liver, toxic K71.6
  tuberculous A18.83
  viral, virus B19.9
    with hepatic coma B19.0
    acute B17.9
    chronic B18.9
      specified NEC B18.8
    type
      B B18.1
        with delta-agent B18.0
      C B18.2
    congenital P35.3
    coxsackie B33.8 *[K77]*
    cytomegalic inclusion B25.1
    in remission, any type - code to Hepatitis, chronic, by type
    non-A, non-B B17.8
    specified type NEC (with or without coma) B17.8
    type
      A B15.9
        with hepatic coma B15.0
      B B19.10
        with hepatic coma B19.11
        acute B16.9
          with
            delta-agent (coinfection) (without hepatic coma) B16.1
              with hepatic coma B16.0
            hepatic coma (without delta-agent coinfection) B16.2
        chronic B18.1
          with delta-agent B18.0
      C B19.20
        with hepatic coma B19.21
        acute B17.10
          with hepatic coma B17.11
        chronic B18.2
      E B17.2
    non-A, non-B B17.8
Hepatization lung (acute) — *see* Pneumonia, lobar
Hepatoblastoma C22.2
Hepatocarcinoma C22.0
Hepatocholangiocarcinoma C22.0
Hepatocholangioma, benign D13.4
Hepatocholangitis K75.89
Hepatolenticular degeneration E83.01
Hepatoma (malignant) C22.0
  benign D13.4
  embryonal C22.0
Hepatomegaly — *see also* Hypertrophy, liver
  with splenomegaly R16.2
  congenital Q44.7
  in mononucleosis
    gammaherpesviral B27.09
    infectious specified NEC B27.89
Hepatoptosis K76.89
Hepatorenal syndrome following labor and delivery O90.4
Hepatosis K76.89
Hepatosplenomegaly R16.2
  hyperlipemic (Bürger-Grütz type) E78.3 *[K77]*
Hereditary — *see* condition
Heredodegeneration, macular — *see* Dystrophy, retina
Heredopathia atactica polyneuritiformis G60.1
Heredosyphilis — *see* Syphilis, congenital
Herlitz' syndrome Q81.1
Hermansky-Pudlak syndrome E70.331
Hermaphrodite, hermaphroditism (true) Q56.0
  46,XX with streak gonads Q99.1
  46,XX/46,XY Q99.0

Hermaphrodite, hermaphroditism (true) - *continued*
  46,XY with streak gonads Q99.1
  chimera 46,XX/46,XY Q99.0
Hernia, hernial (acquired) (recurrent) K46.9
  with
    gangrene — *see* Hernia, by site, with,
      gangrene
    incarceration — *see* Hernia, by site, with,
      obstruction
    irreducible — *see* Hernia, by site, with,
      obstruction
    obstruction — *see* Hernia, by site, with,
      obstruction
    strangulation — *see* Hernia, by site, with,
      obstruction
  abdomen, abdominal K46.9
    with
      gangrene (and obstruction) K46.1
      obstruction K46.0
    femoral — *see* Hernia, femoral
    incisional — *see* Hernia, incisional
    inguinal — *see* Hernia, inguinal
    specified site NEC K45.8
      with
        gangrene (and obstruction) K45.1
        obstruction K45.0
    umbilical — *see* Hernia, umbilical
    wall — *see* Hernia, ventral
  appendix — *see* Hernia, abdomen
  bladder (mucosa) (sphincter)
    congenital (female) (male) Q79.51
    female — *see* Cystocele
    male N32.89
  brain, congenital — *see* Encephalocele
  cartilage, vertebra — *see* Displacement,
    intervertebral disc
  cerebral, congenital — *see also*
    Encephalocele
    endaural Q01.8
  ciliary body (traumatic) S05.2-
  colon — *see* Hernia, abdomen
  Cooper's — *see* Hernia, abdomen, specified
    site NEC
  crural — *see* Hernia, femoral
  diaphragm, diaphragmatic K44.9
    with
      gangrene (and obstruction) K44.1
      obstruction K44.0
    congenital Q79.0
  direct (inguinal) — *see* Hernia, inguinal
  diverticulum, intestine — *see* Hernia,
    abdomen
  double (inguinal) — *see* Hernia, inguinal,
    bilateral
  due to adhesions (with obstruction) K56.50
  epigastric — *see also* Hernia, ventral K43.9
  esophageal hiatus — *see* Hernia, hiatal
  external (inguinal) — *see* Hernia, inguinal
  fallopian tube N83.4-
  fascia M62.89
  femoral K41.90
    with
      gangrene (and obstruction) K41.40
        not specified as recurrent K41.40
        recurrent K41.41
      obstruction K41.30
        not specified as recurrent K41.30
        recurrent K41.31
    bilateral K41.20
      with
        gangrene (and obstruction) K41.10
          not specified as recurrent K41.10
          recurrent K41.11
        obstruction K41.00
          not specified as recurrent K41.00
          recurrent K41.01
      not specified as recurrent K41.20
      recurrent K41.21
    unilateral K41.90
      with
        gangrene (and obstruction) K41.40
          not specified as recurrent K41.40
          recurrent K41.41
        obstruction K41.30

Hernia, hernial (acquired) (recurrent) - *continued*
  femoral - *continued*
    unilateral - *continued*
      with - *continued*
        obstruction - *continued*
          not specified as recurrent K41.30
          recurrent K41.31
      not specified as recurrent K41.90
      recurrent K41.91
    not specified as recurrent K41.90
    recurrent K41.91
  foramen magnum G93.5
    congenital Q01.8
  funicular (umbilical) — *see also* Hernia,
    umbilicus
    spermatic (cord) — *see* Hernia, inguinal
  gastrointestinal tract — *see* Hernia, abdomen
  Hesselbach's — *see* Hernia, femoral,
    specified site NEC
  hiatal (esophageal) (sliding) K44.9
    with
      gangrene (and obstruction) K44.1
      obstruction K44.0
    congenital Q40.1
  hypogastric — *see* Hernia, ventral
  incarcerated — *see also* Hernia, by site, with
    obstruction
    with gangrene — *see* Hernia, by site, with
      gangrene
  incisional K43.2
    with
      gangrene (and obstruction) K43.1
      obstruction K43.0
  indirect (inguinal) — *see* Hernia, inguinal
  inguinal (direct) (external) (funicular)
    (indirect) (internal) (oblique) (scrotal)
    (sliding) K40.90
    with
      gangrene (and obstruction) K40.40
        not specified as recurrent K40.40
        recurrent K40.41
      obstruction K40.30
        not specified as recurrent K40.30
        recurrent K40.31
    not specified as recurrent K40.90
    recurrent K40.91
    bilateral K40.20
      with
        gangrene (and obstruction) K40.10
          not specified as recurrent K40.10
          recurrent K40.11
        obstruction K40.00
          not specified as recurrent K40.00
          recurrent K40.01
      not specified as recurrent K40.20
      recurrent K40.21
    unilateral K40.90
      with
        gangrene (and obstruction) K40.40
          not specified as recurrent K40.40
          recurrent K40.41
        obstruction K40.30
          not specified as recurrent K40.30
          recurrent K40.31
      not specified as recurrent K40.90
      recurrent K40.91
  internal — *see also* Hernia, abdomen
    inguinal — *see* Hernia, inguinal
  interstitial — *see* Hernia, abdomen
  intervertebral cartilage or disc — *see*
    Displacement, intervertebral disc
  intestine, intestinal — *see* Hernia, by site
  intra-abdominal — *see* Hernia, abdomen
  iris (traumatic) S05.2-
  irreducible — *see also* Hernia, by site, with
    obstruction
    with gangrene — *see* Hernia, by site, with
      gangrene
  ischiatic — *see* Hernia, abdomen, specified
    site NEC
  ischiorectal — *see* Hernia, abdomen,
    specified site NEC
  lens (traumatic) S05.2-

Hernia, hernial (acquired) (recurrent) - *continued*
  linea (alba) (semilunaris) — *see* Hernia,
    ventral
  Littre's — *see* Hernia, abdomen
  lumbar — *see* Hernia, abdomen, specified
    site NEC
  lung (subcutaneous) J98.4
  mediastinum J98.59
  mesenteric (internal) — *see* Hernia, abdomen
  midline — *see* Hernia, ventral
  muscle (sheath) M62.89
  nucleus pulposus — *see* Displacement,
    intervertebral disc
  oblique (inguinal) — *see* Hernia, inguinal
  obstructive — *see also* Hernia, by site, with
    obstruction
    with gangrene — *see* Hernia, by site, with
      gangrene
  obturator — *see* Hernia, abdomen, specified
    site NEC
  omental — *see* Hernia, abdomen
  ovary N83.4-
  oviduct N83.4-
  paraesophageal — *see also* Hernia,
    diaphragm
    congenital Q40.1
  parastomal K43.5
    with
      gangrene (and obstruction) K43.4
      obstruction K43.3
  paraumbilical — *see* Hernia, umbilicus
  perineal — *see* Hernia, abdomen, specified
    site NEC
  Petit's — *see* Hernia, abdomen, specified site
    NEC
  postoperative — *see* Hernia, incisional
  pregnant uterus — *see* Abnormal, uterus in
    pregnancy or childbirth
  prevesical N32.89
  properitoneal — *see* Hernia, abdomen,
    specified site NEC
  pudendal — *see* Hernia, abdomen, specified
    site NEC
  rectovaginal N81.6
  retroperitoneal — *see* Hernia, abdomen,
    specified site NEC
  Richter's — *see* Hernia, abdomen, with
    obstruction
  Rieux's, Riex's — *see* Hernia, abdomen,
    specified site NEC
  sac condition (adhesion) (dropsy)
    (inflammation) (laceration)
    (suppuration) - code by site under
    Hernia
  sciatic — *see* Hernia, abdomen, specified site
    NEC
  scrotum, scrotal — *see* Hernia, inguinal
  sliding (inguinal) — *see also* Hernia,
    inguinal
    hiatus — *see* Hernia, hiatal
  spigelian — *see* Hernia, ventral
  spinal — *see* Spina bifida
  strangulated — *see also* Hernia, by site, with
    obstruction
    with gangrene — *see* Hernia, by site, with
      gangrene
  subxiphoid — *see* Hernia, ventral
  supra-umbilicus — *see* Hernia, ventral
  tendon — *see* Disorder, tendon, specified
    type NEC
  Treitz's (fossa) — *see* Hernia, abdomen,
    specified site NEC
  tunica vaginalis Q55.29
  umbilicus, umbilical K42.9
    with
      gangrene (and obstruction) K42.1
      obstruction K42.0
  ureter N28.89
  urethra, congenital Q64.79
  urinary meatus, congenital Q64.79
  uterus N81.4
    pregnant — *see* Abnormal, uterus in
      pregnancy or childbirth
  vaginal (anterior) (wall) — *see* Cystocele

Hernia, hernial (acquired) (recurrent) -
continued
Velpeau's — *see* Hernia, femoral
ventral K43.9
with
gangrene (and obstruction) K43.7
obstruction K43.6
recurrent — *see* Hernia, incisional
incisional K43.2
with
gangrene (and obstruction) K43.1
obstruction K43.0
specified NEC K43.9
with
gangrene (and obstruction) K43.7
obstruction K43.6
vesical
congenital (female) (male) Q79.51
female — *see* Cystocele
male N32.89
vitreous (into wound) S05.2-
into anterior chamber — *see* Prolapse,
vitreous
Herniation — *see also* Hernia
brain (stem) G93.5
cerebral G93.5
mediastinum J98.59
nucleus pulposus — *see* Displacement,
intervertebral disc
Herpangina B08.5
Herpes, herpesvirus, herpetic B00.9
anogenital A60.9
perianal skin A60.1
rectum A60.1
urogenital tract A60.00
cervix A60.03
male genital organ NEC A60.02
penis A60.01
specified site NEC A60.09
vagina A60.04
vulva A60.04
blepharitis (zoster) B02.39
simplex B00.59
circinatus B35.4
bullosus L12.0
conjunctivitis (simplex) B00.53
zoster B02.31
cornea B02.33
encephalitis B00.4
due to herpesvirus 6 B10.01
due to herpesvirus 7 B10.09
specified NEC B10.09
eye (zoster) B02.30
simplex B00.50
eyelid (zoster) B02.39
simplex B00.59
facialis B00.1
febrilis B00.1
geniculate ganglionitis B02.21
genital, genitalis A60.00
female A60.09
male A60.02
gestational, gestationis O26.4-
gingivostomatitis B00.2
human B00.9
1 — *see* Herpes, simplex
2 — *see* Herpes, simplex
3 — *see* Varicella
4 — *see* Mononucleosis, Epstein-Barr
(virus)
5 — *see* Disease, cytomegalic inclusion
(generalized)
6
encephalitis B10.01
specified NEC B10.81
7
encephalitis B10.09
specified NEC B10.82
8 B10.89
infection NEC B10.89
Kaposi's sarcoma associated B10.89
iridocyclitis (simplex) B00.51
zoster B02.32
iris (vesicular erythema multiforme) L51.9
iritis (simplex) B00.51

Herpes, herpesvirus, herpetic - *continued*
Kaposi's sarcoma associated B10.89
keratitis (simplex) (dendritic) (disciform)
(interstitial) B00.52
zoster (interstitial) B02.33
keratoconjunctivitis (simplex) B00.52
zoster B02.33
labialis B00.1
lip B00.1
meningitis (simplex) B00.3
zoster B02.1
ophthalmicus (zoster) NEC B02.30
simplex B00.50
penis A60.01
perianal skin A60.1
pharyngitis, pharyngotonsillitis B00.2
rectum A60.1
scrotum A60.02
sepsis B00.7
simplex B00.9
complicated NEC B00.89
congenital P35.2
conjunctivitis B00.53
external ear B00.1
eyelid B00.59
hepatitis B00.81
keratitis (interstitial) B00.52
myleitis B00.82
specified complication NEC B00.89
visceral B00.89
stomatitis B00.2
tonsurans B35.0
visceral B00.89
vulva A60.04
whitlow B00.89
zoster — *see also* condition B02.9
auricularis B02.21
complicated NEC B02.8
conjunctivitis B02.31
disseminated B02.7
encephalitis B02.0
eye (lid) B02.39
geniculate ganglionitis B02.21
keratitis (interstitial) B02.33
meningitis B02.1
myelitis B02.24
neuritis, neuralgia B02.29
ophthalmicus NEC B02.30
oticus B02.21
polyneuropathy B02.23
specified complication NEC B02.8
trigeminal neuralgia B02.22
Herpesvirus (human) — *see* Herpes
Herpetophobia F40.218
Herrick's anemia — *see* Disease, sickle-cell
Hers' disease E74.09
Herter-Gee syndrome K90.0
Herxheimer's reaction R68.89
Hesitancy
of micturition R39.11
urinary R39.11
Hesselbach's hernia — *see* Hernia, femoral,
specified site NEC
Heterochromia (congenital) Q13.2
cataract — *see* Cataract, complicated
cyclitis (Fuchs) — *see* Cyclitis, Fuchs'
heterochromic
hair L67.1
iritis — *see* Cyclitis, Fuchs' heterochromic
retained metallic foreign body
(nonmagnetic) — *see* Foreign body,
intraocular, old, retained
magnetic — *see* Foreign body, intraocular,
old, retained, magnetic
uveitis — *see* Cyclitis, Fuchs' heterochromic
Heterophoria — *see* Strabismus, heterophoria
**Heterophyes, heterophyiasis (small
intestine)** B66.8
Heterotopia, heterotopic — *see also*
Malposition, congenital
cerebralis Q04.8
Heterotropia — *see* Strabismus
Heubner-Herter disease K90.0
Hexadactylism Q69.9

**HGSIL (cytology finding) (high grade
squamous intraepithelial lesion on
cytologic smear) (Pap smear finding)**
anus R85.613
cervix R87.613
biopsy (histology) finding — *see*
Neoplasia, intraepithelial, cervix,
grade II or grade III
vagina R87.623
biopsy (histology) finding — *see*
Neoplasia, intraepithelial, vagina,
grade II or grade III
Hibernoma — *see* Lipoma
Hiccup, hiccough R06.6
epidemic B33.0
psychogenic F45.8
Hidden penis (congenital) Q55.64
acquired N48.83
Hidradenitis (axillaris) (suppurative) L73.2
Hidradenoma (nodular) — *see also*
Neoplasm, skin, benign
clear cell — *see* Neoplasm, skin, benign
papillary — *see* Neoplasm, skin, benign
Hidrocystoma — *see* Neoplasm, skin, benign
High
altitude effects T70.20
anoxia T70.29
on
ears T70.0
sinuses T70.1
polycythemia D75.1
arch
foot Q66.7-
palate, congenital Q38.5
arterial tension — *see* Hypertension
basal metabolic rate R94.8
blood pressure — *see also* Hypertension
borderline R03.0
reading (incidental) (isolated)
(nonspecific) , without diagnosis of
hypertension R03.0
cholesterol E78.00
with high triglycerides E78.2
diaphragm (congenital) Q79.1
expressed emotional level within
family Z63.8
head at term O32.4
palate, congenital Q38.5
risk
infant NEC Z76.2
sexual behavior (heterosexual) Z72.51
bisexual Z72.53
homosexual Z72.52
scrotal testis, testes
bilateral Q53.23
unilateral Q53.13
temperature (of unknown origin) R50.9
thoracic rib Q76.6
triglycerides E78.1
with high cholesterol E78.2
Hildenbrand's disease A75.0
Hilum — *see* condition
Hip — *see* condition
Hippel's disease Q85.8
Hippophobia F40.218
Hippus H57.09
Hirschsprung's disease or megacolon Q43.1
Hirsutism, hirsuties L68.0
Hirudiniasis
external B88.3
internal B83.4
Hiss-Russell dysentery A03.1
Histidinemia, histidinuria E70.41
Histiocytoma — *see also* Neoplasm, skin,
benign
fibrous — *see also* Neoplasm, skin, benign
atypical — *see* Neoplasm, connective
tissue, uncertain behavior
malignant — *see* Neoplasm, connective
tissue, malignant
Histiocytosis D76.3
acute differentiated progressive C96.0
Langerhans' cell NEC C96.6
multifocal X
multisystemic (disseminated) C96.0

Histiocytosis - *continued*
Langerhans' cell NEC - *continued*
multifocal X - *continued*
unisystemic C96.5
pulmonary, adult (adult PLCH) J84.82
unifocal (X) C96.6
lipid, lipoid D76.3
essential E75.29
malignant C96.A
mononuclear phagocytes NEC D76.1
Langerhans' cells C96.6
non-Langerhans cell D76.3
polyostotic sclerosing D76.3
sinus, with massive lymphadenopathy D76.3
syndrome NEC D76.3
X NEC C96.6
acute (progressive) C96.0
chronic C96.6
multifocal C96.5
multisystemic C96.0
unifocal C96.6
Histoplasmosis B39.9
with pneumonia NEC B39.2
African B39.5
American — *see* Histoplasmosis, capsulati
capsulati B39.4
disseminated B39.3
generalized B39.3
pulmonary B39.2
acute B39.0
chronic B39.1
Darling's B39.4
duboisii B39.5
lung NEC B39.2
History
family (of) — *see also* History, personal (of)
alcohol abuse Z81.1
allergy NEC Z84.89
anemia Z83.2
arthritis Z82.61
asthma Z82.5
blindness Z82.1
cardiac death (sudden) Z82.41
carrier of genetic disease Z84.81
chromosomal anomaly Z82.79
chronic
disabling disease NEC Z82.8
lower respiratory disease Z82.5
colonic polyps Z83.71
congenital malformations and
deformations Z82.79
polycystic kidney Z82.71
consanguinity Z84.3
deafness Z82.2
diabetes mellitus Z83.3
disability NEC Z82.8
disease or disorder (of)
allergic NEC Z84.89
behavioral NEC Z81.8
blood and blood-forming organs Z83.2
cardiovascular NEC Z82.49
chronic disabling NEC Z82.8
digestive Z83.79
ear NEC Z83.52
endocrine NEC Z83.49
elevated lipoprotein (a) (Lp (a))
Z83.430
eye NEC Z83.518
glaucoma Z83.511
familial hypercholesterolemia Z83.42
genitourinary NEC Z84.2
glaucoma Z83.511
hematological Z83.2
immune mechanism Z83.2
infectious NEC Z83.1
ischemic heart Z82.49
kidney Z84.1
lipoprotein metabolism Z83.438
mental NEC Z81.8
metabolic Z83.49
musculoskeletal NEC Z82.69
neurological NEC Z82.0
nutritional Z83.49
parasitic NEC Z83.1
psychiatric NEC Z81.8

History - *continued*
family (of) - *continued*
disease or disorder (of) - *continued*
respiratory NEC Z83.6
skin and subcutaneous tissue NEC Z84.0
specified NEC Z84.89
drug abuse NEC Z81.3
elevated lipoprotein (a) (Lp (a)) Z83.430
epilepsy Z82.0
familial hypercholesterolemia Z83.42
genetic disease carrier Z84.81
glaucoma Z83.511
hearing loss Z82.2
human immunodeficiency virus (HIV)
infection Z83.0
Huntington's chorea Z82.0
hyperlipidemia, familial
combined Z83.438
intellectual disability Z81.0
leukemia Z80.6
lipidemia NEC Z83.438
malignant neoplasm (of) NOS Z80.9
bladder Z80.52
breast Z80.3
bronchus Z80.1
digestive organ Z80.0
gastrointestinal tract Z80.0
genital organ Z80.49
ovary Z80.41
prostate Z80.42
specified organ NEC Z80.49
testis Z80.43
hematopoietic NEC Z80.7
intrathoracic organ NEC Z80.2
kidney Z80.51
lung Z80.1
lymphatic NEC Z80.7
ovary Z80.41
prostate Z80.42
respiratory organ NEC Z80.2
specified site NEC Z80.8
testis Z80.43
trachea Z80.1
urinary organ or tract Z80.59
bladder Z80.52
kidney Z80.51
mental
disorder NEC Z81.8
multiple endocrine neoplasia (MEN)
syndrome Z83.41
osteoporosis Z82.62
polycystic kidney Z82.71
polyps (colon) Z83.71
psychiatric disorder Z81.8
psychoactive substance abuse NEC Z81.3
respiratory condition NEC Z83.6
asthma and other lower respiratory
conditions Z82.5
self-harmful behavior Z81.8
SIDS (sudden infant death
syndrome) Z84.82
skin condition Z84.0
specified condition NEC Z84.89
stroke (cerebrovascular) Z82.3
substance abuse NEC Z81.4
alcohol Z81.1
drug NEC Z81.3
psychoactive NEC Z81.3
tobacco Z81.2
sudden
cardiac death Z82.41
infant death syndrome (SIDS) Z84.82
tobacco abuse Z81.2
violence, violent behavior Z81.8
visual loss Z82.1
personal (of) — *see also* History, family (of)
abuse
adult Z91.419
forced labor or sexual
exploitation Z91.42
physical and sexual Z91.410
psychological Z91.411
childhood Z62.819
forced labor or sexual exploitation in
childhood Z62.813

History - *continued*
personal (of) - *continued*
abuse - *continued*
childhood - *continued*
physical Z62.810
psychological Z62.811
sexual Z62.810
alcohol dependence F10.21
allergy (to) Z88.9
analgesic agent NEC Z88.6
anesthetic Z88.4
antibiotic agent NEC Z88.1
anti-infective agent NEC Z88.3
contrast media Z91.041
drugs, medicaments and biological
substances Z88.9
specified NEC Z88.8
food Z91.018
additives Z91.02
eggs Z91.012
milk products Z91.011
peanuts Z91.010
seafood Z91.013
specified food NEC Z91.018
insect Z91.038
bee Z91.030
latex Z91.040
medicinal agents Z88.9
specified NEC Z88.8
narcotic agent NEC Z88.5
nonmedicinal agents Z91.048
penicillin Z88.0
serum Z88.7
specified NEC Z91.09
sulfonamides Z88.2
vaccine Z88.7
anaphylactic shock Z87.892
anaphylaxis Z87.892
behavioral disorders Z86.59
benign carcinoid tumor Z86.012
benign neoplasm Z86.018
carcinoid Z86.012
brain Z86.011
colonic polyps Z86.010
brain injury (traumatic) Z87.820
breast implant removal Z98.86
calculi, renal Z87.442
cancer — *see* History, personal (of),
malignant neoplasm (of)
cardiac arrest (death) , successfully
resuscitated Z86.74
cerebral infarction without residual
deficit Z86.73
cervical dysplasia Z87.410
chemotherapy for neoplastic
condition Z92.21
childhood abuse — *see* History, personal
(of), abuse
cleft lip (corrected) Z87.730
cleft palate (corrected) Z87.730
collapsed vertebra (healed) Z87.311
due to osteoporosis Z87.310
combat and operational stress
reaction Z86.51
congenital malformation
(corrected) Z87.798
circulatory system (corrected) Z87.74
digestive system (corrected)
NEC Z87.738
ear (corrected) Z87.721
eye (corrected) Z87.720
face and neck (corrected) Z87.790
genitourinary system (corrected)
NEC Z87.718
heart (corrected) Z87.74
integument (corrected) Z87.76
limb (s) (corrected) Z87.76
musculoskeletal system
(corrected) Z87.76
neck (corrected) Z87.790
nervous system (corrected)
NEC Z87.728
respiratory system (corrected) Z87.75
sense organs (corrected) NEC Z87.728
specified NEC Z87.798

History - *continued*
  personal (of) - *continued*
    contraception Z92.0
    deployment (military) Z91.82
    diabetic foot ulcer Z86.31
    disease or disorder (of) Z87.898
      blood and blood-forming organs Z86.2
      circulatory system Z86.79
        specified condition NEC Z86.79
      connective tissue NEC Z87.39
      digestive system Z87.19
        colonic polyp Z86.010
        peptic ulcer disease Z87.11
        specified condition NEC Z87.19
      ear Z86.69
      endocrine Z86.39
        diabetic foot ulcer Z86.31
        gestational diabetes Z86.32
        specified type NEC Z86.39
      eye Z86.69
      genital (track) system NEC
        female Z87.42
        male Z87.438
      hematological Z86.2
      Hodgkin Z85.71
      immune mechanism Z86.2
      infectious Z86.19
        malaria Z86.13
        Methicillin resistant Staphylococcus
          aureus (MRSA) Z86.14
        poliomyelitis Z86.12
        specified NEC Z86.19
        tuberculosis Z86.11
      mental NEC Z86.59
      metabolic Z86.39
        diabetic foot ulcer Z86.31
        gestational diabetes Z86.32
        specified type NEC Z86.39
      musculoskeletal NEC Z87.39
      nervous system Z86.69
      nutritional Z86.39
      parasitic Z86.19
      respiratory system NEC Z87.09
      sense organs Z86.69
      skin Z87.2
      specified site or type NEC Z87.898
      subcutaneous tissue Z87.2
      trophoblastic Z87.59
      urinary system NEC Z87.448
    drug dependence — *see* Dependence, drug,
      by type, in remission
    drug therapy
      antineoplastic chemotherapy Z92.21
      estrogen Z92.23
      immunosupression Z92.25
      inhaled steroids Z92.240
      monoclonal drug Z92.22
      specified NEC Z92.29
      steroid Z92.241
      systemic steroids Z92.241
    dysplasia
      cervical (mild) (moderate) Z87.410
        severe (grade III) Z86.001
      prostatic Z87.430
      vaginal (mild) (moderate) Z87.411
        severe (grade III) Z86.002
      vulvar (mild) (moderate) Z87.412
        severe (grade III) Z86.002
    embolism (venous) Z86.718
      pulmonary Z86.711
    encephalitis Z86.61
    estrogen therapy Z92.23
    extracorporeal membrane oxygenation
      (ECMO) Z92.81
    failed moderate sedation Z92.83
    failed conscious sedation Z92.83
    fall, falling Z91.81
    forced labor or sexual exploitation Z91.42
      in childhood Z62.813
    fracture (healed)
      fatigue Z87.312
      fragility Z87.310
      osteoporosis Z87.310
      pathological NEC Z87.311
      stress Z87.312

History - *continued*
  personal (of) - *continued*
    fracture (healed) - *continued*
      traumatic Z87.81
    gestational diabetes Z86.32
    hepatitis
      B Z86.19
      C Z86.19
    Hodgkin disease Z85.71
    hyperthermia, malignant Z88.4
    hypospadias (corrected) Z87.710
    hysterectomy Z90.710
    immunosupression therapy Z92.25
    in situ neoplasm
      breast Z86.000
      cervix uteri Z86.001
      digestive organs, specified NEC Z86.004
      esophagus Z86.003
      genital organs, specified NEC Z86.002
      melanoma Z86.006
      middle ear Z86.005
      oral cavity Z86.003
      respiratory system Z86.005
      skin Z86.007
      specified NEC Z86.008
      stomach Z86.003
    infection NEC Z86.19
      central nervous system Z86.61
      latent tuberculosis Z86.15
      Methicillin resistant Staphylococcus
        aureus (MRSA) Z86.14
      urinary (recurrent) (tract) Z87.440
    injury NEC Z87.828
    in utero procedure during
        pregnancy Z98.870
    in utero procedure while a fetus Z98.871
    irradiation Z92.3
    kidney stones Z87.442
    latent tuberculosis infection Z86.15
    leukemia Z85.6
    lymphoma (non-Hodgkin) Z85.72
    malignant melanoma (skin) Z85.820
    malignant neoplasm (of) Z85.9
      accessory sinuses Z85.22
      anus NEC Z85.048
        carcinoid Z85.040
      bladder Z85.51
      bone Z85.830
      brain Z85.841
      breast Z85.3
      bronchus NEC Z85.118
        carcinoid Z85.110
      carcinoid — *see* History, personal (of),
        malignant neoplasm, by site,
        carcinioid
      cervix Z85.41
      colon NEC Z85.038
        carcinoid Z85.030
      digestive organ Z85.00
        specified NEC Z85.09
      endocrine gland NEC Z85.858
      epididymis Z85.48
      esophagus Z85.01
      eye Z85.840
      gastrointestinal tract — *see* History,
        malignant neoplasm, digestive
        organ
      genital organ
        female Z85.40
          specified NEC Z85.44
        male Z85.45
          specified NEC Z85.49
      hematopoietic NEC Z85.79
      intrathoracic organ Z85.20
      kidney NEC Z85.528
        carcinoid Z85.520
      large intestine NEC Z85.038
        carcinoid Z85.030
      larynx Z85.21
      liver Z85.05
      lung NEC Z85.118
        carcinoid Z85.110
      mediastinum Z85.29
      Merkel cell Z85.821
      middle ear Z85.22

History - *continued*
  personal (of) - *continued*
    malignant neoplasm (of) - *continued*
      nasal cavities Z85.22
      nervous system NEC Z85.848
      oral cavity Z85.819
        specified site NEC Z85.818
      ovary Z85.43
      pancreas Z85.07
      pharynx Z85.819
        specified site NEC Z85.818
      pelvis Z85.53
      pleura Z85.29
      prostate Z85.46
      rectosigmoid junction NEC Z85.048
        carcinoid Z85.040
      rectum NEC Z85.048
        carcinoid Z85.040
      respiratory organ Z85.20
      sinuses, accessory Z85.22
      skin NEC Z85.828
        melanoma Z85.820
        Merkel cell Z85.821
      small intestine NEC Z85.068
        carcinoid Z85.060
      soft tissue Z85.831
      specified site NEC Z85.89
      stomach NEC Z85.028
        carcinoid Z85.020
      testis Z85.47
      thymus NEC Z85.238
        carcinoid Z85.230
      thyroid Z85.850
      tongue Z85.810
      trachea Z85.12
      ureter Z85.54
      urinary organ or tract Z85.50
        specified NEC Z85.59
      uterus Z85.42
    maltreatment Z91.89
    medical treatment NEC Z92.89
    melanoma Z85.820
      in situ Z86.006
      malignant (skin) Z85.820
    meningitis Z86.61
    mental disorder Z86.59
    Merkel cell carcinoma (skin) Z85.821
    Methicillin resistant Staphylococcus
      aureus (MRSA) Z86.14
    military deployment Z91.82
    military war, peacekeeping and
      humanitarian deployment (current or
      past conflict) Z91.82
    myocardial infarction (old) I25.2
    neglect (in)
      adult Z91.412
      childhood Z62.812
    neoplasia
      anal intraepithelial, III [AIN
        III] Z86.004
      high-grade prostatic intraepithelial, III
        [HGPIN III] Z86.002
      vaginal intraepithelial, III [VAIN
        III] Z86.002
      vulvar intraepithelial, III [VIN
        III] Z86.002
    neoplasm
      benign Z86.018
        brain Z86.011
        colon polyp Z86.010
      in situ
        breast Z86.000
        cervix uteri Z86.001
        digestive organs, specified
          NEC Z86.004
        esophagus Z86.003
        genital organs, specified NEC Z86.002
        melanoma Z86.006
        middle ear Z86.005
        oral cavity Z86.003
        respiratory system Z86.005
        skin Z86.007
        specified NEC Z86.008
        stomach Z86.003

History - *continued*
  personal (of) - *continued*
    neoplasm - *continued*
      malignant — *see* History of, malignant neoplasm
      uncertain behavior Z86.03
    nephrotic syndrome Z87.441
    nicotine dependence Z87.891
    noncompliance with medical treatment or regimen — *see* Noncompliance
    nutritional deficiency Z86.39
    obstetric complications Z87.59
      childbirth Z87.59
      pregnancy Z87.59
      pre-term labor Z87.51
      puerperium Z87.59
    osteoporosis fractures Z87.31
    parasuicide (attempt) Z91.5
    physical trauma NEC Z87.828
      self-harm or suicide attempt Z91.5
    poisoning NEC Z91.89
      self-harm or suicide attempt Z91.5
    poor personal hygiene Z91.89
    pneumonia (recurrent) Z87.01
    preterm labor Z87.51
    prolonged reversible ischemic neurologic deficit (PRIND) Z86.73
    procedure during pregnancy Z98.870
    procedure while a fetus Z98.871
    prostatic dysplasia Z87.430
    psychological
      abuse
        adult Z91.411
        child Z62.811
      trauma, specified NEC Z91.49
    radiation therapy Z92.3
    removal
      implant
        breast Z98.86
    renal calculi Z87.442
    respiratory condition NEC Z87.09
    retained foreign body fully removed Z87.821
    risk factors NEC Z91.89
    self-harm Z91.5
    self-poisoning attempt Z91.5
    sex reassignment Z87.890
    sleep-wake cycle problem Z72.821
    specified NEC Z87.898
    steroid therapy (systemic) Z92.241
      inhaled Z92.240
    stroke without residual deficits Z86.73
    substance abuse NEC F10-F19
    sudden cardiac arrest Z86.74
    sudden cardiac death successfully resuscitated Z86.74
    suicide attempt Z91.5
    surgery NEC Z98.890
      with uterine scar Z98.891
      sex reassignment Z87.890
      transplant — *see* Transplant
    thrombophlebitis Z86.72
    thrombosis (venous) Z86.718
      pulmonary Z86.711
    tobacco dependence Z87.891
    transient ischemic attack (TIA) without residual deficits Z86.73
    trauma (physical) NEC Z87.828
      psychological NEC Z91.49
      self-harm Z91.5
    traumatic brain injury Z87.820
    tuberculosis, latent infection Z86.15
    unhealthy sleep-wake cycle Z72.821
    unintended awareness under general anesthesia Z92.84
    urinary calculi Z87.442
    urinary (recurrent) (tract) infection (s) Z87.440
    uterine scar from previous surgery Z98.891
    vaginal dysplasia Z87.411
    venous thrombosis or embolism Z86.718
      pulmonary Z86.711
    vulvar dysplasia Z87.412
His-Werner disease A79.0

HIV — *see also* Human, immunodeficiency virus B20
  laboratory evidence (nonconclusive) R75
  positive, seropositive Z21
  nonconclusive test (in infants) R75
Hives (bold) — *see* Urticaria
Hoarseness R49.0
Hobo Z59.0
Hodgkin disease — *see* Lymphoma, Hodgkin
Hodgson's disease I71.2
  ruptured I71.1
Hoffa-Kastert disease E88.89
Hoffa's disease E88.89
Hoffmann-Bouveret syndrome I47.9
Hoffmann's syndrome E03.9 *[G73.7]*
Hole (round)
  macula H35.34-
  retina (without detachment) — *see* Break, retina, round hole
    with detachment — *see* Detachment, retina, with retinal, break
Holiday relief care Z75.5
Hollenhorst's plaque — *see* Occlusion, artery, retina
Hollow foot (congenital) Q66.7-
  acquired — *see* Deformity, limb, foot, specified NEC
Holoprosencephaly Q04.2
Holt-Oram syndrome Q87.2
Homelessness Z59.0
Homesickness — *see* Disorder, adjustment
Homocystinemia, homocystinuria E72.11
Homogentisate 1,2-dioxygenase deficiency E70.29
Homologous serum hepatitis (prophylactic) (therapeutic) — *see* Hepatitis, viral, type B
Honeycomb lung J98.4
  congenital Q33.0
Hooded
  clitoris Q52.6
  penis Q55.69
Hookworm (disease) (infection) (infestation) B76.9
  with anemia B76.9 *[D63.8]*
  specified NEC B76.8
Hordeolum (eyelid) (externum) (recurrent) H00.019
  internum H00.029
    left H00.026
      lower H00.025
      upper H00.024
    right H00.023
      lower H00.022
      upper H00.021
  left H00.016
    lower H00.015
    upper H00.014
  right H00.013
    lower H00.012
    upper H00.011
Horn
  cutaneous L85.8
  nail L60.2
    congenital Q84.6
Horner (-Claude Bernard) syndrome G90.2
  traumatic — *see* Injury, nerve, cervical sympathetic
Horseshoe kidney (congenital) Q63.1
Horton's headache or neuralgia G44.099
  intractable G44.091
  not intractable G44.099
Hospital hopper syndrome — *see* Disorder, factitious
Hospitalism in children — *see* Disorder, adjustment
Hostility R45.5
  towards child Z62.3
Hot flashes
  menopausal N95.1
Hourglass (contracture) — *see also* Contraction, hourglass
  stomach K31.89
    congenital Q40.2
    stricture K31.2

Household, housing circumstance affecting care Z59.9
  specified NEC Z59.8
Housemaid's knee — *see* Bursitis, prepatellar
Hudson (-Stähli) line (cornea) — *see* Pigmentation, cornea, anterior
Human
  bite (open wound) — *see also* Bite
    intact skin surface — *see* Bite, superficial
  herpesvirus — *see* Herpes
  immunodeficiency virus (HIV) disease (infection) B20
    asymptomatic status Z21
    contact Z20.6
    counseling Z71.7
    dementia B20 *[F02.80]*
      with behavioral disturbance B20 *[F02.81]*
    exposure to Z20.6
    laboratory evidence R75
    type-2 (HIV 2) as cause of disease classified elsewhere B97.35
  papillomavirus (HPV)
    DNA test positive
      high risk
        cervix R87.810
        vagina R87.811
      low risk
        cervix R87.820
        vagina R87.821
    screening for Z11.51
  T-cell lymphotropic virus
    type-1 (HTLV-I) infection B33.3
      as cause of disease classified elsewhere B97.33
      carrier Z22.6
    type-2 (HTLV-II) as cause of disease classified elsewhere B97.34
Humidifier lung or pneumonitis J67.7
Humiliation (experience) in childhood Z62.898
Humpback (acquired) — *see* Kyphosis
Hunchback (acquired) — *see* Kyphosis
Hunger T73.0
  air, psychogenic F45.8
Hungry bone syndrome E83.81
Hunner's ulcer — *see* Cystitis, chronic, interstitial
Hunter's
  glossitis D51.0
  syndrome E76.1
Huntington's disease or chorea G10
  with dementia G10 *[F02.80]*
    with behavioral disturbance G10 *[F02.81]*
Hunt's
  disease or syndrome (herpetic geniculate ganglionitis) B02.21
  dyssynergia cerebellaris myoclonica G11.1
  neuralgia B02.21
Hurler (-Scheie) disease or syndrome E76.02
Hurst's disease G36.1
Hurthle cell
  adenocarcinoma C73
  adenoma D34
  carcinoma C73
  tumor D34
Hutchinson-Boeck disease or syndrome — *see* Sarcoidosis
Hutchinson-Gilford disease or syndrome E34.8
Hutchinson's
  disease, meaning
    angioma serpiginosum L81.7
    pompholyx (cheiropompholyx) L30.1
    prurigo estivalis L56.4
    summer eruption or summer prurigo L56.4
  melanotic freckle — *see* Melanoma, in situ
    malignant melanoma in — *see* Melanoma
  teeth or incisors (congenital syphilis) A50.52
  triad (congenital syphilis) A50.53
Hyalin plaque, sclera, senile H15.89
Hyaline membrane (disease) (lung) (pulmonary) (newborn) P22.0
Hyalinosis
  cutis (et mucosae) E78.89

Hyalinosis - *continued*
  focal and segmental (glomerular) — *see also*
    N00-N07 with fourth character
    .1 N05.1
Hyalitis, hyalosis, asteroid — *see also*
  Deposit, crystalline
  syphilitic (late) A52.71
Hydatid
  cyst or tumor — *see* Echinococcus
  mole — *see* Hydatidiform mole
  Morgagni
    female Q50.5
    male (epididymal) Q55.4
    testicular Q55.29
Hydatidiform mole (benign) (complicating
  pregnancy) (delivered) (undelivered)
  O01.9
  classical O01.0
  complete O01.0
  incomplete O01.1
  invasive D39.2
  malignant D39.2
  partial O01.1
Hydatidosis — *see* Echinococcus
Hydradenitis (axillaris) (suppurative) L73.2
Hydradenoma — *see* Hidradenoma
Hydramnios O40.-
Hydrancephaly, hydranencephaly Q04.3
  with spina bifida — *see* Spina bifida, with
    hydrocephalus
Hydrargyrism NEC — *see* Poisoning,
  mercury
Hydrarthrosis — *see also* Effusion, joint
  gonococcal A54.42
  intermittent M12.40
    ankle M12.47-
    elbow M12.42-
    foot joint M12.47-
    hand joint M12.44-
    hip M12.45-
    knee M12.46-
    multiple site M12.49
    shoulder M12.41-
    specified joint NEC M12.48
    wrist M12.43-
  of yaws (early) (late) (*see also* subcategory
    M14.8-) A66.6
  syphilitic (late) A52.77
    congenital A50.55 *[M12.80]*
Hydremia D64.89
Hydrencephalocele (congenital) — *see*
  Encephalocele
Hydrencephalomeningocele
  (congenital) — *see* Encephalocele
Hydroa R23.8
  aestivale L56.4
  vacciniforme L56.4
Hydroadenitis (axillaris) (suppurative) L73.2
Hydrocalycosis — *see* Hydronephrosis
Hydrocele (spermatic cord) (testis) (tunica
  vaginalis) N43.3
  canal of Nuck N94.89
  communicating N43.2
    congenital P83.5
  congenital P83.5
  encysted N43.0
  female NEC N94.89
  infected N43.1
  newborn P83.5
  round ligament N94.89
  specified NEC N43.2
  spinalis — *see* Spina bifida
  vulva N90.89
Hydrocephalus (acquired) (external)
  (internal) (malignant) (recurrent) G91.9
  aqueduct Sylvius stricture Q03.0
  causing disproportion O33.6
    with obstructed labor O66.3
  communicating G91.0
  congenital (external) (internal) Q03.9
    with spina bifida Q05.4
      cervical Q05.0
      dorsal Q05.1
      lumbar Q05.2
      lumbosacral Q05.2

Hydrocephalus (acquired) (external)
(internal) (malignant) (recurrent) - *continued*
  congenital (external) (internal) - *continued*
    with spina bifida - *continued*
      sacral Q05.3
      thoracic Q05.1
      thoracolumbar Q05.1
    specified NEC Q03.8
  due to toxoplasmosis (congenital) P37.1
  foramen Magendie block (acquired) G91.1
    congenital — *see also* Hydrocephalus,
      congenital Q03.1
  in (due to)
    infectious disease NEC B89 *[G91.4]*
    neoplastic disease NEC (see also
      Neoplasm) G91.4
    parasitic disease B89 *[G91.4]*
  newborn Q03.9
    with spina bifida — *see* Spina bifida, with
      hydrocephalus
  noncommunicating G91.1
  normal pressure G91.2
    secondary G91.0
  obstructive G91.1
  otitic G93.2
  post-traumatic NEC G91.3
  secondary G91.4
    post-traumatic G91.3
  specified NEC G91.8
  syphilitic, congenital A50.49
Hydrocolpos (congenital) N89.8
Hydrocystoma — *see* Neoplasm, skin, benign
Hydroencephalocele (congenital) — *see*
  Encephalocele
Hydroencephalomeningocele
  (congenital) — *see* Encephalocele
Hydrohematopneumothorax — *see*
  Hemothorax
Hydromeningitis — *see* Meningitis
Hydromeningocele (spinal) — *see also* Spina
  bifida
  cranial — *see* Encephalocele
Hydrometra N85.8
Hydrometrocolpos N89.8
Hydromicrocephaly Q02
Hydromphalos (since birth) Q45.8
Hydromyelia Q06.4
Hydromyelocele — *see* Spina bifida
Hydronephrosis (atrophic) (early)
  (functionless) (intermittent) (primary)
  (secondary) NEC N13.30
  with
    infection N13.6
    obstruction (by) (of)
      renal calculus N13.2
        with infection N13.6
      ureteral NEC N13.1
        with infection N13.6
        calculus N13.2
          with infection N13.6
        ureteropelvic junction
          (congenital) Q62.11
        acquired N13.0
          with infection N13.6
      ureteral stricture NEC N13.1
        with infection N13.6
  congenital Q62.0
    due to acquired occlusion of ureteropelvic
      junction N13.0
  specified type NEC N13.39
  tuberculous A18.11
Hydropericarditis — *see* Pericarditis
Hydropericardium — *see* Pericarditis
Hydroperitoneum R18.8
Hydrophobia — *see* Rabies
Hydrophthalmos Q15.0
Hydropneumohemothorax — *see*
  Hemothorax
Hydropneumopericarditis — *see* Pericarditis
Hydropneumopericardium — *see* Pericarditis
Hydropneumothorax J94.8
  traumatic — *see* Injury, intrathoracic, lung
  tuberculous NEC A15.6
Hydrops R60.9
  abdominis R18.8

Hydrops - *continued*
  articulorum intermittens — *see*
    Hydrarthrosis, intermittent
  cardiac — *see* Failure, heart, congestive
  causing obstructed labor (mother) O66.3
  endolymphatic H81.0-
  fetal — *see* Pregnancy, complicated by,
    hydrops, fetalis
  fetalis P83.2
    due to
      ABO isoimmunization P56.0
      alpha thalassemia D56.0
      hemolytic disease P56.90
        specified NEC P56.99
      isoimmunization (ABO) (Rh) P56.0
      other specified nonhemolytic disease
        NEC P83.2
      Rh incompatibility P56.0
    during pregnancy — *see* Pregnancy,
      complicated by, hydrops, fetalis
  gallbladder K82.1
  joint — *see* Effusion, joint
  labyrinth H81.0-
  newborn (idiopathic) P83.2
    due to
      ABO isoimmunization P56.0
      alpha thalassemia D56.0
      hemolytic disease P56.90
        specified NEC P56.99
      isoimmunization (ABO) (Rh) P56.0
      Rh incompatibility P56.0
  nutritional — *see* Malnutrition, severe
  pericardium — *see* Pericarditis
  pleura — *see* Hydrothorax
  spermatic cord — *see* Hydrocele
Hydropyonephrosis N13.6
Hydrorachis Q06.4
Hydrorrhea (nasal) J34.89
  pregnancy — *see* Rupture, membranes,
    premature
Hydrosadenitis (axillaris)
  (suppurative) L73.2
Hydrosalpinx (fallopian tube)
  (follicularis) N70.11
Hydrothorax (double) (pleura) J94.8
  chylous (nonfilarial) I89.8
    filarial — *see also* Infestation,
      filarial B74.9 *[J91.8]*
  traumatic — *see* Injury, intrathoracic
  tuberculous NEC (non primary) A15.6
Hydroureter — *see also*
  Hydronephrosis N13.4
  with infection N13.6
  congenital Q62.39
Hydroureteronephrosis — *see*
  Hydronephrosis
Hydrourethra N36.8
Hydroxykynureninuria E70.8
Hydroxylysinemia E72.3
Hydroxyprolinemia E72.59
Hygiene, sleep
  abuse Z72.821
  inadequate Z72.821
  poor Z72.821
Hygroma (congenital) (cystic) D18.1
  praepatellare, prepatellar — *see* Bursitis,
    prepatellar
Hymen — *see* condition
Hymenolepis, hymenolepiasis (diminuta)
  (infection) (infestation) (nana) B71.0
Hypalgesia R20.8
Hyperacidity (gastric) K31.89
  psychogenic F45.8
Hyperactive, hyperactivity F90.9
  basal cell, uterine cervix — *see* Dysplasia,
    cervix
  bowel sounds R19.12
  cervix epithelial (basal) — *see* Dysplasia,
    cervix
  child F90.9
    attention deficit — *see* Disorder, attention-
      deficit hyperactivity
  detrusor muscle N32.81
  gastrointestinal K31.89
    psychogenic F45.8

Hyperactive, hyperactivity - continued
  nasal mucous membrane J34.3
  stomach K31.89
  thyroid (gland) — see Hyperthyroidism
Hyperacusis H93.23-
Hyperadrenalism E27.5
Hyperadrenocorticism E24.9
  congenital E25.0
  iatrogenic E24.2
    correct substance properly
      administered — see Table of Drugs
      and Chemicals, by drug, adverse
      effect
    overdose or wrong substance given or
      taken — see Table of Drugs and
      Chemicals, by drug, poisoning
  not associated with Cushing's
    syndrome E27.0
  pituitary-dependent E24.0
Hyperaldosteronism E26.9
  familial (type I) E26.02
  glucocorticoid-remediable E26.02
  primary (due to (bilateral) adrenal
    hyperplasia) E26.09
  primary NEC E26.09
  secondary E26.1
  specified NEC E26.89
Hyperalgesia R20.8
Hyperalimentation R63.2
  carotene, carotin E67.1
  specified NEC E67.8
  vitamin
    A E67.0
    D E67.3
Hyperaminoaciduria
  arginine E72.21
  cystine E72.01
  lysine E72.3
  ornithine E72.4
Hyperammonemia (congenital) E72.20
Hyperazotemia — see Uremia
Hyperbetalipoproteinemia (familial) E78.00
  with prebetalipoproteinemia E78.2
Hyperbicarbonatemia P74.41
Hyperbilirubinemia
  constitutional E80.6
  familial conjugated E80.6
  neonatal (transient) — see Jaundice, newborn
Hypercalcemia, hypocalciuric,
    familial E83.52
Hypercalciuria, idiopathic R82.994
Hypercapnia R06.89
  newborn P84
Hypercarotenemia (dietary) E67.1
Hypercementosis K03.4
Hyperchloremia E87.8
Hyperchlorhydria K31.89
  neurotic F45.8
  psychogenic F45.8
Hypercholesterinemia — see
    Hypercholesterolemia
Hypercholesterolemia (essential) (primary)
    (pure) E78.00
  with hyperglyceridemia, endogenous E78.2
  dietary counseling and surveillance Z71.3
  familial E78.01
  hereditary E78.01
Hyperchylia gastrica, psychogenic F45.8
Hyperchylomicronemia (familial) (primary)
    E78.3
  with hyperbetalipoproteinemia E78.3
Hypercoagulable (state) D68.59
  activated protein C resistance D68.51
  antithrombin (III) deficiency D68.59
  factor V Leiden mutation D68.51
  primary NEC D68.59
  protein C deficiency D68.59
  protein S deficiency D68.59
  prothrombin gene mutation D68.52
  secondary D68.69
  specified NEC D68.69
Hypercoagulation (state) D68.59
Hypercorticalism, pituitary-dependent E24.0
Hypercorticosolism — see Cushing's,
    syndrome

Hypercorticosteronism E24.2
  correct substance properly administered —
    see Table of Drugs and Chemicals, by
    drug, adverse effect
  overdose or wrong substance given or
    taken — see Table of Drugs and
    Chemicals, by drug, poisoning
Hypercortisonism E24.2
  correct substance properly administered —
    see Table of Drugs and Chemicals, by
    drug, adverse effect
  overdose or wrong substance given or
    taken — see Table of Drugs and
    Chemicals, by drug, poisoning
Hyperekplexia Q89.8
Hyperelectrolytemia E87.8
Hyperemesis R11.10
  with nausea R11.2
  gravidarum (mild) O21.0
    with
      carbohydrate depletion O21.1
      dehydration O21.1
      electrolyte imbalance O21.1
      metabolic disturbance O21.1
    severe (with metabolic disturbance) O21.1
  projectile R11.12
  psychogenic F45.8
Hyperemia (acute) (passive) R68.89
  anal mucosa K62.89
  bladder N32.89
  cerebral I67.89
  conjunctiva H11.43-
  ear internal, acute — see subcategory H83.0
  enteric K59.8
  eye — see Hyperemia, conjunctiva
  eyelid (active) (passive) — see Disorder,
    eyelid, specified type NEC
  intestine K59.8
  iris — see Disorder, iris, vascular
  kidney N28.89
  labyrinth — see subcategory H83.0
  liver (active) K76.89
  lung (passive) — see Edema, lung
  pulmonary (passive) — see Edema, lung
  renal N28.89
  retina H35.89
  stomach K31.89
Hyperesthesia (body surface) R20.3
  larynx (reflex) J38.7
    hysterical F44.89
  pharynx (reflex) J39.2
    hysterical F44.89
Hyperestrogenism (drug-induced)
    (iatrogenic) E28.0
Hyperexplexia Q89.8
Hyperfibrinolysis — see Fibrinolysis
Hyperfructosemia E74.19
Hyperfunction
  adrenal cortex, not associated with Cushing's
    syndrome E27.0
  medulla E27.5
    adrenomedullary E27.5
  virilism E25.9
    congenital E25.0
  ovarian E28.8
  pancreas K86.89
  parathyroid (gland) E21.3
  pituitary (gland) (anterior) E22.9
    specified NEC E22.8
  polyglandular E31.1
  testicular E29.0
Hypergammaglobulinemia D89.2
  polyclonal D89.2
  Waldenström D89.0
Hypergastrinemia E16.4
Hyperglobulinemia R77.1
Hyperglycemia, hyperglycemic (transient)
    R73.9
  coma — see Diabetes, by type, with coma
  postpancreatectomy E89.1
Hyperglyceridemia (endogenous) (essential)
    (familial) (hereditary) (pure) E78.1
  mixed E78.3
Hyperglycinemia (non-ketotic) E72.51

Hypergonadism
  ovarian E28.8
  testicular (primary) (infantile) E29.0
Hyperheparinemia D68.32
Hyperhidrosis, hyperidrosis R61
  focal
    primary L74.519
      axilla L74.510
      face L74.511
      palms L74.512
      soles L74.513
    secondary L74.52
  generalized R61
  localized
    primary L74.519
      axilla L74.510
      face L74.511
      palms L74.512
      soles L74.513
    secondary L74.52
  psychogenic F45.8
  secondary R61
    focal L74.52
Hyperhistidinemia E70.41
Hyperhomocysteinemia E72.11
Hyperhydroxyprolinemia E72.59
Hyperinsulinism (functional) E16.1
  with
    coma (hypoglycemic) E15
    encephalopathy E16.1 [G94]
  ectopic E16.1
  therapeutic misadventure (from
    administration of insulin) — see
    subcategory T38.3
Hyperkalemia E87.5
Hyperkeratosis — see also Keratosis L85.9
  cervix N88.0
  due to yaws (early) (late) (palmar or
    plantar) A66.3
  follicularis Q82.8
    penetrans (in cutem) L87.0
  palmoplantaris climacterica L85.1
  pinta A67.1
  senile (with pruritus) L57.0
  universalis congenita Q80.8
  vocal cord J38.3
  vulva N90.4
Hyperkinesia, hyperkinetic (disease)
    (reaction) (syndrome) (childhood)
    (adolescence) — see also Disorder,
    attention-deficit hyperactivity
  heart I51.89
Hyperleucine-isoleucinemia E71.19
Hyperlipemia, hyperlipidemia E78.5
  combined E78.2
    familial E78.49
  group
    A E78.00
    B E78.1
    C E78.2
    D E78.3
  mixed E78.2
  specified NEC E78.49
Hyperlipidosis E75.6
  hereditary NEC E75.5
Hyperlipoproteinemia E78.5
  Fredrickson's type
    I E78.3
    IIa E78.00
    IIb E78.2
    III E78.2
    IV E78.1
    V E78.3
  low-density-lipoprotein-type (LDL) E78.00
  very-low-density-lipoprotein-type
    (VLDL) E78.1
Hyperlucent lung, unilateral J43.0
Hyperlysinemia E72.3
Hypermagnesemia E83.41
  neonatal P71.8
Hypermenorrhea N92.0
Hypermethioninemia E72.19
Hypermetropia (congenital) H52.0-
Hypermobility, hypermotility
  cecum — see Syndrome, irritable bowel

Hypermobility, hypermotility - *continued*
coccyx — *see* subcategory M53.2
colon — *see* Syndrome, irritable bowel
  psychogenic F45.8
ileum K58.9
intestine — *see also* Syndrome, irritable
  bowel K58.9
  psychogenic F45.8
meniscus (knee) — *see* Derangement, knee,
  meniscus
scapula — *see* Instability, joint, shoulder
stomach K31.89
  psychogenic F45.8
syndrome M35.7
urethra N36.41
  with intrinsic sphincter deficiency N36.43
Hypernasality R49.21
Hypernatremia E87.0
Hypernephroma C64.-
Hyperopia — *see* Hypermetropia
Hyperorexia nervosa F50.2
Hyperornithinemia E72.4
Hyperosmia R43.1
Hyperosmolality E87.0
Hyperostosis (monomelic) — *see also*
  Disorder, bone, density and structure,
  specified NEC
ankylosing (spine) M48.10
  cervical region M48.12
  cervicothoracic region M48.13
  lumbar region M48.16
  lumbosacral region M48.17
  multiple sites M48.19
  occipito-atlanto-axial region M48.11
  sacrococcygeal region M48.18
  thoracic region M48.14
  thoracolumbar region M48.15
cortical (skull) M85.2
  infantile M89.8X-
frontal, internal of skull M85.2
interna frontalis M85.2
skeletal, diffuse idiopathic — *see*
  Hyperostosis, ankylosing
skull M85.2
  congenital Q75.8
vertebral, ankylosing — *see* Hyperostosis,
  ankylosing
Hyperovarism E28.8
Hyperoxaluria R82.992
primary E72.53
Hyperparathyroidism E21.3
primary E21.0
secondary (renal) N25.81
  non-renal E21.1
specified NEC E21.2
tertiary E21.2
Hyperpathia R20.8
Hyperperistalsis R19.2
psychogenic F45.8
Hyperpermeability, capillary I78.8
Hyperphagia R63.2
Hyperphenylalaninemia NEC E70.1
Hyperphoria (alternating) H50.53
Hyperphosphatemia E83.39
Hyperpiesis, hyperpiesia — *see* Hypertension
Hyperpigmentation — *see also* Pigmentation
melanin NEC L81.4
postinflammatory L81.0
Hyperpinealism E34.8
Hyperpituitarism E22.9
Hyperplasia, hyperplastic
adenoids J35.2
adrenal (capsule) (cortex) (gland) E27.8
  with
    sexual precocity (male) E25.9
     congenital E25.0
    virilism, adrenal E25.9
     congenital E25.0
    virilization (female) E25.9
     congenital E25.0
  congenital E25.0
  salt-losing E25.0
adrenomedullary E27.5
angiolymphoid, eosinophilia (ALHE) D18.01
appendix (lymphoid) K38.0

Hyperplasia, hyperplastic - *continued*
artery, fibromuscular I77.3
bone — *see also* Hypertrophy, bone
  marrow D75.89
breast — *see also* Hypertrophy, breast
  atypical, atypia N60.9-
    ductal N60.9-
    lobular N60.9-
C-cell, thyroid E07.0
cementation (tooth) (teeth) K03.4
cervical gland R59.0
cervix (uteri) (basal cell) (endometrium)
  (polypoid) — *see also* Dysplasia, cervix
  congenital Q51.828
clitoris, congenital Q52.6
denture K06.2
endocervicitis N72
endometrium, endometrial (adenomatous)
  (cystic) (glandular) (glandular-cystic)
  (polypoid) N85.00
  with atypia N85.02
  benign N85.01
  cervix — *see* Dysplasia, cervix
  complex (without atypia) N85.01
  simple (without atypia) N85.01
epithelial L85.9
  focal, oral, including tongue K13.29
  nipple N62
  skin L85.9
  tongue K13.29
  vaginal wall N89.3
erythroid D75.89
fibromuscular of artery (carotid) (renal) I77.3
genital
  female NEC N94.89
  male N50.89
gingiva K06.1
glandularis cystica uteri (interstitialis) — *see*
  also Hyperplasia, endometrial N85.00-
gum K06.1
hymen, congenital Q52.4
irritative, edentulous (alveolar) K06.2
jaw M26.09
  alveolar M26.79
  lower M26.03
    alveolar M26.72
  upper M26.01
    alveolar M26.71
kidney (congenital) Q63.3
labia N90.69
  epithelial N90.3
liver (congenital) Q44.7
  nodular, focal K76.89
lymph gland or node R59.9
mandible, mandibular M26.03
  alveolar M26.72
  unilateral condylar M27.8
maxilla, maxillary M26.01
  alveolar M26.71
myometrium, myometrial N85.2
neuroendocrine cell, of infancy J84.841
nose
  lymphoid J34.89
  polypoid J33.9
oral mucosa (irritative) K13.6
organ or site, congenital NEC — *see*
  Anomaly, by site
ovary N83.8
palate, papillary (irritative) K13.6
pancreatic islet cells E16.9
  alpha E16.8
    with excess
     gastrin E16.4
     glucagon E16.3
  beta E16.1
parathyroid (gland) E21.0
pharynx (lymphoid) J39.2
prostate (adenofibromatous) (nodular) N40.0
  with lower urinary tract symptoms
    (LUTS) N40.1
  without lower urinary tract symtpoms
    (LUTS) N40.0
renal artery I77.89
reticulo-endothelial (cell) D75.89
salivary gland (any) K11.1

Hyperplasia, hyperplastic - *continued*
Schimmelbusch's — *see* Mastopathy, cystic
suprarenal capsule (gland) E27.8
thymus (gland) (persistent) E32.0
thyroid (gland) — *see* Goiter
tonsils (faucial) (infective) (lingual)
  (lymphoid) J35.1
  with adenoids J35.3
unilateral condylar M27.8
uterus, uterine N85.2
  endometrium (glandular) — *see also*
    Hyperplasia, endometrial N85.00-
vulva N90.69
  epithelial N90.3
Hyperpnea — *see* Hyperventilation
Hyperpotassemia E87.5
**Hyperprebetalipoproteinemia
  (familial)** E78.1
Hyperprolactinemia E22.1
Hyperprolinemia (type I) (type II) E72.59
Hyperproteinemia E88.09
**Hyperprothrombinemia, causing
  coagulation factor deficiency** D68.4
Hyperpyrexia R50.9
heat (effects) T67.01
malignant, due to anesthetic T88.3
rheumatic — *see* Fever, rheumatic
unknown origin R50.9
Hyper-reflexia R29.2
Hypersalivation K11.7
Hypersecretion
ACTH (not associated with Cushing's
  syndrome) E27.0
  pituitary E24.0
adrenaline E27.5
adrenomedullary E27.5
androgen (testicular) E29.0
  ovarian (drug-induced) (iatrogenic) E28.1
calcitonin E07.0
catecholamine E27.5
corticoadrenal E24.9
cortisol E24.9
epinephrine E27.5
estrogen E28.0
gastric K31.89
  psychogenic F45.8
gastrin E16.4
glucagon E16.3
hormone (s)
  ACTH (not associated with Cushing's
    syndrome) E27.0
    pituitary E24.0
  antidiuretic E22.2
  growth E22.0
  intestinal NEC E34.1
  ovarian androgen E28.1
  pituitary E22.9
  testicular E29.0
  thyroid stimulating E05.80
    with thyroid storm E05.81
insulin — *see* Hyperinsulinism
lacrimal glands — *see* Epiphora
medulloadrenal E27.5
milk O92.6
ovarian androgens E28.1
salivary gland (any) K11.7
thyrocalcitonin E07.0
upper respiratory J39.8
**Hypersegmentation, leukocytic,
  hereditary** D72.0
**Hypersensitive, hypersensitiveness,
  hypersensitivity** — *see also* Allergy
carotid sinus G90.01
colon — *see* Irritable, colon
drug T88.7
gastrointestinal K52.29
  immediate K52.29
  psychogenic F45.8
labyrinth — *see* subcategory H83.2
pain R20.8
pneumonitis — *see* Pneumonitis, allergic
reaction T78.40
  upper respiratory tract NEC J39.3
Hypersomnia (organic) G47.10
due to

Hypersomnia (organic) - *continued*
  due to - *continued*
    alcohol
      abuse F10.182
      dependence F10.282
      use F10.982
    amphetamines
      abuse F15.182
      dependence F15.282
      use F15.982
    caffeine
      abuse F15.182
      dependence F15.282
      use F15.982
    cocaine
      abuse F14.182
      dependence F14.282
      use F14.982
    drug NEC
      abuse F19.182
      dependence F19.282
      use F19.982
    medical condition G47.14
    mental disorder F51.13
    opioid
      abuse F11.182
      dependence F11.282
      use F11.982
    psychoactive substance NEC
      abuse F19.182
      dependence F19.282
      use F19.982
    sedative, hypnotic, or anxiolytic
      abuse F13.182
      dependence F13.282
      use F13.982
    stimulant NEC
      abuse F15.182
      dependence F15.282
      use F15.982
  idiopathic G47.11
    with long sleep time G47.11
    without long sleep time G47.12
  menstrual related G47.13
  nonorganic origin F51.11
    specified NEC F51.19
  not due to a substance or known
    physiological condition F51.11
    specified NEC F51.19
  primary F51.11
  recurrent G47.13
  specified NEC G47.19
Hypersplenia, hypersplenism D73.1
Hyperstimulation, ovaries (associated with induced ovulation) N98.1
Hypersusceptibility — *see* Allergy
Hypertelorism (ocular) (orbital) Q75.2
Hypertension, hypertensive (accelerated) (benign) (essential) (idiopathic) (malignant) (systemic) I10
  with
    heart failure (congestive) I11.0
    heart involvement (conditions in I50.-, I51.4- I51.9 due to hypertension) — *see* Hypertension, heart
    kidney involvement — *see* Hypertension, kidney
  benign, intracranial G93.2
  borderline R03.0
  cardiorenal (disease) I13.10
    with heart failure I13.0
      with stage 1 through stage 4 chronic kidney disease I13.0
      with stage 5 or end stage renal disease I13.2
    without heart failure I13.10
      with stage 1 through stage 4 chronic kidney disease I13.10
      with stage 5 or end stage renal disease I13.11
  cardiovascular
    disease (arteriosclerotic) (sclerotic) — *see* Hypertension, heart
    renal (disease) — *see* Hypertension, cardiorenal

Hypertension, hypertensive (accelerated) (benign) (essential) (idiopathic) (malignant) (systemic) - *continued*
  chronic venous — *see* Hypertension, venous (chronic)
  complicating
    childbirth (labor) O16.4
      pre-existing O10.92
        with
          heart disease O10.12
            with renal disease O10.32
          pre-eclampsia O11.4
          renal disease O10.22
            with heart disease O10.32
        essential O10.02
      secondary O10.42
    pregnancy O16.-
      with edema — *see also* Pre-eclampsia O14.9-
      gestational (pregnancy induced) (without proteinuria) O13.-
        with proteinuria O14.9-
          mild pre-eclampsia O14.0-
          moderate pre-eclampsia O14.0-
          severe pre-eclampsia O14.1-
            with hemolysis, elevated liver enzymes and low platelet count (HELLP) O14.2-
      pre-existing O10.91-
        with
          heart disease O10.11-
            with renal disease O10.31-
          pre-eclampsia — *see* category O11
          renal disease O10.21-
            with heart disease O10.31-
        essential O10.01-
        secondary O10.41-
      transient O13.-
    puerperium, pre-existing O16.5
      pre-existing
        with
          heart disease O10.13
            with renal disease O10.33
          pre-eclampsia O11.5
          renal disease O10.23
            with heart disease O10.33
        essential O10.03
      pregnancy-induced O13.9
      secondary O10.43
  crisis I16.9
  due to
    endocrine disorders I15.2
    pheochromocytoma I15.2
    renal disorders NEC I15.1
      arterial I15.0
    renovascular disorders I15.0
    specified disease NEC I15.8
  emergency I16.1
  encephalopathy I67.4
  gestational (without significant proteinuria) (pregnancy-induced) (transient) O13.-
    with significant proteinuria — *see* Pre-eclampsia
    complicating
      delivery O13.4
      puerperium O13.5
  Goldblatt's I70.1
  heart (disease) (conditions in I51.4-I51.9 due to hypertension) I11.9
    with
      heart failure (congestive) I11.0
      kidney disease (chronic) — *see* Hypertension, cardiorenal
  intracranial (benign) G93.2
  kidney I12.9
    with
      heart disease — *see* Hypertension, cardiorenal
      stage 5 chronic kidney disease (CKD) or end stage renal disease (ESRD) I12.0
      stage 1 through stage 4 chronic kidney disease I12.9
  lesser circulation I27.0
  maternal O16.-

Hypertension, hypertensive (accelerated) (benign) (essential) (idiopathic) (malignant) (systemic) - *continued*
  newborn P29.2
    pulmonary (persistent) P29.30
  ocular H40.05-
  pancreatic duct - code to underlying condition
    with chronic pancreatitis K86.1
  portal (due to chronic liver disease) (idiopathic) K76.6
    gastropathy K31.89
    in (due to) schistosomiasis (bilharziasis) B65.9 *[K77]*
  postoperative I97.3
  psychogenic F45.8
  pulmonary I27.20
    with
      cor pulmonale (chronic) I27.29
        acute I26.09
      right heart ventricular strain/failure I27.29
        acute I26.09
      right to left shunt related to congenital heart disease I27.83
      unclear multifactorial mechanisms I27.29
    arterial (associated) (drug-induced) (toxin-induced) I27.21
    chronic thromboembolic I27.24
    due to
      hematologic disorders I27.29
      left heart disease I27.22
      lung diseases and hypoxia I27.23
      metabolic disorders I27.29
      specified systemic disorders NEC I27.29
    group 1 (associated) (drug-induced) (toxin-induced) I27.21
    group 2 I27.22
    group 3 I27.23
    group 4 I27.24
    group 5 I27.29
    of newborn (persistent) P29.30
    primary (idiopathic) I27.0
    secondary
      arterial I27.21
      specified NEC I27.29
  renal — *see* Hypertension, kidney
  renovascular I15.0
  secondary NEC I15.9
    due to
      endocrine disorders I15.2
      pheochromocytoma I15.2
      renal disorders NEC I15.1
        arterial I15.0
      renovascular disorders I15.0
    specified NEC I15.8
  transient R03.0
    of pregnancy O13.-
  urgency I16.0
  venous (chronic)
    due to
      deep vein thrombosis — *see* Syndrome, postthrombotic
    idiopathic I87.309
      with
        inflammation I87.32-
          with ulcer I87.33-
        specified complication NEC I87.39-
        ulcer I87.31-
          with inflammation I87.33-
      asymptomatic I87.30-
Hypertensive urgency — *see* Hypertension
Hyperthecosis ovary E28.8
Hyperthermia (of unknown origin) — *see also* Hyperpyrexia
  malignant, due to anesthesia T88.3
  newborn P81.9
    environmental P81.0
Hyperthyroid (recurrent) — *see* Hyperthyroidism
Hyperthyroidism (latent) (pre-adult) (recurrent) E05.90
  with
    goiter (diffuse) E05.00

Hyperthyroidism (latent) (pre-adult) (recurrent) - *continued*
 with - *continued*
  goiter (diffuse) - *continued*
   with thyroid storm E05.01
   nodular (multinodular) E05.20
    with thyroid storm E05.21
   uninodular E05.10
    with thyroid storm E05.11
   storm E05.91
  due to ectopic thyroid tissue E05.30
   with thyroid storm E05.31
  neonatal, transitory P72.1
  specified NEC E05.80
   with thyroid storm E05.81
Hypertony, hypertonia, hypertonicity
 bladder N31.8
 congenital P94.1
 stomach K31.89
  psychogenic F45.8
 uterus, uterine (contractions) (complicating delivery) O62.4
Hypertrichosis L68.9
 congenital Q84.2
 eyelid H02.869
  left H02.866
   lower H02.865
   upper H02.864
  right H02.863
   lower H02.862
   upper H02.861
 lanuginosa Q84.2
  acquired L68.1
 localized L68.2
 specified NEC L68.8
Hypertriglyceridemia, essential E78.1
Hypertrophy, hypertrophic
 adenofibromatous, prostate — *see* Enlargement, enlarged, prostate
 adenoids (infective) J35.2
  with tonsils J35.3
 adrenal cortex E27.8
 alveolar process or ridge — *see* Anomaly, alveolar
 anal papillae K62.89
 artery I77.89
  congenital NEC Q27.8
   digestive system Q27.8
   lower limb Q27.8
   specified site NEC Q27.8
   upper limb Q27.8
 auricular — *see* Hypertrophy, cardiac
 Bartholin's gland N75.8
 bile duct (common) (hepatic) K83.8
 bladder (sphincter) (trigone) N32.89
 bone M89.30
  carpus M89.34-
  clavicle M89.31-
  femur M89.35-
  fibula M89.36-
  finger M89.34-
  humerus M89.32-
  ilium M89.359
  ischium M89.359
  metacarpus M89.34-
  metatarsus M89.37-
  multiple sites M89.39
  neck M89.38
  radius M89.33-
  rib M89.38
  scapula M89.31-
  skull M89.38
  tarsus M89.37-
  tibia M89.36-
  toe M89.37-
  ulna M89.33-
  vertebra M89.38
 brain G93.89
 breast N62
  cystic — *see* Mastopathy, cystic
  newborn P83.4
  pubertal, massive N62
  puerperal, postpartum — *see* Disorder, breast, specified type NEC
  senile (parenchymatous) N62

Hypertrophy, hypertrophic - *continued*
 cardiac (chronic) (idiopathic) I51.7
  with rheumatic fever (conditions in I00)
   active I01.8
   inactive or quiescent (with chorea) I09.89
  congenital NEC Q24.8
  fatty — *see* Degeneration, myocardial
  hypertensive — *see* Hypertension, heart
  rheumatic (with chorea) I09.89
   active or acute I01.8
    with chorea I02.0
  valve — *see* Endocarditis
 cartilage — *see* Disorder, cartilage, specified type NEC
 cecum — *see* Megacolon
 cervix (uteri) N88.8
  congenital Q51.828
  elongation N88.4
 clitoris (cirrhotic) N90.89
  congenital Q52.6
 colon — *see also* Megacolon
  congenital Q43.2
 conjunctiva, lymphoid H11.89
 corpora cavernosa N48.89
 cystic duct K82.8
 duodenum K31.89
 endometrium (glandular) — *see also* Hyperplasia, endometrial N85.00-
  cervix N88.8
 epididymis N50.89
 esophageal hiatus (congenital) Q79.1
  with hernia — *see* Hernia, hiatal
 eyelid — *see* Disorder, eyelid, specified type NEC
 fat pad E65
  knee (infrapatellar) (popliteal) (prepatellar) (retropatellar) M79.4
 foot (congenital) Q74.2
 frenulum, frenum (tongue) K14.8
  lip K13.0
 gallbladder K82.8
 gastric mucosa K29.60
  with bleeding K29.61
 gland, glandular R59.9
  generalized R59.1
  localized R59.0
 gum (mucous membrane) K06.1
 heart (idiopathic) — *see also* Hypertrophy, cardiac
  valve — *see also* Endocarditis I38
 hemifacial Q67.4
 hepatic — *see* Hypertrophy, liver
 hiatus (esophageal) Q79.1
 hilus gland R59.0
 hymen, congenital Q52.4
 ileum K63.89
 intestine NEC K63.89
 jejunum K63.89
 kidney (compensatory) N28.81
  congenital Q63.3
 labium (majus) (minus) N90.60
 ligament — *see* Disorder, ligament
 lingual tonsil (infective) J35.1
  with adenoids J35.3
 lip K13.0
  congenital Q18.6
 liver R16.0
  acute K76.89
  congenital Q44.7
  cirrhotic — *see* Cirrhosis, liver
  fatty — *see* Fatty, liver
 lymph, lymphatic gland R59.9
  generalized R59.1
  localized R59.0
  tuberculous — *see* Tuberculosis, lymph gland
 mammary gland — *see* Hypertrophy, breast
 Meckel's diverticulum (congenital) Q43.0
  malignant — *see* Table of Neoplasms, small intestine, malignant
 median bar — *see* Hyperplasia, prostate
 meibomian gland — *see* Chalazion
 meniscus, knee, congenital Q74.1

Hypertrophy, hypertrophic - *continued*
 metatarsal head — *see* Hypertrophy, bone, metatarsus
 metatarsus — *see* Hypertrophy, bone, metatarsus
 mucous membrane
  alveolar ridge K06.2
  gum K06.1
  nose (turbinate) J34.3
 muscle M62.89
 muscular coat, artery I77.89
 myocardium — *see also* Hypertrophy, cardiac
  idiopathic I42.2
 myometrium N85.2
 nail L60.2
  congenital Q84.5
 nasal J34.89
  alae J34.89
  bone J34.89
  cartilage J34.89
  mucous membrane (septum) J34.3
  sinus J34.89
  turbinate J34.3
 nasopharynx, lymphoid (infectional) (tissue) (wall) J35.2
 nipple N62
 organ or site, congenital NEC — *see* Anomaly, by site
 ovary N83.8
 palate (hard) M27.8
  soft K13.79
 pancreas, congenital Q45.3
 parathyroid (gland) E21.0
 parotid gland K11.1
 penis N48.89
 pharyngeal tonsil J35.2
 pharynx J39.2
  lymphoid (infectional) (tissue) (wall) J35.2
 pituitary (anterior) (fossa) (gland) E23.6
 prepuce (congenital) N47.8
  female N90.89
 prostate — *see* Enlargement, enlarged, prostate
  congenital Q55.4
 pseudomuscular G71.09
 pylorus (adult) (muscle) (sphincter) K31.1
  congenital or infantile Q40.0
 rectal, rectum (sphincter) K62.89
 rhinitis (turbinate) J31.0
 salivary gland (any) K11.1
  congenital Q38.4
 scaphoid (tarsal) — *see* Hypertrophy, bone, tarsus
 scar L91.0
 scrotum N50.89
 seminal vesicle N50.89
 sigmoid — *see* Megacolon
 skin L91.9
  specified NEC L91.8
 spermatic cord N50.89
 spleen — *see* Splenomegaly
 spondylitis — *see* Spondylosis
 stomach K31.89
 sublingual gland K11.1
 submandibular gland K11.1
 suprarenal cortex (gland) E27.8
 synovial NEC M67.20
  acromioclavicular M67.21-
  ankle M67.27-
  elbow M67.22-
  foot M67.27-
  hand M67.24-
  hip M67.25-
  knee M67.26-
  multiple sites M67.29
  specified site NEC M67.28
  wrist M67.23-
 tendon — *see* Disorder, tendon, specified type NEC
 testis N44.8
  congenital Q55.29
 thymic, thymus (gland) (congenital) E32.0
 thyroid (gland) — *see* Goiter
 toe (congenital) Q74.2

Hypertrophy, hypertrophic - *continued*
  toe (congenital) - *continued*
    acquired — *see also* Deformity, toe,
      specified NEC
  tongue K14.8
    congenital Q38.2
    papillae (foliate) K14.3
  tonsils (faucial) (infective) (lingual)
    (lymphoid) J35.1
    with adenoids J35.3
  tunica vaginalis N50.89
  ureter N28.89
  urethra N36.8
  uterus N85.2
    neck (with elongation) N88.4
    puerperal O90.89
  uvula K13.79
  vagina N89.8
  vas deferens N50.89
  vein I87.8
  ventricle, ventricular (heart) — *see also*
    Hypertrophy, cardiac
    congenital Q24.8
    in tetralogy of Fallot Q21.3
  verumontanum N36.8
  vocal cord J38.3
  vulva N90.60
    stasis (nonfilarial) N90.69
Hypertropia H50.2-
Hypertyrosinemia E70.21
Hyperuricemia (asymptomatic) E79.0
Hyperuricosuria R82.993
Hypervalinemia E71.19
Hyperventilation (tetany) R06.4
  hysterical F45.8
  psychogenic F45.8
  syndrome F45.8
Hypervitaminosis (dietary) NEC E67.8
  A E67.0
    administered as drug (prolonged
      intake) — *see* Table of Drugs and
      Chemicals, vitamins, adverse effect
    overdose or wrong substance given or
      taken — *see* Table of Drugs and
      Chemicals, vitamins, poisoning
  B6 E67.2
  D E67.3
    administered as drug (prolonged
      intake) — *see* Table of Drugs and
      Chemicals, vitamins, adverse effect
    overdose or wrong substance given or
      taken — *see* Table of Drugs and
      Chemicals, vitamins, poisoning
  K E67.8
    administered as drug (prolonged
      intake) — *see* Table of Drugs and
      Chemicals, vitamins, adverse effect
    overdose or wrong substance given or
      taken — *see* Table of Drugs and
      Chemicals, vitamins, poisoning
Hypervolemia E87.70
  specified NEC E87.79
Hypesthesia R20.1
  cornea — *see* Anesthesia, cornea
Hyphema H21.0-
  traumatic S05.1-
Hypoacidity, gastric K31.89
  psychogenic F45.8
Hypoadrenalism, hypoadrenia E27.40
  primary E27.1
  tuberculous A18.7
Hypoadrenocorticism E27.40
  pituitary E23.0
  primary E27.1
Hypoalbuminemia E88.09
Hypoaldosteronism E27.40
Hypoalphalipoproteinemia E78.6
Hypobarism T70.29
Hypobaropathy T70.29
Hypobetalipoproteinemia (familial) E78.6
Hypocalcemia E83.51
  dietary E58
  neonatal P71.1
    due to cow's milk P71.0
    phosphate-loading (newborn) P71.1

Hypochloremia E87.8
Hypochlorhydria K31.89
  neurotic F45.8
  psychogenic F45.8
Hypochondria, hypochondriac,
  hypochondriasis (reaction) F45.21
  sleep F51.03
Hypochondrogenesis Q77.0
Hypochondroplasia Q77.4
Hypochromasia, blood cells D50.8
Hypocitraturia R82.991
Hypodontia — *see* Anodontia
Hypoeosinophilia D72.89
Hypoesthesia R20.1
Hypofibrinogenemia D68.8
  acquired D65
  congenital (hereditary) D68.2
Hypofunction
  adrenocortical E27.40
    drug-induced E27.3
    postprocedural E89.6
    primary E27.1
  adrenomedullary, postprocedural E89.6
  cerebral R29.818
  corticoadrenal NEC E27.40
  intestinal K59.8
  labyrinth — *see* subcategory H83.2
  ovary E28.39
  pituitary (gland) (anterior) E23.0
  testicular E29.1
    postprocedural (postsurgical)
      (postirradiation) (iatrogenic) E89.5
Hypogalactia O92.4
Hypogammaglobulinemia — *see also*
  Agammaglobulinemia D80.1
  hereditary D80.0
  nonfamilial D80.1
  transient, of infancy D80.7
Hypogenitalism (congenital) — *see*
  Hypogonadism
Hypoglossia Q38.3
Hypoglycemia (spontaneous) E16.2
  coma E15
    diabetic — *see* Diabetes, by type, with
      hypoglycemia, with coma
  diabetic — *see* Diabetes, hypoglycemia
  dietary counseling and surveillance Z71.3
  drug-induced E16.0
    with coma (nondiabetic) E15
  due to insulin E16.0
    with coma (nondiabetic) E15
    therapeutic misadventure — *see*
      subcategory T38.3
  functional, nonhyperinsulinemic E16.1
  iatrogenic E16.0
    with coma (nondiabetic) E15
  in infant of diabetic mother P70.1
    gestational diabetes P70.0
  infantile E16.1
  leucine-induced E71.19
  neonatal (transitory) P70.4
    iatrogenic P70.3
  reactive (not drug-induced) E16.1
  transitory neonatal P70.4
Hypogonadism
  female E28.39
  hypogonadotropic E23.0
  male E29.1
  ovarian (primary) E28.39
  pituitary E23.0
  testicular (primary) E29.1
Hypohidrosis, hypoidrosis L74.4
Hypoinsulinemia, postprocedural E89.1
Hypokalemia E87.6
Hypoleukocytosis — *see* Agranulocytosis
Hypolipoproteinemia (alpha) (beta) E78.6
Hypomagnesemia E83.42
  neonatal P71.2
Hypomania, hypomanic reaction F30.8
Hypomenorrhea — *see* Oligomenorrhea
Hypometabolism R63.8
Hypomotility
  gastrointestinal (tract) K31.89
    psychogenic F45.8
  intestine K59.8

Hypomotility - *continued*
  intestine - *continued*
    psychogenic F45.8
  stomach K31.89
    psychogenic F45.8
Hyponasality R49.22
Hyponatremia E87.1
Hypo-osmolality E87.1
Hypo-ovarianism, hypo-ovarism E28.39
Hypoparathyroidism E20.9
  familial E20.8
  idiopathic E20.0
  neonatal, transitory P71.4
  postprocedural E89.2
  specified NEC E20.8
Hypoperfusion (in)
  newborn P96.89
Hypopharyngitis — *see* Laryngopharyngitis
Hypophoria H50.53
Hypophosphatemia, hypophosphatasia
  (acquired) (congenital) (renal) E83.39
  familial E83.31
Hypophyseal, hypophysis — *see also*
  condition
  dwarfism E23.0
  gigantism E22.0
Hypopiesis — *see* Hypotension
Hypopinealism E34.8
Hypopituitarism (juvenile) E23.0
  drug-induced E23.1
  due to
    hypophysectomy E89.3
    radiotherapy E89.3
  iatrogenic NEC E23.1
  postirradiation E89.3
  postpartum O99.285
  postprocedural E89.3
Hypoplasia, hypoplastic
  adrenal (gland) , congenital Q89.1
  alimentary tract, congenital Q45.8
    upper Q40.8
  anus, anal (canal) Q42.3
    with fistula Q42.2
  aorta, aortic Q25.42
    ascending, in hypoplastic left heart
      syndrome Q23.4
    valve Q23.1
      in hypoplastic left heart syndrome Q23.4
  areola, congenital Q83.8
  arm (congenital) — *see* Defect, reduction,
    upper limb
  artery (peripheral) Q27.8
    brain (congenital) Q28.3
    coronary Q24.5
    digestive system Q27.8
    lower limb Q27.8
    pulmonary Q25.79
      functional, unilateral J43.0
    retinal (congenital) Q14.1
    specified site NEC Q27.8
    umbilical Q27.0
    upper limb Q27.8
  auditory canal Q17.8
    causing impairment of hearing Q16.9
  biliary duct or passage Q44.5
  bone NOS Q79.9
    face Q75.8
    marrow D61.9
      megakaryocytic D69.49
    skull — *see* Hypoplasia, skull
  brain Q02
    gyri Q04.3
    part of Q04.3
  breast (areola) N64.82
  bronchus Q32.4
  cardiac Q24.8
  carpus — *see* Defect, reduction, upper limb,
    specified type NEC
  cartilage hair Q78.8
  cecum Q42.8
  cementum K00.4
  cephalic Q02
  cerebellum Q04.3
  cervix (uteri) , congenital Q51.821
  clavicle (congenital) Q74.0

Hypoplasia, hypoplastic - *continued*
coccyx Q76.49
colon Q42.9
  specified NEC Q42.8
corpus callosum Q04.0
cricoid cartilage Q31.2
digestive organ (s) or tract NEC Q45.8
  upper (congenital) Q40.8
ear (auricle) (lobe) Q17.2
  middle Q16.4
enamel of teeth (neonatal) (postnatal)
  (prenatal) K00.4
endocrine (gland) NEC Q89.2
endometrium N85.8
epididymis (congenital) Q55.4
epiglottis Q31.2
erythroid, congenital D61.01
esophagus (congenital) Q39.8
eustachian tube Q17.8
eye Q11.2
eyelid (congenital) Q10.3
face Q18.8
  bone (s) Q75.8
femur (congenital) — *see* Defect, reduction,
  lower limb, specified type NEC
fibula (congenital) — *see* Defect, reduction,
  lower limb, specified type NEC
finger (congenital) — *see* Defect, reduction,
  upper limb, specified type NEC
focal dermal Q82.8
foot — *see* Defect, reduction, lower limb,
  specified type NEC
gallbladder Q44.0
genitalia, genital organ (s)
  female, congenital Q52.8
   external Q52.79
   internal NEC Q52.8
  in adiposogenital dystrophy E23.6
glottis Q31.2
hair Q84.2
hand (congenital) — *see* Defect, reduction,
  upper limb, specified type NEC
heart Q24.8
humerus (congenital) — *see* Defect,
  reduction, upper limb, specified type
  NEC
intestine (small) Q41.9
  large Q42.9
   specified NEC Q42.8
jaw M26.09
  alveolar M26.79
  lower M26.04
   alveolar M26.74
  upper M26.02
   alveolar M26.73
kidney (s) Q60.5
  bilateral Q60.4
  unilateral Q60.3
labium (majus) (minus) , congenital Q52.79
larynx Q31.2
left heart syndrome Q23.4
leg (congenital) — *see* Defect, reduction,
  lower limb
limb Q73.8
  lower (congenital) — *see* Defect,
   reduction, lower limb
  upper (congenital) — *see* Defect,
   reduction, upper limb
liver Q44.7
lung (lobe) (not associated with short
  gestation) Q33.6
  associated with immaturity, low birth
   weight, prematurity, or short
   gestation P28.0
mammary (areola) , congenital Q83.8
mandible, mandibular M26.04
  alveolar M26.74
  unilateral condylar M27.8
maxillary M26.02
  alveolar M26.73
medullary D61.9
megakaryocytic D69.49
metacarpus — *see* Defect, reduction, upper
  limb, specified type NEC

Hypoplasia, hypoplastic - *continued*
metatarsus — *see* Defect, reduction, lower
  limb, specified type NEC
muscle Q79.8
nail (s) Q84.6
nose, nasal Q30.1
optic nerve H47.03-
osseous meatus (ear) Q17.8
ovary, congenital Q50.39
pancreas Q45.0
parathyroid (gland) Q89.2
parotid gland Q38.4
patella Q74.1
pelvis, pelvic girdle Q74.2
penis (congenital) Q55.62
peripheral vascular system Q27.8
  digestive system Q27.8
  lower limb Q27.8
  specified site NEC Q27.8
  upper limb Q27.8
pituitary (gland) (congenital) Q89.2
pulmonary (not associated with short
  gestation) Q33.6
  artery, functional J43.0
  associated with short gestation P28.0
radioulnar — *see* Defect, reduction, upper
  limb, specified type NEC
radius — *see* Defect, reduction, upper limb
rectum Q42.1
  with fistula Q42.0
respiratory system NEC Q34.8
rib Q76.6
right heart syndrome Q22.6
sacrum Q76.49
scapula Q74.0
scrotum Q55.1
shoulder girdle Q74.0
skin Q82.8
skull (bone) Q75.8
  with
   anencephaly Q00.0
   encephalocele — *see* Encephalocele
   hydrocephalus Q03.9
    with spina bifida — *see* Spina bifida,
    by site, with hydrocephalus
   microcephaly Q02
spinal (cord) (ventral horn cell) Q06.1
spine Q76.49
sternum Q76.7
tarsus — *see* Defect, reduction, lower limb,
  specified type NEC
testis Q55.1
thymic, with immunodeficiency D82.1
thymus (gland) Q89.2
  with immunodeficiency D82.1
thyroid (gland) E03.1
  cartilage Q31.2
tibiofibular (congenital) — *see* Defect,
  reduction, lower limb, specified type
  NEC
toe — *see* Defect, reduction, lower limb,
  specified type NEC
tongue Q38.3
Turner's K00.4
ulna (congenital) — *see* Defect, reduction,
  upper limb
umbilical artery Q27.0
unilateral condylar M27.8
ureter Q62.8
uterus, congenital Q51.811
vagina Q52.4
vascular NEC peripheral Q27.8
  brain Q28.3
  digestive system Q27.8
  lower limb Q27.8
  specified site NEC Q27.8
  upper limb Q27.8
vein (s) (peripheral) Q27.8
  brain Q28.3
  digestive system Q27.8
  great Q26.8
  lower limb Q27.8
  specified site NEC Q27.8
  upper limb Q27.8
vena cava (inferior) (superior) Q26.8

Hypoplasia, hypoplastic - *continued*
vertebra Q76.49
vulva, congenital Q52.79
zonule (ciliary) Q12.8
Hypoplasminogenemia E88.02
Hypopnea, obstructive sleep apnea G47.33
Hypopotassemia E87.6
**Hypoproconvertinemia, congenital
  (hereditary)** D68.2
Hypoproteinemia E77.8
**Hypoprothrombinemia (congenital)
  (hereditary) (idiopathic)** D68.2
  acquired D68.4
  newborn, transient P61.6
Hypoptyalism K11.7
Hypopyon (eye) (anterior chamber) — *see*
  Iridocyclitis, acute, hypopyon
Hypopyrexia R68.0
Hyporeflexia R29.2
Hyposecretion
  ACTH E23.0
  antidiuretic hormone E23.2
  ovary E28.39
  salivary gland (any) K11.7
  vasopressin E23.2
**Hyposegmentation, leukocytic,
  hereditary** D72.0
Hyposiderinemia D50.9
Hypospadias Q54.9
  balanic Q54.0
  coronal Q54.0
  glandular Q54.0
  penile Q54.1
  penoscrotal Q54.2
  perineal Q54.3
  specified NEC Q54.8
Hypospermatogenesis — *see* Oligospermia
Hyposplenism D73.0
Hypostasis pulmonary, passive — *see* Edema,
  lung
Hypostatic — *see* condition
Hyposthenuria N28.89
Hypotension (arterial) (constitutional) I95.9
  chronic I95.89
  due to (of) hemodialysis I95.3
  drug-induced I95.2
  iatrogenic I95.89
  idiopathic (permanent) I95.0
  intracranial, following ventricular shunting
   (ventriculostomy) G97.2
  intra-dialytic I95.3
  maternal, syndrome (following labor and
   delivery) O26.5-
  neurogenic, orthostatic G90.3
  orthostatic (chronic) I95.1
   due to drugs I95.2
   neurogenic G90.3
  postoperative I95.81
  postural I95.1
  specified NEC I95.89
Hypothermia (accidental) T68
  due to anesthesia, anesthetic T88.51
  low environmental temperature T68
  neonatal P80.9
   environmental (mild) NEC P80.8
   mild P80.8
   severe (chronic) (cold injury
    syndrome) P80.0
   specified NEC P80.8
  not associated with low environmental
   temperature R68.0
Hypothyroidism (acquired) E03.9
  autoimmune — *see* Thyroiditis, autoimmune
  congenital (without goiter) E03.1
   with goiter (diffuse) E03.0
  due to
   exogenous substance NEC E03.2
   iodine-deficiency, acquired E01.8
    subclinical E02
   irradiation therapy E89.0
   medicament NEC E03.2
   P-aminosalicylic acid (PAS) E03.2
   phenylbutazone E03.2
   resorcinol E03.2
   sulfonamide E03.2

Hypothyroidism (acquired) - *continued*
  due to - *continued*
    surgery E89.0
    thiourea group drugs E03.2
  iatrogenic NEC E03.2
  iodine-deficiency (acquired) E01.8
    congenital — *see* Syndrome, iodine-deficiency, congenital
    subclinical E02
  neonatal, transitory P72.2
  postinfectious E03.3
  postirradiation E89.0
  postprocedural E89.0
  postsurgical E89.0
  specified NEC E03.8
  subclinical, iodine-deficiency related E02
Hypotonia, hypotonicity, hypotony
  bladder N31.2
  congenital (benign) P94.2
  eye — *see* Disorder, globe, hypotony
Hypotrichosis — *see* Alopecia
Hypotropia H50.2-
Hypoventilation R06.89
  congenital central alveolar G47.35
  sleep related
    idiopathic nonobstructive alveolar G47.34
    in conditions classified elsewhere G47.36
Hypovitaminosis — *see* Deficiency, vitamin
Hypovolemia E86.1
  surgical shock T81.19
  traumatic (shock) T79.4
Hypoxemia R09.02
  newborn P84
  sleep related, in conditions classified elsewhere G47.36
Hypoxia — *see also* Anoxia R09.02
  cerebral, during a procedure NEC G97.81
    postprocedural NEC G97.82
  intrauterine P84
  myocardial — *see* Insufficiency, coronary
  newborn P84
  sleep-related G47.34
Hypsarhythmia — *see* Epilepsy, generalized, specified NEC
Hysteralgia, pregnant uterus O26.89-
Hysteria, hysterical (conversion) (dissociative state) F44.9
  anxiety F41.8
  convulsions F44.5
  psychosis, acute F44.9
Hysteroepilepsy F44.5

I

I.Q.
  under 20 F73
  20-34 F72
  35-49 F71
  50-69 F70
IBDU (colonic inflammatory bowel dissease unclassified) K52.3
Ichthyoparasitism due to Vandellia cirrhosa B88.8
Ichthyosis (congenital) Q80.9
  acquired L85.0
  fetalis Q80.4
  hystrix Q80.8
  lamellar Q80.2
  lingual K13.29
  palmaris and plantaris Q82.8
  simplex Q80.0
  vera Q80.8
  vulgaris Q80.0
  X-linked Q80.1
Ichthyotoxism — *see* Poisoning, fish
  bacterial — *see* Intoxication, foodborne
Icteroanemia, hemolytic (acquired) D59.9
  congenital — *see* Spherocytosis
Icterus — *see also* Jaundice
  conjunctiva R17
  newborn P59.9
  gravis, newborn P55.0
  hematogenous (acquired) D59.9
  hemolytic (acquired) D59.9
    congenital — *see* Spherocytosis
  hemorrhagic (acute) (leptospiral) (spirochetal) A27.0

Icterus - *continued*
  hemorrhagic (acute) (leptospiral) (spirochetal) - *continued*
    newborn P53
  infectious B15.9
    with hepatic coma B15.0
    leptospiral A27.0
    spirochetal A27.0
  neonatorum — *see* Jaundice, newborn
  spirochetal A27.0
Ictus solaris, solis T67.01
Id reaction (due to bacteria) L30.2
Ideation
  homicidal R45.850
  suicidal R45.851
Identity disorder (child) F64.9
  gender role F64.2
  psychosexual F64.2
Idioglossia F80.0
Idiopathic — *see* condition
Idiot, idiocy (congenital) F73
  amaurotic (Bielschowsky (-Jansky)) (family) (infantile (late)) (juvenile (late)) (Vogt-Spielmeyer) E75.4
  microcephalic Q02
IgE asthma J45.909
IIAC (idiopathic infantile arterial calcification) Q28.8
Ileitis (chronic) (noninfectious) — *see also* Enteritis K52.9
  backwash — *see* Pancolitis, ulcerative (chronic)
  infectious A09
  regional (ulcerative) — *see* Enteritis, regional, small intestine
  segmental — *see* Enteritis, regional
  terminal (ulcerative) — *see* Enteritis, regional, small intestine
Ileocolitis — *see also* Enteritis K52.9
  infectious A09
  regional — *see* Enteritis, regional
  ulcerative K51.0-
Ileostomy
  attention to Z43.2
  malfunctioning K94.13
  status Z93.2
    with complication — *see* Complications, enterostomy
Ileotyphus — *see* Typhoid
Ileum — *see* condition
Ileus (bowel) (colon) (inhibitory) (intestine) K56.7
  adynamic K56.0
  due to gallstone (in intestine) K56.3
  duodenal (chronic) K31.5
  gallstone K56.3
  mechanical NEC — *see also* Obstruction, intestine, specified NEC K56.699
  meconium P76.0
    in cystic fibrosis E84.11
    meaning meconium plug (without cystic fibrosis) P76.0
  myxedema K59.8
  neurogenic K56.0
    Hirschsprung's disease or megacolon Q43.1
  newborn
    due to meconium P76.0
      in cystic fibrosis E84.11
      meaning meconium plug (without cystic fibrosis) P76.0
    transitory P76.1
  obstructive — *see also* Obstruction, intestine, specified NEC K56.699
  paralytic K56.0
  postoperative K91.89
Iliac — *see* condition
Iliotibial band syndrome M76.3-
Illiteracy Z55.0
Illness — *see also* Disease R69
  manic-depressive — *see* Disorder, bipolar
Imbalance R26.89
  autonomic G90.8
  constituents of food intake E63.1
  electrolyte E87.8

Imbalance - *continued*
  electrolyte - *continued*
    with
      abortion — *see* Abortion by type, complicated by, electrolyte imbalance
      molar pregnancy O08.5
    due to hyperemesis gravidarum O21.1
    following ectopic or molar pregnancy O08.5
    neonatal, transitory NEC P74.49
      potassium
        hyperkalemia P74.31
        hypokalemia P74.32
      sodium
        hypernatremia P74.21
        hyponatremia P74.22
  endocrine E34.9
  eye muscle NOS H50.9
  hormone E34.9
  hysterical F44.4
  labyrinth — *see* subcategory H83.2
  posture R29.3
  protein-energy — *see* Malnutrition
  sympathetic G90.8
Imbecile, imbecility (I.Q.35-49) F71
Imbedding, intrauterine device T83.39
Imbibition, cholesterol (gallbladder) K82.4
Imbrication, teeth,, fully erupted M26.30
Imerslund (-Gräsbeck) syndrome D51.1
Immature — *see also* Immaturity
  birth (less than 37 completed weeks) — *see* Preterm, newborn
  extremely (less than 28 completed weeks) — *see* Immaturity, extreme
  personality F60.89
Immaturity (less than 37 completed weeks) — *see also* Preterm, newborn
  extreme of newborn (less than 28 completed weeks of gestation) (less than 196 completed days of gestation) (unspecified weeks of gestation) P07.20
    gestational age
      23 completed weeks (23 weeks, 0 days through 23 weeks, 6 days) P07.22
      24 completed weeks (24 weeks, 0 days through 24 weeks, 6 days) P07.23
      25 completed weeks (25 weeks, 0 days through 25 weeks, 6 days) P07.24
      26 completed weeks (26 weeks, 0 days through 26 weeks, 6 days) P07.25
      27 completed weeks (27 weeks, 0 days through 27 weeks, 6 days) P07.26
      less than 23 completed weeks P07.21
  fetus or infant light-for-dates — *see* Light-for-dates
  lung, newborn P28.0
  organ or site NEC — *see* Hypoplasia
  pulmonary, newborn P28.0
  reaction F60.89
  sexual (female) (male) , after puberty E30.0
Immersion T75.1
  hand T69.01-
  foot T69.02-
Immobile, immobility
  complete, due to severe physical disability or frailty R53.2
  intestine K59.8
  syndrome (paraplegic) M62.3
Immune reconstitution (inflammatory) syndrome [IRIS] D89.3
Immunization — *see also* Vaccination
  ABO — *see* Incompatibility, ABO
    in newborn P55.1
  appropriate for age
    child (over 28 days old) Z00.129
      with abnormal findings Z00.121
  complication — *see* Complications, vaccination
  encounter for Z23
  not done (not carried out) Z28.9
    because (of)
      acute illness of patient Z28.01
      allergy to vaccine (or component) Z28.04

Immunization - *continued*
  not done (not carried out) - *continued*
    because (of) - *continued*
      caregiver refusal Z28.82
      chronic illness of patient Z28.02
      contraindication NEC Z28.09
      delay in delivery of vaccine Z28.83
      group pressure Z28.1
      guardian refusal Z28.82
      immune compromised state of
        patient Z28.03
      lack of availability of vaccine Z28.83
      manufacturer delay of vaccine Z28.83
      parent refusal Z28.82
      patient's belief Z28.1
      patient had disease being vaccinated
        against Z28.81
      patient refusal Z28.21
      religious beliefs of patient Z28.1
      specified reason NEC Z28.89
        of patient Z28.29
      unavailability of vaccine Z28.83
      unspecified patient reason Z28.20
  Rh factor
    affecting management of pregnancy
      NEC O36.09-
    anti-D antibody O36.01-
    from transfusion — *see* Complication(s),
      transfusion, incompatibility reaction,
      Rh (factor)
Immunocytoma C83.0-
Immunodeficiency D84.9
  with
    adenosine-deaminase deficiency — *see
      also* Deficiency, adenosine
      deaminase D81.30
    antibody defects D80.9
      specified type NEC D80.8
    hyperimmunoglobulinemia D80.6
    increased immunoglobulin M (IgM) D80.5
    major defect D82.9
      specified type NEC D82.8
    partial albinism D82.8
    short-limbed stature D82.2
    thrombocytopenia and eczema D82.0
  antibody with
    hyperimmunoglobulinemia D80.6
    near-normal immunoglobulins D80.6
  autosomal recessive, Swiss type D80.0
  combined D81.9
    biotin-dependent carboxylase D81.819
      biotinidase D81.810
      holocarboxylase synthetase D81.818
      specified type NEC D81.818
    severe (SCID) D81.9
      with
        low or normal B-cell numbers D81.2
        low T- and B-cell numbers D81.1
        reticular dysgenesis D81.0
    specified type NEC D81.89
  common variable D83.9
    with
      abnormalities of B-cell numbers and
        function D83.0
      autoantibodies to B- or T-cells D83.2
      immunoregulatory T-cell
        disorders D83.1
      specified type NEC D83.8
  following hereditary defective response to
    Epstein-Barr virus (EBV) D82.3
  selective, immunoglobulin
    A (IgA) D80.2
    G (IgG) (subclasses) D80.3
    M (IgM) D80.4
  severe combined (SCID) D81.9
    due to adenosine deaminase
      deficiency D81.31
  specified type NEC D84.8
  X-linked, with increased IgM D80.5
Immunotherapy (encounter for)
  antineoplastic Z51.12
Impaction, impacted
  bowel, colon, rectum — *see also* Impaction,
    fecal K56.49
    by gallstone K56.3

Impaction, impacted - *continued*
  calculus — *see* Calculus
  cerumen (ear) (external) H61.2-
  cuspid — *see* Impaction, tooth
  dental (same or adjacent tooth) K01.1
  fecal, feces K56.41
  fracture — *see* Fracture, by site
  gallbladder — *see* Calculus, gallbladder
  gallstone (s) — *see* Calculus, gallbladder
    bile duct (common) (hepatic) — *see*
      Calculus, bile duct
    cystic duct — *see* Calculus, gallbladder
    in intestine, with obstruction (any
      part) K56.3
  intestine (calculous) NEC — *see also*
    Impaction, fecal K56.49
    gallstone, with ileus K56.3
  intrauterine device (IUD) T83.39
  molar — *see* Impaction, tooth
  shoulder, causing obstructed labor O66.0
  tooth, teeth K01.1
  turbinate J34.89
Impaired, impairment (function)
  auditory discrimination — *see* Abnormal,
    auditory perception
  cognitive, mild, so stated G31.84
  dual sensory Z73.82
  fasting glucose R73.01
  glucose tolerance (oral) R73.02
  hearing — *see* Deafness
  heart — *see* Disease, heart
  kidney N28.9
    disorder resulting from N25.9
      specified NEC N25.89
  liver K72.90
    with coma K72.91
  mastication K08.89
  mild cognitive, so stated G31.84
  mobility
    ear ossicles — *see* Ankylosis, ear ossicles
    requiring care provider Z74.09
  myocardium, myocardial — *see*
    Insufficiency, myocardial
  rectal sphincter R19.8
  renal (acute) (chronic) N28.9
    disorder resulting from N25.9
      specified NEC N25.89
  vision NEC H54.7
    both eyes H54.3
Impediment, speech R47.9
  psychogenic (childhood) F98.8
  slurring R47.81
  specified NEC R47.89
Impending
  coronary syndrome I20.0
  delirium tremens F10.239
  myocardial infarction I20.0
Imperception auditory (acquired) — *see also*
  Deafness
  congenital H93.25
Imperfect
  aeration, lung (newborn) NEC — *see*
    Atelectasis
  closure (congenital)
    alimentary tract NEC Q45.8
      lower Q43.8
      upper Q40.8
    atrioventricular ostium Q21.2
    atrium (secundum) Q21.1
    branchial cleft NOS Q18.2
      cyst Q18.0
      fistula Q18.0
      sinus Q18.0
    choroid Q14.3
    cricoid cartilage Q31.8
    cusps, heart valve NEC Q24.8
      pulmonary Q22.3
    ductus
      arteriosus Q25.0
      Botalli Q25.0
    ear drum (causing impairment of
      hearing) Q16.4
    esophagus with communication to
      bronchus or trachea Q39.1
    eyelid Q10.3

Imperfect - *continued*
  closure (congenital) - *continued*
    foramen
      botalli Q21.1
      ovale Q21.1
    genitalia, genital organ (s) or system
      female Q52.8
        external Q52.79
        internal NEC Q52.8
      male Q55.8
    glottis Q31.8
    interatrial ostium or septum Q21.1
    interauricular ostium or septum Q21.1
    interventricular ostium or septum Q21.0
    larynx Q31.8
    lip — *see* Cleft, lip
    nasal septum Q30.3
    nose Q30.2
    omphalomesenteric duct Q43.0
    optic nerve entry Q14.2
    organ or site not listed — *see* Anomaly, by
      site
    ostium
      interatrial Q21.1
      interauricular Q21.1
      interventricular Q21.0
    palate — *see* Cleft, palate
    preauricular sinus Q18.1
    retina Q14.1
    roof of orbit Q75.8
    sclera Q13.5
    septum
      aorticopulmonary Q21.4
      atrial (secundum) Q21.1
      between aorta and pulmonary
        artery Q21.4
      heart Q21.9
      interatrial (secundum) Q21.1
      interauricular (secundum) Q21.1
      interventricular Q21.0
        in tetralogy of Fallot Q21.3
      nasal Q30.3
      ventricular Q21.0
        with pulmonary stenosis or atresia,
          dextraposition of aorta, and
          hypertrophy of right
          ventricle Q21.3
        in tetralogy of Fallot Q21.3
    skull Q75.0
      with
        anencephaly Q00.0
        encephalocele — *see* Encephalocele
        hydrocephalus Q03.9
          with spina bifida — *see* Spina
            bifida, by site, with
            hydrocephalus
        microcephaly Q02
    spine (with meningocele) — *see* Spina
      bifida
    trachea Q32.1
    tympanic membrane (causing impairment
      of hearing) Q16.4
    uterus Q51.818
    vitelline duct Q43.0
  erection — *see* Dysfunction, sexual, male,
    erectile
  fusion — *see* Imperfect, closure
  inflation, lung (newborn) — *see* Atelectasis
  posture R29.3
  rotation, intestine Q43.3
  septum, ventricular Q21.0
Imperfectly descended testis — *see*
  Cryptorchid
Imperforate (congenital) — *see also* Atresia
  anus Q42.3
    with fistula Q42.2
  cervix (uteri) Q51.828
  esophagus Q39.0
    with tracheoesophageal fistula Q39.1
  hymen Q52.3
  jejunum Q41.1
  pharynx Q38.8
  rectum Q42.1
    with fistula Q42.0
  urethra Q64.39

Imperforate (congenital) - *continued*
  vagina Q52.4
Impervious (congenital) — *see also* Atresia
  anus Q42.3
    with fistula Q42.2
  bile duct Q44.2
  esophagus Q39.0
    with tracheoesophageal fistula Q39.1
  intestine (small) Q41.9
    large Q42.9
      specified NEC Q42.8
  rectum Q42.1
    with fistula Q42.0
  ureter — *see* Atresia, ureter
  urethra Q64.39
Impetiginization of dermatoses L01.1
Impetigo (any organism) (any site)
    (circinate) (contagiosa) (simplex)
    (vulgaris) L01.00
  Bockhart's L01.02
  bullous, bullosa L01.03
  external ear L01.00 *[H62.40]*
  follicularis L01.02
  furfuracea L30.5
  herpetiformis L40.1
    nonobstetrical L40.1
  neonatorum L01.03
  nonbullous L01.01
  specified type NEC L01.09
  ulcerative L01.09
Impingement (on teeth)
  joint — *see* Disorder, joint, specified type
    NEC
  soft tissue
    anterior M26.81
    posterior M26.82
Implant, endometrial N80.9
Implantation
  anomalous — *see* Anomaly, by site
    ureter Q62.63
  cyst
    external area or site (skin) NEC L72.0
    iris — *see* Cyst, iris, implantation
    vagina N89.8
    vulva N90.7
  dermoid (cyst) — *see* Implantation, cyst
Impotence (sexual) N52.9
  counseling Z70.1
  organic origin — *see also* Dysfunction,
    sexual, male, erectile N52.9
  psychogenic F52.21
Impression, basilar Q75.8
Imprisonment, anxiety concerning Z65.1
Improper care (child) (newborn) — *see*
  Maltreatment
Improperly tied umbilical cord (causing
  hemorrhage) P51.8
Impulsiveness (impulsive) R45.87
Inability to swallow — *see* Aphagia
Inaccessible, inaccessibility
  health care NEC Z75.3
    due to
      waiting period Z75.2
        for admission to facility
          elsewhere Z75.1
    other helping agencies Z75.4
Inactive — *see* condition
Inadequate, inadequacy
  aesthetics of dental restoration K08.56
  biologic, constitutional, functional, or
    social F60.7
  development
    child R62.50
    genitalia
      after puberty NEC E30.0
      congenital
        female Q52.8
          external Q52.79
          internal Q52.8
        male Q55.8
    lungs Q33.6
      associated with short gestation P28.0
    organ or site not listed — *see* Anomaly, by
      site
  diet (causing nutritional deficiency) E63.9

Inadequate, inadequacy - *continued*
  eating habits Z72.4
  environment, household Z59.1
  family support Z63.8
  food (supply) NEC Z59.4
    hunger effects T73.0
  functional F60.7
  household care, due to
    family member
      handicapped or ill Z74.2
      on vacation Z75.5
      temporarily away from home Z74.2
    technical defects in home Z59.1
    temporary absence from home of person
      rendering care Z74.2
  housing (heating) (space) Z59.1
  income (financial) Z59.6
  intrafamilial communication Z63.8
  material resources Z59.9
  mental — *see* Disability, intellectual
  parental supervision or control of child Z62.0
  personality F60.7
  pulmonary
    function R06.89
      newborn P28.5
    ventilation, newborn P28.5
  sample of cytologic smear
    anus R85.615
    cervix R87.615
    vagina R87.625
  social F60.7
    insurance Z59.7
    skills NEC Z73.4
  supervision of child by parent Z62.0
  teaching affecting education Z55.8
  welfare support Z59.7
Inanition R64
  with edema — *see* Malnutrition, severe
  due to
    deprivation of food T73.0
    malnutrition — *see* Malnutrition
  fever R50.9
Inappropriate
  change in quantitative human chorionic
    gonadotropin (hCG) in early
    pregnancy O02.81
  diet or eating habits Z72.4
  level of quantitative human chorionic
    gonadotropin (hCG) for gestational age
    in early pregnancy O02.81
  secretion
    antidiuretic hormone (ADH)
      (excessive) E22.2
      deficiency E23.2
    pituitary (posterior) E22.2
Inattention at or after birth — *see* Neglect
Incarceration, incarcerated
  enterocele K46.0
    gangrenous K46.1
  epiplocele K46.0
    gangrenous K46.1
  exomphalos K42.0
    gangrenous K42.1
  hernia — *see also* Hernia, by site, with
    obstruction
    with gangrene — *see* Hernia, by site, with
      gangrene
  iris, in wound — *see* Injury, eye, laceration,
    with prolapse
  lens, in wound — *see* Injury, eye, laceration,
    with prolapse
  omphalocele K42.0
  prison, anxiety concerning Z65.1
  rupture — *see* Hernia, by site
  sarcoepiplocele K46.0
    gangrenous K46.1
  sarcoepiplomphalocele K42.0
    with gangrene K42.1
  uterus N85.8
    gravid O34.51-
      causing obstructed labor O65.5
Incised wound
  external — *see* Laceration
  internal organs — *see* Injury, by site

Incision, incisional
  hernia K43.2
    with
      gangrene (and obstruction) K43.1
      obstruction K43.0
  surgical, complication — *see* Complications,
    surgical procedure
  traumatic
    external — *see* Laceration
    internal organs — *see* Injury, by site
Inclusion
  azurophilic leukocytic D72.0
  blennorrhea (neonatal) (newborn) P39.1
  gallbladder in liver (congenital) Q44.1
Incompatibility
  ABO
    affecting management of
      pregnancy O36.11-
      anti-A sensitization O36.11-
      anti-B sensitization O36.19-
      specified NEC O36.19-
    infusion or transfusion reaction — *see*
      Complication(s), transfusion,
      incompatibility reaction, ABO
    newborn P55.1
  blood (group) (Duffy) (K) (Kell) (Kidd)
    (Lewis) (M) (S) NEC
    affecting management of
      pregnancy O36.11-
      anti-A sensitization O36.11-
      anti-B sensitization O36.19-
    infusion or transfusion reaction T80.89
    newborn P55.8
  divorce or estrangement Z63.5
  Rh (blood group) (factor) Z31.82
    affecting management of pregnancy
      NEC O36.09-
      anti-D antibody O36.01-
    infusion or transfusion reaction — *see*
      Complication(s), transfusion,
      incompatibility reaction, Rh (factor)
    newborn P55.0
  rhesus — *see* Incompatibility, Rh
Incompetency, incompetent, incompetence
  annular
    aortic (valve) — *see* Insufficiency, aortic
    mitral (valve) I34.0
    pulmonary valve (heart) I37.1
  aortic (valve) — *see* Insufficiency, aortic
  cardiac valve — *see* Endocarditis
  cervix, cervical (os) N88.3
    in pregnancy O34.3-
  chronotropic I45.89
    with
      autonomic dysfunction G90.8
      ischemic heart disease I25.89
      left ventricular dysfunction I51.89
      sinus node dysfunction I49.8
  esophagogastric (junction) (sphincter) K22.0
  mitral (valve) — *see* Insufficiency, mitral
  pelvic fundus N81.89
  pubocervical tissue N81.82
  pulmonary valve (heart) I37.1
    congenital Q22.3
  rectovaginal tissue N81.83
  tricuspid (annular) (valve) — *see*
    Insufficiency, tricuspid
  valvular — *see* Endocarditis
    congenital Q24.8
  vein, venous (saphenous) (varicose) — *see*
    Varix, leg
Incomplete — *see also* condition
  bladder, emptying R33.9
  defecation R15.0
  expansion lungs (newborn) NEC — *see*
    Atelectasis
  rotation, intestine Q43.3
Inconclusive
  diagnostic imaging due to excess body fat of
    patient R93.9
  findings on diagnostic imaging of breast
    NEC R92.8
  mammogram (due to dense breasts) R92.2
Incontinence R32
  anal sphincter R15.9

Incontinence - *continued*
coital N39.491
feces R15.9
nonorganic origin F98.1
insensible (urinary) N39.42
overflow N39.490
postural (urinary) N39.492
psychogenic F45.8
rectal R15.9
reflex N39.498
stress (female) (male) N39.3
and urge N39.46
urethral sphincter R32
urge N39.41
and stress (female) (male) N39.46
urine (urinary) R32
continuous N39.45
due to cognitive impairment, or severe
physical disability or
immobility R39.81
functional R39.81
insensible N39.42
mixed (stress and urge) N39.46
nocturnal N39.44
nonorganic origin F98.0
overflow N39.490
post dribbling N39.43
postural N39.492
reflex N39.498
specified NEC N39.498
stress (female) (male) N39.3
and urge N39.46
total N39.498
unaware N39.42
urge N39.41
and stress (female) (male) N39.46
Incontinentia pigmenti Q82.3
Incoordinate, incoordination
esophageal-pharyngeal (newborn) — *see*
Dysphagia
muscular R27.8
uterus (action) (contractions) (complicating
delivery) O62.4
Increase, increased
abnormal, in development R63.8
androgens (ovarian) E28.1
anticoagulants (antithrombin) (anti-VIIIa)
(anti-IXa) (anti-Xa) (anti-XIa) — *see*
Circulating anticoagulants
cold sense R20.8
estrogen E28.0
function
adrenal
cortex — *see* Cushing's, syndrome
medulla E27.5
pituitary (gland) (anterior) (lobe) E22.9
posterior E22.2
heat sense R20.8
intracranial pressure (benign) G93.2
permeability, capillaries I78.8
pressure, intracranial G93.2
secretion
gastrin E16.4
glucagon E16.3
pancreas, endocrine E16.9
growth hormone-releasing
hormone E16.8
pancreatic polypeptide E16.8
somatostatin E16.8
vasoactive-intestinal polypeptide E16.8
sphericity, lens Q12.4
splenic activity D73.1
venous pressure I87.8
portal K76.6
Increta placenta O43.22-
**Incrustation, cornea, foreign body (lead)
(zinc)** — *see* Foreign body, cornea
Incyclophoria H50.54
Incyclotropia — *see* Cyclotropia
Indeterminate sex Q56.4
India rubber skin Q82.8
Indigestion (acid) (bilious) (functional) K30
catarrhal K31.89
due to decomposed food NOS A05.9
nervous F45.8

Indigestion (acid) (bilious) (functional) -
continued
psychogenic F45.8
Indirect — *see* condition
Induratio penis plastica N48.6
Induration, indurated
brain G93.89
breast (fibrous) N64.51
puerperal, postpartum O92.29
broad ligament N83.8
chancre
anus A51.1
congenital A50.07
extragenital NEC A51.2
corpora cavernosa (penis) (plastic) N48.6
liver (chronic) K76.89
lung (black) (chronic) (fibroid) — *see also*
Fibrosis, lung J84.10
essential brown J84.03
penile (plastic) N48.6
phlebitic — *see* Phlebitis
skin R23.4
Inebriety (without dependence) — *see*
Alcohol, intoxication
Inefficiency, kidney N28.9
Inelasticity, skin R23.4
Inequality, leg (length) (acquired) — *see also*
Deformity, limb, unequal length
congenital — *see* Defect, reduction, lower
limb
lower leg — *see* Deformity, limb, unequal
length
Inertia
bladder (neurogenic) N31.2
stomach K31.89
psychogenic F45.8
uterus, uterine during labor O62.2
during latent phase of labor O62.0
primary O62.0
secondary O62.1
vesical (neurogenic) N31.2
Infancy, infantile, infantilism — *see also*
condition
celiac K90.0
genitalia, genitals (after puberty) E30.0
Herter's (nontropical sprue) K90.0
intestinal K90.0
Lorain E23.0
pancreatic K86.89
pelvis M95.5
with disproportion (fetopelvic) O33.1
causing obstructed labor O65.1
pituitary E23.0
renal N25.0
uterus — *see* Infantile, genitalia
Infant (s) — *see also* Infancy
excessive crying R68.11
irritable child R68.12
lack of care — *see* Neglect
liveborn (singleton) Z38.2
born in hospital Z38.00
by cesarean Z38.01
born outside hospital Z38.1
multiple NEC Z38.8
born in hospital Z38.68
by cesarean Z38.69
born outside hospital Z38.7
quadruplet Z38.8
born in hospital Z38.63
by cesarean Z38.64
born outside hospital Z38.7
quintuplet Z38.8
born in hospital Z38.65
by cesarean Z38.66
born outside hospital Z38.7
triplet Z38.8
born in hospital Z38.61
by cesarean Z38.62
born outside hospital Z38.7
twin Z38.5
born in hospital Z38.30
by cesarean Z38.31
born outside hospital Z38.4
of diabetic mother (syndrome of) P70.1
gestational diabetes P70.0

Infantile — *see also* condition
genitalia, genitals E30.0
os, uterine E30.0
penis E30.0
testis E29.1
uterus E30.0
Infantilism — *see* Infancy
Infarct, infarction
adrenal (capsule) (gland) E27.49
appendices epiploicae — *see also* Infarct,
intestine K55.069
bowel — *see also* Infarct, intestine K55.069
brain (stem) — *see* Infarct, cerebral
breast N64.89
brewer's (kidney) N28.0
cardiac — *see* Infarct, myocardium
cerebellar — *see* Infarct, cerebral
cerebral (acute) (chronic) — *see also*
Occlusion, artery cerebral or
precerebral, with infarction I63.9-
aborted I63.9
cortical I63.9
due to
cerebral venous thrombosis,
nonpyogenic I63.6
embolism
cerebral arteries I63.4-
precerebral arteries I63.1-
occlusion NEC
cerebral arteries I63.5-
precerebral arteries I63.2-
small artery I63.81
stenosis NEC
cerebral arteries I63.5-
precerebral arteries I63.2-
small artery I63.81
thrombosis
cerebral artery I63.3-
precerebral artery I63.0-
intraoperative
during cardiac surgery I97.810
during other surgery I97.811
postprocedural
following cardiac surgery I97.820
following other surgery I97.821
specified NEC I63.89
colon (acute) (agnogenic) (embolic)
(hemorrhagic) (nonocclusive)
(nonthrombotic) (occlusive) (segmental)
(thrombotic) (with gangrene) — *see
also* Infarct, intestine K55.049
coronary artery — *see* Infarct, myocardium
embolic — *see* Embolism
fallopian tube N83.8
gallbladder K82.8
heart — *see* Infarct, myocardium
hepatic K76.3
hypophysis (anterior lobe) E23.6
impending (myocardium) I20.0
intestine (acute) (agnogenic) (embolic)
(hemorrhagic) (nonocclusive)
(nonthrombotic) (occlusive)
(thrombotic) (with gangrene) K55.069
diffuse K55.062
focal K55.061
large K55.049
diffuse K55.042
focal K55.041
small K55.029
diffuse K55.022
focal K55.021
kidney N28.0
lacunar I63.81
liver K76.3
lung (embolic) (thrombotic) — *see*
Embolism, pulmonary
lymph node I89.8
mesentery, mesenteric (embolic)
(thrombotic) (with gangrene) — *see
also* Infarct, intestine K55.069
muscle (ischemic) M62.20
ankle M62.27-
foot M62.27-
forearm M62.23-
hand M62.24-

Infarct, infarction - *continued*
muscle (ischemic) - *continued*
    lower leg M62.26-
    pelvic region M62.25-
    shoulder region M62.21-
    specified site NEC M62.28
    thigh M62.25-
    upper arm M62.22-
myocardium, myocardial (acute) (with stated
        duration of 4 weeks or less) I21.9
    associated with revascularization
            procedure I21.A9
    diagnosed on ECG, but presenting no
            symptoms I25.2
    due to
        demand ischemia I21.A1
        ischemic imbalance I21.A1
    healed or old I25.2
    intraoperative — *see also* Infarct,
            myocardium, associated with
            revascularization procedure
        during cardiac surgery I97.790
        during other surgery I97.791
    non-Q wave I21.4
    non-ST elevation (NSTEMI) I21.4
        subsequent I22.2
    nontransmural I21.4
    past (diagnosed on ECG or other
            investigation, but currently presenting
            no symptoms) I25.2
    postprocedural — *see also* Infarct,
            myocardium, associated with
            revascularization procedure
        following cardiac surgery surgery — *see
            also* Infarct, myocardium, type 4 or
            type 5 I97.190
        following other surgery I97.191
    Q wave (see also, Infarct, myocardium, by
            site) I21.3
    secondary to
        demand ischemia I21.A1
        ischemic imbalance I21.A1
    ST elevation (STEMI) I21.3
        anterior (anteroapical) (anterolateral)
                (anteroseptal) (Q wave)
                (wall) I21.09
            subsequent I22.0
        inferior (diaphragmatic) (inferolateral)
                (inferoposterior) (wall) NEC I21.19
            subsequent I22.1
        inferoposterior transmural (Q
                wave) I21.11
        involving
            coronary artery of anterior wall
                    NEC I21.09
            coronary artery of inferior wall
                    NEC I21.19
            diagonal coronary artery I21.02
            left anterior descending coronary
                    artery I21.02
            left circumflex coronary artery I21.21
            left main coronary artery I21.01
            oblique marginal coronary
                    artery I21.21
            right coronary artery I21.11
        lateral (apical-lateral) (basal-lateral)
                (high) I21.29
            subsequent I22.8
        posterior (posterobasal) (posterolateral)
                (posteroseptal) (true) I21.29
            subsequent I22.8
        septal I21.29
            subsequent I22.8
        specified NEC I21.29
            subsequent I22.8
        subsequent I22.9
    subsequent (recurrent) (reinfarction) I22.9
        anterior (anteroapical) (anterolateral)
                (anteroseptal) (wall) I22.0
        diaphragmatic (wall) I22.1
        inferior (diaphragmatic) (inferolateral)
                (inferoposterior) (wall) I22.1
        lateral (apical-lateral) (basal-lateral)
                (high) I22.8
        non-ST elevation (NSTEMI) I22.2

Infarct, infarction - *continued*
myocardium, myocardial (acute) (with stated
        duration of 4 weeks or less) - *continued*
    subsequent (recurrent) (reinfarction) -
        continued
        posterior (posterobasal) (posterolateral)
                (posteroseptal) (true) I22.8
        septal I22.8
        specified NEC I22.8
        ST elevation I22.9
            anterior (anteroapical) (anterolateral)
                    (anteroseptal) (wall) I22.0
            inferior (diaphragmatic) (inferolateral)
                    (inferoposterior) (wall) I22.1
            specified NEC I22.8
        subendocardial I22.2
        transmural I22.9
            anterior (anteroapical) (anterolateral)
                    (anteroseptal) (wall) I22.0
            diaphragmatic (wall) I22.1
            inferior (diaphragmatic) (inferolateral)
                    (inferoposterior) (wall) I22.1
            lateral (apical-lateral) (basal-lateral)
                    (high) I22.8
            posterior (posterobasal)
                    (posterolateral) (posteroseptal)
                    (true) I22.8
            specified NEC I22.8
        type 1 — *see also* Infarction,
                myocardial, subsequent, by site, or
                by ST elevation or non-ST
                elevation I22.9
        type 2 I21.A1
        type 3 I21.A9
        type 4 I21.A9
        type 5 I21.A9
    syphilitic A52.06
    transmural I21.9
        anterior (anteroapical) (anterolateral)
                (anteroseptal) (Q wave) (wall)
                NEC I21.09
        inferior (diaphragmatic) (inferolateral)
                (inferoposterior) (Q wave) (wall)
                NEC I21.19
        inferoposterior (Q wave) I21.11
        lateral (apical-lateral) (basal-lateral)
                (high) NEC I21.29
        posterior (posterobasal) (posterolateral)
                (posteroseptal) (true) NEC I21.29
        septal NEC I21.29
        specified NEC I21.29
        type 1 — *see also* Infarction, myocardial,
                by site, or by ST elevation or non-ST
                elevation I21.9
        type 2 I21.A1
        type 3 I21.A9
        type 4 (a) (b) (c) I21.A9
        type 5 I21.A9
    nontransmural I21.4
    omentum — *see also* Infarct,
            intestine K55.069
    ovary N83.8
    pancreas K86.89
    papillary muscle — *see* Infarct, myocardium
    parathyroid gland E21.4
    pituitary (gland) E23.6
    placenta O43.81-
    prostate N42.89
    pulmonary (artery) (vein) (hemorrhagic) —
            see Embolism, pulmonary
    renal (embolic) (thrombotic) N28.0
    retina, retinal (artery) — *see* Occlusion,
            artery, retina
    spinal (cord) (acute) (embolic)
            (nonembolic) G95.11
    spleen D73.5
        embolic or thrombotic I74.8
    subendocardial (acute) (nontransmural) I21.4
    suprarenal (capsule) (gland) E27.49
    testis N50.1
    thrombotic — *see also* Thrombosis
        artery, arterial — *see* Embolism
    thyroid (gland) E07.89
    ventricle (heart) — *see* Infarct, myocardium

Infecting — *see* condition

Infection, infected, infective (opportunistic)
B99.9
with
    drug resistant organism — *see* Resistance
            (to), drug — *see also* specific
            organism
    lymphangitis — *see* Lymphangitis
    organ dysfunction (acute) R65.20
        with septic shock R65.21
abscess (skin) - code by site under Abscess
Absidia — *see* Mucormycosis
Acanthamoeba — *see* Acanthamebiasis
Acanthocheilonema (perstans)
        (streptocerca) B74.4
accessory sinus (chronic) — *see* Sinusitis
achorion — *see* Dermatophytosis
Acremonium falciforme B47.0
acromioclavicular M00.9
Actinobacillus (actinomycetem-
        comitans) A28.8
    mallei A24.0
    muris A25.1
Actinomadura B47.1
Actinomyces (israelii) — *see also*
        Actinomycosis A42.9
Actinomycetales — *see* Actinomycosis
actinomycotic NOS — *see* Actinomycosis
adenoid (and tonsil) J03.90
    chronic J35.02
adenovirus NEC
    as cause of disease classified
            elsewhere B97.0
    unspecified nature or site B34.0
aerogenes capsulatus A48.0
aertrycke — *see* Infection, salmonella
alimentary canal NOS — *see* Enteritis,
        infectious
Allescheria boydii B48.2
Alternaria B48.8
alveolus, alveolar (process) K04.7
Ameba, amebic (histolytica) — *see*
        Amebiasis
amniotic fluid, sac or cavity O41.10-
    chorioamnionitis O41.12-
    placentitis O41.14-
amputation stump (surgical) — *see*
        Complication, amputation stump,
        infection
Ancylostoma (duodenalis) B76.0
Anisakiasis, Anisakis larvae B81.0
anthrax — *see* Anthrax
antrum (chronic) — *see* Sinusitis, maxillary
anus, anal (papillae) (sphincter) K62.89
arbovirus (arbor virus) A94
    specified type NEC A93.8
artificial insemination N98.0
Ascaris lumbricoides — *see* Ascariasis
Ascomycetes B47.0
Aspergillus (flavus) (fumigatus) (terreus) —
        see Aspergillosis
atypical
    acid-fast (bacilli) — *see* Mycobacterium,
            atypical
    mycobacteria — *see* Mycobacterium,
            atypical
    virus A81.9
        specified type NEC A81.89
auditory meatus (external) — *see* Otitis,
        externa, infective
auricle (ear) — *see* Otitis, externa, infective
axillary gland (lymph) L04.2
Bacillus A49.9
    abortus A23.1
    anthracis — *see* Anthrax
    Ducrey's (any location) A57
    Flexner's A03.1
    Friedländer's NEC A49.8
    gas (gangrene) A48.0
    mallei A24.0
    melitensis A23.0
    paratyphoid, paratyphosus A01.4
        A A01.1
        B A01.2
        C A01.3
    Shiga (-Kruse) A03.0

Infection, infected, infective (opportunistic) - *continued*

Bacillus - *continued*
suipestifer — *see* Infection, salmonella
swimming pool A31.1
typhosa A01.00
welchii — *see* Gangrene, gas
bacterial NOS A49.9
as cause of disease classified elsewhere B96.89
Clostridium perfringens [C. perfringens] B96.7
Bacteroides fragilis [B. fragilis] B96.6
Enterobacter sakazakii B96.89
Enterococcus B95.2
Escherichia coli [E. coli] — *see also* Escherichia coli B96.20
Helicobacter pylori [H.pylori] B96.81
Hemophilus influenzae [H. influenzae] B96.3
Klebsiella pneumoniae [K. pneumoniae] B96.1
Mycoplasma pneumoniae [M. pneumoniae] B96.0
Proteus (mirabilis) (morganii) B96.4
Pseudomonas (aeruginosa) (mallei) (pseudomallei) B96.5
Staphylococcus B95.8
aureus (methicillin susceptible) (MSSA) B95.61
methicillin resistant (MRSA) B95.62
specified NEC B95.7
Streptococcus B95.5
group A B95.0
group B B95.1
pneumoniae B95.3
specified NEC B95.4
Vibrio vulnificus B96.82
specified NEC A48.8
Bacterium
paratyphosum A01.4
A A01.1
B A01.2
C A01.3
typhosum A01.00
Bacteroides NEC A49.8
fragilis, as cause of disease classified elsewhere B96.6
Balantidium coli A07.0
Bartholin's gland N75.8
Basidiobolus B46.8
bile duct (common) (hepatic) — *see* Cholangitis
bladder — *see* Cystitis
Blastomyces, blastomycotic — *see also* Blastomycosis
brasiliensis — *see* Paracoccidioidomycosis
dermatitidis — *see* Blastomycosis
European — *see* Cryptococcosis
Loboi B48.0
North American B40.9
South American — *see* Paracoccidioidomycosis
bleb, postprocedure — *see* Blebitis
bone — *see* Osteomyelitis
Bordetella — *see* Whooping cough
Borrelia bergdorfi A69.20
brain — *see also* Encephalitis G04.90
membranes — *see* Meningitis
septic G06.0
meninges — *see* Meningitis, bacterial
branchial cyst Q18.0
breast — *see* Mastitis
bronchus — *see* Bronchitis
Brucella A23.9
abortus A23.1
canis A23.3
melitensis A23.0
mixed A23.8
specified NEC A23.8
suis A23.2
Brugia (malayi) B74.1
timori B74.2
bursa — *see* Bursitis, infective

Infection, infected, infective (opportunistic) - *continued*

buttocks (skin) L08.9
Campylobacter, intestinal A04.5
as cause of disease classified elsewhere B96.81
Candida (albicans) (tropicalis) — *see* Candidiasis
candiru B88.8
Capillaria (intestinal) B81.1
hepatica B83.8
philippinensis B81.1
cartilage — *see* Disorder, cartilage, specified type NEC
catheter-related bloodstream (CRBSI) T80.211
cat liver fluke B66.0
cellulitis - code by site under Cellulitis
central line-associated T80.219
bloodstream (CLABSI) T80.211
specified NEC T80.218
Cephalosporium falciforme B47.0
cerebrospinal — *see* Meningitis
cervical gland (lymph) L04.0
cervix — *see* Cervicitis
cesarean delivery wound (puerperal) O86.00
cestodes — *see* Infestation, cestodes
chest J22
Chilomastix (intestinal) A07.8
Chlamydia, chlamydial A74.9
anus A56.3
genitourinary tract A56.2
lower A56.00
specified NEC A56.19
lymphogranuloma A55
pharynx A56.4
psittaci A70
rectum A56.3
sexually transmitted NEC A56.8
cholera — *see* Cholera
Cladosporium
bantianum (brain abscess) B43.1
carrionii B43.0
castellanii B36.1
trichoides (brain abscess) B43.1
werneckii B36.1
Clonorchis (sinensis) (liver) B66.1
Clostridium NEC
bifermentans A48.0
botulinum (food poisoning) A05.1
infant A48.51
wound A48.52
difficile
as cause of disease classified elsewhere B96.89
foodborne (disease)
not specified as recurrent A04.72
recurrent A04.71
gas gangrene A48.0
necrotizing enterocolitis
not specified as recurrent A04.72
recurrent A04.71
sepsis A41.4
gas-forming NEC A48.0
histolyticum A48.0
novyi, causing gas gangrene A48.0
oedematiens A48.0
perfringens
as cause of disease classified elsewhere B96.7
due to food A05.2
foodborne (disease) A05.2
gas gangrene A48.0
sepsis A41.4
septicum, causing gas gangrene A48.0
sordellii, causing gas gangrene A48.0
welchii
as cause of disease classified elsewhere B96.7
foodborne (disease) A05.2
gas gangrene A48.0
necrotizing enteritis A05.2
sepsis A41.4
Coccidioides (immitis) — *see* Coccidioidomycosis

Infection, infected, infective (opportunistic) - *continued*

colon — *see* Enteritis, infectious
colostomy K94.02
common duct — *see* Cholangitis
congenital P39.9
Candida (albicans) P37.5
cytomegalovirus P35.1
hepatitis, viral P35.3
herpes simplex P35.2
infectious or parasitic disease P37.9
specified NEC P37.8
listeriosis (disseminated) P37.2
malaria NEC P37.4
falciparum P37.3
Plasmodium falciparum P37.3
poliomyelitis P35.8
rubella P35.0
skin P39.4
toxoplasmosis (acute) (subacute) (chronic) P37.1
tuberculosis P37.0
urinary (tract) P39.3
vaccinia P35.8
virus P35.9
specified type NEC P35.8
Conidiobolus B46.8
coronavirus NEC B34.2
as cause of disease classified elsewhere B97.29
severe acute respiratory syndrome (SARS associated) B97.21
corpus luteum — *see* Salpingo-oophoritis
Corynebacterium diphtheriae — *see* Diphtheria
cotia virus B08.8
Coxiella burnetii A78
coxsackie — *see* Coxsackie
Cryptococcus neoformans — *see* Cryptococcosis
Cryptosporidium A07.2
Cunninghamella — *see* Mucormycosis
cyst — *see* Cyst
cystic duct — *see also* Cholecystitis K81.9
Cysticercus cellulosae — *see* Cysticercosis
cytomegalovirus, cytomegaloviral B25.9
congenital P35.1
maternal, maternal care for (suspected) damage to fetus O35.3
mononucleosis B27.10
with
complication NEC B27.19
meningitis B27.12
polyneuropathy B27.11
delta-agent (acute) , in hepatitis B
carrier B17.0
dental (pulpal origin) K04.7
Deuteromycetes B47.0
Dicrocoelium dendriticum B66.2
Dipetalonema (perstans) (streptocerca) B74.4
diphtherial — *see* Diphtheria
Diphyllobothrium (adult) (latum) (pacificum) B70.0
larval B70.1
Diplogonoporus (grandis) B71.8
Dipylidium caninum B67.4
Dirofilaria B74.8
Dracunculus medinensis B72
Drechslera (hawaiiensis) B43.8
Ducrey Haemophilus (any location) A57
due to or resulting from
artificial insemination N98.0
central venous catheter T80.219
bloodstream T80.211
exit or insertion site T80.212
localized T80.212
port or reservoir T80.212
specified NEC T80.218
tunnel T80.212
device, implant or graft — *see also* Complications, by site and type, infection or inflammation T85.79
arterial graft NEC T82.7
breast (implant) T85.79
catheter NEC T85.79

Infection, infected, infective (opportunistic) - *continued*
  due to or resulting from - *continued*
    device, implant or graft - *continued*
      catheter NEC - *continued*
        dialysis (renal) T82.7
          intraperitoneal T85.71
        infusion NEC T82.7
          cranial T85.735
          intrathecal T85.735
          spinal (epidural) (subdural) T85.735
          subarachnoid T85.735
        urinary T83.518
          cystostomy T83.510
          Hopkins T83.518
          ileostomy T83.518
          nephrostomy T83.512
          specified NEC T83.518
          urethral indwelling T83.511
          urostomy T83.518
      electronic (electrode) (pulse generator) (stimulator)
        bone T84.7
        cardiac T82.7
        nervous system T85.738
          brain T85.731
          cranial nerve T85.732
          gastric nerve T85.732
          generator pocket T85.734
          neurostimulator generator T85.734
          peripheral nerve T85.732
          sacral nerve T85.732
          spinal cord T85.733
          vagal nerve T85.732
        urinary T83.590
      fixation, internal (orthopedic) NEC — *see* Complication, fixation device, infection
      gastrointestinal (bile duct) (esophagus) T85.79
        neurostimulator electrode (lead) T85.732
      genital NEC T83.69
      heart NEC T82.7
        valve (prosthesis) T82.6
          graft T82.7
      joint prosthesis — *see* Complication, joint prosthesis, infection
      ocular (corneal graft) (orbital implant) NEC T85.79
      orthopedic NEC T84.7
      penile (cylinder) (pump) (resevoir) T83.61
      specified NEC T85.79
      testicular T83.62
      urinary NEC T83.598
        ileal conduit stent T83.593
        implanted neurostimulation T83.590
        implanted sphincter T83.591
        indwelling ureteral stent T83.592
        nephroureteral stent T83.593
        specified stent NEC T83.593
      vascular NEC T82.7
      ventricular intracranial (communicating) shunt T85.730
    Hickman catheter T80.219
      bloodstream T80.211
      localized T80.212
      specified NEC T80.218
    immunization or vaccination T88.0
    infusion, injection or transfusion NEC T80.29
      acute T80.22
    injury NEC - code by site under Wound, open
    peripherally inserted central catheter (PICC) T80.219
      bloodstream T80.211
      localized T80.212
      specified NEC T80.218
    portacath (port-a-cath) T80.219
      bloodstream T80.211
      localized T80.212
      specified NEC T80.218

Infection, infected, infective (opportunistic) - *continued*
  due to or resulting from - *continued*
    pulmonary artery catheter — *see* Infection, due to or resulting from, central venous catheter
    surgery T81.40
    Swan Ganz catheter — *see* Infection, due to or resulting from, central venous catheter
    triple lumen catheter T80.219
      bloodstream T80.211
      localized T80.212
      specified NEC T80.218
    umbilical venous catheter T80.219
      bloodstream T80.211
      localized T80.212
      specified NEC T80.218
  during labor NEC O75.3
  ear (middle) — *see also* Otitis media
    external — *see* Otitis, externa, infective
    inner — *see* subcategory H83.0
  Eberthella typhosa A01.00
  Echinococcus — *see* Echinococcus
  echovirus
    as cause of disease classified elsewhere B97.12
    unspecified nature or site B34.1
  endocardium I33.0
  endocervix — *see* Cervicitis
  Entamoeba — *see* Amebiasis
  enteric — *see* Enteritis, infectious
  Enterobacter sakazakii B96.89
  Enterobius vermicularis B80
  enterostomy K94.12
  enterovirus B34.1
    as cause of disease classified elsewhere B97.10
      coxsackievirus B97.11
      echovirus B97.12
      specified NEC B97.19
  Entomophthora B46.8
  Epidermophyton — *see* Dermatophytosis
  epididymus — *see* Epididymitis
  episiotomy (puerperal) O86.09
  Erysipelothrix (insidiosa) (rhusiopathiae) — *see* Erysipeloid
  erythema infectiosum B08.3
  Escherichia (E.) coli NEC A49.8
    as cause of disease classified elsewhere — *see also* Escherichia coli B96.20
    congenital P39.8
      sepsis P36.4
    generalized A41.51
    intestinal — *see* Enteritis, infectious, due to, Escherichia coli
  ethmoidal (chronic) (sinus) — *see* Sinusitis, ethmoidal
  eustachian tube (ear) — *see* Salpingitis, eustachian
  external auditory canal (meatus) NEC — *see* Otitis, externa, infective
  eye (purulent) — *see* Endophthalmitis, purulent
  eyelid — *see* Inflammation, eyelid
  fallopian tube — *see* Salpingo-oophoritis
  Fasciola (gigantica) (hepatica) (indica) B66.3
  Fasciolopsis (buski) B66.5
  filarial — *see* Infestation, filarial
  finger (skin) L08.9
    nail L03.01-
      fungus B35.1
  fish tapeworm B70.0
    larval B70.1
  flagellate, intestinal A07.9
  fluke — *see* Infestation, fluke
  focal
    teeth (pulpal origin) K04.7
    tonsils J35.01
  Fonsecaea (compactum) (pedrosoi) B43.0
  food — *see* Intoxication, foodborne
  foot (skin) L08.9
    dermatophytic fungus B35.3
  Francisella tularensis — *see* Tularemia

Infection, infected, infective (opportunistic) - *continued*
  frontal (sinus) (chronic) — *see* Sinusitis, frontal
  fungus NOS B49
    beard B35.0
    dermatophytic — *see* Dermatophytosis
    foot B35.3
    groin B35.6
    hand B35.2
    nail B35.1
    pathogenic to compromised host only B48.8
    perianal (area) B35.6
    scalp B35.0
    skin B36.9
      foot B35.3
      hand B35.2
      toenails B35.1
  Fusarium B48.8
  gallbladder — *see* Cholecystitis
  gas bacillus — *see* Gangrene, gas
  gastrointestinal — *see* Enteritis, infectious
  generalized NEC — *see* Sepsis
  generator pocket, implanted electronic neurostimulator T85.734
  genital organ or tract
    female — *see* Disease, pelvis, inflammatory
    male N49.9
      multiple sites N49.8
      specified NEC N49.8
  Ghon tubercle, primary A15.7
  Giardia lamblia A07.1
  gingiva (chronic) K05.10
    acute K05.00
      nonplaque induced K05.01
      plaque induced K05.00
    nonplaque induced K05.11
    plaque induced K05.10
  glanders A24.0
  glenosporopsis B48.0
  Gnathostoma (spinigerum) B83.1
  Gongylonema B83.8
  gonococcal — *see* Gonococcus
  gram-negative bacilli NOS A49.9
  guinea worm B72
  gum (chronic) K05.10
    acute K05.00
      nonplaque induced K05.01
      plaque induced K05.00
    nonplaque induced K05.11
    plaque induced K05.10
  Haemophilus — *see* Infection, Hemophilus
  heart — *see* Carditis
  Helicobacter pylori A04.8
    as cause of disease classified elsewhere B96.81
  helminths B83.9
    intestinal B82.0
      mixed (types classifiable to more than one of the titles B65.0-B81.3 and B81.8) B81.4
      specified type NEC B81.8
    specified type NEC B83.8
  Hemophilus
    aegyptius, systemic A48.4
    ducrey (any location) A57
    influenzae NEC A49.2
      as cause of disease classified elsewhere B96.3
      generalized A41.3
  herpes (simplex) — *see also* Herpes
    congenital P35.2
    disseminated B00.7
    zoster B02.9
  herpesvirus, herpesviral — *see* Herpes
  hip (joint) NEC M00.9
    due to internal joint prosthesis
      left T84.52
      right T84.51
    skin NEC L08.9
  Heterophyes (heterophyes) B66.8
  Histoplasma — *see* Histoplasmosis
    American B39.4

Infection, infected, infective (opportunistic) -
continued
  Histoplasma - *continued*
    capsulatum B39.4
  hookworm B76.9
  human
    papilloma virus A63.0
    T-cell lymphotropic virus type-1 (HTLV-1) B33.3
  hydrocele N43.0
  Hymenolepis B71.0
  hypopharynx — *see* Pharyngitis
  inguinal (lymph) glands L04.1
    due to soft chancre A57
  intervertebral disc, pyogenic M46.30
    cervical region M46.32
    cervicothoracic region M46.33
    lumbar region M46.36
    lumbosacral region M46.37
    multiple sites M46.39
    occipito-atlanto-axial region M46.31
    sacrococcygeal region M46.38
    thoracic region M46.34
    thoracolumbar region M46.35
  intestine, intestinal — *see* Enteritis, infectious
    specified NEC A08.8
  intra-amniotic affecting newborn NEC P39.2
  Isospora belli or hominis A07.3
  Japanese B encephalitis A83.0
  jaw (bone) (lower) (upper) M27.2
  joint NEC M00.9
    due to internal joint prosthesis T84.50
  kidney (cortex) (hematogenous) N15.9
    with calculus N20.0
      with hydronephrosis N13.6
    following ectopic gestation O08.83
    pelvis and ureter (cystic) N28.85
    puerperal (postpartum) O86.21
    specified NEC N15.8
  Klebsiella (K.) pneumoniae NEC A49.8
    as cause of disease classified elsewhere B96.1
  knee (joint) NEC M00.9
    joint M00.9
      due to internal joint prosthesis
        left T84.54
        right T84.53
    skin L08.9
  Koch's — *see* Tuberculosis
  labia (majora) (minora) (acute) — *see* Vulvitis
  lacrimal
    gland — *see* Dacryoadenitis
    passages (duct) (sac) — *see* Inflammation, lacrimal, passages
  lancet fluke B66.2
  larynx NEC J38.7
  leg (skin) NOS L08.9
  Legionella pneumophila A48.1
    nonpneumonic A48.2
  Leishmania — *see also* Leishmaniasis
    aethiopica B55.1
    braziliensis B55.2
    chagasi B55.0
    donovani B55.0
    infantum B55.0
    major B55.1
    mexicana B55.1
    tropica B55.1
  lentivirus, as cause of disease classified elsewhere B97.31
  Leptosphaeria senegalensis B47.0
  Leptospira interrogans A27.9
    autumnalis A27.89
    canicola A27.89
    hebdomadis A27.89
    icterohaemorrhagiae A27.0
    pomona A27.89
    specified type NEC A27.89
  leptospirochetal NEC — *see* Leptospirosis
  Listeria monocytogenes — *see also* Listeriosis
    congenital P37.2
  Loa loa B74.3

Infection, infected, infective (opportunistic) -
continued
  Loa loa - *continued*
    with conjunctival infestation B74.3
      eyelid B74.3
  Loboa loboi B48.0
  local, skin (staphylococcal) (streptococcal) L08.9
    abscess - code by site under Abscess
    cellulitis - code by site under Cellulitis
    specified NEC L08.89
    ulcer — *see* Ulcer, skin
  Loefflerella mallei A24.0
  lung — *see also* Pneumonia J18.9
    atypical Mycobacterium A31.0
    spirochetal A69.8
    tuberculous — *see* Tuberculosis, pulmonary
    virus — *see* Pneumonia, viral
  lymph gland — *see also* Lymphadenitis, acute
    mesenteric I88.0
  lymphoid tissue, base of tongue or posterior pharynx, NEC (chronic) J35.03
  Madurella (grisea) (mycetomii) B47.0
  major
    following ectopic or molar pregnancy O08.0
    puerperal, postpartum, childbirth O85
  Malassezia furfur B36.0
  Malleomyces
    mallei A24.0
    pseudomallei (whitmori) — *see* Melioidosis
  mammary gland N61.0
  Mansonella (ozzardi) (perstans) (streptocerca) B74.4
  mastoid — *see* Mastoiditis
  maxilla, maxillary M27.2
    sinus (chronic) — *see* Sinusitis, maxillary
  mediastinum J98.51
  Medina (worm) B72
  meibomian cyst or gland — *see* Hordeolum
  meninges — *see* Meningitis, bacterial
  meningococcal — *see also* condition A39.9
    adrenals A39.1
    brain A39.81
    cerebrospinal A39.0
    conjunctiva A39.89
    endocardium A39.51
    heart A39.50
      endocardium A39.51
      myocardium A39.52
      pericardium A39.53
    joint A39.83
    meninges A39.0
    meningococcemia A39.4
      acute A39.2
      chronic A39.3
    myocardium A39.52
    pericardium A39.53
    retrobulbar neuritis A39.82
    specified site NEC A39.89
  mesenteric lymph nodes or glands NEC I88.0
  Metagonimus B66.8
  metatarsophalangeal M00.9
  methicillin
    resistant Staphylococcus aureus (MRSA) A49.02
    susceptible Staphylococcus aureus (MSSA) A49.01
  Microsporum, microsporic — *see* Dermatophytosis
  mixed flora (bacterial) NEC A49.8
  Monilia — *see* Candidiasis
  Monosporium apiospermum B48.2
  mouth, parasitic B37.0
  Mucor — *see* Mucormycosis
  muscle NEC — *see* Myositis, infective
  mycelium NOS B49
  mycetoma B47.9
    actinomycotic NEC B47.1
    mycotic NEC B47.0
  Mycobacterium, mycobacterial — *see* Mycobacterium

Infection, infected, infective (opportunistic) -
continued
  Mycoplasma NEC A49.3
    pneumoniae, as cause of disease classified elsewhere B96.0
  mycotic NOS B49
    pathogenic to compromised host only B48.8
    skin NOS B36.9
  myocardium NEC I40.0
  nail (chronic)
    with lymphangitis — *see* Lymphangitis, acute, digit
    finger L03.01-
      fungus B35.1
    ingrowing L60.0
    toe L03.03-
      fungus B35.1
  nasal sinus (chronic) — *see* Sinusitis
  nasopharynx — *see* Nasopharyngitis
  navel L08.82
  Necator americanus B76.1
  Neisseria — *see* Gonococcus
  Neotestudina rosatii B47.0
  newborn P39.9
    intra-amniotic NEC P39.2
    skin P39.4
    specified type NEC P39.8
  nipple N61.0
    associated with
      lactation O91.03
      pregnancy O91.01-
      puerperium O91.02
  Nocardia — *see* Nocardiosis
  obstetrical surgical wound (puerperal) O86.00
    incisional site
      deep O86.02
      superficial O86.01
    organ and space site O86.03
    surgical site specified NEC O86.09
  Oesophagostomum (apiostomum) B81.8
  Oestrus ovis — *see* Myiasis
  Oidium albicans B37.9
  Onchocerca (volvulus) — *see* Onchocerciasis
  oncovirus, as cause of disease classified elsewhere B97.32
  operation wound T81.49
  Opisthorchis (felineus) (viverrini) B66.0
  orbit, orbital — *see* Inflammation, orbit
  orthopoxvirus NEC B08.09
  ovary — *see* Salpingo-oophoritis
  Oxyuris vermicularis B80
  pancreas (acute) — *see* Pancreatitis, acute
    abscess — *see* Pancreatitis, acute
    specified NEC — *see also* Pancreatitis, acute K85.80
  papillomavirus, as cause of disease classified elsewhere B97.7
  papovavirus NEC B34.4
  Paracoccidioides brasiliensis — *see* Paracoccidioidomycosis
  Paragonimus (westermani) B66.4
  parainfluenza virus B34.8
  parameningococcus NOS A39.9
  parapoxvirus B08.60
    specified NEC B08.69
  parasitic B89
  Parastrongylus
    cantonensis B83.2
    costaricensis B81.3
  paratyphoid A01.4
    Type A A01.1
    Type B A01.2
    Type C A01.3
  paraurethral ducts N34.2
  parotid gland — *see* Sialoadenitis
  parvovirus NEC B34.3
    as cause of disease classified elsewhere B97.6
  Pasteurella NEC A28.0
    multocida A28.0
    pestis — *see* Plague
    pseudotuberculosis A28.0
    septica (cat bite) (dog bite) A28.0

Infection, infected, infective (opportunistic) - *continued*

Pasteurella NEC - *continued*
  tularensis — *see* Tularemia
pelvic, female — *see* Disease, pelvis,
  inflammatory
Penicillium (marneffei) B48.4
penis (glans) (retention) NEC N48.29
periapical K04.5
peridental, periodontal K05.20
  generalized — *see* Periodontitis,
    aggressive, generalized
  localized — *see* Periodontitis, aggressive,
    localized
perinatal period P39.9
  specified type NEC P39.8
perineal repair (puerperal) O86.09
periorbital — *see* Inflammation, orbit
perirectal K62.89
perirenal — *see* Infection, kidney
peritoneal — *see* Peritonitis
periureteral N28.89
Petriellidium boydii B48.2
pharynx — *see also* Pharyngitis
  coxsackievirus B08.5
  posterior, lymphoid (chronic) J35.03
Phialophora
  gougerotii (subcutaneous abscess or
    cyst) B43.2
  jeanselmei (subcutaneous abscess or
    cyst) B43.2
  verrucosa (skin) B43.0
Piedraia hortae B36.3
pinta A67.9
  intermediate A67.1
  late A67.2
  mixed A67.3
  primary A67.0
pinworm B80
pityrosporum furfur B36.0
pleuro-pneumonia-like organism (PPLO)
  NEC A49.3
  as cause of disease classified
    elsewhere B96.0
pneumococcus, pneumococcal NEC A49.1
  as cause of disease classified
    elsewhere B95.3
  generalized (purulent) A40.3
    with pneumonia J13
Pneumocystis carinii (pneumonia) B59
Pneumocystis jiroveci (pneumonia) B59
port or reservoir T80.212
postoperative T81.40
postoperative wound T81.49
  surgical site
    deep incisional T81.42
    organ and space T81.43
    specified NEC T81.49
    superficial incisional T81.41
postprocedural T81.40
postvaccinal T88.0
prepuce NEC N47.7
  with penile inflammation N47.6
prion — *see* Disease, prion, central nervous
  system
prostate (capsule) — *see* Prostatitis
Proteus (mirabilis) (morganii) (vulgaris)
  NEC A49.8
  as cause of disease classified
    elsewhere B96.4
protozoal NEC B64
  intestinal A07.9
    specified NEC A07.8
  specified NEC B60.8
Pseudoallescheria boydii B48.2
Pseudomonas NEC A49.8
  as cause of disease classified
    elsewhere B96.5
  mallei A24.0
  pneumonia J15.1
  pseudomallei — *see* Melioidosis
puerperal O86.4
  genitourinary tract NEC O86.89
  major or generalized O85
  minor O86.4

Infection, infected, infective (opportunistic) - *continued*

puerperal - *continued*
  specified NEC O86.89
pulmonary — *see* Infection, lung
purulent — *see* Abscess
Pyrenochaeta romeroi B47.0
Q fever A78
rectum (sphincter) K62.89
renal — *see also* Infection, kidney
  pelvis and ureter (cystic) N28.85
reovirus, as cause of disease classified
  elsewhere B97.5
respiratory (tract) NEC J98.8
  acute J22
  chronic J98.8
  influenzal (upper) (acute) — *see* Influenza,
    with, respiratory manifestations NEC
  lower (acute) J22
    chronic — *see* Bronchitis, chronic
  rhinovirus J00
  syncytial virus (RSV) — *see* Infection,
    virus, respiratory syncytial (RSV)
  upper (acute) NOS J06.9
    chronic J39.8
    streptococcal J06.9
    viral NOS J06.9
      due to respiratory syncytial virus
        (RSV) J06.9 *[B97.4]*
resulting from
  presence of internal prosthesis, implant,
    graft — *see* Complications, by site
    and type, infection
retortamoniasis A07.8
retroperitoneal NEC K68.9
retrovirus B33.3
  as cause of disease classified
    elsewhere B97.30
  human
    immunodeficiency, type 2 (HIV
      2) B97.35
    T-cell lymphotropic
      type I (HTLV-I) B97.33
      type II (HTLV-II) B97.34
  lentivirus B97.31
  oncovirus B97.32
  specified NEC B97.39
Rhinosporidium (seeberi) B48.1
rhinovirus
  as cause of disease classified
    elsewhere B97.89
  unspecified nature or site B34.8
Rhizopus — *see* Mucormycosis
rickettsial NOS A79.9
roundworm (large) NEC B82.0
  Ascariasis — *see also* Ascariasis B77.9
rubella — *see* Rubella
Saccharomyces — *see* Candidiasis
salivary duct or gland (any) — *see*
  Sialoadenitis
Salmonella (aertrycke) (arizonae)
  (callinarum) (cholerae-suis) (enteritidis)
  (suipestifer) (typhimurium) A02.9
  with
    (gastro) enteritis A02.0
    sepsis A02.1
    specified manifestation NEC A02.8
  due to food (poisoning) A02.9
  hirschfeldii A01.3
  localized A02.20
    arthritis A02.23
    meningitis A02.21
    osteomyelitis A02.24
    pneumonia A02.22
    pyelonephritis A02.25
    specified NEC A02.29
  paratyphi A01.4
    A A01.1
    B A01.2
    C A01.3
  schottmuelleri A01.2
  typhi, typhosa — *see* Typhoid
Sarcocystis A07.8
scabies B86
Schistosoma — *see* Infestation, Schistosoma

Infection, infected, infective (opportunistic) - *continued*

scrotum (acute) NEC N49.2
seminal vesicle — *see* Vesiculitis
septic
  localized, skin — *see* Abscess
sheep liver fluke B66.3
Shigella A03.9
  boydii A03.2
  dysenteriae A03.0
  flexneri A03.1
  group
    A A03.0
    B A03.1
    C A03.2
    D A03.3
  Schmitz (-Stutzer) A03.0
  schmitzii A03.0
  shigae A03.0
  sonnei A03.3
  specified NEC A03.8
shoulder (joint) NEC M00.9
  due to internal joint prosthesis T84.59
  skin NEC L08.9
sinus (accessory) (chronic) (nasal) — *see*
  also Sinusitis
  pilonidal — *see* Sinus, pilonidal
  skin NEC L08.89
Skene's duct or gland — *see* Urethritis
skin (local) (staphylococcal)
  (streptococcal) L08.9
  abscess - code by site under Abscess
  cellulitis - code by site under Cellulitis
  due to fungus B36.9
    specified type NEC B36.8
  mycotic B36.9
    specified type NEC B36.8
  newborn P39.4
  ulcer — *see* Ulcer, skin
slow virus A81.9
  specified NEC A81.89
Sparganum (mansoni) (proliferum)
  (baxteri) B70.1
specific — *see also* Syphilis
  to perinatal period — *see* Infection,
    congenital
specified NEC B99.8
spermatic cord NEC N49.1
sphenoidal (sinus) — *see* Sinusitis,
  sphenoidal
spinal cord NOS — *see also* Myelitis G04.91
  abscess G06.1
  meninges — *see* Meningitis
  streptococcal G04.89
Spirillum A25.0
spirochetal NOS A69.9
  lung A69.8
  specified NEC A69.8
Spirometra larvae B70.1
spleen D73.89
Sporotrichum, Sporothrix (schenckii) — *see*
  Sporotrichosis
staphylococcal, unspecified site
  aureus (methicillin susceptible)
    (MSSA) A49.01
    methicillin resistant (MRSA) A49.02
  as cause of disease classified
    elsewhere B95.8
    aureus (methicillin susceptible)
      (MSSA) B95.61
      methicillin resistant (MRSA) B95.62
    specified NEC B95.7
  food poisoning A05.0
  generalized (purulent) A41.2
  pneumonia — *see* Pneumonia,
    staphylococcal
Stellantchasmus falcatus B66.8
streptobacillus moniliformis A25.1
streptococcal NEC A49.1
  as cause of disease classified
    elsewhere B95.5
  B genitourinary complicating
    childbirth O98.82
    pregnancy O98.81-
    puerperium O98.83

Infection, infected, infective (opportunistic) - *continued*
  streptococcal NEC - *continued*
    congenital
      sepsis P36.10
        group B P36.0
        specified NEC P36.19
      generalized (purulent) A40.9
  Streptomyces B47.1
  Strongyloides (stercoralis) — *see*
      Strongyloidiasis
  stump (amputation) (surgical) — *see*
      Complication, amputation stump,
      infection
  subcutaneous tissue, local L08.9
  suipestifer — *see* Infection, salmonella
  swimming pool bacillus A31.1
  Taenia — *see* Infestation, Taenia
  Taeniarhynchus saginatus B68.1
  tapeworm — *see* Infestation, tapeworm
  tendon (sheath) — *see* Tenosynovitis,
      infective NEC
  Ternidens diminutus B81.8
  testis — *see* Orchitis
  threadworm B80
  throat — *see* Pharyngitis
  thyroglossal duct K14.8
  toe (skin) L08.9
    cellulitis L03.03-
      fungus B35.1
    nail L03.03-
      fungus B35.1
  tongue NEC K14.0
    parasitic B37.0
  tonsil (and adenoid) (faucial) (lingual)
      (pharyngeal) — *see* Tonsillitis
  tooth, teeth K04.7
    periapical K04.7
    peridental, periodontal K05.20
      generalized — *see* Periodontitis,
        aggressive, generalized
      localized — *see* Periodontitis,
        aggressive, localized
    pulp K04.01
      irreversible K04.02
      reversible K04.01
    socket M27.3
  TORCH — *see* Infection, congenital
      without active infection P00.2
  Torula histolytica — *see* Cryptococcosis
  Toxocara (canis) (cati) (felis) B83.0
  Toxoplasma gondii — *see* Toxoplasma
  trachea, chronic J42
  trematode NEC — *see* Infestation, fluke
  trench fever A79.0
  Treponema pallidum — *see* Syphilis
  Trichinella (spiralis) B75
  Trichomonas A59.9
    cervix A59.09
    intestine A07.8
    prostate A59.02
    specified site NEC A59.8
    urethra A59.03
    urogenitalis A59.00
    vagina A59.01
    vulva A59.01
  Trichophyton, trichophytic — *see*
      Dermatophytosis
  Trichosporon (beigelii) cutaneum B36.2
  Trichostrongylus B81.2
  Trichuris (trichiura) B79
  Trombicula (irritans) B88.0
  Trypanosoma
    brucei
      gambiense B56.0
      rhodesiense B56.1
    cruzi — *see* Chagas' disease
  tubal — *see* Salpingo-oophoritis
  tuberculous
    latent (LTBI) Z22.7
    NEC — *see* Tuberculosis
  tubo-ovarian — *see* Salpingo-oophoritis
  tunnel T80.212
  tunica vaginalis N49.1
  tympanic membrane NEC — *see* Myringitis

Infection, infected, infective (opportunistic) - *continued*
  typhoid (abortive) (ambulant) (bacillus) —
      see Typhoid
  typhus A75.9
    flea-borne A75.2
    mite-borne A75.3
    recrudescent A75.1
    tick-borne A77.9
      African A77.1
      North Asian A77.2
  umbilicus L08.82
  ureter — *see* Ureteritis
  urethra — *see* Urethritis
  urinary (tract) N39.0
    bladder — *see* Cystitis
    complicating
      pregnancy O23.4-
        specified type NEC O23.3-
      kidney — *see* Infection, kidney
    newborn P39.3
    puerperal (postpartum) O86.20
    tuberculous A18.13
    urethra — *see* Urethritis
  uterus, uterine — *see* Endometritis
  vaccination T88.0
  vaccinia not from vaccination B08.011
  vagina (acute) — *see* Vaginitis
  varicella B01.9
  varicose veins — *see* Varix
  vas deferens NEC N49.1
  vesical — *see* Cystitis
  Vibrio
    cholerae A00.0
      El Tor A00.1
    parahaemolyticus (food poisoning) A05.3
    vulnificus
      as cause of disease classified
        elsewhere B96.82
      foodborne intoxication A05.5
  Vincent's (gum) (mouth) (tonsil) A69.1
  virus, viral NOS B34.9
    adenovirus
      as cause of disease classified
        elsewhere B97.0
      unspecified nature or site B34.0
    arborvirus, arbovirus arthropod-borne A94
      as cause of disease classified
        elsewhere B97.89
      adenovirus B97.0
      coronavirus B97.29
        SARS-associated B97.21
      coxsackievirus B97.11
      echovirus B97.12
      enterovirus B97.10
        coxsackievirus B97.11
        echovirus B97.12
        specified NEC B97.19
      human
        immunodeficiency, type 2 (HIV
          2) B97.35
        T-cell lymphotropic,
          type I (HTLV-I) B97.33
          type II (HTLV-II) B97.34
        metapneumovirus B97.81
      papillomavirus B97.7
      parvovirus B97.6
      reovirus B97.5
      respiratory syncytial (RSV) — *see*
        Infection, virus, respiratory
        syncytial (RSV)
      retrovirus B97.30
        human
          immunodeficiency, type 2 (HIV
            2) B97.35
          T-cell lymphotropic,
            type I (HTLV-I) B97.33
            type II (HTLV-II) B97.34
        lentivirus B97.31
        oncovirus B97.32
        specified NEC B97.39
      specified NEC B97.89
    central nervous system A89
      atypical A81.9
        specified NEC A81.89

Infection, infected, infective (opportunistic) - *continued*
  virus, viral NOS - *continued*
    central nervous system - *continued*
      enterovirus NEC A88.8
        meningitis A87.0
      slow virus A81.9
        specified NEC A81.89
      specified NEC A88.8
    chest J98.8
    cotia B08.8
    coxsackie — *see also* Infection,
        coxsackie B34.1
      as cause of disease classified
        elsewhere B97.11
    ECHO
      as cause of disease classified
        elsewhere B97.12
      unspecified nature or site B34.1
    encephalitis, tick-borne A84.9
    enterovirus, as cause of disease classified
        elsewhere B97.10
      coxsackievirus B97.11
      echovirus B97.12
      specified NEC B97.19
    exanthem NOS B09
    human papilloma as cause of disease
        classified elsewhere B97.7
    human metapneumovirus as cause of
        disease classified elsewhere B97.81
    intestine — *see* Enteritis, viral
    respiratory syncytial (RSV)
      as cause of disease classified
        elsewhere B97.4
      bronchiolitis J21.0
      bronchitis J20.5
      bronchopneumonia J12.1
      otitis media H65.- *[B97.4]*
      pneumonia J12.1
      upper respiratory infection J06.9 *[B97.4]*
    rhinovirus
      as cause of disease classified
        elsewhere B97.89
      unspecified nature or site B34.8
    slow A81.9
      specified NEC A81.89
    specified type NEC B33.8
      as cause of disease classified
        elsewhere B97.89
      unspecified nature or site B34.8
    unspecified nature or site B34.9
    West Nile — *see* Virus, West Nile
    vulva (acute) — *see* Vulvitis
  West Nile — *see* Virus, West Nile
  whipworm B79
  worms B83.9
    specified type NEC B83.8
  Wuchereria (bancrofti) B74.0
    malayi B74.1
  yatapoxvirus B08.70
    specified NEC B08.79
  yeast — *see also* Candidiasis B37.9
  yellow fever — *see* Fever, yellow
  Yersinia
    enterocolitica (intestinal) A04.6
    pestis — *see* Plague
    pseudotuberculosis A28.2
  Zeis' gland — *see* Hordeolum
  Zika virus A92.5
    congenital P35.4
  zoonotic bacterial NOS A28.9
  Zopfia senegalensis B47.0
Infective, infectious — *see* condition
Infertility
  female N97.9
    age-related N97.8
    associated with
      anovulation N97.0
      cervical (mucus) disease or
        anomaly N88.3
      congenital anomaly
        cervix N88.3
        fallopian tube N97.1
        uterus N97.2
        vagina N97.8

Infertility - *continued*
  female - *continued*
    associated with - *continued*
      dysmucorrhea N88.3
      fallopian tube disease or anomaly N97.1
      pituitary-hypothalamic origin E23.0
      specified origin NEC N97.8
      Stein-Leventhal syndrome E28.2
      uterine disease or anomaly N97.2
      vaginal disease or anomaly N97.8
    due to
      cervical anomaly N88.3
      fallopian tube anomaly N97.1
      ovarian failure E28.39
      Stein-Leventhal syndrome E28.2
      uterine anomaly N97.2
      vaginal anomaly N97.8
    nonimplantation N97.2
    origin
      cervical N88.3
      tubal (block) (occlusion)
        (stenosis) N97.1
      uterine N97.2
      vaginal N97.8
  male N46.9
    azoospermia N46.01
      extratesticular cause N46.029
        drug therapy N46.021
        efferent duct obstruction N46.023
        infection N46.022
        radiation N46.024
        specified cause NEC N46.029
        systemic disease N46.025
    oligospermia N46.11
      extratesticular cause N46.129
        drug therapy N46.121
        efferent duct obstruction N46.123
        infection N46.122
        radiation N46.124
        specified cause NEC N46.129
        systemic disease N46.125
    specified type NEC N46.8
Infestation B88.9
  Acanthocheilonema (perstans)
    (streptocerca) B74.4
  Acariasis B88.0
    demodex folliculorum B88.0
    sarcoptes scabiei B86
    trombiculae B88.0
  Agamofilaria streptocerca B74.4
  Ancylostoma, ankylostoma (braziliense)
    (caninum) (ceylanicum)
    (duodenale) B76.0
    americanum B76.1
    new world B76.1
  Anisakis larvae, anisakiasis B81.0
  arthropod NEC B88.2
  Ascaris lumbricoides — *see* Ascariasis
  Balantidium coli A07.0
  beef tapeworm B68.1
  Bothriocephalus (latus) B70.0
    larval B70.1
  broad tapeworm B70.0
    larval B70.1
  Brugia (malayi) B74.1
    timori B74.2
  candiru B88.8
  Capillaria
    hepatica B83.8
    philippinensis B81.1
  cat liver fluke B66.0
  cestodes B71.9
    diphyllobothrium — *see* Infestation,
      diphyllobothrium
    dipylidiasis B71.1
    hymenolepiasis B71.0
    specified type NEC B71.8
  chigger B88.0
  chigo, chigoe B88.1
  Clonorchis (sinensis) (liver) B66.1
  coccidial A07.3
  crab-lice B85.3
  Cysticercus cellulosae — *see* Cysticercosis
  Demodex (folliculorum) B88.0
  Dermanyssus gallinae B88.0

Infestation - *continued*
  Dermatobia (hominis) — *see* Myiasis
  Dibothriocephalus (latus) B70.0
    larval B70.1
  Dicrocoelium dendriticum B66.2
  Diphyllobothrium (adult) (latum) (intestinal)
    (pacificum) B70.0
    larval B70.1
  Diplogonoporus (grandis) B71.8
  Dipylidium caninum B67.4
  Distoma hepaticum B66.3
  dog tapeworm B67.4
  Dracunculus medinensis B72
  dragon worm B72
  dwarf tapeworm B71.0
  Echinococcus — *see* Echinococcus
  Echinostomum ilocanum B66.8
  Entamoeba (histolytica) — *see* Infection,
    Ameba
  Enterobius vermicularis B80
  eyelid
    in (due to)
      leishmaniasis B55.1
      loiasis B74.3
      onchocerciasis B73.09
      phthiriasis B85.3
      parasitic NOS B89
  eyeworm B74.3
  Fasciola (gigantica) (hepatica) (indica) B66.3
  Fasciolopsis (buski) (intestine) B66.5
  filarial B74.9
    bancroftian B74.0
    conjunctiva B74.9
    due to
      Acanthocheilonema (perstans)
        (streptocerca) B74.4
      Brugia (malayi) B74.1
        timori B74.2
      Dracunculus medinensis B72
      guinea worm B72
      loa loa B74.3
      Mansonella (ozzardi) (perstans)
        (streptocerca) B74.4
      Onchocerca volvulus B73.00
        eye B73.00
        eyelid B73.09
      Wuchereria (bancrofti) B74.0
    Malayan B74.1
    ozzardi B74.4
    specified type NEC B74.8
  fish tapeworm B70.0
    larval B70.1
  fluke B66.9
    blood NOS — *see* Schistosomiasis
    cat liver B66.0
    intestinal B66.5
    liver (sheep) B66.3
      cat B66.0
      Chinese B66.1
      due to clonorchiasis B66.1
      oriental B66.1
    lancet B66.2
    lung (oriental) B66.4
    sheep liver B66.3
    specified type NEC B66.8
  fly larvae — *see* Myiasis
  Gasterophilus (intestinalis) — *see* Myiasis
  Gastrodiscoides hominis B66.8
  Giardia lamblia A07.1
  Gnathostoma (spinigerum) B83.1
  Gongylonema B83.8
  guinea worm B72
  helminth B83.9
    angiostrongyliasis B83.2
      intestinal B81.3
    gnathostomiasis B83.1
    hirudiniasis, internal B83.4
    intestinal B82.0
      angiostrongyliasis B81.3
      anisakiasis B81.0
      ascariasis — *see* Ascariasis
      capillariasis B81.1
      cysticercosis — *see* Cysticercosis
      diphyllobothriasis — *see* Infestation,
        diphyllobothriasis

Infestation - *continued*
  helminth - *continued*
    intestinal - *continued*
      dracunculiasis B72
      echinococcus — *see* Echinococcosis
      enterobiasis B80
      filariasis - — *see* Infestation, filarial
      fluke — *see* Infestation, fluke
      hookworm — *see* Infestation, hookworm
      mixed (types classifiable to more than
        one of the titles B65.0-B81.3 and
        B81.8) B81.4
      onchocerciasis — *see* Onchocerciasis
      schistosomiasis — *see* Infestation,
        schistosoma
      specified
        cestode NEC — *see* Infestation,
          cestode
        type NEC B81.8
      strongyloidiasis — *see* Strongyloidiasis
      taenia — *see* Infestation, taenia
      trichinellosis B75
      trichostrongyliasis B81.2
      trichuriasis B79
    specified type NEC B83.8
    syngamiasis B83.3
    visceral larva migrans B83.0
  Heterophyes (heterophyes) B66.8
  hookworm B76.9
    ancylostomiasis B76.0
    necatoriasis B76.1
    specified type NEC B76.8
  Hymenolepis (diminuta) (nana) B71.0
  intestinal NEC B82.9
  leeches (aquatic) (land) — *see* Hirudiniasis
  Leishmania — *see* Leishmaniasis
  lice, louse — *see* Infestation, Pediculus
  Linguatula B88.8
  Liponyssoides sanguineus B88.0
  Loa loa B74.3
    conjunctival B74.3
    eyelid B74.3
  louse — *see* Infestation, Pediculus
  maggots — *see* Myiasis
  Mansonella (ozzardi) (perstans)
    (streptocerca) B74.4
  Medina (worm) B72
  Metagonimus (yokogawai) B66.8
  microfilaria streptocerca — *see*
    Onchocerciasis
    eye B73.00
    eyelid B73.09
  mites B88.9
    scabic B86
  Monilia (albicans) — *see* Candidiasis
  mouth B37.0
  Necator americanus B76.1
  nematode NEC (intestinal) B82.0
    Ancylostoma B76.0
    conjunctiva NEC B83.9
    Enterobius vermicularis B80
    Gnathostoma spinigerum B83.1
    physaloptera B80
    specified NEC B81.8
    trichostrongylus B81.2
    trichuris (trichuria) B79
  Oesophagostomum (apiostomum) B81.8
  Oestrus ovis — *see also* Myiasis B87.9
  Onchocerca (volvulus) — *see* Onchocerciasis
  Opisthorchis (felineus) (viverrini) B66.0
  orbit, parasitic NOS B89
  Oxyuris vermicularis B80
  Paragonimus (westermani) B66.4
  parasite, parasitic B89
    eyelid B89
    intestinal NOS B82.9
    mouth B37.0
    skin B88.9
    tongue B37.0
  Parastrongylus
    cantonensis B83.2
    costaricensis B81.3
  Pediculus B85.2
    body B85.1
    capitis (humanus) (any site) B85.0

Infestation - *continued*
  Pediculus - *continued*
    corporis (humanus) (any site) B85.1
    head B85.0
    mixed (classifiable to more than one of the titles B85.0-B85.3) B85.4
    pubis (any site) B85.3
  Pentastoma B88.8
  Phthirus (pubis) (any site) B85.3
    with any infestation classifiable to B85.0-B85.2 B85.4
  pinworm B80
  pork tapeworm (adult) B68.0
  protozoal NEC B64
    intestinal A07.9
      specified NEC A07.8
    specified NEC B60.8
  pubic, louse B85.3
  rat tapeworm B71.0
  red bug B88.0
  roundworm (large) NEC B82.0
    Ascariasis — *see also* Ascariasis B77.9
  sandflea B88.1
  Sarcoptes scabiei B86
  scabies B86
  Schistosoma B65.9
    bovis B65.8
    cercariae B65.3
    haematobium B65.0
    intercalatum B65.8
    japonicum B65.2
    mansoni B65.1
    mattheei B65.8
    mekongi B65.8
    specified type NEC B65.8
    spindale B65.8
  screw worms — *see* Myiasis
  skin NOS B88.9
  Sparganum (mansoni) (proliferum) (baxteri) B70.1
    larval B70.1
  specified type NEC B88.8
  Spirometra larvae B70.1
  Stellantchasmus falcatus B66.8
  Strongyloides stercoralis — *see* Strongyloidiasis
  Taenia B68.9
    diminuta B71.0
    echinococcus — *see* Echinococcus
    mediocanellata B68.1
    nana B71.0
    saginata B68.1
    solium (intestinal form) B68.0
      larval form — *see* Cysticercosis
  Taeniarhynchus saginatus B68.1
  tapeworm B71.9
    beef B68.1
    broad B70.0
      larval B70.1
    dog B67.4
    dwarf B71.0
    fish B70.0
      larval B70.1
    pork B68.0
    rat B71.0
  Ternidens diminutus B81.8
  Tetranychus molestissimus B88.0
  threadworm B80
  tongue B37.0
  Toxocara (canis) (cati) (felis) B83.0
  trematode (s) NEC — *see* Infestation, fluke
  Trichinella (spiralis) B75
  Trichocephalus B79
  Trichomonas — *see* Trichomoniasis
  Trichostrongylus B81.2
  Trichuris (trichiura) B79
  Trombicula (irritans) B88.0
  Tunga penetrans B88.1
  Uncinaria americana B76.1
  Vandellia cirrhosa B88.8
  whipworm B79
  worms B83.9
    intestinal B82.0
  Wuchereria (bancrofti) B74.0

Infiltrate, infiltration
  amyloid (generalized) (localized) — *see* Amyloidosis
  calcareous NEC R89.7
    localized — *see* Degeneration, by site
  calcium salt R89.7
  cardiac
    fatty — *see* Degeneration, myocardial
    glycogenic E74.02 *[I43]*
  corneal — *see* Edema, cornea
  eyelid — *see* Inflammation, eyelid
  glycogen, glycogenic — *see* Disease, glycogen storage
  heart, cardiac
    fatty — *see* Degeneration, myocardial
    glycogenic E74.02 *[I43]*
  inflammatory in vitreous H43.89
  kidney N28.89
  leukemic — *see* Leukemia
  liver K76.89
    fatty — *see* Fatty, liver NEC
    glycogen — *see also* Disease, glycogen storage E74.03 *[K77]*
  lung R91.8
    eosinophilic J82
  lymphatic — *see also* Leukemia, lymphatic C91.9-
    gland I88.9
  muscle, fatty M62.89
  myocardium, myocardial
    fatty — *see* Degeneration, myocardial
    glycogenic E74.02 *[I43]*
  on chest x-ray R91.8
  pulmonary R91.8
    with eosinophilia J82
  skin (lymphocytic) L98.6
  thymus (gland) (fatty) E32.8
  urine R39.0
  vesicant agent
    antineoplastic chemotherapy T80.810
    other agent NEC T80.818
  vitreous body H43.89

Infirmity R68.89
  senile R54

Inflammation, inflamed, inflammatory (with exudation)
  abducent (nerve) — *see* Strabismus, paralytic, sixth nerve
  accessory sinus (chronic) — *see* Sinusitis
  adrenal (gland) E27.8
  alveoli, teeth M27.3
    scorbutic E54
  anal canal, anus K62.89
  antrum (chronic) — *see* Sinusitis, maxillary
  appendix — *see* Appendicitis
  arachnoid — *see* Meningitis
  areola N61.0
    puerperal, postpartum or gestational — *see* Infection, nipple
  areolar tissue NOS L08.9
  artery — *see* Arteritis
  auditory meatus (external) — *see* Otitis, externa
  Bartholin's gland N75.8
  bile duct (common) (hepatic) or passage — *see* Cholangitis
  bladder — *see* Cystitis
  bone — *see* Osteomyelitis
  brain — *see also* Encephalitis
    membrane — *see* Meningitis
  breast N61.0
    puerperal, postpartum, gestational — *see* Mastitis, obstetric
  broad ligament — *see* Disease, pelvis, inflammatory
  bronchi — *see* Bronchitis
  catarrhal J00
  cecum — *see* Appendicitis
  cerebral — *see also* Encephalitis
    membrane — *see* Meningitis
  cerebrospinal
    meningococcal A39.0
  cervix (uteri) — *see* Cervicitis
  chest J98.8
  chorioretinal H30.9-

Inflammation, inflamed, inflammatory (with exudation) - *continued*
  chorioretinal - *continued*
    cyclitis — *see* Cyclitis
    disseminated H30.10-
      generalized H30.13-
      peripheral H30.12-
      posterior pole H30.11-
    epitheliopathy — *see* Epitheliopathy
    focal H30.00-
      juxtapapillary H30.01-
      macular H30.04-
      paramacular — *see* Inflammation, chorioretinal, focal, macular
      peripheral H30.03-
      posterior pole H30.02-
    specified type NEC H30.89-
  choroid — *see* Inflammation, chorioretinal
  chronic, postmastoidectomy cavity — *see* Complications, postmastoidectomy, inflammation
  colon — *see* Enteritis
  connective tissue (diffuse) NEC — *see* Disorder, soft tissue, specified type NEC
  cornea — *see* Keratitis
  corpora cavernosa N48.29
  cranial nerve — *see* Disorder, nerve, cranial
  Douglas' cul-de-sac or pouch (chronic) N73.0
  due to device, implant or graft — *see also* Complications, by site and type, infection or inflammation
    arterial graft T82.7
    breast (implant) T85.79
    catheter T85.79
      dialysis (renal) T82.7
        intraperitoneal T85.71
      infusion T82.7
        cranial T85.735
        intrathecal T85.735
        spinal (epidural) (subdural) T85.735
        subarachnoid T85.735
      urinary T83.518
        cystostomy T83.510
        Hopkins T83.518
        ileostomy T83.518
        nephrostomy T83.512
        specified NEC T83.518
        urethral indwelling T83.511
        urostomy T83.518
    electronic (electrode) (pulse generator) (stimulator)
      bone T84.7
      cardiac T82.7
      nervous system T85.738
        brain T85.731
        cranial nerve T85.732
        gastric nerve T85.732
        neurostimulator generator T85.734
        peripheral nerve T85.732
        sacral nerve T85.732
        spinal cord T85.733
        vagal nerve T85.732
      urinary T83.590
    fixation, internal (orthopedic) NEC — *see* Complication, fixation device, infection
    gastrointestinal (bile duct) (esophagus) T85.79
      neurostimulator electrode (lead) T85.732
    genital NEC T83.69
    heart NEC T82.7
      valve (prosthesis) T82.6
        graft T82.7
    joint prosthesis — *see* Complication, joint prosthesis, infection
    ocular (corneal graft) (orbital implant) NEC T85.79
    orthopedic NEC T84.7
    penile (cylinder) (pump) (resevoir) T83.61
    specified NEC T85.79
    testicular T83.62
    urinary NEC T83.598
      ileal conduit stent T83.593
      implanted neurostimulation T83.590

Inflammation, inflamed, inflammatory (with exudation) - *continued*
  due to device, implant or graft - *continued*
    urinary NEC - *continued*
      implanted sphincter T83.591
      indwelling ureteral stent T83.592
      nephroureteral stent T83.593
      specified stent NEC T83.593
    vascular NEC T82.7
    ventricular intracranial (communicating) shunt T85.730
  duodenum K29.80
    with bleeding K29.81
  dura mater — *see* Meningitis
  ear (middle) — *see also* Otitis, media
    external — *see* Otitis, externa
    inner — *see* subcategory H83.0
  epididymis — *see* Epididymitis
  esophagus K20.9
  ethmoidal (sinus) (chronic) — *see* Sinusitis, ethmoidal
  eustachian tube (catarrhal) — *see* Salpingitis, eustachian
  eyelid H01.9
    abscess — *see* Abscess, eyelid
    blepharitis — *see* Blepharitis
    chalazion — *see* Chalazion
    dermatosis (noninfectious) — *see* Dermatosis, eyelid
    hordeolum — *see* Hordeolum
    specified NEC H01.8
  fallopian tube — *see* Salpingo-oophoritis
  fascia — *see* Myositis
  follicular, pharynx J31.2
  frontal (sinus) (chronic) — *see* Sinusitis, frontal
  gallbladder — *see* Cholecystitis
  gastric — *see* Gastritis
  gastrointestinal — *see* Enteritis
  genital organ (internal) (diffuse)
    female — *see* Disease, pelvis, inflammatory
    male N49.9
      multiple sites N49.8
      specified NEC N49.8
  gland (lymph) — *see* Lymphadenitis
  glottis — *see* Laryngitis
  granular, pharynx J31.2
  gum K05.10
    nonplaque induced K05.11
    plaque induced K05.10
  heart — *see* Carditis
  hepatic duct — *see* Cholangitis
  ileoanal (internal) pouch K91.850
  ileum — *see also* Enteritis
    regional or terminal — *see* Enteritis, regional
  intestine (any part) — *see* Enteritis
  intestinal pouch K91.850
  jaw (acute) (bone) (chronic) (lower) (suppurative) (upper) M27.2
  joint NEC — *see* Arthritis
    sacroiliac M46.1
  kidney — *see* Nephritis
  knee (joint) M13.169
    tuberculous A18.02
  labium (majus) (minus) — *see* Vulvitis
  lacrimal
    gland — *see* Dacryoadenitis
    passages (duct) (sac) — *see also* Dacryocystitis
      canaliculitis — *see* Canaliculitis, lacrimal
  larynx — *see* Laryngitis
  leg NOS L08.9
  lip K13.0
  liver (capsule) — *see also* Hepatitis
    chronic K73.9
    suppurative K75.0
  lung (acute) — *see also* Pneumonia
    chronic J98.4
  lymph gland or node — *see* Lymphadenitis
  lymphatic vessel — *see* Lymphangitis
  maxilla, maxillary M27.2
    sinus (chronic) — *see* Sinusitis, maxillary

Inflammation, inflamed, inflammatory (with exudation) - *continued*
  membranes of brain or spinal cord — *see* Meningitis
  meninges — *see* Meningitis
  mouth K12.1
  muscle — *see* Myositis
  myocardium — *see* Myocarditis
  nasal sinus (chronic) — *see* Sinusitis
  nasopharynx — *see* Nasopharyngitis
  navel L08.82
  nerve NEC — *see* Neuralgia
  nipple N61.0
    puerperal, postpartum or gestational — *see* Infection, nipple
  nose — *see* Rhinitis
  oculomotor (nerve) — *see* Strabismus, paralytic, third nerve
  optic nerve — *see* Neuritis, optic
  orbit (chronic) H05.10
    acute H05.00
      abscess — *see* Abscess, orbit
      cellulitis — *see* Cellulitis, orbit
      osteomyelitis — *see* Osteomyelitis, orbit
      periostitis — *see* Periostitis, orbital
      tenonitis — *see* Tenonitis, eye
    granuloma — *see* Granuloma, orbit
    myositis — *see* Myositis, orbital
  ovary — *see* Salpingo-oophoritis
  oviduct — *see* Salpingo-oophoritis
  pancreas (acute) — *see* Pancreatitis
  parametrium N73.0
  parotid region L08.9
  pelvis, female — *see* Disease, pelvis, inflammatory
  penis (corpora cavernosa) N48.29
  perianal K62.89
  pericardium — *see* Pericarditis
  perineum (female) (male) L08.9
  perirectal K62.89
  peritoneum — *see* Peritonitis
  periuterine — *see* Disease, pelvis, inflammatory
  perivesical — *see* Cystitis
  petrous bone (acute) (chronic) — *see* Petrositis
  pharynx (acute) — *see* Pharyngitis
  pia mater — *see* Meningitis
  pleura — *see* Pleurisy
  polyp, colon — *see also* Polyp, colon, inflammatory K51.40
  prostate — *see also* Prostatitis
    specified type NEC N41.8
  rectosigmoid — *see* Rectosigmoiditis
  rectum — *see also* Proctitis K62.89
  respiratory, upper — *see also* Infection, respiratory, upper J06.9
    acute, due to radiation J70.0
    chronic, due to external agent — *see* condition, respiratory, chronic, due to
    due to
      chemicals, gases, fumes or vapors (inhalation) J68.2
      radiation J70.1
  retina — *see* Chorioretinitis
  retrocecal — *see* Appendicitis
  retroperitoneal — *see* Peritonitis
  salivary duct or gland (any) (suppurative) — *see* Sialoadenitis
  scorbutic, alveoli, teeth E54
  scrotum N49.2
  seminal vesicle — *see* Vesiculitis
  sigmoid — *see* Enteritis
  sinus — *see* Sinusitis
  Skene's duct or gland — *see* Urethritis
  skin L08.9
  spermatic cord N49.1
  sphenoidal (sinus) — *see* Sinusitis, sphenoidal
  spinal
    cord — *see* Encephalitis
    membrane — *see* Meningitis
    nerve — *see* Disorder, nerve
  spine — *see* Spondylopathy, inflammatory
  spleen (capsule) D73.89

Inflammation, inflamed, inflammatory (with exudation) - *continued*
  stomach — *see* Gastritis
  subcutaneous tissue L08.9
  suprarenal (gland) E27.8
  synovial — *see* Tenosynovitis
  tendon (sheath) NEC — *see* Tenosynovitis
  testis — *see* Orchitis
  throat (acute) — *see* Pharyngitis
  thymus (gland) E32.8
  thyroid (gland) — *see* Thyroiditis
  tongue K14.0
  tonsil — *see* Tonsillitis
  trachea — *see* Tracheitis
  trochlear (nerve) — *see* Strabismus, paralytic, fourth nerve
  tubal — *see* Salpingo-oophoritis
  tuberculous NEC — *see* Tuberculosis
  tubo-ovarian — *see* Salpingo-oophoritis
  tunica vaginalis N49.1
  tympanic membrane — *see* Tympanitis
  umbilicus, umbilical L08.82
  uterine ligament — *see* Disease, pelvis, inflammatory
  uterus (catarrhal) — *see* Endometritis
  uveal tract (anterior) NOS — *see also* Iridocyclitis
    posterior — *see* Chorioretinitis
  vagina — *see* Vaginitis
  vas deferens N49.1
  vein — *see also* Phlebitis
    intracranial or intraspinal (septic) G08
    thrombotic I80.9
      leg — *see* Phlebitis, leg
      lower extremity — *see* Phlebitis, leg
  vocal cord J38.3
  vulva — *see* Vulvitis
  Wharton's duct (suppurative) — *see* Sialoadenitis
Inflation, lung, imperfect (newborn) — *see* Atelectasis
Influenza (bronchial) (epidemic) (respiratory (upper)) (unidentified influenza virus) J11.1
  with
    digestive manifestations J11.2
    encephalopathy J11.81
    enteritis J11.2
    gastroenteritis J11.2
    gastrointestinal manifestations J11.2
    laryngitis J11.1
    myocarditis J11.82
    otitis media J11.83
    pharyngitis J11.1
    pneumonia J11.00
      specified type J11.08
    respiratory manifestations NEC J11.1
    specified manifestation NEC J11.89
  A/H5N1 — *see also* Influenza, due to, identified novel influenza A virus J09.X2
  avian — *see also* Influenza, due to, identified novel influenza A virus J09.X2
  bird — *see also* Influenza, due to, identified novel influenza A virus J09.X2
  novel (2009) H1N1 influenza — *see also* Influenza, due to, identified influenza virus NEC J10.1
  novel influenza A/H1N1 — *see also* Influenza, due to, identified influenza virus NEC J10.1
  due to
    avian — *see also* Influenza, due to, identified novel influenza A virus J09.X2
    identified influenza virus NEC J10.1
      with
        digestive manifestations J10.2
        encephalopathy J10.81
        enteritis J10.2
        gastroenteritis J10.2
        gastrointestinal manifestations J10.2
        laryngitis J10.1
        myocarditis J10.82
        otitis media J10.83

Influenza (bronchial) (epidemic) (respiratory (upper)) (unidentified influenza virus) - *continued*
  due to - *continued*
    identified influenza virus NEC - *continued*
      with - *continued*
        pharyngitis J10.1
        pneumonia (unspecified type) J10.00
          with same identified influenza virus J10.01
          specified type NEC J10.08
        respiratory manifestations NEC J10.1
        specified manifestation NEC J10.89
    identified novel influenza A virus J09.X2
      with
        digestive manifestations J09.X3
        encephalopathy J09.X9
        enteritis J09.X3
        gastroenteritis J09.X3
        gastrointestinal manifestations J09.X3
        laryngitis J09.X2
        myocarditis J09.X9
        otitis media J09.X9
        pharyngitis J09.X2
        pneumonia J09.X1
        respiratory manifestations NEC J09.X2
        specified manifestation NEC J09.X9
        upper respiratory symptoms J09.X2
    of other animal origin, not bird or swine — *see also* Influenza, due to, identified novel influenza A virus J09.X2
    swine (viruses that normally cause infections in pigs) — *see also* Influenza, due to, identified novel influenza A virus J09.X2
Influenzal — *see* Influenza
Influenza-like disease — *see* Influenza
Infraction, Freiberg's (metatarsal head) — *see* Osteochondrosis, juvenile, metatarsus
Infraeruption of tooth (teeth) M26.34
Infusion complication, misadventure, or reaction — *see* Complications, infusion
Ingestion
  chemical — *see* Table of Drugs and Chemicals, by substance, poisoning
  drug or medicament
    correct substance properly administered — *see* Table of Drugs and Chemicals, by drug, adverse effect
    overdose or wrong substance given or taken — *see* Table of Drugs and Chemicals, by drug, poisoning
  foreign body — *see* Foreign body, alimentary tract
  multiple drug — *see* Table of Drugs and Chemicals, multiple
  tularemia A21.3
Ingrowing
  hair (beard) L73.1
  nail (finger) (toe) L60.0
Inguinal — *see also* condition
  testicle Q53.9
    bilateral Q53.212
    unilateral Q53.112
Inhalant-induced
  anxiety disorder F18.980
  depressive disorder F18.94
  major neurocognitive disorder F18.97
  mild neurocognitive disorder F18.988
  psychotic disorder F18.959
Inhalation
  anthrax A22.1
  flame T27.3
  food or foreign body — *see* Foreign body, by site
  gases, fumes, or vapors NEC T59.9-
    specified agent — *see* Table of Drugs and Chemicals, by substance
  liquid or vomitus — *see* Asphyxia
  meconium (newborn) P24.00
    with
      pneumonia (pneumonitis) P24.01

Inhalation - *continued*
  meconium (newborn) - *continued*
    with - *continued*
      with respiratory symptoms P24.01
  mucus — *see* Asphyxia, mucus
  oil or gasoline (causing suffocation) — *see* Foreign body, by site
  smoke J70.5
    due to chemicals, gases, fumes and vapors J68.9
  steam — *see* Toxicity, vapors
  stomach contents or secretions — *see* Foreign body, by site
    due to anesthesia (general) (local) or other sedation T88.59
      in labor and delivery O74.0
      in pregnancy O29.01-
      postpartum, puerperal O89.01
Inhibition, orgasm
  female F52.31
  male F52.32
Inhibitor, systemic lupus erythematosus (presence of) D68.62
Iniencephalus, iniencephaly Q00.2
Injection, traumatic jet (air) (industrial) (water) (paint or dye) T70.4
Injury — *see also* specified injury type T14.90
  abdomen, abdominal S39.91
    blood vessel — *see* Injury, blood vessel, abdomen
    cavity — *see* Injury, intra-abdominal
    contusion S30.1
    internal — *see* Injury, intra-abdominal
    intra-abdominal organ — *see* Injury, intra-abdominal
    nerve — *see* Injury, nerve, abdomen
    open — *see* Wound, open, abdomen
    specified NEC S39.81
    superficial — *see* Injury, superficial, abdomen
  Achilles tendon S86.00-
    laceration S86.02-
    specified type NEC S86.09-
    strain S86.01-
  acoustic, resulting in deafness — *see* Injury, nerve, acoustic
  adrenal (gland) S37.819
    contusion S37.812
    laceration S37.813
    specified type NEC S37.818
  alveolar (process) S09.93
  ankle S99.91-
    contusion — *see* Contusion, ankle
    dislocation — *see* Dislocation, ankle
    fracture — *see* Fracture, ankle
    nerve — *see* Injury, nerve, ankle
    open — *see* Wound, open, ankle
    specified type NEC S99.81-
    sprain — *see* Sprain, ankle
    superficial — *see* Injury, superficial, ankle
  anterior chamber, eye — *see* Injury, eye, specified site NEC
  anus — *see* Injury, abdomen
  aorta (thoracic) S25.00
    abdominal S35.00
      laceration (minor) (superficial) S35.01
        major S35.02
      specified type NEC S35.09
    laceration (minor) (superficial) S25.01
      major S25.02
    specified type NEC S25.09
  arm (upper) S49.9-
    blood vessel — *see* Injury, blood vessel, arm
    contusion — *see* Contusion, arm, upper
    fracture — *see* Fracture, humerus
    lower — *see* Injury, forearm
    muscle — *see* Injury, muscle, shoulder
    nerve — *see* Injury, nerve, arm
    open — *see* Wound, open, arm
    specified type NEC S49.8-
    superficial — *see* Injury, superficial, arm
  artery (complicating trauma) — *see also* Injury, blood vessel, by site

Injury - *continued*
  artery (complicating trauma) - *continued*
    cerebral or meningeal — *see* Injury, intracranial
  auditory canal (external) (meatus) S09.91
  auricle, auris, ear S09.91
  axilla — *see* Injury, shoulder
  back — *see* Injury, back, lower
  bile duct S36.13
  birth — *see also* Birth, injury P15.9
  bladder (sphincter) S37.20
    at delivery O71.5
    contusion S37.22
    laceration S37.23
    obstetrical trauma O71.5
    specified type NEC S37.29
  blast (air) (hydraulic) (immersion) (underwater) NEC T14.8
    acoustic nerve trauma — *see* Injury, nerve, acoustic
    bladder — *see* Injury, bladder
    brain — *see* Concussion
    colon — *see* Injury, intestine, large, blast injury
    ear (primary) S09.31-
      secondary S09.39-
    generalized T70.8
    lung — *see* Injury, intrathoracic, lung, blast injury
    multiple body organs T70.8
    peritoneum S36.81
    rectum S36.61
    retroperitoneum S36.898
    small intestine S36.419
      duodenum S36.410
      specified site NEC S36.418
    specified
      intra-abdominal organ NEC S36.898
      pelvic organ NEC S37.899
  blood vessel NEC T14.8
    abdomen S35.9-
      aorta — *see* Injury, aorta, abdominal
      celiac artery — *see* Injury, blood vessel, celiac artery
      iliac vessel — *see* Injury, blood vessel, iliac
      laceration S35.91
      mesenteric vessel — *see* Injury, mesenteric
      portal vein — *see* Injury, blood vessel, portal vein
      renal vessel — *see* Injury, blood vessel, renal
      specified vessel NEC S35.8X-
      splenic vessel — *see* Injury, blood vessel, splenic
      vena cava — *see* Injury, vena cava, inferior
    ankle — *see* Injury, blood vessel, foot
    aorta (abdominal) (thoracic) — *see* Injury, aorta
    arm (upper) NEC S45.90-
      forearm — *see* Injury, blood vessel, forearm
      laceration S45.91-
      specified
        site NEC S45.80-
          laceration S45.81-
          specified type NEC S45.89-
        type NEC S45.99-
      superficial vein S45.30-
        laceration S45.31-
        specified type NEC S45.39-
    axillary
      artery S45.00-
        laceration S45.01-
        specified type NEC S45.09-
      vein S45.20-
        laceration S45.21-
        specified type NEC S45.29-
    azygos vein — *see* Injury, blood vessel, thoracic, specified site NEC
    brachial
      artery S45.10-
        laceration S45.11-

Injury - *continued*
blood vessel NEC - *continued*
brachial - *continued*
artery - *continued*
specified type NEC S45.19-
vein S45.20-
laceration S45.219
specified type NEC S45.29-
carotid artery (common) (external)
(internal, extracranial) S15.00-
internal, intracranial S06.8-
laceration (minor) (superficial) S15.01-
major S15.02-
specified type NEC S15.09-
celiac artery S35.219
branch S35.299
laceration (minor)
(superficial) S35.291
major S35.292
specified NEC S35.298
laceration (minor) (superficial) S35.211
major S35.212
specified type NEC S35.218
cerebral — *see* Injury, intracranial
deep plantar — *see* Injury, blood vessel,
plantar artery
digital (hand) — *see* Injury, blood vessel,
finger
dorsal
artery (foot) S95.00-
laceration S95.01-
specified type NEC S95.09-
vein (foot) S95.20-
laceration S95.21-
specified type NEC S95.29-
due to accidental laceration during
procedure — *see* Laceration,
accidental complicating surgery
extremity — *see* Injury, blood vessel, limb
femoral
artery (common) (superficial) S75.00-
laceration (minor)
(superficial) S75.01-
major S75.02-
specified type NEC S75.09-
vein (hip level) (thigh level) S75.10-
laceration (minor)
(superficial) S75.11-
major S75.12-
specified type NEC S75.19-
finger S65.50-
index S65.50-
laceration S65.51-
specified type NEC S65.59-
laceration S65.51-
little S65.50-
laceration S65.51-
specified type NEC S65.59-
middle S65.50-
laceration S65.51-
specified type NEC S65.59-
specified type NEC S65.59-
thumb — *see* Injury, blood vessel, thumb
foot S95.90-
dorsal
artery — *see* Injury, blood vessel,
dorsal, artery
vein — *see* Injury, blood vessel,
dorsal, vein
laceration S95.91-
plantar artery — *see* Injury, blood vessel,
plantar artery
specified
site NEC S95.80-
laceration S95.81-
specified type NEC S95.89-
specified type NEC S95.99-
forearm S55.90-
laceration S55.91-
radial artery — *see* Injury, blood vessel,
radial artery
specified
site NEC S55.80-
laceration S55.81-
specified type NEC S55.89-

Injury - *continued*
blood vessel NEC - *continued*
forearm - *continued*
specified - *continued*
type NEC S55.99-
ulnar artery — *see* Injury, blood vessel,
ulnar artery
vein S55.20-
laceration S55.21-
specified type NEC S55.29-
gastric
artery — *see* Injury, mesenteric, artery,
branch
vein — *see* Injury, blood vessel,
abdomen
gastroduodenal artery — *see* Injury,
mesenteric, artery, branch
greater saphenous vein (lower leg
level) S85.30-
hip (and thigh) level S75.20-
laceration (minor)
(superficial) S75.21-
major S75.22-
specified type NEC S75.29-
laceration S85.31-
specified type NEC S85.39-
hand (level) S65.90-
finger — *see* Injury, blood vessel, finger
laceration S65.91-
palmar arch — *see* Injury, blood vessel,
palmar arch
radial artery — *see* Injury, blood vessel,
radial artery, hand
specified
site NEC S65.80-
laceration S65.81-
specified type NEC S65.89-
type NEC S65.99-
thumb — *see* Injury, blood vessel, thumb
ulnar artery — *see* Injury, blood vessel,
ulnar artery, hand
head S09.0
intracranial — *see* Injury, intracranial
multiple S09.0
hepatic
artery — *see* Injury, mesenteric, artery
vein — *see* Injury, vena cava, inferior
hip S75.90-
femoral artery — *see* Injury, blood
vessel, femoral, artery
femoral vein — *see* Injury, blood vessel,
femoral, vein
greater saphenous vein — *see* Injury,
blood vessel, greater saphenous, hip
level
laceration S75.91-
specified
site NEC S75.80-
laceration S75.81-
specified type NEC S75.89-
type NEC S75.99-
hypogastric (artery) (vein) — *see* Injury,
blood vessel, iliac
iliac S35.5-
artery S35.51-
specified vessel NEC S35.5-
uterine vessel — *see* Injury, blood
vessel, uterine
vein S35.51-
innominate — *see* Injury, blood vessel,
thoracic, innominate
intercostal (artery) (vein) — *see* Injury,
blood vessel, thoracic, intercostal
jugular vein (external) S15.20-
internal S15.30-
laceration (minor)
(superficial) S15.31-
major S15.32-
specified type NEC S15.39-
laceration (minor) (superficial) S15.21-
major S15.22-
specified type NEC S15.29-
leg (level) (lower) S85.90-
greater saphenous — *see* Injury, blood
vessel, greater saphenous

Injury - *continued*
blood vessel NEC - *continued*
leg (level) (lower) - *continued*
laceration S85.91-
lesser saphenous — *see* Injury, blood
vessel, lesser saphenous
peroneal artery — *see* Injury, blood
vessel, peroneal artery
popliteal
artery — *see* Injury, blood vessel,
popliteal, artery
vein — *see* Injury, blood vessel,
popliteal, vein
specified
site NEC S85.80-
laceration S85.81-
specified type NEC S85.89-
type NEC S85.99-
thigh — *see* Injury, blood vessel, hip
tibial artery — *see* Injury, blood vessel,
tibial artery
lesser saphenous vein (lower leg
level) S85.40-
laceration S85.41-
specified type NEC S85.49-
limb
lower — *see* Injury, blood vessel, leg
upper — *see* Injury, blood vessel, arm
lower back — *see* Injury, blood vessel,
abdomen
specified NEC — *see* Injury, blood
vessel, abdomen, specified, site
NEC
mammary (artery) (vein) — *see* Injury,
blood vessel, thoracic, specified site
NEC
mesenteric (inferior) (superior)
artery — *see* Injury, mesenteric, artery
vein — *see* Injury, mesenteric, vein
neck S15.9
specified site NEC S15.8
ovarian (artery) (vein) — *see* subcategory
S35.8
palmar arch (superficial) S65.20-
deep S65.30-
laceration S65.31-
specified type NEC S65.39-
laceration S65.21-
specified type NEC S65.29-
pelvis — *see* Injury, blood vessel,
abdomen
specified NEC — *see* Injury, blood
vessel, abdomen, specified, site
NEC
peroneal artery S85.20-
laceration S85.21-
specified type NEC S85.29-
plantar artery (deep) (foot) S95.10-
laceration S95.11-
specified type NEC S95.19-
popliteal
artery S85.00-
laceration S85.01-
specified type NEC S85.09-
vein S85.50-
laceration S85.51-
specified type NEC S85.59-
portal vein S35.319
laceration S35.311
specified type NEC S35.318
precerebral — *see* Injury, blood vessel,
neck
pulmonary (artery) (vein) — *see* Injury,
blood vessel, thoracic, pulmonary
radial artery (forearm level) S55.10-
hand and wrist (level) S65.10-
laceration S65.11-
specified type NEC S65.19-
laceration S55.11-
specified type NEC S55.19-
renal
artery S35.40-
laceration S35.41-
specified NEC S35.49-
vein S35.40-

Injury - *continued*
  blood vessel NEC - *continued*
    renal - *continued*
      vein - *continued*
        laceration S35.41-
        specified NEC S35.49-
      saphenous vein (greater) (lower leg
          level) — *see* Injury, blood vessel,
          greater saphenous
        hip and thigh level — *see* Injury, blood
            vessel, greater saphenous, hip level
        lesser — *see* Injury, blood vessel, lesser
            saphenous
      shoulder
        specified NEC — *see* Injury, blood
            vessel, arm, specified site NEC
        superficial vein — *see* Injury, blood
            vessel, arm, superficial vein
      specified NEC T14.8
      splenic
        artery — *see* Injury, blood vessel, celiac
            artery, branch
        vein S35.329
          laceration S35.321
          specified NEC S35.328
      subclavian — *see* Injury, blood vessel,
          thoracic, innominate
      thigh — *see* Injury, blood vessel, hip
      thoracic S25.90
        aorta S25.00
          laceration (minor) (superficial) S25.01
          major S25.02
          specified type NEC S25.09
        azygos vein — *see* Injury, blood vessel,
            thoracic, specified, site NEC
        innominate
          artery S25.10-
            laceration (minor)
                (superficial) S25.11-
            major S25.12-
            specified type NEC S25.19-
          vein S25.30-
            laceration (minor)
                (superficial) S25.31-
            major S25.32-
            specified type NEC S25.39-
        intercostal S25.50-
          laceration S25.51-
          specified type NEC S25.59-
        laceration S25.91
        mammary vessel — *see* Injury, blood
            vessel, thoracic, specified, site NEC
        pulmonary S25.40-
          laceration (minor)
              (superficial) S25.41-
          major S25.42-
          specified type NEC S25.49-
        specified
          site NEC S25.80-
            laceration S25.81-
            specified type NEC S25.89-
          type NEC S25.99
        subclavian — *see* Injury, blood vessel,
            thoracic, innominate
        vena cava (superior) S25.20
          laceration (minor) (superficial) S25.21
          major S25.22
          specified type NEC S25.29
      thumb S65.40-
        laceration S65.41-
        specified type NEC S65.49-
      tibial artery S85.10-
        anterior S85.13-
          laceration S85.14-
          specified injury NEC S85.15-
        laceration S85.11-
        posterior S85.16-
          laceration S85.17-
          specified injury NEC S85.18-
        specified injury NEC S85.12-
      ulnar artery (forearm level) S55.00-
        hand and wrist (level) S65.00-
          laceration S65.01-
          specified type NEC S65.09-
        laceration S55.01-

Injury - *continued*
  blood vessel NEC - *continued*
    ulnar artery (forearm level) - *continued*
      specified type NEC S55.09-
    upper arm (level) — *see* Injury, blood
        vessel, arm
      superficial vein — *see* Injury, blood
          vessel, arm, superficial vein
    uterine S35.5-
      artery S35.53-
      vein S35.53-
    vena cava — *see* Injury, vena cava
    vertebral artery S15.10-
      laceration (minor) (superficial) S15.11-
      major S15.12-
      specified type NEC S15.19-
    wrist (level) — *see* Injury, blood vessel,
        hand
  brachial plexus S14.3
    newborn P14.3
  brain (traumatic) S06.9-
    diffuse (axonal) S06.2X-
    focal S06.30-
  brainstem S06.38-
  breast NOS S29.9
  broad ligament — *see* Injury, pelvic organ,
      specified site NEC
  bronchus, bronchi — *see* Injury,
      intrathoracic, bronchus
  brow S09.90
  buttock S39.92
  canthus, eye S05.90
  cardiac plexus — *see* Injury, nerve, thorax,
      sympathetic
  cauda equina S34.3
  cavernous sinus — *see* Injury, intracranial
  cecum — *see* Injury, colon
  celiac ganglion or plexus — *see* Injury,
      nerve, lumbosacral, sympathetic
  cerebellum — *see* Injury, intracranial
  cerebral — *see* Injury, intracranial
  cervix (uteri) — *see* Injury, uterus
  cheek (wall) S09.93
  chest — *see* Injury, thorax
  childbirth (newborn) — *see also* Birth, injury
    maternal NEC O71.9
  chin S09.93
  choroid (eye) — *see* Injury, eye, specified
      site NEC
  clitoris S39.94
  coccyx — *see also* Injury, back, lower
    complicating delivery O71.6
  colon — *see* Injury, intestine, large
  common bile duct — *see* Injury, liver
  conjunctiva (superficial) — *see* Injury, eye,
      conjunctiva
  conus medullaris — *see* Injury, spinal, sacral
      cord
    spermatic (pelvic region) S37.898
      scrotal region S39.848
    spinal — *see* Injury, spinal cord, by region
  cornea — *see* Injury, eye, specified site NEC
    abrasion — *see* Injury, eye, cornea,
        abrasion
  cortex (cerebral) — *see also* Injury,
      intracranial
    visual — *see* Injury, nerve, optic
  costal region NEC S29.9
  costochondral NEC S29.9
  cranial
    cavity — *see* Injury, intracranial
    nerve — *see* Injury, nerve, cranial
  crushing — *see* Crush
  cutaneous sensory nerve
  cystic duct — *see* Injury, liver
  deep tissue — *see* Contusion, by site
    meaning pressure ulcer — *see* Ulcer,
        pressure, unstageable, by site
  delivery (newborn) P15.9
    maternal NEC O71.9
  Descemet's membrane — *see* Injury, eyeball,
      penetrating
  diaphragm — *see* Injury, intrathoracic,
      diaphragm

Injury - *continued*
  duodenum — *see* Injury, intestine, small,
      duodenum
  ear (auricle) (external) (canal) S09.91
    abrasion — *see* Abrasion, ear
    bite — *see* Bite, ear
    blister — *see* Blister, ear
    bruise — *see* Contusion, ear
    contusion — *see* Contusion, ear
    external constriction — *see* Constriction,
        external, ear
    hematoma — *see* Hematoma, ear
    inner — *see* Injury, ear, middle
    laceration — *see* Laceration, ear
    middle S09.30-
      blast — *see* Injury, blast, ear
      specified NEC S09.39-
    puncture — *see* Puncture, ear
    superficial — *see* Injury, superficial, ear
  eighth cranial nerve (acoustic or
      auditory) — *see* Injury, nerve, acoustic
  elbow S59.90-
    contusion — *see* Contusion, elbow
    dislocation — *see* Dislocation, elbow
    fracture — *see* Fracture, ulna, upper end
    open — *see* Wound, open, elbow
    specified NEC S59.80-
    sprain — *see* Sprain, elbow
    superficial — *see* Injury, superficial, elbow
  eleventh cranial nerve (accessory) — *see*
      Injury, nerve, accessory
  epididymis S39.94
  epigastric region S39.91
  epiglottis NEC S19.89
  esophageal plexus — *see* Injury, nerve,
      thorax, sympathetic
  esophagus (thoracic part) — *see also* Injury,
      intrathoracic, esophagus
    cervical NEC S19.85
  eustachian tube S09.30-
  eye S05.9-
    avulsion S05.7-
    ball — *see* Injury, eyeball
    conjunctiva S05.0-
    cornea
      abrasion S05.0-
      laceration S05.3-
        with prolapse S05.2-
    lacrimal apparatus S05.8X-
    orbit penetration S05.4-
    specified site NEC S05.8X-
  eyeball S05.8X-
    contusion S05.1-
    penetrating S05.6-
      with
        foreign body S05.5-
        prolapse or loss of intraocular
            tissue S05.2-
      without prolapse or loss of intraocular
          tissue S05.3-
    specified type NEC S05.8-
  eyebrow S09.93
  eyelid S09.93
    abrasion — *see* Abrasion, eyelid
    contusion — *see* Contusion, eyelid
    open — *see* Wound, open, eyelid
  face S09.93
  fallopian tube S37.509
    bilateral S37.502
      blast injury S37.512
      contusion S37.522
      laceration S37.532
      specified type NEC S37.592
    blast injury (primary) S37.519
      bilateral S37.512
      secondary — *see* Injury, fallopian tube,
          specified type NEC
      unilateral S37.511
    contusion S37.529
      bilateral S37.522
      unilateral S37.521
    laceration S37.539
      bilateral S37.532
      unilateral S37.531
    specified type NEC S37.599

Injury - *continued*
  fallopian tube - *continued*
    specified type NEC - *continued*
      bilateral S37.592
      unilateral S37.591
    unilateral S37.501
      blast injury S37.511
      contusion S37.521
      laceration S37.531
      specified type NEC S37.591
  fascia — *see* Injury, muscle
  fifth cranial nerve (trigeminal) — *see* Injury, nerve, trigeminal
  finger (nail) S69.9-
    blood vessel — *see* Injury, blood vessel, finger
    contusion — *see* Contusion, finger
    dislocation — *see* Dislocation, finger
    fracture — *see* Fracture, finger
    muscle — *see* Injury, muscle, finger
    nerve — *see* Injury, nerve, digital, finger
    open — *see* Wound, open, finger
    specified NEC S69.8-
    sprain — *see* Sprain, finger
    superficial — *see* Injury, superficial, finger
  first cranial nerve (olfactory) — *see* Injury, nerve, olfactory
  flank — *see* Injury, abdomen
  foot S99.92-
    blood vessel — *see* Injury, blood vessel, foot
    contusion — *see* Contusion, foot
    dislocation — *see* Dislocation, foot
    fracture — *see* Fracture, foot
    muscle — *see* Injury, muscle, foot
    open — *see* Wound, open, foot
    specified type NEC S99.82-
    sprain — *see* Sprain, foot
    superficial — *see* Injury, superficial, foot
  forceps NOS P15.9
  forearm S59.91-
    blood vessel — *see* Injury, blood vessel, forearm
    contusion — *see* Contusion, forearm
    fracture — *see* Fracture, forearm
    muscle — *see* Injury, muscle, forearm
    nerve — *see* Injury, nerve, forearm
    open — *see* Wound, open, forearm
    specified NEC S59.81-
    superficial — *see* Injury, superficial, forearm
  forehead S09.90
  fourth cranial nerve (trochlear) — *see* Injury, nerve, trochlear
  gallbladder S36.129
    contusion S36.122
    laceration S36.123
    specified NEC S36.128
  ganglion
    celiac, coeliac — *see* Injury, nerve, lumbosacral, sympathetic
    gasserian — *see* Injury, nerve, trigeminal
    stellate — *see* Injury, nerve, thorax, sympathetic
    thoracic sympathetic — *see* Injury, nerve, thorax, sympathetic
  gasserian ganglion — *see* Injury, nerve, trigeminal
  gastric artery — *see* Injury, blood vessel, celiac artery, branch
  gastroduodenal artery — *see* Injury, blood vessel, celiac artery, branch
  gastrointestinal tract — *see* Injury, intra-abdominal
    with open wound into abdominal cavity — *see* Wound, open, with penetration into peritoneal cavity
    colon — *see* Injury, intestine, large
    rectum — *see* Injury, intestine, large, rectum
      with open wound into abdominal cavity S36.61
    specified site NEC — *see* Injury, intra-abdominal, specified, site NEC
    stomach — *see* Injury, stomach

Injury - *continued*
  gastrointestinal tract - *continued*
    small intestine — *see* Injury, intestine, small
  genital organ (s)
    external S39.94
      specified NEC S39.848
    internal S37.90
      fallopian tube — *see* Injury, fallopian tube
      ovary — *see* Injury, ovary
      prostate — *see* Injury, prostate
      seminal vesicle — *see* Injury, pelvis, organ, specified site NEC
      uterus — *see* Injury, uterus
      vas deferens — *see* Injury, pelvis, organ, specified site NEC
    obstetrical trauma O71.9
  gland
    lacrimal laceration — *see* Injury, eye, specified site NEC
    salivary S09.93
    thyroid S19.84
  globe (eye) S05.90
    specified NEC S05.8X-
  groin — *see* Injury, abdomen
  gum S09.90
  hand S69.9-
    blood vessel — *see* Injury, blood vessel, hand
    contusion — *see* Contusion, hand
    fracture — *see* Fracture, hand
    muscle — *see* Injury, muscle, hand
    nerve — *see* Injury, nerve, hand
    open — *see* Wound, open, hand
    specified NEC S69.8-
    sprain — *see* Sprain, hand
    superficial — *see* Injury, superficial, hand
  head S09.90
    with loss of consciousness S06.9-
    specified NEC S09.8
  heart S26.90
    with hemopericardium S26.00
      contusion S26.01
      laceration (mild) S26.020
        moderate S26.021
        major S26.022
      specified type NEC S26.09
    contusion S26.91
    laceration S26.92
    specified type NEC S26.99
    without hemopericardium S26.10
      contusion S26.11
      laceration S26.12
      specified type NEC S26.19
  heel — *see* Injury, foot
  hepatic
    artery — *see* Injury, blood vessel, celiac artery, branch
    duct — *see* Injury, liver
    vein — *see* Injury, vena cava, inferior
  hip S79.91-
    blood vessel — *see* Injury, blood vessel, hip
    contusion — *see* Contusion, hip
    dislocation — *see* Dislocation, hip
    fracture — *see* Fracture, femur, neck
    muscle — *see* Injury, muscle, hip
    nerve — *see* Injury, nerve, hip
    open — *see* Wound, open, hip
    sprain — *see* Sprain, hip
    superficial — *see* Injury, superficial, hip
    specified NEC S79.81-
  hymen S39.94
  hypogastric
    blood vessel — *see* Injury, blood vessel, iliac
    plexus — *see* Injury, nerve, lumbosacral, sympathetic
  ileum — *see* Injury, intestine, small
  iliac region S39.91
  instrumental (during surgery) — *see* Laceration, accidental complicating surgery
    birth injury — *see* Birth, injury

Injury - *continued*
  instrumental (during surgery) - *continued*
    nonsurgical — *see* Injury, by site
    obstetrical O71.9
      bladder O71.5
      cervix O71.3
      high vaginal O71.4
      perineal NOS O70.9
      urethra O71.5
      uterus O71.5
        with rupture or perforation O71.1
  internal T14.8
    aorta — *see* Injury, aorta
    bladder (sphincter) — *see* Injury, bladder
      with
        ectopic or molar pregnancy O08.6
        following ectopic or molar pregnancy O08.6
      obstetrical trauma O71.5
    bronchus, bronchi — *see* Injury, intrathoracic, bronchus
    cecum — *see* Injury, intestine, large
    cervix (uteri) — *see also* Injury, uterus
      with ectopic or molar pregnancy O08.6
      following ectopic or molar pregnancy O08.6
      obstetrical trauma O71.3
    chest — *see* Injury, intrathoracic
    gastrointestinal tract — *see* Injury, intra-abdominal
    heart — *see* Injury, heart
    intestine NEC — *see* Injury, intestine
    intrauterine — *see* Injury, uterus
    mesentery — *see* Injury, intra-abdominal, specified, site NEC
    pelvis, pelvic (organ) S37.90
      following ectopic or molar pregnancy (subsequent episode) O08.6
      obstetrical trauma NEC O71.5
      rupture or perforation O71.1
      specified NEC S39.83
    rectum — *see* Injury, intestine, large, rectum
    stomach — *see* Injury, stomach
    ureter — *see* Injury, ureter
    urethra (sphincter) following ectopic or molar pregnancy O08.6
    uterus — *see* Injury, uterus
  interscapular area — *see* Injury, thorax
  intestine
    large S36.509
      ascending (right) S36.500
        blast injury (primary) S36.510
          secondary S36.590
        contusion S36.520
        laceration S36.530
        specified type NEC S36.590
      blast injury (primary) S36.519
        ascending (right) S36.510
        descending (left) S36.512
        rectum S36.61
        sigmoid S36.513
        specified site NEC S36.518
        transverse S36.511
      contusion S36.529
        ascending (right) S36.520
        descending (left) S36.522
        rectum S36.62
        sigmoid S36.523
        specified site NEC S36.528
        transverse S36.521
      descending (left) S36.502
        blast injury (primary) S36.512
          secondary S36.592
        contusion S36.522
        laceration S36.532
        specified type NEC S36.592
      laceration S36.539
        ascending (right) S36.530
        descending (left) S36.532
        rectum S36.63
        sigmoid S36.533
        specified site NEC S36.538
        transverse S36.531
      rectum S36.60

Injury - *continued*
intestine - *continued*
  large - *continued*
    rectum - *continued*
      blast injury (primary) S36.61
        secondary S36.69
      contusion S36.62
      laceration S36.63
      specified type NEC S36.69
    sigmoid S36.503
      blast injury (primary) S36.513
        secondary S36.593
      contusion S36.523
      laceration S36.533
      specified type NEC S36.593
    specified
      site NEC S36.508
        blast injury (primary) S36.518
          secondary S36.598
        contusion S36.528
        laceration S36.538
        specified type NEC S36.598
      type NEC S36.599
        ascending (right) S36.590
        descending (left) S36.592
        rectum S36.69
        sigmoid S36.593
        specified site NEC S36.598
        transverse S36.591
    transverse S36.501
      blast injury (primary) S36.511
        secondary S36.591
      contusion S36.521
      laceration S36.531
      specified type NEC S36.591
  small S36.409
    blast injury (primary) S36.419
      duodenum S36.410
        secondary S36.499
          duodenum S36.490
            specified site NEC S36.498
        specified site NEC S36.418
    contusion S36.429
      duodenum S36.420
      specified site NEC S36.428
    duodenum S36.400
      blast injury (primary) S36.410
        secondary S36.490
      contusion S36.420
      laceration S36.430
      specified NEC S36.490
    laceration S36.439
      duodenum S36.430
      specified site NEC S36.438
    specified
      type NEC S36.499
        duodenum S36.490
        specified site NEC S36.498
      site NEC S36.408
intra-abdominal S36.90
  adrenal gland — *see* Injury, adrenal gland
  bladder — *see* Injury, bladder
  colon — *see* Injury, intestine, large
  contusion S36.92
  fallopian tube — *see* Injury, fallopian tube
  gallbladder — *see* Injury, gallbladder
  intestine — *see* Injury, intestine
  laceration S36.93
  liver — *see* Injury, liver
  kidney — *see* Injury, kidney
  ovary — *see* Injury, ovary
  pancreas — *see* Injury, pancreas
  pelvic NOS S37.90
  peritoneum — *see* Injury, intra-abdominal,
    specified, site NEC
  prostate — *see* Injury, prostate
  rectum — *see* Injury, intestine, large,
    rectum
  retroperitoneum — *see* Injury, intra-
    abdominal, specified, site NEC
  seminal vesicle — *see* Injury, pelvis,
    organ, specified site NEC
  small intestine — *see* Injury, intestine,
    small
  specified

Injury - *continued*
intra-abdominal - *continued*
  specified - *continued*
    site NEC S36.899
      contusion S36.892
      laceration S36.893
      specified type NEC S36.898
    type NEC S36.99
  pelvic S37.90
    specified
      site NEC S37.899
        specified type NEC S37.898
      type NEC S37.99
  spleen — *see* Injury, spleen
  stomach — *see* Injury, stomach
  ureter — *see* Injury, ureter
  urethra — *see* Injury, urethra
  uterus — *see* Injury, uterus
  vas deferens — *see* Injury, pelvis, organ,
    specified site NEC
intracranial (traumatic) S06.9-
  cerebellar hemorrhage, traumatic — *see*
    Injury, intracranial, focal
  cerebral edema, traumatic S06.1X-
    diffuse S06.1X-
    focal S06.1X-
  diffuse (axonal) S06.2X-
  epidural hemorrhage (traumatic) S06.4X-
  focal brain injury S06.30-
    contusion — *see* Contusion, cerebral
    laceration — *see* Laceration, cerebral
    intracerebral hemorrhage,
      traumatic S06.36-
      left side S06.35-
      right side S06.34-
    subarachnoid hemorrhage,
      traumatic S06.6X-
    subdural hemorrhage, traumatic S06.5X-
intraocular — *see* Injury, eyeball, penetrating
intrathoracic S27.9
  bronchus S27.409
    bilateral S27.402
    blast injury (primary) S27.419
      bilateral S27.412
      secondary — *see* Injury, intrathoracic,
        bronchus, specified type NEC
      unilateral S27.411
    contusion S27.429
      bilateral S27.422
      unilateral S27.421
    laceration S27.439
      bilateral S27.432
      unilateral S27.431
    specified type NEC S27.499
      bilateral S27.492
      unilateral S27.491
    unilateral S27.401
  diaphragm S27.809
    contusion S27.802
    laceration S27.803
    specified type NEC S27.808
  esophagus (thoracic) S27.819
    contusion S27.812
    laceration S27.813
    specified type NEC S27.818
  heart — *see* Injury, heart
  hemopneumothorax S27.2
  hemothorax S27.1
  lung S27.309
    aspiration J69.0
    bilateral S27.302
    blast injury (primary) S27.319
      bilateral S27.312
      secondary — *see* Injury, intrathoracic,
        lung, specified type NEC
      unilateral S27.311
    contusion S27.329
      bilateral S27.322
      unilateral S27.321
    laceration S27.339
      bilateral S27.332
      unilateral S27.331
    specified type NEC S27.399
      bilateral S27.392
      unilateral S27.391

Injury - *continued*
intrathoracic - *continued*
  lung - *continued*
    unilateral S27.301
  pleura S27.60
    laceration S27.63
    specified type NEC S27.69
  pneumothorax S27.0
  specified organ NEC S27.899
    contusion S27.892
    laceration S27.893
    specified type NEC S27.898
  thoracic duct — *see* Injury, intrathoracic,
    specified organ NEC
  thymus gland — *see* Injury, intrathoracic,
    specified organ NEC
  trachea, thoracic S27.50
    blast (primary) S27.51
    contusion S27.52
    laceration S27.53
    specified type NEC S27.59
iris — *see* Injury, eye, specified site NEC
  penetrating — *see* Injury, eyeball,
    penetrating
jaw S09.93
jejunum — *see* Injury, intestine, small
joint NOS T14.8
  old or residual — *see* Disorder, joint,
    specified type NEC
kidney S37.00-
  acute (nontraumatic) N17.9
  contusion — *see* Contusion, kidney
  laceration — *see* Laceration, kidney
  specified NEC S37.09-
knee S89.9-
  contusion — *see* Contusion, knee
  dislocation — *see* Dislocation, knee
  meniscus (lateral) (medial) — *see* Sprain,
    knee, specified site NEC
  old injury or tear — *see* Derangement,
    knee, meniscus, due to old injury
  open — *see* Wound, open, knee
  specified NEC S89.8-
  sprain — *see* Sprain, knee
  superficial — *see* Injury, superficial, knee
labium (majus) (minus) S39.94
labyrinth, ear S09.30-
lacrimal apparatus, duct, gland, or sac — *see*
  Injury, eye, specified site NEC
larynx NEC S19.81
leg (lower) S89.9-
  blood vessel — *see* Injury, blood vessel,
    leg
  contusion — *see* Contusion, leg
  fracture — *see* Fracture, leg
  muscle — *see* Injury, muscle, leg
  nerve — *see* Injury, nerve, leg
  open — *see* Wound, open, leg
  specified NEC S89.8-
  superficial — *see* Injury, superficial, leg
lens, eye — *see* Injury, eye, specified site
  NEC
  penetrating — *see* Injury, eyeball,
    penetrating
limb NEC T14.8
lip S09.93
liver S36.119
  contusion S36.112
  laceration S36.113
    major (stellate) S36.116
    minor S36.114
    moderate S36.115
    specified NEC S36.118
lower back S39.92
  specified NEC S39.82
lumbar, lumbosacral (region) S39.92
  plexus — *see* Injury, lumbosacral plexus
lumbosacral plexus S34.4
lung — *see also* Injury, intrathoracic, lung
  aspiration J69.0
  transfusion-related (TRALI) J95.84
lymphatic thoracic duct — *see* Injury,
  intrathoracic, specified organ NEC
malar region S09.93
mastoid region S09.90

Injury - *continued*
 maxilla S09.93
 mediastinum — *see* Injury, intrathoracic, specified organ NEC
 membrane, brain — *see* Injury, intracranial
 meningeal artery — *see* Injury, intracranial, subdural hemorrhage
 meninges (cerebral) — *see* Injury, intracranial
 mesenteric
  artery
   branch S35.299
    laceration (minor) (superficial) S35.291
     major S35.292
    specified NEC S35.298
   inferior S35.239
    laceration (minor) (superficial) S35.231
     major S35.232
    specified NEC S35.238
   superior S35.229
    laceration (minor) (superficial) S35.221
     major S35.222
    specified NEC S35.228
   plexus (inferior) (superior) — *see* Injury, nerve, lumbosacral, sympathetic
  vein
   inferior S35.349
    laceration S35.341
    specified NEC S35.348
   superior S35.339
    laceration S35.331
    specified NEC S35.338
 mesentery — *see* Injury, intra-abdominal, specified site NEC
 mesosalpinx — *see* Injury, pelvic organ, specified site NEC
 middle ear S09.30-
 midthoracic region NOS S29.9
 mouth S09.93
 multiple NOS T07
 muscle (and fascia) (and tendon)
  abdomen S39.001
   laceration S39.021
   specified type NEC S39.091
   strain S39.011
  abductor
   thumb, forearm level — *see* Injury, muscle, thumb, abductor
  adductor
   thigh S76.20-
    laceration S76.22-
    specified type NEC S76.29-
    strain S76.21-
  ankle — *see* Injury, muscle, foot
  anterior muscle group, at leg level (lower) S86.20-
   laceration S86.22-
   specified type NEC S86.29-
   strain S86.21-
  arm (upper) — *see* Injury, muscle, shoulder
  biceps (parts NEC) S46.20-
   laceration S46.22-
   long head S46.10-
    laceration S46.12-
    strain S46.11-
   specified type NEC S46.19-
   specified type NEC S46.29-
   strain S46.21-
  extensor
   finger (s) (other than thumb) — *see* Injury, muscle, finger by site, extensor
   forearm level, specified NEC — *see* Injury, muscle, forearm, extensor
   thumb — *see* Injury, muscle, thumb, extensor
   toe (large) (ankle level) (foot level) — *see* Injury, muscle, toe, extensor
  finger
   extensor (forearm level) S56.40-
    hand level S66.309

 muscle (and fascia) (and tendon) - *continued*
  finger - *continued*
   extensor (forearm level) - *continued*
    hand level - *continued*
     laceration S66.329
     specified type NEC S66.399
     strain S66.319
    laceration S56.429
    specified type NEC S56.499
    strain S56.419
   flexor (forearm level) S56.10-
    hand level S66.109
     laceration S66.129
     specified type NEC S66.199
     strain S66.119
    laceration S56.129
    specified type NEC S56.199
    strain S56.119
   intrinsic S66.509
    laceration S66.529
    specified type NEC S66.599
    strain S66.519
  index
   extensor (forearm level)
    hand level S66.308
     laceration S66.32-
     specified type NEC S66.39-
     strain S66.31-
    specified type NEC S56.492-
   flexor (forearm level)
    hand level S66.108
     laceration S66.12-
     specified type NEC S66.19-
     strain S66.11-
    specified type NEC S56.19-
    strain S56.11-
   intrinsic S66.50-
    laceration S66.52-
    specified type NEC S66.59-
    strain S66.51-
  little
   extensor (forearm level)
    hand level S66.30-
     laceration S66.32-
     specified type NEC S66.39-
     strain S66.31-
    laceration S56.42-
    specified type NEC S56.49-
    strain S56.41-
   flexor (forearm level)
    hand level S66.10-
     laceration S66.12-
     specified type NEC S66.19-
     strain S66.11-
    laceration S56.12-
    specified type NEC S56.19-
    strain S56.11-
   intrinsic S66.50-
    laceration S66.52-
    specified type NEC S66.59-
    strain S66.51-
  middle
   extensor (forearm level)
    hand level S66.30-
     laceration S66.32-
     specified type NEC S66.39-
     strain S66.31-
    laceration S56.42-
    specified type NEC S56.49-
    strain S56.41-
   flexor (forearm level)
    hand level S66.10-
     laceration S66.12-
     specified type NEC S66.19-
     strain S66.11-
    laceration S56.12-
    specified type NEC S56.19-
    strain S56.11-
   intrinsic S66.50-
    laceration S66.52-
    specified type NEC S66.59-
    strain S66.51-
  ring
   extensor (forearm level)

 muscle (and fascia) (and tendon) - *continued*
  finger - *continued*
   ring - *continued*
    extensor (forearm level) - *continued*
     hand level S66.30-
      laceration S66.32-
      specified type NEC S66.39-
      strain S66.31-
     laceration S56.42-
     specified type NEC S56.49-
     strain S56.41-
    flexor (forearm level)
     hand level S66.10-
      laceration S66.12-
      specified type NEC S66.19-
      strain S66.11-
     laceration S56.12-
     specified type NEC S56.19-
     strain S56.11-
    intrinsic S66.50-
     laceration S66.52-
     specified type NEC S66.59-
     strain S66.51-
  flexor
   finger (s) (other than thumb) — *see* Injury, muscle, finger
   forearm level, specified NEC — *see* Injury, muscle, forearm, flexor
   thumb — *see* Injury, muscle, thumb, flexor
   toe (long) (ankle level) (foot level) — *see* Injury, muscle, toe, flexor
  foot S96.90-
   intrinsic S96.20-
    laceration S96.22-
    specified type NEC S96.29-
    strain S96.21-
   laceration S96.92-
   long extensor, toe — *see* Injury, muscle, toe, extensor
   long flexor, toe — *see* Injury, muscle, toe, flexor
   specified
    site NEC S96.80-
     laceration S96.82-
     specified type NEC S96.89-
     strain S96.81-
    type NEC S96.99-
   strain S96.91-
  forearm (level) S56.90-
   extensor S56.50-
    laceration S56.52-
    specified type NEC S56.59-
    strain S56.51-
   flexor S56.20-
    laceration S56.22-
    specified type NEC S56.29-
    strain S56.21-
   laceration S56.92-
   specified S56.99-
    site NEC S56.80-
     laceration S56.82-
     strain S56.81-
     type NEC S56.89-
    strain S56.91-
  hand (level) S66.90-
   laceration S66.92-
   specified
    site NEC S66.80-
     laceration S66.82-
     specified type NEC S66.89-
     strain S66.81-
    type NEC S66.99-
   strain S66.91-
  head S09.10
   laceration S09.12
   specified type NEC S09.19
   strain S09.11
  hip NEC S76.00-
   laceration S76.02-
   specified type NEC S76.09-
   strain S76.01-
  intrinsic

Injury - *continued*
muscle (and fascia) (and tendon) - *continued*
intrinsic - *continued*
ankle and foot level — *see* Injury,
muscle, foot, intrinsic
finger (other than thumb) — *see* Injury,
muscle, finger by site, intrinsic
foot (level) — *see* Injury, muscle, foot,
intrinsic
thumb — *see* Injury, muscle, thumb,
intrinsic
leg (level) (lower) S86.90-
Achilles tendon — *see* Injury, Achilles
tendon
anterior muscle group — *see* Injury,
muscle, anterior muscle group
laceration S86.92-
peroneal muscle group — *see* Injury,
muscle, peroneal muscle group
posterior muscle group — *see* Injury,
muscle, posterior muscle group, leg
level
specified
site NEC S86.80-
laceration S86.82-
specified type NEC S86.89-
strain S86.81-
type NEC S86.99-
strain S86.91-
long
extensor toe, at ankle and foot level —
see Injury, muscle, toe, extensor
flexor, toe, at ankle and foot level — *see*
Injury, muscle, toe, flexor
head, biceps — *see* Injury, muscle,
biceps, long head
lower back S39.002
laceration S39.022
specified type NEC S39.092
strain S39.012
neck (level) S16.9
laceration S16.2
specified type NEC S16.8
strain S16.1
pelvis S39.003
laceration S39.023
specified type NEC S39.093
strain S39.013
peroneal muscle group, at leg level
(lower) S86.30-
laceration S86.32-
specified type NEC S86.39-
strain S86.31-
posterior muscle (group)
leg level (lower) S86.10-
laceration S86.12-
specified type NEC S86.19-
strain S86.11-
thigh level S76.30-
laceration S76.32-
specified type NEC S76.39-
strain S76.31-
quadriceps (thigh) S76.10-
laceration S76.12-
specified type NEC S76.19-
strain S76.11-
shoulder S46.90-
laceration S46.92-
rotator cuff — *see* Injury, rotator cuff
specified site NEC S46.80-
laceration S46.82-
strain S46.81-
specified type NEC S46.89-
strain S46.91-
specified type NEC S46.99-
thigh NEC (level) S76.90-
adductor — *see* Injury, muscle, adductor,
thigh
laceration S76.92-
posterior muscle (group) — *see* Injury,
muscle, posterior muscle, thigh
level
quadriceps — *see* Injury, muscle,
quadriceps
specified

Injury - *continued*
muscle (and fascia) (and tendon) - *continued*
thigh NEC (level) - *continued*
specified - *continued*
site NEC S76.80-
laceration S76.82-
specified type NEC S76.89-
strain S76.81-
type NEC S76.99-
strain S76.91-
thorax (level) S29.009
back wall S29.002
front wall S29.001
laceration S29.029
back wall S29.022
front wall S29.021
specified type NEC S29.099
back wall S29.092
front wall S29.091
strain S29.019
back wall S29.012
front wall S29.011
thumb
abductor (forearm level) S56.30-
laceration S56.32-
specified type NEC S56.39-
strain S56.31-
extensor (forearm level) S56.30-
hand level S66.20-
laceration S66.22-
specified type NEC S66.29-
strain S66.21-
laceration S56.32-
specified type NEC S56.39-
strain S56.31-
flexor (forearm level) S56.00-
hand level S66.00-
laceration S66.02-
specified type NEC S66.09-
strain S66.01-
laceration S56.02-
specified type NEC S56.09-
strain S56.01-
wrist level — *see* Injury, muscle,
thumb, flexor, hand level
intrinsic S66.40-
laceration S66.42-
specified type NEC S66.49-
strain S66.41-
toe — *see also* Injury, muscle, foot
extensor, long S96.10-
laceration S96.12-
specified type NEC S96.19-
strain S96.11-
flexor, long S96.00-
laceration S96.02-
specified type NEC S96.09-
strain S96.01-
triceps S46.30-
laceration S46.32-
specified type NEC S46.39-
strain S46.31-
wrist (and hand) level — *see* Injury,
muscle, hand
musculocutaneous nerve — *see* Injury, nerve,
musculocutaneous
myocardium — *see* Injury, heart
nape — *see* Injury, neck
nasal (septum) (sinus) S09.92
nasopharynx S09.92
neck S19.9
specified NEC S19.80
specified site NEC S19.89
nerve NEC T14.8
abdomen S34.9
peripheral S34.6
specified site NEC S34.8
abducens S04.4-
contusion S04.4-
laceration S04.4-
specified type NEC S04.4-
abducent — *see* Injury, nerve, abducens
accessory S04.7-
contusion S04.7-
laceration S04.7-

Injury - *continued*
nerve NEC - *continued*
accessory - *continued*
specified type NEC S04.7-
acoustic S04.6-
contusion S04.6-
laceration S04.6-
specified type NEC S04.6-
ankle S94.9-
cutaneous sensory S94.3-
specified site NEC — *see* subcategory
S94.8
anterior crural, femoral — *see* Injury,
nerve, femoral
arm (upper) S44.9-
axillary — *see* Injury, nerve, axillary
cutaneous — *see* Injury, nerve,
cutaneous, arm
median — *see* Injury, nerve, median,
upper arm
musculocutaneous — *see* Injury, nerve,
musculocutaneous
radial — *see* Injury, nerve, radial, upper
arm
specified site NEC — *see* subcategory
S44.8
ulnar — *see* Injury, nerve, ulnar, arm
auditory — *see* Injury, nerve, acoustic
axillary S44.3-
brachial plexus — *see* Injury, brachial
plexus
cervical sympathetic S14.5
cranial S04.9
contusion S04.9
eighth (acoustic or auditory) — *see*
Injury, nerve, acoustic
eleventh (accessory) — *see* Injury,
nerve, accessory
fifth (trigeminal) — *see* Injury, nerve,
trigeminal
first (olfactory) — *see* Injury, nerve,
olfactory
fourth (trochlear) — *see* Injury, nerve,
trochlear
laceration S04.9
ninth (glossopharyngeal) — *see* Injury,
nerve, glossopharyngeal
second (optic) — *see* Injury, nerve, optic
seventh (facial) — *see* Injury, nerve,
facial
sixth (abducent) — *see* Injury, nerve,
abducens
specified
nerve NEC S04.89-
contusion S04.89-
laceration S04.89-
specified type NEC S04.89-
type NEC S04.9
tenth (pneumogastric or vagus) — *see*
Injury, nerve, vagus
third (oculomotor) — *see* Injury, nerve,
oculomotor
twelfth (hypoglossal) — *see* Injury,
nerve, hypoglossal
cutaneous sensory
ankle (level) S94.3-
arm (upper) (level) S44.5-
foot (level) — *see* Injury, nerve,
cutaneous sensory, ankle
forearm (level) S54.3-
hip (level) S74.2-
leg (lower level) S84.2-
shoulder (level) — *see* Injury, nerve,
cutaneous sensory, arm
thigh (level) — *see* Injury, nerve,
cutaneous sensory, hip
deep peroneal — *see* Injury, nerve,
peroneal, foot
digital
finger S64.4-
index S64.49-
little S64.49-
middle S64.49-
ring S64.49-
thumb S64.3-

Injury - *continued*
  nerve NEC - *continued*
    digital - *continued*
      toe — *see* Injury, nerve, ankle, specified site NEC
    eighth cranial (acoustic or auditory) — *see* Injury, nerve, acoustic
    eleventh cranial (accessory) — *see* Injury, nerve, accessory
    facial S04.5-
      contusion S04.5-
      laceration S04.5-
      newborn P11.3
      specified type NEC S04.5-
    femoral (hip level) (thigh level) S74.1-
    fifth cranial (trigeminal) — *see* Injury, nerve, trigeminal
    finger (digital) — *see* Injury, nerve, digital, finger
    first cranial (olfactory) — *see* Injury, nerve, olfactory
    foot S94.9-
      cutaneous sensory S94.3-
      deep peroneal S94.2-
      lateral plantar S94.0-
      medial plantar S94.1-
      specified site NEC — *see* subcategory S94.8
    forearm (level) S54.9-
      cutaneous sensory — *see* Injury, nerve, cutaneous sensory, forearm
      median — *see* Injury, nerve, median
      radial — *see* Injury, nerve, radial
      specified site NEC — *see* subcategory S54.8
      ulnar — *see* Injury, nerve, ulnar
    fourth cranial (trochlear) — *see* Injury, nerve, trochlear
    glossopharyngeal S04.89-
      specified type NEC S04.89-
    hand S64.9-
      median — *see* Injury, nerve, median, hand
      radial — *see* Injury, nerve, radial, hand
      specified NEC — *see* subcategory S64.8
      ulnar — *see* Injury, nerve, ulnar, hand
    hip (level) S74.9-
      cutaneous sensory — *see* Injury, nerve, cutaneous sensory, hip
      femoral — *see* Injury, nerve, femoral
      sciatic — *see* Injury, nerve, sciatic
      specified site NEC — *see* subcategory S74.8
    hypoglossal S04.89-
      specified type NEC S04.89-
    lateral plantar S94.0-
    leg (lower) S84.9-
      cutaneous sensory — *see* Injury, nerve, cutaneous sensory, leg
      peroneal — *see* Injury, nerve, peroneal
      specified site NEC — *see* subcategory S84.8
      tibial — *see* Injury, nerve, tibial
      upper — *see* Injury, nerve, thigh
    lower
      back — *see* Injury, nerve, abdomen, specified site NEC
        peripheral — *see* Injury, nerve, abdomen, peripheral
      limb — *see* Injury, nerve, leg
    lumbar spinal — *see* Injury, nerve, spinal, lumbar
    lumbar plexus — *see* Injury, nerve, lumbosacral, sympathetic
    lumbosacral
      plexus — *see* Injury, nerve, lumbosacral, sympathetic
      sympathetic S34.5
    medial plantar S94.1-
    median (forearm level) S54.1-
      hand (level) S64.1-
      upper arm (level) S44.1-
      wrist (level) — *see* Injury, nerve, median, hand
    musculocutaneous S44.4-

Injury - *continued*
  nerve NEC - *continued*
    musculospiral (upper arm level) — *see* Injury, nerve, radial, upper arm
    neck S14.9
      peripheral S14.4
      specified site NEC S14.8
      sympathetic S14.5
    ninth cranial (glossopharyngeal) — *see* Injury, nerve, glossopharyngeal
    oculomotor S04.1-
      contusion S04.1-
      laceration S04.1-
      specified type NEC S04.1-
    olfactory S04.81-
      specified type NEC S04.81-
    optic S04.01-
      contusion S04.01-
      laceration S04.01-
      specified type NEC S04.01-
    pelvic girdle — *see* Injury, nerve, hip
    pelvis — *see* Injury, nerve, abdomen, specified site NEC
      peripheral — *see* Injury, nerve, abdomen, peripheral
    peripheral NEC T14.8
      abdomen — *see* Injury, nerve, abdomen, peripheral
      lower back — *see* Injury, nerve, abdomen, peripheral
      neck — *see* Injury, nerve, neck, peripheral
      pelvis — *see* Injury, nerve, abdomen, peripheral
      specified NEC T14.8
    peroneal (lower leg level) S84.1-
      foot S94.2-
    plexus
      brachial — *see* Injury, brachial plexus
      celiac, coeliac — *see* Injury, nerve, lumbosacral, sympathetic
      mesenteric, inferior — *see* Injury, nerve, lumbosacral, sympathetic
      sacral — *see* Injury, lumbosacral plexus
      spinal
        brachial — *see* Injury, brachial plexus
        lumbosacral — *see* Injury, lumbosacral plexus
    pneumogastric — *see* Injury, nerve, vagus
    radial (forearm level) S54.2-
      hand (level) S64.2-
      upper arm (level) S44.2-
      wrist (level) — *see* Injury, nerve, radial, hand
    root — *see* Injury, nerve, spinal, root
    sacral plexus — *see* Injury, lumbosacral plexus
    sacral spinal — *see* Injury, nerve, spinal, sacral
    sciatic (hip level) (thigh level) S74.0-
    second cranial (optic) — *see* Injury, nerve, optic
    seventh cranial (facial) — *see* Injury, nerve, facial
    shoulder — *see* Injury, nerve, arm
    sixth cranial (abducent) — *see* Injury, nerve, abducens
    spinal
      plexus — *see* Injury, nerve, plexus, spinal
      root
        cervical S14.2
        dorsal S24.2
        lumbar S34.21
        sacral S34.22
        thoracic — *see* Injury, nerve, spinal, root, dorsal
      splanchnic — *see* Injury, nerve, lumbosacral, sympathetic
      sympathetic NEC — *see* Injury, nerve, lumbosacral, sympathetic
        cervical — *see* Injury, nerve, cervical sympathetic
    tenth cranial (pneumogastric or vagus) — *see* Injury, nerve, vagus

Injury - *continued*
  nerve NEC - *continued*
    thigh (level) — *see* Injury, nerve, hip
      cutaneous sensory — *see* Injury, nerve, cutaneous sensory, hip
      femoral — *see* Injury, nerve, femoral
      sciatic — *see* Injury, nerve, sciatic
      specified NEC — *see* Injury, nerve, hip
    third cranial (oculomotor) — *see* Injury, nerve, oculomotor
    thorax S24.9
      peripheral S24.3
      specified site NEC S24.8
      sympathetic S24.4
    thumb, digital — *see* Injury, nerve, digital, thumb
    tibial (lower leg level) (posterior) S84.0-
    toe — *see* Injury, nerve, ankle
    trigeminal S04.3-
      contusion S04.3-
      laceration S04.3-
      specified type NEC S04.3-
    trochlear S04.2-
      contusion S04.2-
      laceration S04.2-
      specified type NEC S04.2-
    twelfth cranial (hypoglossal) — *see* Injury, nerve, hypoglossal
    ulnar (forearm level) S54.0-
      arm (upper) (level) S44.0-
      hand (level) S64.0-
      wrist (level) — *see* Injury, nerve, ulnar, hand
    vagus S04.89-
      specified type NEC S04.89-
    wrist (level) — *see* Injury, nerve, hand
  ninth cranial nerve (glossopharyngeal) — *see* Injury, nerve, glossopharyngeal
  nose (septum) S09.92
  obstetrical O71.9
    specified NEC O71.89
  occipital (region) (scalp) S09.90
    lobe — *see* Injury, intracranial
  optic chiasm S04.02
  optic radiation S04.03-
  optic tract and pathways S04.03-
  orbit, orbital (region) — *see* Injury, eye
    penetrating (with foreign body) — *see* Injury, eye, orbit, penetrating
    specified NEC — *see* Injury, eye, specified site NEC
  ovary, ovarian S37.409
    bilateral S37.402
      contusion S37.422
      laceration S37.432
      specified type NEC S37.492
    blood vessel — *see* Injury, blood vessel, ovarian
    contusion S37.429
      bilateral S37.422
      unilateral S37.421
    laceration S37.439
      bilateral S37.432
      unilateral S37.431
    specified type NEC S37.499
      bilateral S37.492
      unilateral S37.491
    unilateral S37.401
      contusion S37.421
      laceration S37.431
      specified type NEC S37.491
  palate (hard) (soft) S09.93
  pancreas S36.209
    body S36.201
      contusion S36.221
      laceration S36.231
        major S36.261
        minor S36.241
        moderate S36.251
      specified type NEC S36.291
    contusion S36.229
    head S36.200
      contusion S36.220
      laceration S36.230
        major S36.260

Injury - *continued*
pancreas - *continued*
  head - *continued*
    laceration - *continued*
      minor S36.240
      moderate S36.250
      specified type NEC S36.290
    laceration S36.239
      major S36.269
      minor S36.249
      moderate S36.259
    specified type NEC S36.299
    tail S36.202
      contusion S36.222
      laceration S36.232
        major S36.262
        minor S36.242
        moderate S36.252
      specified type NEC S36.292
  parietal (region) (scalp) S09.90
    lobe — *see* Injury, intracranial
  patellar ligament (tendon) S76.10-
    laceration S76.12-
    specified NEC S76.19-
    strain S76.11-
  pelvis, pelvic (floor) S39.93
    complicating delivery O70.1
    joint or ligament, complicating
      delivery O71.6
    organ S37.90
      with ectopic or molar pregnancy O08.6
      complication of abortion — *see*
        Abortion
      contusion S37.92
      following ectopic or molar
        pregnancy O08.6
      laceration S37.93
      obstetrical trauma NEC O71.5
      specified
        site NEC S37.899
          contusion S37.892
          laceration S37.893
          specified type NEC S37.898
        type NEC S37.99
    specified NEC S39.83
  penis S39.94
  perineum S39.94
  peritoneum S36.81
    laceration S36.893
  periurethral tissue — *see* Injury, urethra
    complicating delivery O71.82
  phalanges
    foot — *see* Injury, foot
    hand — *see* Injury, hand
  pharynx NEC S19.85
  pleura — *see* Injury, intrathoracic, pleura
  plexus
    brachial — *see* Injury, brachial plexus
    cardiac — *see* Injury, nerve, thorax,
      sympathetic
    celiac, coeliac — *see* Injury, nerve,
      lumbosacral, sympathetic
    esophageal — *see* Injury, nerve, thorax,
      sympathetic
    hypogastric — *see* Injury, nerve,
      lumbosacral, sympathetic
    lumbar, lumbosacral — *see* Injury,
      lumbosacral plexus
    mesenteric — *see* Injury, nerve,
      lumbosacral, sympathetic
    pulmonary — *see* Injury, nerve, thorax,
      sympathetic
  postcardiac surgery (syndrome) I97.0
  prepuce S39.94
  pressure
    injury — *see* Ulcer, pressure, by site
  prostate S37.829
    contusion S37.822
    laceration S37.823
    specified type NEC S37.828
  pubic region S39.94
  pudendum S39.94
  pulmonary plexus — *see* Injury, nerve,
    thorax, sympathetic
  rectovaginal septum NEC S39.83

Injury - *continued*
  rectum — *see* Injury, intestine, large, rectum
  retina — *see* Injury, eye, specified site NEC
    penetrating — *see* Injury, eyeball,
      penetrating
  retroperitoneal — *see* Injury, intra-
    abdominal, specified site NEC
  rotator cuff (muscle (s)) (tendon (s))
    S46.00-
    laceration S46.02-
    specified type NEC S46.09-
    strain S46.01-
  round ligament — *see* Injury, pelvic organ,
    specified site NEC
  sacral plexus — *see* Injury, lumbosacral
    plexus
  salivary duct or gland S09.93
  scalp S09.90
    newborn (birth injury) P12.9
      due to monitoring (electrode) (sampling
        incision) P12.4
      specified NEC P12.89
        caput succedaneum P12.81
  scapular region — *see* Injury, shoulder
  sclera — *see* Injury, eye, specified site NEC
    penetrating — *see* Injury, eyeball,
      penetrating
  scrotum S39.94
  second cranial nerve (optic) — *see* Injury,
    nerve, optic
  seminal vesicle — *see* Injury, pelvic organ,
    specified site NEC
  seventh cranial nerve (facial) — *see* Injury,
    nerve, facial
  shoulder S49.9-
    blood vessel — *see* Injury, blood vessel,
      arm
    contusion — *see* Contusion, shoulder
    dislocation — *see* Dislocation, shoulder
    fracture — *see* Fracture, shoulder
    muscle — *see* Injury, muscle, shoulder
    nerve — *see* Injury, nerve, shoulder
    open — *see* Wound, open, shoulder
    specified type NEC S49.8-
    sprain — *see* Sprain, shoulder girdle
    superficial — *see* Injury, superficial,
      shoulder
  sinus
    cavernous — *see* Injury, intracranial
    nasal S09.92
  sixth cranial nerve (abducent) — *see* Injury,
    nerve, abducens
  skeleton, birth injury P13.9
    specified part NEC P13.8
  skin NEC T14.8
    surface intact — *see* Injury, superficial
  skull NEC S09.90
  specified NEC T14.8
  spermatic cord (pelvic region) S37.898
    scrotal region S39.848
  spinal (cord)
    cervical (neck) S14.109
      anterior cord syndrome S14.139
        C1 level S14.131
        C2 level S14.132
        C3 level S14.133
        C4 level S14.134
        C5 level S14.135
        C6 level S14.136
        C7 level S14.137
        C8 level S14.138
      Brown-Séquard syndrome S14.149
        C1 level S14.141
        C2 level S14.142
        C3 level S14.143
        C4 level S14.144
        C5 level S14.145
        C6 level S14.146
        C7 level S14.147
        C8 level S14.148
      S14.139
        C1 level S14.101
        C2 level S14.102
        C3 level S14.103
        C4 level S14.104
        C5 level S14.105

Injury - *continued*
  spinal (cord) - *continued*
    cervical (neck) - *continued*
      C6 level S14.106
      C7 level S14.107
      C8 level S14.108
      central cord syndrome S14.129
        C1 level S14.121
        C2 level S14.122
        C3 level S14.123
        C4 level S14.124
        C5 level S14.125
        C6 level S14.126
        C7 level S14.127
        C8 level S14.128
      complete lesion S14.119
        C1 level S14.111
        C2 level S14.112
        C3 level S14.113
        C4 level S14.114
        C5 level S14.115
        C6 level S14.116
        C7 level S14.117
        C8 level S14.118
      concussion S14.0
      edema S14.0
      incomplete lesion specified
        NEC S14.159
        C1 level S14.151
        C2 level S14.152
        C3 level S14.153
        C4 level S14.154
        C5 level S14.155
        C6 level S14.156
        C7 level S14.157
        C8 level S14.158
      posterior cord syndrome S14.159
        C1 level S14.151
        C2 level S14.152
        C3 level S14.153
        C4 level S14.154
        C5 level S14.155
        C6 level S14.156
        C7 level S14.157
        C8 level S14.158
      dorsal — *see* Injury, spinal, thoracic
    lumbar S34.109
      complete lesion S34.119
        L1 level S34.111
        L2 level S34.112
        L3 level S34.113
        L4 level S34.114
        L5 level S34.115
      concussion S34.01
      edema S34.01
      incomplete lesion S34.129
        L1 level S34.121
        L2 level S34.122
        L3 level S34.123
        L4 level S34.124
        L5 level S34.125
      L1 level S34.101
      L2 level S34.102
      L3 level S34.103
      L4 level S34.104
      L5 level S34.105
    nerve root NEC
      cervical — *see* Injury, nerve, spinal,
        root, cervical
      dorsal — *see* Injury, nerve, spinal, root,
        dorsal
      lumbar S34.21
      sacral S34.22
      thoracic — *see* Injury, nerve, spinal,
        root, dorsal
    plexus
      brachial — *see* Injury, brachial plexus
      lumbosacral — *see* Injury, lumbosacral
        plexus
    sacral S34.139
      complete lesion S34.131
      incomplete lesion S34.132
    thoracic S24.109
      anterior cord syndrome S24.139
        T1 level S24.131

Injury - *continued*
  spinal (cord) - *continued*
    thoracic - *continued*
      anterior cord syndrome - *continued*
        T2-T6 level S24.132
        T7-T10 level S24.133
        T11-T12 level S24.134
      Brown-Séquard syndrome S24.149
        T1 level S24.141
        T2-T6 level S24.142
        T7-T10 level S24.143
        T11-T12 level S24.144
      complete lesion S24.119
        T1 level S24.111
        T2-T6 level S24.112
        T7-T10 level S24.113
        T11-T12 level S24.114
      concussion S24.0
      edema S24.0
      incomplete lesion specified
        NEC S24.159
        T1 level S24.151
        T2-T6 level S24.152
        T7-T10 level S24.153
        T11-T12 level S24.154
      posterior cord syndrome S24.159
        T1 level S24.151
        T2-T6 level S24.152
        T7-T10 level S24.153
        T11-T12 level S24.154
      T1 level S24.101
      T2-T6 level S24.102
      T7-T10 level S24.103
      T11-T12 level S24.104
  splanchnic nerve — *see* Injury, nerve,
    lumbosacral, sympathetic
  spleen S36.00
    contusion S36.029
      major S36.021
      minor S36.020
    laceration S36.039
      major (massive) (stellate) S36.032
      moderate S36.031
      superficial (capsular) (minor) S36.030
    specified type NEC S36.09
  splenic artery — *see* Injury, blood vessel,
    celiac artery, branch
  stellate ganglion — *see* Injury, nerve, thorax,
    sympathetic
  sternal region S29.9
  stomach S36.30
    contusion S36.32
    laceration S36.33
    specified type NEC S36.39
  subconjunctival — *see* Injury, eye,
    conjunctiva
  subcutaneous NEC T14.8
  submaxillary region S09.93
  submental region S09.93
  subungual
    fingers — *see* Injury, hand
    toes — *see* Injury, foot
  superficial NEC T14.8
    abdomen, abdominal (wall) S30.92
      abrasion S30.811
      bite S30.871
        insect S30.861
      contusion S30.1
      external constriction S30.841
      foreign body S30.851
    abrasion — *see* Abrasion, by site
    adnexa, eye NEC — *see* Injury, eye,
      specified site NEC
    alveolar process — *see* Injury, superficial,
      oral cavity
    ankle S90.91-
      abrasion — *see* Abrasion, ankle
      blister — *see* Blister, ankle
      bite — *see* Bite, ankle
      contusion — *see* Contusion, ankle
      external constriction — *see* Constriction,
        external, ankle
      foreign body — *see* Foreign body,
        superficial, ankle
    anus S30.98

Injury - *continued*
  superficial NEC - *continued*
    arm (upper) S40.92-
      abrasion — *see* Abrasion, arm
      bite — *see* Bite, superficial, arm
      blister — *see* Blister, arm (upper)
      contusion — *see* Contusion, arm
      external constriction — *see* Constriction,
        external, arm
      foreign body — *see* Foreign body,
        superficial, arm
    auditory canal (external) (meatus) — *see*
      Injury, superficial, ear
    auricle — *see* Injury, superficial, ear
    axilla — *see* Injury, superficial, arm
    back — *see also* Injury, superficial, thorax,
      back
      lower S30.91
        abrasion S30.810
        contusion S30.0
        external constriction S30.840
        superficial
          bite NEC S30.870
            insect S30.860
          foreign body S30.850
    bite NEC — *see* Bite, superficial NEC, by
      site
    blister — *see* Blister, by site
    breast S20.10-
      abrasion — *see* Abrasion, breast
      bite — *see* Bite, superficial, breast
      contusion — *see* Contusion, breast
      external constriction — *see* Constriction,
        external, breast
      foreign body — *see* Foreign body,
        superficial, breast
    brow — *see* Injury, superficial, head,
      specified NEC
    buttock S30.91
    calf — *see* Injury, superficial, leg
    canthus, eye — *see* Injury, superficial,
      periocular area
    cheek (external) — *see* Injury, superficial,
      head, specified NEC
      internal — *see* Injury, superficial, oral
        cavity
    chest wall — *see* Injury, superficial, thorax
    chin — *see* Injury, superficial, head NEC
    clitoris S30.95
    conjunctiva — *see* Injury, eye, conjunctiva
      with foreign body (in conjunctival
        sac) — *see* Foreign body,
        conjunctival sac
    contusion — *see* Contusion, by site
    costal region — *see* Injury, superficial,
      thorax
    digit (s)
      hand — *see* Injury, superficial, finger
    ear (auricle) (canal) (external) S00.40-
      abrasion — *see* Abrasion, ear
      bite — *see* Bite, superficial, ear
      contusion — *see* Contusion, ear
      external constriction — *see* Constriction,
        external, ear
      foreign body — *see* Foreign body,
        superficial, ear
    elbow S50.90-
      abrasion — *see* Abrasion, elbow
      bite — *see* Bite, superficial, elbow
      blister — *see* Blister, elbow
      contusion — *see* Contusion, elbow
      external constriction — *see* Constriction,
        external, elbow
      foreign body — *see* Foreign body,
        superficial, elbow
    epididymis S30.94
    epigastric region S30.92
    epiglottis — *see* Injury, superficial, throat
    esophagus
      cervical — *see* Injury, superficial, throat
    external constriction — *see* Constriction,
      external, by site
    extremity NEC T14.8
    eyeball NEC — *see* Injury, eye, specified
      site NEC

Injury - *continued*
  superficial NEC - *continued*
    eyebrow — *see* Injury, superficial,
      periocular area
    eyelid S00.20-
      abrasion — *see* Abrasion, eyelid
      bite — *see* Bite, superficial, eyelid
      contusion — *see* Contusion, eyelid
      external constriction — *see* Constriction,
        external, eyelid
      foreign body — *see* Foreign body,
        superficial, eyelid
    face NEC — *see* Injury, superficial, head,
      specified NEC
    finger (s) S60.949
      abrasion — *see* Abrasion, finger
      bite — *see* Bite, superficial, finger
      blister — *see* Blister, finger
      contusion — *see* Contusion, finger
      external constriction — *see* Constriction,
        external, finger
      foreign body — *see* Foreign body,
        superficial, finger
      insect bite — *see* Bite, by site,
        superficial, insect
      index S60.94-
      little S60.94-
      middle S60.94-
      ring S60.94-
    flank S30.92
    foot S90.92-
      abrasion — *see* Abrasion, foot
      bite — *see* Bite, foot
      blister — *see* Blister, foot
      contusion — *see* Contusion, foot
      external constriction — *see* Constriction,
        external, foot
      foreign body — *see* Foreign body,
        superficial, foot
    forearm S50.91-
      abrasion — *see* Abrasion, forearm
      bite — *see* Bite, forearm, superficial
      blister — *see* Blister, forearm
      contusion — *see* Contusion, forearm
      elbow only — *see* Injury, superficial,
        elbow
      external constriction — *see* Constriction,
        external, forearm
      foreign body — *see* Foreign body,
        superficial, forearm
    forehead — *see* Injury, superficial, head
      NEC
    foreign body — *see* Foreign body,
      superficial
    genital organs, external
      female S30.97
      male S30.96
    globe (eye) — *see* Injury, eye, specified
      site NEC
    groin S30.92
    gum — *see* Injury, superficial, oral cavity
    hand S60.92-
      abrasion — *see* Abrasion, hand
      bite — *see* Bite, superficial, hand
      contusion — *see* Contusion, hand
      external constriction — *see* Constriction,
        external, hand
      foreign body — *see* Foreign body,
        superficial, hand
    head S00.90
      ear — *see* Injury, superficial, ear
      eyelid — *see* Injury, superficial, eyelid
      nose S00.30
      oral cavity S00.502
      scalp S00.00
      specified site NEC S00.80
    heel — *see* Injury, superficial, foot
    hip S70.91-
      abrasion — *see* Abrasion, hip
      bite — *see* Bite, superficial, hip
      blister — *see* Blister, hip
      contusion — *see* Contusion, hip
      external constriction — *see* Constriction,
        external, hip

Injury - *continued*
  superficial NEC - *continued*
    hip - *continued*
      foreign body — *see* Foreign body, superficial, hip
      iliac region — *see* Injury, superficial, abdomen
      inguinal region — *see* Injury, superficial, abdomen
      insect bite — *see* Bite, by site, superficial, insect
      interscapular region — *see* Injury, superficial, thorax, back
      jaw — *see* Injury, superficial, head, specified NEC
      knee S80.91-
        abrasion — *see* Abrasion, knee
        bite — *see* Bite, superficial, knee
        blister — *see* Blister, knee
        contusion — *see* Contusion, knee
        external constriction — *see* Constriction, external, knee
        foreign body — *see* Foreign body, superficial, knee
      labium (majus) (minus) S30.95
      lacrimal (apparatus) (gland) (sac) — *see* Injury, eye, specified site NEC
      larynx — *see* Injury, superficial, throat
      leg (lower) S80.92-
        abrasion — *see* Abrasion, leg
        bite — *see* Bite, superficial, leg
        contusion — *see* Contusion, leg
        external constriction — *see* Constriction, external, leg
        foreign body — *see* Foreign body, superficial, leg
        knee — *see* Injury, superficial, knee
      limb NEC T14.8
      lip S00.501
      lower back S30.91
      lumbar region S30.91
      malar region — *see* Injury, superficial, head, specified NEC
      mammary — *see* Injury, superficial, breast
      mastoid region — *see* Injury, superficial, head, specified NEC
      mouth — *see* Injury, superficial, oral cavity
      muscle NEC T14.8
      nail NEC T14.8
        finger — *see* Injury, superficial, finger
        toe — *see* Injury, superficial, toe
      nasal (septum) — *see* Injury, superficial, nose
      neck S10.90
        specified site NEC S10.80
      nose (septum) S00.30
      occipital region — *see* Injury, superficial, scalp
      oral cavity S00.502
      orbital region — *see* Injury, superficial, periocular area
      palate — *see* Injury, superficial, oral cavity
      palm — *see* Injury, superficial, hand
      parietal region — *see* Injury, superficial, scalp
      pelvis S30.91
        girdle — *see* Injury, superficial, hip
      penis S30.93
      perineum
        female S30.95
        male S30.91
      periocular area S00.20-
        abrasion — *see* Abrasion, eyelid
        bite — *see* Bite, superficial, eyelid
        contusion — *see* Contusion, eyelid
        external constriction — *see* Constriction, external, eyelid
        foreign body — *see* Foreign body, superficial, eyelid
      phalanges
        finger — *see* Injury, superficial, finger
        toe — *see* Injury, superficial, toe
      pharynx — *see* Injury, superficial, throat
      pinna — *see* Injury, superficial, ear

Injury - *continued*
  superficial NEC - *continued*
    popliteal space — *see* Injury, superficial, knee
    prepuce S30.93
    pubic region S30.91
    pudendum
      female S30.97
      male S30.96
    sacral region S30.91
    scalp S00.00
    scapular region — *see* Injury, superficial, shoulder
    sclera — *see* Injury, eye, specified site NEC
    scrotum S30.94
    shin — *see* Injury, superficial, leg
    shoulder S40.91-
      abrasion — *see* Abrasion, shoulder
      bite — *see* Bite, superficial, shoulder
      blister — *see* Blister, shoulder
      contusion — *see* Contusion, shoulder
      external constriction — *see* Constriction, external, shoulder
      foreign body — *see* Foreign body, superficial, shoulder
    skin NEC T14.8
    sternal region — *see* Injury, superficial, thorax, front
    subconjunctival — *see* Injury, eye, specified site NEC
    subcutaneous NEC T14.8
    submaxillary region — *see* Injury, superficial, head, specified NEC
    submental region — *see* Injury, superficial, head, specified NEC
    subungual
      finger (s) — *see* Injury, superficial, finger
      toe (s) — *see* Injury, superficial, toe
    supraclavicular fossa — *see* Injury, superficial, neck
    supraorbital — *see* Injury, superficial, head, specified NEC
    temple — *see* Injury, superficial, head, specified NEC
    temporal region — *see* Injury, superficial, head, specified NEC
    testis S30.94
    thigh S70.92-
      abrasion — *see* Abrasion, thigh
      bite — *see* Bite, superficial, thigh
      blister — *see* Blister, thigh
      contusion — *see* Contusion, thigh
      external constriction — *see* Constriction, external, thigh
      foreign body — *see* Foreign body, superficial, thigh
    thorax, thoracic (wall) S20.90
      abrasion — *see* Abrasion, thorax
      back S20.40-
      bite — *see* Bite, thorax, superficial
      blister — *see* Blister, thorax
      contusion — *see* Contusion, thorax
      external constriction — *see* Constriction, external, thorax
      foreign body — *see* Foreign body, superficial, thorax
      front S20.30-
    throat S10.10
      abrasion S10.11
      bite S10.17
        insect S10.16
      blister S10.12
      contusion S10.0
      external constriction S10.14
      foreign body S10.15
    thumb S60.93-
      abrasion — *see* Abrasion, thumb
      bite — *see* Bite, superficial, thumb
      blister — *see* Blister, thumb
      contusion — *see* Contusion, thumb
      external constriction — *see* Constriction, external, thumb

Injury - *continued*
  superficial NEC - *continued*
    thumb - *continued*
      foreign body — *see* Foreign body, superficial, thumb
      insect bite — *see* Bite, by site, superficial, insect
      specified type NEC S60.39-
    toe (s) S90.93-
      abrasion — *see* Abrasion, toe
      bite — *see* Bite, toe
      blister — *see* Blister, toe
      contusion — *see* Contusion, toe
      external constriction — *see* Constriction, external, toe
      foreign body — *see* Foreign body, superficial, toe
      great S90.93-
    tongue — *see* Injury, superficial, oral cavity
    tooth, teeth — *see* Injury, superficial, oral cavity
    trachea S10.10
    tunica vaginalis S30.94
    tympanum, tympanic membrane — *see* Injury, superficial, ear
    uvula — *see* Injury, superficial, oral cavity
    vagina S30.95
    vocal cords — *see* Injury, superficial, throat
    vulva S30.95
    wrist S60.91-
  supraclavicular region — *see* Injury, neck
  supraorbital S09.93
  suprarenal gland (multiple) — *see* Injury, adrenal
  surgical complication (external or internal site) — *see* Laceration, accidental complicating surgery
  temple S09.90
  temporal region S09.90
  tendon — *see also* Injury, muscle, by site
    abdomen — *see* Injury, muscle, abdomen
    Achilles — *see* Injury, Achilles tendon
    lower back — *see* Injury, muscle, lower back
    pelvic organs — *see* Injury, muscle, pelvis
  tenth cranial nerve (pneumogastric or vagus) — *see* Injury, nerve, vagus
  testis S39.94
  thigh S79.92-
    blood vessel — *see* Injury, blood vessel, hip
    contusion — *see* Contusion, thigh
    fracture — *see* Fracture, femur
    muscle — *see* Injury, muscle, thigh
    nerve — *see* Injury, nerve, thigh
    open — *see* Wound, open, thigh
    specified NEC S79.82-
    superficial — *see* Injury, superficial, thigh
  third cranial nerve (oculomotor) — *see* Injury, nerve, oculomotor
  thorax, thoracic S29.9
    blood vessel — *see* Injury, blood vessel, thorax
    cavity — *see* Injury, intrathoracic
    dislocation — *see* Dislocation, thorax
    external (wall) S29.9
      contusion — *see* Contusion, thorax
      nerve — *see* Injury, nerve, thorax
      open — *see* Wound, open, thorax
      specified NEC S29.8
      sprain — *see* Sprain, thorax
      superficial — *see* Injury, superficial, thorax
    fracture — *see* Fracture, thorax
    internal — *see* Injury, intrathoracic
    intrathoracic organ — *see* Injury, intrathoracic
    sympathetic ganglion — *see* Injury, nerve, thorax, sympathetic
  throat — *see also* Injury, neck S19.9
  thumb S69.9-
    blood vessel — *see* Injury, blood vessel, thumb

Injury - *continued*
thumb - *continued*
contusion — *see* Contusion, thumb
dislocation — *see* Dislocation, thumb
fracture — *see* Fracture, thumb
muscle — *see* Injury, muscle, thumb
nerve — *see* Injury, nerve, digital, thumb
open — *see* Wound, open, thumb
specified NEC S69.8-
sprain — *see* Sprain, thumb
superficial — *see* Injury, superficial,
thumb
thymus (gland) — *see* Injury, intrathoracic,
specified organ NEC
thyroid (gland) NEC S19.84
toe S99.92-
contusion — *see* Contusion, toe
dislocation — *see* Dislocation, toe
fracture — *see* Fracture, toe
muscle — *see* Injury, muscle, toe
open — *see* Wound, open, toe
specified type NEC S99.82-
sprain — *see* Sprain, toe
superficial — *see* Injury, superficial, toe
tongue S09.93
tonsil S09.93
tooth S09.93
trachea (cervical) NEC S19.82
thoracic — *see* Injury, intrathoracic,
trachea, thoracic
transfusion-related acute lung
(TRALI) J95.84
tunica vaginalis S39.94
twelfth cranial nerve (hypoglossal) — *see*
Injury, nerve, hypoglossal
ureter S37.10
contusion S37.12
laceration S37.13
specified type NEC S37.19
urethra (sphincter) S37.30
at delivery O71.5
contusion S37.32
laceration S37.33
specified type NEC S37.39
urinary organ S37.90
contusion S37.92
laceration S37.93
specified
site NEC S37.899
contusion S37.892
laceration S37.893
specified type NEC S37.898
type NEC S37.99
uterus, uterine S37.60
with ectopic or molar pregnancy O08.6
blood vessel — *see* Injury, blood vessel,
iliac
contusion S37.62
laceration S37.63
cervix at delivery O71.3
rupture associated with obstetrics — *see*
Rupture, uterus
specified type NEC S37.69
uvula S09.93
vagina S39.93
abrasion S30.814
bite S31.45
insect S30.864
superficial NEC S30.874
contusion S30.23
crush S38.03
during delivery — *see* Laceration, vagina,
during delivery
external constriction S30.844
insect bite S30.864
laceration S31.41
with foreign body S31.42
open wound S31.40
puncture S31.43
with foreign body S31.44
superficial S30.95
foreign body S30.854
vas deferens — *see* Injury, pelvic organ,
specified site NEC
vascular NEC T14.8

Injury - *continued*
vein — *see* Injury, blood vessel
vena cava (superior) S25.20
inferior S35.10
laceration (minor) (superficial) S35.11
major S35.12
specified type NEC S35.19
laceration (minor) (superficial) S25.21
major S25.22
specified type NEC S25.29
vesical (sphincter) — *see* Injury, bladder
visual cortex S04.04-
vitreous (humor) S05.90
specified NEC S05.8X-
vocal cord NEC S19.83
vulva S39.94
abrasion S30.814
bite S31.45
insect S30.864
superficial NEC S30.874
contusion S30.23
crush S38.03
during delivery — *see* Laceration,
perineum, female, during delivery
external constriction S30.844
insect bite S30.864
laceration S31.41
with foreign body S31.42
open wound S31.40
puncture S31.43
with foreign body S31.44
superficial S30.95
foreign body S30.854
whiplash (cervical spine) S13.4
wrist S69.9-
blood vessel — *see* Injury, blood vessel,
hand
contusion — *see* Contusion, wrist
dislocation — *see* Dislocation, wrist
fracture — *see* Fracture, wrist
muscle — *see* Injury, muscle, hand
nerve — *see* Injury, nerve, hand
open — *see* Wound, open, wrist
specified NEC S69.8-
sprain — *see* Sprain, wrist
superficial — *see* Injury, superficial, wrist
Inoculation — *see also* Vaccination
complication or reaction — *see*
Complications, vaccination
Insanity, insane — *see also* Psychosis
adolescent — *see* Schizophrenia
confusional F28
acute or subacute F05
delusional F22
senile F03
Insect
bite — *see* Bite, by site, superficial, insect
venomous, poisoning NEC (by) — *see*
Venom, arthropod
Insensitivity
adrenocorticotropin hormone
(ACTH) E27.49
androgen E34.50
complete E34.51
partial E34.52
Insertion
cord (umbilical) lateral or
velamentous O43.12-
intrauterine contraceptive device (encounter
for) — *see* Intrauterine contraceptive
device
Insolation (sunstroke) T67.01
Insomnia (organic) G47.00
adjustment F51.02
adjustment disorder F51.02
behavioral, of childhood Z73.819
combined type Z73.812
limit setting type Z73.811
sleep-onset association type Z73.810
childhood Z73.819
chronic F51.04
somatized tension F51.04
conditioned F51.04
due to
alcohol

Insomnia (organic) - *continued*
due to - *continued*
alcohol - *continued*
abuse F10.182
dependence F10.282
use F10.982
amphetamines
abuse F15.182
dependence F15.282
use F15.982
anxiety disorder F51.05
caffeine
abuse F15.182
dependence F15.282
use F15.982
cocaine
abuse F14.182
dependence F14.282
use F14.982
depression F51.05
drug NEC
abuse F19.182
dependence F19.282
use F19.982
medical condition G47.01
mental disorder NEC F51.05
opioid
abuse F11.182
dependence F11.282
use F11.982
psychoactive substance NEC
abuse F19.182
dependence F19.282
use F19.982
sedative, hypnotic, or anxiolytic
abuse F13.182
dependence F13.282
use F13.982
stimulant NEC
abuse F15.182
dependence F15.282
use F15.982
fatal familial (FFI) A81.83
idiopathic F51.01
learned F51.3
nonorganic origin F51.01
not due to a substance or known
physiological condition F51.01
specified NEC F51.09
paradoxical F51.03
primary F51.01
psychiatric F51.05
psychophysiologic F51.04
related to psychopathology F51.05
short-term F51.02
specified NEC G47.09
stress-related F51.02
transient F51.02
without objective findings F51.02
Inspiration
food or foreign body — *see* Foreign body, by
site
mucus — *see* Asphyxia, mucus
Inspissated bile syndrome (newborn) P59.1
Instability
emotional (excessive) F60.3
joint (post-traumatic) M25.30
ankle M25.37-
due to old ligament injury — *see* Disorder,
ligament
elbow M25.32-
flail — *see* Flail, joint
foot M25.37-
hand M25.34-
hip M25.35-
knee M25.36-
lumbosacral — *see* subcategory M53.2
prosthesis — *see* Complications, joint
prosthesis, mechanical, displacement,
by site
sacroiliac — *see* subcategory M53.2
secondary to
old ligament injury — *see* Disorder,
ligament
removal of joint prosthesis M96.89

Instability - *continued*
joint (post-traumatic) - *continued*
shoulder (region) M25.31-
spine — *see* subcategory M53.2
wrist M25.33-
knee (chronic) M23.5-
lumbosacral — *see* subcategory M53.2
nervous F48.8
personality (emotional) F60.3
spine — *see* Instability, joint, spine
vasomotor R55
Institutional syndrome (childhood) F94.2
Institutionalization, affecting child Z62.22
disinhibited attachment F94.2
Insufficiency, insufficient
accommodation, old age H52.4
adrenal (gland) E27.40
primary E27.1
adrenocortical E27.40
drug-induced E27.3
iatrogenic E27.3
primary E27.1
anatomic crown height K08.89
anterior (occlusal) guidance M26.54
anus K62.89
aortic (valve) I35.1
with
mitral (valve) disease I08.0
with tricuspid (valve) disease I08.3
stenosis I35.2
tricuspid (valve) disease I08.2
with mitral (valve) disease I08.3
congenital Q23.1
rheumatic I06.1
with
mitral (valve) disease I08.0
with tricuspid (valve) disease I08.3
stenosis I06.2
with mitral (valve) disease I08.0
with tricuspid (valve)
disease I08.3
tricuspid (valve) disease I08.2
with mitral (valve) disease I08.3
specified cause NEC I35.1
syphilitic A52.03
arterial I77.1
basilar G45.0
carotid (hemispheric) G45.1
cerebral I67.81
coronary (acute or subacute) I24.8
mesenteric K55.1
peripheral I73.9
precerebral (multiple) (bilateral) G45.2
vertebral G45.0
arteriovenous I99.8
biliary K83.8
cardiac — *see also* Insufficiency, myocardial
due to presence of (cardiac)
prosthesis I97.11-
postprocedural I97.11-
cardiorenal, hypertensive I13.2
cardiovascular — *see* Disease,
cardiovascular
cerebrovascular (acute) I67.81
with transient focal neurological signs and
symptoms G45.8
circulatory NEC I99.8
newborn P29.89
clinical crown length K08.89
convergence H51.11
coronary (acute or subacute) I24.8
chronic or with a stated duration of over 4
weeks I25.89
corticoadrenal E27.40
primary E27.1
dietary E63.9
divergence H51.8
food T73.0
gastroesophageal K22.8
gonadal
ovary E28.39
testis E29.1
heart — *see also* Insufficiency, myocardial
newborn P29.0
valve — *see* Endocarditis

Insufficiency, insufficient - *continued*
hepatic — *see* Failure, hepatic
idiopathic autonomic G90.09
interocclusal distance of fully erupted teeth
(ridge) M26.36
kidney N28.9
acute N28.9
chronic N18.9
lacrimal (secretion) H04.12-
passages — *see* Stenosis, lacrimal
liver — *see* Failure, hepatic
lung — *see* Insufficiency, pulmonary
mental (congenital) — *see* Disability,
intellectual
mesenteric K55.1
mitral (valve) I34.0
with
aortic valve disease I08.0
with tricuspid (valve) disease I08.3
obstruction or stenosis I05.2
with aortic valve disease I08.0
tricuspid (valve) disease I08.1
with aortic (valve) disease I08.3
congenital Q23.3
rheumatic I05.1
with
aortic valve disease I08.0
with tricuspid (valve) disease I08.3
obstruction or stenosis I05.2
with aortic valve disease I08.0
with tricuspid (valve)
disease I08.3
tricuspid (valve) disease I08.1
with aortic (valve) disease I08.3
active or acute I01.1
with chorea, rheumatic
(Sydenham's) I02.0
specified cause, except rheumatic I34.0
muscle — *see also* Disease, muscle
heart — *see* Insufficiency, myocardial
ocular NEC H50.9
myocardial, myocardium (with
arteriosclerosis) — *see also* Failure,
heart I50.9
with
rheumatic fever (conditions in I00) I09.0
active, acute or subacute I01.2
with chorea I02.0
inactive or quiescent (with
chorea) I09.0
congenital Q24.8
hypertensive — *see* Hypertension, heart
newborn P29.0
rheumatic I09.0
active, acute, or subacute I01.2
syphilitic A52.06
nourishment T73.0
pancreatic K86.89
exocrine K86.81
parathyroid (gland) E20.9
peripheral vascular (arterial) I73.9
pituitary E23.0
placental (mother) O36.51-
platelets D69.6
prenatal care affecting management of
pregnancy O09.3-
progressive pluriglandular E31.0
pulmonary J98.4
acute, following surgery
(nonthoracic) J95.2
thoracic J95.1
chronic, following surgery J95.3
following
shock J98.4
trauma J98.4
newborn P28.89
valve I37.1
with stenosis I37.2
congenital Q22.2
rheumatic I09.89
with aortic, mitral or tricuspid (valve)
disease I08.8
pyloric K31.89
renal (acute) N28.9
chronic N18.9

Insufficiency, insufficient - *continued*
respiratory R06.89
newborn P28.5
rotation — *see* Malrotation
sleep syndrome F51.12
social insurance Z59.7
suprarenal E27.40
primary E27.1
tarso-orbital fascia, congenital Q10.3
testis E29.1
thyroid (gland) (acquired) E03.9
congenital E03.1
tricuspid (valve) (rheumatic) I07.1
with
aortic (valve) disease I08.2
with mitral (valve) disease I08.3
mitral (valve) disease I08.1
with aortic (valve) disease I08.3
obstruction or stenosis I07.2
with aortic (valve) disease I08.2
with mitral (valve) disease I08.3
congenital Q22.8
nonrheumatic I36.1
with stenosis I36.2
urethral sphincter R32
valve, valvular (heart) I38
aortic — *see* Insufficiency, aortic (valve)
mitral — *see* Insufficiency, mitral (valve)
pulmonary — *see* Insufficiency,
pulmonary, valve
tricuspid — *see* Insufficiency, tricuspid
(valve)
congenital Q24.8
vascular I99.8
intestine K55.9
acute — *see also* Ischemia, intestine,
acute K55.059
mesenteric K55.1
peripheral I73.9
renal — *see* Hypertension, kidney
velopharyngeal
acquired K13.79
congenital Q38.8
venous (chronic) (peripheral) I87.2
ventricular — *see* Insufficiency, myocardial
welfare support Z59.7
Insufflation, fallopian Z31.41
Insular — *see* condition
Insulinoma
pancreas
benign D13.7
malignant C25.4
uncertain behavior D37.8
specified site
benign — *see* Neoplasm, by site, benign
malignant — *see* Neoplasm, by site,
malignant
uncertain behavior — *see* Neoplasm, by
site, uncertain behavior
unspecified site
benign D13.7
malignant C25.4
uncertain behavior D37.8
Insuloma — *see* Insulinoma
Interference
balancing side M26.56
non-working side M26.56
Intermenstrual — *see* condition
Intermittent — *see* condition
Internal — *see* condition
Interrogation
cardiac defibrillator (automatic)
(implantable) Z45.02
cardiac pacemaker Z45.018
cardiac (event) (loop) recorder Z45.09
infusion pump (implanted)
(intrathecal) Z45.1
neurostimulator Z46.2
Interruption
aortic arch Q25.21
bundle of His I44.30
phase-shift, sleep cycle — *see* Disorder,
sleep, circadian rhythm

Interruption - *continued*
  sleep phase-shift, or 24 hour sleep-wake
    cycle — *see* Disorder, sleep, circadian
    rhythm
Interstitial — *see* condition
Intertrigo L30.4
  labialis K13.0
Intervertebral disc — *see* condition
Intestine, intestinal — *see* condition
Intolerance
  carbohydrate K90.49
  disaccharide, hereditary E73.0
  fat NEC K90.49
    pancreatic K90.3
  food K90.49
    dietary counseling and surveillance Z71.3
  fructose E74.10
    hereditary E74.12
  glucose (-galactose) E74.39
  gluten K90.41
  lactose E73.9
    specified NEC E73.8
  lysine E72.3
  milk NEC K90.49
    lactose E73.9
  protein K90.49
  starch NEC K90.49
  sucrose (-isomaltose) E74.31
Intoxicated NEC (without
    dependence) — *see* Alcohol, intoxication
Intoxication
  acid E87.2
  alcoholic (acute) (without dependence) —
    see Alcohol, intoxication
  alimentary canal K52.1
  amphetamine (without dependence) — *see*
    also Abuse, drug, stimulant, with
    intoxication
    with dependence — *see* Dependence, drug,
      stimulant, with intoxication
    stimulant NEC F15.10
      with
        anxiety disorder F15.180
        intoxication F15.129
          with
            delirium F15.121
            perceptual disturbance F15.122
  anxiolytic (acute) (without dependence) —
    see Abuse, drug, sedative, with
    intoxication
    with dependence — *see* Dependence, drug,
      sedative, with intoxication
  caffeine F15.929
    with dependence — *see* Dependence, drug,
      stimulant, with intoxication
  cannabinoids (acute) (without
    dependence) — *see* Use, cannabis, with
    intoxication
    with
      abuse — *see* Abuse, drug, cannabis, with
        intoxication
      dependence — *see* Dependence, drug,
        cannabis, with intoxication
  chemical — *see* Table of Drugs and
    Chemicals
    via placenta or breast milk — *see* -
      Absorption, chemical, through
      placenta
  cocaine (acute) (without dependence) — *see*
    Abuse, drug, cocaine, with intoxication
    with dependence — *see* Dependence, drug,
      cocaine, with intoxication
  drug
    acute (without dependence) — *see* Abuse,
      drug, by type with intoxication
      with dependence — *see* Dependence,
        drug, by type with intoxication
    addictive
      via placenta or breast milk — *see*
        Absorption, drug, addictive,
        through placenta
    newborn P93.8
      gray baby syndrome P93.0

Intoxication - *continued*
  drug - *continued*
    overdose or wrong substance given or
      taken — *see* Table of Drugs and
      Chemicals, by drug, poisoning
  enteric K52.1
  foodborne A05.9
    bacterial A05.9
    classical (Clostridium botulinum) A05.1
    due to
      Bacillus cereus A05.4
      bacterium A05.9
        specified NEC A05.8
      Clostridium
        botulinum A05.1
        perfringens A05.2
        welchii A05.2
      Salmonella A02.9
        with
          (gastro) enteritis A02.0
          localized infection (s) A02.20
            arthritis A02.23
            meningitis A02.21
            osteomyelitis A02.24
            pneumonia A02.22
            pyelonephritis A02.25
            specified NEC A02.29
          sepsis A02.1
          specified manifestation NEC A02.8
      Staphylococcus A05.0
      Vibrio
        parahaemolyticus A05.3
        vulnificus A05.5
    enterotoxin, staphylococcal A05.0
    noxious — *see* Poisoning, food, noxious
  gastrointestinal K52.1
  hallucinogenic (without dependence) — *see*
    Abuse, drug, hallucinogen, with
    intoxication
    with dependence — *see* Dependence, drug,
      hallucinogen, with intoxication
  hypnotic (acute) (without dependence) — *see*
    Abuse, drug, sedative, with intoxication
    with dependence — *see* Dependence, drug,
      sedative, with intoxication
  inhalant (acute) (without dependence) — *see*
    Abuse, drug, inhalant, with intoxication
    with dependence — *see* Dependence, drug,
      inhalant, with intoxication
  meaning
    inebriation — *see* category F10
    poisoning — *see* Table of Drugs and
      Chemicals
  methyl alcohol (acute) (without
    dependence) — *see* Alcohol,
    intoxication
  opioid (acute) (without dependence) — *see*
    Abuse, drug, opioid, with intoxication
    with dependence — *see* Dependence, drug,
      opioid, with intoxication
  pathologic NEC (without dependence) — *see*
    Alcohol, intoxication
  phencyclidine (without dependence) — *see*
    Abuse, drug, hallucinogen, with
    intoxication
    with dependence - — *see* Dependence,
      drug, hallucinogen, with intoxication
  potassium (K) E87.5
  psychoactive substance NEC (without
    dependence) — *see* Abuse, drug,
    psychoactive NEC, with intoxication
    with dependence — *see* Dependence, drug,
      psychoactive NEC, with intoxication
  sedative (acute) (without dependence) — *see*
    Abuse, drug, sedative, with intoxication
    with dependence — *see* Dependence, drug,
      sedative, with intoxication
  serum — *see also* Reaction, serum T80.69
  uremic — *see* Uremia
  volatile solvents (acute) (without
    dependence) — *see* Abuse, drug,
    inhalant, with intoxication
    with dependence — *see* Dependence, drug,
      inhalant, with intoxication
  water E87.79

Intraabdominal testis, testes
  bilateral Q53.211
  unilateral Q53.111
Intracranial — *see* condition
Intrahepatic gallbladder Q44.1
Intraligamentous — *see* condition
Intrathoracic — *see also* condition
  kidney Q63.2
Intrauterine contraceptive device
  checking Z30.431
  insertion Z30.430
    immediately following removal Z30.433
  in situ Z97.5
  management Z30.431
  reinsertion Z30.433
  removal Z30.432
  replacement Z30.433
  retention in pregnancy O26.3-
Intraventricular — *see* condition
Intrinsic deformity — *see* Deformity
Intubation, difficult or failed T88.4
Intumescence, lens (eye) (cataract) — *see*
  Cataract
Intussusception (bowel) (colon) (enteric)
  (ileocecal) (ileocolic) (intestine)
  (rectum) K56.1
  appendix K38.8
  congenital Q43.8
  ureter (with obstruction) N13.5
Invagination (bowel, colon, intestine or
  rectum) K56.1
Inversion
  albumin-globulin (A-G) ratio E88.09
  bladder N32.89
  cecum — *see* Intussusception
  cervix N88.8
  chromosome in normal individual Q95.1
  circadian rhythm — *see* Disorder, sleep,
    circadian rhythm
  nipple N64.59
    congenital Q83.8
    gestational — *see* Retraction, nipple
    puerperal, postpartum — *see* Retraction,
      nipple
  nyctohemeral rhythm — *see* Disorder, sleep,
    circadian rhythm
  optic papilla Q14.2
  organ or site, congenital NEC — *see*
    Anomaly, by site
  sleep rhythm — *see* Disorder, sleep,
    circadian rhythm
  testis (congenital) Q55.29
  uterus (chronic) (postinfectional) (postpartal,
    old) N85.5
    postpartum O71.2
  vagina (posthysterectomy) N99.3
  ventricular Q20.5
Investigation — *see also* Examination Z04.9
  clinical research subject (control) (normal
    comparison) (participant) Z00.6
Involuntary movement, abnormal R25.9
Involution, involutional — *see also* condition
  breast, cystic — *see* Dysplasia, mammary,
    specified type NEC
  depression (single episode) F32.89
    recurrent episode F33.9
  melancholia (single episode) F32.89
    recurrent episode F33.8
  ovary, senile — *see* Atrophy, ovary
  thymus failure E32.8
IRDS (type I) P22.0
  type II P22.1
Irideremia Q13.1
Iridis rubeosis — *see* Disorder, iris, vascular
Iridochoroiditis (panuveitis) — *see*
  Panuveitis
Iridocyclitis H20.9
  acute H20.0-
    hypopyon H20.05-
    primary H20.01-
    recurrent H20.02-
    secondary (noninfectious) H20.04-
      infectious H20.03-
  chronic H20.1-

Iridocyclitis - *continued*
  due to allergy — *see* Iridocyclitis, acute,
    secondary
  endogenous — *see* Iridocyclitis, acute,
    primary
  Fuchs' — *see* Cyclitis, Fuchs' heterochromic
  gonococcal A54.32
  granulomatous — *see* Iridocyclitis, chronic
  herpes, herpetic (simplex) B00.51
    zoster B02.32
  hypopyon — *see* Iridocyclitis, acute,
    hypopyon
  in (due to)
    ankylosing spondylitis M45.9
    gonococcal infection A54.32
    herpes (simplex) virus B00.51
      zoster B02.32
    infectious disease NOS B99
    parasitic disease NOS B89 *[H22]*
    sarcoidosis D86.83
    syphilis A51.43
    tuberculosis A18.54
    zoster B02.32
  lens-induced H20.2-
  nongranulomatous — *see* Iridocyclitis, acute
  recurrent — *see* Iridocyclitis, acute, recurrent
  rheumatic — *see* Iridocyclitis, chronic
  subacute — *see* Iridocyclitis, acute
  sympathetic — *see* Uveitis, sympathetic
  syphilitic (secondary) A51.43
  tuberculous (chronic) A18.54
  Vogt-Koyanagi H20.82-
Iridocyclochoroiditis (panuveitis) — *see*
    Panuveitis
Iridodialysis H21.53-
Iridodonesis H21.89
Iridoplegia (complete) (partial)
    (reflex) H57.09
Iridoschisis H21.25-
Iris — *see also* condition
  bombé — *see* Membrane, pupillary
Iritis — *see also* Iridocyclitis
  chronic — *see* Iridocyclitis, chronic
  diabetic — *see* E08-E13 with .39
  due to
    herpes simplex B00.51
    leprosy A30.9 *[H22]*
  gonococcal A54.32
  gouty — *see also* Gout, by type M10.9
    [H22]
  granulomatous — *see* Iridocyclitis, chronic
  lens induced — *see* Iridocyclitis, lens-
    induced
  papulosa (syphilitic) A52.71
  rheumatic — *see* Iridocyclitis, chronic
  syphilitic (secondary) A51.43
    congenital (early) A50.01
    late A52.71
  tuberculous A18.54
Iron — *see* condition
Iron-miner's lung J63.4
Irradiated enamel (tooth, teeth) K03.89
Irradiation effects, adverse T66
Irreducible, irreducibility — *see* condition
Irregular, irregularity
  action, heart I49.9
  alveolar process K08.89
  bleeding N92.6
  breathing R06.89
  contour of cornea (acquired) — *see*
    Deformity, cornea
    congenital Q13.4
  contour, reconstructed breast N65.0
  dentin (in pulp) K04.3
  eye movements H55.89
    nystagmus — *see* Nystagmus
    saccadic H55.81
  labor O62.2
  menstruation (cause unknown) N92.6
  periods N92.6
  prostate N42.9
  pupil — *see* Abnormality, pupillary
  reconstructed breast N65.0
  respiratory R06.89
  septum (nasal) J34.2

Irregular, irregularity - *continued*
  shape, organ or site, congenital NEC — *see*
    Distortion
  sleep-wake pattern (rhythm) G47.23
Irritable, irritability R45.4
  bladder N32.89
  bowel (syndrome) K58.9
    with
      constipation K58.1
      diarrhea K58.0
      mixed K58.2
      psychogenic F45.8
      specified NEC K58.8
  bronchial — *see* Bronchitis
  cerebral, in newborn P91.3
  colon — *see also* Irritable, bowel K58.9
    with diarrhea K58.0
    psychogenic F45.8
  duodenum K59.8
  heart (psychogenic) F45.8
  hip — *see* Derangement, joint, specified type
    NEC, hip
  ileum K59.8
  infant R68.12
  jejunum K59.8
  rectum K59.8
  stomach K31.89
    psychogenic F45.8
  sympathetic G90.8
  urethra N36.8
Irritation
  anus K62.89
  axillary nerve G54.0
  bladder N32.89
  brachial plexus G54.0
  bronchial — *see* Bronchitis
  cervical plexus G54.2
  cervix — *see* Cervicitis
  choroid, sympathetic — *see* Endophthalmitis
  cranial nerve — *see* Disorder, nerve, cranial
  gastric K31.89
    psychogenic F45.8
  globe, sympathetic — *see* Uveitis,
    sympathetic
  labyrinth — *see* subcategory H83.2
  lumbosacral plexus G54.1
  meninges (traumatic) — *see* Injury,
    intracranial
    nontraumatic — *see* Meningismus
  nerve — *see* Disorder, nerve
  nervous R45.0
  penis N48.89
  perineum NEC L29.3
  peripheral autonomic nervous system G90.8
  peritoneum — *see* Peritonitis
  pharynx J39.2
  plantar nerve — *see* Lesion, nerve, plantar
  spinal (cord) (traumatic) — *see also* Injury,
    spinal cord, by region
    nerve G58.9
      root NEC — *see* Radiculopathy
    nontraumatic — *see* Myelopathy
  stomach K31.89
    psychogenic F45.8
  sympathetic nerve NEC G90.8
  ulnar nerve — *see* Lesion, nerve, ulnar
  vagina N89.8
Ischemia, ischemic I99.8
  brain — *see* Ischemia, cerebral
  bowel (transient)
    acute — *see also* Ischemia, intestine,
      acute K55.059
    chronic K55.1
    due to mesenteric artery
      insufficiency K55.1
  cardiac (see Disease, heart, ischemic)
  cardiomyopathy I25.5
  cerebral (chronic) (generalized) I67.82
    arteriosclerotic I67.2
    intermittent G45.9
    newborn P91.0
    recurrent focal G45.8
    transient G45.9
  colon chronic (due to mesenteric artery
    insufficiency) K55.1

Ischemia, ischemic - *continued*
  coronary — *see* Disease, heart, ischemic
  demand (coronary) — *see also* Angina I24.8
    with myocardial infarction I21.A1
    resulting in myocardial infarction I21.A1
  heart (chronic or with a stated duration of
    over 4 weeks) I25.9
    acute or with a stated duration of 4 weeks
      or less I24.9
    subacute I24.9
  infarction, muscle — *see* Infarct, muscle
  intestine (large) (small) (transient) K55.9
    acute K55.059
      diffuse K55.052
      focal K55.051
      large K55.039
        diffuse K55.032
        focal K55.031
      small K55.019
        diffuse K55.012
        focal K55.011
    chronic K55.1
      due to mesenteric artery
        insufficiency K55.1
  kidney N28.0
  mesenteric, acute — *see also* Ischemia,
    intestine, acute K55.059
  muscle, traumatic T79.6
  myocardium, myocardial (chronic or with a
    stated duration of over 4 weeks) I25.9
    acute, without myocardial infarction I51.3
    silent (asymptomatic) I25.6
    transient of newborn P29.4
  renal N28.0
  retina, retinal — *see* Occlusion, artery, retina
  small bowel
    acute K55.019
      diffuse K55.012
      focal K55.011
    chronic K55.1
      due to mesenteric artery
        insufficiency K55.1
  spinal cord G95.11
  subendocardial — *see* Insufficiency,
    coronary
  supply (coronary) — *see also* Angina I25.9
    due to vasospasm I20.1
Ischial spine — *see* condition
Ischialgia — *see* Sciatica
Ischiopagus Q89.4
Ischium, ischial — *see* condition
Ischuria R34
Iselin's disease or osteochondrosis — *see*
    Osteochondrosis, juvenile, metatarsus
Islands of
  parotid tissue in
    lymph nodes Q38.6
    neck structures Q38.6
  submaxillary glands in
    fascia Q38.6
    lymph nodes Q38.6
    neck muscles Q38.6
Islet cell tumor, pancreas D13.7
Isoimmunization NEC — *see also*
    Incompatibility
  affecting management of pregnancy (ABO)
    (with hydrops fetalis) O36.11-
    anti-A sensitization O36.11-
    anti-B sensitization O36.19-
    anti-c sensitization O36.09-
    anti-C sensitization O36.09-
    anti-e sensitization O36.09-
    anti-E sensitization O36.09-
    Rh NEC O36.09-
      anti-D antibody O36.01-
    specified NEC O36.19-
  newborn P55.9
    with
      hydrops fetalis P56.0
      kernicterus P57.0
    ABO (blood groups) P55.1
    Rhesus (Rh) factor P55.0
    specified type NEC P55.8
Isolation, isolated
  dwelling Z59.8

Isolation, isolated - *continued*
   family Z63.79
   social Z60.4
Isoleucinosis E71.19
Isomerism atrial appendages (with asplenia or polysplenia) Q20.6
Isosporiasis, isosporosis A07.3
Isovaleric acidemia E71.110
Issue of
   medical certificate Z02.79
     for disability determination Z02.71
   repeat prescription (appliance) (glasses) (medicinal substance, medicament, medicine) Z76.0
     contraception — *see* Contraception
Itch, itching — *see also* Pruritus
   baker's L23.6
   barber's B35.0
   bricklayer's L24.5
   cheese B88.0
   clam digger's B65.3
   coolie B76.9
   copra B88.0
   dew B76.9
   dhobi B35.6
   filarial — *see* Infestation, filarial
   grain B88.0
   grocer's B88.0
   ground B76.9
   harvest B88.0
   jock B35.6
   Malabar B35.5
     beard B35.0
     foot B35.3
     scalp B35.0
   meaning scabies B86
   Norwegian B86
   perianal L29.0
   poultrymen's B88.0
   sarcoptic B86
   scabies B86
   scrub B88.0
   straw B88.0
   swimmer's B65.3
   water B76.9
   winter L29.8
Ivemark's syndrome (asplenia with congenital heart disease) Q89.01
Ivory bones Q78.2
Ixodiasis NEC B88.8

J

Jaccoud's syndrome — *see* Arthropathy, postrheumatic, chronic
Jackson's
   membrane Q43.3
   paralysis or syndrome G83.89
   veil Q43.3
Jacquet's dermatitis (diaper dermatitis) L22
Jadassohn-Pellizari's disease or anetoderma L90.2
Jadassohn's
   blue nevus — *see* Nevus
   intraepidermal epithelioma — *see* Neoplasm, skin, benign
Jaffe-Lichtenstein (-Uehlinger) syndrome — *see* Dysplasia, fibrous, bone NEC
Jakob-Creutzfeldt disease or syndrome — *see* Creutzfeldt-Jakob disease or syndrome
Jaksch-Luzet disease D64.89
Jamaican
   neuropathy G92
   paraplegic tropical ataxic-spastic syndrome G92
Janet's disease F48.8
Janiceps Q89.4
Jansky-Bielschowsky amaurotic idiocy E75.4
Japanese
   B-type encephalitis A83.0
   river fever A75.3
Jaundice (yellow) R17
   acholuric (familial) (splenomegalic) — *see also* Spherocytosis
     acquired D59.8

Jaundice (yellow) - *continued*
   breast-milk (inhibitor) P59.3
   catarrhal (acute) B15.9
     with hepatic coma B15.0
   cholestatic (benign) R17
   due to or associated with
     delayed conjugation P59.8
       associated with (due to) preterm delivery P59.0
     preterm delivery P59.0
   epidemic (catarrhal) B15.9
     with hepatic coma B15.0
     leptospiral A27.0
     spirochetal A27.0
   familial nonhemolytic (congenital) (Gilbert) E80.4
     Crigler-Najjar E80.5
   febrile (acute) B15.9
     with hepatic coma B15.0
     leptospiral A27.0
     spirochetal A27.0
   hematogenous D59.9
   hemolytic (acquired) D59.9
     congenital — *see* Spherocytosis
   hemorrhagic (acute) (leptospiral) (spirochetal) A27.0
   infectious (acute) (subacute) B15.9
     with hepatic coma B15.0
     leptospiral A27.0
     spirochetal A27.0
   leptospiral (hemorrhagic) A27.0
   malignant (without coma) K72.90
     with coma K72.91
   newborn P59.9
     due to or associated with
       ABO
         antibodies P55.1
         incompatibility, maternal/fetal P55.1
         isoimmunization P55.1
       absence or deficiency of enzyme system for bilirubin conjugation (congenital) P59.8
       bleeding P58.1
       breast milk inhibitors to conjugation P59.3
        associated with preterm delivery P59.0
       bruising P58.0
       Crigler-Najjar syndrome E80.5
       delayed conjugation P59.8
        associated with preterm delivery P59.0
       drugs or toxins
        given to newborn P58.42
        transmitted from mother P58.41
       excessive hemolysis P58.9
        due to
         bleeding P58.1
         bruising P58.0
         drugs or toxins
          given to newborn P58.42
          transmitted from mother P58.41
         infection P58.2
         polycythemia P58.3
         swallowed maternal blood P58.5
        specified type NEC P58.8
       galactosemia E74.21
       Gilbert syndrome E80.4
       hemolytic disease P55.9
        ABO isoimmunization P55.1
        Rh isoimmunization P55.0
        specified NEC P55.8
       hepatocellular damage P59.20
        specified NEC P59.29
       hereditary hemolytic anemia P58.8
       hypothyroidism, congenital E03.1
       incompatibility, maternal/fetal NOS P55.9
       infection P58.2
       inspissated bile syndrome P59.1
       isoimmunization NOS P55.9
       mucoviscidosis E84.9
       polycythemia P58.3
       preterm delivery P59.0
       Rh
        antibodies P55.0
        incompatibility, maternal/fetal P55.0

Jaundice (yellow) - *continued*
   newborn - *continued*
     due to or associated with - *continued*
       Rh - *continued*
        isoimmunization P55.0
      specified cause NEC P59.8
      swallowed maternal blood P58.5
     spherocytosis (congenital) D58.0
   neonatal — *see* Jaundice, newborn
   nonhemolytic congenital familial (Gilbert) E80.4
   nuclear, newborn — *see also* Kernicterus of newborn P57.9
   obstructive — *see also* Obstruction, bile duct K83.1
   post-immunization — *see* Hepatitis, viral, type, B
   post-transfusion — *see* Hepatitis, viral, type, B
   regurgitation — *see also* Obstruction, bile duct K83.1
   serum (homologous) (prophylactic) (therapeutic) — *see* Hepatitis, viral, type, B
   spirochetal (hemorrhagic) A27.0
   symptomatic R17
     newborn P59.9
Jaw — *see* condition
Jaw-winking phenomenon or syndrome Q07.8
Jealousy
   alcoholic F10.988
   childhood F93.8
   sibling F93.8
Jejunitis — *see* Enteritis
Jejunostomy status Z93.4
Jejunum, jejunal — *see* condition
Jensen's disease — *see* Inflammation, chorioretinal, focal, juxtapapillary
Jerks, myoclonic G25.3
Jervell-Lange-Nielsen syndrome I45.81
Jeune's disease Q77.2
Jigger disease B88.1
Job's syndrome (chronic granulomatous disease) D71
Joint — *see also* condition
   mice — *see* Loose, body, joint
     knee M23.4-
Jordan's anomaly or syndrome D72.0
Joseph-Diamond-Blackfan anemia (congenital hypoplastic) D61.01
Jungle yellow fever A95.0
Jüngling's disease — *see* Sarcoidosis
Juvenile — *see* condition

K

Kahler's disease C90.0-
Kakke E51.11
Kala-azar B55.0
Kallmann's syndrome E23.0
Kanner's syndrome (autism) — *see* Psychosis, childhood
Kaposi's
   dermatosis (xeroderma pigmentosum) Q82.1
   lichen ruber L44.0
     acuminatus L44.0
   sarcoma
     colon C46.4
     connective tissue C46.1
     gastrointestinal organ C46.4
     lung C46.5-
     lymph node (multiple) C46.3
     palate (hard) (soft) C46.2
     rectum C46.4
     skin (multiple sites) C46.0
     specified site NEC C46.7
     stomach C46.4
     unspecified site C46.9
   varicelliform eruption B00.0
     vaccinia T88.1
Kartagener's syndrome or triad (sinusitis, bronchiectasis, situs inversus) Q89.3
Karyotype
   with abnormality except iso (Xq) Q96.2
   45,X Q96.0
   46,X

Karyotype - *continued*
 46,X - *continued*
  iso (Xq) Q96.1
 46,XX Q98.3
  with streak gonads Q50.32
  hermaphrodite (true) Q99.1
  male Q98.3
 46,XY
  with streak gonads Q56.1
  female Q97.3
  hermaphrodite (true) Q99.1
 47,XXX Q97.0
 47,XXY Q98.0
 47,XYY Q98.5
Kaschin-Beck disease — *see* Disease,
  Kaschin-Beck
Katayama's disease or fever B65.2
Kawasaki's syndrome M30.3
Kayser-Fleischer ring (cornea)
  (pseudosclerosis) H18.04-
Kaznelson's syndrome (congenital
  hypoplastic anemia) D61.01
Kearns-Sayre syndrome H49.81-
Kedani fever A75.3
Kelis L91.0
Kelly (-Patterson) syndrome (sideropenic
  dysphagia) D50.1
Keloid, cheloid L91.0
 acne L73.0
 Addison's L94.0
 cornea — *see* Opacity, cornea
 Hawkin's L91.0
 scar L91.0
Keloma L91.0
Kenya fever A77.1
Keratectasia — *see also* Ectasia, cornea
 congenital Q13.4
Keratinization of alveolar ridge mucosa
 excessive K13.23
 minimal K13.22
Keratinized residual ridge mucosa
 excessive K13.23
 minimal K13.22
Keratitis (nodular) (nonulcerative) (simple)
  (zonular) H16.9
 with ulceration (central) (marginal)
   (perforated) (ring) — *see* Ulcer, cornea
 actinic — *see* Photokeratitis
 arborescens (herpes simplex) B00.52
 areolar H16.11-
 bullosa H16.8
 deep H16.309
  specified type NEC H16.399
 dendritic (a) (herpes simplex) B00.52
 disciform (is) (herpes simplex) B00.52
  varicella B01.81
 filamentary H16.12-
 gonococcal (congenital or prenatal) A54.33
 herpes, herpetic (simplex) B00.52
  zoster B02.33
 in (due to)
  acanthamebiasis B60.13
  adenovirus B30.0
  exanthema — *see also* Exanthem B09
  herpes (simplex) virus B00.52
  measles B05.81
  syphilis A50.31
  tuberculosis A18.52
  zoster B02.33
 interstitial (nonsyphilitic) H16.30-
  diffuse H16.32-
  herpes, herpetic (simplex) B00.52
   zoster B02.33
  sclerosing H16.33-
  specified type NEC H16.39-
  syphilitic (congenital) (late) A50.31
  tuberculous A18.52
 macular H16.11-
 nummular H16.11-
 oyster shuckers' H16.8
 parenchymatous — *see* Keratitis, interstitial
 petrificans H16.8
 postmeasles B05.81
 punctata
  leprosa A30.9 *[H16.14-]*

Keratitis (nodular) (nonulcerative) (simple)
 (zonular) - *continued*
 punctata - *continued*
  syphilitic (profunda) A50.31
 punctate H16.14-
 purulent H16.8
 rosacea L71.8
 sclerosing H16.33-
 specified type NEC H16.8
 stellate H16.11-
 striate H16.11-
 superficial H16.10-
  with conjunctivitis — *see*
   Keratoconjunctivitis
  due to light — *see* Photokeratitis
 suppurative H16.8
 syphilitic (congenital) (prenatal) A50.31
 trachomatous A71.1
  sequelae B94.0
 tuberculous A18.52
 vesicular H16.8
 xerotic — *see also* Keratomalacia H16.8
  vitamin A deficiency E50.4
Keratoacanthoma L85.8
Keratocele — *see* Descemetocele
Keratoconjunctivitis H16.20-
 Acanthamoeba B60.13
 adenoviral B30.0
 epidemic B30.0
 exposure H16.21-
 herpes, herpetic (simplex) B00.52
  zoster B02.33
 in exanthema — *see also* Exanthem B09
 infectious B30.0
 lagophthalmic — *see* Keratoconjunctivitis,
  specified type NEC
 neurotrophic H16.23-
 phlyctenular H16.25-
 postmeasles B05.81
 shipyard B30.0
 sicca (Sjogren's) M35.0-
  not Sjogren's H16.22-
 specified type NEC H16.29-
 tuberculous (phlyctenular) A18.52
 vernal H16.26-
Keratoconus H18.60-
 congenital Q13.4
 stable H18.61-
 unstable H18.62-
Keratocyst (dental) (odontogenic) — *see*
  Cyst, calcifying odontogenic
Keratoderma, keratodermia (congenital)
  (palmaris et plantaris) (symmetrical)
  Q82.8
 acquired L85.1
  in diseases classified elsewhere L86
 climactericum L85.1
 gonococcal A54.89
 gonorrheal A54.89
 punctata L85.2
 Reiter's — *see* Reiter's disease
Keratodermatocele — *see* Descemetocele
Keratoglobus H18.79
 congenital Q15.8
  with glaucoma Q15.0
Keratohemia — *see* Pigmentation, cornea,
  stromal
Keratoiritis — *see also* Iridocyclitis
 syphilitic A50.39
 tuberculous A18.54
Keratoma L57.0
 palmaris and plantaris hereditarium Q82.8
 senile L57.0
Keratomalacia H18.44-
 vitamin A deficiency E50.4
Keratomegaly Q13.4
Keratomycosis B49
 nigrans, nigricans (palmaris) B36.1
Keratopathy H18.9
 band H18.42-
 bullous H18.1-
 bullous (aphakic) , following cataract
   surgery H59.01-
Keratoscleritis, tuberculous A18.52

Keratosis L57.0
 actinic L57.0
 arsenical L85.8
 congenital, specified NEC Q80.8
 female genital NEC N94.89
 follicularis Q82.8
  acquired L11.0
  congenita Q82.8
  et parafollicularis in cutem
    penetrans L87.0
  spinulosa (decalvans) Q82.8
  vitamin A deficiency E50.8
 gonococcal A54.89
 male genital (external) N50.89
 nigricans L83
 obturans, external ear (canal) — *see*
   Cholesteatoma, external ear
 palmaris et plantaris (inherited)
   (symmetrical) Q82.8
  acquired L85.1
 penile N48.89
 pharynx J39.2
 pilaris, acquired L85.8
 punctata (palmaris et plantaris) L85.2
 scrotal N50.89
 seborrheic L82.1
  inflamed L82.0
 senile L57.0
 solar L57.0
 tonsillaris J35.8
 vagina N89.4
 vegetans Q82.8
 vitamin A deficiency E50.8
 vocal cord J38.3
Kerato-uveitis — *see* Iridocyclitis
Kerion (celsi) B35.0
Kernicterus of newborn (not due to
  isoimmunization) P57.9
 due to isoimmunization (conditions in P55.0-
   P55.9) P57.0
 specified type NEC P57.8
Kerunoparalysis T75.09
Keshan disease E59
Ketoacidosis E87.2
 diabetic — *see* Diabetes, by type, with
   ketoacidosis
Ketonuria R82.4
Ketosis NEC E88.89
 diabetic — *see* Diabetes, by type, with
   ketoacidosis
Kew Garden fever A79.1
Kidney — *see* condition
Kienböck's disease — *see also*
   Osteochondrosis, juvenile, hand, carpal
   lunate
 adult M93.1
Kimmelstiel (-Wilson) disease — *see*
   Diabetes, Kimmelstiel (-Wilson) disease
Kimura disease D21.9
 specified site (see Neoplasm, connective
   tissue benign)
Kink, kinking
 artery I77.1
 hair (acquired) L67.8
 ileum or intestine — *see* Obstruction,
   intestine
 Lane's — *see* Obstruction, intestine
 organ or site, congenital NEC — *see*
   Anomaly, by site
 ureter (pelvic junction) N13.5
  with
   hydronephrosis N13.1
    with infection N13.6
   pyelonephritis (chronic) N11.1
  congenital Q62.39
 vein (s) I87.8
  caval I87.1
  peripheral I87.1
Kinnier Wilson's disease (hepatolenticular
  degeneration) E83.01
Kissing spine M48.20
 cervical region M48.22
 cervicothoracic region M48.23
 lumbar region M48.26
 lumbosacral region M48.27

Kissing spine - *continued*
  occipito-atlanto-axial region M48.21
  thoracic region M48.24
  thoracolumbar region M48.25
Klatskin's tumor C24.0
Klauder's disease A26.8
Klebs' disease — *see*
  also Glomerulonephritis N05.-
Klebsiella (K.) pneumoniae, as cause of
  disease classified elsewhere B96.1
Klein (e) -Levin syndrome G47.13
Kleptomania F63.2
Klinefelter's syndrome Q98.4
  karyotype 47,XXY Q98.0
  male with more than two X
    chromosomes Q98.1
Klippel-Feil deficiency, disease, or syndrome
  (brevicollis) Q76.1
Klippel's disease I67.2
Klippel-Trenaunay (-Weber)
  syndrome Q87.2
Klumpke (-Déjerine) palsy, paralysis (birth)
  (newborn) P14.1
Knee — *see* condition
Knock knee (acquired) M21.06-
  congenital Q74.1
Knot (s)
  intestinal, syndrome (volvulus) K56.2
  surfer S89.8-
  umbilical cord (true) O69.2
Knotting (of)
  hair L67.8
  intestine K56.2
Knuckle pad (Garrod's) M72.1
Koch's
  infection — *see* Tuberculosis
  relapsing fever A68.9
Koch-Weeks' conjunctivitis — *see*
  Conjunctivitis, acute, mucopurulent
Köebner's syndrome Q81.8
Köenig's disease (osteochondritis
  dissecans) — *see* Osteochondritis,
  dissecans
Köhler-Pellegrini-Steida disease or
  syndrome (calcification, knee
  joint) — *see* Bursitis, tibial collateral
Köhler's disease
  patellar — *see* Osteochondrosis, juvenile,
    patella
  tarsal navicular — *see* Osteochondrosis,
    juvenile, tarsus
Koilonychia L60.3
  congenital Q84.6
Kojevnikov's, epilepsy — *see* Kozhevnikof's
  epilepsy
Koplik's spots B05.9
Kopp's asthma E32.8
Korsakoff's (Wernicke) disease, psychosis or
  syndrome (alcoholic) F10.96
  with dependence F10.26
  drug-induced
    due to drug abuse — *see* Abuse, drug, by
      type, with amnestic disorder
    due to drug dependence — *see*
      Dependence, drug, by type, with
      amnestic disorder
  nonalcoholic F04
Korsakov's disease, psychosis or
  syndrome — *see* Korsakoff's disease
Korsakow's disease, psychosis or
  syndrome — *see* Korsakoff's disease
Kostmann's disease or syndrome (infantile
  genetic agranulocytosis) — *see*
  Agranulocytosis
Kozhevnikof's epilepsy G40.109
  intractable G40.119
    with status epilepticus G40.111
    without status epilepticus G40.119
  not intractable G40.109
    with status epilepticus G40.101
    without status epilepticus G40.109
Krabbe's
  disease E75.23
  syndrome, congenital muscle
    hypoplasia Q79.8

Kraepelin-Morel disease — *see*
  Schizophrenia
Kraft-Weber-Dimitri disease Q85.8
Kraurosis
  ani K62.89
  penis N48.0
  vagina N89.8
  vulva N90.4
Kreotoxism A05.9
Krukenberg's
  spindle — *see* Pigmentation, cornea,
    posterior
  tumor C79.6-
Kufs' disease E75.4
Kugelberg-Welander disease G12.1
Kuhnt-Junius degeneration — *see*
  also Degeneration, macula H35.32-
Kümmell's disease or spondylitis — *see*
  Spondylopathy, traumatic
Kupffer cell sarcoma C22.3
Kuru A81.81
Kussmaul's
  disease M30.0
  respiration E87.2
    in diabetic acidosis — *see* Diabetes, by
      type, with ketoacidosis
Kwashiorkor E40
  marasmic, marasmus type E42
Kyasanur Forest disease A98.2
Kyphoscoliosis, kyphoscoliotic (acquired) —
  see also Scoliosis M41.9
  congenital Q67.5
  heart (disease) I27.1
  sequelae of rickets E64.3
  tuberculous A18.01
Kyphosis, kyphotic (acquired) M40.209
  cervical region M40.202
  cervicothoracic region M40.203
  congenital Q76.419
    cervical region Q76.412
    cervicothoracic region Q76.413
    occipito-atlanto-axial region Q76.411
    thoracic region Q76.414
    thoracolumbar region Q76.415
  Morquio-Brailsford type (spinal) (*see also*
    subcategory M49.8) E76.219
  postlaminectomy M96.3
  postradiation therapy M96.2
  postural (adolescent) M40.00
    cervicothoracic region M40.03
    thoracic region M40.04
    thoracolumbar region M40.05
  secondary NEC M40.10
    cervical region M40.12
    cervicothoracic region M40.13
    thoracic region M40.14
    thoracolumbar region M40.15
  sequelae of rickets E64.3
  specified type NEC M40.299
    cervical region M40.292
    cervicothoracic region M40.293
    thoracic region M40.294
    thoracolumbar region M40.295
  syphilitic, congenital A50.56
  thoracic region M40.204
  thoracolumbar region M40.205
  tuberculous A18.01
Kyrle disease L87.0

L

Labia, labium — *see* condition
Labile
  blood pressure R09.89
  vasomotor system I73.9
Labioglossal paralysis G12.29
Labium leporinum — *see* Cleft, lip
Labor — *see* Delivery
Labored breathing — *see* Hyperventilation
Labyrinthitis (circumscribed) (destructive)
  (diffuse) (inner ear) (latent) (purulent)
  (suppurative) (*see also* subcategory
    H83.0)
  syphilitic A52.79

Laceration
  with abortion — *see* Abortion, by type,
    complicated by laceration of pelvic
    organs
  abdomen, abdominal
    wall S31.119
      with
        foreign body S31.129
        penetration into peritoneal
          cavity S31.619
          with foreign body S31.629
      epigastric region S31.112
        with
          foreign body S31.122
          penetration into peritoneal
            cavity S31.612
            with foreign body S31.622
      left
        lower quadrant S31.114
          with
            foreign body S31.124
            penetration into peritoneal
              cavity S31.614
              with foreign body S31.624
        upper quadrant S31.111
          with
            foreign body S31.121
            penetration into peritoneal
              cavity S31.611
              with foreign body S31.621
      periumbilic region S31.115
        with
          foreign body S31.125
          penetration into peritoneal
            cavity S31.615
            with foreign body S31.625
      right
        lower quadrant S31.113
          with
            foreign body S31.123
            penetration into peritoneal
              cavity S31.613
              with foreign body S31.623
        upper quadrant S31.110
          with
            foreign body S31.120
            penetration into peritoneal
              cavity S31.610
              with foreign body S31.620
  accidental, complicating surgery — *see*
    Complications, surgical, accidental
    puncture or laceration
  Achilles tendon S86.02-
  adrenal gland S37.813
  alveolar (process) — *see* Laceration, oral
    cavity
  ankle S91.01-
    with
      foreign body S91.02-
  antecubital space — *see* Laceration, elbow
  anus (sphincter) S31.831
    with
      ectopic or molar pregnancy O08.6
      foreign body S31.832
    complicating delivery — *see* Delivery,
      complicated, by, laceration, anus
      (sphincter)
    following ectopic or molar
      pregnancy O08.6
    nontraumatic, nonpuerperal — *see* Fissure,
      anus
  arm (upper) S41.11-
    with foreign body S41.12-
    lower — *see* Laceration, forearm
  auditory canal (external) (meatus) — *see*
    Laceration, ear
  auricle, ear — *see* Laceration, ear
  axilla — *see* Laceration, arm
  back — *see also* Laceration, thorax, back
    lower S31.010
      with
        foreign body S31.020
          with penetration into retroperitoneal
            space S31.021

Laceration - *continued*
 back - *continued*
  lower - *continued*
   with - *continued*
    penetration into retroperitoneal
      space S31.011
 bile duct S36.13
 bladder S37.23
  with ectopic or molar pregnancy O08.6
  following ectopic or molar
    pregnancy O08.6
  obstetrical trauma O71.5
 blood vessel — *see* Injury, blood vessel
 bowel — *see also* Laceration, intestine
  with ectopic or molar pregnancy O08.6
  complicating abortion — *see* Abortion, by
    type, complicated by, specified
    condition NEC
  following ectopic or molar
    pregnancy O08.6
  obstetrical trauma O71.5
 brain (any part) (cortex) (diffuse)
   (membrane) — *see also* Injury,
   intracranial, diffuse
  during birth P10.8
   with hemorrhage P10.1
  focal — *see* Injury, intracranial, focal brain
    injury
 brainstem S06.38-
 breast S21.01-
  with foreign body S21.02-
 broad ligament S37.893
  with ectopic or molar pregnancy O08.6
  following ectopic or molar
    pregnancy O08.6
  laceration syndrome N83.8
  obstetrical trauma O71.6
  syndrome (laceration) N83.8
 buttock S31.801
  with foreign body S31.802
  left S31.821
   with foreign body S31.822
  right S31.811
   with foreign body S31.812
 calf — *see* Laceration, leg
 canaliculus lacrimalis — *see* Laceration,
   eyelid
 canthus, eye — *see* Laceration, eyelid
 capsule, joint — *see* Sprain
 causing eversion of cervix uteri (old) N86
 central (perineal) , complicating
   delivery O70.9
 cerebellum, traumatic S06.37-
 cerebral S06.33-
  left side S06.32-
  during birth P10.8
   with hemorrhage P10.1
  right side S06.31-
 cervix (uteri)
  with ectopic or molar pregnancy O08.6
  following ectopic or molar
    pregnancy O08.6
  nonpuerperal, nontraumatic N88.1
  obstetrical trauma (current) O71.3
  old (postpartal) N88.1
  traumatic S37.63
 cheek (external) S01.41-
  with foreign body S01.42-
  internal — *see* Laceration, oral cavity
 chest wall — *see* Laceration, thorax
 chin — *see* Laceration, head, specified site
   NEC
 chordae tendinae NEC I51.1
  concurrent with acute myocardial
    infarction — *see* Infarct, myocardium
  following acute myocardial infarction
    (current complication) I23.4
 clitoris — *see* Laceration, vulva
 colon — *see* Laceration, intestine, large,
   colon
 common bile duct S36.13
 cortex (cerebral) — *see* Injury, intracranial,
   diffuse
 costal region — *see* Laceration, thorax
 cystic duct S36.13

Laceration - *continued*
 diaphragm S27.803
 digit (s)
  hand — *see* Laceration, finger
  foot — *see* Laceration, toe
 duodenum S36.430
 ear (canal) (external) S01.31-
  with foreign body S01.32-
  drum S09.2-
 elbow S51.01-
  with
   foreign body S51.02-
 epididymis — *see* Laceration, testis
 epigastric region — *see* Laceration,
   abdomen, wall, epigastric region
 esophagus K22.8
  traumatic
   cervical S11.21
    with foreign body S11.22
   thoracic S27.813
 eye (ball) S05.3-
  with prolapse or loss of intraocular
    tissue S05.2-
  penetrating S05.6-
 eyebrow — *see* Laceration, eyelid
 eyelid S01.11-
  with foreign body S01.12-
 face NEC — *see* Laceration, head, specified
   site NEC
 fallopian tube S37.539
  bilateral S37.532
  unilateral S37.531
 finger (s) S61.219
  with
   damage to nail S61.319
    with
     foreign body S61.329
   foreign body S61.229
  index S61.218
   with
    damage to nail S61.318
     with
      foreign body S61.328
    foreign body S61.228
   left S61.211
    with
     damage to nail S61.311
      with
       foreign body S61.321
     foreign body S61.221
   right S61.210
    with
     damage to nail S61.310
      with
       foreign body S61.320
     foreign body S61.220
  little S61.218
   with
    damage to nail S61.318
     with
      foreign body S61.328
    foreign body S61.228
   left S61.217
    with
     damage to nail S61.317
      with
       foreign body S61.327
     foreign body S61.227
   right S61.216
    with
     damage to nail S61.316
      with
       foreign body S61.326
     foreign body S61.226
  middle S61.218
   with
    damage to nail S61.318
     with
      foreign body S61.328
    foreign body S61.228
   left S61.213
    with
     damage to nail S61.313
      with
       foreign body S61.323

Laceration - *continued*
 finger (s) - *continued*
  middle - *continued*
   left - *continued*
    with - *continued*
     foreign body S61.223
   right S61.212
    with
     damage to nail S61.312
      with
       foreign body S61.322
     foreign body S61.222
  ring S61.218
   with
    damage to nail S61.318
     with
      foreign body S61.328
    foreign body S61.228
   left S61.215
    with
     damage to nail S61.315
      with
       foreign body S61.325
     foreign body S61.225
   right S61.214
    with
     damage to nail S61.314
      with
       foreign body S61.324
     foreign body S61.224
 flank S31.119
  with foreign body S31.129
 foot (except toe (s) alone) S91.319
  with foreign body S91.329
  left S91.312
   with foreign body S91.322
  right S91.311
   with foreign body S91.321
  toe — *see* Laceration, toe
 forearm S51.819
  with
   foreign body S51.829
  elbow only — *see* Laceration, elbow
  left S51.812
   with
    foreign body S51.822
  right S51.811
   with
    foreign body S51.821
 forehead S01.81
  with foreign body S01.82
 fourchette O70.0
  with ectopic or molar pregnancy O08.6
  complicating delivery O70.0
  following ectopic or molar
    pregnancy O08.6
 gallbladder S36.123
 genital organs, external
  female S31.512
   with foreign body S31.522
   vagina — *see* Laceration, vagina
   vulva — *see* Laceration, vulva
  male S31.511
   with foreign body S31.521
   penis — *see* Laceration, penis
   scrotum — *see* Laceration, scrotum
   testis — *see* Laceration, testis
 groin — *see* Laceration, abdomen, wall
 gum — *see* Laceration, oral cavity
 hand S61.419
  with
   foreign body S61.429
  finger — *see* Laceration, finger
  left S61.412
   with
    foreign body S61.422
  right S61.411
   with
    foreign body S61.421
  thumb — *see* Laceration, thumb
 head S01.91
  with foreign body S01.92
  cheek — *see* Laceration, cheek
  ear — *see* Laceration, ear
  eyelid — *see* Laceration, eyelid

Laceration - *continued*
  head - *continued*
    lip — *see* Laceration, lip
    nose — *see* Laceration, nose
    oral cavity — *see* Laceration, oral cavity
    scalp S01.01
      with foreign body S01.02
    specified site NEC S01.81
      with foreign body S01.82
    temporomandibular area — *see* Laceration, cheek
  heart — *see* Injury, heart, laceration
  heel — *see* Laceration, foot
  hepatic duct S36.13
  hip S71.019
    with foreign body S71.029
    left S71.012
      with foreign body S71.022
    right S71.011
      with foreign body S71.021
  hymen — *see* Laceration, vagina
  hypochondrium — *see* Laceration, abdomen, wall
  hypogastric region — *see* Laceration, abdomen, wall
  ileum S36.438
  inguinal region — *see* Laceration, abdomen, wall
  instep — *see* Laceration, foot
  internal organ — *see* Injury, by site
  interscapular region — *see* Laceration, thorax, back
  intestine
    large
      colon S36.539
        ascending S36.530
        descending S36.532
        sigmoid S36.533
        specified site NEC S36.538
      rectum S36.63
        transverse S36.531
    small S36.439
      duodenum S36.430
      specified site NEC S36.438
  intra-abdominal organ S36.93
    intestine — *see* Laceration, intestine
    liver — *see* Laceration, liver
    pancreas — *see* Laceration, pancreas
    peritoneum S36.81
    specified site NEC S36.893
    spleen — *see* Laceration, spleen
    stomach — *see* Laceration, stomach
  intracranial NEC — *see also* Injury, intracranial, diffuse
    birth injury P10.9
  jaw — *see* Laceration, head, specified site NEC
  jejunum S36.438
  joint capsule — *see* Sprain, by site
  kidney S37.03-
    major (greater than 3 cm) (massive) (stellate) S37.06-
    minor (less than 1 cm) S37.04-
    moderate (1 to 3 cm) S37.05-
      multiple S37.06-
  knee S81.01-
    with foreign body S81.02-
  labium (majus) (minus) — *see* Laceration, vulva
  lacrimal duct — *see* Laceration, eyelid
  large intestine — *see* Laceration, intestine, large
  larynx S11.011
    with foreign body S11.012
  leg (lower) S81.819
    with foreign body S81.829
    foot — *see* Laceration, foot
    knee — *see* Laceration, knee
    left S81.812
      with foreign body S81.822
    right S81.811
      with foreign body S81.821
    upper — *see* Laceration, thigh
  ligament — *see* Sprain
  lip S01.511

Laceration - *continued*
  lip - *continued*
    with foreign body S01.521
  liver S36.113
    major (stellate) S36.116
    minor S36.114
    moderate S36.115
  loin — *see* Laceration, abdomen, wall
  lower back — *see* Laceration, back, lower
  lumbar region — *see* Laceration, back, lower
  lung S27.339
    bilateral S27.332
    unilateral S27.331
  malar region — *see* Laceration, head, specified site NEC
  mammary — *see* Laceration, breast
  mastoid region — *see* Laceration, head, specified site NEC
  meninges — *see* Injury, intracranial, diffuse
  meniscus — *see* Tear, meniscus
  mesentery S36.893
  mesosalpinx S37.893
  mouth — *see* Laceration, oral cavity
  muscle — *see* Injury, muscle, by site, laceration
  nail
    finger — *see* Laceration, finger, with damage to nail
    toe — *see* Laceration, toe, with damage to nail
  nasal (septum) (sinus) — *see* Laceration, nose
  nasopharynx — *see* Laceration, head, specified site NEC
  neck S11.91
    with foreign body S11.92
    involving
      cervical esophagus S11.21
        with foreign body S11.22
      larynx — *see* Laceration, larynx
      pharynx — *see* Laceration, pharynx
      thyroid gland — *see* Laceration, thyroid gland
      trachea — *see* Laceration, trachea
    specified site NEC S11.81
      with foreign body S11.82
  nerve — *see* Injury, nerve
  nose (septum) (sinus) S01.21
    with foreign body S01.22
  ocular NOS S05.3-
    adnexa NOS S01.11-
  oral cavity S01.512
    with foreign body S01.522
  orbit (eye) — *see* Wound, open, ocular, orbit
  ovary S37.439
    bilateral S37.432
    unilateral S37.431
  palate — *see* Laceration, oral cavity
  palm — *see* Laceration, hand
  pancreas S36.239
    body S36.231
      major S36.261
      minor S36.241
      moderate S36.251
    head S36.230
      major S36.260
      minor S36.240
      moderate S36.250
    major S36.269
    minor S36.249
    moderate S36.259
    tail S36.232
      major S36.262
      minor S36.242
      moderate S36.252
  pelvic S31.010
    with
      foreign body S31.020
        penetration into retroperitoneal cavity S31.021
      penetration into retroperitoneal cavity S31.011
    floor — *see also* Laceration, back, lower
      with ectopic or molar pregnancy O08.6
      complicating delivery O70.1

Laceration - *continued*
  pelvic - *continued*
    floor - *continued*
      following ectopic or molar pregnancy O08.6
      old (postpartal) N81.89
    organ S37.93
      with ectopic or molar pregnancy O08.6
      adrenal gland S37.813
      bladder S37.23
      fallopian tube — *see* Laceration, fallopian tube
      following ectopic or molar pregnancy O08.6
      kidney — *see* Laceration, kidney
      obstetrical trauma O71.5
      ovary — *see* Laceration, ovary
      prostate S37.823
      specified site NEC S37.893
      ureter S37.13
      urethra S37.33
      uterus S37.63
  penis S31.21
    with foreign body S31.22
  perineum
    female S31.41
      with
        ectopic or molar pregnancy O08.6
        foreign body S31.42
      during delivery O70.9
        first degree O70.0
        fourth degree O70.3
        second degree O70.1
        third degree — *see also* Delivery, complicated, by, laceration, perineum, third degree O70.20
      old (postpartal) N81.89
      postpartal N81.89
      secondary (postpartal) O90.1
    male S31.119
      with foreign body S31.129
  periocular area (with or without lacrimal passages) — *see* Laceration, eyelid
  peritoneum S36.893
  periumbilic region — *see* Laceration, abdomen, wall, periumbilic
  periurethral tissue — *see* Laceration, urethra
  phalanges
    finger — *see* Laceration, finger
    toe — *see* Laceration, toe
  pharynx S11.21
    with foreign body S11.22
  pinna — *see* Laceration, ear
  popliteal space — *see* Laceration, knee
  prepuce — *see* Laceration, penis
  prostate S37.823
  pubic region S31.119
    with foreign body S31.129
  pudendum — *see* Laceration, genital organs, external
  rectovaginal septum — *see* Laceration, vagina
  rectum S36.63
  retroperitoneum S36.893
  round ligament S37.893
  sacral region — *see* Laceration, back, lower
  sacroiliac region — *see* Laceration, back, lower
  salivary gland — *see* Laceration, oral cavity
  scalp S01.01
    with foreign body S01.02
  scapular region — *see* Laceration, shoulder
  scrotum S31.31
    with foreign body S31.32
  seminal vesicle S37.893
  shin — *see* Laceration, leg
  shoulder S41.019
    with foreign body S41.029
    left S41.012
      with foreign body S41.022
    right S41.011
      with foreign body S41.021
  small intestine — *see* Laceration, intestine, small
  spermatic cord — *see* Laceration, testis

Laceration - *continued*
 spinal cord (meninges) — *see also* Injury,
  spinal cord, by region
  due to injury at birth P11.5
  newborn (birth injury) P11.5
 spleen S36.039
  major (massive) (stellate) S36.032
  moderate S36.031
  superficial (minor) S36.030
 sternal region — *see* Laceration, thorax, front
 stomach S36.33
 submaxillary region — *see* Laceration, head,
  specified site NEC
 submental region — *see* Laceration, head,
  specified site NEC
 subungual
  finger (s) — *see* Laceration, finger, with
   damage to nail
  toe (s) — *see* Laceration, toe, with damage
   to nail
 suprarenal gland — *see* Laceration, adrenal
  gland
 temple, temporal region — *see* Laceration,
  head, specified site NEC
 temporomandibular area — *see* Laceration,
  cheek
 tendon — *see* Injury, muscle, by site,
  laceration
  Achilles S86.02-
 tentorium cerebelli — *see* Injury, intracranial,
  diffuse
 testis S31.31
  with foreign body S31.32
 thigh S71.11-
  with foreign body S71.12-
 thorax, thoracic (wall) S21.91
  with foreign body S21.92
   back S21.22-
    with penetration into thoracic
     cavity S21.42-
   front S21.12-
    with penetration into thoracic
     cavity S21.32-
  back S21.21-
   with
    foreign body S21.22-
     with penetration into thoracic
      cavity S21.42-
    penetration into thoracic
     cavity S21.41-
  breast — *see* Laceration, breast
  front S21.11-
   with
    foreign body S21.12-
     with penetration into thoracic
      cavity S21.32-
    penetration into thoracic
     cavity S21.31-
 thumb S61.019
  with
   damage to nail S61.119
    with
     foreign body S61.129
   foreign body S61.029
  left S61.012
   with
    damage to nail S61.112
     with
      foreign body S61.122
    foreign body S61.022
  right S61.011
   with
    damage to nail S61.111
     with
      foreign body S61.121
    foreign body S61.021
 thyroid gland S11.11
  with foreign body S11.12
 toe (s) S91.119
  with
   damage to nail S91.219
    with
     foreign body S91.229
   foreign body S91.129
  great S91.113

Laceration - *continued*
 toe (s) - *continued*
  great - *continued*
   with
    damage to nail S91.213
     with
      foreign body S91.223
    foreign body S91.123
   left S91.112
    with
     damage to nail S91.212
      with
       foreign body S91.222
     foreign body S91.122
   right S91.111
    with
     damage to nail S91.211
      with
       foreign body S91.221
     foreign body S91.121
  lesser S91.116
   with
    damage to nail S91.216
     with
      foreign body S91.226
    foreign body S91.126
   left S91.115
    with
     damage to nail S91.215
      with
       foreign body S91.225
     foreign body S91.125
   right S91.114
    with
     damage to nail S91.214
      with
       foreign body S91.224
     foreign body S91.124
 tongue — *see* Laceration, oral cavity
 trachea S11.021
  with foreign body S11.022
 tunica vaginalis — *see* Laceration, testis
 tympanum, tympanic membrane — *see*
  Laceration, ear, drum
 umbilical region S31.115
  with foreign body S31.125
 ureter S37.13
 urethra S37.33
  with or following ectopic or molar
   pregnancy O08.6
  obstetrical trauma O71.5
 urinary organ NEC S37.893
 uterus S37.63
  with ectopic or molar pregnancy O08.6
  following ectopic or molar
   pregnancy O08.6
  nonpuerperal, nontraumatic N85.8
  obstetrical trauma NEC O71.81
  old (postpartal) N85.8
 uvula — *see* Laceration, oral cavity
 vagina S31.41
  with
   ectopic or molar pregnancy O08.6
   foreign body S31.42
  during delivery O71.4
   with perineal laceration — *see*
    Laceration, perineum, female,
    during delivery
  following ectopic or molar
   pregnancy O08.6
  nonpuerperal, nontraumatic N89.8
  old (postpartal) N89.8
 vas deferens S37.893
 vesical — *see* Laceration, bladder
 vocal cords S11.031
  with foreign body S11.032
 vulva S31.41
  with
   ectopic or molar pregnancy O08.6
   foreign body S31.42
  complicating delivery O70.0
  following ectopic or molar
   pregnancy O08.6
  nonpuerperal, nontraumatic N90.89
  old (postpartal) N90.89

Laceration - *continued*
 wrist S61.519
  with
   foreign body S61.529
  left S61.512
   with
    foreign body S61.522
  right S61.511
   with
    foreign body S61.521
Lack of
 achievement in school Z55.3
 adequate
  food Z59.4
  intermaxillary vertical dimension of fully
   erupted teeth M26.36
  sleep Z72.820
 appetite (see Anorexia) R63.0
 awareness R41.9
 care
  in home Z74.2
  of infant (at or after birth) T76.02
   confirmed T74.02
 cognitive functions R41.9
 coordination R27.9
  ataxia R27.0
  specified type NEC R27.8
 development (physiological) R62.50
  failure to thrive (child over 28 days
   old) R62.51
  adult R62.7
  newborn P92.6
  short stature R62.52
  specified type NEC R62.59
 energy R53.83
 financial resources Z59.6
 food T73.0
 growth R62.52
 heating Z59.1
 housing (permanent) (temporary) Z59.0
  adequate Z59.1
 learning experiences in childhood Z62.898
 leisure time (affecting life-style) Z73.2
 material resources Z59.9
 memory — *see also* Amnesia
  mild, following organic brain
   damage F06.8
 ovulation N97.0
 parental supervision or control of child Z62.0
 person able to render necessary care Z74.2
 physical exercise Z72.3
 play experience in childhood Z62.898
 posterior occlusal support M26.57
 relaxation (affecting life-style) Z73.2
 sexual
  desire F52.0
  enjoyment F52.1
 shelter Z59.0
 sleep (adequate) Z72.820
 supervision of child by parent Z62.0
 support, posterior occlusal M26.57
 water T73.1
Lacrimal — *see* condition
Lacrimation, abnormal — *see* Epiphora
Lacrimonasal duct — *see* condition
Lactation, lactating (breast) (puerperal,
 postpartum)
 associated
  cracked nipple O92.13
  retracted nipple O92.03
 defective O92.4
 disorder NEC O92.79
 excessive O92.6
 failed (complete) O92.3
  partial O92.4
 mastitis NEC — *see* Mastitis, obstetric
 mother (care and/or examination) Z39.1
 nonpuerperal N64.3
Lacticemia, excessive E87.2
Lacunar skull Q75.8
Laennec's cirrhosis K70.30
 with ascites K70.31
 nonalcoholic K74.69
Lafora's disease — *see* Epilepsy, generalized,
 idiopathic

Lag, lid (nervous) — *see* Retraction, lid
Lagophthalmos (eyelid) (nervous) H02.209
  bilateral, upper and lower eyelids H02.20C
  cicatricial H02.219
    bilateral, upper and lower eyelids H02.21C
    left H02.216
      lower H02.215
      upper H02.214
      upper and lower eyelids H02.21B
    right H02.213
      lower H02.212
      upper H02.211
      upper and lower eyelids H02.21A
  keratoconjunctivitis — *see*
      Keratoconjunctivitis
  left H02.206
    lower H02.205
    upper H02.204
    upper and lower eyelids H02.20B
  mechanical H02.229
    bilateral, upper and lower eyelids H02.22C
    left H02.226
      lower H02.225
      upper H02.224
      upper and lower eyelids H02.22B
    right H02.223
      lower H02.222
      upper H02.221
      upper and lower eyelids H02.22A
  paralytic H02.239
    bilateral, upper and lower eyelids H02.23C
    left H02.236
      lower H02.235
      upper H02.234
      upper and lower eyelids H02.23B
    right H02.233
      lower H02.232
      upper H02.231
      upper and lower eyelids H02.23A
  right H02.203
    lower H02.202
    upper H02.201
    upper and lower eyelids H02.20A
Laki-Lorand factor deficiency — *see* Defect,
    coagulation, specified type NEC
Lalling F80.0
Lambert-Eaton syndrome — *see* Syndrome,
    Lambert-Eaton
Lambliasis, lambliosis A07.1
Landau-Kleffner syndrome — *see* Epilepsy,
    specified NEC
Landouzy-Déjérine dystrophy or
    facioscapulohumeral atrophy G71.02
Landouzy's disease (icterohemorrhagic
    leptospirosis) A27.0
Landry-Guillain-Barré, syndrome or
    paralysis G61.0
Landry's disease or paralysis G61.0
Lane's
  band Q43.3
  kink — *see* Obstruction, intestine
  syndrome K90.2
Langdon Down syndrome — *see* Trisomy, 21
Lapsed immunization schedule status Z28.3
Large
  baby (regardless of gestational age) (4000g
      to 4499g) P08.1
  ear, congenital Q17.1
  physiological cup Q14.2
  stature R68.89
Large-for-dates NEC (infant) (4000g to
    4499g) P08.1
  affecting management of pregnancy O36.6-
  exceptionally (4500g or more) P08.0
Larsen-Johansson disease
    orosteochondrosis — *see*
    Osteochondrosis, juvenile, patella
Larsen's syndrome (flattened facies and
    multiple congenital dislocations) Q74.8
Larva migrans
  cutaneous B76.9
    Ancylostoma B76.0
  visceral B83.0
Laryngeal — *see* condition

Laryngismus (stridulus) J38.5
  congenital P28.89
  diphtheritic A36.2
Laryngitis (acute) (edematous) (fibrinous)
    (infective) (infiltrative) (malignant)
    (membranous) (phlegmonous)
    (pneumococcal) (pseudomembranous)
    (septic) (subglottic) (suppurative)
    (ulcerative) J04.0
  with
    influenza, flu, or grippe — *see* Influenza,
        with, laryngitis
    tracheitis (acute) — *see* Laryngotracheitis
  atrophic J37.0
  catarrhal J37.0
  chronic J37.0
    with tracheitis (chronic) J37.1
  diphtheritic A36.2
  due to external agent — *see* Inflammation,
      respiratory, upper, due to
  Hemophilus influenzae J04.0
  H. influenzae J04.0
  hypertrophic J37.0
  influenzal — *see* Influenza, with, respiratory
      manifestations NEC
  obstructive J05.0
  sicca J37.0
  spasmodic J05.0
    acute J04.0
  streptococcal J04.0
  stridulous J05.0
  syphilitic (late) A52.73
    congenital A50.59 *[J99]*
    early A50.03 *[J99]*
  tuberculous A15.5
  Vincent's A69.1
Laryngocele (congenital) (ventricular) Q31.3
Laryngofissure J38.7
  congenital Q31.8
Laryngomalacia (congenital) Q31.5
Laryngopharyngitis (acute) J06.0
  chronic J37.0
  due to external agent — *see* Inflammation,
      respiratory, upper, due to
Laryngoplegia J38.00
  bilateral J38.02
  unilateral J38.01
Laryngoptosis J38.7
Laryngospasm J38.5
Laryngostenosis J38.6
Laryngotracheitis (acute) (Infectional)
    (infective) (viral) J04.2
  atrophic J37.1
  catarrhal J37.1
  chronic J37.1
  diphtheritic A36.2
  due to external agent — *see* Inflammation,
      respiratory, upper, due to
  Hemophilus influenzae J04.2
  hypertrophic J37.1
  influenzal — *see* Influenza, with, respiratory
      manifestations NEC
  pachydermic J38.7
  sicca J37.1
  spasmodic J38.5
    acute J05.0
  streptococcal J04.2
  stridulous J38.5
  syphilitic (late) A52.73
    congenital A50.59 *[J99]*
    early A50.03 *[J99]*
  tuberculous A15.5
  Vincent's A69.1
Laryngotracheobronchitis — *see* Bronchitis
Larynx, laryngeal — *see* condition
Lassa fever A96.2
Lassitude — *see* Weakness
Late
  talker R62.0
  walker R62.0
Late effect (s) — *see* Sequelae
Latent — *see* condition
Laterocession — *see* Lateroversion
Lateroflexion — *see* Lateroversion

Lateroversion
  cervix — *see* Lateroversion, uterus
  uterus, uterine (cervix) (postinfectional)
      (postpartal, old) N85.4
    congenital Q51.818
    in pregnancy or childbirth O34.59-
Lathyrism — *see* Poisoning, food, noxious,
    plant
Launois' syndrome (pituitary
    gigantism) E22.0
Launois-Bensaude adenolipomatosis E88.89
Laurence-Moon (-Bardet) -Biedl
    syndrome Q87.89
Lax, laxity — *see also* Relaxation
  ligament (ous) — *see also* Disorder, ligament
    familial M35.7
  knee — *see* Derangement, knee
  skin (acquired) L57.4
    congenital Q82.8
Laxative habit F55.2
Lazy leukocyte syndrome D70.8
Lead miner's lung J63.6
Leak, leakage
  air NEC J93.82
    postprocedural J95.812
  amniotic fluid — *see* Rupture, membranes,
      premature
  blood (microscopic) , fetal, into maternal
      circulation affecting management of
      pregnancy — *see* Pregnancy,
      complicated by
  cerebrospinal fluid G96.0
    from spinal (lumbar) puncture G97.0
  device, implant or graft — *see also*
      Complications, by site and type,
      mechanical
    arterial graft NEC — *see* Complication,
        cardiovascular device, mechanical,
        vascular
    breast (implant) T85.43
    catheter NEC T85.638
      urinary T83.038
        cystostomy T83.030
        Hopkins T83.038
        ileostomy T83.038
        indwelling T83.031
        nephrostomy T83.032
        specified NEC T83.038
        urostomy T83.038
      dialysis (renal) T82.43
        intraperitoneal T85.631
      infusion NEC T82.534
        spinal (epidural) (subdural) T85.630
    gastrointestinal — *see* Complications,
        prosthetic device, mechanical,
        gastrointestinal device
    genital NEC T83.498
      penile prosthesis (cylinder) (implanted)
          (pump) (resevoir) T83.490
      testicular prosthesis T83.491
    heart NEC — *see* Complication,
        cardiovascular device, mechanical
    joint prosthesis — *see* Complications, joint
        prosthesis, mechanical, specified
        NEC, by site
    ocular NEC — *see* Complications,
        prosthetic device, mechanical, ocular
        device
    orthopedic NEC — *see* Complication,
        orthopedic, device, mechanical
    persistent air J93.82
    specified NEC T85.638
    urinary NEC — *see also* Complication,
        genitourinary, device, urinary,
        mechanical
      graft T83.23
    vascular NEC — *see* Complication,
        cardiovascular device, mechanical
    ventricular intracranial shunt T85.03
  urine — *see* Incontinence
Leaky heart — *see* Endocarditis
Learning defect (specific) F81.9
Leather bottle stomach C16.9
Leber's
  congenital amaurosis H35.50

DecisionHealth's FY 2020 Complete Home Health ICD-10-CM Diagnosis Coding Manual

Leber's - *continued*
  optic atrophy (hereditary) H47.22
Lederer's anemia D59.1
Leeches (external) — *see* Hirudiniasis
Leg — *see* condition
Legg (-Calvé) -Perthes disease, syndrome or osteochondrosis M91.1-
Legionellosis A48.1
  nonpneumonic A48.2
Legionnaires'
  disease A48.1
    nonpneumonic A48.2
  pneumonia A48.1
Leigh's disease G31.82
Leiner's disease L21.1
Leiofibromyoma — *see* Leiomyoma
Leiomyoblastoma — *see* Neoplasm, connective tissue, benign
Leiomyofibroma — *see also* Neoplasm, connective tissue, benign
  uterus (cervix) (corpus) D25.9
Leiomyoma — *see also* Neoplasm, connective tissue, benign
  bizarre — *see* Neoplasm, connective tissue, benign
  cellular — *see* Neoplasm, connective tissue, benign
  epithelioid — *see* Neoplasm, connective tissue, benign
  uterus (cervix) (corpus) D25.9
    intramural D25.1
    submucous D25.0
    subserosal D25.2
  vascular — *see* Neoplasm, connective tissue, benign
Leiomyoma, leiomyomatosis (intravascular) — *see* Neoplasm, connective tissue, uncertain behavior
Leiomyosarcoma — *see also* Neoplasm, connective tissue, malignant
  epithelioid — *see* Neoplasm, connective tissue, malignant
  myxoid — *see* Neoplasm, connective tissue, malignant
Leishmaniasis B55.9
  American (mucocutaneous) B55.2
    cutaneous B55.1
  Asian Desert B55.1
  Brazilian B55.2
  cutaneous (any type) B55.1
  dermal — *see also* Leishmaniasis, cutaneous
    post-kala-azar B55.0
  eyelid B55.1
  infantile B55.0
  Mediterranean B55.0
  mucocutaneous (American) (New World) B55.2
  naso-oral B55.2
  nasopharyngeal B55.2
  old world B55.1
  tegumentaria diffusa B55.1
  visceral B55.0
Leishmanoid, dermal — *see also* Leishmaniasis, cutaneous
  post-kala-azar B55.0
Lenegre's disease I44.2
Lengthening, leg — *see* Deformity, limb, unequal length
Lennert's lymphoma — *see* Lymphoma, Lennert's
Lennox-Gastaut syndrome G40.812
  intractable G40.814
    with status epilepticus G40.813
    without status epilepticus G40.814
  not intractable G40.812
    with status epilepticus G40.811
    without status epilepticus G40.812
Lens — *see* condition
Lenticonus (anterior) (posterior) (congenital) Q12.8
Lenticular degeneration, progressive E83.01
Lentiglobus (posterior) (congenital) Q12.8
Lentigo (congenital) L81.4
  maligna — *see also* Melanoma, in situ
    melanoma — *see* Melanoma

Lentivirus, as cause of disease classified elsewhere B97.31
Leontiasis
  ossium M85.2
  syphilitic (late) A52.78
    congenital A50.59
Lepothrix A48.8
Lepra — *see* Leprosy
Leprechaunism E34.8
Leprosy A30.-
  with muscle disorder A30.9 *[M63.80]*
    ankle A30.9 *[M63.87-]*
    foot A30.9 *[M63.87-]*
    forearm A30.9 *[M63.83-]*
    hand A30.9 *[M63.84-]*
    lower leg A30.9 *[M63.86-]*
    multiple sites A30.9 *[M63.89]*
    pelvic region A30.9 *[M63.85-]*
    shoulder region A30.9 *[M63.81-]*
    specified site NEC A30.9 *[M63.88]*
    thigh A30.9 *[M63.85-]*
    upper arm A30.9 *[M63.82-]*
  anesthetic A30.9
  BB A30.3
  BL A30.4
  borderline (infiltrated) (neuritic) A30.3
    lepromatous A30.4
    tuberculoid A30.2
  BT A30.2
  dimorphous (infiltrated) (neuritic) A30.3
  I A30.0
  indeterminate (macular) (neuritic) A30.0
  lepromatous (diffuse) (infiltrated) (macular) (neuritic) (nodular) A30.5
  LL A30.5
  macular (early) (neuritic) (simple) A30.9
  maculoanesthetic A30.9
  mixed A30.3
  neural A30.9
  nodular A30.5
  primary neuritic A30.3
  specified type NEC A30.8
  TT A30.1
  tuberculoid (major) (minor) A30.1
Leptocytosis, hereditary D56.9
Leptomeningitis (chronic) (circumscribed) (hemorrhagic) (nonsuppurative) — *see* Meningitis
Leptomeningopathy G96.19
Leptospiral — *see* condition
Leptospirochetal — *see* condition
Leptospirosis A27.9
  canicola A27.89
  due to Leptospira interrogans serovar icterohaemorrhagiae A27.0
  icterohemorrhagica A27.0
  pomona A27.89
  Weil's disease A27.0
Leptus dermatitis B88.0
Leriche's syndrome (aortic bifurcation occlusion) I74.09
Leri's pleonosteosis Q78.8
Leri-Weill syndrome Q77.8
Lermoyez' syndrome — *see* Vertigo, peripheral NEC
Lesch-Nyhan syndrome E79.1
Leser-Trélat disease L82.1
  inflamed L82.0
Lesion (s) (nontraumatic)
  abducens nerve — *see* Strabismus, paralytic, sixth nerve
  alveolar process K08.9
  angiocentric immunoproliferative D47.Z9
  anorectal K62.9
  aortic (valve) I35.9
  auditory nerve — *see* subcategory H93.3
  basal ganglion G25.9
  bile duct — *see* Disease, bile duct
  biomechanical M99.9
    specified type NEC M99.89
      abdomen M99.89
      acromioclavicular M99.87
      cervical region M99.81
      cervicothoracic M99.81
      costochondral M99.88

Lesion (s) (nontraumatic) - *continued*
  biomechanical - *continued*
    specified type NEC - *continued*
      costovertebral M99.88
      head region M99.80
      hip M99.85
      lower extremity M99.86
      lumbar region M99.83
      lumbosacral M99.83
      occipitocervical M99.80
      pelvic region M99.85
      pubic M99.85
      rib cage M99.88
      sacral region M99.84
      sacrococcygeal M99.84
      sacroiliac M99.84
      specified NEC M99.89
      sternochondral M99.88
      sternoclavicular M99.87
      thoracic region M99.82
      thoracolumbar M99.82
      upper extremity M99.87
  bladder N32.9
  bone — *see* Disorder, bone
  brachial plexus G54.0
  brain G93.9
    congenital Q04.9
    vascular I67.9
      degenerative I67.9
      hypertensive I67.4
  buccal cavity K13.79
  calcified — *see* Calcification
  canthus — *see* Disorder, eyelid
  carate — *see* Pinta, lesions
  cardia K31.9
  cardiac — *see also* Disease, heart I51.9
    congenital Q24.9
    valvular — *see* Endocarditis
  cauda equina G83.4
  cecum K63.9
  cerebral — *see* Lesion, brain
  cerebrovascular I67.9
    degenerative I67.9
    hypertensive I67.4
  cervical (nerve) root NEC G54.2
  chiasmal — *see* Disorder, optic, chiasm
  chorda tympani G51.8
  coin, lung R91.1
  colon K63.9
  combined periodontic - endodontic K05.5
  congenital — *see* Anomaly, by site
  conjunctiva H11.9
  conus medullaris — *see* Injury, conus medullaris
  coronary artery — *see* Ischemia, heart
  cranial nerve G52.9
    eighth — *see* Disorder, ear
    eleventh G52.9
    fifth G50.9
    first G52.0
    fourth — *see* Strabismus, paralytic, fourth nerve
    seventh G51.9
    sixth — *see* Strabismus, paralytic, sixth nerve
    tenth G52.2
    twelfth G52.3
  cystic — *see* Cyst
  degenerative — *see* Degeneration
  duodenum K31.9
  edentulous (alveolar) ridge, associated with trauma, due to traumatic occlusion K06.2
  en coup de sabre L94.1
  eyelid — *see* Disorder, eyelid
  gasserian ganglion G50.8
  gastric K31.9
  gastroduodenal K31.9
  gastrointestinal K63.9
  gingiva, associated with trauma K06.2
  glomerular
    focal and segmental — *see also* N00-N07 with fourth character .1 N05.1
    minimal change — *see also* N00-N07 with fourth character .0 N05.0

Lesion (s) (nontraumatic) - *continued*
  heart (organic) — *see* Disease, heart
  hyperchromic, due to pinta (carate) A67.1
  hyperkeratotic — *see* Hyperkeratosis
  hypothalamic E23.7
  ileocecal K63.9
  ileum K63.9
  iliohypogastric nerve G57.8-
  inflammatory — *see* Inflammation
  intestine K63.9
  intracerebral — *see* Lesion, brain
  intrachiasmal (optic) — *see* Disorder, optic, chiasm
  intracranial, space-occupying R90.0
  joint — *see* Disorder, joint
    sacroiliac (old) M53.3
  keratotic — *see* Keratosis
  kidney — *see* Disease, renal
  laryngeal nerve (recurrent) G52.2
  lip K13.0
  liver K76.9
  lumbosacral
    plexus G54.1
    root (nerve) NEC G54.4
  lung (coin) R91.1
  maxillary sinus J32.0
  mitral I05.9
  Morel-Lavallée — *see* Hematoma, by site
  motor cortex NEC G93.89
  mouth K13.79
  nerve G58.9
    femoral G57.2-
    median G56.1-
      carpal tunnel syndrome — *see* Syndrome, carpal tunnel
    plantar G57.6-
    popliteal (lateral) G57.3-
      medial G57.4-
    radial G56.3-
    sciatic G57.0-
    spinal — *see* Injury, nerve, spinal
    ulnar G56.2-
  nervous system, congenital Q07.9
  nonallopathic — *see* Lesion, biomechanical
  nose (internal) J34.89
  obstructive — *see* Obstruction
  obturator nerve G57.8-
  oral mucosa K13.70
  organ or site NEC — *see* Disease, by site
  osteolytic — *see* Osteolysis
  peptic K27.9
  periodontal, due to traumatic occlusion K05.5
  pharynx J39.2
  pigment, pigmented (skin) L81.9
  pinta — *see* Pinta, lesions
  polypoid — *see* Polyp
  prechiasmal (optic) — *see* Disorder, optic, chiasm
  primary — *see also* Syphilis, primary A51.0
    carate A67.0
    pinta A67.0
    yaws A66.0
  pulmonary J98.4
    valve I37.9
  pylorus K31.9
  rectosigmoid K63.9
  retina, retinal H35.9
  sacroiliac (joint) (old) M53.3
  salivary gland K11.9
    benign lymphoepithelial K11.8
  saphenous nerve G57.8-
  sciatic nerve G57.0-
  secondary — *see* Syphilis, secondary
  shoulder (region) M75.9-
    specified NEC M75.8-
  sigmoid K63.9
  sinus (accessory) (nasal) J34.89
  skin L98.9
    suppurative L08.0
  SLAP S43.43-
  spinal cord G95.9
    congenital Q06.9
  spleen D73.89
  stomach K31.9

Lesion (s) (nontraumatic) - *continued*
  superior glenoid labrum S43.43-
  syphilitic — *see* Syphilis
  tertiary — *see* Syphilis, tertiary
  thoracic root (nerve) NEC G54.3
  tonsillar fossa J35.9
  tooth, teeth K08.9
    white spot
      chewing surface K02.51
      pit and fissure surface K02.51
      smooth surface K02.61
  traumatic — *see* specific type of injury by site
  tricuspid (valve) I07.9
    nonrheumatic I36.9
  trigeminal nerve G50.9
  ulcerated or ulcerative — *see* Ulcer, skin
  uterus N85.9
  vagina N89.8
  vulva N90.89
  vagus nerve G52.2
  valvular — *see* Endocarditis
  vascular I99.9
    affecting central nervous system I67.9
    following trauma NEC T14.8
    umbilical cord, complicating delivery O69.5
  warty — *see* Verruca
  white spot (tooth)
    chewing surface K02.51
    pit and fissure surface K02.51
    smooth surface K02.61
Lethargic — *see* condition
Lethargy R53.83
Letterer-Siwe's disease C96.0
Leukemia, leukemic C95.9-
  acute basophilic C94.8-
  acute bilineal C95.0-
  acute erythroid C94.0-
  acute lymphoblastic C91.0-
  acute megakaryoblastic C94.2-
  acute megakaryocytic C94.2-
  acute mixed lineage C95.0-
  acute monoblastic (monoblastic/monocytic) C93.0-
  acute monocytic (monoblastic/monocytic) C93.0-
  acute myeloblastic (minimal differentiation) (with maturation) C92.0-
  acute myeloid, NOS C92.0-
    with
      11q23-abnormality C92.6-
      dysplasia of remaining hematopoesis and/or myelodysplastic disease in its history C92.A-
      multilineage dysplasia C92.A-
      variation of MLL-gene C92.6-
    M6 (a) (b) C94.0-
    M7 C94.2-
  acute myelomonocytic C92.5-
  acute promyelocytic C92.4-
  adult T-cell (HTLV-1-associated) (acute variant) (chronic variant) (lymphomatoid variant) (smouldering variant) C91.5-
  aggressive NK-cell C94.8-
  AML (1/ETO) (M0) (M1) (M2) (without a FAB classification) C92.0-
  AML M3 C92.4-
  AML M4 (Eo with inv (16) or t (16;16)) C92.5-
  AML M5 C93.0-
  AML M5a C93.0-
  AML M5b C93.0-
  AML Me with t (15;17) and variants C92.4-
  atypical chronic myeloid, BCR/ABL-negative C92.2-
  biphenotypic acute C95.0-
  blast cell C95.0-
  Burkitt-type, mature B-cell C91.A-
  chronic lymphocytic, of B-cell type C91.1-
  chronic monocytic C93.1-

Leukemia, leukemic - *continued*
  chronic myelogenous (Philadelphia chromosome (Ph1) positive) (t (9;22)) (q34;q11) (with crisis of blast cells) C92.1-
  chronic myeloid, BCR/ABL-positive C92.1-
    atypical, BCR/ABL-negative C92.2-
  chronic myelomonocytic C93.1-
  chronic neutrophilic D47.1
  CMML (-1) (-2) (with eosinophilia) C93.1-
  granulocytic (*see also* Category C92) C92.9-
  hairy cell C91.4-
  juvenile myelomonocytic C93.3-
  lymphoid C91.9-
    specified NEC C91.Z-
  mast cell C94.3-
  mature B-cell, Burkitt-type C91.A-
  monocytic (subacute) C93.9-
    specified NEC C93.Z-
  myelogenous (*see also* Category C92) C92.9-
  myeloid C92.9-
    acute C92.0-
    specified NEC C92.Z-
  plasma cell C90.1-
  plasmacytic C90.1-
  prolymphocytic
    of B-cell type C91.3-
    of T-cell type C91.6-
  specified NEC C94.8-
  stem cell, of unclear lineage C95.0-
  subacute lymphocytic C91.9-
  T-cell large granular lymphocytic C91.Z-
  unspecified cell type C95.9-
    acute C95.0-
    chronic C95.1-
Leukemoid reaction — *see also* Reaction, leukemoid D72.823-
Leukoaraiosis (hypertensive) I67.81
Leukoariosis — *see* Leukoaraiosis
Leukocoria — *see* Disorder, globe, degenerated condition, leucocoria
Leukocytopenia D72.819
Leukocytosis D72.829
  eosinophilic D72.1
Leukoderma, leukodermia NEC L81.5
  syphilitic A51.39
    late A52.79
Leukodystrophy E75.29
Leukoedema, oral epithelium K13.29
Leukoencephalitis G04.81
  acute (subacute) hemorrhagic G36.1
    postimmunization or postvaccinal G04.02
  postinfectious G04.01
  subacute sclerosing A81.1
  van Bogaert's (sclerosing) A81.1
Leukoencephalopathy — *see also* Encephalopathy G93.49
  Binswanger's I67.3
  heroin vapor G92
  metachromatic E75.25
  multifocal (progressive) A81.2
  postimmunization and postvaccinal G04.02
  progressive multifocal A81.2
  reversible, posterior G93.6
  van Bogaert's (sclerosing) A81.1
  vascular, progressive I67.3
Leukoerythroblastosis D75.9
Leukokeratosis — *see also* Leukoplakia
  mouth K13.21
  nicotina palati K13.24
  oral mucosa K13.21
  tongue K13.21
  vocal cord J38.3
Leukokraurosis vulva (e) N90.4
Leukoma (cornea) — *see also* Opacity, cornea
  adherent H17.0-
  interfering with central vision — *see* Opacity, cornea, central
Leukomalacia, cerebral, newborn P91.2
  periventricular P91.2
Leukomelanopathy, hereditary D72.0
Leukonychia (punctata) (striata) L60.8
  congenital Q84.4
Leukopathia unguium L60.8
  congenital Q84.4

Leukopenia D72.819
  basophilic D72.818
  chemotherapy (cancer) induced D70.1
  congenital D70.0
  cyclic D70.0
  drug induced NEC D70.2
    due to cytoreductive cancer
      chemotherapy D70.1
  eosinophilic D72.818
  familial D70.0
  infantile genetic D70.0
  malignant D70.9
  periodic D70.0
  transitory neonatal P61.5
Leukopenic — *see* condition
Leukoplakia
  anus K62.89
  bladder (postinfectional) N32.89
  buccal K13.21
  cervix (uteri) N88.0
  esophagus K22.8
  gingiva K13.21
  hairy (oral mucosa) (tongue) K13.3
  kidney (pelvis) N28.89
  larynx J38.7
  lip K13.21
  mouth K13.21
  oral epithelium, including tongue
    (mucosa) K13.21
  palate K13.21
  pelvis (kidney) N28.89
  penis (infectional) N48.0
  rectum K62.89
  syphilitic (late) A52.79
  tongue K13.21
  ureter (postinfectional) N28.89
  urethra (postinfectional) N36.8
  uterus N85.8
  vagina N89.4
  vocal cord J38.3
  vulva N90.4
Leukorrhea N89.8
  due to Trichomonas (vaginalis) A59.00
  trichomonal A59.00
Leukosarcoma C85.9-
Levocardia (isolated) Q24.1
  with situs inversus Q89.3
Levotransposition Q20.5
**Lev's disease or syndrome (acquired
  complete heart block)** I44.2
Levulosuria — *see* Fructosuria
Levurid L30.2
Lewy body (ies) (dementia) (disease) G31.83
Leyden-Moebius dystrophy G71.09
Leydig cell
  carcinoma
    specified site — *see* Neoplasm, malignant,
      by site
    unspecified site
      female C56.9
      male C62.9-
  tumor
    benign
      specified site — *see* Neoplasm, benign,
        by site
      unspecified site
        female D27.-
        male D29.2-
    malignant
      specified site — *see* Neoplasm,
        malignant, by site
      unspecified site
        female C56.-
        male C62.9-
    specified site — *see* Neoplasm, uncertain
      behavior, by site
    unspecified site
      female D39.1-
      male D40.1-
Leydig-Sertoli cell tumor
  specified site — *see* Neoplasm, benign, by
    site
  unspecified site
    female D27.-
    male D29.2-

**LGSIL (Low grade squamous intraepithelial
  lesion on cytologic smear of)**
  anus R85.612
  cervix R87.612
  vagina R87.622
Liar, pathologic F60.2
Libido
  decreased R68.82
Libman-Sacks disease M32.11
Lice (infestation) B85.2
  body (Pediculus corporis) B85.1
  crab B85.3
  head (Pediculus capitis) B85.0
  mixed (classifiable to more than one of the
    titles B85.0-B85.3) B85.4
  pubic (Phthirus pubis) B85.3
Lichen L28.0
  albus L90.0
    penis N48.0
    vulva N90.4
  amyloidosis E85.4 *[L99]*
  atrophicus L90.0
    penis N48.0
    vulva N90.4
  congenital Q82.8
  myxedematosus L98.5
  nitidus L44.1
  pilaris Q82.8
    acquired L85.8
  planopilaris L66.1
  planus (chronicus) L43.9
    annularis L43.8
    bullous L43.1
    follicular L66.1
    hypertrophic L43.0
    moniliformis L44.3
    of Wilson L43.9
    specified NEC L43.8
    subacute (active) L43.3
    tropicus L43.3
  ruber
    acuminatus L44.0
    moniliformis L44.3
    planus L43.9
  sclerosus (et atrophicus) L90.0
    penis N48.0
    vulva N90.4
  scrofulosus (primary) (tuberculous) A18.4
  simplex (chronicus) (circumscriptus) L28.0
  striatus L44.2
  urticatus L28.2
Lichenification L28.0
Lichenoides tuberculosis (primary) A18.4
Lichtheim's disease or syndrome D51.0
Lien migrans D73.89
Ligament — *see* condition
Light
  for gestational age — *see* Light for dates
  headedness R42
Light-for-dates (infant) P05.00
  with weight of
    499 grams or less P05.01
    500-749 grams P05.02
    750-999 grams P05.03
    1000-1249 grams P05.04
    1250-1499 grams P05.05
    1500-1749 grams P05.06
    1750-1999 grams P05.07
    2000-2499 grams P05.08
    2500 grams and over P05.09
  specified NEC P05.09
  and small-for-dates — *see* Small for dates
  affecting management of pregnancy O36.59-
Lightning (effects) (stroke) (struck by)
  T75.00
  burn — *see* Burn
  foot E53.8
  shock T75.01
  specified effect NEC T75.09
Lightwood-Albright syndrome N25.89
**Lightwood's disease or syndrome (renal
  tubular acidosis)** N25.89
**Lignac (-de Toni) (-Fanconi) (-Debré) disease
  or syndrome** E72.09
  with cystinosis E72.04

Ligneous thyroiditis E06.5
Likoff's syndrome I20.8
Limb — *see* condition
Limbic epilepsy personality syndrome F07.0
Limitation, limited
  activities due to disability Z73.6
  cardiac reserve — *see* Disease, heart
  eye muscle duction, traumatic — *see*
    Strabismus, mechanical
  mandibular range of motion M26.52
Lindau (-von Hippel) disease Q85.8
Line (s)
  Beau's L60.4
  Harris' — *see* Arrest, epiphyseal
  Hudson's (cornea) — *see* Pigmentation,
    cornea, anterior
  Stähli's (cornea) — *see* Pigmentation, cornea,
    anterior
Linea corneae senilis — *see* Change, cornea,
  senile
Lingua
  geographica K14.1
  nigra (villosa) K14.3
  plicata K14.5
  tylosis K13.29
Lingual — *see* condition
Linguatulosis B88.8
Linitis (gastric) plastica C16.9
Lip — *see* condition
Lipedema — *see* Edema
Lipemia — *see also* Hyperlipidemia
  retina, retinalis E78.3
Lipidosis E75.6
  cerebral (infantile) (juvenile) (late) E75.4
  cerebroretinal E75.4
  cerebroside E75.22
  cholesterol (cerebral) E75.5
  glycolipid E75.21
  hepatosplenomegalic E78.3
  sphingomyelin — *see* Niemann-Pick disease
    or syndrome
  sulfatide E75.29
Lipoadenoma — *see* Neoplasm, benign, by
  site
Lipoblastoma — *see* Lipoma
Lipoblastomatosis — *see* Lipoma
Lipochondrodystrophy E76.01
Lipochrome histiocytosis (familial) D71
Lipodermatosclerosis — *see* Varix, leg, with,
  inflammation
  ulcerated — *see* Varix, leg, with, ulcer, with
    inflammation by site
Lipodystrophia progressiva E88.1
Lipodystrophy (progressive) E88.1
  insulin E88.1
  intestinal K90.81
  mesenteric K65.4
Lipofibroma — *see* Lipoma
**Lipofuscinosis, neuronal (with
  ceroidosis)** E75.4
Lipogranuloma, sclerosing L92.8
Lipogranulomatosis E78.89
Lipoid — *see also* condition
  histiocytosis D76.3
    essential E75.29
  nephrosis N04.9
  proteinosis of Urbach E78.89
Lipoidemia — *see* Hyperlipidemia
Lipoidosis — *see* Lipidosis
Lipoma D17.9
  fetal D17.9
    fat cell D17.9
  infiltrating D17.9
  intramuscular D17.9
  pleomorphic D17.9
  site classification
    arms (skin) (subcutaneous) D17.2-
    connective tissue D17.30
      intra-abdominal D17.5
      intrathoracic D17.4
      peritoneum D17.79
      retroperitoneum D17.79
      specified site NEC D17.39
      spermatic cord D17.6
    face (skin) (subcutaneous) D17.0

Lipoma - *continued*
  site classification - *continued*
    genitourinary organ NEC D17.72
    head (skin) (subcutaneous) D17.0
    intra-abdominal D17.5
    intrathoracic D17.4
    kidney D17.71
    legs (skin) (subcutaneous) D17.2-
    neck (skin) (subcutaneous) D17.0
    peritoneum D17.79
    retroperitoneum D17.79
    skin D17.30
      specified site NEC D17.39
    specified site NEC D17.79
    spermatic cord D17.6
    subcutaneous D17.30
      specified site NEC D17.39
    trunk (skin) (subcutaneous) D17.1
    unspecified D17.9
    spindle cell D17.9
Lipomatosis E88.2
  dolorosa (Dercum) E88.2
  fetal — *see* Lipoma
  Launois-Bensaude E88.89
Lipomyoma — *see* Lipoma
Lipomyxoma — *see* Lipoma
Lipomyxosarcoma — *see* Neoplasm,
  connective tissue, malignant
Lipoprotein metabolism disorder E78.9
Lipoproteinemia E78.5
  broad-beta E78.2
  floating-beta E78.2
  hyper-pre-beta E78.1
Liposarcoma — *see also* Neoplasm,
  connective tissue, malignant
  dedifferentiated — *see* Neoplasm, connective
    tissue, malignant
  differentiated type — *see* Neoplasm,
    connective tissue, malignant
  embryonal — *see* Neoplasm, connective
    tissue, malignant
  mixed type — *see* Neoplasm, connective
    tissue, malignant
  myxoid — *see* Neoplasm, connective tissue,
    malignant
  pleomorphic — *see* Neoplasm, connective
    tissue, malignant
  round cell — *see* Neoplasm, connective
    tissue, malignant
  well differentiated type — *see* Neoplasm,
    connective tissue, malignant
Liposynovitis prepatellaris E88.89
Lipping, cervix N86
Lipschütz disease or ulcer N76.6
Lipuria R82.0
  schistosomiasis (bilharziasis) B65.0
Lisping F80.0
Lissauer's paralysis A52.17
Lissencephalia, lissencephaly Q04.3
Listeriosis, listerellosis A32.9
  congenital (disseminated) P37.2
  cutaneous A32.0
  neonatal, newborn (disseminated) P37.2
  oculoglandular A32.81
  specified NEC A32.89
Lithemia E79.0
Lithiasis — *see* Calculus
Lithosis J62.8
Lithuria R82.998
Litigation, anxiety concerning Z65.3
Little leaguer's elbow — *see* Epicondylitis,
  medial
Little's disease G80.9
Littre's
  gland — *see* condition
  hernia — *see* Hernia, abdomen
Littritis — *see* Urethritis
Livedo (annularis) (racemosa)
  (reticularis) R23.1
Liver — *see* condition
Living alone (problems with) Z60.2
  with handicapped person Z74.2
Lloyd's syndrome — *see* Adenomatosis,
  endocrine
Loa loa, loaiasis, loasis B74.3

Lobar — *see* condition
Lobomycosis B48.0
Lobo's disease B48.0
Lobotomy syndrome F07.0
Lobstein (-Ekman) disease or
  syndrome Q78.0
Lobster-claw hand Q71.6-
Lobulation (congenital) — *see also* Anomaly,
  by site
  kidney, Q63.1
  liver, abnormal Q44.7
  spleen Q89.09
Lobule, lobular — *see* condition
Local, localized — *see* condition
Locked twins causing obstructed
  labor O66.1
Locked-in state G83.5
Locking
  joint — *see* Derangement, joint, specified
    type NEC
  knee — *see* Derangement, knee
Lockjaw — *see* Tetanus
Löffler's
  endocarditis I42.3
  eosinophilia J82
  pneumonia J82
  syndrome (eosinophilic pneumonitis) J82
Loiasis (with conjunctival infestation)
  (eyelid) B74.3
Lone Star fever A77.0
Long
  labor O63.9
    first stage O63.0
    second stage O63.1
  QT syndrome I45.81
Longitudinal stripes or grooves, nails L60.8
  congenital Q84.6
Long-term (current) (prophylactic) drug
  therapy (use of)
  agents affecting estrogen receptors and
    estrogen levels NEC Z79.818
  anastrozole (Arimidex) Z79.811
  antibiotics Z79.2
    short-term use - omit code
  anticoagulants Z79.01
  anti-inflammatory, non-steroidal
    (NSAID) Z79.1
  antiplatelet Z79.02
  antithrombotics Z79.02
  aromatase inhibitors Z79.811
  aspirin Z79.82
  birth control pill or patch Z79.3
  bisphosphonates Z79.83
  contraceptive, oral Z79.3
  drug, specified NEC Z79.899
  estrogen receptor downregulators Z79.818
  Evista Z79.810
  exemestane (Aromasin) Z79.811
  Fareston Z79.810
  fulvestrant (Faslodex) Z79.818
  gonadotropin-releasing hormone (GnRH)
    agonist Z79.818
  goserelin acetate (Zoladex) Z79.818
  hormone replacement Z79.890
  insulin Z79.4
  letrozole (Femara) Z79.811
  leuprolide acetate (leuprorelin)
    (Lupron) Z79.818
  megestrol acetate (Megace) Z79.818
  methadone for pain management Z79.891
  Nolvadex Z79.810
  non-steroidal anti-inflammatories
    (NSAID) Z79.1
  opiate analgesic Z79.891
  oral
    antidiabetic Z79.84
    contraceptive Z79.3
    hypoglycemic Z79.84
  raloxifene (Evista) Z79.810
  selective estrogen receptor modulators
    (SERMs) Z79.810
  steroids
    inhaled Z79.51
    systemic Z79.52
  tamoxifen (Nolvadex) Z79.810

Long-term (current) (prophylactic) drug
therapy (use of) - *continued*
  toremifene (Fareston) Z79.810
Loop
  intestine — *see* Volvulus
  vascular on papilla (optic) Q14.2
Loose — *see also* condition
  body
    joint M24.00
      ankle M24.07-
      elbow M24.02-
      hand M24.04-
      hip M24.05-
      knee M23.4-
      shoulder (region) M24.01-
      specified site NEC M24.08
      vertebra M24.08
      toe M24.07-
      wrist M24.03-
    knee M23.4-
    sheath, tendon — *see* Disorder, tendon,
      specified type NEC
  cartilage — *see* Loose, body, joint
  skin and subcutaneous tissue (following
    bariatric surgery weight loss) (following
    dietary weight loss) L98.7
  tooth, teeth K08.89
Loosening
  aseptic
    joint prosthesis — *see* Complications, joint
      prosthesis, mechanical, loosening, by
      site
  epiphysis — *see* Osteochondropathy
  mechanical
    joint prosthesis — *see* Complications, joint
      prosthesis, mechanical, loosening, by
      site
Looser-Milkman (-Debray) syndrome M83.8
Lop ear (deformity) Q17.3
Lorain (-Levi) short stature syndrome E23.0
Lordosis M40.50
  acquired — *see* Lordosis, specified type
    NEC
  congenital Q76.429
    lumbar region Q76.426
    lumbosacral region Q76.427
    sacral region Q76.428
    sacrococcygeal region Q76.428
    thoracolumbar region Q76.425
  lumbar region M40.56
  lumbosacral region M40.57
  postsurgical M96.4
  postural — *see* Lordosis, specified type NEC
  rachitic (late effect) (sequelae) E64.3
  sequelae of rickets E64.3
  specified type NEC M40.40
    lumbar region M40.46
    lumbosacral region M40.47
    thoracolumbar region M40.45
  thoracolumbar region M40.55
  tuberculous A18.01
Loss (of)
  appetite (see Anorexia) R63.0
    hysterical F50.89
    nonorganic origin F50.89
    psychogenic F50.89
  blood — *see* Hemorrhage
  bone — *see* Loss, substance of, bone
  control, sphincter, rectum R15.9
    nonorganic origin F98.1
  consciousness, transient R55
    traumatic — *see* Injury, intracranial
  elasticity, skin R23.4
  family (member) in childhood Z62.898
  fluid (acute) E86.9
  function of labyrinth — *see* subcategory
    H83.2
  hair, nonscarring — *see* Alopecia
  hearing — *see also* Deafness
    central NOS H90.5
    conductive H90.2
      bilateral H90.0
      unilateral
        with

Loss (of) - *continued*
  hearing - *continued*
    conductive - *continued*
      unilateral - *continued*
        with - *continued*
          restricted hearing on the
            contralateral side H90.A1-
          unrestricted hearing on the
            contralateral side H90.1-
    mixed conductive and sensorineural
      hearing loss H90.8
      bilateral H90.6
      unilateral
        with
          restricted hearing on the
            contralateral side H90.A3-
          unrestricted hearing on the
            contralateral side H90.7-
    neural NOS H90.5
    perceptive NOS H90.5
    sensorineural NOS H90.5
      bilateral H90.3
      unilateral
        with
          restricted hearing on the
            contralateral side H90.A2-
          unrestricted hearing on the
            contralateral side H90.4-
    sensory NOS H90.5
  height R29.890
  limb or member, traumatic, current — *see*
    Amputation, traumatic
  love relationship in childhood Z62.898
  memory — *see also* Amnesia
    mild, following organic brain
      damage F06.8
  mind — *see* Psychosis
  occlusal vertical dimension of fully erupted
    teeth M26.37
  organ or part — *see* Absence, by site,
    acquired
  ossicles, ear (partial) H74.32-
  parent in childhood Z63.4
  pregnancy, recurrent N96
    care in current pregnancy O26.2-
    without current pregnancy N96
  recurrent pregnancy — *see* Loss, pregnancy,
    recurrent
  self-esteem, in childhood Z62.898
  sense of
    smell — *see* Disturbance, sensation, smell
    taste — *see* Disturbance, sensation, taste
    touch R20.8
  sensory R44.9
    dissociative F44.6
  sexual desire F52.0
  sight (acquired) (complete) (congenital) —
    see Blindness
  substance of
    bone — *see* Disorder, bone, density and
      structure, specified NEC
      horizontal alveolar K06.3
    cartilage — *see* Disorder, cartilage,
      specified type NEC
      auricle (ear) — *see* Disorder, pinna,
        specified type NEC
    vitreous (humor) H15.89
  tooth, teeth — *see* Absence, teeth, acquired
  vision, visual H54.7
    both eyes H54.3
    one eye H54.60
      left (normal vision on right) H54.62
      right (normal vision on left) H54.61
    specified as blindness — *see* Blindness
    subjective
      sudden H53.13-
      transient H53.12-
  vitreous — *see* Prolapse, vitreous
  voice — *see* Aphonia
  weight (abnormal) (cause unknown) R63.4
Louis-Bar syndrome (ataxia
  -telangiectasia) G11.3
Louping ill (encephalitis) A84.8
Louse, lousiness — *see* Lice

Low
  achiever, school Z55.3
  back syndrome M54.5
  basal metabolic rate R94.8
  birthweight (2499 grams or less) P07.10
    with weight of
      1000-1249 grams P07.14
      1250-1499 grams P07.15
      1500-1749 grams P07.16
      1750-1999 grams P07.17
      2000-2499 grams P07.18
    extreme (999 grams or less) P07.00
      with weight of
        499 grams or less P07.01
        500-749 grams P07.02
        750-999 grams P07.03
    for gestational age — *see* Light for dates
  blood pressure — *see also* Hypotension
    reading (incidental) (isolated)
      (nonspecific) R03.1
  cardiac reserve — *see* Disease, heart
  function — *see also* Hypofunction
    kidney N28.9
  hematocrit D64.9
  hemoglobin D64.9
  income Z59.6
  level of literacy Z55.0
  lying
    kidney N28.89
    organ or site, congenital — *see*
      Malposition, congenital
  output syndrome (cardiac) — *see* Failure,
    heart
  platelets (blood) — *see* Thrombocytopenia
  reserve, kidney N28.89
  salt syndrome E87.1
  self esteem R45.81
  set ears Q17.4
  vision H54.2X-
    one eye (other eye normal) H54.50
      left (normal vision on right) H54.52A-
      other eye blind — *see* Blindness
      right (normal vision on left) H54.511-
Low-density-lipoprotein-type (LDL)
  hyperlipoproteinemia E78.00
Lowe's syndrome E72.03
Lown-Ganong-Levine syndrome I45.6
LSD reaction (acute) (without dependence)
  F16.90
  with dependence F16.20
L-shaped kidney Q63.8
LTBI (latent tuberculosis infection) Z22.7
Ludwig's angina or disease K12.2
Lues (venerea) , luetic — *see* Syphilis
Luetscher's syndrome (dehydration) E86.0
Lumbago, lumbalgia M54.5
  with sciatica M54.4-
    due to intervertebral disc disorder M51.17
  due to displacement, intervertebral
    disc M51.27
    with sciatica M51.17
Lumbar — *see* condition
Lumbarization, vertebra, congenital Q76.49
Lumbermen's itch B88.0
Lump — *see also* Mass
  breast N63.0
    axillary tail
      left N63.32
      right N63.31
    left
      lower inner quadrant N63.24
      lower outer quadrant N63.23
      overlapping quadrants N63.25
      unspecified quadrant N63.20
      upper inner quadrant N63.22
      upper outer quadrant N63.21
    right
      lower inner quadrant N63.14
      lower outer quadrant N63.13
      overlapping quadrants N63.15
      unspecified quadrant N63.10
      upper inner quadrant N63.12
      upper outer quadrant N63.11
    subareolar
      left N63.42

Lump - *continued*
  breast - *continued*
    subareolar - *continued*
      right N63.41
Lunacy — *see* Psychosis
Lung — *see* condition
Lupoid (miliary) of Boeck D86.3
Lupus
  anticoagulant D68.62
    with
      hemorrhagic disorder D68.312
      hypercoagulable state D68.62
    finding without diagnosis R76.0
  discoid (local) L93.0
  erythematosus (discoid) (local) L93.0
    disseminated — *see* Lupus, erythematosus,
      systemic
    eyelid H01.129
      left H01.126
        lower H01.125
        upper H01.124
      right H01.123
        lower H01.122
        upper H01.121
    profundus L93.2
    specified NEC L93.2
    subacute cutaneous L93.1
    systemic M32.9
      with organ or system
        involvement M32.10
      endocarditis M32.11
      lung M32.13
      pericarditis M32.12
      renal (glomerular) M32.14
        tubulo-interstitial M32.15
      specified organ or system
        NEC M32.19
    drug-induced M32.0
      inhibitor (presence of) D68.62
        with
          hemorrhagic disorder D68.312
          hypercoagulable state D68.62
        finding without diagnosis R76.0
    specified NEC M32.8
  exedens A18.4
  hydralazine M32.0
    correct substance properly
      administered — *see* Table of Drugs
      and Chemicals, by drug, adverse
      effect
    overdose or wrong substance given or
      taken — *see* Table of Drugs and
      Chemicals, by drug, poisoning
  nephritis (chronic) M32.14
  nontuberculous, not disseminated L93.0
  panniculitis L93.2
  pernio (Besnier) D86.3
  systemic — *see* Lupus, erythematosus,
    systemic
  tuberculous A18.4
    eyelid A18.4
  vulgaris A18.4
    eyelid A18.4
Luteinoma D27.-
Lutembacher's disease or syndrome (atrial
  septal defect with mitral stenosis) Q21.1
Luteoma D27.-
Lutz (-Splendore-de Almeida) disease — *see*
  Paracoccidioidomycosis
Luxation — *see also* Dislocation
  eyeball (nontraumatic) — *see* Luxation,
    globe
    birth injury P15.3
  globe, nontraumatic H44.82-
  lacrimal gland — *see* Dislocation, lacrimal
    gland
  lens (old) (partial) (spontaneous)
    congenital Q12.1
    syphilitic A50.39
Lycanthropy F22
Lyell's syndrome L51.2
  due to drug L51.2

Lyell's syndrome - *continued*
  due to drug - *continued*
    correct substance properly
      administered — *see* Table of Drugs
      and Chemicals, by drug, adverse
      effect
    overdose or wrong substance given or
      taken — *see* Table of Drugs and
      Chemicals, by drug, poisoning
Lyme disease A69.20
Lymph
  gland or node — *see* condition
  scrotum — *see* Infestation, filarial
Lymphadenitis I88.9
  with ectopic or molar pregnancy O08.0
  acute L04.9
    axilla L04.2
    face L04.0
    head L04.0
    hip L04.3
    limb
      lower L04.3
      upper L04.2
    neck L04.0
    shoulder L04.2
    specified site NEC L04.8
    trunk L04.1
  anthracosis (occupational) J60
  any site, except mesenteric I88.9
    chronic I88.1
    subacute I88.1
  breast
    gestational — *see* Mastitis, obstetric
    puerperal, postpartum
      (nonpurulent) O91.22
  chancroidal (congenital) A57
  chronic I88.1
    mesenteric I88.0
  due to
    Brugia (malayi) B74.1
      timori B74.2
    chlamydial lymphogranuloma A55
    diphtheria (toxin) A36.89
    lymphogranuloma venereum A55
    Wuchereria bancrofti B74.0
  following ectopic or molar pregnancy O08.0
  gonorrheal A54.89
  infective — *see* Lymphadenitis, acute
  mesenteric (acute) (chronic) (nonspecific)
    (subacute) I88.0
    due to Salmonella typhi A01.09
    tuberculous A18.39
  mycobacterial A31.8
  purulent — *see* Lymphadenitis, acute
  pyogenic — *see* Lymphadenitis, acute
  regional, nonbacterial I88.8
  septic — *see* Lymphadenitis, acute
  subacute, unspecified site I88.1
  suppurative — *see* Lymphadenitis, acute
  syphilitic (early) (secondary) A51.49
    late A52.79
  tuberculous — *see* Tuberculosis, lymph
    gland
  venereal (chlamydial) A55
Lymphadenoid goiter E06.3
Lymphadenopathy (generalized) R59.1
  angioimmunoblastic, with dysproteinemia
    (AILD) C86.5
  due to toxoplasmosis (acquired) B58.89
    congenital (acute) (subacute)
      (chronic) P37.1
  localized R59.0
  syphilitic (early) (secondary) A51.49
Lymphadenosis R59.1
Lymphangiectasis I89.0
  conjunctiva H11.89
  postinfectional I89.0
  scrotum I89.0
**Lymphangiectatic elephantiasis,
  nonfilarial** I89.0
Lymphangioendothelioma D18.1
  malignant — *see* Neoplasm, connective
    tissue, malignant
Lymphangioleiomyomatosis J84.81

Lymphangioma D18.1
  capillary D18.1
  cavernous D18.1
  cystic D18.1
  malignant — *see* Neoplasm, connective
    tissue, malignant
Lymphangiomyoma D18.1
Lymphangiomyomatosis J84.81
Lymphangiosarcoma — *see* Neoplasm,
  connective tissue, malignant
Lymphangitis I89.1
  with
    abscess - code by site under Abscess
    cellulitis - code by site under Cellulitis
    ectopic or molar pregnancy O08.0
  acute L03.91
    abdominal wall L03.321
    ankle — *see* Lymphangitis, acute, lower
      limb
    arm — *see* Lymphangitis, acute, upper
      limb
    auricle (ear) — *see* Lymphangitis, acute,
      ear
    axilla L03.12-
    back (any part) L03.322
    buttock L03.327
    cervical (meaning neck) L03.222
    cheek (external) L03.212
    chest wall L03.323
    digit
      finger — *see* Lymphangitis, acute, finger
      toe — *see* Lymphangitis, acute, toe
    ear (external) H60.1-
    external auditory canal — *see*
      Lymphangitis, acute, ear
    eyelid — *see* Abscess, eyelid
    face NEC L03.212
    finger (intrathecal) (periosteal)
      (subcutaneous) (subcuticular) L03.02-
    foot — *see* Lymphangitis, acute, lower
      limb
    gluteal (region) L03.327
    groin L03.324
    hand — *see* Lymphangitis, acute, upper
      limb
    head NEC L03.891
      face (any part, except ear, eye and
        nose) L03.212
    heel — *see* Lymphangitis, acute, lower
      limb
    hip — *see* Lymphangitis, acute, lower limb
    jaw (region) L03.212
    knee — *see* Lymphangitis, acute, lower
      limb
    leg — *see* Lymphangitis, acute, lower limb
    lower limb L03.12-
      toe — *see* Lymphangitis, acute, toe
    navel L03.326
    neck (region) L03.222
    orbit, orbital — *see* Cellulitis, orbit
    pectoral (region) L03.323
    perineal, perineum L03.325
    scalp (any part) L03.891
    shoulder — *see* Lymphangitis, acute, upper
      limb
    specified site NEC L03.898
    thigh — *see* Lymphangitis, acute, lower
      limb
    thumb (intrathecal) (periosteal)
      (subcutaneous) (subcuticular) — *see*
      Lymphangitis, acute, finger
    toe (intrathecal) (periosteal)
      (subcutaneous) (subcuticular) L03.04-
    trunk L03.329
      abdominal wall L03.321
      back (any part) L03.322
      buttock L03.327
      chest wall L03.323
      groin L03.324
      perineal, perineum L03.325
      umbilicus L03.326
    umbilicus L03.326
    upper limb L03.12-
      axilla — *see* Lymphangitis, acute, axilla
      finger — *see* Lymphangitis, acute, finger

Lymphangitis - *continued*
  acute - *continued*
    upper limb - *continued*
      thumb — *see* Lymphangitis, acute,
        finger
      wrist — *see* Lymphangitis, acute, upper
        limb
  breast
    gestational — *see* Mastitis, obstetric
  chancroidal A57
  chronic (any site) I89.1
  due to
    Brugia (malayi) B74.1
      timori B74.2
    Wuchereria bancrofti B74.0
  following ectopic or molar
    pregnancy O08.89
  penis
    acute N48.29
    gonococcal (acute) (chronic) A54.09
  puerperal, postpartum, childbirth O86.89
  strumous, tuberculous A18.2
  subacute (any site) I89.1
  tuberculous — *see* Tuberculosis, lymph
    gland
Lymphatic (vessel) — *see* condition
Lymphatism E32.8
Lymphectasia I89.0
Lymphedema (acquired) — *see also*
  Elephantiasis
  congenital Q82.0
  hereditary (chronic) (idiopathic) Q82.0
  postmastectomy I97.2
  praecox I89.0
  secondary I89.0
  surgical NEC I97.89
    postmastectomy (syndrome) I97.2
Lymphoblastic — *see* condition
Lymphoblastoma (diffuse) — *see* Lymphoma,
  lymphoblastic (diffuse)
  giant follicular — *see* Lymphoma,
    lymphoblastic (diffuse)
  macrofollicular — *see* Lymphoma,
    lymphoblastic (diffuse)
Lymphocele I89.8
Lymphocytic
  chorioencephalitis (acute) (serous) A87.2
  choriomeningitis (acute) (serous) A87.2
  meningoencephalitis A87.2
Lymphocytoma, benign cutis L98.8
Lymphocytopenia D72.810
Lymphocytosis (symptomatic) D72.820
  infectious (acute) B33.8
Lymphoepithelioma — *see* Neoplasm,
  malignant, by site
Lymphogranuloma (malignant) — *see also*
  Lymphoma, Hodgkin
  chlamydial A55
  inguinale A55
  venereum (any site) (chlamydial) (with
    stricture of rectum) A55
Lymphogranulomatosis (malignant) — *see*
  also Lymphoma, Hodgkin
  benign (Boeck's sarcoid)
    (Schaumann's) D86.1
**Lymphohistiocytosis, hemophagocytic
  (familial)** D76.1
Lymphoid — *see* condition
Lymphoma (of) (malignant) C85.90
  adult T-cell (HTLV-1-associated) (acute
    variant) (chronic variant)
    (lymphomatoid variant) (smouldering
    variant) C91.5-
  anaplastic large cell
    ALK-negative C84.7-
    ALK-positive C84.6-
    CD30-positive C84.6-
    primary cutaneous C86.6
  angioimmunoblastic T-cell C86.5
  BALT C88.4
  B-cell C85.1-
  B-precursor C83.5-
  blastic NK-cell C86.4
  blastic plasmacytoid dendritic cell neoplasm
    (BPDCN) C86.4

Lymphoma (of) (malignant) - *continued*
  bronchial-associated lymphoid tissue [BALT-lymphoma] C88.4
  Burkitt (atypical) C83.7-
  Burkitt-like C83.7-
  centrocytic C83.1-
  cutaneous follicle center C82.6-
  cutaneous T-cell C84.A-
  diffuse follicle center C82.5-
  diffuse large cell C83.3-
    anaplastic C83.3-
    B-cell C83.3-
    CD30-positive C83.3-
    centroblastic C83.3-
    immunoblastic C83.3-
    plasmablastic C83.3-
    subtype not specified C83.3-
    T-cell rich C83.3-
  enteropathy-type (associated) (intestinal) T-cell C86.2
  extranodal NK/T-cell, nasal type C86.0
  extranodal marginal zone B-cell lymphoma of mucosa-associated lymphoid tissue [MALT-lymphoma] C88.4
  follicular C82.9-
    grade
      I C82.0-
      II C82.1-
      III C82.2-
      IIIa C82.3-
      IIIb C82.4-
    specified NEC C82.8-
  hepatosplenic T-cell (alpha-beta) (gamma-delta) C86.1
  histiocytic C85.9-
    true C96.A
  Hodgkin C81.9
    lymphocyte-rich (classical) C81.4-
    lymphocyte depleted (classical) C81.3-
    mixed cellularity (classical) C81.2-
    nodular sclerosis (classical) C81.1-
    specified NEC (classical) C81.7-
    lymphocyte-rich classical C81.4-
    lymphocyte depleted classical C81.3-
    mixed cellularity classical C81.2-
    nodular
      lymphocyte predominant C81.0-
      sclerosis (classical) C81.1-
  intravascular large B-cell C83.8-
  Lennert's C84.4-
  lymphoblastic B-cell C83.5-
  lymphoblastic (diffuse) C83.5-
  lymphoblastic T-cell C83.5-
  lymphoepithelioid C84.4-
  lymphoplasmacytic C83.0-
    with IgM-production C88.0
  MALT C88.4
  mantle cell C83.1-
  mature T-cell NEC C84.4-
  mature T/NK-cell C84.9-
    specified NEC C84.Z-
  mediastinal (thymic) large B-cell C85.2-
  Mediterranean C88.3
  mucosa-associated lymphoid tissue [MALT-lymphoma] C88.4
  NK/T cell C84.9-
  nodal marginal zone C83.0-
  non-follicular (diffuse) C83.9-
    specified NEC C83.8-
  non-Hodgkin — *see also* Lymphoma, by type C85.9-
    specified NEC C85.8-
  non-leukemic variant of B-CLL C83.0-
  peripheral T-cell, not classified C84.4-
  primary cutaneous
    anaplastic large cell C86.6
    CD30-positive large T-cell C86.6
  primary effusion B-cell C83.8-
  SALT C88.4
  skin-associated lymphoid tissue [SALT-lymphoma] C88.4
  small cell B-cell C83.0-
  splenic marginal zone C83.0-
  subcutaneous panniculitis-like T-cell C86.3
  T-precursor C83.5-

Lymphoma (of) (malignant) - *continued*
  true histiocytic C96.A
Lymphomatosis — *see* Lymphoma
Lymphopathia, veneris A55
Lymphopenia D72.810
Lymphoplasmacytic leukemia — *see* Leukemia, chronic lymphocytic, B-cell type
Lymphoproliferation, X-linked disease D82.3
Lymphoreticulosis, benign (of inoculation) A28.1
Lymphorrhea I89.8
Lymphosarcoma (diffuse) — *see also* Lymphoma C85.9-
Lymphostasis I89.8
Lypemania — *see* Melancholia
Lysine and hydroxylysine metabolism disorder E72.3
Lyssa — *see* Rabies

M

Macacus ear Q17.3
Maceration, wet feet, tropical (syndrome) T69.02-
MacLeod's syndrome J43.0
Macrocephalia, macrocephaly Q75.3
Macrocheilia, macrochilia (congenital) Q18.6
Macrocolon — *see also* Megacolon Q43.1
Macrocornea Q15.8
  with glaucoma Q15.0
Macrocytic — *see* condition
Macrocytosis D75.89
Macrodactylia, macrodactylism (fingers) (thumbs) Q74.0
  toes Q74.2
Macrodontia K00.2
Macrogenia M26.05
Macrogenitosomia (adrenal) (male) (praecox) E25.9
  congenital E25.0
Macroglobulinemia (idiopathic) (primary) C88.0
  monoclonal (essential) D47.2
  Waldenström C88.0
Macroglossia (congenital) Q38.2
  acquired K14.8
Macrognathia, macrognathism (congenital) (mandibular) (maxillary) M26.09
Macrogyria (congenital) Q04.8
Macrohydrocephalus — *see* Hydrocephalus
Macromastia — *see* Hypertrophy, breast
Macrophthalmos Q11.3
  in congenital glaucoma Q15.0
Macropsia H53.15
Macrosigmoid K59.39
  congenital Q43.2
Macrospondylitis , acromegalic E22.0
Macrostomia (congenital) Q18.4
Macrotia (external ear) (congenital) Q17.1
Macula
  cornea, corneal — *see* Opacity, cornea
  degeneration (atrophic) (exudative) (senile) — *see also* Degeneration, macula
  hereditary — *see* Dystrophy, retina
Maculae ceruleae -- B85.1
Maculopathy, toxic — *see* Degeneration, macula, toxic
Madarosis (eyelid) H02.729
  left H02.726
    lower H02.725
    upper H02.724
  right H02.723
    lower H02.722
    upper H02.721
Madelung's
  deformity (radius) Q74.0
  disease
    radial deformity Q74.0
    symmetrical lipomas, neck E88.89
Madness — *see* Psychosis
Madura
  foot B47.9
    actinomycotic B47.1
    mycotic B47.0
Maduromycosis B47.0

Maffucci's syndrome Q78.4
Magnesium metabolism disorder — *see* Disorder, metabolism, magnesium
Main en griffe (acquired) — *see also* Deformity, limb, clawhand
  congenital Q74.0
Maintenance (encounter for)
  antineoplastic chemotherapy Z51.11
  antineoplastic radiation therapy Z51.0
  methadone F11.20
Majocchi's
  disease L81.7
  granuloma B35.8
Major — *see* condition
Mal de los pintos — *see* Pinta
Mal de mer T75.3
Malabar itch (any site) B35.5
Malabsorption K90.9
  calcium K90.89
  carbohydrate K90.49
  disaccharide E73.9
  fat K90.49
  galactose E74.20
  glucose (-galactose) E74.39
  intestinal K90.9
    specified NEC K90.89
  isomaltose E74.31
  lactose E73.9
  methionine E72.19
  monosaccharide E74.39
  postgastrectomy K91.2
  postsurgical K91.2
  protein K90.49
  starch K90.49
  sucrose E74.39
  syndrome K90.9
    postsurgical K91.2
Malacia, bone (adult) M83.9
  juvenile — *see* Rickets
Malacoplakia
  bladder N32.89
  pelvis (kidney) N28.89
  ureter N28.89
  urethra N36.8
Malacosteon, juvenile — *see* Rickets
Maladaptation — *see* Maladjustment
Maladie de Roger Q21.0
Maladjustment
  conjugal Z63.0
    involving divorce or estrangement Z63.5
  educational Z55.4
  family Z63.9
  marital Z63.0
    involving divorce or estrangement Z63.5
  occupational NEC Z56.89
  simple, adult — *see* Disorder, adjustment
  situational — *see* Disorder, adjustment
  social Z60.9
    due to
      acculturation difficulty Z60.3
      discrimination and persecution (perceived) Z60.5
      exclusion and isolation Z60.4
      life-cycle (phase of life) transition Z60.0
      rejection Z60.4
      specified reason NEC Z60.8
Malaise R53.81
Malakoplakia — *see* Malacoplakia
Malaria, malarial (fever) B54
  with
    blackwater fever B50.8
      hemoglobinuric (bilious) B50.8
    hemoglobinuria B50.8
  accidentally induced (therapeutically) - code by type under Malaria
  algid B50.9
  cerebral B50.0 *[G94]*
  clinically diagnosed (without parasitological confirmation) B54
  congenital NEC P37.4
    falciparum P37.3
  congestion, congestive B54
  continued (fever) B50.9
  estivo-autumnal B50.9
  falciparum B50.9

Malaria, malarial (fever) - *continued*
falciparum - *continued*
  with complications NEC B50.8
    cerebral B50.0 *[G94]*
    severe B50.8
  hemorrhagic B54
malariae B52.9
  with
    complications NEC B52.8
    glomerular disorder B52.0
  malignant (tertian) — *see* Malaria,
    falciparum
  mixed infections - code to first listed type in
    B50-B53
  ovale B53.0
  parasitologically confirmed NEC B53.8
  pernicious, acute — *see* Malaria, falciparum
  Plasmodium (P.)
    falciparum NEC — *see* Malaria,
      falciparum
    malariae NEC B52.9
      with Plasmodium
        falciparum (and or vivax) — *see*
          Malaria, falciparum
        vivax — *see also* Malaria, vivax
          and falciparum — *see* Malaria,
            falciparum
    ovale B53.0
      with Plasmodium malariae — *see also*
        Malaria, malariae
        and vivax — *see also* Malaria, vivax
          and falciparum — *see* Malaria,
            falciparum
    simian B53.1
      with Plasmodium malariae — *see also*
        Malaria, malariae
        and vivax — *see also* Malaria, vivax
          and falciparum — *see* Malaria,
            falciparum
    vivax NEC B51.9
      with Plasmodium falciparum — *see*
        Malaria, falciparum
  quartan — *see* Malaria, malariae
  quotidian — *see* Malaria, falciparum
  recurrent B54
  remittent B54
  specified type NEC (parasitologically
    confirmed) B53.8
  spleen B54
  subtertian (fever) — *see* Malaria, falciparum
  tertian (benign) — *see also* Malaria, vivax
    malignant B50.9
  tropical B50.9
  typhoid B54
  vivax B51.9
    with
      complications NEC B51.8
      ruptured spleen B51.0
Malassez's disease (cystic) N50.89
Malassimilation K90.9
Maldescent, testis Q53.9
  bilateral Q53.20
    abdominal Q53.211
    perineal Q53.22
  unilateral Q53.10
    abdominal Q53.111
    perineal Q53.12
Maldevelopment — *see also* Anomaly
  brain Q07.9
  colon Q43.9
  hip Q74.2
    congenital dislocation Q65.2
      bilateral Q65.1
      unilateral Q65.0-
  mastoid process Q75.8
  middle ear Q16.4
    except ossicles Q16.4
    ossicles Q16.3
  ossicles Q16.3
  spine Q76.49
  toe Q74.2
Male type pelvis Q74.2
  with disproportion (fetopelvic) O33.3
    causing obstructed labor O65.3

Malformation (congenital) — *see also*
  Anomaly
adrenal gland Q89.1
affecting multiple systems with skeletal
  changes NEC Q87.5
alimentary tract Q45.9
  specified type NEC Q45.8
  upper Q40.9
    specified type NEC Q40.8
aorta Q25.40
  absence Q25.41
  aneurysm, congenital Q25.43
  aplasia Q25.41
  atresia Q25.29
    aortic arch Q25.21
  coarctation (preductal) (postductal) Q25.1
  dilatation, congenital Q25.44
  hypoplasia Q25.42
  patent ductus arteriosus Q25.0
  specified type NEC Q25.49
  stenosis Q25.1
    supravalvular Q25.3
aortic valve Q23.9
  specified NEC Q23.8
arteriovenous, aneurysmatic
  (congenital) Q27.30
  brain Q28.2
    ruptured I60.8
      intracerebral I61.8
      intraparenchymal I61.8
      intraventricular I61.5
      subarachnoid I60.8
  cerebral — *see also* Malformation,
    arteriovenous, brain Q28.2
  peripheral Q27.30
    digestive system — *see* Angiodysplasia
      congenital Q27.33
    lower limb Q27.32
    other specified site Q27.39
    renal vessel Q27.34
    upper limb Q27.31
  precerebral vessels (nonruptured) Q28.0
auricle
  ear (congenital) Q17.3
    acquired H61.119
      left H61.112
        with right H61.113
      right H61.111
        with left H61.113
bile duct Q44.5
bladder Q64.79
  aplasia Q64.5
  diverticulum Q64.6
  exstrophy — *see* Exstrophy, bladder
  neck obstruction Q64.31
bone Q79.9
  face Q75.9
    specified type NEC Q75.8
  skull Q75.9
    specified type NEC Q75.8
brain (multiple) Q04.9
  arteriovenous Q28.2
  specified type NEC Q04.8
branchial cleft Q18.2
breast Q83.9
  specified type NEC Q83.8
broad ligament Q50.6
bronchus Q32.4
bursa Q79.9
cardiac
  chambers Q20.9
    specified type NEC Q20.8
  septum Q21.9
    specified type NEC Q21.8
cerebral Q04.9
  vessels Q28.3
cervix uteri Q51.9
  specified type NEC Q51.828
Chiari
  Type I G93.5
  Type II Q07.01
choroid (congenital) Q14.3
  plexus Q07.8
circulatory system Q28.9
cochlea Q16.5

Malformation (congenital) - *continued*
cornea Q13.4
coronary vessels Q24.5
corpus callosum (congenital) Q04.0
diaphragm Q79.1
digestive system NEC, specified type
  NEC Q45.8
dura Q07.9
  brain Q04.9
  spinal Q06.9
ear Q17.9
  causing impairment of hearing Q16.9
  external Q17.9
    accessory auricle Q17.0
    causing impairment of hearing Q16.9
      absence of
        auditory canal Q16.1
        auricle Q16.0
    macrotia Q17.1
    microtia Q17.2
    misplacement Q17.4
    misshapen NEC Q17.3
    prominence Q17.5
    specified type NEC Q17.8
  inner Q16.5
  middle Q16.4
    absence of eustachian tube Q16.2
    ossicles (fusion) Q16.3
  ossicles Q16.3
  specified type NEC Q17.8
epididymis Q55.4
esophagus Q39.9
  specified type NEC Q39.8
eye Q15.9
  lid Q10.3
  specified NEC Q15.8
fallopian tube Q50.6
genital organ — *see* Anomaly, genitalia
great
  artery Q25.9
    aorta — *see* Malformation, aorta
    pulmonary artery — *see* Malformation,
      pulmonary, artery
    specified type NEC Q25.8
  vein Q26.9
    anomalous
      portal venous connection Q26.5
      pulmonary venous connection Q26.4
        partial Q26.3
        total Q26.2
    persistent left superior vena cava Q26.1
    portal vein-hepatic artery fistula Q26.6
    specified type NEC Q26.8
    vena cava stenosis, congenital Q26.0
gum Q38.6
hair Q84.2
heart Q24.9
  specified type NEC Q24.8
integument Q84.9
  specified type NEC Q84.8
internal ear Q16.5
intestine Q43.9
  specified type NEC Q43.8
iris Q13.2
joint Q74.9
  ankle Q74.2
  lumbosacral Q76.49
  sacroiliac Q74.2
  specified type NEC Q74.8
kidney Q63.9
  accessory Q63.0
  giant Q63.3
  horseshoe Q63.1
  hydronephrosis Q62.0
  malposition Q63.2
  specified type NEC Q63.8
lacrimal apparatus Q10.6
lip Q38.0
lingual Q38.3
liver Q44.7
lung Q33.9
meninges or membrane (congenital) Q07.9
  cerebral Q04.8
  spinal (cord) Q06.9
middle ear Q16.4

Malformation (congenital) - *continued*
  middle ear - *continued*
    ossicles Q16.3
  mitral valve Q23.9
    specified NEC Q23.8
  Mondini's (congenital) (malformation, cochlea) Q16.5
  mouth (congenital) Q38.6
  multiple types NEC Q89.7
  musculoskeletal system Q79.9
  myocardium Q24.8
  nail Q84.6
  nervous system (central) Q07.9
  nose Q30.9
    specified type NEC Q30.8
  optic disc Q14.2
  orbit Q10.7
  ovary Q50.39
  palate Q38.5
  parathyroid gland Q89.2
  pelvic organs or tissues NEC
    in pregnancy or childbirth O34.8-
      causing obstructed labor O65.5
  penis Q55.69
    aplasia Q55.5
    curvature (lateral) Q55.61
    hypoplasia Q55.62
  pericardium Q24.8
  peripheral vascular system Q27.9
    specified type NEC Q27.8
  pharynx Q38.8
  precerebral vessels Q28.1
  prostate Q55.4
  pulmonary
    arteriovenous Q25.72
    artery Q25.9
      atresia Q25.5
      specified type NEC Q25.79
      stenosis Q25.6
    valve Q22.3
  renal artery Q27.2
  respiratory system Q34.9
  retina Q14.1
  scrotum — *see* Malformation, testis and scrotum
  seminal vesicles Q55.4
  sense organs NEC Q07.9
  skin Q82.9
  specified NEC Q89.8
  spinal
    cord Q06.9
    nerve root Q07.8
  spine Q76.49
    kyphosis — *see* Kyphosis, congenital
    lordosis — *see* Lordosis, congenital
  spleen Q89.09
  stomach Q40.3
    specified type NEC Q40.2
  teeth, tooth K00.9
  tendon Q79.9
  testis and scrotum Q55.20
    aplasia Q55.0
    hypoplasia Q55.1
    polyorchism Q55.21
    retractile testis Q55.22
    scrotal transposition Q55.23
    specified NEC Q55.29
  throat Q38.8
  thorax, bony Q76.9
  thyroid gland Q89.2
  tongue (congenital) Q38.3
    hypertrophy Q38.2
    tie Q38.1
  trachea Q32.1
  tricuspid valve Q22.9
    specified type NEC Q22.8
  umbilical cord NEC (complicating delivery) O69.89
  umbilicus Q89.9
  ureter Q62.8
    agenesis Q62.4
    duplication Q62.5
    malposition — *see* Malposition, congenital, ureter

Malformation (congenital) - *continued*
  ureter - *continued*
    obstructive defect — *see* Defect, obstructive, ureter
    vesico-uretero-renal reflux Q62.7
  urethra Q64.79
    aplasia Q64.5
    duplication Q64.74
    posterior valves Q64.2
    prolapse Q64.71
    stricture Q64.32
  urinary system Q64.9
  uterus Q51.9
    specified type NEC Q51.818
  vagina Q52.4
  vascular system, peripheral Q27.9
  vas deferens Q55.4
    atresia Q55.3
  venous — *see* Anomaly, vein(s)
  vulva Q52.70
Malfunction — *see also* Dysfunction
  cardiac electronic device T82.119
    electrode T82.110
    pulse generator T82.111
    specified type NEC T82.118
  catheter device NEC T85.618
    cystostomy T83.010
    dialysis (renal) (vascular) T82.41
      intraperitoneal T85.611
    infusion NEC T82.514
      cranial T85.610
      epidural T85.610
      intrathecal T85.610
      spinal T85.610
      subarachnoid T85.610
      subdural T85.610
    urinary — *see also* Breakdown, device, catheter T83.018
  colostomy K94.03
    valve K94.03
  cystostomy (stoma) N99.512
    catheter T83.010
  enteric stoma K94.13
  enterostomy K94.13
  esophagostomy K94.33
  gastroenteric K31.89
  gastrostomy K94.23
  ileostomy K94.13
    valve K94.13
  intrathecal infusion pump T85.615
  jejunostomy K94.13
  nervous system device, implant or graft, specified NEC T85.615
  pacemaker — *see* Malfunction, cardiac electronic device
  prosthetic device, internal — *see* Complications, prosthetic device, by site, mechanical
  tracheostomy J95.03
  urinary device NEC — *see* Complication, genitourinary, device, urinary, mechanical
  valve
    colostomy K94.03
    heart T82.09
    ileostomy K94.13
  vascular graft or shunt NEC — *see* Complication, cardiovascular device, mechanical, vascular
  ventricular (communicating shunt) T85.01
Malherbe's tumor — *see* Neoplasm, skin, benign
Malibu disease L98.8
Malignancy — *see also* Neoplasm, malignant, by site
  unspecified site (primary) C80.1
Malignant — *see* condition
Malingerer, malingering Z76.5
Mallet finger (acquired) — *see* Deformity, finger, mallet finger
  congenital Q74.0
  sequelae of rickets E64.3
Malleus A24.0
Mallory's bodies R89.7
Mallory-Weiss syndrome K22.6

Malnutrition E46
  degree
    first E44.1
    mild (protein) E44.1
    moderate (protein) E44.0
    second E44.0
    severe (protein-energy) E43
      intermediate form E42
        with
          kwashiorkor (and marasmus) E42
          marasmus E41
    third E43
  following gastrointestinal surgery K91.2
  intrauterine
    light-for-dates — *see* Light for dates
    small-for-dates — *see* Small for dates
  lack of care, or neglect (child) (infant) T76.02
    confirmed T74.02
  malignant E40
  protein E46
    calorie E46
      mild E44.1
      moderate E44.0
      severe E43
        intermediate form E42
          with
            kwashiorkor (and marasmus) E42
            marasmus E41
    energy E46
      mild E44.1
      moderate E44.0
      severe E43
        intermediate form E42
          with
            kwashiorkor (and marasmus) E42
            marasmus E41
  severe (protein-energy) E43
    with
      kwashiorkor (and marasmus) E42
      marasmus E41
Malocclusion (teeth) M26.4
  Angle's M26.219
    class I M26.211
    class II M26.212
    class III M26.213
  due to
    abnormal swallowing M26.59
    mouth breathing M26.59
    tongue, lip or finger habits M26.59
  temporomandibular (joint) M26.69
Malposition
  cervix — *see* Malposition, uterus
  congenital
    adrenal (gland) Q89.1
    alimentary tract Q45.8
      lower Q43.8
      upper Q40.8
    aorta Q25.49
    appendix Q43.8
    arterial trunk Q20.0
    artery (peripheral) Q27.8
      coronary Q24.5
      digestive system Q27.8
      lower limb Q27.8
      pulmonary Q25.79
      specified site NEC Q27.8
      upper limb Q27.8
    auditory canal Q17.8
      causing impairment of hearing Q16.9
    auricle (ear) Q17.4
      causing impairment of hearing Q16.9
      cervical Q18.2
    biliary duct or passage Q44.5
    bladder (mucosa) — *see* Exstrophy, bladder
    brachial plexus Q07.8
    brain tissue Q04.8
    breast Q83.8
    bronchus Q32.4
    cecum Q43.8
    clavicle Q74.0
    colon Q43.8
    digestive organ or tract NEC Q45.8
      lower Q43.8

Malposition - *continued*
  congenital - *continued*
    digestive organ or tract NEC - *continued*
      upper Q40.8
    ear (auricle) (external) Q17.4
      ossicles Q16.3
    endocrine (gland) NEC Q89.2
    epiglottis Q31.8
    eustachian tube Q17.8
    eye Q15.8
    facial features Q18.8
    fallopian tube Q50.6
    finger (s) Q68.1
      supernumerary Q69.0
    foot Q66.9-
    gallbladder Q44.1
    gastrointestinal tract Q45.8
    genitalia, genital organ (s) or tract
      female Q52.8
        external Q52.79
        internal NEC Q52.8
      male Q55.8
    glottis Q31.8
    hand Q68.1
    heart Q24.8
      dextrocardia Q24.0
        with complete transposition of
          viscera Q89.3
    hepatic duct Q44.5
    hip (joint) Q65.89
    intestine (large) (small) Q43.8
      with anomalous adhesions, fixation or
        malrotation Q43.3
    joint NEC Q68.8
    kidney Q63.2
    larynx Q31.8
    limb Q68.8
      lower Q68.8
      upper Q68.8
    liver Q44.7
    lung (lobe) Q33.8
    nail (s) Q84.6
    nerve Q07.8
    nervous system NEC Q07.8
    nose, nasal (septum) Q30.8
    organ or site not listed — *see* Anomaly, by
      site
    ovary Q50.39
    pancreas Q45.3
    parathyroid (gland) Q89.2
    patella Q74.1
    peripheral vascular system Q27.8
    pituitary (gland) Q89.2
    respiratory organ or system NEC Q34.8
    rib (cage) Q76.6
      supernumerary in cervical region Q76.5
    scapula Q74.0
    shoulder Q74.0
    spinal cord Q06.8
    spleen Q89.09
    sternum NEC Q76.7
    stomach Q40.2
    symphysis pubis Q74.2
    thymus (gland) Q89.2
    thyroid (gland) (tissue) Q89.2
      cartilage Q31.8
    toe (s) Q66.9-
      supernumerary Q69.2
    tongue Q38.3
    trachea Q32.1
    ureter Q62.60
      deviation Q62.61
      displacement Q62.62
      ectopia Q62.63
      specified type NEC Q62.69
    uterus Q51.818
    vein (s) (peripheral) Q27.8
      great Q26.8
    vena cava (inferior) (superior) Q26.8
  device, implant or graft — *see also*
    Complications, by site and type,
    mechanical T85.628
    arterial graft NEC — *see* Complication,
      cardiovascular device, mechanical,
      vascular

Malposition - *continued*
  device, implant or graft - *continued*
    breast (implant) T85.42
    catheter NEC T85.628
      cystostomy T83.020
      dialysis (renal) T82.42
        intraperitoneal T85.621
      infusion NEC T82.524
        spinal (epidural) (subdural) T85.620
      urinary — *see also* Displacement,
        device, catheter, urinary T83.028
    electronic (electrode) (pulse generator)
      (stimulator)
      bone T84.320
      cardiac T82.129
        electrode T82.120
        pulse generator T82.121
        specified type NEC T82.128
      nervous system — *see* Complication,
        prosthetic device, mechanical,
        electronic nervous system
        stimulator
      urinary — *see* Complication,
        genitourinary, device, urinary,
        mechanical
    fixation, internal (orthopedic) NEC — *see*
      Complication, fixation device,
      mechanical
    gastrointestinal — *see* Complications,
      prosthetic device, mechanical,
      gastrointestinal device
    genital NEC T83.428
      intrauterine contraceptive device
        (string) T83.32
      penile prosthesis (cylinder) (implanted)
        (pump) (resevoir) T83.420
      testicular prosthesis T83.421
    heart NEC — *see* Complication,
      cardiovascular device, mechanical
    joint prosthesis — *see* Complication, joint
      prosthesis, mechanical
    ocular NEC — *see* Complications,
      prosthetic device, mechanical, ocular
      device
    orthopedic NEC — *see* Complication,
      orthopedic, device, mechanical
    specified NEC T85.628
    urinary NEC — *see also* Complication,
      genitourinary, device, urinary,
      mechanical
      graft T83.22
    vascular NEC — *see* Complication,
      cardiovascular device, mechanical
    ventricular intracranial shunt T85.02
  fetus — *see* Pregnancy, complicated by
    (management affected by), presentation,
    fetal
  gallbladder K82.8
  gastrointestinal tract, congenital Q45.8
  heart, congenital NEC Q24.8
  joint prosthesis — *see* Complications, joint
    prosthesis, mechanical, displacement,
    by site
  stomach K31.89
    congenital Q40.2
  tooth, teeth, fully erupted M26.30
  uterus (acute) (acquired) (adherent)
    (asymptomatic) (postinfectional)
    (postpartal, old) N85.4
    anteflexion or anteversion N85.4
      congenital Q51.818
    flexion N85.4
      lateral — *see* Lateroversion, uterus
    inversion N85.5
    lateral (flexion) (version) — *see*
      Lateroversion, uterus
      in pregnancy or childbirth — *see*
        subcategory O34.5
    retroflexion or retroversion — *see*
      Retroversion, uterus

Malposture R29.3
Malrotation
  cecum Q43.3
  colon Q43.3
  intestine Q43.3

Malrotation - *continued*
  kidney Q63.2
Malta fever — *see* Brucellosis
Maltreatment
  adult
    abandonment
      confirmed T74.01
      suspected T76.01
    bullying
      confirmed T74.31
      suspected T76.31
    confirmed T74.91
    history of Z91.419
    intimidation (through social media)
      confirmed T74.31
      suspected T76.31
    neglect
      confirmed T74.01
      suspected T76.01
    physical abuse
      confirmed T74.11
      suspected T76.11
    psychological abuse
      confirmed T74.31
      suspected T76.31
      history of Z91.411
    sexual abuse
      confirmed T74.21
      suspected T76.21
    suspected T76.91
  child
    abandonment
      confirmed T74.02
      suspected T76.02
    bullying
      confirmed T74.32
      suspected T76.32
    confirmed T74.92
    history of — *see* History, personal (of),
      abuse
    intimidation (through social media)
      confirmed T74.32
      suspected T76.32
    neglect
      confirmed T74.02
      history of — *see* History, personal (of),
        abuse
      suspected T76.02
    physical abuse
      confirmed T74.12
      history of — *see* History, personal (of),
        abuse
      suspected T76.12
    psychological abuse
      confirmed T74.32
      history of — *see* History, personal (of),
        abuse
      suspected T76.32
    sexual abuse
      confirmed T74.22
      history of — *see* History, personal (of),
        abuse
      suspected T76.22
    suspected T76.92
  personal history of Z91.89
Maltworker's lung J67.4
Malunion, fracture — *see* Fracture, by site
Mammillitis N61.0
  puerperal, postpartum O91.02
Mammitis — *see* Mastitis
Mammogram (examination) Z12.39
  routine Z12.31
Mammoplasia N62
Management (of)
  bone conduction hearing device
    (implanted) Z45.320
  cardiac pacemaker NEC Z45.018
  cerebrospinal fluid drainage device Z45.41
  cochlear device (implanted) Z45.321
  contraceptive Z30.9
    specified NEC Z30.8
  implanted device Z45.9
    specified NEC Z45.89
  infusion pump Z45.1
  procreative Z31.9

Management (of) - *continued*
  procreative - *continued*
    male factor infertility in female Z31.81
     specified NEC Z31.89
    prosthesis (external) — *see also*
     Fitting Z44.9
     implanted Z45.9
      specified NEC Z45.89
    renal dialysis catheter Z49.01
    vascular access device Z45.2
Mangled — *see* specified injury by site
Mania (monopolar) — *see also* Disorder, mood, manic episode
  with psychotic symptoms F30.2
  without psychotic symptoms F30.10
   mild F30.11
   moderate F30.12
   severe F30.13
  Bell's F30.8
  chronic (recurrent) F31.89
  hysterical F44.89
  puerperal F30.8
  recurrent F31.89
Manic depression F31.9
Manic-depressive insanity, psychosis, or syndrome — *see* Disorder, bipolar
Mannosidosis E77.1
Mansonelliasis, mansonellosis B74.4
Manson's
  disease B65.1
  schistosomiasis B65.1
Manual — *see* condition
Maple-bark-stripper's lung (disease) J67.6
Maple-syrup-urine disease E71.0
Marable's syndrome (celiac artery compression) I77.4
Marasmus E41
  due to malnutrition E41
  intestinal E41
  nutritional E41
  senile R54
  tuberculous NEC — *see* Tuberculosis
Marble
  bones Q78.2
  skin R23.8
Marburg virus disease A98.3
March
  fracture — *see* Fracture, traumatic, stress, by site
  hemoglobinuria D59.6
Marchesani (-Weill) syndrome Q87.0
Marchiafava (-Bignami) syndrome or disease G37.1
Marchiafava-Micheli syndrome D59.5
Marcus Gunn's syndrome Q07.8
Marfan's syndrome — *see* Syndrome, Marfan's
Marie-Bamberger disease — *see* Osteoarthropathy, hypertrophic, specified NEC
Marie-Charcot-Tooth neuropathic muscular atrophy G60.0
Marie's
  cerebellar ataxia (late-onset) G11.2
  disease or syndrome (acromegaly) E22.0
Marie-Strümpell arthritis, disease or spondylitis — *see* Spondylitis, ankylosing
Marion's disease (bladder neck obstruction) N32.0
Marital conflict Z63.0
Mark
  port wine Q82.5
  raspberry Q82.5
  strawberry Q82.5
  stretch L90.6
  tattoo L81.8
Marker heterochromatin — *see* Extra, marker chromosomes
Maroteaux-Lamy syndrome (mild) (severe) E76.29
Marrow (bone)
  arrest D61.9
  poor function D75.89
Marseilles fever A77.1
Marsh fever — *see* Malaria

Marshall's (hidrotic) ectodermal dysplasia Q82.4
Marsh's disease (exophthalmic goiter) E05.00
  with storm E05.01
Masculinization (female) with adrenal hyperplasia E25.9
  congenital E25.0
Masculinovoblastoma D27.-
Masochism (sexual) F65.51
Mason's lung J62.8
Mass
  abdominal R19.00
   epigastric R19.06
   generalized R19.07
   left lower quadrant R19.04
   left upper quadrant R19.02
   periumbilic R19.05
   right lower quadrant R19.03
   right upper quadrant R19.01
   specified site NEC R19.09
  breast — *see also* Lump, breast N63.0
  chest R22.2
  cystic — *see* Cyst
  ear H93.8-
  head R22.0
  intra-abdominal (diffuse) (generalized) — *see* Mass, abdominal
  kidney N28.89
  liver R16.0
  localized (skin) R22.9
   chest R22.2
   head R22.0
   limb
    lower R22.4-
    upper R22.3-
   neck R22.1
   trunk R22.2
  lung R91.8
  malignant — *see* Neoplasm, malignant, by site
  neck R22.1
  pelvic (diffuse) (generalized) — *see* Mass, abdominal
  specified organ NEC — *see* Disease, by site
  splenic R16.1
  substernal thyroid — *see* Goiter
  superficial (localized) R22.9
  umbilical (diffuse) (generalized) R19.09
Massive — *see* condition
Mast cell
  disease, systemic tissue D47.02
  leukemia C94.3-
  neoplasm
   malignant C96.20
    specified type NEC C96.29
   of uncertain behavior NEC D47.09
  sarcoma C96.22
  tumor D47.09
Mastalgia N64.4
Masters-Allen syndrome N83.8
Mastitis (acute) (diffuse) (nonpuerperal) (subacute) N61.0
  with abscess N61.1
  chronic (cystic) — *see* Mastopathy, cystic
  cystic (Schimmelbusch's type) — *see* Mastopathy, cystic
  fibrocystic — *see* Mastopathy, cystic
  infective N61.0
   newborn P39.0
  interstitial, gestational or puerperal — *see* Mastitis, obstetric
  neonatal (noninfective) P83.4
   infective P39.0
  obstetric (interstitial) (nonpurulent)
   associated with
    lactation O91.23
    pregnancy O91.21-
    puerperium O91.22
   purulent
    associated with
     lactation O91.13
     pregnancy O91.11-
     puerperium O91.12
  periductal — *see* Ectasia, mammary duct

Mastitis (acute) (diffuse) (nonpuerperal) (subacute) - *continued*
  phlegmonous — *see* Mastopathy, cystic
  plasma cell — *see* Ectasia, mammary duct without abscess N61.0
Mastocytoma (extracutaneous) D47.09
  malignant C96.29
  solitary D47.01
Mastocytosis D47.09
  aggressive systemic C96.21
  cutaneous (diffuse) (maculopapular) D47.01
   congenital Q82.2
   of neonatal onset Q82.2
   of newborn onset Q82.2
  indolent systemic D47.02
  isolated bone marrow D47.02
  malignant C96.29
  systemic (indolent) (smoldering)
   with an associated hematological non-mast cell lineage disease (SM-AHNMD) D47.02
Mastodynia N64.4
Mastoid — *see* condition
Mastoidalgia — *see* subcategory H92.0
Mastoiditis (coalescent) (hemorrhagic) (suppurative) H70.9-
  acute, subacute H70.00-
   complicated NEC H70.09-
   subperiosteal H70.01-
  chronic (necrotic) (recurrent) H70.1-
  in (due to)
   infectious disease NEC B99 *[H75.0-]*
   parasitic disease NEC B89 *[H75.0-]*
   tuberculosis A18.03
  petrositis — *see* Petrositis
  postauricular fistula — *see* Fistula, postauricular
  specified NEC H70.89-
  tuberculous A18.03
Mastopathy, mastopathia N64.9
  chronica cystica — *see* Mastopathy, cystic
  cystic (chronic) (diffuse) N60.1-
   with epithelial proliferation N60.3-
  diffuse cystic — *see* Mastopathy, cystic
  estrogenic, oestrogenica N64.89
  ovarian origin N64.89
Mastoplasia, mastoplastia N62
Masturbation (excessive) F98.8
Maternal care (for) — *see* Pregnancy (complicated by) (management affected by)
Matheiu's disease (leptospiral jaundice) A27.0
Mauclaire's disease or osteochondrosis — *see* Osteochondrosis, juvenile, hand, metacarpal
Maxcy's disease A75.2
Maxilla, maxillary — *see* condition
May (-Hegglin) anomaly or syndrome D72.0
McArdle (-Schmid) (-Pearson) disease (glycogen storage) E74.04
McCune-Albright syndrome Q78.1
McQuarrie's syndrome (idiopathic familial hypoglycemia) E16.2
Meadow's syndrome Q86.1
Measles (black) (hemorrhagic) (suppressed) B05.9
  with
   complications NEC B05.89
   encephalitis B05.0
   intestinal complications B05.4
   keratitis (keratoconjunctivitis) B05.81
   meningitis B05.1
   otitis media B05.3
   pneumonia B05.2
  French — *see* Rubella
  German — *see* Rubella
  Liberty — *see* Rubella
Meatitis, urethral — *see* Urethritis
Meatus, meatal — *see* condition
Meat-wrappers' asthma J68.9
Meckel-Gruber syndrome Q61.9

Meckel's diverticulitis, diverticulum
(displaced) (hypertrophic) Q43.0
malignant — *see* Table of Neoplasms, small
intestine, malignant
Meconium
ileus, newborn P76.0
in cystic fibrosis E84.11
meaning meconium plug (without cystic
fibrosis) P76.0
obstruction, newborn P76.0
due to fecaliths P76.0
in mucoviscidosis E84.11
peritonitis P78.0
plug syndrome (newborn) NEC P76.0
Median — *see also* condition
arcuate ligament syndrome I77.4
bar (prostate) (vesical orifice) — *see*
Hyperplasia, prostate
rhomboid glossitis K14.2
Mediastinal shift R93.89
Mediastinitis (acute) (chronic) J98.51
syphilitic A52.73
tuberculous A15.8
Mediastinopericarditis — *see also*
Pericarditis
acute I30.9
adhesive I31.0
chronic I31.8
rheumatic I09.2
Mediastinum, mediastinal — *see* condition
Medicine poisoning — *see* Table of Drugs and
Chemicals, by drug, poisoning
Mediterranean
fever — *see* Brucellosis
familial M04.1
tick A77.1
kala-azar B55.0
leishmaniasis B55.0
tick fever A77.1
Medulla — *see* condition
Medullary cystic kidney Q61.5
Medullated fibers
optic (nerve) Q14.8
retina Q14.1
Medulloblastoma
desmoplastic C71.6
specified site — *see* Neoplasm, malignant,
by site
unspecified site C71.6
Medulloepithelioma — *see also* Neoplasm,
malignant, by site
teratoid — *see* Neoplasm, malignant, by site
Medullomyoblastoma
specified site — *see* Neoplasm, malignant,
by site
unspecified site C71.6
Meekeren-Ehlers-Danlos syndrome — *see*
also Syndrome, Ehlers-Danlos Q79.69
Megacolon (acquired) (functional) (not
Hirschsprung's disease) (in) K59.39
Chagas' disease B57.32
congenital, congenitum (aganglionic) Q43.1
Hirschsprung's (disease) Q43.1
toxic NEC K59.31
due to Clostridium difficile
not specified as recurrent A04.72
recurrent A04.71
Megaesophagus (functional) K22.0
congenital Q39.5
in (due to) Chagas' disease B57.31
Megalencephaly Q04.5
Megalerythema (epidemic) B08.3
Megaloappendix Q43.8
Megalocephalus, megalocephaly NEC Q75.3
Megalocornea Q15.8
with glaucoma Q15.0
Megalocytic anemia D53.1
Megalodactylia (fingers) (thumbs)
(congenital) Q74.0
toes Q74.2
Megaloduodenum Q43.8
Megaloesophagus (functional) K22.0
congenital Q39.5
Megalogastria (acquired) K31.89
congenital Q40.2

Megalophthalmos Q11.3
Megalopsia H53.15
Megalosplenia — *see* Splenomegaly
Megaloureter N28.82
congenital Q62.2
Megarectum K62.89
Megasigmoid K59.39
congenital Q43.2
Megaureter N28.82
congenital Q62.2
Megavitamin-B6 syndrome E67.2
Megrim — *see* Migraine
Meibomian
cyst, infected — *see* Hordeolum
gland — *see* condition
sty, stye — *see* Hordeolum
Meibomitis — *see* Hordeolum
Meige-Milroy disease (chronic hereditary
edema) Q82.0
Meige's syndrome Q82.0
Melalgia, nutritional E53.8
Melancholia F32.9
climacteric (single episode) F32.89
recurrent episode F33.8
hypochondriac F45.29
intermittent (single episode) F32.89
recurrent episode F33.8
involutional (single episode) F32.89
recurrent episode F33.8
menopausal (single episode) F32.89
recurrent episode F33.8
puerperal F32.89
reactive (emotional stress or trauma) F32.3
recurrent F33.9
senile F03
stuporous (single episode) F32.89
recurrent episode F33.8
Melanemia R79.89
Melanoameloblastoma — *see* Neoplasm,
bone, benign
Melanoblastoma — *see* Melanoma
Melanocarcinoma — *see* Melanoma
Melanocytoma, eyeball D31.9-
Melanocytosis, neurocutaneous Q82.8
Melanoderma, melanodermia L81.4
Melanodontia, infantile K03.89
Melanodontoclasia K03.89
Melanoepithelioma — *see* Melanoma
Melanoma (malignant) C43.9
acral lentiginous, malignant — *see*
Melanoma, skin, by site
amelanotic — *see* Melanoma, skin, by site
balloon cell — *see* Melanoma, skin, by site
benign — *see* Nevus
desmoplastic, malignant — *see* Melanoma,
skin, by site
epithelioid cell — *see* Melanoma, skin, by
site
with spindle cell, mixed — *see* Melanoma,
skin, by site
in
giant pigmented nevus — *see* Melanoma,
skin, by site
Hutchinson's melanotic freckle — *see*
Melanoma, skin, by site
junctional nevus — *see* Melanoma, skin,
by site
precancerous melanosis — *see* Melanoma,
skin, by site
in situ D03.9
abdominal wall D03.59
ala nasi D03.39
ankle D03.7-
anus, anal (margin) (skin) D03.51
arm D03.6-
auditory canal D03.2-
auricle (ear) D03.2-
auricular canal (external) D03.2-
axilla, axillary fold D03.59
back D03.59
breast D03.52
brow D03.39
buttock D03.59
canthus (eye) D03.1-
cheek (external) D03.39

Melanoma (malignant) - *continued*
in situ - *continued*
chest wall D03.59
chin D03.39
choroid D03.8
conjunctiva D03.8
ear (external) D03.2-
external meatus (ear) D03.2-
eye D03.8
eyebrow D03.39
eyelid (lower) (upper) D03.1-
face D03.30
specified NEC D03.39
female genital organ (external) NEC D03.8
finger D03.6-
flank D03.59
foot D03.7-
forearm D03.6-
forehead D03.39
foreskin D03.8
gluteal region D03.59
groin D03.59
hand D03.6-
heel D03.7-
helix D03.2-
hip D03.7-
interscapular region D03.59
iris D03.8
jaw D03.39
knee D03.7-
labium (majus) (minus) D03.8
lacrimal gland D03.8
leg D03.7-
lip (lower) (upper) D03.0
lower limb NEC D03.7-
male genital organ (external) NEC D03.8
nail D03.9
finger D03.6-
toe D03.7-
neck D03.4
nose (external) D03.39
orbit D03.8
penis D03.8
perianal skin D03.51
perineum D03.51
pinna D03.2-
popliteal fossa or space D03.7-
prepuce D03.8
pudendum D03.8
retina D03.8
retrobulbar D03.8
scalp D03.4
scrotum D03.8
shoulder D03.6-
specified site NEC D03.8
submammary fold D03.52
temple D03.39
thigh D03.7-
toe D03.7-
trunk NEC D03.59
umbilicus D03.59
upper limb NEC D03.6-
vulva D03.8
juvenile — *see* Nevus
malignant, of soft parts except skin — *see*
Neoplasm, connective tissue, malignant
metastatic
breast C79.81
genital organ C79.82
specified site NEC C79.89
neurotropic, malignant — *see* Melanoma,
skin, by site
nodular — *see* Melanoma, skin, by site
regressing, malignant — *see* Melanoma,
skin, by site
skin C43.9
abdominal wall C43.59
ala nasi C43.31
ankle C43.7-
anus, anal (skin) C43.51
arm C43.6-
auditory canal (external) C43.2-
auricle (ear) C43.2-
auricular canal (external) C43.2-
axilla, axillary fold C43.59

Melanoma (malignant) - *continued*
skin - *continued*
  back C43.59
  breast (female) (male) C43.52
  brow C43.39
  buttock C43.59
  canthus (eye) C43.1-
  cheek (external) C43.39
  chest wall C43.59
  chin C43.39
  ear (external) C43.2-
  elbow C43.6-
  external meatus (ear) C43.2-
  eyebrow C43.39
  eyelid (lower) (upper) C43.1-
  face C43.30
    specified NEC C43.39
  female genital organ (external) NEC C51.9
  finger C43.6-
  flank C43.59
  foot C43.7-
  forearm C43.6-
  forehead C43.39
  foreskin C60.0
  glabella C43.39
  gluteal region C43.59
  groin C43.59
  hand C43.6-
  heel C43.7-
  helix C43.2-
  hip C43.7-
  interscapular region C43.59
  jaw (external) C43.39
  knee C43.7-
  labium C51.9
    majus C51.0
    minus C51.1
  leg C43.7-
  lip (lower) (upper) C43.0
  lower limb NEC C43.7-
  male genital organ (external) NEC C63.9
  nail
    finger C43.6-
    toe C43.7-
  nasolabial groove C43.39
  nates C43.59
  neck C43.4
  nose (external) C43.31
  overlapping site C43.8
  palpebra C43.1-
  penis C60.9
  perianal skin C43.51
  perineum C43.51
  pinna C43.2-
  popliteal fossa or space C43.7-
  prepuce C60.0
  pudendum C51.9
  scalp C43.4
  scrotum C63.2
  shoulder C43.6-
  skin NEC C43.9
  submammary fold C43.52
  temple C43.39
  thigh C43.7-
  toe C43.7-
  trunk NEC C43.59
  umbilicus C43.59
  upper limb NEC C43.6-
  vulva C51.9
    overlapping sites C51.8
spindle cell
  with epithelioid, mixed — *see* Melanoma, skin, by site
  type A C69.4-
  type B C69.4-
superficial spreading — *see* Melanoma, skin, by site
Melanosarcoma — *see also* Melanoma
epithelioid cell — *see* Melanoma
Melanosis L81.4
addisonian E27.1
  tuberculous A18.7
adrenal E27.1
colon K63.89
conjunctiva — *see* Pigmentation, conjunctiva

Melanosis - *continued*
conjunctiva - *continued*
  congenital Q13.89
cornea (presenile) (senile) — *see also* Pigmentation, cornea
  congenital Q13.4
eye NEC H57.89
  congenital Q15.8
lenticularis progressiva Q82.1
liver K76.89
precancerous — *see also* Melanoma, in situ
  malignant melanoma in — *see* Melanoma
Riehl's L81.4
sclera H15.89
  congenital Q13.89
suprarenal E27.1
tar L81.4
toxic L81.4
Melanuria R82.998
MELAS syndrome E88.41
Melasma L81.1
adrenal (gland) E27.1
suprarenal (gland) E27.1
Melena K92.1
with ulcer - code by site under Ulcer, with hemorrhage K27.4
due to swallowed maternal blood P78.2
newborn, neonatal P54.1
  due to swallowed maternal blood P78.2
Meleney's
gangrene (cutaneous) — *see* Ulcer, skin
ulcer (chronic undermining) — *see* Ulcer, skin
Melioidosis A24.9
acute A24.1
chronic A24.2
fulminating A24.1
pneumonia A24.1
pulmonary (chronic) A24.2
  acute A24.1
  subacute A24.2
sepsis A24.1
specified NEC A24.3
subacute A24.2
Melitensis, febris A23.0
Melkersson (-Rosenthal) syndrome G51.2
Mellitus, diabetes — *see* Diabetes
Melorheostosis (bone) — *see* Disorder, bone, density and structure, specified NEC
Meloschisis Q18.4
Melotia Q17.4
Membrana
capsularis lentis posterior Q13.89
epipapillaris Q14.2
Membranacea placenta O43.19-
Membranaceous uterus N85.8
Membrane (s) , membranous — *see also* condition
cyclitic — *see* Membrane, pupillary
folds, congenital — *see* Web
Jackson's Q43.3
over face of newborn P28.9
premature rupture — *see* Rupture, membranes, premature
pupillary H21.4-
  persistent Q13.89
retained (with hemorrhage) (complicating delivery) O72.2
  without hemorrhage O73.1
secondary cataract — *see* Cataract, secondary
unruptured (causing asphyxia) — *see* Asphyxia, newborn
vitreous — *see* Opacity, vitreous, membranes and strands
Membranitis — *see* Chorioamnionitis
Memory disturbance, lack or loss — *see also* Amnesia
mild, following organic brain damage F06.8
Menadione deficiency E56.1
Menarche
delayed E30.0
precocious E30.1
Mendacity, pathologic F60.2

Mendelson's syndrome (due to anesthesia) J95.4
in labor and delivery O74.0
in pregnancy O29.01-
obstetric O74.0
postpartum, puerperal O89.01
Ménétrier's disease or syndrome K29.60
with bleeding K29.61
Ménière's disease, syndrome or vertigo H81.0-
Meninges, meningeal — *see* condition
Meningioma — *see also* Neoplasm, meninges, benign
angioblastic — *see* Neoplasm, meninges, benign
angiomatous — *see* Neoplasm, meninges, benign
endotheliomatous — *see* Neoplasm, meninges, benign
fibroblastic — *see* Neoplasm, meninges, benign
fibrous — *see* Neoplasm, meninges, benign
hemangioblastic — *see* Neoplasm, meninges, benign
hemangiopericytic — *see* Neoplasm, meninges, benign
malignant — *see* Neoplasm, meninges, malignant
meningiothelial — *see* Neoplasm, meninges, benign
meningotheliomatous — *see* Neoplasm, meninges, benign
mixed — *see* Neoplasm, meninges, benign
multiple — *see* Neoplasm, meninges, uncertain behavior
papillary — *see* Neoplasm, meninges, uncertain behavior
psammomatous — *see* Neoplasm, meninges, benign
syncytial — *see* Neoplasm, meninges, benign
transitional — *see* Neoplasm, meninges, benign
Meningiomatosis (diffuse) — *see* Neoplasm, meninges, uncertain behavior
Meningism — *see* Meningismus
Meningismus (infectional) (pneumococcal) R29.1
due to serum or vaccine R29.1
influenzal — *see* Influenza, with, manifestations NEC
Meningitis (basal) (basic) (brain) (cerebral) (cervical) (congestive) (diffuse) (hemorrhagic) (infantile) (membranous) (metastatic) (nonspecific) (pontine) (progressive) (simple) (spinal) (subacute) (sympathetic) (toxic) G03.9
abacterial G03.0
actinomycotic A42.81
adenoviral A87.1
arbovirus A87.8
aseptic (acute) G03.0
bacterial G00.9
  Escherichia coli (E. coli) G00.8
  Friedländer (bacillus) G00.8
  gram-negative G00.9
  H. influenzae G00.0
  Klebsiella G00.8
  pneumococcal G00.1
  specified organism NEC G00.8
  staphylococcal G00.3
  streptococcal (acute) G00.2
benign recurrent (Mollaret) G03.2
candidal B37.5
caseous (tuberculous) A17.0
cerebrospinal A39.0
chronic NEC G03.1
clear cerebrospinal fluid NEC G03.0
coxsackievirus A87.0
cryptococcal B45.1
diplococcal (gram positive) A39.0
echovirus A87.0
enteroviral A87.0
eosinophilic B83.2
epidemic NEC A39.0
Escherichia coli (E. coli) G00.8

Meningitis (basal) (basic) (brain) (cerebral) (cervical) (congestive) (diffuse) (hemorrhagic) (infantile) (membranous) (metastatic) (nonspecific) (pontine) (progressive) (simple) (spinal) (subacute) (sympathetic) (toxic) - *continued*
  fibrinopurulent G00.9
    specified organism NEC G00.8
  Friedländer (bacillus) G00.8
  gonococcal A54.81
  gram-negative cocci G00.9
  gram-positive cocci G00.9
  Haemophilus (influenzae) G00.0
  H. influenzae G00.0
  in (due to)
    adenovirus A87.1
    African trypanosomiasis B56.9 *[G02]*
    anthrax A22.8
    bacterial disease NEC A48.8 *[G01]*
    Chagas' disease (chronic) B57.41
    chickenpox B01.0
    coccidioidomycosis B38.4
    Diplococcus pneumoniae G00.1
    enterovirus A87.0
    herpes (simplex) virus B00.3
      zoster B02.1
    infectious mononucleosis B27.92
    leptospirosis A27.81
    Listeria monocytogenes A32.11
    Lyme disease A69.21
    measles B05.1
    mumps (virus) B26.1
    neurosyphilis (late) A52.13
    parasitic disease NEC B89 *[G02]*
    poliovirus A80.9 *[G02]*
    preventive immunization, inoculation or vaccination G03.8
    rubella B06.02
    Salmonella infection A02.21
    specified cause NEC G03.8
    Streptococcal pneumoniae G00.1
    typhoid fever A01.01
    varicella B01.0
    viral disease NEC A87.8
    whooping cough A37.90
    zoster B02.1
  infectious G00.9
  influenzal (H. influenzae) G00.0
  Klebsiella G00.8
  leptospiral (aseptic) A27.81
  lymphocytic (acute) (benign) (serous) A87.2
  meningococcal A39.0
  Mima polymorpha G00.8
  Mollaret (benign recurrent) G03.2
  monilial B37.5
  mycotic NEC B49 *[G02]*
  Neisseria A39.0
  nonbacterial G03.0
  nonpyogenic NEC G03.0
  ossificans G96.19
  pneumococcal streptococcus pneumoniae G00.1
  poliovirus A80.9 *[G02]*
  postmeasles B05.1
  purulent G00.9
    specified organism NEC G00.8
  pyogenic G00.9
    specified organism NEC G00.8
  Salmonella (arizonae) (Cholerae-Suis) (enteritidis) (typhimurium) A02.21
  septic G00.9
    specified organism NEC G00.8
  serosa circumscripta NEC G03.0
  serous NEC G93.2
  specified organism NEC G00.8
  sporotrichosis B42.81
  staphylococcal G00.3
  sterile G03.0
  Streptococcal (acute) G00.2
    pneumoniae G00.1
  suppurative G00.9
    specified organism NEC G00.8
  syphilitic (late) (tertiary) A52.13
    acute A51.41
    congenital A50.41

Meningitis (basal) (basic) (brain) (cerebral) (cervical) (congestive) (diffuse) (hemorrhagic) (infantile) (membranous) (metastatic) (nonspecific) (pontine) (progressive) (simple) (spinal) (subacute) (sympathetic) (toxic) - *continued*
  syphilitic (late) (tertiary) - *continued*
    secondary A51.41
  Torula histolytica (cryptococcal) B45.1
  traumatic (complication of injury) T79.8
  tuberculous A17.0
  typhoid A01.01
  viral NEC A87.9
  Yersinia pestis A20.3
Meningocele (spinal) — *see also* Spina bifida
  with hydrocephalus — *see* Spina bifida, by site, with hydrocephalus
  acquired (traumatic) G96.19
  cerebral — *see* Encephalocele
Meningocerebritis — *see* Meningoencephalitis
Meningococcemia A39.4
  acute A39.2
  chronic A39.3
Meningococcus, meningococcal — *see also* condition A39.9
  adrenalitis, hemorrhagic A39.1
  carrier (suspected) of Z22.31
  meningitis (cerebrospinal) A39.0
Meningoencephalitis — *see also* Encephalitis G04.90
  acute NEC — *see also* Encephalitis, viral A86
  bacterial NEC G04.2
  California A83.5
  diphasic A84.1
  eosinophilic B83.2
  epidemic A39.81
  herpesviral, herpetic B00.4
    due to herpesvirus 6 B10.01
    due to herpesvirus 7 B10.09
    specified NEC B10.09
  in (due to)
    blastomycosis NEC B40.81
    diseases classified elsewhere G05.3
    free-living amebae B60.2
    Hemophilus influenzae (H .influenzae) G00.0
    herpes B00.4
      due to herpesvirus 6 B10.01
      due to herpesvirus 7 B10.09
      specified NEC B10.09
    H. influenzae G00.0
    Lyme disease A69.22
    mercury — *see* subcategory T56.1
    mumps B26.2
    Naegleria (amebae) (organisms) (fowleri) B60.2
    Parastrongylus cantonensis B83.2
    toxoplasmosis (acquired) B58.2
      congenital P37.1
  infectious (acute) (viral) A86
  influenzal (H. influenzae) G00.0
  Listeria monocytogenes A32.12
  lymphocytic (serous) A87.2
  mumps B26.2
  parasitic NEC B89 *[G05.3]*
  pneumococcal G04.2
  primary ambeic B60.2
  specific (syphilitic) A52.14
  specified organism NEC G04.81
  staphylococcal G04.2
  streptococcal G04.2
  syphilitic A52.14
  toxic NEC G92
    due to mercury — *see* subcategory T56.1
  tuberculous A17.82
  virus NEC A86
Meningoencephalocele — *see also* Encephalocele
  syphilitic A52.19
    congenital A50.49
Meningoencephalomyelitis — *see also* Meningoencephalitis
  acute NEC (viral) A86

Meningoencephalomyelitis - *continued*
  acute NEC (viral) - *continued*
    disseminated G04.00
      postimmunization or postvaccination G04.02
      postinfectious G04.01
  due to
    actinomycosis A42.82
    Torula B45.1
    Toxoplasma or toxoplasmosis (acquired) B58.2
      congenital P37.1
  postimmunization or postvaccination G04.02
Meningoencephalomyelopathy G96.9
Meningoencephalopathy G96.9
Meningomyelitis — *see also* Meningoencephalitis
  bacterial NEC G04.2
  blastomycotic NEC B40.81
  cryptococcal B45.1
  in diseases classified elsewhere G05.4
  meningococcal A39.81
  syphilitic A52.14
  tuberculous A17.82
Meningomyelocele — *see also* Spina bifida
  syphilitic A52.19
Meningomyeloneuritis — *see* Meningoencephalitis
Meningoradiculitis — *see* Meningitis
Meningovascular — *see* condition
Menkes' disease or syndrome E83.09
  meaning maple-syrup-urine disease E71.0
Menometrorrhagia N92.1
Menopause, menopausal (asymptomatic) (state) Z78.0
  arthritis (any site) NEC — *see* Arthritis, specified form NEC
  bleeding N92.4
  depression (single episode) F32.89
    agitated (single episode) F32.2
      recurrent episode F33.9
    psychotic (single episode) F32.89
      recurrent episode F33.9
    recurrent episode F33.8
  melancholia (single episode) F32.89
    recurrent episode F33.8
  paranoid state F22
  premature E28.319
    asymptomatic E28.319
      postirradiation E89.40
      postsurgical E89.40
    symptomatic E28.310
      postirradiation E89.41
      postsurgical E89.41
  psychosis NEC F28
  symptomatic N95.1
  toxic polyarthritis NEC — *see* Arthritis, specified form NEC
Menorrhagia (primary) N92.0
  climacteric N92.4
    menopausal N92.4
  menopausal N92.4
  perimenopausal N92.4
  postclimacteric N95.0
  postmenopausal N95.0
  preclimacteric or premenopausal N92.4
  pubertal (menses retained) N92.2
Menostaxis N92.0
Menses, retention N94.89
Menstrual — *see* Menstruation
Menstruation
  absent — *see* Amenorrhea
  anovulatory N97.0
  cycle, irregular N92.6
  delayed N91.0
  disorder N93.9
    psychogenic F45.8
  during pregnancy O20.8
  excessive (with regular cycle) N92.0
    with irregular cycle N92.1
    at puberty N92.2
  frequent N92.0
  infrequent — *see* Oligomenorrhea
  irregular N92.6
    specified NEC N92.5

Menstruation - *continued*
  latent N92.5
  membranous N92.5
  painful — *see also* Dysmenorrhea N94.6
    primary N94.4
    psychogenic F45.8
    secondary N94.5
  passage of clots N92.0
  precocious E30.1
  protracted N92.5
  rare — *see* Oligomenorrhea
  retained N94.89
  retrograde N92.5
  scanty — *see* Oligomenorrhea
  suppression N94.89
  vicarious (nasal) N94.89
Mental — *see also* condition
  deficiency — *see* Disability, intellectual
  deterioration — *see* Psychosis
  disorder — *see* Disorder, mental
  exhaustion F48.8
  insufficiency (congenital) — *see* Disability,
    intellectual
  observation without need for further medical
    care Z03.89
  retardation — *see* Disability, intellectual
  subnormality — *see* Disability, intellectuall
  upset — *see* Disorder, mental
Meralgia paresthetica G57.1-
Mercurial — *see* condition
Mercurialism — *see* subcategory T56.1
Merkel cell tumor — *see* Carcinoma, Merkel
    cell
Merocele — *see* Hernia, femoral
Meromelia
  lower limb — *see* Defect, reduction, lower
    limb
  intercalary
    femur — *see* Defect, reduction, lower
      limb, specified type NEC
    tibiofibular (complete)
      (incomplete) — *see* Defect,
      reduction, lower limb
  upper limb — *see* Defect, reduction, upper
    limb
    intercalary, humeral, radioulnar — *see*
      Agenesis, arm, with hand present
**MERRF syndrome (myoclonic epilepsy
    associated with ragged-red
    fiber)** E88.42
Merzbacher-Pelizaeus disease E75.29
Mesaortitis — *see* Aortitis
Mesarteritis — *see* Arteritis
Mesencephalitis — *see* Encephalitis
Mesenchymoma — *see also* Neoplasm,
    connective tissue, uncertain behavior
  benign — *see* Neoplasm, connective tissue,
    benign
  malignant — *see* Neoplasm, connective
    tissue, malignant
Mesenteritis
  retractile K65.4
  sclerosing K65.4
Mesentery, mesenteric — *see* condition
Mesiodens, mesiodentes K00.1
Mesio-occlusion M26.213
Mesocolon — *see* condition
Mesonephroma (malignant) — *see*
    Neoplasm, malignant, by site
  benign — *see* Neoplasm, benign, by site
Mesophlebitis — *see* Phlebitis
Mesostromal dysgenesia Q13.89
Mesothelioma (malignant) C45.9
  benign
    mesentery D19.1
    mesocolon D19.1
    omentum D19.1
    peritoneum D19.1
    pleura D19.0
    specified site NEC D19.7
    unspecified site D19.9
  biphasic C45.9
    benign
      mesentery D19.1
      mesocolon D19.1

Mesothelioma (malignant) - *continued*
  biphasic - *continued*
    benign - *continued*
      omentum D19.1
      peritoneum D19.1
      pleura D19.0
      specified site NEC D19.7
      unspecified site D19.9
  cystic D48.4
  epithelioid C45.9
    benign
      mesentery D19.1
      mesocolon D19.1
      omentum D19.1
      peritoneum D19.1
      pleura D19.0
      specified site NEC D19.7
      unspecified site D19.9
  fibrous C45.9
    benign
      mesentery D19.1
      mesocolon D19.1
      omentum D19.1
      peritoneum D19.1
      pleura D19.0
      specified site NEC D19.7
      unspecified site D19.9
  site classification
    liver C45.7
    lung C45.7
    mediastinum C45.7
    mesentery C45.1
    mesocolon C45.1
    omentum C45.1
    pericardium C45.2
    peritoneum C45.1
    pleura C45.0
      parietal C45.0
    retroperitoneum C45.7
    specified site NEC C45.7
    unspecified C45.9
Metabolic syndrome E88.81
Metagonimiasis B66.8
Metagonimus infestation (intestine) B66.8
Metal
  pigmentation L81.8
  polisher's disease J62.8
Metamorphopsia H53.15
Metaplasia
  apocrine (breast) — *see* Dysplasia,
    mammary, specified type NEC
  cervix (squamous) — *see* Dysplasia, cervix
  endometrium (squamous) (uterus) N85.8
  esophagus K22.7-
  kidney (pelvis) (squamous) N28.89
  myelogenous D73.1
  myeloid (agnogenic)
    (megakaryocytic) D73.1
  spleen D73.1
  squamous cell, bladder N32.89
Metastasis, metastatic
  abscess — *see* Abscess
  calcification E83.59
  cancer
    from specified site — *see* Neoplasm,
      malignant, by site
    to specified site — *see* Neoplasm,
      secondary, by site
  deposits (in) — *see* Neoplasm, secondary, by
    site
  disease — *see also* Neoplasm, secondary, by
    site C79.9
  spread (to) — *see* Neoplasm, secondary, by
    site
Metastrongyliasis B83.8
Metatarsalgia M77.4-
  anterior G57.6-
  Morton's G57.6-
Metatarsus, metatarsal — *see also* condition
  adductus, congenital Q66.22-
  valgus (abductus) , congenital Q66.6
  varus (congenital) Q66.22-
    primus Q66.21-
Methadone use — *see* Use, opioid

Methemoglobinemia D74.9
  acquired (with sulfhemoglobinemia) D74.8
  congenital D74.0
  enzymatic (congenital) D74.0
  Hb M disease D74.0
  hereditary D74.0
  toxic D74.8
Methemoglobinuria — *see* Hemoglobinuria
Methioninemia E72.19
Methylmalonic acidemia E71.120
**Metritis (catarrhal) (hemorrhagic) (septic)
    (suppurative)** — *see also* Endometritis
  cervical — *see* Cervicitis
Metropathia hemorrhagica N93.8
Metroperitonitis — *see* Peritonitis, pelvic,
    female
Metrorrhagia N92.1
  climacteric N92.4
  menopausal N92.4
  perimenopausal N92.4
  postpartum NEC (atonic) (following delivery
    of placenta) O72.1
    delayed or secondary O72.2
  preclimacteric or premenopausal N92.4
  psychogenic F45.8
Metrorrhexis — *see* Rupture, uterus
Metrosalpingitis N70.91
Metrostaxis N93.8
Metrovaginitis — *see* Endometritis
**Meyer-Schwickerath and Weyers
    syndrome** Q87.0
Meynert's amentia (nonalcoholic) F04
  alcoholic F10.96
    with dependence F10.26
Mibelli's disease (porokeratosis) Q82.8
Mice, joint — *see* Loose, body, joint
  knee M23.4-
Micrencephalon, micrencephaly Q02
Microalbuminuria R80.9
Microaneurysm, retinal — *see also* Disorder,
    retina, microaneurysms
  diabetic — *see* E08-E13 with .31
Microangiopathy (peripheral) I73.9
  thrombotic M31.1
Microcalcifications, breast R92.0
Microcephalus, microcephalic, microcephaly
    Q02
  due to toxoplasmosis (congenital) P37.1
Microcheilia Q18.7
Microcolon (congenital) Q43.8
Microcornea (congenital) Q13.4
Microcytic — *see* condition
Microdeletions NEC Q93.88
Microdontia K00.2
Microdrepanocytosis D57.40
  with crisis (vasoocclusive pain) D57.419
    with
      acute chest syndrome D57.411
      splenic sequestration D57.412
Microembolism
  atherothrombotic — *see* Atheroembolism
  retinal — *see* Occlusion, artery, retina
Microencephalon Q02
Microfilaria streptocerca infestation — *see*
    Onchocerciasis
Microgastria (congenital) Q40.2
Microgenia M26.06
Microgenitalia, congenital
  female Q52.8
  male Q55.8
Microglioma — *see* Lymphoma, non-Hodgkin,
    specified NEC
Microglossia (congenital) Q38.3
**Micrognathia, micrognathism (congenital)
    (mandibular) (maxillary)** M26.09
Microgyria (congenital) Q04.3
Microinfarct of heart — *see* Insufficiency,
    coronary
Microlentia (congenital) Q12.8
Microlithiasis, alveolar, pulmonary J84.02
Micromastia N64.82
Micromyelia (congenital) Q06.8
Micropenis Q55.62
Microphakia (congenital) Q12.8

Microphthalmos, microphthalmia (congenital) Q11.2
  due to toxoplasmosis P37.1
Micropsia H53.15
Microscopic polyangiitis (polyarteritis) M31.7
Microsporidiosis B60.8
  intestinal A07.8
Microsporon furfur infestation B36.0
Microsporosis — *see also* Dermatophytosis
  nigra B36.1
Microstomia (congenital) Q18.5
Microtia (congenital) (external ear) Q17.2
Microtropia H50.40
Microvillus inclusion disease (MVD) (MVID) Q43.8
Micturition
  disorder NEC — *see also* Difficulty, micturition R39.198
    psychogenic F45.8
  frequency R35.0
    psychogenic F45.8
  hesitancy R39.11
  incomplete emptying R39.14
  nocturnal R35.1
  painful R30.9
    dysuria R30.0
    psychogenic F45.8
    tenesmus R30.1
  poor stream R39.12
  position dependent R39.192
  split stream R39.13
  straining R39.16
  urgency R39.15
Mid plane — *see* condition
Middle
  ear — *see* condition
  lobe (right) syndrome J98.19
Miescher's elastoma L87.2
Mietens' syndrome Q87.2
Migraine (idiopathic) G43.909
  with refractory migraine G43.919
    with status migrainosus G43.911
    without status migrainosus G43.919
  with aura (acute-onset) (prolonged) (typical) (without headache) G43.109
    with refractory migraine G43.119
      with status migrainosus G43.111
      without status migrainosus G43.119
    intractable G43.119
      with status migrainosus G43.111
      without status migrainosus G43.119
    not intractable G43.109
      with status migrainosus G43.101
      without status migrainosus G43.109
    persistent G43.509
      with cerebral infarction G43.609
        with refractory migraine G43.619
          with status migrainosus G43.611
          without status migrainosus G43.619
        intractable G43.619
          with status migrainosus G43.611
          without status migrainosus G43.619
        not intractable G43.609
          with status migrainosus G43.601
          without status migrainosus G43.609
        without refractory migraine G43.609
          with status migrainosus G43.601
          without status migrainosus G43.609
      without cerebral infarction G43.509
        with refractory migraine G43.519
          with status migrainosus G43.511
          without status migrainosus G43.519
        intractable G43.519
          with status migrainosus G43.511
          without status migrainosus G43.519
        not intractable G43.509
          with status migrainosus G43.501
          without status migrainosus G43.509
        without refractory migraine G43.509
          with status migrainosus G43.501
          without status migrainosus G43.509
    without mention of refractory migraine G43.109
      with status migrainosus G43.101

Migraine (idiopathic) - *continued*
  with aura (acute-onset) (prolonged) (typical) (without headache) - *continued*
    without mention of refractory migraine - *continued*
      without status migrainosus G43.109
  abdominal G43.D0
    with refractory migraine G43.D1
    intractable G43.D1
    not intractable G43.D0
    without refractory migraine G43.D0
  basilar — *see* Migraine, with aura
  classical — *see* Migraine, with aura
  common — *see* Migraine, without aura
  complicated G43.109
  equivalents — *see* Migraine, with aura
  familiar — *see* Migraine, hemiplegic
  hemiplegic G43.409
    with refractory migraine G43.419
      with status migrainosus G43.411
      without status migrainosus G43.419
    intractable G43.419
      with status migrainosus G43.411
      without status migrainosus G43.419
    not intractable G43.409
      with status migrainosus G43.401
      without status migrainosus G43.409
    without refractory migraine G43.409
      with status migrainosus G43.401
      without status migrainosus G43.409
  intractable G43.919
    with status migrainosus G43.911
    without status migrainosus G43.919
  menstrual G43.829
    with refractory migraine G43.839
      with status migrainosus G43.831
      without status migrainosus G43.839
    intractable G43.839
      with status migrainosus G43.831
      without status migrainosus G43.839
    not intractable 4G43.829
      with status migrainosus G43.821
      without status migrainosus G43.829
    without refractory migraine G43.829
      with status migrainosus G43.821
      without status migrainosus G43.829
  menstrually related — *see* Migraine, menstrual
  not intractable G43.909
    with status migrainosus G43.901
    without status migrainosus G43.919
  ophthalmoplegic G43.B0
    with refractory migraine G43.B1
    intractable G43.B1
    not intractable G43.B0
    without refractory migraine G43.B0
  persistent aura (with, without) cerebral infarction — *see* Migraine, with aura, persistent
  preceded or accompanied by transient focal neurological phenomena — *see* Migraine, with aura
  pre-menstrual — *see* Migraine, menstrual
  pure menstrual — *see* Migraine, menstrual
  retinal — *see* Migraine, with aura
  specified NEC G43.809
    intractable G43.819
      with status migrainosus G43.811
      without status migrainosus G43.819
    not intractable G43.809
      with status migrainosus G43.801
      without status migrainosus G43.809
  sporadic — *see* Migraine, hemiplegic
  transformed — *see* Migraine, without aura, chronic
  triggered seizures — *see* Migraine, with aura
  without aura G43.009
    with refractory migraine G43.019
      with status migrainosus G43.011
      without status migrainosus G43.019
    chronic G43.709
      with refractory migraine G43.719
        with status migrainosus G43.711
        without status migrainosus G43.719
      intractable

Migraine (idiopathic) - *continued*
  without aura - *continued*
    chronic - *continued*
      intractable - *continued*
        with status migrainosus G43.711
        without status migrainosus G43.719
      not intractable
        with status migrainosus G43.701
        without status migrainosus G43.709
      without refractory migraine G43.709
        with status migrainosus G43.701
        without status migrainosus G43.709
    intractable
      with status migrainosus G43.011
      without status migrainosus G43.019
    not intractable
      with status migrainosus G43.001
      without status migrainosus G43.009
    without mention of refractory migraine G43.009
      with status migrainosus G43.001
      without status migrainosus G43.009
    without refractory migraine G43.909
      with status migrainosus G43.901
      without status migrainosus G43.919
Migrant, social Z59.0
Migration, anxiety concerning Z60.3
Migratory, migrating — *see also* condition
  person Z59.0
  testis Q55.29
Mikity-Wilson disease or syndrome P27.0
Mikulicz' disease or syndrome K11.8
Miliaria L74.3
  alba L74.1
  apocrine L75.2
  crystallina L74.1
  profunda L74.2
  rubra L74.0
  tropicalis L74.2
Miliary — *see* condition
Milium L72.0
  colloid L57.8
Milk
  crust L21.0
  excessive secretion O92.6
  poisoning — *see* Poisoning, food, noxious
  retention O92.79
  sickness — *see* Poisoning, food, noxious
  spots I31.0
Milk-alkali disease or syndrome E83.52
Milk-leg (deep vessels) (nonpuerperal) — *see* Embolism, vein, lower extremity
  complicating pregnancy O22.3-
  puerperal, postpartum, childbirth O87.1
Milkman's disease or syndrome M83.8
Milky urine — *see* Chyluria
Millard-Gubler (-Foville) paralysis or syndrome G46.3
Millar's asthma J38.5
Miller Fisher syndrome G61.0
Mills' disease — *see* Hemiplegia
Millstone maker's pneumoconiosis J62.8
Milroy's disease (chronic hereditary edema) Q82.0
Minamata disease T56.1
Miners' asthma or lung J60
Minkowski-Chauffard syndrome — *see* Spherocytosis
Minor — *see* condition
Minor's disease (hematomyelia) G95.19
Minot's disease (hemorrhagic disease), newborn P53
Minot-von Willebrand-Jurgens disease or syndrome (angiohemophilia) D68.0
Minus (and plus) hand (intrinsic) — *see* Deformity, limb, specified type NEC, forearm
Miosis (pupil) H57.03
Mirizzi's syndrome (hepatic duct stenosis) K83.1
Mirror writing F81.0

**Misadventure (of) (prophylactic)
(therapeutic)** — *see also*
Complications T88.9
administration of insulin (by accident) — *see*
subcategory T38.3
infusion — *see* Complications, infusion
local applications (of fomentations, plasters,
etc.) T88.9
burn or scald — *see* Burn
specified NEC T88.8
medical care (early) (late) T88.9
adverse effect of drugs or chemicals — *see*
Table of Drugs and Chemicals
medical care (early) (late)
burn or scald — *see* Burn
specified NEC T88.8
specified NEC T88.8
surgical procedure (early) (late) — *see*
Complications, surgical procedure
transfusion — *see* Complications, transfusion
vaccination or other immunological
procedure — *see* Complications,
vaccination
Miscarriage O03.9
Misdirection, aqueous H40.83-
Misperception, sleep state F51.02
Misplaced, misplacement
ear Q17.4
kidney (acquired) N28.89
congenital Q63.2
organ or site, congenital NEC — *see*
Malposition, congenital
Missed
abortion O02.1
delivery O36.4
Missing — *see also* Absence
string of intrauterine contraceptive
device T83.32
Misuse of drugs F19.99
Mitchell's disease (erythromelalgia) I73.81
Mite (s) (infestation) B88.9
diarrhea B88.0
grain (itch) B88.0
hair follicle (itch) B88.0
in sputum B88.0
Mitral — *see* condition
Mittelschmerz N94.0
Mixed — *see* condition
MMN (multifocal motor neuropathy) G61.82
**MNGIE (Mitochondrial
Neurogastrointestinal Encephalopathy)
syndrome** E88.49
Mobile, mobility
cecum Q43.3
excessive — *see* Hypermobility
gallbladder, congenital Q44.1
kidney N28.89
organ or site, congenital NEC — *see*
Malposition, congenital
Mobitz heart block (atrioventricular) I44.1
Moebius, Möbius
disease (ophthalmoplegic migraine) — *see*
Migraine, ophthalmoplegic
syndrome Q87.0
congenital oculofacial paralysis (with other
anomalies) Q87.0
ophthalmoplegic migraine — *see*
Migraine, ophthalmoplegic
Moeller's glossitis K14.0
Mohr's syndrome (Types I and II) Q87.0
Mola destruens D39.2
Molar pregnancy O02.0
Molarization of premolars K00.2
Molding, head (during birth) - omit code
Mole (pigmented) — *see also* Nevus
blood O02.0
Breus' O02.0
cancerous — *see* Melanoma
carneous O02.0
destructive D39.2
fleshy O02.0
hydatid, hydatidiform (benign) (complicating
pregnancy) (delivered)
(undelivered) O01.9
classical O01.0

Mole (pigmented) - *continued*
hydatid, hydatidiform (benign) (complicating
pregnancy) (delivered) (undelivered) -
continued
complete O01.0
incomplete O01.1
invasive D39.2
malignant D39.2
partial O01.1
intrauterine O02.0
invasive (hydatidiform) D39.2
malignant
meaning
malignant hydatidiform mole D39.2
melanoma — *see* Melanoma
nonhydatidiform O02.0
nonpigmented — *see* Nevus
pregnancy NEC O02.0
skin — *see* Nevus
tubal O00.10-
with intrauterine pregnancy O00.11-
vesicular — *see* Mole, hydatidiform
Molimen, molimina (menstrual) N94.3
Molluscum contagiosum (epitheliale) B08.1
**Mönckeberg's arteriosclerosis, disease, or
sclerosis** — *see* Arteriosclerosis,
extremities
Mondini's malformation (cochlea) Q16.5
Mondor's disease I80.8
Monge's disease T70.29
Monilethrix (congenital) Q84.1
Moniliasis — *see also* Candidiasis B37.9
neonatal P37.5
Monitoring (encounter for)
therapeutic drug level Z51.81
Monkey malaria B53.1
Monkeypox B04
Monoarthritis M13.10
ankle M13.17-
elbow M13.12-
foot joint M13.17-
hand joint M13.14-
hip M13.15-
knee M13.16-
shoulder M13.11-
wrist M13.13-
Monoblastic — *see* condition
**Monochromat (ism) , monochromatopsia
(acquired) (congenital)** H53.51
Monocytic — *see* condition
Monocytopenia D72.818
Monocytosis (symptomatic) D72.821
Monomania — *see* Psychosis
Mononeuritis G58.9
cranial nerve — *see* Disorder, nerve, cranial
femoral nerve G57.2-
lateral
cutaneous nerve of thigh G57.1-
popliteal nerve G57.3-
lower limb G57.9-
specified nerve NEC G57.8-
medial popliteal nerve G57.4-
median nerve G56.1-
multiplex G58.7
plantar nerve G57.6-
posterior tibial nerve G57.5-
radial nerve G56.3-
sciatic nerve G57.0-
specified NEC G58.8
tibial nerve G57.4-
ulnar nerve G56.2-
upper limb G56.9-
specified nerve NEC G56.8-
vestibular — *see* subcategory H93.3
Mononeuropathy G58.9
carpal tunnel syndrome — *see* Syndrome,
carpal tunnel
diabetic NEC — *see* E08-E13 with .41
femoral nerve — *see* Lesion, nerve, femoral
ilioinguinal nerve G57.8-
in diseases classified elsewhere — *see*
category G59
intercostal G58.0
lower limb G57.9-
causalgia — *see* Causalgia, lower limb

Mononeuropathy - *continued*
lower limb - *continued*
femoral nerve — *see* Lesion, nerve,
femoral
meralgia paresthetica G57.1-
plantar nerve — *see* Lesion, nerve, plantar
popliteal nerve — *see* Lesion, nerve,
popliteal
sciatic nerve — *see* Lesion, nerve, sciatic
specified NEC G57.8-
tarsal tunnel syndrome — *see* Syndrome,
tarsal tunnel
median nerve — *see* Lesion, nerve, median
multiplex G58.7
obturator nerve G57.8-
popliteal nerve — *see* Lesion, nerve,
popliteal
radial nerve — *see* Lesion, nerve, radial
saphenous nerve G57.8-
specified NEC G58.8
tarsal tunnel syndrome — *see* Syndrome,
tarsal tunnel
tuberculous A17.83
ulnar nerve — *see* Lesion, nerve, ulnar
upper limb G56.9-
carpal tunnel syndrome — *see* Syndrome,
carpal tunnel
causalgia — *see* Causalgia
median nerve — *see* Lesion, nerve, median
radial nerve — *see* Lesion, nerve, radial
specified site NEC G56.8-
ulnar nerve — *see* Lesion, nerve, ulnar
Mononucleosis, infectious B27.90
with
complication NEC B27.99
meningitis B27.92
polyneuropathy B27.91
cytomegaloviral B27.10
with
complication NEC B27.19
meningitis B27.12
polyneuropathy B27.11
Epstein-Barr (virus) B27.00
with
complication NEC B27.09
meningitis B27.02
polyneuropathy B27.01
gammaherpesviral B27.00
with
complication NEC B27.09
meningitis B27.02
polyneuropathy B27.01
specified NEC B27.80
with
complication NEC B27.89
meningitis B27.82
polyneuropathy B27.81
Monoplegia G83.3-
congenital (cerebral) G80.8
spastic G80.1
embolic (current episode) I63.4-
following
cerebrovascular disease
cerebral infarction
lower limb I69.34-
upper limb I69.33-
intracerebral hemorrhage
lower limb I69.14-
upper limb I69.13-
lower limb I69.94-
nontraumatic intracranial hemorrhage
NEC
lower limb I69.24-
upper limb I69.23-
specified disease NEC
lower limb I69.84-
upper limb I69.83-
stroke NOS
lower limb I69.34-
upper limb I69.33-
subarachnoid hemorrhage
lower limb I69.04-
upper limb I69.03-
upper limb I69.93-
hysterical (transient) F44.4

Monoplegia - *continued*
lower limb G83.1-
psychogenic (conversion reaction) F44.4
thrombotic (current episode) I63.3-
transient R29.818
upper limb G83.2-
Monorchism, monorchidism Q55.0
Monosomy — *see also* Deletion,
chromosome Q93.9
specified NEC Q93.89
whole chromosome
meiotic nondisjunction Q93.0
mitotic nondisjunction Q93.1
mosaicism Q93.1
X Q96.9
Monster, monstrosity (single) Q89.7
acephalic Q00.0
twin Q89.4
Monteggia's fracture (-dislocation) S52.27-
Mooren's ulcer (cornea) — *see* Ulcer, cornea,
Mooren's
Moore's syndrome — *see* Epilepsy, specified
NEC
Mooser-Neill reaction A75.2
Mooser's bodies A75.2
Morbidity not stated or unknown R69
Morbilli — *see* Measles
Morbus — *see also* Disease
angelicus, anglorum E55.0
Beigel B36.2
caducus — *see* Epilepsy
celiacus K90.0
comitialis — *see* Epilepsy
cordis — *see also* Disease, heart I51.9
valvulorum — *see* Endocarditis
coxae senilis M16.9
tuberculous A18.02
hemorrhagicus neonatorum P53
maculosus neonatorum P54.5
Morel (-Stewart) (-Morgagni)
syndrome M85.2
Morel-Kraepelin disease — *see*
Schizophrenia
Morel-Moore syndrome M85.2
Morgagni's
cyst, organ, hydatid, or appendage
female Q50.5
male (epididymal) Q55.4
testicular Q55.29
syndrome M85.2
Morgagni-Stewart-Morel syndrome M85.2
Morgagni-Stokes-Adams syndrome I45.9
Morgagni-Turner (-Albright)
syndrome Q96.9
Moria F07.0
Moron (I.Q.50-69) F70
Morphea L94.0
Morphinism (without remission) F11.20
with remission F11.21
Morphinomania (without remission) F11.20
with remission F11.21
Morquio (-Ullrich) (-Brailsford) disease or
syndrome — *see* Mucopolysaccharidosis
Mortification (dry) (moist) — *see* Gangrene
Morton's metatarsalgia (neuralgia)
(neuroma) (syndrome) G57.6-
Morvan's disease or syndrome G60.8
Mosaicism, mosaic (autosomal)
(chromosomal)
45,X/other cell lines NEC with abnormal sex
chromosome Q96.4
45,X/46,XX Q96.3
sex chromosome
female Q97.8
lines with various numbers of X
chromosomes Q97.2
male Q98.7
XY Q96.3
Moschowitz' disease M31.1
Mother yaw A66.0
Motion sickness (from travel, any vehicle)
(from roundabouts or swings) T75.3
Mottled, mottling, teeth (enamel) (endemic)
(nonendemic) K00.3

Mounier-Kuhn syndrome Q32.4
with bronchiectasis J47.9
exacerbation (acute) J47.1
lower respiratory infection J47.0
acquired J98.09
with bronchiectasis J47.9
with
exacerbation (acute) J47.1
lower respiratory infection J47.0
Mountain
sickness T70.29
with polycythemia , acquired
(acute) D75.1
tick fever A93.2
Mouse, joint — *see* Loose, body, joint
knee M23.4-
Mouth — *see* condition
Movable
coccyx — *see* subcategory M53.2
kidney N28.89
congenital Q63.8
spleen D73.89
Movements, dystonic R25.8
Moyamoya disease I67.5
MRSA (Methicillin resistant Staphylococcus
aureus)
infection A49.02
as the cause of diseases classified
elsewhere B95.62
sepsis A41.02
MSD (multiple sulfatase deficiency) E75.26
MSSA (Methicillin susceptible
Staphylococcus aureus)
infection A49.01
as the cause of diseases classified
elsewhere B95.61
sepsis A41.01
Mucha-Habermann disease L41.0
Mucinosis (cutaneous) (focal) (papular)
(reticular erythematous) (skin) L98.5
oral K13.79
Mucocele
appendix K38.8
buccal cavity K13.79
gallbladder K82.1
lacrimal sac, chronic H04.43-
nasal sinus J34.1
nose J34.1
salivary gland (any) K11.6
sinus (accessory) (nasal) J34.1
turbinate (bone) (middle) (nasal) J34.1
uterus N85.8
Mucolipidosis
I E77.1
II, III E77.0
IV E75.11
Mucopolysaccharidosis E76.3
beta-gluduronidase deficiency E76.29
cardiopathy E76.3 *[I52]*
Hunter's syndrome E76.1
Hurler's syndrome E76.01
Hurler-Scheie syndrome E76.02
Maroteaux-Lamy syndrome E76.29
Morquio syndrome E76.219
A E76.210
B E76.211
classic E76.210
Sanfilippo syndrome E76.22
Scheie's syndrome E76.03
specified NEC E76.29
type
I
Hurler's syndrome E76.01
Hurler-Scheie syndrome E76.02
Scheie's syndrome E76.03
II E76.1
III E76.22
IV E76.219
IVA E76.210
IVB E76.211
VI E76.29
VII E76.29
Mucormycosis B46.5
cutaneous B46.3
disseminated B46.4

Mucormycosis - *continued*
gastrointestinal B46.2
generalized B46.4
pulmonary B46.0
rhinocerebral B46.1
skin B46.3
subcutaneous B46.3
Mucositis (ulcerative) K12.30
due to drugs NEC K12.32
gastrointestinal K92.81
mouth (oral) (oropharyngeal) K12.30
due to antineoplastic therapy K12.31
due to drugs NEC K12.32
due to radiation K12.33
specified NEC K12.39
viral K12.39
nasal J34.81
oral cavity — *see* Mucositis, mouth
oral soft tissues — *see* Mucositis, mouth
vagina and vulva N76.81
Mucosis necroticans agranulocytica — *see*
Agranulocytosis
Mucous — *see also* condition
patches (syphilitic) A51.39
congenital A50.07
Mucoviscidosis E84.9
with meconium obstruction E84.11
Mucus
asphyxia or suffocation — *see* Asphyxia,
mucus
in stool R19.5
plug — *see* Asphyxia, mucus
Muguet B37.0
Mulberry molars (congenital
syphilis) A50.52
Müllerian mixed tumor
specified site — *see* Neoplasm, malignant,
by site
unspecified site C54.9
Multicystic kidney (development) Q61.4
Multiparity (grand) Z64.1
affecting management of pregnancy, labor
and delivery (supervision only) O09.4-
requiring contraceptive management — *see*
Contraception
Multipartita placenta O43.19-
Multiple, multiplex — *see also* condition
digits (congenital) Q69.9
endocrine neoplasia — *see* Neoplasia,
endocrine, multiple (MEN)
personality F44.81
Mumps B26.9
arthritis B26.85
complication NEC B26.89
encephalitis B26.2
hepatitis B26.81
meningitis (aseptic) B26.1
meningoencephalitis B26.2
myocarditis B26.82
oophoritis B26.89
orchitis B26.0
pancreatitis B26.3
polyneuropathy B26.84
Mumu — *see also* Infestation,
filarial B74.9 *[N51]*
Münchhausen's syndrome — *see* Disorder,
factitious
Münchmeyer's syndrome — *see* Myositis,
ossificans, progressiva
Mural — *see* condition
Murmur (cardiac) (heart) (organic) R01.1
abdominal R19.15
aortic (valve) — *see* Endocarditis, aortic
benign R01.0
diastolic — *see* Endocarditis
Flint I35.1
functional R01.0
Graham Steell I37.1
innocent R01.0
mitral (valve) — *see* Insufficiency, mitral
nonorganic R01.0
presystolic, mitral — *see* Insufficiency,
mitral
pulmonic (valve) I37.8
systolic R01.1

Murmur (cardiac) (heart) (organic) -
continued
    tricuspid (valve) I07.9
    valvular — *see* Endocarditis
Murri's disease (intermittent hemoglobinuria) D59.6
Muscle, muscular — *see also* condition
    carnitine (palmityltransferase)
      deficiency E71.314
Musculoneuralgia — *see* Neuralgia
Mushrooming hip — *see* Derangement, joint, specified NEC, hip
Mushroom-workers' (pickers') disease or lung J67.5
Mutation (s)
    factor V Leiden D68.51
    surfactant, of lung J84.83
    prothrombin gene D68.52
Mutism — *see also* Aphasia
    deaf (acquired) (congenital) NEC H91.3
    elective (adjustment reaction)
      (childhood) F94.0
    hysterical F44.4
    selective (childhood) F94.0
MVD (microvillus inclusion disease) Q43.8
MVID (microvillus inclusion disease) Q43.8
Myalgia M79.10
    auxiliary muscles, head and neck M79.12
    epidemic (cervical) B33.0
    mastication muscle M79.11
    site specified NEC M79.18
    traumatic NEC T14.8
Myasthenia G70.9
    congenital G70.2
    cordis — *see* Failure, heart
    developmental G70.2
    gravis G70.00
      with exacerbation (acute) G70.01
      in crisis G70.01
      neonatal, transient P94.0
      pseudoparalytica G70.00
        with exacerbation (acute) G70.01
        in crisis G70.01
    stomach, psychogenic F45.8
    syndrome
      in
        diabetes mellitus — *see* E08-E13 with
          .44
        neoplastic disease — *see also*
          Neoplasm D49.9 *[G73.3]*
        pernicious anemia D51.0 *[G73.3]*
        thyrotoxicosis E05.90 *[G73.3]*
          with thyroid storm E05.91 *[G73.3]*
Myasthenic M62.81
Mycelium infection B49
Mycetismus — *see* Poisoning, food, noxious, mushroom
Mycetoma B47.9
    actinomycotic B47.1
    bone (mycotic) B47.9 *[M90.80]*
    eumycotic B47.0
    foot B47.9
      actinomycotic B47.1
      mycotic B47.0
    madurae NEC B47.9
      mycotic B47.0
    maduromycotic B47.0
    mycotic B47.0
    nocardial B47.1
Mycobacteriosis — *see* Mycobacterium
Mycobacterium, mycobacterial (infection) A31.9
    anonymous A31.9
    atypical A31.9
      cutaneous A31.1
      pulmonary A31.0
        tuberculous — *see* Tuberculosis,
          pulmonary
      specified site NEC A31.8
    avium (intracellulare complex) A31.0
    balnei A31.1
    Battey A31.0
    chelonei A31.8
    cutaneous A31.1
    extrapulmonary systemic A31.8

Mycobacterium, mycobacterial (infection) -
continued
    fortuitum A31.8
    intracellulare (Battey bacillus) A31.0
    kansasii (yellow bacillus) A31.0
    kakaferifu A31.8
    kasongo A31.8
    leprae — *see also* Leprosy A30.9
    luciflavum A31.1
    marinum (M. balnei) A31.1
    nonspecific — *see* Mycobacterium, atypical
    pulmonary (atypical) A31.0
      tuberculous — *see* Tuberculosis,
        pulmonary
    scrofulaceum A31.8
    simiae A31.8
    systemic, extrapulmonary A31.8
    szulgai A31.8
    terrae A31.8
    triviale A31.8
    tuberculosis (human, bovine) -
      seeTuberculosis
    ulcerans A31.1
    xenopi A31.8
Mycoplasma (M.) pneumoniae, as cause of disease classified elsewhere B96.0
Mycosis, mycotic B49
    cutaneous NEC B36.9
    ear B36.9
      in
        aspergillosis B44.89
        candidiasis B37.84
        moniliasis B37.84
    fungoides (extranodal) (solid organ) C84.0-
    mouth B37.0
    nails B35.1
    opportunistic B48.8
    skin NEC B36.9
    specified NEC B48.8
    stomatitis B37.0
    vagina, vaginitis (candidal) B37.3
Mydriasis (pupil) H57.04
Myelatelia Q06.1
Myelinolysis, pontine, central G37.2
Myelitis (acute) (ascending) (childhood) (chronic) (descending) (diffuse) (disseminated) (idiopathic) (pressure) (progressive) (spinal cord) (subacute) — *see also* Encephalitis G04.91
    herpes simplex B00.82
    herpes zoster B02.24
    in diseases classified elsewhere G05.4
    necrotizing, subacute G37.4
    optic neuritis in G36.0
    postchickenpox B01.12
    postherpetic B02.24
    postimmunization G04.02
    postinfectious NEC G04.89
    postvaccinal G04.02
    specified NEC G04.89
    syphilitic (transverse) A52.14
    toxic G92
    transverse (in demyelinating diseases of
      central nervous system) G37.3
    tuberculous A17.82
    varicella B01.12
Myeloblastic — *see* condition
Myeloblastoma
    granular cell — *see also* Neoplasm,
      connective tissue
    malignant — *see* Neoplasm, connective
      tissue, malignant
    tongue D10.1
Myelocele — *see* Spina bifida
Myelocystocele — *see* Spina bifida
Myelocytic — *see* condition
Myelodysplasia D46.9
    specified NEC D46.Z
    spinal cord (congenital) Q06.1
Myelodysplastic syndrome D46.9
    with
      5q deletion D46.C
      isolated del (5q) chromosomal
        abnormality D46.C
    specified NEC D46.Z

Myeloencephalitis — *see* Encephalitis
Myelofibrosis D75.81
    with myeloid metaplasia D47.4
    acute C94.4-
    idiopathic (chronic) D47.4
    primary D47.1
    secondary D75.81
      in myeloproliferative disease D47.4
Myelogenous — *see* condition
Myeloid — *see* condition
Myelokathexis D70.9
Myeloleukodystrophy E75.29
Myelolipoma — *see* Lipoma
Myeloma (multiple) C90.0-
    monostotic C90.3
      plasma cell C90.0-
    plasma cell C90.0-
    solitary — *see also* Plasmacytoma,
      solitary C90.3-
Myelomalacia G95.89
Myelomatosis C90.0-
Myelomeningitis — *see* Meningoencephalitis
Myelomeningocele (spinal cord) — *see* Spina bifida
Myelo-osteo-musculodysplasia hereditaria Q79.8
Myelopathic
    anemia D64.89
    muscle atrophy — *see* Atrophy, muscle,
      spinal
    pain syndrome G89.0
Myelopathy (spinal cord) G95.9
    drug-induced G95.89
    in (due to)
      degeneration or displacement,
        intervertebral disc NEC — *see*
        Disorder, disc, with, myelopathy
      infection — *see* Encephalitis
      intervertebral disc disorder — *see also*
        Disorder, disc, with, myelopathy
      mercury — *see* subcategory T56.1
      neoplastic disease — *see also*
        Neoplasm D49.9 *[G99.2]*
      pernicious anemia D51.0 *[G99.2]*
      spondylosis — *see* Spondylosis, with
        myelopathy NEC
    necrotic (subacute) (vascular) G95.19
    radiation-induced G95.89
    spondylogenic NEC — *see* Spondylosis, with
      myelopathy NEC
    toxic G95.89
    transverse, acute G37.3
    vascular G95.19
    vitamin B12 E53.8 *[G32.0]*
Myelophthisis D61.82
Myeloradiculitis G04.91
Myeloradiculodysplasia (spinal) Q06.1
Myelosarcoma C92.3-
Myelosclerosis D75.89
    with myeloid metaplasia D47.4
    disseminated, of nervous system G35
    megakaryocytic D47.4
      with myeloid metaplasia D47.4
Myelosis
    acute C92.0-
    aleukemic C92.9-
    chronic D47.1
    erythremic (acute) C94.0-
    megakaryocytic C94.2-
    nonleukemic D72.828
    subacute C92.9-
Myiasis (cavernous) B87.9
    aural B87.4
    creeping B87.0
    cutaneous B87.0
    dermal B87.0
    ear (external) (middle) B87.4
    eye B87.2
    genitourinary B87.81
    intestinal B87.82
    laryngeal B87.3
    nasopharyngeal B87.3
    ocular B87.2
    orbit B87.2
    skin B87.0

Myiasis (cavernous) - *continued*
  specified site NEC B87.89
  traumatic B87.1
  wound B87.1
Myoadenoma, prostate — *see* Hyperplasia,
  prostate
Myoblastoma
  granular cell — *see also* Neoplasm,
    connective tissue, benign
    malignant — *see* Neoplasm, connective
     tissue, malignant
  tongue D10.1
Myocardial — *see* condition
Myocardiopathy (congestive) (constrictive)
  (familial) (hypertrophic nonobstructive)
  (idiopathic) (infiltrative) (obstructive)
  (primary) (restrictive) (sporadic) — *see*
  also Cardiomyopathy I42.9
  alcoholic I42.6
  cobalt-beer I42.6
  glycogen storage E74.02 *[I43]*
  hypertrophic obstructive I42.1
  in (due to)
    beriberi E51.12
    cardiac glycogenosis E74.02 *[I43]*
    Friedreich's ataxia G11.1 *[I43]*
    myotonia atrophica G71.11 *[I43]*
    progressive muscular dystrophy G71.09
     [I43]
  obscure (African) I42.8
  secondary I42.9
  thyrotoxic E05.90 *[I43]*
    with storm E05.91 *[I43]*
  toxic NEC I42.7
Myocarditis (with arteriosclerosis) (chronic)
  (fibroid) (interstitial) (old) (progressive)
  (senile) I51.4
  with
    rheumatic fever (conditions in I00) I09.0
     active — *see* Myocarditis, acute,
      rheumatic
     inactive or quiescent (with chorea) I09.0
  active I40.9
    rheumatic I01.2
     with chorea (acute) (rheumatic)
      (Sydenham's) I02.0
  acute or subacute (interstitial) I40.9
    due to
     streptococcus (beta-hemolytic) I01.2
    idiopathic I40.1
    rheumatic I01.2
     with chorea (acute) (rheumatic)
      (Sydenham's) I02.0
    specified NEC I40.8
  aseptic of newborn B33.22
  bacterial (acute) I40.0
  Coxsackie (virus) B33.22
  diphtheritic A36.81
  eosinophilic I40.1
  epidemic of newborn (Coxsackie) B33.22
  Fiedler's (acute) (isolated) I40.1
  giant cell (acute) (subacute) I40.1
  gonococcal A54.83
  granulomatous (idiopathic) (isolated)
    (nonspecific) I40.1
  hypertensive — *see* Hypertension, heart
  idiopathic (granulomatous) I40.1
  in (due to)
    diphtheria A36.81
    epidemic louse-borne typhus A75.0 *[I41]*
    Lyme disease A69.29
    sarcoidosis D86.85
    scarlet fever A38.1
    toxoplasmosis (acquired) B58.81
    typhoid A01.02
    typhus NEC A75.9 *[I41]*
  infective I40.0
  influenzal — *see* Influenza, with,
    myocarditis
  isolated (acute) I40.1
  meningococcal A39.52
  mumps B26.82
  nonrheumatic, active I40.9
  parenchymatous I40.9
  pneumococcal I40.0

Myocarditis (with arteriosclerosis) (chronic)
(fibroid) (interstitial) (old) (progressive)
(senile) - *continued*
  rheumatic (chronic) (inactive) (with
    chorea) I09.0
    active or acute I01.2
     with chorea (acute) (rheumatic)
      (Sydenham's) I02.0
  rheumatoid — *see* Rheumatoid, carditis
  septic I40.0
  staphylococcal I40.0
  suppurative I40.0
  syphilitic (chronic) A52.06
  toxic I40.8
    rheumatic — *see* Myocarditis, acute,
     rheumatic
  tuberculous A18.84
  typhoid A01.02
  valvular — *see* Endocarditis
  virus, viral I40.0
    of newborn (Coxsackie) B33.22
Myocardium, myocardial — *see* condition
Myocardosis — *see* Cardiomyopathy
Myoclonus, myoclonic, myoclonia (familial)
  (essential) (multifocal) (simplex) G25.3
  drug-induced G25.3
  epilepsy — *see also* Epilepsy, generalized,
    specified NEC G40.4-
    familial (progressive) G25.3
  epileptica G40.409
    with status epilepticus G40.401
  facial G51.3-
  familial progressive G25.3
  Friedreich's G25.3
  jerks G25.3
  massive G25.3
  palatal G25.3
  pharyngeal G25.3
Myocytolysis I51.5
Myodiastasis — *see* Diastasis, muscle
Myoendocarditis — *see* Endocarditis
Myoepithelioma — *see* Neoplasm, benign, by
  site
Myofasciitis (acute) — *see* Myositis
Myofibroma — *see also* Neoplasm,
  connective tissue, benign
  uterus (cervix) (corpus) — *see* Leiomyoma
Myofibromatosis D48.1
  infantile Q89.8
Myofibrosis M62.89
  heart — *see* Myocarditis
  scapulohumeral — *see* Lesion, shoulder,
    specified NEC
Myofibrositis M79.7
  scapulohumeral — *see* Lesion, shoulder,
    specified NEC
Myoglobulinuria, myoglobinuria
  (primary) R82.1
Myokymia, facial G51.4
Myolipoma — *see* Lipoma
Myoma — *see also* Neoplasm, connective
  tissue, benign
  malignant — *see* Neoplasm, connective
    tissue, malignant
  prostate D29.1
  uterus (cervix) (corpus) — *see* Leiomyoma
Myomalacia M62.89
Myometritis — *see* Endometritis
Myometrium — *see* condition
Myonecrosis, clostridial A48.0
Myopathy G72.9
  acute
    necrotizing G72.81
    quadriplegic G72.81
  alcoholic G72.1
  benign congenital G71.2
  central core G71.2
  centronuclear G71.2
  congenital (benign) G71.2
  critical illness G72.81
  distal G71.09
  drug-induced G72.0
  endocrine NEC E34.9 *[G73.7]*
  extraocular muscles H05.82-
  facioscapulohumeral G71.02

Myopathy - *continued*
  hereditary G71.9
    specified NEC G71.8
  immune NEC G72.49
  in (due to)
    Addison's disease E27.1 *[G73.7]*
    alcohol G72.1
    amyloidosis E85.0 *[G73.7]*
    cretinism E00.9 *[G73.7]*
    Cushing's syndrome E24.9 *[G73.7]*
    drugs G72.0
    endocrine disease NEC E34.9 *[G73.7]*
    giant cell arteritis M31.6 *[G73.7]*
    glycogen storage disease E74.00 *[G73.7]*
    hyperadrenocorticism E24.9 *[G73.7]*
    hyperparathyroidism NEC E21.3 *[G73.7]*
    hypoparathyroidism E20.9 *[G73.7]*
    hypopituitarism E23.0 *[G73.7]*
    hypothyroidism E03.9 *[G73.7]*
    infectious disease NEC B99 *[G73.7]*
    lipid storage disease E75.6 *[G73.7]*
    metabolic disease NEC E88.9 *[G73.7]*
    myxedema E03.9 *[G73.7]*
    parasitic disease NEC B89 *[G73.7]*
    polyarteritis nodosa M30.0 *[G73.7]*
    rheumatoid arthritis — *see* Rheumatoid,
     myopathy
    sarcoidosis D86.87
    scleroderma M34.82
    sicca syndrome M35.03
    Sjögren's syndrome M35.03
    systemic lupus erythematosus M32.19
    thyrotoxicosis (hyperthyroidism) E05.90
     [G73.7]
     with thyroid storm E05.91 *[G73.7]*
    toxic agent NEC G72.2
  inflammatory NEC G72.49
  intensive care (ICU) G72.81
  limb-girdle G71.09
  mitochondrial NEC G71.3
  mytonic, proximal (PROMM) G71.11
  myotubular G71.2
  nemaline G71.2
  ocular G71.09
  oculopharyngeal G71.09
  of critical illness G72.81
  primary G71.9
    specified NEC G71.8
  progressive NEC G72.89
  proximal myotonic (PROMM) G71.11
  rod G71.2
  scapulohumeral G71.02
  specified NEC G72.89
  toxic G72.2
Myopericarditis — *see also* Pericarditis
  chronic rheumatic I09.2
Myopia (axial) (congenital) H52.1-
  degenerative (malignant) H44.20
    with
     choroidal neovascularization H44.2A-
     foveoschisis H44.2D-
     macular hole H44.2B-
     retinal detachment H44.2C-
     specified maculopathy NEC H44.2E-
    bilateral H44.23
    left eye H44.22
    right eye H44.21
  malignant — *see also* Myopia,
    degenerative H44.2-
  pernicious — *see also* Myopia,
    degenerative H44.2-
  progressive high (degenerative) — *see also*
    Myopia, degenerative H44.2-
Myosarcoma — *see* Neoplasm, connective
  tissue, malignant
Myosis (pupil) H57.03
  stromal (endolymphatic) D39.0
Myositis M60.9
  clostridial A48.0
  due to posture — *see* Myositis, specified type
    NEC
  epidemic B33.0
  fibrosa or fibrous (chronic) ,
    Volkmann's T79.6

Myositis - *continued*
foreign body granuloma — *see* Granuloma,
 foreign body
 in (due to)
 bilharziasis B65.9 *[M63.8-]*
 cysticercosis B69.81
 leprosy A30.9 *[M63.8-]*
 mycosis B49 *[M63.8-]*
 sarcoidosis D86.87
 schistosomiasis B65.9 *[M63.8-]*
 syphilis
 late A52.78
 secondary A51.49
 toxoplasmosis (acquired) B58.82
 trichinellosis B75 *[M63.8-]*
 tuberculosis A18.09
 inclusion body [IBM] G72.41
 infective M60.009
 arm M60.002
 left M60.001
 right M60.000
 leg M60.005
 left M60.004
 right M60.003
 lower limb M60.005
 ankle M60.07-
 foot M60.07-
 lower leg M60.06-
 thigh M60.05-
 toe M60.07-
 multiple sites M60.09
 specified site NEC M60.08
 upper limb M60.002
 finger M60.04-
 forearm M60.03-
 hand M60.04-
 shoulder region M60.01-
 upper arm M60.02-
 interstitial M60.10
 ankle M60.17-
 foot M60.17-
 forearm M60.13-
 hand M60.14-
 lower leg M60.16-
 multiple sites M60.19
 shoulder region M60.11-
 specified site NEC M60.18
 thigh M60.15-
 upper arm M60.12-
 mycotic B49 *[M63.8-]*
 orbital, chronic H05.12-
 ossificans or ossifying (circumscripta) — *see*
 also Ossification, muscle, specified
 NEC
 in (due to)
 burns M61.30
 ankle M61.37-
 foot M61.37-
 forearm M61.33-
 hand M61.34-
 lower leg M61.36-
 multiple sites M61.39
 pelvic region M61.35-
 shoulder region M61.31-
 specified site NEC M61.38
 thigh M61.35-
 upper arm M61.32-
 quadriplegia or paraplegia M61.20
 ankle M61.27-
 foot M61.27-
 forearm M61.23-
 hand M61.24-
 lower leg M61.26-
 multiple sites M61.29
 pelvic region M61.25-
 shoulder region M61.21-
 specified site NEC M61.28
 thigh M61.25-
 upper arm M61.22-
 progressiva M61.10
 ankle M61.17-
 finger M61.14-
 foot M61.17-
 forearm M61.13-
 hand M61.14-

Myositis - *continued*
 ossificans or ossifying (circumscripta) -
 continued
 progressiva - *continued*
 lower leg M61.16-
 multiple sites M61.19
 pelvic region M61.15-
 shoulder region M61.11-
 specified site NEC M61.18
 thigh M61.15-
 toe M61.17-
 upper arm M61.12-
 traumatica M61.00
 ankle M61.07-
 foot M61.07-
 forearm M61.03-
 hand M61.04-
 lower leg M61.06-
 multiple sites M61.09
 pelvic region M61.05-
 shoulder region M61.01-
 specified site NEC M61.08
 thigh M61.05-
 upper arm M61.02-
 purulent — *see* Myositis, infective
 specified type NEC M60.80
 ankle M60.87-
 foot M60.87-
 forearm M60.83-
 hand M60.84-
 lower leg M60.86-
 multiple sites M60.89
 pelvic region M60.85-
 shoulder region M60.81-
 specified site NEC M60.88
 thigh M60.85-
 upper arm M60.82-
 suppurative — *see* Myositis, infective
 traumatic (old) — *see* Myositis, specified
 type NEC
Myospasia impulsiva F95.2
Myotonia (acquisita) (intermittens) M62.89
 atrophica G71.11
 chondrodystrophic G71.13
 congenita (acetazolamide responsive)
 (dominant) (recessive) G71.12
 drug-induced G71.14
 dystrophica G71.11
 fluctuans G71.19
 levior G71.12
 permanens G71.19
 symptomatic G71.19
Myotonic pupil — *see* Anomaly, pupil,
 function, tonic pupil
Myriapodiasis B88.2
Myringitis H73.2-
 with otitis media — *see* Otitis, media
 acute H73.00-
 bullous H73.01-
 specified NEC H73.09-
 bullous — *see* Myringitis, acute, bullous
 chronic H73.1-
Mysophobia F40.228
Mytilotoxism — *see* Poisoning, fish
Myxadenitis labialis K13.0
Myxedema (adult) (idiocy) (infantile)
 (juvenile) — *see also*
 Hypothyroidism E03.9
 circumscribed E05.90
 with storm E05.91
 coma E03.5
 congenital E00.1
 cutis L98.5
 localized (pretibial) E05.90
 with storm E05.91
 papular L98.5
Myxochondrosarcoma — *see* Neoplasm,
 cartilage, malignant
Myxofibroma — *see* Neoplasm, connective
 tissue, benign
 odontogenic — *see* Cyst, calcifying
 odontogenic
Myxofibrosarcoma — *see* Neoplasm,
 connective tissue, malignant
Myxolipoma D17.9

Myxoliposarcoma — *see* Neoplasm,
 connective tissue, malignant
Myxoma — *see also* Neoplasm, connective
 tissue, benign
 nerve sheath — *see* Neoplasm, nerve, benign
 odontogenic — *see* Cyst, calcifying
 odontogenic
Myxosarcoma — *see* Neoplasm, connective
 tissue, malignant

N

Naegeli's
 disease Q82.8
 leukemia, monocytic C93.1-
Naegleriasis (with
 meningoencephalitis) B60.2
Naffziger's syndrome G54.0
Naga sore — *see* Ulcer, skin
Nägele's pelvis M95.5
 with disproportion (fetopelvic) O33.0
 causing obstructed labor O65.0
Nail — *see also* condition
 biting F98.8
 patella syndrome Q87.2
Nanism, nanosomia — *see* Dwarfism
Nanophyetiasis B66.8
Nanukayami A27.89
Napkin rash L22
Narcolepsy G47.419
 with cataplexy G47.411
 in conditions classified elsewhere G47.429
 with cataplexy G47.421
Narcosis R06.89
Narcotism — *see* Dependence
NARP (Neuropathy, Ataxia and Retinitis
 pigmentosa) syndrome E88.49
Narrow
 anterior chamber angle H40.03-
 gingival width (of periodontal soft
 tissue) K05.5
 pelvis — *see* Contraction, pelvis
Narrowing — *see also* Stenosis
 artery I77.1
 auditory, internal I65.8
 basilar — *see* Occlusion, artery, basilar
 carotid — *see* Occlusion, artery, carotid
 cerebellar — *see* Occlusion, artery,
 cerebellar
 cerebral — *see* Occlusion artery, cerebral
 choroidal — *see* Occlusion, artery,
 precerebral, specified NEC
 communicating posterior — *see* Occlusion,
 artery, precerebral, specified NEC
 coronary — *see also* Disease, heart,
 ischemic, atherosclerotic
 congenital Q24.5
 syphilitic A50.54 *[I52]*
 due to syphilis NEC A52.06
 hypophyseal — *see* Occlusion, artery,
 precerebral, specified NEC
 pontine — *see* Occlusion, artery,
 precerebral, specified NEC
 precerebral — *see* Occlusion, artery,
 precerebral
 vertebral — *see* Occlusion, artery,
 vertebral
 auditory canal (external) — *see* Stenosis,
 external ear canal
 eustachian tube — *see* Obstruction,
 eustachian tube
 eyelid — *see* Disorder, eyelid function
 larynx J38.6
 mesenteric artery — *see also* Ischemia,
 intestine, acute K55.059
 palate M26.89
 palpebral fissure — *see* Disorder, eyelid
 function
 ureter N13.5
 with infection N13.6
 urethra — *see* Stricture, urethra
Narrowness, abnormal, eyelid Q10.3
Nasal — *see* condition
Nasolachrymal, nasolacrimal — *see*
 condition
Nasopharyngeal — *see also* condition
 pituitary gland Q89.2

Nasopharyngeal - *continued*
torticollis M43.6
Nasopharyngitis (acute) (infective)
(streptococcal) (subacute) J00
chronic (suppurative) (ulcerative) J31.1
Nasopharynx, nasopharyngeal — *see*
condition
Natal tooth, teeth K00.6
Nausea (without vomiting) R11.0
with vomiting R11.2
gravidarum — *see* Hyperemesis, gravidarum
marina T75.3
navalis T75.3
Navel — *see* condition
Neapolitan fever — *see* Brucellosis
Near drowning T75.1
Nearsightedness — *see* Myopia
Near-syncope R55
Nebula, cornea — *see* Opacity, cornea
Necator americanus infestation B76.1
Necatoriasis B76.1
Neck — *see* condition
Necrobiosis R68.89
lipoidica NEC L92.1
with diabetes — *see* E08-E13 with .620
Necrolysis, toxic epidermal L51.2
due to drug
correct substance properly
administered — *see* Table of Drugs
and Chemicals, by drug, adverse
effect
overdose or wrong substance given or
taken — *see* Table of Drugs and
Chemicals, by drug, poisoning
Necrophilia F65.89
Necrosis, necrotic (ischemic) — *see also*
Gangrene
adrenal (capsule) (gland) E27.49
amputation stump (surgical) (late) T87.50
arm T87.5-
leg T87.5-
antrum J32.0
aorta (hyaline) — *see also* Aneurysm, aorta
cystic medial — *see* Dissection, aorta
artery I77.5
bladder (aseptic) (sphincter) N32.89
bone — *see also* Osteonecrosis M87.9
aseptic or avascular — *see* Osteonecrosis
idiopathic M87.00
ethmoid J32.2
jaw M27.2
tuberculous — *see* Tuberculosis, bone
brain I67.89
breast (aseptic) (fat) (segmental) N64.1
bronchus J98.09
central nervous system NEC I67.89
cerebellar I67.89
cerebral I67.89
colon — *see also* Infarct, intestine K55.049
cornea H18.89-
cortical (acute) (renal) N17.1
cystic medial (aorta) — *see* Dissection, aorta
dental pulp K04.1
esophagus K22.8
ethmoid (bone) J32.2
eyelid — *see* Disorder, eyelid, degenerative
fat, fatty (generalized) — *see also* Disorder,
soft tissue, specified type NEC
abdominal wall K65.4
breast (aseptic) (segmental) N64.1
localized — *see* Degeneration, by site,
fatty
mesentery K65.4
omentum K65.4
pancreas K86.89
peritoneum K65.4
skin (subcutaneous) , newborn P83.0
subcutaneous, due to birth injury P15.6
gallbladder — *see* Cholecystitis, acute
heart — *see* Infarct, myocardium
hip, aseptic or avascular — *see*
Osteonecrosis, by type, femur
intestine (acute) (hemorrhagic) (massive) —
see also Infarct, intestine K55.069
jaw M27.2

Necrosis, necrotic (ischemic) - *continued*
kidney (bilateral) N28.0
acute N17.9
cortical (acute) (bilateral) N17.1
with ectopic or molar pregnancy O08.4
medullary (bilateral) (in acute renal
failure) (papillary) N17.2
papillary (bilateral) (in acute renal
failure) N17.2
tubular N17.0
with ectopic or molar pregnancy O08.4
complicating
abortion — *see* Abortion, by type,
complicated by, tubular necrosis
ectopic or molar pregnancy O08.4
pregnancy — *see* Pregnancy,
complicated by, diseases of,
specified type or system NEC
following ectopic or molar
pregnancy O08.4
traumatic T79.5
larynx J38.7
liver (with hepatic failure) (cell) — *see*
Failure, hepatic
hemorrhagic, central K76.2
lung J85.0
lymphatic gland — *see* Lymphadenitis, acute
mammary gland (fat) (segmental) N64.1
mastoid (chronic) — *see* Mastoiditis, chronic
medullary (acute) (renal) N17.2
mesentery — *see also* Infarct,
intestine K55.069
fat K65.4
mitral valve — *see* Insufficiency, mitral
myocardium, myocardial — *see* Infarct,
myocardium
nose J34.0
omentum (with mesenteric infarction) — *see
also* Infarct, intestine K55.069
fat K65.4
orbit, orbital — *see* Osteomyelitis, orbit
ossicles, ear — *see* Abnormal, ear ossicles
ovary (N70.92
pancreas (aseptic) (duct) (fat) K86.89
acute (infective) — *see* Pancreatitis, acute
infective — *see* Pancreatitis, acute
papillary (acute) (renal) N17.2
perineum N90.89
peritoneum (with mesenteric infarction) —
see also Infarct, intestine K55.069
fat K65.4
pharynx J02.9
in granulocytopenia — *see* Neutropenia
Vincent's A69.1
phosphorus — *see* subcategory T54.2
pituitary (gland) E23.0
postpartum O99.285
Sheehan O99.285
pressure — *see* Ulcer, pressure, by site
pulmonary J85.0
pulp (dental) K04.1
radiation — *see* Necrosis, by site
radium — *see* Necrosis, by site
renal — *see* Necrosis, kidney
sclera H15.89
scrotum N50.89
skin or subcutaneous tissue NEC I96
spine, spinal (column) — *see also*
Osteonecrosis, by type, vertebra
cord G95.19
spleen D73.5
stomach K31.89
stomatitis (ulcerative) A69.0
subcutaneous fat, newborn P83.88
subendocardial (acute) I21.4
chronic I25.89
suprarenal (capsule) (gland) E27.49
testis N50.89
thymus (gland) E32.8
tonsil J35.8
trachea J39.8
tuberculous NEC — *see* Tuberculosis
tubular (acute) (anoxic) (renal) (toxic) N17.0
postprocedural N99.0
vagina N89.8

Necrosis, necrotic (ischemic) - *continued*
vertebra — *see also* Osteonecrosis, by type,
vertebra
tuberculous A18.01
vulva N90.89
X-ray — *see* Necrosis, by site
Necrospermia — *see* Infertility, male
Need (for)
care provider because (of)
assistance with personal care Z74.1
continuous supervision required Z74.3
impaired mobility Z74.09
no other household member able to render
care Z74.2
specified reason NEC Z74.8
immunization — *see* Vaccination
vaccination — *see* Vaccination
Neglect
adult
confirmed T74.01
history of Z91.412
suspected T76.01
child (childhood)
confirmed T74.02
history of Z62.812
suspected T76.02
emotional, in childhood Z62.898
hemispatial R41.4
left-sided R41.4
sensory R41.4
visuospatial R41.4
Neisserian infection NEC — *see* Gonococcus
Nelaton's syndrome G60.8
Nelson's syndrome E24.1
Nematodiasis (intestinal) B82.0
Ancylostoma B76.0
Neonatal — *see also* Newborn
acne L70.4
bradycardia P29.12
tachycardia P29.11
screening, abnormal findings on P09
tooth, teeth K00.6
Neonatorum — *see* condition
Neoplasia
endocrine, multiple (MEN) E31.20
type I E31.21
type IIA E31.22
type IIB E31.23
intraepithelial (histologically confirmed)
anal (AIN) (histologically
confirmed) K62.82
grade I K62.82
grade II K62.82
severe D01.3
cervical glandular (histologically
confirmed) D06.9
cervix (uteri) (CIN) (histologically
confirmed) N87.9
glandular D06.9
grade I N87.0
grade II N87.1
grade III (severe dysplasia) — *see also*
Carcinoma, cervix uteri, in
situ D06.9
prostate (histologically confirmed)
(PIN) N42.31
grade I N42.31
grade II N42.31
grade III (severe dysplasia) D07.5
vagina (histologically confirmed)
(VAIN) N89.3
grade I N89.0
grade II N89.1
grade III (severe dysplasia) D07.2
vulva (histologically confirmed)
(VIN) N90.3
grade I N90.0
grade II N90.1
grade III (severe dysplasia) D07.1
Neoplasm, neoplastic — *see also* Table of
Neoplasms
lipomatous, benign — *see* Lipoma
malignant mast cell C96.20
specified type NEC C96.29
mast cell, of uncertain behavior NEC D47.09

Neovascularization
  ciliary body — *see* Disorder, iris, vascular
  cornea H16.40-
    deep H16.44-
    ghost vessels — *see* Ghost, vessels
    localized H16.43-
    pannus — *see* Pannus
  iris — *see* Disorder, iris, vascular
  retina H35.05-
Nephralgia N23
Nephritis, nephritic (albuminuric)
    (azotemic) (congenital) (disseminated)
    (epithelial) (familial) (focal)
    (granulomatous) (hemorrhagic)
    (infantile) (nonsuppurative, excretory)
    (uremic) N05.9
  with
    dense deposit disease N05.6
    diffuse
      crescentic glomerulonephritis N05.7
      endocapillary proliferative
        glomerulonephritis N05.4
      membranous glomerulonephritis N05.2
      mesangial proliferative
        glomerulonephritis N05.3
      mesangiocapillary
        glomerulonephritis N05.5
    edema — *see* Nephrosis
    focal and segmental glomerular
      lesions N05.1
    foot process disease N04.9
    glomerular lesion
      diffuse sclerosing N05.8
      hypocomplementemic — *see* Nephritis,
        membranoproliferative
      IgA — *see* Nephropathy, IgA
      lobular, lobulonodular — *see* Nephritis,
        membranoproliferative
      nodular — *see* Nephritis,
        membranoproliferative
    lesion of
      glomerulonephritis, proliferative N05.8
    renal necrosis N05.9
    minor glomerular abnormality N05.0
    specified morphological changes
      NEC N05.8
  acute N00.9
    with
      dense deposit disease N00.6
      diffuse
        crescentic glomerulonephritis N00.7
        endocapillary proliferative
          glomerulonephritis N00.4
        membranous
          glomerulonephritis N00.2
        mesangial proliferative
          glomerulonephritis N00.3
        mesangiocapillary
          glomerulonephritis N00.5
      focal and segmental glomerular
        lesions N00.1
      minor glomerular abnormality N00.0
      specified morphological changes
        NEC N00.8
  amyloid E85.4 *[N08]*
  antiglomerular basement membrane (anti-
    GBM) antibody NEC
    in Goodpasture's syndrome M31.0
  antitubular basement membrane (tubulo-
    interstitial) NEC N12
  toxic — *see* Nephropathy, toxic
  arteriolar — *see* Hypertension, kidney
  arteriosclerotic — *see* Hypertension, kidney
  ascending — *see* Nephritis, tubulo-interstitial
  atrophic N03.9
  Balkan (endemic) N15.0
  calculous, calculus — *see* Calculus, kidney
  cardiac — *see* Hypertension, kidney
  cardiovascular — *see* Hypertension, kidney
  chronic N03.9
    with
      dense deposit disease N03.6
      diffuse
        crescentic glomerulonephritis N03.7

Nephritis, nephritic (albuminuric)
    (azotemic) (congenital) (disseminated)
    (epithelial) (familial) (focal) (granulomatous)
    (hemorrhagic) (infantile) (nonsuppurative,
    excretory) (uremic) - *continued*
  chronic - *continued*
    with - *continued*
      diffuse - *continued*
        endocapillary proliferative
          glomerulonephritis N03.4
        membranous
          glomerulonephritis N03.2
        mesangial proliferative
          glomerulonephritis N03.3
        mesangiocapillary
          glomerulonephritis N03.5
      focal and segmental glomerular
        lesions N03.1
      minor glomerular abnormality N03.0
      specified morphological changes
        NEC N03.8
  arteriosclerotic — *see* Hypertension,
    kidney
  cirrhotic N26.9
  complicating pregnancy O26.83-
  croupous N00.9
  degenerative — *see* Nephrosis
  diffuse sclerosing N05.8
  due to
    diabetes mellitus — *see* E08-E13 with .21
    subacute bacterial endocarditis I33.0
    systemic lupus erythematosus
      (chronic) M32.14
    typhoid fever A01.09
  gonococcal (acute) (chronic) A54.21
  hypocomplementemic — *see* Nephritis,
    membranoproliferative
  IgA — *see* Nephropathy, IgA
  immune complex (circulating) NEC N05.8
  infective — *see* Nephritis, tubulo-interstitial
  interstitial — *see* Nephritis, tubulo-interstitial
  lead N14.3
  membranoproliferative (diffuse) (type 1 or
    3) — *see also* N00-N07 with fourth
    character .5 N05.5
    type 2 — *see also* N00-N07 with fourth
      character .6 N05.6
  minimal change N05.0
  necrotic, necrotizing NEC — *see also* N00-
    N07 with fourth character .8 N05.8
  nephrotic — *see* Nephrosis
  nodular — *see* Nephritis,
    membranoproliferative
  polycystic Q61.3
    adult type Q61.2
    autosomal
      dominant Q61.2
      recessive NEC Q61.19
    childhood type NEC Q61.19
    infantile type NEC Q61.19
  poststreptococcal N05.9
    acute N00.9
    chronic N03.9
    rapidly progressive N01.9
  proliferative NEC — *see also* N00-N07 with
    fourth character .8 N05.8
  purulent — *see* Nephritis, tubulo-interstitial
  rapidly progressive N01.9
    with
      dense deposit disease N01.6
      diffuse
        crescentic glomerulonephritis N01.7
        endocapillary proliferative
          glomerulonephritis N01.4
        membranous
          glomerulonephritis N01.2
        mesangial proliferative
          glomerulonephritis N01.3
        mesangiocapillary
          glomerulonephritis N01.5
      focal and segmental glomerular
        lesions N01.1
      minor glomerular abnormality N01.0
      specified morphological changes
        NEC N01.8

Nephritis, nephritic (albuminuric)
    (azotemic) (congenital) (disseminated)
    (epithelial) (familial) (focal) (granulomatous)
    (hemorrhagic) (infantile) (nonsuppurative,
    excretory) (uremic) - *continued*
  salt losing or wasting NEC N28.89
  saturnine N14.3
  sclerosing, diffuse N05.8
  septic — *see* Nephritis, tubulo-interstitial
  specified pathology NEC — *see also* N00-
    N07 with fourth character .8 N05.8
  subacute N01.9
  suppurative — *see* Nephritis, tubulo-
    interstitial
  syphilitic (late) A52.75
    congenital A50.59 *[N08]*
    early (secondary) A51.44
  toxic — *see* Nephropathy, toxic
  tubal, tubular — *see* Nephritis, tubulo-
    interstitial
  tuberculous A18.11
  tubulo-interstitial (in) N12
    acute (infectious) N10
    chronic (infectious) N11.9
      nonobstructive N11.8
        reflux-associated N11.0
      obstructive N11.1
      specified NEC N11.8
    due to
      brucellosis A23.9 *[N16]*
      cryoglobulinemia D89.1 *[N16]*
      glycogen storage disease E74.00 *[N16]*
    Sjögren's syndrome M35.04
  vascular — *see* Hypertension, kidney
  war N00.9
Nephroblastoma (epithelial)
    (mesenchymal) C64-
Nephrocalcinosis E83.59 *[N29]*
Nephrocystitis, pustular — *see* Nephritis,
    tubulo-interstitial
Nephrolithiasis (congenital) (pelvis)
    (recurrent) — *see also* Calculus, kidney
Nephroma C64-
  mesoblastic D41.0-
Nephronephritis — *see* Nephrosis
Nephronophthisis Q61.5
Nephropathia epidemica A98.5
Nephropathy — *see also* Nephritis N28.9
  with
    edema — *see* Nephrosis
    glomerular lesion — *see*
      Glomerulonephritis
  amyloid, hereditary E85.0
  analgesic N14.0
    with medullary necrosis, acute N17.2
  Balkan (endemic) N15.0
  chemical — *see* Nephropathy, toxic
  diabetic — *see* E08-E13 with .21
  drug-induced N14.2
    specified NEC N14.1
  focal and segmental hyalinosis or
    sclerosis N02.1
  heavy metal-induced N14.3
  hereditary NEC N07.9
    with
      dense deposit disease N07.6
      diffuse
        crescentic glomerulonephritis N07.7
        endocapillary proliferative
          glomerulonephritis N07.4
        membranous
          glomerulonephritis N07.2
        mesangial proliferative
          glomerulonephritis N07.3
        mesangiocapillary
          glomerulonephritis N07.5
      focal and segmental glomerular
        lesions N07.1
      minor glomerular abnormality N07.0
      specified morphological changes
        NEC N07.8
  hypercalcemic N25.89
  hypertensive — *see* Hypertension, kidney
  hypokalemic (vacuolar) N25.89
  IgA N02.8

Nephropathy - *continued*
  IgA - *continued*
    with glomerular lesion N02.9
      focal and segmental hyalinosis or
        sclerosis N02.1
      membranoproliferative (diffuse) N02.5
      membranous (diffuse) N02.2
      mesangial proliferative (diffuse) N02.3
      mesangiocapillary (diffuse) N02.5
      proliferative NEC N02.8
      specified pathology NEC N02.8
  lead N14.3
  membranoproliferative (diffuse) N02.5
  membranous (diffuse) N02.2
  mesangial (IgA/IgG) — *see* Nephropathy, IgA
    proliferative (diffuse) N02.3
  mesangiocapillary (diffuse) N02.5
  obstructive N13.8
  phenacetin N17.2
  phosphate-losing N25.0
  potassium depletion N25.89
  pregnancy-related O26.83-
  proliferative NEC — *see also* N00-N07 with fourth character .8 N05.8
  protein-losing N25.89
  saturnine N14.3
  sickle-cell D57.- *[N08]*
  toxic NEC N14.4
    due to
      drugs N14.2
        analgesic N14.0
        specified NEC N14.1
      heavy metals N14.3
  vasomotor N17.0
  water-losing N25.89
Nephroptosis N28.83
Nephropyosis — *see* Abscess, kidney
Nephrorrhagia N28.89
Nephrosclerosis (arteriolar) (arteriosclerotic) (chronic) (hyaline) — *see also* Hypertension, kidney
  hyperplastic — *see* Hypertension, kidney
  senile N26.9
Nephrosis, nephrotic (Epstein's) (syndrome) (congenital) N04.9
  with
    foot process disease N04.9
    glomerular lesion N04.1
    hypocomplementemic N04.5
  acute N04.9
  anoxic — *see* Nephrosis, tubular
  chemical — *see* Nephrosis, tubular
  cholemic K76.7
  diabetic — *see* E08-E13 with .21
  Finnish type (congenital) Q89.8
  hemoglobin N10
  hemoglobinuric — *see* Nephrosis, tubular
  in
    amyloidosis E85.4 *[N08]*
    diabetes mellitus — *see* E08-E13 with .21
    epidemic hemorrhagic fever A98.5
    malaria (malariae) B52.0
  ischemic — *see* Nephrosis, tubular
  lipoid N04.9
  lower nephron — *see* Nephrosis, tubular
  malarial (malariae) B52.0
  minimal change N04.0
  myoglobin N10
  necrotizing — *see* Nephrosis, tubular
  osmotic (sucrose) N25.89
  radiation N04.9
  syphilitic (late) A52.75
  toxic — *see* Nephrosis, tubular
  tubular (acute) N17.0
    postprocedural N99.0
    radiation N04.9
Nephrosonephritis, hemorrhagic (endemic) A98.5
Nephrostomy
  attention to Z43.6
  status Z93.6
Nerve — *see also* condition
  injury — *see* Injury, nerve, by body site
Nerves R45.0

Nervous — *see also* condition R45.0
  heart F45.8
  stomach F45.8
  tension R45.0
Nervousness R45.0
Nesidioblastoma
  pancreas D13.7
  specified site NEC — *see* Neoplasm, benign, by site
  unspecified site D13.7
Nettleship's syndrome — *see* Urticaria pigmentosa
Neumann's disease or syndrome L10.1
Neuralgia, neuralgic (acute) M79.2
  accessory (nerve) G52.8
  acoustic (nerve) — *see* subcategory H93.3
  auditory (nerve) — *see* subcategory H93.3
  ciliary G44.009
    intractable G44.001
    not intractable G44.009
  cranial
    nerve — *see also* Disorder, nerve, cranial
      fifth or trigeminal — *see* Neuralgia, trigeminal
    postherpetic, postzoster B02.29
  ear — *see* subcategory H92.0
  facialis vera G51.1
  Fothergill's — *see* Neuralgia, trigeminal
  glossopharyngeal (nerve) G52.1
  Horton's G44.099
    intractable G44.091
    not intractable G44.099
  Hunt's B02.21
  hypoglossal (nerve) G52.3
  infraorbital — *see* Neuralgia, trigeminal
  malarial — *see* Malaria
  migrainous G44.009
    intractable G44.001
    not intractable G44.009
  Morton's G57.6-
  nerve, cranial — *see* Disorder, nerve, cranial
  nose G52.0
  occipital M54.81
  olfactory G52.0
  penis N48.9
  perineum R10.2
  postherpetic NEC B02.29
    trigeminal B02.22
  pubic region R10.2
  scrotum R10.2
  Sluder's G44.89
  specified nerve NEC G58.8
  spermatic cord R10.2
  sphenopalatine (ganglion) G90.09
  trifacial — *see* Neuralgia, trigeminal
  trigeminal G50.0
    postherpetic, postzoster B02.22
  vagus (nerve) G52.2
  writer's F48.8
    organic G25.89
Neurapraxia — *see* Injury, nerve
Neurasthenia F48.8
  cardiac F45.8
  gastric F45.8
  heart F45.8
Neurilemmoma — *see also* Neoplasm, nerve, benign
  acoustic (nerve) D33.3
  malignant — *see also* Neoplasm, nerve, malignant
    acoustic (nerve) C72.4-
Neurilemmosarcoma — *see* Neoplasm, nerve, malignant
Neurinoma — *see* Neoplasm, nerve, benign
Neurinomatosis — *see* Neoplasm, nerve, uncertain behavior
Neuritis (rheumatoid) M79.2
  abducens (nerve) — *see* Strabismus, paralytic, sixth nerve
  accessory (nerve) G52.8
  acoustic (nerve) (*see also* subcategory H93.3)
    in (due to)
      infectious disease NEC B99 *[H94.0-]*
      parasitic disease NEC B89 *[H94.0-]*
      syphilitic A52.15

Neuritis (rheumatoid) - *continued*
  alcoholic G62.1
    with psychosis — *see* Psychosis, alcoholic
  amyloid, any site E85.4 *[G63]*
  auditory (nerve) — *see* subcategory H93.3
  brachial — *see* Radiculopathy
    due to displacement, intervertebral disc — *see* Disorder, disc, cervical, with neuritis
  cranial nerve
    due to Lyme disease A69.22
    eighth or acoustic or auditory — *see* subcategory H93.3
    eleventh or accessory G52.8
    fifth or trigeminal G51.0
    first or olfactory G52.0
    fourth or trochlear — *see* Strabismus, paralytic, fourth nerve
    second or optic — *see* Neuritis, optic
    seventh or facial G51.8
      newborn (birth injury) P11.3
    sixth or abducent — *see* Strabismus, paralytic, sixth nerve
    tenth or vagus G52.2
    third or oculomotor — *see* Strabismus, paralytic, third nerve
    twelfth or hypoglossal G52.3
  Déjérine-Sottas G60.0
  diabetic (mononeuropathy) — *see* E08-E13 with .41
    polyneuropathy — *see* E08-E13 with .42
  due to
    beriberi E51.11
    displacement, prolapse or rupture, intervertebral disc — *see* Disorder, disc, with, radiculopathy
    herniation, nucleus pulposus M51.9 *[G55]*
  endemic E51.11
  facial G51.8
    newborn (birth injury) P11.3
  general — *see* Polyneuropathy
  geniculate ganglion G51.1
    due to herpes (zoster) B02.21
  gouty — *see also* Gout, by type M10.9 *[G63]*
  hypoglossal (nerve) G52.3
  ilioinguinal (nerve) G57.9-
  infectious (multiple) NEC G61.0
  interstitial hypertrophic progressive G60.0
  lumbar M54.16
  lumbosacral M54.17
  multiple — *see also* Polyneuropathy
    endemic E51.11
    infective, acute G61.0
  multiplex endemica E51.11
  nerve root — *see* Radiculopathy
  oculomotor (nerve) — *see* Strabismus, paralytic, third nerve
  olfactory nerve G52.0
  optic (nerve) (hereditary) (sympathetic) H46.9
    with demyelination G36.0
    in myelitis G36.0
    nutritional H46.2
    papillitis — *see* Papillitis, optic
    retrobulbar H46.1-
    specified type NEC H46.8
    toxic H46.3
  peripheral (nerve) G62.9
    multiple — *see* Polyneuropathy
    single — *see* Mononeuritis
  pneumogastric (nerve) G52.2
  postherpetic, postzoster B02.29
  progressive hypertrophic interstitial G60.0
  retrobulbar — *see also* Neuritis, optic, retrobulbar
  in (due to)
    late syphilis A52.15
    meningococcal infection A39.82
    meningococcal A39.82
    syphilitic A52.15
  sciatic (nerve) — *see also* Sciatica
    due to displacement of intervertebral disc — *see* Disorder, disc, with, radiculopathy

Neuritis (rheumatoid) - *continued*
  serum — *see also* Reaction, serum T80.69
  shoulder-girdle G54.5
  specified nerve NEC G58.8
  spinal (nerve) root — *see* Radiculopathy
  syphilitic A52.15
  thenar (median) G56.1-
  thoracic M54.14
  toxic NEC G62.2
  trochlear (nerve) — *see* Strabismus,
    paralytic, fourth nerve
  vagus (nerve) G52.2
Neuroastrocytoma — *see* Neoplasm,
    uncertain behavior, by site
Neuroavitaminosis E56.9 *[G99.8]*
Neuroblastoma
  olfactory C30.0
  specified site — *see* Neoplasm, malignant,
    by site
  unspecified site C74.90
Neurochorioretinitis — *see* Chorioretinitis
Neurocirculatory asthenia F45.8
Neurocysticercosis B69.0
Neurocytoma — *see* Neoplasm, benign, by
    site
Neurodermatitis (circumscribed)
    (circumscripta) (local) L28.0
  atopic L20.81
  diffuse (Brocq) L20.81
  disseminated L20.81
Neuroencephalomyelopathy, optic G36.0
Neuroepithelioma — *see also* Neoplasm,
    malignant, by site
  olfactory C30.0
Neurofibroma — *see also* Neoplasm, nerve,
    benign
  melanotic — *see* Neoplasm, nerve, benign
  multiple — *see* Neurofibromatosis
  plexiform — *see* Neoplasm, nerve, benign
Neurofibromatosis (multiple)
    (nonmalignant) Q85.00
  acoustic Q85.02
  malignant — *see* Neoplasm, nerve,
    malignant
  specified NEC Q85.09
  type 1 (von Recklinghausen) Q85.01
  type 2 Q85.02
Neurofibrosarcoma — *see* Neoplasm, nerve,
    malignant
Neurogenic — *see also* condition
  bladder — *see also* Dysfunction, bladder,
    neuromuscular N31.9
    cauda equina syndrome G83.4
  bowel NEC K59.2
  heart F45.8
Neuroglioma — *see* Neoplasm, uncertain
    behavior, by site
Neurolabyrinthitis (of Dix and
    Hallpike) — *see* Neuronitis, vestibular
Neurolathyrism — *see* Poisoning, food,
    noxious, plant
Neuroleprosy A30.9
Neuroma — *see also* Neoplasm, nerve, benign
  acoustic (nerve) D33.3
  amputation (stump) (traumatic) (surgical
    complication) (late) T87.3-
    arm T87.3-
    leg T87.3-
  digital (toe) G57.6-
  interdigital G58.8
    lower limb (toe) G57.8-
    upper limb G56.8-
  intermetatarsal G57.8-
  Morton's G57.6-
  nonneoplastic
    arm G56.9-
    leg G57.9-
    lower extremity G57.9-
    upper extremity G56.9-
  optic (nerve) D33.3
  plantar G57.6-
  plexiform — *see* Neoplasm, nerve, benign
  surgical (nonneoplastic)
    arm G56.9-
    leg G57.9-

Neuroma - *continued*
  surgical (nonneoplastic) - *continued*
    lower extremity G57.9-
    upper extremity G56.9-
Neuromyalgia — *see* Neuralgia
Neuromyasthenia (epidemic)
    (postinfectious) G93.3
Neuromyelitis G36.9
  ascending G61.0
  optica G36.0
Neuromyopathy G70.9
  paraneoplastic D49.9 *[G13.0]*
Neuromyotonia (Isaacs) G71.19
Neuronevus — *see* Nevus
Neuronitis G58.9
  ascending (acute) G57.2-
  vestibular H81.2-
Neuroparalytic — *see* condition
Neuropathy, neuropathic G62.9
  acute motor G62.81
  alcoholic G62.1
    with psychosis — *see* Psychosis, alcoholic
  arm G56.9-
  autonomic, peripheral — *see* Neuropathy,
    peripheral, autonomic
  axillary G56.9-
  bladder N31.9
    atonic (motor) (sensory) N31.2
    autonomous N31.2
    flaccid N31.2
    nonreflex N31.2
    reflex N31.1
    uninhibited N31.0
  brachial plexus G54.0
  cervical plexus G54.2
  chronic
    progressive segmentally
      demyelinating G62.89
    relapsing demyelinating G62.89
  Déjérine-Sottas G60.0
  diabetic — *see* E08-E13 with .40
    mononeuropathy — *see* E08-E13 with .41
    polyneuropathy — *see* E08-E13 with .42
  entrapment G58.9
    iliohypogastric nerve G57.8-
    ilioinguinal nerve G57.8-
    lateral cutaneous nerve of thigh G57.1-
    median nerve G56.0-
    obturator nerve G57.8-
    peroneal nerve G57.3-
    posterior tibial nerve G57.5-
    saphenous nerve G57.8-
    ulnar nerve G56.2-
  facial nerve G51.9
  hereditary G60.9
    motor and sensory (types I-IV) G60.0
    sensory G60.8
    specified NEC G60.8
  hypertrophic G60.0
    Charcot-Marie-Tooth G60.0
    Déjérine-Sottas G60.0
    interstitial progressive G60.0
    of infancy G60.0
    Refsum G60.1
  idiopathic G60.9
    progressive G60.3
    specified NEC G60.8
  in association with hereditary ataxia G60.2
  intercostal G58.0
  ischemic — *see* Disorder, nerve
  Jamaica (ginger) G62.2
  leg NEC G57.9-
  lower extremity G57.9-
  lumbar plexus G54.1
  median nerve G56.1-
  motor and sensory — *see also*
    Polyneuropathy
    hereditary (types I-IV) G60.0
  multifocal motor (MMN) G61.82
  multiple (acute) (chronic) — *see*
    Polyneuropathy
  optic (nerve) — *see also* Neuritis, optic
    ischemic H47.01-
  paraneoplastic (sensorial) (Denny
    Brown) D49.9 *[G13.0]*

Neuropathy, neuropathic - *continued*
  peripheral (nerve) — *see also*
    Polyneuropathy G62.9
  autonomic G90.9
    idiopathic G90.09
    in (due to)
      amyloidosis E85.4 *[G99.0]*
      diabetes mellitus — *see* E08-E13 with
        .43
      endocrine disease NEC E34.9 *[G99.0]*
      gout M10.00 *[G99.0]*
      hyperthyroidism E05.90 *[G99.0]*
        with thyroid storm E05.91 *[G99.0]*
      metabolic disease NEC E88.9 *[G99.0]*
  idiopathic G60.9
    progressive G60.3
  in (due to)
    antitetanus serum G62.0
    arsenic G62.2
    drugs NEC G62.0
    lead G62.2
    organophosphate compounds G62.2
    toxic agent NEC G62.2
  plantar nerves G57.6-
  progressive
    hypertrophic interstitial G60.0
    inflammatory G62.81
  radicular NEC — *see* Radiculopathy
  sacral plexus G54.1
  sciatic G57.0-
  serum G61.1
  toxic NEC G62.2
  trigeminal sensory G50.8
  ulnar nerve G56.2-
  uremic N18.9 *[G63]*
  vitamin B12 E53.8 *[G63]*
    with anemia (pernicious) D51.0 *[G63]*
    due to dietary deficiency D51.3 *[G63]*
Neurophthisis — *see also* Disorder, nerve
  peripheral, diabetic — *see* E08-E13 with .42
Neuroretinitis — *see* Chorioretinitis
Neuroretinopathy, hereditary optic H47.22
Neurosarcoma — *see* Neoplasm, nerve,
    malignant
Neurosclerosis — *see* Disorder, nerve
Neurosis, neurotic F48.9
  anankastic F42.8
  anxiety (state) F41.1
    panic type F41.0
  asthenic F48.8
  bladder F45.8
  cardiac (reflex) F45.8
  cardiovascular F45.8
  character F60.9
  colon F45.8
  compensation F68.10
  compulsive, compulsion F42.8
  conversion F44.9
  craft F48.8
  cutaneous F45.8
  depersonalization F48.1
  depressive (reaction) (type) F34.1
  environmental F48.8
  excoriation L98.1
  fatigue F48.8
  functional — *see* Disorder, somatoform
  gastric F45.8
  gastrointestinal F45.8
  heart F45.8
  hypochondriacal F45.21
  hysterical F44.9
  incoordination F45.8
    larynx F45.8
    vocal cord F45.8
  intestine F45.8
  larynx (sensory) F45.8
    hysterical F44.4
  mixed NEC F48.8
  musculoskeletal F45.8
  obsessional F42.8
  obsessive-compulsive F42.8
  occupational F48.8
  ocular NEC F45.8
  organ — *see* Disorder, somatoform
  pharynx F45.8

Neurosis, neurotic - *continued*
  phobic F40.9
  posttraumatic (situational) F43.10
    acute F43.11
    chronic F43.12
  psychasthenic (type) F48.8
  railroad F48.8
  rectum F45.8
  respiratory F45.8
  rumination F45.8
  sexual F65.9
  situational F48.8
  social F40.10
    generalized F40.11
  specified type NEC F48.8
  state F48.9
    with depersonalization episode F48.1
  stomach F45.8
  traumatic F43.10
    acute F43.11
    chronic F43.12
  vasomotor F45.8
  visceral F45.8
  war F48.8
Neurospongioblastosis diffusa Q85.1
Neurosyphilis (arrested) (early) (gumma) (late) (latent) (recurrent) (relapse) A52.3
  with ataxia (cerebellar) (locomotor) (spastic) (spinal) A52.19
  aneurysm (cerebral) A52.05
  arachnoid (adhesive) A52.13
  arteritis (any artery) (cerebral) A52.04
  asymptomatic A52.2
  congenital A50.40
  dura (mater) A52.13
  general paresis A52.17
  hemorrhagic A52.05
  juvenile (asymptomatic) (meningeal) A50.40
  leptomeninges (aseptic) A52.13
  meningeal, meninges (adhesive) A52.13
  meningitis A52.13
  meningovascular (diffuse) A52.13
  optic atrophy A52.15
  parenchymatous (degenerative) A52.19
  paresis, paretic A52.17
    juvenile A50.45
  remission in (sustained) A52.3
  serological (without symptoms) A52.2
  specified nature or site NEC A52.19
  tabes, tabetic (dorsalis) A52.11
    juvenile A50.45
  taboparesis A52.17
    juvenile A50.45
  thrombosis (cerebral) A52.05
  vascular (cerebral) NEC A52.05
Neurothekeoma — *see* Neoplasm, nerve, benign
Neurotic — *see* Neurosis
Neurotoxemia — *see* Toxemia
Neutroclusion M26.211
Neutropenia, neutropenic (chronic) (genetic) (idiopathic) (immune) (infantile) (malignant) (pernicious) (splenic) D70.9
  congenital (primary) D70.0
  cyclic D70.4
  cytoreductive cancer chemotherapy sequela D70.1
  drug-induced D70.2
    due to cytoreductive cancer chemotherapy D70.1
  due to infection D70.3
  fever D70.9
  neonatal, transitory (isoimmune) (maternal transfer) P61.5
  periodic D70.4
  secondary (cyclic) (periodic) (splenic) D70.4
    drug-induced D70.2
      due to cytoreductive cancer chemotherapy D70.1
  toxic D70.8
Neutrophilia, hereditary giant D72.0
Nevocarcinoma — *see* Melanoma
Nevus D22.9
  achromic — *see* Neoplasm, skin, benign

Nevus - *continued*
  amelanotic — *see* Neoplasm, skin, benign
  angiomatousD18.00
    intra-abdominal D18.03
    intracranial D18.02
    skin D18.01
    specified site NEC D18.09
  araneus I78.1
  balloon cell — *see* Neoplasm, skin, benign
  bathing trunk D48.5
  blue — *see* Neoplasm, skin, benign
    cellular — *see* Neoplasm, skin, benign
    giant — *see* Neoplasm, skin, benign
    Jadassohn's — *see* Neoplasm, skin, benign
    malignant — *see* Melanoma
  capillary D18.00
    intra-abdominal D18.03
    intracranial D18.02
    skin D18.01
    specified site NEC D18.09
  cavernous D18.00
    intra-abdominal D18.03
    intracranial D18.02
    skin D18.01
    specified site NEC D18.09
  cellular — *see* Neoplasm, skin, benign
    blue — *see* Neoplasm, skin, benign
  choroid D31.3-
  comedonicus Q82.5
  conjunctiva D31.0-
  dermal — *see* Neoplasm, skin, benign
    with epidermal nevus — *see* Neoplasm, skin, benign
  dysplastic — *see* Neoplasm, skin, benign
  eye D31.9-
  flammeus Q82.5
  hemangiomatous D18.00
    intra-abdominal D18.03
    intracranial D18.02
    skin D18.01
    specified site NEC D18.09
  iris D31.4-
  lacrimal gland D31.5-
  lymphatic D18.1
  magnocellular
    specified site — *see* Neoplasm, benign, by site
    unspecified site D31.40
  malignant — *see* Melanoma
  meaning hemangioma D18.00
    intra-abdominal D18.03
    intracranial D18.02
    skin D18.01
    specified site NEC D18.09
  mouth (mucosa) D10.30
    specified site NEC D10.39
    white sponge Q38.6
  multiplex Q85.1
  non-neoplastic I78.1
  oral mucosa D10.30
    specified site NEC D10.39
    white sponge Q38.6
  orbit D31.6-
  pigmented
    giant — *see also* Neoplasm, skin, uncertain behavior D48.5
      malignant melanoma in — *see* Melanoma
  portwine Q82.5
  retina D31.2-
  retrobulbar D31.6-
  sanguineous Q82.5
  senile I78.1
  skin D22.9
    abdominal wall D22.5
    ala nasi D22.39
    ankle D22.7-
    anus, anal D22.5
    arm D22.6-
    auditory canal (external) D22.2-
    auricle (ear) D22.2-
    auricular canal (external) D22.2-
    axilla, axillary fold D22.5
    back D22.5
    breast D22.5

Nevus - *continued*
  skin - *continued*
    brow D22.39
    buttock D22.5
    canthus (eye) D22.1-
    cheek (external) D22.39
    chest wall D22.5
    chin D22.39
    ear (external) D22.2-
    external meatus (ear) D22.2-
    eyebrow D22.39
    eyelid (lower) (upper) D22.1-
    face D22.30
      specified NEC D22.39
    female genital organ (external) NEC D28.0
    finger D22.6-
    flank D22.5
    foot D22.7-
    forearm D22.6-
    forehead D22.39
    foreskin D29.0
    genital organ (external) NEC
      female D28.0
      male D29.9
    gluteal region D22.5
    groin D22.5
    hand D22.6-
    heel D22.7-
    helix D22.2-
    hip D22.7-
    interscapular region D22.5
    jaw D22.39
    knee D22.7-
    labium (majus) (minus) D28.0
    leg D22.7-
    lip (lower) (upper) D22.0
    lower limb D22.7-
    male genital organ (external) D29.9
    nail D22.9
      finger D22.6-
      toe D22.7-
    nasolabial groove D22.39
    nates D22.5
    neck D22.4
    nose (external) D22.39
    palpebra D22.1-
    penis D29.0
    perianal skin D22.5
    perineum D22.5
    pinna D22.2-
    popliteal fossa or space D22.7-
    prepuce D29.0
    pudendum D28.0
    scalp D22.4
    scrotum D29.4
    shoulder D22.6-
    submammary fold D22.5
    temple D22.39
    thigh D22.7-
    toe D22.7-
    trunk NEC D22.5
    umbilicus D22.5
    upper limb D22.6-
    vulva D28.0
  specified site NEC — *see* Neoplasm, by site, benign
  spider I78.1
  stellar I78.1
  strawberry Q82.5
  Sutton's benign D22.9
  unius lateris Q82.5
  Unna's Q82.5
  vascular Q82.5
  verrucous Q82.5
Newborn (infant) (liveborn) (singleton) Z38.2
  acne L70.4
  abstinence syndrome P96.1
  affected by
    abnormalities of membranes P02.9
      specified NEC P02.8
    abruptio placenta P02.1
    amino-acid metabolic disorder, transitory P74.8
    amniocentesis (while in utero) P00.6

Newborn (infant) (liveborn) (singleton) - *continued*
- affected by - *continued*
  - amnionitis P02.78
  - apparent life threatening event (ALTE) R68.13
  - bleeding (into)
    - cerebral cortex P52.22
    - germinal matrix P52.0
    - ventricles P52.1
  - breech delivery P03.0
  - cardiac arrest P29.81
  - cardiomyopathy I42.8
    - congenital I42.4
  - cerebral ischemia P91.0
  - Cesarean delivery P03.4
  - chemotherapy agents P04.11
  - chorioamnionitis P02.78
  - cocaine (crack) P04.41
  - complications of labor and delivery P03.9
    - specified NEC P03.89
  - compression of umbilical cord NEC P02.5
  - contracted pelvis P03.1
  - cyanosis P28.2
  - delivery P03.9
    - Cesarean P03.4
    - forceps P03.2
    - vacuum extractor P03.3
  - drugs of addiction P04.40
    - cocaine P04.41
    - hallucinogens P04.42
    - specified drug NEC P04.49
  - environmental chemicals P04.6
  - entanglement (knot) in umbilical cord P02.5
  - fetal (intrauterine)
    - growth retardation P05.9
    - inflammatory response syndrome (FIRS) P02.70
    - malnutrition not light or small for gestational age P05.2
  - FIRS (fetal inflammatory response syndrome) P02.70
  - forceps delivery P03.2
  - heart rate abnormalities
    - bradycardia P29.12
    - intrauterine P03.819
      - before onset of labor P03.810
      - during labor P03.811
    - tachycardia P29.11
  - hemorrhage (antepartum) P02.1
    - cerebellar (nontraumatic) P52.6
    - intracerebral (nontraumatic) P52.4
    - intracranial (nontraumatic) P52.9
      - specified NEC P52.8
    - intraventricular (nontraumatic) P52.3
      - grade 1 P52.0
      - grade 2 P52.1
      - grade 3 P52.21
      - grade 4 P52.22
    - posterior fossa (nontraumatic) P52.6
    - subarachnoid (nontraumatic) P52.5
    - subependymal P52.0
      - with intracerebral extension P52.22
      - with intraventricular extension P52.1
        - with enlargment of ventricles P52.21
      - without intraventricular extension P52.0
  - hypoxic ischemic encephalopathy [HIE] P91.60
    - mild P91.61
    - moderate P91.62
    - severe P91.63
  - induction of labor P03.89
  - intestinal perforation P78.0
  - intrauterine (fetal) blood loss P50.9
    - due to (from)
      - cut end of co-twin cord P50.5
      - hemorrhage into
        - co-twin P50.3
        - maternal circulation P50.4
      - placenta P50.2
      - ruptured cord blood P50.1
      - vasa previa P50.0

Newborn (infant) (liveborn) (singleton) - *continued*
- affected by - *continued*
  - intrauterine (fetal) blood loss - *continued*
    - specified NEC P50.8
  - intrauterine (fetal) hemorrhage P50.9
  - intrauterine (in utero) procedure P96.5
  - malpresentation (malposition) NEC P03.1
  - maternal (complication of) (use of)
    - alcohol P04.3
    - amphetamines P04.16
    - analgesia (maternal) P04.0
    - anesthesia (maternal) P04.0
    - anticonvulsants P04.13
    - antidepressants P04.15
    - antineoplastic chemotherapy P04.11
    - anxiolytics P04.1A
    - blood loss P02.1
    - cannabis P04.81
    - circulatory disease P00.3
    - condition P00.9
      - specified NEC P00.89
    - cytotoxic drugs P04.12
    - delivery P03.9
      - Cesarean P03.4
      - forceps P03.2
      - vacuum extractor P03.3
    - diabetes mellitus (pre-existing) P70.1
    - disorder P00.9
      - specified NEC P00.89
    - drugs (addictive) (illegal) NEC P04.49
    - ectopic pregnancy P01.4
    - gestational diabetes P70.0
    - hemorrhage P02.1
    - hypertensive disorder P00.0
    - incompetent cervix P01.0
    - infectious disease P00.2
    - injury P00.5
    - labor and delivery P03.9
    - malpresentation before labor P01.7
    - maternal death P01.6
    - medical procedure P00.7
    - medication P04.19
      - specified type NEC P04.18
    - multiple pregnancy P01.5
    - nutritional disorder P00.4
    - oligohydramnios P01.2
    - opiates P04.14
      - administered for procedures during pregnancy or labor and delivery P04.0
    - parasitic disease P00.2
    - periodontal disease P00.81
    - placenta previa P02.0
    - polyhydramnios P01.3
    - precipitate delivery P03.5
    - pregnancy P01.9
      - specified P01.8
    - premature rupture of membranes P01.1
    - renal disease P00.1
    - respiratory disease P00.3
    - sedative-hypnotics P04.17
    - surgical procedure P00.6
    - tranquilizers administered for procedures during pregnancy or labor and delivery P04.0
    - urinary tract disease P00.1
    - uterine contraction (abnormal) P03.6
  - meconium peritonitis P78.0
  - medication (legal) (maternal use) (prescribed) P04.19
  - membrane abnormalities P02.9
    - specified NEC P02.8
  - membranitis P02.78
  - methamphetamine (s) P04.49
  - mixed metabolic and respiratory acidosis P84
  - neonatal abstinence syndrome P96.1
  - noxious substances transmitted via placenta or breast milk P04.9
    - cannabis P04.81
    - specified NEC P04.89
  - nutritional supplements P04.5
  - placenta previa P02.0
  - placental

Newborn (infant) (liveborn) (singleton) - *continued*
- affected by - *continued*
  - placental - *continued*
    - abnormality (functional) (morphological) P02.20
      - specified NEC P02.29
    - dysfunction P02.29
    - infarction P02.29
    - insufficiency P02.29
    - separation NEC P02.1
    - transfusion syndromes P02.3
  - placentitis P02.78
  - precipitate delivery P03.5
  - prolapsed cord P02.4
  - respiratory arrest P28.81
  - slow intrauterine growth P05.9
  - tobacco P04.2
  - twin to twin transplacental transfusion P02.3
  - umbilical cord (tightly) around neck P02.5
  - umbilical cord condition P02.60
    - short cord P02.69
    - specified NEC P02.69
  - uterine contractions (abnormal) P03.6
  - vasa previa P02.69
    - from intrauterine blood loss P50.0
- apnea P28.4
  - primary P28.3
  - obstructive P28.4
  - sleep (central) (obstructive) (primary) P28.3
- born in hospital Z38.00
  - by cesarean Z38.01
- born outside hospital Z38.1
- breast buds P96.89
- breast engorgement P83.4
- check-up — *see* Newborn, examination
- convulsion P90
- dehydration P74.1
- examination
  - 8 to 28 days old Z00.111
  - under 8 days old Z00.110
- fever P81.9
  - environmentally-induced P81.0
- hyperbilirubinemia P59.9
  - of prematurity P59.0
- hypernatremia P74.21
- hyponatremia P74.22
- infection P39.9
  - candidal P37.5
  - specified NEC P39.8
  - urinary tract P39.3
- jaundice P59.9
  - due to
    - breast milk inhibitor P59.3
    - hepatocellular damage P59.20
      - specified NEC P59.29
    - preterm delivery P59.0
  - of prematurity P59.0
  - specified NEC P59.8
- late metabolic acidosis P74.0
- mastitis P39.0
  - infective P39.0
  - noninfective P83.4
- multiple born NEC Z38.8
  - born in hospital Z38.68
    - by cesarean Z38.69
  - born outside hospital Z38.7
- omphalitis P38.9
  - with mild hemorrhage P38.1
  - without hemorrhage P38.9
- post-term P08.21
- prolonged gestation (over 42 completed weeks) P08.22
- quadruplet Z38.8
  - born in hospital Z38.63
    - by cesarean Z38.64
  - born outside hospital Z38.7
- quintuplet Z38.8
  - born in hospital Z38.65
    - by cesarean Z38.66
  - born outside hospital Z38.7
- seizure P90
- sepsis (congenital) P36.9

Newborn (infant) (liveborn) (singleton) - *continued*
  sepsis (congenital) - *continued*
    due to
      anaerobes NEC P36.5
      Escherichia coli P36.4
      Staphylococcus P36.30
        aureus P36.2
        specified NEC P36.39
      Streptococcus P36.10
        group B P36.0
        specified NEC P36.19
      specified NEC P36.8
  triplet Z38.8
    born in hospital Z38.61
      by cesarean Z38.62
    born outside hospital Z38.7
  twin Z38.5
    born in hospital Z38.30
      by cesarean Z38.31
    born outside hospital Z38.4
  vomiting P92.09
    bilious P92.01
  weight check Z00.111
Newcastle conjunctivitis or disease B30.8
Nezelof's syndrome (pure alymphocytosis) D81.4
Niacin (amide) deficiency E52
Nicolas (-Durand) -Favre disease A55
Nicotine — *see* Tobacco
Nicotinic acid deficiency E52
Niemann-Pick disease or syndrome E75.249
  specified NEC E75.248
  type
    A E75.240
    B E75.241
    C E75.242
    D E75.243
Night
  blindness — *see* Blindness, night
  sweats R61
  terrors (child) F51.4
Nightmares (REM sleep type) F51.5
NIHSS (National Institutes of Health Stroke Scale) score R29.7-
Nipple — *see* condition
Nisbet's chancre A57
Nishimoto (-Takeuchi) disease I67.5
Nitritoid crisis or reaction — *see* Crisis, nitritoid
Nitrosohemoglobinemia D74.8
Njovera A65
Nocardiosis, nocardiasis A43.9
  cutaneous A43.1
  lung A43.0
  pneumonia A43.0
  pulmonary A43.0
  specified site NEC A43.8
Nocturia R35.1
  psychogenic F45.8
Nocturnal — *see* condition
Nodal rhythm I49.8
Node (s) — *see also* Nodule
  Bouchard's (with arthropathy) M15.2
  Haygarth's M15.8
  Heberden's (with arthropathy) M15.1
  larynx J38.7
  lymph — *see* condition
  milker's B08.03
  Osler's I33.0
  Schmorl's — *see* Schmorl's disease
  singer's J38.2
  teacher's J38.2
  tuberculous — *see* Tuberculosis, lymph gland
  vocal cord J38.2
Nodule (s) , nodular
  actinomycotic — *see* Actinomycosis
  breast NEC — *see also* Lump, breast N63.0
  colloid (cystic) , thyroid E04.1
  cutaneous — *see* Swelling, localized
  endometrial (stromal) D26.1
  Haygarth's M15.8
  inflammatory — *see* Inflammation
  juxta-articular

Nodule (s) , nodular - *continued*
  juxta-articular - *continued*
    syphilitic A52.77
    yaws A66.7
  larynx J38.7
  lung, solitary (subsegmental branch of the bronchial tree) R91.1
    multiple R91.8
  milker's B08.03
  prostate N40.2
    with lower urinary tract symptoms (LUTS) N40.3
    without lower urinary tract symtpoms (LUTS) N40.2
  pulmonary, solitary (subsegmental branch of the bronchial tree) R91.1
  retrocardiac R09.89
  rheumatoid M06.30
    ankle M06.37-
    elbow M06.32-
    foot joint M06.37-
    hand joint M06.34-
    hip M06.35-
    knee M06.36-
    multiple site M06.39
    shoulder M06.31-
    vertebra M06.38
    wrist M06.33-
  scrotum (inflammatory) N49.2
  singer's J38.2
  solitary, lung (subsegmental branch of the bronchial tree) R91.1
    multiple R91.8
  subcutaneous — *see* Swelling, localized
  teacher's J38.2
  thyroid (cold) (gland) (nontoxic) E04.1
    with thyrotoxicosis E05.20
      with thyroid storm E05.21
    toxic or with hyperthyroidism E05.20
      with thyroid storm E05.21
  vocal cord J38.2
Noma (gangrenous) (hospital) (infective) A69.0
  auricle I96
  mouth A69.0
  pudendi N76.89
  vulvae N76.89
Nomad, nomadism Z59.0
NOMID (neonatal onset multisystemic inflammatory disorder) M04.2
Nonadherence to medical treatment Z91.19
Nonautoimmune hemolytic anemia D59.4
  drug-induced D59.2
Nonclosure — *see also* Imperfect, closure
  ductus arteriosus (Botallo's) Q25.0
  foramen
    botalli Q21.1
    ovale Q21.1
Noncompliance Z91.19
  with
    dietary regimen Z91.11
    dialysis Z91.15
    medical treatment Z91.19
    medication regimen NEC Z91.14
      underdosing — *see also* Table of Drugs and Chemicals, categories T36-T50, with final character 6 Z91.14
      intentional NEC Z91.128
        due to financial hardship of patient Z91.120
      unintentional NEC Z91.138
        due to patient's age related debility Z91.130
    renal dialysis Z91.15
Nondescent (congenital) — *see also* Malposition, congenital
  cecum Q43.3
  colon Q43.3
  testicle Q53.9
    bilateral Q53.20
      abdominal Q53.211
      perineal Q53.22
    unilateral Q53.10
      abdominal Q53.111
      perineal Q53.12

Nondevelopment
  brain Q02
    part of Q04.3
  heart Q24.8
  organ or site, congenital NEC — *see* Hypoplasia
Nonengagement
  head NEC O32.4
    in labor, causing obstructed labor O64.8
Nonexanthematous tick fever A93.2
Nonexpansion, lung (newborn) P28.0
Nonfunctioning
  cystic duct — *see also* Disease, gallbladder K82.8
  gallbladder — *see also* Disease, gallbladder K82.8
  kidney N28.9
  labyrinth — *see* subcategory H83.2
Non-Hodgkin lymphoma NEC — *see* Lymphoma, non-Hodgkin
Nonimplantation, ovum N97.2
Noninsufflation, fallopian tube N97.1
Non-ketotic hyperglycinemia E72.51
Nonne-Milroy syndrome Q82.0
Nonovulation N97.0
Non-palpable testicle (s)
  bilateral R39.84
  unilateral R39.83
Nonpatent fallopian tube N97.1
Nonpneumatization, lung NEC P28.0
Nonrotation — *see* Malrotation
Nonsecretion, urine — *see* Anuria
Nonunion
  fracture — *see* Fracture, by site
  joint, following fusion or arthrodesis M96.0
  organ or site, congenital NEC — *see* Imperfect, closure
  symphysis pubis, congenital Q74.2
Nonvisualization, gallbladder R93.2
Nonvital, nonvitalized tooth K04.99
Non-working side interference M26.56
Noonan's syndrome Q87.19
Normocytic anemia (infectional) due to blood loss (chronic) D50.0
  acute D62
Norrie's disease (congenital) Q15.8
North American blastomycosis B40.9
Norwegian itch B86
Nose, nasal — *see* condition
Nosebleed R04.0
Nose-picking F98.8
Nosomania F45.21
Nosophobia F45.22
Nostalgia F43.20
Notch of iris Q13.2
Notching nose, congenital (tip) Q30.2
Nothnagel's
  syndrome — *see* Strabismus, paralytic, third nerve
  vasomotor acroparesthesia I73.89
Novy's relapsing fever A68.9
  louse-borne A68.0
  tick-borne A68.1
Noxious
  foodstuffs, poisoning by — *see* Poisoning, food, noxious, plant
  substances transmitted through placenta or breast milk P04.9
Nucleus pulposus — *see* condition
Numbness R20.0
Nuns' knee — *see* Bursitis, prepatellar
Nursemaid's elbow S53.03-
Nutcracker esophagus K22.4
Nutmeg liver K76.1
Nutrient element deficiency E61.9
  specified NEC E61.8
Nutrition deficient or insufficient — *see also* Malnutrition E46
  due to
    insufficient food T73.0
    lack of
      care (child) T76.02
        adult T76.01
      food T73.0
Nutritional stunting E45

Nyctalopia (night blindness) — *see*
  Blindness, night
Nycturia R35.1
  psychogenic F45.8
Nymphomania F52.8
Nystagmus H55.00
  benign paroxysmal — *see* Vertigo, benign
    paroxysmal
  central positional H81.4
  congenital H55.01
  dissociated H55.04
  latent H55.02
  miners' H55.09
  positional
    benign paroxysmal H81.4
    central H81.4
  specified form NEC H55.09
  visual deprivation H55.03

O

**Obermeyer's relapsing fever
  (European)** A68.0
Obesity E66.9
  with alveolar hypoventilation E66.2
  adrenal E27.8
  complicating
    childbirth O99.214
    pregnancy O99.21-
    puerperium O99.215
  constitutional E66.8
  dietary counseling and surveillance Z71.3
  drug-induced E66.1
  due to
    drug E66.1
    excess calories E66.09
      morbid E66.01
      severe E66.01
  endocrine E66.8
  endogenous E66.8
  exogenous E66.09
  familial E66.8
  glandular E66.8
  hypothyroid — *see* Hypothyroidism
  hypoventilation syndrome (OHS) E66.2
  morbid E66.01
    with
      alveolar hypoventilation E66.2
      obesity hypoventilation syndrome
        (OHS) E66.2
    due to excess calories E66.01
  nutritional E66.09
  pituitary E23.6
  severe E66.01
  specified type NEC E66.8
Oblique — *see* condition
Obliteration
  appendix (lumen) K38.8
  artery I77.1
  bile duct (noncalculous) K83.1
  common duct (noncalculous) K83.1
  cystic duct — *see* Obstruction, gallbladder
  disease, arteriolar I77.1
  endometrium N85.8
  eye, anterior chamber — *see* Disorder, globe,
    hypotony
  fallopian tube N97.1
  lymphatic vessel I89.0
    due to mastectomy I97.2
  organ or site, congenital NEC — *see* Atresia,
    by site
  ureter N13.5
    with infection N13.6
  urethra — *see* Stricture, urethra
  vein I87.8
  vestibule (oral) K08.89
**Observation (following) (for) (without need
  for further medical care)** Z04.9
  accident NEC Z04.3
    at work Z04.2
    transport Z04.1
  adverse effect of drug Z03.6
  alleged rape or sexual assault (victim) , ruled
    out
    adult Z04.41
    child Z04.42
  criminal assault Z04.89

**Observation (following) (for) (without need
  for further medical care)** - *continued*
  development state
    adolescent Z00.3
    period of rapid growth in childhood Z00.2
    puberty Z00.3
  disease, specified NEC Z03.89
  following work accident Z04.2
  forced sexual exploitation Z04.81
  forced labor exploitation Z04.82
  growth and development state — *see*
    Observation, development state
  injuries (accidental) NEC — *see also*
    Observation, accident
  newborn (for)
    suspected condition, related to exposure
      from the mother or birth process —
      see - Newborn, affected by, maternal
    ruled out Z05.9
      cardiac Z05.0
      connective tissue Z05.73
      gastrointestinal Z05.5
      genetic Z05.41
      genitourinary Z05.6
      immunologic Z05.43
      infectious Z05.1
      metabolic Z05.42
      musculoskeletal Z05.72
      neurological Z05.2
      respiratory Z05.3
      skin and subcutaneous tissue Z05.71
      specified condition NEC Z05.8
  postpartum
    immediately after delivery Z39.0
    routine follow-up Z39.2
  pregnancy (normal) (without
    complication) Z34.9-
    high risk O09.9-
  suicide attempt, alleged NEC Z03.89
    self-poisoning Z03.6
  suspected, ruled out — *see also* Suspected
    condition, ruled out
    abuse, physical
      adult Z04.71
      child Z04.72
    accident at work Z04.2
    adult battering victim Z04.71
    child battering victim Z04.72
    condition NEC Z03.89
      newborn — *see also* Observation,
        newborn (for), suspected condition,
        ruled out Z05.9
    drug poisoning or adverse effect Z03.6
    exposure (to)
      anthrax Z03.810
      biological agent NEC Z03.818
    inflicted injury NEC Z04.89
    suicide attempt, alleged Z03.89
      self-poisoning Z03.6
    toxic effects from ingested substance
      (drug) (poison) Z03.6
  toxic effects from ingested substance (drug)
    (poison) Z03.6
Obsession, obsessional state F42.8
  mixed thoughts and acts F42.2
**Obsessive-compulsive neurosis or
  reaction** F42.8
Obstetric embolism, septic — *see* Embolism,
  obstetric, septic
Obstetrical trauma (complicating delivery)
  O71.9
  with or following ectopic or molar
    pregnancy O08.6
  specified type NEC O71.89
Obstipation — *see* Constipation
Obstruction, obstructed, obstructive
  airway J98.8
    with
      allergic alveolitis J67.9
      asthma J45.909
        with
          exacerbation (acute) J45.901
          status asthmaticus J45.902
      bronchiectasis J47.9
        with

Obstruction, obstructed, obstructive -
continued
  airway - *continued*
    with - *continued*
      bronchiectasis - *continued*
        with - *continued*
          exacerbation (acute) J47.1
          lower respiratory infection J47.0
      bronchitis (chronic) J44.9
      emphysema J43.9
    chronic J44.9
      with
        allergic alveolitis — *see* Pneumonitis,
          hypersensitivity
        bronchiectasis J47.9
          with
            exacerbation (acute) J47.1
            lower respiratory infection J47.0
    due to
      foreign body — *see* Foreign body, by
        site, causing asphyxia
      inhalation of fumes or vapors J68.9
      laryngospasm J38.5
  ampulla of Vater K83.1
  aortic (heart) (valve) — *see* Stenosis, aortic
  aortoiliac I74.09
  aqueduct of Sylvius G91.1
    congenital Q03.0
      with spina bifida — *see* Spina bifida, by
        site, with hydrocephalus
  Arnold-Chiari — *see* Arnold-Chiari disease
  artery — *see also* Atherosclerosis,
    artery I70.9
    stent — *see* Restenosis, stent
    basilar (complete) (partial) — *see*
      Occlusion, artery, basilar
    carotid (complete) (partial) — *see*
      Occlusion, artery, carotid
    cerebellar — *see* Occlusion, artery,
      cerebellar
    cerebral (anterior) (middle) (posterior) —
      see Occlusion, artery, cerebral
    precerebral — *see* Occlusion, artery,
      precerebral
    renal N28.0
    retinal NEC — *see* Occlusion, artery,
      retina
    vertebral (complete) (partial) — *see*
      Occlusion, artery, vertebral
  band (intestinal) — *see also* Obstruction,
    intestine, specified NEC K56.699
  bile duct or passage (common) (hepatic)
    (noncalculus) K83.1
    with calculus K80.51
    congenital (causing jaundice) Q44.3
  biliary (duct) (tract) K83.1
    gallbladder K82.0
  bladder-neck (acquired) N32.0
    congenital Q64.31
    due to hyperplasia (hypertrophy) of
      prostate — *see* Hyperplasia, prostate
  bowel — *see* Obstruction, intestine
  bronchus J98.09
  canal, ear — *see* Stenosis, external ear canal
  cardia K22.2
  caval veins (inferior) (superior) I87.1
  cecum — *see* Obstruction, intestine
  circulatory I99.8
  colon — *see* Obstruction, intestine
  common duct (noncalculous) K83.1
  coronary (artery) — *see* Occlusion, coronary
  cystic duct — *see also* Obstruction,
    gallbladder
    with calculus K80.21
  device, implant or graft — *see also*
    Complications, by site and type,
    mechanical T85.698
    arterial graft NEC — *see* Complication,
      cardiovascular device, mechanical,
      vascular
    catheter NEC T85.628
      cystostomy T83.090
      dialysis (renal) T82.49
        intraperitoneal T85.691
      Hopkins T83.098

Obstruction, obstructed, obstructive - *continued*
  device, implant or graft - *continued*
    catheter NEC - *continued*
      ileostomy T83.098
      infusion NEC T82.594
        spinal (epidural) (subdural) T85.690
      nephrostomy T83.092
      urethral indwelling T83.091
      urinary T83.098
      urostomy T83.098
      due to infection T85.79
    gastrointestinal — *see* Complications, prosthetic device, mechanical, gastrointestinal device
    genital NEC T83.498
      intrauterine contraceptive device T83.39
      penile prosthesis (cylinder) (implanted) (pump) (resevoir) T83.490
      testicular prosthesis T83.491
    heart NEC — *see* Complication, cardiovascular device, mechanical
    joint prosthesis — *see* Complications, joint prosthesis, mechanical, specified NEC, by site
    orthopedic NEC — *see* Complication, orthopedic, device, mechanical
    specified NEC T85.628
    urinary NEC — *see also* Complication, genitourinary, device, urinary, mechanical
      graft T83.29
    vascular NEC — *see* Complication, cardiovascular device, mechanical
    ventricular intracranial shunt T85.09
  due to foreign body accidentally left in operative wound T81.529
  duodenum K31.5
  ejaculatory duct N50.89
  esophagus K22.2
  eustachian tube (complete) (partial) H68.10-
    cartilagenous (extrinsic) H68.13-
      intrinsic H68.12-
    osseous H68.11-
  fallopian tube (bilateral) N97.1
  fecal K56.41
    with hernia — *see* Hernia, by site, with obstruction
  foramen of Monro (congenital) Q03.8
    with spina bifida — *see* Spina bifida, by site, with hydrocephalus
  foreign body — *see* Foreign body
  gallbladder K82.0
    with calculus, stones K80.21
    congenital Q44.1
  gastric outlet K31.1
  gastrointestinal — *see* Obstruction, intestine
  hepatic K76.89
    duct (noncalculous) K83.1
  hepatobiliary K83.1
  ileum — *see* Obstruction, intestine
  iliofemoral (artery) I74.5
  intestine K56.609
    complete K56.601
    incomplete K56.600
    partial K56.600
    with
      adhesions (intestinal) (peritoneal) K56.50
        complete K56.52
        incomplete K56.51
        partial K56.51
    adynamic K56.0
    by gallstone K56.3
    congenital (small) Q41.9
      large Q42.9
        specified part NEC Q42.8
    neurogenic K56.0
      Hirschsprung's disease or megacolon Q43.1
    newborn P76.9
      due to
        fecaliths P76.8
        inspissated milk P76.2
        meconium (plug) P76.0

Obstruction, obstructed, obstructive - *continued*
  intestine - *continued*
    newborn - *continued*
      due to - *continued*
        meconium (plug) - *continued*
          in mucoviscidosis E84.11
        specified NEC P76.8
    postoperative K91.30
      complete K91.32
      incomplete K91.31
      partial K91.31
    reflex K56.0
    specified NEC K56.699
      complete K56.691
      incomplete K56.690
      partial K56.690
    volvulus K56.2
  intracardiac ball valve prosthesis T82.09
  jejunum — *see* Obstruction, intestine
  joint prosthesis — *see* Complications, joint prosthesis, mechanical, specified NEC, by site
  kidney (calices) N28.89
  labor — *see* Delivery
  lacrimal (passages) (duct)
    by
      dacryolith — *see* Dacryolith
      stenosis — *see* Stenosis, lacrimal
    congenital Q10.5
    neonatal H04.53-
  lacrimonasal duct — *see* Obstruction, lacrimal
  lacteal, with steatorrhea K90.2
  laryngitis — *see* Laryngitis
  larynx NEC J38.6
    congenital Q31.8
  lung J98.4
    disease, chronic J44.9
  lymphatic I89.0
  meconium (plug)
    newborn P76.0
      due to fecaliths P76.0
      in mucoviscidosis E84.11
  mitral — *see* Stenosis, mitral
  nasal J34.89
  nasolacrimal duct — *see also* Obstruction, lacrimal
    congenital Q10.5
  nasopharynx J39.2
  nose J34.89
  organ or site, congenital NEC — *see* Atresia, by site
  pancreatic duct K86.89
  parotid duct or gland K11.8
  pelviureteral junction N13.5
    with hydronephrosis N13.0
    congenital Q62.39
  pharynx J39.2
  portal (circulation) (vein) I81
  prostate — *see also* Hyperplasia, prostate
    valve (urinary) N32.0
  pulmonary valve (heart) I37.0
  pyelonephritis (chronic) N11.1
  pylorus
    adult K31.1
    congenital or infantile Q40.0
  rectosigmoid — *see* Obstruction, intestine
  rectum K62.4
  renal N28.89
    outflow N13.8
    pelvis, congenital Q62.39
  respiratory J98.8
    chronic J44.9
  retinal (vessels) H34.9
  salivary duct (any) K11.8
    with calculus K11.5
  sigmoid — *see* Obstruction, intestine
  sinus (accessory) (nasal) J34.89
  Stensen's duct K11.8
  stomach NEC K31.89
    acute K31.0
    congenital Q40.2
    due to pylorospasm K31.3
  submandibular duct K11.8

Obstruction, obstructed, obstructive - *continued*
  submaxillary gland K11.8
    with calculus K11.5
  thoracic duct I89.0
  thrombotic — *see* Thrombosis
  trachea J39.8
  tracheostomy airway J95.03
  tricuspid (valve) — *see* Stenosis, tricuspid
  upper respiratory, congenital Q34.8
  ureter (functional) (pelvic junction) NEC N13.5
    with
      hydronephrosis N13.1
        with infection N13.6
      pyelonephritis (chronic) N11.1
    congenital Q62.39
    due to calculus — *see* Calculus, ureter
  urethra NEC N36.8
    congenital Q64.39
  urinary (moderate) N13.9
    due to hyperplasia (hypertrophy) of prostate — *see* Hyperplasia, prostate
    organ or tract (lower) N13.9
    prostatic valve N32.0
    specified NEC N13.8
  uropathy N13.9
  uterus N85.8
  vagina N89.5
  valvular — *see* Endocarditis
  vein, venous I87.1
    caval (inferior) (superior) I87.1
    thrombotic — *see* Thrombosis
  vena cava (inferior) (superior) I87.1
  vesical NEC N32.0
  vesicourethral orifice N32.0
    congenital Q64.31
  vessel NEC I99.8
    stent — *see* Restenosis, stent
Obturator — *see* condition
Occlusal wear, teeth K03.0
Occlusio pupillae — *see* Membrane, pupillary
Occlusion, occluded
  anus K62.4
    congenital Q42.3
      with fistula Q42.2
  aortoiliac (chronic) I74.09
  aqueduct of Sylvius G91.1
    congenital Q03.0
      with spina bifida — *see* Spina bifida, by site, with hydrocephalus
  artery — *see also* Atherosclerosis, artery I70.9
    auditory, internal I65.8
    basilar I65.1
      with
        infarction I63.22
          due to
            embolism I63.12
            thrombosis I63.02
    brain or cerebral I66.9
      with infarction (due to) I63.5-
        embolism I63.4-
        thrombosis I63.3-
    carotid I65.2-
      with
        infarction I63.23-
          due to
            embolism I63.13-
            thrombosis I63.03-
    cerebellar (anterior inferior) (posterior inferior) (superior) I66.3
      with infarction I63.54-
        due to
          embolism I63.44-
          thrombosis I63.34-
    cerebral I66.9
      with infarction I63.50
        due to
          embolism I63.40
            specified NEC I63.49
          thrombosis I63.30
            specified NEC I63.39
      anterior I66.1-
        with infarction I63.52-

Occlusion, occluded - *continued*
artery - *continued*
cerebral - *continued*
anterior - *continued*
with infarction - *continued*
due to
embolism I63.42-
thrombosis I63.32-
middle I66.0-
with infarction I63.51-
due to
embolism I63.41-
thrombosis I63.31-
posterior I66.2-
with infarction I63.53-
due to
embolism I63.43-
thrombosis I63.33-
specified NEC I66.8
with infarction I63.59
due to
embolism I63.4-
thrombosis I63.3-
choroidal (anterior) — *see* Occlusion,
artery, precerebral, specified NEC
communicating posterior — *see* Occlusion,
artery, precerebral, specified NEC
complete
coronary I25.82
extremities I70.92
coronary (acute) (thrombotic) (without
myocardial infarction) I24.0
with myocardial infarction — *see*
Infarction, myocardium
chronic total I25.82
complete I25.82
healed or old I25.2
total (chronic) I25.82
hypophyseal — *see* Occlusion, artery,
precerebral, specified NEC
iliac I74.5
lower extremities due to stenosis or
stricture I77.1
mesenteric (embolic) (thrombotic) — *see*
also Infarct, intestine K55.069
perforating — *see* Occlusion, artery,
cerebral, specified NEC
peripheral I77.9
thrombotic or embolic I74.4
pontine — *see* Occlusion, artery,
precerebral, specified NEC
precerebral I65.9
with infarction I63.20
specified NEC I63.29
due to
embolism I63.10
specified NEC I63.19
thrombosis I63.00
specified NEC I63.09
basilar — *see* Occlusion, artery, basilar
carotid — *see* Occlusion, artery, carotid
puerperal O88.23
specified NEC I65.8
with infarction I63.29
due to
embolism I63.19
thrombosis I63.09
vertebral — *see* Occlusion, artery,
vertebral
renal N28.0
retinal
central H34.1-
partial H34.21-
branch H34.23-
transient H34.0-
spinal — *see* Occlusion, artery,
precerebral, vertebral
total (chronic)
coronary I25.82
extremities I70.92
vertebral I65.0-
with
infarction I63.21-
due to
embolism I63.11-

Occlusion, occluded - *continued*
artery - *continued*
vertebral - *continued*
with - *continued*
infarction - *continued*
due to - *continued*
thrombosis I63.01-
basilar artery — *see* Occlusion, artery, basilar
bile duct (common) (hepatic)
(noncalculous) K83.1
bowel — *see* Obstruction, intestine
carotid (artery) (common) (internal) — *see*
Occlusion, artery, carotid
centric (of teeth) M26.59
maximum intercuspation
discrepancy M26.55
cerebellar (artery) — *see* Occlusion, artery,
cerebellar
cerebral (artery) — *see* Occlusion, artery,
cerebral
cerebrovascular — *see also* Occlusion,
artery, cerebral
with infarction I63.5-
cervical canal — *see* Stricture, cervix
cervix (uteri) — *see* Stricture, cervix
choanal Q30.0
choroidal (artery) — *see* Occlusion, artery,
precerebral, specified NEC
colon — *see* Obstruction, intestine
communicating posterior artery — *see*
Occlusion, artery, precerebral, specified
NEC
coronary (artery) (vein) (thrombotic) — *see*
also Infarct, myocardium
chronic total I25.82
healed or old I25.2
not resulting in infarction I24.0
total (chronic) I25.82
cystic duct — *see* Obstruction, gallbladder
embolic — *see* Embolism
fallopian tube N97.1
congenital Q50.6
gallbladder — *see also* Obstruction,
gallbladder
congenital (causing jaundice) Q44.1
gingiva, traumatic K06.2
hymen N89.6
congenital Q52.3
hypophyseal (artery) — *see* Occlusion,
artery, precerebral, specified NEC
iliac artery I74.5
intestine — *see* Obstruction, intestine
lacrimal passages — *see* Obstruction,
lacrimal
lung J98.4
lymph or lymphatic channel I89.0
mammary duct N64.89
mesenteric artery (embolic) (thrombotic) —
see also Infarct, intestine K55.069
nose J34.89
congenital Q30.0
organ or site, congenital NEC — *see* Atresia,
by site
oviduct N97.1
congenital Q50.6
peripheral arteries
due to stricture or stenosis I77.1
upper extremity I74.2
pontine (artery) — *see* Occlusion, artery,
precerebral, specified NEC
posterior lingual, of mandibular
teeth M26.29
precerebral artery — *see* Occlusion, artery,
precerebral
punctum lacrimale — *see* Obstruction,
lacrimal
pupil — *see* Membrane, pupillary
pylorus, adult — *see also* Stricture,
pylorus K31.1
renal artery N28.0
retina, retinal
artery — *see* Occlusion, artery, retinal
vein (central) H34.81-
engorgement H34.82-
tributary H34.83-

Occlusion, occluded - *continued*
retina, retinal - *continued*
vessels H34.9
spinal artery — *see* Occlusion, artery,
precerebral, vertebral
teeth (mandibular) (posterior
lingual) M26.29
thoracic duct I89.0
thrombotic — *see* Thrombosis, artery
traumatic
edentulous (alveolar) ridge K06.2
gingiva K06.2
periodontal K05.5
tubal N97.1
ureter (complete) (partial) N13.5
congenital Q62.10
ureteropelvic junction N13.5
congenital Q62.11
ureterovesical orifice N13.5
congenital Q62.12
urethra — *see* Stricture, urethra
uterus N85.8
vagina N89.5
vascular NEC I99.8
vein — *see* Thrombosis
retinal — *see* Occlusion, retinal, vein
vena cava (inferior) (superior) — *see*
Embolism, vena cava
ventricle (brain) NEC G91.1
vertebral (artery) — *see* Occlusion, artery,
vertebral
vessel (blood) I99.8
vulva N90.5
Occult
blood in feces (stools) R19.5
Occupational
problems NEC Z56.89
Ochlophobia — *see* Agoraphobia
Ochronosis (endogenous) E70.29
Ocular muscle — *see* condition
Oculogyric crisis or disturbance H51.8
psychogenic F45.8
Oculomotor syndrome H51.9
Oculopathy
syphilitic NEC A52.71
congenital
early A50.01
late A50.30
early (secondary) A51.43
late A52.71
Oddi's sphincter spasm K83.4
Odontalgia K08.89
Odontoameloblastoma — *see* Cyst, calcifying
odontogenic
Odontoclasia K03.89
Odontodysplasia, regional K00.4
Odontogenesis imperfecta K00.5
Odontoma (ameloblastic) (complex)
(compound) (fibroameloblastic) — *see*
Cyst, calcifying odontogenic
Odontomyelitis (closed) (open) K04.01
irreversible K04.02
reversible K04.01
Odontorrhagia K08.89
Odontosarcoma, ameloblastic C41.1
upper jaw (bone) C41.0
Oestriasis — *see* Myiasis
Oguchi's disease H53.63
Ohara's disease — *see* Tularemia
OHS (obesity hypoventilation
syndrome) E66.2
Oidiomycosis — *see* Candidiasis
Oidium albicans infection — *see* Candidiasis
Old age (without mention of debility) R54
dementia F03
Old (previous) myocardial infarction I25.2
Olfactory — *see* condition
Oligemia — *see* Anemia
Oligoastrocytoma
specified site — *see* Neoplasm, malignant,
by site
unspecified site C71.9
Oligocythemia D64.9
Oligodendroblastoma
specified site — *see* Neoplasm, malignant

Oligodendroblastoma - *continued*
  unspecified site C71.9
Oligodendroglioma
  anaplastic type
    specified site — *see* Neoplasm, malignant,
      by site
    unspecified site C71.9
  specified site — *see* Neoplasm, malignant,
    by site
  unspecified site C71.9
Oligodontia — *see* Anodontia
Oligoencephalon Q02
Oligohidrosis L74.4
Oligohydramnios O41.0-
Oligohydrosis L74.4
Oligomenorrhea N91.5
  primary N91.3
  secondary N91.4
Oligophrenia — *see also* Disability,
    intellectual
  phenylpyruvic E70.0
Oligospermia N46.11
  due to
    drug therapy N46.121
    efferent duct obstruction N46.123
    infection N46.122
    radiation N46.124
    specified cause NEC N46.129
    systemic disease N46.125
Oligotrichia — *see* Alopecia
Oliguria R34
  with, complicating or following ectopic or
    molar pregnancy O08.4
  postprocedural N99.0
Ollier's disease Q78.4
Omenotocele — *see* Hernia, abdomen,
    specified site NEC
Omentitis — *see* Peritonitis
Omentum, omental — *see* condition
Omphalitis (congenital) (newborn) P38.9
  with mild hemorrhage P38.1
  without hemorrhage P38.9
  not of newborn L08.82
  tetanus A33
Omphalocele Q79.2
Omphalomesenteric duct, persistent Q43.0
Omphalorrhagia, newborn P51.9
Omsk hemorrhagic fever A98.1
Onanism (excessive) F98.8
Onchocerciasis, onchocercosis B73.1
  with
    eye disease B73.00
      endophthalmitis B73.01
      eyelid B73.09
      glaucoma B73.02
      specified NEC B73.09
    eye NEC B73.00
    eyelid B73.09
Oncocytoma — *see* Neoplasm, benign, by site
**Oncovirus, as cause of disease classified
    elsewhere** B97.32
Ondine's curse — *see* Apnea, sleep
Oneirophrenia F23
Onychauxis L60.2
  congenital Q84.5
Onychia — *see also* Cellulitis, digit
  with lymphangitis — *see* Lymphangitis,
    acute, digit
  candidal B37.2
  dermatophytic B35.1
Onychitis — *see also* Cellulitis, digit
  with lymphangitis — *see* Lymphangitis,
    acute, digit
Onychocryptosis L60.0
Onychodystrophy L60.3
  congenital Q84.6
Onychogryphosis, onychogryposis L60.2
Onycholysis L60.1
Onychomadesis L60.8
Onychomalacia L60.3
Onychomycosis (finger) (toe) B35.1
Onycho-osteodysplasia Q87.2
Onychophagia F98.8
Onychophosis L60.8
Onychoptosis L60.8

Onychorrhexis L60.3
  congenital Q84.6
Onychoschizia L60.3
Onyxis (finger) (toe) L60.0
Onyxitis — *see also* Cellulitis, digit
  with lymphangitis — *see* Lymphangitis,
    acute, digit
Oophoritis (cystic) (infectional) (interstitial)
    N70.92
  with salpingitis N70.93
  acute N70.02
    with salpingitis N70.03
  chronic N70.12
    with salpingitis N70.13
  complicating abortion — *see* Abortion, by
    type, complicated by, oophoritis
Oophorocele N83.4-
Opacity, opacities
  cornea H17.-
    central H17.1-
    congenital Q13.3
    degenerative — *see* Degeneration, cornea
    hereditary — *see* Dystrophy, cornea
    inflammatory — *see* Keratitis
    minor H17.81-
    peripheral H17.82-
    sequelae of trachoma (healed) B94.0
    specified NEC H17.89
  enamel (teeth) (fluoride) (nonfluoride) K00.3
  lens — *see* Cataract
  snowball — *see* Deposit, crystalline
  vitreous (humor) NEC H43.39-
    congenital Q14.0
    membranes and strands H43.31-
Opalescent dentin (hereditary) K00.5
Open, opening
  abnormal, organ or site, congenital — *see*
    Imperfect, closure
  angle with
    borderline
      findings
        high risk H40.02-
        low risk H40.01-
      intraocular pressure H40.00-
    cupping of discs H40.01-
    glaucoma (primary) — *see* Glaucoma,
      open angle
  bite
    anterior M26.220
    posterior M26.221
  false — *see* Imperfect, closure
  margin on tooth restoration K08.51
  restoration margins of tooth K08.51
  wound — *see* Wound, open
Operational fatigue F48.8
Operative — *see* condition
Operculitis — *see* Periodontitis
Operculum — *see* Break, retina
Ophiasis L63.2
Ophthalmia — *see also* Conjunctivitis H10.9
  actinic rays — *see* Photokeratitis
  allergic (acute) — *see* Conjunctivitis, acute,
    atopic
  blennorrhagic (gonococcal)
    (neonatorum) A54.31
  diphtheritic A36.86
  Egyptian A71.1
  electrica — *see* Photokeratitis
  gonococcal (neonatorum) A54.31
  metastatic — *see* Endophthalmitis, purulent
  migraine — *see* Migraine, ophthalmoplegic
  neonatorum, newborn P39.1
    gonococcal A54.31
  nodosa H16.24-
  purulent — *see* Conjunctivitis, acute,
    mucopurulent
  spring — *see* Conjunctivitis, acute, atopic
  sympathetic — *see* Uveitis, sympathetic
Ophthalmitis — *see* Ophthalmia
Ophthalmocele (congenital) Q15.8
Ophthalmoneuromyelitis G36.0
Ophthalmoplegia — *see also* Strabismus,
    paralytic
  anterior internuclear — *see*
    Ophthalmoplegia, internuclear

Ophthalmoplegia - *continued*
  ataxia-areflexia G61.0
  diabetic — *see* E08-E13 with .39
  exophthalmic E05.00
    with thyroid storm E05.01
  external H49.88-
    progressive H49.4-
      with pigmentary retinopathy — *see*
        Kearns-Sayre syndrome
    total H49.3-
  internal (complete) (total) H52.51-
  internuclear H51.2-
  migraine — *see* Migraine, ophthalmoplegic
  Parinaud's H49.88-
  progressive external — *see*
    Ophthalmoplegia, external, progressive
  supranuclear, progressive G23.1
  total (external) — *see* Ophthalmoplegia,
    external, total
Opioid (s)
  abuse — *see* Abuse, drug, opioids
  dependence — *see* Dependence, drug,
    opioids
  induced, without use disorder
    anxiety disorder F11.988
    delirium F11.921
    depressive disorder F11.94
    sexual dysfunction F11.981
    sleep disorder F11.982
Opisthognathism M26.09
Opisthorchiasis (felineus) (viverrini) B66.0
Opitz' disease D73.2
Opiumism — *see* Dependence, drug, opioid
Oppenheim's disease G70.2
**Oppenheim-Urbach disease (necrobiosis
    lipoidica diabeticorum)** — *see* E08-E13
    with .620
Optic nerve — *see* condition
Orbit — *see* condition
Orchioblastoma C62.9-
**Orchitis (gangrenous) (nonspecific) (septic)
    (suppurative)** N45.2
  blennorrhagic (gonococcal) (acute)
    (chronic) A54.23
  chlamydial A56.19
  filarial — *see also* Infestation, filarial B74.9
    [N51]
  gonococcal (acute) (chronic) A54.23
  mumps B26.0
  syphilitic A52.76
  tuberculous A18.15
Orf (virus disease) B08.02
Organic — *see also* condition
  brain syndrome F09
  heart — *see* Disease, heart
  mental disorder F09
  psychosis F09
Orgasm
  anejaculatory N53.13
Oriental
  bilharziasis B65.2
  schistosomiasis B65.2
Orifice — *see* condition
**Origin of both great vessels from right
    ventricle** Q20.1
**Ormond's disease (with ureteral
    obstruction)** N13.5
  with infection N13.6
Ornithine metabolism disorder E72.4
Ornithinemia (Type I) (Type II) E72.4
Ornithosis A70
**Orotaciduria, oroticaciduria (congenital)
    (hereditary) (pyrimidine deficiency)**
    E79.8
  anemia D53.0
Orthodontics
  adjustment Z46.4
  fitting Z46.4
Orthopnea R06.01
Orthopoxvirus B08.09
Os, uterus — *see* condition
**Osgood-Schlatter disease or
    osteochondrosis** — *see* Osteochondrosis,
    juvenile, tibia
Osler (-Weber) -Rendu disease I78.0

Osler's nodes I33.0
Osmidrosis L75.0
Osseous — *see* condition
Ossification
  artery — *see* Arteriosclerosis
  auricle (ear) — *see* Disorder, pinna, specified
    type NEC
  bronchial J98.09
  cardiac — *see* Degeneration, myocardial
  cartilage (senile) — *see* Disorder, cartilage,
    specified type NEC
  coronary (artery) — *see* Disease, heart,
    ischemic, atherosclerotic
  diaphragm J98.6
  ear, middle — *see* Otosclerosis
  falx cerebri G96.19
  fontanel, premature Q75.0
  heart — *see also* Degeneration, myocardial
    valve — *see* Endocarditis
  larynx J38.7
  ligament — *see* Disorder, tendon, specified
    type NEC
    posterior longitudinal — *see*
      Spondylopathy, specified NEC
  meninges (cerebral) (spinal) G96.19
  multiple, eccentric centers — *see* Disorder,
    bone, development or growth
  muscle — *see also* Calcification, muscle
    due to burns — *see* Myositis, ossificans,
      in, burns
    paralytic — *see* Myositis, ossificans, in,
      quadriplegia
    progressive — *see* Myositis, ossificans,
      progressiva
    specified NEC M61.50
      ankle M61.57-
      foot M61.57-
      forearm M61.53-
      hand M61.54-
      lower leg M61.56-
      multiple sites M61.59
      pelvic region M61.55-
      shoulder region M61.51-
      specified site NEC M61.58
      thigh M61.55-
      upper arm M61.52-
    traumatic — *see* Myositis, ossificans,
      traumatica
  myocardium, myocardial — *see*
    Degeneration, myocardial
  penis N48.89
  periarticular — *see* Disorder, joint, specified
    type NEC
  pinna — *see* Disorder, pinna, specified type
    NEC
  rider's bone — *see* Ossification, muscle,
    specified NEC
  sclera H15.89
  subperiosteal, post-traumatic M89.8X-
  tendon — *see* Disorder, tendon, specified
    type NEC
  trachea J39.8
  tympanic membrane — *see* Disorder,
    tympanic membrane, specified NEC
  vitreous (humor) — *see* Deposit, crystalline
Osteitis — *see also* Osteomyelitis
  alveolar M27.3
  condensans M85.30
    ankle M85.37-
    foot M85.37-
    forearm M85.33-
    hand M85.34-
    lower leg M85.36-
    multiple site M85.39
    neck M85.38
    rib M85.38
    shoulder M85.31-
    skull M85.38
    specified site NEC M85.38
    thigh M85.35-
    toe M85.37-
    upper arm M85.32-
    vertebra M85.38
  deformans M88.9
    in (due to)

Osteitis - *continued*
  deformans - *continued*
    in (due to) - *continued*
      malignant neoplasm of bone C41.9
        [M90.60]
      neoplastic disease — *see also*
        Neoplasm D49.9 *[M90.60]*
        carpus D49.9 *[M90.64-]*
        clavicle D49.9 *[M90.61-]*
        femur D49.9 *[M90.65-]*
        fibula D49.9 *[M90.66-]*
        finger D49.9 *[M90.64-]*
        humerus D49.9 *[M90.62-]*
        ilium D49.9 *[M90.65-]*
        ischium D49.9 *[M90.65-]*
        metacarpus D49.9 *[M90.64-]*
        metatarsus D49.9 *[M90.67-]*
        multiple sites D49.9 *[M90.69]*
        neck D49.9 *[M90.68]*
        radius D49.9 *[M90.63-]*
        rib D49.9 *[M90.68]*
        scapula D49.9 *[M90.61-]*
        skull D49.9 *[M90.68]*
        tarsus D49.9 *[M90.67-]*
        tibia D49.9 *[M90.66-]*
        toe D49.9 *[M90.67-]*
        ulna D49.9 *[M90.63-]*
        vertebra D49.9 *[M90.68]*
      skull M88.0
      specified NEC — *see* Paget's disease,
        bone, by site
      vertebra M88.1
    due to yaws A66.6
    fibrosa NEC — *see* Cyst, bone, by site
      circumscripta — *see* Dysplasia, fibrous,
        bone NEC
      cystica (generalisata) E21.0
      disseminata Q78.1
      osteoplastica E21.0
    fragilitans Q78.0
    Garr's (sclerosing) — *see* Osteomyelitis,
      specified type NEC
    jaw (acute) (chronic) (lower) (suppurative)
      (upper) M27.2
    parathyroid E21.0
    petrous bone (acute) (chronic) — *see*
      Petrositis
    sclerotic, nonsuppurative — *see*
      Osteomyelitis, specified type NEC
    tuberculosa A18.09
      cystica D86.89
      multiplex cystoides D86.89
Osteoarthritis M19.90
  ankle M19.07-
  elbow M19.02-
  foot joint M19.07-
  generalized M15.9
    erosive M15.4
    primary M15.0
    specified NEC M15.8
  hand joint M19.04-
    first carpometacarpal joint M18.9
  hip M16.1-
    bilateral M16.0
    due to hip dysplasia (unilateral) M16.3-
      bilateral M16.2
  interphalangeal
    distal (Heberden) M15.1
    proximal (Bouchard) M15.2
  knee M17.1-
    bilateral M17.0
  shoulder M19.01-
  spine — *see* Spondylosis
  wrist M19.03-
  post-traumatic NEC M19.92
    ankle M19.17-
    elbow M19.12-
    foot joint M19.17-
    hand joint M19.14-
      first carpometacarpal joint M18.3-
        bilateral M18.2
    hip M16.5-
      bilateral M16.4
    knee M17.3-
      bilateral M17.2

Osteoarthritis - *continued*
  post-traumatic NEC - *continued*
    shoulder M19.11-
    wrist M19.13-
  primary M19.91
    ankle M19.07-
    elbow M19.02-
    foot joint M19.07-
    hand joint M19.04-
      first carpometacarpal joint M18.1-
        bilateral M18.0
    hip M16.1-
      bilateral M16.0
    knee M17.1-
      bilateral M17.0
    multiple sites M89.49
    shoulder M19.01-
    spine — *see* Spondylosis
    wrist M19.03-
  secondary M19.93
    ankle M19.27-
    elbow M19.22-
    foot joint M19.27-
    hand joint M19.24-
      first carpometacarpal joint M18.5-
        bilateral M18.4
    hip M16.7
      bilateral M16.6
    knee M17.5
      bilateral M17.4
    multiple M15.3
    shoulder M19.21-
    spine — *see* Spondylosis
    wrist M19.23-
Osteoarthropathy (hypertrophic) M19.90
  ankle — *see* Osteoarthritis, primary, ankle
  elbow — *see* Osteoarthritis, primary, elbow
  foot joint — *see* Osteoarthritis, primary, foot
  hand joint — *see* Osteoarthritis, primary,
    hand joint
  knee joint — *see* Osteoarthritis, primary,
    knee
  multiple site — *see* Osteoarthritis, primary,
    multiple joint
  pulmonary — *see also* Osteoarthropathy,
    specified type NEC
    hypertrophic — *see* Osteoarthropathy,
      hypertrophic, specified type NEC
  secondary hypertrophic — *see*
    Osteoarthropathy, specified type NEC
  shoulder — *see* Osteoarthritis, primary,
    shoulder
  specified joint NEC — *see* Osteoarthritis,
    primary, specified joint NEC
  specified type NEC M89.40
    carpus M89.44-
    clavicle M89.41-
    femur M89.45-
    fibula M89.46-
    finger M89.44-
    humerus M89.42-
    ilium M89.459
    ischium M89.459
    metacarpus M89.44-
    metatarsus M89.47-
    multiple sites M89.49
    neck M89.48
    radius M89.43-
    rib M89.48
    scapula M89.41-
    skull M89.48
    tarsus M89.47-
    tibia M89.46-
    toe M89.47-
    ulna M89.43-
    vertebra M89.48
  secondary — *see* Osteoarthropathy, specified
    type NEC
  spine — *see* Spondylosis
  wrist — *see* Osteoarthritis, primary, wrist
Osteoarthrosis (degenerative) (hypertrophic)
  (joint) — *see also* Osteoarthritis
  deformans alkaptonurica E70.29 *[M36.8]*
  erosive M15.4
  generalized M15.9

Osteoarthrosis (degenerative) (hypertrophic) (joint) - *continued*
  generalized - *continued*
    primary M15.0
    polyarticular M15.9
    spine — *see* Spondylosis
Osteoblastoma — *see* Neoplasm, bone, benign
  aggressive — *see* Neoplasm, bone, uncertain behavior
Osteochondritis — *see also*
    Osteochondropathy, by site
  Brailsford's — *see* Osteochondrosis, juvenile, radius
  dissecans M93.20
    ankle M93.27-
    elbow M93.22-
    foot M93.27-
    hand M93.24-
    hip M93.25-
    knee M93.26-
    multiple sites M93.29
    shoulder joint M93.21-
    specified site NEC M93.28
    wrist M93.23-
  juvenile M92.9
    patellar — *see* Osteochondrosis, juvenile, patella
  syphilitic (congenital) (early) A50.02 *[M90.80]*
    ankle A50.02 *[M90.87-]*
    elbow A50.02 *[M90.82-]*
    foot A50.02 *[M90.87-]*
    forearm A50.02 *[M90.83-]*
    hand A50.02 *[M90.84-]*
    hip A50.02 *[M90.85-]*
    knee A50.02 *[M90.86-]*
    multiple sites A50.02 *[M90.89]*
    shoulder joint A50.02 *[M90.81-]*
    specified site NEC A50.02 *[M90.88]*
Osteochondroarthrosis deformans endemica — *see* Disease, Kaschin-Beck
Osteochondrodysplasia Q78.9
  with defects of growth of tubular bones and spine Q77.9
    specified NEC Q77.8
  specified NEC Q78.8
Osteochondrodystrophy E78.9
Osteochondrolysis — *see* Osteochondritis, dissecans
Osteochondroma — *see* Neoplasm, bone, benign
Osteochondromatosis D48.0
  syndrome Q78.4
Osteochondromyxosarcoma — *see* Neoplasm, bone, malignant
Osteochondropathy M93.90
  ankle M93.97-
  elbow M93.92-
  foot M93.97-
  hand M93.94-
  hip M93.95-
  Kienböck's disease of adults M93.1
  knee M93.96-
  multiple joints M93.99
  osteochondritis dissecans — *see* Osteochondritis, dissecans
  osteochondrosis — *see* Osteochondrosis
  shoulder region M93.91-
  slipped upper femoral epiphysis — *see* Slipped, epiphysis, upper femoral
  specified joint NEC M93.98
  specified type NEC M93.80
    ankle M93.87-
    elbow M93.82-
    foot M93.87-
    hand M93.84-
    hip M93.85-
    knee M93.86-
    multiple joints M93.89
    shoulder region M93.81-
    specified joint NEC M93.88
    wrist M93.83-
  syphilitic, congenital
    early A50.02 *[M90.80]*
    late A50.56 *[M90.80]*

Osteochondropathy - *continued*
  wrist M93.93-
Osteochondrosarcoma — *see* Neoplasm, bone, malignant
Osteochondrosis — *see also*
    Osteochondropathy, by site
  acetabulum (juvenile) M91.0
  adult — *see* Osteochondropathy, specified type NEC, by site
  astragalus (juvenile) — *see* Osteochondrosis, juvenile, tarsus
  Blount's — *see* Osteochondrosis, juvenile, tibia
  Buchanan's M91.0
  Burns' — *see* Osteochondrosis, juvenile, ulna
  calcaneus (juvenile) — *see* Osteochondrosis, juvenile, tarsus
  capitular epiphysis (femur) (juvenile) — *see* Legg-Calvé-Perthes disease
  carpal (juvenile) (lunate) (scaphoid) — *see* Osteochondrosis, juvenile, hand, carpal lunate
    adult M93.1
  coxae juvenilis — *see* Legg-Calvé-Perthes disease
  deformans juvenilis, coxae — *see* Legg-Calvé-Perthes disease
  Diaz' — *see* Osteochondrosis, juvenile, tarsus
  dissecans (knee) (shoulder) — *see* Osteochondritis, dissecans
  femoral capital epiphysis (juvenile) — *see* Legg-Calvé-Perthes disease
  femur (head) , juvenile — *see* Legg-Calvé-Perthes disease
  fibula (juvenile) — *see* Osteochondrosis, juvenile, fibula
  foot NEC (juvenile) M92.8
  Freiberg's — *see* Osteochondrosis, juvenile, metatarsus
  Haas' (juvenile) — *see* Osteochondrosis, juvenile, humerus
  Haglund's — *see* Osteochondrosis, juvenile, tarsus
  hip (juvenile) — *see* Legg-Calvé-Perthes disease
  humerus (capitulum) (head) (juvenile) — *see* Osteochondrosis, juvenile, humerus
  ilium, iliac crest (juvenile) M91.0
  ischiopubic synchondrosis M91.0
  Iselin's — *see* Osteochondrosis, juvenile, metatarsus
  juvenile, juvenilis M92.9
    after congenital dislocation of hip reduction — *see* Osteochondrosis, juvenile, hip, specified NEC
    arm — *see* Osteochondrosis, juvenile, upper limb NEC
    capitular epiphysis (femur) — *see* Legg-Calvé-Perthes disease
    clavicle, sternal epiphysis — *see* Osteochondrosis, juvenile, upper limb NEC
    coxae — *see* Legg-Calvé-Perthes disease
    deformans M92.9
    fibula M92.5-
    foot NEC M92.8
    hand M92.20-
      carpal lunate M92.21-
      metacarpal head M92.22-
      specified site NEC M92.29-
    head of femur — *see* Legg-Calvé-Perthes disease
    hip and pelvis M91.9-
      coxa plana — *see* Coxa, plana
      femoral head — *see* Legg-Calvé-Perthes disease
      pelvis M91.0
      pseudocoxalgia — *see* Pseudocoxalgia
      specified NEC M91.8-
    humerus M92.0-
    limb
      lower NEC M92.8
      upper NEC — *see* Osteochondrosis, juvenile, upper limb NEC

Osteochondrosis - *continued*
  juvenile, juvenilis - *continued*
    medial cuneiform bone — *see* Osteochondrosis, juvenile, tarsus
    metatarsus M92.7-
    patella M92.4-
    radius M92.1-
    specified site NEC M92.8
    spine M42.00
      cervical region M42.02
      cervicothoracic region M42.03
      lumbar region M42.06
      lumbosacral region M42.07
      multiple sites M42.09
      occipito-atlanto-axial region M42.01
      sacrococcygeal region M42.08
      thoracic region M42.04
      thoracolumbar region M42.05
    tarsus M92.6-
    tibia M92.5-
    ulna M92.1-
    upper limb NEC M92.3-
    vertebra (body) (epiphyseal plates) (Calvé's) (Scheuermann's) — *see* Osteochondrosis, juvenile, spine
  Kienböck's — *see* Osteochondrosis, juvenile, hand, carpal lunate
    adult M93.1
  Köhler's
    patellar — *see* Osteochondrosis, juvenile, patella
    tarsal navicular — *see* Osteochondrosis, juvenile, tarsus
  Legg-Perthes (-Calvé) (-Waldenström) — *see* Legg-Calvé-Perthes disease
  limb
    lower NEC (juvenile) M92.8
    upper NEC (juvenile) — *see* Osteochondrosis, juvenile, upper limb NEC
  lunate bone (carpal) (juvenile) — *see also* Osteochondrosis, juvenile, hand, carpal lunate
    adult M93.1
  Mauclaire's — *see* Osteochondrosis, juvenile, hand, metacarpal
  metacarpal (head) (juvenile) — *see* Osteochondrosis, juvenile, hand, metacarpal
  metatarsus (fifth) (head) (juvenile) (second) — *see* Osteochondrosis, juvenile, metatarsus
  navicular (juvenile) — *see* Osteochondrosis, juvenile, tarsus
  os
    calcis (juvenile) — *see* Osteochondrosis, juvenile, tarsus
    tibiale externum (juvenile) — *see* Osteochondrosis, juvenile, tarsus
  Osgood-Schlatter — *see* Osteochondrosis, juvenile, tibia
  Panner's — *see* Osteochondrosis, juvenile, humerus
  patellar center (juvenile) (primary) (secondary) — *see* Osteochondrosis, juvenile, patella
  pelvis (juvenile) M91.0
  Pierson's M91.0
  radius (head) (juvenile) — *see* Osteochondrosis, juvenile, radius
  Scheuermann's — *see* Osteochondrosis, juvenile, spine
  Sever's — *see* Osteochondrosis, juvenile, tarsus
  Sinding-Larsen — *see* Osteochondrosis, juvenile, patella
  spine M42.9
    adult M42.10
      cervical region M42.12
      cervicothoracic region M42.13
      lumbar region M42.16
      lumbosacral region M42.17
      multiple sites M42.19
      occipito-atlanto-axial region M42.11
      sacrococcygeal region M42.18

Osteochondrosis - *continued*
  spine - *continued*
    adult - *continued*
      thoracic region M42.14
      thoracolumbar region M42.15
    juvenile — *see* Osteochondrosis, juvenile, spine
  symphysis pubis (juvenile) M91.0
  syphilitic (congenital) A50.02
  talus (juvenile) — *see* Osteochondrosis, juvenile, tarsus
  tarsus (navicular) (juvenile) — *see* Osteochondrosis, juvenile, tarsus
  tibia (proximal) (tubercle) (juvenile) — *see* Osteochondrosis, juvenile, tibia
  tuberculous — *see* Tuberculosis, bone
  ulna (lower) (juvenile) — *see* Osteochondrosis, juvenile, ulna
  van Neck's M91.0
  vertebral — *see* Osteochondrosis, spine
Osteoclastoma D48.0
  malignant — *see* Neoplasm, bone, malignant
Osteodynia — *see* Disorder, bone, specified type NEC
Osteodystrophy Q78.9
  azotemic N25.0
  congenital Q78.9
  parathyroid, secondary E21.1
  renal N25.0
Osteofibroma — *see* Neoplasm, bone, benign
Osteofibrosarcoma — *see* Neoplasm, bone, malignant
Osteogenesis imperfecta Q78.0
Osteogenic — *see* condition
Osteolysis M89.50
  carpus M89.54-
  clavicle M89.51-
  femur M89.55-
  fibula M89.56-
  finger M89.54-
  humerus M89.52-
  ilium M89.559
  ischium M89.559
  joint prosthesis (periprosthetic) — *see* Complications, joint prosthesis, mechanical, periprosthetic, osteolysis, by site
  metacarpus M89.54-
  metatarsus M89.57-
  multiple sites M89.59
  neck M89.58
  periprosthetic — *see* Complications, joint prosthesis, mechanical, periprosthetic, osteolysis, by site
  radius M89.53-
  rib M89.58
  scapula M89.51-
  skull M89.58
  tarsus M89.57-
  tibia M89.56-
  toe M89.57-
  ulna M89.53-
  vertebra M89.58
Osteoma — *see also* Neoplasm, bone, benign
  osteoid — *see also* Neoplasm, bone, benign
    giant — *see* Neoplasm, bone, benign
Osteomalacia M83.9
  adult M83.9
    drug-induced NEC M83.5
    due to
      malabsorption (postsurgical) M83.2
      malnutrition M83.3
    specified NEC M83.8
  aluminium-induced M83.4
  infantile — *see* Rickets
  juvenile — *see* Rickets
  oncogenic E83.89
  pelvis M83.8
  puerperal M83.0
  senile M83.1
  vitamin-D-resistant in adults E83.31 *[M90.8-]*
    carpus E83.31 *[M90.84-]*
    clavicle E83.31 *[M90.81-]*
    femur E83.31 *[M90.85-]*

Osteomalacia - *continued*
  vitamin-D-resistant in adults - *continued*
    fibula E83.31 *[M90.86-]*
    finger E83.31 *[M90.84-]*
    humerus E83.31 *[M90.82-]*
    ilium E83.31 *[M90.859]*
    ischium E83.31 *[M90.859]*
    metacarpus E83.31 *[M90.84-]*
    metatarsus E83.31 *[M90.87-]*
    multiple sites E83.31 *[M90.89]*
    neck E83.31 *[M90.88]*
    radius E83.31 *[M90.83-]*
    rib E83.31 *[M90.88]*
    scapula E83.31 *[M90.819]*
    skull E83.31 *[M90.88]*
    tarsus E83.31 *[M90.879]*
    tibia E83.31 *[M90.869]*
    toe E83.31 *[M90.879]*
    ulna E83.31 *[M90.839]*
    vertebra E83.31 *[M90.88]*
Osteomyelitis (general) (infective) (localized) (neonatal) (purulent) (septic) (staphylococcal) (streptococcal) (suppurative) (with periostitis) M86.9
  acute M86.10
    carpus M86.14-
    clavicle M86.11-
    femur M86.15-
    fibula M86.16-
    finger M86.14-
    hematogenous M86.00
      carpus M86.04-
      clavicle M86.01-
      femur M86.05-
      fibula M86.06-
      finger M86.04-
      humerus M86.02-
      ilium M86.059
      ischium M86.059
      mandible M27.2
      metacarpus M86.04-
      metatarsus M86.07-
      multiple sites M86.09
      neck M86.08
      orbit H05.02-
      petrous bone — *see* Petrositis
      radius M86.03-
      rib M86.08
      scapula M86.01-
      skull M86.08
      tarsus M86.07-
      tibia M86.06-
      toe M86.07-
      ulna M86.03-
      vertebra — *see* Osteomyelitis, vertebra
    humerus M86.12-
    ilium M86.18
    ischium M86.18
    mandible M27.2
    metacarpus M86.14-
    metatarsus M86.17-
    multiple sites M86.19
    neck M86.18
    orbit H05.02-
    petrous bone — *see* Petrositis
    radius M86.13-
    rib M86.18
    scapula M86.11-
    skull M86.18
    tarsus M86.17-
    tibia M86.16-
    toe M86.17-
    ulna M86.13-
    vertebra — *see* Osteomyelitis, vertebra
  chronic (or old) M86.60
    with draining sinus M86.40
      carpus M86.44-
      clavicle M86.41-
      femur M86.45-
      fibula M86.46-
      finger M86.44-
      humerus M86.42-
      ilium M86.459
      ischium M86.459
      mandible M27.2

Osteomyelitis (general) (infective) (localized) (neonatal) (purulent) (septic) (staphylococcal) (streptococcal) (suppurative) (with periostitis) - *continued*
  chronic (or old) - *continued*
    with draining sinus - *continued*
      metacarpus M86.44-
      metatarsus M86.47-
      multiple sites M86.49
      neck M86.48
      orbit H05.02-
      petrous bone — *see* Petrositis
      radius M86.43-
      rib M86.48
      scapula M86.41-
      skull M86.48
      tarsus M86.47-
      tibia M86.46-
      toe M86.47-
      ulna M86.43-
      vertebra — *see* Osteomyelitis, vertebra
    carpus M86.64-
    clavicle M86.61-
    femur M86.65-
    fibula M86.66-
    finger M86.64-
    hematogenous NEC M86.50
      carpus M86.54-
      clavicle M86.51-
      femur M86.55-
      fibula M86.56-
      finger M86.54-
      humerus M86.52-
      ilium M86.559
      ischium M86.559
      mandible M27.2
      metacarpus M86.54-
      metatarsus M86.57-
      multifocal M86.30
        carpus M86.34-
        clavicle M86.31-
        femur M86.35-
        fibula M86.36-
        finger M86.34-
        humerus M86.32-
        ilium M86.359
        ischium M86.359
        metacarpus M86.34-
        metatarsus M86.37-
        multiple sites M86.39
        neck M86.38
        radius M86.33-
        rib M86.38
        scapula M86.31-
        skull M86.38
        tarsus M86.37-
        tibia M86.36-
        toe M86.37-
        ulna M86.33-
        vertebra — *see* Osteomyelitis, vertebra
      multiple sites M86.59
      neck M86.58
      orbit H05.02-
      petrous bone — *see* Petrositis
      radius M86.53-
      rib M86.58
      scapula M86.51-
      skull M86.58
      tarsus M86.57-
      tibia M86.56-
      toe M86.57-
      ulna M86.53-
      vertebra — *see* Osteomyelitis, vertebra
    humerus M86.62-
    ilium M86.659
    ischium M86.659
    mandible M27.2
    metacarpus M86.64-
    metatarsus M86.67-
    multifocal — *see* Osteomyelitis, chronic, hematogenous, multifocal
    multiple sites M86.69
    neck M86.68
    orbit H05.02-

Osteomyelitis (general) (infective) (localized) (neonatal) (purulent) (septic) (staphylococcal) (streptococcal) (suppurative) (with periostitis) - *continued*
  chronic (or old) - *continued*
    petrous bone — *see* Petrositis
    radius M86.63-
    rib M86.68
    scapula M86.61-
    skull M86.68
    tarsus M86.67-
    tibia M86.66-
    toe M86.67-
    ulna M86.63-
    vertebra — *see* Osteomyelitis, vertebra
  echinococcal B67.2
  Garr's — *see* Osteomyelitis, specified type NEC
  in diabetes mellitus — *see* E08-E13 with .69
  jaw (acute) (chronic) (lower) (neonatal) (suppurative) (upper) M27.2
  nonsuppurating — *see* Osteomyelitis, specified type NEC
  orbit H05.02-
  petrous bone — *see* Petrositis
  Salmonella (arizonae) (cholerae-suis) (enteritidis) (typhimurium) A02.24
  sclerosing, nonsuppurative — *see* Osteomyelitis, specified type NEC
  specified type NEC (*see also* subcategory M86.8X-)
    mandible M27.2
    orbit H05.02-
    petrous bone — *see* Petrositis
    vertebra — *see* Osteomyelitis, vertebra
  subacute M86.20
    carpus M86.24-
    clavicle M86.21-
    femur M86.25-
    fibula M86.26-
    finger M86.24-
    humerus M86.22-
    mandible M27.2
    metacarpus M86.24-
    metatarsus M86.27-
    multiple sites M86.29
    neck M86.28
    orbit H05.02-
    petrous bone — *see* Petrositis
    radius M86.23-
    rib M86.28
    scapula M86.21-
    skull M86.28
    tarsus M86.27-
    tibia M86.26-
    toe M86.27-
    ulna M86.23-
    vertebra — *see* Osteomyelitis, vertebra
  syphilitic A52.77
    congenital (early) A50.02 *[M90.80]*
  tuberculous — *see* Tuberculosis, bone
  typhoid A01.05
  vertebra M46.20
    cervical region M46.22
    cervicothoracic region M46.23
    lumbar region M46.26
    lumbosacral region M46.27
    occipito-atlanto-axial region M46.21
    sacrococcygeal region M46.28
    thoracic region M46.24
    thoracolumbar region M46.25
Osteomyelofibrosis D47.4
Osteomyelosclerosis D75.89
Osteonecrosis M87.9
  due to
    drugs — *see* Osteonecrosis, secondary, due to, drugs
    trauma — *see* Osteonecrosis, secondary, due to, trauma
  idiopathic aseptic M87.00
    ankle M87.07-
    carpus M87.03-
    clavicle M87.01-
    femur M87.05-
    fibula M87.06-

Osteonecrosis - *continued*
  idiopathic aseptic - *continued*
    finger M87.04-
    humerus M87.02-
    ilium M87.050
    ischium M87.050
    metacarpus M87.04-
    metatarsus M87.07-
    multiple sites M87.09
    neck M87.08
    pelvis M87.050
    radius M87.03-
    rib M87.08
    scapula M87.01-
    skull M87.08
    tarsus M87.07-
    tibia M87.06-
    toe M87.07-
    ulna M87.03-
    vertebra M87.08
  secondary NEC M87.30
    carpus M87.33-
    clavicle M87.31-
    due to
      drugs M87.10
        carpus M87.13-
        clavicle M87.11-
        femur M87.15-
        fibula M87.16-
        finger M87.14-
        humerus M87.12-
        ilium M87.159
        ischium M87.159
        jaw M87.180
        metacarpus M87.14-
        metatarsus M87.17-
        multiple sites M87.19
        neck M87.18
        radius M87.13-
        rib M87.18
        scapula M87.11-
        skull M87.18
        tarsus M87.17-
        tibia M87.16-
        toe M87.17-
        ulna M87.13-
        vertebra M87.18
      hemoglobinopathy NEC D58.2 *[M90.50]*
        carpus D58.2 *[M90.54-]*
        clavicle D58.2 *[M90.51-]*
        femur D58.2 *[M90.55-]*
        fibula D58.2 *[M90.56-]*
        finger D58.2 *[M90.54-]*
        humerus D58.2 *[M90.52-]*
        ilium D58.2 *[M90.55-]*
        ischium D58.2 *[M90.55-]*
        metacarpus D58.2 *[M90.54-]*
        metatarsus D58.2 *[M90.57-]*
        multiple sites D58.2 *[M90.58]*
        neck D58.2 *[M90.58]*
        radius D58.2 *[M90.53-]*
        rib D58.2 *[M90.58]*
        scapula D58.2 *[M90.51-]*
        skull D58.2 *[M90.58]*
        tarsus D58.2 *[M90.57-]*
        tibia D58.2 *[M90.56-]*
        toe D58.2 *[M90.57-]*
        ulna D58.2 *[M90.53-]*
        vertebra D58.2 *[M90.58]*
      trauma (previous) M87.20
        carpus M87.23-
        clavicle M87.21-
        femur M87.25-
        fibula M87.26-
        finger M87.24-
        humerus M87.22-
        ilium M87.25-
        ischium M87.25-
        metacarpus M87.24-
        metatarsus M87.27-
        multiple sites M87.29
        neck M87.28
        radius M87.23-
        rib M87.28

Osteonecrosis - *continued*
  secondary NEC - *continued*
    due to - *continued*
      trauma (previous) - *continued*
        scapula M87.21-
        skull M87.28
        tarsus M87.27-
        tibia M87.26-
        toe M87.27-
        ulna M87.23-
        vertebra M87.28
    femur M87.35-
    fibula M87.36-
    finger M87.34-
    humerus M87.32-
    ilium M87.350
    in
      caisson disease T70.3 *[M90.50]*
        carpus T70.3 *[M90.54-]*
        clavicle T70.3 *[M90.51-]*
        femur T70.3 *[M90.55-]*
        fibula T70.3 *[M90.56-]*
        finger T70.3 *[M90.54-]*
        humerus T70.3 *[M90.52-]*
        ilium T70.3 *[M90.55-]*
        ischium T70.3 *[M90.55-]*
        metacarpus T70.3 *[M90.54-]*
        metatarsus T70.3 *[M90.57-]*
        multiple sites T70.3 *[M90.59]*
        neck T70.3 *[M90.58]*
        radius T70.3 *[M90.53-]*
        rib T70.3 *[M90.58]*
        scapula T70.3 *[M90.51-]*
        skull T70.3 *[M90.58]*
        tarsus T70.3 *[M90.57-]*
        tibia T70.3 *[M90.56-]*
        toe T70.3 *[M90.57-]*
        ulna T70.3 *[M90.53-]*
        vertebra T70.3 *[M90.58]*
    ischium M87.350
    metacarpus M87.34-
    metatarsus M87.37-
    multiple site M87.39
    neck M87.38
    radius M87.33-
    rib M87.38
    scapula M87.319
    skull M87.38
    tarsus M87.379
    tibia M87.366
    toe M87.379
    ulna M87.33-
    vertebra M87.38
  specified type NEC M87.80
    carpus M87.83-
    clavicle M87.81-
    femur M87.85-
    fibula M87.86-
    finger M87.84-
    humerus M87.82-
    ilium M87.85-
    ischium M87.85-
    metacarpus M87.84-
    metatarsus M87.87-
    multiple sites M87.89
    neck M87.88
    radius M87.83-
    rib M87.88
    scapula M87.81-
    skull M87.88
    tarsus M87.87-
    tibia M87.86-
    toe M87.87-
    ulna M87.83-
    vertebra M87.88
Osteo-onycho-arthro-dysplasia Q87.2
Osteo-onychodysplasia, hereditary Q87.2
Osteopathia condensans disseminata Q78.8
Osteopathy — *see also* Osteomyelitis, Osteonecrosis, Osteoporosis
  after poliomyelitis M89.60
    carpus M89.64-
    clavicle M89.61-
    femur M89.65-
    fibula M89.66-

Osteopathy - *continued*
  after poliomyelitis - *continued*
    finger M89.64-
    humerus M89.62-
    ilium M89.659
    ischium M89.659
    metacarpus M89.64-
    metatarsus M89.67-
    multiple sites M89.69
    neck M89.68
    radius M89.63-
    rib M89.68
    scapula M89.61-
    skull M89.68
    tarsus M89.67-
    tibia M89.66-
    toe M89.67-
    ulna M89.63-
    vertebra M89.68
  in (due to)
    renal osteodystrophy N25.0
    specified diseases classified elsewhere —
      see subcategory M90.8
Osteopenia M85.8-
  borderline M85.8-
Osteoperiostitis — *see* Osteomyelitis,
    specified type NEC
Osteopetrosis (familial) Q78.2
Osteophyte M25.70
  ankle M25.77-
  elbow M25.72-
  foot joint M25.77-
  hand joint M25.74-
  hip M25.75-
  knee M25.76-
  shoulder M25.71-
  spine M25.78
  vertebrae M25.78
  wrist M25.73-
Osteopoikilosis Q78.8
Osteoporosis (female) (male) M81.0
  with current pathological fracture M80.00
  age-related M81.0
    with current pathologic fracture M80.00
      carpus M80.04-
      clavicle M80.01-
      fibula M80.06-
      finger M80.04-
      humerus M80.02-
      ilium M80.05-
      ischium M80.05-
      metacarpus M80.04-
      metatarsus M80.07-
      pelvis M80.05-
      radius M80.03-
      scapula M80.01-
      tarsus M80.07-
      tibia M80.06-
      toe M80.07-
      ulna M80.03-
      vertebra M80.08
  disuse M81.8
    with current pathological fracture M80.80
      carpus M80.84-
      clavicle M80.81-
      fibula M80.86-
      finger M80.84-
      humerus M80.82-
      ilium M80.85-
      ischium M80.85-
      metacarpus M80.84-
      metatarsus M80.87-
      pelvis M80.85-
      radius M80.83-
      scapula M80.81-
      tarsus M80.87-
      tibia M80.86-
      toe M80.87-
      ulna M80.83-
      vertebra M80.88
  drug-induced — *see* Osteoporosis, specified
    type NEC
  idiopathic — *see* Osteoporosis, specified
    type NEC
  involutional — *see* Osteoporosis, age-related

Osteoporosis (female) (male) - *continued*
  Lequesne M81.6
  localized M81.6
  postmenopausal M81.0
    with pathological fracture M80.00
      carpus M80.04-
      clavicle M80.01-
      fibula M80.06-
      finger M80.04-
      humerus M80.02-
      ilium M80.05-
      ischium M80.05-
      metacarpus M80.04-
      metatarsus M80.07-
      pelvis M80.05-
      radius M80.03-
      scapula M80.01-
      tarsus M80.07-
      tibia M80.06-
      toe M80.07-
      ulna M80.03-
      vertebra M80.08
  postoophorectomy — *see* Osteoporosis,
    specified type NEC
  postsurgical malabsorption — *see*
    Osteoporosis, specified type NEC
  post-traumatic — *see* Osteoporosis, specified
    type NEC
  senile — *see* Osteoporosis, age-related
  specified type NEC M81.8
    with pathological fracture M80.80
      carpus M80.84-
      clavicle M80.81-
      fibula M80.86-
      finger M80.84-
      humerus M80.82-
      ilium M80.85-
      ischium M80.85-
      metacarpus M80.84-
      metatarsus M80.87-
      pelvis M80.85-
      radius M80.83-
      scapula M80.81-
      tarsus M80.87-
      tibia M80.86-
      toe M80.87-
      ulna M80.83-
      vertebra M80.88
Osteopsathyrosis (idiopathica) Q78.0
Osteoradionecrosis, jaw (acute) (chronic)
    (lower) (suppurative) (upper) M27.2
Osteosarcoma (any form) — *see* Neoplasm,
    bone, malignant
Osteosclerosis Q78.2
  acquired M85.8-
  congenita Q77.4
  fragilitas (generalisata) Q78.2
  myelofibrosis D75.81
Osteosclerotic anemia D64.89
Osteosis
  cutis L94.2
  renal fibrocystic N25.0
Österreicher-Turner syndrome Q87.2
Ostium
  atrioventriculare commune Q21.2
  primum (arteriosum) (defect)
    (persistent) Q21.2
  secundum (arteriosum) (defect) (patent)
    (persistent) Q21.1
Ostrum-Furst syndrome Q75.8
Otalgia — *see* subcategory H92.0
Otitis (acute) H66.90
  with effusion — *see also* Otitis, media,
    nonsuppurative
    purulent — *see* Otitis, media, suppurative
  adhesive — *see* subcategory H74.1
  chronic — *see also* Otitis, media, chronic
    with effusion — *see also* Otitis, media,
      nonsuppurative, chronic
  externa H60.9-
    abscess — *see* Abscess, ear, external
    acute (noninfective) H60.50-
      actinic H60.51-
      chemical H60.52-
      contact H60.53-

Otitis (acute) - *continued*
  externa - *continued*
    acute (noninfective) - *continued*
      eczematoid H60.54-
      infective — *see* Otitis, externa, infective
      reactive H60.55-
      specified NEC H60.59-
    cellulitis — *see* Cellulitis, ear
    chronic H60.6-
    diffuse — *see* Otitis, externa, infective,
      diffuse
    hemorrhagic — *see* Otitis, externa,
      infective, hemorrhagic
    in (due to)
      aspergillosis B44.89
      candidiasis B37.84
      erysipelas A46 *[H62.40]*
      herpes (simplex) virus infection B00.1
        zoster B02.8
      impetigo L01.00 *[H62.40]*
      infectious disease NEC B99 *[H62.4-]*
      mycosis NEC B36.9 *[H62.40]*
      parasitic disease NEC B89 *[H62.40]*
      viral disease NEC B34.9 *[H62.40]*
        zoster B02.8
    infective NEC H60.39-
      abscess — *see* Abscess, ear, external
      cellulitis — *see* Cellulitis, ear
      diffuse H60.31-
      hemorrhagic H60.32-
      swimmer's ear — *see* Swimmer's, ear
    malignant H60.2-
    mycotic NEC B36.9 *[H62.40]*
      in
        aspergillosis B44.89
        candidiasis B37.84
        moniliasis B37.84
    necrotizing — *see* Otitis, externa,
      malignant
    Pseudomonas aeruginosa — *see* Otitis,
      externa, malignant
    reactive — *see* Otitis, externa, acute,
      reactive
    specified NEC — *see* subcategory H60.8
    tropical NEC B36.9 *[H62.40]*
      in
        aspergillosis B44.89
        candidiasis B37.84
        moniliasis B37.84
  insidiosa — *see* Otosclerosis
  interna — *see* subcategory H83.0
  media (hemorrhagic) (staphylococcal)
    (streptococcal) H66.9-
    with effusion (nonpurulent) — *see* Otitis,
      media, nonsuppurative
    acute, subacute H66.90
      allergic — *see* Otitis, media,
        nonsuppurative, acute, allergic
      exudative — *see* Otitis, media,
        suppurative, acute
      mucoid — *see* Otitis, media,
        nonsuppurative, acute
      necrotizing — *see also* Otitis, media,
        suppurative, acute
        in
          measles B05.3
          scarlet fever A38.0
      nonsuppurative NEC — *see* Otitis,
        media, nonsuppurative, acute
      purulent — *see* Otitis, media,
        suppurative, acute
      sanguinous — *see* Otitis, media,
        nonsuppurative, acute
      secretory — *see* Otitis, media,
        nonsuppurative, acute, serous
      seromucinous — *see* Otitis, media,
        nonsuppurative, acute
      serous — *see* Otitis, media,
        nonsuppurative, acute, serous
      suppurative — *see* Otitis, media,
        suppurative, acute
      allergic — *see* Otitis, media,
        nonsuppurative
      catarrhal — *see* Otitis, media,
        nonsuppurative

Otitis (acute) - *continued*
  media (hemorrhagic) (staphylococcal)
  (streptococcal) - *continued*
    chronic H66.90
      with effusion (nonpurulent) — *see*
        Otitis, media, nonsuppurative,
        chronic
      allergic — *see* Otitis, media,
        nonsuppurative, chronic, allergic
      benign suppurative — *see* Otitis, media,
        suppurative, chronic, tubotympanic
      catarrhal — *see* Otitis, media,
        nonsuppurative, chronic, serous
      exudative — *see* Otitis, media,
        nonsuppurative, chronic
      mucinous — *see* Otitis, media,
        nonsuppurative, chronic, mucoid
      mucoid — *see* Otitis, media,
        nonsuppurative, chronic, mucoid
      nonsuppurative NEC — *see* Otitis,
        media, nonsuppurative, chronic
      purulent — *see* Otitis, media,
        suppurative, chronic
      secretory — *see* Otitis, media,
        nonsuppurative, chronic, mucoid
      seromucinous — *see* Otitis, media,
        nonsuppurative, chronic
      serous — *see* Otitis, media,
        nonsuppurative, chronic, serous
      suppurative — *see* Otitis, media,
        suppurative, chronic
      transudative — *see* Otitis, media,
        nonsuppurative, chronic, mucoid
    exudative — *see* Otitis, media, suppurative
    in (due to) (with)
      influenza — *see* Influenza, with, otitis
        media
      measles B05.3
      scarlet fever A38.0
      tuberculosis A18.6
      viral disease NEC B34.- *[H67.-]*
    mucoid — *see* Otitis, media,
      nonsuppurative
    nonsuppurative H65.9-
      acute or subacute NEC H65.19-
        allergic H65.11-
          recurrent H65.11-
        recurrent H65.19-
        secretory — *see* Otitis, media,
          nonsuppurative, serous
        serous H65.0-
          recurrent H65.0-
      chronic H65.49-
        allergic H65.41-
        mucoid H65.3-
        serous H65.2-
      postmeasles B05.3
    purulent — *see* Otitis, media, suppurative
    secretory — *see* Otitis, media,
      nonsuppurative
    seromucinous — *see* Otitis, media,
      nonsuppurative
    serous — *see* Otitis, media,
      nonsuppurative
    suppurative H66.4-
      acute H66.00-
        with rupture of ear drum H66.01-
        recurrent H66.00-
          with rupture of ear drum H66.01-
      chronic (*see also* subcategory H66.3)
        atticoantral H66.2-
        benign — *see* Otitis, media,
          suppurative, chronic,
          tubotympanic
        tubotympanic H66.1-
    transudative — *see* Otitis, media,
      nonsuppurative
    tuberculous A18.6
Otocephaly Q18.2
Otolith syndrome — *see* subcategory H81.8
Otomycosis (diffuse) NEC B36.9 *[H62.40]*
  in
    aspergillosis B44.89
    candidiasis B37.84
    moniliasis B37.84

Otoporosis — *see* Otosclerosis
Otorrhagia (nontraumatic) H92.2-
  traumatic - code by Type of injury
Otorrhea H92.1-
  cerebrospinal G96.0
Otosclerosis (general) H80.9-
  cochlear (endosteal) H80.2-
  involving
    otic capsule — *see* Otosclerosis, cochlear
    oval window
      nonobliterative H80.0-
      obliterative H80.1-
    round window — *see* Otosclerosis,
      cochlear
  nonobliterative — *see* Otosclerosis,
    involving, oval window, nonobliterative
  obliterative — *see* Otosclerosis, involving,
    oval window, obliterative
  specified NEC H80.8-
Otospongiosis — *see* Otosclerosis
Otto's disease or pelvis M24.7
Outcome of delivery Z37.9
  multiple births Z37.9
    all liveborn Z37.50
      quadruplets Z37.52
      quintuplets Z37.53
      sextuplets Z37.54
      specified number NEC Z37.59
      triplets Z37.51
    all stillborn Z37.7
    some liveborn Z37.60
      quadruplets Z37.62
      quintuplets Z37.63
      sextuplets Z37.64
      specified number NEC Z37.69
      triplets Z37.61
  single NEC Z37.9
    liveborn Z37.0
    stillborn Z37.1
  twins NEC Z37.9
    both liveborn Z37.2
    both stillborn Z37.4
    one liveborn, one stillborn Z37.3
Outlet — *see* condition
Ovalocytosis (congenital) (hereditary) — *see*
  Elliptocytosis
Ovarian — *see* Condition
Ovariocele N83.4-
Ovaritis (cystic) — *see* Oophoritis
Ovary, ovarian — *see also* condition
  resistant syndrome E28.39
  vein syndrome N13.8
Overactive — *see also* Hyperfunction
  adrenal cortex NEC E27.0
  bladder N32.81
  hypothalamus E23.3
  thyroid — *see* Hyperthyroidism
Overactivity R46.3
  child — *see* Disorder, attention-deficit
    hyperactivity
Overbite (deep) (excessive) (horizontal)
  (vertical) M26.29
Overbreathing — *see* Hyperventilation
Overconscientious personality F60.5
Overdevelopment — *see* Hypertrophy
Overdistension — *see* Distension
Overdose, overdosage (drug) — *see* Table of
  Drugs and Chemicals, by drug, poisoning
Overeating R63.2
  nonorganic origin F50.89
  psychogenic F50.89
Overexertion (effects) (exhaustion) T73.3
Overexposure (effects) T73.9
  exhaustion T73.2
Overfeeding — *see* Overeating
  newborn P92.4
Overfill, endodontic M27.52
Overgrowth, bone — *see* Hypertrophy, bone
Overhanging of dental restorative material
  (unrepairable) K08.52
Overheated (places) (effects) — *see* Heat
Overjet (excessive horizontal) M26.23
Overlaid, overlying (suffocation) — *see*
  Asphyxia, traumatic, due to mechanical
  threat

Overlap, excessive horizontal (teeth) M26.23
Overlapping toe (acquired) — *see also*
  Deformity, toe, specified NEC
  congenital (fifth toe) Q66.89
Overload
  circulatory, due to transfusion (blood) (blood
    components) (TACO) E87.71
  fluid E87.70
    due to transfusion (blood) (blood
      components) E87.71
    specified NEC E87.79
  iron, due to repeated red blood cell
    transfusions E83.111
  potassium (K) E87.5
  sodium (Na) E87.0
Overnutrition — *see* Hyperalimentation
Overproduction — *see also* Hypersecretion
  ACTH E27.0
  catecholamine E27.5
  growth hormone E22.0
Overprotection, child by parent Z62.1
Overriding
  aorta Q25.49
  finger (acquired) — *see* Deformity, finger
    congenital Q68.1
  toe (acquired) — *see also* Deformity, toe,
    specified NEC
    congenital Q66.89
Overstrained R53.83
  heart — *see* Hypertrophy, cardiac
Overuse, muscle NEC M70.8-
Overweight E66.3
Overworked R53.83
Oviduct — *see* condition
Ovotestis Q56.0
Ovulation (cycle)
  failure or lack of N97.0
  pain N94.0
Ovum — *see* condition
Owren's disease or syndrome
  (parahemophilia) D68.2
Ox heart — *see* Hypertrophy, cardiac
Oxalosis E72.53
Oxaluria E72.53
Oxycephaly, oxycephalic Q75.0
  syphilitic, congenital A50.02
Oxyuriasis B80
Oxyuris vermicularis (infestation) B80
Ozena J31.0

P

Pachyderma, pachydermia L85.9
  larynx (verrucosa) J38.7
Pachydermatocele (congenital) Q82.8
Pachydermoperiostosis — *see also*
  Osteoarthropathy, hypertrophic, specified
  type NEC
  clubbed nail M89.40 *[L62]*
Pachygyria Q04.3
Pachymeningitis (adhesive) (basal) (brain)
  (cervical) (chronic) (circumscribed)
  (external) (fibrous) (hemorrhagic)
  (hypertrophic) (internal) (purulent)
  (spinal) (suppurative) — *see* Meningitis
Pachyonychia (congenital) Q84.5
Pacinian tumor — *see* Neoplasm, skin, benign
Pad, knuckle or Garrod's M72.1
Paget's disease
  with infiltrating duct carcinoma — *see*
    Neoplasm, breast, malignant
  bone M88.9
    carpus M88.84-
    clavicle M88.81-
    femur M88.85-
    fibula M88.86-
    finger M88.84-
    humerus M88.82-
    ilium M88.85-
    in neoplastic disease — *see* Osteitis,
      deformans, in neoplastic disease
    ischium M88.85-
    metacarpus M88.84-
    metatarsus M88.87-
    multiple sites M88.89
    neck M88.88
    radius M88.83-

Paget's disease - *continued*
  bone - *continued*
    rib M88.88
    scapula M88.81-
    skull M88.0
    specified NEC M88.88
    tarsus M88.87-
    tibia M88.86-
    toe M88.87-
    ulna M88.83-
    vertebra M88.1
  breast (female) C50.01-
    male C50.02-
  extramammary — *see also* Neoplasm, skin,
    malignant
    anus C21.0
      margin C44.590
      skin C44.590
  intraductal carcinoma — *see* Neoplasm,
    breast, malignant
  malignant — *see* Neoplasm, skin, malignant
    breast (female) C50.01-
      male C50.02-
    unspecified site (female) C50.01-
      male C50.02-
  mammary — *see* Paget's disease, breast
  nipple — *see* Paget's disease, breast
  osteitis deformans — *see* Paget's disease,
    bone
Paget-Schroetter syndrome I82.890
Pain (s) — *see also* Painful R52
  abdominal R10.9
    colic R10.83
    generalized R10.84
      with acute abdomen R10.0
    lower R10.30
      left quadrant R10.32
      pelvic or perineal R10.2
      periumbilical R10.33
      right quadrant R10.31
    rebound — *see* Tenderness, abdominal,
      rebound
    severe with abdominal rigidity R10.0
    tenderness — *see* Tenderness, abdominal
    upper R10.10
      epigastric R10.13
      left quadrant R10.12
      right quadrant R10.11
  acute R52
    due to trauma G89.11
    neoplasm related G89.3
    postprocedural NEC G89.18
    post-thoracotomy G89.12
    specified by site - code to Pain, by site
  adnexa (uteri) R10.2
  anginoid — *see* Pain, precordial
  anus K62.89
  arm — *see* Pain, limb, upper
  axillary (axilla) M79.62-
  back (postural) M54.9
  bladder R39.89
    associated with micturition — *see*
      Micturition, painful
    chronic R39.82
  bone — *see* Disorder, bone, specified type
    NEC
  breast N64.4
  broad ligament R10.2
  cancer associated (acute) (chronic) G89.3
  cecum — *see* Pain, abdominal
  cervicobrachial M53.1
  chest (central) R07.9
    anterior wall R07.89
    atypical R07.89
    ischemic I20.9
    musculoskeletal R07.89
    non-cardiac R07.89
    on breathing R07.1
    pleurodynia R07.81
    precordial R07.2
    wall (anterior) R07.89
  chronic G89.29
    associated with significant psychosocial
      dysfunction G89.4
    due to trauma G89.21

Pain (s) - *continued*
  chronic - *continued*
    neoplasm related G89.3
    postoperative NEC G89.28
    postprocedural NEC G89.28
    post-thoracotomy G89.22
    specified NEC G89.29
  coccyx M53.3
  colon — *see* Pain, abdominal
  coronary — *see* Angina
  costochondral R07.1
  diaphragm R07.1
  due to cancer G89.3
  due to device, implant or graft — *see also*
    Complications, by site and type,
    specified NEC T85.848
    arterial graft NEC T82.848
    breast (implant) T85.848
    catheter NEC T85.848
      dialysis (renal) T82.848
        intraperitoneal T85.848
      infusion NEC T82.848
        spinal (epidural) (subdural) T85.840
      urinary (indwelling) T83.84
    electronic (electrode) (pulse generator)
      (stimulator)
      bone T84.84
      cardiac T82.847
      nervous system (brain) (peripheral
        nerve) (spinal) T85.840
      urinary T83.84
    fixation, internal (orthopedic) NEC T84.84
    gastrointestinal (bile duct)
      (esophagus) T85.848
    genital NEC T83.84
    heart NEC T82.847
      infusion NEC T85.848
    joint prosthesis T84.84
    ocular (corneal graft) (orbital implant)
      NEC T85.848
    orthopedic NEC T84.84
    specified NEC T85.848
    urinary NEC T83.84
    vascular NEC T82.848
    ventricular intracranial shunt T85.840
  due to malignancy (primary)
    (secondary) G89.3
  ear — *see* subcategory H92.0
  epigastric, epigastrium R10.13
  eye — *see* Pain, ocular
  face, facial R51
    atypical G50.1
  female genital organs NEC N94.89
  finger — *see* Pain, limb, upper
  flank — *see* Pain, abdominal
  foot — *see* Pain, limb, lower
  gallbladder K82.9
  gas (intestinal) R14.1
  gastric — *see* Pain, abdominal
  generalized NOS R52
  genital organ
    female N94.89
    male N50.89
  groin — *see* Pain, abdominal, lower
  hand — *see* Pain, limb, upper
  head — *see* Headache
  heart — *see* Pain, precordial
  infra-orbital — *see* Neuralgia, trigeminal
  intercostal R07.82
  intermenstrual N94.0
  jaw R68.84
  joint M25.50
    ankle M25.57-
    elbow M25.52-
    finger M25.54-
    foot M25.57-
    hand M25.54-
    hip M25.55-
    knee M25.56-
    shoulder M25.51-
    toe M25.57-
    wrist M25.53-
  kidney N23
  laryngeal R07.0
  leg — *see* Pain, limb, lower

Pain (s) - *continued*
  limb M79.609
    lower M79.60-
      foot M79.67-
      lower leg M79.66-
      thigh M79.65-
      toe M79.67-
    upper M79.60-
      axilla M79.62-
      finger M79.64-
      forearm M79.63-
      hand M79.64-
      upper arm M79.62-
  loin M54.5
  low back M54.5
  lumbar region M54.5
  mandibular R68.84
  mastoid — *see* subcategory H92.0
  maxilla R68.84
  menstrual — *see also* Dysmenorrhea N94.6
  metacarpophalangeal (joint) — *see* Pain,
    joint, hand
  metatarsophalangeal (joint) — *see* Pain,
    joint, foot
  mouth K13.79
  muscle — *see* Myalgia
  musculoskeletal — *see also* Pain, by
    site M79.18
  myofascial M79.18
  nasal J34.89
  nasopharynx J39.2
  neck NEC M54.2
  nerve NEC — *see* Neuralgia
  neuromuscular — *see* Neuralgia
  nose J34.89
  ocular H57.1-
  ophthalmic — *see* Pain, ocular
  orbital region — *see* Pain, ocular
  ovary N94.89
  over heart — *see* Pain, precordial
  ovulation N94.0
  pelvic (female) R10.2
  penis N48.89
  pericardial — *see* Pain, precordial
  perineal, perineum R10.2
  pharynx J39.2
  pleura, pleural, pleuritic R07.81
  postoperative NOS G89.18
  postprocedural NOS G89.18
  post-thoracotomy G89.12
  precordial (region) R07.2
  premenstrual N94.3
  psychogenic (persistent) (any site) F45.41
  radicular (spinal) — *see* Radiculopathy
  rectum K62.89
  respiration R07.1
  retrosternal R07.2
  rheumatoid, muscular — *see* Myalgia
  rib R07.81
  root (spinal) — *see* Radiculopathy
  round ligament (stretch) R10.2
  sacroiliac M53.3
  sciatic — *see* Sciatica
  scrotum N50.82
  seminal vesicle N50.89
  shoulder M25.51-
  spermatic cord N50.89
  spinal root — *see* Radiculopathy
  spine M54.9
    cervical M54.2
    low back M54.5
      with sciatica M54.4-
    thoracic M54.6
  stomach — *see* Pain, abdominal
  substernal R07.2
  temporomandibular (joint) M26.62-
  testis N50.81-
  thoracic spine M54.6
    with radicular and visceral pain M54.14
  throat R07.0
  tibia — *see* Pain, limb, lower
  toe — *see* Pain, limb, lower
  tongue K14.6
  tooth K08.89
  trigeminal — *see* Neuralgia, trigeminal

Pain (s) - *continued*
tumor associated G89.3
ureter N23
urinary (organ) (system) N23
uterus NEC N94.89
vagina R10.2
vertebrogenic (syndrome) M54.89
vesical R39.89
associated with micturition — *see*
Micturition, painful
vulva R10.2
Painful — *see also* Pain
coitus
female N94.10
male N53.12
psychogenic F52.6
ejaculation (semen) N53.12
psychogenic F52.6
erection — *see* Priapism
feet syndrome E53.8
joint replacement (hip) (knee) T84.84
menstruation — *see* Dysmenorrhea
psychogenic F45.8
micturition — *see* Micturition, painful
respiration R07.1
scar NEC L90.5
wire sutures T81.89
Painter's colic — *see* subcategory T56.0
Palate — *see* condition
Palatoplegia K13.79
Palatoschisis — *see* Cleft, palate
Palilalia R48.8
Palliative care Z51.5
Pallor R23.1
optic disc, temporal — *see* Atrophy, optic
Palmar — *see also* condition
fascia — *see* condition
Palpable
cecum K63.89
kidney N28.89
ovary N83.8
prostate N42.9
spleen — *see* Splenomegaly
Palpitations (heart) R00.2
psychogenic F45.8
Palsy — *see also* Paralysis G83.9
atrophic diffuse (progressive) G12.22
Bell's — *see also* Palsy, facial
newborn P11.3
brachial plexus NEC G54.0
newborn (birth injury) P14.3
brain — *see* Palsy, cerebral
bulbar (progressive) (chronic) G12.22
of childhood (Fazio-Londe) G12.1
pseudo NEC G12.29
supranuclear (progressive) G23.1
cerebral (congenital) G80.9
ataxic G80.4
athetoid G80.3
choreathetoid G80.3
diplegic G80.8
spastic G80.1
dyskinetic G80.3
athetoid G80.3
choreathetoid G80.3
distonic G80.3
dystonic G80.3
hemiplegic G80.8
spastic G80.2
mixed G80.8
monoplegic G80.8
spastic G80.1
paraplegic G80.8
spastic G80.1
quadriplegic G80.8
spastic G80.0
spastic G80.1
diplegic G80.1
hemiplegic G80.2
monoplegic G80.1
quadriplegic G80.0
specified NEC G80.1
tetrapelgic G80.0
specified NEC G80.8
syphilitic A52.12

Palsy - *continued*
cerebral (congenital) - *continued*
syphilitic - *continued*
congenital A50.49
tetraplegic G80.8
spastic G80.0
cranial nerve — *see also* Disorder, nerve,
cranial
multiple G52.7
in
infectious disease B99 *[G53]*
neoplastic disease — *see also*
Neoplasm D49.9 *[G53]*
parasitic disease B89 *[G53]*
sarcoidosis D86.82
creeping G12.22
diver's T70.3
Erb's P14.0
facial G51.0
newborn (birth injury) P11.3
glossopharyngeal G52.1
Klumpke (-Déjérine) P14.1
lead — *see* subcategory T56.0
median nerve (tardy) G56.1-
nerve G58.9
specified NEC G58.8
peroneal nerve (acute) (tardy) G57.3-
progressive supranuclear G23.1
pseudobulbar NEC G12.29
radial nerve (acute) G56.3-
seventh nerve — *see also* Palsy, facial
newborn P11.3
shaking — *see* Parkinsonism
spastic (cerebral) (spinal) G80.1
ulnar nerve (tardy) G56.2-
wasting G12.29
Paludism — *see* Malaria
Panangiitis M30.0
Panaris, panaritium — *see also* Cellulitis,
digit
with lymphangitis — *see* Lymphangitis,
acute, digit
Panarteritis nodosa M30.0
brain or cerebral I67.7
Pancake heart R93.1
with cor pulmonale (chronic) I27.81
Pancarditis (acute) (chronic) I51.89
rheumatic I09.89
active or acute I01.8
Pancoast's syndrome or tumor C34.1-
Pancolitis, ulcerative (chronic) K51.00
with
complication K51.019
abscess K51.014
fistula K51.013
obstruction K51.012
rectal bleeding K51.011
specified complication NEC K51.018
Pancreas, pancreatic — *see* condition
Pancreatitis (annular) (apoplectic)
(calcareous) (edematous) (hemorrhagic)
(malignant) (recurrent) (subacute)
(suppurative) K85.90
with necrosis (uninfected) K85.91
infected K85.92
acute (without necrosis or infection) K85.90
with necrosis (uninfected) K85.91
infected K85.92
alcohol induced (without necrosis or
infection) K85.20
with necrosis (uninfected) K85.21
infected K85.22
biliary (without necrosis or
infection) K85.10
with necrosis (uninfected) K85.11
infected K85.12
drug induced (without necrosis or
infection) K85.30
with necrosis (uninfected) K85.31
infected K85.32
gallstone (without necrosis or
infection) K85.10
with necrosis (uninfected) K85.11
infected K85.12

Pancreatitis (annular) (apoplectic)
(calcareous) (edematous) (hemorrhagic)
(malignant) (recurrent) (subacute)
(suppurative) - *continued*
acute (without necrosis or infection) -
continued
idiopathic (without necrosis or
infection) K85.00
with necrosis (uninfected) K85.01
infected K85.02
specified NEC (without necrosis or
infection) K85.80
with necrosis (uninfected) K85.81
infected K85.82
chronic (infectious) K86.1
alcohol-induced K86.0
recurrent K86.1
relapsing K86.1
cystic (chronic) K86.1
cytomegaloviral B25.2
fibrous (chronic) K86.1
gangrenous — *see* Pancreatitis, acute
gallstone (without necrosis or
infection) K85.10
with necrosis (uninfected) K85.11
infected K85.12
interstitial (chronic) K86.1
acute — *see also* Pancreatitis,
acute K85.80
mumps B26.3
recurrent (chronic) K86.1
relapsing, chronic K86.1
syphilitic A52.74
Pancreatoblastoma — *see* Neoplasm,
pancreas, malignant
Pancreolithiasis K86.89
Pancytolysis D75.89
Pancytopenia (acquired) D61.818
with
malformations D61.09
myelodysplastic syndrome — *see*
Syndrome, myelodysplastic
antineoplastic chemotherapy
induced D61.810
congenital D61.09
drug-induced NEC D61.811
PANDAS (pediatric autoimmune
neuropsychiatric disorders associated
with streptococcal infections
syndrome) D89.89
Panencephalitis, subacute, sclerosing A81.1
Panhematopenia D61.9
congenital D61.09
constitutional D61.09
splenic, primary D73.1
Panhemocytopenia D61.9
congenital D61.09
constitutional D61.09
Panhypogonadism E29.1
Panhypopituitarism E23.0
prepubertal E23.0
Panic (attack) (state) F41.0
reaction to exceptional stress
(transient) F43.0
Panmyelopathy, familial,
constitutional D61.09
Panmyelophthisis D61.82
congenital D61.09
Panmyelosis (acute) (with
myelofibrosis) C94.4-
Panner's disease — *see* Osteochondrosis,
juvenile, humerus
Panneuritis endemica E51.11
Panniculitis (nodular) (nonsuppurative)
M79.3
back M54.00
cervical region M54.02
cervicothoracic region M54.03
lumbar region M54.06
lumbosacral region M54.07
multiple sites M54.09
occipito-atlanto-axial region M54.01
sacrococcygeal region M54.08
thoracic region M54.04
thoracolumbar region M54.05

Panniculitis (nodular) (nonsuppurative) - *continued*
  lupus L93.2
  mesenteric K65.4
  neck M54.02
    cervicothoracic region M54.03
    occipito-atlanto-axial region M54.01
  relapsing M35.6
Panniculus adiposus (abdominal) E65
Pannus (allergic) (cornea) (degenerativus)
  (keratic) H16.42-
  abdominal (symptomatic) E65
  trachomatosus, trachomatous (active) A71.1
Panophthalmitis H44.01-
Pansinusitis (chronic) (hyperplastic)
  (nonpurulent) (purulent) J32.4
  acute J01.40
    recurrent J01.41
  tuberculous A15.8
Panuveitis (sympathetic) H44.11-
Panvalvular disease I08.9
  specified NEC I08.8
PAPA (pyogenic arthritis, pyoderma
  gangrenosum, and acne
  syndrome) M04.8
Papanicolaou smear, cervix Z12.4
  as part of routine gynecological
    examination Z01.419
    with abnormal findings Z01.411
  for suspected neoplasm Z12.4
  nonspecific abnormal finding R87.619
  routine Z01.419
    with abnormal findings Z01.411
Papilledema (choked disc) H47.10
  associated with
    decreased ocular pressure H47.12
    increased intracranial pressure H47.11
    retinal disorder H47.13
  Foster-Kennedy syndrome H47.14-
Papillitis H46.00
  anus K62.89
  chronic lingual K14.4
  necrotizing, kidney N17.2
  optic H46.0-
  rectum K62.89
  renal, necrotizing N17.2
  tongue K14.0
Papilloma — *see also* Neoplasm, benign, by
  site
  acuminatum (female) (male)
    (anogenital) A63.0
  basal cell L82.1
    inflamed L82.0
  benign pinta (primary) A67.0
  bladder (urinary) (transitional cell) D41.4
  choroid plexus (lateral ventricle) (third
    ventricle) D33.0
    anaplastic C71.5
    fourth ventricle D33.1
    malignant C71.5
  renal pelvis (transitional cell) D41.1-
    benign D30.1-
  Schneiderian
    specified site — *see* Neoplasm, benign, by
      site
    unspecified site D14.0
  serous surface
    borderline malignancy
      specified site — *see* Neoplasm,
        uncertain behavior, by site
      unspecified site D39.10
    specified site — *see* Neoplasm, benign, by
      site
    unspecified site D27.9
  transitional (cell)
    bladder (urinary) D41.4
    inverted type — *see* Neoplasm, uncertain
      behavior, by site
    renal pelvis D41.1-
    ureter D41.2-
  ureter (transitional cell) D41.2-
    benign D30.2-
  urothelial — *see* Neoplasm, uncertain
    behavior, by site

Papilloma - *continued*
  villous — *see* Neoplasm, uncertain behavior,
    by site
    adenocarcinoma in — *see* Neoplasm,
      malignant, by site
    in situ — *see* Neoplasm, in situ
  yaws, plantar or palmar A66.1
Papillomata, multiple, of yaws A66.1
Papillomatosis — *see also* Neoplasm, benign,
  by site
  confluent and reticulated L83
  cystic, breast — *see* Mastopathy, cystic
  ductal, breast — *see* Mastopathy, cystic
  intraductal (diffuse) — *see* Neoplasm,
    benign, by site
  subareolar duct D24-
Papillomavirus, as cause of disease classified
  elsewhere B97.7
Papillon-Léage and Psaume syndrome Q87.0
Papule (s) R23.8
  carate (primary) A67.0
  fibrous, of nose D22.39
  Gottron's L94.4
  pinta (primary) A67.0
Papulosis
  lymphomatoid C86.6
  malignant I77.89
Papyraceous fetus O31.0-
Para-albuminemia E88.09
Paracephalus Q89.7
Parachute mitral valve Q23.2
Paracoccidioidomycosis B41.9
  disseminated B41.7
  generalized B41.7
  mucocutaneous-lymphangitic B41.8
  pulmonary B41.0
  specified NEC B41.8
  visceral B41.8
Paradentosis K05.4
Paraffinoma T88.8
Paraganglioma D44.7
  adrenal D35.0-
    malignant C74.1-
  aortic body D44.7
    malignant C75.5
  carotid body D44.6
    malignant C75.4
  chromaffin — *see also* Neoplasm, benign, by
    site
    malignant — *see* Neoplasm, malignant, by
      site
  extra-adrenal D44.7
    malignant C75.5
      specified site — *see* Neoplasm,
        malignant, by site
      unspecified site C75.5
    specified site — *see* Neoplasm, uncertain
      behavior, by site
    unspecified site D44.7
  gangliocytic D13.2
    specified site — *see* Neoplasm, benign, by
      site
    unspecified site D13.2
  glomus jugulare D44.7
    malignant C75.5
  jugular D44.7
  malignant C75.5
    specified site — *see* Neoplasm, malignant,
      by site
    unspecified site C75.5
  nonchromaffin D44.7
    malignant C75.5
      specified site — *see* Neoplasm,
        malignant, by site
      unspecified site C75.5
    specified site — *see* Neoplasm, uncertain
      behavior, by site
    unspecified site D44.7
  parasympathetic D44.7
    specified site — *see* Neoplasm, uncertain
      behavior, by site
    unspecified site D44.7
  specified site — *see* Neoplasm, uncertain
    behavior, by site
  sympathetic D44.7

Paraganglioma - *continued*
  sympathetic - *continued*
    specified site — *see* Neoplasm, uncertain
      behavior, by site
    unspecified site D44.7
  unspecified site D44.7
Parageusia R43.2
  psychogenic F45.8
Paragonimiasis B66.4
Paragranuloma, Hodgkin — *see* Lymphoma,
  Hodgkin, specified NEC
Parahemophilia — *see also* Defect,
  coagulation D68.2
Parakeratosis R23.4
  variegata L41.0
Paralysis, paralytic (complete) (incomplete)
  G83.9
  with
    syphilis A52.17
  abducens, abducent (nerve) — *see*
    Strabismus, paralytic, sixth nerve
  abductor, lower extremity G57.9-
  accessory nerve G52.8
  accommodation — *see also* Paresis, of
    accommodation
    hysterical F44.89
  acoustic nerve (except Deafness) — *see*
    subcategory H93.3
  agitans — *see also* Parkinsonism G20
    arteriosclerotic G21.4
  alternating (oculomotor) G83.89
  amyotrophic G12.21
  ankle G57.9-
  anus (sphincter) K62.89
  arm — *see* Monoplegia, upper limb
  ascending (spinal) , acute G61.0
  association G12.29
  asthenic bulbar G70.00
    with exacerbation (acute) G70.01
    in crisis G70.01
  ataxic (hereditary) G11.9
    general (syphilitic) A52.17
  atrophic G58.9
    infantile, acute — *see* Poliomyelitis,
      paralytic
    progressive G12.22
    spinal (acute) — *see* Poliomyelitis,
      paralytic
  axillary G54.0
  Babinski-Nageotte's G83.89
  Bell's G51.0
    newborn P11.3
  Benedikt's G46.3
  birth injury P14.9
    spinal cord P11.5
  bladder (neurogenic) (sphincter) N31.2
  bowel, colon or intestine K56.0
  brachial plexus G54.0
    birth injury P14.3
    newborn (birth injury) P14.3
  brain G83.9
    diplegia G83.0
    triplegia G83.89
  bronchial J98.09
  Brown-Séquard G83.81
  bulbar (chronic) (progressive) G12.22
    infantile — *see* Poliomyelitis, paralytic
    poliomyelitic — *see* Poliomyelitis,
      paralytic
    pseudo G12.29
  bulbospinal G70.00
    with exacerbation (acute) G70.01
    in crisis G70.01
  cardiac — *see also* Failure, heart I50.9
  cerebrocerebellar, diplegic G80.1
  cervical
    plexus G54.2
    sympathetic G90.09
  Céstan-Chenais G46.3
  Charcot-Marie-Tooth type G60.0
  Clark's G80.2
  colon K56.0
  compressed air T70.3
  compression
    arm G56.9-

Paralysis, paralytic (complete) (incomplete) - *continued*

compression - *continued*
  leg G57.9-
    lower extremity G57.9-
    upper extremity G56.9-
  congenital (cerebral) — *see* Palsy, cerebral
  conjugate movement (gaze) (of eye) H51.0
    cortical (nuclear) (supranuclear) H51.0
  cordis — *see* Failure, heart
  cranial or cerebral nerve G52.9
  creeping G12.22
  crossed leg G83.89
  crutch — *see* Injury, brachial plexus
  deglutition R13.0
    hysterical F44.4
  dementia A52.17
  descending (spinal) NEC G12.29
  diaphragm (flaccid) J98.6
    due to accidental dissection of phrenic
      nerve during procedure — *see*
      Puncture, accidental complicating
      surgery
  digestive organs NEC K59.8
  diplegic — *see* Diplegia
  divergence (nuclear) H51.8
  diver's T70.3
  Duchenne's
    birth injury P14.0
    due to or associated with
      motor neuron disease G12.22
      muscular dystrophy G71.01
    due to intracranial or spinal birth injury —
      see Palsy, cerebral
  embolic (current episode) I63.4-
  Erb (-Duchenne) (birth) (newborn) P14.0
  Erb's syphilitic spastic spinal A52.17
  esophagus K22.8
  eye muscle (extrinsic) H49.9
    intrinsic — *see also* Paresis, of
      accommodation
  facial (nerve) G51.0
    birth injury P11.3
    congenital P11.3
    following operation NEC — *see* Puncture,
      accidental complicating surgery
    newborn (birth injury) P11.3
  familial (recurrent) (periodic) G72.3
    spastic G11.4
  fauces J39.2
  finger G56.9-
  gait R26.1
  gastric nerve (nondiabetic) G52.2
  gaze, conjugate H51.0
  general (progressive) (syphilitic) A52.17
    juvenile A50.45
  glottis J38.00
    bilateral J38.02
    unilateral J38.01
  gluteal G54.1
  Gubler (-Millard) G46.3
  hand — *see* Monoplegia, upper limb
  heart — *see* Arrest, cardiac
  hemiplegic — *see* Hemiplegia
  hyperkalemic periodic (familial) G72.3
  hypoglossal (nerve) G52.3
  hypokalemic periodic G72.3
  hysterical F44.4
  ileus K56.0
  infantile — *see also* Poliomyelitis,
      paralytic A80.30
    bulbar — *see* Poliomyelitis, paralytic
    cerebral — *see* Palsy, cerebral
    spastic — *see* Palsy, cerebral, spastic
  infective — *see* Poliomyelitis, paralytic
  inferior nuclear G83.9
  internuclear — *see* Ophthalmoplegia,
      internuclear
  intestine K56.0
  iris H57.09
    due to diphtheria (toxin) A36.89
  ischemic, Volkmann's (complicating
      trauma) T79.6
  Jackson's G83.89
  jake — *see* Poisoning, food, noxious, plant

Paralysis, paralytic (complete) (incomplete) - *continued*

Jamaica ginger (jake) G62.2
juvenile general A50.45
Klumpke (-Déjérine) (birth) (newborn) P14.1
labioglossal (laryngeal) (pharyngeal) G12.29
Landry's G61.0
laryngeal nerve (recurrent) (superior)
    (unilateral) J38.00
  bilateral J38.02
  unilateral J38.01
larynx J38.00
  bilateral J38.02
  due to diphtheria (toxin) A36.2
  unilateral J38.01
lateral G12.23
lead — *see* subcategory T56.0
left side — *see* Hemiplegia
leg G83.1-
  both — *see* Paraplegia
  crossed G83.89
  hysterical F44.4
  psychogenic F44.4
  transient or transitory R29.818
    traumatic NEC — *see* Injury, nerve, leg
levator palpebrae superioris — *see*
    Blepharoptosis, paralytic
limb — *see* Monoplegia
lip K13.0
Lissauer's A52.17
lower limb — *see* Monoplegia, lower limb
  both — *see* Paraplegia
lung J98.4
median nerve G56.1-
medullary (tegmental) G83.89
mesencephalic NEC G83.89
  tegmental G83.89
middle alternating G83.89
Millard-Gubler-Foville G46.3
monoplegic — *see* Monoplegia
motor G83.9
muscle, muscular NEC G72.89
  due to nerve lesion G58.9
  eye (extrinsic) H49.9
    intrinsic — *see* Paresis, of
      accommodation
    oblique — *see* Strabismus, paralytic,
      fourth nerve
  iris sphincter H21.9
  ischemic (Volkmann's) (complicating
      trauma) T79.6
  progressive G12.21
  progressive, spinal G12.25
  spinal progressive G12.25
  pseudohypertrophic G71.02
musculocutaneous nerve G56.9-
musculospiral G56.9-
nerve — *see also* Disorder, nerve
  abducent — *see* Strabismus, paralytic,
      sixth nerve
  accessory G52.8
  auditory (except Deafness) — *see*
      subcategory H93.3
  birth injury P14.9
  cranial or cerebral G52.9
  facial G51.0
    birth injury P11.3
    congenital P11.3
    newborn (birth injury) P11.3
  fourth or trochlear — *see* Strabismus,
      paralytic, fourth nerve
  newborn (birth injury) P14.9
  oculomotor — *see* Strabismus, paralytic,
      third nerve
  phrenic (birth injury) P14.2
  radial G56.3-
  seventh or facial G51.0
    newborn (birth injury) P11.3
  sixth or abducent — *see* Strabismus,
      paralytic, sixth nerve
  syphilitic A52.15
  third or oculomotor — *see* Strabismus,
      paralytic, third nerve
  trigeminal G50.9

Paralysis, paralytic (complete) (incomplete) - *continued*

nerve - *continued*
  trochlear — *see* Strabismus, paralytic,
      fourth nerve
  ulnar G56.2-
normokalemic periodic G72.3
ocular H49.9
  alternating G83.89
oculofacial, congenital (Moebius) Q87.0
oculomotor (external bilateral) (nerve) — *see*
    Strabismus, paralytic, third nerve
palate (soft) K13.79
paratrigeminal G50.9
periodic (familial) (hyperkalemic)
    (hypokalemic) (myotonic)
    (normokalemic) (potassium sensitive)
    (secondary) G72.3
peripheral autonomic nervous system — *see*
    Neuropathy, peripheral, autonomic
peroneal (nerve) G57.3-
pharynx J39.2
phrenic nerve G56.8-
plantar nerve (s) G57.6-
pneumogastric nerve G52.2
poliomyelitis (current) — *see* Poliomyelitis,
    paralytic
popliteal nerve G57.3-
postepileptic transitory G83.84
progressive (atrophic) (bulbar)
    (spinal) G12.22
  general A52.17
  infantile acute — *see* Poliomyelitis,
    paralytic
  supranuclear G23.1
pseudobulbar G12.29
pseudohypertrophic (muscle) G71.09
psychogenic F44.4
quadriceps G57.9-
quadriplegic — *see* Tetraplegia
radial nerve G56.3-
rectus muscle (eye) H49.9
recurrent isolated sleep G47.53
respiratory (muscle) (system) (tract) R06.81
  center NEC G93.89
  congenital P28.89
  newborn P28.89
right side — *see* Hemiplegia
saturnine — *see* subcategory T56.0
sciatic nerve G57.0-
senile G83.9
shaking — *see* Parkinsonism
shoulder G56.9-
sleep, recurrent isolated G47.53
spastic G83.9
  cerebral — *see* Palsy, cerebral, spastic
  congenital (cerebral) — *see* Palsy,
    cerebral, spastic
  familial G11.4
  hereditary G11.4
  quadriplegic G80.0
  syphilitic (spinal) A52.17
sphincter, bladder — *see* Paralysis, bladder
spinal (cord) G83.9
  accessory nerve G52.8
  acute — *see* Poliomyelitis, paralytic
  ascending acute G61.0
  atrophic (acute) — *see also* Poliomyelitis,
    paralytic
    spastic, syphilitic A52.17
  congenital NEC — *see* Palsy, cerebral
  infantile — *see* Poliomyelitis, paralytic
  hereditary G95.89
  progressive G12.21
    muscle G12.25
  sequelae NEC G83.89
sternomastoid G52.8
stomach K31.84
  diabetic — *see* Diabetes, by type, with
    gastroparesis
  nerve G52.2
    diabetic — *see* Diabetes, by type, with
      gastroparesis
stroke — *see* Infarct, brain
subcapsularis G56.8-

Paralysis, paralytic (complete) (incomplete) - continued
supranuclear (progressive) G23.1
sympathetic G90.8
cervical G90.09
nervous system — see Neuropathy,
peripheral, autonomic
syndrome G83.9
specified NEC G83.89
syphilitic spastic spinal (Erb's) A52.17
thigh G57.9-
throat J39.2
diphtheritic A36.0
muscle J39.2
thrombotic (current episode) I63.3-
thumb G56.9-
tick — see Toxicity, venom, arthropod,
specified NEC
Todd's (postepileptic transitory
paralysis) G83.84
toe G57.6-
tongue K14.8
transient R29.5
arm or leg NEC R29.818
traumatic NEC — see Injury, nerve
trapezius G52.8
traumatic, transient NEC — see Injury, nerve
trembling — see Parkinsonism
triceps brachii G56.9-
trigeminal nerve G50.9
trochlear (nerve) — see Strabismus,
paralytic, fourth nerve
ulnar nerve G56.2-
upper limb — see Monoplegia, upper limb
uremic N18.9 [G99.8]
uveoparotitic D86.89
uvula K13.79
postdiphtheritic A36.0
vagus nerve G52.2
vasomotor NEC G90.8
velum palati K13.79
vesical — see Paralysis, bladder
vestibular nerve (except Vertigo) — see
subcategory H93.3
vocal cords J38.00
bilateral J38.02
unilateral J38.01
Volkmann's (complicating trauma) T79.6
wasting G12.29
Weber's G46.3
wrist G56.9-
Paramedial urethrovesical orifice Q64.79
Paramenia N92.6
Parametritis — see also Disease, pelvis,
inflammatory N73.2
acute N73.0
complicating abortion — see Abortion, by
type, complicated by, parametritis
Parametrium, parametric — see condition
Paramnesia — see Amnesia
Paramolar K00.1
Paramyloidosis E85.89
Paramyoclonus multiplex G25.3
Paramyotonia (congenita) G71.19
Parangi — see Yaws
Paranoia (querulans) F22
senile F03
Paranoid
dementia (senile) F03
praecox — see Schizophrenia
personality F60.0
psychosis (climacteric) (involutional)
(menopausal) F22
psychogenic (acute) F23
senile F03
reaction (acute) F23
chronic F22
schizophrenia F20.0
state (climacteric) (involutional)
(menopausal) (simple) F22
senile F03
tendencies F60.0
traits F60.0
trends F60.0
type, psychopathic personality F60.0

Paraparesis — see Paraplegia
Paraphasia R47.02
Paraphilia F65.9
Paraphimosis (congenital) N47.2
chancroidal A57
Paraphrenia, paraphrenic (late) F22
schizophrenia F20.0
Paraplegia (lower) G82.20
ataxic — see Degeneration, combined, spinal
cord
complete G82.21
congenital (cerebral) G80.8
spastic G80.1
familial spastic G11.4
functional (hysterical) F44.4
hereditary, spastic G11.4
hysterical F44.4
incomplete G82.22
Pott's A18.01
psychogenic F44.4
spastic
Erb's spinal, syphilitic A52.17
hereditary G11.4
tropical G04.1
syphilitic (spastic) A52.17
traumatic
current injury - code to injury with seventh
character A
sequela of previous injury - code to
injury with seventh character S
tropical spastic G04.1
Parapoxvirus B08.60
specified NEC B08.69
Paraproteinemia D89.2
benign (familial) D89.2
monoclonal D47.2
secondary to malignant disease D47.2
Parapsoriasis L41.9
en plaques L41.4
guttata L41.1
large plaque L41.4
retiform, retiformis L41.5
small plaque L41.3
specified NEC L41.8
varioliformis (acuta) L41.0
Parasitic — see also condition
disease NEC B89
stomatitis B37.0
sycosis (beard) (scalp) B35.0
twin Q89.4
Parasitism B89
intestinal B82.9
skin B88.9
specified — see Infestation
Parasitophobia F40.218
Parasomnia G47.50
due to
alcohol
abuse F10.182
dependence F10.282
use F10.982
amphetamines
abuse F15.182
dependence F15.282
use F15.982
caffeine
abuse F15.182
dependence F15.282
use F15.982
cocaine
abuse F14.182
dependence F14.282
use F14.982
drug NEC
abuse F19.182
dependence F19.282
use F19.982
opioid
abuse F11.182
dependence F11.282
use F11.982
psychoactive substance NEC
abuse F19.182
dependence F19.282
use F19.982

Parasomnia - continued
due to - continued
sedative, hypnotic, or anxiolytic
abuse F13.182
dependence F13.282
use F13.982
stimulant NEC
abuse F15.182
dependence F15.282
use F15.982
in conditions classified elsewhere G47.54
nonorganic origin F51.8
organic G47.50
specified NEC G47.59
Paraspadias Q54.9
Paraspasmus facialis G51.8
Parasuicide (attempt)
history of (personal) Z91.5
in family Z81.8
Parathyroid gland — see condition
Parathyroid tetany E20.9
Paratrachoma A74.0
Paratyphilitis — see Appendicitis
Paratyphoid (fever) — see Fever, paratyphoid
Paratyphus — see Fever, paratyphoid
Paraurethral duct Q64.79
Paraurethritis — see also Urethritis
gonococcal (acute) (chronic) (with
abscess) A54.1
Paravaccinia NEC B08.04
Paravaginitis — see Vaginitis
Parencephalitis — see also Encephalitis
sequelae G09
Parent-child conflict — see Conflict, parent-
child
estrangement NEC Z62.890
Paresis — see also Paralysis
accommodation — see Paresis, of
accommodation
Bernhardt's G57.1-
bladder (sphincter) — see also Paralysis,
bladder
tabetic A52.17
bowel, colon or intestine K56.0
extrinsic muscle, eye H49.9
general (progressive) (syphilitic) A52.17
juvenile A50.45
heart — see Failure, heart
insane (syphilitic) A52.17
juvenile (general) A50.45
of accommodation H52.52-
peripheral progressive (idiopathic) G60.3
pseudohypertrophic G71.09
senile G83.9
syphilitic (general) A52.17
congenital A50.45
vesical NEC N31.2
Paresthesia — see also Disturbance, sensation,
skin R20.2
Bernhardt G57.1-
Paretic — see condition
Parinaud's
conjunctivitis H10.89
oculoglandular syndrome H10.89
ophthalmoplegia H49.88-
Parkinsonism (idiopathic) (primary) G20
with neurogenic orthostatic hypotension
(symptomatic) G90.3
arteriosclerotic G21.4
dementia G31.83 [F02.80]
with behavioral disturbance G31.83
[F02.81]
due to
drugs NEC G21.19
neuroleptic G21.11
medication-induced NEC G21.19
neuroleptic induced G21.11
postencephalitic G21.3
secondary G21.9
due to
arteriosclerosis G21.4
drugs NEC G21.19
neuroleptic G21.11
encephalitis G21.3
external agents NEC G21.2

Parkinsonism (idiopathic) (primary) - *continued*
  secondary - *continued*
    due to - *continued*
      syphilis A52.19
    specified NEC G21.8
    syphilitic A52.19
    treatment-induced NEC G21.19
    vascular G21.4
Parkinson's disease, syndrome or tremor — *see* Parkinsonism
Parodontitis — *see* Periodontitis
Parodontosis K05.4
Paronychia — *see also* Cellulitis, digit
  with lymphangitis — *see* Lymphangitis, acute, digit
  candidal (chronic) B37.2
  tuberculous (primary) A18.4
Parorexia (psychogenic) F50.89
Parosmia R43.1
  psychogenic F45.8
Parotid gland — *see* condition
Parotitis, parotiditis (allergic) (nonspecific toxic) (purulent) (septic) (suppurative) — *see also* Sialoadenitis
  epidemic — *see* Mumps
  infectious — *see* Mumps
  postoperative K91.89
  surgical K91.89
Parrot fever A70
Parrot's disease (early congenital syphilitic pseudoparalysis) A50.02
Parry-Romberg syndrome G51.8
Parry's disease or syndrome E05.00
  with thyroid storm E05.01
Pars planitis — *see* Cyclitis
Parsonage (-Aldren) -Turner syndrome G54.5
Parson's disease (exophthalmic goiter) E05.00
  with thyroid storm E05.01
Particolored infant Q82.8
Parturition — *see* Delivery
Parulis K04.7
  with sinus K04.6
Parvovirus, as cause of disease classified elsewhere B97.6
Pasini and Pierini's atrophoderma L90.3
Passage
  false, urethra N36.5
  meconium (newborn) during delivery P03.82
  of sounds or bougies — *see* Attention to, artificial, opening
Passive — *see* condition
  smoking Z77.22
Pasteurella septica A28.0
Pasteurellosis — *see* Infection, Pasteurella
PAT (paroxysmal atrial tachycardia) I47.1
Patau's syndrome — *see* Trisomy, 13
Patches
  mucous (syphilitic) A51.39
    congenital A50.07
  smokers' (mouth) K13.24
Patellar — *see* condition
Patent — *see also* Imperfect, closure
  canal of Nuck Q52.4
  cervix N88.3
  ductus arteriosus or Botallo's Q25.0
  foramen
    botalli Q21.1
    ovale Q21.1
  interauricular septum Q21.1
  interventricular septum Q21.0
  omphalomesenteric duct Q43.0
  os (uteri) — *see* Patent, cervix
  ostium secundum Q21.1
  urachus Q64.4
  vitelline duct Q43.0
Paterson (-Brown) (-Kelly) syndrome or web D50.1
Pathologic, pathological — *see also* condition
  asphyxia R09.01
  fire-setting F63.1
  gambling F63.0
  ovum O02.0

Pathologic, pathological - *continued*
  resorption, tooth K03.3
  stealing F63.2
Pathology (of) — *see* Disease
  periradicular, associated with previous endodontic treatment NEC M27.59
Pattern, sleep-wake, irregular G47.23
Patulous — *see also* Imperfect, closure (congenital)
  alimentary tract Q45.8
    lower Q43.8
    upper Q40.8
  eustachian tube H69.0-
Pause, sinoatrial I49.5
Paxton's disease B36.2
Pearl (s)
  enamel K00.2
  Epstein's K09.8
Pearl-worker's disease — *see* Osteomyelitis, specified type NEC
Pectenosis K62.4
Pectoral — *see* condition
Pectus
  carinatum (congenital) Q67.7
    acquired M95.4
    rachitic sequelae (late effect) E64.3
  excavatum (congenital) Q67.6
    acquired M95.4
    rachitic sequelae (late effect) E64.3
  recurvatum (congenital) Q67.6
Pedatrophia E41
Pederosis F65.4
Pediculosis (infestation) B85.2
  capitis (head-louse) (any site) B85.0
  corporis (body-louse) (any site) B85.1
  eyelid B85.0
  mixed (classifiable to more than one of the titles B85.0-B85.3) B85.4
  pubis (pubic louse) (any site) B85.3
  vestimenti B85.1
  vulvae B85.3
Pediculus (infestation) — *see* Pediculosis
Pedophilia F65.4
Peg-shaped teeth K00.2
Pelade — *see* Alopecia, areata
Pelger-Huët anomaly or syndrome D72.0
Peliosis (rheumatica) D69.0
  hepatis K76.4
    with toxic liver disease K71.8
Pelizaeus-Merzbacher disease E75.29
Pellagra (alcoholic) (with polyneuropathy) E52
Pellagra-cerebellar-ataxia-renal aminoaciduria syndrome E72.02
Pellegrini (-Stieda) disease or syndrome — *see* Bursitis, tibial collateral
Pellizzi's syndrome E34.8
Pel's crisis A52.11
Pelvic — *see also* condition
  examination (periodic) (routine) Z01.419
    with abnormal findings Z01.411
  kidney, congenital Q63.2
Pelviolithiasis — *see* Calculus, kidney
Pelviperitonitis — *see also* Peritonitis, pelvic
  gonococcal A54.24
  puerperal O85
Pelvis — *see* condition or type
Pemphigoid L12.9
  benign, mucous membrane L12.1
  bullous L12.0
  cicatricial L12.1
  juvenile L12.2
  ocular L12.1
  specified NEC L12.8
Pemphigus L10.9
  benign familial (chronic) Q82.8
  Brazilian L10.3
  circinatus L13.0
  conjunctiva L12.1
  drug-induced L10.5
  erythematosus L10.4
  foliaceus L10.2
  gangrenous — *see* Gangrene
  neonatorum L01.03
  ocular L12.1

Pemphigus - *continued*
  paraneoplastic L10.81
  specified NEC L10.89
  syphilitic (congenital) A50.06
  vegetans L10.1
  vulgaris L10.0
  wildfire L10.3
Pendred's syndrome E07.1
Pendulous
  abdomen, in pregnancy — *see* Pregnancy, complicated by, abnormal, pelvic organs or tissues NEC
  breast N64.89
Penetrating wound — *see also* Puncture
  with internal injury — *see* Injury, by site
  eyeball — *see* Puncture, eyeball
  orbit (with or without foreign body) — *see* Puncture, orbit
  uterus by instrument with or following ectopic or molar pregnancy O08.6
Penicillosis B48.4
Penis — *see* condition
Penitis N48.29
Pentalogy of Fallot Q21.8
Pentasomy X syndrome Q97.1
Pentosuria (essential) E74.8
Percreta placenta O43.23-
Peregrinating patient — *see* Disorder, factitious
Perforation, perforated (nontraumatic) (of)
  accidental during procedure (blood vessel) (nerve) (organ) — *see* Complication, accidental puncture or laceration
  antrum — *see* Sinusitis, maxillary
  appendix K35.32
    with localized peritonitis K35.32
  atrial septum, multiple Q21.1
  attic, ear — *see* Perforation, tympanum, attic
  bile duct (common) (hepatic) K83.2
    cystic K82.2
  bladder (urinary)
    with or following ectopic or molar pregnancy O08.6
    obstetrical trauma O71.5
    traumatic S37.29
      at delivery O71.5
  bowel K63.1
    with or following ectopic or molar pregnancy O08.6
    newborn P78.0
    obstetrical trauma O71.5
    traumatic — *see* Laceration, intestine
  broad ligament N83.8
    with or following ectopic or molar pregnancy O08.6
    obstetrical trauma O71.6
  by
    device, implant or graft — *see also* Complications, by site and type, mechanical T85.628
      arterial graft NEC — *see* Complication, cardiovascular device, mechanical, vascular
      breast (implant) T85.49
      catheter NEC T85.698
        cystostomy T83.090
        dialysis (renal) T82.49
          intraperitoneal T85.691
        infusion NEC T82.594
          spinal (epidural) (subdural) T85.690
        urinary — *see also* Complications, catheter, urinary T83.098
      electronic (electrode) (pulse generator) (stimulator)
        bone T84.390
        cardiac T82.199
          electrode T82.190
          pulse generator T82.191
          specified type NEC T82.198
        nervous system — *see* Complication, prosthetic device, mechanical, electronic nervous system stimulator

Perforation, perforated (nontraumatic) (of) - *continued*

by - *continued*

device, implant or graft - *continued*

electronic (electrode) (pulse generator) (stimulator) - *continued*

urinary — *see* Complication, genitourinary, device, urinary, mechanical

fixation, internal (orthopedic) NEC — *see* Complication, fixation device, mechanical

gastrointestinal — *see* Complications, prosthetic device, mechanical, gastrointestinal device

genital NEC T83.498

intrauterine contraceptive device T83.39

penile prosthesis T83.490

heart NEC — *see* Complication, cardiovascular device, mechanical

joint prosthesis — *see* Complications, joint prosthesis, mechanical, specified NEC, by site

ocular NEC — *see* Complications, prosthetic device, mechanical, ocular device

orthopedic NEC — *see* Complication, orthopedic, device, mechanical

specified NEC T85.628

urinary NEC — *see also* Complication, genitourinary, device, urinary, mechanical

graft T83.29

vascular NEC — *see* Complication, cardiovascular device, mechanical

ventricular intracranial shunt T85.09

foreign body left accidentally in operative wound T81.539

instrument (any) during a procedure, accidental — *see* Puncture, accidental complicating surgery

cecum K35.32

with localized peritonitis K35.32

cervix (uteri) N88.8

with or following ectopic or molar pregnancy O08.6

obstetrical trauma O71.3

colon K63.1

newborn P78.0

obstetrical trauma O71.5

traumatic — *see* Laceration, intestine, large

common duct (bile) K83.2

cornea (due to ulceration) — *see* Ulcer, cornea, perforated

cystic duct K82.2

diverticulum (intestine) K57.80

with bleeding K57.81

large intestine K57.20

with

bleeding K57.21

small intestine K57.40

with bleeding K57.41

small intestine K57.00

with

bleeding K57.01

large intestine K57.40

with bleeding K57.41

ear drum — *see* Perforation, tympanum

esophagus K22.3

ethmoidal sinus — *see* Sinusitis, ethmoidal

frontal sinus — *see* Sinusitis, frontal

gallbladder K82.2

heart valve — *see* Endocarditis

ileum K63.1

newborn P78.0

obstetrical trauma O71.5

traumatic — *see* Laceration, intestine, small

instrumental, surgical (accidental) (blood vessel) (nerve) (organ) — *see* Puncture, accidental complicating surgery

intestine NEC K63.1

with ectopic or molar pregnancy O08.6

Perforation, perforated (nontraumatic) (of) - *continued*

intestine NEC - *continued*

newborn P78.0

obstetrical trauma O71.5

traumatic — *see* Laceration, intestine

ulcerative NEC K63.1

newborn P78.0

jejunum, jejunal K63.1

obstetrical trauma O71.5

traumatic — *see* Laceration, intestine, small

ulcer — *see* Ulcer, gastrojejunal, with perforation

joint prosthesis — *see* Complications, joint prosthesis, mechanical, specified NEC, by site

mastoid (antrum) (cell) — *see* Disorder, mastoid, specified NEC

maxillary sinus — *see* Sinusitis, maxillary

membrana tympani — *see* Perforation, tympanum

nasal

septum J34.89

congenital Q30.3

syphilitic A52.73

sinus J34.89

congenital Q30.8

due to sinusitis — *see* Sinusitis

palate — *see also* Cleft, palate Q35.9

syphilitic A52.79

palatine vault — *see also* Cleft, palate, hard Q35.1

syphilitic A52.79

congenital A50.59

pars flaccida (ear drum) — *see* Perforation, tympanum, attic

pelvic

floor S31.030

with

ectopic or molar pregnancy O08.6

penetration into retroperitoneal space S31.031

retained foreign body S31.040

with penetration into retroperitoneal space S31.041

following ectopic or molar pregnancy O08.6

obstetrical trauma O70.1

organ S37.99

adrenal gland S37.818

bladder — *see* Perforation, bladder

fallopian tube S37.599

bilateral S37.592

unilateral S37.591

kidney S37.09-

obstetrical trauma O71.5

ovary S37.499

bilateral S37.492

unilateral S37.491

prostate S37.828

specified organ NEC S37.898

ureter — *see* Perforation, ureter

urethra — *see* Perforation, urethra

uterus — *see* Perforation, uterus

perineum — *see* Laceration, perineum

pharynx J39.2

rectum K63.1

newborn P78.0

obstetrical trauma O71.5

traumatic S36.63

root canal space due to endodontic treatment M27.51

sigmoid K63.1

newborn P78.0

obstetrical trauma O71.5

traumatic S36.533

sinus (accessory) (chronic) (nasal) J34.89

sphenoidal sinus — *see* Sinusitis, sphenoidal

surgical (accidental) (by instrument) (blood vessel) (nerve) (organ) — *see* Puncture, accidental complicating surgery

traumatic

external — *see* Puncture

eye — *see* Puncture, eyeball

Perforation, perforated (nontraumatic) (of) - *continued*

traumatic - *continued*

internal organ — *see* Injury, by site

tympanum, tympanic (membrane) (persistent post-traumatic) (postinflammatory) H72.9-

attic H72.1-

multiple — *see* Perforation, tympanum, multiple

total — *see* Perforation, tympanum, total

central H72.0-

multiple — *see* Perforation, tympanum, multiple

total — *see* Perforation, tympanum, total

marginal NEC — *see* subcategory H72.2

multiple H72.81-

pars flaccida — *see* Perforation, tympanum, attic

total H72.82-

traumatic, current episode S09.2-

typhoid, gastrointestinal — *see* Typhoid

ulcer — *see* Ulcer, by site, with perforation

ureter N28.89

traumatic S37.19

urethra N36.8

with ectopic or molar pregnancy O08.6

following ectopic or molar pregnancy O08.6

obstetrical trauma O71.5

traumatic S37.39

at delivery O71.5

uterus

with ectopic or molar pregnancy O08.6

by intrauterine contraceptive device T83.39

following ectopic or molar pregnancy O08.6

obstetrical trauma O71.1

traumatic S37.69

obstetric O71.1

uvula K13.79

syphilitic A52.79

vagina

obstetrical trauma O71.4

other trauma — *see* Puncture, vagina

Periadenitis mucosa necrotica recurrens K12.0

Periappendicitis (acute) — *see* Appendicitis

Periarteritis nodosa (disseminated) (infectious) (necrotizing) M30.0

Periarthritis (joint) — *see also* Enthesopathy

Duplay's M75.0-

gonococcal A54.42

humeroscapularis — *see* Capsulitis, adhesive

scapulohumeral — *see* Capsulitis, adhesive

shoulder — *see* Capsulitis, adhesive

wrist M77.2-

Periarthrosis (angioneural) — *see* Enthesopathy

Pericapsulitis, adhesive (shoulder) — *see* Capsulitis, adhesive

Pericarditis (with decompensation) (with effusion) I31.9

with rheumatic fever (conditions in I00)

active — *see* Pericarditis, rheumatic

inactive or quiescent I09.2

acute (hemorrhagic) (nonrheumatic) (Sicca) I30.9

with chorea (acute) (rheumatic) (Sydenham's) I02.0

benign I30.8

nonspecific I30.0

rheumatic I01.0

with chorea (acute) (Sydenham's) I02.0

adhesive or adherent (chronic) (external) (internal) I31.0

acute — *see* Pericarditis, acute

rheumatic I09.2

bacterial (acute) (subacute) (with serous or seropurulent effusion) I30.1

calcareous I31.1

cholesterol (chronic) I31.8

acute I30.9

chronic (nonrheumatic) I31.9

Pericarditis (with decompensation) (with effusion) - *continued*
  chronic (nonrheumatic) - *continued*
    rheumatic I09.2
  constrictive (chronic) I31.1
  coxsackie B33.23
  fibrinocaseous (tuberculous) A18.84
  fibrinopurulent I30.1
  fibrinous I30.8
  fibrous I31.0
  gonococcal A54.83
  idiopathic I30.0
  in systemic lupus erythematosus M32.12
  infective I30.1
  meningococcal A39.53
  neoplastic (chronic) I31.8
    acute I30.9
  obliterans, obliterating I31.0
  plastic I31.0
  pneumococcal I30.1
  postinfarction I24.1
  purulent I30.1
  rheumatic (active) (acute) (with effusion) (with pneumonia) I01.0
    with chorea (acute) (rheumatic) (Sydenham's) I02.0
    chronic or inactive (with chorea) I09.2
  rheumatoid — *see* Rheumatoid, carditis
  septic I30.1
  serofibrinous I30.8
  staphylococcal I30.1
  streptococcal I30.1
  suppurative I30.1
  syphilitic A52.06
  tuberculous A18.84
  uremic N18.9 *[I32]*
  viral I30.1
Pericardium, pericardial — *see* condition
Pericellulitis — *see* Cellulitis
Pericementitis (chronic) (suppurative) — *see also* Periodontitis
  acute K05.20
    generalized — *see* Periodontitis, aggressive, generalized
    localized — *see* Periodontitis, aggressive, localized
Perichondritis
  auricle — *see* Perichondritis, ear
  bronchus J98.09
  ear (external) H61.00-
    acute H61.01-
    chronic H61.02-
  external auditory canal — *see* Perichondritis, ear
  larynx J38.7
    syphilitic A52.73
    typhoid A01.09
  nose J34.89
  pinna — *see* Perichondritis, ear
  trachea J39.8
Periclasia K05.4
Pericoronitis — *see* Periodontitis
Pericystitis N30.90
  with hematuria N30.91
Peridiverticulitis (intestine) K57.92
  cecum — *see* Diverticulitis, intestine, large
  colon — *see* Diverticulitis, intestine, large
  duodenum — *see* Diverticulitis, intestine, small
  intestine — *see* Diverticulitis, intestine
  jejunum — *see* Diverticulitis, intestine, small
  rectosigmoid — *see* Diverticulitis, intestine, large
  rectum — *see* Diverticulitis, intestine, large
  sigmoid — *see* Diverticulitis, intestine, large
Periendocarditis — *see* Endocarditis
Periepididymitis N45.1
Perifolliculitis L01.02
  abscedens, caput, scalp L66.3
  capitis, abscedens (et suffodiens) L66.3
  superficial pustular L01.02
Perihepatitis K65.8
Perilabyrinthitis (acute) — *see* subcategory H83.0
Perimeningitis — *see* Meningitis

Perimetritis — *see* Endometritis
Perimetrosalpingitis — *see* Salpingo-oophoritis
Perineocele N81.81
Perinephric, perinephritic — *see* condition
Perinephritis — *see also* Infection, kidney
  purulent — *see* Abscess, kidney
Perineum, perineal — *see* condition
Perineuritis NEC — *see* Neuralgia
Periodic — *see* condition
Periodontitis (chronic) (complex) (compound) (local) (simplex) K05.30
  acute K05.20
    generalized K05.229
      moderate K05.222
      severe K05.223
      slight K05.221
    localized K05.219
      moderate K05.212
      severe K05.213
      slight K05.211
  apical K04.5
    acute (pulpal origin) K04.4
  generalized K05.329
    moderate K05.322
    severe K05.323
    slight K05.321
  localized K05.319
    moderate K05.312
    severe K05.313
    slight K05.311
Periodontoclasia K05.4
Periodontosis (juvenile) K05.4
Periods — *see also* Menstruation
  heavy N92.0
  irregular N92.6
  shortened intervals (irregular) N92.1
Perionychia — *see also* Cellulitis, digit
  with lymphangitis — *see* Lymphangitis, acute, digit
Perioophoritis — *see* Salpingo-oophoritis
Periorchitis N45.2
Periosteum, periosteal — *see* condition
Periostitis (albuminosa) (circumscribed) (diffuse) (infective) (monomelic) — *see also* Osteomyelitis
  alveolar M27.3
  alveolodental M27.3
  dental M27.3
  gonorrheal A54.43
  jaw (lower) (upper) M27.2
  orbit H05.03-
  syphilitic A52.77
    congenital (early) A50.02 *[M90.80]*
    secondary A51.46
  tuberculous — *see* Tuberculosis, bone
  yaws (hypertrophic) (early) (late) A66.6 *[M90.80]*
Periostosis (hyperplastic) — *see also* Disorder, bone, specified type NEC
  with osteomyelitis — *see* Osteomyelitis, specified type NEC
Peripartum
  cardiomyopathy O90.3
Periphlebitis — *see* Phlebitis
Periproctitis K62.89
Periprostatitis — *see* Prostatitis
Perirectal — *see* condition
Perirenal — *see* condition
Perisalpingitis — *see* Salpingo-oophoritis
Perisplenitis (infectional) D73.89
Peristalsis, visible or reversed R19.2
Peritendinitis — *see* Enthesopathy
Peritoneum, peritoneal — *see* condition
Peritonitis (adhesive) (bacterial) (fibrinous) (hemorrhagic) (idiopathic) (localized) (perforative) (primary) (with adhesions) (with effusion) K65.9
  with or following
    abscess K65.1
    appendicitis
      with perforation or rupture K35.32
      generalized — *see also* Appendicitis K35.20

Peritonitis (adhesive) (bacterial) (fibrinous) (hemorrhagic) (idiopathic) (localized) (perforative) (primary) (with adhesions) (with effusion) - *continued*
  with or following - *continued*
    appendicitis - *continued*
      localized — *see also* Appendicitis K35.30
    diverticular disease (intestine) K57.80
      with bleeding K57.81
      large intestine K57.20
        with
          bleeding K57.21
          small intestine K57.40
            with bleeding K57.41
      small intestine K57.00
        with
          bleeding K57.01
          large intestine K57.40
            with bleeding K57.41
    ectopic or molar pregnancy O08.0
  acute (generalized) K65.0
  aseptic T81.61
  bile, biliary K65.3
  chemical T81.61
  chlamydial A74.81
  complicating abortion — *see* Abortion, by type, complicated by, pelvic peritonitis
  congenital P78.1
  chronic proliferative K65.8
  diaphragmatic K65.0
  diffuse K65.0
  diphtheritic A36.89
  disseminated K65.0
  due to
    bile K65.3
    foreign
      body or object accidentally left during a procedure (instrument) (sponge) (swab) T81.599
      substance accidentally left during a procedure (chemical) (powder) (talc) T81.61
    talc T81.61
    urine K65.8
  eosinophilic K65.8
    acute K65.0
  fibrocaseous (tuberculous) A18.31
  fibropurulent K65.0
  following ectopic or molar pregnancy O08.0
  general (ized) K65.0
  gonococcal A54.85
  meconium (newborn) P78.0
  neonatal P78.1
    meconium P78.0
  pancreatic K65.0
  paroxysmal, familial E85.0
    benign E85.0
  pelvic
    female N73.5
      acute N73.3
      chronic N73.4
        with adhesions N73.6
    male K65.0
  periodic, familial E85.0
  proliferative, chronic K65.8
  puerperal, postpartum, childbirth O85
  purulent K65.0
  septic K65.0
  specified NEC K65.8
  spontaneous bacterial K65.2
  subdiaphragmatic K65.0
  subphrenic K65.0
  suppurative K65.0
  syphilitic A52.74
    congenital (early) A50.08 *[K67]*
  talc T81.61
  tuberculous A18.31
  urine K65.8
Peritonsillar — *see* condition
Peritonsillitis J36
Perityphlitis K37
Periureteritis N28.89
Periurethral — *see* condition
Periurethritis (gangrenous) — *see* Urethritis

Periuterine — *see* condition
Perivaginitis — *see* Vaginitis
Perivasculitis, retinal H35.06-
Perivasitis (chronic) N49.1
Perivesiculitis (seminal) — *see* Vesiculitis
Perlèche NEC K13.0
  due to
    candidiasis B37.83
    moniliasis B37.83
    riboflavin deficiency E53.0
    vitamin B2 (riboflavin) deficiency E53.0
Pernicious — *see* condition
Pernio, perniosis T69.1
Perpetrator (of abuse) — *see* Index to
    External Causes of Injury, Perpetrator
Persecution
  delusion F22
  social Z60.5
Perseveration (tonic) R48.8
Persistence, persistent (congenital)
  anal membrane Q42.3
    with fistula Q42.2
  arteria stapedia Q16.3
  atrioventricular canal Q21.2
  branchial cleft NOS Q18.2
    cyst Q18.0
    fistula Q18.0
    sinus Q18.0
  bulbus cordis in left ventricle Q21.8
  canal of Cloquet Q14.0
  capsule (opaque) Q12.8
  cilioretinal artery or vein Q14.8
  cloaca Q43.7
  communication — *see* Fistula, congenital
  convolutions
    aortic arch Q25.46
    fallopian tube Q50.6
    oviduct Q50.6
    uterine tube Q50.6
  double aortic arch Q25.45
  ductus arteriosus (Botalli) Q25.0
  fetal
    circulation P29.38
    form of cervix (uteri) Q51.828
    hemoglobin, hereditary (HPFH) D56.4
  foramen
    Botalli Q21.1
    ovale Q21.1
  Gartner's duct Q52.4
  hemoglobin, fetal (hereditary) (HPFH) D56.4
  hyaloid
    artery (generally incomplete) Q14.0
    system Q14.8
  hymen, in pregnancy or childbirth — *see*
      Pregnancy, complicated by, abnormal,
      vulva
  lanugo Q84.2
  left
    posterior cardinal vein Q26.8
    root with right arch of aorta Q25.49
    superior vena cava Q26.1
  Meckel's diverticulum Q43.0
    malignant — *see* Table of Neoplasms,
        small intestine, malignant
  mucosal disease (middle ear) — *see* Otitis,
      media, suppurative, chronic,
      tubotympanic
  nail (s) , anomalous Q84.6
  omphalomesenteric duct Q43.0
  organ or site not listed — *see* Anomaly, by
      site
  ostium
    atrioventriculare commune Q21.2
    primum Q21.2
    secundum Q21.1
  ovarian rests in fallopian tube Q50.6
  pancreatic tissue in intestinal tract Q43.8
  primary (deciduous)
    teeth K00.6
    vitreous hyperplasia Q14.0
  pupillary membrane Q13.89
  right aortic arch Q25.47
  rhesus (Rh) titer — *see* Complication(s),
      transfusion, incompatibility reaction, Rh
      (factor)

Persistence, persistent (congenital) -
continued
  sinus
    urogenitalis
      female Q52.8
      male Q55.8
    venosus with imperfect incorporation in
        right auricle Q26.8
  thymus (gland) (hyperplasia) E32.0
  thyroglossal duct Q89.2
  thyrolingual duct Q89.2
  truncus arteriosus or communis Q20.0
  tunica vasculosa lentis Q12.2
  umbilical sinus Q64.4
  urachus Q64.4
  vitelline duct Q43.0
Person (with)
  admitted for clinical research, as a control
      subject (normal comparison)
      (participant) Z00.6
  awaiting admission to adequate facility
      elsewhere Z75.1
  concern (normal) about sick person in
      family Z63.6
  consulting on behalf of another Z71.0
  feigning illness Z76.5
  living (in)
    alone Z60.2
    boarding school Z59.3
    residential institution Z59.3
    without
      adequate housing (heating)
          (space) Z59.1
      housing (permanent) (temporary) Z59.0
      person able to render necessary
          care Z74.2
      shelter Z59.0
  on waiting list Z75.1
  sick or handicapped in family Z63.6
Personality (disorder) F60.9
  accentuation of traits (type A pattern) Z73.1
  affective F34.0
  aggressive F60.3
  amoral F60.2
  anacastic, anankastic F60.5
  antisocial F60.2
  anxious F60.6
  asocial F60.2
  asthenic F60.7
  avoidant F60.6
  borderline F60.3
  change due to organic condition
      (enduring) F07.0
  compulsive F60.5
  cycloid F34.0
  cyclothymic F34.0
  dependent F60.7
  depressive F34.1
  dissocial F60.2
  dual F44.81
  eccentric F60.89
  emotionally unstable F60.3
  expansive paranoid F60.0
  explosive F60.3
  fanatic F60.0
  haltose type F60.89
  histrionic F60.4
  hyperthymic F34.0
  hypothymic F34.1
  hysterical F60.4
  immature F60.89
  inadequate F60.7
  labile (emotional) F60.3
  mixed (nonspecific) F60.89
  morally defective F60.2
  multiple F44.81
  narcissistic F60.81
  obsessional F60.5
  obsessive (-compulsive) F60.5
  organic F07.0
  overconscientious F60.5
  paranoid F60.0
  passive (-dependent) F60.7
  passive-aggressive F60.89
  pathologic F60.9

Personality (disorder) - *continued*
  pattern defect or disturbance F60.9
  pseudopsychopathic (organic) F07.0
  pseudoretarded (organic) F07.0
  psychoinfantile F60.4
  psychoneurotic NEC F60.89
  psychopathic F60.2
  querulant F60.0
  sadistic F60.89
  schizoid F60.1
  self-defeating F60.89
  sensitive paranoid F60.0
  sociopathic (amoral) (antisocial) (asocial)
      (dissocial) F60.2
  specified NEC F60.89
  type A Z73.1
  unstable (emotional) F60.3
Perthes' disease — *see* Legg-Calvé-Perthes
    disease
Pertussis — *see also* Whooping cough A37.90
Perversion, perverted
  appetite F50.89
    psychogenic F50.89
  function
    pituitary gland E23.2
      posterior lobe E22.2
  sense of smell and taste R43.8
    psychogenic F45.8
  sexual — *see* Deviation, sexual
Pervious, congenital — *see also* Imperfect,
    closure
  ductus arteriosus Q25.0
Pes (congenital) — *see also* Talipes
  acquired — *see also* Deformity, limb, foot,
      specified NEC
    planus — *see* Deformity, limb, flat foot
  adductus Q66.89
  cavus Q66.7-
  deformity NEC, acquired — *see* Deformity,
      limb, foot, specified NEC
  planus (acquired) (any degree) — *see also*
      Deformity, limb, flat foot
  rachitic sequelae (late effect) E64.3
  valgus Q66.6
Pest, pestis — *see* Plague
Petechia, petechiae R23.3
  newborn P54.5
Petechial typhus A75.9
Peter's anomaly Q13.4
Petit mal seizure — *see* Epilepsy, childhood,
    absence
Petit's hernia — *see* Hernia, abdomen,
    specified site NEC
Petrellidosis B48.2
Petrositis H70.20-
  acute H70.21-
  chronic H70.22-
Peutz-Jeghers disease or syndrome Q85.8
Peyronie's disease N48.6
PFAPA (periodic fever, aphthous stomatitis,
    pharyngitis, and adenopathy
    syndrome) M04.8
Pfeiffer's disease — *see* Mononucleosis,
    infectious
Phagedena (dry) (moist) (sloughing) — *see*
    also Gangrene
  geometric L88
  penis N48.29
  tropical — *see* Ulcer, skin
  vulva N76.6
Phagedenic — *see* condition
Phakoma H35.89
Phakomatosis — *see also* specific eponymous
    syndromes Q85.9
  Bourneville's Q85.1
  specified NEC Q85.8
Phantom limb syndrome (without pain)
    G54.7
  with pain G54.6
Pharyngeal pouch syndrome D82.1

Pharyngitis (acute) (catarrhal) (gangrenous) (infective) (malignant) (membranous) (phlegmonous) (pseudomembranous) (simple) (subacute) (suppurative) (ulcerative) (viral) J02.9
  with influenza, flu, or grippe — *see* Influenza, with, pharyngitis
  aphthous B08.5
  atrophic J31.2
  chlamydial A56.4
  chronic (atrophic) (granular) (hypertrophic) J31.2
  coxsackievirus B08.5
  diphtheritic A36.0
  enteroviral vesicular B08.5
  follicular (chronic) J31.2
  fusospirochetal A69.1
  gonococcal A54.5
  granular (chronic) J31.2
  herpesviral B00.2
  hypertrophic J31.2
  infectional, chronic J31.2
  influenzal — *see* Influenza, with, respiratory manifestations NEC
  lymphonodular, acute (enteroviral) B08.8
  pneumococcal J02.8
  purulent J02.9
  putrid J02.9
  septic J02.0
  sicca J31.2
  specified organism NEC J02.8
  staphylococcal J02.8
  streptococcal J02.0
  syphilitic, congenital (early) A50.03
  tuberculous A15.8
  vesicular, enteroviral B08.5
  viral NEC J02.8
Pharyngoconjunctivitis, viral B30.2
Pharyngolaryngitis (acute) J06.0
  chronic J37.0
Pharyngoplegia J39.2
Pharyngotonsillitis, herpesviral B00.2
Pharyngotracheitis, chronic J42
Pharynx, pharyngeal — *see* condition
Phencyclidine-induced
  anxiety disorder F16.980
  bipolar and related disorder F16.94
  depressive disorder F16.94
  psychotic disorder F16.959
Phenomenon
  Arthus' — *see* Arthus' phenomenon
  jaw-winking Q07.8
  lupus erythematosus (LE) cell M32.9
  Raynaud's (secondary) I73.00
    with gangrene I73.01
  vasomotor R55
  vasospastic I73.9
  vasovagal R55
  Wenckebach's I44.1
Phenylketonuria E70.1
  classical E70.0
  maternal E70.1
Pheochromoblastoma
  specified site — *see* Neoplasm, malignant, by site
  unspecified site C74.10
Pheochromocytoma
  malignant
    specified site — *see* Neoplasm, malignant, by site
    unspecified site C74.10
  specified site — *see* Neoplasm, benign, by site
  unspecified site D35.00
Pheohyphomycosis — *see* Chromomycosis
Pheomycosis — *see* Chromomycosis
Phimosis (congenital) (due to infection) N47.1
  chancroidal A57
Phlebectasia — *see also* Varix
  congenital Q27.4
Phlebitis (infective) (pyemic) (septic) (suppurative) I80.9
  antepartum — *see* Thrombophlebitis, antepartum

Phlebitis (infective) (pyemic) (septic) (suppurative) - *continued*
  blue — *see* Phlebitis, leg, deep
  breast, superficial I80.8
  cavernous (venous) sinus — *see* Phlebitis, intracranial (venous) sinus
  calf muscular vein (NOS) I80.25-
  cerebral (venous) sinus — *see* Phlebitis, intracranial (venous) sinus
  chest wall, superficial I80.8
  cranial (venous) sinus — *see* Phlebitis, intracranial (venous) sinus
  deep (vessels) — *see* Phlebitis, leg, deep
  due to implanted device — *see* Complications, by site and type, specified NEC
  during or resulting from a procedure T81.72
  femoral vein (superficial) I80.1-
  femoropopliteal vein I80.0-
  gastrocnemial vein I80.25-
  gestational — *see* Phlebopathy, gestational
  hepatic veins I80.8
  iliac vein (common) (external) (internal) I80.21-
  iliofemoral — *see* Phlebitis, femoral vein
  intracranial (venous) sinus (any) G08
    nonpyogenic I67.6
  intraspinal venous sinuses and veins G08
    nonpyogenic G95.19
  lateral (venous) sinus — *see* Phlebitis, intracranial (venous) sinus
  leg I80.3
    antepartum — *see* Thrombophlebitis, antepartum
    deep (vessels) NEC I80.20-
      iliac I80.21-
      popliteal vein I80.22-
      specified vessel NEC I80.29-
      tibial vein (anterior) (posterior) I80.23-
    femoral vein (superficial) I80.1-
    superficial (vessels) I80.0-
  longitudinal sinus — *see* Phlebitis, intracranial (venous) sinus
  lower limb — *see* Phlebitis, leg
  migrans, migrating (superficial) I82.1
  pelvic
    with ectopic or molar pregnancy O08.0
    following ectopic or molar pregnancy O08.0
    puerperal, postpartum O87.1
  peroneal vein I80.24-
  popliteal vein — *see* Phlebitis, leg, deep, popliteal
  portal (vein) K75.1
  postoperative T81.72
  pregnancy — *see* Thrombophlebitis, antepartum
  puerperal, postpartum, childbirth O87.0
    deep O87.1
    pelvic O87.1
    superficial O87.0
  retina — *see* Vasculitis, retina
  saphenous (accessory) (great) (long) (small) — *see* Phlebitis, leg, superficial
  sinus (meninges) — *see* Phlebitis, intracranial (venous) sinus
  soleal vein I80.25-
  specified site NEC I80.8
  syphilitic A52.09
  tibial vein — *see* Phlebitis, leg, deep, tibial
  ulcerative I80.9
    leg — *see* Phlebitis, leg
  umbilicus I80.8
  uterus (septic) — *see* Endometritis
  varicose (leg) (lower limb) — *see* Varix, leg, with, inflammation
Phlebofibrosis I87.8
Phleboliths I87.8
Phlebopathy,
  gestational O22.9-
  puerperal O87.9
Phlebosclerosis I87.8
Phlebothrombosis — *see also* Thrombosis
  antepartum — *see* Thrombophlebitis, antepartum

Phlebothrombosis - *continued*
  pregnancy — *see* Thrombophlebitis, antepartum
  puerperal — *see* Thrombophlebitis, puerperal
Phlebotomus fever A93.1
Phlegmasia
  alba dolens O87.1
    nonpuerperal — *see* Phlebitis, femoral vein
  cerulea dolens — *see* Phlebitis, leg, deep
Phlegmon — *see* Abscess
Phlegmonous — *see* condition
Phlyctenulosis (allergic) (keratoconjunctivitis) (nontuberculous) — *see also* Keratoconjunctivitis
  cornea — *see* Keratoconjunctivitis
  tuberculous A18.52
Phobia, phobic F40.9
  animal F40.218
    spiders F40.210
  examination F40.298
  reaction F40.9
  simple F40.298
  social F40.10
    generalized F40.11
  specific (isolated) F40.298
    animal F40.218
      spiders F40.210
    blood F40.230
    injection F40.231
    injury F40.233
    men F40.290
    natural environment F40.228
      thunderstorms F40.220
    situational F40.248
      bridges F40.242
      closed in spaces F40.240
      flying F40.243
      heights F40.241
    specified focus NEC F40.298
    transfusion F40.231
    women F40.291
  specified NEC F40.8
    medical care NEC F40.232
  state F40.9
Phocas' disease — *see* Mastopathy, cystic
Phocomelia Q73.1
  lower limb — *see* Agenesis, leg, with foot present
  upper limb — *see* Agenesis, arm, with hand present
Phoria H50.50
Phosphate-losing tubular disorder N25.0
Phosphatemia E83.39
Phosphaturia E83.39
Photodermatitis (sun) L56.8
  chronic L57.8
  due to drug L56.8
  light other than sun L59.8
Photokeratitis H16.13-
Photophobia H53.14-
Photophthalmia — *see* Photokeratitis
Photopsia H53.19
Photoretinitis — *see* Retinopathy, solar
Photosensitivity, photosensitization (sun) skin L56.8
  light other than sun L59.8
Phrenitis — *see* Encephalitis
Phrynoderma (vitamin A deficiency) E50.8
Phthiriasis (pubis) B85.3
  with any infestation classifiable to B85.0-B85.2 B85.4
Phthirus infestation — *see* Phthiriasis
Phthisis — *see also* Tuberculosis
  bulbi (infectional) — *see* Disorder, globe, degenerated condition, atrophy
  eyeball (due to infection) — *see* Disorder, globe, degenerated condition, atrophy
Phycomycosis — *see* Zygomycosis
Physalopteriasis B81.8
Physical restraint status Z78.1
Phytobezoar T18.9
  intestine T18.3
  stomach T18.2
Pian — *see* Yaws
Pianoma A66.1

Pica F50.89
  in adults F50.89
  infant or child F98.3
Picking, nose F98.8
Pick-Niemann disease — *see* Niemann-Pick
    disease or syndrome
Pick's
  cerebral atrophy G31.01 *[F02.80]*
    with behavioral disturbance G31.01
      [F02.81]
  disease or syndrome (brain) G31.01 *[F02.80]*
    with behavioral disturbance G31.01
      [F02.81]
    brain G31.01 *[F02.80]*
      with behavioral disturbance G31.01
        [F02.81]
    pericardium (pericardial pseudocirrhosis of
      liver) I31.1
  syndrome
    brain G31.01 *[F02.80]*
      with behavioral disturbance G31.01
        [F02.81]
    of heart (pericardial pseudocirrhosis of
      liver) I31.1
Pickwickian syndrome E66.2
Piebaldism E70.39
Piedra (beard) (scalp) B36.8
  black B36.3
  white B36.2
Pierre Robin deformity or syndrome Q87.0
Pierson's disease or osteochondrosis M91.0
Pig-bel A05.2
Pigeon
  breast or chest (acquired) M95.4
    congenital Q67.7
    rachitic sequelae (late effect) E64.3
  breeder's disease or lung J67.2
  fancier's disease or lung J67.2
  toe — *see* Deformity, toe, specified NEC
Pigmentation (abnormal) (anomaly) L81.9
  conjunctiva H11.13-
  cornea (anterior) H18.01-
    posterior H18.05-
    stromal H18.06-
  diminished melanin formation NEC L81.6
  iron L81.8
  lids, congenital Q82.8
  limbus corneae — *see* Pigmentation, cornea
  metals L81.8
  optic papilla, congenital Q14.2
  retina, congenital (grouped) (nevoid) Q14.1
  scrotum, congenital Q82.8
  tattoo L81.8
Piles — *see also* Hemorrhoids K64.9
Pili
  annulati or torti (congenital) Q84.1
  incarnati L73.1
Pill roller hand (intrinsic) — *see*
    Parkinsonism
Pilomatrixoma — *see* Neoplasm, skin, benign
  malignant — *see* Neoplasm, skin, malignant
Pilonidal — *see* condition
Pimple R23.8
PIN — *see* Neoplasia, intraepithelial, prostate
Pinched nerve — *see* Neuropathy, entrapment
Pindborg tumor — *see* Cyst, calcifying
    odontogenic
Pineal body or gland — *see* condition
Pinealoblastoma C75.3
Pinealoma D44.5
  malignant C75.3
Pineoblastoma C75.3
Pineocytoma D44.5
Pinguecula H11.15-
Pingueculitis H10.81-
Pinhole meatus — *see also* Stricture,
    urethra N35.919
Pink
  disease — *see* subcategory T56.1
  eye — *see* Conjunctivitis, acute,
    mucopurulent
Pinkus' disease (lichen nitidus) L44.1
Pinpoint
  meatus — *see* Stricture, urethra
  os (uteri) — *see* Stricture, cervix

Pins and needles R20.2
Pinta A67.9
  cardiovascular lesions A67.2
  chancre (primary) A67.0
  erythematous plaques A67.1
  hyperchromic lesions A67.1
  hyperkeratosis A67.1
  lesions A67.9
    cardiovascular A67.2
    hyperchromic A67.1
    intermediate A67.1
    late A67.2
    mixed A67.3
    primary A67.0
    skin (achromic) (cicatricial)
      (dyschromic) A67.2
      hyperchromic A67.1
      mixed (achromic and
        hyperchromic) A67.3
  papule (primary) A67.0
  skin lesions (achromic) (cicatricial)
    (dyschromic) A67.2
    hyperchromic A67.1
    mixed (achromic and hyperchromic) A67.3
  vitiligo A67.2
Pintids A67.1
Pinworm (disease) (infection)
    (infestation) B80
Piroplasmosis B60.0
Pistol wound — *see* Gunshot wound
Pitcher's elbow — *see* Derangement, joint,
    specified type NEC, elbow
Pithecoid pelvis Q74.2
  with disproportion (fetopelvic) O33.0
    causing obstructed labor O65.0
Pithiatism F48.8
Pitted — *see* Pitting
Pitting — *see also* Edema R60.9
  lip R60.0
  nail L60.8
  teeth K00.4
Pituitary gland — *see* condition
Pituitary-snuff-taker's disease J67.8
Pityriasis (capitis) L21.0
  alba L30.5
  circinata (et maculata) L42
  furfuracea L21.0
  Hebra's L26
  lichenoides L41.0
    chronica L41.1
    et varioliformis (acuta) L41.0
  maculata (et circinata) L30.5
  nigra B36.1
  pilaris, Hebra's L44.0
  rosea L42
  rotunda L44.8
  rubra (Hebra) pilaris L44.0
  simplex L30.5
  specified type NEC L30.5
  streptogenes L30.5
  versicolor (scrotal) B36.0
Placenta, placental — *see* Pregnancy,
    complicated by (care of) (management
    affected by), specified condition
Placentitis O41.14-
Plagiocephaly Q67.3
Plague A20.9
  abortive A20.8
  ambulatory A20.8
  asymptomatic A20.8
  bubonic A20.0
  cellulocutaneous A20.1
  cutaneobubonic A20.1
  lymphatic gland A20.0
  meningitis A20.3
  pharyngeal A20.8
  pneumonic (primary) (secondary) A20.2
  pulmonary, pulmonic A20.2
  septicemic A20.7
  tonsillar A20.8
    septicemic A20.7
Planning, family
  contraception Z30.9
  procreation Z31.69

Plaque (s)
  artery, arterial — *see* Arteriosclerosis
  calcareous — *see* Calcification
  coronary, lipid rich I25.83
  epicardial I31.8
  erythematous, of pinta A67.1
  Hollenhorst's — *see* Occlusion, artery, retina
  lipid rich, coronary I25.83
  pleural (without asbestos) J92.9
    with asbestos J92.0
  tongue K13.29
Plasmacytoma C90.3-
  extramedullary C90.2-
  medullary C90.0-
  solitary C90.3-
Plasmacytopenia D72.818
Plasmacytosis D72.822
Plaster ulcer — *see* Ulcer, pressure, by site
Plateau iris syndrome (post-iridectomy)
    (postprocedural) (without glaucoma)
    H21.82
  with glaucoma H40.22-
Platybasia Q75.8
Platyonychia (congenital) Q84.6
  acquired L60.8
Platypelloid pelvis M95.5
  with disproportion (fetopelvic) O33.0
    causing obstructed labor O65.0
  congenital Q74.2
Platyspondylisis Q76.49
Plaut (-Vincent) disease — *see*
    also Vincent's A69.1
Plethora R23.2
  newborn P61.1
Pleura, pleural — *see* condition
Pleuralgia R07.81
Pleurisy (acute) (adhesive) (chronic) (costal)
    (diaphragmatic) (double) (dry)
    (fibrinous) (fibrous) (interlobar) (latent)
    (plastic) (primary) (residual) (sicca)
    (sterile) (subacute) (unresolved) R09.1
  with
    adherent pleura J86.0
    effusion J90
      chylous, chyliform J94.0
      tuberculous (non primary) A15.6
        primary (progressive) A15.7
      tuberculosis — *see* Pleurisy, tuberculous
        (non primary)
  encysted — *see* Pleurisy, with effusion
  exudative — *see* Pleurisy, with effusion
  fibrinopurulent, fibropurulent — *see*
      Pyothorax
  hemorrhagic — *see* Hemothorax
  pneumococcal J90
  purulent — *see* Pyothorax
  septic — *see* Pyothorax
  serofibrinous — *see* Pleurisy, with effusion
  seropurulent — *see* Pyothorax
  serous — *see* Pleurisy, with effusion
  staphylococcal J86.9
  streptococcal J90
  suppurative — *see* Pyothorax
  traumatic (post) (current) — *see* Injury,
      intrathoracic, pleura
  tuberculous (with effusion) (non
      primary) A15.6
    primary (progressive) A15.7
Pleuritis sicca — *see* Pleurisy
Pleurobronchopneumonia — *see* Pneumonia,
    broncho-
Pleurodynia R07.81
  epidemic B33.0
  viral B33.0
Pleuropericarditis — *see also* Pericarditis
  acute I30.9
Pleuropneumonia (acute) (bilateral) (double)
    (septic) — *see also* Pneumonia J18.8
  chronic — *see* Fibrosis, lung
Pleuro-pneumonia-like-organism (PPLO) ,
    as cause of disease classified
    elsewhere B96.0
Pleurorrhea — *see* Pleurisy, with effusion
Plexitis, brachial G54.0

Plica
  polonica B85.0
  syndrome, knee M67.5-
  tonsil J35.8
Plicated tongue K14.5
Plug
  bronchus NEC J98.09
  meconium (newborn) NEC syndrome P76.0
  mucus — *see* Asphyxia, mucus
Plumbism — *see* subcategory T56.0
Plummer's disease E05.20
  with thyroid storm E05.21
Plummer-Vinson syndrome D50.1
Pluricarential syndrome of infancy E40
Plus (and minus) hand (intrinsic) — *see*
  Deformity, limb, specified type NEC,
  forearm
Pneumathemia — *see* Air, embolism
Pneumatic hammer (drill) syndrome T75.21
Pneumatocele (lung) J98.4
  intracranial G93.89
  tension J44.9
Pneumatosis
  cystoides intestinalis K63.89
  intestinalis K63.89
  peritonei K66.8
Pneumaturia R39.89
Pneumoblastoma — *see* Neoplasm, lung,
  malignant
Pneumocephalus G93.89
Pneumococcemia A40.3
Pneumococcus, pneumococcal — *see*
  condition
Pneumoconiosis (due to) (inhalation of) J64
  with tuberculosis (any type in A15) J65
  aluminum J63.0
  asbestos J61
  bagasse, bagassosis J67.1
  bauxite J63.1
  beryllium J63.2
  coal miners' (simple) J60
  coalworkers' (simple) J60
  collier's J60
  cotton dust J66.0
  diatomite (diatomaceous earth) J62.8
  dust
    inorganic NEC J63.6
    lime J62.8
    marble J62.8
    organic NEC J66.8
  fumes or vapors (from silo) J68.9
  graphite J63.3
  grinder's J62.8
  kaolin J62.8
  mica J62.8
  millstone maker's J62.8
  mineral fibers NEC J61
  miner's J60
  moldy hay J67.0
  potter's J62.8
  rheumatoid — *see* Rheumatoid, lung
  sandblaster's J62.8
  silica, silicate NEC J62.8
    with carbon J60
  stonemason's J62.8
  talc (dust) J62.0
Pneumocystis carinii pneumonia B59
Pneumocystis jiroveci (pneumonia) B59
Pneumocystosis (with pneumonia) B59
Pneumohemopericardium I31.2
Pneumohemothorax J94.2
  traumatic S27.2
Pneumohydropericardium — *see* Pericarditis
Pneumohydrothorax — *see* Hydrothorax
Pneumomediastinum J98.2
  congenital or perinatal P25.2
Pneumomycosis B49 *[J99]*
Pneumonia (acute) (double) (migratory)
  (purulent) (septic) (unresolved) J18.9
  with
    lung abscess J85.1
      due to specified organism — *see*
        Pneumonia, in (due to)
    influenza — *see* Influenza, with,
      pneumonia

**Pneumonia (acute) (double) (migratory)
(purulent) (septic) (unresolved)** - *continued*
  adenoviral J12.0
  adynamic J18.2
  alba A50.04
  allergic (eosinophilic) J82
  alveolar — *see* Pneumonia, lobar
  anaerobes J15.8
  anthrax A22.1
  apex, apical — *see* Pneumonia, lobar
  Ascaris B77.81
  aspiration J69.0
    due to
      aspiration of microorganisms
        bacterial J15.9
        viral J12.9
      food (regurgitated) J69.0
      gastric secretions J69.0
      milk (regurgitated) J69.0
      oils, essences J69.1
      solids, liquids NEC J69.8
      vomitus J69.0
    newborn P24.81
      amniotic fluid (clear) P24.11
      blood P24.21
      liquor (amnii) P24.11
      meconium P24.01
      milk P24.31
      mucus P24.11
      food (regurgitated) P24.31
      specified NEC P24.81
      stomach contents P24.31
    postprocedural J95.4
  atypical NEC J18.9
  bacillus J15.9
    specified NEC J15.8
  bacterial J15.9
    specified NEC J15.8
  Bacteroides (fragilis) (oralis)
    (melaninogenicus) J15.8
  basal, basic, basilar — *see* Pneumonia, by
    type
  bronchiolitis obliterans organized
    (BOOP) J84.89
  broncho-, bronchial (confluent) (croupous)
    (diffuse) (disseminated) (hemorrhagic)
    (involving lobes) (lobar)
    (terminal) J18.0
    allergic (eosinophilic) J82
    aspiration — *see* Pneumonia, aspiration
    bacterial J15.9
      specified NEC J15.8
    chronic — *see* Fibrosis, lung
    diplococcal J13
    Eaton's agent J15.7
    Escherichia coli (E. coli) J15.5
    Friedländer's bacillus J15.0
    Hemophilus influenzae J14
    hypostatic J18.2
    inhalation — *see also* Pneumonia,
      aspiration
      due to fumes or vapors (chemical) J68.0
      of oils or essences J69.1
    Klebsiella (pneumoniae) J15.0
    lipid, lipoid J69.1
      endogenous J84.89
    Mycoplasma (pneumoniae) J15.7
    pleuro-pneumonia-like-organisms
      (PPLO) J15.7
    pneumococcal J13
    Proteus J15.6
    Pseudomonas J15.1
    Serratia marcescens J15.6
    specified organism NEC J16.8
    staphylococcal — *see* Pneumonia,
      staphylococcal
    streptococcal NEC J15.4
      group B J15.3
      pneumoniae J13
    viral, virus — *see* Pneumonia, viral
  Butyrivibrio (fibrisolvens) J15.8
  Candida B37.1
  caseous — *see* Tuberculosis, pulmonary
  catarrhal — *see* Pneumonia, broncho
  chlamydial J16.0

**Pneumonia (acute) (double) (migratory)
(purulent) (septic) (unresolved)** - *continued*
  chlamydial - *continued*
    congenital P23.1
  cholesterol J84.89
  cirrhotic (chronic) — *see* Fibrosis, lung
  Clostridium (haemolyticum) (novyi) J15.8
  confluent — *see* Pneumonia, broncho
  congenital (infective) P23.9
    due to
      bacterium NEC P23.6
      Chlamydia P23.1
      Escherichia coli P23.4
      Haemophilus influenzae P23.6
      infective organism NEC P23.8
      Klebsiella pneumoniae P23.6
      Mycoplasma P23.6
      Pseudomonas P23.5
      Staphylococcus P23.2
      Streptococcus (except group B) P23.6
        group B P23.3
      viral agent P23.0
    specified NEC P23.8
  croupous — *see* Pneumonia, lobar
  cryptogenic organizing J84.116
  cytomegalic inclusion B25.0
  cytomegaloviral B25.0
  deglutition — *see* Pneumonia, aspiration
  desquamative interstitial J84.117
  diffuse — *see* Pneumonia, broncho
  diplococcal, diplococcus (broncho-)
    (lobar) J13
  disseminated (focal) — *see* Pneumonia,
    broncho
  Eaton's agent J15.7
  embolic, embolism — *see* Embolism,
    pulmonary
  Enterobacter J15.6
  eosinophilic J82
  Escherichia coli (E. coli) J15.5
  Eubacterium J15.8
  fibrinous — *see* Pneumonia, lobar
  fibroid, fibrous (chronic) — *see* Fibrosis,
    lung
  Friedländer's bacillus J15.0
  Fusobacterium (nucleatum) J15.8
  gangrenous J85.0
  giant cell (measles) B05.2
  gonococcal A54.84
  gram-negative bacteria NEC J15.6
    anaerobic J15.8
  Hemophilus influenzae (broncho) (lobar) J14
  human metapneumovirus J12.3
  hypostatic (broncho) (lobar) J18.2
  in (due to)
    actinomycosis A42.0
    adenovirus J12.0
    anthrax A22.1
    ascariasis B77.81
    aspergillosis B44.9
    Bacillus anthracis A22.1
    Bacterium anitratum J15.6
    candidiasis B37.1
    chickenpox B01.2
    Chlamydia J16.0
      neonatal P23.1
    coccidioidomycosis B38.2
      acute B38.0
      chronic B38.1
    cytomegalovirus disease B25.0
    Diplococcus (pneumoniae) J13
    Eaton's agent J15.7
    Enterobacter J15.6
    Escherichia coli (E. coli) J15.5
    Friedländer's bacillus J15.0
    fumes and vapors (chemical)
      (inhalation) J68.0
    gonorrhea A54.84
    Hemophilus influenzae (H. influenzae) J14
    Herellea J15.6
    histoplasmosis B39.2
      acute B39.0
      chronic B39.1
    human metapneumovirus J12.3
    Klebsiella (pneumoniae) J15.0

Pneumonia (acute) (double) (migratory)
(purulent) (septic) (unresolved) - *continued*
in (due to) - *continued*
  measles B05.2
  Mycoplasma (pneumoniae) J15.7
  nocardiosis, nocardiasis A43.0
  ornithosis A70
  parainfluenza virus J12.2
  pleuro-pneumonia-like-organism
    (PPLO) J15.7
  pneumococcus J13
  pneumocystosis (Pneumocystis carinii)
    (Pneumocystis jiroveci) B59
  Proteus J15.6
  Pseudomonas NEC J15.1
    pseudomallei A24.1
  psittacosis A70
  Q fever A78
  respiratory syncytial virus (RSV) J12.1
  rheumatic fever I00 *[J17]*
  rubella B06.81
  Salmonella (infection) A02.22
    typhi A01.03
  schistosomiasis B65.9 *[J17]*
  Serratia marcescens J15.6
  specified
    bacterium NEC J15.8
    organism NEC J16.8
  spirochetal NEC A69.8
  Staphylococcus J15.20
    aureus (methicillin susceptible)
      (MSSA) J15.211
      methicillin resistant (MRSA) J15.212
    specified NEC J15.29
  Streptococcus J15.4
    group B J15.3
    pneumoniae J13
    specified NEC J15.4
  toxoplasmosis B58.3
  tularemia A21.2
  typhoid (fever) A01.03
  varicella B01.2
  virus — *see* Pneumonia, viral
  whooping cough A37.91
    due to
      Bordetella parapertussis A37.11
      Bordetella pertussis A37.01
      specified NEC A37.81
  Yersinia pestis A20.2
inhalation of food or vomit — *see*
  Pneumonia, aspiration
interstitial J84.9
  chronic J84.111
  desquamative J84.117
  due to
    collagen vascular disease J84.17
    known underlying cause J84.17
  idiopathic NOS J84.111
  in disease classified elsewhere J84.17
  lymphocytic (due to collagen vascular
    disease) (in diseases classified
    elsewhere) J84.17
  lymphoid J84.2
  non-specific J84.89
    due to
      collagen vascular disease J84.17
      known underlying cause J84.17
    idiopathic J84.113
    in diseases classified elsewhere J84.17
  plasma cell B59
  pseudomonas J15.1
  usual J84.112
    due to collagen vascular disease J84.17
    idiopathic J84.112
    in diseases classified elsewhere J84.17
Klebsiella (pneumoniae) J15.0
lipid, lipoid (exogenous) J69.1
  endogenous J84.89
lobar (disseminated) (double)
  (interstitial) J18.1
  bacterial J15.9
    specified NEC J15.8
  chronic — *see* Fibrosis, lung
  Escherichia coli (E. coli) J15.5
  Friedländer's bacillus J15.0

Pneumonia (acute) (double) (migratory)
(purulent) (septic) (unresolved) - *continued*
lobar (disseminated) (double) (interstitial) -
  continued
  Hemophilus influenzae J14
  hypostatic J18.2
  Klebsiella (pneumoniae) J15.0
  pneumococcal J13
  Proteus J15.6
  Pseudomonas J15.1
  specified organism NEC J16.8
  staphylococcal — *see* Pneumonia,
    staphylococcal
  streptococcal NEC J15.4
  Streptococcus pneumoniae J13
  viral, virus — *see* Pneumonia, viral
lobular — *see* Pneumonia, broncho
Löffler's J82
lymphoid interstitial J84.2
massive — *see* Pneumonia, lobar
meconium P24.01
MRSA (Methicillin resistant Staphylococcus
  aureus) J15.212
MSSA (methicillin susceptible
  Staphylococcus aureus) J15.211
multilobar — *see* Pneumonia, by type
Mycoplasma (pneumoniae) J15.7
necrotic J85.0
neonatal P23.9
  aspiration — *see* Aspiration, by substance,
    with pneumonia
nitrogen dioxide J68.0
organizing J84.89
  due to
    collagen vascular disease J84.17
    known underlying cause J84.17
  in diseases classified elsewhere J84.17
orthostatic J18.2
parainfluenza virus J12.2
parenchymatous — *see* Fibrosis, lung
passive J18.2
patchy — *see* Pneumonia, broncho
Peptococcus J15.8
Peptostreptococcus J15.8
plasma cell (of infants) B59
pleurolobar — *see* Pneumonia, lobar
pleuro-pneumonia-like organism
  (PPLO) J15.7
pneumococcal (broncho) (lobar) J13
Pneumocystis (carinii) (jiroveci) B59
postinfectional NEC B99 *[J17]*
postmeasles B05.2
Proteus J15.6
Pseudomonas J15.1
psittacosis A70
radiation J70.0
respiratory syncytial virus (RSV) J12.1
resulting from a procedure J95.89
rheumatic I00 *[J17]*
Salmonella (arizonae) (cholerae-suis)
  (enteritidis) (typhimurium) A02.22
  typhi A01.03
  typhoid fever A01.03
SARS-associated coronavirus J12.81
segmented, segmental — *see* Pneumonia,
  broncho-
Serratia marcescens J15.6
specified NEC J18.8
  bacterium NEC J15.8
  organism NEC J16.8
  virus NEC J12.89
spirochetal NEC A69.8
staphylococcal (broncho) (lobar) J15.20
  aureus (methicillin susceptible)
    (MSSA) J15.211
    methicillin resistant (MRSA) J15.212
  specified NEC J15.29
static, stasis J18.2
streptococcal NEC (broncho) (lobar) J15.4
  group
    A J15.4
    B J15.3
    specified NEC J15.4
  Streptococcus pneumoniae J13
syphilitic, congenital (early) A50.04

Pneumonia (acute) (double) (migratory)
(purulent) (septic) (unresolved) - *continued*
traumatic (complication) (early)
  (secondary) T79.8
tuberculous (any) — *see* Tuberculosis,
  pulmonary
tularemic A21.2
varicella B01.2
Veillonella J15.8
ventilator associated J95.851
viral, virus (broncho) (interstitial)
  (lobar) J12.9
  adenoviral J12.0
  congenital P23.0
  human metapneumovirus J12.3
  parainfluenza J12.2
  respiratory syncytial (RSV) J12.1
  SARS-associated coronavirus J12.81
  specified NEC J12.89
white (congenital) A50.04
Pneumonic — *see* condition
Pneumonitis (acute) (primary) — *see also*
  Pneumonia
air-conditioner J67.7
allergic (due to) J67.9
  organic dust NEC J67.8
  red cedar dust J67.8
  sequoiosis J67.8
  wood dust J67.8
aspiration J69.0
  due to
    anesthesia J95.4
      during
        labor and delivery O74.0
        pregnancy O29.01-
        puerperium O89.01
    fumes or gases J68.0
    obstetric O74.0
chemical (due to gases, fumes or vapors)
  (inhalation) J68.0
  due to anesthesia J95.4
cholesterol J84.89
crack (cocaine) J68.0
chronic — *see* Fibrosis, lung
congenital rubella P35.0
due to
  beryllium J68.0
  cadmium J68.0
  crack (cocaine) J68.0
  detergent J69.8
  fluorocarbon-polymer J68.0
  food, vomit (aspiration) J69.0
  fumes or vapors J68.0
  gases, fumes or vapors (inhalation) J68.0
  inhalation
    blood J69.8
    essences J69.1
    food (regurgitated) , milk, vomit J69.0
    oils, essences J69.1
    saliva J69.0
    solids, liquids NEC J69.8
  manganese J68.0
  nitrogen dioxide J68.0
  oils, essences J69.1
  solids, liquids NEC J69.8
  toxoplasmosis (acquired) B58.3
    congenital P37.1
  vanadium J68.0
  ventilator J95.851
eosinophilic J82
hypersensitivity J67.9
  air conditioner lung J67.7
  bagassosis J67.1
  bird fancier's lung J67.2
  farmer's lung J67.0
  maltworker's lung J67.4
  maple bark-stripper's lung J67.6
  mushroom worker's lung J67.5
  specified organic dust NEC J67.8
  suberosis J67.3
interstitial (chronic) J84.89
  acute J84.114
  lymphoid J84.2
  non-specific J84.89
    idiopathic J84.113

Pneumonitis (acute) (primary) - *continued*
  lymphoid, interstitial J84.2
  meconium P24.01
  postanesthetic J95.4
    correct substance properly
      administered — *see* Table of Drugs
      and Chemicals, by drug, adverse
      effect
    in labor and delivery O74.0
    in pregnancy O29.01-
    obstetric O74.0
    overdose or wrong substance given or
      taken (by accident) — *see* Table of
      Drugs and Chemicals, by drug,
      poisoning
    postpartum, puerperal O89.01
  postoperative J95.4
    obstetric O74.0
  radiation J70.0
  rubella, congenital P35.0
  ventilation (air-conditioning) J67.7
  ventilator associated J95.851
  wood-dust J67.8
Pneumonoconiosis — *see* Pneumoconiosis
Pneumoparotid K11.8
Pneumopathy NEC J98.4
  alveolar J84.09
  due to organic dust NEC J66.8
  parietoalveolar J84.09
Pneumopericarditis — *see also* Pericarditis
  acute I30.9
Pneumopericardium — *see also* Pericarditis
  congenital P25.3
  newborn P25.3
  traumatic (post) — *see* Injury, heart
Pneumophagia (psychogenic) F45.8
Pneumopleurisy, pneumopleuritis — *see
  also* Pneumonia J18.8
Pneumopyopericardium I30.1
Pneumopyothorax — *see* Pyopneumothorax
  with fistula J86.0
Pneumorrhagia — *see also* Hemorrhage, lung
  tuberculous — *see* Tuberculosis, pulmonary
Pneumothorax NOS J93.9
  acute J93.83
  chronic J93.81
  congenital P25.1
  perinatal period P25.1
  postprocedural J95.811
  specified NEC J93.83
  spontaneous NOS J93.83
    newborn P25.1
    primary J93.11
    secondary J93.12
    tension J93.0
  tense valvular, infectional J93.0
  tension (spontaneous) J93.0
  traumatic S27.0
    with hemothorax S27.2
  tuberculous — *see* Tuberculosis, pulmonary
Podagra — *see also* Gout M10.9
Podencephalus Q01.9
Poikilocytosis R71.8
Poikiloderma L81.6
  Civatte's L57.3
  congenital Q82.8
  vasculare atrophicans L94.5
Poikilodermatomyositis M33.10
  with
    myopathy M33.12
    respiratory involvement M33.11
    specified organ involvement NEC M33.19
Pointed ear (congenital) Q17.3
**Poison ivy, oak, sumac or other plant
  dermatitis (allergic) (contact)** L23.7
Poisoning (acute) — *see also* Table of Drugs
  and Chemicals
  algae and toxins T65.82-
  Bacillus B (aertrycke) (cholerae (suis))
    (paratyphosus) (suipestifer) A02.9
    botulinus A05.1
  bacterial toxins A05.9
  berries, noxious — *see* Poisoning, food,
    noxious, berries
  botulism A05.1

Poisoning (acute) - *continued*
  ciguatera fish T61.0-
  Clostridium botulinum A05.1
  death-cap (Amanita phalloides) (Amanita
    verna) — *see* Poisoning, food, noxious,
    mushrooms
  drug — *see* Table of Drugs and Chemicals,
    by drug, poisoning
  epidemic, fish (noxious) — *see* Poisoning,
    seafood
    bacterial A05.9
  fava bean D55.0
  fish (noxious) T61.9-
    bacterial — *see* Intoxication, foodborne,
      by agent
    ciguatera fish — *see* Poisoning, ciguatera
      fish
    scombroid fish — *see* Poisoning,
      scombroid fish
    specified type NEC T61.77-
  food NEC A05.9
    bacterial — *see* Intoxication, foodborne,
      by agent
    due to
      Bacillus (aertrycke) (choleraesuis)
        (paratyphosus) (suipestifer) A02.9
        botulinus A05.1
      Clostridium (perfringens)
        (Welchii) A05.2
      salmonella (aertrycke) (callinarum)
        (choleraesuis) (enteritidis)
        (paratyphi) (suipestifer) A02.9
        with
          gastroenteritis A02.0
          sepsis A02.1
      staphylococcus A05.0
      Vibrio
        parahaemolyticus A05.3
        vulnificus A05.5
    noxious or naturally toxic T62.9-
      berries — *see* subcategory T62.1-
      fish — *see* Poisoning, seafood
      mushrooms — *see* subcategory T62.0X-
      plants NEC — *see* subcategory T62.2X-
      seafood — *see* Poisoning, seafood
      specified NEC — *see* subcategory
        T62.8X-
  ichthyotoxism — *see* Poisoning, seafood
  kreotoxism, food A05.9
  latex T65.81-
  lead T56.0-
  mushroom — *see* Poisoning, food, noxious,
    mushroom
  mussels — *see also* Poisoning, shellfish
    bacterial — *see* Intoxication, foodborne,
      by agent
  nicotine (tobacco) T65.2-
  noxious foodstuffs — *see* Poisoning, food,
    noxious
  plants, noxious — *see* Poisoning, food,
    noxious, plants NEC
  ptomaine — *see* Poisoning, food
  radiation J70.0
  Salmonella (arizonae) (cholerae-suis)
    (enteritidis) (typhimurium) A02.9
  scombroid fish T61.1-
  seafood (noxious) T61.9-
    bacterial — *see* Intoxication, foodborne,
      by agent
    fish — *see* Poisoning, fish
    shellfish — *see* Poisoning, shellfish
    specified NEC — *see* subcategory T61.8X-
  shellfish (amnesic) (azaspiracid) (diarrheic)
    (neurotoxic) (noxious)
    (paralytic) T61.78-
    bacterial — *see* Intoxication, foodborne,
      by agent
    ciguatera mollusk — *see* Poisoning,
      ciguatera fish
  specified substance NEC T65.891
  Staphylococcus, food A05.0
  tobacco (nicotine) T65.2-
  water E87.79
Poker spine — *see* Spondylitis, ankylosing
Poland syndrome Q79.8

Polioencephalitis (acute) (bulbar) A80.9
  inferior G12.22
  influenzal — *see* Influenza, with,
    encephalopathy
  superior hemorrhagic (acute)
    (Wernicke's) E51.2
  Wernicke's E51.2
Polioencephalomyelitis (acute) (anterior)
  A80.9
  with beriberi E51.2
Polioencephalopathy, superior hemorrhagic
  E51.2
  with
    beriberi E51.11
    pellagra E52
Poliomeningoencephalitis — *see*
  Meningoencephalitis
Poliomyelitis (acute) (anterior) (epidemic)
  A80.9
  with paralysis (bulbar) — *see* Poliomyelitis,
    paralytic
  abortive A80.4
  ascending (progressive) — *see* Poliomyelitis,
    paralytic
  bulbar (paralytic) — *see* Poliomyelitis,
    paralytic
  congenital P35.8
  nonepidemic A80.9
  nonparalytic A80.4
  paralytic A80.30
    specified NEC A80.39
    vaccine-associated A80.0
    wild virus
      imported A80.1
      indigenous A80.2
  spinal, acute A80.9
Poliosis (eyebrow) (eyelashes) L67.1
  circumscripta, acquired L67.1
Pollakiuria R35.0
  psychogenic F45.8
Pollinosis J30.1
Pollitzer's disease L73.2
Polyadenitis — *see also* Lymphadenitis
  malignant A20.0
Polyalgia M79.89
Polyangiitis M30.0
  microscopic M31.7
  overlap syndrome M30.8
Polyarteritis
  microscopic M31.7
  nodosa M30.0
    with lung involvement M30.1
    juvenile M30.2
    related condition NEC M30.8
Polyarthralgia — *see* Pain, joint
Polyarthritis, polyarthropathy — *see also*
  Arthritis M13.0
  due to or associated with other specified
    conditions — *see* Arthritis
  epidemic (Australian) (with
    exanthema) B33.1
  infective — *see* Arthritis, pyogenic or
    pyemic
  inflammatory M06.4
  juvenile (chronic) (seronegative) M08.3
  migratory M13.8-
  rheumatic, acute — *see* Fever, rheumatic
Polyarthrosis M15.9
  post-traumatic M15.3
  primary M15.0
  specified NEC M15.8
Polycarential syndrome of infancy E40
Polychondritis (atrophic) (chronic) — *see
  also* Disorder, cartilage, specified type
  NEC
  relapsing M94.1
Polycoria Q13.2
Polycystic (disease)
  degeneration, kidney Q61.3
    autosomal dominant (adult type) Q61.2
    autosomal recessive (infantile type)
      NEC Q61.19
  kidney Q61.3
    autosomal
      dominant Q61.2

Polycystic (disease) - *continued*
  kidney - *continued*
    autosomal - *continued*
      recessive NEC Q61.19
    autosomal dominant (adult type) Q61.2
    autosomal recessive (childhood type)
        NEC Q61.19
    infantile type NEC Q61.19
  liver Q44.6
  lung J98.4
    congenital Q33.0
  ovary, ovaries E28.2
  spleen Q89.09
Polycythemia (secondary) D75.1
  acquired D75.1
  benign (familial) D75.0
  due to
    donor twin P61.1
    erythropoietin D75.1
    fall in plasma volume D75.1
    high altitude D75.1
    maternal-fetal transfusion P61.1
    stress D75.1
  emotional D75.1
  erythropoietin D75.1
  familial (benign) D75.0
  Gaisböck's (hypertonica) D75.1
  high altitude D75.1
  hypertonica D75.1
  hypoxemic D75.1
  neonatorum P61.1
  nephrogenous D75.1
  relative D75.1
  secondary D75.1
  spurious D75.1
  stress D75.1
  vera D45
Polycytosis cryptogenica D75.1
Polydactylism, polydactyly Q69.9
  toes Q69.2
Polydipsia R63.1
Polydystrophy, pseudo-Hurler E77.0
Polyembryoma — *see* Neoplasm, malignant,
    by site
Polyglandular
  deficiency E31.0
  dyscrasia E31.9
  dysfunction E31.9
  syndrome E31.8
Polyhydramnios O40.-
Polymastia Q83.1
Polymenorrhea N92.0
Polymyalgia M35.3
  arteritica, giant cell M31.5
  rheumatica M35.3
    with giant cell arteritis M31.5
Polymyositis (acute) (chronic) (hemorrhagic)
    M33.20
  with
    myopathy M33.22
    respiratory involvement M33.21
    skin involvement — *see*
        Dermatopolymyositis
    specified organ involvement NEC M33.29
  ossificans (generalisata) (progressiva) — *see*
      Myositis, ossificans, progressiva
Polyneuritis, polyneuritic — *see also*
      Polyneuropathy
  acute (post-) infective G61.0
  alcoholic G62.1
  cranialis G52.7
  demyelinating, chronic inflammatory
      (CIDP) G61.81
  diabetic — *see* Diabetes, polyneuropathy
  diphtheritic A36.83
  due to lack of vitamin NEC E56.9 *[G63]*
  endemic E51.11
  erythredema — *see* subcategory T56.1
  febrile, acute G61.0
  hereditary ataxic G60.1
  idiopathic, acute G61.0
  infective (acute) G61.0
  inflammatory, chronic demyelinating
      (CIDP) G61.81
  nutritional E63.9 *[G63]*

Polyneuritis, polyneuritic - *continued*
  postinfective (acute) G61.0
  specified NEC G62.89
Polyneuropathy (peripheral) G62.9
  alcoholic G62.1
  amyloid (Portuguese) E85.1 *[G63]*
    transthyretin-related (ATTR)
        familial E85.1 *[G63]*
  arsenical G62.2
  critical illness G62.81
  demyelinating, chronic inflammatory
      (CIDP) G61.81
  diabetic — *see* Diabetes, polyneuropathy
  drug-induced G62.0
  hereditary G60.9
    specified NEC G60.8
  idiopathic G60.9
    progressive G60.3
  in (due to)
    alcohol G62.1
      sequelae G65.2
    amyloidosis, familial (Portuguese) E85.1
        [G63]
    antitetanus serum G61.1
    arsenic G62.2
      sequelae G65.2
    avitaminosis NEC E56.9 *[G63]*
    beriberi E51.11
    collagen vascular disease NEC M35.9
        [G63]
    deficiency (of)
      B (-complex) vitamins E53.9 *[G63]*
      vitamin B6 E53.1 *[G63]*
    diabetes — *see* Diabetes, polyneuropathy
    diphtheria A36.83
    drug or medicament G62.0
      correct substance properly
          administered — *see* Table of Drugs
          and Chemicals, by drug, adverse
          effect
      overdose or wrong substance given or
          taken — *see* Table of Drugs and
          Chemicals, by drug, poisoning
    endocrine disease NEC E34.9 *[G63]*
    herpes zoster B02.23
    hypoglycemia E16.2 *[G63]*
    infectious
      disease NEC B99 *[G63]*
      mononucleosis B27.91
    lack of vitamin NEC E56.9 *[G63]*
    lead G62.2
      sequelae G65.2
    leprosy A30.9 *[G63]*
    Lyme disease A69.22
    metabolic disease NEC E88.9 *[G63]*
    microscopic polyangiitis M31.7 *[G63]*
    mumps B26.84
    neoplastic disease — *see also*
        Neoplasm D49.9 *[G63]*
    nutritional deficiency NEC E63.9 *[G63]*
    organophosphate compounds G62.2
      sequelae G65.2
    parasitic disease NEC B89 *[G63]*
    pellagra E52 *[G63]*
    polyarteritis nodosa M30.0
    porphyria E80.20 *[G63]*
    radiation G62.82
    rheumatoid arthritis — *see* Rheumatoid,
        polyneuropathy
    sarcoidosis D86.89
    serum G61.1
    syphilis (late) A52.15
      congenital A50.43
    systemic
      connective tissue disorder M35.9 *[G63]*
      lupus erythematosus M32.19
    toxic agent NEC G62.2
      sequelae G65.2
    transthyretin-related (ATTR) familial
        amyloid E85.1
    triorthocresyl phosphate G62.2
      sequelae G65.2
    tuberculosis A17.89
    uremia N18.9 *[G63]*
    vitamin B12 deficiency E53.8 *[G63]*

Polyneuropathy (peripheral) - *continued*
  transthyretin-related (ATTR) familial
    amyloid - *continued*
      vitamin B12 deficiency - *continued*
        with anemia (pernicious) D51.0 *[G63]*
          due to dietary deficiency D51.3 *[G63]*
      zoster B02.23
  inflammatory G61.9
    chronic demyelinating (CIDP) G61.81
    sequelae G65.1
    specified NEC G61.89
  lead G62.2
    sequelae G65.2
  nutritional NEC E63.9 *[G63]*
  postherpetic (zoster) B02.23
  progressive G60.3
  radiation-induced G62.82
  sensory (hereditary) (idiopathic) G60.8
  specified NEC G62.89
  syphilitic (late) A52.15
    congenital A50.43
Polyopia H53.8
Polyorchism, polyorchidism Q55.21
Polyosteoarthritis — *see also* Osteoarthritis,
    generalized M15.9-
  post-traumatic M15.3
  specified NEC M15.8
Polyostotic fibrous dysplasia Q78.1
Polyotia Q17.0
Polyp, polypus
  accessory sinus J33.8
  adenocarcinoma in — *see* Neoplasm,
    malignant, by site
  adenocarcinoma in situ in — *see* Neoplasm,
    in situ, by site
  adenoid tissue J33.0
  adenomatous — *see also* Neoplasm, benign,
    by site
    adenocarcinoma in — *see* Neoplasm,
      malignant, by site
    adenocarcinoma in situ in — *see*
      Neoplasm, in situ, by site
    carcinoma in — *see* Neoplasm, malignant,
      by site
    carcinoma in situ in — *see* Neoplasm, in
      situ, by site
    multiple — *see* Neoplasm, benign
      adenocarcinoma in — *see* Neoplasm,
        malignant, by site
      adenocarcinoma in situ in — *see*
        Neoplasm, in situ, by site
  antrum J33.8
  anus, anal (canal) K62.0
  Bartholin's gland N84.3
  bladder D41.4
  carcinoma in — *see* Neoplasm, malignant, by
    site
  carcinoma in situ in — *see* Neoplasm, in situ,
    by site
  cecum D12.0
  cervix (uteri) N84.1
    in pregnancy or childbirth — *see*
      Pregnancy, complicated by, abnormal,
      cervix
    mucous N84.1
    nonneoplastic N84.1
  choanal J33.0
  cholesterol K82.4
  clitoris N84.3
  colon K63.5
    adenomatous D12.6
      ascending D12.2
      cecum D12.0
      descending D12.4
    hyperplastic, (any site) K63.5
    inflammatory K51.40
      with
        abscess K51.414
        complication K51.419
          specified NEC K51.418
        fistula K51.413
        intestinal obstruction K51.412
        rectal bleeding K51.411
    sigmoid D12.5
    transverse D12.3

Polyp, polypus - *continued*
  corpus uteri N84.0
  dental K04.01
    irreversible K04.02
    reversible K04.01
  duodenum K31.7
  ear (middle) H74.4-
  endometrium N84.0
  ethmoidal (sinus) J33.8
  fallopian tube N84.8
  female genital tract N84.9
    specified NEC N84.8
  frontal (sinus) J33.8
  gallbladder K82.4
  gingiva, gum K06.8
  labia, labium (majus) (minus) N84.3
  larynx (mucous) J38.1
    adenomatous D14.1
  malignant — *see* Neoplasm, malignant, by
      site
  maxillary (sinus) J33.8
  middle ear — *see* Polyp, ear (middle)
  myometrium N84.0
  nares
      anterior J33.9
      posterior J33.0
  nasal (mucous) J33.9
      cavity J33.0
      septum J33.0
  nasopharyngeal J33.0
  nose (mucous) J33.9
  oviduct N84.8
  pharynx J39.2
  placenta O90.89
  prostate — *see* Enlargement, enlarged,
      prostate
  pudenda, pudendum N84.3
  pulpal (dental) K04.01
    irreversible K04.02
    reversible K04.01
  rectum (nonadenomatous) K62.1
    adenomatous — *see* Polyp, adenomatous
  septum (nasal) J33.0
  sinus (accessory) (ethmoidal) (frontal)
      (maxillary) (sphenoidal) J33.8
  sphenoidal (sinus) J33.8
  stomach K31.7
    adenomatous D13.1
  tube, fallopian N84.8
  turbinate, mucous membrane J33.8
  umbilical, newborn P83.6
  ureter N28.89
  urethra N36.2
  uterus (body) (corpus) (mucous) N84.0
    cervix N84.1
    in pregnancy or childbirth — *see*
        Pregnancy, complicated by, tumor,
        uterus
  vagina N84.2
  vocal cord (mucous) J38.1
  vulva N84.3
Polyphagia R63.2
Polyploidy Q92.7
Polypoid — *see* condition
Polyposis — *see also* Polyp
  coli (adenomatous) D12.6
    adenocarcinoma in C18.9
    adenocarcinoma in situ in — *see*
        Neoplasm, in situ, by site
    carcinoma in C18.9
  colon (adenomatous) D12.6
  familial D12.6
    adenocarcinoma in situ in — *see*
        Neoplasm, in situ, by site
  intestinal (adenomatous) D12.6
  malignant lymphomatous C83.1-
  multiple, adenomatous — *see also*
      Neoplasm, benign D36.9
Polyradiculitis — *see* Polyneuropathy
**Polyradiculoneuropathy (acute)
  (postinfective) (segmentally
  demyelinating)** G61.0
Polyserositis
  due to pericarditis I31.1
  pericardial I31.1

Polyserositis - *continued*
  periodic, familial E85.0
  tuberculous A19.9
    acute A19.1
    chronic A19.8
Polysplenia syndrome Q89.09
Polysyndactyly — *see also* Syndactylism,
      syndactyly Q70.4
Polytrichia L68.3
Polyunguia Q84.6
Polyuria R35.8
  nocturnal R35.1
  psychogenic F45.8
Pompe's disease (glycogen storage) E74.02
Pompholyx L30.1
**Poncet's disease (tuberculous
  rheumatism)** A18.09
Pond fracture — *see* Fracture, skull
Ponos B55.0
Pons, pontine — *see* condition
Poor
  aesthetic of existing restoration of
      tooth K08.56
  contractions, labor O62.2
  gingival margin to tooth restoration K08.51
  personal hygiene R46.0
  prenatal care, affecting management of
      pregnancy — *see* Pregnancy,
      complicated by, insufficient, prenatal
      care
  sucking reflex (newborn) R29.2
  urinary stream R39.12
  vision NEC H54.7
**Poradenitis, nostras inguinalis or
  venerea** A55
**Porencephaly (congenital) (developmental)
  (true)** Q04.6
  acquired G93.0
  nondevelopmental G93.0
  traumatic (post) F07.89
Porocephaliasis B88.8
Porokeratosis Q82.8
Poroma, eccrine — *see* Neoplasm, skin,
      benign
Porphyria (South African) E80.20
  acquired E80.20
  acute intermittent (hepatic) (Swedish) E80.21
  cutanea tarda (hereditary)
      (symptomatic) E80.1
  due to drugs E80.20
    correct substance properly
        administered — *see* Table of Drugs
        and Chemicals, by drug, adverse
        effect
    overdose or wrong substance given or
        taken — *see* Table of Drugs and
        Chemicals, by drug, poisoning
  erythropoietic (congenital) (hereditary) E80.0
  hepatocutaneous type E80.1
  secondary E80.20
  toxic NEC E80.20
  variegata E80.20
Porphyrinuria — *see* Porphyria
Porphyruria — *see* Porphyria
Port wine nevus, mark, or stain Q82.5
Portal — *see* condition
Posadas-Wernicke disease B38.9
Positive
  culture (nonspecific)
    blood R78.81
    bronchial washings R84.5
    cerebrospinal fluid R83.5
    cervix uteri R87.5
    nasal secretions R84.5
    nipple discharge R89.5
    nose R84.5
      staphylococcus (Methicillin
          susceptible) Z22.321
      Methicillin resistant Z22.322
    peritoneal fluid R85.5
    pleural fluid R84.5
    prostatic secretions R86.5
    saliva R85.5
    seminal fluid R86.5
    sputum R84.5

Positive - *continued*
  culture (nonspecific) - *continued*
    synovial fluid R89.5
    throat scrapings R84.5
    urine R82.79
    vagina R87.5
    vulva R87.5
    wound secretions R89.5
  PPD (skin test) R76.11
  serology for syphilis A53.0
    false R76.8
    with signs or symptoms - code as Syphilis,
        by site and stage
  skin test, tuberculin (without active
      tuberculosis) R76.11
  test, human immunodeficiency virus
      (HIV) R75
  VDRL A53.0
    with signs or symptoms - code by site and
        stage under Syphilis A53.9
  Wassermann reaction A53.0
Postcardiotomy syndrome I97.0
Postcaval ureter Q62.62
Postcholecystectomy syndrome K91.5
Postclimacteric bleeding N95.0
Postcommissurotomy syndrome I97.0
Postconcussional syndrome F07.81
Postcontusional syndrome F07.81
Postcricoid region — *see* condition
**Post-dates (40-42 weeks) (pregnancy)
  (mother)** O48.0
  more than 42 weeks gestation O48.1
Postencephalitic syndrome F07.89
Posterior — *see* condition
Posterolateral sclerosis (spinal cord) — *see*
      Degeneration, combined
Postexanthematous — *see* condition
Postfebrile — *see* condition
Postgastrectomy dumping syndrome K91.1
Posthemiplegic chorea — *see* Monoplegia
Posthemorrhagic anemia (chronic) D50.0
  acute D62
  newborn P61.3
Postherpetic neuralgia (zoster) B02.29
  trigeminal B02.22
Posthitis N47.7
**Postimmunization complication or
  reaction** — *see* Complications,
      vaccination
Postinfectious — *see* condition
Postlaminectomy syndrome NEC M96.1
Postleukotomy syndrome F07.0
**Postmastectomy lymphedema
  (syndrome)** I97.2
Postmaturity, postmature (over 42 weeks)
  maternal (over 42 weeks gestation) O48.1
  newborn P08.22
Postmeasles complication NEC — *see
      also* condition B05.89
Postmenopausal
  endometrium (atrophic) N95.8
    suppurative — *see also*
        Endometritis N71.9
  osteoporosis — *see* Osteoporosis,
      postmenopausal
Postnasal drip R09.82
  due to
    allergic rhinitis — *see* Rhinitis, allergic
    common cold J00
    gastroesophageal reflux — *see* Reflux,
        gastroesophageal
    nasopharyngitis — *see* Nasopharyngitis
    other know condition - code to condition
    sinusitis — *see* Sinusitis
Postnatal — *see* condition
Postoperative (postprocedural) — *see*
      Complication, postoperative
  pneumothorax, therapeutic Z98.3
  state NEC Z98.890
Postpancreatectomy hyperglycemia E89.1
Postpartum — *see* Puerperal
Postphlebitic syndrome — *see* Syndrome,
      postthrombotic
Postpolio (myelitic) syndrome G14

Postpoliomyelitic — *see also* condition
  osteopathy — *see* Osteopathy, after
    poliomyelitis
Postprocedural — *see also* Postoperative
  hypoinsulinemia E89.1
Postschizophrenic depression F32.89
Postsurgery status — *see also* Status (post)
  pneumothorax, therapeutic Z98.3
Post-term (40-42 weeks) (pregnancy)
  (mother) O48.0
  infant P08.21
  more than 42 weeks gestation
    (mother) O48.1
Post-traumatic brain syndrome,
  nonpsychotic F07.81
Post-typhoid abscess A01.09
Postures, hysterical F44.2
Postvaccinal reaction or complication — *see*
  Complications, vaccination
Postvalvulotomy syndrome I97.0
Potain's
  disease (pulmonary edema) — *see* Edema,
    lung
  syndrome (gastrectasis with
    dyspepsia) K31.0
Potter's
  asthma J62.8
  facies Q60.6
  lung J62.8
  syndrome (with renal agenesis) Q60.6
Pott's
  curvature (spinal) A18.01
  disease or paraplegia A18.01
  spinal curvature A18.01
  tumor, puffy — *see* Osteomyelitis, specified
    type NEC
Pouch
  bronchus Q32.4
  Douglas' — *see* condition
  esophagus, esophageal, congenital Q39.6
    acquired K22.5
  gastric K31.4
  Hartmann's K82.8
  pharynx, pharyngeal (congenital) Q38.7
Pouchitis K91.850
Poultrymen's itch B88.0
Poverty NEC Z59.6
  extreme Z59.5
Poxvirus NEC B08.8
Prader-Willi syndrome Q87.11
Prader-Willi-like syndrome Q87.19
Preauricular appendage or tag Q17.0
Prebetalipoproteinemia (acquired)
  (essential) (familial) (hereditary)
  (primary) (secondary) E78.1
  with chylomicronemia E78.3
Precipitate labor or delivery O62.3
Preclimacteric bleeding
  (menorrhagia) N92.4
Precocious
  adrenarche E30.1
  menarche E30.1
  menstruation E30.1
  pubarche E30.1
  puberty E30.1
    central E22.8
  sexual development NEC E30.1
  thelarche E30.8
Precocity, sexual (constitutional)
  (cryptogenic) (female) (idiopathic)
  (male) E30.1
  with adrenal hyperplasia E25.9
    congenital E25.0
Precordial pain R07.2
Predeciduous teeth K00.2
Prediabetes, prediabetic R73.03
  complicating
    pregnancy — *see* Pregnancy, complicated
     by, diseases of, specified type or
     system NEC
    puerperium O99.89
Predislocation status of hip at birth Q65.6

Pre-eclampsia O14.9-
  with pre-existing hypertension — *see* Hyperte
    nsion, complicating pregnancy, pre-
    existing, with, pre-eclampsia
  complicating
    childbirth O14.94
    puerperium O14.95
  mild O14.0-
    complicating
     childbirth O14.04
     puerperium O14.05
  moderate O14.0-
    complicating
     childbirth O14.04
     puerperium O14.05
  severe O14.1-
    with hemolysis, elevated liver enzymes
     and low platelet count
     (HELLP) O14.2-
    complicating
     childbirth O14.24
     puerperium O14.25
    complicating
     childbirth O14.14
     puerperium O14.15
Pre-eruptive color change, teeth, tooth K00.8
Pre-excitation atrioventricular
  conduction I45.6
Preglaucoma H40.00-
Pregnancy (single) (uterine) — *see also*
  Delivery and Puerperal
  Note: The Tabular must be reviewed for
    assignment of the appropriate character
    indicating the trimester of the pregnancy
  Note: The Tabular must be reviewed for
    assignment of appropriate seventh
    character for multiple gestation codes in
    Chapter 15
  abdominal (ectopic) O00.00
    with intrauterine pregnancy O00.01
    with viable fetus O36.7-
  ampullar O00.10-
    with intrauterine pregnancy O00.11-
  biochemical O02.81
  broad ligament O00.80
    with intrauterine pregnancy O00.81
  cervical O00.80
    with intrauterine pregnancy O00.81
  chemical O02.81
  complicated NOS O26.9-
  complicated by (care of) (management
    affected by)
    abnormal, abnormality
     cervix O34.4-
      causing obstructed labor O65.5
     cord (umbilical) O69.9
     fetal heart rate or rhythm O36.83-
     findings on antenatal screening of
      mother O28.9
      biochemical O28.1
      cytological O28.2
      chromosomal O28.5
      genetic O28.5
      hematological O28.0
      radiological O28.4
      specified NEC O28.8
      ultrasonic O28.3
     glucose (tolerance) NEC O99.810
     pelvic organs O34.9-
      specified NEC O34.8-
       causing obstructed labor O65.5
     pelvis (bony) (major) NEC O33.0
     perineum O34.7-
     position
      placenta O44.0-
       with hemorrhage O44.1-
      uterus O34.59-
     uterus O34.59-
      causing obstructed labor O65.5
      congenital O34.0-
     vagina O34.6-
      causing obstructed labor O65.5
     vulva O34.7-
      causing obstructed labor O65.5

Pregnancy (single) (uterine) - *continued*
  complicated by (care of) (management
    affected by) - *continued*
    abruptio placentae — *see* Abruptio
     placentae
    abscess or cellulitis
     bladder O23.1-
     breast O91.11-
     genital organ or tract O23.9-
    abuse
     physical O9A.31-
     psychological O9A.51-
     sexual O9A.41-
    adverse effect anesthesia O29.9-
     aspiration pneumonitis O29.01-
     cardiac arrest O29.11-
     cardiac complication NEC O29.19-
     cardiac failure O29.12-
     central nervous system complication
      NEC O29.29-
     cerebral anoxia O29.21-
     failed or difficult intubation O29.6-
     inhalation of stomach contents or
      secretions NOS O29.01-
     local, toxic reaction O29.3X
     Mendelson's syndrome O29.01-
     pressure collapse of lung O29.02-
     pulmonary complications NEC O29.09-
     specified NEC O29.8X-
     spinal and epidural type NEC O29.5X
      induced headache O29.4-
    albuminuria — *see also* Proteinuria,
     gestational O12.1-
    alcohol use O99.31-
    amnionitis O41.12-
    anaphylactoid syndrome of
     pregnancy O88.01-
    anemia (conditions in D50-D64) (pre-
     existing) O99.01-
     complicating the puerperium O99.03
    antepartum hemorrhage O46.9-
     with coagulation defect — *see*
      Hemorrhage, antepartum, with
      coagulation defect
     specified NEC O46.8X-
    appendicitis O99.61-
    atrophy (yellow) (acute) liver
     (subacute) O26.61-
    bariatric surgery status O99.84-
    bicornis or bicornuate uterus O34.0-
    biliary tract problems O26.61-
    breech presentation O32.1
    cardiovascular diseases (conditions in I00-
     I09, I20-I52, I70-I99) O99.41-
    cerebrovascular disorders (conditions in
     I60-I69) O99.41-
    cervical shortening O26.87-
    cervicitis O23.51-
    chloasma (gravidarum) O26.89-
    cholestasis (intrahepatic) O26.61-
    cholecystitis O99.61-
    chorioamnionitis O41.12-
    circulatory system disorder (conditions in
     I00-I09, I20-I99, O99.41-)
    compound presentation O32.6
    conjoined twins O30.02-
    connective system disorders (conditions in
     M00-M99) O99.89
    contracted pelvis (general) O33.1
     inlet O33.2
     outlet O33.3
    convulsions (eclamptic) (uremic) — *see*
     also Eclampsia O15.9-
    cracked nipple O92.11-
    cystitis O23.1-
    cystocele O34.8-
    death of fetus (near term) O36.4
     early pregnancy O02.1
     of one fetus or more in multiple
      gestation O31.2-
    deciduitis O41.14-
    decreased fetal movement O36.81-
    dental problems O99.61-
    diabetes (mellitus) O24.91-

Pregnancy (single) (uterine) - *continued*
complicated by (care of) (management
affected by) - *continued*
diabetes (mellitus) - *continued*
gestational (pregnancy induced) — *see*
Diabetes, gestational
pre-existing O24.31-
specified NEC O24.81-
type 1 O24.01-
type 2 O24.11-
digestive system disorders (conditions in
K00-K93) O99.61-
diseases of — *see* Pregnancy, complicated
by, specified body system disease
biliary tract O26.61-
blood NEC (conditions in D65-
D77) O99.11-
liver O26.61-
specified NEC O99.89
disorders of — *see* Pregnancy, complicated
by, specified body system disorder
amniotic fluid and membranes O41.9-
specified NEC O41.8X-
biliary tract O26.61-
ear and mastoid process (conditions in
H60-H95) O99.89
eye and adnexa (conditions in H00-
H59) O99.89
liver O26.61-
skin (conditions in L00-L99) O99.71-
specified NEC O99.89
displacement, uterus NEC O34.59-
causing obstructed labor O65.5
disproportion (due to) O33.9
fetal (ascites) (hydrops)
(meningomyelocele) (sacral
teratoma) (tumor) deformities
NEC O33.7
generally contracted pelvis O33.1
hydrocephalic fetus O33.6
inlet contraction of pelvis O33.2
mixed maternal and fetal origin O33.4
specified NEC O33.8
double uterus O34.0-
causing obstructed labor O65.5
drug use (conditions in F11-F19) O99.32-
eclampsia, eclamptic (coma) (convulsions)
(delirium) (nephritis) (uremia) — *see
also* Eclampsia O15.-
ectopic pregnancy — *see* Pregnancy,
ectopic
edema O12.0-
with
gestational hypertension, mild — *see
also* Pre-eclampsia O14.0-
proteinuria O12.2-
effusion, amniotic fluid — *see* Pregnancy,
complicated by, premature rupture of
membranes
elderly
multigravida O09.52-
primigravida O09.51-
embolism — *see also* Embolism, obstetric,
pregnancy O88.-
endocrine diseases NEC O99.28-
endometritis O86.12
excessive weight gain O26.0-
exhaustion O26.81-
during labor and delivery O75.81
face presentation O32.3
failed induction of labor O61.9
instrumental O61.1
mechanical O61.1
medical O61.0
specified NEC O61.8
surgical O61.1
failed or difficult intubation for
anesthesia O29.6-
false labor (pains) O47.9
at or after 37 completed weeks of
pregnancy O47.1
before 37 completed weeks of
pregnancy O47.0-
fatigue O26.81-
during labor and delivery O75.81

Pregnancy (single) (uterine) - *continued*
complicated by (care of) (management
affected by) - *continued*
fatty metamorphosis of liver O26.61-
female genital mutilation O34.8- *[N90.81-]*
fetal (maternal care for)
abnormality or damage O35.9
acid-base balance O68
specified type NEC O35.8
acidemia O68
acidosis O68
alkalosis O68
anemia and thrombocytopenia O36.82-
anencephaly O35.0
bradycardia O36.83-
chromosomal abnormality (conditions in
Q90-Q99) O35.1
conjoined twins O30.02-
damage from
amniocentesis O35.7
biopsy procedures O35.7
drug addiction O35.5
hematological investigation O35.7
intrauterine contraceptive
device O35.7
maternal
alcohol addiction O35.4
cytomegalovirus infection O35.3
disease NEC O35.8
drug addiction O35.5
listeriosis O35.3
rubella O35.3
toxoplasmosis O35.8
viral infection O35.3
medical procedure NEC O35.7
radiation O35.6
death (near term) O36.4
early pregnancy O02.1
decreased movement O36.81-
depressed heart rate tones O36.83-
disproportion due to deformity
(fetal) O33.7
excessive growth (large for
dates) O36.6-
growth retardation O36.59-
light for dates O36.59-
small for dates O36.59-
heart rate irregularity (abnormal
variability) (bradycardia)
(decelerations)
(tachycardia) O36.83-
hereditary disease O35.2
hydrocephalus O35.0
intrauterine death O36.4
non-reassuring heart rate or
rhythm O36.83-
poor growth O36.59-
light for dates O36.59-
small for dates O36.59-
problem O36.9-
specified NEC O36.89-
reduction (elective) O31.3-
selective termination O31.3-
spina bifida O35.0
thrombocytopenia O36.82-
fibroid (tumor) (uterus) O34.1-
fissure of nipple O92.11-
gallstones O99.61-
gastric banding status O99.84-
gastric bypass status O99.84-
genital herpes (asymptomatic) (history of)
(inactive) O98.3-
genital tract infection O23.9-
glomerular diseases (conditions in N00-
N07) O26.83-
with hypertension, pre-existing — *see*
Hypertension, complicating,
pregnancy, pre-existing, with, renal
disease
gonorrhea O98.21-
grand multiparity O09.4
habitual aborter — *see* Pregnancy,
complicated by, recurrent pregnancy
loss

Pregnancy (single) (uterine) - *continued*
complicated by (care of) (management
affected by) - *continued*
HELLP syndrome (hemolysis, elevated
liver enzymes and low platelet
count) O14.2-
hemorrhage
antepartum — *see* Hemorrhage,
antepartum
before 20 completed weeks
gestation O20.9
specified NEC O20.8
due to premature separation, placenta —
see also Abruptio placentae O45.9-
early O20.9
specified NEC O20.8
threatened abortion O20.0
hemorrhoids O22.4-
hepatitis (viral) O98.41-
herniation of uterus O34.59-
high
head at term O32.4
risk — *see* Supervision (of) (for), high-
risk
history of in utero procedure during
previous pregnancy O09.82-
HIV O98.71-
human immunodeficiency virus (HIV)
disease O98.71-
hydatidiform mole — *see also* Mole,
hydatidiform O01.9-
hydramnios O40.-
hydrocephalic fetus (disproportion) O33.6
hydrops
amnii O40.-
fetalis O36.2-
associated with isoimmunization —
see also Pregnancy, complicated
by, isoimmunization O36.11-
hydrorrhea O42.90
hyperemesis (gravidarum) (mild) — *see
also* Hyperemesis, gravidarum O21.0-
hypertension — *see* Hypertension,
complicating pregnancy
hypertensive
heart and renal disease, pre-existing —
see Hypertension, complicating,
pregnancy, pre-existing, with, heart
disease, with renal disease
heart disease, pre-existing — *see*
Hypertension, complicating,
pregnancy, pre-existing, with, heart
disease
renal disease, pre-existing — *see*
Hypertension, complicating,
pregnancy, pre-existing, with, renal
disease
hypotension O26.5-
immune disorders NEC (conditions in
D80-D89) O99.11-
incarceration, uterus O34.51-
incompetent cervix O34.3-
inconclusive fetal viability O36.80
infection (s) O98.91-
amniotic fluid or sac O41.10-
bladder O23.1-
carrier state NEC O99.830
streptococcus B O99.820
genital organ or tract O23.9-
specified NEC O23.59-
genitourinary tract O23.9-
gonorrhea O98.21-
hepatitis (viral) O98.41-
HIV O98.71-
human immunodeficiency virus
(HIV) O98.71-
kidney O23.0-
nipple O91.01-
parasitic disease O98.91-
specified NEC O98.81-
protozoal disease O98.61-
sexually transmitted NEC O98.31-
specified type NEC O98.81-
syphilis O98.11-
tuberculosis O98.01-

Pregnancy (single) (uterine) - *continued*
complicated by (care of) (management
affected by) - *continued*
  infection (s) - *continued*
    urethra O23.2-
    urinary (tract) O23.4-
      specified NEC O23.3-
    viral disease O98.51-
  injury or poisoning (conditions in S00-
    T88) O9A.21-
    due to abuse
      physical O9A.31-
      psychological O9A.51-
      sexual O9A.41-
  insufficient
    prenatal care O09.3-
    weight gain O26.1-
  insulin resistance O26.89
  intrauterine fetal death (near term) O36.4
    early pregnancy O02.1
    multiple gestation (one fetus or
      more) O31.2-
  isoimmunization O36.11-
    anti-A sensitization O36.11-
    anti-B sensitization O36.19-
    Rh O36.09-
      anti-D antibody O36.01-
    specified NEC O36.19-
  laceration of uterus NEC O71.81
  malformation
    placenta, placental (vessel) O43.10-
      specified NEC O43.19-
    uterus (congenital) O34.0-
  malnutrition (conditions in E40-
    E46) O25.1-
  maternal hypotension syndrome O26.5-
  mental disorders (conditions in F01-F09,
    F20-F99) O99.34-
    alcohol use O99.31-
    drug use O99.32-
    smoking O99.33-
  mentum presentation O32.3
  metabolic disorders O99.28-
  missed
    abortion O02.1
    delivery O36.4
  multiple gestations O30.9-
    conjoined twins O30.02-
    specified number of multiples NEC —
      see Pregnancy, multiple (gestation),
      specified NEC
    quadruplet — *see* Pregnancy, quadruplet
    specified complication NEC O31.8X-
    triplet — *see* Pregnancy, triplet
    twin — *see* Pregnancy, twin
  musculoskeletal condition (conditions is
    M00-M99) O99.89
  necrosis, liver (conditions in K72) O26.61-
  neoplasm
    benign
      cervix O34.4-
      corpus uteri O34.1-
      uterus O34.1-
    malignant O9A.11-
  nephropathy NEC O26.83-
  nervous system condition (conditions in
    G00-G99) O99.35-
  nutritional diseases NEC O99.28-
  obesity (pre-existing) O99.21-
  obesity surgery status O99.84-
  oblique lie or presentation O32.2
  older mother — *see* Pregnancy,
    complicated by, elderly
  oligohydramnios O41.0-
    with premature rupture of
      membranes — *see also* Pregnancy,
      complicated by, premature rupture
      of membranes O42.-
  onset (spontaneous) of labor after 37
    completed weeks of gestation but
    before 39 completed weeks gestation,
    with delivery by (planned) cesarean
    section O75.82
  oophoritis O23.52-

Pregnancy (single) (uterine) - *continued*
complicated by (care of) (management
affected by) - *continued*
  overdose, drug — *see also* Table of Drugs
    and Chemicals, by drug,
    poisoning O9A.21-
  oversize fetus O33.5
  papyraceous fetus O31.0-
  pelvic inflammatory disease O99.89
  periodontal disease O99.61-
  peripheral neuritis O26.82-
  peritoneal (pelvic) adhesions O99.89
  phlebitis O22.9-
  phlebopathy O22.9-
  phlebothrombosis (superficial) O22.2-
    deep O22.3-
  placenta accreta O43.21-
  placenta increta O43.22-
  placenta percreta O43.23-
  placenta previa O44.0-
    complete O44.0-
      with hemorrhage O44.1-
    marginal O44.2-
      with hemorrhage O44.3-
    partial O44.2-
      with hemorrhage O44.3-
  placental disorder O43.9-
    specified NEC O43.89-
  placental dysfunction O43.89-
  placental infarction O43.81-
  placental insufficiency O36.51-
  placental transfusion syndromes
    fetomaternal O43.01-
    fetus to fetus O43.02-
    maternofetal O43.01-
  placentitis O41.14-
  pneumonia O99.51-
  poisoning — *see also* Table of Drugs and
    Chemicals O9A.21-
  polyhydramnios O40-
  polymorphic eruption of
    pregnancy O26.86
  poor obstetric history NEC O09.29-
  postmaturity (post-term) (40 to 42
    weeks) O48.0
    more than 42 completed weeks gestation
      (prolonged) O48.1
  pre-eclampsia O14.9-
    mild O14.0-
    moderate O14.0-
    severe O14.1-
      with hemolysis, elevated liver
        enzymes and low platelet count
        (HELLP) O14.2-
  premature labor — *see* Pregnancy,
    complicated by, preterm labor
  premature rupture of membranes O42.90
    full-term, unspecified as to length of
      time between rupture and onset of
      labor O42.92
    with onset of labor
      within 24 hours O42.00
        at or after 37 weeks gestation, onset
          of labor within 24 hours of
          rupture O42.02
        pre-term (before 37 completed
          weeks of gestation) O42.01-
      after 24 hours O42.10
        at or after 37 weeks gestation, onset
          of labor more than 24 hours
          following rupture O42.12
        pre-term (before 37 completed
          weeks of gestation) O42.11-
      at or after 37 weeks gestation,
        unspecified as to length of time
        between rupture and onset of
        labor O42.92
      pre-term (before 37 completed weeks of
        gestation) O42.91-
  premature separation of placenta — *see
    also* Abruptio placentae O45.9-
  presentation, fetal — *see* Delivery,
    complicated by, malposition
  preterm delivery O60.10
  preterm labor

Pregnancy (single) (uterine) - *continued*
complicated by (care of) (management
affected by) - *continued*
  preterm labor - *continued*
    with delivery O60.10
      preterm O60.10
      term O60.20
    second trimester
      with term delivery O60.22
      without delivery O60.02
      with preterm delivery
        second trimester O60.12
        third trimester O60.13
    third trimester
      with term delivery O60.23
      without delivery O60.03
      with third trimester preterm
        delivery O60.14
    without delivery O60.00
      second trimester O60.02
      third trimester O60.03
  previous history of — *see* Pregnancy,
    supervision of, high-risk
  prolapse, uterus O34.52-
  proteinuria (gestational) — *see also*
    Proteinuria, gestational O12.1-
    with edema O12.2-
  pruritic urticarial papules and plaques of
    pregnancy (PUPPP) O26.86
  pruritus (neurogenic) O26.89-
  psychosis or psychoneurosis
    (puerperal) F53.1
  ptyalism O26.89-
  PUPPP (pruritic urticarial papules and
    plaques of pregnancy) O26.86
  pyelitis O23.0-
  recurrent pregnancy loss O26.2-
  renal disease or failure NEC O26.83-
    with secondary hypertension, pre-
      existing — *see* Hypertension,
      complicating, pregnancy, pre-
      existing, secondary
    hypertensive, pre-existing — *see*
      Hypertension, complicating,
      pregnancy, pre-existing, with, renal
      disease
  respiratory condition (conditions in J00-
    J99) O99.51-
  retained, retention
    dead ovum O02.0
    intrauterine contraceptive device O26.3-
  retroversion, uterus O34.53-
  Rh immunization, incompatibility or
    sensitization NEC O36.09-
    anti-D antibody O36.01-
  rupture
    amnion (premature) — *see also*
      Pregnancy, complicated by,
      premature rupture of
      membranes O42-
    membranes (premature) — *see also*
      Pregnancy, complicated by,
      premature rupture of
      membranes O42-
    uterus (during labor) O71.1
      before onset of labor O71.0-
  salivation (excessive) O26.89-
  salpingitis O23.52-
  salpingo-oophoritis O23.52-
  sepsis (conditions in A40, A41) O98.81-
  size date discrepancy (uterine) O26.84-
  skin condition (conditions in L00-
    L99) O99.71-
  smoking (tobacco) O99.33-
  social problem O09.7-
  specified condition NEC O26.89-
  spotting O26.85-
  streptococcus group B (GBS) carrier
    state O99.820
  subluxation of symphysis (pubis) O26.71-
  syphilis (conditions in A50-A53) O98.11-
  threatened
    abortion O20.0
    labor O47.9

Pregnancy (single) (uterine) - *continued*
complicated by (care of) (management
affected by) - *continued*
  threatened - *continued*
    labor - *continued*
      at or after 37 completed weeks of
        gestation O47.1
      before 37 completed weeks of
        gestation O47.0-
  thrombophlebitis (superficial) O22.2-
  thrombosis O22.9-
    cerebral venous O22.5-
    cerebrovenous sinus O22.5-
    deep O22.3-
  tobacco use disorder (smoking) O99.33-
  torsion of uterus O34.59-
  toxemia O14.9-
  transverse lie or presentation O32.2
  tuberculosis (conditions in A15-
    A19) O98.01-
  tumor (benign)
    cervix O34.4-
    malignant O9A.11-
    uterus O34.1-
  unstable lie O32.0
  upper respiratory infection O99.51-
  urethritis O23.2-
  uterine size date discrepancy O26.84-
  vaginitis or vulvitis O23.59-
  varicose veins (lower extremities) O22.0-
    genitals O22.1-
    legs O22.0-
    perineal O22.1-
    vaginal or vulval O22.1-
  venereal disease NEC (conditions in
    A63.8) O98.31-
  venous disorders O22.9-
    specified NEC O22.8X-
  viral diseases (conditions in A80-B09,
    B25-B34) O98.51-
  very young mother — *see* Pregnancy,
    complicated by, young mother
  vomiting O21.9
    due to diseases classified
      elsewhere O21.8
    hyperemesis gravidarum (mild) — *see
      also* Hyperemesis,
      gravidarum O21.0-
    late (occurring after 20 weeks of
      gestation) O21.2
  young mother
    multigravida O09.62-
    primigravida O09.61-
concealed O09.3-
continuing following
  elective fetal reduction of one or more
    fetus O31.3-
  intrauterine death of one or more
    fetus O31.2-
  spontaneous abortion of one or more
    fetus O31.1-
cornual O00.80
  with intrauterine pregnancy O00.81
ectopic (ruptured) O00.90
  with intrauterine pregnancy O00.91
  abdominal O00.00
    with
      intrauterine pregnancy O00.01
      viable fetus O36.7-
  cervical O00.80
    with intrauterine pregnancy O00.81
  complicated (by) O08.9
    afibrinogenemia O08.1
    cardiac arrest O08.81
    chemical damage of pelvic organ
      (s) O08.6
    circulatory collapse O08.3
    defibrination syndrome O08.1
    electrolyte imbalance O08.5
    embolism (amniotic fluid) (blood clot)
      (pulmonary) (septic) O08.2
    endometritis O08.0
    genital tract and pelvic infection O08.0
    hemorrhage (delayed) (excessive) O08.1
    infection

Pregnancy (single) (uterine) - *continued*
ectopic (ruptured) - *continued*
  complicated (by) - *continued*
    infection - *continued*
      genital tract or pelvic O08.0
      kidney 008.83
      urinary tract O08.83
    intravascular coagulation O08.1
    laceration of pelvic organ (s) O08.6
    metabolic disorder O08.5
    oliguria O08.4
    oophoritis O08.0
    parametritis O08.0
    pelvic peritonitis O08.0
    perforation of pelvic organ (s) O08.6
    renal failure or shutdown O08.4
    salpingitis or salpingo-oophoritis O08.0
    sepsis O08.82
    shock O08.83
      septic O08.82
    specified condition NEC O08.89
    tubular necrosis (renal) O08.4
    uremia O08.4
    urinary infection O08.83
    venous complication NEC O08.7
      embolism O08.2
  cornual O00.80
    with intrauterine pregnancy O00.81
  intraligamentous O00.80
    with intrauterine pregnancy O00.81
  mural O00.80
    with intrauterine pregnancy O00.81
  ovarian O00.20-
    with intrauterine pregnancy O00.21-
  specified site NEC O00.80
    with intrauterine pregnancy O00.81
  tubal (ruptured) O00.10-
    with intrauterine pregnancy O00.11-
examination (normal) Z34.9-
  high-risk — *see* Pregnancy, supervision of,
    high-risk
  first Z34.0-
  specified Z34.8-
extrauterine — *see* Pregnancy, ectopic
fallopian O00.10-
  with intrauterine pregnancy O00.11-
false F45.8
gestational carrier Z33.3
heptachorionic, hepta-amniotic
  (septuplets) O30.83-
hexachorionic, hexa-amniotic
  (sextuplets) O30.83-
hidden O09.3-
high-risk — *see* Pregnancy, supervision of,
  high-risk
incidental finding Z33.1
interstitial O00.80
  with intrauterine pregnancy O00.81
intraligamentous O00.80
  with intrauterine pregnancy O00.81
intramural O00.80
  with intrauterine pregnancy O00.81
intraperitoneal O00.00
  with intrauterine pregnancy O00.01
isthmian O00.10-
  with intrauterine pregnancy O00.11-
mesometric (mural) O00.80
  with intrauterine pregnancy O00.81
molar NEC O02.0
  complicated (by) O08.9
    afibrinogenemia O08.1
    cardiac arrest O08.81
    chemical damage of pelvic organ
      (s) O08.6
    circulatory collapse O08.3
    defibrination syndrome O08.1
    electrolyte imbalance O08.5
    embolism (amniotic fluid) (blood clot)
      (pulmonary) (septic) O08.2
    endometritis O08.0
    genital tract and pelvic infection O08.0
    hemorrhage (delayed) (excessive) O08.1
    infection
      genital tract or pelvic O08.0
      kidney O08.83

Pregnancy (single) (uterine) - *continued*
molar NEC - *continued*
  complicated (by) - *continued*
    infection - *continued*
      urinary tract O08.83
    intravascular coagulation O08.1
    laceration of pelvic organ (s) O08.6
    metabolic disorder O08.5
    oliguria O08.4
    oophoritis O08.0
    parametritis O08.0
    pelvic peritonitis O08.0
    perforation of pelvic organ (s) O08.6
    renal failure or shutdown O08.4
    salpingitis or salpingo-oophoritis O08.0
    sepsis O08.82
    shock O08.3
      septic O08.82
    specified condition NEC O08.89
    tubular necrosis (renal) O08.4
    uremia O08.4
    urinary infection O08.83
    venous complication NEC O08.7
      embolism O08.2
  hydatidiform — *see also* Mole,
    hydatidiform O01.9-
multiple (gestation) O30.9-
  greater than quadruplets — *see* Pregnancy,
    multiple (gestation), specified NEC
  specified NEC O30.80-
    with
      two or more monoamniotic
        fetuses O30.82
      two or more monochorionic
        fetuses O30.81-
    number of chorions and amnions are
      both equal to the number of
      fetuses O30.83-
    two or more monoamniotic
      fetuses O30.82
    two or more monochorionic
      fetuses O30.81-
    unable to determine number of placenta
      and number of amniotic
      sacs O30.89-
    unspecified number of placenta and
      unspecified number of amniotic
      sacs O30.80-
  mural O00.80
    with intrauterine pregnancy O00.81
normal (supervision of) Z34.9-
  high-risk — *see* Pregnancy, supervision of,
    high-risk
  first Z34.0-
  specified Z34.8-
ovarian O00.20-
  with intrauterine pregnancy O00.21-
pentachorionic, penta-amniotic
  (quintuplets) O30.83-
postmature (40 to 42 weeks) O48.0
  more than 42 weeks gestation O48.1
post-term (40 to 42 weeks) O48.0
prenatal care only Z34.9-
  high-risk — *see* Pregnancy, supervision of,
    high-risk
  first Z34.0-
  specified Z34.8-
prolonged (more than 42 weeks
  gestation) O48.1
quadruplet O30.20-
  with
    two or more monoamniotic
      fetuses O30.22-
    two or more monochorionic
      fetuses O30.21-
  quadrachorionic/quadra-amniotic O30.23-
  two or more monoamniotic
    fetuses O30.22-
  two or more monochorionic
    fetuses O30.21-
  unable to determine number of placenta
    and number of amniotic sacs O30.29-
  unspecified number of placenta and
    unspecified number of amniotic
    sacs O30.20-

Pregnancy (single) (uterine) - *continued*
quintuplet — *see* Pregnancy, multiple
(gestation), specified NEC
sextuplet — *see* Pregnancy, multiple
(gestation), specified NEC
supervision of
concealed pregnancy O09.3-
elderly mother
multigravida O09.52-
primigravida O09.51-
hidden pregnancy O09.3-
high-risk O09.9-
due to (history of)
ectopic pregnancy O09.1-
elderly — *see* Pregnancy, supervision,
elderly mother
grand multiparity O09.4
infertility O09.0-
insufficient prenatal care O09.3-
in utero procedure during previous
pregnancy O09.82-
in vitro fertilization O09.81-
molar pregnancy O09.A-
multiple previous pregnancies O09.4-
older mother — *see* Pregnancy,
supervision of, elderly mother
poor reproductive or obstetric history
NEC O09.29-
pre-term labor O09.21-
previous
neonatal death O09.29-
social problems O09.7-
specified NEC O09.89-
very young mother — *see* Pregnancy,
supervision, young mother
resulting from in vitro
fertilization O09.81-
normal Z34.9-
first Z34.0-
specified NEC Z34.8-
young mother
multigravida O09.62-
primigravida O09.61-
triplet O30.10-
with
two or more monoamniotic
fetuses O30.12-
two or more monochorionic
fetuses O30.11-
trichorionic/triamniotic O30.13-
two or more monoamniotic
fetuses O30.12-
two or more monochorionic
fetuses O30.11-
unable to determine number of placenta
and number of amniotic sacs O30.19-
unspecified number of placenta and
unspecified number of amniotic
sacs O30.10-
tubal (with abortion) (with rupture) O00.10-
with intrauterine pregnancy O00.11-
twin O30.00-
conjoined O30.02-
dichorionic/diamniotic (two placenta, two
amniotic sacs) O30.04-
monochorionic/diamniotic (one placenta,
two amniotic sacs) O30.03-
monochorionic/monoamniotic (one
placenta, one amniotic sac) O30.01-
unable to determine number of placenta
and number of amniotic sacs O30.09-
unspecified number of placenta and
unspecified number of amniotic
sacs O30.00-
unwanted Z64.0
weeks of gestation
8 weeks Z3A.08
9 weeks Z3A.09
10 weeks Z3A.10
11 weeks Z3A.11
12 weeks Z3A.12
13 weeks Z3A.13
14 weeks Z3A.14
15 weeks Z3A.15
16 weeks Z3A.16

Pregnancy (single) (uterine) - *continued*
weeks of gestation - *continued*
17 weeks Z3A.17
18 weeks Z3A.18
19 weeks Z3A.19
20 weeks Z3A.20
21 weeks Z3A.21
22 weeks Z3A.22
23 weeks Z3A.23
24 weeks Z3A.24
25 weeks Z3A.25
26 weeks Z3A.26
27 weeks Z3A.27
28 weeks Z3A.28
29 weeks Z3A.29
30 weeks Z3A.30
31 weeks Z3A.31
32 weeks Z3A.32
33 weeks Z3A.33
34 weeks Z3A.34
35 weeks Z3A.35
36 weeks Z3A.36
37 weeks Z3A.37
38 weeks Z3A.38
39 weeks Z3A.39
40 weeks Z3A.40
41 weeks Z3A.41
42 weeks Z3A.42
greater than 42 weeks Z3A.49
less than 8 weeks Z3A.01
not specified Z3A.00
Preiser's disease — *see* Osteonecrosis,
secondary, due to, trauma, metacarpus
Pre-kwashiorkor — *see* Malnutrition, severe
Preleukemia (syndrome) D46.9
Preluxation, hip, congenital Q65.6
Premature — *see also* condition
adrenarche E27.0
aging E34.8
beats I49.40
atrial I49.1
auricular I49.1
supraventricular I49.1
birth NEC — *see* Preterm, newborn
closure, foramen ovale Q21.8
contraction
atrial I49.1
atrioventricular I49.2
auricular I49.1
auriculoventricular I49.49
heart (extrasystole) I49.49
junctional I49.2
ventricular I49.3
delivery — *see also* Pregnancy, complicated
by, preterm labor O60.10
ejaculation F52.4
infant NEC — *see* Preterm, newborn
light-for-dates — *see* Light for dates
labor — *see* Pregnancy, complicated by,
preterm labor
lungs P28.0
menopause E28.319
asymptomatic E28.319
symptomatic E28.310
newborn
extreme (less than 28 completed
weeks) — *see* Immaturity, extreme
less than 37 completed weeks — *see*
Preterm, newborn
puberty E30.1
rupture membranes or amnion — *see*
Pregnancy, complicated by, premature
rupture of membranes
senility E34.8
thelarche E30.8
ventricular systole I49.3
**Prematurity NEC (less than 37 completed
weeks)** — *see* Preterm, newborn
extreme (less than 28 completed weeks) —
see Immaturity, extreme
Premenstrual
dysphoric disorder (PMDD) F32.81
tension (syndrome) N94.3
Premolarization, cuspids K00.2

Prenatal
care, normal pregnancy — *see* Pregnancy,
normal
screening of mother — *see also* Encounter,
antenatal screening Z36.9
teeth K00.6
**Preparatory care for subsequent treatment
NEC**
for dialysis Z49.01
peritoneal Z49.02
Prepartum — *see* condition
**Preponderance, left or right
ventricular** I51.7
Prepuce — *see* condition
**PRES (posterior reversible encephalopathy
syndrome)** I67.83
Presbycardia R54
Presbycusis, presbyacusia H91.1-
Presbyesophagus K22.8
Presbyophrenia F03
Presbyopia H52.4
Prescription of contraceptives (initial)
Z30.019
barrier Z30.018
diaphragm Z30.018
emergency (postcoital) Z30.012
implantable subdermal Z30.017
injectable Z30.013
intrauterine contraceptive device Z30.014
pills Z30.011
postcoital (emergency) Z30.012
repeat Z30.40
barrier Z30.49
diaphragm Z30.49
implantable subdermal Z30.46
injectable Z30.42
pills Z30.41
specified type NEC Z30.49
transdermal patch hormonal Z30.45
vaginal ring hormonal Z30.44
specified type NEC Z30.018
transdermal patch hormonal Z30.016
vaginal ring hormonal Z30.015
Presence (of)
ankle-joint implant (functional)
(prosthesis) Z96.66-
aortocoronary (bypass) graft Z95.1
arterial-venous shunt (dialysis) Z99.2
artificial
eye (globe) Z97.0
heart (fully implantable)
(mechanical) Z95.812
valve Z95.2
larynx Z96.3
lens (intraocular) Z96.1
limb (complete) (partial) Z97.1-
arm Z97.1-
bilateral Z97.15
leg Z97.1-
bilateral Z97.16
audiological implant (functional) Z96.29
bladder implant (functional) Z96.0
bone
conduction hearing device Z96.29
implant (functional) NEC Z96.7
joint (prosthesis) — *see* Presence, joint
implant
cardiac
defibrillator (functional) (with
synchronous cardiac
pacemaker) Z95.810
implant or graft Z95.9
specified type NEC Z95.818
pacemaker Z95.0
resynchronization therapy
defibrillator Z95.810
pacemaker Z95.0
cerebrospinal fluid drainage device Z98.2
cochlear implant (functional) Z96.21
contact lens (es) Z97.3
coronary artery graft or prosthesis Z95.5
CRT-D (cardiac resynchronization therapy
defibrillator) Z95.810
CRT-P (cardiac resynchronization therapy
pacemaker) Z95.0

Presence (of) - *continued*
  cardioverter-defibrillator (ICD) Z95.810
  CSF shunt Z98.2
  dental prosthesis device Z97.2
  dentures Z97.2
  device (external) NEC Z97.8
    cardiac NEC Z95.818
    heart assist Z95.811
    implanted (functional) Z96.9
      specified NEC Z96.89
    prosthetic Z97.8
  ear implant Z96.20
    cochlear implant Z96.21
    myringotomy tube Z96.22
    specified type NEC Z96.29
  elbow-joint implant (functional)
    (prosthesis) Z96.62-
  endocrine implant (functional) NEC Z96.49
  eustachian tube stent or device
    (functional) Z96.29
  external hearing-aid or device Z97.4
  finger-joint implant (functional)
    (prosthetic) Z96.69-
  functional implant Z96.9
    specified NEC Z96.89
  graft
    cardiac NEC Z95.818
    vascular NEC Z95.828
  hearing-aid or device (external) Z97.4
    implant (bone) (cochlear)
      (functional) Z96.21
  heart assist device Z95.811
  heart valve implant (functional) Z95.2
    prosthetic Z95.2
    specified type NEC Z95.4
    xenogenic Z95.3
  hip-joint implant (functional)
    (prosthesis) Z96.64-
  ICD (cardioverter-defibrillator) Z95.810
  implanted device (artificial) (functional)
    (prosthetic) Z96.9
    automatic cardiac defibrillator (with
      synchronous cardiac
      pacemaker) Z95.810
    cardiac pacemaker Z95.0
    cochlear Z96.21
    dental Z96.5
    heart Z95.812
    heart valve Z95.2
      prosthetic Z95.2
      specified NEC Z95.4
      xenogenic Z95.3
    insulin pump Z96.41
    intraocular lens Z96.1
    joint Z96.60
      ankle Z96.66-
      elbow Z96.62-
      finger Z96.69-
      hip Z96.64-
      knee Z96.65-
      shoulder Z96.61-
      specified NEC Z96.698
      wrist Z96.63-
    larynx Z96.3
    myringotomy tube Z96.22
    otological Z96.20
      cochlear Z96.21
      eustachian stent Z96.29
      myringotomy Z96.22
      specified NEC Z96.29
      stapes Z96.29
    skin Z96.81
    skull plate Z96.7
    specified NEC Z96.89
    urogenital Z96.0
  insulin pump (functional) Z96.41
  intestinal bypass or anastomosis Z98.0
  intraocular lens (functional) Z96.1
  intrauterine contraceptive device
    (IUD) Z97.5
  intravascular implant (functional)
    (prosthetic) NEC Z95.9
    coronary artery Z95.5
    defibrillator (with synchronous cardiac
      pacemaker) Z95.810

Presence (of) - *continued*
  intravascular implant (functional)
    (prosthetic) NEC - *continued*
    peripheral vessel (with
      angioplasty) Z95.820
  joint implant (prosthetic) (any) Z96.60
    ankle — *see* Presence, ankle joint implant
    elbow — *see* Presence, elbow joint implant
    finger — *see* Presence, finger joint implant
    hip — *see* Presence, hip joint implant
    knee — *see* Presence, knee joint implant
    shoulder — *see* Presence, shoulder joint
      implant
    specified joint NEC Z96.698
    wrist — *see* Presence, wrist joint implant
  knee-joint implant (functional)
    (prosthesis) Z96.65-
  laryngeal implant (functional) Z96.3
  mandibular implant (dental) Z96.5
  myringotomy tube (s) Z96.22
  neurostimulator (brain) (gastric) (peripheral
    nerve) (sacral nerve) (spinal cord)
    (vagus nerve) Z96.82
  orthopedic-joint implant (prosthetic)
    (any) — *see* Presence, joint implant
  otological implant (functional) Z96.29
  shoulder-joint implant (functional)
    (prosthesis) Z96.61-
  skull-plate implant Z96.7
  spectacles Z97.3
  stapes implant (functional) Z96.29
  systemic lupus erythematosus [SLE]
    inhibitor D68.62
  tendon implant (functional) (graft) Z96.7
  tooth root (s) implant Z96.5
  ureteral stent Z96.0
  urethral stent Z96.0
  urogenital implant (functional) Z96.0
  vascular implant or device Z95.9
    access port device Z95.828
    specified type NEC Z95.828
  wrist-joint implant (functional)
    (prosthesis) Z96.63-
Presenile — *see also* condition
  dementia F03
  premature aging E34.8
Presentation, fetal — *see* Delivery ,
  complicated by, malposition
Prespondylolisthesis (congenital) Q76.2
Pressure
  area, skin — *see* Ulcer, pressure, by site
  brachial plexus G54.0
  brain G93.5
    injury at birth NEC P11.1
  cerebral — *see* Pressure, brain
  chest R07.89
  cone, tentorial G93.5
  hyposystolic — *see also* Hypotension
    incidental reading, without diagnosis of
      hypotension R03.1
  increased
    intracranial (benign) G93.2
      injury at birth P11.0
    intraocular H40.05-
  injury — *see* Ulcer, pressure, by site
  lumbosacral plexus G54.1
  mediastinum J98.59
  necrosis (chronic) — *see* Ulcer, pressure, by
    site
  parental, inappropriate (excessive) Z62.6
  sore — *see* Ulcer, pressure, by site
  spinal cord G95.20
  ulcer (chronic) — *see* Ulcer, pressure, by site
  venous, increased I87.8
Pre-syncope R55
Preterm
  delivery — *see also* Pregnancy, complicated
    by, preterm labor O60.10
  labor — *see* Pregnancy, complicated by,
    preterm labor
  newborn (infant) P07.30
    gestational age
      28 completed weeks (28 weeks, 0 days
        through 28 weeks, 6 days) P07.31

Preterm - *continued*
  newborn (infant) - *continued*
    gestational age - *continued*
      29 completed weeks (29 weeks, 0 days
        through 29 weeks, 6 days) P07.32
      30 completed weeks (30 weeks, 0 days
        through 30 weeks, 6 days) P07.33
      31 completed weeks (31 weeks, 0 days
        through 31 weeks, 6 days) P07.34
      32 completed weeks (32 weeks, 0 days
        through 32 weeks, 6 days) P07.35
      33 completed weeks (33 weeks, 0 days
        through 33 weeks, 6 days) P07.36
      34 completed weeks (34 weeks, 0 days
        through 34 weeks, 6 days) P07.37
      35 completed weeks (35 weeks, 0 days
        through 35 weeks, 6 days) P07.38
      36 completed weeks (36 weeks, 0 days
        through 36 weeks, 6 days) P07.39
Previa
  placenta (total) (without hemorrhage) O44.0-
    with hemorrhage O44.1-
    complete O44.0-
      with hemorrhage O44.1-
    low — *see also* Delivery, complicated, by,
      placenta, low O44.4-
      with hemorrhage O44.5-
    marginal O44.2-
      with hemorrhage O44.3-
    partial O44.2-
      with hemorrhage O44.3-
  vasa O69.4
Priapism N48.30
  due to
    disease classified elsewhere N48.32
    drug N48.33
    specified cause NEC N48.39
    trauma N48.31
Prickling sensation (skin) R20.2
Prickly heat L74.0
Primary — *see* condition
Primigravida
  elderly, affecting management of pregnancy,
    labor and delivery (supervision
    only) — *see* Pregnancy, complicated by,
    elderly, primigravida
  older, affecting management of pregnancy,
    labor and delivery (supervision
    only) — *see* Pregnancy, complicated by,
    elderly, primigravida
  very young, affecting management of
    pregnancy, labor and delivery
    (supervision only) — *see* Pregnancy,
    complicated by, young mother,
    primigravida
Primipara
  elderly, affecting management of pregnancy,
    labor and delivery (supervision
    only) — *see* Pregnancy, complicated by,
    elderly, primigravida
  older, affecting management of pregnancy,
    labor and delivery (supervision
    only) — *see* Pregnancy, complicated by,
    elderly, primigravida
  very young, affecting management of
    pregnancy, labor and delivery
    (supervision only) — *see* Pregnancy,
    complicated by, young mother,
    primigravida
Primus varus Q66.21-
**PRIND (Prolonged reversible ischemic
  neurologic deficit)** I63.9
Pringle's disease (tuberous sclerosis) Q85.1
Prinzmetal angina I20.1
Prizefighter ear — *see* Cauliflower ear
Problem (with) (related to)
  academic Z55.8
  acculturation Z60.3
  adjustment (to)
    change of job Z56.1
    life-cycle transition Z60.0
    pension Z60.0
    retirement Z60.0
  adopted child Z62.821
  alcoholism in family Z63.72

Problem (with) (related to) - *continued*
  atypical parenting situation Z62.9
  bankruptcy Z59.8
  behavioral (adult) F69
    drug seeking Z76.5
  birth of sibling affecting child Z62.898
  care (of)
    provider dependency Z74.9
      specified NEC Z74.8
    sick or handicapped person in family or
      household Z63.6
  child
    abuse (affecting the child) — *see*
      Maltreatment, child
    custody or support proceedings Z65.3
    in welfare custody Z62.21
    in care of non-parental family
      member Z62.21
    in foster care Z62.21
    living in orphanage or group home Z62.22
  child-rearing Z62.9
    specified NEC Z62.898
  communication (developmental) F80.9
  conflict or discord (with)
    boss Z56.4
    classmates Z55.4
    counselor Z64.4
    employer Z56.4
    family Z63.9
      specified NEC Z63.8
    probation officer Z64.4
    social worker Z64.4
    teachers Z55.4
    workmates Z56.4
  conviction in legal proceedings Z65.0
    with imprisonment Z65.1
  counselor Z64.4
  creditors Z59.8
  digestive K92.9
  drug addict in family Z63.72
  ear — *see* Disorder, ear
  economic Z59.9
    affecting care Z59.9
    specified NEC Z59.8
  education Z55.9
    specified NEC Z55.8
  employment Z56.9
    change of job Z56.1
    discord Z56.4
    environment Z56.5
    sexual harassment Z56.81
    specified NEC Z56.89
    stress NEC Z56.6
    stressful schedule Z56.3
    threat of job loss Z56.2
    unemployment Z56.0
  enuresis, child F98.0
  eye H57.9
  failed examinations (school) Z55.2
  falling Z91.81
  family — *see also* Disruption, family Z63.9-
    specified NEC Z63.8
  feeding (elderly) (infant) R63.3
    newborn P92.9
      breast P92.5
      overfeeding P92.4
      slow P92.2
      specified NEC P92.8
      underfeeding P92.3
    nonorganic F50.89
  finance Z59.9
    specified NEC Z59.8
  foreclosure on loan Z59.8
  foster child Z62.822
  frightening experience (s) in
    childhood Z62.898
  genital NEC
    female N94.9
    male N50.9
  health care Z75.9
    specified NEC Z75.8
  hearing — *see* Deafness
  homelessness Z59.0
  housing Z59.9
    inadequate Z59.1

Problem (with) (related to) - *continued*
  housing - *continued*
    isolated Z59.8
    specified NEC Z59.8
  identity (of childhood) F93.8
  illegitimate pregnancy (unwanted) Z64.0
  illiteracy Z55.0
  impaired mobility Z74.09
  imprisonment or incarceration Z65.1
  inadequate teaching affecting
    education Z55.8
  inappropriate (excessive) parental
    pressure Z62.6
  influencing health status NEC Z78.9
  in-law Z63.1
  institutionalization, affecting child Z62.22
  intrafamilial communication Z63.8
  jealousy, child F93.8
  landlord Z59.2
  language (developmental) F80.9
  learning (developmental) F81.9
  legal Z65.3
    conviction without imprisonment Z65.0
    imprisonment Z65.1
    release from prison Z65.2
  life-management Z73.9
    specified NEC Z73.89
  life-style Z72.9
    gambling Z72.6
    high-risk sexual behavior
      (heterosexual) Z72.51
      bisexual Z72.53
      homosexual Z72.52
    inappropriate eating habits Z72.4
    self-damaging behavior NEC Z72.89
    specified NEC Z72.89
    tobacco use Z72.0
  literacy Z55.9
    low level Z55.0
    specified NEC Z55.8
  living alone Z60.2
  lodgers Z59.2
  loss of love relationship in
    childhood Z62.898
  marital Z63.0
    involving
      divorce Z63.5
      estrangement Z63.5
      gender identity F66
  mastication K08.89
  medical
    care, within family Z63.6
    facilities Z75.9
      specified NEC Z75.8
  mental F48.9
  multiparity Z64.1
  negative life events in childhood Z62.9
    altered pattern of family
      relationships Z62.898
    frightening experience Z62.898
    loss of
      love relationship Z62.898
      self-esteem Z62.898
    physical abuse (alleged) — *see*
      Maltreatment, child
    removal from home Z62.29
    specified event NEC Z62.898
  neighbor Z59.2
  neurological NEC R29.818
  new step-parent affecting child Z62.898
  none (feared complaint unfounded) Z71.1
  occupational NEC Z56.89
  parent-child — *see* Conflict, parent-child
  personal hygiene Z91.89
  personality F69
  phase-of-life transition, adjustment Z60.0
  presence of sick or disabled person in family
    or household Z63.79
    needing care Z63.6
  primary support group (family) Z63.9
    specified NEC Z63.8
  probation officer Z64.4
  psychiatric F99
  psychosexual (development) F66
  psychosocial Z65.9

Problem (with) (related to) - *continued*
  psychosocial - *continued*
    religious or spiritual Z65.8
    specified NEC Z65.8
  relationship Z63.9
    childhood F93.8
  release from prison Z65.2
    religious or spiritual Z65.8
  removal from home affecting child Z62.29
  seeking and accepting known hazardous and
    harmful
    behavioral or psychological
      interventions Z65.8
    chemical, nutritional or physical
      interventions Z65.8
  sexual function (nonorganic) F52.9
  sight H54.7
  sleep disorder, child F51.9
  smell — *see* Disturbance, sensation, smell
  social
    environment Z60.9
      specified NEC Z60.8
    exclusion and rejection Z60.4
    worker Z64.4
  speech R47.9
    developmental F80.9
    specified NEC R47.89
  swallowing — *see* Dysphagia
  taste — *see* Disturbance, sensation, taste
  tic, child F95.0
  underachievement in school Z55.3
  unemployment Z56.0
    threatened Z56.2
  unwanted pregnancy Z64.0
  upbringing Z62.9
    specified NEC Z62.898
  urinary N39.9
  voice production R47.89
  work schedule (stressful) Z56.3
Procedure (surgical)
  converted
    arthroscopic to open Z53.33
    laparoscopic to open Z53.31
    specified procedure NEC to open Z53.39
    thoracoscopic to open Z53.32
  for purpose other than remedying health
    state Z41.9
    specified NEC Z41.8
  not done Z53.9
    because of
      administrative reasons Z53.8
      contraindication Z53.09
        smoking Z53.01
      patient's decision Z53.20
        for reasons of belief or group
          pressure Z53.1
        left against medical advice
          (AMA) Z53.21
        specified reason NEC Z53.29
      specified reason NEC Z53.8
Procidentia (uteri) N81.3
Proctalgia K62.89
  fugax K59.4
  spasmodic K59.4
Proctitis K62.89
  amebic (acute) A06.0
  chlamydial A56.3
  gonococcal A54.6
  granulomatous — *see* Enteritis, regional,
    large intestine
  herpetic A60.1
  radiation K62.7
  tuberculous A18.32
  ulcerative (chronic) K51.20
    with
      complication K51.219
        abscess K51.214
        fistula K51.213
        obstruction K51.212
        rectal bleeding K51.211
        specified NEC K51.218
Proctocele
  female (without uterine prolapse) N81.6
    with uterine prolapse N81.2
      complete N81.3

Proctocele - *continued*
male K62.3
Proctocolitis
food-induced eosinophilic K52.82
food protein-induced K52.82
milk protein-induced K52.82
mucosal — *see* Rectosigmoiditis, ulcerative
Proctoptosis K62.3
Proctorrhagia K62.5
Proctosigmoiditis K63.89
ulcerative (chronic) — *see* Rectosigmoiditis, ulcerative
Proctospasm K59.4
psychogenic F45.8
Profichet's disease — *see* Disorder, soft tissue, specified type NEC
Progeria E34.8
Prognathism (mandibular) (maxillary) M26.19
Progonoma (melanotic) — *see* Neoplasm, benign, by site
Progressive — *see* condition
Prolactinoma
specified site — *see* Neoplasm, benign, by site
unspecified site D35.2
Prolapse, prolapsed
anus, anal (canal) (sphincter) K62.2
arm or hand O32.2
causing obstructed labor O64.4
bladder (mucosa) (sphincter) (acquired)
congenital Q79.4
female — *see* Cystocele
male N32.89
breast implant (prosthetic) T85.49
cecostomy K94.09
cecum K63.4
cervix, cervical (hypertrophied) N81.2
anterior lip, obstructing labor O65.5
congenital Q51.828
postpartal, old N81.2
stump N81.85
ciliary body (traumatic) — *see* Laceration, eye(ball), with prolapse or loss of interocular tissue
colon (pedunculated) K63.4
colostomy K94.09
disc (intervertebral) — *see* Displacement, intervertebral disc
eye implant (orbital) T85.398
lens (ocular) — *see* Complications, intraocular lens
fallopian tube N83.4-
gastric (mucosa) K31.89
genital, female N81.9
specified NEC N81.89
globe, nontraumatic — *see* Luxation, globe
ileostomy bud K94.19
intervertebral disc — *see* Displacement, intervertebral disc
intestine (small) K63.4
iris (traumatic) — *see* Laceration, eye(ball), with prolapse or loss of interocular tissue
nontraumatic H21.89
kidney N28.83
congenital Q63.2
laryngeal muscles or ventricle J38.7
liver K76.89
meatus urinarius N36.8
mitral (valve) I34.1
ocular lens implant — *see* Complications, intraocular lens
organ or site, congenital NEC — *see* Malposition, congenital
ovary N83.4-
pelvic floor, female N81.89
perineum, female N81.89
rectum (mucosa) (sphincter) K62.3
due to trichuris trichuria B79
spleen D73.89
stomach K31.89
umbilical cord
complicating delivery O69.0
urachus, congenital Q64.4

Prolapse, prolapsed - *continued*
ureter N28.89
with obstruction N13.5
with infection N13.6
ureterovesical orifice N28.89
urethra (acquired) (infected) (mucosa) N36.8
congenital Q64.71
urinary meatus N36.8
congenital Q64.72
uterovaginal N81.4
complete N81.3
incomplete N81.2
uterus (with prolapse of vagina) N81.4
complete N81.3
congenital Q51.818
first degree N81.2
in pregnancy or childbirth — *see* Pregnancy, complicated by, abnormal, uterus
incomplete N81.2
postpartal (old) N81.4
second degree N81.3
third degree N81.3
uveal (traumatic) — *see* Laceration, eye(ball), with prolapse or loss of interocular tissue
vagina (anterior) (wall) — *see* Cystocele
with prolapse of uterus N81.4
complete N81.3
incomplete N81.2
posterior wall N81.6
posthysterectomy N99.3
vitreous (humor) H43.0-
in wound — *see* Laceration, eye(ball), with prolapse or loss of interocular tissue
womb — *see* Prolapse, uterus
Prolapsus, female N81.9
specified NEC N81.89
Proliferation (s)
prostate, atypical small acinar N42.32
primary cutaneous CD30-positive large T-cell C86.6
Proliferative — *see* condition
Prolonged, prolongation (of)
bleeding (time) (idiopathic) R79.1
coagulation (time) R79.1
gestation (over 42 completed weeks)
mother O48.1
newborn P08.22
interval I44.0
labor O63.9
first stage O63.0
second stage O63.1
partial thromboplastin time (PTT) R79.1
pregnancy (more than 42 weeks gestation) O48.1
prothrombin time R79.1
QT interval R94.31
uterine contractions in labor O62.4
Prominence, prominent
auricle (congenital) (ear) Q17.5
ischial spine or sacral promontory
with disproportion (fetopelvic) O33.0
causing obstructed labor O65.5
nose (congenital) acquired M95.0
Promiscuity — *see* High, risk, sexual behavior
Pronation
ankle — *see* Deformity, limb, foot, specified NEC
foot — *see also* Deformity, limb, foot, specified NEC
congenital Q74.2
Prophylactic
administration of
antibiotics, long-term Z79.2
short-term use - omit code
drug — *see also* Long-term (current) drug therapy (use of) Z79.899-
medication Z79.899
organ removal (for neoplasia management) Z40.00
breast Z40.01
fallopian tube (s) Z40.03
with ovary (s) Z40.02
ovary (s) Z40.02

Prophylactic - *continued*
organ removal (for neoplasia management) - *continued*
specified site NEC Z40.09
surgery Z40.9
for risk factors related to malignant neoplasm — *see* Prophylactic, organ removal
specified NEC Z40.8
vaccination Z23
Propionic acidemia E71.121
Proptosis (ocular) — *see also* Exophthalmos
thyroid — *see* Hyperthyroidism, with goiter
Prosecution, anxiety concerning Z65.3
Prosopagnosia R48.3
Prostadynia N42.81
Prostate, prostatic — *see* condition
Prostatism — *see* Hyperplasia, prostate
Prostatitis (congestive) (suppurative) (with cystitis) N41.9
acute N41.0
cavitary N41.8
chronic N41.1
diverticular N41.8
due to Trichomonas (vaginalis) A59.02
fibrous N41.1
gonococcal (acute) (chronic) A54.22
granulomatous N41.4
hypertrophic N41.1
subacute N41.1
trichomonal A59.02
tuberculous A18.14
Prostatocystitis N41.3
Prostatorrhea N42.89
Prostatosis N42.82
Prostration R53.83
heat — *see also* Heat, exhaustion
anhydrotic T67.3
due to
salt (and water) depletion T67.4
water depletion T67.3
nervous F48.8
senile R54
Protanomaly (anomalous trichromat) H53.54
Protanopia (complete) (incomplete) H53.54
Protection (against) (from) — *see* Prophylactic
Protein
deficiency NEC — *see* Malnutrition
malnutrition — *see* Malnutrition
sickness — *see also* Reaction, serum T80.69
Proteinemia R77.9
Proteinosis
alveolar (pulmonary) J84.01
lipid or lipoid (of Urbach) E78.89
Proteinuria R80.9
Bence Jones R80.3
complicating pregnancy — *see* Proteinuria, gestational
gestational
complicating
childbirth O12.14
pregnancy O12.1-
with edema O12.2-
puerperium O12.15
idiopathic R80.0
isolated R80.0
with glomerular lesion N06.9
dense deposit disease N06.6
diffuse
crescentic glomerulonephritis N06.7
endocapillary proliferative glomerulonephritis N06.4
mesangiocapillary glomerulonephritis N06.5
focal and segmental hyalinosis or sclerosis N06.1
membranous (diffuse) N06.2
mesangial proliferative (diffuse) N06.3
minimal change N06.0
specified pathology NEC N06.8
orthostatic R80.2
with glomerular lesion — *see* Proteinuria, isolated, with glomerular lesion
persistent R80.1

Proteinuria - *continued*
  persistent - *continued*
    with glomerular lesion — *see* Proteinuria, isolated, with glomerular lesion
    postural R80.2
      with glomerular lesion — *see* Proteinuria, isolated, with glomerular lesion
    pre-eclamptic — *see* Pre-eclampsia
    puerperal O12.15
    specified type NEC R80.8
Proteolysis, pathologic D65
Proteus (mirabilis) (morganii) , as cause of disease classified elsewhere B96.4
Prothrombin gene mutation D68.52
Protoporphyria, erythropoietic E80.0
Protozoal — *see also* condition
  disease B64
    specified NEC B60.8
Protrusion, protrusio
  acetabuli M24.7
  acetabulum (into pelvis) M24.7
  device, implant or graft — *see also* Complications, by site and type, mechanical T85.698
    arterial graft NEC — *see* Complication, cardiovascular device, mechanical, vascular
    breast (implant) T85.49
    catheter NEC T85.698
      cystostomy T83.090
      dialysis (renal) T82.49
        intraperitoneal T85.691
      infusion NEC T82.594
        spinal (epidural) (subdural) T85.690
      urinary — *see also* Complications, catheter, urinary T83.098
    electronic (electrode) (pulse generator) (stimulator)
      bone T84.390
      nervous system — *see* Complication, prosthetic device, mechanical, electronic nervous system stimulator
    fixation, internal (orthopedic) NEC — *see* Complication, fixation device, mechanical
    gastrointestinal — *see* Complications, prosthetic device, mechanical, gastrointestinal device
    genital NEC T83.498
      intrauterine contraceptive device T83.39
      penile prosthesis (cylinder) (implanted) (pump) (resevoir) T83.490
      testicular prosthesis T83.491
    heart NEC — *see* Complication, cardiovascular device, mechanical
    joint prosthesis — *see* Complications, joint prosthesis, mechanical, specified NEC, by site
    ocular NEC — *see* Complications, prosthetic device, mechanical, ocular device
    orthopedic NEC — *see* Complication, orthopedic, device, mechanical
    specified NEC T85.628
    urinary NEC — *see also* Complication, genitourinary, device, urinary, mechanical
      graft T83.29
    vascular NEC — *see* Complication, cardiovascular device, mechanical
    ventricular intracranial shunt T85.09
  intervertebral disc — *see* Displacement, intervertebral disc
  joint prosthesis — *see* Complications, joint prosthesis, mechanical, specified NEC, by site
  nucleus pulposus — *see* Displacement, intervertebral disc
Prune belly (syndrome) Q79.4
Prurigo (ferox) (gravis) (Hebrae) (Hebra's) (mitis) (simplex) L28.2
  Besnier's L20.0
  estivalis L56.4
  nodularis L28.1

Prurigo (ferox) (gravis) (Hebrae) (Hebra's) (mitis) (simplex) - *continued*
  psychogenic F45.8
Pruritus, pruritic (essential) L29.9
  ani, anus L29.0
    psychogenic F45.8
  anogenital L29.3
    psychogenic F45.8
  due to onchocerca volvulus B73.1
  gravidarum — *see* Pregnancy, complicated by, specified pregnancy-related condition NEC
  hiemalis L29.8
  neurogenic (any site) F45.8
  perianal L29.0
  psychogenic (any site) F45.8
  scroti, scrotum L29.1
    psychogenic F45.8
  senile, senilis L29.8
  specified NEC L29.8
    psychogenic F45.8
  Trichomonas A59.9
  vulva, vulvae L29.2
    psychogenic F45.8
Pseudarthrosis, pseudoarthrosis (bone) — *see* Nonunion, fracture
  clavicle, congenital Q74.0
  joint, following fusion or arthrodesis M96.0
Pseudoaneurysm — *see* Aneurysm
Pseudoangina (pectoris) — *see* Angina
Pseudoangioma I81
Pseudoarteriosus Q28.8
Pseudoarthrosis — *see* Pseudarthrosis
Pseudobulbar affect (PBA) F48.2
Pseudochromhidrosis L67.8
Pseudocirrhosis, liver, pericardial I31.1
Pseudocowpox B08.03
Pseudocoxalgia M91.3-
Pseudocroup J38.5
Pseudo-Cushing's syndrome, alcohol-induced E24.4
Pseudocyesis F45.8
Pseudocyst
  lung J98.4
  pancreas K86.3
  retina — *see* Cyst, retina
Pseudoelephantiasis neuroarthritica Q82.0
Pseudoexfoliation, capsule (lens) — *see* Cataract, specified NEC
Pseudofolliculitis barbae L73.1
Pseudoglioma H44.89
Pseudohemophilia (Bernuth's) (hereditary) (type B) D68.0
  Type A D69.8
  vascular D69.8
Pseudohermaphroditism Q56.3
  adrenal E25.8
  female Q56.2
    with adrenocortical disorder E25.8
    without adrenocortical disorder Q56.2
    adrenal (congenital) E25.0
    unspecified E25.9
  male Q56.1
    with
      adrenocortical disorder E25.8
      androgen resistance E34.51
      cleft scrotum Q56.1
      feminizing testis E34.51
      5-alpha-reductase deficiency E29.1
    without gonadal disorder Q56.1
    adrenal E25.8
    unspecified E25.9
Pseudo-Hurler's polydystrophy E77.0
Pseudohydrocephalus G93.2
Pseudohypertrophic muscular dystrophy (Erb's) G71.02
Pseudohypertrophy, muscle G71.09
Pseudohypoparathyroidism E20.1
Pseudoinsomnia F51.03
Pseudoleukemia, infantile D64.89
Pseudomembranous — *see* condition
Pseudomeningocele (cerebral) (infective) (post-traumatic) G96.19
  postprocedural (spinal) G97.82
Pseudomenses (newborn) P54.6

Pseudomenstruation (newborn) P54.6
Pseudomonas
  aeruginosa, as cause of disease classified elsewhere B96.5
  mallei infection A24.0
    as cause of disease classified elsewhere B96.5
  pseudomallei, as cause of disease classified elsewhere B96.5
Pseudomyotonia G71.19
Pseudomyxoma peritonei C78.6
Pseudoneuritis, optic (nerve) (disc) (papilla) , congenital Q14.2
Pseudo-obstruction intestine (acute) (chronic) (idiopathic) (intermittent secondary) (primary) K59.8
Pseudopapilledema H47.33-
  congenital Q14.2
Pseudoparalysis
  arm or leg R29.818
  atonic, congenital P94.2
Pseudopelade L66.0
Pseudophakia Z96.1
Pseudopolyarthritis, rhizomelic M35.3
Pseudopolycythemia D75.1
Pseudopseudohypoparathyroidism E20.1
Pseudopterygium H11.81-
Pseudoptosis (eyelid) — *see* Blepharochalasis
Pseudopuberty, precocious
  female heterosexual E25.8
  male isosexual E25.8
Pseudorickets (renal) N25.0
Pseudorubella B08.20
Pseudosclerema, newborn P83.88
Pseudosclerosis (brain)
  of Westphal (Strümpell) E83.01
  Jakob's — *see* Creutzfeldt-Jakob disease or syndrome
  spastic — *see* Creutzfeldt-Jakob disease or syndrome
Pseudotetanus — *see* Convulsions
Pseudotetany R29.0
  hysterical F44.5
Pseudotruncus arteriosus Q25.49
Pseudotuberculosis A28.2
  enterocolitis A04.8
  pasteurella (infection) A28.0
Pseudotumor
  cerebri G93.2
  orbital H05.11-
Pseudoxanthoma elasticum Q82.8
Psilosis (sprue) (tropical) K90.1
  nontropical K90.0
Psittacosis A70
Psoitis M60.88
Psoriasis L40.9
  arthropathic L40.50
    arthritis mutilans L40.52
    distal interphalangeal L40.51
    juvenile L40.54
    other specified L40.59
    spondylitis L40.53
  buccal K13.29
  flexural L40.8
  guttate L40.4
  mouth K13.29
  nummular L40.0
  plaque L40.0
  psychogenic F54
  pustular (generalized) L40.1
    palmaris et plantaris L40.3
  specified NEC L40.8
  vulgaris L40.0
Psychasthenia F48.8
Psychiatric disorder or problem F99
Psychogenic — *see also* condition
  factors associated with physical conditions F54
Psychological and behavioral factors affecting medical condition F59
Psychoneurosis, psychoneurotic — *see also* Neurosis
  anxiety (state) F41.1
  depersonalization F48.1
  hypochondriacal F45.21

Psychoneurosis, psychoneurotic - *continued*
  hysteria F44.9
  neurasthenic F48.8
  personality NEC F60.89
Psychopathy, psychopathic
  affectionless F94.2
  autistic F84.5
  constitution, post-traumatic F07.81
  personality — *see* Disorder, personality
  sexual — *see* Deviation, sexual
  state F60.2
Psychosexual identity disorder of
  childhood F64.2
Psychosis, psychotic F29
  acute (transient) F23
    hysterical F44.9
  affective — *see* Disorder, mood
  alcoholic F10.959
    with
      abuse F10.159
      anxiety disorder F10.980
        with
          abuse F10.180
          dependence F10.280
      delirium tremens F10.231
      delusions F10.950
        with
          abuse F10.150
          dependence F10.250
      dementia F10.97
        with dependence F10.27
      dependence F10.259
      hallucinosis F10.951
        with
          abuse F10.151
          dependence F10.251
      mood disorder F10.94
        with
          abuse F10.14
          dependence F10.24
      paranoia F10.950
        with
          abuse F10.150
          dependence F10.250
      persisting amnesia F10.96
        with dependence F10.26
      amnestic confabulatory F10.96
        with dependence F10.26
      delirium tremens F10.231
      Korsakoff's, Korsakov's,
        Korsakow's F10.26
      paranoid type F10.950
        with
          abuse F10.150
          dependence F10.250
  anergastic — *see* Psychosis, organic
  arteriosclerotic (simple type)
    (uncomplicated) F01.50
    with behavioral disturbance F01.51
  childhood F84.0
    atypical F84.8
  climacteric — *see* Psychosis, involutional
  confusional F29
    acute or subacute F05
    reactive F23
  cycloid F23
  depressive — *see* Disorder, depressive
  disintegrative (childhood) F84.3
  drug-induced — *see* F11-F19 with .x59
    paranoid and hallucinatory states — *see*
      F11-F19 with .x50 or .x51
  due to or associated with
    addiction, drug — *see* F11-F19 with .x59
    dependence
      alcohol F10.259
      drug — *see* F11-F19 with .x59
    epilepsy F06.8
    Huntington's chorea F06.8
    ischemia, cerebrovascular
      (generalized) F06.8
    multiple sclerosis F06.8
    physical disease F06.8
    presenile dementia F03
    senile dementia F03

Psychosis, psychotic - *continued*
  due to or associated with - *continued*
    vascular disease (arteriosclerotic)
      (cerebral) F01.50
      with behavioral disturbance F01.51
  epileptic F06.8
  episode F23
    due to or associated with physical
      condition F06.8
  exhaustive F43.0
  hallucinatory, chronic F28
  hypomanic F30.8
  hysterical (acute) F44.9
  induced F24
  infantile F84.0
    atypical F84.8
  infective (acute) (subacute) F05
  involutional F28
    depressive — *see* Disorder, depressive
    melancholic — *see* Disorder, depressive
    paranoid (state) F22
  Korsakoff's, Korsakov's, Korsakow's
    (nonalcoholic) F04
    alcoholic F10.96
      in dependence F10.26
    induced by other psychoactive
      substance — *see* categories F11-F19
      with .x5x
  mania, manic (single episode) F30.2
    recurrent type F31.89
  manic-depressive — *see* Disorder, bipolar
  menopausal — *see* Psychosis, involutional
  mixed schizophrenic and affective F25.8
  multi-infarct (cerebrovascular) F01.50
    with behavioral disturbance F01.51
  nonorganic F29
    specified NEC F28
  organic F09
    due to or associated with
      arteriosclerosis (cerebral) — *see*
        Psychosis, arteriosclerotic
      cerebrovascular disease,
        arteriosclerotic — *see* Psychosis,
        arteriosclerotic
      childbirth — *see* Psychosis, puerperal
      Creutzfeldt-Jakob disease or
        syndrome — *see* Creutzfeldt-Jakob
        disease or syndrome
      dependence, alcohol F10.259
      disease
        alcoholic liver F10.259
        brain, arteriosclerotic — *see*
          Psychosis, arteriosclerotic
        cerebrovascular F01.50
          with behavioral disturbance F01.51
        Creutzfeldt-Jakob — *see* Creutzfeldt-
          Jakob disease or syndrome
        endocrine or metabolic F06.8
          acute or subacute F05
        liver, alcoholic F10.259
      epilepsy transient (acute) F05
      infection
        brain (intracranial) F06.8
          acute or subacute F05
      intoxication
        alcoholic (acute) F10.259
        drug F11-F19 with .x59
      ischemia, cerebrovascular
        (generalized) — *see* Psychosis,
        arteriosclerotic
      puerperium — *see* Psychosis, puerperal
      trauma, brain (birth) (from electric
        current) (surgical) F06.8
        acute or subacute F05
    infective F06.8
      acute or subacute F05
    post-traumatic F06.8
      acute or subacute F05
  paranoiac F22
  paranoid (climacteric) (involutional)
    (menopausal) F22
    psychogenic (acute) F23
    schizophrenic F20.0
    senile F03
  postpartum (NOS) F53.1

Psychosis, psychotic - *continued*
  presbyophrenic (type) F03
  presenile F03
  psychogenic (paranoid) F23
    depressive F32.3
  puerperal (NOS) F53.1
    specified type — *see* Psychosis, by type
  reactive (brief) (transient) (emotional stress)
    (psychological trauma) F23
    depressive F32.3
      recurrent F33.3
    excitative type F30.8
  schizoaffective F25.9
    depressive type F25.1
    manic type F25.0
  schizophrenia, schizophrenic — *see*
    Schizophrenia
  schizophrenia-like, in epilepsy F06.2
  schizophreniform F20.81
    affective type F25.9
    brief F23
    confusional type F23
    mixed type F25.0
  senile NEC F03
    depressed or paranoid type F03
    simple deterioration F03
    specified type - code to condition
  shared F24
  situational (reactive) F23
  symbiotic (childhood) F84.3
  symptomatic F09
Psychosomatic — *see* Disorder,
  psychosomatic
Psychosyndrome, organic F07.9
Psychotic episode due to or associated with
  physical condition F06.8
Pterygium (eye) H11.00-
  amyloid H11.01-
  central H11.02-
  colli Q18.3
  double H11.03-
  peripheral
    progressive H11.05-
    stationary H11.04-
  recurrent H11.06-
Ptilosis (eyelid) — *see* Madarosis
Ptomaine (poisoning) — *see* Poisoning, food
Ptosis — *see also* Blepharoptosis
  adiposa (false) — *see* Blepharoptosis
  breast N64.81
  brow H57.81-
  cecum K63.4
  colon K63.4
  congenital (eyelid) Q10.0
    specified site NEC — *see* Anomaly, by site
  eyebrow H57.81-
  eyelid — *see* Blepharoptosis
    congenital Q10.0
  gastric K31.89
  intestine K63.4
  kidney N28.83
  liver K76.89
  renal N28.83
  splanchnic K63.4
  spleen D73.89
  stomach K31.89
  viscera K63.4
PTP D69.51
Ptyalism (periodic) K11.7
  hysterical F45.8
  pregnancy — *see* Pregnancy, complicated by,
    specified pregnancy-related condition
    NEC
  psychogenic F45.8
Ptyalolithiasis K11.5
Pubarche, precocious E30.1
Pubertas praecox E30.1
Puberty (development state) Z00.3
  bleeding (excessive) N92.2
  delayed E30.0
  precocious (constitutional) (cryptogenic)
    (idiopathic) E30.1
    central E22.8
    due to
      ovarian hyperfunction E28.1

Puberty (development state) - *continued*
  precocious (constitutional) (cryptogenic) (idiopathic) - *continued*
    due to - *continued*
      ovarian hyperfunction - *continued*
        estrogen E28.0
      testicular hyperfunction E29.0
    premature E30.1
      due to
        adrenal cortical hyperfunction E25.8
        pineal tumor E34.8
        pituitary (anterior) hyperfunction E22.8
Puckering, macula — *see* Degeneration, macula, puckering
Pudenda, pudendum — *see* condition
Puente's disease (simple glandular cheilitis) K13.0
Puerperal, puerperium (complicated by, complications)
  abnormal glucose (tolerance test) O99.815
  abscess
    areola O91.02
      associated with lactation O91.03
    Bartholin's gland O86.19
    breast O91.12
      associated with lactation O91.13
    cervix (uteri) O86.11
    genital organ NEC O86.19
    kidney O86.21
    mammary O91.12
      associated with lactation O91.13
    nipple O91.02
      associated with lactation O91.03
    peritoneum O85
    subareolar O91.12
      associated with lactation O91.13
    urinary tract — *see* Puerperal, infection, urinary
    uterus O86.12
    vagina (wall) O86.13
    vaginorectal O86.13
    vulvovaginal gland O86.13
  adnexitis O86.19
  afibrinogenemia, or other coagulation defect O72.3
  albuminuria (acute) (subacute) — *see* Proteinuria, gestational
  alcohol use O99.315
  anemia O90.81
    pre-existing (pre-pregnancy) O99.03
  anesthetic death O89.8
  apoplexy O99.43
  bariatric surgery status O99.845
  blood disorder NEC O99.13
  blood dyscrasia O72.3
  cardiomyopathy O90.3
  cerebrovascular disorder (conditions in I60-I69) O99.43
  cervicitis O86.11
  circulatory system disorder O99.43
  coagulopathy (any) O99.13
    with hemorrhage O72.3
  complications O90.9
    specified NEC O90.89
  convulsions — *see* Eclampsia
  cystitis O86.22
  cystopyelitis O86.29
  delirium NEC F05
  diabetes O24.93
    gestational — *see* Puerperal, gestational diabetes
    pre-existing O24.33
      specified NEC O24.83
      type 1 O24.03
      type 2 O24.13
  digestive system disorder O99.63
  disease O90.9
    breast NEC O92.29
    cerebrovascular (acute) O99.43
    nonobstetric NEC O99.89
    tubo-ovarian O86.19
    Valsuani's O99.03
  disorder O90.9
    biliary tract O26.63
    lactation O92.70

Puerperal, puerperium (complicated by, complications) - *continued*
  disorder - *continued*
    liver O26.63
    nonobstetric NEC O99.89
  disruption
    cesarean wound O90.0
    episiotomy wound O90.1
    perineal laceration wound O90.1
  drug use O99.325
  eclampsia (with pre-existing hypertension) O15.2
  embolism (pulmonary) (blood clot) — *see* Embolism, obstetric, puerperal
  endocrine, nutritional or metabolic disease NEC O99.285
  endophlebitis — *see* Puerperal, phlebitis
  endotrachelitis O86.11
  failure
    lactation (complete) O92.3
      partial O92.4
    renal, acute O90.4
  fever (of unknown origin) O86.4
    septic O85
  fissure, nipple O92.12
    associated with lactation O92.13
  fistula
    breast (due to mastitis) O91.12
      associated with lactation O91.13
    nipple O91.02
      associated with lactation O91.03
  galactophoritis O91.22
    associated with lactation O91.23
  galactorrhea O92.6
  gastric banding status O99.845
  gastric bypass status O99.845
  gastrointestinal disease NEC O99.63
  gestational
    diabetes O24.439
      diet controlled O24.430
      insulin (and diet) controlled O24.434
      oral drug controlled (antidiabetic) (hypoglycemic) O24.435
    edema O12.05
      with proteinuria O12.25
    proteinuria O12.15
  gonorrhea O98.23
  hematoma, subdural O99.43
  hemiplegia, cerebral O99.355
    due to cerbrovascular disorder O99.43
  hemorrhage O72.1
    brain O99.43
    bulbar O99.43
    cerebellar O99.43
    cerebral O99.43
    cortical O99.43
    delayed or secondary O72.2
    extradural O99.43
    internal capsule O99.43
    intracranial O99.43
    intrapontine O99.43
    meningeal O99.43
    pontine O99.43
    retained placenta O72.0
    subarachnoid O99.43
    subcortical O99.43
    subdural O99.43
    third stage O72.0
    uterine, delayed O72.2
    ventricular O99.43
  hemorrhoids O87.2
  hepatorenal syndrome O90.4
  hypertension — *see* Hypertension, complicating, puerperium
  hypertrophy, breast O92.29
  induration breast (fibrous) O92.29
  infection O86.4
    cervix O86.11
    generalized O85
    genital tract NEC O86.19
      obstetric surgical wound O86.09
    kidney (bacillus coli) O86.21
    maternal O98.93
      carrier state NEC O99.835
      gonorrhea O98.23

Puerperal, puerperium (complicated by, complications) - *continued*
  infection - *continued*
    maternal - *continued*
      human immunodeficiency virus (HIV) O98.73
      protozoal O98.63
      sexually transmitted NEC O98.33
      specified NEC O98.83
      streptococcus group B (GBS) carrier state O99.825
      syphilis O98.13
      tuberculosis O98.03
      viral hepatitis O98.43
      viral NEC O98.53
    nipple O91.02
      associated with lactation O91.03
    peritoneum O85
    renal O86.21
    specified NEC O86.89
    urinary (asymptomatic) (tract) NEC O86.20
      bladder O86.22
      kidney O86.21
      specified site NEC O86.29
      urethra O86.22
    vagina O86.13
    vein — *see* Puerperal, phlebitis
  ischemia, cerebral O99.43
  lymphangitis O86.89
    breast O91.22
      associated with lactation O91.23
  malignancy O9A.13
  malnutrition O25.3
  mammillitis O91.02
    associated with lactation O91.03
  mammitis O91.22
    associated with lactation O91.23
  mania F30.8
  mastitis O91.22
    associated with lactation O91.23
    purulent O91.12
      associated with lactation O91.13
  melancholia — *see* Disorder, depressive
  mental disorder NEC O99.345
  metroperitonitis O85
  metrorrhagia — *see* Hemorrhage, postpartum
  metrosalpingitis O86.19
  metrovaginitis O86.13
  milk leg O87.1
  monoplegia, cerebral O99.43
  mood disturbance O90.6
  necrosis, liver (acute) (subacute) (conditions in subcategory K72.0) O26.63
    with renal failure O90.4
  nervous system disorder O99.355
  neuritis O90.89
  obesity (pre-existing prior to pregnancy) O99.215
  obesity surgery status O99.845
  occlusion, precerebral artery O99.43
  paralysis
    bladder (sphincter) O90.89
    cerebral O99.43
  paralytic stroke O99.43
  parametritis O85
  paravaginitis O86.13
  pelviperitonitis O85
  perimetritis O86.12
  perimetrosalpingitis O86.19
  perinephritis O86.21
  periphlebitis — *see* Puerperal phlebitis
  peritoneal infection O85
  peritonitis (pelvic) O85
  perivaginitis O86.13
  phlebitis O87.0
    deep O87.1
    pelvic O87.1
    superficial O87.0
  phlebothrombosis, deep O87.1
  phlegmasia alba dolens O87.1
  placental polyp O90.89
  pneumonia, embolic — *see* Embolism, obstetric, puerperal
  pre-eclampsia — *see* Pre-eclampsia

Puerperal, puerperium (complicated by, complications) - continued

psychosis (NOS) F53.1
pyelitis O86.21
pyelocystitis O86.29
pyelonephritis O86.21
pyelonephrosis O86.21
pyemia O85
pyocystitis O86.29
pyohemia O85
pyometra O86.12
pyonephritis O86.21
pyosalpingitis O86.19
pyrexia (of unknown origin) O86.4
renal
  disease NEC O90.89
  failure O90.4
respiratory disease NEC O99.53
retention
  decidua — see Retention, decidua
  placenta O72.0
  secundines — see Retention, secundines
retrated nipple O92.02
salpingo-ovaritis O86.19
salpingoperitonitis O85
secondary perineal tear O90.1
sepsis (pelvic) O85
sepsis O85
septic thrombophlebitis O86.81
skin disorder NEC O99.73
specified condition NEC O99.89
stroke O99.43
subinvolution (uterus) O90.89
subluxation of symphysis (pubis) O26.73
suppuration — see Puerperal, abscess
tetanus A34
thelitis O91.02
  associated with lactation O91.03
thrombocytopenia O72.3
thrombophlebitis (superficial) O87.0
  deep O87.1
  pelvic O87.1
  septic O86.81
thrombosis (venous) — see Thrombosis, puerperal
thyroiditis O90.5
toxemia (eclamptic) (pre-eclamptic) (with convulsions) O15.2
trauma, non-obstetric O9A.23
  caused by abuse (physical) (suspected) O9A.33
    confirmed O9A.33
    psychological (suspected) O9A.53
     confirmed O9A.53
    sexual (suspected) O9A.43
     confirmed O9A.43
uremia (due to renal failure) O90.4
urethritis O86.22
vaginitis O86.13
varicose veins (legs) O87.4
  vulva or perineum O87.8
venous O87.9
vulvitis O86.19
vulvovaginitis O86.13
white leg O87.1

Puerperium — see Puerperal
Pulmolithiasis J98.4
Pulmonary — see condition
Pulpitis (acute) (anachoretic) (chronic) (hyperplastic) (putrescent) (suppurative) (ulcerative) K04.01
  irreversible K04.02
  reversible K04.01
Pulpless tooth K04.99
Pulse
  alternating R00.8
  bigeminal R00.8
  fast R00.0
  feeble, rapid due to shock following injury T79.4
  rapid R00.0
  weak R09.89
Pulsus alternans or trigeminus R00.8
Punch drunk F07.81

Punctum lacrimale occlusion — see Obstruction, lacrimal

Puncture

abdomen, abdominal
  wall S31.139
    with
      foreign body S31.149
      penetration into peritoneal cavity S31.639
        with foreign body S31.649
    epigastric region S31.132
      with
        foreign body S31.142
        penetration into peritoneal cavity S31.632
          with foreign body S31.642
    left
      lower quadrant S31.134
        with
          foreign body S31.144
          penetration into peritoneal cavity S31.634
            with foreign body S31.644
      upper quadrant S31.131
        with
          foreign body S31.141
          penetration into peritoneal cavity S31.631
            with foreign body S31.641
    periumbilic region S31.135
      with
        foreign body S31.145
        penetration into peritoneal cavity S31.635
          with foreign body S31.645
    right
      lower quadrant S31.133
        with
          foreign body S31.143
          penetration into peritoneal cavity S31.633
            with foreign body S31.643
      upper quadrant S31.130
        with
          foreign body S31.140
          penetration into peritoneal cavity S31.630
            with foreign body S31.640
accidental, complicating surgery — see Complication, accidental puncture or laceration
alveolar (process) — see Puncture, oral cavity
ankle S91.039
  with
    foreign body S91.049
  left S91.032
    with
      foreign body S91.042
  right S91.031
    with
      foreign body S91.041
anus S31.833
  with foreign body S31.834
arm (upper) S41.139
  with foreign body S41.149
  left S41.132
    with foreign body S41.142
  lower — see Puncture, forearm
  right S41.131
    with foreign body S41.141
auditory canal (external) (meatus) — see Puncture, ear
auricle, ear — see Puncture, ear
axilla — see Puncture, arm
back — see also Puncture, thorax, back
  lower S31.030
    with
      foreign body S31.040
        with penetration into retroperitoneal space S31.041
      penetration into retroperitoneal space S31.031
bladder (traumatic) S37.29
  nontraumatic N32.89

Puncture - continued

breast S21.039
  with foreign body S21.049
  left S21.032
    with foreign body S21.042
  right S21.031
    with foreign body S21.041
buttock S31.803
  with foreign body S31.804
  left S31.823
    with foreign body S31.824
  right S31.813
    with foreign body S31.814
by
  device, implant or graft — see Complications, by site and type, mechanical
  foreign body left accidentally in operative wound T81.539
  instrument (any) during a procedure, accidental — see Puncture, accidental complicating surgery
calf — see Puncture, leg
canaliculus lacrimalis — see Puncture, eyelid
canthus, eye — see Puncture, eyelid
cervical esophagus S11.23
  with foreign body S11.24
cheek (external) S01.439
  with foreign body S01.449
  left S01.432
    with foreign body S01.442
  right S01.431
    with foreign body S01.441
  internal — see Puncture, oral cavity
chest wall — see Puncture, thorax
chin — see Puncture, head, specified site NEC
clitoris — see Puncture, vulva
costal region — see Puncture, thorax
digit (s)
  hand — see Puncture, finger
  foot — see Puncture, toe
ear (canal) (external) S01.339
  with foreign body S01.349
  left S01.332
    with foreign body S01.342
  right S01.331
    with foreign body S01.341
  drum S09.2-
elbow S51.039
  with
    foreign body S51.049
  left S51.032
    with
      foreign body S51.042
  right S51.031
    with
      foreign body S51.041
epididymis — see Puncture, testis
epigastric region — see Puncture, abdomen, wall, epigastric
epiglottis S11.83
  with foreign body S11.84
esophagus
  cervical S11.23
    with foreign body S11.24
  thoracic S27.818
eyeball S05.6-
  with foreign body S05.5-
eyebrow — see Puncture, eyelid
eyelid S01.13-
  with foreign body S01.14-
  left S01.132
    with foreign body S01.142
  right S01.131
    with foreign body S01.141
face NEC — see Puncture, head, specified site NEC
finger (s) S61.239
  with
    damage to nail S61.339
      with
        foreign body S61.349
    foreign body S61.249
  index S61.238

Puncture - *continued*
finger (s) - *continued*
index - *continued*
with
damage to nail S61.338
with
foreign body S61.348
foreign body S61.248
left S61.231
with
damage to nail S61.331
with
foreign body S61.341
foreign body S61.241
right S61.230
with
damage to nail S61.330
with
foreign body S61.340
foreign body S61.240
little S61.238
with
damage to nail S61.338
with
foreign body S61.348
foreign body S61.248
left S61.237
with
damage to nail S61.337
with
foreign body S61.347
foreign body S61.247
right S61.236
with
damage to nail S61.336
with
foreign body S61.346
foreign body S61.246
middle S61.238
with
damage to nail S61.338
with
foreign body S61.348
foreign body S61.248
left S61.233
with
damage to nail S61.333
with
foreign body S61.343
foreign body S61.243
right S61.232
with
damage to nail S61.332
with
foreign body S61.342
foreign body S61.242
ring S61.238
with
damage to nail S61.338
with
foreign body S61.348
foreign body S61.248
left S61.235
with
damage to nail S61.335
with
foreign body S61.345
foreign body S61.245
right S61.234
with
damage to nail S61.334
with
foreign body S61.344
foreign body S61.244
flank S31.139
with foreign body S31.149
foot (except toe (s) alone) S91.339
with foreign body S91.349
left S91.332
with foreign body S91.342
right S91.331
with foreign body S91.341
toe — *see* Puncture, toe
forearm S51.839
with

Puncture - *continued*
forearm - *continued*
with - *continued*
foreign body S51.849
elbow only — *see* Puncture, elbow
left S51.832
with
foreign body S51.842
right S51.831
with
foreign body S51.841
forehead — *see* Puncture, head, specified site
NEC
genital organs, external
female S31.532
with foreign body S31.542
vagina — *see* Puncture, vagina
vulva — *see* Puncture, vulva
male S31.531
with foreign body S31.541
penis — *see* Puncture, penis
scrotum — *see* Puncture, scrotum
testis — *see* Puncture, testis
groin — *see* Puncture, abdomen, wall
gum — *see* Puncture, oral cavity
hand S61.439
with
foreign body S61.449
finger — *see* Puncture, finger
left S61.432
with
foreign body S61.442
right S61.431
with
foreign body S61.441
thumb — *see* Puncture, thumb
head S01.93
with foreign body S01.94
cheek — *see* Puncture, cheek
ear — *see* Puncture, ear
eyelid — *see* Puncture, eyelid
lip — *see* Puncture, oral cavity
nose — *see* Puncture, nose
oral cavity — *see* Puncture, oral cavity
scalp S01.03
with foreign body S01.04
specified site NEC S01.83
with foreign body S01.84
temporomandibular area — *see* Puncture,
cheek
heart S26.99
with hemopericardium S26.09
without hemopericardium S26.19
heel — *see* Puncture, foot
hip S71.039
with foreign body S71.049
left S71.032
with foreign body S71.042
right S71.031
with foreign body S71.041
hymen — *see* Puncture, vagina
hypochondrium — *see* Puncture, abdomen,
wall
hypogastric region — *see* Puncture,
abdomen, wall
inguinal region — *see* Puncture, abdomen,
wall
instep — *see* Puncture, foot
internal organs — *see* Injury, by site
interscapular region — *see* Puncture, thorax,
back
intestine
large
colon S36.599
ascending S36.590
descending S36.592
sigmoid S36.593
specified site NEC S36.598
transverse S36.591
rectum S36.69
small S36.499
duodenum S36.490
specified site NEC S36.498
intra-abdominal organ S36.99
gallbladder S36.128

Puncture - *continued*
intra-abdominal organ - *continued*
intestine — *see* Puncture, intestine
liver S36.118
pancreas — *see* Puncture, pancreas
peritoneum S36.81
specified site NEC S36.898
spleen S36.09
stomach S36.39
jaw — *see* Puncture, head, specified site
NEC
knee S81.039
with foreign body S81.049
left S81.032
with foreign body S81.042
right S81.031
with foreign body S81.041
labium (majus) (minus) — *see* Puncture,
vulva
lacrimal duct — *see* Puncture, eyelid
larynx S11.013
with foreign body S11.014
leg (lower) S81.839
with foreign body S81.849
foot — *see* Puncture, foot
knee — *see* Puncture, knee
left S81.832
with foreign body S81.842
right S81.831
with foreign body S81.841
upper — *see* Puncture, thigh
lip S01.531
with foreign body S01.541
loin — *see* Puncture, abdomen, wall
lower back — *see* Puncture, back, lower
lumbar region — *see* Puncture, back, lower
malar region — *see* Puncture, head, specified
site NEC
mammary — *see* Puncture, breast
mastoid region — *see* Puncture, head,
specified site NEC
mouth — *see* Puncture, oral cavity
nail
finger — *see* Puncture, finger, with
damage to nail
toe — *see* Puncture, toe, with damage to
nail
nasal (septum) (sinus) — *see* Puncture, nose
nasopharynx — *see* Puncture, head, specified
site NEC
neck S11.93
with foreign body S11.94
involving
cervical esophagus — *see* Puncture,
cervical esophagus
larynx — *see* Puncture, larynx
pharynx — *see* Puncture, pharynx
thyroid gland — *see* Puncture, thyroid
gland
trachea — *see* Puncture, trachea
specified site NEC S11.83
with foreign body S11.84
nose (septum) (sinus) S01.23
with foreign body S01.24
ocular — *see* Puncture, eyeball
oral cavity S01.532
with foreign body S01.542
orbit S05.4-
palate — *see* Puncture, oral cavity
palm — *see* Puncture, hand
pancreas S36.299
body S36.291
head S36.290
tail S36.292
pelvis — *see* Puncture, back, lower
penis S31.23
with foreign body S31.24
perineum
female S31.43
with foreign body S31.44
male S31.139
with foreign body S31.149
periocular area (with or without lacrimal
passages) — *see* Puncture, eyelid
phalanges

Puncture - *continued*
　phalanges - *continued*
　　finger — *see* Puncture, finger
　　toe — *see* Puncture, toe
　pharynx S11.23
　　with foreign body S11.24
　pinna — *see* Puncture, ear
　popliteal space — *see* Puncture, knee
　prepuce — *see* Puncture, penis
　pubic region S31.139
　　with foreign body S31.149
　pudendum — *see* Puncture, genital organs,
　　external
　rectovaginal septum — *see* Puncture, vagina
　sacral region — *see* Puncture, back, lower
　sacroiliac region — *see* Puncture, back,
　　lower
　salivary gland — *see* Puncture, oral cavity
　scalp S01.03
　　with foreign body S01.04
　scapular region — *see* Puncture, shoulder
　scrotum S31.33
　　with foreign body S31.34
　shin — *see* Puncture, leg
　shoulder S41.039
　　with foreign body S41.049
　　left S41.032
　　　with foreign body S41.042
　　right S41.031
　　　with foreign body S41.041
　spermatic cord — *see* Puncture, testis
　sternal region — *see* Puncture, thorax, front
　submaxillary region — *see* Puncture, head,
　　specified site NEC
　submental region — *see* Puncture, head,
　　specified site NEC
　subungual
　　finger (s) — *see* Puncture, finger, with
　　　damage to nail
　　toe — *see* Puncture, toe, with damage to
　　　nail
　supraclavicular fossa — *see* Puncture, neck,
　　specified site NEC
　temple, temporal region — *see* Puncture,
　　head, specified site NEC
　temporomandibular area — *see* Puncture,
　　cheek
　testis S31.33
　　with foreign body S31.34
　thigh S71.139
　　with foreign body S71.149
　　left S71.132
　　　with foreign body S71.142
　　right S71.131
　　　with foreign body S71.141
　thorax, thoracic (wall) S21.93
　　with foreign body S21.94
　　back S21.23-
　　　with
　　　　foreign body S21.24-
　　　　　with penetration S21.44
　　　　penetration S21.43
　　breast — *see* Puncture, breast
　　front S21.13-
　　　with
　　　　foreign body S21.14-
　　　　　with penetration S21.34
　　　　penetration S21.33
　throat — *see* Puncture, neck
　thumb S61.039
　　with
　　　damage to nail S61.139
　　　　with
　　　　　foreign body S61.149
　　　foreign body S61.049
　　left S61.032
　　　with
　　　　damage to nail S61.132
　　　　　with
　　　　　　foreign body S61.142
　　　　foreign body S61.042
　　right S61.031
　　　with
　　　　damage to nail S61.131
　　　　　with

Puncture - *continued*
　thumb - *continued*
　　right - *continued*
　　　with - *continued*
　　　　damage to nail - *continued*
　　　　　with - *continued*
　　　　　　foreign body S61.141
　　　　foreign body S61.041
　thyroid gland S11.13
　　with foreign body S11.14
　toe (s) S91.139
　　with
　　　damage to nail S91.239
　　　　with
　　　　　foreign body S91.249
　　　foreign body S91.149
　　great S91.133
　　　with
　　　　damage to nail S91.233
　　　　　with
　　　　　　foreign body S91.243
　　　　foreign body S91.143
　　　left S91.132
　　　　with
　　　　　damage to nail S91.232
　　　　　　with
　　　　　　　foreign body S91.242
　　　　　foreign body S91.142
　　　right S91.131
　　　　with
　　　　　damage to nail S91.231
　　　　　　with
　　　　　　　foreign body S91.241
　　　　　foreign body S91.141
　　lesser S91.136
　　　with
　　　　damage to nail S91.236
　　　　　with
　　　　　　foreign body S91.246
　　　　foreign body S91.146
　　　left S91.135
　　　　with
　　　　　damage to nail S91.235
　　　　　　with
　　　　　　　foreign body S91.245
　　　　　foreign body S91.145
　　　right S91.134
　　　　with
　　　　　damage to nail S91.234
　　　　　　with
　　　　　　　foreign body S91.244
　　　　　foreign body S91.144
　tongue — *see* Puncture, oral cavity
　trachea S11.023
　　with foreign body S11.024
　tunica vaginalis — *see* Puncture, testis
　tympanum, tympanic membrane S09.2-
　umbilical region S31.135
　　with foreign body S31.145
　uvula — *see* Puncture, oral cavity
　vagina S31.43
　　with foreign body S31.44
　vocal cords S11.033
　　with foreign body S11.034
　vulva S31.43
　　with foreign body S31.44
　wrist S61.539
　　with
　　　foreign body S61.549
　　left S61.532
　　　with
　　　　foreign body S61.542
　　right S61.531
　　　with
　　　　foreign body S61.541
PUO (pyrexia of unknown origin) R50.9
Pupillary membrane (persistent) Q13.89
Pupillotonia — *see* Anomaly, pupil, function,
　tonic pupil
Purpura D69.2
　abdominal D69.0
　allergic D69.0
　anaphylactoid D69.0
　annularis telangiectodes L81.7
　arthritic D69.0

Purpura - *continued*
　autoerythrocyte sensitization D69.2
　autoimmune D69.0
　bacterial D69.0
　Bateman's (senile) D69.2
　capillary fragility (hereditary)
　　(idiopathic) D69.8
　cryoglobulinemic D89.1
　Devil's pinches D69.2
　fibrinolytic — *see* Fibrinolysis
　fulminans, fulminous D65
　gangrenous D65
　hemorrhagic, hemorrhagica D69.3
　　not due to thrombocytopenia D69.0
　Henoch (-Schönlein) (allergic) D69.0
　hypergammaglobulinemic (benign)
　　(Waldenström) D89.0
　idiopathic (thrombocytopenic) D69.3
　　nonthrombocytopenic D69.0
　immune thrombocytopenic D69.3
　infectious D69.0
　malignant D69.0
　neonatorum P54.5
　nervosa D69.0
　newborn P54.5
　nonthrombocytopenic D69.2
　　hemorrhagic D69.0
　　idiopathic D69.0
　nonthrombopenic D69.2
　peliosis rheumatica D69.0
　posttransfusion (post-transfusion) (from
　　(fresh) whole blood or blood
　　products) D69.51
　primary D69.49
　red cell membrane sensitivity D69.2
　rheumatica D69.0
　Schönlein (-Henoch) (allergic) D69.0
　scorbutic E54 *[D77]*
　senile D69.2
　simplex D69.2
　symptomatica D69.0
　telangiectasia annularis L81.7
　thrombocytopenic D69.49
　　congenital D69.42
　　hemorrhagic D69.3
　　hereditary D69.42
　　idiopathic D69.3
　　immune D69.3
　　neonatal, transitory P61.0
　　thrombotic M31.1
　thrombohemolytic — *see* Fibrinolysis
　thrombolytic — *see* Fibrinolysis
　thrombopenic D69.49
　thrombotic, thrombocytopenic M31.1
　toxic D69.0
　vascular D69.0
　visceral symptoms D69.0
Purpuric spots R23.3
Purulent — *see* condition
Pus
　in
　　stool R19.5
　　urine N39.0
　tube (rupture) — *see* Salpingo-oophoritis
Pustular rash L08.0
Pustule (nonmalignant) L08.9
　malignant A22.0
Pustulosis palmaris et plantaris L40.3
Putnam (-Dana) disease or syndrome — *see*
　Degeneration, combined
Putrescent pulp (dental) K04.1
Pyarthritis, pyarthrosis — *see* Arthritis,
　pyogenic or pyemic
　tuberculous — *see* Tuberculosis, joint
Pyelectasis — *see* Hydronephrosis
Pyelitis (congenital) (uremic) — *see also*
　　Pyelonephritis
　with
　　calculus — *see* category N20
　　　with hydronephrosis N13.6
　　contracted kidney N11.9
　acute N10
　chronic N11.9
　　with calculus — *see* category N20
　　　with hydronephrosis N13.6

Pyelitis (congenital) (uremic) - *continued*
  cystica N28.84
  puerperal (postpartum) O86.21
  tuberculous A18.11
Pyelocystitis — *see* Pyelonephritis
Pyelonephritis — *see also* Nephritis, tubulo-
  interstitial
  with
    calculus — *see* category N20
      with hydronephrosis N13.6
    contracted kidney N11.9
  acute N10
    calculous — *see* category N20
      with hydronephrosis N13.6
  chronic N11.9
    with calculus — *see* category N20
      with hydronephrosis N13.6
    associated with ureteral obstruction or
      stricture N11.1
    nonobstructive N11.8
      with reflux (vesicoureteral) N11.0
    obstructive N11.1
    specified NEC N11.8
  in (due to)
    brucellosis A23.9 *[N16]*
    cryoglobulinemia (mixed) D89.1 *[N16]*
    cystinosis E72.04
    diphtheria A36.84
    glycogen storage disease E74.09 *[N16]*
    leukemia NEC C95.9- *[N16]*
    lymphoma NEC C85.90 *[N16]*
    multiple myeloma C90.0- *[N16]*
    obstruction N11.1
    Salmonella infection A02.25
    sarcoidosis D86.84
    sepsis A41.9 *[N16]*
    Sjögren's disease M35.04
    toxoplasmosis B58.83
    transplant rejection T86.91 *[N16]*
    Wilson's disease E83.01 *[N16]*
  nonobstructive N12
    with reflux (vesicoureteral) N11.0
    chronic N11.8
  syphilitic A52.75
Pyelonephrosis (obstructive) N11.1
  chronic N11.9
Pyelophlebitis I80.8
Pyeloureteritis cystica N28.85
Pyemia, pyemic (fever) (infection) (purulent)
  — *see also* Sepsis
  joint — *see* Arthritis, pyogenic or pyemic
  liver K75.1
  pneumococcal A40.3
  portal K75.1
  postvaccinal T88.0
  puerperal, postpartum, childbirth O85
  specified organism NEC A41.89
  tuberculous — *see* Tuberculosis, miliary
Pygopagus Q89.4
Pyknoepilepsy (idiopathic) — *see* Pyknolepsy
Pyknolepsy G40.A09
  intractable G40.A19
    with status epilepticus G40.A11
    without status epilepticus G40.A19
  not intractable G40.A09
    with status epilepticus G40.A01
    without status epilepticus G40.A09
Pylephlebitis K75.1
Pyle's syndrome Q78.5
Pylethrombophlebitis K75.1
Pylethrombosis K75.1
Pyloritis K29.90
  with bleeding K29.91
Pylorospasm (reflex) NEC K31.3
  congenital or infantile Q40.0
  newborn Q40.0
  neurotic F45.8
  psychogenic F45.8
Pylorus, pyloric — *see* condition
Pyoarthrosis — *see* Arthritis, pyogenic or
  pyemic
Pyocele
  mastoid — *see* Mastoiditis, acute
  sinus (accessory) — *see* Sinusitis
  turbinate (bone) J32.9

Pyocele - *continued*
  urethra — *see also* Urethritis N34.0
Pyocolpos — *see* Vaginitis
Pyocystitis N30.80
  with hematuria N30.81
Pyoderma, pyodermia L08.0
  gangrenosum L88
  newborn P39.4
  phagedenic L88
  vegetans L08.81
Pyodermatitis L08.0
  vegetans L08.81
Pyogenic — *see* condition
Pyohydronephrosis N13.6
Pyometra, pyometrium, pyometritis — *see*
  Endometritis
Pyomyositis (tropical) — *see* Myositis,
  infective
Pyonephritis N12
Pyonephrosis N13.6
  tuberculous A18.11
Pyo-oophoritis — *see* Salpingo-oophoritis
Pyo-ovarium — *see* Salpingo-oophoritis
Pyopericarditis, pyopericardium I30.1
Pyophlebitis — *see* Phlebitis
Pyopneumopericardium I30.1
Pyopneumothorax (infective) J86.9
  with fistula J86.0
  tuberculous NEC A15.6
Pyosalpinx, pyosalpingitis — *see*
  also Salpingo-oophoritis
Pyothorax J86.9
  with fistula J86.0
  tuberculous NEC A15.6
Pyoureter N28.89
  tuberculous A18.11
Pyramidopallidonigral syndrome G20
Pyrexia (of unknown origin) R50.9
  atmospheric T67.01
  during labor NEC O75.2
  heat T67.01
  newborn P81.9
    environmentally-induced P81.0
  persistent R50.9
  puerperal O86.4
Pyroglobulinemia NEC E88.09
Pyromania F63.1
Pyrosis R12
Pyuria (bacterial) (sterile) R82.81

Q

Q fever A78
  with pneumonia A78
Quadricuspid aortic valve Q23.8
Quadrilateral fever A78
Quadriparesis — *see* Quadriplegia
  meaning muscle weakness M62.81
Quadriplegia G82.50
  complete
    C1-C4 level G82.51
    C5-C7 level G82.53
  congenital (cerebral) (spinal) G80.8
    spastic G80.0
  embolic (current episode) I63.4-
  functional R53.2
  incomplete
    C1-C4 level G82.52
    C5-C7 level G82.54
  thrombotic (current episode) I63.3-
  traumatic -- code to injury with seventh
    character S
    current episode — *see* Injury, spinal (cord),
      cervical
Quadruplet, pregnancy — *see* Pregnancy,
  quadruplet
Quarrelsomeness F60.3
Queensland fever A77.3
Quervain's disease M65.4
  thyroid E06.1
Queyrat's erythroplasia D07.4
  penis D07.4
  specified site — *see* Neoplasm, skin, in situ
  unspecified site D07.4
Quincke's disease or edema T78.3
  hereditary D84.1
Quinsy (gangrenous) J36

Quintan fever A79.0
Quintuplet, pregnancy — *see* Pregnancy,
  quintuplet

R

Rabbit fever — *see* Tularemia
Rabies A82.9
  contact Z20.3
  exposure to Z20.3
  inoculation reaction — *see* Complications,
    vaccination
  sylvatic A82.0
  urban A82.1
Rachischisis — *see* Spina bifida
Rachitic — *see also* condition
  deformities of spine (late effect)
    (sequelae) E64.3
  pelvis (late effect) (sequelae) E64.3
    with disproportion (fetopelvic) O33.0
      causing obstructed labor O65.0
Rachitis, rachitism (acute) (tarda) — *see*
  also Rickets
  renalis N25.0
  sequelae E64.3
Radial nerve — *see* condition
Radiation
  burn — *see* Burn
  effects NOS T66
  sickness NOS T66
  therapy, encounter for Z51.0
Radiculitis (pressure) (vertebrogenic) — *see*
  Radiculopathy
Radiculomyelitis — *see also* Encephalitis
  toxic, due to
    Clostridium tetani A35
    Corynebacterium diphtheriae A36.82
Radiculopathy M54.10
  cervical region M54.12
  cervicothoracic region M54.13
  due to
    disc disorder
      C3 M50.11
      C4 M50.11
      C5 M50.121
      C6 M50.122
      C7 M50.123
      C8 M50.13
    displacement of intervertebral disc — *see*
      Disorder, disc, with, radiculopathy
  leg M54.1-
  lumbar region M54.16
  lumbosacral region M54.17
  occipito-atlanto-axial region M54.11
  postherpetic B02.29
  sacrococcygeal region M54.18
  syphilitic A52.11
  thoracic region (with visceral pain) M54.14
  thoracolumbar region M54.15
Radiodermal burns (acute, chronic, or
  occupational) — *see* Burn
Radiodermatitis L58.9
  acute L58.0
  chronic L58.1
Radiotherapy session Z51.0
RAEB (refractory anemia with excess
  blasts) D46.2-
Rage, meaning rabies — *see* Rabies
Ragpicker's disease A22.1
Ragsorter's disease A22.1
Raillietiniasis B71.8
Railroad neurosis F48.8
Railway spine F48.8
Raised — *see also* Elevated
  antibody titer R76.0
Rake teeth, tooth M26.39
Rales R09.89
Ramifying renal pelvis Q63.8
Ramsay-Hunt disease or syndrome — *see*
  also Hunt's disease B02.21
  meaning dyssynergia cerebellaris
    myoclonica G11.1
Ranula K11.6
  congenital Q38.4
Rape
  adult
    confirmed T74.21

Rape - *continued*
  adult - *continued*
    suspected T76.21
    alleged, observation or examination, ruled out
      adult Z04.41
      child Z04.42
    child
      confirmed T74.22
      suspected T76.22
Rapid
  feeble pulse, due to shock, following injury T79.4
  heart (beat) R00.0
    psychogenic F45.8
  second stage (delivery) O62.3
  time-zone change syndrome G47.25
Rarefaction, bone — *see* Disorder, bone, density and structure, specified NEC
Rash (toxic) R21
  canker A38.9
  diaper L22
  drug (internal use) L27.0
    contact — *see also* Dermatitis, due to, drugs, external L25.1
  following immunization T88.1
  food — *see* Dermatitis, due to, food
  heat L74.0
  napkin (psoriasiform) L22
  nettle — *see* Urticaria
  pustular L08.0
  rose R21
    epidemic B06.9
  scarlet A38.9
  serum — *see also* Reaction, serum T80.69
  wandering tongue K14.1
Rasmussen aneurysm — *see* Tuberculosis, pulmonary
Rasmussen encephalitis G04.81
Rat-bite fever A25.9
  due to Streptobacillus moniliformis A25.1
  spirochetal (morsus muris) A25.0
Rathke's pouch tumor D44.3
Raymond (-Céstan) syndrome I65.8
Raynaud's disease, phenomenon or syndrome (secondary) I73.00
  with gangrene (symmetric) I73.01
RDS (newborn) (type I) P22.0
  type II P22.1
Reaction — *see also* Disorder
  adaptation — *see* Disorder, adjustment
  adjustment (anxiety) (conduct disorder) (depressiveness) (distress) — *see* Disorder, adjustment
    with
      mutism, elective (child) (adolescent) F94.0
  adverse
    food (any) (ingested) NEC T78.1
      anaphylactic — *see* Shock, anaphylactic, due to food
  affective — *see* Disorder, mood
  allergic — *see* Allergy
  anaphylactic — *see* Shock, anaphylactic
  anaphylactoid — *see* Shock, anaphylactic
  anesthesia — *see* Anesthesia, complication
  antitoxin (prophylactic) (therapeutic) — *see* Complications, vaccination
  anxiety F41.1
  Arthus — *see* Arthus' phenomenon
  asthenic F48.8
  combat and operational stress F43.0
  compulsive F42.8
  conversion F44.9
  crisis, acute F43.0
  deoxyribonuclease (DNA) (DNase) hypersensitivity D69.2
  depressive (single episode) F32.9
    affective (single episode) F31.4
      recurrent episode F33.9
    neurotic F34.1
    psychoneurotic F34.1
    psychotic F32.3
    recurrent — *see* Disorder, depressive, recurrent

Reaction - *continued*
  dissociative F44.9
  drug NEC T88.7
    addictive — *see* Dependence, drug
      transmitted via placenta or breast milk — *see* Absorption, drug, addictive, through placenta
    allergic — *see* Allergy, drug
    lichenoid L43.2
    newborn P93.8
      gray baby syndrome P93.0
    overdose or poisoning (by accident) — *see* Table of Drugs and Chemicals, by drug, poisoning
    photoallergic L56.1
    phototoxic L56.0
    withdrawal — *see* Dependence, by drug, with, withdrawal
      infant of dependent mother P96.1
      newborn P96.1
    wrong substance given or taken (by accident) — *see* Table of Drugs and Chemicals, by drug, poisoning
  fear F40.9
    child (abnormal) F93.8
  febrile nonhemolytic transfusion (FNHTR) R50.84
  fluid loss, cerebrospinal G97.1
  foreign
    body NEC — *see* Granuloma, foreign body
    in operative wound (inadvertently left) — *see* Foreign body, accidentally left during a procedure
    substance accidentally left during a procedure (chemical) (powder) (talc) T81.60
      aseptic peritonitis T81.61
      body or object (instrument) (sponge) (swab) — *see* Foreign body, accidentally left during a procedure
      specified reaction NEC T81.69
  grief — *see* Disorder, adjustment
  Herxheimer's R68.89
  hyperkinetic — *see* Hyperkinesia
  hypochondriacal F45.20
  hypoglycemic, due to insulin E16.0
    with coma (diabetic) — *see* Diabetes, coma
      nondiabetic E15
    therapeutic misadventure — *see* subcategory T38.3
  hypomanic F30.8
  hysterical F44.9
  immunization — *see* Complications, vaccination
  incompatibility
    ABO blood group (infusion) (transfusion) — *see* Complication(s), transfusion, incompatibility reaction, ABO
      delayed serologic T80.39
    minor blood group (Duffy) (E) (K) (Kell) (Kidd) (Lewis) (M) (N) (P) (S) T80.89
    Rh (factor) (infusion) (transfusion) — *see* Complication(s), transfusion, incompatibility reaction, Rh (factor)
  inflammatory — *see* Infection
  infusion — *see* Complications, infusion
  inoculation (immune serum) — *see* Complications, vaccination
  insulin T38.3-
  involutional psychotic — *see* Disorder, depressive
  leukemoid D72.823
    basophilic D72.823
    lymphocytic D72.823
    monocytic D72.823
    myelocytic D72.823
    neutrophilic D72.823
  LSD (acute)
    due to drug abuse — *see* Abuse, drug, hallucinogen

Reaction - *continued*
  LSD (acute) - *continued*
    due to drug dependence — *see* Dependence, drug, hallucinogen
  lumbar puncture G97.1
  manic-depressive — *see* Disorder, bipolar
  neurasthenic F48.8
  neurogenic — *see* Neurosis
  neurotic F48.9
  neurotic-depressive F34.1
  nitritoid — *see* Crisis, nitritoid
  nonspecific
    to
      cell mediated immunity measurement of gamma interferon antigen response without active tuberculosis R76.12
      QuantiFERON-TB test (QFT) without active tuberculosis R76.12
      tuberculin test — *see also* Reaction, tuberculin skin test R76.11
  obsessive-compulsive F42.8
  organic, acute or subacute — *see* Delirium
  paranoid (acute) F23
    chronic F22
    senile F03
  passive dependency F60.7
  phobic F40.9
  post-traumatic stress, uncomplicated Z73.3
  psychogenic F99
  psychoneurotic — *see also* Neurosis
    compulsive F42.8
    depersonalization F48.1
    depressive F34.1
    hypochondriacal F45.20
    neurasthenic F48.8
    obsessive F42.8
  psychophysiologic — *see* Disorder, somatoform
  psychosomatic — *see* Disorder, somatoform
  psychotic — *see* Psychosis
  scarlet fever toxin — *see* Complications, vaccination
  schizophrenic F23
    acute (brief) (undifferentiated) F23
    latent F21
    undifferentiated (acute) (brief) F23
  serological for syphilis — *see* Serology for syphilis
  serum T80.69
    anaphylactic (immediate) — *see also* Shock, anaphylactic T80.59
    specified reaction NEC
      due to
        administration of blood and blood products T80.61
        immunization T80.62
        serum specified NEC T80.69
        vaccination T80.62
  situational — *see* Disorder, adjustment
  somatization — *see* Disorder, somatoform
  spinal puncture G97.1
  stress (severe) F43.9
    acute (agitation) ("daze") (disorientation) (disturbance of consciousness) (flight reaction) (fugue) F43.0
    specified NEC F43.8
  surgical procedure — *see* Complications, surgical procedure
  tetanus antitoxin — *see* Complications, vaccination
  toxic, to local anesthesia T88.59
    in labor and delivery O74.4
    in pregnancy O29.3X-
    postpartum, puerperal O89.3
  toxin-antitoxin — *see* Complications, vaccination
  transfusion (blood) (bone marrow) (lymphocytes) (allergic) — *see* Complications, transfusion
  tuberculin skin test, abnormal R76.11
  vaccination (any) — *see* Complications, vaccination
  withdrawing, child or adolescent F93.8
Reactive airway disease — *see* Asthma

Reactive depression — *see* Reaction, depressive
Rearrangement
chromosomal
balanced (in) Q95.9
abnormal individual (autosomal) Q95.2
non-sex (autosomal)
chromosomes Q95.2
sex/non-sex chromosomes Q95.3
specified NEC Q95.8
Recalcitrant patient — *see* Noncompliance
Recanalization, thrombus — *see* Thrombosis
Recession, receding
chamber angle (eye) H21.55-
chin M26.09
gingival (postinfective) (postoperative)
generalized K06.020
minimal K06.021
moderate K06.022
severe K06.023
localized K06.010
minimal K06.011
moderate K06.012
severe K06.013
Recklinghausen disease Q85.01
bones E21.0
Reclus' disease (cystic) — *see* Mastopathy, cystic
Recrudescent typhus (fever) A75.1
Recruitment, auditory H93.21-
Rectalgia K62.89
Rectitis K62.89
Rectocele
female (without uterine prolapse) N81.6
with uterine prolapse N81.4
incomplete N81.2
in pregnancy — *see* Pregnancy, complicated
by, abnormal, pelvic organs or tissues
NEC
male K62.3
Rectosigmoid junction — *see* condition
Rectosigmoiditis K63.89
ulcerative (chronic) K51.30
with
complication K51.319
abscess K51.314
fistula K51.313
obstruction K51.312
rectal bleeding K51.311
specified NEC K51.318
Rectourethral — *see* condition
Rectovaginal — *see* condition
Rectovesical — *see* condition
Rectum, rectal — *see* condition
Recurrent — *see* condition
pregnancy loss — *see* Loss (of), pregnancy, recurrent
Red bugs B88.0
Red tide — *see also* Table of Drugs and Chemicals T65.82-
Red-cedar lung or pneumonitis J67.8
Reduced
mobility Z74.09
ventilatory or vital capacity R94.2
Redundant, redundancy
anus (congenital) Q43.8
clitoris N90.89
colon (congenital) Q43.8
foreskin (congenital) N47.8
intestine (congenital) Q43.8
labia N90.69
organ or site, congenital NEC — *see* Accessory
panniculus (abdominal) E65
prepuce (congenital) N47.8
pylorus K31.89
rectum (congenital) Q43.8
scrotum N50.89
sigmoid (congenital) Q43.8
skin L98.7
and subcutaneous tissue L98.7
of face L57.4
eyelids — *see* Blepharochalasis
stomach K31.89
Reduplication — *see* Duplication

Reflex R29.2
hyperactive gag J39.2
pupillary, abnormal — *see* Anomaly, pupil, function
vasoconstriction I73.9
vasovagal R55
Reflux K21.9
acid K21.9
esophageal K21.9
with esophagitis K21.0
newborn P78.83
gastroesophageal K21.9
with esophagitis K21.0
mitral — *see* Insufficiency, mitral
ureteral — *see* Reflux, vesicoureteral
vesicoureteral (with scarring) N13.70
with
nephropathy N13.729
with hydroureter N13.739
bilateral N13.732
unilateral N13.731
bilateral N13.722
unilateral N13.721
without hydroureter N13.729
bilateral N13.722
unilateral N13.721
pyelonephritis (chronic) N11.0
congenital Q62.7
without nephropathy N13.71
Reforming, artificial openings — *see*
Attention to, artificial, opening
Refractive error — *see* Disorder, refraction
Refsum's disease or syndrome G60.1
Refusal of
food, psychogenic F50.89
treatment (because of) Z53.20
left against medical advice (AMA) Z53.21
patient's decision NEC Z53.29
reasons of belief or group pressure Z53.1
Regional — *see* condition
Regurgitation R11.10
aortic (valve) — *see* Insufficiency, aortic
food — *see also* Vomiting
with reswallowing — *see* Rumination
newborn P92.1
gastric contents — *see* Vomiting
heart — *see* Endocarditis
mitral (valve) — *see* Insufficiency, mitral
congenital Q23.3
myocardial — *see* Endocarditis
pulmonary (valve) (heart) I37.1
congenital Q22.2
syphilitic A52.03
tricuspid — *see* Insufficiency, tricuspid
valve, valvular — *see* Endocarditis
congenital Q24.8
vesicoureteral — *see* Reflux, vesicoureteral
Reichmann's disease or syndrome K31.89
Reifenstein syndrome E34.52
Reinsertion
implantable subdermal contraceptive Z30.46
intrauterine contraceptive device Z30.433
Reiter's disease, syndrome, or urethritis
M02.30
ankle M02.37-
elbow M02.32-
foot joint M02.37-
hand joint M02.34-
hip M02.35-
knee M02.36-
multiple site M02.39
shoulder M02.31-
vertebra M02.38
wrist M02.33-
Rejection
food, psychogenic F50.89
transplant T86.91
bone T86.830
marrow T86.01
cornea T86.840
heart T86.21
with lung (s) T86.31
intestine T86.850
kidney T86.11
liver T86.41

Rejection - *continued*
transplant - *continued*
lung (s) T86.810
with heart T86.31
organ (immune or nonimmune
cause) T86.91
pancreas T86.890
skin (allograft) (autograft) T86.820
specified NEC T86.890
stem cell (peripheral blood) (umbilical
cord) T86.5
Relapsing fever A68.9
Carter's (Asiatic) A68.1
Dutton's (West African) A68.1
Koch's A68.9
louse-borne (epidemic) A68.0
Novy's (American) A68.1
Obermeyers's (European) A68.0
Spirillum A68.9
tick-borne (endemic) A68.1
Relationship
occlusal
open anterior M26.220
open posterior M26.221
Relaxation
anus (sphincter) K62.89
psychogenic F45.8
arch (foot) — *see also* Deformity, limb, flat
foot
back ligaments — *see* Instability, joint, spine
bladder (sphincter) N31.2
cardioesophageal K21.9
cervix — *see* Incompetency, cervix
diaphragm J98.6
joint (capsule) (ligament) (paralytic) — *see*
Flail, joint
congenital NEC Q74.8
lumbosacral (joint) — *see* subcategory
M53.2
pelvic floor N81.89
perineum N81.89
posture R29.3
rectum (sphincter) K62.89
sacroiliac (joint) — *see* subcategory M53.2
scrotum N50.89
urethra (sphincter) N36.44
vesical N31.2
**Release from prison, anxiety
concerning** Z65.2
Remains
canal of Cloquet Q14.0
capsule (opaque) Q14.8
Remittent fever (malarial) B54
Remnant
canal of Cloquet Q14.0
capsule (opaque) Q14.8
cervix, cervical stump (acquired)
(postoperative) N88.8
cystic duct, postcholecystectomy K91.5
fingernail L60.8
congenital Q84.6
meniscus, knee — *see* Derangement, knee,
meniscus, specified NEC
thyroglossal duct Q89.2
tonsil J35.8
infected (chronic) J35.01
urachus Q64.4
Removal (from) (of)
artificial
arm Z44.00-
complete Z44.01-
partial Z44.02-
eye Z44.2-
leg Z44.10-
complete Z44.11-
partial Z44.12-
breast implant Z45.81
cardiac pulse generator (battery) (end-of-
life) Z45.010
catheter (urinary) (indwelling) Z46.6
from artificial opening — *see* Attention to,
artificial, opening
non-vascular Z46.82
vascular NEC Z45.2
drains Z48.03

Removal (from) (of) - *continued*
device Z46.9
  contraceptive Z30.432
    implantable subdermal Z30.46
  implanted NEC Z45.89
  specified NEC Z46.89
dressing (nonsurgical) Z48.00
  surgical Z48.01
external
  fixation device - code to fracture with
    seventh character D
  prosthesis, prosthetic device Z44.9
    breast Z44.3-
    specified NEC Z44.8
home in childhood (to foster home or
  institution) Z62.29
ileostomy Z43.2
insulin pump Z46.81
myringotomy device (stent) (tube) Z45.82
nervous system device NEC Z46.2
  brain neuropacemaker Z46.2
  visual substitution device Z46.2
    implanted Z45.31
non-vascular catheter Z46.82
orthodontic device Z46.4
organ, prophylactic (for neoplasia
  management) — *see* Prophylactic,
  organ removal
staples Z48.02
stent
  ureteral Z46.6
suture Z48.02
urinary device Z46.6
vascular access device or catheter Z45.2
Ren
arcuatus Q63.1
mobile, mobilis N28.89
  congenital Q63.8
unguliformis Q63.1
Renal — *see* condition
Rendu-Osler-Weber disease or
  syndrome I78.0
Reninoma D41.0-
Renon-Delille syndrome E23.3
Reovirus, as cause of disease classified
  elsewhere B97.5
Repeated falls NEC R29.6
Replaced chromosome by dicentric
  ring Q93.2
Replacement by artificial or mechanical
  device or prosthesis of
bladder Z96.0
blood vessel NEC Z95.828
bone NEC Z96.7
cochlea Z96.21
coronary artery Z95.5
eustachian tube Z96.29
eye globe Z97.0
heart Z95.812
  valve Z95.2
    prosthetic Z95.2
    specified NEC Z95.4
    xenogenic Z95.3
intestine Z96.89
joint Z96.60
  hip — *see* Presence, hip joint implant
  knee — *see* Presence, knee joint implant
  specified site NEC Z96.698
larynx Z96.3
lens Z96.1
limb (s) — *see* Presence, artificial, limb
mandible NEC (for tooth root implant (s))
  Z96.5
organ NEC Z96.89
peripheral vessel NEC Z95.828
stapes Z96.29
teeth Z97.2
tendon Z96.7
tissue NEC Z96.89
tooth root (s) Z96.5
vessel NEC Z95.828
  coronary (artery) Z95.5
Request for expert evidence Z04.89
Reserve, decreased or low
cardiac — *see* Disease, heart

Reserve, decreased or low - *continued*
kidney N28.89
Residual — *see also* condition
ovary syndrome N99.83
state, schizophrenic F20.5
urine R39.198
Resistance, resistant (to)
activated protein C D68.51
complicating pregnancy O26.89
insulin E88.81
organism (s)
  to
    drug Z16.30
      aminoglycosides Z16.29
      amoxicillin Z16.11
      ampicillin Z16.11
      antibiotic (s) Z16.20
        multiple Z16.24
        specified NEC Z16.29
      antifungal Z16.32
      antimicrobial (single) Z16.30
        multiple Z16.35
        specified NEC Z16.39
      antimycobacterial (single) Z16.341
        multiple Z16.342
      antiparasitic Z16.31
      antiviral Z16.33
      beta lactam antibiotics Z16.10
        specified NEC Z16.19
      cephalosporins Z16.19
      extended beta lactamase
        (ESBL) Z16.12
      fluoroquinolones Z16.23
      macrolides Z16.29
      methicillin — *see* MRSA
      multiple drugs (MDRO)
        antibiotics Z16.24
        antimicrobial Z16.35
        antimycobacterials Z16.342
      penicillins Z16.11
      quinine (and related
        compounds) Z16.31
      quinolones Z16.23
      sulfonamides Z16.29
      tetracyclines Z16.29
      tuberculostatics (single) Z16.341
        multiple Z16.342
      vancomycin Z16.21
        related antibiotics Z16.22
thyroid hormone E07.89
Resorption
dental (roots) K03.3
  alveoli M26.79
teeth (external) (internal) (pathological)
  (roots) K03.3
Respiration
Cheyne-Stokes R06.3
decreased due to shock, following
  injury T79.4
disorder of, psychogenic F45.8
insufficient, or poor R06.89
  newborn P28.5
painful R07.1
sighing, psychogenic F45.8
Respiratory — *see also* condition
distress syndrome (newborn) (type I) P22.0
  type II P22.1
syncytial virus, as cause of disease classified
  elsewhere — *see also* Virus, respiratory
  syncytial (RSV) B97.4
Respite care Z75.5
Response (drug)
photoallergic L56.1
phototoxic L56.0
Restenosis
stent
  vascular
    end stent
      adjacent to stent — *see*
        Arteriosclerosis
      within the stent
        coronary T82.855
        peripheral T82.856
    in stent
      coronary vessel T82.855

Restenosis - *continued*
stent - *continued*
  vascular - *continued*
    in stent - *continued*
      peripheral vessel T82.856
Restless legs (syndrome) G25.81
Restlessness R45.1
Restoration (of)
dental
  aesthetically inadequate or
    displeasing K08.56
  defective K08.50
    specified NEC K08.59
  failure of marginal integrity K08.51
  failure of periodontal anatomical
    intergrity K08.54
organ continuity from previous sterilization
  (tuboplasty) (vasoplasty) Z31.0
  aftercare Z31.42
tooth (existing)
  contours biologically incompatible with
    oral health K08.54
  open margins K08.51
  overhanging K08.52
  poor aesthetic K08.56
  poor gingival margins K08.51
  unsatisfactory, of tooth K08.50
    specified NEC K08.59
Restorative material (dental)
allergy to K08.55
fractured K08.539
  with loss of material K08.531
  without loss of material K08.530
unrepairable overhanging of K08.52
Restriction of housing space Z59.1
Rests, ovarian, in fallopian tube Q50.6
Restzustand (schizophrenic) F20.5
Retained — *see also* Retention
cholelithiasis following
  cholecystectomy K91.86
foreign body fragments (type of) Z18.9
  acrylics Z18.2
  animal quill (s) or spines Z18.31
  cement Z18.83
  concrete Z18.83
  crystalline Z18.83
  depleted isotope Z18.09
  depleted uranium Z18.01
  diethylhexyl phthalates Z18.2
  glass Z18.81
  isocyanate Z18.2
  magnetic metal Z18.11
  metal Z18.10
  nonmagnectic metal Z18.12
  nontherapeutic radioactive Z18.09
  organic NEC Z18.39
  plastic Z18.2
  quill (s) (animal) Z18.31
  radioactive (nontherapeutic) NEC Z18.09
  specified NEC Z18.89
  spine (s) (animal) Z18.31
  stone Z18.83
  tooth (teeth) Z18.32
  wood Z18.33
fragments (type of) Z18.9
  acrylics Z18.2
  animal quill (s) or spines Z18.31
  cement Z18.83
  concrete Z18.83
  crystalline Z18.83
  depleted isotope Z18.09
  depleted uranium Z18.01
  diethylhexyl phthalates Z18.2
  glass Z18.81
  isocyanate Z18.2
  magnetic metal Z18.11
  metal Z18.10
  nonmagnectic metal Z18.12
  nontherapeutic radioactive Z18.09
  organic NEC Z18.39
  plastic Z18.2
  quill (s) (animal) Z18.31
  radioactive (nontherapeutic) NEC Z18.09
  specified NEC Z18.89
  spine (s) (animal) Z18.31

Retained - *continued*
  fragments (type of) - *continued*
    stone Z18.83
    tooth (teeth) Z18.32
    wood Z18.33
    gallstones, following
      cholecystectomy K91.86
Retardation
  development, developmental, specific — *see*
    Disorder, developmental
  endochondral bone growth — *see* Disorder,
    bone, development or growth
  growth R62.50
    due to malnutrition E45
  mental — *see* Disability, intellectual
  motor function, specific F82
  physical (child) R62.52
    due to malnutrition E45
  reading (specific) F81.0
  spelling (specific) (without reading
    disorder) F81.81
Retching — *see* Vomiting
Retention — *see also* Retained
  bladder — *see* Retention, urine
  carbon dioxide E87.2
  cholelithiasis following
    cholecystectomy K91.86
  cyst — *see* Cyst
  dead
    fetus (at or near term) (mother) O36.4
      early fetal death O02.1
    ovum O02.0
  decidua (fragments) (following delivery)
    (with hemorrhage) O72.2
    without hemorrhage O73.1
  deciduous tooth K00.6
  dental root K08.3
  fecal — *see* Constipation
  fetus
    dead O36.4
    early O02.1
  fluid R60.9
  foreign body — *see also* Foreign body,
    retained
    current trauma - code as Foreign body, by
      site or type
  gallstones, following
    cholecystectomy K91.86
  gastric K31.89
  intrauterine contraceptive device, in
    pregnancy — *see* Pregnancy,
    complicated by, retention, intrauterine
    device
  membranes (complicating delivery) (with
    hemorrhage) O72.2
    with abortion — *see* Abortion, by type
    without hemorrhage O73.1
  meniscus — *see* Derangement, meniscus
  menses N94.89
  milk (puerperal, postpartum) O92.79
  nitrogen, extrarenal R39.2
  ovary syndrome N99.83
  placenta (total) (with hemorrhage) O72.0
    without hemorrhage O73.0
    portions or fragments (with
      hemorrhage) O72.2
      without hemorrhage O73.1
  products of conception
    early pregnancy (dead fetus) O02.1
    following
      delivery (with hemorrhage) O72.2
      without hemorrhage O73.1
  secundines (following delivery) (with
    hemorrhage) O72.0
    without hemorrhage O73.0
    complicating puerperium (delayed
      hemorrhage) O72.2
    partial O72.2
    without hemorrhage O73.1
  smegma, clitoris N90.89
  urine R33.9
    due to hyperplasia (hypertrophy) of
      prostate — *see* Hyperplasia, prostate
    drug-induced R33.0
    organic R33.8

Retention - *continued*
  urine - *continued*
    organic - *continued*
      drug-induced R33.0
      psychogenic F45.8
      specified NEC R33.8
    water (in tissues) — *see* Edema
Reticular erythematous mucinosis L98.5
Reticulation, dust — *see* Pneumoconiosis
Reticulocytosis R70.1
Reticuloendotheliosis
  acute infantile C96.0
  leukemic C91.4-
  nonlipid C96.0
Reticulohistiocytoma (giant-cell) D76.3
Reticuloid, actinic L57.1
Reticulosis (skin)
  acute of infancy C96.0
  hemophagocytic, familial D76.1
  histiocytic medullary C96.A
  lipomelanotic I89.8
  malignant (midline) C86.0
  polymorphic C86.0
  Sézary — *see* Sézary disease
Retina, retinal — *see also* condition
  dark area D49.81
Retinitis — *see also* Inflammation,
  chorioretinal
  albuminurica N18.9 *[H32]*
  diabetic — *see* Diabetes, retinitis
  disciformis — *see* Degeneration, macula
  focal — *see* Inflammation, chorioretinal,
    focal
  gravidarum — *see* Pregnancy, complicated
    by, specified pregnancy-related
    condition NEC
  juxtapapillaris — *see* Inflammation,
    chorioretinal, focal, juxtapapillary
  luetic — *see* Retinitis, syphilitic
  pigmentosa H35.52
  proliferans — *see* Disorder, globe,
    degenerative, specified type NEC
  proliferating — *see* Disorder, globe,
    degenerative, specified type NEC
  renal N18.9 *[H32]*
  syphilitic (early) (secondary) A51.43
    central, recurrent A52.71
    congenital (early) A50.01 *[H32]*
    late A52.71
  tuberculous A18.53
Retinoblastoma C69.2-
  differentiated C69.2-
  undifferentiated C69.2-
Retinochoroiditis — *see also* Inflammation,
  chorioretinal
  disseminated — *see* Inflammation,
    chorioretinal, disseminated
    syphilitic A52.71
  focal — *see* Inflammation, chorioretinal
  juxtapapillaris — *see* Inflammation,
    chorioretinal, focal, juxtapapillary
Retinopathy (background) H35.00
  arteriosclerotic I70.8 *[H35.0-]*
  atherosclerotic I70.8 *[H35.0-]*
  central serous — *see* Chorioretinopathy,
    central serous
  Coats H35.02-
  diabetic — *see* Diabetes, retinopathy
  exudative H35.02-
  hypertensive H35.03-
  in (due to)
    diabetes — *see* Diabetes, retinopathy
    sickle-cell disorders D57.- *[H36]*
  of prematurity H35.10-
    stage 0 H35.11-
    stage 1 H35.12-
    stage 2 H35.13-
    stage 3 H35.14-
    stage 4 H35.15-
    stage 5 H35.16-
  pigmentary, congenital — *see* Dystrophy,
    retina
  proliferative NEC H35.2-
    diabetic — *see* Diabetes, retinopathy,
      proliferative

Retinopathy (background) - *continued*
  proliferative NEC - *continued*
    sickle-cell D57.- *[H36]*
  solar H31.02-
Retinoschisis H33.10-
  congenital Q14.1
  specified type NEC H33.19-
Retortamoniasis A07.8
Retractile testis Q55.22
Retraction
  cervix — *see* Retroversion, uterus
  drum (membrane) — *see* Disorder, tympanic
    membrane, specified NEC
  finger — *see* Deformity, finger
  lid H02.539
    left H02.536
      lower H02.535
      upper H02.534
    right H02.533
      lower H02.532
      upper H02.531
  lung J98.4
  mediastinum J98.59
  nipple N64.53
    associated with
      lactation O92.03
      pregnancy O92.01-
      puerperium O92.02
    congenital Q83.8
  palmar fascia M72.0
  pleura — *see* Pleurisy
  ring, uterus (Bandl's) (pathological) O62.4
  sternum (congenital) Q76.7
    acquired M95.4
  uterus — *see* Retroversion, uterus
  valve (heart) — *see* Endocarditis
Retrobulbar — *see* condition
Retrocecal — *see* condition
Retrocession — *see* Retroversion
Retrodisplacement — *see* Retroversion
Retroflection, retroflexion — *see*
  Retroversion
Retrognathia, retrognathism (mandibular)
  (maxillary) M26.19
Retrograde menstruation N92.5
Retroperineal — *see* condition
Retroperitoneal — *see* condition
Retroperitonitis K68.9
Retropharyngeal — *see* condition
Retroplacental — *see* condition
Retroposition — *see* Retroversion
Retroprosthetic membrane T85.398
Retrosternal thyroid (congenital) Q89.2
Retroversion, retroverted
  cervix — *see* Retroversion, uterus
  female NEC — *see* Retroversion, uterus
  iris H21.89
  testis (congenital) Q55.29
  uterus (acquired) (acute) (any degree)
    (asymptomatic) (cervix)
    (postinfectional) (postpartal, old) N85.4
    congenital Q51.818
    in pregnancy O34.53-
Retrovirus, as cause of disease classified
  elsewhere B97.30
  human
    immunodeficiency, type 2 (HIV 2) B97.35
    T-cell lymphotropic
      type I (HTLV-I) B97.33
      type II (HTLV-II) B97.34
  lentivirus B97.31
  oncovirus B97.32
  specified NEC B97.39
Retrusion, premaxilla
  (developmental) M26.09
Rett's disease or syndrome F84.2
Reverse peristalsis R19.2
Reye's syndrome G93.7
Rh (factor)
  hemolytic disease (newborn) P55.0
  incompatibility, immunization or
    sensitization
    affecting management of pregnancy
      NEC O36.09-
      anti-D antibody O36.01-

Rh (factor) - *continued*
  incompatibility, immunization or
      sensitization - *continued*
    newborn P55.0
    transfusion reaction — *see*
        Complication(s), transfusion,
        incompatibility reaction, Rh (factor)
  negative mother affecting newborn P55.0
  titer elevated — *see* Complication(s),
      transfusion, incompatibility reaction, Rh
      (factor)
  transfusion reaction — *see* Complication(s),
      transfusion, incompatibility reaction, Rh
      (factor)
Rhabdomyolysis (idiopathic) NEC M62.82
  traumatic T79.6
Rhabdomyoma — *see also* Neoplasm,
      connective tissue, benign
  adult — *see* Neoplasm, connective tissue,
      benign
  fetal — *see* Neoplasm, connective tissue,
      benign
  glycogenic — *see* Neoplasm, connective
      tissue, benign
Rhabdomyosarcoma (any type) — *see*
      Neoplasm, connective tissue, malignant
Rhabdosarcoma — *see* Rhabdomyosarcoma
Rhesus (factor) incompatibility — *see* Rh,
      incompatibility
Rheumatic (acute) (subacute)
  adherent pericardium I09.2
  chronic I09.89
  coronary arteritis I01.8
  degeneration, myocardium I09.0
  fever (acute) — *see* Fever, rheumatic
  heart — *see* Disease, heart, rheumatic
  myocardial degeneration — *see*
      Degeneration, myocardium
  myocarditis (chronic) (inactive) (with
      chorea) I09.0
    active or acute I01.2
      with chorea (acute) (rheumatic)
          (Sydenham's) I02.0
  pancarditis, acute I01.8
    with chorea (acute (rheumatic)
        Sydenham's) I02.0
  pericarditis (active) (acute) (with effusion)
      (with pneumonia) I01.0
    with chorea (acute) (rheumatic)
        (Sydenham's) I02.0
    chronic or inactive I09.2
  pneumonia I00 *[J17]*
  torticollis M43.6
  typhoid fever A01.09
Rheumatism (articular) (neuralgic)
      (nonarticular) M79.0
  gout — *see* Arthritis, rheumatoid
  intercostal, meaning Tietze's disease M94.0
  palindromic (any site) M12.30
    ankle M12.37-
    elbow M12.32-
    foot joint M12.37-
    hand joint M12.34-
    hip M12.35-
    knee M12.36-
    multiple site M12.39
    shoulder M12.31-
    specified joint NEC M12.38
    vertebrae M12.38
    wrist M12.33-
  sciatic M54.4-
Rheumatoid — *see also* condition
  arthritis — *see also* Arthritis, rheumatoid
    with involvement of organs NEC M05.60
      ankle M05.67-
      elbow M05.62-
      foot joint M05.67-
      hand joint M05.64-
      hip M05.65-
      knee M05.66-
      multiple site M05.69
      shoulder M05.61-
      vertebra — *see* Spondylitis, ankylosing
      wrist M05.63-

Rheumatoid - *continued*
  arthritis - *continued*
    seronegative — *see* Arthritis, rheumatoid,
        seronegative
    seropositive — *see* Arthritis, rheumatoid,
        seropositive
  carditis M05.30
    ankle M05.37-
    elbow M05.32-
    foot joint M05.37-
    hand joint M05.34-
    hip M05.35-
    knee M05.36-
    multiple site M05.39
    shoulder M05.31-
    vertebra — *see* Spondylitis, ankylosing
    wrist M05.33-
  endocarditis — *see* Rheumatoid, carditis
  lung (disease) M05.10
    ankle M05.17-
    elbow M05.12-
    foot joint M05.17-
    hand joint M05.14-
    hip M05.15-
    knee M05.16-
    multiple site M05.19
    shoulder M05.11-
    vertebra — *see* Spondylitis, ankylosing
    wrist M05.13-
  myocarditis — *see* Rheumatoid, carditis
  myopathy M05.40
    ankle M05.47-
    elbow M05.42-
    foot joint M05.47-
    hand joint M05.44-
    hip M05.45-
    knee M05.46-
    multiple site M05.49
    shoulder M05.41-
    vertebra — *see* Spondylitis, ankylosing
    wrist M05.43-
  pericarditis — *see* Rheumatoid, carditis
  polyarthritis — *see* Arthritis, rheumatoid
  polyneuropathy M05.50
    ankle M05.57-
    elbow M05.52-
    foot joint M05.57-
    hand joint M05.54-
    hip M05.55-
    knee M05.56-
    multiple site M05.59
    shoulder M05.51-
    vertebra — *see* Spondylitis, ankylosing
    wrist M05.53-
  vasculitis M05.20
    ankle M05.27-
    elbow M05.22-
    foot joint M05.27-
    hand joint M05.24-
    hip M05.25-
    knee M05.26-
    multiple site M05.29
    shoulder M05.21-
    vertebra — *see* Spondylitis, ankylosing
    wrist M05.23-
Rhinitis (atrophic) (catarrhal) (chronic)
      (croupous) (fibrinous) (granulomatous)
      (hyperplastic) (hypertrophic)
      (membranous) (obstructive) (purulent)
      (suppurative) (ulcerative) J31.0
  with
    sore throat — *see* Nasopharyngitis
  acute J00
  allergic J30.9
    with asthma J45.909
      with
        exacerbation (acute) J45.901
        status asthmaticus J45.902
      due to
        food J30.5
        pollen J30.1
    nonseasonal J30.89
    perennial J30.89
    seasonal NEC J30.2
    specified NEC J30.89

Rhinitis (atrophic) (catarrhal) (chronic)
      (croupous) (fibrinous) (granulomatous)
      (hyperplastic) (hypertrophic) (membranous)
      (obstructive) (purulent) (suppurative)
      (ulcerative) - *continued*
  infective J00
  pneumococcal J00
  syphilitic A52.73
    congenital A50.05 *[J99]*
  tuberculous A15.8
  vasomotor J30.0
Rhinoantritis (chronic) — *see* Sinusitis,
      maxillary
Rhinodacryolith — *see* Dacryolith
Rhinolith (nasal sinus) J34.89
Rhinomegaly J34.89
Rhinopharyngitis (acute) (subacute) — *see*
      also Nasopharyngitis
  chronic J31.1
  destructive ulcerating A66.5
  mutilans A66.5
Rhinophyma L71.1
Rhinorrhea J34.89
  cerebrospinal (fluid) G96.0
  paroxysmal — *see* Rhinitis, allergic
  spasmodic — *see* Rhinitis, allergic
Rhinosalpingitis — *see* Salpingitis, eustachian
Rhinoscleroma A48.8
Rhinosporidiosis B48.1
Rhinovirus infection NEC B34.8
Rhizomelic chondrodysplasia
      punctata E71.540
Rhythm
  atrioventricular nodal I49.8
  disorder I49.9
    coronary sinus I49.8
    ectopic I49.8
    nodal I49.8
  escape I49.9
  heart, abnormal I49.9
  idioventricular I44.2
  nodal I49.8
  sleep, inversion G47.2-
    nonorganic origin — *see* Disorder, sleep,
        circadian rhythm, psychogenic
Rhytidosis facialis L98.8
Rib — *see also* condition
  cervical Q76.5
Riboflavin deficiency E53.0
Rice bodies — *see also* Loose, body, joint
  knee M23.4-
Richter syndrome — *see* Leukemia, chronic
      lymphocytic, B-cell type
Richter's hernia — *see* Hernia, abdomen, with
      obstruction
Ricinism — *see* Poisoning, food, noxious,
      plant
Rickets (active) (acute) (adolescent) (chest
      wall) (congenital) (current) (infantile)
      (intestinal) E55.0
  adult — *see* Osteomalacia
  celiac K90.0
  hypophosphatemic with nephrotic-glycosuric
      dwarfism E72.09
  inactive E64.3
  kidney N25.0
  renal N25.0
  sequelae, any E64.3
  vitamin-D-resistant E83.31 *[M90.80]*
Rickettsial disease A79.9
  specified type NEC A79.89
Rickettsialpox (Rickettsia akari) A79.1
Rickettsiosis A79.9
  due to
    Ehrlichia sennetsu A79.81
    Rickettsia akari (rickettsialpox) A79.1
  specified type NEC A79.89
  tick-borne A77.9
  vesicular A79.1
Rider's bone — *see* Ossification, muscle,
      specified NEC
Ridge, alveolus — *see also* condition
  flabby K06.8
Ridged ear, congenital Q17.3

Riedel's
  lobe, liver Q44.7
  struma, thyroiditis or disease E06.5
Rieger's anomaly or syndrome Q13.81
Riehl's melanosis L81.4
Rietti-Greppi-Micheli anemia D56.9
Rieux's hernia — *see* Hernia, abdomen,
    specified site NEC
Riga (-Fede) disease K14.0
Riggs' disease — *see* Periodontitis
Right aortic arch Q25.47
Right middle lobe syndrome J98.11
Rigid, rigidity — *see also* condition
  abdominal R19.30
    with severe abdominal pain R10.0
    epigastric R19.36
    generalized R19.37
    left lower quadrant R19.34
    left upper quadrant R19.32
    periumbilic R19.35
    right lower quadrant R19.33
    right upper quadrant R19.31
  articular, multiple, congenital Q68.8
  cervix (uteri) in pregnancy — *see* Pregnancy,
    complicated by, abnormal, cervix
  hymen (acquired) (congenital) N89.6
  nuchal R29.1
  pelvic floor in pregnancy — *see* Pregnancy,
    complicated by, abnormal, pelvic organs
    or tissues NEC
  perineum or vulva in pregnancy — *see*
    Pregnancy, complicated by, abnormal,
    vulva
  spine — *see* Dorsopathy, specified NEC
  vagina in pregnancy — *see* Pregnancy,
    complicated by, abnormal, vagina
Rigors R68.89
  with fever R50.9
Riley-Day syndrome G90.1
**RIND (reversible ischemic neurologic
  deficit)** I63.9
Ring (s)
  aorta (vascular) Q25.45
  Bandl's O62.4
  contraction, complicating delivery O62.4
  esophageal, lower (muscular) K22.2
  Fleischer's (cornea) H18.04-
  hymenal, tight (acquired) (congenital) N89.6
  Kayser-Fleischer (cornea) H18.04-
  retraction, uterus, pathological O62.4
  Schatzki's (esophagus) (lower) K22.2
    congenital Q39.3
  Soemmerring's — *see* Cataract, secondary
  vascular (congenital) Q25.8
    aorta Q25.45
Ringed hair (congenital) Q84.1
Ringworm B35.9
  beard B35.0
  black dot B35.0
  body B35.4
  Burmese B35.5
  corporeal B35.4
  foot B35.3
  groin B35.6
  hand B35.2
  honeycomb B35.0
  nails B35.1
  perianal (area) B35.6
  scalp B35.0
  specified NEC B35.8
  Tokelau B35.5
Rise, venous pressure I87.8
**Rising, PSA following treatment for
  malignant neoplasm of prostate** R97.21
Risk
  for
    dental caries Z91.849
      high Z91.843
      low Z91.841
      moderate Z91.842
    suicidal
      meaning personal history of attempted
        suicide Z91.5
      meaning suicidal ideation — *see* Ideation,
        suicidal

Ritter's disease L00
Rivalry, sibling Z62.891
Rivalta's disease A42.2
River blindness B73.01
Robert's pelvis Q74.2
  with disproportion (fetopelvic) O33.0
    causing obstructed labor O65.0
Robin (-Pierre) syndrome Q87.0
**Robinow-Silvermann-Smith
  syndrome** Q87.19
**Robinson's (hidrotic) ectodermal dysplasia
  or syndrome** Q82.4
Robles' disease B73.01
Rocky Mountain (spotted) fever A77.0
Roetheln — *see* Rubella
Roger's disease Q21.0
**Rokitansky-Aschoff sinuses
  (gallbladder)** K82.8
Rolando's fracture (displaced) S62.22-
  nondisplaced S62.22-
**Romano-Ward (prolonged QT interval)
  syndrome** I45.81
Romberg's disease or syndrome G51.8
Roof, mouth — *see* condition
Rosacea L71.9
  acne L71.9
  keratitis L71.8
  specified NEC L71.8
Rosary, rachitic E55.0
Rose
  cold J30.1
  fever J30.1
  rash R21
    epidemic B06.9
Rosenbach's erysipeloid A26.0
Rosenthal's disease or syndrome D68.1
Roseola B09
  infantum B08.20
    due to human herpesvirus 6 B08.21
    due to human herpesvirus 7 B08.22
Ross River disease or fever B33.1
Rossbach's disease K31.89
  psychogenic F45.8
Rostan's asthma (cardiac) — *see* Failure,
  ventricular, left
Rotation
  anomalous, incomplete or insufficient,
    intestine Q43.3
  cecum (congenital) Q43.3
  colon (congenital) Q43.3
  spine, incomplete or insufficient — *see*
    Dorsopathy, deforming, specified NEC
  tooth, teeth, fully erupted M26.35
  vertebra, incomplete or insufficient — *see*
    Dorsopathy, deforming, specified NEC
Rotes Quérol disease or syndrome — *see*
  Hyperostosis, ankylosing
**Roth (-Bernhardt) disease or
  syndrome** — *see* Meralgia paraesthetica
Rothmund (-Thomson) syndrome Q82.8
Rotor's disease or syndrome E80.6
Round
  back (with wedging of vertebrae) — *see*
    Kyphosis
    sequelae (late effect) of rickets E64.3
  worms (large) (infestation) NEC B82.0
    Ascariasis — *see also* Ascariasis B77.9
Roussy-Lévy syndrome G60.0
Rubella (German measles) B06.9
  complication NEC B06.09
    neurological B06.00
  congenital P35.0
  contact Z20.4
  exposure to Z20.4
  maternal
    manifest rubella in infant P35.0
    care for (suspected) damage to fetus O35.3
    suspected damage to fetus affecting
      management of pregnancy O35.3
  specified complications NEC B06.89
Rubeola (meaning measles) — *see* Measles
  meaning rubella — *see* Rubella
Rubeosis, iris — *see* Disorder, iris, vascular
Rubinstein-Taybi syndrome Q87.2

Rudimentary (congenital) — *see also*
  Agenesis
  arm — *see* Defect, reduction, upper limb
  bone Q79.9
  cervix uteri Q51.828
  eye Q11.2
  lobule of ear Q17.3
  patella Q74.1
  respiratory organs in thoracopagus Q89.4
  tracheal bronchus Q32.4
  uterus Q51.818
    in male Q56.1
  vagina Q52.0
Ruled out condition — *see* Observation,
  suspected
Rumination R11.10
  with nausea R11.2
  disorder of infancy F98.21
  neurotic F42.8
  newborn P92.1
  obsessional F42.8
  psychogenic F42.8
Runeberg's disease D51.0
Runny nose R09.89
Rupia (syphilitic) A51.39
  congenital A50.06
  tertiary A52.79
Rupture, ruptured
  abscess (spontaneous) - code by site under
    Abscess
  aneurysm — *see* Aneurysm
  anus (sphincter) — *see* Laceration, anus
  aorta, aortic I71.8
    abdominal I71.3
    arch I71.1
    ascending I71.1
    descending I71.8
      abdominal I71.3
      thoracic I71.1
    syphilitic A52.01
    thoracoabdominal I71.5
    thorax, thoracic I71.1
    transverse I71.1
    traumatic — *see* Injury, aorta, laceration,
      major
    valve or cusp — *see also* Endocarditis,
      aortic I35.8
  appendix (with peritonitis) — *see also*
    Appendicitis K35.32
    with localized peritonitis — *see also*
      Appendicitis K35.32
  arteriovenous fistula, brain — *see* Fistula,
    arteriovenous, brain, ruptured
  artery I77.2
    brain — *see* Hemorrhage, intracranial,
      intracerebral
    coronary — *see* Infarct, myocardium
    heart — *see* Infarct, myocardium
    pulmonary I28.8
    traumatic (complication) — *see* Injury,
      blood vessel
  bile duct (common) (hepatic) K83.2
    cystic K82.8
  bladder (sphincter) (nontraumatic)
    (spontaneous) N32.89
    following ectopic or molar
      pregnancy O08.6
    obstetrical trauma O71.5
    traumatic S37.29
  blood vessel — *see also* Hemorrhage
    brain — *see* Hemorrhage, intracranial,
      intracerebral
    heart — *see* Infarct, myocardium
    traumatic (complication) — *see* Injury,
      blood vessel, laceration, major, by site
  bone — *see* Fracture
  bowel (nontraumatic) K63.1
  brain
    aneurysm (congenital) — *see also*
      Hemorrhage, intracranial,
      subarachnoid
    syphilitic A52.05
    hemorrhagic — *see* Hemorrhage,
      intracranial, intracerebral
  capillaries I78.8

Rupture, ruptured - *continued*
cardiac (auricle) (ventricle) (wall) I23.3
with hemopericardium I23.0
infectional I40.9
traumatic — *see* Injury, heart
cartilage (articular) (current) — *see also*
Sprain
knee S83.3-
semilunar — *see* Tear, meniscus
cecum (with peritonitis) K65.0
with peritoneal abscess K35.33
traumatic S36.598
celiac artery, traumatic — *see* Injury, blood
vessel, celiac artery, laceration, major
cerebral aneurysm (congenital) (see
Hemorrhage, intracranial, subarachnoid)
cervix (uteri)
with ectopic or molar pregnancy O08.6
following ectopic or molar
pregnancy O08.6
obstetrical trauma O71.3
traumatic S37.69
chordae tendineae NEC I51.1
concurrent with acute myocardial
infarction — *see* Infarct, myocardium
following acute myocardial infarction
(current complication) I23.4
choroid (direct) (indirect)
(traumatic) H31.32-
circle of Willis I60.6
colon (nontraumatic) K63.1
traumatic — *see* Injury, intestine, large
cornea (traumatic) — *see* Injury, eye,
laceration
coronary (artery) (thrombotic) — *see* Infarct,
myocardium
corpus luteum (infected) (ovary) N83.1-
cyst — *see* Cyst
cystic duct K82.2
Descemet's membrane — *see* Change,
corneal membrane, Descemet's, rupture
traumatic — *see* Injury, eye, laceration
diaphragm, traumatic — *see* Injury,
intrathoracic, diaphragm
disc — *see* Rupture, intervertebral disc
diverticulum (intestine) K57.80
with bleeding K57.81
bladder N32.3
large intestine K57.20
with
bleeding K57.21
small intestine K57.40
with bleeding K57.41
small intestine K57.00
with
bleeding K57.01
large intestine K57.40
with bleeding K57.41
duodenal stump K31.89
ear drum (nontraumatic) — *see also*
Perforation, tympanum
traumatic S09.2-
due to blast injury — *see* Injury, blast,
ear
esophagus K22.3
eye (without prolapse or loss of intraocular
tissue) — *see* Injury, eye, laceration
fallopian tube NEC (nonobstetric)
(nontraumatic) N83.8
due to pregnancy O00.10-
with intrauterine pregnancy O00.11-
fontanel P13.1
gallbladder K82.2
traumatic S36.128
gastric — *see also* Rupture, stomach
vessel K92.2
globe (eye) (traumatic) — *see* Injury, eye,
laceration
graafian follicle (hematoma) N83.0-
heart — *see* Rupture, cardiac
hymen (nontraumatic)
(nonintentional) N89.8
internal organ, traumatic — *see* Injury, by
site

Rupture, ruptured - *continued*
intervertebral disc — *see* Displacement,
intervertebral disc
traumatic — *see* Rupture, traumatic,
intervertebral disc
intestine NEC (nontraumatic) K63.1
traumatic — *see* Injury, intestine
iris — *see also* Abnormality, pupillary
traumatic — *see* Injury, eye, laceration
joint capsule, traumatic — *see* Sprain
kidney (traumatic) S37.06-
birth injury P15.8
nontraumatic N28.89
lacrimal duct (traumatic) — *see* Injury, eye,
specified site NEC
lens (cataract) (traumatic) — *see* Cataract,
traumatic
ligament, traumatic — *see* Rupture,
traumatic, ligament, by site
liver S36.116
birth injury P15.0
lymphatic vessel I89.8
marginal sinus (placental) (with
hemorrhage) — *see* Hemorrhage,
antepartum, specified cause NEC
membrana tympani (nontraumatic) — *see*
Perforation, tympanum
membranes (spontaneous)
artificial
delayed delivery following O75.5
delayed delivery following — *see*
Pregnancy, complicated by, premature
rupture of membranes
meningeal artery I60.8
meniscus (knee) — *see also* Tear, meniscus
old — *see* Derangement, meniscus
site other than knee - code as Sprain
mesenteric artery, traumatic — *see* Injury,
mesenteric, artery, laceration, major
mesentery (nontraumatic) K66.8
traumatic — *see* Injury, intra-abdominal,
specified, site NEC
mitral (valve) I34.8
muscle (traumatic) — *see also* Strain
diastasis — *see* Diastasis, muscle
nontraumatic M62.10
ankle M62.17-
foot M62.17-
forearm M62.13-
hand M62.14-
lower leg M62.16-
pelvic region M62.15-
shoulder region M62.11-
specified site NEC M62.18
thigh M62.15-
upper arm M62.12-
traumatic — *see* Strain, by site
musculotendinous junction NEC,
nontraumatic — *see* Rupture, tendon,
spontaneous
mycotic aneurysm causing cerebral
hemorrhage — *see* Hemorrhage,
intracranial, subarachnoid
myocardium, myocardial — *see* Rupture,
cardiac
traumatic — *see* Injury, heart
nontraumatic, meaning hernia — *see* Hernia
obstructed — *see* Hernia, by site, obstructed
operation wound — *see* Disruption, wound,
operation
ovary, ovarian N83.8
corpus luteum cyst N83.1-
follicle (graafian) N83.0-
oviduct (nonobstetric) (nontraumatic) N83.8
due to pregnancy O00.10-
with intrauterine pregnancy O00.11-
pancreas (nontraumatic) K86.89
traumatic S36.299
papillary muscle NEC I51.2
following acute myocardial infarction
(current complication) I23.5
pelvic
floor, complicating delivery O70.1
organ NEC, obstetrical trauma O71.5

Rupture, ruptured - *continued*
perineum (nonobstetric)
(nontraumatic) N90.89
complicating delivery — *see* Delivery,
complicated, by, laceration, anus
(sphincter)
postoperative wound — *see* Disruption,
wound, operation
prostate (traumatic) S37.828
pulmonary
artery I28.8
valve (heart) I37.8
vein I28.8
vessel I28.8
pus tube — *see* Salpingitis
pyosalpinx — *see* Salpingitis
rectum (nontraumatic) K63.1
traumatic S36.69
retina, retinal (traumatic) (without
detachment) — *see also* Break, retina
with detachment — *see* Detachment,
retina, with retinal, break
rotator cuff (nontraumatic) M75.10-
complete M75.12-
incomplete M75.11-
sclera — *see* Injury, eye, laceration
sigmoid (nontraumatic) K63.1
traumatic S36.593
spinal cord — *see also* Injury, spinal cord, by
region
due to injury at birth P11.5
newborn (birth injury) P11.5
spleen (traumatic) S36.09
birth injury P15.1
congenital (birth injury) P15.1
due to P. vivax malaria B51.0
nontraumatic D73.5
spontaneous D73.5
splenic vein R58
traumatic — *see* Injury, blood vessel,
splenic vein
stomach (nontraumatic)
(spontaneous) K31.89
traumatic S36.39
supraspinatus (complete) (incomplete)
(nontraumatic) — *see* Tear, rotator cuff
symphysis pubis
obstetric O71.6
traumatic S33.4
synovium (cyst) M66.10
ankle M66.17-
elbow M66.12-
finger M66.14-
foot M66.17-
forearm M66.13-
hand M66.14-
pelvic region M66.15-
shoulder region M66.11-
specified site NEC M66.18
thigh M66.15-
toe M66.17-
upper arm M66.12-
wrist M66.13-
tendon (traumatic) — *see* Strain
nontraumatic (spontaneous) M66.9
ankle M66.87-
extensor M66.20
ankle M66.27-
foot M66.27-
forearm M66.23-
hand M66.24-
lower leg M66.26-
multiple sites M66.29
pelvic region M66.25-
shoulder region M66.21-
specified site NEC M66.28
thigh M66.25-
upper arm M66.22-
flexor M66.30
ankle M66.37-
foot M66.37-
forearm M66.33-
hand M66.34-
lower leg M66.36-
multiple sites M66.39

Rupture, ruptured - *continued*
  tendon (traumatic) - *continued*
    nontraumatic (spontaneous) - *continued*
      flexor - *continued*
        pelvic region M66.35-
        shoulder region M66.31-
        specified site NEC M66.38
        thigh M66.35-
        upper arm M66.32-
      foot M66.87-
      forearm M66.83-
      hand M66.84-
      lower leg M66.86-
      multiple sites M66.89
      pelvic region M66.85-
      shoulder region M66.81-
      specified
        site NEC M66.88
        tendon M66.80
      thigh M66.85-
      upper arm M66.82-
  thoracic duct I89.8
  tonsil J35.8
  traumatic
    aorta — *see* Injury, aorta, laceration, major
    diaphragm — *see* Injury, intrathoracic, diaphragm
    external site — *see* Wound, open, by site
    eye — *see* Injury, eye, laceration
    internal organ — *see* Injury, by site
    intervertebral disc
      cervical S13.0
      lumbar S33.0
      thoracic S23.0
    kidney S37.06-
    ligament — *see also* Sprain
      ankle — *see* Sprain, ankle
      carpus — *see* Rupture, traumatic, ligament, wrist
      collateral (hand) — *see* Rupture, traumatic, ligament, finger, collateral
      finger (metacarpophalangeal) (interphalangeal) S63.40-
        collateral S63.41-
          index S63.41-
          little S63.41-
          middle S63.41-
          ring S63.41-
        index S63.40-
        little S63.40-
        middle S63.40-
        palmar S63.42-
          index S63.42-
          little S63.42-
          middle S63.42-
          ring S63.42-
        ring S63.40-
        specified site NEC S63.499
          index S63.49-
          little S63.49-
          middle S63.49-
          ring S63.49-
        volar plate S63.43-
          index S63.43-
          little S63.43-
          middle S63.43-
          ring S63.43-
      foot — *see* Sprain, foot
      radial collateral S53.2-
      radiocarpal — *see* Rupture, traumatic, ligament, wrist, radiocarpal
      ulnar collateral S53.3-
      ulnocarpal — *see* Rupture, traumatic, ligament, wrist, ulnocarpal
      wrist S63.30-
        collateral S63.31-
        radiocarpal S63.32-
        specified site NEC S63.39-
        ulnocarpal (palmar) S63.33-
    liver S36.116
    membrana tympani — *see* Rupture, ear drum, traumatic
    muscle or tendon — *see* Strain
    myocardium — *see* Injury, heart

Rupture, ruptured - *continued*
  traumatic - *continued*
    pancreas S36.299
    rectum S36.69
    sigmoid S36.593
    spleen S36.09
    stomach S36.39
    symphysis pubis S33.4
    tympanum, tympanic (membrane) — *see* Rupture, ear drum, traumatic
    ureter S37.19
    uterus S37.69
    vagina — *see* Injury, vagina
    vena cava — *see* Injury, vena cava, laceration, major
  tricuspid (heart) (valve) I07.8
  tube, tubal (nonobstetric) (nontraumatic) N83.8
    abscess — *see* Salpingitis
    due to pregnancy O00.10-
      with intrauterine pregnancy O00.11-
  tympanum, tympanic (membrane) (nontraumatic) — *see also* Perforation, tympanic membrane H72.9-
    traumatic — *see* Rupture, ear drum, traumatic
  umbilical cord, complicating delivery O69.89
  ureter (traumatic) S37.19
    nontraumatic N28.89
  urethra (nontraumatic) N36.8
    with ectopic or molar pregnancy O08.6
    following ectopic or molar pregnancy O08.6
    obstetrical trauma O71.5
    traumatic S37.39
  uterosacral ligament (nonobstetric) (nontraumatic) N83.8
  uterus (traumatic) S37.69
    before labor O71.0-
    during or after labor O71.1
    nonpuerperal, nontraumatic N85.8
    pregnant (during labor) O71.1
      before labor O71.0-
  vagina — *see* Injury, vagina
  valve, valvular (heart) — *see* Endocarditis
  varicose vein — *see* Varix
  varix — *see* Varix
  vena cava R58
    traumatic — *see* Injury, vena cava, laceration, major
  vesical (urinary) N32.89
  vessel (blood) R58
    pulmonary I28.8
    traumatic — *see* Injury, blood vessel
  viscus R19.8
  vulva complicating delivery O70.0
Russell-Silver syndrome Q87.19
Russian spring-summer type encephalitis A84.0
Rust's disease (tuberculous cervical spondylitis) A18.01
Ruvalcaba-Myhre-Smith syndrome E71.440
Rytand-Lipsitch syndrome I44.2

S

Saber, sabre shin or tibia (syphilitic) A50.56 *[M90.8-]*
Sac lacrimal — *see* condition
Saccharomyces infection B37.9
Saccharopinuria E72.3
Saccular — *see* condition
Sacculation
  aorta (nonsyphilitic) — *see* Aneurysm, aorta
  bladder N32.3
  intralaryngeal (congenital) (ventricular) Q31.3
  larynx (congenital) (ventricular) Q31.3
  organ or site, congenital — *see* Distortion
  pregnant uterus — *see* Pregnancy, complicated by, abnormal, uterus
  ureter N28.89
  urethra N36.1
  vesical N32.3
Sachs' amaurotic familial idiocy or disease E75.02
Sachs-Tay disease E75.02

Sacks-Libman disease M32.11
Sacralgia M53.3
Sacralization Q76.49
Sacrodynia M53.3
Sacroiliac joint — *see* condition
Sacroiliitis NEC M46.1
Sacrum — *see* condition
Saddle
  back — *see* Lordosis
  embolus
    abdominal aorta I74.01
    pulmonary artery I26.92
      with acute cor pulmonale I26.02
  injury - code to condition
  nose M95.0
    due to syphilis A50.57
Sadism (sexual) F65.52
Sadness, postpartal O90.6
Sadomasochism F65.50
Saemisch's ulcer (cornea) — *see* Ulcer, cornea, central
Sagging
  skin and subcutaneous tissue (following bariatric surgery weight loss) (following dietary weight loss) L98.7
Sahib disease B55.0
Sailors' skin L57.8
Saint
  Anthony's fire — *see* Erysipelas
  triad — *see* Hernia, diaphragm
  Vitus' dance — *see* Chorea, Sydenham's
Salaam
  attack (s) — *see* Epilepsy, spasms
  tic R25.8
Salicylism
  abuse F55.8
  overdose or wrong substance given — *see* Table of Drugs and Chemicals, by drug, poisoning
Salivary duct or gland — *see* condition
Salivation, excessive K11.7
Salmonella — *see* Infection, Salmonella
Salmonellosis A02.0
Salpingitis (catarrhal) (fallopian tube) (nodular) (pseudofollicular) (purulent) (septic) N70.91
  with oophoritis N70.93
  acute N70.01
    with oophoritis N70.03
  chlamydial A56.11
  chronic N70.11
    with oophoritis N70.13
  complicating abortion — *see* Abortion, by type, complicated by, salpingitis
  ear — *see* Salpingitis, eustachian
  eustachian (tube) H68.00-
    acute H68.01-
    chronic H68.02-
  follicularis N70.11
    with oophoritis N70.13
  gonococcal (acute) (chronic) A54.24
  interstitial, chronic N70.11
    with oophoritis N70.13
  isthmica nodosa N70.11
    with oophoritis N70.13
  specific (gonococcal) (acute) (chronic) A54.24
  tuberculous (acute) (chronic) A18.17
  venereal (gonococcal) (acute) (chronic) A54.24
Salpingocele N83.4-
Salpingo-oophoritis (catarrhal) (purulent) (ruptured) (septic) (suppurative) N70.93
  acute N70.03
    with ectopic or molar pregnancy O08.0
    following ectopic or molar pregnancy O08.0
    gonococcal A54.24
  chronic N70.13
  following ectopic or molar pregnancy O08.0
  gonococcal (acute) (chronic) A54.24
  puerperal O86.19
  specific (gonococcal) (acute) (chronic) A54.24
  subacute N70.03

Salpingo-oophoritis (catarrhal) (purulent) (ruptured) (septic) (suppurative) - *continued*
  tuberculous (acute) (chronic) A18.17
  venereal (gonococcal) (acute)
    (chronic) A54.24
Salpingo-ovaritis — *see* Salpingo-oophoritis
Salpingoperitonitis — *see* Salpingo-oophoritis
Salzmann's nodular dystrophy — *see*
    Degeneration, cornea, nodular
Sampson's cyst or tumor N80.1
San Joaquin (Valley) fever B38.0
**Sandblaster's asthma, lung or
    pneumoconiosis** J62.8
Sander's disease (paranoia) F22
Sandfly fever A93.1
Sandhoff's disease E75.01
**Sanfilippo (Type B) (Type C) (Type D)
    syndrome** E76.22
Sanger-Brown ataxia G11.2
Sao Paulo fever or typhus A77.0
Saponification, mesenteric K65.8
Sarcocele (benign)
  syphilitic A52.76
    congenital A50.59
Sarcocystosis A07.8
Sarcoepiplocele — *see* Hernia
Sarcoepiplomphalocele Q79.2
Sarcoid — *see also* Sarcoidosis
  arthropathy D86.86
  Boeck's D86.9
  Darier-Roussy D86.3
  iridocyclitis D86.83
  meningitis D86.81
  myocarditis D86.85
  myositis D86.87
  pyelonephritis D86.84
  Spiegler-Fendt L08.89
Sarcoidosis D86.9
  with
    cranial nerve palsies D86.82
    hepatic granuloma D86.89
    polyarthritis D86.86
    tubulo-interstitial nephropathy D86.84
  combined sites NEC D86.89
  lung D86.0
    and lymph nodes D86.2
  lymph nodes D86.1
    and lung D86.2
  meninges D86.81
  skin D86.3
  specified type NEC D86.89
Sarcoma (of) — *see also* Neoplasm,
    connective tissue, malignant
  alveolar soft part — *see* Neoplasm,
    connective tissue, malignant
  ameloblastic C41.1
    upper jaw (bone) C41.0
  botryoid — *see* Neoplasm, connective tissue,
    malignant
  botryoides — *see* Neoplasm, connective
    tissue, malignant
  cerebellar C71.6
    circumscribed (arachnoidal) C71.6
  circumscribed (arachnoidal) cerebellar C71.6
  clear cell — *see also* Neoplasm, connective
    tissue, malignant
    kidney C64.-
  dendritic cells (accessory cells) C96.4
  embryonal — *see* Neoplasm, connective
    tissue, malignant
  endometrial (stromal) C54.1
    isthmus C54.0
  epithelioid (cell) — *see* Neoplasm,
    connective tissue, malignant
  Ewing's — *see* Neoplasm, bone, malignant
  follicular dendritic cell C96.4
  germinoblastic (diffuse) — *see* Lymphoma,
    diffuse large cell
    follicular — *see* Lymphoma, follicular,
      specified NEC
  giant cell (except of bone) — *see also*
    Neoplasm, connective tissue, malignant
    bone — *see* Neoplasm, bone, malignant
  glomoid — *see* Neoplasm, connective tissue,
    malignant

Sarcoma (of) - *continued*
  granulocytic C92.3-
  hemangioendothelial — *see* Neoplasm,
    connective tissue, malignant
  hemorrhagic, multiple — *see* Sarcoma,
    Kaposi's
  histiocytic C96.A
  Hodgkin — *see* Lymphoma, Hodgkin
  immunoblastic (diffuse) — *see* Lymphoma,
    diffuse large cell
  interdigitating dendritic cell C96.4
  Kaposi's
    colon C46.4
    connective tissue C46.1
    gastrointestinal organ C46.4
    lung C46.5-
    lymph node (s) C46.3
    palate (hard) (soft) C46.2
    rectum C46.4
    skin C46.0
    specified site NEC C46.7
    stomach C46.4
    unspecified site C46.9
  Kupffer cell C22.3
  Langerhans cell C96.4
  leptomeningeal — *see* Neoplasm, meninges,
    malignant
  liver NEC C22.4
  lymphangioendothelial — *see* Neoplasm,
    connective tissue, malignant
  lymphoblastic — *see* Lymphoma,
    lymphoblastic (diffuse)
  lymphocytic — *see* Lymphoma, small cell B-
    cell
  mast cell C96.22
  melanotic — *see* Melanoma
  meningeal — *see* Neoplasm, meninges,
    malignant
  meningothelial — *see* Neoplasm, meninges,
    malignant
  mesenchymal — *see also* Neoplasm,
    connective tissue, malignant
    mixed — *see* Neoplasm, connective tissue,
      malignant
  mesothelial — *see* Mesothelioma
  monstrocellular
    specified site — *see* Neoplasm, malignant,
      by site
    unspecified site C71.9
  myeloid C92.3-
  neurogenic — *see* Neoplasm, nerve,
    malignant
  odontogenic C41.1
    upper jaw (bone) C41.0
  osteoblastic — *see* Neoplasm, bone,
    malignant
  osteogenic — *see also* Neoplasm, bone,
    malignant
    juxtacortical — *see* Neoplasm, bone,
      malignant
    periosteal — *see* Neoplasm, bone,
      malignant
  periosteal — *see also* Neoplasm, bone,
    malignant
    osteogenic — *see* Neoplasm, bone,
      malignant
  pleomorphic cell — *see* Neoplasm,
    connective tissue, malignant
  reticulum cell (diffuse) — *see* Lymphoma,
    diffuse large cell
    nodular — *see* Lymphoma, follicular
    pleomorphic cell type — *see* Lymphoma,
      diffuse large cell
  rhabdoid — *see* Neoplasm, malignant, by site
  round cell — *see* Neoplasm, connective
    tissue, malignant
  small cell — *see* Neoplasm, connective
    tissue, malignant
  soft tissue — *see* Neoplasm, connective
    tissue, malignant
  spindle cell — *see* Neoplasm, connective
    tissue, malignant
  stromal (endometrial) C54.1
    isthmus C54.0

Sarcoma (of) - *continued*
  synovial — *see also* Neoplasm, connective
    tissue, malignant
    biphasic — *see* Neoplasm, connective
      tissue, malignant
    epithelioid cell — *see* Neoplasm,
      connective tissue, malignant
    spindle cell — *see* Neoplasm, connective
      tissue, malignant
Sarcomatosis
  meningeal — *see* Neoplasm, meninges,
    malignant
  specified site NEC — *see* Neoplasm,
    connective tissue, malignant
  unspecified site C80.1
Sarcopenia (age-related) M62.84
Sarcosinemia E72.59
Sarcosporidiosis (intestinal) A07.8
Satiety, early R68.81
Saturnine — *see* condition
Saturnism
  overdose or wrong substance given or
    taken — *see* Table of Drugs and
    Chemicals, by drug, poisoning
Satyriasis F52.8
Sauriasis — *see* Ichthyosis
SBE (subacute bacterial endocarditis) I33.0
Scabies (any site) B86
Scabs R23.4
Scaglietti-Dagnini syndrome E22.0
Scald — *see* Burn
Scalenus anticus (anterior) syndrome G54.0
Scales R23.4
Scaling, skin R23.4
Scalp — *see* condition
Scapegoating affecting child Z62.3
Scaphocephaly Q75.0
Scapulalgia M89.8X1
Scapulohumeral myopathy G71.02
Scar, scarring — *see also* Cicatrix L90.5
  adherent L90.5
  atrophic L90.5
  cervix
    in pregnancy or childbirth — *see*
      Pregnancy, complicated by, abnormal
      cervix
  cheloid L91.0
  chorioretinal H31.00-
    posterior pole macula H31.01-
    postsurgical H59.81-
    solar retinopathy H31.02-
    specified type NEC H31.09-
  choroid — *see* Scar, chorioretinal
  conjunctiva H11.24-
  cornea H17.9
    xerophthalmic — *see also* Opacity, cornea
      vitamin A deficiency E50.6
  duodenum, obstructive K31.5
  hypertrophic L91.0
  keloid L91.0
  labia N90.89
  lung (base) J98.4
  macula — *see* Scar, chorioretinal, posterior
    pole
  muscle M62.89
  myocardium, myocardial I25.2
  painful L90.5
  posterior pole (eye) — *see* Scar,
    chorioretinal, posterior pole
  retina — *see* Scar, chorioretinal
  trachea J39.8
  transmural uterine, in pregnancy O34.29
  uterus N85.8
    in pregnancy O34.29
  vagina N89.8
    postoperative N99.2
  vulva N90.89
Scarabiasis B88.2
Scarlatina (anginosa) (maligna) A38.9
  myocarditis (acute) A38.1
  old — *see* Myocarditis
  otitis media A38.0
  ulcerosa A38.8
Scarlet fever (albuminuria) (angina) A38.9

Schamberg's disease (progressive pigmentary dermatosis) L81.7
Schatzki's ring (acquired) (esophagus) (lower) K22.2
  congenital Q39.3
Schaufenster krankheit I20.8
Schaumann's
  benign lymphogranulomatosis D86.1
  disease or syndrome — *see* Sarcoidosis
Scheie's syndrome E76.03
Schenck's disease B42.1
Scheuermann's disease or osteochondrosis — *see* Osteochondrosis, juvenile, spine
Schilder (-Flatau) disease G37.0
Schilling-type monocytic leukemia C93.0-
Schimmelbusch's disease, cystic mastitis, or hyperplasia — *see* Mastopathy, cystic
Schistosoma infestation — *see* Infestation, Schistosoma
Schistosomiasis B65.9
  with muscle disorder B65.9 *[M63.80]*
    ankle B65.9 *[M63.87-]*
    foot B65.9 *[M63.87-]*
    forearm B65.9 *[M63.83-]*
    hand B65.9 *[M63.84-]*
    lower leg B65.9 *[M63.86-]*
    multiple sites B65.9 *[M63.89]*
    pelvic region B65.9 *[M63.85-]*
    shoulder region B65.9 *[M63.81-]*
    specified site NEC B65.9 *[M63.88]*
    thigh B65.9 *[M63.85-]*
    upper arm B65.9 *[M63.82-]*
  Asiatic B65.2
  bladder B65.0
  chestermani B65.8
  colon B65.1
  cutaneous B65.3
  due to
    S. haematobium B65.0
    S. japonicum B65.2
    S. mansoni B65.1
    S. mattheii B65.8
  Eastern B65.2
  genitourinary tract B65.0
  intestinal B65.1
  lung NEC B65.9 *[J99]*
    pneumonia B65.9 *[J17]*
  Manson's (intestinal) B65.1
  oriental B65.2
  pulmonary NEC B65.9 *[J99]*
    pneumonia B65.9
  Schistosoma
    haematobium B65.0
    japonicum B65.2
    mansoni B65.1
  specified type NEC B65.8
  urinary B65.0
  vesical B65.0
Schizencephaly Q04.6
Schizoaffective psychosis F25.9
Schizodontia K00.2
Schizoid personality F60.1
Schizophrenia, schizophrenic F20.9
  acute (brief) (undifferentiated) F23
  atypical (form) F20.3
  borderline F21
  catalepsy F20.2
  catatonic (type) (excited) (withdrawn) F20.2
  cenesthopathic, cenesthesiopathic F20.89
  childhood type F84.5
  chronic undifferentiated F20.5
  cyclic F25.0
  disorganized (type) F20.1
  flexibilitas cerea F20.2
  hebephrenic (type) F20.1
  incipient F21
  latent F21
  negative type F20.5
  paranoid (type) F20.0
  paraphrenic F20.0
  post-psychotic depression F32.89
  prepsychotic F21
  prodromal F21
  pseudoneurotic F21

Schizophrenia, schizophrenic - *continued*
  pseudopsychopathic F21
  reaction F23
  residual (state) (type) F20.5
  restzustand F20.5
  schizoaffective (type) — *see* Psychosis, schizoaffective
  simple (type) F20.89
  simplex F20.89
  specified type NEC F20.89
  spectrum and other psychotic disorder F29
    specified NEC F28
  stupor F20.2
  syndrome of childhood F84.5
  undifferentiated (type) F20.3
    chronic F20.5
Schizothymia (persistent) F60.1
Schlatter-Osgood disease or osteochondrosis — *see* Osteochondrosis, juvenile, tibia
Schlatter's tibia — *see* Osteochondrosis, juvenile, tibia
Schmidt's syndrome (polyglandular, autoimmune) E31.0
Schmincke's carcinoma or tumor — *see* Neoplasm, nasopharynx, malignant
Schmitz (-Stutzer) dysentery A03.0
Schmorl's disease or nodes
  lumbar region M51.46
  lumbosacral region M51.47
  sacrococcygeal region M53.3
  thoracic region M51.44
  thoracolumbar region M51.45
Schneiderian
  papilloma — *see* Neoplasm, nasopharynx, benign
    specified site — *see* Neoplasm, benign, by site
    unspecified site D14.0
  specified site — *see* Neoplasm, malignant, by site
    unspecified site C30.0
Scholte's syndrome (malignant carcinoid) E34.0
Scholz (-Bielchowsky-Henneberg) disease or syndrome E75.25
Schönlein (-Henoch) disease or purpura (primary) (rheumatic) D69.0
Schottmuller's disease A01.4
Schroeder's syndrome (endocrine hypertensive) E27.0
Schüller-Christian disease or syndrome C96.5
Schultze's type acroparesthesia, simple I73.89
Schultz's disease or syndrome — *see* Agranulocytosis
Schwalbe-Ziehen-Oppenheim disease G24.1
Schwannoma — *see also* Neoplasm, nerve, benign
  malignant — *see also* Neoplasm, nerve, malignant
    with rhabdomyoblastic differentiation — *see* Neoplasm, nerve, malignant
  melanocytic — *see* Neoplasm, nerve, benign
  pigmented — *see* Neoplasm, nerve, benign
Schwannomatosis Q85.03
Schwartz (-Jampel) syndrome G71.13
Schwartz-Bartter syndrome E22.2
Schweniger-Buzzi anetoderma L90.1
Sciatic — *see* condition
Sciatica (infective)
  with lumbago M54.4-
    due to intervertebral disc disorder — *see* Disorder, disc, with, radiculopathy
  due to displacement of intervertebral disc (with lumbago) — *see* Disorder, disc, with, radiculopathy
  wallet M54.3-
Scimitar syndrome Q26.8
Sclera — *see* condition
Sclerectasia H15.84-
Scleredema
  adultorum — *see* Sclerosis, systemic
  Buschke's — *see* Sclerosis, systemic

Scleredema - *continued*
  newborn P83.0
Sclerema (adiposum) (edematosum) (neonatorum) (newborn) P83.0
  adultorum — *see* Sclerosis, systemic
Scleriasis — *see* Scleroderma
Scleritis H15.00-
  with corneal involvement H15.04-
  anterior H15.01-
  brawny H15.02-
  in (due to) zoster B02.34
  posterior H15.03-
  specified type NEC H15.09-
  syphilitic A52.71
  tuberculous (nodular) A18.51
Sclerochoroiditis H31.8
Scleroconjunctivitis — *see* Scleritis
Sclerocystic ovary syndrome E28.2
Sclerodactyly, sclerodactylia L94.3
Scleroderma, sclerodermia (acrosclerotic) (diffuse) (generalized) (progressive) (pulmonary) — *see also* Sclerosis, systemic M34.9-
  circumscribed L94.0
  linear L94.1
  localized L94.0
  newborn P83.88
  systemic M34.9
Sclerokeratitis H16.8
  tuberculous A18.52
Scleroma nasi A48.8
Scleromalacia (perforans) H15.05-
Scleromyxedema L98.5
Sclérose en plaques G35
Sclerosis, sclerotic
  adrenal (gland) E27.8
  Alzheimer's — *see* Disease, Alzheimer's
  amyotrophic (lateral) G12.21
  aorta, aortic I70.0
    valve — *see* Endocarditis, aortic
  artery, arterial, arteriolar, arteriovascular — *see* Arteriosclerosis
  ascending multiple G35
  brain (generalized) (lobular) G37.9
    artery, arterial I67.2
    diffuse G37.0
    disseminated G35
    insular G35
    Krabbe's E75.23
    miliary G35
    multiple G35
    presenile (Alzheimer's) — *see* Disease, Alzheimer's, early onset
    senile (arteriosclerotic) I67.2
    stem, multiple G35
    tuberous Q85.1
  bulbar, multiple G35
  bundle of His I44.39
  cardiac — *see* Disease, heart, ischemic, atherosclerotic
  cardiorenal — *see* Hypertension, cardiorenal
  cardiovascular — *see also* Disease, cardiovascular
    renal — *see* Hypertension, cardiorenal
  cerebellar — *see* Sclerosis, brain
  cerebral — *see* Sclerosis, brain
  cerebrospinal (disseminated) (multiple) G35
  cerebrovascular I67.2
  choroid — *see* Degeneration, choroid
  combined (spinal cord) — *see also* Degeneration, combined
    multiple G35
  concentric (Balo) G37.5
  cornea — *see* Opacity, cornea
  coronary (artery) I25.10
    with angina pectoris — *see* Arteriosclerosis, coronary (artery),
  corpus cavernosum
    female N90.89
    male N48.6
  diffuse (brain) (spinal cord) G37.0
  disseminated G35
  dorsal G35
  dorsolateral (spinal cord) — *see* Degeneration, combined

Sclerosis, sclerotic - *continued*
  endometrium N85.5
  extrapyramidal G25.9
  eye, nuclear (senile) — *see* Cataract, senile,
    nuclear
  focal and segmental (glomerular) — *see also*
    N00-N07 with fourth character
    .1 N05.1
  Friedreich's (spinal cord) G11.1
  funicular (spermatic cord) N50.89
  general (vascular) — *see* Arteriosclerosis
  gland (lymphatic) I89.8
  hepatic K74.1
    alcoholic K70.2
  hereditary
    cerebellar G11.9
    spinal (Friedreich's ataxia) G11.1
  hippocampal G93.81
  insular G35
  kidney — *see* Sclerosis, renal
  larynx J38.7
  lateral (amyotrophic) (descending)
    (spinal) G12.21
    primary G12.23
  lens, senile nuclear — *see* Cataract, senile,
    nuclear
  liver K74.1
    with fibrosis K74.2
      alcoholic K70.2
    alcoholic K70.2
    cardiac K76.1
  lung — *see* Fibrosis, lung
  mastoid — *see* Mastoiditis, chronic
  mesial temporal G93.81
  mitral I05.8
  Mönckeberg's (medial) — *see*
    Arteriosclerosis, extremities
  multiple (brain stem) (cerebral) (generalized)
    (spinal cord) G35
  myocardium, myocardial — *see* Disease,
    heart, ischemic, atherosclerotic
  nuclear (senile) , eye — *see* Cataract, senile,
    nuclear
  ovary N83.8
  pancreas K86.89
  penis N48.6
  peripheral arteries — *see* Arteriosclerosis,
    extremities
  plaques G35
  pluriglandular E31.8
  polyglandular E31.8
  posterolateral (spinal cord) — *see*
    Degeneration, combined
  presenile (Alzheimer's) — *see* Disease,
    Alzheimer's, early onset
  primary, lateral G12.23
  progressive, systemic M34.0
  pulmonary — *see* Fibrosis, lung
    artery I27.0
    valve (heart) — *see* Endocarditis,
      pulmonary
  renal N26.9
    with
      cystine storage disease E72.09
      hypertensive heart disease (conditions in
        I11) — *see* Hypertension,
        cardiorenal
    arteriolar (hyaline) (hyperplastic) — *see*
      Hypertension, kidney
  retina (senile) (vascular) H35.00
  senile (vascular) — *see* Arteriosclerosis
  spinal (cord) (progressive) G95.89
    ascending G61.0
    combined — *see also* Degeneration,
      combined
      multiple G35
      syphilitic A52.11
    disseminated G35
    dorsolateral — *see* Degeneration,
      combined
    hereditary (Friedreich's) (mixed
      form) G11.1
    lateral (amyotrophic) G12.21
      progressive G12.23
    multiple G35

Sclerosis, sclerotic - *continued*
  spinal (cord) (progressive) - *continued*
    posterior (syphilitic) A52.11
  stomach K31.89
  subendocardial, congenital I42.4
  systemic M34.9
    with
      lung involvement M34.81
      myopathy M34.82
      polyneuropathy M34.83
    drug-induced M34.2
    due to chemicals NEC M34.2
    progressive M34.0
    specified NEC M34.89
  temporal (mesial) G93.81
  tricuspid (heart) (valve) I07.8
  tuberous (brain) Q85.1
  tympanic membrane — *see* Disorder,
    tympanic membrane, specified NEC
  valve, valvular (heart) — *see* Endocarditis
  vascular — *see* Arteriosclerosis
  vein I87.8
Scoliosis (acquired) (postural) M41.9
  adolescent (idiopathic) — *see* Scoliosis,
    idiopathic, adolescent
  congenital Q67.5
    due to bony malformation Q76.3
    failure of segmentation
      (hemivertebra) Q76.3
    hemivertebra fusion Q76.3
    postural Q67.5
  idiopathic M41.20
    adolescent M41.129
      cervical region M41.122
      cervicothoracic region M41.123
      lumbar region M41.126
      lumbosacral region M41.127
      thoracic region M41.124
      thoracolumbar region M41.125
    cervical region M41.22
    cervicothoracic region M41.23
    infantile M41.00
      cervical region M41.02
      cervicothoracic region M41.03
      lumbar region M41.06
      lumbosacral region M41.07
      sacrococcygeal region M41.08
      thoracic region M41.04
      thoracolumbar region M41.05
    juvenile M41.119
      cervical region M41.112
      cervicothoracic region M41.113
      lumbar region M41.116
      lumbosacral region M41.117
      thoracic region M41.114
      thoracolumbar region M41.115
    lumbar region M41.26
    lumbosacral region M41.27
    thoracic region M41.24
    thoracolumbar region M41.25
  infantile — *see* Scoliosis, idiopathic,
    infantile
  neuromuscular M41.40
    cervical region M41.42
    cervicothoracic region M41.43
    lumbar region M41.46
    lumbosacral region M41.47
    occipito-atlanto-axial region M41.41
    thoracic region M41.44
    thoracolumbar region M41.45
  paralytic — *see* Scoliosis, neuromuscular
  postradiation therapy M96.5
  rachitic (late effect or sequelae) E64.3
    [M49.80]
    cervical region E64.3 *[M49.82]*
    cervicothoracic region E64.3 *[M49.83]*
    lumbar region E64.3 *[M49.86]*
    lumbosacral region E64.3 *[M49.87]*
    multiple sites E64.3 *[M49.89]*
    occipito-atlanto-axial region E64.3
      [M49.81]
    sacrococcygeal region E64.3 *[M49.88]*
    thoracic region E64.3 *[M49.84]*
    thoracolumbar region E64.3 *[M49.85]*
  sciatic M54.4-

Scoliosis (acquired) (postural) - *continued*
  secondary (to) NEC M41.50
    cerebral palsy, Friedreich's ataxia,
      poliomyelitis, neuromuscular
      disorders — *see* Scoliosis,
      neuromuscular
    cervical region M41.52
    cervicothoracic region M41.53
    lumbar region M41.56
    lumbosacral region M41.57
    thoracic region M41.54
    thoracolumbar region M41.55
  specified form NEC M41.80
    cervical region M41.82
    cervicothoracic region M41.83
    lumbar region M41.86
    lumbosacral region M41.87
    thoracic region M41.84
    thoracolumbar region M41.85
  thoracogenic M41.30
    thoracic region M41.34
    thoracolumbar region M41.35
  tuberculous A18.01
Scoliotic pelvis
  with disproportion (fetopelvic) O33.0
    causing obstructed labor O65.0
Scorbutus, scorbutic — *see also* Scurvy
  anemia D53.2
**Score, NIHSS (National Institutes of Health
  Stroke Scale)** R29.7-
Scotoma (arcuate) (Bjerrum) (central) (ring)
    — *see also* Defect, visual field, localized,
    scotoma
  scintillating H53.19
Scratch — *see* Abrasion
Scratchy throat R09.89
Screening (for) Z13.9
  alcoholism Z13.39
  anemia Z13.0
  anomaly, congenital Z13.89
  antenatal, of mother — *see also* Encounter,
    antenatal screening Z36.9
  arterial hypertension Z13.6
  arthropod-borne viral disease NEC Z11.59
  autism Z13.41
  bacteriuria, asymptomatic Z13.89
  behavioral disorder Z13.30
    specified NEC Z13.39
  brain injury, traumatic Z13.850
  bronchitis, chronic Z13.83
  brucellosis Z11.2
  cardiovascular disorder Z13.6
  cataract Z13.5
  chlamydial diseases Z11.8
  cholera Z11.0
  chromosomal abnormalities (nonprocreative)
    NEC Z13.79
  colonoscopy Z12.11
  congenital
    dislocation of hip Z13.89
    eye disorder Z13.5
    malformation or deformation Z13.89
  contamination NEC Z13.88
  cystic fibrosis Z13.228
  dengue fever Z11.59
  dental disorder Z13.84
  depression (adult) (adolescent)
    (child) Z13.31
    maternal Z13.32
    perinatal Z13.32
  developmental
    delays Z13.40
      global (milestones) Z13.42
      specified NEC Z13.49
    handicap Z13.42
      in early childhood Z13.42
  diabetes mellitus Z13.1
  diphtheria Z11.2
  disability, intellectual Z13.39
  disease or disorder Z13.9
    bacterial NEC Z11.2
      intestinal infectious Z11.0
      respiratory tuberculosis Z11.1
    behavioral Z13.30
      specified NEC Z13.39

Screening (for) - *continued*
  disease or disorder - *continued*
    blood or blood-forming organ Z13.0
    cardiovascular Z13.6
    Chagas' Z11.6
    chlamydial Z11.8
    dental Z13.89
    developmental delays Z13.40
      global (milestones) Z13.42
      specified NEC Z13.49
    digestive tract NEC Z13.818
      lower GI Z13.811
      upper GI Z13.810
    ear Z13.5
    endocrine Z13.29
    eye Z13.5
    genitourinary Z13.89
    heart Z13.6
    human immunodeficiency virus (HIV)
        infection Z11.4
    immunity Z13.0
    infection
      intestinal Z11.0
      specified NEC Z11.6
    infectious Z11.9
    mental health and behavioral Z13.30
      specified NEC Z13.39
    metabolic Z13.228
    neurological Z13.89
    nutritional Z13.21
      metabolic Z13.228
        lipoid disorders Z13.220
    protozoal Z11.6
      intestinal Z11.0
    respiratory Z13.83
    rheumatic Z13.828
    rickettsial Z11.8
    sexually-transmitted NEC Z11.3
      human immunodeficiency virus
        (HIV) Z11.4
    sickle-cell (trait) Z13.0
    skin Z13.89
    specified NEC Z13.89
    spirochetal Z11.8
    thyroid Z13.29
    vascular Z13.6
    venereal Z11.3
    viral NEC Z11.59
      human immunodeficiency virus
        (HIV) Z11.4
      intestinal Z11.0
  elevated titer Z13.89
  emphysema Z13.83
  encephalitis, viral (mosquito- or tick-
      borne) Z11.59
  exposure to contaminants (toxic) Z13.88
  fever
    dengue Z11.59
    hemorrhagic Z11.59
    yellow Z11.59
  filariasis Z11.6
  galactosemia Z13.228
  gastrointestinal condition Z13.818
  genetic (nonprocreative) - for procreative
      management — *see* Testing, genetic, for
      procreative management
    disease carrier status
        (nonprocreative) Z13.71
      specified NEC (nonprocreative) Z13.79
  genitourinary condition Z13.89
  glaucoma Z13.5
  gonorrhea Z11.3
  gout Z13.89
  helminthiasis (intestinal) Z11.6
  hematopoietic malignancy Z12.89
  hemoglobinopathies NEC Z13.0
  hemorrhagic fever Z11.59
  Hodgkin disease Z12.89
  human immunodeficiency virus (HIV) Z11.4
  human papillomavirus Z11.51
  hypertension Z13.6
  immunity disorders Z13.0
  infant or child (over 28 days old) Z00.129
    with abnormal findings Z00.121
  infection

Screening (for) - *continued*
  infection - *continued*
    mycotic Z11.8
    parasitic Z11.8
  ingestion of radioactive substance Z13.88
  intellectual disability Z13.39
  intestinal
    helminthiasis Z11.6
    infectious disease Z11.0
  leishmaniasis Z11.6
  leprosy Z11.2
  leptospirosis Z11.8
  leukemia Z12.89
  lymphoma Z12.89
  malaria Z11.6
  malnutrition Z13.29
    metabolic Z13.228
    nutritional Z13.21
  measles Z11.59
  mental health disorder Z13.30
    specified NEC Z13.39
  metabolic errors, inborn Z13.228
  multiphasic Z13.89
  musculoskeletal disorder Z13.828
    osteoporosis Z13.820
  mycoses Z11.8
  myocardial infarction (acute) Z13.6
  neoplasm (malignant) (of) Z12.9
    bladder Z12.6
    blood Z12.89
    breast Z12.39
      routine mammogram Z12.31
    cervix Z12.4
    colon Z12.11
    genitourinary organs NEC Z12.79
      bladder Z12.6
      cervix Z12.4
      ovary Z12.73
      prostate Z12.5
      testis Z12.71
      vagina Z12.72
    hematopoietic system Z12.89
    intestinal tract Z12.10
      colon Z12.11
      rectum Z12.12
      small intestine Z12.13
    lung Z12.2
    lymph (glands) Z12.89
    nervous system Z12.82
    oral cavity Z12.81
    prostate Z12.5
    rectum Z12.12
    respiratory organs Z12.2
    skin Z12.83
    small intestine Z12.13
    specified site NEC Z12.89
    stomach Z12.0
  nephropathy Z13.89
  nervous system disorders NEC Z13.858
  neurological condition Z13.89
  osteoporosis Z13.820
  parasitic infestation Z11.9
    specified NEC Z11.8
  phenylketonuria Z13.228
  plague Z11.2
  poisoning (chemical) (heavy metal) Z13.88
  poliomyelitis Z11.59
  postnatal, chromosomal
      abnormalities Z13.89
  prenatal, of mother — *see also* Encounter,
      antenatal screening Z36.9
  protozoal disease Z11.6
    intestinal Z11.0
  pulmonary tuberculosis Z11.1
  radiation exposure Z13.88
  respiratory condition Z13.83
  respiratory tuberculosis Z11.1
  rheumatoid arthritis Z13.828
  rubella Z11.59
  schistosomiasis Z11.6
  sexually-transmitted disease NEC Z11.3
    human immunodeficiency virus
        (HIV) Z11.4
  sickle-cell disease or trait Z13.0
  skin condition Z13.89

Screening (for) - *continued*
  sleeping sickness Z11.6
  special Z13.9
    specified NEC Z13.89
  syphilis Z11.3
  tetanus Z11.2
  trachoma Z11.8
  traumatic brain injury Z13.850
  trypanosomiasis Z11.6
  tuberculosis, respiratory Z11.1
    active Z11.1
    latent Z11.7
  venereal disease Z11.3
  viral encephalitis (mosquito- or tick-
      borne) Z11.59
  whooping cough Z11.2
  worms, intestinal Z11.6
  yaws Z11.8
  yellow fever Z11.59
**Scrofula, scrofulosis (tuberculosis of cervical
    lymph glands)** A18.2
Scrofulide (primary) (tuberculous) A18.4
**Scrofuloderma, scrofulodermia (any site)
    (primary)** A18.4
**Scrofulosus lichen (primary)
    (tuberculous)** A18.4
Scrofulous — *see* condition
Scrotal tongue K14.5
Scrotum — *see* condition
Scurvy, scorbutic E54
  anemia D53.2
  gum E54
  infantile E54
  rickets E55.0 *[M90.80]*
Sealpox B08.62
Seasickness T75.3
Seatworm (infection) (infestation) B80
Sebaceous — *see also* condition
  cyst — *see* Cyst, sebaceous
Seborrhea, seborrheic L21.9
  capillitii R23.8
  capitis L21.0
  dermatitis L21.9
    infantile L21.1
  eczema L21.9
    infantile L21.1
  sicca L21.0
Seckel's syndrome Q87.19
Seclusion, pupil — *see* Membrane, pupillary
**Second hand tobacco smoke exposure
    (acute) (chronic)** Z77.22
  in the perinatal period P96.81
Secondary
  dentin (in pulp) K04.3
  neoplasm, secondaries — *see* Table of
      Neoplasms, secondary
Secretion
  antidiuretic hormone, inappropriate E22.2
  catecholamine, by pheochromocytoma E27.5
  hormone
    antidiuretic, inappropriate
        (syndrome) E22.2
    by
      carcinoid tumor E34.0
      pheochromocytoma E27.5
    ectopic NEC E34.2
  urinary
    excessive R35.8
    suppression R34
Section
  nerve, traumatic — *see* Injury, nerve
Sedative, hypnotic, or anxiolytic-induced
  anxiety disorder F13.980
  bipolar and related disorder F13.94
  delirium F13.921
  depressive disorder F13.94
  major neurocognitive disorder F13.97
  mild neurocognitive disorder F13.988
  psychotic disorder F13.959
  sexual dysfunction F13.981
  sleep disorder F13.982
Segmentation, incomplete (congenital) — *see
    also* Fusion
  bone NEC Q78.8
  lumbosacral (joint) (vertebra) Q76.49

Seitelberger's syndrome (infantile neuraxonal dystrophy) G31.89
Seizure (s) — *see also* Convulsions R56.9
absence G40.A-
akinetic — *see* Epilepsy, generalized, specified NEC
atonic — *see* Epilepsy, generalized, specified NEC
autonomic (hysterical) F44.5
convulsive — *see* Convulsions
cortical (focal) (motor) — *see* Epilepsy, localization-related, symptomatic, with simple partial seizures
disorder — *see also* Epilepsy G40.909
due to stroke — *see* Sequelae (of), disease, cerebrovascular, by type, specified NEC
epileptic — *see* Epilepsy
febrile (simple) R56.00
with status epilepticus G40.901
complex (atypical) (complicated) R56.01
with status epilepticus G40.901
grand mal G40.409
intractable G40.419
with status epilepticus G40.411
without status epilepticus G40.419
not intractable G40.409
with status epilepticus G40.401
without status epilepticus G40.409
heart — *see* Disease, heart
hysterical F44.5
intractable G40.919
with status epilepticus G40.911
Jacksonian (focal) (motor type) (sensory type) — *see* Epilepsy, localization-related, symptomatic, with simple partial seizures
newborn P90
nonspecific epileptic
atonic — *see* Epilepsy, generalized, specified NEC
clonic — *see* Epilepsy, generalized, specified NEC
myoclonic — *see* Epilepsy, generalized, specified NEC
tonic — *see* Epilepsy, generalized, specified NEC
tonic-clonic — *see* Epilepsy, generalized, specified NEC
partial, developing into secondarily generalized seizures
complex — *see* Epilepsy, localization-related, symptomatic, with complex partial seizures
simple — *see* Epilepsy, localization-related, symptomatic, with simple partial seizures
petit mal G40.A-
intractable G40.419
with status epilepticus G40.411
without status epilepticus G40.419
not intractable G40.409
with status epilepticus G40.401
without status epilepticus G40.409
post traumatic R56.1
recurrent G40.909
specified NEC G40.89
uncinate — *see* Epilepsy, localization-related, symptomatic, with complex partial seizures
Selenium deficiency, dietary E59
Self-damaging behavior (life-style) Z72.89
Self-harm (attempted)
history (personal) Z91.5
in family Z81.8
Self-mutilation (attempted)
history (personal) Z91.5
in family Z81.8
Self-poisoning
history (personal) Z91.5
in family Z81.8
observation following (alleged) attempt Z03.6
Semicoma R40.1
Seminal vesiculitis N49.0

Seminoma C62.9-
specified site — *see* Neoplasm, malignant, by site
Senear-Usher disease or syndrome L10.4
Senectus R54
Senescence (without mention of psychosis) R54
Senile, senility — *see also* condition R41.81
with
acute confusional state F05
mental changes NOS F03
psychosis NEC — *see* Psychosis, senile
asthenia R54
cervix (atrophic) N88.8
debility R54
endometrium (atrophic) N85.8
fallopian tube (atrophic) — *see* Atrophy, fallopian tube
heart (failure) R54
ovary (atrophic) — *see* Atrophy, ovary
premature E34.8
vagina, vaginitis (atrophic) N95.2
wart L82.1
Sensation
burning (skin) R20.8
tongue K14.6
loss of R20.8
prickling (skin) R20.2
tingling (skin) R20.2
Sense loss
smell — *see* Disturbance, sensation, smell
taste — *see* Disturbance, sensation, taste
touch R20.8
Sensibility disturbance (cortical) (deep) (vibratory) R20.9
Sensitive, sensitivity — *see also* Allergy
carotid sinus G90.01
child (excessive) F93.8
cold, autoimmune D59.1
dentin K03.89
gluten (non-celiac) K90.41
latex Z91.040
methemoglobin D74.8
tuberculin, without clinical or radiological symptoms R76.11
visual
glare H53.71
impaired contrast H53.72
Sensitiver Beziehungswahn F22
Sensitization, auto-erythrocytic D69.2
Separation
anxiety, abnormal (of childhood) F93.0
apophysis, traumatic - code as Fracture, by site
choroid — *see* Detachment, choroid
epiphysis, epiphyseal
nontraumatic — *see also* Osteochondropathy, specified type NEC
upper femoral — *see* Slipped, epiphysis, upper femoral
traumatic - code as Fracture, by site
fracture — *see* Fracture
infundibulum cardiac from right ventricle by a partition Q24.3
joint (traumatic) (current) - code by site under Dislocation
muscle (nontraumatic) — *see* Diastasis, muscle
pubic bone, obstetrical trauma O71.6
retina, retinal — *see* Detachment, retina
symphysis pubis, obstetrical trauma O71.6
tracheal ring, incomplete, congenital Q32.1
Sepsis (generalized) (unspecified organism) A41.9
with
organ dysfunction (acute) (multiple) R65.20
with septic shock R65.21
actinomycotic A42.7
adrenal hemorrhage syndrome (meningococcal) A39.1
anaerobic A41.4
Bacillus anthracis A22.7
Brucella — *see also* Brucellosis A23.9

Sepsis (generalized) (unspecified organism) - *continued*
candidal B37.7
cryptogenic A41.9
due to device, implant or graft T85.79
arterial graft NEC T82.7
breast (implant) T85.79
catheter NEC T85.79
dialysis (renal) T82.7
intraperitoneal T85.71
infusion NEC T82.7
spinal (cranial) (epidural) (intrathecal) (spinal) (subarachnoid) (subdural) T85.735
urethral indwelling T83.511
urinary T83.518
ectopic or molar pregnancy O08.82
electronic (electrode) (pulse generator) (stimulator)
bone T84.7
cardiac T82.7
nervous system T85.738
brain T85.731
neurostimulator generator T85.734
peripheral nerve T85.732
spinal cord T85.733
urinary T83.590
fixation, internal (orthopedic) — *see* Complication, fixation device, infection
gastrointestinal (bile duct) (esophagus) T85.79
neurostimulator electrode (lead) T85.732
genital T83.69
heart NEC T82.7
valve (prosthesis) T82.6
graft T82.7
joint prosthesis — *see* Complication, joint prosthesis, infection
ocular (corneal graft) (orbital implant) T85.79
orthopedic NEC T84.7
fixation device, internal — *see* Complication, fixation device, infection
specified NEC T85.79
vascular T82.7
ventricular intracranial (communicating) shunt T85.730
during labor O75.3
Enterococcus A41.81
Erysipelothrix (rhusiopathiae) (erysipeloid) A26.7
Escherichia coli (E. coli) A41.5
extraintestinal yersiniosis A28.2
following
abortion (subsequent episode) O08.0
current episode — *see* Abortion
ectopic or molar pregnancy O08.82
immunization T88.0
infusion, therapeutic injection or transfusion NEC T80.29
obstetrical procedure O86.04
gangrenous A41.9
gonococcal A54.86
Gram-negative (organism) A41.5
anaerobic A41.4
Haemophilus influenzae A41.3
herpesviral B00.7
intra-abdominal K65.1
intraocular — *see* Endophthalmitis, purulent
Listeria monocytogenes A32.7
localized - code to specific localized infection
in operation wound T81.49
skin — *see* Abscess
malleus A24.0
melioidosis A24.1
meningeal — *see* Meningitis
meningococcal A39.4
acute A39.2
chronic A39.3
MSSA (Methicillin susceptible Staphylococcus aureus) A41.01
newborn P36.9

Sepsis (generalized) (unspecified organism) - *continued*
  newborn - *continued*
    due to
      anaerobes NEC P36.5
      Escherichia coli P36.4
      Staphylococcus P36.30
        aureus P36.2
        specified NEC P36.39
      Streptococcus P36.10
        group B P36.0
        specified NEC P36.19
      specified NEC P36.8
    Pasteurella multocida A28.0
    pelvic, puerperal, postpartum, childbirth O85
    postprocedural T81.44
    pneumococcal A40.3
    puerperal, postpartum, childbirth
      (pelvic) O85
    Salmonella (arizonae) (cholerae-suis)
      (enteritidis) (typhimurium) A02.1
    severe R65.20
      with septic shock R65.21
    skin, localized — *see* Abscess
    Shigella — *see also* Dysentery,
      bacillary A03.9
    specified organism NEC A41.89
    Staphylococcus, staphylococcal A41.2
      aureus (methicillin susceptible)
        (MSSA) A41.01
        methicillin resistant (MRSA) A41.02
      coagulase-negative A41.1
      specified NEC A41.1
    Streptococcus, streptococcal A40.9
      agalactiae A40.1
      group
        A A40.0
        B A40.1
        D A41.81
      neonatal P36.10
        group B P36.0
        specified NEC P36.19
      pneumoniae A40.3
      pyogenes A40.0
      specified NEC A40.8
    tracheostomy stoma J95.02
    tularemic A21.7
    umbilical, umbilical cord (newborn) — *see*
      Sepsis, newborn
    Yersinia pestis A20.7
Septate — *see* Septum
Septic — *see* condition
  arm — *see* Cellulitis, upper limb
    with lymphangitis — *see* Lymphangitis,
      acute, upper limb
  embolus — *see* Embolism
  finger — *see* Cellulitis, digit
    with lymphangitis — *see* Lymphangitis,
      acute, digit
  foot — *see* Cellulitis, lower limb
    with lymphangitis — *see* Lymphangitis,
      acute, lower limb
  gallbladder (acute) K81.0
  hand — *see* Cellulitis, upper limb
    with lymphangitis — *see* Lymphangitis,
      acute, upper limb
  joint — *see* Arthritis, pyogenic or pyemic
  leg — *see* Cellulitis, lower limb
    with lymphangitis — *see* Lymphangitis,
      acute, lower limb
  nail — *see also* Cellulitis, digit
    with lymphangitis — *see* Lymphangitis,
      acute, digit
  sore — *see also* Abscess
    throat J02.0
      streptococcal J02.0
  spleen (acute) D73.89
  teeth, tooth (pulpal origin) K04.4
  throat — *see* Pharyngitis
  thrombus — *see* Thrombosis
  toe — *see* Cellulitis, digit
    with lymphangitis — *see* Lymphangitis,
      acute, digit
  tonsils, chronic J35.01
    with adenoiditis J35.03

Septic - *continued*
  uterus — *see* Endometritis
Septicemia A41.9
  meaning sepsis — *see* Sepsis
Septum, septate (congenital) — *see also*
  Anomaly, by site
  anal Q42.3
    with fistula Q42.2
  aqueduct of Sylvius Q03.0
    with spina bifida — *see* Spina bifida, by
      site, with hydrocephalus
  uterus Q51.20
    complete Q51.21
    partial Q51.22
    specified NEC Q51.28
  vagina Q52.10
    in pregnancy — *see* Pregnancy,
      complicated by, abnormal vagina
      causing obstructed labor O65.5
    longitudinal Q52.129
      microperforate
        left side Q52.124
        right side Q52.123
      nonobstruction Q52.120
      obstructing Q52.129
        left side Q52.122
        right side Q52.121
    transverse Q52.11
Sequelae (of) — *see also* condition
  abscess, intracranial or intraspinal
    (conditions in G06) G09
  amputation -- code to injury with seventh
    character S
  ·burn and corrosion -- code to injury with
    seventh character S
  calcium deficiency E64.8
  cerebrovascular disease — *see* Sequelae,
    disease, cerebrovascular
  childbirth O94
  contusion -- code to injury with seventh
    character S
  corrosion — *see* Sequelae, burn and
    corrosion
  crushing injury -- code to injury with seventh
    character S
  disease
    cerebrovascular I69.90
      alteration of sensation I69.998
      aphasia I69.920
      apraxia I69.990
      ataxia I69.993
      cognitive deficits I69.91
      disturbance of vision I69.998
      dysarthria I69.922
      dysphagia I69.991
      dysphasia I69.921
      facial droop I69.992
      facial weakness I69.992
      fluency disorder I69.923
      hemiplegia I69.95-
      hemorrhage
        intracerebral — *see* Sequelae,
          hemorrhage, intracerebral
        intracranial, nontraumatic NEC — *see*
          Sequelae, hemorrhage,
          intracranial, nontraumatic
        subarachnoid — *see* Sequelae,
          hemorrhage, subarachnoid
      language deficit I69.928
      monoplegia
        lower limb I69.94-
        upper limb I69.93-
      paralytic syndrome I69.96-
      specified effect NEC I69.998
      specified type NEC I69.80
        alteration of sensation I69.898
        aphasia I69.890
        apraxia I69.890
        ataxia I69.893
        cognitive deficits I69.81
        disturbance of vision I69.898
        dysarthria I69.822
        dysphagia I69.891
        dysphasia I69.821
        facial droop I69.892

Sequelae (of) - *continued*
  disease - *continued*
    cerebrovascular - *continued*
      specified type NEC - *continued*
        facial weakness I69.892
        fluency disorder I69.823
        hemiplegia I69.85-
        language deficit I69.828
        monoplegia
          lower limb I69.84-
          upper limb I69.83-
        paralytic syndrome I69.86-
        specified effect NEC I69.898
        speech deficit I69.928
      speech deficit I69.828
      stroke NOS — *see* Sequelae, stroke
        NOS
  dislocation -- code to injury with seventh
    character S
  encephalitis or encephalomyelitis (conditions
    in G04) G09
    in infectious disease NEC B94.8
    viral B94.1
  external cause -- code to injury with seventh
    character S
  foreign body entering natural orifice -- code
    to injury with seventh character S
  fracture -- code to injury with seventh
    character S
  frostbite -- code to injury with seventh
    character S
  Hansen's disease B92
  hemorrhage
    intracerebral I69.10
      alteration of sensation I69.198
      aphasia I69.120
      apraxia I69.190
      ataxia I69.193
      cognitive deficits I69.11
      disturbance of vision I69.198
      dysarthria I69.122
      dysphagia I69.191
      dysphasia I69.121
      facial droop I69.192
      facial weakness I69.192
      fluency disorder I69.123
      hemiplegia I69.15-
      language deficit NEC I69.128
      monoplegia
        lower limb I69.14-
        upper limb I69.13-
      paralytic syndrome I69.16-
      specified effect NEC I69.198
      speech deficit NEC I69.128
    intracranial, nontraumatic NEC I69.20
      alteration of sensation I69.298
      aphasia I69.220
      apraxia I69.290
      ataxia I69.293
      cognitive deficits I69.21
      disturbance of vision I69.298
      dysarthria I69.222
      dysphagia I69.291
      dysphasia I69.221
      facial droop I69.292
      facial weakness I69.292
      fluency disorder I69.223
      hemiplegia I69.25-
      language deficit NEC I69.228
      monoplegia
        lower limb I69.24-
        upper limb I69.23-
      paralytic syndrome I69.26-
      specified effect NEC I69.298
      speech deficit NEC I69.228
    subarachnoid I69.00
      alteration of sensation I69.098
      aphasia I69.020
      apraxia I69.090
      ataxia I69.093
      cognitive deficits — *see* subcategory
        I69.01-
      disturbance of vision I69.098
      dysarthria I69.022
      dysphagia I69.091

Sequelae (of) - *continued*
  hemorrhage - *continued*
    subarachnoid - *continued*
      dysphasia I69.021
      facial droop I69.092
      facial weakness I69.092
      fluency disorder I69.023
      hemiplegia I69.05-
      language deficit NEC I69.028
      monoplegia
        lower limb I69.04-
        upper limb I69.03-
      paralytic syndrome I69.06-
      specified effect NEC I69.098
      speech deficit NEC I69.028
  hepatitis, viral B94.2
  hyperalimentation E68
  infarction
    cerebral I69.30
      alteration of sensation I69.398
      aphasia I69.320
      apraxia I69.390
      ataxia I69.393
      cognitive deficits I69.31
      disturbance of vision I69.398
      dysarthria I69.322
      dysphagia I69.391
      dysphasia I69.321
      facial droop I69.392
      facial weakness I69.392
      fluency disorder I69.323
      hemiplegia I69.35-
      language deficit NEC I69.328
      monoplegia
        lower limb I69.34-
        upper limb I69.33-
      paralytic syndrome I69.36-
      specified effect NEC I69.398
      speech deficit NEC I69.328
  infection, pyogenic, intracranial or
    intraspinal G09
  infectious disease B94.9
    specified NEC B94.8
  injury -- code to injury with seventh
    character S
  leprosy B92
  meningitis
    bacterial (conditions in G00) G09
    other or unspecified cause (conditions in
      G03) G09
  muscle (and tendon) injury -- code to injury
    with seventh character S
  myelitis — *see* Sequelae, encephalitis
  niacin deficiency E64.8
  nutritional deficiency E64.9
    specified NEC E64.8
  obstetrical condition O94
  parasitic disease B94.9
  phlebitis or thrombophlebitis of intracranial
    or intraspinal venous sinuses and veins
    (conditions in G08) G09
  poisoning -- code to poisoning with seventh
    character S
    nonmedicinal substance — *see* Sequelae,
      toxic effect, nonmedicinal substance
  poliomyelitis (acute) B91
  pregnancy O94
  protein-energy malnutrition E64.0
  puerperium O94
  rickets E64.3
  selenium deficiency E64.8
  sprain and strain -- code to injury with
    seventh character S
  stroke NOS I69.30
    alteration in sensation I69.398
    aphasia I69.320
    apraxia I69.390
    ataxia I69.393
    cognitive deficits I69.31
    disturbance of vision I69.398
    dysarthria I69.322
    dysphagia I69.391
    dysphasia I69.321
    facial droop I69.392
    facial weakness I69.392

Sequelae (of) - *continued*
  stroke NOS - *continued*
    hemiplegia I69.35-
    language deficit NEC I69.328
    monoplegia
      lower limb I69.34-
      upper limb I69.33-
    paralytic syndrome I69.36-
    specified effect NEC I69.398
    speech deficit NEC I69.328
  tendon and muscle injury -- code to injury
    with seventh character S
  thiamine deficiency E64.8
  trachoma B94.0
  tuberculosis B90.9
    bones and joints B90.2
    central nervous system B90.0
    genitourinary B90.1
    pulmonary (respiratory) B90.9
    specified organs NEC B90.8
  viral
    encephalitis B94.1
    hepatitis B94.2
  vitamin deficiency NEC E64.8
    A E64.1
    B E64.8
    C E64.2
  wound, open -- code to injury with seventh
    character S
Sequestration — *see also* Sequestrum
  disk — *see* Displacement, intervertebral disk
  lung, congenital Q33.2
Sequestrum
  bone — *see* Osteomyelitis, chronic
  dental M27.2
  jaw bone M27.2
  orbit — *see* Osteomyelitis, orbit
  sinus (accessory) (nasal) — *see* Sinusitis
Sequoiosis lung or pneumonitis J67.8
Serology for syphilis
  doubtful
    with signs or symptoms - code by site and
      stage under Syphilis
    follow-up of latent syphilis — *see*
      Syphilis, latent
  negative, with signs or symptoms - code by
    site and stage under Syphilis
  positive A53.0
    with signs or symptoms - code by site and
      stage under Syphilis
  reactivated A53.0
Seroma — *see also* Hematoma
  postprocedural — *see* Complication,
    postprocedural, seroma
  traumatic, secondary and recurrent T79.2
Seropurulent — *see* condition
Serositis, multiple K65.8
  pericardial I31.1
  peritoneal K65.8
Serous — *see* condition
Sertoli cell
  adenoma
    specified site — *see* Neoplasm, benign, by
      site
    unspecified site
      female D27.9
      male D29.20
  carcinoma
    specified site — *see* Neoplasm, malignant,
      by site
    unspecified site (male) C62.9-
      female C56.9
  tumor
    with lipid storage
      specified site — *see* Neoplasm, benign,
        by site
      unspecified site
        female D27.9
        male D29.20
    specified site — *see* Neoplasm, benign, by
      site
    unspecified site
      female D27.9
      male D29.20

Sertoli-Leydig cell tumor — *see* Neoplasm,
  benign, by site
  specified site — *see* Neoplasm, benign, by
    site
  unspecified site
    female D27.9
    male D29.20
Serum
  allergy, allergic reaction — *see also*
    Reaction, serum T80.69
    shock — *see also* Shock,
      anaphylactic T80.59
  arthritis — *see also* Reaction, serum T80.69
  complication or reaction NEC — *see also*
    Reaction, serum T80.69
  disease NEC — *see also* Reaction,
    serum T80.69
  hepatitis — *see also* Hepatitis, viral, type B
    carrier (suspected) of B18.1
  intoxication — *see also* Reaction,
    serum T80.69
  neuritis — *see also* Reaction, serum T80.69
  neuropathy G61.1
  poisoning NEC — *see also* Reaction,
    serum T80.69
  rash NEC — *see also* Reaction,
    serum T80.69
  reaction NEC — *see also* Reaction,
    serum T80.69
  sickness NEC — *see also* Reaction,
    serum T80.69
  urticaria — *see also* Reaction, serum T80.69
Sesamoiditis M25.8-
Severe sepsis R65.20
  with septic shock R65.21
Sever's disease or osteochondrosis — *see*
  Osteochondrosis, juvenile, tarsus
Sex
  chromosome mosaics Q97.8
    lines with various numbers of X
      chromosomes Q97.2
  education Z70.8
  reassignment surgery status Z87.890
Sextuplet pregnancy — *see* Pregnancy,
  sextuplet
Sexual
  function, disorder of (psychogenic) F52.9
  immaturity (female) (male) E30.0
  impotence (psychogenic) organic origin
    NEC — *see* Dysfunction, sexual, male
  precocity (constitutional) (cryptogenic)
    (female) (idiopathic) (male) E30.1
Sexuality, pathologic — *see* Deviation, sexual
Sézary disease C84.1-
Shadow, lung R91.8
Shaking palsy or paralysis — *see*
  Parkinsonism
Shallowness, acetabulum — *see*
  Derangement, joint, specified type NEC,
  hip
Shaver's disease J63.1
Sheath (tendon) — *see* condition
Sheathing, retinal vessels H35.01-
Shedding
  nail L60.8
  premature, primary (deciduous) teeth K00.6
Sheehan's disease or syndrome E23.0
Shelf, rectal K62.89
Shell teeth K00.5
Shellshock (current) F43.0
  lasting state — *see* Disorder, post-traumatic
    stress
Shield kidney Q63.1
Shift
  auditory threshold (temporary) H93.24-
  mediastinal R93.89
**Shifting sleep-work schedule (affecting
  sleep)** G47.26
Shiga (-Kruse) dysentery A03.0
Shiga's bacillus A03.0
Shigella (dysentery) — *see* Dysentery,
  bacillary
Shigellosis A03.9
  Group A A03.0
  Group B A03.1

Shigellosis - *continued*
  Group C A03.2
  Group D A03.3
Shin splints S86.89
Shingles — *see* Herpes, zoster
Shipyard disease or eye B30.0
Shirodkar suture, in pregnancy — *see*
  Pregnancy, complicated by, incompetent
  cervix
Shock R57.9
  with ectopic or molar pregnancy O08.3
  adrenal (cortical) (Addisonian) E27.2
  adverse food reaction (anaphylactic) — *see*
    Shock, anaphylactic, due to food
  allergic — *see* Shock, anaphylactic
  anaphylactic T78.2
    chemical — *see* Table of Drugs and
      Chemicals
    due to drug or medicinal substance
      correct substance properly
        administered T88.6
      overdose or wrong substance given or
        taken (by accident) — *see* Table of
        Drugs and Chemicals, by drug,
        poisoning
    due to food (nonpoisonous) T78.00
      additives T78.06
      dairy products T78.07
      eggs T78.08
      fish T78.03
        shellfish T78.02
      fruit T78.04
      milk T78.07
      nuts T78.05
        multiple types T78.05
        peanuts T78.01
      peanuts T78.01
      seeds T78.05
      specified type NEC T78.09
      vegetable T78.04
    following sting (s) — *see* Venom
    immunization T80.52
    serum T80.59
      blood and blood products T80.51
      immunization T80.52
      specified NEC T80.59
      vaccination T80.52
  anaphylactoid — *see* Shock, anaphylactic
  anesthetic
    correct substance properly
      administered T88.2
    overdose or wrong substance given or
      taken — *see* Table of Drugs and
      Chemicals, by drug, poisoning
    specified anesthetic — *see* Table of
      Drugs and Chemicals, by drug,
      poisoning
  cardiogenic R57.0
  chemical substance — *see* Table of Drugs
    and Chemicals
  complicating ectopic or molar
    pregnancy O08.3
  culture — *see* Disorder, adjustment
  drug
    due to correct substance properly
      administered T88.6
    overdose or wrong substance given or
      taken (by accident) — *see* Table of
      Drugs and Chemicals, by drug,
      poisoning
  during or after labor and delivery O75.1
  electric T75.4
    (taser) T75.4
  endotoxic R65.21
    postprocedural (resulting from a
      procedure, not elsewhere
      classified) T81.12
  following
    ectopic or molar pregnancy O08.3
    injury (immediate) (delayed) T79.4
    labor and delivery O75.1
  food (anaphylactic) — *see* Shock,
    anaphylactic, due to food
  from electroshock gun (taser) T75.4
  gram-negative R65.21

Shock - *continued*
  gram-negative - *continued*
    postprocedural (resulting from a
      procedure, not elsewhere
      classified) T81.12
  hematologic R57.8
  hemorrhagic R57.8
    surgery (intraoperative)
      (postoperative) T81.19
    trauma T79.4
  hypovolemic R57.1
    surgical T81.19
    traumatic T79.4
  insulin E15
    therapeutic misadventure — *see*
      subcategory T38.3
  kidney N17.0
    traumatic (following crushing) T79.5
  liver K72.00
  lightning T75.01
  lung J80
  obstetric O75.1
    with ectopic or molar pregnancy O08.3
    following ectopic or molar
      pregnancy O08.3
  pleural (surgical) T81.19
    due to trauma T79.4
  postprocedural (postoperative) T81.10
    with ectopic or molar pregnancy O08.3
    cardiogenic T81.11
    endotoxic T81.12
      following ectopic or molar
        pregnancy O08.3
    gram-negative T81.12
    hypovolemic T81.19
    septic T81.12
    specified type NEC T81.19
  psychic F43.0
  septic (due to severe sepsis) R65.21
  specified NEC R57.8
  surgical T81.10
  taser gun (taser) T75.4
  therapeutic misadventure NEC T81.10
  thyroxin
    overdose or wrong substance given or
      taken — *see* Table of Drugs and
      Chemicals, by drug, poisoning
  toxic, syndrome A48.3
  transfusion — *see* Complications, transfusion
  traumatic (immediate) (delayed) T79.4
Shoemaker's chest M95.4
Short, shortening, shortness
  arm (acquired) — *see also* Deformity, limb,
    unequal length
    congenital Q71.81-
    forearm — *see* Deformity, limb, unequal
      length
  bowel syndrome K91.2
  breath R06.02
  cervical (complicating pregnancy) O26.87-
    non-gravid uterus N88.3
  common bile duct, congenital Q44.5
  cord (umbilical) , complicating
    delivery O69.3
  cystic duct, congenital Q44.5
  esophagus (congenital) Q39.8
  femur (acquired) — *see* Deformity, limb,
    unequal length, femur
    congenital — *see* Defect, reduction, lower
      limb, longitudinal, femur
  frenum, frenulum, linguae
    (congenital) Q38.1
  hip (acquired) — *see also* Deformity, limb,
    unequal length
    congenital Q65.89
  leg (acquired) — *see also* Deformity, limb,
    unequal length
    congenital Q72.81-
    lower leg — *see also* Deformity, limb,
      unequal length
  limbed stature, with
    immunodeficiency D82.2
  lower limb (acquired) — *see also* Deformity,
    limb, unequal length
    congenital Q72.81-

Short, shortening, shortness - *continued*
  organ or site, congenital NEC — *see*
    Distortion
  palate, congenital Q38.5
  radius (acquired) — *see also* Deformity,
    limb, unequal length
    congenital — *see* Defect, reduction, upper
      limb, longitudinal, radius
  rib syndrome Q77.2
  stature (child) (hereditary) (idiopathic)
    NEC R62.52
    constitutional E34.3
    due to endocrine disorder E34.3
    Laron-type E34.3
  tendon — *see also* Contraction, tendon
    with contracture of joint — *see*
      Contraction, joint
    Achilles (acquired) M67.0-
      congenital Q66.89
    congenital Q79.8
  thigh (acquired) — *see also* Deformity, limb,
    unequal length, femur
    congenital — *see* Defect, reduction, lower
      limb, longitudinal, femur
  tibialis anterior (tendon) — *see* Contraction,
    tendon
  umbilical cord
    complicating delivery O69.3
  upper limb, congenital — *see* Defect,
    reduction, upper limb, specified type
    NEC
  urethra N36.8
  uvula, congenital Q38.5
  vagina (congenital) Q52.4
Shortsightedness — *see* Myopia
Shoshin (acute fulminating beriberi) E51.11
Shoulder — *see* condition
Shovel-shaped incisors K00.2
Shower, thromboembolic — *see* Embolism
Shunt
  arterial-venous (dialysis) Z99.2
  arteriovenous, pulmonary (acquired) I28.0
    congenital Q25.72
  cerebral ventricle (communicating) in
    situ Z98.2
  surgical, prosthetic, with complications —
    see Complications, cardiovascular,
    device or implant
Shutdown, renal N28.9
Shy-Drager syndrome G90.3
Sialadenitis, sialadenosis (any gland)
  (chronic) (periodic) (suppurative) — *see*
    Sialoadenitis
Sialectasia K11.8
Sialidosis E77.1
Sialitis, silitis (any gland) (chronic)
  (suppurative) — *see* Sialoadenitis
Sialoadenitis (any gland) (periodic)
  (suppurative) K11.20
    acute K11.21
      recurrent K11.22
    chronic K11.23
Sialoadenopathy K11.9
Sialoangitis — *see* Sialoadenitis
Sialodochitis (fibrinosa) — *see* Sialoadenitis
Sialodocholithiasis K11.5
Sialolithiasis K11.5
Sialometaplasia, necrotizing K11.8
Sialorrhea — *see also* Ptyalism
  periodic — *see* Sialoadenitis
Sialosis K11.7
Siamese twin Q89.4
Sibling rivalry Z62.891
Sicard's syndrome G52.7
Sicca syndrome M35.00
  with
    keratoconjunctivitis M35.01
    lung involvement M35.02
    myopathy M35.03
    renal tubulo-interstitial disorders M35.04
    specified organ involvement NEC M35.09
Sick R69
  or handicapped person in family Z63.79
    needing care at home Z63.6
  sinus (syndrome) I49.5

Sick-euthyroid syndrome E07.81
Sickle-cell
  anemia — *see* Disease, sickle-cell
  trait D57.3
Sicklemia — *see also* Disease, sickle-cell
  trait D57.3
Sickness
  air (travel) T75.3
  airplane T75.3
  alpine T70.29
  altitude T70.20
  Andes T70.29
  aviator's T70.29
  balloon T70.29
  car T75.3
  compressed air T70.3
  decompression T70.3
  green D50.8
  milk — *see* Poisoning, food, noxious
  motion T75.3
  mountain T70.29
    acute D75.1
  protein — *see also* Reaction, serum T80.69
  radiation T66
  roundabout (motion) T75.3
  sea T75.3
  serum NEC — *see also* Reaction,
    serum T80.69
  sleeping (African) B56.9
    by Trypanosoma B56.9
      brucei
        gambiense B56.0
        rhodesiense B56.1
      East African B56.1
      Gambian B56.0
      Rhodesian B56.1
      West African B56.0
  swing (motion) T75.3
  train (railway) (travel) T75.3
  travel (any vehicle) T75.3
Sideropenia — *see* Anemia, iron deficiency
Siderosilicosis J62.8
Siderosis (lung) J63.4
. eye (globe) — *see* Disorder, globe,
    degenerative, siderosis
Siemens' syndrome (ectodermal
    dysplasia) Q82.8
Sighing R06.89
  psychogenic F45.8
Sigmoid — *see also* condition
  flexure — *see* condition
  kidney Q63.1
Sigmoiditis — *see also* Enteritis K52.9
  infectious A09
  noninfectious K52.9
Silfversköld's syndrome Q78.9
Silicosiderosis J62.8
Silicosis, silicotic (simple) (complicated)
    J62.8
  with tuberculosis J65
Silicotuberculosis J65
Silo-fillers' disease J68.8
  bronchitis J68.0
  pneumonitis J68.0
  pulmonary edema J68.1
Silver's syndrome Q87.19
Simian malaria B53.1
Simmonds' cachexia or disease E23.0
Simons' disease or syndrome (progressive
    lipodystrophy) E88.1
Simple, simplex — *see* condition
Simulation, conscious (of illness) Z76.5
Simultanagnosia (asimultagnosia) R48.3
Sin Nombre virus disease (Hantavirus)
    (cardio) -pulmonary syndrome) B33.4
Sinding-Larsen disease or
    osteochondrosis — *see* Osteochondrosis,
    juvenile, patella
Singapore hemorrhagic fever A91
Singer's node or nodule J38.2
Single
  atrium Q21.2
  coronary artery Q24.5
  umbilical artery Q27.0
  ventricle Q20.4

Singultus R06.6
  epidemicus B33.0
Sinus — *see also* Fistula
  abdominal K63.89
  arrest I45.5
  arrhythmia I49.8
  bradycardia R00.1
  branchial cleft (internal) (external) Q18.0
  coccygeal — *see* Sinus, pilonidal
  dental K04.6
  dermal (congenital) Q06.8
    with abscess Q06.8
    coccygeal, pilonidal — *see* Sinus,
      coccygeal
  infected, skin NEC L08.89
  marginal, ruptured or bleeding — *see*
    Hemorrhage, antepartum, specified
    cause NEC
  medial, face and neck Q18.8
  pause I45.5
  pericranii Q01.9
  pilonidal (infected) (rectum) L05.92
    with abscess L05.02
  preauricular Q18.1
  rectovaginal N82.3
  Rokitansky-Aschoff (gallbladder) K82.8
  sacrococcygeal (dermoid) (infected) — *see*
    Sinus, pilonidal
  tachycardia R00.0
    paroxysmal I47.1
  tarsi syndrome M25.57-
  testis N50.89
  tract (postinfective) — *see* Fistula
  urachus Q64.4
Sinusitis (accessory) (chronic) (hyperplastic)
    (nasal) (nonpurulent) (purulent) J32.9
  acute J01.90
    ethmoidal J01.20
      recurrent J01.21
    frontal J01.10
      recurrent J01.11
    involving more than one sinus, other than
      pansinusitis J01.80
      recurrent J01.81
    maxillary J01.00
      recurrent J01.01
    pansinusitis J01.40
      recurrent J01.41
    recurrent J01.91
    specified NEC J01.80
      recurrent J01.81
    sphenoidal J01.30
      recurrent J01.31
  allergic — *see* Rhinitis, allergic
  due to high altitude T70.1
  ethmoidal J32.2
    acute J01.20
      recurrent J01.21
  frontal J32.1
    acute J01.10
      recurrent J01.11
  influenzal — *see* Influenza, with, respiratory
    manifestations NEC
  involving more than one sinus but not
    pansinusitis J32.8
    acute J01.80
      recurrent J01.81
  maxillary J32.0
    acute J01.00
      recurrent J01.01
  sphenoidal J32.3
    acute J01.30
      recurrent J01.31
  tuberculous, any sinus A15.8
Sinusitis-bronchiectasis-situs inversus
    (syndrome) (triad) Q89.3
Sipple's syndrome E31.22
Sirenomelia (syndrome) Q87.2
Siriasis T67.01
Sirkari's disease B55.0
Siti A65
Situation, psychiatric F99
Situational
  disturbance (transient) — *see* Disorder,
    adjustment

Situational - *continued*
  disturbance (transient) - *continued*
    acute F43.0
    maladjustment — *see* Disorder, adjustment
    reaction — *see* Disorder, adjustment
      acute F43.0
Situs inversus or transversus (abdominalis)
    (thoracis) Q89.3
Sixth disease B08.20
  due to human herpesvirus 6 B08.21
  due to human herpesvirus 7 B08.22
Sjögren-Larsson syndrome Q87.19
Sjögren's syndrome or disease — *see* Sicca
    syndrome
Skeletal — *see* condition
Skene's gland — *see* condition
Skenitis — *see* Urethritis
Skerljevo A65
Skevas-Zerfus disease — *see* Toxicity, venom,
    marine animal, sea anemone
Skin — *see also* condition
  clammy R23.1
  donor — *see* Donor, skin
  hidebound M35.9
Slate-dressers' or slate-miners' lung J62.8
Sleep
  apnea — *see* Apnea, sleep
  deprivation Z72.820
  disorder or disturbance G47.9
    child F51.9
    nonorganic origin F51.9
    specified NEC G47.8
  disturbance G47.9
    nonorganic origin F51.9
  drunkenness F51.9
  rhythm inversion G47.2-
  terrors F51.4
  walking F51.3
    hysterical F44.89
Sleep hygiene
  abuse Z72.821
  inadequate Z72.821
  poor Z72.821
Sleeping sickness — *see* Sickness, sleeping
Sleeplessness — *see* Insomnia
  menopausal N95.1
Sleep-wake schedule disorder G47.20
Slim disease (in HIV infection) B20
Slipped, slipping
  epiphysis (traumatic) — *see also*
    Osteochondropathy, specified type
    NEC
    capital femoral (traumatic)
      acute (on chronic) S79.01-
      current traumatic - code as Fracture, by site
    upper femoral (nontraumatic) M93.00-
      acute M93.01-
      on chronic M93.03-
      chronic M93.02-
  intervertebral disc — *see* Displacement,
    intervertebral disc
  ligature, umbilical P51.8
  patella — *see* Disorder, patella, derangement
    NEC
  rib M89.8X8
  sacroiliac joint — *see* subcategory M53.2
  tendon — *see* Disorder, tendon
  ulnar nerve, nontraumatic — *see* Lesion,
    nerve, ulnar
  vertebra NEC — *see* Spondylolisthesis
Slocumb's syndrome E27.0
Sloughing (multiple) (phagedena) (skin) —
    see also Gangrene
  abscess — *see* Abscess
  appendix K38.8
  fascia — *see* Disorder, soft tissue, specified
    type NEC
  scrotum N50.89
  tendon — *see* Disorder, tendon
  transplanted organ — *see* Rejection,
    transplant
  ulcer — *see* Ulcer, skin
Slow
  feeding, newborn P92.2
  flow syndrome, coronary I20.8

Slow - *continued*
  heart (beat) R00.1
Slowing, urinary stream R39.198
Sluder's neuralgia (syndrome) G44.89
Slurred, slurring speech R47.81
Small (ness)
  for gestational age — *see* Small for dates
  introitus, vagina N89.6
  kidney (unknown cause) N27.9
    bilateral N27.1
    unilateral N27.0
  ovary (congenital) Q50.39
  pelvis
    with disproportion (fetopelvic) O33.1
      causing obstructed labor O65.1
  uterus N85.8
  white kidney N03.9
Small-and-light-for-dates — *see* Small for dates
Small-for-dates (infant) P05.10
  with weight of
    499 grams or less P05.11
    500-749 grams P05.12
    750-999 grams P05.13
    1000-1249 grams P05.14
    1250-1499 grams P05.15
    1500-1749 grams P05.16
    1750-1999 grams P05.17
    2000-2499 grams P05.18
    2500 grams and over P05.19
  specified NEC P05.19
Smallpox B03
Smearing, fecal R15.1
Smith-Lemli-Opitz syndrome E78.72
Smith's fracture S52.54-
Smoker — *see* Dependence, drug, nicotine
Smoker's
  bronchitis J41.0
  cough J41.0
  palate K13.24
  throat J31.2
  tongue K13.24
Smoking
  passive Z77.22
Smothering spells R06.81
Snaggle teeth, tooth M26.39
Snapping
  finger — *see* Trigger finger
  hip — *see* Derangement, joint, specified type NEC, hip
    involving the iliotiblial band M76.3-
  knee — *see* Derangement, knee
    involving the iliotiblial band M76.3-
Sneddon-Wilkinson disease or syndrome (sub-corneal pustular dermatosis) L13.1
Sneezing (intractable) R06.7
Sniffing
  cocaine
    abuse — *see* Abuse, drug, cocaine
    dependence — *see* Dependence, drug, cocaine
  gasoline
    abuse — *see* Abuse, drug, inhalant
    dependence — *see* Dependence, drug, inhalant
  glue (airplane)
    abuse — *see* Abuse, drug, inhalant
    drug dependence — *see* Dependence, drug, inhalant
Sniffles
  newborn P28.89
Snoring R06.83
Snow blindness — *see* Photokeratitis
Snuffles (non-syphilitic) R06.5
  newborn P28.89
  syphilitic (infant) A50.05 *[J99]*
Social
  exclusion Z60.4
    due to discrimination or persecution (perceived) Z60.5
  migrant Z59.0
  acculturation difficulty Z60.3
  rejection Z60.4
    due to discrimination or persecution Z60.5
  role conflict NEC Z73.5

Social - *continued*
  skills inadequacy NEC Z73.4
  transplantation Z60.3
Sodoku A25.0
Soemmerring's ring — *see* Cataract, secondary
Soft — *see also* condition
  nails L60.3
Softening
  bone — *see* Osteomalacia
  brain (necrotic) (progressive) G93.89
    congenital Q04.8
    embolic I63.4-
    hemorrhagic — *see* Hemorrhage, intracranial, intracerebral
    occlusive I63.5-
    thrombotic I63.3-
  cartilage M94.2-
    patella M22.4-
  cerebellar — *see* Softening, brain
  cerebral — *see* Softening, brain
  cerebrospinal — *see* Softening, brain
  myocardial, heart — *see* Degeneration, myocardial
  spinal cord G95.89
  stomach K31.89
Soldier's
  heart F45.8
  patches I31.0
Solitary
  cyst, kidney N28.1
  kidney, congenital Q60.0
Solvent abuse — *see* Abuse, drug, inhalant
  dependence — *see* Dependence, drug, inhalant
Somatization reaction, somatic reaction — *see* Disorder, somatoform
Somnambulism F51.3
  hysterical F44.89
Somnolence R40.0
  nonorganic origin F51.11
Sonne dysentery A03.3
Soor B37.0
Sore
  bed — *see* Ulcer, pressure, by site
  chiclero B55.1
  Delhi B55.1
  desert — *see* Ulcer, skin
  eye H57.1-
  Lahore B55.1
  mouth K13.79
    canker K12.0
  muscle M79.10
  Naga — *see* Ulcer, skin
  of skin — *see* Ulcer, skin
  oriental B55.1
  pressure — *see* Ulcer, pressure, by site
  skin L98.9
  soft A57
  throat (acute) — *see also* Pharyngitis
    with influenza, flu, or grippe — *see* Influenza, with, respiratory manifestations NEC
    chronic J31.2
    coxsackie (virus) B08.5
    diphtheritic A36.0
    herpesviral B00.2
    influenzal — *see* Influenza, with, respiratory manifestations NEC
    septic J02.0
    streptococcal (ulcerative) J02.0
    viral NEC J02.8
      coxsackie B08.5
  tropical — *see* Ulcer, skin
  veldt — *see* Ulcer, skin
Soto's syndrome (cerebral gigantism) Q87.3
South African cardiomyopathy syndrome I42.8
Southeast Asian hemorrhagic fever A91
Spacing
  abnormal, tooth, teeth, fully erupted M26.30
  excessive, tooth, fully erupted M26.32
Spade-like hand (congenital) Q68.1
Spading nail L60.8
  congenital Q84.6

Spanish collar N47.1
Sparganosis B70.1
Spasm (s) , spastic, spasticity — *see also* condition R25.2
  accommodation — *see* Spasm, of accommodation
  ampulla of Vater K83.4
  anus, ani (sphincter) (reflex) K59.4
    psychogenic F45.8
  artery I73.9
    cerebral G45.9
  Bell's G51.3-
  bladder (sphincter, external or internal) N32.89
    psychogenic F45.8
  bronchus, bronchiole J98.01
  cardia K22.0
  cardiac I20.1
  carpopedal — *see* Tetany
  cerebral (arteries) (vascular) G45.9
  cervix, complicating delivery O62.4
  ciliary body (of accommodation) — *see* Spasm, of accommodation
  colon — *see also* Irritable, bowel K58.9
    with diarrhea K58.0
    psychogenic F45.8
  common duct K83.8
  compulsive — *see* Tic
  conjugate H51.8
  coronary (artery) I20.1
  diaphragm (reflex) R06.6
    epidemic B33.0
    psychogenic F45.8
  duodenum K59.8
  epidemic diaphragmatic (transient) B33.0
  esophagus (diffuse) K22.4
    psychogenic F45.8
  facial G51.3-
  fallopian tube N83.8
  gastrointestinal (tract) K31.89
    psychogenic F45.8
  glottis J38.5
    hysterical F44.4
    psychogenic F45.8
      conversion reaction F44.4
    reflex through recurrent laryngeal nerve J38.5
  habit — *see* Tic
  heart I20.1
  hemifacial (clonic) G51.3-
  hourglass — *see* Contraction, hourglass
  hysterical F44.4
  infantile — *see* Epilepsy, spasms
  inferior oblique, eye H51.8
  intestinal — *see also* Syndrome, irritable bowel K58.9
    psychogenic F45.8
  larynx, laryngeal J38.5
    hysterical F44.4
    psychogenic F45.8
      conversion reaction F44.4
  levator palpebrae superioris — *see* Disorder, eyelid function
  muscle NEC M62.838
    back M62.830
  nerve, trigeminal G51.0
  nervous F45.8
  nodding F98.4
  occupational F48.8
  oculogyric H51.8
    psychogenic F45.8
  of accommodation H52.53-
  ophthalmic artery — *see* Occlusion, artery, retina
  perineal, female N94.89
  peroneo-extensor — *see also* Deformity, limb, flat foot
  pharynx (reflex) J39.2
    hysterical F45.8
    psychogenic F45.8
  psychogenic F45.8
  pylorus NEC K31.3
    adult hypertrophic K31.89
    congenital or infantile Q40.0
    psychogenic F45.8

Spasm (s) , spastic, spasticity - *continued*
  rectum (sphincter) K59.4
    psychogenic F45.8
  retinal (artery) — *see* Occlusion, artery,
    retina
  sigmoid — *see also* Syndrome, irritable
    bowel K58.9
    psychogenic F45.8
  sphincter of Oddi K83.4
  stomach K31.89
    neurotic F45.8
  throat J39.2
    hysterical F45.8
    psychogenic F45.8
  tic F95.9
    chronic F95.1
    transient of childhood F95.0
  tongue K14.8
  torsion (progressive) G24.1
  trigeminal nerve — *see* Neuralgia, trigeminal
  ureter N13.5
  urethra (sphincter) N35.919
  uterus N85.8
    complicating labor O62.4
  vagina N94.2
    psychogenic F52.5
  vascular I73.9
  vasomotor I73.9
  vein NEC I87.8
  viscera — *see* Pain, abdominal
Spasmodic — *see* condition
Spasmophilia — *see* Tetany
Spasmus nutans F98.4
Spastic, spasticity — *see also* Spasm
  child (cerebral) (congenital)
    (paralysis) G80.1
Speaker's throat R49.8
Specific, specified — *see* condition
Speech
  defect, disorder, disturbance,
    impediment R47.9
    psychogenic, in childhood and
      adolescence F98.8
    slurring R47.81
    specified NEC R47.89
Spencer's disease A08.19
**Spens' syndrome (syncope with heart
  block)** I45.9
Sperm counts (fertility testing) Z31.41
  postvasectomy Z30.8
    reversal Z31.42
Spermatic cord — *see* condition
Spermatocele N43.40
  congenital Q55.4
  multiple N43.42
  single N43.41
Spermatocystitis N49.0
Spermatocytoma C62.9-
  specified site — *see* Neoplasm, malignant,
    by site
Spermatorrhea N50.89
Sphacelus — *see* Gangrene
Sphenoidal — *see* condition
Sphenoiditis (chronic) — *see* Sinusitis,
  sphenoidal
Sphenopalatine ganglion neuralgia G90.09
Sphericity, increased, lens (congenital) Q12.4
**Spherocytosis (congenital) (familial)
  (hereditary)** D58.0
  hemoglobin disease D58.0
  sickle-cell (disease) D57.8-
Spherophakia Q12.4
Sphincter — *see* condition
Sphincteritis, sphincter of Oddi — *see*
  Cholangitis
Sphingolipidosis E75.3
  specified NEC E75.29
Sphingomyelinosis E75.3
Spicule tooth K00.2
Spider
  bite — *see* Toxicity, venom, spider
  fingers — *see* Syndrome, Marfan's
  nevus I78.1
  toes — *see* Syndrome, Marfan's
  vascular I78.1

Spiegler-Fendt
  benign lymphocytoma L98.8
  sarcoid L08.89
Spielmeyer-Vogt disease E75.4
Spina bifida (aperta) Q05.9
  with hydrocephalus NEC Q05.4
  cervical Q05.5
    with hydrocephalus Q05.0
  dorsal Q05.6
    with hydrocephalus Q05.1
  lumbar Q05.7
    with hydrocephalus Q05.2
  lumbosacral Q05.7
    with hydrocephalus Q05.2
  occulta Q76.0
  sacral Q05.8
    with hydrocephalus Q05.3
  thoracic Q05.6
    with hydrocephalus Q05.1
  thoracolumbar Q05.6
    with hydrocephalus Q05.1
Spindle, Krukenberg's — *see* Pigmentation,
  cornea, posterior
Spine, spinal — *see* condition
Spiradenoma (eccrine) — *see* Neoplasm,
  skin, benign
Spirillosis A25.0
Spirillum
  minus A25.0
  obermeieri infection A68.0
Spirochetal — *see* condition
Spirochetosis A69.9
  arthritic, arthritica A69.9
  bronchopulmonary A69.8
  icterohemorrhagic A27.0
  lung A69.8
Spirometrosis B70.1
Spitting blood — *see* Hemoptysis
Splanchnoptosis K63.4
Spleen, splenic — *see* condition
Splenectasis — *see* Splenomegaly
**Splenitis (interstitial) (malignant)
  (nonspecific)** D73.89
  malarial — *see also* Malaria B54 *[D77]*
  tuberculous A18.85
Splenocele D73.89
**Splenomegaly, splenomegalia (Bengal)
  (cryptogenic) (idiopathic) (tropical)**
  R16.1
  with hepatomegaly R16.2
  cirrhotic D73.2
  congenital Q89.09
  congestive, chronic D73.2
  Egyptian B65.1
  Gaucher's E75.22
  malarial — *see also* Malaria B54 *[D77]*
  neutropenic D73.81
  Niemann-Pick — *see* Niemann-Pick disease
    or syndrome
  siderotic D73.2
  syphilitic A52.79
    congenital (early) A50.08 *[D77]*
Splenopathy D73.9
Splenoptosis D73.89
Splenosis D73.89
Splinter — *see* Foreign body, superficial, by
  site
Split, splitting
  foot Q72.7-
  hand Q71.6
  heart sounds R01.2
  lip, congenital — *see* Cleft, lip
  nails L60.3
  urinary stream R39.13
Spondylarthrosis — *see* Spondylosis
Spondylitis (chronic) — *see also*
  Spondylopathy, inflammatory
  ankylopoietica — *see* Spondylitis,
    ankylosing
  ankylosing (chronic) M45.9
    with lung involvement M45.9 *[J99]*
    cervical region M45.2
    cervicothoracic region M45.3
    juvenile M08.1
    lumbar region M45.6

Spondylitis (chronic) - *continued*
  ankylosing (chronic) - *continued*
    lumbosacral region M45.7
    multiple sites M45.0
    occipito-atlanto-axial region M45.1
    sacrococcygeal region M45.8
    thoracic region M45.4
    thoracolumbar region M45.5
  atrophic (ligamentous) — *see* Spondylitis,
    ankylosing
  deformans (chronic) — *see* Spondylosis
  gonococcal A54.41
  gouty — *see also* Gout, by type,
    vertebrae M10.08
  in (due to)
    brucellosis A23.9 *[M49.80]*
      cervical region A23.9 *[M49.82]*
      cervicothoracic region A23.9 *[M49.83]*
      lumbar region A23.9 *[M49.86]*
      lumbosacral region A23.9 *[M49.87]*
      multiple sites A23.9 *[M49.89]*
      occipito-atlanto-axial region A23.9
        [M49.81]
      sacrococcygeal region A23.9 *[M49.88]*
      thoracic region A23.9 *[M49.84]*
      thoracolumbar region A23.9 *[M49.85]*
    enterobacteria (*see also* subcategory
      M49.8) A04.9
    tuberculosis A18.01
  infectious NEC — *see* Spondylopathy,
    infective
  juvenile ankylosing (chronic) M08.1
  Kümmell's — *see* Spondylopathy, traumatic
  Marie-Strümpell — *see* Spondylitis,
    ankylosing
  muscularis — *see* Spondylopathy, specified
    NEC
  psoriatic L40.53
  rheumatoid — *see* Spondylitis, ankylosing
  rhizomelica — *see* Spondylitis, ankylosing
  sacroiliac NEC M46.1
  senescent, senile — *see* Spondylosis
  traumatic (chronic) or post-traumatic — *see*
    Spondylopathy, traumatic
  tuberculous A18.01
  typhosa A01.05
Spondylolisthesis (acquired) (degenerative)
  M43.10
  with disproportion (fetopelvic) O33.0
    causing obstructed labor O65.0
  cervical region M43.12
  cervicothoracic region M43.13
  congenital Q76.2
  lumbar region M43.16
  lumbosacral region M43.17
  multiple sites M43.19
  occipito-atlanto-axial region M43.11
  sacrococcygeal region M43.18
  thoracic region M43.14
  thoracolumbar region M43.15
  traumatic (old) M43.10
    acute
      fifth cervical (displaced) S12.430
        nondisplaced S12.431
        specified type NEC
          (displaced) S12.450
          nondisplaced S12.451
        type III S12.44
      fourth cervical (displaced) S12.330
        nondisplaced S12.331
        specified type NEC
          (displaced) S12.350
          nondisplaced S12.351
        type III S12.34
      second cervical (displaced) S12.130
        nondisplaced S12.131
        specified type NEC
          (displaced) S12.150
          nondisplaced S12.151
        type III S12.14
      seventh cervical (displaced) S12.630
        nondisplaced S12.631
        specified type NEC
          (displaced) S12.650
          nondisplaced S12.651

Spondylolisthesis (acquired) (degenerative) - *continued*
  traumatic (old) - *continued*
    acute - *continued*
      seventh cervical (displaced) - *continued*
        type III S12.64
      sixth cervical (displaced) S12.530
        nondisplaced S12.531
        specified type NEC
          (displaced) S12.550
          nondisplaced S12.551
        type III S12.54
      third cervical (displaced) S12.230
        nondisplaced S12.231
        specified type NEC
          (displaced) S12.250
          nondisplaced S12.251
        type III S12.24
Spondylolysis (acquired) M43.00
  cervical region M43.02
  cervicothoracic region M43.03
  congenital Q76.2
  lumbar region M43.06
  lumbosacral region M43.07
    with disproportion (fetopelvic) O33.0
      causing obstructed labor O65.8
  multiple sites M43.09
  occipito-atlanto-axial region M43.01
  sacrococcygeal region M43.08
  thoracic region M43.04
  thoracolumbar region M43.05
Spondylopathy M48.9
  infective NEC M46.50
    cervical region M46.52
    cervicothoracic region M46.53
    lumbar region M46.56
    lumbosacral region M46.57
    multiple sites M46.59
    occipito-atlanto-axial region M46.51
    sacrococcygeal region M46.58
    thoracic region M46.54
    thoracolumbar region M46.55
  inflammatory M46.90
    cervical region M46.92
    cervicothoracic region M46.93
    lumbar region M46.96
    lumbosacral region M46.97
    multiple sites M46.99
    occipito-atlanto-axial region M46.91
    sacrococcygeal region M46.98
    specified type NEC M46.80
      cervical region M46.82
      cervicothoracic region M46.83
      lumbar region M46.86
      lumbosacral region M46.87
      multiple sites M46.89
      occipito-atlanto-axial region M46.81
      sacrococcygeal region M46.88
      thoracic region M46.84
      thoracolumbar region M46.85
    thoracic region M46.94
    thoracolumbar region M46.95
  neuropathic, in
    syringomyelia and syringobulbia G95.0
    tabes dorsalis A52.11
  specified NEC — *see* subcategory M48.8
  traumatic M48.30
    cervical region M48.32
    cervicothoracic region M48.33
    lumbar region M48.36
    lumbosacral region M48.37
    occipito-atlanto-axial region M48.31
    sacrococcygeal region M48.38
    thoracic region M48.34
    thoracolumbar region M48.35
Spondylosis M47.9
  with
    disproportion (fetopelvic) O33.0
      causing obstructed labor O65.0
    myelopathy NEC M47.10
      cervical region M47.12
      cervicothoracic region M47.13
      lumbar region M47.16
      occipito-atlanto-axial region M47.11
      thoracic region M47.14

Spondylosis - *continued*
  with - *continued*
    myelopathy NEC - *continued*
      thoracolumbar region M47.15
    radiculopathy M47.20
      cervical region M47.22
      cervicothoracic region M47.23
      lumbar region M47.26
      lumbosacral region M47.27
      occipito-atlanto-axial region M47.21
      sacrococcygeal region M47.28
      thoracic region M47.24
      thoracolumbar region M47.25
  specified NEC M47.899
    cervical region M47.892
    cervicothoracic region M47.893
    lumbar region M47.896
    lumbosacral region M47.897
    occipito-atlanto-axial region M47.891
    sacrococcygeal region M47.898
    thoracic region M47.894
    thoracolumbar region M47.895
  traumatic — *see* Spondylopathy, traumatic
  without myelopathy or
    radiculopathy M47.819
    cervical region M47.812
    cervicothoracic region M47.813
    lumbar region M47.816
    lumbosacral region M47.817
    occipito-atlanto-axial region M47.811
    sacrococcygeal region M47.818
    thoracic region M47.814
    thoracolumbar region M47.815
Sponge
  inadvertently left in operation wound — *see*
    Foreign body, accidentally left during a
    procedure
  kidney (medullary) Q61.5
Sponge-diver's disease — *see* Toxicity,
  venom, marine animal, sea anemone
Spongioblastoma (any type) — *see*
  Neoplasm, malignant, by site
  specified site — *see* Neoplasm, malignant,
    by site
  unspecified site C71.9
Spongioneuroblastoma — *see* Neoplasm,
  malignant, by site
Spontaneous — *see also* condition
  fracture (cause unknown) — *see* Fracture,
    pathological
Spoon nail L60.3
  congenital Q84.6
Sporadic — *see* condition
Sporothrix schenckii infection — *see*
  Sporotrichosis
Sporotrichosis B42.9
  arthritis B42.82
  disseminated B42.7
  generalized B42.7
  lymphocutaneous (fixed) (progressive) B42.1
  pulmonary B42.0
  specified NEC B42.89
Spots, spotting (in) (of)
  Bitot's — *see also* Pigmentation, conjunctiva
    in the young child E50.1
    vitamin A deficiency E50.1
  café, au lait L81.3
  Cayenne pepper I78.1
  cotton wool, retina — *see* Occlusion, artery,
    retina
  de Morgan's (senile angiomas) I78.1
  Fuchs' black (myopic) — *see also* Myopia,
    degenerative H44.2-
  intermenstrual (regular) N92.0
    irregular N92.1
  Koplik's B05.9
  liver L81.4
  pregnancy O26.85-
  purpuric R23.3
  ruby I78.1
Spotted fever — *see* Fever, spotted N92.3
Sprain (joint) (ligament)
  acromioclavicular joint or ligament S43.5-
  ankle S93.40-
    calcaneofibular ligament S93.41-

Sprain (joint) (ligament) - *continued*
  ankle - *continued*
    deltoid ligament S93.42-
    internal collateral ligament — *see* Sprain,
      ankle, specified ligament NEC
    specified ligament NEC S93.49-
    talofibular ligament — *see* Sprain, ankle,
      specified ligament NEC
    tibiofibular ligament S93.43-
  anterior longitudinal, cervical S13.4
  atlas, atlanto-axial, atlanto-occipital S13.4
  breast bone — *see* Sprain, sternum
  calcaneofibular — *see* Sprain, ankle
  carpal — *see* Sprain, wrist
  carpometacarpal — *see* Sprain, hand,
    specified site NEC
  cartilage
    costal S23.41
    semilunar (knee) — *see* Sprain, knee,
      specified site NEC
      with current tear — *see* Tear, meniscus
    thyroid region S13.5
    xiphoid — *see* Sprain, sternum
  cervical, cervicodorsal, cervicothoracic S13.4
  chondrosternal S23.421
  coracoclavicular S43.8-
  coracohumeral S43.41-
  coronary, knee — *see* Sprain, knee, specified
    site NEC
  costal cartilage S23.41
  cricoarytenoid articulation or ligament S13.5
  cricothyroid articulation S13.5
  cruciate, knee — *see* Sprain, knee, cruciate
  deltoid, ankle — *see* Sprain, ankle
  dorsal (spine) S23.3
  elbow S53.40-
    radial collateral ligament S53.43-
    radiohumeral S53.41-
    rupture
      radial collateral ligament — *see*
        Rupture, traumatic, ligament, radial
        collateral
      ulnar collateral ligament — *see* Rupture,
        traumatic, ligament, ulnar collateral
    specified type NEC S53.49-
    ulnar collateral ligament S53.44-
    ulnohumeral S53.42-
  femur, head — *see* Sprain, hip
  fibular collateral, knee — *see* Sprain, knee,
    collateral
  fibulocalcaneal — *see* Sprain, ankle
  finger (s) S63.61-
    index S63.61-
    interphalangeal (joint) S63.63-
      index S63.63-
      little S63.63-
      middle S63.63-
      ring S63.63-
    little S63.61-
    middle S63.61-
    ring S63.61-
    metacarpophalangeal (joint) S63.65-
    specified site NEC S63.69-
      index S63.69-
      little S63.69-
      middle S63.69-
      ring S63.69-
  foot S93.60-
    specified ligament NEC S93.69-
    tarsal ligament S93.61-
    tarsometatarsal ligament S93.62-
    toe — *see* Sprain, toe
  hand S63.9-
    finger — *see* Sprain, finger
    specified site NEC — *see* subcategory
      S63.8
    thumb — *see* Sprain, thumb
  head S03.9
  hip S73.10-
    iliofemoral ligament S73.11-
    ischiocapsular (ligament) S73.12-
    specified NEC S73.19-
  iliofemoral — *see* Sprain, hip
  innominate
    acetabulum — *see* Sprain, hip

Sprain (joint) (ligament) - *continued*
  innominate - *continued*
    sacral junction S33.6
  internal
    collateral, ankle — *see* Sprain, ankle
    semilunar cartilage — *see* Sprain, knee,
      specified site NEC
  interphalangeal
    finger — *see* Sprain, finger,
      interphalangeal (joint)
    toe — *see* Sprain, toe, interphalangeal joint
  ischiocapsular — *see* Sprain, hip
  ischiofemoral — *see* Sprain, hip
  jaw (articular disc) (cartilage)
    (meniscus) S03.4-
    old M26.69
  knee S83.9-
    collateral ligament S83.40-
      lateral (fibular) S83.42-
      medial (tibial) S83.41-
    cruciate ligament S83.50-
      anterior S83.51-
      posterior S83.52-
    lateral (fibular) collateral ligament S83.42-
    medial (tibial) collateral ligament S83.41-
    patellar ligament S76.11-
    specified site NEC S83.8X-
    superior tibiofibular joint
      (ligament) S83.6-
  lateral collateral, knee — *see* Sprain, knee,
    collateral
  lumbar (spine) S33.5
  lumbosacral S33.9
  mandible (articular disc) S03.4-
    old M26.69
  medial collateral, knee — *see* Sprain, knee,
    collateral
  meniscus
    jaw S03.4-
      old M26.69
    knee — *see* Sprain, knee, specified site
      NEC
      with current tear — *see* Tear, meniscus
      old — *see* Derangement, knee,
        meniscus, due to old tear
    mandible S03.4-
      old M26.69
  metacarpal (distal) (proximal) — *see* Sprain,
    hand, specified site NEC
  metacarpophalangeal — *see* Sprain, finger,
    metacarpophalangeal (joint)
  metatarsophalangeal — *see* Sprain, toe,
    metatarsophalangeal joint
  midcarpal — *see* Sprain, hand, specified site
    NEC
  midtarsal — *see* Sprain, foot, specified site
    NEC
  neck S13.9
    anterior longitudinal cervical
      ligament S13.4
    atlanto-axial joint S13.4
    atlanto-occipital joint S13.4
    cervical spine S13.4
    cricoarytenoid ligament S13.5
    cricothyroid ligament S13.5
    specified site NEC S13.8
    thyroid region (cartilage) S13.5
  nose S03.8
  orbicular, hip — *see* Sprain, hip
  patella — *see* Sprain, knee, specified site
    NEC
  patellar ligament S76.11-
  pelvis NEC S33.8
  phalanx
    finger — *see* Sprain, finger
    toe — *see* Sprain, toe
  pubofemoral — *see* Sprain, hip
  radiocarpal — *see* Sprain, wrist
  radiohumeral — *see* Sprain, elbow
  radius, collateral — *see* Rupture, traumatic,
    ligament, radial collateral
  rib (cage) S23.41
  rotator cuff (capsule) S43.42-
  sacroiliac (region)
    chronic or old — *see* subcategory M53.2

Sprain (joint) (ligament) - *continued*
  sacroiliac (region) - *continued*
    joint S33.6
  scaphoid (hand) — *see* Sprain, hand,
    specified site NEC
  scapula (r) — *see* Sprain, shoulder girdle,
    specified site NEC
  semilunar cartilage (knee) — *see* Sprain,
    knee, specified site NEC
    with current tear — *see* Tear, meniscus
    old — *see* Derangement, knee,
      meniscus, due to old tear
  shoulder joint S43.40-
    acromioclavicular joint (ligament) — *see*
      Sprain, acromioclavicular joint
    blade — *see* Sprain, shoulder, girdle,
      specified site NEC
    coracoclavicular joint (ligament) — *see*
      Sprain, coracoclavicular joint
    coracohumeral ligament — *see* Sprain,
      coracohumeral joint
    girdle S43.9-
      specified site NEC S43.8-
    rotator cuff — *see* Sprain, rotator cuff
    specified site NEC S43.49-
    sternoclavicular joint (ligament) — *see*
      Sprain, sternoclavicular joint
  spine
    cervical S13.4
    lumbar S33.5
    thoracic S23.3
  sternoclavicular joint S43.6-
  sternum S23.429
    chondrosternal joint S23.421
    specified site NEC S23.428
    sternoclavicular (joint) (ligament) S23.420
  symphysis
    jaw S03.4-
      old M26.69
    mandibular S03.4-
      old M26.69
  talofibular — *see* Sprain, ankle
  tarsal — *see* Sprain, foot, specified site NEC
  tarsometatarsal — *see* Sprain, foot, specified
    site NEC
  temporomandibular S03.4-
    old M26.69
  thorax S23.9
    ribs S23.41
    specified site NEC S23.8
    spine S23.3
    sternum — *see* Sprain, sternum
  thumb S63.60-
    interphalangeal (joint) S63.62-
    metacarpophalangeal (joint) S63.64-
    specified site NEC S63.68-
  thyroid cartilage or region S13.5
  tibia (proximal end) — *see* Sprain, knee,
    specified site NEC
  tibial collateral, knee — *see* Sprain, knee,
    collateral
  tibiofibular
    distal — *see* Sprain, ankle
    superior — *see* Sprain, knee, specified site
      NEC
  toe (s) S93.50-
    great S93.50-
    interphalangeal joint S93.51-
      great S93.51-
      lesser S93.51-
    lesser S93.50-
    metatarsophalangeal joint S93.52-
      great S93.52-
      lesser S93.52-
  ulna, collateral — *see* Rupture, traumatic,
    ligament, ulnar collateral
  ulnohumeral — *see* Sprain, elbow
  wrist S63.50-
    carpal S63.51-
    radiocarpal S63.52-
    specified site NEC S63.59-
  xiphoid cartilage — *see* Sprain, sternum
Sprengel's deformity (congenital) Q74.0
Sprue (tropical) K90.1
  celiac K90.0

Sprue (tropical) - *continued*
  idiopathic K90.49
  meaning thrush B37.0
  nontropical K90.0
Spur, bone — *see also* Enthesopathy
  calcaneal M77.3-
  iliac crest M76.2-
  nose (septum) J34.89
Spurway's syndrome Q78.0
Sputum
  abnormal (amount) (color) (odor)
    (purulent) R09.3
  blood-stained R04.2
  excessive (cause unknown) R09.3
Squamous — *see also* condition
  epithelium in
    cervical canal (congenital) Q51.828
    uterine mucosa (congenital) Q51.818
Squashed nose M95.0
  congenital Q67.4
Squeeze, diver's T70.3
Squint — *see also* Strabismus
  accommodative — *see* Strabismus,
    convergent concomitant
**SSADHD (succinic semialdehyde
  dehydrogenase deficiency)** E72.81
St. Hubert's disease A82.9
Stab — *see also* Laceration
  internal organs — *see* Injury, by site
Stafne's cyst or cavity M27.0
Staggering gait R26.0
  hysterical F44.4
Staghorn calculus — *see* Calculus, kidney
Stähli's line (cornea) (pigment) — *see*
  Pigmentation, cornea, anterior
Stain, staining
  meconium (newborn) P96.83
  port wine Q82.5
  tooth, teeth (hard tissues) (extrinsic) K03.6
    due to
      accretions K03.6
      deposits (betel) (black) (green) (materia
        alba) (orange) (soft)
        (tobacco) K03.6
      metals (copper) (silver) K03.7
      nicotine K03.6
      pulpal bleeding K03.7
      tobacco K03.6
    intrinsic K00.8
Stammering — *see also* Disorder,
  fluency F80.81
Standstill
  auricular I45.5
  cardiac — *see* Arrest, cardiac
  sinoatrial I45.5
  ventricular — *see* Arrest, cardiac
Stannosis J63.5
Stanton's disease — *see* Melioidosis
**Staphylitis (acute) (catarrhal) (chronic)
  (gangrenous) (membranous)
  (suppurative) (ulcerative)** K12.2
Staphylococcal scalded skin syndrome L00
Staphylococcemia A41.2
Staphylococcus, staphylococcal — *see also*
  condition
  as cause of disease classified
    elsewhere B95.8
    aureus (methicillin susceptible)
      (MSSA) B95.61
      methicillin resistant (MRSA) B95.62
    specified NEC, as cause of disease classified
      elsewhere B95.7
Staphyloma (sclera)
  cornea H18.72-
  equatorial H15.81-
  localized (anterior) H15.82-
  posticum H15.83-
  ring H15.85-
Stargardt's disease — *see* Dystrophy, retina
Starvation (inanition) (due to lack of food)
  T73.0
  edema — *see* Malnutrition, severe
Stasis
  bile (noncalculous) K83.1
  bronchus J98.09

Stasis - *continued*
  bronchus - *continued*
    with infection — *see* Bronchitis
  cardiac — *see* Failure, heart, congestive
  cecum K59.8
  colon K59.8
  dermatitis I87.2
    with
        varicose ulcer — *see* Varix, leg, with
            ulcer, with inflammation
        varicose veins — *see* Varix, leg, with,
            inflammation
        due to postthrombotic syndrome — *see*
            Syndrome, postthrombotic
  duodenal K31.5
  eczema — *see* Varix, leg, with, inflammation
  edema — *see* Hypertension, venous
        (chronic), idiopathic
  foot T69.0-
  ileocecal coil K59.8
  ileum K59.8
  intestinal K59.8
  jejunum K59.8
  kidney N19
  liver (cirrhotic) K76.1
  lymphatic I89.8
  pneumonia J18.2
  pulmonary — *see* Edema, lung
  rectal K59.8
  renal N19
    tubular N17.0
  ulcer — *see* Varix, leg, with, ulcer
        without varicose veins I87.2
  urine — *see* Retention, urine
  venous I87.8
State (of)
  affective and paranoid, mixed, organic
        psychotic F06.8
  agitated R45.1
    acute reaction to stress F43.0
  anxiety (neurotic) F41.1
  apprehension F41.1
  burn-out Z73.0
  climacteric, female Z78.0
    symptomatic N95.1
  compulsive F42.8
    mixed with obsessional thoughts F42.2
  confusional (psychogenic) F44.89
    acute — *see also* Delirium
        with
            arteriosclerotic dementia F01.50
                with behavioral disturbance F01.51
            senility or dementia F05
        alcoholic F10.231
        epileptic F05
        reactive (from emotional stress,
            psychological trauma) F44.89
    subacute — *see* Delirium
  convulsive — *see* Convulsions
  crisis F43.0
  depressive F32.9
    neurotic F34.1
  dissociative F44.9
  emotional shock (stress) R45.7
  hypercoagulation — *see* Hypercoagulable
  locked-in G83.5
  menopausal Z78.0
    symptomatic N95.1
  neurotic F48.9
    with depersonalization F48.1
  obsessional F42.8
  oneiroid (schizophrenia-like) F23
  organic
    hallucinatory (nonalcoholic) F06.0
    paranoid (-hallucinatory) F06.2
  panic F41.0
  paranoid F22
    climacteric F22
    involutional F22
    menopausal F22
    organic F06.2
    senile F03
    simple F22
  persistent vegetative R40.3
  phobic F40.9

State (of) - *continued*
  postleukotomy F07.0
  pregnant
    gestational carrier Z33.3
    incidental Z33.1
  psychogenic, twilight F44.89
  psychopathic (constitutional) F60.2
  psychotic, organic — *see also* Psychosis,
        organic
    mixed paranoid and affective F06.8
    senile or presenile F03
    transient NEC F06.8
        with
            hallucinations F06.0
            depression F06.31
  residual schizophrenic F20.5
  restlessness R45.1
  stress (emotional) R45.7
  tension (mental) F48.9
    specified NEC F48.8
  transient organic psychotic NEC F06.8
    depressive type F06.31
    hallucinatory type F06.0
  twilight
    epileptic F05
    psychogenic F44.89
  vegetative, persistent R40.3
  vital exhaustion Z73.0
  withdrawal, — *see* Withdrawal, state
Status (post) — *see also* Presence (of)
  absence, epileptic — *see* Epilepsy, by type,
        with status epilepticus
  administration of tPA (rtPA) in a different
        facility within the last 24 hours prior to
        admission to current facility Z92.82
  adrenalectomy (unilateral) (bilateral) E89.6
  anastomosis Z98.0
  angioplasty (peripheral) Z98.62
    with implant Z95.820
    coronary artery Z98.61
        with implant Z95.5
  anginosus I20.9
  aortocoronary bypass Z95.1
  arthrodesis Z98.1
  artificial opening (of) Z93.9
    gastrointestinal tract Z93.4
    specified NEC Z93.8
    urinary tract Z93.6
    vagina Z93.8
  asthmaticus — *see* Asthma, by type, with
        status asthmaticus
  awaiting organ transplant Z76.82
  bariatric surgery Z98.84
  bed confinement Z74.01
  bleb, filtering (vitreous) , after glaucoma
        surgery Z98.83
  breast implant Z98.82
    removal Z98.86
  cataract extraction Z98.4-
  cholecystectomy Z90.49
  clitorectomy N90.811
    with excision of labia minora N90.812
  colectomy (complete) (partial) Z90.49
  colonization — *see* Carrier (suspected) of
  colostomy Z93.3
  convulsivus idiopathicus — *see* Epilepsy, by
        type, with status epilepticus
  coronary artery angioplasty — *see* Status,
        angioplasty, coronary artery
  coronary artery bypass graft Z95.1
  cystectomy (urinary bladder) Z90.6
  cystostomy Z93.50
    appendico-vesicostomy Z93.52
    cutaneous Z93.51
    specified NEC Z93.59
  delinquent immunization Z28.3
  dental Z98.818
    crown Z98.811
    fillings Z98.811
    restoration Z98.811
    sealant Z98.810
    specified NEC Z98.818
  deployment (current) (military) Z56.82
  dialysis (hemodialysis) (peritoneal) Z99.2
  do not resuscitate (DNR) Z66

Status (post) - *continued*
  donor — *see* Donor
  embedded fragments — *see* Retained,
        foreign body fragments (type of)
  embedded splinter — *see* Retained, foreign
        body fragments (type of)
  enterostomy Z93.4
  epileptic, epilepticus — *see also* Epilepsy, by
        type, with status epilepticus G40.901
  estrogen receptor
    negative Z17.1
    positive Z17.0
  female genital cutting — *see* Female genital
        mutilation status
  female genital mutilation — *see* Female
        genital mutilation status
  filtering (vitreous) bleb after glaucoma
        surgery Z98.83
  gastrectomy (complete) (partial) Z90.3
  gastric banding Z98.84
  gastric bypass for obesity Z98.84
  gastrostomy Z93.1
  human immunodeficiency virus (HIV)
        infection, asymptomatic Z21
  hysterectomy (complete) (total) Z90.710
    partial (with remaining cervial
        stump) Z90.711
  ileostomy Z93.2
  implant
    breast Z98.82
  infibulation N90.813
  intestinal bypass Z98.0
  jejunostomy Z93.4
  laryngectomy Z90.02
  lapsed immunization schedule Z28.3
  lymphaticus E32.8
  malignancy
    castrate resistant prostate Z19.2
    hormone resistant Z19.2
    hormone sensitive Z19.1
  marmoratus G80.3
  mastectomy (unilateral) (bilateral) Z90.1-
  military deployment status (current) Z56.82
    in theater or in support of military war,
        peacekeeping and humanitarian
        operations Z56.82
  nephrectomy (unilateral) (bilateral) Z90.5
  nephrostomy Z93.6
  obesity surgery Z98.84
  oophorectomy
    bilateral Z90.722
    unilateral Z90.721
  organ replacement
    by artificial or mechanical device or
        prosthesis of
        artery Z95.828
        bladder Z96.0
        blood vessel Z95.828
        breast Z97.8
        eye globe Z97.0
        heart Z95.812
            valve Z95.2
        intestine Z97.8
        joint Z96.60
            hip — *see* Presence, hip joint implant
            knee — *see* Presence, knee joint
                implant
            specified site NEC Z96.698
        kidney Z97.8
        larynx Z96.3
        lens Z96.1
        limbs — *see* Presence, artificial, limb
        liver Z97.8
        lung Z97.8
        pancreas Z97.8
    by organ transplant (heterologous)
        (homologous) — *see* Transplant
  pacemaker
    brain Z96.89
    cardiac Z95.0
    specified NEC Z96.89
  pancreatectomy Z90.410
    complete Z90.410
    partial Z90.411
    total Z90.410

Status (post) - *continued*
  physical restraint Z78.1
  pneumonectomy (complete) (partial) Z90.2
  pneumothorax, therapeutic Z98.3
  postcommotio cerebri F07.81
  postoperative (postprocedural) NEC Z98.890
    breast implant Z98.82
    dental Z98.818
      crown Z98.811
      fillings Z98.811
      restoration Z98.811
      sealant Z98.810
      specified NEC Z98.818
    uterine scar Z98.891
    pneumothorax, therapeutic Z98.3
  postpartum (routine follow-up) Z39.2
    care immediately after delivery Z39.0
  postsurgical (postprocedural) NEC Z98.890
    pneumothorax, therapeutic Z98.3
  pregnancy, incidental Z33.1
  prosthesis coronary angioplasty Z95.5
  pseudophakia Z96.1
  renal dialysis (hemodialysis)
    (peritoneal) Z99.2
  retained foreign body — *see* Retained,
    foreign body fragments (type of)
  reversed jejunal transposition (for
    bypass) Z98.0
  salpingo-oophorectomy
    bilateral Z90.722
    unilateral Z90.721
  sex reassignment surgery status Z87.890
  shunt
    arteriovenous (for dialysis) Z99.2
    cerebrospinal fluid Z98.2
    ventricular (communicating) (for
      drainage) Z98.2
  splenectomy Z90.81
  thymicolymphaticus E32.8
  thymicus E32.8
  thymolymphaticus E32.8
  thyroidectomy (hypothyroidism) E89.0
  tooth (teeth) extraction — *see also* Absence,
    teeth, acquired K08.409
  tPA (rtPA) administration in a different
    facility within the last 24 hours prior to
    admission to current facility Z92.82
  tracheostomy Z93.0
  transplant — *see* Transplant
    organ removed Z98.85
  tubal ligation Z98.51
  underimmunization Z28.3
  ureterostomy Z93.6
  urethrostomy Z93.6
  vagina, artificial Z93.8
  vasectomy Z98.52
  wheelchair confinement Z99.3
Stealing
  child problem F91.8
  in company with others Z72.810
  pathological (compulsive) F63.2
Steam burn — *see* Burn
Steatocystoma multiplex L72.2
Steatohepatitis (nonalcoholic)
  (NASH) K75.81
Steatoma L72.3
  eyelid (cystic) — *see* Dermatosis, eyelid
  infected — *see* Hordeolum
Steatorrhea (chronic) K90.9
  with lacteal obstruction K90.2
  idiopathic (adult) (infantile) K90.9
  pancreatic K90.3
  primary K90.0
  tropical K90.1
Steatosis E88.89
  heart — *see* Degeneration, myocardial
  kidney N28.89
  liver NEC K76.0
Steele-Richardson-Olszewski disease or
  syndrome G23.1
Steinbrocker's syndrome G90.8
Steinert's disease G71.11
Stein-Leventhal syndrome E28.2
Stein's syndrome E28.2

STEMI — *see also* - Infarct, myocardium, ST
  elevation I21.3
Stenocardia I20.8
Stenocephaly Q75.8
Stenosis, stenotic (cicatricial) — *see also*
  Stricture
  ampulla of Vater K83.1
  anus, anal (canal) (sphincter) K62.4
    and rectum K62.4
    congenital Q42.3
      with fistula Q42.2
  aorta (ascending) (supraventricular)
    (congenital) Q25.1
    arteriosclerotic I70.0
    calcified I70.0
    supravalvular Q25.3
  aortic (valve) I35.0
    with insufficiency I35.2
    congenital Q23.0
    rheumatic I06.0
      with
        incompetency, insufficiency or
          regurgitation I06.2
          with mitral (valve) disease I08.0
            with tricuspid (valve)
              disease I08.3
        mitral (valve) disease I08.0
          with tricuspid (valve) disease I08.3
        tricuspid (valve) disease I08.2
          with mitral (valve) disease I08.3
    specified cause NEC I35.0
    syphilitic A52.03
  aqueduct of Sylvius (congenital) Q03.0
    with spina bifida — *see* Spina bifida, by
      site, with hydrocephalus
    acquired G91.1
  artery NEC — *see also* Arteriosclerosis I77.1
    celiac I77.4
    cerebral — *see* Occlusion, artery, cerebral
    extremities — *see* Arteriosclerosis,
      extremities
    precerebral — *see* Occlusion, artery,
      precerebral
    pulmonary (congenital) Q25.6
      acquired I28.8
    renal I70.1
    stent
      coronary T82.855
      peripheral T82.856
  bile duct (common) (hepatic) K83.1
    congenital Q44.3
  bladder-neck (acquired) N32.0
    congenital Q64.31
  brain G93.89
  bronchus J98.09
    congenital Q32.3
    syphilitic A52.72
  cardia (stomach) K22.2
    congenital Q39.3
  cardiovascular — *see* Disease,
    cardiovascular
  caudal M48.08
  cervix, cervical (canal) N88.2
    congenital Q51.828
    in pregnancy or childbirth — *see*
      Pregnancy, complicated by, abnormal
      cervix
  colon — *see also* Obstruction, intestine
    congenital Q42.9
      specified NEC Q42.8
  colostomy K94.03
  common (bile) duct K83.1
    congenital Q44.3
  coronary (artery) — *see* Disease, heart,
    ischemic, atherosclerotic
  cystic duct — *see* Obstruction, gallbladder
  due to presence of device, implant or
    graft — *see also* Complications, by site
    and type, specified NEC T85.858
    arterial graft NEC T82.858
    breast (implant) T85.858
    catheter T85.858
      dialysis (renal) T82.858
        intraperitoneal T85.858
      infusion NEC T82.858

Stenosis, stenotic (cicatricial) - *continued*
  due to presence of device, implant or graft -
    continued
    catheter - *continued*
      infusion NEC - *continued*
        spinal (epidural) (subdural) T85.850
      urinary (indwelling) T83.85
    fixation, internal (orthopedic) NEC T84.85
    gastrointestinal (bile duct)
      (esophagus) T85.858
    genital NEC T83.85
    heart NEC T82.857
    joint prosthesis T84.85
    ocular (corneal graft) (orbital implant)
      NEC T85.858
    orthopedic NEC T84.85
    specified NEC T85.858
    urinary NEC T83.85
    vascular NEC T82.858
    ventricular intracranial shunt T85.850
  duodenum K31.5
    congenital Q41.0
  ejaculatory duct NEC N50.89
  endocervical os — *see* Stenosis, cervix
  enterostomy K94.13
  esophagus K22.2
    congenital Q39.3
    syphilitic A52.79
      congenital A50.59 *[K23]*
  eustachian tube — *see* Obstruction,
    eustachian tube
  external ear canal (acquired) H61.30-
    congenital Q16.1
    due to
      inflammation H61.32-
      trauma H61.31-
    postprocedural H95.81-
    specified cause NEC H61.39-
  gallbladder — *see* Obstruction, gallbladder
  glottis J38.6
  heart valve (congenital) Q24.8
    aortic Q23.0
    mitral Q23.2
    pulmonary Q22.1
    tricuspid Q22.4
  hepatic duct K83.1
  hymen N89.6
  hypertrophic subaortic (idiopathic) I42.1
  ileum — *see also* Obstruction, intestine,
    specified NEC K56.699
    congenital Q41.2
  infundibulum cardia Q24.3
  intervertebral foramina — *see also* Lesion,
    biomechanical, specified NEC
    connective tissue M99.79
      abdomen M99.79
      cervical region M99.71
      cervicothoracic M99.71
      head region M99.70
      lumbar region M99.73
      lumbosacral M99.73
      occipitocervical M99.70
      sacral region M99.74
      sacrococcygeal M99.74
      sacroiliac M99.74
      specified NEC M99.79
      thoracic region M99.72
      thoracolumbar M99.72
    disc M99.79
      abdomen M99.79
      cervical region M99.71
      cervicothoracic M99.71
      head region M99.70
      lower extremity M99.76
      lumbar region M99.73
      lumbosacral M99.73
      occipitocervical M99.70
      pelvic M99.75
      rib cage M99.78
      sacral region M99.74
      sacrococcygeal M99.74
      sacroiliac M99.74
      specified NEC M99.79
      thoracic region M99.72
      thoracolumbar M99.72

Stenosis, stenotic (cicatricial) - *continued*
  intervertebral foramina - *continued*
    disc - *continued*
      upper extremity M99.77
    osseous M99.69
      abdomen M99.69
      cervical region M99.61
      cervicothoracic M99.61
      head region M99.60
      lower extremity M99.66
      lumbar region M99.63
      lumbosacral M99.63
      occipitocervical M99.60
      pelvic M99.65
      rib cage M99.68
      sacral region M99.64
      sacrococcygeal M99.64
      sacroiliac M99.64
      specified NEC M99.69
      thoracic region M99.62
      thoracolumbar M99.62
      upper extremity M99.67
    subluxation — *see* Stenosis, intervertebral
        foramina, osseous
  intestine — *see also* Obstruction, intestine
    congenital (small) Q41.9
      large Q42.9
        specified NEC Q42.8
      specified NEC Q41.8
  jejunum — *see also* Obstruction, intestine,
      specified NEC K56.699
    congenital Q41.1
  lacrimal (passage)
    canaliculi H04.54-
    congenital Q10.5
    duct H04.55-
    punctum H04.56-
    sac H04.57-
  lacrimonasal duct — *see* Stenosis, lacrimal,
      duct
    congenital Q10.5
  larynx J38.6
    congenital NEC Q31.8
      subglottic Q31.1
    syphilitic A52.73
      congenital A50.59 *[J99]*
  mitral (chronic) (inactive) (valve) I05.0
    with
      aortic valve disease I08.0
      incompetency, insufficiency or
          regurgitation I05.2
    active or acute I01.1
      with rheumatic or Sydenham's
          chorea I02.0
    congenital Q23.2
    specified cause, except rheumatic I34.2
    syphilitic A52.03
  myocardium, myocardial — *see also*
      Degeneration, myocardial
    hypertrophic subaortic (idiopathic) I42.1
  nares (anterior) (posterior) J34.89
    congenital Q30.0
  nasal duct — *see also* Stenosis, lacrimal,
      duct
    congenital Q10.5
  nasolacrimal duct — *see also* Stenosis,
      lacrimal, duct
    congenital Q10.5
  neural canal — *see also* Lesion,
      biomechanical, specified NEC
    connective tissue M99.49
      abdomen M99.49
      cervical region M99.41
      cervicothoracic M99.41
      head region M99.40
      lower extremity M99.46
      lumbar region M99.43
      lumbosacral M99.43
      occipitocervical M99.40
      pelvic M99.45
      rib cage M99.48
      sacral region M99.44
      sacrococcygeal M99.44
      sacroiliac M99.44
      specified NEC M99.49

Stenosis, stenotic (cicatricial) - *continued*
  neural canal - *continued*
    connective tissue - *continued*
      thoracic region M99.42
      thoracolumbar M99.42
      upper extremity M99.47
    intervertebral disc M99.59
      abdomen M99.59
      cervical region M99.51
      cervicothoracic M99.51
      head region M99.50
      lower extremity M99.56
      lumbar region M99.53
      lumbosacral M99.53
      occipitocervical M99.50
      pelvic M99.55
      rib cage M99.58
      sacral region M99.54
      sacrococcygeal M99.54
      sacroiliac M99.54
      specified NEC M99.59
      thoracic region M99.52
      thoracolumbar M99.52
      upper extremity M99.57
    osseous M99.39
      abdomen M99.39
      cervical region M99.31
      cervicothoracic M99.31
      head region M99.30
      lower extremity M99.36
      lumbar region M99.33
      lumbosacral M99.33
      pelvic M99.35
      rib cage M99.38
      occipitocervical M99.30
      sacral region M99.34
      sacrococcygeal M99.34
      sacroiliac M99.34
      specified NEC M99.39
      thoracic region M99.32
      thoracolumbar M99.32
      upper extremity M99.37
    subluxation M99.29
      cervical region M99.21
      cervicothoracic M99.21
      head region M99.20
      lower extremity M99.26
      lumbar region M99.23
      lumbosacral M99.23
      occipitocervical M99.20
      pelvic M99.25
      rib cage M99.28
      sacral region M99.24
      sacrococcygeal M99.24
      sacroiliac M99.24
      specified NEC M99.29
      thoracic region M99.22
      thoracolumbar M99.22
      upper extremity M99.27
  organ or site, congenital NEC — *see* Atresia,
      by site
  papilla of Vater K83.1
  pulmonary (artery) (congenital) Q25.6
    with ventricular septal defect, transposition
        of aorta, and hypertrophy of right
        ventricle Q21.3
    acquired I28.8
    in tetralogy of Fallot Q21.3
    infundibular Q24.3
    subvalvular Q24.3
    supravalvular Q25.6
    valve I37.0
      with insufficiency I37.2
      congenital Q22.1
      rheumatic I09.89
        with aortic, mitral or tricuspid (valve)
            disease I08.8
    vein, acquired I28.8
    vessel NEC I28.8
  pulmonic (congenital) Q22.1
    infundibular Q24.3
    subvalvular Q24.3
  pylorus (hypertrophic) (acquired) K31.1
    adult K31.1
    congenital Q40.0

Stenosis, stenotic (cicatricial) - *continued*
  pylorus (hypertrophic) (acquired) - *continued*
    infantile Q40.0
  rectum (sphincter) — *see* Stricture, rectum
  renal artery I70.1
    congenital Q27.1
  salivary duct (any) K11.8
  sphincter of Oddi K83.1
  spinal M48.00
    cervical region M48.02
    cervicothoracic region M48.03
    lumbar region (NOS) (without neurogenic
        claudication) M48.061
      with neurogenic claudication M48.062
    lumbosacral region M48.07
    occipito-atlanto-axial region M48.01
    sacrococcygeal region M48.08
    thoracic region M48.04
    thoracolumbar region M48.05
  stent
    vascular
      end stent
        adjacent to stent — *see*
            Arteriosclerosis
        within the stent
          coronary T82.855
          peripheral T82.856
      in stent
        coronary vessel T82.855
        peripheral vessel T82.856
  stomach, hourglass K31.2
  subaortic (congenital) Q24.4
    hypertrophic (idiopathic) I42.1
  subglottic J38.6
    congenital Q31.1
    postprocedural J95.5
  trachea J39.8
    congenital Q32.1
    syphilitic A52.73
    tuberculous NEC A15.5
  tracheostomy J95.03
  tricuspid (valve) I07.0
    with
      aortic (valve) disease I08.2
      incompetency, insufficiency or
          regurgitation I07.2
        with aortic (valve) disease I08.2
          with mitral (valve) disease I08.3
      mitral (valve) disease I08.1
        with aortic (valve) disease I08.3
    congenital Q22.4
    nonrheumatic I36.0
      with insufficiency I36.2
  tubal N97.1
  ureter — *see* Atresia, ureter
  ureteropelvic junction, congenital Q62.11
  ureterovesical orifice, congenital Q62.12
  urethra (valve) — *see also* Stricture, urethra
    congenital Q64.32
  urinary meatus, congenital Q64.33
  vagina N89.5
    congenital Q52.4
    in pregnancy — *see* Pregnancy,
        complicated by, abnormal vagina
        causing obstructed labor O65.5
  valve (cardiac) (heart) — *see also*
      Endocarditis I38
    congenital Q24.8
      aortic Q23.0
      mitral Q23.2
      pulmonary Q22.1
      tricuspid Q22.4
  vena cava (inferior) (superior) I87.1
    congenital Q26.0
  vesicourethral orifice Q64.31
  vulva N90.5
Stent jail T82.897
Stercolith (impaction) K56.41
  appendix K38.1
Stercoraceous, stercoral ulcer K63.3
  anus or rectum K62.6
Stereotypies NEC F98.4
Sterility — *see* Infertility
Sterilization — *see* Encounter (for),
    sterilization

Sternalgia — *see* Angina
Sternopagus Q89.4
Sternum bifidum Q76.7
Steroid
  effects (adverse) (adrenocortical) (iatrogenic)
    cushingoid E24.2
      correct substance properly
        administered — *see* Table of Drugs
        and Chemicals, by drug, adverse
        effect
      overdose or wrong substance given or
        taken — *see* Table of Drugs and
        Chemicals, by drug, poisoning
    diabetes — *see* category E09
      correct substance properly
        administered — *see* Table of Drugs
        and Chemicals, by drug, adverse
        effect
      overdose or wrong substance given or
        taken — *see* Table of Drugs and
        Chemicals, by drug, poisoning
    fever R50.2
    insufficiency E27.3
      correct substance properly
        administered — *see* Table of Drugs
        and Chemicals, by drug, adverse
        effect
      overdose or wrong substance given or
        taken — *see* Table of Drugs and
        Chemicals, by drug, poisoning
    responder H40.04-
Stevens-Johnson disease or syndrome L51.1
  toxic epidermal necrolysis overlap L51.3
Stewart-Morel syndrome M85.2
Sticker's disease B08.3
Sticky eye — *see* Conjunctivitis, acute,
  mucopurulent
Stieda's disease — *see* Bursitis, tibial
  collateral
Stiff neck — *see* Torticollis
Stiff-man syndrome G25.82
Stiffness, joint NEC M25.60-
  ankle M25.67-
  ankylosis — *see* Ankylosis, joint
  contracture — *see* Contraction, joint
  elbow M25.62-
  foot M25.67-
  hand M25.64-
  hip M25.65-
  knee M25.66-
  shoulder M25.61-
  wrist M25.63-
Stigmata congenital syphilis A50.59
Stillbirth P95
Still-Felty syndrome — *see* Felty's syndrome
Still's disease or syndrome (juvenile) M08.20
  adult-onset M06.1
  ankle M08.27-
  elbow M08.22-
  foot joint M08.27-
  hand joint M08.24-
  hip M08.25-
  knee M08.26-
  multiple site M08.29
  shoulder M08.21-
  vertebra M08.28
  wrist M08.23-
Stimulation, ovary E28.1
**Sting (venomous) (with allergic or
anaphylactic shock)** — *see* Table of
  Drugs and Chemicals, by animal or
  substance, poisoning
Stippled epiphyses Q78.8
Stitch
  abscess T81.41
  burst (in operation wound) — *see* Disruption,
    wound, operation
Stokes' disease E05.00
  with thyroid storm E05.01
Stokes-Adams disease or syndrome I45.9
Stokvis (-Talma) disease D74.8
Stoma malfunction
  colostomy K94.03
  enterostomy K94.13
  gastrostomy K94.23

Stoma malfunction - *continued*
  ileostomy K94.13
  tracheostomy J95.03
Stomach — *see* condition
Stomatitis (denture) (ulcerative) K12.1
  angular K13.0
    due to dietary or vitamin deficiency E53.0
  aphthous K12.0
  bovine B08.61
  candidal B37.0
  catarrhal K12.1
  diphtheritic A36.89
  due to
    dietary deficiency E53.0
    thrush B37.0
    vitamin deficiency
      B group NEC E53.9
      B2 (riboflavin) E53.0
  epidemic B08.8
  epizootic B08.8
  follicular K12.1
  gangrenous A69.0
  Geotrichum B48.3
  herpesviral, herpetic B00.2
  herpetiformis K12.0
  malignant K12.1
  membranous acute K12.1
  monilial B37.0
  mycotic B37.0
  necrotizing ulcerative A69.0
  parasitic B37.0
  septic K12.1
  spirochetal A69.1
  suppurative (acute) K12.2
  ulceromembranous A69.1
  vesicular K12.1
    with exanthem (enteroviral) B08.4
    virus disease A93.8
  Vincent's A69.1
Stomatocytosis D58.8
Stomatomycosis B37.0
Stomatorrhagia K13.79
Stone (s) — *see also* Calculus
  bladder (diverticulum) N21.0
  cystine E72.09
  heart syndrome I50.1
  kidney N20.0
  prostate N42.0
  pulpal (dental) K04.2
  renal N20.0
  salivary gland or duct (any) K11.5
  urethra (impacted) N21.1
  urinary (duct) (impacted) (passage) N20.9
    bladder (diverticulum) N21.0
    lower tract N21.9
    specified NEC N21.8
  xanthine E79.8 *[N22]*
Stonecutter's lung J62.8
**Stonemason's asthma, disease, lung or
pneumoconiosis** J62.8
Stoppage
  heart — *see* Arrest, cardiac
  urine — *see* Retention, urine
Storm, thyroid — *see* Thyrotoxicosis
Strabismus (congenital) (nonparalytic)
  H50.9
  concomitant H50.40
    convergent — *see* Strabismus, convergent
      concomitant
    divergent — *see* Strabismus, divergent
      concomitant
  convergent concomitant H50.00
    accommodative component H50.43
    alternating H50.05
      with
        A pattern H50.06
        specified nonconcomitances
          NEC H50.08
        V pattern H50.07
    monocular H50.01-
      with
        A pattern H50.02-
        specified nonconcomitances
          NEC H50.04-
        V pattern H50.03-

Strabismus (congenital) (nonparalytic) -
continued
  convergent concomitant - *continued*
    monocular - *continued*
      intermittent H50.31-
        alternating H50.32
    cyclotropia H50.41
  divergent concomitant H50.10
    alternating H50.15
      with
        A pattern H50.16
        specified noncomitances NEC H50.18
        V pattern H50.17
    monocular H50.11-
      with
        A pattern H50.12-
        specified noncomitances
          NEC H50.14-
        V pattern H50.13-
      intermittent H50.33
        alternating H50.34
  Duane's syndrome H50.81-
  due to adhesions, scars H50.69
  heterophoria H50.50
    alternating H50.55
    cyclophoria H50.54
    esophoria H50.51
    exophoria H50.52
    vertical H50.53
  heterotropia H50.40
    intermittent H50.30
  hypertropia H50.2-
  hypotropia — *see* Hypertropia
  latent H50.50
  mechanical H50.60
    Brown's sheath syndrome H50.61-
    specified type NEC H50.69
  monofixation syndrome H50.42
  paralytic H49.9
    abducens nerve H49.2-
    fourth nerve H49.1-
    Kearns-Sayre syndrome H49.81-
    ophthalmoplegia (external)
      progressive H49.4-
        with pigmentary retinopathy H49.81-
      total H49.3-
    sixth nerve H49.2-
    specified type NEC H49.88-
    third nerve H49.0-
    trochlear nerve H49.1-
  specified type NEC H50.89
  vertical H50.2-
Strain
  back S39.012
  cervical S16.1
  eye NEC — *see* Disturbance, vision,
    subjective
  heart — *see* Disease, heart
  low back S39.012
  mental NOS Z73.3
    work-related Z56.6
  muscle (tendon) — *see* Injury, muscle, by
    site, strain
  neck S16.1
  postural — *see also* Disorder, soft tissue, due
    to use
  physical NOS Z73.3
    work-related Z56.6
  psychological NEC Z73.3
  tendon — *see* Injury, muscle, by site, strain
Straining, on urination R39.16
Strand, vitreous — *see* Opacity, vitreous,
  membranes and strands
Strangulation, strangulated — *see also*
  Asphyxia, traumatic
  appendix K38.8
  bladder-neck N32.0
  bowel or colon K56.2
  food or foreign body — *see* Foreign body, by
    site
  hemorrhoids — *see* Hemorrhoids, with
    complication
  hernia — *see also* Hernia, by site, with
    obstruction

Strangulation, strangulated - *continued*
  hernia - *continued*
    with gangrene — *see* Hernia, by site, with
      gangrene
    intestine (large) (small) K56.2
      with hernia — *see also* Hernia, by site,
        with obstruction
        with gangrene — *see* Hernia, by site,
          with gangrene
    mesentery K56.2
    mucus — *see* Asphyxia, mucus
    omentum K56.2
    organ or site, congenital NEC — *see* Atresia,
      by site
    ovary — *see* Torsion, ovary
    penis N48.89
      foreign body T19.4
    rupture — *see* Hernia, by site, with
      obstruction
    stomach due to hernia — *see also* Hernia, by
      site, with obstruction
      with gangrene — *see* Hernia, by site, with
        gangrene
    vesicourethral orifice N32.0
Strangury R30.0
Straw itch B88.0
Strawberry
  gallbladder K82.4
  mark Q82.5
  tongue (red) (white) K14.3
Streak (s)
  macula, angioid H35.33
  ovarian Q50.32
Strephosymbolia F81.0
  secondary to organic lesion R48.8
Streptobacillary fever A25.1
Streptobacillosis A25.1
Streptobacillus moniliformis A25.1
Streptococcus, streptococcal — *see also*
    condition
  as cause of disease classified
    elsewhere B95.5
  group
    A, as cause of disease classified
      elsewhere B95.0
    B, as cause of disease classified
      elsewhere B95.1
    D, as cause of disease classified
      elsewhere B95.2
    pneumoniae, as cause of disease classified
      elsewhere B95.3
    specified NEC, as cause of disease classified
      elsewhere B95.4
Streptomycosis B47.1
Streptotrichosis A48.8
Stress F43.9
  family — *see* Disruption, family
  fetal P84
    complicating pregnancy O77.9
    due to drug administration O77.1
  mental NEC Z73.3
    work-related Z56.6
  physical NEC Z73.3
    work-related Z56.6
  polycythemia D75.1
  reaction — *see also* Reaction, stress F43.9
  work schedule Z56.3
Stretching, nerve — *see* Injury, nerve
Striae albicantes, atrophicae or distensae
  (cutis) L90.6
Stricture — *see also* Stenosis
  ampulla of Vater K83.1
  anus (sphincter) K62.4
    congenital Q42.3
      with fistula Q42.2
    infantile Q42.3
      with fistula Q42.2
  aorta (ascending) (congenital) Q25.1
    arteriosclerotic I70.0
    calcified I70.0
    supravalvular, congenital Q25.3
  aortic (valve) — *see* Stenosis, aortic
  aqueduct of Sylvius (congenital) Q03.0
    with spina bifida — *see* Spina bifida, by
      site, with hydrocephalus

Stricture - *continued*
  aqueduct of Sylvius (congenital) - *continued*
    acquired G91.1
  artery I77.1
    basilar — *see* Occlusion, artery, basilar
    carotid — *see* Occlusion, artery, carotid
    celiac I77.4
    congenital (peripheral) Q27.8
      cerebral Q28.3
      coronary Q24.5
      digestive system Q27.8
      lower limb Q27.8
      retinal Q14.1
      specified site NEC Q27.8
      umbilical Q27.0
      upper limb Q27.8
    coronary — *see* Disease, heart, ischemic,
      atherosclerotic
      congenital Q24.5
    precerebral — *see* Occlusion, artery,
      precerebral
    pulmonary (congenital) Q25.6
      acquired I28.8
    renal I70.1
    vertebral — *see* Occlusion, artery,
      vertebral
  auditory canal (external) (congenital)
    acquired — *see* Stenosis, external ear canal
  bile duct (common) (hepatic) K83.1
    congenital Q44.3
    postoperative K91.89
  bladder N32.89
    neck N32.0
  bowel — *see* Obstruction, intestine
  brain G93.89
  bronchus J98.09
    congenital Q32.3
    syphilitic A52.72
  cardia (stomach) K22.2
    congenital Q39.3
  cardiac — *see also* Disease, heart
    orifice (stomach) K22.2
  cecum — *see* Obstruction, intestine
  cervix, cervical (canal) N88.2
    congenital Q51.828
    in pregnancy — *see* Pregnancy,
      complicated by, abnormal cervix
      causing obstructed labor O65.5
  colon — *see also* Obstruction, intestine
    congenital Q42.9
      specified NEC Q42.8
  colostomy K94.03
  common (bile) duct K83.1
  coronary (artery) — *see* Disease, heart,
    ischemic, atherosclerotic
  cystic duct — *see* Obstruction, gallbladder
  digestive organs NEC, congenital Q45.8
  duodenum K31.5
    congenital Q41.0
  ear canal (external) (congenital) Q16.1
    acquired — *see* Stricture, auditory canal,
      acquired
  ejaculatory duct N50.89
  enterostomy K94.13
  esophagus K22.2
    congenital Q39.3
    syphilitic A52.79
      congenital A50.59 *[K23]*
  eustachian tube — *see also* Obstruction,
    eustachian tube
    congenital Q17.8
  fallopian tube N97.1
    gonococcal A54.24
    tuberculous A18.17
  gallbladder — *see* Obstruction, gallbladder
  glottis J38.6
  heart — *see also* Disease, heart
    valve — *see also* Endocarditis I38
      aortic Q23.0
      mitral Q23.2
      pulmonary Q22.1
      tricuspid Q22.4
  hepatic duct K83.1
  hourglass, of stomach K31.2
  hymen N89.6

Stricture - *continued*
  hypopharynx J39.2
  ileum — *see also* Obstruction, intestine,
    specified NEC K56.699
    congenital Q41.2
  intestine — *see also* Obstruction, intestine
    congenital (small) Q41.9
      large Q42.9
        specified NEC Q42.8
      specified NEC Q41.8
    ischemic K55.1
  jejunum — *see also* Obstruction, intestine,
    specified NEC K56.699
    congenital Q41.1
  lacrimal passages — *see also* Stenosis,
    lacrimal
    congenital Q10.5
  larynx J38.6
    congenital NEC Q31.8
      subglottic Q31.1
    syphilitic A52.73
      congenital A50.59 *[J99]*
  meatus
    ear (congenital) Q16.1
      acquired — *see* Stricture, auditory canal,
        acquired
    osseous (ear) (congenital) Q16.1
      acquired — *see* Stricture, auditory canal,
        acquired
    urinarius — *see also* Stricture, urethra
      congenital Q64.33
  mitral (valve) — *see* Stenosis, mitral
  myocardium, myocardial I51.5
    hypertrophic subaortic (idiopathic) I42.1
  nares (anterior) (posterior) J34.89
    congenital Q30.0
  nasal duct — *see also* Stenosis, lacrimal,
    duct
    congenital Q10.5
  nasolacrimal duct — *see also* Stenosis,
    lacrimal, duct
    congenital Q10.5
  nasopharynx J39.2
    syphilitic A52.73
  nose J34.89
    congenital Q30.0
  nostril (anterior) (posterior) J34.89
    congenital Q30.0
    syphilitic A52.73
      congenital A50.59 *[J99]*
  organ or site, congenital NEC — *see* Atresia,
    by site
  os uteri — *see* Stricture, cervix
  osseous meatus (ear) (congenital) Q16.1
    acquired — *see* Stricture, auditory canal,
      acquired
  oviduct — *see* Stricture, fallopian tube
  pelviureteric junction (congenital) Q62.11
    acquired, with hydronephrosis N13.0
  penis, by foreign body T19.4
  pharynx J39.2
  prostate N42.89
  pulmonary, pulmonic
    artery (congenital) Q25.6
      acquired I28.8
      noncongenital I28.8
    infundibulum (congenital) Q24.3
    valve I37.0
      congenital Q22.1
    vein, acquired I28.8
    vessel NEC I28.8
  punctum lacrimale — *see also* Stenosis,
    lacrimal, punctum
    congenital Q10.5
  pylorus (hypertrophic) K31.1
    adult K31.1
    congenital Q40.0
    infantile Q40.0
  rectosigmoid — *see also* Obstruction,
    intestine, specified NEC K56.699
  rectum (sphincter) K62.4
    congenital Q42.1
      with fistula Q42.0
    due to
      chlamydial lymphogranuloma A55

Stricture - *continued*
  rectum (sphincter) - *continued*
    due to - *continued*
      irradiation K91.89
      lymphogranuloma venereum A55
     gonococcal A54.6
     inflammatory (chlamydial) A55
     syphilitic A52.74
     tuberculous A18.32
  renal artery I70.1
    congenital Q27.1
  salivary duct or gland (any) K11.8
  sigmoid (flexure) — *see* Obstruction,
    intestine
  spermatic cord N50.89
  stoma (following) (of)
    colostomy K94.03
    enterostomy K94.13
    gastrostomy K94.23
    ileostomy K94.13
    tracheostomy J95.03
  stomach K31.89
    congenital Q40.2
    hourglass K31.2
  subaortic Q24.4
    hypertrophic (acquired) (idiopathic) I42.1
  subglottic J38.6
  syphilitic NEC A52.79
  trachea J39.8
    congenital Q32.1
    syphilitic A52.73
    tuberculous NEC A15.5
  tracheostomy J95.03
  tricuspid (valve) — *see* Stenosis, tricuspid
  tunica vaginalis N50.89
  ureter (postoperative) N13.5
    with
      hydronephrosis N13.1
        with infection N13.6
      pyelonephritis (chronic) N11.1
    congenital — *see* Atresia, ureter
    tuberculous A18.11
  ureteropelvic junction (congenital) Q62.11
    acquired, with hydronephrosis N13.0
  ureterovesical orifice N13.5
    with infection N13.6
  urethra (organic) (spasmodic) — *see also*
    Stricture, urethra, male N35.919
    associated with schistosomiasis B65.0
      [N37]
    congenital Q64.39
      valvular (posterior) Q64.2
    due to
      infection — *see* Stricture, urethra,
        postinfective
      trauma — *see* Stricture, urethra, post-
        traumatic
    female N35.92
    gonococcal, gonorrheal A54.01
    infective NEC — *see* Stricture, urethra,
      postinfective
    late effect (sequelae) of injury — *see*
      Stricture, urethra, post-traumatic
    male N35.919
      anterior urethra N35.914
      bulbous urethra N35.912
      meatal N35.911
      membranous urethra N35.913
      overlapping sites N35.916
    postcatheterization — *see* Stricture,
      urethra, postprocedural
    postinfective NEC
      female N35.12
      male N35.119
        anterior urethra N35.114
        bulbous urethra N35.112
        meatal N35.111
        membranous urethra N35.113
        overlapping sites N35.116
    postobstetric N35.021
    postoperative — *see* Stricture, urethra,
      postprocedural
    postprocedural
      female N99.12
      male N99.114

Stricture - *continued*
  urethra (organic) (spasmodic) - *continued*
    postprocedural - *continued*
      male - *continued*
        anterior bulbous urethra N99.113
        bulbous urethra N99.111
        fossa navicularis N99.115
        meatal N99.110
        membranous urethra N99.112
        overlapping sites N99.116
    post-traumatic
      female N35.028
        due to childbirth N35.021
      male N35.014
        anterior urethra N35.013
        bulbous urethra N35.011
        meatal N35.010
        membranous urethra N35.012
        overlapping sites N35.016
    sequela (late effect) of
      childbirth N35.021
      injury — *see* Stricture, urethra, post-
        traumatic
    specified cause NEC
      female N35.82
      male N35.819
        anterior urethra N35.814
        bulbous urethra N35.812
        meatal N35.811
        membranous urethra N35.813
        overlapping sites N35.816
    syphilitic A52.76
    traumatic — *see* Stricture, urethra, post-
      traumatic
    valvular (posterior) , congenital Q64.2
  urinary meatus — *see* Stricture, urethra
  uterus, uterine (synechiae) N85.6
    os (external) (internal) — *see* Stricture,
      cervix
  vagina (outlet) — *see* Stenosis, vagina
  valve (cardiac) (heart) — *see also*
    Endocarditis
    congenital
      aortic Q23.0
      mitral Q23.2
      pulmonary Q22.1
      tricuspid Q22.4
  vas deferens N50.89
    congenital Q55.4
  vein I87.1
  vena cava (inferior) (superior) NEC I87.1
    congenital Q26.0
  vesicourethral orifice N32.0
    congenital Q64.31
  vulva (acquired) N90.5
Stridor R06.1
  congenital (larynx) P28.89
Stridulous — *see* condition
Stroke (apoplectic) (brain) (embolic)
  (ischemic) (paralytic) (thrombotic) I63.9
  cryptogenic — *see also* infarction,
    cerebral I63.9
  epileptic — *see* Epilepsy
  heat T67.01
    exertional T67.02
    specified NEC T67.09
  in evolution I63.9
  intraoperative
    during cardiac surgery I97.810
    during other surgery I97.811
  lightning — *see* Lightning
  meaning
    cerebral hemorrhage - code to
      Hemorrhage, intracranial
    cerebral infarction - code to Infarction,
      cerebral
  postprocedural
    following cardiac surgery I97.820
    following other surgery I97.821
  sun T67.01
    specified NEC T67.09
  unspecified (NOS) I63.9
Stromatosis, endometrial D39.0
Strongyloidiasis, strongyloidosis B78.9
  cutaneous B78.1

Strongyloidiasis, strongyloidosis - *continued*
  disseminated B78.7
  intestinal B78.0
Strophulus pruriginosus L28.2
Struck by lightning — *see* Lightning
Struma — *see also* Goiter
  Hashimoto E06.3
  lymphomatosa E06.3
  nodosa (simplex) E04.9
    endemic E01.2
      multinodular E01.1
    multinodular E04.2
      iodine-deficiency related E01.1
    toxic or with hyperthyroidism E05.20
      with thyroid storm E05.21
      multinodular E05.20
        with thyroid storm E05.21
      uninodular E05.10
        with thyroid storm E05.11
    toxicosa E05.20
      with thyroid storm E05.21
      multinodular E05.20
        with thyroid storm E05.21
      uninodular E05.10
        with thyroid storm E05.11
    uninodular E04.1
  ovarii D27.-
  Riedel's E06.5
Strumipriva cachexia E03.4
Strümpell-Marie spine — *see* Spondylitis,
  ankylosing
Strümpell-Westphal pseudosclerosis E83.01
Stuart deficiency disease (factor X) D68.2
Stuart-Prower factor deficiency (factor
  X) D68.2
Student's elbow — *see* Bursitis, elbow,
  olecranon
Stump — *see* Amputation
Stunting, nutritional E45
Stupor (catatonic) R40.1
  depressive (single episode) F32.89
    recurrent episode F33.8
  dissociative F44.2
  manic F30.2
  manic-depressive F31.89
  psychogenic (anergic) F44.2
  reaction to exceptional stress
    (transient) F43.0
Sturge (-Weber) (-Dimitri) (-Kalischer)
  disease or syndrome Q85.8
Stuttering F80.81
  adult onset F98.5
  childhood onset F80.81
  following cerebrovascular disease — *see*
    Disorder, fluency. following
    cerebrovascular disease
  in conditions classified elsewhere R47.82
Sty, stye (external) (internal) (meibomian)
  (zeisian) — *see* Hordeolum
Subacidity, gastric K31.89
  psychogenic F45.8
Subacute — *see* condition
Subarachnoid — *see* condition
Subcortical — *see* condition
Subcostal syndrome, nerve
  compression — *see* Mononeuropathy,
  upper limb, specified site NEC
Subcutaneous, subcuticular — *see* condition
Subdural — *see* condition
Subendocardium — *see* condition
Subependymoma
  specified site — *see* Neoplasm, uncertain
    behavior, by site
  unspecified site D43.2
Suberosis J67.3
Subglossitis — *see* Glossitis
Subhemophilia D66
Subinvolution
  breast (postlactational)
    (postpuerperal) N64.89
    puerperal O90.89
  uterus (chronic) (nonpuerperal) N85.3
    puerperal O90.89
Sublingual — *see* condition
Sublinguitis — *see* Sialoadenitis

Subluxatable hip Q65.6
Subluxation — *see also* Dislocation
  acromioclavicular S43.11-
  ankle S93.0-
  atlantoaxial, recurrent M43.4
    with myelopathy M43.3
  carpometacarpal (joint) NEC S63.05-
    thumb S63.04-
  complex, vertebral — *see* Complex,
    subluxation
  congenital — *see also* Malposition,
    congenital
    hip — *see* Dislocation, hip, congenital,
      partial
    joint (excluding hip)
      lower limb Q68.8
      shoulder Q68.8
      upper limb Q68.8
  elbow (traumatic) S53.10-
    anterior S53.11-
    lateral S53.14-
    medial S53.13-
    posterior S53.12-
    specified type NEC S53.19-
  finger S63.20-
    index S63.20-
    interphalangeal S63.22-
      distal S63.24-
        index S63.24-
        little S63.24-
        middle S63.24-
        ring S63.24-
      index S63.22-
      little S63.22-
      middle S63.22-
      proximal S63.23-
        index S63.23-
        little S63.23-
        middle S63.23-
        ring S63.23-
      ring S63.22-
    little S63.20-
    metacarpophalangeal S63.21-
      index S63.21-
      little S63.21-
      middle S63.21-
      ring S63.21-
    middle S63.20-
    ring S63.20-
  foot S93.30-
    specified site NEC S93.33-
    tarsal joint S93.31-
    tarsometatarsal joint S93.32-
    toe — *see* Subluxation, toe
  hip S73.00-
    anterior S73.03-
      obturator S73.02-
    central S73.04-
    posterior S73.01-
  interphalangeal (joint)
    finger S63.22-
      distal joint S63.24-
        index S63.24-
        little S63.24-
        middle S63.24-
        ring S63.24-
      index S63.22-
      little S63.22-
      middle S63.22-
      proximal joint S63.23-
        index S63.23-
        little S63.23-
        middle S63.23-
        ring S63.23-
      ring S63.22-
    thumb S63.12-
    toe S93.13-
      great S93.13-
      lesser S93.13-
  joint prosthesis — *see* Complications, joint
    prosthesis, mechanical, displacement,
    by site
  knee S83.10-
    cap — *see* Subluxation, patella
    patella — *see* Subluxation, patella

Subluxation - *continued*
  knee - *continued*
    proximal tibia
      anteriorly S83.11-
      laterally S83.14-
      medially S83.13-
      posteriorly S83.12-
      specified type NEC S83.19-
  lens — *see* Dislocation, lens, partial
  ligament, traumatic — *see* Sprain, by site
  metacarpal (bone)
    proximal end S63.06-
  metacarpophalangeal (joint)
    finger S63.21-
      index S63.21-
      little S63.21-
      middle S63.21-
      ring S63.21-
      thumb S63.11-
  metatarsophalangeal joint S93.14-
    great toe S93.14-
    lesser toe S93.14-
  midcarpal (joint) S63.03-
  patella S83.00-
    lateral S83.01-
    recurrent (nontraumatic) — *see*
      Dislocation, patella, recurrent,
      incomplete
    specified type NEC S83.09-
  pathological — *see* Dislocation, pathological
  radial head S53.00-
    anterior S53.01-
    nursemaid's elbow S53.03-
    posterior S53.02-
    specified type NEC S53.09-
  radiocarpal (joint) S63.02-
  radioulnar (joint)
    distal S63.01-
    proximal — *see* Subluxation, elbow
  shoulder
    congenital Q68.8
    girdle S43.30-
      scapula S43.31-
      specified site NEC S43.39-
    traumatic S43.00-
      anterior S43.01-
      inferior S43.03-
      posterior S43.02-
      specified type NEC S43.08-
  sternoclavicular (joint) S43.20-
    anterior S43.21-
    posterior S43.22-
  symphysis (pubis)
  thumb S63.103
    interphalangeal joint — *see* Subluxation,
      interphalangeal (joint), thumb
    metacarpophalangeal joint — *see*
      Subluxation, metacarpophalangeal
      (joint), thumb
  toe (s) S93.10-
    great S93.10-
      interphalangeal joint S93.13-
      metatarsophalangeal joint S93.14-
    interphalangeal joint S93.13-
    lesser S93.10-
      interphalangeal joint S93.13-
      metatarsophalangeal joint S93.14-
    metatarsophalangeal joint S93.149
  ulnohumeral joint — *see* Subluxation, elbow
  vertebral
    recurrent NEC — *see* subcategory M43.5
    traumatic
      cervical S13.100
        atlantoaxial joint S13.120
        atlantooccipital joint S13.110
        atloidooccipital joint S13.110
        joint between
          C0 and C1 S13.110
          C1 and C2 S13.120
          C2 and C3 S13.130
          C3 and C4 S13.140
          C4 and C5 S13.150
          C5 and C6 S13.160
          C6 and C7 S13.170
          C7 and T1 S13.180

Subluxation - *continued*
  vertebral - *continued*
    traumatic - *continued*
      cervical - *continued*
        occipitoatloid joint S13.110
      lumbar S33.100
        joint between
          L1 and L2 S33.110
          L2 and L3 S33.120
          L3 and L4 S33.130
          L4 and L5 S33.140
      thoracic S23.100
        joint between
          T1 and T2 S23.110
          T2 and T3 S23.120
          T3 and T4 S23.122
          T4 and T5 S23.130
          T5 and T6 S23.132
          T6 and T7 S23.140
          T7 and T8 S23.142
          T8 and T9 S23.150
          T9 and T10 S23.152
          T10 and T11 S23.160
          T11 and T12 S23.162
          T12 and L1 S23.170
  ulna
    distal end S63.07-
    proximal end — *see* Subluxation, elbow
  wrist (carpal bone) S63.00-
    carpometacarpal joint — *see* Subluxation,
      carpometacarpal (joint)
    distal radioulnar joint — *see* Subluxation,
      radioulnar (joint), distal
    metacarpal bone, proximal — *see*
      Subluxation, metacarpal (bone),
      proximal end
    midcarpal — *see* Subluxation, midcarpal
      (joint)
    radiocarpal joint — *see* Subluxation,
      radiocarpal (joint)
    recurrent — *see* Dislocation, recurrent,
      wrist
    specified site NEC S63.09-
    ulna — *see* Subluxation, ulna, distal end
Submaxillary — *see* condition
Submersion (fatal) (nonfatal) T75.1
Submucous — *see* condition
Subnormal, subnormality
  accommodation (old age) H52.4
  mental — *see* Disability, intellectual
  temperature (accidental) T68
Subphrenic — *see* condition
Subscapular nerve — *see* condition
Subseptus uterus Q51.28
Subsiding appendicitis K36
Substance (other psychoactive) -induced
  anxiety disorder F19.980
  bipolar and related disorder F19.94
  delirium F19.921
  depressive disorder F19.94
  major neurocognitive disorder F19.97
  mild neurocognitive disorder F19.988
  obsessive-compulsive and related
    disorder F19.988
  psychotic disorder F19.959
  sexual dysfunction F19.981
  sleep disorder F19.982
Substernal thyroid E04.9
  congenital Q89.2
Substitution disorder F44.9
Subtentorial — *see* condition
Subthyroidism (acquired) — *see also*
  Hypothyroidism
  congenital E03.1
Succenturiate placenta O43.19-
Sucking thumb, child (excessive) F98.8
Sudamen, sudamina L74.1
Sudanese kala-azar B55.0
Sudden
  heart failure — *see* Failure, heart
  hearing loss — *see* Deafness, sudden
Sudeck's atrophy, disease, or
  syndrome — *see* Algoneurodystrophy
Suffocation — *see* Asphyxia, traumatic

Sugar
blood
high (transient) R73.9
low (transient) E16.2
in urine R81
Suicide, suicidal (attempted) T14.91
by poisoning — *see* Table of Drugs and Chemicals
history of (personal) Z91.5
in family Z81.8
ideation — *see* Ideation, suicidal
risk
meaning personal history of attempted suicide Z91.5
meaning suicidal ideation — *see* Ideation, suicidal
tendencies
meaning personal history of attempted suicide Z91.5
meaning suicidal ideation — *see* Ideation, suicidal
trauma — *see* nature of injury by site
Suipestifer infection — *see* Infection, salmonella
Sulfhemoglobinemia, sulphemoglobinemia (acquired) (with methemoglobinemia) D74.8
Sumatran mite fever A75.3
Summer — *see* condition
Sunburn L55.9
due to
tanning bed (acute) L56.8
chronic L57.8
ultraviolet radiation (acute) L56.8
chronic L57.8
first degree L55.0
second degree L55.1
third degree L55.2
SUNCT (short lasting unilateral neuralgiform headache with conjunctival injection and tearing) G44.059
intractable G44.051
not intractable G44.059
Sundowning F05
Sunken acetabulum — *see* Derangement, joint, specified type NEC, hip
Sunstroke T67.01
specified NEC T67.09
Superfecundation — *see* Pregnancy, multiple
Superfetation — *see* Pregnancy, multiple
Superinvolution (uterus) N85.8
Supernumerary (congenital)
aortic cusps Q23.8
auditory ossicles Q16.3
bone Q79.8
breast Q83.1
carpal bones Q74.0
cusps, heart valve NEC Q24.8
aortic Q23.8
mitral Q23.2
pulmonary Q22.3
digit (s) Q69.9
ear (lobule) Q17.0
fallopian tube Q50.6
finger Q69.0
hymen Q52.4
kidney Q63.0
lacrimonasal duct Q10.6
lobule (ear) Q17.0
mitral cusps Q23.2
muscle Q79.8
nipple (s) Q83.3
organ or site not listed — *see* Accessory
ossicles, auditory Q16.3
ovary Q50.31
oviduct Q50.6
pulmonary, pulmonic cusps Q22.3
rib Q76.6
cervical or first (syndrome) Q76.5
roots (of teeth) K00.2
spleen Q89.09
tarsal bones Q74.2
teeth K00.1
testis Q55.29

Supernumerary (congenital) - *continued*
thumb Q69.1
toe Q69.2
uterus Q51.28
vagina Q52.1
vertebra Q76.49
Supervision (of)
contraceptive — *see* Prescription, contraceptives
dietary (for) Z71.3
allergy (food) Z71.3
colitis Z71.3
diabetes mellitus Z71.3
food allergy or intolerance Z71.3
gastritis Z71.3
hypercholesterolemia Z71.3
hypoglycemia Z71.3
intolerance (food) Z71.3
obesity Z71.3
specified NEC Z71.3
healthy infant or child Z76.2
foundling Z76.1
high-risk pregnancy — *see* Pregnancy, complicated by, high, risk
lactation Z39.1
pregnancy — *see* Pregnancy, supervision of
Supplemental teeth K00.1
Suppression
binocular vision H53.34
lactation O92.5
menstruation N94.89
ovarian secretion E28.39
renal N28.9
urine, urinary secretion R34
Suppuration, suppurative — *see also* condition
accessory sinus (chronic) — *see* Sinusitis
adrenal gland
antrum (chronic) — *see* Sinusitis, maxillary
bladder — *see* Cystitis
brain G06.0
sequelae G09
breast N61.1
puerperal, postpartum or gestational — *see* Mastitis, obstetric, purulent
dental periosteum M27.3
ear (middle) — *see also* Otitis, media
external NEC — *see* Otitis, externa, infective
internal — *see* subcategory H83.0
ethmoidal (chronic) (sinus) — *see* Sinusitis, ethmoidal
fallopian tube — *see* Salpingo-oophoritis
frontal (chronic) (sinus) — *see* Sinusitis, frontal
gallbladder (acute) K81.0
gum K05.20
generalized — *see* Periodontitis, aggressive, generalized
localized — *see* Periodontitis, aggressive, localized
intracranial G06.0
joint — *see* Arthritis, pyogenic or pyemic
labyrinthine — *see* subcategory H83.0
lung — *see* Abscess, lung
mammary gland N61.1
puerperal, postpartum O91.12
associated with lactation O91.13
maxilla, maxillary M27.2
sinus (chronic) — *see* Sinusitis, maxillary
muscle — *see* Myositis, infective
nasal sinus (chronic) — *see* Sinusitis
pancreas, acute — *see also* Pancreatitis, acute K85.80
parotid gland — *see* Sialoadenitis
pelvis, pelvic
female — *see* Disease, pelvis, inflammatory
male K65.0
pericranial — *see* Osteomyelitis
salivary duct or gland (any) — *see* Sialoadenitis
sinus (accessory) (chronic) (nasal) — *see* Sinusitis

Suppuration, suppurative - *continued*
sphenoidal sinus (chronic) — *see* Sinusitis, sphenoidal
thymus (gland) E32.1
thyroid (gland) E06.0
tonsil — *see* Tonsillitis
uterus — *see* Endometritis
Supraeruption of tooth (teeth) M26.34
Supraglottitis J04.30
with obstruction J04.31
Suprarenal (gland) — *see* condition
Suprascapular nerve — *see* condition
Suprasellar — *see* condition
Surfer's knots or nodules S89.8-
Surgical
emphysema T81.82
procedures, complication or misadventure — *see* Complications, surgical procedures
shock T81.10
Surveillance (of) (for) — *see also* Observation
alcohol abuse Z71.41
contraceptive — *see* Prescription, contraceptives
dietary Z71.3
drug abuse Z71.51
Susceptibility to disease, genetic Z15.89
malignant neoplasm Z15.09
breast Z15.01
endometrium Z15.04 ·
ovary Z15.02
prostate Z15.03
specified NEC Z15.09
multiple endocrine neoplasia Z15.81
Suspected condition, ruled out — *see also* Observation, suspected
amniotic cavity and membrane Z03.71
cervical shortening Z03.75
fetal anomaly Z03.73
fetal growth Z03.74
maternal and fetal conditions NEC Z03.79
newborn — *see also* Observation, newborn, suspected condition ruled out Z05.9
oligohydramnios Z03.71
placental problem Z03.72
polyhydramnios Z03.71
Suspended uterus
in pregnancy or childbirth — *see* Pregnancy, complicated by, abnormal uterus
Sutton's nevus D22.9
Suture
burst (in operation wound) T81.31
external operation wound T81.31
internal operation wound T81.32
inadvertently left in operation wound — *see* Foreign body, accidentally left during a procedure
removal Z48.02
Swab inadvertently left in operation wound — *see* Foreign body, accidentally left during a procedure
Swallowed, swallowing
difficulty — *see* Dysphagia
foreign body — *see* Foreign body, alimentary tract
Swan-neck deformity (finger) — *see* Deformity, finger, swan-neck
Swearing, compulsive F42.8
in Gilles de la Tourette's syndrome F95.2
Sweat, sweats
fetid L75.0
night R61
Sweating, excessive R61
Sweeley-Klionsky disease E75.21
Sweet's disease or dermatosis L98.2
Swelling (of) R60.9
abdomen, abdominal (not referable to any particular organ) — *see* Mass, abdominal
ankle — *see* Effusion, joint, ankle
arm M79.89
forearm M79.89
breast — *see also* Lump, breast N63.0
Calabar B74.3
cervical gland R59.0

Swelling (of) - *continued*
  chest, localized R22.2
  ear H93.8-
  extremity (lower) (upper) — *see* Disorder,
      soft tissue, specified type NEC
  finger M79.89
  foot M79.89
  glands R59.9
    generalized R59.1
    localized R59.0
  hand M79.89
  head (localized) R22.0
  inflammatory — *see* Inflammation
  intra-abdominal — *see* Mass, abdominal
  joint — *see* Effusion, joint
  leg M79.89
    lower M79.89
  limb — *see* Disorder, soft tissue, specified
      type NEC
  localized (skin) R22.9
    chest R22.2
    head R22.0
    limb
      lower — *see* Mass, localized, limb,
          lower
      upper — *see* Mass, localized, limb,
          upper
    neck R22.1
    trunk R22.2
  neck (localized) R22.1
  pelvic — *see* Mass, abdominal
  scrotum N50.89
  splenic — *see* Splenomegaly
  testis N50.89
  toe M79.89
  umbilical R19.09
  wandering, due to Gnathostoma
      (spinigerum) B83.1
  white — *see* Tuberculosis, arthritis
Swift (-Feer) disease
  overdose or wrong substance given or
      taken — *see* Table of Drugs and
      Chemicals, by drug, poisoning
Swimmer's
  cramp T75.1
  ear H60.33-
  itch B65.3
Swimming in the head R42
Swollen — *see* Swelling
Swyer syndrome Q99.1
Sycosis L73.8
  barbae (not parasitic) L73.8
  contagiosa (mycotic) B35.0
  lupoides L73.8
  mycotic B35.0
  parasitic B35.0
  vulgaris L73.8
Sydenham's chorea — *see* Chorea,
  Sydenham's
Sylvatic yellow fever A95.0
Sylvest's disease B33.0
Symblepharon H11.23-
  congenital Q10.3
Symond's syndrome G93.2
Sympathetic — *see* condition
Sympatheticotonia G90.8
Sympathicoblastoma
  specified site — *see* Neoplasm, malignant,
      by site
  unspecified site C74.90
Sympathogonioma — *see*
  Sympathicoblastoma
Symphalangy (fingers) (toes) Q70.9
Symptoms NEC R68.89
  breast NEC N64.59
  cold J00
  development NEC R63.8
  factitious, self-induced — *see* Disorder,
      factitious
  genital organs, female R10.2
  involving
    abdomen NEC R19.8
    appearance NEC R46.89
    awareness R41.9
      altered mental status R41.82

Symptoms NEC - *continued*
  involving - *continued*
    awareness - *continued*
      amnesia — *see* Amnesia
      borderline intellectual
          functioning R41.83
      coma — *see* Coma
      disorientation R41.0
      neurologic neglect syndrome R41.4
      senile cognitive decline R41.81
      specified symptom NEC R41.89
    behavior NEC R46.89
    cardiovascular system NEC R09.89
    chest NEC R09.89
    circulatory system NEC R09.89
    cognitive functions R41.9
      altered mental status R41.82
      amnesia — *see* Amnesia
      borderline intellectual
          functioning R41.83
      coma — *see* Coma
      disorientation R41.0
      neurologic neglect syndrome R41.4
      senile cognitive decline R41.81
      specified symptom NEC R41.89
    development NEC R62.50
    digestive system NEC R19.8
    emotional state NEC R45.89
      emotional lability R45.86
    food and fluid intake R63.8
    general perceptions and sensations R44.9
      specified NEC R44.8
    musculoskeletal system R29.91
      specified NEC R29.898
    nervous system R29.90
      specified NEC R29.818
    pelvis NEC R19.8
    respiratory system NEC R09.89
    skin and integument R23.9
    urinary system R39.9
  menopausal N95.1
  metabolism NEC R63.8
  neurotic F48.8
  of infancy R68.19
  pelvis NEC, female R10.2
  skin and integument NEC R23.9
  subcutaneous tissue NEC R23.9
  viral cold J00
Sympus Q74.2
Syncephalus Q89.4
Synchondrosis
  abnormal (congenital) Q78.8
  ischiopubic M91.0
**Synchysis (scintillans) (senile) (vitreous
  body)** H43.89
Syncope (near) (pre-) R55
  anginosa I20.8
  bradycardia R00.1
  cardiac R55
  carotid sinus G90.01
  due to spinal (lumbar) puncture G97.1
  heart R55
  heat T67.1
  laryngeal R05
  psychogenic F48.8
  tussive R05
  vasoconstriction R55
  vasodepressor R55
  vasomotor R55
  vasovagal R55
Syndactylism, syndactyly Q70.9
  complex (with synostosis)
    fingers Q70.0-
    toes Q70.2-
  simple (without synostosis)
    fingers Q70.1-
    toes Q70.3-
Syndrome — *see also* Disease
  5q minus NOS D46.C
  48,XXXX Q97.1
  49,XXXXX Q97.1
  abdominal
    acute R10.0
    muscle deficiency Q79.4
  abnormal innervation H02.519

Syndrome - *continued*
  abnormal innervation - *continued*
    left H02.516
      lower H02.515
      upper H02.514
    right H02.513
      lower H02.512
      upper H02.511
  abstinence, neonatal P96.1
  acid pulmonary aspiration, obstetric O74.0
  acquired immunodeficiency — *see* Human,
      immunodeficiency virus (HIV) disease
  acute abdominal R10.0
  acute respiratory distress (adult) (child) J80
    idiopathic J84.114
  Adair-Dighton Q78.0
  Adams-Stokes (-Morgagni) I45.9
  adiposogenital E23.6
  adrenal
    hemorrhage (meningococcal) A39.1
    meningococcic A39.1
  adrenocortical — *see* Cushing's, syndrome
  adrenogenital E25.9
    congenital, associated with enzyme
        deficiency E25.0
  afferent loop NEC K91.89
  Alagille's Q44.7
  alcohol withdrawal (without convulsions) —
      see Dependence, alcohol, with,
      withdrawal
  Alder's D72.0
  Aldrich (-Wiskott) D82.0
  alien hand R41.4
  Alport Q87.81
  alveolar hypoventilation E66.2
  alveolocapillary block J84.10
  amnesic, amnestic (confabulatory) (due
      to) — *see* Disorder, amnesic
  amyostatic (Wilson's disease) E83.01
  androgen insensitivity E34.50
    complete E34.51
    partial E34.52
  androgen resistance — *see also* Syndrome,
      androgen insensitivity E34.50
  Angelman Q93.51
  anginal — *see* Angina
  ankyloglossia superior Q38.1
  anterior
    chest wall R07.89
    cord G83.82
    spinal artery G95.19
      compression M47.019
        cervical region M47.012
        cervicothoracic region M47.013
        lumbar region M47.016
        occipito-atlanto-axial region M47.011
        thoracic region M47.014
        thoracolumbar region M47.015
    tibial M76.81-
  antibody deficiency D80.9
    agammaglobulinemic D80.1
      hereditary D80.0
    congenital D80.0
    hypogammaglobulinemic D80.1
      hereditary D80.0
  anticardiolipin (-antibody) D68.61
  antidepressant discontinuation T43.205
  antiphospholipid (-antibody) D68.61
  aortic
    arch M31.4
    bifurcation I74.09
  aortomesenteric duodenum occlusion K31.5
  apical ballooning (transient left
      ventricular) I51.81
  arcuate ligament I77.4
  argentaffin, argintaffinoma E34.0
  Arnold-Chiari — *see* Arnold-Chiari disease
  Arrillaga-Ayerza I27.0
  arterial tortuosity Q87.82
  arteriovenous steal T82.898-
  Asherman's N85.6
  aspiration, of newborn — *see* Aspiration, by
      substance, with pneumonia
    meconium P24.01
  ataxia-telangiectasia G11.3

Syndrome - *continued*
auriculotemporal G50.8
autoerythrocyte sensitization (Gardner-Diamond) D69.2
autoimmune polyglandular E31.0
autoimmune lymphoproliferative [ALPS] D89.82
autoinflammatory M04.9
  specified type NEC M04.8
autosomal — *see* Abnormal, autosomes
Avellis' G46.8
Ayerza (-Arrillaga) I27.0
Babinski-Nageotte G83.89
Bakwin-Krida Q78.5
bare lymphocyte D81.6
Barré-Guillain G61.0
Barré-Liéou M53.0
Barrett's — *see* Barrett's, esophagus
Barsony-Polgar K22.4
Barsony-Teschendorf K22.4
Barth E78.71
Bartter's E26.81
basal cell nevus Q87.89
Basedow's E05.00
  with thyroid storm E05.01
basilar artery G45.0
Batten-Steinert G71.11
battered
  baby or child — *see* Maltreatment, child, physical abuse
  spouse — *see* Maltreatment, adult, physical abuse
Beals Q87.40
Beau's I51.5
Beck's I65.8
Benedikt's G46.3
Béquez César (-Steinbrinck-Chédiak-Higashi) E70.330
Bernhardt-Roth — *see* Meralgia paresthetica
Bernheim's — *see* Failure, heart, right
big spleen D73.1
bilateral polycystic ovarian E28.2
Bing-Horton's — *see* Horton's headache
Birt-Hogg-Dube syndrome Q87.89
Björck (-Thorsen) E34.0
black
  lung J60
  widow spider bite — *see* Toxicity, venom, spider, black widow
Blackfan-Diamond D61.01
Blau M04.8
blind loop K90.2
  congenital Q43.8
  postsurgical K91.2
blue sclera Q78.0
blue toe I75.02-
Boder-Sedgewick G11.3
Boerhaave's K22.3
Borjeson Forssman Lehmann Q89.8
Bouillaud's I01.9
Bourneville (-Pringle) Q85.1
Bouveret (-Hoffman) I47.9
brachial plexus G54.0
bradycardia-tachycardia I49.5
brain (nonpsychotic) F09
  with psychosis, psychotic reaction F09
  acute or subacute — *see* Delirium
  congenital — *see* Disability, intellectual
  organic F09
    post-traumatic (nonpsychotic) F07.81
      psychotic F09
    personality change F07.0
    postcontusional F07.81
    post-traumatic, nonpsychotic F07.81
    psycho-organic F09
    psychotic F06.8
brain stem stroke G46.3
Brandt's (acrodermatitis enteropathica) E83.2
broad ligament laceration N83.8
Brock's J98.11
bronze baby P83.88
Brown-Sequard G83.81
Brugada I49.8
bubbly lung P27.0
Buchem's M85.2

Syndrome - *continued*
Budd-Chiari I82.0
bulbar (progressive) G12.22
Bürger-Grütz E78.3
Burke's K86.89
Burnett's (milk-alkali) E83.52
burning feet E53.9
Bywaters' T79.5
Call-Fleming I67.841
carbohydrate-deficient glycoprotein (CDGS) E77.8
carcinogenic thrombophlebitis I82.1
carcinoid E34.0
cardiac asthma I50.1
cardiacos negros I27.0
cardiofaciocutaneous Q87.89
cardiopulmonary-obesity E66.2
cardiorenal — *see* Hypertension, cardiorenal
cardiorespiratory distress (idiopathic) , newborn P22.0
cardiovascular renal — *see* Hypertension, cardiorenal
carotid
  artery (hemispheric) (internal) G45.1
  body G90.01
  sinus G90.01
carpal tunnel G56.0-
Cassidy (-Scholte) E34.0
cat cry Q93.4
cat eye Q92.8
cauda equina G83.4
causalgia — *see* Causalgia
celiac K90.0
  artery compression I77.4
  axis I77.4
central pain G89.0
cerebellar
  hereditary G11.9
  stroke G46.4
cerebellomedullary malformation — *see* Spina bifida
cerebral
  artery
    anterior G46.1
    middle G46.0
    posterior G46.2
  gigantism E22.0
cervical (root) M53.1
  disc — *see* Disorder, disc, cervical, with neuritis
  fusion Q76.1
  posterior, sympathicus M53.0
  rib Q76.5
  sympathetic paralysis G90.2
cervicobrachial (diffuse) M53.1
cervicocranial M53.0
cervicodorsal outlet G54.2
cervicothoracic outlet G54.0
Céstan (-Raymond) I65.8
Charcot's (angina cruris) (intermittent claudication) I73.9
Charcot-Weiss-Baker G90.09
CHARGE Q89.8
Chédiak-Higashi (-Steinbrinck) E70.330
chest wall R07.1
Chiari's (hepatic vein thrombosis) I82.0
Chilaiditi's Q43.3
child maltreatment — *see* Maltreatment, child
chondrocostal junction M94.0
chondroectodermal dysplasia Q77.6
chromosome 4 short arm deletion Q93.3
chromosome 5 short arm deletion Q93.4
chronic
  infantile neurological, cutaneous and articular (CINCA) M04.2
  pain G89.4
    personality F68.8
Churg-Strauss M30.1
Clarke-Hadfield K86.89
Clerambault's automatism G93.89
Clouston's (hidrotic ectodermal dysplasia) Q82.4
clumsiness, clumsy child F82
cluster headache G44.009

Syndrome - *continued*
cluster headache - *continued*
  intractable G44.001
  not intractable G44.009
Coffin-Lowry Q89.8
cold injury (newborn) P80.0
combined immunity deficiency D81.9
compartment (deep) (posterior) (traumatic) T79.A0
  abdomen T79.A3
  lower extremity (hip, buttock, thigh, leg, foot, toes) T79.A2
  nontraumatic
    abdomen M79.A3
    lower extremity (hip, buttock, thigh, leg, foot, toes) M79.A2-
    specified site NEC M79.A9
    upper extremity (shoulder, arm, forearm, wrist, hand, fingers) M79.A1-
  postprocedural — *see* Syndrome, compartment, nontraumatic
  specified site NEC T79.A9
  upper extremity (shoulder, arm, forearm, wrist, hand, fingers) T79.A1
complex regional pain — *see* Syndrome, pain, complex regional
compression T79.5
  anterior spinal — *see* Syndrome, anterior, spinal artery, compression
  cauda equina G83.4
  celiac artery I77.4
  vertebral artery M47.029
    occipito-atlanto-axial region M47.021
    cervical region M47.022
concussion F07.81
congenital
  affecting multiple systems NEC Q87.89
  central alveolar hypoventilation G47.35
  facial diplegia Q87.0
  muscular hypertrophy-cerebral Q87.89
  oculo-auriculovertebral Q87.0
  oculofacial diplegia (Moebius) Q87.0
  rubella (manifest) P35.0
congestion-fibrosis (pelvic) , female N94.89
congestive dysmenorrhea N94.6
Conn's E26.01
connective tissue M35.9
  overlap NEC M35.1
conus medullaris G95.81
cord
  anterior G83.82
  posterior G83.83
coronary
  acute NEC I24.9
  insufficiency or intermediate I20.0
  slow flow I20.8
Costen's (complex) M26.69
costochondral junction M94.0
costoclavicular G54.0
costovertebral E22.0
Cowden Q85.8
craniovertebral M53.0
Creutzfeldt-Jakob — *see* Creutzfeldt-Jakob disease or syndrome
cri-du-chat Q93.4
crib death R99
cricopharyngeal — *see* Dysphagia
croup J05.0
CRPS I — *see* Syndrome, pain, complex regional I
crush T79.5
cubital tunnel — *see* Lesion, nerve, ulnar
Curschmann (-Batten) (-Steinert) G71.11
Cushing's E24.9
  alcohol-induced E24.4
  due to
    alcohol
    drugs E24.2
    ectopic ACTH E24.3
    overproduction of pituitary ACTH E24.0
  drug-induced E24.2
  overdose or wrong substance given or taken — *see* Table of Drugs and Chemicals, by drug, poisoning
  pituitary-dependent E24.0

Syndrome - *continued*
  Cushing's - *continued*
    specified type NEC E24.8
  cryopyrin-associated periodic M04.2
  cryptophthalmos Q87.0
  cystic duct stump K91.5
  Dana-Putnam D51.0
  Danbolt (-Cross) (acrodermatitis
    enteropathica) E83.2
  Dandy-Walker Q03.1
    with spina bifida Q07.01
  Danlos' — *see also* Syndrome, Ehlers-
    Danlos Q79.60
  defibrination — *see also* Fibrinolysis
    with
      antepartum hemorrhage — *see*
        Hemorrhage, antepartum, with
        coagulation defect
      intrapartum hemorrhage — *see*
        Hemorrhage, complicating,
        delivery
    newborn P60
    postpartum O72.3
  Degos' I77.89
  Déjérine-Roussy G89.0
  delayed sleep phase G47.21
  demyelinating G37.9
  dependence — *see* F10-F19 with fourth
    character .2
  depersonalization (-derealization) F48.1
  De Quervain E34.51
  de Toni-Fanconi (-Debré) E72.09
    with cystinosis E72.04
  diabetes mellitus-hypertension-nephrosis —
    see Diabetes, nephrosis
  diabetes mellitus in newborn infant P70.2
  diabetes-nephrosis — *see* Diabetes,
    nephrosis
  diabetic amyotrophy — *see* Diabetes,
    amyotrophy
  dialysis associated steal T82.898-
  Diamond-Blackfan D61.01
  Diamond-Gardener D69.2
  DIC (diffuse or disseminated intravascular
    coagulopathy) D65
  di George's D82.1
  Dighton's Q78.0
  disequilibrium E87.8
  Döhle body-panmyelopathic D72.0
  dorsolateral medullary G46.4
  double athetosis G80.3
  Down — *see also* Down syndrome Q90.9
  Dresbach's (elliptocytosis) D58.1
  Dressler's (postmyocardial infarction) I24.1
    postcardiotomy I97.0
  drug withdrawal, infant of dependent
    mother P96.1
  dry eye H04.12-
  due to abnormality
    chromosomal Q99.9
      sex
        female phenotype Q97.9
        male phenotype Q98.9
        specified NEC Q99.8
  dumping (postgastrectomy) K91.1
    nonsurgical K31.89
  Dupré's (meningism) R29.1
  dysmetabolic X E88.81
  dyspraxia, developmental F82
  Eagle-Barrett Q79.4
  Eaton-Lambert — *see* Syndrome, Lambert-
    Eaton
  Ebstein's Q22.5
  ectopic ACTH E24.3
  eczema-thrombocytopenia D82.0
  Eddowes' Q78.0
  effort (psychogenic) F45.8
  Eisenmenger's I27.83
  Ehlers-Danlos Q79.60
    classical (cEDS) (classical EDS) Q79.61
    hypermobile (hEDS) (hypermobile
      EDS) Q79.62
    specified NEC Q79.69
    vascular (vascular EDS) (vEDS) Q79.63
  Ekman's Q78.0

Syndrome - *continued*
  electric feet E53.8
  Ellis-van Creveld Q77.6
  empty nest Z60.0
  endocrine-hypertensive E27.0
  entrapment — *see* Neuropathy, entrapment
  eosinophilia-myalgia M35.8
  epileptic — *see also* Epilepsy, by type
    absence G40.A09
      intractable G40.A19
        with status epilepticus G40.A11
        without status epilepticus G40.A19
      not intractable G40.A09
        with status epilepticus G40.A01
        without status epilepticus G40.A09
  Erdheim-Chester (ECD) E88.89
  Erdheim's E22.0
  erythrocyte fragmentation D59.4
  Evans D69.41
  exhaustion F48.8
  extrapyramidal G25.9
    specified NEC G25.89
  eye retraction — *see* Strabismus
  eyelid-malar-mandible Q87.0
  Faber's D50.9
  facial pain, paroxysmal G50.0
  Fallot's Q21.3
  familial cold autoinflammatory M04.2
  familial eczema-thrombocytopenia (Wiskott-
    Aldrich) D82.0
  Fanconi (-de Toni) (-Debré) E72.09
    with cystinosis E72.04
  Fanconi's (anemia) (congenital
    pancytopenia) D61.09
  fatigue
    chronic R53.82
    psychogenic F48.8
  faulty bowel habit K59.39
  Feil-Klippel (brevicollis) Q76.1
  Felty's — *see* Felty's syndrome
  fertile eunuch E23.0
  fetal
    alcohol (dysmorphic) Q86.0
    hydantoin Q86.1
  Fiedler's I40.1
  first arch Q87.0
  fish odor E72.89
  Fisher's G61.0
  Fitzhugh-Curtis
    due to
      Chlamydia trachomatis A74.81
      Neisseria gonorrhorea (gonococcal
        peritonitis) A54.85
  Fitz's — *see also* Pancreatitis, acute K85.80
  Flajani (-Basedow) E05.00
    with thyroid storm E05.01
  flatback — *see* Flatback syndrome
  floppy
    baby P94.2
    iris (intraoeprative) (IFIS) H21.81
    mitral valve I34.1
  flush E34.0
  Foix-Alajouanine G95.19
  Fong's Q87.2
  food protein-induced enterocolitis
    (FPIES) K52.21
  foramen magnum G93.5
  Foster-Kennedy H47.14-
  Foville's (peduncular) G46.3
  fragile X Q99.2
  Franceschetti Q75.4
  Frey's
    auriculotemporal G50.8
    hyperhidrosis L74.52
  Friderichsen-Waterhouse A39.1
  Froin's G95.89
  frontal lobe F07.0
  Fukuhara E88.49
  functional
    bowel K59.9
    prepubertal castrate E29.1
  Gaisböck's D75.1
  ganglion (basal ganglia brain) G25.9
    geniculi G51.1
  Gardner-Diamond D69.2

Syndrome - *continued*
  gastroesophageal
    junction K22.0
    laceration-hemorrhage K22.6
  gastrojejunal loop obstruction K91.89
  Gee-Herter-Heubner K90.0
  Gelineau's G47.419
    with cataplexy G47.411
  genito-anorectal A55
  Gerstmann-Sträussler-Scheinker
    (GSS) A81.82
  Gianotti-Crosti L44.4
  giant platelet (Bernard-Soulier) D69.1
  Gilles de la Tourette's F95.2
  Glass Q87.89
  goiter-deafness E07.1
  Goldberg Q89.8
  Goldberg-Maxwell E34.51
  Good's D83.8
  Gopalan' (burning feet) E53.8
  Gorlin's Q87.89
  Gougerot-Blum L81.7
  Gouley's I31.1
  Gower's R55
  gray or grey (newborn) P93.0
    platelet D69.1
  Gubler-Millard G46.3
  Guillain-Barré (-Strohl) G61.0
  gustatory sweating G50.8
  Hadfield-Clarke K86.89
  hair tourniquet — *see* Constriction, external,
    by site
  Hamman's J98.19
  hand-foot L27.1
  hand-shoulder G90.8
  hantavirus (cardio) -pulmonary (HPS)
    (HCPS) B33.4
  happy puppet Q93.51
  Harada's H30.81-
  Hayem-Faber D50.9
  headache NEC G44.89
    complicated NEC G44.59
  Heberden's I20.8
  Hedinger's E34.0
  Hegglin's D72.0
  HELLP (hemolysis, elevated liver enzymes
    and low platelet count) O14.2-
    complicating
      childbirth O14.24
      puerperium O14.25
  hemolytic-uremic D59.3
  hemophagocytic, infection-associated D76.2
  Henoch-Schönlein D69.0
  hepatic flexure K59.8
  hepatopulmonary K76.81
  hepatorenal K76.7
    following delivery O90.4
    postoperative or postprocedural K91.83
    postpartum, puerperal O90.4
  hepatourologic K76.7
  Herter (-Gee) (nontropical sprue) K90.0
  Heubner-Herter K90.0
  Heyd's K76.7
  Hilger's G90.09
  histamine-like (fish poisoning) — *see*
    Poisoning, fish
  histiocytic D76.3
  histiocytosis NEC D76.3
  HIV infection, acute B20
  Hoffmann-Werdnig G12.0
  Hollander-Simons E88.1
  Hoppe-Goldflam G70.00
    with exacerbation (acute) G70.01
    in crisis G70.01
  Horner's G90.2
  hungry bone E83.81
  hunterian glossitis D51.0
  Hutchinson's triad A50.53
  hyperabduction G54.0
  hyperammonemia-hyperornithinemia-
    homocitrullinemia E72.4
  hypereosinophilic (idiopathic) D72.1
  hyperimmunoglobulin D M04.1
  hyperimmunoglobulin E (IgE) D82.4
  hyperkalemic E87.5

Syndrome - *continued*

hyperkinetic — *see* Hyperkinesia
hypermobility M35.7
hypernatremia E87.0
hyperosmolarity E87.0
hyperperfusion G97.82
hypersplenic D73.1
hypertransfusion, newborn P61.1
hyperventilation F45.8
hyperviscosity (of serum)
   polycythemic D75.1
   sclerothymic D58.8
hypoglycemic (familial) (neonatal) E16.2
hypokalemic E87.6
hyponatremic E87.1
hypopituitarism E23.0
hypoplastic left-heart Q23.4
hypopotassemia E87.6
hyposmolality E87.1
hypotension, maternal O26.5-
hypothenar hammer I73.89
hypoventilation, obesity (OHS) E66.2
ICF (intravascular coagulation-
   fibrinolysis) D65
idiopathic
   cardiorespiratory distress, newborn P22.0
   nephrotic (infantile) N04.9
iliotibial band M76.3-
immobility, immobilization
   (paraplegic) M62.3
immune reconstitution D89.3
immune reconstitution inflammatory
   [IRIS] D89.3
immunity deficiency, combined D81.9
immunodeficiency
   acquired — *see* Human,
      immunodeficiency virus (HIV)
      disease
   combined D81.9
impending coronary I20.0
impingement, shoulder M75.4-
inappropriate secretion of antidiuretic
   hormone E22.2
infant
   of diabetic mother P70.1
   gestational diabetes P70.0
infantilism (pituitary) E23.0
inferior vena cava I87.1
inspissated bile (newborn) P59.1
institutional (childhood) F94.2
insufficient sleep F51.12
intermediate coronary (artery) I20.0
interspinous ligament — *see* Spondylopathy,
   specified NEC
intestinal
   carcinoid E34.0
   knot K56.2
intravascular coagulation-fibrinolysis
   (ICF) D65
iodine-deficiency, congenital E00.9
   type
      mixed E00.2
      myxedematous E00.1
      neurological E00.0
IRDS (idiopathic respiratory distress,
   newborn) P22.0
irritable
   bowel K58.9
      with
         constipation K58.1
         diarrhea K58.0
      mixed K58.2
      psychogenic F45.8
      specified NEC K58.8
   heart (psychogenic) F45.8
   weakness F48.8
ischemic
   bowel (transient) K55.9
      chronic K55.1
      due to mesenteric artery
         insufficiency K55.1
   steal T82.898
IVC (intravascular coagulopathy) D65
Ivemark's Q89.01

Syndrome - *continued*

Jaccoud's — *see* Arthropathy, postrheumatic,
   chronic
Jackson's G83.89
Jakob-Creutzfeldt — *see* Creutzfeldt-Jakob
   disease or syndrome
jaw-winking Q07.8
Jervell-Lange-Nielsen I45.81
jet lag G47.25
Job's D71
Joseph-Diamond-Blackfan D61.01
jugular foramen G52.7
Kabuki Q89.8
Kanner's (autism) F84.0
Kartagener's Q89.3
Kelly's D50.1
Kimmelsteil-Wilson — *see* Diabetes,
   specified type, with Kimmelstiel-Wilson
   disease
Klein (e) -Levine G47.13
Klippel-Feil (brevicollis) Q76.1
Köhler-Pellegrini-Steida — *see* Bursitis,
   tibial collateral
König's K59.8
Korsakoff (-Wernicke) (nonalcoholic) F04
   alcoholic F10.26
Kostmann's D70.0
Krabbe's congenital muscle
   hypoplasia Q79.8
labyrinthine — *see* subcategory H83.2
lacunar NEC G46.7
Lambert-Eaton G70.80
   in
      neoplastic disease G73.1
      specified disease NEC G70.81
Landau-Kleffner — *see* Epilepsy, specified
   NEC
Larsen's Q74.8
lateral
   cutaneous nerve of thigh G57.1-
   medullary G46.4
Launois' E22.0
lazy
   leukocyte D70.8
   posture M62.3
Lemiere I80.8
Lennox-Gastaut G40.812
   intractable G40.814
      with status epilepticus G40.813
      without status epilepticus G40.814
   not intractable G40.812
      with status epilepticus G40.811
      without status epilepticus G40.812
lenticular, progressive E83.01
Leopold-Levi's E05.90
Lev's I44.2
Li-Fraumeni Z15.01
Lichtheim's D51.0
Lightwood's N25.89
Lignac (de Toni) (-Fanconi) (-Debré) E72.09
   with cystinosis E72.04
Likoff's I20.8
limbic epilepsy personality F07.0
liver-kidney K76.7
lobotomy F07.0
Loffler's J82
long arm 18 or 21 deletion Q93.89
long QT I45.81
Louis-Barré G11.3
low
   atmospheric pressure T70.29
   back M54.5
   output (cardiac) I50.9
lower radicular, newborn (birth injury) P14.8
Luetscher's (dehydration) E86.0
Lupus anticoagulant D68.62
Lutembacher's Q21.1
macrophage activation D76.1
   due to infection D76.2
magnesium-deficiency R29.0
Majeed M04.8
Mal de Debarquement R42
malabsorption K90.9
   postsurgical K91.2
malformation, congenital, due to

Syndrome - *continued*

malformation, congenital, due to - *continued*
   alcohol Q86.0
   exogenous cause NEC Q86.8
   hydantoin Q86.1
   warfarin Q86.2
malignant
   carcinoid E34.0
   neuroleptic G21.0
Mallory-Weiss K22.6
mandibulofacial dysostosis Q75.4
manic-depressive — *see* Disorder, bipolar
maple-syrup-urine E71.0
Marable's I77.4
Marfan's Q87.40
   with
      cardiovascular manifestations Q87.418
         aortic dilation Q87.410
      ocular manifestations Q87.42
      skeletal manifestations Q87.43
Marie's (acromegaly) E22.0
mast cell activation — *see* Activation, mast
   cell
maternal hypotension — *see* Syndrome,
   hypotension, maternal
May (-Hegglin) D72.0
McArdle (-Schmidt) (-Pearson) E74.04
McQuarrie's E16.2
meconium plug (newborn) P76.0
median arcuate ligament I77.4
Meekeren-Ehlers-Danlos Q79.6
megavitamin-B6 E67.2
Meige G24.4
MELAS E88.41
Mendelson's O74.0
MERRF (myoclonic epilepsy associated with
   ragged-red fibers) E88.42
mesenteric
   artery (superior) K55.1
   vascular insufficiency K55.1
metabolic E88.81
metastatic carcinoid E34.0
micrognathia-glossoptosis Q87.0
midbrain NEC G93.89
middle lobe (lung) J98.19
middle radicular G54.0
migraine — *see also* Migraine G43.909-
Mikulicz' K11.8
milk-alkali E83.52
Millard-Gubler G46.3
Miller-Dieker Q93.88
Miller-Fisher G61.0
Minkowski-Chauffard D58.0
Mirizzi's K83.1
MNGIE (Mitochondrial
   Neurogastrointestinal
   Encephalopathy) E88.49
Möbius, ophthalmoplegic migraine — *see*
   Migraine, ophthalmoplegic
monofixation H50.42
Morel-Moore M85.2
Morel-Morgagni M85.2
Morgagni (-Morel) (-Stewart) M85.2
Morgagni-Adams-Stokes I45.9
Muckle-Wells M04.2
mucocutaneous lymph node (acute febrile)
   (MCLS) M30.3
multiple endocrine neoplasia (MEN) — *see*
   Neoplasia, endocrine, multiple (MEN)
multiple operations — *see* Disorder,
   factitious
Mounier-Kuhn Q32.4
   with bronchiectasis J47.9
      with
         exacerbation (acute) J47.1
         lower respiratory infection J47.0
   acquired J98.09
      with bronchiectasis J47.9
         with
            exacerbation (acute) J47.1
            lower respiratory infection J47.0
myasthenic G70.9
   in
      diabetes mellitus — *see* Diabetes,
         amyotrophy

Syndrome - *continued*
myasthenic - *continued*
  in - *continued*
    endocrine disease NEC E34.9 *[G73.3]*
    neoplastic disease — *see also*
      Neoplasm D49.9 *[G73.3]*
    thyrotoxicosis
      (hyperthyroidism) E05.90 *[G73.3]*
      with thyroid storm E05.91 *[G73.3]*
myelodysplastic D46.9
  with
    5q deletion D46.C
    isolated del (5q) chromosomal
      abnormality D46.C
    lesions, low grade D46.20
    specified NEC D46.Z
myelopathic pain G89.0
myeloproliferative (chronic) D47.1
myofascial pain M79.18
Naffziger's G54.0
nail patella Q87.2
NARP (Neuropathy, Ataxia and Retinitis
  pigmentosa) E88.49
neonatal abstinence P96.1
nephritic — *see also* Nephritis
  with edema — *see* Nephrosis
  acute N00.9
  chronic N03.9
  rapidly progressive N01.9
nephrotic (congenital) — *see also*
  Nephrosis N04.9
  with
    dense deposit disease N04.6
    diffuse
      crescentic glomerulonephritis N04.7
      endocapillary proliferative
        glomerulonephritis N04.4
      membranous
        glomerulonephritis N04.2
      mesangial proliferative
        glomerulonephritis N04.3
      mesangiocapillary
        glomerulonephritis N04.5
    focal and segmental glomerular
      lesions N04.1
    minor glomerular abnormality N04.0
    specified morphological changes
      NEC N04.8
  diabetic — *see* Diabetes, nephrosis
neurologic neglect R41.4
Nezelof's D81.4
Nonne-Milroy-Meige Q82.0
Nothnagel's vasomotor
  acroparesthesia I73.89
obesity hypoventilation (OHS) E66.2
oculomotor H51.9
ophthalmoplegia-cerebellar ataxia — *see*
  Strabismus, paralytic, third nerve
oral allergy T78.1
oral-facial-digital Q87.0
organic
  affective F06.30
  amnesic (not alcohol- or drug-
    induced) F04
  brain F09
  depressive F06.31
  hallucinosis F06.0
  personality F07.0
Ormond's N13.5
oro-facial-digital Q87.0
os trigonum Q68.8
Osler-Weber-Rendu I78.0
osteoporosis-osteomalacia M83.8
Osterreicher-Turner Q87.2
otolith — *see* subcategory H81.8
oto-palatal-digital Q87.0
outlet (thoracic) G54.0
ovary
  polycystic E28.2
  resistant E28.39
  sclerocystic E28.2
Owren's D68.2
Paget-Schroetter I82.890
pain — *see also* Pain
  complex regional I G90.50

Syndrome - *continued*
pain - *continued*
  complex regional I - *continued*
    lower limb G90.52-
      specified site NEC G90.59
      upper limb G90.51-
  complex regional II — *see* Causalgia
painful
  bruising D69.2
  feet E53.8
  prostate N42.81
paralysis agitans — *see* Parkinsonism
paralytic G83.9
  specified NEC G83.89
Parinaud's H51.0
parkinsonian — *see* Parkinsonism
Parkinson's — *see* Parkinsonism
paroxysmal facial pain G50.0
Parry's E05.00
  with thyroid storm E05.01
Parsonage (-Aldren) -Turner G54.5
patella clunk M25.86-
Paterson (-Brown) (-Kelly) D50.1
pectoral girdle I77.89
pectoralis minor I77.89
pediatric autoimmune neuropsychiatric
    disorders associated with streptococcal
    infections (PANDAS) D89.89
Pelger-Huet D72.0
pellagra-cerebellar ataxia-renal
    aminoaciduria E72.02
pellagroid E52
Pellegrini-Stieda — *see* Bursitis, tibial
    collateral
pelvic congestion-fibrosis, female N94.89
penta X Q97.1
peptic ulcer — *see* Ulcer, peptic
perabduction I77.89
periodic fever M04.1
periodic fever, aphthous stomatitis,
    pharyngitis, and adenopathy
    [PFAPA] M04.8
periodic headache, in adults and children —
    see Headache, periodic syndromes in
    adults and children
periurethral fibrosis N13.5
phantom limb (without pain) G54.7
  with pain G54.6
pharyngeal pouch D82.1
Pick's — *see* Disease, Pick's
Pickwickian E66.2
PIE (pulmonary infiltration with
    eosinophilia) J82
pigmentary pallidal degeneration
    (progressive) G23.0
pineal E34.8
pituitary E22.0
plantar fascia M72.2
placental transfusion — *see* Pregnancy,
    complicated by, placental transfusion
    syndromes
plateau iris (post-iridectomy)
    (postprocedural) H21.82
Plummer-Vinson D50.1
pluricarential of infancy E40
plurideficiency E40
pluriglandular (compensatory) E31.8
  autoimmune E31.0
pneumatic hammer T75.21
polyangiitis overlap M30.8
polycarential of infancy E40
polyglandular E31.8
  autoimmune E31.0
polysplenia Q89.09
pontine NEC G93.89
popliteal
  artery entrapment I77.89
  web Q87.89
  post endometrial ablation N99.85
postcardiac injury
  postcardiotomy I97.0
  postmyocardial infarction I24.1
postcardiotomy I97.0
post chemoembolization - code to associated
    conditions

Syndrome - *continued*
postcholecystectomy K91.5
postcommissurotomy I97.0
postconcussional F07.81
postcontusional F07.81
postencephalitic F07.89
posterior
  cervical sympathetic M53.0
  cord G83.83
  fossa compression G93.5
  reversible encephalopathy (PRES) I67.83
postgastrectomy (dumping) K91.1
postgastric surgery K91.1
postinfarction I24.1
postlaminectomy NEC M96.1
postleukotomy F07.0
postmastectomy lymphedema I97.2
postmyocardial infarction I24.1
postoperative NEC T81.9
  blind loop K90.2
postpartum panhypopituitary
    (Sheehan) E23.0
postpolio (myelitic) G14
postthrombotic I87.009
  with
    inflammation I87.02-
      with ulcer I87.03-
    specified complication NEC I87.09-
    ulcer I87.01-
      with inflammation I87.03-
  asymptomatic I87.00-
postvagotomy K91.1
postvalvulotomy I97.0
postviral NEC G93.3
  fatigue G93.3
Potain's K31.0
potassium intoxication E87.5
Prader-Willi Q87.11
Prader-Willi-like Q87.19
precerebral artery (multiple) (bilateral) G45.2
preinfarction I20.0
preleukemic D46.9
premature senility E34.8
premenstrual dysphoric F32.81
premenstrual tension N94.3
Prinzmetal-Massumi R07.1
prune belly Q79.4
pseudocarpal tunnel (sublimis) — *see*
    Syndrome, carpal tunnel
pseudoparalytica G70.00
  with exacerbation (acute) G70.01
  in crisis G70.01
pseudo -Turner's Q87.19
psycho-organic (nonpsychotic
    severity) F07.9
  acute or subacute F05
  depressive type F06.31
  hallucinatory type F06.0
  nonpsychotic severity F07.0
  specified NEC F07.89
pulmonary
  arteriosclerosis I27.0
  dysmaturity (Wilson-Mikity) P27.0
  hypoperfusion (idiopathic) P22.0
  renal (hemorrhagic)
    (Goodpasture's) M31.0
pure
  motor lacunar G46.5
  sensory lacunar G46.6
Putnam-Dana D51.0
pyogenic arthritis, pyoderma gangrenosum,
    and acne [PAPA] M04.8
pyramidopallidonigral G20
pyriformis — *see* Lesion, nerve, sciatic
QT interval prolongation I45.81
radicular NEC — *see* Radiculopathy
  upper limbs, newborn (birth injury) P14.3
rapid time-zone change G47.25
Rasmussen G04.81
Raymond (-Céstan) I65.8
Raynaud's I73.00
  with gangrene I73.01
RDS (respiratory distress syndrome,
    newborn) P22.0
reactive airways dysfunction J68.3

Syndrome - *continued*
Refsum's G60.1
Reifenstein E34.52
renal glomerulohyalinosis-diabetic — *see*
        Diabetes, nephrosis
Rendu-Osler-Weber I78.0
residual ovary N99.83
resistant ovary E28.39
respiratory
    distress
        acute J80
            adult J80
            child J80
            idiopathic J84.114
        newborn (idiopathic) (type I) P22.0
            type II P22.1
restless legs G25.81
retinoblastoma (familial) C69.2
retroperitoneal fibrosis N13.5
retroviral seroconversion (acute) Z21
Reye's G93.7
Richter — *see* Leukemia, chronic
        lymphocytic, B-cell type
Ridley's I50.1
right
    heart, hypoplastic Q22.6
    ventricular obstruction — *see* Failure,
            heart, right
Romano-Ward (prolonged QT
        interval) I45.81
rotator cuff, shoulder — *see also* Tear, rotator
        cuff M75.10-
Rotes Quérol — *see* Hyperostosis,
        ankylosing
Roth — *see* Meralgia paresthetica
rubella (congenital) P35.0
Ruvalcaba-Myhre-Smith E71.440
Rytand-Lipsitch I44.2
salt
    depletion E87.1
        due to heat NEC T67.8
            causing heat exhaustion or
                    prostration T67.4
        low E87.1
salt-losing N28.89
SATB2-associated Q87.89
Scaglietti-Dagnini E22.0
scalenus anticus (anterior) G54.0
scapulocostal — *see* Mononeuropathy, upper
        limb, specified site NEC
scapuloperoneal G71.09
schizophrenic, of childhood NEC F84.5
Schnitzler D47.2
Scholte's E34.0
Schroeder's E27.0
Schüller-Christian C96.5
Schwachman's — *see* Syndrome,
        Shwachman's
Schwartz (-Jampel) G71.13
Schwartz-Bartter E22.2
scimitar Q26.8
sclerocystic ovary E28.2
Seitelberger's G31.89
septicemic adrenal hemorrhage A39.1
seroconversion, retroviral (acute) Z21
serous meningitis G93.2
severe acute respiratory (SARS) J12.81
shaken infant T74.4
shock (traumatic) T79.4
    kidney N17.0
        following crush injury T79.5
    toxic A48.3
shock-lung J80
Shone's - code to specific anomalies
short
    bowel K91.2
    rib Q77.2
shoulder-hand — *see* Algoneurodystrophy
Shwachman's D70.4
sicca — *see* Sicca syndrome
sick
    cell E87.1
    sinus I49.5
sick-euthyroid E07.81
sideropenic D50.1

Syndrome - *continued*
Siemens' ectodermal dysplasia Q82.4
Silfversköld's Q78.9
Simons' E88.1
sinus tarsi M25.57-
sinusitis-bronchiectasis-situs inversus Q89.3
Sipple's E31.22
sirenomelia Q87.2
Slocumb's E27.0
slow flow, coronary I20.8
Sluder's G44.89
Smith-Magenis Q93.88
Sneddon-Wilkinson L13.1
Soto's Q87.3
South African cardiomyopathy I42.8
spasmodic
    upward movement, eyes H51.8
    winking F95.8
Spen's I45.9
splenic
    agenesis Q89.01
    flexure K59.8
    neutropenia D73.81
Spurway's Q78.0
staphylococcal scalded skin L00
steal
    arteriovenous T82.898-
    ischemic T82.898-
    subclavian G45.8
Stein-Leventhal E28.2
Stein's E28.2
Stevens-Johnson syndrome L51.1
    toxic epidermal necrolysis overlap L51.3
Stewart-Morel M85.2
Stickler Q89.8
stiff baby Q89.8
stiff man G25.82
Still-Felty — *see* Felty's syndrome
Stokes (-Adams) I45.9
stone heart I50.1
straight back, congenital Q76.49
subclavian steal G45.8
subcoracoid-pectoralis minor G54.0
subcostal nerve compression I77.89
subphrenic interposition Q43.3
superior
    cerebellar artery I63.89
    mesenteric artery K55.1
    semi-circular canal dehiscence H83.8X-
    vena cava I87.1
supine hypotensive (maternal) — *see*
        Syndrome, hypotension, maternal
suprarenal cortical E27.0
supraspinatus — *see also* Tear, rotator
        cuff M75.10-
Susac G93.49
swallowed blood P78.2
sweat retention L74.0
Swyer Q99.1
Symond's G93.2
sympathetic
    cervical paralysis G90.2
    pelvic, female N94.89
systemic inflammatory response (SIRS) , of
        non-infectious origin (without organ
        dysfunction) R65.10
    with acute organ dysfunction R65.11
tachycardia-bradycardia I49.5
takotsubo I51.81
TAR (thrombocytopenia with absent
        radius) Q87.2
tarsal tunnel G57.5-
teething K00.7
tegmental G93.89
telangiectasic-pigmentation-cataract Q82.8
temporal pyramidal apex — *see* Otitis,
        media, suppurative, acute
temporomandibular joint-pain-
        dysfunction M26.62-
Terry's — *see also* Myopia,
        degenerative H44.2-
testicular feminization — *see also* Syndrome,
        androgen insensitivity E34.51
thalamic pain (hyperesthetic) G89.0
thoracic outlet (compression) G54.0

Syndrome - *continued*
Thorson-Björck E34.0
thrombocytopenia with absent radius
        (TAR) Q87.2
thyroid-adrenocortical insufficiency E31.0
tibial
    anterior M76.81-
    posterior M76.82-
Tietze's M94.0
time-zone (rapid) G47.25
Toni-Fanconi E72.09
    with cystinosis E72.04
Touraine's Q79.8
tourniquet — *see* Constriction, external, by
        site
toxic shock A48.3
transient left ventricular apical
        ballooning I51.81
traumatic vasospastic T75.22
Treacher Collins Q75.4
triple X, female Q97.0
trisomy Q92.9
    13 Q91.7
        meiotic nondisjunction Q91.4
        mitotic nondisjunction Q91.5
        mosaicism Q91.5
        translocation Q91.6
    18 Q91.3
        meiotic nondisjunction Q91.0
        mitotic nondisjunction Q91.1
        mosaicism Q91.1
        translocation Q91.2
    20 (q) (p) Q92.8
    21 Q90.9
        meiotic nondisjunction Q90.0
        mitotic nondisjunction Q90.1
        mosaicism Q90.1
        translocation Q90.2
    22 Q92.8
tropical wet feet T69.0-
Trousseau's I82.1
tumor lysis (following antineoplastic
        chemotherapy) (spontaneous)
        NEC E88.3
tumor necrosis factor receptor associated
        periodic (TRAPS) M04.1
Twiddler's (due to)
    automatic implantable
            defibrillator T82.198
    cardiac pacemaker T82.198
Unverricht (-Lundborg) — *see* Epilepsy,
        generalized, idiopathic
upward gaze H51.8
uremia, chronic — *see also* Disease, kidney,
        chronic N18.9
urethral N34.3
urethro-oculo-articular — *see* Reiter's disease
urohepatic K76.7
vago-hypoglossal G52.7
vascular NEC in cerebrovascular
        disease G46.8
vasoconstriction, reversible
        cerebrovascular I67.841
vasomotor I73.9
vasospastic (traumatic) T75.22
vasovagal R55
van Buchem's M85.2
van der Hoeve's Q78.0
VATER Q87.2
velo-cardio-facial Q93.81
vena cava (inferior) (superior)
        (obstruction) I87.1
vertebral
    artery G45.0
        compression — *see* Syndrome, anterior,
                spinal artery, compression
        steal G45.0
vertebro-basilar artery G45.0
vertebrogenic (pain) M54.89
vertiginous — *see* Disorder, vestibular
        function
Vinson-Plummer D50.1
virus B34.9
visceral larva migrans B83.0
visual disorientation H53.8

Syndrome - *continued*
  vitamin B6 deficiency E53.1
  vitreal corneal H59.01-
  vitreous (touch) H59.01-
  Vogt-Koyanagi H20.82-
  Volkmann's T79.6
  von Schroetter's I82.890
  von Willebrand (-Jürgen) D68.0
  Waldenström-Kjellberg D50.1
  Wallenberg's G46.3
  water retention E87.79
  Waterhouse (-Friderichsen) A39.1
  Weber-Gubler G46.3
  Weber-Leyden G46.3
  Weber's G46.3
  Wegener's M31.30
    with
      kidney involvement M31.31
      lung involvement M31.30
        with kidney involvement M31.31
  Weingarten's (tropical eosinophilia) J82
  Weiss-Baker G90.09
  Werdnig-Hoffman G12.0
  Werner's E31.21
  Werner's E34.8
  Wernicke-Korsakoff (nonalcoholic) F04
    alcoholic F10.26
  West's — *see* Epilepsy, spasms
  Westphal-Strümpell E83.01
  wet
    feet (maceration) (tropical) T69.0-
    lung, newborn P22.1
  whiplash S13.4
  whistling face Q87.0
  Wilkie's K55.1
  Wilkinson-Sneddon L13.1
  Williams Q93.82
  Willebrand (-Jürgens) D68.0
  Wilson's (hepatolenticular
    degeneration) E83.01
  Wiskott-Aldrich D82.0
  withdrawal — *see* Withdrawal, state
    drug
      infant of dependent mother P96.1
      therapeutic use, newborn P96.2
  Woakes' (ethmoiditis) J33.1
  Wright's (hyperabduction) G54.0
  X I20.9
  XXXX Q97.1
  XXXXX Q97.1
  XXXXY Q98.1
  XXY Q98.0
  Yao M04.8
  yellow nail L60.5
  Zahorsky's B08.5
  Zellweger syndrome E71.510
  Zellweger-like syndrome E71.541
Synechia (anterior) (iris) (posterior) (pupil)
  — *see also* Adhesions, iris
  intra-uterine (traumatic) N85.6
Synesthesia R20.8
Syngamiasis, syngamosis B83.3
Synodontia K00.2
Synorchidism, synorchism Q55.1
Synostosis (congenital) Q78.8
  astragalo-scaphoid Q74.2
  radioulnar Q74.0
Synovial sarcoma — *see* Neoplasm,
  connective tissue, malignant
Synovioma (malignant) — *see also*
  Neoplasm, connective tissue, malignant
  benign — *see* Neoplasm, connective tissue,
    benign
Synoviosarcoma — *see* Neoplasm, connective
  tissue, malignant
Synovitis — *see also* Tenosynovitis M65.9
  crepitant
    hand M70.0-
    wrist M70.03-
  gonococcal A54.49
  gouty — *see* Gout
  in (due to)
    crystals M65.8-
    gonorrhea A54.49
    syphilis (late) A52.78

Synovitis - *continued*
  in (due to) - *continued*
    use, overuse, pressure — *see* Disorder, soft
      tissue, due to use
    infective NEC — *see* Tenosynovitis,
      infective NEC
    specified NEC — *see* Tenosynovitis,
      specified type NEC
  syphilitic A52.78
    congenital (early) A50.02
  toxic — *see* Synovitis, transient
  transient M67.3-
    ankle M67.37-
    elbow M67.32-
    foot joint M67.37-
    hand joint M67.34-
    hip M67.35-
    knee M67.36-
    multiple site M67.39
    pelvic region M67.35-
    shoulder M67.31-
    specified joint NEC M67.38
    wrist M67.33-
  traumatic, current — *see* Sprain
  tuberculous — *see* Tuberculosis, synovitis
  villonodular (pigmented) M12.2-
    ankle M12.27-
    elbow M12.22-
    foot joint M12.27-
    hand joint M12.24-
    hip M12.25-
    knee M12.26-
    multiple site M12.29
    pelvic region M12.25-
    shoulder M12.21-
    specified joint NEC M12.28
    vertebrae M12.28
    wrist M12.23-
Syphilid A51.39
  congenital A50.06
  newborn A50.06
  tubercular (late) A52.79
Syphilis, syphilitic (acquired) A53.9
  abdomen (late) A52.79
  acoustic nerve A52.15
  adenopathy (secondary) A51.49
  adrenal (gland) (with cortical
    hypofunction) A52.79
  age under 2 years NOS — *see also* Syphilis,
    congenital, early
    acquired A51.9
  alopecia (secondary) A51.32
  anemia (late) A52.79 *[D63.8]*
  aneurysm (aorta) (ruptured) A52.01
    central nervous system A52.05
    congenital A50.54 *[I79.0]*
  anus (late) A52.74
    primary A51.1
    secondary A51.39
  aorta (arch) (abdominal) (thoracic) A52.02
    aneurysm A52.01
  aortic (insufficiency) (regurgitation)
    (stenosis) A52.03
    aneurysm A52.01
  arachnoid (adhesive) (cerebral)
    (spinal) A52.13
  asymptomatic — *see* Syphilis, latent
  ataxia (locomotor) A52.11
  atrophoderma maculatum A51.39
  auricular fibrillation A52.06
  bladder (late) A52.76
  bone A52.77
    secondary A51.46
  brain A52.17
  breast (late) A52.79
  bronchus (late) A52.72
  bubo (primary) A51.0
  bulbar palsy A52.19
  bursa (late) A52.78
  cardiac decompensation A52.06
  cardiovascular A52.00
  central nervous system (late) (recurrent)
    (relapse) (tertiary) A52.3
    with
      ataxia A52.11

Syphilis, syphilitic (acquired) - *continued*
  central nervous system (late) (recurrent)
    (relapse) (tertiary) - *continued*
    with - *continued*
      general paralysis A52.17
        juvenile A50.45
      paresis (general) A52.17
        juvenile A50.45
      tabes (dorsalis) A52.11
        juvenile A50.45
      taboparesis A52.17
        juvenile A50.45
    aneurysm A52.05
      congenital A50.40
      juvenile A50.40
    remission in (sustained) A52.3
    serology doubtful, negative, or
      positive A52.3
    specified nature or site NEC A52.19
    vascular A52.05
  cerebral A52.17
    meningovascular A52.13
    nerves (multiple palsies) A52.15
    sclerosis A52.17
    thrombosis A52.05
  cerebrospinal (tabetic type) A52.12
  cerebrovascular A52.05
  cervix (late) A52.76
  chancre (multiple) A51.0
    extragenital A51.2
    Rollet's A51.0
  Charcot's joint A52.16
  chorioretinitis A51.43
    congenital A50.01
    late A52.71
    prenatal A50.01
  choroiditis — *see* Syphilitic chorioretinitis
  choroidoretinitis — *see* Syphilitic
    chorioretinitis
  ciliary body (secondary) A51.43
    late A52.71
  colon (late) A52.74
  combined spinal sclerosis A52.11
  condyloma (latum) A51.31
  congenital A50.9
    with
      paresis (general) A50.45
      tabes (dorsalis) A50.45
      taboparesis A50.45
    chorioretinitis, choroiditis A50.01 *[H32]*
    early, or less than 2 years after birth
      NEC A50.2
      with manifestations — *see* Syphilis,
        congenital, early, symptomatic
      latent (without manifestations) A50.1
        negative spinal fluid test A50.1
        serology positive A50.1
      symptomatic A50.09
        cutaneous A50.06
        mucocutaneous A50.07
        oculopathy A50.01
        osteochondropathy A50.02
        pharyngitis A50.03
        pneumonia A50.04
        rhinitis A50.05
        visceral A50.08
      interstitial keratitis A50.31
      juvenile neurosyphilis A50.45
    late, or 2 years or more after birth
      NEC A50.7
      chorioretinitis, choroiditis A50.32
      interstitial keratitis A50.31
      juvenile neurosyphilis A50.45
      latent (without manifestations) A50.6
        negative spinal fluid test A50.6
        serology positive A50.6
      symptomatic or with manifestations
        NEC A50.59
        arthropathy A50.55
        cardiovascular A50.54
        Clutton's joints A50.51
        Hutchinson's teeth A50.52
        Hutchinson's triad A50.53
        osteochondropathy A50.56
        saddle nose A50.57

Syphilis, syphilitic (acquired) - *continued*
  conjugal A53.9
    tabes A52.11
  conjunctiva (late) A52.71
  contact Z20.2
  cord bladder A52.19
  cornea, late A52.71
  coronary (artery) (sclerosis) A52.06
  coryza, congenital A50.05
  cranial nerve A52.15
    multiple palsies A52.15
  cutaneous — *see* Syphilis, skin
  dacryocystitis (late) A52.71
  degeneration, spinal cord A52.12
  dementia paralytica A52.17
    juvenilis A50.45
  destruction of bone A52.77
  dilatation, aorta A52.01
  due to blood transfusion A53.9
  dura mater A52.13
  ear A52.79
    inner A52.79
      nerve (eighth) A52.15
      neurorecurrence A52.15
  early A51.9
    cardiovascular A52.00
    central nervous system A52.3
    latent (without manifestations) (less than 2
        years after infection) A51.5
      negative spinal fluid test A51.5
      serological relapse after treatment A51.5
      serology positive A51.5
    relapse (treated, untreated) A51.9
    skin A51.39
    symptomatic A51.9
      extragenital chancre A51.2
      primary, except extragenital
          chancre A51.0
      secondary — *see also* Syphilis,
          secondary A51.39
        relapse (treated, untreated) A51.49
    ulcer A51.39
  eighth nerve (neuritis) A52.15
  endemic A65
  endocarditis A52.03
    aortic A52.03
    pulmonary A52.03
  epididymis (late) A52.76
  epiglottis (late) A52.73
  epiphysitis (congenital) (early) A50.02
  episcleritis (late) A52.71
  esophagus A52.79
  eustachian tube A52.73
  exposure to Z20.2
  eye A52.71
  eyelid (late) (with gumma) A52.71
  fallopian tube (late) A52.76
  fracture A52.77
  gallbladder (late) A52.74
  gastric (polyposis) (late) A52.74
  general A53.9
    paralysis A52.17
      juvenile A50.45
  genital (primary) A51.0
  glaucoma A52.71
  gumma NEC A52.79
    cardiovascular system A52.00
    central nervous system A52.3
    congenital A50.59
  heart (block) (decompensation) (disease)
      (failure) A52.06 *[I52]*
    valve NEC A52.03
  hemianesthesia A52.19
  hemianopsia A52.71
  hemiparesis A52.17
  hemiplegia A52.17
  hepatic artery A52.09
  hepatis A52.74
  hepatomegaly, congenital A50.08
  hereditaria tarda — *see* Syphilis, congenital,
      late
  hereditary — *see* Syphilis, congenital
  Hutchinson's teeth A50.52
  hyalitis A52.71
  inactive — *see* Syphilis, latent

Syphilis, syphilitic (acquired) - *continued*
  infantum — *see* Syphilis, congenital
  inherited — *see* Syphilis, congenital
  internal ear A52.79
  intestine (late) A52.74
  iris, iritis (secondary) A51.43
    late A52.71
  joint (late) A52.77
  keratitis (congenital) (interstitial)
      (late) A50.31
  kidney (late) A52.75
  lacrimal passages (late) A52.71
  larynx (late) A52.73
  late A52.9
    cardiovascular A52.00
    central nervous system A52.3
    kidney A52.75
    latent or 2 years or more after infection
        (without manifestations) A52.8
      negative spinal fluid test A52.8
      serology positive A52.8
    paresis A52.17
    specified site NEC A52.79
    symptomatic or with
        manifestations A52.79
    tabes A52.11
  latent A53.0
    with signs or symptoms - code by site and
        stage under Syphilis
    central nervous system A52.2
    date of infection unspecified A53.0
    early, or less than 2 years after
        infection A51.5
    follow-up of latent syphilis A53.0
      date of infection unspecified A53.0
      late, or 2 years or more after
          infection A52.8
    late, or 2 years or more after
        infection A52.8
    positive serology (only finding) A53.0
      date of infection unspecified A53.0
      early, or less than 2 years after
          infection A51.5
      late, or 2 years or more after
          infection A52.8
  lens (late) A52.71
  leukoderma A51.39
    late A52.79
  lienitis A52.79
  lip A51.39
    chancre (primary) A51.2
    late A52.79
  Lissauer's paralysis A52.17
  liver A52.74
  locomotor ataxia A52.11
  lung A52.72
  lymph gland (early) (secondary) A51.49
    late A52.79
  lymphadenitis (secondary) A51.49
  macular atrophy of skin A51.39
    striated A52.79
  mediastinum (late) A52.73
  meninges (adhesive) (brain) (spinal
      cord) A52.13
  meningitis A52.13
    acute (secondary) A51.41
    congenital A50.41
  meningoencephalitis A52.14
  meningovascular A52.13
    congenital A50.41
  mesarteritis A52.09
    brain A52.04
  middle ear A52.77
  mitral stenosis A52.03
  monoplegia A52.17
  mouth (secondary) A51.39
    late A52.79
  mucocutaneous (secondary) A51.39
    late A52.79
  mucous
    membrane (secondary) A51.39
      late A52.79
    patches A51.39
      congenital A50.07
  mulberry molars A50.52

Syphilis, syphilitic (acquired) - *continued*
  muscle A52.78
  myocardium A52.06
  nasal sinus (late) A52.73
  neonatorum — *see* Syphilis, congenital
  nephrotic syndrome (secondary) A51.44
  nerve palsy (any cranial nerve) A52.15
    multiple A52.15
  nervous system, central A52.3
  neuritis A52.15
    acoustic A52.15
  neurorecidive of retina A52.19
  neuroretinitis A52.19
  newborn — *see* Syphilis, congenital
  nodular superficial (late) A52.79
  nonvenereal A65
  nose (late) A52.73
    saddle back deformity A50.57
  occlusive arterial disease A52.09
  oculopathy A52.71
  ophthalmic (late) A52.71
  optic nerve (atrophy) (neuritis)
      (papilla) A52.15
  orbit (late) A52.71
  organic A53.9
  osseous (late) A52.77
  osteochondritis (congenital) (early) A50.02
      [M90.80]
  osteoporosis A52.77
  ovary (late) A52.76
  oviduct (late) A52.76
  palate (late) A52.79
  pancreas (late) A52.74
  paralysis A52.17
    general A52.17
      juvenile A50.45
  paresis (general) A52.17
    juvenile A50.45
  paresthesia A52.19
  Parkinson's disease or syndrome A52.19
  paroxysmal tachycardia A52.06
  pemphigus (congenital) A50.06
  penis (chancre) A51.0
    late A52.76
  pericardium A52.06
  perichondritis, larynx (late) A52.73
  periosteum (late) A52.77
    congenital (early) A50.02 *[M90.80]*
    early (secondary) A51.46
  peripheral nerve A52.79
  petrous bone (late) A52.77
  pharynx (late) A52.73
    secondary A51.39
  pituitary (gland) A52.79
  pleura (late) A52.73
  pneumonia, white A50.04
  pontine lesion A52.17
  portal vein A52.09
  primary A51.0
    anal A51.1
    and secondary — *see* Syphilis, secondary
    central nervous system A52.3
    extragenital chancre NEC A51.2
    fingers A51.2
    genital A51.0
    lip A51.2
    specified site NEC A51.2
    tonsils A51.2
  prostate (late) A52.76
  ptosis (eyelid) A52.71
  pulmonary (late) A52.72
    artery A52.09
  pyelonephritis (late) A52.75
  recently acquired, symptomatic A51.9
  rectum (late) A52.74
  respiratory tract (late) A52.73
  retina, late A52.71
  retrobulbar neuritis A52.15
  salpingitis A52.76
  sclera (late) A52.71
  sclerosis
    cerebral A52.17
    coronary A52.06
    multiple A52.11
  scotoma (central) A52.71

Syphilis, syphilitic (acquired) - *continued*
  scrotum (late) A52.76
  secondary (and primary) A51.49
    adenopathy A51.49
    anus A51.39
    bone A51.46
    chorioretinitis, choroiditis A51.43
    hepatitis A51.45
    liver A51.45
    lymphadenitis A51.49
    meningitis (acute) A51.41
    mouth A51.39
    mucous membranes A51.39
    periosteum, periostitis A51.46
    pharynx A51.39
    relapse (treated, untreated) A51.49
    skin A51.39
    specified form NEC A51.49
    tonsil A51.39
    ulcer A51.39
    viscera NEC A51.49
    vulva A51.39
  seminal vesicle (late) A52.76
  seronegative with signs or symptoms - code by site and stage under Syphilis
  seropositive
    with signs or symptoms - code by site and stage under Syphilis
    follow-up of latent syphilis — *see* Syphilis, latent
    only finding — *see* Syphilis, latent
  seventh nerve (paralysis) A52.15
  sinus, sinusitis (late) A52.73
  skeletal system A52.77
  skin (with ulceration) (early) (secondary) A51.39
    late or tertiary A52.79
  small intestine A52.74
  spastic spinal paralysis A52.17
  spermatic cord (late) A52.76
  spinal (cord) A52.12
  spleen A52.79
  splenomegaly A52.79
  spondylitis A52.77
  staphyloma A52.71
  stigmata (congenital) A50.59
  stomach A52.74
  synovium A52.78
  tabes dorsalis (late) A52.11
    juvenile A50.45
  tabetic type A52.11
    juvenile A50.45
  taboparesis A52.17
    juvenile A50.45
  tachycardia A52.06
  tendon (late) A52.78
  tertiary A52.9
    with symptoms NEC A52.79
    cardiovascular A52.00
    central nervous system A52.3
    multiple NEC A52.79
    specified site NEC A52.79
  testis A52.76
  thorax A52.73
  throat A52.73
  thymus (gland) (late) A52.79
  thyroid (late) A52.79
  tongue (late) A52.79
  tonsil (lingual) (late) A52.73
    primary A51.2
    secondary A51.39
  trachea (late) A52.73
  tunica vaginalis (late) A52.76
  ulcer (any site) (early) (secondary) A51.39
    late A52.79
    perforating A52.79
      foot A52.11
  urethra (late) A52.76
  urogenital (late) A52.76
  uterus (late) A52.76
  uveal tract (secondary) A51.43
    late A52.71
  uveitis (secondary) A51.43
    late A52.71
  uvula (late) (perforated) A52.79

Syphilis, syphilitic (acquired) - *continued*
  vagina A51.0
    late A52.76
  valvulitis NEC A52.03
  vascular A52.00
    brain (cerebral) A52.05
  ventriculi A52.74
  vesicae urinariae (late) A52.76
  viscera (abdominal) (late) A52.74
    secondary A51.49
  vitreous (opacities) (late) A52.71
    hemorrhage A52.71
  vulva A51.0
    late A52.76
    secondary A51.39
Syphiloma A52.79
  cardiovascular system A52.00
  central nervous system A52.3
  circulatory system A52.00
  congenital A50.59
Syphilophobia F45.29
Syringadenoma — *see also* Neoplasm, skin, benign
  papillary — *see* Neoplasm, skin, benign
Syringobulbia G95.0
Syringocystadenoma — *see* Neoplasm, skin, benign
  papillary — *see* Neoplasm, skin, benign
Syringoma — *see also* Neoplasm, skin, benign
  chondroid — *see* Neoplasm, skin, benign
Syringomyelia G95.0
Syringomyelitis — *see* Encephalitis
Syringomyelocele — *see* Spina bifida
Syringopontia G95.0
System, systemic — *see also* condition
  disease, combined — *see* Degeneration, combined
  inflammatory response syndrome (SIRS) of non-infectious origin (without organ dysfunction) R65.10
    with acute organ dysfunction R65.11
  lupus erythematosus M32.9
    inhibitor present D68.62

T

Tabacism, tabacosis, tabagism — *see also* Poisoning, tobacco
  meaning dependence (without remission) F17.200
    with
      disorder F17.299
        in remission F17.211
        specified disorder NEC F17.298
        withdrawal F17.203
Tabardillo A75.9
  flea-borne A75.2
  louse-borne A75.0
Tabes, tabetic A52.10
  with
    central nervous system syphilis A52.10
    Charcot's joint A52.16
    cord bladder A52.19
    crisis, viscera (any) A52.19
    paralysis, general A52.17
    paresis (general) A52.17
    perforating ulcer (foot) A52.19
  arthropathy (Charcot) A52.16
  bladder A52.19
  bone A52.11
  cerebrospinal A52.12
  congenital A50.45
  conjugal A52.10
  dorsalis A52.11
    juvenile A50.49
  juvenile A50.49
  latent A52.19
  mesenterica A18.39
  paralysis, insane, general A52.17
  spasmodic A52.17
  syphilis (cerebrospinal) A52.12
Taboparalysis A52.17
Taboparesis (remission) A52.17
  juvenile A50.45
TAC (trigeminal autonomic cephalgia) NEC G44.099
  intractable G44.091

TAC (trigeminal autonomic cephalgia) NEC - *continued*
  not intractable G44.099
Tache noir S60.22-
Tachyalimentation K91.2
Tachyarrhythmia, tachyrhythmia — *see* Tachycardia
Tachycardia R00.0
  atrial (paroxysmal) I47.1
  auricular I47.1
  AV nodal re-entry (re-entrant) I47.1
  junctional (paroxysmal) I47.1
  newborn P29.11
  nodal (paroxysmal) I47.1
  non-paroxysmal AV nodal I45.89
  paroxysmal (sustained) (nonsustained) I47.9
    with sinus bradycardia I49.5
    atrial (PAT) I47.1
    atrioventricular (AV) (re-entrant) I47.1
      psychogenic F54
    junctional I47.1
      ectopic I47.1
    nodal I47.1
    psychogenic (atrial) (supraventricular) (ventricular) F54
    supraventricular (sustained) I47.1
      psychogenic F54
    ventricular I47.2
      psychogenic F54
  psychogenic F45.8
  sick sinus I49.5
  sinoauricular NOS R00.0
    paroxysmal I47.1
  sinus [sinusal] NOS R00.0
    paroxysmal I47.1
  supraventricular I47.1
  ventricular (paroxysmal) (sustained) I47.2
    psychogenic F54
Tachygastria K31.89
Tachypnea R06.82
  hysterical F45.8
  newborn (idiopathic) (transitory) P22.1
  psychogenic F45.8
  transitory, of newborn P22.1
TACO (transfusion associated circulatory overload) E87.71
Taenia (infection) (infestation) B68.9
  diminuta B71.0
  echinococcal infestation B67.90
  mediocanellata B68.1
  nana B71.0
  saginata B68.1
  solium (intestinal form) B68.0
    larval form — *see* Cysticercosis
Taeniasis (intestine) — *see* Taenia
Tag (hypertrophied skin) (infected) L91.8
  adenoid J35.8
  anus K64.4
  hemorrhoidal K64.4
  hymen N89.8
  perineal N90.89
  preauricular Q17.0
  sentinel K64.4
  skin L91.8
    accessory (congenital) Q82.8
    anus K64.4
    congenital Q82.8
    preauricular Q17.0
  tonsil J35.8
  urethra, urethral N36.8
  vulva N90.89
Tahyna fever B33.8
Takahara's disease E80.3
Takayasu's disease or syndrome M31.4
Talcosis (pulmonary) J62.0
Talipes (congenital) Q66.89
  acquired, planus — *see* Deformity, limb, flat foot
  asymmetric Q66.89
  calcaneovalgus Q66.4-
  calcaneovarus Q66.1-
  calcaneus Q66.89
  cavus Q66.7-
  equinovalgus Q66.6
  equinovarus Q66.0-

Talipes (congenital) - *continued*
equinus Q66.89
percavus Q66.7-
planovalgus Q66.6
planus (acquired) (any degree) — *see also*
Deformity, limb, flat foot
congenital Q66.5-
due to rickets (sequelae) E64.3
valgus Q66.6
varus Q66.3-
Tall stature, constitutional E34.4
Talma's disease M62.89
Talon noir S90.3-
hand S60.22-
heel S90.3-
toe S90.1-
Tamponade, heart I31.4
Tanapox (virus disease) B08.71
Tangier disease E78.6
Tantrum, child problem F91.8
Tapeworm (infection) (infestation) — *see*
Infestation, tapeworm
Tapia's syndrome G52.7
**TAR (thrombocytopenia with absent radius)
syndrome** Q87.2
Tarral-Besnier disease L44.0
Tarsal tunnel syndrome — *see* Syndrome,
tarsal tunnel
Tarsalgia — *see* Pain, limb, lower
Tarsitis (eyelid) H01.8
syphilitic A52.71
tuberculous A18.4
Tartar (teeth) (dental calculus) K03.6
Tattoo (mark) L81.8
Tauri's disease E74.09
Taurodontism K00.2
Taussig-Bing syndrome Q20.1
Taybi's syndrome Q87.2
**Tay-Sachs amaurotic familial idiocy or
disease** E75.02
TBI (traumatic brain injury) S06.9
Teacher's node or nodule J38.2
Tear, torn (traumatic) — *see also* Laceration
with abortion — *see* Abortion
annular fibrosis M51.35
anus, anal (sphincter) S31.831
complicating delivery
with third degree perineal laceration —
see also Delivery, complicated, by,
laceration, perineum, third
degree O70.20
with mucosa O70.3
without third degree perineal
laceration O70.4
nontraumatic (healed) (old) K62.81
articular cartilage, old — *see* Derangement,
joint, articular cartilage, by site
bladder
with ectopic or molar pregnancy O08.6
following ectopic or molar
pregnancy O08.6
obstetrical O71.5
traumatic — *see* Injury, bladder
bowel
with ectopic or molar pregnancy O08.6
following ectopic or molar
pregnancy O08.6
obstetrical trauma O71.5
broad ligament
with ectopic or molar pregnancy O08.6
following ectopic or molar
pregnancy O08.6
obstetrical trauma O71.6
bucket handle (knee) (meniscus) — *see* Tear,
meniscus
capsule, joint — *see* Sprain
cartilage — *see also* Sprain
articular, old — *see* Derangement, joint,
articular cartilage, by site
cervix
with ectopic or molar pregnancy O08.6
following ectopic or molar
pregnancy O08.6
obstetrical trauma (current) O71.3
old N88.1

Tear, torn (traumatic) - *continued*
cervix - *continued*
traumatic — *see* Injury, uterus
dural G97.41
nontraumatic G96.11
internal organ — *see* Injury, by site
knee cartilage
articular (current) S83.3-
old — *see* Derangement, knee, meniscus,
due to old tear
ligament — *see* Sprain
meniscus (knee) (current injury) S83.209
bucket-handle S83.20-
lateral
bucket-handle S83.25-
complex S83.27-
peripheral S83.26-
specified type NEC S83.28-
medial
bucket-handle S83.21-
complex S83.23-
peripheral S83.22-
specified type NEC S83.24-
old — *see* Derangement, knee, meniscus,
due to old tear
site other than knee - code as Sprain
specified type NEC S83.20-
muscle — *see* Strain
pelvic
floor, complicating delivery O70.1
organ NEC, obstetrical trauma O71.5
with ectopic or molar pregnancy O08.6
following ectopic or molar
pregnancy O08.6
perineal, secondary O90.1
periurethral tissue, obstetrical trauma O71.82
with ectopic or molar pregnancy O08.6
following ectopic or molar
pregnancy O08.6
rectovaginal septum — *see* Laceration,
vagina
retina, retinal (without detachment)
(horseshoe) — *see also* Break, retina,
horseshoe
with detachment — *see* Detachment,
retina, with retinal, break
rotator cuff (nontraumatic) M75.10-
complete M75.12-
incomplete M75.11-
traumatic S46.01-
capsule S43.42-
semilunar cartilage, knee — *see* Tear,
meniscus
supraspinatus (complete) (incomplete)
(nontraumatic) — *see also* Tear, rotator
cuff M75.10-
tendon — *see* Strain
tentorial, at birth P10.4
umbilical cord
complicating delivery O69.89
urethra
with ectopic or molar pregnancy O08.6
following ectopic or molar
pregnancy O08.6
obstetrical trauma O71.5
uterus — *see* Injury, uterus
vagina — *see* Laceration, vagina
vessel, from catheter — *see* Puncture,
accidental complicating surgery
vulva, complicating delivery O70.0
Tear-stone — *see* Dacryolith
Teeth — *see also* condition
grinding
psychogenic F45.8
sleep related G47.63
Teething (syndrome) K00.7
Telangiectasia, telangiectasis (verrucous)
I78.1
ataxic (cerebellar) (Louis-Bar) G11.3
familial I78.0
hemorrhagic, hereditary (congenital)
(senile) I78.0
hereditary, hemorrhagic (congenital)
(senile) I78.0
juxtafoveal H35.07-

Telangiectasia, telangiectasis (verrucous) -
continued
macular H35.07-
macularis eruptiva perstans D47.01
parafoveal H35.07-
retinal (idiopathic) (juxtafoveal) (macular)
(parafoveal) H35.07-
spider I78.1
Telephone scatologia F65.89
Telescoped bowel or intestine K56.1
congenital Q43.8
Temperature
body, high (of unknown origin) R50.9
cold, trauma from T69.9
newborn P80.0
specified effect NEC T69.8
Temple — *see* condition
Temporal — *see* condition
**Temporomandibular joint pain-dysfunction
syndrome** M26.62-
Temporosphenoidal — *see* condition
Tendency
bleeding — *see* Defect, coagulation
suicide
meaning personal history of attempted
suicide Z91.5
meaning suicidal ideation — *see* Ideation,
suicidal
to fall R29.6
Tenderness, abdominal R10.819
epigastric R10.816
generalized R10.817
left lower quadrant R10.814
left upper quadrant R10.812
periumbilic R10.815
right lower quadrant R10.813
right upper quadrant R10.811
rebound R10.829
epigastric R10.826
generalized R10.827
left lower quadrant R10.824
left upper quadrant R10.822
periumbilic R10.825
right lower quadrant R10.823
right upper quadrant R10.821
Tendinitis, tendonitis — *see also*
Enthesopathy
Achilles M76.6-
adhesive — *see* Tenosynovitis, specified type
NEC
shoulder — *see* Capsulitis, adhesive
bicipital M75.2-
calcific M65.2-
ankle M65.27-
foot M65.27-
forearm M65.23-
hand M65.24-
lower leg M65.26-
multiple sites M65.29
pelvic region M65.25-
shoulder M75.3-
specified site NEC M65.28
thigh M65.25-
upper arm M65.22-
due to use, overuse, pressure — *see also*
Disorder, soft tissue, due to use
specified NEC — *see* Disorder, soft tissue,
due to use, specified NEC
gluteal M76.0-
patellar M76.5-
peroneal M76.7-
psoas M76.1-
tibial (posterior) M76.82-
anterior M76.81-
trochanteric — *see* Bursitis, hip, trochanteric
Tendon — *see* condition
Tendosynovitis — *see* Tenosynovitis
Tenesmus (rectal) R19.8
vesical R30.1
Tennis elbow — *see* Epicondylitis, lateral
Tenonitis — *see also* Tenosynovitis
eye (capsule) H05.04-
Tenontosynovitis — *see* Tenosynovitis
Tenontothecitis — *see* Tenosynovitis

Tenophyte — *see* Disorder, synovium, specified type NEC
Tenosynovitis — *see also* Synovitis M65.9
  adhesive — *see* Tenosynovitis, specified type NEC
    shoulder — *see* Capsulitis, adhesive
  bicipital (calcifying) — *see* Tendinitis, bicipital
  gonococcal A54.49
  in (due to)
    crystals M65.8-
    gonorrhea A54.49
    syphilis (late) A52.78
    use, overuse, pressure — *see also* Disorder, soft tissue, due to use
      specified NEC — *see* Disorder, soft tissue, due to use, specified NEC
  infective NEC M65.1-
    ankle M65.17-
    foot M65.17-
    forearm M65.13-
    hand M65.14-
    lower leg M65.16-
    multiple sites M65.19
    pelvic region M65.15-
    shoulder region M65.11-
    specified site NEC M65.18
    thigh M65.15-
    upper arm M65.12-
  radial styloid M65.4
  shoulder region M65.81-
    adhesive — *see* Capsulitis, adhesive
  specified type NEC M65.88
    ankle M65.87-
    foot M65.87-
    forearm M65.83-
    hand M65.84-
    lower leg M65.86-
    multiple sites M65.89
    pelvic region M65.85-
    shoulder region M65.81-
    specified site NEC M65.88
    thigh M65.85-
    upper arm M65.82-
  tuberculous — *see* Tuberculosis, tenosynovitis
Tenovaginitis — *see* Tenosynovitis
Tension
  arterial, high — *see also* Hypertension
    without diagnosis of hypertension R03.0
  headache G44.209
    intractable G44.201
    not intractable G44.209
  nervous R45.0
  pneumothorax J93.0
  premenstrual N94.3
  state (mental) F48.9
Tentorium — *see* condition
Teratencephalus Q89.8
Teratism Q89.7
Teratoblastoma (malignant) — *see* Neoplasm, malignant, by site
Teratocarcinoma — *see also* Neoplasm, malignant, by site
  liver C22.7
Teratoma (solid) — *see also* Neoplasm, uncertain behavior, by site
  with embryonal carcinoma, mixed — *see* Neoplasm, malignant, by site
  with malignant transformation — *see* Neoplasm, malignant, by site
  adult (cystic) — *see* Neoplasm, benign, by site
  benign — *see* Neoplasm, benign, by site
  combined with choriocarcinoma — *see* Neoplasm, malignant, by site
  cystic (adult) — *see* Neoplasm, benign, by site
  differentiated — *see* Neoplasm, benign, by site
  embryonal — *see also* Neoplasm, malignant, by site
    liver C22.7
  immature — *see* Neoplasm, malignant, by site

Teratoma (solid) - *continued*
  liver C22.7
    adult, benign, cystic, differentiated type or mature D13.4
  malignant — *see also* Neoplasm, malignant, by site
    anaplastic — *see* Neoplasm, malignant, by site
    intermediate — *see* Neoplasm, malignant, by site
    specified site — *see* Neoplasm, malignant, by site
    unspecified site C62.90
    undifferentiated — *see* Neoplasm, malignant, by site
  mature — *see* Neoplasm, uncertain behavior, by site
    malignant — *see* Neoplasm, by site, malignant, by site
  ovary D27.-
    embryonal, immature or malignant C56-
  solid — *see* Neoplasm, uncertain behavior, by site
  testis C62.9-
    adult, benign, cystic, differentiated type or mature D29.2-
    scrotal C62.1-
    undescended C62.0-
Termination
  anomalous — *see also* Malposition, congenital
    right pulmonary vein Q26.3
  pregnancy, elective Z33.2
Ternidens diminutus infestation B81.8
Ternidensiasis B81.8
Terror (s) night (child) F51.4
Terrorism, victim of Z65.4
Terry's syndrome — *see also* Myopia, degenerative H44.2-
Tertiary — *see* condition
Test, tests, testing (for)
  adequacy (for dialysis)
    hemodialysis Z49.31
    peritoneal Z49.32
  blood-alcohol Z04.89
    positive — *see* Findings, abnormal, in blood
  blood-drug Z04.89
    positive — *see* Findings, abnormal, in blood
  blood pressure Z01.30
    abnormal reading — *see* Blood, pressure
  blood typing Z01.83
    Rh typing Z01.83
  cardiac pulse generator (battery) Z45.010
  fertility Z31.41
  genetic
    disease carrier status for procreative management
      female Z31.430
      male Z31.440
    male partner of patient with recurrent pregnancy loss Z31.441
    procreative management NEC
      female Z31.438
      male Z31.448
  hearing Z01.10
    with abnormal findings NEC Z01.118
    infant or child (over 28 days old) Z00.129
      with abnormal findings Z00.121
  HIV (human immunodeficiency virus)
    nonconclusive (in infants) R75
    positive Z21
    seropositive Z21
  immunity status Z01.84
  intelligence NEC Z01.89
  laboratory (as part of a general medical examination) Z00.00
    with abnormal finding Z00.01
    for medicolegal reason NEC Z04.89
  male partner of patient with recurrent pregnancy loss Z31.441
  Mantoux (for tuberculosis) Z11.1
    abnormal result R76.11

Test, tests, testing (for) - *continued*
  pregnancy, positive first pregnancy — *see* Pregnancy, normal, first
  procreative Z31.49
    fertility Z31.41
  skin, diagnostic
    allergy Z01.82
      special screening examination — *see* Screening, by name of disease
    Mantoux Z11.1
    tuberculin Z11.1
  specified NEC Z01.89
  tuberculin Z11.1
    abnormal result R76.11
  vision Z01.00
    with abnormal findings Z01.01
    following failed vision screening Z01.020
      with abnormal findings Z01.021
    infant or child (over 28 days old) Z00.129
      with abnormal findings Z00.121
  Wassermann Z11.3
    positive — *see* Serology for syphilis, positive
Testicle, testicular, testis — *see also* condition
  feminization syndrome — *see also* Syndrome, androgen insensitivity E34.51
  migrans Q55.29
Tetanus, tetanic (cephalic) (convulsions) A35
  with
    abortion A34
    ectopic or molar pregnancy O08.0
  following ectopic or molar pregnancy O08.0
  inoculation reaction (due to serum) — *see* Complications, vaccination
  neonatorum A33
  obstetrical A34
  puerperal, postpartum, childbirth A34
Tetany (due to) R29.0
  alkalosis E87.3
  associated with rickets E55.0
  convulsions R29.0
    hysterical F44.5
  functional (hysterical) F44.5
  hyperkinetic R29.0
    hysterical F44.5
  hyperpnea R06.4
    hysterical F44.5
    psychogenic F45.8
  hyperventilation — *see also* Hyperventilation R06.4
    hysterical F44.5
  neonatal (without calcium or magnesium deficiency) P71.3
  parathyroid (gland) E20.9
  parathyroprival E89.2
  post- (para) thyroidectomy E89.2
  postoperative E89.2
  pseudotetany R29.0
  psychogenic (conversion reaction) F44.5
Tetralogy of Fallot Q21.3
Tetraplegia (chronic) — *see also* Quadriplegia G82.50
Thailand hemorrhagic fever A91
Thalassanemia — *see* Thalassemia
Thalassemia (anemia) (disease) D56.9
  with other hemoglobinopathy D56.8
  alpha (major) (severe) (triple gene defect) D56.0
    minor D56.3
    silent carrier D56.3
    trait D56.3
  beta (severe) D56.1
    homozygous D56.1
    major D56.1
    minor D56.3
    trait D56.3
  delta-beta (homozygous) D56.2
    minor D56.3
    trait D56.3
  dominant D56.8
  hemoglobin
    C D56.8
    E-beta D56.5
  intermedia D56.1

Thalassemia (anemia) (disease) - *continued*
  major D56.1
  minor D56.3
  mixed D56.8
  sickle-cell — *see* Disease, sickle-cell,
      thalassemia
  specified type NEC D56.8
  trait D56.3
  variants D56.8
**Thanatophoric dwarfism or short
    stature** Q77.1
**Thaysen-Gee disease (nontropical
    sprue)** K90.0
Thaysen's disease K90.0
Thecoma D27-
  luteinized D27-
  malignant C56-
Thelarche, premature E30.8
Thelaziasis B83.8
Thelitis N61.0
  puerperal, postpartum or gestational — *see*
      Infection, nipple
Therapeutic — *see* condition
Therapy
  drug, long-term (current) (prophylactic)
      agents affecting estrogen receptors and
          estrogen levels NEC Z79.818
      anastrozole (Arimidex) Z79.811
      antibiotics Z79.2
          short-term use - omit code
      anticoagulants Z79.01
      anti-inflammatory Z79.1
      antiplatelet Z79.02
      antithrombotics Z79.02
      aromatase inhibitors Z79.811
      aspirin Z79.82
      birth control pill or patch Z79.3
      bisphosphonates Z79.83
      contraceptive, oral Z79.3
      drug, specified NEC Z79.899
      estrogen receptor downregulators Z79.818
      Evista Z79.810
      exemestane (Aromasin) Z79.811
      Fareston Z79.810
      fulvestrant (Faslodex) Z79.818
      gonadotropin-releasing hormone (GnRH)
          agonist Z79.818
      goserelin acetate (Zoladex) Z79.818
      hormone replacement Z79.890
      insulin Z79.4
      letrozole (Femara) Z79.811
      leuprolide acetate (leuprorelin)
          (Lupron) Z79.818
      megestrol acetate (Megace) Z79.818
      methadone
          for pain management Z79.891
          maintenance therapy F11.20
      Nolvadex Z79.810
      opiate analgesic Z79.891
      oral contraceptive Z79.3
      raloxifene (Evista) Z79.810
      selective estrogen receptor modulators
          (SERMs) Z79.810
      short term - omit code
      steroids
          inhaled Z79.51
          systemic Z79.52
      tamoxifen (Nolvadex) Z79.810
      toremifene (Fareston) Z79.810
Thermic — *see* condition
Thermography (abnormal) — *see also*
      Abnormal, diagnostic imaging R93.89
  breast R92.8
Thermoplegia T67.01
Thesaurismosis, glycogen — *see* Disease,
      glycogen storage
Thiamin deficiency E51.9
  specified NEC E51.8
Thiaminic deficiency with beriberi E51.11
Thibierge-Weissenbach syndrome — *see*
      Sclerosis, systemic
Thickening
  bone — *see* Hypertrophy, bone
  breast N64.59
  endometrium R93.89

Thickening - *continued*
  epidermal L85.9
      specified NEC L85.8
  hymen N89.6
  larynx J38.7
  nail L60.2
      congenital Q84.5
  periosteal — *see* Hypertrophy, bone
  pleura J92.9
      with asbestos J92.0
  skin R23.4
  subepiglottic J38.7
  tongue K14.8
  valve, heart — *see* Endocarditis
Thigh — *see* condition
Thinning vertebra — *see* Spondylopathy,
      specified NEC
Thirst, excessive R63.1
  due to deprivation of water T73.1
Thomsen disease G71.12
Thoracic — *see also* condition
  kidney Q63.2
  outlet syndrome G54.0
Thoracogastroschisis (congenital) Q79.8
Thoracopagus Q89.4
Thorax — *see* condition
Thorn's syndrome N28.89
Thorson-Björck syndrome E34.0
Threadworm (infection) (infestation) B80
Threatened
  abortion O20.0
      with subsequent abortion O03.9
  job loss, anxiety concerning Z56.2
  labor (without delivery) O47.9
      at or after 37 completed weeks of
          gestation O47.1
      before 37 completed weeks of
          gestation O47.0-
  loss of job, anxiety concerning Z56.2
  miscarriage O20.0
  unemployment, anxiety concerning Z56.2
Three-day fever A93.1
Threshers' lung J67.0
Thrix annulata (congenital) Q84.1
Throat — *see* condition
**Thrombasthenia (Glanzmann)
    (hemorrhagic) (hereditary)** D69.1
Thromboangiitis I73.1
  obliterans (general) I73.1
      cerebral I67.89
      vessels
          brain I67.89
          spinal cord I67.89
Thromboarteritis — *see* Arteritis
**Thromboasthenia (Glanzmann)
    (hemorrhagic) (hereditary)** D69.1
Thrombocytasthenia (Glanzmann) D69.1
**Thrombocythemia (essential) (hemorrhagic)
    (idiopathic) (primary)** D47.3
**Thrombocytopathy (dystrophic)
    (granulopenic)** D69.1
Thrombocytopenia, thrombocytopenic D69.6
  with absent radius (TAR) Q87.2
  congenital D69.42
  dilutional D69.59
  due to
      drugs D69.59
      extracorporeal circulation of blood D69.59
      (massive) blood transfusion D69.59
      platelet alloimmunization D69.59
  essential D69.3
  heparin induced (HIT) D75.82
  hereditary D69.42
  idiopathic D69.3
  neonatal, transitory P61.0
      due to
          exchange transfusion P61.0
          idiopathic maternal
              thrombocytopenia P61.0
          isoimmunization P61.0
  primary NEC D69.49
      idiopathic D69.3
  puerperal, postpartum O72.3
  secondary D69.59
  transient neonatal P61.0

Thrombocytosis, essential D47.3
  primary D47.3
Thromboembolism — *see* Embolism
Thrombopathy (Bernard-Soulier) D69.1
  constitutional D68.0
  Willebrand-Jurgens D68.0
Thrombopenia — *see* Thrombocytopenia
Thrombophilia D68.59
  primary NEC D68.59
  secondary NEC D68.69
  specified NEC D68.69
Thrombophlebitis I80.9
  antepartum O22.2-
      deep O22.3-
      superficial O22.2-
  calf muscular vein (NOS) I80.25-
  cavernous (venous) sinus G08
      complicating pregnancy O22.5-
      nonpyogenic I67.6
  cerebral (sinus) (vein) G08
      nonpyogenic I67.6
      sequelae G09
  due to implanted device — *see*
      Complications, by site and type,
      specified NEC
  during or resulting from a procedure
      NEC T81.72
  femoral vein (superficial) I80.1-
  femoropopliteal vein I80.0-
  gastrocnemial vein I80.25-
  hepatic (vein) I80.8
  idiopathic, recurrent I82.1
  iliac vein (common) (external)
      (internal) I80.21-
  iliofemoral I80.1-
  intracranial venous sinus (any) G08
      nonpyogenic I67.6
      sequelae G09
  intraspinal venous sinuses and veins G08
      nonpyogenic G95.19
  lateral (venous) sinus G08
      nonpyogenic I67.6
  leg I80.3
      superficial I80.0-
  longitudinal (venous) sinus G08
      nonpyogenic I67.6
  lower extremity I80.299
  migrans, migrating I82.1
  pelvic
      with ectopic or molar pregnancy O08.0
      following ectopic or molar
          pregnancy O08.0
      puerperal O87.1
  peroneal vein I80.24-
  popliteal vein — *see* Phlebitis, leg, deep,
      popliteal
  portal (vein) K75.1
  postoperative T81.72
  pregnancy — *see* Thrombophlebitis,
      antepartum
  puerperal, postpartum, childbirth O87.0
      deep O87.1
      pelvic O87.1
      septic O86.81
      superficial O87.0
  saphenous (greater) (lesser) I80.0-
  sinus (intracranial) G08
      nonpyogenic I67.6
  soleal vein I80.25-
  specified site NEC I80.8
  tibial vein (anterior) (posterior) I80.23-
**Thrombosis, thrombotic (bland) (multiple)
    (progressive) (silent) (vessel)** I82.90
  anal K64.5
  antepartum — *see* Thrombophlebitis,
      antepartum
  aorta, aortic I74.10
      abdominal I74.09
          saddle I74.01
      bifurcation I74.09
          saddle I74.01
      specified site NEC I74.19
      terminal I74.09
      thoracic I74.11
      valve — *see* Endocarditis, aortic

Thrombosis, thrombotic (bland) (multiple) (progressive) (silent) (vessel) - *continued*
  apoplexy I63.3-
  artery, arteries (postinfectional) I74.9
    auditory, internal — *see* Occlusion, artery, precerebral, specified NEC
    basilar — *see* Occlusion, artery, basilar
    carotid (common) (internal) — *see* Occlusion, artery, carotid
    cerebellar (anterior inferior) (posterior inferior) (superior) — *see* Occlusion, artery, cerebellar
    cerebral — *see* Occlusion, artery, cerebral
    choroidal (anterior) — *see* Occlusion, artery, precerebral, specified NEC
    communicating, posterior — *see* Occlusion, artery, precerebral, specified NEC
    coronary — *see also* Infarct, myocardium
      not resulting in infarction I24.0
    hepatic I74.8
    hypophyseal — *see* Occlusion, artery, precerebral, specified NEC
    iliac I74.5
    limb I74.4
      lower I74.3
      upper I74.2
    meningeal, anterior or posterior — *see* Occlusion, artery, cerebral, specified NEC
    mesenteric (with gangrene) — *see also* Infarct, intestine K55.069
    ophthalmic — *see* Occlusion, artery, retina
    pontine — *see* Occlusion, artery, precerebral, specified NEC
    precerebral — *see* Occlusion, artery, precerebral
    pulmonary (iatrogenic) — *see* Embolism, pulmonary
    renal N28.0
    retinal — *see* Occlusion, artery, retina
    spinal, anterior or posterior G95.11
    traumatic NEC T14.8
    vertebral — *see* Occlusion, artery, vertebral
  atrium, auricular — *see also* Infarct, myocardium
    following acute myocardial infarction (current complication) I23.6
    not resulting in infarction I51.3
    old I51.3
  basilar (artery) — *see* Occlusion, artery, basilar
  brain (artery) (stem) — *see also* Occlusion, artery, cerebral
    due to syphilis A52.05
    puerperal O99.43
    sinus — *see* Thrombosis, intracranial venous sinus
  capillary I78.8
  cardiac — *see also* Infarct, myocardium
    not resulting in infarction I51.3
    old I51.3
    valve — *see* Endocarditis
  carotid (artery) (common) (internal) — *see* Occlusion, artery, carotid
  cavernous (venous) sinus — *see* Thrombosis, intracranial venous sinus
  cerebellar artery (anterior inferior) (posterior inferior) (superior) I66.3
  cerebral (artery) — *see* Occlusion, artery, cerebral
  cerebrovenous sinus — *see also* Thrombosis, intracranial venous sinus
    puerperium O87.3
  chronic I82.91
  coronary (artery) (vein) — *see also* Infarct, myocardium
    not resulting in infarction I24.0
  corpus cavernosum N48.89
  cortical I66.9
  deep — *see* Embolism, vein, lower extremity
  due to device, implant or graft — *see also* Complications, by site and type, specified NEC T85.868

Thrombosis, thrombotic (bland) (multiple) (progressive) (silent) (vessel) - *continued*
  due to device, implant or graft - *continued*
    arterial graft NEC T82.868
    breast (implant) T85.868
    catheter NEC T85.868
      dialysis (renal) T82.868
        intraperitoneal T85.868
      infusion NEC T82.868
        spinal (epidural) (subdural) T85.860
      urinary (indwelling) T83.86
    electronic (electrode) (pulse generator) (stimulator)
      bone T84.86
      cardiac T82.867
      nervous system (brain) (peripheral nerve) (spinal) T85.860
      urinary T83.86
    fixation, internal (orthopedic) NEC T84.86
    gastrointestinal (bile duct) (esophagus) T85.868
    genital NEC T83.86
    heart T82.867
    joint prosthesis T84.86
    ocular (corneal graft) (orbital implant) NEC T85.868
    orthopedic NEC T84.86
    specified NEC T85.868
    urinary NEC T83.86
    vascular NEC T82.868
    ventricular intracranial shunt T85.860
  during the puerperium — *see* Thrombosis, puerperal
  endocardial — *see also* Infarct, myocardium
    not resulting in infarction I51.3
  eye — *see* Occlusion, retina
  genital organ
    female NEC N94.89
      pregnancy — *see* Thrombophlebitis, antepartum
    male N50.1
  gestational — *see* Phlebopathy, gestational
  heart (chamber) — *see also* Infarct, myocardium
    not resulting in infarction I51.3
    old I51.3
  hepatic (vein) I82.0
    artery I74.8
  history (of) Z86.718
  intestine (with gangrene) — *see also* Infarct, intestine K55.069
  intracardiac NEC (apical) (atrial) (auricular) (ventricular) (old) I51.3
  intracranial (arterial) I66.9
    venous sinus (any) G08
      nonpyogenic origin I67.6
      puerperium O87.3
  intramural — *see also* Infarct, myocardium
    not resulting in infarction I51.3
    old I51.3
  intraspinal venous sinuses and veins G08
    nonpyogenic G95.19
  kidney (artery) N28.0
  lateral (venous) sinus — *see* Thrombosis, intracranial venous sinus
  leg — *see* Thrombosis, vein, lower extremity
    arterial I74.3
  liver (venous) I82.0
    artery I74.8
    portal vein I81
  longitudinal (venous) sinus — *see* Thrombosis, intracranial venous sinus
  lower limb — *see* Thrombosis, vein, lower extremity
  lung (iatrogenic) (postoperative) — *see* Embolism, pulmonary
  meninges (brain) (arterial) I66.8
  mesenteric (artery) (with gangrene) — *see also* Infarct, intestine K55.069
    vein (inferior) (superior) K55.0
  mitral I34.8
  mural — *see also* Infarct, myocardium
    due to syphilis A52.06
    not resulting in infarction I51.3
    old I51.3

Thrombosis, thrombotic (bland) (multiple) (progressive) (silent) (vessel) - *continued*
  omentum (with gangrene) — *see also* Infarct, intestine K55.069
  ophthalmic — *see* Occlusion, retina
  pampiniform plexus (male) N50.1
  parietal — *see also* Infarct, myocardium
    not resulting in infarction I24.0
  penis, superficial vein N48.81
  perianal venous K64.5
  peripheral arteries I74.4
    upper I74.2
  personal history (of) Z86.718
  portal I81
    due to syphilis A52.09
  precerebral artery — *see* Occlusion, artery, precerebral
  puerperal, postpartum O87.0
    brain (artery) O99.43
      venous (sinus) O87.3
    cardiac O99.43
    cerebral (artery) O99.43
      venous (sinus) O87.3
    superficial O87.0
  pulmonary (artery) (iatrogenic) (postoperative) (vein) — *see* Embolism, pulmonary
  renal (artery) N28.0
    vein I82.3
  resulting from presence of device, implant or graft — *see* Complications, by site and type, specified NEC
  retina, retinal — *see* Occlusion, retina
  scrotum N50.1
  seminal vesicle N50.1
  sigmoid (venous) sinus — *see* Thrombosis, intracranial venous sinus
  sinus, intracranial (any) — *see* Thrombosis, intracranial venous sinus
  specified site NEC I82.890
    chronic I82.891
  spermatic cord N50.1
  spinal cord (arterial) G95.11
    due to syphilis A52.09
    pyogenic origin G06.1
  spleen, splenic D73.5
    artery I74.8
  testis N50.1
  tumor — *see* Neoplasm, unspecified behavior, by site
  traumatic NEC T14.8
  tricuspid I07.8
  tunica vaginalis N50.1
  umbilical cord (vessels) , complicating delivery O69.5
  vas deferens N50.1
  vein (acute) I82.90
    antecubital I82.61-
      chronic I82.71-
    axillary I82.A1-
      chronic I82.A2-
    basilic I82.61-
      chronic I82.71-
    brachial I82.62-
      chronic I82.72-
    brachiocephalic (innominate) I82.290
      chronic I82.291
    cerebral, nonpyogenic I67.6
    cephalic I82.61-
      chronic I82.71-
    chronic I82.91
    deep (DVT) I82.40-
      calf I82.4Z-
        chronic I82.5Z-
      lower leg I82.4Z-
        chronic I82.5Z-
      thigh I82.4Y-
        chronic I82.5Y-
      upper leg I82.4Y
        chronic I82.5y--
    femoral I82.41-
      chronic I82.51-
    iliac (iliofemoral) I82.42-
      chronic I82.52-
    innominate I82.290

Thrombosis, thrombotic (bland) (multiple) (progressive) (silent) (vessel) - *continued*
  vein (acute) - *continued*
    innominate - *continued*
      chronic I82.291
     internal jugular I82.C1-
      chronic I82.C2-
     lower extremity
      deep I82.40-
       chronic I82.50-
        specified NEC I82.49-
         chronic NEC I82.59-
      distal
       deep I82.4Z-
      proximal
       deep I82.4Y-
        chronic I82.5Y-
      superficial I82.81-
     perianal K64.5
     popliteal I82.43-
      chronic I82.53-
     radial I82.62-
      chronic I82.72-
     renal I82.3
     saphenous (greater) (lesser) I82.81-
     specified NEC I82.890
      chronic NEC I82.891
     subclavian I82.B1-
      chronic I82.B2-
     thoracic NEC I82.290
      chronic I82.291
     tibial I82.44-
      chronic I82.54-
     ulnar I82.62-
      chronic I82.72-
     upper extremity I82.60-
      chronic I82.70-
      deep I82.62-
       chronic I82.72-
      superficial I82.61-
       chronic I82.71-
    vena cava
     inferior I82.220
      chronic I82.221
     superior I82.210
      chronic I82.211
   venous, perianal K64.5
   ventricle — *see also* Infarct, myocardium
    following acute myocardial infarction
     (current complication) I23.6
    not resulting in infarction I24.0
    old I51.3
Thrombus — *see* Thrombosis
Thrush — *see also* Candidiasis
  oral B37.0
  newborn P37.5
  vaginal B37.3
Thumb — *see also* condition
  sucking (child problem) F98.8
Thymitis E32.8
Thymoma (benign) D15.0
  malignant C37
Thymus, thymic (gland) — *see* condition
Thyrocele — *see* Goiter
Thyroglossal — *see also* condition
  cyst Q89.2
  duct, persistent Q89.2
Thyroid (gland) (body) — *see also* condition
  hormone resistance E07.89
  lingual Q89.2
  nodule (cystic) (nontoxic) (single) E04.1
Thyroiditis E06.9
  acute (nonsuppurative) (pyogenic) (suppurative) E06.0
  autoimmune E06.3
  chronic (nonspecific) (sclerosing) E06.5
   with thyrotoxicosis, transient E06.2
   fibrous E06.5
   lymphadenoid E06.3
   lymphocytic E06.3
   lymphoid E06.3
  de Quervain's E06.1
  drug-induced E06.4
  fibrous (chronic) E06.5
  giant-cell (follicular) E06.1

Thyroiditis - *continued*
  granulomatous (de Quervain) (subacute) E06.1
  Hashimoto's (struma lymphomatosa) E06.3
  iatrogenic E06.4
  ligneous E06.5
  lymphocytic (chronic) E06.3
  lymphoid E06.3
  lymphomatous E06.3
  nonsuppurative E06.1
  postpartum, puerperal O90.5
  pseudotuberculous E06.1
  pyogenic E06.0
  radiation E06.4
  Riedel's E06.5
  subacute (granulomatous) E06.1
  suppurative E06.0
  tuberculous A18.81
  viral E06.1
  woody E06.5
Thyrolingual duct, persistent Q89.2
Thyromegaly E01.0
Thyrotoxic
  crisis — *see* Thyrotoxicosis
  heart disease or failure — *see also* Thyrotoxicosis E05.90 *[143]*
   with thyroid storm E05.91 *[143]*
  storm — *see* Thyrotoxicosis
Thyrotoxicosis (recurrent) E05.90
  with
   goiter (diffuse) E05.00
    with thyroid storm E05.01
    adenomatous uninodular E05.10
     with thyroid storm E05.11
    multinodular E05.20
     with thyroid storm E05.21
    nodular E05.20
     with thyroid storm E05.21
    uninodular E05.10
     with thyroid storm E05.11
   infiltrative
    dermopathy E05.00
     with thyroid storm E05.01
    ophthalmopathy E05.00
     with thyroid storm E05.01
   single thyroid nodule E05.10
    with thyroid storm E05.11
   thyroid storm E05.91
  due to
   ectopic thyroid nodule or tissue E05.30
    with thyroid storm E05.31
   ingestion of (excessive) thyroid material E05.40
    with thyroid storm E05.41
   overproduction of thyroid-stimulating hormone E05.80
    with thyroid storm E05.81
   specified cause NEC E05.80
    with thyroid storm E05.81
  factitia E05.40
   with thyroid storm E05.41
  heart — *see also* Failure, heart, high-output E05.90 *[143]*
   with thyroid storm — *see also* Failure, heart, high-output E05.91 *[143]*
   failure — *see also* Failure, heart, high-output E05.90 *[143]*
  neonatal (transient) P72.1
  transient with chronic thyroiditis E06.2
Tibia vara — *see* Osteochondrosis, juvenile, tibia
Tic (disorder) F95.9
  breathing F95.8
  child problem F95.0
  compulsive F95.1
  de la Tourette F95.2
  degenerative (generalized) (localized) G25.69
   facial G25.69
  disorder
   chronic
    motor F95.1
    vocal F95.1
   combined vocal and multiple motor F95.2
   transient F95.0

Tic (disorder) - *continued*
  douloureux G50.0
   atypical G50.1
   postherpetic, postzoster B02.22
  drug-induced G25.61
  eyelid F95.8
  habit F95.9
   chronic F95.1
   transient of childhood F95.0
  lid, transient of childhood F95.0
  motor-verbal F95.2
  occupational F48.8
  orbicularis F95.8
   transient of childhood F95.0
  organic origin G25.69
  provisional F95.0
  postchoreic G25.69
  psychogenic, compulsive F95.1
  salaam R25.8
  spasm (motor or vocal) F95.9
   chronic F95.1
   transient of childhood F95.0
  specified NEC F95.8
Tick-borne — *see* condition
Tietze's disease or syndrome M94.0
Tight, tightness
  anus K62.89
  chest R07.89
  fascia (lata) M62.89
  foreskin (congenital) N47.1
  hymen, hymenal ring N89.6
  introitus (acquired) (congenital) N89.6
  rectal sphincter K62.89
  tendon — *see* Short, tendon
  urethral sphincter N35.919
Tilting vertebra — *see* Dorsopathy, deforming, specified NEC
Timidity, child F93.8
Tinea (intersecta) (tarsi) B35.9
  amiantacea L44.8
  asbestina B35.0
  barbae B35.0
  beard B35.0
  black dot B35.0
  blanca B36.2
  capitis B35.0
  corporis B35.4
  cruris B35.6
  flava B36.0
  foot B35.3
  furfuracea B36.0
  imbricata (Tokelau) B35.5
  kerion B35.0
  manuum B35.2
  microsporic — *see* Dermatophytosis
  nigra B36.1
  nodosa — *see* Piedra
  pedis B35.3
  scalp B35.0
  specified NEC B35.8
  sycosis B35.0
  tonsurans B35.0
  trichophytic — *see* Dermatophytosis
  unguium B35.1
  versicolor B36.0
Tingling sensation (skin) R20.2
Tin-miner's lung J63.5
Tinnitus NOS H93.1-
  audible H93.1-
  aurium H93.1-
  pulsatile H93.A-
  subjective H93.1-
Tipped tooth (teeth) M26.33
Tipping
  pelvis M95.5
   with disproportion (fetopelvic) O33.0
    causing obstructed labor O65.0
  tooth (teeth) , fully erupted M26.33
Tiredness R53.83
Tissue — *see* condition
Tobacco (nicotine)
  abuse — *see* Tobacco, use
  dependence — *see* Dependence, drug, nicotine
  harmful use Z72.0

Tobacco (nicotine) - *continued*
  heart — *see* Tobacco, toxic effect
  maternal use, affecting newborn P04.2
  toxic effect — *see* Table of Drugs and
    Chemicals, by substance, poisoning
    chewing tobacco — *see* Table of Drugs
      and Chemicals, by substance,
      poisoning
    cigarettes — *see* Table of Drugs and
      Chemicals, by substance, poisoning
  use Z72.0
    complicating
      childbirth O99.334
      pregnancy O99.33-
      puerperium O99.335
    counseling and surveillance Z71.6
    history Z87.891
    withdrawal state — *see also* Dependence,
      drug, nicotine F17.203
Tocopherol deficiency E56.0
Todd's
  cirrhosis K74.3
  paralysis (postepileptic) (transitory) G83.84
Toe — *see* condition
Toilet, artificial opening — *see* Attention to,
  artificial, opening
Tokelau (ringworm) B35.5
Tollwut — *see* Rabies
Tommaselli's disease R31.9
  correct substance properly administered —
    see Table of Drugs and Chemicals, by
    drug, adverse effect
  overdose or wrong substance given or
    taken — *see* Table of Drugs and
    Chemicals, by drug, poisoning
Tongue — *see also* condition
  tie Q38.1
Tonic pupil — *see* Anomaly, pupil, function,
  tonic pupil
Toni-Fanconi syndrome (cystinosis) E72.09
  with cystinosis E72.04
Tonsil — *see* condition
Tonsillitis (acute) (catarrhal) (croupous)
  (follicular) (gangrenous) (infective)
  (lacunar) (lingual) (malignant)
  (membranous) (parenchymatous)
  (phlegmonous) (pseudomembranous)
  (purulent) (septic) (subacute)
  (suppurative) (toxic) (ulcerative)
  (vesicular) (viral) J03.90
  chronic J35.01
    with adenoiditis J35.03
  diphtheritic A36.0
  hypertrophic J35.01
    with adenoiditis J35.03
  recurrent J03.91
  specified organism NEC J03.80
    recurrent J03.81
  staphylococcal J03.80
    recurrent J03.81
  streptococcal J03.00
    recurrent J03.01
  tuberculous A15.8
  Vincent's A69.1
Tooth, teeth — *see* condition
Toothache K08.89
Topagnosis R20.8
Tophi — *see* Gout, chronic
TORCH infection — *see* Infection, congenital
  without active infection P00.2
Torn — *see* Tear
Tornwaldt's cyst or disease J39.2
Torsion
  accessory tube — *see* Torsion, fallopian tube
  adnexa (female) — *see* Torsion, fallopian
    tube
  aorta, acquired I77.1
  appendix epididymis N44.04
  appendix testis N44.03
  bile duct (common) (hepatic) K83.8
    congenital Q44.5
  bowel, colon or intestine K56.2
  cervix — *see* Malposition, uterus
  cystic duct K82.8
  dystonia — *see* Dystonia, torsion

Torsion - *continued*
  epididymis (appendix) N44.04
  fallopian tube N83.52-
    with ovary N83.53
  gallbladder K82.8
    congenital Q44.1
  hydatid of Morgagni
    female N83.52-
    male N44.03
  kidney (pedicle) (leading to infarction) N28.0
  Meckel's diverticulum (congenital) Q43.0
    malignant — *see* Table of Neoplasms,
      small intestine, malignant
  mesentery K56.2
  omentum K56.2
  organ or site, congenital NEC — *see*
    Anomaly, by site
  ovary (pedicle) N83.51-
    with fallopian tube N83.53
    congenital Q50.2
  oviduct — *see* Torsion, fallopian tube
  penis (acquired) N48.82
    congenital Q55.63
  spasm — *see* Dystonia, torsion
  spermatic cord N44.02
    extravaginal N44.01
    intravaginal N44.02
  spleen D73.5
  testis, testicle N44.00
    appendix N44.03
  tibia — *see* Deformity, limb, specified type
    NEC, lower leg
  uterus — *see* Malposition, uterus
Torticollis (intermittent) (spastic) M43.6
  congenital (sternomastoid) Q68.0
  due to birth injury P15.8
  hysterical F44.4
  ocular R29.891
  psychogenic F45.8
    conversion reaction F44.4
  rheumatic M43.6
  rheumatoid M06.88
  spasmodic G24.3
  traumatic, current S13.4
Tortipelvis G24.1
Tortuous
  aortic arch Q25.46
  artery I77.1
  organ or site, congenital NEC — *see*
    Distortion
  retinal vessel, congenital Q14.1
  ureter N13.8
  urethra N36.8
  vein — *see* Varix
Torture, victim of Z65.4
Torula, torular (histolytica) (infection) — *see*
  Cryptococcosis
Torulosis — *see* Cryptococcosis
Torus (mandibularis) (palatinus) M27.0
  fracture — *see* Fracture, by site, torus
Touraine's syndrome Q79.8
Tourette's syndrome F95.2
Tourniquet syndrome — *see* Constriction,
  external, by site
Tower skull Q75.0
  with exophthalmos Q87.0
Toxemia R68.89
  bacterial — *see* Sepsis
  burn — *see* Burn
  eclamptic (with pre-existing
    hypertension) — *see* Eclampsia
  erysipelatous — *see* Erysipelas
  fatigue R68.89
  food — *see* Poisoning, food
  gastrointestinal K52.1
  intestinal K52.1
  kidney — *see* Uremia
  malarial — *see* Malaria
  myocardial — *see* Myocarditis, toxic
  of pregnancy — *see* Pre-eclampsia
  pre-eclamptic — *see* Pre-eclampsia
  small intestine K52.1
  staphylococcal, due to food A05.0
  stasis R68.89
  uremic — *see* Uremia

Toxemia - *continued*
  urinary — *see* Uremia
Toxemica cerebropathia psychica
  (nonalcoholic) F04
  alcoholic — *see* Alcohol, amnestic disorder
Toxic (poisoning) — *see also* condition T65.91
  effect — *see* Table of Drugs and Chemicals,
    by substance, poisoning
  shock syndrome A48.3
  thyroid (gland) — *see* Thyrotoxicosis
Toxicemia — *see* Toxemia
Toxicity — *see* Table of Drugs and Chemicals,
  by substance, poisoning
  fava bean D55.0
  food, noxious — *see* Poisoning, food
  from drug or nonmedicinal substance — *see*
    Table of Drugs and Chemicals, by drug
Toxicosis — *see also* Toxemia
  capillary, hemorrhagic D69.0
Toxinfection, gastrointestinal K52.1
Toxocariasis B83.0
Toxoplasma, toxoplasmosis (acquired) B58.9
  with
    hepatitis B58.1
    meningoencephalitis B58.2
    ocular involvement B58.00
    other organ involvement B58.89
    pneumonia, pneumonitis B58.3
  congenital (acute) (subacute) (chronic) P37.1
  maternal, manifest toxoplasmosis in infant
    (acute) (subacute) (chronic) P37.1
tPA (rtPA) administation in a different
  facility within the last 24 hours prior to
  admission to current facility Z92.82
Trabeculation, bladder N32.89
Trachea — *see* condition
Tracheitis (catarrhal) (infantile)
  (membranous) (plastic) (septal)
  (suppurative) (viral) J04.10
  with
    bronchitis (15 years of age and above) J40
      acute or subacute — *see* Bronchitis,
        acute
      chronic J42
      tuberculous NEC A15.5
      under 15 years of age J20.9
    laryngitis (acute) J04.2
      chronic J37.1
      tuberculous NEC A15.5
  acute J04.10
    with obstruction J04.11
  chronic J42
    with
      bronchitis (chronic) J42
      laryngitis (chronic) J37.1
  diphtheritic (membranous) A36.89
  due to external agent — *see* Inflammation,
    respiratory, upper, due to
  syphilitic A52.73
  tuberculous A15.5
Trachelitis (nonvenereal) — *see* Cervicitis
Tracheobronchial — *see* condition
Tracheobronchitis (15 years of age and
  above) — *see also* Bronchitis
  due to
    Bordetella bronchiseptica A37.80
      with pneumonia A37.81
    Francisella tularensis A21.8
Tracheobronchomegaly Q32.4
  with bronchiectasis J47.9
    with
      exacerbation (acute) J47.1
      lower respiratory infection J47.0
  acquired J98.09
    with bronchiectasis J47.9
      with
        exacerbation (acute) J47.1
        lower respiratory infection J47.0
Tracheobronchopneumonitis — *see*
  Pneumonia, broncho-
Tracheocele (external) (internal) J39.8
  congenital Q32.1
Tracheomalacia J39.8
  congenital Q32.0

Tracheopharyngitis (acute) J06.9
  chronic J42
  due to external agent — *see* Inflammation,
    respiratory, upper, due to
Tracheostenosis J39.8
Tracheostomy
  complication — *see* Complication,
    tracheostomy
  status Z93.0
    attention to Z43.0
    malfunctioning J95.03
Trachoma, trachomatous A71.9
  active (stage) A71.1
  contraction of conjunctiva A71.1
  dubium A71.0
  initial (stage) A71.0
  healed or sequelae B94.0
  pannus A71.1
  Türck's J37.0
Traction, vitreomacular H43.82-
Train sickness T75.3
Trait (s)
  Hb-S D57.3
  hemoglobin
    abnormal NEC D58.2
      with thalassemia D56.3
    C — *see* Disease, hemoglobin C
    S (Hb-S) D57.3
  Lepore D56.3
  personality, accentuated Z73.1
  sickle-cell D57.3
    with elliptocytosis or spherocytosis D57.3
  type A personality Z73.1
Tramp Z59.0
Trance R41.89
  hysterical F44.89
Transaminasemia R74.0
Transection
  abdomen (partial) S38.3
  aorta (incomplete) — *see also* Injury, aorta
    complete — *see* Injury, aorta, laceration,
      major
  carotid artery (incomplete) — *see also* Injury,
    blood vessel, carotid, laceration
    complete — *see* Injury, blood vessel,
      carotid, laceration, major
  celiac artery (incomplete) S35.211
    branch (incomplete) S35.291
      complete S35.292
    complete S35.212
  innominate
    artery (incomplete) — *see also* Injury,
      blood vessel, thoracic, innominate,
      artery, laceration
      complete — *see* Injury, blood vessel,
        thoracic, innominate, artery,
        laceration, major
    vein (incomplete) — *see also* Injury, blood
      vessel, thoracic, innominate, vein,
      laceration
      complete — *see* Injury, blood vessel,
        thoracic, innominate, vein,
        laceration, major
  jugular vein (external) (incomplete) — *see*
    also Injury, blood vessel, jugular vein,
    laceration
    complete — *see* Injury, blood vessel,
      jugular vein, laceration, major
    internal (incomplete) — *see also* Injury,
      blood vessel, jugular vein, internal,
      laceration
      complete — *see* Injury, blood vessel,
        jugular vein, internal, laceration,
        major
  mesenteric artery (incomplete) — *see also*
    Injury, mesenteric, artery, laceration
    complete — *see* Injury, mesenteric artery,
      laceration, major
  pulmonary vessel (incomplete) — *see also*
    Injury, blood vessel, thoracic,
    pulmonary, laceration
    complete — *see* Injury, blood vessel,
      thoracic, pulmonary, laceration, major
  subclavian — *see* Transection, innominate

Transection - *continued*
  vena cava (incomplete) — *see also* Injury,
    vena cava
    complete — *see* Injury, vena cava,
      laceration, major
  vertebral artery (incomplete) — *see also*
    Injury, blood vessel, vertebral,
    laceration
    complete — *see* Injury, blood vessel,
      vertebral, laceration, major
Transfusion
  associated (red blood cell)
    hemochromatosis E83.111
  blood
    ABO incompatible — *see* Complication(s),
      transfusion, incompatibility reaction,
      ABO
    minor blood group (Duffy) (E) (K) (Kell)
      (Kidd) (Lewis) (M) (N) (P)
      (S) T80.89
    reaction or complication — *see*
      Complications, transfusion
  fetomaternal (mother) — *see* Pregnancy,
    complicated by, placenta, transfusion
    syndrome
  maternofetal (mother) — *see* Pregnancy,
    complicated by, placenta, transfusion
    syndrome
  placental (syndrome) (mother) — *see*
    Pregnancy, complicated by, placenta,
    transfusion syndrome
  reaction (adverse) — *see* Complications,
    transfusion
  related acute lung injury (TRALI) J95.84
  twin-to-twin — *see* Pregnancy, complicated
    by, placenta, transfusion syndrome,
    fetus to fetus
Transient (meaning homeless) — *see*
  also condition Z59.0
Translocation
  balanced autosomal Q95.9
    in normal individual Q95.0
  chromosomes NEC Q99.8
    balanced and insertion in normal
      individual Q95.0
  Down syndrome Q90.2
  trisomy
    13 Q91.6
    18 Q91.2
    21 Q90.2
Translucency, iris — *see* Degeneration, iris
Transmission of chemical substances
  through the placenta — *see* Absorption,
    chemical, through placenta
Transparency, lung, unilateral J43.0
Transplant (ed) (status) Z94.9
  awaiting organ Z76.82
  bone Z94.6
    marrow Z94.81
  candidate Z76.82
  complication — *see* Complication, transplant
  cornea Z94.7
  heart Z94.1
    and lung (s) Z94.3
    valve Z95.2
      prosthetic Z95.2
      specified NEC Z95.4
      xenogenic Z95.3
  intestine Z94.82
  kidney Z94.0
  liver Z94.4
  lung (s) Z94.2
    and heart Z94.3
  organ (failure) (infection) (rejection) Z94.9
    removal status Z98.85
  pancreas Z94.83
  skin Z94.5
  social Z60.3
  specified organ or tissue NEC Z94.89
  stem cells Z94.84
  tissue Z94.9
Transplants, ovarian, endometrial N80.1
Transposed — *see* Transposition

Transposition (congenital) — *see also*
  Malposition, congenital
  abdominal viscera Q89.3
  aorta (dextra) Q20.3
  appendix Q43.8
  colon Q43.8
  corrected Q20.5
  great vessels (complete) (partial) Q20.3
  heart Q24.0
    with complete transposition of
      viscera Q89.3
  intestine (large) (small) Q43.8
  reversed jejunal (for bypass) (status) Z98.0
  scrotum Q55.23
  stomach Q40.2
    with general transposition of viscera Q89.3
  tooth, teeth, fully erupted M26.30
  vessels, great (complete) (partial) Q20.3
  viscera (abdominal) (thoracic) Q89.3
Transsexualism F64.0
Transverse — *see also* condition
  arrest (deep) , in labor O64.0
  lie (mother) O32.2
    causing obstructed labor O64.8
Transvestism, transvestitism (dual-role)
  F64.1
  fetishistic F65.1
Trapped placenta (with hemorrhage) O72.0
  without hemorrhage O73.0
TRAPS (tumor necrosis factor receptor
  associated periodic syndrome) M04.1
Trauma, traumatism — *see also* Injury
  acoustic — *see* subcategory H83.3
  birth — *see* Birth, injury
  complicating ectopic or molar
    pregnancy O08.6
  during delivery O71.9
  following ectopic or molar pregnancy O08.6
  obstetric O71.9
    specified NEC O71.89
  occlusal
    primary K08.81
    secondary K08.82
Traumatic — *see also* condition
  brain injury S06.9
Treacher Collins syndrome Q75.4
Treitz's hernia — *see* Hernia, abdomen,
  specified site NEC
Trematode infestation — *see* Infestation,
  fluke
Trematodiasis — *see* Infestation, fluke
Trembling paralysis — *see* Parkinsonism
Tremor (s) R25.1
  drug induced G25.1
  essential (benign) G25.0
  familial G25.0
  hereditary G25.0
  hysterical F44.4
  intention G25.2
  medication induced postural G25.1
  mercurial — *see* subcategory T56.1
  Parkinson's — *see* Parkinsonism
  psychogenic (conversion reaction) F44.4
  senilis R54
  specified type NEC G25.2
Trench
  fever A79.0
  foot — *see* Immersion, foot
  mouth A69.1
Treponema pallidum infection — *see*
  Syphilis
Treponematosis
  due to
    T. pallidum — *see* Syphilis
    T. pertenue — *see* Yaws
Triad
  Hutchinson's (congenital syphilis) A50.53
  Kartagener's Q89.3
  Saint's — *see* Hernia, diaphragm
Trichiasis (eyelid) H02.059
  with entropion — *see* Entropion
  left H02.056
    lower H02.055
    upper H02.054
  right H02.053

Trichiasis (eyelid) - *continued*
   right - *continued*
      lower H02.052
      upper H02.051
Trichinella spiralis (infection)
   (infestation) B75
Trichinellosis, trichiniasis, trichinelliasis,
   trichinosis B75
   with muscle disorder B75 *[M63.80]*
      ankle B75 *[M63.87-]*
      foot B75 *[M63.87-]*
      forearm B75 *[M63.83-]*
      hand B75 *[M63.84-]*
      lower leg B75 *[M63.86-]*
      multiple sites B75 *[M63.89]*
      pelvic region B75 *[M63.85-]*
      shoulder region B75 *[M63.81-]*
      specified site NEC B75 *[M63.88]*
      thigh B75 *[M63.85-]*
      upper arm B75 *[M63.82-]*
Trichobezoar T18.9
   intestine T18.3
   stomach T18.2
Trichocephaliasis, trichocephalosis B79
Trichocephalus infestation B79
Trichoclasis L67.8
Trichoepithelioma — *see also* Neoplasm,
   skin, benign
   malignant — *see* Neoplasm, skin, malignant
Trichofolliculoma — *see* Neoplasm, skin,
   benign
Tricholemmoma — *see* Neoplasm, skin,
   benign
Trichomoniasis A59.9
   bladder A59.03
   cervix A59.09
   intestinal A07.8
   prostate A59.02
   seminal vesicles A59.09
   specified site NEC A59.8
   urethra A59.03
   urogenitalis A59.00
   vagina A59.01
   vulva A59.01
Trichomycosis
   axillaris A48.8
   nodosa, nodularis B36.8
Trichonodosis L67.8
Trichophytid, trichophyton infection — *see*
   Dermatophytosis
Trichophytobezoar T18.9
   intestine T18.3
   stomach T18.2
Trichophytosis — *see* Dermatophytosis
Trichoptilosis L67.8
Trichorrhexis (nodosa) (invaginata) L67.0
Trichosis axillaris A48.8
Trichosporosis nodosa B36.2
Trichostasis spinulosa (congenital) Q84.1
Trichostrongyliasis, trichostrongylosis (small
   intestine) B81.2
Trichostrongylus infection B81.2
Trichotillomania F63.3
Trichromat, trichromatopsia, anomalous
   (congenital) H53.55
Trichuriasis B79
Trichuris trichiura (infection) (infestation)
   (any site) B79
Tricuspid (valve) — *see* condition
Trifid — *see also* Accessory
   kidney (pelvis) Q63.8
   tongue Q38.3
Trigeminal neuralgia — *see* Neuralgia,
   trigeminal
Trigeminy R00.8
Trigger finger (acquired) M65.30
   congenital Q74.0
   index finger M65.32-
   little finger M65.35-
   middle finger M65.33-
   ring finger M65.34-
   thumb M65.31-
Trigonitis (bladder) (chronic)
   (pseudomembranous) N30.30
   with hematuria N30.31

Trigonocephaly Q75.0
Trilocular heart — *see* Cor triloculare
Trimethylaminuria E72.52
Tripartite placenta O43.19-
Triphalangeal thumb Q74.0
Triple — *see also* Accessory
   kidneys Q63.0
   uteri Q51.818
   X, female Q97.0
Triplegia G83.89
   congenital G80.8
Triplet (newborn) — *see also* Newborn, triplet
   complicating pregnancy — *see* Pregnancy,
      triplet
Triplication — *see* Accessory
Triploidy Q92.7
Trismus R25.2
   neonatorum A33
   newborn A33
Trisomy (syndrome) Q92.9
   autosomes Q92.9
   chromosome specified NEC Q92.8
      partial Q92.2
         due to unbalanced translocation Q92.5
      whole (nonsex chromosome)
         meiotic nondisjunction Q92.0
         mitotic nondisjunction Q92.1
         mosaicism Q92.1
      specified NEC Q92.8
   due to
      dicentrics — *see* Extra, marker
         chromosomes
      extra rings — *see* Extra, marker
         chromosomes
      isochromosomes — *see* Extra, marker
         chromosomes
   specified NEC Q92.8
   whole chromosome Q92.9
      meiotic nondisjunction Q92.0
      mitotic nondisjunction Q92.1
      mosaicism Q92.1
      partial Q92.9
      specified NEC Q92.8
   13 (partial) Q91.7
      meiotic nondisjunction Q91.4
      mitotic nondisjunction Q91.5
      mosaicism Q91.5
      translocation Q91.6
   18 (partial) Q91.3
      meiotic nondisjunction Q91.0
      mitotic nondisjunction Q91.1
      mosaicism Q91.1
      translocation Q91.2
   20 Q92.8
   21 (partial) Q90.9
      meiotic nondisjunction Q90.0
      mitotic nondisjunction Q90.1
      mosaicism Q90.1
      translocation Q90.2
   22 Q92.8
Tritanomaly, tritanopia H53.55
Trombiculosis, trombiculiasis,
   trombidiosis B88.0
Trophedema (congenital) (hereditary) Q82.0
Trophoblastic disease — *see also* Mole,
   hydatidiform O01.9
Tropholymphedema Q82.0
Trophoneurosis NEC G96.8
   disseminated M34.9
Tropical — *see* condition
Trouble — *see also* Disease
   heart — *see* Disease, heart
   kidney — *see* Disease, renal
   nervous R45.0
   sinus — *see* Sinusitis
Trousseau's syndrome (thrombophlebitis
   migrans) I82.1
Truancy, childhood
   from school Z72.810
Truncus
   arteriosus (persistent) Q20.0
   communis Q20.0
Trunk — *see* condition
Trypanosomiasis
   African B56.9

Trypanosomiasis - *continued*
   African - *continued*
      by Trypanosoma brucei
         gambiense B56.0
         rhodesiense B56.1
      American — *see* Chagas' disease
      Brazilian — *see* Chagas' disease
      by Trypanosoma
         brucei gambiense B56.0
         brucei rhodesiense B56.1
         cruzi — *see* Chagas' disease
      gambiensis, Gambian B56.0
      rhodesiensis, Rhodesian B56.1
      South American — *see* Chagas' disease
      where
         African trypanosomiasis is prevalent B56.9
         Chagas' disease is prevalent B57.2
T-shaped incisors K00.2
Tsutsugamushi (disease) (fever) A75.3
Tube, tubal, tubular — *see* condition
Tubercle — *see also* Tuberculosis
   brain, solitary A17.81
   Darwin's Q17.8
   Ghon, primary infection A15.7
Tuberculid, tuberculide (indurating,
   subcutaneous) (lichenoid) (miliary)
   (papulonecrotic) (primary) (skin) A18.4
Tuberculoma — *see also* Tuberculosis
   brain A17.81
   meninges (cerebral) (spinal) A17.1
   spinal cord A17.81
Tuberculosis, tubercular, tuberculous
   (calcification) (calcified) (caseous)
   (chromogenic acid-fast bacilli)
   (degeneration) (fibrocaseous) (fistula)
   (interstitial) (isolated circumscribed
   lesions) (necrosis) (parenchymatous)
   (ulcerative) A15.9
   with pneumoconiosis (any condition in J60-
      J64) J65
   abdomen (lymph gland) A18.39
   abscess (respiratory) A15.9
      bone A18.03
         hip A18.02
         knee A18.02
         sacrum A18.01
         specified site NEC A18.03
         spinal A18.01
         vertebra A18.01
      brain A17.81
      breast A18.89
      Cowper's gland A18.15
      dura (mater) (cerebral) (spinal) A17.81
      epidural (cerebral) (spinal) A17.81
      female pelvis A18.17
      frontal sinus A15.8
      genital organs NEC A18.10
      genitourinary A18.10
      gland (lymphatic) — *see* Tuberculosis,
         lymph gland
      hip A18.02
      intestine A18.32
      ischiorectal A18.32
      joint NEC A18.02
         hip A18.02
         knee A18.02
         specified NEC A18.02
         vertebral A18.01
      kidney A18.11
      knee A18.02
      latent Z22.7
      lumbar (spine) A18.01
      lung — *see* Tuberculosis, pulmonary
      meninges (cerebral) (spinal) A17.0
      muscle A18.09
      perianal (fistula) A18.32
      perinephritic A18.11
      perirectal A18.32
      rectum A18.32
      retropharyngeal A15.8
      sacrum A18.01
      scrofulous A18.2
      scrotum A18.15
      skin (primary) A18.4
      spinal cord A17.81

Tuberculosis, tubercular, tuberculous (calcification) (calcified) (caseous) (chromogenic acid-fast bacilli) (degeneration) (fibrocaseous) (fistula) (interstitial) (isolated circumscribed lesions) (necrosis) (parenchymatous) (ulcerative) - *continued*
  abscess (respiratory) - *continued*
    spine or vertebra (column) A18.01
      subdiaphragmatic A18.31
      testis A18.15
      urinary A18.13
      uterus A18.17
  accessory sinus — *see* Tuberculosis, sinus
  Addison's disease A18.7
  adenitis — *see* Tuberculosis, lymph gland
  adenoids A15.8
  adenopathy — *see* Tuberculosis, lymph gland
  adherent pericardium A18.84
  adnexa (uteri) A18.17
  adrenal (capsule) (gland) A18.7
  alimentary canal A18.32
  anemia A18.89
  ankle (joint) (bone) A18.02
  anus A18.32
  apex, apical — *see* Tuberculosis, pulmonary
  appendicitis, appendix A18.32
  arachnoid A17.0
  artery, arteritis A18.89
    cerebral A18.89
  arthritis (chronic) (synovial) A18.02
    spine or vertebra (column) A18.01
  articular — *see* Tuberculosis, joint
  ascites A18.31
  asthma — *see* Tuberculosis, pulmonary
  axilla, axillary (gland) A18.2
  bladder A18.12
  bone A18.03
    hip A18.02
    knee A18.02
    limb NEC A18.03
    sacrum A18.01
    spine or vertebral column A18.01
  bowel (miliary) A18.32
  brain A17.81
  breast A18.89
  broad ligament A18.17
  bronchi, bronchial, bronchus A15.5
    ectasia, ectasis (bronchiectasis) — *see* Tuberculosis, pulmonary
    fistula A15.5
      primary (progressive) A15.7
    gland or node A15.4
      primary (progressive) A15.7
    lymph gland or node A15.4
      primary (progressive) A15.7
  bronchiectasis — *see* Tuberculosis, pulmonary
  bronchitis A15.5
  bronchopleural A15.6
  bronchopneumonia, bronchopneumonic — *see* Tuberculosis, pulmonary
  bronchorrhagia A15.5
  bronchotracheal A15.5
  bronze disease A18.7
  buccal cavity A18.83
  bulbourethral gland A18.15
  bursa A18.09
  cachexia A15.9
  cardiomyopathy A18.84
  caries — *see* Tuberculosis, bone
  cartilage A18.02
    intervertebral A18.01
  catarrhal — *see* Tuberculosis, respiratory
  cecum A18.32
  cellulitis (primary) A18.4
  cerebellum A17.81
  cerebral, cerebrum A17.81
  cerebrospinal A17.81
    meninges A17.0
  cervical (lymph gland or node) A18.2
  cervicitis, cervix (uteri) A18.16
  chest — *see* Tuberculosis, respiratory
  chorioretinitis A18.53

Tuberculosis, tubercular, tuberculous (calcification) (calcified) (caseous) (chromogenic acid-fast bacilli) (degeneration) (fibrocaseous) (fistula) (interstitial) (isolated circumscribed lesions) (necrosis) (parenchymatous) (ulcerative) - *continued*
  choroid, choroiditis A18.53
  ciliary body A18.54
  colitis A18.32
  collier's J65
  colliquativa (primary) A18.4
  colon A18.32
  complex, primary A15.7
  congenital P37.0
  conjunctiva A18.59
  connective tissue (systemic) A18.89
  contact Z20.1
  cornea (ulcer) A18.52
  Cowper's gland A18.15
  coxae A18.02
  coxalgia A18.02
  cul-de-sac of Douglas A18.17
  curvature, spine A18.01
  cutis (colliquativa) (primary) A18.4
  cyst, ovary A18.18
  cystitis A18.12
  dactylitis A18.03
  diarrhea A18.32
  diffuse — *see* Tuberculosis, miliary
  digestive tract A18.32
  disseminated — *see* Tuberculosis, miliary
  duodenum A18.32
  dura (mater) (cerebral) (spinal) A17.0
    abscess (cerebral) (spinal) A17.81
  dysentery A18.32
  ear (inner) (middle) A18.6
    bone A18.03
    external (primary) A18.4
    skin (primary) A18.4
  elbow A18.02
  emphysema — *see* Tuberculosis, pulmonary
  empyema A15.6
  encephalitis A17.82
  endarteritis A18.89
  endocarditis A18.84
    aortic A18.84
    mitral A18.84
    pulmonary A18.84
    tricuspid A18.84
  endocrine glands NEC A18.82
  endometrium A18.17
  enteric, enterica, enteritis A18.32
  enterocolitis A18.32
  epididymis, epididymitis A18.15
  epidural abscess (cerebral) (spinal) A17.81
  epiglottis A15.5
  episcleritis A18.51
  erythema (induratum) (nodosum) (primary) A18.4
  esophagus A18.83
  eustachian tube A18.6
  exposure (to) Z20.1
  exudative — *see* Tuberculosis, pulmonary
  eye A18.50
  eyelid (primary) (lupus) A18.4
  fallopian tube (acute) (chronic) A18.17
  fascia A18.09
  fauces A15.8
  female pelvic inflammatory disease A18.17
  finger A18.03
  first infection A15.7
  gallbladder A18.83
  ganglion A18.09
  gastritis A18.83
  gastrocolic fistula A18.32
  gastroenteritis A18.32
  gastrointestinal tract A18.32
  general, generalized — *see* Tuberculosis, miliary
  genital organs A18.10
  genitourinary A18.10
  genu A18.02
  glandula suprarenalis A18.7
  glandular, general A18.2

Tuberculosis, tubercular, tuberculous (calcification) (calcified) (caseous) (chromogenic acid-fast bacilli) (degeneration) (fibrocaseous) (fistula) (interstitial) (isolated circumscribed lesions) (necrosis) (parenchymatous) (ulcerative) - *continued*
  glottis A15.5
  grinder's J65
  gum A18.83
  hand A18.03
  heart A18.84
  hematogenous — *see* Tuberculosis, miliary
  hemoptysis — *see* Tuberculosis, pulmonary
  hemorrhage NEC — *see* Tuberculosis, pulmonary
  hemothorax A15.6
  hepatitis A18.83
  hilar lymph nodes A15.4
    primary (progressive) A15.7
  hip (joint) (disease) (bone) A18.02
  hydropneumothorax A15.6
  hydrothorax A15.6
  hypoadrenalism A18.7
  hypopharynx A15.8
  ileocecal (hyperplastic) A18.32
  ileocolitis A18.32
  ileum A18.32
  iliac spine (superior) A18.03
  immunological findings only A15.7
  indurativa (primary) A18.4
  infantile A15.7
  infection A15.9
    without clinical manifestations A15.7
  infraclavicular gland A18.2
  inguinal gland A18.2
  inguinalis A18.2
  intestine (any part) A18.32
  iridocyclitis A18.54
  iris, iritis A18.54
  ischiorectal A18.32
  jaw A18.03
  jejunum A18.32
  joint A18.02
    vertebral A18.01
  keratitis (interstitial) A18.52
  keratoconjunctivitis A18.52
  kidney A18.11
  knee (joint) A18.02
  kyphosis, kyphoscoliosis A18.01
  laryngitis A15.5
  larynx A15.5
  latent Z22.7
  leptomeninges, leptomeningitis (cerebral) (spinal) A17.0
  lichenoides (primary) A18.4
  linguae A18.83
  lip A18.83
  liver A18.83
  lordosis A18.01
  lung — *see* Tuberculosis, pulmonary
  lupus vulgaris A18.4
  lymph gland or node (peripheral) A18.2
    abdomen A18.39
    bronchial A15.4
      primary (progressive) A15.7
    cervical A18.2
    hilar A15.4
      primary (progressive) A15.7
    intrathoracic A15.4
      primary (progressive) A15.7
    mediastinal A15.4
      primary (progressive) A15.7
    mesenteric A18.39
    retroperitoneal A18.39
    tracheobronchial A15.4
      primary (progressive) A15.7
  lymphadenitis — *see* Tuberculosis, lymph gland
  lymphangitis — *see* Tuberculosis, lymph gland
  lymphatic (gland) (vessel) — *see* Tuberculosis, lymph gland
  mammary gland A18.89
  marasmus A15.9

Tuberculosis, tubercular, tuberculous (calcification) (calcified) (caseous) (chromogenic acid-fast bacilli) (degeneration) (fibrocaseous) (fistula) (interstitial) (isolated circumscribed lesions) (necrosis) (parenchymatous) (ulcerative) - *continued*

mastoiditis A18.03
mediastinal lymph gland or node A15.4
  primary (progressive) A15.7
mediastinitis A15.8
  primary (progressive) A15.7
mediastinum A15.8
  primary (progressive) A15.7
medulla A17.81
melanosis, Addisonian A18.7
meninges, meningitis (basilar) (cerebral) (cerebrospinal) (spinal) A17.0
meningoencephalitis A17.82
mesentery, mesenteric (gland or node) A18.39
miliary A19.9
  acute A19.2
    multiple sites A19.1
    single specified site A19.0
  chronic A19.8
  specified NEC A19.8
millstone makers' J65
miner's J65
molder's J65
mouth A18.83
multiple A19.9
  acute A19.1
  chronic A19.8
muscle A18.09
myelitis A17.82
myocardium, myocarditis A18.84
nasal (passage) (sinus) A15.8
nasopharynx A15.8
neck gland A18.2
nephritis A18.11
nerve (mononeuropathy) A17.83
nervous system A17.9
nose (septum) A15.8
ocular A18.50
omentum A18.31
oophoritis (acute) (chronic) A18.17
optic (nerve trunk) (papilla) A18.59
orbit A18.59
orchitis A18.15
organ, specified NEC A18.89
osseous — *see* Tuberculosis, bone
osteitis — *see* Tuberculosis, bone
osteomyelitis — *see* Tuberculosis, bone
otitis media A18.6
ovary, ovaritis (acute) (chronic) A18.17
oviduct (acute) (chronic) A18.17
pachymeningitis A17.0
palate (soft) A18.83
pancreas A18.83
papulonecrotic (a) (primary) A18.4
parathyroid glands A18.82
paronychia (primary) A18.4
parotid gland or region A18.83
pelvis (bony) A18.03
penis A18.15
peribronchitis A15.5
pericardium, pericarditis A18.84
perichondritis, larynx A15.5
periostitis — *see* Tuberculosis, bone
perirectal fistula A18.32
peritoneum NEC A18.31
peritonitis A18.31
pharynx, pharyngitis A15.8
phlyctenulosis (keratoconjunctivitis) A18.52
phthisis NEC — *see* Tuberculosis, pulmonary
pituitary gland A18.82
pleura, pleural, pleurisy, pleuritis (fibrinous) (obliterative) (purulent) (simple plastic) (with effusion) A15.6
  primary (progressive) A15.7
pneumonia, pneumonic — *see* Tuberculosis, pulmonary

pneumothorax (spontaneous) (tense valvular) — *see* Tuberculosis, pulmonary
polyneuropathy A17.89
polyserositis A19.9
  acute A19.1
  chronic A19.8
potter's J65
prepuce A18.15
primary (complex) A15.7
proctitis A18.32
prostate, prostatitis A18.14
pulmonalis — *see* Tuberculosis, pulmonary
pulmonary (cavitated) (fibrotic) (infiltrative) (nodular) A15.0
  childhood type or first infection A15.7
  primary (complex) A15.7
pyelitis A18.11
pyelonephritis A18.11
pyemia — *see* Tuberculosis, miliary
pyonephrosis A18.11
pyopneumothorax A15.6
pyothorax A15.6
rectum (fistula) (with abscess) A18.32
reinfection stage — *see* Tuberculosis, pulmonary
renal A18.11
renis A18.11
respiratory A15.9
  primary A15.7
  specified site NEC A15.8
retina, retinitis A18.53
retroperitoneal (lymph gland or node) A18.39
rheumatism NEC A18.09
rhinitis A15.8
sacroiliac (joint) A18.01
sacrum A18.01
salivary gland A18.83
salpingitis (acute) (chronic) A18.17
sandblaster's J65
sclera A18.51
scoliosis A18.01
scrofulous A18.2
scrotum A18.15
seminal tract or vesicle A18.15
senile A15.9
septic — *see* Tuberculosis, miliary
shoulder (joint) A18.02
  blade A18.03
sigmoid A18.32
sinus (any nasal) A15.8
  bone A18.03
  epididymis A18.15
skeletal NEC A18.03
skin (any site) (primary) A18.4
small intestine A18.32
soft palate A18.83
spermatic cord A18.15
spine, spinal (column) A18.01
  cord A17.81
  medulla A17.81
  membrane A17.0
  meninges A17.0
spleen, splenitis A18.85
spondylitis A18.01
sternoclavicular joint A18.02
stomach A18.83
stonemason's J65
subcutaneous tissue (cellular) (primary) A18.4
subcutis (primary) A18.4
subdeltoid bursa A18.83
submaxillary (region) A18.83
supraclavicular gland A18.2
suprarenal (capsule) (gland) A18.7
swelling, joint (see also category M01) — *see also* Tuberculosis, joint A18.02
symphysis pubis A18.02

synovitis A18.09
  articular A18.02
  spine or vertebra A18.01
systemic — *see* Tuberculosis, miliary
tarsitis A18.4
tendon (sheath) — *see* Tuberculosis, tenosynovitis
tenosynovitis A18.09
  spine or vertebra A18.01
testis A18.15
throat A15.8
thymus gland A18.82
thyroid gland A18.81
tongue A18.83
tonsil, tonsillitis A15.8
trachea, tracheal A15.5
  lymph gland or node A15.4
    primary (progressive) A15.7
tracheobronchial A15.5
  lymph gland or node A15.4
    primary (progressive) A15.7
tubal (acute) (chronic) A18.17
tunica vaginalis A18.15
ulcer (skin) (primary) A18.4
  bowel or intestine A18.32
  specified NEC - code under Tuberculosis, by site
unspecified site A15.9
ureter A18.11
urethra, urethral (gland) A18.13
urinary organ or tract A18.13
uterus A18.17
uveal tract A18.54
uvula A18.83
vagina A18.18
vas deferens A18.15
verruca, verrucosa (cutis) (primary) A18.4
vertebra (column) A18.01
vesiculitis A18.15
vulva A18.18
wrist (joint) A18.02
Tuberculum
  Carabelli — *see* Note at K00.2
  occlusal — *see* Note at K00.2
  paramolare K00.2
Tuberosity, enitre maxillary M26.07
Tuberous sclerosis (brain) Q85.1
Tubo-ovarian — *see* condition
Tuboplasty, after previous sterilization Z31.0
  aftercare Z31.42
Tubotympanitis, catarrhal (chronic) — *see* Otitis, media, nonsuppurative, chronic, serous
Tularemia A21.9
  with
    conjunctivitis A21.1
    pneumonia A21.2
  abdominal A21.3
  bronchopneumonic A21.2
  conjunctivitis A21.1
  cryptogenic A21.3
  enteric A21.3
  gastrointestinal A21.3
  generalized A21.7
  ingestion A21.3
  intestinal A21.3
  oculoglandular A21.1
  ophthalmic A21.1
  pneumonia (any) , pneumonic A21.2
  pulmonary A21.2
  sepsis A21.7
  specified NEC A21.8
  typhoidal A21.7
  ulceroglandular A21.0
Tularensis conjunctivitis A21.1
Tumefaction — *see also* Swelling
  liver — *see* Hypertrophy, liver

Tumor — *see also* Neoplasm, unspecified
   behavior, by site
  acinar cell — *see* Neoplasm, uncertain
   behavior, by site
  acinic cell — *see* Neoplasm, uncertain
   behavior, by site
  adenocarcinoid — *see* Neoplasm, malignant,
   by site
  adenomatoid — *see also* Neoplasm, benign,
   by site
   odontogenic — *see* Cyst, calcifying
    odontogenic
  adnexal (skin) — *see* Neoplasm, skin,
   benign, by site
  adrenal
   cortical (benign) D35.0-
    malignant C74.0-
   rest — *see* Neoplasm, benign, by site
  alpha-cell
   malignant
    pancreas C25.4
    specified site NEC — *see* Neoplasm,
     malignant, by site
    unspecified site C25.4
   pancreas D13.7
   specified site NEC — *see* Neoplasm,
    benign, by site
   unspecified site D13.7
  aneurysmal — *see* Aneurysm
  aortic body D44.7
   malignant C75.5
  Askin's — *see* Neoplasm, connective tissue,
   malignant
  basal cell — *see also* Neoplasm, skin,
   uncertain behavior D48.5
  Bednar — *see* Neoplasm, skin, malignant
  benign (unclassified) — *see* Neoplasm,
   benign, by site
  beta-cell
   malignant
    pancreas C25.4
    specified site NEC — *see* Neoplasm,
     malignant, by site
    unspecified site C25.4
   pancreas D13.7
   specified site NEC — *see* Neoplasm,
    benign, by site
   unspecified site D13.7
  Brenner D27.9
   borderline malignancy D39.1-
   malignant C56-
   proliferating D39.1-
  bronchial alveolar, intravascular D38.1
  Brooke's — *see* Neoplasm, skin, benign
  brown fat — *see* Lipoma
  Burkitt — *see* Lymphoma, Burkitt
  calcifying epithelial odontogenic — *see* Cyst,
   calcifying odontogenic
  carcinoid D3A.00
   benign D3A.00
    appendix D3A.020
    ascending colon D3A.022
    bronchus (lung) D3A.090
    cecum D3A.021
    colon D3A.029
    descending colon D3A.024
    duodenum D3A.010
    foregut NOS D3A.094
    hindgut NOS D3A.096
    ileum D3A.012
    jejunum D3A.011
    kidney D3A.093
    large intestine D3A.029
    lung (bronchus) D3A.090
    midgut NOS D3A.095
    rectum D3A.026
    sigmoid colon D3A.025
    small intestine D3A.019
    specified NEC D3A.098
    stomach D3A.092
    thymus D3A.091
    transverse colon D3A.023
   malignant C7A.00
    appendix C7A.020
    ascending colon C7A.022

Tumor - *continued*
  carcinoid - *continued*
   malignant - *continued*
    bronchus (lung) C7A.090
    cecum C7A.021
    colon C7A.029
    descending colon C7A.024
    duodenum C7A.010
    foregut NOS C7A.094
    hindgut NOS C7A.096
    ileum C7A.012
    jejunum C7A.011
    kidney C7A.093
    large intestine C7A.029
    lung (bronchus) C7A.090
    midgut NOS C7A.095
    rectum C7A.026
    sigmoid colon C7A.025
    small intestine C7A.019
    specified NEC C7A.098
    stomach C7A.092
    thymus C7A.091
    transverse colon C7A.023
   mesentary metastasis C7B.04
   secondary C7B.00
    bone C7B.03
    distant lymph nodes C7B.01
    liver C7B.02
    peritoneum C7B.04
    specified NEC C7B.09
  carotid body D44.6
   malignant C75.4
  cells — *see also* Neoplasm, unspecified
   behavior, by site
   benign — *see* Neoplasm, benign, by site
   malignant — *see* Neoplasm, malignant, by
    site
   uncertain whether benign or malignant —
    see Neoplasm, uncertain behavior, by
    site
  cervix, in pregnancy or childbirth — *see*
   Pregnancy, complicated by, tumor,
   cervix
  chondromatous giant cell — *see* Neoplasm,
   bone, benign
  chromaffin — *see also* Neoplasm, benign, by
   site
   malignant — *see* Neoplasm, malignant, by
    site
  Cock's peculiar L72.3
  Codman's — *see* Neoplasm, bone, benign
  dentigerous, mixed — *see* Cyst, calcifying
   odontogenic
  dermoid — *see* Neoplasm, benign, by site
   with malignant transformation C56-
  desmoid (extra-abdominal) — *see also*
   Neoplasm, connective tissue, uncertain
   behavior
   abdominal — *see* Neoplasm, connective
    tissue, uncertain behavior
  embolus — *see* Neoplasm, secondary, by site
  embryonal (mixed) — *see also* Neoplasm,
   uncertain behavior, by site
   liver C22.7
  endodermal sinus
   specified site — *see* Neoplasm, malignant,
    by site
   unspecified site
    female C56.-
    male C62.90
  epithelial
   benign — *see* Neoplasm, benign, by site
   malignant — *see* Neoplasm, malignant, by
    site
  Ewing's — *see* Neoplasm, bone, malignant,
   by site
  fatty — *see* Lipoma
  fibroid — *see* Leiomyoma
  G cell
   malignant
    pancreas C25.4
    specified site NEC — *see* Neoplasm,
     malignant, by site
    unspecified site C25.4

Tumor - *continued*
  G cell - *continued*
   specified site — *see* Neoplasm, uncertain
    behavior, by site
   unspecified site D37.8
  germ cell — *see also* Neoplasm, malignant,
   by site
   mixed — *see* Neoplasm, malignant, by site
  ghost cell, odontogenic — *see* Cyst,
   calcifying odontogenic
  giant cell — *see also* Neoplasm, uncertain
   behavior, by site
   bone D48.0
    malignant — *see* Neoplasm, bone,
     malignant
   chondromatous — *see* Neoplasm, bone,
    benign
   malignant — *see* Neoplasm, malignant, by
    site
   soft parts — *see* Neoplasm, connective
    tissue, uncertain behavior
    malignant — *see* Neoplasm, connective
     tissue, malignant
  glomus D18.00
   intra-abdominal D18.03
   intracranial D18.02
   jugulare D44.7
    malignant C75.5
   skin D18.01
   specified site NEC D18.09
  gonadal stromal — *see* Neoplasm, uncertain
   behavior, by site
  granular cell — *see also* Neoplasm,
   connective tissue, benign
   malignant — *see* Neoplasm, connective
    tissue, malignant
  granulosa cell D39.1-
   juvenile D39.1-
   malignant C56-
  granulosa cell-theca cell D39.1-
   malignant C56-
  Grawitz's C64-
  hemorrhoidal — *see* Hemorrhoids
  hilar cell D27-
  hilus cell D27-
  Hurthle cell (benign) D34
   malignant C73
  hydatid — *see* Echinococcus
  hypernephroid — *see also* Neoplasm,
   uncertain behavior, by site
  interstitial cell — *see also* Neoplasm,
   uncertain behavior, by site
   benign — *see* Neoplasm, benign, by site
   malignant — *see* Neoplasm, malignant, by
    site
  intravascular bronchial alveolar D38.1
  islet cell — *see* Neoplasm, benign, by site
   malignant — *see* Neoplasm, malignant, by
    site
    pancreas C25.4
    specified site NEC — *see* Neoplasm,
     malignant, by site
    unspecified site C25.4
   pancreas D13.7
   specified site NEC — *see* Neoplasm,
    benign, by site
   unspecified site D13.7
  juxtaglomerular D41.0-
  Klatskin's C24.0
  Krukenberg's C79.6-
  Leydig cell — *see also* Neoplasm, uncertain
   behavior, by site
   benign — *see* Neoplasm, benign, by site
    specified site — *see* Neoplasm, benign,
     by site
    unspecified site
     female D27.9
     male D29.20
   malignant — *see* Neoplasm, malignant, by
    site
    specified site — *see* Neoplasm,
     malignant, by site
    unspecified site
     female C56.9
     male C62.90

TUMOR - TUMOR

Tumor - *continued*
  Leydig cell - *continued*
    specified site — *see* Neoplasm, uncertain behavior, by site
    unspecified site
      female D39.10
      male D40.10
  lipid cell, ovary D27-
  lipoid cell, ovary D27-
  malignant — *see also* Neoplasm, malignant, by site C80.1
    fusiform cell (type) C80.1
    giant cell (type) C80.1
    localized, plasma cell — *see* Plasmacytoma, solitary
    mixed NEC C80.1
    small cell (type) C80.1
    spindle cell (type) C80.1
    unclassified C80.1
  mast cell D47.09
  melanotic, neuroectodermal — *see* Neoplasm, benign, by site
  Merkel cell — *see* Carcinoma, Merkel cell
  mesenchymal
    malignant — *see* Neoplasm, connective tissue, malignant
    mixed — *see* Neoplasm, connective tissue, uncertain behavior
  mesodermal, mixed — *see also* Neoplasm, malignant, by site
    liver C22.4
  mesonephric — *see also* Neoplasm, uncertain behavior, by site
    malignant — *see* Neoplasm, malignant, by site
  metastatic
    from specified site — *see* Neoplasm, malignant, by site
    of specified site — *see* Neoplasm, malignant, by site
    to specified site — *see* Neoplasm, secondary, by site
  mixed NEC — *see also* Neoplasm, benign, by site
    malignant — *see* Neoplasm, malignant, by site
  mucinous of low malignant potential
    specified site — *see* Neoplasm, malignant, by site
    unspecified site C56.9
  mucocarcinoid
    specified site — *see* Neoplasm, malignant, by site
    unspecified site C18.1
  mucoepidermoid — *see* Neoplasm, uncertain behavior, by site
  Müllerian, mixed
    specified site — *see* Neoplasm, malignant, by site
    unspecified site C54.9
  myoepithelial — *see* Neoplasm, benign, by site
  neuroectodermal (peripheral) — *see* Neoplasm, malignant, by site
    primitive
      specified site — *see* Neoplasm, malignant, by site
      unspecified site C71.9
  neuroendocrine D3A.8
    malignant poorly differentiated C7A.1
    secondary NEC C7B.8
    specified NEC C7A.8
  neurogenic olfactory C30.0
  nonencapsulated sclerosing C73
  odontogenic (adenomatoid) (benign) (calcifying epithelial) (keratocystic) (squamous) — *see* Cyst, calcifying odontogenic
    malignant C41.1
    upper jaw (bone) C41.0
  ovarian stromal D39.1-
  ovary, in pregnancy — *see* Pregnancy, complicated by
  pacinian — *see* Neoplasm, skin, benign
  Pancoast's — *see* Pancoast's syndrome

Tumor - *continued*
  papillary — *see also* Papilloma
    cystic D37.9
    mucinous of low malignant potential C56-
      specified site — *see* Neoplasm, malignant, by site
      unspecified site C56.9
    serous of low malignant potential
      specified site — *see* Neoplasm, malignant, by site
      unspecified site C56.9
  pelvic, in pregnancy or childbirth — *see* Pregnancy, complicated by
  phantom F45.8
  phyllodes D48.6-
    benign D24-
    malignant — *see* Neoplasm, breast, malignant
  Pindborg — *see* Cyst, calcifying odontogenic
  placental site trophoblastic D39.2
  plasma cell (malignant) (localized) — *see* Plasmacytoma, solitary
  polyvesicular vitelline
    specified site — *see* Neoplasm, malignant, by site
    unspecified site
      female C56.9
      male C62.90
  Pott's puffy — *see* Osteomyelitis, specified NEC
  Rathke's pouch D44.3
  retinal anlage — *see* Neoplasm, benign, by site
  salivary gland type, mixed — *see* Neoplasm, salivary gland, benign
    malignant — *see* Neoplasm, salivary gland, malignant
  Sampson's N80.1
  Schmincke's — *see* Neoplasm, nasopharynx, malignant
  sclerosing stromal D27-
  sebaceous — *see* Cyst, sebaceous
  secondary — *see* Neoplasm, secondary, by site
    carcinoid C7B.00
      bone C7B.03
      distant lymph nodes C7B.01
      liver C7B.02
      peritoneum C7B.04
      specified NEC C7B.09
    neuroendocrine NEC C7B.8
  serous of low malignant potential
    specified site — *see* Neoplasm, malignant, by site
    unspecified site C56.9
  Sertoli cell — *see* Neoplasm, benign, by site
    with lipid storage
      specified site — *see* Neoplasm, benign, by site
      unspecified site
        female D27.9
        male D29.20
    specified site — *see* Neoplasm, benign, by site
    unspecified site
      female D27.9
      male D29.20
  Sertoli-Leydig cell — *see* Neoplasm, benign, by site
    specified site — *see* Neoplasm, benign, by site
    unspecified site
      female D27.9
      male D29.20
  sex cord (-stromal) — *see* Neoplasm, uncertain behavior, by site
    with annular tubules D39.1-
  skin appendage — *see* Neoplasm, skin, benign
  smooth muscle — *see* Neoplasm, connective tissue, uncertain behavior
  soft tissue
    benign — *see* Neoplasm, connective tissue, benign

Tumor - *continued*
  soft tissue - *continued*
    malignant — *see* Neoplasm, connective tissue, malignant
  sternomastoid (congenital) Q68.0
  stromal
    endometrial D39.0
    gastric D48.1
      benign D21.4
      malignant C16.9
      uncertain behavior D48.1
    gastrointestinal C49.A-
      benign D21.4
      esophagus C49.A1
      large intestine C49.A4
      malignant C49.A0
        colon C49.A4
        duodenum C49.A3
        esophagus C49.A1
        ileum C49.A3
        jejunum C49.A3
        large intestine C49.A4
        Meckel diverticulum C49.A3
        omentum C49.A9
        peritoneum C49.A9
        rectum C49.A5
        small intestine C49.A3
        specified site NEC C49.A9
        stomach C49.A2
      rectum C49.A5
      small intestine C49.A3
      specified site NEC C49.A9
      stomach C49.A2
      uncertain behavior D48.1
    intestine
      benign D21.4
      malignant
        large C49.A4
        small C49.A3
      uncertain behavior D48.1
    ovarian D39.1-
    stomach C49.A2
      benign D21.4
      malignant C49.A2
      uncertain behavior D48.1
  testicular D40.10
  sweat gland — *see also* Neoplasm, skin, uncertain behavior
    benign — *see* Neoplasm, skin, benign
    malignant — *see* Neoplasm, skin, malignant
  syphilitic, brain A52.17
  testicular stromal D40.1-
  theca cell D27.-
  theca cell-granulosa cell D39.1-
  Triton, malignant — *see* Neoplasm, nerve, malignant
  trophoblastic, placental site D39.2
  turban D23.4
  uterus (body), in pregnancy or childbirth — *see* Pregnancy, complicated by, tumor, uterus
  vagina, in pregnancy or childbirth — *see* Pregnancy, complicated by
  varicose — *see* Varix
  von Recklinghausen's — *see* Neurofibromatosis
  vulva or perineum, in pregnancy or childbirth — *see* Pregnancy, complicated by
    causing obstructed labor O65.5
  Warthin's — *see* Neoplasm, salivary gland, benign
  Wilms' C64-
  yolk sac — *see* Neoplasm, malignant, by site
    specified site — *see* Neoplasm, malignant, by site
    unspecified site
      female C56.9
      male C62.90
Tumor lysis syndrome (following antineoplastic chemotherapy) (spontaneous) NEC E88.3
Tumorlet — *see* Neoplasm, uncertain behavior, by site

Tungiasis B88.1
Tunica vasculosa lentis Q12.2
Turban tumor D23.4
Türck's trachoma J37.0
Turner-Kieser syndrome Q87.2
Turner-like syndrome Q87.19
Turner's
  hypoplasia (tooth) K00.4
  syndrome Q96.9
    specified NEC Q96.8
  tooth K00.4
Turner-Ullrich syndrome Q96.9
Tussis convulsiva — *see* Whooping cough
Twiddler's syndrome (due to)
  automatic implantable defibrillator T82.198
  cardiac pacemaker T82.198
Twilight state
  epileptic F05
  psychogenic F44.89
Twin (newborn) — *see also* Newborn, twin
  conjoined Q89.4
  pregnancy — *see* Pregnancy, twin
Twinning, teeth K00.2
Twist, twisted
  bowel, colon or intestine K56.2
  hair (congenital) Q84.1
  mesentery K56.2
  omentum K56.2
  organ or site, congenital NEC — *see*
    Anomaly, by site
  ovarian pedicle — *see* Torsion, ovary
Twitching R25.3
Tylosis (acquired) L84
  buccalis K13.29
  linguae K13.29
  palmaris et plantaris (congenital)
    (inherited) Q82.8
    acquired L85.1
Tympanism R14.0
Tympanites (abdominal) (intestinal) R14.0
Tympanitis — *see* Myringitis
Tympanosclerosis — *see* subcategory H74.0
Tympanum — *see* condition
Tympany
  abdomen R14.0
  chest R09.89
Type A behavior pattern Z73.1
Typhlitis — *see* Appendicitis
Typhoenteritis — *see* Typhoid
Typhoid (abortive) (ambulant) (any site)
    (clinical) (fever) (hemorrhagic)
    (infection) (intermittent) (malignant)
    (rheumatic) (Widal negative) A01.00
  with pneumonia A01.03
  abdominal A01.09
  arthritis A01.04
  carrier (suspected) of Z22.0
  cholecystitis (current) A01.09
  endocarditis A01.02
  heart involvement A01.02
  inoculation reaction — *see* Complications,
    vaccination
  meningitis A01.01
  mesenteric lymph nodes A01.09
  myocarditis A01.02
  osteomyelitis A01.05
  perichondritis, larynx A01.09
  pneumonia A01.03
  spine A01.05
  specified NEC A01.09
  ulcer (perforating) A01.09
Typhomalaria (fever) — *see* Malaria
Typhomania A01.00
Typhoperitonitis A01.09
Typhus (fever) A75.9
  abdominal, abdominalis — *see* Typhoid
  African tick A77.1
  amarillic A95.9
  brain A75.9 *[G94]*
  cerebral A75.9 *[G94]*
  classical A75.0
  due to Rickettsia
    prowazekii A75.0
      recrudescent A75.1
    tsutsugamushi A75.3

Typhus (fever) - *continued*
  due to Rickettsia - *continued*
    typhi A75.2
  endemic (flea-borne) A75.2
  epidemic (louse-borne) A75.0
  exanthematic NEC A75.0
  exanthematicus SAI A75.0
    brillii SAI A75.1
    mexicanus SAI A75.2
    typhus murinus A75.2
  flea-borne A75.2
  India tick A77.1
  Kenya (tick) A77.1
  louse-borne A75.0
  Mexican A75.2
  mite-borne A75.3
  murine A75.2
  North Asian tick-borne A77.2
  petechial A75.9
  Queensland tick A77.3
  rat A75.2
  recrudescent A75.1
  recurrens — *see* Fever, relapsing
  Sao Paulo A77.0
  scrub (China) (India) (Malaysia) (New
    Guinea) A75.3
  shop (of Malaysia) A75.2
  Siberian tick A77.2
  tick-borne A77.9
  tropical (mite-borne) A75.3
Tyrosinemia E70.21
  newborn, transitory P74.5
Tyrosinosis E70.21
Tyrosinuria E70.29

U

Uhl's anomaly or disease Q24.8
Ulcer, ulcerated, ulcerating, ulceration,
    ulcerative
  alveolar process M27.3
  amebic (intestine) A06.1
    skin A06.7
  anastomotic — *see* Ulcer, gastrojejunal
  anorectal K62.6
  antral — *see* Ulcer, stomach
  anus (sphincter) (solitary) K62.6
  aorta — *see* Aneurysm
  aphthous (oral) (recurrent) K12.0
    genital organ (s)
      female N76.6
      male N50.89
  artery I77.2
  atrophic — *see* Ulcer, skin
    decubitus — *see* Ulcer, pressure, by site
  back L98.429
    with
      bone involvement without evidence of
        necrosis L98.426
      bone necrosis L98.424
      exposed fat layer L98.422
      muscle involvement without evidence of
        necrosis L98.425
      muscle necrosis L98.423
      skin breakdown only L98.421
      specified severity NEC L98.428
  Barrett's (esophagus) K22.10
    with bleeding K22.11
  bile duct (common) (hepatic) K83.8
  bladder (solitary) (sphincter) NEC N32.89
    bilharzial B65.9 *[N33]*
    in schistosomiasis (bilharzial) B65.9 *[N33]*
    submucosal — *see* Cystitis, interstitial
    tuberculous A18.12
  bleeding K27.4
  bone — *see* Osteomyelitis, specified type
    NEC
  bowel — *see* Ulcer, intestine
  breast N61.1
  bronchus J98.09
  buccal (cavity) (traumatic) K12.1
  Buruli A31.1
  buttock L98.419
    with
      bone involvement without evidence of
        necrosis L98.416
      bone necrosis L98.414

Ulcer, ulcerated, ulcerating, ulceration,
    ulcerative - *continued*
  buttock - *continued*
    with - *continued*
      exposed fat layer L98.412
      muscle involvement without evidence of
        necrosis L98.415
      muscle necrosis L98.413
      skin breakdown only L98.411
      specified severity NEC L98.418
  cancerous — *see* Neoplasm, malignant, by
    site
  cardia K22.10
    with bleeding K22.11
  cardioesophageal (peptic) K22.10
    with bleeding K22.11
  cecum — *see* Ulcer, intestine
  cervix (uteri) (decubitus) (trophic) N86
    with cervicitis N72
  chancroidal A57
  chiclero B55.1
  chronic (cause unknown) — *see* Ulcer, skin
  Cochin-China B55.1
  colon — *see* Ulcer, intestine
  conjunctiva H10.89
  cornea H16.00-
    with hypopyon H16.03-
    central H16.01-
    dendritic (herpes simplex) B00.52
    marginal H16.04-
    Mooren's H16.05-
    mycotic H16.06-
    perforated H16.07-
    ring H16.02-
    tuberculous (phlyctenular) A18.52
  corpus cavernosum (chronic) N48.5
  crural — *see* Ulcer, lower limb
  Curling's — *see* Ulcer, peptic, acute
  Cushing's — *see* Ulcer, peptic, acute
  cystic duct K82.8
  cystitis (interstitial) — *see* Cystitis,
    interstitial
  decubitus — *see* Ulcer, pressure, by site
  dendritic, cornea (herpes simplex) B00.52
  diabetes, diabetic — *see* Diabetes, ulcer
  Dieulafoy's K25.0
  due to
    infection NEC — *see* Ulcer, skin
    radiation NEC L59.8
    trophic disturbance (any region) — *see*
      Ulcer, skin
    X-ray L58.1
  duodenum, duodenal (eroded) (peptic) K26.9
    with
      hemorrhage K26.4
        and perforation K26.6
      perforation K26.5
    acute K26.3
      with
        hemorrhage K26.0
          and perforation K26.2
        perforation K26.1
    chronic K26.7
      with
        hemorrhage K26.4
          and perforation K26.6
        perforation K26.5
  dysenteric A09
  elusive — *see* Cystitis, interstitial
  endocarditis (acute) (chronic)
    (subacute) I28.8
  epiglottis J38.7
  esophagus (peptic) K22.10
    with bleeding K22.11
    due to
      aspirin K22.10
        with bleeding K22.11
      gastrointestinal reflux disease K21.0
      ingestion of chemical or
        medicament K22.10
        with bleeding K22.11
    fungal K22.10
      with bleeding K22.11
    infective K22.10
      with bleeding K22.11

Ulcer, ulcerated, ulcerating, ulceration, ulcerative - *continued*
  esophagus (peptic) - *continued*
    varicose — *see* Varix, esophagus
  eyelid (region) H01.8
  fauces J39.2
  Fenwick (-Hunner) (solitary) — *see* Cystitis, interstitial
  fistulous — *see* Ulcer, skin
  foot (indolent) (trophic) — *see* Ulcer, lower limb
  frambesial, initial A66.0
  frenum (tongue) K14.0
  gallbladder or duct K82.8
  gangrenous — *see* Gangrene
  gastric — *see* Ulcer, stomach
  gastrocolic — *see* Ulcer, gastrojejunal
  gastroduodenal — *see* Ulcer, peptic
  gastroesophageal — *see* Ulcer, stomach
  gastrointestinal — *see* Ulcer, gastrojejunal
  gastrojejunal (peptic) K28.9
    with
      hemorrhage K28.4
        and perforation K28.6
      perforation K28.5
    acute K28.3
      with
        hemorrhage K28.0
          and perforation K28.2
        perforation K28.1
    chronic K28.7
      with
        hemorrhage K28.4
          and perforation K28.6
        perforation K28.5
  gastrojejunocolic — *see* Ulcer, gastrojejunal
  gingiva K06.8
  gingivitis K05.10
    nonplaque induced K05.11
    plaque induced K05.10
  glottis J38.7
  granuloma of pudenda A58
  gum K06.8
  gumma, due to yaws A66.4
  heel — *see* Ulcer, lower limb
  hemorrhoid — *see also* Hemorrhoids, by degree K64.8
  Hunner's — *see* Cystitis, interstitial
  hypopharynx J39.2
  hypopyon (chronic) (subacute) — *see* Ulcer, cornea, with hypopyon
  hypostaticum — *see* Ulcer, varicose
  ileum — *see* Ulcer, intestine
  intestine, intestinal K63.3
    with perforation K63.1
    amebic A06.1
    duodenal — *see* Ulcer, duodenum
    granulocytopenic (with hemorrhage) — *see* Neutropenia
    marginal — *see* Ulcer, gastrojejunal
    perforating K63.1
      newborn P78.0
    primary, small intestine K63.3
    rectum K62.6
    stercoraceous, stercoral K63.3
    tuberculous A18.32
    typhoid (fever) — *see* Typhoid
    varicose I86.8
  jejunum, jejunal — *see* Ulcer, gastrojejunal
  keratitis — *see* Ulcer, cornea
  knee — *see* Ulcer, lower limb
  labium (majus) (minus) N76.6
  laryngitis — *see* Laryngitis
  larynx (aphthous) (contact) J38.7
    diphtheritic A36.2
  leg — *see* Ulcer, lower limb
  lip K13.0
  Lipschütz's N76.6
  lower limb (atrophic) (chronic) (neurogenic) (perforating) (pyogenic) (trophic) (tropical) L97.909
    with
      bone involvement without evidence of necrosis L97.906
      bone necrosis L97.904

Ulcer, ulcerated, ulcerating, ulceration, ulcerative - *continued*
  lower limb (atrophic) (chronic) (neurogenic) (perforating) (pyogenic) (trophic) (tropical) - *continued*
    with - *continued*
      exposed fat layer L97.902
      muscle involvement without evidence of necrosis L97.905
      muscle necrosis L97.903
      skin breakdown only L97.901
      specified severity NEC L97.908
    ankle L97.309
      with
        bone involvement without evidence of necrosis L97.306
        bone necrosis L97.304
        exposed fat layer L97.302
        muscle involvement without evidence of necrosis L97.305
        muscle necrosis L97.303
        skin breakdown only L97.301
        specified severity NEC L97.308
      left L97.329
        with
          bone involvement without evidence of necrosis L97.326
          bone necrosis L97.324
          exposed fat layer L97.322
          muscle involvement without evidence of necrosis L97.325
          muscle necrosis L97.323
          skin breakdown only L97.321
          specified severity NEC L97.328
      right L97.319
        with
          bone involvement without evidence of necrosis L97.316
          bone necrosis L97.314
          exposed fat layer L97.312
          muscle involvement without evidence of necrosis L97.315
          muscle necrosis L97.313
          skin breakdown only L97.311
          specified severity NEC L97.318
    calf L97.209
      with
        bone involvement without evidence of necrosis L97.206
        bone necrosis L97.204
        exposed fat layer L97.202
        muscle involvement without evidence of necrosis L97.205
        muscle necrosis L97.203
        skin breakdown only L97.201
        specified severity NEC L97.208
      left L97.229
        with
          bone involvement without evidence of necrosis L97.226
          bone necrosis L97.224
          exposed fat layer L97.222
          muscle involvement without evidence of necrosis L97.225
          muscle necrosis L97.223
          skin breakdown only L97.221
          specified severity NEC L97.228
      right L97.219
        with
          bone involvement without evidence of necrosis L97.216
          bone necrosis L97.214
          exposed fat layer L97.212
          muscle involvement without evidence of necrosis L97.215
          muscle necrosis L97.213
          skin breakdown only L97.211
          specified severity NEC L97.218
    decubitus — *see* Ulcer, pressure, by site
    foot specified NEC L97.509
      with
        bone involvement without evidence of necrosis L97.506
        bone necrosis L97.504
        exposed fat layer L97.502

Ulcer, ulcerated, ulcerating, ulceration, ulcerative - *continued*
  lower limb (atrophic) (chronic) (neurogenic) (perforating) (pyogenic) (trophic) (tropical) - *continued*
    foot specified NEC - *continued*
      with - *continued*
        muscle involvement without evidence of necrosis L97.505
        muscle necrosis L97.503
        skin breakdown only L97.501
        specified severity NEC L97.508
      left L97.529
        with
          bone involvement without evidence of necrosis L97.526
          bone necrosis L97.524
          exposed fat layer L97.522
          muscle involvement without evidence of necrosis L97.525
          muscle necrosis L97.523
          skin breakdown only L97.521
          specified severity NEC L97.528
      right L97.519
        with
          bone involvement without evidence of necrosis L97.516
          bone necrosis L97.514
          exposed fat layer L97.512
          muscle involvement without evidence of necrosis L97.515
          muscle necrosis L97.513
          skin breakdown only L97.511
          specified severity NEC L97.518
    heel L97.409
      with
        bone involvement without evidence of necrosis L97.406
        bone necrosis L97.404
        exposed fat layer L97.402
        muscle involvement without evidence of necrosis L97.405
        muscle necrosis L97.403
        skin breakdown only L97.401
        specified severity NEC L97.408
      left L97.429
        with
          bone involvement without evidence of necrosis L97.426
          bone necrosis L97.424
          exposed fat layer L97.422
          muscle involvement without evidence of necrosis L97.425
          muscle necrosis L97.423
          skin breakdown only L97.421
          specified severity NEC L97.428
      right L97.419
        with
          bone involvement without evidence of necrosis L97.416
          bone necrosis L97.414
          exposed fat layer L97.412
          muscle involvement without evidence of necrosis L97.415
          muscle necrosis L97.413
          skin breakdown only L97.411
          specified severity NEC L97.418
    left L97.929
      with
        bone involvement without evidence of necrosis L97.926
        bone necrosis L97.924
        exposed fat layer L97.922
        muscle involvement without evidence of necrosis L97.925
        muscle necrosis L97.923
        skin breakdown only L97.921
        specified severity NEC L97.928
    lower leg NOS L97.909
      with
        bone involvement without evidence of necrosis L97.906
        bone necrosis L97.904
        exposed fat layer L97.902

Ulcer, ulcerated, ulcerating, ulceration, ulcerative - *continued*
  lower limb (atrophic) (chronic) (neurogenic) (perforating) (pyogenic) (trophic) (tropical) - *continued*
    lower leg NOS - *continued*
      with - *continued*
        muscle involvement without evidence of necrosis L97.905
        muscle necrosis L97.903
        skin breakdown only L97.901
        specified severity NEC L97.908
      left L97.929
        with
          bone involvement without evidence of necrosis L97.926
          bone necrosis L97.924
          exposed fat layer L97.922
          muscle involvement without evidence of necrosis L97.925
          muscle necrosis L97.923
          skin breakdown only L97.921
          specified severity NEC L97.928
      right L97.919
        with
          bone involvement without evidence of necrosis L97.916
          bone necrosis L97.914
          exposed fat layer L97.912
          muscle involvement without evidence of necrosis L97.915
          muscle necrosis L97.913
          skin breakdown only L97.911
          specified severity NEC L97.918
    specified site NEC L97.809
      with
        bone involvement without evidence of necrosis L97.806
        bone necrosis L97.804
        exposed fat layer L97.802
        muscle involvement without evidence of necrosis L97.805
        muscle necrosis L97.803
        skin breakdown only L97.801
        specified severity NEC L97.808
      left L97.829
        with
          bone involvement without evidence of necrosis L97.826
          bone necrosis L97.824
          exposed fat layer L97.822
          muscle involvement without evidence of necrosis L97.825
          muscle necrosis L97.823
          skin breakdown only L97.821
          specified severity NEC L97.828
      right L97.819
        with
          bone involvement without evidence of necrosis L97.816
          bone necrosis L97.814
          exposed fat layer L97.812
          muscle involvement without evidence of necrosis L97.815
          muscle necrosis L97.813
          skin breakdown only L97.811
          specified severity NEC L97.818
    midfoot L97.409
      with
        bone involvement without evidence of necrosis L97.406
        bone necrosis L97.404
        exposed fat layer L97.402
        muscle involvement without evidence of necrosis L97.405
        muscle necrosis L97.403
        skin breakdown only L97.401
        specified severity NEC L97.408
      left L97.429
        with

Ulcer, ulcerated, ulcerating, ulceration, ulcerative - *continued*
  lower limb (atrophic) (chronic) (neurogenic) (perforating) (pyogenic) (trophic) (tropical) - *continued*
    midfoot - *continued*
      left - *continued*
        with - *continued*
          bone involvement without evidence of necrosis L97.426
          bone necrosis L97.424
          exposed fat layer L97.422
          muscle involvement without evidence of necrosis L97.425
          muscle necrosis L97.423
          skin breakdown only L97.421
          specified severity NEC L97.428
      right L97.419
        with
          bone involvement without evidence of necrosis L97.416
          bone necrosis L97.414
          exposed fat layer L97.412
          muscle involvement without evidence of necrosis L97.415
          muscle necrosis L97.413
          skin breakdown only L97.411
          specified severity NEC L97.418
    right L97.919
      with
        bone involvement without evidence of necrosis L97.916
        bone necrosis L97.914
        exposed fat layer L97.912
        muscle involvement without evidence of necrosis L97.915
        muscle necrosis L97.913
        skin breakdown only L97.911
        specified severity NEC L97.918
    thigh L97.109
      with
        bone involvement without evidence of necrosis L97.106
        bone necrosis L97.104
        muscle involvement without evidence of necrosis L97.105
        exposed fat layer L97.102
        muscle necrosis L97.103
        skin breakdown only L97.101
        specified severity NEC L97.108
      left L97.129
        with
          bone involvement without evidence of necrosis L97.126
          bone necrosis L97.124
          exposed fat layer L97.122
          muscle involvement without evidence of necrosis L97.125
          muscle necrosis L97.123
          skin breakdown only L97.121
          specified severity NEC L97.128
      right L97.119
        with
          bone involvement without evidence of necrosis L97.116
          bone necrosis L97.114
          exposed fat layer L97.112
          muscle involvement without evidence of necrosis L97.115
          muscle necrosis L97.113
          skin breakdown only L97.111
          specified severity NEC L97.118
    toe L97.509
      with
        bone involvement without evidence of necrosis L97.506
        bone necrosis L97.504
        exposed fat layer L97.502
        muscle involvement without evidence of necrosis L97.505
        muscle necrosis L97.503
        skin breakdown only L97.501
        specified severity NEC L97.508
      left L97.529
        with

Ulcer, ulcerated, ulcerating, ulceration, ulcerative - *continued*
  lower limb (atrophic) (chronic) (neurogenic) (perforating) (pyogenic) (trophic) (tropical) - *continued*
    toe - *continued*
      left - *continued*
        with - *continued*
          bone involvement without evidence of necrosis L97.526
          bone necrosis L97.524
          exposed fat layer L97.522
          muscle involvement without evidence of necrosis L97.525
          muscle necrosis L97.523
          skin breakdown only L97.521
          specified severity NEC L97.528
      right L97.519
        with
          bone involvement without evidence of necrosis L97.516
          bone necrosis L97.514
          exposed fat layer L97.512
          muscle involvement without evidence of necrosis L97.515
          muscle necrosis L97.513
          skin breakdown only L97.511
          specified severity NEC L97.518
    leprous A30.1
    syphilitic A52.19
    varicose — *see* Varix, leg, with, ulcer
  luetic — *see* Ulcer, syphilitic
  lung J98.4
    tuberculous — *see* Tuberculosis, pulmonary
  malignant — *see* Neoplasm, malignant, by site
  marginal NEC — *see* Ulcer, gastrojejunal
  meatus (urinarius) N34.2
  Meckel's diverticulum Q43.0
    malignant — *see* Table of Neoplasms, small intestine, malignant
  Meleney's (chronic undermining) — *see* Ulcer, skin
  Mooren's (cornea) — *see* Ulcer, cornea, Mooren's
  mycobacterial (skin) A31.1
  nasopharynx J39.2
  neck, uterus N86
  neurogenic NEC — *see* Ulcer, skin
  nose, nasal (passage) (infective) (septum) J34.0
    skin — *see* Ulcer, skin
    spirochetal A69.8
    varicose (bleeding) I86.8
  oral mucosa (traumatic) K12.1
  palate (soft) K12.1
  penis (chronic) N48.5
  peptic (site unspecified) K27.9
    with
      hemorrhage K27.4
        and perforation K27.6
      perforation K27.5
    acute K27.3
      with
        hemorrhage K27.0
          and perforation K27.2
        perforation K27.1
    chronic K27.7
      with
        hemorrhage K27.4
          and perforation K27.6
        perforation K27.5
  esophagus K22.10
    with bleeding K22.11
  newborn P78.82
  perforating K27.5
    skin — *see* Ulcer, skin
  peritonsillar J35.8
  phagedenic (tropical) — *see* Ulcer, skin
  pharynx J39.2
  phlebitis — *see* Phlebitis
  plaster — *see* Ulcer, pressure, by site
  popliteal space — *see* Ulcer, lower limb
  postpyloric — *see* Ulcer, duodenum

Ulcer, ulcerated, ulcerating, ulceration, ulcerative - *continued*

prepuce N47.7

prepyloric — *see* Ulcer, stomach

pressure (pressure area) L89.9-
- ankle L89.5-
- back L89.1-
- buttock L89.3-
- coccyx L89.15-
- contiguous site of back, buttock, hip L89.4-
- elbow L89.0-
- face L89.81-
- head L89.81-
- heel L89.6-
- hip L89.2-
- sacral region (tailbone) L89.15-
- specified site NEC L89.89-
- stage 1 (healing) (pre-ulcer skin changes limited to persistent focal edema)
  - ankle L89.5-
  - back L89.1-
  - buttock L89.3-
  - coccyx L89.15-
  - contiguous site of back, buttock, hip L89.4-
  - elbow L89.0-
  - face L89.81-
  - head L89.81-
  - heel L89.6-
  - hip L89.2-
  - sacral region (tailbone) L89.15-
  - specified site NEC L89.89-
- stage 2 (healing) (abrasion, blister, partial thickness skin loss involving epidermis and/or dermis)
  - ankle L89.5-
  - back L89.1-
  - buttock L89.3-
  - coccyx L89.15-
  - contiguous site of back, buttock, hip L89.4-
  - elbow L89.0-
  - face L89.81-
  - head L89.81-
  - heel L89.6-
  - hip L89.2-
  - sacral region (tailbone) L89.15-
  - specified site NEC L89.89-
- stage 3 (healing) (full thickness skin loss involving damage or necrosis of subcutaneous tissue)
  - ankle L89.5-
  - back L89.1-
  - buttock L89.3-
  - coccyx L89.15-
  - contiguous site of back, buttock, hip L89.4-
  - elbow L89.0-
  - face L89.81-
  - head L89.81-
  - heel L89.6-
  - hip L89.2-
  - sacral region (tailbone) L89.15-
  - specified site NEC L89.89-
- stage 4 (healing) (necrosis of soft tissues through to underlying muscle, tendon, or bone)
  - ankle L89.5-
  - back L89.1-
  - buttock L89.3-
  - coccyx L89.15-
  - contiguous site of back, buttock, hip L89.4-
  - elbow L89.0-
  - face L89.81-
  - head L89.81-
  - heel L89.6-
  - hip L89.2-
  - sacral region (tailbone) L89.15-
  - specified site NEC L89.89-
- unspecified stage
  - ankle L89.5-
  - back L89.1-
  - buttock L89.3-

Ulcer, ulcerated, ulcerating, ulceration, ulcerative - *continued*

pressure (pressure area) - *continued*
- unspecified stage - *continued*
  - coccyx L89.15-
  - contiguous site of back, buttock, hip L89.4-
  - elbow L89.0-
  - face L89.81-
  - head L89.81-
  - heel L89.6-
  - hip L89.2-
  - sacral region (tailbone) L89.15-
  - specified site NEC L89.89-
- unstageable
  - ankle L89.5-
  - back L89.1-
  - buttock L89.3-
  - coccyx L89.15-
  - contiguous site of back, buttock, hip L89.4-
  - elbow L89.0-
  - face L89.81-
  - head L89.81-
  - heel L89.6-
  - hip L89.2-
  - sacral region (tailbone) L89.15-
  - specified site NEC L89.89-

primary of intestine K63.3
- with perforation K63.1

prostate N41.9

pyloric — *see* Ulcer, stomach

rectosigmoid K63.3
- with perforation K63.1

rectum (sphincter) (solitary) K62.6
- stercoraceous, stercoral K62.6

retina — *see* Inflammation, chorioretinal

rodent — *see also* Neoplasm, skin, malignant

sclera — *see* Scleritis

scrofulous (tuberculous) A18.2

scrotum N50.89
- tuberculous A18.15
- varicose I86.1

seminal vesicle N50.89

sigmoid — *see* Ulcer, intestine

skin (atrophic) (chronic) (neurogenic) (non-healing) (perforating) (pyogenic) (trophic) (tropical) L98.499
- with gangrene — *see* Gangrene
- amebic A06.7
- back — *see* Ulcer, back
- buttock — *see* Ulcer, buttock
- decubitus — *see* Ulcer, pressure
- lower limb — *see* Ulcer, lower limb
- mycobacterial A31.1
- specified site NEC L98.499
  - with
    - bone involvement without evidence of necrosis L98.496
    - bone necrosis L98.494
    - exposed fat layer L98.492
    - muscle involvement without evidence of necrosis L98.495
    - muscle necrosis L98.493
    - skin breakdown only L98.491
    - specified severity NEC L98.498
- tuberculous (primary) A18.4
- varicose — *see* Ulcer, varicose

sloughing — *see* Ulcer, skin

solitary, anus or rectum (sphincter) K62.6

sore throat J02.9
- streptococcal J02.0

spermatic cord N50.89

spine (tuberculous) A18.01

stasis (venous) — *see* Varix, leg, with, ulcer
- without varicose veins I87.2

stercoraceous, stercoral K63.3
- with perforation K63.1
- anus or rectum K62.6

stoma, stomal — *see* Ulcer, gastrojejunal

stomach (eroded) (peptic) (round) K25.9
- with
  - hemorrhage K25.4
    - and perforation K25.6
  - perforation K25.5

Ulcer, ulcerated, ulcerating, ulceration, ulcerative - *continued*

stomach (eroded) (peptic) (round) - *continued*
- acute K25.3
  - with
    - hemorrhage K25.0
      - and perforation K25.2
    - perforation K25.1
- chronic K25.7
  - with
    - hemorrhage K25.4
      - and perforation K25.6
    - perforation K25.5

stomal — *see* Ulcer, gastrojejunal

stomatitis K12.1

stress — *see* Ulcer, peptic

strumous (tuberculous) A18.2

submucosal, bladder — *see* Cystitis, interstitial

syphilitic (any site) (early) (secondary) A51.39
- late A52.79
- perforating A52.79
  - foot A52.11

testis N50.89

thigh — *see* Ulcer, lower limb

throat J39.2
- diphtheritic A36.0

toe — *see* Ulcer, lower limb

tongue (traumatic) K14.0

tonsil J35.8
- diphtheritic A36.0

trachea J39.8

trophic — *see* Ulcer, skin

tropical — *see* Ulcer, skin

tuberculous — *see* Tuberculosis, ulcer

tunica vaginalis N50.89

turbinate J34.89

typhoid (perforating) — *see* Typhoid

unspecified site — *see* Ulcer, skin

urethra (meatus) — *see* Urethritis

uterus N85.8
- cervix N86
  - with cervicitis N72
- neck N86
  - with cervicitis N72

vagina N76.5
- in Behçet's disease M35.2 *[N77.0]*
- pessary N89.8

valve, heart I33.0

varicose (lower limb, any part) — *see also* Varix, leg, with, ulcer
- broad ligament I86.2
- esophagus — *see* Varix, esophagus
- inflamed or infected — *see* Varix, leg, with, ulcer, with inflammation
- nasal septum I86.8
- perineum I86.3
- scrotum I86.1
- specified site NEC I86.8
- sublingual I86.0
- vulva I86.3

vas deferens N50.89

vulva (acute) (infectional) N76.6
- in (due to)
  - Behçet's disease M35.2 *[N77.0]*
  - herpesviral (herpes simplex) infection A60.04
  - tuberculosis A18.18

vulvobuccal, recurring N76.6

X-ray L58.1

yaws A66.4

Ulcerosa scarlatina A38.8

Ulcus — *see also* Ulcer
- cutis tuberculosum A18.4
- duodeni — *see* Ulcer, duodenum
- durum (syphilitic) A51.0
  - extragenital A51.2
- gastrojejunale — *see* Ulcer, gastrojejunal
- hypostaticum — *see* Ulcer, varicose
- molle (cutis) (skin) A57
- serpens corneae — *see* Ulcer, cornea, central
- ventriculi — *see* Ulcer, stomach

Ulegyria Q04.8

Ulerythema

ophryogenes, congenital Q84.2
sycosiforme L73.8

Ullrich (-Bonnevie) (-Turner) syndrome — *see also* Turner's syndrome Q87.19

Ullrich-Feichtiger syndrome Q87.0

Ulnar — *see* condition

Ulorrhagia, ulorrhea K06.8

Umbilicus, umbilical — *see* condition

Unacceptable

contours of tooth K08.54
morphology of tooth K08.54

Unavailability (of)

bed at medical facility Z75.1
health service-related agencies Z75.4
medical facilities (at) Z75.3
due to
investigation by social service agency Z75.2
lack of services at home Z75.0
remoteness from facility Z75.3
waiting list Z75.1
home Z75.0
outpatient clinic Z75.3
schooling Z55.1
social service agencies Z75.4

Uncinaria americana infestation B76.1

Uncinariasis B76.9

Uncongenial work Z56.5

Unconscious (ness) — *see* Coma

Under observation — *see* Observation

Underachievement in school Z55.3

Underdevelopment — *see also* Undeveloped
nose Q30.1
sexual E30.0

Underdosing — *see also* Table of Drugs and Chemicals, categories T36-T50, with final character 6 Z91.14
intentional NEC Z91.128
due to financial hardship of patient Z91.120
unintentional NEC Z91.138
due to patient's age related debility Z91.130

Underfeeding, newborn P92.3

Underfill, endodontic M27.53

Underimmunization status Z28.3

Undernourishment — *see* Malnutrition

Undernutrition — *see* Malnutrition

Underweight R63.6
for gestational age — *see* Light for dates

Underwood's disease P83.0

Undescended — *see also* Malposition, congenital
cecum Q43.3
colon Q43.3
testicle — *see* Cryptorchid

Undeveloped, undevelopment — *see also* Hypoplasia
brain (congenital) Q02
cerebral (congenital) Q02
heart Q24.8
lung Q33.6
testis E29.1
uterus E30.0

Undiagnosed (disease) R69

Undulant fever — *see* Brucellosis

Unemployment, anxiety concerning Z56.0
threatened Z56.2

Unequal length (acquired) (limb) — *see also* Deformity, limb, unequal length
leg — *see also* Deformity, limb, unequal length
congenital Q72.9-

Unextracted dental root K08.3

Unguis incarnatus L60.0

Unhappiness R45.2

Unicornate uterus Q51.4
in pregnancy or childbirth O34.00

Unilateral — *see also* condition
development, breast N64.89
organ or site, congenital NEC — *see* Agenesis, by site

Unilocular heart Q20.8

Union, abnormal — *see also* Fusion
larynx and trachea Q34.8

Universal mesentery Q43.3

Unrepairable overhanging of dental restorative materials K08.52

Unsatisfactory

restoration of tooth K08.50
specified NEC K08.59
sample of cytologic smear
anus R85.615
cervix R87.615
vagina R87.625
surroundings Z59.1
work Z56.5

Unsoundness of mind — *see* Psychosis

Unstable

back NEC — *see* Instability, joint, spine
hip (congenital) Q65.6
acquired — *see* Derangement, joint, specified type NEC, hip
joint — *see* Instability, joint
secondary to removal of joint prosthesis M96.89
lie (mother) O32.0
lumbosacral joint (congenital) — *see* subcategory M53.2
sacroiliac — *see* subcategory M53.2
spine NEC — *see* Instability, joint, spine

Unsteadiness on feet R26.81

Untruthfulness, child problem F91.8

Unverricht (-Lundborg) disease or epilepsy — *see* Epilepsy, generalized, idiopathic

Unwanted pregnancy Z64.0

Upbringing, institutional Z62.22
away from parents NEC Z62.29
in care of non-parental family member Z62.21
in foster care Z62.21
in orphanage or group home Z62.22
in welfare custody Z62.21

Upper respiratory — *see* condition

Upset

gastric K30
gastrointestinal K30
psychogenic F45.8
intestinal (large) (small) K59.9
psychogenic F45.8
menstruation N93.9
mental F48.9
stomach K30
psychogenic F45.8

Urachus — *see also* condition
patent or persistent Q64.4

Urbach-Oppenheim disease (necrobiosis lipoidica diabeticorum) — *see* E08-E13 with .620

Urbach's lipoid proteinosis E78.89

Urbach-Wiethe disease E78.89

Urban yellow fever A95.1

Urea

blood, high — *see* Uremia
cycle metabolism disorder — *see* Disorder, urea cycle metabolism

Uremia, uremic N19

with
ectopic or molar pregnancy O08.4
polyneuropathy N18.9 *[G63]*
chronic NOS — *see also* Disease, kidney, chronic N18.9
due to hypertension — *see* Hypertensive, kidney
complicating
ectopic or molar pregnancy O08.4
congenital P96.0
extrarenal R39.2
following ectopic or molar pregnancy O08.4
newborn P96.0
prerenal R39.2

Ureter, ureteral — *see* condition

Ureteralgia N23

Ureterectasis — *see* Hydroureter

Ureteritis N28.89

cystica N28.86
due to calculus N20.1

Ureteritis - *continued*
due to calculus - *continued*
with calculus, kidney N20.2
with hydronephrosis N13.2
gonococcal (acute) (chronic) A54.21
nonspecific N28.89

Ureterocele N28.89
congenital (orthotopic) Q62.31
ectopic Q62.32

Ureterolith, ureterolithiasis — *see* Calculus, ureter

Ureterostomy

attention to Z43.6
status Z93.6

Urethra, urethral — *see* condition

Urethralgia R39.89

Urethritis (anterior) (posterior) N34.2
calculous N21.1
candidal B37.41
chlamydial A56.01
diplococcal (gonococcal) A54.01
with abscess (accessory gland) (periurethral) A54.1
gonococcal A54.01
with abscess (accessory gland) (periurethral) A54.1
nongonococcal N34.1
Reiter's — *see* Reiter's disease
nonspecific N34.1
nonvenereal N34.1
postmenopausal N34.2
puerperal O86.22
Reiter's — *see* Reiter's disease
specified NEC N34.2
trichomonal or due to Trichomonas (vaginalis) A59.03

Urethrocele N81.0
with
cystocele — *see* Cystocele
prolapse of uterus — *see* Prolapse, uterus

Urethrolithiasis (with colic or infection) N21.1

Urethrorectal — *see* condition

Urethrorrhagia N36.8

Urethrorrhea R36.9

Urethrostomy

attention to Z43.6
status Z93.6

Urethrotrigonitis — *see* Trigonitis

Urethrovaginal — *see* condition

Urgency

fecal R15.2
hypertensive — *see* Hypertension
urinary R39.15

Urhidrosis, uridrosis L74.8

Uric acid in blood (increased) E79.0

Uricacidemia (asymptomatic) E79.0

Uricemia (asymptomatic) E79.0

Uricosuria R82.998

Urinary — *see* condition

Urination

frequent R35.0
painful R30.9

Urine

blood in — *see* Hematuria
discharge, excessive R35.8
enuresis, nonorganic origin F98.0
extravasation R39.0
frequency R35.0
incontinence R32
nonorganic origin F98.0
intermittent stream R39.198
pus in N39.0
retention or stasis R33.9
organic R33.8
drug-induced R33.0
psychogenic F45.8
secretion
deficient R34
excessive R35.8
frequency R35.0
stream
intermittent R39.198
slowing R39.198
splitting R39.13

Urine - *continued*
  stream - *continued*
    weak R39.12
Urinemia — *see* Uremia
Urinoma, urethra N36.8
Uroarthritis, infectious (Reiter's) — *see*
    Reiter's disease
Urodialysis R34
Urolithiasis — *see* Calculus, urinary
Uronephrosis — *see* Hydronephrosis
Uropathy N39.9
  obstructive N13.9
    specified NEC N13.8
  reflux N13.9
    specified NEC N13.8
  vesicoureteral reflux-associated — *see*
    Reflux, vesicoureteral
Urosepsis - code to condition
Urticaria L50.9
  with angioneurotic edema T78.3
    hereditary D84.1
  allergic L50.0
  cholinergic L50.5
  chronic L50.8
  cold, familial L50.2
  contact L50.6
  dermatographic L50.3
  due to
    cold or heat L50.2
    drugs L50.0
    food L50.0
    inhalants L50.0
    plants L50.6
    serum — *see also* Reaction, serum T80.69
  factitial L50.3
  familial cold M04.2
  giant T78.3
    hereditary D84.1
  gigantea T78.3
  idiopathic L50.1
  larynx T78.3
    hereditary D84.1
  neonatorum P83.88
  nonallergic L50.1
  papulosa (Hebra) L28.2
  pigmentosa D47.01
    congenital Q82.2
    of neonatal onset Q82.2
    of newborn onset Q82.2
  recurrent periodic L50.8
  serum — *see also* Reaction, serum T80.69
  solar L56.3
  specified type NEC L50.8
  thermal (cold) (heat) L50.2
  vibratory L50.4
  xanthelasmoidea — *see* Urticaria pigmentosa
Use (of)
  alcohol Z72.89
    with
      intoxication F10.929
      sleep disorder F10.982
    harmful — *see* Abuse, alcohol
  amphetamines — *see* Use, stimulant NEC
  caffeine — *see* Use, stimulant NEC
  cannabis F12.90
    with
      anxiety disorder F12.980
      intoxication F12.929
        with
          delirium F12.921
          perceptual disturbance F12.922
        uncomplicated F12.920
      other specified disorder F12.988
      psychosis F12.959
        delusions F12.950
        hallucinations F12.951
      unspecified disorder F12.99
      withdrawal F12.93
  cocaine F14.90
    with
      anxiety disorder F14.980
      intoxication F14.929
        with
          delirium F14.921
          perceptual disturbance F14.922

Use (of) - *continued*
  cocaine - *continued*
    with - *continued*
      intoxication - *continued*
        uncomplicated F14.920
      other specified disorder F14.988
      psychosis F14.959
        delusions F14.950
        hallucinations F14.951
      sexual dysfunction F14.981
      sleep disorder F14.982
      unspecified disorder F14.99
    harmful — *see* Abuse, drug, cocaine
  drug (s) NEC F19.90
    with sleep disorder F19.982
    harmful — *see* Abuse, drug, by type
  hallucinogen NEC F16.90
    with
      anxiety disorder F16.980
      intoxication F16.929
        with
          delirium F16.921
          uncomplicated F16.920
      mood disorder F16.94
      other specified disorder F16.988
      perception disorder (flashbacks) F16.983
      psychosis F16.959
        delusions F16.950
        hallucinations F16.951
      unspecified disorder F16.99
    harmful — *see* Abuse, drug, hallucinogen
      NEC
  inhalants F18.90
    with
      anxiety disorder F18.980
      intoxication F18.929
        with delirium F18.921
        uncomplicated F18.920
      mood disorder F18.94
      other specified disorder F18.988
      persisting dementia F18.97
      psychosis F18.959
        delusions F18.950
        hallucinations F18.951
      unspecified disorder F18.99
    harmful — *see* Abuse, drug, inhalant
  methadone — *see* Use, opioid
  nonprescribed drugs F19.90
    harmful — *see* Abuse, non-psychoactive
      substance
  opioid F11.90
    with
      disorder F11.99
        mood F11.94
        sleep F11.982
        specified type NEC F11.988
      intoxication F11.929
        with
          delirium F11.921
          perceptual disturbance F11.922
        uncomplicated F11.920
      withdrawal F11.93
    harmful — *see* Abuse, drug, opioid
  patent medicines F19.90
    harmful — *see* Abuse, non-psychoactive
      substance
  psychoactive drug NEC F19.90
    with
      anxiety disorder F19.980
      intoxication F19.929
        with
          delirium F19.921
          perceptual disturbance F19.922
        uncomplicated F19.920
      mood disorder F19.94
      other specified disorder F19.988
      persisting
        amnestic disorder F19.96
        dementia F19.97
      psychosis F19.959
        delusions F19.950
        hallucinations F19.951
      sexual dysfunction F19.981
      sleep disorder F19.982
      unspecified disorder F19.99

Use (of) - *continued*
  psychoactive drug NEC - *continued*
    with - *continued*
      withdrawal F19.939
        with
          delirium F19.931
          perceptual disturbance F19.932
        uncomplicated F19.930
      harmful — *see* Abuse, drug NEC,
        psychoactive NEC
  sedative, hypnotic, or anxiolytic F13.90
    with
      anxiety disorder F13.980
      intoxication F13.929
        with
          delirium F13.921
        uncomplicated F13.920
      other specified disorder F13.988
      persisting
        amnestic disorder F13.96
        dementia F13.97
      psychosis F13.959
        delusions F13.950
        hallucinations F13.951
      sexual dysfunction F13.981
      sleep disorder F13.982
      unspecified disorder F13.99
    harmful — *see* Abuse, drug, sedative,
      hypnotic, or anxiolytic
  stimulant NEC F15.90
    with
      anxiety disorder F15.980
      intoxication F15.929
        with
          delirium F15.921
          perceptual disturbance F15.922
        uncomplicated F15.920
      mood disorder F15.94
      other specified disorder F15.988
      psychosis F15.959
        delusions F15.950
        hallucinations F15.951
      sexual dysfunction F15.981
      sleep disorder F15.982
      unspecified disorder F15.99
      withdrawal F15.93
    harmful — *see* Abuse, drug, stimulant
      NEC
  tobacco Z72.0
    with dependence — *see* Dependence, drug,
      nicotine
  volatile solvents — *see also* Use,
    inhalant F18.90
    harmful — *see* Abuse, drug, inhalant
Usher-Senear disease or syndrome L10.4
Uta B55.1
Uteromegaly N85.2
Uterovaginal — *see* condition
Uterovesical — *see* condition
Uveal — *see* condition
Uveitis (anterior) — *see also* Iridocyclitis
  acute — *see* Iridocyclitis, acute
  chronic — *see* Iridocyclitis, chronic
  due to toxoplasmosis (acquired) B58.09
    congenital P37.1
  granulomatous — *see* Iridocyclitis, chronic
  heterochromic — *see* Cyclitis, Fuchs'
    heterochromic
  lens-induced — *see* Iridocyclitis, lens-
    induced
  posterior — *see* Chorioretinitis
  sympathetic H44.13-
  syphilitic (secondary) A51.43
    congenital (early) A50.01
    late A52.71
  tuberculous A18.54
Uveoencephalitis — *see* Inflammation,
    chorioretinal
Uveokeratitis — *see* Iridocyclitis
Uveoparotitis D86.89
Uvula — *see* condition
Uvulitis (acute) (catarrhal) (chronic)
    (membranous) (suppurative)
    (ulcerative) K12.2

Vaccination (prophylactic)
  complication or reaction — *see*
    Complications, vaccination
  delayed Z28.9
  encounter for Z23
  not done — *see* Immunization, not done,
    because of)
Vaccinia (generalized) (localized) T88.1
  congenital P35.8
  without vaccination B08.011
Vacuum, in sinus (accessory) (nasal) J34.89
Vagabond, vagabondage Z59.0
Vagabond's disease B85.1
Vagina, vaginal — *see* condition
Vaginalitis (tunica) (testis) N49.1
Vaginismus (reflex) N94.2
  functional F52.5
  nonorganic F52.5
  psychogenic F52.5
  secondary N94.2
Vaginitis (acute) (circumscribed) (diffuse)
  (emphysematous) (nonvenereal)
  (ulcerative) N76.0
  with ectopic or molar pregnancy O08.0
  amebic A06.82
  atrophic, postmenopausal N95.2
  bacterial N76.0
  blennorrhagic (gonococcal) A54.02
  candidal B37.3
  chlamydial A56.02
  chronic N76.1
  due to Trichomonas (vaginalis) A59.01
  following ectopic or molar pregnancy O08.0
  gonococcal A54.02
    with abscess (accessory gland)
      (periurethral) A54.1
  granuloma A58
  in (due to)
    candidiasis B37.3
    herpesviral (herpes simplex)
      infection A60.04
    pinworm infection B80 *[N77.1]*
  monilial B37.3
  mycotic (candidal) B37.3
  postmenopausal atrophic N95.2
  puerperal (postpartum) O86.13
  senile (atrophic) N95.2
  subacute or chronic N76.1
  syphilitic (early) A51.0
    late A52.76
  trichomonal A59.01
  tuberculous A18.18
Vaginosis — *see* Vaginitis
Vagotonia G52.2
Vagrancy Z59.0
VAIN — *see* Neoplasia, intraepithelial, vagina
Vallecula — *see* condition
Valley fever B38.0
Valsuani's disease — *see* Anemia, obstetric
Valve, valvular (formation) — *see also*
  condition
  cerebral ventricle (communicating) in
    situ Z98.2
  cervix, internal os Q51.828
  congenital NEC — *see* Atresia, by site
  ureter (pelvic junction) (vesical
    orifice) Q62.39
  urethra (congenital) (posterior) Q64.2
Valvulitis (chronic) — *see* Endocarditis
Valvulopathy — *see* Endocarditis
Van Bogaert's leukoencephalopathy
  (sclerosing) (subacute) A81.1
Van Bogaert-Scherer-Epstein disease or
  syndrome E75.5
Van Buchem's syndrome M85.2
Van Creveld-von Gierke disease E74.01
Van der Hoeve (-de Kleyn) syndrome Q78.0
Van der Woude's syndrome Q38.0
Van Neck's disease or osteochondrosis M91.0
Vanishing lung J44.9
Vapor asphyxia or suffocation T59.9
  specified agent — *see* Table of Drugs and
    Chemicals

Variance, lethal ball, prosthetic heart
  valve T82.09
Variants, thalassemic D56.8
Variations in hair color L67.1
Varicella B01.9
  with
    complications NEC B01.89
    encephalitis B01.11
    encephalomyelitis B01.11
    meningitis B01.0
    myelitis B01.12
    pneumonia B01.2
  congenital P35.8
Varices — *see* Varix
Varicocele (scrotum) (thrombosed) I86.1
  ovary I86.2
  perineum I86.3
  spermatic cord (ulcerated) I86.1
Varicose
  aneurysm (ruptured) I77.0
  dermatitis — *see* Varix, leg, with,
    inflammation
  eczema — *see* Varix, leg, with, inflammation
  phlebitis — *see* Varix, with, inflammation
  tumor — *see* Varix
  ulcer (lower limb, any part) — *see also*
    Varix, leg, with, ulcer
    anus — *see also* Hemorrhoids K64.8
    esophagus — *see* Varix, esophagus
    inflamed or infected — *see* Varix, leg, with
      ulcer, with inflammation
    nasal septum I86.8
    perineum I86.3
    scrotum I86.1
    specified site NEC I86.8
  vein — *see* Varix
  vessel — *see* Varix, leg
Varicosis, varicosities, varicosity — *see* Varix
Variola (major) (minor) B03
Varioloid B03
Varix (lower limb) I83.90
  with
    bleeding I83.899
    edema I83.899
    inflammation I83.10
      with ulcer (venous) I83.209
    pain I83.819
    rupture I83.899
    specified complication NEC I83.899
    stasis dermatitis I83.10
      with ulcer (venous) I83.209
    swelling I83.899
    ulcer I83.009
      with inflammation I83.209
  aneurysmal I77.0
  asymptomatic I83.9-
  bladder I86.2
  broad ligament I86.2
  complicating
    childbirth (lower extremity) O87.4
      anus or rectum O87.2
      genital (vagina, vulva or
        perineum) O87.8
    pregnancy (lower extremity) O22.0-
      anus or rectum O22.4-
      genital (vagina, vulva or
        perineum) O22.1-
    puerperium (lower extremity) O87.4
      anus or rectum O87.2
      genital (vagina, vulva, perineum) O87.8
  congenital (any site) Q27.8
  esophagus (idiopathic) (primary)
    (ulcerated) I85.00
    bleeding I85.01
    congenital Q27.8
    in (due to)
      alcoholic liver disease I85.10
        bleeding I85.11
      cirrhosis of liver I85.10
        bleeding I85.11
      portal hypertension I85.10
        bleeding I85.11
      schistosomiasis I85.10
        bleeding I85.11
      toxic liver disease I85.10

Varix (lower limb) - *continued*
  esophagus (idiopathic) (primary) (ulcerated)
   - *continued*
    in (due to) - *continued*
      toxic liver disease - *continued*
        bleeding I85.11
      secondary I85.10
        bleeding I85.11
  gastric I86.4
  inflamed or infected I83.10
    ulcerated I83.209
  labia (majora) I86.3
  leg (asymptomatic) I83.90
    with
      edema I83.899
      inflammation I83.10
        with ulcer — *see* Varix, leg, with,
          ulcer, with inflammation by site
      pain I83.819
      specified complication NEC I83.899
      swelling I83.899
      ulcer I83.009
        with inflammation I83.209
        ankle I83.003
          with inflammation I83.203
        calf I83.002
          with inflammation I83.202
        foot NEC I83.005
          with inflammation I83.205
        heel I83.004
          with inflammation I83.204
        lower leg NEC I83.008
          with inflammation I83.208
        midfoot I83.004
          with inflammation I83.204
        thigh I83.001
          with inflammation I83.201
    bilateral (asymptomatic) I83.93
      with
        edema I83.893
        pain I83.813
        specified complication NEC I83.893
        swelling I83.893
        ulcer I83.0-
          with inflammation I83.209
    left (asymptomatic) I83.92
      with
        edema I83.892
        pain I83.812
        specified complication NEC I83.892
        swelling I83.892
        inflammation I83.12
          with ulcer — *see* Varix, leg, with,
            ulcer, with inflammation by
            site
        ulcer I83.029
          with inflammation I83.229
          ankle I83.023
            with inflammation I83.223
          calf I83.022
            with inflammation I83.222
          foot NEC I83.025
            with inflammation I83.225
          heel I83.024
            with inflammation I83.224
          lower leg NEC I83.028
            with inflammation I83.228
          midfoot I83.024
            with inflammation I83.224
          thigh I83.021
            with inflammation I83.221
    right (asymptomatic) I83.91
      with
        edema I83.891
        pain I83.811
        specified complication NEC I83.891
        swelling I83.891
        inflammation I83.11
          with ulcer — *see* Varix, leg, with,
            ulcer, with inflammation by
            site
        ulcer I83.019
          with inflammation I83.219
          ankle I83.013
            with inflammation I83.213

Varix (lower limb) - *continued*
  leg (asymptomatic) - *continued*
    right (asymptomatic) - *continued*
      with - *continued*
        ulcer - *continued*
          calf I83.012
            with inflammation I83.212
          foot NEC I83.015
            with inflammation I83.215
          heel I83.014
            with inflammation I83.214
          lower leg NEC I83.018
            with inflammation I83.218
          midfoot I83.014
            with inflammation I83.214
          thigh I83.011
            with inflammation I83.211
  nasal septum I86.8
  orbit I86.8
    congenital Q27.8
  ovary I86.2
  papillary I78.1
  pelvis I86.2
  perineum I86.3
  pharynx I86.8
  placenta O43.89-
  renal papilla I86.8
  retina H35.09
  scrotum (ulcerated) I86.1
  sigmoid colon I86.8
  specified site NEC I86.8
  spinal (cord) (vessels) I86.8
  spleen, splenic (vein) (with phlebolith) I86.8
  stomach I86.4
  sublingual I86.0
  ulcerated I83.009
    inflamed or infected I83.209
  uterine ligament I86.2
  vagina I86.8
  vocal cord I86.8
  vulva I86.3
Vas deferens — *see* condition
Vas deferentitis N49.1
Vasa previa O69.4
  hemorrhage from, affecting newborn P50.0
Vascular — *see also* condition
  loop on optic papilla Q14.2
  spasm I73.9
  spider I78.1
Vascularization, cornea — *see*
  Neovascularization, cornea
Vasculitis I77.6
  allergic D69.0
  cryoglobulinemic D89.1
  disseminated I77.6
  hypocomplementemic M31.8
  kidney I77.89
  livedoid L95.0
  nodular L95.8
  retina H35.06-
  rheumatic — *see* Fever, rheumatic
  rheumatoid — *see* Rheumatoid, vasculitis
  skin (limited to) L95.9
    specified NEC L95.8
  systemic M31.8
Vasculopathy, necrotizing M31.9
  cardiac allograft T86.290
  specified NEC M31.8
Vasitis (nodosa) N49.1
  tuberculous A18.15
Vasodilation I73.9
Vasomotor — *see* condition
Vasoplasty, after previous sterilization Z31.0
  aftercare Z31.42
Vasospasm (vasoconstriction) I73.9
  cerebral (cerebrovascular) (artery) I67.848
    reversible I67.841
  coronary I20.1
  nerve
    arm — *see* Mononeuropathy, upper limb
    brachial plexus G54.0
    cervical plexus G54.2
    leg — *see* Mononeuropathy, lower limb
  peripheral NOS I73.9
  retina (artery) — *see* Occlusion, artery, retina

Vasospastic — *see* condition
Vasovagal attack (paroxysmal) R55
  psychogenic F45.8
VATER syndrome Q87.2
Vater's ampulla — *see* condition
Vegetation, vegetative
  adenoid (nasal fossa) J35.8
  endocarditis (acute) (any valve)
    (subacute) I33.0
  heart (mycotic) (valve) I33.0
Veil
  Jackson's Q43.3
Vein, venous — *see* condition
Veldt sore — *see* Ulcer, skin
Velpeau's hernia — *see* Hernia, femoral
Venereal
  bubo A55
  disease A64
  granuloma inguinale A58
  lymphogranuloma (Durand-Nicolas-
    Favre) A55
Venofibrosis I87.8
Venom, venomous — *see* Table of Drugs and
  Chemicals, by animal or substance,
  poisoning
Venous — *see* condition
Ventilator lung, newborn P27.8
Ventral — *see* condition
Ventricle, ventricular — *see also* condition
  escape I49.3
  inversion Q20.5
Ventriculitis (cerebral) — *see*
  also Encephalitis G04.90
Ventriculostomy status Z98.2
Vernet's syndrome G52.7
Verneuil's disease (syphilitic bursitis) A52.78
Verruca (due to HPV) (filiformis) (simplex)
  (viral) (vulgaris) B07.9
  acuminata A63.0
  necrogenica (primary) (tuberculosa) A18.4
  plana B07.8
  plantaris B07.0
  seborrheica L82.1
    inflamed L82.0
  senile (seborrheic) L82.1
    inflamed L82.0
  tuberculosa (primary) A18.4
  venereal A63.0
Verrucosities — *see* Verruca
Verruga peruana, peruviana A44.1
Version
  with extraction
    cervix — *see* Malposition, uterus
    uterus (postinfectional) (postpartal, old) —
      see Malposition, uterus
Vertebra, vertebral — *see* condition
Vertical talus (congenital) Q66.80
  left foot Q66.82
  right foot Q66.81
Vertigo R42
  auditory — *see* Vertigo, aural
  aural H81.31-
  benign paroxysmal (positional) H81.1-
  central (origin) H81.4
  cerebral H81.4
  Dix and Hallpike (epidemic) — *see*
    Neuronitis, vestibular
  due to infrasound T75.23
  epidemic A88.1
    Dix and Hallpike — *see* Neuronitis,
      vestibular
    Pedersen's — *see* Neuronitis, vestibular
    vestibular neuronitis — *see* Neuronitis,
      vestibular
  hysterical F44.89
  infrasound T75.23
  labyrinthine — *see* subcategory H81.0
  laryngeal R05
  malignant positional H81.4
  Ménière's — *see* subcategory H81.0
  menopausal N95.1
  otogenic — *see* Vertigo, aural
  paroxysmal positional, benign — *see*
    Vertigo, benign paroxysmal

Vertigo - *continued*
  Pedersen's (epidemic) — *see* Neuronitis,
    vestibular
  peripheral NEC H81.39-
  positional
    benign paroxysmal — *see* Vertigo, benign
      paroxysmal
    malignant H81.4
Very-low-density-lipoprotein-type (VLDL)
  hyperlipoproteinemia E78.1
Vesania — *see* Psychosis
Vesical — *see* condition
Vesicle
  cutaneous R23.8
  seminal — *see* condition
  skin R23.8
Vesicocolic — *see* condition
Vesicoperineal — *see* condition
Vesicorectal — *see* condition
Vesicourethrorectal — *see* condition
Vesicovaginal — *see* condition
Vesicular — *see* condition
Vesiculitis (seminal) N49.0
  amebic A06.82
  gonorrheal (acute) (chronic) A54.23
  trichomonal A59.09
  tuberculous A18.15
Vestibulitis (ear) (*see also* subcategory H83.0)
  nose (external) J34.89
  vulvar N94.810
Vestibulopathy , acute peripheral
  (recurrent) — *see* Neuronitis, vestibular
Vestige, vestigial — *see also* Persistence
  branchial Q18.0
  structures in vitreous Q14.0
Vibration
  adverse effects T75.20
    pneumatic hammer syndrome T75.21
    specified effect NEC T75.29
    vasospastic syndrome T75.22
    vertigo from infrasound T75.23
  exposure (occupational) Z57.7
  vertigo T75.23
Vibriosis A28.9
Victim (of)
  crime Z65.4
  disaster Z65.5
  terrorism Z65.4
  torture Z65.4
  war Z65.5
Vidal's disease L28.0
Villaret's syndrome G52.7
Villous — *see* condition
VIN — *see* Neoplasia, intraepithelial, vulva
Vincent's infection (angina) (gingivitis)
  A69.1
  stomatitis NEC A69.1
Vinson-Plummer syndrome D50.1
Violence, physical R45.6
Viosterol deficiency — *see* Deficiency,
  calciferol
Vipoma — *see* Neoplasm, malignant, by site
Viremia B34.9
Virilism (adrenal) E25.9
  congenital E25.0
Virilization (female) (suprarenal) E25.9
  congenital E25.0
  isosexual E28.2
Virulent bubo A57
Virus, viral — *see also* condition
  as cause of disease classified
    elsewhere B97.89
      respiratory syncytial virus (RSV) — *see*
        Virus, infection, respiratory syncytial
        (RSV)
  cytomegalovirus B25.9
  human immunodeficiency (HIV) — *see*
    Human, immunodeficiency virus (HIV)
    disease
  infection — *see* Infection, virus
  respiratory syncytial (RSV)
    as cause of disease classified
      elsewhere B97.4
    bronchiolitis J21.0
    bronchitis J20.5

Virus, viral - *continued*
  respiratory syncytial (RSV) - *continued*
    bronchopneumonia J12.1
    otitis media H65.- *[B97.4]*
    pneumonia J12.1
    upper respiratory infection J06.9 *[B97.4]*
    specified NEC B34.8
  swine influenza (viruses that normally cause
    infections in pigs) — *see also* Influenza,
    due to, identified novel influenza A
    virus J09.X2
  West Nile (fever) A92.30
    with
      complications NEC A92.39
      cranial nerve disorders A92.32
      encephalitis A92.31
      encephalomyelitis A92.31
      neurologic manifestation NEC A92.32
      optic neuritis A92.32
      polyradiculitis A92.32
Viscera, visceral — *see* condition
Visceroptosis K63.4
Visible peristalsis R19.2
Vision, visual
  binocular, suppression H53.34
  blurred, blurring H53.8
    hysterical F44.6
  defect, defective NEC H54.7
  disorientation (syndrome) H53.8
  disturbance H53.9
    hysterical F44.6
  double H53.2
  examination Z01.00
    with abnormal findings Z01.01
    following failed vision screening Z01.020
      with abnormal findings Z01.021
  field, limitation (defect) — *see* Defect, visual
    field
  hallucinations R44.1
  halos H53.19
  loss — *see* Loss, vision
    sudden — *see* Disturbance, vision,
      subjective, loss, sudden
  low (both eyes) — *see* Low, vision
  perception, simultaneous without
    fusion H53.33
Vitality, lack or want of R53.83
  newborn P96.89
Vitamin deficiency — *see* Deficiency, vitamin
Vitelline duct, persistent Q43.0
Vitiligo L80
  eyelid H02.739
    left H02.736
      lower H02.735
      upper H02.734
    right H02.733
      lower H02.732
      upper H02.731
  pinta A67.2
  vulva N90.89
Vitreal corneal syndrome H59.01-
Vitreoretinopathy, proliferative — *see also*
  Retinopathy, proliferative
  with retinal detachment — *see* Detachment,
    retina, traction
Vitreous — *see also* condition
  touch syndrome — *see* Complication,
    postprocedural, following cataract
    surgery
Vocal cord — *see* condition
Vogt-Koyanagi syndrome H20.82-
Vogt's disease or syndrome G80.3
Vogt-Spielmeyer amaurotic idiocy or
  disease E75.4
Voice
  change R49.9
    specified NEC R49.8
  loss — *see* Aphonia
Volhynian fever A79.0
Volkmann's ischemic contracture or
  paralysis (complicating trauma) T79.6
Volvulus (bowel) (colon) (intestine) K56.2
  with perforation K56.2
  congenital Q43.8
  duodenum K31.5

Volvulus (bowel) (colon) (intestine) -
continued
  fallopian tube — *see* Torsion, fallopian tube
  oviduct — *see* Torsion, fallopian tube
  stomach (due to absence of gastrocolic
    ligament) K31.89
Vomiting R11.10
  with nausea R11.2
  asphyxia — *see* Foreign body, by site,
    causing asphyxia, gastric contents
  bilious (cause unknown) R11.14
    in newborn P92.01
    following gastro-intestinal surgery K91.0
  blood — *see* Hematemesis
  causing asphyxia, choking, or suffocation —
    see Foreign body, by site
  cyclical, in migraine, G43.A0
    with refractory migraine G43.A1
    intractable G43.A1
    not intractable G43.A0
    psychogenic F50.89
    without refractory migraine G43.A0
  cyclical syndrome NOS (unrelated to
    migraine) R11.15
  fecal mater R11.13
  following gastrointestinal surgery K91.0
    psychogenic F50.89
  functional K31.89
  hysterical F50.89
  nervous F50.89
  neurotic F50.89
  newborn NEC P92.09
    bilious P92.01
  periodic R11.10
    psychogenic F50.89
  persistent R11.15
  projectile R11.12
  psychogenic F50.89
  uremic — *see* Uremia
  without nausea R11.11
Vomito negro — *see* Fever, yellow
Von Bezold's abscess — *see* Mastoiditis, acute
Von Economo-Cruchet disease A85.8
Von Eulenburg's disease G71.19
Von Gierke's disease E74.01
Von Hippel (-Lindau) disease or
  syndrome Q85.8
Von Jaksch's anemia or disease D64.89
Von Recklinghausen
  disease (neurofibromatosis) Q85.01
    bones E21.0
Von Schroetter's syndrome I82.890
Von Willebrand (-Jurgens) (-Minot) disease
  or syndrome D68.0
Von Zumbusch's disease L40.1
Voyeurism F65.3
Vrolik's disease Q78.0
Vulva — *see* condition
Vulvismus N94.2
Vulvitis (acute) (allergic) (atrophic)
  (hypertrophic) (intertriginous) (senile)
  N76.2
  with ectopic or molar pregnancy O08.0
  adhesive, congenital Q52.79
  blennorrhagic (gonococcal) A54.02
  candidal B37.3
  chlamydial A56.02
  due to Haemophilus ducreyi A57
  following ectopic or molar pregnancy O08.0
  gonococcal A54.02
    with abscess (accessory gland)
      (periurethral) A54.1
  herpesviral A60.04
  leukoplakic N90.4
  monilial B37.3
  puerperal (postpartum) O86.19
  subacute or chronic N76.3
  syphilitic (early) A51.0
    late A52.76
  trichomonal A59.01
  tuberculous A18.18
Vulvodynia N94.819
  specified NEC N94.818
Vulvorectal — *see* condition
Vulvovaginitis (acute) — *see* Vaginitis

W

Waiting list, person on Z75.1
  for organ transplant Z76.82
  undergoing social agency investigation Z75.2
Waldenström
  hypergammaglobulinemia D89.0
  syndrome or macroglobulinemia C88.0
Waldenström-Kjellberg syndrome D50.1
Walking
  difficulty R26.2
    psychogenic F44.4
  sleep F51.3
    hysterical F44.89
Wall, abdominal — *see* condition
Wallenberg's disease or syndrome G46.3
Wallgren's disease I87.8
Wandering
  gallbladder, congenital Q44.1
  in diseases classified elsewhere Z91.83
  kidney, congenital Q63.8
  organ or site, congenital NEC — *see*
    Malposition, congenital, by site
  pacemaker (heart) I49.8
  spleen D73.89
War neurosis F48.8
Wart (due to HPV) (filiform) (infectious)
  (viral) B07.9
  anogenital region (venereal) A63.0
  common B07.8
  external genital organs (venereal) A63.0
  flat B07.8
  Hassal-Henle's (of cornea) H18.49
  Peruvian A44.1
  plantar B07.0
  prosector (tuberculous) A18.4
  seborrheic L82.1
    inflamed L82.0
  senile (seborrheic) L82.1
    inflamed L82.0
  tuberculous A18.4
  venereal A63.0
Warthin's tumor — *see* Neoplasm, salivary
  gland, benign
Wassilieff's disease A27.0
Wasting
  disease R64
    due to malnutrition E41
  extreme (due to malnutrition) E41
  muscle NEC — *see* Atrophy, muscle
Water
  clefts (senile cataract) — *see* Cataract, senile,
    incipient
  deprivation of T73.1
  intoxication E87.79
  itch B76.9
  lack of T73.1
  loading E87.70
  on
    brain — *see* Hydrocephalus
    chest J94.8
  poisoning E87.79
Waterbrash R12
Waterhouse (-Friderichsen) syndrome or
  disease (meningococcal) A39.1
Water-losing nephritis N25.89
Watermelon stomach K31.819
  with hemorrhage K31.811
  without hemorrhage K31.819
Watsoniasis B66.8
Wax in ear — *see* Impaction, cerumen
Weak, weakening, weakness (generalized)
  R53.1
  arches (acquired) — *see also* Deformity,
    limb, flat foot
  bladder (sphincter) R32
  facial R29.810
    following
      cerebrovascular disease I69.992
        cerebral infarction I69.392
        intracerebral hemorrhage I69.192
        nontraumatic intracranial hemorrhage
          NEC I69.292
        specified disease NEC I69.892
        stroke I69.392
        subarachnoid hemorrhage I69.092

Weak, weakening, weakness (generalized) - *continued*
  foot (double) — *see also* Weak, arches
  heart, cardiac — *see* Failure, heart
  mind F70
  muscle M62.81
  myocardium — *see* Failure, heart
  newborn P96.89
  pelvic fundus N81.89
  pubocervical tissue N81.82
  senile R54
  rectovaginal tissue N81.83
  urinary stream R39.12
  valvular — *see* Endocarditis
Wear, worn (with normal or routine use)
  articular bearing surface of internal joint
    prosthesis — *see* Complications, joint
    prosthesis, mechanical, wear of articular
    bearing surfaces, by site
  device, implant or graft — *see*
    Complications, by site, mechanical
    complication
  tooth, teeth (approximal) (hard tissues)
    (interproximal) (occlusal) K03.0
Weather, weathered
  effects of
    cold T69.9
      specified effect NEC T69.8
    hot — *see* Heat
    skin L57.8
Weaver's syndrome Q87.3
Web, webbed (congenital)
  duodenal Q43.8
  esophagus Q39.4
  fingers Q70.1-
  larynx (glottic) (subglottic) Q31.0
  neck (pterygium colli) Q18.3
  Paterson-Kelly D50.1
  popliteal syndrome Q87.89
  toes Q70.3-
Weber-Christian disease M35.6
Weber-Cockayne syndrome (epidermolysis bullosa) Q81.8
Weber-Gubler syndrome G46.3
Weber-Leyden syndrome G46.3
Weber-Osler syndrome I78.0
Weber's paralysis or syndrome G46.3
Wedge-shaped or wedging vertebra — *see* Collapse, vertebra NEC
Wegener's granulomatosis or syndrome M31.30
  with
    kidney involvement M31.31
    lung involvement M31.30
      with kidney involvement M31.31
Wegner's disease A50.02
Weight
  1000-2499 grams at birth (low) — *see* Low, birthweight
  999 grams or less at birth (extremely low) — *see* Low, birthweight, extreme
  and length below 10th percentile for gestational age P05.1-
  below but length above 10th percentile for gestational age P05.0-
  gain (abnormal) (excessive) R63.5
    in pregnancy — *see* Pregnancy, complicated by, excessive weight gain
    low — *see* Pregnancy, complicated by, insufficient, weight gain
  loss (abnormal) (cause unknown) R63.4
Weightlessness (effect of) T75.82
Weil (l) -Marchesani syndrome Q87.19
Weil's disease A27.0
Weingarten's syndrome J82
Weir Mitchell's disease I73.81
Weiss-Baker syndrome G90.09
Wells' disease L98.3
Wen — *see* Cyst, sebaceous
Wenckebach's block or phenomenon I44.1
Werdnig-Hoffmann syndrome (muscular atrophy) G12.0
Werlhof's disease D69.3
Wermer's disease or syndrome E31.21
Werner-His disease A79.0

Werner's disease or syndrome E34.8
Wernicke-Korsakoff's syndrome or psychosis (alcoholic) F10.96
  with dependence F10.26
  drug-induced
    due to drug abuse — *see* Abuse, drug, by type, with amnestic disorder
    due to drug dependence — *see* Dependence, drug, by type, with amnestic disorder
  nonalcoholic F04
Wernicke-Posadas disease B38.9
Wernicke's
  developmental aphasia F80.2
  disease or syndrome E51.2
  encephalopathy E51.2
  polioencephalitis, superior E51.2
West African fever B50.8
Westphal-Strümpell syndrome E83.01
West's syndrome — *see* Epilepsy, spasms
Wet
  feet, tropical (maceration) (syndrome) — *see* Immersion, foot
  lung (newborn) , newborn P22.1
Wharton's duct — *see* condition
Wheal — *see* Urticaria
Wheezing R06.2
Whiplash injury S13.4
Whipple's disease (*see also* subcategory · M14.8-) K90.81
Whipworm (disease) (infection) (infestation) B79
Whistling face Q87.0
White — *see also* condition
  kidney, small N03.9
  leg, puerperal, postpartum, childbirth O87.1
  mouth B37.0
  patches of mouth K13.29
  spot lesions, teeth
    chewing surface K02.51
    pit and fissure surface K02.51
    smooth surface K02.61
Whitehead L70.0
Whitlow — *see also* Cellulitis, digit
  with lymphangitis — *see* Lymphangitis, acute, digit
  herpesviral B00.89
Whitmore's disease or fever — *see* Melioidosis
Whooping cough A37.90
  with pneumonia A37.91
    due to Bordetella
      bronchiseptica A37.81
      parapertussis A37.11
      pertussis A37.01
      specified organism NEC A37.81
  due to
    Bordetella
      bronchiseptica A37.80
        with pneumonia A37.81
      parapertussis A37.10
        with pneumonia A37.11
      pertussis A37.00
        with pneumonia A37.01
      specified NEC A37.80
        with pneumonia A37.81
Wichman's asthma J38.5
Wide cranial sutures, newborn P96.3
Widening aorta — *see* Ectasia, aorta
  with aneurysm — *see* Aneurysm, aorta
Wilkie's disease or syndrome K55.1
Wilkinson-Sneddon disease or syndrome L13.1
Willebrand (-Jürgens) thrombopathy D68.0
Williams syndrome Q93.82
Willige-Hunt disease or syndrome G23.1
Wilms' tumor C64-
Wilson-Mikity syndrome P27.0
Wilson's
  disease or syndrome E83.01
  hepatolenticular degeneration E83.01
  lichen ruber L43.9
Window — *see also* Imperfect, closure
  aorticopulmonary Q21.4
Winter — *see* condition

Wiskott-Aldrich syndrome D82.0
Withdrawal state — *see also* Dependence, drug by type, with withdrawal
  alcohol
    with perceptual disturbances F10.232
    without perceptual disturbances F10.239
  caffeine F15.93
  cannabis F12.23
  newborn
    correct therapeutic substance properly administered P96.2
    infant of dependent mother P96.1
  therapeutic substance, neonatal P96.2
Witts' anemia D50.8
Witzelsucht F07.0
Woakes' ethmoiditis or syndrome J33.1
Wolff-Hirschorn syndrome Q93.3
Wolff-Parkinson-White syndrome I45.6
Wolhynian fever A79.0
Wolman's disease E75.5
Wood lung or pneumonitis J67.8
Woolly, wooly hair (congenital) (nevus) Q84.1
Woolsorter's disease A22.1
Word
  blindness (congenital) (developmental) F81.0
  deafness (congenital) (developmental) H93.25
Worm (s) (infection) (infestation) — *see also* Infestation, helminth
  guinea B72
  in intestine NEC B82.0
Worm-eaten soles A66.3
Worn out — *see* Exhaustion
  cardiac
    defibrillator (with synchronous cardiac pacemaker) Z45.02
    pacemaker
      battery Z45.010
      lead Z45.018
  device, implant or graft — *see* Complications, by site, mechanical
Worried well Z71.1
Worries R45.82
Wound check Z48.0-
  due to injury - code to Injury, by site, using appropriate seventh character for subsequent encounter
Wound, open T14.8-
  abdomen, abdominal
    wall S31.109
      with penetration into peritoneal cavity S31.609
      bite — *see* Bite, abdomen, wall
      epigastric region S31.102
        with penetration into peritoneal cavity S31.602
        bite — *see* Bite, abdomen, wall, epigastric region
        laceration — *see* Laceration, abdomen, wall, epigastric region
        puncture — *see* Puncture, abdomen, wall, epigastric region
      laceration — *see* Laceration, abdomen, wall
      left
        lower quadrant S31.104
          with penetration into peritoneal cavity S31.604
          bite — *see* Bite, abdomen, wall, left, lower quadrant
          laceration — *see* Laceration, abdomen, wall, left, lower quadrant
          puncture — *see* Puncture, abdomen, wall, left, lower quadrant
        upper quadrant S31.101
          with penetration into peritoneal cavity S31.601
          bite — *see* Bite, abdomen, wall, left, upper quadrant
          laceration — *see* Laceration, abdomen, wall, left, upper quadrant

Wound, open - *continued*
abdomen, abdominal - *continued*
   wall - *continued*
     left - *continued*
       upper quadrant - *continued*
         puncture — *see* Puncture, abdomen, wall, left, upper quadrant
      periumbilic region S31.105
        with penetration into peritoneal cavity S31.605
        bite — *see* Bite, abdomen, wall, periumbilic region
        laceration — *see* Laceration, abdomen, wall, periumbilic region
        puncture — *see* Puncture, abdomen, wall, periumbilic region
      puncture — *see* Puncture, abdomen, wall
     right
       lower quadrant S31.103
         with penetration into peritoneal cavity S31.603
         bite — *see* Bite, abdomen, wall, right, lower quadrant
         laceration — *see* Laceration, abdomen, wall, right, lower quadrant
         puncture — *see* Puncture, abdomen, wall, right, lower quadrant
       upper quadrant S31.100
         with penetration into peritoneal cavity S31.600
         bite — *see* Bite, abdomen, wall, right, upper quadrant
         laceration — *see* Laceration, abdomen, wall, right, upper quadrant
         puncture — *see* Puncture, abdomen, wall, right, upper quadrant
alveolar (process) — *see* Wound, open, oral cavity
ankle S91.00-
   bite — *see* Bite, ankle
   laceration — *see* Laceration, ankle
   puncture — *see* Puncture, ankle
antecubital space — *see* Wound, open, elbow
anterior chamber, eye — *see* Wound, open, ocular
anus S31.839
   bite S31.835
   laceration — *see* Laceration, anus
   puncture — *see* Puncture, anus
arm (upper) S41.10-
   with amputation — *see* Amputation, traumatic, arm
   bite — *see* Bite, arm
   forearm — *see* Wound, open, forearm
   laceration — *see* Laceration, arm
   puncture — *see* Puncture, arm
auditory canal (external) (meatus) — *see* Wound, open, ear
auricle, ear — *see* Wound, open, ear
axilla — *see* Wound, open, arm
back — *see also* Wound, open, thorax, back
   lower S31.000
     with penetration into retroperitoneal space S31.001
     bite — *see* Bite, back, lower
     laceration — *see* Laceration, back, lower
     puncture — *see* Puncture, back, lower
bite — *see* Bite
blood vessel — *see* Injury, blood vessel
breast S21.00-
   with amputation — *see* Amputation, traumatic, breast
   bite — *see* Bite, breast
   laceration — *see* Laceration, breast
   puncture — *see* Puncture, breast
buttock S31.809
   bite — *see* Bite, buttock
   laceration — *see* Laceration, buttock
   left S31.829
   puncture — *see* Puncture, buttock
   right S31.819
calf — *see* Wound, open, leg

Wound, open - *continued*
canaliculus lacrimalis — *see* Wound, open, eyelid
canthus, eye — *see* Wound, open, eyelid
cervical esophagus S11.20
   bite S11.25
   laceration — *see* Laceration, esophagus, traumatic, cervical
   puncture — *see* Puncture, cervical esophagus
cheek (external) S01.40-
   bite — *see* Bite, cheek
   laceration — *see* Laceration, cheek
   puncture — *see* Puncture, cheek
   internal — *see* Wound, open, oral cavity
chest wall — *see* Wound, open, thorax
chin — *see* Wound, open, head, specified site NEC
choroid — *see* Wound, open, ocular
ciliary body (eye) — *see* Wound, open, ocular
clitoris S31.40
   with amputation — *see* Amputation, traumatic, clitoris
   bite S31.45
   laceration — *see* Laceration, vulva
   puncture — *see* Puncture, vulva
conjunctiva — *see* Wound, open, ocular
cornea — *see* Wound, open, ocular
costal region — *see* Wound, open, thorax
Descemet's membrane — *see* Wound, open, ocular
digit (s)
   foot — *see* Wound, open, toe
   hand — *see* Wound, open, finger
ear (canal) (external) S01.30-
   with amputation — *see* Amputation, traumatic, ear
   bite — *see* Bite, ear
   laceration — *see* Laceration, ear
   puncture — *see* Puncture, ear
   drum S09.2-
elbow S51.00-
   bite — *see* Bite, elbow
   laceration — *see* Laceration, elbow
   puncture — *see* Puncture, elbow
epididymis — *see* Wound, open, testis
epigastric region S31.102
   with penetration into peritoneal cavity S31.602
   bite — *see* Bite, abdomen, wall, epigastric region
   laceration — *see* Laceration, abdomen, wall, epigastric region
   puncture — *see* Puncture, abdomen, wall, epigastric region
epiglottis — *see* Wound, open, neck, specified site NEC
esophagus (thoracic) S27.819
   cervical — *see* Wound, open, cervical esophagus
   laceration S27.813
   specified type NEC S27.818
eye — *see* Wound, open, ocular
eyeball — *see* Wound, open, ocular
eyebrow — *see* Wound, open, eyelid
eyelid S01.10-
   bite — *see* Bite, eyelid
   laceration — *see* Laceration, eyelid
   puncture — *see* Puncture, eyelid
face NEC — *see* Wound, open, head, specified site NEC
finger (s) S61.209
   with
     amputation — *see* Amputation, traumatic, finger
     damage to nail S61.309
   bite — *see* Bite, finger
   index S61.208
     with
       damage to nail S61.308
     left S61.201
       with
         damage to nail S61.301
     right S61.200

Wound, open - *continued*
finger (s) - *continued*
   index - *continued*
     right - *continued*
       with
         damage to nail S61.300
   laceration — *see* Laceration, finger
   little S61.208
     with
       damage to nail S61.308
     left S61.207
       with damage to nail S61.307
     right S61.206
       with damage to nail S61.306
   middle S61.208
     with
       damage to nail S61.308
     left S61.203
       with damage to nail S61.303
     right S61.202
       with damage to nail S61.302
   puncture — *see* Puncture, finger
   ring S61.208
     with
       damage to nail S61.308
     left S61.205
       with damage to nail S61.305
     right S61.204
       with damage to nail S61.304
flank — *see* Wound, open, abdomen, wall
foot (except toe (s) alone) S91.30-
   with amputation — *see* Amputation, traumatic, foot
   bite — *see* Bite, foot
   laceration — *see* Laceration, foot
   puncture — *see* Puncture, foot
   toe — *see* Wound, open, toe
forearm S51.80-
   with
     amputation — *see* Amputation, traumatic, forearm
   bite — *see* Bite, forearm
   elbow only — *see* Wound, open, elbow
   laceration — *see* Laceration, forearm
   puncture — *see* Puncture, forearm
forehead — *see* Wound, open, head, specified site NEC
genital organs, external
   with amputation — *see* Amputation, traumatic, genital organs
   bite — *see* Bite, genital organ
   female S31.502
     vagina S31.40
     vulva S31.40
   laceration — *see* Laceration, genital organ
   male S31.501
     penis S31.20
     scrotum S31.30
     testes S31.30
   puncture — *see* Puncture, genital organ
globe (eye) — *see* Wound, open, ocular
groin — *see* Wound, open, abdomen, wall
gum — *see* Wound, open, oral cavity
hand S61.40-
   with
     amputation — *see* Amputation, traumatic, hand
   bite — *see* Bite, hand
   finger (s) — *see* Wound, open, finger
   laceration — *see* Laceration, hand
   puncture — *see* Puncture, hand
   thumb — *see* Wound, open, thumb
head S01.90
   bite — *see* Bite, head
   cheek — *see* Wound, open, cheek
   ear — *see* Wound, open, ear
   eyelid — *see* Wound, open, eyelid
   laceration — *see* Laceration, head
   lip — *see* Wound, open, lip
   nose S01.20
   oral cavity — *see* Wound, open, oral cavity
   puncture — *see* Puncture, head
   scalp — *see* Wound, open, scalp
   specified site NEC S01.80

Wound, open - *continued*

head - *continued*
temporomandibular area — *see* Wound, open, cheek
heel — *see* Wound, open, foot
hip S71.00-
with amputation — *see* Amputation, traumatic, hip
bite — *see* Bite, hip
laceration — *see* Laceration, hip
puncture — *see* Puncture, hip
hymen S31.40
bite — *see* Bite, vulva
laceration — *see* Laceration, vagina
puncture — *see* Puncture, vagina
hypochondrium S31.109
bite — *see* Bite, hypochondrium
laceration — *see* Laceration, hypochondrium
puncture — *see* Puncture, hypochondrium
hypogastric region S31.109
bite — *see* Bite, hypogastric region
laceration — *see* Laceration, hypogastric region
puncture — *see* Puncture, hypogastric region
iliac (region) — *see* Wound, open, inguinal region
inguinal region S31.109
bite — *see* Bite, abdomen, wall, lower quadrant
laceration — *see* Laceration, inguinal region
puncture — *see* Puncture, inguinal region
instep — *see* Wound, open, foot
interscapular region — *see* Wound, open, thorax, back
intraocular — *see* Wound, open, ocular
iris — *see* Wound, open, ocular
jaw — *see* Wound, open, head, specified site NEC
knee S81.00-
bite — *see* Bite, knee
laceration — *see* Laceration, knee
puncture — *see* Puncture, knee
labium (majus) (minus) — *see* Wound, open, vulva
laceration — *see* Laceration, by site
lacrimal duct — *see* Wound, open, eyelid
larynx S11.019
bite — *see* Bite, larynx
laceration — *see* Laceration, larynx
puncture — *see* Puncture, larynx
left
lower quadrant S31.104
with penetration into peritoneal cavity S31.604
bite — *see* Bite, abdomen, wall, left, lower quadrant
laceration — *see* Laceration, abdomen, wall, left, lower quadrant
puncture — *see* Puncture, abdomen, wall, left, lower quadrant
upper quadrant S31.101
with penetration into peritoneal cavity S31.601
bite — *see* Bite, abdomen, wall, left, upper quadrant
laceration — *see* Laceration, abdomen, wall, left, upper quadrant
puncture — *see* Puncture, abdomen, wall, left, upper quadrant
leg (lower) S81.80-
with amputation — *see* Amputation, traumatic, leg
ankle — *see* Wound, open, ankle
bite — *see* Bite, leg
foot — *see* Wound, open, foot
knee — *see* Wound, open, knee
laceration — *see* Laceration, leg
puncture — *see* Puncture, leg
toe — *see* Wound, open, toe
upper — *see* Wound, open, thigh
lip S01.501
bite — *see* Bite, lip

Wound, open - *continued*

lip - *continued*
laceration — *see* Laceration, lip
puncture — *see* Puncture, lip
loin S31.109
bite — *see* Bite, abdomen, wall
laceration — *see* Laceration, loin
puncture — *see* Puncture, loin
lower back — *see* Wound, open, back, lower
lumbar region — *see* Wound, open, back, lower
malar region — *see* Wound, open, head, specified site NEC
mammary — *see* Wound, open, breast
mastoid region — *see* Wound, open, head, specified site NEC
mouth — *see* Wound, open, oral cavity
nail
finger — *see* Wound, open, finger, with damage to nail
toe — *see* Wound, open, toe, with damage to nail
nape (neck) — *see* Wound, open, neck
nasal (septum) (sinus) — *see* Wound, open, nose
nasopharynx — *see* Wound, open, head, specified site NEC
neck S11.90
bite — *see* Bite, neck
involving
cervical esophagus S11.20
larynx — *see* Wound, open, larynx
pharynx S11.20
thyroid S11.10
trachea (cervical) S11.029
bite — *see* Bite, trachea
laceration S11.021
with foreign body S11.022
puncture S11.023
with foreign body S11.024
laceration — *see* Laceration, neck
puncture — *see* Puncture, neck
specified site NEC S11.80
specified type NEC S11.89
nose (septum) (sinus) S01.20
with amputation — *see* Amputation, traumatic, nose
bite — *see* Bite, nose
laceration — *see* Laceration, nose
puncture — *see* Puncture, nose
ocular S05.90
avulsion (traumatic enucleation) S05.7-
eyeball S05.6-
with foreign body S05.5-
eyelid — *see* Wound, open, eyelid
laceration and rupture S05.3-
with prolapse or loss of intraocular tissue S05.2-
orbit (penetrating) (with or without foreign body) S05.4-
periocular area — *see* Wound, open, eyelid
specified NEC S05.8X-
oral cavity S01.502
bite S01.552
laceration — *see* Laceration, oral cavity
puncture — *see* Puncture, oral cavity
orbit — *see* Wound, open, ocular, orbit
palate — *see* Wound, open, oral cavity
palm — *see* Wound, open, hand
pelvis, pelvic — *see also* Wound, open, back, lower
girdle — *see* Wound, open, hip
penetrating — *see* Puncture, by site
penis S31.20
with amputation — *see* Amputation, traumatic, penis
bite S31.25
laceration — *see* Laceration, penis
puncture — *see* Puncture, penis
perineum
bite — *see* Bite, perineum
female S31.502
laceration — *see* Laceration, perineum
male S31.501
puncture — *see* Puncture, perineum

Wound, open - *continued*

periocular area (with or without lacrimal passages) — *see* Wound, open, eyelid
periumbilic region S31.105
with penetration into peritoneal cavity S31.605
bite — *see* Bite, abdomen, wall, periumbilic region
laceration — *see* Laceration, abdomen, wall, periumbilic region
puncture — *see* Puncture, abdomen, wall, periumbilic region
phalanges
finger — *see* Wound, open, finger
toe — *see* Wound, open, toe
pharynx S11.20
pinna — *see* Wound, open, ear
popliteal space — *see* Wound, open, knee
prepuce — *see* Wound, open, penis
pubic region — *see* Wound, open, back, lower
pudendum — *see* Wound, open, genital organs, external
puncture wound — *see* Puncture
rectovaginal septum — *see* Wound, open, vagina
right
lower quadrant S31.103
with penetration into peritoneal cavity S31.603
bite — *see* Bite, abdomen, wall, right, lower quadrant
laceration — *see* Laceration, abdomen, wall, right, lower quadrant
puncture — *see* Puncture, abdomen, wall, right, lower quadrant
upper quadrant S31.100
with penetration into peritoneal cavity S31.600
bite — *see* Bite, abdomen, wall, right, upper quadrant
laceration — *see* Laceration, abdomen, wall, right, upper quadrant
puncture — *see* Puncture, abdomen, wall, right, upper quadrant
sacral region — *see* Wound, open, back, lower
sacroiliac region — *see* Wound, open, back, lower
salivary gland — *see* Wound, open, oral cavity
scalp S01.00
bite S01.05
laceration — *see* Laceration, scalp
puncture — *see* Puncture, scalp
scalpel, newborn (birth injury) P15.8
scapular region — *see* Wound, open, shoulder
sclera — *see* Wound, open, ocular
scrotum S31.30
with amputation — *see* Amputation, traumatic, scrotum
bite S31.35
laceration — *see* Laceration, scrotum
puncture — *see* Puncture, scrotum
shin — *see* Wound, open, leg
shoulder S41.00-
with amputation — *see* Amputation, traumatic, arm
bite — *see* Bite, shoulder
laceration — *see* Laceration, shoulder
puncture — *see* Puncture, shoulder
skin NOS T14.8
spermatic cord — *see* Wound, open, testis
sternal region — *see* Wound, open, thorax, front wall
submaxillary region — *see* Wound, open, head, specified site NEC
submental region — *see* Wound, open, head, specified site NEC
subungual
finger (s) — *see* Wound, open, finger
toe (s) — *see* Wound, open, toe
supraclavicular region — *see* Wound, open, neck, specified site NEC

WOUND, OPEN - WOUND, OPEN

Wound, open - *continued*
  temple, temporal region — *see* Wound, open, head, specified site NEC
  temporomandibular area — *see* Wound, open, cheek
  testis S31.30
    with amputation — *see* Amputation, traumatic, testes
    bite S31.35
    laceration — *see* Laceration, testis
    puncture — *see* Puncture, testis
  thigh S71.10-
    with amputation — *see* Amputation, traumatic, hip
    bite — *see* Bite, thigh
    laceration — *see* Laceration, thigh
    puncture — *see* Puncture, thigh
  thorax, thoracic (wall) S21.90
    back S21.20-
      with penetration S21.40
    bite — *see* Bite, thorax
    breast — *see* Wound, open, breast
    front S21.10-
      with penetration S21.30
    laceration — *see* Laceration, thorax
    puncture — *see* Puncture, thorax
  throat — *see* Wound, open, neck
  thumb S61.009
    with
      amputation — *see* Amputation, traumatic, thumb
      damage to nail S61.109
    bite — *see* Bite, thumb
    laceration — *see* Laceration, thumb
    left S61.002
      with
        damage to nail S61.102
    puncture — *see* Puncture, thumb
    right S61.001
      with
        damage to nail S61.101
  thyroid (gland) — *see* Wound, open, neck, thyroid
  toe (s) S91.109
    with
      amputation — *see* Amputation, traumatic, toe
      damage to nail S91.209
    bite — *see* Bite, toe
    great S91.103
      with
        damage to nail S91.203
      left S91.102
        with
          damage to nail S91.202
      right S91.101
        with
          damage to nail S91.201
    laceration — *see* Laceration, toe
    lesser S91.106
      with
        damage to nail S91.206
      left S91.105
        with
          damage to nail S91.205
      right S91.104
        with
          damage to nail S91.204
    puncture — *see* Puncture, toe
  tongue — *see* Wound, open, oral cavity
  trachea (cervical region) — *see* Wound, open, neck, trachea
  tunica vaginalis — *see* Wound, open, testis
  tympanum, tympanic membrane S09.2-
    laceration — *see* Laceration, ear, drum
    puncture — *see* Puncture, tympanum
  umbilical region — *see* Wound, open, abdomen, wall, periumbilic region
  uvula — *see* Wound, open, oral cavity
  vagina S31.40
    bite S31.45
    laceration — *see* Laceration, vagina
    puncture — *see* Puncture, vagina
  vocal cord S11.039
    bite — *see* Bite, vocal cord

Wound, open - *continued*
  vocal cord - *continued*
    laceration S11.031
      with foreign body S11.032
    puncture S11.033
      with foreign body S11.034
    vitreous (humor) — *see* Wound, open, ocular
  vulva S31.40
    with amputation — *see* Amputation, traumatic, vulva
    bite S31.45
    laceration — *see* Laceration, vulva
    puncture — *see* Puncture, vulva
  wrist S61.50-
    bite — *see* Bite, wrist
    laceration — *see* Laceration, wrist
    puncture — *see* Puncture, wrist
Wound, superficial — *see* Injury — *see also* specified injury type
Wright's syndrome G54.0
Wrist — *see* condition
Wrong drug (by accident) (given in error) — *see* Table of Drugs and Chemicals, by drug, poisoning
Wry neck — *see* Torticollis
Wuchereria (bancrofti) infestation B74.0
Wuchereriasis B74.0
Wuchernde Struma Langhans C73

X

Xanthelasma (eyelid) (palpebrarum) H02.60
  left H02.66
    lower H02.65
    upper H02.64
  right H02.63
    lower H02.62
    upper H02.61
Xanthelasmatosis (essential) E78.2
Xanthinuria, hereditary E79.8
Xanthoastrocytoma
  specified site — *see* Neoplasm, malignant, by site
  unspecified site C71.9
Xanthofibroma — *see* Neoplasm, connective tissue, benign
Xanthogranuloma D76.3
Xanthoma (s) , xanthomatosis (primary) (familial) (hereditary) E75.5
  with
    hyperlipoproteinemia
      Type I E78.3
      Type III E78.2
      Type IV E78.1
      Type V E78.3
  bone (generalisata) C96.5
  cerebrotendinous E75.5
  cutaneotendinous E75.5
  disseminatum (skin) E78.2
  eruptive E78.2
  hypercholesterinemic E78.00
  hypercholesterolemic E78.00
  hyperlipidemic E78.5
  joint E75.5
  multiple (skin) E78.2
  tendon (sheath) E75.5
  tubo-eruptive E78.2
  tuberosum E78.2
  tuberous E78.2
  verrucous, oral mucosa K13.4
Xanthosis R23.8
Xenophobia F40.10
Xeroderma — *see also* Ichthyosis
  acquired L85.0
    eyelid H01.149
      left H01.146
        lower H01.145
        upper H01.144
      right H01.143
        lower H01.142
        upper H01.141
  pigmentosum Q82.1
  vitamin A deficiency E50.8
Xerophthalmia (vitamin A deficiency) E50.7
  unrelated to vitamin A deficiency — *see* Keratoconjunctivitis

Xerosis
  conjunctiva H11.14-
    with Bitot's spots — *see also* Pigmentation, conjunctiva
    vitamin A deficiency E50.1
    vitamin A deficiency E50.0
  cornea H18.89-
    with ulceration — *see* Ulcer, cornea
    vitamin A deficiency E50.3
    vitamin A deficiency E50.2
  cutis L85.3
  skin L85.3
Xerostomia K11.7
Xiphopagus Q89.4
XO syndrome Q96.9
X-ray (of)
  abnormal findings — *see* Abnormal, diagnostic imaging
  breast (mammogram) (routine) Z12.31
  chest
    routine (as part of a general medical examination) Z00.00
      with abnormal findings Z00.01
  routine (as part of a general medical examination) Z00.00
    with abnormal findings Z00.01
XXXXY syndrome Q98.1
XXY syndrome Q98.0

Y

Yaba pox (virus disease) B08.72
Yatapoxvirus B08.70
  specified NEC B08.79
Yawning R06.89
  psychogenic F45.8
Yaws A66.9
  bone lesions A66.6
  butter A66.1
  chancre A66.0
  cutaneous, less than five years after infection A66.2
  early (cutaneous) (macular) (maculopapular) (micropapular) (papular) A66.2
    frambeside A66.2
    skin lesions NEC A66.2
  eyelid A66.2
  ganglion A66.6
  gangosis, gangosa A66.5
  gumma, gummata A66.4
    bone A66.6
  gummatous
    frambeside A66.4
    osteitis A66.6
    periostitis A66.6
  hydrarthrosis (*see also* subcategory M14.8-) A66.6
  hyperkeratosis (early) (late) A66.3
  initial lesions A66.0
  joint lesions (*see also* subcategory M14.8-) A66.6
  juxta-articular nodules A66.7
  late nodular (ulcerated) A66.4
  latent (without clinical manifestations) (with positive serology) A66.8
  mother A66.0
  mucosal A66.7
  multiple papillomata A66.1
  nodular, late (ulcerated) A66.4
  osteitis A66.6
  papilloma, plantar or palmar A66.1
  periostitis (hypertrophic) A66.6
  specified NEC A66.7
  ulcers A66.4
  wet crab A66.1
Yeast infection — *see also* Candidiasis B37.9
Yellow
  atrophy (liver) — *see* Failure, hepatic
  fever — *see* Fever, yellow
  jack — *see* Fever, yellow
  jaundice — *see* Jaundice
  nail syndrome L60.5
Yersiniosis — *see also* Infection, Yersinia
  extraintestinal A28.2
  intestinal A04.6

Z

Zahorsky's syndrome (herpangina) B08.5

Zellweger's syndrome E71.510
Zenker's diverticulum (esophagus) K22.5
Ziehen-Oppenheim disease G24.1
Zieve's syndrome K70.0
Zika NOS A92.5
    congenital P35.4
Zinc
    deficiency, dietary E60
    metabolism disorder E83.2
Zollinger-Ellison syndrome E16.4
Zona — *see* Herpes, zoster
Zoophobia F40.218
Zoster (herpes) — *see* Herpes, zoster
Zygomycosis B46.9
    specified NEC B46.8
Zymotic — *see* condition

Neoplasm Table

1. The list below gives the code numbers for neoplasms by anatomical site. For each site there are six possible code numbers according to whether the neoplasm in question is malignant, benign, in situ, of uncertain behavior, or of unspecified nature. The description of the neoplasm will often indicate which of the six columns is appropriate; e.g., malignant melanoma of skin, benign fibroadenoma of breast, carcinoma in situ of cervix uteri. Where such descriptors are not present, the remainder of the Index should be consulted where guidance is given to the appropriate column for each morphological (histological) variety listed; e.g., Mesonephroma -- see Neoplasm, malignant; Embryoma -- see also Neoplasm, uncertain behavior; Disease, Bowen's -- see Neoplasm, skin, in situ. However, the guidance in the Index can be overridden if one of the descriptors mentioned above is present; e.g., malignant adenoma of colon to C18.9 and not to D12.6 as the adjective "malignant" overrides the Index entry "Adenoma - see also Neoplasm, benign."

2. Codes listed with a dash -, following the code have a required additional character for laterality. The tabular must be reviewed for the complete code.

Neoplasm, neoplastic	Malignant Primary	Malignant Secondary	Ca in situ	Benign	Uncertain Behavior	Unspecified Behavior
	C80.1	**C79.9**	**D09.9**	**D36.9**	**D48.9**	**D49.9**
abdomen, abdominal	C76.2	C79.8-	D09.8	D36.7	D48.7	D49.89
cavity	C76.2	C79.8-	D09.8	D36.7	D48.7	D49.89
organ	C76.2	C79.8-	D09.8	D36.7	D48.7	D49.89
viscera	C76.2	C79.8-	D09.8	D36.7	D48.7	D49.89
wall — *see also Neoplasm, abdomen, wall, skin*	C44.509	C79.2-	D04.5	D23.5	D48.5	D49.2
connective tissue	C49.4	C79.8-	-	D21.4	D48.1	D49.2
skin	C44.509					
basal cell carcinoma	C44.519	-	-	-	-	-
specified type NEC	C44.599	-	-	-	-	-
squamous cell carcinoma	C44.529	-	-	-	-	-
abdominopelvic	C76.8	C79.8-	-	D36.7	D48.7	D49.89
accessory sinus — *see Neoplasm, sinus*						
acoustic nerve	C72.4-	C79.49	-	D33.3	D43.3	D49.7
adenoid (pharynx) (tissue)	C11.1	C79.89	D00.08	D10.6	D37.05	D49.0
adipose tissue — *see also Neoplasm, connective tissue*	C49.4	C79.89	-	D21.9	D48.1	D49.2
adnexa (uterine)	C57.4	C79.89	D07.39	D28.7	D39.8	D49.59
adrenal	C74.9-	C79.7-	D09.3	D35.0-	D44.1-	D49.7
capsule	C74.9-	C79.7-	D09.3	D35.0-	D44.1-	D49.7
cortex	C74.0-	C79.7-	D09.3	D35.0-	D44.1-	D49.7
gland	C74.9-	C79.7-	D09.3	D35.0-	D44.1-	D49.7
medulla	C74.1-	C79.7-	D09.3	D35.0-	D44.1-	D49.7
ala nasi (external) — *see also Neoplasm, skin, nose*	C44.301	C79.2	D04.39	D23.39	D48.5	D49.2
alimentary canal or tract NEC	C26.9	C78.80	D01.9	D13.9	D37.9	D49.0
alveolar	C03.9	C79.89	D00.03	D10.39	D37.09	D49.0
mucosa	C03.9	C79.89	D00.03	D10.39	D37.09	D49.0
lower	C03.1	C79.89	D00.03	D10.39	D37.09	D49.0
upper	C03.0	C79.89	D00.03	D10.39	D37.09	D49.0
ridge or process	C41.1	C79.51	-	D16.5-	D48.0	D49.2
carcinoma	C03.9	C79.8-	-	-	-	-
lower	C03.1	C79.8-	-	-	-	-
upper	C03.0	C79.8-	-	-	-	-
lower	C41.1	C79.51	-	D16.5-	D48.0	D49.2
mucosa	C03.9	C79.89	D00.03	D10.39	D37.09	D49.0
lower	C03.1	C79.89	D00.03	D10.39	D37.09	D49.0
upper	C03.0	C79.89	D00.03	D10.39	D37.09	D49.0
upper	C41.0	C79.51	-	D16.4-	D48.0	D49.2
sulcus	C06.1	C79.89	D00.02	D10.39	D37.09	D49.0
alveolus	C03.9	C79.89	D00.03	D10.39	D37.09	D49.0
lower	C03.1	C79.89	D00.03	D10.39	D37.09	D49.0
upper	C03.0	C79.89	D00.03	D10.39	D37.09	D49.0
ampulla of Vater	C24.1	C78.89	D01.5	D13.5	D37.6	D49.0
ankle NEC	C76.5-	C79.89	D04.7-	D36.7	D48.7	D49.89
anorectum, anorectal (junction)	C21.8	C78.5	D01.3	D12.9	D37.8	D49.0
antecubital fossa or space	C76.4-	C79.89	D04.6-	D36.7	D48.7	D49.89
antrum (Highmore) (maxillary)	C31.0	C78.39	D02.3	D14.0	D38.5	D49.1

Neoplasm, neoplastic	Malignant Primary	Malignant Secondary	Ca in situ	Benign	Uncertain Behavior	Unspecified Behavior
pyloric	C16.3	C78.89	D00.2	D13.1	D37.1	D49.0
tympanicum	C30.1	C78.39	D02.3	D14.0	D38.5	D49.1
anus, anal	C21.0	C78.5	D01.3	D12.9	D37.8	D49.0
canal	C21.1	C78.5	D01.3	D12.9	D37.8	D49.0
cloacogenic zone	C21.2	C78.5	D01.3	D12.9	D37.8	D49.0
margin — see also Neoplasm, anus, skin	C44.500	C79.2	D04.5	D23.5	D48.5	D49.2
overlapping lesion with rectosigmoid junction or rectum	C21.8	-	-	-	-	-
skin	C44.500	C79.2	D04.5	D23.5	D48.5	D49.2
basal cell carcinoma	C44.510	-	-	-	-	-
specified type NEC	C44.590	-	-	-	-	-
squamous cell carcinoma	C44.520	-	-	-	-	-
sphincter	C21.1	C78.5	D01.3	D12.9	D37.8	D49.0
aorta (thoracic)	C49.3	C79.89	-	D21.3	D48.1	D49.2
abdominal	C49.4	C79.89	-	D21.4	D48.1	D49.2
aortic body	C75.5	C79.89	-	D35.6	D44.7	D49.7
aponeurosis	C49.9	C79.89	-	D21.9	D48.1	D49.2
palmar	C49.1-	C79.89	-	D21.1-	D48.1	D49.2
plantar	C49.2-	C79.89	-	D21.2-	D48.1	D49.2
appendix	C18.1	C78.5	D01.0	D12.1	D37.3	D49.0
arachnoid	C70.9	C79.49	-	D32.9	D42.9	D49.7
cerebral	C70.0	C79.32	-	D32.0	D42.0	D49.7
spinal	C70.1	C79.49	-	D32.1	D42.1	D49.7
areola	C50.0-	C79.81	D05.-	D24.-	D48.6-	D49.3
arm NEC	C76.4-	C79.89	D04.6-	D36.7	D48.7	D49.89
artery — see Neoplasm, connective tissue						
aryepiglottic fold	C13.1	C79.89	D00.08	D10.7	D37.05	D49.0
hypopharyngeal aspect	C13.1	C79.89	D00.08	D10.7	D37.05	D49.0
laryngeal aspect	C32.1	C78.39	D02.0	D14.1	D38.0	D49.1
marginal zone	C13.1	C79.89	D00.08	D10.7	D37.05	D49.0
arytenoid (cartilage)	C32.3	C78.39	D02.0	D14.1	D38.0	D49.1
fold — see Neoplasm, aryepiglottic						
associated with transplanted organ	C80.2	-	-	-	-	-
atlas	C41.2	C79.51	-	D16.6	D48.0	D49.2
atrium, cardiac	C38.0	C79.89	-	D15.1	D48.7	D49.89
auditory						
canal (external) (skin)	C44.20-	C79.2	D04.2-	D23.2-	D48.5	D49.2
internal	C30.1	C78.39	D02.3	D14.0	D38.5	D49.1
nerve	C72.4-	C79.49	-	D33.3	D43.3	D49.7
tube	C30.1	C78.39	D02.3	D14.0	D38.5	D49.1
opening	C11.2	C79.89	D00.08	D10.6	D37.05	D49.0
auricle, ear — see also Neoplasm, skin, ear	C44.20-	C79.2	D04.2-	D23.2-	D48.5	D49.2
auricular canal (external) — see also Neoplasm, skin, ear	C44.20-	C79.2	D04.2-	D23.2-	D48.5	D49.2
internal	C30.1	C78.39	D02.3	D14.0	D38.5	D49.2
autonomic nerve or nervous system NEC (see Neoplasm, nerve, peripheral)						
axilla, axillary	C76.1	C79.89	D09.8	D36.7	D48.7	D49.89
fold — see also Neoplasm, skin, trunk	C44.509	C79.2	D04.5	D23.5	D48.5	D49.2
back NEC	C76.8	C79.89	D04.5	D36.7	D48.7	D49.89
Bartholin's gland	C51.0	C79.82	D07.1	D28.0	D39.8	D49.59
basal ganglia	C71.0	C79.31	-	D33.0	D43.0	D49.6
basis pedunculi	C71.7	C79.31	-	D33.1	D43.1	D49.6
bile or biliary (tract)	C24.9	C78.89	D01.5	D13.5	D37.6	D49.0
canaliculi (biliferi) (intrahepatic)	C22.1	C78.7	D01.5	D13.4	D37.6	D49.0
canals, interlobular	C22.1	C78.89	D01.5	D13.4	D37.6	D49.0

Neoplasm, neoplastic	Malignant Primary	Malignant Secondary	Ca in situ	Benign	Uncertain Behavior	Unspecified Behavior
duct or passage (common) (cystic) (extrahepatic)	C24.0	C78.89	D01.5	D13.5	D37.6	D49.0
interlobular	C22.1	C78.89	D01.5	D13.4	D37.6	D49.0
intrahepatic	C22.1	C78.7	D01.5	D13.4	D37.6	D49.0
and extrahepatic	C24.8	C78.89	D01.5	D13.5	D37.6	D49.0
bladder (urinary)	C67.9	C79.11	D09.0	D30.3	D41.4	D49.4
dome	C67.1	C79.11	D09.0	D30.3	D41.4	D49.4
neck	C67.5	C79.11	D09.0	D30.3	D41.4	D49.4
orifice	C67.9	C79.11	D09.0	D30.3	D41.4	D49.4
ureteric	C67.6	C79.11	D09.0	D30.3	D41.4	D49.4
urethral	C67.5	C79.11	D09.0	D30.3	D41.4	D49.4
overlapping lesion	C67.8	-	-	-	-	-
sphincter	C67.8	C79.11	D09.0	D30.3	D41.4	D49.4
trigone	C67.0	C79.11	D09.0	D30.3	D41.4	D49.4
urachus	C67.7	C79.11	D09.0	D30.3	D41.4	D49.4
wall	C67.9	C79.11	D09.0	D30.3	D41.4	D49.4
anterior	C67.3	C79.11	D09.0	D30.3	D41.4	D49.4
lateral	C67.2	C79.11	D09.0	D30.3	D41.4	D49.4
posterior	C67.4	C79.11	D09.0	D30.3	D41.4	D49.4
blood vessel — *see Neoplasm, connective tissue*						
bone (periosteum)	C41.9	C79.51	-	D16.9-	D48.0	D49.2
acetabulum	C41.4	C79.51	-	D16.8-	D48.0	D49.2
ankle	C40.3-	C79.51	-	D16.3-	-	-
arm NEC	C40.0-	C79.51	-	D16.0-	-	-
astragalus	C40.3-	C79.51	-	D16.3-	-	-
atlas	C41.2	C79.51	-	D16.6-	D48.0	D49.2
axis	C41.2	C79.51	-	D16.6-	D48.0	D49.2
back NEC	C41.2	C79.51	-	D16.6-	D48.0	D49.2
calcaneus	C40.3-	C79.51	-	D16.3-	-	-
calvarium	C41.0	C79.51	-	D16.4-	D48.0	D49.2
carpus (any)	C40.1-	C79.51	-	D16.1-	-	-
cartilage NEC	C41.9	C79.51	-	D16.9-	D48.0	D49.2
clavicle	C41.3	C79.51	-	D16.7-	D48.0	D49.2
clivus	C41.0	C79.51	-	D16.4-	D48.0	D49.2
coccygeal vertebra	C41.4	C79.51	-	D16.8-	D48.0	D49.2
coccyx	C41.4	C79.51	-	D16.8-	D48.0	D49.2
costal cartilage	C41.3	C79.51	-	D16.7-	D48.0	D49.2
costovertebral joint	C41.3	C79.51	-	D16.7-	D48.0	D49.2
cranial	C41.0	C79.51	-	D16.4-	D48.0	D49.2
cuboid	C40.3-	C79.51	-	D16.3-	-	-
cuneiform	C41.9	C79.51	-	D16.9-	D48.0	D49.2
elbow	C40.0-	C79.51	-	D16.0-	-	-
ethmoid (labyrinth)	C41.0	C79.51	-	D16.4-	D48.0	D49.2
face	C41.0	C79.51	-	D16.4-	D48.0	D49.2
femur (any part)	C40.2-	C79.51	-	D16.2-	-	-
fibula (any part)	C40.2-	C79.51	-	D16.2-	-	-
finger (any)	C40.1-	C79.51	-	D16.1-	-	-
foot	C40.3-	C79.51	-	D16.3-	-	-
forearm	C40.0-	C79.51	-	D16.0-	-	-
frontal	C41.0	C79.51	-	D16.4-	D48.0	D49.2
hand	C40.1-	C79.51	-	D16.1-	-	-
heel	C40.3-	C79.51	-	D16.3-	-	-
hip	C41.4	C79.51	-	D16.8-	D48.0	D49.2
humerus (any part)	C40.0-	C79.51	-	D16.0-	-	-
hyoid	C41.0	C79.51	-	D16.4-	D48.0	D49.2
ilium	C41.4	C79.51	-	D16.8-	D48.0	D49.2
innominate	C41.4	C79.51	-	D16.8-	D48.0	D49.2
intervertebral cartilage or disc	C41.2	C79.51	-	D16.6-	D48.0	D49.2
ischium	C41.4	C79.51	-	D16.8-	D48.0	D49.2

Neoplasm, neoplastic	Malignant Primary	Malignant Secondary	Ca in situ	Benign	Uncertain Behavior	Unspecified Behavior
jaw (lower)	C41.1	C79.51	-	D16.5-	D48.0	D49.2
knee	C40.2-	C79.51	-	D16.2-	-	-
leg NEC	C40.2-	C79.51	-	D16.2-	-	-
limb NEC	C40.9-	C79.51	-	D16.9-	-	-
lower (long bones)	C40.2-	C79.51	-	D16.2-	-	-
short bones	C40.3-	C79.51	-	D16.3-	-	-
upper (long bones)	C40.0-	C79.51	-	D16.0-	-	-
short bones	C40.1-	C79.51	-	D16.1-	-	-
malar	C41.0	C79.51	-	D16.4-	D48.0	D49.2
mandible	C41.1	C79.51	-	D16.5-	D48.0	D49.2
marrow NEC (any bone)	C96.9	C79.52	-	-	D47.9	D49.89
mastoid	C41.0	C79.51	-	D16.4-	D48.0	D49.2
maxilla, maxillary (superior)	C41.0	C79.51	-	D16.4-	D48.0	D49.2
inferior	C41.1	C79.51	-	D16.5-	D48.0	D49.2
metacarpus (any)	C40.1-	C79.51	-	D16.1-	-	-
metatarsus (any)	C40.3-	C79.51	-	D16.3-	-	-
overlapping sites	C40.8-	-	-	-	-	-
navicular						
ankle	C40.3-	C79.51	-	-	-	-
hand	C40.1-	C79.51	-	-	-	-
nose, nasal	C41.0	C79.51	-	D16.4-	D48.0	D49.2
occipital	C41.0	C79.51	-	D16.4-	D48.0	D49.2
orbit	C41.0	C79.51	-	D16.4-	D48.0	D49.2
parietal	C41.0	C79.51	-	D16.4-	D48.0	D49.2
patella	C40.2-	C79.51	-	-	-	-
pelvic	C41.4	C79.51	-	D16.8	D48.0	D49.2
phalanges						
foot	C40.3-	C79.51	-	-	-	-
hand	C40.1-	C79.51	-	-	-	-
pubic	C41.4	C79.51	-	D16.8	D48.0	D49.2
radius (any part)	C40.0-	C79.51	-	D16.0-	-	-
rib	C41.3	C79.51	-	D16.7	D48.0	D49.2
sacral vertebra	C41.4	C79.51	-	D16.8	D48.0	D49.2
sacrum	C41.4	C79.51	-	D16.8	D48.0	D49.2
scaphoid						
of ankle	C40.3-	C79.51	-	-	-	-
of hand	C40.1-	C79.51	-	-	-	-
scapula (any part)	C40.0-	C79.51	-	D16.0-	-	-
sella turcica	C41.0	C79.51	-	D16.4-	D48.0	D49.2
shoulder	C40.0-	C79.51	-	D16.0-	-	-
skull	C41.0	C79.51	-	D16.4-	D48.0	D49.2
sphenoid	C41.0	C79.51	-	D16.4-	D48.0	D49.2
spine, spinal (column)	C41.2	C79.51	-	D16.6	D48.0	D49.2
coccyx	C41.4	C79.51	-	D16.8	D48.0	D49.2
sacrum	C41.4	C79.51	-	D16.8	D48.0	D49.2
sternum	C41.3	C79.51	-	D16.7	D48.0	D49.2
tarsus (any)	C40.3-	C79.51	-	-	-	-
temporal	C41.0	C79.51	-	D16.4-	D48.0	D49.2
thumb	C40.1-	C79.51	-	-	-	-
tibia (any part)	C40.2-	C79.51	-	-	-	-
toe (any)	C40.3-	C79.51	-	-	-	-
trapezium	C40.1-	C79.51	-	-	-	-
trapezoid	C40.1-	C79.51	-	-	-	-
turbinate	C41.0	C79.51	-	D16.4-	D48.0	D49.2
ulna (any part)	C40.0-	C79.51	-	D16.0-	-	-
unciform	C40.1-	C79.51	-	-	-	-
vertebra (column)	C41.2	C79.51	-	D16.6	D48.0	D49.2
coccyx	C41.4	C79.51	-	D16.8	D48.0	D49.2
sacrum	C41.4	C79.51	-	D16.8	D48.0	D49.2

Neoplasm, neoplastic	Malignant Primary	Malignant Secondary	Ca in situ	Benign	Uncertain Behavior	Unspecified Behavior
vomer	C41.0	C79.51	-	D16.4-	D48.0	D49.2
wrist	C40.1-	C79.51	-	-	-	-
xiphoid process	C41.3	C79.51	-	D16.7	D48.0	D49.2
zygomatic	C41.0	C79.51	-	D16.4-	D48.0	D49.2
book-leaf (mouth)	C06.89	C79.89	D00.00	D10.39	D37.09	D49.0
bowel — *see Neoplasm, intestine*						
brachial plexus	C47.1-	C79.89	-	D36.12	D48.2	D49.2
brain NEC	C71.9	C79.31	-	D33.2	D43.2	D49.6
basal ganglia	C71.0	C79.31	-	D33.0	D43.0	D49.6
cerebellopontine angle	C71.6	C79.31	-	D33.1	D43.1	D49.6
cerebellum NOS	C71.6	C79.31	-	D33.1	D43.1	D49.6
cerebrum	C71.0	C79.31	-	D33.0	D43.0	D49.6
choroid plexus	C71.7	C79.31	-	D33.1	D43.1	D49.6
corpus callosum	C71.8	C79.31	-	D33.2	D43.2	D49.6
corpus striatum	C71.0	C79.31	-	D33.0	D43.0	D49.6
cortex (cerebral)	C71.0	C79.31	-	D33.0	D43.0	D49.6
frontal lobe	C71.1	C79.31	-	D33.0	D43.0	D49.6
globus pallidus	C71.0	C79.31	-	D33.0	D43.0	D49.6
hippocampus	C71.2	C79.31	-	D33.0	D43.0	D49.6
hypothalamus	C71.0	C79.31	-	D33.0	D43.0	D49.6
internal capsule	C71.0	C79.31	-	D33.0	D43.0	D49.6
medulla oblongata	C71.7	C79.31	-	D33.1	D43.1	D49.6
meninges	C70.0	C79.32	-	D32.0	D42.0	D49.7
midbrain	C71.7	C79.31	-	D33.1	D43.1	D49.6
occipital lobe	C71.4	C79.31	-	D33.0	D43.0	D49.6
overlapping lesion	C71.8	C79.31	-	-	-	-
parietal lobe	C71.3	C79.31	-	D33.0	D43.0	D49.6
peduncle	C71.7	C79.31	-	D33.1	D43.1	D49.6
pons	C71.7	C79.31	-	D33.1	D43.1	D49.6
stem	C71.7	C79.31	-	D33.1	D43.1	D49.6
tapetum	C71.8	C79.31	-	D33.2	D43.2	D49.6
temporal lobe	C71.2	C79.31	-	D33.0	D43.0	D49.6
thalamus	C71.0	C79.31	-	D33.0	D43.0	D49.6
uncus	C71.2	C79.31	-	D33.0	D43.0	D49.6
ventricle (floor)	C71.5	C79.31	-	D33.0	D43.0	D49.6
fourth	C71.7	C79.31	-	D33.1	D43.1	D49.6
branchial (cleft) (cyst) (vestiges)	C10.4	C79.89	D00.08	D10.5	D37.05	D49.0
breast (connective tissue) (glandular tissue) (soft parts)	C50.9-	C79.81	D05.-	D24.-	D48.6-	D49.3
areola	C50.0-	C79.81	D05.-	D24.-	D48.6-	D49.3
axillary tail	C50.6-	C79.81	D05.-	D24.-	D48.6-	D49.3
central portion	C50.1-	C79.81	D05.-	D24.-	D48.6-	D49.3
inner	C50.8-	C79.81	D05.-	D24.-	D48.6-	D49.3
lower	C50.8-	C79.81	D05.-	D24.-	D48.6-	D49.3
lower-inner quadrant	C50.3-	C79.81	D05.-	D24.-	D48.6-	D49.3
lower-outer quadrant	C50.5-	C79.81	D05.-	D24.-	D48.6-	D49.3
mastectomy site (skin) — *see also Neoplasm, breast, skin*	C44.501	C79.2	-	-	-	-
specified as breast tissue	C50.8-	C79.81	-	-	-	-
midline	C50.8-	C79.81	D05.-	D24.-	D48.6-	D49.3
nipple	C50.0-	C79.81	D05.-	D24.-	D48.6-	D49.3
outer	C50.8-	C79.81	D05.-	D24.-	D48.6-	D49.3
overlapping lesion	C50.8-	-	-	-	-	-
skin	C44.501	C79.2	D04.5	D23.5	D48.5	D49.2
basal cell carcinoma	C44.511	-	-	-	-	-
specified type NEC	C44.591	-	-	-	-	-
squamous cell carcinoma	C44.521	-	-	-	-	-
tail (axillary)	C50.6-	C79.81	D05.-	D24.-	D48.6-	D49.3
upper	C50.8-	C79.81	D05.-	D24.-	D48.6-	D49.3
upper-inner quadrant	C50.2-	C79.81	D05.-	D24.-	D48.6-	D49.3

Neoplasm, neoplastic	Malignant Primary	Malignant Secondary	Ca in situ	Benign	Uncertain Behavior	Unspecified Behavior
upper-outer quadrant	C50.4-	C79.81	D05.-	D24.-	D48.6-	D49.3
broad ligament	C57.1	C79.82	D07.39	D28.2	D39.8	D49.59
bronchiogenic, bronchogenic (lung)	C34.9-	C78.0-	D02.2-	D14.3-	D38.1	D49.1
bronchiole	C34.9-	C78.0-	D02.2-	D14.3-	D38.1	D49.1
bronchus	C34.9-	C78.0-	D02.2-	D14.3-	D38.1	D49.1
carina	C34.0-	C78.0-	D02.2-	D14.3-	D38.1	D49.1
lower lobe of lung	C34.3-	C78.0-	D02.2-	D14.3-	D38.1	D49.1
main	C34.0-	C78.0-	D02.2-	D14.3-	D38.1	D49.1
middle lobe of lung	C34.2	C78.0-	D02.21	D14.31	D38.1	D49.1
overlapping lesion	C34.8-	-	-	-	-	-
upper lobe of lung	C34.1-	C78.0-	D02.2-	D14.3-	D38.1	D49.1
brow	C44.309	C79.2	D04.39	D23.39	D48.5	D49.2
basal cell carcinoma	C44.319	-	-	-	-	-
specified type NEC	C44.399	-	-	-	-	-
squamous cell carcinoma	C44.329	-	-	-	-	-
buccal (cavity)	C06.9	C79.89	D00.00	D10.39	D37.09	D49.0
commissure	C06.0	C79.89	D00.02	D10.39	D37.09	D49.0
groove (lower) (upper)	C06.1	C79.89	D00.02	D10.39	D37.09	D49.0
mucosa	C06.0	C79.89	D00.02	D10.39	D37.09	D49.0
sulcus (lower) (upper)	C06.1	C79.89	D00.02	D10.39	D37.09	D49.0
bulbourethral gland	C68.0	C79.19	D09.19	D30.4	D41.3	D49.59
bursa — *see* Neoplasm, connective tissue						
buttock NEC	C76.3	C79.89	D04.5	D36.7	D48.7	D49.89
calf	C76.5-	C79.89	D04.7-	D36.7	D48.7	D49.89
calvarium	C41.0	C79.51	-	D16.4-	D48.0	D49.2
calyx, renal	C65.-	C79.0-	D09.19	D30.1-	D41.1-	D49.51-
canal						
anal	C21.1	C78.5	D01.3	D12.9	D37.8	D49.0
auditory (external) — *see also* Neoplasm, skin, ear	C44.20-	C79.2	D04.2-	D23.2-	D48.5	D49.2
auricular (external) — *see also* Neoplasm, skin, ear	C44.20-	C79.2	D04.2-	D23.2-	D48.5	D49.2
canaliculi, biliary (biliferi) (intrahepatic)	C22.1	C78.7	D01.5	D13.4	D37.6	D49.0
canthus (eye) (inner) (outer)	C44.10-	C79.2	D04.1-	D23.1-	D48.5	D49.2
basal cell carcinoma	C44.11-	-	-	-	-	-
sebaceous cell	C44.13-	-	-	-	-	-
specified type NEC	C44.19-	-	-	-	-	-
squamous cell carcinoma	C44.12-	-	-	-	-	-
capillary — *see* Neoplasm, connective tissue						
caput coli	C18.0	C78.5	D01.0	D12.0	D37.4	D49.0
carcinoid — *see* Tumor, carcinoid						
cardia (gastric)	C16.0	C78.89	D00.2	D13.1	D37.1	D49.0
cardiac orifice (stomach)	C16.0	C78.89	D00.2	D13.1	D37.1	D49.0
cardio-esophageal junction	C16.0	C78.89	D00.2	D13.1	D37.1	D49.0
cardio-esophagus	C16.0	C78.89	D00.2	D13.1	D37.1	D49.0
carina (bronchus)	C34.0-	C78.0-	D02.2-	D14.3-	D38.1	D49.1
carotid (artery)	C49.0	C79.89	-	D21.0	D48.1	D49.2
body	C75.4	C79.89	-	D35.5	D44.6	D49.7
carpus (any bone)	C40.1-	C79.51	-	D16.1-	-	-
cartilage (articular) (joint) NEC — *see also* Neoplasm, bone	C41.9	C79.51	-	D16.9-	D48.0	D49.2
arytenoid	C32.3	C78.39	D02.0	D14.1	D38.0	D49.1
auricular	C49.0	C79.89	-	D21.0	D48.1	D49.2
bronchi	C34.0-	C78.39	-	D14.3-	D38.1	D49.1
costal	C41.3	C79.51	-	D16.7	D48.0	D49.2
cricoid	C32.3	C78.39	D02.0	D14.1	D38.0	D49.1
cuneiform	C32.3	C78.39	D02.0	D14.1	D38.0	D49.1
ear (external)	C49.0	C79.89	-	D21.0	D48.1	D49.2

Neoplasm, neoplastic	Malignant Primary	Malignant Secondary	Ca in situ	Benign	Uncertain Behavior	Unspecified Behavior
ensiform	C41.3	C79.51	-	D16.7	D48.0	D49.2
epiglottis	C32.1	C78.39	D02.0	D14.1	D38.0	D49.1
anterior surface	C10.1	C79.89	D00.08	D10.5	D37.05	D49.0
eyelid	C49.0	C79.89	-	D21.0	D48.1	D49.2
intervertebral	C41.2	C79.51	-	D16.6	D48.0	D49.2
larynx, laryngeal	C32.3	C78.39	D02.0	D14.1	D38.0	D49.1
nose, nasal	C30.0	C78.39	D02.3	D14.0	D38.5	D49.1
pinna	C49.0	C79.89	-	D21.0	D48.1	D49.2
rib	C41.3	C79.51	-	D16.7	D48.0	D49.2
semilunar (knee)	C40.2-	C79.51	-	D16.2-	D48.0	D49.2
thyroid	C32.3	C78.39	D02.0	D14.1	D38.0	D49.1
trachea	C33	C78.39	D02.1	D14.2	D38.1	D49.1
cauda equina	C72.1	C79.49	-	D33.4	D43.4	D49.7
cavity						
buccal	C06.9	C79.89	D00.00	D10.30	D37.09	D49.0
nasal	C30.0	C78.39	D02.3	D14.0	D38.5	D49.1
oral	C06.9	C79.89	D00.00	D10.30	D37.09	D49.0
peritoneal	C48.2	C78.6	-	D20.1	D48.4	D49.0
tympanic	C30.1	C78.39	D02.3	D14.0	D38.5	D49.1
cecum	C18.0	C78.5	D01.0	D12.0	D37.4	D49.0
central nervous system	C72.9	C79.40	-	-	-	-
cerebellopontine (angle)	C71.6	C79.31	-	D33.1	D43.1	D49.6
cerebellum, cerebellar	C71.6	C79.31	-	D33.1	D43.1	D49.6
cerebrum, cerebra (cortex) (hemisphere) (white matter)	C71.0	C79.31	-	D33.0	D43.0	D49.6
meninges	C70.0	C79.32	-	D32.0	D42.0	D49.7
peduncle	C71.7	C79.31	-	D33.1	D43.1	D49.6
ventricle	C71.5	C79.31	-	D33.0	D43.0	D49.6
fourth	C71.7	C79.31	-	D33.1	D43.1	D49.6
cervical region	C76.0	C79.89	D09.8	D36.7	D48.7	D49.89
cervix (cervical) (uteri) (uterus)	C53.9	C79.82	D06.9	D26.0	D39.0	D49.59
canal	C53.0	C79.82	D06.0	D26.0	D39.0	D49.59
endocervix (canal) (gland)	C53.0	C79.82	D06.0	D26.0	D39.0	D49.59
exocervix	C53.1	C79.82	D06.1	D26.0	D39.0	D49.59
external os	C53.1	C79.82	D06.1	D26.0	D39.0	D49.59
internal os	C53.0	C79.82	D06.0	D26.0	D39.0	D49.59
nabothian gland	C53.0	C79.82	D06.0	D26.0	D39.0	D49.59
overlapping lesion	C53.8	-	-	-	-	-
squamocolumnar junction	C53.8	C79.82	D06.7	D26.0	D39.0	D49.59
stump	C53.8	C79.82	D06.7	D26.0	D39.0	D49.59
cheek	C76.0	C79.89	D09.8	D36.7	D48.7	D49.89
external	C44.309	C79.2	D04.39	D23.39	D48.5	D49.2
basal cell carcinoma	C44.319	-	-	-	-	-
specified type NEC	C44.399	-	-	-	-	-
squamous cell carcinoma	C44.329	-	-	-	-	-
inner aspect	C06.0	C79.89	D00.02	D10.39	D37.09	D49.0
internal	C06.0	C79.89	D00.02	D10.39	D37.09	D49.0
mucosa	C06.0	C79.89	D00.02	D10.39	D37.09	D49.0
chest (wall) NEC	C76.1	C79.89	D09.8	D36.7	D48.7	D49.89
chiasma opticum	C72.3-	C79.49	-	D33.3	D43.3	D49.7
chin	C44.309	C79.2	D04.39	D23.39	D48.5	D49.2
basal cell carcinoma	C44.319	-	-	-	-	-
specified type NEC	C44.399	-	-	-	-	-
squamous cell carcinoma	C44.329	-	-	-	-	-
choana	C11.3	C79.89	D00.08	D10.6	D37.05	D49.0
cholangiole	C22.1	C78.89	D01.5	D13.4	D37.6	D49.0
choledochal duct	C24.0	C78.89	D01.5	D13.5	D37.6	D49.0
choroid	C69.3-	C79.49	D09.2-	D31.3-	D48.7	D49.81
plexus	C71.5	C79.31	-	D33.0	D43.0	D49.6
ciliary body	C69.4-	C79.49	D09.2-	D31.4-	D48.7	D49.89

Neoplasm, neoplastic	Malignant Primary	Malignant Secondary	Ca in situ	Benign	Uncertain Behavior	Unspecified Behavior
clavicle	C41.3	C79.51	-	D16.7	D48.0	D49.2
clitoris	C51.2	C79.82	D07.1	D28.0	D39.8	D49.59
clivus	C41.0	C79.51	-	D16.4-	D48.0	D49.2
cloacogenic zone	C21.2	C78.5	D01.3	D12.9	D37.8	D49.0
coccygeal						
body or glomus	C49.5	C79.89	-	D21.5	D48.1	D49.2
vertebra	C41.4	C79.51	-	D16.8	D48.0	D49.2
coccyx	C41.4	C79.51	-	D16.8	D48.0	D49.2
colon — *see also Neoplasm, intestine, large*	C18.9	C78.5	-	-	-	-
with rectum	C19	C78.5	D01.1	D12.7	D37.5	D49.0
column, spinal — *see Neoplasm, spine*						
columnella — *see also Neoplasm, skin, face*	C44.390	C79.2	D04.39	D23.39	D48.5	D49.2
commissure						
labial, lip	C00.6	C79.89	D00.01	D10.39	D37.01	D49.0
laryngeal	C32.0	C78.39	D02.0	D14.1	D38.0	D49.1
common (bile) duct	C24.0	C78.89	D01.5	D13.5	D37.6	D49.0
concha — *see also Neoplasm, skin, ear*	C44.20-	C79.2	D04.2-	D23.2-	D48.5	D49.2
nose	C30.0	C78.39	D02.3	D14.0	D38.5	D49.1
conjunctiva	C69.0-	C79.49	D09.2-	D31.0-	D48.7	D49.89
connective tissue NEC	C49.9	C79.89	-	D21.9	D48.1	D49.2
Note: For neoplasms of connective tissue (blood vessel, bursa, fascia, ligament, muscle, peripheral nerves, sympathetic and parasympathetic nerves and ganglia, synovia, tendon, etc.) or of morphological types that indicate connective tissue, code according to the list under "Neoplasm, connective tissue". For sites that do not appear in this list, code to neoplasm of that site; e.g., fibrosarcoma, pancreas (C25.9)						
Note: Morphological types that indicate connective tissue appear in their proper place in the alphabetic index with the instruction "see Neoplasm, connective tissue ...."						
abdomen	C49.4	C79.89	-	D21.4	D48.1	D49.2
abdominal wall	C49.4	C79.89	-	D21.4	D48.1	D49.2
ankle	C49.2-	C79.89	-	D21.2-	D48.1	D49.2
antecubital fossa or space	C49.1-	C79.89	-	D21.1-	D48.1	D49.2
arm	C49.1-	C79.89	-	D21.1-	D48.1	D49.2
auricle (ear)	C49.0	C79.89	-	D21.0	D48.1	D49.2
axilla	C49.3	C79.89	-	D21.3	D48.1	D49.2
back	C49.6	C79.89	-	D21.6	D48.1	D49.2
breast — *see Neoplasm, breast*						
buttock	C49.5	C79.89	-	D21.5	D48.1	D49.2
calf	C49.2-	C79.89	-	D21.2-	D48.1	D49.2
cervical region	C49.0	C79.89	-	D21.0	D48.1	D49.2
cheek	C49.0	C79.89	-	D21.0	D48.1	D49.2
chest (wall)	C49.3	C79.89	-	D21.3	D48.1	D49.2
chin	C49.0	C79.89	-	D21.0	D48.1	D49.2
diaphragm	C49.3	C79.89	-	D21.3	D48.1	D49.2
ear (external)	C49.0	C79.89	-	D21.0	D48.1	D49.2
elbow	C49.1-	C79.89	-	D21.1-	D48.1	D49.2
extrarectal	C49.5	C79.89	-	D21.5	D48.1	D49.2
extremity	C49.9	C79.89	-	D21.9	D48.1	D49.2
lower	C49.2-	C79.89	-	D21.2-	D48.1	D49.2
upper	C49.1-	C79.89	-	D21.1-	D48.1	D49.2
eyelid	C49.0	C79.89	-	D21.0	D48.1	D49.2

Neoplasm, neoplastic	Malignant Primary	Malignant Secondary	Ca in situ	Benign	Uncertain Behavior	Unspecified Behavior
face	C49.0	C79.89	-	D21.0	D48.1	D49.2
finger	C49.1-	C79.89	-	D21.1-	D48.1	D49.2
flank	C49.6	C79.89	-	D21.6	D48.1	D49.2
foot	C49.2-	C79.89	-	D21.2-	D48.1	D49.2
forearm	C49.1-	C79.89	-	D21.1-	D48.1	D49.2
forehead	C49.0	C79.89	-	D21.0	D48.1	D49.2
gastric	C49.4	C79.89	-	D21.4	D48.1	D49.2
gastrointestinal	C49.4	C79.89	-	D21.4	D48.1	D49.2
gluteal region	C49.5	C79.89	-	D21.5	D48.1	D49.2
great vessels NEC	C49.3	C79.89	-	D21.3	D48.1	D49.2
groin	C49.5	C79.89	-	D21.5	D48.1	D49.2
hand	C49.1-	C79.89	-	D21.1-	D48.1	D49.2
head	C49.0	C79.89	-	D21.0	D48.1	D49.2
heel	C49.2-	C79.89	-	D21.2-	D48.1	D49.2
hip	C49.2-	C79.89	-	D21.2-	D48.1	D49.2
hypochondrium	C49.4	C79.89	-	D21.4	D48.1	D49.2
iliopsoas muscle	C49.5	C79.89	-	D21.5	D48.1	D49.2
infraclavicular region	C49.3	C79.89	-	D21.3	D48.1	D49.2
inguinal (canal) (region)	C49.5	C79.89	-	D21.5	D48.1	D49.2
intestinal	C49.4	C79.89	-	D21.4	D48.1	D49.2
intrathoracic	C49.3	C79.89	-	D21.3	D48.1	D49.2
ischiorectal fossa	C49.5	C79.89	-	D21.5	D48.1	D49.2
jaw	C03.9	C79.89	D00.03	D10.39	D48.1	D49.0
knee	C49.2-	C79.89	-	D21.2-	D48.1	D49.2
leg	C49.2-	C79.89	-	D21.2-	D48.1	D49.2
limb NEC	C49.9	C79.89	-	D21.9	D48.1	D49.2
lower	C49.2-	C79.89	-	D21.2-	D48.1	D49.2
upper	C49.1-	C79.89	-	D21.1-	D48.1	D49.2
nates	C49.5	C79.89	-	D21.5	D48.1	D49.2
neck	C49.0	C79.89	-	D21.0	D48.1	D49.2
orbit	C69.6-	C79.49	D09.2-	D31.6-	D48.1	D49.89
overlapping lesion	C49.8	-	-	-	-	-
pararectal	C49.5	C79.89	-	D21.5	D48.1	D49.2
para-urethral	C49.5	C79.89	-	D21.5	D48.1	D49.2
paravaginal	C49.5	C79.89	-	D21.5	D48.1	D49.2
pelvis (floor)	C49.5	C79.89	-	D21.5	D48.1	D49.2
pelvo-abdominal	C49.8	C79.89	-	D21.6	D48.1	D49.2
perineum	C49.5	C79.89	-	D21.5	D48.1	D49.2
perirectal (tissue)	C49.5	C79.89	-	D21.5	D48.1	D49.2
periurethral (tissue)	C49.5	C79.89	-	D21.5	D48.1	D49.2
popliteal fossa or space	C49.2-	C79.89	-	D21.2-	D48.1	D49.2
presacral	C49.5	C79.89	-	D21.5	D48.1	D49.2
psoas muscle	C49.4	C79.89	-	D21.4	D48.1	D49.2
pterygoid fossa	C49.0	C79.89	-	D21.0	D48.1	D49.2
rectovaginal septum or wall	C49.5	C79.89	-	D21.5	D48.1	D49.2
rectovesical	C49.5	C79.89	-	D21.5	D48.1	D49.2
retroperitoneum	C48.0	C78.6	-	D20.0	D48.3	D49.0
sacrococcygeal region	C49.5	C79.89	-	D21.5	D48.1	D49.2
scalp	C49.0	C79.89	-	D21.0	D48.1	D49.2
scapular region	C49.3	C79.89	-	D21.3	D48.1	D49.2
shoulder	C49.1-	C79.89	-	D21.1-	D48.1	D49.2
skin (dermis) NEC — see also Neoplasm, skin, by site	C44.90	C79.2	D04.9	D23.9	D48.5	D49.2
stomach	C49.4	C79.89	-	D21.4	D48.1	D49.2
submental	C49.0	C79.89	-	D21.0	D48.1	D49.2
supraclavicular region	C49.0	C79.89	-	D21.0	D48.1	D49.2
temple	C49.0	C79.89	-	D21.0	D48.1	D49.2
temporal region	C49.0	C79.89	-	D21.0	D48.1	D49.2
thigh	C49.2-	C79.89	-	D21.2-	D48.1	D49.2
thoracic (duct) (wall)	C49.3	C79.89	-	D21.3	D48.1	D49.2

Neoplasm, neoplastic	Malignant Primary	Malignant Secondary	Ca in situ	Benign	Uncertain Behavior	Unspecified Behavior
thorax	C49.3	C79.89	-	D21.3	D48.1	D49.2
thumb	C49.1-	C79.89	-	D21.1-	D48.1	D49.2
toe	C49.2-	C79.89	-	D21.2-	D48.1	D49.2
trunk	C49.6	C79.89	-	D21.6	D48.1	D49.2
umbilicus	C49.4	C79.89	-	D21.4	D48.1	D49.2
vesicorectal	C49.5	C79.89	-	D21.5	D48.1	D49.2
wrist	C49.1-	C79.89	-	D21.1-	D48.1	D49.2
conus medullaris	C72.0	C79.49	-	D33.4	D43.4	D49.7
cord (true) (vocal)	C32.0	C78.39	D02.0	D14.1	D38.0	D49.1
false	C32.1	C78.39	D02.0	D14.1	D38.0	D49.1
spermatic	C63.1-	C79.82	D07.69	D29.8	D40.8	D49.59
spinal (cervical) (lumbar) (thoracic)	C72.0	C79.49	-	D33.4	D43.4	D49.7
cornea (limbus)	C69.1-	C79.49	D09.2-	D31.1-	D48.7	D49.89
corpus						
albicans	C56.-	C79.6-	D07.39	D27.-	D39.1-	D49.59
callosum, brain	C71.0	C79.31	-	D33.2	D43.2	D49.6
cavernosum	C60.2	C79.82	D07.4	D29.0	D40.8	D49.59
gastric	C16.2	C78.89	D00.2	D13.1	D37.1	D49.0
overlapping sites	C54.8	-	-	-	-	-
penis	C60.2	C79.82	D07.4	D29.0	D40.8	D49.59
striatum, cerebrum	C71.0	C79.31	-	D33.0	D43.0	D49.6
uteri	C54.9	C79.82	D07.0	D26.1	D39.0	D49.59
isthmus	C54.0	C79.82	D07.0	D26.1	D39.0	D49.59
cortex						
adrenal	C74.0-	C79.7-	D09.3	D35.0-	D44.1-	D49.7
cerebral	C71.0	C79.31	-	D33.0	D43.0	D49.6
costal cartilage	C41.3	C79.51	-	D16.7	D48.0	D49.2
costovertebral joint	C41.3	C79.51	-	D16.7	D48.0	D49.2
Cowper's gland	C68.0	C79.19	D09.19	D30.4	D41.3	D49.59
cranial (fossa, any)	C71.9	C79.31	-	D33.2	D43.2	D49.6
meninges	C70.0	C79.32	-	D32.0	D42.0	D49.7
nerve	C72.50	C79.49	-	D33.3	D43.3	D49.7
specified NEC	C72.59	C79.49	-	D33.3	D43.3	D49.7
craniobuccal pouch	C75.2	C79.89	D09.3	D35.2	D44.3	D49.7
craniopharyngeal (duct) (pouch)	C75.2	C79.89	D09.3	D35.3	D44.4	D49.7
cricoid	C13.0	C79.89	D00.08	D10.7	D37.05	D49.0
cartilage	C32.3	C78.39	D02.0	D14.1	D38.0	D49.1
cricopharynx	C13.0	C79.89	D00.08	D10.7	D37.05	D49.0
crypt of Morgagni	C21.8	C78.5	D01.3	D12.9	D37.8	D49.0
crystalline lens	C69.4-	C79.49	D09.2-	D31.4-	D48.7	D49.89
cul-de-sac (Douglas')	C48.1	C78.6	-	D20.1	D48.4	D49.0
cuneiform cartilage	C32.3	C78.39	D02.0	D14.1	D38.0	D49.1
cutaneous — *see Neoplasm, skin*						
cutis — *see Neoplasm, skin*						
cystic (bile) duct (common)	C24.0	C78.89	D01.5	D13.5	D37.6	D49.0
dermis — *see Neoplasm, skin*						
diaphragm	C49.3	C79.89	-	D21.3	D48.1	D49.2
digestive organs, system, tube, or tract NEC	C26.9	C78.89	D01.9	D13.9	D37.9	D49.0
disc, intervertebral	C41.2	C79.51	-	D16.6	D48.0	D49.2
disease, generalized	C80.0	-	-	-	-	-
disseminated	C80.0	-	-	-	-	-
Douglas' cul-de-sac or pouch	C48.1	C78.6	-	D20.1	D48.4	D49.0
duodenojejunal junction	C17.8	C78.4	D01.49	D13.39	D37.2	D49.0
duodenum	C17.0	C78.4	D01.49	D13.2	D37.2	D49.0
dura (cranial) (mater)	C70.9	C79.49	-	D32.9	D42.9	D49.7
cerebral	C70.0	C79.32	-	D32.0	D42.0	D49.7
spinal	C70.1	C79.49	-	D32.1	D42.1	D49.7
ear (external) — *see also Neoplasm, skin, ear*	C44.20-	C79.2	D04.2-	D23.2-	D48.5	D49.2

Neoplasm, neoplastic	Malignant Primary	Malignant Secondary	Ca in situ	Benign	Uncertain Behavior	Unspecified Behavior
auricle or auris — see also Neoplasm, skin, ear	C44.20-	C79.2	D04.2-	D23.2-	D48.5	D49.2
canal, external — see also Neoplasm, skin, ear	C44.20-	C79.2	D04.2-	D23.2-	D48.5	D49.2
cartilage	C49.0	C79.89	-	D21.0	D48.1	D49.2
external meatus — see also Neoplasm, skin, ear	C44.20-	C79.2	D04.2-	D23.2-	D48.5	D49.2
inner	C30.1	C78.39	D02.3	D14.0	D38.5	D49.1
lobule — see also Neoplasm, skin, ear	C44.20-	C79.2	D04.2-	D23.2-	D48.5	D49.2
middle	C30.1	C78.39	D02.3	D14.0	D38.5	D49.1
overlapping lesion with accessory sinuses	C31.8	-	-	-	-	-
skin	C44.20-	C79.2	D04.2-	D23.2-	D48.5	D49.2
basal cell carcinoma	C44.21-	-	-	-	-	-
specified type NEC	C44.29-	-	-	-	-	-
squamous cell carcinoma	C44.22-	-	-	-	-	-
earlobe	C44.20-	C79.2	D04.2-	D23.2-	D48.5	D49.2
basal cell carcinoma	C44.21-	-	-	-	-	-
specified type NEC	C44.29-	-	-	-	-	-
squamous cell carcinoma	C44.22-	-	-	-	-	-
ejaculatory duct	C63.7	C79.82	D07.69	D29.8	D40.8	D49.59
elbow NEC	C76.4-	C79.89	D04.6-	D36.7	D48.7	D49.89
endocardium	C38.0	C79.89	-	D15.1	D48.7	D49.89
endocervix (canal) (gland)	C53.0	C79.82	D06.0	D26.0	D39.0	D49.59
endocrine gland NEC	C75.9	C79.89	D09.3	D35.9	D44.9	D49.7
pluriglandular	C75.8	C79.89	D09.3	D35.7	D44.9	D49.7
endometrium (gland) (stroma)	C54.1	C79.82	D07.0	D26.1	D39.0	D49.59
ensiform cartilage	C41.3	C79.51	-	D16.7	D48.0	D49.2
enteric — see Neoplasm, intestine						
ependyma (brain)	C71.5	C79.31	-	D33.0	D43.0	D49.6
fourth ventricle	C71.7	C79.31	-	D33.1	D43.1	D49.6
epicardium	C38.0	C79.89	-	D15.1	D48.7	D49.89
epididymis	C63.0-	C79.82	D07.69	D29.3-	D40.8	D49.59
epidural	C72.9	C79.49	-	D33.9	D43.9	D49.7
epiglottis	C32.1	C78.39	D02.0	D14.1	D38.0	D49.1
anterior aspect or surface	C10.1	C79.89	D00.08	D10.5	D37.05	D49.0
cartilage	C32.3	C78.39	D02.0	D14.1	D38.0	D49.1
free border (margin)	C10.1	C79.89	D00.08	D10.5	D37.05	D49.0
junctional region	C10.8	C79.89	D00.08	D10.5	D37.05	D49.0
posterior (laryngeal) surface	C32.1	C78.39	D02.0	D14.1	D38.0	D49.1
suprahyoid portion	C32.1	C78.39	D02.0	D14.1	D38.0	D49.1
esophagogastric junction	C16.0	C78.89	D00.2	D13.1	D37.1	D49.0
esophagus	C15.9	C78.89	D00.1	D13.0	D37.8	D49.0
abdominal	C15.5	C78.89	D00.1	D13.0	D37.8	D49.0
cervical	C15.3	C78.89	D00.1	D13.0	D37.8	D49.0
distal (third)	C15.5	C78.89	D00.1	D13.0	D37.8	D49.0
lower (third)	C15.5	C78.89	D00.1	D13.0	D37.8	D49.0
middle (third)	C15.4	C78.89	D00.1	D13.0	D37.8	D49.0
overlapping lesion	C15.8	-	-	-	-	-
proximal (third)	C15.3	C78.89	D00.1	D13.0	D37.8	D49.0
thoracic	C15.4	C78.89	D00.1	D13.0	D37.8	D49.0
upper (third)	C15.3	C78.89	D00.1	D13.0	D37.8	D49.0
ethmoid (sinus)	C31.1	C78.39	D02.3	D14.0	D38.5	D49.1
bone or labyrinth	C41.0	C79.51	-	D16.4-	D48.0	D49.2
eustachian tube	C30.1	C78.39	D02.3	D14.0	D38.5	D49.1
exocervix	C53.1	C79.82	D06.1	D26.0	D39.0	D49.59
external						
meatus (ear) — see also Neoplasm, skin, ear	C44.20-	C79.2	D04.2-	D23.2-	D48.5	D49.2
os, cervix uteri	C53.1	C79.82	D06.1	D26.0	D39.0	D49.59

	Malignant Primary	Malignant Secondary	Ca in situ	Benign	Uncertain Behavior	Unspecified Behavior
Neoplasm, neoplastic						
extradural	C72.9	C79.49	-	D33.9	D43.9	D49.7
extrahepatic (bile) duct	C24.0	C78.89	D01.5	D13.5	D37.6	D49.0
overlapping lesion with gallbladder	C24.8	-	-	-	-	-
extraocular muscle	C69.6-	C79.49	D09.2-	D31.6-	D48.7	D49.89
extrarectal	C76.3	C79.89	D09.8	D36.7	D48.7	D49.89
extremity	C76.8	C79.89	D04.8	D36.7	D48.7	D49.89
lower	C76.5-	C79.89	D04.7-	D36.7	D48.7	D49.89
upper	C76.4-	C79.89	D04.6-	D36.7	D48.7	D49.89
eye NEC	C69.9-	C79.49	D09.2	D31.9	D48.7	D49.89
overlapping sites	C69.8	-	-	-	-	-
eyeball	C69.9-	C79.49	D09.2-	D31.9-	D48.7	D49.89
eyebrow	C44.309	C79.2	D04.39	D23.39	D48.5	D49.2
basal cell carcinoma	C44.319	-	-	-	-	-
specified type NEC	C44.399	-	-	-	-	-
squamous cell carcinoma	C44.329	-	-	-	-	-
eyelid (lower) (skin) (upper)	C44.10-	-	-	-	-	-
basal cell carcinoma	C44.11-	-	-	-	-	-
sebaceous cell	C44.13-	-	-	-	-	-
specified type NEC	C44.19-	-	-	-	-	-
squamous cell carcinoma	C44.12-	-	-	-	-	-
cartilage	C49.0	C79.89	-	D21.0	D48.1	D49.2
face NEC	C76.0	C79.89	D04.39	D36.7	D48.7	D49.89
fallopian tube (accessory)	C57.0-	C79.82	D07.39	D28.2	D39.8	D49.59
falx (cerebella) (cerebri)	C70.0	C79.32	-	D32.0	D42.0	D49.7
fascia — *see also Neoplasm, connective tissue*						
palmar	C49.1-	C79.89	-	D21.1-	D48.1	D49.2
plantar	C49.2-	C79.89	-	D21.2-	D48.1	D49.2
fatty tissue — *see Neoplasm, connective tissue*						
fauces, faucial NEC	C10.9	C79.89	D00.08	D10.5	D37.05	D49.0
pillars	C09.1	C79.89	D00.08	D10.5	D37.05	D49.0
tonsil	C09.9	C79.89	D00.08	D10.4	D37.05	D49.0
femur (any part)	C40.2-	-	-	D16.2-	-	-
fetal membrane	C58	C79.82	D07.0	D26.7	D39.2	D49.59
fibrous tissue — *see Neoplasm, connective tissue*						
fibula (any part)	C40.2-	C79.51	-	D16.2-	-	-
filum terminale	C72.0	C79.49	-	D33.4	D43.4	D49.7
finger NEC	C76.4-	C79.89	D04.6-	D36.7	D48.7	D49.89
flank NEC	C76.8	C79.89	D04.5	D36.7	D48.7	D49.89
follicle, nabothian	C53.0	C79.82	D06.0	D26.0	D39.0	D49.59
foot NEC	C76.5-	C79.89	D04.7-	D36.7	D48.7	D49.89
forearm NEC	C76.4-	C79.89	D04.6-	D36.7	D48.7	D49.89
forehead (skin)	C44.309	C79.2	D04.39	D23.39	D48.5	D49.2
basal cell carcinoma	C44.319	-	-	-	-	-
specified type NEC	C44.399	-	-	-	-	-
squamous cell carcinoma	C44.329	-	-	-	-	-
foreskin	C60.0	C79.82	D07.4	D29.0	D40.8	D49.59
fornix						
pharyngeal	C11.3	C79.89	D00.08	D10.6	D37.05	D49.0
vagina	C52	C79.82	D07.2	D28.1	D39.8	D49.59
fossa (of)						
anterior (cranial)	C71.9	C79.31	-	D33.2	D43.2	D49.6
cranial	C71.9	C79.31	-	D33.2	D43.2	D49.6
ischiorectal	C76.3	C79.89	D09.8	D36.7	D48.7	D49.89
middle (cranial)	C71.9	C79.31	-	D33.2	D43.2	D49.6
piriform	C12	C79.89	D00.08	D10.7	D37.05	D49.0
pituitary	C75.1	C79.89	D09.3	D35.2	D44.3	D49.7
posterior (cranial)	C71.9	C79.31	-	D33.2	D43.2	D49.6

Neoplasm, neoplastic	Malignant Primary	Malignant Secondary	Ca in situ	Benign	Uncertain Behavior	Unspecified Behavior
pterygoid	C49.0	C79.89	-	D21.0	D48.1	D49.2
pyriform	C12	C79.89	D00.08	D10.7	D37.05	D49.0
Rosenmuller	C11.2	C79.89	D00.08	D10.6	D37.05	D49.0
tonsillar	C09.0	C79.89	D00.08	D10.5	D37.05	D49.0
fourchette	C51.9	C79.82	D07.1	D28.0	D39.8	D49.59
frenulum						
labii — *see Neoplasm, lip, internal*						
linguae	C02.2	C79.89	D00.07	D10.1	D37.02	D49.0
frontal						
bone	C41.0	C79.51	-	D16.4-	D48.0	D49.2
lobe, brain	C71.1	C79.31	-	D33.0	D43.0	D49.6
pole	C71.1	C79.31	-	D33.0	D43.0	D49.6
sinus	C31.2	C78.39	D02.3	D14.0	D38.5	D49.1
fundus						
stomach	C16.1	C78.89	D00.2	D13.1	D37.1	D49.0
uterus	C54.3	C79.82	D07.0	D26.1	D39.0	D49.59
gall duct (extrahepatic)	C24.0	C78.89	D01.5	D13.5	D37.6	D49.0
intrahepatic	C22.1	C78.7	D01.5	D13.4	D37.6	D49.0
gallbladder	C23	C78.89	D01.5	D13.5	D37.6	D49.0
overlapping lesion with extrahepatic bile ducts	C24.8	-	-	-	-	-
ganglia — *see also Neoplasm, nerve, peripheral*	C47.9	C79.89	-	D36.10	D48.2	D49.2
basal	C71.0	C79.31	-	D33.0	D43.0	D49.6
cranial nerve	C72.50	C79.49	-	D33.3	D43.3	D49.7
Gartner's duct	C52	C79.82	D07.2	D28.1	D39.8	D49.59
gastric — *see Neoplasm, stomach*						
gastrocolic	C26.9	C78.89	D01.9	D13.9	D37.9	D49.0
gastroesophageal junction	C16.0	C78.89	D00.2	D13.1	D37.1	D49.0
gastrointestinal (tract) NEC	C26.9	C78.89	D01.9	D13.9	D37.9	D49.0
generalized	C80.0	-	-	-	-	-
genital organ or tract						
female NEC	C57.9	C79.82	D07.30	D28.9	D39.9	D49.59
overlapping lesion	C57.8	-	-	-	-	-
specified site NEC	C57.7	C79.82	D07.39	D28.7	D39.8	D49.59
male NEC	C63.9	C79.82	D07.60	D29.9	D40.9	D49.59
overlapping lesion	C63.8	-	-	-	-	-
specified site NEC	C63.7	C79.82	D07.69	D29.8	D40.8	D49.59
genitourinary tract						
female	C57.9	C79.82	D07.30	D28.9	D39.9	D49.59
male	C63.9	C79.82	D07.60	D29.9	D40.9	D49.59
gingiva (alveolar) (marginal)	C03.9	C79.89	D00.03	D10.39	D37.09	D49.0
lower	C03.1	C79.89	D00.03	D10.39	D37.09	D49.0
mandibular	C03.1	C79.89	D00.03	D10.39	D37.09	D49.0
maxillary	C03.0	C79.89	D00.03	D10.39	D37.09	D49.0
upper	C03.0	C79.89	D00.03	D10.39	D37.09	D49.0
gland, glandular (lymphatic) (system) — *see also Neoplasm, lymph gland*						
endocrine NEC	C75.9	C79.89	D09.3	D35.9	D44.9	D49.7
salivary — *see Neoplasm, salivary gland*						
glans penis	C60.1	C79.82	D07.4	D29.0	D40.8	D49.59
globus pallidus	C71.0	C79.31	-	D33.0	D43.0	D49.6
glomus						
coccygeal	C49.5	C79.89	-	D21.5	D48.1	D49.2
jugularis	C75.5	C79.89	-	D35.6	D44.7	D49.7
glosso-epiglottic fold (s)	C10.1	C79.89	D00.08	D10.5	D37.05	D49.0
glossopalatine fold	C09.1	C79.89	D00.08	D10.5	D37.05	D49.0
glossopharyngeal sulcus	C09.0	C79.89	D00.08	D10.5	D37.05	D49.0
glottis	C32.0	C78.39	D02.0	D14.1	D38.0	D49.1

Neoplasm, neoplastic	Malignant Primary	Malignant Secondary	Ca in situ	Benign	Uncertain Behavior	Unspecified Behavior
gluteal region	C76.3	C79.89	D04.5	D36.7	D48.7	D49.89
great vessels NEC	C49.3	C79.89	-	D21.3	D48.1	D49.2
groin NEC	C76.3	C79.89	D04.5	D36.7	D48.7	D49.89
gum	C03.9	C79.89	D00.03	D10.39	D37.09	D49.0
lower	C03.1	C79.89	D00.03	D10.39	D37.09	D49.0
upper	C03.0	C79.89	D00.03	D10.39	D37.09	D49.0
hand NEC	C76.4-	C79.89	D04.6-	D36.7	D48.7	D49.89
head NEC	C76.0	C79.89	D04.4	D36.7	D48.7	D49.89
heart	C38.0	C79.89	-	D15.1	D48.7	D49.89
heel NEC	C76.5-	C79.89	D04.7-	D36.7	D48.7	D49.89
helix — *see also Neoplasm, skin, ear*	C44.20-	C79.2	D04.2-	D23.2-	D48.5	D49.2
hematopoietic, hemopoietic tissue NEC	C96.9	-	-	-	-	-
specified NEC	C96.Z	-	-	-	-	-
hemisphere, cerebral	C71.0	C79.31	-	D33.0	D43.0	D49.6
hemorrhoidal zone	C21.1	C78.5	D01.3	D12.9	D37.8	D49.0
hepatic — *see also Index to disease, by histology*	C22.9	C78.7	D01.5	D13.4	D37.6	D49.0
duct (bile)	C24.0	C78.89	D01.5	D13.5	D37.6	D49.0
flexure (colon)	C18.3	C78.5	D01.0	D12.3	D37.4	D49.0
primary	C22.8	C78.7	D01.5	D13.4	D37.6	D49.0
hepatobiliary	C24.9	C78.89	D01.5	D13.5	D37.6	D49.0
hepatoblastoma	C22.2	C78.7	D01.5	D13.4	D37.6	D49.0
hepatoma	C22.0	C78.7	D01.5	D13.4	D37.6	D49.0
hilus of lung	C34.0-	C78.0-	D02.2-	D14.3-	D38.1	D49.1
hip NEC	C76.5-	C79.89	D04.7-	D36.7	D48.7	D49.89
hippocampus, brain	C71.2	C79.31	-	D33.0	D43.0	D49.6
humerus (any part)	C40.0-	C79.51	-	D16.0-	-	-
hymen	C52	C79.82	D07.2	D28.1	D39.8	D49.59
hypopharynx, hypopharyngeal NEC	C13.9	C79.89	D00.08	D10.7	D37.05	D49.0
overlapping lesion	C13.8	-	-	-	-	-
postcricoid region	C13.0	C79.89	D00.08	D10.7	D37.05	D49.0
posterior wall	C13.2	C79.89	D00.08	D10.7	D37.05	D49.0
pyriform fossa (sinus)	C12	C79.89	D00.08	D10.7	D37.05	D49.0
hypophysis	C75.1	C79.89	D09.3	D35.2	D44.3	D49.7
hypothalamus	C71.0	C79.31	-	D33.0	D43.0	D49.6
ileocecum, ileocecal (coil) (junction) (valve)	C18.0	C78.5	D01.0	D12.0	D37.4	D49.0
ileum	C17.2	C78.4	D01.49	D13.39	D37.2	D49.0
ilium	C41.4	C79.51	-	D16.8	D48.0	D49.2
immunoproliferative NEC	C88.9	-	-	-	-	-
infraclavicular (region)	C76.1	C79.89	D04.5	D36.7	D48.7	D49.89
inguinal (region)	C76.3	C79.89	D04.5	D36.7	D48.7	D49.89
insula	C71.0	C79.31	-	D33.0	D43.0	D49.6
insular tissue (pancreas)	C25.4	C78.89	D01.7	D13.7	D37.8	D49.0
brain	C71.0	C79.31	-	D33.0	D43.0	D49.6
interarytenoid fold	C13.1	C79.89	D00.08	D10.7	D37.05	D49.0
hypopharyngeal aspect	C13.1	C79.89	D00.08	D10.7	D37.05	D49.0
laryngeal aspect	C32.1	C78.39	D02.0	D14.1	D38.0	D49.1
marginal zone	C13.1	C79.89	D00.08	D10.7	D37.05	D49.0
interdental papillae	C03.9	C79.89	D00.03	D10.39	D37.09	D49.0
lower	C03.1	C79.89	D00.03	D10.39	D37.09	D49.0
upper	C03.0	C79.89	D00.03	D10.39	D37.09	D49.0
internal						
capsule	C71.0	C79.31	-	D33.0	D43.0	D49.6
os (cervix)	C53.0	C79.82	D06.0	D26.0	D39.0	D49.59
intervertebral cartilage or disc	C41.2	C79.51	-	D16.6	D48.0	D49.2
intestine, intestinal	C26.0	C78.80	D01.40	D13.9	D37.8	D49.0
large	C18.9	C78.5	D01.0	D12.6	D37.4	D49.0
appendix	C18.1	C78.5	D01.0	D12.1	D37.3	D49.0

	Malignant Primary	Malignant Secondary	Ca in situ	Benign	Uncertain Behavior	Unspecified Behavior
Neoplasm, neoplastic						
caput coli	C18.0	C78.5	D01.0	D12.0	D37.4	D49.0
cecum	C18.0	C78.5	D01.0	D12.0	D37.4	D49.0
colon	C18.9	C78.5	D01.0	D12.6	D37.4	D49.0
and rectum	C19	C78.5	D01.1	D12.7	D37.5	D49.0
ascending	C18.2	C78.5	D01.0	D12.2	D37.4	D49.0
caput	C18.0	C78.5	D01.0	D12.0	D37.4	D49.0
descending	C18.6	C78.5	D01.0	D12.4	D37.4	D49.0
distal	C18.6	C78.5	D01.0	D12.4	D37.4	D49.0
left	C18.6	C78.5	D01.0	D12.4	D37.4	D49.0
overlapping lesion	C18.8	-	-	-	-	-
pelvic	C18.7	C78.5	D01.0	D12.5	D37.4	D49.0
right	C18.2	C78.5	D01.0	D12.2	D37.4	D49.0
sigmoid (flexure)	C18.7	C78.5	D01.0	D12.5	D37.4	D49.0
transverse	C18.4	C78.5	D01.0	D12.3	D37.4	D49.0
hepatic flexure	C18.3	C78.5	D01.0	D12.3	D37.4	D49.0
ileocecum, ileocecal (coil) (valve)	C18.0	C78.5	D01.0	D12.0	D37.4	D49.0
overlapping lesion	C18.8	-	-	-	-	-
sigmoid flexure (lower) (upper)	C18.7	C78.5	D01.0	D12.5	D37.4	D49.0
splenic flexure	C18.5	C78.5	D01.0	D12.3	D37.4	D49.0
small	C17.9	C78.4	D01.40	D13.30	D37.2	D49.0
duodenum	C17.0	C78.4	D01.49	D13.2	D37.2	D49.0
ileum	C17.2	C78.4	D01.49	D13.39	D37.2	D49.0
jejunum	C17.1	C78.4	D01.49	D13.39	D37.2	D49.0
overlapping lesion	C17.8	-	-	-	-	-
tract NEC	C26.0	C78.89	D01.40	D13.9	D37.8	D49.0
intra-abdominal	C76.2	C79.89	D09.8	D36.7	D48.7	D49.89
intracranial NEC	C71.9	C79.31	-	D33.2	D43.2	D49.6
intrahepatic (bile) duct	C22.1	C78.7	D01.5	D13.4	D37.6	D49.0
intraocular	C69.9-	C79.49	D09.2-	D31.9-	D48.7	D49.89
intraorbital	C69.6-	C79.49	D09.2-	D31.6-	D48.7	D49.89
intrasellar	C75.1	C79.89	D09.3	D35.2	D44.3	D49.7
intrathoracic (cavity) (organs)	C76.1	C79.89	D09.8	D15.9	D48.7	D49.89
specified NEC	C76.1	C79.89	D09.8	D15.7	-	-
iris	C69.4-	C79.49	D09.2-	D31.4-	D48.7	D49.89
ischiorectal (fossa)	C76.3	C79.89	D09.8	D36.7	D48.7	D49.89
ischium	C41.4	C79.51	-	D16.8	D48.0	D49.2
island of Reil	C71.0	C79.31	-	D33.0	D43.0	D49.6
islands or islets of Langerhans	C25.4	C78.89	D01.7	D13.7	D37.8	D49.0
isthmus uteri	C54.0	C79.82	D07.0	D26.1	D39.0	D49.59
jaw	C76.0	C79.89	D09.8	D36.7	D48.7	D49.89
bone	C41.1	C79.51	-	D16.5-	D48.0	D49.2
lower	C41.1	C79.51	-	D16.5-	-	-
upper	C41.0	C79.51	-	D16.4-	-	-
carcinoma (any type) (lower) (upper)	C76.0	C79.89	-	-	-	-
skin — *see also Neoplasm, skin, face*	C44.309	C79.2	D04.39	D23.39	D48.5	D49.2
soft tissues	C03.9	C79.89	D00.03	D10.39	D37.09	D49.0
lower	C03.1	C79.89	D00.03	D10.39	D37.09	D49.0
upper	C03.0	C79.89	D00.03	D10.39	D37.09	D49.0
jejunum	C17.1	C78.4	D01.49	D13.39	D37.2	D49.0
joint NEC — *see also Neoplasm, bone*	C41.9	C79.51	-	D16.9-	D48.0	D49.2
acromioclavicular	C40.0-	C79.51	-	D16.0-	-	-
bursa or synovial membrane — *see Neoplasm, connective tissue*						
costovertebral	C41.3	C79.51	-	D16.7	D48.0	D49.2
sternocostal	C41.3	C79.51	-	D16.7	D48.0	D49.2
temporomandibular	C41.1	C79.51	-	D16.5-	D48.0	D49.2
junction						
anorectal	C21.8	C78.5	D01.3	D12.9	D37.8	D49.0
cardioesophageal	C16.0	C78.89	D00.2	D13.1	D37.1	D49.0

Neoplasm, neoplastic

	Malignant Primary	Malignant Secondary	Ca in situ	Benign	Uncertain Behavior	Unspecified Behavior
esophagogastric	C16.0	C78.89	D00.2	D13.1	D37.1	D49.0
gastroesophageal	C16.0	C78.89	D00.2	D13.1	D37.1	D49.0
hard and soft palate	C05.9	C79.89	D00.00	D10.39	D37.09	D49.0
ileocecal	C18.0	C78.5	D01.0	D12.0	D37.4	D49.0
pelvirectal	C19	C78.5	D01.1	D12.7	D37.5	D49.0
pelviureteric	C65.-	C79.0-	D09.19	D30.1-	D41.1-	D49.59
rectosigmoid	C19	C78.5	D01.1	D12.7	D37.5	D49.0
squamocolumnar, of cervix	C53.8	C79.82	D06.7	D26.0	D39.0	D49.59
Kaposi's sarcoma — see Kaposi's, sarcoma						
kidney (parenchymal)	C64.-	C79.0-	D09.19	D30.0-	D41.0-	D49.51-
calyx	C65.-	C79.0-	D09.19	D30.1-	D41.1-	D49.51-
hilus	C65.-	C79.0-	D09.19	D30.1-	D41.1-	D49.51-
pelvis	C65.-	C79.0-	D09.19	D30.1-	D41.1-	D49.51-
knee NEC	C76.5-	C79.89	D04.7-	D36.7	D48.7	D49.89
labia (skin)	C51.9	C79.82	D07.1	D28.0	D39.8	D49.59
majora	C51.0	C79.82	D07.1	D28.0	D39.8	D49.59
minora	C51.1	C79.82	D07.1	D28.0	D39.8	D49.59
labial — see also Neoplasm, lip	C00.9	C79.89	D00.01	D10.0	D37.01	D49.0
sulcus (lower) (upper)	C06.1	C79.89	D00.02	D10.39	D37.09	D49.0
labium (skin)	C51.9	C79.82	D07.1	D28.0	D39.8	D49.59
majus	C51.0	C79.82	D07.1	D28.0	D39.8	D49.59
minus	C51.1	C79.82	D07.1	D28.0	D39.8	D49.59
lacrimal						
canaliculi	C69.5-	C79.49	D09.2-	D31.5-	D48.7	D49.89
duct (nasal)	C69.5-	C79.49	D09.2-	D31.5-	D48.7	D49.89
gland	C69.5-	C79.49	D09.2-	D31.5-	D48.7	D49.89
punctum	C69.5-	C79.49	D09.2-	D31.5-	D48.7	D49.89
sac	C69.5-	C79.49	D09.2-	D31.5-	D48.7	D49.89
Langerhans, islands or islets	C25.4	C78.89	D01.7	D13.7	D37.8	D49.0
laryngopharynx	C13.9	C79.89	D00.08	D10.7	D37.05	D49.0
larynx, laryngeal NEC	C32.9	C78.39	D02.0	D14.1	D38.0	D49.1
aryepiglottic fold	C32.1	C78.39	D02.0	D14.1	D38.0	D49.1
cartilage (arytenoid) (cricoid) (cuneiform) (thyroid)	C32.3	C78.39	D02.0	D14.1	D38.0	D49.1
commissure (anterior) (posterior)	C32.0	C78.39	D02.0	D14.1	D38.0	D49.1
extrinsic NEC	C32.1	C78.39	D02.0	D14.1	D38.0	D49.1
meaning hypopharynx	C13.9	C79.89	D00.08	D10.7	D37.05	D49.0
interarytenoid fold	C32.1	C78.39	D02.0	D14.1	D38.0	D49.1
intrinsic	C32.0	C78.39	D02.0	D14.1	D38.0	D49.1
overlapping lesion	C32.8	-	-	-	-	-
ventricular band	C32.1	C78.39	D02.0	D14.1	D38.0	D49.1
leg NEC	C76.5-	C79.89	D04.7-	D36.7	D48.7	D49.89
lens, crystalline	C69.4-	C79.49	D09.2-	D31.4-	D48.7	D49.89
lid (lower) (upper)	C44.10-	C79.2	D04.1-	D23.1-	D48.5	D49.2
basal cell carcinoma	C44.11-	-	-	-	-	-
sebaceous cell	C44.13-	-	-	-	-	-
specified type NEC	C44.19-	-	-	-	-	-
squamous cell carcinoma	C44.12-	-	-	-	-	-
ligament — see also Neoplasm, connective tissue						
broad	C57.1	C79.82	D07.39	D28.2	D39.8	D49.59
Mackenrodt's	C57.7	C79.82	D07.39	D28.7	D39.8	D49.59
non-uterine — see Neoplasm, connective tissue						
round	C57.2	C79.82	-	D28.2	D39.8	D49.59
sacro-uterine	C57.3	C79.82	-	D28.2	D39.8	D49.59
uterine	C57.3	C79.82	-	D28.2	D39.8	D49.59
utero-ovarian	C57.7	C79.82	D07.39	D28.2	D39.8	D49.59
uterosacral	C57.3	C79.82	-	D28.2	D39.8	D49.59

Neoplasm, neoplastic	Malignant Primary	Malignant Secondary	Ca in situ	Benign	Uncertain Behavior	Unspecified Behavior
limb	C76.8	C79.89	D04.8	D36.7	D48.7	D49.89
lower	C76.5-	C79.89	D04.7-	D36.7	D48.7	D49.89
upper	C76.4-	C79.89	D04.6-	D36.7	D48.7	D49.89
limbus of cornea	C69.1-	C79.49	D09.2-	D31.1-	D48.7	D49.89
lingual NEC — see also Neoplasm, tongue	C02.9	C79.89	D00.07	D10.1	D37.02	D49.0
lingula, lung	C34.1-	C78.0-	D02.2-	D14.3-	D38.1	D49.1
lip	C00.9	C79.89	D00.01	D10.0	D37.01	D49.0
buccal aspect — see Neoplasm, lip, internal						
commissure	C00.6	C79.89	D00.01	D10.0	D37.01	D49.0
external	C00.2	C79.89	D00.01	D10.0	D37.01	D49.0
lower	C00.1	C79.89	D00.01	D10.0	D37.01	D49.0
upper	C00.0	C79.89	D00.01	D10.0	D37.01	D49.0
frenulum — see Neoplasm, lip, internal						
inner aspect — see Neoplasm, lip, internal						
internal	C00.5	C79.89	D00.01	D10.0	D37.01	D49.0
lower	C00.4	C79.89	D00.01	D10.0	D37.01	D49.0
upper	C00.3	C79.89	D00.01	D10.0	D37.01	D49.0
lipstick area	C00.2	C79.89	D00.01	D10.0	D37.01	D49.0
lower	C00.1	C79.89	D00.01	D10.0	D37.01	D49.0
upper	C00.0	C79.89	D00.01	D10.0	D37.01	D49.0
lower	C00.1	C79.89	D00.01	D10.0	D37.01	D49.0
internal	C00.4	C79.89	D00.01	D10.0	D37.01	D49.0
mucosa — see Neoplasm, lip, internal						
oral aspect — see Neoplasm, lip, internal						
overlapping lesion	C00.8	-	-	-	-	-
with oral cavity or pharynx	C14.8	-	-	-	-	-
skin (commissure) (lower) (upper)	C44.00	C79.2	D04.0	D23.0	D48.5	D49.2
basal cell carcinoma	C44.01	-	-	-	-	-
specified type NEC	C44.09	-	-	-	-	-
squamous cell carcinoma	C44.02	-	-	-	-	-
upper	C00.0	C79.89	D00.01	D10.0	D37.01	D49.0
internal	C00.3	C79.89	D00.01	D10.0	D37.01	D49.0
vermilion border	C00.2	C79.89	D00.01	D10.0	D37.01	D49.0
lower	C00.1	C79.89	D00.01	D10.0	D37.01	D49.0
upper	C00.0	C79.89	D00.01	D10.0	D37.01	D49.0
lipomatous — see Lipoma, by site						
liver — see also Index to disease, by histology	C22.9	C78.7	D01.5	D13.4	D37.6	D49.0
primary	C22.8	C78.7	D01.5	D13.4	D37.6	D49.0
lumbosacral plexus	C47.5	C79.89	-	D36.16	D48.2	D49.2
lung	C34.9-	C78.0-	D02.2-	D14.3-	D38.1	D49.1
azygos lobe	C34.1-	C78.0-	D02.2-	D14.3-	D38.1	D49.1
carina	C34.0-	C78.0-	D02.2-	D14.3-	D38.1	D49.1
hilus	C34.0-	C78.0-	D02.2-	D14.3-	D38.1	D49.1
linqula	C34.1-	C78.0-	D02.2-	D14.3-	D38.1	D49.1
lobe NEC	C34.9-	C78.0-	D02.2-	D14.3-	D38.1	D49.1
lower lobe	C34.3-	C78.0-	D02.2-	D14.3-	D38.1	D49.1
main bronchus	C34.0-	C78.0-	D02.2-	D14.3-	D38.1	D49.1
mesothelioma — see Mesothelioma						
middle lobe	C34.2	C78.0-	D02.21	D14.31	D38.1	D49.1
overlapping lesion	C34.8-	-	-	-	-	-
upper lobe	C34.1-	C78.0-	D02.2-	D14.3-	D38.1	D49.1
lymph, lymphatic channel NEC	C49.9	C79.89	-	D21.9	D48.1	D49.2
gland (secondary)	-	C77.9	-	D36.0	D48.7	D49.89
abdominal	-	C77.2	-	D36.0	D48.7	D49.89

	Malignant Primary	Malignant Secondary	Ca in situ	Benign	Uncertain Behavior	Unspecified Behavior
Neoplasm, neoplastic						
aortic	-	C77.2	-	D36.0	D48.7	D49.89
arm	-	C77.3	-	D36.0	D48.7	D49.89
auricular (anterior) (posterior)	-	C77.0	-	D36.0	D48.7	D49.89
axilla, axillary	-	C77.3	-	D36.0	D48.7	D49.89
brachial	-	C77.3	-	D36.0	D48.7	D49.89
bronchial	-	C77.1	-	D36.0	D48.7	D49.89
bronchopulmonary	-	C77.1	-	D36.0	D48.7	D49.89
celiac	-	C77.2	-	D36.0	D48.7	D49.89
cervical	-	C77.0	-	D36.0	D48.7	D49.89
cervicofacial	-	C77.0	-	D36.0	D48.7	D49.89
Cloquet	-	C77.4	-	D36.0	D48.7	D49.89
colic	-	C77.2	-	D36.0	D48.7	D49.89
common duct	-	C77.2	-	D36.0	D48.7	D49.89
cubital	-	C77.3	-	D36.0	D48.7	D49.89
diaphragmatic	-	C77.1	-	D36.0	D48.7	D49.89
epigastric, inferior	-	C77.1	-	D36.0	D48.7	D49.89
epitrochlear	-	C77.3	-	D36.0	D48.7	D49.89
esophageal	-	C77.1	-	D36.0	D48.7	D49.89
face	-	C77.0	-	D36.0	D48.7	D49.89
femoral	-	C77.4	-	D36.0	D48.7	D49.89
gastric	-	C77.2	-	D36.0	D48.7	D49.89
groin	-	C77.4	-	D36.0	D48.7	D49.89
head	-	C77.0	-	D36.0	D48.7	D49.89
hepatic	-	C77.2	-	D36.0	D48.7	D49.89
hilar (pulmonary)	-	C77.1	-	D36.0	D48.7	D49.89
splenic	-	C77.2	-	D36.0	D48.7	D49.89
hypogastric	-	C77.5	-	D36.0	D48.7	D49.89
ileocolic	-	C77.2	-	D36.0	D48.7	D49.89
iliac	-	C77.5	-	D36.0	D48.7	D49.89
infraclavicular	-	C77.3	-	D36.0	D48.7	D49.89
inguina, inguinal	-	C77.4	-	D36.0	D48.7	D49.89
innominate	-	C77.1	-	D36.0	D48.7	D49.89
intercostal	-	C77.1	-	D36.0	D48.7	D49.89
intestinal	-	C77.2	-	D36.0	D48.7	D49.89
intrabdominal	-	C77.2	-	D36.0	D48.7	D49.89
intrapelvic	-	C77.5	-	D36.0	D48.7	D49.89
intrathoracic	-	C77.1	-	D36.0	D48.7	D49.89
jugular	-	C77.0	-	D36.0	D48.7	D49.89
leg	-	C77.4	-	D36.0	D48.7	D49.89
limb						
lower	-	C77.4	-	D36.0	D48.7	D49.89
upper	-	C77.3	-	D36.0	D48.7	D49.89
lower limb	-	C77.4	-	D36.0	D48.7	D49.89
lumbar	-	C77.2	-	D36.0	D48.7	D49.89
mandibular	-	C77.0	-	D36.0	D48.7	D49.89
mediastinal	-	C77.1	-	D36.0	D48.7	D49.89
mesenteric (inferior) (superior)	-	C77.2	-	D36.0	D48.7	D49.89
midcolic	-	C77.2	-	D36.0	D48.7	D49.89
multiple sites in categories C77.0 - C77.5	-	C77.8	-	D36.0	D48.7	D49.89
neck	-	C77.0	-	D36.0	D48.7	D49.89
obturator	-	C77.5	-	D36.0	D48.7	D49.89
occipital	-	C77.0	-	D36.0	D48.7	D49.89
pancreatic	-	C77.2	-	D36.0	D48.7	D49.89
para-aortic	-	C77.2	-	D36.0	D48.7	D49.89
paracervical	-	C77.5	-	D36.0	D48.7	D49.89
parametrial	-	C77.5	-	D36.0	D48.7	D49.89
parasternal	-	C77.1	-	D36.0	D48.7	D49.89
parotid	-	C77.0	-	D36.0	D48.7	D49.89
pectoral	-	C77.3	-	D36.0	D48.7	D49.89

Neoplasm, neoplastic	Malignant Primary	Malignant Secondary	Ca in situ	Benign	Uncertain Behavior	Unspecified Behavior
pelvic	-	C77.5	-	D36.0	D48.7	D49.89
peri-aortic	-	C77.2	-	D36.0	D48.7	D49.89
peripancreatic	-	C77.2	-	D36.0	D48.7	D49.89
popliteal	-	C77.4	-	D36.0	D48.7	D49.89
porta hepatis	-	C77.2	-	D36.0	D48.7	D49.89
portal	-	C77.2	-	D36.0	D48.7	D49.89
preauricular	-	C77.0	-	D36.0	D48.7	D49.89
prelaryngeal	-	C77.0	-	D36.0	D48.7	D49.89
presymphysial	-	C77.5	-	D36.0	D48.7	D49.89
pretracheal	-	C77.0	-	D36.0	D48.7	D49.89
primary (any site) NEC	C96.9	-	-	-	-	-
pulmonary (hiler)	-	C77.1	-	D36.0	D48.7	D49.89
pyloric	-	C77.2	-	D36.0	D48.7	D49.89
retroperitoneal	-	C77.2	-	D36.0	D48.7	D49.89
retropharyngeal	-	C77.0	-	D36.0	D48.7	D49.89
Rosenmuller's	-	C77.4	-	D36.0	D48.7	D49.89
sacral	-	C77.5	-	D36.0	D48.7	D49.89
scalene	-	C77.0	-	D36.0	D48.7	D49.89
site NEC	-	C77.9	-	D36.0	D48.7	D49.89
splenic (hilar)	-	C77.2	-	D36.0	D48.7	D49.89
subclavicular	-	C77.3	-	D36.0	D48.7	D49.89
subinguinal	-	C77.4	-	D36.0	D48.7	D49.89
sublingual	-	C77.0	-	D36.0	D48.7	D49.89
submandibular	-	C77.0	-	D36.0	D48.7	D49.89
submaxillary	-	C77.0	-	D36.0	D48.7	D49.89
submental	-	C77.0	-	D36.0	D48.7	D49.89
subscapular	-	C77.3	-	D36.0	D48.7	D49.89
supraclavicular	-	C77.0	-	D36.0	D48.7	D49.89
thoracic	-	C77.1	-	D36.0	D48.7	D49.89
tibial	-	C77.4	-	D36.0	D48.7	D49.89
tracheal	-	C77.1	-	D36.0	D48.7	D49.89
tracheobronchial	-	C77.1	-	D36.0	D48.7	D49.89
upper limb	-	C77.3	-	D36.0	D48.7	D49.89
Virchow's	-	C77.0	-	D36.0	D48.7	D49.89
node — *see also Neoplasm, lymph gland*						
primary NEC	C96.9	-	-	-	-	-
vessel — *see also Neoplasm, connective tissue*	C49.9	C79.89	-	D21.9	D48.1	D49.2
Mackenrodt's ligament	C57.7	C79.82	D07.39	D28.7	D39.8	D49.59
malar	C41.0	C79.51	-	D16.4-	D48.0	D49.2
region — *see Neoplasm, cheek*						
mammary gland — *see Neoplasm, breast*						
mandible	C41.1	C79.51	-	D16.5-	D48.0	D49.2
alveolar						
mucosa (carcinoma)	C03.1	C79.89	D00.03	D10.39	D37.09	D49.0
ridge or process	C41.1	C79.51	-	D16.5-	D48.0	D49.2
marrow (bone) NEC	C96.9	C79.52	-	-	D47.9	D49.89
mastectomy site (skin) — *see also Neoplasm, breast, skin*	C44.501	C79.2	-	-	-	-
specified as breast tissue	C50.8-	C79.81	-	-	-	-
mastoid (air cells) (antrum) (cavity)	C30.1	C78.39	D02.3	D14.0	D38.5	D49.1
bone or process	C41.0	C79.51	-	D16.4-	D48.0	D49.2
maxilla, maxillary (superior)	C41.0	C79.51	-	D16.4-	D48.0	D49.2
alveolar						
mucosa	C03.0	C79.89	D00.03	D10.39	D37.09	D49.0
ridge or process (carcinoma)	C41.0	C79.51	-	D16.4-	D48.0	D49.2
antrum	C31.0	C78.39	D02.3	D14.0	D38.5	D49.1
carcinoma	C03.0	C79.51	-	-	-	-

Neoplasm, neoplastic	Malignant Primary	Malignant Secondary	Ca in situ	Benign	Uncertain Behavior	Unspecified Behavior
inferior — *see Neoplasm, mandible*						
sinus	C31.0	C78.39	D02.3	D14.0	D38.5	D49.1
meatus external (ear) — *see also Neoplasm, skin, ear*	C44.20-	C79.2	D04.2-	D23.2-	D48.5	D49.2
Meckel diverticulum, malignant	C17.3	C78.4	D01.49	D13.39	D37.2	D49.0
mediastinum, mediastinal	C38.3	C78.1	-	D15.2	D38.3	D49.89
anterior	C38.1	C78.1		D15.2	D38.3	D49.89
posterior	C38.2	C78.1	-	D15.2	D38.3	D49.89
medulla						
adrenal	C74.1-	C79.7-	D09.3	D35.0-	D44.1-	D49.7
oblongata	C71.7	C79.31	-	D33.1	D43.1	D49.6
meibomian gland	C44.10-	C79.2	D04.1-	D23.1-	D48.5	D49.2
basal cell carcinoma	C44.11-	-	-	-	-	-
sebaceous cell	C44.13-	-	-	-	-	-
specified type NEC	C44.19-	-	-	-	-	-
squamous cell carcinoma	C44.12-	-	-	-	-	-
melanoma — *see Melanoma*						
meninges	C70.9	C79.49	-	D32.9	D42.9	D49.7
brain	C70.0	C79.32	-	D32.0	D42.0	D49.7
cerebral	C70.0	C79.32	-	D32.0	D42.0	D49.7
crainial	C70.0	C79.32	-	D32.0	D42.0	D49.7
intracranial	C70.0	C79.32	-	D32.0	D42.0	D49.7
spinal (cord)	C70.1	C79.49	-	D32.1	D42.1	D49.7
meniscus, knee joint (lateral) (medial)	C40.2-	C79.51	-	D16.2-	D48.0	D49.2
Merkel cell — *see Carcinoma, Merkel cell*						
mesentery, mesenteric	C48.1	C78.6	-	D20.1	D48.4	D49.0
mesoappendix	C48.1	C78.6	-	D20.1	D48.4	D49.0
mesocolon	C48.1	C78.6	-	D20.1	D48.4	D49.0
mesopharynx — *see Neoplasm, oropharynx*						
mesosalpinx	C57.1	C79.82	D07.39	D28.2	D39.8	D49.59
mesothelial tissue — *see Mesothelioma*						
mesothelioma — *see Mesothelioma*						
mesovarium	C57.1	C79.82	D07.39	D28.2	D39.8	D49.59
metacarpus (any bone)	C40.1-	C79.51	-	D16.1-	-	-
metastatic NEC — *see also Neoplasm, by site, secondary*	-	C79.9	-	-	-	-
metatarsus (any bone)	C40.3-	C79.51	-	D16.3-	-	-
midbrain	C71.7	C79.31	-	D33.1	D43.1	D49.6
milk duct — *see Neoplasm, breast*						
mons						
pubis	C51.9	C79.82	D07.1	D28.0	D39.8	D49.59
veneris	C51.9	C79.82	D07.1	D28.0	D39.8	D49.59
motor tract	C72.9	C79.49	-	D33.9	D43.9	D49.7
brain	C71.9	C79.31	-	D33.2	D43.2	D49.6
cauda equina	C72.1	C79.49	-	D33.4	D43.4	D49.7
spinal	C72.0	C79.49	-	D33.4	D43.4	D49.7
mouth	C06.9	C79.89	D00.00	D10.30	D37.09	D49.0
book-leaf	C06.89	C79.89	-	-	-	-
floor	C04.9	C79.89	D00.06	D10.2	D37.09	D49.0
anterior portion	C04.0	C79.89	D00.06	D10.2	D37.09	D49.0
lateral portion	C04.1	C79.89	D00.06	D10.2	D37.09	D49.0
overlapping lesion	C04.8	-	-	-	-	-
overlapping NEC	C06.80	-	-	-	-	-
roof	C05.9	C79.89	D00.00	D10.39	D37.09	D49.0
specified part NEC	C06.89	C79.89	D00.00	D10.39	D37.09	D49.0
vestibule	C06.1	C79.89	D00.00	D10.39	D37.09	D49.0
mucosa						
alveolar (ridge or process)	C03.9	C79.89	D00.03	D10.39	D37.09	D49.0

Neoplasm, neoplastic	Malignant Primary	Malignant Secondary	Ca in situ	Benign	Uncertain Behavior	Unspecified Behavior
lower	C03.1	C79.89	D00.03	D10.39	D37.09	D49.0
upper	C03.0	C79.89	D00.03	D10.39	D37.09	D49.0
buccal	C06.0	C79.89	D00.02	D10.39	D37.09	D49.0
cheek	C06.0	C79.89	D00.02	D10.39	D37.09	D49.0
lip — see Neoplasm, lip, internal						
nasal	C30.0	C78.39	D02.3	D14.0	D38.5	D49.1
oral	C06.0	C79.89	D00.02	D10.39	D37.09	D49.0
Mullerian duct						
female	C57.7	C79.82	D07.39	D28.7	D39.8	D49.59
male	C63.7	C79.82	D07.69	D29.8	D40.8	D49.59
muscle — see also Neoplasm, connective tissue						
extraocular	C69.6-	C79.49	D09.2-	D31.6-	D48.7	D49.89
myocardium	C38.0	C79.89	-	D15.1	D48.7	D49.89
myometrium	C54.2	C79.82	D07.0	D26.1	D39.0	D49.59
myopericardium	C38.0	C79.89	-	D15.1	D48.7	D49.89
nabothian gland (follicle)	C53.0	C79.82	D06.0	D26.0	D39.0	D49.59
nail — see also Neoplasm, skin, limb	C44.90	C79.2	D04.9	D23.9	D48.5	D49.2
finger — see also Neoplasm, skin, limb, upper	C44.60-	C79.2	D04.6-	D23.6-	D48.5	D49.2
toe — see also Neoplasm, skin, limb, lower	C44.70-	C79.2	D04.7-	D23.7-	D48.5	D49.2
nares, naris (anterior) (posterior)	C30.0	C78.39	D02.3	D14.0	D38.5	D49.1
nasal — see Neoplasm, nose						
nasolabial groove — see also Neoplasm, skin, face	C44.309	C79.2	D04.39	D23.39	D48.5	D49.2
nasolacrimal duct	C69.5-	C79.49	D09.2-	D31.5-	D48.7	D49.89
nasopharynx, nasopharyngeal	C11.9	C79.89	D00.08	D10.6	D37.05	D49.0
floor	C11.3	C79.89	D00.08	D10.6	D37.05	D49.0
overlapping lesion	C11.8	-	-	-	-	-
roof	C11.0	C79.89	D00.08	D10.6	D37.05	D49.0
wall	C11.9	C79.89	D00.08	D10.6	D37.05	D49.0
anterior	C11.3	C79.89	D00.08	D10.6	D37.05	D49.0
lateral	C11.2	C79.89	D00.08	D10.6	D37.05	D49.0
posterior	C11.1	C79.89	D00.08	D10.6	D37.05	D49.0
superior	C11.0	C79.89	D00.08	D10.6	D37.05	D49.0
nates — see also Neoplasm, skin, trunk	C44.509	C79.2	D04.5	D23.5	D48.5	D49.2
neck NEC	C76.0	C79.89	D09.8	D36.7	D48.7	D49.89
skin	C44.40	-	-	-	-	-
basal cell carcinoma	C44.41	-	-	-	-	-
specified type NEC	C44.49	-	-	-	-	-
squamous cell carcinoma	C44.42	-	-	-	-	-
nerve (ganglion)	C47.9	C79.89	-	D36.10	D48.2	D49.2
abducens	C72.59	C79.49	-	D33.3	D43.3	D49.7
accessory (spinal)	C72.59	C79.49	-	D33.3	D43.3	D49.7
acoustic	C72.4-	C79.49	-	D33.3	D43.3	D49.7
auditory	C72.4-	C79.49	-	D33.3	D43.3	D49.7
autonomic NEC — see also Neoplasm, nerve, peripheral	C47.9	C79.89	-	D36.10	D48.2	D49.2
brachial	C47.1-	C79.89	-	D36.12	D48.2	D49.2
cranial	C72.50	C79.49	-	D33.3	D43.3	D49.7
specified NEC	C72.59	C79.49	-	D33.3	D43.3	D49.7
facial	C72.59	C79.49	-	D33.3	D43.3	D49.7
femoral	C47.2-	C79.89	-	D36.13	D48.2	D49.2
ganglion NEC — see also Neoplasm, nerve, peripheral	C47.9	C79.89	-	D36.10	D48.2	D49.2
glossopharyngeal	C72.59	C79.49	-	D33.3	D43.3	D49.7
hypoglossal	C72.59	C79.49	-	D33.3	D43.3	D49.7
intercostal	C47.3	C79.89	-	D36.14	D48.2	D49.2
lumbar	C47.6	C79.89	-	D36.17	D48.2	D49.2

	Malignant Primary	Malignant Secondary	Ca in situ	Benign	Uncertain Behavior	Unspecified Behavior
Neoplasm, neoplastic						
median	C47.1-	C79.89	-	D36.12	D48.2	D49.2
obturator	C47.2-	C79.89	-	D36.13	D48.2	D49.2
oculomotor	C72.59	C79.49	-	D33.3	D43.3	D49.7
olfactory	C47.2-	C79.49	-	D33.3	D43.3	D49.7
optic	C72.3-	C79.49	-	D33.3	D43.3	D49.7
parasympathetic NEC	C47.9	C79.89	-	D36.10	D48.2	D49.2
peripheral NEC	C47.9	C79.89	-	D36.10	D48.2	D49.2
abdomen	C47.4	C79.89	-	D36.15	D48.2	D49.2
abdominal wall	C47.4	C79.89	-	D36.15	D48.2	D49.2
ankle	C47.2-	C79.89	-	D36.13	D48.2	D49.2
antecubital fossa or space	C47.1-	C79.89	-	D36.12	D48.2	D49.2
arm	C47.1-	C79.89	-	D36.12	D48.2	D49.2
auricle (ear)	C47.0	C79.89	-	D36.11	D48.2	D49.2
axilla	C47.3	C79.89	-	D36.12	D48.2	D49.2
back	C47.6	C79.89	-	D36.17	D48.2	D49.2
buttock	C47.5	C79.89	-	D36.16	D48.2	D49.2
calf	C47.2-	C79.89	-	D36.13	D48.2	D49.2
cervical region	C47.0	C79.89	-	D36.11	D48.2	D49.2
cheek	C47.0	C79.89	-	D36.11	D48.2	D49.2
chest (wall)	C47.3	C79.89	-	D36.14	D48.2	D49.2
chin	C47.0	C79.89	-	D36.11	D48.2	D49.2
ear (external)	C47.0	C79.89	-	D36.11	D48.2	D49.2
elbow	C47.1-	C79.89	-	D36.12	D48.2	D49.2
extrarectal	C47.5	C79.89	-	D36.16	D48.2	D49.2
extremity	C47.9	C79.89	-	D36.10	D48.2	D49.2
lower	C47.2-	C79.89	-	D36.13	D48.2	D49.2
upper	C47.1-	C79.89	-	D36.12	D48.2	D49.2
eyelid	C47.0	C79.89	-	D36.11	D48.2	D49.2
face	C47.0	C79.89	-	D36.11	D48.2	D49.2
finger	C47.1-	C79.89	-	D36.12	D48.2	D49.2
flank	C47.6	C79.89	-	D36.17	D48.2	D49.2
foot	C47.2-	C79.89	-	D36.13	D48.2	D49.2
forearm	C47.1-	C79.89	-	D36.12	D48.2	D49.2
forehead	C47.0	C79.89	-	D36.11	D48.2	D49.2
gluteal region	C47.5	C79.89	-	D36.16	D48.2	D49.2
groin	C47.5	C79.89	-	D36.16	D48.2	D49.2
hand	C47.1-	C79.89	-	D36.12	D48.2	D49.2
head	C47.0	C79.89	-	D36.11	D48.2	D49.2
heel	C47.2-	C79.89	-	D36.13	D48.2	D49.2
hip	C47.2-	C79.89	-	D36.13	D48.2	D49.2
infraclavicular region	C47.3	C79.89	-	D36.14	D48.2	D49.2
inguinal (canal) (region)	C47.5	C79.89	-	D36.16	D48.2	D49.2
intrathoracic	C47.3	C79.89	-	D36.14	D48.2	D49.2
ischiorectal fossa	C47.5	C79.89	-	D36.16	D48.2	D49.2
knee	C47.2-	C79.89	-	D36.13	D48.2	D49.2
leg	C47.2-	C79.89	-	D36.13	D48.2	D49.2
limb NEC	C47.9	C79.89	-	D36.10	D48.2	D49.2
lower	C47.2-	C79.89	-	D36.13	D48.2	D49.2
upper	C47.1-	C79.89	-	D36.12	D48.2	D49.2
nates	C47.5	C79.89	-	D36.16	D48.2	D49.2
neck	C47.0	C79.89	-	D36.11	D48.2	D49.2
orbit	C69.6-	C79.49	-	D31.6-	D48.7	D49.2
pararectal	C47.5	C79.89	-	D36.16	D48.2	D49.2
paraurethral	C47.5	C79.89	-	D36.16	D48.2	D49.2
paravaginal	C47.5	C79.89	-	D36.16	D48.2	D49.2
pelvis (floor)	C47.5	C79.89	-	D36.16	D48.2	D49.2
pelvoabdominal	C47.8	C79.89	-	D36.17	D48.2	D49.2
perineum	C47.5	C79.89	-	D36.16	D48.2	D49.2
perirectal (tissue)	C47.5	C79.89	-	D36.16	D48.2	D49.2

Neoplasm, neoplastic	Malignant Primary	Malignant Secondary	Ca in situ	Benign	Uncertain Behavior	Unspecified Behavior
periurethral (tissue)	C47.5	C79.89	-	D36.16	D48.2	D49.2
popliteal fossa or space	C47.2-	C79.89	-	D36.13	D48.2	D49.2
presacral	C47.5	C79.89	-	D36.16	D48.2	D49.2
pterygoid fossa	C47.0	C79.89	-	D36.11	D48.2	D49.2
rectovaginal septum or wall	C47.5	C79.89	-	D36.16	D48.2	D49.2
rectovesical	C47.5	C79.89	-	D36.16	D48.2	D49.2
sacrococcygeal region	C47.5	C79.89	-	D36.16	D48.2	D49.2
scalp	C47.0	C79.89	-	D36.11	D48.2	D49.2
scapular region	C47.3	C79.89	-	D36.14	D48.2	D49.2
shoulder	C47.1-	C79.89	-	D36.12	D48.2	D49.2
submental	C47.0	C79.89	-	D36.11	D48.2	D49.2
supraclavicular region	C47.0	C79.89	-	D36.11	D48.2	D49.2
temple	C47.0	C79.89	-	D36.11	D48.2	D49.2
temporal region	C47.0	C79.89	-	D36.11	D48.2	D49.2
thigh	C47.2-	C79.89	-	D36.13	D48.2	D49.2
thoracic (duct) (wall)	C47.3	C79.89	-	D36.14	D48.2	D49.2
thorax	C47.3	C79.89	-	D36.14	D48.2	D49.2
thumb	C47.1-	C79.89	-	D36.12	D48.2	D49.2
toe	C47.2-	C79.89	-	D36.13	D48.2	D49.2
trunk	C47.6	C79.89	-	D36.17	D48.2	D49.2
umbilicus	C47.4	C79.89	-	D36.15	D48.2	D49.2
vesicorectal	C47.5	C79.89	-	D36.16	D48.2	D49.2
wrist	C47.1-	C79.89	-	D36.12	D48.2	D49.2
radial	C47.1-	C79.89	-	D36.12	D48.2	D49.2
sacral	C47.5	C79.89	-	D36.16	D48.2	D49.2
sciatic	C47.2-	C79.89	-	D36.13	D48.2	D49.2
spinal NEC	C47.9	C79.89	-	D36.10	D48.2	D49.2
accessory	C72.59	C79.49	-	D33.3	D43.3	D49.7
sympathetic NEC — see also Neoplasm, nerve, peripheral	C47.9	C79.89	-	D36.10	D48.2	D49.2
trigeminal	C72.59	C79.49	-	D33.3	D43.3	D49.7
trochlear	C72.59	C79.49	-	D33.3	D43.3	D49.7
ulnar	C47.1-	C79.89	-	D36.12	D48.2	D49.2
vagus	C72.59	C79.49	-	D33.3	D43.3	D49.7
nervous system (central)	C72.9	C79.40	-	D33.9	D43.9	D49.7
autonomic — see Neoplasm, nerve, peripheral						
parasympathetic — see Neoplasm, nerve, peripheral						
specified site NEC	-	C79.49	-	D33.7	D43.8	-
sympathetic — see Neoplasm, nerve, peripheral						
nevus — see Nevus						
nipple	C50.0-	C79.81	D05.-	D24.-	-	-
nose, nasal	C76.0	C79.89	D09.8	D36.7	D48.7	D49.89
ala (external) (nasi) — see also Neoplasm, nose, skin	C44.301	C79.2	D04.39	D23.39	D48.5	D49.2
bone	C41.0	C79.51	-	D16.4-	D48.0	D49.2
cartilage	C30.0	C78.39	D02.3	D14.0	D38.5	D49.1
cavity	C30.0	C78.39	D02.3	D14.0	D38.5	D49.1
choana	C11.3	C79.89	D00.08	D10.6	D37.05	D49.0
external (skin) — see also Neoplasm, nose, skin	C44.301	C79.2	D04.39	D23.39	D48.5	D49.2
fossa	C30.0	C78.39	D02.3	D14.0	D38.5	D49.1
internal	C30.0	C78.39	D02.3	D14.0	D38.5	D49.1
mucosa	C30.0	C78.39	D02.3	D14.0	D38.5	D49.1
septum	C30.0	C78.39	D02.3	D14.0	D38.5	D49.1
posterior margin	C11.3	C79.89	D00.08	D10.6	D37.05	D49.0
sinus — see Neoplasm, sinus						
skin	C44.301	C79.2	D04.39	D23.39	D48.5	D49.2

	Malignant Primary	Malignant Secondary	Ca in situ	Benign	Uncertain Behavior	Unspecified Behavior
Neoplasm, neoplastic						
basal cell carcinoma	C44.311	-	-	-	-	-
specified type NEC	C44.391	-	-	-	-	-
squamous cell carcinoma	C44.321	-	-	-	-	-
turbinate (mucosa)	C30.0	C78.39	D02.3	D14.0	D38.5	D49.1
bone	C41.0	C79.51	-	D16.4-	D48.0	D49.2
vestibule	C30.0	C78.39	D02.3	D14.0	D38.5	D49.1
nostril	C30.0	C78.39	D02.3	D14.0	D38.5	D49.1
nucleus pulposus	C41.2	C79.51	-	D16.6	D48.0	D49.2
occipital						
bone	C41.0	C79.51	-	D16.4-	D48.0	D49.2
lobe or pole, brain	C71.4	C79.31	-	D33.0	D43.0	D49.6
odontogenic — *see Neoplasm, jaw bone*						
olfactory nerve or bulb	C72.2-	C79.49	-	D33.3	D43.3	D49.7
olive (brain)	C71.7	C79.31	-	D33.1	D43.1	D49.6
omentum	C48.1	C78.6	-	D20.1	D48.4	D49.0
operculum (brain)	C71.0	C79.31	-	D33.0	D43.0	D49.6
optic nerve, chiasm, or tract	C72.3-	C79.49	-	D33.3	D43.3	D49.7
oral (cavity)	C06.9	C79.89	D00.00	D10.30	D37.09	D49.0
ill-defined	C14.8	C79.89	D00.00	D10.30	D37.09	D49.0
mucosa	C06.0	C79.89	D00.02	D10.39	D37.09	D49.0
orbit	C69.6-	C79.49	D09.2-	D31.6-	D48.7	D49.89
autonomic nerve	C69.6-	C79.49	-	D31.6-	D48.7	D49.2
bone	C41.0	C79.51	-	D16.4-	D48.0	D49.2
eye	C69.6-	C79.49	D09.2-	D31.6-	D48.7	D49.89
peripheral nerves	C69.6-	C79.49	-	D31.6-	D48.7	D49.2
soft parts	C69.6-	C79.49	D09.2-	D31.6-	D48.7	D49.89
organ of Zuckerkandl	C75.5	C79.89	-	D35.6	D44.7	D49.7
oropharynx	C10.9	C79.89	D00.08	D10.5	D37.05	D49.0
branchial cleft (vestige)	C10.4	C79.89	D00.08	D10.5	D37.05	D49.0
junctional region	C10.8	C79.89	D00.08	D10.5	D37.05	D49.0
lateral wall	C10.2	C79.89	D00.08	D10.5	D37.05	D49.0
overlapping lesion	C10.8	-	-	-	-	-
pillars or fauces	C09.1	C79.89	D00.08	D10.5	D37.05	D49.0
posterior wall	C10.3	C79.89	D00.08	D10.5	D37.05	D49.0
vallecula	C10.0	C79.89	D00.08	D10.5	D37.05	D49.0
os						
external	C53.1	C79.82	D06.1	D26.0	D39.0	D49.59
internal	C53.0	C79.82	D06.0	D26.0	D39.0	D49.59
ovary	C56.-	C79.6-	D07.39	D27.-	D39.1-	D49.59
oviduct	C57.0-	C79.82	D07.39	D28.2	D39.8	D49.59
palate	C05.9	C79.89	D00.00	D10.39	D37.09	D49.0
hard	C05.0	C79.89	D00.05	D10.39	D37.09	D49.0
junction of hard and soft palate	C05.9	C79.89	D00.00	D10.39	D37.09	D49.0
overlapping lesions	C05.8	-	-	-	-	-
soft	C05.1	C79.89	D00.04	D10.39	D37.09	D49.0
nasopharyngeal surface	C11.3	C79.89	D00.08	D10.6	D37.05	D49.0
posterior surface	C11.3	C79.89	D00.08	D10.6	D37.05	D49.0
superior surface	C11.3	C79.89	D00.08	D10.6	D37.05	D49.0
palatoglossal arch	C09.1	C79.89	D00.00	D10.5	D37.09	D49.0
palatopharyngeal arch	C09.1	C79.89	D00.00	D10.5	D37.09	D49.0
pallium	C71.0	C79.31	-	D33.0	D43.0	D49.6
palpebra	C44.10-	C79.2	D04.1-	D23.1-	D48.5	D49.2
basal cell carcinoma	C44.11-	-	-	-	-	-
sebaceous cell	C44.13-	-	-	-	-	-
specified type NEC	C44.19-	-	-	-	-	-
squamous cell carcinoma	C44.12-	-	-	-	-	-
pancreas	C25.9	C78.89	D01.7	D13.6	D37.8	D49.0
body	C25.1	C78.89	D01.7	D13.6	D37.8	D49.0
duct (of Santorini) (of Wirsung)	C25.3	C78.89	D01.7	D13.6	D37.8	D49.0

NOSE, NASAL - PANCREAS

NEOPLASM

Neoplasm, neoplastic	Malignant Primary	Malignant Secondary	Ca in situ	Benign	Uncertain Behavior	Unspecified Behavior
ectopic tissue	C25.7	C78.89	-	D13.6	D37.8	D49.0
head	C25.0	C78.89	D01.7	D13.6	D37.8	D49.0
islet cells	C25.4	C78.89	D01.7	D13.7	D37.8	D49.0
neck	C25.7	C78.89	D01.7	D13.6	D37.8	D49.0
overlapping lesion	C25.8	-	-	-	-	-
tail	C25.2	C78.89	D01.7	D13.6	D37.8	D49.0
para-aortic body	C75.5	C79.89	-	D35.6	D44.7	D49.7
paraganglion NEC	C75.5	C79.89	-	D35.6	D44.7	D49.7
parametrium	C57.3	C79.82	-	D28.2	D39.8	D49.59
paranephric	C48.0	C78.6	-	D20.0	D48.3	D49.0
pararectal	C76.3	C79.89	-	D36.7	D48.7	D49.89
parasagittal (region)	C76.0	C79.89	D09.8	D36.7	D48.7	D49.89
parasellar	C72.9	C79.49	-	D33.9	D43.8	D49.7
parathyroid (gland)	C75.0	C79.89	D09.3	D35.1	D44.2	D49.7
paraurethral	C76.3	C79.89	-	D36.7	D48.7	D49.89
gland	C68.1	C79.19	D09.19	D30.8	D41.8	D49.59
paravaginal	C76.3	C79.89	-	D36.7	D48.7	D49.89
parenchyma, kidney	C64.-	C79.0-	D09.19	D30.0-	D41.0-	D49.51-
parietal						
bone	C41.0	C79.51	-	D16.4-	D48.0	D49.2
lobe, brain	C71.3	C79.31	-	D33.0	D43.0	D49.6
paroophoron	C57.1	C79.82	D07.39	D28.2	D39.8	D49.59
parotid (duct) (gland)	C07	C79.89	D00.00	D11.0	D37.030	D49.0
parovarium	C57.1	C79.82	D07.39	D28.2	D39.8	D49.59
patella	C40.20	C79.51	-	-	-	-
peduncle, cerebral	C71.7	C79.31	-	D33.1	D43.1	D49.6
pelvirectal junction	C19	C78.5	D01.1	D12.7	D37.5	D49.0
pelvis, pelvic	C76.3	C79.89	D09.8	D36.7	D48.7	D49.89
bone	C41.4	C79.51	-	D16.8	D48.0	D49.2
floor	C76.3	C79.89	D09.8	D36.7	D48.7	D49.89
renal	C65.-	C79.0-	D09.19	D30.1-	D41.1-	D49.51-
viscera	C76.3	C79.89	D09.8	D36.7	D48.7	D49.89
wall	C76.3	C79.89	D09.8	D36.7	D48.7	D49.89
pelvo-abdominal	C76.8	C79.89	D09.8	D36.7	D48.7	D49.89
penis	C60.9	C79.82	D07.4	D29.0	D40.8	D49.59
body	C60.2	C79.82	D07.4	D29.0	D40.8	D49.59
corpus (cavernosum)	C60.2	C79.82	D07.4	D29.0	D40.8	D49.59
glans	C60.1	C79.82	D07.4	D29.0	D40.8	D49.59
overlapping sites	C60.8	-	-	-	-	-
skin NEC	C60.9	C79.82	D07.4	D29.0	D40.8	D49.59
periadrenal (tissue)	C48.0	C78.6	-	D20.0	D48.3	D49.0
perianal (skin) — *see also Neoplasm, anus, skin*	C44.500	C79.2	D04.5	D23.5	D48.5	D49.2
pericardium	C38.0	C79.89	-	D15.1	D48.7	D49.89
perinephric	C48.0	C78.6	-	D20.0	D48.3	D49.0
perineum	C76.3	C79.89	D09.8	D36.7	D48.7	D49.89
periodontal tissue NEC	C03.9	C79.89	D00.03	D10.39	D37.09	D49.0
periosteum — *see Neoplasm, bone*						
peripancreatic	C48.0	C78.6	-	D20.0	D48.3	D49.0
peripheral nerve NEC	C47.9	C79.89	-	D36.10	D48.2	D49.2
perirectal (tissue)	C76.3	C79.89	-	D36.7	D48.7	D49.89
perirenal (tissue)	C48.0	C78.6	-	D20.0	D48.3	D49.0
peritoneum, peritoneal (cavity)	C48.2	C78.6	-	D20.1	D48.4	D49.0
benign mesothelial tissue — *see Mesothelioma, benign*						
overlapping lesion	C48.8	-	-	-	-	-
with digestive organs	C26.9	-	-	-	-	-
parietal	C48.1	C78.6	-	D20.1	D48.4	D49.0
pelvic	C48.1	C78.6	-	D20.1	D48.4	D49.0

	Malignant Primary	Malignant Secondary	Ca in situ	Benign	Uncertain Behavior	Unspecified Behavior
Neoplasm, neoplastic						
specified part NEC	C48.1	C78.6	-	D20.1	D48.4	D49.0
peritonsillar (tissue)	C76.0	C79.89	D09.8	D36.7	D48.7	D49.89
periurethral tissue	C76.3	C79.89	-	D36.7	D48.7	D49.89
phalanges						
foot	C40.3-	C79.51	-	D16.3-	-	-
hand	C40.1-	C79.51	-	D16.1-	-	-
pharynx, pharyngeal	C14.0	C79.89	D00.08	D10.9	D37.05	D49.0
bursa	C11.1	C79.89	D00.08	D10.6	D37.05	D49.0
fornix	C11.3	C79.89	D00.08	D10.6	D37.05	D49.0
recess	C11.2	C79.89	D00.08	D10.6	D37.05	D49.0
region	C14.0	C79.89	D00.08	D10.9	D37.05	D49.0
tonsil	C11.1	C79.89	D00.08	D10.6	D37.05	D49.0
wall (lateral) (posterior)	C14.0	C79.89	D00.08	D10.9	D37.05	D49.0
pia mater	C70.9	C79.40	-	D32.9	D42.9	D49.7
cerebral	C70.0	C79.32	-	D32.0	D42.0	D49.7
cranial	C70.0	C79.32	-	D32.0	D42.0	D49.7
spinal	C70.1	C79.49	-	D32.1	D42.1	D49.7
pillars of fauces	C09.1	C79.89	D00.08	D10.5	D37.05	D49.0
pineal (body) (gland)	C75.3	C79.89	D09.3	D35.4	D44.5	D49.7
pinna (ear) NEC — *see also Neoplasm, skin, ear*	C44.20-	C79.2	D04.2-	D23.2-	D48.5	D49.2
piriform fossa or sinus	C12	C79.89	D00.08	D10.7	D37.05	D49.0
pituitary (body) (fossa) (gland) (lobe)	C75.1	C79.89	D09.3	D35.2	D44.3	D49.7
placenta	C58	C79.82	D07.0	D26.7	D39.2	D49.59
pleura, pleural (cavity)	C38.4	C78.2	-	D19.0	D38.2	D49.1
overlapping lesion with heart or mediastinum	C38.8	-	-	-	-	-
parietal	C38.4	C78.2	-	D19.0	D38.2	D49.1
visceral	C38.4	C78.2	-	D19.0	D38.2	D49.1
plexus						
brachial	C47.1-	C79.89	-	D36.12	D48.2	D49.2
cervical	C47.0	C79.89	-	D36.11	D48.2	D49.2
choroid	C71.5	C79.31	-	D33.0	D43.0	D49.6
lumbosacral	C47.5	C79.89	-	D36.16	D48.2	D49.2
sacral	C47.5	C79.89	-	D36.16	D48.2	D49.2
pluriendocrine	C75.8	C79.89	D09.3	D35.7	D44.9	D49.7
pole						
frontal	C71.1	C79.31	-	D33.0	D43.0	D49.6
occipital	C71.4	C79.31	-	D33.0	D43.0	D49.6
pons (varolii)	C71.7	C79.31	-	D33.1	D43.1	D49.6
popliteal fossa or space	C76.5-	C79.89	D04.7-	D36.7	D48.7	D49.89
postcricoid (region)	C13.0	C79.89	D00.08	D10.7	D37.05	D49.0
posterior fossa (cranial)	C71.9	C79.31	-	D33.2	D43.2	D49.6
postnasal space	C11.9	C79.89	D00.08	D10.6	D37.05	D49.0
prepuce	C60.0	C79.82	D07.4	D29.0	D40.8	D49.59
prepylorus	C16.4	C78.89	D00.2	D13.1	D37.1	D49.0
presacral (region)	C76.3	C79.89	-	D36.7	D48.7	D49.89
prostate (gland)	C61	C79.82	D07.5	D29.1	D40.0	D49.59
utricle	C68.0	C79.19	D09.19	D30.4	D41.3	D49.59
pterygoid fossa	C49.0	C79.89	-	D21.0	D48.1	D49.2
pubic bone	C41.4	C79.51	-	D16.8	D48.0	D49.2
pudenda, pudendum (femaie)	C51.9	C79.82	D07.1	D28.0	D39.8	D49.59
pulmonary — *see also Neoplasm, lung*	C34.9-	C78.0-	D02.2-	D14.3-	D38.1	D49.1
putamen	C71.0	C79.31	-	D33.0	D43.0	D49.6
pyloric						
antrum	C16.3	C78.89	D00.2	D13.1	D37.1	D49.0
canal	C16.4	C78.89	D00.2	D13.1	D37.1	D49.0
pylorus	C16.4	C78.89	D00.2	D13.1	D37.1	D49.0
pyramid (brain)	C71.7	C79.31	-	D33.1	D43.1	D49.6
pyriform fossa or sinus	C12	C79.89	D00.08	D10.7	D37.05	D49.0

PERITONEUM, PERITONEAL - PYRIFORM FOSSA OR SINUS

NEOPLASM

Neoplasm, neoplastic	Malignant Primary	Malignant Secondary	Ca in situ	Benign	Uncertain Behavior	Unspecified Behavior
radius (any part)	C40.0-	C79.51	-	D16.0-	-	-
Rathke's pouch	C75.1	C79.89	D09.3	D35.2	D44.3	D49.7
rectosigmoid (junction)	C19	C78.5	D01.1	D12.7	D37.5	D49.0
overlapping lesion with anus or rectum	C21.8	-	-	-	-	-
rectouterine pouch	C48.1	C78.6	-	D20.1	D48.4	D49.0
rectovaginal septum or wall	C76.3	C79.89	D09.8	D36.7	D48.7	D49.89
rectovesical septum	C76.3	C79.89	D09.8	D36.7	D48.7	D49.89
rectum (ampulla)	C20	C78.5	D01.2	D12.8	D37.5	D49.0
and colon	C19	C78.5	D01.1	D12.7	D37.5	D49.0
overlapping lesion with anus or rectosigmoid junction	C21.8	-	-	-	-	-
renal	C64.-	C79.0-	D09.19	D30.0-	D41.0-	D49.51-
calyx	C65.-	C79.0-	D09.19	D30.1-	D41.1-	D49.51-
hilus	C65.-	C79.0-	D09.19	D30.1-	D41.1-	D49.51-
parenchyma	C64.-	C79.0-	D09.19	D30.0-	D41.0-	D49.51-
pelvis	C65.-	C79.0-	D09.19	D30.1-	D41.1-	D49.51-
respiratory						
organs or system NEC	C39.9	C78.30	D02.4	D14.4	D38.6	D49.1
tract NEC	C39.9	C78.30	D02.4	D14.4	D38.5	D49.1
upper	C39.0	C78.30	D02.4	D14.4	D38.5	D49.1
retina	C69.2-	C79.49	D09.2-	D31.2-	D48.7	D49.81
retrobulbar	C69.6-	C79.49	-	D31.6-	D48.7	D49.89
retrocecal	C48.0	C78.6	-	D20.0	D48.3	D49.0
retromolar (area) (triangle) (trigone)	C06.2	C79.89	D00.00	D10.39	D37.09	D49.0
retro-orbital	C76.0	C79.89	D09.8	D36.7	D48.7	D49.89
retroperitoneal (space) (tissue)	C48.0	C78.6	-	D20.0	D48.3	D49.0
retroperitoneum	C48.0	C78.6	-	D20.0	D48.3	D49.0
retropharyngeal	C14.0	C79.89	D00.08	D10.9	D37.05	D49.0
retrovesical (septum)	C76.3	C79.89	D09.8	D36.7	D48.7	D49.89
rhinencephalon	C71.0	C79.31	-	D33.0	D43.0	D49.6
rib	C41.3	C79.51	-	D16.7	D48.0	D49.2
Rosenmuller's fossa	C11.2	C79.89	D00.08	D10.6	D37.05	D49.0
round ligament	C57.2	C79.82	-	D28.2	D39.8	D49.59
sacrococcyx, sacrococcygeal	C41.4	C79.51	-	D16.8	D48.0	D49.2
region	C76.3	C79.89	D09.8	D36.7	D48.7	D49.89
sacrouterine ligament	C57.3	C79.82	-	D28.2	D39.8	D49.59
sacrum, sacral (vertebra)	C41.4	C79.51	-	D16.8	D48.0	D49.2
salivary gland or duct (major)	C08.9	C79.89	D00.00	D11.9	D37.039	D49.0
minor NEC	C06.9	C79.89	D00.00	D10.39	D37.04	D49.0
overlapping lesion	C08.9	-	-	-	-	-
parotid	C07	C79.89	D00.00	D11.0	D37.030	D49.0
pluriglandular	C08.9	C79.89	D00.00	D11.9	D37.039	D49.0
sublingual	C08.1	C79.89	D00.00	D11.7	D37.031	D49.0
submandibular	C08.0	C79.89	D00.00	D11.7	D37.032	D49.0
submaxillary	C08.0	C79.89	D00.00	D11.7	D37.032	D49.0
salpinx (uterine)	C57.0-	C79.82	D07.39	D28.2	D39.8	D49.59
Santorini's duct	C25.3	C78.89	D01.7	D13.6	D37.8	D49.0
scalp	C44.40	C79.2	D04.4	D23.4	D48.5	D49.2
basal cell carcinoma	C44.41	-	-	-	-	-
specified type NEC	C44.49	-	-	-	-	-
squamous cell carcinoma	C44.42	-	-	-	-	-
scapula (any part)	C40.0-	C79.51	-	D16.0-	-	-
scapular region	C76.1	C79.89	D09.8	D36.7	D48.7	D49.89
scar NEC — *see also Neoplasm, skin, by site*	C44.90	C79.2	D04.9	D23.9	D48.5	D49.2
sciatic nerve	C47.2-	C79.89	-	D36.13	D48.2	D49.2
sclera	C69.4-	C79.49	D09.2-	D31.4-	D48.7	D49.89
scrotum (skin)	C63.2	C79.82	D07.61	D29.4	D40.8	D49.59
sebaceous gland — *see Neoplasm, skin*						

Neoplasm, neoplastic	Malignant Primary	Malignant Secondary	Ca in situ	Benign	Uncertain Behavior	Unspecified Behavior
sella turcica	C75.1	C79.89	D09.3	D35.2	D44.3	D49.7
bone	C41.0	C79.51	-	D16.4-	D48.0	D49.2
semilunar cartilage (knee)	C40.2-	C79.51	-	D16.2-	D48.0	D49.2
seminal vesicle	C63.7	C79.82	D07.69	D29.8	D40.8	D49.59
septum						
nasal	C30.0	C78.39	D02.3	D14.0	D38.5	D49.1
posterior margin	C11.3	C79.89	D00.08	D10.6	D37.05	D49.0
rectovaginal	C76.3	C79.89	D09.8	D36.7	D48.7	D49.89
rectovesical	C76.3	C79.89	D09.8	D36.7	D48.7	D49.89
urethrovaginal	C57.9	C79.82	D07.30	D28.9	D39.9	D49.59
vesicovaginal	C57.9	C79.82	D07.30	D28.9	D39.9	D49.59
shoulder NEC	C76.4-	C79.89	D04.6-	D36.7	D48.7	D49.89
sigmoid flexure (lower) (upper)	C18.7	C78.5	D01.0	D12.5	D37.4	D49.0
sinus (accessory)	C31.9	C78.39	D02.3	D14.0	D38.5	D49.1
bone (any)	C41.0	C79.51	-	D16.4-	D48.0	D49.2
ethmoidal	C31.1	C78.39	D02.3	D14.0	D38.5	D49.1
frontal	C31.2	C78.39	D02.3	D14.0	D38.5	D49.1
maxillary	C31.0	C78.39	D02.3	D14.0	D38.5	D49.1
nasal, paranasal NEC	C31.9	C78.39	D02.3	D14.0	D38.5	D49.1
overlapping lesion	C31.8	-	-	-	-	-
pyriform	C12	C79.89	D00.08	D10.7	D37.05	D49.0
sphenoid	C31.3	C78.39	D02.3	D14.0	D38.5	D49.1
skeleton, skeletal NEC	C41.9	C79.51	-	D16.9-	D48.0	D49.2
Skene's gland	C68.1	C79.19	D09.19	D30.8	D41.8	D49.59
skin NOS	C44.90	C79.2	D04.9	D23.9	D48.5	D49.2
abdominal wall	C44.509	C79.2	D04.5	D23.5	D48.5	D49.2
basal cell carcinoma	C44.519	-	-	-	-	-
specified type NEC	C44.599	-	-	-	-	-
squamous cell carcinoma	C44.529	-	-	-	-	-
ala nasi — *see also Neoplasm, nose, skin*	C44.301	C79.2	D04.39	D23.39	D48.5	D49.2
ankle — *see also Neoplasm, skin, limb, lower*	C44.70-	C79.2	D04.7-	D23.7-	D48.5	D49.2
antecubital space — *see also Neoplasm, skin, limb, upper*	C44.60-	C79.2	D04.6-	D23.6-	D48.5	D49.2
anus	C44.500	C79.2	D04.5	D23.5	D48.5	D49.2
basal cell carcinoma	C44.510	-	-	-	-	-
specified type NEC	C44.590	-	-	-	-	-
squamous cell carcinoma	C44.520	-	-	-	-	-
arm — *see also Neoplasm, skin, limb, upper*	C44.60-	C79.2	D04.6-	D23.6-	D48.5	D49.2
auditory canal (external) — *see also Neoplasm, skin, ear*	C44.20-	C79.2	D04.2-	D23.2-	D48.5	D49.2
auricle (ear) — *see also Neoplasm, skin, ear*	C44.20-	C79.2	D04.2-	D23.2-	D48.5	D49.2
auricular canal (external) — *see also Neoplasm, skin, ear*	C44.20-	C79.2	D04.2-	D23.2-	D48.5	D49.2
axilla, axillary fold — *see also Neoplasm, skin, trunk*	C44.509	C79.2	D04.5	D23.5	D48.5	D49.2
back — *see also Neoplasm, skin, trunk*	C44.509	C79.2	D04.5	D23.5	D48.5	D49.2
basal cell carcinoma	C44.91					
breast	C44.501	C79.2	D04.5	D23.5	D48.5	D49.2
basal cell carcinoma	C44.511	-	-	-	-	-
specified type NEC	C44.591	-	-	-	-	-
squamous cell carcinoma	C44.521	-	-	-	-	-
brow — *see also Neoplasm, skin, face*	C44.309	C79.2	D04.39	D23.39	D48.5	D49.2
buttock — *see also Neoplasm, skin, trunk*	C44.509	C79.2	D04.5	D23.5	D48.5	D49.2
calf — *see also Neoplasm, skin, limb, lower*	C44.70-	C79.2	D04.7-	D23.7-	D48.5	D49.2

Neoplasm, neoplastic	Malignant Primary	Malignant Secondary	Ca in situ	Benign	Uncertain Behavior	Unspecified Behavior
canthus (eye) (inner) (outer)	C44.10-	C79.2	D04.1-	D23.1-	D48.5	D49.2
basal cell carcinoma	C44.11-	-	-	-	-	-
sebaceous cell	C44.13-	-	-	-	-	-
specified type NEC	C44.19-	-	-	-	-	-
squamous cell carcinoma	C44.12-	-	-	-	-	-
cervical region — see also Neoplasm, skin, neck	C44.40	C79.2	D04.4	D23.4	D48.5	D49.2
cheek (external) — see also Neoplasm, skin, face	C44.309	C79.2	D04.39	D23.39	D48.5	D49.2
chest (wall) — see also Neoplasm, skin, trunk	C44.509	C79.2	D04.5	D23.5	D48.5	D49.2
chin — see also Neoplasm, skin, face	C44.309	C79.2	D04.39	D23.39	D48.5	D49.2
clavicular area — see also Neoplasm, skin, trunk	C44.509	C79.2	D04.5	D23.5	D48.5	D49.2
clitoris	C51.2	C79.82	D07.1	D28.0	D39.8	D49.59
columnella — see also Neoplasm, skin, face	C44.309	C79.2	D04.39	D23.39	D48.5	D49.2
concha — see also Neoplasm, skin, ear	C44.20-	C79.2	D04.2-	D23.2-	D48.5	D49.2
ear (external)	C44.20-	C79.2	D04.2-	D23.2-	D48.5	D49.2
basal cell carcinoma	C44.21-	-	-	-	-	-
specified type NEC	C44.29-	-	-	-	-	-
squamous cell carcinoma	C44.22-	-	-	-	-	-
elbow — see also Neoplasm, skin, limb, upper	C44.60-	C79.2	D04.6-	D23.6-	D48.5	D49.2
eyebrow — see also Neoplasm, skin, face	C44.309	C79.2	D04.39	D23.39	D48.5	D49.2
eyelid	C44.10-	C79.2	D04.1-	D23.1-	D48.5	D49.2
basal cell carcinoma	C44.11-	-	-	-	-	-
sebaceous cell	C44.13-	-	-	-	-	-
specified type NEC	C44.19-	-	-	-	-	-
squamous cell carcinoma	C44.12-	-	-	-	-	-
face NOS	C44.300	C79.2	D04.30	D23.30	D48.5	D49.2
basal cell carcinoma	C44.310	-	-	-	-	-
specified type NEC	C44.390	-	-	-	-	-
squamous cell carcinoma	C44.320	-	-	-	-	-
female genital organs (external)	C51.9	C79.82	D07.1	D28.0	D39.8	D49.59
clitoris	C51.2	C79.82	D07.1	D28.0	D39.8	D49.59
labium NEC	C51.9	C79.82	D07.1	D28.0	D39.8	D49.59
majus	C51.0	C79.82	D07.1	D28.0	D39.8	D49.59
minus	C51.1	C79.82	D07.1	D28.0	D39.8	D49.59
pudendum	C51.9	C79.82	D07.1	D28.0	D39.8	D49.59
vulva	C51.9	C79.82	D07.1	D28.0	D39.8	D49.59
finger — see also Neoplasm, skin, limb, upper	C44.60-	C79.2	D04.6-	D23.6-	D48.5	D49.2
flank — see also Neoplasm, skin, trunk	C44.509	C79.2	D04.5	D23.5	D48.5	D49.2
foot — see also Neoplasm, skin, limb, lower	C44.70-	C79.2	D04.7-	D23.7-	D48.5	D49.2
forearm — see also Neoplasm, skin, limb, upper	C44.60-	C79.2	D04.6-	D23.6-	D48.5	D49.2
forehead — see also Neoplasm, skin, face	C44.309	C79.2	D04.39	D23.39	D48.5	D49.2
glabella — see also Neoplasm, skin, face	C44.309	C79.2	D04.39	D23.39	D48.5	D49.2
gluteal region — see also Neoplasm, skin, trunk	C44.509	C79.2	D04.5	D23.5	D48.5	D49.2
groin — see also Neoplasm, skin, trunk	C44.509	C79.2	D04.5	D23.5	D48.5	D49.2
hand — see also Neoplasm, skin, limb, upper	C44.60-	C79.2	D04.6-	D23.6-	D48.5	D49.2
head NEC — see also Neoplasm, skin, scalp	C44.40	C79.2	D04.4	D23.4	D48.5	D49.2

Neoplasm, neoplastic	Malignant Primary	Malignant Secondary	Ca in situ	Benign	Uncertain Behavior	Unspecified Behavior
heel — *see also Neoplasm, skin, limb, lower*	C44.70-	C79.2	D04.7-	D23.7-	D48.5	D49.2
helix — *see also Neoplasm, skin, ear*	C44.20-	C79.2	D04.2-	D23.2-	D48.5	D49.2
hip — *see also Neoplasm, skin, limb, lower*	C44.70-	C79.2	D04.7-	D23.7-	D48.5	D49.2
infraclavicular region — *see also Neoplasm, skin, trunk*	C44.509	C79.2	D04.5	D23.5	D48.5	D49.2
inguinal region — *see also Neoplasm, skin, trunk*	C44.509	C79.2	D04.5	D23.5	D48.5	D49.2
jaw — *see also Neoplasm, skin, face*	C44.309	C79.2	D04.39	D23.39	D48.5	D49.2
Kaposi's sarcoma — *see Kaposi's, sarcoma, skin*						
knee — *see also Neoplasm, skin, limb, lower*	C44.70-	C79.2	D04.7-	D23.7-	D48.5	D49.2
labia						
majora	C51.0	C79.82	D07.1	D28.0	D39.8	D49.59
minora	C51.1	C79.82	D07.1	D28.0	D39.8	D49.59
leg — *see also Neoplasm, skin, limb, lower*	C44.70-	C79.2	D04.7-	D23.7-	D48.5	D49.2
lid (lower) (upper)	C44.10-	C79.2	D04.1-	D23.1-	D48.5	D49.2
basal cell carcinoma	C44.11-	-	-	-	-	-
sebaceous cell	C44.13-	-	-	-	-	-
specified type NEC	C44.19-	-	-	-	-	-
squamous cell carcinoma	C44.12-	-	-	-	-	-
limb NEC	C44.90	C79.2	D04.9	D23.9	D48.5	D49.2
basal cell carcinoma	C44.91					
lower	C44.70-	C79.2	D04.7-	D23.7-	D48.5	D49.2
basal cell carcinoma	C44.71-	-	-	-	-	-
specified type NEC	C44.79-	-	-	-	-	-
squamous cell carcinoma	C44.72-	-	-	-	-	-
upper	C44.60-	C79.2	D04.6-	D23.6-	D48.5	D49.2
basal cell carcinoma	C44.61-	-	-	-	-	-
specified type NEC	C44.69-	-	-	-	-	-
squamous cell carcinoma	C44.62-	-	-	-	-	-
lip (lower) (upper)	C44.00	C79.2	D04.0	D23.0	D48.5	D49.2
basal cell carcinoma	C44.01	-	-	-	-	-
specified type NEC	C44.09	-	-	-	-	-
squamous cell carcinoma	C44.02	-	-	-	-	-
male genital organs	C63.9	C79.82	D07.60	D29.9	D40.8	D49.59
penis	C60.9	C79.82	D07.4	D29.0	D40.8	D49.59
prepuce	C60.0	C79.82	D07.4	D29.0	D40.8	D49.59
scrotum	C63.2	C79.82	D07.61	D29.4	D40.8	D49.59
mastectomy site (skin) — *see also Neoplasm, skin, breast*	C44.501	C79.2	-	-	-	-
specified as breast tissue	C50.8-	C79.81	-	-	-	-
meatus, acoustic (external) — *see also Neoplasm, skin, ear*	C44.20-	C79.2	D04.2-	D23.2-	D48.5	D49.2
melanotic — *see Melanoma*						
Merkel cell — *see Carcinoma, Merkel cell*						
nates — *see also Neoplasm, skin, trunk*	C44.509	C79.2	D04.5	D23.5	D48.5	D49.2
neck	C44.40	C79.2	D04.4	D23.4	D48.5	D49.2
basal cell carcinoma	C44.41	-	-	-	-	-
specified type NEC	C44.49	-	-	-	-	-
squamous cell carcinoma	C44.42	-	-	-	-	-
nevus — *see Nevus, skin*						
nose (external) — *see also Neoplasm, nose, skin*	C44.301	C79.2	D04.39	D23.39	D48.5	D49.2
overlapping lesion	C44.80	-	-	-	-	-
basal cell carcinoma	C44.81	-	-	-	-	-
specified type NEC	C44.89	-	-	-	-	-
squamous cell carcinoma	C44.82	-	-	-	-	-

SKIN NOS - SKIN NOS

NEOPLASM

Neoplasm, neoplastic	Malignant Primary	Malignant Secondary	Ca in situ	Benign	Uncertain Behavior	Unspecified Behavior
palm — *see also Neoplasm, skin, limb, upper*	C44.60-	C79.2	D04.6-	D23.6-	D48.5	D49.2
palpebra	C44.10-	C79.2	D04.1-	D23.1-	D48.5	D49.2
basal cell carcinoma	C44.11-	-	-	-	-	-
sebaceous cell	C44.13-	-	-	-	-	-
specified type NEC	C44.19-	-	-	-	-	-
squamous cell carcinoma	C44.12-	-	-	-	-	-
penis NEC	C60.9	C79.82	D07.4	D29.0	D40.8	D49.59
perianal — *see also Neoplasm, skin, anus*	C44.500	C79.2	D04.5	D23.5	D48.5	D49.2
perineum — *see also Neoplasm, skin, anus*	C44.500	C79.2	D04.5	D23.5	D48.5	D49.2
pinna — *see also Neoplasm, skin, ear*	C44.20-	C79.2	D04.2-	D23.2-	D48.5	D49.2
plantar — *see also Neoplasm, skin, limb, lower*	C44.70-	C79.2	D04.7-	D23.7-	D48.5	D49.2
popliteal fossa or space — *see also Neoplasm, skin, limb, lower*	C44.70-	C79.2	D04.7-	D23.7-	D48.5	D49.2
prepuce	C60.0	C79.82	D07.4	D29.0	D40.8	D49.59
pubes — *see also Neoplasm, skin, trunk*	C44.509	C79.2	D04.5	D23.5	D48.5	D49.2
sacrococcygeal region — *see also Neoplasm, skin, trunk*	C44.509	C79.2	D04.5	D23.5	D48.5	D49.2
scalp	C44.40	C79.2	D04.4	D23.4	D48.5	D49.2
basal cell carcinoma	C44.41	-	-	-	-	-
specified type NEC	C44.49	-	-	-	-	-
squamous cell carcinoma	C44.42	-	-	-	-	-
scapular region — *see also Neoplasm, skin, trunk*	C44.509	C79.2	D04.5	D23.5	D48.5	D49.2
scrotum	C63.2	C79.82	D07.61	D29.4	D40.8	D49.59
shoulder — *see also Neoplasm, skin, limb, upper*	C44.60-	C79.2	D04.6-	D23.6-	D48.5	D49.2
sole (foot) — *see also Neoplasm, skin, limb, lower*	C44.70-	C79.2	D04.7-	D23.7-	D48.5	D49.2
specified sites NEC	C44.80	C79.2	D04.8	D23.9	D48.5	D49.2
basal cell carcinoma	C44.81	-	-	-	-	-
specified type NEC	C44.89	-	-	-	-	-
squamous cell carcinoma	C44.82	-	-	-	-	-
specified type NEC	C44.99	-	-	-	-	-
squamous cell carcinoma	C44.92	-	-	-	-	-
submammary fold — *see also Neoplasm, skin, trunk*	C44.509	C79.2	D04.5	D23.5	D48.5	D49.2
supraclavicular region — *see also Neoplasm, skin, neck*	C44.40	C79.2	D04.4	D23.4	D48.5	D49.2
temple — *see also Neoplasm, skin, face*	C44.309	C79.2	D04.39	D23.39	D48.5	D49.2
thigh — *see also Neoplasm, skin, limb, lower*	C44.70-	C79.2	D04.7-	D23.7-	D48.5	D49.2
thoracic wall — *see also Neoplasm, skin, trunk*	C44.509	C79.2	D04.5	D23.5	D48.5	D49.2
thumb — *see also Neoplasm, skin, limb, upper*	C44.60-	C79.2	D04.6-	D23.6-	D48.5	D49.2
toe — *see also Neoplasm, skin, limb, lower*	C44.70-	C79.2	D04.7-	D23.7-	D48.5	D49.2
tragus — *see also Neoplasm, skin, ear*	C44.20-	C79.2	D04.2-	D23.2-	D48.5	D49.2
trunk	C44.509	C79.2	D04.5	D23.5	D48.5	D49.2
basal cell carcinoma	C44.519	-	-	-	-	-
specified type NEC	C44.599	-	-	-	-	-
squamous cell carcinoma	C44.529	-	-	-	-	-
umbilicus — *see also Neoplasm, skin, trunk*	C44.509	C79.2	D04.5	D23.5	D48.5	D49.2
vulva	C51.9	C79.82	D07.1	D28.0	D39.8	D49.59
overlapping lesion	C51.8	-	-	-	-	-

Neoplasm, neoplastic	Malignant Primary	Malignant Secondary	Ca in situ	Benign	Uncertain Behavior	Unspecified Behavior
wrist — *see also Neoplasm, skin, limb, upper*	C44.60-	C79.2	D04.6-	D23.6-	D48.5	D49.2
skull	C41.0	C79.51	-	D16.4-	D48.0	D49.2
soft parts or tissues — *see Neoplasm, connective tissue*						
specified site NEC	C76.8	C79.89	D09.8	D36.7	D48.7	D49.89
spermatic cord	C63.1-	C79.82	D07.69	D29.8	D40.8	D49.59
sphenoid	C31.3	C78.39	D02.3	D14.0	D38.5	D49.1
bone	C41.0	C79.51	-	D16.4-	D48.0	D49.2
sinus	C31.3	C78.39	D02.3	D14.0	D38.5	D49.1
sphincter						
anal	C21.1	C78.5	D01.3	D12.9	D37.8	D49.0
of Oddi	C24.0	C78.89	D01.5	D13.5	D37.6	D49.0
spine, spinal (column)	C41.2	C79.51	-	D16.6	D48.0	D49.2
bulb	C71.7	C79.31	-	D33.1	D43.1	D49.6
coccyx	C41.4	C79.51	-	D16.8	D48.0	D49.2
cord (cervical) (lumbar) (sacral) (thoracic)	C72.0	C79.49	-	D33.4	D43.4	D49.7
dura mater	C70.1	C79.49	-	D32.1	D42.1	D49.7
lumbosacral	C41.2	C79.51	-	D16.6	D48.0	D49.2
marrow NEC	C96.9	C79.52	-	-	D47.9	D49.89
membrane	C70.1	C79.49	-	D32.1	D42.1	D49.7
meninges	C70.1	C79.49	-	D32.1	D42.1	D49.7
nerve (root)	C47.9	C79.89	-	D36.10	D48.2	D49.2
pia mater	C70.1	C79.49	-	D32.1	D42.1	D49.7
root	C47.9	C79.89	-	D36.10	D48.2	D49.2
sacrum	C41.4	C79.51	-	D16.8	D48.0	D49.2
spleen, splenic NEC	C26.1	C78.89	D01.7	D13.9	D37.8	D49.0
flexure (colon)	C18.5	C78.5	D01.0	D12.3	D37.4	D49.0
stem, brain	C71.7	C79.31	-	D33.1	D43.1	D49.6
Stensen's duct	C07	C79.89	D00.00	D11.0	D37.030	D49.0
sternum	C41.3	C79.51	-	D16.7	D48.0	D49.2
stomach	C16.9	C78.89	D00.2	D13.1	D37.1	D49.0
antrum (pyloric)	C16.3	C78.89	D00.2	D13.1	D37.1	D49.0
body	C16.2	C78.89	D00.2	D13.1	D37.1	D49.0
cardia	C16.0	C78.89	D00.2	D13.1	D37.1	D49.0
cardiac orifice	C16.0	C78.89	D00.2	D13.1	D37.1	D49.0
corpus	C16.2	C78.89	D00.2	D13.1	D37.1	D49.0
fundus	C16.1	C78.89	D00.2	D13.1	D37.1	D49.0
greater curvature NEC	C16.6	C78.89	D00.2	D13.1	D37.1	D49.0
lesser curvature NEC	C16.5	C78.89	D00.2	D13.1	D37.1	D49.0
overlapping lesion	C16.8	-	-	-	-	-
prepylorus	C16.4	C78.89	D00.2	D13.1	D37.1	D49.0
pylorus	C16.4	C78.89	D00.2	D13.1	D37.1	D49.0
wall NEC	C16.9	C78.89	D00.2	D13.1	D37.1	D49.0
anterior NEC	C16.8	C78.89	D00.2	D13.1	D37.1	D49.0
posterior NEC	C16.8	C78.89	D00.2	D13.1	D37.1	D49.0
stroma, endometrial	C54.1	C79.82	D07.0	D26.1	D39.0	D49.59
stump, cervical	C53.8	C79.82	D06.7	D26.0	D39.0	D49.59
subcutaneous (nodule) (tissue) NEC — *see Neoplasm, connective tissue*						
subdural	C70.9	C79.32	-	D32.9	D42.9	D49.7
subglottis, subglottic	C32.2	C78.39	D02.0	D14.1	D38.0	D49.1
sublingual	C04.9	C79.89	D00.06	D10.2	D37.09	D49.0
gland or duct	C08.1	C79.89	D00.00	D11.7	D37.031	D49.0
submandibular gland	C08.0	C79.89	D00.00	D11.7	D37.032	D49.0
submaxillary gland or duct	C08.0	C79.89	D00.00	D11.7	D37.032	D49.0
submental	C76.0	C79.89	D09.8	D36.7	D48.7	D49.89
subpleural	C34.9-	C78.0-	D02.2-	D14.3-	D38.1	D49.1
substernal	C38.1	C78.1	-	D15.2	D38.3	D49.89

Neoplasm, neoplastic	Malignant Primary	Malignant Secondary	Ca in situ	Benign	Uncertain Behavior	Unspecified Behavior
sudoriferous, sudoriparous gland, site unspecified	C44.90	C79.2	D04.9	D23.9	D48.5	D49.2
specified site — *see Neoplasm, skin*						
supraclavicular region	C76.0	C79.89	D09.8	D36.7	D48.7	D49.89
supraglottis	C32.1	C78.39	D02.0	D14.1	D38.0	D49.1
suprarenal	C74.9-	C79.7-	D09.3	D35.0-	D44.1-	D49.7
capsule	C74.9-	C79.7-	D09.3	D35.0-	D44.1-	D49.7
cortex	C74.0-	C79.7-	D09.3	D35.0-	D44.1-	D49.7
gland	C74.9-	C79.7-	D09.3	D35.0-	D44.1-	D49.7
medulla	C74.1-	C79.7-	D09.3	D35.0-	D44.1-	D49.7
suprasellar (region)	C71.9	C79.31	-	D33.2	D43.2	D49.6
supratentorial (brain) NEC	C71.0	C79.31	-	D33.0	D43.0	D49.6
sweat gland (apocrine) (eccrine) , site unspecified	C44.90	C79.2	D04.9	D23.9	D48.5	D49.2
specified site — *see Neoplasm, skin*						
sympathetic nerve or nervous system NEC	C47.9	C79.89	-	D36.10	D48.2	D49.2
symphysis pubis	C41.4	C79.51	-	D16.8	D48.0	D49.2
synovial membrane — *see Neoplasm, connective tissue*						
tapetum, brain	C71.8	C79.31	-	D33.2	D43.2	D49.6
tarsus (any bone)	C40.3-	C79.51	-	D16.3-	-	-
temple (skin) — *see also Neoplasm, skin, face*	C44.309	C79.2	D04.39	D23.39	D48.5	D49.2
temporal						
bone	C41.0	C79.51	-	D16.4-	D48.0	D49.2
lobe or pole	C71.2	C79.31	-	D33.0	D43.0	D49.6
region	C76.0	C79.89	D09.8	D36.7	D48.7	D49.89
skin — *see also Neoplasm, skin, face*	C44.309	C79.2	D04.39	D23.39	D48.5	D49.2
tendon (sheath) — *see Neoplasm, connective tissue*						
tentorium (cerebelli)	C70.0	C79.32	-	D32.0	D42.0	D49.7
testis, testes	C62.9-	C79.82	D07.69	D29.2-	D40.1-	D49.59
descended	C62.1-	C79.82	D07.69	D29.2-	D40.1-	D49.59
ectopic	C62.0-	C79.82	D07.69	D29.2-	D40.1-	D49.59
retained	C62.0-	C79.82	D07.69	D29.2-	D40.1-	D49.59
scrotal	C62.1-	C79.82	D07.69	D29.2-	D40.1-	D49.59
undescended	C62.0-	C79.82	D07.69	D29.2-	D40.1-	D49.59
unspecified whether descended or undescended	C62.9-	C79.82	D07.69	D29.2-	D40.1-	D49.59
thalamus	C71.0	C79.31	-	D33.0	D43.0	D49.6
thigh NEC	C76.5-	C79.89	D04.7-	D36.7	D48.7	D49.89
thorax, thoracic (cavity) (organs NEC)	C76.1	C79.89	D09.8	D36.7	D48.7	D49.89
duct	C49.3	C79.89	-	D21.3	D48.1	D49.2
wall NEC	C76.1	C79.89	D09.8	D36.7	D48.7	D49.89
throat	C14.0	C79.89	D00.08	D10.9	D37.05	D49.0
thumb NEC	C76.4-	C79.89	D04.6-	D36.7	D48.7	D49.89
thymus (gland)	C37	C79.89	D09.3	D15.0	D38.4	D49.89
thyroglossal duct	C73	C79.89	D09.3	D34	D44.0	D49.7
thyroid (gland)	C73	C79.89	D09.3	D34	D44.0	D49.7
cartilage	C32.3	C78.39	D02.0	D14.1	D38.0	D49.1
tibia (any part)	C40.2-	C79.51	-	D16.2-	-	-
toe NEC	C76.5-	C79.89	D04.7-	D36.7	D48.7	D49.89
tongue	C02.9	C79.89	D00.07	D10.1	D37.02	D49.0
anterior (two-thirds) NEC	C02.3	C79.89	D00.07	D10.1	D37.02	D49.0
dorsal surface	C02.0	C79.89	D00.07	D10.1	D37.02	D49.0
ventral surface	C02.2	C79.89	D00.07	D10.1	D37.02	D49.0
base (dorsal surface)	C01	C79.89	D00.07	D10.1	D37.02	D49.0
border (lateral)	C02.1	C79.89	D00.07	D10.1	D37.02	D49.0
dorsal surface NEC	C02.0	C79.89	D00.07	D10.1	D37.02	D49.0
fixed part NEC	C01	C79.89	D00.07	D10.1	D37.02	D49.0

	Malignant Primary	Malignant Secondary	Ca in situ	Benign	Uncertain Behavior	Unspecified Behavior
Neoplasm, neoplastic						
foreamen cecum	C02.0	C79.89	D00.07	D10.1	D37.02	D49.0
frenulum linguae	C02.2	C79.89	D00.07	D10.1	D37.02	D49.0
junctional zone	C02.8	C79.89	D00.07	D10.1	D37.02	D49.0
margin (lateral)	C02.1	C79.89	D00.07	D10.1	D37.02	D49.0
midline NEC	C02.0	C79.89	D00.07	D10.1	D37.02	D49.0
mobile part NEC	C02.3	C79.89	D00.07	D10.1	D37.02	D49.0
overlapping lesion	C02.8	-	-	-	-	-
posterior (third)	C01	C79.89	D00.07	D10.1	D37.02	D49.0
root	C01	C79.89	D00.07	D10.1	D37.02	D49.0
surface (dorsal)	C02.0	C79.89	D00.07	D10.1	D37.02	D49.0
base	C01	C79.89	D00.07	D10.1	D37.02	D49.0
ventral	C02.2	C79.89	D00.07	D10.1	D37.02	D49.0
tip	C02.1	C79.89	D00.07	D10.1	D37.02	D49.0
tonsil	C02.4	C79.89	D00.07	D10.1	D37.02	D49.0
tonsil	C09.9	C79.89	D00.08	D10.4	D37.05	D49.0
fauces, faucial	C09.9	C79.89	D00.08	D10.4	D37.05	D49.0
lingual	C02.4	C79.89	D00.07	D10.1	D37.02	D49.0
overlapping sites	C09.8	-	-	-	-	-
palatine	C09.9	C79.89	D00.08	D10.4	D37.05	D49.0
pharyngeal	C11.1	C79.89	D00.08	D10.6	D37.05	D49.0
pillar (anterior) (posterior)	C09.1	C79.89	D00.08	D10.5	D37.05	D49.0
tonsillar fossa	C09.0	C79.89	D00.08	D10.5	D37.05	D49.0
tooth socket NEC	C03.9	C79.89	D00.03	D10.39	D37.09	D49.0
trachea (cartilage) (mucosa)	C33	C78.39	D02.1	D14.2	D38.1	D49.1
overlapping lesion with bronchus or lung	C34.8-	-	-	-	-	-
tracheobronchial	C34.8-	C78.39	D02.1	D14.2	D38.1	D49.1
overlapping lesion with lung	C34.8-	-	-	-	-	-
tragus — *see also Neoplasm, skin, ear*	C44.20-	C79.2	D04.2-	D23.2-	D48.5	D49.2
trunk NEC	C76.8	C79.89	D04.5	D36.7	D48.7	D49.89
tubo-ovarian	C57.8	C79.82	D07.39	D28.7	D39.8	D49.59
tunica vaginalis	C63.7	C79.82	D07.69	D29.8	D40.8	D49.59
turbinate (bone)	C41.0	C79.51	-	D16.4-	D48.0	D49.2
nasal	C30.0	C78.39	D02.3	D14.0	D38.5	D49.1
tympanic cavity	C30.1	C78.39	D02.3	D14.0	D38.5	D49.1
ulna (any part)	C40.0-	C79.51	-	D16.0-	-	-
umbilicus, umbilical — *see also Neoplasm, skin, trunk*	C44.509	C79.2	D04.5	D23.5	D48.5	D49.2
uncus, brain	C71.2	C79.31	-	D33.0	D43.0	D49.6
unknown site or unspecified	C80.1	C79.9	D09.9	D36.9	D48.9	D49.9
urachus	C67.7	C79.11	D09.0	D30.3	D41.4	D49.4
ureter, ureteral	C66.-	C79.19	D09.19	D30.2-	D41.2-	D49.59
orifice (bladder)	C67.6	C79.11	D09.0	D30.3	D41.4	D49.4
ureter-bladder (junction)	C67.6	C79.11	D09.0	D30.3	D41.4	D49.4
urethra, urethral (gland)	C68.0	C79.19	D09.19	D30.4	D41.3	D49.59
orifice, internal	C67.5	C79.11	D09.0	D30.3	D41.4	D49.4
urethrovaginal (septum)	C57.9	C79.82	D07.30	D28.9	D39.8	D49.59
urinary organ or system	C68.9	C79.10	D09.10	D30.9	D41.9	D49.59
bladder — *see Neoplasm, bladder*						
overlapping lesion	C68.8	-	-	-	-	-
specified sites NEC	C68.8	C79.19	D09.19	D30.8	D41.8	D49.59
utero-ovarian	C57.8	C79.82	D07.39	D28.7	D39.8	D49.59
ligament	C57.1	C79.82	D07.39	D28.2	D39.8	D49.59
uterosacral ligament	C57.3	C79.82	-	D28.2	D39.8	D49.59
uterus, uteri, uterine	C55	C79.82	D07.0	D26.9	D39.0	D49.59
adnexa NEC	C57.4	C79.82	D07.39	D28.7	D39.8	D49.59
body	C54.9	C79.82	D07.0	D26.1	D39.0	D49.59
cervix	C53.9	C79.82	D06.9	D26.0	D39.0	D49.59
cornu	C54.9	C79.82	D07.0	D26.1	D39.0	D49.59
corpus	C54.9	C79.82	D07.0	D26.1	D39.0	D49.59

Neoplasm, neoplastic	Malignant Primary	Malignant Secondary	Ca in situ	Benign	Uncertain Behavior	Unspecified Behavior
endocervix (canal) (gland)	C53.0	C79.82	D06.0	D26.0	D39.0	D49.59
endometrium	C54.1	C79.82	D07.0	D26.1	D39.0	D49.59
exocervix	C53.1	C79.82	D06.1	D26.0	D39.0	D49.59
external os	C53.1	C79.82	D06.1	D26.0	D39.0	D49.59
fundus	C54.3	C79.82	D07.0	D26.1	D39.0	D49.59
internal os	C53.0	C79.82	D06.0	D26.0	D39.0	D49.59
isthmus	C54.0	C79.82	D07.0	D26.1	D39.0	D49.59
ligament	C57.3	C79.82	-	D28.2	D39.8	D49.59
broad	C57.1	C79.82	D07.39	D28.2	D39.8	D49.59
round	C57.2	C79.82	-	D28.2	D39.8	D49.59
lower segment	C54.0	C79.82	D07.0	D26.1	D39.0	D49.59
myometrium	C54.2	C79.82	D07.0	D26.1	D39.0	D49.59
overlapping sites	C54.8	-	-	-	-	-
squamocolumnar junction	C53.8	C79.82	D06.7	D26.0	D39.0	D49.59
tube	C57.0-	C79.82	D07.39	D28.2	D39.8	D49.59
utricle, prostatic	C68.0	C79.19	D09.19	D30.4	D41.3	D49.59
uveal tract	C69.4-	C79.49	D09.2-	D31.4-	D48.7	D49.89
uvula	C05.2	C79.89	D00.04	D10.39	D37.09	D49.0
vagina, vaginal (fornix) (vault) (wall)	C52	C79.82	D07.2	D28.1	D39.8	D49.59
vaginovesical	C57.9	C79.82	D07.30	D28.9	D39.9	D49.59
septum	C57.9	C79.82	D07.30	D28.9	D39.9	D49.59
vallecula (epigiottis)	C10.0	C79.89	D00.08	D10.5	D37.05	D49.0
vas deferens	C63.1-	C79.82	D07.69	D29.8	D40.8	D49.59
vascular — *see Neoplasm, connective tissue*						
Vater's ampulla	C24.1	C78.89	D01.5	D13.5	D37.6	D49.0
vein, venous — *see Neoplasm, connective tissue*						
vena cava (abdominal) (inferior)	C49.4	C79.89	-	D21.4	D48.1	D49.2
superior	C49.3	C79.89	-	D21.3	D48.1	D49.2
ventricle (cerebral) (floor) (lateral) (third)	C71.5	C79.31	-	D33.0	D43.0	D49.6
cardiac (left) (right)	C38.0	C79.89	-	D15.1	D48.7	D49.89
fourth	C71.7	C79.31	-	D33.1	D43.1	D49.6
ventricular band of larynx	C32.1	C78.39	D02.0	D14.1	D38.0	D49.1
ventriculus — *see Neoplasm, stomach*						
vermillion border — *see Neoplasm, lip*						
vermis, cerebellum	C71.6	C79.31	-	D33.1	D43.1	D49.6
vertebra (column)	C41.2	C79.51	-	D16.6	D48.0	D49.2
coccyx	C41.4	C79.51	-	D16.8-	D48.0	D49.2
marrow NEC	C96.9	C79.52	-	-	D47.9	D49.89
sacrum	C41.4	C79.51	-	D16.8-	D48.0	D49.2
vesical — *see Neoplasm, bladder*						
vesicle, seminal	C63.7	C79.82	D07.69	D29.8	D40.8	D49.59
vesicocervical tissue	C57.9	C79.82	D07.30	D28.9	D39.9	D49.59
vesicorectal	C76.3	C79.82	D09.8	D36.7	D48.7	D49.89
vesicovaginal	C57.9	C79.82	D07.30	D28.9	D39.9	D49.59
septum	C57.9	C79.82	D07.30	D28.9	D39.8	D49.59
vessel (blood) — *see Neoplasm, connective tissue*						
vestibular gland, greater	C51.0	C79.82	D07.1	D28.0	D39.8	D49.59
vestibule						
mouth	C06.1	C79.89	D00.00	D10.39	D37.09	D49.0
nose	C30.0	C78.39	D02.3	D14.0	D38.5	D49.1
Virchow's gland	C77.0	C77.0	-	D36.0	D48.7	D49.89
viscera NEC	C76.8	C79.89	D09.8	D36.7	D48.7	D49.89
vocal cords (true)	C32.0	C78.39	D02.0	D14.1	D38.0	D49.1
false	C32.1	C78.39	D02.0	D14.1	D38.0	D49.1
vomer	C41.0	C79.51	-	D16.4-	D48.0	D49.2
vulva	C51.9	C79.82	D07.1	D28.0	D39.8	D49.59

Neoplasm, neoplastic

	Malignant Primary	Malignant Secondary	Ca in situ	Benign	Uncertain Behavior	Unspecified Behavior
vulvovaginal gland	C51.0	C79.82	D07.1	D28.0	D39.8	D49.59
Waldeyer's ring	C14.2	C79.89	D00.08	D10.9	D37.05	D49.0
Wharton's duct	C08.0	C79.89	D00.00	D11.7	D37.032	D49.0
white matter (central) (cerebral)	C71.0	C79.31	-	D33.0	D43.0	D49.6
windpipe	C33	C78.39	D02.1	D14.2	D38.1	D49.1
Wirsung's duct	C25.3	C78.89	D01.7	D13.6	D37.8	D49.0
wolffian (body) (duct)						
female	C57.7	C79.82	D07.39	D28.7	D39.8	D49.59
male	C63.7	C79.82	D07.69	D29.8	D40.8	D49.59
womb — *see Neoplasm, uterus*						
wrist NEC	C76.4-	C79.89	D04.6-	D36.7	D48.7	D49.89
xiphoid process	C41.3	C79.51	-	D16.7	D48.0	D49.2
Zuckerkandl organ	C75.5	C79.89	-	D35.6	D44.7	D49.7

Table of Drugs and Chemicals

Substance	Poisoning Accidental (unintentional)	Poisoning Intentional self-harm	Poisoning Assault	Poisoning Undetermined	Adverse effect	Underdosing
1-propanol	T51.3X1-	T51.3X2-	T51.3X3-	T51.3X4-	-	-
2-propanol	T51.2X1-	T51.2X2-	T51.2X3-	T51.2X4-	-	-
2,4-D (dichlorophen-oxyacetic acid)	T60.3X1-	T60.3X2-	T60.3X3-	T60.3X4-	-	-
2,4-toluene diisocyanate	T65.0X1-	T65.0X2-	T65.0X3-	T65.0X4-	-	-
2,4,5-T (trichloro-phenoxyacetic acid)	T60.1X1-	T60.1X2-	T60.1X3-	T60.1X4-	-	-
3,4-methylenedioxymethamphetamine	T43.641-	T43.642-	T43.643-	T43.644-	-	-
14-hydroxydihydro-morphinone	T40.2X1-	T40.2X2-	T40.2X3-	T40.2X4-	T40.2X5-	T40.2X6-
ABOB	T37.5X1-	T37.5X2-	T37.5X3-	T37.5X4-	T37.5X5-	T37.5X6-
Abrine	T62.2X1-	T62.2X2-	T62.2X3-	T62.2X4-	-	-
Abrus (seed)	T62.2X1-	T62.2X2-	T62.2X3-	T62.2X4-	-	-
Absinthe	T51.0X1-	T51.0X2-	T51.0X3-	T51.0X4-	-	-
beverage	T51.0X1-	T51.0X2-	T51.0X3-	T51.0X4-	-	-
Acaricide	T60.8X1-	T60.8X2-	T60.8X3-	T60.8X4-	-	-
Acebutolol	T44.7X1-	T44.7X2-	T44.7X3-	T44.7X4-	T44.7X5-	T44.7X6-
Acecarbromal	T42.6X1-	T42.6X2-	T42.6X3-	T42.6X4-	T42.6X5-	T42.6X6-
Aceclidine	T44.1X1-	T44.1X2-	T44.1X3-	T44.1X4-	T44.1X5-	T44.1X6-
Acedapsone	T37.0X1-	T37.0X2-	T37.0X3-	T37.0X4-	T37.0X5-	T37.0X6-
Acefylline piperazine	T48.6X1-	T48.6X2-	T48.6X3-	T48.6X4-	T48.6X5-	T48.6X6-
Acemorphan	T40.2X1-	T40.2X2-	T40.2X3-	T40.2X4-	T40.2X5-	T40.2X6-
Acenocoumarin	T45.511-	T45.512-	T45.513-	T45.514-	T45.515-	T45.516-
Acenocoumarol	T45.511-	T45.512-	T45.513-	T45.514-	T45.515-	T45.516-
Acepifylline	T48.6X1-	T48.6X2-	T48.6X3-	T48.6X4-	T48.6X5-	T48.6X6-
Acepromazine	T43.3X1-	T43.3X2-	T43.3X3-	T43.3X4-	T43.3X5-	T43.3X6-
Acesulfamethoxypyridazine	T37.0X1-	T37.0X2-	T37.0X3-	T37.0X4-	T37.0X5-	T37.0X6-
Acetal	T52.8X1-	T52.8X2-	T52.8X3-	T52.8X4-	-	-
Acetaldehyde (vapor)	T52.8X1-	T52.8X2-	T52.8X3-	T52.8X4-	-	-
liquid	T65.891-	T65.892-	T65.893-	T65.894-	-	-
P-Acetamidophenol	T39.1X1-	T39.1X2-	T39.1X3-	T39.1X4-	T39.1X5-	T39.1X6-
Acetaminophen	T39.1X1-	T39.1X2-	T39.1X3-	T39.1X4-	T39.1X5-	T39.1X6-
Acetaminosalol	T39.1X1-	T39.1X2-	T39.1X3-	T39.1X4-	T39.1X5-	T39.1X6-
Acetanilide	T39.1X1-	T39.1X2-	T39.1X3-	T39.1X4-	T39.1X5-	T39.1X6-
Acetarsol	T37.3X1-	T37.3X2-	T37.3X3-	T37.3X4-	T37.3X5-	T37.3X6-
Acetazolamide	T50.2X1-	T50.2X2-	T50.2X3-	T50.2X4-	T50.2X5-	T50.2X6-
Acetiamine	T45.2X1-	T45.2X2-	T45.2X3-	T45.2X4-	T45.2X5-	T45.2X6-
Acetic						
acid	T54.2X1-	T54.2X2-	T54.2X3-	T54.2X4-	-	-
with sodium acetate (ointment)	T49.3X1-	T49.3X2-	T49.3X3-	T49.3X4-	T49.3X5-	T49.3X6-
ester (solvent) (vapor)	T52.8X1-	T52.8X2-	T52.8X3-	T52.8X4-	-	-
irrigating solution	T50.3X1-	T50.3X2-	T50.3X3-	T50.3X4-	T50.3X5-	T50.3X6-
medicinal (lotion)	T49.2X1-	T49.2X2-	T49.2X3-	T49.2X4-	T49.2X5-	T49.2X6-
anhydride	T65.891-	T65.892-	T65.893-	T65.894-	-	-
ether (vapor)	T52.8X1-	T52.8X2-	T52.8X3-	T52.8X4-	-	-
Acetohexamide	T38.3X1-	T38.3X2-	T38.3X3-	T38.3X4-	T38.3X5-	T38.3X6-
Acetohydroxamic acid	T50.991-	T50.992-	T50.993-	T50.994-	T50.995-	T50.996-
Acetomenaphthone	T45.7X1-	T45.7X2-	T45.7X3-	T45.7X4-	T45.7X5-	T45.7X6-
Acetomorphine	T40.1X1-	T40.1X2-	T40.1X3-	T40.1X4-	-	-
Acetone (oils)	T52.4X1-	T52.4X2-	T52.4X3-	T52.4X4-	-	-
chlorinated	T52.4X1-	T52.4X2-	T52.4X3-	T52.4X4-	-	-
vapor	T52.4X1-	T52.4X2-	T52.4X3-	T52.4X4-	-	-
Acetonitrile	T52.8X1-	T52.8X2-	T52.8X3-	T52.8X4-	-	-
Acetophenazine	T43.3X1-	T43.3X2-	T43.3X3-	T43.3X4-	T43.3X5-	T43.3X6-
Acetophenetedin	T39.1X1-	T39.1X2-	T39.1X3-	T39.1X4-	T39.1X5-	T39.1X6-
Acetophenone	T52.4X1-	T52.4X2-	T52.4X3-	T52.4X4-	-	-
Acetorphine	T40.2X1-	T40.2X2-	T40.2X3-	T40.2X4-	-	-
Acetosulfone (sodium)	T37.1X1-	T37.1X2-	T37.1X3-	T37.1X4-	T37.1X5-	T37.1X6-
Acetrizoate (sodium)	T50.8X1-	T50.8X2-	T50.8X3-	T50.8X4-	T50.8X5-	T50.8X6-

Substance	Poisoning Accidental (unintentional)	Poisoning Intentional self-harm	Poisoning Assault	Poisoning Undetermined	Adverse effect	Underdosing
Acetrizoic acid	T50.8X1-	T50.8X2-	T50.8X3-	T50.8X4-	T50.8X5-	T50.8X6-
Acetyl						
bromide	T53.6X1-	T53.6X2-	T53.6X3-	T53.6X4-	-	-
chloride	T53.6X1-	T53.6X2-	T53.6X3-	T53.6X4-	-	-
Acetylcarbromal	T42.6X1-	T42.6X2-	T42.6X3-	T42.6X4-	T42.6X5-	T42.6X6-
Acetylcholine						
chloride	T44.1X1-	T44.1X2-	T44.1X3-	T44.1X4-	T44.1X5-	T44.1X6-
derivative	T44.1X1-	T44.1X2-	T44.1X3-	T44.1X4-	T44.1X5-	T44.1X6-
Acetylcysteine	T48.4X1-	T48.4X2-	T48.4X3-	T48.4X4-	T48.4X5-	T48.4X6-
Acetyldigitoxin	T46.0X1-	T46.0X2-	T46.0X3-	T46.0X4-	T46.0X5-	T46.0X6-
Acetyldigoxin	T46.0X1-	T46.0X2-	T46.0X3-	T46.0X4-	T46.0X5-	T46.0X6-
Acetyldihydrocodeine	T40.2X1-	T40.2X2-	T40.2X3-	T40.2X4-	-	-
Acetyldihydrocodeinone	T40.2X1-	T40.2X2-	T40.2X3-	T40.2X4-	-	-
Acetylene (gas)	T59.891-	T59.892-	T59.893-	T59.894-		
dichloride	T53.6X1-	T53.6X2-	T53.6X3-	T53.6X4-	-	-
incomplete combustion of	T58.11X-	T58.12X-	T58.13X-	T58.14X-	-	-
industrial	T59.891-	T59.892-	T59.893-	T59.894-	-	-
tetrachloride	T53.6X1-	T53.6X2-	T53.6X3-	T53.6X4-	-	-
vapor	T53.6X1-	T53.6X2-	T53.6X3-	T53.6X4-	-	-
Acetylpheneturide	T42.6X1-	T42.6X2-	T42.6X3-	T42.6X4-	T42.6X5-	T42.6X6-
Acetylphenylhydrazine	T39.8X1-	T39.8X2-	T39.8X3-	T39.8X4-	T39.8X5-	T39.8X6-
Acetylsalicylic acid (salts)	T39.011-	T39.012-	T39.013-	T39.014-	T39.015-	T39.016-
enteric coated	T39.011-	T39.012-	T39.013-	T39.014-	T39.015-	T39.016-
Acetylsulfamethoxypyridazine	T37.0X1-	T37.0X2-	T37.0X3-	T37.0X4-	T37.0X5-	T37.0X6-
Achromycin	T36.4X1-	T36.4X2-	T36.4X3-	T36.4X4-	T36.4X5-	T36.4X6-
ophthalmic preparation	T49.5X1-	T49.5X2-	T49.5X3-	T49.5X4-	T49.5X5-	T49.5X6-
topical NEC	T49.0X1-	T49.0X2-	T49.0X3-	T49.0X4-	T49.0X5-	T49.0X6-
Aciclovir	T37.5X1-	T37.5X2-	T37.5X3-	T37.5X4-	T37.5X5-	T37.5X6-
Acid (corrosive) NEC	T54.2X1-	T54.2X2-	T54.2X3-	T54.2X4-	-	-
Acidifying agent NEC	T50.901-	T50.902-	T50.903-	T50.904-	T50.905-	T50.906-
Acipimox	T46.6X1-	T46.6X2-	T46.6X3-	T46.6X4-	T46.6X5-	T46.6X6-
Acitretin	T50.991-	T50.992-	T50.993-	T50.994-	T50.995-	T50.996-
Aclarubicin	T45.1X1-	T45.1X2-	T45.1X3-	T45.1X4-	T45.1X5-	T45.1X6-
Aclatonium napadisilate	T48.1X1-	T48.1X2-	T48.1X3-	T48.1X4-	T48.1X5-	T48.1X6-
Aconite (wild)	T46.991-	T46.992-	T46.993-	T46.994-	T46.995-	T46.996-
Aconitine	T46.991-	T46.992-	T46.993-	T46.994-	T46.995-	T46.996-
Aconitum ferox	T46.991-	T46.992-	T46.993-	T46.994-	T46.995-	T46.996-
Acridine	T65.6X1-	T65.6X2-	T65.6X3-	T65.6X4-	-	-
vapor	T59.891-	T59.892-	T59.893-	T59.894-	-	-
Acriflavine	T37.91X-	T37.92X-	T37.93X-	T37.94X-	T37.95X-	T37.96X-
Acriflavinium chloride	T49.0X1-	T49.0X2-	T49.0X3-	T49.0X4-	T49.0X5-	T49.0X6-
Acrinol	T49.0X1-	T49.0X2-	T49.0X3-	T49.0X4-	T49.0X5-	T49.0X6-
Acrisorcin	T49.0X1-	T49.0X2-	T49.0X3-	T49.0X4-	T49.0X5-	T49.0X6-
Acrivastine	T45.0X1-	T45.0X2-	T45.0X3-	T45.0X4-	T45.0X5-	T45.0X6-
Acrolein (gas)	T59.891-	T59.892-	T59.893-	T59.894-	-	-
liquid	T54.1X1-	T54.1X2-	T54.1X3-	T54.1X4-	-	-
Acrylamide	T65.891-	T65.892-	T65.893-	T65.894-	-	-
Acrylic resin	T49.3X1-	T49.3X2-	T49.3X3-	T49.3X4-	T49.3X5-	T49.3X6-
Acrylonitrile	T65.891-	T65.892-	T65.893-	T65.894-	-	-
Actaea spicata	T62.2X1-	T62.2X2-	T62.2X3-	T62.2X4-	-	-
berry	T62.1X1-	T62.1X2-	T62.1X3-	T62.1X4-	-	-
Acterol	T37.3X1-	T37.3X2-	T37.3X3-	T37.3X4-	T37.3X5-	T37.3X6-
ACTH	T38.811-	T38.812-	T38.813-	T38.814-	T38.815-	T38.816-
Actinomycin C	T45.1X1-	T45.1X2-	T45.1X3-	T45.1X4-	T45.1X5-	T45.1X6-
Actinomycin D	T45.1X1-	T45.1X2-	T45.1X3-	T45.1X4-	T45.1X5-	T45.1X6-
Activated charcoal — *see also Charcoal, medicinal*	T47.6X1-	T47.6X2-	T47.6X3-	T47.6X4-	T47.6X5-	T47.6X6-
Acyclovir	T37.5X1-	T37.5X2-	T37.5X3-	T37.5X4-	T37.5X5-	T37.5X6-

Substance	Poisoning Accidental (unintentional)	Poisoning Intentional self-harm	Poisoning Assault	Poisoning Undetermined	Adverse effect	Underdosing
Adenine	T45.2X1-	T45.2X2-	T45.2X3-	T45.2X4-	T45.2X5-	T45.2X6-
arabinoside	T37.5X1-	T37.5X2-	T37.5X3-	T37.5X4-	T37.5X5-	T37.5X6-
Adenosine (phosphate)	T46.2X1-	T46.2X2-	T46.2X3-	T46.2X4-	T46.2X5-	T46.2X6-
ADH	T38.891-	T38.892-	T38.893-	T38.894-	T38.895-	T38.896-
Adhesive NEC	T65.891-	T65.892-	T65.893-	T65.894-	-	-
Adicillin	T36.0X1-	T36.0X2-	T36.0X3-	T36.0X4-	T36.0X5-	T36.0X6-
Adiphenine	T44.3X1-	T44.3X2-	T44.3X3-	T44.3X4-	T44.3X5-	T44.3X6-
Adipiodone	T50.8X1-	T50.8X2-	T50.8X3-	T50.8X4-	T50.8X5-	T50.8X6-
Adjunct, pharmaceutical	T50.901-	T50.902-	T50.903-	T50.904-	T50.905-	T50.906-
Adrenal (extract, cortex or medulla) (glucocorticoids) (hormones) (mineralocorticoids)	T38.0X1-	T38.0X2-	T38.0X3-	T38.0X4-	T38.0X5-	T38.0X6-
ENT agent	T49.6X1-	T49.6X2-	T49.6X3-	T49.6X4-	T49.6X5-	T49.6X6-
ophthalmic preparation	T49.5X1-	T49.5X2-	T49.5X3-	T49.5X4-	T49.5X5-	T49.5X6-
topical NEC	T49.0X1-	T49.0X2-	T49.0X3-	T49.0X4-	T49.0X5-	T49.0X6-
Adrenaline	T44.5X1-	T44.5X2-	T44.5X3-	T44.5X4-	T44.5X5-	T44.5X6-
Adrenalin — *see Adrenaline*						
Adrenergic NEC	T44.901-	T44.902-	T44.903-	T44.904-	T44.905-	T44.906-
blocking agent NEC	T44.8X1-	T44.8X2-	T44.8X3-	T44.8X4-	T44.8X5-	T44.8X6-
beta, heart	T44.7X1-	T44.7X2-	T44.7X3-	T44.7X4-	T44.7X5-	T44.7X6-
specified NEC	T44.991-	T44.992-	T44.993-	T44.994-	T44.995-	T44.996-
Adrenochrome						
(mono) semicarbazone	T46.991-	T46.992-	T46.993-	T46.994-	T46.995-	T46.996-
derivative	T46.991-	T46.992-	T46.993-	T46.994-	T46.995-	T46.996-
Adrenocorticotrophic hormone	T38.811-	T38.812-	T38.813-	T38.814-	T38.815-	T38.816-
Adrenocorticotrophin	T38.811-	T38.812-	T38.813-	T38.814-	T38.815-	T38.816-
Adriamycin	T45.1X1-	T45.1X2-	T45.1X3-	T45.1X4-	T45.1X5-	T45.1X6-
Aerosol spray NEC	T65.91X-	T65.92X-	T65.93X-	T65.94X-	-	-
Aerosporin	T36.8X1-	T36.8X2-	T36.8X3-	T36.8X4-	T36.8X5-	T36.8X6-
ENT agent	T49.6X1-	T49.6X2-	T49.6X3-	T49.6X4-	T49.6X5-	T49.6X6-
ophthalmic preparation	T49.5X1-	T49.5X2-	T49.5X3-	T49.5X4-	T49.5X5-	T49.5X6-
topical NEC	T49.0X1-	T49.0X2-	T49.0X3-	T49.0X4-	T49.0X5-	T49.0X6-
Aethusa cynapium	T62.2X1-	T62.2X2-	T62.2X3-	T62.2X4-	-	-
Afghanistan black	T40.7X1-	T40.7X2-	T40.7X3-	T40.7X4-	T40.7X5-	T40.7X6-
Aflatoxin	T64.01X-	T64.02X-	T64.03X-	T64.04X-	-	-
Afloqualone	T42.8X1-	T42.8X2-	T42.8X3-	T42.8X4-	T42.8X5-	T42.8X6-
African boxwood	T62.2X1-	T62.2X2-	T62.2X3-	T62.2X4-	-	-
Agar	T47.4X1-	T47.4X2-	T47.4X3-	T47.4X4-	T47.4X5-	T47.4X6-
Agonist						
predominantly						
alpha-adrenoreceptor	T44.4X1-	T44.4X2-	T44.4X3-	T44.4X4-	T44.4X5-	T44.4X6-
beta-adrenoreceptor	T44.5X1-	T44.5X2-	T44.5X3-	T44.5X4-	T44.5X5-	T44.5X6-
Agricultural agent NEC	T65.91X-	T65.92X-	T65.93X-	T65.94X-	-	-
Agrypnal	T42.3X1-	T42.3X2-	T42.3X3-	T42.3X4-	T42.3X5-	T42.3X6-
AHLG	T50.Z11-	T50.Z12-	T50.Z13-	T50.Z14-	T50.Z15-	T50.Z16-
Air contaminant (s) , source/type NOS	T65.91X-	T65.92X-	T65.93X-	T65.94X-	-	-
Ajmaline	T46.2X1-	T46.2X2-	T46.2X3-	T46.2X4-	T46.2X5-	T46.2X6-
Akee	T62.1X1-	T62.1X2-	T62.1X3-	T62.1X4-	-	-
Akrinol	T49.0X1-	T49.0X2-	T49.0X3-	T49.0X4-	T49.0X5-	T49.0X6-
Akritoin	T37.8X1-	T37.8X2-	T37.8X3-	T37.8X4-	T37.8X5-	T37.8X6-
Alacepril	T46.4X1-	T46.4X2-	T46.4X3-	T46.4X4-	T46.4X5-	T46.4X6-
Alantolactone	T37.4X1-	T37.4X2-	T37.4X3-	T37.4X4-	T37.4X5-	T37.4X6-
Albamycin	T36.8X1-	T36.8X2-	T36.8X3-	T36.8X4-	T36.8X5-	T36.8X6-
Albendazole	T37.4X1-	T37.4X2-	T37.4X3-	T37.4X4-	T37.4X5-	T37.4X6-
Albumin						
bovine	T45.8X1-	T45.8X2-	T45.8X3-	T45.8X4-	T45.8X5-	T45.8X6-
human serum	T45.8X1-	T45.8X2-	T45.8X3-	T45.8X4-	T45.8X5-	T45.8X6-
salt-poor	T45.8X1-	T45.8X2-	T45.8X3-	T45.8X4-	T45.8X5-	T45.8X6-

Substance	Poisoning Accidental (unintentional)	Poisoning Intentional self-harm	Poisoning Assault	Poisoning Undetermined	Adverse effect	Underdosing
Albumin (*continued*)						
normal human serum	T45.8X1-	T45.8X2-	T45.8X3-	T45.8X4-	T45.8X5-	T45.8X6-
Albuterol	T48.6X1-	T48.6X2-	T48.6X3-	T48.6X4-	T48.6X5-	T48.6X6-
Albutoin	T42.0X1-	T42.0X2-	T42.0X3-	T42.0X4-	T42.0X5-	T42.0X6-
Alclometasone	T49.0X1-	T49.0X2-	T49.0X3-	T49.0X4-	T49.0X5-	T49.0X6-
Alcohol	T51.91X-	T51.92X-	T51.93X-	T51.94X-	-	-
absolute	T51.0X1-	T51.0X2-	T51.0X3-	T51.0X4-	-	-
beverage	T51.0X1-	T51.0X2-	T51.0X3-	T51.0X4-	-	-
allyl	T51.8X1-	T51.8X2-	T51.8X3-	T51.8X4-	-	-
amyl	T51.3X1-	T51.3X2-	T51.3X3-	T51.3X4-	-	-
antifreeze	T51.1X1-	T51.1X2-	T51.1X3-	T51.1X4-	-	-
beverage	T51.0X1-	T51.0X2-	T51.0X3-	T51.0X4-	-	-
butyl	T51.3X1-	T51.3X2-	T51.3X3-	T51.3X4-	-	-
dehydrated	T51.0X1-	T51.0X2-	T51.0X3-	T51.0X4-	-	-
beverage	T51.0X1-	T51.0X2-	T51.0X3-	T51.0X4-	-	-
denatured	T51.0X1-	T51.0X2-	T51.0X3-	T51.0X4-	-	-
deterrent NEC	T50.6X1-	T50.6X2-	T50.6X3-	T50.6X4-	T50.6X5-	T50.6X6-
diagnostic (gastric function)	T50.8X1-	T50.8X2-	T50.8X3-	T50.8X4-	T50.8X5-	T50.8X6-
ethyl	T51.0X1-	T51.0X2-	T51.0X3-	T51.0X4-	-	-
beverage	T51.0X1-	T51.0X2-	T51.0X3-	T51.0X4-	-	-
grain	T51.0X1-	T51.0X2-	T51.0X3-	T51.0X4-	-	-
beverage	T51.0X1-	T51.0X2-	T51.0X3-	T51.0X4-	-	-
industrial	T51.0X1-	T51.0X2-	T51.0X3-	T51.0X4-	-	-
isopropyl	T51.2X1-	T51.2X2-	T51.2X3-	T51.2X4-	-	-
methyl	T51.1X1-	T51.1X2-	T51.1X3-	T51.1X4-	-	-
preparation for consumption	T51.0X1-	T51.0X2-	T51.0X3-	T51.0X4-	-	-
propyl	T51.3X1-	T51.3X2-	T51.3X3-	T51.3X4-	-	-
secondary	T51.2X1-	T51.2X2-	T51.2X3-	T51.2X4-	-	-
radiator	T51.1X1-	T51.1X2-	T51.1X3-	T51.1X4-	-	-
rubbing	T51.2X1-	T51.2X2-	T51.2X3-	T51.2X4-	-	-
specified type NEC	T51.8X1-	T51.8X2-	T51.8X3-	T51.8X4-	-	-
surgical	T51.0X1-	T51.0X2-	T51.0X3-	T51.0X4-	-	-
vapor (from any type of Alcohol)	T59.891-	T59.892-	T59.893-	T59.894-	-	-
wood	T51.1X1-	T51.1X2-	T51.1X3-	T51.1X4-	-	-
Alcuronium (chloride)	T48.1X1-	T48.1X2-	T48.1X3-	T48.1X4-	T48.1X5-	T48.1X6-
Aldactone	T50.0X1-	T50.0X2-	T50.0X3-	T50.0X4-	T50.0X5-	T50.0X6-
Aldesulfone sodium	T37.1X1-	T37.1X2-	T37.1X3-	T37.1X4-	T37.1X5-	T37.1X6-
Aldicarb	T60.0X1-	T60.0X2-	T60.0X3-	T60.0X4-	-	-
Aldomet	T46.5X1-	T46.5X2-	T46.5X3-	T46.5X4-	T46.5X5-	T46.5X6-
Aldosterone	T50.0X1-	T50.0X2-	T50.0X3-	T50.0X4-	T50.0X5-	T50.0X6-
Aldrin (dust)	T60.1X1-	T60.1X2-	T60.1X3-	T60.1X4-	-	-
Aleve — *see Naproxen*						
Alexitol sodium	T47.1X1-	T47.1X2-	T47.1X3-	T47.1X4-	T47.1X5-	T47.1X6-
Alfacalcidol	T45.2X1-	T45.2X2-	T45.2X3-	T45.2X4-	T45.2X5-	T45.2X6-
Alfadolone	T41.1X1-	T41.1X2-	T41.1X3-	T41.1X4-	T41.1X5-	T41.1X6-
Alfaxalone	T41.1X1-	T41.1X2-	T41.1X3-	T41.1X4-	T41.1X5-	T41.1X6-
Alfentanil	T40.4X1-	T40.4X2-	T40.4X3-	T40.4X4-	T40.4X5-	T40.4X6-
Alfuzosin (hydrochloride)	T44.8X1-	T44.8X2-	T44.8X3-	T44.8X4-	T44.8X5-	T44.8X6-
Algae (harmful) (toxin)	T65.821-	T65.822-	T65.823-	T65.824-	-	-
Algeldrate	T47.1X1-	T47.1X2-	T47.1X3-	T47.1X4-	T47.1X5-	T47.1X6-
Algin	T47.8X1-	T47.8X2-	T47.8X3-	T47.8X4-	T47.8X5-	T47.8X6-
Alglucerase	T45.3X1-	T45.3X2-	T45.3X3-	T45.3X4-	T45.3X5-	T45.3X6-
Alidase	T45.3X1-	T45.3X2-	T45.3X3-	T45.3X4-	T45.3X5-	T45.3X6-
Alimemazine	T43.3X1-	T43.3X2-	T43.3X3-	T43.3X4-	T43.3X5-	T43.3X6-
Aliphatic thiocyanates	T65.0X1-	T65.0X2-	T65.0X3-	T65.0X4-	-	-
Alizapride	T45.0X1-	T45.0X2-	T45.0X3-	T45.0X4-	T45.0X5-	T45.0X6-
Alkali (caustic)	T54.3X1-	T54.3X2-	T54.3X3-	T54.3X4-	-	-
Alkaline antiseptic solution (aromatic)	T49.6X1-	T49.6X2-	T49.6X3-	T49.6X4-	T49.6X5-	T49.6X6-
Alkalinizing agents (medicinal)	T50.901-	T50.902-	T50.903-	T50.904-	T50.905-	T50.906-

Substance	Poisoning Accidental (unintentional)	Poisoning Intentional self-harm	Poisoning Assault	Poisoning Undetermined	Adverse effect	Underdosing
Alkalizing agent NEC	T50.901-	T50.902-	T50.903-	T50.904-	T50.905-	T50.906-
Alka-seltzer	T39.011-	T39.012-	T39.013-	T39.014-	T39.015-	T39.016-
Alkavervir	T46.5X1-	T46.5X2-	T46.5X3-	T46.5X4-	T46.5X5-	T46.5X6-
Alkonium (bromide)	T49.0X1-	T49.0X2-	T49.0X3-	T49.0X4-	T49.0X5-	T49.0X6-
Alkylating drug NEC	T45.1X1-	T45.1X2-	T45.1X3-	T45.1X4-	T45.1X5-	T45.1X6-
antimyeloproliferative	T45.1X1-	T45.1X2-	T45.1X3-	T45.1X4-	T45.1X5-	T45.1X6-
lymphatic	T45.1X1-	T45.1X2-	T45.1X3-	T45.1X4-	T45.1X5-	T45.1X6-
Alkylisocyanate	T65.0X1-	T65.0X2-	T65.0X3-	T65.0X4-	-	-
Allantoin	T49.4X1-	T49.4X2-	T49.4X3-	T49.4X4-	T49.4X5-	T49.4X6-
Allegron	T43.011-	T43.012-	T43.013-	T43.014-	T43.015-	T43.016-
Allethrin	T49.0X1-	T49.0X2-	T49.0X3-	T49.0X4-	T49.0X5-	T49.0X6-
Allobarbital	T42.3X1-	T42.3X2-	T42.3X3-	T42.3X4-	T42.3X5-	T42.3X6-
Allopurinol	T50.4X1-	T50.4X2-	T50.4X3-	T50.4X4-	T50.4X5-	T50.4X6-
Allyl						
Alcohol	T51.8X1-	T51.8X2-	T51.8X3-	T51.8X4-	-	-
disulfide	T46.6X1-	T46.6X2-	T46.6X3-	T46.6X4-	T46.6X5-	T46.6X6-
Allylestrenol	T38.5X1-	T38.5X2-	T38.5X3-	T38.5X4-	T38.5X5-	T38.5X6-
Allylisopropylacetylurea	T42.6X1-	T42.6X2-	T42.6X3-	T42.6X4-	T42.6X5-	T42.6X6-
Allylisopropylmalonylurea	T42.3X1-	T42.3X2-	T42.3X3-	T42.3X4-	T42.3X5-	T42.3X6-
Allylthiourea	T49.3X1-	T49.3X2-	T49.3X3-	T49.3X4-	T49.3X5-	T49.3X6-
Allyltribromide	T42.6X1-	T42.6X2-	T42.6X3-	T42.6X4-	T42.6X5-	T42.6X6-
Allypropymal	T42.3X1-	T42.3X2-	T42.3X3-	T42.3X4-	T42.3X5-	T42.3X6-
Almagate	T47.1X1-	T47.1X2-	T47.1X3-	T47.1X4-	T47.1X5-	T47.1X6-
Almasilate	T47.1X1-	T47.1X2-	T47.1X3-	T47.1X4-	T47.1X5-	T47.1X6-
Almitrine	T50.7X1-	T50.7X2-	T50.7X3-	T50.7X4-	T50.7X5-	T50.7X6-
Aloes	T47.2X1-	T47.2X2-	T47.2X3-	T47.2X4-	T47.2X5-	T47.2X6-
Aloglutamol	T47.1X1-	T47.1X2-	T47.1X3-	T47.1X4-	T47.1X5-	T47.1X6-
Aloin	T47.2X1-	T47.2X2-	T47.2X3-	T47.2X4-	T47.2X5-	T47.2X6-
Aloxidone	T42.2X1-	T42.2X2-	T42.2X3-	T42.2X4-	T42.2X5-	T42.2X6-
Alpha						
acetyldigoxin	T46.0X1-	T46.0X2-	T46.0X3-	T46.0X4-	T46.0X5-	T46.0X6-
adrenergic blocking drug	T44.6X1-	T44.6X2-	T44.6X3-	T44.6X4-	T44.6X5-	T44.6X6-
amylase	T45.3X1-	T45.3X2-	T45.3X3-	T45.3X4-	T45.3X5-	T45.3X6-
tocoferol (acetate)	T45.2X1-	T45.2X2-	T45.2X3-	T45.2X4-	T45.2X5-	T45.2X6-
tocopherol	T45.2X1-	T45.2X2-	T45.2X3-	T45.2X4-	T45.2X5-	T45.2X6-
Alphadolone	T41.1X1-	T41.1X2-	T41.1X3-	T41.1X4-	T41.1X5-	T41.1X6-
Alphaprodine	T40.4X1-	T40.4X2-	T40.4X3-	T40.4X4-	T40.4X5-	T40.4X6-
Alphaxalone	T41.1X1-	T41.1X2-	T41.1X3-	T41.1X4-	T41.1X5-	T41.1X6-
Alprazolam	T42.4X1-	T42.4X2-	T42.4X3-	T42.4X4-	T42.4X5-	T42.4X6-
Alprenolol	T44.7X1-	T44.7X2-	T44.7X3-	T44.7X4-	T44.7X5-	T44.7X6-
Alprostadil	T46.7X1-	T46.7X2-	T46.7X3-	T46.7X4-	T46.7X5-	T46.7X6-
Alsactide	T38.811-	T38.812-	T38.813-	T38.814-	T38.815-	T38.816-
Alseroxylon	T46.5X1-	T46.5X2-	T46.5X3-	T46.5X4-	T46.5X5-	T46.5X6-
Alteplase	T45.611-	T45.612-	T45.613-	T45.614-	T45.615-	T45.616-
Altizide	T50.2X1-	T50.2X2-	T50.2X3-	T50.2X4-	T50.2X5-	T50.2X6-
Altretamine	T45.1X1-	T45.1X2-	T45.1X3-	T45.1X4-	T45.1X5-	T45.1X6-
Alum (medicinal)	T49.4X1-	T49.4X2-	T49.4X3-	T49.4X4-	T49.4X5-	T49.4X6-
nonmedicinal (ammonium) (potassium)	T56.891-	T56.892-	T56.893-	T56.894-	-	-
Aluminium, aluminum						
acetate	T49.2X1-	T49.2X2-	T49.2X3-	T49.2X4-	T49.2X5-	T49.2X6-
solution	T49.0X1-	T49.0X2-	T49.0X3-	T49.0X4-	T49.0X5-	T49.0X6-
aspirin	T39.011-	T39.012-	T39.013-	T39.014-	T39.015-	T39.016-
bis (acetylsalicylate)	T39.011-	T39.012-	T39.013-	T39.014-	T39.015-	T39.016-
carbonate (gel, basic)	T47.1X1-	T47.1X2-	T47.1X3-	T47.1X4-	T47.1X5-	T47.1X6-
chlorhydroxide-complex	T47.1X1-	T47.1X2-	T47.1X3-	T47.1X4-	T47.1X5-	T47.1X6-
chloride	T49.2X1-	T49.2X2-	T49.2X3-	T49.2X4-	T49.2X5-	T49.2X6-
clofibrate	T46.6X1-	T46.6X2-	T46.6X3-	T46.6X4-	T46.6X5-	T46.6X6-
diacetate	T49.2X1-	T49.2X2-	T49.2X3-	T49.2X4-	T49.2X5-	T49.2X6-

Substance	Poisoning Accidental (unintentional)	Poisoning Intentional self-harm	Poisoning Assault	Poisoning Undetermined	Adverse effect	Underdosing
Aluminium, aluminum (continued)						
glycinate	T47.1X1-	T47.1X2-	T47.1X3-	T47.1X4-	T47.1X5-	T47.1X6-
hydroxide (gel)	T47.1X1-	T47.1X2-	T47.1X3-	T47.1X4-	T47.1X5-	T47.1X6-
hydroxide-magnesium carb. gel	T47.1X1-	T47.1X2-	T47.1X3-	T47.1X4-	T47.1X5-	T47.1X6-
magnesium silicate	T47.1X1-	T47.1X2-	T47.1X3-	T47.1X4-	T47.1X5-	T47.1X6-
nicotinate	T46.7X1-	T46.7X2-	T46.7X3-	T46.7X4-	T46.7X5-	T46.7X6-
ointment (surgical) (topical)	T49.3X1-	T49.3X2-	T49.3X3-	T49.3X4-	T49.3X5-	T49.3X6-
phosphate	T47.1X1-	T47.1X2-	T47.1X3-	T47.1X4-	T47.1X5-	T47.1X6-
salicylate	T39.091-	T39.092-	T39.093-	T39.094-	T39.095-	T39.096-
silicate	T47.1X1-	T47.1X2-	T47.1X3-	T47.1X4-	T47.1X5-	T47.1X6-
sodium silicate	T47.1X1-	T47.1X2-	T47.1X3-	T47.1X4-	T47.1X5-	T47.1X6-
subacetate	T49.2X1-	T49.2X2-	T49.2X3-	T49.2X4-	T49.2X5-	T49.2X6-
sulfate	T49.0X1-	T49.0X2-	T49.0X3-	T49.0X4-	T49.0X5-	T49.0X6-
tannate	T47.6X1-	T47.6X2-	T47.6X3-	T47.6X4-	T47.6X5-	T47.6X6-
topical NEC	T49.3X1-	T49.3X2-	T49.3X3-	T49.3X4-	T49.3X5-	T49.3X6-
Alurate	T42.3X1-	T42.3X2-	T42.3X3-	T42.3X4-	T42.3X5-	T42.3X6-
Alverine	T44.3X1-	T44.3X2-	T44.3X3-	T44.3X4-	T44.3X5-	T44.3X6-
Alvodine	T40.2X1-	T40.2X2-	T40.2X3-	T40.2X4-	T40.2X5-	T40.2X6-
Amanita phalloides	T62.0X1-	T62.0X2-	T62.0X3-	T62.0X4-	-	-
Amanitine	T62.0X1-	T62.0X2-	T62.0X3-	T62.0X4-	-	-
Amantadine	T42.8X1-	T42.8X2-	T42.8X3-	T42.8X4-	T42.8X5-	T42.8X6-
Ambazone	T49.6X1-	T49.6X2-	T49.6X3-	T49.6X4-	T49.6X5-	T49.6X6-
Ambenonium (chloride)	T44.0X1-	T44.0X2-	T44.0X3-	T44.0X4-	T44.0X5-	T44.0X6-
Ambroxol	T48.4X1-	T48.4X2-	T48.4X3-	T48.4X4-	T48.4X5-	T48.4X6-
Ambuphylline	T48.6X1-	T48.6X2-	T48.6X3-	T48.6X4-	T48.6X5-	T48.6X6-
Ambutonium bromide	T44.3X1-	T44.3X2-	T44.3X3-	T44.3X4-	T44.3X5-	T44.3X6-
Amcinonide	T49.0X1-	T49.0X2-	T49.0X3-	T49.0X4-	T49.0X5-	T49.0X6-
Amdinocilline	T36.0X1-	T36.0X2-	T36.0X3-	T36.0X4-	T36.0X5-	T36.0X6-
Ametazole	T50.8X1-	T50.8X2-	T50.8X3-	T50.8X4-	T50.8X5-	T50.8X6-
Amethocaine	T41.3X1-	T41.3X2-	T41.3X3-	T41.3X4-	T41.3X5-	T41.3X6-
regional	T41.3X1-	T41.3X2-	T41.3X3-	T41.3X4-	T41.3X5-	T41.3X6-
spinal	T41.3X1-	T41.3X2-	T41.3X3-	T41.3X4-	T41.3X5-	T41.3X6-
Amethopterin	T45.1X1-	T45.1X2-	T45.1X3-	T45.1X4-	T45.1X5-	T45.1X6-
Amezinium metilsulfate	T44.991-	T44.992-	T44.993-	T44.994-	T44.995-	T44.996-
Amfebutamone	T43.291-	T43.292-	T43.293-	T43.294-	T43.295-	T43.296-
Amfepramone	T50.5X1-	T50.5X2-	T50.5X3-	T50.5X4-	T50.5X5-	T50.5X6-
Amfetamine	T43.621-	T43.622-	T43.623-	T43.624-	T43.625-	T43.626-
Amfetaminil	T43.621-	T43.622-	T43.623-	T43.624-	T43.625-	T43.626-
Amfomycin	T36.8X1-	T36.8X2-	T36.8X3-	T36.8X4-	T36.8X5-	T36.8X6-
Amidefrine mesilate	T48.5X1-	T48.5X2-	T48.5X3-	T48.5X4-	T48.5X5-	T48.5X6-
Amidone	T40.3X1-	T40.3X2-	T40.3X3-	T40.3X4-	T40.3X5-	T40.3X6-
Amidopyrine	T39.2X1-	T39.2X2-	T39.2X3-	T39.2X4-	T39.2X5-	T39.2X6-
Amidotrizoate	T50.8X1-	T50.8X2-	T50.8X3-	T50.8X4-	T50.8X5-	T50.8X6-
Amiflamine	T43.1X1-	T43.1X2-	T43.1X3-	T43.1X4-	T43.1X5-	T43.1X6-
Amikacin	T36.5X1-	T36.5X2-	T36.5X3-	T36.5X4-	T36.5X5-	T36.5X6-
Amikhelline	T46.3X1-	T46.3X2-	T46.3X3-	T46.3X4-	T46.3X5-	T46.3X6-
Amiloride	T50.2X1-	T50.2X2-	T50.2X3-	T50.2X4-	T50.2X5-	T50.2X6-
Aminacrine	T49.0X1-	T49.0X2-	T49.0X3-	T49.0X4-	T49.0X5-	T49.0X6-
Amineptine	T43.011-	T43.012-	T43.013-	T43.014-	T43.015-	T43.016-
Aminitrozole	T37.3X1-	T37.3X2-	T37.3X3-	T37.3X4-	T37.3X5-	T37.3X6-
Amino acids	T50.3X1-	T50.3X2-	T50.3X3-	T50.3X4-	T50.3X5-	T50.3X6-
Aminoacetic acid (derivatives)	T50.3X1-	T50.3X2-	T50.3X3-	T50.3X4-	T50.3X5-	T50.3X6-
Aminoacridine	T49.0X1-	T49.0X2-	T49.0X3-	T49.0X4-	T49.0X5-	T49.0X6-
Aminobenzoic acid (-p)	T49.3X1-	T49.3X2-	T49.3X3-	T49.3X4-	T49.3X5-	T49.3X6-
4-Aminobutyric acid	T43.8X1-	T43.8X2-	T43.8X3-	T43.8X4-	T43.8X5-	T43.8X6-
Aminocaproic acid	T45.621-	T45.622-	T45.623-	T45.624-	T45.625-	T45.626-
Aminoethylisothiourium	T45.8X1-	T45.8X2-	T45.8X3-	T45.8X4-	T45.8X5-	T45.8X6-
Aminofenazone	T39.2X1-	T39.2X2-	T39.2X3-	T39.2X4-	T39.2X5-	T39.2X6-
Aminoglutethimide	T45.1X1-	T45.1X2-	T45.1X3-	T45.1X4-	T45.1X5-	T45.1X6-

Substance	Poisoning Accidental (unintentional)	Poisoning Intentional self-harm	Poisoning Assault	Poisoning Undetermined	Adverse effect	Underdosing
Aminohippuric acid	T50.8X1-	T50.8X2-	T50.8X3-	T50.8X4-	T50.8X5-	T50.8X6-
Aminomethylbenzoic acid	T45.691-	T45.692-	T45.693-	T45.694-	T45.695-	T45.696-
Aminometradine	T50.2X1-	T50.2X2-	T50.2X3-	T50.2X4-	T50.2X5-	T50.2X6-
Aminopentamide	T44.3X1-	T44.3X2-	T44.3X3-	T44.3X4-	T44.3X5-	T44.3X6-
Aminophenazone	T39.2X1-	T39.2X2-	T39.2X3-	T39.2X4-	T39.2X5-	T39.2X6-
Aminophenol	T54.0X1-	T54.0X2-	T54.0X3-	T54.0X4-	-	-
4-Aminophenol derivatives	T39.1X1-	T39.1X2-	T39.1X3-	T39.1X4-	T39.1X5-	T39.1X6-
Aminophenylpyridone	T43.591-	T43.592-	T43.593-	T43.594-	T43.595-	T43.596-
Aminophylline	T48.6X1-	T48.6X2-	T48.6X3-	T48.6X4-	T48.6X5-	T48.6X6-
Aminopterin sodium	T45.1X1-	T45.1X2-	T45.1X3-	T45.1X4-	T45.1X5-	T45.1X6-
Aminopyrine	T39.2X1-	T39.2X2-	T39.2X3-	T39.2X4-	T39.2X5-	T39.2X6-
8-Aminoquinoline drugs	T37.2X1-	T37.2X2-	T37.2X3-	T37.2X4-	T37.2X5-	T37.2X6-
Aminorex	T50.5X1-	T50.5X2-	T50.5X3-	T50.5X4-	T50.5X5-	T50.5X6-
Aminosalicylic acid	T37.1X1-	T37.1X2-	T37.1X3-	T37.1X4-	T37.1X5-	T37.1X6-
Aminosalylum	T37.1X1-	T37.1X2-	T37.1X3-	T37.1X4-	T37.1X5-	T37.1X6-
Amiodarone	T46.2X1-	T46.2X2-	T46.2X3-	T46.2X4-	T46.2X5-	T46.2X6-
Amiphenazole	T50.7X1-	T50.7X2-	T50.7X3-	T50.7X4-	T50.7X5-	T50.7X6-
Amiquinsin	T46.5X1-	T46.5X2-	T46.5X3-	T46.5X4-	T46.5X5-	T46.5X6-
Amisometradine	T50.2X1-	T50.2X2-	T50.2X3-	T50.2X4-	T50.2X5-	T50.2X6-
Amisulpride	T43.591-	T43.592-	T43.593-	T43.594-	T43.595-	T43.596-
Amitriptyline	T43.011-	T43.012-	T43.013-	T43.014-	T43.015-	T43.016-
Amitriptylinoxide	T43.011-	T43.012-	T43.013-	T43.014-	T43.015-	T43.016-
Amlexanox	T48.6X1-	T48.6X2-	T48.6X3-	T48.6X4-	T48.6X5-	T48.6X6-
Ammonia (fumes) (gas) (vapor)	T59.891-	T59.892-	T59.893-	T59.894-	-	-
aromatic spirit	T48.991-	T48.992-	T48.993-	T48.994-	T48.995-	T48.996-
liquid (household)	T54.3X1-	T54.3X2-	T54.3X3-	T54.3X4-	-	-
Ammoniated mercury	T49.0X1-	T49.0X2-	T49.0X3-	T49.0X4-	T49.0X5-	T49.0X6-
Ammonium						
acid tartrate	T49.5X1-	T49.5X2-	T49.5X3-	T49.5X4-	T49.5X5-	T49.5X6-
bromide	T42.6X1-	T42.6X2-	T42.6X3-	T42.6X4-	T42.6X5-	T42.6X6-
carbonate	T54.3X1-	T54.3X2-	T54.3X3-	T54.3X4-	-	-
chloride	T50.991-	T50.992-	T50.993-	T50.994-	T50.995-	T50.996-
expectorant	T48.4X1-	T48.4X2-	T48.4X3-	T48.4X4-	T48.4X5-	T48.4X6-
compounds (household) NEC	T54.3X1-	T54.3X2-	T54.3X3-	T54.3X4-	-	-
fumes (any usage)	T59.891-	T59.892-	T59.893-	T59.894-	-	-
industrial	T54.3X1-	T54.3X2-	T54.3X3-	T54.3X4-	-	-
ichthyosulronate	T49.4X1-	T49.4X2-	T49.4X3-	T49.4X4-	T49.4X5-	T49.4X6-
mandelate	T37.91X-	T37.92X-	T37.93X-	T37.94X-	T37.95X-	T37.96X-
sulfamate	T60.3X1-	T60.3X2-	T60.3X3-	T60.3X4-	-	-
sulfonate resin	T47.8X1-	T47.8X2-	T47.8X3-	T47.8X4-	T47.8X5-	T47.8X6-
Amobarbital (sodium)	T42.3X1-	T42.3X2-	T42.3X3-	T42.3X4-	T42.3X5-	T42.3X6-
Amodiaquine	T37.2X1-	T37.2X2-	T37.2X3-	T37.2X4-	T37.2X5-	T37.2X6-
Amopyroquin (e)	T37.2X1-	T37.2X2-	T37.2X3-	T37.2X4-	T37.2X5-	T37.2X6-
Amoxapine	T43.011-	T43.012-	T43.013-	T43.014-	T43.015-	T43.016-
Amoxicillin	T36.0X1-	T36.0X2-	T36.0X3-	T36.0X4-	T36.0X5-	T36.0X6-
Amperozide	T43.591-	T43.592-	T43.593-	T43.594-	T43.595-	T43.596-
Amphenidone	T43.591-	T43.592-	T43.593-	T43.594-	T43.595-	T43.596-
Amphetamine NEC	T43.621-	T43.622-	T43.623-	T43.624-	T43.625-	T43.626-
Amphomycin	T36.8X1-	T36.8X2-	T36.8X3-	T36.8X4-	T36.8X5-	T36.8X6-
Amphotalide	T37.4X1-	T37.4X2-	T37.4X3-	T37.4X4-	T37.4X5-	T37.4X6-
Amphotericin B	T36.7X1-	T36.7X2-	T36.7X3-	T36.7X4-	T36.7X5-	T36.7X6-
topical	T49.0X1-	T49.0X2-	T49.0X3-	T49.0X4-	T49.0X5-	T49.0X6-
Ampicillin	T36.0X1-	T36.0X2-	T36.0X3-	T36.0X4-	T36.0X5-	T36.0X6-
Amprotropine	T44.3X1-	T44.3X2-	T44.3X3-	T44.3X4-	T44.3X5-	T44.3X6-
Amsacrine	T45.1X1-	T45.1X2-	T45.1X3-	T45.1X4-	T45.1X5-	T45.1X6-
Amygdaline	T62.2X1-	T62.2X2-	T62.2X3-	T62.2X4-	-	-
Amyl						
acetate	T52.8X1-	T52.8X2-	T52.8X3-	T52.8X4-	-	-
vapor	T59.891-	T59.892-	T59.893-	T59.894-	-	-

AMINOHIPPURIC ACID - AMYL

Substance	Poisoning Accidental (unintentional)	Poisoning Intentional self-harm	Poisoning Assault	Poisoning Undetermined	Adverse effect	Underdosing
Amyl (*continued*)						
alcohol	T51.3X1-	T51.3X2-	T51.3X3-	T51.3X4-	-	-
chloride	T53.6X1-	T53.6X2-	T53.6X3-	T53.6X4-	-	-
formate	T52.8X1-	T52.8X2-	T52.8X3-	T52.8X4-	-	-
nitrite	T46.3X1-	T46.3X2-	T46.3X3-	T46.3X4-	T46.3X5-	T46.3X6-
propionate	T65.891-	T65.892-	T65.893-	T65.894-	-	-
Amylase	T47.5X1-	T47.5X2-	T47.5X3-	T47.5X4-	T47.5X5-	T47.5X6-
Amyleine, regional	T41.3X1-	T41.3X2-	T41.3X3-	T41.3X4-	T41.3X5-	T41.3X6-
Amylene						
dichloride	T53.6X1-	T53.6X2-	T53.6X3-	T53.6X4-	-	-
hydrate	T51.3X1-	T51.3X2-	T51.3X3-	T51.3X4-	-	-
Amylmetacresol	T49.6X1-	T49.6X2-	T49.6X3-	T49.6X4-	T49.6X5-	T49.6X6-
Amylobarbitone	T42.3X1-	T42.3X2-	T42.3X3-	T42.3X4-	T42.3X5-	T42.3X6-
Amylocaine, regional	T41.3X1-	T41.3X2-	T41.3X3-	T41.3X4-	T41.3X5-	T41.3X6-
infiltration (subcutaneous)	T41.3X1-	T41.3X2-	T41.3X3-	T41.3X4-	T41.3X5-	T41.3X6-
nerve block (peripheral) (plexus)	T41.3X1-	T41.3X2-	T41.3X3-	T41.3X4-	T41.3X5-	T41.3X6-
spinal	T41.3X1-	T41.3X2-	T41.3X3-	T41.3X4-	T41.3X5-	T41.3X6-
topical (surface)	T41.3X1-	T41.3X2-	T41.3X3-	T41.3X4-	T41.3X5-	T41.3X6-
Amylopectin	T47.6X1-	T47.6X2-	T47.6X3-	T47.6X4-	T47.6X5-	T47.6X6-
Amytal (sodium)	T42.3X1-	T42.3X2-	T42.3X3-	T42.3X4-	T42.3X5-	T42.3X6-
Anabolic steroid	T38.7X1-	T38.7X2-	T38.7X3-	T38.7X4-	T38.7X5-	T38.7X6-
Analeptic NEC	T50.7X1-	T50.7X2-	T50.7X3-	T50.7X4-	T50.7X5-	T50.7X6-
Analgesic	T39.91X-	T39.92X-	T39.93X-	T39.94X-	T39.95X-	T39.96X-
anti-inflammatory NEC	T39.91X-	T39.92X-	T39.93X-	T39.94X-	T39.95X-	T39.96X-
propionic acid derivative	T39.311-	T39.312-	T39.313-	T39.314-	T39.315-	T39.316-
antirheumatic NEC	T39.4X1-	T39.4X2-	T39.4X3-	T39.4X4-	T39.4X5-	T39.4X6-
aromatic NEC	T39.1X1-	T39.1X2-	T39.1X3-	T39.1X4-	T39.1X5-	T39.1X6-
narcotic NEC	T40.601-	T40.602-	T40.603-	T40.604-	T40.605-	T40.606-
combination	T40.601-	T40.602-	T40.603-	T40.604-	T40.605-	T40.606-
obstetric	T40.601-	T40.602-	T40.603-	T40.604-	T40.605-	T40.606-
non-narcotic NEC	T39.91X-	T39.92X-	T39.93X-	T39.94X-	T39.95X-	T39.96X-
combination	T39.91X-	T39.92X-	T39.93X-	T39.94X-	T39.95X-	T39.96X-
pyrazole	T39.2X1-	T39.2X2-	T39.2X3-	T39.2X4-	T39.2X5-	T39.2X6-
specified NEC	T39.8X1-	T39.8X2-	T39.8X3-	T39.8X4-	T39.8X5-	T39.8X6-
Analgin	T39.2X1-	T39.2X2-	T39.2X3-	T39.2X4-	T39.2X5-	T39.2X6-
Anamirta cocculus	T62.1X1-	T62.1X2-	T62.1X3-	T62.1X4-	-	-
Ancillin	T36.0X1-	T36.0X2-	T36.0X3-	T36.0X4-	T36.0X5-	T36.0X6-
Ancrod	T45.691-	T45.692-	T45.693-	T45.694-	T45.695-	T45.696-
Androgen	T38.7X1-	T38.7X2-	T38.7X3-	T38.7X4-	T38.7X5-	T38.7X6-
Androgen-estrogen mixture	T38.7X1-	T38.7X2-	T38.7X3-	T38.7X4-	T38.7X5-	T38.7X6-
Androstalone	T38.7X1-	T38.7X2-	T38.7X3-	T38.7X4-	T38.7X5-	T38.7X6-
Androstanolone	T38.7X1-	T38.7X2-	T38.7X3-	T38.7X4-	T38.7X5-	T38.7X6-
Androsterone	T38.7X1-	T38.7X2-	T38.7X3-	T38.7X4-	T38.7X5-	T38.7X6-
Anemone pulsatilla	T62.2X1-	T62.2X2-	T62.2X3-	T62.2X4-	-	-
Anesthesia						
caudal	T41.3X1-	T41.3X2-	T41.3X3-	T41.3X4-	T41.3X5-	T41.3X6-
endotracheal	T41.0X1-	T41.0X2-	T41.0X3-	T41.0X4-	T41.0X5-	T41.0X6-
epidural	T41.3X1-	T41.3X2-	T41.3X3-	T41.3X4-	T41.3X5-	T41.3X6-
inhalation	T41.0X1-	T41.0X2-	T41.0X3-	T41.0X4-	T41.0X5-	T41.0X6-
local	T41.3X1-	T41.3X2-	T41.3X3-	T41.3X4-	T41.3X5-	T41.3X6-
mucosal	T41.3X1-	T41.3X2-	T41.3X3-	T41.3X4-	T41.3X5-	T41.3X6-
muscle relaxation	T48.1X1-	T48.1X2-	T48.1X3-	T48.1X4-	T48.1X5-	T48.1X6-
nerve blocking	T41.3X1-	T41.3X2-	T41.3X3-	T41.3X4-	T41.3X5-	T41.3X6-
plexus blocking	T41.3X1-	T41.3X2-	T41.3X3-	T41.3X4-	T41.3X5-	T41.3X6-
potentiated	T41.201-	T41.202-	T41.203-	T41.204-	T41.205-	T41.206-
rectal	T41.201-	T41.202-	T41.203-	T41.204-	T41.205-	T41.206-
general	T41.201-	T41.202-	T41.203-	T41.204-	T41.205-	T41.206-
local	T41.3X1-	T41.3X2-	T41.3X3-	T41.3X4-	T41.3X5-	T41.3X6-
regional	T41.3X1-	T41.3X2-	T41.3X3-	T41.3X4-	T41.3X5-	T41.3X6-

AMYL - ANESTHESIA

Substance	Poisoning Accidental (unintentional)	Poisoning Intentional self-harm	Poisoning Assault	Poisoning Undetermined	Adverse effect	Underdosing
Anesthesia (continued)						
surface	T41.3X1-	T41.3X2-	T41.3X3-	T41.3X4-	T41.3X5-	T41.3X6-
Anesthetic NEC — *see also Anesthesia*	T41.41X-	T41.42X-	T41.43X-	T41.44X-	T41.45X-	T41.46X-
with muscle relaxant	T41.201-	T41.202-	T41.203-	T41.204-	T41.205-	T41.206-
general	T41.201-	T41.202-	T41.203-	T41.204-	T41.205-	T41.206-
local	T41.3X1-	T41.3X2-	T41.3X3-	T41.3X4-	T41.3X5-	T41.3X6-
gaseous NEC	T41.0X1-	T41.0X2-	T41.0X3-	T41.0X4-	T41.0X5-	T41.0X6-
general NEC	T41.201-	T41.202-	T41.203-	T41.204-	T41.205-	T41.206-
halogenated hydrocarbon derivatives NEC	T41.0X1-	T41.0X2-	T41.0X3-	T41.0X4-	T41.0X5-	T41.0X6-
infiltration NEC	T41.3X1-	T41.3X2-	T41.3X3-	T41.3X4-	T41.3X5-	T41.3X6-
intravenous NEC	T41.1X1-	T41.1X2-	T41.1X3-	T41.1X4-	T41.1X5-	T41.1X6-
local NEC	T41.3X1-	T41.3X2-	T41.3X3-	T41.3X4-	T41.3X5-	T41.3X6-
rectal	T41.201-	T41.202-	T41.203-	T41.204-	T41.205-	T41.206-
general	T41.201-	T41.202-	T41.203-	T41.204-	T41.205-	T41.206-
local	T41.3X1-	T41.3X2-	T41.3X3-	T41.3X4-	T41.3X5-	T41.3X6-
regional NEC	T41.3X1-	T41.3X2-	T41.3X3-	T41.3X4-	T41.3X5-	T41.3X6-
spinal NEC	T41.3X1-	T41.3X2-	T41.3X3-	T41.3X4-	T41.3X5-	T41.3X6-
thiobarbiturate	T41.1X1-	T41.1X2-	T41.1X3-	T41.1X4-	T41.1X5-	T41.1X6-
topical	T41.3X1-	T41.3X2-	T41.3X3-	T41.3X4-	T41.3X5-	T41.3X6-
Aneurine	T45.2X1-	T45.2X2-	T45.2X3-	T45.2X4-	T45.2X5-	T45.2X6-
Angio-Conray	T50.8X1-	T50.8X2-	T50.8X3-	T50.8X4-	T50.8X5-	T50.8X6-
Angiotensin	T44.5X1-	T44.5X2-	T44.5X3-	T44.5X4-	T44.5X5-	T44.5X6-
Angiotensinamide	T44.991-	T44.992-	T44.993-	T44.994-	T44.995-	T44.996-
Anhydrohydroxy-progesterone	T38.5X1-	T38.5X2-	T38.5X3-	T38.5X4-	T38.5X5-	T38.5X6-
Anhydron	T50.2X1-	T50.2X2-	T50.2X3-	T50.2X4-	T50.2X5-	T50.2X6-
Anileridine	T40.4X1-	T40.4X2-	T40.4X3-	T40.4X4-	T40.4X5-	T40.4X6-
Aniline (dye) (liquid)	T65.3X1-	T65.3X2-	T65.3X3-	T65.3X4-	-	-
analgesic	T39.1X1-	T39.1X2-	T39.1X3-	T39.1X4-	T39.1X5-	T39.1X6-
derivatives, therapeutic NEC	T39.1X1-	T39.1X2-	T39.1X3-	T39.1X4-	T39.1X5-	T39.1X6-
vapor	T65.3X1-	T65.3X2-	T65.3X3-	T65.3X4-	-	-
Aniscoropine	T44.3X1-	T44.3X2-	T44.3X3-	T44.3X4-	T44.3X5-	T44.3X6-
Anise oil	T47.5X1-	T47.5X2-	T47.5X3-	T47.5X4-	T47.5X5-	T47.5X6-
Anisidine	T65.3X1-	T65.3X2-	T65.3X3-	T65.3X4-	-	-
Anisindione	T45.511-	T45.512-	T45.513-	T45.514-	T45.515-	T45.516-
Anisotropine methyl-bromide	T44.3X1-	T44.3X2-	T44.3X3-	T44.3X4-	T44.3X5-	T44.3X6-
Anistreplase	T45.611-	T45.612-	T45.613-	T45.614-	T45.615-	T45.616-
Anorexiant (central)	T50.5X1-	T50.5X2-	T50.5X3-	T50.5X4-	T50.5X5-	T50.5X6-
Anorexic agents	T50.5X1-	T50.5X2-	T50.5X3-	T50.5X4-	T50.5X5-	T50.5X6-
Ansamycin	T36.6X1-	T36.6X2-	T36.6X3-	T36.6X4-	T36.6X5-	T36.6X6-
Ant (bite) (sting)	T63.421-	T63.422-	T63.423-	T63.424-	-	-
Ant poison — *see Insecticide*						
Antabuse	T50.6X1-	T50.6X2-	T50.6X3-	T50.6X4-	T50.6X5-	T50.6X6-
Antacid NEC	T47.1X1-	T47.1X2-	T47.1X3-	T47.1X4-	T47.1X5-	T47.1X6-
Antagonist						
Aldosterone	T50.0X1-	T50.0X2-	T50.0X3-	T50.0X4-	T50.0X5-	T50.0X6-
alpha-adrenoreceptor	T44.6X1-	T44.6X2-	T44.6X3-	T44.6X4-	T44.6X5-	T44.6X6-
anticoagulant	T45.7X1-	T45.7X2-	T45.7X3-	T45.7X4-	T45.7X5-	T45.7X6-
beta-adrenoreceptor	T44.7X1-	T44.7X2-	T44.7X3-	T44.7X4-	T44.7X5-	T44.7X6-
extrapyramidal NEC	T44.3X1-	T44.3X2-	T44.3X3-	T44.3X4-	T44.3X5-	T44.3X6-
folic acid	T45.1X1-	T45.1X2-	T45.1X3-	T45.1X4-	T45.1X5-	T45.1X6-
H2 receptor	T47.0X1-	T47.0X2-	T47.0X3-	T47.0X4-	T47.0X5-	T47.0X6-
heavy metal	T45.8X1-	T45.8X2-	T45.8X3-	T45.8X4-	T45.8X5-	T45.8X6-
narcotic analgesic	T50.7X1-	T50.7X2-	T50.7X3-	T50.7X4-	T50.7X5-	T50.7X6-
opiate	T50.7X1-	T50.7X2-	T50.7X3-	T50.7X4-	T50.7X5-	T50.7X6-
pyrimidine	T45.1X1-	T45.1X2-	T45.1X3-	T45.1X4-	T45.1X5-	T45.1X6-
serotonin	T46.5X1-	T46.5X2-	T46.5X3-	T46.5X4-	T46.5X5-	T46.5X6-
Antazolin (e)	T45.0X1-	T45.0X2-	T45.0X3-	T45.0X4-	T45.0X5-	T45.0X6-
Anterior pituitary hormone NEC	T38.811-	T38.812-	T38.813-	T38.814-	T38.815-	T38.816-

Substance	Poisoning Accidental (unintentional)	Poisoning Intentional self-harm	Poisoning Assault	Poisoning Undetermined	Adverse effect	Underdosing
Anthelmintic NEC	T37.4X1-	T37.4X2-	T37.4X3-	T37.4X4-	T37.4X5-	T37.4X6-
Anthiolimine	T37.4X1-	T37.4X2-	T37.4X3-	T37.4X4-	T37.4X5-	T37.4X6-
Anthralin	T49.4X1-	T49.4X2-	T49.4X3-	T49.4X4-	T49.4X5-	T49.4X6-
Anthramycin	T45.1X1-	T45.1X2-	T45.1X3-	T45.1X4-	T45.1X5-	T45.1X6-
Antiadrenergic NEC	T44.8X1-	T44.8X2-	T44.8X3-	T44.8X4-	T44.8X5-	T44.8X6-
Antiallergic NEC	T45.0X1-	T45.0X2-	T45.0X3-	T45.0X4-	T45.0X5-	T45.0X6-
Anti-anemic (drug) (preparation)	T45.8X1-	T45.8X2-	T45.8X3-	T45.8X4-	T45.8X5-	T45.8X6-
Antiandrogen NEC	T38.6X1-	T38.6X2-	T38.6X3-	T38.6X4-	T38.6X5-	T38.6X6-
Antianxiety drug NEC	T43.501-	T43.502-	T43.503-	T43.504-	T43.505-	T43.506-
Antiaris toxicaria	T65.891-	T65.892-	T65.893-	T65.894-	-	-
Antiarteriosclerotic drug	T46.6X1-	T46.6X2-	T46.6X3-	T46.6X4-	T46.6X5-	T46.6X6-
Antiasthmatic drug NEC	T48.6X1-	T48.6X2-	T48.6X3-	T48.6X4-	T48.6X5-	T48.6X6-
Antibiotic NEC	T36.91X-	T36.92X-	T36.93X-	T36.94X-	T36.95X-	T36.96X-
aminoglycoside	T36.5X1-	T36.5X2-	T36.5X3-	T36.5X4-	T36.5X5-	T36.5X6-
anticancer	T45.1X1-	T45.1X2-	T45.1X3-	T45.1X4-	T45.1X5-	T45.1X6-
antifungal	T36.7X1-	T36.7X2-	T36.7X3-	T36.7X4-	T36.7X5-	T36.7X6-
antimycobacterial	T36.5X1-	T36.5X2-	T36.5X3-	T36.5X4-	T36.5X5-	T36.5X6-
antineoplastic	T45.1X1-	T45.1X2-	T45.1X3-	T45.1X4-	T45.1X5-	T45.1X6-
cephalosporin (group)	T36.1X1-	T36.1X2-	T36.1X3-	T36.1X4-	T36.1X5-	T36.1X6-
chloramphenicol (group)	T36.2X1-	T36.2X2-	T36.2X3-	T36.2X4-	T36.2X5-	T36.2X6-
ENT	T49.6X1-	T49.6X2-	T49.6X3-	T49.6X4-	T49.6X5-	T49.6X6-
eye	T49.5X1-	T49.5X2-	T49.5X3-	T49.5X4-	T49.5X5-	T49.5X6-
fungicidal (local)	T49.0X1-	T49.0X2-	T49.0X3-	T49.0X4-	T49.0X5-	T49.0X6-
intestinal	T36.8X1-	T36.8X2-	T36.8X3-	T36.8X4-	T36.8X5-	T36.8X6-
b-lactam NEC	T36.1X1-	T36.1X2-	T36.1X3-	T36.1X4-	T36.1X5-	T36.1X6-
local	T49.0X1-	T49.0X2-	T49.0X3-	T49.0X4-	T49.0X5-	T49.0X6-
macrolides	T36.3X1-	T36.3X2-	T36.3X3-	T36.3X4-	T36.3X5-	T36.3X6-
polypeptide	T36.8X1-	T36.8X2-	T36.8X3-	T36.8X4-	T36.8X5-	T36.8X6-
specified NEC	T36.8X1-	T36.8X2-	T36.8X3-	T36.8X4-	T36.8X5-	T36.8X6-
tetracycline (group)	T36.4X1-	T36.4X2-	T36.4X3-	T36.4X4-	T36.4X5-	T36.4X6-
throat	T49.6X1-	T49.6X2-	T49.6X3-	T49.6X4-	T49.6X5-	T49.6X6-
Anticancer agents NEC	T45.1X1-	T45.1X2-	T45.1X3-	T45.1X4-	T45.1X5-	T45.1X6-
Anticholesterolemic drug NEC	T46.6X1-	T46.6X2-	T46.6X3-	T46.6X4-	T46.6X5-	T46.6X6-
Anticholinergic NEC	T44.3X1-	T44.3X2-	T44.3X3-	T44.3X4-	T44.3X5-	T44.3X6-
Anticholinesterase	T44.0X1-	T44.0X2-	T44.0X3-	T44.0X4-	T44.0X5-	T44.0X6-
organophosphorus	T44.0X1-	T44.0X2-	T44.0X3-	T44.0X4-	T44.0X5-	T44.0X6-
insecticide	T60.0X1-	T60.0X2-	T60.0X3-	T60.0X4-	-	-
nerve gas	T59.891-	T59.892-	T59.893-	T59.894-	-	-
reversible	T44.0X1-	T44.0X2-	T44.0X3-	T44.0X4-	T44.0X5-	T44.0X6-
ophthalmological	T49.5X1-	T49.5X2-	T49.5X3-	T49.5X4-	T49.5X5-	T49.5X6-
Anticoagulant NEC	T45.511-	T45.512-	T45.513-	T45.514-	T45.515-	T45.516-
Antagonist	T45.7X1-	T45.7X2-	T45.7X3-	T45.7X4-	T45.7X5-	T45.7X6-
Anti-common-cold drug NEC	T48.5X1-	T48.5X2-	T48.5X3-	T48.5X4-	T48.5X5-	T48.5X6-
Anticonvulsant	T42.71X-	T42.72X-	T42.73X-	T42.74X-	T42.75X-	T42.76X-
barbiturate	T42.3X1-	T42.3X2-	T42.3X3-	T42.3X4-	T42.3X5-	T42.3X6-
combination (with barbiturate)	T42.3X1-	T42.3X2-	T42.3X3-	T42.3X4-	T42.3X5-	T42.3X6-
hydantoin	T42.0X1-	T42.0X2-	T42.0X3-	T42.0X4-	T42.0X5-	T42.0X6-
hypnotic NEC	T42.6X1-	T42.6X2-	T42.6X3-	T42.6X4-	T42.6X5-	T42.6X6-
oxazolidinedione	T42.2X1-	T42.2X2-	T42.2X3-	T42.2X4-	T42.2X5-	T42.2X6-
pyrimidinedione	T42.6X1-	T42.6X2-	T42.6X3-	T42.6X4-	T42.6X5-	T42.6X6-
specified NEC	T42.6X1-	T42.6X2-	T42.6X3-	T42.6X4-	T42.6X5-	T42.6X6-
succinimide	T42.2X1-	T42.2X2-	T42.2X3-	T42.2X4-	T42.2X5-	T42.2X6-
Anti-D immunoglobulin (human)	T50.Z11-	T50.Z12-	T50.Z13-	T50.Z14-	T50.Z15-	T50.Z16-
Antidepressant	T43.201-	T43.202-	T43.203-	T43.204-	T43.205-	T43.206-
monoamine oxidase inhibitor	T43.1X1-	T43.1X2-	T43.1X3-	T43.1X4-	T43.1X5-	T43.1X6-
selective serotonin norepinephrine reuptake inhibitor	T43.211-	T43.212-	T43.213-	T43.214-	T43.215-	T43.216-
selective serotonin reuptake inhibitor	T43.221-	T43.222-	T43.223-	T43.224-	T43.225-	T43.226-
specified NEC	T43.291-	T43.292-	T43.293-	T43.294-	T43.295-	T43.296-

Substance	Poisoning Accidental (unintentional)	Poisoning Intentional self-harm	Poisoning Assault	Poisoning Undetermined	Adverse effect	Underdosing
Antidepressant (continued)						
tetracyclic	T43.021-	T43.022-	T43.023-	T43.024-	T43.025-	T43.026-
triazolopyridine	T43.211-	T43.212-	T43.213-	T43.214-	T43.215-	T43.216-
tricyclic	T43.011-	T43.012-	T43.013-	T43.014-	T43.015-	T43.016-
Antidiabetic NEC	T38.3X1-	T38.3X2-	T38.3X3-	T38.3X4-	T38.3X5-	T38.3X6-
biguanide	T38.3X1-	T38.3X2-	T38.3X3-	T38.3X4-	T38.3X5-	T38.3X6-
and sulfonyl combined	T38.3X1-	T38.3X2-	T38.3X3-	T38.3X4-	T38.3X5-	T38.3X6-
combined	T38.3X1-	T38.3X2-	T38.3X3-	T38.3X4-	T38.3X5-	T38.3X6-
sulfonylurea	T38.3X1-	T38.3X2-	T38.3X3-	T38.3X4-	T38.3X5-	T38.3X6-
Antidiarrheal drug NEC	T47.6X1-	T47.6X2-	T47.6X3-	T47.6X4-	T47.6X5-	T47.6X6-
absorbent	T47.6X1-	T47.6X2-	T47.6X3-	T47.6X4-	T47.6X5-	T47.6X6-
Antidiphtheria serum	T50.Z11-	T50.Z12-	T50.Z13-	T50.Z14-	T50.Z15-	T50.Z16-
Antidiuretic hormone	T38.891-	T38.892-	T38.893-	T38.894-	T38.895-	T38.896-
Antidote NEC	T50.6X1-	T50.6X2-		T50.6X4-	T50.6X5-	T50.6X6-
heavy metal	T45.8X1-	T45.8X2-	T45.8X3-	T45.8X4-	T45.8X5-	T45.8X6-
Antidysrhythmic NEC	T46.2X1-	T46.2X2-	T46.2X3-	T46.2X4-	T46.2X5-	T46.2X6-
Antiemetic drug	T45.0X1-	T45.0X2-	T45.0X3-	T45.0X4-	T45.0X5-	T45.0X6-
Antiepilepsy agent	T42.71X-	T42.72X-	T42.73X-	T42.74X-	T42.75X-	T42.76X-
combination	T42.5X1-	T42.5X2-	T42.5X3-	T42.5X4-	T42.5X5-	T42.5X6-
mixed	T42.5X1-	T42.5X2-	T42.5X3-	T42.5X4-	T42.5X5-	T42.5X6-
specified, NEC	T42.6X1-	T42.6X2-	T42.6X3-	T42.6X4-	T42.6X5-	T42.6X6-
Antiestrogen NEC	T38.6X1-	T38.6X2-	T38.6X3-	T38.6X4-	T38.6X5-	T38.6X6-
Antifertility pill	T38.4X1-	T38.4X2-	T38.4X3-	T38.4X4-	T38.4X5-	T38.4X6-
Antifibrinolytic drug	T45.621-	T45.622-	T45.623-	T45.624-	T45.625-	T45.626-
Antifilarial drug	T37.4X1-	T37.4X2-	T37.4X3-	T37.4X4-	T37.4X5-	T37.4X6-
Antiflatulent	T47.5X1-	T47.5X2-	T47.5X3-	T47.5X4-	T47.5X5-	T47.5X6-
Antifreeze	T65.91X-	T65.92X-	T65.93X-	T65.94X-	-	-
alcohol	T51.1X1-	T51.1X2-	T51.1X3-	T51.1X4-	-	-
ethylene glycol	T51.8X1-	T51.8X2-	T51.8X3-	T51.8X4-	-	-
Antifungal						
antibiotic (systemic)	T36.7X1-	T36.7X2-	T36.7X3-	T36.7X4-	T36.7X5-	T36.7X6-
anti-infective NEC	T37.91X-	T37.92X-	T37.93X-	T37.94X-	T37.95X-	T37.96X-
disinfectant, local	T49.0X1-	T49.0X2-	T49.0X3-	T49.0X4-	T49.0X5-	T49.0X6-
nonmedicinal (spray)	T60.3X1-	T60.3X2-	T60.3X3-	T60.3X4-	-	-
topical	T49.0X1-	T49.0X2-	T49.0X3-	T49.0X4-	T49.0X5-	T49.0X6-
Anti-gastric-secretion drug NEC	T47.1X1-	T47.1X2-	T47.1X3-	T47.1X4-	T47.1X5-	T47.1X6-
Antigonadotrophin NEC	T38.6X1-	T38.6X2-	T38.6X3-	T38.6X4-	T38.6X5-	T38.6X6-
Antihallucinogen	T43.501-	T43.502-	T43.503-	T43.504-	T43.505-	T43.506-
Antihelmintics	T37.4X1-	T37.4X2-	T37.4X3-	T37.4X4-	T37.4X5-	T37.4X6-
Antihemophilic						
factor	T45.8X1-	T45.8X2-	T45.8X3-	T45.8X4-	T45.8X5-	T45.8X6-
fraction	T45.8X1-	T45.8X2-	T45.8X3-	T45.8X4-	T45.8X5-	T45.8X6-
globulin concentrate	T45.7X1-	T45.7X2-	T45.7X3-	T45.7X4-	T45.7X5-	T45.7X6-
human plasma	T45.8X1-	T45.8X2-	T45.8X3-	T45.8X4-	T45.8X5-	T45.8X6-
plasma, dried	T45.7X1-	T45.7X2-	T45.7X3-	T45.7X4-	T45.7X5-	T45.7X6-
Antihemorrhoidal preparation	T49.2X1-	T49.2X2-	T49.2X3-	T49.2X4-	T49.2X5-	T49.2X6-
Antiheparin drug	T45.7X1-	T45.7X2-	T45.7X3-	T45.7X4-	T45.7X5-	T45.7X6-
Antihistamine	T45.0X1-	T45.0X2-	T45.0X3-	T45.0X4-	T45.0X5-	T45.0X6-
Antihookworm drug	T37.4X1-	T37.4X2-	T37.4X3-	T37.4X4-	T37.4X5-	T37.4X6-
Anti-human lymphocytic globulin	T50.Z11-	T50.Z12-	T50.Z13-	T50.Z14-	T50.Z15-	T50.Z16-
Antihyperlipidemic drug	T46.6X1-	T46.6X2-	T46.6X3-	T46.6X4-	T46.6X5-	T46.6X6-
Antihypertensive drug NEC	T46.5X1-	T46.5X2-	T46.5X3-	T46.5X4-	T46.5X5-	T46.5X6-
Anti-infective NEC	T37.91X-	T37.92X-	T37.93X-	T37.94X-	T37.95X-	T37.96X-
anthelmintic	T37.4X1-	T37.4X2-	T37.4X3-	T37.4X4-	T37.4X5-	T37.4X6-
antibiotics	T36.91X-	T36.92X-	T36.93X-	T36.94X-	T36.95X-	T36.96X-
specified NEC	T36.8X1-	T36.8X2-	T36.8X3-	T36.8X4-	T36.8X5-	T36.8X6-
antimalarial	T37.2X1-	T37.2X2-	T37.2X3-	T37.2X4-	T37.2X5-	T37.2X6-
antimycobacterial NEC	T37.1X1-	T37.1X2-	T37.1X3-	T37.1X4-	T37.1X5-	T37.1X6-

Substance	Poisoning Accidental (unintentional)	Poisoning Intentional self-harm	Poisoning Assault	Poisoning Undetermined	Adverse effect	Underdosing
Anti-infective NEC (continued)						
antibiotics	T36.5X1-	T36.5X2-	T36.5X3-	T36.5X4-	T36.5X5-	T36.5X6-
antiprotozoal NEC	T37.3X1-	T37.3X2-	T37.3X3-	T37.3X4-	T37.3X5-	T37.3X6-
blood	T37.2X1-	T37.2X2-	T37.2X3-	T37.2X4-	T37.2X5-	T37.2X6-
antiviral	T37.5X1-	T37.5X2-	T37.5X3-	T37.5X4-	T37.5X5-	T37.5X6-
arsenical	T37.8X1-	T37.8X2-	T37.8X3-	T37.8X4-	T37.8X5-	T37.8X6-
bismuth, local	T49.0X1-	T49.0X2-	T49.0X3-	T49.0X4-	T49.0X5-	T49.0X6-
ENT	T49.6X1-	T49.6X2-	T49.6X3-	T49.6X4-	T49.6X5-	T49.6X6-
eye NEC	T49.5X1-	T49.5X2-	T49.5X3-	T49.5X4-	T49.5X5-	T49.5X6-
heavy metals NEC	T37.8X1-	T37.8X2-	T37.8X3-	T37.8X4-	T37.8X5-	T37.8X6-
local NEC	T49.0X1-	T49.0X2-	T49.0X3-	T49.0X4-	T49.0X5-	T49.0X6-
specified NEC	T49.0X1-	T49.0X2-	T49.0X3-	T49.0X4-	T49.0X5-	T49.0X6-
mixed	T37.91X-	T37.92X-	T37.93X-	T37.94X-	T37.95X-	T37.96X-
ophthalmic preparation	T49.5X1-	T49.5X2-	T49.5X3-	T49.5X4-	T49.5X5-	T49.5X6-
topical NEC	T49.0X1-	T49.0X2-	T49.0X3-	T49.0X4-	T49.0X5-	T49.0X6-
Anti-inflammatory drug NEC	T39.391-	T39.392-	T39.393-	T39.394-	T39.395-	T39.396-
local	T49.0X1-	T49.0X2-	T49.0X3-	T49.0X4-	T49.0X5-	T49.0X6-
nonsteroidal NEC	T39.391-	T39.392-	T39.393-	T39.394-	T39.395-	T39.396-
propionic acid derivative	T39.311-	T39.312-	T39.313-	T39.314-	T39.315-	T39.316-
specified NEC	T39.391-	T39.392-	T39.393-	T39.394-	T39.395-	T39.396-
Antikaluretic	T50.3X1-	T50.3X2-	T50.3X3-	T50.3X4-	T50.3X5-	T50.3X6-
Antiknock (tetraethyl lead)	T56.0X1-	T56.0X2-	T56.0X3-	T56.0X4-	-	-
Antilipemic drug NEC	T46.6X1-	T46.6X2-	T46.6X3-	T46.6X4-	T46.6X5-	T46.6X6-
Antimalarial	T37.2X1-	T37.2X2-	T37.2X3-	T37.2X4-	T37.2X5-	T37.2X6-
prophylactic NEC	T37.2X1-	T37.2X2-	T37.2X3-	T37.2X4-	T37.2X5-	T37.2X6-
pyrimidine derivative	T37.2X1-	T37.2X2-	T37.2X3-	T37.2X4-	T37.2X5-	T37.2X6-
Antimetabolite	T45.1X1-	T45.1X2-	T45.1X3-	T45.1X4-	T45.1X5-	T45.1X6-
Antimitotic agent	T45.1X1-	T45.1X2-	T45.1X3-	T45.1X4-	T45.1X5-	T45.1X6-
Antimony (compounds) (vapor) NEC	T56.891-	T56.892-	T56.893-	T56.894-	-	-
anti-infectives	T37.8X1-	T37.8X2-	T37.8X3-	T37.8X4-	T37.8X5-	T37.8X6-
dimercaptosuccinate	T37.3X1-	T37.3X2-	T37.3X3-	T37.3X4-	T37.3X5-	T37.3X6-
hydride	T56.891-	T56.892-	T56.893-	T56.894-	-	-
pesticide (vapor)	T60.8X1-	T60.8X2-	T60.8X3-	T60.8X4-	-	-
potassium (sodium) tartrate	T37.8X1-	T37.8X2-	T37.8X3-	T37.8X4-	T37.8X5-	T37.8X6-
sodium dimercaptosuccinate	T37.3X1-	T37.3X2-	T37.3X3-	T37.3X4-	T37.3X5-	T37.3X6-
tartrated	T37.8X1-	T37.8X2-	T37.8X3-	T37.8X4-	T37.8X5-	T37.8X6-
Antimuscarinic NEC	T44.3X1-	T44.3X2-	T44.3X4-	T44.3X4-	T44.3X5-	T44.3X6-
Antimycobacterial drug NEC	T37.1X1-	T37.1X2-	T37.1X3-	T37.1X4-	T37.1X5-	T37.1X6-
antibiotics	T36.5X1-	T36.5X2-	T36.5X3-	T36.5X4-	T36.5X5-	T36.5X6-
combination	T37.1X1-	T37.1X2-	T37.1X3-	T37.1X4-	T37.1X5-	T37.1X6-
Antinausea drug	T45.0X1-	T45.0X2-	T45.0X3-	T45.0X4-	T45.0X5-	T45.0X6-
Antinematode drug	T37.4X1-	T37.4X2-	T37.4X3-	T37.4X4-	T37.4X5-	T37.4X6-
Antineoplastic NEC	T45.1X1-	T45.1X2-	T45.1X3-	T45.1X4-	T45.1X5-	T45.1X6-
alkaloidal	T45.1X1-	T45.1X2-	T45.1X3-	T45.1X4-	T45.1X5-	T45.1X6-
antibiotics	T45.1X1-	T45.1X2-	T45.1X3-	T45.1X4-	T45.1X5-	T45.1X6-
combination	T45.1X1-	T45.1X2-	T45.1X3-	T45.1X4-	T45.1X5-	T45.1X6-
estrogen	T38.5X1-	T38.5X2-	T38.5X3-	T38.5X4-	T38.5X5-	T38.5X6-
steroid	T38.7X1-	T38.7X2-	T38.7X3-	T38.7X4-	T38.7X5-	T38.7X6-
Antiparasitic drug (systemic)	T37.91X-	T37.92X-	T37.93X-	T37.94X-	T37.95X-	T37.96X-
local	T49.0X1-	T49.0X2-	T49.0X3-	T49.0X4-	T49.0X5-	T49.0X6-
specified NEC	T37.8X1-	T37.8X2-	T37.8X3-	T37.8X4-	T37.8X5-	T37.8X6-
Antiparkinsonism drug NEC	T42.8X1-	T42.8X2-	T42.8X3-	T42.8X4-	T42.8X5-	T42.8X6-
Antiperspirant NEC	T49.2X1-	T49.2X2-	T49.2X3-	T49.2X4-	T49.2X5-	T49.2X6-
Antiphlogistic NEC	T39.4X1-	T39.4X2-	T39.4X3-	T39.4X4-	T39.4X5-	T39.4X6-
Antiplatyhelmintic drug	T37.4X1-	T37.4X2-	T37.4X3-	T37.4X4-	T37.4X5-	T37.4X6-
Antiprotozoal drug NEC	T37.3X1-	T37.3X2-	T37.3X3-	T37.3X4-	T37.3X5-	T37.3X6-
blood	T37.2X1-	T37.2X2-	T37.2X3-	T37.2X4-	T37.2X5-	T37.2X6-
local	T49.0X1-	T49.0X2-	T49.0X3-	T49.0X4-	T49.0X5-	T49.0X6-

Substance	Poisoning Accidental (unintentional)	Poisoning Intentional self-harm	Poisoning Assault	Poisoning Undetermined	Adverse effect	Underdosing
Antipruritic drug NEC	T49.1X1-	T49.1X2-	T49.1X3-	T49.1X4-	T49.1X5-	T49.1X6-
Antipsychotic drug	T43.501-	T43.502-	T43.503-	T43.504-	T43.505-	T43.506-
specified NEC	T43.591-	T43.592-	T43.593-	T43.594-	T43.595-	T43.596-
Antipyretic	T39.91X-	T39.92X-	T39.93X-	T39.94X-	T39.95X-	T39.96X-
specified NEC	T39.8X1-	T39.8X2-	T39.8X3-	T39.8X4-	T39.8X5-	T39.8X6-
Antipyrine	T39.2X1-	T39.2X2-	T39.2X3-	T39.2X4-	T39.2X5-	T39.2X6-
Antirabies hyperimmune serum	T50.Z11-	T50.Z12-	T50.Z13-	T50.Z14-	T50.Z15-	T50.Z16-
Antirheumatic NEC	T39.4X1-	T39.4X2-	T39.4X3-	T39.4X4-	T39.4X5-	T39.4X6-
Antirigidity drug NEC	T42.8X1-	T42.8X2-	T42.8X3-	T42.8X4-	T42.8X5-	T42.8X6-
Antischistosomal drug	T37.4X1-	T37.4X2-	T37.4X3-	T37.4X4-	T37.4X5-	T37.4X6-
Antiscorpion sera	T50.Z11-	T50.Z12-	T50.Z13-	T50.Z14-	T50.Z15-	T50.Z16-
Antiseborrheics	T49.4X1-	T49.4X2-	T49.4X3-	T49.4X4-	T49.4X5-	T49.4X6-
Antiseptics (external) (medicinal)	T49.0X1-	T49.0X2-	T49.0X3-	T49.0X4-	T49.0X5-	T49.0X6-
Antistine	T45.0X1-	T45.0X2-	T45.0X3-	T45.0X4-	T45.0X5-	T45.0X6-
Antitapeworm drug	T37.4X1-	T37.4X2-	T37.4X3-	T37.4X4-	T37.4X5-	T37.4X6-
Antitetanus immunoglobulin	T50.Z11-	T50.Z12-	T50.Z13-	T50.Z14-	T50.Z15-	T50.Z16-
Antithrombotic	T45.521-	T45.522-	T45.523-	T45.524-	T45.525-	T45.526-
Antithyroid drug NEC	T38.2X1-	T38.2X2-	T38.2X3-	T38.2X4-	T38.2X5-	T38.2X6-
Antitoxin	T50.Z11-	T50.Z12-	T50.Z13-	T50.Z14-	T50.Z15-	T50.Z16-
diphtheria	T50.Z11-	T50.Z12-	T50.Z13-	T50.Z14-	T50.Z15-	T50.Z16-
gas gangrene	T50.Z11-	T50.Z12-	T50.Z13-	T50.Z14-	T50.Z15-	T50.Z16-
tetanus	T50.Z11-	T50.Z12-	T50.Z13-	T50.Z14-	T50.Z15-	T50.Z16-
Antitrichomonal drug	T37.3X1-	T37.3X2-	T37.3X3-	T37.3X4-	T37.3X5-	T37.3X6-
Antituberculars	T37.1X1-	T37.1X2-	T37.1X3-	T37.1X4-	T37.1X5-	T37.1X6-
antibiotics	T36.5X1-	T36.5X2-	T36.5X3-	T36.5X4-	T36.5X5-	T36.5X6-
Antitussive NEC	T48.3X1-	T48.3X2-	T48.3X3-	T48.3X4-	T48.3X5-	T48.3X6-
codeine mixture	T40.2X1-	T40.2X2-	T40.2X3-	T40.2X4-	T40.2X5-	T40.2X6-
opiate	T40.2X1-	T40.2X2-	T40.2X3-	T40.2X4-	T40.2X5-	T40.2X6-
Antivaricose drug	T46.8X1-	T46.8X2-	T46.8X3-	T46.8X4-	T46.8X5-	T46.8X6-
Antivenin, antivenom (sera)	T50.Z11-	T50.Z12-	T50.Z13-	T50.Z14-	T50.Z15-	T50.Z16-
crotaline	T50.Z11-	T50.Z12-	T50.Z13-	T50.Z14-	T50.Z15-	T50.Z16-
spider bite	T50.Z11-	T50.Z12-	T50.Z13-	T50.Z14-	T50.Z15-	T50.Z16-
Antivertigo drug	T45.0X1-	T45.0X2-	T45.0X3-	T45.0X4-	T45.0X5-	T45.0X6-
Antiviral drug NEC	T37.5X1-	T37.5X2-	T37.5X3-	T37.5X4-	T37.5X5-	T37.5X6-
eye	T49.5X1-	T49.5X2-	T49.5X3-	T49.5X4-	T49.5X5-	T49.5X6-
Antiwhipworm drug	T37.4X1-	T37.4X2-	T37.4X3-	T37.4X4-	T37.4X5-	T37.4X6-
Antrol — *see also by specific chemical substance*	T60.91X-	T60.92X-	T60.93X-	T60.94X-	-	
fungicide	T60.91X-	T60.92X-	T60.93X-	T60.94X-	-	-
ANTU (alpha naphthylthiourea)	T60.4X1-	T60.4X2-	T60.4X3-	T60.4X4-	-	-
Apalcillin	T36.0X1-	T36.0X2-	T36.0X3-	T36.0X4-	T36.0X5-	T36.0X6-
APC	T48.5X1-	T48.5X2-	T48.5X3-	T48.5X4-	T48.5X5-	T48.5X6-
Aplonidine	T44.4X1-	T44.4X2-	T44.4X3-	T44.4X4-	T44.4X5-	T44.4X6-
Apomorphine	T47.7X1-	T47.7X2-	T47.7X3-	T47.7X4-	T47.7X5-	T47.7X6-
Appetite depressants, central	T50.5X1-	T50.5X2-	T50.5X3-	T50.5X4-	T50.5X5-	T50.5X6-
Apraclonidine (hydrochloride)	T44.4X1-	T44.4X2-	T44.4X3-	T44.4X4-	T44.4X5-	T44.4X6-
Apresoline	T46.5X1-	T46.5X2-	T46.5X3-	T46.5X4-	T46.5X5-	T46.5X6-
Aprindine	T46.2X1-	T46.2X2-	T46.2X3-	T46.2X4-	T46.2X5-	T46.2X6-
Aprobarbital	T42.3X1-	T42.3X2-	T42.3X3-	T42.3X4-	T42.3X5-	T42.3X6-
Apronalide	T42.6X1-	T42.6X2-	T42.6X3-	T42.6X4-	T42.6X5-	T42.6X6-
Aprotinin	T45.621-	T45.622-	T45.623-	T45.624-	T45.625-	T45.626-
Aptocaine	T41.3X1-	T41.3X2-	T41.3X3-	T41.3X4-	T41.3X5-	T41.3X6-
Aqua fortis	T54.2X1-	T54.2X2-	T54.2X3-	T54.2X4-	-	-
Ara-A	T37.5X1-	T37.5X2-	T37.5X3-	T37.5X4-	T37.5X5-	T37.5X6-
Ara-C	T45.1X1-	T45.1X2-	T45.1X3-	T45.1X4-	T45.1X5-	T45.1X6-
Arachis oil	T49.3X1-	T49.3X2-	T49.3X3-	T49.3X4-	T49.3X5-	T49.3X6-
cathartic	T47.4X1-	T47.4X2-	T47.4X3-	T47.4X4-	T47.4X5-	T47.4X6-
Aralen	T37.2X1-	T37.2X2-	T37.2X3-	T37.2X4-	T37.2X5-	T37.2X6-

Substance	Poisoning Accidental (unintentional)	Poisoning Intentional self-harm	Poisoning Assault	Poisoning Undetermined	Adverse effect	Underdosing
Arecoline	T44.1X1-	T44.1X2-	T44.1X3-	T44.1X4-	T44.1X5-	T44.1X6-
Arginine	T50.991-	T50.992-	T50.993-	T50.994-	T50.995-	T50.996-
glutamate	T50.991-	T50.992-	T50.993-	T50.994-	T50.995-	T50.996-
Argyrol	T49.0X1-	T49.0X2-	T49.0X3-	T49.0X4-	T49.0X5-	T49.0X6-
ENT agent	T49.6X1-	T49.6X2-	T49.6X3-	T49.6X4-	T49.6X5-	T49.6X6-
ophthalmic preparation	T49.5X1-	T49.5X2-	T49.5X3-	T49.5X4-	T49.5X5-	T49.5X6-
Aristocort	T38.0X1-	T38.0X2-	T38.0X3-	T38.0X4-	T38.0X5-	T38.0X6-
ENT agent	T49.6X1-	T49.6X2-	T49.6X3-	T49.6X4-	T49.6X5-	T49.6X6-
ophthalmic preparation	T49.5X1-	T49.5X2-	T49.5X3-	T49.5X4-	T49.5X5-	T49.5X6-
topical NEC	T49.0X1-	T49.0X2-	T49.0X3-	T49.0X4-	T49.0X5-	T49.0X6-
Aromatics, corrosive	T54.1X1-	T54.1X2-	T54.1X3-	T54.1X4-	-	-
disinfectants	T54.1X1-	T54.1X2-	T54.1X3-	T54.1X4-	-	-
Arsenate of lead	T57.0X1-	T57.0X2-	T57.0X3-	T57.0X4-	-	-
herbicide	T57.0X1-	T57.0X2-	T57.0X3-	T57.0X4-	-	-
Arsenic, arsenicals (compounds) (dust) (vapor) NEC	T57.0X1-	T57.0X2-	T57.0X3-	T57.0X4-	-	-
anti-infectives	T37.8X1-	T37.8X2-	T37.8X3-	T37.8X4-	T37.8X5-	T37.8X6-
pesticide (dust) (fumes)	T57.0X1-	T57.0X2-	T57.0X3-	T57.0X4-	-	-
Arsine (gas)	T57.0X1-	T57.0X2-	T57.0X3-	T57.0X4-	-	-
Arsphenamine (silver)	T37.8X1-	T37.8X2-	T37.8X3-	T37.8X4-	T37.8X5-	T37.8X6-
Arsthinol	T37.3X1-	T37.3X2-	T37.3X3-	T37.3X4-	T37.3X5-	T37.3X6-
Artane	T44.3X1-	T44.3X2-	T44.3X3-	T44.3X4-	T44.3X5-	T44.3X6-
Arthropod (venomous) NEC	T63.481-	T63.482-	T63.483-	T63.484-	-	-
Articaine	T41.3X1-	T41.3X2-	T41.3X3-	T41.3X4-	T41.3X5-	T41.3X6-
Asbestos	T57.8X1-	T57.8X2-	T57.8X3-	T57.8X4-	-	-
Ascaridole	T37.4X1-	T37.4X2-	T37.4X3-	T37.4X4-	T37.4X5-	T37.4X6-
Ascorbic acid	T45.2X1-	T45.2X2-	T45.2X3-	T45.2X4-	T45.2X5-	T45.2X6-
Asiaticoside	T49.0X1-	T49.0X2-	T49.0X3-	T49.0X4-	T49.0X5-	T49.0X6-
Asparaginase	T45.1X1-	T45.1X2-	T45.1X3-	T45.1X4-	T45.1X5-	T45.1X6-
Aspidium (oleoresin)	T37.4X1-	T37.4X2-	T37.4X3-	T37.4X4-	T37.4X5-	T37.4X6-
Aspirin (aluminum) (soluble)	T39.011-	T39.012-	T39.013-	T39.014-	T39.015-	T39.016-
Aspoxicillin	T36.0X1-	T36.0X2-	T36.0X3-	T36.0X4-	T36.0X5-	T36.0X6-
Astemizole	T45.0X1-	T45.0X2-	T45.0X3-	T45.0X4-	T45.0X5-	T45.0X6-
Astringent (local)	T49.2X1-	T49.2X2-	T49.2X3-	T49.2X4-	T49.2X5-	T49.2X6-
specified NEC	T49.2X1-	T49.2X2-	T49.2X3-	T49.2X4-	T49.2X5-	T49.2X6-
Astromicin	T36.5X1-	T36.5X2-	T36.5X3-	T36.5X4-	T36.5X5-	T36.5X6-
Ataractic drug NEC	T43.501-	T43.502-	T43.503-	T43.504-	T43.505-	T43.506-
Atenolol	T44.7X1-	T44.7X2-	T44.7X3-	T44.7X4-	T44.7X5-	T44.7X6-
Atonia drug, intestinal	T47.4X1-	T47.4X2-	T47.4X3-	T47.4X4-	T47.4X5-	T47.4X6-
Atophan	T50.4X1-	T50.4X2-	T50.4X3-	T50.4X4-	T50.4X5-	T50.4X6-
Atracurium besilate	T48.1X1-	T48.1X2-	T48.1X3-	T48.1X4-	T48.1X5-	T48.1X6-
Atropine	T44.3X1-	T44.3X2-	T44.3X3-	T44.3X4-	T44.3X5-	T44.3X6-
derivative	T44.3X1-	T44.3X2-	T44.3X3-	T44.3X4-	T44.3X5-	T44.3X6-
methonitrate	T44.3X1-	T44.3X2-	T44.3X3-	T44.3X4-	T44.3X5-	T44.3X6-
Attapulgite	T47.6X1-	T47.6X2-	T47.6X3-	T47.6X4-	T47.6X5-	T47.6X6-
Auramine	T65.891-	T65.892-	T65.893-	T65.894-	-	-
dye	T65.6X1-	T65.6X2-	T65.6X3-	T65.6X4-	-	-
fungicide	T60.3X1-	T60.3X2-	T60.3X3-	T60.3X4-	-	-
Auranofin	T39.4X1-	T39.4X2-	T39.4X3-	T39.4X4-	T39.4X5-	T39.4X6-
Aurantiin	T46.991-	T46.992-	T46.993-	T46.994-	T46.995-	T46.996-
Aureomycin	T36.4X1-	T36.4X2-	T36.4X3-	T36.4X4-	T36.4X5-	T36.4X6-
ophthalmic preparation	T49.5X1-	T49.5X2-	T49.5X3-	T49.5X4-	T49.5X5-	T49.5X6-
topical NEC	T49.0X1-	T49.0X2-	T49.0X3-	T49.0X4-	T49.0X5-	T49.0X6-
Aurothioglucose	T39.4X1-	T39.4X2-	T39.4X3-	T39.4X4-	T39.4X5-	T39.4X6-
Aurothioglycanide	T39.4X1-	T39.4X2-	T39.4X3-	T39.4X4-	T39.4X5-	T39.4X6-
Aurothiomalate sodium	T39.4X1-	T39.4X2-	T39.4X3-	T39.4X4-	T39.4X5-	T39.4X6-
Aurotioprol	T39.4X1-	T39.4X2-	T39.4X3-	T39.4X4-	T39.4X5-	T39.4X6-

Substance	Poisoning Accidental (unintentional)	Poisoning Intentional self-harm	Poisoning Assault	Poisoning Undetermined	Adverse effect	Underdosing
Automobile fuel	T52.0X1-	T52.0X2-	T52.0X3-	T52.0X4-	-	-
Autonomic nervous system agent NEC	T44.901-	T44.902-	T44.903-	T44.904-	T44.905-	T44.906-
Avlosulfon	T37.1X1-	T37.1X2-	T37.1X3-	T37.1X4-	T37.1X5-	T37.1X6-
Avomine	T42.6X1-	T42.6X2-	T42.6X3-	T42.6X4-	T42.6X5-	T42.6X6-
Axerophthol	T45.2X1-	T45.2X2-	T45.2X3-	T45.2X4-	T45.2X5-	T45.2X6-
Azacitidine	T45.1X1-	T45.1X2-	T45.1X3-	T45.1X4-	T45.1X5-	T45.1X6-
Azacyclonol	T43.591-	T43.592-	T43.593-	T43.594-	T43.595-	T43.596-
Azadirachta	T60.2X1-	T60.2X2-	T60.2X3-	T60.2X4-	-	-
Azanidazole	T37.3X1-	T37.3X2-	T37.3X3-	T37.3X4-	T37.3X5-	T37.3X6-
Azapetine	T46.7X1-	T46.7X2-	T46.7X3-	T46.7X4-	T46.7X5-	T46.7X6-
Azapropazone	T39.2X1-	T39.2X2-	T39.2X3-	T39.2X4-	T39.2X5-	T39.2X6-
Azaribine	T45.1X1-	T45.1X2-	T45.1X3-	T45.1X4-	T45.1X5-	T45.1X6-
Azaserine	T45.1X1-	T45.1X2-	T45.1X3-	T45.1X4-	T45.1X5-	T45.1X6-
Azatadine	T45.0X1-	T45.0X2-	T45.0X3-	T45.0X4-	T45.0X5-	T45.0X6-
Azatepa	T45.1X1-	T45.1X2-	T45.1X3-	T45.1X4-	T45.1X5-	T45.1X6-
Azathioprine	T45.1X1-	T45.1X2-	T45.1X3-	T45.1X4-	T45.1X5-	T45.1X6-
Azelaic acid	T49.0X1-	T49.0X2-	T49.0X3-	T49.0X4-	T49.0X5-	T49.0X6-
Azelastine	T45.0X1-	T45.0X2-	T45.0X3-	T45.0X4-	T45.0X5-	T45.0X6-
Azidocillin	T36.0X1-	T36.0X2-	T36.0X3-	T36.0X4-	T36.0X5-	T36.0X6-
Azidothymidine	T37.5X1-	T37.5X2-	T37.5X3-	T37.5X4-	T37.5X5-	T37.5X6-
Azinphos (ethyl) (methyl)	T60.0X1-	T60.0X2-	T60.0X3-	T60.0X4-	-	-
Aziridine (chelating)	T54.1X1-	T54.1X2-	T54.1X3-	T54.1X4-	-	-
Azithromycin	T36.3X1-	T36.3X2-	T36.3X3-	T36.3X4-	T36.3X5-	T36.3X6-
Azlocillin	T36.0X1-	T36.0X2-	T36.0X3-	T36.0X4-	T36.0X5-	T36.0X6-
Azobenzene smoke	T65.3X1-	T65.3X2-	T65.3X3-	T65.3X4-	-	-
acaricide	T60.8X1-	T60.8X2-	T60.8X3-	T60.8X4-	-	-
Azosulfamide	T37.0X1-	T37.0X2-	T37.0X3-	T37.0X4-	T37.0X5-	T37.0X6-
AZT	T37.5X1-	T37.5X2-	T37.5X3-	T37.5X4-	T37.5X5-	T37.5X6-
Aztreonam	T36.1X1-	T36.1X2-	T36.1X3-	T36.1X4-	T36.1X5-	T36.1X6-
Azulfidine	T37.0X1-	T37.0X2-	T37.0X3-	T37.0X4-	T37.0X5-	T37.0X6-
Azuresin	T50.8X1-	T50.8X2-	T50.8X3-	T50.8X4-	T50.8X5-	T50.8X6-
Bacampicillin	T36.0X1-	T36.0X2-	T36.0X3-	T36.0X4-	T36.0X5-	T36.0X6-
Bacillus						
lactobacillus	T47.8X1-	T47.8X2-	T47.8X3-	T47.8X4-	T47.8X5-	T47.8X6-
subtilis	T47.6X1-	T47.6X2-	T47.6X3-	T47.6X4-	T47.6X5-	T47.6X6-
Bacimycin	T49.0X1-	T49.0X2-	T49.0X3-	T49.0X4-	T49.0X5-	T49.0X6-
ophthalmic preparation	T49.5X1-	T49.5X2-	T49.5X3-	T49.5X4-	T49.5X5-	T49.5X6-
Bacitracin zinc	T49.0X1-	T49.0X2-	T49.0X3-	T49.0X4-	T49.0X5-	T49.0X6-
with neomycin	T49.0X1-	T49.0X2-	T49.0X3-	T49.0X4-	T49.0X5-	T49.0X6-
ENT agent	T49.6X1-	T49.6X2-	T49.6X3-	T49.6X4-	T49.6X5-	T49.6X6-
ophthalmic preparation	T49.5X1-	T49.5X2-	T49.5X3-	T49.5X4-	T49.5X5-	T49.5X6-
topical NEC	T49.0X1-	T49.0X2-	T49.0X3-	T49.0X4-	T49.0X5-	T49.0X6-
Baclofen	T42.8X1-	T42.8X2-	T42.8X3-	T42.8X4-	T42.8X5-	T42.8X6-
Baking soda	T50.991-	T50.992-	T50.993-	T50.994-	T50.995-	T50.996-
BAL	T45.8X1-	T45.8X2-	T45.8X3-	T45.8X4-	T45.8X5-	T45.8X6-
Bambuterol	T48.6X1-	T48.6X2-	T48.6X3-	T48.6X4-	T48.6X5-	T48.6X6-
Bamethan (sulfate)	T46.7X1-	T46.7X2-	T46.7X3-	T46.7X4-	T46.7X5-	T46.7X6-
Bamifylline	T48.6X1-	T48.6X2-	T48.6X3-	T48.6X4-	T48.6X5-	T48.6X6-
Bamipine	T45.0X1-	T45.0X2-	T45.0X3-	T45.0X4-	T45.0X5-	T45.0X6-
Baneberry — *see Actaea spicata*						
Banewort — *see Belladonna*						
Barbenyl	T42.3X1-	T42.3X2-	T42.3X3-	T42.3X4-	T42.3X5-	T42.3X6-
Barbexaclone	T42.6X1-	T42.6X2-	T42.6X3-	T42.6X4-	T42.6X5-	T42.6X6-
Barbital	T42.3X1-	T42.3X2-	T42.3X3-	T42.3X4-	T42.3X5-	T42.3X6-
sodium	T42.3X1-	T42.3X2-	T42.3X3-	T42.3X4-	T42.3X5-	T42.3X6-
Barbitone	T42.3X1-	T42.3X2-	T42.3X3-	T42.3X4-	T42.3X5-	T42.3X6-
Barbiturate NEC	T42.3X1-	T42.3X2-	T42.3X3-	T42.3X4-	T42.3X5-	T42.3X6-
with tranquilizer	T42.3X1-	T42.3X2-	T42.3X3-	T42.3X4-	T42.3X5-	T42.3X6-

Substance	Poisoning Accidental (unintentional)	Poisoning Intentional self-harm	Poisoning Assault	Poisoning Undetermined	Adverse effect	Underdosing
Barbiturate NEC (*continued*)						
anesthetic (intravenous)	T41.1X1-	T41.1X2-	T41.1X3-	T41.1X4-	T41.1X5-	T41.1X6-
Barium (carbonate) (chloride) (sulfite)	T57.8X1-	T57.8X2-	T57.8X3-	T57.8X4-	-	-
diagnostic agent	T50.8X1-	T50.8X2-	T50.8X3-	T50.8X4-	T50.8X5-	T50.8X6-
pesticide	T60.4X1-	T60.4X2-	T60.4X3-	T60.4X4-	-	-
rodenticide	T60.4X1-	T60.4X2-	T60.4X3-	T60.4X4-	-	-
sulfate (medicinal)	T50.8X1-	T50.8X2-	T50.8X3-	T50.8X4-	T50.8X5-	T50.8X6-
Barrier cream	T49.3X1-	T49.3X2-	T49.3X3-	T49.3X4-	T49.3X5-	T49.3X6-
Basic fuchsin	T49.0X1-	T49.0X2-	T49.0X3-	T49.0X4-	T49.0X5-	T49.0X6-
Battery acid or fluid	T54.2X1-	T54.2X2-	T54.2X3-	T54.2X4-	-	-
Bay rum	T51.8X1-	T51.8X2-	T51.8X3-	T51.8X4-	-	-
BCG (vaccine)	T50.A91-	T50.A92-	T50.A93-	T50.A94-	T50.A95-	T50.A96-
BCNU	T45.1X1-	T45.1X2-	T45.1X3-	T45.1X4-	T45.1X5-	T45.1X6-
Bearsfoot	T62.2X1-	T62.2X2-	T62.2X3-	T62.2X4-	-	-
Beclamide	T42.6X1-	T42.6X2-	T42.6X3-	T42.6X4-	T42.6X5-	T42.6X6-
Beclomethasone	T44.5X1-	T44.5X2-	T44.5X3-	T44.5X4-	T44.5X5-	T44.5X6-
Bee (sting) (venom)	T63.441-	T63.442-	T63.443-	T63.444-	-	-
Befunolol	T49.5X1-	T49.5X2-	T49.5X3-	T49.5X4-	T49.5X5-	T49.5X6-
Bekanamycin	T36.5X1-	T36.5X2-	T36.5X3-	T36.5X4-	T36.5X5-	T36.5X6-
Belladonna — *see also Nightshade*						
alkaloids	T44.3X1-	T44.3X2-	T44.3X3-	T44.3X4-	T44.3X5-	T44.3X6-
extract	T44.3X1-	T44.3X2-	T44.3X3-	T44.3X4-	T44.3X5-	T44.3X6-
herb	T44.3X1-	T44.3X2-	T44.3X3-	T44.3X4-	T44.3X5-	T44.3X6-
Bemegride	T50.7X1-	T50.7X2-	T50.7X3-	T50.7X4-	T50.7X5-	T50.7X6-
Benactyzine	T44.3X1-	T44.3X2-	T44.3X3-	T44.3X4-	T44.3X5-	T44.3X6-
Benadryl	T45.0X1-	T45.0X2-	T45.0X3-	T45.0X4-	T45.0X5-	T45.0X6-
Benaprizine	T44.3X1-	T44.3X2-	T44.3X3-	T44.3X4-	T44.3X5-	T44.3X6-
Benazepril	T46.4X1-	T46.4X2-	T46.4X3-	T46.4X4-	T46.4X5-	T46.4X6-
Bencyclane	T46.7X1-	T46.7X2-	T46.7X3-	T46.7X4-	T46.7X5-	T46.7X6-
Bendazol	T46.3X1-	T46.3X2-	T46.3X3-	T46.3X4-	T46.3X5-	T46.3X6-
Bendrofluazide	T50.2X1-	T50.2X2-	T50.2X3-	T50.2X4-	T50.2X5-	T50.2X6-
Bendroflumethiazide	T50.2X1-	T50.2X2-	T50.2X3-	T50.2X4-	T50.2X5-	T50.2X6-
Benemid	T50.4X1-	T50.4X2-	T50.4X3-	T50.4X4-	T50.4X5-	T50.4X6-
Benethamine penicillin	T36.0X1-	T36.0X2-	T36.0X3-	T36.0X4-	T36.0X5-	T36.0X6-
Benexate	T47.1X1-	T47.1X2-	T47.1X3-	T47.1X4-	T47.1X5-	T47.1X6-
Benfluorex	T46.6X1-	T46.6X2-	T46.6X3-	T46.6X4-	T46.6X5-	T46.6X6-
Benfotiamine	T45.2X1-	T45.2X2-	T45.2X3-	T45.2X4-	T45.2X5-	T45.2X6-
Benisone	T49.0X1-	T49.0X2-	T49.0X3-	T49.0X4-	T49.0X5-	T49.0X6-
Benomyl	T60.0X1-	T60.0X2-	T60.0X3-	T60.0X4-	-	-
Benoquin	T49.8X1-	T49.8X2-	T49.8X3-	T49.8X4-	T49.8X5-	T49.8X6-
Benoxinate	T41.3X1-	T41.3X2-	T41.3X3-	T41.3X4-	T41.3X5-	T41.3X6-
Benperidol	T43.4X1-	T43.4X2-	T43.4X3-	T43.4X4-	T43.4X5-	T43.4X6-
Benproperine	T48.3X1-	T48.3X2-	T48.3X3-	T48.3X4-	T48.3X5-	T48.3X6-
Benserazide	T42.8X1-	T42.8X2-	T42.8X3-	T42.8X4-	T42.8X5-	T42.8X6-
Bentazepam	T42.4X1-	T42.4X2-	T42.4X3-	T42.4X4-	T42.4X5-	T42.4X6-
Bentiromide	T50.8X1-	T50.8X2-	T50.8X3-	T50.8X4-	T50.8X5-	T50.8X6-
Bentonite	T49.3X1-	T49.3X2-	T49.3X3-	T49.3X4-	T49.3X5-	T49.3X6-
Benzalbutyramide	T46.6X1-	T46.6X2-	T46.6X3-	T46.6X4-	T46.6X5-	T46.6X6-
Benzalkonium (chloride)	T49.0X1-	T49.0X2-	T49.0X3-	T49.0X4-	T49.0X5-	T49.0X6-
ophthalmic preparation	T49.5X1-	T49.5X2-	T49.5X3-	T49.5X4-	T49.5X5-	T49.5X6-
Benzamidosalicylate (calcium)	T37.1X1-	T37.1X2-	T37.1X3-	T37.1X4-	T37.1X5-	T37.1X6-
Benzamine	T41.3X1-	T41.3X2-	T41.3X3-	T41.3X4-	T41.3X5-	T41.3X6-
lactate	T49.1X1-	T49.1X2-	T49.1X3-	T49.1X4-	T49.1X5-	T49.1X6-
Benzamphetamine	T50.5X1-	T50.5X2-	T50.5X3-	T50.5X4-	T50.5X5-	T50.5X6-
Benzapril hydrochloride	T46.5X1-	T46.5X2-	T46.5X3-	T46.5X4-	T46.5X5-	T46.5X6-
Benzathine benzylpenicillin	T36.0X1-	T36.0X2-	T36.0X3-	T36.0X4-	T36.0X5-	T36.0X6-
Benzathine penicillin	T36.0X1-	T36.0X2-	T36.0X3-	T36.0X4-	T36.0X5-	T36.0X6-
Benzatropine	T42.8X1-	T42.8X2-	T42.8X3-	T42.8X4-	T42.8X5-	T42.8X6-
Benzbromarone	T50.4X1-	T50.4X2-	T50.4X3-	T50.4X4-	T50.4X5-	T50.4X6-

Substance	Poisoning Accidental (unintentional)	Poisoning Intentional self-harm	Poisoning Assault	Poisoning Undetermined	Adverse effect	Underdosing
Benzcarbimine	T45.1X1-	T45.1X2-	T45.1X3-	T45.1X4-	T45.1X5-	T45.1X6-
Benzedrex	T44.991-	T44.992-	T44.993-	T44.994-	T44.995-	T44.996-
Benzedrine (amphetamine)	T43.621-	T43.622-	T43.623-	T43.624-	T43.625-	T43.626-
Benzenamine	T65.3X1-	T65.3X2-	T65.3X3-	T65.3X4-	-	-
Benzene	T52.1X1-	T52.1X2-	T52.1X3-	T52.1X4-	-	-
homologues (acetyl) (dimethyl) (methyl) (solvent)	T52.2X1-	T52.2X2-	T52.2X3-	T52.2X4-	-	-
Benzethonium (chloride)	T49.0X1-	T49.0X2-	T49.0X3-	T49.0X4-	T49.0X5-	T49.0X6-
Benzfetamine	T50.5X1-	T50.5X2-	T50.5X3-	T50.5X4-	T50.5X5-	T50.5X6-
Benzhexol	T44.3X1-	T44.3X2-	T44.3X3-	T44.3X4-	T44.3X5-	T44.3X6-
Benzhydramine (chloride)	T45.0X1-	T45.0X2-	T45.0X3-	T45.0X4-	T45.0X5-	T45.0X6-
Benzidine	T65.891-	T65.892-	T65.893-	T65.894-	-	-
Benzilonium bromide	T44.3X1-	T44.3X2-	T44.3X3-	T44.3X4-	T44.3X5-	T44.3X6-
Benzimidazole	T60.3X1-	T60.3X2-	T60.3X3-	T60.3X4-	-	-
Benzin (e) — *see* Ligroin						
Benziodarone	T46.3X1-	T46.3X2-	T46.3X3-	T46.3X4-	T46.3X5-	T46.3X6-
Benznidazole	T37.3X1-	T37.3X2-	T37.3X3-	T37.3X4-	T37.3X5-	T37.3X6-
Benzocaine	T41.3X1-	T41.3X2-	T41.3X3-	T41.3X4-	T41.3X5-	T41.3X6-
Benzodiapin	T42.4X1-	T42.4X2-	T42.4X3-	T42.4X4-	T42.4X5-	T42.4X6-
Benzodiazepine NEC	T42.4X1-	T42.4X2-	T42.4X3-	T42.4X4-	T42.4X5-	T42.4X6-
Benzoic acid	T49.0X1-	T49.0X2-	T49.0X3-	T49.0X4-	T49.0X5-	T49.0X6-
with salicylic acid	T49.0X1-	T49.0X2-	T49.0X3-	T49.0X4-	T49.0X5-	T49.0X6-
Benzoin (tincture)	T48.5X1-	T48.5X2-	T48.5X3-	T48.5X4-	T48.5X5-	T48.5X6-
Benzol (benzene)	T52.1X1-	T52.1X2-	T52.1X3-	T52.1X4-	-	-
vapor	T52.0X1-	T52.0X2-	T52.0X3-	T52.0X4-	-	-
Benzomorphan	T40.2X1-	T40.2X2-	T40.2X3-	T40.2X4-	T40.2X5-	T40.2X6-
Benzonatate	T48.3X1-	T48.3X2-	T48.3X3-	T48.3X4-	T48.3X5-	T48.3X6-
Benzophenones	T49.3X1-	T49.3X2-	T49.3X3-	T49.3X4-	T49.3X5-	T49.3X6-
Benzopyrone	T46.991-	T46.992-	T46.993-	T46.994-	T46.995-	T46.996-
Benzothiadiazides	T50.2X1-	T50.2X2-	T50.2X3-	T50.2X4-	T50.2X5-	T50.2X6-
Benzoxonium chloride	T49.0X1-	T49.0X2-	T49.0X3-	T49.0X4-	T49.0X5-	T49.0X6-
Benzoyl peroxide	T49.0X1-	T49.0X2-	T49.0X3-	T49.0X4-	T49.0X5-	T49.0X6-
Benzoylpas calcium	T37.1X1-	T37.1X2-	T37.1X3-	T37.1X4-	T37.1X5-	T37.1X6-
Benzperidin	T43.591-	T43.592-	T43.593-	T43.594-	T43.595-	T43.596-
Benzperidol	T43.591-	T43.592-	T43.593-	T43.594-	T43.595-	T43.596-
Benzphetamine	T50.5X1-	T50.5X2-	T50.5X3-	T50.5X4-	T50.5X5-	T50.5X6-
Benzpyrinium bromide	T44.1X1-	T44.1X2-	T44.1X3-	T44.1X4-	T44.1X5-	T44.1X6-
Benzquinamide	T45.0X1-	T45.0X2-	T45.0X3-	T45.0X4-	T45.0X5-	T45.0X6-
Benzthiazide	T50.2X1-	T50.2X2-	T50.2X3-	T50.2X4-	T50.2X5-	T50.2X6-
Benztropine						
anticholinergic	T44.3X1-	T44.3X2-	T44.3X3-	T44.3X4-	T44.3X5-	T44.3X6-
antiparkinson	T42.8X1-	T42.8X2-	T42.8X3-	T42.8X4-	T42.8X5-	T42.8X6-
Benzydamine	T49.0X1-	T49.0X2-	T49.0X3-	T49.0X4-	T49.0X5-	T49.0X6-
Benzyl						
acetate	T52.8X1-	T52.8X2-	T52.8X3-	T52.8X4-	-	-
alcohol	T49.0X1-	T49.0X2-	T49.0X3-	T49.0X4-	T49.0X5-	T49.0X6-
benzoate	T49.0X1-	T49.0X2-	T49.0X3-	T49.0X4-	T49.0X5-	T49.0X6-
Benzoic acid	T49.0X1-	T49.0X2-	T49.0X3-	T49.0X4-	T49.0X5-	T49.0X6-
morphine	T40.2X1-	T40.2X2-	T40.2X3-	T40.2X4-	-	-
nicotinate	T46.6X1-	T46.6X2-	T46.6X3-	T46.6X4-	T46.6X5-	T46.6X6-
penicillin	T36.0X1-	T36.0X2-	T36.0X3-	T36.0X4-	T36.0X5-	T36.0X6-
Benzylhydrochlorthia-zide	T50.2X1-	T50.2X2-	T50.2X3-	T50.2X4-	T50.2X5-	T50.2X6-
Benzylpenicillin	T36.0X1-	T36.0X2-	T36.0X3-	T36.0X4-	T36.0X5-	T36.0X6-
Benzylthiouracil	T38.2X1-	T38.2X2-	T38.2X3-	T38.2X4-	T38.2X5-	T38.2X6-
Bephenium hydroxy-naphthoate	T37.4X1-	T37.4X2-	T37.4X3-	T37.4X4-	T37.4X5-	T37.4X6-
Bepridil	T46.1X1-	T46.1X2-	T46.1X3-	T46.1X4-	T46.1X5-	T46.1X6-
Bergamot oil	T65.891-	T65.892-	T65.893-	T65.894-	-	-
Bergapten	T50.991-	T50.992-	T50.993-	T50.994-	T50.995-	T50.996-
Berries, poisonous	T62.1X1-	T62.1X2-	T62.1X3-	T62.1X4-	-	-

Substance	Poisoning Accidental (unintentional)	Poisoning Intentional self-harm	Poisoning Assault	Poisoning Undetermined	Adverse effect	Underdosing
Beryllium (compounds)	T56.7X1-	T56.7X2-	T56.7X3-	T56.7X4-	-	-
b-acetyldigoxin	T46.0X1-	T46.0X2-	T46.0X3-	T46.0X4-	T46.0X5-	T46.0X6-
beta adrenergic blocking agent, heart	T44.7X1-	T44.7X2-	T44.7X3-	T44.7X4-	T44.7X5-	T44.7X6-
b-benzalbutyramide	T46.6X1-	T46.6X2-	T46.6X3-	T46.6X4-	T46.6X5-	T46.6X6-
Betacarotene	T45.2X1-	T45.2X2-	T45.2X3-	T45.2X4-	T45.2X5-	T45.2X6-
b-eucaine	T49.1X1-	T49.1X2-	T49.1X3-	T49.1X4-	T49.1X5-	T49.1X6-
Beta-Chlor	T42.6X1-	T42.6X2-	T42.6X3-	T42.6X4-	T42.6X5-	T42.6X6-
b-galactosidase	T47.5X1-	T47.5X2-	T47.5X3-	T47.5X4-	T47.5X5-	T47.5X6-
Betahistine	T46.7X1-	T46.7X2-	T46.7X3-	T46.7X4-	T46.7X5-	T46.7X6-
Betaine	T47.5X1-	T47.5X2-	T47.5X3-	T47.5X4-	T47.5X5-	T47.5X6-
Betamethasone	T49.0X1-	T49.0X2-	T49.0X3-	T49.0X4-	T49.0X5-	T49.0X6-
topical	T49.0X1-	T49.0X2-	T49.0X3-	T49.0X4-	T49.0X5-	T49.0X6-
Betamicin	T36.8X1-	T36.8X2-	T36.8X3-	T36.8X4-	T36.8X5-	T36.8X6-
Betanidine	T46.5X1-	T46.5X2-	T46.5X3-	T46.5X4-	T46.5X5-	T46.5X6-
b-sitosterol (s)	T46.6X1-	T46.6X2-	T46.6X3-	T46.6X4-	T46.6X5-	T46.6X6-
Betaxolol	T44.7X1-	T44.7X2-	T44.7X3-	T44.7X4-	T44.7X5-	T44.7X6-
Betazole	T50.8X1-	T50.8X2-	T50.8X3-	T50.8X4-	T50.8X5-	T50.8X6-
Bethanechol	T44.1X1-	T44.1X2-	T44.1X3-	T44.1X4-	T44.1X5-	T44.1X6-
chloride	T44.1X1-	T44.1X2-	T44.1X3-	T44.1X4-	T44.1X5-	T44.1X6-
Bethanidine	T46.5X1-	T46.5X2-	T46.5X3-	T46.5X4-	T46.5X5-	T46.5X6-
Betoxycaine	T41.3X1-	T41.3X2-	T41.3X3-	T41.3X4-	T41.3X5-	T41.3X6-
Betula oil	T49.3X1-	T49.3X2-	T49.3X3-	T49.3X4-	T49.3X5-	T49.3X6-
Bevantolol	T44.7X1-	T44.7X2-	T44.7X3-	T44.7X4-	T44.7X5-	T44.7X6-
Bevonium metilsulfate	T44.3X1-	T44.3X2-	T44.3X3-	T44.3X4-	T44.3X5-	T44.3X6-
Bezafibrate	T46.6X1-	T46.6X2-	T46.6X3-	T46.6X4-	T46.6X5-	T46.6X6-
Bezitramide	T40.4X1-	T40.4X2-	T40.4X3-	T40.4X4-	T40.4X5-	T40.4X6-
BHA	T50.991-	T50.992-	T50.993-	T50.994-	T50.995-	T50.996-
Bhang	T40.7X1-	T40.7X2-	T40.7X3-	T40.7X4-	T40.7X5-	T40.7X6-
BHC (medicinal)	T49.0X1-	T49.0X2-	T49.0X3-	T49.0X4-	T49.0X5-	T49.0X6-
nonmedicinal (vapor)	T53.6X1-	T53.6X2-	T53.6X3-	T53.6X4-	-	-
Bialamicol	T37.3X1-	T37.3X2-	T37.3X3-	T37.3X4-	T37.3X5-	T37.3X6-
Bibenzonium bromide	T48.3X1-	T48.3X2-	T48.3X3-	T48.3X4-	T48.3X5-	T48.3X6-
Bibrocathol	T49.5X1-	T49.5X2-	T49.5X3-	T49.5X4-	T49.5X5-	T49.5X6-
Bichloride of mercury — *see Mercury, chloride*						
Bichromates (calcium) (potassium) (sodium) (crystals)	T57.8X1-	T57.8X2-	T57.8X3-	T57.8X4-	-	-
fumes	T56.2X1-	T56.2X2-	T56.2X3-	T56.2X4-	-	-
Biclotymol	T49.6X1-	T49.6X2-	T49.6X3-	T49.6X4-	T49.6X5-	T49.6X6-
Bicucculine	T50.7X1-	T50.7X2-	T50.7X3-	T50.7X4-	T50.7X5-	T50.7X6-
Bifemelane	T43.291-	T43.292-	T43.293-	T43.294-	T43.295-	T43.296-
Biguanide derivatives, oral	T38.3X1-	T38.3X2-	T38.3X3-	T38.3X4-	T38.3X5-	T38.3X6-
Bile salts	T47.5X1-	T47.5X2-	T47.5X3-	T47.5X4-	T47.5X5-	T47.5X6-
Biligrafin	T50.8X1-	T50.8X2-	T50.8X3-	T50.8X4-	T50.8X5-	T50.8X6-
Bilopaque	T50.8X1-	T50.8X2-	T50.8X3-	T50.8X4-	T50.8X5-	T50.8X6-
Binifibrate	T46.6X1-	T46.6X2-	T46.6X3-	T46.6X4-	T46.6X5-	T46.6X6-
Binitrobenzol	T65.3X1-	T65.3X2-	T65.3X3-	T65.3X4-	-	-
Bioflavonoid (s)	T46.991-	T46.992-	T46.993-	T46.994-	T46.995-	T46.996-
Biological substance NEC	T50.901-	T50.902-	T50.903-	T50.904-	T50.905-	T50.906-
Biotin	T45.2X1-	T45.2X2-	T45.2X3-	T45.2X4-	T45.2X5-	T45.2X6-
Biperiden	T44.3X1-	T44.3X2-	T44.3X3-	T44.3X4-	T44.3X5-	T44.3X6-
Bisacodyl	T47.2X1-	T47.2X2-	T47.2X3-	T47.2X4-	T47.2X5-	T47.2X6-
Bisbentiamine	T45.2X1-	T45.2X2-	T45.2X3-	T45.2X4-	T45.2X5-	T45.2X6-
Bisbutiamine	T45.2X1-	T45.2X2-	T45.2X3-	T45.2X4-	T45.2X5-	T45.2X6-
Bisdequalinium (salts) (diacetate)	T49.6X1-	T49.6X2-	T49.6X3-	T49.6X4-	T49.6X5-	T49.6X6-
Bishydroxycoumarin	T45.511-	T45.512-	T45.513-	T45.514-	T45.515-	T45.516-
Bismarsen	T37.8X1-	T37.8X2-	T37.8X3-	T37.8X4-	T37.8X5-	T37.8X6-
Bismuth salts	T47.6X1-	T47.6X2-	T47.6X3-	T47.6X4-	T47.6X5-	T47.6X6-
aluminate	T47.1X1-	T47.1X2-	T47.1X3-	T47.1X4-	T47.1X5-	T47.1X6-

Substance	Poisoning Accidental (unintentional)	Poisoning Intentional self-harm	Poisoning Assault	Poisoning Undetermined	Adverse effect	Underdosing
Bismuth salts (continued)						
anti-infectives	T37.8X1-	T37.8X2-	T37.8X3-	T37.8X4-	T37.8X5-	T37.8X6-
formic iodide	T49.0X1-	T49.0X2-	T49.0X3-	T49.0X4-	T49.0X5-	T49.0X6-
glycolylarsenate	T49.0X1-	T49.0X2-	T49.0X3-	T49.0X4-	T49.0X5-	T49.0X6-
nonmedicinal (compounds) NEC	T65.91X-	T65.92X-	T65.93X-	T65.94X-	-	-
subcarbonate	T47.6X1-	T47.6X2-	T47.6X3-	T47.6X4-	T47.6X5-	T47.6X6-
subsalicylate	T37.8X1-	T37.8X2-	T37.8X3-	T37.8X4-	T37.8X5-	T37.8X6-
sulfarsphenamine	T37.8X1-	T37.8X2-	T37.8X3-	T37.8X4-	T37.8X5-	T37.8X6-
Bisoprolol	T44.7X1-	T44.7X2-	T44.7X3-	T44.7X4-	T44.7X5-	T44.7X6-
Bisoxatin	T47.2X1-	T47.2X2-	T47.2X3-	T47.2X4-	T47.2X5-	T47.2X6-
Bisulepin (hydrochloride)	T45.0X1-	T45.0X2-	T45.0X3-	T45.0X4-	T45.0X5-	T45.0X6-
Bithionol	T37.8X1-	T37.8X2-	T37.8X3-	T37.8X4-	T37.8X5-	T37.8X6-
anthelminthic	T37.4X1-	T37.4X2-	T37.4X3-	T37.4X4-	T37.4X5-	T37.4X6-
Bitolterol	T48.6X1-	T48.6X2-	T48.6X3-	T48.6X4-	T48.6X5-	T48.6X6-
Bitoscanate	T37.4X1-	T37.4X2-	T37.4X3-	T37.4X4-	T37.4X5-	T37.4X6-
Bitter almond oil	T62.8X1-	T62.8X2-	T62.8X3-	T62.8X4-	-	-
Bittersweet	T62.2X1-	T62.2X2-	T62.2X3-	T62.2X4-	-	-
Black						
flag	T60.91X-	T60.92X-	T60.93X-	T60.94X-	-	-
henbane	T62.2X1-	T62.2X2-	T62.2X3-	T62.2X4-	-	-
leaf (40)	T60.91X-	T60.92X-	T60.93X-	T60.94X-	-	-
widow spider (bite)	T63.311-	T63.312-	T63.313-	T63.314-	-	-
antivenin	T50.Z11-	T50.Z12-	T50.Z13-	T50.Z14-	T50.Z15-	T50.Z16-
Blast furnace gas (carbon monoxide from)	T58.8X1-	T58.8X2-	T58.8X3-	T58.8X4-	-	-
Bleach	T54.91X-	T54.92X-	T54.93X-	T54.94X-	-	-
Bleaching agent (medicinal)	T49.4X1-	T49.4X2-	T49.4X3-	T49.4X4-	T49.4X5-	T49.4X6-
Bleomycin	T45.1X1-	T45.1X2-	T45.1X3-	T45.1X4-	T45.1X5-	T45.1X6-
Blockain	T41.3X1-	T41.3X2-	T41.3X3-	T41.3X4-	T41.3X5-	T41.3X6-
infiltration (subcutaneous)	T41.3X1-	T41.3X2-	T41.3X3-	T41.3X4-	T41.3X5-	T41.3X6-
nerve block (peripheral) (plexus)	T41.3X1-	T41.3X2-	T41.3X3-	T41.3X4-	T41.3X5-	T41.3X6-
topical (surface)	T41.3X1-	T41.3X2-	T41.3X3-	T41.3X4-	T41.3X5-	T41.3X6-
Blockers, calcium channel	T46.1X1-	T46.1X2-	T46.1X3-	T46.1X4-	T46.1X5-	T46.1X6-
Blood (derivatives) (natural) (plasma) (whole)	T45.8X1-	T45.8X2-	T45.8X3-	T45.8X4-	T45.8X5-	T45.8X6-
dried	T45.8X1-	T45.8X2-	T45.8X3-	T45.8X4-	T45.8X5-	T45.8X6-
drug affecting NEC	T45.91X-	T45.92X-	T45.93X-	T45.94X-	T45.95X-	T45.96X-
expander NEC	T45.8X1-	T45.8X2-	T45.8X3-	T45.8X4-	T45.8X5-	T45.8X6-
fraction NEC	T45.8X1-	T45.8X2-	T45.8X3-	T45.8X4-	T45.8X5-	T45.8X6-
substitute (macromolecular)	T45.8X1-	T45.8X2-	T45.8X3-	T45.8X4-	T45.8X5-	T45.8X6-
Blue velvet	T40.2X1-	T40.2X2-	T40.2X3-	T40.2X4-	-	-
Bone meal	T62.8X1-	T62.8X2-	T62.8X3-	T62.8X4-	-	-
Bonine	T45.0X1-	T45.0X2-	T45.0X3-	T45.0X4-	T45.0X5-	T45.0X6-
Bopindolol	T44.7X1-	T44.7X2-	T44.7X3-	T44.7X4-	T44.7X5-	T44.7X6-
Boracic acid	T49.0X1-	T49.0X2-	T49.0X3-	T49.0X4-	T49.0X5-	T49.0X6-
ENT agent	T49.6X1-	T49.6X2-	T49.6X3-	T49.6X4-	T49.6X5-	T49.6X6-
ophthalmic preparation	T49.5X1-	T49.5X2-	T49.5X3-	T49.5X4-	T49.5X5-	T49.5X6-
Borane complex	T57.8X1-	T57.8X2-	T57.8X3-	T57.8X4-	-	-
Borate (s)	T57.8X1-	T57.8X2-	T57.8X3-	T57.8X4-	-	-
buffer	T50.991-	T50.992-	T50.993-	T50.994-	T50.995-	T50.996-
cleanser	T54.91X-	T54.92X-	T54.93X-	T54.94X-	-	-
sodium	T57.8X1-	T57.8X2-	T57.8X3-	T57.8X4-	-	-
Borax (cleanser)	T54.91X-	T54.92X-	T54.93X-	T54.94X-	-	-
Bordeaux mixture	T60.3X1-	T60.3X2-	T60.3X3-	T60.3X4-	-	-
Boric acid	T49.0X1-	T49.0X2-	T49.0X3-	T49.0X4-	T49.0X5-	T49.0X6-
ENT agent	T49.6X1-	T49.6X2-	T49.6X3-	T49.6X4-	T49.6X5-	T49.6X6-
ophthalmic preparation	T49.5X1-	T49.5X2-	T49.5X3-	T49.5X4-	T49.5X5-	T49.5X6-
Bornaprine	T44.3X1-	T44.3X2-	T44.3X3-	T44.3X4-	T44.3X5-	T44.3X6-

Substance	Poisoning Accidental (unintentional)	Poisoning Intentional self-harm	Poisoning Assault	Poisoning Undetermined	Adverse effect	Underdosing
Boron	T57.8X1-	T57.8X2-	T57.8X3-	T57.8X4-	-	-
hydride NEC	T57.8X1-	T57.8X2-	T57.8X3-	T57.8X4-	-	-
fumes or gas	T57.8X1-	T57.8X2-	T57.8X3-	T57.8X4-	-	-
trifluoride	T59.891-	T59.892-	T59.893-	T59.894-	-	-
Botox	T48.291-	T48.292-	T48.293-	T48.294-	T48.295-	T48.296-
Botulinus anti-toxin (type A, B)	T50.Z11-	T50.Z12-	T50.Z13-	T50.Z14-	T50.Z15-	T50.Z16-
Brake fluid vapor	T59.891-	T59.892-	T59.893-	T59.894-	-	-
Brallobarbital	T42.3X1-	T42.3X2-	T42.3X3-	T42.3X4-	T42.3X5-	T42.3X6-
Bran (wheat)	T47.4X1-	T47.4X2-	T47.4X3-	T47.4X4-	T47.4X5-	T47.4X6-
Brass (fumes)	T56.891-	T56.892-	T56.893-	T56.894-	-	-
Brasso	T52.0X1-	T52.0X2-	T52.0X3-	T52.0X4-	-	-
Bretylium tosilate	T46.2X1-	T46.2X2-	T46.2X3-	T46.2X4-	T46.2X5-	T46.2X6-
Brevital (sodium)	T41.1X1-	T41.1X2-	T41.1X3-	T41.1X4-	T41.1X5-	T41.1X6-
Brinase	T45.3X1-	T45.3X2-	T45.3X3-	T45.3X4-	T45.3X5-	T45.3X6-
British antilewisite	T45.8X1-	T45.8X2-	T45.8X3-	T45.8X4-	T45.8X5-	T45.8X6-
Brodifacoum	T60.4X1-	T60.4X2-	T60.4X3-	T60.4X4-	-	-
Bromal (hydrate)	T42.6X1-	T42.6X2-	T42.6X3-	T42.6X4-	T42.6X5-	T42.6X6-
Bromazepam	T42.4X1-	T42.4X2-	T42.4X3-	T42.4X4-	T42.4X5-	T42.4X6-
Bromazine	T45.0X1-	T45.0X2-	T45.0X3-	T45.0X4-	T45.0X5-	T45.0X6-
Brombenzylcyanide	T59.3X1-	T59.3X2-	T59.3X3-	T59.3X4-	-	-
Bromelains	T45.3X1-	T45.3X2-	T45.3X3-	T45.3X4-	T45.3X5-	T45.3X6-
Bromethalin	T60.4X1-	T60.4X2-	T60.4X3-	T60.4X4-	-	-
Bromhexine	T48.4X1-	T48.4X2-	T48.4X3-	T48.4X4-	T48.4X5-	T48.4X6-
Bromide salts	T42.6X1-	T42.6X2-	T42.6X3-	T42.6X4-	T42.6X5-	T42.6X6-
Bromindione	T45.511-	T45.512-	T45.513-	T45.514-	T45.515-	T45.516-
Bromine						
compounds (medicinal)	T42.6X1-	T42.6X2-	T42.6X3-	T42.6X4-	T42.6X5-	T42.6X6-
sedative	T42.6X1-	T42.6X2-	T42.6X3-	T42.6X4-	T42.6X5-	T42.6X6-
vapor	T59.891-	T59.892-	T59.893-	T59.894-	-	-
Bromisoval	T42.6X1-	T42.6X2-	T42.6X3-	T42.6X4-	T42.6X5-	T42.6X6-
Bromisovalum	T42.6X1-	T42.6X2-	T42.6X3-	T42.6X4-	T42.6X5-	T42.6X6-
Bromobenzylcyanide	T59.3X1-	T59.3X2-	T59.3X3-	T59.3X4-	-	-
Bromochlorosalicylani-lide	T49.0X1-	T49.0X2-	T49.0X3-	T49.0X4-	T49.0X5-	T49.0X6-
Bromocriptine	T42.8X1-	T42.8X2-	T42.8X3-	T42.8X4-	T42.8X5-	T42.8X6-
Bromodiphenhydramine	T45.0X1-	T45.0X2-	T45.0X3-	T45.0X4-	T45.0X5-	T45.0X6-
Bromoform	T42.6X1-	T42.6X2-	T42.6X3-	T42.6X4-	T42.6X5-	T42.6X6-
Bromophenol blue reagent	T50.991-	T50.992-	T50.993-	T50.994-	T50.995-	T50.996-
Bromopride	T47.8X1-	T47.8X2-	T47.8X3-	T47.8X4-	T47.8X5-	T47.8X6-
Bromosalicylchloranitide	T49.0X1-	T49.0X2-	T49.0X3-	T49.0X4-	T49.0X5-	T49.0X6-
Bromosalicylhydroxamic acid	T37.1X1-	T37.1X2-	T37.1X3-	T37.1X4-	T37.1X5-	T37.1X6-
Bromo-seltzer	T39.1X1-	T39.1X2-	T39.1X3-	T39.1X4-	T39.1X5-	T39.1X6-
Bromoxynil	T60.3X1-	T60.3X2-	T60.3X3-	T60.3X4-	-	-
Bromperidol	T43.4X1-	T43.4X2-	T43.4X3-	T43.4X4-	T43.4X5-	T43.4X6-
Brompheniramine	T45.0X1-	T45.0X2-	T45.0X3-	T45.0X4-	T45.0X5-	T45.0X6-
Bromsulfophthalein	T50.8X1-	T50.8X2-	T50.8X3-	T50.8X4-	T50.8X5-	T50.8X6-
Bromural	T42.6X1-	T42.6X2-	T42.6X3-	T42.6X4-	T42.6X5-	T42.6X6-
Bromvaletone	T42.6X1-	T42.6X2-	T42.6X3-	T42.6X4-	T42.6X5-	T42.6X6-
Bronchodilator NEC	T48.6X1-	T48.6X2-	T48.6X3-	T48.6X4-	T48.6X5-	T48.6X6-
Brotizolam	T42.4X1-	T42.4X2-	T42.4X3-	T42.4X4-	T42.4X5-	T42.4X6-
Brovincamine	T46.7X1-	T46.7X2-	T46.7X3-	T46.7X4-	T46.7X5-	T46.7X6-
Brown recluse spider (bite) (venom)	T63.331-	T63.332-	T63.333-	T63.334-	-	-
Brown spider (bite) (venom)	T63.391-	T63.392-	T63.393-	T63.394-	-	-
Broxaterol	T48.6X1-	T48.6X2-	T48.6X3-	T48.6X4-	T48.6X5-	T48.6X6-
Broxuridine	T45.1X1-	T45.1X2-	T45.1X3-	T45.1X4-	T45.1X5-	T45.1X6-
Broxyquinoline	T37.8X1-	T37.8X2-	T37.8X3-	T37.8X4-	T37.8X5-	T37.8X6-
Bruceine	T48.291-	T48.292-	T48.293-	T48.294-	T48.295-	T48.296-
Brucia	T62.2X1-	T62.2X2-	T62.2X3-	T62.2X4-	-	-
Brucine	T65.1X1-	T65.1X2-	T65.1X3-	T65.1X4-	-	-
Brunswick green — *see Copper*						

Substance	Poisoning Accidental (unintentional)	Poisoning Intentional self-harm	Poisoning Assault	Poisoning Undetermined	Adverse effect	Underdosing
Bruten — *see Ibuprofen*						
Bryonia	T47.2X1-	T47.2X2-	T47.2X3-	T47.2X4-	T47.2X5-	T47.2X6-
Buclizine	T45.0X1-	T45.0X2-	T45.0X3-	T45.0X4-	T45.0X5-	T45.0X6-
Buclosamide	T49.0X1-	T49.0X2-	T49.0X3-	T49.0X4-	T49.0X5-	T49.0X6-
Budesonide	T44.5X1-	T44.5X2-	T44.5X3-	T44.5X4-	T44.5X5-	T44.5X6-
Budralazine	T46.5X1-	T46.5X2-	T46.5X3-	T46.5X4-	T46.5X5-	T46.5X6-
Bufferin	T39.011-	T39.012-	T39.013-	T39.014-	T39.015-	T39.016-
Buflomedil	T46.7X1-	T46.7X2-	T46.7X3-	T46.7X4-	T46.7X5-	T46.7X6-
Buformin	T38.3X1-	T38.3X2-	T38.3X3-	T38.3X4-	T38.3X5-	T38.3X6-
Bufotenine	T40.991-	T40.992-	T40.993-	T40.994-	-	-
Bufrolin	T48.6X1-	T48.6X2-	T48.6X3-	T48.6X4-	T48.6X5-	T48.6X6-
Bufylline	T48.6X1-	T48.6X2-	T48.6X3-	T48.6X4-	T48.6X5-	T48.6X6-
Bulk filler	T50.5X1-	T50.5X2-	T50.5X3-	T50.5X4-	T50.5X5-	T50.5X6-
cathartic	T47.4X1-	T47.4X2-	T47.4X3-	T47.4X4-	T47.4X5-	T47.4X6-
Bumetanide	T50.1X1-	T50.1X2-	T50.1X3-	T50.1X4-	T50.1X5-	T50.1X6-
Bunaftine	T46.2X1-	T46.2X2-	T46.2X3-	T46.2X4-	T46.2X5-	T46.2X6-
Bunamiodyl	T50.8X1-	T50.8X2-	T50.8X3-	T50.8X4-	T50.8X5-	T50.8X6-
Bunazosin	T44.6X1-	T44.6X2-	T44.6X3-	T44.6X4-	T44.6X5-	T44.6X6-
Bunitrolol	T44.7X1-	T44.7X2-	T44.7X3-	T44.7X4-	T44.7X5-	T44.7X6-
Buphenine	T46.7X1-	T46.7X2-	T46.7X3-	T46.7X4-	T46.7X5-	T46.7X6-
Bupivacaine	T41.3X1-	T41.3X2-	T41.3X3-	T41.3X4-	T41.3X5-	T41.3X6-
infiltration (subcutaneous)	T41.3X1-	T41.3X2-	T41.3X3-	T41.3X4-	T41.3X5-	T41.3X6-
nerve block (peripheral) (plexus)	T41.3X1-	T41.3X2-	T41.3X3-	T41.3X4-	T41.3X5-	T41.3X6-
spinal	T41.3X1-	T41.3X2-	T41.3X3-	T41.3X4-	T41.3X5-	T41.3X6-
Bupranolol	T44.7X1-	T44.7X2-	T44.7X3-	T44.7X4-	T44.7X5-	T44.7X6-
Buprenorphine	T40.4X1-	T40.4X2-	T40.4X3-	T40.4X4-	T40.4X5-	T40.4X6-
Bupropion	T43.291-	T43.292-	T43.293-	T43.294-	T43.295-	T43.296-
Burimamide	T47.1X1-	T47.1X2-	T47.1X3-	T47.1X4-	T47.1X5-	T47.1X6-
Buserelin	T38.891-	T38.892-	T38.893-	T38.894-	T38.895-	T38.896-
Buspirone	T43.591-	T43.592-	T43.593-	T43.594-	T43.595-	T43.596-
Busulfan, busulphan	T45.1X1-	T45.1X2-	T45.1X3-	T45.1X4-	T45.1X5-	T45.1X6-
Butabarbital (sodium)	T42.3X1-	T42.3X2-	T42.3X3-	T42.3X4-	T42.3X5-	T42.3X6-
Butabarbitone	T42.3X1-	T42.3X2-	T42.3X3-	T42.3X4-	T42.3X5-	T42.3X6-
Butabarpal	T42.3X1-	T42.3X2-	T42.3X3-	T42.3X4-	T42.3X5-	T42.3X6-
Butacaine	T41.3X1-	T41.3X2-	T41.3X3-	T41.3X4-	T41.3X5-	T41.3X6-
Butalamine	T46.7X1-	T46.7X2-	T46.7X3-	T46.7X4-	T46.7X5-	T46.7X6-
Butalbital	T42.3X1-	T42.3X2-	T42.3X3-	T42.3X4-	T42.3X5-	T42.3X6-
Butallylonal	T42.3X1-	T42.3X2-	T42.3X3-	T42.3X4-	T42.3X5-	T42.3X6-
Butamben	T41.3X1-	T41.3X2-	T41.3X3-	T41.3X4-	T41.3X5-	T41.3X6-
Butamirate	T48.3X1-	T48.3X2-	T48.3X3-	T48.3X4-	T48.3X5-	T48.3X6-
Butane (distributed in mobile container)	T59.891-	T59.892-	T59.893-	T59.894-	-	-
distributed through pipes	T59.891-	T59.892-	T59.893-	T59.894-	-	-
incomplete combustion	T58.11X-	T58.12X-	T58.13X-	T58.14X-	-	-
Butanilicaine	T41.3X1-	T41.3X2-	T41.3X3-	T41.3X4-	T41.3X5-	T41.3X6-
Butanol	T51.3X1-	T51.3X2-	T51.3X3-	T51.3X4-	-	
Butanone, 2-butanone	T52.4X1-	T52.4X2-	T52.4X3-	T52.4X4-	-	
Butantrone	T49.4X1-	T49.4X2-	T49.4X3-	T49.4X4-	T49.4X5-	T49.4X6-
Butaperazine	T43.3X1-	T43.3X2-	T43.3X3-	T43.3X4-	T43.3X5-	T43.3X6-
Butazolidin	T39.2X1-	T39.2X2-	T39.2X3-	T39.2X4-	T39.2X5-	T39.2X6-
Butetamate	T48.6X1-	T48.6X2-	T48.6X3-	T48.6X4-	T48.6X5-	T48.6X6-
Butethal	T42.3X1-	T42.3X2-	T42.3X3-	T42.3X4-	T42.3X5-	T42.3X6-
Butethamate	T44.3X1-	T44.3X2-	T44.3X3-	T44.3X4-	T44.3X5-	T44.3X6-
Buthalitone (sodium)	T41.1X1-	T41.1X2-	T41.1X3-	T41.1X4-	T41.1X5-	T41.1X6-
Butisol (sodium)	T42.3X1-	T42.3X2-	T42.3X3-	T42.3X4-	T42.3X5-	T42.3X6-
Butizide	T50.2X1-	T50.2X2-	T50.2X3-	T50.2X4-	T50.2X5-	T50.2X6-
Butobarbital	T42.3X1-	T42.3X2-	T42.3X3-	T42.3X4-	T42.3X5-	T42.3X6-
sodium	T42.3X1-	T42.3X2-	T42.3X3-	T42.3X4-	T42.3X5-	T42.3X6-
Butobarbitone	T42.3X1-	T42.3X2-	T42.3X3-	T42.3X4-	T42.3X5-	T42.3X6-

Substance	Poisoning Accidental (unintentional)	Poisoning Intentional self-harm	Poisoning Assault	Poisoning Undetermined	Adverse effect	Underdosing
Butoconazole (nitrate)	T49.0X1-	T49.0X2-	T49.0X3-	T49.0X4-	T49.0X5-	T49.0X6-
Butorphanol	T40.4X1-	T40.4X2-	T40.4X3-	T40.4X4-	T40.4X5-	T40.4X6-
Butriptyline	T43.011-	T43.012-	T43.013-	T43.014-	T43.015-	T43.016-
Butropium bromide	T44.3X1-	T44.3X2-	T44.3X3-	T44.3X4-	T44.3X5-	T44.3X6-
Butter of antimony — *see Antimony*						
Buttercups	T62.2X1-	T62.2X2-	T62.2X3-	T62.2X4-	-	-
Butyl						
acetate (secondary)	T52.8X1-	T52.8X2-	T52.8X3-	T52.8X4-	-	-
alcohol	T51.3X1-	T51.3X2-	T51.3X3-	T51.3X4-	-	-
aminobenzoate	T41.3X1-	T41.3X2-	T41.3X3-	T41.3X4-	T41.3X5-	T41.3X6-
butyrate	T52.8X1-	T52.8X2-	T52.8X3-	T52.8X4-	-	-
carbinol	T51.3X1-	T51.3X2-	T51.3X3-	T51.3X4-	-	-
carbitol	T52.3X1-	T52.3X2-	T52.3X3-	T52.3X4-	-	-
cellosolve	T52.3X1-	T52.3X2-	T52.3X3-	T52.3X4-	-	-
chloral (hydrate)	T42.6X1-	T42.6X2-	T42.6X3-	T42.6X4-	T42.6X5-	T42.6X6-
formate	T52.8X1-	T52.8X2-	T52.8X3-	T52.8X4-	-	-
lactate	T52.8X1-	T52.8X2-	T52.8X3-	T52.8X4-	-	-
propionate	T52.8X1-	T52.8X2-	T52.8X3-	T52.8X4-	-	-
scopolamine bromide	T44.3X1-	T44.3X2-	T44.3X3-	T44.3X4-	T44.3X5-	T44.3X6-
thiobarbital sodium	T41.1X1-	T41.1X2-	T41.1X3-	T41.1X4-	T41.1X5-	T41.1X6-
Butylated hydroxy-anisole	T50.991-	T50.992-	T50.993-	T50.994-	T50.995-	T50.996-
Butylchloral hydrate	T42.6X1-	T42.6X2-	T42.6X3-	T42.6X4-	T42.6X5-	T42.6X6-
Butyltoluene	T52.2X1-	T52.2X2-	T52.2X3-	T52.2X4-	-	-
Butyn	T41.3X1-	T41.3X2-	T41.3X3-	T41.3X4-	T41.3X5-	T41.3X6-
Butyrophenone (-based tranquilizers)	T43.4X1-	T43.4X2-	T43.4X3-	T43.4X4-	T43.4X5-	T43.4X6-
Cabergoline	T42.8X1-	T42.8X2-	T42.8X3-	T42.8X4-	T42.8X5-	T42.8X6-
Cacodyl, cacodylic acid	T57.0X1-	T57.0X2-	T57.0X3-	T57.0X4-	-	-
Cactinomycin	T45.1X1-	T45.1X2-	T45.1X3-	T45.1X4-	T45.1X5-	T45.1X6-
Cade oil	T49.4X1-	T49.4X2-	T49.4X3-	T49.4X4-	T49.4X5-	T49.4X6-
Cadexomer iodine	T49.0X1-	T49.0X2-	T49.0X3-	T49.0X4-	T49.0X5-	T49.0X6-
Cadmium (chloride) (fumes) (oxide)	T56.3X1-	T56.3X2-	T56.3X3-	T56.3X4-	-	-
sulfide (medicinal) NEC	T49.4X1-	T49.4X2-	T49.4X3-	T49.4X4-	T49.4X5-	T49.4X6-
Cadralazine	T46.5X1-	T46.5X2-	T46.5X3-	T46.5X4-	T46.5X5-	T46.5X6-
Caffeine	T43.611-	T43.612-	T43.613-	T43.614-	T43.615-	T43.616-
Calabar bean	T62.2X1-	T62.2X2-	T62.2X3-	T62.2X4-	-	-
Caladium seguinum	T62.2X1-	T62.2X2-	T62.2X3-	T62.2X4-	-	-
Calamine (lotion)	T49.3X1-	T49.3X2-	T49.3X3-	T49.3X4-	T49.3X5-	T49.3X6-
Calcifediol	T45.2X1-	T45.2X2-	T45.2X3-	T45.2X4-	T45.2X5-	T45.2X6-
Calciferol	T45.2X1-	T45.2X2-	T45.2X3-	T45.2X4-	T45.2X5-	T45.2X6-
Calcitonin	T50.991-	T50.992-	T50.993-	T50.994-	T50.995-	T50.996-
Calcitriol	T45.2X1-	T45.2X2-	T45.2X3-	T45.2X4-	T45.2X5-	T45.2X6-
Calcium	T50.3X1-	T50.3X2-	T50.3X3-	T50.3X4-	T50.3X5-	T50.3X6-
actylsalicylate	T39.011-	T39.012-	T39.013-	T39.014-	T39.015-	T39.016-
benzamidosalicylate	T37.1X1-	T37.1X2-	T37.1X3-	T37.1X4-	T37.1X5-	T37.1X6-
bromide	T42.6X1-	T42.6X2-	T42.6X3-	T42.6X4-	T42.6X5-	T42.6X6-
bromolactobionate	T42.6X1-	T42.6X2-	T42.6X3-	T42.6X4-	T42.6X5-	T42.6X6-
carbaspirin	T39.011-	T39.012-	T39.013-	T39.014-	T39.015-	T39.016-
carbimide	T50.6X1-	T50.6X2-	T50.6X3-	T50.6X4-	T50.6X5-	T50.6X6-
carbonate	T47.1X1-	T47.1X2-	T47.1X3-	T47.1X4-	T47.1X5-	T47.1X6-
chloride	T50.991-	T50.992-	T50.993-	T50.994-	T50.995-	T50.996-
anhydrous	T50.991-	T50.992-	T50.993-	T50.994-	T50.995-	T50.996-
cyanide	T57.8X1-	T57.8X2-	T57.8X3-	T57.8X4-	-	-
dioctyl sulfosuccinate	T47.4X1-	T47.4X2-	T47.4X3-	T47.4X4-	T47.4X5-	T47.4X6-
disodium edathamil	T45.8X1-	T45.8X2-	T45.8X3-	T45.8X4-	T45.8X5-	T45.8X6-
disodium edetate	T45.8X1-	T45.8X2-	T45.8X3-	T45.8X4-	T45.8X5-	T45.8X6-
dobesilate	T46.991-	T46.992-	T46.993-	T46.994-	T46.995-	T46.996-
EDTA	T45.8X1-	T45.8X2-	T45.8X3-	T45.8X4-	T45.8X5-	T45.8X6-
ferrous citrate	T45.4X1-	T45.4X2-	T45.4X3-	T45.4X4-	T45.4X5-	T45.4X6-
folinate	T45.8X1-	T45.8X2-	T45.8X3-	T45.8X4-	T45.8X5-	T45.8X6-

Substance	Poisoning Accidental (unintentional)	Poisoning Intentional self-harm	Poisoning Assault	Poisoning Undetermined	Adverse effect	Underdosing
Calcium (continued)						
glubionate	T50.3X1-	T50.3X2-	T50.3X3-	T50.3X4-	T50.3X5-	T50.3X6-
gluconate	T50.3X1-	T50.3X2-	T50.3X3-	T50.3X4-	T50.3X5-	T50.3X6-
gluconogalactogluc-onate	T50.3X1-	T50.3X2-	T50.3X3-	T50.3X4-	T50.3X5-	T50.3X6-
hydrate, hydroxide	T54.3X1-	T54.3X2-	T54.3X3-	T54.3X4-	-	-
hypochlorite	T54.3X1-	T54.3X2-	T54.3X3-	T54.3X4-	-	-
iodide	T48.4X1-	T48.4X2-	T48.4X3-	T48.4X4-	T48.4X5-	T48.4X6-
ipodate	T50.8X1-	T50.8X2-	T50.8X3-	T50.8X4-	T50.8X5-	T50.8X6-
lactate	T50.3X1-	T50.3X2-	T50.3X3-	T50.3X4-	T50.3X5-	T50.3X6-
leucovorin	T45.8X1-	T45.8X2-	T45.8X3-	T45.8X4-	T45.8X5-	T45.8X6-
mandelate	T37.91X-	T37.92X-	T37.93X-	T37.94X-	T37.95X-	T37.96X-
oxide	T54.3X1-	T54.3X2-	T54.3X3-	T54.3X4-	-	-
pantothenate	T45.2X1-	T45.2X2-	T45.2X3-	T45.2X4-	T45.2X5-	T45.2X6-
phosphate	T50.3X1-	T50.3X2-	T50.3X3-	T50.3X4-	T50.3X5-	T50.3X6-
salicylate	T39.091-	T39.092-	T39.093-	T39.094-	T39.095-	T39.096-
salts	T50.3X1-	T50.3X2-	T50.3X3-	T50.3X4-	T50.3X5-	T50.3X6-
Calculus-dissolving drug	T50.991-	T50.992-	T50.993-	T50.994-	T50.995-	T50.996-
Calomel	T49.0X1-	T49.0X2-	T49.0X3-	T49.0X4-	T49.0X5-	T49.0X6-
Caloric agent	T50.3X1-	T50.3X2-	T50.3X3-	T50.3X4-	T50.3X5-	T50.3X6-
Calusterone	T38.7X1-	T38.7X2-	T38.7X3-	T38.7X4-	T38.7X5-	T38.7X6-
Camazepam	T42.4X1-	T42.4X2-	T42.4X3-	T42.4X4-	T42.4X5-	T42.4X6-
Camomile	T49.0X1-	T49.0X2-	T49.0X3-	T49.0X4-	T49.0X5-	T49.0X6-
Camoquin	T37.2X1-	T37.2X2-	T37.2X3-	T37.2X4-	T37.2X5-	T37.2X6-
Camphor						
insecticide	T60.2X1-	T60.2X2-	T60.2X3-	T60.2X4-	-	-
medicinal	T49.8X1-	T49.8X2-	T49.8X3-	T49.8X4-	T49.8X5-	T49.8X6-
Camylofin	T44.3X1-	T44.3X2-	T44.3X3-	T44.3X4-	T44.3X5-	T44.3X6-
Cancer chemotherapy drug regimen	T45.1X1-	T45.1X2-	T45.1X3-	T45.1X4-	T45.1X5-	T45.1X6-
Candeptin	T49.0X1-	T49.0X2-	T49.0X3-	T49.0X4-	T49.0X5-	T49.0X6-
Candicidin	T49.0X1-	T49.0X2-	T49.0X3-	T49.0X4-	T49.0X5-	T49.0X6-
Cannabinol	T40.7X1-	T40.7X2-	T40.7X3-	T40.7X4-	T40.7X5-	T40.7X6-
Cannabis (derivatives)	T40.7X1-	T40.7X2-	T40.7X3-	T40.7X4-	T40.7X5-	T40.7X6-
Canned heat	T51.1X1-	T51.1X2-	T51.1X3-	T51.1X4-	-	-
Canrenoic acid	T50.0X1-	T50.0X2-	T50.0X3-	T50.0X4-	T50.0X5-	T50.0X6-
Canrenone	T50.0X1-	T50.0X2-	T50.0X3-	T50.0X4-	T50.0X5-	T50.0X6-
Cantharides, cantharidin, cantharis	T49.8X1-	T49.8X2-	T49.8X3-	T49.8X4-	T49.8X5-	T49.8X6-
Canthaxanthin	T50.991-	T50.992-	T50.993-	T50.994-	T50.995-	T50.996-
Capillary-active drug NEC	T46.901-	T46.902-	T46.903-	T46.904-	T46.905-	T46.906-
Capreomycin	T36.8X1-	T36.8X2-	T36.8X3-	T36.8X4-	T36.8X5-	T36.8X6-
Capsicum	T49.4X1-	T49.4X2-	T49.4X3-	T49.4X4-	T49.4X5-	T49.4X6-
Captafol	T60.3X1-	T60.3X2-	T60.3X3-	T60.3X4-	-	-
Captan	T60.3X1-	T60.3X2-	T60.3X3-	T60.3X4-	-	-
Captodiame, captodiamine	T43.591-	T43.592-	T43.593-	T43.594-	T43.595-	T43.596-
Captopril	T46.4X1-	T46.4X2-	T46.4X3-	T46.4X4-	T46.4X5-	T46.4X6-
Caramiphen	T44.3X1-	T44.3X2-	T44.3X3-	T44.3X4-	T44.3X5-	T44.3X6-
Carazolol	T44.7X1-	T44.7X2-	T44.7X3-	T44.7X4-	T44.7X5-	T44.7X6-
Carbachol	T44.1X1-	T44.1X2-	T44.1X3-	T44.1X4-	T44.1X5-	T44.1X6-
Carbacrylamine (resin)	T50.3X1-	T50.3X2-	T50.3X3-	T50.3X4-	T50.3X5-	T50.3X6-
Carbamate (insecticide)	T60.0X1-	T60.0X2-	T60.0X3-	T60.0X4-	-	-
Carbamate (sedative)	T42.6X1-	T42.6X2-	T42.6X3-	T42.6X4-	T42.6X5-	T42.6X6-
herbicide	T60.0X1-	T60.0X2-	T60.0X3-	T60.0X4-	-	-
insecticide	T60.0X1-	T60.0X2-	T60.0X3-	T60.0X4-	-	-
Carbamazepine	T42.1X1-	T42.1X2-	T42.1X3-	T42.1X4-	T42.1X5-	T42.1X6-
Carbamide	T47.3X1-	T47.3X2-	T47.3X3-	T47.3X4-	T47.3X5-	T47.3X6-
peroxide	T49.0X1-	T49.0X2-	T49.0X3-	T49.0X4-	T49.0X5-	T49.0X6-
topical	T49.8X1-	T49.8X2-	T49.8X3-	T49.8X4-	T49.8X5-	T49.8X6-
Carbamylcholine chloride	T44.1X1-	T44.1X2-	T44.1X3-	T44.1X4-	T44.1X5-	T44.1X6-
Carbaril	T60.0X1-	T60.0X2-	T60.0X3-	T60.0X4-	-	-
Carbarsone	T37.3X1-	T37.3X2-	T37.3X3-	T37.3X4-	T37.3X5-	T37.3X6-

Substance	Poisoning Accidental (unintentional)	Poisoning Intentional self-harm	Poisoning Assault	Poisoning Undetermined	Adverse effect	Underdosing
Carbaryl	T60.0X1-	T60.0X2-	T60.0X3-	T60.0X4-	-	-
Carbaspirin	T39.011-	T39.012-	T39.013-	T39.014-	T39.015-	T39.016-
Carbazochrome (salicylate) (sodium sulfonate)	T49.4X1-	T49.4X2-	T49.4X3-	T49.4X4-	T49.4X5-	T49.4X6-
Carbenicillin	T36.0X1-	T36.0X2-	T36.0X3-	T36.0X4-	T36.0X5-	T36.0X6-
Carbenoxolone	T47.1X1-	T47.1X2-	T47.1X3-	T47.1X4-	T47.1X5-	T47.1X6-
Carbetapentane	T48.3X1-	T48.3X2-	T48.3X3-	T48.3X4-	T48.3X5-	T48.3X6-
Carbethyl salicylate	T39.091-	T39.092-	T39.093-	T39.094-	T39.095-	T39.096-
Carbidopa (with levodopa)	T42.8X1-	T42.8X2-	T42.8X3-	T42.8X4-	T42.8X5-	T42.8X6-
Carbimazole	T38.2X1-	T38.2X2-	T38.2X3-	T38.2X4-	T38.2X5-	T38.2X6-
Carbinol	T51.1X1-	T51.1X2-	T51.1X3-	T51.1X4-	-	-
Carbinoxamine	T45.0X1-	T45.0X2-	T45.0X3-	T45.0X4-	T45.0X5-	T45.0X6-
Carbiphene	T39.8X1-	T39.8X2-	T39.8X3-	T39.8X4-	T39.8X5-	T39.8X6-
Carbitol	T52.3X1-	T52.3X2-	T52.3X3-	T52.3X4-	-	-
Carbo medicinalis	T47.6X1-	T47.6X2-	T47.6X3-	T47.6X4-	T47.6X5-	T47.6X6-
Carbocaine	T41.3X1-	T41.3X2-	T41.3X3-	T41.3X4-	T41.3X5-	T41.3X6-
infiltration (subcutaneous)	T41.3X1-	T41.3X2-	T41.3X3-	T41.3X4-	T41.3X5-	T41.3X6-
nerve block (peripheral) (plexus)	T41.3X1-	T41.3X2-	T41.3X3-	T41.3X4-	T41.3X5-	T41.3X6-
topical (surface)	T41.3X1-	T41.3X2-	T41.3X3-	T41.3X4-	T41.3X5-	T41.3X6-
Carbocisteine	T48.4X1-	T48.4X2-	T48.4X3-	T48.4X4-	T48.4X5-	T48.4X6-
Carbocromen	T46.3X1-	T46.3X2-	T46.3X3-	T46.3X4-	T46.3X5-	T46.3X6-
Carbol fuchsin	T49.0X1-	T49.0X2-	T49.0X3-	T49.0X4-	T49.0X5-	T49.0X6-
Carbolic acid — *see also* Phenol	T54.0X1-	T54.0X2-	T54.0X3-	T54.0X4-	-	-
Carbolonium (bromide)	T48.1X1-	T48.1X2-	T48.1X3-	T48.1X4-	T48.1X5-	T48.1X6-
Carbomycin	T36.8X1-	T36.8X2-	T36.8X3-	T36.8X4-	T36.8X5-	T36.8X6-
Carbon						
bisulfide (liquid)	T65.4X1-	T65.4X2-	T65.4X3-	T65.4X4-	-	-
vapor	T65.4X1-	T65.4X2-	T65.4X3-	T65.4X4-	-	-
dioxide (gas)	T59.7X1-	T59.7X2-	T59.7X3-	T59.7X4-	-	-
medicinal	T41.5X1-	T41.5X2-	T41.5X3-	T41.5X4-	T41.5X5-	T41.5X6-
nonmedicinal	T59.7X1-	T59.7X2-	T59.7X3-	T59.7X4-	-	-
snow	T49.4X1-	T49.4X2-	T49.4X3-	T49.4X4-	T49.4X5-	T49.4X6-
disulfide (liquid)	T65.4X1-	T65.4X2-	T65.4X3-	T65.4X4-	-	-
vapor	T65.4X1-	T65.4X2-	T65.4X3-	T65.4X4-	-	-
monoxide (from incomplete combustion)	T58.91X-	T58.92X-	T58.93X-	T58.94X-	-	-
blast furnace gas	T58.8X1-	T58.8X2-	T58.8X3-	T58.8X4-	-	-
butane (distributed in mobile container)	T58.11X-	T58.12X-	T58.13X-	T58.14X-	-	-
distributed through pipes	T58.11X-	T58.12X-	T58.13X-	T58.14X-	-	-
charcoal fumes	T58.2X1-	T58.2X2-	T58.2X3-	T58.2X4-	-	-
coal	T58.2X1-	T58.2X2-	T58.2X3-	T58.2X4-	-	-
coke (in domestic stoves, fireplaces)	T58.2X1-	T58.2X2-	T58.2X3-	T58.2X4-	-	-
gas (piped)	T58.11X-	T58.12X-	T58.13X-	T58.14X-	-	-
solid (in domestic stoves, fireplaces)	T58.2X1-	T58.2X2-	T58.2X3-	T58.2X4-	-	-
exhaust gas (motor) not in transit	T58.01X-	T58.02X-	T58.03X-	T58.04X-	-	-
combustion engine, any not in watercraft	T58.01X-	T58.02X-	T58.03X-	T58.04X-	-	-
farm tractor, not in transit	T58.01X-	T58.02X-	T58.03X-	T58.04X-	-	-
gas engine	T58.01X-	T58.02X-	T58.03X-	T58.04X-	-	-
motor pump	T58.01X-	T58.02X-	T58.03X-	T58.04X-	-	-
motor vehicle, not in transit	T58.01X-	T58.02X-	T58.03X-	T58.04X-	-	-
fuel (in domestic use)	T58.2X1-	T58.2X2-	T58.2X3-	T58.2X4-	-	-
gas (piped)	T58.11X-	T58.12X-	T58.13X-	T58.14X-	-	-
in mobile container	T58.11X-	T58.12X-	T58.13X-	T58.14X-	-	-
piped (natural)	T58.11X-	T58.12X-	T58.13X-	T58.14X-	-	-
utility	T58.11X-	T58.12X-	T58.13X-	T58.14X-	-	-
in mobile container	T58.11X-	T58.12X-	T58.13X-	T58.14X-	-	-
illuminating gas	T58.11X-	T58.12X-	T58.13X-	T58.14X-	-	-
industrial fuels or gases, any	T58.8X1-	T58.8X2-	T58.8X3-	T58.8X4-	-	-

Substance	Poisoning Accidental (unintentional)	Poisoning Intentional self-harm	Poisoning Assault	Poisoning Undetermined	Adverse effect	Underdosing
Carbon (continued)						
kerosene (in domestic stoves, fireplaces)	T58.2X1-	T58.2X2-	T58.2X3-	T58.2X4-	-	-
kiln gas or vapor	T58.8X1-	T58.8X2-	T58.8X3-	T58.8X4-	-	-
motor exhaust gas, not in transit	T58.01X-	T58.02X-	T58.03X-	T58.04X-	-	-
piped gas (manufactured) (natural)	T58.11X-	T58.12X-	T58.13X-	T58.14X-	-	-
producer gas	T58.8X1-	T58.8X2-	T58.8X3-	T58.8X4-	-	-
propane (distributed in mobile container)	T58.11X-	T58.12X-	T58.13X-	T58.14X-	-	-
distributed through pipes	T58.11X-	T58.12X-	T58.13X-	T58.14X-	-	-
specified source NEC	T58.8X1-	T58.8X2-	T58.8X3-	T58.8X4-	-	-
stove gas	T58.11X-	T58.12X-	T58.13X-	T58.14X-	-	-
piped	T58.11X-	T58.12X-	T58.13X-	T58.14X-	-	-
utility gas	T58.11X-	T58.12X-	T58.13X-	T58.14X-	-	-
piped	T58.11X-	T58.12X-	T58.13X-	T58.14X-	-	-
water gas	T58.11X-	T58.12X-	T58.13X-	T58.14X-	-	-
wood (in domestic stoves, fireplaces)	T58.2X1-	T58.2X2-	T58.2X3-	T58.2X4-	-	-
tetrachloride (vapor) NEC	T53.0X1-	T53.0X2-	T53.0X3-	T53.0X4-	-	-
liquid (cleansing agent) NEC	T53.0X1-	T53.0X2-	T53.0X3-	T53.0X4-	-	-
solvent	T53.0X1-	T53.0X2-	T53.0X3-	T53.0X4-	-	-
Carbonic acid gas	T59.7X1-	T59.7X2-	T59.7X3-	T59.7X4-	-	-
anhydrase inhibitor NEC	T50.2X1-	T50.2X2-	T50.2X3-	T50.2X4-	T50.2X5-	T50.2X6-
Carbophenothion	T60.0X1-	T60.0X2-	T60.0X3-	T60.0X4-	-	-
Carboplatin	T45.1X1-	T45.1X2-	T45.1X3-	T45.1X4-	T45.1X5-	T45.1X6-
Carboprost	T48.0X1-	T48.0X2-	T48.0X3-	T48.0X4-	T48.0X5-	T48.0X6-
Carboquone	T45.1X1-	T45.1X2-	T45.1X3-	T45.1X4-	T45.1X5-	T45.1X6-
Carbowax	T49.3X1-	T49.3X2-	T49.3X3-	T49.3X4-	T49.3X5-	T49.3X6-
Carboxymethyl-cellulose	T47.4X1-	T47.4X2-	T47.4X3-	T47.4X4-	T47.4X5-	T47.4X6-
S-Carboxymethyl-cysteine	T48.4X1-	T48.4X2-	T48.4X3-	T48.4X4-	T48.4X5-	T48.4X6-
Carbrital	T42.3X1-	T42.3X2-	T42.3X3-	T42.3X4-	T42.3X5-	T42.3X6-
Carbromal	T42.6X1-	T42.6X2-	T42.6X3-	T42.6X4-	T42.6X5-	T42.6X6-
Carbutamide	T38.3X1-	T38.3X2-	T38.3X3-	T38.3X4-	T38.3X5-	T38.3X6-
Carbuterol	T48.6X1-	T48.6X2-	T48.6X3-	T48.6X4-	T48.6X5-	T48.6X6-
Cardiac						
depressants	T46.2X1-	T46.2X2-	T46.2X3-	T46.2X4-	T46.2X5-	T46.2X6-
rhythm regulator	T46.2X1-	T46.2X2-	T46.2X3-	T46.2X4-	T46.2X5-	T46.2X6-
specified NEC	T46.2X1-	T46.2X2-	T46.2X3-	T46.2X4-	T46.2X5-	T46.2X6-
Cardiografin	T50.8X1-	T50.8X2-	T50.8X3-	T50.8X4-	T50.8X5-	T50.8X6-
Cardio-green	T50.8X1-	T50.8X2-	T50.8X3-	T50.8X4-	T50.8X5-	T50.8X6-
Cardiotonic (glycoside) NEC	T46.0X1-	T46.0X2-	T46.0X3-	T46.0X4-	T46.0X5-	T46.0X6-
Cardiovascular drug NEC	T46.901-	T46.902-	T46.903-	T46.904-	T46.905-	T46.906-
Cardrase	T50.2X1-	T50.2X2-	T50.2X3-	T50.2X4-	T50.2X5-	T50.2X6-
Carfecillin	T36.0X1-	T36.0X2-	T36.0X3-	T36.0X4-	T36.0X5-	T36.0X6-
Carfenazine	T43.3X1-	T43.3X2-	T43.3X3-	T43.3X4-	T43.3X5-	T43.3X6-
Carfusin	T49.0X1-	T49.0X2-	T49.0X3-	T49.0X4-	T49.0X5-	T49.0X6-
Carindacillin	T36.0X1-	T36.0X2-	T36.0X3-	T36.0X4-	T36.0X5-	T36.0X6-
Carisoprodol	T42.8X1-	T42.8X2-	T42.8X3-	T42.8X4-	T42.8X5-	T42.8X6-
Carmellose	T47.4X1-	T47.4X2-	T47.4X3-	T47.4X4-	T47.4X5-	T47.4X6-
Carminative	T47.5X1-	T47.5X2-	T47.5X3-	T47.5X4-	T47.5X5-	T47.5X6-
Carmofur	T45.1X1-	T45.1X2-	T45.1X3-	T45.1X4-	T45.1X5-	T45.1X6-
Carmustine	T45.1X1-	T45.1X2-	T45.1X3-	T45.1X4-	T45.1X5-	T45.1X6-
Carotene	T45.2X1-	T45.2X2-	T45.2X3-	T45.2X4-	T45.2X5-	T45.2X6-
Carphenazine	T43.3X1-	T43.3X2-	T43.3X3-	T43.3X4-	T43.3X5-	T43.3X6-
Carpipramine	T42.4X1-	T42.4X2-	T42.4X3-	T42.4X4-	T42.4X5-	T42.4X6-
Carprofen	T39.311-	T39.312-	T39.313-	T39.314-	T39.315-	T39.316-
Carpronium chloride	T44.3X1-	T44.3X2-	T44.3X3-	T44.3X4-	T44.3X5-	T44.3X6-
Carrageenan	T47.8X1-	T47.8X2-	T47.8X3-	T47.8X4-	T47.8X5-	T47.8X6-
Carteolol	T44.7X1-	T44.7X2-	T44.7X3-	T44.7X4-	T44.7X5-	T44.7X6-
Carter's Little Pills	T47.2X1-	T47.2X2-	T47.2X3-	T47.2X4-	T47.2X5-	T47.2X6-
Cascara (sagrada)	T47.2X1-	T47.2X2-	T47.2X3-	T47.2X4-	T47.2X5-	T47.2X6-

CARBON - CASCARA

Substance	Poisoning Accidental (unintentional)	Poisoning Intentional self-harm	Poisoning Assault	Poisoning Undetermined	Adverse effect	Underdosing
Cassava	T62.2X1-	T62.2X2-	T62.2X3-	T62.2X4-	-	-
Castellani's paint	T49.0X1-	T49.0X2-	T49.0X3-	T49.0X4-	T49.0X5-	T49.0X6-
Castor						
bean	T62.2X1-	T62.2X2-	T62.2X3-	T62.2X4-	-	-
oil	T47.2X1-	T47.2X2-	T47.2X3-	T47.2X4-	T47.2X5-	T47.2X6-
Catalase	T45.3X1-	T45.3X2-	T45.3X3-	T45.3X4-	T45.3X5-	T45.3X6-
Caterpillar (sting)	T63.431-	T63.432-	T63.433-	T63.434-	-	-
Catha (edulis) (tea)	T43.691-	T43.692-	T43.693-	T43.694-	-	-
Cathartic NEC	T47.4X1-	T47.4X2-	T47.4X3-	T47.4X4-	T47.4X5-	T47.4X6-
anthacene derivative	T47.2X1-	T47.2X2-	T47.2X3-	T47.2X4-	T47.2X5-	T47.2X6-
bulk	T47.4X1-	T47.4X2-	T47.4X3-	T47.4X4-	T47.4X5-	T47.4X6-
contact	T47.2X1-	T47.2X2-	T47.2X3-	T47.2X4-	T47.2X5-	T47.2X6-
emollient NEC	T47.4X1-	T47.4X2-	T47.4X3-	T47.4X4-	T47.4X5-	T47.4X6-
irritant NEC	T47.2X1-	T47.2X2-	T47.2X3-	T47.2X4-	T47.2X5-	T47.2X6-
mucilage	T47.4X1-	T47.4X2-	T47.4X3-	T47.4X4-	T47.4X5-	T47.4X6-
saline	T47.3X1-	T47.3X2-	T47.3X3-	T47.3X4-	T47.3X5-	T47.3X6-
vegetable	T47.2X1-	T47.2X2-	T47.2X3-	T47.2X4-	T47.2X5-	T47.2X6-
Cathine	T50.5X1-	T50.5X2-	T50.5X3-	T50.5X4-	T50.5X5-	T50.5X6-
Cathomycin	T36.8X1-	T36.8X2-	T36.8X3-	T36.8X4-	T36.8X5-	T36.8X6-
Cation exchange resin	T50.3X1-	T50.3X2-	T50.3X3-	T50.3X4-	T50.3X5-	T50.3X6-
Caustic (s) NEC	T54.91X-	T54.92X-	T54.93X-	T54.94X-	-	-
alkali	T54.3X1-	T54.3X2-	T54.3X3-	T54.3X4-	-	-
hydroxide	T54.3X1-	T54.3X2-	T54.3X3-	T54.3X4-	-	-
potash	T54.3X1-	T54.3X2-	T54.3X3-	T54.3X4-	-	-
soda	T54.3X1-	T54.3X2-	T54.3X3-	T54.3X4-	-	-
specified NEC	T54.91X-	T54.92X-	T54.93X-	T54.94X-	-	-
Ceepryn	T49.0X1-	T49.0X2-	T49.0X3-	T49.0X4-	T49.0X5-	T49.0X6-
ENT agent	T49.6X1-	T49.6X2-	T49.6X3-	T49.6X4-	T49.6X5-	T49.6X6-
lozenges	T49.6X1-	T49.6X2-	T49.6X3-	T49.6X4-	T49.6X5-	T49.6X6-
Cefacetrile	T36.1X1-	T36.1X2-	T36.1X3-	T36.1X4-	T36.1X5-	T36.1X6-
Cefaclor	T36.1X1-	T36.1X2-	T36.1X3-	T36.1X4-	T36.1X5-	T36.1X6-
Cefadroxil	T36.1X1-	T36.1X2-	T36.1X3-	T36.1X4-	T36.1X5-	T36.1X6-
Cefalexin	T36.1X1-	T36.1X2-	T36.1X3-	T36.1X4-	T36.1X5-	T36.1X6-
Cefaloglycin	T36.1X1-	T36.1X2-	T36.1X3-	T36.1X4-	T36.1X5-	T36.1X6-
Cefaloridine	T36.1X1-	T36.1X2-	T36.1X3-	T36.1X4-	T36.1X5-	T36.1X6-
Cefalosporins	T36.1X1-	T36.1X2-	T36.1X3-	T36.1X4-	T36.1X5-	T36.1X6-
Cefalotin	T36.1X1-	T36.1X2-	T36.1X3-	T36.1X4-	T36.1X5-	T36.1X6-
Cefamandole	T36.1X1-	T36.1X2-	T36.1X3-	T36.1X4-	T36.1X5-	T36.1X6-
Cefamycin antibiotic	T36.1X1-	T36.1X2-	T36.1X3-	T36.1X4-	T36.1X5-	T36.1X6-
Cefapirin	T36.1X1-	T36.1X2-	T36.1X3-	T36.1X4-	T36.1X5-	T36.1X6-
Cefatrizine	T36.1X1-	T36.1X2-	T36.1X3-	T36.1X4-	T36.1X5-	T36.1X6-
Cefazedone	T36.1X1-	T36.1X2-	T36.1X3-	T36.1X4-	T36.1X5-	T36.1X6-
Cefazolin	T36.1X1-	T36.1X2-	T36.1X3-	T36.1X4-	T36.1X5-	T36.1X6-
Cefbuperazone	T36.1X1-	T36.1X2-	T36.1X3-	T36.1X4-	T36.1X5-	T36.1X6-
Cefetamet	T36.1X1-	T36.1X2-	T36.1X3-	T36.1X4-	T36.1X5-	T36.1X6-
Cefixime	T36.1X1-	T36.1X2-	T36.1X3-	T36.1X4-	T36.1X5-	T36.1X6-
Cefmenoxime	T36.1X1-	T36.1X2-	T36.1X3-	T36.1X4-	T36.1X5-	T36.1X6-
Cefmetazole	T36.1X1-	T36.1X2-	T36.1X3-	T36.1X4-	T36.1X5-	T36.1X6-
Cefminox	T36.1X1-	T36.1X2-	T36.1X3-	T36.1X4-	T36.1X5-	T36.1X6-
Cefonicid	T36.1X1-	T36.1X2-	T36.1X3-	T36.1X4-	T36.1X5-	T36.1X6-
Cefoperazone	T36.1X1-	T36.1X2-	T36.1X3-	T36.1X4-	T36.1X5-	T36.1X6-
Ceforanide	T36.1X1-	T36.1X2-	T36.1X3-	T36.1X4-	T36.1X5-	T36.1X6-
Cefotaxime	T36.1X1-	T36.1X2-	T36.1X3-	T36.1X4-	T36.1X5-	T36.1X6-
Cefotetan	T36.1X1-	T36.1X2-	T36.1X3-	T36.1X4-	T36.1X5-	T36.1X6-
Cefotiam	T36.1X1-	T36.1X2-	T36.1X3-	T36.1X4-	T36.1X5-	T36.1X6-
Cefoxitin	T36.1X1-	T36.1X2-	T36.1X3-	T36.1X4-	T36.1X5-	T36.1X6-
Cefpimizole	T36.1X1-	T36.1X2-	T36.1X3-	T36.1X4-	T36.1X5-	T36.1X6-
Cefpiramide	T36.1X1-	T36.1X2-	T36.1X3-	T36.1X4-	T36.1X5-	T36.1X6-
Cefradine	T36.1X1-	T36.1X2-	T36.1X3-	T36.1X4-	T36.1X5-	T36.1X6-

Substance	Poisoning Accidental (unintentional)	Poisoning Intentional self-harm	Poisoning Assault	Poisoning Undetermined	Adverse effect	Underdosing
Cefroxadine	T36.1X1-	T36.1X2-	T36.1X3-	T36.1X4-	T36.1X5-	T36.1X6-
Cefsulodin	T36.1X1-	T36.1X2-	T36.1X3-	T36.1X4-	T36.1X5-	T36.1X6-
Ceftazidime	T36.1X1-	T36.1X2-	T36.1X3-	T36.1X4-	T36.1X5-	T36.1X6-
Cefteram	T36.1X1-	T36.1X2-	T36.1X3-	T36.1X4-	T36.1X5-	T36.1X6-
Ceftezole	T36.1X1-	T36.1X2-	T36.1X3-	T36.1X4-	T36.1X5-	T36.1X6-
Ceftizoxime	T36.1X1-	T36.1X2-	T36.1X3-	T36.1X4-	T36.1X5-	T36.1X6-
Ceftriaxone	T36.1X1-	T36.1X2-	T36.1X3-	T36.1X4-	T36.1X5-	T36.1X6-
Cefuroxime	T36.1X1-	T36.1X2-	T36.1X3-	T36.1X4-	T36.1X5-	T36.1X6-
Cefuzonam	T36.1X1-	T36.1X2-	T36.1X3-	T36.1X4-	T36.1X5-	T36.1X6-
Celestone	T38.0X1-	T38.0X2-	T38.0X3-	T38.0X4-	T38.0X5-	T38.0X6-
topical	T49.0X1-	T49.0X2-	T49.0X3-	T49.0X4-	T49.0X5-	T49.0X6-
Celiprolol	T44.7X1-	T44.7X2-	T44.7X3-	T44.7X4-	T44.7X5-	T44.7X6-
Cell stimulants and proliferants	T49.8X1-	T49.8X2-	T49.8X3-	T49.8X4-	T49.8X5-	T49.8X6-
Cellosolve	T52.91X-	T52.92X-	T52.93X-	T52.94X-	-	-
Cellulose						
cathartic	T47.4X1-	T47.4X2-	T47.4X3-	T47.4X4-	T47.4X5-	T47.4X6-
hydroxyethyl	T47.4X1-	T47.4X2-	T47.4X3-	T47.4X4-	T47.4X5-	T47.4X6-
nitrates (topical)	T49.3X1-	T49.3X2-	T49.3X3-	T49.3X4-	T49.3X5-	T49.3X6-
oxidized	T49.4X1-	T49.4X2-	T49.4X3-	T49.4X4-	T49.4X5-	T49.4X6-
Centipede (bite)	T63.411-	T63.412-	T63.413-	T63.414-	-	-
Central nervous system						
depressants	T42.71X-	T42.72X-	T42.73X-	T42.74X-	T42.75X-	T42.76X-
anesthetic (general) NEC	T41.201-	T41.202-	T41.203-	T41.204-	T41.205-	T41.206-
gases NEC	T41.0X1-	T41.0X2-	T41.0X3-	T41.0X4-	T41.0X5-	T41.0X6-
intravenous	T41.1X1-	T41.1X2-	T41.1X3-	T41.1X4-	T41.1X5-	T41.1X6-
barbiturates	T42.3X1-	T42.3X2-	T42.3X3-	T42.3X4-	T42.3X5-	T42.3X6-
benzodiazepines	T42.4X1-	T42.4X2-	T42.4X3-	T42.4X4-	T42.4X5-	T42.4X6-
bromides	T42.6X1-	T42.6X2-	T42.6X3-	T42.6X4-	T42.6X5-	T42.6X6-
cannabis sativa	T40.7X1-	T40.7X2-	T40.7X3-	T40.7X4-	T40.7X5-	T40.7X6-
chloral hydrate	T42.6X1-	T42.6X2-	T42.6X3-	T42.6X4-	T42.6X5-	T42.6X6-
ethanol	T51.0X1-	T51.0X2-	T51.0X3-	T51.0X4-	-	-
hallucinogenics	T40.901-	T40.902-	T40.903-	T40.904-	T40.905-	T40.906-
hypnotics	T42.71X-	T42.72X-	T42.73X-	T42.74X-	T42.75X-	T42.76X-
specified NEC	T42.6X1-	T42.6X2-	T42.6X3-	T42.6X4-	T42.6X5-	T42.6X6-
muscle relaxants	T42.8X1-	T42.8X2-	T42.8X3-	T42.8X4-	T42.8X5-	T42.8X6-
paraldehyde	T42.6X1-	T42.6X2-	T42.6X3-	T42.6X4-	T42.6X5-	T42.6X6-
sedatives; sedative-hypnotics	T42.71X-	T42.72X-	T42.73X-	T42.74X-	T42.75X-	T42.76X-
mixed NEC	T42.6X1-	T42.6X2-	T42.6X3-	T42.6X4-	T42.6X5-	T42.6X6-
specified NEC	T42.6X1-	T42.6X2-	T42.6X3-	T42.6X4-	T42.6X5-	T42.6X6-
muscle-tone depressants	T42.8X1-	T42.8X2-	T42.8X3-	T42.8X4-	T42.8X5-	T42.8X6-
stimulants	T43.601-	T43.602-	T43.603-	T43.604-	T43.605-	T43.606-
amphetamines	T43.621-	T43.622-	T43.623-	T43.624-	T43.625-	T43.626-
analeptics	T50.7X1-	T50.7X2-	T50.7X3-	T50.7X4-	T50.7X5-	T50.7X6-
antidepressants	T43.201-	T43.202-	T43.203-	T43.204-	T43.205-	T43.206-
opiate antagonists	T50.7X1-	T50.7X2-	T50.7X3-	T50.7X4-	T50.7X5-	T50.7X6-
specified NEC	T43.691-	T43.692-	T43.693-	T43.694-	T43.695-	T43.696-
Cephalexin	T36.1X1-	T36.1X2-	T36.1X3-	T36.1X4-	T36.1X5-	T36.1X6-
Cephaloglycin	T36.1X1-	T36.1X2-	T36.1X3-	T36.1X4-	T36.1X5-	T36.1X6-
Cephaloridine	T36.1X1-	T36.1X2-	T36.1X3-	T36.1X4-	T36.1X5-	T36.1X6-
Cephalosporins	T36.1X1-	T36.1X2-	T36.1X3-	T36.1X4-	T36.1X5-	T36.1X6-
N (adicillin)	T36.0X1-	T36.0X2-	T36.0X3-	T36.0X4-	T36.0X5-	T36.0X6-
Cephalothin	T36.1X1-	T36.1X2-	T36.1X3-	T36.1X4-	T36.1X5-	T36.1X6-
Cephalotin	T36.1X1-	T36.1X2-	T36.1X3-	T36.1X4-	T36.1X5-	T36.1X6-
Cephradine	T36.1X1-	T36.1X2-	T36.1X3-	T36.1X4-	T36.1X5-	T36.1X6-
Cerbera (odallam)	T62.2X1-	T62.2X2-	T62.2X3-	T62.2X4-	-	-
Cerberin	T46.0X1-	T46.0X2-	T46.0X3-	T46.0X4-	T46.0X5-	T46.0X6-
Cerebral stimulants	T43.601-	T43.602-	T43.603-	T43.604-	T43.605-	T43.606-
psychotherapeutic	T43.601-	T43.602-	T43.603-	T43.604-	T43.605-	T43.606-

CEFROXADINE - CEREBRAL STIMULANTS

Substance	Poisoning Accidental (unintentional)	Poisoning Intentional self-harm	Poisoning Assault	Poisoning Undetermined	Adverse effect	Underdosing
Cerebral stimulants (continued)						
specified NEC	T43.691-	T43.692-	T43.693-	T43.694-	T43.695-	T43.696-
Cerium oxalate	T45.0X1-	T45.0X2-	T45.0X3-	T45.0X4-	T45.0X5-	T45.0X6-
Cerous oxalate	T45.0X1-	T45.0X2-	T45.0X3-	T45.0X4-	T45.0X5-	T45.0X6-
Ceruletide	T50.8X1-	T50.8X2-	T50.8X3-	T50.8X4-	T50.8X5-	T50.8X6-
Cetalkonium (chloride)	T49.0X1-	T49.0X2-	T49.0X3-	T49.0X4-	T49.0X5-	T49.0X6-
Cethexonium chloride	T49.0X1-	T49.0X2-	T49.0X3-	T49.0X4-	T49.0X5-	T49.0X6-
Cetiedil	T46.7X1-	T46.7X2-	T46.7X3-	T46.7X4-	T46.7X5-	T46.7X6-
Cetirizine	T45.0X1-	T45.0X2-	T45.0X3-	T45.0X4-	T45.0X5-	T45.0X6-
Cetomacrogol	T50.991-	T50.992-	T50.993-	T50.994-	T50.995-	T50.996-
Cetotiamine	T45.2X1-	T45.2X2-	T45.2X3-	T45.2X4-	T45.2X5-	T45.2X6-
Cetoxime	T45.0X1-	T45.0X2-	T45.0X3-	T45.0X4-	T45.0X5-	T45.0X6-
Cetraxate	T47.1X1-	T47.1X2-	T47.1X3-	T47.1X4-	T47.1X5-	T47.1X6-
Cetrimide	T49.0X1-	T49.0X2-	T49.0X3-	T49.0X4-	T49.0X5-	T49.0X6-
Cetrimonium (bromide)	T49.0X1-	T49.0X2-	T49.0X3-	T49.0X4-	T49.0X5-	T49.0X6-
Cetylpyridinium chloride	T49.0X1-	T49.0X2-	T49.0X3-	T49.0X4-	T49.0X5-	T49.0X6-
ENT agent	T49.6X1-	T49.6X2-	T49.6X3-	T49.6X4-	T49.6X5-	T49.6X6-
lozenges	T49.6X1-	T49.6X2-	T49.6X3-	T49.6X4-	T49.6X5-	T49.6X6-
Cevadilla — *see Sabadilla*						
Cevitamic acid	T45.2X1-	T45.2X2-	T45.2X3-	T45.2X4-	T45.2X5-	T45.2X6-
Chalk, precipitated	T47.1X1-	T47.1X2-	T47.1X3-	T47.1X4-	T47.1X5-	T47.1X6-
Chamomile	T49.0X1-	T49.0X2-	T49.0X3-	T49.0X4-	T49.0X5-	T49.0X6-
Ch'an su	T46.0X1-	T46.0X2-	T46.0X3-	T46.0X4-	T46.0X5-	T46.0X6-
Charcoal	T47.6X1-	T47.6X2-	T47.6X3-	T47.6X4-	T47.6X5-	T47.6X6-
activated — *see also Charcoal, medicinal*	T47.6X1-	T47.6X2-	T47.6X3-	T47.6X4-	T47.6X5-	T47.6X6-
fumes (Carbon monoxide)	T58.2X1-	T58.2X2-	T58.2X3-	T58.2X4-	-	-
industrial	T58.8X1-	T58.8X2-	T58.8X3-	T58.8X4-	-	-
medicinal (activated)	T47.6X1-	T47.6X2-	T47.6X3-	T47.6X4-	T47.6X5-	T47.6X6-
antidiarrheal	T47.6X1-	T47.6X2-	T47.6X3-	T47.6X4-	T47.6X5-	T47.6X6-
poison control	T47.8X1-	T47.8X2-	T47.8X3-	T47.8X4-	T47.8X5-	T47.8X6-
specified use other than for diarrhea	T47.8X1-	T47.8X2-	T47.8X3-	T47.8X4-	T47.8X5-	T47.8X6-
topical	T49.8X1-	T49.8X2-	T49.8X3-	T49.8X4-	T49.8X5-	T49.8X6-
Chaulmosulfone	T37.1X1-	T37.1X2-	T37.1X3-	T37.1X4-	T37.1X5-	T37.1X6-
Chelating agent NEC	T50.6X1-	T50.6X2-	T50.6X3-	T50.6X4-	T50.6X5-	T50.6X6-
Chelidonium majus	T62.2X1-	T62.2X2-	T62.2X3-	T62.2X4-	-	-
Chemical substance NEC	T65.91X-	T65.92X-	T65.93X-	T65.94X-	-	-
Chenodeoxycholic acid	T47.5X1-	T47.5X2-	T47.5X3-	T47.5X4-	T47.5X5-	T47.5X6-
Chenodiol	T47.5X1-	T47.5X2-	T47.5X3-	T47.5X4-	T47.5X5-	T47.5X6-
Chenopodium	T37.4X1-	T37.4X2-	T37.4X3-	T37.4X4-	T37.4X5-	T37.4X6-
Cherry laurel	T62.2X1-	T62.2X2-	T62.2X3-	T62.2X4-	-	-
Chinidin (e)	T46.2X1-	T46.2X2-	T46.2X3-	T46.2X4-	T46.2X5-	T46.2X6-
Chiniofon	T37.8X1-	T37.8X2-	T37.8X3-	T37.8X4-	T37.8X5-	T37.8X6-
Chlophedianol	T48.3X1-	T48.3X2-	T48.3X3-	T48.3X4-	T48.3X5-	T48.3X6-
Chloral	T42.6X1-	T42.6X2-	T42.6X3-	T42.6X4-	T42.6X5-	T42.6X6-
derivative	T42.6X1-	T42.6X2-	T42.6X3-	T42.6X4-	T42.6X5-	T42.6X6-
hydrate	T42.6X1-	T42.6X2-	T42.6X3-	T42.6X4-	T42.6X5-	T42.6X6-
Chloralamide	T42.6X1-	T42.6X2-	T42.6X3-	T42.6X4-	T42.6X5-	T42.6X6-
Chloralodol	T42.6X1-	T42.6X2-	T42.6X3-	T42.6X4-	T42.6X5-	T42.6X6-
Chloralose	T60.4X1-	T60.4X2-	T60.4X3-	T60.4X4-	-	-
Chlorambucil	T45.1X1-	T45.1X2-	T45.1X3-	T45.1X4-	T45.1X5-	T45.1X6-
Chloramine	T57.8X1-	T57.8X2-	T57.8X3-	T57.8X4-	-	-
T	T49.0X1-	T49.0X2-	T49.0X3-	T49.0X4-	T49.0X5-	T49.0X6-
topical	T49.0X1-	T49.0X2-	T49.0X3-	T49.0X4-	T49.0X5-	T49.0X6-
Chloramphenicol	T36.2X1-	T36.2X2-	T36.2X3-	T36.2X4-	T36.2X5-	T36.2X6-
ENT agent	T49.6X1-	T49.6X2-	T49.6X3-	T49.6X4-	T49.6X5-	T49.6X6-
ophthalmic preparation	T49.5X1-	T49.5X2-	T49.5X3-	T49.5X4-	T49.5X5-	T49.5X6-
topical NEC	T49.0X1-	T49.0X2-	T49.0X3-	T49.0X4-	T49.0X5-	T49.0X6-

Substance	Poisoning Accidental (unintentional)	Poisoning Intentional self-harm	Poisoning Assault	Poisoning Undetermined	Adverse effect	Underdosing
Chlorate (potassium) (sodium) NEC	T60.3X1-	T60.3X2-	T60.3X3-	T60.3X4-	-	-
herbicide	T60.3X1-	T60.3X2-	T60.3X3-	T60.3X4-	-	-
Chlorazanil	T50.2X1-	T50.2X2-	T50.2X3-	T50.2X4-	T50.2X5-	T50.2X6-
Chlorbenzene, chlorbenzol	T53.7X1-	T53.7X2-	T53.7X3-	T53.7X4-	-	-
Chlorbenzoxamine	T44.3X1-	T44.3X2-	T44.3X3-	T44.3X4-	T44.3X5-	T44.3X6-
Chlorbutol	T42.6X1-	T42.6X2-	T42.6X3-	T42.6X4-	T42.6X5-	T42.6X6-
Chlorcyclizine	T45.0X1-	T45.0X2-	T45.0X3-	T45.0X4-	T45.0X5-	T45.0X6-
Chlordan (e) (dust)	T60.1X1-	T60.1X2-	T60.1X3-	T60.1X4-	-	-
Chlordantoin	T49.0X1-	T49.0X2-	T49.0X3-	T49.0X4-	T49.0X5-	T49.0X6-
Chlordiazepoxide	T42.4X1-	T42.4X2-	T42.4X3-	T42.4X4-	T42.4X5-	T42.4X6-
Chlordiethyl benzamide	T49.3X1-	T49.3X2-	T49.3X3-	T49.3X4-	T49.3X5-	T49.3X6-
Chloresium	T49.8X1-	T49.8X2-	T49.8X3-	T49.8X4-	T49.8X5-	T49.8X6-
Chlorethiazol	T42.6X1-	T42.6X2-	T42.6X3-	T42.6X4-	T42.6X5-	T42.6X6-
Chlorethyl — see Ethyl chloride						
Chloretone	T42.6X1-	T42.6X2-	T42.6X3-	T42.6X4-	T42.6X5-	T42.6X6-
Chlorex	T53.6X1-	T53.6X2-	T53.6X3-	T53.6X4-	-	-
insecticide	T60.1X1-	T60.1X2-	T60.1X3-	T60.1X4-	-	-
Chlorfenvinphos	T60.0X1-	T60.0X2-	T60.0X3-	T60.0X4-	-	-
Chlorhexadol	T42.6X1-	T42.6X2-	T42.6X3-	T42.6X4-	T42.6X5-	T42.6X6-
Chlorhexamide	T45.1X1-	T45.1X2-	T45.1X3-	T45.1X4-	T45.1X5-	T45.1X6-
Chlorhexidine	T49.0X1-	T49.0X2-	T49.0X3-	T49.0X4-	T49.0X5-	T49.0X6-
Chlorhydroxyquinolin	T49.0X1-	T49.0X2-	T49.0X3-	T49.0X4-	T49.0X5-	T49.0X6-
Chloride of lime (bleach)	T54.3X1-	T54.3X2-	T54.3X3-	T54.3X4-	-	-
Chlorimipramine	T43.011-	T43.012-	T43.013-	T43.014-	T43.015-	T43.016-
Chlorinated						
camphene	T53.6X1-	T53.6X2-	T53.6X3-	T53.6X4-	-	-
diphenyl	T53.7X1-	T53.7X2-	T53.7X3-	T53.7X4-	-	-
hydrocarbons NEC	T53.91X-	T53.92X-	T53.93X-	T53.94X-	-	-
solvents	T53.91X-	T53.92X-	T53.93X-	T53.94X-	-	-
lime (bleach)	T54.3X1-	T54.3X2-	T54.3X3-	T54.3X4-	-	-
and boric acid solution	T49.0X1-	T49.0X2-	T49.0X3-	T49.0X4-	T49.0X5-	T49.0X6-
naphthalene (insecticide)	T60.1X1-	T60.1X2-	T60.1X3-	T60.1X4-	-	-
industrial (non-pesticide)	T53.7X1-	T53.7X2-	T53.7X3-	T53.7X4-	-	-
pesticide NEC	T60.8X1-	T60.8X2-	T60.8X3-	T60.8X4-	-	-
soda — see also sodium hypochlorite						
solution	T49.0X1-	T49.0X2-	T49.0X3-	T49.0X4-	T49.0X5-	T49.0X6-
Chlorine (fumes) (gas)	T59.4X1-	T59.4X2-	T59.4X3-	T59.4X4-	-	-
bleach	T54.3X1-	T54.3X2-	T54.3X3-	T54.3X4-	-	-
compound gas NEC	T59.4X1-	T59.4X2-	T59.4X3-	T59.4X4-	-	-
disinfectant	T59.4X1-	T59.4X2-	T59.4X3-	T59.4X4-	-	-
releasing agents NEC	T59.4X1-	T59.4X2-	T59.4X3-	T59.4X4-	-	-
Chlorisondamine chloride	T46.991-	T46.992-	T46.993-	T46.994-	T46.995-	T46.996-
Chlormadinone	T38.5X1-	T38.5X2-	T38.5X3-	T38.5X4-	T38.5X5-	T38.5X6-
Chlormephos	T60.0X1-	T60.0X2-	T60.0X3-	T60.0X4-	-	-
Chlormerodrin	T50.2X1-	T50.2X2-	T50.2X3-	T50.2X4-	T50.2X5-	T50.2X6-
Chlormethiazole	T42.6X1-	T42.6X2-	T42.6X3-	T42.6X4-	T42.6X5-	T42.6X6-
Chlormethine	T45.1X1-	T45.1X2-	T45.1X3-	T45.1X4-	T45.1X5-	T45.1X6-
Chlormethylenecycline	T36.4X1-	T36.4X2-	T36.4X3-	T36.4X4-	T36.4X5-	T36.4X6-
Chlormezanone	T42.6X1-	T42.6X2-	T42.6X3-	T42.6X4-	T42.6X5-	T42.6X6-
Chloroacetic acid	T60.3X1-	T60.3X2-	T60.3X3-	T60.3X4-	-	-
Chloroacetone	T59.3X1-	T59.3X2-	T59.3X3-	T59.3X4-	-	-
Chloroacetophenone	T59.3X1-	T59.3X2-	T59.3X3-	T59.3X4-	-	-
Chloroaniline	T53.7X1-	T53.7X2-	T53.7X3-	T53.7X4-	-	-
Chlorobenzene, chlorobenzol	T53.7X1-	T53.7X2-	T53.7X3-	T53.7X4-	-	-
Chlorobromomethane (fire extinguisher)	T53.6X1-	T53.6X2-	T53.6X3-	T53.6X4-	-	-
Chlorobutanol	T49.0X1-	T49.0X2-	T49.0X3-	T49.0X4-	T49.0X5-	T49.0X6-
Chlorocresol	T49.0X1-	T49.0X2-	T49.0X3-	T49.0X4-	T49.0X5-	T49.0X6-
Chlorodehydro-methyltestosterone	T38.7X1-	T38.7X2-	T38.7X3-	T38.7X4-	T38.7X5-	T38.7X6-

Substance	Poisoning Accidental (unintentional)	Poisoning Intentional self-harm	Poisoning Assault	Poisoning Undetermined	Adverse effect	Underdosing
Chlorodinitrobenzene	T53.7X1-	T53.7X2-	T53.7X3-	T53.7X4-	-	-
dust or vapor	T53.7X1-	T53.7X2-	T53.7X3-	T53.7X4-	-	-
Chlorodiphenyl	T53.7X1-	T53.7X2-	T53.7X3-	T53.7X4-	-	-
Chloroethane — *see Ethyl chloride*						
Chloroethylene	T53.6X1-	T53.6X2-	T53.6X3-	T53.6X4-	-	-
Chlorofluorocarbons	T53.5X1-	T53.5X2-	T53.5X3-	T53.5X4-	-	-
Chloroform (fumes) (vapor)	T53.1X1-	T53.1X2-	T53.1X3-	T53.1X4-	-	-
anesthetic	T41.0X1-	T41.0X2-	T41.0X3-	T41.0X4-	T41.0X5-	T41.0X6-
solvent	T53.1X1-	T53.1X2-	T53.1X3-	T53.1X4-	-	-
water, concentrated	T41.0X1-	T41.0X2-	T41.0X3-	T41.0X4-	T41.0X5-	T41.0X6-
Chloroguanide	T37.2X1-	T37.2X2-	T37.2X3-	T37.2X4-	T37.2X5-	T37.2X6-
Chloromycetin	T36.2X1-	T36.2X2-	T36.2X3-	T36.2X4-	T36.2X5-	T36.2X6-
ENT agent	T49.6X1-	T49.6X2-	T49.6X3-	T49.6X4-	T49.6X5-	T49.6X6-
ophthalmic preparation	T49.5X1-	T49.5X2-	T49.5X3-	T49.5X4-	T49.5X5-	T49.5X6-
otic solution	T49.6X1-	T49.6X2-	T49.6X3-	T49.6X4-	T49.6X5-	T49.6X6-
topical NEC	T49.0X1-	T49.0X2-	T49.0X3-	T49.0X4-	T49.0X5-	T49.0X6-
Chloronitrobenzene	T53.7X1-	T53.7X2-	T53.7X3-	T53.7X4-	-	-
dust or vapor	T53.7X1-	T53.7X2-	T53.7X3-	T53.7X4-	-	-
Chlorophacinone	T60.4X1-	T60.4X2-	T60.4X3-	T60.4X4-	-	-
Chlorophenol	T53.7X1-	T53.7X2-	T53.7X3-	T53.7X4-	-	-
Chlorophenothane	T60.1X1-	T60.1X2-	T60.1X3-	T60.1X4-	-	-
Chlorophyll	T50.991-	T50.992-	T50.993-	T50.994-	T50.995-	T50.996-
Chloropicrin (fumes)	T53.6X1-	T53.6X2-	T53.6X3-	T53.6X4-	-	-
fumigant	T60.8X1-	T60.8X2-	T60.8X3-	T60.8X4-	-	-
fungicide	T60.3X1-	T60.3X2-	T60.3X3-	T60.3X4-	-	-
pesticide	T60.8X1-	T60.8X2-	T60.8X3-	T60.8X4-	-	-
Chloroprocaine	T41.3X1-	T41.3X2-	T41.3X3-	T41.3X4-	T41.3X5-	T41.3X6-
infiltration (subcutaneous)	T41.3X1-	T41.3X2-	T41.3X3-	T41.3X4-	T41.3X5-	T41.3X6-
nerve block (peripheral) (plexus)	T41.3X1-	T41.3X2-	T41.3X3-	T41.3X4-	T41.3X5-	T41.3X6-
spinal	T41.3X1-	T41.3X2-	T41.3X3-	T41.3X4-	T41.3X5-	T41.3X6-
Chloroptic	T49.5X1-	T49.5X2-	T49.5X3-	T49.5X4-	T49.5X5-	T49.5X6-
Chloropurine	T45.1X1-	T45.1X2-	T45.1X3-	T45.1X4-	T45.1X5-	T45.1X6-
Chloropyramine	T45.0X1-	T45.0X2-	T45.0X3-	T45.0X4-	T45.0X5-	T45.0X6-
Chloropyrifos	T60.0X1-	T60.0X2-	T60.0X3-	T60.0X4-	-	-
Chloropyrilene	T45.0X1-	T45.0X2-	T45.0X3-	T45.0X4-	T45.0X5-	T45.0X6-
Chloroquine	T37.2X1-	T37.2X2-	T37.2X3-	T37.2X4-	T37.2X5-	T37.2X6-
Chlorothalonil	T60.3X1-	T60.3X2-	T60.3X3-	T60.3X4-	-	-
Chlorothen	T45.0X1-	T45.0X2-	T45.0X3-	T45.0X4-	T45.0X5-	T45.0X6-
Chlorothiazide	T50.2X1-	T50.2X2-	T50.2X3-	T50.2X4-	T50.2X5-	T50.2X6-
Chlorothymol	T49.4X1-	T49.4X2-	T49.4X3-	T49.4X4-	T49.4X5-	T49.4X6-
Chlorotrianisene	T38.5X1-	T38.5X2-	T38.5X3-	T38.5X4-	T38.5X5-	T38.5X6-
Chlorovinyldichloro-arsine, not in war	T57.0X1-	T57.0X2-	T57.0X3-	T57.0X4-	-	-
Chloroxine	T49.4X1-	T49.4X2-	T49.4X3-	T49.4X4-	T49.4X5-	T49.4X6-
Chloroxylenol	T49.0X1-	T49.0X2-	T49.0X3-	T49.0X4-	T49.0X5-	T49.0X6-
Chlorphenamine	T45.0X1-	T45.0X2-	T45.0X3-	T45.0X4-	T45.0X5-	T45.0X6-
Chlorphenesin	T42.8X1-	T42.8X2-	T42.8X3-	T42.8X4-	T42.8X5-	T42.8X6-
topical (antifungal)	T49.0X1-	T49.0X2-	T49.0X3-	T49.0X4-	T49.0X5-	T49.0X6-
Chlorpheniramine	T45.0X1-	T45.0X2-	T45.0X3-	T45.0X4-	T45.0X5-	T45.0X6-
Chlorphenoxamine	T45.0X1-	T45.0X2-	T45.0X3-	T45.0X4-	T45.0X5-	T45.0X6-
Chlorphentermine	T50.5X1-	T50.5X2-	T50.5X3-	T50.5X4-	T50.5X5-	T50.5X6-
Chlorprocaine — *see Chloroprocaine*						
Chlorproguanil	T37.2X1-	T37.2X2-	T37.2X3-	T37.2X4-	T37.2X5-	T37.2X6-
Chlorpromazine	T43.3X1-	T43.3X2-	T43.3X3-	T43.3X4-	T43.3X5-	T43.3X6-
Chlorpropamide	T38.3X1-	T38.3X2-	T38.3X3-	T38.3X4-	T38.3X5-	T38.3X6-
Chlorprothixene	T43.4X1-	T43.4X2-	T43.4X3-	T43.4X4-	T43.4X5-	T43.4X6-
Chlorquinaldol	T49.0X1-	T49.0X2-	T49.0X3-	T49.0X4-	T49.0X5-	T49.0X6-
Chlorquinol	T49.0X1-	T49.0X2-	T49.0X3-	T49.0X4-	T49.0X5-	T49.0X6-
Chlortalidone	T50.2X1-	T50.2X2-	T50.2X3-	T50.2X4-	T50.2X5-	T50.2X6-

Substance	Poisoning Accidental (unintentional)	Poisoning Intentional self-harm	Poisoning Assault	Poisoning Undetermined	Adverse effect	Underdosing
Chlortetracycline	T36.4X1-	T36.4X2-	T36.4X3-	T36.4X4-	T36.4X5-	T36.4X6-
Chlorthalidone	T50.2X1-	T50.2X2-	T50.2X3-	T50.2X4-	T50.2X5-	T50.2X6-
Chlorthiophos	T60.0X1-	T60.0X2-	T60.0X3-	T60.0X4-	-	-
Chlortrianisene	T38.5X1-	T38.5X2-	T38.5X3-	T38.5X4-	T38.5X5-	T38.5X6-
Chlor-Trimeton	T45.0X1-	T45.0X2-	T45.0X3-	T45.0X4-	T45.0X5-	T45.0X6-
Chlorthion	T60.0X1-	T60.0X2-	T60.0X3-	T60.0X4-	-	-
Chlorzoxazone	T42.8X1-	T42.8X2-	T42.8X3-	T42.8X4-	T42.8X5-	T42.8X6-
Choke damp	T59.7X1-	T59.7X2-	T59.7X3-	T59.7X4-	-	-
Cholagogues	T47.5X1-	T47.5X2-	T47.5X3-	T47.5X4-	T47.5X5-	T47.5X6-
Cholebrine	T50.8X1-	T50.8X2-	T50.8X3-	T50.8X4-	T50.8X5-	T50.8X6-
Cholecalciferol	T45.2X1-	T45.2X2-	T45.2X3-	T45.2X4-	T45.2X5-	T45.2X6-
Cholecystokinin	T50.8X1-	T50.8X2-	T50.8X3-	T50.8X4-	T50.8X5-	T50.8X6-
Cholera vaccine	T50.A91-	T50.A92-	T50.A93-	T50.A94-	T50.A95-	T50.A96-
Choleretic	T47.5X1-	T47.5X2-	T47.5X3-	T47.5X4-	T47.5X5-	T47.5X6-
Cholesterol-lowering agents	T46.6X1-	T46.6X2-	T46.6X3-	T46.6X4-	T46.6X5-	T46.6X6-
Cholestyramine (resin)	T46.6X1-	T46.6X2-	T46.6X3-	T46.6X4-	T46.6X5-	T46.6X6-
Cholic acid	T47.5X1-	T47.5X2-	T47.5X3-	T47.5X4-	T47.5X5-	T47.5X6-
Choline	T48.6X1-	T48.6X2-	T48.6X3-	T48.6X4-	T48.6X5-	T48.6X6-
chloride	T50.991-	T50.992-	T50.993-	T50.994-	T50.995-	T50.996-
dihydrogen citrate	T50.991-	T50.992-	T50.993-	T50.994-	T50.995-	T50.996-
salicylate	T39.091-	T39.092-	T39.093-	T39.094-	T39.095-	T39.096-
theophyllinate	T48.6X1-	T48.6X2-	T48.6X3-	T48.6X4-	T48.6X5-	T48.6X6-
Cholinergic (drug) NEC	T44.1X1-	T44.1X2-	T44.1X3-	T44.1X4-	T44.1X5-	T44.1X6-
muscle tone enhancer	T44.1X1-	T44.1X2-	T44.1X3-	T44.1X4-	T44.1X5-	T44.1X6-
organophosphorus	T44.0X1-	T44.0X2-	T44.0X3-	T44.0X4-	T44.0X5-	T44.0X6-
insecticide	T60.0X1-	T60.0X2-	T60.0X3-	T60.0X4-	-	-
nerve gas	T59.891-	T59.892-	T59.893-	T59.894-	-	-
trimethyl ammonium propanediol	T44.1X1-	T44.1X2-	T44.1X3-	T44.1X4-	T44.1X5-	T44.1X6-
Cholinesterase reactivator	T50.6X1-	T50.6X2-	T50.6X3-	T50.6X4-	T50.6X5-	T50.6X6-
Cholografin	T50.8X1-	T50.8X2-	T50.8X3-	T50.8X4-	T50.8X5-	T50.8X6-
Chorionic gonadotropin	T38.891-	T38.892-	T38.893-	T38.894-	T38.895-	T38.896-
Chromate	T56.2X1-	T56.2X2-	T56.2X3-	T56.2X4-	-	-
dust or mist	T56.2X1-	T56.2X2-	T56.2X3-	T56.2X4-	-	-
lead — *see also lead*	T56.0X1-	T56.0X2-	T56.0X3-	T56.0X4-	-	-
paint	T56.0X1-	T56.0X2-	T56.0X3-	T56.0X4-	-	-
Chromic						
acid	T56.2X1-	T56.2X2-	T56.2X3-	T56.2X4-	-	-
dust or mist	T56.2X1-	T56.2X2-	T56.2X3-	T56.2X4-	-	-
phosphate 32P	T45.1X1-	T45.1X2-	T45.1X3-	T45.1X4-	T45.1X5-	T45.1X6-
Chromium	T56.2X1-	T56.2X2-	T56.2X3-	T56.2X4-	-	-
compounds — *see Chromate*						
sesquioxide	T50.8X1-	T50.8X2-	T50.8X3-	T50.8X4-	T50.8X5-	T50.8X6-
Chromomycin A3	T45.1X1-	T45.1X2-	T45.1X3-	T45.1X4-	T45.1X5-	T45.1X6-
Chromonar	T46.3X1-	T46.3X2-	T46.3X3-	T46.3X4-	T46.3X5-	T46.3X6-
Chromyl chloride	T56.2X1-	T56.2X2-	T56.2X3-	T56.2X4-	-	-
Chrysarobin	T49.4X1-	T49.4X2-	T49.4X3-	T49.4X4-	T49.4X5-	T49.4X6-
Chrysazin	T47.2X1-	T47.2X2-	T47.2X3-	T47.2X4-	T47.2X5-	T47.2X6-
Chymar	T45.3X1-	T45.3X2-	T45.3X3-	T45.3X4-	T45.3X5-	T45.3X6-
ophthalmic preparation	T49.5X1-	T49.5X2-	T49.5X3-	T49.5X4-	T49.5X5-	T49.5X6-
Chymopapain	T45.3X1-	T45.3X2-	T45.3X3-	T45.3X4-	T45.3X5-	T45.3X6-
Chymotrypsin	T45.3X1-	T45.3X2-	T45.3X3-	T45.3X4-	T45.3X5-	T45.3X6-
ophthalmic preparation	T49.5X1-	T49.5X2-	T49.5X3-	T49.5X4-	T49.5X5-	T49.5X6-
Cianidanol	T50.991-	T50.992-	T50.993-	T50.994-	T50.995-	T50.996-
Cianopramine	T43.011-	T43.012-	T43.013-	T43.014-	T43.015-	T43.016-
Cibenzoline	T46.2X1-	T46.2X2-	T46.2X3-	T46.2X4-	T46.2X5-	T46.2X6-
Ciclacillin	T36.0X1-	T36.0X2-	T36.0X3-	T36.0X4-	T36.0X5-	T36.0X6-
Ciclobarbital — *see Hexobarbital*						
Ciclonicate	T46.7X1-	T46.7X2-	T46.7X3-	T46.7X4-	T46.7X5-	T46.7X6-

CICLOPIROX - CLOFENOTANE

Substance	Poisoning Accidental (unintentional)	Poisoning Intentional self-harm	Poisoning Assault	Poisoning Undetermined	Adverse effect	Underdosing
Ciclopirox (olamine)	T49.0X1-	T49.0X2-	T49.0X3-	T49.0X4-	T49.0X5-	T49.0X6-
Ciclosporin	T45.1X1-	T45.1X2-	T45.1X3-	T45.1X4-	T45.1X5-	T45.1X6-
Cicuta maculata or virosa	T62.2X1-	T62.2X2-	T62.2X3-	T62.2X4-	-	-
Cicutoxin	T62.2X1-	T62.2X2-	T62.2X3-	T62.2X4-	-	-
Cigarette lighter fluid	T52.0X1-	T52.0X2-	T52.0X3-	T52.0X4-	-	-
Cigarettes (tobacco)	T65.221-	T65.222-	T65.223-	T65.224-	-	-
Ciguatoxin	T61.01X-	T61.02X-	T61.03X-	T61.04X-	-	-
Cilazapril	T46.4X1-	T46.4X2-	T46.4X3-	T46.4X4-	T46.4X5-	T46.4X6-
Cimetidine	T47.0X1-	T47.0X2-	T47.0X3-	T47.0X4-	T47.0X5-	T47.0X6-
Cimetropium bromide	T44.3X1-	T44.3X2-	T44.3X3-	T44.3X4-	T44.3X5-	T44.3X6-
Cinchocaine	T41.3X1-	T41.3X2-	T41.3X3-	T41.3X4-	T41.3X5-	T41.3X6-
topical (surface)	T41.3X1-	T41.3X2-	T41.3X3-	T41.3X4-	T41.3X5-	T41.3X6-
Cinchona	T37.2X1-	T37.2X2-	T37.2X3-	T37.2X4-	T37.2X5-	T37.2X6-
Cinchonine alkaloids	T37.2X1-	T37.2X2-	T37.2X3-	T37.2X4-	T37.2X5-	T37.2X6-
Cinchophen	T50.4X1-	T50.4X2-	T50.4X3-	T50.4X4-	T50.4X5-	T50.4X6-
Cinepazide	T46.7X1-	T46.7X2-	T46.7X3-	T46.7X4-	T46.7X5-	T46.7X6-
Cinnamedrine	T48.5X1-	T48.5X2-	T48.5X3-	T48.5X4-	T48.5X5-	T48.5X6-
Cinnarizine	T45.0X1-	T45.0X2-	T45.0X3-	T45.0X4-	T45.0X5-	T45.0X6-
Cinoxacin	T37.8X1-	T37.8X2-	T37.8X3-	T37.8X4-	T37.8X5-	T37.8X6-
Ciprofibrate	T46.6X1-	T46.6X2-	T46.6X3-	T46.6X4-	T46.6X5-	T46.6X6-
Ciprofloxacin	T36.8X1-	T36.8X2-	T36.8X3-	T36.8X4-	T36.8X5-	T36.8X6-
Cisapride	T47.8X1-	T47.8X2-	T47.8X3-	T47.8X4-	T47.8X5-	T47.8X6-
Cisplatin	T45.1X1-	T45.1X2-	T45.1X3-	T45.1X4-	T45.1X5-	T45.1X6-
Citalopram	T43.221-	T43.222-	T43.223-	T43.224-	T43.225-	T43.226-
Citanest	T41.3X1-	T41.3X2-	T41.3X3-	T41.3X4-	T41.3X5-	T41.3X6-
infiltration (subcutaneous)	T41.3X1-	T41.3X2-	T41.3X3-	T41.3X4-	T41.3X5-	T41.3X6-
nerve block (peripheral) (plexus)	T41.3X1-	T41.3X2-	T41.3X3-	T41.3X4-	T41.3X5-	T41.3X6-
Citric acid	T47.5X1-	T47.5X2-	T47.5X3-	T47.5X4-	T47.5X5-	T47.5X6-
Citrovorum (factor)	T45.8X1-	T45.8X2-	T45.8X3-	T45.8X4-	T45.8X5-	T45.8X6-
Claviceps purpurea	T62.2X1-	T62.2X2-	T62.2X3-	T62.2X4-	-	-
Clavulanic acid	T36.1X1-	T36.1X2-	T36.1X3-	T36.1X4-	T36.1X5-	T36.1X6-
Cleaner, cleansing agent, type not specified	T65.891-	T65.892-	T65.893-	T65.894-	-	-
of paint or varnish	T52.91X-	T52.92X-	T52.93X-	T52.94X-	-	-
specified type NEC	T65.891-	T65.892-	T65.893-	T65.894-	-	-
Clebopride	T47.8X1-	T47.8X2-	T47.8X3-	T47.8X4-	T47.8X5-	T47.8X6-
Clefamide	T37.3X1-	T37.3X2-	T37.3X3-	T37.3X4-	T37.3X5-	T37.3X6-
Clemastine	T45.0X1-	T45.0X2-	T45.0X3-	T45.0X4-	T45.0X5-	T45.0X6-
Clematis vitalba	T62.2X1-	T62.2X2-	T62.2X3-	T62.2X4-	-	-
Clemizole	T45.0X1-	T45.0X2-	T45.0X3-	T45.0X4-	T45.0X5-	T45.0X6-
penicillin	T36.0X1-	T36.0X2-	T36.0X3-	T36.0X4-	T36.0X5-	T36.0X6-
Clenbuterol	T48.6X1-	T48.6X2-	T48.6X3-	T48.6X4-	T48.6X5-	T48.6X6-
Clidinium bromide	T44.3X1-	T44.3X2-	T44.3X3-	T44.3X4-	T44.3X5-	T44.3X6-
Clindamycin	T36.8X1-	T36.8X2-	T36.8X3-	T36.8X4-	T36.8X5-	T36.8X6-
Clinofibrate	T46.6X1-	T46.6X2-	T46.6X3-	T46.6X4-	T46.6X5-	T46.6X6-
Clioquinol	T37.8X1-		T37.8X3-	T37.8X4-	T37.8X5-	T37.8X6-
Cliradon	T40.2X1-	T40.2X2-	T40.2X3-	T40.2X4-	-	-
Clobazam	T42.4X1-	T42.4X2-	T42.4X3-	T42.4X4-	T42.4X5-	T42.4X6-
Clobenzorex	T50.5X1-	T50.5X2-	T50.5X3-	T50.5X4-	T50.5X5-	T50.5X6-
Clobetasol	T49.0X1-	T49.0X2-	T49.0X3-	T49.0X4-	T49.0X5-	T49.0X6-
Clobetasone	T49.0X1-	T49.0X2-	T49.0X3-	T49.0X4-	T49.0X5-	T49.0X6-
Clobutinol	T48.3X1-	T48.3X2-	T48.3X3-	T48.3X4-	T48.3X5-	T48.3X6-
Clocortolone	T38.0X1-	T38.0X2-	T38.0X3-	T38.0X4-	T38.0X5-	T38.0X6-
Clodantoin	T49.0X1-	T49.0X2-	T49.0X3-	T49.0X4-	T49.0X5-	T49.0X6-
Clodronic acid	T50.991-	T50.992-	T50.993-	T50.994-	T50.995-	T50.996-
Clofazimine	T37.1X1-	T37.1X2-	T37.1X3-	T37.1X4-	T37.1X5-	T37.1X6-
Clofedanol	T48.3X1-	T48.3X2-	T48.3X3-	T48.3X4-	T48.3X5-	T48.3X6-
Clofenamide	T50.2X1-	T50.2X2-	T50.2X3-	T50.2X4-	T50.2X5-	T50.2X6-
Clofenotane	T49.0X1-	T49.0X2-	T49.0X3-	T49.0X4-	T49.0X5-	T49.0X6-

Substance	Poisoning Accidental (unintentional)	Poisoning Intentional self-harm	Poisoning Assault	Poisoning Undetermined	Adverse effect	Underdosing
Clofezone	T39.2X1-	T39.2X2-	T39.2X3-	T39.2X4-	T39.2X5-	T39.2X6-
Clofibrate	T46.6X1-	T46.6X2-	T46.6X3-	T46.6X4-	T46.6X5-	T46.6X6-
Clofibride	T46.6X1-	T46.6X2-	T46.6X3-	T46.6X4-	T46.6X5-	T46.6X6-
Cloforex	T50.5X1-	T50.5X2-	T50.5X3-	T50.5X4-	T50.5X5-	T50.5X6-
Clomethiazole	T42.6X1-	T42.6X2-	T42.6X3-	T42.6X4-	T42.6X5-	T42.6X6-
Clometocillin	T36.0X1-	T36.0X2-	T36.0X3-	T36.0X4-	T36.0X5-	T36.0X6-
Clomifene	T38.5X1-	T38.5X2-	T38.5X3-	T38.5X4-	T38.5X5-	T38.5X6-
Clomiphene	T38.5X1-	T38.5X2-	T38.5X3-	T38.5X4-	T38.5X5-	T38.5X6-
Clomipramine	T43.011-	T43.012-	T43.013-	T43.014-	T43.015-	T43.016-
Clomocycline	T36.4X1-	T36.4X2-	T36.4X3-	T36.4X4-	T36.4X5-	T36.4X6-
Clonazepam	T42.4X1-	T42.4X2-	T42.4X3-	T42.4X4-	T42.4X5-	T42.4X6-
Clonidine	T46.5X1-	T46.5X2-	T46.5X3-	T46.5X4-	T46.5X5-	T46.5X6-
Clonixin	T39.8X1-	T39.8X2-	T39.8X3-	T39.8X4-	T39.8X5-	T39.8X6-
Clopamide	T50.2X1-	T50.2X2-	T50.2X3-	T50.2X4-	T50.2X5-	T50.2X6-
Clopenthixol	T43.4X1-	T43.4X2-	T43.4X3-	T43.4X4-	T43.4X5-	T43.4X6-
Cloperastine	T48.3X1-	T48.3X2-	T48.3X3-	T48.3X4-	T48.3X5-	T48.3X6-
Clophedianol	T48.3X1-	T48.3X2-	T48.3X3-	T48.3X4-	T48.3X5-	T48.3X6-
Cloponone	T36.2X1-	T36.2X2-	T36.2X3-	T36.2X4-	T36.2X5-	T36.2X6-
Cloprednol	T38.0X1-	T38.0X2-	T38.0X3-	T38.0X4-	T38.0X5-	T38.0X6-
Cloral betaine	T42.6X1-	T42.6X2-	T42.6X3-	T42.6X4-	T42.6X5-	T42.6X6-
Cloramfenicol	T36.2X1-	T36.2X2-	T36.2X3-	T36.2X4-	T36.2X5-	T36.2X6-
Clorazepate (dipotassium)	T42.4X1-	T42.4X2-	T42.4X3-	T42.4X4-	T42.4X5-	T42.4X6-
Clorexolone	T50.2X1-	T50.2X2-	T50.2X3-	T50.2X4-	T50.2X5-	T50.2X6-
Clorfenamine	T45.0X1-	T45.0X2-	T45.0X3-	T45.0X4-	T45.0X5-	T45.0X6-
Clorgiline	T43.1X1-	T43.1X2-	T43.1X3-	T43.1X4-	T43.1X5-	T43.1X6-
Clorotepine	T44.3X1-	T44.3X2-	T44.3X3-	T44.3X4-	T44.3X5-	T44.3X6-
Clorox (bleach)	T54.91X-	T54.92X-	T54.93X-	T54.94X-	-	-
Clorprenaline	T48.6X1-	T48.6X2-	T48.6X3-	T48.6X4-	T48.6X5-	T48.6X6-
Clortermine	T50.5X1-	T50.5X2-	T50.5X3-	T50.5X4-	T50.5X5-	T50.5X6-
Clotiapine	T43.591-	T43.592-	T43.593-	T43.594-	T43.595-	T43.596-
Clotiazepam	T42.4X1-	T42.4X2-	T42.4X3-	T42.4X4-	T42.4X5-	T42.4X6-
Clotibric acid	T46.6X1-	T46.6X2-	T46.6X3-	T46.6X4-	T46.6X5-	T46.6X6-
Clotrimazole	T49.0X1-	T49.0X2-	T49.0X3-	T49.0X4-	T49.0X5-	T49.0X6-
Cloxacillin	T36.0X1-	T36.0X2-	T36.0X3-	T36.0X4-	T36.0X5-	T36.0X6-
Cloxazolam	T42.4X1-	T42.4X2-	T42.4X3-	T42.4X4-	T42.4X5-	T42.4X6-
Cloxiquine	T49.0X1-	T49.0X2-	T49.0X3-	T49.0X4-	T49.0X5-	T49.0X6-
Clozapine	T42.4X1-	T42.4X2-	T42.4X3-	T42.4X4-	T42.4X5-	T42.4X6-
Coagulant NEC	T45.7X1-	T45.7X2-	T45.7X3-	T45.7X4-	T45.7X5-	T45.7X6-
Coal (carbon monoxide from) — see also Carbon, monoxide, coal	T58.2X1-	T58.2X2-	T58.2X3-	T58.2X4-	-	-
oil — see Kerosene						
tar	T49.1X1-	T49.1X2-	T49.1X3-	T49.1X4-	T49.1X5-	T49.1X6-
fumes	T59.891-	T59.892-	T59.893-	T59.894-	-	-
medicinal (ointment)	T49.4X1-	T49.4X2-	T49.4X3-	T49.4X4-	T49.4X5-	T49.4X6-
analgesics NEC	T39.2X1-	T39.2X2-	T39.2X3-	T39.2X4-	T39.2X5-	T39.2X6-
naphtha (solvent)	T52.0X1-	T52.0X2-	T52.0X3-	T52.0X4-	-	-
Cobalamine	T45.2X1-	T45.2X2-	T45.2X3-	T45.2X4-	T45.2X5-	T45.2X6-
Cobalt (nonmedicinal) (fumes) (industrial)	T56.891-	T56.892-	T56.893-	T56.894-	-	-
medicinal (trace) (chloride)	T45.8X1-	T45.8X2-	T45.8X3-	T45.8X4-	T45.8X5-	T45.8X6-
Cobra (venom)	T63.041-	T63.042-	T63.043-	T63.044-	-	-
Coca (leaf)	T40.5X1-	T40.5X2-	T40.5X3-	T40.5X4-	T40.5X5-	T40.5X6-
Cocaine	T40.5X1-	T40.5X2-	T40.5X3-	T40.5X4-	T40.5X5-	T40.5X6-
topical anesthetic	T41.3X1-	T41.3X2-	T41.3X3-	T41.3X4-	T41.3X5-	T41.3X6-
Cocarboxylase	T45.3X1-	T45.3X2-	T45.3X3-	T45.3X4-	T45.3X5-	T45.3X6-
Coccidioidin	T50.8X1-	T50.8X2-	T50.8X3-	T50.8X4-	T50.8X5-	T50.8X6-
Cocculus indicus	T62.1X1-	T62.1X2-	T62.1X3-	T62.1X4-	-	-
Cochineal	T65.6X1-	T65.6X2-	T65.6X3-	T65.6X4-	-	-
medicinal products	T50.991-	T50.992-	T50.993-	T50.994-	T50.995-	T50.996-

Substance	Poisoning Accidental (unintentional)	Poisoning Intentional self-harm	Poisoning Assault	Poisoning Undetermined	Adverse effect	Underdosing
Codeine	T40.2X1-	T40.2X2-	T40.2X3-	T40.2X4-	T40.2X5-	T40.2X6-
Cod-liver oil	T45.2X1-	T45.2X2-	T45.2X3-	T45.2X4-	T45.2X5-	T45.2X6-
Coenzyme A	T50.991-	T50.992-	T50.993-	T50.994-	T50.995-	T50.996-
Coffee	T62.8X1-	T62.8X2-	T62.8X3-	T62.8X4-	-	-
Cogalactoiso-merase	T50.991-	T50.992-	T50.993-	T50.994-	T50.995-	T50.996-
Cogentin	T44.3X1-	T44.3X2-	T44.3X3-	T44.3X4-	T44.3X5-	T44.3X6-
Coke fumes or gas (carbon monoxide)	T58.2X1-	T58.2X2-	T58.2X3-	T58.2X4-	-	-
industrial use	T58.8X1-	T58.8X2-	T58.8X3-	T58.8X4-	-	-
Colace	T47.4X1-	T47.4X2-	T47.4X3-	T47.4X4-	T47.4X5-	T47.4X6-
Colaspase	T45.1X1-	T45.1X2-	T45.1X3-	T45.1X4-	T45.1X5-	T45.1X6-
Colchicine	T50.4X1-	T50.4X2-	T50.4X3-	T50.4X4-	T50.4X5-	T50.4X6-
Colchicum	T62.2X1-	T62.2X2-	T62.2X3-	T62.2X4-	-	-
Cold cream	T49.3X1-	T49.3X2-	T49.3X3-	T49.3X4-	T49.3X5-	T49.3X6-
Colecalciferol	T45.2X1-	T45.2X2-	T45.2X3-	T45.2X4-	T45.2X5-	T45.2X6-
Colestipol	T46.6X1-	T46.6X2-	T46.6X3-	T46.6X4-	T46.6X5-	T46.6X6-
Colestyramine	T46.6X1-	T46.6X2-	T46.6X3-	T46.6X4-	T46.6X5-	T46.6X6-
Colimycin	T36.8X1-	T36.8X2-	T36.8X3-	T36.8X4-	T36.8X5-	T36.8X6-
Colistimethate	T36.8X1-	T36.8X2-	T36.8X3-	T36.8X4-	T36.8X5-	T36.8X6-
Colistin	T36.8X1-	T36.8X2-	T36.8X3-	T36.8X4-	T36.8X5-	T36.8X6-
sulfate (eye preparation)	T49.5X1-	T49.5X2-	T49.5X3-	T49.5X4-	T49.5X5-	T49.5X6-
Collagen	T50.991-	T50.992-	T50.993-	T50.994-	T50.995-	T50.996-
Collagenase	T49.4X1-	T49.4X2-	T49.4X3-	T49.4X4-	T49.4X5-	T49.4X6-
Collodion	T49.3X1-	T49.3X2-	T49.3X3-	T49.3X4-	T49.3X5-	T49.3X6-
Colocynth	T47.2X1-	T47.2X2-	T47.2X3-	T47.2X4-	T47.2X5-	T47.2X6-
Colophony adhesive	T49.3X1-	T49.3X2-	T49.3X3-	T49.3X4-	T49.3X5-	T49.3X6-
Colorant — see also Dye	T50.991-	T50.992-	T50.993-	T50.994-	T50.995-	T50.996-
Coloring matter — see Dye(s)						
Combustion gas (after combustion) — see Carbon, monoxide						
prior to combustion	T59.891-	T59.892-	T59.893-	T59.894-	-	-
Compazine	T43.3X1-	T43.3X2-	T43.3X3-	T43.3X4-	T43.3X5-	T43.3X6-
Compound						
42 (warfarin)	T60.4X1-	T60.4X2-	T60.4X3-	T60.4X4-	-	-
269 (endrin)	T60.1X1-	T60.1X2-	T60.1X3-	T60.1X4-	-	-
497 (dieldrin)	T60.1X1-	T60.1X2-	T60.1X3-	T60.1X4-	-	-
1080 (sodium fluoroacetate)	T60.4X1-	T60.4X2-	T60.4X3-	T60.4X4-	-	-
3422 (parathion)	T60.0X1-	T60.0X2-	T60.0X3-	T60.0X4-	-	-
3911 (phorate)	T60.0X1-	T60.0X2-	T60.0X3-	T60.0X4-	-	-
3956 (toxaphene)	T60.1X1-	T60.1X2-	T60.1X3-	T60.1X4-	-	-
4049 (malathion)	T60.0X1-	T60.0X2-	T60.0X3-	T60.0X4-	-	-
4069 (malathion)	T60.0X1-	T60.0X2-	T60.0X3-	T60.0X4-	-	-
4124 (dicapthon)	T60.0X1-	T60.0X2-	T60.0X3-	T60.0X4-	-	-
E (cortisone)	T38.0X1-	T38.0X2-	T38.0X3-	T38.0X4-	T38.0X5-	T38.0X6-
F (hydrocortisone)	T38.0X1-	T38.0X2-	T38.0X3-	T38.0X4-	T38.0X5-	T38.0X6-
Congener, anabolic	T38.7X1-	T38.7X2-	T38.7X3-	T38.7X4-	T38.7X5-	T38.7X6-
Congo red	T50.8X1-	T50.8X2-	T50.8X3-	T50.8X4-	T50.8X5-	T50.8X6-
Coniine, conine	T62.2X1-	T62.2X2-	T62.2X3-	T62.2X4-	-	-
Conium (maculatum)	T62.2X1-	T62.2X2-	T62.2X3-	T62.2X4-	-	-
Conjugated estrogenic substances	T38.5X1-	T38.5X2-	T38.5X3-	T38.5X4-	T38.5X5-	T38.5X6-
Contac	T48.5X1-	T48.5X2-	T48.5X3-	T48.5X4-	T48.5X5-	T48.5X6-
Contact lens solution	T49.5X1-	T49.5X2-	T49.5X3-	T49.5X4-	T49.5X5-	T49.5X6-
Contraceptive (oral)	T38.4X1-	T38.4X2-	T38.4X3-	T38.4X4-	T38.4X5-	T38.4X6-
vaginal	T49.8X1-	T49.8X2-	T49.8X3-	T49.8X4-	T49.8X5-	T49.8X6-
Contrast medium, radiography	T50.8X1-	T50.8X2-	T50.8X3-	T50.8X4-	T50.8X5-	T50.8X6-
Convallaria glycosides	T46.0X1-	T46.0X2-	T46.0X3-	T46.0X4-	T46.0X5-	T46.0X6-
Convallaria majalis	T62.2X1-	T62.2X2-	T62.2X3-	T62.2X4-	-	-
berry	T62.1X1-	T62.1X2-	T62.1X3-	T62.1X4-	-	-

Substance	Poisoning Accidental (unintentional)	Poisoning Intentional self-harm	Poisoning Assault	Poisoning Undetermined	Adverse effect	Underdosing
Copper (dust) (fumes) (nonmedicinal) NEC	T56.4X1-	T56.4X2-	T56.4X3-	T56.4X4-	-	-
arsenate, arsenite	T57.0X1-	T57.0X2-	T57.0X3-	T57.0X4-	-	-
insecticide	T60.2X1-	T60.2X2-	T60.2X3-	T60.2X4-	-	-
emetic	T47.7X1-	T47.7X2-	T47.7X3-	T47.7X4-	T47.7X5-	T47.7X6-
fungicide	T60.3X1-	T60.3X2-	T60.3X3-	T60.3X4-	-	-
gluconate	T49.0X1-	T49.0X2-	T49.0X3-	T49.0X4-	T49.0X5-	T49.0X6-
insecticide	T60.2X1-	T60.2X2-	T60.2X3-	T60.2X4-	-	-
medicinal (trace)	T45.8X1-	T45.8X2-	T45.8X3-	T45.8X4-	T45.8X5-	T45.8X6-
oleate	T49.0X1-	T49.0X2-	T49.0X3-	T49.0X4-	T49.0X5-	T49.0X6-
sulfate	T56.4X1-	T56.4X2-	T56.4X3-	T56.4X4-	-	-
cupric	T56.4X1-	T56.4X2-	T56.4X3-	T56.4X4-	-	-
fungicide	T60.3X1-	T60.3X2-	T60.3X3-	T60.3X4-	-	-
medicinal						
ear	T49.6X1-	T49.6X2-	T49.6X3-	T49.6X4-	T49.6X5-	T49.6X6-
emetic	T47.7X1-	T47.7X2-	T47.7X3-	T47.7X4-	T47.7X5-	T47.7X6-
eye	T49.5X1-	T49.5X2-	T49.5X3-	T49.5X4-	T49.5X5-	T49.5X6-
cuprous	T56.4X1-	T56.4X2-	T56.4X3-	T56.4X4-	-	-
fungicide	T60.3X1-	T60.3X2-	T60.3X3-	T60.3X4-	-	-
medicinal						
ear	T49.6X1-	T49.6X2-	T49.6X3-	T49.6X4-	T49.6X5-	T49.6X6-
emetic	T47.7X1-	T47.7X2-	T47.7X3-	T47.7X4-	T47.7X5-	T47.7X6-
eye	T49.5X1-	T49.5X2-	T49.5X3-	T49.5X4-	T49.5X5-	T49.5X6-
Copperhead snake (bite) (venom)	T63.061-	T63.062-	T63.063-	T63.064-	-	-
Coral (sting)	T63.691-	T63.692-	T63.693-	T63.694-	-	-
snake (bite) (venom)	T63.021-	T63.022-	T63.023-	T63.024-	-	-
Corbadrine	T49.6X1-	T49.6X2-	T49.6X3-	T49.6X4-	T49.6X5-	T49.6X6-
Cordite	T65.891-	T65.892-	T65.893-	T65.894-	-	-
vapor	T59.891-	T59.892-	T59.893-	T59.894-	-	-
Cordran	T49.0X1-	T49.0X2-	T49.0X3-	T49.0X4-	T49.0X5-	T49.0X6-
Corn cures	T49.4X1-	T49.4X2-	T49.4X3-	T49.4X4-	T49.4X5-	T49.4X6-
Corn starch	T49.3X1-	T49.3X2-	T49.3X3-	T49.3X4-	T49.3X5-	T49.3X6-
Cornhusker's lotion	T49.3X1-	T49.3X2-	T49.3X3-	T49.3X4-	T49.3X5-	T49.3X6-
Coronary vasodilator NEC	T46.3X1-	T46.3X2-	T46.3X3-	T46.3X4-	T46.3X5-	T46.3X6-
Corrosive NEC	T54.91X-	T54.92X-	T54.93X-	T54.94X-	-	-
acid NEC	T54.2X1-	T54.2X2-	T54.2X3-	T54.2X4-	-	-
aromatics	T54.1X1-	T54.1X2-	T54.1X3-	T54.1X4-	-	-
disinfectant	T54.1X1-	T54.1X2-	T54.1X3-	T54.1X4-	-	-
fumes NEC	T54.91X-	T54.92X-	T54.93X-	T54.94X-	-	-
specified NEC	T54.91X-	T54.92X-	T54.93X-	T54.94X-	-	-
sublimate	T56.1X1-	T56.1X2-	T56.1X3-	T56.1X4-	-	-
Cortate	T38.0X1-	T38.0X2-	T38.0X3-	T38.0X4-	T38.0X5-	T38.0X6-
Cort-Dome	T38.0X1-	T38.0X2-	T38.0X3-	T38.0X4-	T38.0X5-	T38.0X6-
ENT agent	T49.6X1-	T49.6X2-	T49.6X3-	T49.6X4-	T49.6X5-	T49.6X6-
ophthalmic preparation	T49.5X1-	T49.5X2-	T49.5X3-	T49.5X4-	T49.5X5-	T49.5X6-
topical NEC	T49.0X1-	T49.0X2-	T49.0X3-	T49.0X4-	T49.0X5-	T49.0X6-
Cortef	T38.0X1-	T38.0X2-	T38.0X3-	T38.0X4-	T38.0X5-	T38.0X6-
ENT agent	T49.6X1-	T49.6X2-	T49.6X3-	T49.6X4-	T49.6X5-	T49.6X6-
ophthalmic preparation	T49.5X1-	T49.5X2-	T49.5X3-	T49.5X4-	T49.5X5-	T49.5X6-
topical NEC	T49.0X1-	T49.0X2-	T49.0X3-	T49.0X4-	T49.0X5-	T49.0X6-
Corticosteroid	T38.0X1-	T38.0X2-	T38.0X3-	T38.0X4-	T38.0X5-	T38.0X6-
ENT agent	T49.6X1-	T49.6X2-	T49.6X3-	T49.6X4-	T49.6X5-	T49.6X6-
mineral	T50.0X1-	T50.0X2-	T50.0X3-	T50.0X4-	T50.0X5-	T50.0X6-
ophthalmic	T49.5X1-	T49.5X2-	T49.5X3-	T49.5X4-	T49.5X5-	T49.5X6-
topical NEC	T49.0X1-	T49.0X2-	T49.0X3-	T49.0X4-	T49.0X5-	T49.0X6-
Corticotropin	T38.811-	T38.812-	T38.813-	T38.814-	T38.815-	T38.816-
Cortisol	T49.0X1-	T49.0X2-	T49.0X3-	T49.0X4-	T49.0X5-	T49.0X6-
ENT agent	T49.6X1-	T49.6X2-	T49.6X3-	T49.6X4-	T49.6X5-	T49.6X6-

COPPER - CORTISOL

Substance	Poisoning Accidental (unintentional)	Poisoning Intentional self-harm	Poisoning Assault	Poisoning Undetermined	Adverse effect	Underdosing
Cortisol *(continued)*						
ophthalmic preparation	T49.5X1-	T49.5X2-	T49.5X3-	T49.5X4-	T49.5X5-	T49.5X6-
topical NEC	T49.0X1-	T49.0X2-	T49.0X3-	T49.0X4-	T49.0X5-	T49.0X6
Cortisone (acetate)	T38.0X1-	T38.0X2-	T38.0X3-	T38.0X4-	T38.0X5-	T38.0X6-
ENT agent	T49.6X1-	T49.6X2-	T49.6X3-	T49.6X4-	T49.6X5-	T49.6X6-
ophthalmic preparation	T49.5X1-	T49.5X2-	T49.5X3-	T49.5X4-	T49.5X5-	T49.5X6-
topical NEC	T49.0X1-	T49.0X2-	T49.0X3-	T49.0X4-	T49.0X5-	T49.0X6-
Cortivazol	T38.0X1-	T38.0X2-	T38.0X3-	T38.0X4-	T38.0X5-	T38.0X6-
Cortogen	T38.0X1-	T38.0X2-	T38.0X3-	T38.0X4-	T38.0X5-	T38.0X6-
ENT agent	T49.6X1-	T49.6X2-	T49.6X3-	T49.6X4-	T49.6X5-	T49.6X6-
ophthalmic preparation	T49.5X1-	T49.5X2-	T49.5X3-	T49.5X4-	T49.5X5-	T49.5X6-
Cortone	T38.0X1-	T38.0X2-	T38.0X3-	T38.0X4-	T38.0X5-	T38.0X6-
ENT agent	T49.6X1-	T49.6X2-	T49.6X3-	T49.6X4-	T49.6X5-	T49.6X6-
ophthalmic preparation	T49.5X1-	T49.5X2-	T49.5X3-	T49.5X4-	T49.5X5-	T49.5X6-
Cortril	T38.0X1-	T38.0X2-	T38.0X3-	T38.0X4-	T38.0X5-	T38.0X6-
ENT agent	T49.6X1-	T49.6X2-	T49.6X3-	T49.6X4-	T49.6X5-	T49.6X6-
ophthalmic preparation	T49.5X1-	T49.5X2-	T49.5X3-	T49.5X4-	T49.5X5-	T49.5X6-
topical NEC	T49.0X1-	T49.0X2-	T49.0X3-	T49.0X4-	T49.0X5-	T49.0X6-
Corynebacterium parvum	T45.1X1-	T45.1X2-	T45.1X3-	T45.1X4-	T45.1X5-	T45.1X6-
Cosmetic preparation	T49.8X1-	T49.8X2-	T49.8X3-	T49.8X4-	T49.8X5-	T49.8X6-
Cosmetics	T49.8X1-	T49.8X2-	T49.8X3-	T49.8X4-	T49.8X5-	T49.8X6-
Cosyntropin	T38.811-	T38.812-	T38.813-	T38.814-	T38.815-	T38.816-
Cotarnine	T45.7X1-	T45.7X2-	T45.7X3-	T45.7X4-	T45.7X5-	T45.7X6-
Co-trimoxazole	T36.8X1-	T36.8X2-	T36.8X3-	T36.8X4-	T36.8X5-	T36.8X6-
Cottonseed oil	T49.3X1-	T49.3X2-	T49.3X3-	T49.3X4-	T49.3X5-	T49.3X6-
Cough mixture (syrup)	T48.4X1-	T48.4X2-	T48.4X3-	T48.4X4-	T48.4X5-	T48.4X6-
containing opiates	T40.2X1-	T40.2X2-	T40.2X3-	T40.2X4-	T40.2X5-	T40.2X6-
expectorants	T48.4X1-	T48.4X2-	T48.4X3-	T48.4X4-	T48.4X5-	T48.4X6-
Coumadin	T45.511-	T45.512-	T45.513-	T45.514-	T45.515-	T45.516-
rodenticide	T60.4X1-	T60.4X2-	T60.4X3-	T60.4X4-	-	-
Coumaphos	T60.0X1-	T60.0X2-	T60.0X3-	T60.0X4-	-	-
Coumarin	T45.511-	T45.512-	T45.513-	T45.514-	T45.515-	T45.516-
Coumetarol	T45.511-	T45.512-	T45.513-	T45.514-	T45.515-	T45.516-
Cowbane	T62.2X1-	T62.2X2-	T62.2X3-	T62.2X4-	-	-
Cozyme	T45.2X1-	T45.2X2-	T45.2X3-	T45.2X4-	T45.2X5-	T45.2X6-
Crack	T40.5X1-	T40.5X2-	T40.5X3-	T40.5X4-	-	-
Crataegus extract	T46.0X1-	T46.0X2-	T46.0X3-	T46.0X4-	T46.0X5-	T46.0X6-
Creolin	T54.1X1-	T54.1X2-	T54.1X3-	T54.1X4-	-	-
disinfectant	T54.1X1-	T54.1X2-	T54.1X3-	T54.1X4-	-	-
Creosol (compound)	T49.0X1-	T49.0X2-	T49.0X3-	T49.0X4-	T49.0X5-	T49.0X6-
Creosote (coal tar) (beechwood)	T49.0X1-	T49.0X2-	T49.0X3-	T49.0X4-	T49.0X5-	T49.0X6-
medicinal (expectorant)	T48.4X1-	T48.4X2-	T48.4X3-	T48.4X4-	T48.4X5-	T48.4X6-
syrup	T48.4X1-	T48.4X2-	T48.4X3-	T48.4X4-	T48.4X5-	T48.4X6-
Cresol (s)	T49.0X1-	T49.0X2-	T49.0X3-	T49.0X4-	T49.0X5-	T49.0X6-
and soap solution	T49.0X1-	T49.0X2-	T49.0X3-	T49.0X4-	T49.0X5-	T49.0X6-
Cresyl acetate	T49.0X1-	T49.0X2-	T49.0X3-	T49.0X4-	T49.0X5-	T49.0X6-
Cresylic acid	T49.0X1-	T49.0X2-	T49.0X3-	T49.0X4-	T49.0X5-	T49.0X6-
Crimidine	T60.4X1-	T60.4X2-	T60.4X3-	T60.4X4-	-	-
Croconazole	T37.8X1-	T37.8X2-	T37.8X3-	T37.8X4-	T37.8X5-	T37.8X6-
Cromoglicic acid	T48.6X1-	T48.6X2-	T48.6X3-	T48.6X4-	T48.6X5-	T48.6X6-
Cromolyn	T48.6X1-	T48.6X2-	T48.6X3-	T48.6X4-	T48.6X5-	T48.6X6-
Cromonar	T46.3X1-	T46.3X2-	T46.3X3-	T46.3X4-	T46.3X5-	T46.3X6-
Cropropamide	T39.8X1-	T39.8X2-	T39.8X3-	T39.8X4-	T39.8X5-	T39.8X6-
with crotethamide	T50.7X1-	T50.7X2-	T50.7X3-	T50.7X4-	T50.7X5-	T50.7X6-
Crotamiton	T49.0X1-	T49.0X2-	T49.0X3-	T49.0X4-	T49.0X5-	T49.0X6-
Crotethamide	T39.8X1-	T39.8X2-	T39.8X3-	T39.8X4-	T39.8X5-	T39.8X6-
with cropropamide	T50.7X1-	T50.7X2-	T50.7X3-	T50.7X4-	T50.7X5-	T50.7X6-

Substance	Poisoning Accidental (unintentional)	Poisoning Intentional self-harm	Poisoning Assault	Poisoning Undetermined	Adverse effect	Underdosing
Croton (oil)	T47.2X1-	T47.2X2-	T47.2X3-	T47.2X4-	T47.2X5-	T47.2X6-
chloral	T42.6X1-	T42.6X2-	T42.6X3-	T42.6X4-	T42.6X5-	T42.6X6-
Crude oil	T52.0X1-	T52.0X2-	T52.0X3-	T52.0X4-	-	-
Cryogenine	T39.8X1-	T39.8X2-	T39.8X3-	T39.8X4-	T39.8X5-	T39.8X6-
Cryolite (vapor)	T60.1X1-	T60.1X2-	T60.1X3-	T60.1X4-	-	-
insecticide	T60.1X1-	T60.1X2-	T60.1X3-	T60.1X4-	-	-
Cryptenamine (tannates)	T46.5X1-	T46.5X2-	T46.5X3-	T46.5X4-	T46.5X5-	T46.5X6-
Crystal violet	T49.0X1-	T49.0X2-	T49.0X3-	T49.0X4-	T49.0X5-	T49.0X6-
Cuckoopint	T62.2X1-	T62.2X2-	T62.2X3-	T62.2X4-	-	-
Cumetharol	T45.511-	T45.512-	T45.513-	T45.514-	T45.515-	T45.516-
Cupric						
acetate	T60.3X1-	T60.3X2-	T60.3X3-	T60.3X4-	-	-
acetoarsenite	T57.0X1-	T57.0X2-	T57.0X3-	T57.0X4-	-	-
arsenate	T57.0X1-	T57.0X2-	T57.0X3-	T57.0X4-	-	-
gluconate	T49.0X1-	T49.0X2-	T49.0X3-	T49.0X4-	T49.0X5-	T49.0X6-
oleate	T49.0X1-	T49.0X2-	T49.0X3-	T49.0X4-	T49.0X5-	T49.0X6-
sulfate	T56.4X1-	T56.4X2-	T56.4X3-	T56.4X4-	-	-
Cuprous sulfate — *see also Copper sulfate*	T56.4X1-	T56.4X2-	T56.4X3-	T56.4X4-	-	-
Curare, curarine	T48.1X1-	T48.1X2-	T48.1X3-	T48.1X4-	T48.1X5-	T48.1X6-
Cyamemazine	T43.3X1-	T43.3X2-	T43.3X3-	T43.3X4-	T43.3X5-	T43.3X6-
Cyamopsis tetragono-loba	T46.6X1-	T46.6X2-	T46.6X3-	T46.6X4-	T46.6X5-	T46.6X6-
Cyanacetyl hydrazide	T37.1X1-	T37.1X2-	T37.1X3-	T37.1X4-	T37.1X5-	T37.1X6-
Cyanic acid (gas)	T59.891-	T59.892-	T59.893-	T59.894-	-	-
Cyanide (s) (compounds) (potassium) (sodium) NEC	T65.0X1-	T65.0X2-	T65.0X3-	T65.0X4-	-	-
dust or gas (inhalation) NEC	T57.3X1-	T57.3X2-	T57.3X3-	T57.3X4-	-	-
fumigant	T65.0X1-	T65.0X2-	T65.0X3-	T65.0X4-	-	-
hydrogen	T57.3X1-	T57.3X2-	T57.3X3-	T57.3X4-	-	-
mercuric — *see Mercury*						
pesticide (dust) (fumes)	T65.0X1-	T65.0X2-	T65.0X3-	T65.0X4-	-	-
Cyanoacrylate adhesive	T49.3X1-	T49.3X2-	T49.3X3-	T49.3X4-	T49.3X5-	T49.3X6-
Cyanocobalamin	T45.8X1-	T45.8X2-	T45.8X3-	T45.8X4-	T45.8X5-	T45.8X6-
Cyanogen (chloride) (gas) NEC	T59.891-	T59.892-	T59.893-	T59.894-	-	-
Cyclacillin	T36.0X1-	T36.0X2-	T36.0X3-	T36.0X4-	T36.0X5-	T36.0X6-
Cyclaine	T41.3X1-	T41.3X2-	T41.3X3-	T41.3X4-	T41.3X5-	T41.3X6-
Cyclamate	T50.991-	T50.992-	T50.993-	T50.994-	T50.995-	T50.996-
Cyclamen europaeum	T62.2X1-	T62.2X2-	T62.2X3-	T62.2X4-	-	-
Cyclandelate	T46.7X1-	T46.7X2-	T46.7X3-	T46.7X4-	T46.7X5-	T46.7X6-
Cyclazocine	T50.7X1-	T50.7X2-	T50.7X3-	T50.7X4-	T50.7X5-	T50.7X6-
Cyclizine	T45.0X1-	T45.0X2-	T45.0X3-	T45.0X4-	T45.0X5-	T45.0X6-
Cyclobarbital	T42.3X1-	T42.3X2-	T42.3X3-	T42.3X4-	T42.3X5-	T42.3X6-
Cyclobarbitone	T42.3X1-	T42.3X2-	T42.3X3-	T42.3X4-	T42.3X5-	T42.3X6-
Cyclobenzaprine	T48.1X1-	T48.1X2-	T48.1X3-	T48.1X4-	T48.1X5-	T48.1X6-
Cyclodrine	T44.3X1-	T44.3X2-	T44.3X3-	T44.3X4-	T44.3X5-	T44.3X6-
Cycloguanil embonate	T37.2X1-	T37.2X2-	T37.2X3-	T37.2X4-	T37.2X5-	T37.2X6-
Cyclohexane	T52.8X1-	T52.8X2-	T52.8X3-	T52.8X4-	-	-
Cyclohexanol	T51.8X1-	T51.8X2-	T51.8X3-	T51.8X4-	-	-
Cyclohexanone	T52.4X1-	T52.4X2-	T52.4X3-	T52.4X4-	-	-
Cycloheximide	T60.3X1-	T60.3X2-	T60.3X3-	T60.3X4-	-	-
Cyclohexyl acetate	T52.8X1-	T52.8X2-	T52.8X3-	T52.8X4-	-	-
Cycloleucin	T45.1X1-	T45.1X2-	T45.1X3-	T45.1X4-	T45.1X5-	T45.1X6-
Cyclomethycaine	T41.3X1-	T41.3X2-	T41.3X3-	T41.3X4-	T41.3X5-	T41.3X6-
Cyclopentamine	T44.4X1-	T44.4X2-	T44.4X3-	T44.4X4-	T44.4X5-	T44.4X6-
Cyclopenthiazide	T50.2X1-	T50.2X2-	T50.2X3-	T50.2X4-	T50.2X5-	T50.2X6-
Cyclopentolate	T44.3X1-	T44.3X2-	T44.3X3-	T44.3X4-	T44.3X5-	T44.3X6-
Cyclophosphamide	T45.1X1-	T45.1X2-	T45.1X3-	T45.1X4-	T45.1X5-	T45.1X6-
Cycloplegic drug	T49.5X1-	T49.5X2-	T49.5X3-	T49.5X4-	T49.5X5-	T49.5X6-
Cyclopropane	T41.291-	T41.292-	T41.293-	T41.294-	T41.295-	T41.296-

Substance	Poisoning Accidental (unintentional)	Poisoning Intentional self-harm	Poisoning Assault	Poisoning Undetermined	Adverse effect	Underdosing
Cyclopyrabital	T39.8X1-	T39.8X2-	T39.8X3-	T39.8X4-	T39.8X5-	T39.8X6-
Cycloserine	T37.1X1-	T37.1X2-	T37.1X3-	T37.1X4-	T37.1X5-	T37.1X6-
Cyclosporin	T45.1X1-	T45.1X2-	T45.1X3-	T45.1X4-	T45.1X5-	T45.1X6-
Cyclothiazide	T50.2X1-	T50.2X2-	T50.2X3-	T50.2X4-	T50.2X5-	T50.2X6-
Cycrimine	T44.3X1-	T44.3X2-	T44.3X3-	T44.3X4-	T44.3X5-	T44.3X6-
Cyhalothrin	T60.1X1-	T60.1X2-	T60.1X3-	T60.1X4-	-	-
Cymarin	T46.0X1-	T46.0X2-	T46.0X3-	T46.0X4-	T46.0X5-	T46.0X6-
Cypermethrin	T60.1X1-	T60.1X2-	T60.1X3-	T60.1X4-	-	-
Cyphenothrin	T60.2X1-	T60.2X2-	T60.2X3-	T60.2X4-	-	-
Cyproheptadine	T45.0X1-	T45.0X2-	T45.0X3-	T45.0X4-	T45.0X5-	T45.0X6-
Cyproterone	T38.6X1-	T38.6X2-	T38.6X3-	T38.6X4-	T38.6X5-	T38.6X6-
Cysteamine	T50.6X1-	T50.6X2-	T50.6X3-	T50.6X4-	T50.6X5-	T50.6X6-
Cytarabine	T45.1X1-	T45.1X2-	T45.1X3-	T45.1X4-	T45.1X5-	T45.1X6-
Cytisus						
laburnum	T62.2X1-	T62.2X2-	T62.2X3-	T62.2X4-	-	-
scoparius	T62.2X1-	T62.2X2-	T62.2X3-	T62.2X4-	-	-
Cytochrome C	T47.5X1-	T47.5X2-	T47.5X3-	T47.5X4-	T47.5X5-	T47.5X6-
Cytomel	T38.1X1-	T38.1X2-	T38.1X3-	T38.1X4-	T38.1X5-	T38.1X6-
Cytosine arabinoside	T45.1X1-	T45.1X2-	T45.1X3-	T45.1X4-	T45.1X5-	T45.1X6-
Cytoxan	T45.1X1-	T45.1X2-	T45.1X3-	T45.1X4-	T45.1X5-	T45.1X6-
Cytozyme	T45.7X1-	T45.7X2-	T45.7X3-	T45.7X4-	T45.7X5-	T45.7X6-
2,4-D	T60.3X1-	T60.3X2-	T60.3X3-	T60.3X4-	-	-
Dacarbazine	T45.1X1-	T45.1X2-	T45.1X3-	T45.1X4-	T45.1X5-	T45.1X6-
Dactinomycin	T45.1X1-	T45.1X2-	T45.1X3-	T45.1X4-	T45.1X5-	T45.1X6-
DADPS	T37.1X1-	T37.1X2-	T37.1X3-	T37.1X4-	T37.1X5-	T37.1X6-
Dakin's solution	T49.0X1-	T49.0X2-	T49.0X3-	T49.0X4-	T49.0X5-	T49.0X6-
Dalapon (sodium)	T60.3X1-	T60.3X2-	T60.3X3-	T60.3X4-	-	-
Dalmane	T42.4X1-	T42.4X2-	T42.4X3-	T42.4X4-	T42.4X5-	T42.4X6-
Danazol	T38.6X1-	T38.6X2-	T38.6X3-	T38.6X4-	T38.6X5-	T38.6X6-
Danilone	T45.511-	T45.512-	T45.513-	T45.514-	T45.515-	T45.516-
Danthron	T47.2X1-	T47.2X2-	T47.2X3-	T47.2X4-	T47.2X5-	T47.2X6-
Dantrolene	T42.8X1-	T42.8X2-	T42.8X3-	T42.8X4-	T42.8X5-	T42.8X6-
Dantron	T47.2X1-	T47.2X2-	T47.2X3-	T47.2X4-	T47.2X5-	T47.2X6-
Daphne (gnidium) (mezereum)	T62.2X1-	T62.2X2-	T62.2X3-	T62.2X4-	-	-
berry	T62.1X1-	T62.1X2-	T62.1X3-	T62.1X4-	-	-
Dapsone	T37.1X1-	T37.1X2-	T37.1X3-	T37.1X4-	T37.1X5-	T37.1X6-
Daraprim	T37.2X1-	T37.2X2-	T37.2X3-	T37.2X4-	T37.2X5-	T37.2X6-
Darnel	T62.2X1-	T62.2X2-	T62.2X3-	T62.2X4-	-	-
Darvon	T39.8X1-	T39.8X2-	T39.8X3-	T39.8X4-	T39.8X5-	T39.8X6-
Daunomycin	T45.1X1-	T45.1X2-	T45.1X3-	T45.1X4-	T45.1X5-	T45.1X6-
Daunorubicin	T45.1X1-	T45.1X2-	T45.1X3-	T45.1X4-	T45.1X5-	T45.1X6-
DBI	T38.3X1-	T38.3X2-	T38.3X3-	T38.3X4-	T38.3X5-	T38.3X6-
D-Con	T60.91X-	T60.92X-	T60.93X-	T60.94X-	-	-
insecticide	T60.2X1-	T60.2X2-	T60.2X3-	T60.2X4-	-	-
rodenticide	T60.4X1-	T60.4X2-	T60.4X3-	T60.4X4-	-	-
DDAVP	T38.891-	T38.892-	T38.893-	T38.894-	T38.895-	T38.896-
DDE (bis (chlorophenyl) -dichloroethylene)	T60.2X1-	T60.2X2-	T60.2X3-	T60.2X4-		
DDS	T37.1X1-	T37.1X2-	T37.1X3-	T37.1X4-	T37.1X5-	T37.1X6-
DDT (dust)	T60.1X1-	T60.1X2-	T60.1X3-	T60.1X4-	-	-
Deadly nightshade — see also Belladonna	T62.2X1-	T62.2X2-	T62.2X3-	T62.2X4-	-	-
berry	T62.1X1-	T62.1X2-	T62.1X3-	T62.1X4-	-	-
Deamino-D-arginine vasopressin	T38.891-	T38.892-	T38.893-	T38.894-	T38.895-	T38.896-
Deanol (aceglumate)	T50.991-	T50.992-	T50.993-	T50.994-	T50.995-	T50.996-
Debrisoquine	T46.5X1-	T46.5X2-	T46.5X3-	T46.5X4-	T46.5X5-	T46.5X6-
Decaborane	T57.8X1-	T57.8X2-	T57.8X3-	T57.8X4-		
fumes	T59.891-	T59.892-	T59.893-	T59.894-	-	-

Substance	Poisoning Accidental (unintentional)	Poisoning Intentional self-harm	Poisoning Assault	Poisoning Undetermined	Adverse effect	Underdosing
Decadron	T38.0X1-	T38.0X2-	T38.0X3-	T38.0X4-	T38.0X5-	T38.0X6-
ENT agent	T49.6X1-	T49.6X2-	T49.6X3-	T49.6X4-	T49.6X5-	T49.6X6-
ophthalmic preparation	T49.5X1-	T49.5X2-	T49.5X3-	T49.5X4-	T49.5X5-	T49.5X6-
topical NEC	T49.0X1-	T49.0X2-	T49.0X3-	T49.0X4-	T49.0X5-	T49.0X6-
Decahydronaphthalene	T52.8X1-	T52.8X2-	T52.8X3-	T52.8X4-	-	-
Decalin	T52.8X1-	T52.8X2-	T52.8X3-	T52.8X4-	-	-
Decamethonium (bromide)	T48.1X1-	T48.1X2-	T48.1X3-	T48.1X4-	T48.1X5-	T48.1X6-
Decholin	T47.5X1-	T47.5X2-	T47.5X3-	T47.5X4-	T47.5X5-	T47.5X6-
Declomycin	T36.4X1-	T36.4X2-	T36.4X3-	T36.4X4-	T36.4X5-	T36.4X6-
Decongestant, nasal (mucosa)	T48.5X1-	T48.5X2-	T48.5X3-	T48.5X4-	T48.5X5-	T48.5X6-
combination	T48.5X1-	T48.5X2-	T48.5X3-	T48.5X4-	T48.5X5-	T48.5X6-
Deet	T60.8X1-	T60.8X2-	T60.8X3-	T60.8X4-	-	-
Deferoxamine	T45.8X1-	T45.8X2-	T45.8X3-	T45.8X4-	T45.8X5-	T45.8X6-
Deflazacort	T38.0X1-	T38.0X2-	T38.0X3-	T38.0X4-	T38.0X5-	T38.0X6-
Deglycyrrhizinized extract of licorice	T48.4X1-	T48.4X2-	T48.4X3-	T48.4X4-	T48.4X5-	T48.4X6-
Dehydrocholic acid	T47.5X1-	T47.5X2-	T47.5X3-	T47.5X4-	T47.5X5-	T47.5X6-
Dehydroemetine	T37.3X1-	T37.3X2-	T37.3X3-	T37.3X4-	T37.3X5-	T37.3X6-
Dekalin	T52.8X1-	T52.8X2-	T52.8X3-	T52.8X4-	-	-
Delalutin	T38.5X1-	T38.5X2-	T38.5X3-	T38.5X4-	T38.5X5-	T38.5X6-
Delorazepam	T42.4X1-	T42.4X2-	T42.4X3-	T42.4X4-	T42.4X5-	T42.4X6-
Delphinium	T62.2X1-	T62.2X2-	T62.2X3-	T62.2X4-	-	-
Deltamethrin	T60.1X1-	T60.1X2-	T60.1X3-	T60.1X4-	-	-
Deltasone	T38.0X1-	T38.0X2-	T38.0X3-	T38.0X4-	T38.0X5-	T38.0X6-
Deltra	T38.0X1-	T38.0X2-	T38.0X3-	T38.0X4-	T38.0X5-	T38.0X6-
Delvinal	T42.3X1-	T42.3X2-	T42.3X3-	T42.3X4-	T42.3X5-	T42.3X6-
Demecarium (bromide)	T49.5X1-	T49.5X2-	T49.5X3-	T49.5X4-	T49.5X5-	T49.5X6-
Demeclocycline	T36.4X1-	T36.4X2-	T36.4X3-	T36.4X4-	T36.4X5-	T36.4X6-
Demecolcine	T45.1X1-	T45.1X2-	T45.1X3-	T45.1X4-	T45.1X5-	T45.1X6-
Demegestone	T38.5X1-	T38.5X2-	T38.5X3-	T38.5X4-	T38.5X5-	T38.5X6-
Demelanizing agents	T49.8X1-	T49.8X2-	T49.8X3-	T49.8X4-	T49.8X5-	T49.8X6-
Demephion -O and -S	T60.0X1-	T60.0X2-	T60.0X3-	T60.0X4-	-	-
Demerol	T40.2X1-	T40.2X2-	T40.2X3-	T40.2X4-	T40.2X5-	T40.2X6-
Demethylchlortetracycline	T36.4X1-	T36.4X2-	T36.4X3-	T36.4X4-	T36.4X5-	T36.4X6-
Demethyltetracycline	T36.4X1-	T36.4X2-	T36.4X3-	T36.4X4-	T36.4X5-	T36.4X6-
Demeton -O and -S	T60.0X1-	T60.0X2-	T60.0X3-	T60.0X4-		
Demulcent (external)	T49.3X1-	T49.3X2-	T49.3X3-	T49.3X4-	T49.3X5-	T49.3X6-
specified NEC	T49.3X1-	T49.3X2-	T49.3X3-	T49.3X4-	T49.3X5-	T49.3X6-
Demulen	T38.4X1-	T38.4X2-	T38.4X3-	T38.4X4-	T38.4X5-	T38.4X6-
Denatured alcohol	T51.0X1-	T51.0X2-	T51.0X3-	T51.0X4-	-	-
Dendrid	T49.5X1-	T49.5X2-	T49.5X3-	T49.5X4-	T49.5X5-	T49.5X6-
Dental drug, topical application NEC	T49.7X1-	T49.7X2-	T49.7X3-	T49.7X4-	T49.7X5-	T49.7X6-
Dentifrice	T49.7X1-	T49.7X2-	T49.7X3-	T49.7X4-	T49.7X5-	T49.7X6-
Deodorant spray (feminine hygiene)	T49.8X1-	T49.8X2-	T49.8X3-	T49.8X4-	T49.8X5-	T49.8X6-
Deoxycortone	T50.0X1-	T50.0X2-	T50.0X3-	T50.0X4-	T50.0X5-	T50.0X6-
2-Deoxy-5-fluorouridine	T45.1X1-	T45.1X2-	T45.1X3-	T45.1X4-	T45.1X5-	T45.1X6-
5-Deoxy-5-fluorouridine	T45.1X1-	T45.1X2-	T45.1X3-	T45.1X4-	T45.1X5-	T45.1X6-
Deoxyribonuclease (pancreatic)	T45.3X1-	T45.3X2-	T45.3X3-	T45.3X4-	T45.3X5-	T45.3X6-
Depilatory	T49.4X1-	T49.4X2-	T49.4X3-	T49.4X4-	T49.4X5-	T49.4X6-
Deprenalin	T42.8X1-	T42.8X2-	T42.8X3-	T42.8X4-	T42.8X5-	T42.8X6-
Deprenyl	T42.8X1-	T42.8X2-	T42.8X3-	T42.8X4-	T42.8X5-	T42.8X6-
Depressant, appetite	T50.5X1-	T50.5X2-	T50.5X3-	T50.5X4-	T50.5X5-	T50.5X6-
Depressant						
appetite (central)	T50.5X1-	T50.5X2-	T50.5X3-	T50.5X4-	T50.5X5-	T50.5X6-
cardiac	T46.2X1-	T46.2X2-	T46.2X3-	T46.2X4-	T46.2X5-	T46.2X6-
central nervous system (anesthetic) — *see also Central nervous system, depressants*	T42.71X-	T42.72X-	T42.73X-	T42.74X-	T42.75X-	T42.76X-
general anesthetic	T41.201-	T41.202-	T41.203-	T41.204-	T41.205-	T41.206-
muscle tone	T42.8X1-	T42.8X2-	T42.8X3-	T42.8X4-	T42.8X5-	T42.8X6-

DEPRESSANT - DFP

Substance	Poisoning Accidental (unintentional)	Poisoning Intentional self-harm	Poisoning Assault	Poisoning Undetermined	Adverse effect	Underdosing
Depressant (continued)						
muscle tone, central	T42.8X1-	T42.8X2-	T42.8X3-	T42.8X4-	T42.8X5-	T42.8X6-
psychotherapeutic	T43.501-	T43.502-	T43.503-	T43.504-	T43.505-	T43.506-
Deptropine	T45.0X1-	T45.0X2-	T45.0X3-	T45.0X4-	T45.0X5-	T45.0X6-
Dequalinium (chloride)	T49.0X1-	T49.0X2-	T49.0X3-	T49.0X4-	T49.0X5-	T49.0X6-
Derris root	T60.2X1-	T60.2X2-	T60.2X3-	T60.2X4-	-	-
Deserpidine	T46.5X1-	T46.5X2-	T46.5X3-	T46.5X4-	T46.5X5-	T46.5X6-
Desferrioxamine	T45.8X1-	T45.8X2-	T45.8X3-	T45.8X4-	T45.8X5-	T45.8X6-
Desipramine	T43.011-	T43.012-	T43.013-	T43.014-	T43.015-	T43.016-
Deslanoside	T46.0X1-	T46.0X2-	T46.0X3-	T46.0X4-	T46.0X5-	T46.0X6-
Desloughing agent	T49.4X1-	T49.4X2-	T49.4X3-	T49.4X4-	T49.4X5-	T49.4X6-
Desmethylimipramine	T43.011-	T43.012-	T43.013-	T43.014-	T43.015-	T43.016-
Desmopressin	T38.891-	T38.892-	T38.893-	T38.894-	T38.895-	T38.896-
Desocodeine	T40.2X1-	T40.2X2-	T40.2X3-	T40.2X4-	T40.2X5-	T40.2X6-
Desogestrel	T38.5X1-	T38.5X2-	T38.5X3-	T38.5X4-	T38.5X5-	T38.5X6-
Desomorphine	T40.2X1-	T40.2X2-	T40.2X3-	T40.2X4-	-	-
Desonide	T49.0X1-	T49.0X2-	T49.0X3-	T49.0X4-	T49.0X5-	T49.0X6-
Desoximetasone	T49.0X1-	T49.0X2-	T49.0X3-	T49.0X4-	T49.0X5-	T49.0X6-
Desoxycorticosteroid	T50.0X1-	T50.0X2-	T50.0X3-	T50.0X4-	T50.0X5-	T50.0X6-
Desoxycortone	T50.0X1-	T50.0X2-	T50.0X3-	T50.0X4-	T50.0X5-	T50.0X6-
Desoxyephedrine	T43.621-	T43.622-	T43.623-	T43.624-	T43.625-	T43.626-
Detaxtran	T46.6X1-	T46.6X2-	T46.6X3-	T46.6X4-	T46.6X5-	T46.6X6-
Detergent	T49.2X1-	T49.2X2-	T49.2X3-	T49.2X4-	T49.2X5-	T49.2X6-
external medication	T49.2X1-	T49.2X2-	T49.2X3-	T49.2X4-	T49.2X5-	T49.2X6-
local	T49.2X1-	T49.2X2-	T49.2X3-	T49.2X4-	T49.2X5-	T49.2X6-
medicinal	T49.2X1-	T49.2X2-	T49.2X3-	T49.2X4-	T49.2X5-	T49.2X6-
nonmedicinal	T55.1X1-	T55.1X2-	T55.1X3-	T55.1X4-	-	-
specified NEC	T55.1X1-	T55.1X2-	T55.1X3-	T55.1X4-	-	-
Deterrent, alcohol	T50.6X1-	T50.6X2-	T50.6X3-	T50.6X4-	T50.6X5-	T50.6X6-
Detoxifying agent	T50.6X1-	T50.6X2-	T50.6X3-	T50.6X4-	T50.6X5-	T50.6X6-
Detrothyronine	T38.1X1-	T38.1X2-	T38.1X3-	T38.1X4-	T38.1X5-	T38.1X6-
Dettol (external medication)	T49.0X1-	T49.0X2-	T49.0X3-	T49.0X4-	T49.0X5-	T49.0X6-
Dexamethasone	T38.0X1-	T38.0X2-	T38.0X3-	T38.0X4-	T38.0X5-	T38.0X6-
ENT agent	T49.6X1-	T49.6X2-	T49.6X3-	T49.6X4-	T49.6X5-	T49.6X6-
ophthalmic preparation	T49.5X1-	T49.5X2-	T49.5X3-	T49.5X4-	T49.5X5-	T49.5X6-
topical NEC	T49.0X1-	T49.0X2-	T49.0X3-	T49.0X4-	T49.0X5-	T49.0X6-
Dexamfetamine	T43.621-	T43.622-	T43.623-	T43.624-	T43.625-	T43.626-
Dexamphetamine	T43.621-	T43.622-	T43.623-	T43.624-	T43.625-	T43.626-
Dexbrompheniramine	T45.0X1-	T45.0X2-	T45.0X3-	T45.0X4-	T45.0X5-	T45.0X6-
Dexchlorpheniramine	T45.0X1-	T45.0X2-	T45.0X3-	T45.0X4-	T45.0X5-	T45.0X6-
Dexedrine	T43.621-	T43.622-	T43.623-	T43.624-	T43.625-	T43.626-
Dexetimide	T44.3X1-	T44.3X2-	T44.3X3-	T44.3X4-	T44.3X5-	T44.3X6-
Dexfenfluramine	T50.5X1-	T50.5X2-	T50.5X3-	T50.5X4-	T50.5X5-	T50.5X6-
Dexpanthenol	T45.2X1-	T45.2X2-	T45.2X3-	T45.2X4-	T45.2X5-	T45.2X6-
Dextran (40) (70) (150)	T45.8X1-	T45.8X2-	T45.8X3-	T45.8X4-	T45.8X5-	T45.8X6-
Dextriferron	T45.4X1-	T45.4X2-	T45.4X3-	T45.4X4-	T45.4X5-	T45.4X6-
Dextro calcium pantothenate	T45.2X1-	T45.2X2-	T45.2X3-	T45.2X4-	T45.2X5-	T45.2X6-
Dextro pantothenyl alcohol	T45.2X1-	T45.2X2-	T45.2X3-	T45.2X4-	T45.2X5-	T45.2X6-
Dextroamphetamine	T43.621-	T43.622-	T43.623-	T43.624-	T43.625-	T43.626-
Dextromethorphan	T48.3X1-	T48.3X2-	T48.3X3-	T48.3X4-	T48.3X5-	T48.3X6-
Dextromoramide	T40.4X1-	T40.4X2-	T40.4X3-	T40.4X4-	-	-
topical	T49.8X1-	T49.8X2-	T49.8X3-	T49.8X4-	T49.8X5-	T49.8X6-
Dextropropoxyphene	T40.4X1-	T40.4X2-	T40.4X3-	T40.4X4-	T40.4X5-	T40.4X6-
Dextrorphan	T40.2X1-	T40.2X2-	T40.2X3-	T40.2X4-	T40.2X5-	T40.2X6-
Dextrose	T50.3X1-	T50.3X2-	T50.3X3-	T50.3X4-	T50.3X5-	T50.3X6-
concentrated solution, intravenous	T46.8X1-	T46.8X2-	T46.8X3-	T46.8X4-	T46.8X5-	T46.8X6-
Dextrothyroxin	T38.1X1-	T38.1X2-	T38.1X3-	T38.1X4-	T38.1X5-	T38.1X6-
Dextrothyroxine sodium	T38.1X1-	T38.1X2-	T38.1X3-	T38.1X4-	T38.1X5-	T38.1X6-
DFP	T44.0X1-	T44.0X2-	T44.0X3-	T44.0X4-	T44.0X5-	T44.0X6-

Substance	Poisoning Accidental (unintentional)	Poisoning Intentional self-harm	Poisoning Assault	Poisoning Undetermined	Adverse effect	Underdosing
DHE	T37.3X1-	T37.3X2-	T37.3X3-	T37.3X4-	T37.3X5-	T37.3X6-
45	T46.5X1-	T46.5X2-	T46.5X3-	T46.5X4-	T46.5X5-	T46.5X6-
Diabinese	T38.3X1-	T38.3X2-	T38.3X3-	T38.3X4-	T38.3X5-	T38.3X6-
Diacetone alcohol	T52.4X1-	T52.4X2-	T52.4X3-	T52.4X4-	-	-
Diacetyl monoxime	T50.991-	T50.992-	T50.993-	T50.994-	-	-
Diacetylmorphine	T40.1X1-	T40.1X2-	T40.1X3-	T40.1X4-	-	-
Diachylon plaster	T49.4X1-	T49.4X2-	T49.4X3-	T49.4X4-	T49.4X5-	T49.4X6-
Diaethylstilboestrolum	T38.5X1-	T38.5X2-	T38.5X3-	T38.5X4-	T38.5X5-	T38.5X6-
Diagnostic agent NEC	T50.8X1-	T50.8X2-	T50.8X3-	T50.8X4-	T50.8X5-	T50.8X6-
Dial (soap)	T49.2X1-	T49.2X2-	T49.2X3-	T49.2X4-	T49.2X5-	T49.2X6-
sedative	T42.3X1-	T42.3X2-	T42.3X3-	T42.3X4-	T42.3X5-	T42.3X6-
Dialkyl carbonate	T52.91X-	T52.92X-	T52.93X-	T52.94X-	-	-
Diallylbarbituric acid	T42.3X1-	T42.3X2-	T42.3X3-	T42.3X4-	T42.3X5-	T42.3X6-
Diallymal	T42.3X1-	T42.3X2-	T42.3X3-	T42.3X4-	T42.3X5-	T42.3X6-
Dialysis solution (intraperitoneal)	T50.3X1-	T50.3X2-	T50.3X3-	T50.3X4-	T50.3X5-	T50.3X6-
Diaminodiphenylsulfone	T37.1X1-	T37.1X2-	T37.1X3-	T37.1X4-	T37.1X5-	T37.1X6-
Diamorphine	T40.1X1-	T40.1X2-	T40.1X3-	T40.1X4-	-	-
Diamox	T50.2X1-	T50.2X2-	T50.2X3-	T50.2X4-	T50.2X5-	T50.2X6-
Diamthazole	T49.0X1-	T49.0X2-	T49.0X3-	T49.0X4-	T49.0X5-	T49.0X6-
Dianthone	T47.2X1-	T47.2X2-	T47.2X3-	T47.2X4-	T47.2X5-	T47.2X6-
Diaphenylsulfone	T37.0X1-	T37.0X2-	T37.0X3-	T37.0X4-	T37.0X5-	T37.0X6-
Diasone (sodium)	T37.1X1-	T37.1X2-	T37.1X3-	T37.1X4-	T37.1X5-	T37.1X6-
Diastase	T47.5X1-	T47.5X2-	T47.5X3-	T47.5X4-	T47.5X5-	T47.5X6-
Diatrizoate	T50.8X1-	T50.8X2-	T50.8X3-	T50.8X4-	T50.8X5-	T50.8X6-
Diazepam	T42.4X1-	T42.4X2-	T42.4X3-	T42.4X4-	T42.4X5-	T42.4X6-
Diazinon	T60.0X1-	T60.0X2-	T60.0X3-	T60.0X4-	-	-
Diazomethane (gas)	T59.891-	T59.892-	T59.893-	T59.894-	-	-
Diazoxide	T46.5X1-	T46.5X2-	T46.5X3-	T46.5X4-	T46.5X5-	T46.5X6-
Dibekacin	T36.5X1-	T36.5X2-	T36.5X3-	T36.5X4-	T36.5X5-	T36.5X6-
Dibenamine	T44.6X1-	T44.6X2-	T44.6X3-	T44.6X4-	T44.6X5-	T44.6X6-
Dibenzepin	T43.011-	T43.012-	T43.013-	T43.014-	T43.015-	T43.016-
Dibenzheptropine	T45.0X1-	T45.0X2-	T45.0X3-	T45.0X4-	T45.0X5-	T45.0X6-
Dibenzyline	T44.6X1-	T44.6X2-	T44.6X3-	T44.6X4-	T44.6X5-	T44.6X6-
Diborane (gas)	T59.891-	T59.892-	T59.893-	T59.894-	-	-
Dibromochloropropane	T60.8X1-	T60.8X2-	T60.8X3-	T60.8X4-	-	-
Dibromodulcitol	T45.1X1-	T45.1X2-	T45.1X3-	T45.1X4-	T45.1X5-	T45.1X6-
Dibromoethane	T53.6X1-	T53.6X2-	T53.6X3-	T53.6X4-	-	-
Dibromomannitol	T45.1X1-	T45.1X2-	T45.1X3-	T45.1X4-	T45.1X5-	T45.1X6-
Dibromopropamidine isethionate	T49.0X1-	T49.0X2-	T49.0X3-	T49.0X4-	T49.0X5-	T49.0X6-
Dibrompropamidine	T49.0X1-	T49.0X2-	T49.0X3-	T49.0X4-	T49.0X5-	T49.0X6-
Dibucaine	T41.3X1-	T41.3X2-	T41.3X3-	T41.3X4-	T41.3X5-	T41.3X6-
topical (surface)	T41.3X1-	T41.3X2-	T41.3X3-	T41.3X4-	T41.3X5-	T41.3X6-
Dibunate sodium	T48.3X1-	T48.3X2-	T48.3X3-	T48.3X4-	T48.3X5-	T48.3X6-
Dibutoline sulfate	T44.3X1-	T44.3X2-	T44.3X3-	T44.3X4-	T44.3X5-	T44.3X6-
Dicamba	T60.3X1-	T60.3X2-	T60.3X3-	T60.3X4-	-	-
Dicapthon	T60.0X1-	T60.0X2-	T60.0X3-	T60.0X4-	-	-
Dichlobenil	T60.3X1-	T60.3X2-	T60.3X3-	T60.3X4-	-	-
Dichlone	T60.3X1-	T60.3X2-	T60.3X3-	T60.3X4-	-	-
Dichloralphenozone	T42.6X1-	T42.6X2-	T42.6X3-	T42.6X4-	T42.6X5-	T42.6X6-
Dichlorbenzidine	T65.3X1-	T65.3X2-	T65.3X3-	T65.3X4-	-	-
Dichlorhydrin	T52.8X1-	T52.8X2-	T52.8X3-	T52.8X4-	-	-
Dichlorhydroxyquinoline	T37.8X1-	T37.8X2-	T37.8X3-	T37.8X4-	T37.8X5-	T37.8X6-
Dichlorobenzene	T53.7X1-	T53.7X2-	T53.7X3-	T53.7X4-	-	-
Dichlorobenzyl alcohol	T49.6X1-	T49.6X2-	T49.6X3-	T49.6X4-	T49.6X5-	T49.6X6-
Dichlorodifluoromethane	T53.5X1-	T53.5X2-	T53.5X3-	T53.5X4-	-	-
Dichloroethane	T52.8X1-	T52.8X2-	T52.8X3-	T52.8X4-	-	-
Sym-Dichloroethyl ether	T53.6X1-	T53.6X2-	T53.6X3-	T53.6X4-	-	-
Dichloroethyl sulfide, not in war	T59.891-	T59.892-	T59.893-	T59.894-	-	-
Dichloroethylene	T53.6X1-	T53.6X2-	T53.6X3-	T53.6X4-	-	-

Substance	Poisoning Accidental (unintentional)	Poisoning Intentional self-harm	Poisoning Assault	Poisoning Undetermined	Adverse effect	Underdosing
Dichloroformoxine, not in war	T59.891-	T59.892-	T59.893-	T59.894-	-	-
Dichlorohydrin, alpha-dichlorohydrin	T52.8X1-	T52.8X2-	T52.8X3-	T52.8X4-	-	-
Dichloromethane (solvent)	T53.4X1-	T53.4X2-	T53.4X3-	T53.4X4-	-	-
vapor	T53.4X1-	T53.4X2-	T53.4X3-	T53.4X4-	-	-
Dichloronaphthoquinone	T60.3X1-	T60.3X2-	T60.3X3-	T60.3X4-	-	-
Dichlorophen	T37.4X1-	T37.4X2-	T37.4X3-	T37.4X4-	T37.4X5-	T37.4X6-
2,4-Dichlorophenoxyacetic acid	T60.3X1-	T60.3X2-	T60.3X3-	T60.3X4-	-	-
Dichloropropene	T60.3X1-	T60.3X2-	T60.3X3-	T60.3X4-	-	-
Dichloropropionic acid	T60.3X1-	T60.3X2-	T60.3X3-	T60.3X4-	-	-
Dichlorphenamide	T50.2X1-	T50.2X2-	T50.2X3-	T50.2X4-	T50.2X5-	T50.2X6-
Dichlorvos	T60.0X1-	T60.0X2-	T60.0X3-	T60.0X4-	-	-
Diclofenac	T39.391-	T39.392-	T39.393-	T39.394-	T39.395-	T39.396-
Diclofenamide	T50.2X1-	T50.2X2-	T50.2X3-	T50.2X4-	T50.2X5-	T50.2X6-
Diclofensine	T43.291-	T43.292-	T43.293-	T43.294-	T43.295-	T43.296-
Diclonixine	T39.8X1-	T39.8X2-	T39.8X3-	T39.8X4-	T39.8X5-	T39.8X6-
Dicloxacillin	T36.0X1-	T36.0X2-	T36.0X3-	T36.0X4-	T36.0X5-	T36.0X6-
Dicophane	T49.0X1-	T49.0X2-	T49.0X3-	T49.0X4-	T49.0X5-	T49.0X6-
Dicoumarol, dicoumarin, dicumarol	T45.511-	T45.512-	T45.513-	T45.514-	T45.515-	T45.516-
Dicrotophos	T60.0X1-	T60.0X2-	T60.0X3-	T60.0X4-	-	-
Dicyanogen (gas)	T65.0X1-	T65.0X2-	T65.0X3-	T65.0X4-	-	-
Dicyclomine	T44.3X1-	T44.3X2-	T44.3X3-	T44.3X4-	T44.3X5-	T44.3X6-
Dicycloverine	T44.3X1-	T44.3X2-	T44.3X3-	T44.3X4-	T44.3X5-	T44.3X6-
Dideoxycytidine	T37.5X1-	T37.5X2-	T37.5X3-	T37.5X4-	T37.5X5-	T37.5X6-
Dideoxyinosine	T37.5X1-	T37.5X2-	T37.5X3-	T37.5X4-	T37.5X5-	T37.5X6-
Dieldrin (vapor)	T60.1X1-	T60.1X2-	T60.1X3-	T60.1X4-	-	-
Diemal	T42.3X1-	T42.3X2-	T42.3X3-	T42.3X4-	T42.3X5-	T42.3X6-
Dienestrol	T38.5X1-	T38.5X2-	T38.5X3-	T38.5X4-	T38.5X5-	T38.5X6-
Dienoestrol	T38.5X1-	T38.5X2-	T38.5X3-	T38.5X4-	T38.5X5-	T38.5X6-
Dietetic drug NEC	T50.901-	T50.902-	T50.903-	T50.904-	T50.905-	T50.906-
Diethazine	T42.8X1-	T42.8X2-	T42.8X3-	T42.8X4-	T42.8X5-	T42.8X6-
Diethyl						
barbituric acid	T42.3X1-	T42.3X2-	T42.3X3-	T42.3X4-	T42.3X5-	T42.3X6-
carbamazine	T37.4X1-	T37.4X2-	T37.4X3-	T37.4X4-	T37.4X5-	T37.4X6-
carbinol	T51.3X1-	T51.3X2-	T51.3X3-	T51.3X4-	-	-
carbonate	T52.8X1-	T52.8X2-	T52.8X3-	T52.8X4-	-	-
ether (vapor) — *see also ether*	T41.0X1-	T41.0X2-	T41.0X3-	T41.0X4-	T41.0X5-	T41.0X6-
oxide	T52.8X1-	T52.8X2-	T52.8X3-	T52.8X4-	-	-
propion	T50.5X1-	T50.5X2-	T50.5X3-	T50.5X4-	T50.5X5-	T50.5X6-
stilbestrol	T38.5X1-	T38.5X2-	T38.5X3-	T38.5X4-	T38.5X5-	T38.5X6-
toluamide (nonmedicinal)	T60.8X1-	T60.8X2-	T60.8X3-	T60.8X4-	-	-
medicinal	T49.3X1-	T49.3X2-	T49.3X3-	T49.3X4-	T49.3X5-	T49.3X6-
Diethylcarbamazine	T37.4X1-	T37.4X2-	T37.4X3-	T37.4X4-	T37.4X5-	T37.4X6-
Diethylene						
dioxide	T52.8X1-	T52.8X2-	T52.8X3-	T52.8X4-	-	-
glycol (monoacetate) (monobutyl ether) (monoethyl ether)	T52.3X1-	T52.3X2-	T52.3X3-	T52.3X4-	-	-
Diethylhexylphthalate	T65.891-	T65.892-	T65.893-	T65.894-	-	-
Diethylpropion	T50.5X1-	T50.5X2-	T50.5X3-	T50.5X4-	T50.5X5-	T50.5X6-
Diethylstilbestrol	T38.5X1-	T38.5X2-	T38.5X3-	T38.5X4-	T38.5X5-	T38.5X6-
Diethylstilboestrol	T38.5X1-	T38.5X2-	T38.5X3-	T38.5X4-	T38.5X5-	T38.5X6-
Diethylsulfone-diethylmethane	T42.6X1-	T42.6X2-	T42.6X3-	T42.6X4-	T42.6X5-	T42.6X6-
Diethyltoluamide	T49.0X1-	T49.0X2-	T49.0X3-	T49.0X4-	T49.0X5-	T49.0X6-
Diethyltryptamine (DET)	T40.991-	T40.992-	T40.993-	T40.994-	-	-
Difebarbamate	T42.3X1-	T42.3X2-	T42.3X3-	T42.3X4-	T42.3X5-	T42.3X6-
Difencloxazine	T40.2X1-	T40.2X2-	T40.2X3-	T40.2X4-	T40.2X5-	T40.2X6-
Difenidol	T45.0X1-	T45.0X2-	T45.0X3-	T45.0X4-	T45.0X5-	T45.0X6-
Difenoxin	T47.6X1-	T47.6X2-	T47.6X3-	T47.6X4-	T47.6X5-	T47.6X6-
Difetarsone	T37.3X1-	T37.3X2-	T37.3X3-	T37.3X4-	T37.3X5-	T37.3X6-
Diffusin	T45.3X1-	T45.3X2-	T45.3X3-	T45.3X4-	T45.3X5-	T45.3X6-

Substance	Poisoning Accidental (unintentional)	Poisoning Intentional self-harm	Poisoning Assault	Poisoning Undetermined	Adverse effect	Underdosing
Diflorasone	T49.0X1-	T49.0X2-	T49.0X3-	T49.0X4-	T49.0X5-	T49.0X6-
Diflos	T44.0X1-	T44.0X2-	T44.0X3-	T44.0X4-	T44.0X5-	T44.0X6-
Diflubenzuron	T60.1X1-	T60.1X2-	T60.1X3-	T60.1X4-	-	-
Diflucortolone	T49.0X1-	T49.0X2-	T49.0X3-	T49.0X4-	T49.0X5-	T49.0X6-
Diflunisal	T39.091-	T39.092-	T39.093-	T39.094-	T39.095-	T39.096-
Difluoromethyldopa	T42.8X1-	T42.8X2-	T42.8X3-	T42.8X4-	T42.8X5-	T42.8X6-
Difluorophate	T44.0X1-	T44.0X2-	T44.0X3-	T44.0X4-	T44.0X5-	T44.0X6-
Digestant NEC	T47.5X1-	T47.5X2-	T47.5X3-	T47.5X4-	T47.5X5-	T47.5X6-
Digitalin (e)	T46.0X1-	T46.0X2-	T46.0X3-	T46.0X4-	T46.0X5-	T46.0X6-
Digitalis (leaf) (glycoside)	T46.0X1-	T46.0X2-	T46.0X3-	T46.0X4-	T46.0X5-	T46.0X6-
lanata	T46.0X1-	T46.0X2-	T46.0X3-	T46.0X4-	T46.0X5-	T46.0X6-
purpurea	T46.0X1-	T46.0X2-	T46.0X3-	T46.0X4-	T46.0X5-	T46.0X6-
Digitoxin	T46.0X1-	T46.0X2-	T46.0X3-	T46.0X4-	T46.0X5-	T46.0X6-
Digitoxose	T46.0X1-	T46.0X2-	T46.0X3-	T46.0X4-	T46.0X5-	T46.0X6-
Digoxin	T46.0X1-	T46.0X2-	T46.0X3-	T46.0X4-	T46.0X5-	T46.0X6-
Digoxine	T46.0X1-	T46.0X2-	T46.0X3-	T46.0X4-	T46.0X5-	T46.0X6-
Dihydralazine	T46.5X1-	T46.5X2-	T46.5X3-	T46.5X4-	T46.5X5-	T46.5X6-
Dihydrazine	T46.5X1-	T46.5X2-	T46.5X3-	T46.5X4-	T46.5X5-	T46.5X6-
Dihydrocodeine	T40.2X1-	T40.2X2-	T40.2X3-	T40.2X4-	T40.2X5-	T40.2X6-
Dihydrocodeinone	T40.2X1-	T40.2X2-	T40.2X3-	T40.2X4-	T40.2X5-	T40.2X6-
Dihydroergocornine	T46.7X1-	T46.7X2-	T46.7X3-	T46.7X4-	T46.7X5-	T46.7X6-
Dihydroergocristine (mesilate)	T46.7X1-	T46.7X2-	T46.7X3-	T46.7X4-	T46.7X5-	T46.7X6-
Dihydroergokryptine	T46.7X1-	T46.7X2-	T46.7X3-	T46.7X4-	T46.7X5-	T46.7X6-
Dihydroergotamine	T46.5X1-	T46.5X2-	T46.5X3-	T46.5X4-	T46.5X5-	T46.5X6-
Dihydroergotoxine	T46.7X1-	T46.7X2-	T46.7X3-	T46.7X4-	T46.7X5-	T46.7X6-
mesilate	T46.7X1-	T46.7X2-	T46.7X3-	T46.7X4-	T46.7X5-	T46.7X6-
Dihydrohydroxycodeinone	T40.2X1-	T40.2X2-	T40.2X3-	T40.2X4-	T40.2X5-	T40.2X6-
Dihydrohydroxymorphinone	T40.2X1-	T40.2X2-	T40.2X3-	T40.2X4-	T40.2X5-	T40.2X6-
Dihydroisocodeine	T40.2X1-	T40.2X2-	T40.2X3-	T40.2X4-	T40.2X5-	T40.2X6-
Dihydromorphine	T40.2X1-	T40.2X2-	T40.2X3-	T40.2X4-	-	-
Dihydromorphinone	T40.2X1-	T40.2X2-	T40.2X3-	T40.2X4-	T40.2X5-	T40.2X6-
Dihydrostreptomycin	T36.5X1-	T36.5X2-	T36.5X3-	T36.5X4-	T36.5X5-	T36.5X6-
Dihydrotachysterol	T45.2X1-	T45.2X2-	T45.2X3-	T45.2X4-	T45.2X5-	T45.2X6-
Dihydroxyaluminum aminoacetate	T47.1X1-	T47.1X2-	T47.1X3-	T47.1X4-	T47.1X5-	T47.1X6-
Dihydroxyaluminum sodium carbonate	T47.1X1-	T47.1X2-	T47.1X3-	T47.1X4-	T47.1X5-	T47.1X6-
Dihydroxyanthraquinone	T47.2X1-	T47.2X2-	T47.2X3-	T47.2X4-	T47.2X5-	T47.2X6-
Dihydroxycodeinone	T40.2X1-	T40.2X2-	T40.2X3-	T40.2X4-	T40.2X5-	T40.2X6-
Dihydroxypropyl theophylline	T50.2X1-	T50.2X2-	T50.2X3-	T50.2X4-	T50.2X5-	T50.2X6-
Diiodohydroxyquin	T37.8X1-	T37.8X2-	T37.8X3-	T37.8X4-	T37.8X5-	T37.8X6-
topical	T49.0X1-	T49.0X2-	T49.0X3-	T49.0X4-	T49.0X5-	T49.0X6-
Diiodohydroxyquinoline	T37.8X1-	T37.8X2-	T37.8X3-	T37.8X4-	T37.8X5-	T37.8X6-
Diiodotyrosine	T38.2X1-	T38.2X2-	T38.2X3-	T38.2X4-	T38.2X5-	T38.2X6-
Diisopromine	T44.3X1-	T44.3X2-	T44.3X3-	T44.3X4-	T44.3X5-	T44.3X6-
Diisopropylamine	T46.3X1-	T46.3X2-	T46.3X3-	T46.3X4-	T46.3X5-	T46.3X6-
Diisopropylfluorophos-phonate	T44.0X1-	T44.0X2-	T44.0X3-	T44.0X4-	T44.0X5-	T44.0X6-
Dilantin	T42.0X1-	T42.0X2-	T42.0X3-	T42.0X4-	T42.0X5-	T42.0X6-
Dilaudid	T40.2X1-	T40.2X2-	T40.2X3-	T40.2X4-	T40.2X5-	T40.2X6-
Dilazep	T46.3X1-	T46.3X2-	T46.3X3-	T46.3X4-	T46.3X5-	T46.3X6-
Dill	T47.5X1-	T47.5X2-	T47.5X3-	T47.5X4-	T47.5X5-	T47.5X6-
Diloxanide	T37.3X1-	T37.3X2-	T37.3X3-	T37.3X4-	T37.3X5-	T37.3X6-
Diltiazem	T46.1X1-	T46.1X2-	T46.1X3-	T46.1X4-	T46.1X5-	T46.1X6-
Dimazole	T49.0X1-	T49.0X2-	T49.0X3-	T49.0X4-	T49.0X5-	T49.0X6-
Dimefline	T50.7X1-	T50.7X2-	T50.7X3-	T50.7X4-	T50.7X5-	T50.7X6-
Dimefox	T60.0X1-	T60.0X2-	T60.0X3-	T60.0X4-	-	-
Dimemorfan	T48.3X1-	T48.3X2-	T48.3X3-	T48.3X4-	T48.3X5-	T48.3X6-
Dimenhydrinate	T45.0X1-	T45.0X2-	T45.0X3-	T45.0X4-	T45.0X5-	T45.0X6-
Dimercaprol (British anti-lewisite)	T45.8X1-	T45.8X2-	T45.8X3-	T45.8X4-	T45.8X5-	T45.8X6-
Dimercaptopropanol	T45.8X1-	T45.8X2-	T45.8X3-	T45.8X4-	T45.8X5-	T45.8X6-

Substance	Poisoning Accidental (unintentional)	Poisoning Intentional self-harm	Poisoning Assault	Poisoning Undetermined	Adverse effect	Underdosing
Dimestrol	T38.5X1-	T38.5X2-	T38.5X3-	T38.5X4-	T38.5X5-	T38.5X6-
Dimetane	T45.0X1-	T45.0X2-	T45.0X3-	T45.0X4-	T45.0X5-	T45.0X6-
Dimethicone	T47.1X1-	T47.1X2-	T47.1X3-	T47.1X4-	T47.1X5-	T47.1X6-
Dimethindene	T45.0X1-	T45.0X2-	T45.0X3-	T45.0X4-	T45.0X5-	T45.0X6-
Dimethisoquin	T49.1X1-	T49.1X2-	T49.1X3-	T49.1X4-	T49.1X5-	T49.1X6-
Dimethisterone	T38.5X1-	T38.5X2-	T38.5X3-	T38.5X4-	T38.5X5-	T38.5X6-
Dimethoate	T60.0X1-	T60.0X2-	T60.0X3-	T60.0X4-	-	-
Dimethocaine	T41.3X1-	T41.3X2-	T41.3X3-	T41.3X4-	T41.3X5-	T41.3X6-
Dimethoxanate	T48.3X1-	T48.3X2-	T48.3X3-	T48.3X4-	T48.3X5-	T48.3X6-
Dimethyl						
arsine, arsinic acid	T57.0X1-	T57.0X2-	T57.0X3-	T57.0X4-	-	-
carbinol	T51.2X1-	T51.2X2-	T51.2X3-	T51.2X4-	-	-
carbonate	T52.8X1-	T52.8X2-	T52.8X3-	T52.8X4-	-	-
diguanide	T38.3X1-	T38.3X2-	T38.3X3-	T38.3X4-	T38.3X5-	T38.3X6-
ketone	T52.4X1-	T52.4X2-	T52.4X3-	T52.4X4-	-	-
vapor	T52.4X1-	T52.4X2-	T52.4X3-	T52.4X4-	-	-
meperidine	T40.2X1-	T40.2X2-	T40.2X3-	T40.2X4-	T40.2X5-	T40.2X6-
parathion	T60.0X1-	T60.0X2-	T60.0X3-	T60.0X4-	-	-
phthlate	T49.3X1-	T49.3X2-	T49.3X3-	T49.3X4-	T49.3X5-	T49.3X6-
polysiloxane	T47.8X1-	T47.8X2-	T47.8X3-	T47.8X4-	T47.8X5-	T47.8X6-
sulfate (fumes)	T59.891-	T59.892-	T59.893-	T59.894-	-	-
liquid	T65.891-	T65.892-	T65.893-	T65.894-	-	-
sulfoxide (nonmedicinal)	T52.8X1-	T52.8X2-	T52.8X3-	T52.8X4-	-	-
medicinal	T49.4X1-	T49.4X2-	T49.4X3-	T49.4X4-	-	T49.4X6-
tryptamine	T40.991-	T40.992-	T40.993-	T40.994-	-	-
tubocurarine	T48.1X1-	T48.1X2-	T48.1X3-	T48.1X4-	T48.1X5-	T48.1X6-
Dimethylamine sulfate	T49.4X1-	T49.4X2-	T49.4X3-	T49.4X4-	T49.4X5-	T49.4X6-
Dimethylformamide	T52.8X1-	T52.8X2-	T52.8X3-	T52.8X4-	-	-
Dimethyltubocurarinium chloride	T48.1X1-	T48.1X2-	T48.1X3-	T48.1X4-	T48.1X5-	T48.1X6-
Dimeticone	T47.1X1-	T47.1X2-	T47.1X3-	T47.1X4-	T47.1X5-	T47.1X6-
Dimetilan	T60.0X1-	T60.0X2-	T60.0X3-	T60.0X4-	-	-
Dimetindene	T45.0X1-	T45.0X2-	T45.0X3-	T45.0X4-	T45.0X5-	T45.0X6-
Dimetotiazine	T43.3X1-	T43.3X2-	T43.3X3-	T43.3X4-	T43.3X5-	T43.3X6-
Dimorpholamine	T50.7X1-	T50.7X2-	T50.7X3-	T50.7X4-	T50.7X5-	T50.7X6-
Dimoxyline	T46.3X1-	T46.3X2-	T46.3X3-	T46.3X4-	T46.3X5-	T46.3X6-
Dinitrobenzene	T65.3X1-	T65.3X2-	T65.3X3-	T65.3X4-	-	-
vapor	T59.891-	T59.892-	T59.893-	T59.894-	-	-
Dinitrobenzol	T65.3X1-	T65.3X2-	T65.3X3-	T65.3X4-	-	-
vapor	T59.891-	T59.892-	T59.893-	T59.894-	-	-
Dinitrobutylphenol	T65.3X1-	T65.3X2-	T65.3X3-	T65.3X4-	-	-
Dinitro (-ortho-) cresol (pesticide) (spray)	T65.3X1-	T65.3X2-	T65.3X3-	T65.3X4-	-	-
Dinitrocyclohexylphenol	T65.3X1-	T65.3X2-	T65.3X3-	T65.3X4-	-	-
Dinitrophenol	T65.3X1-	T65.3X2-	T65.3X3-	T65.3X4-	-	-
Dinoprost	T48.0X1-	T48.0X2-	T48.0X3-	T48.0X4-	T48.0X5-	T48.0X6-
Dinoprostone	T48.0X1-	T48.0X2-	T48.0X3-	T48.0X4-	T48.0X5-	T48.0X6-
Dinoseb	T60.3X1-	T60.3X2-	T60.3X3-	T60.3X4-	-	-
Dioctyl sulfosuccinate (calcium) (sodium)	T47.4X1-	T47.4X2-	T47.4X3-	T47.4X4-	T47.4X5-	T47.4X6-
Diodone	T50.8X1-	T50.8X2-	T50.8X3-	T50.8X4-	T50.8X5-	T50.8X6-
Diodoquin	T37.8X1-	T37.8X2-	T37.8X3-	T37.8X4-	T37.8X5-	T37.8X6-
Dionin	T40.2X1-	T40.2X2-	T40.2X3-	T40.2X4-	T40.2X5-	T40.2X6-
Diosmin	T46.991-	T46.992-	T46.993-	T46.994-	T46.995-	T46.996-
Dioxane	T52.8X1-	T52.8X2-	T52.8X3-	T52.8X4-	-	-
Dioxathion	T60.0X1-	T60.0X2-	T60.0X3-	T60.0X4-	-	-
Dioxin	T53.7X1-	T53.7X2-	T53.7X3-	T53.7X4-	-	-
Dioxopromethazine	T43.3X1-	T43.3X2-	T43.3X3-	T43.3X4-	T43.3X5-	T43.3X6-
Dioxyline	T46.3X1-	T46.3X2-	T46.3X3-	T46.3X4-	T46.3X5-	T46.3X6-
Dipentene	T52.8X1-	T52.8X2-	T52.8X3-	T52.8X4-	-	-

Substance	Poisoning Accidental (unintentional)	Poisoning Intentional self-harm	Poisoning Assault	Poisoning Undetermined	Adverse effect	Underdosing
Diperodon	T41.3X1-	T41.3X2-	T41.3X3-	T41.3X4-	T41.3X5-	T41.3X6-
Diphacinone	T60.4X1-	T60.4X2-	T60.4X3-	T60.4X4-	-	-
Diphemanil	T44.3X1-	T44.3X2-	T44.3X3-	T44.3X4-	T44.3X5-	T44.3X6-
metilsulfate	T44.3X1-	T44.3X2-	T44.3X3-	T44.3X4-	T44.3X5-	T44.3X6-
Diphenadione	T45.511-	T45.512-	T45.513-	T45.514-	T45.515-	T45.516-
rodenticide	T60.4X1-	T60.4X2-	T60.4X3-	T60.4X4-	-	-
Diphenhydramine	T45.0X1-	T45.0X2-	T45.0X3-	T45.0X4-	T45.0X5-	T45.0X6-
Diphenidol	T45.0X1-	T45.0X2-	T45.0X3-	T45.0X4-	T45.0X5-	T45.0X6-
Diphenoxylate	T47.6X1-	T47.6X2-	T47.6X3-	T47.6X4-	T47.6X5-	T47.6X6-
Diphenylamine	T65.3X1-	T65.3X2-	T65.3X3-	T65.3X4-	-	-
Diphenylbutazone	T39.2X1-	T39.2X2-	T39.2X3-	T39.2X4-	T39.2X5-	T39.2X6-
Diphenylchloroarsine, not in war	T57.0X1-	T57.0X2-	T57.0X3-	T57.0X4-	-	-
Diphenylhydantoin	T42.0X1-	T42.0X2-	T42.0X3-	T42.0X4-	T42.0X5-	T42.0X6-
Diphenylmethane dye	T52.1X1-	T52.1X2-	T52.1X3-	T52.1X4-	-	-
Diphenylpyraline	T45.0X1-	T45.0X2-	T45.0X3-	T45.0X4-	T45.0X5-	T45.0X6-
Diphtheria						
antitoxin	T50.Z11-	T50.Z12-	T50.Z13-	T50.Z14-	T50.Z15-	T50.Z16-
toxoid	T50.A91-	T50.A92-	T50.A93-	T50.A94-	T50.A95-	T50.A96-
with tetanus toxoid	T50.A21-	T50.A22-	T50.A23-	T50.A24-	T50.A25-	T50.A26-
with pertussis component	T50.A11-	T50.A12-	T50.A13-	T50.A14-	T50.A15-	T50.A16-
vaccine	T50.A91-	T50.A92-	T50.A93-	T50.A94-	T50.A95-	T50.A96-
combination						
including pertussis	T50.A11-	T50.A12-	T50.A13-	T50.A14-	T50.A15-	T50.A16-
without pertussis	T50.A21-	T50.A22-	T50.A23-	T50.A24-	T50.A25-	T50.A26-
Diphylline	T50.2X1-	T50.2X2-	T50.2X3-	T50.2X4-	T50.2X5-	T50.2X6-
Dipipanone	T40.4X1-	T40.4X2-	T40.4X3-	T40.4X4-	-	-
Dipivefrine	T49.5X1-	T49.5X2-	T49.5X3-	T49.5X4-	T49.5X5-	T49.5X6-
Diplovax	T50.B91-	T50.B92-	T50.B93-	T50.B94-	T50.B95-	T50.B96-
Diprophylline	T50.2X1-	T50.2X2-	T50.2X3-	T50.2X4-	T50.2X5-	T50.2X6-
Dipropyline	T48.291-	T48.292-	T48.293-	T48.294-	T48.295-	T48.296-
Dipyridamole	T46.3X1-	T46.3X2-	T46.3X3-	T46.3X4-	T46.3X5-	T46.3X6-
Dipyrone	T39.2X1-	T39.2X2-	T39.2X3-	T39.2X4-	T39.2X5-	T39.2X6-
Diquat (dibromide)	T60.3X1-	T60.3X2-	T60.3X3-	T60.3X4-	-	-
Disinfectant	T65.891-	T65.892-	T65.893-	T65.894-	-	-
alkaline	T54.3X1-	T54.3X2-	T54.3X3-	T54.3X4-	-	-
aromatic	T54.1X1-	T54.1X2-	T54.1X3-	T54.1X4-	-	-
intestinal	T37.8X1-	T37.8X2-	T37.8X3-	T37.8X4-	T37.8X5-	T37.8X6-
Disipal	T42.8X1-	T42.8X2-	T42.8X3-	T42.8X4-	T42.8X5-	T42.8X6-
Disodium edetate	T50.6X1-	T50.6X2-	T50.6X3-	T50.6X4-	T50.6X5-	T50.6X6-
Disoprofol	T41.291-	T41.292-	T41.293-	T41.294-	T41.295-	T41.296-
Disopyramide	T46.2X1-	T46.2X2-	T46.2X3-	T46.2X4-	T46.2X5-	T46.2X6-
Distigmine (bromide)	T44.0X1-	T44.0X2-	T44.0X3-	T44.0X4-	T44.0X5-	T44.0X6-
Disulfamide	T50.2X1-	T50.2X2-	T50.2X3-	T50.2X4-	T50.2X5-	T50.2X6-
Disulfanilamide	T37.0X1-	T37.0X2-	T37.0X3-	T37.0X4-	T37.0X5-	T37.0X6-
Disulfiram	T50.6X1-	T50.6X2-	T50.6X3-	T50.6X4-	T50.6X5-	T50.6X6-
Disulfoton	T60.0X1-	T60.0X2-	T60.0X3-	T60.0X4-	-	-
Dithiazanine iodide	T37.4X1-	T37.4X2-	T37.4X3-	T37.4X4-	T37.4X5-	T37.4X6-
Dithiocarbamate	T60.0X1-	T60.0X2-	T60.0X3-	T60.0X4-	-	-
Dithranol	T49.4X1-	T49.4X2-	T49.4X3-	T49.4X4-	T49.4X5-	T49.4X6-
Diucardin	T50.2X1-	T50.2X2-	T50.2X3-	T50.2X4-	T50.2X5-	T50.2X6-
Diupres	T50.2X1-	T50.2X2-	T50.2X3-	T50.2X4-	T50.2X5-	T50.2X6-
Diuretic NEC	T50.2X1-	T50.2X2-	T50.2X3-	T50.2X4-	T50.2X5-	T50.2X6-
benzothiadiazine	T50.2X1-	T50.2X2-	T50.2X3-	T50.2X4-	T50.2X5-	T50.2X6-
carbonic acid anhydrase inhibitors	T50.2X1-	T50.2X2-	T50.2X3-	T50.2X4-	T50.2X5-	T50.2X6-
furfuryl NEC	T50.2X1-	T50.2X2-	T50.2X3-	T50.2X4-	T50.2X5-	T50.2X6-
loop (high-ceiling)	T50.1X1-	T50.1X2-	T50.1X3-	T50.1X4-	T50.1X5-	T50.1X6-
mercurial NEC	T50.2X1-	T50.2X2-	T50.2X3-	T50.2X4-	T50.2X5-	T50.2X6-
osmotic	T50.2X1-	T50.2X2-	T50.2X3-	T50.2X4-	T50.2X5-	T50.2X6-

Substance	Poisoning Accidental (unintentional)	Poisoning Intentional self-harm	Poisoning Assault	Poisoning Undetermined	Adverse effect	Underdosing
Diuretic NEC *(continued)*						
purine NEC	T50.2X1-	T50.2X2-	T50.2X3-	T50.2X4-	T50.2X5-	T50.2X6-
saluretic NEC	T50.2X1-	T50.2X2-	T50.2X3-	T50.2X4-	T50.2X5-	T50.2X6-
sulfonamide	T50.2X1-	T50.2X2-	T50.2X3-	T50.2X4-	T50.2X5-	T50.2X6-
thiazide NEC	T50.2X1-	T50.2X2-	T50.2X3-	T50.2X4-	T50.2X5-	T50.2X6-
xanthine	T50.2X1-	T50.2X2-	T50.2X3-	T50.2X4-	T50.2X5-	T50.2X6-
Diurgin	T50.2X1-	T50.2X2-	T50.2X3-	T50.2X4-	T50.2X5-	T50.2X6-
Diuril	T50.2X1-	T50.2X2-	T50.2X3-	T50.2X4-	T50.2X5-	T50.2X6-
Diuron	T60.3X1-	T60.3X2-	T60.3X3-	T60.3X4-	-	-
Divalproex	T42.6X1-	T42.6X2-	T42.6X3-	T42.6X4-	T42.6X5-	T42.6X6-
Divinyl ether	T41.0X1-	T41.0X2-	T41.0X3-	T41.0X4-	T41.0X5-	T41.0X6-
Dixanthogen	T49.0X1-	T49.0X2-	T49.0X3-	T49.0X4-	T49.0X5-	T49.0X6-
Dixyrazine	T43.3X1-	T43.3X2-	T43.3X3-	T43.3X4-	T43.3X5-	T43.3X6-
D-lysergic acid diethylamide	T40.8X1-	T40.8X2-	T40.8X3-	T40.8X4-	-	-
DMCT	T36.4X1-	T36.4X2-	T36.4X3-	T36.4X4-	T36.4X5-	T36.4X6-
DMSO — *see Dimethyl sulfoxide*						
DNBP	T60.3X1-	T60.3X2-	T60.3X3-	T60.3X4-	-	-
DNOC	T65.3X1-	T65.3X2-	T65.3X3-	T65.3X4-	-	-
Dobutamine	T44.5X1-	T44.5X2-	T44.5X3-	T44.5X4-	T44.5X5-	T44.5X6-
DOCA	T38.0X1-	T38.0X2-	T38.0X3-	T38.0X4-	T38.0X5-	T38.0X6-
Docusate sodium	T47.4X1-	T47.4X2-	T47.4X3-	T47.4X4-	T47.4X5-	T47.4X6-
Dodicin	T49.0X1-	T49.0X2-	T49.0X3-	T49.0X4-	T49.0X5-	T49.0X6-
Dofamium chloride	T49.0X1-	T49.0X2-	T49.0X3-	T49.0X4-	T49.0X5-	T49.0X6-
Dolophine	T40.3X1-	T40.3X2-	T40.3X3-	T40.3X4-	T40.3X5-	T40.3X6-
Doloxene	T39.8X1-	T39.8X2-	T39.8X3-	T39.8X4-	T39.8X5-	T39.8X6-
Domestic gas (after combustion) — *see Gas, utility*						
prior to combustion	T59.891-	T59.892-	T59.893-	T59.894-	-	-
Domiodol	T48.4X1-	T48.4X2-	T48.4X3-	T48.4X4-	T48.4X5-	T48.4X6-
Domiphen (bromide)	T49.0X1-	T49.0X2-	T49.0X3-	T49.0X4-	T49.0X5-	T49.0X6-
Domperidone	T45.0X1-	T45.0X2-	T45.0X3-	T45.0X4-	T45.0X5-	T45.0X6-
Dopa	T42.8X1-	T42.8X2-	T42.8X3-	T42.8X4-	T42.8X5-	T42.8X6-
Dopamine	T44.991-	T44.992-	T44.993-	T44.994-	T44.995-	T44.996-
Doriden	T42.6X1-	T42.6X2-	T42.6X3-	T42.6X4-	T42.6X5-	T42.6X6-
Dormiral	T42.3X1-	T42.3X2-	T42.3X3-	T42.3X4-	T42.3X5-	T42.3X6-
Dormison	T42.6X1-	T42.6X2-	T42.6X3-	T42.6X4-	T42.6X5-	T42.6X6-
Dornase	T48.4X1-	T48.4X2-	T48.4X3-	T48.4X4-	T48.4X5-	T48.4X6-
Dorsacaine	T41.3X1-	T41.3X2-	T41.3X3-	T41.3X4-	T41.3X5-	T41.3X6-
Dosulepin	T43.011-	T43.012-	T43.013-	T43.014-	T43.015-	T43.016-
Dothiepin	T43.011-	T43.012-	T43.013-	T43.014-	T43.015-	T43.016-
Doxantrazole	T48.6X1-	T48.6X2-	T48.6X3-	T48.6X4-	T48.6X5-	T48.6X6-
Doxapram	T50.7X1-	T50.7X2-	T50.7X3-	T50.7X4-	T50.7X5-	T50.7X6-
Doxazosin	T44.6X1-	T44.6X2-	T44.6X3-	T44.6X4-	T44.6X5-	T44.6X6-
Doxepin	T43.011-	T43.012-	T43.013-	T43.014-	T43.015-	T43.016-
Doxifluridine	T45.1X1-	T45.1X2-	T45.1X3-	T45.1X4-	T45.1X5-	T45.1X6-
Doxorubicin	T45.1X1-	T45.1X2-	T45.1X3-	T45.1X4-	T45.1X5-	T45.1X6-
Doxycycline	T36.4X1-	T36.4X2-	T36.4X3-	T36.4X4-	T36.4X5-	T36.4X6-
Doxylamine	T45.0X1-	T45.0X2-	T45.0X3-	T45.0X4-	T45.0X5-	T45.0X6-
Dramamine	T45.0X1-	T45.0X2-	T45.0X3-	T45.0X4-	T45.0X5-	T45.0X6-
Drano (drain cleaner)	T54.3X1-	T54.3X2-	T54.3X3-	T54.3X4-	-	-
Dressing, live pulp	T49.7X1-	T49.7X2-	T49.7X3-	T49.7X4-	T49.7X5-	T49.7X6-
Drocode	T40.2X1-	T40.2X2-	T40.2X3-	T40.2X4-	T40.2X5-	T40.2X6-
Dromoran	T40.2X1-	T40.2X2-	T40.2X3-	T40.2X4-	T40.2X5-	T40.2X6-
Dromostanolone	T38.7X1-	T38.7X2-	T38.7X3-	T38.7X4-	T38.7X5-	T38.7X6-
Dronabinol	T40.7X1-	T40.7X2-	T40.7X3-	T40.7X4-	T40.7X5-	T40.7X6-
Droperidol	T43.591-	T43.592-	T43.593-	T43.594-	T43.595-	T43.596-
Dropropizine	T48.3X1-	T48.3X2-	T48.3X3-	T48.3X4-	T48.3X5-	T48.3X6-
Drostanolone	T38.7X1-	T38.7X2-	T38.7X3-	T38.7X4-	T38.7X5-	T38.7X6-
Drotaverine	T44.3X1-	T44.3X2-	T44.3X3-	T44.3X4-	T44.3X5-	T44.3X6-
Drotrecogin alfa	T45.511-	T45.512-	T45.513-	T45.514-	T45.515-	T45.516-

Substance	Poisoning Accidental (unintentional)	Poisoning Intentional self-harm	Poisoning Assault	Poisoning Undetermined	Adverse effect	Underdosing
Drug NEC	T50.901-	T50.902-	T50.903-	T50.904-	T50.905-	T50.906-
specified NEC	T50.991-	T50.992-	T50.993-	T50.994-	T50.995-	T50.996-
DTIC	T45.1X1-	T45.1X2-	T45.1X3-	T45.1X4-	T45.1X5-	T45.1X6-
Duboisine	T44.3X1-	T44.3X2-	T44.3X3-	T44.3X4-	T44.3X5-	T44.3X6-
Dulcolax	T47.2X1-	T47.2X2-	T47.2X3-	T47.2X4-	T47.2X5-	T47.2X6-
Duponol (C) (EP)	T49.2X1-	T49.2X2-	T49.2X3-	T49.2X4-	T49.2X5-	T49.2X6-
Durabolin	T38.7X1-	T38.7X2-	T38.7X3-	T38.7X4-	T38.7X5-	T38.7X6-
Dyclone	T41.3X1-	T41.3X2-	T41.3X3-	T41.3X4-	T41.3X5-	T41.3X6-
Dyclonine	T41.3X1-	T41.3X2-	T41.3X3-	T41.3X4-	T41.3X5-	T41.3X6-
Dydrogesterone	T38.5X1-	T38.5X2-	T38.5X3-	T38.5X4-	T38.5X5-	T38.5X6-
Dye NEC	T65.6X1-	T65.6X2-	T65.6X3-	T65.6X4-	-	-
antiseptic	T49.0X1-	T49.0X2-	T49.0X3-	T49.0X4-	T49.0X5-	T49.0X6-
diagnostic agents	T50.8X1-	T50.8X2-	T50.8X3-	T50.8X4-	T50.8X5-	T50.8X6-
pharmaceutical NEC	T50.901-	T50.902-	T50.903-	T50.904-	T50.905-	T50.906-
Dyflos	T44.0X1-	T44.0X2-	T44.0X3-	T44.0X4-	T44.0X5-	T44.0X6-
Dymelor	T38.3X1-	T38.3X2-	T38.3X3-	T38.3X4-	T38.3X5-	T38.3X6-
Dynamite	T65.3X1-	T65.3X2-	T65.3X3-	T65.3X4-	-	-
fumes	T59.891-	T59.892-	T59.893-	T59.894-	-	-
Dyphylline	T44.3X1-	T44.3X2-	T44.3X3-	T44.3X4-	T44.3X5-	T44.3X6-
Ear drug NEC	T49.6X1-	T49.6X2-	T49.6X3-	T49.6X4-	T49.6X5-	T49.6X6-
Ear preparations	T49.6X1-	T49.6X2-	T49.6X3-	T49.6X4-	T49.6X5-	T49.6X6-
Echothiophate, echothiopate, ecothiophate	T49.5X1-	T49.5X2-	T49.5X3-	T49.5X4-	T49.5X5-	T49.5X6-
Econazole	T49.0X1-	T49.0X2-	T49.0X3-	T49.0X4-	T49.0X5-	T49.0X6-
Ecothiopate iodide	T49.5X1-	T49.5X2-	T49.5X3-	T49.5X4-	T49.5X5-	T49.5X6-
Ecstasy	T43.641-	T43.642-	T43.643-	T43.644-	-	-
Ectylurea	T42.6X1-	T42.6X2-	T42.6X3-	T42.6X4-	T42.6X5-	T42.6X6-
Edathamil disodium	T45.8X1-	T45.8X2-	T45.8X3-	T45.8X4-	T45.8X5-	T45.8X6-
Edecrin	T50.1X1-	T50.1X2-	T50.1X3-	T50.1X4-	T50.1X5-	T50.1X6-
Edetate, disodium (calcium)	T45.8X1-	T45.8X2-	T45.8X3-	T45.8X4-	T45.8X5-	T45.8X6-
Edoxudine	T49.5X1-	T49.5X2-	T49.5X3-	T49.5X4-	T49.5X5-	T49.5X6-
Edrophonium	T44.0X1-	T44.0X2-	T44.0X3-	T44.0X4-	T44.0X5-	T44.0X6-
chloride	T44.0X1-	T44.0X2-	T44.0X3-	T44.0X4-	T44.0X5-	T44.0X6-
EDTA	T50.6X1-	T50.6X2-	T50.6X3-	T50.6X4-	T50.6X5-	T50.6X6-
Eflornithine	T37.2X1-	T37.2X2-	T37.2X3-	T37.2X4-	T37.2X5-	T37.2X6-
Efloxate	T46.3X1-	T46.3X2-	T46.3X3-	T46.3X4-	T46.3X5-	T46.3X6-
Elase	T49.8X1-	T49.8X2-	T49.8X3-	T49.8X4-	T49.8X5-	T49.8X6-
Elastase	T47.5X1-	T47.5X2-	T47.5X3-	T47.5X4-	T47.5X5-	T47.5X6-
Elaterium	T47.2X1-	T47.2X2-	T47.2X3-	T47.2X4-	T47.2X5-	T47.2X6-
Elcatonin	T50.991-	T50.992-	T50.993-	T50.994-	T50.995-	T50.996-
Elder	T62.2X1-	T62.2X2-	T62.2X3-	T62.2X4-	-	-
berry, (unripe)	T62.1X1-	T62.1X2-	T62.1X3-	T62.1X4-	-	-
Electrolyte balance drug	T50.3X1-	T50.3X2-	T50.3X3-	T50.3X4-	T50.3X5-	T50.3X6-
Electrolytes NEC	T50.3X1-	T50.3X2-	T50.3X3-	T50.3X4-	T50.3X5-	T50.3X6-
Electrolytic agent NEC	T50.3X1-	T50.3X2-	T50.3X3-	T50.3X4-	T50.3X5-	T50.3X6-
Elemental diet	T50.901-	T50.902-	T50.903-	T50.904-	T50.905-	T50.906-
Elliptinium acetate	T45.1X1-	T45.1X2-	T45.1X3-	T45.1X4-	T45.1X5-	T45.1X6-
Embramine	T45.0X1-	T45.0X2-	T45.0X3-	T45.0X4-	T45.0X5-	T45.0X6-
Emepronium (salts)	T44.3X1-	T44.3X2-	T44.3X3-	T44.3X4-	T44.3X5-	T44.3X6-
bromide	T44.3X1-	T44.3X2-	T44.3X3-	T44.3X4-	T44.3X5-	T44.3X6-
Emetic NEC	T47.7X1-	T47.7X2-	T47.7X3-	T47.7X4-	T47.7X5-	T47.7X6-
Emetine	T37.3X1-	T37.3X2-	T37.3X3-	T37.3X4-	T37.3X5-	T37.3X6-
Emollient NEC	T49.3X1-	T49.3X2-	T49.3X3-	T49.3X4-	T49.3X5-	T49.3X6-
Emorfazone	T39.8X1-	T39.8X2-	T39.8X3-	T39.8X4-	T39.8X5-	T39.8X6-
Emylcamate	T43.591-	T43.592-	T43.593-	T43.594-	T43.595-	T43.596-
Enalapril	T46.4X1-	T46.4X2-	T46.4X3-	T46.4X4-	T46.4X5-	T46.4X6-
Enalaprilat	T46.4X1-	T46.4X2-	T46.4X3-	T46.4X4-	T46.4X5-	T46.4X6-
Encainide	T46.2X1-	T46.2X2-	T46.2X3-	T46.2X4-	T46.2X5-	T46.2X6-

DRUG NEC - ENCAINIDE

Substance	Poisoning Accidental (unintentional)	Poisoning Intentional self-harm	Poisoning Assault	Poisoning Undetermined	Adverse effect	Underdosing
Endocaine	T41.3X1-	T41.3X2-	T41.3X3-	T41.3X4-	T41.3X5-	T41.3X6-
Endosulfan	T60.2X1-	T60.2X2-	T60.2X3-	T60.2X4-	-	-
Endothall	T60.3X1-	T60.3X2-	T60.3X3-	T60.3X4-	-	-
Endralazine	T46.5X1-	T46.5X2-	T46.5X3-	T46.5X4-	T46.5X5-	T46.5X6-
Endrin	T60.1X1-	T60.1X2-	T60.1X3-	T60.1X4-	-	-
Enflurane	T41.0X1-	T41.0X2-	T41.0X3-	T41.0X4-	T41.0X5-	T41.0X6-
Enhexymal	T42.3X1-	T42.3X2-	T42.3X3-	T42.3X4-	T42.3X5-	T42.3X6-
Enocitabine	T45.1X1-	T45.1X2-	T45.1X3-	T45.1X4-	T45.1X5-	T45.1X6-
Enovid	T38.4X1-	T38.4X2-	T38.4X3-	T38.4X4-	T38.4X5-	T38.4X6-
Enoxacin	T36.8X1-	T36.8X2-	T36.8X3-	T36.8X4-	T36.8X5-	T36.8X6-
Enoxaparin (sodium)	T45.511-	T45.512-	T45.513-	T45.514-	T45.515-	T45.516-
Enpiprazole	T43.591-	T43.592-	T43.593-	T43.594-	T43.595-	T43.596-
Enprofylline	T48.6X1-	T48.6X2-	T48.6X3-	T48.6X4-	T48.6X5-	T48.6X6-
Enprostil	T47.1X1-	T47.1X2-	T47.1X3-	T47.1X4-	T47.1X5-	T47.1X6-
ENT preparations (anti-infectives)	T49.6X1-	T49.6X2-	T49.6X3-	T49.6X4-	T49.6X5-	T49.6X6-
Enterogastrone	T38.891-	T38.892-	T38.893-	T38.894-	T38.895-	T38.896-
Enviomycin	T36.8X1-	T36.8X2-	T36.8X3-	T36.8X4-	T36.8X5-	T36.8X6-
Enzodase	T45.3X1-	T45.3X2-	T45.3X3-	T45.3X4-	T45.3X5-	T45.3X6-
Enzyme NEC	T45.3X1-	T45.3X2-	T45.3X3-	T45.3X4-	T45.3X5-	T45.3X6-
depolymerizing	T49.8X1-	T49.8X2-	T49.8X3-	T49.8X4-	T49.8X5-	T49.8X6-
fibrolytic	T45.3X1-	T45.3X2-	T45.3X3-	T45.3X4-	T45.3X5-	T45.3X6-
gastric	T47.5X1-	T47.5X2-	T47.5X3-	T47.5X4-	T47.5X5-	T47.5X6-
intestinal	T47.5X1-	T47.5X2-	T47.5X3-	T47.5X4-	T47.5X5-	T47.5X6-
local action	T49.4X1-	T49.4X2-	T49.4X3-	T49.4X4-	T49.4X5-	T49.4X6-
proteolytic	T49.4X1-	T49.4X2-	T49.4X3-	T49.4X4-	T49.4X5-	T49.4X6-
thrombolytic	T45.3X1-	T45.3X2-	T45.3X3-	T45.3X4-	T45.3X5-	T45.3X6-
EPAB	T41.3X1-	T41.3X2-	T41.3X3-	T41.3X4-	T41.3X5-	T41.3X6-
Epanutin	T42.0X1-	T42.0X2-	T42.0X3-	T42.0X4-	T42.0X5-	T42.0X6-
Ephedra	T44.991-	T44.992-	T44.993-	T44.994-	T44.995-	T44.996-
Ephedrine	T44.991-	T44.992-	T44.993-	T44.994-	T44.995-	T44.996-
Epichlorhydrin, epichlorohydrin	T52.8X1-	T52.8X2-	T52.8X3-	T52.8X4-	-	-
Epicillin	T36.0X1-	T36.0X2-	T36.0X3-	T36.0X4-	T36.0X5-	T36.0X6-
Epiestriol	T38.5X1-	T38.5X2-	T38.5X3-	T38.5X4-	T38.5X5-	T38.5X6-
Epilim — see Sodium valproate						
Epimestrol	T38.5X1-	T38.5X2-	T38.5X3-	T38.5X4-	T38.5X5-	T38.5X6-
Epinephrine	T44.5X1-	T44.5X2-	T44.5X3-	T44.5X4-	T44.5X5-	T44.5X6-
Epirubicin	T45.1X1-	T45.1X2-	T45.1X3-	T45.1X4-	T45.1X5-	T45.1X6-
Epitiostanol	T38.7X1-	T38.7X2-	T38.7X3-	T38.7X4-	T38.7X5-	T38.7X6-
Epitizide	T50.2X1-	T50.2X2-	T50.2X3-	T50.2X4-	T50.2X5-	T50.2X6-
EPN	T60.0X1-	T60.0X2-	T60.0X3-	T60.0X4-	-	-
EPO	T45.8X1-	T45.8X2-	T45.8X3-	T45.8X4-	T45.8X5-	T45.8X6-
Epoetin alpha	T45.8X1-	T45.8X2-	T45.8X3-	T45.8X4-	T45.8X5-	T45.8X6-
Epomediol	T50.991-	T50.992-	T50.993-	T50.994-	T50.995-	T50.996-
Epoprostenol	T45.521-	T45.522-	T45.523-	T45.524-	T45.525-	T45.526-
Epoxy resin	T65.891-	T65.892-	T65.893-	T65.894-	-	-
Eprazinone	T48.4X1-	T48.4X2-	T48.4X3-	T48.4X4-	T48.4X5-	T48.4X6-
Epsilon amino-caproic acid	T45.621-	T45.622-	T45.623-	T45.624-	T45.625-	T45.626-
Epsom salt	T47.3X1-	T47.3X2-	T47.3X3-	T47.3X4-	T47.3X5-	T47.3X6-
Eptazocine	T40.4X1-	T40.4X2-	T40.4X3-	T40.4X4-	T40.4X5-	T40.4X6-
Equanil	T43.591-	T43.592-	T43.593-	T43.594-	T43.595-	T43.596-
Equisetum	T62.2X1-	T62.2X2-	T62.2X3-	T62.2X4-	-	-
diuretic	T50.2X1-	T50.2X2-	T50.2X3-	T50.2X4-	T50.2X5-	T50.2X6-
Ergobasine	T48.0X1-	T48.0X2-	T48.0X3-	T48.0X4-	T48.0X5-	T48.0X6-
Ergocalciferol	T45.2X1-	T45.2X2-	T45.2X3-	T45.2X4-	T45.2X5-	T45.2X6-
Ergoloid mesylates	T46.7X1-	T46.7X2-	T46.7X3-	T46.7X4-	T46.7X5-	T46.7X6-
Ergometrine	T48.0X1-	T48.0X2-	T48.0X3-	T48.0X4-	T48.0X5-	T48.0X6-
Ergonovine	T48.0X1-	T48.0X2-	T48.0X3-	T48.0X4-	T48.0X5-	T48.0X6-
Ergot NEC	T64.81X-	T64.82X-	T64.83X-	T64.84X-	-	-
derivative	T48.0X1-	T48.0X2-	T48.0X3-	T48.0X4-	T48.0X5-	T48.0X6-

Substance	Poisoning Accidental (unintentional)	Poisoning Intentional self-harm	Poisoning Assault	Poisoning Undetermined	Adverse effect	Underdosing
Ergot NEC (continued)						
medicinal (alkaloids)	T48.0X1-	T48.0X2-	T48.0X3-	T48.0X4-	T48.0X5-	T48.0X6-
prepared	T48.0X1-	T48.0X2-	T48.0X3-	T48.0X4-	T48.0X5-	T48.0X6-
Ergotamine	T46.5X1-	T46.5X2-	T46.5X3-	T46.5X4-	T46.5X5-	T46.5X6-
Ergotocine	T48.0X1-	T48.0X2-	T48.0X3-	T48.0X4-	T48.0X5-	T48.0X6-
Ergotrate	T48.0X1-	T48.0X2-	T48.0X3-	T48.0X4-	T48.0X5-	T48.0X6-
Eritrityl tetranitrate	T46.3X1-	T46.3X2-	T46.3X3-	T46.3X4-	T46.3X5-	T46.3X6-
Erythrityl tetranitrate	T46.3X1-	T46.3X2-	T46.3X3-	T46.3X4-	T46.3X5-	T46.3X6-
Erythrol tetranitrate	T46.3X1-	T46.3X2-	T46.3X3-	T46.3X4-	T46.3X5-	T46.3X6-
Erythromycin (salts)	T36.3X1-	T36.3X2-	T36.3X3-	T36.3X4-	T36.3X5-	T36.3X6-
ophthalmic preparation	T49.5X1-	T49.5X2-	T49.5X3-	T49.5X4-	T49.5X5-	T49.5X6-
topical NEC	T49.0X1-	T49.0X2-	T49.0X3-	T49.0X4-	T49.0X5-	T49.0X6-
Erythropoietin	T45.8X1-	T45.8X2-	T45.8X3-	T45.8X4-	T45.8X5-	T45.8X6-
human	T45.8X1-	T45.8X2-	T45.8X3-	T45.8X4-	T45.8X5-	T45.8X6-
Escin	T46.991-	T46.992-	T46.993-	T46.994-	T46.995-	T46.996-
Esculin	T45.2X1-	T45.2X2-	T45.2X3-	T45.2X4-	T45.2X5-	T45.2X6-
Esculoside	T45.2X1-	T45.2X2-	T45.2X3-	T45.2X4-	T45.2X5-	T45.2X6-
ESDT (ether-soluble tar distillate)	T49.1X1-	T49.1X2-	T49.1X3-	T49.1X4-	T49.1X5-	T49.1X6-
Eserine	T49.5X1-	T49.5X2-	T49.5X3-	T49.5X4-	T49.5X5-	T49.5X6-
Esflurbiprofen	T39.311-	T39.312-	T39.313-	T39.314-	T39.315-	T39.316-
Eskabarb	T42.3X1-	T42.3X2-	T42.3X3-	T42.3X4-	T42.3X5-	T42.3X6-
Eskalith	T43.8X1-	T43.8X2-	T43.8X3-	T43.8X4-	T43.8X5-	T43.8X6-
Esmolol	T44.7X1-	T44.7X2-	T44.7X3-	T44.7X4-	T44.7X5-	T44.7X6-
Estanozolol	T38.7X1-	T38.7X2-	T38.7X3-	T38.7X4-	T38.7X5-	T38.7X6-
Estazolam	T42.4X1-	T42.4X2-	T42.4X3-	T42.4X4-	T42.4X5-	T42.4X6-
Estradiol	T38.5X1-	T38.5X2-	T38.5X3-	T38.5X4-	T38.5X5-	T38.5X6-
with testosterone	T38.7X1-	T38.7X2-	T38.7X3-	T38.7X4-	T38.7X5-	T38.7X6-
benzoate	T38.5X1-	T38.5X2-	T38.5X3-	T38.5X4-	T38.5X5-	T38.5X6-
Estramustine	T45.1X1-	T45.1X2-	T45.1X3-	T45.1X4-	T45.1X5-	T45.1X6-
Estriol	T38.5X1-	T38.5X2-	T38.5X3-	T38.5X4-	T38.5X5-	T38.5X6-
Estrogen	T38.5X1-	T38.5X2-	T38.5X3-	T38.5X4-	T38.5X5-	T38.5X6-
with progesterone	T38.5X1-	T38.5X2-	T38.5X3-	T38.5X4-	T38.5X5-	T38.5X6-
conjugated	T38.5X1-	T38.5X2-	T38.5X3-	T38.5X4-	T38.5X5-	T38.5X6-
Estrone	T38.5X1-	T38.5X2-	T38.5X3-	T38.5X4-	T38.5X5-	T38.5X6-
Estropipate	T38.5X1-	T38.5X2-	T38.5X3-	T38.5X4-	T38.5X5-	T38.5X6-
Etacrynate sodium	T50.1X1-	T50.1X2-	T50.1X3-	T50.1X4-	T50.1X5-	T50.1X6-
Etacrynic acid	T50.1X1-	T50.1X2-	T50.1X3-	T50.1X4-	T50.1X5-	T50.1X6-
Etafedrine	T48.6X1-	T48.6X2-	T48.6X3-	T48.6X4-	T48.6X5-	T48.6X6-
Etafenone	T46.3X1-	T46.3X2-	T46.3X3-	T46.3X4-	T46.3X5-	T46.3X6-
Etambutol	T37.1X1-	T37.1X2-	T37.1X3-	T37.1X4-	T37.1X5-	T37.1X6-
Etamiphyllin	T48.6X1-	T48.6X2-	T48.6X3-	T48.6X4-	T48.6X5-	T48.6X6-
Etamivan	T50.7X1-	T50.7X2-	T50.7X3-	T50.7X4-	T50.7X5-	T50.7X6-
Etamsylate	T45.7X1-	T45.7X2-	T45.7X3-	T45.7X4-	T45.7X5-	T45.7X6-
Etebenecid	T50.4X1-	T50.4X2-	T50.4X3-	T50.4X4-	T50.4X5-	T50.4X6-
Ethacridine	T49.0X1-	T49.0X2-	T49.0X3-	T49.0X4-	T49.0X5-	T49.0X6-
Ethacrynic acid	T50.1X1-	T50.1X2-	T50.1X3-	T50.1X4-	T50.1X5-	T50.1X6-
Ethadione	T42.2X1-	T42.2X2-	T42.2X3-	T42.2X4-	T42.2X5-	T42.2X6-
Ethambutol	T37.1X1-	T37.1X2-	T37.1X3-	T37.1X4-	T37.1X5-	T37.1X6-
Ethamide	T50.2X1-	T50.2X2-	T50.2X3-	T50.2X4-	T50.2X5-	T50.2X6-
Ethamivan	T50.7X1-	T50.7X2-	T50.7X3-	T50.7X4-	T50.7X5-	T50.7X6-
Ethamsylate	T45.7X1-	T45.7X2-	T45.7X3-	T45.7X4-	T45.7X5-	T45.7X6-
Ethanol	T51.0X1-	T51.0X2-	T51.0X3-	T51.0X4-	-	-
beverage	T51.0X1-	T51.0X2-	T51.0X3-	T51.0X4-	-	-
Ethanolamine oleate	T46.8X1-	T46.8X2-	T46.8X3-	T46.8X4-	T46.8X5-	T46.8X6-
Ethaverine	T44.3X1-	T44.3X2-	T44.3X3-	T44.3X4-	T44.3X5-	T44.3X6-
Ethchlorvynol	T42.6X1-	T42.6X2-	T42.6X3-	T42.6X4-	T42.6X5-	T42.6X6-
Ethebenecid	T50.4X1-	T50.4X2-	T50.4X3-	T50.4X4-	T50.4X5-	T50.4X6-

ERGOT NEC - ETHEBENECID

Substance	Poisoning Accidental (unintentional)	Poisoning Intentional self-harm	Poisoning Assault	Poisoning Undetermined	Adverse effect	Underdosing
Ether (vapor)	T41.0X1-	T41.0X2-	T41.0X3-	T41.0X4-	T41.0X5-	T41.0X6-
anesthetic	T41.0X1-	T41.0X2-	T41.0X3-	T41.0X4-	T41.0X5-	T41.0X6-
divinyl	T41.0X1-	T41.0X2-	T41.0X3-	T41.0X4-	T41.0X5-	T41.0X6-
ethyl (medicinal)	T41.0X1-	T41.0X2-	T41.0X3-	T41.0X4-	T41.0X5-	T41.0X6-
nonmedicinal	T52.8X1-	T52.8X2-	T52.8X3-	T52.8X4-	-	-
petroleum — *see Ligroin*						
solvent	T52.8X1-	T52.8X2-	T52.8X3-	T52.8X4-	-	-
Ethiazide	T50.2X1-	T50.2X2-	T50.2X3-	T50.2X4-	T50.2X5-	T50.2X6-
Ethidium chloride (vapor)	T59.891-	T59.892-	T59.893-	T59.894-	-	-
Ethinamate	T42.6X1-	T42.6X2-	T42.6X3-	T42.6X4-	T42.6X5-	T42.6X6-
Ethinylestradiol, ethinyloestradiol	T38.5X1-	T38.5X2-	T38.5X3-	T38.5X4-	T38.5X5-	T38.5X6-
with						
levonorgestrel	T38.4X1-	T38.4X2-	T38.4X3-	T38.4X4-	T38.4X5-	T38.4X6-
norethisterone	T38.4X1-	T38.4X2-	T38.4X3-	T38.4X4-	T38.4X5-	T38.4X6-
Ethiodized oil (131 I)	T50.8X1-	T50.8X2-	T50.8X3-	T50.8X4-	T50.8X5-	T50.8X6-
Ethion	T60.0X1-	T60.0X2-	T60.0X3-	T60.0X4-	-	-
Ethionamide	T37.1X1-	T37.1X2-	T37.1X3-	T37.1X4-	T37.1X5-	T37.1X6-
Ethioniamide	T37.1X1-	T37.1X2-	T37.1X3-	T37.1X4-	T37.1X5-	T37.1X6-
Ethisterone	T38.5X1-	T38.5X2-	T38.5X3-	T38.5X4-	T38.5X5-	T38.5X6-
Ethobral	T42.3X1-	T42.3X2-	T42.3X3-	T42.3X4-	T42.3X5-	T42.3X6-
Ethocaine (infiltration) (topical)	T41.3X1-	T41.3X2-	T41.3X3-	T41.3X4-	T41.3X5-	T41.3X6-
nerve block (peripheral) (plexus)	T41.3X1-	T41.3X2-	T41.3X3-	T41.3X4-	T41.3X5-	T41.3X6-
spinal	T41.3X1-	T41.3X2-	T41.3X3-	T41.3X4-	T41.3X5-	T41.3X6-
Ethoheptazine	T40.4X1-	T40.4X2-	T40.4X3-	T40.4X4-	T40.4X5-	T40.4X6-
Ethopropazine	T44.3X1-	T44.3X2-	T44.3X3-	T44.3X4-	T44.3X5-	T44.3X6-
Ethosuximide	T42.2X1-	T42.2X2-	T42.2X3-	T42.2X4-	T42.2X5-	T42.2X6-
Ethotoin	T42.0X1-	T42.0X2-	T42.0X3-	T42.0X4-	T42.0X5-	T42.0X6-
Ethoxazene	T37.91X-	T37.92X-	T37.93X-	T37.94X-	T37.95X-	T37.96X-
Ethoxazorutoside	T46.991-	T46.992-	T46.993-	T46.994-	T46.995-	T46.996-
2-Ethoxyethanol	T52.3X1-	T52.3X2-	T52.3X3-	T52.3X4-	-	-
Ethoxzolamide	T50.2X1-	T50.2X2-	T50.2X3-	T50.2X4-	T50.2X5-	T50.2X6-
Ethyl						
acetate	T52.8X1-	T52.8X2-	T52.8X3-	T52.8X4-	-	-
alcohol	T51.0X1-	T51.0X2-	T51.0X3-	T51.0X4-	-	-
beverage	T51.0X1-	T51.0X2-	T51.0X3-	T51.0X4-	-	-
aldehyde (vapor)	T59.891-	T59.892-	T59.893-	T59.894-	-	-
liquid	T52.8X1-	T52.8X2-	T52.8X3-	T52.8X4-	-	-
aminobenzoate	T41.3X1-	T41.3X2-	T41.3X3-	T41.3X4-	T41.3X5-	T41.3X6-
aminophenothiazine	T43.3X1-	T43.3X2-	T43.3X3-	T43.3X4-	T43.3X5-	T43.3X6-
benzoate	T52.8X1-	T52.8X2-	T52.8X3-	T52.8X4-	-	-
biscoumacetate	T45.511-	T45.512-	T45.513-	T45.514-	T45.515-	T45.516-
bromide (anesthetic)	T41.0X1-	T41.0X2-	T41.0X3-	T41.0X4-	T41.0X5-	T41.0X6-
carbamate	T45.1X1-	T45.1X2-	T45.1X3-	T45.1X4-	T45.1X5-	T45.1X6-
carbinol	T51.3X1-	T51.3X2-	T51.3X3-	T51.3X4-	-	-
carbonate	T52.8X1-	T52.8X2-	T52.8X3-	T52.8X4-	-	-
chaulmoograte	T37.1X1-	T37.1X2-	T37.1X3-	T37.1X4-	T37.1X5-	T37.1X6-
chloride (anesthetic)	T41.0X1-	T41.0X2-	T41.0X3-	T41.0X4-	T41.0X5-	T41.0X6-
anesthetic (local)	T41.3X1-	T41.3X2-	T41.3X3-	T41.3X4-	T41.3X5-	T41.3X6-
inhaled	T41.0X1-	T41.0X2-	T41.0X3-	T41.0X4-	T41.0X5-	T41.0X6-
local	T49.4X1-	T49.4X2-	T49.4X3-	T49.4X4-	T49.4X5-	T49.4X6-
solvent	T53.6X1-	T53.6X2-	T53.6X3-	T53.6X4-	-	-
dibunate	T48.3X1-	T48.3X2-	T48.3X3-	T48.3X4-	T48.3X5-	T48.3X6-
dichloroarsine (vapor)	T57.0X1-	T57.0X2-	T57.0X3-	T57.0X4-	-	-
estranol	T38.7X1-	T38.7X2-	T38.7X3-	T38.7X4-	T38.7X5-	T38.7X6-
ether — *see also ether*	T52.8X1-	T52.8X2-	T52.8X3-	T52.8X4-	-	-
formate NEC (solvent)	T52.0X1-	T52.0X2-	T52.0X3-	T52.0X4-	-	-
fumarate	T49.4X1-	T49.4X2-	T49.4X3-	T49.4X4-	T49.4X5-	T49.4X6-
hydroxyisobutyrate NEC (solvent)	T52.8X1-	T52.8X2-	T52.8X3-	T52.8X4-	-	-
iodoacetate	T59.3X1-	T59.3X2-	T59.3X3-	T59.3X4-	-	-

Substance	Poisoning Accidental (unintentional)	Poisoning Intentional self-harm	Poisoning Assault	Poisoning Undetermined	Adverse effect	Underdosing
Ethyl *(continued)*						
lactate NEC (solvent)	T52.8X1-	T52.8X2-	T52.8X3-	T52.8X4-	-	-
loflazepate	T42.4X1-	T42.4X2-	T42.4X3-	T42.4X4-	T42.4X5-	T42.4X6-
mercuric chloride	T56.1X1-	T56.1X2-	T56.1X3-	T56.1X4-	-	-
methylcarbinol	T51.8X1-	T51.8X2-	T51.8X3-	T51.8X4-	-	-
morphine	T40.2X1-	T40.2X2-	T40.2X3-	T40.2X4-	T40.2X5-	T40.2X6-
noradrenaline	T48.6X1-	T48.6X2-	T48.6X3-	T48.6X4-	T48.6X5-	T48.6X6-
oxybutyrate NEC (solvent)	T52.8X1-	T52.8X2-	T52.8X3-	T52.8X4-	-	-
Ethylene (gas)	T59.891-	T59.892-	T59.893-	T59.894-	-	-
anesthetic (general)	T41.0X1-	T41.0X2-	T41.0X3-	T41.0X4-	T41.0X5-	T41.0X6-
chlorohydrin	T52.8X1-	T52.8X2-	T52.8X3-	T52.8X4-	-	-
vapor	T53.6X1-	T53.6X2-	T53.6X3-	T53.6X4-	-	-
dichloride	T52.8X1-	T52.8X2-	T52.8X3-	T52.8X4-	-	-
vapor	T53.6X1-	T53.6X2-	T53.6X3-	T53.6X4-	-	-
dinitrate	T52.3X1-	T52.3X2-	T52.3X3-	T52.3X4-	-	-
glycol (s)	T52.8X1-	T52.8X2-	T52.8X3-	T52.8X4-	-	-
dinitrate	T52.3X1-	T52.3X2-	T52.3X3-	T52.3X4-	-	-
monobutyl ether	T52.3X1-	T52.3X2-	T52.3X3-	T52.3X4-	-	-
imine	T54.1X1-	T54.1X2-	T54.1X3-	T54.1X4-	-	-
oxide (fumigant) (nonmedicinal)	T59.891-	T59.892-	T59.893-	T59.894-	-	-
medicinal	T49.0X1-	T49.0X2-	T49.0X3-	T49.0X4-	T49.0X5-	T49.0X6-
Ethylenediamine theophylline	T48.6X1-	T48.6X2-	T48.6X3-	T48.6X4-	T48.6X5-	T48.6X6-
Ethylenediaminetetra-acetic acid	T50.6X1-	T50.6X2-	T50.6X3-	T50.6X4-	T50.6X5-	T50.6X6-
Ethylenedinitrilotetra-acetate	T50.6X1-	T50.6X2-	T50.6X3-	T50.6X4-	T50.6X5-	T50.6X6-
Ethylestrenol	T38.7X1-	T38.7X2-	T38.7X3-	T38.7X4-	T38.7X5-	T38.7X6-
Ethylhydroxycellulose	T47.4X1-	T47.4X2-	T47.4X3-	T47.4X4-	T47.4X5-	T47.4X6-
Ethylidene						
chloride NEC	T53.6X1-	T53.6X2-	T53.6X3-	T53.6X4-	-	-
diacetate	T60.3X1-	T60.3X2-	T60.3X3-	T60.3X4-	-	-
dicoumarin	T45.511-	T45.512-	T45.513-	T45.514-	T45.515-	T45.516-
dicoumarol	T45.511-	T45.512-	T45.513-	T45.514-	T45.515-	T45.516-
diethyl ether	T52.0X1-	T52.0X2-	T52.0X3-	T52.0X4-	-	-
Ethylmorphine	T40.2X1-	T40.2X2-	T40.2X3-	T40.2X4-	T40.2X5-	T40.2X6-
Ethylnorepinephrine	T48.6X1-	T48.6X2-	T48.6X3-	T48.6X4-	T48.6X5-	T48.6X6-
Ethylparachlorophen-oxyisobutyrate	T46.6X1-	T46.6X2-	T46.6X3-	T46.6X4-	T46.6X5-	T46.6X6-
Ethynodiol	T38.4X1-	T38.4X2-	T38.4X3-	T38.4X4-	T38.4X5-	T38.4X6-
with mestranol diacetate	T38.4X1-	T38.4X2-	T38.4X3-	T38.4X4-	T38.4X5-	T38.4X6-
Etidocaine	T41.3X1-	T41.3X2-	T41.3X3-	T41.3X4-	T41.3X5-	T41.3X6-
infiltration (subcutaneous)	T41.3X1-	T41.3X2-	T41.3X3-	T41.3X4-	T41.3X5-	T41.3X6-
nerve (peripheral) (plexus)	T41.3X1-	T41.3X2-	T41.3X3-	T41.3X4-	T41.3X5-	T41.3X6-
Etidronate	T50.991-	T50.992-	T50.993-	T50.994-	T50.995-	T50.996-
Etidronic acid (disodium salt)	T50.991-	T50.992-	T50.993-	T50.994-	T50.995-	T50.996-
Etifoxine	T42.6X1-	T42.6X2-	T42.6X3-	T42.6X4-	T42.6X5-	T42.6X6-
Etilefrine	T44.4X1-	T44.4X2-	T44.4X3-	T44.4X4-	T44.4X5-	T44.4X6-
Etilfen	T42.3X1-	T42.3X2-	T42.3X3-	T42.3X4-	T42.3X5-	T42.3X6-
Etinodiol	T38.4X1-	T38.4X2-	T38.4X3-	T38.4X4-	T38.4X5-	T38.4X6-
Etiroxate	T46.6X1-	T46.6X2-	T46.6X3-	T46.6X4-	T46.6X5-	T46.6X6-
Etizolam	T42.4X1-	T42.4X2-	T42.4X3-	T42.4X4-	T42.4X5-	T42.4X6-
Etodolac	T39.391-	T39.392-	T39.393-	T39.394-	T39.395-	T39.396-
Etofamide	T37.3X1-	T37.3X2-	T37.3X3-	T37.3X4-	T37.3X5-	T37.3X6-
Etofibrate	T46.6X1-	T46.6X2-	T46.6X3-	T46.6X4-	T46.6X5-	T46.6X6-
Etofylline	T46.7X1-	T46.7X2-	T46.7X3-	T46.7X4-	T46.7X5-	T46.7X6-
clofibrate	T46.6X1-	T46.6X2-	T46.6X3-	T46.6X4-	T46.6X5-	T46.6X6-
Etoglucid	T45.1X1-	T45.1X2-	T45.1X3-	T45.1X4-	T45.1X5-	T45.1X6-
Etomidate	T41.1X1-	T41.1X2-	T41.1X3-	T41.1X4-	T41.1X5-	T41.1X6-
Etomide	T39.8X1-	T39.8X2-	T39.8X3-	T39.8X4-	T39.8X5-	T39.8X6-
Etomidoline	T44.3X1-	T44.3X2-	T44.3X3-	T44.3X4-	T44.3X5-	T44.3X6-
Etoposide	T45.1X1-	T45.1X2-	T45.1X3-	T45.1X4-	T45.1X5-	T45.1X6-

Substance	Poisoning Accidental (unintentional)	Poisoning Intentional self-harm	Poisoning Assault	Poisoning Undetermined	Adverse effect	Underdosing
Etorphine	T40.2X1-	T40.2X2-	T40.2X3-	T40.2X4-	T40.2X5-	T40.2X6-
Etoval	T42.3X1-	T42.3X2-	T42.3X3-	T42.3X4-	T42.3X5-	T42.3X6-
Etozolin	T50.1X1-	T50.1X2-	T50.1X3-	T50.1X4-	T50.1X5-	T50.1X6-
Etretinate	T50.991-	T50.992-	T50.993-	T50.994-	T50.995-	T50.996-
Etryptamine	T43.691-	T43.692-	T43.693-	T43.694-	T43.695-	T43.696-
Etybenzatropine	T44.3X1-	T44.3X2-	T44.3X3-	T44.3X4-	T44.3X5-	T44.3X6-
Etynodiol	T38.4X1-	T38.4X2-	T38.4X3-	T38.4X4-	T38.4X5-	T38.4X6-
Eucaine	T41.3X1-	T41.3X2-	T41.3X3-	T41.3X4-	T41.3X5-	T41.3X6-
Eucalyptus oil	T49.7X1-	T49.7X2-	T49.7X3-	T49.7X4-	T49.7X5-	T49.7X6-
Eucatropine	T49.5X1-	T49.5X2-	T49.5X3-	T49.5X4-	T49.5X5-	T49.5X6-
Eucodal	T40.2X1-	T40.2X2-	T40.2X3-	T40.2X4-	T40.2X5-	T40.2X6-
Euneryl	T42.3X1-	T42.3X2-	T42.3X3-	T42.3X4-	T42.3X5-	T42.3X6-
Euphthalmine	T44.3X1-	T44.3X2-	T44.3X3-	T44.3X4-	T44.3X5-	T44.3X6-
Eurax	T49.0X1-	T49.0X2-	T49.0X3-	T49.0X4-	T49.0X5-	T49.0X6-
Euresol	T49.4X1-	T49.4X2-	T49.4X3-	T49.4X4-	T49.4X5-	T49.4X6-
Euthroid	T38.1X1-	T38.1X2-	T38.1X3-	T38.1X4-	T38.1X5-	T38.1X6-
Evans blue	T50.8X1-	T50.8X2-	T50.8X3-	T50.8X4-	T50.8X5-	T50.8X6-
Evipal	T42.3X1-	T42.3X2-	T42.3X3-	T42.3X4-	T42.3X5-	T42.3X6-
sodium	T41.1X1-	T41.1X2-	T41.1X3-	T41.1X4-	T41.1X5-	T41.1X6-
Evipan	T42.3X1-	T42.3X2-	T42.3X3-	T42.3X4-	T42.3X5-	T42.3X6-
sodium	T41.1X1-	T41.1X2-	T41.1X3-	T41.1X4-	T41.1X5-	T41.1X6-
Exalamide	T49.0X1-	T49.0X2-	T49.0X3-	T49.0X4-	T49.0X5-	T49.0X6-
Exalgin	T39.1X1-	T39.1X2-	T39.1X3-	T39.1X4-	T39.1X5-	T39.1X6-
Excipients, pharmaceutical	T50.901-	T50.902-	T50.903-	T50.904-	T50.905-	T50.906-
Exhaust gas (engine) (motor vehicle)	T58.01X-	T58.02X-	T58.03X-	T58.04X-	-	-
Ex-Lax (phenolphthalein)	T47.2X1-	T47.2X2-	T47.2X3-	T47.2X4-	T47.2X5-	T47.2X6-
Expectorant NEC	T48.4X1-	T48.4X2-	T48.4X3-	T48.4X4-	T48.4X5-	T48.4X6-
Extended insulin zinc suspension	T38.3X1-	T38.3X2-	T38.3X3-	T38.3X4-	T38.3X5-	T38.3X6-
External medications (skin) (mucous membrane)	T49.91X-	T49.92X-	T49.93X-	T49.94X-	T49.95X-	T49.96X-
dental agent	T49.7X1-	T49.7X2-	T49.7X3-	T49.7X4-	T49.7X5-	T49.7X6-
ENT agent	T49.6X1-	T49.6X2-	T49.6X3-	T49.6X4-	T49.6X5-	T49.6X6-
ophthalmic preparation	T49.5X1-	T49.5X2-	T49.5X3-	T49.5X4-	T49.5X5-	T49.5X6-
specified NEC	T49.8X1-	T49.8X2-	T49.8X3-	T49.8X4-	T49.8X5-	T49.8X6-
Extrapyramidal antagonist NEC	T44.3X1-	T44.3X2-	T44.3X3-	T44.3X4-	T44.3X5-	T44.3X6-
Eye agents (anti-infective)	T49.5X1-	T49.5X2-	T49.5X3-	T49.5X4-	T49.5X5-	T49.5X6-
Eye drug NEC	T49.5X1-	T49.5X2-	T49.5X3-	T49.5X4-	T49.5X5-	T49.5X6-
FAC (fluorouracil + doxorubicin + cyclophosphamide)	T45.1X1-	T45.1X2-	T45.1X3-	T45.1X4-	T45.1X5-	T45.1X6-
Factor						
I (fibrinogen)	T45.8X1-	T45.8X2-	T45.8X3-	T45.8X4-	T45.8X5-	T45.8X6-
III (thromboplastin)	T45.8X1-	T45.8X2-	T45.8X3-	T45.8X4-	T45.8X5-	T45.8X6-
VIII (antihemophilic Factor) (concentrate)	T45.8X1-	T45.8X2-	T45.8X3-	T45.8X4-	T45.8X5-	T45.8X6-
IX complex	T45.7X1-	T45.7X2-	T45.7X3-	T45.7X4-	T45.7X5-	T45.7X6-
human	T45.8X1-	T45.8X2-	T45.8X3-	T45.8X4-	T45.8X5-	T45.8X6-
Famotidine	T47.0X1-	T47.0X2-	T47.0X3-	T47.0X4-	T47.0X5-	T47.0X6-
Fat suspension, intravenous	T50.991-	T50.992-	T50.993-	T50.994-	T50.995-	T50.996-
Fazadinium bromide	T48.1X1-	T48.1X2-	T48.1X3-	T48.1X4-	T48.1X5-	T48.1X6-
Febarbamate	T42.3X1-	T42.3X2-	T42.3X3-	T42.3X4-	T42.3X5-	T42.3X6-
Fecal softener	T47.4X1-	T47.4X2-	T47.4X3-	T47.4X4-	T47.4X5-	T47.4X6-
Fedrilate	T48.3X1-	T48.3X2-	T48.3X3-	T48.3X4-	T48.3X5-	T48.3X6-
Felodipine	T46.1X1-	T46.1X2-	T46.1X3-	T46.1X4-	T46.1X5-	T46.1X6-
Felypressin	T38.891-	T38.892-	T38.893-	T38.894-	T38.895-	T38.896-
Femoxetine	T43.221-	T43.222-	T43.223-	T43.224-	T43.225-	T43.226-
Fenalcomine	T46.3X1-	T46.3X2-	T46.3X3-	T46.3X4-	T46.3X5-	T46.3X6-
Fenamisal	T37.1X1-	T37.1X2-	T37.1X3-	T37.1X4-	T37.1X5-	T37.1X6-
Fenazone	T39.2X1-	T39.2X2-	T39.2X3-	T39.2X4-	T39.2X5-	T39.2X6-
Fenbendazole	T37.4X1-	T37.4X2-	T37.4X3-	T37.4X4-	T37.4X5-	T37.4X6-

Substance	Poisoning Accidental (unintentional)	Poisoning Intentional self-harm	Poisoning Assault	Poisoning Undetermined	Adverse effect	Underdosing
Fenbutrazate	T50.5X1-	T50.5X2-	T50.5X3-	T50.5X4-	T50.5X5-	T50.5X6-
Fencamfamine	T43.691-	T43.692-	T43.693-	T43.694-	T43.695-	T43.696-
Fendiline	T46.1X1-	T46.1X2-	T46.1X3-	T46.1X4-	T46.1X5-	T46.1X6-
Fenetylline	T43.691-	T43.692-	T43.693-	T43.694-	T43.695-	T43.696-
Fenflumizole	T39.391-	T39.392-	T39.393-	T39.394-	T39.395-	T39.396-
Fenfluramine	T50.5X1-	T50.5X2-	T50.5X3-	T50.5X4-	T50.5X5-	T50.5X6-
Fenobarbital	T42.3X1-	T42.3X2-	T42.3X3-	T42.3X4-	T42.3X5-	T42.3X6-
Fenofibrate	T46.6X1-	T46.6X2-	T46.6X3-	T46.6X4-	T46.6X5-	T46.6X6-
Fenoprofen	T39.311-	T39.312-	T39.313-	T39.314-	T39.315-	T39.316-
Fenoterol	T48.6X1-	T48.6X2-	T48.6X3-	T48.6X4-	T48.6X5-	T48.6X6-
Fenoverine	T44.3X1-	T44.3X2-	T44.3X3-	T44.3X4-	T44.3X5-	T44.3X6-
Fenoxazoline	T48.5X1-	T48.5X2-	T48.5X3-	T48.5X4-	T48.5X5-	T48.5X6-
Fenproporex	T50.5X1-	T50.5X2-	T50.5X3-	T50.5X4-	T50.5X5-	T50.5X6-
Fenquizone	T50.2X1-	T50.2X2-	T50.2X3-	T50.2X4-	T50.2X5-	T50.2X6-
Fentanyl	T40.4X1-	T40.4X2-	T40.4X3-	T40.4X4-	T40.4X5-	T40.4X6-
Fentazin	T43.3X1-	T43.3X2-	T43.3X3-	T43.3X4-	T43.3X5-	T43.3X6-
Fenthion	T60.0X1-	T60.0X2-	T60.0X3-	T60.0X4-	-	-
Fenticlor	T49.0X1-	T49.0X2-	T49.0X3-	T49.0X4-	T49.0X5-	T49.0X6-
Fenylbutazone	T39.2X1-	T39.2X2-	T39.2X3-	T39.2X4-	T39.2X5-	T39.2X6-
Feprazone	T39.2X1-	T39.2X2-	T39.2X3-	T39.2X4-	T39.2X5-	T39.2X6-
Fer de lance (bite) (venom)	T63.061-	T63.062-	T63.063-	T63.064-		
Ferric — see also Iron						
chloride	T45.4X1-	T45.4X2-	T45.4X3-	T45.4X4-	T45.4X5-	T45.4X6-
citrate	T45.4X1-	T45.4X2-	T45.4X3-	T45.4X4-	T45.4X5-	T45.4X6-
hydroxide						
colloidal	T45.4X1-	T45.4X2-	T45.4X3-	T45.4X4-	T45.4X5-	T45.4X6-
polymaltose	T45.4X1-	T45.4X2-	T45.4X3-	T45.4X4-	T45.4X5-	T45.4X6-
pyrophosphate	T45.4X1-	T45.4X2-	T45.4X3-	T45.4X4-	T45.4X5-	T45.4X6-
Ferritin	T45.4X1-	T45.4X2-	T45.4X3-	T45.4X4-	T45.4X5-	T45.4X6-
Ferrocholinate	T45.4X1-	T45.4X2-	T45.4X3-	T45.4X4-	T45.4X5-	T45.4X6-
Ferrodextrane	T45.4X1-	T45.4X2-	T45.4X3-	T45.4X4-	T45.4X5-	T45.4X6-
Ferropolimaler	T45.4X1-	T45.4X2-	T45.4X3-	T45.4X4-	T45.4X5-	T45.4X6-
Ferrous — see also Iron						
phosphate	T45.4X1-	T45.4X2-	T45.4X3-	T45.4X4-	T45.4X5-	T45.4X6-
salt	T45.4X1-	T45.4X2-	T45.4X3-	T45.4X4-	T45.4X5-	T45.4X6-
with folic acid	T45.4X1-	T45.4X2-	T45.4X3-	T45.4X4-	T45.4X5-	T45.4X6-
Ferrous fumerate, gluconate, lactate, salt NEC, sulfate (medicinal)	T45.4X1-	T45.4X2-	T45.4X3-	T45.4X4-	T45.4X5-	T45.4X6-
Ferrovanadium (fumes)	T59.891-	T59.892-	T59.893-	T59.894-	-	-
Ferrum — see Iron						
Fertilizers NEC	T65.891-	T65.892-	T65.893-	T65.894-	-	-
with herbicide mixture	T60.3X1-	T60.3X2-	T60.3X3-	T60.3X4-	-	-
Fetoxilate	T47.6X1-	T47.6X2-	T47.6X3-	T47.6X4-	T47.6X5-	T47.6X6-
Fiber, dietary	T47.4X1-	T47.4X2-	T47.4X3-	T47.4X4-	T47.4X5-	T47.4X6-
Fiberglass	T65.831-	T65.832-	T65.833-	T65.834-	-	-
Fibrinogen (human)	T45.8X1-	T45.8X2-	T45.8X3-	T45.8X4-	T45.8X5-	T45.8X6-
Fibrinolysin (human)	T45.691-	T45.692-	T45.693-	T45.694-	T45.695-	T45.696-
Fibrinolysis						
affecting drug	T45.601-	T45.602-	T45.603-	T45.604-	T45.605-	T45.606-
inhibitor NEC	T45.621-	T45.622-	T45.623-	T45.624-	T45.625-	T45.626-
Fibrinolytic drug	T45.611-	T45.612-	T45.613-	T45.614-	T45.615-	T45.616-
Filix mas	T37.4X1-	T37.4X2-	T37.4X3-	T37.4X4-	T37.4X5-	T37.4X6-
Filtering cream	T49.3X1-	T49.3X2-	T49.3X3-	T49.3X4-	T49.3X5-	T49.3X6-
Fiorinal	T39.011-	T39.012-	T39.013-	T39.014-	T39.015-	T39.016-
Firedamp	T59.891-	T59.892-	T59.893-	T59.894-	-	-
Fish, noxious, nonbacterial	T61.91X-	T61.92X-	T61.93X-	T61.94X-	-	-
ciguatera	T61.01X-	T61.02X-	T61.03X-	T61.04X-	-	-
scombroid	T61.11X-	T61.12X-	T61.13X-	T61.14X-	-	-
shell	T61.781-	T61.782-	T61.783-	T61.784-	-	-

Substance	Poisoning Accidental (unintentional)	Poisoning Intentional self-harm	Poisoning Assault	Poisoning Undetermined	Adverse effect	Underdosing
Fish, noxious, nonbacterial (continued)						
specified NEC	T61.771-	T61.772-	T61.773-	T61.774-	-	-
Flagyl	T37.3X1-	T37.3X2-	T37.3X3-	T37.3X4-	T37.3X5-	T37.3X6-
Flavine adenine dinucleotide	T45.2X1-	T45.2X2-	T45.2X3-	T45.2X4-	T45.2X5-	T45.2X6-
Flavodic acid	T46.991-	T46.992-	T46.993-	T46.994-	T46.995-	T46.996-
Flavoxate	T44.3X1-	T44.3X2-	T44.3X3-	T44.3X4-	T44.3X5-	T44.3X6-
Flaxedil	T48.1X1-	T48.1X2-	T48.1X3-	T48.1X4-	T48.1X5-	T48.1X6-
Flaxseed (medicinal)	T49.3X1-	T49.3X2-	T49.3X3-	T49.3X4-	T49.3X5-	T49.3X6-
Flecainide	T46.2X1-	T46.2X2-	T46.2X3-	T46.2X4-	T46.2X5-	T46.2X6-
Fleroxacin	T36.8X1-	T36.8X2-	T36.8X3-	T36.8X4-	T36.8X5-	T36.8X6-
Floctafenine	T39.8X1-	T39.8X2-	T39.8X3-	T39.8X4-	T39.8X5-	T39.8X6-
Flomax	T44.6X1-	T44.6X2-	T44.6X3-	T44.6X4-	T44.6X5-	T44.6X6-
Flomoxef	T36.1X1-	T36.1X2-	T36.1X3-	T36.1X4-	T36.1X5-	T36.1X6-
Flopropione	T44.3X1-	T44.3X2-	T44.3X3-	T44.3X4-	T44.3X5-	T44.3X6-
Florantyrone	T47.5X1-	T47.5X2-	T47.5X3-	T47.5X4-	T47.5X5-	T47.5X6-
Floraquin	T37.8X1-	T37.8X2-	T37.8X3-	T37.8X4-	T37.8X5-	T37.8X6-
Florinef	T38.0X1-	T38.0X2-	T38.0X3-	T38.0X4-	T38.0X5-	T38.0X6-
ENT agent	T49.6X1-	T49.6X2-	T49.6X3-	T49.6X4-	T49.6X5-	T49.6X6-
ophthalmic preparation	T49.5X1-	T49.5X2-	T49.5X3-	T49.5X4-	T49.5X5-	T49.5X6-
topical NEC	T49.0X1-	T49.0X2-	T49.0X3-	T49.0X4-	T49.0X5-	T49.0X6-
Flowers of sulfur	T49.4X1-	T49.4X2-	T49.4X3-	T49.4X4-	T49.4X5-	T49.4X6-
Floxuridine	T45.1X1-	T45.1X2-	T45.1X3-	T45.1X4-	T45.1X5-	T45.1X6-
Fluanisone	T43.4X1-	T43.4X2-	T43.4X3-	T43.4X4-	T43.4X5-	T43.4X6-
Flubendazole	T37.4X1-	T37.4X2-	T37.4X3-	T37.4X4-	T37.4X5-	T37.4X6-
Fluclorolone acetonide	T49.0X1-	T49.0X2-	T49.0X3-	T49.0X4-	T49.0X5-	T49.0X6-
Flucloxacillin	T36.0X1-	T36.0X2-	T36.0X3-	T36.0X4-	T36.0X5-	T36.0X6-
Fluconazole	T37.8X1-	T37.8X2-	T37.8X3-	T37.8X4-	T37.8X5-	T37.8X6-
Flucytosine	T37.8X1-	T37.8X2-	T37.8X3-	T37.8X4-	T37.8X5-	T37.8X6-
Fludeoxyglucose (18F)	T50.8X1-	T50.8X2-	T50.8X3-	T50.8X4-	T50.8X5-	T50.8X6-
Fludiazepam	T42.4X1-	T42.4X2-	T42.4X3-	T42.4X4-	T42.4X5-	T42.4X6-
Fludrocortisone	T50.0X1-	T50.0X2-	T50.0X3-	T50.0X4-	T50.0X5-	T50.0X6-
ENT agent	T49.6X1-	T49.6X2-	T49.6X3-	T49.6X4-	T49.6X5-	T49.6X6-
ophthalmic preparation	T49.5X1-	T49.5X2-	T49.5X3-	T49.5X4-	T49.5X5-	T49.5X6-
topical NEC	T49.0X1-	T49.0X2-	T49.0X3-	T49.0X4-	T49.0X5-	T49.0X6-
Fludroxycortide	T49.0X1-	T49.0X2-	T49.0X3-	T49.0X4-	T49.0X5-	T49.0X6-
Flufenamic acid	T39.391-	T39.392-	T39.393-	T39.394-	T39.395-	T39.396-
Fluindione	T45.511-	T45.512-	T45.513-	T45.514-	T45.515-	T45.516-
Flumequine	T37.8X1-	T37.8X2-	T37.8X3-	T37.8X4-	T37.8X5-	T37.8X6-
Flumethasone	T49.0X1-	T49.0X2-	T49.0X3-	T49.0X4-	T49.0X5-	T49.0X6-
Flumethiazide	T50.2X1-	T50.2X2-	T50.2X3-	T50.2X4-	T50.2X5-	T50.2X6-
Flumidin	T37.5X1-	T37.5X2-	T37.5X3-	T37.5X4-	T37.5X5-	T37.5X6-
Flunarizine	T46.7X1-	T46.7X2-	T46.7X3-	T46.7X4-	T46.7X5-	T46.7X6-
Flunidazole	T37.8X1-	T37.8X2-	T37.8X3-	T37.8X4-	T37.8X5-	T37.8X6-
Flunisolide	T48.6X1-	T48.6X2-	T48.6X3-	T48.6X4-	T48.6X5-	T48.6X6-
Flunitrazepam	T42.4X1-	T42.4X2-	T42.4X3-	T42.4X4-	T42.4X5-	T42.4X6-
Fluocinolone (acetonide)	T49.0X1-	T49.0X2-	T49.0X3-	T49.0X4-	T49.0X5-	T49.0X6-
Fluocinonide	T49.0X1-	T49.0X2-	T49.0X3-	T49.0X4-	T49.0X5-	T49.0X6-
Fluocortin (butyl)	T49.0X1-	T49.0X2-	T49.0X3-	T49.0X4-	T49.0X5-	T49.0X6-
Fluocortolone	T49.0X1-	T49.0X2-	T49.0X3-	T49.0X4-	T49.0X5-	T49.0X6-
Fluohydrocortisone	T38.0X1-	T38.0X2-	T38.0X3-	T38.0X4-	T38.0X5-	T38.0X6-
ENT agent	T49.6X1-	T49.6X2-	T49.6X3-	T49.6X4-	T49.6X5-	T49.6X6-
ophthalmic preparation	T49.5X1-	T49.5X2-	T49.5X3-	T49.5X4-	T49.5X5-	T49.5X6-
topical NEC	T49.0X1-	T49.0X2-	T49.0X3-	T49.0X4-	T49.0X5-	T49.0X6-
Fluonid	T49.0X1-	T49.0X2-	T49.0X3-	T49.0X4-	T49.0X5-	T49.0X6-
Fluopromazine	T43.3X1-	T43.3X2-	T43.3X3-	T43.3X4-	T43.3X5-	T43.3X6-
Fluoracetate	T60.8X1-	T60.8X2-	T60.8X3-	T60.8X4-	-	-
Fluorescein	T50.8X1-	T50.8X2-	T50.8X3-	T50.8X4-	T50.8X5-	T50.8X6-
Fluorhydrocortisone	T50.0X1-	T50.0X2-	T50.0X3-	T50.0X4-	T50.0X5-	T50.0X6-

Substance	Poisoning Accidental (unintentional)	Poisoning Intentional self-harm	Poisoning Assault	Poisoning Undetermined	Adverse effect	Underdosing
Fluoride (nonmedicinal) (pesticide) (sodium) NEC	T60.8X1-	T60.8X2-	T60.8X3-	T60.8X4-	-	-
hydrogen — *see Hydrofluoric acid*						
medicinal NEC	T50.991-	T50.992-	T50.993-	T50.994-	T50.995-	T50.996-
dental use	T49.7X1-	T49.7X2-	T49.7X3-	T49.7X4-	T49.7X5-	T49.7X6-
not pesticide NEC	T54.91X-	T54.92X-	T54.93X-	T54.94X-	-	-
stannous	T49.7X1-	T49.7X2-	T49.7X3-	T49.7X4-	T49.7X5-	T49.7X6-
Fluorinated corticosteroids	T38.0X1-	T38.0X2-	T38.0X3-	T38.0X4-	T38.0X5-	T38.0X6-
Fluorine (gas)	T59.5X1-	T59.5X2-	T59.5X3-	T59.5X4-	-	-
salt — *see Fluoride(s)*						
Fluoristan	T49.7X1-	T49.7X2-	T49.7X3-	T49.7X4-	T49.7X5-	T49.7X6-
Fluormetholone	T49.0X1-	T49.0X2-	T49.0X3-	T49.0X4-	T49.0X5-	T49.0X6-
Fluoroacetate	T60.8X1-	T60.8X2-	T60.8X3-	T60.8X4-	-	-
Fluorocarbon monomer	T53.6X1-	T53.6X2-	T53.6X3-	T53.6X4-	-	-
Fluorocytosine	T37.8X1-	T37.8X2-	T37.8X3-	T37.8X4-	T37.8X5-	T37.8X6-
Fluorodeoxyuridine	T45.1X1-	T45.1X2-	T45.1X3-	T45.1X4-	T45.1X5-	T45.1X6-
Fluorometholone	T49.0X1-	T49.0X2-	T49.0X3-	T49.0X4-	T49.0X5-	T49.0X6-
ophthalmic preparation	T49.5X1-	T49.5X2-	T49.5X3-	T49.5X4-	T49.5X5-	T49.5X6-
Fluorophosphate insecticide	T60.0X1-	T60.0X2-	T60.0X3-	T60.0X4-	-	-
Fluorosol	T46.3X1-	T46.3X2-	T46.3X3-	T46.3X4-	T46.3X5-	T46.3X6-
Fluorouracil	T45.1X1-	T45.1X2-	T45.1X3-	T45.1X4-	T45.1X5-	T45.1X6-
Fluorphenylalanine	T49.5X1-	T49.5X2-	T49.5X3-	T49.5X4-	T49.5X5-	T49.5X6-
Fluothane	T41.0X1-	T41.0X2-	T41.0X3-	T41.0X4-	T41.0X5-	T41.0X6-
Fluoxetine	T43.221-	T43.222-	T43.223-	T43.224-	T43.225-	T43.226-
Fluoxymesterone	T38.7X1-	T38.7X2-	T38.7X3-	T38.7X4-	T38.7X5-	T38.7X6-
Flupenthixol	T43.4X1-	T43.4X2-	T43.4X3-	T43.4X4-	T43.4X5-	T43.4X6-
Flupentixol	T43.4X1-	T43.4X2-	T43.4X3-	T43.4X4-	T43.4X5-	T43.4X6-
Fluphenazine	T43.3X1-	T43.3X2-	T43.3X3-	T43.3X4-	T43.3X5-	T43.3X6-
Fluprednidene	T49.0X1-	T49.0X2-	T49.0X3-	T49.0X4-	T49.0X5-	T49.0X6-
Fluprednisolone	T38.0X1-	T38.0X2-	T38.0X3-	T38.0X4-	T38.0X5-	T38.0X6-
Fluradoline	T39.8X1-	T39.8X2-	T39.8X3-	T39.8X4-	T39.8X5-	T39.8X6-
Flurandrenolide	T49.0X1-	T49.0X2-	T49.0X3-	T49.0X4-	T49.0X5-	T49.0X6-
Flurandrenolone	T49.0X1-	T49.0X2-	T49.0X3-	T49.0X4-	T49.0X5-	T49.0X6-
Flurazepam	T42.4X1-	T42.4X2-	T42.4X3-	T42.4X4-	T42.4X5-	T42.4X6-
Flurbiprofen	T39.311-	T39.312-	T39.313-	T39.314-	T39.315-	T39.316-
Flurobate	T49.0X1-	T49.0X2-	T49.0X3-	T49.0X4-	T49.0X5-	T49.0X6-
Fluroxene	T41.0X1-	T41.0X2-	T41.0X3-	T41.0X4-	T41.0X5-	T41.0X6-
Fluspirilene	T43.591-	T43.592-	T43.593-	T43.594-	T43.595-	T43.596-
Flutamide	T38.6X1-	T38.6X2-	T38.6X3-	T38.6X4-	T38.6X5-	T38.6X6-
Flutazolam	T42.4X1-	T42.4X2-	T42.4X3-	T42.4X4-	T42.4X5-	T42.4X6-
Fluticasone propionate	T38.0X1-	T38.0X2-	T38.0X3-	T38.0X4-	T38.0X5-	T38.0X6-
Flutoprazepam	T42.4X1-	T42.4X2-	T42.4X3-	T42.4X4-	T42.4X5-	T42.4X6-
Flutropium bromide	T48.6X1-	T48.6X2-	T48.6X3-	T48.6X4-	T48.6X5-	T48.6X6-
Fluvoxamine	T43.221-	T43.222-	T43.223-	T43.224-	T43.225-	T43.226-
Folacin	T45.8X1-	T45.8X2-	T45.8X3-	T45.8X4-	T45.8X5-	T45.8X6-
Folic acid	T45.8X1-	T45.8X2-	T45.8X3-	T45.8X4-	T45.8X5-	T45.8X6-
with ferrous salt	T45.2X1-	T45.2X2-	T45.2X3-	T45.2X4-	T45.2X5-	T45.2X6-
antagonist	T45.1X1-	T45.1X2-	T45.1X3-	T45.1X4-	T45.1X5-	T45.1X6-
Folinic acid	T45.8X1-	T45.8X2-	T45.8X3-	T45.8X4-	T45.8X5-	T45.8X6-
Folium stramoniae	T48.6X1-	T48.6X2-	T48.6X3-	T48.6X4-	T48.6X5-	T48.6X6-
Follicle-stimulating hormone, human	T38.811-	T38.812-	T38.813-	T38.814-	T38.815-	T38.816-
Folpet	T60.3X1-	T60.3X2-	T60.3X3-	T60.3X4-	-	-
Fominoben	T48.3X1-	T48.3X2-	T48.3X3-	T48.3X4-	T48.3X5-	T48.3X6-
Food, foodstuffs, noxious, nonbacterial, NEC	T62.91X-	T62.92X-	T62.93X-	T62.94X-	-	-
berries	T62.1X1-	T62.1X2-	T62.1X3-	T62.1X4-	-	-
fish — *see also Fish*	T61.91X-	T61.92X-	T61.93X-	T61.94X-	-	-
mushrooms	T62.0X1-	T62.0X2-	T62.0X3-	T62.0X4-	-	-
plants	T62.2X1-	T62.2X2-	T62.2X3-	T62.2X4-	-	-

Substance	Poisoning Accidental (unintentional)	Poisoning Intentional self-harm	Poisoning Assault	Poisoning Undetermined	Adverse effect	Underdosing
Food, foodstuffs, noxious, nonbacterial, NEC (continued)						
seafood	T61.91X-	T61.92X-	T61.93X-	T61.94X-	-	-
specified NEC	T61.8X1-	T61.8X2-	T61.8X3-	T61.8X4-	-	-
seeds	T62.2X1-	T62.2X2-	T62.2X3-	T62.2X4-	-	-
shellfish	T61.781-	T61.782-	T61.783-	T61.784-	-	-
specified NEC	T62.8X1-	T62.8X2-	T62.8X3-	T62.8X4-	-	-
Fool's parsley	T62.2X1-	T62.2X2-	T62.2X3-	T62.2X4-	-	-
Formaldehyde (solution) , gas or vapor	T59.2X1-	T59.2X2-	T59.2X3-	T59.2X4-	-	-
fungicide	T60.3X1-	T60.3X2-	T60.3X3-	T60.3X4-	-	-
Formalin	T59.2X1-	T59.2X2-	T59.2X3-	T59.2X4-	-	-
fungicide	T60.3X1-	T60.3X2-	T60.3X3-	T60.3X4-	-	-
vapor	T59.2X1-	T59.2X2-	T59.2X3-	T59.2X4-	-	-
Formic acid	T54.2X1-	T54.2X2-	T54.2X3-	T54.2X4-	-	-
vapor	T59.891-	T59.892-	T59.893-	T59.894-	-	-
Foscarnet sodium	T37.5X1-	T37.5X2-	T37.5X3-	T37.5X4-	T37.5X5-	T37.5X6-
Fosfestrol	T38.5X1-	T38.5X2-	T38.5X3-	T38.5X4-	T38.5X5-	T38.5X6-
Fosfomycin	T36.8X1-	T36.8X2-	T36.8X3-	T36.8X4-	T36.8X5-	T36.8X6-
Fosfonet sodium	T37.5X1-	T37.5X2-	T37.5X3-	T37.5X4-	T37.5X5-	T37.5X6-
Fosinopril	T46.4X1-	T46.4X2-	T46.4X3-	T46.4X4-	T46.4X5-	T46.4X6-
sodium	T46.4X1-	T46.4X2-	T46.4X3-	T46.4X4-	T46.4X5-	T46.4X6-
Fowler's solution	T57.0X1-	T57.0X2-	T57.0X3-	T57.0X4-	-	-
Foxglove	T62.2X1-	T62.2X2-	T62.2X3-	T62.2X4-	-	-
Framycetin	T36.5X1-	T36.5X2-	T36.5X3-	T36.5X4-	T36.5X5-	T36.5X6-
Frangula	T47.2X1-	T47.2X2-	T47.2X3-	T47.2X4-	T47.2X5-	T47.2X6-
extract	T47.2X1-	T47.2X2-	T47.2X3-	T47.2X4-	T47.2X5-	T47.2X6-
Frei antigen	T50.8X1-	T50.8X2-	T50.8X3-	T50.8X4-	T50.8X5-	T50.8X6-
Freon	T53.5X1-	T53.5X2-	T53.5X3-	T53.5X4-	-	-
Fructose	T50.3X1-	T50.3X2-	T50.3X3-	T50.3X4-	T50.3X5-	T50.3X6-
Frusemide	T50.1X1-	T50.1X2-	T50.1X3-	T50.1X4-	T50.1X5-	T50.1X6-
FSH	T38.811-	T38.812-	T38.813-	T38.814-	T38.815-	T38.816-
Ftorafur	T45.1X1-	T45.1X2-	T45.1X3-	T45.1X4-	T45.1X5-	T45.1X6-
Fuel						
automobile	T52.0X1-	T52.0X2-	T52.0X3-	T52.0X4-	-	-
exhaust gas, not in transit	T58.01X-	T58.02X-	T58.03X-	T58.04X-	-	-
vapor NEC	T52.0X1-	T52.0X2-	T52.0X3-	T52.0X4-	-	-
gas (domestic use) — *see also Carbon, monoxide, fuel, utility*	T59.891-	T59.892-	T59.893-	T59.894-	-	-
utility	T59.891-	T59.892-	T59.893-	T59.894-	-	-
in mobile container	T59.891-	T59.892-	T59.893-	T59.894-	-	-
incomplete combustion of — *see Carbon, monoxide, fuel, utility*						
piped (natural)	T59.891-	T59.892-	T59.893-	T59.894-	-	-
industrial, incomplete combustion	T58.8X1-	T58.8X2-	T58.8X3-	T58.8X4-	-	-
Fugillin	T36.8X1-	T36.8X2-	T36.8X3-	T36.8X4-	T36.8X5-	T36.8X6-
Fulminate of mercury	T56.1X1-	T56.1X2-	T56.1X3-	T56.1X4-	-	-
Fulvicin	T36.7X1-	T36.7X2-	T36.7X3-	T36.7X4-	T36.7X5-	T36.7X6-
Fumadil	T36.8X1-	T36.8X2-	T36.8X3-	T36.8X4-	T36.8X5-	T36.8X6-
Fumagillin	T36.8X1-	T36.8X2-	T36.8X3-	T36.8X4-	T36.8X5-	T36.8X6-
Fumaric acid	T49.4X1-	T49.4X2-	T49.4X3-	T49.4X4-	T49.4X5-	T49.4X6-
Fumes (from)	T59.91X-	T59.92X-	T59.93X-	T59.94X-	-	-
carbon monoxide — *see Carbon, monoxide*						
charcoal (domestic use) — *see Charcoal, fumes*						
chloroform — *see Chloroform*						
coke (in domestic stoves, fireplaces) — *see Coke fumes*						
corrosive NEC	T54.91X-	T54.92X-	T54.93X-	T54.94X-	-	-

Substance	Poisoning Accidental (unintentional)	Poisoning Intentional self-harm	Poisoning Assault	Poisoning Undetermined	Adverse effect	Underdosing
Fumes (from) *(continued)*						
ether — *see* ether						
freons	T53.5X1-	T53.5X2-	T53.5X3-	T53.5X4-	-	-
hydrocarbons	T59.891-	T59.892-	T59.893-	T59.894-	-	-
petroleum (liquefied)	T59.891-	T59.892-	T59.893-	T59.894-	-	-
distributed through pipes (pure or mixed with air)	T59.891-	T59.892-	T59.893-	T59.894-	-	-
lead — *see* lead						
metal — *see* Metals, or the specified metal						
nitrogen dioxide	T59.0X1-	T59.0X2-	T59.0X3-	T59.0X4-	-	-
pesticides — *see* Pesticides						
petroleum (liquefied)	T59.891-	T59.892-	T59.893-	T59.894-	-	-
distributed through pipes (pure or mixed with air)	T59.891-	T59.892-	T59.893-	T59.894-	-	-
polyester	T59.891-	T59.892-	T59.893-	T59.894-	-	-
specified source NEC — *see also* substance specified	T59.891-	T59.892-	T59.893-	T59.894-	-	-
sulfur dioxide	T59.1X1-	T59.1X2-	T59.1X3-	T59.1X4-	-	-
Fumigant NEC	T60.91X-	T60.92X-	T60.93X-	T60.94X-	-	-
Fungi, noxious, used as food	T62.0X1-	T62.0X2-	T62.0X3-	T62.0X4-	-	-
Fungicide NEC (nonmedicinal)	T60.3X1-	T60.3X2-	T60.3X3-	T60.3X4-	-	-
Fungizone	T36.7X1-	T36.7X2-	T36.7X3-	T36.7X4-	T36.7X5-	T36.7X6-
topical	T49.0X1-	T49.0X2-	T49.0X3-	T49.0X4-	T49.0X5-	T49.0X6-
Furacin	T49.0X1-	T49.0X2-	T49.0X3-	T49.0X4-	T49.0X5-	T49.0X6-
Furadantin	T37.91X-	T37.92X-	T37.93X-	T37.94X-	T37.95X-	T37.96X-
Furazolidone	T37.8X1-	T37.8X2-	T37.8X3-	T37.8X4-	T37.8X5-	T37.8X6-
Furazolium chloride	T49.0X1-	T49.0X2-	T49.0X3-	T49.0X4-	T49.0X5-	T49.0X6-
Furfural	T52.8X1-	T52.8X2-	T52.8X3-	T52.8X4-	-	-
Furnace (coal burning) (domestic) , gas from	T58.2X1-	T58.2X2-	T58.2X3-	T58.2X4-	-	-
industrial	T58.8X1-	T58.8X2-	T58.8X3-	T58.8X4-	-	-
Furniture polish	T65.891-	T65.892-	T65.893-	T65.894-	-	-
Furosemide	T50.1X1-	T50.1X2-	T50.1X3-	T50.1X4-	T50.1X5-	T50.1X6-
Furoxone	T37.91X-	T37.92X-	T37.93X-	T37.94X-	T37.95X-	T37.96X-
Fursultiamine	T45.2X1-	T45.2X2-	T45.2X3-	T45.2X4-	T45.2X5-	T45.2X6-
Fusafungine	T36.8X1-	T36.8X2-	T36.8X3-	T36.8X4-	T36.8X5-	T36.8X6-
Fusel oil (any) (amyl) (butyl) (propyl) , vapor	T51.3X1-	T51.3X2-	T51.3X3-	T51.3X4-	-	-
Fusidate (ethanolamine) (sodium)	T36.8X1-	T36.8X2-	T36.8X3-	T36.8X4-	T36.8X5-	T36.8X6-
Fusidic acid	T36.8X1-	T36.8X2-	T36.8X3-	T36.8X4-	T36.8X5-	T36.8X6-
Fytic acid, nonasodium	T50.6X1-	T50.6X2-	T50.6X3-	T50.6X4-	T50.6X5-	T50.6X6-
GABA	T43.8X1-	T43.8X2-	T43.8X3-	T43.8X4-	T43.8X5-	T43.8X6-
Gadopentetic acid	T50.8X1-	T50.8X2-	T50.8X3-	T50.8X4-	T50.8X5-	T50.8X6-
Galactose	T50.3X1-	T50.3X2-	T50.3X3-	T50.3X4-	T50.3X5-	T50.3X6-
b-Galactosidase	T47.5X1-	T47.5X2-	T47.5X3-	T47.5X4-	T47.5X5-	T47.5X6-
Galantamine	T44.0X1-	T44.0X2-	T44.0X3-	T44.0X4-	T44.0X5-	T44.0X6-
Gallamine (triethiodide)	T48.1X1-	T48.1X2-	T48.1X3-	T48.1X4-	T48.1X5-	T48.1X6-
Gallium citrate	T50.991-	T50.992-	T50.993-	T50.994-	T50.995-	T50.996-
Gallopamil	T46.1X1-	T46.1X2-	T46.1X3-	T46.1X4-	T46.1X5-	T46.1X6-
Gamboge	T47.2X1-	T47.2X2-	T47.2X3-	T47.2X4-	T47.2X5-	T47.2X6-
Gamimune	T50.Z11-	T50.Z12-	T50.Z13-	T50.Z14-	T50.Z15-	T50.Z16-
Gamma globulin	T50.Z11-	T50.Z12-	T50.Z13-	T50.Z14-	T50.Z15-	T50.Z16-
Gamma-aminobutyric acid	T43.8X1-	T43.8X2-	T43.8X3-	T43.8X4-	T43.8X5-	T43.8X6-
Gamma-benzene hexachloride (medicinal)	T49.0X1-	T49.0X2-	T49.0X3-	T49.0X4-	T49.0X5-	T49.0X6-
nonmedicinal, vapor	T53.6X1-	T53.6X2-	T53.6X3-	T53.6X4-	-	-
Gamma-BHC (medicinal) — *see also Gamma-benzene hexachloride*	T49.0X1-	T49.0X2-	T49.0X3-	T49.0X4-	T49.0X5-	T49.0X6-
Gamulin	T50.Z11-	T50.Z12-	T50.Z13-	T50.Z14-	T50.Z15-	T50.Z16-
Ganciclovir (sodium)	T37.5X1-	T37.5X2-	T37.5X3-	T37.5X4-	T37.5X5-	T37.5X6-

Substance	Poisoning Accidental (unintentional)	Poisoning Intentional self-harm	Poisoning Assault	Poisoning Undetermined	Adverse effect	Underdosing
Ganglionic blocking drug NEC	T44.2X1-	T44.2X2-	T44.2X3-	T44.2X4-	T44.2X5-	T44.2X6-
specified NEC	T44.2X1-	T44.2X2-	T44.2X3-	T44.2X4-	T44.2X5-	T44.2X6-
Ganja	T40.7X1-	T40.7X2-	T40.7X3-	T40.7X4-	T40.7X5-	T40.7X6-
Garamycin	T36.5X1-	T36.5X2-	T36.5X3-	T36.5X4-	T36.5X5-	T36.5X6-
ophthalmic preparation	T49.5X1-	T49.5X2-	T49.5X3-	T49.5X4-	T49.5X5-	T49.5X6-
topical NEC	T49.0X1-	T49.0X2-	T49.0X3-	T49.0X4-	T49.0X5-	T49.0X6-
Gardenal	T42.3X1-	T42.3X2-	T42.3X3-	T42.3X4-	T42.3X5-	T42.3X6-
Gardepanyl	T42.3X1-	T42.3X2-	T42.3X3-	T42.3X4-	T42.3X5-	T42.3X6-
Gas NEC	T59.91X-	T59.92X-	T59.93X-	T59.94X-	-	-
acetylene	T59.891-	T59.892-	T59.893-	T59.894-	-	-
incomplete combustion of	T58.11X-	T58.12X-	T58.13X-	T58.14X-	-	-
air contaminants, source or type not specified	T59.91X-	T59.92X-	T59.93X-	T59.94X-	-	-
anesthetic	T41.0X1-	T41.0X2-	T41.0X3-	T41.0X4-	T41.0X5-	T41.0X6-
blast furnace	T58.8X1-	T58.8X2-	T58.8X3-	T58.8X4-	-	-
butane — *see butane*						
carbon monoxide — *see Carbon, monoxide*						
chlorine	T59.4X1-	T59.4X2-	T59.4X3-	T59.4X4-	-	-
coal	T58.2X1-	T58.2X2-	T58.2X3-	T58.2X4-	-	-
cyanide	T57.3X1-	T57.3X2-	T57.3X3-	T57.3X4-	-	-
dicyanogen	T65.0X1-	T65.0X2-	T65.0X3-	T65.0X4-	-	-
domestic — *see Domestic gas*						
exhaust	T58.01X-	T58.02X-	T58.03X-	T58.04X-	-	-
from utility (for cooking, heating, or lighting) (after combustion) — *see Carbon, monoxide, fuel, utility*						
prior to combustion	T59.891-	T59.892-	T59.893-	T59.894-	-	-
from wood- or coal-burning stove or fireplace	T58.2X1-	T58.2X2-	T58.2X3-	T58.2X4-	-	-
fuel (domestic use) (after combustion) — *see also Carbon, monoxide, fuel*						
industrial use	T58.8X1-	T58.8X2-	T58.8X3-	T58.8X4-	-	-
prior to combustion	T59.891-	T59.892-	T59.893-	T59.894-	-	-
utility	T59.891-	T59.892-	T59.893-	T59.894-	-	-
in mobile container	T59.891-	T59.892-	T59.893-	T59.894-	-	-
incomplete combustion of — *see Carbon, monoxide, fuel, utility*						
piped (natural)	T59.891-	T59.892-	T59.893-	T59.894-	-	-
garage	T58.01X-	T58.02X-	T58.03X-	T58.04X-	-	-
hydrocarbon NEC	T59.891-	T59.892-	T59.893-	T59.894-	-	-
incomplete combustion of — *see Carbon, monoxide, fuel, utility*						
liquefied — *see butane*						
piped	T59.891-	T59.892-	T59.893-	T59.894-	-	-
hydrocyanic acid	T65.0X1-	T65.0X2-	T65.0X3-	T65.0X4-	-	-
illuminating (after combustion)	T58.11X-	T58.12X-	T58.13X-	T58.14X-	-	-
prior to combustion	T59.891-	T59.892-	T59.893-	T59.894-	-	-
incomplete combustion, any — *see Carbon, monoxide*						
kiln	T58.8X1-	T58.8X2-	T58.8X3-	T58.8X4-	-	-
lacrimogenic	T59.3X1-	T59.3X2-	T59.3X3-	T59.3X4-	-	-
liquefied petroleum — *see butane*						
marsh	T59.891-	T59.892-	T59.893-	T59.894-	-	-
motor exhaust, not in transit	T58.01X-	T58.02X-	T58.03X-	T58.04X-	-	-
mustard, not in war	T59.891-	T59.892-	T59.893-	T59.894-	-	-
natural	T59.891-	T59.892-	T59.893-	T59.894-	-	-
nerve, not in war	T59.91X-	T59.92X-	T59.93X-	T59.94X-	-	-

Substance	Poisoning Accidental (unintentional)	Poisoning Intentional self-harm	Poisoning Assault	Poisoning Undetermined	Adverse effect	Underdosing
Gas NEC *(continued)*						
oil	T52.0X1-	T52.0X2-	T52.0X3-	T52.0X4-	-	-
petroleum (liquefied) (distributed in mobile containers)	T59.891-	T59.892-	T59.893-	T59.894-	-	-
piped (pure or mixed with air)	T59.891-	T59.892-	T59.893-	T59.894-	-	-
piped (manufactured) (natural) NEC	T59.891-	T59.892-	T59.893-	T59.894-	-	-
producer	T58.8X1-	T58.8X2-	T58.8X3-	T58.8X4-	-	-
propane — *see propane*						
refrigerant (chlorofluoro-carbon)	T53.5X1-	T53.5X2-	T53.5X3-	T53.5X4-	-	-
not chlorofluoro-carbon	T59.891-	T59.892-	T59.893-	T59.894-	-	-
sewer	T59.91X-	T59.92X-	T59.93X-	T59.94X-	-	-
specified source NEC	T59.91X-	T59.92X-	T59.93X-	T59.94X-	-	-
stove (after combustion)	T58.11X-	T58.12X-	T58.13X-	T58.14X-	-	-
prior to combustion	T59.891-	T59.892-	T59.893-	T59.894-	-	-
tear	T59.3X1-	T59.3X2-	T59.3X3-	T59.3X4-	-	-
therapeutic	T41.5X1-	T41.5X2-	T41.5X3-	T41.5X4-	T41.5X5-	T41.5X6-
utility (for cooking, heating, or lighting) (piped) NEC	T59.891-	T59.892-	T59.893-	T59.894-	-	-
in mobile container	T59.891-	T59.892-	T59.893-	T59.894-	-	-
incomplete combustion of — *see Carbon, monoxide, fuel, utilty*						
piped (natural)	T59.891-	T59.892-	T59.893-	T59.894-	-	-
water	T58.11X-	T58.12X-	T58.13X-	T58.14X-	-	-
incomplete combustion of — *see Carbon, monoxide, fuel, utility*						
Gaseous substance — *see Gas*						
Gasoline	T52.0X1-	T52.0X2-	T52.0X3-	T52.0X4-	-	-
vapor	T52.0X1-	T52.0X2-	T52.0X3-	T52.0X4-	-	-
Gastric enzymes	T47.5X1-	T47.5X2-	T47.5X3-	T47.5X4-	T47.5X5-	T47.5X6-
Gastrografin	T50.8X1-	T50.8X2-	T50.8X3-	T50.8X4-	T50.8X5-	T50.8X6-
Gastrointestinal drug	T47.91X-	T47.92X-	T47.93X-	T47.94X-	T47.95X-	T47.96X-
biological	T47.8X1-	T47.8X2-	T47.8X3-	T47.8X4-	T47.8X5-	T47.8X6-
specified NEC	T47.8X1-	T47.8X2-	T47.8X3-	T47.8X4-	T47.8X5-	T47.8X6-
Gaultheria procumbens	T62.2X1-	T62.2X2-	T62.2X3-	T62.2X4-	-	-
Gefarnate	T44.3X1-	T44.3X2-	T44.3X3-	T44.3X4-	T44.3X5-	T44.3X6-
Gelatin (intravenous)	T45.8X1-	T45.8X2-	T45.8X3-	T45.8X4-	T45.8X5-	T45.8X6-
absorbable (sponge)	T45.7X1-	T45.7X2-	T45.7X3-	T45.7X4-	T45.7X5-	T45.7X6-
Gelfilm	T49.8X1-	T49.8X2-	T49.8X3-	T49.8X4-	T49.8X5-	T49.8X6-
Gelfoam	T45.7X1-	T45.7X2-	T45.7X3-	T45.7X4-	T45.7X5-	T45.7X6-
Gelsemine	T50.991-	T50.992-	T50.993-	T50.994-	T50.995-	T50.996-
Gelsemium (sempervirens)	T62.2X1-	T62.2X2-	T62.2X3-	T62.2X4-	-	-
Gemeprost	T48.0X1-	T48.0X2-	T48.0X3-	T48.0X4-	T48.0X5-	T48.0X6-
Gemfibrozil	T46.6X1-	T46.6X2-	T46.6X3-	T46.6X4-	T46.6X5-	T46.6X6-
Gemonil	T42.3X1-	T42.3X2-	T42.3X3-	T42.3X4-	T42.3X5-	T42.3X6-
Gentamicin	T36.5X1-	T36.5X2-	T36.5X3-	T36.5X4-	T36.5X5-	T36.5X6-
ophthalmic preparation	T49.5X1-	T49.5X2-	T49.5X3-	T49.5X4-	T49.5X5-	T49.5X6-
topical NEC	T49.0X1-	T49.0X2-	T49.0X3-	T49.0X4-	T49.0X5-	T49.0X6-
Gentian	T47.5X1-	T47.5X2-	T47.5X3-	T47.5X4-	T47.5X5-	T47.5X6-
violet	T49.0X1-	T49.0X2-	T49.0X3-	T49.0X4-	T49.0X5-	T49.0X6-
Gepefrine	T44.4X1-	T44.4X2-	T44.4X3-	T44.4X4-	T44.4X5-	T44.4X6-
Gestonorone caproate	T38.5X1-	T38.5X2-	T38.5X3-	T38.5X4-	T38.5X5-	T38.5X6-
Gexane	T49.0X1-	T49.0X2-	T49.0X3-	T49.0X4-	T49.0X5-	T49.0X6-
Gila monster (venom)	T63.111-	T63.112-	T63.113-	T63.114-	-	-
Ginger	T47.5X1-	T47.5X2-	T47.5X3-	T47.5X4-	T47.5X5-	T47.5X6-
Jamaica — *see Jamaica, ginger*						
Gitalin	T46.0X1-	T46.0X2-	T46.0X3-	T46.0X4-	T46.0X5-	T46.0X6-
amorphous	T46.0X1-	T46.0X2-	T46.0X3-	T46.0X4-	T46.0X5-	T46.0X6-

Substance	Poisoning Accidental (unintentional)	Poisoning Intentional self-harm	Poisoning Assault	Poisoning Undetermined	Adverse effect	Underdosing
Gitaloxin	T46.0X1-	T46.0X2-	T46.0X3-	T46.0X4-	T46.0X5-	T46.0X6-
Gitoxin	T46.0X1-	T46.0X2-	T46.0X3-	T46.0X4-	T46.0X5-	T46.0X6-
Glafenine	T39.8X1-	T39.8X2-	T39.8X3-	T39.8X4-	T39.8X5-	T39.8X6-
Glandular extract (medicinal) NEC	T50.Z91-	T50.Z92-	T50.Z93-	T50.Z94-	T50.Z95-	T50.Z96-
Glaucarubin	T37.3X1-	T37.3X2-	T37.3X3-	T37.3X4-	T37.3X5-	T37.3X6-
Glibenclamide	T38.3X1-	T38.3X2-	T38.3X3-	T38.3X4-	T38.3X5-	T38.3X6-
Glibornuride	T38.3X1-	T38.3X2-	T38.3X3-	T38.3X4-	T38.3X5-	T38.3X6-
Gliclazide	T38.3X1-	T38.3X2-	T38.3X3-	T38.3X4-	T38.3X5-	T38.3X6-
Glimidine	T38.3X1-	T38.3X2-	T38.3X3-	T38.3X4-	T38.3X5-	T38.3X6-
Glipizide	T38.3X1-	T38.3X2-	T38.3X3-	T38.3X4-	T38.3X5-	T38.3X6-
Gliquidone	T38.3X1-	T38.3X2-	T38.3X3-	T38.3X4-	T38.3X5-	T38.3X6-
Glisolamide	T38.3X1-	T38.3X2-	T38.3X3-	T38.3X4-	T38.3X5-	T38.3X6-
Glisoxepide	T38.3X1-	T38.3X2-	T38.3X3-	T38.3X4-	T38.3X5-	T38.3X6-
Globin zinc insulin	T38.3X1-	T38.3X2-	T38.3X3-	T38.3X4-	T38.3X5-	T38.3X6-
Globulin						
antilymphocytic	T50.Z11-	T50.Z12-	T50.Z13-	T50.Z14-	T50.Z15-	T50.Z16-
antirhesus	T50.Z11-	T50.Z12-	T50.Z13-	T50.Z14-	T50.Z15-	T50.Z16-
antivenin	T50.Z11-	T50.Z12-	T50.Z13-	T50.Z14-	T50.Z15-	T50.Z16-
antiviral	T50.Z11-	T50.Z12-	T50.Z13-	T50.Z14-	T50.Z15-	T50.Z16-
Glucagon	T38.3X1-	T38.3X2-	T38.3X3-	T38.3X4-	T38.3X5-	T38.3X6-
Glucocorticoids	T38.0X1-	T38.0X2-	T38.0X3-	T38.0X4-	T38.0X5-	T38.0X6-
Glucocorticosteroid	T38.0X1-	T38.0X2-	T38.0X3-	T38.0X4-	T38.0X5-	T38.0X6-
Gluconic acid	T50.991-	T50.992-	T50.993-	T50.994-	T50.995-	T50.996-
Glucosamine sulfate	T39.4X1-	T39.4X2-	T39.4X3-	T39.4X4-	T39.4X5-	T39.4X6-
Glucose	T50.3X1-	T50.3X2-	T50.3X3-	T50.3X4-	T50.3X5-	T50.3X6-
with sodium chloride	T50.3X1-	T50.3X2-	T50.3X3-	T50.3X4-	T50.3X5-	T50.3X6-
Glucosulfone sodium	T37.1X1-	T37.1X2-	T37.1X3-	T37.1X4-	T37.1X5-	T37.1X6-
Glucurolactone	T47.8X1-	T47.8X2-	T47.8X3-	T47.8X4-	T47.8X5-	T47.8X6-
Glue NEC	T52.8X1-	T52.8X2-	T52.8X3-	T52.8X4-	-	-
Glutamic acid	T47.5X1-	T47.5X2-	T47.5X3-	T47.5X4-	T47.5X5-	T47.5X6-
Glutaral (medicinal)	T49.0X1-	T49.0X2-	T49.0X3-	T49.0X4-	T49.0X5-	T49.0X6-
nonmedicinal	T65.891-	T65.892-	T65.893-	T65.894-	-	-
Glutaraldehyde (nonmedicinal)	T65.891-	T65.892-	T65.893-	T65.894-	-	-
medicinal	T49.0X1-	T49.0X2-	T49.0X3-	T49.0X4-	T49.0X5-	T49.0X6-
Glutathione	T50.6X1-	T50.6X2-	T50.6X3-	T50.6X4-	T50.6X5-	T50.6X6-
Glutethimide	T42.6X1-	T42.6X2-	T42.6X3-	T42.6X4-	T42.6X5-	T42.6X6-
Glyburide	T38.3X1-	T38.3X2-	T38.3X3-	T38.3X4-	T38.3X5-	T38.3X6-
Glycerin	T47.4X1-	T47.4X2-	T47.4X3-	T47.4X4-	T47.4X5-	T47.4X6-
Glycerol	T47.4X1-	T47.4X2-	T47.4X3-	T47.4X4-	T47.4X5-	T47.4X6-
borax	T49.6X1-	T49.6X2-	T49.6X3-	T49.6X4-	T49.6X5-	T49.6X6-
intravenous	T50.3X1-	T50.3X2-	T50.3X3-	T50.3X4-	T50.3X5-	T50.3X6-
iodinated	T48.4X1-	T48.4X2-	T48.4X3-	T48.4X4-	T48.4X5-	T48.4X6-
Glycerophosphate	T50.991-	T50.992-	T50.993-	T50.994-	T50.995-	T50.996-
Glyceryl						
gualacolate	T48.4X1-	T48.4X2-	T48.4X3-	T48.4X4-	T48.4X5-	T48.4X6-
nitrate	T46.3X1-	T46.3X2-	T46.3X3-	T46.3X4-	T46.3X5-	T46.3X6-
triacetate (topical)	T49.0X1-	T49.0X2-	T49.0X3-	T49.0X4-	T49.0X5-	T49.0X6-
trinitrate	T46.3X1-	T46.3X2-	T46.3X3-	T46.3X4-	T46.3X5-	T46.3X6-
Glycine	T50.3X1-	T50.3X2-	T50.3X3-	T50.3X4-	T50.3X5-	T50.3X6-
Glyclopyramide	T38.3X1-	T38.3X2-	T38.3X3-	T38.3X4-	T38.3X5-	T38.3X6-
Glycobiarsol	T37.3X1-	T37.3X2-	T37.3X3-	T37.3X4-	T37.3X5-	T37.3X6-
Glycols (ether)	T52.3X1-	T52.3X2-	T52.3X3-	T52.3X4-	-	-
Glyconiazide	T37.1X1-	T37.1X2-	T37.1X3-	T37.1X4-	T37.1X5-	T37.1X6-
Glycopyrrolate	T44.3X1-	T44.3X2-	T44.3X3-	T44.3X4-	T44.3X5-	T44.3X6-
Glycopyrronium	T44.3X1-	T44.3X2-	T44.3X3-	T44.3X4-	T44.3X5-	T44.3X6-
bromide	T44.3X1-	T44.3X2-	T44.3X3-	T44.3X4-	T44.3X5-	T44.3X6-
Glycoside, cardiac (stimulant)	T46.0X1-	T46.0X2-	T46.0X3-	T46.0X4-	T46.0X5-	T46.0X6-
Glycyclamide	T38.3X1-	T38.3X2-	T38.3X3-	T38.3X4-	T38.3X5-	T38.3X6-

Substance	Poisoning Accidental (unintentional)	Poisoning Intentional self-harm	Poisoning Assault	Poisoning Undetermined	Adverse effect	Underdosing
Glycyrrhiza extract	T48.4X1-	T48.4X2-	T48.4X3-	T48.4X4-	T48.4X5-	T48.4X6-
Glycyrrhizic acid	T48.4X1-	T48.4X2-	T48.4X3-	T48.4X4-	T48.4X5-	T48.4X6-
Glycyrrhizinate potassium	T48.4X1-	T48.4X2-	T48.4X3-	T48.4X4-	T48.4X5-	T48.4X6-
Glymidine sodium	T38.3X1-	T38.3X2-	T38.3X3-	T38.3X4-	T38.3X5-	T38.3X6-
Glyphosate	T60.3X1-	T60.3X2-	T60.3X3-	T60.3X4-	-	-
Glyphylline	T48.6X1-	T48.6X2-	T48.6X3-	T48.6X4-	T48.6X5-	T48.6X6-
Gold						
colloidal (l98Au)	T45.1X1-	T45.1X2-	T45.1X3-	T45.1X4-	T45.1X5-	T45.1X6-
salts	T39.4X1-	T39.4X2-	T39.4X3-	T39.4X4-	T39.4X5-	T39.4X6-
Golden sulfide of antimony	T56.891-	T56.892-	T56.893-	T56.894-	-	-
Goldylocks	T62.2X1-	T62.2X2-	T62.2X3-	T62.2X4-	-	-
Gonadal tissue extract	T38.901-	T38.902-	T38.903-	T38.904-	T38.905-	T38.906-
female	T38.5X1-	T38.5X2-	T38.5X3-	T38.5X4-	T38.5X5-	T38.5X6-
male	T38.7X1-	T38.7X2-	T38.7X3-	T38.7X4-	T38.7X5-	T38.7X6-
Gonadorelin	T38.891-	T38.892-	T38.893-	T38.894-	T38.895-	T38.896-
Gonadotropin	T38.891-	T38.892-	T38.893-	T38.894-	T38.895-	T38.896-
chorionic	T38.891-	T38.892-	T38.893-	T38.894-	T38.895-	T38.896-
pituitary	T38.811-	T38.812-	T38.813-	T38.814-	T38.815-	T38.816-
Goserelin	T45.1X1-	T45.1X2-	T45.1X3-	T45.1X4-	T45.1X5-	T45.1X6-
Grain alcohol	T51.0X1-	T51.0X2-	T51.0X3-	T51.0X4-	-	-
Gramicidin	T49.0X1-	T49.0X2-	T49.0X3-	T49.0X4-	T49.0X5-	T49.0X6-
Granisetron	T45.0X1-	T45.0X2-	T45.0X3-	T45.0X4-	T45.0X5-	T45.0X6-
Gratiola officinalis	T62.2X1-	T62.2X2-	T62.2X3-	T62.2X4-	-	-
Grease	T65.891-	T65.892-	T65.893-	T65.894-	-	-
Green hellebore	T62.2X1-	T62.2X2-	T62.2X3-	T62.2X4-	-	-
Green soap	T49.2X1-	T49.2X2-	T49.2X3-	T49.2X4-	T49.2X5-	T49.2X6-
Grifulvin	T36.7X1-	T36.7X2-	T36.7X3-	T36.7X4-	T36.7X5-	T36.7X6-
Griseofulvin	T36.7X1-	T36.7X2-	T36.7X3-	T36.7X4-	T36.7X5-	T36.7X6-
Growth hormone	T38.811-	T38.812-	T38.813-	T38.814-	T38.815-	T38.816-
Guaiac reagent	T50.991-	T50.992-	T50.993-	T50.994-	T50.995-	T50.996-
Guaiacol derivatives	T48.4X1-	T48.4X2-	T48.4X3-	T48.4X4-	T48.4X5-	T48.4X6-
Guaifenesin	T48.4X1-	T48.4X2-	T48.4X3-	T48.4X4-	T48.4X5-	T48.4X6-
Guaimesal	T48.4X1-	T48.4X2-	T48.4X3-	T48.4X4-	T48.4X5-	T48.4X6-
Guaiphenesin	T48.4X1-	T48.4X2-	T48.4X3-	T48.4X4-	T48.4X5-	T48.4X6-
Guamecycline	T36.4X1-	T36.4X2-	T36.4X3-	T36.4X4-	T36.4X5-	T36.4X6-
Guanabenz	T46.5X1-	T46.5X2-	T46.5X3-	T46.5X4-	T46.5X5-	T46.5X6-
Guanacline	T46.5X1-	T46.5X2-	T46.5X3-	T46.5X4-	T46.5X5-	T46.5X6-
Guanadrel	T46.5X1-	T46.5X2-	T46.5X3-	T46.5X4-	T46.5X5-	T46.5X6-
Guanatol	T37.2X1-	T37.2X2-	T37.2X3-	T37.2X4-	T37.2X5-	T37.2X6-
Guanethidine	T46.5X1-	T46.5X2-	T46.5X3-	T46.5X4-	T46.5X5-	T46.5X6-
Guanfacine	T46.5X1-	T46.5X2-	T46.5X3-	T46.5X4-	T46.5X5-	T46.5X6-
Guano	T65.891-	T65.892-	T65.893-	T65.894-	-	-
Guanochlor	T46.5X1-	T46.5X2-	T46.5X3-	T46.5X4-	T46.5X5-	T46.5X6-
Guanoclor	T46.5X1-	T46.5X2-	T46.5X3-	T46.5X4-	T46.5X5-	T46.5X6-
Guanoctine	T46.5X1-	T46.5X2-	T46.5X3-	T46.5X4-	T46.5X5-	T46.5X6-
Guanoxabenz	T46.5X1-	T46.5X2-	T46.5X3-	T46.5X4-	T46.5X5-	T46.5X6-
Guanoxan	T46.5X1-	T46.5X2-	T46.5X3-	T46.5X4-	T46.5X5-	T46.5X6-
Guar gum (medicinal)	T46.6X1-	T46.6X2-	T46.6X3-	T46.6X4-	T46.6X5-	T46.6X6-
Hachimycin	T36.7X1-	T36.7X2-	T36.7X3-	T36.7X4-	T36.7X5-	T36.7X6-
Hair						
dye	T49.4X1-	T49.4X2-	T49.4X3-	T49.4X4-	T49.4X5-	T49.4X6-
preparation NEC	T49.4X1-	T49.4X2-	T49.4X3-	T49.4X4-	T49.4X5-	T49.4X6-
Halazepam	T42.4X1-	T42.4X2-	T42.4X3-	T42.4X4-	T42.4X5-	T42.4X6-
Halcinolone	T49.0X1-	T49.0X2-	T49.0X3-	T49.0X4-	T49.0X5-	T49.0X6-
Halcinonide	T49.0X1-	T49.0X2-	T49.0X3-	T49.0X4-	T49.0X5-	T49.0X6-
Halethazole	T49.0X1-	T49.0X2-	T49.0X3-	T49.0X4-	T49.0X5-	T49.0X6-
Hallucinogen NOS	T40.901-	T40.902-	T40.903-	T40.904-	T40.905-	T40.906-
specified NEC	T40.991-	T40.992-	T40.993-	T40.994-	T40.995-	T40.996-

HALOFANTRINE - HESPERIDIN

Substance	Poisoning Accidental (unintentional)	Poisoning Intentional self-harm	Poisoning Assault	Poisoning Undetermined	Adverse effect	Underdosing
Halofantrine	T37.2X1-	T37.2X2-	T37.2X3-	T37.2X4-	T37.2X5-	T37.2X6-
Halofenate	T46.6X1-	T46.6X2-	T46.6X3-	T46.6X4-	T46.6X5-	T46.6X6-
Halometasone	T49.0X1-	T49.0X2-	T49.0X3-	T49.0X4-	T49.0X5-	T49.0X6-
Haloperidol	T43.4X1-	T43.4X2-	T43.4X3-	T43.4X4-	T43.4X5-	T43.4X6-
Haloprogin	T49.0X1-	T49.0X2-	T49.0X3-	T49.0X4-	T49.0X5-	T49.0X6-
Halotex	T49.0X1-	T49.0X2-	T49.0X3-	T49.0X4-	T49.0X5-	T49.0X6-
Halothane	T41.0X1-	T41.0X2-	T41.0X3-	T41.0X4-	T41.0X5-	T41.0X6-
Haloxazolam	T42.4X1-	T42.4X2-	T42.4X3-	T42.4X4-	T42.4X5-	T42.4X6-
Halquinols	T49.0X1-	T49.0X2-	T49.0X3-	T49.0X4-	T49.0X5-	T49.0X6-
Hamamelis	T49.2X1-	T49.2X2-	T49.2X3-	T49.2X4-	T49.2X5-	T49.2X6-
Haptendextran	T45.8X1-	T45.8X2-	T45.8X3-	T45.8X4-	T45.8X5-	T45.8X6-
Harmonyl	T46.5X1-	T46.5X2-	T46.5X3-	T46.5X4-	T46.5X5-	T46.5X6-
Hartmann's solution	T50.3X1-	T50.3X2-	T50.3X3-	T50.3X4-	T50.3X5-	T50.3X6-
Hashish	T40.7X1-	T40.7X2-	T40.7X3-	T40.7X4-	T40.7X5-	T40.7X6-
Hawaiian Woodrose seeds	T40.991-	T40.992-	T40.993-	T40.994-	-	-
HCB	T60.3X1-	T60.3X2-	T60.3X3-	T60.3X4-	-	-
HCH	T53.6X1-	T53.6X2-	T53.6X3-	T53.6X4-	-	-
medicinal	T49.0X1-	T49.0X2-	T49.0X3-	T49.0X4-	T49.0X5-	T49.0X6-
HCN	T57.3X1-	T57.3X2-	T57.3X3-	T57.3X4-	-	-
Headache cures, drugs, powders NEC	T50.901-	T50.902-	T50.903-	T50.904-	T50.905-	T50.906-
Heavenly Blue (morning glory)	T40.991-	T40.992-	T40.993-	T40.994-	-	-
Heavy metal antidote	T45.8X1-	T45.8X2-	T45.8X3-	T45.8X4-	T45.8X5-	T45.8X6-
Hedaquinium	T49.0X1-	T49.0X2-	T49.0X3-	T49.0X4-	T49.0X5-	T49.0X6-
Hedge hyssop	T62.2X1-	T62.2X2-	T62.2X3-	T62.2X4-	-	-
Heet	T49.8X1-	T49.8X2-	T49.8X3-	T49.8X4-	T49.8X5-	T49.8X6-
Helenin	T37.4X1-	T37.4X2-	T37.4X3-	T37.4X4-	T37.4X5-	T37.4X6-
Helium (nonmedicinal) NEC	T59.891-	T59.892-	T59.893-	T59.894-	-	-
medicinal	T48.991-	T48.992-	T48.993-	T48.994-	T48.995-	T48.996-
Hellebore (black) (green) (white)	T62.2X1-	T62.2X2-	T62.2X3-	T62.2X4-	-	-
Hematin	T45.8X1-	T45.8X2-	T45.8X3-	T45.8X4-	T45.8X5-	T45.8X6-
Hematinic preparation	T45.8X1-	T45.8X2-	T45.8X3-	T45.8X4-	T45.8X5-	T45.8X6-
Hematological agent	T45.91X-	T45.92X-	T45.93X-	T45.94X-	T45.95X-	T45.96X-
specified NEC	T45.8X1-	T45.8X2-	T45.8X3-	T45.8X4-	T45.8X5-	T45.8X6-
Hemlock	T62.2X1-	T62.2X2-	T62.2X3-	T62.2X4-	-	-
Hemostatic	T45.621-	T45.622-	T45.623-	T45.624-	T45.625-	T45.626-
drug, systemic	T45.621-	T45.622-	T45.623-	T45.624-	T45.625-	T45.626-
Hemostyptic	T49.4X1-	T49.4X2-	T49.4X3-	T49.4X4-	T49.4X5-	T49.4X6-
Henbane	T62.2X1-	T62.2X2-	T62.2X3-	T62.2X4-	-	-
Heparin (sodium)	T45.511-	T45.512-	T45.513-	T45.514-	T45.515-	T45.516-
action reverser	T45.7X1-	T45.7X2-	T45.7X3-	T45.7X4-	T45.7X5-	T45.7X6-
Heparin-fraction	T45.511-	T45.512-	T45.513-	T45.514-	T45.515-	T45.516-
Heparinoid (systemic)	T45.511-	T45.512-	T45.513-	T45.514-	T45.515-	T45.516-
Hepatic secretion stimulant	T47.8X1-	T47.8X2-	T47.8X3-	T47.8X4-	T47.8X5-	T47.8X6-
Hepatitis B						
immune globulin	T50.Z11-	T50.Z12-	T50.Z13-	T50.Z14-	T50.Z15-	T50.Z16-
vaccine	T50.B91-	T50.B92-	T50.B93-	T50.B94-	T50.B95-	T50.B96-
Hepronicate	T46.7X1-	T46.7X2-	T46.7X3-	T46.7X4-	T46.7X5-	T46.7X6-
Heptabarb	T42.3X1-	T42.3X2-	T42.3X3-	T42.3X4-	T42.3X5-	T42.3X6-
Heptabarbital	T42.3X1-	T42.3X2-	T42.3X3-	T42.3X4-	T42.3X5-	T42.3X6-
Heptabarbitone	T42.3X1-	T42.3X2-	T42.3X3-	T42.3X4-	T42.3X5-	T42.3X6-
Heptachlor	T60.1X1-	T60.1X2-	T60.1X3-	T60.1X4-	-	-
Heptalgin	T40.2X1-	T40.2X2-	T40.2X3-	T40.2X4-	T40.2X5-	T40.2X6-
Heptaminol	T46.3X1-	T46.3X2-	T46.3X3-	T46.3X4-	T46.3X5-	T46.3X6-
Herbicide NEC	T60.3X1-	T60.3X2-	T60.3X3-	T60.3X4-	-	-
Heroin	T40.1X1-	T40.1X2-	T40.1X3-	T40.1X4-	-	-
Herplex	T49.5X1-	T49.5X2-	T49.5X3-	T49.5X4-	T49.5X5-	T49.5X6-
HES	T45.8X1-	T45.8X2-	T45.8X3-	T45.8X4-	T45.8X5-	T45.8X6-
Hesperidin	T46.991-	T46.992-	T46.993-	T46.994-	T46.995-	T46.996-

Substance	Poisoning Accidental (unintentional)	Poisoning Intentional self-harm	Poisoning Assault	Poisoning Undetermined	Adverse effect	Underdosing
Hetacillin	T36.0X1-	T36.0X2-	T36.0X3-	T36.0X4-	T36.0X5-	T36.0X6-
Hetastarch	T45.8X1-	T45.8X2-	T45.8X3-	T45.8X4-	T45.8X5-	T45.8X6-
HETP	T60.0X1-	T60.0X2-	T60.0X3-	T60.0X4-	-	-
Hexachlorobenzene (vapor)	T60.3X1-	T60.3X2-	T60.3X3-	T60.3X4-	-	-
Hexachlorocyclohexane	T53.6X1-	T53.6X2-	T53.6X3-	T53.6X4-	-	-
Hexachlorophene	T49.0X1-	T49.0X2-	T49.0X3-	T49.0X4-	T49.0X5-	T49.0X6-
Hexadiline	T46.3X1-	T46.3X2-	T46.3X3-	T46.3X4-	T46.3X5-	T46.3X6-
Hexadimethrine (bromide)	T45.7X1-	T45.7X2-	T45.7X3-	T45.7X4-	T45.7X5-	T45.7X6-
Hexadylamine	T46.3X1-	T46.3X2-	T46.3X3-	T46.3X4-	T46.3X5-	T46.3X6-
Hexaethyl tetraphos-phate	T60.0X1-	T60.0X2-	T60.0X3-	T60.0X4-	-	-
Hexafluorenium bromide	T48.1X1-	T48.1X2-	T48.1X3-	T48.1X4-	T48.1X5-	T48.1X6-
Hexafluronium (bromide)	T48.1X1-	T48.1X2-	T48.1X3-	T48.1X4-	T48.1X5-	T48.1X6-
Hexa-germ	T49.2X1-	T49.2X2-	T49.2X3-	T49.2X4-	T49.2X5-	T49.2X6-
Hexahydrobenzol	T52.8X1-	T52.8X2-	T52.8X3-	T52.8X4-	-	-
Hexahydrocresol (s)	T51.8X1-	T51.8X2-	T51.8X3-	T51.8X4-	-	-
arsenide	T57.0X1-	T57.0X2-	T57.0X3-	T57.0X4-	-	-
arseniurated	T57.0X1-	T57.0X2-	T57.0X3-	T57.0X4-	-	-
cyanide	T57.3X1-	T57.3X2-	T57.3X3-	T57.3X4-	-	-
gas	T59.891-	T59.892-	T59.893-	T59.894-	-	-
Fluoride (liquid)	T57.8X1-	T57.8X2-	T57.8X3-	T57.8X4-	-	-
vapor	T59.891-	T59.892-	T59.893-	T59.894-	-	-
phophorated	T60.0X1-	T60.0X2-	T60.0X3-	T60.0X4-	-	-
sulfate	T57.8X1-	T57.8X2-	T57.8X3-	T57.8X4-	-	-
sulfide (gas)	T59.6X1-	T59.6X2-	T59.6X3-	T59.6X4-	-	-
arseniurated	T57.0X1-	T57.0X2-	T57.0X3-	T57.0X4-	-	-
sulfurated	T57.8X1-	T57.8X2-	T57.8X3-	T57.8X4-	-	-
Hexahydrophenol	T51.8X1-	T51.8X2-	T51.8X3-	T51.8X4-	-	-
Hexalen	T51.8X1-	T51.8X2-	T51.8X3-	T51.8X4-	-	-
Hexamethonium bromide	T44.2X1-	T44.2X2-	T44.2X3-	T44.2X4-	T44.2X5-	T44.2X6-
Hexamethylene	T52.8X1-	T52.8X2-	T52.8X3-	T52.8X4-	-	-
Hexamethylmelamine	T45.1X1-	T45.1X2-	T45.1X3-	T45.1X4-	T45.1X5-	T45.1X6-
Hexamidine	T49.0X1-	T49.0X2-	T49.0X3-	T49.0X4-	T49.0X5-	T49.0X6-
Hexamine (mandelate)	T37.8X1-	T37.8X2-	T37.8X3-	T37.8X4-	T37.8X5-	T37.8X6-
Hexanone, 2-hexanone	T52.4X1-	T52.4X2-	T52.4X3-	T52.4X4-	-	-
Hexanuorenium	T48.1X1-	T48.1X2-	T48.1X3-	T48.1X4-	T48.1X5-	T48.1X6-
Hexapropymate	T42.6X1-	T42.6X2-	T42.6X3-	T42.6X4-	T42.6X5-	T42.6X6-
Hexasonium iodide	T44.3X1-	T44.3X2-	T44.3X3-	T44.3X4-	T44.3X5-	T44.3X6-
Hexcarbacholine bromide	T48.1X1-	T48.1X2-	T48.1X3-	T48.1X4-	T48.1X5-	T48.1X6-
Hexemal	T42.3X1-	T42.3X2-	T42.3X3-	T42.3X4-	T42.3X5-	T42.3X6-
Hexestrol	T38.5X1-	T38.5X2-	T38.5X3-	T38.5X4-	T38.5X5-	T38.5X6-
Hexethal (sodium)	T42.3X1-	T42.3X2-	T42.3X3-	T42.3X4-	T42.3X5-	T42.3X6-
Hexetidine	T37.8X1-	T37.8X2-	T37.8X3-	T37.8X4-	T37.8X5-	T37.8X6-
Hexobarbital	T42.3X1-	T42.3X2-	T42.3X3-	T42.3X4-	T42.3X5-	T42.3X6-
rectal	T41.291-	T41.292-	T41.293-	T41.294-	T41.295-	T41.296-
sodium	T41.1X1-	T41.1X2-	T41.1X3-	T41.1X4-	T41.1X5-	T41.1X6-
Hexobendine	T46.3X1-	T46.3X2-	T46.3X3-	T46.3X4-	T46.3X5-	T46.3X6-
Hexocyclium	T44.3X1-	T44.3X2-	T44.3X3-	T44.3X4-	T44.3X5-	T44.3X6-
metilsulfate	T44.3X1-	T44.3X2-	T44.3X3-	T44.3X4-	T44.3X5-	T44.3X6-
Hexoestrol	T38.5X1-	T38.5X2-	T38.5X3-	T38.5X4-	T38.5X5-	T38.5X6-
Hexone	T52.4X1-	T52.4X2-	T52.4X3-	T52.4X4-	-	-
Hexoprenaline	T48.6X1-	T48.6X2-	T48.6X3-	T48.6X4-	T48.6X5-	T48.6X6-
Hexylcaine	T41.3X1-	T41.3X2-	T41.3X3-	T41.3X4-	T41.3X5-	T41.3X6-
Hexylresorcinol	T52.2X1-	T52.2X2-	T52.2X3-	T52.2X4-	-	-
HGH (human growth hormone)	T38.811-	T38.812-	T38.813-	T38.814-	T38.815-	T38.816-
Hinkle's pills	T47.2X1-	T47.2X2-	T47.2X3-	T47.2X4-	T47.2X5-	T47.2X6-
Histalog	T50.8X1-	T50.8X2-	T50.8X3-	T50.8X4-	T50.8X5-	T50.8X6-
Histamine (phosphate)	T50.8X1-	T50.8X2-	T50.8X3-	T50.8X4-	T50.8X5-	T50.8X6-
Histoplasmin	T50.8X1-	T50.8X2-	T50.8X3-	T50.8X4-	T50.8X5-	T50.8X6-
Holly berries	T62.2X1-	T62.2X2-	T62.2X3-	T62.2X4-	-	-

HETACILLIN - HOLLY BERRIES

Substance	Poisoning Accidental (unintentional)	Poisoning Intentional self-harm	Poisoning Assault	Poisoning Undetermined	Adverse effect	Underdosing
Homatropine	T44.3X1-	T44.3X2-	T44.3X3-	T44.3X4-	T44.3X5-	T44.3X6-
methylbromide	T44.3X1-	T44.3X2-	T44.3X3-	T44.3X4-	T44.3X5-	T44.3X6-
Homochlorcyclizine	T45.0X1-	T45.0X2-	T45.0X3-	T45.0X4-	T45.0X5-	T45.0X6-
Homosalate	T49.3X1-	T49.3X2-	T49.3X3-	T49.3X4-	T49.3X5-	T49.3X6-
Homo-tet	T50.Z11-	T50.Z12-	T50.Z13-	T50.Z14-	T50.Z15-	T50.Z16-
Hormone	T38.801-	T38.802-	T38.803-	T38.804-	T38.805-	T38.806-
adrenal cortical steroids	T38.0X1-	T38.0X2-	T38.0X3-	T38.0X4-	T38.0X5-	T38.0X6-
androgenic	T38.7X1-	T38.7X2-	T38.7X3-	T38.7X4-	T38.7X5-	T38.7X6-
anterior pituitary NEC	T38.811-	T38.812-	T38.813-	T38.814-	T38.815-	T38.816-
antidiabetic agents	T38.3X1-	T38.3X2-	T38.3X3-	T38.3X4-	T38.3X5-	T38.3X6-
antidiuretic	T38.891-	T38.892-	T38.893-	T38.894-	T38.895-	T38.896-
cancer therapy	T45.1X1-	T45.1X2-	T45.1X3-	T45.1X4-	T45.1X5-	T45.1X6-
follicle stimulating	T38.811-	T38.812-	T38.813-	T38.814-	T38.815-	T38.816-
gonadotropic	T38.891-	T38.892-	T38.893-	T38.894-	T38.895-	T38.896-
pituitary	T38.811-	T38.812-	T38.813-	T38.814-	T38.815-	T38.816-
growth	T38.811-	T38.812-	T38.813-	T38.814-	T38.815-	T38.816-
luteinizing	T38.811-	T38.812-	T38.813-	T38.814-	T38.815-	T38.816-
ovarian	T38.5X1-	T38.5X2-	T38.5X3-	T38.5X4-	T38.5X5-	T38.5X6-
oxytocic	T48.0X1-	T48.0X2-	T48.0X3-	T48.0X4-	T48.0X5-	T48.0X6-
parathyroid (derivatives)	T50.991-	T50.992-	T50.993-	T50.994-	T50.995-	T50.996-
pituitary (posterior) NEC	T38.891-	T38.892-	T38.893-	T38.894-	T38.895-	T38.896-
anterior	T38.811-	T38.812-	T38.813-	T38.814-	T38.815-	T38.816-
specified, NEC	T38.891-	T38.892-	T38.893-	T38.894-	T38.895-	T38.896-
thyroid	T38.1X1-	T38.1X2-	T38.1X3-	T38.1X4-	T38.1X5-	T38.1X6-
Hornet (sting)	T63.451-	T63.452-	T63.453-	T63.454-	-	-
Horse anti-human lymphocytic serum	T50.Z11-	T50.Z12-	T50.Z13-	T50.Z14-	T50.Z15-	T50.Z16-
Horticulture agent NEC	T65.91X-	T65.92X-	T65.93X-	T65.94X-	-	-
with pesticide	T60.91X-	T60.92X-	T60.93X-	T60.94X-	-	-
Human						
albumin	T45.8X1-	T45.8X2-	T45.8X3-	T45.8X4-	T45.8X5-	T45.8X6-
growth hormone (HGH)	T38.811-	T38.812-	T38.813-	T38.814-	T38.815-	T38.816-
immune serum	T50.Z11-	T50.Z12-	T50.Z13-	T50.Z14-	T50.Z15-	T50.Z16-
Hyaluronidase	T45.3X1-	T45.3X2-	T45.3X3-	T45.3X4-	T45.3X5-	T45.3X6-
Hyazyme	T45.3X1-	T45.3X2-	T45.3X3-	T45.3X4-	T45.3X5-	T45.3X6-
Hycodan	T40.2X1-	T40.2X2-	T40.2X3-	T40.2X4-	T40.2X5-	T40.2X6-
Hydantoin derivative NEC	T42.0X1-	T42.0X2-	T42.0X3-	T42.0X4-	T42.0X5-	T42.0X6-
Hydeltra	T38.0X1-	T38.0X2-	T38.0X3-	T38.0X4-	T38.0X5-	T38.0X6-
Hydergine	T44.6X1-	T44.6X2-	T44.6X3-	T44.6X4-	T44.6X5-	T44.6X6-
Hydrabamine penicillin	T36.0X1-	T36.0X2-	T36.0X3-	T36.0X4-	T36.0X5-	T36.0X6-
Hydralazine	T46.5X1-	T46.5X2-	T46.5X3-	T46.5X4-	T46.5X5-	T46.5X6-
Hydrargaphen	T49.0X1-	T49.0X2-	T49.0X3-	T49.0X4-	T49.0X5-	T49.0X6-
Hydrargyri amino-chloridum	T49.0X1-	T49.0X2-	T49.0X3-	T49.0X4-	T49.0X5-	T49.0X6-
Hydrastine	T48.291-	T48.292-	T48.293-	T48.294-	T48.295-	T48.296-
Hydrazine	T54.1X1-	T54.1X2-	T54.1X3-	T54.1X4-	-	-
monoamine oxidase inhibitors	T43.1X1-	T43.1X2-	T43.1X3-	T43.1X4-	T43.1X5-	T43.1X6-
Hydrazoic acid, azides	T54.2X1-	T54.2X2-	T54.2X3-	T54.2X4-	-	-
Hydriodic acid	T48.4X1-	T48.4X2-	T48.4X3-	T48.4X4-	T48.4X5-	T48.4X6-
Hydrocarbon gas	T59.891-	T59.892-	T59.893-	T59.894-	-	-
incomplete combustion of — *see Carbon, monoxide, fuel, utility*						
liquefied (mobile container)	T59.891-	T59.892-	T59.893-	T59.894-	-	-
piped (natural)	T59.891-	T59.892-	T59.893-	T59.894-	-	-
Hydrochloric acid (liquid)	T54.2X1-	T54.2X2-	T54.2X3-	T54.2X4-	-	-
medicinal (digestant)	T47.5X1-	T47.5X2-	T47.5X3-	T47.5X4-	T47.5X5-	T47.5X6-
vapor	T59.891-	T59.892-	T59.893-	T59.894-	-	-
Hydrochlorothiazide	T50.2X1-	T50.2X2-	T50.2X3-	T50.2X4-	T50.2X5-	T50.2X6-
Hydrocodone	T40.2X1-	T40.2X2-	T40.2X3-	T40.2X4-	T40.2X5-	T40.2X6-

Substance	Poisoning Accidental (unintentional)	Poisoning Intentional self-harm	Poisoning Assault	Poisoning Undetermined	Adverse effect	Underdosing
Hydrocortisone (derivatives)	T38.0X1-	T38.0X2-	T38.0X3-	T38.0X4-	T38.0X5-	T38.0X6-
aceponate	T49.0X1-	T49.0X2-	T49.0X3-	T49.0X4-	T49.0X5-	T49.0X6-
ENT agent	T49.6X1-	T49.6X2-	T49.6X3-	T49.6X4-	T49.6X5-	T49.6X6-
ophthalmic preparation	T49.5X1-	T49.5X2-	T49.5X3-	T49.5X4-	T49.5X5-	T49.5X6-
topical NEC	T49.0X1-	T49.0X2-	T49.0X3-	T49.0X4-	T49.0X5-	T49.0X6-
Hydrocortone	T38.0X1-	T38.0X2-	T38.0X3-	T38.0X4-	T38.0X5-	T38.0X6-
ENT agent	T49.6X1-	T49.6X2-	T49.6X3-	T49.6X4-	T49.6X5-	T49.6X6-
ophthalmic preparation	T49.5X1-	T49.5X2-	T49.5X3-	T49.5X4-	T49.5X5-	T49.5X6-
topical NEC	T49.0X1-	T49.0X2-	T49.0X3-	T49.0X4-	T49.0X5-	T49.0X6-
Hydrocyanic acid (liquid)	T57.3X1-	T57.3X2-	T57.3X3-	T57.3X4-	-	-
gas	T65.0X1-	T65.0X2-	T65.0X3-	T65.0X4-	-	-
Hydroflumethiazide	T50.2X1-	T50.2X2-	T50.2X3-	T50.2X4-	T50.2X5-	T50.2X6-
Hydrofluoric acid (liquid)	T54.2X1-	T54.2X2-	T54.2X3-	T54.2X4-	-	-
vapor	T59.891-	T59.892-	T59.893-	T59.894-	-	-
Hydrogen	T59.891-	T59.892-	T59.893-	T59.894-	-	-
arsenide	T57.0X1-	T57.0X2-	T57.0X3-	T57.0X4-	-	-
arseniureted	T57.0X1-	T57.0X2-	T57.0X3-	T57.0X4-	-	-
chloride	T57.8X1-	T57.8X2-	T57.8X3-	T57.8X4-	-	-
cyanide (salts)	T57.3X1-	T57.3X2-	T57.3X3-	T57.3X4-	-	-
gas	T57.3X1-	T57.3X2-	T57.3X3-	T57.3X4-	-	-
Fluoride	T59.5X1-	T59.5X2-	T59.5X3-	T59.5X4-	-	-
vapor	T59.5X1-	T59.5X2-	T59.5X3-	T59.5X4-	-	-
peroxide	T49.0X1-	T49.0X2-	T49.0X3-	T49.0X4-	T49.0X5-	T49.0X6-
phosphureted	T57.1X1-	T57.1X2-	T57.1X3-	T57.1X4-	-	-
sulfide	T59.6X1-	T59.6X2-	T59.6X3-	T59.6X4-	-	-
arseniureted	T57.0X1-	T57.0X2-	T57.0X3-	T57.0X4-	-	-
sulfureted	T59.6X1-	T59.6X2-	T59.6X3-	T59.6X4-	-	-
Hydromethylpyridine	T46.7X1-	T46.7X2-	T46.7X3-	T46.7X4-	T46.7X5-	T46.7X6-
Hydromorphinol	T40.2X1-	T40.2X2-	T40.2X3-	T40.2X4-	-	-
Hydromorphinone	T40.2X1-	T40.2X2-	T40.2X3-	T40.2X4-	T40.2X5-	T40.2X6-
Hydromorphone	T40.2X1-	T40.2X2-	T40.2X3-	T40.2X4-	T40.2X5-	T40.2X6-
Hydromox	T50.2X1-	T50.2X2-	T50.2X3-	T50.2X4-	T50.2X5-	T50.2X6-
Hydrophilic lotion	T49.3X1-	T49.3X2-	T49.3X3-	T49.3X4-	T49.3X5-	T49.3X6-
Hydroquinidine	T46.2X1-	T46.2X2-	T46.2X3-	T46.2X4-	T46.2X5-	T46.2X6-
Hydroquinone	T52.2X1-	T52.2X2-	T52.2X3-	T52.2X4-	-	-
vapor	T59.891-	T59.892-	T59.893-	T59.894-	-	-
Hydrosulfuric acid (gas)	T59.6X1-	T59.6X2-	T59.6X3-	T59.6X4-	-	-
Hydrotalcite	T47.1X1-	T47.1X2-	T47.1X3-	T47.1X4-	T47.1X5-	T47.1X6-
Hydrous wool fat	T49.3X1-	T49.3X2-	T49.3X3-	T49.3X4-	T49.3X5-	T49.3X6-
Hydroxide, caustic	T54.3X1-	T54.3X2-	T54.3X3-	T54.3X4-	-	-
Hydroxocobalamin	T45.8X1-	T45.8X2-	T45.8X3-	T45.8X4-	T45.8X5-	T45.8X6-
Hydroxyamphetamine	T49.5X1-	T49.5X2-	T49.5X3-	T49.5X4-	T49.5X5-	T49.5X6-
Hydroxycarbamide	T45.1X1-	T45.1X2-	T45.1X3-	T45.1X4-	T45.1X5-	T45.1X6-
Hydroxychloroquine	T37.8X1-	T37.8X2-	T37.8X3-	T37.8X4-	T37.8X5-	T37.8X6-
Hydroxydihydrocodeinone	T40.2X1-	T40.2X2-	T40.2X3-	T40.2X4-	T40.2X5-	T40.2X6-
Hydroxyestrone	T38.5X1-	T38.5X2-	T38.5X3-	T38.5X4-	T38.5X5-	T38.5X6-
Hydroxyethyl starch	T45.8X1-	T45.8X2-	T45.8X3-	T45.8X4-	T45.8X5-	T45.8X6-
Hydroxymethylpenta-none	T52.4X1-	T52.4X2-	T52.4X3-	T52.4X4-	-	-
Hydroxyphenamate	T43.591-	T43.592-	T43.593-	T43.594-	T43.595-	T43.596-
Hydroxyphenylbutazone	T39.2X1-	T39.2X2-	T39.2X3-	T39.2X4-	T39.2X5-	T39.2X6-
Hydroxyprogesterone	T38.5X1-	T38.5X2-	T38.5X3-	T38.5X4-	T38.5X5-	T38.5X6-
caproate	T38.5X1-	T38.5X2-	T38.5X3-	T38.5X4-	T38.5X5-	T38.5X6-
Hydroxyquinoline (derivatives) NEC	T37.8X1-	T37.8X2-	T37.8X3-	T37.8X4-	T37.8X5-	T37.8X6-
Hydroxystilbamidine	T37.3X1-	T37.3X2-	T37.3X3-	T37.3X4-	T37.3X5-	T37.3X6-
Hydroxytoluene (nonmedicinal)	T54.0X1-	T54.0X2-	T54.0X3-	T54.0X4-	-	-
medicinal	T49.0X1-	T49.0X2-	T49.0X3-	T49.0X4-	T49.0X5-	T49.0X6-
Hydroxyurea	T45.1X1-	T45.1X2-	T45.1X3-	T45.1X4-	T45.1X5-	T45.1X6-
Hydroxyzine	T43.591-	T43.592-	T43.593-	T43.594-	T43.595-	T43.596-

Substance	Poisoning Accidental (unintentional)	Poisoning Intentional self-harm	Poisoning Assault	Poisoning Undetermined	Adverse effect	Underdosing
Hyoscine	T44.3X1-	T44.3X2-	T44.3X3-	T44.3X4-	T44.3X5-	T44.3X6-
Hyoscyamine	T44.3X1-	T44.3X2-	T44.3X3-	T44.3X4-	T44.3X5-	T44.3X6-
Hyoscyamus	T44.3X1-	T44.3X2-	T44.3X3-	T44.3X4-	T44.3X5-	T44.3X6-
dry extract	T44.3X1-	T44.3X2-	T44.3X3-	T44.3X4-	T44.3X5-	T44.3X6-
Hypaque	T50.8X1-	T50.8X2-	T50.8X3-	T50.8X4-	T50.8X5-	T50.8X6-
Hypertussis	T50.Z11-	T50.Z12-	T50.Z13-	T50.Z14-	T50.Z15-	T50.Z16-
Hypnotic	T42.71X-	T42.72X-	T42.73X-	T42.74X-	T42.75X-	T42.76X-
anticonvulsant	T42.71X-	T42.72X-	T42.73X-	T42.74X-	T42.75X-	T42.76X-
specified NEC	T42.6X1-	T42.6X2-	T42.6X3-	T42.6X4-	T42.6X5-	T42.6X6-
Hypochlorite	T49.0X1-	T49.0X2-	T49.0X3-	T49.0X4-	T49.0X5-	T49.0X6-
Hypophysis, posterior	T38.891-	T38.892-	T38.893-	T38.894-	T38.895-	T38.896-
Hypotensive NEC	T46.5X1-	T46.5X2-	T46.5X4-	T46.5X4-	T46.5X5-	T46.5X6-
Hypromellose	T49.5X1-	T49.5X2-	T49.5X3-	T49.5X4-	T49.5X5-	T49.5X6-
Ibacitabine	T37.5X1-	T37.5X2-	T37.5X3-	T37.5X4-	T37.5X5-	T37.5X6-
Ibopamine	T44.991-	T44.992-	T44.993-	T44.994-	T44.995-	T44.996-
Ibufenac	T39.311-	T39.312-	T39.313-	T39.314-	T39.315-	T39.316-
Ibuprofen	T39.311-	T39.312-	T39.313-	T39.314-	T39.315-	T39.316-
Ibuproxam	T39.311-	T39.312-	T39.313-	T39.314-	T39.315-	T39.316-
Ibuterol	T48.6X1-	T48.6X2-	T48.6X3-	T48.6X4-	T48.6X5-	T48.6X6-
Ichthammol	T49.0X1-	T49.0X2-	T49.0X3-	T49.0X4-	T49.0X5-	T49.0X6-
Ichthyol	T49.4X1-	T49.4X2-	T49.4X3-	T49.4X4-	T49.4X5-	T49.4X6-
Idarubicin	T45.1X1-	T45.1X2-	T45.1X3-	T45.1X4-	T45.1X5-	T45.1X6-
Idrocilamide	T42.8X1-	T42.8X2-	T42.8X3-	T42.8X4-	T42.8X5-	T42.8X6-
Ifenprodil	T46.7X1-	T46.7X2-	T46.7X3-	T46.7X4-	T46.7X5-	T46.7X6-
Ifosfamide	T45.1X1-	T45.1X2-	T45.1X3-	T45.1X4-	T45.1X5-	T45.1X6-
Iletin	T38.3X1-	T38.3X2-	T38.3X3-	T38.3X4-	T38.3X5-	T38.3X6-
Ilex	T62.2X1-	T62.2X2-	T62.2X3-	T62.2X4-	-	-
Illuminating gas (after combustion)	T58.11X-	T58.12X-	T58.13X-	T58.14X-	-	-
prior to combustion	T59.891-	T59.892-	T59.893-	T59.894-	-	-
Ilopan	T45.2X1-	T45.2X2-	T45.2X3-	T45.2X4-	T45.2X5-	T45.2X6-
Iloprost	T46.7X1-	T46.7X2-	T46.7X3-	T46.7X4-	T46.7X5-	T46.7X6-
Ilotycin	T36.3X1-	T36.3X2-	T36.3X3-	T36.3X4-	T36.3X5-	T36.3X6-
ophthalmic preparation	T49.5X1-	T49.5X2-	T49.5X3-	T49.5X4-	T49.5X5-	T49.5X6-
topical NEC	T49.0X1-	T49.0X2-	T49.0X3-	T49.0X4-	T49.0X5-	T49.0X6-
Imidazole-4-carboxamide	T45.1X1-	T45.1X2-	T45.1X3-	T45.1X4-	T45.1X5-	T45.1X6-
Imipenem	T36.0X1-	T36.0X2-	T36.0X3-	T36.0X4-	T36.0X5-	T36.0X6-
Imipramine	T43.011-	T43.012-	T43.013-	T43.014-	T43.015-	T43.016-
Iminostilbene	T42.1X1-	T42.1X2-	T42.1X3-	T42.1X4-	T42.1X5-	T42.1X6-
Immu-G	T50.Z11-	T50.Z12-	T50.Z13-	T50.Z14-	T50.Z15-	T50.Z16-
Immuglobin	T50.Z11-	T50.Z12-	T50.Z13-	T50.Z14-	T50.Z15-	T50.Z16-
Immune						
globulin	T50.Z11-	T50.Z12-	T50.Z13-	T50.Z14-	T50.Z15-	T50.Z16-
serum globulin	T50.Z11-	T50.Z12-	T50.Z13-	T50.Z14-	T50.Z15-	T50.Z16-
Immunoglobin human (intravenous) (normal)	T50.Z11-	T50.Z12-	T50.Z13-	T50.Z14-	T50.Z15-	T50.Z16-
unmodified	T50.Z11-	T50.Z12-	T50.Z13-	T50.Z14-	T50.Z15-	T50.Z16-
Immunosuppressive drug	T45.1X1-	T45.1X2-	T45.1X3-	T45.1X4-	T45.1X5-	T45.1X6-
Immu-tetanus	T50.Z11-	T50.Z12-	T50.Z13-	T50.Z14-	T50.Z15-	T50.Z16-
Indalpine	T43.221-	T43.222-	T43.223-	T43.224-	T43.225-	T43.226-
Indanazoline	T48.5X1-	T48.5X2-	T48.5X3-	T48.5X4-	T48.5X5-	T48.5X6-
Indandione (derivatives)	T45.511-	T45.512-	T45.513-	T45.514-	T45.515-	T45.516-
Indapamide	T46.5X1-	T46.5X2-	T46.5X3-	T46.5X4-	T46.5X5-	T46.5X6-
Indendione (derivatives)	T45.511-	T45.512-	T45.513-	T45.514-	T45.515-	T45.516-
Indenolol	T44.7X1-	T44.7X2-	T44.7X3-	T44.7X4-	T44.7X5-	T44.7X6-
Inderal	T44.7X1-	T44.7X2-	T44.7X3-	T44.7X4-	T44.7X5-	T44.7X6-
Indian						
hemp	T40.7X1-	T40.7X2-	T40.7X3-	T40.7X4-	T40.7X5-	T40.7X6-
tobacco	T62.2X1-	T62.2X2-	T62.2X3-	T62.2X4-	-	-

Substance	Poisoning Accidental (unintentional)	Poisoning Intentional self-harm	Poisoning Assault	Poisoning Undetermined	Adverse effect	Underdosing
Indigo carmine	T50.8X1-	T50.8X2-	T50.8X3-	T50.8X4-	T50.8X5-	T50.8X6-
Indobufen	T45.521-	T45.522-	T45.523-	T45.524-	T45.525-	T45.526-
Indocin	T39.2X1-	T39.2X2-	T39.2X3-	T39.2X4-	T39.2X5-	T39.2X6-
Indocyanine green	T50.8X1-	T50.8X2-	T50.8X3-	T50.8X4-	T50.8X5-	T50.8X6-
Indometacin	T39.391-	T39.392-	T39.393-	T39.394-	T39.395-	T39.396-
Indomethacin	T39.391-	T39.392-	T39.393-	T39.394-	T39.395-	T39.396-
farnesil	T39.4X1-	T39.4X2-	T39.4X3-	T39.4X4-	T39.4X5-	T39.4X6-
Indoramin	T44.6X1-	T44.6X2-	T44.6X3-	T44.6X4-	T44.6X5-	T44.6X6-
Industrial						
alcohol	T51.0X1-	T51.0X2-	T51.0X3-	T51.0X4-	-	-
fumes	T59.891-	T59.892-	T59.893-	T59.894-	-	-
solvents (fumes) (vapors)	T52.91X-	T52.92X-	T52.93X-	T52.94X-	-	-
Influenza vaccine	T50.B91-	T50.B92-	T50.B93-	T50.B94-	T50.B95-	T50.B96-
Ingested substance NEC	T65.91X-	T65.92X-	T65.93X-	T65.94X-	-	-
INH	T37.1X1-	T37.1X2-	T37.1X3-	T37.1X4-	T37.1X5-	T37.1X6-
Inhalation, gas (noxious) — *see Gas*						
Inhibitor						
angiotensin-converting enzyme	T46.4X1-	T46.4X2-	T46.4X3-	T46.4X4-	T46.4X5-	T46.4X6-
carbonic anhydrase	T50.2X1-	T50.2X2-	T50.2X3-	T50.2X4-	T50.2X5-	T50.2X6-
fibrinolysis	T45.621-	T45.622-	T45.623-	T45.624-	T45.625-	T45.626-
monoamine oxidase NEC	T43.1X1-	T43.1X2-	T43.1X3-	T43.1X4-	T43.1X5-	T43.1X6-
hydrazine	T43.1X1-	T43.1X2-	T43.1X3-	T43.1X4-	T43.1X5-	T43.1X6-
postsynaptic	T43.8X1-	T43.8X2-	T43.8X3-	T43.8X4-	T43.8X5-	T43.8X6-
prothrombin synthesis	T45.511-	T45.512-	T45.513-	T45.514-	T45.515-	T45.516-
Ink	T65.891-	T65.892-	T65.893-	T65.894-	-	-
Inorganic substance NEC	T57.91X-	T57.92X-	T57.93X-	T57.94X-	-	-
Inosine pranobex	T37.5X1-	T37.5X2-	T37.5X3-	T37.5X4-	T37.5X5-	T37.5X6-
Inositol	T50.991-	T50.992-	T50.993-	T50.994-	T50.995-	T50.996-
nicotinate	T46.7X1-	T46.7X2-	T46.7X3-	T46.7X4-	T46.7X5-	T46.7X6-
Inproquone	T45.1X1-	T45.1X2-	T45.1X3-	T45.1X4-	T45.1X5-	T45.1X6-
Insect (sting) , venomous	T63.481-	T63.482-	T63.483-	T63.484-	-	-
ant	T63.421-	T63.422-	T63.423-	T63.424-	-	-
bee	T63.441-	T63.442-	T63.443-	T63.444-	-	-
caterpillar	T63.431-	T63.432-	T63.433-	T63.434-	-	-
hornet	T63.451-	T63.452-	T63.453-	T63.454-	-	-
wasp	T63.461-	T63.462-	T63.463-	T63.464-	-	-
Insecticide NEC	T60.91X-	T60.92X-	T60.93X-	T60.94X-	-	-
carbamate	T60.0X1-	T60.0X2-	T60.0X3-	T60.0X4-	-	-
chlorinated	T60.1X1-	T60.1X2-	T60.1X3-	T60.1X4-	-	-
mixed	T60.91X-	T60.92X-	T60.93X-	T60.94X-	-	-
organochlorine	T60.1X1-	T60.1X2-	T60.1X3-	T60.1X4-	-	-
organophosphorus	T60.0X1-	T60.0X2-	T60.0X3-	T60.0X4-	-	-
Insular tissue extract	T38.3X1-	T38.3X2-	T38.3X3-	T38.3X4-	T38.3X5-	T38.3X6-
Insulin (amorphous) (globin) (isophane) (Lente) (NPH) (Semilente) (Ultralente)	T38.3X1-	T38.3X2-	T38.3X3-	T38.3X4-	T38.3X5-	T38.3X6-
defalan	T38.3X1-	T38.3X2-	T38.3X3-	T38.3X4-	T38.3X5-	T38.3X6-
human	T38.3X1-	T38.3X2-	T38.3X3-	T38.3X4-	T38.3X5-	T38.3X6-
injection, soluble	T38.3X1-	T38.3X2-	T38.3X3-	T38.3X4-	T38.3X5-	T38.3X6-
biphasic	T38.3X1-	T38.3X2-	T38.3X3-	T38.3X4-	T38.3X5-	T38.3X6-
intermediate acting	T38.3X1-	T38.3X2-	T38.3X3-	T38.3X4-	T38.3X5-	T38.3X6-
protamine zinc	T38.3X1-	T38.3X2-	T38.3X3-	T38.3X4-	T38.3X5-	T38.3X6-
slow acting	T38.3X1-	T38.3X2-	T38.3X3-	T38.3X4-	T38.3X5-	T38.3X6-
zinc						
protamine injection	T38.3X1-	T38.3X2-	T38.3X3-	T38.3X4-	T38.3X5-	T38.3X6-
suspension (amorphous) (crystalline)	T38.3X1-	T38.3X2-	T38.3X3-	T38.3X4-	T38.3X5-	T38.3X6-
Interferon (alpha) (beta) (gamma)	T37.5X1-	T37.5X2-	T37.5X3-	T37.5X4-	T37.5X5-	T37.5X6-

INDIGO CARMINE - INTERFERON

Substance	Poisoning Accidental (unintentional)	Poisoning Intentional self-harm	Poisoning Assault	Poisoning Undetermined	Adverse effect	Underdosing
Intestinal motility control drug	T47.6X1-	T47.6X2-	T47.6X3-	T47.6X4-	T47.6X5-	T47.6X6-
biological	T47.8X1-	T47.8X2-	T47.8X3-	T47.8X4-	T47.8X5-	T47.8X6-
Intranarcon	T41.1X1-	T41.1X2-	T41.1X3-	T41.1X4-	T41.1X5-	T41.1X6-
Intravenous						
amino acids	T50.991-	T50.992-	T50.993-	T50.994-	T50.995-	T50.996-
fat suspension	T50.991-	T50.992-	T50.993-	T50.994-	T50.995-	T50.996-
Inulin	T50.8X1-	T50.8X2-	T50.8X3-	T50.8X4-	T50.8X5-	T50.8X6-
Invert sugar	T50.3X1-	T50.3X2-	T50.3X3-	T50.3X4-	T50.3X5-	T50.3X6-
Inza — *see Naproxen*						
Iobenzamic acid	T50.8X1-	T50.8X2-	T50.8X3-	T50.8X4-	T50.8X5-	T50.8X6-
Iocarmic acid	T50.8X1-	T50.8X2-	T50.8X3-	T50.8X4-	T50.8X5-	T50.8X6-
Iocetamic acid	T50.8X1-	T50.8X2-	T50.8X3-	T50.8X4-	T50.8X5-	T50.8X6-
Iodamide	T50.8X1-	T50.8X2-	T50.8X3-	T50.8X4-	T50.8X5-	T50.8X6-
Iodide NEC — *see also Iodine*	T49.0X1-	T49.0X2-	T49.0X3-	T49.0X4-	T49.0X5-	T49.0X6-
mercury (ointment)	T49.0X1-	T49.0X2-	T49.0X3-	T49.0X4-	T49.0X5-	T49.0X6-
methylate	T49.0X1-	T49.0X2-	T49.0X3-	T49.0X4-	T49.0X5-	T49.0X6-
potassium (expectorant) NEC	T48.4X1-	T48.4X2-	T48.4X3-	T48.4X4-	T48.4X5-	T48.4X6-
Iodinated						
contrast medium	T50.8X1-	T50.8X2-	T50.8X3-	T50.8X4-	T50.8X5-	T50.8X6-
glycerol	T48.4X1-	T48.4X2-	T48.4X3-	T48.4X4-	T48.4X5-	T48.4X6-
human serum albumin (131I)	T50.8X1-	T50.8X2-	T50.8X3-	T50.8X4-	T50.8X5-	T50.8X6-
Iodine (antiseptic, external) (tincture) NEC	T49.0X1-	T49.0X2-	T49.0X3-	T49.0X4-	T49.0X5-	T49.0X6-
125 — *see also Radiation sickness, and Exposure to radioactivce isotopes*	T50.8X1-	T50.8X2-	T50.8X3-	T50.8X4-	T50.8X5-	T50.8X6-
therapeutic	T50.991-	T50.992-	T50.993-	T50.994-	T50.995-	T50.996-
131 — *see also Radiation sickness, and Exposure to radioactivce isotopes*	T50.8X1-	T50.8X2-	T50.8X3-	T50.8X4-	T50.8X5-	T50.8X6-
therapeutic	T38.2X1-	T38.2X2-	T38.2X3-	T38.2X4-	T38.2X5-	T38.2X6-
diagnostic	T50.8X1-	T50.8X2-	T50.8X3-	T50.8X4-	T50.8X5-	T50.8X6-
for thyroid conditions (antithyroid)	T38.2X1-	T38.2X2-	T38.2X3-	T38.2X4-	T38.2X5-	T38.2X6-
solution	T49.0X1-	T49.0X2-	T49.0X3-	T49.0X4-	T49.0X5-	T49.0X6-
vapor	T59.891-	T59.892-	T59.893-	T59.894-	-	-
Iodipamide	T50.8X1-	T50.8X2-	T50.8X3-	T50.8X4-	T50.8X5-	T50.8X6-
Iodized (poppy seed) oil	T50.8X1-	T50.8X2-	T50.8X3-	T50.8X4-	T50.8X5-	T50.8X6-
Iodobismitol	T37.8X1-	T37.8X2-	T37.8X3-	T37.8X4-	T37.8X5-	T37.8X6-
Iodochlorhydroxyquin	T37.8X1-	T37.8X2-	T37.8X3-	T37.8X4-	T37.8X5-	T37.8X6-
topical	T49.0X1-	T49.0X2-	T49.0X3-	T49.0X4-	T49.0X5-	T49.0X6-
Iodochlorhydroxyquinoline	T37.8X1-	T37.8X2-	T37.8X3-	T37.8X4-	T37.8X5-	T37.8X6-
Iodocholesterol (131I)	T50.8X1-	T50.8X2-	T50.8X3-	T50.8X4-	T50.8X5-	T50.8X6-
Iodoform	T49.0X1-	T49.0X2-	T49.0X3-	T49.0X4-	T49.0X5-	T49.0X6-
Iodohippuric acid	T50.8X1-	T50.8X2-	T50.8X3-	T50.8X4-	T50.8X5-	T50.8X6-
Iodopanoic acid	T50.8X1-	T50.8X2-	T50.8X3-	T50.8X4-	T50.8X5-	T50.8X6-
Iodophthalein (sodium)	T50.8X1-	T50.8X2-	T50.8X3-	T50.8X4-	T50.8X5-	T50.8X6-
Iodopyracet	T50.8X1-	T50.8X2-	T50.8X3-	T50.8X4-	T50.8X5-	T50.8X6-
Iodoquinol	T37.8X1-	T37.8X2-	T37.8X3-	T37.8X4-	T37.8X5-	T37.8X6-
Iodoxamic acid	T50.8X1-	T50.8X2-	T50.8X3-	T50.8X4-	T50.8X5-	T50.8X6-
Iofendylate	T50.8X1-	T50.8X2-	T50.8X3-	T50.8X4-	T50.8X5-	T50.8X6-
Ioglycamic acid	T50.8X1-	T50.8X2-	T50.8X3-	T50.8X4-	T50.8X5-	T50.8X6-
Iohexol	T50.8X1-	T50.8X2-	T50.8X3-	T50.8X4-	T50.8X5-	T50.8X6-
Ion exchange resin						
anion	T47.8X1-	T47.8X2-	T47.8X3-	T47.8X4-	T47.8X5-	T47.8X6-
cation	T50.3X1-	T50.3X2-	T50.3X3-	T50.3X4-	T50.3X5-	T50.3X6-
cholestyramine	T46.6X1-	T46.6X2-	T46.6X3-	T46.6X4-	T46.6X5-	T46.6X6-
intestinal	T47.8X1-	T47.8X2-	T47.8X3-	T47.8X4-	T47.8X5-	T47.8X6-
Iopamidol	T50.8X1-	T50.8X2-	T50.8X3-	T50.8X4-	T50.8X5-	T50.8X6-
Iopanoic acid	T50.8X1-	T50.8X2-	T50.8X3-	T50.8X4-	T50.8X5-	T50.8X6-
Iophenoic acid	T50.8X1-	T50.8X2-	T50.8X3-	T50.8X4-	T50.8X5-	T50.8X6-
Iopodate, sodium	T50.8X1-	T50.8X2-	T50.8X3-	T50.8X4-	T50.8X5-	T50.8X6-

Substance	Poisoning Accidental (unintentional)	Poisoning Intentional self-harm	Poisoning Assault	Poisoning Undetermined	Adverse effect	Underdosing
Iopodic acid	T50.8X1-	T50.8X2-	T50.8X3-	T50.8X4-	T50.8X5-	T50.8X6-
Iopromide	T50.8X1-	T50.8X2-	T50.8X3-	T50.8X4-	T50.8X5-	T50.8X6-
Iopydol	T50.8X1-	T50.8X2-	T50.8X3-	T50.8X4-	T50.8X5-	T50.8X6-
Iotalamic acid	T50.8X1-	T50.8X2-	T50.8X3-	T50.8X4-	T50.8X5-	T50.8X6-
Iothalamate	T50.8X1-	T50.8X2-	T50.8X3-	T50.8X4-	T50.8X5-	T50.8X6-
Iothiouracil	T38.2X1-	T38.2X2-	T38.2X3-	T38.2X4-	T38.2X5-	T38.2X6-
Iotrol	T50.8X1-	T50.8X2-	T50.8X3-	T50.8X4-	T50.8X5-	T50.8X6-
Iotrolan	T50.8X1-	T50.8X2-	T50.8X3-	T50.8X4-	T50.8X5-	T50.8X6-
Iotroxate	T50.8X1-	T50.8X2-	T50.8X3-	T50.8X4-	T50.8X5-	T50.8X6-
Iotroxic acid	T50.8X1-	T50.8X2-	T50.8X3-	T50.8X4-	T50.8X5-	T50.8X6-
Ioversol	T50.8X1-	T50.8X2-	T50.8X3-	T50.8X4-	T50.8X5-	T50.8X6-
Ioxaglate	T50.8X1-	T50.8X2-	T50.8X3-	T50.8X4-	T50.8X5-	T50.8X6-
Ioxaglic acid	T50.8X1-	T50.8X2-	T50.8X3-	T50.8X4-	T50.8X5-	T50.8X6-
Ioxitalamic acid	T50.8X1-	T50.8X2-	T50.8X3-	T50.8X4-	T50.8X5-	T50.8X6-
Ipecac	T47.7X1-	T47.7X2-	T47.7X3-	T47.7X4-	T47.7X5-	T47.7X6-
Ipecacuanha	T48.4X1-	T48.4X2-	T48.4X3-	T48.4X4-	T48.4X5-	T48.4X6-
Ipodate, calcium	T50.8X1-	T50.8X2-	T50.8X3-	T50.8X4-	T50.8X5-	T50.8X6-
Ipral	T42.3X1-	T42.3X2-	T42.3X3-	T42.3X4-	T42.3X5-	T42.3X6-
Ipratropium (bromide)	T48.6X1-	T48.6X2-	T48.6X3-	T48.6X4-	T48.6X5-	T48.6X6-
Ipriflavone	T46.3X1-	T46.3X2-	T46.3X3-	T46.3X4-	T46.3X5-	T46.3X6-
Iprindole	T43.011-	T43.012-	T43.013-	T43.014-	T43.015-	T43.016-
Iproclozide	T43.1X1-	T43.1X2-	T43.1X3-	T43.1X4-	T43.1X5-	T43.1X6-
Iprofenin	T50.8X1-	T50.8X2-	T50.8X3-	T50.8X4-	T50.8X5-	T50.8X6-
Iproheptine	T49.2X1-	T49.2X2-	T49.2X3-	T49.2X4-	T49.2X5-	T49.2X6-
Iproniazid	T43.1X1-	T43.1X2-	T43.1X3-	T43.1X4-	T43.1X5-	T43.1X6-
Iproplatin	T45.1X1-	T45.1X2-	T45.1X3-	T45.1X4-	T45.1X5-	T45.1X6-
Iproveratril	T46.1X1-	T46.1X2-	T46.1X3-	T46.1X4-	T46.1X5-	T46.1X6-
Iron (compounds) (medicinal) NEC	T45.4X1-	T45.4X2-	T45.4X3-	T45.4X4-	T45.4X5-	T45.4X6-
ammonium	T45.4X1-	T45.4X2-	T45.4X3-	T45.4X4-	T45.4X5-	T45.4X6-
dextran injection	T45.4X1-	T45.4X2-	T45.4X3-	T45.4X4-	T45.4X5-	T45.4X6-
nonmedicinal	T56.891-	T56.892-	T56.893-	T56.894-	-	-
salts	T45.4X1-	T45.4X2-	T45.4X3-	T45.4X4-	T45.4X5-	T45.4X6-
sorbitex	T45.4X1-	T45.4X2-	T45.4X3-	T45.4X4-	T45.4X5-	T45.4X6-
sorbitol citric acid complex	T45.4X1-	T45.4X2-	T45.4X3-	T45.4X4-	T45.4X5-	T45.4X6-
Irrigating fluid (vaginal)	T49.8X1-	T49.8X2-	T49.8X3-	T49.8X4-	T49.8X5-	T49.8X6-
eye	T49.5X1-	T49.5X2-	T49.5X3-	T49.5X4-	T49.5X5-	T49.5X6-
Isepamicin	T36.5X1-	T36.5X2-	T36.5X3-	T36.5X4-	T36.5X5-	T36.5X6-
Isoaminile (citrate)	T48.3X1-	T48.3X2-	T48.3X3-	T48.3X4-	T48.3X5-	T48.3X6-
Isoamyl nitrite	T46.3X1-	T46.3X2-	T46.3X3-	T46.3X4-	T46.3X5-	T46.3X6-
Isobenzan	T60.1X1-	T60.1X2-	T60.1X3-	T60.1X4-	-	-
Isobutyl acetate	T52.8X1-	T52.8X2-	T52.8X3-	T52.8X4-	-	-
Isocarboxazid	T43.1X1-	T43.1X2-	T43.1X3-	T43.1X4-	T43.1X5-	T43.1X6-
Isoconazole	T49.0X1-	T49.0X2-	T49.0X3-	T49.0X4-	T49.0X5-	T49.0X6-
Isocyanate	T65.0X1-	T65.0X2-	T65.0X3-	T65.0X4-	-	-
Isoephedrine	T44.991-	T44.992-	T44.993-	T44.994-	T44.995-	T44.996-
Isoetarine	T48.6X1-	T48.6X2-	T48.6X3-	T48.6X4-	T48.6X5-	T48.6X6-
Isoethadione	T42.2X1-	T42.2X2-	T42.2X3-	T42.2X4-	T42.2X5-	T42.2X6-
Isoetharine	T44.5X1-	T44.5X2-	T44.5X3-	T44.5X4-	T44.5X5-	T44.5X6-
Isoflurane	T41.0X1-	T41.0X2-	T41.0X3-	T41.0X4-	T41.0X5-	T41.0X6-
Isoflurophate	T44.0X1-	T44.0X2-	T44.0X3-	T44.0X4-	T44.0X5-	T44.0X6-
Isomaltose, ferric complex	T45.4X1-	T45.4X2-	T45.4X3-	T45.4X4-	T45.4X5-	T45.4X6-
Isometheptene	T44.3X1-	T44.3X2-	T44.3X3-	T44.3X4-	T44.3X5-	T44.3X6-
Isoniazid	T37.1X1-	T37.1X2-	T37.1X3-	T37.1X4-	T37.1X5-	T37.1X6-
with						
rifampicin	T36.6X1-	T36.6X2-	T36.6X3-	T36.6X4-	T36.6X5-	T36.6X6-
thioacetazone	T37.1X1-	T37.1X2-	T37.1X3-	T37.1X4-	T37.1X5-	T37.1X6-
Isonicotinic acid hydrazide	T37.1X1-	T37.1X2-	T37.1X3-	T37.1X4-	T37.1X5-	T37.1X6-
Isonipecaine	T40.4X1-	T40.4X2-	T40.4X3-	T40.4X4-	T40.4X5-	T40.4X6-
Isopentaquine	T37.2X1-	T37.2X2-	T37.2X3-	T37.2X4-	T37.2X5-	T37.2X6-

Substance	Poisoning Accidental (unintentional)	Poisoning Intentional self-harm	Poisoning Assault	Poisoning Undetermined	Adverse effect	Underdosing
Isophane insulin	T38.3X1-	T38.3X2-	T38.3X3-	T38.3X4-	T38.3X5-	T38.3X6-
Isophorone	T65.891-	T65.892-	T65.893-	T65.894-	-	-
Isophosphamide	T45.1X1-	T45.1X2-	T45.1X3-	T45.1X4-	T45.1X5-	T45.1X6-
Isopregnenone	T38.5X1-	T38.5X2-	T38.5X3-	T38.5X4-	T38.5X5-	T38.5X6-
Isoprenaline	T48.6X1-	T48.6X2-	T48.6X3-	T48.6X4-	T48.6X5-	T48.6X6-
Isopromethazine	T43.3X1-	T43.3X2-	T43.3X3-	T43.3X4-	T43.3X5-	T43.3X6-
Isopropamide	T44.3X1-	T44.3X2-	T44.3X3-	T44.3X4-	T44.3X5-	T44.3X6-
iodide	T44.3X1-	T44.3X2-	T44.3X3-	T44.3X4-	T44.3X5-	T44.3X6-
Isopropanol	T51.2X1-	T51.2X2-	T51.2X3-	T51.2X4-	-	-
Isopropyl						
acetate	T52.8X1-	T52.8X2-	T52.8X3-	T52.8X4-	-	-
alcohol	T51.2X1-	T51.2X2-	T51.2X3-	T51.2X4-	-	-
medicinal	T49.4X1-	T49.4X2-	T49.4X3-	T49.4X4-	T49.4X5-	T49.4X6-
ether	T52.8X1-	T52.8X2-	T52.8X3-	T52.8X4-	-	-
Isopropylaminophenazone	T39.2X1-	T39.2X2-	T39.2X3-	T39.2X4-	T39.2X5-	T39.2X6-
Isoproterenol	T48.6X1-	T48.6X2-	T48.6X3-	T48.6X4-	T48.6X5-	T48.6X6-
Isosorbide dinitrate	T46.3X1-	T46.3X2-	T46.3X3-	T46.3X4-	T46.3X5-	T46.3X6-
Isothipendyl	T45.0X1-	T45.0X2-	T45.0X3-	T45.0X4-	T45.0X5-	T45.0X6-
Isotretinoin	T50.991-	T50.992-	T50.993-	T50.994-	T50.995-	T50.996-
Isoxazolyl penicillin	T36.0X1-	T36.0X2-	T36.0X3-	T36.0X4-	T36.0X5-	T36.0X6-
Isoxicam	T39.391-	T39.392-	T39.393-	T39.394-	T39.395-	T39.396-
Isoxsuprine	T46.7X1-	T46.7X2-	T46.7X3-	T46.7X4-	T46.7X5-	T46.7X6-
Ispagula	T47.4X1-	T47.4X2-	T47.4X3-	T47.4X4-	T47.4X5-	T47.4X6-
husk	T47.4X1-	T47.4X2-	T47.4X3-	T47.4X4-	T47.4X5-	T47.4X6-
Isradipine	T46.1X1-	T46.1X2-	T46.1X3-	T46.1X4-	T46.1X5-	T46.1X6-
I-thyroxine sodium	T38.1X1-	T38.1X2-	T38.1X3-	T38.1X4-	T38.1X5-	T38.1X6-
Itraconazole	T37.8X1-	T37.8X2-	T37.8X3-	T37.8X4-	T37.8X5-	T37.8X6-
Itramin tosilate	T46.3X1-	T46.3X2-	T46.3X3-	T46.3X4-	T46.3X5-	T46.3X6-
Ivermectin	T37.4X1-	T37.4X2-	T37.4X3-	T37.4X4-	T37.4X5-	T37.4X6-
Izoniazid	T37.1X1-	T37.1X2-	T37.1X3-	T37.1X4-	T37.1X5-	T37.1X6-
with thioacetazone	T37.1X1-	T37.1X2-	T37.1X3-	T37.1X4-	T37.1X5-	T37.1X6-
Jalap	T47.2X1-	T47.2X2-	T47.2X3-	T47.2X4-	T47.2X5-	T47.2X6-
Jamaica						
dogwood (bark)	T39.8X1-	T39.8X2-	T39.8X3-	T39.8X4-	T39.8X5-	T39.8X6-
ginger	T65.891-	T65.892-	T65.893-	T65.894-	-	-
root	T62.2X1-	T62.2X2-	T62.2X3-	T62.2X4-	-	-
Jatropha	T62.2X1-	T62.2X2-	T62.2X3-	T62.2X4-	-	-
curcas	T62.2X1-	T62.2X2-	T62.2X3-	T62.2X4-	-	-
Jectofer	T45.4X1-	T45.4X2-	T45.4X3-	T45.4X4-	T45.4X5-	T45.4X6-
Jellyfish (sting)	T63.621-	T63.622-	T63.623-	T63.624-	-	-
Jequirity (bean)	T62.2X1-	T62.2X2-	T62.2X3-	T62.2X4-	-	-
Jimson weed (stramonium)	T62.2X1-	T62.2X2-	T62.2X3-	T62.2X4-	-	-
seeds	T62.2X1-	T62.2X2-	T62.2X3-	T62.2X4-	-	-
Josamycin	T36.3X1-	T36.3X2-	T36.3X3-	T36.3X4-	T36.3X5-	T36.3X6-
Juniper tar	T49.1X1-	T49.1X2-	T49.1X3-	T49.1X4-	T49.1X5-	T49.1X6-
Kallidinogenase	T46.7X1-	T46.7X2-	T46.7X3-	T46.7X4-	T46.7X5-	T46.7X6-
Kallikrein	T46.7X1-	T46.7X2-	T46.7X3-	T46.7X4-	T46.7X5-	T46.7X6-
Kanamycin	T36.5X1-	T36.5X2-	T36.5X3-	T36.5X4-	T36.5X5-	T36.5X6-
Kantrex	T36.5X1-	T36.5X2-	T36.5X3-	T36.5X4-	T36.5X5-	T36.5X6-
Kaolin	T47.6X1-	T47.6X2-	T47.6X3-	T47.6X4-	T47.6X5-	T47.6X6-
light	T47.6X1-	T47.6X2-	T47.6X3-	T47.6X4-	T47.6X5-	T47.6X6-
Karaya (gum)	T47.4X1-	T47.4X2-	T47.4X3-	T47.4X4-	T47.4X5-	T47.4X6-
Kebuzone	T39.2X1-	T39.2X2-	T39.2X3-	T39.2X4-	T39.2X5-	T39.2X6-
Kelevan	T60.1X1-	T60.1X2-	T60.1X3-	T60.1X4-	-	-
Kemithal	T41.1X1-	T41.1X2-	T41.1X3-	T41.1X4-	T41.1X5-	T41.1X6-
Kenacort	T38.0X1-	T38.0X2-	T38.0X3-	T38.0X4-	T38.0X5-	T38.0X6-

ISOPHANE INSULIN - KENACORT

Substance	Poisoning Accidental (unintentional)	Poisoning Intentional self-harm	Poisoning Assault	Poisoning Undetermined	Adverse effect	Underdosing
Keratolytic drug NEC	T49.4X1-	T49.4X2-	T49.4X3-	T49.4X4-	T49.4X5-	T49.4X6-
anthracene	T49.4X1-	T49.4X2-	T49.4X3-	T49.4X4-	T49.4X5-	T49.4X6-
Keratoplastic NEC	T49.4X1-	T49.4X2-	T49.4X3-	T49.4X4-	T49.4X5-	T49.4X6-
Kerosene, kerosine (fuel) (solvent) NEC	T52.0X1-	T52.0X2-	T52.0X3-	T52.0X4-	-	-
insecticide	T52.0X1-	T52.0X2-	T52.0X3-	T52.0X4-	-	-
vapor	T52.0X1-	T52.0X2-	T52.0X3-	T52.0X4-	-	-
Ketamine	T41.291-	T41.292-	T41.293-	T41.294-	T41.295-	T41.296-
Ketazolam	T42.4X1-	T42.4X2-	T42.4X3-	T42.4X4-	T42.4X5-	T42.4X6-
Ketazon	T39.2X1-	T39.2X2-	T39.2X3-	T39.2X4-	T39.2X5-	T39.2X6-
Ketobemidone	T40.4X1-	T40.4X2-	T40.4X3-	T40.4X4-	-	-
Ketoconazole	T49.0X1-	T49.0X2-	T49.0X3-	T49.0X4-	T49.0X5-	T49.0X6-
Ketols	T52.4X1-	T52.4X2-	T52.4X3-	T52.4X4-	-	-
Ketone oils	T52.4X1-	T52.4X2-	T52.4X3-	T52.4X4-	-	-
Ketoprofen	T39.311-	T39.312-	T39.313-	T39.314-	T39.315-	T39.316-
Ketorolac	T39.8X1-	T39.8X2-	T39.8X3-	T39.8X4-	T39.8X5-	T39.8X6-
Ketotifen	T45.0X1-	T45.0X2-	T45.0X3-	T45.0X4-	T45.0X5-	T45.0X6-
Khat	T43.691-	T43.692-	T43.693-	T43.694-	-	-
Khellin	T46.3X1-	T46.3X2-	T46.3X3-	T46.3X4-	T46.3X5-	T46.3X6-
Khelloside	T46.3X1-	T46.3X2-	T46.3X3-	T46.3X4-	T46.3X5-	T46.3X6-
Kiln gas or vapor (carbon monoxide)	T58.8X1-	T58.8X2-	T58.8X3-	T58.8X4-	-	-
Kitasamycin	T36.3X1-	T36.3X2-	T36.3X3-	T36.3X4-	T36.3X5-	T36.3X6-
Konsyl	T47.4X1-	T47.4X2-	T47.4X3-	T47.4X4-	T47.4X5-	T47.4X6-
Kosam seed	T62.2X1-	T62.2X2-	T62.2X3-	T62.2X4-	-	-
Krait (venom)	T63.091-	T63.092-	T63.093-	T63.094-	-	-
Kwell (insecticide)	T60.1X1-	T60.1X2-	T60.1X3-	T60.1X4-	-	-
anti-infective (topical)	T49.0X1-	T49.0X2-	T49.0X3-	T49.0X4-	T49.0X5-	T49.0X6-
Labetalol	T44.8X1-	T44.8X2-	T44.8X3-	T44.8X4-	T44.8X5-	T44.8X6-
Laburnum (seeds)	T62.2X1-	T62.2X2-	T62.2X3-	T62.2X4-	-	-
leaves	T62.2X1-	T62.2X2-	T62.2X3-	T62.2X4-	-	-
Lachesine	T49.5X1-	T49.5X2-	T49.5X3-	T49.5X4-	T49.5X5-	T49.5X6-
Lacidipine	T46.5X1-	T46.5X2-	T46.5X3-	T46.5X4-	T46.5X5-	T46.5X6-
Lacquer	T65.6X1-	T65.6X2-	T65.6X3-	T65.6X4-	-	-
Lacrimogenic gas	T59.3X1-	T59.3X2-	T59.3X3-	T59.3X4-	-	-
Lactated potassic saline	T50.3X1-	T50.3X2-	T50.3X3-	T50.3X4-	T50.3X5-	T50.3X6-
Lactic acid	T49.8X1-	T49.8X2-	T49.8X3-	T49.8X4-	T49.8X5-	T49.8X6-
Lactobacillus						
acidophilus	T47.6X1-	T47.6X2-	T47.6X3-	T47.6X4-	T47.6X5-	T47.6X6-
compound	T47.6X1-	T47.6X2-	T47.6X3-	T47.6X4-	T47.6X5-	T47.6X6-
bifidus, lyophilized	T47.6X1-	T47.6X2-	T47.6X3-	T47.6X4-	T47.6X5-	T47.6X6-
bulgaricus	T47.6X1-	T47.6X2-	T47.6X3-	T47.6X4-	T47.6X5-	T47.6X6-
sporogenes	T47.6X1-	T47.6X2-	T47.6X3-	T47.6X4-	T47.6X5-	T47.6X6-
Lactoflavin	T45.2X1-	T45.2X2-	T45.2X3-	T45.2X4-	T45.2X5-	T45.2X6-
Lactose (as excipient)	T50.901-	T50.902-	T50.903-	T50.904-	T50.905-	T50.906-
Lactuca (virosa) (extract)	T42.6X1-	T42.6X2-	T42.6X3-	T42.6X4-	T42.6X5-	T42.6X6-
Lactucarium	T42.6X1-	T42.6X2-	T42.6X3-	T42.6X4-	T42.6X5-	T42.6X6-
Lactulose	T47.3X1-	T47.3X2-	T47.3X3-	T47.3X4-	T47.3X5-	T47.3X6-
Laevo — *see Levo-*						
Lanatosides	T46.0X1-	T46.0X2-	T46.0X3-	T46.0X4-	T46.0X5-	T46.0X6-
Lanolin	T49.3X1-	T49.3X2-	T49.3X3-	T49.3X4-	T49.3X5-	T49.3X6-
Largactil	T43.3X1-	T43.3X2-	T43.3X3-	T43.3X4-	T43.3X5-	T43.3X6-
Larkspur	T62.2X1-	T62.2X2-	T62.2X3-	T62.2X4-	-	-
Laroxyl	T43.011-	T43.012-	T43.013-	T43.014-	T43.015-	T43.016-
Lasix	T50.1X1-	T50.1X2-	T50.1X3-	T50.1X4-	T50.1X5-	T50.1X6-
Lassar's paste	T49.4X1-	T49.4X2-	T49.4X3-	T49.4X4-	T49.4X5-	T49.4X6-
Latamoxef	T36.1X1-	T36.1X2-	T36.1X3-	T36.1X4-	T36.1X5-	T36.1X6-
Latex	T65.811-	T65.812-	T65.813-	T65.814-	-	-
Lathyrus (seed)	T62.2X1-	T62.2X2-	T62.2X3-	T62.2X4-	-	-
Laudanum	T40.0X1-	T40.0X2-	T40.0X3-	T40.0X4-	T40.0X5-	T40.0X6-

Substance	Poisoning Accidental (unintentional)	Poisoning Intentional self-harm	Poisoning Assault	Poisoning Undetermined	Adverse effect	Underdosing
Laudexium	T48.1X1-	T48.1X2-	T48.1X3-	T48.1X4-	T48.1X5-	T48.1X6-
Laughing gas	T41.0X1-	T41.0X2-	T41.0X3-	T41.0X4-	T41.0X5-	T41.0X6-
Laurel, black or cherry	T62.2X1-	T62.2X2-	T62.2X3-	T62.2X4-	-	-
Laurolinium	T49.0X1-	T49.0X2-	T49.0X3-	T49.0X4-	T49.0X5-	T49.0X6-
Lauryl sulfoacetate	T49.2X1-	T49.2X2-	T49.2X3-	T49.2X4-	T49.2X5-	T49.2X6-
Laxative NEC	T47.4X1-	T47.4X2-	T47.4X3-	T47.4X4-	T47.4X5-	T47.4X6-
osmotic	T47.3X1-	T47.3X2-	T47.3X3-	T47.3X4-	T47.3X5-	T47.3X6-
saline	T47.3X1-	T47.3X2-	T47.3X3-	T47.3X4-	T47.3X5-	T47.3X6-
stimulant	T47.2X1-	T47.2X2-	T47.2X3-	T47.2X4-	T47.2X5-	T47.2X6-
L-dopa	T42.8X1-	T42.8X2-	T42.8X3-	T42.8X4-	T42.8X5-	T42.8X6-
Lead (dust) (fumes) (vapor) NEC	T56.0X1-	T56.0X2-	T56.0X3-	T56.0X4-	-	-
acetate	T49.2X1-	T49.2X2-	T49.2X3-	T49.2X4-	T49.2X5-	T49.2X6-
alkyl (fuel additive)	T56.0X1-	T56.0X2-	T56.0X3-	T56.0X4-	-	-
anti-infectives	T37.8X1-	T37.8X2-	T37.8X3-	T37.8X4-	T37.8X5-	T37.8X6-
antiknock compound (tetraethyl)	T56.0X1-	T56.0X2-	T56.0X3-	T56.0X4-	-	-
arsenate, arsenite (dust) (herbicide) (insecticide) (vapor)	T57.0X1-	T57.0X2-	T57.0X3-	T57.0X4-	-	-
carbonate	T56.0X1-	T56.0X2-	T56.0X3-	T56.0X4-	-	-
paint	T56.0X1-	T56.0X2-	T56.0X3-	T56.0X4-	-	-
chromate	T56.0X1-	T56.0X2-	T56.0X3-	T56.0X4-	-	-
paint	T56.0X1-	T56.0X2-	T56.0X3-	T56.0X4-	-	-
dioxide	T56.0X1-	T56.0X2-	T56.0X3-	T56.0X4-	-	-
inorganic	T56.0X1-	T56.0X2-	T56.0X3-	T56.0X4-	-	-
iodide	T56.0X1-	T56.0X2-	T56.0X3-	T56.0X4-	-	-
pigment (paint)	T56.0X1-	T56.0X2-	T56.0X3-	T56.0X4-	-	-
monoxide (dust)	T56.0X1-	T56.0X2-	T56.0X3-	T56.0X4-	-	-
paint	T56.0X1-	T56.0X2-	T56.0X3-	T56.0X4-	-	-
organic	T56.0X1-	T56.0X2-	T56.0X3-	T56.0X4-	-	-
oxide	T56.0X1-	T56.0X2-	T56.0X3-	T56.0X4-	-	-
paint	T56.0X1-	T56.0X2-	T56.0X3-	T56.0X4-	-	-
paint	T56.0X1-	T56.0X2-	T56.0X3-	T56.0X4-	-	-
salts	T56.0X1-	T56.0X2-	T56.0X3-	T56.0X4-	-	-
specified compound NEC	T56.0X1-	T56.0X2-	T56.0X3-	T56.0X4-	-	-
tetra-ethyl	T56.0X1-	T56.0X2-	T56.0X3-	T56.0X4-	-	-
Lebanese red	T40.7X1-	T40.7X2-	T40.7X3-	T40.7X4-	T40.7X5-	T40.7X6-
Lefetamine	T39.8X1-	T39.8X2-	T39.8X3-	T39.8X4-	T39.8X5-	T39.8X6-
Lenperone	T43.4X1-	T43.4X2-	T43.4X3-	T43.4X4-	T43.4X5-	T43.4X6-
Lente lietin (insulin)	T38.3X1-	T38.3X2-	T38.3X3-	T38.3X4-	T38.3X5-	T38.3X6-
Leptazol	T50.7X1-	T50.7X2-	T50.7X3-	T50.7X4-	T50.7X5-	T50.7X6-
Leptophos	T60.0X1-	T60.0X2-	T60.0X3-	T60.0X4-	-	-
Leritine	T40.2X1-	T40.2X2-	T40.2X3-	T40.2X4-	T40.2X5-	T40.2X6-
Letosteine	T48.4X1-	T48.4X2-	T48.4X3-	T48.4X4-	T48.4X5-	T48.4X6-
Letter	T38.1X1-	T38.1X2-	T38.1X3-	T38.1X4-	T38.1X5-	T38.1X6-
Lettuce opium	T42.6X1-	T42.6X2-	T42.6X3-	T42.6X4-	T42.6X5-	T42.6X6-
Leucinocaine	T41.3X1-	T41.3X2-	T41.3X3-	T41.3X4-	T41.3X5-	T41.3X6-
Leucocianidol	T46.991-	T46.992-	T46.993-	T46.994-	T46.995-	T46.996-
Leucovorin (factor)	T45.8X1-	T45.8X2-	T45.8X3-	T45.8X4-	T45.8X5-	T45.8X6-
Leukeran	T45.1X1-	T45.1X2-	T45.1X3-	T45.1X4-	T45.1X5-	T45.1X6-
Leuprolide	T38.891-	T38.892-	T38.893-	T38.894-	T38.895-	T38.896-
Levalbuterol	T48.6X1-	T48.6X2-	T48.6X3-	T48.6X4-	T48.6X5-	T48.6X6-
Levallorphan	T50.7X1-	T50.7X2-	T50.7X3-	T50.7X4-	T50.7X5-	T50.7X6-
Levamisole	T37.4X1-	T37.4X2-	T37.4X3-	T37.4X4-	T37.4X5-	T37.4X6-
Levanil	T42.6X1-	T42.6X2-	T42.6X3-	T42.6X4-	T42.6X5-	T42.6X6-
Levarterenol	T44.4X1-	T44.4X2-	T44.4X3-	T44.4X4-	T44.4X5-	T44.4X6-
Levdropropizine	T48.3X1-	T48.3X2-	T48.3X3-	T48.3X4-	T48.3X5-	T48.3X6-
Levobunolol	T49.5X1-	T49.5X2-	T49.5X3-	T49.5X4-	T49.5X5-	T49.5X6-
Levocabastine (hydrochloride)	T45.0X1-	T45.0X2-	T45.0X3-	T45.0X4-	T45.0X5-	T45.0X6-
Levocarnitine	T50.991-	T50.992-	T50.993-	T50.994-	T50.995-	T50.996-

Substance	Poisoning Accidental (unintentional)	Poisoning Intentional self-harm	Poisoning Assault	Poisoning Undetermined	Adverse effect	Underdosing
Levodopa	T42.8X1-	T42.8X2-	T42.8X3-	T42.8X4-	T42.8X5-	T42.8X6-
with carbidopa	T42.8X1-	T42.8X2-	T42.8X3-	T42.8X4-	T42.8X5-	T42.8X6-
Levo-dromoran	T40.2X1-	T40.2X2-	T40.2X3-	T40.2X4-	T40.2X5-	T40.2X6-
Levoglutamide	T50.991-	T50.992-	T50.993-	T50.994-	T50.995-	T50.996-
Levoid	T38.1X1-	T38.1X2-	T38.1X3-	T38.1X4-	T38.1X5-	T38.1X6-
Levo-iso-methadone	T40.3X1-	T40.3X2-	T40.3X3-	T40.3X4-	T40.3X5-	T40.3X6-
Levomepromazine	T43.3X1-	T43.3X2-	T43.3X3-	T43.3X4-	T43.3X5-	T43.3X6-
Levonordefrin	T49.6X1-	T49.6X2-	T49.6X3-	T49.6X4-	T49.6X5-	T49.6X6-
Levonorgestrel	T38.4X1-	T38.4X2-	T38.4X3-	T38.4X4-	T38.4X5-	T38.4X6-
with ethinylestradiol	T38.5X1-	T38.5X2-	T38.5X3-	T38.5X4-	T38.5X5-	T38.5X6-
Levopromazine	T43.3X1-	T43.3X2-	T43.3X3-	T43.3X4-	T43.3X5-	T43.3X6-
Levoprome	T42.6X1-	T42.6X2-	T42.6X3-	T42.6X4-	T42.6X5-	T42.6X6-
Levopropoxyphene	T40.4X1-	T40.4X2-	T40.4X3-	T40.4X4-	T40.4X5-	T40.4X6-
Levopropylhexedrine	T50.5X1-	T50.5X2-	T50.5X3-	T50.5X4-	T50.5X5-	T50.5X6-
Levoproxyphylline	T48.6X1-	T48.6X2-	T48.6X3-	T48.6X4-	T48.6X5-	T48.6X6-
Levorphanol	T40.4X1-	T40.4X2-	T40.4X3-	T40.4X4-	T40.4X5-	T40.4X6-
Levothyroxine	T38.1X1-	T38.1X2-	T38.1X3-	T38.1X4-	T38.1X5-	T38.1X6-
sodium	T38.1X1-	T38.1X2-	T38.1X3-	T38.1X4-	T38.1X5-	T38.1X6-
Levsin	T44.3X1-	T44.3X2-	T44.3X3-	T44.3X4-	T44.3X5-	T44.3X6-
Levulose	T50.3X1-	T50.3X2-	T50.3X3-	T50.3X4-	T50.3X5-	T50.3X6-
Lewisite (gas) , not in war	T57.0X1-	T57.0X2-	T57.0X3-	T57.0X4-	-	-
Librium	T42.4X1-	T42.4X2-	T42.4X3-	T42.4X4-	T42.4X5-	T42.4X6-
Lidex	T49.0X1-	T49.0X2-	T49.0X3-	T49.0X4-	T49.0X5-	T49.0X6-
Lidocaine	T41.3X1-	T41.3X2-	T41.3X3-	T41.3X4-	T41.3X5-	T41.3X6-
regional	T41.3X1-	T41.3X2-	T41.3X3-	T41.3X4-	T41.3X5-	T41.3X6-
spinal	T41.3X1-	T41.3X2-	T41.3X3-	T41.3X4-	T41.3X5-	T41.3X6-
Lidofenin	T50.8X1-	T50.8X2-	T50.8X3-	T50.8X4-	T50.8X5-	T50.8X6-
Lidoflazine	T46.1X1-	T46.1X2-	T46.1X3-	T46.1X4-	T46.1X5-	T46.1X6-
Lighter fluid	T52.0X1-	T52.0X2-	T52.0X3-	T52.0X4-	-	-
Lignin hemicellulose	T47.6X1-	T47.6X2-	T47.6X3-	T47.6X4-	T47.6X5-	T47.6X6-
Lignocaine	T41.3X1-	T41.3X2-	T41.3X3-	T41.3X4-	T41.3X5-	T41.3X6-
regional	T41.3X1-	T41.3X2-	T41.3X3-	T41.3X4-	T41.3X5-	T41.3X6-
spinal	T41.3X1-	T41.3X2-	T41.3X3-	T41.3X4-	T41.3X5-	T41.3X6-
Ligroin (e) (solvent)	T52.0X1-	T52.0X2-	T52.0X3-	T52.0X4-	-	-
vapor	T59.891-	T59.892-	T59.893-	T59.894-	-	-
Ligustrum vulgare	T62.2X1-	T62.2X2-	T62.2X3-	T62.2X4-	-	-
Lily of the valley	T62.2X1-	T62.2X2-	T62.2X3-	T62.2X4-	-	-
Lime (chloride)	T54.3X1-	T54.3X2-	T54.3X3-	T54.3X4-	-	-
Limonene	T52.8X1-	T52.8X2-	T52.8X3-	T52.8X4-	-	-
Lincomycin	T36.8X1-	T36.8X2-	T36.8X3-	T36.8X4-	T36.8X5-	T36.8X6-
Lindane (insecticide) (nonmedicinal) (vapor)	T53.6X1-	T53.6X2-	T53.6X3-	T53.6X4-	-	-
medicinal	T49.0X1-	T49.0X2-	T49.0X3-	T49.0X4-	T49.0X5-	T49.0X6-
Liniments NEC	T49.91X-	T49.92X-	T49.93X-	T49.94X-	T49.95X-	T49.96X-
Linoleic acid	T46.6X1-	T46.6X2-	T46.6X3-	T46.6X4-	T46.6X5-	T46.6X6-
Linolenic acid	T46.6X1-	T46.6X2-	T46.6X3-	T46.6X4-	T46.6X5-	T46.6X6-
Linseed	T47.4X1-	T47.4X2-	T47.4X3-	T47.4X4-	T47.4X5-	T47.4X6-
Liothyronine	T38.1X1-	T38.1X2-	T38.1X3-	T38.1X4-	T38.1X5-	T38.1X6-
Liotrix	T38.1X1-	T38.1X2-	T38.1X3-	T38.1X4-	T38.1X5-	T38.1X6-
Lipancreatin	T47.5X1-	T47.5X2-	T47.5X3-	T47.5X4-	T47.5X5-	T47.5X6-
Lipo-alprostadil	T46.7X1-	T46.7X2-	T46.7X3-	T46.7X4-	T46.7X5-	T46.7X6-
Lipo-Lutin	T38.5X1-	T38.5X2-	T38.5X3-	T38.5X4-	T38.5X5-	T38.5X6-
Lipotropic drug NEC	T50.901-	T50.902-	T50.903-	T50.904-	T50.905-	T50.906-
Liquefied petroleum gases	T59.891-	T59.892-	T59.893-	T59.894-	-	-
piped (pure or mixed with air)	T59.891-	T59.892-	T59.893-	T59.894-	-	-
Liquid						
paraffin	T47.4X1-	T47.4X2-	T47.4X3-	T47.4X4-	T47.4X5-	T47.4X6-
petrolatum	T47.4X1-	T47.4X2-	T47.4X3-	T47.4X4-	T47.4X5-	T47.4X6-

LEVODOPA - LIQUID

Substance	Poisoning Accidental (unintentional)	Poisoning Intentional self-harm	Poisoning Assault	Poisoning Undetermined	Adverse effect	Underdosing
Liquid *(continued)*						
topical	T49.3X1-	T49.3X2-	T49.3X3-	T49.3X4-	T49.3X5-	T49.3X6-
specified NEC	T65.891-	T65.892-	T65.893-	T65.894-	-	-
substance	T65.91X-	T65.92X-	T65.93X-	T65.94X-	-	-
Liquor creosolis compositus	T65.891-	T65.892-	T65.893-	T65.894-	-	-
Liquorice	T48.4X1-	T48.4X2-	T48.4X3-	T48.4X4-	T48.4X5-	T48.4X6-
extract	T47.8X1-	T47.8X2-	T47.8X3-	T47.8X4-	T47.8X5-	T47.8X6-
Lisinopril	T46.4X1-	T46.4X2-	T46.4X3-	T46.4X4-	T46.4X5-	T46.4X6-
Lisuride	T42.8X1-	T42.8X2-	T42.8X3-	T42.8X4-	T42.8X5-	T42.8X6-
Lithane	T43.8X1-	T43.8X2-	T43.8X3-	T43.8X4-	T43.8X5-	T43.8X6-
Lithium	T56.891-	T56.892-	T56.893-	T56.894-	-	-
gluconate	T43.591-	T43.592-	T43.593-	T43.594-	T43.595-	T43.596-
salts (carbonate)	T43.591-	T43.592-	T43.593-	T43.594-	T43.595-	T43.596-
Lithonate	T43.8X1-	T43.8X2-	T43.8X3-	T43.8X4-	T43.8X5-	T43.8X6-
Liver						
extract	T45.8X1-	T45.8X2-	T45.8X3-	T45.8X4-	T45.8X5-	T45.8X6-
for parenteral use	T45.8X1-	T45.8X2-	T45.8X3-	T45.8X4-	T45.8X5-	T45.8X6-
fraction 1	T45.8X1-	T45.8X2-	T45.8X3-	T45.8X4-	T45.8X5-	T45.8X6-
hydrolysate	T45.8X1-	T45.8X2-	T45.8X3-	T45.8X4-	T45.8X5-	T45.8X6-
Lizard (bite) (venom)	T63.121-	T63.122-	T63.123-	T63.124-	-	-
LMD	T45.8X1-	T45.8X2-	T45.8X3-	T45.8X4-	T45.8X5-	T45.8X6-
Lobelia	T62.2X1-	T62.2X2-	T62.2X3-	T62.2X4-	-	-
Lobeline	T50.7X1-	T50.7X2-	T50.7X3-	T50.7X4-	T50.7X5-	T50.7X6-
Local action drug NEC	T49.8X1-	T49.8X2-	T49.8X3-	T49.8X4-	T49.8X5-	T49.8X6-
Locorten	T49.0X1-	T49.0X2-	T49.0X3-	T49.0X4-	T49.0X5-	T49.0X6-
Lofepramine	T43.011-	T43.012-	T43.013-	T43.014-	T43.015-	T43.016-
Lolium temulentum	T62.2X1-	T62.2X2-	T62.2X3-	T62.2X4-	-	-
Lomotil	T47.6X1-	T47.6X2-	T47.6X3-	T47.6X4-	T47.6X5-	T47.6X6-
Lomustine	T45.1X1-	T45.1X2-	T45.1X3-	T45.1X4-	T45.1X5-	T45.1X6-
Lonidamine	T45.1X1-	T45.1X2-	T45.1X3-	T45.1X4-	T45.1X5-	T45.1X6-
Loperamide	T47.6X1-	T47.6X2-	T47.6X3-	T47.6X4-	T47.6X5-	T47.6X6-
Loprazolam	T42.4X1-	T42.4X2-	T42.4X3-	T42.4X4-	T42.4X5-	T42.4X6-
Lorajmine	T46.2X1-	T46.2X2-	T46.2X3-	T46.2X4-	T46.2X5-	T46.2X6-
Loratidine	T45.0X1-	T45.0X2-	T45.0X3-	T45.0X4-	T45.0X5-	T45.0X6-
Lorazepam	T42.4X1-	T42.4X2-	T42.4X3-	T42.4X4-	T42.4X5-	T42.4X6-
Lorcainide	T46.2X1-	T46.2X2-	T46.2X3-	T46.2X4-	T46.2X5-	T46.2X6-
Lormetazepam	T42.4X1-	T42.4X2-	T42.4X3-	T42.4X4-	T42.4X5-	T42.4X6-
Lotions NEC	T49.91X-	T49.92X-	T49.93X-	T49.94X-	T49.95X-	T49.96X-
Lotusate	T42.3X1-	T42.3X2-	T42.3X3-	T42.3X4-	T42.3X5-	T42.3X6-
Lovastatin	T46.6X1-	T46.6X2-	T46.6X3-	T46.6X4-	T46.6X5-	T46.6X6-
Lowila	T49.2X1-	T49.2X2-	T49.2X3-	T49.2X4-	T49.2X5-	T49.2X6-
Loxapine	T43.591-	T43.592-	T43.593-	T43.594-	T43.595-	T43.596-
Lozenges (throat)	T49.6X1-	T49.6X2-	T49.6X3-	T49.6X4-	T49.6X5-	T49.6X6-
LSD	T40.8X1-	T40.8X2-	T40.8X3-	T40.8X4-	-	-
L-Tryptophan — *see amino acid*						
Lubricant, eye	T49.5X1-	T49.5X2-	T49.5X3-	T49.5X4-	T49.5X5-	T49.5X6-
Lubricating oil NEC	T52.0X1-	T52.0X2-	T52.0X3-	T52.0X4-	-	-
Lucanthone	T37.4X1-	T37.4X2-	T37.4X3-	T37.4X4-	T37.4X5-	T37.4X6-
Luminal	T42.3X1-	T42.3X2-	T42.3X3-	T42.3X4-	T42.3X5-	T42.3X6-
Lung irritant (gas) NEC	T59.91X-	T59.92X-	T59.93X-	T59.94X-	-	-
Luteinizing hormone	T38.811-	T38.812-	T38.813-	T38.814-	T38.815-	T38.816-
Lutocylol	T38.5X1-	T38.5X2-	T38.5X3-	T38.5X4-	T38.5X5-	T38.5X6-
Lutromone	T38.5X1-	T38.5X2-	T38.5X3-	T38.5X4-	T38.5X5-	T38.5X6-
Lututrin	T48.291-	T48.292-	T48.293-	T48.294-	T48.295-	T48.296-
Lye (concentrated)	T54.3X1-	T54.3X2-	T54.3X3-	T54.3X4-	-	-
Lygranum (skin test)	T50.8X1-	T50.8X2-	T50.8X3-	T50.8X4-	T50.8X5-	T50.8X6-
Lymecycline	T36.4X1-	T36.4X2-	T36.4X3-	T36.4X4-	T36.4X5-	T36.4X6-
Lymphogranuloma venereum antigen	T50.8X1-	T50.8X2-	T50.8X3-	T50.8X4-	T50.8X5-	T50.8X6-
Lynestrenol	T38.4X1-	T38.4X2-	T38.4X3-	T38.4X4-	T38.4X5-	T38.4X6-

Substance	Poisoning Accidental (unintentional)	Poisoning Intentional self-harm	Poisoning Assault	Poisoning Undetermined	Adverse effect	Underdosing
Lyovac Sodium Edecrin	T50.1X1-	T50.1X2-	T50.1X3-	T50.1X4-	T50.1X5-	T50.1X6-
Lypressin	T38.891-	T38.892-	T38.893-	T38.894-	T38.895-	T38.896-
Lysergic acid diethylamide	T40.8X1-	T40.8X2-	T40.8X3-	T40.8X4-	-	-
Lysergide	T40.8X1-	T40.8X2-	T40.8X3-	T40.8X4-	-	-
Lysine vasopressin	T38.891-	T38.892-	T38.893-	T38.894-	T38.895-	T38.896-
Lysol	T54.1X1-	T54.1X2-	T54.1X3-	T54.1X4-	-	-
Lysozyme	T49.0X1-	T49.0X2-	T49.0X3-	T49.0X4-	T49.0X5-	T49.0X6-
Lytta (vitatta)	T49.8X1-	T49.8X2-	T49.8X3-	T49.8X4-	T49.8X5-	T49.8X6-
Mace	T59.3X1-	T59.3X2-	T59.3X3-	T59.3X4-	-	-
Macrogol	T50.991-	T50.992-	T50.993-	T50.994-	T50.995-	T50.996-
Macrolide						
anabolic drug	T38.7X1-	T38.7X2-	T38.7X3	T38.7X4-	T38.7X5-	T38.7X6-
antibiotic	T36.3X1-	T36.3X2-	T36.3X3-	T36.3X4-	T36.3X5-	T36.3X6-
Mafenide	T49.0X1-	T49.0X2-	T49.0X3-	T49.0X4-	T49.0X5-	T49.0X6-
Magaldrate	T47.1X1-	T47.1X2-	T47.1X3-	T47.1X4-	T47.1X5-	T47.1X6-
Magic mushroom	T40.991-	T40.992-	T40.993-	T40.994-	-	-
Magnamycin	T36.8X1-	T36.8X2-	T36.8X3-	T36.8X4-	T36.8X5-	T36.8X6-
Magnesia magma	T47.1X1-	T47.1X2-	T47.1X3-	T47.1X4-	T47.1X5-	T47.1X6-
Magnesium NEC	T56.891-	T56.892-	T56.893-	T56.894-	-	-
carbonate	T47.1X1-	T47.1X2-	T47.1X3-	T47.1X4-	T47.1X5-	T47.1X6-
citrate	T47.4X1-	T47.4X2-	T47.4X3-	T47.4X4-	T47.4X5-	T47.4X6-
hydroxide	T47.1X1-	T47.1X2-	T47.1X3-	T47.1X4-	T47.1X5-	T47.1X6-
oxide	T47.1X1-	T47.1X2-	T47.1X3-	T47.1X4-	T47.1X5-	T47.1X6-
peroxide	T49.0X1-	T49.0X2-	T49.0X3-	T49.0X4-	T49.0X5-	T49.0X6-
salicylate	T39.091-	T39.092-	T39.093-	T39.094-	T39.095-	T39.096-
silicofluoride	T50.3X1-	T50.3X2-	T50.3X3-	T50.3X4-	T50.3X5-	T50.3X6-
sulfate	T47.4X1-	T47.4X2-	T47.4X3-	T47.4X4-	T47.4X5-	T47.4X6-
thiosulfate	T45.0X1-	T45.0X2-	T45.0X3-	T45.0X4-	T45.0X5-	T45.0X6-
trisilicate	T47.1X1-	T47.1X2-	T47.1X3-	T47.1X4-	T47.1X5-	T47.1X6-
Malathion (medicinal)	T49.0X1-	T49.0X2-	T49.0X3-	T49.0X4-	T49.0X5-	T49.0X6-
insecticide	T60.0X1-	T60.0X2-	T60.0X3-	T60.0X4-	-	-
Male fern extract	T37.4X1-	T37.4X2-	T37.4X3-	T37.4X4-	T37.4X5-	T37.4X6-
M-AMSA	T45.1X1-	T45.1X2-	T45.1X3-	T45.1X4-	T45.1X5-	T45.1X6-
Mandelic acid	T37.8X1-	T37.8X2-	T37.8X3-	T37.8X4-	T37.8X5-	T37.8X6-
Manganese (dioxide) (salts)	T57.2X1-	T57.2X2-	T57.2X3-	T57.2X4-	-	-
medicinal	T50.991-	T50.992-	T50.993-	T50.994-	T50.995-	T50.996-
Mannitol	T47.3X1-	T47.3X2-	T47.3X3-	T47.3X4-	T47.3X5-	T47.3X6-
hexanitrate	T46.3X1-	T46.3X2-	T46.3X3-	T46.3X4-	T46.3X5-	T46.3X6-
Mannomustine	T45.1X1-	T45.1X2-	T45.1X3-	T45.1X4-	T45.1X5-	T45.1X6-
MAO inhibitors	T43.1X1-	T43.1X2-	T43.1X3-	T43.1X4-	T43.1X5-	T43.1X6-
Mapharsen	T37.8X1-	T37.8X2-	T37.8X3-	T37.8X4-	T37.8X5-	T37.8X6-
Maphenide	T49.0X1-	T49.0X2-	T49.0X3-	T49.0X4-	T49.0X5-	T49.0X6-
Maprotiline	T43.021-	T43.022-	T43.023-	T43.024-	T43.025-	T43.026-
Marcaine	T41.3X1-	T41.3X2-	T41.3X3-	T41.3X4-	T41.3X5-	T41.3X6-
infiltration (subcutaneous)	T41.3X1-	T41.3X2-	T41.3X3-	T41.3X4-	T41.3X5-	T41.3X6-
nerve block (peripheral) (plexus)	T41.3X1-	T41.3X2-	T41.3X3-	T41.3X4-	T41.3X5-	T41.3X6-
Marezine	T45.0X1-	T45.0X2-	T45.0X3-	T45.0X4-	T45.0X5-	T45.0X6-
Marihuana	T40.7X1-	T40.7X2-	T40.7X3-	T40.7X4-	T40.7X5-	T40.7X6-
Marijuana	T40.7X1-	T40.7X2-	T40.7X3-	T40.7X4-	T40.7X5-	T40.7X6-
Marine (sting)	T63.691-	T63.692-	T63.693-	T63.694-	-	-
animals (sting)	T63.691-	T63.692-	T63.693-	T63.694-	-	-
plants (sting)	T63.711-	T63.712-	T63.713-	T63.714-	-	-
Marplan	T43.1X1-	T43.1X2-	T43.1X3-	T43.1X4-	T43.1X5-	T43.1X6-
Marsh gas	T59.891-	T59.892-	T59.893-	T59.894-	-	-
Marsilid	T43.1X1-	T43.1X2-	T43.1X3-	T43.1X4-	T43.1X5-	T43.1X6-
Matulane	T45.1X1-	T45.1X2-	T45.1X3-	T45.1X4-	T45.1X5-	T45.1X6-
Mazindol	T50.5X1-	T50.5X2-	T50.5X3-	T50.5X4-	T50.5X5-	T50.5X6-
MCPA	T60.3X1-	T60.3X2-	T60.3X3-	T60.3X4-	-	-

Substance	Poisoning Accidental (unintentional)	Poisoning Intentional self-harm	Poisoning Assault	Poisoning Undetermined	Adverse effect	Underdosing
MDMA	T43.641-	T43.642-	T43.643-	T43.644-	-	-
Meadow saffron	T62.2X1-	T62.2X2-	T62.2X3-	T62.2X4-	-	-
Measles virus vaccine (attenuated)	T50.B91-	T50.B92-	T50.B93-	T50.B94-	T50.B95-	T50.B96-
Meat, noxious	T62.8X1-	T62.8X2-	T62.8X3-	T62.8X4-	-	-
Meballymal	T42.3X1-	T42.3X2-	T42.3X3-	T42.3X4-	T42.3X5-	T42.3X6-
Mebanazine	T43.1X1-	T43.1X2-	T43.1X3-	T43.1X4-	T43.1X5-	T43.1X6-
Mebaral	T42.3X1-	T42.3X2-	T42.3X3-	T42.3X4-	T42.3X5-	T42.3X6-
Mebendazole	T37.4X1-	T37.4X2-	T37.4X3-	T37.4X4-	T37.4X5-	T37.4X6-
Mebeverine	T44.3X1-	T44.3X2-	T44.3X3-	T44.3X4-	T44.3X5-	T44.3X6-
Mebhydrolin	T45.0X1-	T45.0X2-	T45.0X3-	T45.0X4-	T45.0X5-	T45.0X6-
Mebumal	T42.3X1-	T42.3X2-	T42.3X3-	T42.3X4-	T42.3X5-	T42.3X6-
Mebutamate	T43.591-	T43.592-	T43.593-	T43.594-	T43.595-	T43.596-
Mecamylamine	T44.2X1-	T44.2X2-	T44.2X3-	T44.2X4-	T44.2X5-	T44.2X6-
Mechlorethamine	T45.1X1-	T45.1X2-	T45.1X3-	T45.1X4-	T45.1X5-	T45.1X6-
Mecillinam	T36.0X1-	T36.0X2-	T36.0X3-	T36.0X4-	T36.0X5-	T36.0X6-
Meclizine (hydrochloride)	T45.0X1-	T45.0X2-	T45.0X3-	T45.0X4-	T45.0X5-	T45.0X6-
Meclocycline	T36.4X1-	T36.4X2-	T36.4X3-	T36.4X4-	T36.4X5-	T36.4X6-
Meclofenamate	T39.391-	T39.392-	T39.393-	T39.394-	T39.395-	T39.396-
Meclofenamic acid	T39.391-	T39.392-	T39.393-	T39.394-	T39.395-	T39.396-
Meclofenoxate	T43.691-	T43.692-	T43.693-	T43.694-	T43.695-	T43.696-
Meclozine	T45.0X1-	T45.0X2-	T45.0X3-	T45.0X4-	T45.0X5-	T45.0X6-
Mecobalamin	T45.8X1-	T45.8X2-	T45.8X3-	T45.8X4-	T45.8X5-	T45.8X6-
Mecoprop	T60.3X1-	T60.3X2-	T60.3X3-	T60.3X4-	-	-
Mecrilate	T49.3X1-	T49.3X2-	T49.3X3-	T49.3X4-	T49.3X5-	T49.3X6-
Mecysteine	T48.4X1-	T48.4X2-	T48.4X3-	T48.4X4-	T48.4X5-	T48.4X6-
Medazepam	T42.4X1-	T42.4X2-	T42.4X3-	T42.4X4-	T42.4X5-	T42.4X6-
Medicament NEC	T50.901-	T50.902-	T50.903-	T50.904-	T50.905-	T50.906-
Medinal	T42.3X1-	T42.3X2-	T42.3X3-	T42.3X4-	T42.3X5-	T42.3X6-
Medomin	T42.3X1-	T42.3X2-	T42.3X3-	T42.3X4-	T42.3X5-	T42.3X6-
Medrogestone	T38.5X1-	T38.5X2-	T38.5X3-	T38.5X4-	T38.5X5-	T38.5X6-
Medroxalol	T44.8X1-	T44.8X2-	T44.8X3-	T44.8X4-	T44.8X5-	T44.8X6-
Medroxyprogesterone acetate (depot)	T38.5X1-	T38.5X2-	T38.5X3-	T38.5X4-	T38.5X5-	T38.5X6-
Medrysone	T49.0X1-	T49.0X2-	T49.0X3-	T49.0X4-	T49.0X5-	T49.0X6-
Mefenamic acid	T39.391-	T39.392-	T39.393-	T39.394-	T39.395-	T39.396-
Mefenorex	T50.5X1-	T50.5X2-	T50.5X3-	T50.5X4-	T50.5X5-	T50.5X6-
Mefloquine	T37.2X1-	T37.2X2-	T37.2X3-	T37.2X4-	T37.2X5-	T37.2X6-
Mefruside	T50.2X1-	T50.2X2-	T50.2X3-	T50.2X4-	T50.2X5-	T50.2X6-
Megahallucinogen	T40.901-	T40.902-	T40.903-	T40.904-	T40.905-	T40.906-
Megestrol	T38.5X1-	T38.5X2-	T38.5X3-	T38.5X4-	T38.5X5-	T38.5X6-
Meglumine						
antimoniate	T37.8X1-	T37.8X2-	T37.8X3-	T37.8X4-	T37.8X5-	T37.8X6-
diatrizoate	T50.8X1-	T50.8X2-	T50.8X3-	T50.8X4-	T50.8X5-	T50.8X6-
iodipamide	T50.8X1-	T50.8X2-	T50.8X3-	T50.8X4-	T50.8X5-	T50.8X6-
iotroxate	T50.8X1-	T50.8X2-	T50.8X3-	T50.8X4-	T50.8X5-	T50.8X6-
MEK (methyl ethyl ketone)	T52.4X1-	T52.4X2-	T52.4X3-	T52.4X4-	-	-
Meladinin	T49.3X1-	T49.3X2-	T49.3X3-	T49.3X4-	T49.3X5-	T49.3X6-
Meladrazine	T44.3X1-	T44.3X2-	T44.3X3-	T44.3X4-	T44.3X5-	T44.3X6-
Melaleuca alternifolia oil	T49.0X1-	T49.0X2-	T49.0X3-	T49.0X4-	T49.0X5-	T49.0X6-
Melanizing agents	T49.3X1-	T49.3X2-	T49.3X3-	T49.3X4-	T49.3X5-	T49.3X6-
Melanocyte-stimulating hormone	T38.891-	T38.892-	T38.893-	T38.894-	T38.895-	T38.896-
Melarsonyl potassium	T37.3X1-	T37.3X2-	T37.3X3-	T37.3X4-	T37.3X5-	T37.3X6-
Melarsoprol	T37.3X1-	T37.3X2-	T37.3X3-	T37.3X4-	T37.3X5-	T37.3X6-
Melia azedarach	T62.2X1-	T62.2X2-	T62.2X3-	T62.2X4-	-	-
Melitracen	T43.011-	T43.012-	T43.013-	T43.014-	T43.015-	T43.016-
Mellaril	T43.3X1-	T43.3X2-	T43.3X3-	T43.3X4-	T43.3X5-	T43.3X6-
Meloxine	T49.3X1-	T49.3X2-	T49.3X3-	T49.3X4-	T49.3X5-	T49.3X6-
Melperone	T43.4X1-	T43.4X2-	T43.4X3-	T43.4X4-	T43.4X5-	T43.4X6-
Melphalan	T45.1X1-	T45.1X2-	T45.1X3-	T45.1X4-	T45.1X5-	T45.1X6-
Memantine	T43.8X1-	T43.8X2-	T43.8X3-	T43.8X4-	T43.8X5-	T43.8X6-

Substance	Poisoning Accidental (unintentional)	Poisoning Intentional self-harm	Poisoning Assault	Poisoning Undetermined	Adverse effect	Underdosing
Menadiol	T45.7X1-	T45.7X2-	T45.7X3-	T45.7X4-	T45.7X5-	T45.7X6-
sodium sulfate	T45.7X1-	T45.7X2-	T45.7X3-	T45.7X4-	T45.7X5-	T45.7X6-
Menadione	T45.7X1-	T45.7X2-	T45.7X3-	T45.7X4-	T45.7X5-	T45.7X6-
sodium bisulfite	T45.7X1-	T45.7X2-	T45.7X3-	T45.7X4-	T45.7X5-	T45.7X6-
Menaphthone	T45.7X1-	T45.7X2-	T45.7X3-	T45.7X4-	T45.7X5-	T45.7X6-
Menaquinone	T45.7X1-	T45.7X2-	T45.7X3-	T45.7X4-	T45.7X5-	T45.7X6-
Menatetrenone	T45.7X1-	T45.7X2-	T45.7X3-	T45.7X4-	T45.7X5-	T45.7X6-
Meningococcal vaccine	T50.A91-	T50.A92-	T50.A93-	T50.A94-	T50.A95-	T50.A96-
Menningovax (-AC) (-C)	T50.A91-	T50.A92-	T50.A93-	T50.A94-	T50.A95-	T50.A96-
Menotropins	T38.811-	T38.812-	T38.813-	T38.814-	T38.815-	T38.816-
Menthol	T48.5X1-	T48.5X2-	T48.5X3-	T48.5X4-	T48.5X5-	T48.5X6-
Mepacrine	T37.2X1-	T37.2X2-	T37.2X3-	T37.2X4-	T37.2X5-	T37.2X6-
Meparfynol	T42.6X1-	T42.6X2-	T42.6X3-	T42.6X4-	T42.6X5-	T42.6X6-
Mepartricin	T36.7X1-	T36.7X2-	T36.7X3-	T36.7X4-	T36.7X5-	T36.7X6-
Mepazine	T43.3X1-	T43.3X2-	T43.3X3-	T43.3X4-	T43.3X5-	T43.3X6-
Mepenzolate	T44.3X1-	T44.3X2-	T44.3X3-	T44.3X4-	T44.3X5-	T44.3X6-
bromide	T44.3X1-	T44.3X2-	T44.3X3-	T44.3X4-	T44.3X5-	T44.3X6-
Meperidine	T40.4X1-	T40.4X2-	T40.4X3-	T40.4X4-	T40.4X5-	T40.4X6-
Mephebarbital	T42.3X1-	T42.3X2-	T42.3X3-	T42.3X4-	T42.3X5-	T42.3X6-
Mephenamin (e)	T42.8X1-	T42.8X2-	T42.8X3-	T42.8X4-	T42.8X5-	T42.8X6-
Mephenesin	T42.8X1-	T42.8X2-	T42.8X3-	T42.8X4-	T42.8X5-	T42.8X6-
Mephenhydramine	T45.0X1-	T45.0X2-	T45.0X3-	T45.0X4-	T45.0X5-	T45.0X6-
Mephenoxalone	T42.8X1-	T42.8X2-	T42.8X3-	T42.8X4-	T42.8X5-	T42.8X6-
Mephentermine	T44.991-	T44.992-	T44.993-	T44.994-	T44.995-	T44.996-
Mephenytoin	T42.0X1-	T42.0X2-	T42.0X3-	T42.0X4-	T42.0X5-	T42.0X6-
with phenobarbital	T42.3X1-	T42.3X2-	T42.3X3-	T42.3X4-	T42.3X5-	T42.3X6-
Mephobarbital	T42.3X1-	T42.3X2-	T42.3X3-	T42.3X4-	T42.3X5-	T42.3X6-
Mephosfolan	T60.0X1-	T60.0X2-	T60.0X3-	T60.0X4-	-	-
Mepindolol	T44.7X1-	T44.7X2-	T44.7X3-	T44.7X4-	T44.7X5-	T44.7X6-
Mepiperphenidol	T44.3X1-	T44.3X2-	T44.3X3-	T44.3X4-	T44.3X5-	T44.3X6-
Mepitiostane	T38.7X1-	T38.7X2-	T38.7X3-	T38.7X4-	T38.7X5-	T38.7X6-
Mepivacaine	T41.3X1-	T41.3X2-	T41.3X3-	T41.3X4-	T41.3X5-	T41.3X6-
epidural	T41.3X1-	T41.3X2-	T41.3X3-	T41.3X4-	T41.3X5-	T41.3X6-
Meprednisone	T38.0X1-	T38.0X2-	T38.0X3-	T38.0X4-	T38.0X5-	T38.0X6-
Meprobam	T43.591-	T43.592-	T43.593-	T43.594-	T43.595-	T43.596-
Meprobamate	T43.591-	T43.592-	T43.593-	T43.594-	T43.595-	T43.596-
Meproscillarin	T46.0X1-	T46.0X2-	T46.0X3-	T46.0X4-	T46.0X5-	T46.0X6-
Meprylcaine	T41.3X1-	T41.3X2-	T41.3X3-	T41.3X4-	T41.3X5-	T41.3X6-
Meptazinol	T39.8X1-	T39.8X2-	T39.8X3-	T39.8X4-	T39.8X5-	T39.8X6-
Mepyramine	T45.0X1-	T45.0X2-	T45.0X3-	T45.0X4-	T45.0X5-	T45.0X6-
Mequitazine	T43.3X1-	T43.3X2-	T43.3X3-	T43.3X4-	T43.3X5-	T43.3X6-
Meralluride	T50.2X1-	T50.2X2-	T50.2X3-	T50.2X4-	T50.2X5-	T50.2X6-
Merbaphen	T50.2X1-	T50.2X2-	T50.2X3-	T50.2X4-	T50.2X5-	T50.2X6-
Merbromin	T49.0X1-	T49.0X2-	T49.0X3-	T49.0X4-	T49.0X5-	T49.0X6-
Mercaptobenzothiazole salts	T49.0X1-	T49.0X2-	T49.0X3-	T49.0X4-	T49.0X5-	T49.0X6-
Mercaptomerin	T50.2X1-	T50.2X2-	T50.2X3-	T50.2X4-	T50.2X5-	T50.2X6-
Mercaptopurine	T45.1X1-	T45.1X2-	T45.1X3-	T45.1X4-	T45.1X5-	T45.1X6-
Mercumatilin	T50.2X1-	T50.2X2-	T50.2X3-	T50.2X4-	T50.2X5-	T50.2X6-
Mercuramide	T50.2X1-	T50.2X2-	T50.2X3-	T50.2X4-	T50.2X5-	T50.2X6-
Mercurochrome	T49.0X1-	T49.0X2-	T49.0X3-	T49.0X4-	T49.0X5-	T49.0X6-
Mercurophylline	T50.2X1-	T50.2X2-	T50.2X3-	T50.2X4-	T50.2X5-	
Mercury, mercurial, mercuric, mercurous (compounds) (cyanide) (fumes) (nonmedicinal) (vapor) NEC	T56.1X1-	T56.1X2-	T56.1X3-	T56.1X4-	-	-
ammoniated	T49.0X1-	T49.0X2-	T49.0X3-	T49.0X4-	T49.0X5-	T49.0X6-
anti-infective						
local	T49.0X1-	T49.0X2-	T49.0X3-	T49.0X4-	T49.0X5-	T49.0X6-
systemic	T37.8X1-	T37.8X2-	T37.8X3-	T37.8X4-	T37.8X5-	T37.8X6-

Substance	Poisoning Accidental (unintentional)	Poisoning Intentional self-harm	Poisoning Assault	Poisoning Undetermined	Adverse effect	Underdosing
Mercury, mercurial, mercuric, mercurous (compounds) (cyanide) (fumes) (nonmedicinal) (vapor) NEC (continued)						
topical	T49.0X1-	T49.0X2-	T49.0X3-	T49.0X4-	T49.0X5-	T49.0X6-
chloride (ammoniated)	T49.0X1-	T49.0X2-	T49.0X3-	T49.0X4-	T49.0X5-	T49.0X6-
fungicide	T56.1X1-	T56.1X2-	T56.1X3-	T56.1X4-	-	-
diuretic NEC	T50.2X1-	T50.2X2-	T50.2X3-	T50.2X4-	T50.2X5-	T50.2X6-
fungicide	T56.1X1-	T56.1X2-	T56.1X3-	T56.1X4-	-	-
organic (fungicide)	T56.1X1-	T56.1X2-	T56.1X3-	T56.1X4-	-	-
oxide, yellow	T49.0X1-	T49.0X2-	T49.0X3-	T49.0X4-	T49.0X5-	T49.0X6-
Mersalyl	T50.2X1-	T50.2X2-	T50.2X3-	T50.2X4-	T50.2X5-	T50.2X6-
Merthiolate	T49.0X1-	T49.0X2-	T49.0X3-	T49.0X4-	T49.0X5-	T49.0X6-
ophthalmic preparation	T49.5X1-	T49.5X2-	T49.5X3-	T49.5X4-	T49.5X5-	T49.5X6-
Meruvax	T50.B91-	T50.B92-	T50.B93-	T50.B94-	T50.B95-	T50.B96-
Mesalazine	T47.8X1-	T47.8X2-	T47.8X3-	T47.8X4-	T47.8X5-	T47.8X6-
Mescal buttons	T40.991-	T40.992-	T40.993-	T40.994-	-	-
Mescaline	T40.991-	T40.992-	T40.993-	T40.994-	-	-
Mesna	T48.4X1-	T48.4X2-	T48.4X3-	T48.4X4-	T48.4X5-	T48.4X6-
Mesoglycan	T46.6X1-	T46.6X2-	T46.6X3-	T46.6X4-	T46.6X5-	T46.6X6-
Mesoridazine	T43.3X1-	T43.3X2-	T43.3X3-	T43.3X4-	T43.3X5-	T43.3X6-
Mestanolone	T38.7X1-	T38.7X2-	T38.7X3-	T38.7X4-	T38.7X5-	T38.7X6-
Mesterolone	T38.7X1-	T38.7X2-	T38.7X3-	T38.7X4-	T38.7X5-	T38.7X6-
Mestranol	T38.5X1-	T38.5X2-	T38.5X3-	T38.5X4-	T38.5X5-	T38.5X6-
Mesulergine	T42.8X1-	T42.8X2-	T42.8X3-	T42.8X4-	T42.8X5-	T42.8X6-
Mesulfen	T49.0X1-	T49.0X2-	T49.0X3-	T49.0X4-	T49.0X5-	T49.0X6-
Mesuximide	T42.2X1-	T42.2X2-	T42.2X3-	T42.2X4-	T42.2X5-	T42.2X6-
Metabutethamine	T41.3X1-	T41.3X2-	T41.3X3-	T41.3X4-	T41.3X5-	T41.3X6-
Metactesylacetate	T49.0X1-	T49.0X2-	T49.0X3-	T49.0X4-	T49.0X5-	T49.0X6-
Metacycline	T36.4X1-	T36.4X2-	T36.4X3-	T36.4X4-	T36.4X5-	T36.4X6-
Metaldehyde (snail killer) NEC	T60.8X1-	T60.8X2-	T60.8X3-	T60.8X4-	-	-
Metals (heavy) (nonmedicinal)	T56.91X-	T56.92X-	T56.93X-	T56.94X-	-	-
dust, fumes, or vapor NEC	T56.91X-	T56.92X-	T56.93X-	T56.94X-	-	-
light NEC	T56.91X-	T56.92X-	T56.93X-	T56.94X-	-	-
dust, fumes, or vapor NEC	T56.91X-	T56.92X-	T56.93X-	T56.94X-	-	-
specified NEC	T56.891-	T56.892-	T56.893-	T56.894-	-	-
thallium	T56.811-	T56.812-	T56.813-	T56.814-	-	-
Metamfetamine	T43.621-	T43.622-	T43.623-	T43.624-	T43.625-	T43.626-
Metamizole sodium	T39.2X1-	T39.2X2-	T39.2X3-	T39.2X4-	T39.2X5-	T39.2X6-
Metampicillin	T36.0X1-	T36.0X2-	T36.0X3-	T36.0X4-	T36.0X5-	T36.0X6-
Metamucil	T47.4X1-	T47.4X2-	T47.4X3-	T47.4X4-	T47.4X5-	T47.4X6-
Metandienone	T38.7X1-	T38.7X2-	T38.7X3-	T38.7X4-	T38.7X5-	T38.7X6-
Metandrostenolone	T38.7X1-	T38.7X2-	T38.7X3-	T38.7X4-	T38.7X5-	T38.7X6-
Metaphen	T49.0X1-	T49.0X2-	T49.0X3-	T49.0X4-	T49.0X5-	T49.0X6-
Metaphos	T60.0X1-	T60.0X2-	T60.0X3-	T60.0X4-	-	-
Metapramine	T43.011-	T43.012-	T43.013-	T43.014-	T43.015-	T43.016-
Metaproterenol	T48.291-	T48.292-	T48.293-	T48.294-	T48.295-	T48.296-
Metaraminol	T44.4X1-	T44.4X2-	T44.4X3-	T44.4X4-	T44.4X5-	T44.4X6-
Metaxalone	T42.8X1-	T42.8X2-	T42.8X3-	T42.8X4-	T42.8X5-	T42.8X6-
Metenolone	T38.7X1-	T38.7X2-	T38.7X3-	T38.7X4-	T38.7X5-	T38.7X6-
Metergoline	T42.8X1-	T42.8X2-	T42.8X3-	T42.8X4-	T42.8X5-	T42.8X6-
Metescufylline	T46.991-	T46.992-	T46.993-	T46.994-	T46.995-	T46.996-
Metetoin	T42.0X1-	T42.0X2-	T42.0X3-	T42.0X4-	T42.0X5-	T42.0X6-
Metformin	T38.3X1-	T38.3X2-	T38.3X3-	T38.3X4-	T38.3X5-	T38.3X6-
Methacholine	T44.1X1-	T44.1X2-	T44.1X3-	T44.1X4-	T44.1X5-	T44.1X6-
Methacycline	T36.4X1-	T36.4X2-	T36.4X3-	T36.4X4-	T36.4X5-	T36.4X6-
Methadone	T40.3X1-	T40.3X2-	T40.3X3-	T40.3X4-	T40.3X5-	T40.3X6-
Methallenestril	T38.5X1-	T38.5X2-	T38.5X3-	T38.5X4-	T38.5X5-	T38.5X6-
Methallenoestril	T38.5X1-	T38.5X2-	T38.5X3-	T38.5X4-	T38.5X5-	T38.5X6-
Methamphetamine	T43.621-	T43.622-	T43.623-	T43.624-	T43.625-	T43.626-

Substance	Poisoning Accidental (unintentional)	Poisoning Intentional self-harm	Poisoning Assault	Poisoning Undetermined	Adverse effect	Underdosing
Methampyrone	T39.2X1-	T39.2X2-	T39.2X3-	T39.2X4-	T39.2X5-	T39.2X6-
Methandienone	T38.7X1-	T38.7X2-	T38.7X3-	T38.7X4-	T38.7X5-	T38.7X6-
Methandriol	T38.7X1-	T38.7X2-	T38.7X3-	T38.7X4-	T38.7X5-	T38.7X6-
Methandrostenolone	T38.7X1-	T38.7X2-	T38.7X3-	T38.7X4-	T38.7X5-	T38.7X6-
Methane	T59.891-	T59.892-	T59.893-	T59.894-	-	-
Methanethiol	T59.891-	T59.892-	T59.893-	T59.894-	-	-
Methaniazide	T37.1X1-	T37.1X2-	T37.1X3-	T37.1X4-	T37.1X5-	T37.1X6-
Methanol (vapor)	T51.1X1-	T51.1X2-	T51.1X3-	T51.1X4-	-	-
Methantheline	T44.3X1-	T44.3X2-	T44.3X3-	T44.3X4-	T44.3X5-	T44.3X6-
Methanthelinium bromide	T44.3X1-	T44.3X2-	T44.3X3-	T44.3X4-	T44.3X5-	T44.3X6-
Methaphenilene	T45.0X1-	T45.0X2-	T45.0X3-	T45.0X4-	T45.0X5-	T45.0X6-
Methapyrilene	T45.0X1-	T45.0X2-	T45.0X3-	T45.0X4-	T45.0X5-	T45.0X6-
Methaqualone (compound)	T42.6X1-	T42.6X2-	T42.6X3-	T42.6X4-	T42.6X5-	T42.6X6-
Metharbital	T42.3X1-	T42.3X2-	T42.3X3-	T42.3X4-	T42.3X5-	T42.3X6-
Methazolamide	T50.2X1-	T50.2X2-	T50.2X3-	T50.2X4-	T50.2X5-	T50.2X6-
Methdilazine	T43.3X1-	T43.3X2-	T43.3X3-	T43.3X4-	T43.3X5-	T43.3X6-
Methedrine	T43.621-	T43.622-	T43.623-	T43.624-	T43.625-	T43.626-
Methenamine (mandelate)	T37.8X1-	T37.8X2-	T37.8X3-	T37.8X4-	T37.8X5-	T37.8X6-
Methenolone	T38.7X1-	T38.7X2-	T38.7X3-	T38.7X4-	T38.7X5-	T38.7X6-
Methergine	T48.0X1-	T48.0X2-	T48.0X3-	T48.0X4-	T48.0X5-	T48.0X6-
Methetoin	T42.0X1-	T42.0X2-	T42.0X3-	T42.0X4-	T42.0X5-	T42.0X6-
Methiacil	T38.2X1-	T38.2X2-	T38.2X3-	T38.2X4-	T38.2X5-	T38.2X6-
Methicillin	T36.0X1-	T36.0X2-	T36.0X3-	T36.0X4-	T36.0X5-	T36.0X6-
Methimazole	T38.2X1-	T38.2X2-	T38.2X3-	T38.2X4-	T38.2X5-	T38.2X6-
Methiodal sodium	T50.8X1-	T50.8X2-	T50.8X3-	T50.8X4-	T50.8X5-	T50.8X6-
Methionine	T50.991-	T50.992-	T50.993-	T50.994-	T50.995-	T50.996-
Methisazone	T37.5X1-	T37.5X2-	T37.5X3-	T37.5X4-	T37.5X5-	T37.5X6-
Methisoprinol	T37.5X1-	T37.5X2-	T37.5X3-	T37.5X4-	T37.5X5-	T37.5X6-
Methitural	T42.3X1-	T42.3X2-	T42.3X3-	T42.3X4-	T42.3X5-	T42.3X6-
Methixene	T44.3X1-	T44.3X2-	T44.3X3-	T44.3X4-	T44.3X5-	T44.3X6-
Methobarbital, methobarbitone	T42.3X1-	T42.3X2-	T42.3X3-	T42.3X4-	T42.3X5-	T42.3X6-
Methocarbamol	T42.8X1-	T42.8X2-	T42.8X3-	T42.8X4-	T42.8X5-	T42.8X6-
skeletal muscle relaxant	T48.1X1-	T48.1X2-	T48.1X3-	T48.1X4-	T48.1X5-	T48.1X6-
Methohexital	T41.1X1-	T41.1X2-	T41.1X3-	T41.1X4-	T41.1X5-	T41.1X6-
Methohexitone	T41.1X1-	T41.1X2-	T41.1X3-	T41.1X4-	T41.1X5-	T41.1X6-
Methoin	T42.0X1-	T42.0X2-	T42.0X3-	T42.0X4-	T42.0X5-	T42.0X6-
Methopholine	T39.8X1-	T39.8X2-	T39.8X3-	T39.8X4-	T39.8X5-	T39.8X6-
Methopromazine	T43.3X1-	T43.3X2-	T43.3X3-	T43.3X4-	T43.3X5-	T43.3X6-
Methorate	T48.3X1-	T48.3X2-	T48.3X3-	T48.3X4-	T48.3X5-	T48.3X6-
Methoserpidine	T46.5X1-	T46.5X2-	T46.5X3-	T46.5X4-	T46.5X5-	T46.5X6-
Methotrexate	T45.1X1-	T45.1X2-	T45.1X3-	T45.1X4-	T45.1X5-	T45.1X6-
Methotrimeprazine	T43.3X1-	T43.3X2-	T43.3X3-	T43.3X4-	T43.3X5-	T43.3X6-
Methoxa-Dome	T49.3X1-	T49.3X2-	T49.3X3-	T49.3X4-	T49.3X5-	T49.3X6-
Methoxamine	T44.4X1-	T44.4X2-	T44.4X3-	T44.4X4-	T44.4X5-	T44.4X6-
Methoxsalen	T50.991-	T50.992-	T50.993-	T50.994-	T50.995-	T50.996-
Methoxyaniline	T65.3X1-	T65.3X2-	T65.3X3-	T65.3X4-	-	-
Methoxybenzyl penicillin	T36.0X1-	T36.0X2-	T36.0X3-	T36.0X4-	T36.0X5-	T36.0X6-
Methoxychlor	T53.7X1-	T53.7X2-	T53.7X3-	T53.7X4-	-	-
Methoxy-DDT	T53.7X1-	T53.7X2-	T53.7X3-	T53.7X4-	-	-
2-Methoxyethanol	T52.3X1-	T52.3X2-	T52.3X3-	T52.3X4-	-	-
Methoxyflurane	T41.0X1-	T41.0X2-	T41.0X3-	T41.0X4-	T41.0X5-	T41.0X6-
Methoxyphenamine	T48.6X1-	T48.6X2-	T48.6X3-	T48.6X4-	T48.6X5-	T48.6X6-
Methoxypromazine	T43.3X1-	T43.3X2-	T43.3X3-	T43.3X4-	T43.3X5-	T43.3X6-
5-Methoxypsoralen (5-MOP)	T50.991-	T50.992-	T50.993-	T50.994-	T50.995-	T50.996-
8-Methoxypsoralen (8-MOP)	T50.991-	T50.992-	T50.993-	T50.994-	T50.995-	T50.996-
Methscopolamine bromide	T44.3X1-	T44.3X2-	T44.3X3-	T44.3X4-	T44.3X5-	T44.3X6-
Methsuximide	T42.2X1-	T42.2X2-	T42.2X3-	T42.2X4-	T42.2X5-	T42.2X6-
Methyclothiazide	T50.2X1-	T50.2X2-	T50.2X3-	T50.2X4-	T50.2X5-	T50.2X6-

METHYL - METHYLATROPINE NITRATE

Substance	Poisoning Accidental (unintentional)	Poisoning Intentional self-harm	Poisoning Assault	Poisoning Undetermined	Adverse effect	Underdosing
Methyl						
acetate	T52.4X1-	T52.4X2-	T52.4X3-	T52.4X4-	-	-
acetone	T52.4X1-	T52.4X2-	T52.4X3-	T52.4X4-	-	-
acrylate	T65.891-	T65.892-	T65.893-	T65.894-	-	-
alcohol	T51.1X1-	T51.1X2-	T51.1X3-	T51.1X4-	-	-
aminophenol	T65.3X1-	T65.3X2-	T65.3X3-	T65.3X4-	-	-
amphetamine	T43.621-	T43.622-	T43.623-	T43.624-	T43.625-	T43.626-
androstanolone	T38.7X1-	T38.7X2-	T38.7X3-	T38.7X4-	T38.7X5-	T38.7X6-
atropine	T44.3X1-	T44.3X2-	T44.3X3-	T44.3X4-	T44.3X5-	T44.3X6-
benzene	T52.2X1-	T52.2X2-	T52.2X3-	T52.2X4-	-	-
benzoate	T52.8X1-	T52.8X2-	T52.8X3-	T52.8X4-	-	-
benzol	T52.2X1-	T52.2X2-	T52.2X3-	T52.2X4-	-	-
bromide (gas)	T59.891-	T59.892-	T59.893-	T59.894-	-	-
fumigant	T60.8X1-	T60.8X2-	T60.8X3-	T60.8X4-	-	-
butanol	T51.3X1-	T51.3X2-	T51.3X3-	T51.3X4-	-	-
carbinol	T51.1X1-	T51.1X2-	T51.1X3-	T51.1X4-	-	-
carbonate	T52.8X1-	T52.8X2-	T52.8X3-	T52.8X4-	-	-
CCNU	T45.1X1-	T45.1X2-	T45.1X3-	T45.1X4-	T45.1X5-	T45.1X6-
cellosolve	T52.91X-	T52.92X-	T52.93X-	T52.94X-	-	-
cellulose	T47.4X1-	T47.4X2-	T47.4X3-	T47.4X4-	T47.4X5-	T47.4X6-
chloride (gas)	T59.891-	T59.892-	T59.893-	T59.894-	-	-
chloroformate	T59.3X1-	T59.3X2-	T59.3X3-	T59.3X4-	-	-
cyclohexane	T52.8X1-	T52.8X2-	T52.8X3-	T52.8X4-	-	-
cyclohexanol	T51.8X1-	T51.8X2-	T51.8X3-	T51.8X4-	-	-
cyclohexanone	T52.8X1-	T52.8X2-	T52.8X3-	T52.8X4-	-	-
cyclohexyl acetate	T52.8X1-	T52.8X2-	T52.8X3-	T52.8X4-	-	-
demeton	T60.0X1-	T60.0X2-	T60.0X3-	T60.0X4-	-	-
dihydromorphinone	T40.2X1-	T40.2X2-	T40.2X3-	T40.2X4-	T40.2X5-	T40.2X6-
ergometrine	T48.0X1-	T48.0X2-	T48.0X3-	T48.0X4-	T48.0X5-	T48.0X6-
ergonovine	T48.0X1-	T48.0X2-	T48.0X3-	T48.0X4-	T48.0X5-	T48.0X6-
ethyl ketone	T52.4X1-	T52.4X2-	T52.4X3-	T52.4X4-	-	-
glucamine antimonate	T37.8X1-	T37.8X2-	T37.8X3-	T37.8X4-	T37.8X5-	T37.8X6-
hydrazine	T65.891-	T65.892-	T65.893-	T65.894-	-	-
iodide	T65.891-	T65.892-	T65.893-	T65.894-	-	-
isobutyl ketone	T52.4X1-	T52.4X2-	T52.4X3-	T52.4X4-	-	-
isothiocyanate	T60.3X1-	T60.3X2-	T60.3X3-	T60.3X4-	-	-
mercaptan	T59.891-	T59.892-	T59.893-	T59.894-	-	-
morphine NEC	T40.2X1-	T40.2X2-	T40.2X3-	T40.2X4-	T40.2X5-	T40.2X6-
nicotinate	T49.4X1-	T49.4X2-	T49.4X3-	T49.4X4-	T49.4X5-	T49.4X6-
paraben	T49.0X1-	T49.0X2-	T49.0X3-	T49.0X4-	T49.0X5-	T49.0X6-
parafynol	T42.6X1-	T42.6X2-	T42.6X3-	T42.6X4-	T42.6X5-	T42.6X6-
parathion	T60.0X1-	T60.0X2-	T60.0X3-	T60.0X4-	-	-
peridol	T43.4X1-	T43.4X2-	T43.4X3-	T43.4X4-	T43.4X5-	T43.4X6-
phenidate	T43.631-	T43.632-	T43.633-	T43.634-	T43.635-	T43.636-
prednisolone	T38.0X1-	T38.0X2-	T38.0X3-	T38.0X4-	T38.0X5-	T38.0X6-
ENT agent	T49.6X1-	T49.6X2-	T49.6X3-	T49.6X4-	T49.6X5-	T49.6X6-
ophthalmic preparation	T49.5X1-	T49.5X2-	T49.5X3-	T49.5X4-	T49.5X5-	T49.5X6-
topical NEC	T49.0X1-	T49.0X2-	T49.0X3-	T49.0X4-	T49.0X5-	T49.0X6-
propylcarbinol	T51.3X1-	T51.3X2-	T51.3X3-	T51.3X4-	-	-
rosaniline NEC	T49.0X1-	T49.0X2-	T49.0X3-	T49.0X4-	T49.0X5-	T49.0X6-
salicylate	T49.2X1-	T49.2X2-	T49.2X3-	T49.2X4-	T49.2X5-	T49.2X6-
sulfate (fumes)	T59.891-	T59.892-	T59.893-	T59.894-	-	-
liquid	T52.8X1-	T52.8X2-	T52.8X3-	T52.8X4-	-	-
sulfonal	T42.6X1-	T42.6X2-	T42.6X3-	T42.6X4-	T42.6X5-	T42.6X6-
testosterone	T38.7X1-	T38.7X2-	T38.7X3-	T38.7X4-	T38.7X5-	T38.7X6-
thiouracil	T38.2X1-	T38.2X2-	T38.2X3-	T38.2X4-	T38.2X5-	T38.2X6-
Methylamphetamine	T43.621-	T43.622-	T43.623-	T43.624-	T43.625-	T43.626-
Methylated spirit	T51.1X1-	T51.1X2-	T51.1X3-	T51.1X4-	-	-
Methylatropine nitrate	T44.3X1-	T44.3X2-	T44.3X3-	T44.3X4-	T44.3X5-	T44.3X6-

Substance	Poisoning Accidental (unintentional)	Poisoning Intentional self-harm	Poisoning Assault	Poisoning Undetermined	Adverse effect	Underdosing
Methylbenactyzium bromide	T44.3X1-	T44.3X2-	T44.3X3-	T44.3X4-	T44.3X5-	T44.3X6-
Methylbenzethonium chloride	T49.0X1-	T49.0X2-	T49.0X3-	T49.0X4-	T49.0X5-	T49.0X6-
Methylcellulose	T47.4X1-	T47.4X2-	T47.4X3-	T47.4X4-	T47.4X5-	T47.4X6-
laxative	T47.4X1-	T47.4X2-	T47.4X3-	T47.4X4-	T47.4X5-	T47.4X6-
Methylchlorophenoxy-acetic acid	T60.3X1-	T60.3X2-	T60.3X3-	T60.3X4-	-	-
Methyldopa	T46.5X1-	T46.5X2-	T46.5X3-	T46.5X4-	T46.5X5-	T46.5X6-
Methyldopate	T46.5X1-	T46.5X2-	T46.5X3-	T46.5X4-	T46.5X5-	T46.5X6-
Methylene						
blue	T50.6X1-	T50.6X2-	T50.6X3-	T50.6X4-	T50.6X5-	T50.6X6-
chloride or dichloride (solvent) NEC	T53.4X1-	T53.4X2-	T53.4X3-	T53.4X4-	-	-
Methylenedioxyamphetamine	T43.621-	T43.622-	T43.623-	T43.624-	T43.625-	T43.626-
Methylenedioxymethamphetamine	T43.641-	T43.642-	T43.643-	T43.644-	-	-
Methylergometrine	T48.0X1-	T48.0X2-	T48.0X3-	T48.0X4-	T48.0X5-	T48.0X6-
Methylergonovine	T48.0X1-	T48.0X2-	T48.0X3-	T48.0X4-	T48.0X5-	T48.0X6-
Methylestrenolone	T38.5X1-	T38.5X2-	T38.5X3-	T38.5X4-	T38.5X5-	T38.5X6-
Methylethyl cellulose	T50.991-	T50.992-	T50.993-	T50.994-	T50.995-	T50.996-
Methylhexabital	T42.3X1-	T42.3X2-	T42.3X3-	T42.3X4-	T42.3X5-	T42.3X6-
Methylmorphine	T40.2X1-	T40.2X2-	T40.2X3-	T40.2X4-	T40.2X5-	T40.2X6-
Methylparaben (ophthalmic)	T49.5X1-	T49.5X2-	T49.5X3-	T49.5X4-	T49.5X5-	T49.5X6-
Methylparafynol	T42.6X1-	T42.6X2-	T42.6X3-	T42.6X4-	T42.6X5-	T42.6X6-
Methylpentynol, methylpenthynol	T42.6X1-	T42.6X2-	T42.6X3-	T42.6X4-	T42.6X5-	T42.6X6-
Methylphenidate	T43.631-	T43.632-	T43.633-	T43.634-	T43.635-	T43.636-
Methylphenobarbital	T42.3X1-	T42.3X2-	T42.3X3-	T42.3X4-	T42.3X5-	T42.3X6-
Methylpolysiloxane	T47.1X1-	T47.1X2-	T47.1X3-	T47.1X4-	T47.1X5-	T47.1X6-
Methylprednisolone — *see Methyl, prednisolone*						
Methylrosaniline	T49.0X1-	T49.0X2-	T49.0X3-	T49.0X4-	T49.0X5-	T49.0X6-
Methylrosanilinium chloride	T49.0X1-	T49.0X2-	T49.0X3-	T49.0X4-	T49.0X5-	T49.0X6-
Methyltestosterone	T38.7X1-	T38.7X2-	T38.7X3-	T38.7X4-	T38.7X5-	T38.7X6-
Methylthionine chloride	T50.6X1-	T50.6X2-	T50.6X3-	T50.6X4-	T50.6X5-	T50.6X6-
Methylthioninium chloride	T50.6X1-	T50.6X2-	T50.6X3-	T50.6X4-	T50.6X5-	T50.6X6-
Methylthiouracil	T38.2X1-	T38.2X2-	T38.2X3-	T38.2X4-	T38.2X5-	T38.2X6-
Methyprylon	T42.6X1-	T42.6X2-	T42.6X3-	T42.6X4-	T42.6X5-	T42.6X6-
Methysergide	T46.5X1-	T46.5X2-	T46.5X3-	T46.5X4-	T46.5X5-	T46.5X6-
Metiamide	T47.1X1-	T47.1X2-	T47.1X3-	T47.1X4-	T47.1X5-	T47.1X6-
Meticillin	T36.0X1-	T36.0X2-	T36.0X3-	T36.0X4-	T36.0X5-	T36.0X6-
Meticrane	T50.2X1-	T50.2X2-	T50.2X3-	T50.2X4-	T50.2X5-	T50.2X6-
Metildigoxin	T46.0X1-	T46.0X2-	T46.0X3-	T46.0X4-	T46.0X5-	T46.0X6-
Metipranolol	T49.5X1-	T49.5X2-	T49.5X3-	T49.5X4-	T49.5X5-	T49.5X6-
Metirosine	T46.5X1-	T46.5X2-	T46.5X3-	T46.5X4-	T46.5X5-	T46.5X6-
Metisazone	T37.5X1-	T37.5X2-	T37.5X3-	T37.5X4-	T37.5X5-	T37.5X6-
Metixene	T44.3X1-	T44.3X2-	T44.3X3-	T44.3X4-	T44.3X5-	T44.3X6-
Metizoline	T48.5X1-	T48.5X2-	T48.5X3-	T48.5X4-	T48.5X5-	T48.5X6-
Metoclopramide	T45.0X1-	T45.0X2-	T45.0X3-	T45.0X4-	T45.0X5-	T45.0X6-
Metofenazate	T43.3X1-	T43.3X2-	T43.3X3-	T43.3X4-	T43.3X5-	T43.3X6-
Metofoline	T39.8X1-	T39.8X2-	T39.8X3-	T39.8X4-	T39.8X5-	T39.8X6-
Metolazone	T50.2X1-	T50.2X2-	T50.2X3-	T50.2X4-	T50.2X5-	T50.2X6-
Metopon	T40.2X1-	T40.2X2-	T40.2X3-	T40.2X4-	T40.2X5-	T40.2X6-
Metoprine	T45.1X1-	T45.1X2-	T45.1X3-	T45.1X4-	T45.1X5-	T45.1X6-
Metoprolol	T44.7X1-	T44.7X2-	T44.7X3-	T44.7X4-	T44.7X5-	T44.7X6-
Metrifonate	T60.0X1-	T60.0X2-	T60.0X3-	T60.0X4-	-	-
Metrizamide	T50.8X1-	T50.8X2-	T50.8X3-	T50.8X4-	T50.8X5-	T50.8X6-
Metrizoic acid	T50.8X1-	T50.8X2-	T50.8X3-	T50.8X4-	T50.8X5-	T50.8X6-
Metronidazole	T37.8X1-	T37.8X2-	T37.8X3-	T37.8X4-	T37.8X5-	T37.8X6-
Metycaine	T41.3X1-	T41.3X2-	T41.3X3-	T41.3X4-	T41.3X5-	T41.3X6-
infiltration (subcutaneous)	T41.3X1-	T41.3X2-	T41.3X3-	T41.3X4-	T41.3X5-	T41.3X6-
nerve block (peripheral) (plexus)	T41.3X1-	T41.3X2-	T41.3X3-	T41.3X4-	T41.3X5-	T41.3X6-
topical (surface)	T41.3X1-	T41.3X2-	T41.3X3-	T41.3X4-	T41.3X5-	T41.3X6-
Metyrapone	T50.8X1-	T50.8X2-	T50.8X3-	T50.8X4-	T50.8X5-	T50.8X6-

Substance	Poisoning Accidental (unintentional)	Poisoning Intentional self-harm	Poisoning Assault	Poisoning Undetermined	Adverse effect	Underdosing
Mevinphos	T60.0X1-	T60.0X2-	T60.0X3-	T60.0X4-	-	-
Mexazolam	T42.4X1-	T42.4X2-	T42.4X3-	T42.4X4-	T42.4X5-	T42.4X6-
Mexenone	T49.3X1-	T49.3X2-	T49.3X3-	T49.3X4-	T49.3X5-	T49.3X6-
Mexiletine	T46.2X1-	T46.2X2-	T46.2X3-	T46.2X4-	T46.2X5-	T46.2X6-
Mezereon	T62.2X1-	T62.2X2-	T62.2X3-	T62.2X4-	-	-
berries	T62.1X1-	T62.1X2-	T62.1X3-	T62.1X4-	-	-
Mezlocillin	T36.0X1-	T36.0X2-	T36.0X3-	T36.0X4-	T36.0X5-	T36.0X6-
Mianserin	T43.021-	T43.022-	T43.023-	T43.024-	T43.025-	T43.026-
Micatin	T49.0X1-	T49.0X2-	T49.0X3-	T49.0X4-	T49.0X5-	T49.0X6-
Miconazole	T49.0X1-	T49.0X2-	T49.0X3-	T49.0X4-	T49.0X5-	T49.0X6-
Micronomicin	T36.5X1-	T36.5X2-	T36.5X3-	T36.5X4-	T36.5X5-	T36.5X6-
Midazolam	T42.4X1-	T42.4X2-	T42.4X3-	T42.4X4-	T42.4X5-	T42.4X6-
Midecamycin	T36.3X1-	T36.3X2-	T36.3X3-	T36.3X4-	T36.3X5-	T36.3X6-
Mifepristone	T38.6X1-	T38.6X2-	T38.6X3-	T38.6X4-	T38.6X5-	T38.6X6-
Milk of magnesia	T47.1X1-	T47.1X2-	T47.1X3-	T47.1X4-	T47.1X5-	T47.1X6-
Millipede (tropical) (venomous)	T63.411-	T63.412-	T63.413-	T63.414-	-	-
Miltown	T43.591-	T43.592-	T43.593-	T43.594-	T43.595-	T43.596-
Milverine	T44.3X1-	T44.3X2-	T44.3X3-	T44.3X4-	T44.3X5-	T44.3X6-
Minaprine	T43.291-	T43.292-	T43.293-	T43.294-	T43.295-	T43.296-
Minaxolone	T41.291-	T41.292-	T41.293-	T41.294-	T41.295-	T41.296-
Mineral						
acids	T54.2X1-	T54.2X2-	T54.2X3-	T54.2X4-	-	-
oil (laxative) (medicinal)	T47.4X1-	T47.4X2-	T47.4X3-	T47.4X4-	T47.4X5-	T47.4X6-
emulsion	T47.2X1-	T47.2X2-	T47.2X3-	T47.2X4-	T47.2X5-	T47.2X6-
nonmedicinal	T52.0X1-	T52.0X2-	T52.0X3-	T52.0X4-	-	-
topical	T49.3X1-	T49.3X2-	T49.3X3-	T49.3X4-	T49.3X5-	T49.3X6-
salt NEC	T50.3X1-	T50.3X2-	T50.3X3-	T50.3X4-	T50.3X5-	T50.3X6-
spirits	T52.0X1-	T52.0X2-	T52.0X3-	T52.0X4-	-	-
Mineralocorticosteroid	T50.0X1-	T50.0X2-	T50.0X3-	T50.0X4-	T50.0X5-	T50.0X6-
Minocycline	T36.4X1-	T36.4X2-	T36.4X3-	T36.4X4-	T36.4X5-	T36.4X6-
Minoxidil	T46.7X1-	T46.7X2-	T46.7X3-	T46.7X4-	T46.7X5-	T46.7X6-
Miokamycin	T36.3X1-	T36.3X2-	T36.3X3-	T36.3X4-	T36.3X5-	T36.3X6-
Miotic drug	T49.5X1-	T49.5X2-	T49.5X3-	T49.5X4-	T49.5X5-	T49.5X6-
Mipafox	T60.0X1-	T60.0X2-	T60.0X3-	T60.0X4-	-	-
Mirex	T60.1X1-	T60.1X2-	T60.1X3-	T60.1X4-	-	-
Mirtazapine	T43.021-	T43.022-	T43.023-	T43.024-	T43.025-	T43.026-
Misonidazole	T37.3X1-	T37.3X2-	T37.3X3-	T37.3X4-	T37.3X5-	T37.3X6-
Misoprostol	T47.1X1-	T47.1X2-	T47.1X3-	T47.1X4-	T47.1X5-	T47.1X6-
Mithramycin	T45.1X1-	T45.1X2-	T45.1X3-	T45.1X4-	T45.1X5-	T45.1X6-
Mitobronitol	T45.1X1-	T45.1X2-	T45.1X3-	T45.1X4-	T45.1X5-	T45.1X6-
Mitoguazone	T45.1X1-	T45.1X2-	T45.1X3-	T45.1X4-	T45.1X5-	T45.1X6-
Mitolactol	T45.1X1-	T45.1X2-	T45.1X3-	T45.1X4-	T45.1X5-	T45.1X6-
Mitomycin	T45.1X1-	T45.1X2-	T45.1X3-	T45.1X4-	T45.1X5-	T45.1X6-
Mitopodozide	T45.1X1-	T45.1X2-	T45.1X3-	T45.1X4-	T45.1X5-	T45.1X6-
Mitotane	T45.1X1-	T45.1X2-	T45.1X3-	T45.1X4-	T45.1X5-	T45.1X6-
Mitoxantrone	T45.1X1-	T45.1X2-	T45.1X3-	T45.1X4-	T45.1X5-	T45.1X6-
Mivacurium chloride	T48.1X1-	T48.1X2-	T48.1X3-	T48.1X4-	T48.1X5-	T48.1X6-
Miyari bacteria	T47.6X1-	T47.6X2-	T47.6X3-	T47.6X4-	T47.6X5-	T47.6X6-
Moclobemide	T43.1X1-	T43.1X2-	T43.1X3-	T43.1X4-	T43.1X5-	T43.1X6-
Moderil	T46.5X1-	T46.5X2-	T46.5X3-	T46.5X4-	T46.5X5-	T46.5X6-
Mofebutazone	T39.2X1-	T39.2X2-	T39.2X3-	T39.2X4-	T39.2X5-	
Mogadon — *see Nitrazepam*						
Molindone	T43.591-	T43.592-	T43.593-	T43.594-	T43.595-	T43.596-
Molsidomine	T46.3X1-	T46.3X2-	T46.3X3-	T46.3X4-	T46.3X5-	T46.3X6-
Mometasone	T49.0X1-	T49.0X2-	T49.0X3-	T49.0X4-	T49.0X5-	T49.0X6-
Monistat	T49.0X1-	T49.0X2-	T49.0X3-	T49.0X4-	T49.0X5-	
Monkshood	T62.2X1-	T62.2X2-	T62.2X3-	T62.2X4-	-	-
Monoamine oxidase inhibitor NEC	T43.1X1-	T43.1X2-	T43.1X3-	T43.1X4-	T43.1X5-	T43.1X6-
hydrazine	T43.1X1-	T43.1X2-	T43.1X3-	T43.1X4-	T43.1X5-	T43.1X6-

Substance	Poisoning Accidental (unintentional)	Poisoning Intentional self-harm	Poisoning Assault	Poisoning Undetermined	Adverse effect	Underdosing
Monobenzone	T49.4X1-	T49.4X2-	T49.4X3-	T49.4X4-	T49.4X5-	T49.4X6-
Monochloroacetic acid	T60.3X1-	T60.3X2-	T60.3X3-	T60.3X4-	-	-
Monochlorobenzene	T53.7X1-	T53.7X2-	T53.7X3-	T53.7X4-	-	-
Monoethanolamine	T46.8X1-	T46.8X2-	T46.8X3-	T46.8X4-	T46.8X5-	T46.8X6-
oleate	T46.8X1-	T46.8X2-	T46.8X3-	T46.8X4-	T46.8X5-	T46.8X6-
Monooctanoin	T50.991-	T50.992-	T50.993-	T50.994-	T50.995-	T50.996-
Monophenylbutazone	T39.2X1-	T39.2X2-	T39.2X3-	T39.2X4-	T39.2X5-	T39.2X6-
Monosodium glutamate	T65.891-	T65.892-	T65.893-	T65.894-	-	-
Monosulfiram	T49.0X1-	T49.0X2-	T49.0X3-	T49.0X4-·	T49.0X5-	T49.0X6-
Monoxide, carbon — *see Carbon, monoxide*						
Monoxidine hydrochloride	T46.1X1-	T46.1X2-	T46.1X3-	T46.1X4-	T46.1X5-	T46.1X6-
Monuron	T60.3X1-	T60.3X2-	T60.3X3-	T60.3X4-	-	-
Moperone	T43.4X1-	T43.4X2-	T43.4X3-	T43.4X4-	T43.4X5-	T43.4X6-
Mopidamol	T45.1X1-	T45.1X2-	T45.1X3-	T45.1X4-	T45.1X5-	T45.1X6-
MOPP (mechloreth-amine + vincristine + prednisone + procarba-zine)	T45.1X1-	T45.1X2-	T45.1X3-	T45.1X4-	T45.1X5-	T45.1X6-
Morfin	T40.2X1-	T40.2X2-	T40.2X3-	T40.2X4-	T40.2X5-	T40.2X6-
Morinamide	T37.1X1-	T37.1X2-	T37.1X3-	T37.1X4-	T37.1X5-	T37.1X6-
Morning glory seeds	T40.991-	T40.992-	T40.993-	T40.994-	-	-
Moroxydine	T37.5X1-	T37.5X2-	T37.5X3-	T37.5X4-	T37.5X5-	T37.5X6-
Morphazinamide	T37.1X1-	T37.1X2-	T37.1X3-	T37.1X4-	T37.1X5-	T37.1X6-
Morphine	T40.2X1-	T40.2X2-	T40.2X3-	T40.2X4-	T40.2X5-	T40.2X6-
antagonist	T50.7X1-	T50.7X2-	T50.7X3-	T50.7X4-	T50.7X5-	T50.7X6-
Morpholinylethylmorphine	T40.2X1-	T40.2X2-	T40.2X3-	T40.2X4-	-	-
Morsuximide	T42.2X1-	T42.2X2-	T42.2X3-	T42.2X4-	T42.2X5-	T42.2X6-
Mosapramine	T43.591-	T43.592-	T43.593-	T43.594-	T43.595-	T43.596-
Moth balls — *see also Pesticides*	T60.2X1-	T60.2X2-	T60.2X3-	T60.2X4-	-	-
naphthalene	T60.2X1-	T60.2X2-	T60.2X3-	T60.2X4-	-	-
paradichlorobenzene	T60.1X1-	T60.1X2-	T60.1X3-	T60.1X4-	-	-
Motor exhaust gas	T58.01X-	T58.02X-	T58.03X-	T58.04X-	-	-
Mouthwash (antiseptic) (zinc chloride)	T49.6X1-	T49.6X2-	T49.6X3-	T49.6X4-	T49.6X5-	T49.6X6-
Moxastine	T45.0X1-	T45.0X2-	T45.0X3-	T45.0X4-	T45.0X5-	T45.0X6-
Moxaverine	T44.3X1-	T44.3X2-	T44.3X3-	T44.3X4-	T44.3X5-	T44.3X6-
Moxisylyte	T46.7X1-	T46.7X2-	T46.7X3-	T46.7X4-	T46.7X5-	T46.7X6-
Mucilage, plant	T47.4X1-	T47.4X2-	T47.4X3-	T47.4X4-	T47.4X5-	T47.4X6-
Mucolytic drug	T48.4X1-	T48.4X2-	T48.4X3-	T48.4X4-	T48.4X5-	T48.4X6-
Mucomyst	T48.4X1-	T48.4X2-	T48.4X3-	T48.4X4-	T48.4X5-	T48.4X6-
Mucous membrane agents (external)	T49.91X-	T49.92X-	T49.93X-	T49.94X-	T49.95X-	T49.96X-
specified NEC	T49.8X1-	T49.8X2-	T49.8X3-	T49.8X4-	T49.8X5-	T49.8X6-
Multiple unspecified drugs, medicaments and biological substances	T50.911-	T50.912-	T50.913-	T50.914-	T50.915-	T50.916-
Mumps						
immune globulin (human)	T50.Z11-	T50.Z12-	T50.Z13-	T50.Z14-	T50.Z15-	T50.Z16-
skin test antigen	T50.8X1-	T50.8X2-	T50.8X3-	T50.8X4-	T50.8X5-	T50.8X6-
vaccine	T50.B91-	T50.B92-	T50.B93-	T50.B94-	T50.B95-	T50.B96-
Mumpsvax	T50.B91-	T50.B92-	T50.B93-	T50.B94-	T50.B95-	T50.B96-
Mupirocin	T49.0X1-	T49.0X2-	T49.0X3-	T49.0X4-	T49.0X5-	T49.0X6-
Muriatic acid — *see Hydrochloric acid*						
Muromonab-CD3	T45.1X1-	T45.1X2-	T45.1X3-	T45.1X4-	T45.1X5-	T45.1X6-
Muscle-action drug NEC	T48.201-	T48.202-	T48.203-	T48.204-	T48.205-	T48.206-
Muscle affecting agents NEC	T48.201-	T48.202-	T48.203-	T48.204-	T48.205-	T48.206-
oxytocic	T48.0X1-	T48.0X2-	T48.0X3-	T48.0X4-	T48.0X5-	T48.0X6-
relaxants	T48.201-	T48.202-	T48.203-	T48.204-	T48.205-	T48.206-
central nervous system	T42.8X1-	T42.8X2-	T42.8X3-	T42.8X4-	T42.8X5-	T42.8X6-
skeletal	T48.1X1-	T48.1X2-	T48.1X3-	T48.1X4-	T48.1X5-	T48.1X6-
smooth	T44.3X1-	T44.3X2-	T44.3X3-	T44.3X4-	T44.3X5-	T44.3X6-

Substance	Poisoning Accidental (unintentional)	Poisoning Intentional self-harm	Poisoning Assault	Poisoning Undetermined	Adverse effect	Underdosing
Muscle relaxant — *see Relaxant, muscle*						
Muscle-tone depressant, central NEC	T42.8X1-	T42.8X2-	T42.8X3-	T42.8X4-	T42.8X5-	T42.8X6-
specified NEC	T42.8X1-	T42.8X2-	T42.8X3-	T42.8X4-	T42.8X5-	T42.8X6-
Mushroom, noxious	T62.0X1-	T62.0X2-	T62.0X3-	T62.0X4-	-	-
Mussel, noxious	T61.781-	T61.782-	T61.783-	T61.784-	-	-
Mustard (emetic)	T47.7X1-	T47.7X2-	T47.7X3-	T47.7X4-	T47.7X5-	T47.7X6-
black	T47.7X1-	T47.7X2-	T47.7X3-	T47.7X4-	T47.7X5-	T47.7X6-
gas, not in war	T59.91X-	T59.92X-	T59.93X-	T59.94X-	-	-
nitrogen	T45.1X1-	T45.1X2-	T45.1X3-	T45.1X4-	T45.1X5-	T45.1X6-
Mustine	T45.1X1-	T45.1X2-	T45.1X3-	T45.1X4-	T45.1X5-	T45.1X6-
M-vac	T45.1X1-	T45.1X2-	T45.1X3-	T45.1X4-	T45.1X5-	T45.1X6-
Mycifradin	T36.5X1-	T36.5X2-	T36.5X3-	T36.5X4-	T36.5X5-	T36.5X6-
topical	T49.0X1-	T49.0X2-	T49.0X3-	T49.0X4-	T49.0X5-	T49.0X6-
Mycitracin	T36.8X1-	T36.8X2-	T36.8X3-	T36.8X4-	T36.8X5-	T36.8X6-
ophthalmic preparation	T49.5X1-	T49.5X2-	T49.5X3-	T49.5X4-	T49.5X5-	T49.5X6-
Mycostatin	T36.7X1-	T36.7X2-	T36.7X3-	T36.7X4-	T36.7X5-	T36.7X6-
topical	T49.0X1-	T49.0X2-	T49.0X3-	T49.0X4-	T49.0X5-	T49.0X6-
Mycotoxins	T64.81X-	T64.82X-	T64.83X-	T64.84X-	-	-
aflatoxin	T64.01X-	T64.02X-	T64.03X-	T64.04X-	-	-
specified NEC	T64.81X-	T64.82X-	T64.83X-	T64.84X-	-	-
Mydriacyl	T44.3X1-	T44.3X2-	T44.3X3-	T44.3X4-	T44.3X5-	T44.3X6-
Mydriatic drug	T49.5X1-	T49.5X2-	T49.5X3-	T49.5X4-	T49.5X5-	T49.5X6-
Myelobromal	T45.1X1-	T45.1X2-	T45.1X3-	T45.1X4-	T45.1X5-	T45.1X6-
Myleran	T45.1X1-	T45.1X2-	T45.1X3-	T45.1X4-	T45.1X5-	T45.1X6-
Myochrysin (e)	T39.2X1-	T39.2X2-	T39.2X3-	T39.2X4-	T39.2X5-	T39.2X6-
Myoneural blocking agents	T48.1X1-	T48.1X2-	T48.1X3-	T48.1X4-	T48.1X5-	T48.1X6-
Myralact	T49.0X1-	T49.0X2-	T49.0X3-	T49.0X4-	T49.0X5-	T49.0X6-
Myristica fragrans	T62.2X1-	T62.2X2-	T62.2X3-	T62.2X4-	-	-
Myristicin	T65.891-	T65.892-	T65.893-	T65.894-	-	-
Mysoline	T42.3X1-	T42.3X2-	T42.3X3-	T42.3X4-	T42.3X5-	T42.3X6-
Nabilone	T40.7X1-	T40.7X2-	T40.7X3-	T40.7X4-	T40.7X5-	T40.7X6-
Nabumetone	T39.391-	T39.392-	T39.393-	T39.394-	T39.395-	T39.396-
Nadolol	T44.7X1-	T44.7X2-	T44.7X3-	T44.7X4-	T44.7X5-	T44.7X6-
Nafcillin	T36.0X1-	T36.0X2-	T36.0X3-	T36.0X4-	T36.0X5-	T36.0X6-
Nafoxidine	T38.6X1-	T38.6X2-	T38.6X3-	T38.6X4-	T38.6X5-	T38.6X6-
Naftazone	T46.991-	T46.992-	T46.993-	T46.994-	T46.995-	T46.996-
Naftidrofuryl (oxalate)	T46.7X1-	T46.7X2-	T46.7X3-	T46.7X4-	T46.7X5-	T46.7X6-
Naftifine	T49.0X1-	T49.0X2-	T49.0X3-	T49.0X4-	T49.0X5-	T49.0X6-
Nail polish remover	T52.91X-	T52.92X-	T52.93X-	T52.94X-	-	-
Nalbuphine	T40.4X1-	T40.4X2-	T40.4X3-	T40.4X4-	T40.4X5-	T40.4X6-
Naled	T60.0X1-	T60.0X2-	T60.0X3-	T60.0X4-	-	-
Nalidixic acid	T37.8X1-	T37.8X2-	T37.8X3-	T37.8X4-	T37.8X5-	T37.8X6-
Nalorphine	T50.7X1-	T50.7X2-	T50.7X3-	T50.7X4-	T50.7X5-	T50.7X6-
Naloxone	T50.7X1-	T50.7X2-	T50.7X3-	T50.7X4-	T50.7X5-	T50.7X6-
Naltrexone	T50.7X1-	T50.7X2-	T50.7X3-	T50.7X4-	T50.7X5-	T50.7X6-
Namenda	T43.8X1-	T43.8X2-	T43.8X3-	T43.8X4-	T43.8X5-	T43.8X6-
Nandrolone	T38.7X1-	T38.7X2-	T38.7X3-	T38.7X4-	T38.7X5-	T38.7X6-
Naphazoline	T48.5X1-	T48.5X2-	T48.5X3-	T48.5X4-	T48.5X5-	T48.5X6-
Naphtha (painters') (petroleum)	T52.0X1-	T52.0X2-	T52.0X3-	T52.0X4-	-	-
solvent	T52.0X1-	T52.0X2-	T52.0X3-	T52.0X4-	-	-
vapor	T52.0X1-	T52.0X2-	T52.0X3-	T52.0X4-	-	-
Naphthalene (non-chlorinated)	T60.2X1-	T60.2X2-	T60.2X3-	T60.2X4-	-	-
chlorinated	T60.1X1-	T60.1X2-	T60.1X3-	T60.1X4-	-	-
vapor	T60.1X1-	T60.1X2-	T60.1X3-	T60.1X4-	-	-
insecticide or moth repellent	T60.2X1-	T60.2X2-	T60.2X3-	T60.2X4-	-	-
chlorinated	T60.1X1-	T60.1X2-	T60.1X3-	T60.1X4-	-	-
vapor	T60.2X1-	T60.2X2-	T60.2X3-	T60.2X4-	-	-
chlorinated	T60.1X1-	T60.1X2-	T60.1X3-	T60.1X4-	-	-

Substance	Poisoning Accidental (unintentional)	Poisoning Intentional self-harm	Poisoning Assault	Poisoning Undetermined	Adverse effect	Underdosing
Naphthol	T65.891-	T65.892-	T65.893-	T65.894-	-	-
Naphthylamine	T65.891-	T65.892-	T65.893-	T65.894-	-	-
Naphthylthiourea (ANTU)	T60.4X1-	T60.4X2-	T60.4X3-	T60.4X4-	-	-
Naprosyn — *see Naproxen*						
Naproxen	T39.311-	T39.312-	T39.313-	T39.314-	T39.315-	T39.316-
Narcotic (drug)	T40.601-	T40.602-	T40.603-	T40.604-	T40.605-	T40.606-
analgesic NEC	T40.601-	T40.602-	T40.603-	T40.604-	T40.605-	T40.606-
antagonist	T50.7X1-	T50.7X2-	T50.7X3-	T50.7X4-	T50.7X5-	T50.7X6-
specified NEC	T40.691-	T40.692-	T40.693-	T40.694-	T40.695-	T40.696-
synthetic	T40.4X1-	T40.4X2-	T40.4X3-	T40.4X4-	T40.4X5-	T40.4X6-
Narcotine	T48.3X1-	T48.3X2-	T48.3X3-	T48.3X4-	T48.3X5-	T48.3X6-
Nardil	T43.1X1-	T43.1X2-	T43.1X3-	T43.1X4-	T43.1X5-	T43.1X6-
Nasal drug NEC	T49.6X1-	T49.6X2-	T49.6X3-	T49.6X4-	T49.6X5-	T49.6X6-
Natamycin	T49.0X1-	T49.0X2-	T49.0X3-	T49.0X4-	T49.0X5-	T49.0X6-
Natrium cyanide — *see Cyanide(s)*						
Natural						
blood (product)	T45.8X1-	T45.8X2-	T45.8X3-	T45.8X4-	T45.8X5-	T45.8X6-
gas (piped)	T59.891-	T59.892-	T59.893-	T59.894-	-	-
incomplete combustion	T58.11X-	T58.12X-	T58.13X-	T58.14X-	-	-
Nealbarbital	T42.3X1-	T42.3X2-	T42.3X3-	T42.3X4-	T42.3X5-	T42.3X6-
Nectadon	T48.3X1-	T48.3X2-	T48.3X3-	T48.3X4-	T48.3X5-	T48.3X6-
Nedocromil	T48.6X1-	T48.6X2-	T48.6X3-	T48.6X4-	T48.6X5-	T48.6X6-
Nefopam	T39.8X1-	T39.8X2-	T39.8X3-	T39.8X4-	T39.8X5-	T39.8X6-
Nematocyst (sting)	T63.691-	T63.692-	T63.693-	T63.694-	-	-
Nembutal	T42.3X1-	T42.3X2-	T42.3X3-	T42.3X4-	T42.3X5-	T42.3X6-
Nemonapride	T43.591-	T43.592-	T43.593-	T43.594-	T43.595-	T43.596-
Neoarsphenamine	T37.8X1-	T37.8X2-	T37.8X3-	T37.8X4-	T37.8X5-	T37.8X6-
Neocinchophen	T50.4X1-	T50.4X2-	T50.4X3-	T50.4X4-	T50.4X5-	T50.4X6-
Neomycin (derivatives)	T36.5X1-	T36.5X2-	T36.5X3-	T36.5X4-	T36.5X5-	T36.5X6-
with						
bacitracin	T49.0X1-	T49.0X2-	T49.0X3-	T49.0X4-	T49.0X5-	T49.0X6-
neostigmine	T44.0X1-	T44.0X2-	T44.0X3-	T44.0X4-	T44.0X5-	T44.0X6-
ENT agent	T49.6X1-	T49.6X2-	T49.6X3-	T49.6X4-	T49.6X5-	T49.6X6-
ophthalmic preparation	T49.5X1-	T49.5X2-	T49.5X3-	T49.5X4-	T49.5X5-	T49.5X6-
topical NEC	T49.0X1-	T49.0X2-	T49.0X3-	T49.0X4-	T49.0X5-	T49.0X6-
Neonal	T42.3X1-	T42.3X2-	T42.3X3-	T42.3X4-	T42.3X5-	T42.3X6-
Neoprontosil	T37.0X1-	T37.0X2-	T37.0X3-	T37.0X4-	T37.0X5-	T37.0X6-
Neosalvarsan	T37.8X1-	T37.8X2-	T37.8X3-	T37.8X4-	T37.8X5-	T37.8X6-
Neosilversalvarsan	T37.8X1-	T37.8X2-	T37.8X3-	T37.8X4-	T37.8X5-	T37.8X6-
Neosporin	T36.8X1-	T36.8X2-	T36.8X3-	T36.8X4-	T36.8X5-	T36.8X6-
ENT agent	T49.6X1-	T49.6X2-	T49.6X3-	T49.6X4-	T49.6X5-	T49.6X6-
opthalmic preparation	T49.5X1-	T49.5X2-	T49.5X3-	T49.5X4-	T49.5X5-	T49.5X6-
topical NEC	T49.0X1-	T49.0X2-	T49.0X3-	T49.0X4-	T49.0X5-	T49.0X6-
Neostigmine bromide	T44.0X1-	T44.0X2-	T44.0X3-	T44.0X4-	T44.0X5-	T44.0X6-
Neraval	T42.3X1-	T42.3X2-	T42.3X3-	T42.3X4-	T42.3X5-	T42.3X6-
Neravan	T42.3X1-	T42.3X2-	T42.3X3-	T42.3X4-	T42.3X5-	T42.3X6-
Nerium oleander	T62.2X1-	T62.2X2-	T62.2X3-	T62.2X4-	-	-
Nerve gas, not in war	T59.91X-	T59.92X-	T59.93X-	T59.94X-	-	-
Nesacaine	T41.3X1-	T41.3X2-	T41.3X3-	T41.3X4-	T41.3X5-	T41.3X6-
infiltration (subcutaneous)	T41.3X1-	T41.3X2-	T41.3X3-	T41.3X4-	T41.3X5-	T41.3X6-
nerve block (peripheral) (plexus)	T41.3X1-	T41.3X2-	T41.3X3-	T41.3X4-	T41.3X5-	T41.3X6-
Netilmicin	T36.5X1-	T36.5X2-	T36.5X3-	T36.5X4-	T36.5X5-	T36.5X6-
Neurobarb	T42.3X1-	T42.3X2-	T42.3X3-	T42.3X4-	T42.3X5-	T42.3X6-
Neuroleptic drug NEC	T43.501-	T43.502-	T43.503-	T43.504-	T43.505-	T43.506-
Neuromuscular blocking drug	T48.1X1-	T48.1X2-	T48.1X3-	T48.1X4-	T48.1X5-	T48.1X6-
Neutral insulin injection	T38.3X1-	T38.3X2-	T38.3X3-	T38.3X4-	T38.3X5-	T38.3X6-
Neutral spirits	T51.0X1-	T51.0X2-	T51.0X3-	T51.0X4-	-	-
beverage	T51.0X1-	T51.0X2-	T51.0X3-	T51.0X4-	-	-

Substance	Poisoning Accidental (unintentional)	Poisoning Intentional self-harm	Poisoning Assault	Poisoning Undetermined	Adverse effect	Underdosing
Niacin	T46.7X1-	T46.7X2-	T46.7X3-	T46.7X4-	T46.7X5-	T46.7X6-
Niacinamide	T45.2X1-	T45.2X2-	T45.2X3-	T45.2X4-	T45.2X5-	T45.2X6-
Nialamide	T43.1X1-	T43.1X2-	T43.1X3-	T43.1X4-	T43.1X5-	T43.1X6-
Niaprazine	T42.6X1-	T42.6X2-	T42.6X3-	T42.6X4-	T42.6X5-	T42.6X6-
Nicametate	T46.7X1-	T46.7X2-	T46.7X3-	T46.7X4-	T46.7X5-	T46.7X6-
Nicardipine	T46.1X1-	T46.1X2-	T46.1X3-	T46.1X4-	T46.1X5-	T46.1X6-
Nicergoline	T46.7X1-	T46.7X2-	T46.7X3-	T46.7X4-	T46.7X5-	T46.7X6-
Nickel (carbonyl) (tetra-carbonyl) (fumes) (vapor)	T56.891-	T56.892-	T56.893-	T56.894-	-	-
Nickelocene	T56.891-	T56.892-	T56.893-	T56.894-	-	-
Niclosamide	T37.4X1-	T37.4X2-	T37.4X3-	T37.4X4-	T37.4X5-	T37.4X6-
Nicofuranose	T46.7X1-	T46.7X2-	T46.7X3-	T46.7X4-	T46.7X5-	T46.7X6-
Nicomorphine	T40.2X1-	T40.2X2-	T40.2X3-	T40.2X4-	-	-
Nicorandil	T46.3X1-	T46.3X2-	T46.3X3-	T46.3X4-	T46.3X5-	T46.3X6-
Nicotiana (plant)	T62.2X1-	T62.2X2-	T62.2X3-	T62.2X4-	-	-
Nicotinamide	T45.2X1-	T45.2X2-	T45.2X3-	T45.2X4-	T45.2X5-	T45.2X6-
Nicotine (insecticide) (spray) (sulfate) NEC	T60.2X1-	T60.2X2-	T60.2X3-	T60.2X4-	-	-
from tobacco	T65.291-	T65.292-	T65.293-	T65.294-	-	-
cigarettes	T65.221-	T65.222-	T65.223-	T65.224-	-	-
not insecticide	T65.291-	T65.292-	T65.293-	T65.294-	-	-
Nicotinic acid	T46.7X1-	T46.7X2-	T46.7X3-	T46.7X4-	T46.7X5-	T46.7X6-
Nicotinyl alcohol	T46.7X1-	T46.7X2-	T46.7X3-	T46.7X4-	T46.7X5-	T46.7X6-
Nicoumalone	T45.511-	T45.512-	T45.513-	T45.514-	T45.515-	T45.516-
Nifedipine	T46.1X1-	T46.1X2-	T46.1X3-	T46.1X4-	T46.1X5-	T46.1X6-
Nifenazone	T39.2X1-	T39.2X2-	T39.2X3-	T39.2X4-	T39.2X5-	T39.2X6-
Nifuraldezone	T37.91X-	T37.92X-	T37.93X-	T37.94X-	T37.95X-	T37.96X-
Nifuratel	T37.8X1-	T37.8X2-	T37.8X3-	T37.8X4-	T37.8X5-	T37.8X6-
Nifurtimox	T37.3X1-	T37.3X2-	T37.3X3-	T37.3X4-	T37.3X5-	T37.3X6-
Nifurtoinol	T37.8X1-	T37.8X2-	T37.8X3-	T37.8X4-	T37.8X5-	T37.8X6-
Nightshade, deadly (solanum) — see also Belladonna	T62.2X1-	T62.2X2-	T62.2X3-	T62.2X4-	-	-
berry	T62.1X1-	T62.1X2-	T62.1X3-	T62.1X4-	-	-
Nikethamide	T50.7X1-	T50.7X2-	T50.7X3-	T50.7X4-	T50.7X5-	T50.7X6-
Nilstat	T36.7X1-	T36.7X2-	T36.7X3-	T36.7X4-	T36.7X5-	T36.7X6-
topical	T49.0X1-	T49.0X2-	T49.0X3-	T49.0X4-	T49.0X5-	T49.0X6-
Nilutamide	T38.6X1-	T38.6X2-	T38.6X3-	T38.6X4-	T38.6X5-	T38.6X6-
Nimesulide	T39.391-	T39.392-	T39.393-	T39.394-	T39.395-	T39.396-
Nimetazepam	T42.4X1-	T42.4X2-	T42.4X3-	T42.4X4-	T42.4X5-	T42.4X6-
Nimodipine	T46.1X1-	T46.1X2-	T46.1X3-	T46.1X4-	T46.1X5-	T46.1X6-
Nimorazole	T37.3X1-	T37.3X2-	T37.3X3-	T37.3X4-	T37.3X5-	T37.3X6-
Nimustine	T45.1X1-	T45.1X2-	T45.1X3-	T45.1X4-	T45.1X5-	T45.1X6-
Niridazole	T37.4X1-	T37.4X2-	T37.4X3-	T37.4X4-	T37.4X5-	T37.4X6-
Nisentil	T40.2X1-	T40.2X2-	T40.2X3-	T40.2X4-	T40.2X5-	T40.2X6-
Nisoldipine	T46.1X1-	T46.1X2-	T46.1X3-	T46.1X4-	T46.1X5-	T46.1X6-
Nitramine	T65.3X1-	T65.3X2-	T65.3X3-	T65.3X4-	-	-
Nitrate, organic	T46.3X1-	T46.3X2-	T46.3X3-	T46.3X4-	T46.3X5-	T46.3X6-
Nitrazepam	T42.4X1-	T42.4X2-	T42.4X3-	T42.4X4-	T42.4X5-	T42.4X6-
Nitrefazole	T50.6X1-	T50.6X2-	T50.6X3-	T50.6X4-	T50.6X5-	T50.6X6-
Nitrendipine	T46.1X1-	T46.1X2-	T46.1X3-	T46.1X4-	T46.1X5-	T46.1X6-
Nitric						
acid (liquid)	T54.2X1-	T54.2X2-	T54.2X3-	T54.2X4-		
vapor	T59.891-	T59.892-	T59.893-	T59.894-	-	-
oxide (gas)	T59.0X1-	T59.0X2-	T59.0X3-	T59.0X4-	-	-
Nitrimidazine	T37.3X1-	T37.3X2-	T37.3X3-	T37.3X4-	T37.3X5-	T37.3X6-
Nitrite, amyl (medicinal) (vapor)	T46.3X1-	T46.3X2-	T46.3X3-	T46.3X4-	T46.3X5-	T46.3X6-
Nitroaniline	T65.3X1-	T65.3X2-	T65.3X3-	T65.3X4-	-	-
vapor	T59.891-	T59.892-	T59.893-	T59.894-	-	-

NIACIN - NITROANILINE

Substance	Poisoning Accidental (unintentional)	Poisoning Intentional self-harm	Poisoning Assault	Poisoning Undetermined	Adverse effect	Underdosing
Nitrobenzene, nitrobenzol	T65.3X1-	T65.3X2-	T65.3X3-	T65.3X4-	-	-
vapor	T65.3X1-	T65.3X2-	T65.3X3-	T65.3X4-	-	-
Nitrocellulose	T65.891-	T65.892-	T65.893-	T65.894-	-	-
lacquer	T65.891-	T65.892-	T65.893-	T65.894-	-	-
Nitrodiphenyl	T65.3X1-	T65.3X2-	T65.3X3-	T65.3X4-	-	-
Nitrofural	T49.0X1-	T49.0X2-	T49.0X3-	T49.0X4-	T49.0X5-	T49.0X6-
Nitrofurantoin	T37.8X1-	T37.8X2-	T37.8X3-	T37.8X4-	T37.8X5-	T37.8X6-
Nitrofurazone	T49.0X1-	T49.0X2-	T49.0X3-	T49.0X4-	T49.0X5-	T49.0X6-
Nitrogen	T59.0X1-	T59.0X2-	T59.0X3-	T59.0X4-	-	-
mustard	T45.1X1-	T45.1X2-	T45.1X3-	T45.1X4-	T45.1X5-	T45.1X6-
Nitroglycerin, nitro-glycerol (medicinal)	T46.3X1-	T46.3X2-	T46.3X3-	T46.3X4-	T46.3X5-	T46.3X6-
nonmedicinal	T65.5X1-	T65.5X2-	T65.5X3-	T65.5X4-	-	-
fumes	T65.5X1-	T65.5X2-	T65.5X3-	T65.5X4-	-	-
Nitroglycol	T52.3X1-	T52.3X2-	T52.3X3-	T52.3X4-	-	-
Nitrohydrochloric acid	T54.2X1-	T54.2X2-	T54.2X3-	T54.2X4-	-	-
Nitromersol	T49.0X1-	T49.0X2-	T49.0X3-	T49.0X4-	T49.0X5-	T49.0X6-
Nitronaphthalene	T65.891-	T65.892-	T65.893-	T65.894-	-	-
Nitrophenol	T54.0X1-	T54.0X2-	T54.0X3-	T54.0X4-	-	-
Nitropropane	T52.8X1-	T52.8X2-	T52.8X3-	T52.8X4-	-	-
Nitroprusside	T46.5X1-	T46.5X2-	T46.5X3-	T46.5X4-	T46.5X5-	T46.5X6-
Nitrosodimethylamine	T65.3X1-	T65.3X2-	T65.3X3-	T65.3X4-	-	-
Nitrothiazol	T37.4X1-	T37.4X2-	T37.4X3-	T37.4X4-	T37.4X5-	T37.4X6-
Nitrotoluene, nitrotoluol	T65.3X1-	T65.3X2-	T65.3X3-	T65.3X4-	-	-
vapor	T65.3X1-	T65.3X2-	T65.3X3-	T65.3X4-	-	-
Nitrous						
acid (liquid)	T54.2X1-	T54.2X2-	T54.2X3-	T54.2X4-	-	-
fumes	T59.891-	T59.892-	T59.893-	T59.894-	-	-
ether spirit	T46.3X1-	T46.3X2-	T46.3X3-	T46.3X4-	T46.3X5-	T46.3X6-
oxide	T41.0X1-	T41.0X2-	T41.0X3-	T41.0X4-	T41.0X5-	T41.0X6-
Nitroxoline	T37.8X1-	T37.8X2-	T37.8X3-	T37.8X4-	T37.8X5-	T37.8X6-
Nitrozone	T49.0X1-	T49.0X2-	T49.0X3-	T49.0X4-	T49.0X5-	T49.0X6-
Nizatidine	T47.0X1-	T47.0X2-	T47.0X3-	T47.0X4-	T47.0X5-	T47.0X6-
Nizofenone	T43.8X1-	T43.8X2-	T43.8X3-	T43.8X4-	T43.8X5-	T43.8X6-
Noctec	T42.6X1-	T42.6X2-	T42.6X3-	T42.6X4-	T42.6X5-	T42.6X6-
Noludar	T42.6X1-	T42.6X2-	T42.6X3-	T42.6X4-	T42.6X5-	T42.6X6-
Nomegestrol	T38.5X1-	T38.5X2-	T38.5X3-	T38.5X4-	T38.5X5-	T38.5X6-
Nomifensine	T43.291-	T43.292-	T43.293-	T43.294-	T43.295-	T43.296-
Nonoxinol	T49.8X1-	T49.8X2-	T49.8X3-	T49.8X4-	T49.8X5-	T49.8X6-
Nonylphenoxy (polyethoxy-ethanol)	T49.8X1-	T49.8X2-	T49.8X3-	T49.8X4-	T49.8X5-	T49.8X6-
Noptil	T42.3X1-	T42.3X2-	T42.3X3-	T42.3X4-	T42.3X5-	T42.3X6-
Noradrenaline	T44.4X1-	T44.4X2-	T44.4X3-	T44.4X4-	T44.4X5-	T44.4X6-
Noramidopyrine	T39.2X1-	T39.2X2-	T39.2X3-	T39.2X4-	T39.2X5-	T39.2X6-
methanesulfonate sodium	T39.2X1-	T39.2X2-	T39.2X3-	T39.2X4-	T39.2X5-	T39.2X6-
Norbormide	T60.4X1-	T60.4X2-	T60.4X3-	T60.4X4-	-	-
Nordazepam	T42.4X1-	T42.4X2-	T42.4X3-	T42.4X4-	T42.4X5-	T42.4X6-
Norepinephrine	T44.4X1-	T44.4X2-	T44.4X3-	T44.4X4-	T44.4X5-	T44.4X6-
Norethandrolone	T38.7X1-	T38.7X2-	T38.7X3-	T38.7X4-	T38.7X5-	T38.7X6-
Norethindrone	T38.4X1-	T38.4X2-	T38.4X3-	T38.4X4-	T38.4X5-	T38.4X6-
Norethisterone (acetate) (enantate)	T38.4X1-	T38.4X2-	T38.4X3-	T38.4X4-	T38.4X5-	T38.4X6-
with ethinylestradiol	T38.5X1-	T38.5X2-	T38.5X3-	T38.5X4-	T38.5X5-	T38.5X6-
Noretynodrel	T38.5X1-	T38.5X2-	T38.5X3-	T38.5X4-	T38.5X5-	T38.5X6-
Norfenefrine	T44.4X1-	T44.4X2-	T44.4X3-	T44.4X4-	T44.4X5-	T44.4X6-
Norfloxacin	T36.8X1-	T36.8X2-	T36.8X3-	T36.8X4-	T36.8X5-	T36.8X6-
Norgestrel	T38.4X1-	T38.4X2-	T38.4X3-	T38.4X4-	T38.4X5-	T38.4X6-
Norgestrienone	T38.4X1-	T38.4X2-	T38.4X3-	T38.4X4-	T38.4X5-	T38.4X6-
Norlestrin	T38.4X1-	T38.4X2-	T38.4X3-	T38.4X4-	T38.4X5-	T38.4X6-
Norlutin	T38.4X1-	T38.4X2-	T38.4X3-	T38.4X4-	T38.4X5-	T38.4X6-

NITROBENZENE, NITROBENZOL - NORLUTIN

Substance	Poisoning Accidental (unintentional)	Poisoning Intentional self-harm	Poisoning Assault	Poisoning Undetermined	Adverse effect	Underdosing
Normal serum albumin (human) , salt-poor	T45.8X1-	T45.8X2-	T45.8X3-	T45.8X4-	T45.8X5-	T45.8X6-
Normethandrone	T38.5X1-	T38.5X2-	T38.5X3-	T38.5X4-	T38.5X5-	T38.5X6-
Normison — *see Benzodiazepines*						
Normorphine	T40.2X1-	T40.2X2-	T40.2X3-	T40.2X4-	-	-
Norpseudoephedrine	T50.5X1-	T50.5X2-	T50.5X3-	T50.5X4-	T50.5X5-	T50.5X6-
Nortestosterone (furanpropionate)	T38.7X1-	T38.7X2-	T38.7X3-	T38.7X4-	T38.7X5-	T38.7X6-
Nortriptyline	T43.011-	T43.012-	T43.013-	T43.014-	T43.015-	T43.016-
Noscapine	T48.3X1-	T48.3X2-	T48.3X3-	T48.3X4-	T48.3X5-	T48.3X6-
Nose preparations	T49.6X1-	T49.6X2-	T49.6X3-	T49.6X4-	T49.6X5-	T49.6X6-
Novobiocin	T36.5X1-	T36.5X2-	T36.5X3-	T36.5X4-	T36.5X5-	T36.5X6-
Novocain (infiltration) (topical)	T41.3X1-	T41.3X2-	T41.3X3-	T41.3X4-	T41.3X5-	T41.3X6-
nerve block (peripheral) (plexus)	T41.3X1-	T41.3X2-	T41.3X3-	T41.3X4-	T41.3X5-	T41.3X6-
spinal	T41.3X1-	T41.3X2-	T41.3X3-	T41.3X4-	T41.3X5-	T41.3X6-
Noxious foodstuff	T62.91X-	T62.92X-	T62.93X-	T62.94X-	-	-
specified NEC	T62.8X1-	T62.8X2-	T62.8X3-	T62.8X4-	-	-
Noxiptiline	T43.011-	T43.012-	T43.013-	T43.014-	T43.015-	T43.016-
Noxytiolin	T49.0X1-	T49.0X2-	T49.0X3-	T49.0X4-	T49.0X5-	T49.0X6-
NPH Iletin (insulin)	T38.3X1-	T38.3X2-	T38.3X3-	T38.3X4-	T38.3X5-	T38.3X6-
Numorphan	T40.2X1-	T40.2X2-	T40.2X3-	T40.2X4-	T40.2X5-	T40.2X6-
Nunol	T42.3X1-	T42.3X2-	T42.3X3-	T42.3X4-	T42.3X5-	T42.3X6-
Nupercaine (spinal anesthetic)	T41.3X1-	T41.3X2-	T41.3X3-	T41.3X4-	T41.3X5-	T41.3X6-
topical (surface)	T41.3X1-	T41.3X2-	T41.3X3-	T41.3X4-	T41.3X5-	T41.3X6-
Nutmeg oil (liniment)	T49.3X1-	T49.3X2-	T49.3X3-	T49.3X4-	T49.3X5-	T49.3X6-
Nutritional supplement	T50.901-	T50.902-	T50.903-	T50.904-	T50.905-	T50.906-
Nux vomica	T65.1X1-	T65.1X2-	T65.1X3-	T65.1X4-	-	-
Nydrazid	T37.1X1-	T37.1X2-	T37.1X3-	T37.1X4-	T37.1X5-	T37.1X6-
Nylidrin	T46.7X1-	T46.7X2-	T46.7X3-	T46.7X4-	T46.7X5-	T46.7X6-
Nystatin	T36.7X1-	T36.7X2-	T36.7X3-	T36.7X4-	T36.7X5-	T36.7X6-
topical	T49.0X1-	T49.0X2-	T49.0X3-	T49.0X4-	T49.0X5-	T49.0X6-
Nytol	T45.0X1-	T45.0X2-	T45.0X3-	T45.0X4-	T45.0X5-	T45.0X6-
Obidoxime chloride	T50.6X1-	T50.6X2-	T50.6X3-	T50.6X4-	T50.6X5-	T50.6X6-
Octafonium (chloride)	T49.3X1-	T49.3X2-	T49.3X3-	T49.3X4-	T49.3X5-	T49.3X6-
Octamethyl pyrophos-phoramide	T60.0X1-	T60.0X2-	T60.0X3-	T60.0X4-	-	-
Octanoin	T50.991-	T50.992-	T50.993-	T50.994-	T50.995-	T50.996-
Octatropine methyl-bromide	T44.3X1-	T44.3X2-	T44.3X3-	T44.3X4-	T44.3X5-	T44.3X6-
Octotiamine	T45.2X1-	T45.2X2-	T45.2X3-	T45.2X4-	T45.2X5-	T45.2X6-
Octoxinol (9)	T49.8X1-	T49.8X2-	T49.8X3-	T49.8X4-	T49.8X5-	T49.8X6-
Octreotide	T38.991-	T38.992-	T38.993-	T38.994-	T38.995-	T38.996-
Octyl nitrite	T46.3X1-	T46.3X2-	T46.3X3-	T46.3X4-	T46.3X5-	T46.3X6-
Oestradiol	T38.5X1-	T38.5X2-	T38.5X3-	T38.5X4-	T38.5X5-	T38.5X6-
Oestriol	T38.5X1-	T38.5X2-	T38.5X3-	T38.5X4-	T38.5X5-	T38.5X6-
Oestrogen	T38.5X1-	T38.5X2-	T38.5X3-	T38.5X4-	T38.5X5-	T38.5X6-
Oestrone	T38.5X1-	T38.5X2-	T38.5X3-	T38.5X4-	T38.5X5-	T38.5X6-
Ofloxacin	T36.8X1-	T36.8X2-	T36.8X3-	T36.8X4-	T36.8X5-	T36.8X6-
Oil (of)	T65.891-	T65.892-	T65.893-	T65.894-	-	-
bitter almond	T62.8X1-	T62.8X2-	T62.8X3-	T62.8X4-	-	-
cloves	T49.7X1-	T49.7X2-	T49.7X3-	T49.7X4-	T49.7X5-	T49.7X6-
colors	T65.6X1-	T65.6X2-	T65.6X3-	T65.6X4-	-	-
fumes	T59.891-	T59.892-	T59.893-	T59.894-	-	-
lubricating	T52.0X1-	T52.0X2-	T52.0X3-	T52.0X4-	-	-
Niobe	T52.8X1-	T52.8X2-	T52.8X3-	T52.8X4-	-	-
vitriol (liquid)	T54.2X1-	T54.2X2-	T54.2X3-	T54.2X4-	-	-
fumes	T54.2X1-	T54.2X2-	T54.2X3-	T54.2X4-	-	-
wintergreen (bitter) NEC	T49.3X1-	T49.3X2-	T49.3X3-	T49.3X4-	T49.3X5-	T49.3X6-
Oily preparation (for skin)	T49.3X1-	T49.3X2-	T49.3X3-	T49.3X4-	T49.3X5-	T49.3X6-
Ointment NEC	T49.3X1-	T49.3X2-	T49.3X3-	T49.3X4-	T49.3X5-	T49.3X6-
Olanzapine	T43.591-	T43.592-	T43.593-	T43.594-	T43.595-	T43.596-
Oleander	T62.2X1-	T62.2X2-	T62.2X3-	T62.2X4-	-	-

Substance	Poisoning Accidental (unintentional)	Poisoning Intentional self-harm	Poisoning Assault	Poisoning Undetermined	Adverse effect	Underdosing
Oleandomycin	T36.3X1-	T36.3X2-	T36.3X3-	T36.3X4-	T36.3X5-	T36.3X6-
Oleandrin	T46.0X1-	T46.0X2-	T46.0X3-	T46.0X4-	T46.0X5-	T46.0X6-
Oleic acid	T46.6X1-	T46.6X2-	T46.6X3-	T46.6X4-	T46.6X5-	T46.6X6-
Oleovitamin A	T45.2X1-	T45.2X2-	T45.2X3-	T45.2X4-	T45.2X5-	T45.2X6-
Oleum ricini	T47.2X1-	T47.2X2-	T47.2X3-	T47.2X4-	T47.2X5-	T47.2X6-
Olive oil (medicinal) NEC	T47.4X1-	T47.4X2-	T47.4X3-	T47.4X4-	T47.4X5-	T47.4X6-
Olivomycin	T45.1X1-	T45.1X2-	T45.1X3-	T45.1X4-	T45.1X5-	T45.1X6-
Olsalazine	T47.8X1-	T47.8X2-	T47.8X3-	T47.8X4-	T47.8X5-	T47.8X6-
Omeprazole	T47.1X1-	T47.1X2-	T47.1X3-	T47.1X4-	T47.1X5-	T47.1X6-
OMPA	T60.0X1	T60.0X2-	T60.0X3-	T60.0X4-	-	-
Oncovin	T45.1X1-	T45.1X2-	T45.1X3-	T45.1X4-	T45.1X5-	T45.1X6-
Ondansetron	T45.0X1-	T45.0X2-	T45.0X3-	T45.0X4-	T45.0X5-	T45.0X6-
Ophthaine	T41.3X1-	T41.3X2-	T41.3X3-	T41.3X4-	T41.3X5-	T41.3X6-
Ophthetic	T41.3X1-	T41.3X2-	T41.3X3-	T41.3X4-	T41.3X5-	T41.3X6-
Opiate NEC	T40.601-	T40.602-	T40.603-	T40.604-	T40.605-	T40.606-
antagonists	T50.7X1-	T50.7X2-	T50.7X3-	T50.7X4-	T50.7X5-	T50.7X6-
Opioid NEC	T40.2X1-	T40.2X2-	T40.2X3-	T40.2X4-	T40.2X5-	T40.2X6-
Opipramol	T43.011-	T43.012-	T43.013-	T43.014-	T43.015-	T43.016-
Opium alkaloids (total)	T40.0X1-	T40.0X2-	T40.0X3-	T40.0X4-	T40.0X5-	T40.0X6-
standardized powdered	T40.0X1-	T40.0X2-	T40.0X3-	T40.0X4-	T40.0X5-	T40.0X6-
tincture (camphorated)	T40.0X1-	T40.0X2-	T40.0X3-	T40.0X4-	T40.0X5-	T40.0X6-
Oracon	T38.4X1-	T38.4X2-	T38.4X3-	T38.4X4-	T38.4X5-	T38.4X6-
Oragrafin	T50.8X1-	T50.8X2-	T50.8X3-	T50.8X4-	T50.8X5-	T50.8X6-
Oral contraceptives	T38.4X1-	T38.4X2-	T38.4X3-	T38.4X4-	T38.4X5-	T38.4X6-
Oral rehydration salts	T50.3X1-	T50.3X2-	T50.3X3-	T50.3X4-	T50.3X5-	T50.3X6-
Orazamide	T50.991-	T50.992-	T50.993-	T50.994-	T50.995-	T50.996-
Orciprenaline	T48.291-	T48.292-	T48.293-	T48.294-	T48.295-	T48.296-
Organidin	T48.4X1-	T48.4X2-	T48.4X3-	T48.4X4-	T48.4X5-	T48.4X6-
Organonitrate NEC	T46.3X1-	T46.3X2-	T46.3X3-	T46.3X4-	T46.3X5-	T46.3X6-
Organophosphates	T60.0X1-	T60.0X2-	T60.0X3-	T60.0X4-	-	-
Orimune	T50.B91-	T50.B92-	T50.B93-	T50.B94-	T50.B95-	T50.B96-
Orinase	T38.3X1-	T38.3X2-	T38.3X3-	T38.3X4-	T38.3X5-	T38.3X6-
Ormeloxifene	T38.6X1-	T38.6X2-	T38.6X3-	T38.6X4-	T38.6X5-	T38.6X6-
Ornidazole	T37.3X1-	T37.3X2-	T37.3X3-	T37.3X4-	T37.3X5-	T37.3X6-
Ornithine aspartate	T50.991-	T50.992-	T50.993-	T50.994-	T50.995-	T50.996-
Ornoprostil	T47.1X1-	T47.1X2-	T47.1X3-	T47.1X4-	T47.1X5-	T47.1X6-
Orphenadrine (hydrochloride)	T42.8X1-	T42.8X2-	T42.8X3-	T42.8X4-	T42.8X5-	T42.8X6-
Ortal (sodium)	T42.3X1-	T42.3X2-	T42.3X3-	T42.3X4-	T42.3X5-	T42.3X6-
Orthoboric acid	T49.0X1-	T49.0X2-	T49.0X3-	T49.0X4-	T49.0X5-	T49.0X6-
ENT agent	T49.6X1-	T49.6X2-	T49.6X3-	T49.6X4-	T49.6X5-	T49.6X6-
ophthalmic preparation	T49.5X1-	T49.5X2-	T49.5X3-	T49.5X4-	T49.5X5-	T49.5X6-
Orthocaine	T41.3X1-	T41.3X2-	T41.3X3-	T41.3X4-	T41.3X5-	T41.3X6-
Orthodichlorobenzene	T53.7X1-	T53.7X2-	T53.7X3-	T53.7X4-	-	-
Ortho-Novum	T38.4X1-	T38.4X2-	T38.4X3-	T38.4X4-	T38.4X5-	T38.4X6-
Orthotolidine (reagent)	T54.2X1-	T54.2X2-	T54.2X3-	T54.2X4-	-	-
Osmic acid (liquid)	T54.2X1-	T54.2X2-	T54.2X3-	T54.2X4-	-	-
fumes	T54.2X1-	T54.2X2-	T54.2X3-	T54.2X4-	-	-
Osmotic diuretics	T50.2X1-	T50.2X2-	T50.2X3-	T50.2X4-	T50.2X5-	T50.2X6-
Otilonium bromide	T44.3X1-	T44.3X2-	T44.3X3-	T44.3X4-	T44.3X5-	T44.3X6-
Otorhinolaryngological drug NEC	T49.6X1-	T49.6X2-	T49.6X3-	T49.6X4-	T49.6X5-	T49.6X6-
Ouabain (e)	T46.0X1-	T46.0X2-	T46.0X3-	T46.0X4-	T46.0X5-	T46.0X6-
Ovarian						
hormone	T38.5X1-	T38.5X2-	T38.5X3-	T38.5X4-	T38.5X5-	T38.5X6-
stimulant	T38.5X1-	T38.5X2-	T38.5X3-	T38.5X4-	T38.5X5-	T38.5X6-
Ovral	T38.4X1-	T38.4X2-	T38.4X3-	T38.4X4-	T38.4X5-	T38.4X6-
Ovulen	T38.4X1-	T38.4X2-	T38.4X3-	T38.4X4-	T38.4X5-	T38.4X6-
Oxacillin	T36.0X1-	T36.0X2-	T36.0X3-	T36.0X4-	T36.0X5-	T36.0X6-

OLEANDOMYCIN - OXACILLIN

Substance	Poisoning Accidental (unintentional)	Poisoning Intentional self-harm	Poisoning Assault	Poisoning Undetermined	Adverse effect	Underdosing
Oxalic acid	T54.2X1-	T54.2X2-	T54.2X3-	T54.2X4-	-	-
ammonium salt	T50.991-	T50.992-	T50.993-	T50.994-	T50.995-	T50.996-
Oxamniquine	T37.4X1-	T37.4X2-	T37.4X3-	T37.4X4-	T37.4X5-	T37.4X6-
Oxanamide	T43.591-	T43.592-	T43.593-	T43.594-	T43.595-	T43.596-
Oxandrolone	T38.7X1-	T38.7X2-	T38.7X3-	T38.7X4-	T38.7X5-	T38.7X6-
Oxantel	T37.4X1-	T37.4X2-	T37.4X3-	T37.4X4-	T37.4X5-	T37.4X6-
Oxapium iodide	T44.3X1-	T44.3X2-	T44.3X3-	T44.3X4-	T44.3X5-	T44.3X6-
Oxaprotiline	T43.021-	T43.022-	T43.023-	T43.024-	T43.025-	T43.026-
Oxaprozin	T39.311-	T39.312-	T39.313-	T39.314-	T39.315-	T39.316-
Oxatomide	T45.0X1-	T45.0X2-	T45.0X3-	T45.0X4-	T45.0X5-	T45.0X6-
Oxazepam	T42.4X1-	T42.4X2-	T42.4X3-	T42.4X4-	T42.4X5-	T42.4X6-
Oxazimedrine	T50.5X1-	T50.5X2-	T50.5X3-	T50.5X4-	T50.5X5-	T50.5X6-
Oxazolam	T42.4X1-	T42.4X2-	T42.4X3-	T42.4X4-	T42.4X5-	T42.4X6-
Oxazolidine derivatives	T42.2X1-	T42.2X2-	T42.2X3-	T42.2X4-	T42.2X5-	T42.2X6-
Oxazolidinedione (derivative)	T42.2X1-	T42.2X2-	T42.2X3-	T42.2X4-	T42.2X5-	T42.2X6-
Ox bile extract	T47.5X1-	T47.5X2-	T47.5X3-	T47.5X4-	T47.5X5-	T47.5X6-
Oxcarbazepine	T42.1X1-	T42.1X2-	T42.1X3-	T42.1X4-	T42.1X5-	T42.1X6-
Oxedrine	T44.4X1-	T44.4X2-	T44.4X3-	T44.4X4-	T44.4X5-	T44.4X6-
Oxeladin (citrate)	T48.3X1-	T48.3X2-	T48.3X3-	T48.3X4-	T48.3X5-	T48.3X6-
Oxendolone	T38.5X1-	T38.5X2-	T38.5X3-	T38.5X4-	T38.5X5-	T38.5X6-
Oxetacaine	T41.3X1-	T41.3X2-	T41.3X3-	T41.3X4-	T41.3X5-	T41.3X6-
Oxethazine	T41.3X1-	T41.3X2-	T41.3X3-	T41.3X4-	T41.3X5-	T41.3X6-
Oxetorone	T39.8X1-	T39.8X2-	T39.8X3-	T39.8X4-	T39.8X5-	T39.8X6-
Oxiconazole	T49.0X1-	T49.0X2-	T49.0X3-	T49.0X4-	T49.0X5-	T49.0X6-
Oxidizing agent NEC	T54.91X-	T54.92X-	T54.93X-	T54.94X-	-	-
Oxipurinol	T50.4X1-	T50.4X2-	T50.4X3-	T50.4X4-	T50.4X5-	T50.4X6-
Oxitriptan	T43.291-	T43.292-	T43.293-	T43.294-	T43.295-	T43.296-
Oxitropium bromide	T48.6X1-	T48.6X2-	T48.6X3-	T48.6X4-	T48.6X5-	T48.6X6-
Oxodipine	T46.1X1-	T46.1X2-	T46.1X3-	T46.1X4-	T46.1X5-	T46.1X6-
Oxolamine	T48.3X1-	T48.3X2-	T48.3X3-	T48.3X4-	T48.3X5-	T48.3X6-
Oxolinic acid	T37.8X1-	T37.8X2-	T37.8X3-	T37.8X4-	T37.8X5-	T37.8X6-
Oxomemazine	T43.3X1-	T43.3X2-	T43.3X3-	T43.3X4-	T43.3X5-	T43.3X6-
Oxophenarsine	T37.3X1-	T37.3X2-	T37.3X3-	T37.3X4-	T37.3X5-	T37.3X6-
Oxprenolol	T44.7X1-	T44.7X2-	T44.7X3-	T44.7X4-	T44.7X5-	T44.7X6-
Oxsoralen	T49.3X1-	T49.3X2-	T49.3X3-	T49.3X4-	T49.3X5-	T49.3X6-
Oxtriphylline	T48.6X1-	T48.6X2-	T48.6X3-	T48.6X4-	T48.6X5-	T48.6X6-
Oxybate sodium	T41.291-	T41.292-	T41.293-	T41.294-	T41.295-	T41.296-
Oxybuprocaine	T41.3X1-	T41.3X2-	T41.3X3-	T41.3X4-	T41.3X5-	T41.3X6-
Oxybutynin	T44.3X1-	T44.3X2-	T44.3X3-	T44.3X4-	T44.3X5-	T44.3X6-
Oxychlorosene	T49.0X1-	T49.0X2-	T49.0X3-	T49.0X4-	T49.0X5-	T49.0X6-
Oxycodone	T40.2X1-	T40.2X2-	T40.2X3-	T40.2X4-	T40.2X5-	T40.2X6-
Oxyfedrine	T46.3X1-	T46.3X2-	T46.3X3-	T46.3X4-	T46.3X5-	T46.3X6-
Oxygen	T41.5X1-	T41.5X2-	T41.5X3-	T41.5X4-	T41.5X5-	T41.5X6-
Oxylone	T49.0X1-	T49.0X2-	T49.0X3-	T49.0X4-	T49.0X5-	T49.0X6-
ophthalmic preparation	T49.5X1-	T49.5X2-	T49.5X3-	T49.5X4-	T49.5X5-	T49.5X6-
Oxymesterone	T38.7X1-	T38.7X2-	T38.7X3-	T38.7X4-	T38.7X5-	T38.7X6-
Oxymetazoline	T48.5X1-	T48.5X2-	T48.5X3-	T48.5X4-	T48.5X5-	T48.5X6-
Oxymetholone	T38.7X1-	T38.7X2-	T38.7X3-	T38.7X4-	T38.7X5-	T38.7X6-
Oxymorphone	T40.2X1-	T40.2X2-	T40.2X3-	T40.2X4-	T40.2X5-	T40.2X6-
Oxypertine	T43.591-	T43.592-	T43.593-	T43.594-	T43.595-	T43.596-
Oxyphenbutazone	T39.2X1-	T39.2X2-	T39.2X3-	T39.2X4-	T39.2X5-	T39.2X6-
Oxyphencyclimine	T44.3X1-	T44.3X2-	T44.3X3-	T44.3X4-	T44.3X5-	T44.3X6-
Oxyphenisatine	T47.2X1-	T47.2X2-	T47.2X3-	T47.2X4-	T47.2X5-	T47.2X6-
Oxyphenonium bromide	T44.3X1-	T44.3X2-	T44.3X3-	T44.3X4-	T44.3X5-	T44.3X6-
Oxypolygelatin	T45.8X1-	T45.8X2-	T45.8X3-	T45.8X4-	T45.8X5-	T45.8X6-
Oxyquinoline (derivatives)	T37.8X1-	T37.8X2-	T37.8X3-	T37.8X4-	T37.8X5-	T37.8X6-
Oxytetracycline	T36.4X1-	T36.4X2-	T36.4X3-	T36.4X4-	T36.4X5-	T36.4X6-
Oxytocic drug NEC	T48.0X1-	T48.0X2-	T48.0X3-	T48.0X4-	T48.0X5-	T48.0X6-
Oxytocin (synthetic)	T48.0X1-	T48.0X2-	T48.0X3-	T48.0X4-	T48.0X5-	T48.0X6-

Substance	Poisoning Accidental (unintentional)	Poisoning Intentional self-harm	Poisoning Assault	Poisoning Undetermined	Adverse effect	Underdosing
Ozone	T59.891-	T59.892-	T59.893-	T59.894-	-	-
PABA	T49.3X1-	T49.3X2-	T49.3X3-	T49.3X4-	T49.3X5-	T49.3X6-
Packed red cells	T45.8X1-	T45.8X2-	T45.8X3-	T45.8X4-	T45.8X5-	T45.8X6-
Padimate	T49.3X1-	T49.3X2-	T49.3X3-	T49.3X4-	T49.3X5-	T49.3X6-
Paint NEC	T65.6X1-	T65.6X2-	T65.6X3-	T65.6X4-	-	-
cleaner	T52.91X-	T52.92X-	T52.93X-	T52.94X-	-	-
fumes NEC	T59.891-	T59.892-	T59.893-	T59.894-	-	-
lead (fumes)	T56.0X1-	T56.0X2-	T56.0X3-	T56.0X4-	-	-
solvent NEC	T52.8X1-	T52.8X2-	T52.8X3-	T52.8X4-	-	-
stripper	T52.8X1-	T52.8X2-	T52.8X3-	T52.8X4-	-	-
Palfium	T40.2X1-	T40.2X2-	T40.2X3-	T40.2X4-	-	-
Palm kernel oil	T50.991-	T50.992-	T50.993-	T50.994-	T50.995-	T50.996-
Paludrine	T37.2X1-	T37.2X2-	T37.2X3-	T37.2X4-	T37.2X5-	T37.2X6-
PAM (pralidoxime)	T50.6X1-	T50.6X2-	T50.6X3-	T50.6X4-	T50.6X5-	T50.6X6-
Pamaquine (naphthoute)	T37.2X1-	T37.2X2-	T37.2X3-	T37.2X4-	T37.2X5-	T37.2X6-
Panadol	T39.1X1-	T39.1X2-	T39.1X3-	T39.1X4-	T39.1X5-	T39.1X6-
Pancreatic						
digestive secretion stimulant	T47.8X1-	T47.8X2-	T47.8X3-	T47.8X4-	T47.8X5-	T47.8X6-
dornase	T45.3X1-	T45.3X2-	T45.3X3-	T45.3X4-	T45.3X5-	T45.3X6-
Pancreatin	T47.5X1-	T47.5X2-	T47.5X3-	T47.5X4-	T47.5X5-	T47.5X6-
Pancrelipase	T47.5X1-	T47.5X2-	T47.5X3-	T47.5X4-	T47.5X5-	T47.5X6-
Pancuronium (bromide)	T48.1X1-	T48.1X2-	T48.1X3-	T48.1X4-	T48.1X5-	T48.1X6-
Pangamic acid	T45.2X1-	T45.2X2-	T45.2X3-	T45.2X4-	T45.2X5-	T45.2X6-
Panthenol	T45.2X1-	T45.2X2-	T45.2X3-	T45.2X4-	T45.2X5-	T45.2X6-
topical	T49.8X1-	T49.8X2-	T49.8X3-	T49.8X4-	T49.8X5-	T49.8X6-
Pantopon	T40.0X1-	T40.0X2-	T40.0X3-	T40.0X4-	T40.0X5-	T40.0X6-
Pantothenic acid	T45.2X1-	T45.2X2-	T45.2X3-	T45.2X4-	T45.2X5-	T45.2X6-
Panwarfin	T45.511-	T45.512-	T45.513-	T45.514-	T45.515-	T45.516-
Papain	T47.5X1-	T47.5X2-	T47.5X3-	T47.5X4-	T47.5X5-	T47.5X6-
digestant	T47.5X1-	T47.5X2-	T47.5X3-	T47.5X4-	T47.5X5-	T47.5X6-
Papaveretum	T40.0X1-	T40.0X2-	T40.0X3-	T40.0X4-	T40.0X5-	T40.0X6-
Papaverine	T44.3X1-	T44.3X2-	T44.3X3-	T44.3X4-	T44.3X5-	T44.3X6-
Para-acetamidophenol	T39.1X1-	T39.1X2-	T39.1X3-	T39.1X4-	T39.1X5-	T39.1X6-
Para-aminobenzoic acid	T49.3X1-	T49.3X2-	T49.3X3-	T49.3X4-	T49.3X5-	T49.3X6-
Para-aminophenol derivatives	T39.1X1-	T39.1X2-	T39.1X3-	T39.1X4-	T39.1X5-	T39.1X6-
Para-aminosalicylic acid	T37.1X1-	T37.1X2-	T37.1X3-	T37.1X4-	T37.1X5-	T37.1X6-
Paracetaldehyde	T42.6X1-	T42.6X2-	T42.6X3-	T42.6X4-	T42.6X5-	T42.6X6-
Paracetamol	T39.1X1-	T39.1X2-	T39.1X3-	T39.1X4-	T39.1X5-	T39.1X6-
Parachlorophenol (camphorated)	T49.0X1-	T49.0X2-	T49.0X3-	T49.0X4-	T49.0X5-	T49.0X6-
Paracodin	T40.2X1-	T40.2X2-	T40.2X3-	T40.2X4-	T40.2X5-	T40.2X6-
Paradione	T42.2X1-	T42.2X2-	T42.2X3-	T42.2X4-	T42.2X5-	T42.2X6-
Paraffin (s) (wax)	T52.0X1-	T52.0X2-	T52.0X3-	T52.0X4-	-	-
liquid (medicinal)	T47.4X1-	T47.4X2-	T47.4X3-	T47.4X4-	T47.4X5-	T47.4X6-
nonmedicinal	T52.0X1-	T52.0X2-	T52.0X3-	T52.0X4-	-	-
Paraformaldehyde	T60.3X1-	T60.3X2-	T60.3X3-	T60.3X4-	-	-
Paraldehyde	T42.6X1-	T42.6X2-	T42.6X3-	T42.6X4-	T42.6X5-	T42.6X6-
Paramethadione	T42.2X1-	T42.2X2-	T42.2X3-	T42.2X4-	T42.2X5-	T42.2X6-
Paramethasone	T38.0X1-	T38.0X2-	T38.0X3-	T38.0X4-	T38.0X5-	T38.0X6-
acetate	T49.0X1-	T49.0X2-	T49.0X3-	T49.0X4-	T49.0X5-	T49.0X6-
Paraoxon	T60.0X1-	T60.0X2-	T60.0X3-	T60.0X4-	-	-
Paraquat	T60.3X1-	T60.3X2-	T60.3X3-	T60.3X4-	-	-
Parasympatholytic NEC	T44.3X1-	T44.3X2-	T44.3X3-	T44.3X4-	T44.3X5-	T44.3X6-
Parasympathomimetic drug NEC	T44.1X1-	T44.1X2-	T44.1X3-	T44.1X4-	T44.1X5-	T44.1X6-
Parathion	T60.0X1-	T60.0X2-	T60.0X3-	T60.0X4-	-	-
Parathormone	T50.991-	T50.992-	T50.993-	T50.994-	T50.995-	T50.996-
Parathyroid extract	T50.991-	T50.992-	T50.993-	T50.994-	T50.995-	T50.996-
Paratyphoid vaccine	T50.A91-	T50.A92-	T50.A93-	T50.A94-	T50.A95-	T50.A96-
Paredrine	T44.4X1-	T44.4X2-	T44.4X3-	T44.4X4-	T44.4X5-	T44.4X6-

Substance	Poisoning Accidental (unintentional)	Poisoning Intentional self-harm	Poisoning Assault	Poisoning Undetermined	Adverse effect	Underdosing
Paregoric	T40.0X1-	T40.0X2-	T40.0X3-	T40.0X4-	T40.0X5-	T40.0X6-
Pargyline	T46.5X1-	T46.5X2-	T46.5X3-	T46.5X4-	T46.5X5-	T46.5X6-
Paris green	T57.0X1-	T57.0X2-	T57.0X3-	T57.0X4-	-	-
insecticide	T57.0X1-	T57.0X2-	T57.0X3-	T57.0X4-	-	-
Parnate	T43.1X1-	T43.1X2-	T43.1X3-	T43.1X4-	T43.1X5-	T43.1X6-
Paromomycin	T36.5X1-	T36.5X2-	T36.5X3-	T36.5X4-	T36.5X5-	T36.5X6-
Paroxypropione	T45.1X1-	T45.1X2-	T45.1X3-	T45.1X4-	T45.1X5-	T45.1X6-
Parzone	T40.2X1-	T40.2X2-	T40.2X3-	T40.2X4-	T40.2X5-	T40.2X6-
PAS	T37.1X1-	T37.1X2-	T37.1X3-	T37.1X4-	T37.1X5-	T37.1X6-
Pasiniazid	T37.1X1-	T37.1X2-	T37.1X3-	T37.1X4-	T37.1X5-	T37.1X6-
PBB (polybrominated biphenyls)	T65.891-	T65.892-	T65.893-	T65.894-	-	-
PCB	T65.891-	T65.892-	T65.893-	T65.894-	-	-
PCP						
meaning pentachlorophenol	T60.1X1-	T60.1X2-	T60.1X3-	T60.1X4-	-	-
fungicide	T60.3X1-	T60.3X2-	T60.3X3-	T60.3X4-	-	-
herbicide	T60.3X1-	T60.3X2-	T60.3X3-	T60.3X4-	-	-
insecticide	T60.1X1-	T60.1X2-	T60.1X3-	T60.1X4-	-	-
meaning phencyclidine	T40.991-	T40.992-	T40.993-	T40.994-	-	-
Peach kernel oil (emulsion)	T47.4X1-	T47.4X2-	T47.4X3-	T47.4X4-	T47.4X5-	T47.4X6-
Peanut oil (emulsion) NEC	T47.4X1-	T47.4X2-	T47.4X3-	T47.4X4-	T47.4X5-	T47.4X6-
topical	T49.3X1-	T49.3X2-	T49.3X3-	T49.3X4-	T49.3X5-	T49.3X6-
Pearly Gates (morning glory seeds)	T40.991-	T40.992-	T40.993-	T40.994-	-	-
Pecazine	T43.3X1-	T43.3X2-	T43.3X3-	T43.3X4-	T43.3X5-	T43.3X6-
Pectin	T47.6X1-	T47.6X2-	T47.6X3-	T47.6X4-	T47.6X5-	T47.6X6-
Pefloxacin	T37.8X1-	T37.8X2-	T37.8X3-	T37.8X4-	T37.8X5-	T37.8X6-
Pegademase, bovine	T50.Z91-	T50.Z92-	T50.Z93-	T50.Z94-	T50.Z95-	T50.Z96-
Pelletierine tannate	T37.4X1-	T37.4X2-	T37.4X3-	T37.4X4-	T37.4X5-	T37.4X6-
Pemirolast (potassium)	T48.6X1-	T48.6X2-	T48.6X3-	T48.6X4-	T48.6X5-	T48.6X6-
Pemoline	T50.7X1-	T50.7X2-	T50.7X3-	T50.7X4-	T50.7X5-	T50.7X6-
Pempidine	T44.2X1-	T44.2X2-	T44.2X3-	T44.2X4-	T44.2X5-	T44.2X6-
Penamecillin	T36.0X1-	T36.0X2-	T36.0X3-	T36.0X4-	T36.0X5-	T36.0X6-
Penbutolol	T44.7X1-	T44.7X2-	T44.7X3-	T44.7X4-	T44.7X5-	T44.7X6-
Penethamate	T36.0X1-	T36.0X2-	T36.0X3-	T36.0X4-	T36.0X5-	T36.0X6-
Penfluridol	T43.591-	T43.592-	T43.593-	T43.594-	T43.595-	T43.596-
Penflutizide	T50.2X1-	T50.2X2-	T50.2X3-	T50.2X4-	T50.2X5-	T50.2X6-
Pengitoxin	T46.0X1-	T46.0X2-	T46.0X3-	T46.0X4-	T46.0X5-	T46.0X6-
Penicillamine	T50.6X1-	T50.6X2-	T50.6X3-	T50.6X4-	T50.6X5-	T50.6X6-
Penicillin (any)	T36.0X1-	T36.0X2-	T36.0X3-	T36.0X4-	T36.0X5-	T36.0X6-
Penicillinase	T45.3X1-	T45.3X2-	T45.3X3-	T45.3X4-	T45.3X5-	T45.3X6-
Penicilloyl polylysine	T50.8X1-	T50.8X2-	T50.8X3-	T50.8X4-	T50.8X5-	T50.8X6-
Penimepicycline	T36.4X1-	T36.4X2-	T36.4X3-	T36.4X4-	T36.4X5-	T36.4X6-
Pentachloroethane	T53.6X1-	T53.6X2-	T53.6X3-	T53.6X4-	-	-
Pentachloronaphthalene	T53.7X1-	T53.7X2-	T53.7X3-	T53.7X4-	-	-
Pentachlorophenol (pesticide)	T60.1X1-	T60.1X2-	T60.1X3-	T60.1X4-	-	-
fungicide	T60.3X1-	T60.3X2-	T60.3X3-	T60.3X4-	-	-
herbicide	T60.3X1-	T60.3X2-	T60.3X3-	T60.3X4-	-	-
insecticide	T60.1X1-	T60.1X2-	T60.1X3-	T60.1X4-	-	-
Pentaerythritol	T46.3X1-	T46.3X2-	T46.3X3-	T46.3X4-	T46.3X5-	T46.3X6-
chloral	T42.6X1-	T42.6X2-	T42.6X3-	T42.6X4-	T42.6X5-	T42.6X6-
tetranitrate NEC	T46.3X1-	T46.3X2-	T46.3X3-	T46.3X4-	T46.3X5-	T46.3X6-
Pentaerythrityl tetranitrate	T46.3X1-	T46.3X2-	T46.3X3-	T46.3X4-	T46.3X5-	T46.3X6-
Pentagastrin	T50.8X1-	T50.8X2-	T50.8X3-	T50.8X4-	T50.8X5-	T50.8X6-
Pentalin	T53.6X1-	T53.6X2-	T53.6X3-	T53.6X4-	-	-
Pentamethonium bromide	T44.2X1-	T44.2X2-	T44.2X3-	T44.2X4-	T44.2X5-	T44.2X6-
Pentamidine	T37.3X1-	T37.3X2-	T37.3X3-	T37.3X4-	T37.3X5-	T37.3X6-
Pentanol	T51.3X1-	T51.3X2-	T51.3X3-	T51.3X4-	-	-
Pentapyrrolinium (bitartrate)	T44.2X1-	T44.2X2-	T44.2X3-	T44.2X4-	T44.2X5-	T44.2X6-
Pentaquine	T37.2X1-	T37.2X2-	T37.2X3-	T37.2X4-	T37.2X5-	T37.2X6-

Substance	Poisoning Accidental (unintentional)	Poisoning Intentional self-harm	Poisoning Assault	Poisoning Undetermined	Adverse effect	Underdosing
Pentazocine	T40.4X1-	T40.4X2-	T40.4X3-	T40.4X4-	T40.4X5-	T40.4X6-
Pentetrazole	T50.7X1-	T50.7X2-	T50.7X3-	T50.7X4-	T50.7X5-	T50.7X6-
Penthienate bromide	T44.3X1-	T44.3X2-	T44.3X3-	T44.3X4-	T44.3X5-	T44.3X6-
Pentifylline	T46.7X1-	T46.7X2-	T46.7X3-	T46.7X4-	T46.7X5-	T46.7X6-
Pentobarbital	T42.3X1-	T42.3X2-	T42.3X3-	T42.3X4-	T42.3X5-	T42.3X6-
sodium	T42.3X1-	T42.3X2-	T42.3X3-	T42.3X4-	T42.3X5-	T42.3X6-
Pentobarbitone	T42.3X1-	T42.3X2-	T42.3X3-	T42.3X4-	T42.3X5-	T42.3X6-
Pentolonium tartrate	T44.2X1-	T44.2X2-	T44.2X3-	T44.2X4-	T44.2X5-	T44.2X6-
Pentosan polysulfate (sodium)	T39.8X1-	T39.8X2-	T39.8X3-	T39.8X4-	T39.8X5-	T39.8X6-
Pentostatin	T45.1X1-	T45.1X2-	T45.1X3-	T45.1X4-	T45.1X5-	T45.1X6-
Pentothal	T41.1X1-	T41.1X2-	T41.1X3-	T41.1X4-	T41.1X5-	T41.1X6-
Pentoxifylline	T46.7X1-	T46.7X2-	T46.7X3-	T46.7X4-	T46.7X5-	T46.7X6-
Pentoxyverine	T48.3X1-	T48.3X2-	T48.3X3-	T48.3X4-	T48.3X5-	T48.3X6-
Pentrinat	T46.3X1-	T46.3X2-	T46.3X3-	T46.3X4-	T46.3X5-	T46.3X6-
Pentylenetetrazole	T50.7X1-	T50.7X2-	T50.7X3-	T50.7X4-	T50.7X5-	T50.7X6-
Pentylsalicylamide	T37.1X1-	T37.1X2-	T37.1X3-	T37.1X4-	T37.1X5-	T37.1X6-
Pentymal	T42.3X1-	T42.3X2-	T42.3X3-	T42.3X4-	T42.3X5-	T42.3X6-
Peplomycin	T45.1X1-	T45.1X2-	T45.1X3-	T45.1X4-	T45.1X5-	T45.1X6-
Peppermint (oil)	T47.5X1-	T47.5X2-	T47.5X3-	T47.5X4-	T47.5X5-	T47.5X6-
Pepsin	T47.5X1-	T47.5X2-	T47.5X3-	T47.5X4-	T47.5X5-	T47.5X6-
digestant	T47.5X1-	T47.5X2-	T47.5X3-	T47.5X4-	T47.5X5-	T47.5X6-
Pepstatin	T47.1X1-	T47.1X2-	T47.1X3-	T47.1X4-	T47.1X5-	T47.1X6-
Peptavlon	T50.8X1-	T50.8X2-	T50.8X3-	T50.8X4-	T50.8X5-	T50.8X6-
Perazine	T43.3X1-	T43.3X2-	T43.3X3-	T43.3X4-	T43.3X5-	T43.3X6-
Percaine (spinal)	T41.3X1-	T41.3X2-	T41.3X3-	T41.3X4-	T41.3X5-	T41.3X6-
topical (surface)	T41.3X1-	T41.3X2-	T41.3X3-	T41.3X4-	T41.3X5-	T41.3X6-
Perchloroethylene	T53.3X1-	T53.3X2-	T53.3X3-	T53.3X4-	-	-
medicinal	T37.4X1-	T37.4X2-	T37.4X3-	T37.4X4-	T37.4X5-	T37.4X6-
vapor	T53.3X1-	T53.3X2-	T53.3X3-	T53.3X4-	-	-
Percodan	T40.2X1-	T40.2X2-	T40.2X3-	T40.2X4-	T40.2X5-	T40.2X6-
Percogesic — see also acetaminophen	T45.0X1-	T45.0X2-	T45.0X3-	T45.0X4-	T45.0X5-	T45.0X6-
Percorten	T38.0X1-	T38.0X2-	T38.0X3-	T38.0X4-	T38.0X5-	T38.0X6-
Pergolide	T42.8X1-	T42.8X2-	T42.8X3-	T42.8X4-	T42.8X5-	T42.8X6-
Pergonal	T38.811-	T38.812-	T38.813-	T38.814-	T38.815-	T38.816-
Perhexilene	T46.3X1-	T46.3X2-	T46.3X3-	T46.3X4-	T46.3X5-	T46.3X6-
Perhexiline (maleate)	T46.3X1-	T46.3X2-	T46.3X3-	T46.3X4-	T46.3X5-	T46.3X6-
Periactin	T45.0X1-	T45.0X2-	T45.0X3-	T45.0X4-	T45.0X5-	T45.0X6-
Periciazine	T43.3X1-	T43.3X2-	T43.3X3-	T43.3X4-	T43.3X5-	T43.3X6-
Periclor	T42.6X1-	T42.6X2-	T42.6X3-	T42.6X4-	T42.6X5-	T42.6X6-
Perindopril	T46.4X1-	T46.4X2-	T46.4X3-	T46.4X4-	T46.4X5-	T46.4X6-
Perisoxal	T39.8X1-	T39.8X2-	T39.8X3-	T39.8X4-	T39.8X5-	T39.8X6-
Peritoneal dialysis solution	T50.3X1-	T50.3X2-	T50.3X3-	T50.3X4-	T50.3X5-	T50.3X6-
Peritrate	T46.3X1-	T46.3X2-	T46.3X3-	T46.3X4-	T46.3X5-	T46.3X6-
Perlapine	T42.4X1-	T42.4X2-	T42.4X3-	T42.4X4-	T42.4X5-	T42.4X6-
Permanganate	T65.891-	T65.892-	T65.893-	T65.894-	-	-
Permethrin	T60.1X1-	T60.1X2-	T60.1X3-	T60.1X4-	-	-
Pernocton	T42.3X1-	T42.3X2-	T42.3X3-	T42.3X4-	T42.3X5-	T42.3X6-
Pernoston	T42.3X1-	T42.3X2-	T42.3X3-	T42.3X4-	T42.3X5-	T42.3X6-
Peronine	T40.2X1-	T40.2X2-	T40.2X3-	T40.2X4-	-	-
Perphenazine	T43.3X1-	T43.3X2-	T43.3X3-	T43.3X4-	T43.3X5-	T43.3X6-
Pertofrane	T43.011-	T43.012-	T43.013-	T43.014-	T43.015-	T43.016-
Pertussis						
immune serum (human)	T50.Z11-	T50.Z12-	T50.Z13-	T50.Z14-	T50.Z15-	T50.Z16-
vaccine (with diphtheria toxoid) (with tetanus toxoid)	T50.A11-	T50.A12-	T50.A13-	T50.A14-	T50.A15-	T50.A16-
Peruvian balsam	T49.0X1-	T49.0X2-	T49.0X3-	T49.0X4-	T49.0X5-	T49.0X6-
Peruvoside	T46.0X1-	T46.0X2-	T46.0X3-	T46.0X4-	T46.0X5-	T46.0X6-

PENTAZOCINE - PERUVOSIDE

Substance	Poisoning Accidental (unintentional)	Poisoning Intentional self-harm	Poisoning Assault	Poisoning Undetermined	Adverse effect	Underdosing
Pesticide (dust) (fumes) (vapor) NEC	T60.91X-	T60.92X-	T60.93X-	T60.94X-	-	-
arsenic	T57.0X1-	T57.0X2-	T57.0X3-	T57.0X4-	-	-
chlorinated	T60.1X1-	T60.1X2-	T60.1X3-	T60.1X4-	-	-
cyanide	T65.0X1-	T65.0X2-	T65.0X3-	T65.0X4-	-	-
kerosene	T52.0X1-	T52.0X2-	T52.0X3-	T52.0X4-	-	-
mixture (of compounds)	T60.91X-	T60.92X-	T60.93X-	T60.94X-	-	-
naphthalene	T60.2X1-	T60.2X2-	T60.2X3-	T60.2X4-	-	-
organochlorine (compounds)	T60.1X1-	T60.1X2-	T60.1X3-	T60.1X4-	-	-
petroleum (distillate) (products) NEC	T60.8X1-	T60.8X2-	T60.8X3-	T60.8X4-	-	-
specified ingredient NEC	T60.8X1-	T60.8X2-	T60.8X3-	T60.8X4-	-	-
strychnine	T65.1X1-	T65.1X2-	T65.1X3-	T65.1X4-	-	-
thallium	T60.4X1-	T60.4X2-	T60.4X3-	T60.4X4-	-	-
Pethidine	T40.4X1-	T40.4X2-	T40.4X3-	T40.4X4-	T40.4X5-	T40.4X6-
Petrichloral	T42.6X1-	T42.6X2-	T42.6X3-	T42.6X4-	T42.6X5-	T42.6X6-
Petrol	T52.0X1-	T52.0X2-	T52.0X3-	T52.0X4-	-	-
vapor	T52.0X1-	T52.0X2-	T52.0X3-	T52.0X4-	-	-
Petrolatum	T49.3X1-	T49.3X2-	T49.3X3-	T49.3X4-	T49.3X5-	T49.3X6-
hydrophilic	T49.3X1-	T49.3X2-	T49.3X3-	T49.3X4-	T49.3X5-	T49.3X6-
liquid	T47.4X1-	T47.4X2-	T47.4X3-	T47.4X4-	T47.4X5-	T47.4X6-
topical	T49.3X1-	T49.3X2-	T49.3X3-	T49.3X4-	T49.3X5-	T49.3X6-
nonmedicinal	T52.0X1-	T52.0X2-	T52.0X3-	T52.0X4-	-	-
red veterinary	T49.3X1-	T49.3X2-	T49.3X3-	T49.3X4-	T49.3X5-	T49.3X6-
white	T49.3X1-	T49.3X2-	T49.3X3-	T49.3X4-	T49.3X5-	T49.3X6-
Petroleum (products) NEC	T52.0X1-	T52.0X2-	T52.0X3-	T52.0X4-	-	-
benzine (s) — see Ligroin						
ether — see Ligroin						
jelly — see Petrolatum						
naphtha — see Ligroin						
pesticide	T60.8X1-	T60.8X2-	T60.8X3-	T60.8X4-	-	-
solids	T52.0X1-	T52.0X2-	T52.0X3-	T52.0X4-	-	-
solvents	T52.0X1-	T52.0X2-	T52.0X3-	T52.0X4-	-	-
vapor	T52.0X1-	T52.0X2-	T52.0X3-	T52.0X4-	-	-
Peyote	T40.991-	T40.992-	T40.993-	T40.994-	-	-
Phanodorm, phanodorn	T42.3X1-	T42.3X2-	T42.3X3-	T42.3X4-	T42.3X5-	T42.3X6-
Phanquinone	T37.3X1-	T37.3X2-	T37.3X3-	T37.3X4-	T37.3X5-	T37.3X6-
Phanquone	T37.3X1-	T37.3X2-	T37.3X3-	T37.3X4-	T37.3X5-	T37.3X6-
Pharmaceutical						
adjunct NEC	T50.901-	T50.902-	T50.903-	T50.904-	T50.905-	T50.906-
excipient NEC	T50.901-	T50.902-	T50.903-	T50.904-	T50.905-	T50.906-
sweetener	T50.901-	T50.902-	T50.903-	T50.904-	T50.905-	T50.906-
viscous agent	T50.901-	T50.902-	T50.903-	T50.904-	T50.905-	T50.906-
Phemitone	T42.3X1-	T42.3X2-	T42.3X3-	T42.3X4-	T42.3X5-	T42.3X6-
Phenacaine	T41.3X1-	T41.3X2-	T41.3X3-	T41.3X4-	T41.3X5-	T41.3X6-
Phenacemide	T42.6X1-	T42.6X2-	T42.6X3-	T42.6X4-	T42.6X5-	T42.6X6-
Phenacetin	T39.1X1-	T39.1X2-	T39.1X3-	T39.1X4-	T39.1X5-	T39.1X6-
Phenadoxone	T40.2X1-	T40.2X2-	T40.2X3-	T40.2X4-	-	-
Phenaglycodol	T43.591-	T43.592-	T43.593-	T43.594-	T43.595-	T43.596-
Phenantoin	T42.0X1-	T42.0X2-	T42.0X3-	T42.0X4-	T42.0X5-	T42.0X6-
Phenaphthazine reagent	T50.991-	T50.992-	T50.993-	T50.994-	T50.995-	T50.996-
Phenazocine	T40.4X1-	T40.4X2-	T40.4X3-	T40.4X4-	T40.4X5-	T40.4X6-
Phenazone	T39.2X1-	T39.2X2-	T39.2X3-	T39.2X4-	T39.2X5-	T39.2X6-
Phenazopyridine	T39.8X1-	T39.8X2-	T39.8X3-	T39.8X4-	T39.8X5-	T39.8X6-
Phenbenicillin	T36.0X1-	T36.0X2-	T36.0X3-	T36.0X4-	T36.0X5-	T36.0X6-
Phenbutrazate	T50.5X1-	T50.5X2-	T50.5X3-	T50.5X4-	T50.5X5-	T50.5X6-
Phencyclidine	T40.991-	T40.992-	T40.993-	T40.994-	T40.995-	T40.996-
Phendimetrazine	T50.5X1-	T50.5X2-	T50.5X3-	T50.5X4-	T50.5X5-	T50.5X6-
Phenelzine	T43.1X1-	T43.1X2-	T43.1X3-	T43.1X4-	T43.1X5-	T43.1X6-
Phenemal	T42.3X1-	T42.3X2-	T42.3X3-	T42.3X4-	T42.3X5-	T42.3X6-

Substance	Poisoning Accidental (unintentional)	Poisoning Intentional self-harm	Poisoning Assault	Poisoning Undetermined	Adverse effect	Underdosing
Phenergan	T42.6X1-	T42.6X2-	T42.6X3-	T42.6X4-	T42.6X5-	T42.6X6-
Pheneticillin	T36.0X1-	T36.0X2-	T36.0X3-	T36.0X4-	T36.0X5-	T36.0X6-
Pheneturide	T42.6X1-	T42.6X2-	T42.6X3-	T42.6X4-	T42.6X5-	T42.6X6-
Phenformin	T38.3X1-	T38.3X2-	T38.3X3-	T38.3X4-	T38.3X5-	T38.3X6-
Phenglutarimide	T44.3X1-	T44.3X2-	T44.3X3-	T44.3X4-	T44.3X5-	T44.3X6-
Phenicarbazide	T39.8X1-	T39.8X2-	T39.8X3-	T39.8X4-	T39.8X5-	T39.8X6-
Phenindamine	T45.0X1-	T45.0X2-	T45.0X3-	T45.0X4-	T45.0X5-	T45.0X6-
Phenindione	T45.511-	T45.512-	T45.513-	T45.514-	T45.515-	T45.516-
Pheniprazine	T43.1X1-	T43.1X2-	T43.1X3-	T43.1X4-	T43.1X5-	T43.1X6-
Pheniramine	T45.0X1-	T45.0X2-	T45.0X3-	T45.0X4-	T45.0X5-	T45.0X6-
Phenisatin	T47.2X1-	T47.2X2-	T47.2X3-	T47.2X4-	T47.2X5-	T47.2X6-
Phenmetrazine	T50.5X1-	T50.5X2-	T50.5X3-	T50.5X4-	T50.5X5-	T50.5X6-
Phenobal	T42.3X1-	T42.3X2-	T42.3X3-	T42.3X4-	T42.3X5-	T42.3X6-
Phenobarbital	T42.3X1-	T42.3X2-	T42.3X3-	T42.3X4-	T42.3X5-	T42.3X6-
with						
mephenytoin	T42.3X1-	T42.3X2-	T42.3X3-	T42.3X4-	T42.3X5-	T42.3X6-
phenytoin	T42.3X1-	T42.3X2-	T42.3X3-	T42.3X4-	T42.3X5-	T42.3X6-
sodium	T42.3X1-	T42.3X2-	T42.3X3-	T42.3X4-	T42.3X5-	T42.3X6-
Phenobarbitone	T42.3X1-	T42.3X2-	T42.3X3-	T42.3X4-	T42.3X5-	T42.3X6-
Phenobutiodil	T50.8X1-	T50.8X2-	T50.8X3-	T50.8X4-	T50.8X5-	T50.8X6-
Phenoctide	T49.0X1-	T49.0X2-	T49.0X3-	T49.0X4-	T49.0X5-	T49.0X6-
Phenol	T49.0X1-	T49.0X2-	T49.0X3-	T49.0X4-	T49.0X5-	T49.0X6-
disinfectant	T54.0X1-	T54.0X2-	T54.0X3-	T54.0X4-	-	-
in oil injection	T46.8X1-	T46.8X2-	T46.8X3-	T46.8X4-	T46.8X5-	T46.8X6-
medicinal	T49.1X1-	T49.1X2-	T49.1X3-	T49.1X4-	T49.1X5-	T49.1X6-
nonmedicinal NEC	T54.0X1-	T54.0X2-	T54.0X3-	T54.0X4-	-	-
pesticide	T60.8X1-	T60.8X2-	T60.8X3-	T60.8X4-	-	-
red	T50.8X1-	T50.8X2-	T50.8X3-	T50.8X4-	T50.8X5-	T50.8X6-
Phenolic preparation	T49.1X1-	T49.1X2-	T49.1X3-	T49.1X4-	T49.1X5-	T49.1X6-
Phenolphthalein	T47.2X1-	T47.2X2-	T47.2X3-	T47.2X4-	T47.2X5-	T47.2X6-
Phenolsulfonphthalein	T50.8X1-	T50.8X2-	T50.8X3-	T50.8X4-	T50.8X5-	T50.8X6-
Phenomorphan	T40.2X1-	T40.2X2-	T40.2X3-	T40.2X4-	-	-
Phenonyl	T42.3X1-	T42.3X2-	T42.3X3-	T42.3X4-	T42.3X5-	T42.3X6-
Phenoperidine	T40.4X1-	T40.4X2-	T40.4X3-	T40.4X4-	-	-
Phenopyrazone	T46.991-	T46.992-	T46.993-	T46.994-	T46.995-	T46.996-
Phenoquin	T50.4X1-	T50.4X2-	T50.4X3-	T50.4X4-	T50.4X5-	T50.4X6-
Phenothiazine (psychotropic) NEC	T43.3X1-	T43.3X2-	T43.3X3-	T43.3X4-	T43.3X5-	T43.3X6-
insecticide	T60.2X1-	T60.2X2-	T60.2X3-	T60.2X4-	-	-
Phenothrin	T49.0X1-	T49.0X2-	T49.0X3-	T49.0X4-	T49.0X5-	T49.0X6-
Phenoxybenzamine	T46.7X1-	T46.7X2-	T46.7X3-	T46.7X4-	T46.7X5-	T46.7X6-
Phenoxyethanol	T49.0X1-	T49.0X2-	T49.0X3-	T49.0X4-	T49.0X5-	T49.0X6-
Phenoxymethyl penicillin	T36.0X1-	T36.0X2-	T36.0X3-	T36.0X4-	T36.0X5-	T36.0X6-
Phenprobamate	T42.8X1-	T42.8X2-	T42.8X3-	T42.8X4-	T42.8X5-	T42.8X6-
Phenprocoumon	T45.511-	T45.512-	T45.513-	T45.514-	T45.515-	T45.516-
Phensuximide	T42.2X1-	T42.2X2-	T42.2X3-	T42.2X4-	T42.2X5-	T42.2X6-
Phentermine	T50.5X1-	T50.5X2-	T50.5X3-	T50.5X4-	T50.5X5-	T50.5X6-
Phenthicillin	T36.0X1-	T36.0X2-	T36.0X3-	T36.0X4-	T36.0X5-	T36.0X6-
Phentolamine	T46.7X1-	T46.7X2-	T46.7X3-	T46.7X4-	T46.7X5-	T46.7X6-
Phenyl						
butazone	T39.2X1-	T39.2X2-	T39.2X3-	T39.2X4-	T39.2X5-	T39.2X6-
enediamine	T65.3X1-	T65.3X2-	T65.3X3-	T65.3X4-	-	-
hydrazine	T65.3X1-	T65.3X2-	T65.3X3-	T65.3X4-	-	-
antineoplastic	T45.1X1-	T45.1X2-	T45.1X3-	T45.1X4-	T45.1X5-	T45.1X6-
mercuric compounds — *see Mercury*						
salicylate	T49.3X1-	T49.3X2-	T49.3X3-	T49.3X4-	T49.3X5-	T49.3X6-
Phenylalanine mustard	T45.1X1-	T45.1X2-	T45.1X3-	T45.1X4-	T45.1X5-	T45.1X6-
Phenylbutazone	T39.2X1-	T39.2X2-	T39.2X3-	T39.2X4-	T39.2X5-	T39.2X6-
Phenylenediamine	T65.3X1-	T65.3X2-	T65.3X3-	T65.3X4-	-	-
Phenylephrine	T44.4X1-	T44.4X2-	T44.4X3-	T44.4X4-	T44.4X5-	T44.4X6-

Substance	Poisoning Accidental (unintentional)	Poisoning Intentional self-harm	Poisoning Assault	Poisoning Undetermined	Adverse effect	Underdosing
Phenylethylbiguanide	T38.3X1-	T38.3X2-	T38.3X3-	T38.3X4-	T38.3X5-	T38.3X6-
Phenylmercuric						
acetate	T49.0X1-	T49.0X2-	T49.0X3-	T49.0X4-	T49.0X5-	T49.0X6-
borate	T49.0X1-	T49.0X2-	T49.0X3-	T49.0X4-	T49.0X5-	T49.0X6-
nitrate	T49.0X1-	T49.0X2-	T49.0X3-	T49.0X4-	T49.0X5-	T49.0X6-
Phenylmethylbarbitone	T42.3X1-	T42.3X2-	T42.3X3-	T42.3X4-	T42.3X5-	T42.3X6-
Phenylpropanol	T47.5X1-	T47.5X2-	T47.5X3-	T47.5X4-	T47.5X5-	T47.5X6-
Phenylpropanolamine	T44.991-	T44.992-	T44.993-	T44.994-	T44.995-	T44.996-
Phenylsulfthion	T60.0X1-	T60.0X2-	T60.0X3-	T60.0X4-	-	-
Phenyltoloxamine	T45.0X1-	T45.0X2-	T45.0X3-	T45.0X4-	T45.0X5-	T45.0X6-
Phenyramidol, phenyramidon	T39.8X1-	T39.8X2-	T39.8X3-	T39.8X4-	T39.8X5-	T39.8X6-
Phenytoin	T42.0X1-	T42.0X2-	T42.0X3-	T42.0X4-	T42.0X5-	T42.0X6-
with Phenobarbital	T42.3X1-	T42.3X2-	T42.3X3-	T42.3X4-	T42.3X5-	T42.3X6-
pHisoHex	T49.2X1-	T49.2X2-	T49.2X3-	T49.2X4-	T49.2X5-	T49.2X6-
Pholcodine	T48.3X1-	T48.3X2-	T48.3X3-	T48.3X4-	T48.3X5-	T48.3X6-
Pholedrine	T46.991-	T46.992-	T46.993-	T46.994-	T46.995-	T46.996-
Phorate	T60.0X1-	T60.0X2-	T60.0X3-	T60.0X4-	-	-
Phosdrin	T60.0X1-	T60.0X2-	T60.0X3-	T60.0X4-	-	-
Phosfolan	T60.0X1-	T60.0X2-	T60.0X3-	T60.0X4-	-	-
Phosgene (gas)	T59.891-	T59.892-	T59.893-	T59.894-	-	-
Phosphamidon	T60.0X1-	T60.0X2-	T60.0X3-	T60.0X4-	-	-
Phosphate	T65.891-	T65.892-	T65.893-	T65.894-	-	-
laxative	T47.4X1-	T47.4X2-	T47.4X3-	T47.4X4-	T47.4X5-	T47.4X6-
organic	T60.0X1-	T60.0X2-	T60.0X3-	T60.0X4-	-	-
solvent	T52.91X-	T52.92X-	T52.93X-	T52.94X-	-	-
tricresyl	T65.891-	T65.892-	T65.893-	T65.894-	-	-
Phosphine	T57.1X1-	T57.1X2-	T57.1X3-	T57.1X4-	-	-
fumigant	T57.1X1-	T57.1X2-	T57.1X3-	T57.1X4-	-	-
Phospholine	T49.5X1-	T49.5X2-	T49.5X3-	T49.5X4-	T49.5X5-	T49.5X6-
Phosphoric acid	T54.2X1-	T54.2X2-	T54.2X3-	T54.2X4-	-	-
Phosphorus (compound) NEC	T57.1X1-	T57.1X2-	T57.1X3-	T57.1X4-	-	-
pesticide	T60.0X1-	T60.0X2-	T60.0X3-	T60.0X4-	-	-
Phthalates	T65.891-	T65.892-	T65.893-	T65.894-	-	-
Phthalic anhydride	T65.891-	T65.892-	T65.893-	T65.894-	-	-
Phthalimidoglutarimide	T42.6X1-	T42.6X2-	T42.6X3-	T42.6X4-	T42.6X5-	T42.6X6-
Phthalylsulfathiazole	T37.0X1-	T37.0X2-	T37.0X3-	T37.0X4-	T37.0X5-	T37.0X6-
Phylloquinone	T45.7X1-	T45.7X2-	T45.7X3-	T45.7X4-	T45.7X5-	T45.7X6-
Physeptone	T40.3X1-	T40.3X2-	T40.3X3-	T40.3X4-	T40.3X5-	T40.3X6-
Physostigma venenosum	T62.2X1-	T62.2X2-	T62.2X3-	T62.2X4-	-	-
Physostigmine	T49.5X1-	T49.5X2-	T49.5X3-	T49.5X4-	T49.5X5-	T49.5X6-
Phytolacca decandra	T62.2X1-	T62.2X2-	T62.2X3-	T62.2X4-	-	-
berries	T62.1X1-	T62.1X2-	T62.1X3-	T62.1X4-	-	-
Phytomenadione	T45.7X1-	T45.7X2-	T45.7X3-	T45.7X4-	T45.7X5-	T45.7X6-
Phytonadione	T45.7X1-	T45.7X2-	T45.7X3-	T45.7X4-	T45.7X5-	T45.7X6-
Picoperine	T48.3X1-	T48.3X2-	T48.3X3-	T48.3X4-	T48.3X5-	T48.3X6-
Picosulfate (sodium)	T47.2X1-	T47.2X2-	T47.2X3-	T47.2X4-	T47.2X5-	T47.2X6-
Picric (acid)	T54.2X1-	T54.2X2-	T54.2X3-	T54.2X4-	-	-
Picrotoxin	T50.7X1-	T50.7X2-	T50.7X3-	T50.7X4-	T50.7X5-	T50.7X6-
Piketoprofen	T49.0X1-	T49.0X2-	T49.0X3-	T49.0X4-	T49.0X5-	T49.0X6-
Pilocarpine	T44.1X1-	T44.1X2-	T44.1X3-	T44.1X4-	T44.1X5-	T44.1X6-
Pilocarpus (jaborandi) extract	T44.1X1-	T44.1X2-	T44.1X3-	T44.1X4-	T44.1X5-	T44.1X6-
Pilsicainide (hydrochloride)	T46.2X1-	T46.2X2-	T46.2X3-	T46.2X4-	T46.2X5-	T46.2X6-
Pimaricin	T36.7X1-	T36.7X2-	T36.7X3-	T36.7X4-	T36.7X5-	T36.7X6-
Pimeclone	T50.7X1-	T50.7X2-	T50.7X3-	T50.7X4-	T50.7X5-	T50.7X6-
Pimelic ketone	T52.8X1-	T52.8X2-	T52.8X3-	T52.8X4-	-	-
Pimethixene	T45.0X1-	T45.0X2-	T45.0X3-	T45.0X4-	T45.0X5-	T45.0X6-
Piminodine	T40.2X1-	T40.2X2-	T40.2X3-	T40.2X4-	T40.2X5-	T40.2X6-
Pimozide	T43.591-	T43.592-	T43.593-	T43.594-	T43.595-	T43.596-

Substance	Poisoning Accidental (unintentional)	Poisoning Intentional self-harm	Poisoning Assault	Poisoning Undetermined	Adverse effect	Underdosing
Pinacidil	T46.5X1-	T46.5X2-	T46.5X3-	T46.5X4-	T46.5X5-	T46.5X6-
Pinaverium bromide	T44.3X1-	T44.3X2-	T44.3X3-	T44.3X4-	T44.3X5-	T44.3X6-
Pinazepam	T42.4X1-	T42.4X2-	T42.4X3-	T42.4X4-	T42.4X5-	T42.4X6-
Pindolol	T44.7X1-	T44.7X2-	T44.7X3-	T44.7X4-	T44.7X5-	T44.7X6-
Pindone	T60.4X1-	T60.4X2-	T60.4X3-	T60.4X4-	-	-
Pine oil (disinfectant)	T65.891-	T65.892-	T65.893-	T65.894-	-	-
Pinkroot	T37.4X1-	T37.4X2-	T37.4X3-	T37.4X4-	T37.4X5-	T37.4X6-
Pipadone	T40.2X1-	T40.2X2-	T40.2X3-	T40.2X4-	-	-
Pipamazine	T45.0X1-	T45.0X2-	T45.0X3-	T45.0X4-	T45.0X5-	T45.0X6-
Pipamperone	T43.4X1-	T43.4X2-	T43.4X3-	T43.4X4-	T43.4X5-	T43.4X6-
Pipazetate	T48.3X1-	T48.3X2-	T48.3X3-	T48.3X4-	T48.3X5-	T48.3X6-
Pipemidic acid	T37.8X1-	T37.8X2-	T37.8X3-	T37.8X4-	T37.8X5-	T37.8X6-
Pipenzolate bromide	T44.3X1-	T44.3X2-	T44.3X3-	T44.3X4-	T44.3X5-	T44.3X6-
Piperacetazine	T43.3X1-	T43.3X2-	T43.3X3-	T43.3X4-	T43.3X5-	T43.3X6-
Piperacillin	T36.0X1-	T36.0X2-	T36.0X3-	T36.0X4-	T36.0X5-	T36.0X6-
Piperazine	T37.4X1-	T37.4X2-	T37.4X3-	T37.4X4-	T37.4X5-	T37.4X6-
estrone sulfate	T38.5X1-	T38.5X2-	T38.5X3-	T38.5X4-	T38.5X5-	T38.5X6-
Piper cubeba	T62.2X1-	T62.2X2-	T62.2X3-	T62.2X4-	-	-
Piperidione	T48.3X1-	T48.3X2-	T48.3X3-	T48.3X4-	T48.3X5-	T48.3X6-
Piperidolate	T44.3X1-	T44.3X2-	T44.3X3-	T44.3X4-	T44.3X5-	T44.3X6-
Piperocaine	T41.3X1-	T41.3X2-	T41.3X3-	T41.3X4-	T41.3X5-	T41.3X6-
infiltration (subcutaneous)	T41.3X1-	T41.3X2-	T41.3X3-	T41.3X4-	T41.3X5-	T41.3X6-
nerve block (peripheral) (plexus)	T41.3X1-	T41.3X2-	T41.3X3-	T41.3X4-	T41.3X5-	T41.3X6-
topical (surface)	T41.3X1-	T41.3X2-	T41.3X3-	T41.3X4-	T41.3X5-	T41.3X6-
Piperonyl butoxide	T60.8X1-	T60.8X2-	T60.8X3-	T60.8X4-	-	-
Pipethanate	T44.3X1-	T44.3X2-	T44.3X3-	T44.3X4-	T44.3X5-	T44.3X6-
Pipobroman	T45.1X1-	T45.1X2-	T45.1X3-	T45.1X4-	T45.1X5-	T45.1X6-
Pipotiazine	T43.3X1-	T43.3X2-	T43.3X3-	T43.3X4-	T43.3X5-	T43.3X6-
Pipoxizine	T45.0X1-	T45.0X2-	T45.0X3-	T45.0X4-	T45.0X5-	T45.0X6-
Pipradrol	T43.691-	T43.692-	T43.693-	T43.694-	T43.695-	T43.696-
Piprinhydrinate	T45.0X1-	T45.0X2-	T45.0X3-	T45.0X4-	T45.0X5-	T45.0X6-
Pirarubicin	T45.1X1-	T45.1X2-	T45.1X3-	T45.1X4-	T45.1X5-	T45.1X6-
Pirazinamide	T37.1X1-	T37.1X2-	T37.1X3-	T37.1X4-	T37.1X5-	T37.1X6-
Pirbuterol	T48.6X1-	T48.6X2-	T48.6X3-	T48.6X4-	T48.6X5-	T48.6X6-
Pirenzepine	T47.1X1-	T47.1X2-	T47.1X3-	T47.1X4-	T47.1X5-	T47.1X6-
Piretanide	T50.1X1-	T50.1X2-	T50.1X3-	T50.1X4-	T50.1X5-	T50.1X6-
Piribedil	T42.8X1-	T42.8X2-	T42.8X3-	T42.8X4-	T42.8X5-	T42.8X6-
Piridoxilate	T46.3X1-	T46.3X2-	T46.3X3-	T46.3X4-	T46.3X5-	T46.3X6-
Piritramide	T40.4X1-	T40.4X2-	T40.4X3-	T40.4X4-	-	-
Piromidic acid	T37.8X1-	T37.8X2-	T37.8X3-	T37.8X4-	T37.8X5-	T37.8X6-
Piroxicam	T39.391-	T39.392-	T39.393-	T39.394-	T39.395-	T39.396-
beta-cyclodextrin complex	T39.8X1-	T39.8X2-	T39.8X3-	T39.8X4-	T39.8X5-	T39.8X6-
Pirozadil	T46.6X1-	T46.6X2-	T46.6X3-	T46.6X4-	T46.6X5-	T46.6X6-
Piscidia (bark) (erythrina)	T39.8X1-	T39.8X2-	T39.8X3-	T39.8X4-	T39.8X5-	T39.8X6-
Pitch	T65.891-	T65.892-	T65.893-	T65.894-	-	-
Pitkin's solution	T41.3X1-	T41.3X2-	T41.3X3-	T41.3X4-	T41.3X5-	T41.3X6-
Pitocin	T48.0X1-	T48.0X2-	T48.0X3-	T48.0X4-	T48.0X5-	T48.0X6-
Pitressin (tannate)	T38.891-	T38.892-	T38.893-	T38.894-	T38.895-	T38.896-
Pituitary extracts (posterior)	T38.891-	T38.892-	T38.893-	T38.894-	T38.895-	T38.896-
anterior	T38.811-	T38.812-	T38.813-	T38.814-	T38.815-	T38.816-
Pituitrin	T38.891-	T38.892-	T38.893-	T38.894-	T38.895-	T38.896-
Pivampicillin	T36.0X1-	T36.0X2-	T36.0X3-	T36.0X4-	T36.0X5-	T36.0X6-
Pivmecillinam	T36.0X1-	T36.0X2-	T36.0X3-	T36.0X4-	T36.0X5-	T36.0X6-
Placental hormone	T38.891-	T38.892-	T38.893-	T38.894-	T38.895-	T38.896-
Placidyl	T42.6X1-	T42.6X2-	T42.6X3-	T42.6X4-	T42.6X5-	T42.6X6-
Plague vaccine	T50.A91-	T50.A92-	T50.A93-	T50.A94-	T50.A95-	T50.A96-
Plant						
food or fertilizer NEC	T65.891-	T65.892-	T65.893-	T65.894-	-	-

PINACIDIL - PLANT

Substance	Poisoning Accidental (unintentional)	Poisoning Intentional self-harm	Poisoning Assault	Poisoning Undetermined	Adverse effect	Underdosing
Plant (continued)						
containing herbicide	T60.3X1-	T60.3X2-	T60.3X3-	T60.3X4-	-	-
noxious, used as food	T62.2X1-	T62.2X2-	T62.2X3-	T62.2X4-	-	-
berries	T62.1X1-	T62.1X2-	T62.1X3-	T62.1X4-	-	-
seeds	T62.2X1-	T62.2X2-	T62.2X3-	T62.2X4-	-	-
specified type NEC	T62.2X1-	T62.2X2-	T62.2X3-	T62.2X4-	-	-
Plasma	T45.8X1-	T45.8X2-	T45.8X3-	T45.8X4-	T45.8X5-	T45.8X6-
expander NEC	T45.8X1-	T45.8X2-	T45.8X3-	T45.8X4-	T45.8X5-	T45.8X6-
protein fraction (human)	T45.8X1-	T45.8X2-	T45.8X3-	T45.8X4-	T45.8X5-	T45.8X6-
Plasmanate	T45.8X1-	T45.8X2-	T45.8X3-	T45.8X4-	T45.8X5-	T45.8X6-
Plasminogen (tissue) activator	T45.611-	T45.612-	T45.613-	T45.614-	T45.615-	T45.616-
Plaster dressing	T49.3X1-	T49.3X2-	T49.3X3-	T49.3X4-	T49.3X5-	T49.3X6-
Plastic dressing	T49.3X1-	T49.3X2-	T49.3X3-	T49.3X4-	T49.3X5-	T49.3X6-
Plegicil	T43.3X1-	T43.3X2-	T43.3X3-	T43.3X4-	T43.3X5-	T43.3X6-
Plicamycin	T45.1X1-	T45.1X2-	T45.1X3-	T45.1X4-	T45.1X5-	T45.1X6-
Podophyllotoxin	T49.8X1-	T49.8X2-	T49.8X3-	T49.8X4-	T49.8X5-	T49.8X6-
Podophyllum (resin)	T49.4X1-	T49.4X2-	T49.4X3-	T49.4X4-	T49.4X5-	T49.4X6-
Poison NEC	T65.91X-	T65.92X-	T65.93X-	T65.94X-	-	-
Poisonous berries	T62.1X1-	T62.1X2-	T62.1X3-	T62.1X4-	-	-
Pokeweed (any part)	T62.2X1-	T62.2X2-	T62.2X3-	T62.2X4-	-	-
Poldine metilsulfate	T44.3X1-	T44.3X2-	T44.3X3-	T44.3X4-	T44.3X5-	T44.3X6-
Polidexide (sulfate)	T46.6X1-	T46.6X2-	T46.6X3-	T46.6X4-	T46.6X5-	T46.6X6-
Polidocanol	T46.8X1-	T46.8X2-	T46.8X3-	T46.8X4-	T46.8X5-	T46.8X6-
Poliomyelitis vaccine	T50.B91-	T50.B92-	T50.B93-	T50.B94-	T50.B95-	T50.B96-
Polish (car) (floor) (furni-ture) (metal) (porcelain) (silver)	T65.891-	T65.892-	T65.893-	T65.894-	-	-
abrasive	T65.891-	T65.892-	T65.893-	T65.894-	-	-
porcelain	T65.891-	T65.892-	T65.893-	T65.894-	-	-
Poloxalkol	T47.4X1-	T47.4X2-	T47.4X3-	T47.4X4-	T47.4X5-	T47.4X6-
Poloxamer	T47.4X1-	T47.4X2-	T47.4X3-	T47.4X4-	T47.4X5-	T47.4X6-
Polyaminostyrene resins	T50.3X1-	T50.3X2-	T50.3X3-	T50.3X4-	T50.3X5-	T50.3X6-
Polycarbophil	T47.4X1-	T47.4X2-	T47.4X3-	T47.4X4-	T47.4X5-	T47.4X6-
Polychlorinated biphenyl	T65.891-	T65.892-	T65.893-	T65.894-	-	-
Polycycline	T36.4X1-	T36.4X2-	T36.4X3-	T36.4X4-	T36.4X5-	T36.4X6-
Polyester fumes	T59.891-	T59.892-	T59.893-	T59.894-	-	-
Polyester resin hardener	T52.91X-	T52.92X-	T52.93X-	T52.94X-	-	-
fumes	T59.891-	T59.892-	T59.893-	T59.894-	-	-
Polyestradiol phosphate	T38.5X1-	T38.5X2-	T38.5X3-	T38.5X4-	T38.5X5-	T38.5X6-
Polyethanolamine alkyl sulfate	T49.2X1-	T49.2X2-	T49.2X3-	T49.2X4-	T49.2X5-	T49.2X6-
Polyethylene adhesive	T49.3X1-	T49.3X2-	T49.3X3-	T49.3X4-	T49.3X5-	T49.3X6-
Polyferose	T45.4X1-	T45.4X2-	T45.4X3-	T45.4X4-	T45.4X5-	T45.4X6-
Polygeline	T45.8X1-	T45.8X2-	T45.8X3-	T45.8X4-	T45.8X5-	T45.8X6-
Polymyxin	T36.8X1-	T36.8X2-	T36.8X3-	T36.8X4-	T36.8X5-	T36.8X6-
B	T36.8X1-	T36.8X2-	T36.8X3-	T36.8X4-	T36.8X5-	T36.8X6-
ENT agent	T49.6X1-	T49.6X2-	T49.6X3-	T49.6X4-	T49.6X5-	T49.6X6-
ophthalmic preparation	T49.5X1-	T49.5X2-	T49.5X3-	T49.5X4-	T49.5X5-	T49.5X6-
topical NEC	T49.0X1-	T49.0X2-	T49.0X3-	T49.0X4-	T49.0X5-	T49.0X6-
E sulfate (eye preparation)	T49.5X1-	T49.5X2-	T49.5X3-	T49.5X4-	T49.5X5-	T49.5X6-
Polynoxylin	T49.0X1-	T49.0X2-	T49.0X3-	T49.0X4-	T49.0X5-	T49.0X6-
Polyoestradiol phosphate	T38.5X1-	T38.5X2-	T38.5X3-	T38.5X4-	T38.5X5-	T38.5X6-
Polyoxymethyleneurea	T49.0X1-	T49.0X2-	T49.0X3-	T49.0X4-	T49.0X5-	T49.0X6-
Polysilane	T47.8X1-	T47.8X2-	T47.8X3-	T47.8X4-	T47.8X5-	T47.8X6-
Polytetrafluoroethylene (inhaled)	T59.891-	T59.892-	T59.893-	T59.894-	-	-
Polythiazide	T50.2X1-	T50.2X2-	T50.2X3-	T50.2X4-	T50.2X5-	T50.2X6-
Polyvidone	T45.8X1-	T45.8X2-	T45.8X3-	T45.8X4-	T45.8X5-	T45.8X6-
Polyvinylpyrrolidone	T45.8X1-	T45.8X2-	T45.8X3-	T45.8X4-	T45.8X5-	T45.8X6-
Pontocaine (hydrochloride) (infiltration) (topical)	T41.3X1-	T41.3X2-	T41.3X3-	T41.3X4-	T41.3X5-	T41.3X6-
nerve block (peripheral) (plexus)	T41.3X1-	T41.3X2-	T41.3X3-	T41.3X4-	T41.3X5-	T41.3X6-

Substance	Poisoning Accidental (unintentional)	Poisoning Intentional self-harm	Poisoning Assault	Poisoning Undetermined	Adverse effect	Underdosing
Pontocaine (hydrochloride) (infiltration) (topical) (continued)						
spinal	T41.3X1-	T41.3X2-	T41.3X3-	T41.3X4-	T41.3X5-	T41.3X6-
Porfiromycin	T45.1X1-	T45.1X2-	T45.1X3-	T45.1X4-	T45.1X5-	T45.1X6-
Posterior pituitary hormone NEC	T38.891-	T38.892-	T38.893-	T38.894-	T38.895-	T38.896-
Pot	T40.7X1-	T40.7X2-	T40.7X3-	T40.7X4-	T40.7X5-	T40.7X6-
Potash (caustic)	T54.3X1-	T54.3X2-	T54.3X3-	T54.3X4-	-	-
Potassic saline injection (lactated)	T50.3X1-	T50.3X2-	T50.3X3-	T50.3X4-	T50.3X5-	T50.3X6-
Potassium (salts) NEC	T50.3X1-	T50.3X2-	T50.3X3-	T50.3X4-	T50.3X5-	T50.3X6-
aminobenzoate	T45.8X1-	T45.8X2-	T45.8X3-	T45.8X4-	T45.8X5-	T45.8X6-
aminosalicylate	T37.1X1-	T37.1X2-	T37.1X3-	T37.1X4-	T37.1X5-	T37.1X6-
antimony ' tartrate'	T37.8X1-	T37.8X2-	T37.8X3-	T37.8X4-	T37.8X5-	T37.8X6-
arsenite (solution)	T57.0X1-	T57.0X2-	T57.0X3-	T57.0X4-	-	-
bichromate	T56.2X1-	T56.2X2-	T56.2X3-	T56.2X4-	-	-
bisulfate	T47.3X1-	T47.3X2-	T47.3X3-	T47.3X4-	T47.3X5-	T47.3X6-
bromide	T42.6X1-	T42.6X2-	T42.6X3-	T42.6X4-	T42.6X5-	T42.6X6-
canrenoate	T50.0X1-	T50.0X2-	T50.0X3-	T50.0X4-	T50.0X5-	T50.0X6-
carbonate	T54.3X1-	T54.3X2-	T54.3X3-	T54.3X4-	-	-
chlorate NEC	T65.891-	T65.892-	T65.893-	T65.894-	-	-
chloride	T50.3X1-	T50.3X2-	T50.3X3-	T50.3X4-	T50.3X5-	T50.3X6-
citrate	T50.991-	T50.992-	T50.993-	T50.994-	T50.995-	T50.996-
cyanide	T65.0X1-	T65.0X2-	T65.0X3-	T65.0X4-	-	-
ferric hexacyanoferrate (medicinal)	T50.6X1-	T50.6X2-	T50.6X3-	T50.6X4-	T50.6X5-	T50.6X6-
nonmedicinal	T65.891-	T65.892-	T65.893-	T65.894-	-	-
Fluoride	T57.8X1-	T57.8X2-	T57.8X3-	T57.8X4-	-	-
glucaldrate	T47.1X1-	T47.1X2-	T47.1X3-	T47.1X4-	T47.1X5-	T47.1X6-
hydroxide	T54.3X1-	T54.3X2-	T54.3X3-	T54.3X4-	-	-
iodate	T49.0X1-	T49.0X2-	T49.0X3-	T49.0X4-	T49.0X5-	T49.0X6-
iodide	T48.4X1-	T48.4X2-	T48.4X3-	T48.4X4-	T48.4X5-	T48.4X6-
nitrate	T57.8X1-	T57.8X2-	T57.8X3-	T57.8X4-	-	-
oxalate	T65.891-	T65.892-	T65.893-	T65.894-	-	-
perchlorate (nonmedicinal) NEC	T65.891-	T65.892-	T65.893-	T65.894-	-	-
antithyroid	T38.2X1-	T38.2X2-	T38.2X3-	T38.2X4-	T38.2X5-	T38.2X6-
medicinal	T38.2X1-	T38.2X2-	T38.2X3-	T38.2X4-	T38.2X5-	T38.2X6-
Permanganate (nonmedicinal)	T65.891-	T65.892-	T65.893-	T65.894-	-	-
medicinal	T49.0X1-	T49.0X2-	T49.0X3-	T49.0X4-	T49.0X5-	T49.0X6-
sulfate	T47.2X1-	T47.2X2-	T47.2X3-	T47.2X4-	T47.2X5-	T47.2X6-
Potassium-removing resin	T50.3X1-	T50.3X2-	T50.3X3-	T50.3X4-	T50.3X5-	T50.3X6-
Potassium-retaining drug	T50.3X1-	T50.3X2-	T50.3X3-	T50.3X4-	T50.3X5-	T50.3X6-
Povidone	T45.8X1-	T45.8X2-	T45.8X3-	T45.8X4-	T45.8X5-	T45.8X6-
iodine	T49.0X1-	T49.0X2-	T49.0X3-	T49.0X4-	T49.0X5-	T49.0X6-
Practolol	T44.7X1-	T44.7X2-	T44.7X3-	T44.7X4-	T44.7X5-	T44.7X6-
Prajmalium bitartrate	T46.2X1-	T46.2X2-	T46.2X3-	T46.2X4-	T46.2X5-	T46.2X6-
Pralidoxime (iodide)	T50.6X1-	T50.6X2-	T50.6X3-	T50.6X4-	T50.6X5-	T50.6X6-
chloride	T50.6X1-	T50.6X2-	T50.6X3-	T50.6X4-	T50.6X5-	T50.6X6-
Pramiverine	T44.3X1-	T44.3X2-	T44.3X3-	T44.3X4-	T44.3X5-	T44.3X6-
Pramocaine	T49.1X1-	T49.1X2-	T49.1X3-	T49.1X4-	T49.1X5-	T49.1X6-
Pramoxine	T49.1X1-	T49.1X2-	T49.1X3-	T49.1X4-	T49.1X5-	T49.1X6-
Prasterone	T38.7X1-	T38.7X2-	T38.7X3-	T38.7X4-	T38.7X5-	T38.7X6-
Pravastatin	T46.6X1-	T46.6X2-	T46.6X3-	T46.6X4-	T46.6X5-	T46.6X6-
Prazepam	T42.4X1-	T42.4X2-	T42.4X3-	T42.4X4-	T42.4X5-	T42.4X6-
Praziquantel	T37.4X1-	T37.4X2-	T37.4X3-	T37.4X4-	T37.4X5-	T37.4X6-
Prazitone	T43.291-	T43.292-	T43.293-	T43.294-	T43.295-	T43.296-
Prazosin	T44.6X1-	T44.6X2-	T44.6X3-	T44.6X4-	T44.6X5-	T44.6X6-
Prednicarbate	T49.0X1-	T49.0X2-	T49.0X3-	T49.0X4-	T49.0X5-	T49.0X6-
Prednimustine	T45.1X1-	T45.1X2-	T45.1X3-	T45.1X4-	T45.1X5-	T45.1X6-
Prednisolone	T38.0X1-	T38.0X2-	T38.0X3-	T38.0X4-	T38.0X5-	T38.0X6-
ENT agent	T49.6X1-	T49.6X2-	T49.6X3-	T49.6X4-	T49.6X5-	T49.6X6-
ophthalmic preparation	T49.5X1-	T49.5X2-	T49.5X3-	T49.5X4-	T49.5X5-	T49.5X6-

PONTOCAINE - PREDNISOLONE

Substance	Poisoning Accidental (unintentional)	Poisoning Intentional self-harm	Poisoning Assault	Poisoning Undetermined	Adverse effect	Underdosing
Prednisolone (continued)						
steaglate	T49.0X1-	T49.0X2-	T49.0X3-	T49.0X4-	T49.0X5-	T49.0X6-
topical NEC	T49.0X1-	T49.0X2-	T49.0X3-	T49.0X4-	T49.0X5-	T49.0X6-
Prednisone	T38.0X1-	T38.0X2-	T38.0X3-	T38.0X4-	T38.0X5-	T38.0X6-
Prednylidene	T38.0X1-	T38.0X2-	T38.0X3-	T38.0X4-	T38.0X5-	T38.0X6-
Pregnandiol	T38.5X1-	T38.5X2-	T38.5X3-	T38.5X4-	T38.5X5-	T38.5X6-
Pregneninolone	T38.5X1-	T38.5X2-	T38.5X3-	T38.5X4-	T38.5X5-	T38.5X6-
Preludin	T43.691-	T43.692-	T43.693-	T43.694-	T43.695-	T43.696-
Premarin	T38.5X1-	T38.5X2-	T38.5X3-	T38.5X4-	T38.5X5-	T38.5X6-
Premedication anesthetic	T41.201-	T41.202-	T41.203-	T41.204-	T41.205-	T41.206-
Prenalterol	T44.5X1-	T44.5X2-	T44.5X3-	T44.5X4-	T44.5X5-	T44.5X6-
Prenoxdiazine	T48.3X1-	T48.3X2-	T48.3X3-	T48.3X4-	T48.3X5-	T48.3X6-
Prenylamine	T46.3X1-	T46.3X2-	T46.3X3-	T46.3X4-	T46.3X5-	T46.3X6-
Preparation H	T49.8X1-	T49.8X2-	T49.8X3-	T49.8X4-	T49.8X5-	T49.8X6-
Preparation, local	T49.4X1-	T49.4X2-	T49.4X3-	T49.4X4-	T49.4X5-	T49.4X6-
Preservative (nonmedicinal)	T65.891-	T65.892-	T65.893-	T65.894-	-	-
medicinal	T50.901-	T50.902-	T50.903-	T50.904-	T50.905-	T50.906-
wood	T60.91X-	T60.92X-	T60.93X-	T60.94X-	-	-
Prethcamide	T50.7X1-	T50.7X2-	T50.7X3-	T50.7X4-	T50.7X5-	T50.7X6-
Pride of China	T62.2X1-	T62.2X2-	T62.2X3-	T62.2X4-	-	-
Pridinol	T44.3X1-	T44.3X2-	T44.3X3-	T44.3X4-	T44.3X5-	T44.3X6-
Prifinium bromide	T44.3X1-	T44.3X2-	T44.3X3-	T44.3X4-	T44.3X5-	T44.3X6-
Prilocaine	T41.3X1-	T41.3X2-	T41.3X3-	T41.3X4-	T41.3X5-	T41.3X6-
infiltration (subcutaneous)	T41.3X1-	T41.3X2-	T41.3X3-	T41.3X4-	T41.3X5-	T41.3X6-
nerve block (peripheral) (plexus)	T41.3X1-	T41.3X2-	T41.3X3-	T41.3X4-	T41.3X5-	T41.3X6-
regional	T41.3X1-	T41.3X2-	T41.3X3-	T41.3X4-	T41.3X5-	T41.3X6-
Primaquine	T37.2X1-	T37.2X2-	T37.2X3-	T37.2X4-	T37.2X5-	T37.2X6-
Primidone	T42.6X1-	T42.6X2-	T42.6X3-	T42.6X4-	T42.6X5-	T42.6X6-
Primula (veris)	T62.2X1-	T62.2X2-	T62.2X3-	T62.2X4-	-	-
Prinadol	T40.2X1-	T40.2X2-	T40.2X3-	T40.2X4-	T40.2X5-	T40.2X6-
Priscol, Priscoline	T44.6X1-	T44.6X2-	T44.6X3-	T44.6X4-	T44.6X5-	T44.6X6-
Pristinamycin	T36.3X1-	T36.3X2-	T36.3X3-	T36.3X4-	T36.3X5-	T36.3X6-
Privet	T62.2X1-	T62.2X2-	T62.2X3-	T62.2X4-	-	-
berries	T62.1X1-	T62.1X2-	T62.1X3-	T62.1X4-	-	-
Privine	T44.4X1-	T44.4X2-	T44.4X3-	T44.4X4-	T44.4X5-	T44.4X6-
Pro-Banthine	T44.3X1-	T44.3X2-	T44.3X3-	T44.3X4-	T44.3X5-	T44.3X6-
Probarbital	T42.3X1-	T42.3X2-	T42.3X3-	T42.3X4-	T42.3X5-	T42.3X6-
Probenecid	T50.4X1-	T50.4X2-	T50.4X3-	T50.4X4-	T50.4X5-	T50.4X6-
Probucol	T46.6X1-	T46.6X2-	T46.6X3-	T46.6X4-	T46.6X5-	T46.6X6-
Procainamide	T46.2X1-	T46.2X2-	T46.2X3-	T46.2X4-	T46.2X5-	T46.2X6-
Procaine	T41.3X1-	T41.3X2-	T41.3X3-	T41.3X4-	T41.3X5-	T41.3X6-
benzylpenicillin	T36.0X1-	T36.0X2-	T36.0X3-	T36.0X4-	T36.0X5-	T36.0X6-
nerve block (periphreal) (plexus)	T41.3X1-	T41.3X2-	T41.3X3-	T41.3X4-	T41.3X5-	T41.3X6-
penicillin G	T36.0X1-	T36.0X2-	T36.0X3-	T36.0X4-	T36.0X5-	T36.0X6-
regional	T41.3X1-	T41.3X2-	T41.3X3-	T41.3X4-	T41.3X5-	T41.3X6-
spinal	T41.3X1-	T41.3X2-	T41.3X3-	T41.3X4-	T41.3X5-	T41.3X6-
Procalmidol	T43.591-	T43.592-	T43.593-	T43.594-	T43.595-	T43.596-
Procarbazine	T45.1X1-	T45.1X2-	T45.1X3-	T45.1X4-	T45.1X5-	T45.1X6-
Procaterol	T44.5X1-	T44.5X2-	T44.5X3-	T44.5X4-	T44.5X5-	T44.5X6-
Prochlorperazine	T43.3X1-	T43.3X2-	T43.3X3-	T43.3X4-	T43.3X5-	T43.3X6-
Procyclidine	T44.3X1-	T44.3X2-	T44.3X3-	T44.3X4-	T44.3X5-	T44.3X6-
Producer gas	T58.8X1-	T58.8X2-	T58.8X3-	T58.8X4-	-	-
Profadol	T40.4X1-	T40.4X2-	T40.4X3-	T40.4X4-	T40.4X5-	T40.4X6-
Profenamine	T44.3X1-	T44.3X2-	T44.3X3-	T44.3X4-	T44.3X5-	T44.3X6-
Profenil	T44.3X1-	T44.3X2-	T44.3X3-	T44.3X4-	T44.3X5-	T44.3X6-
Proflavine	T49.0X1-	T49.0X2-	T49.0X3-	T49.0X4-	T49.0X5-	T49.0X6-
Progabide	T42.6X1-	T42.6X2-	T42.6X3-	T42.6X4-	T42.6X5-	T42.6X6-
Progesterone	T38.5X1-	T38.5X2-	T38.5X3-	T38.5X4-	T38.5X5-	T38.5X6-

Substance	Poisoning Accidental (unintentional)	Poisoning Intentional self-harm	Poisoning Assault	Poisoning Undetermined	Adverse effect	Underdosing
Progestin	T38.5X1-	T38.5X2-	T38.5X3-	T38.5X4-	T38.5X5-	T38.5X6-
oral contraceptive	T38.4X1-	T38.4X2-	T38.4X3-	T38.4X4-	T38.4X5-	T38.4X6-
Progestogen NEC	T38.5X1-	T38.5X2-	T38.5X3-	T38.5X4-	T38.5X5-	T38.5X6-
Progestone	T38.5X1-	T38.5X2-	T38.5X3-	T38.5X4-	T38.5X5-	T38.5X6-
Proglumide	T47.1X1-	T47.1X2-	T47.1X3-	T47.1X4-	T47.1X5-	T47.1X6-
Proguanil	T37.2X1-	T37.2X2-	T37.2X3-	T37.2X4-	T37.2X5-	T37.2X6-
Prolactin	T38.811-	T38.812-	T38.813-	T38.814-	T38.815-	T38.816-
Prolintane	T43.691-	T43.692-	T43.693-	T43.694-	T43.695-	T43.696-
Proloid	T38.1X1-	T38.1X2-	T38.1X3-	T38.1X4-	T38.1X5-	T38.1X6-
Proluton	T38.5X1-	T38.5X2-	T38.5X3-	T38.5X4-	T38.5X5-	T38.5X6-
Promacetin	T37.1X1-	T37.1X2-	T37.1X3-	T37.1X4-	T37.1X5-	T37.1X6-
Promazine	T43.3X1-	T43.3X2-	T43.3X3-	T43.3X4-	T43.3X5-	T43.3X6-
Promedol	T40.2X1-	T40.2X2-	T40.2X3-	T40.2X4-	-	-
Promegestone	T38.5X1-	T38.5X2-	T38.5X3-	T38.5X4-	T38.5X5-	T38.5X6-
Promethazine (teoclate)	T43.3X1-	T43.3X2-	T43.3X3-	T43.3X4-	T43.3X5-	T43.3X6-
Promin	T37.1X1-	T37.1X2-	T37.1X3-	T37.1X4-	T37.1X5-	T37.1X6-
Pronase	T45.3X1-	T45.3X2-	T45.3X3-	T45.3X4-	T45.3X5-	T45.3X6-
Pronestyl (hydrochloride)	T46.2X1-	T46.2X2-	T46.2X3-	T46.2X4-	T46.2X5-	T46.2X6-
Pronetalol	T44.7X1-	T44.7X2-	T44.7X3-	T44.7X4-	T44.7X5-	T44.7X6-
Prontosil	T37.0X1-	T37.0X2-	T37.0X3-	T37.0X4-	T37.0X5-	T37.0X6-
Propachlor	T60.3X1-	T60.3X2-	T60.3X3-	T60.3X4-	-	-
Propafenone	T46.2X1-	T46.2X2-	T46.2X3-	T46.2X4-	T46.2X5-	T46.2X6-
Propallylonal	T42.3X1-	T42.3X2-	T42.3X3-	T42.3X4-	T42.3X5-	T42.3X6-
Propamidine	T49.0X1-	T49.0X2-	T49.0X3-	T49.0X4-	T49.0X5-	T49.0X6-
Propane (distributed in mobile container)	T59.891-	T59.892-	T59.893-	T59.894-	-	-
distributed through pipes	T59.891-	T59.892-	T59.893-	T59.894-	-	-
incomplete combustion	T58.11X-	T58.12X-	T58.13X-	T58.14X-	-	-
Propanidid	T41.291-	T41.292-	T41.293-	T41.294-	T41.295-	T41.296-
Propanil	T60.3X1-	T60.3X2-	T60.3X3-	T60.3X4-	-	-
1-Propanol	T51.3X1-	T51.3X2-	T51.3X3-	T51.3X4-	-	-
2-Propanol	T51.2X1-	T51.2X2-	T51.2X3-	T51.2X4-	-	-
Propantheline	T44.3X1-	T44.3X2-	T44.3X3-	T44.3X4-	T44.3X5-	T44.3X6-
bromide	T44.3X1-	T44.3X2-	T44.3X3-	T44.3X4-	T44.3X5-	T44.3X6-
Proparacaine	T41.3X1-	T41.3X2-	T41.3X3-	T41.3X4-	T41.3X5-	T41.3X6-
Propatylnitrate	T46.3X1-	T46.3X2-	T46.3X3-	T46.3X4-	T46.3X5-	T46.3X6-
Propicillin	T36.0X1-	T36.0X2-	T36.0X3-	T36.0X4-	T36.0X5-	T36.0X6-
Propiolactone	T49.0X1-	T49.0X2-	T49.0X3-	T49.0X4-	T49.0X5-	T49.0X6-
Propiomazine	T45.0X1-	T45.0X2-	T45.0X3-	T45.0X4-	T45.0X5-	T45.0X6-
Propionaldehyde (medicinal)	T42.6X1-	T42.6X2-	T42.6X3-	T42.6X4-	T42.6X5-	T42.6X6-
Propionate (calcium) (sodium)	T49.0X1-	T49.0X2-	T49.0X3-	T49.0X4-	T49.0X5-	T49.0X6-
Propion gel	T49.0X1-	T49.0X2-	T49.0X3-	T49.0X4-	T49.0X5-	T49.0X6-
Propitocaine	T41.3X1-	T41.3X2-	T41.3X3-	T41.3X4-	T41.3X5-	T41.3X6-
infiltration (subcutaneous)	T41.3X1-	T41.3X2-	T41.3X3-	T41.3X4-	T41.3X5-	T41.3X6-
nerve block (peripheral) (plexus)	T41.3X1-	T41.3X2-	T41.3X3-	T41.3X4-	T41.3X5-	T41.3X6-
Propofol	T41.291-	T41.292-	T41.293-	T41.294-	T41.295-	T41.296-
Propoxur	T60.0X1-	T60.0X2-	T60.0X3-	T60.0X4-	-	-
Propoxycaine	T41.3X1-	T41.3X2-	T41.3X3-	T41.3X4-	T41.3X5-	T41.3X6-
infiltration (subcutaneous)	T41.3X1-	T41.3X2-	T41.3X3-	T41.3X4-	T41.3X5-	T41.3X6-
nerve block (peripheral) (plexus)	T41.3X1-	T41.3X2-	T41.3X3-	T41.3X4-	T41.3X5-	T41.3X6-
topical (surface)	T41.3X1-	T41.3X2-	T41.3X3-	T41.3X4-	T41.3X5-	T41.3X6-
Propoxyphene	T40.4X1-	T40.4X2-	T40.4X3-	T40.4X4-	T40.4X5-	T40.4X6-
Propranolol	T44.7X1-	T44.7X2-	T44.7X3-	T44.7X4-	T44.7X5-	T44.7X6-
Propyl						
alcohol	T51.3X1-	T51.3X2-	T51.3X3-	T51.3X4-	-	-
carbinol	T51.3X1-	T51.3X2-	T51.3X3-	T51.3X4-	-	-
hexadrine	T44.4X1-	T44.4X2-	T44.4X3-	T44.4X4-	T44.4X5-	T44.4X6-
iodone	T50.8X1-	T50.8X2-	T50.8X3-	T50.8X4-	T50.8X5-	T50.8X6-

PROPYL - PSP

Substance	Poisoning Accidental (unintentional)	Poisoning Intentional self-harm	Poisoning Assault	Poisoning Undetermined	Adverse effect	Underdosing
Propyl (continued)						
thiouracil	T38.2X1-	T38.2X2-	T38.2X3-	T38.2X4-	T38.2X5-	T38.2X6-
Propylaminopheno-thiazine	T43.3X1-	T43.3X2-	T43.3X3-	T43.3X4-	T43.3X5-	T43.3X6-
Propylene	T59.891-	T59.892-	T59.893-	T59.894-	-	-
Propylhexedrine	T48.5X1-	T48.5X2-	T48.5X3-	T48.5X4-	T48.5X5-	T48.5X6-
Propyliodone	T50.8X1-	T50.8X2-	T50.8X3-	T50.8X4-	T50.8X5-	T50.8X6-
Propylparaben (ophthalmic)	T49.5X1-	T49.5X2-	T49.5X3-	T49.5X4-	T49.5X5-	T49.5X6-
Propylthiouracil	T38.2X1-	T38.2X2-	T38.2X3-	T38.2X4-	T38.2X5-	T38.2X6-
Propyphenazone	T39.2X1-	T39.2X2-	T39.2X3-	T39.2X4-	T39.2X5-	T39.2X6-
Proquazone	T39.391-	T39.392-	T39.393-	T39.394-	T39.395-	T39.396-
Proscillaridin	T46.0X1-	T46.0X2-	T46.0X3-	T46.0X4-	T46.0X5-	T46.0X6-
Prostacyclin	T45.521-	T45.522-	T45.523-	T45.524-	T45.525-	T45.526-
Prostaglandin (I2)	T45.521-	T45.522-	T45.523-	T45.524-	T45.525-	T45.526-
E1	T46.7X1-	T46.7X2-	T46.7X3-	T46.7X4-	T46.7X5-	T46.7X6-
E2	T48.0X1-	T48.0X2-	T48.0X3-	T48.0X4-	T48.0X5-	T48.0X6-
F2 alpha	T48.0X1-	T48.0X2-	T48.0X3-	T48.0X4-	T48.0X5-	T48.0X6-
Prostigmin	T44.0X1-	T44.0X2-	T44.0X3-	T44.0X4-	T44.0X5-	T44.0X6-
Prosultiamine	T45.2X1-	T45.2X2-	T45.2X3-	T45.2X4-	T45.2X5-	T45.2X6-
Protamine sulfate	T45.7X1-	T45.7X2-	T45.7X3-	T45.7X4-	T45.7X5-	T45.7X6-
zinc insulin	T38.3X1-	T38.3X2-	T38.3X3-	T38.3X4-	T38.3X5-	T38.3X6-
Protease	T47.5X1-	T47.5X2-	T47.5X3-	T47.5X4-	T47.5X5-	T47.5X6-
Protectant, skin NEC	T49.3X1-	T49.3X2-	T49.3X3-	T49.3X4-	T49.3X5-	T49.3X6-
Protein hydrolysate	T50.991-	T50.992-	T50.993-	T50.994-	T50.995-	T50.996-
Prothiaden — *see Dothiepin hydrochloride*						
Prothionamide	T37.1X1-	T37.1X2-	T37.1X3-	T37.1X4-	T37.1X5-	T37.1X6-
Prothipendyl	T43.591-	T43.592-	T43.593-	T43.594-	T43.595-	T43.596-
Prothoate	T60.0X1-	T60.0X2-	T60.0X3-	T60.0X4-	-	-
Prothrombin						
activator	T45.7X1-	T45.7X2-	T45.7X3-	T45.7X4-	T45.7X5-	T45.7X6-
synthesis inhibitor	T45.511-	T45.512-	T45.513-	T45.514-	T45.515-	T45.516-
Protionamide	T37.1X1-	T37.1X2-	T37.1X3-	T37.1X4-	T37.1X5-	T37.1X6-
Protirelin	T38.891-	T38.892-	T38.893-	T38.894-	T38.895-	T38.896-
Protokylol	T48.6X1-	T48.6X2-	T48.6X3-	T48.6X4-	T48.6X5-	T48.6X6-
Protopam	T50.6X1-	T50.6X2-	T50.6X3-	T50.6X4-	T50.6X5-	T50.6X6-
Protoveratrine (s) (A) (B)	T46.5X1-	T46.5X2-	T46.5X3-	T46.5X4-	T46.5X5-	T46.5X6-
Protriptyline	T43.011-	T43.012-	T43.013-	T43.014-	T43.015-	T43.016-
Provera	T38.5X1-	T38.5X2-	T38.5X3-	T38.5X4-	T38.5X5-	T38.5X6-
Provitamin A	T45.2X1-	T45.2X2-	T45.2X3-	T45.2X4-	T45.2X5-	T45.2X6-
Proxibarbal	T42.3X1-	T42.3X2-	T42.3X3-	T42.3X4-	T42.3X5-	T42.3X6-
Proxymetacaine	T41.3X1-	T41.3X2-	T41.3X3-	T41.3X4-	T41.3X5-	T41.3X6-
Proxyphylline	T48.6X1-	T48.6X2-	T48.6X3-	T48.6X4-	T48.6X5-	T48.6X6-
Prozac — *see Fluoxetine hydrochloride*						
Prunus						
laurocerasus	T62.2X1-	T62.2X2-	T62.2X3-	T62.2X4-	-	-
virginiana	T62.2X1-	T62.2X2-	T62.2X3-	T62.2X4-	-	-
Prussian blue						
commercial	T65.891-	T65.892-	T65.893-	T65.894-	-	-
therapeutic	T50.6X1-	T50.6X2-	T50.6X3-	T50.6X4-	T50.6X5-	T50.6X6-
Prussic acid	T65.0X1-	T65.0X2-	T65.0X3-	T65.0X4-	-	-
vapor	T57.3X1-	T57.3X2-	T57.3X3-	T57.3X4-	-	-
Pseudoephedrine	T44.991-	T44.992-	T44.993-	T44.994-	T44.995-	T44.996-
Psilocin	T40.991-	T40.992-	T40.993-	T40.994-	-	-
Psilocybin	T40.991-	T40.992-	T40.993-	T40.994-	-	-
Psilocybine	T40.991-	T40.992-	T40.993-	T40.994-	-	-
Psoralene (nonmedicinal)	T65.891-	T65.892-	T65.893-	T65.894-	-	-
Psoralens (medicinal)	T50.991-	T50.992-	T50.993-	T50.994-	T50.995-	T50.996-
PSP (phenolsulfonphthalein)	T50.8X1-	T50.8X2-	T50.8X3-	T50.8X4-	T50.8X5-	T50.8X6-

Substance	Poisoning Accidental (unintentional)	Poisoning Intentional self-harm	Poisoning Assault	Poisoning Undetermined	Adverse effect	Underdosing
Psychodysleptic drug NOS	T40.901-	T40.902-	T40.903-	T40.904-	T40.905-	T40.906-
specified NEC	T40.991-	T40.992-	T40.993-	T40.994-	T40.995-	T40.996-
Psychostimulant	T43.601-	T43.602-	T43.603-	T43.604-	T43.605-	T43.606-
amphetamine	T43.621-	T43.622-	T43.623-	T43.624-	T43.625-	T43.626-
caffeine	T43.611-	T43.612-	T43.613-	T43.614-	T43.615-	T43.616-
methylphenidate	T43.631-	T43.632-	T43.633-	T43.634-	T43.635-	T43.636-
specified NEC	T43.691-	T43.692-	T43.693-	T43.694-	T43.695-	T43.696-
Psychotherapeutic drug NEC	T43.91X-	T43.92X-	T43.93X-	T43.94X-	T43.95X-	T43.96X-
antidepressants — *see also Antidepressant*	T43.201-	T43.202-	T43.203-	T43.204-	T43.205-	T43.206-
specified NEC	T43.8X1-	T43.8X2-	T43.8X3-	T43.8X4-	T43.8X5-	T43.8X6-
tranquilizers NEC	T43.501-	T43.502-	T43.503-	T43.504-	T43.505-	T43.506-
Psychotomimetic agents	T40.901-	T40.902-	T40.903-	T40.904-	T40.905-	T40.906-
Psychotropic drug NEC	T43.91X-	T43.92X-	T43.93X-	T43.94X-	T43.95X-	T43.96X-
specified NEC	T43.8X1-	T43.8X2-	T43.8X3-	T43.8X4-	T43.8X5-	T43.8X6-
Psyllium hydrophilic mucilloid	T47.4X1-	T47.4X2-	T47.4X3-	T47.4X4-	T47.4X5-	T47.4X6-
Pteroylglutamic acid	T45.8X1-	T45.8X2-	T45.8X3-	T45.8X4-	T45.8X5-	T45.8X6-
Pteroyltriglutamate	T45.1X1-	T45.1X2-	T45.1X3-	T45.1X4-	T45.1X5-	T45.1X6-
PTFE — *see Polytetrafluoroethylene*						
Pulp						
devitalizing paste	T49.7X1-	T49.7X2-	T49.7X3-	T49.7X4-	T49.7X5-	T49.7X6-
dressing	T49.7X1-	T49.7X2-	T49.7X3-	T49.7X4-	T49.7X5-	T49.7X6-
Pulsatilla	T62.2X1-	T62.2X2-	T62.2X3-	T62.2X4-	-	-
Pumpkin seed extract	T37.4X1-	T37.4X2-	T37.4X3-	T37.4X4-	T37.4X5-	T37.4X6-
Purex (bleach)	T54.91X-	T54.92X-	T54.93X-	T54.94X-	-	-
Purgative NEC — *see also Cathartic*	T47.4X1-	T47.4X2-	T47.4X3-	T47.4X4-	T47.4X5-	T47.4X6-
Purine analogue (antineoplastic)	T45.1X1-	T45.1X2-	T45.1X3-	T45.1X4-	T45.1X5-	T45.1X6-
Purine diuretics	T50.2X1-	T50.2X2-	T50.2X3-	T50.2X4-	T50.2X5-	T50.2X6-
Purinethol	T45.1X1-	T45.1X2-	T45.1X3-	T45.1X4-	T45.1X5-	T45.1X6-
PVP	T45.8X1	T45.8X2-	T45.8X3-	T45.8X4-	T45.8X5-	T45.8X6-
Pyrabital	T39.8X1-	T39.8X2-	T39.8X3-	T39.8X4-	T39.8X5-	T39.8X6-
Pyramidon	T39.2X1-	T39.2X2-	T39.2X3-	T39.2X4-	T39.2X5-	T39.2X6-
Pyrantel	T37.4X1-	T37.4X2-	T37.4X3-	T37.4X4-	T37.4X5-	T37.4X6-
Pyrathiazine	T45.0X1-	T45.0X2-	T45.0X3-	T45.0X4-	T45.0X5-	T45.0X6-
Pyrazinamide	T37.1X1-	T37.1X2-	T37.1X3-	T37.1X4-	T37.1X5-	T37.1X6-
Pyrazinoic acid (amide)	T37.1X1-	T37.1X2-	T37.1X3-	T37.1X4-	T37.1X5-	T37.1X6-
Pyrazole (derivatives)	T39.2X1-	T39.2X2-	T39.2X3-	T39.2X4-	T39.2X5-	T39.2X6-
Pyrazolone analgesic NEC	T39.2X1-	T39.2X2-	T39.2X3-	T39.2X4-	T39.2X5-	T39.2X6-
Pyrethrin, pyrethrum (nonmedicinal)	T60.2X1-	T60.2X2-	T60.2X3-	T60.2X4-	-	-
Pyrethrum extract	T49.0X1-	T49.0X2-	T49.0X3-	T49.0X4-	T49.0X5-	T49.0X6-
Pyribenzamine	T45.0X1-	T45.0X2-	T45.0X3-	T45.0X4-	T45.0X5-	T45.0X6-
Pyridine	T52.8X1-	T52.8X2-	T52.8X3-	T52.8X4-	-	-
aldoxime methiodide	T50.6X1-	T50.6X2-	T50.6X3-	T50.6X4-	T50.6X5-	T50.6X6-
aldoxime methyl chloride	T50.6X1-	T50.6X2-	T50.6X3-	T50.6X4-	T50.6X5-	T50.6X6-
vapor	T59.891-	T59.892-	T59.893-	T59.894-	-	-
Pyridium	T39.8X1-	T39.8X2-	T39.8X3-	T39.8X4-	T39.8X5-	T39.8X6-
Pyridostigmine bromide	T44.0X1-	T44.0X2-	T44.0X3-	T44.0X4-	T44.0X5-	T44.0X6-
Pyridoxal phosphate	T45.2X1-	T45.2X2-	T45.2X3-	T45.2X4-	T45.2X5-	T45.2X6-
Pyridoxine	T45.2X1-	T45.2X2-	T45.2X3-	T45.2X4-	T45.2X5-	T45.2X6-
Pyrilamine	T45.0X1-	T45.0X2-	T45.0X3-	T45.0X4-	T45.0X5-	T45.0X6-
Pyrimethamine	T37.2X1-	T37.2X2-	T37.2X3-	T37.2X4-	T37.2X5-	T37.2X6-
with sulfadoxine	T37.2X1-	T37.2X2-	T37.2X3-	T37.2X4-	T37.2X5-	T37.2X6-
Pyrimidine antagonist	T45.1X1-	T45.1X2-	T45.1X3-	T45.1X4-	T45.1X5-	T45.1X6-
Pyriminil	T60.4X1-	T60.4X2-	T60.4X3-	T60.4X4-	-	-
Pyrithione zinc	T49.4X1-	T49.4X2-	T49.4X3-	T49.4X4-	T49.4X5-	T49.4X6-
Pyrithyldione	T42.6X1-	T42.6X2-	T42.6X3-	T42.6X4-	T42.6X5-	T42.6X6-
Pyrogallic acid	T49.0X1-	T49.0X2-	T49.0X3-	T49.0X4-	T49.0X5-	T49.0X6-
Pyrogallol	T49.0X1-	T49.0X2-	T49.0X3-	T49.0X4-	T49.0X5-	T49.0X6-

Substance	Poisoning Accidental (unintentional)	Poisoning Intentional self-harm	Poisoning Assault	Poisoning Undetermined	Adverse effect	Underdosing
Pyroxylin	T49.3X1-	T49.3X2-	T49.3X3-	T49.3X4-	T49.3X5-	T49.3X6-
Pyrrobutamine	T45.0X1-	T45.0X2-	T45.0X3-	T45.0X4-	T45.0X5-	T45.0X6-
Pyrrolizidine alkaloids	T62.8X1-	T62.8X2-	T62.8X3-	T62.8X4-	-	-
Pyrvinium chloride	T37.4X1-	T37.4X2-	T37.4X3-	T37.4X4-	T37.4X5-	T37.4X6-
PZI	T38.3X1-	T38.3X2-	T38.3X3-	T38.3X4-	T38.3X5-	T38.3X6-
Quaalude	T42.6X1-	T42.6X2-	T42.6X3-	T42.6X4-	T42.6X5-	T42.6X6-
Quarternary ammonium						
anti-infective	T49.0X1-	T49.0X2-	T49.0X3-	T49.0X4-	T49.0X5-	T49.0X6-
ganglion blocking	T44.2X1-	T44.2X2-	T44.2X3-	T44.2X4-	T44.2X5-	T44.2X6-
parasympatholytic	T44.3X1-	T44.3X2-	T44.3X3-	T44.3X4-	T44.3X5-	T44.3X6-
Quazepam	T42.4X1-	T42.4X2-	T42.4X3-	T42.4X4-	T42.4X5-	T42.4X6-
Quicklime	T54.3X1-	T54.3X2-	T54.3X3-	T54.3X4-	-	-
Quillaja extract	T48.4X1-	T48.4X2-	T48.4X3-	T48.4X4-	T48.4X5-	T48.4X6-
Quinacrine	T37.2X1-	T37.2X2-	T37.2X3-	T37.2X4-	T37.2X5-	T37.2X6-
Quinaglute	T46.2X1-	T46.2X2-	T46.2X3-	T46.2X4-	T46.2X5-	T46.2X6-
Quinalbarbital	T42.3X1-	T42.3X2-	T42.3X3-	T42.3X4-	T42.3X5-	T42.3X6-
Quinalbarbitone sodium	T42.3X1-	T42.3X2-	T42.3X3-	T42.3X4-	T42.3X5-	T42.3X6-
Quinalphos	T60.0X1-	T60.0X2-	T60.0X3-	T60.0X4-	-	-
Quinapril	T46.4X1-	T46.4X2-	T46.4X3-	T46.4X4-	T46.4X5-	T46.4X6-
Quinestradiol	T38.5X1-	T38.5X2-	T38.5X3-	T38.5X4-	T38.5X5-	T38.5X6-
Quinestradol	T38.5X1-	T38.5X2-	T38.5X3-	T38.5X4-	T38.5X5-	T38.5X6-
Quinestrol	T38.5X1-	T38.5X2-	T38.5X3-	T38.5X4-	T38.5X5-	T38.5X6-
Quinethazone	T50.2X1-	T50.2X2-	T50.2X3-	T50.2X4-	T50.2X5-	T50.2X6-
Quingestanol	T38.4X1-	T38.4X2-	T38.4X3-	T38.4X4-	T38.4X5-	T38.4X6-
Quinidine	T46.2X1-	T46.2X2-	T46.2X3-	T46.2X4-	T46.2X5-	T46.2X6-
Quinine	T37.2X1-	T37.2X2-	T37.2X3-	T37.2X4-	T37.2X5-	T37.2X6-
Quiniobine	T37.8X1-	T37.8X2-	T37.8X3-	T37.8X4-	T37.8X5-	T37.8X6-
Quinisocaine	T49.1X1-	T49.1X2-	T49.1X3-	T49.1X4-	T49.1X5-	T49.1X6-
Quinocide	T37.2X1-	T37.2X2-	T37.2X3-	T37.2X4-	T37.2X5-	T37.2X6-
Quinoline (derivatives) NEC	T37.8X1-	T37.8X2-	T37.8X3-	T37.8X4-	T37.8X5-	T37.8X6-
Quinupramine	T43.011-	T43.012-	T43.013-	T43.014-	T43.015-	T43.016-
Quotane	T41.3X1-	T41.3X2-	T41.3X3-	T41.3X4-	T41.3X5-	T41.3X6-
Rabies						
immune globulin (human)	T50.Z11-	T50.Z12-	T50.Z13-	T50.Z14-	T50.Z15-	T50.Z16-
vaccine	T50.B91-	T50.B92-	T50.B93-	T50.B94-	T50.B95-	T50.B96-
Racemoramide	T40.2X1-	T40.2X2-	T40.2X3-	T40.2X4-	-	-
Racemorphan	T40.2X1-	T40.2X2-	T40.2X3-	T40.2X4-	T40.2X5-	T40.2X6-
Racepinefrin	T44.5X1-	T44.5X2-	T44.5X3-	T44.5X4-	T44.5X5-	T44.5X6-
Raclopride	T43.591-	T43.592-	T43.593-	T43.594-	T43.595-	T43.596-
Radiator alcohol	T51.1X1-	T51.1X2-	T51.1X3-	T51.1X4-	-	-
Radioactive drug NEC	T50.8X1-	T50.8X2-	T50.8X3-	T50.8X4-	T50.8X5-	T50.8X6-
Radio-opaque (drugs) (materials)	T50.8X1-	T50.8X2-	T50.8X3-	T50.8X4-	T50.8X5-	T50.8X6-
Ramifenazone	T39.2X1-	T39.2X2-	T39.2X3-	T39.2X4-	T39.2X5-	T39.2X6-
Ramipril	T46.4X1-	T46.4X2-	T46.4X3-	T46.4X4-	T46.4X5-	T46.4X6-
Ranitidine	T47.0X1-	T47.0X2-	T47.0X3-	T47.0X4-	T47.0X5-	T47.0X6-
Ranunculus	T62.2X1-	T62.2X2-	T62.2X3-	T62.2X4-	-	-
Rat poison NEC	T60.4X1-	T60.4X2-	T60.4X3-	T60.4X4-	-	-
Rattlesnake (venom)	T63.011-	T63.012-	T63.013-	T63.014-	-	-
Raubasine	T46.7X1-	T46.7X2-	T46.7X3-	T46.7X4-	T46.7X5-	T46.7X6-
Raudixin	T46.5X1-	T46.5X2-	T46.5X3-	T46.5X4-	T46.5X5-	T46.5X6-
Rautensin	T46.5X1-	T46.5X2-	T46.5X3-	T46.5X4-	T46.5X5-	T46.5X6-
Rautina	T46.5X1-	T46.5X2-	T46.5X3-	T46.5X4-	T46.5X5-	T46.5X6-
Rautotal	T46.5X1-	T46.5X2-	T46.5X3-	T46.5X4-	T46.5X5-	T46.5X6-
Rauwiloid	T46.5X1-	T46.5X2-	T46.5X3-	T46.5X4-	T46.5X5-	T46.5X6-
Rauwoldin	T46.5X1-	T46.5X2-	T46.5X3-	T46.5X4-	T46.5X5-	T46.5X6-
Rauwolfia (alkaloids)	T46.5X1-	T46.5X2-	T46.5X3-	T46.5X4-	T46.5X5-	T46.5X6-
Razoxane	T45.1X1-	T45.1X2-	T45.1X3-	T45.1X4-	T45.1X5-	T45.1X6-
Realgar	T57.0X1-	T57.0X2-	T57.0X3-	T57.0X4-	-	-
Recombinant (R) — *see specific protein*						

Substance	Poisoning Accidental (unintentional)	Poisoning Intentional self-harm	Poisoning Assault	Poisoning Undetermined	Adverse effect	Underdosing
Red blood cells, packed	T45.8X1-	T45.8X2-	T45.8X3-	T45.8X4-	T45.8X5-	T45.8X6-
Red squill (scilliroside)	T60.4X1-	T60.4X2-	T60.4X3-	T60.4X4-	-	-
Reducing agent, industrial NEC	T65.891-	T65.892-	T65.893-	T65.894-	-	-
Refrigerant gas (chlorofluoro-carbon)	T53.5X1-	T53.5X2-	T53.5X3-	T53.5X4-	-	-
not chlorofluoro-carbon	T59.891-	T59.892-	T59.893-	T59.894-	-	-
Regroton	T50.2X1-	T50.2X2-	T50.2X3-	T50.2X4-	T50.2X5-	T50.2X6-
Rehydration salts (oral)	T50.3X1-	T50.3X2-	T50.3X3-	T50.3X4-	T50.3X5-	T50.3X6-
Rela	T42.8X1-	T42.8X2-	T42.8X3-	T42.8X4-	T42.8X5-	T42.8X6-
Relaxant, muscle						
anesthetic	T48.1X1-	T48.1X2-	T48.1X3-	T48.1X4-	T48.1X5-	T48.1X6-
central nervous system	T42.8X1-	T42.8X2-	T42.8X3-	T42.8X4-	T42.8X5-	T42.8X6-
skeletal NEC	T48.1X1-	T48.1X2-	T48.1X3-	T48.1X4-	T48.1X5-	T48.1X6-
smooth NEC	T44.3X1-	T44.3X2-	T44.3X3-	T44.3X4-	T44.3X5-	T44.3X6-
Remoxipride	T43.591-	T43.592-	T43.593-	T43.594-	T43.595-	T43.596-
Renese	T50.2X1-	T50.2X2-	T50.2X3-	T50.2X4-	T50.2X5-	T50.2X6-
Renografin	T50.8X1-	T50.8X2-	T50.8X3-	T50.8X4-	T50.8X5-	T50.8X6-
Replacement solution	T50.3X1-	T50.3X2-	T50.3X3-	T50.3X4-	T50.3X5-	T50.3X6-
Reproterol	T48.6X1-	T48.6X2-	T48.6X3-	T48.6X4-	T48.6X5-	T48.6X6-
Rescinnamine	T46.5X1-	T46.5X2-	T46.5X3-	T46.5X4-	T46.5X5-	T46.5X6-
Reserpin (e)	T46.5X1-	T46.5X2-	T46.5X3-	T46.5X4-	T46.5X5-	T46.5X6-
Resorcin, resorcinol (nonmedicinal)	T65.891-	T65.892-	T65.893-	T65.894-	-	-
medicinal	T49.4X1-	T49.4X2-	T49.4X3-	T49.4X4-	T49.4X5-	T49.4X6-
Respaire	T48.4X1-	T48.4X2-	T48.4X3-	T48.4X4-	T48.4X5-	T48.4X6-
Respiratory drug NEC	T48.901-	T48.902-	T48.903-	T48.904-	T48.905-	T48.906-
antiasthmatic NEC	T48.6X1-	T48.6X2-	T48.6X3-	T48.6X4-	T48.6X5-	T48.6X6-
anti-common-cold NEC	T48.5X1-	T48.5X2-	T48.5X3-	T48.5X4-	T48.5X5-	T48.5X6-
expectorant NEC	T48.4X1-	T48.4X2-	T48.4X3-	T48.4X4-	T48.4X5-	T48.4X6-
stimulant	T48.901-	T48.902-	T48.903-	T48.904-	T48.905-	T48.906-
Retinoic acid	T49.0X1-	T49.0X2-	T49.0X3-	T49.0X4-	T49.0X5-	T49.0X6-
Retinol	T45.2X1-	T45.2X2-	T45.2X3-	T45.2X4-	T45.2X5-	T45.2X6-
Rh (D) immune globulin (human)	T50.Z11-	T50.Z12-	T50.Z13-	T50.Z14-	T50.Z15-	T50.Z16-
Rhodine	T39.011-	T39.012-	T39.013-	T39.014-	T39.015-	T39.016-
RhoGAM	T50.Z11-	T50.Z12-	T50.Z13-	T50.Z14-	T50.Z15-	T50.Z16-
Rhubarb						
dry extract	T47.2X1-	T47.2X2-	T47.2X3-	T47.2X4-	T47.2X5-	T47.2X6-
tincture, compound	T47.2X1-	T47.2X2-	T47.2X3-	T47.2X4-	T47.2X5-	T47.2X6-
Ribavirin	T37.5X1-	T37.5X2-	T37.5X3-	T37.5X4-	T37.5X5-	T37.5X6-
Riboflavin	T45.2X1-	T45.2X2-	T45.2X3-	T45.2X4-	T45.2X5-	T45.2X6-
Ribostamycin	T36.5X1-	T36.5X2-	T36.5X3-	T36.5X4-	T36.5X5-	T36.5X6-
Ricin	T62.2X1-	T62.2X2-	T62.2X3-	T62.2X4-	-	-
Ricinus communis	T62.2X1-	T62.2X2-	T62.2X3-	T62.2X4-	-	-
Rickettsial vaccine NEC	T50.A91-	T50.A92-	T50.A93-	T50.A94-	T50.A95-	T50.A96-
Rifabutin	T36.6X1-	T36.6X2-	T36.6X3-	T36.6X4-	T36.6X5-	T36.6X6-
Rifamide	T36.6X1-	T36.6X2-	T36.6X3-	T36.6X4-	T36.6X5-	T36.6X6-
Rifampicin	T36.6X1-	T36.6X2-	T36.6X3-	T36.6X4-	T36.6X5-	T36.6X6-
with isoniazid	T37.1X1-	T37.1X2-	T37.1X3-	T37.1X4-	T37.1X5-	T37.1X6-
Rifampin	T36.6X1-	T36.6X2-	T36.6X3-	T36.6X4-	T36.6X5-	T36.6X6-
Rifamycin	T36.6X1-	T36.6X2-	T36.6X3-	T36.6X4-	T36.6X5-	T36.6X6-
Rifaximin	T36.6X1-	T36.6X2-	T36.6X3-	T36.6X4-	T36.6X5-	T36.6X6-
Rimantadine	T37.5X1-	T37.5X2-	T37.5X3-	T37.5X4-	T37.5X5-	T37.5X6-
Rimazolium metilsulfate	T39.8X1-	T39.8X2-	T39.8X3-	T39.8X4-	T39.8X5-	T39.8X6-
Rimifon	T37.1X1-	T37.1X2-	T37.1X3-	T37.1X4-	T37.1X5-	T37.1X6-
Rimiterol	T48.6X1-	T48.6X2-	T48.6X3-	T48.6X4-	T48.6X5-	T48.6X6-
Ringer (lactate) solution	T50.3X1-	T50.3X2-	T50.3X3-	T50.3X4-	T50.3X5-	T50.3X6-
Ristocetin	T36.8X1-	T36.8X2-	T36.8X3-	T36.8X4-	T36.8X5-	T36.8X6-
Ritalin	T43.631-	T43.632-	T43.633-	T43.634-	T43.635-	T43.636-
Ritodrine	T44.5X1-	T44.5X2-	T44.5X3-	T44.5X4-	T44.5X5-	T44.5X6-
Roach killer — *see* Insecticide						

Substance	Poisoning Accidental (unintentional)	Poisoning Intentional self-harm	Poisoning Assault	Poisoning Undetermined	Adverse effect	Underdosing
Rociverine	T44.3X1-	T44.3X2-	T44.3X3-	T44.3X4-	T44.3X5-	T44.3X6-
Rocky Mountain spotted fever vaccine	T50.A91-	T50.A92-	T50.A93-	T50.A94-	T50.A95-	T50.A96-
Rodenticide NEC	T60.4X1-	T60.4X2-	T60.4X3-	T60.4X4-	-	-
Rohypnol	T42.4X1-	T42.4X2-	T42.4X3-	T42.4X4-	T42.4X5-	T42.4X6-
Rokitamycin	T36.3X1-	T36.3X2-	T36.3X3-	T36.3X4-	T36.3X5-	T36.3X6-
Rolaids	T47.1X1-	T47.1X2-	T47.1X3-	T47.1X4-	T47.1X5-	T47.1X6-
Rolitetracycline	T36.4X1-	T36.4X2-	T36.4X3-	T36.4X4-	T36.4X5-	T36.4X6-
Romilar	T48.3X1-	T48.3X2-	T48.3X3-	T48.3X4-	T48.3X5-	T48.3X6-
Ronifibrate	T46.6X1-	T46.6X2-	T46.6X3-	T46.6X4-	T46.6X5-	T46.6X6-
Rosaprostol	T47.1X1-	T47.1X2-	T47.1X3-	T47.1X4-	T47.1X5-	T47.1X6-
Rose bengal sodium (131I)	T50.8X1-	T50.8X2-	T50.8X3-	T50.8X4-	T50.8X5-	T50.8X6-
Rose water ointment	T49.3X1-	T49.3X2-	T49.3X3-	T49.3X4-	T49.3X5-	T49.3X6-
Rosoxacin	T37.8X1-	T37.8X2-	T37.8X3-	T37.8X4-	T37.8X5-	T37.8X6-
Rotenone	T60.2X1-	T60.2X2-	T60.2X3-	T60.2X4-	-	-
Rotoxamine	T45.0X1-	T45.0X2-	T45.0X3-	T45.0X4-	T45.0X5-	T45.0X6-
Rough-on-rats	T60.4X1-	T60.4X2-	T60.4X3-	T60.4X4-	-	-
Roxatidine	T47.0X1-	T47.0X2-	T47.0X3-	T47.0X4-	T47.0X5-	T47.0X6-
Roxithromycin	T36.3X1-	T36.3X2-	T36.3X3-	T36.3X4-	T36.3X5-	T36.3X6-
Rt-PA	T45.611-	T45.612-	T45.613-	T45.614-	T45.615-	T45.616-
Rubbing alcohol	T51.2X1-	T51.2X2-	T51.2X3-	T51.2X4-	-	-
Rubefacient	T49.4X1-	T49.4X2-	T49.4X3-	T49.4X4-	T49.4X5-	T49.4X6-
Rubella vaccine	T50.B91-	T50.B92-	T50.B93-	T50.B94-	T50.B95-	T50.B96-
Rubeola vaccine	T50.B91-	T50.B92-	T50.B93-	T50.B94-	T50.B95-	T50.B96-
Rubidium chloride Rb82	T50.8X1-	T50.8X2-	T50.8X3-	T50.8X4-	T50.8X5-	T50.8X6-
Rubidomycin	T45.1X1-	T45.1X2-	T45.1X3-	T45.1X4-	T45.1X5-	T45.1X6-
Rue	T62.2X1-	T62.2X2-	T62.2X3-	T62.2X4-	-	-
Rufocromomycin	T45.1X1-	T45.1X2-	T45.1X3-	T45.1X4-	T45.1X5-	T45.1X6-
Russel's viper venin	T45.7X1-	T45.7X2-	T45.7X3-	T45.7X4-	T45.7X5-	T45.7X6-
Ruta (graveolens)	T62.2X1-	T62.2X2-	T62.2X3-	T62.2X4-	-	-
Rutinum	T46.991-	T46.992-	T46.993-	T46.994-	T46.995-	T46.996-
Rutoside	T46.991-	T46.992-	T46.993-	T46.994-	T46.995-	T46.996-
Sabadilla (plant)	T62.2X1-	T62.2X2-	T62.2X3-	T62.2X4-	-	-
pesticide	T60.2X1-	T60.2X2-	T60.2X3-	T60.2X4-	-	-
Saccharated iron oxide	T45.8X1-	T45.8X2-	T45.8X3-	T45.8X4-	T45.8X5-	T45.8X6-
Saccharin	T50.901-	T50.902-	T50.903-	T50.904-	T50.905-	T50.906-
Saccharomyces boulardii	T47.6X1-	T47.6X2-	T47.6X3-	T47.6X4-	T47.6X5-	T47.6X6-
Safflower oil	T46.6X1-	T46.6X2-	T46.6X3-	T46.6X4-	T46.6X5-	T46.6X6-
Safrazine	T43.1X1-	T43.1X2-	T43.1X3-	T43.1X4-	T43.1X5-	T43.1X6-
Salazosulfapyridine	T37.0X1-	T37.0X2-	T37.0X3-	T37.0X4-	T37.0X5-	T37.0X6-
Salbutamol	T48.6X1-	T48.6X2-	T48.6X3-	T48.6X4-	T48.6X5-	T48.6X6-
Salicylamide	T39.091-	T39.092-	T39.093-	T39.094-	T39.095-	T39.096-
Salicylate NEC	T39.091-	T39.092-	T39.093-	T39.094-	T39.095-	T39.096-
methyl	T49.3X1-	T49.3X2-	T49.3X3-	T49.3X4-	T49.3X5-	T49.3X6-
theobromine calcium	T50.2X1-	T50.2X2-	T50.2X3-	T50.2X4-	T50.2X5-	T50.2X6-
Salicylazosulfapyridine	T37.0X1-	T37.0X2-	T37.0X3-	T37.0X4-	T37.0X5-	T37.0X6-
Salicylhydroxamic acid	T49.0X1-	T49.0X2-	T49.0X3-	T49.0X4-	T49.0X5-	T49.0X6-
Salicylic acid	T49.4X1-	T49.4X2-	T49.4X3-	T49.4X4-	T49.4X5-	T49.4X6-
with benzoic acid	T49.4X1-	T49.4X2-	T49.4X3-	T49.4X4-	T49.4X5-	T49.4X6-
congeners	T39.091-	T39.092-	T39.093-	T39.094-	T39.095-	T39.096-
derivative	T39.091-	T39.092-	T39.093-	T39.094-	T39.095-	T39.096-
salts	T39.091-	T39.092-	T39.093-	T39.094-	T39.095-	T39.096-
Salinazid	T37.1X1-	T37.1X2-	T37.1X3-	T37.1X4-	T37.1X5-	T37.1X6-
Salmeterol	T48.6X1-	T48.6X2-	T48.6X3-	T48.6X4-	T48.6X5-	T48.6X6-
Salol	T49.3X1-	T49.3X2-	T49.3X3-	T49.3X4-	T49.3X5-	T49.3X6-
Salsalate	T39.091-	T39.092-	T39.093-	T39.094-	T39.095-	T39.096-
Salt substitute	T50.901-	T50.902-	T50.903-	T50.904-	T50.905-	T50.906-
Salt-replacing drug	T50.901-	T50.902-	T50.903-	T50.904-	T50.905-	T50.906-
Salt-retaining mineralocorticoid	T50.0X1-	T50.0X2-	T50.0X3-	T50.0X4-	T50.0X5-	T50.0X6-
Saluretic NEC	T50.2X1-	T50.2X2-	T50.2X3-	T50.2X4-	T50.2X5-	T50.2X6-

Substance	Poisoning Accidental (unintentional)	Poisoning Intentional self-harm	Poisoning Assault	Poisoning Undetermined	Adverse effect	Underdosing
Saluron	T50.2X1-	T50.2X2-	T50.2X3-	T50.2X4-	T50.2X5-	T50.2X6-
Salvarsan 606 (neosilver) (silver)	T37.8X1-	T37.8X2-	T37.8X3-	T37.8X4-	T37.8X5-	T37.8X6-
Sambucus canadensis	T62.2X1-	T62.2X2-	T62.2X3-	T62.2X4-	-	-
berry	T62.1X1-	T62.1X2-	T62.1X3-	T62.1X4-	-	-
Sandril	T46.5X1-	T46.5X2-	T46.5X3-	T46.5X4-	T46.5X5-	T46.5X6-
Sanguinaria canadensis	T62.2X1-	T62.2X2-	T62.2X3-	T62.2X4-	-	-
Saniflush (cleaner)	T54.2X1-	T54.2X2-	T54.2X3-	T54.2X4-	-	-
Santonin	T37.4X1-	T37.4X2-	T37.4X3-	T37.4X4-	T37.4X5-	T37.4X6-
Santyl	T49.8X1-	T49.8X2-	T49.8X3-	T49.8X4-	T49.8X5-	T49.8X6-
Saralasin	T46.5X1-	T46.5X2-	T46.5X3-	T46.5X4-	T46.5X5-	T46.5X6-
Sarcolysin	T45.1X1-	T45.1X2-	T45.1X3-	T45.1X4-	T45.1X5-	T45.1X6-
Sarkomycin	T45.1X1-	T45.1X2-	T45.1X3-	T45.1X4-	T45.1X5-	T45.1X6-
Saroten	T43.011-	T43.012-	T43.013-	T43.014-	T43.015-	T43.016-
Saturnine — *see Lead*						
Savin (oil)	T49.4X1-	T49.4X2-	T49.4X3-	T49.4X4-	T49.4X5-	T49.4X6-
Scammony	T47.2X1-	T47.2X2-	T47.2X3-	T47.2X4-	T47.2X5-	T47.2X6-
Scarlet red	T49.8X1-	T49.8X2-	T49.8X3-	T49.8X4-	T49.8X5-	T49.8X6-
Scheele's green	T57.0X1-	T57.0X2-	T57.0X3-	T57.0X4-	-	-
insecticide	T57.0X1-	T57.0X2-	T57.0X3-	T57.0X4-	-	-
Schizontozide (blood) (tissue)	T37.2X1-	T37.2X2-	T37.2X3-	T37.2X4-	T37.2X5-	T37.2X6-
Schradan	T60.0X1-	T60.0X2-	T60.0X3-	T60.0X4-	-	-
Schweinfurth green	T57.0X1-	T57.0X2-	T57.0X3-	T57.0X4-	-	-
insecticide	T57.0X1-	T57.0X2-	T57.0X3-	T57.0X4-	-	-
Scilla, rat poison	T60.4X1-	T60.4X2-	T60.4X3-	T60.4X4-	-	-
Scillaren	T60.4X1-	T60.4X2-	T60.4X3-	T60.4X4-	-	-
Sclerosing agent	T46.8X1-	T46.8X2-	T46.8X3-	T46.8X4-	T46.8X5-	T46.8X6-
Scombrotoxin	T61.11X-	T61.12X-	T61.13X-	T61.14X-	-	-
Scopolamine	T44.3X1-	T44.3X2-	T44.3X3-	T44.3X4-	T44.3X5-	T44.3X6-
Scopolia extract	T44.3X1-	T44.3X2-	T44.3X3-	T44.3X4-	T44.3X5-	T44.3X6-
Scouring powder	T65.891-	T65.892-	T65.893-	T65.894-	-	-
Sea						
anemone (sting)	T63.631-	T63.632-	T63.633-	T63.634-	-	-
cucumber (sting)	T63.691-	T63.692-	T63.693-	T63.694-	-	-
snake (bite) (venom)	T63.091-	T63.092-	T63.093-	T63.094-	-	-
urchin spine (puncture)	T63.691-	T63.692-	T63.693-	T63.694-	-	-
Seafood	T61.91X-	T61.92X-	T61.93X-	T61.94X-	-	-
specified NEC	T61.8X1-	T61.8X2-	T61.8X3-	T61.8X4-	-	-
Secbutabarbital	T42.3X1-	T42.3X2-	T42.3X3-	T42.3X4-	T42.3X5-	T42.3X6-
Secbutabarbitone	T42.3X1-	T42.3X2-	T42.3X3-	T42.3X4-	T42.3X5-	T42.3X6-
Secnidazole	T37.3X1-	T37.3X2-	T37.3X3-	T37.3X4-	T37.3X5-	T37.3X6-
Secobarbital	T42.3X1-	T42.3X2-	T42.3X3-	T42.3X4-	T42.3X5-	T42.3X6-
Seconal	T42.3X1-	T42.3X2-	T42.3X3-	T42.3X4-	T42.3X5-	T42.3X6-
Secretin	T50.8X1-	T50.8X2-	T50.8X3-	T50.8X4-	T50.8X5-	T50.8X6-
Sedative NEC	T42.71X-	T42.72X-	T42.73X-	T42.74X-	T42.75X-	T42.76X-
mixed NEC	T42.6X1-	T42.6X2-	T42.6X3-	T42.6X4-	T42.6X5-	T42.6X6-
Sedormid	T42.6X1-	T42.6X2-	T42.6X3-	T42.6X4-	T42.6X5-	T42.6X6-
Seed disinfectant or dressing	T60.8X1-	T60.8X2-	T60.8X3-	T60.8X4-		
Seeds (poisonous)	T62.2X1-	T62.2X2-	T62.2X3-	T62.2X4-	-	-
Selegiline	T42.8X1-	T42.8X2-	T42.8X3-	T42.8X4-	T42.8X5-	T42.8X6-
Selenium NEC	T56.891-	T56.892-	T56.893-	T56.894-	-	-
disulfide or sulfide	T49.4X1-	T49.4X2-	T49.4X3-	T49.4X4-	T49.4X5-	T49.4X6-
fumes	T59.891-	T59.892-	T59.893-	T59.894-	-	-
sulfide	T49.4X1-	T49.4X2-	T49.4X3-	T49.4X4-	T49.4X5-	T49.4X6-
Selenomethionine (75Se)	T50.8X1-	T50.8X2-	T50.8X3-	T50.8X4-	T50.8X5-	T50.8X6-
Selsun	T49.4X1-	T49.4X2-	T49.4X3-	T49.4X4-	T49.4X5-	T49.4X6-
Semustine	T45.1X1-	T45.1X2-	T45.1X3-	T45.1X4-	T45.1X5-	T45.1X6-
Senega syrup	T48.4X1-	T48.4X2-	T48.4X3-	T48.4X4-	T48.4X5-	T48.4X6-
Senna	T47.2X1-	T47.2X2-	T47.2X3-	T47.2X4-	T47.2X5-	T47.2X6-

Substance	Poisoning Accidental (unintentional)	Poisoning Intentional self-harm	Poisoning Assault	Poisoning Undetermined	Adverse effect	Underdosing
Sennoside A+B	T47.2X1-	T47.2X2-	T47.2X3-	T47.2X4-	T47.2X5-	T47.2X6-
Septisol	T49.2X1-	T49.2X2-	T49.2X3-	T49.2X4-	T49.2X5-	T49.2X6-
Seractide	T38.811-	T38.812-	T38.813-	T38.814-	T38.815-	T38.816-
Serax	T42.4X1-	T42.4X2-	T42.4X3-	T42.4X4-	T42.4X5-	T42.4X6-
Serenesil	T42.6X1-	T42.6X2-	T42.6X3-	T42.6X4-	T42.6X5-	T42.6X6-
Serenium (hydrochloride)	T37.91X-	T37.92X-	T37.93X-	T37.94X-	T37.95X-	T37.96X-
Serepax — *see Oxazepam*						
Sermorelin	T38.891-	T38.892-	T38.893-	T38.894-	T38.895-	T38.896-
Sernyl	T41.1X1-	T41.1X2-	T41.1X3-	T41.1X4-	T41.1X5-	T41.1X6-
Serotonin	T50.991-	T50.992-	T50.993-	T50.994-	T50.995-	T50.996-
Serpasil	T46.5X1-	T46.5X2-	T46.5X3-	T46.5X4-	T46.5X5-	T46.5X6-
Serrapeptase	T45.3X1-	T45.3X2-	T45.3X3-	T45.3X4-	T45.3X5-	T45.3X6-
Serum						
antibotulinus	T50.Z11-	T50.Z12-	T50.Z13-	T50.Z14-	T50.Z15-	T50.Z16-
anticytotoxic	T50.Z11-	T50.Z12-	T50.Z13-	T50.Z14-	T50.Z15-	T50.Z16-
antidiphtheria	T50.Z11-	T50.Z12-	T50.Z13-	T50.Z14-	T50.Z15-	T50.Z16-
antimeningococcus	T50.Z11-	T50.Z12-	T50.Z13-	T50.Z14-	T50.Z15-	T50.Z16-
anti-Rh	T50.Z11-	T50.Z12-	T50.Z13-	T50.Z14-	T50.Z15-	T50.Z16-
anti-snake-bite	T50.Z11-	T50.Z12-	T50.Z13-	T50.Z14-	T50.Z15-	T50.Z16-
antitetanic	T50.Z11-	T50.Z12-	T50.Z13-	T50.Z14-	T50.Z15-	T50.Z16-
antitoxic	T50.Z11-	T50.Z12-	T50.Z13-	T50.Z14-	T50.Z15-	T50.Z16-
complement (inhibitor)	T45.8X1-	T45.8X2-	T45.8X3-	T45.8X4-	T45.8X5-	T45.8X6-
convalescent	T50.Z11-	T50.Z12-	T50.Z13-	T50.Z14-	T50.Z15-	T50.Z16-
hemolytic complement	T45.8X1-	T45.8X2-	T45.8X3-	T45.8X4-	T45.8X5-	T45.8X6-
immune (human)	T50.Z11-	T50.Z12-	T50.Z13-	T50.Z14-	T50.Z15-	T50.Z16-
protective NEC	T50.Z11-	T50.Z12-	T50.Z13-	T50.Z14-	T50.Z15-	T50.Z16-
Setastine	T45.0X1-	T45.0X2-	T45.0X3-	T45.0X4-	T45.0X5-	T45.0X6-
Setoperone	T43.591-	T43.592-	T43.593-	T43.594-	T43.595-	T43.596-
Sewer gas	T59.91X-	T59.92X-	T59.93X-	T59.94X-	-	-
Shampoo	T55.0X1-	T55.0X2-	T55.0X3-	T55.0X4-	-	-
Shellfish, noxious, nonbacterial	T61.781-	T61.782-	T61.783-	T61.784-	-	-
Sildenafil	T46.7X1-	T46.7X2-	T46.7X3-	T46.7X4-	T46.7X5-	T46.7X6-
Silibinin	T50.991-	T50.992-	T50.993-	T50.994-	T50.995-	T50.996-
Silicone NEC	T65.891-	T65.892-	T65.893-	T65.894-	-	-
medicinal	T49.3X1-	T49.3X2-	T49.3X3-	T49.3X4-	T49.3X5-	T49.3X6-
Silvadene	T49.0X1-	T49.0X2-	T49.0X3-	T49.0X4-	T49.0X5-	T49.0X6-
Silver	T49.0X1-	T49.0X2-	T49.0X3-	T49.0X4-	T49.0X5-	T49.0X6-
anti-infectives	T49.0X1-	T49.0X2-	T49.0X3-	T49.0X4-	T49.0X5-	T49.0X6-
arsphenamine	T37.8X1-	T37.8X2-	T37.8X3-	T37.8X4-	T37.8X5-	T37.8X6-
colloidal	T49.0X1-	T49.0X2-	T49.0X3-	T49.0X4-	T49.0X5-	T49.0X6-
nitrate	T49.0X1-	T49.0X2-	T49.0X3-	T49.0X4-	T49.0X5-	T49.0X6-
ophthalmic preparation	T49.5X1-	T49.5X2-	T49.5X3-	T49.5X4-	T49.5X5-	T49.5X6-
toughened (keratolytic)	T49.4X1-	T49.4X2-	T49.4X3-	T49.4X4-	T49.4X5-	T49.4X6-
nonmedicinal (dust)	T56.891-	T56.892-	T56.893-	T56.894-	-	-
protein	T49.5X1-	T49.5X2-	T49.5X3-	T49.5X4-	T49.5X5-	T49.5X6-
salvarsan	T37.8X1-	T37.8X2-	T37.8X3-	T37.8X4-	T37.8X5-	T37.8X6-
sulfadiazine	T49.4X1-	T49.4X2-	T49.4X3-	T49.4X4-	T49.4X5-	T49.4X6-
Silymarin	T50.991-	T50.992-	T50.993-	T50.994-	T50.995-	T50.996-
Simaldrate	T47.1X1-	T47.1X2-	T47.1X3-	T47.1X4-	T47.1X5-	T47.1X6-
Simazine	T60.3X1-	T60.3X2-	T60.3X3-	T60.3X4-	-	-
Simethicone	T47.1X1-	T47.1X2-	T47.1X3-	T47.1X4-	T47.1X5-	T47.1X6-
Simfibrate	T46.6X1-	T46.6X2-	T46.6X3-	T46.6X4-	T46.6X5-	T46.6X6-
Simvastatin	T46.6X1-	T46.6X2-	T46.6X3-	T46.6X4-	T46.6X5-	T46.6X6-
Sincalide	T50.8X1-	T50.8X2-	T50.8X3-	T50.8X4-	T50.8X5-	T50.8X6-
Sinequan	T43.011-	T43.012-	T43.013-	T43.014-	T43.015-	T43.016-
Singoserp	T46.5X1-	T46.5X2-	T46.5X3-	T46.5X4-	T46.5X5-	T46.5X6-
Sintrom	T45.511-	T45.512-	T45.513-	T45.514-	T45.515-	T45.516-
Sisomicin	T36.5X1-	T36.5X2-	T36.5X3-	T36.5X4-	T36.5X5-	T36.5X6-
Sitosterols	T46.6X1-	T46.6X2-	T46.6X3-	T46.6X4-	T46.6X5-	T46.6X6-

Substance	Poisoning Accidental (unintentional)	Poisoning Intentional self-harm	Poisoning Assault	Poisoning Undetermined	Adverse effect	Underdosing
Skeletal muscle relaxants	T48.1X1-	T48.1X2-	T48.1X3-	T48.1X4-	T48.1X5-	T48.1X6-
Skin						
agents (external)	T49.91X-	T49.92X-	T49.93X-	T49.94X-	T49.95X-	T49.96X-
specified NEC	T49.8X1-	T49.8X2-	T49.8X3-	T49.8X4-	T49.8X5-	T49.8X6-
test antigen	T50.8X1-	T50.8X2-	T50.8X3-	T50.8X4-	T50.8X5-	T50.8X6-
Sleep-eze	T45.0X1-	T45.0X2-	T45.0X3-	T45.0X4-	T45.0X5-	T45.0X6-
Sleeping draught, pill	T42.71X-	T42.72X-	T42.73X-	T42.74X-	T42.75X-	T42.76X-
Smallpox vaccine	T50.B11-	T50.B12-	T50.B13-	T50.B14-	T50.B15-	T50.B16-
Smelter fumes NEC	T56.91X-	T56.92X-	T56.93X-	T56.94X-	-	-
Smog	T59.1X1-	T59.1X2-	T59.1X3-	T59.1X4-	-	-
Smoke NEC	T59.811-	T59.812-	T59.813-	T59.814-	-	-
Smooth muscle relaxant	T44.3X1-	T44.3X2-	T44.3X3-	T44.3X4-	T44.3X5-	T44.3X6-
Snail killer NEC	T60.8X1-	T60.8X2-	T60.8X3-	T60.8X4-	-	-
Snake venom or bite	T63.001-	T63.002-	T63.003-	T63.004-	-	-
hemocoagulase	T45.7X1-	T45.7X2-	T45.7X3-	T45.7X4-	T45.7X5-	T45.7X6-
Snuff	T65.211-	T65.212-	T65.213-	T65.214-	-	-
Soap (powder) (product)	T55.0X1-	T55.0X2-	T55.0X3-	T55.0X4-	-	-
enema	T47.4X1-	T47.4X2-	T47.4X3-	T47.4X4-	T47.4X5-	T47.4X6-
medicinal, soft	T49.2X1-	T49.2X2-	T49.2X3-	T49.2X4-	T49.2X5-	T49.2X6-
superfatted	T49.2X1-	T49.2X2-	T49.2X3-	T49.2X4-	T49.2X5-	T49.2X6-
Sobrerol	T48.4X1-	T48.4X2-	T48.4X3-	T48.4X4-	T48.4X5-	T48.4X6-
Soda (caustic)	T54.3X1-	T54.3X2-	T54.3X3-	T54.3X4-	-	-
bicarb	T47.1X1-	T47.1X2-	T47.1X3-	T47.1X4-	T47.1X5-	T47.1X6-
chlorinated — *see Sodium, hypochlorite*						
Sodium						
acetosulfone	T37.1X1-	T37.1X2-	T37.1X3-	T37.1X4-	T37.1X5-	T37.1X6-
acetrizoate	T50.8X1-	T50.8X2-	T50.8X3-	T50.8X4-	T50.8X5-	T50.8X6-
acid phosphate	T50.3X1-	T50.3X2-	T50.3X3-	T50.3X4-	T50.3X5-	T50.3X6-
alginate	T47.8X1-	T47.8X2-	T47.8X3-	T47.8X4-	T47.8X5-	T47.8X6-
amidotrizoate	T50.8X1-	T50.8X2-	T50.8X3-	T50.8X4-	T50.8X5-	T50.8X6-
aminopterin	T45.1X1-	T45.1X2-	T45.1X3-	T45.1X4-	T45.1X5-	T45.1X6-
amylosulfate	T47.8X1-	T47.8X2-	T47.8X3-	T47.8X4-	T47.8X5-	T47.8X6-
amytal	T42.3X1-	T42.3X2-	T42.3X3-	T42.3X4-	T42.3X5-	T42.3X6-
antimony gluconate	T37.3X1-	T37.3X2-	T37.3X3-	T37.3X4-	T37.3X5-	T37.3X6-
arsenate	T57.0X1-	T57.0X2-	T57.0X3-	T57.0X4-	-	-
aurothiomalate	T39.4X1-	T39.4X2-	T39.4X3-	T39.4X4-	T39.4X5-	T39.4X6-
aurothiosulfate	T39.4X1-	T39.4X2-	T39.4X3-	T39.4X4-	T39.4X5-	T39.4X6-
barbiturate	T42.3X1-	T42.3X2-	T42.3X3-	T42.3X4-	T42.3X5-	T42.3X6-
basic phosphate	T47.4X1-	T47.4X2-	T47.4X3-	T47.4X4-	T47.4X5-	T47.4X6-
bicarbonate	T47.1X1-	T47.1X2-	T47.1X3-	T47.1X4-	T47.1X5-	T47.1X6-
bichromate	T57.8X1-	T57.8X2-	T57.8X3-	T57.8X4-	-	-
biphosphate	T50.3X1-	T50.3X2-	T50.3X3-	T50.3X4-	T50.3X5-	T50.3X6-
bisulfate	T65.891-	T65.892-	T65.893-	T65.894-	-	-
borate						
cleanser	T57.8X1-	T57.8X2-	T57.8X3-	T57.8X4-	-	-
eye	T49.5X1-	T49.5X2-	T49.5X3-	T49.5X4-	T49.5X5-	T49.5X6-
therapeutic	T49.8X1-	T49.8X2-	T49.8X3-	T49.8X4-	T49.8X5-	T49.8X6-
bromide	T42.6X1-	T42.6X2-	T42.6X3-	T42.6X4-	T42.6X5-	T42.6X6-
cacodylate (nonmedicinal) NEC	T50.8X1-	T50.8X2-	T50.8X3-	T50.8X4-	T50.8X5-	T50.8X6-
anti-infective	T37.8X1-	T37.8X2-	T37.8X3-	T37.8X4-	T37.8X5-	T37.8X6-
herbicide	T60.3X1-	T60.3X2-	T60.3X3-	T60.3X4-	-	-
calcium edetate	T45.8X1-	T45.8X2-	T45.8X3-	T45.8X4-	T45.8X5-	T45.8X6-
carbonate NEC	T54.3X1-	T54.3X2-	T54.3X3-	T54.3X4-	-	-
chlorate NEC	T65.891-	T65.892-	T65.893-	T65.894-	-	-
herbicide	T54.91X-	T54.92X-	T54.93X-	T54.94X-	-	-
chloride	T50.3X1-	T50.3X2-	T50.3X3-	T50.3X4-	T50.3X5-	T50.3X6-
with glucose	T50.3X1-	T50.3X2-	T50.3X3-	T50.3X4-	T50.3X5-	T50.3X6-
chromate	T65.891-	T65.892-	T65.893-	T65.894-	-	-

Substance	Poisoning Accidental (unintentional)	Poisoning Intentional self-harm	Poisoning Assault	Poisoning Undetermined	Adverse effect	Underdosing
Sodium (continued)						
citrate	T50.991-	T50.992-	T50.993-	T50.994-	T50.995-	T50.996-
cromoglicate	T48.6X1-	T48.6X2-	T48.6X3-	T48.6X4-	T48.6X5-	T48.6X6-
cyanide	T65.0X1-	T65.0X2-	T65.0X3-	T65.0X4-	-	-
cyclamate	T50.3X1-	T50.3X2-	T50.3X3-	T50.3X4-	T50.3X5-	T50.3X6-
dehydrocholate	T45.8X1-	T45.8X2-	T45.8X3-	T45.8X4-	T45.8X5-	T45.8X6-
diatrizoate	T50.8X1-	T50.8X2-	T50.8X3-	T50.8X4-	T50.8X5-	T50.8X6-
dibunate	T48.4X1-	T48.4X2-	T48.4X3-	T48.4X4-	T48.4X5-	T48.4X6-
dioctyl sulfosuccinate	T47.4X1-	T47.4X2-	T47.4X3-	T47.4X4-	T47.4X5-	T47.4X6-
dipantoyl ferrate	T45.8X1-	T45.8X2-	T45.8X3-	T45.8X4-	T45.8X5-	T45.8X6-
edetate	T45.8X1-	T45.8X2-	T45.8X3-	T45.8X4-	T45.8X5-	T45.8X6-
ethacrynate	T50.1X1-	T50.1X2-	T50.1X3-	T50.1X4-	T50.1X5-	T50.1X6-
feredetate	T45.8X1-	T45.8X2-	T45.8X3-	T45.8X4-	T45.8X5-	T45.8X6-
Fluoride — *see Fluoride*						
fluoroacetate (dust) (pesticide)	T60.4X1-	T60.4X2-	T60.4X3-	T60.4X4-	-	-
free salt	T50.3X1-	T50.3X2-	T50.3X3-	T50.3X4-	T50.3X5-	T50.3X6-
fusidate	T36.8X1-	T36.8X2-	T36.8X3-	T36.8X4-	T36.8X5-	T36.8X6-
glucaldrate	T47.1X1-	T47.1X2-	T47.1X3-	T47.1X4-	T47.1X5-	T47.1X6-
glucosulfone	T37.1X1-	T37.1X2-	T37.1X3-	T37.1X4-	T37.1X5-	T37.1X6-
glutamate	T45.8X1-	T45.8X2-	T45.8X3-	T45.8X4-	T45.8X5-	T45.8X6-
hydrogen carbonate	T50.3X1-	T50.3X2-	T50.3X3-	T50.3X4-	T50.3X5-	T50.3X6-
hydroxide	T54.3X1-	T54.3X2-	T54.3X3-	T54.3X4-	-	-
hypochlorite (bleach) NEC	T54.3X1-	T54.3X2-	T54.3X3-	T54.3X4-	-	-
disinfectant	T54.3X1-	T54.3X2-	T54.3X3-	T54.3X4-	-	-
medicinal (anti-infective) (external)	T49.0X1-	T49.0X2-	T49.0X3-	T49.0X4-	T49.0X5-	T49.0X6-
vapor	T54.3X1-	T54.3X2-	T54.3X3-	T54.3X4-	-	-
hyposulfite	T49.0X1-	T49.0X2-	T49.0X3-	T49.0X4-	T49.0X5-	T49.0X6-
indigotin disulfonate	T50.8X1-	T50.8X2-	T50.8X3-	T50.8X4-	T50.8X5-	T50.8X6-
iodide	T50.991-	T50.992-	T50.993-	T50.994-	T50.995-	T50.996-
I-131	T50.8X1-	T50.8X2-	T50.8X3-	T50.8X4-	T50.8X5-	T50.8X6-
therapeutic	T38.2X1-	T38.2X2-	T38.2X3-	T38.2X4-	T38.2X5-	T38.2X6-
iodohippurate (131I)	T50.8X1-	T50.8X2-	T50.8X3-	T50.8X4-	T50.8X5-	T50.8X6-
iopodate	T50.8X1-	T50.8X2-	T50.8X3-	T50.8X4-	T50.8X5-	T50.8X6-
iothalamate	T50.8X1-	T50.8X2-	T50.8X3-	T50.8X4-	T50.8X5-	T50.8X6-
iron edetate	T45.4X1-	T45.4X2-	T45.4X3-	T45.4X4-	T45.4X5-	T45.4X6-
lactate (compound solution)	T45.8X1-	T45.8X2-	T45.8X3-	T45.8X4-	T45.8X5-	T45.8X6-
lauryl (sulfate)	T49.2X1-	T49.2X2-	T49.2X3-	T49.2X4-	T49.2X5-	T49.2X6-
L-triiodothyronine	T38.1X1-	T38.1X2-	T38.1X3-	T38.1X4-	T38.1X5-	T38.1X6-
magnesium citrate	T50.991-	T50.992-	T50.993-	T50.994-	T50.995-	T50.996-
mersalate	T50.2X1-	T50.2X2-	T50.2X3-	T50.2X4-	T50.2X5-	T50.2X6-
metasilicate	T65.891-	T65.892-	T65.893-	T65.894-	-	-
metrizoate	T50.8X1-	T50.8X2-	T50.8X3-	T50.8X4-	T50.8X5-	T50.8X6-
monofluoroacetate (pesticide)	T60.1X1-	T60.1X2-	T60.1X3-	T60.1X4-	-	-
morrhuate	T46.8X1-	T46.8X2-	T46.8X3-	T46.8X4-	T46.8X5-	T46.8X6-
nafcillin	T36.0X1-	T36.0X2-	T36.0X3-	T36.0X4-	T36.0X5-	T36.0X6-
nitrate (oxidizing agent)	T65.891-	T65.892-	T65.893-	T65.894-	-	-
nitrite	T50.6X1-	T50.6X2-	T50.6X3-	T50.6X4-	T50.6X5-	T50.6X6-
nitroferricyanide	T46.5X1-	T46.5X2-	T46.5X3-	T46.5X4-	T46.5X5-	T46.5X6-
nitroprusside	T46.5X1-	T46.5X2-	T46.5X3-	T46.5X4-	T46.5X5-	T46.5X6-
oxalate	T65.891-	T65.892-	T65.893-	T65.894-	-	-
oxide/peroxide	T65.891-	T65.892-	T65.893-	T65.894-	-	-
oxybate	T41.291-	T41.292-	T41.293-	T41.294-	T41.295-	T41.296-
para-aminohippurate	T50.8X1-	T50.8X2-	T50.8X3-	T50.8X4-	T50.8X5-	T50.8X6-
perborate (nonmedicinal) NEC	T65.891-	T65.892-	T65.893-	T65.894-	-	-
medicinal	T49.0X1-	T49.0X2-	T49.0X3-	T49.0X4-	T49.0X5-	T49.0X6-
soap	T55.0X1-	T55.0X2-	T55.0X3-	T55.0X4-	-	-
percarbonate — *see Sodium, perborate*						
pertechnetate Tc99m	T50.8X1-	T50.8X2-		T50.8X4-	T50.8X5-	T50.8X6-
phosphate						
cellulose	T45.8X1-	T45.8X2-	T45.8X3-	T45.8X4-	T45.8X5-	T45.8X6-

Substance	Poisoning Accidental (unintentional)	Poisoning Intentional self-harm	Poisoning Assault	Poisoning Undetermined	Adverse effect	Underdosing
Sodium (continued)						
dibasic	T47.2X1-	T47.2X2-	T47.2X3-	T47.2X4-	T47.2X5-	T47.2X6-
monobasic	T47.2X1-	T47.2X2-	T47.2X3-	T47.2X4-	T47.2X5-	T47.2X6-
phytate	T50.6X1-	T50.6X2-	T50.6X3-	T50.6X4-	T50.6X5-	T50.6X6-
picosulfate	T47.2X1-	T47.2X2-	T47.2X3-	T47.2X4-	T47.2X5-	T47.2X6-
polyhydroxyaluminium monocarbonate	T47.1X1-	T47.1X2-	T47.1X3-	T47.1X4-	T47.1X5-	T47.1X6-
polystyrene sulfonate	T50.3X1-	T50.3X2-	T50.3X3-	T50.3X4-	T50.3X5-	T50.3X6-
propionate	T49.0X1-	T49.0X2-	T49.0X3-	T49.0X4-	T49.0X5-	T49.0X6-
propyl hydroxybenzoate	T50.991-	T50.992-	T50.993-	T50.994-	T50.995-	T50.996-
psylliate	T46.8X1-	T46.8X2-	T46.8X3-	T46.8X4-	T46.8X5-	T46.8X6-
removing resins	T50.3X1-	T50.3X2-	T50.3X3-	T50.3X4-	T50.3X5-	T50.3X6-
salicylate	T39.091-	T39.092-	T39.093-	T39.094-	T39.095-	T39.096-
salt NEC	T50.3X1-	T50.3X2-	T50.3X3-	T50.3X4-	T50.3X5-	T50.3X6-
selenate	T60.2X1-	T60.2X2-	T60.2X3-	T60.2X4-	-	-
stibogluconate	T37.3X1-	T37.3X2-	T37.3X3-	T37.3X4-	T37.3X5-	T37.3X6-
sulfate	T47.4X1-	T47.4X2-	T47.4X3-	T47.4X4-	T47.4X5-	T47.4X6-
sulfoxone	T37.1X1-	T37.1X2-	T37.1X3-	T37.1X4-	T37.1X5-	T37.1X6-
tetradecyl sulfate	T46.8X1-	T46.8X2-	T46.8X3-	T46.8X4-	T46.8X5-	T46.8X6-
thiopental	T41.1X1-	T41.1X2-	T41.1X3-	T41.1X4-	T41.1X5-	T41.1X6-
thiosalicylate	T39.091-	T39.092-	T39.093-	T39.094-	T39.095-	T39.096-
thiosulfate	T50.6X1-	T50.6X2-	T50.6X3-	T50.6X4-	T50.6X5-	T50.6X6-
tolbutamide	T38.3X1-	T38.3X2-	T38.3X3-	T38.3X4-	T38.3X5-	T38.3X6-
(L) -triiodothyronine	T38.1X1-	T38.1X2-	T38.1X3-	T38.1X4-	T38.1X5-	T38.1X6-
tyropanoate	T50.8X1-	T50.8X2-	T50.8X3-	T50.8X4-	T50.8X5-	T50.8X6-
valproate	T42.6X1-	T42.6X2-	T42.6X3-	T42.6X4-	T42.6X5-	T42.6X6-
versenate	T50.6X1-	T50.6X2-	T50.6X3-	T50.6X4-	T50.6X5-	T50.6X6-
Sodium-free salt	T50.901-	T50.902-	T50.903-	T50.904-	T50.905-	T50.906-
Sodium-removing resin	T50.3X1-	T50.3X2-	T50.3X3-	T50.3X4-	T50.3X5-	T50.3X6-
Soft soap	T55.0X1-	T55.0X2-	T55.0X3-	T55.0X4-	-	-
Solanine	T62.2X1-	T62.2X2-	T62.2X3-	T62.2X4-	-	-
berries	T62.1X1-	T62.1X2-	T62.1X3-	T62.1X4-	-	-
Solanum dulcamara	T62.2X1-	T62.2X2-	T62.2X3-	T62.2X4-	-	-
berries	T62.1X1-	T62.1X2-	T62.1X3-	T62.1X4-	-	-
Solapsone	T37.1X1-	T37.1X2-	T37.1X3-	T37.1X4-	T37.1X5-	T37.1X6-
Solar lotion	T49.3X1-	T49.3X2-	T49.3X3-	T49.3X4-	T49.3X5-	T49.3X6-
Solasulfone	T37.1X1-	T37.1X2-	T37.1X3-	T37.1X4-	T37.1X5-	T37.1X6-
Soldering fluid	T65.891-	T65.892-	T65.893-	T65.894-	-	-
Solid substance	T65.91X-	T65.92X-	T65.93X-	T65.94X-	-	-
specified NEC	T65.891-	T65.892-	T65.893-	T65.894-	-	-
Solvent, industrial NEC	T52.91X-	T52.92X-	T52.93X-	T52.94X-	-	-
naphtha	T52.0X1-	T52.0X2-	T52.0X3-	T52.0X4-	-	-
petroleum	T52.0X1-	T52.0X2-	T52.0X3-	T52.0X4-	-	-
specified NEC	T52.8X1-	T52.8X2-	T52.8X3-	T52.8X4-	-	-
Soma	T42.8X1-	T42.8X2-	T42.8X3-	T42.8X4-	T42.8X5-	T42.8X6-
Somatorelin	T38.891-	T38.892-	T38.893-	T38.894-	T38.895-	T38.896-
Somatostatin	T38.991-	T38.992-	T38.993-	T38.994-	T38.995-	T38.996-
Somatotropin	T38.811-	T38.812-	T38.813-	T38.814-	T38.815-	T38.816-
Somatrem	T38.811-	T38.812-	T38.813-	T38.814-	T38.815-	T38.816-
Somatropin	T38.811-	T38.812-	T38.813-	T38.814-	T38.815-	T38.816-
Sominex	T45.0X1-	T45.0X2-	T45.0X3-	T45.0X4-	T45.0X5-	T45.0X6-
Somnos	T42.6X1-	T42.6X2-	T42.6X3-	T42.6X4-	T42.6X5-	T42.6X6-
Somonal	T42.3X1-	T42.3X2-	T42.3X3-	T42.3X4-	T42.3X5-	T42.3X6-
Soneryl	T42.3X1-	T42.3X2-	T42.3X3-	T42.3X4-	T42.3X5-	T42.3X6-
Soothing syrup	T50.901-	T50.902-	T50.903-	T50.904-	T50.905-	T50.906-
Sopor	T42.6X1-	T42.6X2-	T42.6X3-	T42.6X4-	T42.6X5-	T42.6X6-
Soporific	T42.71X-	T42.72X-	T42.73X-	T42.74X-	T42.75X-	T42.76X-
Soporific drug	T42.71X-	T42.72X-	T42.73X-	T42.74X-	T42.75X-	T42.76X-
specified type NEC	T42.6X1-	T42.6X2-	T42.6X3-	T42.6X4-	T42.6X5-	T42.6X6-

Substance	Poisoning Accidental (unintentional)	Poisoning Intentional self-harm	Poisoning Assault	Poisoning Undetermined	Adverse effect	Underdosing
Sorbide nitrate	T46.3X1-	T46.3X2-	T46.3X3-	T46.3X4-	T46.3X5-	T46.3X6-
Sorbitol	T47.4X1-	T47.4X2-	T47.4X3-	T47.4X4-	T47.4X5-	T47.4X6-
Sotalol	T44.7X1-	T44.7X2-	T44.7X3-	T44.7X4-	T44.7X5-	T44.7X6-
Sotradecol	T46.8X1-	T46.8X2-	T46.8X3-	T46.8X4-	T46.8X5-	T46.8X6-
Soysterol	T46.6X1-	T46.6X2-	T46.6X3-	T46.6X4-	T46.6X5-	T46.6X6-
Spacoline	T44.3X1-	T44.3X2-	T44.3X3-	T44.3X4-	T44.3X5-	T44.3X6-
Spanish fly	T49.8X1-	T49.8X2-	T49.8X3-	T49.8X4-	T49.8X5-	T49.8X6-
Sparine	T43.3X1-	T43.3X2-	T43.3X3-	T43.3X4-	T43.3X5-	T43.3X6-
Sparteine	T48.0X1-	T48.0X2-	T48.0X3-	T48.0X4-	T48.0X5-	T48.0X6-
Spasmolytic						
anticholinergics	T44.3X1-	T44.3X2-	T44.3X3-	T44.3X4-	T44.3X5-	T44.3X6-
autonomic	T44.3X1-	T44.3X2-	T44.3X3-	T44.3X4-	T44.3X5-	T44.3X6-
bronchial NEC	T48.6X1-	T48.6X2-	T48.6X3-	T48.6X4-	T48.6X5-	T48.6X6-
quaternary ammonium	T44.3X1-	T44.3X2-	T44.3X3-	T44.3X4-	T44.3X5-	T44.3X6-
skeletal muscle NEC	T48.1X1-	T48.1X2-	T48.1X3-	T48.1X4-	T48.1X5-	T48.1X6-
Spectinomycin	T36.5X1-	T36.5X2-	T36.5X3-	T36.5X4-	T36.5X5-	T36.5X6-
Speed	T43.621-	T43.622-	T43.623-	T43.624-	T43.625-	T43.626-
Spermicide	T49.8X1-	T49.8X2-	T49.8X3-	T49.8X4-	T49.8X5-	T49.8X6-
Spider (bite) (venom)	T63.391-	T63.392-	T63.393-	T63.394-	-	-
antivenin	T50.Z11-	T50.Z12-	T50.Z13-	T50.Z14-	T50.Z15-	T50.Z16-
Spigelia (root)	T37.4X1-	T37.4X2-	T37.4X3-	T37.4X4-	T37.4X5-	T37.4X6-
Spindle inactivator	T50.4X1-	T50.4X2-	T50.4X3-	T50.4X4-	T50.4X5-	T50.4X6-
Spiperone	T43.4X1-	T43.4X2-	T43.4X3-	T43.4X4-	T43.4X5-	T43.4X6-
Spiramycin	T36.3X1-	T36.3X2-	T36.3X3-	T36.3X4-	T36.3X5-	T36.3X6-
Spirapril	T46.4X1-	T46.4X2-	T46.4X3-	T46.4X4-	T46.4X5-	T46.4X6-
Spirilene	T43.591-	T43.592-	T43.593-	T43.594-	T43.595-	T43.596-
Spirit (s) (neutral) NEC	T51.0X1-	T51.0X2-	T51.0X3-	T51.0X4-	-	-
beverage	T51.0X1-	T51.0X2-	T51.0X3-	T51.0X4-	-	-
industrial	T51.0X1-	T51.0X2-	T51.0X3-	T51.0X4-	-	-
mineral	T52.0X1-	T52.0X2-	T52.0X3-	T52.0X4-	-	-
of salt — *see Hydrochloric acid*						
surgical	T51.0X1-	T51.0X2-	T51.0X3-	T51.0X4-	-	-
Spironolactone	T50.0X1-	T50.0X2-	T50.0X3-	T50.0X4-	T50.0X5-	T50.0X6-
Spiroperidol	T43.4X1-	T43.4X2-	T43.4X3-	T43.4X4-	T43.4X5-	T43.4X6-
Sponge, absorbable (gelatin)	T45.7X1-	T45.7X2-	T45.7X3-	T45.7X4-	T45.7X5-	T45.7X6-
Sporostacin	T49.0X1-	T49.0X2-	T49.0X3-	T49.0X4-	T49.0X5-	T49.0X6-
Spray (aerosol)	T65.91X-	T65.92X-	T65.93X-	T65.94X-	-	-
cosmetic	T65.891-	T65.892-	T65.893-	T65.894-	-	-
medicinal NEC	T50.901-	T50.902-	T50.903-	T50.904-	T50.905-	T50.906-
pesticides — *see Pesticides*						
specified content — *see specific substance*						
Spurge flax	T62.2X1-	T62.2X2-	T62.2X3-	T62.2X4-	-	-
Spurges	T62.2X1-	T62.2X2-	T62.2X3-	T62.2X4-	-	-
Sputum viscosity-lowering drug	T48.4X1-	T48.4X2-	T48.4X3-	T48.4X4-	T48.4X5-	T48.4X6-
Squill	T46.0X1-	T46.0X2-	T46.0X3-	T46.0X4-	T46.0X5-	T46.0X6-
rat poison	T60.4X1-	T60.4X2-	T60.4X3-	T60.4X4-	-	-
Squirting cucumber (cathartic)	T47.2X1-	T47.2X2-	T47.2X3-	T47.2X4-	T47.2X5-	T47.2X6-
Stains	T65.6X1-	T65.6X2-	T65.6X3-	T65.6X4-	-	-
Stannous fluoride	T49.7X1-	T49.7X2-	T49.7X3-	T49.7X4-	T49.7X5-	T49.7X6-
Stanolone	T38.7X1-	T38.7X2-	T38.7X3-	T38.7X4-	T38.7X5-	T38.7X6-
Stanozolol	T38.7X1-	T38.7X2-	T38.7X3-	T38.7X4-	T38.7X5-	T38.7X6-
Staphisagria or stavesacre (pediculicide)	T49.0X1-	T49.0X2-	T49.0X3-	T49.0X4-	T49.0X5-	T49.0X6-
Starch	T50.901-	T50.902-	T50.903-	T50.904-	T50.905-	T50.906-
Stelazine	T43.3X1-	T43.3X2-	T43.3X3-	T43.3X4-	T43.3X5-	T43.3X6-
Stemetil	T43.3X1-	T43.3X2-	T43.3X3-	T43.3X4-	T43.3X5-	T43.3X6-
Stepronin	T48.4X1-	T48.4X2-	T48.4X3-	T48.4X4-	T48.4X5-	T48.4X6-
Sterculia	T47.4X1-	T47.4X2-	T47.4X3-	T47.4X4-	T47.4X5-	T47.4X6-

Substance	Poisoning Accidental (unintentional)	Poisoning Intentional self-harm	Poisoning Assault	Poisoning Undetermined	Adverse effect	Underdosing
Sternutator gas	T59.891-	T59.892-	T59.893-	T59.894-	-	-
Steroid	T38.0X1-	T38.0X2-	T38.0X3-	T38.0X4-	T38.0X5-	T38.0X6-
anabolic	T38.7X1-	T38.7X2-	T38.7X3-	T38.7X4-	T38.7X5-	T38.7X6-
androgenic	T38.7X1-	T38.7X2-	T38.7X3-	T38.7X4-	T38.7X5-	T38.7X6-
antineoplastic, hormone	T38.7X1-	T38.7X2-	T38.7X3-	T38.7X4-	T38.7X5-	T38.7X6-
estrogen	T38.5X1-	T38.5X2-	T38.5X3-	T38.5X4-	T38.5X5-	T38.5X6-
ENT agent	T49.6X1-	T49.6X2-	T49.6X3-	T49.6X4-	T49.6X5-	T49.6X6-
ophthalmic preparation	T49.5X1-	T49.5X2-	T49.5X3-	T49.5X4-	T49.5X5-	T49.5X6-
topical NEC	T49.0X1-	T49.0X2-	T49.0X3-	T49.0X4-	T49.0X5-	T49.0X6-
Stibine	T56.891-	T56.892-	T56.893-	T56.894-	-	-
Stibogluconate	T37.3X1-	T37.3X2-	T37.3X3-	T37.3X4-	T37.3X5-	T37.3X6-
Stibophen	T37.4X1-	T37.4X2-	T37.4X3-	T37.4X4-	T37.4X5-	T37.4X6-
Stilbamidine (isetionate)	T37.3X1-	T37.3X2-	T37.3X3-	T37.3X4-	T37.3X5-	T37.3X6-
Stilbestrol	T38.5X1-	T38.5X2-	T38.5X3-	T38.5X4-	T38.5X5-	T38.5X6-
Stilboestrol	T38.5X1-	T38.5X2-	T38.5X3-	T38.5X4-	T38.5X5-	T38.5X6-
Stimulant						
central nervous system — *see also Psychostimulant*	T43.601-	T43.602-	T43.603-	T43.604-	T43.605-	T43.606-
analeptics	T50.7X1-	T50.7X2-	T50.7X3-	T50.7X4-	T50.7X5-	T50.7X6-
opiate antagonist	T50.7X1-	T50.7X2-	T50.7X3-	T50.7X4-	T50.7X5-	T50.7X6-
psychotherapeutic NEC — *see also Psychotherapeutic drug*	T43.601-	T43.602-	T43.603-	T43.604-	T43.605-	T43.606-
specified NEC	T43.691-	T43.692-	T43.693-	T43.694-	T43.695-	T43.696-
respiratory	T48.901-	T48.902-	T48.903-	T48.904-	T48.905-	T48.906-
Stone-dissolving drug	T50.901-	T50.902-	T50.903-	T50.904-	T50.905-	T50.906-
Storage battery (cells) (acid)	T54.2X1-	T54.2X2-	T54.2X3-	T54.2X4-	-	-
Stovaine	T41.3X1-	T41.3X2-	T41.3X3-	T41.3X4-	T41.3X5-	T41.3X6-
infiltration (subcutaneous)	T41.3X1-	T41.3X2-	T41.3X3-	T41.3X4-	T41.3X5-	T41.3X6-
nerve block (peripheral) (plexus)	T41.3X1-	T41.3X2-	T41.3X3-	T41.3X4-	T41.3X5-	T41.3X6-
spinal	T41.3X1-	T41.3X2-	T41.3X3-	T41.3X4-	T41.3X5-	T41.3X6-
topical (surface)	T41.3X1-	T41.3X2-	T41.3X3-	T41.3X4-	T41.3X5-	T41.3X6-
Stovarsal	T37.8X1-	T37.8X2-	T37.8X3-	T37.8X4-	T37.8X5-	T37.8X6-
Stove gas — *see Gas, stove*						
Stoxil	T49.5X1-	T49.5X2-	T49.5X3-	T49.5X4-	T49.5X5-	T49.5X6-
Stramonium	T48.6X1-	T48.6X2-	T48.6X3-	T48.6X4-	T48.6X5-	T48.6X6-
natural state	T62.2X1-	T62.2X2-	T62.2X3-	T62.2X4-	-	-
Streptodornase	T45.3X1-	T45.3X2-	T45.3X3-	T45.3X4-	T45.3X5-	T45.3X6-
Streptoduocin	T36.5X1-	T36.5X2-	T36.5X3-	T36.5X4-	T36.5X5-	T36.5X6-
Streptokinase	T45.611-	T45.612-	T45.613-	T45.614-	T45.615-	T45.616-
Streptomycin (derivative)	T36.5X1-	T36.5X2-	T36.5X3-	T36.5X4-	T36.5X5-	T36.5X6-
Streptonivicin	T36.5X1-	T36.5X2-	T36.5X3-	T36.5X4-	T36.5X5-	T36.5X6-
Streptovarycin	T36.5X1-	T36.5X2-	T36.5X3-	T36.5X4-	T36.5X5-	T36.5X6-
Streptozocin	T45.1X1-	T45.1X2-	T45.1X3-	T45.1X4-	T45.1X5-	T45.1X6-
Streptozotocin	T45.1X1-	T45.1X2-	T45.1X3-	T45.1X4-	T45.1X5-	T45.1X6-
Stripper (paint) (solvent)	T52.8X1-	T52.8X2-	T52.8X3-	T52.8X4-	-	-
Strobane	T60.1X1-	T60.1X2-	T60.1X3-	T60.1X4-	-	-
Strofantina	T46.0X1-	T46.0X2-	T46.0X3-	T46.0X4-	T46.0X5-	T46.0X6-
Strophanthin (g) (k)	T46.0X1-	T46.0X2-	T46.0X3-	T46.0X4-	T46.0X5-	T46.0X6-
Strophanthus	T46.0X1-	T46.0X2-	T46.0X3-	T46.0X4-	T46.0X5-	T46.0X6-
Strophantin	T46.0X1-	T46.0X2-	T46.0X3-	T46.0X4-	T46.0X5-	T46.0X6-
Strophantin-g	T46.0X1-	T46.0X2-	T46.0X3-	T46.0X4-	T46.0X5-	T46.0X6-
Strychnine (nonmedicinal) (pesticide) (salts)	T65.1X1-	T65.1X2-	T65.1X3-	T65.1X4-	-	-
medicinal	T48.291-	T48.292-	T48.293-	T48.294-	T48.295-	T48.296-
Strychnos (ignatii) — *see Strychnine*						
Styramate	T42.8X1-	T42.8X2-	T42.8X3-	T42.8X4-	T42.8X5-	T42.8X6-
Styrene	T65.891-	T65.892-	T65.893-	T65.894-	-	-

Substance	Poisoning Accidental (unintentional)	Poisoning Intentional self-harm	Poisoning Assault	Poisoning Undetermined	Adverse effect	Underdosing
Succinimide, antiepileptic or anticonvulsant	T42.2X1-	T42.2X2-	T42.2X3-	T42.2X4-	T42.2X5-	T42.2X6-
mercuric — *see Mercury*						
Succinylcholine	T48.1X1-	T48.1X2-	T48.1X3-	T48.1X4-	T48.1X5-	T48.1X6-
Succinylsulfathiazole	T37.0X1-	T37.0X2-	T37.0X3-	T37.0X4-	T37.0X5-	T37.0X6-
Sucralfate	T47.1X1-	T47.1X2-	T47.1X3-	T47.1X4-	T47.1X5-	T47.1X6-
Sucrose	T50.3X1-	T50.3X2-	T50.3X3-	T50.3X4-	T50.3X5-	T50.3X6-
Sufentanil	T40.4X1-	T40.4X2-	T40.4X3-	T40.4X4-	T40.4X5-	T40.4X6-
Sulbactam	T36.0X1-	T36.0X2-	T36.0X3-	T36.0X4-	T36.0X5-	T36.0X6-
Sulbenicillin	T36.0X1-	T36.0X2-	T36.0X3-	T36.0X4-	T36.0X5-	T36.0X6-
Sulbentine	T49.0X1-	T49.0X2-	T49.0X3-	T49.0X4-	T49.0X5-	T49.0X6-
Sulfacetamide	T49.0X1-	T49.0X2-	T49.0X3-	T49.0X4-	T49.0X5-	T49.0X6-
ophthalmic preparation	T49.5X1-	T49.5X2-	T49.5X3-	T49.5X4-	T49.5X5-	T49.5X6-
Sulfachlorpyridazine	T37.0X1-	T37.0X2-	T37.0X3-	T37.0X4-	T37.0X5-	T37.0X6-
Sulfacitine	T37.0X1-	T37.0X2-	T37.0X3-	T37.0X4-	T37.0X5-	T37.0X6-
Sulfadiasulfone sodium	T37.0X1-	T37.0X2-	T37.0X3-	T37.0X4-	T37.0X5-	T37.0X6-
Sulfadiazine	T37.0X1-	T37.0X2-	T37.0X3-	T37.0X4-	T37.0X5-	T37.0X6-
silver (topical)	T49.0X1-	T49.0X2-	T49.0X3-	T49.0X4-	T49.0X5-	T49.0X6-
Sulfadimethoxine	T37.0X1-	T37.0X2-	T37.0X3-	T37.0X4-	T37.0X5-	T37.0X6-
Sulfadimidine	T37.0X1-	T37.0X2-	T37.0X3-	T37.0X4-	T37.0X5-	T37.0X6-
Sulfadoxine	T37.0X1-	T37.0X2-	T37.0X3-	T37.0X4-	T37.0X5-	T37.0X6-
with pyrimethamine	T37.2X1-	T37.2X2-	T37.2X3-	T37.2X4-	T37.2X5-	T37.2X6-
Sulfaethidole	T37.0X1-	T37.0X2-	T37.0X3-	T37.0X4-	T37.0X5-	T37.0X6-
Sulfafurazole	T37.0X1-	T37.0X2-	T37.0X3-	T37.0X4-	T37.0X5-	T37.0X6-
Sulfaguanidine	T37.0X1-	T37.0X2-	T37.0X3-	T37.0X4-	T37.0X5-	T37.0X6-
Sulfalene	T37.0X1-	T37.0X2-	T37.0X3-	T37.0X4-	T37.0X5-	T37.0X6-
Sulfaloxate	T37.0X1-	T37.0X2-	T37.0X3-	T37.0X4-	T37.0X5-	T37.0X6-
Sulfaloxic acid	T37.0X1-	T37.0X2-	T37.0X3-	T37.0X4-	T37.0X5-	T37.0X6-
Sulfamazone	T39.2X1-	T39.2X2-	T39.2X3-	T39.2X4-	T39.2X5-	T39.2X6-
Sulfamerazine	T37.0X1-	T37.0X2-	T37.0X3-	T37.0X4-	T37.0X5-	T37.0X6-
Sulfameter	T37.0X1-	T37.0X2-	T37.0X3-	T37.0X4-	T37.0X5-	T37.0X6-
Sulfamethazine	T37.0X1-	T37.0X2-	T37.0X3-	T37.0X4-	T37.0X5-	T37.0X6-
Sulfamethizole	T37.0X1-	T37.0X2-	T37.0X3-	T37.0X4-	T37.0X5-	T37.0X6-
Sulfamethoxazole	T37.0X1-	T37.0X2-	T37.0X3-	T37.0X4-	T37.0X5-	T37.0X6-
with trimethoprim	T36.8X1-	T36.8X2-	T36.8X3-	T36.8X4-	T36.8X5-	T36.8X6-
Sulfamethoxydiazine	T37.0X1-	T37.0X2-	T37.0X3-	T37.0X4-	T37.0X5-	T37.0X6-
Sulfamethoxypyridazine	T37.0X1-	T37.0X2-	T37.0X3-	T37.0X4-	T37.0X5-	T37.0X6-
Sulfamethylthiazole	T37.0X1-	T37.0X2-	T37.0X3-	T37.0X4-	T37.0X5-	T37.0X6-
Sulfametoxydiazine	T37.0X1-	T37.0X2-	T37.0X3-	T37.0X4-	T37.0X5-	T37.0X6-
Sulfamidopyrine	T39.2X1-	T39.2X2-	T39.2X3-	T39.2X4-	T39.2X5-	T39.2X6-
Sulfamonomethoxine	T37.0X1-	T37.0X2-	T37.0X3-	T37.0X4-	T37.0X5-	T37.0X6-
Sulfamoxole	T37.0X1-	T37.0X2-	T37.0X3-	T37.0X4-	T37.0X5-	T37.0X6-
Sulfamylon	T49.0X1-	T49.0X2-	T49.0X3-	T49.0X4-	T49.0X5-	T49.0X6-
Sulfan blue (diagnostic dye)	T50.8X1-	T50.8X2-	T50.8X3-	T50.8X4-	T50.8X5-	T50.8X6-
Sulfanilamide	T37.0X1-	T37.0X2-	T37.0X3-	T37.0X4-	T37.0X5-	T37.0X6-
Sulfanilylguanidine	T37.0X1-	T37.0X2-	T37.0X3-	T37.0X4-	T37.0X5-	T37.0X6-
Sulfaperin	T37.0X1-	T37.0X2-	T37.0X3-	T37.0X4-	T37.0X5-	T37.0X6-
Sulfaphenazole	T37.0X1-	T37.0X2-	T37.0X3-	T37.0X4-	T37.0X5-	T37.0X6-
Sulfaphenylthiazole	T37.0X1-	T37.0X2-	T37.0X3-	T37.0X4-	T37.0X5-	T37.0X6-
Sulfaproxyline	T37.0X1-	T37.0X2-	T37.0X3-	T37.0X4-	T37.0X5-	T37.0X6-
Sulfapyridine	T37.0X1-	T37.0X2-	T37.0X3-	T37.0X4-	T37.0X5-	T37.0X6-
Sulfapyrimidine	T37.0X1-	T37.0X2-	T37.0X3-	T37.0X4-	T37.0X5-	T37.0X6-
Sulfarsphenamine	T37.8X1-	T37.8X2-	T37.8X3-	T37.8X4-	T37.8X5-	T37.8X6-
Sulfasalazine	T37.0X1-	T37.0X2-	T37.0X3-	T37.0X4-	T37.0X5-	T37.0X6-
Sulfasuxidine	T37.0X1-	T37.0X2-	T37.0X3-	T37.0X4-	T37.0X5-	T37.0X6-
Sulfasymazine	T37.0X1-	T37.0X2-	T37.0X3-	T37.0X4-	T37.0X5-	T37.0X6-
Sulfated amylopectin	T47.8X1-	T47.8X2-	T47.8X3-	T47.8X4-	T47.8X5-	T47.8X6-
Sulfathiazole	T37.0X1-	T37.0X2-	T37.0X3-	T37.0X4-	T37.0X5-	T37.0X6-
Sulfatostearate	T49.2X1-	T49.2X2-	T49.2X3-	T49.2X4-	T49.2X5-	T49.2X6-

Substance	Poisoning Accidental (unintentional)	Poisoning Intentional self-harm	Poisoning Assault	Poisoning Undetermined	Adverse effect	Underdosing
Sulfinpyrazone	T50.4X1-	T50.4X2-	T50.4X3-	T50.4X4-	T50.4X5-	T50.4X6-
Sulfiram	T49.0X1-	T49.0X2-	T49.0X3-	T49.0X4-	T49.0X5-	T49.0X6-
Sulfisomidine	T37.0X1-	T37.0X2-	T37.0X3-	T37.0X4-	T37.0X5-	T37.0X6-
Sulfisoxazole	T37.0X1-	T37.0X2-	T37.0X3-	T37.0X4-	T37.0X5-	T37.0X6-
ophthalmic preparation	T49.5X1-	T49.5X2-	T49.5X3-	T49.5X4-	T49.5X5-	T49.5X6-
Sulfobromophthalein (sodium)	T50.8X1-	T50.8X2-	T50.8X3-	T50.8X4-	T50.8X5-	T50.8X6-
Sulfobromphthalein	T50.8X1-	T50.8X2-	T50.8X3-	T50.8X4-	T50.8X5-	T50.8X6-
Sulfogaiacol	T48.4X1-	T48.4X2-	T48.4X3-	T48.4X4-	T48.4X5-	T48.4X6-
Sulfomyxin	T36.8X1-	T36.8X2-	T36.8X3-	T36.8X4-	T36.8X5-	T36.8X6-
Sulfonal	T42.6X1-	T42.6X2-	T42.6X3-	T42.6X4-	T42.6X5-	T42.6X6-
Sulfonamide NEC	T37.0X1-	T37.0X2-	T37.0X3-	T37.0X4-	T37.0X5-	T37.0X6-
eye	T49.5X1-	T49.5X2-	T49.5X3-	T49.5X4-	T49.5X5-	T49.5X6-
Sulfonazide	T37.1X1-	T37.1X2-	T37.1X3-	T37.1X4-	T37.1X5-	T37.1X6-
Sulfones	T37.1X1-	T37.1X2-	T37.1X3-	T37.1X4-	T37.1X5-	T37.1X6-
Sulfonethylmethane	T42.6X1-	T42.6X2-	T42.6X3-	T42.6X4-	T42.6X5-	T42.6X6-
Sulfonmethane	T42.6X1-	T42.6X2-	T42.6X3-	T42.6X4-	T42.6X5-	T42.6X6-
Sulfonphthal, sulfonphthol	T50.8X1-	T50.8X2-	T50.8X3-	T50.8X4-	T50.8X5-	T50.8X6-
Sulfonylurea derivatives, oral	T38.3X1-	T38.3X2-	T38.3X3-	T38.3X4-	T38.3X5-	T38.3X6-
Sulforidazine	T43.3X1-	T43.3X2-	T43.3X3-	T43.3X4-	T43.3X5-	T43.3X6-
Sulfoxone	T37.1X1-	T37.1X2-	T37.1X3-	T37.1X4-	T37.1X5-	T37.1X6-
Sulfur, sulfurated, sulfuric, sulfurous, sulfuryl (compounds NEC) (medicinal)	T49.4X1-	T49.4X2-	T49.4X3-	T49.4X4-	T49.4X5-	T49.4X6-
acid	T54.2X1-	T54.2X2-	T54.2X3-	T54.2X4-	-	-
dioxide (gas)	T59.1X1-	T59.1X2-	T59.1X3-	T59.1X4-	-	-
ether — *see Ether(s)*						
hydrogen	T59.6X1-	T59.6X2-	T59.6X3-	T59.6X4-	-	-
medicinal (keratolytic) (ointment) NEC	T49.4X1-	T49.4X2-	T49.4X3-	T49.4X4-	T49.4X5-	T49.4X6-
ointment	T49.0X1-	T49.0X2-	T49.0X3-	T49.0X4-	T49.0X5-	T49.0X6-
pesticide (vapor)	T60.91X-	T60.92X-	T60.93X-	T60.94X-	-	-
vapor NEC	T59.891-	T59.892-	T59.893-	T59.894-	-	-
Sulfuric acid	T54.2X1-	T54.2X2-	T54.2X3-	T54.2X4-	-	-
Sulglicotide	T47.1X1-	T47.1X2-	T47.1X3-	T47.1X4-	T47.1X5-	T47.1X6-
Sulindac	T39.391-	T39.392-	T39.393-	T39.394-	T39.395-	T39.396-
Sulisatin	T47.2X1-	T47.2X2-	T47.2X3-	T47.2X4-	T47.2X5-	T47.2X6-
Sulisobenzone	T49.3X1-	T49.3X2-	T49.3X3-	T49.3X4-	T49.3X5-	T49.3X6-
Sulkowitch's reagent	T50.8X1-	T50.8X2-	T50.8X3-	T50.8X4-	T50.8X5-	T50.8X6-
Sulmetozine	T44.3X1-	T44.3X2-	T44.3X3-	T44.3X4-	T44.3X5-	T44.3X6-
Suloctidil	T46.7X1-	T46.7X2-	T46.7X3-	T46.7X4-	T46.7X5-	T46.7X6-
Sulph- — *see also Sulf-*						
Sulphadiazine	T37.0X1-	T37.0X2-	T37.0X3-	T37.0X4-	T37.0X5-	T37.0X6-
Sulphadimethoxine	T37.0X1-	T37.0X2-	T37.0X3-	T37.0X4-	T37.0X5-	T37.0X6-
Sulphadimidine	T37.0X1-	T37.0X2-	T37.0X3-	T37.0X4-	T37.0X5-	T37.0X6-
Sulphadione	T37.1X1-	T37.1X2-	T37.1X3-	T37.1X4-	T37.1X5-	T37.1X6-
Sulphafurazole	T37.0X1-	T37.0X2-	T37.0X3-	T37.0X4-	T37.0X5-	T37.0X6-
Sulphamethizole	T37.0X1-	T37.0X2-	T37.0X3-	T37.0X4-	T37.0X5-	T37.0X6-
Sulphamethoxazole	T37.0X1-	T37.0X2-	T37.0X3-	T37.0X4-	T37.0X5-	T37.0X6-
Sulphan blue	T50.8X1-	T50.8X2-	T50.8X3-	T50.8X4-	T50.8X5-	T50.8X6-
Sulphaphenazole	T37.0X1-	T37.0X2-	T37.0X3-	T37.0X4-	T37.0X5-	T37.0X6-
Sulphapyridine	T37.0X1-	T37.0X2-	T37.0X3-	T37.0X4-	T37.0X5-	T37.0X6-
Sulphasalazine	T37.0X1-	T37.0X2-	T37.0X3-	T37.0X4-	T37.0X5-	T37.0X6-
Sulphinpyrazone	T50.4X1-	T50.4X2-	T50.4X3-	T50.4X4-	T50.4X5-	T50.4X6-
Sulpiride	T43.591-	T43.592-	T43.593-	T43.594-	T43.595-	T43.596-
Sulprostone	T48.0X1-	T48.0X2-	T48.0X3-	T48.0X4-	T48.0X5-	T48.0X6-
Sulpyrine	T39.2X1-	T39.2X2-	T39.2X3-	T39.2X4-	T39.2X5-	T39.2X6-
Sultamicillin	T36.0X1-	T36.0X2-	T36.0X3-	T36.0X4-	T36.0X5-	T36.0X6-
Sulthiame	T42.6X1-	T42.6X2-	T42.6X3-	T42.6X4-	T42.6X5-	T42.6X6-
Sultiame	T42.6X1-	T42.6X2-	T42.6X3-	T42.6X4-	T42.6X5-	T42.6X6-
Sultopride	T43.591-	T43.592-	T43.593-	T43.594-	T43.595-	T43.596-

Substance	Poisoning Accidental (unintentional)	Poisoning Intentional self-harm	Poisoning Assault	Poisoning Undetermined	Adverse effect	Underdosing
Sumatriptan	T39.8X1-	T39.8X2-	T39.8X3-	T39.8X4-	T39.8X5-	T39.8X6-
Sunflower seed oil	T46.6X1-	T46.6X2-	T46.6X3-	T46.6X4-	T46.6X5-	T46.6X6-
Superinone	T48.4X1-	T48.4X2-	T48.4X3-	T48.4X4-	T48.4X5-	T48.4X6-
Suprofen	T39.311-	T39.312-	T39.313-	T39.314-	T39.315-	T39.316-
Suramin (sodium)	T37.4X1-	T37.4X2-	T37.4X3-	T37.4X4-	T37.4X5-	T37.4X6-
Surfacaine	T41.3X1-	T41.3X2-	T41.3X3-	T41.3X4-	T41.3X5-	T41.3X6-
Surital	T41.1X1-	T41.1X2-	T41.1X3-	T41.1X4-	T41.1X5-	T41.1X6-
Sutilains	T45.3X1-	T45.3X2-	T45.3X3-	T45.3X4-	T45.3X5-	T45.3X6-
Suxamethonium (chloride)	T48.1X1-	T48.1X2-	T48.1X3-	T48.1X4-	T48.1X5-	T48.1X6-
Suxethonium (chloride)	T48.1X1-	T48.1X2-	T48.1X3-	T48.1X4-	T48.1X5-	T48.1X6-
Suxibuzone	T39.2X1-	T39.2X2-	T39.2X3-	T39.2X4-	T39.2X5-	T39.2X6-
Sweet niter spirit	T46.3X1-	T46.3X2-	T46.3X3-	T46.3X4-	T46.3X5-	T46.3X6-
Sweet oil (birch)	T49.3X1-	T49.3X2-	T49.3X3-	T49.3X4-	T49.3X5-	T49.3X6-
Sweetener	T50.901-	T50.902-	T50.903-	T50.904-	T50.905-	T50.906-
Sym-dichloroethyl ether	T53.6X1-	T53.6X2-	T53.6X3-	T53.6X4-	-	-
Sympatholytic NEC	T44.8X1-	T44.8X2-	T44.8X3-	T44.8X4-	T44.8X5-	T44.8X6-
haloalkylamine	T44.8X1-	T44.8X2-	T44.8X3-	T44.8X4-	T44.8X5-	T44.8X6-
Sympathomimetic NEC	T44.901-	T44.902-	T44.903-	T44.904-	T44.905-	T44.906-
anti-common-cold	T48.5X1-	T48.5X2-	T48.5X3-	T48.5X4-	T48.5X5-	T48.5X6-
bronchodilator	T48.6X1-	T48.6X2-	T48.6X3-	T48.6X4-	T48.6X5-	T48.6X6-
specified NEC	T44.991-	T44.992-	T44.993-	T44.994-	T44.995-	T44.996-
Synagis	T50.B91-	T50.B92-	T50.B93-	T50.B94-	T50.B95-	T50.B96-
Synalar	T49.0X1-	T49.0X2-	T49.0X3-	T49.0X4-	T49.0X5-	T49.0X6-
Synthroid	T38.1X1-	T38.1X2-	T38.1X3-	T38.1X4-	T38.1X5-	T38.1X6-
Syntocinon	T48.0X1-	T48.0X2-	T48.0X3-	T48.0X4-	T48.0X5-	T48.0X6-
Syrosingopine	T46.5X1-	T46.5X2-	T46.5X3-	T46.5X4-	T46.5X5-	T46.5X6-
Systemic drug	T45.91X-	T45.92X-	T45.93X-	T45.94X-	T45.95X-	T45.96X-
specified NEC	T45.8X1-	T45.8X2-	T45.8X3-	T45.8X4-	T45.8X5-	T45.8X6-
2,4,5-T	T60.3X1-	T60.3X2-	T60.3X3-	T60.3X4-	-	-
Tablets — *see also specified substance*	T50.901-	T50.902-	T50.903-	T50.904-	T50.905-	T50.906-
Tace	T38.5X1-	T38.5X2-	T38.5X3-	T38.5X4-	T38.5X5-	T38.5X6-
Tacrine	T44.0X1-	T44.0X2-	T44.0X3-	T44.0X4-	T44.0X5-	T44.0X6-
Tadalafil	T46.7X1-	T46.7X2-	T46.7X3-	T46.7X4-	T46.7X5-	T46.7X6-
Talampicillin	T36.0X1-	T36.0X2-	T36.0X3-	T36.0X4-	T36.0X5-	T36.0X6-
Talbutal	T42.3X1-	T42.3X2-	T42.3X3-	T42.3X4-	T42.3X5-	T42.3X6-
Talc powder	T49.3X1-	T49.3X2-	T49.3X3-	T49.3X4-	T49.3X5-	T49.3X6-
Talcum	T49.3X1-	T49.3X2-	T49.3X3-	T49.3X4-	T49.3X5-	T49.3X6-
Taleranol	T38.6X1-	T38.6X2-	T38.6X3-	T38.6X4-	T38.6X5-	T38.6X6-
Tamoxifen	T38.6X1-	T38.6X2-	T38.6X3-	T38.6X4-	T38.6X5-	T38.6X6-
Tamsulosin	T44.6X1-	T44.6X2-	T44.6X3-	T44.6X4-	T44.6X5-	T44.6X6-
Tandearil, tanderil	T39.2X1-	T39.2X2-	T39.2X3-	T39.2X4-	T39.2X5-	T39.2X6-
Tannic acid	T49.2X1-	T49.2X2-	T49.2X3-	T49.2X4-	T49.2X5-	T49.2X6-
medicinal (astringent)	T49.2X1-	T49.2X2-	T49.2X3-	T49.2X4-	T49.2X5-	T49.2X6-
Tannin — *see Tannic acid*						
Tansy	T62.2X1-	T62.2X2-	T62.2X3-	T62.2X4-	-	-
TAO	T36.3X1-	T36.3X2-	T36.3X3-	T36.3X4-	T36.3X5-	T36.3X6-
Tapazole	T38.2X1-	T38.2X2-	T38.2X3-	T38.2X4-	T38.2X5-	T38.2X6-
Tar NEC	T52.0X1-	T52.0X2-	T52.0X3-	T52.0X4-	-	-
camphor	T60.1X1-	T60.1X2-	T60.1X3-	T60.1X4-	-	-
distillate	T49.1X1-	T49.1X2-	T49.1X3-	T49.1X4-	T49.1X5-	T49.1X6-
fumes	T59.891-	T59.892-	T59.893-	T59.894-	-	-
medicinal	T49.1X1-	T49.1X2-	T49.1X3-	T49.1X4-	T49.1X5-	T49.1X6-
ointment	T49.1X1-	T49.1X2-	T49.1X3-	T49.1X4-	T49.1X5-	T49.1X6-
Taractan	T43.591-	T43.592-	T43.593-	T43.594-	T43.595-	T43.596-
Tarantula (venomous)	T63.321-	T63.322-	T63.323-	T63.324-	-	-
Tartar emetic	T37.8X1-	T37.8X2-	T37.8X3-	T37.8X4-	T37.8X5-	T37.8X6-
Tartaric acid	T65.891-	T65.892-	T65.893-	T65.894-	-	-
Tartrate, laxative	T47.4X1-	T47.4X2-	T47.4X3-	T47.4X4-	T47.4X5-	T47.4X6-

Substance	Poisoning Accidental (unintentional)	Poisoning Intentional self-harm	Poisoning Assault	Poisoning Undetermined	Adverse effect	Underdosing
Tartrated antimony (anti-infective)	T37.8X1-	T37.8X2-	T37.8X3-	T37.8X4-	T37.8X5-	T37.8X6-
Tauromustine	T45.1X1-	T45.1X2-	T45.1X3-	T45.1X4-	T45.1X5-	T45.1X6-
TCA — *see Trichloroacetic acid*						
TCDD	T53.7X1-	T53.7X2-	T53.7X3-	T53.7X4-	-	-
TDI (vapor)	T65.0X1-	T65.0X2-	T65.0X3-	T65.0X4-	-	-
Tear						
gas	T59.3X1-	T59.3X2-	T59.3X3-	T59.3X4-	-	-
solution	T49.5X1-	T49.5X2-	T49.5X3-	T49.5X4-	T49.5X5-	T49.5X6-
Teclothiazide	T50.2X1-	T50.2X2-	T50.2X3-	T50.2X4-	T50.2X5-	T50.2X6-
Teclozan	T37.3X1-	T37.3X2-	T37.3X3-	T37.3X4-	T37.3X5-	T37.3X6-
Tegafur	T45.1X1-	T45.1X2-	T45.1X3-	T45.1X4-	T45.1X5-	T45.1X6-
Tegretol	T42.1X1-	T42.1X2-	T42.1X3-	T42.1X4-	T42.1X5-	T42.1X6-
Teicoplanin	T36.8X1-	T36.8X2-	T36.8X3-	T36.8X4-	T36.8X5-	T36.8X6-
Telepaque	T50.8X1-	T50.8X2-	T50.8X3-	T50.8X4-	T50.8X5-	T50.8X6-
Tellurium	T56.891-	T56.892-	T56.893-	T56.894-	-	-
fumes	T56.891-	T56.892-	T56.893-	T56.894-	-	-
TEM	T45.1X1-	T45.1X2-	T45.1X3-	T45.1X4-	T45.1X5-	T45.1X6-
Temazepam	T42.4X1-	T42.4X2-	T42.4X3-	T42.4X4-	T42.4X5-	T42.4X6-
Temocillin	T36.0X1-	T36.0X2-	T36.0X3-	T36.0X4-	T36.0X5-	T36.0X6-
Tenamfetamine	T43.621-	T43.622-	T43.623-	T43.624-	T43.625-	T43.626-
Teniposide	T45.1X1-	T45.1X2-	T45.1X3-	T45.1X4-	T45.1X5-	T45.1X6-
Tenitramine	T46.3X1-	T46.3X2-	T46.3X3-	T46.3X4-	T46.3X5-	T46.3X6-
Tenoglicin	T48.4X1-	T48.4X2-	T48.4X3-	T48.4X4-	T48.4X5-	T48.4X6-
Tenonitrozole	T37.3X1-	T37.3X2-	T37.3X3-	T37.3X4-	T37.3X5-	T37.3X6-
Tenoxicam	T39.391-	T39.392-	T39.393-	T39.394-	T39.395-	T39.396-
TEPA	T45.1X1-	T45.1X2-	T45.1X3-	T45.1X4-	T45.1X5-	T45.1X6-
TEPP	T60.0X1-	T60.0X2-	T60.0X3-	T60.0X4-	-	-
Teprotide	T46.5X1-	T46.5X2-	T46.5X3-	T46.5X4-	T46.5X5-	T46.5X6-
Terazosin	T44.6X1-	T44.6X2-	T44.6X3-	T44.6X4-	T44.6X5-	T44.6X6-
Terbufos	T60.0X1-	T60.0X2-	T60.0X3-	T60.0X4-	-	-
Terbutaline	T48.6X1-	T48.6X2-	T48.6X3-	T48.6X4-	T48.6X5-	T48.6X6-
Terconazole	T49.0X1-	T49.0X2-	T49.0X3-	T49.0X4-	T49.0X5-	T49.0X6-
Terfenadine	T45.0X1-	T45.0X2-	T45.0X3-	T45.0X4-	T45.0X5-	T45.0X6-
Teriparatide (acetate)	T50.991-	T50.992-	T50.993-	T50.994-	T50.995-	T50.996-
Terizidone	T37.1X1-	T37.1X2-	T37.1X3-	T37.1X4-	T37.1X5-	T37.1X6-
Terlipressin	T38.891-	T38.892-	T38.893-	T38.894-	T38.895-	T38.896-
Terodiline	T46.3X1-	T46.3X2-	T46.3X3-	T46.3X4-	T46.3X5-	T46.3X6-
Teroxalene	T37.4X1-	T37.4X2-	T37.4X3-	T37.4X4-	T37.4X5-	T37.4X6-
Terpin (cis) hydrate	T48.4X1-	T48.4X2-	T48.4X3-	T48.4X4-	T48.4X5-	T48.4X6-
Terramycin	T36.4X1-	T36.4X2-	T36.4X3-	T36.4X4-	T36.4X5-	T36.4X6-
Tertatolol	T44.7X1-	T44.7X2-	T44.7X3-	T44.7X4-	T44.7X5-	T44.7X6-
Tessalon	T48.3X1-	T48.3X2-	T48.3X3-	T48.3X4-	T48.3X5-	T48.3X6-
Testolactone	T38.7X1-	T38.7X2-	T38.7X3-	T38.7X4-	T38.7X5-	T38.7X6-
Testosterone	T38.7X1-	T38.7X2-	T38.7X3-	T38.7X4-	T38.7X5-	T38.7X6-
Tetanus toxoid or vaccine	T50.A91-	T50.A92-	T50.A93-	T50.A94-	T50.A95-	T50.A96-
antitoxin	T50.Z11-	T50.Z12-	T50.Z13-	T50.Z14-	T50.Z15-	T50.Z16-
immune globulin (human)	T50.Z11-	T50.Z12-	T50.Z13-	T50.Z14-	T50.Z15-	T50.Z16-
toxoid	T50.A91-	T50.A92-	T50.A93-	T50.A94-	T50.A95-	T50.A96-
with diphtheria toxoid	T50.A21-	T50.A22-	T50.A23-	T50.A24-	T50.A25-	T50.A26-
with pertussis	T50.A11-	T50.A12-	T50.A13-	T50.A14-	T50.A15-	T50.A16-
Tetrabenazine	T43.591-	T43.592-	T43.593-	T43.594-	T43.595-	T43.596-
Tetracaine	T41.3X1-	T41.3X2-	T41.3X3-	T41.3X4-	T41.3X5-	T41.3X6-
nerve block (peripheral) (plexus)	T41.3X1-	T41.3X2-	T41.3X3-	T41.3X4-	T41.3X5-	T41.3X6-
regional	T41.3X1-	T41.3X2-	T41.3X3-	T41.3X4-	T41.3X5-	T41.3X6-
spinal	T41.3X1-	T41.3X2-	T41.3X3-	T41.3X4-	T41.3X5-	T41.3X6-
Tetrachlorethylene — *see Tetrachloroethylene*						
Tetrachlormethiazide	T50.2X1-	T50.2X2-	T50.2X3-	T50.2X4-	T50.2X5-	T50.2X6-
2,3,7,8-Tetrachlorodibenzo-p-dioxin	T53.7X1-	T53.7X2-	T53.7X3-	T53.7X4-	-	-

Substance	Poisoning Accidental (unintentional)	Poisoning Intentional self-harm	Poisoning Assault	Poisoning Undetermined	Adverse effect	Underdosing
Tetrachloroethane	T53.6X1-	T53.6X2-	T53.6X3-	T53.6X4-	-	-
vapor	T53.6X1-	T53.6X2-	T53.6X3-	T53.6X4-	-	-
paint or varnish	T53.6X1-	T53.6X2-	T53.6X3-	T53.6X4-	-	-
Tetrachloroethylene (liquid)	T53.3X1-	T53.3X2-	T53.3X3-	T53.3X4-	-	-
medicinal	T37.4X1-	T37.4X2-	T37.4X3-	T37.4X4-	T37.4X5-	T37.4X6-
vapor	T53.3X1-	T53.3X2-	T53.3X3-	T53.3X4-		
Tetrachloromethane — *see Carbon tetrachloride*						
Tetracosactide	T38.811-	T38.812-	T38.813-	T38.814-	T38.815-	T38.816-
Tetracosactrin	T38.811-	T38.812-	T38.813-	T38.814-	T38.815-	T38.816-
Tetracycline	T36.4X1-	T36.4X2-	T36.4X3-	T36.4X4-	T36.4X5-	T36.4X6-
ophthalmic preparation	T49.5X1-	T49.5X2-	T49.5X3-	T49.5X4-	T49.5X5-	T49.5X6-
topical NEC	T49.0X1-	T49.0X2-	T49.0X3-	T49.0X4-	T49.0X5-	T49.0X6-
Tetradifon	T60.8X1-	T60.8X2-	T60.8X3-	T60.8X4-	-	-
Tetradotoxin	T61.771-	T61.772-	T61.773-	T61.774-	-	-
Tetraethyl						
lead	T56.0X1-	T56.0X2-	T56.0X3-	T56.0X4-	-	-
pyrophosphate	T60.0X1-	T60.0X2-	T60.0X3-	T60.0X4-	-	-
Tetraethylammonium chloride	T44.2X1-	T44.2X2-	T44.2X3-	T44.2X4-	T44.2X5-	T44.2X6-
Tetraethylthiuram disulfide	T50.6X1-	T50.6X2-	T50.6X3-	T50.6X4-	T50.6X5-	T50.6X6-
Tetrahydroaminoacridine	T44.0X1-	T44.0X2-	T44.0X3-	T44.0X4-	T44.0X5-	T44.0X6-
Tetrahydrocannabinol	T40.7X1-	T40.7X2-	T40.7X3-	T40.7X4-	T40.7X5-	T40.7X6-
Tetrahydrofuran	T52.8X1-	T52.8X2-	T52.8X3-	T52.8X4-	-	-
Tetrahydronaphthalene	T52.8X1-	T52.8X2-	T52.8X3-	T52.8X4-	-	-
Tetrahydrozoline	T49.5X1-	T49.5X2-	T49.5X3-	T49.5X4-	T49.5X5-	T49.5X6-
Tetralin	T52.8X1-	T52.8X2-	T52.8X3-	T52.8X4-	-	-
Tetramethrin	T60.2X1-	T60.2X2-	T60.2X3-	T60.2X4-	-	-
Tetramethylthiuram (disulfide) NEC	T60.3X1-	T60.3X2-	T60.3X3-	T60.3X4-	-	-
medicinal	T49.0X1-	T49.0X2-	T49.0X3-	T49.0X4-	T49.0X5-	T49.0X6-
Tetramisole	T37.4X1-	T37.4X2-	T37.4X3-	T37.4X4-	T37.4X5-	T37.4X6-
Tetranicotinoyl fructose	T46.7X1-	T46.7X2-	T46.7X3-	T46.7X4-	T46.7X5-	T46.7X6-
Tetrazepam	T42.4X1-	T42.4X2-	T42.4X3-	T42.4X4-	T42.4X5-	T42.4X6-
Tetronal	T42.6X1-	T42.6X2-	T42.6X3-	T42.6X4-	T42.6X5-	T42.6X6-
Tetryl	T65.3X1-	T65.3X2-	T65.3X3-	T65.3X4-	-	-
Tetrylammonium chloride	T44.2X1-	T44.2X2-	T44.2X3-	T44.2X4-	T44.2X5-	T44.2X6-
Tetryzoline	T49.5X1-	T49.5X2-	T49.5X3-	T49.5X4-	T49.5X5-	T49.5X6-
Thalidomide	T45.1X1-	T45.1X2-	T45.1X3-	T45.1X4-	T45.1X5-	T45.1X6-
Thallium (compounds) (dust) NEC	T56.811-	T56.812-	T56.813-	T56.814-	-	-
pesticide	T60.4X1-	T60.4X2-	T60.4X3-	T60.4X4-	-	-
THC	T40.7X1-	T40.7X2-	T40.7X3-	T40.7X4-	T40.7X5-	T40.7X6-
Thebacon	T48.3X1-	T48.3X2-	T48.3X3-	T48.3X4-	T48.3X5-	T48.3X6-
Thebaine	T40.2X1-	T40.2X2-	T40.2X3-	T40.2X4-	T40.2X5-	T40.2X6-
Thenoic acid	T49.6X1-	T49.6X2-	T49.6X3-	T49.6X4-	T49.6X5-	T49.6X6-
Thenyldiamine	T45.0X1-	T45.0X2-	T45.0X3-	T45.0X4-	T45.0X5-	T45.0X6-
Theobromine (calcium salicylate)	T48.6X1-	T48.6X2-	T48.6X3-	T48.6X4-	T48.6X5-	T48.6X6-
sodium salicylate	T48.6X1-	T48.6X2-	T48.6X3-	T48.6X4-	T48.6X5-	T48.6X6-
Theophyllamine	T48.6X1-	T48.6X2-	T48.6X3-	T48.6X4-	T48.6X5-	T48.6X6-
Theophylline	T48.6X1-	T48.6X2-	T48.6X3-	T48.6X4-	T48.6X5-	T48.6X6-
aminobenzoic acid	T48.6X1-	T48.6X2-	T48.6X3-	T48.6X4-	T48.6X5-	T48.6X6-
ethylenediamine	T48.6X1-	T48.6X2-	T48.6X3-	T48.6X4-	T48.6X5-	T48.6X6-
piperazine p-amino-benzoate	T48.6X1-	T48.6X2-	T48.6X3-	T48.6X4-	T48.6X5-	T48.6X6-
Thiabendazole	T37.4X1-	T37.4X2-	T37.4X3-	T37.4X4-	T37.4X5-	T37.4X6-
Thialbarbital	T41.1X1-	T41.1X2-	T41.1X3-	T41.1X4-	T41.1X5-	T41.1X6-
Thiamazole	T38.2X1-	T38.2X2-	T38.2X3-	T38.2X4-	T38.2X5-	T38.2X6-
Thiambutosine	T37.1X1-	T37.1X2-	T37.1X3-	T37.1X4-	T37.1X5-	T37.1X6-
Thiamine	T45.2X1-	T45.2X2-	T45.2X3-	T45.2X4-	T45.2X5-	T45.2X6-
Thiamphenicol	T36.2X1-	T36.2X2-	T36.2X3-	T36.2X4-	T36.2X5-	T36.2X6-

Substance	Poisoning Accidental (unintentional)	Poisoning Intentional self-harm	Poisoning Assault	Poisoning Undetermined	Adverse effect	Underdosing
Thiamylal	T41.1X1-	T41.1X2-	T41.1X3-	T41.1X4-	T41.1X5-	T41.1X6-
sodium	T41.1X1-	T41.1X2-	T41.1X3-	T41.1X4-	T41.1X5-	T41.1X6-
Thiazesim	T43.291-	T43.292-	T43.293-	T43.294-	T43.295-	T43.296-
Thiazides (diuretics)	T50.2X1-	T50.2X2-	T50.2X3-	T50.2X4-	T50.2X5-	T50.2X6-
Thiazinamium metilsulfate	T43.3X1-	T43.3X2-	T43.3X3-	T43.3X4-	T43.3X5-	T43.3X6-
Thiethylperazine	T43.3X1-	T43.3X2-	T43.3X3-	T43.3X4-	T43.3X5-	T43.3X6-
Thimerosal	T49.0X1-	T49.0X2-	T49.0X3-	T49.0X4-	T49.0X5-	T49.0X6-
ophthalmic preparation	T49.5X1-	T49.5X2-	T49.5X3-	T49.5X4-	T49.5X5-	T49.5X6-
Thioacetazone	T37.1X1-	T37.1X2-	T37.1X3-	T37.1X4-	T37.1X5-	T37.1X6-
with isoniazid	T37.1X1-	T37.1X2-	T37.1X3-	T37.1X4-	T37.1X5-	T37.1X6-
Thiobarbital sodium	T41.1X1-	T41.1X2-	T41.1X3-	T41.1X4-	T41.1X5-	T41.1X6-
Thiobarbiturate anesthetic	T41.1X1-	T41.1X2-	T41.1X3-	T41.1X4-	T41.1X5-	T41.1X6-
Thiobismol	T37.8X1-	T37.8X2-	T37.8X3-	T37.8X4-	T37.8X5-	T37.8X6-
Thiobutabarbital sodium	T41.1X1-	T41.1X2-	T41.1X3-	T41.1X4-	T41.1X5-	T41.1X6-
Thiocarbamate (insecticide)	T60.0X1-	T60.0X2-	T60.0X3-	T60.0X4-	-	-
Thiocarbamide	T38.2X1-	T38.2X2-	T38.2X3-	T38.2X4-	T38.2X5-	T38.2X6-
Thiocarbarsone	T37.8X1-	T37.8X2-	T37.8X3-	T37.8X4-	T37.8X5-	T37.8X6-
Thiocarlide	T37.1X1-	T37.1X2-	T37.1X3-	T37.1X4-	T37.1X5-	T37.1X6-
Thioctamide	T50.991-	T50.992-	T50.993-	T50.994-	T50.995-	T50.996-
Thioctic acid	T50.991-	T50.992-	T50.993-	T50.994-	T50.995-	T50.996-
Thiofos	T60.0X1-	T60.0X2-	T60.0X3-	T60.0X4-	-	-
Thioglycolate	T49.4X1-	T49.4X2-	T49.4X3-	T49.4X4-	T49.4X5-	T49.4X6-
Thioglycolic acid	T65.891-	T65.892-	T65.893-	T65.894-	-	-
Thioguanine	T45.1X1-	T45.1X2-	T45.1X3-	T45.1X4-	T45.1X5-	T45.1X6-
Thiomercaptomerin	T50.2X1-	T50.2X2-	T50.2X3-	T50.2X4-	T50.2X5-	T50.2X6-
Thiomerin	T50.2X1-	T50.2X2-	T50.2X3-	T50.2X4-	T50.2X5-	T50.2X6-
Thiomersal	T49.0X1-	T49.0X2-	T49.0X3-	T49.0X4-	T49.0X5-	T49.0X6-
Thionazin	T60.0X1-	T60.0X2-	T60.0X3-	T60.0X4-	-	-
Thiopental (sodium)	T41.1X1-	T41.1X2-	T41.1X3-	T41.1X4-	T41.1X5-	T41.1X6-
Thiopentone (sodium)	T41.1X1-	T41.1X2-	T41.1X3-	T41.1X4-	T41.1X5-	T41.1X6-
Thiopropazate	T43.3X1-	T43.3X2-	T43.3X3-	T43.3X4-	T43.3X5-	T43.3X6-
Thioproperazine	T43.3X1-	T43.3X2-	T43.3X3-	T43.3X4-	T43.3X5-	T43.3X6-
Thioridazine	T43.3X1-	T43.3X2-	T43.3X3-	T43.3X4-	T43.3X5-	T43.3X6-
Thiosinamine	T49.3X1-	T49.3X2-	T49.3X3-	T49.3X4-	T49.3X5-	T49.3X6-
Thiotepa	T45.1X1-	T45.1X2-	T45.1X3-	T45.1X4-	T45.1X5-	T45.1X6-
Thiothixene	T43.4X1-	T43.4X2-	T43.4X3-	T43.4X4-	T43.4X5-	T43.4X6-
Thiouracil (benzyl) (methyl) (propyl)	T38.2X1-	T38.2X2-	T38.2X3-	T38.2X4-	T38.2X5-	T38.2X6-
Thiourea	T38.2X1-	T38.2X2-	T38.2X3-	T38.2X4-	T38.2X5-	T38.2X6-
Thiphenamil	T44.3X1-	T44.3X2-	T44.3X3-	T44.3X4-	T44.3X5-	T44.3X6-
Thiram	T60.3X1-	T60.3X2-	T60.3X3-	T60.3X4-	-	-
medicinal	T49.2X1-	T49.2X2-	T49.2X3-	T49.2X4-	T49.2X5-	T49.2X6-
Thonzylamine (systemic)	T45.0X1-	T45.0X2-	T45.0X3-	T45.0X4-	T45.0X5-	T45.0X6-
mucosal decongestant	T48.5X1-	T48.5X2-	T48.5X3-	T48.5X4-	T48.5X5-	T48.5X6-
Thorazine	T43.3X1-	T43.3X2-	T43.3X3-	T43.3X4-	T43.3X5-	T43.3X6-
Thorium dioxide suspension	T50.8X1-	T50.8X2-	T50.8X3-	T50.8X4-	T50.8X5-	T50.8X6-
Thornapple	T62.2X1-	T62.2X2-	T62.2X3-	T62.2X4-	-	-
Throat drug NEC	T49.6X1-	T49.6X2-	T49.6X3-	T49.6X4-	T49.6X5-	T49.6X6-
Thrombin	T45.7X1-	T45.7X2-	T45.7X3-	T45.7X4-	T45.7X5-	T45.7X6-
Thrombolysin	T45.611-	T45.612-	T45.613-	T45.614-	T45.615-	T45.616-
Thromboplastin	T45.7X1-	T45.7X2-	T45.7X3-	T45.7X4-	T45.7X5-	T45.7X6-
Thurfyl nicotinate	T46.7X1-	T46.7X2-	T46.7X3-	T46.7X4-	T46.7X5-	T46.7X6-
Thymol	T49.0X1-	T49.0X2-	T49.0X3-	T49.0X4-	T49.0X5-	T49.0X6-
Thymopentin	T37.5X1-	T37.5X2-	T37.5X3-	T37.5X4-	T37.5X5-	T37.5X6-
Thymoxamine	T46.7X1-	T46.7X2-	T46.7X3-	T46.7X4-	T46.7X5-	T46.7X6-
Thymus extract	T38.891-	T38.892-	T38.893-	T38.894-	T38.895-	T38.896-
Thyreotrophic hormone	T38.811-	T38.812-	T38.813-	T38.814-	T38.815-	T38.816-
Thyroglobulin	T38.1X1-	T38.1X2-	T38.1X3-	T38.1X4-	T38.1X5-	T38.1X6-
Thyroid (hormone)	T38.1X1-	T38.1X2-	T38.1X3-	T38.1X4-	T38.1X5-	T38.1X6-

Substance	Poisoning Accidental (unintentional)	Poisoning Intentional self-harm	Poisoning Assault	Poisoning Undetermined	Adverse effect	Underdosing
Thyrolar	T38.1X1-	T38.1X2-	T38.1X3-	T38.1X4-	T38.1X5-	T38.1X6-
Thyrotrophin	T38.811-	T38.812-	T38.813-	T38.814-	T38.815-	T38.816-
Thyrotropic hormone	T38.811-	T38.812-	T38.813-	T38.814-	T38.815-	T38.816-
Thyroxine	T38.1X1-	T38.1X2-	T38.1X3-	T38.1X4-	T38.1X5-	T38.1X6-
Tiabendazole	T37.4X1-	T37.4X2-	T37.4X3-	T37.4X4-	T37.4X5-	T37.4X6-
Tiamizide	T50.2X1-	T50.2X2-	T50.2X3-	T50.2X4-	T50.2X5-	T50.2X6-
Tianeptine	T43.291-	T43.292-	T43.293-	T43.294-	T43.295-	T43.296-
Tiapamil	T46.1X1-	T46.1X2-	T46.1X3-	T46.1X4-	T46.1X5-	T46.1X6-
Tiapride	T43.591-	T43.592-	T43.593-	T43.594-	T43.595-	T43.596-
Tiaprofenic acid	T39.311-	T39.312-	T39.313-	T39.314-	T39.315-	T39.316-
Tiaramide	T39.8X1-	T39.8X2-	T39.8X3-	T39.8X4-	T39.8X5-	T39.8X6-
Ticarcillin	T36.0X1-	T36.0X2-	T36.0X3-	T36.0X4-	T36.0X5-	T36.0X6-
Ticlatone	T49.0X1-	T49.0X2-	T49.0X3-	T49.0X4-	T49.0X5-	T49.0X6-
Ticlopidine	T45.521-	T45.522-	T45.523-	T45.524-	T45.525-	T45.526-
Ticrynafen	T50.1X1-	T50.1X2-	T50.1X3-	T50.1X4-	T50.1X5-	T50.1X6-
Tidiacic	T50.991-	T50.992-	T50.993-	T50.994-	T50.995-	T50.996-
Tiemonium	T44.3X1-	T44.3X2-	T44.3X3-	T44.3X4-	T44.3X5-	T44.3X6-
iodide	T44.3X1-	T44.3X2-	T44.3X3-	T44.3X4-	T44.3X5-	T44.3X6-
Tienilic acid	T50.1X1-	T50.1X2-	T50.1X3-	T50.1X4-	T50.1X5-	T50.1X6-
Tifenamil	T44.3X1-	T44.3X2-	T44.3X3-	T44.3X4-	T44.3X5-	T44.3X6-
Tigan	T45.0X1-	T45.0X2-	T45.0X3-	T45.0X4-	T45.0X5-	T45.0X6-
Tigloidine	T44.3X1-	T44.3X2-	T44.3X3-	T44.3X4-	T44.3X5-	T44.3X6-
Tilactase	T47.5X1-	T47.5X2-	T47.5X3-	T47.5X4-	T47.5X5-	T47.5X6-
Tiletamine	T41.291-	T41.292-	T41.293-	T41.294-	T41.295-	T41.296-
Tilidine	T40.4X1-	T40.4X2-	T40.4X3-	T40.4X4-	-	-
Timepidium bromide	T44.3X1-	T44.3X2-	T44.3X3-	T44.3X4-	T44.3X5-	T44.3X6-
Timiperone	T43.4X1-	T43.4X2-	T43.4X3-	T43.4X4-	T43.4X5-	T43.4X6-
Timolol	T44.7X1-	T44.7X2-	T44.7X3-	T44.7X4-	T44.7X5-	T44.7X6-
Tin (chloride) (dust) (oxide) NEC	T56.6X1-	T56.6X2-	T56.6X3-	T56.6X4-	-	-
anti-infectives	T37.8X1-	T37.8X2-	T37.8X3-	T37.8X4-	T37.8X5-	T37.8X6-
Tincture, iodine — *see Iodine*						
Tindal	T43.3X1-	T43.3X2-	T43.3X3-	T43.3X4-	T43.3X5-	T43.3X6-
Tinidazole	T37.3X1-	T37.3X2-	T37.3X3-	T37.3X4-	T37.3X5-	T37.3X6-
Tinoridine	T39.8X1-	T39.8X2-	T39.8X3-	T39.8X4-	T39.8X5-	T39.8X6-
Tiocarlide	T37.1X1-	T37.1X2-	T37.1X3-	T37.1X4-	T37.1X5-	T37.1X6-
Tioclomarol	T45.511-	T45.512-	T45.513-	T45.514-	T45.515-	T45.516-
Tioconazole	T49.0X1-	T49.0X2-	T49.0X3-	T49.0X4-	T49.0X5-	T49.0X6-
Tioguanine	T45.1X1-	T45.1X2-	T45.1X3-	T45.1X4-	T45.1X5-	T45.1X6-
Tiopronin	T50.991-	T50.992-	T50.993-	T50.994-	T50.995-	T50.996-
Tiotixene	T43.4X1-	T43.4X2-	T43.4X3-	T43.4X4-	T43.4X5-	T43.4X6-
Tioxolone	T49.4X1-	T49.4X2-	T49.4X3-	T49.4X4-	T49.4X5-	T49.4X6-
Tipepidine	T48.3X1-	T48.3X2-	T48.3X3-	T48.3X4-	T48.3X5-	T48.3X6-
Tiquizium bromide	T44.3X1-	T44.3X2-	T44.3X3-	T44.3X4-	T44.3X5-	T44.3X6-
Tiratricol	T38.1X1-	T38.1X2-	T38.1X3-	T38.1X4-	T38.1X5-	T38.1X6-
Tisopurine	T50.4X1-	T50.4X2-	T50.4X3-	T50.4X4-	T50.4X5-	T50.4X6-
Titanium (compounds) (vapor)	T56.891-	T56.892-	T56.893-	T56.894-	-	-
dioxide	T49.3X1-	T49.3X2-	T49.3X3-	T49.3X4-	T49.3X5-	T49.3X6-
ointment	T49.3X1-	T49.3X2-	T49.3X3-	T49.3X4-	T49.3X5-	T49.3X6-
oxide	T49.3X1-	T49.3X2-	T49.3X3-	T49.3X4-	T49.3X5-	T49.3X6-
tetrachloride	T56.891-	T56.892-	T56.893-	T56.894-	-	-
Titanocene	T56.891-	T56.892-	T56.893-	T56.894-	-	-
Titroid	T38.1X1-	T38.1X2-	T38.1X3-	T38.1X4-	T38.1X5-	T38.1X6-
Tizanidine	T42.8X1-	T42.8X2-	T42.8X3-	T42.8X4-	T42.8X5-	T42.8X6-
TMTD	T60.3X1-	T60.3X2-	T60.3X3-	T60.3X4-	-	-
TNT (fumes)	T65.3X1-	T65.3X2-	T65.3X3-	T65.3X4-	-	-
Toadstool	T62.0X1-	T62.0X2-	T62.0X3-	T62.0X4-	-	-
Tobacco NEC	T65.291-	T65.292-	T65.293-	T65.294-	-	-
cigarettes	T65.221-	T65.222-	T65.223-	T65.224-	-	-
Indian	T62.2X1-	T62.2X2-	T62.2X3-	T62.2X4-	-	-

Substance	Poisoning Accidental (unintentional)	Poisoning Intentional self-harm	Poisoning Assault	Poisoning Undetermined	Adverse effect	Underdosing
Tobacco NEC (continued)						
smoke, second-hand	T65.221-	T65.222-	T65.223-	T65.224-	-	-
Tobramycin	T36.5X1-	T36.5X2-	T36.5X3-	T36.5X4-	T36.5X5-	T36.5X6-
Tocainide	T46.2X1-	T46.2X2-	T46.2X3-	T46.2X4-	T46.2X5-	T46.2X6-
Tocoferol	T45.2X1-	T45.2X2-	T45.2X3-	T45.2X4-	T45.2X5-	T45.2X6-
Tocopherol	T45.2X1-	T45.2X2-	T45.2X3-	T45.2X4-	T45.2X5-	T45.2X6-
acetate	T45.2X1-	T45.2X2-	T45.2X3-	T45.2X4-	T45.2X5-	T45.2X6-
Tocosamine	T48.0X1-	T48.0X2-	T48.0X3-	T48.0X4-	T48.0X5-	T48.0X6-
Todralazine	T46.5X1-	T46.5X2-	T46.5X3-	T46.5X4-	T46.5X5-	T46.5X6-
Tofisopam	T42.4X1-	T42.4X2-	T42.4X3-	T42.4X4-	T42.4X5-	T42.4X6-
Tofranil	T43.011-	T43.012-	T43.013-	T43.014-	T43.015-	T43.016-
Toilet deodorizer	T65.891-	T65.892-	T65.893-	T65.894-	-	-
Tolamolol	T44.7X1-	T44.7X2-	T44.7X3-	T44.7X4-	T44.7X5-	T44.7X6-
Tolazamide	T38.3X1-	T38.3X2-	T38.3X3-	T38.3X4-	T38.3X5-	T38.3X6-
Tolazoline	T46.7X1-	T46.7X2-	T46.7X3-	T46.7X4-	T46.7X5-	T46.7X6-
Tolbutamide (sodium)	T38.3X1-	T38.3X2-	T38.3X3-	T38.3X4-	T38.3X5-	T38.3X6-
Tolciclate	T49.0X1-	T49.0X2-	T49.0X3-	T49.0X4-	T49.0X5-	T49.0X6-
Tolmetin	T39.391-	T39.392-	T39.393-	T39.394-	T39.395-	T39.396-
Tolnaftate	T49.0X1-	T49.0X2-	T49.0X3-	T49.0X4-	T49.0X5-	T49.0X6-
Tolonidine	T46.5X1-	T46.5X2-	T46.5X3-	T46.5X4-	T46.5X5-	T46.5X6-
Toloxatone	T42.6X1-	T42.6X2-	T42.6X3-	T42.6X4-	T42.6X5-	T42.6X6-
Tolperisone	T44.3X1-	T44.3X2-	T44.3X3-	T44.3X4-	T44.3X5-	T44.3X6-
Tolserol	T42.8X1-	T42.8X2-	T42.8X3-	T42.8X4-	T42.8X5-	T42.8X6-
Toluene (liquid)	T52.2X1-	T52.2X2-	T52.2X3-	T52.2X4-	-	-
diisocyanate	T65.0X1-	T65.0X2-	T65.0X3-	T65.0X4-	-	-
Toluidine	T65.891-	T65.892-	T65.893-	T65.894-	-	-
vapor	T59.891-	T59.892-	T59.893-	T59.894-	-	-
Toluol (liquid)	T52.2X1-	T52.2X2-	T52.2X3-	T52.2X4-	-	-
vapor	T52.2X1-	T52.2X2-	T52.2X3-	T52.2X4-	-	-
Toluylenediamine	T65.3X1-	T65.3X2-	T65.3X3-	T65.3X4-	-	-
Tolylene-2,4-diisocyanate	T65.0X1-	T65.0X2-	T65.0X3-	T65.0X4-	-	-
Tonic NEC	T50.901-	T50.902-	T50.903-	T50.904-	T50.905-	T50.906-
Topical action drug NEC	T49.91X-	T49.92X-	T49.93X-	T49.94X-	T49.95X-	T49.96X-
ear, nose or throat	T49.6X1-	T49.6X2-	T49.6X3-	T49.6X4-	T49.6X5-	T49.6X6-
eye	T49.5X1-	T49.5X2-	T49.5X3-	T49.5X4-	T49.5X5-	T49.5X6-
skin	T49.91X-	T49.92X-	T49.93X-	T49.94X-	T49.95X-	T49.96X-
specified NEC	T49.8X1-	T49.8X2-	T49.8X3-	T49.8X4-	T49.8X5-	T49.8X6-
Toquizine	T44.3X1-	T44.3X2-	T44.3X3-	T44.3X4-	T44.3X5-	T44.3X6-
Toremifene	T38.6X1-	T38.6X2-	T38.6X3-	T38.6X4-	T38.6X5-	T38.6X6-
Tosylchloramide sodium	T49.8X1-	T49.8X2-	T49.8X3-	T49.8X4-	T49.8X5-	T49.8X6-
Toxaphene (dust) (spray)	T60.1X1-	T60.1X2-	T60.1X3-	T60.1X4-	-	-
Toxin, diphtheria (Schick Test)	T50.8X1-	T50.8X2-	T50.8X3-	T50.8X4-	T50.8X5-	T50.8X6-
Toxoid						
combined	T50.A21-	T50.A22-	T50.A23-	T50.A24-	T50.A25-	T50.A26-
diphtheria	T50.A91-	T50.A92-	T50.A93-	T50.A94-	T50.A95-	T50.A96-
tetanus	T50.A91-	T50.A92-	T50.A93-	T50.A94-	T50.A95-	T50.A96-
Trace element NEC	T45.8X1-	T45.8X2-	T45.8X3-	T45.8X4-	T45.8X5-	T45.8X6-
Tractor fuel NEC	T52.0X1-	T52.0X2-	T52.0X3-	T52.0X4-	-	-
Tragacanth	T50.991-	T50.992-	T50.993-	T50.994-	T50.995-	T50.996-
Tramadol	T40.4X1-	T40.4X2-	T40.4X3-	T40.4X4-	T40.4X5-	T40.4X6-
Tramazoline	T48.5X1-	T48.5X2-	T48.5X3-	T48.5X4-	T48.5X5-	T48.5X6-
Tranexamic acid	T45.621-	T45.622-	T45.623-	T45.624-	T45.625-	T45.626-
Tranilast	T45.0X1-	T45.0X2-	T45.0X3-	T45.0X4-	T45.0X5-	T45.0X6-
Tranquilizer NEC	T43.501-	T43.502-	T43.503-	T43.504-	T43.505-	T43.506-
with hypnotic or sedative	T42.6X1-	T42.6X2-	T42.6X3-	T42.6X4-	T42.6X5-	T42.6X6-
benzodiazepine NEC	T42.4X1-	T42.4X2-	T42.4X3-	T42.4X4-	T42.4X5-	T42.4X6-
butyrophenone NEC	T43.4X1-	T43.4X2-	T43.4X3-	T43.4X4-	T43.4X5-	T43.4X6-
carbamate	T43.591-	T43.592-	T43.593-	T43.594-	T43.595-	T43.596-

Substance	Poisoning Accidental (unintentional)	Poisoning Intentional self-harm	Poisoning Assault	Poisoning Undetermined	Adverse effect	Underdosing
Tranquilizer NEC (continued)						
dimethylamine	T43.3X1-	T43.3X2-	T43.3X3-	T43.3X4-	T43.3X5-	T43.3X6-
ethylamine	T43.3X1-	T43.3X2-	T43.3X3-	T43.3X4-	T43.3X5-	T43.3X6-
hydroxyzine	T43.591-	T43.592-	T43.593-	T43.594-	T43.595-	T43.596-
major NEC	T43.501-	T43.502-	T43.503-	T43.504-	T43.505-	T43.506-
penothiazine NEC	T43.3X1-	T43.3X2-	T43.3X3-	T43.3X4-	T43.3X5-	T43.3X6-
phenothiazine-based	T43.3X1-	T43.3X2-	T43.3X3-	T43.3X4-	T43.3X5-	T43.3X6-
piperazine NEC	T43.3X1-	T43.3X2-	T43.3X3-	T43.3X4-	T43.3X5-	T43.3X6-
piperidine	T43.3X1-	T43.3X2-	T43.3X3-	T43.3X4-	T43.3X5-	T43.3X6-
propylamine	T43.3X1-	T43.3X2-	T43.3X3-	T43.3X4-	T43.3X5-	T43.3X6-
specified NEC	T43.591-	T43.592-	T43.593-	T43.594-	T43.595-	T43.596-
thioxanthene NEC	T43.591-	T43.592-	T43.593-	T43.594-	T43.595-	T43.596-
Tranxene	T42.4X1-	T42.4X2-	T42.4X3-	T42.4X4-	T42.4X5-	T42.4X6-
Tranylcypromine	T43.1X1-	T43.1X2-	T43.1X3-	T43.1X4-	T43.1X5-	T43.1X6-
Trapidil	T46.3X1-	T46.3X2-	T46.3X3-	T46.3X4-	T46.3X5-	T46.3X6-
Trasentine	T44.3X1-	T44.3X2-	T44.3X3-	T44.3X4-	T44.3X5-	T44.3X6-
Travert	T50.3X1-	T50.3X2-	T50.3X3-	T50.3X4-	T50.3X5-	T50.3X6-
Trazodone	T43.211-	T43.212-	T43.213-	T43.214-	T43.215-	T43.216-
Trecator	T37.1X1-	T37.1X2-	T37.1X3-	T37.1X4-	T37.1X5-	T37.1X6-
Treosulfan	T45.1X1-	T45.1X2-	T45.1X3-	T45.1X4-	T45.1X5-	T45.1X6-
Tretamine	T45.1X1-	T45.1X2-	T45.1X3-	T45.1X4-	T45.1X5-	T45.1X6-
Tretinoin	T49.0X1-	T49.0X2-	T49.0X3-	T49.0X4-	T49.0X5-	T49.0X6-
Tretoquinol	T48.6X1-	T48.6X2-	T48.6X3-	T48.6X4-	T48.6X5-	T48.6X6-
Triacetin	T49.0X1-	T49.0X2-	T49.0X3-	T49.0X4-	T49.0X5-	T49.0X6-
Triacetoxyanthracene	T49.4X1-	T49.4X2-	T49.4X3-	T49.4X4-	T49.4X5-	T49.4X6-
Triacetyloleandomycin	T36.3X1-	T36.3X2-	T36.3X3-	T36.3X4-	T36.3X5-	T36.3X6-
Triamcinolone	T38.0X1-	T38.0X2-	T38.0X3-	T38.0X4-	T38.0X5-	T38.0X6-
ENT agent	T49.6X1-	T49.6X2-	T49.6X3-	T49.6X4-	T49.6X5-	T49.6X6-
hexacetonide	T49.0X1-	T49.0X2-	T49.0X3-	T49.0X4-	T49.0X5-	T49.0X6-
ophthalmic preparation	T49.5X1-	T49.5X2-	T49.5X3-	T49.5X4-	T49.5X5-	T49.5X6-
topical NEC	T49.0X1-	T49.0X2-	T49.0X3-	T49.0X4-	T49.0X5-	T49.0X6-
Triampyzine	T44.3X1-	T44.3X2-	T44.3X3-	T44.3X4-	T44.3X5-	T44.3X6-
Triamterene	T50.2X1-	T50.2X2-	T50.2X3-	T50.2X4-	T50.2X5-	T50.2X6-
Triazine (herbicide)	T60.3X1-	T60.3X2-	T60.3X3-	T60.3X4-	-	-
Triaziquone	T45.1X1-	T45.1X2-	T45.1X3-	T45.1X4-	T45.1X5-	T45.1X6-
Triazolam	T42.4X1-	T42.4X2-	T42.4X3-	T42.4X4-	T42.4X5-	T42.4X6-
Triazole (herbicide)	T60.3X1-	T60.3X2-	T60.3X3-	T60.3X4-	-	-
Tribenoside	T46.991-	T46.992-	T46.993-	T46.994-	T46.995-	T46.996-
Tribromacetaldehyde	T42.6X1-	T42.6X2-	T42.6X3-	T42.6X4-	T42.6X5-	T42.6X6-
Tribromoethanol, rectal	T41.291-	T41.292-	T41.293-	T41.294-	T41.295-	T41.296-
Tribromomethane	T42.6X1-	T42.6X2-	T42.6X3-	T42.6X4-	T42.6X5-	T42.6X6-
Trichlorethane	T53.2X1-	T53.2X2-	T53.2X3-	T53.2X4-	-	-
Trichlorethylene	T53.2X1-	T53.2X2-	T53.2X3-	T53.2X4-	-	-
Trichlorfon	T60.0X1-	T60.0X2-	T60.0X3-	T60.0X4-	-	-
Trichlormethiazide	T50.2X1-	T50.2X2-	T50.2X3-	T50.2X4-	T50.2X5-	T50.2X6-
Trichlormethine	T45.1X1-	T45.1X2-	T45.1X3-	T45.1X4-	T45.1X5-	T45.1X6-
Trichloroacetic acid, Trichloracetic acid	T54.2X1-	T54.2X2-	T54.2X3-	T54.2X4-	-	-
medicinal	T49.4X1-	T49.4X2-	T49.4X3-	T49.4X4-	T49.4X5-	T49.4X6-
Trichloroethane	T53.2X1-	T53.2X2-	T53.2X3-	T53.2X4-	-	-
Trichloroethanol	T42.6X1-	T42.6X2-	T42.6X3-	T42.6X4-	T42.6X5-	T42.6X6-
Trichloroethyl phosphate	T42.6X1-	T42.6X2-	T42.6X3-	T42.6X4-	T42.6X5-	T42.6X6-
Trichloroethylene (liquid) (vapor)	T53.2X1-	T53.2X2-	T53.2X3-	T53.2X4-	-	-
anesthetic (gas)	T41.0X1-	T41.0X2-	T41.0X3-	T41.0X4-	T41.0X5-	T41.0X6-
vapor NEC	T53.2X1-	T53.2X2-	T53.2X3-	T53.2X4-	-	-
Trichlorofluoromethane NEC	T53.5X1-	T53.5X2-	T53.5X3-	T53.5X4-	-	-
Trichloronate	T60.0X1-	T60.0X2-	T60.0X3-	T60.0X4-	-	-
2,4,5-Trichlorophen-oxyacetic acid	T60.3X1-	T60.3X2-	T60.3X3-	T60.3X4-	-	-
Trichloropropane	T53.6X1-	T53.6X2-	T53.6X3-	T53.6X4-	-	-

Substance	Poisoning Accidental (unintentional)	Poisoning Intentional self-harm	Poisoning Assault	Poisoning Undetermined	Adverse effect	Underdosing
Trichlorotriethylamine	T45.1X1-	T45.1X2-	T45.1X3-	T45.1X4-	T45.1X5-	T45.1X6-
Trichomonacides NEC	T37.3X1-	T37.3X2-	T37.3X3-	T37.3X4-	T37.3X5-	T37.3X6-
Trichomycin	T36.7X1-	T36.7X2-	T36.7X3-	T36.7X4-	T36.7X5-	T36.7X6-
Triclobisonium chloride	T49.0X1-	T49.0X2-	T49.0X3-	T49.0X4-	T49.0X5-	T49.0X6-
Triclocarban	T49.0X1-	T49.0X2-	T49.0X3-	T49.0X4-	T49.0X5-	T49.0X6-
Triclofos	T42.6X1-	T42.6X2-	T42.6X3-	T42.6X4-	T42.6X5-	T42.6X6-
Triclosan	T49.0X1-	T49.0X2-	T49.0X3-	T49.0X4-	T49.0X5-	T49.0X6-
Tricresyl phosphate	T65.891-	T65.892-	T65.893-	T65.894-	-	-
solvent	T52.91X-	T52.92X-	T52.93X-	T52.94X-	-	-
Tricyclamol chloride	T44.3X1-	T44.3X2-	T44.3X3-	T44.3X4-	T44.3X5-	T44.3X6-
Tridesilon	T49.0X1-	T49.0X2-	T49.0X3-	T49.0X4-	T49.0X5-	T49.0X6-
Tridihexethyl iodide	T44.3X1-	T44.3X2-	T44.3X3-	T44.3X4-	T44.3X5-	T44.3X6-
Tridione	T42.2X1-	T42.2X2-	T42.2X3-	T42.2X4-	T42.2X5-	T42.2X6-
Trientine	T45.8X1-	T45.8X2-	T45.8X3-	T45.8X4-	T45.8X5-	T45.8X6-
Triethanolamine NEC	T54.3X1-	T54.3X2-	T54.3X3-	T54.3X4-	-	-
detergent	T54.3X1-	T54.3X2-	T54.3X3-	T54.3X4-	-	-
trinitrate (biphosphate)	T46.3X1-	T46.3X2-	T46.3X3-	T46.3X4-	T46.3X5-	T46.3X6-
Triethanomelamine	T45.1X1-	T45.1X2-	T45.1X3-	T45.1X4-	T45.1X5-	T45.1X6-
Triethylenemelamine	T45.1X1-	T45.1X2-	T45.1X3-	T45.1X4-	T45.1X5-	T45.1X6-
Triethylenephosphoramide	T45.1X1-	T45.1X2-	T45.1X3-	T45.1X4-	T45.1X5-	T45.1X6-
Triethylenethiophosphoramide	T45.1X1-	T45.1X2-	T45.1X3-	T45.1X4-	T45.1X5-	T45.1X6-
Trifluoperazine	T43.3X1-	T43.3X2-	T43.3X3-	T43.3X4-	T43.3X5-	T43.3X6-
Trifluoroethyl vinyl ether	T41.0X1-	T41.0X2-	T41.0X3-	T41.0X4-	T41.0X5-	T41.0X6-
Trifluperidol	T43.4X1-	T43.4X2-	T43.4X3-	T43.4X4-	T43.4X5-	T43.4X6-
Triflupromazine	T43.3X1-	T43.3X2-	T43.3X3-	T43.3X4-	T43.3X5-	T43.3X6-
Trifluridine	T37.5X1-	T37.5X2-	T37.5X3-	T37.5X4-	T37.5X5-	T37.5X6-
Triflusal	T45.521-	T45.522-	T45.523-	T45.524-	T45.525-	T45.526-
Trihexyphenidyl	T44.3X1-	T44.3X2-	T44.3X3-	T44.3X4-	T44.3X5-	T44.3X6-
Triiodothyronine	T38.1X1-	T38.1X2-	T38.1X3-	T38.1X4-	T38.1X5-	T38.1X6-
Trilene	T41.0X1-	T41.0X2-	T41.0X3-	T41.0X4-	T41.0X5-	T41.0X6-
Trilostane	T38.991-	T38.992-	T38.993-	T38.994-	T38.995-	T38.996-
Trimebutine	T44.3X1-	T44.3X2-	T44.3X3-	T44.3X4-	T44.3X5-	T44.3X6-
Trimecaine	T41.3X1-	T41.3X2-	T41.3X3-	T41.3X4-	T41.3X5-	T41.3X6-
Trimeprazine (tartrate)	T44.3X1-	T44.3X2-	T44.3X3-	T44.3X4-	T44.3X5-	T44.3X6-
Trimetaphan camsilate	T44.2X1-	T44.2X2-	T44.2X3-	T44.2X4-	T44.2X5-	T44.2X6-
Trimetazidine	T46.7X1-	T46.7X2-	T46.7X3-	T46.7X4-	T46.7X5-	T46.7X6-
Trimethadione	T42.2X1-	T42.2X2-	T42.2X3-	T42.2X4-	T42.2X5-	T42.2X6-
Trimethaphan	T44.2X1-	T44.2X2-	T44.2X3-	T44.2X4-	T44.2X5-	T44.2X6-
Trimethidinium	T44.2X1-	T44.2X2-	T44.2X3-	T44.2X4-	T44.2X5-	T44.2X6-
Trimethobenzamide	T45.0X1-	T45.0X2-	T45.0X3-	T45.0X4-	T45.0X5-	T45.0X6-
Trimethoprim	T37.8X1-	T37.8X2-	T37.8X3-	T37.8X4-	T37.8X5-	T37.8X6-
with sulfamethoxazole	T36.8X1-	T36.8X2-	T36.8X3-	T36.8X4-	T36.8X5-	T36.8X6-
Trimethylcarbinol	T51.3X1-	T51.3X2-	T51.3X3-	T51.3X4-	-	-
Trimethylpsoralen	T49.3X1-	T49.3X2-	T49.3X3-	T49.3X4-	T49.3X5-	T49.3X6-
Trimeton	T45.0X1-	T45.0X2-	T45.0X3-	T45.0X4-	T45.0X5-	T45.0X6-
Trimetrexate	T45.1X1-	T45.1X2-	T45.1X3-	T45.1X4-	T45.1X5-	T45.1X6-
Trimipramine	T43.011-	T43.012-	T43.013-	T43.014-	T43.015-	T43.016-
Trimustine	T45.1X1-	T45.1X2-	T45.1X3-	T45.1X4-	T45.1X5-	T45.1X6-
Trinitrine	T46.3X1-	T46.3X2-	T46.3X3-	T46.3X4-	T46.3X5-	T46.3X6-
Trinitrobenzol	T65.3X1-	T65.3X2-	T65.3X3-	T65.3X4-	-	-
Trinitrophenol	T65.3X1-	T65.3X2-	T65.3X3-	T65.3X4-	-	-
Trinitrotoluene (fumes)	T65.3X1-	T65.3X2-	T65.3X3-	T65.3X4-	-	-
Trional	T42.6X1-	T42.6X2-	T42.6X3-	T42.6X4-	T42.6X5-	T42.6X6-
Triorthocresyl phosphate	T65.891-	T65.892-	T65.893-	T65.894-	-	-
Trioxide of arsenic	T57.0X1-	T57.0X2-	T57.0X3-	T57.0X4-	-	-
Trioxysalen	T49.4X1-	T49.4X2-	T49.4X3-	T49.4X4-	T49.4X5-	T49.4X6-
Tripamide	T50.2X1-	T50.2X2-	T50.2X3-	T50.2X4-	T50.2X5-	T50.2X6-
Triparanol	T46.6X1-	T46.6X2-	T46.6X3-	T46.6X4-	T46.6X5-	T46.6X6-
Tripelennamine	T45.0X1-	T45.0X2-	T45.0X3-	T45.0X4-	T45.0X5-	T45.0X6-

Substance	Poisoning Accidental (unintentional)	Poisoning Intentional self-harm	Poisoning Assault	Poisoning Undetermined	Adverse effect	Underdosing
Triperiden	T44.3X1-	T44.3X2-	T44.3X3-	T44.3X4-	T44.3X5-	T44.3X6-
Triperidol	T43.4X1-	T43.4X2-	T43.4X3-	T43.4X4-	T43.4X5-	T43.4X6-
Triphenylphosphate	T65.891-	T65.892-	T65.893-	T65.894-	-	-
Triple						
bromides	T42.6X1-	T42.6X2-	T42.6X3-	T42.6X4-	T42.6X5-	T42.6X6-
carbonate	T47.1X1-	T47.1X2-	T47.1X3-	T47.1X4-	T47.1X5-	T47.1X6-
vaccine						
DPT	T50.A11-	T50.A12-	T50.A13-	T50.A14-	T50.A15-	T50.A16-
including pertussis	T50.A11-	T50.A12-	T50.A13-	T50.A14-	T50.A15-	T50.A16-
MMR	T50.B91-	T50.B92-	T50.B93-	T50.B94-	T50.B95-	T50.B96-
Triprolidine	T45.0X1-	T45.0X2-	T45.0X3-	T45.0X4-	T45.0X5-	T45.0X6-
Trisodium hydrogen edetate	T50.6X1-	T50.6X2-	T50.6X3-	T50.6X4-	T50.6X5-	T50.6X6-
Trisoralen	T49.3X1-	T49.3X2-	T49.3X3-	T49.3X4-	T49.3X5-	T49.3X6-
Trisulfapyrimidines	T37.0X1-	T37.0X2-	T37.0X3-	T37.0X4-	T37.0X5-	T37.0X6-
Trithiozine	T44.3X1-	T44.3X2-	T44.3X3-	T44.3X4-	T44.3X5-	T44.3X6-
Tritiozine	T44.3X1-	T44.3X2-	T44.3X3-	T44.3X4-	T44.3X5-	T44.3X6-
Tritoqualine	T45.0X1-	T45.0X2-	T45.0X3-	T45.0X4-	T45.0X5-	T45.0X6-
Trofosfamide	T45.1X1-	T45.1X2-	T45.1X3-	T45.1X4-	T45.1X5-	T45.1X6-
Troleandomycin	T36.3X1-	T36.3X2-	T36.3X3-	T36.3X4-	T36.3X5-	T36.3X6-
Trolnitrate (phosphate)	T46.3X1-	T46.3X2-	T46.3X3-	T46.3X4-	T46.3X5-	T46.3X6-
Tromantadine	T37.5X1-	T37.5X2-	T37.5X3-	T37.5X4-	T37.5X5-	T37.5X6-
Trometamol	T50.2X1-	T50.2X2-	T50.2X3-	T50.2X4-	T50.2X5-	T50.2X6-
Tromethamine	T50.2X1-	T50.2X2-	T50.2X3-	T50.2X4-	T50.2X5-	T50.2X6-
Tronothane	T41.3X1-	T41.3X2-	T41.3X3-	T41.3X4-	T41.3X5-	T41.3X6-
Tropacine	T44.3X1-	T44.3X2-	T44.3X3-	T44.3X4-	T44.3X5-	T44.3X6-
Tropatepine	T44.3X1-	T44.3X2-	T44.3X3-	T44.3X4-	T44.3X5-	T44.3X6-
Tropicamide	T44.3X1-	T44.3X2-	T44.3X3-	T44.3X4-	T44.3X5-	T44.3X6-
Trospium chloride	T44.3X1-	T44.3X2-	T44.3X3-	T44.3X4-	T44.3X5-	T44.3X6-
Troxerutin	T46.991-	T46.992-	T46.993-	T46.994-	T46.995-	T46.996-
Troxidone	T42.2X1-	T42.2X2-	T42.2X3-	T42.2X4-	T42.2X5-	T42.2X6-
Tryparsamide	T37.3X1-	T37.3X2-	T37.3X3-	T37.3X4-	T37.3X5-	T37.3X6-
Trypsin	T45.3X1-	T45.3X2-	T45.3X3-	T45.3X4-	T45.3X5-	T45.3X6-
Tryptizol	T43.011-	T43.012-	T43.013-	T43.014-	T43.015-	T43.016-
TSH	T38.811-	T38.812-	T38.813-	T38.814-	T38.815-	T38.816-
Tuaminoheptane	T48.5X1-	T48.5X2-	T48.5X3-	T48.5X4-	T48.5X5-	T48.5X6-
Tuberculin, purified protein derivative (PPD)	T50.8X1-	T50.8X2-	T50.8X3-	T50.8X4-	T50.8X5-	T50.8X6-
Tubocurare	T48.1X1-	T48.1X2-	T48.1X3-	T48.1X4-	T48.1X5-	T48.1X6-
Tubocurarine (chloride)	T48.1X1-	T48.1X2-	T48.1X3-	T48.1X4-	T48.1X5-	T48.1X6-
Tulobuterol	T48.6X1-	T48.6X2-	T48.6X3-	T48.6X4-	T48.6X5-	T48.6X6-
Turpentine (spirits of)	T52.8X1-	T52.8X2-	T52.8X3-	T52.8X4-	-	-
vapor	T52.8X1-	T52.8X2-	T52.8X3-	T52.8X4-	-	-
Tybamate	T43.591-	T43.592-	T43.593-	T43.594-	T43.595-	T43.596-
Tyloxapol	T48.4X1-	T48.4X2-	T48.4X3-	T48.4X4-	T48.4X5-	T48.4X6-
Tymazoline	T48.5X1-	T48.5X2-	T48.5X3-	T48.5X4-	T48.5X5-	T48.5X6-
Typhoid-paratyphoid vaccine	T50.A91-	T50.A92-	T50.A93-	T50.A94-	T50.A95-	T50.A96-
Typhus vaccine	T50.A91-	T50.A92-	T50.A93-	T50.A94-	T50.A95-	T50.A96-
Tyropanoate	T50.8X1-	T50.8X2-	T50.8X3-	T50.8X4-	T50.8X5-	T50.8X6-
Tyrothricin	T49.6X1-	T49.6X2-	T49.6X3-	T49.6X4-	T49.6X5-	T49.6X6-
ENT agent	T49.6X1-	T49.6X2-	T49.6X3-	T49.6X4-	T49.6X5-	T49.6X6-
ophthalmic preparation	T49.5X1-	T49.5X2-	T49.5X3-	T49.5X4-	T49.5X5-	T49.5X6-
Ufenamate	T39.391-	T39.392-	T39.393-	T39.394-	T39.395-	T39.396-
Ultraviolet light protectant	T49.3X1-	T49.3X2-	T49.3X3-	T49.3X4-	T49.3X5-	T49.3X6-
Undecenoic acid	T49.0X1-	T49.0X2-	T49.0X3-	T49.0X4-	T49.0X5-	T49.0X6-
Undecoylium	T49.0X1-	T49.0X2-	T49.0X3-	T49.0X4-	T49.0X5-	T49.0X6-
Undecylenic acid (derivatives)	T49.0X1-	T49.0X2-	T49.0X3-	T49.0X4-	T49.0X5-	T49.0X6-
Unna's boot	T49.3X1-	T49.3X2-	T49.3X3-	T49.3X4-	T49.3X5-	T49.3X6-
Unsaturated fatty acid	T46.6X1-	T46.6X2-	T46.6X3-	T46.6X4-	T46.6X5-	T46.6X6-
Uracil mustard	T45.1X1-	T45.1X2-	T45.1X3-	T45.1X4-	T45.1X5-	T45.1X6-

Substance	Poisoning Accidental (unintentional)	Poisoning Intentional self-harm	Poisoning Assault	Poisoning Undetermined	Adverse effect	Underdosing
Uramustine	T45.1X1-	T45.1X2-	T45.1X3-	T45.1X4-	T45.1X5-	T45.1X6-
Urapidil	T46.5X1-	T46.5X2-	T46.5X3-	T46.5X4-	T46.5X5-	T46.5X6-
Urari	T48.1X1-	T48.1X2-	T48.1X3-	T48.1X4-	T48.1X5-	T48.1X6-
Urate oxidase	T50.4X1-	T50.4X2-	T50.4X3-	T50.4X4-	T50.4X5-	T50.4X6-
Urea	T47.3X1-	T47.3X2-	T47.3X3-	T47.3X4-	T47.3X5-	T47.3X6-
peroxide	T49.0X1-	T49.0X2-	T49.0X3-	T49.0X4-	T49.0X5-	T49.0X6-
stibamine	T37.4X1-	T37.4X2-	T37.4X3-	T37.4X4-	T37.4X5-	T37.4X6-
topical	T49.8X1-	T49.8X2-	T49.8X3-	T49.8X4-	T49.8X5-	T49.8X6-
Urethane	T45.1X1-	T45.1X2-	T45.1X3-	T45.1X4-	T45.1X5-	T45.1X6-
Urginea (maritima) (scilla) — *see Squill*						
Uric acid metabolism drug NEC	T50.4X1-	T50.4X2-	T50.4X3-	T50.4X4-	T50.4X5-	T50.4X6-
Uricosuric agent	T50.4X1-	T50.4X2-	T50.4X3-	T50.4X4-	T50.4X5-	T50.4X6-
Urinary anti-infective	T37.8X1-	T37.8X2-	T37.8X3-	T37.8X4-	T37.8X5-	T37.8X6-
Urofollitropin	T38.811-	T38.812-	T38.813-	T38.814-	T38.815-	T38.816-
Urokinase	T45.611-	T45.612-	T45.613-	T45.614-	T45.615-	T45.616-
Urokon	T50.8X1-	T50.8X2-	T50.8X3-	T50.8X4-	T50.8X5-	T50.8X6-
Ursodeoxycholic acid	T50.991-	T50.992-	T50.993-	T50.994-	T50.995-	T50.996-
Ursodiol	T50.991-	T50.992-	T50.993-	T50.994-	T50.995-	T50.996-
Urtica	T62.2X1-	T62.2X2-	T62.2X3-	T62.2X4-	-	-
Utility gas — *see Gas, utility*						
Vaccine NEC	T50.Z91-	T50.Z92-	T50.Z93-	T50.Z94-	T50.Z95-	T50.Z96-
antineoplastic	T50.Z91-	T50.Z92-	T50.Z93-	T50.Z94-	T50.Z95-	T50.Z96-
bacterial NEC	T50.A91-	T50.A92-	T50.A93-	T50.A94-	T50.A95-	T50.A96-
with						
other bacterial component	T50.A21-	T50.A22-	T50.A23-	T50.A24-	T50.A25-	T50.A26-
pertussis component	T50.A11-	T50.A12-	T50.A13-	T50.A14-	T50.A15-	T50.A16-
viral-rickettsial component	T50.A21-	T50.A22-	T50.A23-	T50.A24-	T50.A25-	T50.A26-
mixed NEC	T50.A21-	T50.A22-	T50.A23-	T50.A24-	T50.A25-	T50.A26-
BCG	T50.A91-	T50.A92-	T50.A93-	T50.A94-	T50.A95-	T50.A96-
cholera	T50.A91-	T50.A92-	T50.A93-	T50.A94-	T50.A95-	T50.A96-
diphtheria	T50.A91-	T50.A92-	T50.A93-	T50.A94-	T50.A95-	T50.A96-
with tetanus	T50.A21-	T50.A22-	T50.A23-	T50.A24-	T50.A25-	T50.A26-
and pertussis	T50.A11-	T50.A12-	T50.A13-	T50.A14-	T50.A15-	T50.A16-
influenza	T50.B91-	T50.B92-	T50.B93-	T50.B94-	T50.B95-	T50.B96-
measles	T50.B91-	T50.B92-	T50.B93-	T50.B94-	T50.B95-	T50.B96-
with mumps and rubella	T50.B91-	T50.B92-	T50.B93-	T50.B94-	T50.B95-	T50.B96-
meningococcal	T50.A91-	T50.A92-	T50.A93-	T50.A94-	T50.A95-	T50.A96-
mumps	T50.B91-	T50.B92-	T50.B93-	T50.B94-	T50.B95-	T50.B96-
paratyphoid	T50.A91-	T50.A92-	T50.A93-	T50.A94-	T50.A95-	T50.A96-
pertussis	T50.A11-	T50.A12-	T50.A13-	T50.A14-	T50.A15-	T50.A16-
with diphtheria	T50.A11-	T50.A12-	T50.A13-	T50.A14-	T50.A15-	T50.A16-
and tetanus	T50.A11-	T50.A12-	T50.A13-	T50.A14-	T50.A15-	T50.A16-
with other component	T50.A11-	T50.A12-	T50.A13-	T50.A14-	T50.A15-	T50.A16-
plague	T50.A91-	T50.A92-	T50.A93-	T50.A94-	T50.A95-	T50.A96-
poliomyelitis	T50.B91-	T50.B92-	T50.B93-	T50.B94-	T50.B95-	T50.B96-
poliovirus	T50.B91-	T50.B92-	T50.B93-	T50.B94-	T50.B95-	T50.B96-
rabies	T50.B91-	T50.B92-	T50.B93-	T50.B94-	T50.B95-	T50.B96-
respiratory syncytial virus	T50.B91-	T50.B92-	T50.B93-	T50.B94-	T50.B95-	T50.B96-
rickettsial NEC	T50.A91-	T50.A92-	T50.A93-	T50.A94-	T50.A95-	T50.A96-
with						
bacterial component	T50.A21-	T50.A22-	T50.A23-	T50.A24-	T50.A25-	T50.A26-
Rocky Mountain spotted fever	T50.A91-	T50.A92-	T50.A93-	T50.A94-	T50.A95-	T50.A96-
rubella	T50.B91-	T50.B92-	T50.B93-	T50.B94-	T50.B95-	T50.B96-
sabin oral	T50.B91-	T50.B92-	T50.B93-	T50.B94-	T50.B95-	T50.B96-
smallpox	T50.B11-	T50.B12-	T50.B13-	T50.B14-	T50.B15-	T50.B16-
TAB	T50.A91-	T50.A92-	T50.A93-	T50.A94-	T50.A95-	T50.A96-
tetanus	T50.A91-	T50.A92-	T50.A93-	T50.A94-	T50.A95-	T50.A96-
typhoid	T50.A91-	T50.A92-	T50.A93-	T50.A94-	T50.A95-	T50.A96-

URAMUSTINE - VACCINE NEC

Substance	Poisoning Accidental (unintentional)	Poisoning Intentional self-harm	Poisoning Assault	Poisoning Undetermined	Adverse effect	Underdosing
Vaccine NEC (continued)						
typhus	T50.A91-	T50.A92-	T50.A93-	T50.A94-	T50.A95-	T50.A96-
viral NEC	T50.B91-	T50.B92-	T50.B93-	T50.B94-	T50.B95-	T50.B96-
yellow fever	T50.B91-	T50.B92-	T50.B93-	T50.B94-	T50.B95-	T50.B96-
Vaccinia immune globulin	T50.Z11-	T50.Z12-	T50.Z13-	T50.Z14-	T50.Z15-	T50.Z16-
Vaginal contraceptives	T49.8X1-	T49.8X2-	T49.8X3-	T49.8X4-	T49.8X5-	T49.8X6-
Valerian						
root	T42.6X1-	T42.6X2-	T42.6X3-	T42.6X4-	T42.6X5-	T42.6X6-
tincture	T42.6X1-	T42.6X2-	T42.6X3-	T42.6X4-	T42.6X5-	T42.6X6-
Valethamate bromide	T44.3X1-	T44.3X2-	T44.3X3-	T44.3X4-	T44.3X5-	T44.3X6-
Valisone	T49.0X1-	T49.0X2-	T49.0X3-	T49.0X4-	T49.0X5-	T49.0X6-
Valium	T42.4X1-	T42.4X2-	T42.4X3-	T42.4X4-	T42.4X5-	T42.4X6-
Valmid	T42.6X1-	T42.6X2-	T42.6X3-	T42.6X4-	T42.6X5-	T42.6X6-
Valnoctamide	T42.6X1-	T42.6X2-	T42.6X3-	T42.6X4-	T42.6X5-	T42.6X6-
Valproate (sodium)	T42.6X1-	T42.6X2-	T42.6X3-	T42.6X4-	T42.6X5-	T42.6X6-
Valproic acid	T42.6X1-	T42.6X2-	T42.6X3-	T42.6X4-	T42.6X5-	T42.6X6-
Valpromide	T42.6X1-	T42.6X2-	T42.6X3-	T42.6X4-	T42.6X5-	T42.6X6-
Vanadium	T56.891-	T56.892-	T56.893-	T56.894-	-	-
Vancomycin	T36.8X1-	T36.8X2-	T36.8X3-	T36.8X4-	T36.8X5-	T36.8X6-
Vapor — *see also Gas*	T59.91X-	T59.92X-	T59.93X-	T59.94X-	-	-
kiln (carbon monoxide)	T58.8X1-	T58.8X2-	T58.8X3-	T58.8X4-	-	-
lead — *see lead*						
specified source NEC	T59.891-	T59.892-	T59.893-	T59.894-	-	-
Vardenafil	T46.7X1-	T46.7X2-	T46.7X3-	T46.7X4-	T46.7X5-	T46.7X6-
Varicose reduction drug	T46.8X1-	T46.8X2-	T46.8X3-	T46.8X4-	T46.8X5-	T46.8X6-
Varnish	T65.4X1-	T65.4X2-	T65.4X3-	T65.4X4-	-	-
cleaner	T52.91X-	T52.92X-	T52.93X-	T52.94X-	-	-
Vaseline	T49.3X1-	T49.3X2-	T49.3X3-	T49.3X4-	T49.3X5-	T49.3X6-
Vasodilan	T46.7X1-	T46.7X2-	T46.7X3-	T46.7X4-	T46.7X5-	T46.7X6-
Vasodilator						
coronary NEC	T46.3X1-	T46.3X2-	T46.3X3-	T46.3X4-	T46.3X5-	T46.3X6-
peripheral NEC	T46.7X1-	T46.7X2-	T46.7X3-	T46.7X4-	T46.7X5-	T46.7X6-
Vasopressin	T38.891-	T38.892-	T38.893-	T38.894-	T38.895-	T38.896-
Vasopressor drugs	T38.891-	T38.892-	T38.893-	T38.894-	T38.895-	T38.896-
Vecuronium bromide	T48.1X1-	T48.1X2-	T48.1X3-	T48.1X4-	T48.1X5-	T48.1X6-
Vegetable extract, astringent	T49.2X1-	T49.2X2-	T49.2X3-	T49.2X4-	T49.2X5-	T49.2X6-
Venlafaxine	T43.211-	T43.212-	T43.213-	T43.214-	T43.215-	T43.216-
Venom, venomous (bite) (sting)	T63.91X-	T63.92X-	T63.93X-	T63.94X-	-	-
amphibian NEC	T63.831-	T63.832-	T63.833-	T63.834-	-	-
animal NEC	T63.891-	T63.892-	T63.893-	T63.894-	-	-
ant	T63.421-	T63.422-	T63.423-	T63.424-	-	-
arthropod NEC	T63.481-	T63.482-	T63.483-	T63.484-	-	-
bee	T63.441-	T63.442-	T63.443-	T63.444-	-	-
centipede	T63.411-	T63.412-	T63.413-	T63.414-	-	-
fish	T63.591-	T63.592-	T63.593-	T63.594-	-	-
frog	T63.811-	T63.812-	T63.813-	T63.814-	-	-
hornet	T63.451-	T63.452-	T63.453-	T63.454-	-	-
insect NEC	T63.481-	T63.482-	T63.483-	T63.484-	-	-
lizard	T63.121-	T63.122-	T63.123-	T63.124-	-	-
marine						
animals	T63.691-	T63.692-	T63.693-	T63.694-	-	-
bluebottle	T63.611-	T63.612-	T63.613-	T63.614-	-	-
jellyfish NEC	T63.621-	T63.622-	T63.623-	T63.624-	-	-
Portugese Man-o-war	T63.611-	T63.612-	T63.613-	T63.614-	-	-
sea anemone	T63.631-	T63.632-	T63.633-	T63.634-	-	-
specified NEC	T63.691-	T63.692-	T63.693-	T63.694-	-	-
fish	T63.591-	T63.592-	T63.593-	T63.594-	-	-
plants	T63.711-	T63.712-	T63.713-	T63.714-	-	-

Substance	Poisoning Accidental (unintentional)	Poisoning Intentional self-harm	Poisoning Assault	Poisoning Undetermined	Adverse effect	Underdosing
Venom, venomous (bite) (sting) (continued)						
sting ray	T63.511-	T63.512-	T63.513-	T63.514-	-	-
millipede (tropical)	T63.411-	T63.412-	T63.413-	T63.414-	-	-
plant NEC	T63.791-	T63.792-	T63.793-	T63.794-	-	-
marine	T63.711-	T63.712-	T63.713-	T63.714-	-	-
reptile	T63.191-	T63.192-	T63.193-	T63.194-	-	-
gila monster	T63.111-	T63.112-	T63.113-	T63.114-	-	-
lizard NEC	T63.121-	T63.122-	T63.123-	T63.124-	-	-
scorpion	T63.2X1-	T63.2X2-	T63.2X3-	T63.2X4-	-	-
snake	T63.001-	T63.002-	T63.003-	T63.004-	-	-
African NEC	T63.081-	T63.082-	T63.083-	T63.084-	-	-
American (North) (South) NEC	T63.061-	T63.062-	T63.063-	T63.064-	-	-
Asian	T63.081-	T63.082-	T63.083-	T63.084-	-	-
Australian	T63.071-	T63.072-	T63.073-	T63.074-	-	-
cobra	T63.041-	T63.042-	T63.043-	T63.044-	-	-
coral snake	T63.021-	T63.022-	T63.023-	T63.024-	-	-
rattlesnake	T63.011-	T63.012-	T63.013-	T63.014-	-	-
specified NEC	T63.091-	T63.092-	T63.093-	T63.094-	-	-
taipan	T63.031-	T63.032-	T63.033-	T63.034-	-	-
specified NEC	T63.891-	T63.892-	T63.893-	T63.894-	-	-
spider	T63.301-	T63.302-	T63.303-	T63.304-	-	-
black widow	T63.311-	T63.312-	T63.313-	T63.314-	-	-
brown recluse	T63.331-	T63.332-	T63.333-	T63.334-	-	-
specified NEC	T63.391-	T63.392-	T63.393-	T63.394-	-	-
tarantula	T63.321-	T63.322-	T63.323-	T63.324-	-	-
sting ray	T63.511-	T63.512-	T63.513-	T63.514-	-	-
toad	T63.821-	T63.822-	T63.823-	T63.824-	-	-
wasp	T63.461-	T63.462-	T63.463-	T63.464-	-	-
Venous sclerosing drug NEC	T46.8X1-	T46.8X2-	T46.8X3-	T46.8X4-	T46.8X5-	T46.8X6-
Ventolin — *see Albuterol*						
Veramon	T42.3X1-	T42.3X2-	T42.3X3-	T42.3X4-	T42.3X5-	T42.3X6-
Verapamil	T46.1X1-	T46.1X2-	T46.1X3-	T46.1X4-	T46.1X5-	T46.1X6-
Veratrine	T46.5X1-	T46.5X2-	T46.5X3-	T46.5X4-	T46.5X5-	T46.5X6-
Veratrum						
album	T62.2X1-	T62.2X2-	T62.2X3-	T62.2X4-	-	-
alkaloids	T46.5X1-	T46.5X2-	T46.5X3-	T46.5X4-	T46.5X5-	T46.5X6-
viride	T62.2X1-	T62.2X2-	T62.2X3-	T62.2X4-	-	-
Verdigris	T60.3X1-	T60.3X2-	T60.3X3-	T60.3X4-	-	-
Veronal	T42.3X1-	T42.3X2-	T42.3X3-	T42.3X4-	T42.3X5-	T42.3X6-
Veroxil	T37.4X1-	T37.4X2-	T37.4X3-	T37.4X4-	T37.4X5-	T37.4X6-
Versenate	T50.6X1-	T50.6X2-	T50.6X3-	T50.6X4-	T50.6X5-	T50.6X6-
Versidyne	T39.8X1-	T39.8X2-	T39.8X3-	T39.8X4-	T39.8X5-	T39.8X6-
Vetrabutine	T48.0X1-	T48.0X2-	T48.0X3-	T48.0X4-	T48.0X5-	T48.0X6-
Vidarabine	T37.5X1-	T37.5X2-	T37.5X3-	T37.5X4-	T37.5X5-	T37.5X6-
Vienna						
green	T57.0X1-	T57.0X2-	T57.0X3-	T57.0X4-	-	-
insecticide	T60.2X1-	T60.2X2-	T60.2X3-	T60.2X4-	-	-
red	T57.0X1-	T57.0X2-	T57.0X3-	T57.0X4-	-	-
pharmaceutical dye	T50.991-	T50.992-	T50.993-	T50.994-	T50.995-	T50.996-
Vigabatrin	T42.6X1-	T42.6X2-	T42.6X3-	T42.6X4-	T42.6X5-	T42.6X6-
Viloxazine	T43.291-	T43.292-	T43.293-	T43.294-	T43.295-	T43.296-
Viminol	T39.8X1-	T39.8X2-	T39.8X3-	T39.8X4-	T39.8X5-	T39.8X6-
Vinbarbital, vinbarbitone	T42.3X1-	T42.3X2-	T42.3X3-	T42.3X4-	T42.3X5-	T42.3X6-
Vinblastine	T45.1X1-	T45.1X2-	T45.1X3-	T45.1X4-	T45.1X5-	T45.1X6-
Vinburnine	T46.7X1-	T46.7X2-	T46.7X3-	T46.7X4-	T46.7X5-	T46.7X6-
Vincamine	T45.1X1-	T45.1X2-	T45.1X3-	T45.1X4-	T45.1X5-	T45.1X6-
Vincristine	T45.1X1-	T45.1X2-	T45.1X3-	T45.1X4-	T45.1X5-	T45.1X6-
Vindesine	T45.1X1-	T45.1X2-	T45.1X3-	T45.1X4-	T45.1X5-	T45.1X6-

Substance	Poisoning Accidental (unintentional)	Poisoning Intentional self-harm	Poisoning Assault	Poisoning Undetermined	Adverse effect	Underdosing
Vinesthene, vinethene	T41.0X1-	T41.0X2-	T41.0X3-	T41.0X4-	T41.0X5-	T41.0X6-
Vinorelbine tartrate	T45.1X1-	T45.1X2-	T45.1X3-	T45.1X4-	T45.1X5-	T45.1X6-
Vinpocetine	T46.7X1-	T46.7X2-	T46.7X3-	T46.7X4-	T46.7X5-	T46.7X6-
Vinyl						
acetate	T65.891-	T65.892-	T65.893-	T65.894-	-	-
bital	T42.3X1-	T42.3X2-	T42.3X3-	T42.3X4-	T42.3X5-	T42.3X6-
bromide	T65.891-	T65.892-	T65.893-	T65.894-	-	-
chloride	T59.891-	T59.892-	T59.893-	T59.894-	-	-
ether	T41.0X1-	T41.0X2-	T41.0X3-	T41.0X4-	T41.0X5-	T41.0X6-
Vinylbital	T42.3X1-	T42.3X2-	T42.3X3-	T42.3X4-	T42.3X5-	T42.3X6-
Vinylidene chloride	T65.891-	T65.892-	T65.893-	T65.894-	-	-
Vioform	T37.8X1-	T37.8X2-	T37.8X3-	T37.8X4-	T37.8X5-	T37.8X6-
topical	T49.0X1-	T49.0X2-	T49.0X3-	T49.0X4-	T49.0X5-	T49.0X6-
Viomycin	T36.8X1-	T36.8X2-	T36.8X3-	T36.8X4-	T36.8X5-	T36.8X6-
Viosterol	T45.2X1-	T45.2X2-	T45.2X3-	T45.2X4-	T45.2X5-	T45.2X6-
Viper (venom)	T63.091-	T63.092-	T63.093-	T63.094-	-	-
Viprynium	T37.4X1-	T37.4X2-	T37.4X3-	T37.4X4-	T37.4X5-	T37.4X6-
Viquidil	T46.7X1-	T46.7X2-	T46.7X3-	T46.7X4-	T46.7X5-	T46.7X6-
Viral vaccine NEC	T50.B91-	T50.B92-	T50.B93-	T50.B94-	T50.B95-	T50.B96-
Virginiamycin	T36.8X1-	T36.8X2-	T36.8X3-	T36.8X4-	T36.8X5-	T36.8X6-
Virugon	T37.5X1-	T37.5X2-	T37.5X3-	T37.5X4-	T37.5X5-	T37.5X6-
Viscous agent	T50.901-	T50.902-	T50.903-	T50.904-	T50.905-	T50.906-
Visine	T49.5X1-	T49.5X2-	T49.5X3-	T49.5X4-	T49.5X5-	T49.5X6-
Visnadine	T46.3X1-	T46.3X2-	T46.3X3-	T46.3X4-	T46.3X5-	T46.3X6-
Vitamin NEC	T45.2X1-	T45.2X2-	T45.2X3-	T45.2X4-	T45.2X5-	T45.2X6-
A	T45.2X1-	T45.2X2-	T45.2X3-	T45.2X4-	T45.2X5-	T45.2X6-
B NEC	T45.2X1-	T45.2X2-	T45.2X3-	T45.2X4-	T45.2X5-	T45.2X6-
nicotinic acid	T46.7X1-	T46.7X2-	T46.7X3-	T46.7X4-	T46.7X5-	T46.7X6-
B1	T45.2X1-	T45.2X2-	T45.2X3-	T45.2X4-	T45.2X5-	T45.2X6-
B2	T45.2X1-	T45.2X2-	T45.2X3-	T45.2X4-	T45.2X5-	T45.2X6-
B6	T45.2X1-	T45.2X2-	T45.2X3-	T45.2X4-	T45.2X5-	T45.2X6-
B12	T45.2X1-	T45.2X2-	T45.2X3-	T45.2X4-	T45.2X5-	T45.2X6-
B15	T45.2X1-	T45.2X2-	T45.2X3-	T45.2X4-	T45.2X5-	T45.2X6-
C	T45.2X1-	T45.2X2-	T45.2X3-	T45.2X4-	T45.2X5-	T45.2X6-
D	T45.2X1-	T45.2X2-	T45.2X3-	T45.2X4-	T45.2X5-	T45.2X6-
D2	T45.2X1-	T45.2X2-	T45.2X3-	T45.2X4-	T45.2X5-	T45.2X6-
D3	T45.2X1-	T45.2X2-	T45.2X3-	T45.2X4-	T45.2X5-	T45.2X6-
E	T45.2X1-	T45.2X2-	T45.2X3-	T45.2X4-	T45.2X5-	T45.2X6-
E acetate	T45.2X1-	T45.2X2-	T45.2X3-	T45.2X4-	T45.2X5-	T45.2X6-
hematopoietic	T45.8X1-	T45.8X2-	T45.8X3-	T45.8X4-	T45.8X5-	T45.8X6-
K NEC	T45.7X1-	T45.7X2-	T45.7X3-	T45.7X4-	T45.7X5-	T45.7X6-
K1	T45.7X1-	T45.7X2-	T45.7X3-	T45.7X4-	T45.7X5-	T45.7X6-
K2	T45.7X1-	T45.7X2-	T45.7X3-	T45.7X4-	T45.7X5-	T45.7X6-
PP	T45.2X1-	T45.2X2-	T45.2X3-	T45.2X4-	T45.2X5-	T45.2X6-
ulceroprotectant	T47.1X1-	T47.1X2-	T47.1X3-	T47.1X4-	T47.1X5-	T47.1X6-
Vleminckx's solution	T49.4X1-	T49.4X2-	T49.4X3-	T49.4X4-	T49.4X5-	T49.4X6-
Voltaren — *see Diclofenac sodium*						
Warfarin	T45.511-	T45.512-	T45.513-	T45.514-	T45.515-	T45.516-
rodenticide	T60.4X1-	T60.4X2-	T60.4X3-	T60.4X4-	-	-
sodium	T45.511-	T45.512-	T45.513-	T45.514-	T45.515-	T45.516-
Wasp (sting)	T63.461-	T63.462-	T63.463-	T63.464-	-	-
Water						
balance drug	T50.3X1-	T50.3X2-	T50.3X3-	T50.3X4-	T50.3X5-	T50.3X6-
distilled	T50.3X1-	T50.3X2-	T50.3X3-	T50.3X4-	T50.3X5-	T50.3X6-
gas — *see Gas, water*						
incomplete combustion of — *see Carbon, monoxide, fuel, utility*						
hemlock	T62.2X1-	T62.2X2-	T62.2X3-	T62.2X4-	-	-

Substance	Poisoning Accidental (unintentional)	Poisoning Intentional self-harm	Poisoning Assault	Poisoning Undetermined	Adverse effect	Underdosing
Water (continued)						
moccasin (venom)	T63.061-	T63.062-	T63.063-	T63.064-	-	-
purified	T50.3X1-	T50.3X2-	T50.3X3-	T50.3X4-	T50.3X5-	T50.3X6-
Wax (paraffin) (petroleum)	T52.0X1-	T52.0X2-	T52.0X3-	T52.0X4-	-	-
automobile	T65.891-	T65.892-	T65.893-	T65.894-	-	-
floor	T52.0X1-	T52.0X2-	T52.0X3-	T52.0X4-	-	-
Weed killers NEC	T60.3X1-	T60.3X2-	T60.3X3-	T60.3X4-	-	-
Welldorm	T42.6X1-	T42.6X2-	T42.6X3-	T42.6X4-	T42.6X5-	T42.6X6-
White						
arsenic	T57.0X1-	T57.0X2-	T57.0X3-	T57.0X4-	-	-
hellebore	T62.2X1-	T62.2X2-	T62.2X3-	T62.2X4-	-	-
lotion (keratolytic)	T49.4X1-	T49.4X2-	T49.4X3-	T49.4X4-	T49.4X5-	T49.4X6-
spirit	T52.0X1-	T52.0X2-	T52.0X3-	T52.0X4-	-	-
Whitewash	T65.891-	T65.892-	T65.893-	T65.894-	-	-
Whole blood (human)	T45.8X1-	T45.8X2-	T45.8X3-	T45.8X4-	T45.8X5-	T45.8X6-
Wild						
black cherry	T62.2X1-	T62.2X2-	T62.2X3-	T62.2X4-	-	-
poisonous plants NEC	T62.2X1-	T62.2X2-	T62.2X3-	T62.2X4-	-	-
Window cleaning fluid	T65.891-	T65.892-	T65.893-	T65.894-	-	-
Wintergreen (oil)	T49.3X1-	T49.3X2-	T49.3X3-	T49.3X4-	T49.3X5-	T49.3X6-
Wisterine	T62.2X1-	T62.2X2-	T62.2X3-	T62.2X4-	-	-
Witch hazel	T49.2X1-	T49.2X2-	T49.2X3-	T49.2X4-	T49.2X5-	T49.2X6-
Wood alcohol or spirit	T51.1X1-	T51.1X2-	T51.1X3-	T51.1X4-	-	-
Wool fat (hydrous)	T49.3X1-	T49.3X2-	T49.3X3-	T49.3X4-	T49.3X5-	T49.3X6-
Woorali	T48.1X1-	T48.1X2-	T48.1X3-	T48.1X4-	T48.1X5-	T48.1X6-
Wormseed, American	T37.4X1-	T37.4X2-	T37.4X3-	T37.4X4-	T37.4X5-	T37.4X6-
Xamoterol	T44.5X1-	T44.5X2-	T44.5X3-	T44.5X4-	T44.5X5-	T44.5X6-
Xanthine diuretics	T50.2X1-	T50.2X2-	T50.2X3-	T50.2X4-	T50.2X5-	T50.2X6-
Xanthinol nicotinate	T46.7X1-	T46.7X2-	T46.7X3-	T46.7X4-	T46.7X5-	T46.7X6-
Xanthotoxin	T49.3X1-	T49.3X2-	T49.3X3-	T49.3X4-	T49.3X5-	T49.3X6-
Xantinol nicotinate	T46.7X1-	T46.7X2-	T46.7X3-	T46.7X4-	T46.7X5-	T46.7X6-
Xantocillin	T36.0X1-	T36.0X2-	T36.0X3-	T36.0X4-	T36.0X5-	T36.0X6-
Xenon (127Xe) (133Xe)	T50.8X1-	T50.8X2-	T50.8X3-	T50.8X4-	T50.8X5-	T50.8X6-
Xenysalate	T49.4X1-	T49.4X2-	T49.4X3-	T49.4X4-	T49.4X5-	T49.4X6-
Xibornol	T37.8X1-	T37.8X2-	T37.8X3-	T37.8X4-	T37.8X5-	T37.8X6-
Xigris	T45.511-	T45.512-	T45.513-	T45.514-	T45.515-	T45.516-
Xipamide	T50.2X1-	T50.2X2-	T50.2X3-	T50.2X4-	T50.2X5-	T50.2X6-
Xylene (vapor)	T52.2X1-	T52.2X2-	T52.2X3-	T52.2X4-	-	-
Xylocaine (infiltration) (topical)	T41.3X1-	T41.3X2-	T41.3X3-	T41.3X4-	T41.3X5-	T41.3X6-
nerve block (peripheral) (plexus)	T41.3X1-	T41.3X2-	T41.3X3-	T41.3X4-	T41.3X5-	T41.3X6-
spinal	T41.3X1-	T41.3X2-	T41.3X3-	T41.3X4-	T41.3X5-	T41.3X6-
Xylol (vapor)	T52.2X1-	T52.2X2-	T52.2X3-	T52.2X4-	-	-
Xylometazoline	T48.5X1-	T48.5X2-	T48.5X3-	T48.5X4-	T48.5X5-	T48.5X6-
Yeast	T45.2X1-	T45.2X2-	T45.2X3-	T45.2X4-	T45.2X5-	T45.2X6-
dried	T45.2X1-	T45.2X2-	T45.2X3-	T45.2X4-	T45.2X5-	T45.2X6-
Yellow						
fever vaccine	T50.B91-	T50.B92-	T50.B93-	T50.B94-	T50.B95-	T50.B96-
jasmine	T62.2X1-	T62.2X2-	T62.2X3-	T62.2X4-	-	-
phenolphthalein	T47.2X1-	T47.2X2-	T47.2X3-	T47.2X4-	T47.2X5-	T47.2X6-
Yew	T62.2X1-	T62.2X2-	T62.2X3-	T62.2X4-	-	-
Yohimbic acid	T40.991-	T40.992-	T40.993-	T40.994-	T40.995-	T40.996-
Zactane	T39.8X1-	T39.8X2-	T39.8X3-	T39.8X4-	T39.8X5-	T39.8X6-
Zalcitabine	T37.5X1-	T37.5X2-	T37.5X3-	T37.5X4-	T37.5X5-	T37.5X6-
Zaroxolyn	T50.2X1-	T50.2X2-	T50.2X3-	T50.2X4-	T50.2X5-	T50.2X6-
Zephiran (topical)	T49.0X1-	T49.0X2-	T49.0X3-	T49.0X4-	T49.0X5-	T49.0X6-
ophthalmic preparation	T49.5X1-	T49.5X2-	T49.5X3-	T49.5X4-	T49.5X5-	T49.5X6-
Zeranol	T38.7X1-	T38.7X2-	T38.7X3-	T38.7X4-	T38.7X5-	T38.7X6-
Zerone	T51.1X1-	T51.1X2-	T51.1X3-	T51.1X4-	-	-

WATER - ZERONE

Substance	Poisoning Accidental (unintentional)	Poisoning Intentional self-harm	Poisoning Assault	Poisoning Undetermined	Adverse effect	Underdosing
Zidovudine	T37.5X1-	T37.5X2-	T37.5X3-	T37.5X4-	T37.5X5-	T37.5X6-
Zimeldine	T43.221-	T43.222-	T43.223-	T43.224-	T43.225-	T43.226-
Zinc (compounds) (fumes) (vapor) NEC	T56.5X1-	T56.5X2-	T56.5X3-	T56.5X4-	-	-
anti-infectives	T49.0X1-	T49.0X2-	T49.0X3-	T49.0X4-	T49.0X5-	T49.0X6-
antivaricose	T46.8X1-	T46.8X2-	T46.8X3-	T46.8X4-	T46.8X5-	T46.8X6-
bacitracin	T49.0X1-	T49.0X2-	T49.0X3-	T49.0X4-	T49.0X5-	T49.0X6-
chloride (mouthwash)	T49.6X1-	T49.6X2-	T49.6X3-	T49.6X4-	T49.6X5-	T49.6X6-
chromate	T56.5X1-	T56.5X2-	T56.5X3-	T56.5X4-	-	-
gelatin	T49.3X1-	T49.3X2-	T49.3X3-	T49.3X4-	T49.3X5-	T49.3X6-
oxide	T49.3X1-	T49.3X2-	T49.3X3-	T49.3X4-	T49.3X5-	T49.3X6-
plaster	T49.3X1-	T49.3X2-	T49.3X3-	T49.3X4-	T49.3X5-	T49.3X6-
peroxide	T49.0X1-	T49.0X2-	T49.0X3-	T49.0X4-	T49.0X5-	T49.0X6-
pesticides	T56.5X1-	T56.5X2-	T56.5X3-	T56.5X4-	-	-
phosphide	T60.4X1-	T60.4X2-	T60.4X3-	T60.4X4-	-	-
pyrithionate	T49.4X1-	T49.4X2-	T49.4X3-	T49.4X4-	T49.4X5-	T49.4X6-
stearate	T49.3X1-	T49.3X2-	T49.3X3-	T49.3X4-	T49.3X5-	T49.3X6-
sulfate	T49.5X1-	T49.5X2-	T49.5X3-	T49.5X4-	T49.5X5-	T49.5X6-
ENT agent	T49.6X1-	T49.6X2-	T49.6X3-	T49.6X4-	T49.6X5-	T49.6X6-
ophthalmic solution	T49.5X1-	T49.5X2-	T49.5X3-	T49.5X4-	T49.5X5-	T49.5X6-
topical NEC	T49.0X1-	T49.0X2-	T49.0X3-	T49.0X4-	T49.0X5-	T49.0X6-
undecylenate	T49.0X1-	T49.0X2-	T49.0X3-	T49.0X4-	T49.0X5-	T49.0X6-
Zineb	T60.0X1-	T60.0X2-	T60.0X3-	T60.0X4-	-	-
Zinostatin	T45.1X1-	T45.1X2-	T45.1X3-	T45.1X4-	T45.1X5-	T45.1X6-
Zipeprol	T48.3X1-	T48.3X2-	T48.3X3-	T48.3X4-	T48.3X5-	T48.3X6-
Zofenopril	T46.4X1-	T46.4X2-	T46.4X3-	T46.4X4-	T46.4X5-	T46.4X6-
Zolpidem	T42.6X1-	T42.6X2-	T42.6X3-	T42.6X4-	T42.6X5-	T42.6X6-
Zomepirac	T39.391-	T39.392-	T39.393-	T39.394-	T39.395-	T39.396-
Zopiclone	T42.6X1-	T42.6X2-	T42.6X3-	T42.6X4-	T42.6X5-	T42.6X6-
Zorubicin	T45.1X1-	T45.1X2-	T45.1X3-	T45.1X4-	T45.1X5-	T45.1X6-
Zotepine	T43.591-	T43.592-	T43.593-	T43.594-	T43.595-	T43.596-
Zovant	T45.511-	T45.512-	T45.513-	T45.514-	T45.515-	T45.516-
Zoxazolamine	T42.8X1-	T42.8X2-	T42.8X3-	T42.8X4-	T42.8X5-	T42.8X6-
Zuclopenthixol	T43.4X1-	T43.4X2-	T43.4X3-	T43.4X4-	T43.4X5-	T43.4X6-
Zygadenus (venenosus)	T62.2X1-	T62.2X2-	T62.2X3-	T62.2X4-	-	-
Zyprexa	T43.591-	T43.592-	T43.593-	T43.594-	T43.595-	T43.596-

Index to External Cause of Injuries

The final section of the Alphabetic Index is the Index to External Cause of Injuries. This section classifies environmental events, circumstances, and conditions as the ***cause of*** injury, poisoning and other adverse effects. The Index to External Cause of Injuries is organized by main terms that describe the accident, circumstance, event, or specific agent causing the injury or other adverse effect.

External cause codes are intended to provide data for injury research and evaluation of injury prevention strategies. These codes capture how the injury or health condition happened (cause), the intent (unintentional or accidental; or intentional, such as suicide or assault), the place where the event occurred, the activity of the patient at the time of the event, and the person's status (e.g., civilian, military).

An external cause code may be used with any code in the range of A00.0 – T88.9, Z00 – Z99, classification that is a health condition due to an external cause. Though they are most applicable to injuries, they are also valid for use with such things as infections or diseases due to an external source, and other health conditions, such as a heart attack that occurs during strenuous physical activity.

Important: An external cause code can never be a principal (**first-listed**) diagnosis.

The selection of the appropriate external cause code is guided by the Alphabetic Index of External Causes and by Inclusion and Exclusion notes in the Tabular List.

A

Abandonment (causing exposure to weather conditions) (with intent to injure or kill) NEC X58

Abuse (adult) (child) (mental) (physical) (sexual) X58

Accident (to) X58
  aircraft (in transit) (powered) — *see also* Accident, transport, aircraft
    due to, caused by cataclysm — *see* Forces of nature, by type
  animal-rider — *see* Accident, transport, animal-rider
  animal-drawn vehicle — *see* Accident, transport, animal-drawn vehicle occupant
  automobile — *see* Accident, transport, car occupant
  bare foot water skiier V94.4
  boat, boating — *see also* Accident, watercraft
    striking swimmer
      powered V94.11
      unpowered V94.12
  bus — *see* Accident, transport, bus occupant
  cable car, not on rails V98.0
    on rails — *see* Accident, transport, streetcar occupant
  car — *see* Accident, transport, car occupant
  caused by, due to
    animal NEC W64
    chain hoist W24.0
    cold (excessive) — *see* Exposure, cold
    corrosive liquid, substance — *see* Table of Drugs and Chemicals
    cutting or piercing instrument — *see* Contact, with, by type of instrument
    drive belt W24.0
    electric
      current — *see* Exposure, electric current
      motor — *see also* Contact, with, by type of machine W31.3
        current (of) W86.8
    environmental factor NEC X58
    explosive material — *see* Explosion
    fire, flames — *see* Exposure, fire
    firearm missile — *see* Discharge, firearm by type
    heat (excessive) — *see* Heat
    hot — *see* Contact, with, hot
    ignition — *see* Ignition
    lifting device W24.0
    lightning — *see* subcategory T75.0
      causing fire — *see* Exposure, fire
    machine, machinery — *see* Contact, with, by type of machine
    natural factor NEC X58
    pulley (block) W24.0
    radiation — *see* Radiation
    steam X13.1
      inhalation X13.0
      pipe X16
    thunderbolt — *see* subcategory T75.0
      causing fire — *see* Exposure, fire
    transmission device W24.1
  coach — *see* Accident, transport, bus occupant
  coal car — *see* Accident, transport, industrial vehicle occupant
  diving — *see also* Fall, into, water
    with
      drowning or submersion — *see* Drowning
  forklift — *see* Accident, transport, industrial vehicle occupant
  heavy transport vehicle NOS — *see* Accident, transport, truck occupant
  ice yacht V98.2
  in
    medical, surgical procedure
      as, or due to misadventure — *see* Misadventure

Accident (to) - *continued*
  in - *continued*
    medical, surgical procedure - *continued*
      causing an abnormal reaction or later complication without mention of misadventure — *see also* Complication of or following, by type of procedure Y84.9
  land yacht V98.1
  late effect of — *see* W00-X58 with 7th character S
  logging car — *see* Accident, transport, industrial vehicle occupant
  machine, machinery — *see also* Contact, with, by type of machine
    on board watercraft V93.69
      explosion — *see* Explosion, in, watercraft
      fire — *see* Burn, on board watercraft
      powered craft V93.63
        ferry boat V93.61
        fishing boat V93.62
        jetskis V93.63
        liner V93.61
        merchant ship V93.60
        passenger ship V93.61
        sailboat V93.64
  mine tram — *see* Accident, transport, industrial vehicle occupant
  mobility scooter (motorized) — *see* Accident, transport, pedestrian, conveyance, specified type NEC
  motor scooter — *see* Accident, transport, motorcyclist
  motor vehicle NOS (traffic) — *see also* Accident, transport V89.2
    nontraffic V89.0
    three-wheeled NOS — *see* Accident, transport, three-wheeled motor vehicle occupant
  motorcycle NOS — *see* Accident, transport, motorcyclist
  nonmotor vehicle NOS (nontraffic) — *see also* Accident, transport V89.1
    traffic NOS V89.3
  nontraffic (victim's mode of transport NOS) V88.9
    collision (between) V88.7
      bus and truck V88.5
      car and:
        bus V88.3
        pickup V88.2
        three-wheeled motor vehicle V88.0
        train V88.6
        truck V88.4
        two-wheeled motor vehicle V88.0
        van V88.2
      specified vehicle NEC and:
        three-wheeled motor vehicle V88.1
        two-wheeled motor vehicle V88.1
      known mode of transport — *see* Accident, transport, by type of vehicle
    noncollision V88.8
  on board watercraft V93.89
    powered craft V93.83
      ferry boat V93.81
      fishing boat V93.82
      jetskis V93.83
      liner V93.81
      merchant ship V93.80
      passenger ship V93.81
    unpowered craft V93.88
      canoe V93.85
      inflatable V93.86
        in tow
          recreational V94.31
          specified NEC V94.32
      kayak V93.85
      sailboat V93.84
      surf-board V93.88
      water skis V93.87
      windsurfer V93.88
  parachutist V97.29
    entangled in object V97.21
    injured on landing V97.22

Accident (to) - *continued*
  pedal cycle — *see* Accident, transport, pedal cyclist
  pedestrian (on foot)
    with
      another pedestrian W51
        with fall W03
          due to ice or snow W00.0
      on pedestrian conveyance NEC V00.09
      roller skater (in-line) V00.01
      skate boarder V00.02
      transport vehicle — *see* Accident, transport
      on pedestrian conveyance — *see* Accident, transport, pedestrian, conveyance
  pick-up truck or van — *see* Accident, transport, pickup truck occupant
  quarry truck — *see* Accident, transport, industrial vehicle occupant
  railway vehicle (any) (in motion) — *see* Accident, transport, railway vehicle occupant
    due to cataclysm — *see* Forces of nature, by type
  scooter (non-motorized) — *see* Accident, transport, pedestrian, conveyance, scooter
  sequelae of — *see* W00-X58 with 7th character S
  skateboard — *see* Accident, transport, pedestrian, conveyance, skateboard
  ski (ing) — *see* Accident, transport, pedestrian, conveyance
    lift V98.3
  specified cause NEC X58
  streetcar — *see* Accident, transport, streetcar occupant
  traffic (victim's mode of transport NOS) V87.9
    collision (between) V87.7
      bus and truck V87.5
      car and:
        bus V87.3
        pickup V87.2
        three-wheeled motor vehicle V87.0
        train V87.6
        truck V87.4
        two-wheeled motor vehicle V87.0
        van V87.2
      specified vehicle NEC V86.39
        and
          three-wheeled motor vehicle V87.1
          two-wheeled motor vehicle V87.1
        driver V86.09
        person on outside V86.29
        passenger V86.19
        while boarding or alighting V86.49
      known mode of transport — *see* Accident, transport, by type of vehicle
    noncollision V87.8
  transport (involving injury to) V99
    18 wheeler — *see* Accident, transport, truck occupant
    agricultural vehicle occupant (nontraffic) V84.9
      driver V84.5
      hanger-on V84.7
      passenger V84.6
      traffic V84.3
        driver V84.0
        hanger-on V84.2
        passenger V84.1
      while boarding or alighting V84.4
    aircraft NEC V97.89
      military NEC V97.818
        with civilian aircraft V97.810
        civilian injured by V97.811
      occupant injured (in)
        nonpowered craft accident V96.9
          balloon V96.00
            collision V96.03
            crash V96.01
            explosion V96.05
            fire V96.04

Accident (to) - *continued*
transport (involving injury to) - *continued*
  aircraft NEC - *continued*
    occupant injured (in) - *continued*
      nonpowered craft accident - *continued*
        balloon - *continued*
          forced landing V96.02
          specified type NEC V96.09
        glider V96.20
          collision V96.23
          crash V96.21
          explosion V96.25
          fire V96.24
          forced landing V96.22
          specified type NEC V96.29
        hang glider V96.10
          collision V96.13
          crash V96.11
          explosion V96.15
          fire V96.14
          forced landing V96.12
          specified type NEC V96.19
        specified craft NEC V96.8
      powered craft accident V95.9
        fixed wing NEC
          commercial V95.30
            collision V95.33
            crash V95.31
            explosion V95.35
            fire V95.34
            forced landing V95.32
            specified type NEC V95.39
          private V95.20
            collision V95.23
            crash V95.21
            explosion V95.25
            fire V95.24
            forced landing V95.22
            specified type NEC V95.29
        glider V95.10
          collision V95.13
          crash V95.11
          explosion V95.15
          fire V95.14
          forced landing V95.12
          specified type NEC V95.19
        helicopter V95.00
          collision V95.03
          crash V95.01
          explosion V95.05
          fire V95.04
          forced landing V95.02
          specified type NEC V95.09
        spacecraft V95.40
          collision V95.43
          crash V95.41
          explosion V95.45
          fire V95.44
          forced landing V95.42
          specified type NEC V95.49
        specified craft NEC V95.8
        ultralight V95.10
          collision V95.13
          crash V95.11
          explosion V95.15
          fire V95.14
          forced landing V95.12
          specified type NEC V95.19
      specified accident NEC V97.0
      while boarding or alighting V97.1
    person (injured by)
      falling from, in or on aircraft V97.0
      machinery on aircraft V97.89
      on ground with aircraft
        involvement V97.39
      rotating propeller V97.32
      struck by object falling from
        aircraft V97.31
      sucked into aircraft jet V97.33
      while boarding or alighting
        aircraft V97.1
  airport (battery-powered) passenger
    vehicle — *see* Accident, transport,
    industrial vehicle occupant

Accident (to) - *continued*
transport (involving injury to) - *continued*
  all-terrain vehicle occupant
    (nontraffic) V86.95
    driver V86.55
    dune buggy — *see* Accident, transport,
      dune buggy occupant
    hanger-on V86.75
    passenger V86.65
    snowmobile — *see* Accident, transport,
      snowmobile occupant
    specified type NEC V86.99
      driver V86.59
      passenger V86.69
      person on outside V86.79
    traffic V86.35
      driver V86.05
      hanger-on V86.25
      passenger V86.15
    while boarding or alighting V86.45
  ambulance occupant (traffic) V86.31
    driver V86.01
    hanger-on V86.21
    nontraffic V86.91
      driver V86.51
      hanger-on V86.71
      passenger V86.61
    passenger V86.11
    while boarding or alighting V86.41
  animal-drawn vehicle occupant
    (in) V80.929
    collision (with)
      animal V80.12
        being ridden V80.711
      animal-drawn vehicle V80.721
      bus V80.42
      car V80.42
      fixed or stationary object V80.82
      military vehicle V80.920
      nonmotor vehicle V80.791
      pedal cycle V80.22
      pedestrian V80.12
      pickup V80.42
      railway train or vehicle V80.62
      specified motor vehicle NEC V80.52
      streetcar V80.731
      truck V80.42
      two- or three-wheeled motor
        vehicle V80.32
      van V80.42
    noncollision V80.02
    specified circumstance NEC V80.928
  animal-rider V80.919
    collision (with)
      animal V80.11
        being ridden V80.710
      animal-drawn vehicle V80.720
      bus V80.41
      car V80.41
      fixed or stationary object V80.81
      military vehicle V80.910
      nonmotor vehicle V80.790
      pedal cycle V80.21
      pedestrian V80.11
      pickup V80.41
      railway train or vehicle V80.61
      specified motor vehicle NEC V80.51
      streetcar V80.730
      truck V80.41
      two- or three-wheeled motor
        vehicle V80.31
      van V80.41
    noncollision V80.018
      specified as horse rider V80.010
    specified circumstance NEC V80.918
  armored car — *see* Accident, transport,
    truck occupant
  battery-powered truck (baggage) (mail) —
    see Accident, transport, industrial
    vehicle occupant
  bus occupant V79.9
    collision (with)
      animal (traffic) V70.9
        being ridden (traffic) V76.9
          nontraffic V76.3

Accident (to) - *continued*
transport (involving injury to) - *continued*
  bus occupant - *continued*
    collision (with) - *continued*
      animal (traffic) - *continued*
        being ridden (traffic) - *continued*
          while boarding or alighting V76.4
        nontraffic V70.3
        while boarding or alighting V70.4
      animal-drawn vehicle (traffic) V76.9
        nontraffic V76.3
        while boarding or alighting V76.4
      bus (traffic) V74.9
        nontraffic V74.3
        while boarding or alighting V74.4
      car (traffic) V73.9
        nontraffic V73.3
        while boarding or alighting V73.4
      motor vehicle NOS (traffic) V79.60
        nontraffic V79.20
        specified type NEC (traffic) V79.69
          nontraffic V79.29
      pedal cycle (traffic) V71.9
        nontraffic V71.3
        while boarding or alighting V71.4
      pickup truck (traffic) V73.9
        nontraffic V73.3
        while boarding or alighting V73.4
      railway vehicle (traffic) V75.9
        nontraffic V75.3
        while boarding or alighting V75.4
      specified vehicle NEC (traffic) V76.9
        nontraffic V76.3
        while boarding or alighting V76.4
      stationary object (traffic) V77.9
        nontraffic V77.3
        while boarding or alighting V77.4
      streetcar (traffic) V76.9
        nontraffic V76.3
        while boarding or alighting V76.4
      three wheeled motor vehicle
        (traffic) V72.9
        nontraffic V72.3
        while boarding or alighting V72.4
      truck (traffic) V74.9
        nontraffic V74.3
        while boarding or alighting V74.4
      two wheeled motor vehicle
        (traffic) V72.9
        nontraffic V72.3
        while boarding or alighting V72.4
      van (traffic) V73.9
        nontraffic V73.3
        while boarding or alighting V73.4
    driver
      collision (with)
        animal (traffic) V70.5
          being ridden (traffic) V76.5
            nontraffic V76.0
          nontraffic V70.0
        animal-drawn vehicle
          (traffic) V76.5
          nontraffic V76.0
        bus (traffic) V74.5
          nontraffic V74.0
        car (traffic) V73.5
          nontraffic V73.0
        motor vehicle NOS (traffic) V79.40
          nontraffic V79.00
          specified type NEC
            (traffic) V79.49
            nontraffic V79.09
        pedal cycle (traffic) V71.5
          nontraffic V71.0
        pickup truck (traffic) V73.5
          nontraffic V73.0
        railway vehicle (traffic) V75.5
          nontraffic V75.0
        specified vehicle NEC
          (traffic) V76.5
          nontraffic V76.0
        stationary object (traffic) V77.5
          nontraffic V77.0
        streetcar (traffic) V76.5
          nontraffic V76.0

Accident (to) - *continued*
　transport (involving injury to) - *continued*
　　bus occupant - *continued*
　　　driver - *continued*
　　　　collision (with) - *continued*
　　　　　three wheeled motor vehicle
　　　　　　(traffic) V72.5
　　　　　　nontraffic V72.0
　　　　　truck (traffic) V74.5
　　　　　　nontraffic V74.0
　　　　　two wheeled motor vehicle
　　　　　　(traffic) V72.5
　　　　　　nontraffic V72.0
　　　　　van (traffic) V73.5
　　　　　　nontraffic V73.0
　　　　　noncollision accident (traffic) V78.5
　　　　　　nontraffic V78.0
　　　　noncollision accident (traffic) V78.9
　　　　　nontraffic V78.3
　　　　　while boarding or alighting V78.4
　　　　nontraffic V79.3
　　　hanger-on
　　　　collision (with)
　　　　　animal (traffic) V70.7
　　　　　　being ridden (traffic) V76.7
　　　　　　　nontraffic V76.2
　　　　　　nontraffic V70.2
　　　　　animal-drawn vehicle
　　　　　　(traffic) V76.7
　　　　　　nontraffic V76.2
　　　　　bus (traffic) V74.7
　　　　　　nontraffic V74.2
　　　　　car (traffic) V73.7
　　　　　　nontraffic V73.2
　　　　　pedal cycle (traffic) V71.7
　　　　　　nontraffic V71.2
　　　　　pickup truck (traffic) V73.7
　　　　　　nontraffic V73.2
　　　　　railway vehicle (traffic) V75.7
　　　　　　nontraffic V75.2
　　　　　specified vehicle NEC
　　　　　　(traffic) V76.7
　　　　　　nontraffic V76.2
　　　　　stationary object (traffic) V77.7
　　　　　　nontraffic V77.2
　　　　　streetcar (traffic) V76.7
　　　　　　nontraffic V76.2
　　　　　three wheeled motor vehicle
　　　　　　(traffic) V72.7
　　　　　　nontraffic V72.2
　　　　　truck (traffic) V74.7
　　　　　　nontraffic V74.2
　　　　　two wheeled motor vehicle
　　　　　　(traffic) V72.7
　　　　　　nontraffic V72.2
　　　　　van (traffic) V73.7
　　　　　　nontraffic V73.2
　　　　noncollision accident (traffic) V78.7
　　　　　nontraffic V78.2
　　　passenger
　　　　collision (with)
　　　　　animal (traffic) V70.6
　　　　　　being ridden (traffic) V76.6
　　　　　　　nontraffic V76.1
　　　　　　nontraffic V70.1
　　　　　animal-drawn vehicle
　　　　　　(traffic) V76.6
　　　　　　nontraffic V76.1
　　　　　bus (traffic) V74.6
　　　　　　nontraffic V74.1
　　　　　car (traffic) V73.6
　　　　　　nontraffic V73.1
　　　　　motor vehicle NOS (traffic) V79.50
　　　　　　nontraffic V79.10
　　　　　　specified type NEC
　　　　　　　(traffic) V79.59
　　　　　　　nontraffic V79.19
　　　　　pedal cycle (traffic) V71.6
　　　　　　nontraffic V71.1
　　　　　pickup truck (traffic) V73.6
　　　　　　nontraffic V73.1
　　　　　railway vehicle (traffic) V75.6
　　　　　　nontraffic V75.1
　　　　　specified vehicle NEC
　　　　　　(traffic) V76.6

Accident (to) - *continued*
　transport (involving injury to) - *continued*
　　bus occupant - *continued*
　　　passenger - *continued*
　　　　collision (with) - *continued*
　　　　　specified vehicle NEC (traffic) -
　　　　　　continued
　　　　　　nontraffic V76.1
　　　　　stationary object (traffic) V77.6
　　　　　　nontraffic V77.1
　　　　　streetcar (traffic) V76.6
　　　　　　nontraffic V76.1
　　　　　three wheeled motor vehicle
　　　　　　(traffic) V72.6
　　　　　　nontraffic V72.1
　　　　　truck (traffic) V74.6
　　　　　　nontraffic V74.1
　　　　　two wheeled motor vehicle
　　　　　　(traffic) V72.6
　　　　　　nontraffic V72.1
　　　　　van (traffic) V73.6
　　　　　　nontraffic V73.1
　　　　noncollision accident (traffic) V78.6
　　　　　nontraffic V78.1
　　　specified type NEC V79.88
　　　　military vehicle V79.81
　　cable car, not on rails V98.0
　　　on rails — *see* Accident, transport,
　　　　streetcar occupant
　　car occupant V49.9
　　　ambulance occupant — *see* Accident,
　　　　transport, ambulance occupant
　　　collision (with)
　　　　animal (traffic) V40.9
　　　　　being ridden (traffic) V46.9
　　　　　　nontraffic V46.3
　　　　　　while boarding or alighting V46.4
　　　　　nontraffic V40.3
　　　　　while boarding or alighting V40.4
　　　　animal-drawn vehicle (traffic) V46.9
　　　　　nontraffic V46.3
　　　　　while boarding or alighting V46.4
　　　　bus (traffic) V44.9
　　　　　nontraffic V44.3
　　　　　while boarding or alighting V44.4
　　　　car (traffic) V43.92
　　　　　nontraffic V43.32
　　　　　while boarding or alighting V43.42
　　　　motor vehicle NOS (traffic) V49.60
　　　　　nontraffic V49.20
　　　　　specified type NEC (traffic) V49.69
　　　　　　nontraffic V49.29
　　　　pedal cycle (traffic) V41.9
　　　　　nontraffic V41.3
　　　　　while boarding or alighting V41.4
　　　　pickup truck (traffic) V43.93
　　　　　nontraffic V43.33
　　　　　while boarding or alighting V43.43
　　　　railway vehicle (traffic) V45.9
　　　　　nontraffic V45.3
　　　　　while boarding or alighting V45.4
　　　　specified vehicle NEC (traffic) V46.9
　　　　　nontraffic V46.3
　　　　　while boarding or alighting V46.4
　　　　sport utility vehicle (traffic) V43.91
　　　　　nontraffic V43.31
　　　　　while boarding or alighting V43.41
　　　　stationary object (traffic) V47.9
　　　　　nontraffic V47.3
　　　　　while boarding or alighting V47.4
　　　　streetcar (traffic) V46.9
　　　　　nontraffic V46.3
　　　　　while boarding or alighting V46.4
　　　　three wheeled motor vehicle
　　　　　(traffic) V42.9
　　　　　nontraffic V42.3
　　　　　while boarding or alighting V42.4
　　　　truck (traffic) V44.9
　　　　　nontraffic V44.3
　　　　　while boarding or alighting V44.4
　　　　two wheeled motor vehicle
　　　　　(traffic) V42.9
　　　　　nontraffic V42.3
　　　　　while boarding or alighting V42.4
　　　　van (traffic) V43.94

Accident (to) - *continued*
　transport (involving injury to) - *continued*
　　car occupant - *continued*
　　　collision (with) - *continued*
　　　　van (traffic) - *continued*
　　　　　nontraffic V43.34
　　　　　while boarding or alighting V43.44
　　　driver
　　　　collision (with)
　　　　　animal (traffic) V40.5
　　　　　　being ridden (traffic) V46.5
　　　　　　　nontraffic V46.0
　　　　　　nontraffic V40.0
　　　　　animal-drawn vehicle
　　　　　　(traffic) V46.5
　　　　　　nontraffic V46.0
　　　　　bus (traffic) V44.5
　　　　　　nontraffic V44.0
　　　　　car (traffic) V43.52
　　　　　　nontraffic V43.02
　　　　　motor vehicle NOS (traffic) V49.40
　　　　　　nontraffic V49.00
　　　　　　specified type NEC
　　　　　　　(traffic) V49.49
　　　　　　　nontraffic V49.09
　　　　　pedal cycle (traffic) V41.5
　　　　　　nontraffic V41.0
　　　　　pickup truck (traffic) V43.53
　　　　　　nontraffic V43.03
　　　　　railway vehicle (traffic) V45.5
　　　　　　nontraffic V45.0
　　　　　specified vehicle NEC
　　　　　　(traffic) V46.5
　　　　　　nontraffic V46.0
　　　　　sport utility vehicle (traffic) V43.51
　　　　　　nontraffic V43.01
　　　　　stationary object (traffic) V47.5
　　　　　　nontraffic V47.0
　　　　　streetcar (traffic) V46.5
　　　　　　nontraffic V46.0
　　　　　three wheeled motor vehicle
　　　　　　(traffic) V42.5
　　　　　　nontraffic V42.0
　　　　　truck (traffic) V44.5
　　　　　　nontraffic V44.0
　　　　　two wheeled motor vehicle
　　　　　　(traffic) V42.5
　　　　　　nontraffic V42.0
　　　　　van (traffic) V43.54
　　　　　　nontraffic V43.04
　　　　noncollision accident (traffic) V48.5
　　　　　nontraffic V48.0
　　　noncollision accident (traffic) V48.9
　　　　nontraffic V48.3
　　　　while boarding or alighting V48.4
　　　nontraffic V49.3
　　　hanger-on
　　　　collision (with)
　　　　　animal (traffic) V40.7
　　　　　　being ridden (traffic) V46.7
　　　　　　　nontraffic V46.2
　　　　　　nontraffic V40.2
　　　　　animal-drawn vehicle
　　　　　　(traffic) V46.7
　　　　　　nontraffic V46.2
　　　　　bus (traffic) V44.7
　　　　　　nontraffic V44.2
　　　　　car (traffic) V43.72
　　　　　　nontraffic V43.22
　　　　　pedal cycle (traffic) V41.7
　　　　　　nontraffic V41.2
　　　　　pickup truck (traffic) V43.73
　　　　　　nontraffic V43.23
　　　　　railway vehicle (traffic) V45.7
　　　　　　nontraffic V45.2
　　　　　specified vehicle NEC
　　　　　　(traffic) V46.7
　　　　　　nontraffic V46.2
　　　　　sport utility vehicle (traffic) V43.71
　　　　　　nontraffic V43.21
　　　　　stationary object (traffic) V47.7
　　　　　　nontraffic V47.2
　　　　　streetcar (traffic) V46.7
　　　　　　nontraffic V46.2

Accident (to) - *continued*
transport (involving injury to) - *continued*
car occupant - *continued*
hanger-on - *continued*
collision (with) - *continued*
three wheeled motor vehicle
(traffic) V42.7
nontraffic V42.2
truck (traffic) V44.7
nontraffic V44.2
two wheeled motor vehicle
(traffic) V42.7
nontraffic V42.2
van (traffic) V43.74
nontraffic V43.24
noncollision accident (traffic) V48.7
nontraffic V48.2
passenger
collision (with)
animal (traffic) V40.6
being ridden (traffic) V46.6
nontraffic V46.1
nontraffic V40.1
animal-drawn vehicle
(traffic) V46.6
nontraffic V46.1
bus (traffic) V44.6
nontraffic V44.1
car (traffic) V43.62
nontraffic V43.12
motor vehicle NOS (traffic) V49.50
nontraffic V49.10
specified type NEC
(traffic) V49.59
nontraffic V49.19
pedal cycle (traffic) V41.6
nontraffic V41.1
pickup truck (traffic) V43.63
nontraffic V43.13
railway vehicle (traffic) V45.6
nontraffic V45.1
specified vehicle NEC
(traffic) V46.6
nontraffic V46.1
sport utility vehicle (traffic) V43.61
nontraffic V43.11
stationary object (traffic) V47.6
nontraffic V47.1
streetcar (traffic) V46.6
nontraffic V46.1
three wheeled motor vehicle
(traffic) V42.6
nontraffic V42.1
truck (traffic) V44.6
nontraffic V44.1
two wheeled motor vehicle
(traffic) V42.6
nontraffic V42.1
van (traffic) V43.64
nontraffic V43.14
noncollision accident (traffic) V48.6
nontraffic V48.1
specified type NEC V49.88
military vehicle V49.81
coal car — *see* Accident, transport,
industrial vehicle occupant
construction vehicle occupant
(nontraffic) V85.9
driver V85.5
hanger-on V85.7
passenger V85.6
traffic V85.3
driver V85.0
hanger-on V85.2
passenger V85.1
while boarding or alighting V85.4
dirt bike rider (nontraffic) V86.96
driver V86.56
hanger-on V86.76
passenger V86.66
traffic V86.36
driver V86.06
hanger-on V86.26
passenger V86.16
while boarding or alighting V86.46

Accident (to) - *continued*
transport (involving injury to) - *continued*
due to cataclysm — *see* Forces of nature,
by type
dune buggy occupant (nontraffic) V86.93
driver V86.53
hanger-on V86.73
passenger V86.63
traffic V86.33
driver V86.03
hanger-on V86.23
passenger V86.13
while boarding or alighting V86.43
forklift — *see* Accident, transport,
industrial vehicle occupant
go cart — *see* Accident, transport, all-
terrain vehicle occupant
golf cart — *see* Accident, transport, all-
terrain vehicle occupant
heavy transport vehicle occupant — *see*
Accident, transport, truck occupant
ice yacht V98.2
industrial vehicle occupant
(nontraffic) V83.9
driver V83.5
hanger-on V83.7
passenger V83.6
traffic V83.3
driver V83.0
hanger-on V83.2
passenger V83.1
while boarding or alighting V83.4
interurban electric car — *see* Accident,
transport, streetcar
land yacht V98.1
logging car — *see* Accident, transport,
industrial vehicle occupant
military vehicle occupant (traffic) V86.34
driver V86.04
hanger-on V86.24
nontraffic V86.94
driver V86.54
hanger-on V86.74
passenger V86.64
passenger V86.14
while boarding or alighting V86.44
mine tram — *see* Accident, transport,
industrial vehicle occupant
motorcoach — *see* Accident, transport, bus
occupant
motor/cross bike rider — *see also*
Accident, transport, dirt bike
rider V86.96
motorcyclist V29.9
collision (with)
animal (traffic) V20.9
being ridden (traffic) V26.9
nontraffic V26.2
while boarding or alighting V26.3
nontraffic V20.2
while boarding or alighting V20.3
animal-drawn vehicle (traffic) V26.9
nontraffic V26.2
while boarding or alighting V26.3
bus (traffic) V24.9
nontraffic V24.2
while boarding or alighting V24.3
car (traffic) V23.9
nontraffic V23.2
while boarding or alighting V23.3
motor vehicle NOS (traffic) V29.60
nontraffic V29.20
specified type NEC (traffic) V29.69
nontraffic V29.29
pedal cycle (traffic) V21.9
nontraffic V21.2
while boarding or alighting V21.3
pickup truck (traffic) V23.9
nontraffic V23.2
while boarding or alighting V23.3
railway vehicle (traffic) V25.9
nontraffic V25.2
while boarding or alighting V25.3
specified vehicle NEC (traffic) V26.9
nontraffic V26.2

Accident (to) - *continued*
transport (involving injury to) - *continued*
motorcyclist - *continued*
collision (with) - *continued*
specified vehicle NEC (traffic) -
continued
while boarding or alighting V26.3
stationary object (traffic) V27.9
nontraffic V27.2
while boarding or alighting V27.3
streetcar (traffic) V26.9
nontraffic V26.2
while boarding or alighting V26.3
three wheeled motor vehicle
(traffic) V22.9
nontraffic V22.2
while boarding or alighting V22.3
truck (traffic) V24.9
nontraffic V24.2
while boarding or alighting V24.3
two wheeled motor vehicle
(traffic) V22.9
nontraffic V22.2
while boarding or alighting V22.3
van (traffic) V23.9
nontraffic V23.2
while boarding or alighting V23.3
driver
collision (with)
animal (traffic) V20.4
being ridden (traffic) V26.4
nontraffic V26.0
nontraffic V20.0
animal-drawn vehicle
(traffic) V26.4
nontraffic V26.0
bus (traffic) V24.4
nontraffic V24.0
car (traffic) V23.4
nontraffic V23.0
motor vehicle NOS (traffic) V29.40
nontraffic V29.00
specified type NEC
(traffic) V29.49
nontraffic V29.09
pedal cycle (traffic) V21.4
nontraffic V21.0
pickup truck (traffic) V23.4
nontraffic V23.0
railway vehicle (traffic) V25.4
nontraffic V25.0
specified vehicle NEC
(traffic) V26.4
nontraffic V26.0
stationary object (traffic) V27.4
nontraffic V27.0
streetcar (traffic) V26.4
nontraffic V26.0
three wheeled motor vehicle
(traffic) V22.4
nontraffic V22.0
truck (traffic) V24.4
nontraffic V24.0
two wheeled motor vehicle
(traffic) V22.4
nontraffic V22.0
van (traffic) V23.4
nontraffic V23.0
noncollision accident (traffic) V28.4
nontraffic V28.0
noncollision accident (traffic) V28.9
nontraffic V28.2
while boarding or alighting V28.3
nontraffic V29.3
passenger
collision (with)
animal (traffic) V20.5
being ridden (traffic) V26.5
nontraffic V26.1
nontraffic V20.1
animal-drawn vehicle
(traffic) V26.5
nontraffic V26.1
bus (traffic) V24.5
nontraffic V24.1

ACCIDENT - ACCIDENT

Accident (to) - *continued*
  transport (involving injury to) - *continued*
    motorcyclist - *continued*
      passenger - *see continued*
        collision (with) - *continued*
          car (traffic) V23.5
            nontraffic V23.1
          motor vehicle NOS (traffic) V29.50
            nontraffic V29.10
            specified type NEC
              (traffic) V29.59
              nontraffic V29.19
          pedal cycle (traffic) V21.5
            nontraffic V21.1
          pickup truck (traffic) V23.5
            nontraffic V23.1
          railway vehicle (traffic) V25.5
            nontraffic V25.1
          specified vehicle NEC
            (traffic) V26.5
            nontraffic V26.1
          stationary object (traffic) V27.5
            nontraffic V27.1
          streetcar (traffic) V26.5
            nontraffic V26.1
          three wheeled motor vehicle
            (traffic) V22.5
            nontraffic V22.1
          truck (traffic) V24.5
            nontraffic V24.1
          two wheeled motor vehicle
            (traffic) V22.5
            nontraffic V22.1
          van (traffic) V23.5
            nontraffic V23.1
        noncollision accident (traffic) V28.5
          nontraffic V28.1
        specified type NEC V29.88
        military vehicle V29.81
      motor vehicle NEC occupant
        (traffic) V89.2
    occupant (of)
      aircraft (powered) V95.9
        fixed wing
          commercial — *see* Accident,
            transport, aircraft, occupant,
            powered, fixed wing,
            commercial
          private — *see* Accident, transport,
            aircraft, occupant, powered,
            fixed wing, private
        nonpowered V96.9
        specified NEC V95.8
      airport battery-powered vehicle — *see*
        Accident, transport, industrial
        vehicle occupant
      all-terrain vehicle (ATV) — *see*
        Accident, transport, all-terrain
        vehicle occupant
      animal-drawn vehicle — *see* Accident,
        transport, animal-drawn vehicle
        occupant
      automobile — *see* Accident, transport,
        car occupant
      balloon V96.00
      battery-powered vehicle — *see*
        Accident, transport, industrial
        vehicle occupant
      bicycle — *see* Accident, transport, pedal
        cyclist
        motorized — *see* Accident, transport,
          motorcycle rider
      boat NEC — *see* Accident, watercraft
      bulldozer — *see* Accident, transport,
        construction vehicle occupant
      bus — *see* Accident, transport, bus
        occupant
      cable car (on rails) — *see also* Accident,
        transport, streetcar occupant
        not on rails V98.0
      car — *see also* Accident, transport, car
        occupant
        cable (on rails) — *see also* Accident,
          transport, streetcar occupant
          not on rails V98.0

Accident (to) - *continued*
  transport (involving injury to) - *continued*
    occupant (of) - *continued*
      coach — *see* Accident, transport, bus
        occupant
      coal-car — *see* Accident, transport,
        industrial vehicle occupant
      digger — *see* Accident, transport,
        construction vehicle occupant
      dump truck — *see* Accident, transport,
        construction vehicle occupant
      earth-leveler — *see* Accident, transport,
        construction vehicle occupant
      farm machinery (self-propelled) — *see*
        Accident, transport, agricultural
        vehicle occupant
      forklift — *see* Accident, transport,
        industrial vehicle occupant
      glider (unpowered) V96.20
        hang V96.10
        powered (microlight) (ultralight) —
          see Accident, transport, aircraft,
          occupant, powered, glider
      glider (unpowered) NEC V96.20
      hang-glider V96.10
      harvester — *see* Accident, transport,
        agricultural vehicle occupant
      heavy (transport) vehicle — *see*
        Accident, transport, truck occupant
      helicopter — *see* Accident, transport,
        aircraft, occupant, helicopter
      ice-yacht V98.2
      kite (carrying person) V96.8
      land-yacht V98.1
      logging car — *see* Accident, transport,
        industrial vehicle occupant
      mechanical shovel — *see* Accident,
        transport, construction vehicle
        occupant
      microlight — *see* Accident, transport,
        aircraft, occupant, powered, glider
      minibus — *see* Accident, transport,
        pickup truck occupant
      minivan — *see* Accident, transport,
        pickup truck occupant
      moped — *see* Accident, transport,
        motorcycle
      motor scooter — *see* Accident, transport,
        motorcycle
      motorcycle (with sidecar) — *see*
        Accident, transport, motorcycle
      off-road motor-vehicle — *see also*
        Accident, transport, all-terrain
        vehicle occupant V86.99
      pedal cycle — *see also* Accident,
        transport, pedal cyclist
      pick-up (truck) — *see* Accident,
        transport, pickup truck occupant
      railway (train) (vehicle) (subterranean)
        (elevated) — *see* Accident,
        transport, railway vehicle occupant
      rickshaw — *see* Accident, transport,
        pedal cycle
        motorized — *see* Accident, transport,
          three-wheeled motor vehicle
        pedal driven — *see* Accident,
          transport, pedal cyclist
      road-roller — *see* Accident, transport,
        construction vehicle occupant
      ship NOS V94.9
      ski-lift (chair) (gondola) V98.3
      snowmobile — *see* Accident, transport,
        snowmobile occupant
      spacecraft, spaceship — *see* Accident,
        transport, aircraft, occupant,
        spacecraft
      sport utility vehicle — *see* Accident,
        transport, pickup truck occupant
      streetcar (interurban) (operating on
        public street or highway) — *see*
        Accident, transport, streetcar
        occupant
      SUV — *see* Accident, transport, pickup
        truck occupant
      téléférique V98.0

Accident (to) - *continued*
  transport (involving injury to) - *continued*
    occupant (of) - *continued*
      three-wheeled vehicle (motorized) —
        see also Accident, transport, three-
        wheeled motor vehicle occupant
        nonmotorized — *see* Accident,
          transport, pedal cycle
      tractor (farm) (and trailer) — *see*
        Accident, transport, agricultural
        vehicle occupant
      train — *see* Accident, transport, railway
        vehicle occupant
      tram — *see* Accident, transport, streetcar
        occupant
        in mine or quarry — *see* Accident,
          transport, industrial vehicle
          occupant
      tricycle — *see* Accident, transport, pedal
        cycle
        motorized — *see* Accident, transport,
          three-wheeled motor vehicle
      trolley — *see* Accident, transport,
        streetcar occupant
        in mine or quarry — *see* Accident,
          transport, industrial vehicle
          occupant
      tub, in mine or quarry — *see* Accident,
        transport, industrial vehicle
        occupant
      ultralight — *see* Accident, transport,
        aircraft, occupant, powered, glider
      van — *see* Accident, transport, van
        occupant
      vehicle NEC V89.9
        heavy transport — *see* Accident,
          transport, truck occupant
        motor (traffic) NEC V89.2
          nontraffic NEC V89.0
      watercraft NOS V94.9
        causing drowning — *see* Drowning,
          resulting from accident to boat
      off-road motor-vehicle — *see also*
        Accident, transport, all-terrain
        vehicle occupant V86.99
    parachutist V97.29
      after accident to aircraft — *see* Accident,
        transport, aircraft
      entangled in object V97.21
      injured on landing V97.22
    pedal cyclist V19.9
      collision (with)
        animal (traffic) V10.9
          being ridden (traffic) V16.9
            nontraffic V16.2
              while boarding or alighting V16.3
          nontraffic V10.2
            while boarding or alighting V10.3
        animal-drawn vehicle (traffic) V16.9
          nontraffic V16.2
            while boarding or alighting V16.3
        bus (traffic) V14.9
          nontraffic V14.2
            while boarding or alighting V14.3
        car (traffic) V13.9
          nontraffic V13.2
            while boarding or alighting V13.3
        motor vehicle NOS (traffic) V19.60
          nontraffic V19.20
          specified type NEC (traffic) V19.69
            nontraffic V19.29
        pedal cycle (traffic) V11.9
          nontraffic V11.2
            while boarding or alighting V11.3
        pickup truck (traffic) V13.9
          nontraffic V13.2
            while boarding or alighting V13.3
        railway vehicle (traffic) V15.9
          nontraffic V15.2
            while boarding or alighting V15.3
        specified vehicle NEC (traffic) V16.9
          nontraffic V16.2
            while boarding or alighting V16.3
        stationary object (traffic) V17.9
          nontraffic V17.2

Accident (to) - *continued*
transport (involving injury to) - *continued*
pedal cyclist - *continued*
collision (with) - *continued*
stationary object (traffic) - *continued*
while boarding or alighting V17.3
streetcar (traffic) V16.9
nontraffic V16.2
while boarding or alighting V16.3
three wheeled motor vehicle
(traffic) V12.9
nontraffic V12.2
while boarding or alighting V12.3
truck (traffic) V14.9
nontraffic V14.2
while boarding or alighting V14.3
two wheeled motor vehicle
(traffic) V12.9
nontraffic V12.2
while boarding or alighting V12.3
van (traffic) V13.9
nontraffic V13.2
while boarding or alighting V13.3
driver
collision (with)
animal (traffic) V10.4
being ridden (traffic) V16.4
nontraffic V16.0
nontraffic V10.0
animal-drawn vehicle
(traffic) V16.4
nontraffic V16.0
bus (traffic) V14.4
nontraffic V14.0
car (traffic) V13.4
nontraffic V13.0
motor vehicle NOS (traffic) V19.40
nontraffic V19.00
specified type NEC
(traffic) V19.49
nontraffic V19.09
pedal cycle (traffic) V11.4
nontraffic V11.0
pickup truck (traffic) V13.4
nontraffic V13.0
railway vehicle (traffic) V15.4
nontraffic V15.0
specified vehicle NEC
(traffic) V16.4
nontraffic V16.0
stationary object (traffic) V17.4
nontraffic V17.0
streetcar (traffic) V16.4
nontraffic V16.0
three wheeled motor vehicle
(traffic) V12.4
nontraffic V12.0
truck (traffic) V14.4
nontraffic V14.0
two wheeled motor vehicle
(traffic) V12.4
nontraffic V12.0
van (traffic) V13.4
nontraffic V13.0
noncollision accident (traffic) V18.4
nontraffic V18.0
noncollision accident (traffic) V18.9
nontraffic V18.2
while boarding or alighting V18.3
nontraffic V19.3
passenger
collision (with)
animal (traffic) V10.5
being ridden (traffic) V16.5
nontraffic V16.1
nontraffic V10.1
animal-drawn vehicle
(traffic) V16.5
nontraffic V16.1
bus (traffic) V14.5
nontraffic V14.1
car (traffic) V13.5
nontraffic V13.1
motor vehicle NOS (traffic) V19.50
nontraffic V19.10

Accident (to) - *continued*
transport (involving injury to) - *continued*
pedal cyclist - *continued*
passenger - *continued*
collision (with) - *continued*
motor vehicle NOS (traffic) -
continued
specified type NEC
(traffic) V19.59
nontraffic V19.19
pedal cycle (traffic) V11.5
nontraffic V11.1
pickup truck (traffic) V13.5
nontraffic V13.1
railway vehicle (traffic) V15.5
nontraffic V15.1
specified vehicle NEC
(traffic) V16.5
nontraffic V16.1
stationary object (traffic) V17.5
nontraffic V17.1
streetcar (traffic) V16.5
nontraffic V16.1
three wheeled motor vehicle
(traffic) V12.5
nontraffic V12.1
truck (traffic) V14.5
nontraffic V14.1
two wheeled motor vehicle
(traffic) V12.5
nontraffic V12.1
van (traffic) V13.5
nontraffic V13.1
noncollision accident (traffic) V18.5
nontraffic V18.1
specified type NEC V19.88
military vehicle V19.81
pedestrian
conveyance (occupant) V09.9
baby stroller V00.828
collision (with) V09.9
animal being ridden or animal
drawn vehicle V06.99
nontraffic V06.09
traffic V06.19
bus or heavy transport V04.99
nontraffic V04.09
traffic V04.19
car V03.99
nontraffic V03.09
traffic V03.19
pedal cycle V01.99
nontraffic V01.09
traffic V01.19
pick-up truck or van V03.99
nontraffic V03.09
traffic V03.19
railway (train) (vehicle) V05.99
nontraffic V05.09
traffic V05.19
streetcar V06.99
nontraffic V06.09
traffic V06.19
stationary object V00.822
two- or three-wheeled motor
vehicle V02.99
nontraffic V02.09
traffic V02.19
vehicle V09.9
animal-drawn V06.99
nontraffic V06.09
traffic V06.19
motor
nontraffic V09.00
traffic V09.20
fall V00.821
nontraffic V09.1
involving motor vehicle
NEC V09.00
traffic V09.3
involving motor vehicle
NEC V09.20
flat-bottomed NEC V00.388
collision (with) V09.9

Accident (to) - *continued*
transport (involving injury to) - *continued*
pedestrian - *continued*
conveyance (occupant) - *continued*
flat-bottomed NEC - *continued*
collision (with) - *continued*
animal being ridden or animal
drawn vehicle V06.99
nontraffic V06.09
traffic V06.19
bus or heavy transport V04.99
nontraffic V04.09
traffic V04.19
car V03.99
nontraffic V03.09
traffic V03.19
pedal cycle V01.99
nontraffic V01.09
traffic V01.19
pick-up truck or van V03.99
nontraffic V03.09
traffic V03.19
railway (train) (vehicle) V05.99
nontraffic V05.09
traffic V05.19
stationary object V00.382
streetcar V06.99
nontraffic V06.09
traffic V06.19
two- or three-wheeled motor
vehicle V02.99
nontraffic V02.09
traffic V02.19
vehicle V09.9
animal-drawn V06.99
nontraffic V06.09
traffic V06.19
motor
nontraffic V09.00
traffic V09.20
fall V00.381
nontraffic V09.1
involving motor vehicle
NEC V09.00
snow
board — *see* Accident, transport,
pedestrian, conveyance,
snow board
ski- — *see* Accident, transport,
pedestrian, conveyance, skis
(snow)
traffic V09.3
involving motor vehicle
NEC V09.20
gliding type NEC V00.288
collision (with) V09.9
animal being ridden or animal
drawn vehicle V06.99
nontraffic V06.09
traffic V06.19
bus or heavy transport V04.99
nontraffic V04.09
traffic V04.19
car V03.99
nontraffic V03.09
traffic V03.19
pedal cycle V01.99
nontraffic V01.09
traffic V01.19
pick-up truck or van V03.99
nontraffic V03.09
traffic V03.19
railway (train) (vehicle) V05.99
nontraffic V05.09
traffic V05.19
stationary object V00.282
streetcar V06.99
nontraffic V06.09
traffic V06.19
two- or three-wheeled motor
vehicle V02.99
nontraffic V02.09
traffic V02.19
vehicle V09.9
animal-drawn V06.99

Accident (to) - *continued*
  transport (involving injury to) - *continued*
    pedestrian - *continued*
      conveyance (occupant) - *continued*
        gliding type NEC - *continued*
          collision (with) - *continued*
            vehicle - *continued*
              animal-drawn - *continued*
                nontraffic V06.09
                traffic V06.19
              motor
                nontraffic V09.00
                traffic V09.20
          fall V00.281
          heelies — *see* Accident, transport,
            pedestrian, conveyance, heelies
          ice skate — *see* Accident, transport,
            pedestrian, conveyance, ice
            skate
          nontraffic V09.1
            involving motor vehicle
              NEC V09.00
          sled — *see* Accident, transport,
            pedestrian, conveyance, sled
          traffic V09.3
            involving motor vehicle
              NEC V09.20
          wheelies — *see* Accident,
            transport, pedestrian,
            conveyance, heelies
        heelies V00.158
          colliding with stationary
            object V00.152
          fall V00.151
        ice skates V00.218
          collision (with) V09.9
            animal being ridden or animal
              drawn vehicle V06.99
              nontraffic V06.09
              traffic V06.19
            bus or heavy transport V04.99
              nontraffic V04.09
              traffic V04.19
            car V03.99
              nontraffic V03.09
              traffic V03.19
            pedal cycle V01.99
              nontraffic V01.09
              traffic V01.19
            pick-up truck or van V03.99
              nontraffic V03.09
              traffic V03.19
            railway (train) (vehicle) V05.99
              nontraffic V05.09
              traffic V05.19
            streetcar V06.99
              nontraffic V06.09
              traffic V06.19
            stationary object V00.212
            two- or three-wheeled motor
              vehicle V02.99
              nontraffic V02.09
              traffic V02.19
            vehicle V09.9
              animal-drawn V06.99
                nontraffic V06.09
                traffic V06.19
              motor
                nontraffic V09.00
                traffic V09.20
          fall V00.211
          nontraffic V09.1
            involving motor vehicle
              NEC V09.00
          traffic V09.3
            involving motor vehicle
              NEC V09.20
        motorized mobility scooter V00.838
          collision with stationary
            object V00.832
          fall from V00.831
          nontraffic V09.1
            involving motor vehicle V09.00
              military V09.01
              specified type NEC V09.09

Accident (to) - *continued*
  transport (involving injury to) - *continued*
    pedestrian - *continued*
      conveyance (occupant) - *continued*
        roller skates (non in-line) V00.128
          collision (with) V09.9
            animal being ridden or animal
              drawn vehicle V06.91
              nontraffic V06.01
              traffic V06.11
            bus or heavy transport V04.91
              nontraffic V04.01
              traffic V04.11
            car V03.91
              nontraffic V03.01
              traffic V03.11
            pedal cycle V01.91
              nontraffic V01.01
              traffic V01.11
            pick-up truck or van V03.91
              nontraffic V03.01
              traffic V03.11
            railway (train) (vehicle) V05.91
              nontraffic V05.01
              traffic V05.11
            streetcar V06.91
              nontraffic V06.01
              traffic V06.11
            stationary object V00.122
            two- or three-wheeled motor
              vehicle V02.91
              nontraffic V02.01
              traffic V02.11
            vehicle V09.9
              animal-drawn V06.91
                nontraffic V06.01
                traffic V06.11
              motor
                nontraffic V09.00
                traffic V09.20
          fall V00.121
          in-line V00.118
            collision- — *see also* Accident,
              transport, pedestrian,
              conveyance occupant, roller
              skates, collision
            with stationary object V00.112
            fall V00.111
            nontraffic V09.1
              involving motor vehicle
                NEC V09.00
            traffic V09.3
              involving motor vehicle
                NEC V09.20
        rolling shoes V00.158
          colliding with stationary
            object V00.152
          fall V00.151
        rolling type NEC V00.188
          collision (with) V09.9
            animal being ridden or animal
              drawn vehicle V06.99
              nontraffic V06.09
              traffic V06.19
            bus or heavy transport V04.99
              nontraffic V04.09
              traffic V04.19
            car V03.99
              nontraffic V03.09
              traffic V03.19
            pedal cycle V01.99
              nontraffic V01.09
              traffic V01.19
            pick-up truck or van V03.99
              nontraffic V03.09
              traffic V03.19
            railway (train) (vehicle) V05.99
              nontraffic V05.09
              traffic V05.19
            stationary object V00.182
            streetcar V06.99
              nontraffic V06.09
              traffic V06.19
            two- or three-wheeled motor
              vehicle V02.99

Accident (to) - *continued*
  transport (involving injury to) - *continued*
    pedestrian - *continued*
      conveyance (occupant) - *continued*
        rolling type NEC - *continued*
          collision (with) - *continued*
            two- or three-wheeled motor
              vehicle - *continued*
                nontraffic V02.09
                traffic V02.19
            vehicle V09.9
              animal-drawn V06.99
                nontraffic V06.09
                traffic V06.19
              motor
                nontraffic V09.00
                traffic V09.20
          fall V00.181
          in-line roller skate — *see* Accident,
            transport, pedestrian,
            conveyance, roller skate, in-
            line
          nontraffic V09.1
            involving motor vehicle
              NEC V09.00
          roller skate — *see* Accident,
            transport, pedestrian,
            conveyance, roller skate
          scooter (non-motorized) — *see*
            Accident, transport, pedestrian,
            conveyance, scooter
          skateboard — *see* Accident,
            transport, pedestrian,
            conveyance, skateboard
          traffic V09.3
            involving motor vehicle
              NEC V09.20
        scooter (non-motorized) V00.148
          collision (with) V09.9
            animal being ridden or animal
              drawn vehicle V06.99
              nontraffic V06.09
              traffic V06.19
            bus or heavy transport V04.99
              nontraffic V04.09
              traffic V04.19
            car V03.99
              nontraffic V03.09
              traffic V03.19
            pedal cycle V01.99
              nontraffic V01.09
              traffic V01.19
            pick-up truck or van V03.99
              nontraffic V03.09
              traffic V03.19
            railway (train) (vehicle) V05.99
              nontraffic V05.09
              traffic V05.19
            streetcar V06.99
              nontraffic V06.09
              traffic V06.19
            stationary object V00.142
            two- or three-wheeled motor
              vehicle V02.99
              nontraffic V02.09
              traffic V02.19
            vehicle V09.9
              animal-drawn V06.99
                nontraffic V06.09
                traffic V06.19
              motor
                nontraffic V09.00
                traffic V09.20
          fall V00.141
          nontraffic V09.1
            involving motor vehicle
              NEC V09.00
          traffic V09.3
            involving motor vehicle
              NEC V09.20
        skate board V00.138
          collision (with) V09.9
            animal being ridden or animal
              drawn vehicle V06.92
              nontraffic V06.02

Accident (to) - *continued*
 transport (involving injury to) - *continued*
  pedestrian - *continued*
   conveyance (occupant) - *continued*
    skate board - *continued*
     collision (with) - *continued*
      animal being ridden or animal
        drawn vehicle - *continued*
       traffic V06.12
       bus or heavy transport V04.92
        nontraffic V04.02
        traffic V04.12
       car V03.92
        nontraffic V03.02
        traffic V03.12
       pedal cycle V01.92
        nontraffic V01.02
        traffic V01.12
       pick-up truck or van V03.92
        nontraffic V03.02
        traffic V03.12
       railway (train) (vehicle) V05.92
        nontraffic V05.02
        traffic V05.12
       streetcar V06.92
        nontraffic V06.02
        traffic V06.12
       stationary object V00.132
       two- or three-wheeled motor
         vehicle V02.92
        nontraffic V02.02
        traffic V02.12
       vehicle V09.9
        animal-drawn V06.92
         nontraffic V06.02
         traffic V06.12
        motor
         nontraffic V09.00
         traffic V09.20
      fall V00.131
      nontraffic V09.1
       involving motor vehicle
         NEC V09.00
      traffic V09.3
       involving motor vehicle
         NEC V09.20
     sled V00.228
      collision (with) V09.9
       animal being ridden or animal
         drawn vehicle V06.99
        nontraffic V06.09
        traffic V06.19
       bus or heavy transport V04.99
        nontraffic V04.09
        traffic V04.19
       car V03.99
        nontraffic V03.09
        traffic V03.19
       pedal cycle V01.99
        nontraffic V01.09
        traffic V01.19
       pick-up truck or van V03.99
        nontraffic V03.09
        traffic V03.19
       railway (train) (vehicle) V05.99
        nontraffic V05.09
        traffic V05.19
       streetcar V06.99
        nontraffic V06.09
        traffic V06.19
       stationary object V00.222
       two- or three-wheeled motor
         vehicle V02.99
        nontraffic V02.09
        traffic V02.19
       vehicle V09.9
        animal-drawn V06.99
         nontraffic V06.09
         traffic V06.19
        motor
         nontraffic V09.00
         traffic V09.20
      fall V00.221
      nontraffic V09.1

Accident (to) - *continued*
 transport (involving injury to) - *continued*
  pedestrian - *continued*
   conveyance (occupant) - *continued*
    sled - *continued*
     nontraffic - *continued*
      involving motor vehicle
        NEC V09.00
     traffic V09.3
      involving motor vehicle
        NEC V09.20
    skis (snow) V00.328
     collision (with) V09.9
      animal being ridden or animal
        drawn vehicle V06.99
       nontraffic V06.09
       traffic V06.19
      bus or heavy transport V04.99
       nontraffic V04.09
       traffic V04.19
      car V03.99
       nontraffic V03.09
       traffic V03.19
      pedal cycle V01.99
       nontraffic V01.09
       traffic V01.19
      pick-up truck or van V03.99
       nontraffic V03.09
       traffic V03.19
      railway (train) (vehicle) V05.99
       nontraffic V05.09
       traffic V05.19
      streetcar V06.99
       nontraffic V06.09
       traffic V06.19
      stationary object V00.322
      two- or three-wheeled motor
        vehicle V02.99
       nontraffic V02.09
       traffic V02.19
      vehicle V09.9
       animal-drawn V06.99
        nontraffic V06.09
        traffic V06.19
       motor
        nontraffic V09.00
        traffic V09.20
     fall V00.321
     nontraffic V09.1
      involving motor vehicle
        NEC V09.00
     traffic V09.3
      involving motor vehicle
        NEC V09.20
    snow board V00.318
     collision (with) V09.9
      animal being ridden or animal
        drawn vehicle V06.99
       nontraffic V06.09
       traffic V06.19
      bus or heavy transport V04.99
       nontraffic V04.09
       traffic V04.19
      car V03.99
       nontraffic V03.09
       traffic V03.19
      pedal cycle V01.99
       nontraffic V01.09
       traffic V01.19
      pick-up truck or van V03.99
       nontraffic V03.09
       traffic V03.19
      railway (train) (vehicle) V05.99
       nontraffic V05.09
       traffic V05.19
      streetcar V06.99
       nontraffic V06.09
       traffic V06.19
      stationary object V00.312
      two- or three-wheeled motor
        vehicle V02.99
       nontraffic V02.09
       traffic V02.19
      vehicle V09.9
       animal-drawn V06.99

Accident (to) - *continued*
 transport (involving injury to) - *continued*
  pedestrian - *continued*
   conveyance (occupant) - *continued*
    snow board - *continued*
     collision (with) - *continued*
      vehicle - *continued*
       animal-drawn - *continued*
        nontraffic V06.09
        traffic V06.19
       motor
        nontraffic V09.00
        traffic V09.20
     fall V00.311
     nontraffic V09.1
      involving motor vehicle
        NEC V09.00
     traffic V09.3
      involving motor vehicle
        NEC V09.20
    specified type NEC V00.898
     collision (with) V09.9
      animal being ridden or animal
        drawn vehicle V06.99
       nontraffic V06.09
       traffic V06.19
      bus or heavy transport V04.99
       nontraffic V04.09
       traffic V04.19
      car V03.99
       nontraffic V03.09
       traffic V03.19
      pedal cycle V01.99
       nontraffic V01.09
       traffic V01.19
      pick-up truck or van V03.99
       nontraffic V03.09
       traffic V03.19
      railway (train) (vehicle) V05.99
       nontraffic V05.09
       traffic V05.19
      streetcar V06.99
       nontraffic V06.09
       traffic V06.19
      stationary object V00.892
      two- or three-wheeled motor
        vehicle V02.99
       nontraffic V02.09
       traffic V02.19
      vehicle V09.9
       animal-drawn V06.99
        nontraffic V06.09
        traffic V06.19
       motor
        nontraffic V09.00
        traffic V09.20
     fall V00.891
     nontraffic V09.1
      involving motor vehicle
        NEC V09.00
     traffic V09.3
      involving motor vehicle
        NEC V09.20
    traffic V09.3
     involving motor vehicle V09.20
      military V09.21
      specified type NEC V09.29
    wheelchair (powered) V00.818
     collision (with) V09.9
      animal being ridden or animal
        drawn vehicle V06.99
       nontraffic V06.09
       traffic V06.19
      bus or heavy transport V04.99
       nontraffic V04.09
       traffic V04.19
      car V03.99
       nontraffic V03.09
       traffic V03.19
      pedal cycle V01.99
       nontraffic V01.09
       traffic V01.19
      pick-up truck or van V03.99
       nontraffic V03.09
       traffic V03.19

Accident (to) - *continued*
  transport (involving injury to) - *continued*
    pedestrian - *continued*
      conveyance (occupant) - *continued*
        wheelchair (powered) - *continued*
          collision (with) - *continued*
            railway (train) (vehicle) V05.99
              nontraffic V05.09
              traffic V05.19
            streetcar V06.99
              nontraffic V06.09
              traffic V06.19
            stationary object V00.812
            two- or three-wheeled motor
              vehicle V02.99
              nontraffic V02.09
              traffic V02.19
            vehicle V09.9
              animal-drawn V06.99
                nontraffic V06.09
                traffic V06.19
              motor
                nontraffic V09.00
                traffic V09.20
          fall V00.811
          nontraffic V09.1
            involving motor vehicle
              NEC V09.00
          traffic V09.3
            involving motor vehicle
              NEC V09.20
        wheeled shoe V00.158
          colliding with stationary
            object V00.152
          fall V00.151
      on foot — *see also* Accident, pedestrian
        collision (with)
          animal being ridden or animal
            drawn vehicle V06.90
            nontraffic V06.00
            traffic V06.10
          bus or heavy transport V04.90
            nontraffic V04.00
            traffic V04.10
          car V03.90
            nontraffic V03.00
            traffic V03.10
          pedal cycle V01.90
            nontraffic V01.00
            traffic V01.10
          pick-up truck or van V03.90
            nontraffic V03.00
            traffic V03.10
          railway (train) (vehicle) V05.90
            nontraffic V05.00
            traffic V05.10
          streetcar V06.90
            nontraffic V06.00
            traffic V06.10
          two- or three-wheeled motor
            vehicle V02.90
            nontraffic V02.00
            traffic V02.10
          vehicle V09.9
            animal-drawn V06.90
              nontraffic V06.00
              traffic V06.10
            motor
              nontraffic V09.00
              traffic V09.20
         nontraffic V09.1
          involving motor vehicle V09.00
            military V09.01
            specified type NEC V09.09
        traffic V09.3
          involving motor vehicle V09.20
            military V09.21
            specified type NEC V09.29
      person NEC (unknown way or
        transportation) V99
      collision (between)
        bus (with)
          heavy transport vehicle
            (traffic) V87.5
            nontraffic V88.5

Accident (to) - *continued*
  transport (involving injury to) - *continued*
    person NEC (unknown way or
      transportation) - *continued*
      collision (between) - *continued*
        car (with)
          nontraffic V88.5
          bus (traffic) V87.3
            nontraffic V88.3
          heavy transport vehicle
            (traffic) V87.4
            nontraffic V88.4
          pick-up truck or van (traffic) V87.2
            nontraffic V88.2
          train or railway vehicle
            (traffic) V87.6
            nontraffic V88.6
          two-or three-wheeled motor vehicle
            (traffic) V87.0
            nontraffic V88.0
          motor vehicle (traffic) NEC V87.7
            nontraffic V88.7
        two-or three-wheeled vehicle (with)
          (traffic)
          motor vehicle NEC V87.1
            nontraffic V88.1
        nonmotor vehicle (collision)
          (noncollision) (traffic) V87.9
          nontraffic V88.9
    pickup truck occupant V59.9
      collision (with)
        animal (traffic) V50.9
          being ridden (traffic) V56.9
            nontraffic V56.3
            while boarding or alighting V56.4
          nontraffic V50.3
          while boarding or alighting V50.4
        animal-drawn vehicle (traffic) V56.9
          nontraffic V56.3
          while boarding or alighting V56.4
        bus (traffic) V54.9
          nontraffic V54.3
          while boarding or alighting V54.4
        car (traffic) V53.9
          nontraffic V53.3
          while boarding or alighting V53.4
        motor vehicle NOS (traffic) V59.60
          nontraffic V59.20
          specified type NEC (traffic) V59.69
            nontraffic V59.29
        pedal cycle (traffic) V51.9
          nontraffic V51.3
          while boarding or alighting V51.4
        pickup truck (traffic) V53.9
          nontraffic V53.3
          while boarding or alighting V53.4
        railway vehicle (traffic) V55.9
          nontraffic V55.3
          while boarding or alighting V55.4
        specified vehicle NEC (traffic) V56.9
          nontraffic V56.3
          while boarding or alighting V56.4
        stationary object (traffic) V57.9
          nontraffic V57.3
          while boarding or alighting V57.4
        streetcar (traffic) V56.9
          nontraffic V56.3
          while boarding or alighting V56.4
        three wheeled motor vehicle
          (traffic) V52.9
          nontraffic V52.3
          while boarding or alighting V52.4
        truck (traffic) V54.9
          nontraffic V54.3
          while boarding or alighting V54.4
        two wheeled motor vehicle
          (traffic) V52.9
          nontraffic V52.3
          while boarding or alighting V52.4
        van (traffic) V53.9
          nontraffic V53.3
          while boarding or alighting V53.4
      driver
        collision (with)
          animal (traffic) V50.5

Accident (to) - *continued*
  transport (involving injury to) - *continued*
    pickup truck occupant - *continued*
      driver - *continued*
        collision (with) - *continued*
          animal (traffic) - *continued*
            being ridden (traffic) V56.5
              nontraffic V56.0
            nontraffic V50.0
          animal-drawn vehicle
            (traffic) V56.5
            nontraffic V56.0
          bus (traffic) V54.5
            nontraffic V54.0
          car (traffic) V53.5
            nontraffic V53.0
          motor vehicle NOS (traffic) V59.40
            nontraffic V59.00
            specified type NEC
              (traffic) V59.49
              nontraffic V59.09
          pedal cycle (traffic) V51.5
            nontraffic V51.0
          pickup truck (traffic) V53.5
            nontraffic V53.0
          railway vehicle (traffic) V55.5
            nontraffic V55.0
          specified vehicle NEC
            (traffic) V56.5
            nontraffic V56.0
          stationary object (traffic) V57.5
            nontraffic V57.0
          streetcar (traffic) V56.5
            nontraffic V56.0
          three wheeled motor vehicle
            (traffic) V52.5
            nontraffic V52.0
          truck (traffic) V54.5
            nontraffic V54.0
          two wheeled motor vehicle
            (traffic) V52.5
            nontraffic V52.0
          van (traffic) V53.5
            nontraffic V53.0
        noncollision accident (traffic) V58.5
          nontraffic V58.0
      noncollision accident (traffic) V58.9
        nontraffic V58.3
        while boarding or alighting V58.4
      nontraffic V59.3
      hanger-on
        collision (with)
          animal (traffic) V50.7
            being ridden (traffic) V56.7
              nontraffic V56.2
            nontraffic V50.2
          animal-drawn vehicle
            (traffic) V56.7
            nontraffic V56.2
          bus (traffic) V54.7
            nontraffic V54.2
          car (traffic) V53.7
            nontraffic V53.2
          pedal cycle (traffic) V51.7
            nontraffic V51.2
          pickup truck (traffic) V53.7
            nontraffic V53.2
          railway vehicle (traffic) V55.7
            nontraffic V55.2
          specified vehicle NEC
            (traffic) V56.7
            nontraffic V56.2
          stationary object (traffic) V57.7
            nontraffic V57.2
          streetcar (traffic) V56.7
            nontraffic V56.2
          three wheeled motor vehicle
            (traffic) V52.7
            nontraffic V52.2
          truck (traffic) V54.7
            nontraffic V54.2
          two wheeled motor vehicle
            (traffic) V52.7
            nontraffic V52.2
          van (traffic) V53.7

Accident (to) - *continued*
transport (involving injury to) - *continued*
pickup truck occupant - *continued*
hanger-on - *continued*
collision (with) - *continued*
van (traffic) - *continued*
nontraffic V53.2
noncollision accident (traffic) V58.7
nontraffic V58.2
passenger
collision (with)
animal (traffic) V50.6
being ridden (traffic) V56.6
nontraffic V56.1
nontraffic V50.1
animal-drawn vehicle
(traffic) V56.6
nontraffic V56.1
bus (traffic) V54.6
nontraffic V54.1
car (traffic) V53.6
nontraffic V53.1
motor vehicle NOS (traffic) V59.50
nontraffic V59.10
specified type NEC
(traffic) V59.59
nontraffic V59.19
pedal cycle (traffic) V51.6
nontraffic V51.1
pickup truck (traffic) V53.6
nontraffic V53.1
railway vehicle (traffic) V55.6
nontraffic V55.1
specified vehicle NEC
(traffic) V56.6
nontraffic V56.1
stationary object (traffic) V57.6
nontraffic V57.1
streetcar (traffic) V56.6
nontraffic V56.1
three wheeled motor vehicle
(traffic) V52.6
nontraffic V52.1
truck (traffic) V54.6
nontraffic V54.1
two wheeled motor vehicle
(traffic) V52.6
nontraffic V52.1
van (traffic) V53.6
nontraffic V53.1
noncollision accident (traffic) V58.6
nontraffic V58.1
specified type NEC V59.88
military vehicle V59.81
quarry truck — *see* Accident, transport,
industrial vehicle occupant
race car — *see* Accident, transport, motor
vehicle NEC occupant
railway vehicle occupant V81.9
collision (with) V81.3
motor vehicle (non-military)
(traffic) V81.1
military V81.83
nontraffic V81.0
rolling stock V81.2
specified object NEC V81.3
during derailment V81.7
with antecedent collision — *see*
Accident, transport, railway
vehicle occupant, collision
explosion V81.81
fall (in railway vehicle) V81.5
during derailment V81.7
with antecedent collision — *see*
Accident, transport, railway
vehicle occupant, collision
from railway vehicle V81.6
during derailment V81.7
with antecedent collision — *see*
Accident, transport, railway
vehicle occupant, collision
while boarding or alighting V81.4
fire V81.81
object falling onto train V81.82
specified type NEC V81.89

Accident (to) - *continued*
transport (involving injury to) - *continued*
railway vehicle occupant - *continued*
while boarding or alighting V81.4
ski lift V98.3
snowmobile occupant (nontraffic) V86.92
driver V86.52
hanger-on V86.72
passenger V86.62
traffic V86.32
driver V86.02
hanger-on V86.22
passenger V86.12
while boarding or alighting V86.42
specified NEC V98.8
sport utility vehicle occupant — *see also*
Accident, transport, pickup truck
occupant
streetcar occupant V82.9
collision (with) V82.3
motor vehicle (traffic) V82.1
nontraffic V82.0
rolling stock V82.2
during derailment V82.7
with antecedent collision — *see*
Accident, transport, streetcar
occupant, collision
fall (in streetcar) V82.5
during derailment V82.7
with antecedent collision — *see*
Accident, transport, streetcar
occupant, collision
from streetcar V82.6
during derailment V82.7
with antecedent collision — *see*
Accident, transport, streetcar
occupant, collision
while boarding or alighting V82.4
while boarding or alighting V82.4
specified type NEC V82.8
while boarding or alighting V82.4
three-wheeled motor vehicle
occupant V39.9
collision (with)
animal (traffic) V30.9
being ridden (traffic) V36.9
nontraffic V36.3
while boarding or alighting V36.4
nontraffic V30.3
while boarding or alighting V30.4
animal-drawn vehicle (traffic) V36.9
nontraffic V36.3
while boarding or alighting V36.4
bus (traffic) V34.9
nontraffic V34.3
while boarding or alighting V34.4
car (traffic) V33.9
nontraffic V33.3
while boarding or alighting V33.4
motor vehicle NOS (traffic) V39.60
nontraffic V39.20
specified type NEC (traffic) V39.69
nontraffic V39.29
pedal cycle (traffic) V31.9
nontraffic V31.3
while boarding or alighting V31.4
pickup truck (traffic) V33.9
nontraffic V33.3
while boarding or alighting V33.4
railway vehicle (traffic) V35.9
nontraffic V35.3
while boarding or alighting V35.4
specified vehicle NEC (traffic) V36.9
nontraffic V36.3
while boarding or alighting V36.4
stationary object (traffic) V37.9
nontraffic V37.3
while boarding or alighting V37.4
streetcar (traffic) V36.9
nontraffic V36.3
while boarding or alighting V36.4
three wheeled motor vehicle
(traffic) V32.9
nontraffic V32.3
while boarding or alighting V32.4

Accident (to) - *continued*
transport (involving injury to) - *continued*
three-wheeled motor vehicle occupant -
continued
collision (with) - *continued*
truck (traffic) V34.9
nontraffic V34.3
while boarding or alighting V34.4
two wheeled motor vehicle
(traffic) V32.9
nontraffic V32.3
while boarding or alighting V32.4
van (traffic) V33.9
nontraffic V33.3
while boarding or alighting V33.4
driver
collision (with)
animal (traffic) V30.5
being ridden (traffic) V36.5
nontraffic V36.0
nontraffic V30.0
animal-drawn vehicle
(traffic) V36.5
nontraffic V36.0
bus (traffic) V34.5
nontraffic V34.0
car (traffic) V33.5
nontraffic V33.0
motor vehicle NOS (traffic) V39.40
nontraffic V39.00
specified type NEC
(traffic) V39.49
nontraffic V39.09
pedal cycle (traffic) V31.5
nontraffic V31.0
pickup truck (traffic) V33.5
nontraffic V33.0
railway vehicle (traffic) V35.5
nontraffic V35.0
specified vehicle NEC
(traffic) V36.5
nontraffic V36.0
stationary object (traffic) V37.5
nontraffic V37.0
streetcar (traffic) V36.5
nontraffic V36.0
three wheeled motor vehicle
(traffic) V32.5
nontraffic V32.0
truck (traffic) V34.5
nontraffic V34.0
two wheeled motor vehicle
(traffic) V32.5
nontraffic V32.0
van (traffic) V33.5
nontraffic V33.0
noncollision accident (traffic) V38.5
nontraffic V38.0
continued
noncollision accident (traffic) V38.9
nontraffic V38.3
while boarding or alighting V38.4
nontraffic V39.3
hanger-on
collision (with)
animal (traffic) V30.7
being ridden (traffic) V36.7
nontraffic V36.2
nontraffic V30.2
animal-drawn vehicle
(traffic) V36.7
nontraffic V36.2
bus (traffic) V34.7
nontraffic V34.2
car (traffic) V33.7
nontraffic V33.2
pedal cycle (traffic) V31.7
nontraffic V31.2
pickup truck (traffic) V33.7
nontraffic V33.2
railway vehicle (traffic) V35.7
nontraffic V35.2
specified vehicle NEC
(traffic) V36.7
nontraffic V36.2
stationary object (traffic) V37.7

Accident (to) - *continued*
transport (involving injury to) - *continued*
three-wheeled motor vehicle occupant -
continued
hanger-on - *continued*
collision (with) - *continued*
stationary object (traffic) -
continued
nontraffic V37.2
streetcar (traffic) V36.7
nontraffic V36.2
three wheeled motor vehicle
(traffic) V32.7
nontraffic V32.2
truck (traffic) V34.7
nontraffic V34.2
two wheeled motor vehicle
(traffic) V32.7
nontraffic V32.2
van (traffic) V33.7
nontraffic V33.2
noncollision accident (traffic) V38.7
nontraffic V38.2
passenger
collision (with)
animal (traffic) V30.6
being ridden (traffic) V36.6
nontraffic V36.1
nontraffic V30.1
animal-drawn vehicle
(traffic) V36.6
nontraffic V36.1
bus (traffic) V34.6
nontraffic V34.1
car (traffic) V33.6
nontraffic V33.1
motor vehicle NOS (traffic) V39.50
nontraffic V39.10
specified type NEC
(traffic) V39.59
nontraffic V39.19
pedal cycle (traffic) V31.6
nontraffic V31.1
pickup truck (traffic) V33.6
nontraffic V33.1
railway vehicle (traffic) V35.6
nontraffic V35.1
specified vehicle NEC
(traffic) V36.6
nontraffic V36.1
stationary object (traffic) V37.6
nontraffic V37.1
streetcar (traffic) V36.6
nontraffic V36.1
three wheeled motor vehicle
(traffic) V32.6
nontraffic V32.1
truck (traffic) V34.6
nontraffic V34.1
two wheeled motor vehicle
(traffic) V32.6
nontraffic V32.1
van (traffic) V33.6
nontraffic V33.1
noncollision accident (traffic) V38.6
nontraffic V38.1
specified type NEC V39.89
military vehicle V39.81
tractor (farm) (and trailer) — *see* Accident,
transport, agricultural vehicle
occupant
tram — *see* Accident, transport, streetcar
in mine or quarry — *see* Accident,
transport, industrial vehicle
occupant
trolley — *see* Accident, transport, streetcar
in mine or quarry — *see* Accident,
transport, industrial vehicle
occupant
truck (heavy) occupant V69.9
collision (with)
animal (traffic) V60.9
being ridden (traffic) V66.9
nontraffic V66.3
while boarding or alighting V66.4

Accident (to) - *continued*
transport (involving injury to) - *continued*
truck (heavy) occupant - *continued*
collision (with) - *continued*
animal (traffic) - *continued*
nontraffic V60.3
while boarding or alighting V60.4
animal-drawn vehicle (traffic) V66.9
nontraffic V66.3
while boarding or alighting V66.4
bus (traffic) V64.9
nontraffic V64.3
while boarding or alighting V64.4
car (traffic) V63.9
nontraffic V63.3
while boarding or alighting V63.4
motor vehicle NOS (traffic) V69.60
nontraffic V69.20
specified type NEC (traffic) V69.69
nontraffic V69.29
pedal cycle (traffic) V61.9
nontraffic V61.3
while boarding or alighting V61.4
pickup truck (traffic) V63.9
nontraffic V63.3
while boarding or alighting V63.4
railway vehicle (traffic) V65.9
nontraffic V65.3
while boarding or alighting V65.4
specified vehicle NEC (traffic) V66.9
nontraffic V66.3
while boarding or alighting V66.4
stationary object (traffic) V67.9
nontraffic V67.3
while boarding or alighting V67.4
streetcar (traffic) V66.9
nontraffic V66.3
while boarding or alighting V66.4
three wheeled motor vehicle
(traffic) V62.9
nontraffic V62.3
while boarding or alighting V62.4
truck (traffic) V64.9
nontraffic V64.3
while boarding or alighting V64.4
two wheeled motor vehicle
(traffic) V62.9
nontraffic V62.3
while boarding or alighting V62.4
van (traffic) V63.9
nontraffic V63.3
while boarding or alighting V63.4
driver
collision (with)
animal (traffic) V60.5
being ridden (traffic) V66.5
nontraffic V66.0
nontraffic V60.0
animal-drawn vehicle
(traffic) V66.5
nontraffic V66.0
bus (traffic) V64.5
nontraffic V64.0
car (traffic) V63.5
nontraffic V63.0
motor vehicle NOS (traffic) V69.40
nontraffic V69.00
specified type NEC
(traffic) V69.49
nontraffic V69.09
pedal cycle (traffic) V61.5
nontraffic V61.0
pickup truck (traffic) V63.5
nontraffic V63.0
railway vehicle (traffic) V65.5
nontraffic V65.0
specified vehicle NEC
(traffic) V66.5
nontraffic V66.0
stationary object (traffic) V67.5
nontraffic V67.0
streetcar (traffic) V66.5
nontraffic V66.0
three wheeled motor vehicle
(traffic) V62.5

Accident (to) - *continued*
transport (involving injury to) - *continued*
truck (heavy) occupant - *continued*
driver - *continued*
collision (with) - *continued*
three wheeled motor vehicle
(traffic) - *continued*
nontraffic V62.0
truck (traffic) V64.5
nontraffic V64.0
two wheeled motor vehicle
(traffic) V62.5
nontraffic V62.0
van (traffic) V63.5
nontraffic V63.0
noncollision accident (traffic) V68.5
nontraffic V68.0
dump — *see* Accident, transport,
construction vehicle occupant
hanger-on
collision (with)
animal (traffic) V60.7
being ridden (traffic) V66.7
nontraffic V66.2
nontraffic V60.2
animal-drawn vehicle
(traffic) V66.7
nontraffic V66.2
bus (traffic) V64.7
nontraffic V64.2
car (traffic) V63.7
nontraffic V63.2
pedal cycle (traffic) V61.7
nontraffic V61.2
pickup truck (traffic) V63.7
nontraffic V63.2
railway vehicle (traffic) V65.7
nontraffic V65.2
specified vehicle NEC
(traffic) V66.7
nontraffic V66.2
stationary object (traffic) V67.7
nontraffic V67.2
streetcar (traffic) V66.7
nontraffic V66.2
three wheeled motor vehicle
(traffic) V62.7
nontraffic V62.2
truck (traffic) V64.7
nontraffic V64.2
two wheeled motor vehicle
(traffic) V62.7
nontraffic V62.2
van (traffic) V63.7
nontraffic V63.2
noncollision accident (traffic) V68.7
nontraffic V68.2
noncollision accident (traffic) V68.9
nontraffic V68.3
while boarding or alighting V68.4
nontraffic V69.3
passenger
collision (with)
animal (traffic) V60.6
being ridden (traffic) V66.6
nontraffic V66.1
nontraffic V60.1
animal-drawn vehicle
(traffic) V66.6
nontraffic V66.1
bus (traffic) V64.6
nontraffic V64.1
car (traffic) V63.6
nontraffic V63.1
motor vehicle NOS (traffic) V69.50
nontraffic V69.10
specified type NEC
(traffic) V69.59
nontraffic V69.19
pedal cycle (traffic) V61.6
nontraffic V61.1
pickup truck (traffic) V63.6
nontraffic V63.1
railway vehicle (traffic) V65.6
nontraffic V65.1

Accident (to) - *continued*
transport (involving injury to) - *continued*
truck (heavy) occupant - *continued*
passenger - *continued*
collision (with) - *continued*
specified vehicle NEC
(traffic) V66.6
nontraffic V66.1
stationary object (traffic) V67.6
nontraffic V67.1
streetcar (traffic) V66.6
nontraffic V66.1
three wheeled motor vehicle
(traffic) V62.6
nontraffic V62.1
truck (traffic) V64.6
nontraffic V64.1
two wheeled motor vehicle
(traffic) V62.6
nontraffic V62.1
van (traffic) V63.6
nontraffic V63.1
noncollision accident (traffic) V68.6
nontraffic V68.1
pickup — *see* Accident, transport,
pickup truck occupant
specified type NEC V69.88
military vehicle V69.81
van occupant V59.9
collision (with)
animal (traffic) V50.9
being ridden (traffic) V56.9
nontraffic V56.3
while boarding or alighting V56.4
nontraffic V50.3
while boarding or alighting V50.4
animal-drawn vehicle (traffic) V56.9
nontraffic V56.3
while boarding or alighting V56.4
bus (traffic) V54.9
nontraffic V54.3
while boarding or alighting V54.4
car (traffic) V53.9
nontraffic V53.3
while boarding or alighting V53.4
motor vehicle NOS (traffic) V59.60
nontraffic V59.20
specified type NEC (traffic) V59.69
nontraffic V59.29
pedal cycle (traffic) V51.9
nontraffic V51.3
while boarding or alighting V51.4
pickup truck (traffic) V53.9
nontraffic V53.3
while boarding or alighting V53.4
railway vehicle (traffic) V55.9
nontraffic V55.3
while boarding or alighting V55.4
specified vehicle NEC (traffic) V56.9
nontraffic V56.3
while boarding or alighting V56.4
stationary object (traffic) V57.9
nontraffic V57.3
while boarding or alighting V57.4
streetcar (traffic) V56.9
nontraffic V56.3
while boarding or alighting V56.4
three wheeled motor vehicle
(traffic) V52.9
nontraffic V52.3
while boarding or alighting V52.4
truck (traffic) V54.9
nontraffic V54.3
while boarding or alighting V54.4
two wheeled motor vehicle
(traffic) V52.9
nontraffic V52.3
while boarding or alighting V52.4
van (traffic) V53.9
nontraffic V53.3
while boarding or alighting V53.4
driver
collision (with)
animal (traffic) V50.5
being ridden (traffic) V56.5

Accident (to) - *continued*
transport (involving injury to) - *continued*
van occupant - *continued*
driver - *continued*
collision (with) - *continued*
animal (traffic) - *continued*
being ridden (traffic) - *continued*
nontraffic V56.0
nontraffic V50.0
animal-drawn vehicle
(traffic) V56.5
nontraffic V56.0
bus (traffic) V54.5
nontraffic V54.0
car (traffic) V53.5
nontraffic V53.0
motor vehicle NOS (traffic) V59.40
nontraffic V59.00
specified type NEC
(traffic) V59.49
nontraffic V59.09
pedal cycle (traffic) V51.5
nontraffic V51.0
pickup truck (traffic) V53.5
nontraffic V53.0
railway vehicle (traffic) V55.5
nontraffic V55.0
specified vehicle NEC
(traffic) V56.5
nontraffic V56.0
stationary object (traffic) V57.5
nontraffic V57.0
streetcar (traffic) V56.5
nontraffic V56.0
three wheeled motor vehicle
(traffic) V52.5
nontraffic V52.0
truck (traffic) V54.5
nontraffic V54.0
two wheeled motor vehicle
(traffic) V52.5
nontraffic V52.0
van (traffic) V53.5
nontraffic V53.0
noncollision accident (traffic) V58.5
nontraffic V58.0
noncollision accident (traffic) V58.9
nontraffic V58.3
while boarding or alighting V58.4
nontraffic V59.3
hanger-on
collision (with)
animal (traffic) V50.7
being ridden (traffic) V56.7
nontraffic V56.2
nontraffic V50.2
animal-drawn vehicle
(traffic) V56.7
nontraffic V56.2
bus (traffic) V54.7
nontraffic V54.2
car (traffic) V53.7
nontraffic V53.2
pedal cycle (traffic) V51.7
nontraffic V51.2
pickup truck (traffic) V53.7
nontraffic V53.2
railway vehicle (traffic) V55.7
nontraffic V55.2
specified vehicle NEC
(traffic) V56.7
nontraffic V56.2
stationary object (traffic) V57.7
nontraffic V57.2
streetcar (traffic) V56.7
nontraffic V56.2
three wheeled motor vehicle
(traffic) V52.7
nontraffic V52.2
truck (traffic) V54.7
nontraffic V54.2
two wheeled motor vehicle
(traffic) V52.7
nontraffic V52.2
van (traffic) V53.7

Accident (to) - *continued*
transport (involving injury to) - *continued*
van occupant - *continued*
hanger-on - *continued*
collision (with) - *continued*
van (traffic) - *continued*
nontraffic V53.2
noncollision accident (traffic) V58.7
nontraffic V58.2
passenger
collision (with)
animal (traffic) V50.6
being ridden (traffic) V56.6
nontraffic V56.1
nontraffic V50.1
animal-drawn vehicle
(traffic) V56.6
nontraffic V56.1
bus (traffic) V54.6
nontraffic V54.1
car (traffic) V53.6
nontraffic V53.1
motor vehicle NOS (traffic) V59.50
nontraffic V59.10
specified type NEC
(traffic) V59.59
nontraffic V59.19
pedal cycle (traffic) V51.6
nontraffic V51.1
pickup truck (traffic) V53.6
nontraffic V53.1
railway vehicle (traffic) V55.6
nontraffic V55.1
specified vehicle NEC
(traffic) V56.6
nontraffic V56.1
stationary object (traffic) V57.6
nontraffic V57.1
streetcar (traffic) V56.6
nontraffic V56.1
three wheeled motor vehicle
(traffic) V52.6
nontraffic V52.1
truck (traffic) V54.6
nontraffic V54.1
two wheeled motor vehicle
(traffic) V52.6
nontraffic V52.1
van (traffic) V53.6
nontraffic V53.1
noncollision accident (traffic) V58.6
nontraffic V58.1
specified type NEC V59.88
military vehicle V59.81
watercraft occupant — *see* Accident,
watercraft
vehicle NEC V89.9
animal-drawn NEC — *see* Accident,
transport, animal-drawn vehicle
occupant
special
agricultural — *see* Accident, transport,
agricultural vehicle occupant
construction — *see* Accident, transport,
construction vehicle occupant
industrial — *see* Accident, transport,
industrial vehicle occupant
three-wheeled NEC (motorized) — *see*
Accident, transport, three-wheeled
motor vehicle occupant
watercraft V94.9
causing
drowning — *see* Drowning, due to,
accident to, watercraft
injury NEC V91.89
crushed between craft and
object V91.19
powered craft V91.13
ferry boat V91.11
fishing boat V91.12
jetskis V91.13
liner V91.11
merchant ship V91.10
passenger ship V91.11
unpowered craft V91.18

ACCIDENT - ACCIDENT

Accident (to) - *continued*
  watercraft - *continued*
    causing - *continued*
      injury NEC - *continued*
        crushed between craft and object - *continued*
          unpowered craft - *continued*
            canoe V91.15
            inflatable V91.16
            kayak V91.15
            sailboat V91.14
            surf-board V91.18
            windsurfer V91.18
        fall on board V91.29
          powered craft V91.23
            ferry boat V91.21
            fishing boat V91.22
            jetskis V91.23
            liner V91.21
            merchant ship V91.20
            passenger ship V91.21
          unpowered craft
            canoe V91.25
            inflatable V91.26
            kayak V91.25
            sailboat V91.24
        fire on board causing burn V91.09
          powered craft V91.03
            ferry boat V91.01
            fishing boat V91.02
            jetskis V91.03
            liner V91.01
            merchant ship V91.00
            passenger ship V91.01
          unpowered craft V91.08
            canoe V91.05
            inflatable V91.06
            kayak V91.05
            sailboat V91.04
            surf-board V91.08
            water skis V91.07
            windsurfer V91.08
        hit by falling object V91.39
          powered craft V91.33
            ferry boat V91.31
            fishing boat V91.32
            jetskis V91.33
            liner V91.31
            merchant ship V91.30
            passenger ship V91.31
          unpowered craft V91.38
            canoe V91.35
            inflatable V91.36
            kayak V91.35
            sailboat V91.34
            surf-board V91.38
            water skis V91.37
            windsurfer V91.38
        specified type NEC V91.89
          powered craft V91.83
            ferry boat V91.81
            fishing boat V91.82
            jetskis V91.83
            liner V91.81
            merchant ship V91.80
            passenger ship V91.81
          unpowered craft V91.88
            canoe V91.85
            inflatable V91.86
            kayak V91.85
            sailboat V91.84
            surf-board V91.88
            water skis V91.87
            windsurfer V91.88
      due to, caused by cataclysm — *see* Forces of nature, by type
    military NEC V94.818
      with civilian watercraft V94.810
      civilian in water injured by V94.811
    nonpowered, struck by
      nonpowered vessel V94.22
      powered vessel V94.21
    specified type NEC V94.89
    striking swimmer
      powered V94.11

Accident (to) - *continued*
  watercraft - *continued*
    striking swimmer - *continued*
      unpowered V94.12
Acid throwing (assault) Y08.89
Activity (involving) (of victim at time of event) Y93.9
  aerobic and step exercise (class) Y93.A3
  alpine skiing Y93.23
  animal care NEC Y93.K9
  arts and handcrafts NEC Y93.D9
  athletics NEC Y93.79
  athletics played as a team or group NEC Y93.69
  athletics played individually NEC Y93.59
  baking Y93.G3
  ballet Y93.41
  barbells Y93.B3
  BASE (Building, Antenna, Span, Earth) jumping Y93.33
  baseball Y93.64
  basketball Y93.67
  bathing (personal) Y93.E1
  beach volleyball Y93.68
  bike riding Y93.55
  blackout game Y93.85
  boogie boarding Y93.18
  bowling Y93.54
  boxing Y93.71
  brass instrument playing Y93.J4
  building construction Y93.H3
  bungee jumping Y93.34
  calisthenics Y93.A2
  canoeing (in calm and turbulent water) Y93.16
  capture the flag Y93.6A
  cardiorespiratory exercise NEC Y93.A9
  caregiving (providing) NEC Y93.F9
    bathing Y93.F1
    lifting Y93.F2
  cellular
    communication device Y93.C2
    telephone Y93.C2
  challenge course Y93.A5
  cheerleading Y93.45
  choking game Y93.85
  circuit training Y93.A4
  cleaning
    floor Y93.E5
  climbing NEC Y93.39
    mountain Y93.31
    rock Y93.31
    wall Y93.31
  clothing care and maintenance NEC Y93.E9
  combatives Y93.75
  computer
    keyboarding Y93.C1
    technology NEC Y93.C9
  confidence course Y93.A5
  construction (building) Y93.H3
  cooking and baking Y93.G3
  cool down exercises Y93.A2
  cricket Y93.69
  crocheting Y93.D1
  cross country skiing Y93.24
  dancing (all types) Y93.41
  digging
    dirt Y93.H1
  dirt digging Y93.H1
  dishwashing Y93.G1
  diving (platform) (springboard) Y93.12
    underwater Y93.15
  dodge ball Y93.6A
  downhill skiing Y93.23
  drum playing Y93.J2
  dumbbells Y93.B3
  electronic
    devices NEC Y93.C9
      hand held interactive Y93.C2
    game playing (using) (with)
      interactive device Y93.C2
      keyboard or other stationary device Y93.C1
  elliptical machine Y93.A1
  exercise (s)

Activity (involving) (of victim at time of event) - *continued*
  exercise (s) - *continued*
    machines ((primarily) for)
      cardiorespiratory conditioning Y93.A1
      muscle strengthening Y93.B1
      muscle strengthening (non-machine) NEC Y93.B9
    external motion NEC Y93.I9
      rollercoaster Y93.I1
    fainting game Y93.85
    field hockey Y93.65
    figure skating (pairs) (singles) Y93.21
    flag football Y93.62
    floor mopping and cleaning Y93.E5
    food preparation and clean up Y93.G1
    football (American) NOS Y93.61
      flag Y93.62
      tackle Y93.61
      touch Y93.62
    four square Y93.6A
    free weights Y93.B3
    frisbee (ultimate) Y93.74
    furniture
      building Y93.D3
      finishing Y93.D3
      repair Y93.D3
    game playing (electronic)
      using keyboard or other stationary device Y93.C1
      using interactive device Y93.C2
    gardening Y93.H2
    golf Y93.53
    grass drills Y93.A6
    grilling and smoking food Y93.G2
    grooming and shearing an animal Y93.K3
    guerilla drills Y93.A6
    gymnastics (rhythmic) Y93.43
    handball Y93.73
    handcrafts NEC Y93.D9
    hand held interactive electronic device Y93.C2
    hang gliding Y93.35
    hiking (on level or elevated terrain) Y93.01
    hockey (ice) Y93.22
      field Y93.65
    horseback riding Y93.52
    household (interior) maintenance NEC Y93.E9
    ice NEC Y93.29
      dancing Y93.21
      hockey Y93.22
      skating Y93.21
    inline roller skating Y93.51
    ironing Y93.E4
    judo Y93.75
    jumping (off) NEC Y93.39
      BASE (Building, Antenna, Span, Earth) Y93.33
      bungee Y93.34
      jacks Y93.A2
      rope Y93.56
    jumping jacks Y93.A2
    jumping rope Y93.56
    karate Y93.75
    kayaking (in calm and turbulent water) Y93.16
    keyboarding (computer) Y93.C1
    kickball Y93.6A
    knitting Y93.D1
    lacrosse Y93.65
    land maintenance NEC Y93.H9
    landscaping Y93.H2
    laundry Y93.E2
    machines (exercise)
      primarily for cardiorespiratory conditioning Y93.A1
      primarily for muscle strengthening Y93.B1
    maintenance
      exterior building NEC Y93.H9
      household (interior) NEC Y93.E9
      land Y93.H9
      property Y93.H9
    marching (on level or elevated terrain) Y93.01

Activity (involving) (of victim at time of event) - *continued*
  martial arts Y93.75
  microwave oven Y93.G3
  milking an animal Y93.K2
  mopping (floor) Y93.E5
  mountain climbing Y93.31
  muscle strengthening
    exercises (non-machine) NEC Y93.B9
    machines Y93.B1
  musical keyboard (electronic) playing Y93.J1
  nordic skiing Y93.24
  obstacle course Y93.A5
  oven (microwave) Y93.G3
  packing up and unpacking in moving to a
      new residence Y93.E6
  parasailing Y93.19
  pass out game Y93.85
  percussion instrument playing NEC Y93.J2
  personal
    bathing and showering Y93.E1
    hygiene NEC Y93.E8
    showering Y93.E1
  physical games generally associated with
      school recess, summer camp and
      children Y93.6A
  physical training NEC Y93.A9
  piano playing Y93.J1
  pilates Y93.B4
  platform diving Y93.12
  playing musical instrument
    brass instrument Y93.J4
    drum Y93.J2
    musical keyboard (electronic) Y93.J1
    percussion instrument NEC Y93.J2
    piano Y93.J1
    string instrument Y93.J3
    winds instrument Y93.J4
  property maintenance
    exterior NEC Y93.H9
    interior NEC Y93.E9
  pruning (garden and lawn) Y93.H2
  pull-ups Y93.B2
  push-ups Y93.B2
  racquetball Y93.73
  rafting (in calm and turbulent water) Y93.16
  raking (leaves) Y93.H1
  rappelling Y93.32
  refereeing a sports activity Y93.81
  residential relocation Y93.E6
  rhythmic gymnastics Y93.43
  rhythmic movement NEC Y93.49
  riding
    horseback Y93.52
    rollercoaster Y93.I1
  rock climbing Y93.31
  rollercoaster riding Y93.I1
  roller skating (inline) Y93.51
  rough housing and horseplay Y93.83
  rowing (in calm and turbulent water) Y93.16
  rugby Y93.63
  running Y93.02
  SCUBA diving Y93.15
  sewing Y93.D2
  shoveling Y93.H1
    dirt Y93.H1
    snow Y93.H1
  showering (personal) Y93.E1
  sit-ups Y93.B2
  skateboarding Y93.51
  skating (ice) Y93.21
    roller Y93.51
  skiing (alpine) (downhill) Y93.23
    cross country Y93.24
    nordic Y93.24
    water Y93.17
  sledding (snow) Y93.23
  sleeping (sleep) Y93.84
  smoking and grilling food Y93.G2
  snorkeling Y93.15
  snow NEC Y93.29
    boarding Y93.23
    shoveling Y93.H1
    sledding Y93.23
    tubing Y93.23

Activity (involving) (of victim at time of event) - *continued*
  soccer Y93.66
  softball Y93.64
  specified NEC Y93.89
  spectator at an event Y93.82
  sports NEC Y93.79
    sports played as a team or group
        NEC Y93.69
    sports played individually NEC Y93.59
  springboard diving Y93.12
  squash Y93.73
  stationary bike Y93.A1
  step (stepping) exercise (class) Y93.A3
  stepper machine Y93.A1
  stove Y93.G3
  string instrument playing Y93.J3
  surfing Y93.18
    wind Y93.18
  swimming Y93.11
  tackle football Y93.61
  tap dancing Y93.41
  tennis Y93.73
  tobogganing Y93.23
  touch football Y93.62
  track and field events (non-running) Y93.57
    running Y93.02
  trampoline Y93.44
  treadmill Y93.A1
  trimming shrubs Y93.H2
  tubing (in calm and turbulent water) Y93.16
    snow Y93.23
  ultimate frisbee Y93.74
  underwater diving Y93.15
  unpacking in moving to a new
      residence Y93.E6
  use of stove, oven and microwave
      oven Y93.G3
  vacuuming Y93.E3
  volleyball (beach) (court) Y93.68
  wake boarding Y93.17
  walking an animal Y93.K1
  walking (on level or elevated terrain) Y93.01
    an animal Y93.K1
  wall climbing Y93.31
  warm up and cool down exercises Y93.A2
  water NEC Y93.19
    aerobics Y93.14
    craft NEC Y93.19
    exercise Y93.14
    polo Y93.13
    skiing Y93.17
    sliding Y93.18
    survival training and testing Y93.19
  weeding (garden and lawn) Y93.H2
  wind instrument playing Y93.J4
  windsurfing Y93.18
  wrestling Y93.72
  yoga Y93.42
Adverse effect of drugs — *see* Table of Drugs
    and Chemicals
Aerosinusitis - — *see* Air, pressure
After-effect, late — *see* Sequelae
Air
  blast in war operations — *see* War
      operations, air blast
  pressure
    change, rapid
      during
        ascent W94.29
          while (in) (surfacing from)
            aircraft W94.23
            deep water diving W94.21
            underground W94.22
        descent W94.39
          in
            aircraft W94.31
            water W94.32
        high, prolonged W94.0
        low, prolonged W94.12
        due to residence or long visit at high
            altitude W94.11
Alpine sickness W94.11
Altitude sickness W94.11

Anaphylactic shock, anaphylaxis — *see*
    Table of Drugs and Chemicals
Andes disease W94.11
Arachnidism, arachnoidism X58
Arson (with intent to injure or kill) X97
Asphyxia, asphyxiation
  by
    food (bone) (seed) — *see* categories T17
        and T18
    gas — *see also* Table of Drugs and
        Chemicals
      legal
        execution — *see* Legal, intervention,
            gas
        intervention — *see* Legal,
            intervention, gas
  from
    fire — *see also* Exposure, fire
      in war operations — *see* War operations,
          fire
    ignition — *see* Ignition
    vomitus T17.81
  in war operations — *see* War operations,
      restriction of airway
Aspiration
  food (any type) (into respiratory tract) (with
      asphyxia, obstruction respiratory tract,
      suffocation) — *see* categories T17
      and T18
  foreign body — *see* Foreign body, aspiration
  vomitus (with asphyxia, obstruction
      respiratory tract, suffocation) T17.81
Assassination (attempt) — *see* Assault
Assault (homicidal) (by) (in) Y09
  arson X97
  bite (of human being) Y04.1
  bodily force Y04.8
    bite Y04.1
    bumping into Y04.2
    sexual — *see* subcategories T74.0, T76.0
    unarmed fight Y04.0
  bomb X96.9
    antipersonnel X96.0
    fertilizer X96.3
    gasoline X96.1
    letter X96.2
    petrol X96.1
    pipe X96.3
    specified NEC X96.8
  brawl (hand) (fists) (foot) (unarmed) Y04.0
  burning, burns (by fire) NEC X97
    acid Y08.89
    caustic, corrosive substance Y08.89
    chemical from swallowing caustic,
        corrosive substance — *see* Table of
        Drugs and Chemicals
    cigarette (s) X97
    hot object X98.9
      fluid NEC X98.2
      household appliance X98.3
      specified NEC X98.8
      steam X98.0
      tap water X98.1
      vapors X98.0
    scalding — *see* Assault, burning
    steam X98.0
    vitriol Y08.89
  caustic, corrosive substance (gas) Y08.89
  crashing of
    aircraft Y08.81
    motor vehicle Y03.8
      pushed in front of Y02.0
      run over Y03.0
      specified NEC Y03.8
  cutting or piercing instrument X99.9
    dagger X99.2
    glass X99.0
    knife X99.1
    specified NEC X99.8
    sword X99.2
  dagger X99.2
  drowning (in) X92.9
    bathtub X92.0
    natural water X92.3
    specified NEC X92.8

Assault (homicidal) (by) (in) - *continued*
  drowning (in) - *continued*
    swimming pool X92.1
      following fall X92.2
  dynamite X96.8
  explosive (s) (material) X96.9
  fight (hand) (fists) (foot) (unarmed) Y04.0
    with weapon — *see* Assault, by type of
      weapon
  fire X97
  firearm X95.9
    airgun X95.01
    handgun X93
    hunting rifle X94.1
    larger X94.9
      specified NEC X94.8
    machine gun X94.2
    shotgun X94.0
    specified NEC X95.8
  gunshot (wound) NEC — *see* Assault,
    firearm, by type
  incendiary device X97
  injury Y09
    to child due to criminal abortion attempt
      NEC Y08.89
  knife X99.1
  late effect of — *see* X92-Y08 with 7th
    character S
  placing before moving object NEC Y02.8
    motor vehicle Y02.0
  poisoning — *see* categories T36-T65 with
    7th character S
  puncture, any part of body — *see* Assault,
    cutting or piercing instrument
  pushing
    before moving object NEC Y02.8
      motor vehicle Y02.0
      subway train Y02.1
      train Y02.1
  from high place Y01
  rape T74.2-
  scalding — *see* Assault, burning
  sequelae of — *see* X92-Y08 with 7th
    character S
  sexual (by bodily force) T74.2-
  shooting — *see* Assault, firearm
  specified means NEC Y08.89
  stab, any part of body — *see* Assault, cutting
    or piercing instrument
  steam X98.0
  striking against
    other person Y04.2
    sports equipment Y08.09
      baseball bat Y08.02
      hockey stick Y08.01
  struck by
    sports equipment Y08.09
      baseball bat Y08.02
      hockey stick Y08.01
  submersion — *see* Assault, drowning
  violence Y09
  weapon Y09
    blunt Y00
    cutting or piercing — *see* Assault, cutting
      or piercing instrument
    firearm — *see* Assault, firearm
  wound Y09
    cutting — *see* Assault, cutting or piercing
      instrument
    gunshot — *see* Assault, firearm
    knife X99.1
    piercing — *see* Assault, cutting or piercing
      instrument
    puncture — *see* Assault, cutting or
      piercing instrument
    stab — *see* Assault, cutting or piercing
      instrument
Attack by mammals NEC W55.89
Avalanche — *see* Landslide
Aviator's disease - — *see* Air, pressure

B

Barotitis, barodontalgia, barosinusitis,
  barotrauma (otitic) (sinus) - — *see* Air,
    pressure

Battered (baby) (child) (person)
  (syndrome) X58
Bayonet wound W26.1
  in
    legal intervention — *see* Legal,
      intervention, sharp object, bayonet
    war operations — *see* War operations,
      combat
  stated as undetermined whether accidental or
    intentional Y28.8
  suicide (attempt) X78.2
Bean in nose — *see* categories T17 and T18
Bed set on fire NEC — *see* Exposure, fire,
  uncontrolled, building, bed
Beheading (by guillotine)
  homicide X99.9
  legal execution — *see* Legal, intervention
Bending, injury in (prolonged) (static) X50.1
Bends - — *see* Air, pressure, change
Bite, bitten by
  alligator W58.01
  arthropod (nonvenomous) NEC W57
  bull W55.21
  cat W55.01
  cow W55.21
  crocodile W58.11
  dog W54.0
  goat W55.31
  hoof stock NEC W55.31
  horse W55.11
  human being (accidentally) W50.3
    with intent to injure or kill Y04.1
    as, or caused by, a crowd or human
      stampede (with fall) W52
    assault Y04.1
    homicide (attempt) Y04.1
    in
      fight Y04.1
  insect (nonvenomous) W57
  lizard (nonvenomous) W59.01
  mammal NEC W55.81
    marine W56.31
  marine animal (nonvenomous) W56.81
  millipede W57
  moray eel W56.51
  mouse W53.01
  person (s) (accidentally) W50.3
    with intent to injure or kill Y04.1
    as, or caused by, a crowd or human
      stampede (with fall) W52
    assault Y04.1
    homicide (attempt) Y04.1
    in
      fight Y04.1
  pig W55.41
  raccoon W55.51
  rat W53.11
  reptile W59.81
    lizard W59.01
    snake W59.11
    turtle W59.21
    terrestrial W59.81
  rodent W53.81
    mouse W53.01
    rat W53.11
    specified NEC W53.81
    squirrel W53.21
  shark W56.41
  sheep W55.31
  snake (nonvenomous) W59.11
  spider (nonvenomous) W57
  squirrel W53.21
Blast (air) in war operations — *see* War
  operations, blast
Blizzard X37.2
Blood alcohol level Y90.9
  less than 20mg/100ml Y90.0
  presence in blood, level not specified Y90.9
  20-39mg/100ml Y90.1
  40-59mg/100ml Y90.2
  60-79mg/100ml Y90.3
  80-99mg/100ml Y90.4
  100-119mg/100ml Y90.5
  120-199mg/100ml Y90.6
  200-239mg/100ml Y90.7

Blow X58
  by law-enforcing agent, police (on duty) —
    see Legal, intervention, manhandling
    blunt object — *see* Legal, intervention,
      blunt object
Blowing up — *see* Explosion
Brawl (hand) (fists) (foot) Y04.0
Breakage (accidental) (part of)
  ladder (causing fall) W11
  scaffolding (causing fall) W12
Broken
  glass, contact with — *see* Contact, with,
    glass
  power line (causing electric shock) W85
Bumping against, into (accidentally)
  object NEC W22.8
    with fall — *see* Fall, due to, bumping
      against, object
    caused by crowd or human stampede (with
      fall) W52
    sports equipment W21.9
  person (s) W51
    with fall W03
      due to ice or snow W00.0
    assault Y04.2
    caused by, a crowd or human stampede
      (with fall) W52
    homicide (attempt) Y04.2
  sports equipment W21.9
Burn, burned, burning (accidental) (by)
  (from) (on)
  acid NEC — *see* Table of Drugs and
    Chemicals
  bed linen — *see* Exposure, fire, uncontrolled,
    in building, bed
  blowtorch X08.8
    with ignition of clothing NEC X06.2
      nightwear X05
  bonfire, campfire (controlled) — *see also*
    Exposure, fire, controlled, not in
    building
    uncontrolled — *see* Exposure, fire,
      uncontrolled, not in building
  candle X08.8
    with ignition of clothing NEC X06.2
      nightwear X05
  caustic liquid, substance (external) (internal)
    NEC — *see* Table of Drugs and
    Chemicals
  chemical (external) (internal) — *see also*
    Table of Drugs and Chemicals
    in war operations — *see* War operations.
      fire
  cigar (s) or cigarette (s) X08.8
    with ignition of clothing NEC X06.2
      nightwear X05
  clothes, clothing NEC (from controlled
    fire) X06.2
    with conflagration — *see* Exposure, fire,
      uncontrolled, building
    not in building or structure — *see*
      Exposure, fire, uncontrolled, not in
      building
  cooker (hot) X15.8
    stated as undetermined whether accidental
      or intentional Y27.3
    suicide (attempt) X77.3
  electric blanket X16
  engine (hot) X17
  fire, flames — *see* Exposure, fire
  flare, Very pistol — *see* Discharge, firearm
    NEC
  heat
    from appliance (electrical)
      (household) X15.8
      cooker X15.8
      hotplate X15.2
      kettle X15.8
      light bulb X15.8
      saucepan X15.3
      skillet X15.3
      stove X15.0
        stated as undetermined whether
          accidental or intentional Y27.3
        suicide (attempt) X77.3

Burn, burned, burning (accidental) (by) (from) (on) - *continued*
heat - *continued*
from appliance (electrical) (household) - *continued*
toaster X15.1
in local application or packing during medical or surgical procedure Y63.5
heating
appliance, radiator or pipe X16
homicide (attempt) — *see* Assault, burning
hot
air X14.1
cooker X15.8
drink X10.0
engine X17
fat X10.2
fluid NEC X12
food X10.1
gases X14.1
heating appliance X16
household appliance NEC X15.8
kettle X15.8
liquid NEC X12
machinery X17
metal (molten) (liquid) NEC X18
object (not producing fire or flames) NEC X19
oil (cooking) X10.2
pipe (s) X16
radiator X16
saucepan (glass) (metal) X15.3
stove (kitchen) X15.0
substance NEC X19
caustic or corrosive NEC — *see* Table of Drugs and Chemicals
toaster X15.1
tool X17
vapor X13.1
water (tap) — *see* Contact, with, hot, tap water
hotplate X15.2
suicide (attempt) X77.3
ignition — *see* Ignition
in war operations — *see* War operations, fire
inflicted by other person X97
by hot objects, hot vapor, and steam — *see* Assault, burning, hot object
internal, from swallowed caustic, corrosive liquid, substance — *see* Table of Drugs and Chemicals
iron (hot) X15.8
stated as undetermined whether accidental or intentional Y27.3
suicide (attempt) X77.3
kettle (hot) X15.8
stated as undetermined whether accidental or intentional Y27.3
suicide (attempt) X77.3
lamp (flame) X08.8
with ignition of clothing NEC X06.2
nightwear X05
lighter (cigar) (cigarette) X08.8
with ignition of clothing NEC X06.2
nightwear X05
lightning — *see* subcategory T75.0
causing fire — *see* Exposure, fire
liquid (boiling) (hot) NEC X12
stated as undetermined whether accidental or intentional Y27.2
suicide (attempt) X77.2
local application of externally applied substance in medical or surgical care Y63.5
on board watercraft
due to
accident to watercraft V91.09
powered craft V91.03
ferry boat V91.01
fishing boat V91.02
jetskis V91.03
liner V91.01
merchant ship V91.00
passenger ship V91.01
unpowered craft V91.08

Burn, burned, burning (accidental) (by) (from) (on) - *continued*
on board watercraft - *continued*
due to - *continued*
accident to watercraft - *continued*
unpowered craft - *continued*
canoe V91.05
inflatable V91.06
kayak V91.05
sailboat V91.04
surf-board V91.08
water skis V91.07
windsurfer V91.08
fire on board V93.09
ferry boat V93.01
fishing boat V93.02
jetskis V93.03
liner V93.01
merchant ship V93.00
passenger ship V93.01
powered craft NEC V93.03
sailboat V93.04
specified heat source NEC on board V93.19
ferry boat V93.11
fishing boat V93.12
jetskis V93.13
liner V93.11
merchant ship V93.10
passenger ship V93.11
powered craft NEC V93.13
sailboat V93.14
machinery (hot) X17
matches X08.8
with ignition of clothing NEC X06.2
nightwear X05
mattress — *see* Exposure, fire, uncontrolled, building, bed
medicament, externally applied Y63.5
metal (hot) (liquid) (molten) NEC X18
nightwear (nightclothes, nightdress, gown, pajamas, robe) X05
object (hot) NEC X19
pipe (hot) X16
smoking X08.8
with ignition of clothing NEC X06.2
nightwear X05
powder — *see* Powder burn
radiator X16
saucepan (hot) (glass) (metal) X15.3
stated as undetermined whether accidental or intentional Y27.3
suicide (attempt) X77.3
self-inflicted X76
stated as undetermined whether accidental or intentional Y26
steam X13.1
pipe X16
stated as undetermined whether accidental or intentional Y27.8
stated as undetermined whether accidental or intentional Y27.0
suicide (attempt) X77.0
stove (hot) (kitchen) X15.0
stated as undetermined whether accidental or intentional Y27.3
suicide (attempt) X77.3
substance (hot) NEC X19
boiling X12
stated as undetermined whether accidental or intentional Y27.2
suicide (attempt) X77.2
molten (metal) X18
suicide (attempt) NEC X76
hot
household appliance X77.3
object X77.9
stated as undetermined whether accidental or intentional Y27.0
therapeutic misadventure
heat in local application or packing during medical or surgical procedure Y63.5
overdose of radiation Y63.2
toaster (hot) X15.1

Burn, burned, burning (accidental) (by) (from) (on) - *continued*
toaster (hot) - *continued*
stated as undetermined whether accidental or intentional Y27.3
suicide (attempt) X77.3
tool (hot) X17
torch, welding X08.8
with ignition of clothing NEC X06.2
nightwear X05
trash fire (controlled) — *see* Exposure, fire, controlled, not in building
uncontrolled — *see* Exposure, fire, uncontrolled, not in building
vapor (hot) X13.1
stated as undetermined whether accidental or intentional Y27.0
suicide (attempt) X77.0
Very pistol — *see* Discharge, firearm NEC
Butted by animal W55.82
bull W55.22
cow W55.22
goat W55.32
horse W55.12
pig W55.42
sheep W55.32

C

Caisson disease - — *see* Air, pressure, change
Campfire (exposure to) (controlled) — *see also* Exposure, fire, controlled, not in building
uncontrolled — *see* Exposure, fire, uncontrolled, not in building
Capital punishment (any means) — *see* Legal, intervention
Car sickness T75.3
Casualty (not due to war) NEC X58
war — *see* War operations
Cat
bite W55.01
scratch W55.03
Cataclysm, cataclysmic (any injury) NEC — *see* Forces of nature
Catching fire — *see* Exposure, fire
Caught
between
folding object W23.0
objects (moving) (stationary and moving) W23.0
and machinery — *see* Contact, with, by type of machine
stationary W23.1
sliding door and door frame W23.0
by, in
machinery (moving parts of) — *see* Contact, with, by type of machine
washing-machine wringer W23.0
under packing crate (due to losing grip) W23.1
Cave-in caused by cataclysmic earth surface movement or eruption — *see* Landslide
Change (s) in air pressure - — *see* Air, pressure, change
Choked, choking (on) (any object except food or vomitus)
food (bone) (seed) — *see* categories T17 and T18
vomitus T17.81-
Civil insurrection — *see* War operations
Cloudburst (any injury) X37.8
Cold, exposure to (accidental) (excessive) (extreme) (natural) (place) NEC — *see* Exposure, cold
Collapse
building W20.1
burning (uncontrolled fire) X00.2
dam or man-made structure (causing earth movement) X36.0
machinery — *see* Contact, with, by type of machine
structure W20.1
burning (uncontrolled fire) X00.2
Collision (accidental) NEC — *see also* Accident, transport V89.9
pedestrian W51

Collision (accidental) NEC - *continued*
  pedestrian - *continued*
    with fall W03
      due to ice or snow W00.0
      involving pedestrian conveyance — *see* Accident, transport, pedestrian, conveyance
    and
      crowd or human stampede (with fall) W52
      object W22.8
        with fall — *see* Fall, due to, bumping against, object
  person (s) — *see* Collision, pedestrian
  transport vehicle NEC V89.9
    and
      avalanche, fallen or not moving — *see* Accident, transport
      falling or moving — *see* Landslide
      landslide, fallen or not moving — *see* Accident, transport
      falling or moving — *see* Landslide
    due to cataclysm — *see* Forces of nature, by type
    intentional, purposeful suicide (attempt) — *see* Suicide, collision
Combustion, spontaneous — *see* Ignition
Complication (delayed) of or following (medical or surgical procedure) Y84.9
  with misadventure — *see* Misadventure
  amputation of limb (s) Y83.5
  anastomosis (arteriovenous) (blood vessel) (gastrojejunal) (tendon) (natural or artificial material) Y83.2
  aspiration (of fluid) Y84.4
    tissue Y84.8
  biopsy Y84.8
  blood
    sampling Y84.7
    transfusion
      procedure Y84.8
  bypass Y83.2
  catheterization (urinary) Y84.6
    cardiac Y84.0
  colostomy Y83.3
  cystostomy Y83.3
  dialysis (kidney) Y84.1
  drug — *see* Table of Drugs and Chemicals
  due to misadventure — *see* Misadventure
  duodenostomy Y83.3
  electroshock therapy Y84.3
  external stoma, creation of Y83.3
  formation of external stoma Y83.3
  gastrostomy Y83.3
  graft Y83.2
  hypothermia (medically-induced) Y84.8
  implant, implantation (of)
    artificial
      internal device (cardiac pacemaker) (electrodes in brain) (heart valve prosthesis) (orthopedic) Y83.1
      material or tissue (for anastomosis or bypass) Y83.2
        with creation of external stoma Y83.3
    natural tissues (for anastomosis or bypass) Y83.2
      with creation of external stoma Y83.3
  infusion
    procedure Y84.8
  injection — *see* Table of Drugs and Chemicals
    procedure Y84.8
  insertion of gastric or duodenal sound Y84.5
  insulin-shock therapy Y84.3
  paracentesis (abdominal) (thoracic) (aspirative) Y84.4
  procedures other than surgical operation — *see* Complication of or following, by type of procedure
  radiological procedure or therapy Y84.2
  removal of organ (partial) (total) NEC Y83.6
  sampling
    blood Y84.7
    fluid NEC Y84.4
    tissue Y84.8

Complication (delayed) of or following (medical or surgical procedure) - *continued*
  shock therapy Y84.3
  surgical operation NEC — *see also* Complication of or following, by type of operation Y83.9
    reconstructive NEC Y83.4
      with
        anastomosis, bypass or graft Y83.2
        formation of external stoma Y83.3
    specified NEC Y83.8
  transfusion — *see also* Table of Drugs and Chemicals
    procedure Y84.8
  transplant, transplantation (heart) (kidney) (liver) (whole organ, any) Y83.0
    partial organ Y83.4
  ureterostomy Y83.3
  vaccination — *see also* Table of Drugs and Chemicals
    procedure Y84.8
Compression
  divers' squeeze - — *see* Air, pressure, change
  trachea by
    food (lodged in esophagus) — *see* categories T17 and T18
    vomitus (lodged in esophagus) T17.81-
Conflagration — *see* Exposure, fire, uncontrolled
Constriction (external)
  hair W49.01
  jewelry W49.04
  ring W49.04
  rubber band W49.03
  specified item NEC W49.09
  string W49.02
  thread W49.02
Contact (accidental)
  with
    abrasive wheel (metalworking) W31.1
    alligator W58.09
      bite W58.01
      crushing W58.03
      strike W58.02
    amphibian W62.9
      frog W62.0
      toad W62.1
    animal (nonvenomous) NEC W64
      marine W56.89
        bite W56.81
        dolphin — *see* Contact, with, dolphin
        fish NEC — *see* Contact, with, fish
        mammal — *see* Contact, with, mammal, marine
        orca — *see* Contact, with, orca
        sea lion — *see* Contact, with, sea lion
        shark — *see* Contact, with, shark
        strike W56.82
    animate mechanical force NEC W64
    arrow W21.89
      not thrown, projected or falling W45.8
    arthropods (nonvenomous) W57
    axe W27.0
    band-saw (industrial) W31.2
    bayonet — *see* Bayonet wound
    bee (s) X58
    bench-saw (industrial) W31.2
    bird W61.99
      bite W61.91
      chicken — *see* Contact, with, chicken
      duck — *see* Contact, with, duck
      goose — *see* Contact, with, goose
      macaw — *see* Contact, with, macaw
      parrot — *see* Contact, with, parrot
      psittacine — *see* Contact, with, psittacine
      strike W61.92
      turkey — *see* Contact, with, turkey
    blender W29.0
    boiling water X12
      stated as undetermined whether accidental or intentional Y27.2
      suicide (attempt) X77.2
    bore, earth-drilling or mining (land) (seabed) W31.0

Contact (accidental) - *continued*
  with - *continued*
    buffalo — *see* Contact, with, hoof stock NEC
    bull W55.29
      bite W55.21
      gored W55.22
      strike W55.22
    bumper cars W31.81
    camel — *see* Contact, with, hoof stock NEC
    can
      lid W26.8
      opener W27.4
        powered W29.0
    cat W55.09
      bite W55.01
      scratch W55.03
    caterpillar (venomous) X58
    centipede (venomous) X58
    chain
      hoist W24.0
        agricultural operations W30.89
      saw W29.3
    chicken W61.39
      peck W61.33
      strike W61.32
    chisel W27.0
    circular saw W31.2
    cobra X58
    combine (harvester) W30.0
    conveyer belt W24.1
    cooker (hot) X15.8
      stated as undetermined whether accidental or intentional Y27.3
      suicide (attempt) X77.3
    coral X58
    cotton gin W31.82
    cow W55.29
      bite W55.21
      strike W55.22
    crane W24.0
      agricultural operations W30.89
    crocodile W58.19
      bite W58.11
      crushing W58.13
      strike W58.12
    dagger W26.1
      stated as undetermined whether accidental or intentional Y28.2
      suicide (attempt) X78.2
    dairy equipment W31.82
    dart W21.89
      not thrown, projected or falling W45.8
    deer — *see* Contact, with, hoof stock NEC
    derrick W24.0
      agricultural operations W30.89
      hay W30.2
    dog W54.8
      bite W54.0
      strike W54.1
    dolphin W56.09
      bite W56.01
      strike W56.02
    donkey — *see* Contact, with, hoof stock NEC
    drill (powered) W29.8
      earth (land) (seabed) W31.0
      nonpowered W27.8
    drive belt W24.0
      agricultural operations W30.89
    dry ice — *see* Exposure, cold, man-made
    dryer (clothes) (powered) (spin) W29.2
    duck W61.69
      bite W61.61
      strike W61.62
    earth (-)
      drilling machine (industrial) W31.0
      scraping machine in stationary use W31.83
    edge of stiff paper W26.2
    electric
      beater W29.0
      blanket X16
      fan W29.2

Contact (accidental) - *continued*
  with - *continued*
    electric - *continued*
      fan - *continued*
        commercial W31.82
      knife W29.1
      mixer W29.0
    elevator (building) W24.0
      agricultural operations W30.89
        grain W30.3
    engine (s) , hot NEC X17
    excavating machine W31.0
    farm machine W30.9
    feces — *see* Contact, with, by type of
        animal
    fer de lance X58
    fish W56.59
      bite W56.51
      shark — *see* Contact, with, shark
      strike W56.52
    flying horses W31.81
    forging (metalworking) machine W31.1
    fork W27.4
    forklift (truck) W24.0
      agricultural operations W30.89
    frog W62.0
    garden
      cultivator (powered) W29.3
        riding W30.89
      fork W27.1
    gas turbine W31.3
    Gila monster X58
    giraffe — *see* Contact, with, hoof stock
        NEC
    glass (sharp) (broken) W25
      with subsequent fall W18.02
      assault X99.0
      due to fall — *see* Fall, by type
      stated as undetermined whether
        accidental or intentional Y28.0
      suicide (attempt) X78.0
    goat W55.39
      bite W55.31
      strike W55.32
    goose W61.59
      bite W61.51
      strike W61.52
    hand
      saw W27.0
      tool (not powered) NEC W27.8
        powered W29.8
    harvester W30.0
    hay-derrick W30.2
    heat NEC X19
      from appliance (electrical)
        (household) — *see* Contact, with,
        hot, household appliance
      heating appliance X16
    heating
      appliance (hot) X16
      pad (electric) X16
    hedge-trimmer (powered) W29.3
    hoe W27.1
    hoist (chain) (shaft) NEC W24.0
      agricultural W30.89
    hoof stock NEC W55.39
      bite W55.31
      strike W55.32
    hornet (s) X58
    horse W55.19
      bite W55.11
      strike W55.12
    hot
      air X14.1
        inhalation X14.0
      cooker X15.8
      drinks X10.0
      engine X17
      fats X10.2
      fluids NEC X12
        assault X98.2
        suicide (attempt) X77.2
        undetermined whether accidental or
          intentional Y27.2
      food X10.1

Contact (accidental) - *continued*
  with - *continued*
    hot - *continued*
      gases X14.1
        inhalation X14.0
      heating appliance X16
      household appliance X15.8
        assault X98.3
        cooker X15.8
        hotplate X15.2
        kettle X15.8
        light bulb X15.8
        object NEC X19
          assault X98.8
          stated as undetermined whether
            accidental or intentional Y27.9
          suicide (attempt) X77.8
        saucepan X15.3
        skillet X15.3
        stove X15.0
        stated as undetermined whether
          accidental or intentional Y27.3
        suicide (attempt) X77.3
        toaster X15.1
      kettle X15.8
      light bulb X15.8
      liquid NEC — *see also* Burn X12
        drinks X10.0
        stated as undetermined whether
          accidental or intentional Y27.2
        suicide (attempt) X77.2
        tap water X11.8
          stated as undetermined whether
            accidental or intentional Y27.1
          suicide (attempt) X77.1
      machinery X17
      metal (molten) (liquid) NEC X18
      object (not producing fire or flames)
        NEC X19
      oil (cooking) X10.2
      pipe X16
      plate X15.2
      radiator X16
      saucepan (glass) (metal) X15.3
      skillet X15.3
      stove (kitchen) X15.0
      substance NEC X19
      tap-water X11.8
        assault X98.1
        heated on stove X12
          stated as undetermined whether
            accidental or intentional Y27.2
          suicide (attempt) X77.2
        in bathtub X11.0
        running X11.1
        stated as undetermined whether
          accidental or intentional Y27.1
        suicide (attempt) X77.1
      toaster X15.1
      tool X17
      vapors X13.1
        inhalation X13.0
      water (tap) X11.8
        boiling X12
          stated as undetermined whether
            accidental or intentional Y27.2
          suicide (attempt) X77.2
        heated on stove X12
          stated as undetermined whether
            accidental or intentional Y27.2
          suicide (attempt) X77.2
        in bathtub X11.0
        running X11.1
        stated as undetermined whether
          accidental or intentional Y27.1
        suicide (attempt) X77.1
    hotplate X15.2
    ice-pick W27.4
    insect (nonvenomous) NEC W57
    kettle (hot) X15.8
    knife W26.0
      assault X99.1
      electric W29.1
      stated as undetermined whether
        accidental or intentional Y28.1

Contact (accidental) - *continued*
  with - *continued*
    knife - *continued*
      suicide (attempt) X78.1
    lathe (metalworking) W31.1
      turnings W45.8
      woodworking W31.2
    lawnmower (powered) (ridden) W28
      causing electrocution W86.8
        suicide (attempt) X83.1
      unpowered W27.1
    lift, lifting (devices) W24.0
      agricultural operations W30.89
      shaft W24.0
    liquefied gas — *see* Exposure, cold, man-
        made
    liquid air, hydrogen, nitrogen — *see*
        Exposure, cold, man-made
    lizard (nonvenomous) W59.09
      bite W59.01
      strike W59.02
    llama — *see* Contact, with, hoof stock
        NEC
    macaw W61.19
      bite W61.11
      strike W61.12
    machine, machinery W31.9
      abrasive wheel W31.1
      agricultural including animal-
        powered W30.9
        combine harvester W30.0
        grain storage elevator W30.3
        hay derrick W30.2
        power take-off device W30.1
        reaper W30.0
        specified NEC W30.89
        thresher W30.0
        transport vehicle, stationary W30.81
      band saw W31.2
      bench saw W31.2
      circular saw W31.2
      commercial NEC W31.82
      drilling, metal (industrial) W31.1
      earth-drilling W31.0
      earthmoving or scraping W31.89
      excavating W31.89
      forging machine W31.1
      gas turbine W31.3
      hot X17
      internal combustion engine W31.3
      land drill W31.0
      lathe W31.1
      lifting (devices) W24.0
      metal drill W31.1
      metalworking (industrial) W31.1
      milling, metal W31.1
      mining W31.0
      molding W31.2
      overhead plane W31.2
      power press, metal W31.1
      prime mover W31.3
      printing W31.89
      radial saw W31.2
      recreational W31.81
      roller-coaster W31.81
      rolling mill, metal W31.1
      sander W31.2
      seabed drill W31.0
      shaft
        hoist W31.0
        lift W31.0
      specified NEC W31.89
      spinning W31.89
      steam engine W31.3
      transmission W24.1
      undercutter W31.0
      water driven turbine W31.3
      weaving W31.89
      woodworking or forming
        (industrial) W31.2
    mammal (feces) (urine) W55.89
      bull — *see* Contact, with, bull
      cat — *see* Contact, with, cat
      cow — *see* Contact, with, cow
      goat — *see* Contact, with, goat

Contact (accidental) - *continued*
  with - *continued*
    mammal (feces) (urine) - *continued*
      hoof stock — *see* Contact, with, hoof stock
      horse — *see* Contact, with, horse
      marine W56.39
        dolphin — *see* Contact, with, dolphin
        orca — *see* Contact, with, orca
        sea lion — *see* Contact, with, sea lion
        specified NEC W56.39
          bite W56.31
          strike W56.32
      pig — *see* Contact, with, pig
      raccoon — *see* Contact, with, raccoon
      rodent — *see* Contact, with, rodent
      sheep — *see* Contact, with, sheep
      specified NEC W55.89
        bite W55.81
        strike W55.82
    marine
      animal W56.89
        bite W56.81
        dolphin — *see* Contact, with, dolphin
        fish NEC — *see* Contact, with, fish
        mammal — *see* Contact, with, mammal, marine
        orca — *see* Contact, with, orca
        sea lion — *see* Contact, with, sea lion
        shark — *see* Contact, with, shark
        strike W56.82
    meat
      grinder (domestic) W29.0
        industrial W31.82
        nonpowered W27.4
      slicer (domestic) W29.0
        industrial W31.82
    merry go round W31.81
    metal, hot (liquid) (molten) NEC X18
    millipede W57
    nail W45.0
      gun W29.4
    needle (sewing) W27.3
      hypodermic W46.0
        contaminated W46.1
    object (blunt) NEC
      hot NEC X19
      legal intervention — *see* Legal, intervention, blunt object
      sharp NEC W45.8
        inflicted by other person NEC W45.8
          stated as
            intentional homicide (attempt) — *see* Assault, cutting or piercing instrument
        legal intervention — *see* Legal, intervention, sharp object
        self-inflicted X78.9
    orca W56.29
      bite W56.21
      strike W56.22
    overhead plane W31.2
    paper (as sharp object) W26.2
    paper-cutter W27.5
    parrot W61.09
      bite W61.01
      strike W61.02
    pig W55.49
      bite W55.41
      strike W55.42
    pipe, hot X16
    pitchfork W27.1
    plane (metal) (wood) W27.0
      overhead W31.2
    plant thorns, spines, sharp leaves or other mechanisms W60
    powered
      garden cultivator W29.3
      household appliance, implement, or machine W29.8
      saw (industrial) W31.2
        hand W29.8
    printing machine W31.89
    psittacine bird W61.29
      bite W61.21

Contact (accidental) - *continued*
  with - *continued*
    psittacine bird - *continued*
      macaw — *see* Contact, with, macaw
      parrot — *see* Contact, with, parrot
      strike W61.22
    pulley (block) (transmission) W24.0
      agricultural operations W30.89
    raccoon W55.59
      bite W55.51
      strike W55.52
    radial-saw (industrial) W31.2
    radiator (hot) X16
    rake W27.1
    rattlesnake X58
    reaper W30.0
    reptile W59.89
      lizard — *see* Contact, with, lizard
      snake — *see* Contact, with, snake
      specified NEC W59.89
        bite W59.81
        crushing W59.83
        strike W59.82
      turtle — *see* Contact, with, turtle
    rivet gun (powered) W29.4
    road scraper — *see* Accident, transport, construction vehicle
    rodent (feces) (urine) W53.89
      bite W53.81
      mouse W53.09
        bite W53.01
      rat W53.19
        bite W53.11
      specified NEC W53.89
        bite W53.81
      squirrel W53.29
        bite W53.21
    roller coaster W31.81
    rope NEC W24.0
      agricultural operations W30.89
    saliva — *see* Contact, with, by type of animal
    sander W29.8
      industrial W31.2
    saucepan (hot) (glass) (metal) X15.3
    saw W27.0
      band (industrial) W31.2
      bench (industrial) W31.2
      chain W29.3
      hand W27.0
    sawing machine, metal W31.1
    scissors W27.2
    scorpion X58
    screwdriver W27.0
      powered W29.8
    sea
      anemone, cucumber or urchin (spine) X58
      lion W56.19
        bite W56.11
        strike W56.12
    serpent — *see* Contact, with, snake, by type
    sewing-machine (electric) (powered) W29.2
      not powered W27.8
    shaft (hoist) (lift) (transmission) NEC W24.0
      agricultural W30.89
    shark W56.49
      bite W56.41
      strike W56.42
    sharp object (s) W26.9
      specified NEC W26.8
    shears (hand) W27.2
      powered (industrial) W31.1
        domestic W29.2
    sheep W55.39
      bite W55.31
      strike W55.32
    shovel W27.8
      steam — *see* Accident, transport, construction vehicle
    snake (nonvenomous) W59.19
      bite W59.11

Contact (accidental) - *continued*
  with - *continued*
    snake (nonvenomous) - *continued*
      crushing W59.13
      strike W59.12
    spade W27.1
    spider (venomous) X58
    spin-drier W29.2
    spinning machine W31.89
    splinter W45.8
    sports equipment W21.9
    staple gun (powered) W29.8
    steam X13.1
      engine W31.3
      inhalation X13.0
      pipe X16
      shovel W31.89
    stove (hot) (kitchen) X15.0
    substance, hot NEC X19
      molten (metal) X18
    sword W26.1
      assault X99.2
      stated as undetermined whether accidental or intentional Y28.2
      suicide (attempt) X78.2
    tarantula X58
    thresher W30.0
    tin can lid W26.8
    toad W62.1
    toaster (hot) X15.1
    tool W27.8
      hand (not powered) W27.8
        auger W27.0
        axe W27.0
        can opener W27.4
        chisel W27.0
        fork W27.4
        garden W27.1
        handsaw W27.0
        hoe W27.1
        ice-pick W27.4
        kitchen utensil W27.4
        manual
          lawn mower W27.1
          sewing machine W27.8
        meat grinder W27.4
        needle (sewing) W27.3
          hypodermic W46.0
            contaminated W46.1
        paper cutter W27.5
        pitchfork W27.1
        rake W27.1
        scissors W27.2
        screwdriver W27.0
        specified NEC W27.8
        workbench W27.0
      hot X17
      powered W29.8
        blender W29.0
          commercial W31.82
        can opener W29.0
          commercial W31.82
        chainsaw W29.3
        clothes dryer W29.2
          commercial W31.82
        dishwasher W29.2
          commercial W31.82
        edger W29.3
        electric fan W29.2
          commercial W31.82
        electric knife W29.1
        food processor W29.0
          commercial W31.82
        garbage disposal W29.0
          commercial W31.82
        garden tool W29.3
        hedge trimmer W29.3
        ice maker W29.0
          commercial W31.82
        kitchen appliance W29.0
          commercial W31.82
        lawn mower W28
        meat grinder W29.0
          commercial W31.82
        mixer W29.0

Contact (accidental) - *continued*
  with - *continued*
    tool - *continued*
      powered - *continued*
        mixer - *continued*
          commercial W31.82
        rototiller W29.3
        sewing machine W29.2
          commercial W31.82
        washing machine W29.2
          commercial W31.82
      transmission device (belt, cable, chain, gear, pinion, shaft) W24.1
        agricultural operations W30.89
      turbine (gas) (water-driven) W31.3
      turkey W61.49
        peck W61.43
        strike W61.42
      turtle (nonvenomous) W59.29
        bite W59.21
        strike W59.22
        terrestrial W59.89
          bite W59.81
          crushing W59.83
          strike W59.82
      under-cutter W31.0
      urine — *see* Contact, with, by type of animal
      vehicle
        agricultural use (transport) — *see* Accident, transport, agricultural vehicle
          not on public highway W30.81
        industrial use (transport) — *see* Accident, transport, industrial vehicle
          not on public highway W31.83
        off-road use (transport) — *see* Accident, transport, all-terrain or off-road vehicle
          not on public highway W31.83
        special construction use (transport) — *see* Accident, transport, construction vehicle
          not on public highway W31.83
      venomous
        animal X58
        arthropods X58
        lizard X58
        marine animal NEC X58
        marine plant NEC X58
        millipedes (tropical) X58
        plant (s) X58
        snake X58
        spider X58
        viper X58
      washing-machine (powered) W29.2
      wasp X58
      weaving-machine W31.89
      winch W24.0
        agricultural operations W30.89
      wire NEC W24.0
        agricultural operations W30.89
      wood slivers W45.8
      yellow jacket X58
      zebra — *see* Contact, with, hoof stock NEC
  pressure X50.9
  stress X50.9
Coup de soleil X32
Crash
  aircraft (in transit) (powered) V95.9
    balloon V96.01
    fixed wing NEC (private) V95.21
      commercial V95.31
    glider V96.21
      hang V96.11
      powered V95.11
    helicopter V95.01
    in war operations — *see* War operations, destruction of aircraft
    microlight V95.11
    nonpowered V96.9
      specified NEC V96.8
    powered NEC V95.8

Crash - *continued*
  aircraft (in transit) (powered) - *continued*
    stated as
      homicide (attempt) Y08.81
      suicide (attempt) X83.0
    ultralight V95.11
  spacecraft V95.41
  transport vehicle NEC — *see also* Accident, transport V89.9
    homicide (attempt) Y03.8
    motor NEC (traffic) V89.2
      homicide (attempt) Y03.8
    suicide (attempt) — *see* Suicide, collision
Cruelty (mental) (physical) (sexual) X58
Crushed (accidentally) X58
  between objects (moving) (stationary and moving) W23.0
    stationary W23.1
  by
    alligator W58.03
    avalanche NEC — *see* Landslide
    cave-in W20.0
      caused by cataclysmic earth surface movement — *see* Landslide
    crocodile W58.13
    crowd or human stampede W52
    falling
      aircraft V97.39
        in war operations — *see* War operations, destruction of aircraft
      earth, material W20.0
        caused by cataclysmic earth surface movement — *see* Landslide
      object NEC W20.8
    landslide NEC — *see* Landslide
    lizard (nonvenomous) W59.09
    machinery — *see* Contact, with, by type of machine
    reptile NEC W59.89
    snake (nonvenomous) W59.13
  in
    machinery — *see* Contact, with, by type of machine
Cut, cutting (any part of body) (accidental) — *see also* Contact, with, by object or machine
  during medical or surgical treatment as misadventure — *see* Index to Diseases and Injuries, Complications
  homicide (attempt) — *see* Assault, cutting or piercing instrument
  inflicted by other person — *see* Assault, cutting or piercing instrument
  legal
    execution — *see* Legal, intervention
    intervention — *see* Legal, intervention, sharp object
  machine NEC — *see also* Contact, with, by type of machine W31.9
  self-inflicted — *see* Suicide, cutting or piercing instrument
  suicide (attempt) — *see* Suicide, cutting or piercing instrument
Cyclone (any injury) X37.1

D

Decapitation (accidental circumstances) NEC X58
  homicide X99.9
  legal execution — *see* Legal, intervention
Dehydration from lack of water X58
Deprivation X58
Derailment (accidental)
  railway (rolling stock) (train) (vehicle) (without antecedent collision) V81.7
    with antecedent collision — *see* Accident, transport, railway vehicle occupant
  streetcar (without antecedent collision) V82.7
    with antecedent collision — *see* Accident, transport, streetcar occupant
Descent
  parachute (voluntary) (without accident to aircraft) V97.29
    due to accident to aircraft — *see* Accident, transport, aircraft

Desertion X58
Destitution X58
Disability, late effect or sequela of injury — *see* Sequelae
Discharge (accidental)
  airgun W34.010
    assault X95.01
    homicide (attempt) X95.01
    stated as undetermined whether accidental or intentional Y24.0
    suicide (attempt) X74.01
  BB gun — *see* Discharge, airgun
  firearm (accidental) W34.00
    assault X95.9
    handgun (pistol) (revolver) W32.0
      assault X93
      homicide (attempt) X93
      legal intervention — *see* Legal, intervention, firearm, handgun
      stated as undetermined whether accidental or intentional Y22
      suicide (attempt) X72
    homicide (attempt) X95.9
    hunting rifle W33.02
      assault X94.1
      homicide (attempt) X94.1
      legal intervention
        injuring
          bystander Y35.032
          law enforcement personnel Y35.031
          suspect Y35.033
          unspecified person Y35.039
      stated as undetermined whether accidental or intentional Y23.1
      suicide (attempt) X73.1
    larger W33.00
      assault X94.9
      homicide (attempt) X94.9
      hunting rifle — *see* Discharge, firearm, hunting rifle
      legal intervention — *see* Legal, intervention, firearm by type of firearm
      machine gun — *see* Discharge, firearm, machine gun
      shotgun — *see* Discharge, firearm, shotgun
      specified NEC W33.09
        assault X94.8
        homicide (attempt) X94.8
        legal intervention
          injuring
            bystander Y35.092
            law enforcement personnel Y35.091
            suspect Y35.093
            unspecified person Y35.099
        stated as undetermined whether accidental or intentional Y23.8
        suicide (attempt) X73.8
      stated as undetermined whether accidental or intentional Y23.9
      suicide (attempt) X73.9
    legal intervention
      injuring
        bystander Y35.002
        law enforcement personnel Y35.001
        suspect Y35.03
        unspecified person Y35.009
      using rubber bullet
        injuring
          bystander Y35.042
          law enforcement personnel Y35.041
          suspect Y35.043
          unspecified person Y35.049
    machine gun W33.03
      assault X94.2
      homicide (attempt) X94.2
      legal intervention — *see* Legal, intervention, firearm, machine gun
      stated as undetermined whether accidental or intentional Y23.3
      suicide (attempt) X73.2
    pellet gun — *see* Discharge, airgun
    shotgun W33.01

DISCHARGE - DROWNING

Discharge (accidental) - *continued*
  firearm (accidental) - *continued*
    shotgun - *continued*
      assault X94.0
      homicide (attempt) X94.0
      legal intervention — *see* Legal,
        intervention, firearm, specified
        NEC
      stated as undetermined whether
        accidental or intentional Y23.0
      suicide (attempt) X73.0
    specified NEC W34.09
      assault X95.8
      homicide (attempt) X95.8
      legal intervention — *see* Legal,
        intervention, firearm, specified
        NEC
      stated as undetermined whether
        accidental or intentional Y24.8
      suicide (attempt) X74.8
    stated as undetermined whether accidental
      or intentional Y24.9
    suicide (attempt) X74.9
    Very pistol W34.09
      assault X95.8
      homicide (attempt) X95.8
      stated as undetermined whether
        accidental or intentional Y24.8
      suicide (attempt) X74.8
  firework (s) W39
    stated as undetermined whether accidental
      or intentional Y25
  gas-operated gun NEC W34.018
    airgun — *see* Discharge, airgun
    assault X95.09
    homicide (attempt) X95.09
    paintball gun — *see* Discharge, paintball
      gun
    stated as undetermined whether accidental
      or intentional Y24.8
    suicide (attempt) X74.09
  gun NEC — *see also* Discharge, firearm
    NEC
    air — *see* Discharge, airgun
    BB — *see* Discharge, airgun
    for single hand use — *see* Discharge,
      firearm, handgun
    hand — *see* Discharge, firearm, handgun
    machine — *see* Discharge, firearm,
      machine gun
    other specified — *see* Discharge, firearm
      NEC
    paintball — *see* Discharge, paintball gun
    pellet — *see* Discharge, airgun
  handgun — *see* Discharge, firearm, handgun
  machine gun — *see* Discharge, firearm,
    machine gun
  paintball gun W34.011
    assault X95.02
    homicide (attempt) X95.02
    stated as undetermined whether accidental
      or intentional Y24.8
    suicide (attempt) X74.02
  pistol — *see* Discharge, firearm, handgun
    flare — *see* Discharge, firearm, Very pistol
    pellet — *see* Discharge, airgun
    Very — *see* Discharge, firearm, Very pistol
  revolver — *see* Discharge, firearm, handgun
  rifle (hunting) — *see* Discharge, firearm,
    hunting rifle
  shotgun — *see* Discharge, firearm, shotgun
  spring-operated gun NEC W34.018
    assault X95.09
    homicide (attempt) X95.09
    stated as undetermined whether
      or intentional Y24.8
    suicide (attempt) X74.09
Disease
  Andes W94.11
  aviator's - — *see* Air, pressure
  range W94.11

    Diver's disease, palsy, paralysis, squeeze
    - — *see* Air, pressure
Diving (into water) — *see* Accident, diving

Dog bite W54.0
Dragged by transport vehicle NEC — *see*
  also Accident, transport V09.9
Drinking poison (accidental) — *see* Table of
  Drugs and Chemicals
**Dropped (accidentally) while being carried
  or supported by other person** W04
Drowning (accidental) W74
  assault X92.9
  due to
    accident (to)
      machinery — *see* Contact, with, by type
        of machine
      watercraft V90.89
        burning V90.29
          powered V90.23
            merchant ship V90.20
            passenger ship V90.21
            fishing boat V90.22
            jetskis V90.23
          unpowered V90.28
            canoe V90.25
            inflatable V90.26
            kayak V90.25
            sailboat V90.24
            water skis V90.27
        crushed V90.39
          powered V90.33
            merchant ship V90.30
            passenger ship V90.31
            fishing boat V90.32
            jetskis V90.33
          unpowered V90.38
            canoe V90.35
            inflatable V90.36
            kayak V90.35
            sailboat V90.34
            water skis V90.37
        overturning V90.09
          powered V90.03
            merchant ship V90.00
            passenger ship V90.01
            fishing boat V90.02
            jetskis V90.03
          unpowered V90.08
            canoe V90.05
            inflatable V90.06
            kayak V90.05
            sailboat V90.04
        sinking V90.19
          powered V90.13
            merchant ship V90.10
            passenger ship V90.11
            fishing boat V90.12
            jetskis V90.13
          unpowered V90.18
            canoe V90.15
            inflatable V90.16
            kayak V90.15
            sailboat V90.14
        specified type NEC V90.89
          powered V90.83
            merchant ship V90.80
            passenger ship V90.81
            fishing boat V90.82
            jetskis V90.83
          unpowered V90.88
            canoe V90.85
            inflatable V90.86
            kayak V90.85
            sailboat V90.84
            water skis V90.87
    avalanche — *see* Landslide
    cataclysmic
      earth surface movement NEC — *see*
        Forces of nature, earth movement
      storm — *see* Forces of nature,
        cataclysmic storm
    cloudburst X37.8
    cyclone X37.1
    fall overboard (from) V92.09
      powered craft V92.03
        ferry boat V92.01
        liner V92.01
        merchant ship V92.00

Drowning (accidental) - *continued*
  due to - *continued*
    fall overboard (from) - *continued*
      powered craft - *continued*
        passenger ship V92.01
        fishing boat V92.02
        jetskis V92.03
      unpowered craft V92.08
        canoe V92.05
        inflatable V92.06
        kayak V92.05
        sailboat V92.04
        surf-board V92.08
        water skis V92.07
        windsurfer V92.08
    resulting from
      accident to watercraft — *see*
        Drowning, due to, accident to,
        watercraft
      being washed overboard
        (from) V92.29
        powered craft V92.23
          ferry boat V92.21
          liner V92.21
          merchant ship V92.20
          passenger ship V92.21
          fishing boat V92.22
          jetskis V92.23
        unpowered craft V92.28
          canoe V92.25
          inflatable V92.26
          kayak V92.25
          sailboat V92.24
          surf-board V92.28
          water skis V92.27
          windsurfer V92.28
      motion of watercraft V92.19
        powered craft V92.13
          ferry boat V92.11
          liner V92.11
          merchant ship V92.10
          passenger ship V92.11
          fishing boat V92.12
          jetskis V92.13
        unpowered craft
          canoe V92.15
          inflatable V92.16
          kayak V92.15
          sailboat V92.14
    hurricane X37.0
    jumping into water from watercraft
      (involved in accident) — *see also*
      Drowning, due to, accident to,
      watercraft
      without accident to or on
        watercraft W16.711
    tidal wave NEC — *see* Forces of nature,
      tidal wave
    torrential rain X37.8
  following
    fall
      into
        bathtub W16.211
        bucket W16.221
        fountain — *see* Drowning, following,
          fall, into, water, specified NEC
        quarry — *see* Drowning, following,
          fall, into, water, specified NEC
        reservoir — *see* Drowning, following,
          fall, into, water, specified NEC
        swimming-pool W16.011
          striking
            bottom W16.021
            wall W16.031
          stated as undetermined whether
            accidental or intentional Y21.3
          suicide (attempt) X71.2
        water NOS W16.41
          natural (lake) (open sea) (river)
            (stream) (pond) W16.111
            striking
              bottom W16.121
              side W16.131
          specified NEC W16.311
            striking

Drowning (accidental) - *continued*
  following - *continued*
    fall - *continued*
      into - *continued*
        water NOS - *continued*
          specified NEC - *continued*
            striking - *continued*
              bottom W16.321
              wall W16.331
      overboard NEC — *see* Drowning, due
          to, fall overboard
    jump or dive
      from boat W16.711
        striking bottom W16.721
      into
        fountain — *see* Drowning, following,
            jump or dive, into, water,
            specified NEC
        quarry — *see* Drowning, following,
            jump or dive, into, water,
            specified NEC
        reservoir — *see* Drowning, following,
            jump or dive, into, water,
            specified NEC
        swimming-pool W16.511
          striking
            bottom W16.521
            wall W16.531
          suicide (attempt) X71.2
        water NOS W16.91
          natural (lake) (open sea) (river)
              (stream) (pond) W16.611
          specified NEC W16.811
            striking
              bottom W16.821
              wall W16.831
            striking bottom W16.621
  homicide (attempt) X92.9
  in
    bathtub (accidental) W65
      assault X92.0
      following fall W16.211
        stated as undetermined whether
            accidental or intentional Y21.1
      stated as undetermined whether
          accidental or intentional Y21.0
      suicide (attempt) X71.0
    lake — *see* Drowning, in, natural water
    natural water (lake) (open sea) (river)
        (stream) (pond) W69
      assault X92.3
      following
        dive or jump W16.611
          striking bottom W16.621
        fall W16.111
          striking
            bottom W16.121
            side W16.131
      stated as undetermined whether
          accidental or intentional Y21.4
      suicide (attempt) X71.3
    quarry — *see* Drowning, in, specified
        place NEC
    quenching tank — *see* Drowning, in,
        specified place NEC
    reservoir — *see* Drowning, in, specified
        place NEC
    river — *see* Drowning, in, natural water
    sea — *see* Drowning, in, natural water
    specified place NEC W73
      assault X92.8
      following
        dive or jump W16.811
          striking
            bottom W16.821
            wall W16.831
        fall W16.311
          striking
            bottom W16.321
            wall W16.331
      stated as undetermined whether
          accidental or intentional Y21.8
      suicide (attempt) X71.8
    stream — *see* Drowning, in, natural water
    swimming-pool W67

Drowning (accidental) - *continued*
  in - *continued*
    swimming-pool - *continued*
      assault X92.1
        following fall X92.2
      following
        dive or jump W16.511
          striking
            bottom W16.521
            wall W16.531
        fall W16.011
          striking
            bottom W16.021
            wall W16.031
      stated as undetermined whether
          accidental or intentional Y21.2
        following fall Y21.3
      suicide (attempt) X71.1
        following fall X71.2
    war operations — *see* War operations,
        restriction of airway
  resulting from accident to watercraftCsee
      Drowning, due to, accident, watercraft
  self-inflicted X71.9
  stated as undetermined whether accidental or
      intentional Y21.9
  suicide (attempt) X71.9

E

Earth falling (on) W20.0
  caused by cataclysmic earth surface
      movement or eruption — *see* Landslide
Earth (surface) movement NEC — *see*
    Forces of nature, earth movement
Earthquake (any injury) X34
Effect (s) (adverse) of
  air pressure (any) - — *see* Air, pressure
  cold, excessive (exposure to) — *see*
      Exposure, cold
  heat (excessive) — *see* Heat
  hot place (weather) — *see* Heat
  insolation X30
  late — *see* Sequelae
  motion — *see* Motion
  nuclear explosion or weapon in war
      operations — *see* War operations,
      nuclear weapon
  radiation — *see* Radiation
  travel — *see* Travel
Electric shock (accidental) (by) (in) — *see*
    Exposure, electric current
Electrocution (accidental) — *see* Exposure,
    electric current
**Endotracheal tube wrongly placed during
    anesthetic procedure**
Entanglement
  in
    bed linen, causing suffocation — *see*
        category T71
    wheel of pedal cycle V19.88
Entry of foreign body or material — *see*
    Foreign body
Environmental pollution related condition-
    see Z57
Execution, legal (any method) — *see* Legal,
    intervention
Exhaustion
  cold — *see* Exposure, cold
  due to excessive exertion — *see also*
      Overexertion X50.9
  heat — *see* Heat
**Explosion (accidental) (of) (with secondary
    fire)** W40.9
  acetylene W40.1
  aerosol can W36.1
  air tank (compressed) (in machinery) W36.2
  aircraft (in transit) (powered) NEC V95.9
    balloon V96.05
    fixed wing NEC (private) V95.25
      commercial V95.35
    glider V96.25
      hang V96.15
      powered V95.15
    helicopter V95.05
    in war operations — *see* War operations,
        destruction of aircraft

**Explosion (accidental) (of) (with secondary
    fire)** - *continued*
  aircraft (in transit) (powered) NEC -
      continued
    microlight V95.15
    nonpowered V96.9
      specified NEC V96.8
    powered NEC V95.8
    stated as
      homicide (attempt) Y03.8
      suicide (attempt) X83.0
    ultralight V95.15
  anesthetic gas in operating room W40.1
  antipersonnel bomb W40.8
    assault X96.0
    homicide (attempt) X96.0
    suicide (attempt) X75
  assault X96.9
  bicycle tire W37.0
  blasting (cap) (materials) W40.0
  boiler (machinery) , not on transport
      vehicle W35
    on watercraft — *see* Explosion, in,
        watercraft
  butane W40.1
  caused by other person X96.9
  coal gas W40.1
  detonator W40.0
  dump (munitions) W40.8
  dynamite W40.0
    in
      assault X96.8
      homicide (attempt) X96.8
      legal intervention
        injuring
          bystander Y35.112
          law enforcement personnel Y35.111
          suspect Y35.113
          unspecified person Y35.119
      suicide (attempt) X75
  explosive (material) W40.9
    gas W40.1
    in blasting operation W40.0
    specified NEC W40.8
      in
        assault X96.8
        homicide (attempt) X96.8
        legal intervention
          injuring
            bystander Y35.192
            law enforcement
                personnel Y35.191
            suspect Y35.193
            unspecified person Y35.199
        suicide (attempt) X75
  factory (munitions) W40.8
  fertilizer bomb W40.8
    assault X96.3
    homicide (attempt) X96.3
    suicide (attempt) X75
  firearm (parts) NEC W34.19
    airgun W34.110
    BB gun W34.110
    gas, air or spring-operated gun
        NEC W34.118
    hangun W32.1
    hunting rifle W33.12
    larger firearm W33.10
      specified NEC W33.19
    machine gun W33.13
    paintball gun W34.111
    pellet gun W34.110
    shotgun W33.11
    Very pistol [flare] W34.19
  fire-damp W40.1
  fireworks W39
  gas (coal) (explosive) W40.1
    cylinder W36.9
      aerosol can W36.1
      air tank W36.2
      pressurized W36.3
      specified NEC W36.8
  gasoline (fumes) (tank) not in moving motor
      vehicle W40.1
    bomb W40.8

Explosion (accidental) (of) (with secondary fire) - *continued*
  gasoline (fumes) (tank) not in moving motor vehicle - *continued*
    bomb - *continued*
      assault X96.1
        homicide (attempt) X96.1
        suicide (attempt) X75
      in motor vehicle — *see* Accident, transport, by type of vehicle
  grain store W40.8
  grenade W40.8
    in
      assault X96.8
      homicide (attempt) X96.8
      legal intervention
        injuring
          bystander Y35.192
          law enforcement personnel Y35.191
          suspect Y35.193
          unspecified person Y35.199
      suicide (attempt) X75
  handgun (parts) — *see* Explosion, firearm, hangun (parts)
  homicide (attempt) X96.9
    antipersonnel bomb — *see* Explosion, antipersonnel bomb
    fertilizer bomb — *see* Explosion, fertilizer bomb
    gasoline bomb — *see* Explosion, gasoline bomb
    letter bomb — *see* Explosion, letter bomb
    pipe bomb — *see* Explosion, pipe bomb
    specified NEC X96.8
  hose, pressurized W37.8
  hot water heater, tank (in machinery) W35
    on watercraft — *see* Explosion, in, watercraft
  in, on
    dump W40.8
    factory W40.8
    mine (of explosive gases) NEC W40.1
    watercraft V93.59
      powered craft V93.53
        ferry boat V93.51
        fishing boat V93.52
        jetskis V93.53
        liner V93.51
        merchant ship V93.50
        passenger ship V93.51
        sailboat V93.54
  letter bomb W40.8
    assault X96.2
    homicide (attempt) X96.2
    suicide (attempt) X75
  machinery — *see also* Contact, with, by type of machine
    on board watercraft — *see* Explosion, in, watercraft
    pressure vessel — *see* Explosion, by type of vessel
  methane W40.1
  mine W40.1
  missile NEC W40.8
  mortar bomb W40.8
    in
      assault X96.8
      homicide (attempt) X96.8
      legal intervention
        injuring
          bystander Y35.192
          law enforcement personnel Y35.191
          suspect Y35.193
          unspecified person Y35.199
      suicide (attempt) X75
  munitions (dump) (factory) W40.8
  pipe, pressurized W37.8
    bomb W40.8
      assault X96.4
      homicide (attempt) X96.4
      suicide (attempt) X75
  pressure, pressurized
    cooker W38
    gas tank (in machinery) W36.3
    hose W37.8

Explosion (accidental) (of) (with secondary fire) - *continued*
  pressure, pressurized - *continued*
    pipe W37.8
    specified device NEC W38
    tire W37.8
      bicycle W37.0
    vessel (in machinery) W38
  propane W40.1
  self-inflicted X75
  shell (artillery) NEC W40.8
    during war operations — *see* War operations, explosion
    in
      legal intervention
        injuring
          bystander Y35.122
          law enforcement personnel Y35.121
          suspect Y35.123
          unspecified person Y35.129
    war — *see* War operations, explosion
  spacecraft V95.45
  steam or water lines (in machinery) W37.8
  stove W40.9
  stated as undetermined whether accidental or intentional Y25
  suicide (attempt) X75
  tire, pressurized W37.8
    bicycle W37.0
  undetermined whether accidental or intentional Y25
  vehicle tire NEC W37.8
    bicycle W37.0
  war operations — *see* War operations, explosion

Exposure (to) X58
  air pressure change — *see* Air, pressure
  cold (accidental) (excessive) (extreme) (natural) (place) X31
    assault Y08.89
    due to
      man-made conditions W93.8
        dry ice (contact) W93.01
          inhalation W93.02
        liquid air (contact) (hydrogen) (nitrogen) W93.11
          inhalation W93.12
        refrigeration unit (deep freeze) W93.2
        suicide (attempt) X83.2
      weather (conditions) X31
    homicide (attempt) Y08.89
    self-inflicted X83.2
  due to abandonment or neglect X58
  electric current W86.8
    appliance (faulty) W86.8
      domestic W86.0
    caused by other person Y08.89
    conductor (faulty) W86.1
    control apparatus (faulty) W86.1
    electric power generating plant, distribution station W86.1
    electroshock gun — *see* Exposure, electric current, taser
    high-voltage cable W85
    homicide (attempt) Y08.89
    legal execution — *see* Legal, intervention, specified means NEC
    lightning — *see* subcategory T75.0
    live rail W86.8
    misadventure in medical or surgical procedure in electroshock therapy Y63.4
    motor (electric) (faulty) W86.8
      domestic W86.0
    self-inflicted X83.1
    specified NEC W86.8
      domestic W86.0
    stun gun — *see* Exposure, electric current, taser
    suicide (attempt) X83.1
    taser W86.8
      assault Y08.89
      legal intervention — *see* category Y35
      self-harm (intentional) X83.8
      undetermined intent Y33

Exposure (to) - *continued*
  electric current - *continued*
    third rail W86.8
    transformer (faulty) W86.1
    transmission lines W85
  environmental tobacco smoke X58
  excessive
    cold — *see* Exposure, cold
    heat (natural) NEC X30
      man-made W92
  factor (s) NOS X58
    environmental NEC X58
    man-made NEC W99
    natural NEC — *see* Forces of nature
    specified NEC X58
  fire, flames (accidental) X08.8
    assault X97
    campfire — *see* Exposure, fire, controlled, not in building
    controlled (in)
      with ignition (of) clothing — *see also* Ignition, clothes X06.2
        nightwear X05
      bonfire — *see* Exposure, fire, controlled, not in building
      brazier (in building or structure) — *see also* Exposure, fire, controlled, building
        not in building or structure — *see* Exposure, fire, controlled, not in building
      building or structure X02.0
        with
          fall from building X02.3
          injury due to building collapse X02.2
          from building X02.5
          smoke inhalation X02.1
        hit by object from building X02.4
        specified mode of injury NEC X02.8
      fireplace, furnace or stove — *see* Exposure, fire, controlled, building
      not in building or structure X03.0
        with
          fall X03.3
          smoke inhalation X03.1
        hit by object X03.4
        specified mode of injury NEC X03.8
      trash — *see* Exposure, fire, controlled, not in building
    fireplace — *see* Exposure, fire, controlled, building
    fittings or furniture (in building or structure) (uncontrolled) — *see* Exposure, fire, uncontrolled, building
    forest (uncontrolled) — *see* Exposure, fire, uncontrolled, not in building
    grass (uncontrolled) — *see* Exposure, fire, uncontrolled, not in building
    hay (uncontrolled) — *see* Exposure, fire, uncontrolled, not in building
    homicide (attempt) X97
    ignition of highly flammable material X04
    in, of, on, starting in
      machinery — *see* Contact, with, by type of machine
      motor vehicle (in motion) — *see also* Accident, transport, occupant by type of vehicle V87.8
        with collision — *see* Collision
      railway rolling stock, train, vehicle V81.81
        with collision — *see* Accident, transport, railway vehicle occupant
      street car (in motion) V82.8
        with collision — *see* Accident, transport, streetcar occupant
      transport vehicle NEC — *see also* Accident, transport
        with collision — *see* Collision
      war operations — *see also* War operations, fire
        from nuclear explosion — *see* War operations, nuclear weapons

Exposure (to) - *continued*
  fire, flames (accidental) - *continued*
    in, of, on, starting in - *continued*
      watercraft (in transit) (not in
          transit) V91.09
        localized — *see* Burn, on board
            watercraft, due to, fire on board
        powered craft V91.03
          ferry boat V91.01
          fishing boat V91.02
          jet skis V91.03
          liner V91.01
          merchant ship V91.00
          passenger ship V91.01
        unpowered craft V91.08
          canoe V91.05
          inflatable V91.06
          kayak V91.05
          sailboat V91.04
          surf-board V91.08
          waterskis V91.07
          windsurfer V91.08
  lumber (uncontrolled) — *see* Exposure,
      fire, uncontrolled, not in building
  mine (uncontrolled) — *see* Exposure, fire,
      uncontrolled, not in building
  prairie (uncontrolled) — *see* Exposure,
      fire, uncontrolled, not in building
  resulting from
    explosion — *see* Explosion
    lightning X08.8
  self-inflicted X76
  specified NEC X08.8
  started by other person X97
  stove — *see* Exposure, fire, controlled,
      building
  stated as undetermined whether accidental
      or intentional Y26
  suicide (attempt) X76
  tunnel (uncontrolled) — *see* Exposure,
      fire, uncontrolled, not in building
  uncontrolled
    in building or structure X00.0
      with
        fall from building X00.3
        injury due to building
            collapse X00.2
        jump from building X00.5
        smoke inhalation X00.1
      bed X08.00
        due to
          cigarette X08.01
          specified material NEC X08.09
      furniture NEC X08.20
        due to
          cigarette X08.21
          specified material NEC X08.29
      hit by object from building X00.4
      sofa X08.10
        due to
          cigarette X08.11
          specified material NEC X08.19
      specified mode of injury NEC X00.8
    not in building or structure (any) X01.0
      with
        fall X01.3
        smoke inhalation X01.1
      hit by object X01.4
      specified mode of injury NEC X01.8
    undetermined whether accidental or
        intentional Y26
  forces of nature NEC — *see* Forces of nature
  G-forces (abnormal) W49.9
  gravitational forces (abnormal) W49.9
  heat (natural) NEC — *see* Heat
  high-pressure jet (hydraulic)
      (pneumatic) W49.9
  hydraulic jet W49.9
  inanimate mechanical force W49.9
  jet, high-pressure (hydraulic)
      (pneumatic) W49.9
  lightning — *see* subcategory T75.0
    causing fire — *see* Exposure, fire
  mechanical forces NEC W49.9
    animate NEC W64

Exposure (to) - *continued*
  mechanical forces NEC - *continued*
    inanimate NEC W49.9
  noise W42.9
    supersonic W42.0
  noxious substance — *see* Table of Drugs and
      Chemicals
  pneumatic jet W49.9
  prolonged in deep-freeze unit or
      refrigerator W93.2
  radiation — *see* Radiation
  smoke — *see also* Exposure, fire
    tobacco, second hand Z77.22
  specified factors NEC X58
  sunlight X32
    man-made (sun lamp) W89.8
    tanning bed W89.1
  supersonic waves W42.0
  transmission line (s) , electric W85
  vibration W49.9
  waves
    infrasound W49.9
    sound W42.9
    supersonic W42.0
  weather NEC — *see* Forces of nature
External cause status Y99.9
  child assisting in compensated work for
      family Y99.8
  civilian activity done for financial or other
      compensation Y99.0
  civilian activity done for income or
      pay Y99.0
  family member assisting in compensated
      work for other family member Y99.8
  hobby not done for income Y99.8
  leisure activity Y99.8
  military activity Y99.1
  off-duty activity of military personnel Y99.8
  recreation or sport not for income or while a
      student Y99.8
  specified NEC Y99.8
  student activity Y99.8
  volunteer activity Y99.2

F

Factors, supplemental
  alcohol
    blood level
      less than 20mg/100ml Y90.0
      presence in blood, level not
          specified Y90.9
      20-39mg/100ml Y90.1
      40-59mg/100ml Y90.2
      60-79mg/100ml Y90.3
      80-99mg/100ml Y90.4
      100-119mg/100ml Y90.5
      120-199mg/100ml Y90.6
      200-239mg/100ml Y90.7
      240mg/100ml or more Y90.8
    presence in blood, but level not
        specified Y90.9
  environmental-pollution-related condition-
      see Z57
  nosocomial condition Y95
  work-related condition Y99.0
Failure
  in suture or ligature during surgical
      procedure Y65.2
  mechanical, of instrument or apparatus (any)
      (during any medical or surgical
      procedure) Y65.8
  sterile precautions (during medical and
      surgical care) — *see* Misadventure,
      failure, sterile precautions, by type of
      procedure
  to
    introduce tube or instrument Y65.4
      endotracheal tube during
          anesthesia Y65.3
    make curve (transport vehicle) NEC — *see*
        Accident, transport
    remove tube or instrument Y65.4
Fall, falling (accidental) W19
  building W20.1
    burning (uncontrolled fire) X00.3
  down

Fall, falling (accidental) - *continued*
  down - *continued*
    embankment W17.81
    escalator W10.0
    hill W17.81
    ladder W11
    ramp W10.2
    stairs, steps W10.9
  due to
    bumping against
      object W18.00
        sharp glass W18.02
        specified NEC W18.09
        sports equipment W18.01
      person W03
        due to ice or snow W00.0
        on pedestrian conveyance — *see*
            Accident, transport, pedestrian,
            conveyance
    collision with another person W03
      due to ice or snow W00.0
      involving pedestrian conveyance — *see*
          Accident, transport, pedestrian,
          conveyance
    grocery cart tipping over W17.82
    ice or snow W00.9
      from one level to another W00.2
      on stairs or steps W00.1
      involving pedestrian conveyance — *see*
          Accident, transport, pedestrian,
          conveyance
      on same level W00.0
    slipping (on moving sidewalk) W01.0
      with subsequent striking against
          object W01.10
        furniture W01.190
        sharp object W01.119
          glass W01.110
          power tool or machine W01.111
          specified NEC W01.118
        specified NEC W01.198
    striking against
      object W18.00
        sharp glass W18.02
        specified NEC W18.09
        sports equipment W18.01
      person W03
        due to ice or snow W00.0
        on pedestrian conveyance — *see*
            Accident, transport, pedestrian,
            conveyance
  earth (with asphyxia or suffocation (by
      pressure)) — *see* Earth, falling
  from, off, out of
    aircraft NEC (with accident to aircraft
        NEC) V97.0
      while boarding or alighting V97.1
    balcony W13.0
    bed W06
    boat, ship, watercraft NEC (with drowning
        or submersion) — *see* Drowning, due
        to, fall overboard
      with hitting bottom or object V94.0
    bridge W13.1
    building W13.9
      burning (uncontrolled fire) X00.3
    cavity W17.2
    chair W07
    cherry picker W17.89
    cliff W15
    dock W17.4
    embankment W17.81
    escalator W10.0
    flagpole W13.8
    furniture NEC W08
    grocery cart W17.82
    haystack W17.89
    high place NEC W17.89
      stated as undetermined whether
          accidental or intentional Y30
    hole W17.2
    incline W10.2
    ladder W11
    lifting device W17.89

FALL, FALLING - FALL, FALLING

Fall, falling (accidental) - *continued*
 from, off, out of - *continued*
  machine, machinery — *see also* Contact,
   with, by type of machine
   not in operation W17.89
  manhole W17.1
  mobile elevated work platform
   [MEWP] W17.89
  motorized mobility scooter W05.2
  one level to another NEC W17.89
   intentional, purposeful, suicide
    (attempt) X80
   stated as undetermined whether
    accidental or intentional Y30
  pit W17.2
  playground equipment W09.8
   jungle gym W09.2
   slide W09.0
   swing W09.1
  quarry W17.89
  railing W13.9
  ramp W10.2
  roof W13.2
  scaffolding W12
  scooter (nonmotorized) W05.1
   motorized mobility W05.2
  sky lift W17.89
  stairs, steps W10.9
   curb W10.1
   due to ice or snow W00.1
   escalator W10.0
   incline W10.2
   ramp W10.2
   sidewalk curb W10.1
   specified NEC W10.8
  stepladder W11
  storm drain W17.1
  streetcar NEC V82.6
   with antecedent collision — *see*
    Accident, transport, streetcar
    occupant
   while boarding or alighting V82.4
  structure NEC W13.8
   burning (uncontrolled fire) X00.3
  table W08
  toilet W18.11
   with subsequent striking against
    object W18.12
  train NEC V81.6
   during derailment (without antecedent
    collision) V81.7
   with antecedent collision — *see*
    Accident, transport, railway
    vehicle occupant
   while boarding or alighting V81.4
  transport vehicle after collision — *see*
   Accident, transport, by type of
   vehicle, collision
  tree W14
  vehicle (in motion) NEC — *see also*
   Accident, transport V89.9
   motor NEC — *see also* Accident,
    transport, occupant, by type of
    vehicle V87.8
   stationary W17.89
    while boarding or alighting — *see*
     Accident, transport, by type of
     vehicle, while boarding or
     alighting
  viaduct W13.8
  wall W13.8
  watercraft — *see also* Drowning, due to,
   fall overboard
   with hitting bottom or object V94.0
  well W17.0
  wheelchair, non-moving W05.0
   powered — *see* Accident, transport,
    pedestrian, conveyance occupant,
    specified type NEC
  window W13.4
 in, on
  aircraft NEC V97.0
   with accident to aircraft V97.0
   while boarding or alighting V97.1
  bathtub (empty) W18.2

Fall, falling (accidental) - *continued*
 in, on - *continued*
  bathtub (empty) - *continued*
   filled W16.212
    causing drowning W16.211
  escalator W10.0
  incline W10.2
  ladder W11
  machine, machinery — *see* Contact, with,
   by type of machine
  object, edged, pointed or sharp (with
   cut) — *see* Fall, by type
  playground equipment W09.8
   jungle gym W09.2
   slide W09.0
   swing W09.1
  ramp W10.2
  scaffolding W12
  shower W18.2
   causing drowning W16.211
  staircase, stairs, steps W10.9
   curb W10.1
   due to ice or snow W00.1
   escalator W10.0
   incline W10.2
   specified NEC W10.8
  streetcar (without antecedent
   collision) V82.5
   with antecedent collision — *see*
    Accident, transport, streetcar
    occupant
   while boarding or alighting V82.4
  train (without antecedent collision) V81.5
   with antecedent collision — *see*
    Accident, transport, railway vehicle
    occupant
   during derailment (without antecedent
    collision) V81.7
   with antecedent collision — *see*
    Accident, transport, railway
    vehicle occupant
   while boarding or alighting V81.4
  transport vehicle after collision — *see*
   Accident, transport, by type of
   vehicle, collision
  watercraft V93.39
   due to
    accident to craft V91.29
     powered craft V91.23
      ferry boat V91.21
      fishing boat V91.22
      jetskis V91.23
      liner V91.21
      merchant ship V91.20
      passenger ship V91.21
     unpowered craft
      canoe V91.25
      inflatable V91.26
      kayak V91.25
      sailboat V91.24
    powered craft V93.33
     ferry boat V93.31
     fishing boat V93.32
     jetskis V93.33
     liner V93.31
     merchant ship V93.30
     passenger ship V93.31
    unpowered craft V93.38
     canoe V93.35
     inflatable V93.36
     kayak V93.35
     sailboat V93.34
     surf-board V93.38
     windsurfer V93.38
 into
  cavity W17.2
  dock W17.4
  fire — *see* Exposure, fire, by type
  haystack W17.89
  hole W17.2
  lake — *see* Fall, into, water
  manhole W17.1
  moving part of machinery — *see* Contact,
   with, by type of machine
  ocean — *see* Fall, into, water

Fall, falling (accidental) - *continued*
 into - *continued*
  opening in surface NEC W17.89
  pit W17.2
  pond — *see* Fall, into, water
  quarry W17.89
  river — *see* Fall, into, water
  shaft W17.89
  storm drain W17.1
  stream — *see* Fall, into, water
  swimming pool — *see also* Fall, into,
   water, in, swimming pool
   empty W17.3
  tank W17.89
  water W16.42
   causing drowning W16.41
   from watercraft — *see* Drowning, due
    to, fall overboard
   hitting diving board W21.4
   in
    bathtub W16.212
     causing drowning W16.211
    bucket W16.222
     causing drowning W16.221
    natural body of water W16.112
     causing drowning W16.111
     striking
      bottom W16.122
       causing drowning W16.121
      side W16.132
       causing drowning W16.131
    specified water NEC W16.312
     causing drowning W16.311
     striking
      bottom W16.322
       causing drowning W16.321
      wall W16.332
       causing drowning W16.331
    swimming pool W16.012
     causing drowning W16.011
     striking
      bottom W16.022
       causing drowning W16.021
      wall W16.032
       causing drowning W16.031
    utility bucket W16.222
     causing drowning W16.221
   well W17.0
 involving
  bed W06
  chair W07
  furniture NEC W08
  glass — *see* Fall, by type
  playground equipment W09.8
   jungle gym W09.2
   slide W09.0
   swing W09.1
  roller blades — *see* Accident, transport,
   pedestrian, conveyance
  skateboard (s) — *see* Accident, transport,
   pedestrian, conveyance
  skates (ice) (in line) (roller) — *see*
   Accident, transport, pedestrian,
   conveyance
  skis — *see* Accident, transport, pedestrian,
   conveyance
  table W08
  wheelchair, non-moving W05.0
   powered — *see* Accident, transport,
    pedestrian, conveyance, specified
    type NEC
 object — *see* Struck by, object, falling
 off
  toilet W18.11
   with subsequent striking against
    object W18.12
 on same level W18.30
  due to
   specified NEC W18.39
   stepping on an object W18.31
 out of
  bed W06
  building NEC W13.8
  chair W07
  furniture NEC W08

Fall, falling (accidental) - *continued*
  out of - *continued*
    wheelchair, non-moving W05.0
      powered — *see* Accident, transport, pedestrian, conveyance, specified type NEC
    window W13.4
  over
    animal W01.0
    cliff W15
    embankment W17.81
    small object W01.0
  rock W20.8
  same level W18.30
    from
      being crushed, pushed, or stepped on by a crowd or human stampede W52
      collision, pushing, shoving, by or with other person W03
      slipping, stumbling, tripping W01.0
    involving ice or snow W00.0
      involving skates (ice) (roller) , skateboard, skis — *see* Accident, transport, pedestrian, conveyance
  snowslide (avalanche) — *see* Landslide
  stone W20.8
  structure W20.1
    burning (uncontrolled fire) X00.3
  through
    bridge W13.1
    floor W13.3
    roof W13.2
    wall W13.8
    window W13.4
  timber W20.8
  tree (caused by lightning) W20.8
  while being carried or supported by other person (s) W04
Fallen on by
  animal (not being ridden) NEC W55.89
Felo-de-se — *see* Suicide
Fight (hand) (fists) (foot) — *see* Assault, fight
Fire (accidental) — *see* Exposure, fire
Firearm discharge — *see* Discharge, firearm
Fireball effects from nuclear explosion in war operations — *see* War operations, nuclear weapons
Fireworks (explosion) W39
Flash burns from explosion — *see* Explosion
Flood (any injury) (caused by) X38
  collapse of man-made structure causing earth movement X36.0
  tidal wave — *see* Forces of nature, tidal wave
Food (any type) in
  air passages (with asphyxia, obstruction, or suffocation) — *see* categories T17 and T18
  alimentary tract causing asphyxia (due to compression of trachea) — *see* categories T17 and T18
Forces of nature X39.8
  avalanche X36.1
    causing transport accident — *see* Accident, transport, by type of vehicle
  blizzard X37.2
  cataclysmic storm X37.9
    with flood X38
    blizzard X37.2
    cloudburst X37.8
    cyclone X37.1
    dust storm X37.3
    hurricane X37.0
    specified storm NEC X37.8
    storm surge X37.0
    tornado X37.1
    twister X37.1
    typhoon X37.0
  cloudburst X37.8
  cold (natural) X31
  cyclone X37.1
  dam collapse causing earth movement X36.0
  dust storm X37.3
  earth movement X36.1
    earthquake X34

Forces of nature - *continued*
  earth movement - *continued*
    caused by dam or structure collapse X36.0
  earthquake X34
  flood (caused by) X38
    dam collapse X36.0
    tidal wave — *see* Forces of nature, tidal wave
  heat (natural) X30
  hurricane X37.0
  landslide X36.1
    causing transport accident — *see* Accident, transport, by type of vehicle
  lightning — *see* subcategory T75.0
    causing fire — *see* Exposure, fire
  mudslide X36.1
    causing transport accident — *see* Accident, transport, by type of vehicle
  radiation (natural) X39.08
    radon X39.01
  radon X39.01
  specified force NEC X39.8
  storm surge X37.0
  structure collapse causing earth movement X36.0
  sunlight X32
  tidal wave X37.41
    due to
      earthquake X37.41
      landslide X37.43
      storm X37.42
      volcanic eruption X37.41
  tornado X37.1
  tsunami X37.41
  twister X37.1
  typhoon X37.0
  volcanic eruption X35
Foreign body
  aspiration — *see* Index to Diseases and Injuries, Foreign body, respiratory tract
  embedded in skin W45
  entering through skin W45.8
    can lid W26.8
    nail W45.0
    paper W26.2
    specified NEC W45.8
    splinter W45.8
Forest fire (exposure to) — *see* Exposure, fire, uncontrolled, not in building
Found injured X58
  from exposure (to) — *see* Exposure
  on
    highway, road (way) , street V89.9
    railway right of way V81.9
Fracture (circumstances unknown or unspecified) X58
  due to specified cause NEC X58
Freezing — *see* Exposure, cold
Frostbite X31
  due to man-made conditions — *see* Exposure, cold, man-made
Frozen — *see* Exposure, cold

G

Gored by bull W55.22
Gunshot wound W34.00

H

Hailstones, injured by X39.8
Hanged herself or himself — *see* Hanging, self-inflicted
Hanging (accidental) (*see also* category T71)
  legal execution — *see* Legal, intervention, specified means NEC
Heat (effects of) (excessive) X30
  due to
    man-made conditions W92
      on board watercraft V93.29
        fishing boat V93.22
        merchant ship V93.20
        passenger ship V93.21
        sailboat V93.24
        specified powered craft NEC V93.23
    weather (conditions) X30
  from
    electric heating apparatus causing burning X16

Heat (effects of) (excessive) - *continued*
  from - *continued*
    nuclear explosion in war operations — *see* War operations, nuclear weapons
  inappropriate in local application or packing in medical or surgical procedure Y63.5
Hemorrhage
  delayed following medical or surgical treatment without mention of misadventure — *see* Index to Diseases and Injuries, Complication(s)
  during medical or surgical treatment as misadventure — *see* Index to Diseases and Injuries, Complication(s)
High
  altitude (effects) - — *see* Air, pressure, low
  level of radioactivity, effects — *see* Radiation
  pressure (effects) - — *see* Air, pressure, high
  temperature, effects — *see* Heat
Hit, hitting (accidental) by — *see* Struck by
Hitting against — *see* Striking against
Homicide (attempt) (justifiable) — *see* Assault
Hot
  place, effects — *see also* Heat
  weather, effects X30
House fire (uncontrolled) — *see* Exposure, fire, uncontrolled, building
Humidity, causing problem X39.8
Hunger X58
Hurricane (any injury) X37.0
Hypobarism, hypobaropathy - — *see* Air, pressure, low

I

Ictus
  caloris — *see also* Heat
  solaris X30
Ignition (accidental) — *see also* Exposure, fire X08.8
  anesthetic gas in operating room W40.1
  apparel X06.2
    from highly flammable material X04
    nightwear X05
  bed linen (sheets) (spreads) (pillows) (mattress) — *see* Exposure, fire, uncontrolled, building, bed
  benzine X04
  clothes, clothing NEC (from controlled fire) X06.2
    from
      highly flammable material X04
  ether X04
    in operating room W40.1
  explosive material — *see* Explosion
  gasoline X04
  jewelry (plastic) (any) X06.0
  kerosene X04
  material
    explosive — *see* Explosion
    highly flammable with secondary explosion X04
  nightwear X05
  paraffin X04
  petrol X04
Immersion (accidental) — *see also* Drowning
  hand or foot due to cold (excessive) X31
Implantation of quills of porcupine W55.89
Inanition (from) (hunger) X58
  thirst X58
Inappropriate operation performed
  correct operation on wrong side or body part (wrong side) (wrong site) Y65.53
  operation intended for another patient done on wrong patient Y65.52
  wrong operation performed on correct patient Y65.51
Inattention after, at birth (homicidal intent) (infanticidal intent) X58
Incident, adverse
  device
    anesthesiology Y70.8
      accessory Y70.2
      diagnostic Y70.0
      miscellaneous Y70.8

Incident, adverse - *continued*
  device - *continued*
    anesthesiology - *continued*
      monitoring Y70.0
      prosthetic Y70.2
      rehabilitative Y70.1
      surgical Y70.3
      therapeutic Y70.1
    cardiovascular Y71.8
      accessory Y71.2
      diagnostic Y71.0
      miscellaneous Y71.8
      monitoring Y71.0
      prosthetic Y71.2
      rehabilitative Y71.1
      surgical Y71.3
      therapeutic Y71.1
    gastroenterology Y73.8
      accessory Y73.2
      diagnostic Y73.0
      miscellaneous Y73.8
      monitoring Y73.0
      prosthetic Y73.2
      rehabilitative Y73.1
      surgical Y73.3
      therapeutic Y73.1
    general
      hospital Y74.8
        accessory Y74.2
        diagnostic Y74.0
        miscellaneous Y74.8
        monitoring Y74.0
        prosthetic Y74.2
        rehabilitative Y74.1
        surgical Y74.3
        therapeutic Y74.1
      surgical Y81.8
        accessory Y81.2
        diagnostic Y81.0
        miscellaneous Y81.8
        monitoring Y81.0
        prosthetic Y81.2
        rehabilitative Y81.1
        surgical Y81.3
        therapeutic Y81.1
    gynecological Y76.8
      accessory Y76.2
      diagnostic Y76.0
      miscellaneous Y76.8
      monitoring Y76.0
      prosthetic Y76.2
      rehabilitative Y76.1
      surgical Y76.3
      therapeutic Y76.1
    medical Y82.9
      specified type NEC Y82.8
    neurological Y75.8
      accessory Y75.2
      diagnostic Y75.0
      miscellaneous Y75.8
      monitoring Y75.0
      prosthetic Y75.2
      rehabilitative Y75.1
      surgical Y75.3
      therapeutic Y75.1
    obstetrical Y76.8
      accessory Y76.2
      diagnostic Y76.0
      miscellaneous Y76.8
      monitoring Y76.0
      prosthetic Y76.2
      rehabilitative Y76.1
      surgical Y76.3
      therapeutic Y76.1
    ophthalmic Y77.8
      accessory Y77.2
      diagnostic Y77.0
      miscellaneous Y77.8
      monitoring Y77.0
      prosthetic Y77.2
      rehabilitative Y77.1
      surgical Y77.3
      therapeutic Y77.1
    orthopedic Y79.8
      accessory Y79.2

Incident, adverse - *continued*
  device - *continued*
    orthopedic - *continued*
      diagnostic Y79.0
      miscellaneous Y79.8
      monitoring Y79.0
      prosthetic Y79.2
      rehabilitative Y79.1
      surgical Y79.3
      therapeutic Y79.1
    otorhinolaryngological Y72.8
      accessory Y72.2
      diagnostic Y72.0
      miscellaneous Y72.8
      monitoring Y72.0
      prosthetic Y72.2
      rehabilitative Y72.1
      surgical Y72.3
      therapeutic Y72.1
    personal use Y74.8
      accessory Y74.2
      diagnostic Y74.0
      miscellaneous Y74.8
      monitoring Y74.0
      prosthetic Y74.2
      rehabilitative Y74.1
      surgical Y74.3
      therapeutic Y74.1
    physical medicine Y80.8
      accessory Y80.2
      diagnostic Y80.0
      miscellaneous Y80.8
      monitoring Y80.0
      prosthetic Y80.2
      rehabilitative Y80.1
      surgical Y80.3
      therapeutic Y80.1
    plastic surgical Y81.8
      accessory Y81.2
      diagnostic Y81.0
      miscellaneous Y81.8
      monitoring Y81.0
      prosthetic Y81.2
      rehabilitative Y81.1
      surgical Y81.3
      therapeutic Y81.1
    radiological Y78.8
      accessory Y78.2
      diagnostic Y78.0
      miscellaneous Y78.8
      monitoring Y78.0
      prosthetic Y78.2
      rehabilitative Y78.1
      surgical Y78.3
      therapeutic Y78.1
    urology Y73.8
      accessory Y73.2
      diagnostic Y73.0
      miscellaneous Y73.8
      monitoring Y73.0
      prosthetic Y73.2
      rehabilitative Y73.1
      surgical Y73.3
      therapeutic Y73.1
Incineration (accidental) — *see* Exposure, fire
Infanticide — *see* Assault
Infrasound waves (causing injury) W49.9
Ingestion
  foreign body (causing injury) (with obstruction) — *see* Foreign body, alimentary canal
  poisonous
    plant (s) X58
    substance NEC — *see* Table of Drugs and Chemicals
Inhalation
  excessively cold substance, man-made — *see* Exposure, cold, man-made
  food (any type) (into respiratory tract) (with asphyxia, obstruction respiratory tract, suffocation) — *see* categories T17 and T18
  foreign body — *see* Foreign body, aspiration

Inhalation - *continued*
  gastric contents (with asphyxia, obstruction respiratory passage, suffocation) T17.81-
  hot air or gases X14.0
  liquid air, hydrogen, nitrogen W93.12
    suicide (attempt) X83.2
  steam X13.0
    assault X98.0
    stated as undetermined whether accidental or intentional Y27.0
    suicide (attempt) X77.0
  toxic gas — *see* Table of Drugs and Chemicals
  vomitus (with asphyxia, obstruction respiratory passage, suffocation) T17.81-
Injury, injured (accidental (ly)) NOS X58
  by, caused by, from
    assault — *see* Assault
    law-enforcing agent, police, in course of legal intervention — *see* Legal intervention
    suicide (attempt) X83.8
  due to, in
    civil insurrection — *see* War operations
    fight — *see also* Assault, fight Y04.0
    war operations — *see* War operations
  homicide — *see also* Assault Y09
  inflicted (by)
    in course of arrest (attempted) , suppression of disturbance, maintenance of order, by law-enforcing agents — *see* Legal intervention
    other person
      stated as
        accidental X58
        intentional, homicide (attempt) — *see* Assault
        undetermined whether accidental or intentional Y33
  purposely (inflicted) by other person (s) — *see* Assault
  self-inflicted X83.8
    stated as accidental X58
  specified cause NEC X58
  undetermined whether accidental or intentional Y33
Insolation, effects X30
Insufficient nourishment X58
Interruption of respiration (by)
  food (lodged in esophagus) — *see* categories T17 and T18
  vomitus (lodged in esophagus) T17.81-
Intervention, legal — *see* Legal intervention
Intoxication
  drug — *see* Table of Drugs and Chemicals
  poison — *see* Table of Drugs and Chemicals

J

Jammed (accidentally)
  between objects (moving) (stationary and moving) W23.0
    stationary W23.1
Jumped, jumping
  before moving object NEC X81.8
    motor vehicle X81.0
    subway train X81.1
    train X81.1
    undetermined whether accidental or intentional Y31
  from
    boat (into water) voluntarily, without accident (to or on boat) W16.712
      with
        accident to or on boat — *see* Accident, watercraft
        drowning or submersion W16.711
          suicide (attempt) X71.3
        striking bottom W16.722
          causing drowning W16.721
    building — *see also* Jumped, from, high place W13.9
      burning (uncontrolled fire) X00.5
    high place NEC W17.89

Jumped, jumping - *continued*
  from - *continued*
    high place NEC - *continued*
      suicide (attempt) X80
      undetermined whether accidental or
        intentional Y30
      structure — *see also* Jumped, from, high
        place W13.9
        burning (uncontrolled fire) X00.5
    into water W16.92
    causing drowning W16.91
    from, off watercraft — *see* Jumped, from,
      boat
    in
      natural body W16.612
        causing drowning W16.611
        striking bottom W16.622
          causing drowning W16.621
      specified place NEC W16.812
        causing drowning W16.811
        striking
          bottom W16.822
            causing drowning W16.821
          wall W16.832
            causing drowning W16.831
      swimming pool W16.512
        causing drowning W16.511
        striking
          bottom W16.522
            causing drowning W16.521
          wall W16.532
            causing drowning W16.531
  suicide (attempt) X71.3

K

Kicked by
  animal NEC W55.82
  person (s) (accidentally) W50.1
    with intent to injure or kill Y04.0
  as, or caused by, a crowd or human
    stampede (with fall) W52
  assault Y04.0
  homicide (attempt) Y04.0
  in
    fight Y04.0
    legal intervention
      injuring
        bystander Y35.812
        law enforcement personnel Y35.811
        suspect Y35.813
        unspecified person Y35.819

Kicking
  against
    object W22.8
      sports equipment W21.9
      stationary W22.09
        sports equipment W21.89
    person — *see* Striking against, person
  sports equipment W21.9
  carpet stretcher with knee X50.3
Killed, killing (accidentally) NOS — *see also*
  Injury X58
  in
    action — *see* War operations
    brawl, fight (hand) (fists) (foot) Y04.0
      by weapon — *see also* Assault
        cutting, piercing — *see* Assault,
          cutting or piercing instrument
        firearm — *see* Discharge, firearm, by
          type, homicide
  self
    stated as
      accident NOS X58
      suicide — *see* Suicide
      undetermined whether accidental or
        intentional Y33
Kneeling (prolonged) (static) X50.1
Knocked down (accidentally) (by) NOS X58
  animal (not being ridden) NEC — *see also*
    Struck by, by type of animal
  crowd or human stampede W52
  person W51
    in brawl, fight Y04.0
  transport vehicle NEC — *see also* Accident,
    transport V09.9

L

Laceration NEC — *see* Injury
Lack of
  care (helpless person) (infant)
    (newborn) X58
  food except as result of abandonment or
    neglect X58
    due to abandonment or neglect X58
  water except as result of transport
    accident X58
    due to transport accident — *see* Accident,
      transport, by type
  helpless person, infant, newborn X58
Landslide (falling on transport vehicle)
  X36.1
  caused by collapse of man-made
    structure X36.0
Late effect — *see* Sequelae
Legal
  execution (any method) — *see* Legal,
    intervention
  intervention (by)
    baton — *see* Legal, intervention, blunt
      object, baton
    bayonet — *see* Legal, intervention, sharp
      object, bayonet
    blow — *see* Legal, intervention,
      manhandling
    blunt object
      baton
        injuring
          bystander Y35.312
          law enforcement personnel Y35.311
          suspect Y35.313
          unspecified person Y35.319
      injuring
        bystander Y35.302
        law enforcement personnel Y35.301
        suspect Y35.303
        unspecified person Y35.309
      specified NEC
        injuring
          bystander Y35.392
          law enforcement personnel Y35.391
          suspect Y35.393
          unspecified person Y35.399
      stave
        injuring
          bystander Y35.392
          law enforcement personnel Y35.391
          suspect Y35.393
          unspecified person Y35.399
    bomb — *see* Legal, intervention, explosive
    conducted energy device
      injuring
        bystander Y35.832
        law enforcement personnel Y35.831
        suspect Y35.833
        unspecified person Y35.839
    cutting or piercing instrument — *see*
      Legal, intervention, sharp object
    dynamite — *see* Legal, intervention,
      explosive, dynamite
    electroshock device (taser)
      injuring
        bystander Y35.832
        law enforcement personnel Y35.831
        suspect Y35.833
        unspecified person Y35.839
    explosive (s)
      dynamite
        injuring
          bystander Y35.112
          law enforcement personnel Y35.111
          suspect Y35.113
          unspecified person Y35.119
      grenade
        injuring
          bystander Y35.192
          law enforcement personnel Y35.191
          suspect Y35.193
          unspecified person Y35.199
      injuring
        bystander Y35.102
        law enforcement personnel Y35.101

Legal - *continued*
  intervention (by) - *continued*
    explosive (s) - *continued*
      injuring - *continued*
        suspect Y35.103
        unspecified person Y35.109
      mortar bomb
        injuring
          bystander Y35.192
          law enforcement personnel Y35.191
          suspect Y35.193
          unspecified person Y35.199
      shell
        injuring
          bystander Y35.122
          law enforcement personnel Y35.121
          suspect Y35.123
          unspecified person Y35.129
      specified NEC
        injuring
          bystander Y35.192
          law enforcement personnel Y35.191
          suspect Y35.193
          unspecified person Y35.199
    firearm (s) (discharge)
      handgun
        injuring
          bystander Y35.022
          law enforcement personnel Y35.021
          suspect Y35.023
          unspecified person Y35.029
      injuring
        bystander Y35.002
        law enforcement personnel Y35.001
        suspect Y35.003
        unspecified person Y35.009
      machine gun
        injuring
          bystander Y35.012
          law enforcement personnel Y35.011
          suspect Y35.013
          unspecified person Y35.019
      rifle pellet
        injuring
          bystander Y35.032
          law enforcement personnel Y35.031
          suspect Y35.033
          unspecified person Y35.039
      rubber bullet
        injuring
          bystander Y35.042
          law enforcement personnel Y35.041
          suspect Y35.043
          unspecified person Y35.049
      shotgun — *see* Legal, intervention,
        firearm, specified NEC
      specified NEC
        injuring
          bystander Y35.092
          law enforcement personnel Y35.091
          suspect Y35.093
          unspecified person Y35.099
    gas (asphyxiation) (poisoning)
      injuring
        bystander Y35.202
        law enforcement personnel Y35.201
        suspect Y35.203
        unspecified person Y35.209
      specified NEC
        injuring
          bystander Y35.292
          law enforcement personnel Y35.291
          suspect Y35.293
          unspecified person Y35.299
      tear gas
        injuring
          bystander Y35.212
          law enforcement personnel Y35.211
          suspect Y35.213
          unspecified person Y35.219
    grenade — *see* Legal, intervention,
      explosive, grenade
    injuring
      bystander Y35.92
      law enforcement personnel Y35.91

LEGAL - MILITARY OPERATIONS

Legal - *continued*
intervention (by) - *continued*
injuring - *continued*
suspect Y35.93
unspecified person Y35.99
late effect (of) — *see* with 7th character
S Y35
manhandling
injuring
bystander Y35.812
law enforcement personnel Y35.811
suspect Y35.813
unspecified person Y35.819
sequelae (of) — *see* with 7th character
S Y35
sharp objects
bayonet
injuring
bystander Y35.412
law enforcement personnel Y35.411
suspect Y35.413
unspecified person Y35.419
injuring
bystander Y35.402
law enforcement personnel Y35.401
suspect Y35.403
unspecified person Y35.409
specified NEC
injuring
bystander Y35.492
law enforcement personnel Y35.491
suspect Y35.493
unspecified person Y35.499
specified means NEC
injuring
bystander Y35.892
law enforcement personnel Y35.891
suspect Y35.893
stabbing — *see* Legal, intervention, sharp
object
stave — *see* Legal, intervention, blunt
object, stave
stun gun
injuring
bystander Y35.832
law enforcement personnel Y35.831
suspect Y35.833
unspecified person Y35.839
taser
injuring
bystander Y35.832
law enforcement personnel Y35.831
suspect Y35.833
unspecified person Y35.839
tear gas — *see* Legal, intervention, gas,
tear gas
truncheon — *see* Legal, intervention, blunt
object, stave
Lifting — *see also* Overexertion
heavy objects X50.0
weights X50.0
Lightning (shock) (stroke) (struck by) — *see*
subcategory T75.0
causing fire — *see* Exposure, fire
Loss of control (transport vehicle)
NEC — *see* Accident, transport
Lost at sea NOS — *see* Drowning, due to, fall
overboard
Low
pressure (effects) - — *see* Air, pressure, low
temperature (effects) — *see* Exposure, cold
Lying before train, vehicle or other moving
object X81.8
subway train X81.1
train X81.1
undetermined whether accidental or
intentional Y31
Lynching — *see* Assault

M

Malfunction (mechanism or component) (of)
firearm W34.10
airgun W34.110
BB gun W34.110
gas, air or spring-operated gun
NEC W34.118

Malfunction (mechanism or component) (of)
- *continued*
firearm - *continued*
handgun W32.1
hunting rifle W33.12
larger firearm W33.10
specified NEC W33.19
machine gun W33.13
paintball gun W34.111
pellet gun W34.110
shotgun W33.11
specified NEC W34.19
Very pistol [flare] W34.19
handgun — *see* Malfunction, firearm,
handgun
Maltreatment — *see* Perpetrator
Mangled (accidentally) NOS X58
Manhandling (in brawl, fight) Y04.0
legal intervention — *see* Legal, intervention,
manhandling
Manslaughter (nonaccidental) — *see* Assault
Mauled by animal NEC W55.89
Medical procedure, complication of (delayed
or as an abnormal reaction without
mention of misadventure) — *see*
Complication of or following, by specified
type of procedure
due to or as a result of misadventure — *see*
Misadventure
Melting (due to fire) — *see also* Exposure,
fire
apparel NEC X06.3
clothes, clothing NEC X06.3
nightwear X05
fittings or furniture (burning building)
(uncontrolled fire) X00.8
nightwear X05
plastic jewelry X06.1
Mental cruelty X58
Military operations (injuries to military and
civilians occuring during peacetime on
military property and during routine
military exercises and operations) (by)
(from) (involving) Y37.90-
air blast Y37.20-
aircraft
destruction — *see* Military operations,
destruction of aircraft
airway restriction — *see* Military operations,
restriction of airways
asphyxiation — *see* Military operations,
restriction of airways
biological weapons Y37.6X-
blast Y37.20-
blast fragments Y37.20-
blast wave Y37.20-
blast wind Y37.20-
bomb Y37.20-
dirty Y37.50-
gasoline Y37.31-
incendiary Y37.31-
petrol Y37.31-
bullet Y37.43-
incendiary Y37.32-
rubber Y37.41-
chemical weapons Y37.7X-
combat
hand to hand (unarmed) combat Y37.44-
using blunt or piercing object Y37.45-
conflagration — *see* Military operations, fire
conventional warfare NEC Y37.49-
depth-charge Y37.01-
destruction of aircraft Y37.10-
due to
air to air missile Y37.11-
collision with other aircraft Y37.12-
detonation (accidental) of onboard
munitions and explosives Y37.14-
enemy fire or explosives Y37.11-
explosive placed on aircraft Y37.11-
onboard fire Y37.13-
rocket propelled grenade [RPG] Y37.11-
small arms fire Y37.11-
surface to air missile Y37.11-
specified NEC Y37.19-

Military operations (injuries to military and
civilians occuring during peacetime on
military property and during routine
military exercises and operations) (by)
(from) (involving) - *continued*
detonation (accidental) of
onboard marine weapons Y37.05-
own munitions or munitions launch
device Y37.24-
dirty bomb Y37.50-
explosion (of) Y37.20-
aerial bomb Y37.21-
bomb NOS — *see also* Military
operations, bomb(s) Y37.20-
own munitions or munitions launch device
(accidental) Y37.24-
fragments Y37.20-
grenade Y37.29-
guided missile Y37.22-
improvised explosive device [IED]
(person-borne) (roadside) (vehicle-
borne) Y37.23-
land mine Y37.29-
marine mine (at sea) (in harbor) Y37.02-
marine weapon Y37.00-
specified NEC Y37.09-
sea-based artillery shell Y37.03-
specified NEC Y37.29-
torpedo Y37.04-
fire Y37.30-
specified NEC Y37.39-
firearms
discharge Y37.43-
pellets Y37.42-
flamethrower Y37.33-
fragments (from) (of)
improvised explosive device [IED]
(person-borne) (roadside) (vehicle-
borne) Y37.26-
munitions Y37.25-
specified NEC Y37.29-
weapons Y37.27-
friendly fire Y37.92-
hand to hand (unarmed) combat Y37.44-
hot substances — *see* Military operations,
fire
incendiary bullet Y37.32-
nuclear weapon (effects of) Y37.50-
acute radiation exposure Y37.54-
blast pressure Y37.51-
direct blast Y37.51-
direct heat Y37.53-
fallout exposure Y37.54-
fireball Y37.53-
indirect blast (struck or crushed by blast
debris) (being thrown by
blast) Y37.52-
ionizing radiation (immediate
exposure) Y37.54-
nuclear radiation Y37.54-
radiation
ionizing (immediate exposure) Y37.54-
nuclear Y37.54-
thermal Y37.53-
specified NEC Y37.59-
secondary effects Y37.54-
thermal radiation Y37.53-
restriction of air (airway)
intentional Y37.46-
unintentional Y37.47-
rubber bullets Y37.41-
shrapnel NOS Y37.29-
suffocation — *see* Military operations,
restriction of airways
unconventional warfare NEC Y37.7X-
underwater blast NOS Y37.00-
warfare
conventional NEC Y37.49-
unconventional NEC Y37.7X-
weapons
biological weapons Y37.6X-
chemical Y37.7X-
nuclear (effects of) Y37.50-
acute radiation exposure Y37.54-
blast pressure Y37.51-

Military operations (injuries to military and civilians occuring during peacetime on military property and during routine military exercises and operations) (by) (from) (involving) - *continued*
 weapons - *continued*
  nuclear (effects of) - *continued*
   direct blast Y37.51-
   direct heat Y37.53-
   fallout exposure Y37.54-
   fireball Y37.53-
   indirect blast (struck or crushed by blast debris) (being thrown by blast) Y37.52-
   radiation
    ionizing (immediate exposure) Y37.54-
     nuclear Y37.54-
     thermal Y37.53-
    secondary effects Y37.54-
    specified NEC Y37.59-
  of mass destruction [WMD] Y37.91-
  weapon of mass destruction [WMD] Y37.91-
Misadventure (s) to patient (s) during surgical or medical care Y69
 contaminated medical or biological substance (blood, drug, fluid) Y64.9
  administered (by) NEC Y64.9
   immunization Y64.1
   infusion Y64.0
   injection Y64.1
   specified means NEC Y64.8
   transfusion Y64.0
   vaccination Y64.1
 excessive amount of blood or other fluid during transfusion or infusion Y63.0
 failure
  in dosage Y63.9
   electroshock therapy Y63.4
   inappropriate temperature (too hot or too cold) in local application and packing Y63.5
   infusion
    excessive amount of fluid Y63.0
    incorrect dilution of fluid Y63.1
   insulin-shock therapy Y63.4
   nonadministration of necessary drug or biological substance Y63.6
   overdose — *see* Table of Drugs and Chemicals
    radiation, in therapy Y63.2
   radiation
    overdose Y63.2
   specified procedure NEC Y63.8
   transfusion
    excessive amount of blood Y63.0
  mechanical, of instrument or apparatus (any) (during any procedure) Y65.8
  sterile precautions (during procedure) Y62.9
   aspiration of fluid or tissue (by puncture or catheterization, except heart) Y62.6
   biopsy (except needle aspiration) Y62.8
    needle (aspirating) Y62.6
   blood sampling Y62.6
   catheterization Y62.6
    heart Y62.5
   dialysis (kidney) Y62.2
   endoscopic examination Y62.4
   enema Y62.8
   immunization Y62.3
   infusion Y62.1
   injection Y62.3
   needle biopsy Y62.6
   paracentesis (abdominal) (thoracic) Y62.6
   perfusion Y62.2
   puncture (lumbar) Y62.6
   removal of catheter or packing Y62.8
   specified procedure NEC Y62.8
   surgical operation Y62.0
   transfusion Y62.1
   vaccination Y62.3

Misadventure (s) to patient (s) during surgical or medical care - *continued*
 failure - *continued*
  suture or ligature during surgical procedure Y65.2
  to introduce or to remove tube or instrument — *see* Failure, to
  hemorrhage — *see* Index to Diseases and Injuries, Complication(s)
  inadvertent exposure of patient to radiation Y63.3
  inappropriate
   operation performed — *see* Inappropriate operation performed
   temperature (too hot or too cold) in local application or packing Y63.5
  infusion — *see also* Misadventure, by type, infusion Y69
   excessive amount of fluid Y63.0
   incorrect dilution of fluid Y63.1
   wrong fluid Y65.1
  mismatched blood in transfusion Y65.0
  nonadministration of necessary drug or biological substance Y63.6
  overdose — *see* Table of Drugs and Chemicals
   radiation (in therapy) Y63.2
  perforation — *see* Index to Diseases and Injuries, Complication(s)
  performance of inappropriate operation — *see* Inappropriate operation performed
  puncture — *see* Index to Diseases and Injuries, Complication(s)
  specified type NEC Y65.8
   failure
    suture or ligature during surgical operation Y65.2
    to introduce or to remove tube or instrument — *see* Failure, to
   infusion of wrong fluid Y65.1
   performance of inappropriate operation — *see* Inappropriate operation performed
   transfusion of mismatched blood Y65.0
   wrong
    fluid in infusion Y65.1
    placement of endotracheal tube during anesthetic procedure Y65.3
  transfusion — *see* Misadventure, by type, transfusion
   excessive amount of blood Y63.0
   mismatched blood Y65.0
  wrong
   drug given in error — *see* Table of Drugs and Chemicals
   fluid in infusion Y65.1
   placement of endotracheal tube during anesthetic procedure Y65.3
Mismatched blood in transfusion Y65.0
Motion sickness T75.3
Mountain sickness W94.11
Mudslide (of cataclysmic nature) — *see* Landslide
Murder (attempt) — *see* Assault

N

Nail
 contact with W45.0
  gun W29.4
 embedded in skin W45.0
Neglect (criminal) (homicidal intent) X58
Noise (causing injury) (pollution) W42.9
 supersonic W42.0
Nonadministration (of)
 drug or biological substance (necessary) Y63.6
 surgical and medical care Y66
Nosocomial condition Y95

O

Object
 falling
  from, in, on, hitting
   machinery — *see* Contact, with, by type of machine
 set in motion by
  accidental explosion or rupture of pressure vessel W38

Object - *continued*
 set in motion by - *continued*
  firearm — *see* Discharge, firearm, by type
  machine (ry) — *see* Contact, with, by type of machine
Overdose (drug) — *see* Table of Drugs and Chemicals
 radiation Y63.2
Overexertion X50.9
 from
  prolonged static or awkward postures X50.1
  repetitive movements X50.3
  specified strenuous movements or postures NEC X50.9
  strenuous movement or load X50.0
Overexposure (accidental) (to)
 cold — *see also* Exposure, cold X31
  due to man-made conditions — *see* Exposure, cold, man-made
 heat — *see also* Heat X30
 radiation — *see* Radiation
 radioactivity W88.0
 sun (sunburn) X32
 weather NEC — *see* Forces of nature
 wind NEC — *see* Forces of nature
Overheated — *see* Heat
Overturning (accidental)
 machinery — *see* Contact, with, by type of machine
 transport vehicle NEC — *see also* Accident, transport V89.9
 watercraft (causing drowning, submersion) — *see also* Drowning, due to, accident to, watercraft, overturning
  causing injury except drowning or submersion — *see* Accident, watercraft, causing, injury NEC

P

Parachute descent (voluntary) (without accident to aircraft) V97.29
 due to accident to aircraft — *see* Accident, transport, aircraft
Pecked by bird W61.99
Perforation during medical or surgical treatment as misadventure — *see* Index to Diseases and Injuries, Complication(s)
Perpetrator, perpetration, of assault, maltreatment and neglect (by) Y07.9
 boyfriend Y07.03
 brother Y07.410
  stepbrother Y07.435
 coach Y07.53
 cousin
  female Y07.491
  male Y07.490
 daycare provider Y07.519
  at-home
   adult care Y07.512
   childcare Y07.510
  care center
   adult care Y07.513
   childcare Y07.511
 family member NEC Y07.499
 father Y07.11
  adoptive Y07.13
  foster Y07.420
  stepfather Y07.430
 foster father Y07.420
 foster mother Y07.421
 girl friend Y07.04
 healthcare provider Y07.529
  mental health Y07.521
  specified NEC Y07.528
 husband Y07.01
 instructor Y07.53
 mother Y07.12
  adoptive Y07.14
  foster Y07.421
  stepmother Y07.433
 multiple perpetrators Y07.6
 nonfamily member Y07.50
  specified NEC Y07.59
 nurse Y07.528
 occupational therapist Y07.528

PERPETRATOR, PERPETRATION, OF ASSAULT, MALTREATMENT AND NEGLECT - PLACE OF OCCURRENCE

Perpetrator, perpetration, of assault, maltreatment and neglect (by) - *continued*
  partner of parent
    female Y07.434
    male Y07.432
  physical therapist Y07.528
  sister Y07.411
  speech therapist Y07.528
  stepbrother Y07.435
  stepfather Y07.430
  stepmother Y07.433
  stepsister Y07.436
  teacher Y07.53
  wife Y07.02
Piercing — *see* Contact, with, by type of object or machine
Pinched
  between objects (moving) (stationary and moving) W23.0
    stationary W23.1
Pinned under machine (ry) — *see* Contact, with, by type of machine
Place of occurrence Y92.9
  abandoned house Y92.89
  airplane Y92.813
  airport Y92.520
  ambulatory health services establishment NEC Y92.538
  ambulatory surgery center Y92.530
  amusement park Y92.831
  apartment (co-op) — *see* Place of occurrence, residence, apartment
  assembly hall Y92.29
  bank Y92.510
  barn Y92.71
  baseball field Y92.320
  basketball court Y92.310
  beach Y92.832
  boarding house — *see* Place of occurrence, residence, boarding house
  boat Y92.814
  bowling alley Y92.39
  bridge Y92.89
  building under construction Y92.61
  bus Y92.811
    station Y92.521
  cafe Y92.511
  campsite Y92.833
  campus — *see* Place of occurrence, school
  canal Y92.89
  car Y92.810
  casino Y92.59
  children's home — *see* Place of occurrence, residence, institutional, orphanage
  church Y92.22
  cinema Y92.26
  clubhouse Y92.29
  coal pit Y92.64
  college (community) Y92.214
  condominium — *see* Place of occurrence, residence, apartment
  construction area — *see* Place of occurrence, industrial and construction area
  convalescent home — *see* Place of occurrence, residence, institutional, nursing home
  court-house Y92.240
  cricket ground Y92.328
  cultural building Y92.258
    art gallery Y92.250
    museum Y92.251
    music hall Y92.252
    opera house Y92.253
    specified NEC Y92.258
    theater Y92.254
  dancehall Y92.252
  day nursery Y92.210
  dentist office Y92.531
  derelict house Y92.89
  desert Y92.820
  dock NOS Y92.89
  dockyard Y92.62
  doctor's office Y92.531

Place of occurrence - *continued*
  dormitory — *see* Place of occurrence, residence, institutional, school dormitory
  dry dock Y92.62
  factory (building) (premises) Y92.63
  farm (land under cultivation) (outbuildings) Y92.79
    barn Y92.71
    chicken coop Y92.72
    field Y92.73
    hen house Y92.72
    house — *see* Place of occurrence, residence, house
    orchard Y92.74
    specified NEC Y92.79
  football field Y92.321
  forest Y92.821
  freeway Y92.411
  gallery Y92.250
  garage (commercial) Y92.59
    boarding house Y92.044
    military base Y92.135
    mobile home Y92.025
    nursing home Y92.124
    orphanage Y92.114
    private house Y92.015
    reform school Y92.155
  gas station Y92.524
  gasworks Y92.69
  golf course Y92.39
  gravel pit Y92.64
  grocery Y92.512
  gymnasium Y92.39
  handball court Y92.318
  harbor Y92.89
  harness racing course Y92.39
  healthcare provider office Y92.531
  highway (interstate) Y92.411
  hill Y92.828
  hockey rink Y92.330
  home — *see* Place of occurrence, residence
  hospice — *see* Place of occurrence, residence, institutional, nursing home
  hospital Y92.239
    cafeteria Y92.233
    corridor Y92.232
    operating room Y92.234
    patient
      bathroom Y92.231
      room Y92.230
    specified NEC Y92.238
  hotel Y92.59
  house — *see also* Place of occurrence, residence
    abandoned Y92.89
    under construction Y92.61
  industrial and construction area (yard) Y92.69
    building under construction Y92.61
    dock Y92.62
    dry dock Y92.62
    factory Y92.63
    gasworks Y92.69
    mine Y92.64
    oil rig Y92.65
    pit Y92.64
    power station Y92.69
    shipyard Y92.62
    specified NEC Y92.69
    tunnel under construction Y92.69
    workshop Y92.69
  kindergarten Y92.211
  lacrosse field Y92.328
  lake Y92.828
  library Y92.241
  mall Y92.59
  market Y92.512
  marsh Y92.828
  military
    base — *see* Place of occurrence, residence, institutional, military base
    training ground Y92.84
  mine Y92.64
  mosque Y92.22

Place of occurrence - *continued*
  motel Y92.59
  motorway (interstate) Y92.411
  mountain Y92.828
  movie-house Y92.26
  museum Y92.251
  music-hall Y92.252
  not applicable Y92.9
  nuclear power station Y92.69
  nursing home — *see* Place of occurrence, residence, institutional, nursing home
  office building Y92.59
  offshore installation Y92.65
  oil rig Y92.65
  old people's home — *see* Place of occurrence, residence, institutional, specified NEC
  opera-house Y92.253
  orphanage — *see* Place of occurrence, residence, institutional, orphanage
  outpatient surgery center Y92.530
  park (public) Y92.830
    amusement Y92.831
  parking garage Y92.89
    lot Y92.481
  pavement Y92.480
  physician office Y92.531
  polo field Y92.328
  pond Y92.828
  post office Y92.242
  power station Y92.69
  prairie Y92.828
  prison — *see* Place of occurrence, residence, institutional, prison
  public
    administration building Y92.248
      city hall Y92.243
      courthouse Y92.240
      library Y92.241
      post office Y92.242
      specified NEC Y92.248
    building NEC Y92.29
    hall Y92.29
    place NOS Y92.89
  race course Y92.39
  radio station Y92.59
  railway line (bridge) Y92.85
  ranch (outbuildings) — *see* Place of occurrence, farm
  recreation area Y92.838
    amusement park Y92.831
    beach Y92.832
    campsite Y92.833
    park (public) Y92.830
    seashore Y92.832
    specified NEC Y92.838
  religious institution Y92.22
  reform school - — *see* Place of occurrence, residence, institutional, reform school
  residence (non-institutional) (private) Y92.009
    apartment Y92.039
      bathroom Y92.031
      bedroom Y92.032
      kitchen Y92.030
      specified NEC Y92.038
    bathroom Y92.002
    bedroom Y92.003
    boarding house Y92.049
      bathroom Y92.041
      bedroom Y92.042
      driveway Y92.043
      garage Y92.044
      garden Y92.046
      kitchen Y92.040
      specified NEC Y92.048
      swimming pool Y92.045
      yard Y92.046
    dining room Y92.001
    garden Y92.007
    home Y92.009
    house, single family Y92.019
      bathroom Y92.012
      bedroom Y92.013
      dining room Y92.011

Poisoning (accidental) (by) — *see also* Table of Drugs and Chemicals
  by plant, thorns, spines, sharp leaves or other mechanisms NEC X58
  carbon monoxide
    generated by
      motor vehicle — *see* Accident, transport
      watercraft (in transit) (not in transit) V93.89
        ferry boat V93.81
        fishing boat V93.82
        jet skis V93.83
        liner V93.81
        merchant ship V93.80
        passenger ship V93.81
        powered craft NEC V93.83
  caused by injection of poisons into skin by plant thorns, spines, sharp leaves X58
  marine or sea plants (venomous) X58
  exhaust gas
    generated by
      motor vehicle — *see* Accident, transport
      watercraft (in transit) (not in transit) V93.89
        ferry boat V93.81
        fishing boat V93.82
        jet skis V93.83
        liner V93.81
        merchant ship V93.80
        passenger ship V93.81
        powered craft NEC V93.83
  fumes or smoke due to
    explosion — *see also* Explosion W40.9
    fire — *see* Exposure, fire
    ignition — *see* Ignition
  gas
    in legal intervention — *see* Legal, intervention, gas
    legal execution — *see* Legal, intervention, gas
    in war operations — *see* War operations
  legal
    execution — *see* Legal, intervention, gas
    intervention
      by gas — *see* Legal, intervention, gas
      other specified means — *see* Legal, intervention, specified means NEC

Powder burn (by) (from)
  airgun W34.110
  BB gun W34.110
  firearm NEC W34.19
  gas, air or spring-operated gun NEC W34.118
  handgun W32.1
  hunting rifle W33.12
  larger firearm W33.10
    specified NEC W33.19
  machine gun W33.13
  paintball gun W34.111
  pellet gun W34.110
  shotgun W33.11
  Very pistol [flare] W34.19

Premature cessation (of) surgical and medical care Y66
Privation (food) (water) X58
Procedure (operation)
  correct, on wrong side or body part (wrong side) (wrong site) Y65.53
  intended for another patient done on wrong patient Y65.52
  performed on patient not scheduled for surgery Y65.52
  performed on wrong patient Y65.52
  wrong, performed on correct patient Y65.51
Prolonged
  sitting in transport vehicle — *see* Travel, by type of vehicle
  stay in
    high altitude as cause of anoxia, barodontalgia, barotitis or hypoxia W94.11
    weightless environment X52
Pulling, excessive — *see also* Overexertion X50.9

Puncture, puncturing — *see also* Contact, with, by type of object or machine
  by
    plant thorns, spines, sharp leaves or other mechanisms NEC W60
  during medical or surgical treatment as misadventure — *see* Index to Diseases and Injuries, Complication(s)
Pushed, pushing (accidental) (injury in)
  by other person (s) (accidental) W51
    with fall W03
      due to ice or snow W00.0
    as, or caused by, a crowd or human stampede (with fall) W52
    before moving object NEC Y02.8
      motor vehicle Y02.0
      subway train Y02.1
      train Y02.1
    from
      high place NEC
        in accidental circumstances W17.89
        stated as
          intentional, homicide (attempt) Y01
          undetermined whether accidental or intentional Y30
      transport vehicle NEC — *see also* Accident, transport V89.9
        stated as
          intentional, homicide (attempt) Y08.89
  overexertion X50.9

R

Radiation (exposure to)
  arc lamps W89.0
  atomic power plant (malfunction) NEC W88.1
  complication of or abnormal reaction to medical radiotherapy Y84.2
  electromagnetic, ionizing W88.0
  gamma rays W88.1
  in
    war operations (from or following nuclear explosion) — *see* War operations
  inadvertent exposure of patient (receiving test or therapy) Y63.3
  infrared (heaters and lamps) W90.1
    excessive heat from W92
  ionized, ionizing (particles, artificially accelerated)
    radioisotopes W88.1
    specified NEC W88.8
    x-rays W88.0
  isotopes, radioactive — *see* Radiation, radioactive isotopes
  laser (s) W90.2
    in war operations — *see* War operations
    misadventure in medical care Y63.2
  light sources (man-made visible and ultraviolet) W89.9
    natural X32
    specified NEC W89.8
    tanning bed W89.1
    welding light W89.0
  man-made visible light W89.9
    specified NEC W89.8
    tanning bed W89.1
    welding light W89.0
  microwave W90.8
  misadventure in medical or surgical procedure Y63.2
  natural NEC X39.08
    radon X39.01
  overdose (in medical or surgical procedure) Y63.2
  radar W90.0
  radioactive isotopes (any) W88.1
    atomic power plant malfunction W88.1
    misadventure in medical or surgical treatment Y63.2
  radiofrequency W90.0
  radium NEC W88.1
  sun X32
  ultraviolet (light) (man-made) W89.9
    natural X32
    specified NEC W89.8

Radiation (exposure to) - *continued*
  ultraviolet (light) (man-made) - *continued*
    tanning bed W89.1
    welding light W89.0
  welding arc, torch, or light W89.0
    excessive heat from W92
  x-rays (hard) (soft) W88.0
Range disease W94.11
Rape (attempted) T74.2-
Rat bite W53.11
Reaching (prolonged) (static) X50.1
Reaction, abnormal to medical procedure — *see also* Complication of or following, by type of procedure Y84.9
  with misadventure — *see* Misadventure
  biologicals — *see* Table of Drugs and Chemicals
  drugs — *see* Table of Drugs and Chemicals
  vaccine — *see* Table of Drugs and Chemicals
Recoil
  airgun W34.110
  BB gun W34.110
  firearm NEC W34.19
  gas, air or spring-operated gun NEC W34.118
  handgun W32.1
  hunting rifle W33.12
  larger firearm W33.10
    specified NEC W33.19
  machine gun W33.13
  paintball gun W34.111
  pellet W34.110
  shotgun W33.11
  Very pistol [flare] W34.19
Reduction in
  atmospheric pressure - — *see* Air, pressure, change
Rock falling on or hitting (accidentally) (person) W20.8
  in cave-in W20.0
Run over (accidentally) (by)
  animal (not being ridden) NEC W55.89
  machinery — *see* Contact, with, by specified type of machine
  transport vehicle NEC — *see also* Accident, transport V09.9
    intentional homicide (attempt) Y03.0
    motor NEC V09.20
      intentional homicide (attempt) Y03.0
Running
  before moving object X81.8
    motor vehicle X81.0
Running off, away
  animal (being ridden) — *see also* Accident, transport V80.918
    not being ridden W55.89
  animal-drawn vehicle NEC — *see also* Accident, transport V80.928
  highway, road (way) , street
    transport vehicle NEC — *see also* Accident, transport V89.9
Rupture pressurized devices — *see* Explosion, by type of device

S

Saturnism — *see* Table of Drugs and Chemicals, lead
Scald, scalding (accidental) (by) (from) (in) X19
  air (hot) X14.1
  gases (hot) X14.1
  homicide (attempt) — *see* Assault, burning, hot object
  inflicted by other person
    stated as intentional, homicide (attempt) — *see* Assault, burning, hot object
  liquid (boiling) (hot) NEC X12
    stated as undetermined whether accidental or intentional Y27.2
    suicide (attempt) X77.2
  local application of externally applied substance in medical or surgical care Y63.5
  metal (molten) (liquid) (hot) NEC X18
  self-inflicted X77.9

Scald, scalding (accidental) (by) (from) (in) - *continued*
 stated as undetermined whether accidental or intentional Y27.8
 steam X13.1
  assault X98.0
  stated as undetermined whether accidental or intentional Y27.0
  suicide (attempt) X77.0
 suicide (attempt) X77.9
 vapor (hot) X13.1
  assault X98.0
  stated as undetermined whether accidental or intentional Y27.0
  suicide (attempt) X77.0
Scratched by
 cat W55.03
 person (s) (accidentally) W50.4
  with intent to injure or kill Y04.0
  as, or caused by, a crowd or human stampede (with fall) W52
  assault Y04.0
  homicide (attempt) Y04.0
  in
   fight Y04.0
   legal intervention
    injuring
     bystander Y35.892
     law enforcement personnel Y35.891
     suspect Y35.893
Seasickness T75.3
Self-harm NEC — *see also* External cause by type, undetermined whether accidental or intentional
 intentional — *see* Suicide
 poisoning NEC — *see* Table of drugs and biologicals, accident
Self-inflicted (injury) NEC — *see also* External cause by type, undetermined whether accidental or intentional
 intentional — *see* Suicide
 poisoning NEC — *see* Table of drugs and biologicals, accident
Sequelae (of)
 accident NEC — *see* W00-X58 with 7th character S
 assault (homicidal) (any means) — *see* X92-Y08 with 7th character S
 homicide, attempt (any means) — *see* X92-Y08 with 7th character S
 injury undetermined whether accidentally or purposely inflicted — *see* Y21-Y33 with 7th character S
 intentional self-harm (classifiable to X71-X83) — *see* X71-X83 with 7th character S
 legal intervention — *see* with 7th character S Y35
 motor vehicle accident — *see* V00-V99 with 7th character S
 suicide, attempt (any means) — *see* X71-X83 with 7th character S
 transport accident — *see* V00-V99 with 7th character S
 war operations — *see* War operations
Shock
 electric — *see* Exposure, electric current
 from electric appliance (any) (faulty) W86.8
  domestic W86.0
  suicide (attempt) X83.1
Shooting, shot (accidental (ly)) — *see also* Discharge, firearm, by type
 herself or himself — *see* Discharge, firearm by type, self-inflicted
 homicide (attempt) — *see* Discharge, firearm by type, homicide
 in war operations — *see* War operations
 inflicted by other person — *see* Discharge, firearm by type, homicide
  accidental — *see* Discharge, firearm, by type of firearm
 legal
  execution — *see* Legal, intervention, firearm

Shooting, shot (accidental (ly)) - *continued*
 legal - *continued*
  intervention — *see* Legal, intervention, firearm
  self-inflicted — *see* Discharge, firearm by type, suicide
  accidental — *see* Discharge, firearm, by type of firearm
 suicide (attempt) — *see* Discharge, firearm by type, suicide
Shoving (accidentally) by other person — *see* Pushed, by other person
Sickness
 alpine W94.11
 motion — *see* Motion
 mountain W94.11
Sinking (accidental)
 watercraft (causing drowning, submersion) — *see also* Drowning, due to, accident to, watercraft, sinking
  causing injury except drowning or submersion — *see* Accident, watercraft, causing, injury NEC
Siriasis X32
Sitting (prolonged) (static) X50.1
Slashed wrists — *see* Cut, self-inflicted
Slipping (accidental) (on same level) (with fall) W01.0
 on
  ice W00.0
   with skates — *see* Accident, transport, pedestrian, conveyance
  mud W01.0
  oil W01.0
  snow W00.0
   with skis — *see* Accident, transport, pedestrian, conveyance
  surface (slippery) (wet) NEC W01.0
 without fall W18.40
  due to
   specified NEC W18.49
   stepping from one level to another W18.43
   stepping into hole or opening W18.42
   stepping on object W18.41
Sliver, wood, contact with W45.8
Smoldering (due to fire) — *see* Exposure, fire
Sodomy (attempted) by force T74.2-
Sound waves (causing injury) W42.9
 supersonic W42.0
Splinter, contact with W45.8
Stab, stabbing — *see* Cut
Standing (prolonged) (static) X50.1
Starvation X58
Status of external cause Y99.9
 child assisting in compensated work for family Y99.8
 civilian activity done for financial or other compensation Y99.0
 civilian activity done for income or pay Y99.0
 family member assisting in compensated work for other family member Y99.8
 hobby not done for income Y99.8
 leisure activity Y99.8
 military activity Y99.1
 off-duty activity of military personnel Y99.8
 recreation or sport not for income or while a student Y99.8
 specified NEC Y99.8
 student activity Y99.8
 volunteer activity Y99.2
Stepped on
 by
  animal (not being ridden) NEC W55.89
  crowd or human stampede W52
  person W50.0
Stepping on
 object W22.8
  with fall W18.31
  sports equipment W21.9
  stationary W22.09
   sports equipment W21.89
 person W51
  by crowd or human stampede W52

Stepping on - *continued*
 sports equipment W21.9
Sting
 arthropod, nonvenomous W57
 insect, nonvenomous W57
Storm (cataclysmic) — *see* Forces of nature, cataclysmic storm
Straining, excessive — *see also* Overexertion X50.9
Strangling — *see* Strangulation
Strangulation (accidental) — *see* category T71
Strenuous movements — *see also* Overexertion X50.9
Striking against
 airbag (automobile) W22.10
  driver side W22.11
  front passenger side W22.12
  specified NEC W22.19
 bottom when
  diving or jumping into water (in) W16.822
   causing drowning W16.821
   from boat W16.722
    causing drowning W16.721
   natural body W16.622
    causing drowning W16.821
   swimming pool W16.522
    causing drowning W16.521
  falling into water (in) W16.322
   causing drowning W16.321
   fountain — *see* Striking against, bottom when, falling into water, specified NEC
   natural body W16.122
    causing drowning W16.121
   reservoir — *see* Striking against, bottom when, falling into water, specified NEC
   specified NEC W16.322
    causing drowning W16.321
   swimming pool W16.022
    causing drowning W16.021
 diving board (swimming-pool) W21.4
 object W22.8
  with
   drowning or submersion — *see* Drowning
   fall — *see* Fall, due to, bumping against, object
  caused by crowd or human stampede (with fall) W52
  furniture W22.03
  lamppost W22.02
  sports equipment W21.9
  stationary W22.09
   sports equipment W21.89
  wall W22.01
 person (s) W51
  with fall W03
   due to ice or snow W00.0
  as, or caused by, a crowd or human stampede (with fall) W52
  assault Y04.2
  homicide (attempt) Y04.2
 sports equipment W21.9
 wall (when) W22.01
  diving or jumping into water (in) W16.832
   causing drowning W16.831
   swimming pool W16.532
    causing drowning W16.531
  falling into water (in) W16.332
   causing drowning W16.331
   fountain — *see* Striking against, wall when, falling into water, specified NEC
   natural body W16.132
    causing drowning W16.131
   reservoir — *see* Striking against, wall when, falling into water, specified NEC
   specified NEC W16.332
    causing drowning W16.331
   swimming pool W16.032
    causing drowning W16.031
  swimming pool (when) W22.042

STRIKING AGAINST - STRUCK BY

Striking against - *continued*
wall (when) - *continued*
swimming pool (when) - *continued*
causing drowning W22.041
diving or jumping into water W16.532
causing drowning W16.531
falling into water W16.032
causing drowning W16.031
Struck (accidentally) by
airbag (automobile) W22.10
driver side W22.11
front passenger side W22.12
specified NEC W22.19
alligator W58.02
animal (not being ridden) NEC W55.89
avalanche — *see* Landslide
ball (hit) (thrown) W21.00
assault Y08.09
baseball W21.03
basketball W21.05
golf ball W21.04
football W21.01
soccer W21.02
softball W21.07
specified NEC W21.09
volleyball W21.06
bat or racquet
baseball bat W21.11
assault Y08.02
golf club W21.13
assault Y08.09
specified NEC W21.19
assault Y08.09
tennis racquet W21.12
assault Y08.09
bullet — *see also* Discharge, firearm by type
in war operations — *see* War operations
crocodile W58.12
dog W54.1
flare, Very pistol — *see* Discharge, firearm NEC
hailstones X39.8
hockey (ice)
field
puck W21.221
stick W21.211
puck W21.220
stick W21.210
assault Y08.01
landslide — *see* Landslide
law-enforcement agent (on duty) — *see* Legal, intervention, manhandling
with blunt object — *see* Legal, intervention, blunt object
lightning — *see* subcategory T75.0
causing fire — *see* Exposure, fire
machine — *see* Contact, with, by type of machine
mammal NEC W55.89
marine W56.32
marine animal W56.82
missile
firearm — *see* Discharge, firearm by type
in war operations — *see* War operations, missile
object W22.8
blunt W22.8
assault Y00
suicide (attempt) X79
undetermined whether accidental or intentional Y29
falling W20.8
from, in, on
building W20.1
burning (uncontrolled fire) X00.4
cataclysmic
earth surface movement NEC — *see* Landslide
storm — *see* Forces of nature, cataclysmic storm
cave-in W20.0
earthquake X34
machine (in operation) — *see* Contact, with, by type of machine
structure W20.1

Struck (accidentally) by - *continued*
object - *continued*
falling - *continued*
from, in, on - *continued*
structure - *continued*
burning X00.4
transport vehicle (in motion) — *see* Accident, transport, by type of vehicle
watercraft V93.49
due to
accident to craft V91.39
powered craft V91.33
ferry boat V91.31
fishing boat V91.32
jetskis V91.33
liner V91.31
merchant ship V91.30
passenger ship V91.31
unpowered craft V91.38
canoe V91.35
inflatable V91.36
kayak V91.35
sailboat V91.34
surf-board V91.38
windsurfer V91.38
powered craft V93.43
ferry boat V93.41
fishing boat V93.42
jetskis V93.43
liner V93.41
merchant ship V93.40
passenger ship V93.41
unpowered craft V93.48
sailboat V93.44
surf-board V93.48
windsurfer V93.48
moving NEC W20.8
projected W20.8
assault Y00
in sports W21.9
assault Y08.09
ball W21.00
baseball W21.03
basketball W21.05
football W21.01
golf ball W21.04
soccer W21.02
softball W21.07
specified NEC W21.09
volleyball W21.06
bat or racquet
baseball bat W21.11
assault Y08.02
golf club W21.13
assault Y08.09
specified NEC W21.19
assault Y08.09
tennis racquet W21.12
assault Y08.09
hockey (ice)
field
puck W21.221
stick W21.211
puck W21.220
stick W21.210
assault Y08.01
specified NEC W21.89
set in motion by explosion — *see* Explosion
thrown W20.8
assault Y00
in sports W21.9
assault Y08.09
ball W21.00
baseball W21.03
basketball W21.05
football W21.01
golf ball W21.04
soccer W21.02
soft ball W21.07
specified NEC W21.09
volleyball W21.06
bat or racquet
baseball bat W21.11

Struck (accidentally) by - *continued*
object - *continued*
thrown - *continued*
in sports - *continued*
bat or racquet - *continued*
baseball bat - *continued*
assault Y08.02
golf club W21.13
assault Y08.09
specified NEC W21.19
assault Y08.09
tennis racquet W21.12
assault Y08.09
hockey (ice)
field
puck W21.221
stick W21.211
puck W21.220
stick W21.210
assault Y08.01
specified NEC W21.89
other person (s) W50.0
with
blunt object W22.8
intentional, homicide (attempt) Y00
sports equipment W21.9
undetermined whether accidental or intentional Y29
fall W03
due to ice or snow W00.0
as, or caused by, a crowd or human stampede (with fall) W52
assault Y04.2
homicide (attempt) Y04.2
in legal intervention
injuring
bystander Y35.812
law enforcement personnel Y35.811
suspect Y35.813
unspecified person Y35.819
sports equipment W21.9
police (on duty) — *see* Legal, intervention, manhandling
with blunt object — *see* Legal, intervention, blunt object
sports equipment W21.9
assault Y08.09
ball W21.00
baseball W21.03
basketball W21.05
football W21.01
golf ball W21.04
soccer W21.02
soft ball W21.07
specified NEC W21.09
volleyball W21.06
bat or racquet
baseball bat W21.11
assault Y08.02
golf club W21.13
assault Y08.09
specified NEC W21.19
tennis racquet W21.12
assault Y08.09
cleats (shoe) W21.31
foot wear NEC W21.39
football helmet W21.81
hockey (ice)
field
puck W21.221
stick W21.211
puck W21.220
stick W21.210
assault Y08.01
skate blades W21.32
specified NEC W21.89
assault Y08.09
thunderbolt — *see* subcategory T75.0
causing fire — *see* Exposure, fire
transport vehicle NEC — *see also* Accident, transport V09.9
intentional, homicide (attempt) Y03.0
motor NEC — *see also* Accident, transport V09.20
homicide Y03.0

Struck (accidentally) by - *continued*
vehicle (transport) NEC — *see* Accident,
transport, by type of vehicle
stationary (falling from jack, hydraulic lift,
ramp) W20.8
Stumbling
over
animal NEC W01.0
with fall W18.09
carpet, rug or (small) object W22.8
with fall W18.09
person W51
with fall W03
due to ice or snow W00.0
without fall W18.40
due to
specified NEC W18.49
stepping from one level to
another W18.43
stepping into hole or opening W18.42
stepping on object W18.41
Submersion (accidental) — *see* Drowning
Suffocation (accidental) (by external means)
(by pressure) (mechanical) (*see also*
category T71)
due to, by
avalanche — *see* Landslide
explosion — *see* Explosion
fire — *see* Exposure, fire
food, any type (aspiration) (ingestion)
(inhalation) — *see* categories T17
and T18
ignition — *see* Ignition
landslide — *see* Landslide
machine (ry) — *see* Contact, with, by type
of machine
vomitus (aspiration) (inhalation) T17.81-
in
burning building X00.8
Suicide, suicidal (attempted) (by) X83.8
blunt object X79
burning, burns X76
hot object X77.9
fluid NEC X77.2
household appliance X77.3
specified NEC X77.8
steam X77.0
tap water X77.1
vapors X77.0
caustic substance — *see* Table of Drugs and
Chemicals
cold, extreme X83.2
collision of motor vehicle with
motor vehicle X82.0
specified NEC X82.8
train X82.1
tree X82.2
crashing of aircraft X83.0
cut (any part of body) X78.9
cutting or piercing instrument X78.9
dagger X78.2
glass X78.0
knife X78.1
specified NEC X78.8
sword X78.2
drowning (in) X71.9
bathtub X71.0
natural water X71.3
specified NEC X71.8
swimming pool X71.1
following fall X71.2
electrocution X83.1
explosive (s) (material) X75
fire, flames X76
firearm X74.9
airgun X74.01
handgun X72
hunting rifle X73.1
larger X73.9
specified NEC X73.8
machine gun X73.2
shotgun X73.0
specified NEC X74.8
hanging X83.8
hot object — *see* Suicide, burning, hot object

Suicide, suicidal (attempted) (by) - *continued*
jumping
before moving object X81.8
motor vehicle X81.0
subway train X81.1
train X81.1
from high place X80
late effect of attempt — *see* X71-X83 with
7th character S
lying before moving object, train,
vehicle X81.8
poisoning — *see* Table of Drugs and
Chemicals
puncture (any part of body) — *see* Suicide,
cutting or piercing instrument
scald — *see* Suicide, burning, hot object
sequelae of attempt — *see* X71-X83 with 7th
character S
sharp object (any) — *see* Suicide, cutting or
piercing instrument
shooting — *see* Suicide, firearm
specified means NEC X83.8
stab (any part of body) — *see* Suicide,
cutting or piercing instrument
steam, hot vapors X77.0
strangulation X83.8
submersion — *see* Suicide, drowning
suffocation X83.8
wound NEC X83.8
Sunstroke X32
Supersonic waves (causing injury) W42.0
Surgical procedure, complication of (delayed
or as an abnormal reaction without
mention of misadventure) — *see also*
Complication of or following, by type of
procedure
due to or as a result of misadventure — *see*
Misadventure
Swallowed, swallowing
foreign body — *see* Foreign body, alimentary
canal
poison — *see* Table of Drugs and Chemicals
substance
caustic or corrosive — *see* Table of Drugs
and Chemicals
poisonous — *see* Table of Drugs and
Chemicals

T

Tackle in sport W03
Terrorism (involving) Y38.80
biological weapons Y38.6X-
chemical weapons Y38.7X-
conflagration Y38.3X-
drowning and submersion Y38.89-
explosion Y38.2X-
destruction of aircraft Y38.1X-
marine weapons Y38.0X-
fire Y38.3X-
firearms Y38.4X-
hot substances Y38.3X-
lasers Y38.89-
nuclear weapons Y38.5X-
piercing or stabbing instruments Y38.89-
secondary effects Y38.9X-
specified method NEC Y38.89-
suicide bomber Y38.81-
Thirst X58
Threat to breathing
aspiration — *see* Aspiration
due to cave-in, falling earth or substance
NEC — *see* category T71
Thrown (accidentally)
against part (any) of or object in transport
vehicle (in motion) NEC — *see also*
Accident, transport
from
high place, homicide (attempt) Y01
machinery — *see* Contact, with, by type of
machine
transport vehicle NEC — *see also*
Accident, transport V89.9
off — *see* Thrown, from
Thunderbolt — *see* subcategory T75.0
causing fire — *see* Exposure, fire

Tidal wave (any injury) NEC — *see* Forces
of nature, tidal wave
Took
overdose (drug) — *see* Table of Drugs and
Chemicals
poison — *see* Table of Drugs and Chemicals
Tornado (any injury) X37.1
Torrential rain (any injury) X37.8
Torture X58
Trampled by animal NEC W55.89
Trapped (accidentally)
between objects (moving) (stationary and
moving) — *see* Caught
by part (any) of
motorcycle V29.88
pedal cycle V19.88
transport vehicle NEC — *see also*
Accident, transport V89.9
Travel (effects) (sickness) T75.3
Tree falling on or hitting (accidentally)
(person) W20.8
Tripping
over
animal W01.0
with fall W01.0
carpet, rug or (small) object W22.8
with fall W18.09
person W51
with fall W03
due to ice or snow W00.0
without fall W18.40
due to
specified NEC W18.49
stepping from one level to
another W18.43
stepping into hole or opening W18.42
stepping on object W18.41
Twisted by person (s) (accidentally) W50.2
with intent to injure or kill Y04.0
as, or caused by, a crowd or human stampede
(with fall) W52
assault Y04.0
homicide (attempt) Y04.0
in
fight Y04.0
legal intervention — *see* Legal,
intervention, manhandling
Twisting (prolonged) (static) X50.1

U

Underdosing of necessary drugs,
medicaments or biological
substances Y63.6
Undetermined intent (contact) (exposure)
automobile collision Y32
blunt object Y29
drowning (submersion) (in) Y21.9
bathtub Y21.0
after fall Y21.1
natural water (lake) (ocean) (pond) (river)
(stream) Y21.4
specified place NEC Y21.8
swimming pool Y21.2
after fall Y21.3
explosive material Y25
fall, jump or push from high place Y30
falling, lying or running before moving
object Y31
fire Y26
firearm discharge Y24.9
airgun (BB) (pellet) Y24.0
handgun (pistol) (revolver) Y22
hunting rifle Y23.1
larger Y23.9
hunting rifle Y23.1
machine gun Y23.3
military Y23.2
shotgun Y23.0
specified type NEC Y23.8
machine gun Y23.3
military Y23.2
shotgun Y23.0
specified type NEC Y24.8
Very pistol Y24.8
hot object Y27.9
fluid NEC Y27.2

Undetermined intent (contact) (exposure) - *continued*
  hot object - *continued*
    household appliance Y27.3
    specified object NEC Y27.8
    steam Y27.0
    tap water Y27.1
    vapor Y27.0
  jump, fall or push from high place Y30
  lying, falling or running before moving object Y31
  motor vehicle crash Y32
  push, fall or jump from high place Y30
  running, falling or lying before moving object Y31
  sharp object Y28.9
    dagger Y28.2
    glass Y28.0
    knife Y28.1
    specified object NEC Y28.8
    sword Y28.2
  smoke Y26
  specified event NEC Y33
Use of hand as hammer X50.3

V

Vibration (causing injury) W49.9
Victim (of)
  avalanche — *see* Landslide
  earth movements NEC — *see* Forces of nature, earth movement
  earthquake X34
  flood — *see* Flood
  landslide — *see* Landslide
  lightning — *see* subcategory T75.0
    causing fire — *see* Exposure, fire
  storm (cataclysmic) NEC — *see* Forces of nature, cataclysmic storm
  volcanic eruption X35
Volcanic eruption (any injury) X35
Vomitus, gastric contents in air passages (with asphyxia, obstruction or suffocation) T17.81-

W

Walked into stationary object (any) W22.09
  furniture W22.03
  lamppost W22.02
  wall W22.01
War operations (injuries to military personnel and civilians during war, civil insurrection and peacekeeping missions) (by) (from) (involving) Y36.90
  after cessation of hostilities Y36.89-
    explosion (of)
      bomb placed during war operations Y36.82-
      mine placed during war operations Y36.81-
    specified NEC Y36.88-
  air blast Y36.20-
  aircraft
    destruction — *see* War operations, destruction of aircraft
    airway restriction — *see* War operations, restriction of airways
    asphyxiation — *see* War operations, restriction of airways
  biological weapons Y36.6X-
  blast Y36.20-
  blast fragments Y36.20-
  blast wave Y36.20-
  blast wind Y36.20-
  bomb Y36.20-
    dirty Y36.50-
    gasoline Y36.31-
    incendiary Y36.31-
    petrol Y36.31-
  bullet Y36.43-
    incendiary Y36.32-
    rubber Y36.41-
  chemical weapons Y36.7X-
  combat
    hand to hand (unarmed) combat Y36.44-
    using blunt or piercing object Y36.45-
  conflagration — *see* War operations, fire
  conventional warfare NEC Y36.49-

War operations (injuries to military personnel and civilians during war, civil insurrection and peacekeeping missions) (by) (from) (involving) - *continued*
  depth-charge Y36.01-
  destruction of aircraft Y36.10-
    due to
      air to air missile Y36.11-
      collision with other aircraft Y36.12-
      detonation (accidental) of onboard munitions and explosives Y36.14-
      enemy fire or explosives Y36.11-
      explosive placed on aircraft Y36.11-
      onboard fire Y36.13-
      rocket propelled grenade [RPG] Y36.11-
      small arms fire Y36.11-
      surface to air missile Y36.11-
    specified NEC Y36.19-
  detonation (accidental) of
    onboard marine weapons Y36.05-
    own munitions or munitions launch device Y36.24-
  dirty bomb Y36.50-
  explosion (of) Y36.20-
    after cessation of hostilities
      bomb placed during war operations Y36.82-
      mine placed during war operations Y36.81-
    aerial bomb Y36.21-
    bomb NOS — *see also* War operations, bomb(s) Y36.20-
    own munitions or munitions launch device (accidental) Y36.24-
    fragments Y36.20-
    grenade Y36.29-
    guided missile Y36.22-
    improvised explosive device [IED] (person-borne) (roadside) (vehicle-borne) Y36.23-
    land mine Y36.29-
    marine mine (at sea) (in harbor) Y36.02-
    marine weapon Y36.00-
      specified NEC Y36.09-
    sea-based artillery shell Y36.03-
    specified NEC Y36.29-
    torpedo Y36.04-
  fire Y36.30-
    specified NEC Y36.39-
  firearms
    discharge Y36.43-
    pellets Y36.42-
  flamethrower Y36.33-
  fragments (from) (of)
    improvised explosive device [IED] (person-borne) (roadside) (vehicle-borne) Y36.26-
    munitions Y36.25-
    specified NEC Y36.29-
    weapons Y36.27-
  friendly fire Y36.92
  hand to hand (unarmed) combat Y36.44-
  hot substances — *see* War operations, fire
  incendiary bullet Y36.32-
  nuclear weapon (effects of) Y36.50-
    acute radiation exposure Y36.54-
    blast pressure Y36.51-
    direct blast Y36.51-
    direct heat Y36.53-
    fallout exposure Y36.54-
    fireball Y36.53-
    indirect blast (struck or crushed by blast debris) (being thrown by blast) Y36.52-
    ionizing radiation (immediate exposure) Y36.54-
    nuclear radiation Y36.54-
    radiation
      ionizing (immediate exposure) Y36.54-
      nuclear Y36.54-
      thermal Y36.53-
    specified NEC Y36.59-
    secondary effects Y36.54-
    thermal radiation Y36.53-
  restriction of air (airway)

War operations (injuries to military personnel and civilians during war, civil insurrection and peacekeeping missions) (by) (from) (involving) - *continued*
  restriction of air (airway) - *continued*
    intentional Y36.46-
    unintentional Y36.47-
  rubber bullets Y36.41-
  shrapnel NOS Y36.29-
  suffocation — *see* War operations, restriction of airways
  unconventional warfare NEC Y36.7X-
  underwater blast NOS Y36.00-
  warfare
    conventional NEC Y36.49-
    unconventional NEC Y36.7X-
  weapons
    biological weapons Y36.6X-
    chemical Y36.7X-
    nuclear (effects of) Y36.50-
      acute radiation exposure Y36.54-
      blast pressure Y36.51-
      direct blast Y36.51-
      direct heat Y36.53-
      fallout exposure Y36.54-
      fireball Y36.53-
      indirect blast (struck or crushed by blast debris) (being thrown by blast) Y36.52-
      radiation
        ionizing (immediate exposure) Y36.54-
        nuclear Y36.54-
        thermal Y36.53-
      secondary effects Y36.54-
      specified NEC Y36.59-
    of mass destruction [WMD] Y36.91
  weapon of mass destruction [WMD] Y36.91
Washed
  away by flood — *see* Flood
  off road by storm (transport vehicle) — *see* Forces of nature, cataclysmic storm
Weather exposure NEC — *see* Forces of nature
Weightlessness (causing injury) (effects of) (in spacecraft, real or simulated) X52
Work related condition Y99.0
Wound (accidental) NEC — *see also* Injury X58
  battle — *see also* War operations Y36.90
  gunshot — *see* Discharge, firearm by type
Wreck transport vehicle NEC — *see also* Accident, transport V89.9
Wrong
  device implanted into correct surgical site Y65.51
  fluid in infusion Y65.1
  procedure (operation) on correct patient Y65.51
  patient, procedure performed on Y65.52

Chapter 1: Infectious and Parasitic Diseases (A00-B99)

In this chapter, code selection usually is determined by the specific organism involved in the disease process. "Infectious" refers to a disease caused by a microorganism, or capable of being communicated by infection (contagious). "Parasitic" refers to a disease caused by a parasite (e.g., a tick).

In home care, it is rare to receive documentation naming the infection-causing organism, but when the information is available from the physician, it should be used when selecting the diagnosis code. It is acceptable to code a diagnosis in a lab or pathology report provided by a physician (such as a pathologist or radiologist) *who has interpreted the results*, per Q1 2017 Coding Clinic. As is always the case, the critical data used to assign codes is in the medical record, the assessment, and the Plan of Care documentation. After selecting the correct codes, proper sequencing is the next concern.

Code categories found in this first chapter include infectious conditions related to specific locations or conditions (such as intestinal infectious diseases, tuberculosis and poliomyelitis), viral infections (such as human immunodeficiency virus), bacterial infections (such as leprosy), diseases caused by parasites (zoonotic bacterial and arthropod-borne viral diseases), venereal diseases, mycoses (fungal infections), helminthiases (intestinal parasites or worms), and the late effects of these conditions.

Certain diseases also have been arranged in Chapter 1 of ICD-10-CM within separate subchapters or blocks that group similar conditions together. Examples include: infections with a predominantly sexual mode of transmission (A50-A64), viral hepatitis (B15-B19), and other viral diseases (B25-B34). Some conditions such as streptococcal sore throat and its inclusion terms previously listed in Chapter 1 have been reclassified in ICD-10-CM to Chapter 10: Diseases of the respiratory system.

Many of the codes in Chapter 1 have been expanded to reflect manifestations of the disease with the use of fourth or fifth characters allowing the infectious disease and manifestation to be now captured with one code instead of two.

Example: A01.0 Typhoid fever

Infection due to Salmonella typhi

A01.00, Typhoid fever, unspecified

A01.01, Typhoid meningitis

A01.02, Typhoid fever with heart involvement

A01.03, Typhoid pneumonia

A01.04, Typhoid arthritis

A01.05, Typhoid osteomyelitis

A01.09, Typhoid fever with other complications

The correct code can be found by looking up the term for the condition in the Alphabetic Index and then look at the subterms listed, which will list possible organisms. For example, to find the code for "encephalitis caused by meningococcus, "look up encephalitis with subterm meningococcal, which leads to A39.81.

Remember that sometimes a Chapter 1 code is not the most appropriate choice. The following are a few situations to watch out for:

- If a patient has a **personal or family history of infectious or parasitic disease** reported in this chapter, it may be more appropriate to use a code from the Z code section, such as Z86.19 (Personal history of infectious and parasitic diseases).

- If the patient has **been exposed to an infectious disease** but does not currently have the disease, refer to 'Exposure (to) or Contact, with' in the Alphabetical Index, which leads to Z20.1 (Contact with tuberculosis).

- If the patient is a **carrier or suspected carrier of an infectious disease**, refer to 'Carrier' in the Alphabetical Index, which will generally direct you to a Z22.- code.

- If the organism causing an infection is **resistant to antibiotics (other than methicillin)**, search under 'Resistance' in the Alphabetical Index, which will refer you to a Z16.- code. MRSA is coded with specific codes MRSA codes, and Z16.- codes are not used for MRSA.

- If an **infection is the result of injury or medical treatment**, a code for the injury or medical complication may be reported with a code from this chapter.

- Watch for **combination codes,** especially with pneumonia and influenza under those main terms in the Alphabetical Index. Then, confirm in the Tabular List (Chapter 10: Respiratory Diseases) where the infectious agent is already included in the disease code. For example, Staphylococcus aureus pneumonia is coded with combination code J15.211 (Methicillin susceptible staphylococcus aureus).

- Although not often coded in home health, if reporting an **infectious or parasitic disease in a pregnant patient**, and the condition is complicating the pregnancy, report first a code from Chapter 15, Pregnancy, Childbirth and the Puerperium, and a code from Chapter 1 as an additional diagnosis.

- For **Zika virus infections**, code only a confirmed diagnosis (A92.5) as documented by the provider. This is an exception to the hospital inpatient guideline. In this context, "confirmation" does not require documentation of the type of test performed; the physician's diagnostic statement that the condition is confirmed is sufficient. If the provider documents "suspected", "possible" or "probable" Zika, do not assign code A92.5. Instead, assign a code(s) explaining the reason for encounter (such as fever, rash, or joint pain) or Z20.828, Contact with and (suspected) exposure to other viral communicable diseases

Multiple Coding and Sequencing

Certain infections are classified in chapters other than Chapter 1 and no organism is identified as part of the infection code. In these instances, it is necessary to use an additional code from Chapter 1 to identify the organism. For example, the following codes are to be used as an additional code to identify the organism: A code from category B95, Streptococcus, Staphylococcus, and Enterococcus, as the cause of the disease classified in other chapters; B96, Other bacterial agents as the cause of diseases classified to other chapters; or B97, Viral agents as the cause of other diseases classified to other chapters. An instructional note will be found at the infection code advising that an additional organism code is required.

For these categories, a code from another chapter is reported first to indicate the condition, and an additional code from Chapter 1 categories B95-B97 is reported to indicate the organism responsible for the condition.

Here are some examples:

- A urinary tract infection due to Escherichia coli (E. coli), site not specified, is reported with code N39.0 for the urinary tract infection, site not specified, from Chapter 14 first followed by (the organism), E. coli (B96.20) from Chapter 1. A note under code N39.0 states "Use additional code to identify organism."

- T87.43 describes an infection of an amputation stump, right lower extremity. If the physician documents the causative organism to be staphylococcus, unspecified, (B95.8), the correct code sequence is T87.43 and then B95.8. If the documentation supports staphylococcus aureus, the correct add-on code is B95.61. If the documentation supports MRSA, the additional code is B95.62. The code from the B95 category should be sequenced right after the code for the condition and never in the primary slot.

- A patient with pulmonary insufficiency as a late effect of tuberculosis is another sequencing exception. This is reported using J98.4 (other pulmonary insufficiency) and an additional code B90.9 (sequelae of respiratory and unspecified tuberculosis).

Always remember that Includes and Excludes notes are crucial, and it is important to follow any other instructions under the code or code category.

Special Issues

HIV

Code only confirmed cases of HIV infection/illness. Human immunodeficiency virus [HIV] disease is only reported if the physician's documentation states that the patient is HIV positive with symptoms, or has an HIV-related illness. If the patient has an HIV-related condition, the principal diagnosis should be B20, Human immunodeficiency virus (HIV), followed by additional diagnosis codes for all related HIV-related conditions. Here are some examples:

- If the patient is being seen for a HIV-related condition, report B20 as the first-listed diagnosis. For example, a patient with Kaposi's sarcoma and HIV/AIDS is reported with B20 as the first-listed diagnosis, and C46.- (Kaposi's sarcoma) as the additional diagnosis.

- If the patient is being seen for a condition unrelated to the HIV, report the other condition as first-listed diagnosis.

- Code Z21 (Asymptomatic human immunodeficiency virus [HIV] infection status) is to be applied when the patient without any documentation of symptoms is listed as being "HIV positive," "known HIV," "HIV test positive," or similar terminology. Do not use this code if "AIDS" is used or is described as having any condition(s) resulting from his/her HIV positive status; use B20 in these cases.

- Patients with inconclusive HIV serology, but no definitive diagnosis or manifestation of the illness, may be assigned code R75, Inconclusive laboratory evidence of human immunodeficiency virus [HIV].

- Patients with any known prior diagnoses of an HIV-related illness should be coded to B20. Once a patient has developed an HIV-related illness, the patient should always be assigned code B20 on every subsequent admission/encounter. Patients previously diagnoses with any HIV illness (B20) should never be assigned to R75 or Z21, Asymptomatic human immunodeficiency virus [HIV] infection status.

- During pregnancy, childbirth or the puerperium, a patient admitted for a health care encounter because of an HIV-related illness should receive a principle diagnosis code of O98.7-, Human immunodeficiency [HIV] disease complicating pregnancy, childbirth and the puerperium, followed by the B20 and the code(s) for the HIV-related illness(es). Codes from Chapter 15, (Pregnancy, Childbirth and the Puerperium) always take sequencing priority.

- Some states and U.S. territories have specific restrictions on the coding of HIV, including Alaska, Arizona, California, Colorado, Connecticut, DC, Delaware, Hawaii, Idaho, Illinois, Iowa, Maryland, Massachusetts, Michigan, Mississippi, Montana, Nevada, New Jersey, New Mexico, North Dakota, Oregon, Puerto Rico, South Carolina, Texas, Utah, Virgin Islands, Washington, West Virginia, Wisconsin and Wyoming. Some of these states restrict the coding of B20 as primary and some prohibit the use of the code. Seek a code for an associated condition in these cases, such as B59, pneumocystosis.

Sepsis, Severe Sepsis and Septic Shock

Sepsis

For a diagnosis of sepsis, assign the appropriate code for the underlying systemic infection. If the type of infection or causal organism is not further specified, assign code A41.9, Sepsis, unspecified organism.

A code from subcategory R65.2, Severe sepsis, should not be assigned unless severe sepsis or an associated acute organ dysfunction is documented. This guideline takes precedence over the fact that acute organ dysfunction is listed under "with" in the alphabetic index listing for "sepsis." [I.C.1.d.1.a]

- **Negative or inconclusive blood cultures** do not preclude a diagnosis of sepsis in patients with clinical evidence of the condition, however, the physician should be queried.

- The term **urosepsis is a nonspecific term and it is not to be considered synonymous with sepsis.** It has no default code in the Alphabetical Index. Should a provider use this term, he/she must be queried for clarification.

- If a patient has sepsis **and** associated acute organ dysfunction or multiple organ dysfunction (MOD), **follow the instructions for coding severe sepsis**.

- If a patient has sepsis and an acute organ dysfunction, but the medical record documentation indicates that the acute organ dysfunction is related to a medical condition other than sepsis, do not assign a code from subcategory R65.2, Severe sepsis. **An acute**

organ dysfunction must be associated with the sepsis in order to assign the severe sepsis code. If the documentation is not clear as to whether the acute organ dysfunction is related to the sepsis or another medical condition, query the physician.

Severe sepsis

The coding of severe sepsis requires a minimum of two codes: first a code for the underlying systemic infection, followed by a code from subcategory R65.2, Severe sepsis. If the causal organism is not documented, assign A41.9, Sepsis, unspecified organism, for the infection. Additional code(s) for the associated acute organ dysfunction are also required.

Due to the complex nature of severe sepsis, some cases may require querying the physician prior to assignment of the codes.

Septic shock

Septic shock generally refers to circulatory failure associated with severe sepsis, and therefore, it represents a type of acute organ dysfunction.

For cases of septic shock, the code for the systemic infection should be sequenced first, followed by code R65.21, Severe sepsis with septic shock or code T81.12, Postprocedural septic shock. Any additional codes for the other acute organ dysfunctions should also be assigned. As noted in the sequencing instructions in the Tabular List, the code for the septic shock cannot be assigned as a principal diagnosis.

Sepsis and severe sepsis with a localized infection

If the reason for admission is both sepsis or severe sepsis and a localized infection, such as pneumonia or cellulitis, a code(s) for the underlying systemic infection should be sequenced first, and the code for the localized infection should be assigned as a secondary diagnosis. If the patient has severe sepsis, a code from subcategory R65.2 should also be assigned as a secondary diagnosis. If the patient is admitted with a localized infection, such as pneumonia, and sepsis/severe sepsis doesn't develop until after admission, the localized infection should be assigned first, followed by the appropriate sepsis/severe sepsis codes.

Sepsis due to a post-procedural infection

In cases of sepsis due to post-procedural infection, base the code assignment **on the provider's documentation of the relationship between the infection and the procedure**.

For such cases, the post-procedural infection code, such as T80.2, Infections following infusion, transfusion and therapeutic injection; T81.44, Sepsis following a procedure; T88.0, Infection following immunization; or O86.0-, Infection of obstetrical surgical wound, should be coded first, followed by the code for the specific infection. If the patient has severe sepsis the appropriate code from subcategory R65.2 should also be assigned with the additional code(s) for any acute organ dysfunction.

Sepsis and severe sepsis associated with a noninfectious process (condition)

If sepsis or severe sepsis is documented as associated with a noninfectious condition, such as a burn or serious injury, and this condition meets the definition for principal diagnosis, the code for the noninfectious process is sequenced first, followed by the code for the resulting infection. If severe sepsis is present, a code from subcategory R65.2 should also be assigned with any associated organ dysfunction(s) codes. It is not necessary to assign a code from R65.1, Systemic inflammatory response syndrome (SIRS) of non-infectious origin, for these cases.

MRSA and MSSA

When a patient is diagnoses with an infection that is due to methicillin resistant Staphylococcus aureus (MRSA) or Methicillin susceptible Staphylococcus aureus (MSSA), and that infection has a combination code that includes the causal organism, assign the appropriate combination code for the condition (e.g., A41.02, Sepsis due to MRSA). Do not assign code B95.62, Methicillin resistant Staphylococcus aureus infection, as the cause of diseases classified elsewhere, or Z16.11, Resistance to penicillins, as additional diagnoses. If a patient has a diagnosis of pneumonia due to Methicillin susceptible Staphylococcus aureus, code only the combination code J15.211 without an additional code from B95.61.

When there is documentation of a current infection (e.g., wound infection, stitch abscess, urinary tract infection) due to MRSA, and that infection does not have a combination code that includes the causal organism, assign the appropriate code to identify the condition along with a code from B95.62, Methicillin Resistant Staphylococcus Aureus (MRSA), or B95.61 Methicillin Susceptible Staphylococcus Aureus (MSSA), as the cause of the diseases classified elsewhere for the MRSA or MSSA infection. Do not assign a code from subcategory Z16.11, Resistance to penicillins, along with the B95.62 code.

The condition or state of being colonized or carrying MSSA or MRSA is called colonization or carriage, while an individual person is described as being colonized or being a carrier. Colonization means that MSSA or MRSA is present on or in the body without necessarily causing illness. A positive MRSA colonization test might be documented by the provider as "MRSA positive screen" or "MRSA nasal swab positive."

Assign code Z22.322, Carrier or suspected carrier of Methicillin resistant Staphylococcus aureus, for patients documented as having MRSA colonization. Assign code Z22.321, Carrier or suspected carrier of Methicillin susceptible Staphylococcus aureus, for patients documented as having MSSA colonization. Colonization is not necessarily indicative of a disease process or as the cause of a specific condition the patient may have unless documented as such by the provider. If the patient is stated to have a history of MRSA, use code Z86.14.

If a patient is documented as having both MRSA colonization **and** infection, you may assign both code Z22.322, Carrier or suspected carrier of MRSA, and a code for the MRSA infection.

CHAPTER 1: CERTAIN INFECTIOUS AND PARASITIC DISEASES (A00-B99)

INCLUDES diseases generally recognized as communicable or transmissible

Use additional code to identify resistance to antimicrobial drugs (Z16.-)

EXCLUDES 1 certain localized infections - see body system-related chapters

EXCLUDES 2 carrier or suspected carrier of infectious disease (Z22.-)

infectious and parasitic diseases complicating pregnancy, childbirth and the puerperium (O98.-)

infectious and parasitic diseases specific to the perinatal period (P35-P39)

influenza and other acute respiratory infections (J00-J22)

This chapter contains the following blocks:

A00-A09	Intestinal infectious diseases
A15-A19	Tuberculosis
A20-A28	Certain zoonotic bacterial diseases
A30-A49	Other bacterial diseases
A50-A64	Infections with a predominantly sexual mode of transmission
A65-A69	Other spirochetal diseases
A70-A74	Other diseases caused by chlamydiae
A75-A79	Rickettsioses
A80-A89	Viral and prion infections of the central nervous system
A90-A99	Arthropod-borne viral fevers and viral hemorrhagic fevers
B00-B09	Viral infections characterized by skin and mucous membrane lesions
B10	Other human herpesviruses
B15-B19	Viral hepatitis
B20	Human immunodeficiency virus [HIV] disease
B25-B34	Other viral diseases
B35-B49	Mycoses
B50-B64	Protozoal diseases
B65-B83	Helminthiases
B85-B89	Pediculosis, acariasis and other infestations
B90-B94	Sequelae of infectious and parasitic diseases
B95-B97	Bacterial and viral infectious agents
B99	Other infectious diseases

Intestinal infectious diseases (A00-A09)

4 **A00** Cholera

SP **A00.0** Cholera due to Vibrio cholerae 01, biovar cholerae
Classical cholera

SP **A00.1** Cholera due to Vibrio cholerae 01, biovar eltor
Cholera eltor

SP **A00.9** Cholera, unspecified

4 **A01** Typhoid and paratyphoid fevers

5 **A01.0** Typhoid fever
Infection due to Salmonella typhi

SP **A01.00** Typhoid fever, unspecified

SP **A01.01** Typhoid meningitis

SP **A01.02** Typhoid fever with heart involvement
Typhoid endocarditis
Typhoid myocarditis

SP **A01.03** Typhoid pneumonia

SP **A01.04** Typhoid arthritis

SP **A01.05** Typhoid osteomyelitis

SP **A01.09** Typhoid fever with other complications

SP **A01.1** Paratyphoid fever A

SP **A01.2** Paratyphoid fever B

SP **A01.3** Paratyphoid fever C

SP **A01.4** Paratyphoid fever, unspecified
Infection due to Salmonella paratyphi NOS

4 **A02** Other salmonella infections

INCLUDES infection or foodborne intoxication due to any Salmonella species other than S. typhi and S. paratyphi

SP **A02.0** Salmonella enteritis
Salmonellosis

SP **A02.1** Salmonella sepsis

5 **A02.2** Localized salmonella infections

SP **A02.20** Localized salmonella infection, unspecified

SP **A02.21** Salmonella meningitis

SP **A02.22** Salmonella pneumonia

SP **A02.23** Salmonella arthritis

CODING TIPS ✓ Salmonella arthritis is a form of reactive arthritis. Code A02.23 indicates the arthritis and its cause. Do not assign an additional code for arthritis.

SP **A02.24** Salmonella osteomyelitis

SP **A02.25** Salmonella pyelonephritis
Salmonella tubulo-interstitial nephropathy

SP **A02.29** Salmonella with other localized infection

SP **A02.8** Other specified salmonella infections

SP **A02.9** Salmonella infection, unspecified

4 **A03** Shigellosis

SP **A03.0** Shigellosis due to Shigella dysenteriae
Group A shigellosis [Shiga-Kruse dysentery]

SP **A03.1** Shigellosis due to Shigella flexneri
Group B shigellosis

SP **A03.2** Shigellosis due to Shigella boydii
Group C shigellosis

SP **A03.3** Shigellosis due to Shigella sonnei
Group D shigellosis

SP **A03.8** Other shigellosis

SP **A03.9** Shigellosis, unspecified
Bacillary dysentery NOS

4 **A04** Other bacterial intestinal infections

EXCLUDES 1 bacterial foodborne intoxications, NEC (A05.-)
tuberculous enteritis (A18.32)

SP **A04.0** Enteropathogenic Escherichia coli infection

SP **A04.1** Enterotoxigenic Escherichia coli infection

SP **A04.2** Enteroinvasive Escherichia coli infection

SP **A04.3** Enterohemorrhagic Escherichia coli infection

SP **A04.4** Other intestinal Escherichia coli infections
Escherichia coli enteritis NOS

★ New ▲ Revised Px Primary SP PDGM Px SL Low CoM SH High CoM IQ Quest. Encounter H Hospice non-cancer Dx | Unspecified | M *Manifestation*

CODING TIPS ✓ This code for E. coli (A04.4) is used when the bacterium causes intestinal infection and is not to be used for other E. coli infections, e.g., UTIs. See B96.2- for other infections caused by E. coli.

SP **A04.5** **Campylobacter enteritis**

SP **A04.6** **Enteritis due to Yersinia enterocolitica**
EXCLUDES 1 extraintestinal yersiniosis (A28.2)
CODING TIPS ✓ Arthropathy associated with Yersinia requires an additional code from M02.-.

5 **A04.7** **Enterocolitis due to Clostridium difficile**
Foodborne intoxication by Clostridium difficile
Pseudomembraneous colitis
DEFINITION Clostridium difficile (C. difficile) is an anaerobic gram-positive, spore-forming, toxin-producing bacillus that is transmitted among humans through the fecal–oral route. C. difficile causes antibiotic associated colitis by colonizing the human intestinal tract after the normal gut flora have been altered due to antibiotic therapy. Recurrence is defined by complete abatement of CDI symptoms while on appropriate therapy, followed by subsequent reappearance of diarrhea and other symptoms after treatment has been stopped. Recurrence typically occurs within one week after treatment cessation, however recurrence may occur up to 8 weeks later.

SP **A04.71** **Enterocolitis due to Clostridium difficile, recurrent**
CODING TIPS ✓ Recurrence is defined by complete abatement of CDI symptoms while on appropriate therapy, followed by subsequent reappearance of diarrhea and other symptoms after treatment has been stopped. Recurrence typically occurs within one week after treatment cessation, however recurrence may occur up to 8 weeks later.

SP **A04.72** **Enterocolitis due to Clostridium difficile, not specified as recurrent**
CODING TIPS ✓ A04.72 is the default code for C. difficile enteritis. Use this code when there is no documentation of recurrence.

SP **A04.8** **Other specified bacterial intestinal infections**

SP **A04.9** **Bacterial intestinal infection, unspecified**
Bacterial enteritis NOS
CODING TIPS ✓ Report A04.9 if the patient is suffering from diarrhea known to be infectious and bacterial, but only if the condition is otherwise unspecified, i.e., if the specific bacterial agent is unknown.

4 **A05** **Other bacterial foodborne intoxications, not elsewhere classified**

EXCLUDES 1 Clostridium difficile foodborne intoxication and infection (A04.7-)
Escherichia coli infection (A04.0-A04.4)
listeriosis (A32.-)
salmonella foodborne intoxication and infection (A02.-)
toxic effect of noxious foodstuffs (T61-T62)

SP **A05.0** **Foodborne staphylococcal intoxication**

SP **A05.1** **Botulism food poisoning**
Botulism NOS
Classical foodborne intoxication due to Clostridium botulinum
EXCLUDES 1 infant botulism (A48.51) wound botulism (A48.52)
DEFINITION Muscle-paralyzing disease caused by ingesting the neurotoxins produced by the bacteria Clostridium botulinum.

SP **A05.2** **Foodborne Clostridium perfringens [Clostridium welchii] intoxication**
Enteritis necroticans
Pig-bel

SP **A05.3** **Foodborne Vibrio parahaemolyticus intoxication**

SP **A05.4** **Foodborne Bacillus cereus intoxication**

SP **A05.5** **Foodborne Vibrio vulnificus intoxication**

SP **A05.8** **Other specified bacterial foodborne intoxications**

SP **A05.9** **Bacterial foodborne intoxication, unspecified**

4 **A06** **Amebiasis**
INCLUDES infection due to Entamoeba histolytica
EXCLUDES 1 other protozoal intestinal diseases (A07.-)
EXCLUDES 2 acanthamebiasis (B60.1-) Naegleriasis (B60.2)

SP **A06.0** **Acute amebic dysentery**
Acute amebiasis
Intestinal amebiasis NOS

SP **A06.1** **Chronic intestinal amebiasis**

SP **A06.2** **Amebic nondysenteric colitis**

SP **A06.3** **Ameboma of intestine**
Ameboma NOS

SP **A06.4** **Amebic liver abscess**
Hepatic amebiasis

SP **A06.5** **Amebic lung abscess**
Amebic abscess of lung (and liver)

SP **A06.6** **Amebic brain abscess**
Amebic abscess of brain (and liver) (and lung)
CODING TIPS ✓ Report A06.6 for an amebic infection of the brain, which may or may not include an infection of the liver and/or lung. Do not report a liver or lung infection separately.

SP **A06.7** **Cutaneous amebiasis**

5 **A06.8** **Amebic infection of other sites**

SP **A06.81** **Amebic cystitis**

SP **A06.82** **Other amebic genitourinary infections**
Amebic balanitis

---

4 4th digit required   **5** 5th digit required   **6** 6th digit required   **7** 7th digit required   **7** 7th digit placeholder   **✚** Additional code   **⊟** Laterality

604   *DecisionHealth's* FY 2020 Complete Home Health ICD-10-CM Diagnosis Coding Manual

Amebic vesiculitis
Amebic vulvovaginitis

SP A06.89 **Other amebic infections**
Amebic appendicitis
Amebic splenic abscess

SP A06.9 **Amebiasis, unspecified**

4 A07 **Other protozoal intestinal diseases**

SP A07.0 **Balantidiasis**
Balantidial dysentery

SP A07.1 **Giardiasis [lambliasis]**

SP A07.2 **Cryptosporidiosis**

SP A07.3 **Isosporiasis**
Infection due to Isospora belli and Isospora hominis
Intestinal coccidiosis
Isosporosis

SP A07.4 **Cyclosporiasis**

SP A07.8 **Other specified protozoal intestinal diseases**
Intestinal microsporidiosis
Intestinal trichomoniasis
Sarcocystosis
Sarcosporidiosis

SP A07.9 **Protozoal intestinal disease, unspecified**
Flagellate diarrhea
Protozoal colitis
Protozoal diarrhea
Protozoal dysentery

4 A08 **Viral and other specified intestinal infections**

> **EXCLUDES 1** influenza with involvement of gastrointestinal tract (J09.X3, J10.2, J11.2)

> **CODING TIPS ✓** Note that an influenza infection that also affects the intestinal tract is reported with J09.x3, J10.2, or J11.2 codes, not A08.

SP A08.0 **Rotaviral enteritis**

5 A08.1 **Acute gastroenteropathy due to Norwalk agent and other small round viruses**

SP A08.11 **Acute gastroenteropathy due to Norwalk agent**
Acute gastroenteropathy due to Norovirus
Acute gastroenteropathy due to Norwalk-like agent

SP A08.19 **Acute gastroenteropathy due to other small round viruses**
Acute gastroenteropathy due to small round virus [SRV] NOS

SP A08.2 **Adenoviral enteritis**

5 A08.3 **Other viral enteritis**

SP A08.31 **Calicivirus enteritis**

SP A08.32 **Astrovirus enteritis**

SP A08.39 **Other viral enteritis**
Coxsackie virus enteritis
Echovirus enteritis
Enterovirus enteritis NEC
Torovirus enteritis

SP A08.4 **Viral intestinal infection, unspecified**
Viral enteritis NOS
Viral gastroenteritis NOS
Viral gastroenteropathy NOS

SP A08.8 **Other specified intestinal infections**

SP A09 **Infectious gastroenteritis and colitis, unspecified**
Infectious colitis NOS
Infectious enteritis NOS
Infectious gastroenteritis NOS

> **EXCLUDES 1** colitis NOS (K52.9)
> diarrhea NOS (R19.7)
> enteritis NOS (K52.9)
> gastroenteritis NOS (K52.9)
> noninfective gastroenteritis and colitis, unspecified (K52.9)

Tuberculosis (A15-A19)

> **INCLUDES** infections due to Mycobacterium tuberculosis and Mycobacterium bovis

> **EXCLUDES 1** congenital tuberculosis (P37.0)
> nonspecific reaction to test for tuberculosis without active tuberculosis (R76.1-)
> pneumoconiosis associated with tuberculosis, any type in A15 (J65)
> positive PPD (R76.11)
> positive tuberculin skin test without active tuberculosis (R76.11)
> sequelae of tuberculosis (B90.-)
> silicotuberculosis (J65)

> **CODING TIPS ✓** Codes from A15-A19 should not be assigned to report a positive PPD (Mantoux) test. A positive PPD (Mantoux) skin test without active tuberculosis should be coded to R76.11.

> **CODING TIPS ✓** These codes are for active TB. See B90 for sequelae of TB and Z86.11 for personal history of TB without residuals.

4 A15 **Respiratory tuberculosis**

SP A15.0 **Tuberculosis of lung**
Tuberculous bronchiectasis
Tuberculous fibrosis of lung
Tuberculous pneumonia
Tuberculous pneumothorax

SP A15.4 **Tuberculosis of intrathoracic lymph nodes**
Tuberculosis of hilar lymph nodes
Tuberculosis of mediastinal lymph nodes
Tuberculosis of tracheobronchial lymph nodes

> **EXCLUDES 1** tuberculosis specified as primary (A15.7)

SP A15.5 **Tuberculosis of larynx, trachea and bronchus**
Tuberculosis of bronchus
Tuberculosis of glottis
Tuberculosis of larynx
Tuberculosis of trachea

SP A15.6 **Tuberculous pleurisy**
Tuberculosis of pleura Tuberculous empyema

> **EXCLUDES 1** primary respiratory tuberculosis (A15.7)

SP A15.7 **Primary respiratory tuberculosis**

SP A15.8 **Other respiratory tuberculosis**
Mediastinal tuberculosis
Nasopharyngeal tuberculosis
Tuberculosis of nose
Tuberculosis of sinus [any nasal]

SP A15.9 **Respiratory tuberculosis unspecified**

4 A17 **Tuberculosis of nervous system**

SP A17.0 **Tuberculous meningitis**

★ New ▲ Revised Px Primary SP PDGM Px SL Low CoM SH High CoM IQ Quest. Encounter H Hospice non-cancer Dx Unspecified M *Manifestation*

DecisionHealth's FY 2020 Complete Home Health ICD-10-CM Diagnosis Coding Manual

605

Tuberculosis of meninges
(cerebral)(spinal)
Tuberculous leptomeningitis
> **EXCLUDES 1**   tuberculous
meningoencephalitis
(A17.82)

SP A17.1   Meningeal tuberculoma
Tuberculoma of meninges (cerebral)
(spinal)
> **EXCLUDES 2**   tuberculoma of brain and
spinal cord   (A17.81)

A17.8   Other tuberculosis of nervous system

**SP A17.81   Tuberculoma of brain and spinal
cord**
Tuberculous abscess of brain and
spinal cord

SP A17.82   Tuberculous meningoencephalitis
Tuberculous myelitis

SP A17.83   Tuberculous neuritis
Tuberculous mononeuropathy

SP A17.89   Other tuberculosis of nervous system
Tuberculous polyneuropathy

**SP A17.9   Tuberculosis of nervous system,
unspecified**

A18   Tuberculosis of other organs

A18.0   Tuberculosis of bones and joints

SP A18.01   Tuberculosis of spine
Pott's disease or curvature of spine
Tuberculous arthritis
Tuberculous osteomyelitis of spine
Tuberculous spondylitis

SP A18.02   Tuberculous arthritis of other joints
Tuberculosis of hip (joint)
Tuberculosis of knee (joint)
> **CODING TIPS ✓**   Report A18.02 for a TB
infection of the hip or knee joint or bone.

SP A18.03   Tuberculosis of other bones
Tuberculous mastoiditis
Tuberculous osteomyelitis
> **CODING TIPS ✓**   Report A18.03 for a TB
infection of bones, except for hip, knee
and spine.

SP A18.09   Other musculoskeletal tuberculosis
Tuberculous myositis
Tuberculous synovitis
Tuberculous tenosynovitis

A18.1   Tuberculosis of genitourinary system

**IQ A18.10   Tuberculosis of genitourinary
system, unspecified**

SP A18.11   Tuberculosis of kidney and ureter

SP A18.12   Tuberculosis of bladder

SP A18.13   Tuberculosis of other urinary organs
Tuberculous urethritis

SP A18.14   Tuberculosis of prostate

**SP A18.15   Tuberculosis of other male genital
organs**

SP A18.16   Tuberculosis of cervix

**SP A18.17   Tuberculous female pelvic
inflammatory disease**
Tuberculous endometritis
Tuberculous oophoritis and salpingitis

**SP A18.18   Tuberculosis of other female genital
organs**
Tuberculous ulceration of vulva

**SP A18.2   Tuberculous peripheral
lymphadenopathy**
Tuberculous adenitis
> **EXCLUDES 2**   tuberculosis of bronchial and
mediastinal lymph nodes
(A15.4)
tuberculosis of mesenteric
and retroperitoneal lymph
nodes   (A18.39)
tuberculous tracheobronchial
adenopathy   (A15.4)

**A18.3   Tuberculosis of intestines, peritoneum
and mesenteric glands**

SP A18.31   Tuberculous peritonitis
Tuberculous ascites

SP A18.32   Tuberculous enteritis
Tuberculosis of anus and rectum
Tuberculosis of intestine (large) (small)

SP A18.39   Retroperitoneal tuberculosis
Tuberculosis of mesenteric glands
Tuberculosis of retroperitoneal (lymph
glands)

**▲ SP A18.4   Tuberculosis of skin and subcutaneous
tissue**
Erythema induratum, tuberculous
Lupus excedens
Lupus vulgaris NOS
Lupus vulgaris of eyelid
Scrofuloderma
Tuberculosis of external ear
> **EXCLUDES 2**   lupus erythematosus   (L93.-)
systemic lupus
erythematosus   (M32.-)

A18.5   Tuberculosis of eye
> **EXCLUDES 2**   lupus vulgaris of eyelid
(A18.4)

SP A18.50   Tuberculosis of eye, unspecified

SP A18.51   Tuberculous episcleritis

SP A18.52   Tuberculous keratitis
Tuberculous interstitial keratitis
Tuberculous keratoconjunctivitis
(interstitial) (phlyctenular)

SP A18.53   Tuberculous chorioretinitis

SP A18.54   Tuberculous iridocyclitis

SP A18.59   Other tuberculosis of eye
Tuberculous conjunctivitis

SP A18.6   Tuberculosis of (inner) (middle) ear
Tuberculous otitis media
> **EXCLUDES 2**   tuberculosis of external ear
(A18.4)
tuberculous mastoiditis
(A18.03)

SP A18.7   Tuberculosis of adrenal glands
Tuberculous Addison's disease

A18.8   Tuberculosis of other specified organs

SP A18.81   Tuberculosis of thyroid gland

**SP A18.82   Tuberculosis of other endocrine
glands**
Tuberculosis of pituitary gland
Tuberculosis of thymus gland

**SP A18.83   Tuberculosis of digestive tract
organs, not elsewhere classified**
> **EXCLUDES 1**   tuberculosis of intestine
(A18.32)

SP A18.84   Tuberculosis of heart
Tuberculous cardiomyopathy
Tuberculous endocarditis

---

4 4th digit required   **5** 5th digit required   **6** 6th digit required   **7** 7th digit required   **7** 7th digit placeholder   **+** Additional code   **⊟** Laterality

606   *DecisionHealth's* FY 2020 Complete Home Health ICD-10-CM Diagnosis Coding Manual

Tuberculous myocarditis
Tuberculous pericarditis

SP A18.85   **Tuberculosis of spleen**

SP A18.89   **Tuberculosis of other sites**
Tuberculosis of muscle
Tuberculous cerebral arteritis

4 A19   **Miliary tuberculosis**

> **INCLUDES**   disseminated tuberculosis
> generalized tuberculosis
> tuberculous polyserositis

> **CODING TIPS ✓**   Miliary tuberculosis (TB) is the widespread dissemination of Mycobacterium tuberculosis via hematogenous spread. Code A19.8 should be used for miliary TB that is documented as chronic.

SP A19.0   **Acute miliary tuberculosis of a single specified site**

SP A19.1   **Acute miliary tuberculosis of multiple sites**

SP A19.2   **Acute miliary tuberculosis, unspecified**

SP A19.8   **Other miliary tuberculosis**

SP A19.9   **Miliary tuberculosis, unspecified**

Certain zoonotic bacterial diseases (A20-A28)

4 A20   **Plague**

> **INCLUDES**   infection due to Yersinia pestis

SP A20.0   **Bubonic plague**

> **DEFINITION**   Infection with the Yersinia pestis bacillus, transmitted via flea, tick, and lice bites and by contact with infected persons or materials, causing severe inflammation and death of skin cells.

SP A20.1   **Cellulocutaneous plague**

SP A20.2   **Pneumonic plague**

> **DEFINITION**   Rapidly progressive, often fatal plague pneumonia caused by direct inhalation of bacteria with severe cough producing frothy, bloody, mucoid sputum.

SP A20.3   **Plague meningitis**

SP A20.7   **Septicemic plague**

> **DEFINITION**   High-density bloodstream infection in acute bubonic plague; may cause death before the appearance of buboes or pulmonary manifestations.

SP A20.8   **Other forms of plague**
Abortive plague
Asymptomatic plague
Pestis minor

SP A20.9   **Plague, unspecified**

4 A21   **Tularemia**

> **INCLUDES**   deer-fly fever
> infection due to Francisella
> tularensis
> rabbit fever

SP A21.0   **Ulceroglandular tularemia**

SP A21.1   **Oculoglandular tularemia**
Ophthalmic tularemia

SP A21.2   **Pulmonary tularemia**

SP A21.3   **Gastrointestinal tularemia**
Abdominal tularemia

SP A21.7   **Generalized tularemia**

SP A21.8   **Other forms of tularemia**

SP A21.9   **Tularemia, unspecified**

4 A22   **Anthrax**

> **INCLUDES**   infection due to Bacillus
> anthracis

SP A22.0   **Cutaneous anthrax**
Malignant carbuncle
Malignant pustule

SP A22.1   **Pulmonary anthrax**
Inhalation anthrax
Ragpicker's disease
Woolsorter's disease

SP A22.2   **Gastrointestinal anthrax**

SP A22.7   **Anthrax sepsis**

SP A22.8   **Other forms of anthrax**
Anthrax meningitis

SP A22.9   **Anthrax, unspecified**

4 A23   **Brucellosis**

> **INCLUDES**   Malta fever
> Mediterranean fever
> undulant fever

SP A23.0   **Brucellosis due to Brucella melitensis**

SP A23.1   **Brucellosis due to Brucella abortus**

SP A23.2   **Brucellosis due to Brucella suis**

SP A23.3   **Brucellosis due to Brucella canis**

SP A23.8   **Other brucellosis**

SP A23.9   **Brucellosis, unspecified**

4 A24   **Glanders and melioidosis**

SP A24.0   **Glanders**
Infection due to Pseudomonas mallei
Malleus

SP A24.1   **Acute and fulminating melioidosis**
Melioidosis pneumonia
Melioidosis sepsis

SP A24.2   **Subacute and chronic melioidosis**

SP A24.3   **Other melioidosis**

SP A24.9   **Melioidosis, unspecified**

Infection due to Pseudomonas
pseudomallei NOS
Whitmore's disease

4 A25   **Rat-bite fevers**

SP A25.0   **Spirillosis**
Sodoku

SP A25.1   **Streptobacillosis**
Epidemic arthritic erythema
Haverhill fever
Streptobacillary rat-bite fever

SP A25.9   **Rat-bite fever, unspecified**

4 A26   **Erysipeloid**

SP A26.0   **Cutaneous erysipeloid**
Erythema migrans

SP A26.7   **Erysipelothrix sepsis**

SP A26.8   **Other forms of erysipeloid**

SP A26.9   **Erysipeloid, unspecified**

4 A27   **Leptospirosis**

SP A27.0   **Leptospirosis icterohemorrhagica**
Leptospiral or spirochetal jaundice
(hemorrhagic)
Weil's disease

5 A27.8   **Other forms of leptospirosis**

SP A27.81   **Aseptic meningitis in leptospirosis**

SP A27.89   **Other forms of leptospirosis**

SP A27.9   **Leptospirosis, unspecified**

★ New ▲ Revised   **Px** Primary   **SP** PDGM Px   **SL** Low CoM   **SH** High CoM   **IQ** Quest. Encounter   **H** Hospice non-cancer Dx   Unspecified   **M** *Manifestation*

4 A28   Other zoonotic bacterial diseases, not elsewhere classified

SP A28.0   Pasteurellosis

SP A28.1   Cat-scratch disease
Cat-scratch fever

SP A28.2   Extraintestinal yersiniosis
> **EXCLUDES 1**   enteritis due to Yersinia enterocolitica (A04.6)
> plague (A20.-)

SP A28.8   Other specified zoonotic bacterial diseases, not elsewhere classified

IQ A28.9   Zoonotic bacterial disease, unspecified

Other bacterial diseases   (A30-A49)

4 A30   Leprosy [Hansen's disease]
> **INCLUDES**   infection due to Mycobacterium leprae
> **EXCLUDES 1**   sequelae of leprosy (B92)
> **CODING TIPS ✓**   Arthropathy associated with leprosy requires an additional code from M01.-.

SP A30.0   Indeterminate leprosy
I leprosy

SP A30.1   Tuberculoid leprosy
TT leprosy

SP A30.2   Borderline tuberculoid leprosy
BT leprosy

SP A30.3   Borderline leprosy
BB leprosy

SP A30.4   Borderline lepromatous leprosy
BL leprosy

SP A30.5   Lepromatous leprosy
LL leprosy

SP A30.8   Other forms of leprosy

SP A30.9   Leprosy, unspecified

4 A31   Infection due to other mycobacteria
> **EXCLUDES 2**   leprosy (A30.-)
> tuberculosis (A15-A19)

SP A31.0   Pulmonary mycobacterial infection
Infection due to Mycobacterium avium
Infection due to Mycobacterium intracellulare [Battey bacillus]
Infection due to Mycobacterium kansasii

SP A31.1   Cutaneous mycobacterial infection
Buruli ulcer
Infection due to Mycobacterium marinum
Infection due to Mycobacterium ulcerans

SP A31.2   Disseminated mycobacterium avium-intracellulare complex (DMAC)
MAC sepsis

SP A31.8   Other mycobacterial infections

SP A31.9   Mycobacterial infection, unspecified
Atypical mycobacterial infection NOS
Mycobacteriosis NOS

4 A32   Listeriosis
> **INCLUDES**   listerial foodborne infection
> **EXCLUDES 1**   neonatal (disseminated) listeriosis (P37.2)

SP A32.0   Cutaneous listeriosis

5 A32.1   Listerial meningitis and meningoencephalitis

SP A32.11   Listerial meningitis

SP A32.12   Listerial meningoencephalitis

SP A32.7   Listerial sepsis

5 A32.8   Other forms of listeriosis

SP A32.81   Oculoglandular listeriosis

SP A32.82   Listerial endocarditis

SP A32.89   Other forms of listeriosis
Listerial cerebral arteritis

SP A32.9   Listeriosis, unspecified

SP A33   Tetanus neonatorum

SP A34   Obstetrical tetanus

SP A35   Other tetanus
Tetanus NOS
> **EXCLUDES 1**   obstetrical tetanus (A34)
> tetanus neonatorum (A33)
> **DEFINITION**   Potentially·fatal disease due to the neurotoxin of Clostridium tetani, entering the body through contaminated wound, burn, or ulcer; causes muscular contractions, hyperreflexia, lockjaw, respiratory spasm, seizures, and paralysis.

4 A36   Diphtheria

SP A36.0   Pharyngeal diphtheria
Diphtheritic membranous angina
Tonsillar diphtheria
> **DEFINITION**   An acute infectious disease usually confined to the upper respiratory tract, caused by toxigenic strains of Corynebacterium dipththeriae, and acquired by contact with an infected person or carrier of the disease.

SP A36.1   Nasopharyngeal diphtheria

SP A36.2   Laryngeal diphtheria
Diphtheritic laryngotracheitis

SP A36.3   Cutaneous diphtheria
> **EXCLUDES 2**   erythrasma (L08.1)

5 A36.8   Other diphtheria

SP A36.81   Diphtheritic cardiomyopathy
Diphtheritic myocarditis

SP A36.82   Diphtheritic radiculomyelitis

SP A36.83   Diphtheritic polyneuritis

SP A36.84   Diphtheritic tubulo-interstitial nephropathy

SP A36.85   Diphtheritic cystitis

SP A36.86   Diphtheritic conjunctivitis

SP A36.89   Other diphtheritic complications
Diphtheritic peritonitis

SP A36.9   Diphtheria, unspecified

4 A37   Whooping cough

5 A37.0   Whooping cough due to Bordetella pertussis
> **DEFINITION**   Infectious disease caused by Bordetella pertussis, marked by inflammation of mucous membranes and cough, ending in a prolonged crowing or whooping respiration.

SP A37.00   Whooping cough due to Bordetella pertussis without pneumonia

SP A37.01   Whooping cough due to Bordetella pertussis with pneumonia

5 A37.1   Whooping cough due to Bordetella parapertussis

SP A37.10   Whooping cough due to Bordetella parapertussis without pneumonia

SP A37.11   Whooping cough due to Bordetella parapertussis with pneumonia

5 A37.8   Whooping cough due to other Bordetella species

---

4 4th digit required   **5** 5th digit required   **6** 6th digit required   **7** 7th digit required   **7** 7th digit placeholder   **+** Additional code   **⊟** Laterality

SP A37.80 Whooping cough due to other Bordetella species without pneumonia

SP A37.81 Whooping cough due to other Bordetella species with pneumonia

5 A37.9 Whooping cough, unspecified species

SP A37.90 Whooping cough, unspecified species without pneumonia

SP A37.91 Whooping cough, unspecified species with pneumonia

4 A38 Scarlet fever

> INCLUDES scarlatina
>
> EXCLUDES 2 streptococcal sore throat (J02.0)

SP A38.0 Scarlet fever with otitis media

> DEFINITION Infection with group A beta-hemolytic streptococcal bacteria causing sore throat, fever, and rough, bright red "sandpaper" rash over most of the body.

SP A38.1 Scarlet fever with myocarditis

SP A38.8 Scarlet fever with other complications

SP A38.9 Scarlet fever, uncomplicated
Scarlet fever, NOS

4 A39 Meningococcal infection

SP A39.0 Meningococcal meningitis

> DEFINITION Inflammation of the membranes (meninges) around the brain or spinal cord causing fever, headache, stiff neck, muscle aches, and skin rashes.

SP A39.1 Waterhouse-Friderichsen syndrome
Meningococcal hemorrhagic adrenalitis
Meningococcic adrenal syndrome

> DEFINITION Syndrome associated with meningococcal meningitis, marked by sudden fever, purple skin discoloration, and hemorrhage into the adrenal glands with cardiovascular collapse.

SP A39.2 Acute meningococcemia

SP A39.3 Chronic meningococcemia

SP A39.4 Meningococcemia, unspecified

5 A39.5 Meningococcal heart disease

SP A39.50 Meningococcal carditis, unspecified

SP A39.51 Meningococcal endocarditis

SP A39.52 Meningococcal myocarditis

SP A39.53 Meningococcal pericarditis

5 A39.8 Other meningococcal infections

SP A39.81 Meningococcal encephalitis

SP A39.82 Meningococcal retrobulbar neuritis

SP A39.83 Meningococcal arthritis

SP A39.84 Postmeningococcal arthritis

SP A39.89 Other meningococcal infections
Meningococcal conjunctivitis

SP A39.9 Meningococcal infection, unspecified
Meningococcal disease NOS

4 A40 Streptococcal sepsis
Code first:
> postprocedural streptococcal sepsis (T81.4-)
> streptococcal sepsis during labor (O75.3)
> streptococcal sepsis following abortion or ectopic or molar pregnancy (O03-O07, O08.0)
> streptococcal sepsis following immunization (T88.0)
> streptococcal sepsis following infusion, transfusion or therapeutic injection (T80.2-)

> EXCLUDES 1 neonatal (P36.0-P36.1)
> puerperal sepsis (O85)
> sepsis due to Streptococcus, group D (A41.81)

> GUIDELINES Section I.C.1.d.1)(a)(i-iii)
Negative or inconclusive blood cultures do not preclude a diagnosis of sepsis in patients with clinical evidence of the condition, however, the provider should be queried.

The term urosepsis is a nonspecific term. It is not to be considered synonymous with sepsis. It has no default code in the Alphabetic Index. Should a provider use this term, he/she must be queried for clarification.

If a patient has sepsis and associated acute organ dysfunction or multiple organ dysfunction (MOD), follow the instructions for coding severe sepsis.

> GUIDELINES Section I.C.1.d.1)(a)(iv)
If a patient has sepsis and an acute organ dysfunction, but the medical record documentation indicates that the acute organ dysfunction is related to a medical condition other than the sepsis, do not assign a code from subcategory R65.2, Severe sepsis. An acute organ dysfunction must be associated with the sepsis in order to assign the severe sepsis code. If the documentation is not clear as to whether an acute organ dysfunction is related to the sepsis or another medical condition, query the provider.

> CODING TIPS ✓ If sepsis is related to a medical or surgical procedure, the specific complication code is sequenced prior to the A40. A41 code. If a surgical wound becomes septic, sequence first T81.4-A for the wound infection, followed by T81.44xA.

> CODING TIPS ✓ When sepsis is present with a localized infection, such as UTI or pneumonia, sequence the sepsis and then the localized infection. The causative organism may be identified in the sepsis code, and therefore doesn't need to be repeated with the localized infection, except in the case of combination codes that identify the organism. Use the combination code for the pneumonia, if the localized infection is pneumonia.

> CODING TIPS ✓ Do not assign a code from A40-A41 to indicate a bacterial infection in conditions classified elsewhere, e.g., a localized infection. Codes classified in A40-A41 are used to indicate systemic infection.

★ New ▲ Revised Px Primary SP PDGM Px SL Low CoM SH High CoM IQ Quest. Encounter H Hospice non-cancer Dx Unspecified M *Manifestation*

CODING TIPS ✓   When assigning a code for sepsis, review clinical documentation to ensure the clinician has provided support for the diagnosis, as well as clearly documented the causative organism. While the organism may be clearly stated in the physician record, and the coder may use this to assign the correct code, the home health record should support the continued treatment of the unresolved infection as well as clearly state the causative organism (when known).

CODING TIPS ✓   Severe sepsis is defined as sepsis resulting in organ dysfunction or failure. If sepsis is associated with organ dysfunction or failure, add R65.2 to indicate severe sepsis. Severe sepsis is a complication ordinarily resolved prior to home care, so query the physician regarding the continued presence of severe sepsis at discharge from the inpatient facility. The organ dysfunction or failure should be added as a third code if organ dysfunction is related to the sepsis. R65.21 indicates the presence of septic shock which is considered organ dysfunction in and of itself.

SP A40.0 Sepsis due to streptococcus, group A

SP A40.1 Sepsis due to streptococcus, group B

SP A40.3 Sepsis due to Streptococcus pneumoniae
Pneumococcal sepsis

SP A40.8 Other streptococcal sepsis

SP A40.9 Streptococcal sepsis, unspecified

4 A41   Other sepsis
Code first:
postprocedural sepsis (T81.4-)
sepsis during labor (O75.3)
sepsis following abortion, ectopic or molar pregnancy (O03-O07, O08.0)
sepsis following immunization (T88.0)
sepsis following infusion, transfusion or therapeutic injection (T80.2-)
EXCLUDES 1 bacteremia NOS (R78.81)
neonatal (P36.-)
puerperal sepsis (O85)
streptococcal sepsis (A40.-)
EXCLUDES 2 sepsis (due to) (in) actinomycotic (A42.7)
sepsis (due to) (in) anthrax (A22.7)
sepsis (due to) (in) candidal (B37.7)
sepsis (due to) (in) Erysipelothrix (A26.7)
sepsis (due to) (in) extraintestinal yersiniosis (A28.2)
sepsis (due to) (in) gonococcal (A54.86)
sepsis (due to) (in) herpesviral (B00.7)
sepsis (due to) (in) listerial (A32.7)
sepsis (due to) (in) melioidosis (A24.1)
sepsis (due to) (in) meningococcal (A39.2-A39.4)
sepsis (due to) (in) plague (A20.7)

sepsis (due to) (in) tularemia (A21.7)
toxic shock syndrome (A48.3)

GUIDELINES   **Section I.C.1.d.1)(a)**
For a diagnosis of sepsis, assign the appropriate code for the underlying systemic infection. If the type of infection or causal organism is not further specified, assign code A41.9, Sepsis, unspecified organism. A code from subcategory R65.2, Severe sepsis, should not be assigned unless severe sepsis or an associated acute organ dysfunction is documented.

GUIDELINES   **Section I.C.1.d.1)(b)**
The coding of severe sepsis requires a minimum of two codes: first a code for the underlying systemic infection, followed by a code from subcategory R65.2, Severe sepsis. If the causal organism is not documented, assign code A41.9, Sepsis, unspecified organism, for the infection. Additional code(s) for the associated acute organ dysfunction are also required. Due to the complex nature of severe sepsis, some cases may require querying the provider prior to assignment of the codes.

CODING TIPS ✓   If sepsis is related to a medical or surgical procedure, the specific complication code is sequenced prior to the A40. A41 code. If a surgical wound becomes septic, sequence first T81.4-A for the wound infection, followed by T81.44xA.

CODING TIPS ✓   When sepsis is present with a localized infection, such as UTI or pneumonia, sequence the sepsis and then the localized infection. The causative organism may be identified in the sepsis code, and therefore doesn't need to be repeated with the localized infection, except in the case of combination codes that identify the organism. Use the combination code for the pneumonia, if the localized infection is pneumonia.

CODING TIPS ✓   When assigning a code for sepsis, review clinical documentation to ensure the clinician has provided support for the diagnosis, as well as clearly documented the causative organism. While the organism may be clearly stated in the physician record, and the coder may use this to assign the correct code, the home health record should support the continued treatment of the unresolved infection as well as clearly state the causative organism (when known).

CODING TIPS ✓   Do not assign a code from A40-A41 to indicate a bacterial infection in conditions classified elsewhere, e.g., a localized infection. Codes classified in A40-A41 are used to indicate systemic infection.

4 4th digit required   **5** 5th digit required   **6** 6th digit required   **7** 7th digit required   **7** 7th digit placeholder   **+** Additional code   **⊟** Laterality

610   *DecisionHealth's* FY 2020 Complete Home Health ICD-10-CM Diagnosis Coding Manual

CODING TIPS ✓ Severe sepsis is defined as sepsis resulting in organ dysfunction or failure. If sepsis is associated with organ dysfunction or failure, add R65.2 to indicate severe sepsis. Severe sepsis is a complication ordinarily resolved prior to home care, so query the physician regarding the continued presence of severe sepsis at discharge from the inpatient facility. The organ dysfunction or failure should be added as a third code if organ dysfunction is related to the sepsis. R65.21 indicates the presence of septic shock which is considered organ dysfunction in and of itself.

⑤ A41.0 **Sepsis due to Staphylococcus aureus**

SP A41.01 **Sepsis due to Methicillin susceptible Staphylococcus aureus**
MSSA sepsis
Staphylococcus aureus sepsis NOS
CODING TIPS ✓ Use this code when the Staph aureus causing the sepsis is not methicillin resistant.

SP A41.02 **Sepsis due to Methicillin resistant Staphylococcus aureus**
GUIDELINES Section I.C.1.e.1)(a). When a patient is diagnosed with an infection that is due to methicillin resistant Staphylococcus aureus (MRSA), and that infection has a combination code that includes the causal organism (e.g., sepsis, pneumonia) assign the appropriate combination code for the condition (e.g., code A41.02 ...). Do not assign code B95.62, Methicillin resistant Staphylococcus aureus infection as the cause of diseases classified elsewhere, as an additional code because the combination code includes the type of infection and the MRSA organism.

CODING TIPS ✓ Do not assign a Z16 code to indicate Staph aureus resistance to penicillins. Z16 codes may be added for other resistance, such as Vancomycin resistance, or when other bacteria other than Staphylococcus aureus are involved.

SP A41.1 **Sepsis due to other specified staphylococcus**
Coagulase negative staphylococcus sepsis

SP A41.2 **Sepsis due to unspecified staphylococcus**
CODING TIPS ✓ Use this code if sepsis is identified as caused by staph without specification as to species.

SP A41.3 **Sepsis due to Hemophilus influenzae**

SP A41.4 **Sepsis due to anaerobes**
EXCLUDES 1 gas gangrene (A48.0)

⑤ A41.5 **Sepsis due to other Gram-negative organisms**
SP A41.50 **Gram-negative sepsis, unspecified**
Gram-negative sepsis NOS
SP A41.51 **Sepsis due to Escherichia coli [E. coli]**
SP A41.52 **Sepsis due to Pseudomonas**
Pseudomonas aeroginosa

SP A41.53 **Sepsis due to Serratia**
SP A41.59 **Other Gram-negative sepsis**
⑤ A41.8 **Other specified sepsis**
SP A41.81 **Sepsis due to Enterococcus**
SP A41.89 **Other specified sepsis**
SP A41.9 **Sepsis, unspecified organism**
Septicemia NOS
CODING TIPS ✓ Septicemia is coded to A41.9 when the bacteria has not been identified. A41.9 is also acceptable for sepsis when the bacteria responsible has not been identified. The physician should be queried.

④ A42 **Actinomycosis**
EXCLUDES 1 actinomycetoma (B47.1)

SP A42.0 **Pulmonary actinomycosis**
SP A42.1 **Abdominal actinomycosis**
SP A42.2 **Cervicofacial actinomycosis**
SP A42.7 **Actinomycotic sepsis**
⑤ A42.8 **Other forms of actinomycosis**
SP A42.81 **Actinomycotic meningitis**
SP A42.82 **Actinomycotic encephalitis**
SP A42.89 **Other forms of actinomycosis**
SP A42.9 **Actinomycosis, unspecified**

④ A43 **Nocardiosis**
SP A43.0 **Pulmonary nocardiosis**
SP A43.1 **Cutaneous nocardiosis**
SP A43.8 **Other forms of nocardiosis**
SP A43.9 **Nocardiosis, unspecified**

④ A44 **Bartonellosis**
SP A44.0 **Systemic bartonellosis**
Oroya fever
SP A44.1 **Cutaneous and mucocutaneous bartonellosis**
Verruga peruana
SP A44.8 **Other forms of bartonellosis**
SP A44.9 **Bartonellosis, unspecified**

SP A46 **Erysipelas**
EXCLUDES 1 postpartum or puerperal erysipelas (O86.89)
DEFINITION Superficial cellulitis with dermal lymphatic involvement, commonly caused by group A beta-hemolytic streptococci; presents with shiny, raised, indurated, tender lesions with distinct margins, commonly on the legs and face.

④ A48 **Other bacterial diseases, not elsewhere classified**
EXCLUDES 1 actinomycetoma (B47.1)

SP A48.0 **Gas gangrene**
Clostridial cellulitis
Clostridial myonecrosis
CODING TIPS ✓ Gas gangrene is a medical emergency and is not the gangrene routinely coded in home care and hospice, known as dry gangrene. If gas gangrene is documented, there is an assumed relationship between diabetes and gas gangrene and A48.0 is coded after the appropriate code for diabetes with gangrene.

★ New ▲ Revised Px Primary **SP** PDGM Px **SL** Low CoM **SH** High CoM **IQ** Quest. Encounter **H** Hospice non-cancer Dx Unspecified **M** *Manifestation*

Chapter 1

A00 - B99

SP **A48.1** **Legionnaires' disease**

SP **A48.2** **Nonpneumonic Legionnaires' disease [Pontiac fever]**

SP ✚ **A48.3** **Toxic shock syndrome**
Use additional code to identify the organism (B95, B96)
> **EXCLUDES 1** endotoxic shock NOS (R57.8)
> sepsis NOS (A41.9)

SP **A48.4** **Brazilian purpuric fever**
Systemic Hemophilus aegyptius infection

5 **A48.5** **Other specified botulism**
Non-foodborne intoxication due to toxins of Clostridium botulinum [C. botulinum]
> **EXCLUDES 1** food poisoning due to toxins of Clostridium botulinum (A05.1)

SP **A48.51** **Infant botulism**

SP ✚ **A48.52** **Wound botulism**
Non-foodborne botulism NOS
Use additional code for associated wound
> **DEFINITION** Wound infection with Clostridium botulinum producing neurological effects of severe hypotonia and paralysis without gastrointestinal symptoms of food poisoning.

SP **A48.8** **Other specified bacterial diseases**

4 **A49** **Bacterial infection of unspecified site**
> **EXCLUDES 1** bacterial agents as the cause of diseases classified elsewhere (B95-B96)
> chlamydial infection NOS (A74.9)
> meningococcal infection NOS (A39.9)
> rickettsial infection NOS (A79.9)
> spirochetal infection NOS (A69.9)

> **CODING TIPS ✓** These codes indicate a bacterial infection in an unknown site. Do not use these codes to indicate bacterial infections. See A40-A41 for sepsis or B95 and B96 for causative organisms for localized infections (if a combination code does not apply).

5 **A49.0** **Staphylococcal infection, unspecified site**

!Q **A49.01** **Methicillin susceptible Staphylococcus aureus infection, unspecified site**
Methicillin susceptible Staphylococcus aureus (MSSA) infection
Staphylococcus aureus infection NOS

!Q **A49.02** **Methicillin resistant Staphylococcus aureus infection, unspecified site**
Methicillin resistant Staphylococcus aureus (MRSA) infection

!Q **A49.1** **Streptococcal infection, unspecified site**

!Q **A49.2** **Hemophilus influenzae infection, unspecified site**

!Q **A49.3** **Mycoplasma infection, unspecified site**

!Q **A49.8** **Other bacterial infections of unspecified site**

!Q **A49.9** **Bacterial infection, unspecified**
> **EXCLUDES 1** bacteremia NOS (R78.81)

Infections with a predominantly sexual mode of transmission (A50-A64)

> **EXCLUDES 1** human immunodeficiency virus [HIV] disease (B20)
> nonspecific and nongonococcal urethritis (N34.1)
> Reiter's disease (M02.3-)

4 **A50** **Congenital syphilis**

5 **A50.0** **Early congenital syphilis, symptomatic**
Any congenital syphilitic condition specified as early or manifest less than two years after birth.

SP **A50.01** **Early congenital syphilitic oculopathy**

SP **A50.02** **Early congenital syphilitic osteochondropathy**

SP **A50.03** **Early congenital syphilitic pharyngitis**
Early congenital syphilitic laryngitis

SP **A50.04** **Early congenital syphilitic pneumonia**

SP **A50.05** **Early congenital syphilitic rhinitis**

SP **A50.06** **Early cutaneous congenital syphilis**

SP **A50.07** **Early mucocutaneous congenital syphilis**

SP **A50.08** **Early visceral congenital syphilis**

SP **A50.09** **Other early congenital syphilis, symptomatic**

SP **A50.1** **Early congenital syphilis, latent**
Congenital syphilis without clinical manifestations, with positive serological reaction and negative spinal fluid test, less than two years after birth.

SP **A50.2** **Early congenital syphilis, unspecified**
Congenital syphilis NOS less than two years after birth.

5 **A50.3** **Late congenital syphilitic oculopathy**
> **EXCLUDES 1** Hutchinson's triad (A50.53)

SP **A50.30** **Late congenital syphilitic oculopathy, unspecified**

SP **A50.31** **Late congenital syphilitic interstitial keratitis**

SP **A50.32** **Late congenital syphilitic chorioretinitis**

SP **A50.39** **Other late congenital syphilitic oculopathy**

✚ **5** **A50.4** **Late congenital neurosyphilis [juvenile neurosyphilis]**
Use additional code to identify any associated mental disorder
> **EXCLUDES 1** Hutchinson's triad (A50.53)

SP ✚ **A50.40** **Late congenital neurosyphilis, unspecified**
Juvenile neurosyphilis NOS

SP ✚ **A50.41** **Late congenital syphilitic meningitis**

SP ✚ **A50.42** **Late congenital syphilitic encephalitis**

SP ✚ **A50.43** **Late congenital syphilitic polyneuropathy**

SP ✚ **A50.44** **Late congenital syphilitic optic nerve atrophy**

---

4 4th digit required   **5** 5th digit required   **6** 6th digit required   **7** 7th digit required   **7** 7th digit placeholder   ✚ Additional code   **⊟** Laterality

612   *DecisionHealth's* FY 2020 Complete Home Health ICD-10-CM Diagnosis Coding Manual

SP **+** **A50.45** **Juvenile general paresis**
Dementia paralytica juvenilis
Juvenile tabetoparetic neurosyphilis

SP **+** **A50.49** **Other late congenital neurosyphilis**
Juvenile tabes dorsalis

⑤ **A50.5** **Other late congenital syphilis, symptomatic**
Any congenital syphilitic condition specified as late or manifest two years or more after birth.

SP **A50.51** **Clutton's joints**

SP **A50.52** **Hutchinson's teeth**

SP **A50.53** **Hutchinson's triad**

SP **A50.54** **Late congenital cardiovascular syphilis**

SP **A50.55** **Late congenital syphilitic arthropathy**

SP **A50.56** **Late congenital syphilitic osteochondropathy**

SP **A50.57** **Syphilitic saddle nose**

SP **A50.59** **Other late congenital syphilis, symptomatic**

SP **A50.6** **Late congenital syphilis, latent**
Congenital syphilis without clinical manifestations, with positive serological reaction and negative spinal fluid test, two years or more after birth.

SP **A50.7** **Late congenital syphilis, unspecified**
Congenital syphilis NOS two years or more after birth.

SP **A50.9** **Congenital syphilis, unspecified**

④ **A51** **Early syphilis**

SP **A51.0** **Primary genital syphilis**
Syphilitic chancre NOS

SP **A51.1** **Primary anal syphilis**

SP **A51.2** **Primary syphilis of other sites**

⑤ **A51.3** **Secondary syphilis of skin and mucous membranes**

SP **A51.31** **Condyloma latum**

SP **A51.32** **Syphilitic alopecia**

SP **A51.39** **Other secondary syphilis of skin**
Syphilitic leukoderma
Syphilitic mucous patch
EXCLUDES 1 late syphilitic leukoderma (A52.79)

⑤ **A51.4** **Other secondary syphilis**

SP **A51.41** **Secondary syphilitic meningitis**

SP **A51.42** **Secondary syphilitic female pelvic disease**

SP **A51.43** **Secondary syphilitic oculopathy**
Secondary syphilitic chorioretinitis
Secondary syphilitic iridocyclitis, iritis
Secondary syphilitic uveitis

SP **A51.44** **Secondary syphilitic nephritis**

SP **A51.45** **Secondary syphilitic hepatitis**

SP **A51.46** **Secondary syphilitic osteopathy**

SP **A51.49** **Other secondary syphilitic conditions**
Secondary syphilitic lymphadenopathy
Secondary syphilitic myositis

SP **A51.5** **Early syphilis, latent**
Syphilis (acquired) without clinical manifestations, with positive serological reaction and negative spinal fluid test, less than two years after infection.

SP **A51.9** **Early syphilis, unspecified**

④ **A52** **Late syphilis**

⑤ **A52.0** **Cardiovascular and cerebrovascular syphilis**

SP **A52.00** **Cardiovascular syphilis, unspecified**

SP **A52.01** **Syphilitic aneurysm of aorta**

SP **A52.02** **Syphilitic aortitis**

SP **A52.03** **Syphilitic endocarditis**
Syphilitic aortic valve incompetence or stenosis
Syphilitic mitral valve stenosis
Syphilitic pulmonary valve regurgitation

SP **A52.04** **Syphilitic cerebral arteritis**

SP **A52.05** **Other cerebrovascular syphilis**
Syphilitic cerebral aneurysm (ruptured) (non-ruptured)
Syphilitic cerebral thrombosis

SP **A52.06** **Other syphilitic heart involvement**
Syphilitic coronary artery disease
Syphilitic myocarditis
Syphilitic pericarditis

SP **A52.09** **Other cardiovascular syphilis**

⑤ **A52.1** **Symptomatic neurosyphilis**

SP **A52.10** **Symptomatic neurosyphilis, unspecified**

SP **A52.11** **Tabes dorsalis**
Locomotor ataxia (progressive)
Tabetic neurosyphilis

SP **A52.12** **Other cerebrospinal syphilis**

SP **A52.13** **Late syphilitic meningitis**

SP **A52.14** **Late syphilitic encephalitis**

SP **A52.15** **Late syphilitic neuropathy**
Late syphilitic acoustic neuritis
Late syphilitic optic (nerve) atrophy
Late syphilitic polyneuropathy
Late syphilitic retrobulbar neuritis

SP **A52.16** **Charcôt's arthropathy (tabetic)**
CODING TIPS ✓ Use this code only for Charcot's foot caused by syphillis. Another code is not used to indicate the joint involved, etc. Do not use this code for Charcot's foot caused by other conditions.

SP **A52.17** **General paresis**
Dementia paralytica

SP **A52.19** **Other symptomatic neurosyphilis**
Syphilitic parkinsonism

SP **A52.2** **Asymptomatic neurosyphilis**

SP **A52.3** **Neurosyphilis, unspecified**
Gumma (syphilitic)
Syphilis (late)
Syphiloma

⑤ **A52.7** **Other symptomatic late syphilis**

SP **A52.71** **Late syphilitic oculopathy**
Late syphilitic chorioretinitis
Late syphilitic episcleritis

SP **A52.72** **Syphilis of lung and bronchus**

SP **A52.73** **Symptomatic late syphilis of other respiratory organs**

SP **A52.74** **Syphilis of liver and other viscera**
Late syphilitic peritonitis

SP **A52.75** **Syphilis of kidney and ureter**
Syphilitic glomerular disease

★ New ▲ Revised Px Primary SP PDGM Px SL Low CoM SH High CoM IQ Quest. Encounter H Hospice non-cancer Dx Unspecified M Manifestation

DecisionHealth's FY 2020 Complete Home Health ICD-10-CM Diagnosis Coding Manual

613

Chapter 1

A00 - B99

SP A52.76 **Other genitourinary symptomatic late syphilis**
Late syphilitic female pelvic inflammatory disease

SP A52.77 **Syphilis of bone and joint**

SP A52.78 **Syphilis of other musculoskeletal tissue**
Late syphilitic bursitis
Syphilis [stage unspecified] of bursa
Syphilis [stage unspecified] of muscle
Syphilis [stage unspecified] of synovium
Syphilis [stage unspecified] of tendon

SP A52.79 **Other symptomatic late syphilis**
Late syphilitic leukoderma
Syphilis of adrenal gland
Syphilis of pituitary gland
Syphilis of thyroid gland
Syphilitic splenomegaly
EXCLUDES 1 syphilitic leukoderma (secondary) (A51.39)

SP A52.8 **Late syphilis, latent**
Syphilis (acquired) without clinical manifestations, with positive serological reaction and negative spinal fluid test, two years or more after infection

SP A52.9 **Late syphilis, unspecified**

4 A53 **Other and unspecified syphilis**

SP A53.0 **Latent syphilis, unspecified as early or late**
Latent syphilis NOS
Positive serological reaction for syphilis

SP A53.9 **Syphilis, unspecified**
Infection due to Treponema pallidum NOS
Syphilis (acquired) NOS
EXCLUDES 1 syphilis NOS under two years of age (A50.2)

4 A54 **Gonococcal infection**

5 A54.0 **Gonococcal infection of lower genitourinary tract without periurethral or accessory gland abscess**
EXCLUDES 1 gonococcal infection with genitourinary gland abscess (A54.1)
gonococcal infection with periurethral abscess (A54.1)

SP A54.00 **Gonococcal infection of lower genitourinary tract, unspecified**

SP A54.01 **Gonococcal cystitis and urethritis, unspecified**

SP A54.02 **Gonococcal vulvovaginitis, unspecified**

SP A54.03 **Gonococcal cervicitis, unspecified**

SP A54.09 **Other gonococcal infection of lower genitourinary tract**

SP A54.1 **Gonococcal infection of lower genitourinary tract with periurethral and accessory gland abscess**
Gonococcal Bartholin's gland abscess

5 A54.2 **Gonococcal pelviperitonitis and other gonococcal genitourinary infection**

SP A54.21 **Gonococcal infection of kidney and ureter**

SP A54.22 **Gonococcal prostatitis**

SP A54.23 **Gonococcal infection of other male genital organs**
Gonococcal epididymitis
Gonococcal orchitis

SP A54.24 **Gonococcal female pelvic inflammatory disease**
Gonococcal pelviperitonitis
EXCLUDES 1 gonococcal peritonitis (A54.85)

SP A54.29 **Other gonococcal genitourinary infections**

5 A54.3 **Gonococcal infection of eye**

SP A54.30 **Gonococcal infection of eye, unspecified**

SP A54.31 **Gonococcal conjunctivitis**
Ophthalmia neonatorum due to gonococcus

SP A54.32 **Gonococcal iridocyclitis**

SP A54.33 **Gonococcal keratitis**

SP A54.39 **Other gonococcal eye infection**
Gonococcal endophthalmia

5 A54.4 **Gonococcal infection of musculoskeletal system**

SP A54.40 **Gonococcal infection of musculoskeletal system, unspecified**

SP A54.41 **Gonococcal spondylopathy**

SP A54.42 **Gonococcal arthritis**
EXCLUDES 2 gonococcal infection of spine (A54.41)

SP A54.43 **Gonococcal osteomyelitis**
EXCLUDES 2 gonococcal infection of spine (A54.41)

SP A54.49 **Gonococcal infection of other musculoskeletal tissue**
Gonococcal bursitis
Gonococcal myositis
Gonococcal synovitis
Gonococcal tenosynovitis

SP A54.5 **Gonococcal pharyngitis**

SP A54.6 **Gonococcal infection of anus and rectum**

5 A54.8 **Other gonococcal infections**

SP A54.81 **Gonococcal meningitis**

SP A54.82 **Gonococcal brain abscess**

SP A54.83 **Gonococcal heart infection**
Gonococcal endocarditis
Gonococcal myocarditis
Gonococcal pericarditis

SP A54.84 **Gonococcal pneumonia**

SP A54.85 **Gonococcal peritonitis**
EXCLUDES 1 gonococcal pelviperitonitis (A54.24)

SP A54.86 **Gonococcal sepsis**

SP A54.89 **Other gonococcal infections**
Gonococcal keratoderma
Gonococcal lymphadenitis

SP A54.9 **Gonococcal infection, unspecified**

SP A55 **Chlamydial lymphogranuloma (venereum)**
Climatic or tropical bubo
Durand-Nicolas-Favre disease
Esthiomene
Lymphogranuloma inguinale

4 4th digit required   **5** 5th digit required   **6** 6th digit required   **7** 7th digit required   **7** 7th digit placeholder   **+** Additional code   **⊟** Laterality

614   *DecisionHealth's* FY 2020 Complete Home Health ICD-10-CM Diagnosis Coding Manual

DEFINITION Sexually transmitted infection by Chlamydia trachomatis, seen in warm climates; presents with primary cutaneous or mucosal lesion at infection site and acute unilateral or bilateral lymphadenopathy.

4 A56 **Other sexually transmitted chlamydial diseases**

> **INCLUDES** sexually transmitted diseases due to Chlamydia trachomatis
>
> **EXCLUDES 1** neonatal chlamydial conjunctivitis (P39.1) neonatal chlamydial pneumonia (P23.1)
>
> **EXCLUDES 2** chlamydial lymphogranuloma (A55) conditions classified to A74.-

5 A56.0 **Chlamydial infection of lower genitourinary tract**

SP A56.00 **Chlamydial infection of lower genitourinary tract, unspecified**

SP A56.01 **Chlamydial cystitis and urethritis**

SP A56.02 **Chlamydial vulvovaginitis**

SP A56.09 **Other chlamydial infection of lower genitourinary tract**
Chlamydial cervicitis

5 A56.1 **Chlamydial infection of pelviperitoneum and other genitourinary organs**

SP A56.11 **Chlamydial female pelvic inflammatory disease**

SP A56.19 **Other chlamydial genitourinary infection**
Chlamydial epididymitis
Chlamydial orchitis

SP A56.2 **Chlamydial infection of genitourinary tract, unspecified**

SP A56.3 **Chlamydial infection of anus and rectum**

SP A56.4 **Chlamydial infection of pharynx**

SP A56.8 **Sexually transmitted chlamydial infection of other sites**

SP A57 **Chancroid**
Ulcus molle
> **DEFINITION** Sexually transmitted disease, characterized by a painful, primary ulcer, usually on the external genitalia.

SP A58 **Granuloma inguinale**
Donovanosis

4 A59 **Trichomoniasis**
> **EXCLUDES 2** intestinal trichomoniasis (A07.8)

5 A59.0 **Urogenital trichomoniasis**

SP A59.00 **Urogenital trichomoniasis, unspecified**
Fluor (vaginalis) due to Trichomonas
Leukorrhea (vaginalis) due to Trichomonas

SP A59.01 **Trichomonal vulvovaginitis**
> **DEFINITION** Sexually transmitted disease caused by the protozoan Trichomonas vaginalis infecting the vagina and external female genitalia.

SP A59.02 **Trichomonal prostatitis**

SP A59.03 **Trichomonal cystitis and urethritis**

SP A59.09 **Other urogenital trichomoniasis**

Trichomonas cervicitis

SP A59.8 **Trichomoniasis of other sites**

SP A59.9 **Trichomoniasis, unspecified**

4 A60 **Anogenital herpesviral [herpes simplex] infections**

5 A60.0 **Herpesviral infection of genitalia and urogenital tract**

SP A60.00 **Herpesviral infection of urogenital system, unspecified**

SP A60.01 **Herpesviral infection of penis**

SP A60.02 **Herpesviral infection of other male genital organs**

SP A60.03 **Herpesviral cervicitis**

SP A60.04 **Herpesviral vulvovaginitis**
Herpesviral [herpes simplex] ulceration
Herpesviral [herpes simplex] vaginitis
Herpesviral [herpes simplex] vulvitis

SP A60.09 **Herpesviral infection of other urogenital tract**

SP A60.1 **Herpesviral infection of perianal skin and rectum**

SP A60.9 **Anogenital herpesviral infection, unspecified**

4 A63 **Other predominantly sexually transmitted diseases, not elsewhere classified**
> **EXCLUDES 2** molluscum contagiosum (B08.1) papilloma of cervix (D26.0)

SP A63.0 **Anogenital (venereal) warts**
Anogenital warts due to (human) papillomavirus [HPV]
Condyloma acuminatum
> **DEFINITION** A wartlike growth on the skin or mucous membrane, in the area of the anus or external genitalia.

SP A63.8 **Other specified predominantly sexually transmitted diseases**

IQ A64 **Unspecified sexually transmitted disease**

Other spirochetal diseases (A65-A69)

> **EXCLUDES 2** leptospirosis (A27.-) syphilis (A50-A53)

SP A65 **Nonvenereal syphilis**
Bejel
Endemic syphilis
Njovera

4 A66 **Yaws**
> **INCLUDES** bouba
> frambesia (tropica)
> pian

SP A66.0 **Initial lesions of yaws**
Chancre of yaws
Frambesia, initial or primary
Initial frambesial ulcer
Mother yaw

SP A66.1 **Multiple papillomata and wet crab yaws**
Frambesioma
Pianoma
Plantar or palmar papilloma of yaws

SP A66.2 **Other early skin lesions of yaws**
Cutaneous yaws, less than five years after infection
Early yaws (cutaneous)(macular)(maculopapular)(micropapular)(papular)
Frambeside of early yaws

★ New ▲ Revised Px Primary SP PDGM Px SL Low CoM SH High CoM IQ Quest. Encounter H Hospice non-cancer Dx Unspecified M *Manifestation*

DecisionHealth's FY 2020 Complete Home Health ICD-10-CM Diagnosis Coding Manual

615

SP A66.3 Hyperkeratosis of yaws
Ghoul hand
Hyperkeratosis, palmar or plantar (early) (late) due to yaws
Worm-eaten soles

SP A66.4 Gummata and ulcers of yaws
Gummatous frambeside
Nodular late yaws (ulcerated)

SP A66.5 Gangosa
Rhinopharyngitis mutilans

SP A66.6 Bone and joint lesions of yaws
Yaws ganglion
Yaws goundou
Yaws gumma, bone
Yaws gummatous osteitis or periostitis
Yaws hydrarthrosis
Yaws osteitis
Yaws periostitis (hypertrophic)

SP A66.7 Other manifestations of yaws
Juxta-articular nodules of yaws
Mucosal yaws

SP A66.8 Latent yaws
Yaws without clinical manifestations, with positive serology

SP A66.9 Yaws, unspecified

4 A67 Pinta [carate]

SP A67.0 Primary lesions of pinta
Chancre (primary) of pinta
Papule (primary) of pinta

SP A67.1 Intermediate lesions of pinta
Erythematous plaques of pinta
Hyperchromic lesions of pinta
Hyperkeratosis of pinta
Pintids

SP A67.2 Late lesions of pinta
Achromic skin lesions of pinta
Cicatricial skin lesions of pinta
Dyschromic skin lesions of pinta

SP A67.3 Mixed lesions of pinta
Achromic with hyperchromic skin lesions of pinta [carate]

SP A67.9 Pinta, unspecified

4 A68 Relapsing fevers
| INCLUDES | recurrent fever |
| EXCLUDES 2 | Lyme disease (A69.2-) |

SP A68.0 Louse-borne relapsing fever
Relapsing fever due to Borrelia recurrentis

SP A68.1 Tick-borne relapsing fever
Relapsing fever due to any Borrelia species other than Borrelia recurrentis

SP A68.9 Relapsing fever, unspecified

4 A69 Other spirochetal infections

SP A69.0 Necrotizing ulcerative stomatitis
Cancrum oris
Fusospirochetal gangrene
Noma
Stomatitis gangrenosa

SP A69.1 Other Vincent's infections
Fusospirochetal pharyngitis
Necrotizing ulcerative (acute) gingivitis
Necrotizing ulcerative (acute) gingivostomatitis
Spirochetal stomatitis
Trench mouth
Vincent's angina
Vincent's gingivitis

5 A69.2 Lyme disease
Erythema chronicum migrans due to Borrelia burgdorferi

CODING TIPS ✓ A69.2 codes include 5th characters to include the complications of Lyme disease, and no additional codes for the assorted complications are necessary.

DEFINITION Tick-transmitted infection caused by Borrelia burgdorferi, manifesting with erythema chronicum migrans, myalgia, arthritis of the large joints, and nervous and cardiovascular system involvement.

SP A69.20 Lyme disease, unspecified

SP A69.21 Meningitis due to Lyme disease

SP A69.22 Other neurologic disorders in Lyme disease
Cranial neuritis
Meningoencephalitis
Polyneuropathy

SP A69.23 Arthritis due to Lyme disease

SP A69.29 Other conditions associated with Lyme disease
Myopericarditis due to Lyme disease

SP A69.8 Other specified spirochetal infections

SP A69.9 Spirochetal infection, unspecified

Other diseases caused by chlamydiae (A70-A74)

| EXCLUDES 1 | sexually transmitted chlamydial diseases (A55-A56) |

SP A70 Chlamydia psittaci infections
Ornithosis
Parrot fever
Psittacosis

4 A71 Trachoma
| EXCLUDES 1 | sequelae of trachoma (B94.0) |

CODING TIPS ✓ When coding category A71, physician notes may state "granular conjunctivitis" or 'Egyptian ophthalmia." Use B94.0 for sequelae of trachoma.

SP A71.0 Initial stage of trachoma
Trachoma dubium

SP A71.1 Active stage of trachoma
Granular conjunctivitis (trachomatous)
Trachomatous follicular conjunctivitis
Trachomatous pannus

SP A71.9 Trachoma, unspecified

4 A74 Other diseases caused by chlamydiae
| EXCLUDES 1 | neonatal chlamydial conjunctivitis (P39.1) neonatal chlamydial pneumonia (P23.1) Reiter's disease (M02.3-) sexually transmitted chlamydial diseases (A55-A56) |
| EXCLUDES 2 | chlamydial pneumonia (J16.0) |

SP A74.0 Chlamydial conjunctivitis
Paratrachoma

5 A74.8 Other chlamydial diseases

SP A74.81 Chlamydial peritonitis

SP A74.89 Other chlamydial diseases

SP A74.9 Chlamydial infection, unspecified
Chlamydiosis NOS

---

4 4th digit required   5 5th digit required   6 6th digit required   7 7th digit required   7 7th digit placeholder   + Additional code   ⊟ Laterality

Rickettsioses (A75-A79)

A75 Typhus fever
> EXCLUDES 1   rickettsiosis due to Ehrlichia sennetsu (A79.81)

SP A75.0 Epidemic louse-borne typhus fever due to Rickettsia prowazekii
Classical typhus (fever)
Epidemic (louse-borne) typhus

SP A75.1 Recrudescent typhus [Brill's disease]
Brill-Zinsser disease

SP A75.2 Typhus fever due to Rickettsia typhi
Murine (flea-borne) typhus

SP A75.3 Typhus fever due to Rickettsia tsutsugamushi
Scrub (mite-borne) typhus
Tsutsugamushi fever

SP A75.9 Typhus fever, unspecified
Typhus (fever) NOS

A77 Spotted fever [tick-borne rickettsioses]

SP A77.0 Spotted fever due to Rickettsia rickettsii
Rocky Mountain spotted fever
Sao Paulo fever

SP A77.1 Spotted fever due to Rickettsia conorii
African tick typhus
Boutonneuse fever
India tick typhus
Kenya tick typhus
Marseilles fever
Mediterranean tick fever

SP A77.2 Spotted fever due to Rickettsia siberica
North Asian tick fever
Siberian tick typhus

SP A77.3 Spotted fever due to Rickettsia australis
Queensland tick typhus

A77.4 Ehrlichiosis
> EXCLUDES 1   Rickettsiosis due to Ehrlichia sennetsu (A79.81)

SP A77.40 Ehrlichiosis, unspecified

SP A77.41 Ehrlichiosis chafeensis [E. chafeensis]

SP A77.49 Other ehrlichiosis

SP A77.8 Other spotted fevers

SP A77.9 Spotted fever, unspecified
Tick-borne typhus NOS

SP A78 Q fever
Infection due to Coxiella burnetii
Nine Mile fever
Quadrilateral fever

A79 Other rickettsioses

SP A79.0 Trench fever
Quintan fever
Wolhynian fever

SP A79.1 Rickettsialpox due to Rickettsia akari
Kew Garden fever
Vesicular rickettsiosis

A79.8 Other specified rickettsioses

SP A79.81 Rickettsiosis due to Ehrlichia sennetsu

SP A79.89 Other specified rickettsioses

SP A79.9 Rickettsiosis, unspecified
Rickettsial infection NOS

Viral and prion infections of the central nervous system (A80-A89)

> EXCLUDES 1   postpolio syndrome (G14)
> sequelae of poliomyelitis (B91)
> sequelae of viral encephalitis (B94.1)

A80 Acute poliomyelitis
> CODING TIPS ✓   Assign a code from category A80 to indicate acute poliomyelitis, not a sequela of polio, or post polio syndrome. A80- codes are used to report acute, active poliomyelitis only. Use B91 for sequelae of polio, or G14 for post polio syndrome, which must be documented by the physician.

SP A80.0 Acute paralytic poliomyelitis, vaccine-associated

SP A80.1 Acute paralytic poliomyelitis, wild virus, imported

SP A80.2 Acute paralytic poliomyelitis, wild virus, indigenous

A80.3 Acute paralytic poliomyelitis, other and unspecified

SP A80.30 Acute paralytic poliomyelitis, unspecified

SP A80.39 Other acute paralytic poliomyelitis

SP A80.4 Acute nonparalytic poliomyelitis

SP A80.9 Acute poliomyelitis, unspecified

+ A81 Atypical virus infections of central nervous system
> INCLUDES   diseases of the central nervous system caused by prions
> Use additional code to identify:
> dementia with behavioral disturbance (F02.81)
> dementia without behavioral disturbance (F02.80)

+ A81.0 Creutzfeldt-Jakob disease
> DEFINITION   Degenerative neural disease caused by a prion (an infectious protein); presents with loss of muscular control, balance, and memory, twitching movements, nervousness and agitation, changes in personality, and dementia.

SP + A81.00 Creutzfeldt-Jakob disease, unspecified
Jakob-Creutzfeldt disease, unspecified

SP + A81.01 Variant Creutzfeldt-Jakob disease
vCJD
> DEFINITION   Rare, transmissible form of fatal Jakob-Creutzfeldt disease, affecting younger people with a longer duration, causing spongiform degeneration of the brain with unusual psychiatric and sensory symptoms.

SP + A81.09 Other Creutzfeldt-Jakob disease
CJD
Familial Creutzfeldt-Jakob disease
Iatrogenic Creutzfeldt-Jakob disease
Sporadic Creutzfeldt-Jakob disease
Subacute spongiform encephalopathy (with dementia)

SP + A81.1 Subacute sclerosing panencephalitis
Dawson's inclusion body encephalitis
Van Bogaert's sclerosing leukoencephalopathy

★ New ▲ Revised   Px Primary   SP PDGM Px   SL Low CoM   SH High CoM   IQ Quest. Encounter   H Hospice non-cancer Dx   Unspecified   M Manifestation

DecisionHealth's FY 2020 Complete Home Health ICD-10-CM Diagnosis Coding Manual   617

Chapter 1

A00 - B99

SP + A81.2 Progressive multifocal leukoencephalopathy
Multifocal leukoencephalopathy NOS

+ 5 A81.8 Other atypical virus infections of central nervous system

SP + A81.81 Kuru

SP + A81.82 Gerstmann-Sträussler-Scheinker syndrome
GSS syndrome

> **DEFINITION**   Extremely rare, inherited, fatal disease of the brain that progresses slowly, causing lack of muscle coordination, unsteady gait, dementia, slurred speech, spasticity, and coma before death.

SP + A81.83 Fatal familial insomnia
FFI

> **DEFINITION**   Very rare, inherited brain disease caused by prion protein mutation from soluble to insoluble, resulting in plaques forming in the thalamus, causing insomnia that progresses to dementia, unresponsiveness, and death.

SP + A81.89 Other atypical virus infections of central nervous system

SP + A81.9 Atypical virus infection of central nervous system, unspecified
Prion diseases of the central nervous system NOS

4 A82 Rabies

SP A82.0 Sylvatic rabies

SP A82.1 Urban rabies

SP A82.9 Rabies, unspecified

4 A83 Mosquito-borne viral encephalitis
> **INCLUDES**   mosquito-borne viral meningoencephalitis
> **EXCLUDES 2**   Venezuelan equine encephalitis (A92.2)
> West Nile fever (A92.3-)
> West Nile virus (A92.3-)

SP A83.0 Japanese encephalitis

SP A83.1 Western equine encephalitis

SP A83.2 Eastern equine encephalitis

SP A83.3 St Louis encephalitis

SP A83.4 Australian encephalitis
Kunjin virus disease

SP A83.5 California encephalitis
California meningoencephalitis
La Crosse encephalitis

SP A83.6 Rocio virus disease

SP A83.8 Other mosquito-borne viral encephalitis

SP A83.9 Mosquito-borne viral encephalitis, unspecified

4 A84 Tick-borne viral encephalitis
> **INCLUDES**   tick-borne viral meningoencephalitis

SP A84.0 Far Eastern tick-borne encephalitis [Russian spring-summer encephalitis]

SP A84.1 Central European tick-borne encephalitis

SP A84.8 Other tick-borne viral encephalitis
Louping ill
Powassan virus disease

SP A84.9 Tick-borne viral encephalitis, unspecified

4 A85 Other viral encephalitis, not elsewhere classified
> **INCLUDES**   specified viral encephalomyelitis NEC
> specified viral meningoencephalitis NEC
> **EXCLUDES 1**   benign myalgic encephalomyelitis (G93.3)
> encephalitis due to cytomegalovirus (B25.8)
> encephalitis due to herpesvirus NEC (B10.0-)
> encephalitis due to herpesvirus [herpes simplex] (B00.4)
> encephalitis due to measles virus (B05.0)
> encephalitis due to mumps virus (B26.2)
> encephalitis due to poliomyelitis virus (A80.-)
> encephalitis due to zoster (B02.0)
> lymphocytic choriomeningitis (A87.2)

SP A85.0 Enteroviral encephalitis
Enteroviral encephalomyelitis

SP A85.1 Adenoviral encephalitis
Adenoviral meningoencephalitis

SP A85.2 Arthropod-borne viral encephalitis, unspecified
> **EXCLUDES 1**   West nile virus with encephalitis (A92.31)

SP A85.8 Other specified viral encephalitis
Encephalitis lethargica
Von Economo-Cruchet disease

SP A86 Unspecified viral encephalitis
Viral encephalomyelitis NOS
Viral meningoencephalitis NOS

4 A87 Viral meningitis
> **EXCLUDES 1**   meningitis due to herpesvirus [herpes simplex] (B00.3)
> meningitis due to herpesvirus [herpes simplex] (B00.3)
> meningitis due to measles virus (B05.1)
> meningitis due to mumps virus (B26.1)
> meningitis due to poliomyelitis virus (A80.-)
> meningitis due to zoster (B02.1)

SP A87.0 Enteroviral meningitis
Coxsackievirus meningitis
Echovirus meningitis

SP A87.1 Adenoviral meningitis

SP A87.2 Lymphocytic choriomeningitis
Lymphocytic meningoencephalitis

SP A87.8 Other viral meningitis

SP A87.9 Viral meningitis, unspecified

4 A88 Other viral infections of central nervous system, not elsewhere classified
> **EXCLUDES 1**   viral encephalitis NOS (A86)
> viral meningitis NOS (A87.9)

SP A88.0 Enteroviral exanthematous fever [Boston exanthem]

---

4 4th digit required   5 5th digit required   6 6th digit required   7 7th digit required   7 7th digit placeholder   + Additional code   5 Laterality

618   *DecisionHealth's* FY 2020 Complete Home Health ICD-10-CM Diagnosis Coding Manual

SP A88.1 Epidemic vertigo

SP A88.8 Other specified viral infections of central nervous system

SP A89 Unspecified viral infection of central nervous system

Arthropod-borne viral fevers and viral hemorrhagic fevers   (A90-A99)

SP A90 Dengue fever [classical dengue]
> **EXCLUDES 1**   dengue hemorrhagic fever (A91)

SP A91 Dengue hemorrhagic fever

4 A92 Other mosquito-borne viral fevers
> **EXCLUDES 1**   Ross River disease (B33.1)

SP A92.0 Chikungunya virus disease
Chikungunya (hemorrhagic) fever

SP A92.1 O'nyong-nyong fever

SP A92.2 Venezuelan equine fever
Venezuelan equine encephalitis
Venezuelan equine encephalomyelitis virus disease

5 A92.3 West Nile virus infection
West Nile fever

SP A92.30 West Nile virus infection, unspecified
West Nile fever NOS
West Nile fever without complications
West Nile virus NOS

SP A92.31 West Nile virus infection with encephalitis
West Nile encephalitis
West Nile encephalomyelitis

SP + A92.32 West Nile virus infection with other neurologic manifestation
Use additional code to specify the neurologic manifestation

SP + A92.39 West Nile virus infection with other complications
Use additional code to specify the other conditions

SP A92.4 Rift Valley fever

SP A92.5 Zika virus disease
Zika virus fever
Zika virus infection
Zika NOS
> **EXCLUDES 1**   congenital Zika virus disease (P35.4)

> **CODING TIPS ✓**   Zika virus must be documented by the physician. Suspected or probable Zika should not be coded as Zika. In that case, code the symptoms/signs experienced by the patient.

> **DEFINITION**   Disease caused by infection with the Zika virus most commonly presents with fever, rash, joint pain, reddening of the eyes, muscle pain, and headache. Zika viral infection is primarily spread by the bite of infected mosquitoes.

SP A92.8 Other specified mosquito-borne viral fevers

SP A92.9 Mosquito-borne viral fever, unspecified

4 A93 Other arthropod-borne viral fevers, not elsewhere classified

SP A93.0 Oropouche virus disease
Oropouche fever

SP A93.1 Sandfly fever
Pappataci fever
Phlebotomus fever

SP A93.2 Colorado tick fever

SP A93.8 Other specified arthropod-borne viral fevers
Piry virus disease
Vesicular stomatitis virus disease [Indiana fever]

SP A94 Unspecified arthropod-borne viral fever
Arboviral fever NOS
Arbovirus infection NOS

4 A95 Yellow fever

SP A95.0 Sylvatic yellow fever
Jungle yellow fever

SP A95.1 Urban yellow fever

SP A95.9 Yellow fever, unspecified

4 A96 Arenaviral hemorrhagic fever

SP A96.0 Junin hemorrhagic fever
Argentinian hemorrhagic fever

SP A96.1 Machupo hemorrhagic fever
Bolivian hemorrhagic fever

SP A96.2 Lassa fever

SP A96.8 Other arenaviral hemorrhagic fevers

SP A96.9 Arenaviral hemorrhagic fever, unspecified

4 A98 Other viral hemorrhagic fevers, not elsewhere classified
> **EXCLUDES 1**   chikungunya hemorrhagic fever (A92.0)
> dengue hemorrhagic fever (A91)

SP A98.0 Crimean-Congo hemorrhagic fever
Central Asian hemorrhagic fever

SP A98.1 Omsk hemorrhagic fever

SP A98.2 Kyasanur Forest disease

SP A98.3 Marburg virus disease

SP A98.4 Ebola virus disease

SP A98.5 Hemorrhagic fever with renal syndrome
Epidemic hemorrhagic fever
Korean hemorrhagic fever
Russian hemorrhagic fever
Hantaan virus disease
Hantavirus disease with renal manifestations
Nephropathia epidemica
Songo fever
> **EXCLUDES 1**   hantavirus (cardio)-pulmonary syndrome (B33.4)

SP A98.8 Other specified viral hemorrhagic fevers

SP A99 Unspecified viral hemorrhagic fever

Viral infections characterized by skin and mucous membrane lesions   (B00-B09)

4 B00 Herpesviral [herpes simplex] infections
> **EXCLUDES 1**   congenital herpesviral infections (P35.2)
> **EXCLUDES 2**   anogenital herpesviral infection (A60.-)
> gammaherpesviral mononucleosis (B27.0-)
> herpangina (B08.5)

★ New ▲ Revised Px Primary **SP** PDGM Px **SL** Low CoM **SH** High CoM **IQ** Quest. Encounter **H** Hospice non-cancer Dx   Unspecified   **M** *Manifestation*

Chapter 1

A00 - B99

CODING TIPS ✓ Conditions classified to B00 are due to herpes simplex virus, not those due to herpes zoster virus (such as shingles). Category B02- includes infections due to herpes zoster virus.

SP B00.0 Eczema herpeticum
Kaposi's varicelliform eruption

DEFINITION Potentially fatal infection with the herpes simplex virus at the site of an existing skin condition, often atopic dermatitis, causing severe rash, fever, and fatigue.

SP B00.1 Herpesviral vesicular dermatitis
Herpes simplex facialis
Herpes simplex labialis
Herpes simplex otitis externa
Vesicular dermatitis of ear
Vesicular dermatitis of lip

SP B00.2 Herpesviral gingivostomatitis and pharyngotonsillitis
Herpesviral pharyngitis

SP B00.3 Herpesviral meningitis

SP B00.4 Herpesviral encephalitis
Herpesviral meningoencephalitis
Simian B disease

EXCLUDES 1 herpesviral encephalitis due to herpesvirus 6 and 7 (B10.01, B10.09)
non-simplex herpesviral encephalitis (B10.0-)

5 B00.5 Herpesviral ocular disease

SP B00.50 Herpesviral ocular disease, unspecified

SP B00.51 Herpesviral iridocyclitis
Herpesviral iritis
Herpesviral uveitis, anterior

SP B00.52 Herpesviral keratitis
Herpesviral keratoconjunctivitis

SP B00.53 Herpesviral conjunctivitis

SP B00.59 Other herpesviral disease of eye
Herpesviral dermatitis of eyelid

SP B00.7 Disseminated herpesviral disease
Herpesviral sepsis

5 B00.8 Other forms of herpesviral infections

SP B00.81 Herpesviral hepatitis

SP B00.82 Herpes simplex myelitis

SP B00.89 Other herpesviral infection
Herpesviral whitlow

DEFINITION Viral infection that results in a painful, blistery eruption on one of the digits.

SP B00.9 Herpesviral infection, unspecified
Herpes simplex infection NOS

4 B01 Varicella [chickenpox]

SP B01.0 Varicella meningitis

5 B01.1 Varicella encephalitis, myelitis and encephalomyelitis
Postchickenpox encephalitis, myelitis and encephalomyelitis

SP B01.11 Varicella encephalitis and encephalomyelitis
Postchickenpox encephalitis and encephalomyelitis

SP B01.12 Varicella myelitis
Postchickenpox myelitis

SP B01.2 Varicella pneumonia

5 B01.8 Varicella with other complications

SP B01.81 Varicella keratitis

SP B01.89 Other varicella complications

SP B01.9 Varicella without complication
Varicella NOS

4 B02 Zoster [herpes zoster]
INCLUDES shingles
zona

SP B02.0 Zoster encephalitis
Zoster meningoencephalitis

SP B02.1 Zoster meningitis

5 B02.2 Zoster with other nervous system involvement

SP B02.21 Postherpetic geniculate ganglionitis

SP B02.22 Postherpetic trigeminal neuralgia

SP B02.23 Postherpetic polyneuropathy

SP B02.24 Postherpetic myelitis
Herpes zoster myelitis

SP B02.29 Other postherpetic nervous system involvement
Postherpetic radiculopathy

5 B02.3 Zoster ocular disease

SP B02.30 Zoster ocular disease, unspecified

SP B02.31 Zoster conjunctivitis

SP B02.32 Zoster iridocyclitis

SP B02.33 Zoster keratitis
Herpes zoster keratoconjunctivitis

SP B02.34 Zoster scleritis

SP B02.39 Other herpes zoster eye disease
Zoster blepharitis

SP B02.7 Disseminated zoster

SP B02.8 Zoster with other complications
Herpes zoster otitis externa

SP B02.9 Zoster without complications
Zoster NOS

IQ B03 Smallpox
Note:
In 1980 the 33rd World Health Assembly declared that smallpox had been eradicated. The classification is maintained for surveillance purposes.

SP B04 Monkeypox

4 B05 Measles
INCLUDES morbilli
EXCLUDES 1 subacute sclerosing panencephalitis (A81.1)

SP B05.0 Measles complicated by encephalitis
Postmeasles encephalitis

SP B05.1 Measles complicated by meningitis
Postmeasles meningitis

SP B05.2 Measles complicated by pneumonia
Postmeasles pneumonia

SP B05.3 Measles complicated by otitis media
Postmeasles otitis media

SP B05.4 Measles with intestinal complications

5 B05.8 Measles with other complications

SP B05.81 Measles keratitis and keratoconjunctivitis

SP B05.89 Other measles complications

SP B05.9 Measles without complication
Measles NOS

4 B06 Rubella [German measles]

---

4 4th digit required **5** 5th digit required **6** 6th digit required **7** 7th digit required **☑** 7th digit placeholder **+** Additional code **⊟** Laterality

EXCLUDES 1 congenital rubella (P35.0)

5 B06.0 Rubella with neurological complications

SP B06.00 Rubella with neurological complication, unspecified

SP B06.01 Rubella encephalitis
Rubella meningoencephalitis

SP B06.02 Rubella meningitis

SP B06.09 Other neurological complications of rubella

5 B06.8 Rubella with other complications

SP B06.81 Rubella pneumonia

SP B06.82 Rubella arthritis

SP B06.89 Other rubella complications

SP B06.9 Rubella without complication
Rubella NOS

4 B07 Viral warts
INCLUDES verruca simplex
verruca vulgaris
viral warts due to human papillomavirus
EXCLUDES 2 anogenital (venereal) warts (A63.0)
papilloma of bladder (D41.4)
papilloma of cervix (D26.0)
papilloma larynx (D14.1)

SP B07.0 Plantar wart
Verruca plantaris
DEFINITION Noncancerous skin growths on the soles of the feet, often under pressure points, caused by the human papilloma virus that enters through tiny cuts or cracks in the skin.

SP B07.8 Other viral warts
Common wart
Flat wart
Verruca plana

SP B07.9 Viral wart, unspecified

4 B08 Other viral infections characterized by skin and mucous membrane lesions, not elsewhere classified
EXCLUDES 1 vesicular stomatitis virus disease (A93.8)

5 B08.0 Other orthopoxvirus infections
EXCLUDES 2 monkeypox (B04)

6 B08.01 Cowpox and vaccinia not from vaccine

SP B08.010 Cowpox

SP B08.011 Vaccinia not from vaccine
EXCLUDES 1 vaccinia (from vaccination) (generalized) (T88.1)

SP B08.02 Orf virus disease
Contagious pustular dermatitis
Ecthyma contagiosum
DEFINITION Skin disease closely related to smallpox, manifesting with localized, small, red, fluid-filled pustules that scab and heal, providing immunity to smallpox.

SP B08.03 Pseudocowpox [milker's node]

SP B08.04 Paravaccinia, unspecified

SP B08.09 Other orthopoxvirus infections
Orthopoxvirus infection NOS

SP B08.1 Molluscum contagiosum

5 B08.2 Exanthema subitum [sixth disease]
Roseola infantum

SP B08.20 Exanthema subitum [sixth disease], unspecified
Roseola infantum, unspecified
DEFINITION Common childhood herpes viral illness of mild upper respiratory symptoms, swollen glands, high fever lasting 3-7 days ending abruptly, followed by a rash.

SP B08.21 Exanthema subitum [sixth disease] due to human herpesvirus 6
Roseola infantum due to human herpesvirus 6

SP B08.22 Exanthema subitum [sixth disease] due to human herpesvirus 7
Roseola infantum due to human herpesvirus 7

SP B08.3 Erythema infectiosum [fifth disease]
DEFINITION A mild infectious disease occurring mainly in early childhood, marked by a rosy-red rash on the cheeks, often spreading to the trunk and limbs. Fever and arthritis may also be present.

SP B08.4 Enteroviral vesicular stomatitis with exanthem
Hand, foot and mouth disease

SP B08.5 Enteroviral vesicular pharyngitis
Herpangina

5 B08.6 Parapoxvirus infections

SP B08.60 Parapoxvirus infection, unspecified

SP B08.61 Bovine stomatitis

SP B08.62 Sealpox

SP B08.69 Other parapoxvirus infections

5 B08.7 Yatapoxvirus infections

SP B08.70 Yatapoxvirus infection, unspecified

SP B08.71 Tanapox virus disease

SP B08.72 Yaba pox virus disease
Yaba monkey tumor disease

SP B08.79 Other yatapoxvirus infections

SP B08.8 Other specified viral infections characterized by skin and mucous membrane lesions
Enteroviral lymphonodular pharyngitis
Foot-and-mouth disease
Poxvirus NEC

SP B09 Unspecified viral infection characterized by skin and mucous membrane lesions
Viral enanthema NOS
Viral exanthema NOS

Other human herpesviruses (B10)

4 B10 Other human herpesviruses
EXCLUDES 2 cytomegalovirus (B25.9)
Epstein-Barr virus (B27.0-)
herpes NOS (B00.9)
herpes simplex (B00.-)
herpes zoster (B02.-)
human herpesvirus NOS (B00.-)
human herpesvirus 1 and 2 (B00.-)

★New ▲Revised Px Primary SP PDGM Px SL Low CoM SH High CoM IQ Quest. Encounter H Hospice non-cancer Dx   Unspecified   M *Manifestation*

Chapter 1

A00 - B99

human herpesvirus 3
(B01.-, B02.-)
human herpesvirus 4 (B27.0-)
human herpesvirus 5 (B25.-)
varicella (B01.-)
zoster (B02.-)

5 B10.0 Other human herpesvirus encephalitis
EXCLUDES 2   herpes encephalitis NOS
(B00.4)
herpes simplex encephalitis
(B00.4)
human herpesvirus
encephalitis (B00.4)
simian B herpes virus
encephalitis (B00.4)

SP B10.01 Human herpesvirus 6 encephalitis

**SP B10.09 Other human herpesvirus
encephalitis**
Human herpesvirus 7 encephalitis

5 B10.8 Other human herpesvirus infection

SP B10.81 Human herpesvirus 6 infection

SP B10.82 Human herpesvirus 7 infection

SP B10.89 Other human herpesvirus infection
Human herpesvirus 8 infection
Kaposi's sarcoma-associated
herpesvirus infection

Viral hepatitis   (B15-B19)

EXCLUDES 1   sequelae of viral hepatitis (B94.2)
EXCLUDES 2   cytomegaloviral hepatitis (B25.1)
herpesviral [herpes simplex] hepatitis (B00.81)

CODING TIPS ✓   When viral hepatitis is also documented as a
confirmed diagnosis in a patient with any diagnosis classifiable
to K74.-, the appropriate code from B15-B19 should also be
assigned. The sequencing of the K74.- and the viral hepatitis
code is according to focus of care.

4 B15   Acute hepatitis A

SP B15.0 Hepatitis A with hepatic coma

SP B15.9 Hepatitis A without hepatic coma
Hepatitis A (acute)(viral) NOS

4 B16   Acute hepatitis B

**SP B16.0 Acute hepatitis B with delta-agent with
hepatic coma**

**SP B16.1 Acute hepatitis B with delta-agent
without hepatic coma**

**SP B16.2 Acute hepatitis B without delta-agent
with hepatic coma**

**SP B16.9 Acute hepatitis B without delta-agent
and without hepatic coma**
Hepatitis B (acute) (viral) NOS

4 B17   Other acute viral hepatitis

**SP B17.0 Acute delta-(super) infection of hepatitis
B carrier**

5 B17.1 Acute hepatitis C

**SP B17.10 Acute hepatitis C without hepatic
coma**
Acute hepatitis C NOS

SP B17.11 Acute hepatitis C with hepatic coma

SP B17.2 Acute hepatitis E

SP B17.8 Other specified acute viral hepatitis
Hepatitis non-A non-B (acute) (viral) NEC

SP B17.9 Acute viral hepatitis, unspecified
Acute hepatitis NOS
Acute infectious hepatitis NOS

4 B18   Chronic viral hepatitis
INCLUDES   Carrier of viral hepatitis

**SP B18.0 Chronic viral hepatitis B with delta-
agent**

**SP B18.1 Chronic viral hepatitis B without delta-
agent**
Carrier of viral hepatitis B
Chronic (viral) hepatitis B

SP B18.2 Chronic viral hepatitis C
Carrier of viral hepatitis C

SP B18.8 Other chronic viral hepatitis
Carrier of other viral hepatitis

SP B18.9 Chronic viral hepatitis, unspecified
Carrier of unspecified viral hepatitis

4 B19   Unspecified viral hepatitis

**SP B19.0 Unspecified viral hepatitis with hepatic
coma**

5 B19.1 Unspecified viral hepatitis B

**SP B19.10 Unspecified viral hepatitis B
without hepatic coma**
Unspecified viral hepatitis B NOS

**SP B19.11 Unspecified viral hepatitis B with
hepatic coma**

5 B19.2 Unspecified viral hepatitis C

**SP B19.20 Unspecified viral hepatitis C
without hepatic coma**
Viral hepatitis C NOS

**SP B19.21 Unspecified viral hepatitis C with
hepatic coma**

**SP B19.9 Unspecified viral hepatitis without
hepatic coma**
Viral hepatitis NOS

Human immunodeficiency virus [HIV]
disease   (B20)

CODING TIPS ✓   B20 is sequenced as primary when the patient is
admitted for conditions related to HIV infection. Sequence the
conditions caused by the HIV next. If the patient is being
admitted for another condition unrelated to HIV, code that
condition first and B20 can be used as a secondary code. If the
patient has had a HIV related condition in the past, continue to
use the B20 code, even if that HIV-related condition is resolved.
Z21 is used only for HIV+ patients who have never had a HIV
related condition. Some states may have a prohibition against
sequencing B20 as primary, or using the code at all. Look for
OASIS error code +150 to indicate that state regulations are
stricter than HIPAA, disallowing the code for AIDS.

**H SP + B20   Human immunodeficiency virus [HIV]
disease**
INCLUDES   acquired immune deficiency
syndrome [AIDS]
AIDS-related complex [ARC]
HIV infection, symptomatic
Code first:
Human immunodeficiency virus [HIV]
disease complicating pregnancy,
childbirth and the puerperium, if
applicable (O98.7-)
Use additional code(s) to identify all
manifestations of HIV infection
EXCLUDES 1   asymptomatic human
immunodeficiency virus
[HIV] infection status (Z21)
exposure to HIV virus (Z20.6)

---

4 4th digit required   5 5th digit required   6 6th digit required   7 7th digit required   7 7th digit placeholder   + Additional code   ⊟ Laterality

622   *DecisionHealth's* FY 2020 Complete Home Health ICD-10-CM Diagnosis Coding Manual

inconclusive serologic evidence of HIV (R75)

GUIDELINES Section I.C.1.a.1)
Code only confirmed cases of HIV infection/illness: This [guideline] is an exception to the hospital inpatient guideline Section II, H. In this context, "confirmation" does not require documentation of positive serology or culture for HIV; the provider's diagnostic statement that the patient is HIV positive, or has an HIV-related illness is sufficient. B20, Human immunideficiency virus (HIV) disease should be assigned.

GUIDELINES Section I.C.1.a.2)(a)
If a patient is admitted for an HIV-related condition, the principal diagnosis should be B20, Human immunodeficiency virus [HIV] disease followed by additional diagnosis codes for all reported HIV-related conditions.

GUIDELINES Section I.C.1.a.2)(b)
If a patient with HIV disease is admitted for an unrelated condition (such as a traumatic injury), the code for the unrelated condition (e.g., the nature of injury code) should be the principal diagnosis. Other diagnoses would be B20 followed by additional diagnosis codes for all reported HIV-related conditions.

GUIDELINES Section I.C.1.a.2)(c)
Whether the patient is newly diagnosed or has had previous admissions/encounters for HIV conditions is irrelevant to the sequencing decision.

GUIDELINES Section I.C.1.a.2)(e)
Patients with inconclusive HIV serology, but no definitive diagnosis or manifestations of the illness, may be assigned code R75, Inconclusive laboratory evidence of human immunodeficiency virus [HIV].

GUIDELINES Section I.C.1.a.2)(f)
Patients with any known prior diagnosis of an HIV-related illness should be coded to B20. Once a patient has developed an HIV-related illness, the patient should always be assigned code B20 on every subsequent admission/encounter. Patients previously diagnosed with any HIV illness (B20) should never be assigned to R75 or Z21, Asymptomatic human immunodeficiency virus [HIV] infection status.

Other viral diseases (B25-B34)

4 **B25   Cytomegaloviral disease**
EXCLUDES 1 congenital cytomegalovirus infection (P35.1)
cytomegaloviral mononucleosis (B27.1-)

SP **B25.0 Cytomegaloviral pneumonitis**

SP **B25.1 Cytomegaloviral hepatitis**

SP **B25.2 Cytomegaloviral pancreatitis**

SP **B25.8 Other cytomegaloviral diseases**
Cytomegaloviral encephalitis

SP **B25.9 Cytomegaloviral disease, unspecified**

4 **B26   Mumps**
INCLUDES epidemic parotitis
infectious parotitis

SP **B26.0 Mumps orchitis**

SP **B26.1   Mumps meningitis**

SP **B26.2   Mumps encephalitis**

SP **B26.3   Mumps pancreatitis**

5 **B26.8   Mumps with other complications**

SP **B26.81   Mumps hepatitis**

SP **B26.82   Mumps myocarditis**

SP **B26.83   Mumps nephritis**

SP **B26.84   Mumps polyneuropathy**

SP **B26.85   Mumps arthritis**

SP **B26.89   Other mumps complications**

SP **B26.9   Mumps without complication**
Mumps NOS
Mumps parotitis NOS

4 **B27   Infectious mononucleosis**
INCLUDES glandular fever
monocytic angina
Pfeiffer's disease

5 **B27.0   Gammaherpesviral mononucleosis**
Mononucleosis due to Epstein-Barr virus

SP **B27.00   Gammaherpesviral mononucleosis without complication**

SP **B27.01   Gammaherpesviral mononucleosis with polyneuropathy**

SP **B27.02   Gammaherpesviral mononucleosis with meningitis**

SP **B27.09   Gammaherpesviral mononucleosis with other complications**
Hepatomegaly in gammaherpesviral mononucleosis

5 **B27.1   Cytomegaloviral mononucleosis**

SP **B27.10   Cytomegaloviral mononucleosis without complications**

SP **B27.11   Cytomegaloviral mononucleosis with polyneuropathy**

SP **B27.12   Cytomegaloviral mononucleosis with meningitis**

SP **B27.19   Cytomegaloviral mononucleosis with other complication**
Hepatomegaly in cytomegaloviral mononucleosis

5 **B27.8   Other infectious mononucleosis**

SP **B27.80   Other infectious mononucleosis without complication**

SP **B27.81   Other infectious mononucleosis with polyneuropathy**

SP **B27.82   Other infectious mononucleosis with meningitis**

SP **B27.89   Other infectious mononucleosis with other complication**
Hepatomegaly in other infectious mononucleosis

5 **B27.9   Infectious mononucleosis, unspecified**

SP **B27.90   Infectious mononucleosis, unspecified without complication**

SP **B27.91   Infectious mononucleosis, unspecified with polyneuropathy**

SP **B27.92   Infectious mononucleosis, unspecified with meningitis**

SP **B27.99   Infectious mononucleosis, unspecified with other complication**

Hepatomegaly in unspecified infectious mononucleosis

4 **B30   Viral conjunctivitis**

★ New ▲ Revised Px Primary SP PDGM Px SL Low CoM SH High CoM IQ Quest. Encounter H Hospice non-cancer Dx Unspecified M *Manifestation*

DecisionHealth's FY 2020 Complete Home Health ICD-10-CM Diagnosis Coding Manual

623

EXCLUDES 1 herpesviral [herpes simplex]
    ocular disease (B00.5)
    ocular zoster (B02.3)

SP **B30.0** **Keratoconjunctivitis due to adenovirus**
    Epidemic keratoconjunctivitis
    Shipyard eye

SP **B30.1** **Conjunctivitis due to adenovirus**
    Acute adenoviral follicular conjunctivitis
    Swimming-pool conjunctivitis

SP **B30.2** **Viral pharyngoconjunctivitis**

SP **B30.3** **Acute epidemic hemorrhagic
conjunctivitis (enteroviral)**
    Conjunctivitis due to coxsackievirus 24
    Conjunctivitis due to enterovirus 70
    Hemorrhagic conjunctivitis
      (acute)(epidemic)

SP **B30.8** **Other viral conjunctivitis**
    Newcastle conjunctivitis

SP **B30.9** **Viral conjunctivitis, unspecified**

B33 **Other viral diseases, not elsewhere
classified**

SP **B33.0** **Epidemic myalgia**
    Bornholm disease

SP **B33.1** **Ross River disease**
    Epidemic polyarthritis and exanthema
    Ross River fever

B33.2 **Viral carditis**
    Coxsackie (virus) carditis

SP **B33.20** **Viral carditis, unspecified**

SP **B33.21** **Viral endocarditis**

SP **B33.22** **Viral myocarditis**

SP **B33.23** **Viral pericarditis**

SP **B33.24** **Viral cardiomyopathy**

SP **B33.3** **Retrovirus infections, not elsewhere
classified**
    Retrovirus infection NOS

SP + **B33.4** **Hantavirus (cardio)-pulmonary
syndrome [HPS] [HCPS]**
    Hantavirus disease with pulmonary
      manifestations
    Sin nombre virus disease
    Use additional code to identify any
      associated acute kidney failure (N17.9)
    EXCLUDES 1 hantavirus disease with renal
        manifestations (A98.5)
        hemorrhagic fever with renal
        manifestations (A98.5)

SP **B33.8** **Other specified viral diseases**
    EXCLUDES 1 anogenital human
        papillomavirus infection
        (A63.0)
        viral warts due to human
        papillomavirus infection
        (B07)

B34 **Viral infection of unspecified site**
    EXCLUDES 1 anogenital human
        papillomavirus infection
        (A63.0)
        cytomegaloviral disease NOS
        (B25.9)
        herpesvirus [herpes simplex]
        infection NOS (B00.9)
        retrovirus infection NOS
        (B33.3)
        viral agents as the cause of
        diseases classified elsewhere
        (B97.-)

        viral warts due to human
        papillomavirus infection
        (B07)

CODING TIPS ✓ Avoid using these codes for
viral-caused infections. Most viral infections
have combination codes.

SP **B34.0** **Adenovirus infection, unspecified**

SP **B34.1** **Enterovirus infection, unspecified**
    Coxsackievirus infection NOS
    Echovirus infection NOS

SP **B34.2** **Coronavirus infection, unspecified**
    EXCLUDES 1 pneumonia due to SARS-
        associated coronavirus
        (J12.81)

SP **B34.3** **Parvovirus infection, unspecified**

SP **B34.4** **Papovavirus infection, unspecified**

IQ **B34.8** **Other viral infections of unspecified
site**

IQ **B34.9** **Viral infection, unspecified**
    Viremia NOS

Mycoses (B35-B49)

EXCLUDES 2 hypersensitivity pneumonitis due to organic dust
    (J67.-)
    mycosis fungoides (C84.0-)

B35 **Dermatophytosis**
    INCLUDES favus
      infections due to species of
      Epidermophyton, Micro-
      sporum and Trichophyton
      tinea, any type except those in
      B36.-

SP **B35.0** **Tinea barbae and tinea capitis**
    Beard ringworm
    Kerion
    Scalp ringworm
    Sycosis, mycotic
    DEFINITION Superficial fungal infections
of the skin of bearded parts of the face and
neck, and the scalp.

SP **B35.1** **Tinea unguium**
    Dermatophytic onychia
    Dermatophytosis of nail
    Onychomycosis
    Ringworm of nails
    DEFINITION Fungal infection of the nails,
first the surface, lateral and distal edges,
and later, the part beneath the nail plate.

SP **B35.2** **Tinea manuum**
    Dermatophytosis of hand
    Hand ringworm

SP **B35.3** **Tinea pedis**
    Athlete's foot
    Dermatophytosis of foot
    Foot ringworm

SP **B35.4** **Tinea corporis**
    Ringworm of the body

SP **B35.5** **Tinea imbricata**
    Tokelau
    DEFINITION A fungal infection which
affects skin with few or no hair follicles,
typically seen in humid climates. The early
lesion is annular with a circle of scales at
the outside boundary.

SP **B35.6** **Tinea cruris**

⬛4 4th digit required   **⬛5** 5th digit required   **⬛6** 6th digit required   **⬛7** 7th digit required   **⬜7** 7th digit placeholder   **+** Additional code   **⊟** Laterality

Dhobi itch
Groin ringworm
Jock itch
DEFINITION Fungal infection of the groin commonly known as jock itch.

SP B35.8 Other dermatophytoses
Disseminated dermatophytosis
Granulomatous dermatophytosis

SP B35.9 Dermatophytosis, unspecified
Ringworm NOS

4 B36 Other superficial mycoses

SP B36.0 Pityriasis versicolor
Tinea flava
Tinea versicolor

SP B36.1 Tinea nigra
Keratomycosis nigricans palmaris
Microsporosis nigra
Pityriasis nigra
DEFINITION A minor fungal infection having dark lesions with the appearance of spattered silver nitrate on the skin.

SP B36.2 White piedra
Tinea blanca
DEFINITION A fungal disease of hair covered skin, marked by pale patches and bald spot where the infection occurred.

SP B36.3 Black piedra

SP B36.8 Other specified superficial mycoses

SP B36.9 Superficial mycosis, unspecified

4 B37 Candidiasis
INCLUDES candidosis
moniliasis
EXCLUDES 1 neonatal candidiasis (P37.5)

SP B37.0 Candidal stomatitis
Oral thrush
DEFINITION Fungal infection located in the mouth.

SP B37.1 Pulmonary candidiasis
Candidal bronchitis
Candidal pneumonia

SP B37.2 Candidiasis of skin and nail
Candidal onychia
Candidal paronychia
EXCLUDES 2 diaper dermatitis (L22)

SP B37.3 Candidiasis of vulva and vagina
Candidal vulvovaginitis
Monilial vulvovaginitis
Vaginal thrush

5 B37.4 Candidiasis of other urogenital sites

SP B37.41 Candidal cystitis and urethritis
CODING TIPS ✓ B37.41 is a combination code that includes both the infection of the urinary tract and candida as the infectious cause. No additional codes should be assigned for urinary infection.

SP B37.42 Candidal balanitis

SP B37.49 Other urogenital candidiasis
Candidal pyelonephritis

SP B37.5 Candidal meningitis

SP B37.6 Candidal endocarditis

SP B37.7 Candidal sepsis
Disseminated candidiasis
Systemic candidiasis

5 B37.8 Candidiasis of other sites

SP B37.81 Candidal esophagitis
DEFINITION Fungal infection of the esophagus, usually occurring in patients with immunocompromised states.

SP B37.82 Candidal enteritis
Candidal proctitis

SP B37.83 Candidal cheilitis

SP B37.84 Candidal otitis externa

SP B37.89 Other sites of candidiasis
Candidal osteomyelitis

SP B37.9 Candidiasis, unspecified
Thrush NOS

4 B38 Coccidioidomycosis

SP B38.0 Acute pulmonary coccidioidomycosis

SP B38.1 Chronic pulmonary coccidioidomycosis

SP B38.2 Pulmonary coccidioidomycosis, unspecified

SP B38.3 Cutaneous coccidioidomycosis

SP B38.4 Coccidioidomycosis meningitis

SP B38.7 Disseminated coccidioidomycosis
Generalized coccidioidomycosis

5 B38.8 Other forms of coccidioidomycosis

SP B38.81 Prostatic coccidioidomycosis

SP B38.89 Other forms of coccidioidomycosis

SP B38.9 Coccidioidomycosis, unspecified

+ 4 B39 Histoplasmosis
Code first:
associated AIDS (B20)
Use additional code for any associated manifestations, such as:
endocarditis (I39)
meningitis (G02)
pericarditis (I32)
retinitis (H32)
CODING TIPS ✓ Histoplasmosis (B39) is usually associated with HIV/AIDS. If so, then B20 is coded prior to using the B39 category code, unless other restrictions apply. (*See coding tip at category B20*).

SP + B39.0 Acute pulmonary histoplasmosis capsulati

SP + B39.1 Chronic pulmonary histoplasmosis capsulati

SP + B39.2 Pulmonary histoplasmosis capsulati, unspecified

SP + B39.3 Disseminated histoplasmosis capsulati
Generalized histoplasmosis capsulati

SP + B39.4 Histoplasmosis capsulati, unspecified
American histoplasmosis

SP + B39.5 Histoplasmosis duboisii
African histoplasmosis

SP + B39.9 Histoplasmosis, unspecified

4 B40 Blastomycosis
EXCLUDES 1 Brazilian blastomycosis (B41.-)
keloidal blastomycosis (B48.0)

SP B40.0 Acute pulmonary blastomycosis

SP B40.1 Chronic pulmonary blastomycosis

SP B40.2 Pulmonary blastomycosis, unspecified

SP B40.3 Cutaneous blastomycosis

SP B40.7 Disseminated blastomycosis
Generalized blastomycosis

5 B40.8 Other forms of blastomycosis

SP B40.81 Blastomycotic meningoencephalitis

★ New ▲ Revised Px Primary SP PDGM Px SL Low CoM SH High CoM IQ Quest. Encounter H Hospice non-cancer Dx Unspecified M *Manifestation*

Meningomyelitis due to blastomycosis

SP B40.89 Other forms of blastomycosis

SP B40.9 Blastomycosis, unspecified

4 B41 Paracoccidioidomycosis

> **INCLUDES** Brazilian blastomycosis
> Lutz' disease

SP B41.0 Pulmonary paracoccidioidomycosis

SP B41.7 Disseminated paracoccidioidomycosis
Generalized paracoccidioidomycosis

SP B41.8 Other forms of paracoccidioidomycosis

SP B41.9 Paracoccidioidomycosis, unspecified

4 B42 Sporotrichosis

SP B42.0 Pulmonary sporotrichosis

SP B42.1 Lymphocutaneous sporotrichosis

SP B42.7 Disseminated sporotrichosis
Generalized sporotrichosis

5 B42.8 Other forms of sporotrichosis

SP B42.81 Cerebral sporotrichosis
Meningitis due to sporotrichosis

SP B42.82 Sporotrichosis arthritis

SP B42.89 Other forms of sporotrichosis

SP B42.9 Sporotrichosis, unspecified

4 B43 Chromomycosis and pheomycotic abscess

SP B43.0 Cutaneous chromomycosis
Dermatitis verrucosa

SP B43.1 Pheomycotic brain abscess
Cerebral chromomycosis

SP B43.2 Subcutaneous pheomycotic abscess and cyst

SP B43.8 Other forms of chromomycosis

SP B43.9 Chromomycosis, unspecified

4 B44 Aspergillosis

> **INCLUDES** aspergilloma

SP B44.0 Invasive pulmonary aspergillosis

SP B44.1 Other pulmonary aspergillosis

SP B44.2 Tonsillar aspergillosis

SP B44.7 Disseminated aspergillosis
Generalized aspergillosis

5 B44.8 Other forms of aspergillosis

SP B44.81 Allergic bronchopulmonary aspergillosis

SP B44.89 Other forms of aspergillosis

SP B44.9 Aspergillosis, unspecified

4 B45 Cryptococcosis

SP B45.0 Pulmonary cryptococcosis
> **DEFINITION** Yeastlike fungus infection, by cryptococcus neoformans, commonly occurring in the soil, which infects via the lungs and may spread to the brain and meninges.

SP B45.1 Cerebral cryptococcosis
Cryptococcal meningitis
Cryptococcosis meningocerebralis
> **DEFINITION** Infection of the brain and/or its surrounding tissues causing hydrocephalus and intracerebral cysts due to infection with cryptococcus fungus.

SP B45.2 Cutaneous cryptococcosis

SP B45.3 Osseous cryptococcosis

SP B45.7 Disseminated cryptococcosis
Generalized cryptococcosis

SP B45.8 Other forms of cryptococcosis

SP B45.9 Cryptococcosis, unspecified

4 B46 Zygomycosis

SP B46.0 Pulmonary mucormycosis

SP B46.1 Rhinocerebral mucormycosis

SP B46.2 Gastrointestinal mucormycosis

SP B46.3 Cutaneous mucormycosis
Subcutaneous mucormycosis

SP B46.4 Disseminated mucormycosis
Generalized mucormycosis

SP B46.5 Mucormycosis, unspecified

SP B46.8 Other zygomycoses
Entomophthoromycosis

SP B46.9 Zygomycosis, unspecified
Phycomycosis NOS

4 B47 Mycetoma

SP B47.0 Eumycetoma
Madura foot, mycotic
Maduromycosis

SP B47.1 Actinomycetoma

SP B47.9 Mycetoma, unspecified
Madura foot NOS
> **DEFINITION** Chronic infection involving the feet, characterized by formation of localized lesions, with swelling and multiple draining sinuses.

4 B48 Other mycoses, not elsewhere classified

SP B48.0 Lobomycosis
Keloidal blastomycosis
Lobo's disease
> **DEFINITION** A fungal infection of the skin caused by Lobo loboi and characterized by keloidal nodular lesions occurring on the face, ears, and extremities.

SP B48.1 Rhinosporidiosis

SP B48.2 Allescheriasis
Infection due to Pseudallescheria boydii
> **EXCLUDES 1** eumycetoma (B47.0)

SP B48.3 Geotrichosis
Geotrichum stomatitis

SP B48.4 Penicillosis

SP B48.8 Other specified mycoses
Adiaspiromycosis
Infection of tissue and organs by Alternaria
Infection of tissue and organs by Drechslera
Infection of tissue and organs by Fusarium
Infection of tissue and organs by saprophytic fungi NEC

SP B49 Unspecified mycosis
Fungemia NOS

Protozoal diseases (B50-B64)

> **EXCLUDES 1** amebiasis (A06.-)
> other protozoal intestinal diseases (A07.-)

4 B50 Plasmodium falciparum malaria
> **INCLUDES** mixed infections of Plasmodium falciparum with any other Plasmodium species

SP B50.0 Plasmodium falciparum malaria with cerebral complications
Cerebral malaria NOS

---

4 4th digit required   5 5th digit required   6 6th digit required   7 7th digit required   7 7th digit placeholder   **+** Additional code   Laterality

Post-kala-azar dermal leishmaniasis

SP B50.8 Other severe and complicated Plasmodium falciparum malaria
Severe or complicated Plasmodium falciparum malaria NOS

SP B50.9 Plasmodium falciparum malaria, unspecified

4 B51 Plasmodium vivax malaria
> **INCLUDES** mixed infections of Plasmodium vivax with other Plasmodium species, except Plasmodium falciparum
> **EXCLUDES 1** plasmodium vivax with Plasmodium falciparum (B50.-)

SP B51.0 Plasmodium vivax malaria with rupture of spleen

SP B51.8 Plasmodium vivax malaria with other complications

SP B51.9 Plasmodium vivax malaria without complication
Plasmodium vivax malaria NOS

4 B52 Plasmodium malariae malaria
> **INCLUDES** mixed infections of Plasmodium malariae with other Plasmodium species, except Plasmodium falciparum and Plasmodium vivax
> **EXCLUDES 1** Plasmodium falciparum (B50.-)
> Plasmodium vivax (B51.-)

SP B52.0 Plasmodium malariae malaria with nephropathy

SP B52.8 Plasmodium malariae malaria with other complications

SP B52.9 Plasmodium malariae malaria without complication
Plasmodium malariae malaria NOS

4 B53 Other specified malaria

SP B53.0 Plasmodium ovale malaria
> **EXCLUDES 1** Plasmodium ovale with Plasmodium falciparum (B50.-)
> Plasmodium ovale with Plasmodium malariae (B52.-)
> Plasmodium ovale with Plasmodium vivax (B51.-)

SP B53.1 Malaria due to simian plasmodia
> **EXCLUDES 1** Malaria due to simian plasmodia with Plasmodium falciparum (B50.-)
> Malaria due to simian plasmodia with Plasmodium malariae (B52.-)
> Malaria due to simian plasmodia with Plasmodium ovale (B53.0)
> Malaria due to simian plasmodia with Plasmodium vivax (B51.-)

SP B53.8 Other malaria, not elsewhere classified

SP B54 Unspecified malaria

4 B55 Leishmaniasis

SP B55.0 Visceral leishmaniasis
Kala-azar

SP B55.1 Cutaneous leishmaniasis

SP B55.2 Mucocutaneous leishmaniasis

SP B55.9 Leishmaniasis, unspecified

4 B56 African trypanosomiasis

SP B56.0 Gambiense trypanosomiasis
Infection due to Trypanosoma brucei gambiense
West African sleeping sickness

SP B56.1 Rhodesiense trypanosomiasis
East African sleeping sickness
Infection due to Trypanosoma brucei rhodesiense

SP B56.9 African trypanosomiasis, unspecified
Sleeping sickness NOS

4 B57 Chagas' disease
> **INCLUDES** American trypanosomiasis infection due to Trypanosoma cruzi

SP B57.0 Acute Chagas' disease with heart involvement
Acute Chagas' disease with myocarditis

SP B57.1 Acute Chagas' disease without heart involvement
Acute Chagas' disease NOS

SP B57.2 Chagas' disease (chronic) with heart involvement
American trypanosomiasis NOS
Chagas' disease (chronic) NOS
Chagas' disease (chronic) with myocarditis
Trypanosomiasis NOS

5 B57.3 Chagas' disease (chronic) with digestive system involvement

SP B57.30 Chagas' disease with digestive system involvement, unspecified

SP B57.31 Megaesophagus in Chagas' disease

SP B57.32 Megacolon in Chagas' disease

SP B57.39 Other digestive system involvement in Chagas' disease

5 B57.4 Chagas' disease (chronic) with nervous system involvement

SP B57.40 Chagas' disease with nervous system involvement, unspecified

SP B57.41 Meningitis in Chagas' disease

SP B57.42 Meningoencephalitis in Chagas' disease

SP B57.49 Other nervous system involvement in Chagas' disease

SP B57.5 Chagas' disease (chronic) with other organ involvement

4 B58 Toxoplasmosis
> **INCLUDES** infection due to Toxoplasma gondii
> **EXCLUDES 1** congenital toxoplasmosis (P37.1)

5 B58.0 Toxoplasma oculopathy

SP B58.00 Toxoplasma oculopathy, unspecified

SP B58.01 Toxoplasma chorioretinitis

SP B58.09 Other toxoplasma oculopathy
Toxoplasma uveitis

SP B58.1 Toxoplasma hepatitis

SP B58.2 Toxoplasma meningoencephalitis

SP B58.3 Pulmonary toxoplasmosis

5 B58.8 Toxoplasmosis with other organ involvement

★ New ▲ Revised Px Primary SP PDGM Px SL Low CoM SH High CoM IQ Quest. Encounter H Hospice non-cancer Dx   Unspecified   M Manifestation

DecisionHealth's FY 2020 Complete Home Health ICD-10-CM Diagnosis Coding Manual   627

SP B58.81 Toxoplasma myocarditis

SP B58.82 Toxoplasma myositis

SP B58.83 Toxoplasma tubulo-interstitial nephropathy
Toxoplasma pyelonephritis

SP B58.89 Toxoplasmosis with other organ involvement

SP B58.9 Toxoplasmosis, unspecified

SP B59 Pneumocystosis
Pneumonia due to Pneumocystis carinii
Pneumonia due to Pneumocystis jiroveci

CODING TIPS ✓ Pneumocystosis is usually associated with HIV/AIDS. If so, then B20 is coded prior to using the B59 category code, unless other restrictions apply. (*See coding tip at category B20.*)

4 B60 Other protozoal diseases, not elsewhere classified
EXCLUDES 1 cryptosporidiosis (A07.2)
intestinal microsporidiosis (A07.8)
isosporiasis (A07.3)

SP B60.0 Babesiosis
Piroplasmosis

5 B60.1 Acanthamebiasis

SP B60.10 Acanthamebiasis, unspecified

SP B60.11 Meningoencephalitis due to Acanthamoeba (culbertsoni)

SP B60.12 Conjunctivitis due to Acanthamoeba

SP B60.13 Keratoconjunctivitis due to Acanthamoeba

SP B60.19 Other acanthamebic disease

SP B60.2 Naegleriasis
Primary amebic meningoencephalitis

SP B60.8 Other specified protozoal diseases
Microsporidiosis

!Q B64 Unspecified protozoal disease

Helminthiases (B65-B83)

4 B65 Schistosomiasis [bilharziasis]
INCLUDES snail fever

SP B65.0 Schistosomiasis due to Schistosoma haematobium [urinary schistosomiasis]

SP B65.1 Schistosomiasis due to Schistosoma mansoni [intestinal schistosomiasis]

SP B65.2 Schistosomiasis due to Schistosoma japonicum
Asiatic schistosomiasis

SP B65.3 Cercarial dermatitis
Swimmer's itch

DEFINITION An itching inflammation of the skin due to penetration of larval forms of schistosomes (parasitic worms), occurring in bathers of infested waters.

SP B65.8 Other schistosomiasis
Infection due to Schistosoma intercalatum
Infection due to Schistosoma mattheei
Infection due to Schistosoma mekongi

SP B65.9 Schistosomiasis, unspecified

4 B66 Other fluke infections

SP B66.0 Opisthorchiasis
Infection due to cat liver fluke
Infection due to Opisthorchis (felineus)(viverrini)

SP B66.1 Clonorchiasis
Chinese liver fluke disease
Infection due to Clonorchis sinensis
Oriental liver fluke disease

SP B66.2 Dicroceliasis
Infection due to Dicrocoelium dendriticum
Lancet fluke infection

SP B66.3 Fascioliasis
Infection due to Fasciola gigantica
Infection due to Fasciola hepatica
Infection due to Fasciola indica
Sheep liver fluke disease

SP B66.4 Paragonimiasis
Infection due to Paragonimus species
Lung fluke disease
Pulmonary distomiasis

SP B66.5 Fasciolopsiasis
Infection due to Fasciolopsis buski
Intestinal distomiasis

SP B66.8 Other specified fluke infections
Echinostomiasis
Heterophyiasis
Metagonimiasis
Nanophyetiasis
Watsoniasis

SP B66.9 Fluke infection, unspecified

4 B67 Echinococcosis
INCLUDES hydatidosis

SP B67.0 Echinococcus granulosus infection of liver
DEFINITION A genus of parasitic tapeworm passed from dogs. The larvae form large cysts in the liver, causing serious and sometimes fatal disease.

SP B67.1 Echinococcus granulosus infection of lung

SP B67.2 Echinococcus granulosus infection of bone

5 B67.3 Echinococcus granulosus infection, other and multiple sites

SP B67.31 Echinococcus granulosus infection, thyroid gland

SP B67.32 Echinococcus granulosus infection, multiple sites

SP B67.39 Echinococcus granulosus infection, other sites

!Q B67.4 Echinococcus granulosus infection, unspecified
Dog tapeworm (infection)

SP B67.5 Echinococcus multilocularis infection of liver

5 B67.6 Echinococcus multilocularis infection, other and multiple sites

SP B67.61 Echinococcus multilocularis infection, multiple sites

SP B67.69 Echinococcus multilocularis infection, other sites

!Q B67.7 Echinococcus multilocularis infection, unspecified

SP B67.8 Echinococcosis, unspecified, of liver

5 B67.9 Echinococcosis, other and unspecified

SP B67.90 Echinococcosis, unspecified
Echinococcosis NOS

SP B67.99 Other echinococcosis

4 B68 Taeniasis
EXCLUDES 1 cysticercosis (B69.-)

---

4 4th digit required   5 5th digit required   6 6th digit required   7 7th digit required   ☑ 7th digit placeholder   ✛ Additional code   ⊟ Laterality

SP B68.0 Taenia solium taeniasis
Pork tapeworm (infection)

SP B68.1 Taenia saginata taeniasis
Beef tapeworm (infection)
Infection due to adult tapeworm Taenia
saginata

SP B68.9 Taeniasis, unspecified

4 B69 Cysticercosis
INCLUDES cysticerciasis infection due to
larval form of Taenia solium

SP B69.0 Cysticercosis of central nervous system

SP B69.1 Cysticercosis of eye

5 B69.8 Cysticercosis of other sites

SP B69.81 Myositis in cysticercosis

SP B69.89 Cysticercosis of other sites

SP B69.9 Cysticercosis, unspecified
DEFINITION Infection caused by the pork
tapeworm when its larvae enter the body
and form cysts.

4 B70 Diphyllobothriasis and sparganosis

SP B70.0 Diphyllobothriasis
Diphyllobothrium (adult) (latum)
(pacificum) infection
Fish tapeworm (infection)
EXCLUDES 2 larval diphyllobothriasis
(B70.1)

SP B70.1 Sparganosis
Infection due to Sparganum (mansoni)
(proliferum)
Infection due to Spirometra larva
Larval diphyllobothriasis
Spirometrosis

4 B71 Other cestode infections

SP B71.0 Hymenolepiasis
Dwarf tapeworm infection
Rat tapeworm (infection)

SP B71.1 Dipylidiasis

SP B71.8 Other specified cestode infections
Coenurosis

SP B71.9 Cestode infection, unspecified
Tapeworm (infection) NOS

SP B72 Dracunculiasis
INCLUDES guinea worm infection
infection due to Dracunculus
medinensis

4 B73 Onchocerciasis
INCLUDES onchocerca volvulus infection
onchocercosis
river blindness

5 B73.0 Onchocerciasis with eye disease

**SP B73.00 Onchocerciasis with eye
involvement, unspecified**

SP B73.01 Onchocerciasis with endophthalmitis

SP B73.02 Onchocerciasis with glaucoma

**SP B73.09 Onchocerciasis with other eye
involvement**
Infestation of eyelid due to
onchocerciasis

SP B73.1 Onchocerciasis without eye disease

4 B74 Filariasis
EXCLUDES 2 onchocerciasis (B73)
tropical (pulmonary)
eosinophilia NOS (J82)

SP B74.0 Filariasis due to Wuchereria bancrofti
Bancroftian elephantiasis
Bancroftian filariasis

SP B74.1 Filariasis due to Brugia malayi

SP B74.2 Filariasis due to Brugia timori

SP B74.3 Loiasis
Calabar swelling
Eyeworm disease of Africa
Loa loa infection

SP B74.4 Mansonelliasis
Infection due to Mansonella ozzardi
Infection due to Mansonella perstans
Infection due to Mansonella streptocerca

SP B74.8 Other filariases
Dirofilariasis

SP B74.9 Filariasis, unspecified

SP B75 Trichinellosis
INCLUDES infection due to Trichinella
species
trichiniasis

4 B76 Hookworm diseases
INCLUDES uncinariasis

SP B76.0 Ancylostomiasis
Infection due to Ancylostoma species

SP B76.1 Necatoriasis
Infection due to Necator americanus

SP B76.8 Other hookworm diseases

SP B76.9 Hookworm disease, unspecified
Cutaneous larva migrans NOS

4 B77 Ascariasis
INCLUDES ascaridiasis
roundworm infection

SP B77.0 Ascariasis with intestinal complications

5 B77.8 Ascariasis with other complications

SP B77.81 Ascariasis pneumonia

SP B77.89 Ascariasis with other complications

SP B77.9 Ascariasis, unspecified

4 B78 Strongyloidiasis
EXCLUDES 1 trichostrongyliasis (B81.2)

SP B78.0 Intestinal strongyloidiasis

SP B78.1 Cutaneous strongyloidiasis

SP B78.7 Disseminated strongyloidiasis

SP B78.9 Strongyloidiasis, unspecified

SP B79 Trichuriasis
INCLUDES trichocephaliasis
whipworm (disease) (infection)

SP B80 Enterobiasis
INCLUDES oxyuriasis
pinworm infection
threadworm infection

**4 B81 Other intestinal helminthiases, not
elsewhere classified**
EXCLUDES 1 angiostrongyliasis due to:
Angiostrongylus cantonensis
(B83.2)
Parastrongylus cantonensis
(B83.2)

SP B81.0 Anisakiasis
Infection due to Anisakis larva

SP B81.1 Intestinal capillariasis
Capillariasis NOS
Infection due to Capillaria philippinensis
EXCLUDES 2 hepatic capillariasis (B83.8)

SP B81.2 Trichostrongyliasis

SP B81.3 Intestinal angiostrongyliasis

★ New ▲ Revised Px Primary SP PDGM Px SL Low CoM SH High CoM IQ Quest. Encounter H Hospice non-cancer Dx Unspecified M *Manifestation*

Angiostrongyliasis due to:
Angiostrongylus costaricensis
Parastrongylus costaricensis

SP B81.4　Mixed intestinal helminthiases
Infection due to intestinal helminths
classified to more than one of the
categories B65.0-B81.3 and B81.8
Mixed helminthiasis NOS

SP B81.8　Other specified intestinal helminthiases
Infection due to Oesophagostomum
species [esophagostomiasis]
Infection due to Ternidens diminutus
[ternidensiasis]

4 B82　Unspecified intestinal parasitism

SP B82.0　Intestinal helminthiasis, unspecified

SP B82.9　Intestinal parasitism, unspecified

4 B83　Other helminthiases
　EXCLUDES 1　capillariasis NOS (B81.1)
　EXCLUDES 2　intestinal capillariasis (B81.1)

SP B83.0　Visceral larva migrans
Toxocariasis

SP B83.1　Gnathostomiasis
Wandering swelling

**SP B83.2　Angiostrongyliasis due to
Parastrongylus cantonensis**
Eosinophilic meningoencephalitis due to
Parastrongylus cantonensis
　EXCLUDES 2　intestinal angiostrongyliasis
(B81.3)

SP B83.3　Syngamiasis
Syngamosis

SP B83.4　Internal hirudiniasis
　EXCLUDES 2　external hirudiniasis (B88.3)

SP B83.8　Other specified helminthiases
Acanthocephaliasis
Gongylonemiasis
Hepatic capillariasis
Metastrongyliasis
Thelaziasis

SP B83.9　Helminthiasis, unspecified
Worms NOS
　EXCLUDES 1　intestinal helminthiasis NOS
(B82.0)

Pediculosis, acariasis and other infestations (B85-B89)

4 B85　Pediculosis and phthiriasis

SP B85.0　Pediculosis due to Pediculus humanus capitis
Head-louse infestation

SP B85.1　Pediculosis due to Pediculus humanus corporis
Body-louse infestation

SP B85.2　Pediculosis, unspecified

SP B85.3　Phthiriasis
Infestation by crab-louse
Infestation by Phthirus pubis

SP B85.4　Mixed pediculosis and phthiriasis
Infestation classifiable to more than one of
the categories B85.0-B85.3

SP B86　Scabies
Sarcoptic itch

4 B87　Myiasis
　INCLUDES　infestation by larva of flies

SP B87.0　Cutaneous myiasis

Creeping myiasis
　DEFINITION　Infestation by the fly larvae
of the genus Oestrus causing inflamed
furuncles where the larvae are maturing
beneath the skin.

SP B87.1　Wound myiasis
Traumatic myiasis

SP B87.2　Ocular myiasis

SP B87.3　Nasopharyngeal myiasis
Laryngeal myiasis

SP B87.4　Aural myiasis

5 B87.8　Myiasis of other sites

SP B87.81　Genitourinary myiasis

SP B87.82　Intestinal myiasis

SP B87.89　Myiasis of other sites

SP B87.9　Myiasis, unspecified

4 B88　Other infestations

SP B88.0　Other acariasis
Acarine dermatitis
Dermatitis due to Demodex species
Dermatitis due to Dermanyssus gallinae
Dermatitis due to Liponyssoides
sanguineus
Trombiculosis
　EXCLUDES 2　scabies (B86)

SP B88.1　Tungiasis [sandflea infestation]

SP B88.2　Other arthropod infestations
Scarabiasis

SP B88.3　External hirudiniasis
Leech infestation NOS
　EXCLUDES 2　internal hirudiniasis (B83.4)

SP B88.8　Other specified infestations
Ichthyoparasitism due to Vandellia cirrhosa
Linguatulosis
Porocephaliasis

IQ B88.9　Infestation, unspecified
Infestation (skin) NOS
Infestation by mites NOS
Skin parasites NOS

IQ B89　Unspecified parasitic disease

Sequelae of infectious and parasitic diseases (B90-B94)

Note:
Categories B90-B94 are to be used to indicate conditions in
categories A00-B89 as the cause of sequelae, which are
themselves classified elsewhere. The 'sequelae' include
conditions specified as such; they also include residuals of
diseases classifiable to the above categories if there is
evidence that the disease itself is no longer present. Codes
from these categories are not to be used for chronic
infections. Code chronic current infections to active
infectious disease as appropriate.
Code first:
condition resulting from (sequela) the infectious or parasitic
disease

4 B90　Sequelae of tuberculosis
　CODING TIPS ✓　Conditions classified here are
specifically reportable as sequelae or late
effects of tuberculosis. The active disease is no
longer present. Acute tuberculosis should be
coded to A15-A19.

---

4 4th digit required　　5 5th digit required　　6 6th digit required　　7 7th digit required　　7 7th digit placeholder　　+ Additional code　　⊟ Laterality

CODING TIPS ✓ Do not use B90 to indicate chronic infection. If there are no residuals of a past infection, use Z86.11.

SP B90.0 Sequelae of central nervous system tuberculosis

SP B90.1 Sequelae of genitourinary tuberculosis

SP B90.2 Sequelae of tuberculosis of bones and joints

SP B90.8 Sequelae of tuberculosis of other organs

> **EXCLUDES 2** sequelae of respiratory tuberculosis (B90.9)

SP B90.9 Sequelae of respiratory and unspecified tuberculosis

Sequelae of tuberculosis NOS

SP B91 Sequelae of poliomyelitis

> **EXCLUDES 1** postpolio syndrome (G14)

CODING TIPS ✓ Conditions classified here are specifically reportable as sequelae of poliomyelitis. Acute poliomyelitis should be coded to A80. When postpolio syndrome is specified, report code G14 rather than B91.

CODING TIPS ✓ The general rule is to code the sequela, or residual, first then B91, unless there is a tabular convention that instructs otherwise. If polio has been resolved and there are no residuals, use Z86.12.

SP B92 Sequelae of leprosy

4 B94 Sequelae of other and unspecified infectious and parasitic diseases

SP B94.0 Sequelae of trachoma

SP B94.1 Sequelae of viral encephalitis

SP B94.2 Sequelae of viral hepatitis

SP B94.8 Sequelae of other specified infectious and parasitic diseases

SP B94.9 Sequelae of unspecified infectious and parasitic disease

Bacterial and viral infectious agents (B95-B97)

Note:

These categories are provided for use as supplementary or additional codes to identify the infectious agent(s) in diseases classified elsewhere.

GUIDELINES Section I.C.1.b

Certain infections are classified in chapters other than Chapter 1 and no organism is identified as part of the infection code. In these instances, it is necessary to use an additional code from Chapter 1 to identify the organism. A code from category B95, Streptococcus, Staphylococcus, and Enterococcus as the cause of diseases classified to other chapters, B96, Other bacterial agents as the cause of diseases classified to other chapters, or B97, Viral agents as the cause of diseases classified to other chapters, is to be used as an additional code to identify the organism. An instructional note will be found at the infection code advising that an additional organism code is required.

Section I.C.1.c

Many bacterial infections are resistant to current antibiotics. It is necessary to identify all infections documented as antibiotic resistant. Assign a code from category Z16, Resistance to antimicrobial drugs, following the infection code only if the infection code does not identify drug resistance.

CODING TIPS ✓ Conditions classified here are specifically reportable as additional codes to identify infectious agents in diseases classified elsewhere. Do not assign codes from B95-B97 without a code for the underlying disease process first.

4 B95 Streptococcus, Staphylococcus, and Enterococcus as the cause of diseases classified elsewhere

CODING TIPS ✓ Use B95 codes to identify the organism causing the infection, if known. B95 codes indicate localized streptococcal infections, staphylococcal infections and enterococcal infections (also known as Strep D). These codes are always coded after the code indicating the type of infection from chapters other than chapter 1, such as UTIs and cellulitis, to identify the causative organism. Watch for combination codes. An infectious process, such as pneumonia, is a combination code, and a B95 code is not to be added.

SP B95.0 Streptococcus, group A, as the cause of diseases classified elsewhere

IQ B95.1 Streptococcus, group B, as the cause of diseases classified elsewhere

IQ B95.2 Enterococcus as the cause of diseases classified elsewhere

IQ B95.3 Streptococcus pneumoniae as the cause of diseases classified elsewhere

IQ B95.4 Other streptococcus as the cause of diseases classified elsewhere

IQ B95.5 Unspecified streptococcus as the cause of diseases classified elsewhere

5 B95.6 Staphylococcus aureus as the cause of diseases classified elsewhere

IQ B95.61 Methicillin susceptible Staphylococcus aureus infection as the cause of diseases classified elsewhere

Methicillin susceptible Staphylococcus aureus (MSSA) infection as the cause of diseases classified elsewhere

Staphylococcus aureus infection NOS as the cause of diseases classified elsewhere

CODING TIPS ✓ B95.61 is used when the bacteria is identified as Staphylococcus aureus or MSSA.

IQ B95.62 Methicillin resistant Staphylococcus aureus infection as the cause of diseases classified elsewhere

Methicillin resistant staphylococcus aureus (MRSA) infection as the cause of diseases classified elsewhere

★ New ▲ Revised Px Primary SP PDGM Px SL Low CoM SH High CoM IQ Quest. Encounter H Hospice non-cancer Dx   Unspecified   M *Manifestation*

DecisionHealth's FY 2020 Complete Home Health ICD-10-CM Diagnosis Coding Manual   631

GUIDELINES   Section I.C.1.e.1)
Selection and sequencing of MRSA codes:

(a) Combination codes for MRSA infection. When a patient is diagnosed with an infection that is due to MRSA, and that infection has a combination code that includes the causal organism (e.g., sepsis, pneumonia) assign the appropriate combination code for the condition (e.g., code A41.02, Sepsis due to Methicillin resistant Staphylococcus aureus or code J15.212, Pneumonia due to Methicillin resistant Staphylococcus aureus). Do not assign code B95.62, Methicillin resistant Staphylococcus aureus infection as the cause of diseases classified elsewhere, as an additional code because the combination code includes the type of infection and the MRSA organism. Do not assign a code from subcategory Z16.11, Resistance to penicillins, as an additional diagnosis.

(b) Other codes for MRSA infection. When there is documentation of a current infection (e.g., wound infection, stitch abscess, urinary tract infection) due to MRSA, and that infection does not have a combination code that includes the causal organism, assign the appropriate code to identify the condition along with code B95.62, Methicillin resistant Staphylococcus aureus infection as the cause of diseases classified elsewhere for the MRSA infection. Do not assign a code from subcategory Z16.11, Resistance to penicillins.

CODING TIPS ✓   B95.62 is used when the organism is identified as methicillin-resistant Staph aureus (MRSA). Do not use a Z16 code to indicate resistance to penicillins. Z16 may be added for other resistance, other than penicillins, such as vancomycin.

IQ B95.7   Other staphylococcus as the cause of diseases classified elsewhere

CODING TIPS ✓   Use this code when another staph is identified, such as Staphyloccus epidermidis.

IQ B95.8   Unspecified staphylococcus as the cause of diseases classified elsewhere

CODING TIPS ✓   Use this code if the organism is identified as "staph" without the species name, such as aureus.

4 B96   Other bacterial agents as the cause of diseases classified elsewhere

CODING TIPS ✓   Use B96 codes to identify the organism causing the localized infection, if known. B96 codes indicate other bacterial infections with the exception of streptococcal, staphylococcal, and enterococcal infections. These codes are always coded after the code indicating the type of infection from chapters other than chapter 1, for example, UTIs and cellulitis, to identify the causative organism. Watch for combination codes. An infectious process, such as pneumonia, is a combination code, and a B96 code is not to be added.

IQ B96.0   Mycoplasma pneumoniae [M. pneumoniae] as the cause of diseases classified elsewhere
Pleuro-pneumonia-like-organism [PPLO]

IQ B96.1   Klebsiella pneumoniae [K. pneumoniae] as the cause of diseases classified elsewhere

5 B96.2   Escherichia coli [E. coli] as the cause of diseases classified elsewhere

IQ B96.20   Unspecified Escherichia coli [E. coli] as the cause of diseases classified elsewhere
Escherichia coli [E. coli] NOS
CODING TIPS ✓   E. coli is the most common bacterial agent identified in UTIs. B96.20 is used when a specific E. coli is not specified by the physician.

▲ IQ B96.21   Shiga toxin-producing Escherichia coli [E. coli] [STEC] O157 as the cause of diseases classified elsewhere
E. coli O157:H- (nonmotile) with confirmation of Shiga toxin
E. coli O157 with confirmation of Shiga toxin when H antigen is unknown, or is not H7
O157:H7 Escherichia coli [E.coli] with or without confirmation of Shiga toxin-production
Shiga toxin-producing Escherichia coli [E.coli] O157:H7 with or without confirmation of Shiga toxin-production
STEC O157:H7 with or without confirmation of Shiga toxin-production

▲ IQ B96.22   Other specified Shiga toxin-producing Escherichia coli [E. coli] [STEC] as the cause of diseases classified elsewhere
Non-O157 Shiga toxin-producing Escherichia coli [E.coli]
Non-O157 Shiga toxin-producing Escherichia coli [E.coli] with known O group

▲ IQ B96.23   Unspecified Shiga toxin-producing Escherichia coli [E. coli] [STEC] as the cause of diseases classified elsewhere
Shiga toxin-producing Escherichia coli [E. coli] with unspecified O group
STEC NOS

IQ B96.29   Other Escherichia coli [E. coli] as the cause of diseases classified elsewhere
Non-Shiga toxin-producing E. coli

---

4 4th digit required   5 5th digit required   6 6th digit required   7 7th digit required   7 7th digit placeholder   + Additional code   = Laterality

632   *DecisionHealth's* FY 2020 Complete Home Health ICD-10-CM Diagnosis Coding Manual

IQ B96.3 Hemophilus influenzae [H. influenzae] as the cause of diseases classified elsewhere

CODING TIPS ✓ Hemophilius influenzae (coded to B96.3) is often confused with the influenza virus. H. influenzae is a bacteria.

IQ B96.4 Proteus (mirabilis) (morganii) as the cause of diseases classified elsewhere

IQ B96.5 Pseudomonas (aeruginosa) (mallei) (pseudomallei) as the cause of diseases classified elsewhere

IQ B96.6 Bacteroides fragilis [B. fragilis] as the cause of diseases classified elsewhere

IQ B96.7 Clostridium perfringens [C. perfringens] as the cause of diseases classified elsewhere

CODING TIPS ✓ Clostridium difficile is coded to A04.7-.

5 B96.8 Other specified bacterial agents as the cause of diseases classified elsewhere

IQ B96.81 Helicobacter pylori [H. pylori] as the cause of diseases classified elsewhere

DEFINITION Common gastric pathogen causing dyspepsia, gastritis, peptic ulcer disease, gastric adenocarcinoma, and gastric lymphoma.

IQ B96.82 Vibrio vulnificus as the cause of diseases classified elsewhere

IQ B96.89 Other specified bacterial agents as the cause of diseases classified elsewhere

CODING TIPS ✓ Do not use to indicate an unknown bacteria causing a localized infection. If the bacteria is unknown, there is no need to add a code for the bacteria.

4 B97 Viral agents as the cause of diseases classified elsewhere

CODING TIPS ✓ Most viral conditions use combination codes. Search the index for the specific condition before choosing B97 codes.

IQ B97.0 Adenovirus as the cause of diseases classified elsewhere

5 B97.1 Enterovirus as the cause of diseases classified elsewhere

IQ B97.10 Unspecified enterovirus as the cause of diseases classified elsewhere

IQ B97.11 Coxsackievirus as the cause of diseases classified elsewhere

IQ B97.12 Echovirus as the cause of diseases classified elsewhere

DEFINITION A group of DNA-containing viruses that affect the tissue linings of the respiratory tract, eyes, intestines, and urinary tract. There are approximately 50 serotypes.

IQ B97.19 Other enterovirus as the cause of diseases classified elsewhere

5 B97.2 Coronavirus as the cause of diseases classified elsewhere

IQ B97.21 SARS-associated coronavirus as the cause of diseases classified elsewhere

EXCLUDES 1 pneumonia due to SARS-associated coronavirus (J12.81)

IQ B97.29 Other coronavirus as the cause of diseases classified elsewhere

5 B97.3 Retrovirus as the cause of diseases classified elsewhere

EXCLUDES 1 Human immunodeficiency virus [HIV] disease (B20)

IQ B97.30 Unspecified retrovirus as the cause of diseases classified elsewhere

IQ B97.31 Lentivirus as the cause of diseases classified elsewhere

IQ B97.32 Oncovirus as the cause of diseases classified elsewhere

IQ B97.33 Human T-cell lymphotrophic virus, type I [HTLV-I] as the cause of diseases classified elsewhere

IQ B97.34 Human T-cell lymphotrophic virus, type II [HTLV-II] as the cause of diseases classified elsewhere

IQ B97.35 Human immunodeficiency virus, type 2 [HIV 2] as the cause of diseases classified elsewhere

IQ B97.39 Other retrovirus as the cause of diseases classified elsewhere

▲ M IQ B97.4 _Respiratory syncytial virus as the cause of diseases classified elsewhere_

RSV as the cause of diseases classified elsewhere

Code first related disorders, such as:
otitis media (H65.-)
upper respiratory infection (J06.9)

EXCLUDES 2 acute bronchiolitis due to respiratory syncytial virus (RSV) (J21.0)
acute bronchitis due to respiratory syncytial virus (RSV) (J20.5)
respiratory syncytial virus (RSV) pneumonia (J12.1)

IQ B97.5 Reovirus as the cause of diseases classified elsewhere

IQ B97.6 Parvovirus as the cause of diseases classified elsewhere

IQ B97.7 Papillomavirus as the cause of diseases classified elsewhere

5 B97.8 Other viral agents as the cause of diseases classified elsewhere

IQ B97.81 Human metapneumovirus as the cause of diseases classified elsewhere

IQ B97.89 Other viral agents as the cause of diseases classified elsewhere

Other infectious diseases (B99)

4 B99 Other and unspecified infectious diseases

CODING TIPS ✓ Do not use to indicate an unknown bacteria causing a localized infection. If the bacteria is unknown, there is no need to add a code for the bacteria.

IQ B99.8 Other infectious disease

IQ B99.9 Unspecified infectious disease

★ New ▲ Revised Px Primary SP PDGM Px SL Low CoM SH High CoM IQ Quest. Encounter H Hospice non-cancer Dx Unspecified M _Manifestation_

Chapter 1 Scenarios: Certain infectious and parasitic diseases (A00-B99)

Streptococcus pneumoniae septicemia

A patient is referred for home health nursing following hospitalization for streptococcus pneumoniae septicemia. She was given IV antibiotics for three days and will be taking oral antibiotics at home for five days.

Description	Code
Primary: Sepsis due to streptococcus pneumoniae	A40.3

There are combination codes for sepsis that include the infection and organism. Thus multiple codes are not needed to describe the problem and the bacterium. Note that the ICD-10 alphabetic index refers the coder to sepsis. No unique code exists for septicemia. A code from subcategory R65.2- (Severe sepsis) should not be assigned, unless severe sepsis or an associated acute organ dysfunction is documented. A code for long-term antibiotic use is not assigned because the length of her antibiotic treatment is brief.

Septic shock due to MSSA

A 72-year-old man was admitted to the hospital with acute renal failure due to septic shock, due to Methicillin susceptible Staphylococcus aureus (MSSA). The patient's renal failure is improving, and he was discharged to home health for observation and assessment of the renal condition until the physician determines it has resolved. He received two weeks of IV antibiotics in the hospital to treat the infection, and the home health nurse will administer the remainder of the eight-week course.

Description	Code
Primary: Sepsis due to Methicillin susceptible Staphylococcus aureus	A41.01
Secondary: Severe sepsis with septic shock	R65.21
Secondary: Acute kidney failure, unspecified	N17.9
Secondary: Long-term (current) use of antibiotics	Z79.2
Secondary: Encounter for adjustment and management of vascular access device	Z45.2

A single combination code (R65.21) captures both severe sepsis and septic shock. Tabular instruction at R65.21 tells the coder to code first the underlying infection, which is MSSA sepsis in this case. The code for the still-resolving acute renal failure is assigning additionally, in accordance with tabular instruction. Note that this scenario identifies an eight-week course of IV antibiotics so Z79.2 is appropriate to code. Code Z45.2 is also assigned for the administration of the IV antibiotics.

HIV, cryptosporidiosis

A patient is admitted with an AIDS-related infection specified as Cryptosporidiosis. His symptoms include dehydration and diarrhea.

Description	Code
Primary: HIV	B20
Secondary: Other protozoal intestinal diseases, cryptosporidiosis	A07.2

Cryptosporidiosis is an infection of the small intestine caused by a protozoal organism and is frequently a complication of HIV and AIDS. The ICD-10 guidelines state that if a patient is admitted for an HIV-related condition, the principal diagnosis should be B20, Human immunodeficiency virus (HIV) disease, followed by additional codes for all reported HIV-related conditions. Note that the Coding Clinic issued guidance on the coding of HIV-related illnesses in its Q1 2019 update, saying that B20 should be assigned only when there is a documented diagnosis of AIDS or the patient's illness is documented as related to or resulting from HIV, and that for patients described as "HIV positive" or having known HIV but no HIV-related illnesses, the correct code is Z21 (Asymptomatic human immunodeficiency virus [HIV] infection status. The patient's symptoms of dehydration and diarrhea are not coded additionally as they are integral to the Cryptosporidiosis infection. Note that many states prohibit reporting HIV as a primary diagnosis or reporting it at all. Check with your state's OASIS coordinator to determine the appropriate sequencing of an HIV diagnosis, based on your state's regulations. If prohibited, report the associated condition(s).

Cellulitis with E. coli

A 73-year-old woman comes to home health with a primary diagnosis of cellulitis on her groin that is infected with E. coli and is being treated with IV antibiotics. She also has diabetes and hypertension.

Description	Code
Primary: Cellulitis of groin	L03.314
Secondary: Unspecified Escherichia coli [E. coli] as the cause of diseases classified elsewhere	B96.20
Secondary: Type 2 diabetes mellitus without complications	E11.9
Secondary: Essential (primary) hypertension	I10
Secondary: Encounter for adjustment and management of vascular access device	Z45.2
Secondary: Long term (current) use of antibiotics	Z79.2

E. coli bacteria is the cause of the cellulitis in the patient's groin, which is classified to Chapter 12 (Diseases of Skin and Subcutaneous Tissue). Therefore, the appropriate code to capture the infecting E. coli organism is B96.20. Code B96.20 is sequenced after the disease that it is causing, the cellulitis, in accordance with coding guidelines. The patient is receiving IV antibiotics and therefore Z45.2 and Z79.2 are coded to capture this. As important comorbidities, her diabetes and hypertension are also coded.

HOME HEALTH CODING SCENARIOS

Infected abdominal surgical wound, IV antibiotics

A 72-year-old woman recently underwent surgery to remove cancer in her sigmoid colon. The surgery completely eradicated the cancer but the surgical wound developed an intramuscular abscess that's infected with E. coli and the patient was admitted to home health to continue treatment with a wound VAC and IV antibiotics for six weeks. The patient is morbidly obese with a BMI of 35.

Description	Code
Primary: Infection following a procedure, deep incisional surgical site, initial encounter	T81.42xA
Secondary: Unspecified Escherichia coli [E. coli] as the cause of diseases classified elsewhere	B96.20
Secondary: Morbid (severe) obesity due to excess calories	E66.01
Secondary: Body mass index (BMI) 35.0-35.9, adult	Z68.35
Secondary: Long term (current) use of antibiotics	Z79.2
Secondary: Encounter for adjustment and management of vascular access device	Z45.2
Secondary: Personal history of other malignant neoplasm of large intestine	Z85.038

The surgical wound is complicated by an intramuscular abscess, which equates to a deep incisional surgical site, and is appropriately coded to T81.42-, according to the inclusion terms on the code. Because the patient is still undergoing active treatment for the infection, with IV antibiotics and a wound VAC, it is considered active care and thus should take the seventh character "A," according to the Coding Clinic. The infecting organism, E. coli, is specified and thus is coded immediately following the infection code, in accordance with tabular instruction. Morbid obesity should always be coded when it's documented, according to Q4 2018 Coding Clinic guidance. Therefore, it is coded along with the specified BMI, in accordance with tabular instruction. The patient is receiving IV antibiotic therapy for six weeks and is thus at risk for complications, making the use of Z79.2 necessary. The code for care of the vascular access device, Z45.2, is also required to capture the administration of the antibiotics. The patient's cancer was said to be eradicated through surgery and thus the personal history code (Z85.038) is assigned, versus a current neoplasm code.

Tuberculosis sequelae

A 75-year-old woman comes to home health with lung calcification secondary to resolved pulmonary tuberculosis when she was a child.

Description	Code
Primary: Sequelae of respiratory and unspecified tuberculosis	B90.9

Code B90.9 captures both the lung calcification and the fact that it's due to a now-resolved tuberculosis infection, according to the alphabetic index. Therefore, an additional code is not required. An active tuberculosis code is not used here because the active infection has resolved.

Recurrent Clostridium difficile

A 79-year-old woman was recently hospitalized for severe colitis due to recurrent Clostridium difficile. During her hospitalization she experienced severe diarrhea and acute kidney failure. The kidney failure resolved prior to discharge but the infection is still resolving and she is still experiencing mild to moderate diarrhea. She has comorbidities of chronic diastolic heart failure and hypertension. Following her discharge, she is admitted to home health to continue her recovery. Skilled nursing will provide instruction to her caregiver on the disease process and management of new medications.

Description	Code
Primary: Enterocolitis due to Clostridium difficile, recurrent	A04.71
Secondary: Hypertensive heart disease with heart failure	I11.0
Secondary: Chronic diastolic (congestive) heart failure	I50.32

With the colitis due to Clostridium difficile infection still resolving and the focus of care, it is appropriately coded in the primary position. Since it's noted as recurrent, A04.71 is assigned. Her moderate diarrhea is not coded as it is inherent to the Clostridium difficile infection. There is an assumed relationship between hypertension and heart failure in the ICD-10 classification, unless the physician says they're unrelated to each other. Therefore, the diagnoses are coded as connected with I11.0 and I50.32.

Sepsis due to E. coli UTI

A 69-year-old woman comes to home health for treatment for sepsis that her record says was caused by an E. coli UTI. She will receive IV antibiotics for six weeks.

Description	Code
Primary: Sepsis due to Escherichia coli [E. coli]	A41.51
Secondary: Urinary tract infection, site not specified	N39.0
Secondary: Encounter for adjustment and management of vascular access device	Z45.2
Secondary: Long term (current) use of antibiotics	Z79.2

Only two codes — A41.51 (Sepsis due to Escherichia coli [E. coli]) and N39.0 (Urinary tract infection, site not specified) — are required to capture a diagnosis of sepsis due to a urinary tract infection that was caused by E. coli bacteria, according to Q1 2018 Coding Clinic guidance. The administration of IV antibiotics is captured with Z45.2 and Z79.2.

HOME HEALTH CODING SCENARIOS

Recurrent pneumonia, HIV status

A 65-year-old man is admitted to home health for treatment with intravenous antibiotics for streptococcus pneumoniae pneumonia, which his medical record states is a recurrent diagnosis. His record also indicates that he is HIV positive, lives alone and has very little support, which prompted his physician to order medical social worker services.

Description	Code
Primary: Pneumonia due to Streptococcus pneumoniae	J13
Secondary: Asymptomatic human immunodeficiency virus [HIV] infection status	Z21
Secondary: Problems related to living alone	Z60.2
Secondary: Personal history of pneumonia (recurrent)	Z87.01
Secondary: Encounter for adjustment and management of vascular access device	Z45.2
Secondary: Long term (current) use of antibiotics	Z79.2

As the focus of care, the patient's pneumonia is coded in the primary position. The type of pneumonia is specified, prompting the assignment of the specific pneumonia code J13. Though the patient has streptococcus pneumoniae pneumonia that is stated as recurrent and is also HIV positive, Z21 must be assigned to capture the patient's HIV status, not B20 (Human immunodeficiency virus [HIV] disease. Neither streptococcus pneumoniae pneumonia nor the recurrent pneumonia can be assumed to be HIV-related illness, which must be diagnosed by the physician in order to use B20, according to Q1 2019 Coding Clinic guidance. Additional status codes are assigned to capture that the patient lives alone (Z60.2) and has a history of recurrent pneumonia (Z87.01). The administration of IV antibiotics is captured with Z45.2 and Z79.2 Note that coding guidelines allow for the assignment of codes between the categories of Z55 and Z65 based on a clinician's documentation.

Chapter 2: Neoplasms (C00- D49)

"Neoplasm" refers to any new, abnormal growth of tissue. The words tumor, fibroid, hyperplasia, mass, or adenoma indicate a neoplasm. However, if documentation states 'mass,' go to 'mass' in the Alphabetic Index. All malignant and most benign neoplasms are classified in this chapter by site (topography) with broad groupings for behavior (malignant, in situ, benign), whether they are functionally active or not. In a few cases, such as malignant melanoma and certain neuroendocrine tumors, the morphology (histologic type) is included in the category and codes. An additional code from Chapter 4, Endocrine, nutritional and metabolic diseases, may be used to identify functional activity associated with any neoplasm.

Code selection in this chapter depends on the physician's description of the neoplasm. If there is not enough information to select a code, query the physician.

Types of neoplasms:

- **Malignant neoplasms** (cancers) (C00-C75) grow uncontrollably and may invade healthy surrounding tissues or spread (metastasize) from the point of origin.

- **A primary malignancy** is the area where the tumor first developed in the body.

- **A secondary malignancy** (metastasis) is an area of the body where the first- listed cancer has metastasized.

- **Benign neoplasms** (noncancerous) (D10-D36) do not invade surrounding tissues or metastasize.

- **Carcinoma in situ** (CIS or ca in situ) (D00-D09) is an early form of carcinoma defined by the non-invasion of surrounding tissues. In other words, the neoplastic cells proliferate in their normal habitat, hence the name 'in situ' (Latin for 'in its place'). CIS is considered a precursor or incipient form of cancer that if left untreated long enough may transform into a malignant neoplasm.

- **Uncertain behavior** (D37-D48) describes a neoplasm that is exhibiting characteristics of both malignant and benign neoplasms. Further study is needed to determine the type of neoplasm.

- **Unspecified behavior** (D49) describes a neoplasm when there is not enough information to select the type of neoplasm. This may occur when the physician is waiting for a pathology report before deciding on the nature of the neoplasm. Ask the physician for more information, if possible. Do not code unspecified behavior just because

it is unknown whether a cancer is primary or secondary. It is important to code cancers to malignant neoplasms when appropriate.

If the medical record states "**metastatic to**," this refers to the secondary site. The primary neoplasm is metastatic to the secondary site.

If the medical record states "**metastatic from**," this refers to the primary site. A secondary site is metastatic from the primary site.

If the medical record states "**contiguous sites**," this refers to primary neoplasms with overlapping boundaries in which the point of origin (primary site) cannot be determined. Therefore, contiguous sites should be classified to fourth character of 8 (overlapping lesion), unless a combination code is specifically indexed elsewhere. For example, a cancer may involve the skin of cheek and nose, but the physician has not documented which neoplasm is primary. In this case, report C44.80 (unspecified malignant neoplasm of overlapping sites of skin).

For multiple neoplasms of the same site that are not contiguous, such as tumors in different quadrants of the same breast, codes for each site should be assigned.

There are some situations in which a code from Chapter 2 is not the most appropriate. Below are a few situations to watch out for:

- If a patient has a **personal or family history of a condition** reported in this chapter, it may be more appropriate to select from the Z code section, such as Z85.- (personal history of malignant neoplasms), or Z80.9 (family history of malignant neoplasm). Remember that personal history codes are used more often in home health than family history codes.

- **Nonspecific neoplasms** are sometimes reported using codes from other chapters. If the documentation uses words such as "mass," "swelling," or "lump," but offers no definitive diagnosis, refer to that word in the Alphabetic Index in order to find the correct code.

For example, a breast mass or lump is reported using code N63 from Chapter 14, Diseases of the genitourinary system. An abdominal mass is reported using code R19.00 from Chapter18, Symptoms, signs and abnormal clinical and laboratory findings, not elsewhere classified. Coders should attempt to obtain more specific information before coding lumps or masses as well as the specific location of the mass or lump.

- Although it is not found often in home health, when a **pregnant woman has a malignant**

neoplasm, a code from subcategory O9A.1-, Malignant neoplasm complicating pregnancy, childbirth, and the puerperium, should be sequenced first, followed by the appropriate code from Chapter 2 to indicate the type of neoplasm.

Neoplasms & the alphabetic index

The Alphabetic Index includes a **Neoplasm Table** that can be used to select the correct code. In the left hand column of the table is a list of locations within the body. In the other columns are codes for the types of neoplasms (malignant, benign, uncertain behavior) in that body area. However, **coders should not go directly to the Neoplasm Table unless the only documentation is something like 'lung cancer.'** If the histological term is present in the medical record, first look up the histological term in the alphabetic index. The index will refer you to the table when appropriate.

Consider the following examples of how to use the Index to find a neoplasm code:

- If the documentation states "hyperplasia, adrenal cortex," the Index refers you to E27.8 (other specified disorders of adrenal glands). The Neoplasm Table is not referenced.

- If the documentation states "dysplasia, high grade, focal," of the colon, the Index refers the coder to D12.6, Benign neoplasm of colon, unspecified.

When using the Neoplasm Table, first find the body site, and then refer to the column for malignant, benign, uncertain behavior, or unspecified codes as appropriate. If the neoplasm is malignant, determine whether it is primary, secondary, or cancer in situ. Be sure to refer to the code in the Tabular List to ensure the listed code is correct; do not code using only the Neoplasm Table. If the site is unknown, refer to Neoplasm, unknown site or unspecified, in the Table. There are specific codes for unknown primary malignant, secondary malignant, Ca in situ, benign, uncertain and unspecified behaviors.

Some codes in the Neoplasm Table are grouped under the heading "connective tissue." This includes tissues such as blood vessels, bursa, fascia, ligaments, muscle, peripheral nerves and tendons in a specific body area. Neoplasms of connective tissue have a separate category (C49.-). For example, malignant neoplasm of the abdominal cavity is listed as C76.2 (malignant neoplasm, abdomen). Malignant neoplasm of connective tissue of the abdomen is listed as C49.4 (malignant neoplasm of connective, and other soft tissue, abdomen).

Multiple Coding and Sequencing

It is important to read the Includes and Excludes notes under codes in this chapter, as well as any other instructions under the code or code category. There are many multiple coding and sequencing issues for codes in this chapter.

Important note: Just because a neoplasm is listed as a primary cancer does not mean it should be reported as the primary diagnosis. Sequencing of codes depends on which neoplasm site is the focus of care for that specific episode. If the primary site of the cancer is still present, it is *usually* sequenced prior to the secondary site. If the focus of care is the secondary site, the secondary site is listed as the primary diagnosis even though the primary malignancy is still present and the primary site is coded as an additional code.

If a primary site is considered eradicated and there is no further treatment directed to that site and no evidence of any existing primary malignancy, use the appropriate Z85 code for personal history of the primary malignant neoplasm.

If the primary or secondary site is unknown, use C80.1 (primary malignant site unknown) or C79.9 (secondary site is unknown).

If no determination of known primary or secondary sites of malignancy for advanced cancer can be made, use code C80.0, Disseminated malignant neoplasm, unspecified.

Special Coding Issues

Postoperative Treatment

A neoplasm is still considered present if the patient is receiving treatment. That is, if the neoplasm has been excised but the patient is still receiving chemotherapy or radiotherapy, report a code for the cancer, not a Z85 code (personal history of malignant neoplasm).

When the admission/encounter is for a complication resulting from a surgical procedure, designate the complication as the principal or first listed diagnosis if treatment is directed at resolving the complication.

If the neoplasm has been excised, and there is no complication, the code for aftercare following surgery for a neoplasm, Z48.3, is used. This will be followed by the code for the neoplasm if it is unknown that the neoplasm is fully eradicated, or if the neoplasm is still receiving treatment. If the neoplasm is known to be fully eradicated by the surgery, and only routine post-surgical aftercare is needed, then the personal history code is used.

Coding and sequencing of complications

When admission/encounter is for **management of anemia associated with the malignancy,** and the treatment is only for the anemia, the appropriate code for the malignancy is sequenced as the principal or first-listed diagnosis followed by the appropriate code for the anemia (such as code D63.0, Anemia in neoplastic disease).

When the admission/encounter is for management of an anemia associated with an adverse effect of the administration of chemotherapy, immunotherapy or radiation and the only treatment is for the anemia, the anemia code is sequenced first.

When the admission/encounter is for the management of dehydration due to the malignancy and only the dehydration is being treated (intravenous hydration), the dehydration is sequenced first, followed by the code(s) for the malignancy.

Pathological fracture due to a neoplasm

When an encounter is for a pathological fracture due to a neoplasm, and the focus of treatment is the fracture, a code from subcategory M84.5, Pathological fracture in neoplastic disease, should be sequenced first, followed by the code for the neoplasm from Chapter 2.

If the focus of care is the neoplasm with an associated pathological fracture, the neoplasm code should be sequenced first, followed by a code from M84.5 for the pathological fracture.

Patients with long-term use of agents affecting estrogen receptors and estrogen levels

Codes revolving around long-term use of agents affecting estrogen receptors and estrogen levels, such as SERMS, aromatase inhibitors and other agents, are found in the Z79.81- subcategory. The use of long-term prophylactic agents to prevent recurrence of disease raises questions as to when treatment is actually complete. Instructions at the Z79.81 subcategory include: 'Code first, if applicable': malignant neoplasm of breast (C50-) or malignant neoplasm of prostate (C61) and 'Use additional code, if applicable, to identify': estrogen receptor positive status (Z17.0); family history of breast cancer (Z80.3); genetic susceptibility to cancer (Z15.0-); personal history of breast cancer (Z85.3); personal history of prostate cancer (Z85.46) and/or postmenopausal status (Z78.0).

Admissions/Encounters involving chemotherapy, immunotherapy or radiation therapy

If a patient's admission/encounter is solely for the administration of chemotherapy, immunotherapy or radiation therapy, assign a code from Z51.- as the first listed or principal diagnosis. The malignancy for which the therapy is being administered should be assigned as a secondary diagnosis.

Malignant neoplasm associated with a transplanted organ

The incidence of cancer in transplanted organs has increased. A malignant neoplasm of a transplanted organ should be coded as a transplant complication. Assign first the appropriate code from category T86.-. Complications of transplanted organs and tissue, followed by code C80.2, Malignant neoplasm associated with transplanted organ. Use an additional code for the specific malignancy.

Leukemia, multiple myeloma and malignant plasma cell neoplasm

The categories for leukemia and category C90, Multiple myeloma and malignant plasma cell neoplasms, have codes indicating whether or not the leukemia has achieved remission. There are also codes Z85.6, Personal history of leukemia, and Z85.79, Personal history of lymphoid, hematopoietic and related tissues. If the documentation is unclear as to whether the leukemia has achieved remission, the provider should be queried.

Chapter 2

C00-D49

CHAPTER 2: NEOPLASMS (C00-D49)

Note:

Functional activity

All neoplasms are classified in this chapter, whether they are functionally active or not. An additional code from Chapter 4 may be used, to identify functional activity associated with any neoplasm.

Morphology [Histology]

Chapter 2 classifies neoplasms primarily by site (topography), with broad groupings for behavior, malignant, in situ, benign, etc. The Table of Neoplasms should be used to identify the correct topography code. In a few cases, such as for malignant melanoma and certain neuroendocrine tumors, the morphology (histologic type) is included in the category and codes.

Primary malignant neoplasms overlapping site boundaries

A primary malignant neoplasm that overlaps two or more contiguous (next to each other) sites should be classified to the subcategory/code .8 ('overlapping lesion'), unless the combination is specifically indexed elsewhere. For multiple neoplasms of the same site that are not contiguous, such as tumors in different quadrants of the same breast, codes for each site should be assigned.

Malignant neoplasm of ectopic tissue

Malignant neoplasms of ectopic tissue are to be coded to the site mentioned, e.g., ectopic pancreatic malignant neoplasms are coded to pancreas, unspecified (C25.9).

GUIDELINES Section I.C.2

Chapter 2 of the ICD-10-CM contains the codes for most benign and all malignant neoplasms. Certain benign neoplasms, such as prostatic adenomas, may be found in the specific body system chapters. To properly code a neoplasm it is necessary to determine from the record if the neoplasm is benign, in-situ, malignant, or of uncertain histologic behavior. If malignant, any secondary (metastatic) sites should also be determined.

GUIDELINES Section I.C.2

The neoplasm table in the Alphabetic Index should be referenced first. However, if the histological term is documented, that term should be referenced first, rather than going immediately to the Neoplasm Table, in order to determine which column in the Neoplasm Table is appropriate. For example, if the documentation indicates "adenoma," refer to the term in the Alphabetic Index to review the entries under this term and the instructional note to "see also neoplasm, by site, benign." The table provides the proper code based on the type of neoplasm and the site.

This chapter contains the following blocks:

C00-C14	Malignant neoplasms of lip, oral cavity and pharynx
C15-C26	Malignant neoplasms of digestive organs
C30-C39	Malignant neoplasms of respiratory and intrathoracic organs
C40-C41	Malignant neoplasms of bone and articular cartilage
C43-C44	Melanoma and other malignant neoplasms of skin
C45-C49	Malignant neoplasms of mesothelial and soft tissue
C50	Malignant neoplasms of breast
C51-C58	Malignant neoplasms of female genital organs
C60-C63	Malignant neoplasms of male genital organs
C64-C68	Malignant neoplasms of urinary tract
C69-C72	Malignant neoplasms of eye, brain and other parts of central nervous system
C73-C75	Malignant neoplasms of thyroid and other endocrine glands
C7A	Malignant neuroendocrine tumors
C7B	Secondary neuroendocrine tumors

C76-C80	Malignant neoplasms of ill-defined, other secondary and unspecified sites
C81-C96	Malignant neoplasms of lymphoid, hematopoietic and related tissue
D00-D09	In situ neoplasms
D10-D36	Benign neoplasms, except benign neuroendocrine tumors
D3A	Benign neuroendocrine tumors
D37-D48	Neoplasms of uncertain behavior, polycythemia vera and myelodysplastic syndromes
D49	Neoplasms of unspecified behavior

Malignant neoplasms (C00-C96)

Malignant neoplasms, stated or presumed to be primary (of specified sites), and certain specified histologies, except neuroendocrine, and of lymphoid, hematopoietic and related tissue (C00-C75)

Malignant neoplasms of lip, oral cavity and pharynx (C00-C14)

CODING TIPS ✓ Codes classifiable to C00-C14 include active cancer. History of cancer to the lip, pharynx, or oral cavity should be coded to Z85.81-.

+ 4 C00 Malignant neoplasm of lip

Use additional code to identify:
alcohol abuse and dependence (F10.-)
history of tobacco dependence (Z87.891)
tobacco dependence (F17.-)
tobacco use (Z72.0)

EXCLUDES 1 malignant melanoma of lip (C43.0)
Merkel cell carcinoma of lip (C4A.0)
other and unspecified malignant neoplasm of skin of lip (C44.0-)

CODING TIPS ✓ C00 indicates active cancer. See Z85.818 for personal history of primary malignancy of lip, oral cavity and pharynx.

CODING TIPS ✓ Area on lip must be specified in documentation to choose an acceptable code.

SP SL + C00.0 Malignant neoplasm of external upper lip

Malignant neoplasm of lipstick area of upper lip
Malignant neoplasm of upper lip NOS
Malignant neoplasm of vermilion border of upper lip

SP SL + C00.1 Malignant neoplasm of external lower lip

Malignant neoplasm of lower lip NOS
Malignant neoplasm of lipstick area of lower lip
Malignant neoplasm of vermilion border of lower lip

IQ + C00.2 Malignant neoplasm of external lip, unspecified

Malignant neoplasm of vermilion border of lip NOS

SP SL + C00.3 Malignant neoplasm of upper lip, inner aspect

---

4 4th digit required   5 5th digit required   6 6th digit required   7 7th digit required   7 7th digit placeholder   + Additional code   ▤ Laterality

642   DecisionHealth's FY 2020 Complete Home Health ICD-10-CM Diagnosis Coding Manual

Malignant neoplasm of buccal aspect of upper lip

Malignant neoplasm of frenulum of upper lip

Malignant neoplasm of mucosa of upper lip

Malignant neoplasm of oral aspect of upper lip

SP **SL** **+ C00.4** **Malignant neoplasm of lower lip, inner aspect**

Malignant neoplasm of buccal aspect of lower lip

Malignant neoplasm of frenulum of lower lip

Malignant neoplasm of mucosa of lower lip

Malignant neoplasm of oral aspect of lower lip

IQ **+ C00.5** **Malignant neoplasm of lip, unspecified, inner aspect**

Malignant neoplasm of buccal aspect of lip, unspecified

Malignant neoplasm of frenulum of lip, unspecified

Malignant neoplasm of mucosa of lip, unspecified

Malignant neoplasm of oral aspect of lip, unspecified

SP **+ C00.6** **Malignant neoplasm of commissure of lip, unspecified**

SP **SL** **+ C00.8** **Malignant neoplasm of overlapping sites of lip**

IQ **+ C00.9** **Malignant neoplasm of lip, unspecified**

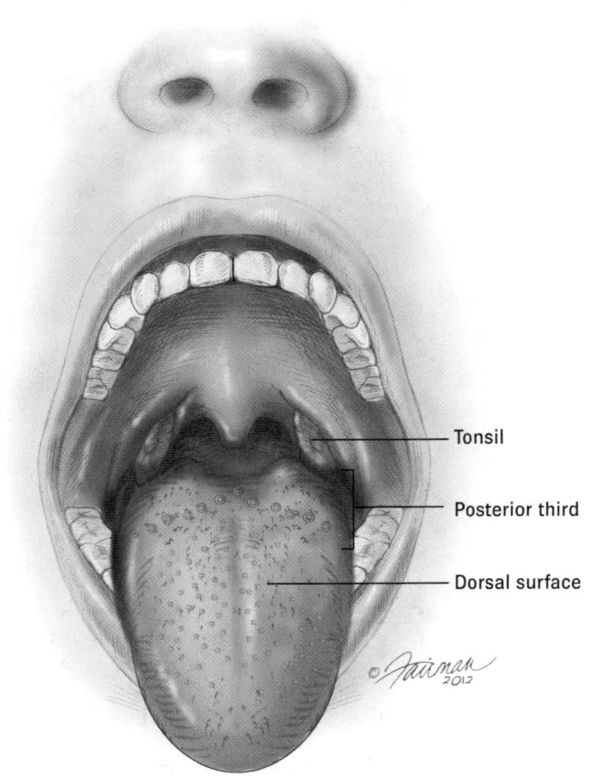

Tonsil

Posterior third

Dorsal surface

©Jarman 2012

SP **SL** **+ C01** **Malignant neoplasm of base of tongue**

Malignant neoplasm of dorsal surface of base of tongue

Malignant neoplasm of fixed part of tongue NOS

Malignant neoplasm of posterior third of tongue

Use additional code to identify:
alcohol abuse and dependence (F10.-)
history of tobacco dependence (Z87.891)
tobacco dependence (F17.-)
tobacco use (Z72.0)

CODING TIPS ✓ C01 codes indicate active cancer. See Z85.810 for personal history of primary malignancy of tongue and Z85.818 for tonsils.

+ 4 C02 **Malignant neoplasm of other and unspecified parts of tongue**

Use additional code to identify:
alcohol abuse and dependence (F10.-)
history of tobacco dependence (Z87.891)
tobacco dependence (F17.-)
tobacco use (Z72.0)

CODING TIPS ✓ C02 codes indicate active cancer. See Z85.810 for personal history of primary malignancy of tongue and Z85.818 for tonsils.

CODING TIPS ✓ Upper or lower gum must be specified in documentation to choose an acceptable code.

SP **SL** **+ C02.0** **Malignant neoplasm of dorsal surface of tongue**

Malignant neoplasm of anterior two-thirds of tongue, dorsal surface

EXCLUDES 2 malignant neoplasm of dorsal surface of base of tongue (C01)

SP **SL** **+ C02.1** **Malignant neoplasm of border of tongue**

Malignant neoplasm of tip of tongue

SP **SL** **+ C02.2** **Malignant neoplasm of ventral surface of tongue**

Malignant neoplasm of anterior two-thirds of tongue, ventral surface

Malignant neoplasm of frenulum linguae

SP **SL** **+ C02.3** **Malignant neoplasm of anterior two-thirds of tongue, part unspecified**

Malignant neoplasm of middle third of tongue NOS

Malignant neoplasm of mobile part of tongue NOS

SP **SL** **+ C02.4** **Malignant neoplasm of lingual tonsil**

EXCLUDES 2 malignant neoplasm of tonsil NOS (C09.9)

SP **SL** **+ C02.8** **Malignant neoplasm of overlapping sites of tongue**

Malignant neoplasm of two or more contiguous sites of tongue

SP **SL** **+ C02.9** **Malignant neoplasm of tongue, unspecified**

+ 4 C03 **Malignant neoplasm of gum**

INCLUDES malignant neoplasm of alveolar (ridge) mucosa
malignant neoplasm of gingiva

Use additional code to identify:
alcohol abuse and dependence (F10.-)
history of tobacco dependence (Z87.891)
tobacco dependence (F17.-)
tobacco use (Z72.0)

EXCLUDES 2 malignant odontogenic neoplasms (C41.0-C41.1)

★ New ▲ Revised Px Primary **SP** PDGM Px **SL** Low CoM **SH** High CoM **IQ** Quest. Encounter **H** Hospice non-cancer Dx Unspecified **M** Manifestation

DecisionHealth's FY 2020 Complete Home Health ICD-10-CM Diagnosis Coding Manual

643

Chapter 2

C00-D49

CODING TIPS ✓ This category indicates active cancer. See Z85.818 for personal history of primary malignancy of lip, oral cavity and pharynx.

SP ✚ **C03.0 Malignant neoplasm of upper gum**

SP SL ✚ **C03.1 Malignant neoplasm of lower gum**

!Q ✚ **C03.9 Malignant neoplasm of gum, unspecified**

✚ **4 C04 Malignant neoplasm of floor of mouth**
Use additional code to identify:
alcohol abuse and dependence (F10.-)
history of tobacco dependence (Z87.891)
tobacco dependence (F17.-)
tobacco use (Z72.0)

CODING TIPS ✓ This category indicates active cancer. See Z85.818 for personal history of primary malignancy of lip, oral cavity and pharynx.

SP SL ✚ **C04.0 Malignant neoplasm of anterior floor of mouth**
Malignant neoplasm of anterior to the premolar-canine junction

SP SL ✚ **C04.1 Malignant neoplasm of lateral floor of mouth**

SP SL ✚ **C04.8 Malignant neoplasm of overlapping sites of floor of mouth**

SP SL ✚ **C04.9 Malignant neoplasm of floor of mouth, unspecified**

✚ **4 C05 Malignant neoplasm of palate**
Use additional code to identify:
alcohol abuse and dependence (F10.-)
history of tobacco dependence (Z87.891)
tobacco dependence (F17.-)
tobacco use (Z72.0)

EXCLUDES 1 Kaposi's sarcoma of palate (C46.2)

CODING TIPS ✓ This category indicates active cancer. See Z85.818 for personal history of primary malignancy of lip, oral cavity and pharynx.

SP SL ✚ **C05.0 Malignant neoplasm of hard palate**

SP SL ✚ **C05.1 Malignant neoplasm of soft palate**

EXCLUDES 2 malignant neoplasm of nasopharyngeal surface of soft palate (C11.3)

SP SL ✚ **C05.2 Malignant neoplasm of uvula**

SP SL ✚ **C05.8 Malignant neoplasm of overlapping sites of palate**

SP SL ✚ **C05.9 Malignant neoplasm of palate, unspecified**
Malignant neoplasm of roof of mouth

✚ **4 C06 Malignant neoplasm of other and unspecified parts of mouth**
Use additional code to identify:
alcohol abuse and dependence (F10.-)
history of tobacco dependence (Z87.891)
tobacco dependence (F17.-)
tobacco use (Z72.0)

CODING TIPS ✓ This category indicates active cancer. See Z85.818 for personal history of primary malignancy of lip, oral cavity and pharynx.

CODING TIPS ✓ Area in mouth should be specified in documentation to choose an acceptable code.

SP SL ✚ **C06.0 Malignant neoplasm of cheek mucosa**
Malignant neoplasm of buccal mucosa NOS
Malignant neoplasm of internal cheek

SP SL ✚ **C06.1 Malignant neoplasm of vestibule of mouth**
Malignant neoplasm of buccal sulcus (upper) (lower)
Malignant neoplasm of labial sulcus (upper) (lower)

SP SL ✚ **C06.2 Malignant neoplasm of retromolar area**

✚ **5 C06.8 Malignant neoplasm of overlapping sites of other and unspecified parts of mouth**

SP SL ✚ **C06.80 Malignant neoplasm of overlapping sites of unspecified parts of mouth**

SP SL ✚ **C06.89 Malignant neoplasm of overlapping sites of other parts of mouth**
'book leaf' neoplasm [ventral surface of tongue and floor of mouth]

!Q SL ✚ **C06.9 Malignant neoplasm of mouth, unspecified**
Malignant neoplasm of minor salivary gland, unspecified site
Malignant neoplasm of oral cavity NOS

SP SL ✚ **C07 Malignant neoplasm of parotid gland**
Use additional code to identify:
alcohol abuse and dependence (F10.-)
exposure to environmental tobacco smoke (Z77.22)
exposure to tobacco smoke in the perinatal period (P96.81)
history of tobacco dependence (Z87.891)
occupational exposure to environmental tobacco smoke (Z57.31)
tobacco dependence (F17.-)
tobacco use (Z72.0)

✚ **4 C08 Malignant neoplasm of other and unspecified major salivary glands**

INCLUDES malignant neoplasm of salivary ducts

Use additional code to identify:
alcohol abuse and dependence (F10.-)
exposure to environmental tobacco smoke (Z77.22)
exposure to tobacco smoke in the perinatal period (P96.81)
history of tobacco dependence (Z87.891)
occupational exposure to environmental tobacco smoke (Z57.31)
tobacco dependence (F17.-)
tobacco use (Z72.0)

EXCLUDES 1 malignant neoplasms of specified minor salivary glands which are classified according to their anatomical location

EXCLUDES 2 malignant neoplasms of minor salivary glands NOS (C06.9)
malignant neoplasm of parotid gland (C07)

SP SL ✚ **C08.0 Malignant neoplasm of submandibular gland**
Malignant neoplasm of submaxillary gland

SP SL ✚ **C08.1 Malignant neoplasm of sublingual gland**

!Q SL ✚ **C08.9 Malignant neoplasm of major salivary gland, unspecified**

---

4 4th digit required   **5** 5th digit required   **6** 6th digit required   **7** 7th digit required   **7** 7th digit placeholder   ✚Additional code   ▱ Laterality

Malignant neoplasm of salivary gland (major) NOS

+ ◪ **C09 Malignant neoplasm of tonsil**
Use additional code to identify:
alcohol abuse and dependence (F10.-)
exposure to environmental tobacco smoke (Z77.22)
exposure to tobacco smoke in the perinatal period (P96.81)
history of tobacco dependence (Z87.891)
occupational exposure to environmental tobacco smoke (Z57.31)
tobacco dependence (F17.-)
tobacco use (Z72.0)
> EXCLUDES 2 malignant neoplasm of lingual tonsil (C02.4)
> malignant neoplasm of pharyngeal tonsil (C11.1)

SP **SL** + **C09.0 Malignant neoplasm of tonsillar fossa**

IQ **SL** + **C09.1 Malignant neoplasm of tonsillar pillar (anterior) (posterior)**

SP **SL** + **C09.8 Malignant neoplasm of overlapping sites of tonsil**

SP **SL** + **C09.9 Malignant neoplasm of tonsil, unspecified**
Malignant neoplasm of tonsil NOS
Malignant neoplasm of faucial tonsils
Malignant neoplasm of palatine tonsils

+ ◪ **C10 Malignant neoplasm of oropharynx**
Use additional code to identify:
alcohol abuse and dependence (F10.-)
exposure to environmental tobacco smoke (Z77.22)
exposure to tobacco smoke in the perinatal period (P96.81)
history of tobacco dependence (Z87.891)
occupational exposure to environmental tobacco smoke (Z57.31)
tobacco dependence (F17.-)
tobacco use (Z72.0)
> EXCLUDES 2 malignant neoplasm of tonsil (C09.-)

SP **SL** + **C10.0 Malignant neoplasm of vallecula**

SP **SL** + **C10.1 Malignant neoplasm of anterior surface of epiglottis**
Malignant neoplasm of epiglottis, free border [margin]
Malignant neoplasm of glossoepiglottic fold(s)
> EXCLUDES 2 malignant neoplasm of epiglottis (suprahyoid portion) NOS (C32.1)

SP **SL** + **C10.2 Malignant neoplasm of lateral wall of oropharynx**

SP **SL** + **C10.3 Malignant neoplasm of posterior wall of oropharynx**

SP **SL** + **C10.4 Malignant neoplasm of branchial cleft**
Malignant neoplasm of branchial cyst [site of neoplasm]

SP **SL** + **C10.8 Malignant neoplasm of overlapping sites of oropharynx**
Malignant neoplasm of junctional region of oropharynx

SP **SL** + **C10.9 Malignant neoplasm of oropharynx, unspecified**

+ ◪ **C11 Malignant neoplasm of nasopharynx**
Use additional code to identify:

exposure to environmental tobacco smoke (Z77.22)
exposure to tobacco smoke in the perinatal period (P96.81)
history of tobacco dependence (Z87.891)
occupational exposure to environmental tobacco smoke (Z57.31)
tobacco dependence (F17.-)
tobacco use (Z72.0)

SP **SL** + **C11.0 Malignant neoplasm of superior wall of nasopharynx**
Malignant neoplasm of roof of nasopharynx

SP **SL** + **C11.1 Malignant neoplasm of posterior wall of nasopharynx**
Malignant neoplasm of adenoid
Malignant neoplasm of pharyngeal tonsil

SP **SL** + **C11.2 Malignant neoplasm of lateral wall of nasopharynx**
Malignant neoplasm of fossa of Rosenmüller
Malignant neoplasm of opening of auditory tube
Malignant neoplasm of pharyngeal recess

SP **SL** + **C11.3 Malignant neoplasm of anterior wall of nasopharynx**
Malignant neoplasm of floor of nasopharynx
Malignant neoplasm of nasopharyngeal (anterior) (posterior) surface of soft palate
Malignant neoplasm of posterior margin of nasal choana
Malignant neoplasm of posterior margin of nasal septum

SP **SL** + **C11.8 Malignant neoplasm of overlapping sites of nasopharynx**

SP + **C11.9 Malignant neoplasm of nasopharynx, unspecified**
Malignant neoplasm of nasopharyngeal wall NOS

SP **SL** + **C12 Malignant neoplasm of pyriform sinus**
Malignant neoplasm of pyriform fossa
Use additional code to identify:
exposure to environmental tobacco smoke (Z77.22)
exposure to tobacco smoke in the perinatal period (P96.81)
history of tobacco dependence (Z87.891)
occupational exposure to environmental tobacco smoke (Z57.31)
tobacco dependence (F17.-)
tobacco use (Z72.0)

+ ◪ **C13 Malignant neoplasm of hypopharynx**
Use additional code to identify:
exposure to environmental tobacco smoke (Z77.22)
exposure to tobacco smoke in the perinatal period (P96.81)
history of tobacco dependence (Z87.891)
occupational exposure to environmental tobacco smoke (Z57.31)
tobacco dependence (F17.-)
tobacco use (Z72.0)
> EXCLUDES 2 malignant neoplasm of pyriform sinus (C12)

SP **SL** + **C13.0 Malignant neoplasm of postcricoid region**

★ New ▲ Revised **Px** Primary **SP** PDGM Px **SL** Low CoM **SH** High CoM **IQ** Quest. Encounter **H** Hospice non-cancer Dx   Unspecified   **M** *Manifestation*

Chapter 2

C00-D49

SP SL ✚ C13.1 Malignant neoplasm of aryepiglottic fold, hypopharyngeal aspect
Malignant neoplasm of aryepiglottic fold, marginal zone
Malignant neoplasm of aryepiglottic fold NOS
Malignant neoplasm of interarytenoid fold, marginal zone
Malignant neoplasm of interarytenoid fold NOS
EXCLUDES 2   malignant neoplasm of aryepiglottic fold or interarytenoid fold, laryngeal aspect (C32.1)

SP SL ✚ C13.2 Malignant neoplasm of posterior wall of hypopharynx

SP SL ✚ C13.8 Malignant neoplasm of overlapping sites of hypopharynx

SP SL ✚ C13.9   Malignant neoplasm of hypopharynx, unspecified
Malignant neoplasm of hypopharyngeal wall NOS

✚ 4 C14 Malignant neoplasm of other and ill-defined sites in the lip, oral cavity and pharynx
Use additional code to identify:
alcohol abuse and dependence (F10.-)
exposure to environmental tobacco smoke (Z77.22)
exposure to tobacco smoke in the perinatal period (P96.81)
history of tobacco dependence (Z87.891)
occupational exposure to environmental tobacco smoke (Z57.31)
tobacco dependence (F17.-)
tobacco use (Z72.0)
EXCLUDES 1   malignant neoplasm of oral cavity NOS (C06.9)

SP SL ✚ C14.0   Malignant neoplasm of pharynx, unspecified

SP SL ✚ C14.2 Malignant neoplasm of Waldeyer's ring

SP SL ✚ C14.8 Malignant neoplasm of overlapping sites of lip, oral cavity and pharynx
Primary malignant neoplasm of two or more contiguous sites of lip, oral cavity and pharynx
EXCLUDES 1   'book leaf' neoplasm [ventral surface of tongue and floor of mouth] (C06.89)

Malignant neoplasms of digestive organs (C15-C26)

EXCLUDES 1   Kaposi's sarcoma of gastrointestinal sites (C46.4)
EXCLUDES 2   gastrointestinal stromal tumors (C49.A-)
CODING TIPS ✓   Codes classifiable to C15-C26 include active cancer. History of cancer to digestive organs should be coded to Z85.0-.

✚ 4 C15 Malignant neoplasm of esophagus
Use additional code to identify:
alcohol abuse and dependence (F10.-)
CODING TIPS ✓   This category indicates active cancer. See Z85.01 for personal history of primary malignancy of esophagus.

SP ✚ C15.3 Malignant neoplasm of upper third of esophagus

SP ✚ C15.4 Malignant neoplasm of middle third of esophagus

SP ✚ C15.5 Malignant neoplasm of lower third of esophagus
EXCLUDES 1   malignant neoplasm of cardio-esophageal junction (C16.0)

SP ✚ C15.8 Malignant neoplasm of overlapping sites of esophagus

SP ✚ C15.9   Malignant neoplasm of esophagus, unspecified

✚ 4 C16 Malignant neoplasm of stomach
Use additional code to identify:
alcohol abuse and dependence (F10.-)
EXCLUDES 2   malignant carcinoid tumor of the stomach (C7A.092)
CODING TIPS ✓   This category indicates active cancer. See Z85.02 for personal history of primary malignancy of stomach.

SP ✚ C16.0 Malignant neoplasm of cardia
Malignant neoplasm of cardiac orifice
Malignant neoplasm of cardio-esophageal junction
Malignant neoplasm of esophagus and stomach
Malignant neoplasm of gastro-esophageal junction

SP ✚ C16.1 Malignant neoplasm of fundus of stomach

SP ✚ C16.2 Malignant neoplasm of body of stomach

SP ✚ C16.3 Malignant neoplasm of pyloric antrum
Malignant neoplasm of gastric antrum

SP ✚ C16.4 Malignant neoplasm of pylorus
Malignant neoplasm of prepylorus
Malignant neoplasm of pyloric canal

SP ✚ C16.5   Malignant neoplasm of lesser curvature of stomach, unspecified
Malignant neoplasm of lesser curvature of stomach, not classifiable to C16.1-C16.4

SP ✚ C16.6   Malignant neoplasm of greater curvature of stomach, unspecified
Malignant neoplasm of greater curvature of stomach, not classifiable to C16.0-C16.4

SP ✚ C16.8 Malignant neoplasm of overlapping sites of stomach

SP ✚ C16.9   Malignant neoplasm of stomach, unspecified
Gastric cancer NOS

4 C17 Malignant neoplasm of small intestine
EXCLUDES 1   malignant carcinoid tumors of the small intestine (C7A.01)
CODING TIPS ✓   This category indicates active cancer. See Z85.068 for personal history of primary malignancy of small intestine.

SP C17.0 Malignant neoplasm of duodenum

SP C17.1 Malignant neoplasm of jejunum

SP C17.2 Malignant neoplasm of ileum
EXCLUDES 1   malignant neoplasm of ileocecal valve (C18.0)

SP C17.3 Meckel's diverticulum, malignant
EXCLUDES 1   Meckel's diverticulum, congenital (Q43.0)

SP C17.8 Malignant neoplasm of overlapping sites of small intestine

---

4 4th digit required   5 5th digit required   6 6th digit required   7 7th digit required   7 7th digit placeholder   ✚ Additional code   ⊟ Laterality

SP C17.9 **Malignant neoplasm of small intestine, unspecified**

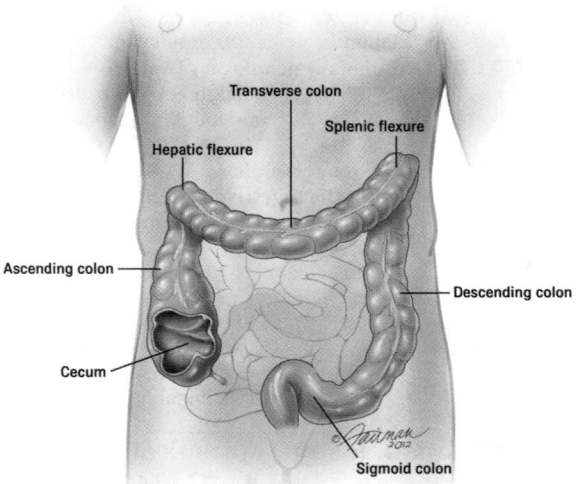

4 C18 **Malignant neoplasm of colon**

> **EXCLUDES 1** malignant carcinoid tumors of the colon (C7A.02-)

> **CODING TIPS ✓** This category indicates active cancer. See Z85.038 for personal history of primary malignancy of large intestine.

SP C18.0 **Malignant neoplasm of cecum**
Malignant neoplasm of ileocecal valve

SP C18.1 **Malignant neoplasm of appendix**

SP C18.2 **Malignant neoplasm of ascending colon**

SP C18.3 **Malignant neoplasm of hepatic flexure**

SP C18.4 **Malignant neoplasm of transverse colon**

SP C18.5 **Malignant neoplasm of splenic flexure**

SP C18.6 **Malignant neoplasm of descending colon**

SP C18.7 **Malignant neoplasm of sigmoid colon**
Malignant neoplasm of sigmoid (flexure)

> **EXCLUDES 1** malignant neoplasm of rectosigmoid junction (C19)

SP C18.8 **Malignant neoplasm of overlapping sites of colon**

SP C18.9 **Malignant neoplasm of colon, unspecified**

Malignant neoplasm of large intestine NOS

SP C19 **Malignant neoplasm of rectosigmoid junction**
Malignant neoplasm of colon with rectum
Malignant neoplasm of rectosigmoid (colon)

> **EXCLUDES 1** malignant carcinoid tumors of the colon (C7A.02-)

> **CODING TIPS ✓** This category indicates active cancer. See Z85.048 for personal history of primary malignancy of rectum, rectosigmoid junction and anus.

SP C20 **Malignant neoplasm of rectum**

Malignant neoplasm of rectal ampulla

> **EXCLUDES 1** malignant carcinoid tumor of the rectum (C7A.026)

> **CODING TIPS ✓** This category indicates active cancer. See Z85.048 for personal history of primary malignancy of rectum, rectosigmoid junction and anus.

4 C21 **Malignant neoplasm of anus and anal canal**

> **EXCLUDES 2** malignant carcinoid tumors of the colon (C7A.02-)
> malignant melanoma of anal margin (C43.51)
> malignant melanoma of anal skin (C43.51)
> malignant melanoma of perianal skin (C43.51)
> other and unspecified malignant neoplasm of anal margin (C44.500, C44.510, C44.520, C44.590)
> other and unspecified malignant neoplasm of anal skin (C44.500, C44.510, C44.520, C44.590)
> other and unspecified malignant neoplasm of perianal skin (C44.500, C44.510, C44.520, C44.590)

> **CODING TIPS ✓** This category indicates active cancer. See Z85.048 for personal history of primary malignancy of rectum, rectosigmoid junction and anus.

SP C21.0 **Malignant neoplasm of anus, unspecified**

SP C21.1 **Malignant neoplasm of anal canal**
Malignant neoplasm of anal sphincter

SP C21.2 **Malignant neoplasm of cloacogenic zone**

SP C21.8 **Malignant neoplasm of overlapping sites of rectum, anus and anal canal**
Malignant neoplasm of anorectal junction
Malignant neoplasm of anorectum
Primary malignant neoplasm of two or more contiguous sites of rectum, anus and anal canal

+ 4 C22 **Malignant neoplasm of liver and intrahepatic bile ducts**
Use additional code to identify:
alcohol abuse and dependence (F10.-)
hepatitis B (B16.-, B18.0-B18.1)
hepatitis C (B17.1-, B18.2)

> **EXCLUDES 1** malignant neoplasm of biliary tract NOS (C24.9)
> secondary malignant neoplasm of liver and intrahepatic bile duct (C78.7)

> **CODING TIPS ✓** This category indicates active cancer. See Z85.05 for personal history of primary malignancy of the liver.

> **CODING TIPS ✓** Primary cancer of the liver (C22) is rare, so look for specific documentation from the physician, such as hepatocellular carcinoma or Kupffer cell sarcoma, before coding primary liver cancer.

H SP + C22.0 **Liver cell carcinoma**
Hepatocellular carcinoma
Hepatoma

SP + C22.1 **Intrahepatic bile duct carcinoma**

★ New ▲ Revised **Px** Primary **SP** PDGM Px **SL** Low CoM **SH** High CoM **IQ** Quest. Encounter **H** Hospice non-cancer Dx ▪ Unspecified **M** *Manifestation*

DecisionHealth's FY 2020 Complete Home Health ICD-10-CM Diagnosis Coding Manual

647

Chapter 2

C00-D49

Cholangiocarcinoma
EXCLUDES 1 malignant neoplasm of
hepatic duct (C24.0)

H **SP** **+** **C22.2 Hepatoblastoma**

H **SP** **+** **C22.3 Angiosarcoma of liver**
Kupffer cell sarcoma

H **SP** **+** **C22.4 Other sarcomas of liver**

H **SP** **+** **C22.7 Other specified carcinomas of liver**

H **SP** **+** **C22.8 Malignant neoplasm of liver, primary,
unspecified as to type**

SP **+** **C22.9 Malignant neoplasm of liver, not
specified as primary or secondary**

SP **C23 Malignant neoplasm of gallbladder**
CODING TIPS ✓ This category indicates active
cancer. See Z85.09 for personal history of
primary malignancy of the other digestive
organs.

4 **C24 Malignant neoplasm of other and
unspecified parts of biliary tract**
EXCLUDES 1 malignant neoplasm of
intrahepatic bile duct (C22.1)

SP **C24.0 Malignant neoplasm of extrahepatic bile
duct**
Malignant neoplasm of biliary duct or
passage NOS
Malignant neoplasm of common bile duct
Malignant neoplasm of cystic duct
Malignant neoplasm of hepatic duct

SP **C24.1 Malignant neoplasm of ampulla of Vater**

SP **C24.8 Malignant neoplasm of overlapping sites
of biliary tract**
Malignant neoplasm involving both
intrahepatic and extrahepatic bile ducts
Primary malignant neoplasm of two or
more contiguous sites of biliary tract

SP **C24.9 Malignant neoplasm of biliary tract,
unspecified**

+ **4** **C25 Malignant neoplasm of pancreas**
Code also:
exocrine pancreatic insufficiency (K86.81)
Use additional code to identify:
alcohol abuse and dependence (F10.-)
CODING TIPS ✓ This category indicates active
cancer. See Z85.07 for personal history of
primary malignancy of the pancreas.

SP **+** **C25.0 Malignant neoplasm of head of pancreas**

SP **+** **C25.1 Malignant neoplasm of body of pancreas**

SP **+** **C25.2 Malignant neoplasm of tail of pancreas**

SP **+** **C25.3 Malignant neoplasm of pancreatic duct**

SP **+** **C25.4 Malignant neoplasm of endocrine
pancreas**
Malignant neoplasm of islets of
Langerhans
Use additional code to identify any
functional activity.
CODING TIPS ✓ Use this code when
malignant neoplasm of the pancreas has
caused diabetes (E08).

SP **+** **C25.7 Malignant neoplasm of other parts of
pancreas**
Malignant neoplasm of neck of pancreas

SP **+** **C25.8 Malignant neoplasm of overlapping sites
of pancreas**

SP **+** **C25.9 Malignant neoplasm of pancreas,
unspecified**

4 **C26 Malignant neoplasm of other and ill-
defined digestive organs**
EXCLUDES 1 malignant neoplasm of
peritoneum and
retroperitoneum (C48.-)

SP **C26.0 Malignant neoplasm of intestinal tract,
part unspecified**
Malignant neoplasm of intestine NOS

SP **C26.1 Malignant neoplasm of spleen**
EXCLUDES 1 Hodgkin lymphoma (C81.-)
non-Hodgkin lymphoma
(C82-C85)

SP **C26.9 Malignant neoplasm of ill-defined sites
within the digestive system**
Malignant neoplasm of alimentary canal or
tract NOS
Malignant neoplasm of gastrointestinal
tract NOS
EXCLUDES 1 malignant neoplasm of
abdominal NOS (C76.2)
malignant neoplasm of intra-
abdominal NOS (C76.2)

Malignant neoplasms of respiratory and intrathoracic organs (C30-C39)

INCLUDES malignant neoplasm of middle ear
EXCLUDES 1 mesothelioma (C45.-)

CODING TIPS ✓ Codes classifiable to C30-C39 include active
cancer. History of cancer to respiratory system and other
intrathoracic organs should be coded using codes from Z85.1-
and Z85.2-.

4 **C30 Malignant neoplasm of nasal cavity and
middle ear**
CODING TIPS ✓ C30 indicates active cancer.
See Z85.22 for personal history of primary
malignancy of the nasal cavities, middle ear
and accessory sinuses.

SP **C30.0 Malignant neoplasm of nasal cavity**
Malignant neoplasm of cartilage of nose
Malignant neoplasm of nasal concha
Malignant neoplasm of internal nose
Malignant neoplasm of septum of nose
Malignant neoplasm of vestibule of nose
EXCLUDES 1 malignant neoplasm of nasal
bone (C41.0)
malignant neoplasm of nose
NOS (C76.0)
malignant neoplasm of
olfactory bulb (C72.2-)
malignant neoplasm of
posterior margin of nasal
septum and choana
(C11.3)
malignant melanoma of skin
of nose (C43.31)
malignant neoplasm of
turbinates (C41.0)
other and unspecified
malignant neoplasm of
skin of nose C44.301,
C44.311, C44.321,
C44.391)

SP **C30.1 Malignant neoplasm of middle ear**
Malignant neoplasm of antrum
tympanicum
Malignant neoplasm of auditory tube
Malignant neoplasm of eustachian tube

---

4 4th digit required   **5** 5th digit required   **6** 6th digit required   **7** 7th digit required   **7** 7th digit placeholder   **+** Additional code   **=** Laterality

Malignant neoplasm of inner ear
Malignant neoplasm of mastoid air cells
Malignant neoplasm of tympanic cavity

EXCLUDES 1 malignant neoplasm of
auricular canal (external)
(C43.2-,C44.2-)
malignant neoplasm of bone
of ear (meatus) (C41.0)
malignant neoplasm of
cartilage of ear (C49.0)
malignant melanoma of skin
of (external) ear (C43.2-)
other and unspecified
malignant neoplasm of
skin of (external) ear
(C44.2-)

◢ C31 Malignant neoplasm of accessory sinuses

CODING TIPS ✓ C31 indicates active cancer.
See Z85.22 for personal history of primary
malignancy of the nasal cavities, middle ear
and accessory sinuses.

SP C31.0 Malignant neoplasm of maxillary sinus
Malignant neoplasm of antrum (Highmore)
(maxillary)

SP C31.1 Malignant neoplasm of ethmoidal sinus

SP C31.2 Malignant neoplasm of frontal sinus

SP C31.3 Malignant neoplasm of sphenoid sinus

**SP C31.8 Malignant neoplasm of overlapping sites
of accessory sinuses**

**SP C31.9 Malignant neoplasm of accessory sinus,
unspecified**

+ ◢ C32 Malignant neoplasm of larynx
Use additional code to identify:
alcohol abuse and dependence (F10.-)
exposure to environmental tobacco smoke
(Z77.22)
exposure to tobacco smoke in the perinatal
period (P96.81)
history of tobacco dependence (Z87.891)
occupational exposure to environmental
tobacco smoke (Z57.31)
tobacco dependence (F17.-)
tobacco use (Z72.0)

CODING TIPS ✓ This code indicates active
cancer. See Z85.21 for history of primary
malignant neoplasm of larynx.

SP + C32.0 Malignant neoplasm of glottis
Malignant neoplasm of intrinsic larynx
Malignant neoplasm of laryngeal
commissure (anterior)(posterior)
Malignant neoplasm of vocal cord (true)
NOS

SP + C32.1 Malignant neoplasm of supraglottis
Malignant neoplasm of aryepiglottic fold
or interarytenoid fold, laryngeal aspect
Malignant neoplasm of epiglottis
(suprahyoid portion) NOS
Malignant neoplasm of extrinsic larynx
Malignant neoplasm of false vocal cord
Malignant neoplasm of posterior
(laryngeal) surface of epiglottis
Malignant neoplasm of ventricular bands

EXCLUDES 2 malignant neoplasm of
anterior surface of
epiglottis (C10.1)

malignant neoplasm of
aryepiglottic fold or
interarytenoid fold,
hypopharyngeal aspect
(C13.1)
malignant neoplasm of
aryepiglottic fold or
interarytenoid fold,
marginal zone (C13.1)
malignant neoplasm of
aryepiglottic fold or
interarytenoid fold NOS
(C13.1)

SP + C32.2 Malignant neoplasm of subglottis

**SP + C32.3 Malignant neoplasm of laryngeal
cartilage**

**SP + C32.8 Malignant neoplasm of overlapping sites
of larynx**

**SP + C32.9 Malignant neoplasm of larynx,
unspecified**

SP + C33 Malignant neoplasm of trachea
Use additional code to identify:
exposure to environmental tobacco smoke
(Z77.22)
exposure to tobacco smoke in the perinatal
period (P96.81)
history of tobacco dependence (Z87.891)
occupational exposure to environmental
tobacco smoke (Z57.31)
tobacco dependence (F17.-)
tobacco use (Z72.0)

+ ◢ C34 Malignant neoplasm of bronchus and lung
Use additional code to identify:
exposure to environmental tobacco smoke
(Z77.22)
exposure to tobacco smoke in the perinatal
period (P96.81)
history of tobacco dependence (Z87.891)
occupational exposure to environmental
tobacco smoke (Z57.31)
tobacco dependence (F17.-)
tobacco use (Z72.0)

EXCLUDES 1 Kaposi's sarcoma of lung
(C46.5-)
malignant carcinoid tumor of
the bronchus and lung
(C7A.090)

CODING TIPS ✓ C34 indicates active cancer in
the lung. Laterality is important. Unspecified
laterality will not be assigned to a Clinical
Grouper in PDGM. Query the physician for
location of tumors in the lung(s). See Z85.118
for personal history of primary malignancy of
the lung and bronchus.

+ ⑤ C34.0 Malignant neoplasm of main bronchus
Malignant neoplasm of carina
Malignant neoplasm of hilus (of lung)

**⊟ SP + C34.00 Malignant neoplasm of unspecified
main bronchus**

**⊟ SP + C34.01 Malignant neoplasm of right main
bronchus**

**⊟ SP + C34.02 Malignant neoplasm of left main
bronchus**

**+ ⑤ C34.1 Malignant neoplasm of upper lobe,
bronchus or lung**

**⊟ IQ + C34.10 Malignant neoplasm of upper lobe,
unspecified bronchus or lung**

★ New ▲ Revised Px Primary SP PDGM Px SL Low CoM SH High CoM IQ Quest. Encounter H Hospice non-cancer Dx Unspecified M Manifestation

DecisionHealth's FY 2020 Complete Home Health ICD-10-CM Diagnosis Coding Manual

649

Chapter 2

C00-D49

⊟ SP ✚ **C34.11 Malignant neoplasm of upper lobe, right bronchus or lung**

⊟ SP ✚ **C34.12 Malignant neoplasm of upper lobe, left bronchus or lung**

SP ✚ **C34.2 Malignant neoplasm of middle lobe, bronchus or lung**

✚ ⑤ **C34.3 Malignant neoplasm of lower lobe, bronchus or lung**

⊟ IQ ✚ **C34.30 Malignant neoplasm of lower lobe, unspecified bronchus or lung**

⊟ SP ✚ **C34.31 Malignant neoplasm of lower lobe, right bronchus or lung**

⊟ SP ✚ **C34.32 Malignant neoplasm of lower lobe, left bronchus or lung**

✚ ⑤ **C34.8 Malignant neoplasm of overlapping sites of bronchus and lung**

⊟ IQ ✚ **C34.80 Malignant neoplasm of overlapping sites of unspecified bronchus and lung**

⊟ SP ✚ **C34.81 Malignant neoplasm of overlapping sites of right bronchus and lung**

⊟ SP ✚ **C34.82 Malignant neoplasm of overlapping sites of left bronchus and lung**

✚ ⑤ **C34.9 Malignant neoplasm of unspecified part of bronchus or lung**

⊟ IQ ✚ **C34.90 Malignant neoplasm of unspecified part of unspecified bronchus or lung**

Lung cancer NOS

⊟ SP ✚ **C34.91 Malignant neoplasm of unspecified part of right bronchus or lung**

⊟ SP ✚ **C34.92 Malignant neoplasm of unspecified part of left bronchus or lung**

SP **C37 Malignant neoplasm of thymus**
> **EXCLUDES 1** malignant carcinoid tumor of the thymus (C7A.091)

④ **C38 Malignant neoplasm of heart, mediastinum and pleura**
> **EXCLUDES 1** mesothelioma (C45.-)

SP **C38.0 Malignant neoplasm of heart**
Malignant neoplasm of pericardium
> **EXCLUDES 1** malignant neoplasm of great vessels (C49.3)

SP **C38.1 Malignant neoplasm of anterior mediastinum**

SP **C38.2 Malignant neoplasm of posterior mediastinum**

SP **C38.3 Malignant neoplasm of mediastinum, part unspecified**

SP **C38.4 Malignant neoplasm of pleura**

SP **C38.8 Malignant neoplasm of overlapping sites of heart, mediastinum and pleura**

✚ ④ **C39 Malignant neoplasm of other and ill-defined sites in the respiratory system and intrathoracic organs**
Use additional code to identify:
exposure to environmental tobacco smoke (Z77.22)
exposure to tobacco smoke in the perinatal period (P96.81)
history of tobacco dependence (Z87.891)
occupational exposure to environmental tobacco smoke (Z57.31)
tobacco dependence (F17.-)
tobacco use (Z72.0)
> **EXCLUDES 1** intrathoracic malignant neoplasm NOS (C76.1)

thoracic malignant neoplasm NOS (C76.1)

IQ ✚ **C39.0 Malignant neoplasm of upper respiratory tract, part unspecified**

IQ ✚ **C39.9 Malignant neoplasm of lower respiratory tract, part unspecified**

Malignant neoplasm of respiratory tract NOS

Malignant neoplasms of bone and articular cartilage   (C40-C41)

INCLUDES malignant neoplasm of cartilage (articular) (joint)
malignant neoplasm of periosteum
EXCLUDES 1 malignant neoplasm of bone marrow NOS (C96.9)
malignant neoplasm of synovia (C49.-)

CODING TIPS ✓ Codes classifiable to C40-C41 include active cancer. History of cancer to bone or soft tissue should be coded to Z85.83-.

✚ ④ **C40 Malignant neoplasm of bone and articular cartilage of limbs**
Use additional code to identify major osseous defect, if applicable (M89.7-)
> **CODING TIPS ✓** If bone cancer is noted in the medical record, confirm with the physician whether the cancer is primary or secondary cancer to the bone. Most commonly, home care agencies care for patients with metastasis to the bone, which is coded C79.51. Category C40 indicates active primary cancer to the bone. See Z85.830 for personal history of primary malignancy of bone.

> **CODING TIPS ✓** Laterality is very important with these codes. Unspecified should not be used and will not be assigned to a Clinical Grouper as primary in PDGM.

✚ ⑤ **C40.0 Malignant neoplasm of scapula and long bones of upper limb**

⊟ IQ ✚ **C40.00 Malignant neoplasm of scapula and long bones of unspecified upper limb**

⊟ SP ✚ **C40.01 Malignant neoplasm of scapula and long bones of right upper limb**

⊟ SP ✚ **C40.02 Malignant neoplasm of scapula and long bones of left upper limb**

✚ ⑤ **C40.1 Malignant neoplasm of short bones of upper limb**

⊟ IQ ✚ **C40.10 Malignant neoplasm of short bones of unspecified upper limb**

⊟ SP ✚ **C40.11 Malignant neoplasm of short bones of right upper limb**

⊟ SP ✚ **C40.12 Malignant neoplasm of short bones of left upper limb**

✚ ⑤ **C40.2 Malignant neoplasm of long bones of lower limb**

⊟ IQ ✚ **C40.20 Malignant neoplasm of long bones of unspecified lower limb**

⊟ SP ✚ **C40.21 Malignant neoplasm of long bones of right lower limb**

⊟ SP ✚ **C40.22 Malignant neoplasm of long bones of left lower limb**

✚ ⑤ **C40.3 Malignant neoplasm of short bones of lower limb**

---

④4th digit required   ⑤5th digit required   ⑥6th digit required   ⑦7th digit required   ⑦7th digit placeholder   ✚Additional code   ⊟Laterality

☐ **IQ** ➕ **C40.30** Malignant neoplasm of short bones of unspecified lower limb

☐ **SP** ➕ **C40.31** Malignant neoplasm of short bones of right lower limb

☐ **SP** ➕ **C40.32** Malignant neoplasm of short bones of left lower limb

➕ 5 **C40.8** Malignant neoplasm of overlapping sites of bone and articular cartilage of limb

☐ **IQ** ➕ **C40.80** Malignant neoplasm of overlapping sites of bone and articular cartilage of unspecified limb

☐ **SP** ➕ **C40.81** Malignant neoplasm of overlapping sites of bone and articular cartilage of right limb

☐ **SP** ➕ **C40.82** Malignant neoplasm of overlapping sites of bone and articular cartilage of left limb

➕ 5 **C40.9** Malignant neoplasm of unspecified bones and articular cartilage of limb

☐ **IQ** ➕ **C40.90** Malignant neoplasm of unspecified bones and articular cartilage of unspecified limb

☐ **SP** ➕ **C40.91** Malignant neoplasm of unspecified bones and articular cartilage of right limb

☐ **SP** ➕ **C40.92** Malignant neoplasm of unspecified bones and articular cartilage of left limb

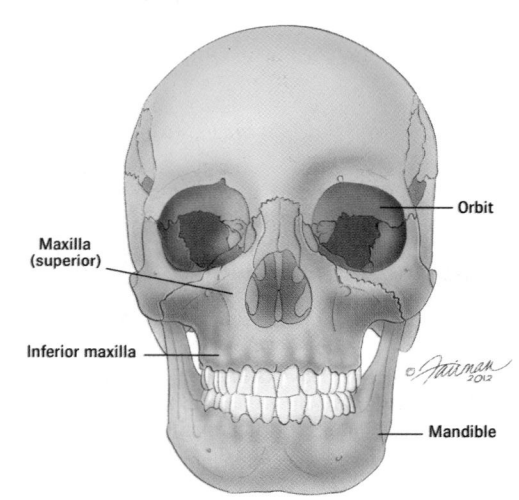

4 **C41** **Malignant neoplasm of bone and articular cartilage of other and unspecified sites**

> **EXCLUDES 1** malignant neoplasm of bones of limbs (C40.-)
> malignant neoplasm of cartilage of ear (C49.0)
> malignant neoplasm of cartilage of eyelid (C49.0)
> malignant neoplasm of cartilage of larynx (C32.3)
> malignant neoplasm of cartilage of limbs (C40.-)
> malignant neoplasm of cartilage of nose (C30.0)

SP **C41.0** **Malignant neoplasm of bones of skull and face**
Malignant neoplasm of maxilla (superior)
Malignant neoplasm of orbital bone

★ New ▲ Revised Px Primary SP PDGM Px SL Low CoM SH High CoM IQ Quest. Encounter H Hospice non-cancer Dx   Unspecified   M *Manifestation*

DecisionHealth's FY 2020 Complete Home Health ICD-10-CM Diagnosis Coding Manual

651

Chapter 2

C00-D49

EXCLUDES 2 carcinoma, any type except
intraosseous or
odontogenic of:
maxillary sinus (C31.0)
upper jaw (C03.0)
malignant neoplasm of jaw
bone (lower) (C41.1)

SP **C41.1 Malignant neoplasm of mandible**
Malignant neoplasm of inferior maxilla
Malignant neoplasm of lower jaw bone
EXCLUDES 2 carcinoma, any type except
intraosseous or
odontogenic of:
jaw NOS (C03.9)
lower (C03.1)
malignant neoplasm of upper
jaw bone (C41.0)

SP **C41.2 Malignant neoplasm of vertebral
column**
EXCLUDES 1 malignant neoplasm of
sacrum and coccyx
(C41.4)

SP **C41.3 Malignant neoplasm of ribs, sternum
and clavicle**

SP **C41.4 Malignant neoplasm of pelvic bones,
sacrum and coccyx**

SP **C41.9 Malignant neoplasm of bone and
articular cartilage, unspecified**

CODING TIPS ✓ Malignant neoplasm of bone,
unspecified is unacceptable. Query the
physician for additional information.

Melanoma and other malignant neoplasms of skin (C43-C44)

CODING TIPS ✓ Codes classifiable to C43-C44 include active
cancer. History of cancer to skin should be coded to Z85.82-.

4 **C43 Malignant melanoma of skin**
EXCLUDES 1 melanoma in situ (D03.-)
EXCLUDES 2 malignant melanoma of skin of
genital organs
(C51-C52, C60.-, C63.-)
Merkel cell carcinoma (C4A.-)
sites other than skin-code to
malignant neoplasm of the
site

CODING TIPS ✓ Malignant melanoma is rapidly
invasive. C43 indicates active cancer. See
Z85.820 for personal history of malignant
melanoma.

CODING TIPS ✓ Laterality is very important with
these codes. Unspecified should not be used
and will not be assigned to a Clinical Grouper
as primary in PDGM.

SP **C43.0 Malignant melanoma of lip**
EXCLUDES 1 malignant neoplasm of
vermilion border of lip
(C00.0-C00.2)

5 **C43.1 Malignant melanoma of eyelid,
including canthus**

IQ **C43.10 Malignant melanoma of unspecified
eyelid, including canthus**

6 **C43.11 Malignant melanoma of right eyelid,
including canthus**

SP **C43.111 Malignant melanoma of right
upper eyelid, including canthus**

SP **C43.112 Malignant melanoma of right
lower eyelid, including canthus**

6 **C43.12 Malignant melanoma of left eyelid,
including canthus**

SP **C43.121 Malignant melanoma of left upper
eyelid, including canthus**

SP **C43.122 Malignant melanoma of left lower
eyelid, including canthus**

5 **C43.2 Malignant melanoma of ear and
external auricular canal**

IQ **C43.20 Malignant melanoma of unspecified
ear and external auricular canal**

SP **C43.21 Malignant melanoma of right ear
and external auricular canal**

SP **C43.22 Malignant melanoma of left ear and
external auricular canal**

5 **C43.3 Malignant melanoma of other and
unspecified parts of face**

IQ **C43.30 Malignant melanoma of unspecified
part of face**

SP **C43.31 Malignant melanoma of nose**

SP **C43.39 Malignant melanoma of other parts
of face**

SP **C43.4 Malignant melanoma of scalp and neck**

5 **C43.5 Malignant melanoma of trunk**
EXCLUDES 2 malignant neoplasm of anus
NOS (C21.0)
malignant neoplasm of
scrotum (C63.2)

SP **C43.51 Malignant melanoma of anal skin**
Malignant melanoma of anal margin
Malignant melanoma of perianal skin

SP **C43.52 Malignant melanoma of skin of
breast**

SP **C43.59 Malignant melanoma of other part
of trunk**

5 **C43.6 Malignant melanoma of upper limb,
including shoulder**

IQ **C43.60 Malignant melanoma of unspecified
upper limb, including shoulder**

SP **C43.61 Malignant melanoma of right upper
limb, including shoulder**

SP **C43.62 Malignant melanoma of left upper
limb, including shoulder**

5 **C43.7 Malignant melanoma of lower limb,
including hip**

IQ **C43.70 Malignant melanoma of unspecified
lower limb, including hip**

SP **C43.71 Malignant melanoma of right lower
limb, including hip**

SP **C43.72 Malignant melanoma of left lower
limb, including hip**

SP **C43.8 Malignant melanoma of overlapping
sites of skin**

IQ **C43.9 Malignant melanoma of skin,
unspecified**
Malignant melanoma of unspecified site of
skin
Melanoma (malignant) NOS

4 **C4A Merkel cell carcinoma**

SP **C4A.0 Merkel cell carcinoma of lip**
EXCLUDES 1 malignant neoplasm of
vermilion border of lip
(C00.0-C00.2)

5 **C4A.1 Merkel cell carcinoma of eyelid,
including canthus**

4 4th digit required   5 5th digit required   6 6th digit required   7 7th digit required   7 7th digit placeholder   + Additional code   ⊟ Laterality

652   *DecisionHealth's* FY 2020 Complete Home Health ICD-10-CM Diagnosis Coding Manual

☐ **IQ** **C4A.10** **Merkel cell carcinoma of unspecified eyelid, including canthus**

⑥ **C4A.11** Merkel cell carcinoma of right eyelid, including canthus

☐ **SP** **C4A.111** Merkel cell carcinoma of right upper eyelid, including canthus

☐ **SP** **C4A.112** Merkel cell carcinoma of right lower eyelid, including canthus

⑥ **C4A.12** Merkel cell carcinoma of left eyelid, including canthus

☐ **SP** **C4A.121** Merkel cell carcinoma of left upper eyelid, including canthus

☐ **SP** **C4A.122** Merkel cell carcinoma of left lower eyelid, including canthus

⑤ **C4A.2** Merkel cell carcinoma of ear and external auricular canal

☐ **IQ** **C4A.20** **Merkel cell carcinoma of unspecified ear and external auricular canal**

☐ **SP** **C4A.21** Merkel cell carcinoma of right ear and external auricular canal

☐ **SP** **C4A.22** Merkel cell carcinoma of left ear and external auricular canal

⑤ **C4A.3** **Merkel cell carcinoma of other and unspecified parts of face**

IQ **C4A.30** **Merkel cell carcinoma of unspecified part of face**

SP **C4A.31** Merkel cell carcinoma of nose

SP **C4A.39** Merkel cell carcinoma of other parts of face

SP **C4A.4** Merkel cell carcinoma of scalp and neck

⑤ **C4A.5** Merkel cell carcinoma of trunk

> **EXCLUDES 2** malignant neoplasm of anus NOS (C21.0)
> malignant neoplasm of scrotum (C63.2)

SP **C4A.51** Merkel cell carcinoma of anal skin
Merkel cell carcinoma of anal margin
Merkel cell carcinoma of perianal skin

SP **C4A.52** Merkel cell carcinoma of skin of breast

SP **C4A.59** Merkel cell carcinoma of other part of trunk

⑤ **C4A.6** Merkel cell carcinoma of upper limb, including shoulder

☐ **IQ** **C4A.60** **Merkel cell carcinoma of unspecified upper limb, including shoulder**

☐ **SP** **C4A.61** Merkel cell carcinoma of right upper limb, including shoulder

☐ **SP** **C4A.62** Merkel cell carcinoma of left upper limb, including shoulder

⑤ **C4A.7** Merkel cell carcinoma of lower limb, including hip

☐ **IQ** **C4A.70** **Merkel cell carcinoma of unspecified lower limb, including hip**

☐ **SP** **C4A.71** Merkel cell carcinoma of right lower limb, including hip

☐ **SP** **C4A.72** Merkel cell carcinoma of left lower limb, including hip

SP **C4A.8** Merkel cell carcinoma of overlapping sites

IQ **C4A.9** **Merkel cell carcinoma, unspecified**
Merkel cell carcinoma of unspecified site

Merkel cell carcinoma NOS

④ **C44** **Other and unspecified malignant neoplasm of skin**

> **INCLUDES** malignant neoplasm of sebaceous glands
> malignant neoplasm of sweat glands

> **EXCLUDES 1** Kaposi's sarcoma of skin (C46.0)
> malignant melanoma of skin (C43.-)
> malignant neoplasm of skin of genital organs (C51-C52, C60.-, C63.2)
> Merkel cell carcinoma (C4A.-)

CODING TIPS✓ C44 is used for squamous cell and basal cell carcinoma of the skin. If malignant melanoma is documented, use C43 instead. See Z85.828 for personal history of skin cancer.

CODING TIPS✓ Do not code Merkel cell carcinoma to C44. See C4A for Merkel cell carcinoma and Z85.821 for personal history of Merkel cell carcinoma.

CODING TIPS✓ Metastasis of common sunlight-induced squamous cell carcinoma is unusual. Lesions more likely to metastasize are lesions of the lip or ear.

⑤ **C44.0** **Other and unspecified malignant neoplasm of skin of lip**

> **EXCLUDES 1** malignant neoplasm of lip (C00.-)

SP **C44.00** **Unspecified malignant neoplasm of skin of lip**

SP **C44.01** Basal cell carcinoma of skin of lip

SP **C44.02** Squamous cell carcinoma of skin of lip

SP **C44.09** Other specified malignant neoplasm of skin of lip

⑤ **C44.1** **Other and unspecified malignant neoplasm of skin of eyelid, including canthus**

> **EXCLUDES 1** connective tissue of eyelid (C49.0)

CODING TIPS✓ Laterality is very important with these codes. Unspecified should not be used and will not be assigned to a Clinical Grouper as primary in PDGM.

⑥ **C44.10** **Unspecified malignant neoplasm of skin of eyelid, including canthus**

☐ **IQ** **C44.101** **Unspecified malignant neoplasm of skin of unspecified eyelid, including canthus**

☐ **SP** ⑦ **C44.102** **Unspecified malignant neoplasm of skin of right eyelid, including canthus**

CODING TIPS✓ There was no 7th character table published with codes C44.102- and C44.109-. A 7th character of 1 denotes "upper" and a 7th character of 2 denotes "lower".

☐ **SP** ⑦ **C44.109** **Unspecified malignant neoplasm of skin of left eyelid, including canthus**

★ New ▲ Revised **Px** Primary **SP** PDGM Px **SL** Low CoM **SH** High CoM **IQ** Quest. Encounter **H** Hospice non-cancer Dx ☐ Unspecified **M** *Manifestation*

DecisionHealth's FY 2020 Complete Home Health ICD-10-CM Diagnosis Coding Manual

653

6 C44.11 Basal cell carcinoma of skin of eyelid, including canthus

⊟ IQ C44.111 Basal cell carcinoma of skin of unspecified eyelid, including canthus

⊟ SP 7 C44.112 Basal cell carcinoma of skin of right eyelid, including canthus

> **CODING TIPS ✓** There was no 7th character table published with codes C44.112- and C44.119-. A 7th character of 1 denotes "upper" and a 7th character of 2 denotes "lower".

⊟ SP 7 C44.119 Basal cell carcinoma of skin of left eyelid, including canthus

6 C44.12 Squamous cell carcinoma of skin of eyelid, including canthus

⊟ IQ C44.121 Squamous cell carcinoma of skin of unspecified eyelid, including canthus

⊟ SP 7 C44.122 Squamous cell carcinoma of skin of right eyelid, including canthus

> **CODING TIPS ✓** There was no 7th character table published with codes C44.122- and C44.129-. A 7th character of 1 denotes "upper" and a 7th character of 2 denotes "lower".

⊟ SP 7 C44.129 Squamous cell carcinoma of skin of left eyelid, including canthus

6 C44.13 Sebaceous cell carcinoma of skin of eyelid, including canthus

⊟ IQ C44.131 Sebaceous cell carcinoma of skin of unspecified eyelid, including canthus

⊟ SP 7 C44.132 Sebaceous cell carcinoma of skin of right eyelid, including canthus

> **CODING TIPS ✓** There was no 7th character table published with codes C44.132- and C44.139-. A 7th character of 1 denotes "upper" and a 7th character of 2 denotes "lower".

⊟ SP 7 C44.139 Sebaceous cell carcinoma of skin of left eyelid, including canthus

6 C44.19 Other specified malignant neoplasm of skin of eyelid, including canthus

⊟ IQ C44.191 Other specified malignant neoplasm of skin of unspecified eyelid, including canthus

⊟ SP 7 C44.192 Other specified malignant neoplasm of skin of right eyelid, including canthus

> **CODING TIPS ✓** There was no 7th character table published with codes C44.192- and C44.199-. A 7th character of 1 denotes "upper" and a 7th character of 2 denotes "lower".

⊟ SP 7 C44.199 Other specified malignant neoplasm of skin of left eyelid, including canthus

5 C44.2 Other and unspecified malignant neoplasm of skin of ear and external auricular canal

> **EXCLUDES 1** connective tissue of ear (C49.0)

6 C44.20 Unspecified malignant neoplasm of skin of ear and external auricular canal

⊟ IQ C44.201 Unspecified malignant neoplasm of skin of unspecified ear and external auricular canal

⊟ SP C44.202 Unspecified malignant neoplasm of skin of right ear and external auricular canal

⊟ IQ C44.209 Unspecified malignant neoplasm of skin of left ear and external auricular canal

6 C44.21 Basal cell carcinoma of skin of ear and external auricular canal

⊟ IQ C44.211 Basal cell carcinoma of skin of unspecified ear and external auricular canal

⊟ SP C44.212 Basal cell carcinoma of skin of right ear and external auricular canal

⊟ SP C44.219 Basal cell carcinoma of skin of left ear and external auricular canal

6 C44.22 Squamous cell carcinoma of skin of ear and external auricular canal

⊟ IQ C44.221 Squamous cell carcinoma of skin of unspecified ear and external auricular canal

⊟ SP C44.222 Squamous cell carcinoma of skin of right ear and external auricular canal

⊟ SP C44.229 Squamous cell carcinoma of skin of left ear and external auricular canal

6 C44.29 Other specified malignant neoplasm of skin of ear and external auricular canal

⊟ IQ C44.291 Other specified malignant neoplasm of skin of unspecified ear and external auricular canal

⊟ SP C44.292 Other specified malignant neoplasm of skin of right ear and external auricular canal

⊟ SP C44.299 Other specified malignant neoplasm of skin of left ear and external auricular canal

5 C44.3 Other and unspecified malignant neoplasm of skin of other and unspecified parts of face

6 C44.30 Unspecified malignant neoplasm of skin of other and unspecified parts of face

IQ C44.300 Unspecified malignant neoplasm of skin of unspecified part of face

SP C44.301 Unspecified malignant neoplasm of skin of nose

SP C44.309 Unspecified malignant neoplasm of skin of other parts of face

6 C44.31 Basal cell carcinoma of skin of other and unspecified parts of face

IQ C44.310 Basal cell carcinoma of skin of unspecified parts of face

SP C44.311 Basal cell carcinoma of skin of nose

SP C44.319 Basal cell carcinoma of skin of other parts of face

6 C44.32 Squamous cell carcinoma of skin of other and unspecified parts of face

IQ C44.320 Squamous cell carcinoma of skin of unspecified parts of face

---

4 4th digit required   5 5th digit required   6 6th digit required   7 7th digit required   7 7th digit placeholder   ✚ Additional code   ⊟ Laterality

654   DecisionHealth's FY 2020 Complete Home Health ICD-10-CM Diagnosis Coding Manual

SP **C44.321** Squamous cell carcinoma of skin of nose

SP **C44.329** Squamous cell carcinoma of skin of other parts of face

6 **C44.39** Other specified malignant neoplasm of skin of other and unspecified parts of face

!Q **C44.390** Other specified malignant neoplasm of skin of unspecified parts of face

SP **C44.391** Other specified malignant neoplasm of skin of nose

SP **C44.399** Other specified malignant neoplasm of skin of other parts of face

5 **C44.4** Other and unspecified malignant neoplasm of skin of scalp and neck

SP **C44.40** Unspecified malignant neoplasm of skin of scalp and neck

SP **C44.41** Basal cell carcinoma of skin of scalp and neck

SP **C44.42** Squamous cell carcinoma of skin of scalp and neck

SP **C44.49** Other specified malignant neoplasm of skin of scalp and neck

5 **C44.5** Other and unspecified malignant neoplasm of skin of trunk

> **EXCLUDES 1** anus NOS (C21.0)
> scrotum (C63.2)

6 **C44.50** Unspecified malignant neoplasm of skin of trunk

SP **C44.500** Unspecified malignant neoplasm of anal skin
Unspecified malignant neoplasm of anal margin
Unspecified malignant neoplasm of perianal skin

SP **C44.501** Unspecified malignant neoplasm of skin of breast

SP **C44.509** Unspecified malignant neoplasm of skin of other part of trunk

6 **C44.51** Basal cell carcinoma of skin of trunk

SP **C44.510** Basal cell carcinoma of anal skin
Basal cell carcinoma of anal margin
Basal cell carcinoma of perianal skin

SP **C44.511** Basal cell carcinoma of skin of breast

SP **C44.519** Basal cell carcinoma of skin of other part of trunk

6 **C44.52** Squamous cell carcinoma of skin of trunk

SP **C44.520** Squamous cell carcinoma of anal skin
Squamous cell carcinoma of anal margin
Squamous cell carcinoma of perianal skin

SP **C44.521** Squamous cell carcinoma of skin of breast

SP **C44.529** Squamous cell carcinoma of skin of other part of trunk

6 **C44.59** Other specified malignant neoplasm of skin of trunk

SP **C44.590** Other specified malignant neoplasm of anal skin
Other specified malignant neoplasm of anal margin
Other specified malignant neoplasm of perianal skin

SP **C44.591** Other specified malignant neoplasm of skin of breast

SP **C44.599** Other specified malignant neoplasm of skin of other part of trunk

5 **C44.6** Other and unspecified malignant neoplasm of skin of upper limb, including shoulder

6 **C44.60** Unspecified malignant neoplasm of skin of upper limb, including shoulder

⊟ !Q **C44.601** Unspecified malignant neoplasm of skin of unspecified upper limb, including shoulder

⊟ SP **C44.602** Unspecified malignant neoplasm of skin of right upper limb, including shoulder

⊟ SP **C44.609** Unspecified malignant neoplasm of skin of left upper limb, including shoulder

6 **C44.61** Basal cell carcinoma of skin of upper limb, including shoulder

⊟ !Q **C44.611** Basal cell carcinoma of skin of unspecified upper limb, including shoulder

⊟ SP **C44.612** Basal cell carcinoma of skin of right upper limb, including shoulder

⊟ SP **C44.619** Basal cell carcinoma of skin of left upper limb, including shoulder

6 **C44.62** Squamous cell carcinoma of skin of upper limb, including shoulder

⊟ !Q **C44.621** Squamous cell carcinoma of skin of unspecified upper limb, including shoulder

⊟ SP **C44.622** Squamous cell carcinoma of skin of right upper limb, including shoulder

⊟ SP **C44.629** Squamous cell carcinoma of skin of left upper limb, including shoulder

6 **C44.69** Other specified malignant neoplasm of skin of upper limb, including shoulder

⊟ !Q **C44.691** Other specified malignant neoplasm of skin of unspecified upper limb, including shoulder

⊟ SP **C44.692** Other specified malignant neoplasm of skin of right upper limb, including shoulder

⊟ SP **C44.699** Other specified malignant neoplasm of skin of left upper limb, including shoulder

5 **C44.7** Other and unspecified malignant neoplasm of skin of lower limb, including hip

6 **C44.70** Unspecified malignant neoplasm of skin of lower limb, including hip

⊟ !Q **C44.701** Unspecified malignant neoplasm of skin of unspecified lower limb, including hip

---

★ New ▲ Revised **Px** Primary **SP** PDGM Px **SL** Low CoM **SH** High CoM **!Q** Quest. Encounter **H** Hospice non-cancer Dx Unspecified **M** *Manifestation*

⊟ **SP** **C44.702** Unspecified malignant neoplasm of skin of right lower limb, including hip

⊟ **SP** **C44.709** Unspecified malignant neoplasm of skin of left lower limb, including hip

6 **C44.71** Basal cell carcinoma of skin of lower limb, including hip

⊟ **IQ** **C44.711** Basal cell carcinoma of skin of unspecified lower limb, including hip

⊟ **SP** **C44.712** Basal cell carcinoma of skin of right lower limb, including hip

⊟ **SP** **C44.719** Basal cell carcinoma of skin of left lower limb, including hip

6 **C44.72** Squamous cell carcinoma of skin of lower limb, including hip

⊟ **IQ** **C44.721** Squamous cell carcinoma of skin of unspecified lower limb, including hip

⊟ **SP** **C44.722** Squamous cell carcinoma of skin of right lower limb, including hip

⊟ **SP** **C44.729** Squamous cell carcinoma of skin of left lower limb, including hip

6 **C44.79** Other specified malignant neoplasm of skin of lower limb, including hip

⊟ **IQ** **C44.791** Other specified malignant neoplasm of skin of unspecified lower limb, including hip

⊟ **SP** **C44.792** Other specified malignant neoplasm of skin of right lower limb, including hip

⊟ **SP** **C44.799** Other specified malignant neoplasm of skin of left lower limb, including hip

5 **C44.8** Other and unspecified malignant neoplasm of overlapping sites of skin

SP **C44.80** Unspecified malignant neoplasm of overlapping sites of skin

SP **C44.81** Basal cell carcinoma of overlapping sites of skin

SP **C44.82** Squamous cell carcinoma of overlapping sites of skin

SP **C44.89** Other specified malignant neoplasm of overlapping sites of skin

5 **C44.9** Other and unspecified malignant neoplasm of skin, unspecified

IQ **C44.90** Unspecified malignant neoplasm of skin, unspecified

Malignant neoplasm of unspecified site of skin

IQ **C44.91** Basal cell carcinoma of skin, unspecified

IQ **C44.92** Squamous cell carcinoma of skin, unspecified

IQ **C44.99** Other specified malignant neoplasm of skin, unspecified

---

Malignant neoplasms of mesothelial and soft tissue (C45-C49)

CODING TIPS ✓ Codes classifiable to C45-C49 include active cancer. History of cancer to soft tissue should be coded to Z85.83-.

4 **C45** Mesothelioma

SP **C45.0** Mesothelioma of pleura
> **EXCLUDES 1** other malignant neoplasm of pleura (C38.4)

SP **C45.1** Mesothelioma of peritoneum
Mesothelioma of cul-de-sac
Mesothelioma of mesentery
Mesothelioma of mesocolon
Mesothelioma of omentum
Mesothelioma of peritoneum (parietal) (pelvic)
> **EXCLUDES 1** other malignant neoplasm of soft tissue of peritoneum (C48.-)

SP **C45.2** Mesothelioma of pericardium
> **EXCLUDES 1** other malignant neoplasm of pericardium (C38.0)

SP **C45.7** Mesothelioma of other sites

IQ **C45.9** Mesothelioma, unspecified

4 **C46** Kaposi's sarcoma
Code first:
any human immunodeficiency virus [HIV] disease (B20)
> **CODING TIPS ✓** Kaposi's sarcoma (C46) is usually associated with HIV/AIDS. If so, then B20 is coded prior to using the C46 category code, unless other restrictions apply. (See coding tip at category B20.)

SP **C46.0** Kaposi's sarcoma of skin

SP **C46.1** Kaposi's sarcoma of soft tissue
Kaposi's sarcoma of blood vessel
Kaposi's sarcoma of connective tissue
Kaposi's sarcoma of fascia
Kaposi's sarcoma of ligament
Kaposi's sarcoma of lymphatic(s) NEC
Kaposi's sarcoma of muscle
> **EXCLUDES 2** Kaposi's sarcoma of lymph glands and nodes (C46.3)

SP **C46.2** Kaposi's sarcoma of palate

SP **C46.3** Kaposi's sarcoma of lymph nodes

SP **C46.4** Kaposi's sarcoma of gastrointestinal sites

5 **C46.5** Kaposi's sarcoma of lung

⊟ **IQ** **C46.50** Kaposi's sarcoma of unspecified lung

⊟ **SP** **C46.51** Kaposi's sarcoma of right lung

⊟ **SP** **C46.52** Kaposi's sarcoma of left lung

SP **C46.7** Kaposi's sarcoma of other sites

IQ **C46.9** Kaposi's sarcoma, unspecified
Kaposi's sarcoma of unspecified site

4 **C47** Malignant neoplasm of peripheral nerves and autonomic nervous system
> **INCLUDES** malignant neoplasm of sympathetic and parasympathetic nerves and ganglia
> **EXCLUDES 1** Kaposi's sarcoma of soft tissue (C46.1)

SP **C47.0** Malignant neoplasm of peripheral nerves of head, face and neck
> **EXCLUDES 1** malignant neoplasm of peripheral nerves of orbit (C69.6-)

5 **C47.1** Malignant neoplasm of peripheral nerves of upper limb, including shoulder

---

4 4th digit required   **5** 5th digit required   **6** 6th digit required   **7** 7th digit required   **7** 7th digit placeholder   **+** Additional code   ⊟ Laterality

656   DecisionHealth's FY 2020 Complete Home Health ICD-10-CM Diagnosis Coding Manual

☐ **IQ** **C47.10** Malignant neoplasm of peripheral nerves of unspecified upper limb, including shoulder

☐ **SP** **C47.11** Malignant neoplasm of peripheral nerves of right upper limb, including shoulder

☐ **SP** **C47.12** Malignant neoplasm of peripheral nerves of left upper limb, including shoulder

5 **C47.2** Malignant neoplasm of peripheral nerves of lower limb, including hip

☐ **IQ** **C47.20** Malignant neoplasm of peripheral nerves of unspecified lower limb, including hip

☐ **SP** **C47.21** Malignant neoplasm of peripheral nerves of right lower limb, including hip

☐ **SP** **C47.22** Malignant neoplasm of peripheral nerves of left lower limb, including hip

SP **C47.3** Malignant neoplasm of peripheral nerves of thorax

SP **C47.4** Malignant neoplasm of peripheral nerves of abdomen

SP **C47.5** Malignant neoplasm of peripheral nerves of pelvis

SP **C47.6** Malignant neoplasm of peripheral nerves of trunk, unspecified

　　　Malignant neoplasm of peripheral nerves of unspecified part of trunk

SP **C47.8** Malignant neoplasm of overlapping sites of peripheral nerves and autonomic nervous system

SP **C47.9** Malignant neoplasm of peripheral nerves and autonomic nervous system, unspecified

　　　Malignant neoplasm of unspecified site of peripheral nerves and autonomic nervous system

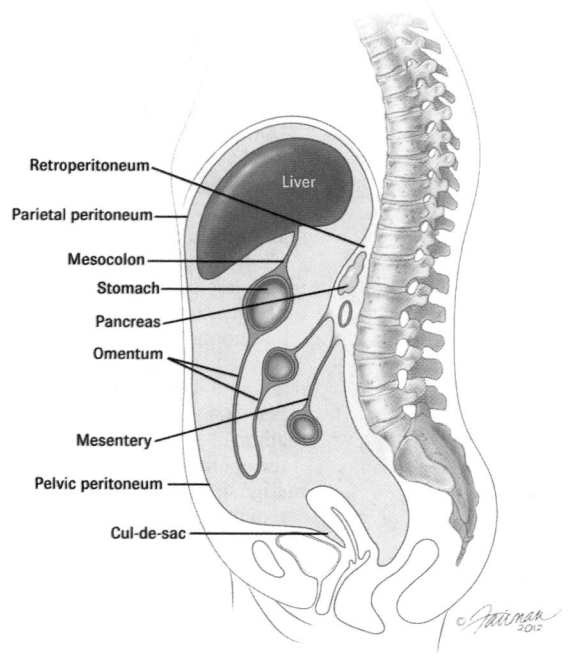

Retroperitoneum
Parietal peritoneum
Mesocolon
Stomach
Pancreas
Omentum
Mesentery
Pelvic peritoneum
Cul-de-sac
Liver

4 **C48** Malignant neoplasm of retroperitoneum and peritoneum

　　EXCLUDES 1 Kaposi's sarcoma of connective tissue (C46.1)
　　　　mesothelioma (C45.-)

　　CODING TIPS ✓ This category indicates active cancer. See Z85.09 for personal history of primary malignancy of the other digestive organs.

SP **C48.0** Malignant neoplasm of retroperitoneum

SP **C48.1** Malignant neoplasm of specified parts of peritoneum

　　　Malignant neoplasm of cul-de-sac
　　　Malignant neoplasm of mesentery
　　　Malignant neoplasm of mesocolon
　　　Malignant neoplasm of omentum
　　　Malignant neoplasm of parietal peritoneum
　　　Malignant neoplasm of pelvic peritoneum

SP **C48.2** Malignant neoplasm of peritoneum, unspecified

SP **C48.8** Malignant neoplasm of overlapping sites of retroperitoneum and peritoneum

4 **C49** Malignant neoplasm of other connective and soft tissue

　　INCLUDES malignant neoplasm of blood vessel
　　　malignant neoplasm of bursa
　　　malignant neoplasm of cartilage
　　　malignant neoplasm of fascia
　　　malignant neoplasm of fat
　　　malignant neoplasm of ligament, except uterine
　　　malignant neoplasm of lymphatic vessel
　　　malignant neoplasm of muscle
　　　malignant neoplasm of synovia

Chapter 2

C00-D49

★ New ▲ Revised **Px** Primary **SP** PDGM Px **SL** Low CoM **SH** High CoM **IQ** Quest. Encounter **H** Hospice non-cancer Dx ☐ Unspecified **M** *Manifestation*

DecisionHealth's FY 2020 Complete Home Health ICD-10-CM Diagnosis Coding Manual

657

malignant neoplasm of tendon
(sheath)

EXCLUDES 1 malignant neoplasm of cartilage
(of) :
articular (C40-C41)
larynx (C32.3)
nose (C30.0)
malignant neoplasm of
connective tissue of breast
(C50.-)

EXCLUDES 2 Kaposi's sarcoma of soft tissue
(C46.1)
malignant neoplasm of heart
(C38.0)
malignant neoplasm of
peripheral nerves and
autonomic nervous system
(C47.-)
malignant neoplasm of
peritoneum (C48.2)
malignant neoplasm of
retroperitoneum (C48.0)
malignant neoplasm of uterine
ligament (C57.3)
mesothelioma (C45.-)

SP C49.0 **Malignant neoplasm of connective and
soft tissue of head, face and neck**
Malignant neoplasm of connective tissue
of ear
Malignant neoplasm of connective tissue
of eyelid
EXCLUDES 1 connective tissue of orbit
(C69.6-)

5 C49.1 **Malignant neoplasm of connective and
soft tissue of upper limb, including
shoulder**

IQ C49.10 Malignant neoplasm of connective
and soft tissue of unspecified upper
limb, including shoulder

SP C49.11 **Malignant neoplasm of connective
and soft tissue of right upper limb,
including shoulder**

SP C49.12 **Malignant neoplasm of connective
and soft tissue of left upper limb,
including shoulder**

5 C49.2 **Malignant neoplasm of connective and
soft tissue of lower limb, including hip**

IQ C49.20 Malignant neoplasm of connective
and soft tissue of unspecified lower
limb, including hip

SP C49.21 **Malignant neoplasm of connective
and soft tissue of right lower limb,
including hip**

SP C49.22 **Malignant neoplasm of connective
and soft tissue of left lower limb,
including hip**

SP C49.3 **Malignant neoplasm of connective and
soft tissue of thorax**
Malignant neoplasm of axilla
Malignant neoplasm of diaphragm
Malignant neoplasm of great vessels
EXCLUDES 1 malignant neoplasm of
breast (C50.-)
malignant neoplasm of heart
(C38.0)
malignant neoplasm of
mediastinum
(C38.1-C38.3)

malignant neoplasm of
thymus (C37)

SP C49.4 **Malignant neoplasm of connective and
soft tissue of abdomen**
Malignant neoplasm of abdominal wall
Malignant neoplasm of hypochondrium

SP C49.5 **Malignant neoplasm of connective and
soft tissue of pelvis**
Malignant neoplasm of buttock
Malignant neoplasm of groin
Malignant neoplasm of perineum

SP C49.6 **Malignant neoplasm of connective and
soft tissue of trunk, unspecified**
Malignant neoplasm of back NOS

SP C49.8 **Malignant neoplasm of overlapping sites
of connective and soft tissue**
Primary malignant neoplasm of two or
more contiguous sites of connective and
soft tissue

IQ C49.9 **Malignant neoplasm of connective and
soft tissue, unspecified**

5 C49.A **Gastrointestinal stromal tumor**

IQ C49.A0 **Gastrointestinal stromal tumor,
unspecified site**

SP C49.A1 **Gastrointestinal stromal tumor of
esophagus**

SP C49.A2 **Gastrointestinal stromal tumor of
stomach**

SP C49.A3 **Gastrointestinal stromal tumor of
small intestine**

SP C49.A4 **Gastrointestinal stromal tumor of
large intestine**

SP C49.A5 **Gastrointestinal stromal tumor of
rectum**

SP C49.A9 **Gastrointestinal stromal tumor of
other sites**

Malignant neoplasms of breast (C50)

CODING TIPS ✓ Code C50 indicates active cancer. History of
cancer to the breast should be coded to Z85.3. Add a Z79.81-
code for treatment agents affecting estrogen receptors and
estrogen levels.

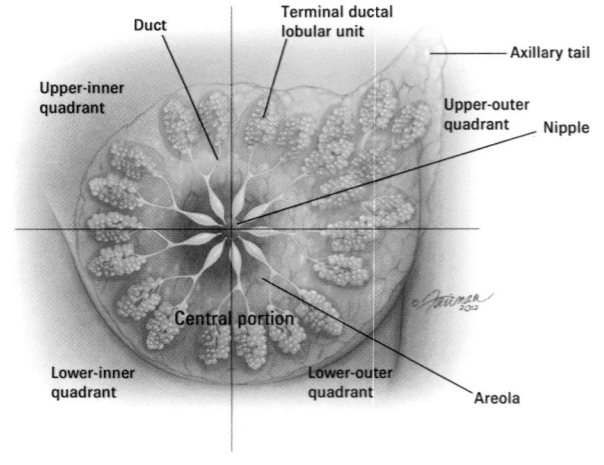

+ 4 C50 Malignant neoplasm of breast

4 4th digit required   **5** 5th digit required   **6** 6th digit required   **7** 7th digit required   **☑** 7th digit placeholder   **+** Additional code   **⊟** Laterality

658   *DecisionHealth's* FY 2020 Complete Home Health ICD-10-CM Diagnosis Coding Manual

INCLUDES connective tissue of breast
Paget's disease of breast
Paget's disease of nipple
Use additional code to identify estrogen
receptor status (Z17.0, Z17.1)
EXCLUDES 1 skin of breast
(C44.501, C44.511, C44.521,
C44.591)

+ 5 **C50.0** Malignant neoplasm of nipple and
areola

+ 6 **C50.01** Malignant neoplasm of nipple and
areola, female

☰ SP + **C50.011** Malignant neoplasm of nipple and
areola, right female breast

☰ SP + **C50.012** Malignant neoplasm of nipple and
areola, left female breast

☰ IQ + **C50.019** Malignant neoplasm of nipple
and areola, unspecified female
breast

+ 6 **C50.02** Malignant neoplasm of nipple and
areola, male

☰ SP + **C50.021** Malignant neoplasm of nipple and
areola, right male breast

☰ SP + **C50.022** Malignant neoplasm of nipple and
areola, left male breast

☰ IQ + **C50.029** Malignant neoplasm of nipple
and areola, unspecified male
breast

+ 5 **C50.1** Malignant neoplasm of central portion
of breast

+ 6 **C50.11** Malignant neoplasm of central
portion of breast, female

☰ SP + **C50.111** Malignant neoplasm of central
portion of right female breast

☰ SP + **C50.112** Malignant neoplasm of central
portion of left female breast

☰ IQ + **C50.119** Malignant neoplasm of central
portion of unspecified female
breast

+ 6 **C50.12** Malignant neoplasm of central
portion of breast, male

☰ SP + **C50.121** Malignant neoplasm of central
portion of right male breast

☰ SP + **C50.122** Malignant neoplasm of central
portion of left male breast

☰ IQ + **C50.129** Malignant neoplasm of central
portion of unspecified male
breast

+ 5 **C50.2** Malignant neoplasm of upper-inner
quadrant of breast

+ 6 **C50.21** Malignant neoplasm of upper-inner
quadrant of breast, female

☰ SP + **C50.211** Malignant neoplasm of upper-
inner quadrant of right female
breast

☰ SP + **C50.212** Malignant neoplasm of upper-
inner quadrant of left female
breast

☰ IQ + **C50.219** Malignant neoplasm of upper-
inner quadrant of unspecified
female breast

+ 6 **C50.22** Malignant neoplasm of upper-inner
quadrant of breast, male

☰ SP + **C50.221** Malignant neoplasm of upper-
inner quadrant of right male
breast

☰ SP + **C50.222** Malignant neoplasm of upper-
inner quadrant of left male breast

☰ IQ + **C50.229** Malignant neoplasm of upper-
inner quadrant of unspecified
male breast

+ 5 **C50.3** Malignant neoplasm of lower-inner
quadrant of breast

+ 6 **C50.31** Malignant neoplasm of lower-inner
quadrant of breast, female

☰ SP + **C50.311** Malignant neoplasm of lower-
inner quadrant of right female
breast

☰ SP + **C50.312** Malignant neoplasm of lower-
inner quadrant of left female
breast

☰ IQ + **C50.319** Malignant neoplasm of lower-
inner quadrant of unspecified
female breast

+ 6 **C50.32** Malignant neoplasm of lower-inner
quadrant of breast, male

☰ SP + **C50.321** Malignant neoplasm of lower-
inner quadrant of right male
breast

☰ SP + **C50.322** Malignant neoplasm of lower-
inner quadrant of left male breast

☰ IQ + **C50.329** Malignant neoplasm of lower-
inner quadrant of unspecified
male breast

+ 5 **C50.4** Malignant neoplasm of upper-outer
quadrant of breast

+ 6 **C50.41** Malignant neoplasm of upper-outer
quadrant of breast, female

☰ SP + **C50.411** Malignant neoplasm of upper-
outer quadrant of right female
breast

☰ SP + **C50.412** Malignant neoplasm of upper-
outer quadrant of left female
breast

☰ IQ + **C50.419** Malignant neoplasm of upper-
outer quadrant of unspecified
female breast

+ 6 **C50.42** Malignant neoplasm of upper-outer
quadrant of breast, male

☰ SP + **C50.421** Malignant neoplasm of upper-
outer quadrant of right male
breast

☰ SP + **C50.422** Malignant neoplasm of upper-
outer quadrant of left male breast

☰ IQ + **C50.429** Malignant neoplasm of upper-
outer quadrant of unspecified
male breast

+ 5 **C50.5** Malignant neoplasm of lower-outer
quadrant of breast

+ 6 **C50.51** Malignant neoplasm of lower-outer
quadrant of breast, female

☰ SP + **C50.511** Malignant neoplasm of lower-
outer quadrant of right female
breast

☰ SP + **C50.512** Malignant neoplasm of lower-
outer quadrant of left female
breast

☰ IQ + **C50.519** Malignant neoplasm of lower-
outer quadrant of unspecified
female breast

+ 6 **C50.52** Malignant neoplasm of lower-outer
quadrant of breast, male

★ New ▲ Revised **Px** Primary **SP** PDGM Px **SL** Low CoM **SH** High CoM **IQ** Quest. Encounter **H** Hospice non-cancer Dx Unspecified **M** *Manifestation*

DecisionHealth's FY 2020 Complete Home Health ICD-10-CM Diagnosis Coding Manual

659

Chapter 2

C00-D49

⊟ SP + **C50.521** Malignant neoplasm of lower-outer quadrant of right male breast

⊟ SP + **C50.522** Malignant neoplasm of lower-outer quadrant of left male breast

⊟ IQ + **C50.529** Malignant neoplasm of lower-outer quadrant of unspecified male breast

+ 5 **C50.6** Malignant neoplasm of axillary tail of breast

   + 6 **C50.61** Malignant neoplasm of axillary tail of breast, female

⊟ SP + **C50.611** Malignant neoplasm of axillary tail of right female breast

⊟ SP + **C50.612** Malignant neoplasm of axillary tail of left female breast

⊟ IQ + **C50.619** Malignant neoplasm of axillary tail of unspecified female breast

   + 6 **C50.62** Malignant neoplasm of axillary tail of breast, male

⊟ SP + **C50.621** Malignant neoplasm of axillary tail of right male breast

⊟ SP + **C50.622** Malignant neoplasm of axillary tail of left male breast

⊟ IQ + **C50.629** Malignant neoplasm of axillary tail of unspecified male breast

+ 5 **C50.8** Malignant neoplasm of overlapping sites of breast

   + 6 **C50.81** Malignant neoplasm of overlapping sites of breast, female

⊟ SP + **C50.811** Malignant neoplasm of overlapping sites of right female breast

⊟ SP + **C50.812** Malignant neoplasm of overlapping sites of left female breast

⊟ IQ + **C50.819** Malignant neoplasm of overlapping sites of unspecified female breast

   + 6 **C50.82** Malignant neoplasm of overlapping sites of breast, male

⊟ SP + **C50.821** Malignant neoplasm of overlapping sites of right male breast

⊟ SP + **C50.822** Malignant neoplasm of overlapping sites of left male breast

⊟ IQ + **C50.829** Malignant neoplasm of overlapping sites of unspecified male breast

+ 5 **C50.9** Malignant neoplasm of breast of unspecified site

   + 6 **C50.91** Malignant neoplasm of breast of unspecified site, female

⊟ SP + **C50.911** Malignant neoplasm of unspecified site of right female breast

⊟ SP + **C50.912** Malignant neoplasm of unspecified site of left female breast

⊟ IQ + **C50.919** Malignant neoplasm of unspecified site of unspecified female breast

CODING TIPS ✓ **Documentation:** If the site is not documented, you **must** query the physician and specify the site with C50.911 (right breast) or C50.912 (left breast). Use an additional code for estrogen receptor status (Z17.0, Z17.1).

+ 6 **C50.92** Malignant neoplasm of breast of unspecified site, male

⊟ SP + **C50.921** Malignant neoplasm of unspecified site of right male breast

⊟ SP + **C50.922** Malignant neoplasm of unspecified site of left male breast

⊟ IQ + **C50.929** Malignant neoplasm of unspecified site of unspecified male breast

Malignant neoplasms of female genital organs (C51-C58)

INCLUDES malignant neoplasm of skin of female genital organs

CODING TIPS ✓ Categories C51-C58 indicate active cancer. See Z85.40-Z85.44 for personal history of primary malignancy of female genital organs and Z85.45-Z85.49 for personal history of primary malignancy of male genital organs.

4 **C51** Malignant neoplasm of vulva

   EXCLUDES 1 carcinoma in situ of vulva (D07.1)

SP **C51.0** Malignant neoplasm of labium majus
   Malignant neoplasm of Bartholin's [greater vestibular] gland

SP **C51.1** Malignant neoplasm of labium minus

SP **C51.2** Malignant neoplasm of clitoris

SP **C51.8** Malignant neoplasm of overlapping sites of vulva

SP **C51.9** Malignant neoplasm of vulva, unspecified

   Malignant neoplasm of external female genitalia NOS
   Malignant neoplasm of pudendum

SP **C52** Malignant neoplasm of vagina

   EXCLUDES 1 carcinoma in situ of vagina (D07.2)

4 **C53** Malignant neoplasm of cervix uteri

   EXCLUDES 1 carcinoma in situ of cervix uteri (D06.-)

SP **C53.0** Malignant neoplasm of endocervix

SP **C53.1** Malignant neoplasm of exocervix

SP **C53.8** Malignant neoplasm of overlapping sites of cervix uteri

SP **C53.9** Malignant neoplasm of cervix uteri, unspecified

4 **C54** Malignant neoplasm of corpus uteri

SP **C54.0** Malignant neoplasm of isthmus uteri
   Malignant neoplasm of lower uterine segment

SP **C54.1** Malignant neoplasm of endometrium

SP **C54.2** Malignant neoplasm of myometrium

SP **C54.3** Malignant neoplasm of fundus uteri

SP **C54.8** Malignant neoplasm of overlapping sites of corpus uteri

4 4th digit required   5 5th digit required   6 6th digit required   7 7th digit required   ☑ 7th digit placeholder   + Additional code   ⊟ Laterality

660   *DecisionHealth's* FY 2020 Complete Home Health ICD-10-CM Diagnosis Coding Manual

SP **C54.9** Malignant neoplasm of corpus uteri, unspecified

SP **C55** Malignant neoplasm of uterus, part unspecified

+ 4 C56 Malignant neoplasm of ovary
Use additional code to identify any functional activity

⊟ SP + **C56.1** Malignant neoplasm of right ovary

⊟ SP + **C56.2** Malignant neoplasm of left ovary

⊟ IQ + **C56.9** Malignant neoplasm of unspecified ovary

4 C57 Malignant neoplasm of other and unspecified female genital organs

5 C57.0 Malignant neoplasm of fallopian tube
Malignant neoplasm of oviduct
Malignant neoplasm of uterine tube

⊟ IQ **C57.00** Malignant neoplasm of unspecified fallopian tube

⊟ SP **C57.01** Malignant neoplasm of right fallopian tube

⊟ SP **C57.02** Malignant neoplasm of left fallopian tube

5 C57.1 Malignant neoplasm of broad ligament

⊟ IQ **C57.10** Malignant neoplasm of unspecified broad ligament

⊟ SP **C57.11** Malignant neoplasm of right broad ligament

⊟ SP **C57.12** Malignant neoplasm of left broad ligament

5 C57.2 Malignant neoplasm of round ligament

⊟ IQ **C57.20** Malignant neoplasm of unspecified round ligament

⊟ SP **C57.21** Malignant neoplasm of right round ligament

⊟ SP **C57.22** Malignant neoplasm of left round ligament

SP **C57.3** Malignant neoplasm of parametrium
Malignant neoplasm of uterine ligament NOS

SP **C57.4** Malignant neoplasm of uterine adnexa, unspecified

SP **C57.7** Malignant neoplasm of other specified female genital organs
Malignant neoplasm of wolffian body or duct

SP **C57.8** Malignant neoplasm of overlapping sites of female genital organs
Primary malignant neoplasm of two or more contiguous sites of the female genital organs whose point of origin cannot be determined
Primary tubo-ovarian malignant neoplasm whose point of origin cannot be determined
Primary utero-ovarian malignant neoplasm whose point of origin cannot be determined

IQ **C57.9** Malignant neoplasm of female genital organ, unspecified
Malignant neoplasm of female genitourinary tract NOS

SP **C58** Malignant neoplasm of placenta
INCLUDES choriocarcinoma NOS
chorionepithelioma NOS
EXCLUDES 1 chorioadenoma (destruens) (D39.2)

hydatidiform mole NOS (O01.9)
invasive hydatidiform mole (D39.2)
male choriocarcinoma NOS (C62.9-)
malignant hydatidiform mole (D39.2)

Malignant neoplasms of male genital organs   (C60-C63)

INCLUDES malignant neoplasm of skin of male genital organs

CODING TIPS ✓ Codes classifiable to C60-C63 include active cancer. History of cancer to the male genital organs should be coded to Z85.4-.

4 C60 Malignant neoplasm of penis

IQ **C60.0** Malignant neoplasm of prepuce
Malignant neoplasm of foreskin

SP **C60.1** Malignant neoplasm of glans penis

SP **C60.2** Malignant neoplasm of body of penis
Malignant neoplasm of corpus cavernosum

SP **C60.8** Malignant neoplasm of overlapping sites of penis

SP **C60.9** Malignant neoplasm of penis, unspecified
Malignant neoplasm of skin of penis NOS

SP + **C61** Malignant neoplasm of prostate
Use additional code to identify:
hormone sensitivity status (Z19.1-Z19.2)
rising PSA following treatment for malignant neoplasm of prostate (R97.21)
EXCLUDES 1 malignant neoplasm of seminal vesicle (C63.7)

+ 4 C62 Malignant neoplasm of testis
Use additional code to identify any functional activity

+ 5 C62.0 Malignant neoplasm of undescended testis
Malignant neoplasm of ectopic testis
Malignant neoplasm of retained testis

⊟ IQ + **C62.00** Malignant neoplasm of unspecified undescended testis

⊟ SP + **C62.01** Malignant neoplasm of undescended right testis

⊟ SP + **C62.02** Malignant neoplasm of undescended left testis

+ 5 C62.1 Malignant neoplasm of descended testis
Malignant neoplasm of scrotal testis

⊟ IQ + **C62.10** Malignant neoplasm of unspecified descended testis

⊟ SP + **C62.11** Malignant neoplasm of descended right testis

⊟ SP + **C62.12** Malignant neoplasm of descended left testis

+ 5 C62.9 Malignant neoplasm of testis, unspecified whether descended or undescended

⊟ IQ + **C62.90** Malignant neoplasm of unspecified testis, unspecified whether descended or undescended
Malignant neoplasm of testis NOS

⊟ SP + **C62.91** Malignant neoplasm of right testis, unspecified whether descended or undescended

★ New ▲ Revised Px Primary **SP** PDGM Px **SL** Low CoM **SH** High CoM **IQ** Quest. Encounter **H** Hospice non-cancer Dx **Unspecified** **M** *Manifestation*

DecisionHealth's FY 2020 Complete Home Health ICD-10-CM Diagnosis Coding Manual

661

Chapter 2

C00-D49

⊟ **SP** ✚ **C62.92** **Malignant neoplasm of left testis, unspecified whether descended or undescended**

4 C63 **Malignant neoplasm of other and unspecified male genital organs**

5 C63.0 Malignant neoplasm of epididymis

⊟ **IQ** **C63.00** **Malignant neoplasm of unspecified epididymis**

⊟ **SP** **C63.01** Malignant neoplasm of right epididymis

⊟ **SP** **C63.02** Malignant neoplasm of left epididymis

5 C63.1 Malignant neoplasm of spermatic cord

⊟ **IQ** **C63.10** **Malignant neoplasm of unspecified spermatic cord**

⊟ **SP** **C63.11** Malignant neoplasm of right spermatic cord

⊟ **SP** **C63.12** Malignant neoplasm of left spermatic cord

SP **C63.2** Malignant neoplasm of scrotum
Malignant neoplasm of skin of scrotum

SP **C63.7** Malignant neoplasm of other specified male genital organs
Malignant neoplasm of seminal vesicle
Malignant neoplasm of tunica vaginalis

SP **C63.8** Malignant neoplasm of overlapping sites of male genital organs
Primary malignant neoplasm of two or more contiguous sites of male genital organs whose point of origin cannot be determined

IQ **C63.9** **Malignant neoplasm of male genital organ, unspecified**
Malignant neoplasm of male genitourinary tract NOS

Malignant neoplasms of urinary tract (C64-C68)

CODING TIPS ✓ Codes classifiable to C64-C68 include active cancer. History of cancer to the urinary tract should be coded to Z85.5-.

4 C64 **Malignant neoplasm of kidney, except renal pelvis**
EXCLUDES 1 malignant carcinoid tumor of the kidney (C7A.093)
malignant neoplasm of renal calyces (C65.-)
malignant neoplasm of renal pelvis (C65.-)
CODING TIPS ✓ This code indicates active cancer. See Z85.52- for personal history of malignant neoplasm of the kidney.

⊟ **SP** **C64.1** Malignant neoplasm of right kidney, except renal pelvis

⊟ **SP** **C64.2** Malignant neoplasm of left kidney, except renal pelvis

⊟ **IQ** **C64.9** **Malignant neoplasm of unspecified kidney, except renal pelvis**

4 C65 **Malignant neoplasm of renal pelvis**
INCLUDES malignant neoplasm of pelviureteric junction
malignant neoplasm of renal calyces

CODING TIPS ✓ This code indicates active cancer. See Z85.53 for personal history of the renal pelvis.

⊟ **SP** **C65.1** Malignant neoplasm of right renal pelvis

⊟ **SP** **C65.2** Malignant neoplasm of left renal pelvis

⊟ **IQ** **C65.9** **Malignant neoplasm of unspecified renal pelvis**

4 C66 **Malignant neoplasm of ureter**
EXCLUDES 1 malignant neoplasm of ureteric orifice of bladder (C67.6)
CODING TIPS ✓ This code indicates active cancer. See Z85.54 for history of primary malignant neoplasm of ureter.

⊟ **SP** **C66.1** Malignant neoplasm of right ureter

⊟ **SP** **C66.2** Malignant neoplasm of left ureter

⊟ **IQ** **C66.9** **Malignant neoplasm of unspecified ureter**

4 C67 **Malignant neoplasm of bladder**
CODING TIPS ✓ This code indicates active cancer. See Z85.51 for personal history of malignant neoplasm of the bladder.

SP **C67.0** Malignant neoplasm of trigone of bladder

SP **C67.1** Malignant neoplasm of dome of bladder

SP **C67.2** Malignant neoplasm of lateral wall of bladder

SP **C67.3** Malignant neoplasm of anterior wall of bladder

SP **C67.4** Malignant neoplasm of posterior wall of bladder

SP **C67.5** Malignant neoplasm of bladder neck
Malignant neoplasm of internal urethral orifice

SP **C67.6** Malignant neoplasm of ureteric orifice

SP **C67.7** Malignant neoplasm of urachus

SP **C67.8** Malignant neoplasm of overlapping sites of bladder

SP **C67.9** **Malignant neoplasm of bladder, unspecified**

4 C68 **Malignant neoplasm of other and unspecified urinary organs**
EXCLUDES 1 malignant neoplasm of female genitourinary tract NOS (C57.9)
malignant neoplasm of male genitourinary tract NOS (C63.9)

SP **C68.0** Malignant neoplasm of urethra
EXCLUDES 1 malignant neoplasm of urethral orifice of bladder (C67.5)

SP **C68.1** Malignant neoplasm of paraurethral glands

SP **C68.8** Malignant neoplasm of overlapping sites of urinary organs
Primary malignant neoplasm of two or more contiguous sites of urinary organs whose point of origin cannot be determined

IQ **C68.9** **Malignant neoplasm of urinary organ, unspecified**
Malignant neoplasm of urinary system NOS

---

4 4th digit required   **5** 5th digit required   **6** 6th digit required   **7** 7th digit required   **☑** 7th digit placeholder   ✚ Additional code   ⊟ Laterality

Malignant neoplasms of eye, brain and other parts of central nervous system (C69-C72)

CODING TIPS ✓ Codes classifiable to C69-C72 include active cancer. History of cancer to eye, brain, or other area of nervous system should be coded to Z85.84-.

4 C69 Malignant neoplasm of eye and adnexa

EXCLUDES 1 malignant neoplasm of connective tissue of eyelid (C49.0)
malignant neoplasm of eyelid (skin) (C43.1-, C44.1-)
malignant neoplasm of optic nerve (C72.3-)

CODING TIPS ✓ This code indicates active cancer. See Z85.840 for personal history of malignant neoplasm of the eye.

5 C69.0 Malignant neoplasm of conjunctiva

▤ IQ C69.00 Malignant neoplasm of unspecified conjunctiva

▤ SP C69.01 Malignant neoplasm of right conjunctiva

▤ SP C69.02 Malignant neoplasm of left conjunctiva

5 C69.1 Malignant neoplasm of cornea

▤ IQ C69.10 Malignant neoplasm of unspecified cornea

▤ SP C69.11 Malignant neoplasm of right cornea

▤ SP C69.12 Malignant neoplasm of left cornea

5 C69.2 Malignant neoplasm of retina

EXCLUDES 1 dark area on retina (D49.81)
neoplasm of unspecified behavior of retina and choroid (D49.81)
retinal freckle (D49.81)

▤ IQ C69.20 Malignant neoplasm of unspecified retina

▤ SP C69.21 Malignant neoplasm of right retina

▤ SP C69.22 Malignant neoplasm of left retina

5 C69.3 Malignant neoplasm of choroid

▤ IQ C69.30 Malignant neoplasm of unspecified choroid

▤ SP C69.31 Malignant neoplasm of right choroid

▤ SP C69.32 Malignant neoplasm of left choroid

5 C69.4 Malignant neoplasm of ciliary body

▤ IQ C69.40 Malignant neoplasm of unspecified ciliary body

▤ SP C69.41 Malignant neoplasm of right ciliary body

▤ SP C69.42 Malignant neoplasm of left ciliary body

5 C69.5 Malignant neoplasm of lacrimal gland and duct
Malignant neoplasm of lacrimal sac
Malignant neoplasm of nasolacrimal duct

▤ IQ C69.50 Malignant neoplasm of unspecified lacrimal gland and duct

▤ SP C69.51 Malignant neoplasm of right lacrimal gland and duct

▤ SP C69.52 Malignant neoplasm of left lacrimal gland and duct

5 C69.6 Malignant neoplasm of orbit
Malignant neoplasm of connective tissue of orbit
Malignant neoplasm of extraocular muscle
Malignant neoplasm of peripheral nerves of orbit
Malignant neoplasm of retrobulbar tissue
Malignant neoplasm of retro-ocular tissue

EXCLUDES 1 malignant neoplasm of orbital bone (C41.0)

▤ IQ C69.60 Malignant neoplasm of unspecified orbit

▤ SP C69.61 Malignant neoplasm of right orbit

▤ SP C69.62 Malignant neoplasm of left orbit

5 C69.8 Malignant neoplasm of overlapping sites of eye and adnexa

▤ IQ C69.80 Malignant neoplasm of overlapping sites of unspecified eye and adnexa

▤ SP C69.81 Malignant neoplasm of overlapping sites of right eye and adnexa

▤ SP C69.82 Malignant neoplasm of overlapping sites of left eye and adnexa

5 C69.9 Malignant neoplasm of unspecified site of eye
Malignant neoplasm of eyeball

▤ IQ C69.90 Malignant neoplasm of unspecified site of unspecified eye

▤ SP C69.91 Malignant neoplasm of unspecified site of right eye

▤ SP C69.92 Malignant neoplasm of unspecified site of left eye

4 C70 Malignant neoplasm of meninges

SP C70.0 Malignant neoplasm of cerebral meninges

SP C70.1 Malignant neoplasm of spinal meninges

SP C70.9 Malignant neoplasm of meninges, unspecified

4 C71 Malignant neoplasm of brain

EXCLUDES 1 malignant neoplasm of cranial nerves (C72.2-C72.5)
retrobulbar malignant neoplasm (C69.6-)

CODING TIPS ✓ C71 indicates active cancer. See Z85.841 for personal history of malignant neoplasm of the brain. Metastasis to the brain is seen more often than a primary lesion. Metastases to the brain are coded with C79.31.

SP C71.0 Malignant neoplasm of cerebrum, except lobes and ventricles
Malignant neoplasm of supratentorial NOS

SP C71.1 Malignant neoplasm of frontal lobe

SP C71.2 Malignant neoplasm of temporal lobe

SP C71.3 Malignant neoplasm of parietal lobe

SP C71.4 Malignant neoplasm of occipital lobe

SP C71.5 Malignant neoplasm of cerebral ventricle

EXCLUDES 1 malignant neoplasm of fourth cerebral ventricle (C71.7)

SP C71.6 Malignant neoplasm of cerebellum

SP C71.7 Malignant neoplasm of brain stem
Malignant neoplasm of fourth cerebral ventricle
Infratentorial malignant neoplasm NOS

★ New ▲ Revised Px Primary SP PDGM Px SL Low CoM SH High CoM IQ Quest. Encounter H Hospice non-cancer Dx Unspecified M *Manifestation*

SP **C71.8** **Malignant neoplasm of overlapping sites of brain**

SP **C71.9** **Malignant neoplasm of brain, unspecified**

4 **C72** **Malignant neoplasm of spinal cord, cranial nerves and other parts of central nervous system**

> **EXCLUDES 1** malignant neoplasm of meninges (C70.-)
> malignant neoplasm of peripheral nerves and autonomic nervous system (C47.-)

> **CODING TIPS ✓** This code indicates active cancer. See Z85.848 for personal history of malignant neoplasm to other parts of the nervous system.

SP **C72.0** **Malignant neoplasm of spinal cord**

SP **C72.1** **Malignant neoplasm of cauda equina**

5 **C72.2** **Malignant neoplasm of olfactory nerve**
> Malignant neoplasm of olfactory bulb

IQ **C72.20** **Malignant neoplasm of unspecified olfactory nerve**

SP **C72.21** **Malignant neoplasm of right olfactory nerve**

SP **C72.22** **Malignant neoplasm of left olfactory nerve**

5 **C72.3** **Malignant neoplasm of optic nerve**

IQ **C72.30** **Malignant neoplasm of unspecified optic nerve**

SP **C72.31** **Malignant neoplasm of right optic nerve**

SP **C72.32** **Malignant neoplasm of left optic nerve**

5 **C72.4** **Malignant neoplasm of acoustic nerve**

IQ **C72.40** **Malignant neoplasm of unspecified acoustic nerve**

SP **C72.41** **Malignant neoplasm of right acoustic nerve**

SP **C72.42** **Malignant neoplasm of left acoustic nerve**

5 **C72.5** **Malignant neoplasm of other and unspecified cranial nerves**

IQ **C72.50** **Malignant neoplasm of unspecified cranial nerve**
> Malignant neoplasm of cranial nerve NOS

SP **C72.59** **Malignant neoplasm of other cranial nerves**

SP **C72.9** **Malignant neoplasm of central nervous system, unspecified**
> Malignant neoplasm of unspecified site of central nervous system
> Malignant neoplasm of nervous system NOS

Malignant neoplasms of thyroid and other endocrine glands (C73-C75)

CODING TIPS ✓ Codes classifiable to C73-C75 include active cancer. History of cancer to endocrine glands should be coded to Z85.85-.

SP **+** **C73** **Malignant neoplasm of thyroid gland**
> Use additional code to identify any functional activity

CODING TIPS ✓ Category C73 indicates active cancer. See Z85.850 for personal history of primary malignancy of the thyroid if the thyroid cancer has been eradicated. If the cancer is being treated, code the cancer. If the malignancy is causing abnormal secretion of thyroid hormones, the effects of the thyroid hormones should also be coded.

4 **C74** **Malignant neoplasm of adrenal gland**

CODING TIPS ✓ This code indicates active cancer. See Z85.858 for personal history of primary history of other endocrine glands if cancer has been eradicated. If cancer is being treated, code the cancer, not the Z code. If the cancer is causing abnormal secretion of hormones, the effects of the hormones should also be coded.

5 **C74.0** **Malignant neoplasm of cortex of adrenal gland**

SP **C74.00** **Malignant neoplasm of cortex of unspecified adrenal gland**

SP **C74.01** **Malignant neoplasm of cortex of right adrenal gland**

SP **C74.02** **Malignant neoplasm of cortex of left adrenal gland**

5 **C74.1** **Malignant neoplasm of medulla of adrenal gland**

IQ **C74.10** **Malignant neoplasm of medulla of unspecified adrenal gland**

SP **C74.11** **Malignant neoplasm of medulla of right adrenal gland**

SP **C74.12** **Malignant neoplasm of medulla of left adrenal gland**

5 **C74.9** **Malignant neoplasm of unspecified part of adrenal gland**

IQ **C74.90** **Malignant neoplasm of unspecified part of unspecified adrenal gland**

SP **C74.91** **Malignant neoplasm of unspecified part of right adrenal gland**

SP **C74.92** **Malignant neoplasm of unspecified part of left adrenal gland**

4 **C75** **Malignant neoplasm of other endocrine glands and related structures**

> **EXCLUDES 1** malignant carcinoid tumors (C7A.0-)
> malignant neoplasm of adrenal gland (C74.-)
> malignant neoplasm of endocrine pancreas (C25.4)
> malignant neoplasm of islets of Langerhans (C25.4)
> malignant neoplasm of ovary (C56.-)
> malignant neoplasm of testis (C62.-)
> malignant neoplasm of thymus (C37)
> malignant neoplasm of thyroid gland (C73)
> malignant neuroendocrine tumors (C7A.-)

---

4 4th digit required   **5** 5th digit required   **6** 6th digit required   **7** 7th digit required   **7** 7th digit placeholder   **+** Additional code   Laterality

CODING TIPS ✓ This code indicates active cancer. See Z85.858 for personal history of primary history of other endocrine glands if cancer has been eradicated. If cancer is being treated, code the cancer, not the Z code. If the cancer is causing abnormal secretion of hormones, the effects of the hormones should also be coded.

SP **C75.0** Malignant neoplasm of parathyroid gland

SP **C75.1** Malignant neoplasm of pituitary gland

SP **C75.2** Malignant neoplasm of craniopharyngeal duct

SP **C75.3** Malignant neoplasm of pineal gland

SP **C75.4** Malignant neoplasm of carotid body

SP **C75.5** Malignant neoplasm of aortic body and other paraganglia

SP **C75.8** Malignant neoplasm with pluriglandular involvement, unspecified

SP **C75.9** Malignant neoplasm of endocrine gland, unspecified

Malignant neuroendocrine tumors (C7A)

CODING TIPS ✓ Codes classifiable to C7A- include primary neuroendocrine tumors, which are considered active malignant carcinoid tumors. A history of any malignant carcinoid tumor (neuroendocrine malignancy) should be coded to the appropriate Z85- code for history of malignant carcinoid tumor of that specific anatomical location.

+ 4 C7A Malignant neuroendocrine tumors
Code also:
any associated multiple endocrine neoplasia [MEN] syndromes (E31.2-)
Use additional code to identify any associated endocrine syndrome, such as:
carcinoid syndrome (E34.0)
EXCLUDES 2 malignant pancreatic islet cell tumors (C25.4)
Merkel cell carcinoma (C4A.-)

+ 5 C7A.0 Malignant carcinoid tumors

IQ + C7A.00 Malignant carcinoid tumor of unspecified site

+ 6 C7A.01 Malignant carcinoid tumors of the small intestine

SP + C7A.010 Malignant carcinoid tumor of the duodenum

SP + C7A.011 Malignant carcinoid tumor of the jejunum

SP + C7A.012 Malignant carcinoid tumor of the ileum

SP + C7A.019 Malignant carcinoid tumor of the small intestine, unspecified portion

+ 6 C7A.02 Malignant carcinoid tumors of the appendix, large intestine, and rectum

SP + C7A.020 Malignant carcinoid tumor of the appendix

SP + C7A.021 Malignant carcinoid tumor of the cecum

SP + C7A.022 Malignant carcinoid tumor of the ascending colon

SP + C7A.023 Malignant carcinoid tumor of the transverse colon

SP + C7A.024 Malignant carcinoid tumor of the descending colon

SP + C7A.025 Malignant carcinoid tumor of the sigmoid colon

SP + C7A.026 Malignant carcinoid tumor of the rectum

SP + C7A.029 Malignant carcinoid tumor of the large intestine, unspecified portion
Malignant carcinoid tumor of the colon NOS

+ 6 C7A.09 Malignant carcinoid tumors of other sites

SP + C7A.090 Malignant carcinoid tumor of the bronchus and lung

SP + C7A.091 Malignant carcinoid tumor of the thymus

SP + C7A.092 Malignant carcinoid tumor of the stomach

SP + C7A.093 Malignant carcinoid tumor of the kidney

SP + C7A.094 Malignant carcinoid tumor of the foregut, unspecified

SP + C7A.095 Malignant carcinoid tumor of the midgut, unspecified

SP + C7A.096 Malignant carcinoid tumor of the hindgut, unspecified

SP + C7A.098 Malignant carcinoid tumors of other sites

SP + C7A.1 Malignant poorly differentiated neuroendocrine tumors
Malignant poorly differentiated neuroendocrine tumor NOS
Malignant poorly differentiated neuroendocrine carcinoma, any site
High grade neuroendocrine carcinoma, any site

SP + C7A.8 Other malignant neuroendocrine tumors

Secondary neuroendocrine tumors (C7B)

CODING TIPS ✓ Codes classifiable to C7B- include secondary (metastases) neuroendocrine tumors, which are considered active malignant carcinoid tumors.

+ 4 C7B Secondary neuroendocrine tumors
Use additional code to identify any functional activity

+ 5 C7B.0 Secondary carcinoid tumors

IQ + C7B.00 Secondary carcinoid tumors, unspecified site

SP + C7B.01 Secondary carcinoid tumors of distant lymph nodes

SP + C7B.02 Secondary carcinoid tumors of liver

SP + C7B.03 Secondary carcinoid tumors of bone

SP + C7B.04 Secondary carcinoid tumors of peritoneum
Mesentary metastasis of carcinoid tumor

SP + C7B.09 Secondary carcinoid tumors of other sites

SP + C7B.1 Secondary Merkel cell carcinoma
Merkel cell carcinoma nodal presentation
Merkel cell carcinoma visceral metastatic presentation

SP + C7B.8 Other secondary neuroendocrine tumors

★ New ▲ Revised **Px** Primary **SP** PDGM Px **SL** Low CoM **SH** High CoM **IQ** Quest. Encounter **H** Hospice non-cancer Dx Unspecified **M** *Manifestation*

Malignant neoplasms of ill-defined, other secondary and unspecified sites (C76-C80)

4 C76 Malignant neoplasm of other and ill-defined sites

EXCLUDES 1 malignant neoplasm of female genitourinary tract NOS (C57.9)

malignant neoplasm of male genitourinary tract NOS (C63.9)

malignant neoplasm of lymphoid, hematopoietic and related tissue (C81-C96)

malignant neoplasm of skin (C44.-)

malignant neoplasm of unspecified site NOS (C80.1)

CODING TIPS ✓ Query the physician before assigning codes from C76. For example, if the documentation indicates cancer of the nose: Is it the nasal passages, skin on the nose, the cartilage of the nose?

SP C76.0 Malignant neoplasm of head, face and neck

Malignant neoplasm of cheek NOS

Malignant neoplasm of nose NOS

SP C76.1 Malignant neoplasm of thorax

Intrathoracic malignant neoplasm NOS

Malignant neoplasm of axilla NOS

Thoracic malignant neoplasm NOS

SP C76.2 Malignant neoplasm of abdomen

SP C76.3 Malignant neoplasm of pelvis

Malignant neoplasm of groin NOS

Malignant neoplasm of sites overlapping systems within the pelvis

Rectovaginal (septum) malignant neoplasm

Rectovesical (septum) malignant neoplasm

5 C76.4 Malignant neoplasm of upper limb

⊟ IQ C76.40 Malignant neoplasm of unspecified upper limb

⊟ SP C76.41 Malignant neoplasm of right upper limb

⊟ SP C76.42 Malignant neoplasm of left upper limb

5 C76.5 Malignant neoplasm of lower limb

⊟ IQ C76.50 Malignant neoplasm of unspecified lower limb

⊟ SP C76.51 Malignant neoplasm of right lower limb

⊟ SP C76.52 Malignant neoplasm of left lower limb

SP C76.8 Malignant neoplasm of other specified ill-defined sites

Malignant neoplasm of overlapping ill-defined sites

4 C77 Secondary and unspecified malignant neoplasm of lymph nodes

EXCLUDES 1 malignant neoplasm of lymph nodes, specified as primary (C81-C86, C88, C96.-)

mesentary metastasis of carcinoid tumor (C7B.04)

secondary carcinoid tumors of distant lymph nodes (C7B.01)

CODING TIPS ✓ Codes classifiable to C77- include neoplasms specified as secondary or metastatic sites of cancer. Primary neoplasms of lymphatic tissue should not be assigned codes from C77-. See C7B for secondary neuroendocrine tumors, such as carcinoid tumors and Merkel cell carcinoma.

SP C77.0 Secondary and unspecified malignant neoplasm of lymph nodes of head, face and neck

Secondary and unspecified malignant neoplasm of supraclavicular lymph nodes

SP C77.1 Secondary and unspecified malignant neoplasm of intrathoracic lymph nodes

SP C77.2 Secondary and unspecified malignant neoplasm of intra-abdominal lymph nodes

SP C77.3 Secondary and unspecified malignant neoplasm of axilla and upper limb lymph nodes

Secondary and unspecified malignant neoplasm of pectoral lymph nodes

SP C77.4 Secondary and unspecified malignant neoplasm of inguinal and lower limb lymph nodes

SP C77.5 Secondary and unspecified malignant neoplasm of intrapelvic lymph nodes

SP C77.8 Secondary and unspecified malignant neoplasm of lymph nodes of multiple regions

IQ C77.9 Secondary and unspecified malignant neoplasm of lymph node, unspecified

4 C78 Secondary malignant neoplasm of respiratory and digestive organs

EXCLUDES 1 secondary carcinoid tumors of liver (C7B.02)

secondary carcinoid tumors of peritoneum (C7B.04)

EXCLUDES 2 lymph node metastases (C77.0)

CODING TIPS ✓ Codes classifiable to C78- include neoplasms specified as secondary or metastatic sites of cancer. Primary neoplasms should not be assigned codes from C78-. See C7B for secondary neuroendocrine tumors, such as carcinoid tumors and Merkel cell carcinoma.

5 C78.0 Secondary malignant neoplasm of lung

⊟ IQ C78.00 Secondary malignant neoplasm of unspecified lung

⊟ SP C78.01 Secondary malignant neoplasm of right lung

⊟ SP C78.02 Secondary malignant neoplasm of left lung

SP C78.1 Secondary malignant neoplasm of mediastinum

SP C78.2 Secondary malignant neoplasm of pleura

5 C78.3 Secondary malignant neoplasm of other and unspecified respiratory organs

---

4 4th digit required   5 5th digit required   6 6th digit required   7 7th digit required   7 7th digit placeholder   ✚ Additional code   ⊟ Laterality

666   DecisionHealth's FY 2020 Complete Home Health ICD-10-CM Diagnosis Coding Manual

IQ C78.30 Secondary malignant neoplasm of unspecified respiratory organ

SP C78.39 Secondary malignant neoplasm of other respiratory organs

SP C78.4 Secondary malignant neoplasm of small intestine

SP C78.5 Secondary malignant neoplasm of large intestine and rectum

SP C78.6 Secondary malignant neoplasm of retroperitoneum and peritoneum

SP C78.7 Secondary malignant neoplasm of liver and intrahepatic bile duct

5 C78.8 Secondary malignant neoplasm of other and unspecified digestive organs

IQ C78.80 Secondary malignant neoplasm of unspecified digestive organ

SP C78.89 Secondary malignant neoplasm of other digestive organs
Code also:
exocrine pancreatic insufficiency (K86.81)

4 C79 Secondary malignant neoplasm of other and unspecified sites

EXCLUDES 1 secondary carcinoid tumors (C7B.-)
secondary neuroendocrine tumors (C7B.-)

CODING TIPS ✓ Codes classifiable to C79- include neoplasms specified as secondary or metastatic sites of cancer. Primary neoplasms should not be assigned codes from C79-. See C7B for secondary neuroendocrine tumors, such as carcinoid tumors and Merkel cell carcinoma.

5 C79.0 Secondary malignant neoplasm of kidney and renal pelvis

IQ C79.00 Secondary malignant neoplasm of unspecified kidney and renal pelvis

SP C79.01 Secondary malignant neoplasm of right kidney and renal pelvis

SP C79.02 Secondary malignant neoplasm of left kidney and renal pelvis

5 C79.1 Secondary malignant neoplasm of bladder and other and unspecified urinary organs

IQ C79.10 Secondary malignant neoplasm of unspecified urinary organs

SP C79.11 Secondary malignant neoplasm of bladder
EXCLUDES 2 lymph node metastases (C77.0)

SP C79.19 Secondary malignant neoplasm of other urinary organs

SP C79.2 Secondary malignant neoplasm of skin
EXCLUDES 1 secondary Merkel cell carcinoma (C7B.1)

5 C79.3 Secondary malignant neoplasm of brain and cerebral meninges

SP C79.31 Secondary malignant neoplasm of brain

SP C79.32 Secondary malignant neoplasm of cerebral meninges

5 C79.4 Secondary malignant neoplasm of other and unspecified parts of nervous system

IQ C79.40 Secondary malignant neoplasm of unspecified part of nervous system

SP C79.49 Secondary malignant neoplasm of other parts of nervous system

5 C79.5 Secondary malignant neoplasm of bone and bone marrow
EXCLUDES 1 secondary carcinoid tumors of bone (C7B.03)

SP C79.51 Secondary malignant neoplasm of bone

SP C79.52 Secondary malignant neoplasm of bone marrow

5 C79.6 Secondary malignant neoplasm of ovary

IQ C79.60 Secondary malignant neoplasm of unspecified ovary

SP C79.61 Secondary malignant neoplasm of right ovary

SP C79.62 Secondary malignant neoplasm of left ovary

5 C79.7 Secondary malignant neoplasm of adrenal gland

IQ C79.70 Secondary malignant neoplasm of unspecified adrenal gland

SP C79.71 Secondary malignant neoplasm of right adrenal gland

SP C79.72 Secondary malignant neoplasm of left adrenal gland

5 C79.8 Secondary malignant neoplasm of other specified sites

SP C79.81 Secondary malignant neoplasm of breast

SP C79.82 Secondary malignant neoplasm of genital organs

SP C79.89 Secondary malignant neoplasm of other specified sites

IQ C79.9 Secondary malignant neoplasm of unspecified site

Metastatic cancer NOS
Metastatic disease NOS
EXCLUDES 1 carcinomatosis NOS (C80.0)
generalized cancer NOS (C80.0)
malignant (primary) neoplasm of unspecified site (C80.1)

CODING TIPS ✓ This code should be reported if the physician documents metastasis but does not indicate the location. Query the physician prior to using this code.

4 C80 Malignant neoplasm without specification of site
EXCLUDES 1 malignant carcinoid tumor of unspecified site (C7A.00)
malignant neoplasm of specified multiple sites- code to each site

SP C80.0 Disseminated malignant neoplasm, unspecified

Carcinomatosis NOS
Generalized cancer, unspecified site (primary) (secondary)
Generalized malignancy, unspecified site (primary) (secondary)

★ New ▲ Revised Px Primary SP PDGM Px SL Low CoM SH High CoM IQ Quest. Encounter H Hospice non-cancer Dx Unspecified M Manifestation

DecisionHealth's FY 2020 Complete Home Health ICD-10-CM Diagnosis Coding Manual

667

Chapter 2

C00-D49

Chapter 2

C00-D49

GUIDELINES Section I.C.2.j
Code C80.0 is for use only in those cases where the patient has advanced metastatic disease and no known primary or secondary sites are specified. It should not be used in place of assigning codes for the primary site and all known secondary sites.

CODING TIPS ✓ This code is used to indicate that the cancer is in multiple locations and no attempt will be made to identify the primary and secondary sites. Advanced metastatic disease may be documented. If there are multiple sites specified, code to each site.

IQ C80.1 Malignant (primary) neoplasm, unspecified
Cancer NOS
Cancer unspecified site (primary)
Carcinoma unspecified site (primary)
Malignancy unspecified site (primary)
EXCLUDES 1 secondary malignant neoplasm of unspecified site (C79.9)
GUIDELINES Section I.C.2.k
Code C80.1 equates to Cancer, unspecified. This code should only be used when no determination can be made as to the primary site of a malignancy. This code should rarely be used in the inpatient setting.

CODING TIPS ✓ When coding a secondary site of the cancer and the primary site is unknown, C80.1 should be added for unknown primary site. A biopsy-proven malignancy for which a primary site cannot be found constitutes 0.5% to 7% of all cancer patients.

IQ + C80.2 Malignant neoplasm associated with transplanted organ
Code first:
    complication of transplanted organ (T86.-)
Use additional code to identify the specific malignancy
GUIDELINES Section I.C.2.r
A malignant neoplasm of a transplanted organ should be coded as a transplant complication. Assign first the appropriate code from category T86.-, Complications of transplanted organs and tissue, followed by code C80.2. Use an additional code for the specific malignancy.

Malignant neoplasms of lymphoid, hematopoietic and related tissue (C81-C96)

EXCLUDES 2 Kaposi's sarcoma of lymph nodes (C46.3)
secondary and unspecified neoplasm of lymph nodes (C77.-)
secondary neoplasm of bone marrow (C79.52)
secondary neoplasm of spleen (C78.89)

CODING TIPS ✓ Codes classifiable to C81-C96 include active malignancy of lymphoid, hematopeotic and related tissues. Secondary neoplastic disease of lymph tissue should not be coded using codes from C81-C96.

4 C81 Hodgkin lymphoma
EXCLUDES 1 personal history of Hodgkin lymphoma (Z85.71)
5 C81.0 Nodular lymphocyte predominant Hodgkin lymphoma
SP C81.00 Nodular lymphocyte predominant Hodgkin lymphoma, unspecified site
SP C81.01 Nodular lymphocyte predominant Hodgkin lymphoma, lymph nodes of head, face, and neck
SP C81.02 Nodular lymphocyte predominant Hodgkin lymphoma, intrathoracic lymph nodes
SP C81.03 Nodular lymphocyte predominant Hodgkin lymphoma, intra-abdominal lymph nodes
SP C81.04 Nodular lymphocyte predominant Hodgkin lymphoma, lymph nodes of axilla and upper limb
SP C81.05 Nodular lymphocyte predominant Hodgkin lymphoma, lymph nodes of inguinal region and lower limb
SP C81.06 Nodular lymphocyte predominant Hodgkin lymphoma, intrapelvic lymph nodes
SP C81.07 Nodular lymphocyte predominant Hodgkin lymphoma, spleen
SP C81.08 Nodular lymphocyte predominant Hodgkin lymphoma, lymph nodes of multiple sites
SP C81.09 Nodular lymphocyte predominant Hodgkin lymphoma, extranodal and solid organ sites
5 C81.1 Nodular sclerosis Hodgkin lymphoma
Nodular sclerosis classical Hodgkin lymphoma
SP C81.10 Nodular sclerosis Hodgkin lymphoma, unspecified site
SP C81.11 Nodular sclerosis Hodgkin lymphoma, lymph nodes of head, face, and neck
SP C81.12 Nodular sclerosis Hodgkin lymphoma, intrathoracic lymph nodes
SP C81.13 Nodular sclerosis Hodgkin lymphoma, intra-abdominal lymph nodes
SP C81.14 Nodular sclerosis Hodgkin lymphoma, lymph nodes of axilla and upper limb
SP C81.15 Nodular sclerosis Hodgkin lymphoma, lymph nodes of inguinal region and lower limb
SP C81.16 Nodular sclerosis Hodgkin lymphoma, intrapelvic lymph nodes
SP C81.17 Nodular sclerosis Hodgkin lymphoma, spleen
SP C81.18 Nodular sclerosis Hodgkin lymphoma, lymph nodes of multiple sites
SP C81.19 Nodular sclerosis Hodgkin lymphoma, extranodal and solid organ sites
5 C81.2 Mixed cellularity Hodgkin lymphoma
Mixed cellularity classical Hodgkin lymphoma

---

4 4th digit required   5 5th digit required   6 6th digit required   7 7th digit required   7 7th digit placeholder   + Additional code   ⊟ Laterality

SP C81.20 Mixed cellularity Hodgkin lymphoma, unspecified site

SP C81.21 Mixed cellularity Hodgkin lymphoma, lymph nodes of head, face, and neck

SP C81.22 Mixed cellularity Hodgkin lymphoma, intrathoracic lymph nodes

SP C81.23 Mixed cellularity Hodgkin lymphoma, intra-abdominal lymph nodes

SP C81.24 Mixed cellularity Hodgkin lymphoma, lymph nodes of axilla and upper limb

SP C81.25 Mixed cellularity Hodgkin lymphoma, lymph nodes of inguinal region and lower limb

SP C81.26 Mixed cellularity Hodgkin lymphoma, intrapelvic lymph nodes

SP C81.27 Mixed cellularity Hodgkin lymphoma, spleen

SP C81.28 Mixed cellularity Hodgkin lymphoma, lymph nodes of multiple sites

SP C81.29 Mixed cellularity Hodgkin lymphoma, extranodal and solid organ sites

5 C81.3 Lymphocyte depleted Hodgkin lymphoma
Lymphocyte depleted classical Hodgkin lymphoma

SP C81.30 Lymphocyte depleted Hodgkin lymphoma, unspecified site

SP C81.31 Lymphocyte depleted Hodgkin lymphoma, lymph nodes of head, face, and neck

SP C81.32 Lymphocyte depleted Hodgkin lymphoma, intrathoracic lymph nodes

SP C81.33 Lymphocyte depleted Hodgkin lymphoma, intra-abdominal lymph nodes

SP C81.34 Lymphocyte depleted Hodgkin lymphoma, lymph nodes of axilla and upper limb

SP C81.35 Lymphocyte depleted Hodgkin lymphoma, lymph nodes of inguinal region and lower limb

SP C81.36 Lymphocyte depleted Hodgkin lymphoma, intrapelvic lymph nodes

SP C81.37 Lymphocyte depleted Hodgkin lymphoma, spleen

SP C81.38 Lymphocyte depleted Hodgkin lymphoma, lymph nodes of multiple sites

SP C81.39 Lymphocyte depleted Hodgkin lymphoma, extranodal and solid organ sites

5 C81.4 Lymphocyte-rich Hodgkin lymphoma
Lymphocyte-rich classical Hodgkin lymphoma
EXCLUDES 1 nodular lymphocyte predominant Hodgkin lymphoma (C81.0-)

SP C81.40 Lymphocyte-rich Hodgkin lymphoma, unspecified site

SP C81.41 Lymphocyte-rich Hodgkin lymphoma, lymph nodes of head, face, and neck

SP C81.42 Lymphocyte-rich Hodgkin lymphoma, intrathoracic lymph nodes

SP C81.43 Lymphocyte-rich Hodgkin lymphoma, intra-abdominal lymph nodes

SP C81.44 Lymphocyte-rich Hodgkin lymphoma, lymph nodes of axilla and upper limb

SP C81.45 Lymphocyte-rich Hodgkin lymphoma, lymph nodes of inguinal region and lower limb

SP C81.46 Lymphocyte-rich Hodgkin lymphoma, intrapelvic lymph nodes

SP C81.47 Lymphocyte-rich Hodgkin lymphoma, spleen

SP C81.48 Lymphocyte-rich Hodgkin lymphoma, lymph nodes of multiple sites

SP C81.49 Lymphocyte-rich Hodgkin lymphoma, extranodal and solid organ sites

5 C81.7 Other Hodgkin lymphoma
Classical Hodgkin lymphoma NOS
Other classical Hodgkin lymphoma

SP C81.70 Other Hodgkin lymphoma, unspecified site

SP C81.71 Other Hodgkin lymphoma, lymph nodes of head, face, and neck

SP C81.72 Other Hodgkin lymphoma, intrathoracic lymph nodes

SP C81.73 Other Hodgkin lymphoma, intra-abdominal lymph nodes

SP C81.74 Other Hodgkin lymphoma, lymph nodes of axilla and upper limb

SP C81.75 Other Hodgkin lymphoma, lymph nodes of inguinal region and lower limb

SP C81.76 Other Hodgkin lymphoma, intrapelvic lymph nodes

SP C81.77 Other Hodgkin lymphoma, spleen

SP C81.78 Other Hodgkin lymphoma, lymph nodes of multiple sites

SP C81.79 Other Hodgkin lymphoma, extranodal and solid organ sites

5 C81.9 Hodgkin lymphoma, unspecified

SP C81.90 Hodgkin lymphoma, unspecified, unspecified site

SP C81.91 Hodgkin lymphoma, unspecified, lymph nodes of head, face, and neck

SP C81.92 Hodgkin lymphoma, unspecified, intrathoracic lymph nodes

SP C81.93 Hodgkin lymphoma, unspecified, intra-abdominal lymph nodes

SP C81.94 Hodgkin lymphoma, unspecified, lymph nodes of axilla and upper limb

SP C81.95 Hodgkin lymphoma, unspecified, lymph nodes of inguinal region and lower limb

SP C81.96 Hodgkin lymphoma, unspecified, intrapelvic lymph nodes

★ New ▲ Revised Px Primary SP PDGM Px SL Low CoM SH High CoM IQ Quest. Encounter H Hospice non-cancer Dx | Unspecified | M *Manifestation*

DecisionHealth's FY 2020 Complete Home Health ICD-10-CM Diagnosis Coding Manual

669

SP C81.97 Hodgkin lymphoma, unspecified, spleen

SP C81.98 Hodgkin lymphoma, unspecified, lymph nodes of multiple sites

SP C81.99 Hodgkin lymphoma, unspecified, extranodal and solid organ sites

4 C82 Follicular lymphoma

> **INCLUDES** follicular lymphoma with or without diffuse areas
>
> **EXCLUDES 1** mature T/NK-cell lymphomas (C84.-)
> personal history of non-Hodgkin lymphoma (Z85.72)

5 C82.0 Follicular lymphoma grade I

SP C82.00 Follicular lymphoma grade I, unspecified site

SP C82.01 Follicular lymphoma grade I, lymph nodes of head, face, and neck

SP C82.02 Follicular lymphoma grade I, intrathoracic lymph nodes

SP C82.03 Follicular lymphoma grade I, intra-abdominal lymph nodes

SP C82.04 Follicular lymphoma grade I, lymph nodes of axilla and upper limb

SP C82.05 Follicular lymphoma grade I, lymph nodes of inguinal region and lower limb

SP C82.06 Follicular lymphoma grade I, intrapelvic lymph nodes

SP C82.07 Follicular lymphoma grade I, spleen

SP C82.08 Follicular lymphoma grade I, lymph nodes of multiple sites

SP C82.09 Follicular lymphoma grade I, extranodal and solid organ sites

5 C82.1 Follicular lymphoma grade II

SP C82.10 Follicular lymphoma grade II, unspecified site

SP C82.11 Follicular lymphoma grade II, lymph nodes of head, face, and neck

SP C82.12 Follicular lymphoma grade II, intrathoracic lymph nodes

SP C82.13 Follicular lymphoma grade II, intra-abdominal lymph nodes

SP C82.14 Follicular lymphoma grade II, lymph nodes of axilla and upper limb

SP C82.15 Follicular lymphoma grade II, lymph nodes of inguinal region and lower limb

SP C82.16 Follicular lymphoma grade II, intrapelvic lymph nodes

SP C82.17 Follicular lymphoma grade II, spleen

SP C82.18 Follicular lymphoma grade II, lymph nodes of multiple sites

SP C82.19 Follicular lymphoma grade II, extranodal and solid organ sites

5 C82.2 Follicular lymphoma grade III, unspecified

SP C82.20 Follicular lymphoma grade III, unspecified, unspecified site

SP C82.21 Follicular lymphoma grade III, unspecified, lymph nodes of head, face, and neck

SP C82.22 Follicular lymphoma grade III, unspecified, intrathoracic lymph nodes

SP C82.23 Follicular lymphoma grade III, unspecified, intra-abdominal lymph nodes

SP C82.24 Follicular lymphoma grade III, unspecified, lymph nodes of axilla and upper limb

SP C82.25 Follicular lymphoma grade III, unspecified, lymph nodes of inguinal region and lower limb

SP C82.26 Follicular lymphoma grade III, unspecified, intrapelvic lymph nodes

SP C82.27 Follicular lymphoma grade III, unspecified, spleen

SP C82.28 Follicular lymphoma grade III, unspecified, lymph nodes of multiple sites

SP C82.29 Follicular lymphoma grade III, unspecified, extranodal and solid organ sites

5 C82.3 Follicular lymphoma grade IIIa

SP C82.30 Follicular lymphoma grade IIIa, unspecified site

SP C82.31 Follicular lymphoma grade IIIa, lymph nodes of head, face, and neck

SP C82.32 Follicular lymphoma grade IIIa, intrathoracic lymph nodes

SP C82.33 Follicular lymphoma grade IIIa, intra-abdominal lymph nodes

SP C82.34 Follicular lymphoma grade IIIa, lymph nodes of axilla and upper limb

SP C82.35 Follicular lymphoma grade IIIa, lymph nodes of inguinal region and lower limb

SP C82.36 Follicular lymphoma grade IIIa, intrapelvic lymph nodes

SP C82.37 Follicular lymphoma grade IIIa, spleen

SP C82.38 Follicular lymphoma grade IIIa, lymph nodes of multiple sites

SP C82.39 Follicular lymphoma grade IIIa, extranodal and solid organ sites

5 C82.4 Follicular lymphoma grade IIIb

SP C82.40 Follicular lymphoma grade IIIb, unspecified site

SP C82.41 Follicular lymphoma grade IIIb, lymph nodes of head, face, and neck

SP C82.42 Follicular lymphoma grade IIIb, intrathoracic lymph nodes

SP C82.43 Follicular lymphoma grade IIIb, intra-abdominal lymph nodes

SP C82.44 Follicular lymphoma grade IIIb, lymph nodes of axilla and upper limb

SP C82.45 Follicular lymphoma grade IIIb, lymph nodes of inguinal region and lower limb

SP C82.46 Follicular lymphoma grade IIIb, intrapelvic lymph nodes

SP C82.47 Follicular lymphoma grade IIIb, spleen

SP C82.48 Follicular lymphoma grade IIIb, lymph nodes of multiple sites

SP C82.49 Follicular lymphoma grade IIIb, extranodal and solid organ sites

---

4 4th digit required   5 5th digit required   6 6th digit required   7 7th digit required   7 7th digit placeholder   ✚ Additional code   ⊟ Laterality

670   *DecisionHealth's* FY 2020 Complete Home Health ICD-10-CM Diagnosis Coding Manual

Chapter 2

C00-D49

⑤ C82.5 Diffuse follicle center lymphoma

SP C82.50 Diffuse follicle center lymphoma, unspecified site

SP C82.51 Diffuse follicle center lymphoma, lymph nodes of head, face, and neck

SP C82.52 Diffuse follicle center lymphoma, intrathoracic lymph nodes

SP C82.53 Diffuse follicle center lymphoma, intra-abdominal lymph nodes

SP C82.54 Diffuse follicle center lymphoma, lymph nodes of axilla and upper limb

SP C82.55 Diffuse follicle center lymphoma, lymph nodes of inguinal region and lower limb

SP C82.56 Diffuse follicle center lymphoma, intrapelvic lymph nodes

SP C82.57 Diffuse follicle center lymphoma, spleen

SP C82.58 Diffuse follicle center lymphoma, lymph nodes of multiple sites

SP C82.59 Diffuse follicle center lymphoma, extranodal and solid organ sites

⑤ C82.6 Cutaneous follicle center lymphoma

SP C82.60 Cutaneous follicle center lymphoma, unspecified site

SP C82.61 Cutaneous follicle center lymphoma, lymph nodes of head, face, and neck

SP C82.62 Cutaneous follicle center lymphoma, intrathoracic lymph nodes

SP C82.63 Cutaneous follicle center lymphoma, intra-abdominal lymph nodes

SP C82.64 Cutaneous follicle center lymphoma, lymph nodes of axilla and upper limb

SP C82.65 Cutaneous follicle center lymphoma, lymph nodes of inguinal region and lower limb

SP C82.66 Cutaneous follicle center lymphoma, intrapelvic lymph nodes

SP C82.67 Cutaneous follicle center lymphoma, spleen

SP C82.68 Cutaneous follicle center lymphoma, lymph nodes of multiple sites

SP C82.69 Cutaneous follicle center lymphoma, extranodal and solid organ sites

⑤ C82.8 Other types of follicular lymphoma

SP C82.80 Other types of follicular lymphoma, unspecified site

SP C82.81 Other types of follicular lymphoma, lymph nodes of head, face, and neck

SP C82.82 Other types of follicular lymphoma, intrathoracic lymph nodes

SP C82.83 Other types of follicular lymphoma, intra-abdominal lymph nodes

SP C82.84 Other types of follicular lymphoma, lymph nodes of axilla and upper limb

SP C82.85 Other types of follicular lymphoma, lymph nodes of inguinal region and lower limb

SP C82.86 Other types of follicular lymphoma, intrapelvic lymph nodes

SP C82.87 Other types of follicular lymphoma, spleen

SP C82.88 Other types of follicular lymphoma, lymph nodes of multiple sites

SP C82.89 Other types of follicular lymphoma, extranodal and solid organ sites

⑤ C82.9 Follicular lymphoma, unspecified

SP C82.90 Follicular lymphoma, unspecified, unspecified site

SP C82.91 Follicular lymphoma, unspecified, lymph nodes of head, face, and neck

SP C82.92 Follicular lymphoma, unspecified, intrathoracic lymph nodes

SP C82.93 Follicular lymphoma, unspecified, intra-abdominal lymph nodes

SP C82.94 Follicular lymphoma, unspecified, lymph nodes of axilla and upper limb

SP C82.95 Follicular lymphoma, unspecified, lymph nodes of inguinal region and lower limb

SP C82.96 Follicular lymphoma, unspecified, intrapelvic lymph nodes

SP C82.97 Follicular lymphoma, unspecified, spleen

SP C82.98 Follicular lymphoma, unspecified, lymph nodes of multiple sites

SP C82.99 Follicular lymphoma, unspecified, extranodal and solid organ sites

④ C83 Non-follicular lymphoma

> **EXCLUDES 1** personal history of non-Hodgkin lymphoma (Z85.72)

⑤ C83.0 Small cell B-cell lymphoma
Lymphoplasmacytic lymphoma
Nodal marginal zone lymphoma
Non-leukemic variant of B-CLL
Splenic marginal zone lymphoma

> **EXCLUDES 1** chronic lymphocytic leukemia (C91.1)
> mature T/NK-cell lymphomas (C84.-)
> Waldenström macroglobulinemia (C88.0)

> **DEFINITION** Uncommon, low-grade, slow-growing B-cell non-Hodgkin's lymphoma involving the marginal, patchy area of the lymph node outside the mantle zone; not very responsive to traditional therapy.

SP C83.00 Small cell B-cell lymphoma, unspecified site

SP C83.01 Small cell B-cell lymphoma, lymph nodes of head, face, and neck

SP C83.02 Small cell B-cell lymphoma, intrathoracic lymph nodes

SP C83.03 Small cell B-cell lymphoma, intra-abdominal lymph nodes

SP C83.04 Small cell B-cell lymphoma, lymph nodes of axilla and upper limb

SP C83.05 Small cell B-cell lymphoma, lymph nodes of inguinal region and lower limb

SP C83.06 Small cell B-cell lymphoma, intrapelvic lymph nodes

SP C83.07 Small cell B-cell lymphoma, spleen

SP C83.08 Small cell B-cell lymphoma, lymph nodes of multiple sites

SP C83.09 Small cell B-cell lymphoma, extranodal and solid organ sites

★New ▲Revised Px Primary SP PDGM Px SL Low CoM SH High CoM IQ Quest. Encounter H Hospice non-cancer Dx Unspecified M *Manifestation*

DecisionHealth's FY 2020 Complete Home Health ICD-10-CM Diagnosis Coding Manual

671

⑤ C83.1 Mantle cell lymphoma
Centrocytic lymphoma
Malignant lymphomatous polyposis

SP C83.10 Mantle cell lymphoma, unspecified site

SP C83.11 Mantle cell lymphoma, lymph nodes of head, face, and neck

SP C83.12 Mantle cell lymphoma, intrathoracic lymph nodes

SP C83.13 Mantle cell lymphoma, intra-abdominal lymph nodes

SP C83.14 Mantle cell lymphoma, lymph nodes of axilla and upper limb

SP C83.15 Mantle cell lymphoma, lymph nodes of inguinal region and lower limb

SP C83.16 Mantle cell lymphoma, intrapelvic lymph nodes

SP C83.17 Mantle cell lymphoma, spleen

SP C83.18 Mantle cell lymphoma, lymph nodes of multiple sites

SP C83.19 Mantle cell lymphoma, extranodal and solid organ sites

⑤ C83.3 Diffuse large B-cell lymphoma
Anaplastic diffuse large B-cell lymphoma
CD30-positive diffuse large B-cell lymphoma
Centroblastic diffuse large B-cell lymphoma
Diffuse large B-cell lymphoma, subtype not specified
Immunoblastic diffuse large B-cell lymphoma
Plasmablastic diffuse large B-cell lymphoma
Diffuse large B-cell lymphoma, subtype not specified
T-cell rich diffuse large B-cell lymphoma
　EXCLUDES 1 mediastinal (thymic) large B-cell lymphoma (C85.2-)
　　　　　mature T/NK-cell lymphomas (C84.-)

SP C83.30 Diffuse large B-cell lymphoma, unspecified site

SP C83.31 Diffuse large B-cell lymphoma, lymph nodes of head, face, and neck

SP C83.32 Diffuse large B-cell lymphoma, intrathoracic lymph nodes

SP C83.33 Diffuse large B-cell lymphoma, intra-abdominal lymph nodes

SP C83.34 Diffuse large B-cell lymphoma, lymph nodes of axilla and upper limb

SP C83.35 Diffuse large B-cell lymphoma, lymph nodes of inguinal region and lower limb

SP C83.36 Diffuse large B-cell lymphoma, intrapelvic lymph nodes

SP C83.37 Diffuse large B-cell lymphoma, spleen

SP C83.38 Diffuse large B-cell lymphoma, lymph nodes of multiple sites

SP C83.39 Diffuse large B-cell lymphoma, extranodal and solid organ sites

⑤ C83.5 Lymphoblastic (diffuse) lymphoma
B-precursor lymphoma
Lymphoblastic B-cell lymphoma
Lymphoblastic lymphoma NOS
Lymphoblastic T-cell lymphoma
T-precursor lymphoma

SP C83.50 Lymphoblastic (diffuse) lymphoma, unspecified site

SP C83.51 Lymphoblastic (diffuse) lymphoma, lymph nodes of head, face, and neck

SP C83.52 Lymphoblastic (diffuse) lymphoma, intrathoracic lymph nodes

SP C83.53 Lymphoblastic (diffuse) lymphoma, intra-abdominal lymph nodes

SP C83.54 Lymphoblastic (diffuse) lymphoma, lymph nodes of axilla and upper limb

SP C83.55 Lymphoblastic (diffuse) lymphoma, lymph nodes of inguinal region and lower limb

SP C83.56 Lymphoblastic (diffuse) lymphoma, intrapelvic lymph nodes

SP C83.57 Lymphoblastic (diffuse) lymphoma, spleen

SP C83.58 Lymphoblastic (diffuse) lymphoma, lymph nodes of multiple sites

SP C83.59 Lymphoblastic (diffuse) lymphoma, extranodal and solid organ sites

⑤ C83.7 Burkitt lymphoma
Atypical Burkitt lymphoma
Burkitt-like lymphoma
　EXCLUDES 1 mature B-cell leukemia Burkitt type (C91.A-)

SP C83.70 Burkitt lymphoma, unspecified site

SP C83.71 Burkitt lymphoma, lymph nodes of head, face, and neck

SP C83.72 Burkitt lymphoma, intrathoracic lymph nodes

SP C83.73 Burkitt lymphoma, intra-abdominal lymph nodes

SP C83.74 Burkitt lymphoma, lymph nodes of axilla and upper limb

SP C83.75 Burkitt lymphoma, lymph nodes of inguinal region and lower limb

SP C83.76 Burkitt lymphoma, intrapelvic lymph nodes

SP C83.77 Burkitt lymphoma, spleen

SP C83.78 Burkitt lymphoma, lymph nodes of multiple sites

SP C83.79 Burkitt lymphoma, extranodal and solid organ sites

⑤ C83.8 Other non-follicular lymphoma
Intravascular large B-cell lymphoma
Lymphoid granulomatosis
Primary effusion B-cell lymphoma
　EXCLUDES 1 mediastinal (thymic) large B-cell lymphoma (C85.2-)
　　　　　T-cell rich B-cell lymphoma (C83.3-)

SP C83.80 Other non-follicular lymphoma, unspecified site

SP C83.81 Other non-follicular lymphoma, lymph nodes of head, face, and neck

SP C83.82 Other non-follicular lymphoma, intrathoracic lymph nodes

SP C83.83 Other non-follicular lymphoma, intra-abdominal lymph nodes

SP C83.84 Other non-follicular lymphoma, lymph nodes of axilla and upper limb

Chapter 2

C00-D49

---

④ 4th digit required　　⑤ 5th digit required　　⑥ 6th digit required　　⑦ 7th digit required　　☑ 7th digit placeholder　　✚ Additional code　　⊟ Laterality

SP C83.85 Other non-follicular lymphoma, lymph nodes of inguinal region and lower limb

SP C83.86 Other non-follicular lymphoma, intrapelvic lymph nodes

SP C83.87 Other non-follicular lymphoma, spleen

SP C83.88 Other non-follicular lymphoma, lymph nodes of multiple sites

SP C83.89 Other non-follicular lymphoma, extranodal and solid organ sites

5 C83.9 Non-follicular (diffuse) lymphoma, unspecified

SP C83.90 Non-follicular (diffuse) lymphoma, unspecified, unspecified site

SP C83.91 Non-follicular (diffuse) lymphoma, unspecified, lymph nodes of head, face, and neck

SP C83.92 Non-follicular (diffuse) lymphoma, unspecified, intrathoracic lymph nodes

SP C83.93 Non-follicular (diffuse) lymphoma, unspecified, intra-abdominal lymph nodes

SP C83.94 Non-follicular (diffuse) lymphoma, unspecified, lymph nodes of axilla and upper limb

SP C83.95 Non-follicular (diffuse) lymphoma, unspecified, lymph nodes of inguinal region and lower limb

SP C83.96 Non-follicular (diffuse) lymphoma, unspecified, intrapelvic lymph nodes

SP C83.97 Non-follicular (diffuse) lymphoma, unspecified, spleen

SP C83.98 Non-follicular (diffuse) lymphoma, unspecified, lymph nodes of multiple sites

SP C83.99 Non-follicular (diffuse) lymphoma, unspecified, extranodal and solid organ sites

4 C84 Mature T/NK-cell lymphomas

> **EXCLUDES 1** personal history of non-Hodgkin lymphoma (Z85.72)

5 C84.0 Mycosis fungoides

> **EXCLUDES 1** peripheral T-cell lymphoma, not classified (C84.4-)

> **DEFINITION** A rare, progressive form of slow-growing cutaneous T-cell lymphoma associated with a chromosome abnormality that evolves into a generalized, high grade, aggressive systemic form of lymphoma.

SP C84.00 Mycosis fungoides, unspecified site

SP C84.01 Mycosis fungoides, lymph nodes of head, face, and neck

SP C84.02 Mycosis fungoides, intrathoracic lymph nodes

SP C84.03 Mycosis fungoides, intra-abdominal lymph nodes

SP C84.04 Mycosis fungoides, lymph nodes of axilla and upper limb

SP C84.05 Mycosis fungoides, lymph nodes of inguinal region and lower limb

SP C84.06 Mycosis fungoides, intrapelvic lymph nodes

SP C84.07 Mycosis fungoides, spleen

SP C84.08 Mycosis fungoides, lymph nodes of multiple sites

SP C84.09 Mycosis fungoides, extranodal and solid organ sites

5 C84.1 Sézary disease

SP C84.10 Sézary disease, unspecified site

SP C84.11 Sézary disease, lymph nodes of head, face, and neck

SP C84.12 Sézary disease, intrathoracic lymph nodes

SP C84.13 Sézary disease, intra-abdominal lymph nodes

SP C84.14 Sézary disease, lymph nodes of axilla and upper limb

SP C84.15 Sézary disease, lymph nodes of inguinal region and lower limb

SP C84.16 Sézary disease, intrapelvic lymph nodes

SP C84.17 Sézary disease, spleen

SP C84.18 Sézary disease, lymph nodes of multiple sites

SP C84.19 Sézary disease, extranodal and solid organ sites

5 C84.4 Peripheral T-cell lymphoma, not classified

Lennert's lymphoma
Lymphoepithelioid lymphoma
Mature T-cell lymphoma, not elsewhere classified

> **DEFINITION** Aggressive, non-Hodgkin's lymphoma derived from mature neoplastic T-cell lymphocytes that have moved to other tissue, causing site-related symptoms and generalized lymphadenopathy.

SP C84.40 Peripheral T-cell lymphoma, not classified, unspecified site

SP C84.41 Peripheral T-cell lymphoma, not classified, lymph nodes of head, face, and neck

SP C84.42 Peripheral T-cell lymphoma, not classified, intrathoracic lymph nodes

SP C84.43 Peripheral T-cell lymphoma, not classified, intra-abdominal lymph nodes

SP C84.44 Peripheral T-cell lymphoma, not classified, lymph nodes of axilla and upper limb

SP C84.45 Peripheral T-cell lymphoma, not classified, lymph nodes of inguinal region and lower limb

SP C84.46 Peripheral T-cell lymphoma, not classified, intrapelvic lymph nodes

SP C84.47 Peripheral T-cell lymphoma, not classified, spleen

SP C84.48 Peripheral T-cell lymphoma, not classified, lymph nodes of multiple sites

SP C84.49 Peripheral T-cell lymphoma, not classified, extranodal and solid organ sites

5 C84.6 Anaplastic large cell lymphoma, ALK-positive

Anaplastic large cell lymphoma, CD30-positive

SP C84.60 Anaplastic large cell lymphoma, ALK-positive, unspecified site

Chapter 2

C00-D49

★ New ▲ Revised Px Primary **SP** PDGM Px **SL** Low CoM **SH** High CoM **IQ** Quest. Encounter **H** Hospice non-cancer Dx Unspecified **M** *Manifestation*

DecisionHealth's FY 2020 Complete Home Health ICD-10-CM Diagnosis Coding Manual

673

SP C84.61 Anaplastic large cell lymphoma, ALK-positive, lymph nodes of head, face, and neck

SP C84.62 Anaplastic large cell lymphoma, ALK-positive, intrathoracic lymph nodes

SP C84.63 Anaplastic large cell lymphoma, ALK-positive, intra-abdominal lymph nodes

SP C84.64 Anaplastic large cell lymphoma, ALK-positive, lymph nodes of axilla and upper limb

SP C84.65 Anaplastic large cell lymphoma, ALK-positive, lymph nodes of inguinal region and lower limb

SP C84.66 Anaplastic large cell lymphoma, ALK-positive, intrapelvic lymph nodes

SP C84.67 Anaplastic large cell lymphoma, ALK-positive, spleen

SP C84.68 Anaplastic large cell lymphoma, ALK-positive, lymph nodes of multiple sites

SP C84.69 Anaplastic large cell lymphoma, ALK-positive, extranodal and solid organ sites

5 C84.7 Anaplastic large cell lymphoma, ALK-negative

> **EXCLUDES 1** primary cutaneous CD30-positive T-cell proliferations (C86.6-)

SP C84.70 Anaplastic large cell lymphoma, ALK-negative, unspecified site

SP C84.71 Anaplastic large cell lymphoma, ALK-negative, lymph nodes of head, face, and neck

SP C84.72 Anaplastic large cell lymphoma, ALK-negative, intrathoracic lymph nodes

SP C84.73 Anaplastic large cell lymphoma, ALK-negative, intra-abdominal lymph nodes

SP C84.74 Anaplastic large cell lymphoma, ALK-negative, lymph nodes of axilla and upper limb

SP C84.75 Anaplastic large cell lymphoma, ALK-negative, lymph nodes of inguinal region and lower limb

SP C84.76 Anaplastic large cell lymphoma, ALK-negative, intrapelvic lymph nodes

SP C84.77 Anaplastic large cell lymphoma, ALK-negative, spleen

SP C84.78 Anaplastic large cell lymphoma, ALK-negative, lymph nodes of multiple sites

SP C84.79 Anaplastic large cell lymphoma, ALK-negative, extranodal and solid organ sites

5 C84.A Cutaneous T-cell lymphoma, unspecified

SP C84.A0 Cutaneous T-cell lymphoma, unspecified, unspecified site

SP C84.A1 Cutaneous T-cell lymphoma, unspecified lymph nodes of head, face, and neck

SP C84.A2 Cutaneous T-cell lymphoma, unspecified, intrathoracic lymph nodes

SP C84.A3 Cutaneous T-cell lymphoma, unspecified, intra-abdominal lymph nodes

SP C84.A4 Cutaneous T-cell lymphoma, unspecified, lymph nodes of axilla and upper limb

SP C84.A5 Cutaneous T-cell lymphoma, unspecified, lymph nodes of inguinal region and lower limb

SP C84.A6 Cutaneous T-cell lymphoma, unspecified, intrapelvic lymph nodes

SP C84.A7 Cutaneous T-cell lymphoma, unspecified, spleen

SP C84.A8 Cutaneous T-cell lymphoma, unspecified, lymph nodes of multiple sites

SP C84.A9 Cutaneous T-cell lymphoma, unspecified, extranodal and solid organ sites

5 C84.Z Other mature T/NK-cell lymphomas

> Note:
> If T-cell lineage or involvement is mentioned in conjunction with a specific lymphoma, code to the more specific description.
>
> **EXCLUDES 1** angioimmunoblastic T-cell lymphoma (C86.5)
> blastic NK-cell lymphoma (C86.4)
> enteropathy-type T-cell lymphoma (C86.2)
> extranodal NK-cell lymphoma, nasal type (C86.0)
> hepatosplenic T-cell lymphoma (C86.1)
> primary cutaneous CD30-positive T-cell proliferations (C86.6)
> subcutaneous panniculitis-like T-cell lymphoma (C86.3)
> T-cell leukemia (C91.1-)

SP C84.Z0 Other mature T/NK-cell lymphomas, unspecified site

SP C84.Z1 Other mature T/NK-cell lymphomas, lymph nodes of head, face, and neck

SP C84.Z2 Other mature T/NK-cell lymphomas, intrathoracic lymph nodes

SP C84.Z3 Other mature T/NK-cell lymphomas, intra-abdominal lymph nodes

SP C84.Z4 Other mature T/NK-cell lymphomas, lymph nodes of axilla and upper limb

SP C84.Z5 Other mature T/NK-cell lymphomas, lymph nodes of inguinal region and lower limb

SP C84.Z6 Other mature T/NK-cell lymphomas, intrapelvic lymph nodes

SP C84.Z7 Other mature T/NK-cell lymphomas, spleen

SP C84.Z8 Other mature T/NK-cell lymphomas, lymph nodes of multiple sites

---

4 4th digit required   5 5th digit required   6 6th digit required   7 7th digit required   7 7th digit placeholder   ✚ Additional code   ⊟ Laterality

674   *DecisionHealth's* FY 2020 Complete Home Health ICD-10-CM Diagnosis Coding Manual

SP C84.Z9 Other mature T/NK-cell lymphomas, extranodal and solid organ sites

⑤ C84.9 Mature T/NK-cell lymphomas, unspecified

NK/T cell lymphoma NOS

EXCLUDES 1 mature T-cell lymphoma, not elsewhere classified (C84.4-)

SP C84.90 Mature T/NK-cell lymphomas, unspecified, unspecified site

SP C84.91 Mature T/NK-cell lymphomas, unspecified, lymph nodes of head, face, and neck

SP C84.92 Mature T/NK-cell lymphomas, unspecified, intrathoracic lymph nodes

SP C84.93 Mature T/NK-cell lymphomas, unspecified, intra-abdominal lymph nodes

SP C84.94 Mature T/NK-cell lymphomas, unspecified, lymph nodes of axilla and upper limb

SP C84.95 Mature T/NK-cell lymphomas, unspecified, lymph nodes of inguinal region and lower limb

SP C84.96 Mature T/NK-cell lymphomas, unspecified, intrapelvic lymph nodes

SP C84.97 Mature T/NK-cell lymphomas, unspecified, spleen

SP C84.98 Mature T/NK-cell lymphomas, unspecified, lymph nodes of multiple sites

SP C84.99 Mature T/NK-cell lymphomas, unspecified, extranodal and solid organ sites

④ C85 Other specified and unspecified types of non-Hodgkin lymphoma

EXCLUDES 1 other specified types of T/NK-cell lymphoma (C86.-)
personal history of non-Hodgkin lymphoma (Z85.72)

⑤ C85.1 Unspecified B-cell lymphoma

Note:

If B-cell lineage or involvement is mentioned in conjunction with a specific lymphoma, code to the more specific description.

SP C85.10 Unspecified B-cell lymphoma, unspecified site

SP C85.11 Unspecified B-cell lymphoma, lymph nodes of head, face, and neck

SP C85.12 Unspecified B-cell lymphoma, intrathoracic lymph nodes

SP C85.13 Unspecified B-cell lymphoma, intra-abdominal lymph nodes

SP C85.14 Unspecified B-cell lymphoma, lymph nodes of axilla and upper limb

SP C85.15 Unspecified B-cell lymphoma, lymph nodes of inguinal region and lower limb

SP C85.16 Unspecified B-cell lymphoma, intrapelvic lymph nodes

SP C85.17 Unspecified B-cell lymphoma, spleen

SP C85.18 Unspecified B-cell lymphoma, lymph nodes of multiple sites

SP C85.19 Unspecified B-cell lymphoma, extranodal and solid organ sites

⑤ C85.2 Mediastinal (thymic) large B-cell lymphoma

SP C85.20 Mediastinal (thymic) large B-cell lymphoma, unspecified site

SP C85.21 Mediastinal (thymic) large B-cell lymphoma, lymph nodes of head, face, and neck

SP C85.22 Mediastinal (thymic) large B-cell lymphoma, intrathoracic lymph nodes

SP C85.23 Mediastinal (thymic) large B-cell lymphoma, intra-abdominal lymph nodes

SP C85.24 Mediastinal (thymic) large B-cell lymphoma, lymph nodes of axilla and upper limb

SP C85.25 Mediastinal (thymic) large B-cell lymphoma, lymph nodes of inguinal region and lower limb

SP C85.26 Mediastinal (thymic) large B-cell lymphoma, intrapelvic lymph nodes

SP C85.27 Mediastinal (thymic) large B-cell lymphoma, spleen

SP C85.28 Mediastinal (thymic) large B-cell lymphoma, lymph nodes of multiple sites

SP C85.29 Mediastinal (thymic) large B-cell lymphoma, extranodal and solid organ sites

⑤ C85.8 Other specified types of non-Hodgkin lymphoma

SP C85.80 Other specified types of non-Hodgkin lymphoma, unspecified site

SP C85.81 Other specified types of non-Hodgkin lymphoma, lymph nodes of head, face, and neck

SP C85.82 Other specified types of non-Hodgkin lymphoma, intrathoracic lymph nodes

SP C85.83 Other specified types of non-Hodgkin lymphoma, intra-abdominal lymph nodes

SP C85.84 Other specified types of non-Hodgkin lymphoma, lymph nodes of axilla and upper limb

SP C85.85 Other specified types of non-Hodgkin lymphoma, lymph nodes of inguinal region and lower limb

SP C85.86 Other specified types of non-Hodgkin lymphoma, intrapelvic lymph nodes

SP C85.87 Other specified types of non-Hodgkin lymphoma, spleen

SP C85.88 Other specified types of non-Hodgkin lymphoma, lymph nodes of multiple sites

SP C85.89 Other specified types of non-Hodgkin lymphoma, extranodal and solid organ sites

⑤ C85.9 Non-Hodgkin lymphoma, unspecified

★ New ▲ Revised Px Primary **SP** PDGM Px **SL** Low CoM **SH** High CoM **IQ** Quest. Encounter ⊞ Hospice non-cancer Dx Unspecified **M** *Manifestation*

Lymphoma NOS
Malignant lymphoma NOS
Non-Hodgkin lymphoma NOS

SP C85.90 **Non-Hodgkin lymphoma, unspecified, unspecified site**

SP C85.91 **Non-Hodgkin lymphoma, unspecified, lymph nodes of head, face, and neck**

SP C85.92 **Non-Hodgkin lymphoma, unspecified, intrathoracic lymph nodes**

SP C85.93 **Non-Hodgkin lymphoma, unspecified, intra-abdominal lymph nodes**

SP C85.94 **Non-Hodgkin lymphoma, unspecified, lymph nodes of axilla and upper limb**

SP C85.95 **Non-Hodgkin lymphoma, unspecified, lymph nodes of inguinal region and lower limb**

SP C85.96 **Non-Hodgkin lymphoma, unspecified, intrapelvic lymph nodes**

SP C85.97 **Non-Hodgkin lymphoma, unspecified, spleen**

SP C85.98 **Non-Hodgkin lymphoma, unspecified, lymph nodes of multiple sites**

SP C85.99 **Non-Hodgkin lymphoma, unspecified, extranodal and solid organ sites**

4 C86 **Other specified types of T/NK-cell lymphoma**
> EXCLUDES 1   anaplastic large cell lymphoma, ALK negative (C84.7-)
> anaplastic large cell lymphoma, ALK positive (C84.6-)
> mature T/NK-cell lymphomas (C84.-)
> other specified types of non-Hodgkin lymphoma (C85.8-)

SP C86.0 **Extranodal NK/T-cell lymphoma, nasal type**

SP C86.1 **Hepatosplenic T-cell lymphoma**
Alpha-beta and gamma delta types

SP C86.2 **Enteropathy-type (intestinal) T-cell lymphoma**
Enteropathy associated T-cell lymphoma

SP C86.3 **Subcutaneous panniculitis-like T-cell lymphoma**

SP C86.4 **Blastic NK-cell lymphoma**
Blastic plasmacytoid dendritic cell neoplasm (BPDCN)

SP C86.5 **Angioimmunoblastic T-cell lymphoma**
Angioimmunoblastic lymphadenopathy with dysproteinemia (AILD)

SP C86.6 **Primary cutaneous CD30-positive T-cell proliferations**
Lymphomatoid papulosis
Primary cutaneous anaplastic large cell lymphoma
Primary cutaneous CD30-positive large T-cell lymphoma

4 C88 **Malignant immunoproliferative diseases and certain other B-cell lymphomas**
> EXCLUDES 1   B-cell lymphoma, unspecified (C85.1-)

personal history of other malignant neoplasms of lymphoid, hematopoietic and related tissues (Z85.79)

SP C88.0 **Waldenström macroglobulinemia**
Lymphoplasmacytic lymphoma with IgM-production
Macroglobulinemia (idiopathic) (primary)
> EXCLUDES 1   small cell B-cell lymphoma (C83.0)

SP C88.2 **Heavy chain disease**
Franklin disease
Gamma heavy chain disease
Mu heavy chain disease

SP C88.3 **Immunoproliferative small intestinal disease**
Alpha heavy chain disease
Mediterranean lymphoma

SP C88.4 **Extranodal marginal zone B-cell lymphoma of mucosa-associated lymphoid tissue [MALT-lymphoma]**
Lymphoma of skin-associated lymphoid tissue [SALT-lymphoma]
Lymphoma of bronchial-associated lymphoid tissue [BALT-lymphoma]
> EXCLUDES 1   high malignant (diffuse large B-cell) lymphoma (C83.3-)

SP C88.8 **Other malignant immunoproliferative diseases**

SP C88.9 **Malignant immunoproliferative disease, unspecified**
Immunoproliferative disease NOS

4 C90 **Multiple myeloma and malignant plasma cell neoplasms**
> EXCLUDES 1   personal history of other malignant neoplasms of lymphoid, hematopoietic and related tissues (Z85.79)

> GUIDELINES   Section I.C.2.n
> The categories for leukemia [C91 - C95], and category C90, Multiple myeloma and malignant plasma cell neoplasms, have codes indicating whether or not the leukemia has achieved remission. There are also codes Z85.6, Personal history of leukemia, and Z85.79, Personal history of other malignant neoplasms of lymphoid, hematopoietic and related tissues. If the documentation is unclear, as to whether the leukemia has achieved remission, the provider should be queried.

> CODING TIPS ✓   Terms such as "in remission" and "in relapse" must be specified by the physician in order to indicate assignment of a code specifying these terms. If the physician has not specified one of these terms, select the code for "not having achieved remission."

5 C90.0 **Multiple myeloma**
Kahler's disease
Medullary plasmacytoma
Myelomatosis
Plasma cell myeloma
> EXCLUDES 1   solitary myeloma (C90.3-)
> solitary plasmactyoma (C90.3-)

SP C90.00 **Multiple myeloma not having achieved remission**

---

4 4th digit required   **5** 5th digit required   **6** 6th digit required   **7** 7th digit required   **7** 7th digit placeholder   ✚ Additional code   ▣ Laterality

676   *DecisionHealth's* FY 2020 Complete Home Health ICD-10-CM Diagnosis Coding Manual

Chapter 2

C00-D49

Multiple myeloma with failed remission

Multiple myeloma NOS

SP C90.01 **Multiple myeloma in remission**

SP C90.02 **Multiple myeloma in relapse**

5 C90.1 **Plasma cell leukemia**

Plasmacytic leukemia

SP C90.10 **Plasma cell leukemia not having achieved remission**

Plasma cell leukemia with failed remission

Plasma cell leukemia NOS

SP C90.11 **Plasma cell leukemia in remission**

SP C90.12 **Plasma cell leukemia in relapse**

5 C90.2 **Extramedullary plasmacytoma**

SP C90.20 **Extramedullary plasmacytoma not having achieved remission**

Extramedullary plasmacytoma with failed remission

Extramedullary plasmacytoma NOS

SP C90.21 **Extramedullary plasmacytoma in remission**

SP C90.22 **Extramedullary plasmacytoma in relapse**

5 C90.3 **Solitary plasmacytoma**

Localized malignant plasma cell tumor NOS

Plasmacytoma NOS

Solitary myeloma

SP C90.30 **Solitary plasmacytoma not having achieved remission**

Solitary plasmacytoma with failed remission

Solitary plasmacytoma NOS

SP C90.31 **Solitary plasmacytoma in remission**

SP C90.32 **Solitary plasmacytoma in relapse**

4 C91 **Lymphoid leukemia**

EXCLUDES 1 personal history of leukemia (Z85.6)

CODING TIPS ✓ Terms such as "in remission" and "in relapse" must be specified by the physician in order to indicate assignment of a code specifying these terms. If the physician has not specified one of these terms, select the code for "not having achieved remission."

▲ 5 C91.0 **Acute lymphoblastic leukemia [ALL]**

Note:

Codes in subcategory C91.0- should only be used for T-cell and B-cell precursor leukemia

SP C91.00 **Acute lymphoblastic leukemia not having achieved remission**

Acute lymphoblastic leukemia with failed remission

Acute lymphoblastic leukemia NOS

SP C91.01 **Acute lymphoblastic leukemia, in remission**

SP C91.02 **Acute lymphoblastic leukemia, in relapse**

5 C91.1 **Chronic lymphocytic leukemia of B-cell type**

Lymphoplasmacytic leukemia

Richter syndrome

EXCLUDES 1 lymphoplasmacytic lymphoma (C83.0-)

SP C91.10 **Chronic lymphocytic leukemia of B-cell type not having achieved remission**

Chronic lymphocytic leukemia of B-cell type with failed remission

Chronic lymphocytic leukemia of B-cell type NOS

SP C91.11 **Chronic lymphocytic leukemia of B-cell type in remission**

SP C91.12 **Chronic lymphocytic leukemia of B-cell type in relapse**

5 C91.3 **Prolymphocytic leukemia of B-cell type**

SP C91.30 **Prolymphocytic leukemia of B-cell type not having achieved remission**

Prolymphocytic leukemia of B-cell type with failed remission

Prolymphocytic leukemia of B-cell type NOS

SP C91.31 **Prolymphocytic leukemia of B-cell type, in remission**

SP C91.32 **Prolymphocytic leukemia of B-cell type, in relapse**

5 C91.4 **Hairy cell leukemia**

Leukemic reticuloendotheliosis

SP C91.40 **Hairy cell leukemia not having achieved remission**

Hairy cell leukemia with failed remission

Hairy cell leukemia NOS

SP C91.41 **Hairy cell leukemia, in remission**

SP C91.42 **Hairy cell leukemia, in relapse**

5 C91.5 **Adult T-cell lymphoma/leukemia (HTLV-1-associated)**

Acute variant of adult T-cell lymphoma/leukemia (HTLV-1-associated)

Chronic variant of adult T-cell lymphoma/leukemia (HTLV-1-associated)

Lymphomatoid variant of adult T-cell lymphoma/leukemia (HTLV-1-associated)

Smouldering variant of adult T-cell lymphoma/leukemia (HTLV-1-associated)

SP C91.50 **Adult T-cell lymphoma/leukemia (HTLV-1-associated) not having achieved remission**

Adult T-cell lymphoma/leukemia (HTLV-1-associated) with failed remission

Adult T-cell lymphoma/leukemia (HTLV-1-associated) NOS

SP C91.51 **Adult T-cell lymphoma/leukemia (HTLV-1-associated), in remission**

SP C91.52 **Adult T-cell lymphoma/leukemia (HTLV-1-associated), in relapse**

5 C91.6 **Prolymphocytic leukemia of T-cell type**

SP C91.60 **Prolymphocytic leukemia of T-cell type not having achieved remission**

Prolymphocytic leukemia of T-cell type with failed remission

Prolymphocytic leukemia of T-cell type NOS

SP C91.61 **Prolymphocytic leukemia of T-cell type, in remission**

SP C91.62 **Prolymphocytic leukemia of T-cell type, in relapse**

★ New ▲ Revised Px Primary **SP** PDGM Px **SL** Low CoM **SH** High CoM **IQ** Quest. Encounter **H** Hospice non-cancer Dx Unspecified **M** *Manifestation*

DecisionHealth's FY 2020 Complete Home Health ICD-10-CM Diagnosis Coding Manual

677

⑤ **C91.A Mature B-cell leukemia Burkitt-type**
> EXCLUDES 1   Burkitt lymphoma (C83.7-)

SP **C91.A0 Mature B-cell leukemia Burkitt-type not having achieved remission**
Mature B-cell leukemia Burkitt-type with failed remission
Mature B-cell leukemia Burkitt-type NOS

SP **C91.A1 Mature B-cell leukemia Burkitt-type, in remission**

SP **C91.A2 Mature B-cell leukemia Burkitt-type, in relapse**

⑤ **C91.Z Other lymphoid leukemia**
T-cell large granular lymphocytic leukemia (associated with rheumatoid arthritis)

SP **C91.Z0 Other lymphoid leukemia not having achieved remission**
Other lymphoid leukemia with failed remission
Other lymphoid leukemia NOS

SP **C91.Z1 Other lymphoid leukemia, in remission**

SP **C91.Z2 Other lymphoid leukemia, in relapse**

⑤ **C91.9 Lymphoid leukemia, unspecified**

SP **C91.90 Lymphoid leukemia, unspecified not having achieved remission**
Lymphoid leukemia with failed remission
Lymphoid leukemia NOS

SP **C91.91 Lymphoid leukemia, unspecified, in remission**

SP **C91.92 Lymphoid leukemia, unspecified, in relapse**

④ **C92   Myeloid leukemia**
> INCLUDES   granulocytic leukemia
> myelogenous leukemia
> EXCLUDES 1   personal history of leukemia (Z85.6)

> CODING TIPS ✓   Coding these types of cancers in remission or in relapse must be based on physician documentation or query. Query the physician to differentiate between leukemia in remission and history of leukemia. History of leukemia is coded to Z85.6. Treatment is different for a patient who has never achieved remission vs. a patient who has achieved remission and then relapsed.

⑤ **C92.0 Acute myeloblastic leukemia**
Acute myeloblastic leukemia, minimal differentiation
Acute myeloblastic leukemia (with maturation)
Acute myeloblastic leukemia 1/ETO
Acute myeloblastic leukemia M0
Acute myeloblastic leukemia M1
Acute myeloblastic leukemia M2
Acute myeloblastic leukemia with t(8;21)
Acute myeloblastic leukemia (without a FAB classification) NOS
Refractory anemia with excess blasts in transformation [RAEB T]
> EXCLUDES 1   acute exacerbation of chronic myeloid leukemia (C92.10)
> refractory anemia with excess of blasts not in transformation (D46.2-)

SP **C92.00 Acute myeloblastic leukemia, not having achieved remission**
Acute myeloblastic leukemia with failed remission
Acute myeloblastic leukemia NOS

SP **C92.01 Acute myeloblastic leukemia, in remission**

SP **C92.02 Acute myeloblastic leukemia, in relapse**

⑤ **C92.1 Chronic myeloid leukemia, BCR/ABL-positive**
Chronic myelogenous leukemia, Philadelphia chromosome (Ph1) positive
Chronic myelogenous leukemia, t(9;22) (q34;q11)
Chronic myelogenous leukemia with crisis of blast cells
> EXCLUDES 1   atypical chronic myeloid leukemia BCR/ABL-negative (C92.2-)
> chronic myelomonocytic leukemia (C93.1-)
> chronic myeloproliferative disease (D47.1)

SP **C92.10 Chronic myeloid leukemia, BCR/ABL-positive, not having achieved remission**
Chronic myeloid leukemia, BCR/ABL-positive with failed remission
Chronic myeloid leukemia, BCR/ABL-positive NOS

SP **C92.11 Chronic myeloid leukemia, BCR/ABL-positive, in remission**

SP **C92.12 Chronic myeloid leukemia, BCR/ABL-positive, in relapse**

⑤ **C92.2 Atypical chronic myeloid leukemia, BCR/ABL-negative**

SP **C92.20 Atypical chronic myeloid leukemia, BCR/ABL-negative, not having achieved remission**
Atypical chronic myeloid leukemia, BCR/ABL-negative with failed remission
Atypical chronic myeloid leukemia, BCR/ABL-negative NOS

SP **C92.21 Atypical chronic myeloid leukemia, BCR/ABL-negative, in remission**

SP **C92.22 Atypical chronic myeloid leukemia, BCR/ABL-negative, in relapse**

⑤ **C92.3 Myeloid sarcoma**
A malignant tumor of immature myeloid cells
Chloroma
Granulocytic sarcoma

SP **C92.30 Myeloid sarcoma, not having achieved remission**
Myeloid sarcoma with failed remission
Myeloid sarcoma NOS

SP **C92.31 Myeloid sarcoma, in remission**

SP **C92.32 Myeloid sarcoma, in relapse**

⑤ **C92.4 Acute promyelocytic leukemia**
AML M3
AML Me with t(15;17) and variants

SP **C92.40 Acute promyelocytic leukemia, not having achieved remission**
Acute promyelocytic leukemia with failed remission
Acute promyelocytic leukemia NOS

---

④ 4th digit required   ⑤ 5th digit required   ⑥ 6th digit required   ⑦ 7th digit required   ⑦ 7th digit placeholder   ✚ Additional code   ⧉ Laterality

678   DecisionHealth's FY 2020 Complete Home Health ICD-10-CM Diagnosis Coding Manual

Chapter 2

C00-D49

SP C92.41 **Acute promyelocytic leukemia, in remission**

SP C92.42 **Acute promyelocytic leukemia, in relapse**

5 C92.5 **Acute myelomonocytic leukemia**
AML M4
AML M4 Eo with inv(16) or t(16;16)

SP C92.50 **Acute myelomonocytic leukemia, not having achieved remission**
Acute myelomonocytic leukemia with failed remission
Acute myelomonocytic leukemia NOS

SP C92.51 **Acute myelomonocytic leukemia, in remission**

SP C92.52 **Acute myelomonocytic leukemia, in relapse**

5 C92.6 **Acute myeloid leukemia with 11q23-abnormality**
Acute myeloid leukemia with variation of MLL-gene

SP C92.60 **Acute myeloid leukemia with 11q23-abnormality not having achieved remission**
Acute myeloid leukemia with 11q23-abnormality with failed remission
Acute myeloid leukemia with 11q23-abnormality NOS

SP C92.61 **Acute myeloid leukemia with 11q23-abnormality in remission**

SP C92.62 **Acute myeloid leukemia with 11q23-abnormality in relapse**

5 C92.A **Acute myeloid leukemia with multilineage dysplasia**
Acute myeloid leukemia with dysplasia of remaining hematopoesis and/or myelodysplastic disease in its history

SP C92.A0 **Acute myeloid leukemia with multilineage dysplasia, not having achieved remission**
Acute myeloid leukemia with multilineage dysplasia with failed remission
Acute myeloid leukemia with multilineage dysplasia NOS

SP C92.A1 **Acute myeloid leukemia with multilineage dysplasia, in remission**

SP C92.A2 **Acute myeloid leukemia with multilineage dysplasia, in relapse**

5 C92.Z **Other myeloid leukemia**

SP C92.Z0 **Other myeloid leukemia not having achieved remission**
Myeloid leukemia NEC with failed remission
Myeloid leukemia NEC

SP C92.Z1 **Other myeloid leukemia, in remission**

SP C92.Z2 **Other myeloid leukemia, in relapse**

5 C92.9 **Myeloid leukemia, unspecified**

SP C92.90 **Myeloid leukemia, unspecified, not having achieved remission**
Myeloid leukemia, unspecified with failed remission
Myeloid leukemia, unspecified NOS

SP C92.91 **Myeloid leukemia, unspecified in remission**

SP C92.92 **Myeloid leukemia, unspecified in relapse**

4 C93 **Monocytic leukemia**
INCLUDES   monocytoid leukemia
EXCLUDES 1   personal history of leukemia (Z85.6)

CODING TIPS ✓   Coding these types of cancers in remission or in relapse must be based on physician documentation or query. Query the physician to differentiate between leukemia in remission and history of leukemia. History of leukemia is coded to Z85.6. Treatment is different for a patient who has never achieved remission vs. a patient who has achieved remission and then relapsed.

5 C93.0 **Acute monoblastic/monocytic leukemia**
AML M5
AML M5a
AML M5b

SP C93.00 **Acute monoblastic/monocytic leukemia, not having achieved remission**
Acute monoblastic/monocytic leukemia with failed remission
Acute monoblastic/monocytic leukemia NOS

SP C93.01 **Acute monoblastic/monocytic leukemia, in remission**

SP C93.02 **Acute monoblastic/monocytic leukemia, in relapse**

5 C93.1 **Chronic myelomonocytic leukemia**
Chronic monocytic leukemia
CMML-1
CMML-2
CMML with eosinophilia

SP C93.10 **Chronic myelomonocytic leukemia not having achieved remission**
Chronic myelomonocytic leukemia with failed remission
Chronic myelomonocytic leukemia NOS

SP C93.11 **Chronic myelomonocytic leukemia, in remission**

SP C93.12 **Chronic myelomonocytic leukemia, in relapse**

5 C93.3 **Juvenile myelomonocytic leukemia**

SP C93.30 **Juvenile myelomonocytic leukemia, not having achieved remission**
Juvenile myelomonocytic leukemia with failed remission
Juvenile myelomonocytic leukemia NOS

SP C93.31 **Juvenile myelomonocytic leukemia, in remission**

SP C93.32 **Juvenile myelomonocytic leukemia, in relapse**

5 C93.Z **Other monocytic leukemia**

SP C93.Z0 **Other monocytic leukemia, not having achieved remission**
Other monocytic leukemia NOS

SP C93.Z1 **Other monocytic leukemia, in remission**

SP C93.Z2 **Other monocytic leukemia, in relapse**

5 C93.9 **Monocytic leukemia, unspecified**

SP C93.90 **Monocytic leukemia, unspecified, not having achieved remission**
Monocytic leukemia, unspecified with failed remission

★ New ▲ Revised Px Primary SP PDGM Px SL Low CoM SH High CoM IQ Quest. Encounter H Hospice non-cancer Dx Unspecified M *Manifestation*

Monocytic leukemia, unspecified NOS

SP **C93.91** **Monocytic leukemia, unspecified in remission**

SP **C93.92** **Monocytic leukemia, unspecified in relapse**

4 **C94** **Other leukemias of specified cell type**

> **EXCLUDES 1** leukemic reticuloendotheliosis (C91.4-)
> myelodysplastic syndromes (D46.-)
> personal history of leukemia (Z85.6)
> plasma cell leukemia (C90.1-)

> **CODING TIPS** ✓ Coding these types of cancers in remission or in relapse must be based on physician documentation or query. Query the physician to differentiate between leukemia in remission and history of leukemia. History of leukemia is coded to Z85.6. Treatment is different for a patient who has never achieved remission vs. a patient who has achieved remission and then relapsed.

5 **C94.0** **Acute erythroid leukemia**
Acute myeloid leukemia M6(a)(b)
Erythroleukemia

SP **C94.00** **Acute erythroid leukemia, not having achieved remission**
Acute erythroid leukemia with failed remission
Acute erythroid leukemia NOS

SP **C94.01** **Acute erythroid leukemia, in remission**

SP **C94.02** **Acute erythroid leukemia, in relapse**

5 **C94.2** **Acute megakaryoblastic leukemia**
Acute myeloid leukemia M7
Acute megakaryocytic leukemia

SP **C94.20** **Acute megakaryoblastic leukemia not having achieved remission**
Acute megakaryoblastic leukemia with failed remission
Acute megakaryoblastic leukemia NOS

SP **C94.21** **Acute megakaryoblastic leukemia, in remission**

SP **C94.22** **Acute megakaryoblastic leukemia, in relapse**

5 **C94.3** **Mast cell leukemia**

SP **C94.30** **Mast cell leukemia not having achieved remission**
Mast cell leukemia with failed remission
Mast cell leukemia NOS

SP **C94.31** **Mast cell leukemia, in remission**

SP **C94.32** **Mast cell leukemia, in relapse**

5 **C94.4** **Acute panmyelosis with myelofibrosis**
Acute myelofibrosis

> **EXCLUDES 1** myelofibrosis NOS (D75.81)
> secondary myelofibrosis NOS (D75.81)

SP **C94.40** **Acute panmyelosis with myelofibrosis not having achieved remission**
Acute myelofibrosis NOS
Acute panmyelosis with myelofibrosis with failed remission
Acute panmyelosis NOS

SP **C94.41** **Acute panmyelosis with myelofibrosis, in remission**

SP **C94.42** **Acute panmyelosis with myelofibrosis, in relapse**

SP **C94.6** **Myelodysplastic disease, not classified**
Myeloproliferative disease, not classified

5 **C94.8** **Other specified leukemias**
Aggressive NK-cell leukemia
Acute basophilic leukemia

SP **C94.80** **Other specified leukemias not having achieved remission**
Other specified leukemia with failed remission
Other specified leukemias NOS

SP **C94.81** **Other specified leukemias, in remission**

SP **C94.82** **Other specified leukemias, in relapse**

4 **C95** **Leukemia of unspecified cell type**

> **EXCLUDES 1** personal history of leukemia (Z85.6)

> **CODING TIPS** ✓ Coding these types of cancers in remission or in relapse must be based on physician documentation or query. Query the physician to differentiate between leukemia in remission and history of leukemia. History of leukemia is coded to Z85.6. Treatment is different for a patient who has never achieved remission vs. a patient who has achieved remission and then relapsed.

5 **C95.0** **Acute leukemia of unspecified cell type**
Acute bilineal leukemia
Acute mixed lineage leukemia
Biphenotypic acute leukemia
Stem cell leukemia of unclear lineage

> **EXCLUDES 1** acute exacerbation of unspecified chronic leukemia (C95.10)

SP **C95.00** **Acute leukemia of unspecified cell type not having achieved remission**
Acute leukemia of unspecified cell type with failed remission
Acute leukemia NOS

SP **C95.01** **Acute leukemia of unspecified cell type, in remission**

SP **C95.02** **Acute leukemia of unspecified cell type, in relapse**

5 **C95.1** **Chronic leukemia of unspecified cell type**

SP **C95.10** **Chronic leukemia of unspecified cell type not having achieved remission**
Chronic leukemia of unspecified cell type with failed remission
Chronic leukemia NOS

SP **C95.11** **Chronic leukemia of unspecified cell type, in remission**

SP **C95.12** **Chronic leukemia of unspecified cell type, in relapse**

5 **C95.9** **Leukemia, unspecified**

SP **C95.90** **Leukemia, unspecified not having achieved remission**
Leukemia, unspecified with failed remission
Leukemia NOS

SP **C95.91** **Leukemia, unspecified, in remission**

SP **C95.92** **Leukemia, unspecified, in relapse**

---

4 4th digit required   **5** 5th digit required   **6** 6th digit required   **7** 7th digit required   ☑ 7th digit placeholder   ✚ Additional code   ⊟ Laterality

680   *DecisionHealth's* FY 2020 Complete Home Health ICD-10-CM Diagnosis Coding Manual

4 C96 Other and unspecified malignant neoplasms of lymphoid, hematopoietic and related tissue

> EXCLUDES 1   personal history of other malignant neoplasms of lymphoid, hematopoietic and related tissues (Z85.79)

SP C96.0 Multifocal and multisystemic (disseminated) Langerhans-cell histiocytosis
Histiocytosis X, multisystemic
Letterer-Siwe disease

> EXCLUDES 1   adult pulmonary Langerhans cell histiocytosis (J84.82)
> multifocal and unisystemic Langerhans-cell histiocytosis (C96.5)
> unifocal Langerhans-cell histiocytosis (C96.6)

5 C96.2 Malignant mast cell neoplasm

> EXCLUDES 1   indolent mastocytosis (D47.02)
> mast cell leukemia (C94.30)
> mastocytosis (congenital) (cutaneous) (Q82.2)

SP C96.20 Malignant mast cell neoplasm, unspecified

SP C96.21 Aggressive systemic mastocytosis

SP C96.22 Mast cell sarcoma

SP C96.29 Other malignant mast cell neoplasm

SP C96.4 Sarcoma of dendritic cells (accessory cells)
Follicular dendritic cell sarcoma
Interdigitating dendritic cell sarcoma
Langerhans cell sarcoma

SP C96.5 Multifocal and unisystemic Langerhans-cell histiocytosis
Hand-Schüller-Christian disease
Histiocytosis X, multifocal

> EXCLUDES 1   multifocal and multisystemic (disseminated) Langerhans-cell histiocytosis (C96.0)
> unifocal Langerhans-cell histiocytosis (C96.6)

SP C96.6 Unifocal Langerhans-cell histiocytosis
Eosinophilic granuloma
Histiocytosis X, unifocal
Histiocytosis X NOS
Langerhans-cell histiocytosis NOS

> EXCLUDES 1   multifocal and multisysemic (disseminated) Langerhans-cell histiocytosis (C96.0)
> multifocal and unisystemic Langerhans-cell histiocytosis (C96.5)

SP C96.A Histiocytic sarcoma
Malignant histiocytosis

SP C96.Z Other specified malignant neoplasms of lymphoid, hematopoietic and related tissue

SP C96.9 Malignant neoplasm of lymphoid, hematopoietic and related tissue, unspecified

In situ neoplasms (D00-D09)

> INCLUDES   Bowen's disease
> erythroplasia
> grade III intraepithelial neoplasia
> Queyrat's erythroplasia

> CODING TIPS ✓   Carcinomas in situ are defined as cancer that has stayed in place in the specific location of origin and not spread or invaded any neighboring tissue. The physician must state "in situ" or pre-cancerous/pre-malignant lesion in order to indicate the correct assignment of any D00-D09 codes.

4 D00 Carcinoma in situ of oral cavity, esophagus and stomach

> EXCLUDES 1   melanoma in situ (D03.-)

+ 5 D00.0 Carcinoma in situ of lip, oral cavity and pharynx
Use additional code to identify:
  exposure to environmental tobacco smoke (Z77.22)
  exposure to tobacco smoke in the perinatal period (P96.81)
  history of tobacco dependence (Z87.891)
  occupational exposure to environmental tobacco smoke (Z57.31)
  tobacco dependence (F17.-)
  tobacco use (Z72.0)

> EXCLUDES 1   carcinoma in situ of aryepiglottic fold or interarytenoid fold, laryngeal aspect (D02.0)
> carcinoma in situ of epiglottis NOS (D02.0)
> carcinoma in situ of epiglottis suprahyoid portion (D02.0)
> carcinoma in situ of skin of lip (D03.0, D04.0)

IQ + D00.00 Carcinoma in situ of oral cavity, unspecified site

SP + D00.01 Carcinoma in situ of labial mucosa and vermilion border

SP + D00.02 Carcinoma in situ of buccal mucosa

SP + D00.03 Carcinoma in situ of gingiva and edentulous alveolar ridge

SP + D00.04 Carcinoma in situ of soft palate

SP + D00.05 Carcinoma in situ of hard palate

SP + D00.06 Carcinoma in situ of floor of mouth

SP + D00.07 Carcinoma in situ of tongue

SP + D00.08 Carcinoma in situ of pharynx
Carcinoma in situ of aryepiglottic fold NOS
Carcinoma in situ of hypopharyngeal aspect of aryepiglottic fold
Carcinoma in situ of marginal zone of aryepiglottic fold

SP D00.1 Carcinoma in situ of esophagus

SP D00.2 Carcinoma in situ of stomach

4 D01 Carcinoma in situ of other and unspecified digestive organs

> EXCLUDES 1   melanoma in situ (D03.-)

SP D01.0 Carcinoma in situ of colon

> EXCLUDES 1   carcinoma in situ of rectosigmoid junction (D01.1)

SP D01.1 Carcinoma in situ of rectosigmoid junction

★ New ▲ Revised   Px Primary   SP PDGM Px   SL Low CoM   SH High CoM   IQ Quest. Encounter   H Hospice non-cancer Dx   Unspecified   M Manifestation

DecisionHealth's FY 2020 Complete Home Health ICD-10-CM Diagnosis Coding Manual   681

Chapter 2

C00-D49

Chapter 2

C00-D49

SP **D01.2** Carcinoma in situ of rectum

SP **D01.3** Carcinoma in situ of anus and anal canal
Anal intraepithelial neoplasia III [AIN III]
Severe dysplasia of anus
> **EXCLUDES 1** anal intraepithelial neoplasia I and II [AIN I and AIN II] (K62.82)
> carcinoma in situ of anal margin (D04.5)
> carcinoma in situ of anal skin (D04.5)
> carcinoma in situ of perianal skin (D04.5)

5 **D01.4** Carcinoma in situ of other and unspecified parts of intestine
> **EXCLUDES 1** carcinoma in situ of ampulla of Vater (D01.5)

IQ **D01.40** Carcinoma in situ of unspecified part of intestine

SP **D01.49** Carcinoma in situ of other parts of intestine

SP **D01.5** Carcinoma in situ of liver, gallbladder and bile ducts
Carcinoma in situ of ampulla of Vater

SP **D01.7** Carcinoma in situ of other specified digestive organs
Carcinoma in situ of pancreas

IQ **D01.9** Carcinoma in situ of digestive organ, unspecified

+ **4** **D02** Carcinoma in situ of middle ear and respiratory system
Use additional code to identify:
exposure to environmental tobacco smoke (Z77.22)
exposure to tobacco smoke in the perinatal period (P96.81)
history of tobacco dependence (Z87.891)
occupational exposure to environmental tobacco smoke (Z57.31)
tobacco dependence (F17.-)
tobacco use (Z72.0)
> **EXCLUDES 1** melanoma in situ (D03.-)

SP **+** **D02.0** Carcinoma in situ of larynx
Carcinoma in situ of aryepiglottic fold or interarytenoid fold, laryngeal aspect
Carcinoma in situ of epiglottis (suprahyoid portion)
> **EXCLUDES 1** carcinoma in situ of aryepiglottic fold or interarytenoid fold NOS (D00.08)
> carcinoma in situ of hypopharyngeal aspect (D00.08)
> carcinoma in situ of marginal zone (D00.08)

SP **+** **D02.1** Carcinoma in situ of trachea

+ **5** **D02.2** Carcinoma in situ of bronchus and lung

≡ **IQ** **+** **D02.20** Carcinoma in situ of unspecified bronchus and lung

≡ **SP** **+** **D02.21** Carcinoma in situ of right bronchus and lung

≡ **SP** **+** **D02.22** Carcinoma in situ of left bronchus and lung

SP **+** **D02.3** Carcinoma in situ of other parts of respiratory system

Carcinoma in situ of accessory sinuses
Carcinoma in situ of middle ear
Carcinoma in situ of nasal cavities
> **EXCLUDES 1** carcinoma in situ of ear (external) (skin) (D04.2-)
> carcinoma in situ of nose NOS D09.8
> carcinoma in situ of skin of nose (D04.3)

IQ **+** **D02.4** Carcinoma in situ of respiratory system, unspecified

4 **D03** Melanoma in situ

SP **D03.0** Melanoma in situ of lip

5 **D03.1** Melanoma in situ of eyelid, including canthus

≡ **IQ** **D03.10** Melanoma in situ of unspecified eyelid, including canthus

6 **D03.11** Melanoma in situ of right eyelid, including canthus

≡ **SP** **D03.111** Melanoma in situ of right upper eyelid, including canthus

≡ **SP** **D03.112** Melanoma in situ of right lower eyelid, including canthus

6 **D03.12** Melanoma in situ of left eyelid, including canthus

≡ **SP** **D03.121** Melanoma in situ of left upper eyelid, including canthus

≡ **SP** **D03.122** Melanoma in situ of left lower eyelid, including canthus

5 **D03.2** Melanoma in situ of ear and external auricular canal

≡ **IQ** **D03.20** Melanoma in situ of unspecified ear and external auricular canal

≡ **SP** **D03.21** Melanoma in situ of right ear and external auricular canal

≡ **SP** **D03.22** Melanoma in situ of left ear and external auricular canal

5 **D03.3** Melanoma in situ of other and unspecified parts of face

IQ **D03.30** Melanoma in situ of unspecified part of face

SP **D03.39** Melanoma in situ of other parts of face

SP **D03.4** Melanoma in situ of scalp and neck

5 **D03.5** Melanoma in situ of trunk

SP **D03.51** Melanoma in situ of anal skin
Melanoma in situ of anal margin
Melanoma in situ of perianal skin

SP **D03.52** Melanoma in situ of breast (skin) (soft tissue)

SP **D03.59** Melanoma in situ of other part of trunk

5 **D03.6** Melanoma in situ of upper limb, including shoulder

≡ **IQ** **D03.60** Melanoma in situ of unspecified upper limb, including shoulder

≡ **SP** **D03.61** Melanoma in situ of right upper limb, including shoulder

≡ **SP** **D03.62** Melanoma in situ of left upper limb, including shoulder

5 **D03.7** Melanoma in situ of lower limb, including hip

≡ **IQ** **D03.70** Melanoma in situ of unspecified lower limb, including hip

≡ **SP** **D03.71** Melanoma in situ of right lower limb, including hip

---

4 4th digit required   **5** 5th digit required   **6** 6th digit required   **7** 7th digit required   **7** 7th digit placeholder   **+** Additional code   **≡** Laterality

⊟ SP **D03.72** **Melanoma in situ of left lower limb, including hip**

SP **D03.8** **Melanoma in situ of other sites**
   Melanoma in situ of scrotum
   > **EXCLUDES 1** carcinoma in situ of scrotum (D07.61)

IQ **D03.9** Melanoma in situ, unspecified

④ **D04** **Carcinoma in situ of skin**
   > **EXCLUDES 1** erythroplasia of Queyrat (penis) NOS (D07.4)
   > melanoma in situ (D03.-)

▲ SP **D04.0** **Carcinoma in situ of skin of lip**
   > **EXCLUDES 2** carcinoma in situ of vermilion border of lip (D00.01)

⑤ **D04.1** **Carcinoma in situ of skin of eyelid, including canthus**

⊟ IQ **D04.10** Carcinoma in situ of skin of unspecified eyelid, including canthus

⑥ **D04.11** **Carcinoma in situ of skin of right eyelid, including canthus**

⊟ SP **D04.111** **Carcinoma in situ of skin of right upper eyelid, including canthus**

⊟ SP **D04.112** **Carcinoma in situ of skin of right lower eyelid, including canthus**

⑥ **D04.12** **Carcinoma in situ of skin of left eyelid, including canthus**

⊟ SP **D04.121** **Carcinoma in situ of skin of left upper eyelid, including canthus**

⊟ SP **D04.122** **Carcinoma in situ of skin of left lower eyelid, including canthus**

⑤ **D04.2** **Carcinoma in situ of skin of ear and external auricular canal**

⊟ IQ **D04.20** Carcinoma in situ of skin of unspecified ear and external auricular canal

⊟ SP **D04.21** **Carcinoma in situ of skin of right ear and external auricular canal**

⊟ SP **D04.22** **Carcinoma in situ of skin of left ear and external auricular canal**

⑤ **D04.3** Carcinoma in situ of skin of other and unspecified parts of face

IQ **D04.30** Carcinoma in situ of skin of unspecified part of face

SP **D04.39** **Carcinoma in situ of skin of other parts of face**

SP **D04.4** **Carcinoma in situ of skin of scalp and neck**

SP **D04.5** **Carcinoma in situ of skin of trunk**
   Carcinoma in situ of anal margin
   Carcinoma in situ of anal skin
   Carcinoma in situ of perianal skin
   Carcinoma in situ of skin of breast
   > **EXCLUDES 1** carcinoma in situ of anus NOS (D01.3)
   > carcinoma in situ of scrotum (D07.61)
   > carcinoma in situ of skin of genital organs (D07.-)

⑤ **D04.6** **Carcinoma in situ of skin of upper limb, including shoulder**

⊟ IQ **D04.60** Carcinoma in situ of skin of unspecified upper limb, including shoulder

⊟ SP **D04.61** **Carcinoma in situ of skin of right upper limb, including shoulder**

⊟ SP **D04.62** **Carcinoma in situ of skin of left upper limb, including shoulder**

⑤ **D04.7** **Carcinoma in situ of skin of lower limb, including hip**

⊟ IQ **D04.70** Carcinoma in situ of skin of unspecified lower limb, including hip

⊟ SP **D04.71** **Carcinoma in situ of skin of right lower limb, including hip**

⊟ SP **D04.72** **Carcinoma in situ of skin of left lower limb, including hip**

SP **D04.8** **Carcinoma in situ of skin of other sites**

IQ **D04.9** Carcinoma in situ of skin, unspecified

④ **D05** **Carcinoma in situ of breast**
   > **EXCLUDES 1** carcinoma in situ of skin of breast (D04.5)
   > melanoma in situ of breast (skin) (D03.5)
   > Paget's disease of breast or nipple (C50.-)

⑤ **D05.0** **Lobular carcinoma in situ of breast**

⊟ IQ **D05.00** Lobular carcinoma in situ of unspecified breast

⊟ SP **D05.01** **Lobular carcinoma in situ of right breast**

⊟ SP **D05.02** **Lobular carcinoma in situ of left breast**

⑤ **D05.1** **Intraductal carcinoma in situ of breast**

⊟ IQ **D05.10** Intraductal carcinoma in situ of unspecified breast

⊟ SP **D05.11** **Intraductal carcinoma in situ of right breast**

⊟ SP **D05.12** **Intraductal carcinoma in situ of left breast**

⑤ **D05.8** **Other specified type of carcinoma in situ of breast**

⊟ IQ **D05.80** Other specified type of carcinoma in situ of unspecified breast

⊟ SP **D05.81** **Other specified type of carcinoma in situ of right breast**

⊟ SP **D05.82** **Other specified type of carcinoma in situ of left breast**

⑤ **D05.9** Unspecified type of carcinoma in situ of breast

⊟ IQ **D05.90** Unspecified type of carcinoma in situ of unspecified breast

⊟ SP **D05.91** Unspecified type of carcinoma in situ of right breast

⊟ SP **D05.92** Unspecified type of carcinoma in situ of left breast

④ **D06** **Carcinoma in situ of cervix uteri**
   > **INCLUDES** cervical adenocarcinoma in situ
   > cervical intraepithelial glandular neoplasia
   > cervical intraepithelial neoplasia III [CIN III]
   > severe dysplasia of cervix uteri
   > **EXCLUDES 1** cervical intraepithelial neoplasia II [CIN II] (N87.1)
   > cytologic evidence of malignancy of cervix without histologic confirmation (R87.614)
   > high grade squamous intraepithelial lesion (HGSIL) of cervix (R87.613)

★ New ▲ Revised Px Primary SP PDGM Px SL Low CoM SH High CoM IQ Quest. Encounter H Hospice non-cancer Dx Unspecified M *Manifestation*

DecisionHealth's FY 2020 Complete Home Health ICD-10-CM Diagnosis Coding Manual   683

Chapter 2

C00-D49

melanoma in situ of cervix
(D03.5)
moderate cervical dysplasia
(N87.1)

CODING TIPS ✓ Class III, or severe dysplasia, is coded to category D06. Mild and moderate dysplasia of the cervix is coded to N87.-

SP **D06.0** Carcinoma in situ of endocervix

SP **D06.1** Carcinoma in situ of exocervix

SP **D06.7** Carcinoma in situ of other parts of cervix

SP **D06.9** Carcinoma in situ of cervix, unspecified

4 **D07** Carcinoma in situ of other and unspecified genital organs

EXCLUDES 1 melanoma in situ of trunk (D03.5)

SP **D07.0** Carcinoma in situ of endometrium

SP **D07.1** Carcinoma in situ of vulva
Severe dysplasia of vulva
Vulvar intraepithelial neoplasia III [VIN III]

EXCLUDES 1 moderate dysplasia of vulva (N90.1)
vulvar intraepithelial neoplasia II [VIN II] (N90.1)

SP **D07.2** Carcinoma in situ of vagina
Severe dysplasia of vagina
Vaginal intraepithelial neoplasia III [VAIN III]

EXCLUDES 1 moderate dysplasia of vagina (N89.1)
vaginal intraepithelial neoplasia II [VIN II] (N89.1)

5 **D07.3** Carcinoma in situ of other and unspecified female genital organs

IQ **D07.30** Carcinoma in situ of unspecified female genital organs

SP **D07.39** Carcinoma in situ of other female genital organs

SP **D07.4** Carcinoma in situ of penis
Erythroplasia of Queyrat NOS

SP **D07.5** Carcinoma in situ of prostate
Prostatic intraepithelial neoplasia III (PIN III)
Severe dysplasia of prostate

EXCLUDES 1 dysplasia (mild) (moderate) of prostate (N42.3-)
prostatic intraepithelial neoplasia II [PIN II] (N42.3-)

5 **D07.6** Carcinoma in situ of other and unspecified male genital organs

IQ **D07.60** Carcinoma in situ of unspecified male genital organs

SP **D07.61** Carcinoma in situ of scrotum

SP **D07.69** Carcinoma in situ of other male genital organs

4 **D09** Carcinoma in situ of other and unspecified sites

EXCLUDES 1 melanoma in situ (D03.-)

SP **D09.0** Carcinoma in situ of bladder

5 **D09.1** Carcinoma in situ of other and unspecified urinary organs

IQ **D09.10** Carcinoma in situ of unspecified urinary organ

SP **D09.19** Carcinoma in situ of other urinary organs

5 **D09.2** Carcinoma in situ of eye
EXCLUDES 1 carcinoma in situ of skin of eyelid (D04.1-)

IQ **D09.20** Carcinoma in situ of unspecified eye

SP **D09.21** Carcinoma in situ of right eye

SP **D09.22** Carcinoma in situ of left eye

SP **D09.3** Carcinoma in situ of thyroid and other endocrine glands
EXCLUDES 1 carcinoma in situ of endocrine pancreas (D01.7),
carcinoma in situ of ovary (D07.39)
carcinoma in situ of testis (D07.69)

SP **D09.8** Carcinoma in situ of other specified sites

IQ **D09.9** Carcinoma in situ, unspecified

Benign neoplasms, except benign neuroendocrine tumors (D10-D36)

4 **D10** Benign neoplasm of mouth and pharynx

SP **D10.0** Benign neoplasm of lip
Benign neoplasm of lip (frenulum) (inner aspect) (mucosa) (vermilion border)
EXCLUDES 1 benign neoplasm of skin of lip (D22.0, D23.0)

SP **D10.1** Benign neoplasm of tongue
Benign neoplasm of lingual tonsil

SP **D10.2** Benign neoplasm of floor of mouth

5 **D10.3** Benign neoplasm of other and unspecified parts of mouth

IQ **D10.30** Benign neoplasm of unspecified part of mouth

SP **D10.39** Benign neoplasm of other parts of mouth
Benign neoplasm of minor salivary gland NOS
EXCLUDES 1 benign odontogenic neoplasms (D16.4-D16.5)
benign neoplasm of mucosa of lip (D10.0)
benign neoplasm of nasopharyngeal surface of soft palate (D10.6)

SP **D10.4** Benign neoplasm of tonsil
Benign neoplasm of tonsil (faucial) (palatine)
EXCLUDES 1 benign neoplasm of lingual tonsil (D10.1)
benign neoplasm of pharyngeal tonsil (D10.6)
benign neoplasm of tonsillar fossa (D10.5)
benign neoplasm of tonsillar pillars (D10.5)

SP **D10.5** Benign neoplasm of other parts of oropharynx
Benign neoplasm of epiglottis, anterior aspect
Benign neoplasm of tonsillar fossa

---

4 4th digit required   **5** 5th digit required   **6** 6th digit required   **7** 7th digit required   **7** 7th digit placeholder   **+** Additional code   **⊟** Laterality

684   *DecisionHealth's* FY 2020 Complete Home Health ICD-10-CM Diagnosis Coding Manual

Benign neoplasm of tonsillar pillars
Benign neoplasm of vallecula

> **EXCLUDES 1**   benign neoplasm of epiglottis NOS (D14.1)
> benign neoplasm of epiglottis, suprahyoid portion (D14.1)

SP D10.6 Benign neoplasm of nasopharynx
Benign neoplasm of pharyngeal tonsil
Benign neoplasm of posterior margin of septum and choanae

SP D10.7 Benign neoplasm of hypopharynx

SP D10.9 Benign neoplasm of pharynx, unspecified

4 D11 Benign neoplasm of major salivary glands

> **EXCLUDES 1**   benign neoplasms of specified minor salivary glands which are classified according to their anatomical location
> benign neoplasms of minor salivary glands NOS (D10.39)

SP D11.0 Benign neoplasm of parotid gland

SP D11.7 Benign neoplasm of other major salivary glands
Benign neoplasm of sublingual salivary gland
Benign neoplasm of submandibular salivary gland

IQ D11.9 Benign neoplasm of major salivary gland, unspecified

▲ 4 D12 Benign neoplasm of colon, rectum, anus and anal canal

> **EXCLUDES 1**   benign carcinoid tumors of the large intestine, and rectum (D3A.02-)
> polyp of colon NOS (K63.5)

> **CODING TIPS ✓**   Adenomatous polyps are coded to D12. Hyperplastic polyps are coded to K63.5.

SP D12.0 Benign neoplasm of cecum
Benign neoplasm of ileocecal valve

SP D12.1 Benign neoplasm of appendix

> **EXCLUDES 1**   benign carcinoid tumor of the appendix (D3A.020)

SP D12.2 Benign neoplasm of ascending colon

SP D12.3 Benign neoplasm of transverse colon
Benign neoplasm of hepatic flexure
Benign neoplasm of splenic flexure

SP D12.4 Benign neoplasm of descending colon

SP D12.5 Benign neoplasm of sigmoid colon

▲ SP D12.6 Benign neoplasm of colon, unspecified
Adenomatosis of colon
Benign neoplasm of large intestine NOS
Polyposis (hereditary) of colon

> **EXCLUDES 1**   inflammatory polyp of colon (K51.4-)

SP D12.7 Benign neoplasm of rectosigmoid junction

SP D12.8 Benign neoplasm of rectum

> **EXCLUDES 1**   benign carcinoid tumor of the rectum (D3A.026)

SP D12.9 Benign neoplasm of anus and anal canal
Benign neoplasm of anus NOS

> **EXCLUDES 1**   benign neoplasm of anal margin (D22.5, D23.5)

benign neoplasm of anal skin (D22.5, D23.5)
benign neoplasm of perianal skin (D22.5, D23.5)

4 D13 Benign neoplasm of other and ill-defined parts of digestive system

> **EXCLUDES 1**   benign stromal tumors of digestive system (D21.4)

SP D13.0 Benign neoplasm of esophagus

SP D13.1 Benign neoplasm of stomach

> **EXCLUDES 1**   benign carcinoid tumor of the stomach (D3A.092)

SP D13.2 Benign neoplasm of duodenum

> **EXCLUDES 1**   benign carcinoid tumor of the duodenum (D3A.010)

5 D13.3 Benign neoplasm of other and unspecified parts of small intestine

> **EXCLUDES 1**   benign carcinoid tumors of the small intestine (D3A.01-)
> benign neoplasm of ileocecal valve (D12.0)

SP D13.30 Benign neoplasm of unspecified part of small intestine

SP D13.39 Benign neoplasm of other parts of small intestine

SP D13.4 Benign neoplasm of liver
Benign neoplasm of intrahepatic bile ducts

SP D13.5 Benign neoplasm of extrahepatic bile ducts

SP D13.6 Benign neoplasm of pancreas

> **EXCLUDES 1**   benign neoplasm of endocrine pancreas (D13.7)

SP ✚ D13.7 Benign neoplasm of endocrine pancreas
Islet cell tumor
Benign neoplasm of islets of Langerhans
Use additional code to identify any functional activity.

SP D13.9 Benign neoplasm of ill-defined sites within the digestive system
Benign neoplasm of digestive system NOS
Benign neoplasm of intestine NOS
Benign neoplasm of spleen

4 D14 Benign neoplasm of middle ear and respiratory system

SP D14.0 Benign neoplasm of middle ear, nasal cavity and accessory sinuses
Benign neoplasm of cartilage of nose

> **EXCLUDES 1**   benign neoplasm of auricular canal (external) (D22.2-, D23.2-)
> benign neoplasm of bone of ear (D16.4)
> benign neoplasm of bone of nose (D16.4)
> benign neoplasm of cartilage of ear (D21.0)
> benign neoplasm of ear (external) (skin) (D22.2-, D23.2-)
> benign neoplasm of nose NOS (D36.7)
> benign neoplasm of skin of nose (D22.39, D23.39)
> benign neoplasm of olfactory bulb (D33.3)

★ New ▲ Revised Px Primary **SP** PDGM Px **SL** Low CoM **SH** High CoM **IQ** Quest. Encounter **H** Hospice non-cancer Dx   Unspecified   **M** *Manifestation*

DecisionHealth's FY 2020 Complete Home Health ICD-10-CM Diagnosis Coding Manual   685

Chapter 2

C00-D49

Chapter 2

C00-D49

benign neoplasm of posterior
margin of septum and
choanae (D10.6)
polyp of accessory sinus
(J33.8)
polyp of ear (middle)
(H74.4)
polyp of nasal (cavity)
(J33.-)

SP **D14.1** **Benign neoplasm of larynx**
Adenomatous polyp of larynx
Benign neoplasm of epiglottis (suprahyoid
portion)
EXCLUDES 1   benign neoplasm of
epiglottis, anterior aspect
(D10.5)
polyp (nonadenomatous) of
vocal cord or larynx
(J38.1)

SP **D14.2** **Benign neoplasm of trachea**

5 **D14.3** **Benign neoplasm of bronchus and lung**
EXCLUDES 1   benign carcinoid tumor of
the bronchus and lung
(D3A.090)

IQ **D14.30** Benign neoplasm of unspecified
bronchus and lung

SP **D14.31** **Benign neoplasm of right bronchus
and lung**

SP **D14.32** **Benign neoplasm of left bronchus
and lung**

IQ **D14.4** Benign neoplasm of respiratory system,
unspecified

4 **D15** Benign neoplasm of other and unspecified
intrathoracic organs
EXCLUDES 1   benign neoplasm of mesothelial
tissue (D19.-)

SP **D15.0** **Benign neoplasm of thymus**
EXCLUDES 1   benign carcinoid tumor of
the thymus (D3A.091)

SP **D15.1** **Benign neoplasm of heart**
EXCLUDES 1   benign neoplasm of great
vessels (D21.3)

SP **D15.2** **Benign neoplasm of mediastinum**

SP **D15.7** **Benign neoplasm of other specified
intrathoracic organs**

IQ **D15.9** Benign neoplasm of intrathoracic
organ, unspecified

4 **D16** Benign neoplasm of bone and articular
cartilage
EXCLUDES 1   benign neoplasm of connective
tissue of ear (D21.0)
benign neoplasm of connective
tissue of eyelid (D21.0)
benign neoplasm of connective
tissue of larynx (D14.1)
benign neoplasm of connective
tissue of nose (D14.0)
benign neoplasm of synovia
(D21.-)

5 **D16.0** **Benign neoplasm of scapula and long
bones of upper limb**

IQ **D16.00** Benign neoplasm of scapula and
long bones of unspecified upper
limb

SP **D16.01** **Benign neoplasm of scapula and long
bones of right upper limb**

SP **D16.02** **Benign neoplasm of scapula and long
bones of left upper limb**

5 **D16.1** **Benign neoplasm of short bones of
upper limb**

IQ **D16.10** Benign neoplasm of short bones of
unspecified upper limb

SP **D16.11** **Benign neoplasm of short bones of
right upper limb**

SP **D16.12** **Benign neoplasm of short bones of
left upper limb**

5 **D16.2** **Benign neoplasm of long bones of lower
limb**

IQ **D16.20** Benign neoplasm of long bones of
unspecified lower limb

SP **D16.21** **Benign neoplasm of long bones of
right lower limb**

SP **D16.22** **Benign neoplasm of long bones of left
lower limb**

5 **D16.3** **Benign neoplasm of short bones of lower
limb**

IQ **D16.30** Benign neoplasm of short bones of
unspecified lower limb

SP **D16.31** **Benign neoplasm of short bones of
right lower limb**

SP **D16.32** **Benign neoplasm of short bones of
left lower limb**

SP **D16.4** **Benign neoplasm of bones of skull and
face**
Benign neoplasm of maxilla (superior)
Benign neoplasm of orbital bone
Keratocyst of maxilla
Keratocystic odontogenic tumor of maxilla
EXCLUDES 2   benign neoplasm of lower
jaw bone (D16.5)

SP **D16.5** **Benign neoplasm of lower jaw bone**
Keratocyst of mandible
Keratocystic odontogenic tumor of
mandible

SP **D16.6** **Benign neoplasm of vertebral column**
EXCLUDES 1   benign neoplasm of sacrum
and coccyx (D16.8)

SP **D16.7** **Benign neoplasm of ribs, sternum and
clavicle**

SP **D16.8** **Benign neoplasm of pelvic bones,
sacrum and coccyx**

IQ **D16.9** Benign neoplasm of bone and articular
cartilage, unspecified

4 **D17** Benign lipomatous neoplasm

SP **D17.0** **Benign lipomatous neoplasm of skin and
subcutaneous tissue of head, face and
neck**

SP **D17.1** **Benign lipomatous neoplasm of skin and
subcutaneous tissue of trunk**

5 **D17.2** **Benign lipomatous neoplasm of skin and
subcutaneous tissue of limb**

IQ **D17.20** Benign lipomatous neoplasm of skin
and subcutaneous tissue of
unspecified limb

SP **D17.21** **Benign lipomatous neoplasm of skin
and subcutaneous tissue of right arm**

SP **D17.22** **Benign lipomatous neoplasm of skin
and subcutaneous tissue of left arm**

SP **D17.23** **Benign lipomatous neoplasm of skin
and subcutaneous tissue of right leg**

SP **D17.24** **Benign lipomatous neoplasm of skin
and subcutaneous tissue of left leg**

---

4 4th digit required   **5** 5th digit required   **6** 6th digit required   **7** 7th digit required   **7** 7th digit placeholder   **+** Additional code   Laterality

5 D17.3 **Benign lipomatous neoplasm of skin and subcutaneous tissue of other and unspecified sites**

IQ D17.30 **Benign lipomatous neoplasm of skin and subcutaneous tissue of unspecified sites**

SP D17.39 **Benign lipomatous neoplasm of skin and subcutaneous tissue of other sites**

SP D17.4 **Benign lipomatous neoplasm of intrathoracic organs**

SP D17.5 **Benign lipomatous neoplasm of intra-abdominal organs**

> EXCLUDES 1   benign lipomatous neoplasm of peritoneum and retroperitoneum (D17.79)

SP D17.6 **Benign lipomatous neoplasm of spermatic cord**

5 D17.7 **Benign lipomatous neoplasm of other sites**

SP D17.71 **Benign lipomatous neoplasm of kidney**

SP D17.72 **Benign lipomatous neoplasm of other genitourinary organ**

SP D17.79 **Benign lipomatous neoplasm of other sites**
Benign lipomatous neoplasm of peritoneum
Benign lipomatous neoplasm of retroperitoneum

IQ D17.9 **Benign lipomatous neoplasm, unspecified**
Lipoma NOS

4 D18 **Hemangioma and lymphangioma, any site**
> EXCLUDES 1   benign neoplasm of glomus jugulare (D35.6)
> blue or pigmented nevus (D22.-)
> nevus NOS (D22.-)
> vascular nevus (Q82.5)

5 D18.0 **Hemangioma**
Angioma NOS
Cavernous nevus

IQ D18.00 **Hemangioma unspecified site**

SP D18.01 **Hemangioma of skin and subcutaneous tissue**

SP D18.02 **Hemangioma of intracranial structures**

SP D18.03 **Hemangioma of intra-abdominal structures**

SP D18.09 **Hemangioma of other sites**

SP D18.1 **Lymphangioma, any site**

4 D19 **Benign neoplasm of mesothelial tissue**

SP D19.0 **Benign neoplasm of mesothelial tissue of pleura**

SP D19.1 **Benign neoplasm of mesothelial tissue of peritoneum**

SP D19.7 **Benign neoplasm of mesothelial tissue of other sites**

IQ D19.9 **Benign neoplasm of mesothelial tissue, unspecified**
Benign mesothelioma NOS

4 D20 **Benign neoplasm of soft tissue of retroperitoneum and peritoneum**
> EXCLUDES 1   benign lipomatous neoplasm of peritoneum and retroperitoneum (D17.79)

benign neoplasm of mesothelial tissue (D19.-)

SP D20.0 **Benign neoplasm of soft tissue of retroperitoneum**

SP D20.1 **Benign neoplasm of soft tissue of peritoneum**

4 D21 **Other benign neoplasms of connective and other soft tissue**
> INCLUDES   benign neoplasm of blood vessel
> benign neoplasm of bursa
> benign neoplasm of cartilage
> benign neoplasm of fascia
> benign neoplasm of fat
> benign neoplasm of ligament, except uterine
> benign neoplasm of lymphatic channel
> benign neoplasm of muscle
> benign neoplasm of synovia
> benign neoplasm of tendon (sheath)
> benign stromal tumors

> EXCLUDES 1   benign neoplasm of articular cartilage (D16.-)
> benign neoplasm of cartilage of larynx (D14.1)
> benign neoplasm of cartilage of nose (D14.0)
> benign neoplasm of connective tissue of breast (D24.-)
> benign neoplasm of peripheral nerves and autonomic nervous system (D36.1-)
> benign neoplasm of peritoneum (D20.1)
> benign neoplasm of retroperitoneum (D20.0)
> benign neoplasm of uterine ligament, any (D28.2)
> benign neoplasm of vascular tissue (D18.-)
> hemangioma (D18.0-)
> lipomatous neoplasm (D17.-)
> lymphangioma (D18.1)
> uterine leiomyoma (D25.-)

SP D21.0 **Benign neoplasm of connective and other soft tissue of head, face and neck**
Benign neoplasm of connective tissue of ear
Benign neoplasm of connective tissue of eyelid
> EXCLUDES 1   benign neoplasm of connective tissue of orbit (D31.6-)

5 D21.1 **Benign neoplasm of connective and other soft tissue of upper limb, including shoulder**

IQ D21.10 **Benign neoplasm of connective and other soft tissue of unspecified upper limb, including shoulder**

SP D21.11 **Benign neoplasm of connective and other soft tissue of right upper limb, including shoulder**

SP D21.12 **Benign neoplasm of connective and other soft tissue of left upper limb, including shoulder**

Chapter 2

C00-D49

★ New ▲ Revised Px Primary SP PDGM Px SL Low CoM SH High CoM IQ Quest. Encounter H Hospice non-cancer Dx   Unspecified   M Manifestation

DecisionHealth's FY 2020 Complete Home Health ICD-10-CM Diagnosis Coding Manual

687

⑤ D21.2 Benign neoplasm of connective and other soft tissue of lower limb, including hip

⊟ IQ D21.20 Benign neoplasm of connective and other soft tissue of unspecified lower limb, including hip

⊟ SP D21.21 Benign neoplasm of connective and other soft tissue of right lower limb, including hip

⊟ SP D21.22 Benign neoplasm of connective and other soft tissue of left lower limb, including hip

SP D21.3 Benign neoplasm of connective and other soft tissue of thorax
Benign neoplasm of axilla
Benign neoplasm of diaphragm
Benign neoplasm of great vessels
> **EXCLUDES 1** benign neoplasm of heart (D15.1)
> benign neoplasm of mediastinum (D15.2)
> benign neoplasm of thymus (D15.0)

SP D21.4 Benign neoplasm of connective and other soft tissue of abdomen
Benign stromal tumors of abdomen

SP D21.5 Benign neoplasm of connective and other soft tissue of pelvis
> **EXCLUDES 1** benign neoplasm of any uterine ligament (D28.2)
> uterine leiomyoma (D25.-)

▲ SP D21.6 Benign neoplasm of connective and other soft tissue of trunk, unspecified
Benign neoplasm of connective and other soft tissue back NOS

IQ D21.9 Benign neoplasm of connective and other soft tissue, unspecified

④ D22 Melanocytic nevi
> **INCLUDES** atypical nevus
> blue hairy pigmented nevus
> nevus NOS

> **CODING TIPS ✓** Melanocytic nevi are also known as moles. These benign neoplasms are generally not treated and pose little threat to individuals. Melanocytic nevi are unlikely to impair patient function in any way and do not support a need for medical necessity under the home health benefit.

SP D22.0 Melanocytic nevi of lip

⑤ D22.1 Melanocytic nevi of eyelid, including canthus

⊟ IQ D22.10 Melanocytic nevi of unspecified eyelid, including canthus

⑥ D22.11 Melanocytic nevi of right eyelid, including canthus

⊟ SP D22.111 Melanocytic nevi of right upper eyelid, including canthus

⊟ SP D22.112 Melanocytic nevi of right lower eyelid, including canthus

⑥ D22.12 Melanocytic nevi of left eyelid, including canthus

⊟ SP D22.121 Melanocytic nevi of left upper eyelid, including canthus

⊟ SP D22.122 Melanocytic nevi of left lower eyelid, including canthus

⑤ D22.2 Melanocytic nevi of ear and external auricular canal

⊟ IQ D22.20 Melanocytic nevi of unspecified ear and external auricular canal

⊟ SP D22.21 Melanocytic nevi of right ear and external auricular canal

⊟ SP D22.22 Melanocytic nevi of left ear and external auricular canal

⑤ D22.3 Melanocytic nevi of other and unspecified parts of face

IQ D22.30 Melanocytic nevi of unspecified part of face

SP D22.39 Melanocytic nevi of other parts of face

SP D22.4 Melanocytic nevi of scalp and neck

SP D22.5 Melanocytic nevi of trunk
Melanocytic nevi of anal margin
Melanocytic nevi of anal skin
Melanocytic nevi of perianal skin
Melanocytic nevi of skin of breast

⑤ D22.6 Melanocytic nevi of upper limb, including shoulder

⊟ IQ D22.60 Melanocytic nevi of unspecified upper limb, including shoulder

⊟ SP D22.61 Melanocytic nevi of right upper limb, including shoulder

⊟ SP D22.62 Melanocytic nevi of left upper limb, including shoulder

⑤ D22.7 Melanocytic nevi of lower limb, including hip

⊟ IQ D22.70 Melanocytic nevi of unspecified lower limb, including hip

⊟ SP D22.71 Melanocytic nevi of right lower limb, including hip

⊟ SP D22.72 Melanocytic nevi of left lower limb, including hip

IQ D22.9 Melanocytic nevi, unspecified

▲ ④ D23 Other benign neoplasms of skin
> **INCLUDES** benign neoplasm of hair follicles
> benign neoplasm of sebaceous glands
> benign neoplasm of sweat glands
> **EXCLUDES 1** benign lipomatous neoplasms of skin (D17.0-D17.3)
> **EXCLUDES 2** melanocytic nevi (D22.-)

SP D23.0 Other benign neoplasm of skin of lip
> **EXCLUDES 1** benign neoplasm of vermilion border of lip (D10.0)

⑤ D23.1 Other benign neoplasm of skin of eyelid, including canthus

⊟ IQ D23.10 Other benign neoplasm of skin of unspecified eyelid, including canthus

⑥ D23.11 Other benign neoplasm of skin of right eyelid, including canthus

⊟ SP D23.111 Other benign neoplasm of skin of right upper eyelid, including canthus

⊟ SP D23.112 Other benign neoplasm of skin of right lower eyelid, including canthus

⑥ D23.12 Other benign neoplasm of skin of left eyelid, including canthus

⊟ SP D23.121 Other benign neoplasm of skin of left upper eyelid, including canthus

---

④4th digit required ⑤5th digit required ⑥6th digit required ⑦7th digit required ⑦7th digit placeholder ✚Additional code ⊟Laterality

☰ **SP** **D23.122** Other benign neoplasm of skin of left lower eyelid, including canthus

5 **D23.2** Other benign neoplasm of skin of ear and external auricular canal

☰ **IQ** **D23.20** Other benign neoplasm of skin of unspecified ear and external auricular canal

☰ **SP** **D23.21** Other benign neoplasm of skin of right ear and external auricular canal

☰ **SP** **D23.22** Other benign neoplasm of skin of left ear and external auricular canal

5 **D23.3** Other benign neoplasm of skin of other and unspecified parts of face

IQ **D23.30** Other benign neoplasm of skin of unspecified part of face

SP **D23.39** Other benign neoplasm of skin of other parts of face

SP **D23.4** Other benign neoplasm of skin of scalp and neck

SP **D23.5** Other benign neoplasm of skin of trunk
Other benign neoplasm of anal margin
Other benign neoplasm of anal skin
Other benign neoplasm of perianal skin
Other benign neoplasm of skin of breast
| EXCLUDES 1 | benign neoplasm of anus NOS (D12.9) |

5 **D23.6** Other benign neoplasm of skin of upper limb, including shoulder

☰ **IQ** **D23.60** Other benign neoplasm of skin of unspecified upper limb, including shoulder

☰ **SP** **D23.61** Other benign neoplasm of skin of right upper limb, including shoulder

☰ **SP** **D23.62** Other benign neoplasm of skin of left upper limb, including shoulder

5 **D23.7** Other benign neoplasm of skin of lower limb, including hip

☰ **IQ** **D23.70** Other benign neoplasm of skin of unspecified lower limb, including hip

☰ **SP** **D23.71** Other benign neoplasm of skin of right lower limb, including hip

☰ **SP** **D23.72** Other benign neoplasm of skin of left lower limb, including hip

IQ **D23.9** Other benign neoplasm of skin, unspecified

4 **D24** Benign neoplasm of breast
INCLUDES	benign neoplasm of connective tissue of breast
	benign neoplasm of soft parts of breast
	fibroadenoma of breast
EXCLUDES 2	adenofibrosis of breast (N60.2)
	benign cyst of breast (N60.-)
	benign mammary dysplasia (N60.-)
	benign neoplasm of skin of breast (D22.5, D23.5)
	fibrocystic disease of breast (N60.-)

☰ **SP** **D24.1** Benign neoplasm of right breast

☰ **SP** **D24.2** Benign neoplasm of left breast

☰ **IQ** **D24.9** Benign neoplasm of unspecified breast

4 **D25** Leiomyoma of uterus

INCLUDES	uterine fibroid
	uterine fibromyoma
	uterine myoma

SP **D25.0** Submucous leiomyoma of uterus

SP **D25.1** Intramural leiomyoma of uterus
Interstitial leiomyoma of uterus

SP **D25.2** Subserosal leiomyoma of uterus
Subperitoneal leiomyoma of uterus

SP **D25.9** Leiomyoma of uterus, unspecified

4 **D26** Other benign neoplasms of uterus

SP **D26.0** Other benign neoplasm of cervix uteri

SP **D26.1** Other benign neoplasm of corpus uteri

SP **D26.7** Other benign neoplasm of other parts of uterus

SP **D26.9** Other benign neoplasm of uterus, unspecified

✚ **4** **D27** Benign neoplasm of ovary
Use additional code to identify any functional activity.
EXCLUDES 2	corpus albicans cyst (N83.2-)
	corpus luteum cyst (N83.1-)
	endometrial cyst (N80.1)
	follicular (atretic) cyst (N83.0-)
	graafian follicle cyst (N83.0-)
	ovarian cyst NEC (N83.2-)
	ovarian retention cyst (N83.2-)

☰ **SP** ✚ **D27.0** Benign neoplasm of right ovary

☰ **SP** ✚ **D27.1** Benign neoplasm of left ovary

☰ **IQ** ✚ **D27.9** Benign neoplasm of unspecified ovary

4 **D28** Benign neoplasm of other and unspecified female genital organs
INCLUDES	adenomatous polyp
	benign neoplasm of skin of female genital organs
	benign teratoma
EXCLUDES 1	epoophoron cyst (Q50.5)
	fimbrial cyst (Q50.4)
	Gartner's duct cyst (Q52.4)
	parovarian cyst (Q50.5)

SP **D28.0** Benign neoplasm of vulva

SP **D28.1** Benign neoplasm of vagina

SP **D28.2** Benign neoplasm of uterine tubes and ligaments
Benign neoplasm of fallopian tube
Benign neoplasm of uterine ligament (broad) (round)

SP **D28.7** Benign neoplasm of other specified female genital organs

IQ **D28.9** Benign neoplasm of female genital organ, unspecified

4 **D29** Benign neoplasm of male genital organs
| INCLUDES | benign neoplasm of skin of male genital organs |

SP **D29.0** Benign neoplasm of penis

SP **D29.1** Benign neoplasm of prostate
| EXCLUDES 1 | enlarged prostate (N40.-) |

✚ **5** **D29.2** Benign neoplasm of testis
Use additional code to identify any functional activity.

☰ **IQ** ✚ **D29.20** Benign neoplasm of unspecified testis

☰ **SP** ✚ **D29.21** Benign neoplasm of right testis

☰ **SP** ✚ **D29.22** Benign neoplasm of left testis

★ New ▲ Revised **Px** Primary **SP** PDGM Px **SL** Low CoM **SH** High CoM **IQ** Quest. Encounter **H** Hospice non-cancer Dx | Unspecified | **M** *Manifestation*

DecisionHealth's FY 2020 Complete Home Health ICD-10-CM Diagnosis Coding Manual

689

⑤ **D29.3** Benign neoplasm of epididymis

⊟ **IQ** **D29.30** **Benign neoplasm of unspecified epididymis**

⊟ **SP** **D29.31** Benign neoplasm of right epididymis

⊟ **SP** **D29.32** Benign neoplasm of left epididymis

SP **D29.4** Benign neoplasm of scrotum
Benign neoplasm of skin of scrotum

SP **D29.8** Benign neoplasm of other specified male genital organs
Benign neoplasm of seminal vesicle
Benign neoplasm of spermatic cord
Benign neoplasm of tunica vaginalis

IQ **D29.9** **Benign neoplasm of male genital organ, unspecified**

④ **D30** **Benign neoplasm of urinary organs**

⑤ **D30.0** Benign neoplasm of kidney
EXCLUDES 1 benign carcinoid tumor of the kidney (D3A.093)
benign neoplasm of renal calyces (D30.1-)
benign neoplasm of renal pelvis (D30.1-)

⊟ **IQ** **D30.00** **Benign neoplasm of unspecified kidney**

⊟ **SP** **D30.01** Benign neoplasm of right kidney

⊟ **SP** **D30.02** Benign neoplasm of left kidney

⑤ **D30.1** Benign neoplasm of renal pelvis

⊟ **IQ** **D30.10** **Benign neoplasm of unspecified renal pelvis**

⊟ **SP** **D30.11** Benign neoplasm of right renal pelvis

⊟ **SP** **D30.12** Benign neoplasm of left renal pelvis

⑤ **D30.2** Benign neoplasm of ureter
EXCLUDES 1 benign neoplasm of ureteric orifice of bladder (D30.3)

⊟ **IQ** **D30.20** **Benign neoplasm of unspecified ureter**

⊟ **SP** **D30.21** Benign neoplasm of right ureter

⊟ **SP** **D30.22** Benign neoplasm of left ureter

SP **D30.3** Benign neoplasm of bladder
Benign neoplasm of ureteric orifice of bladder
Benign neoplasm of urethral orifice of bladder

SP **D30.4** Benign neoplasm of urethra
EXCLUDES 1 benign neoplasm of urethral orifice of bladder (D30.3)

SP **D30.8** Benign neoplasm of other specified urinary organs
Benign neoplasm of paraurethral glands

IQ **D30.9** **Benign neoplasm of urinary organ, unspecified**
Benign neoplasm of urinary system NOS

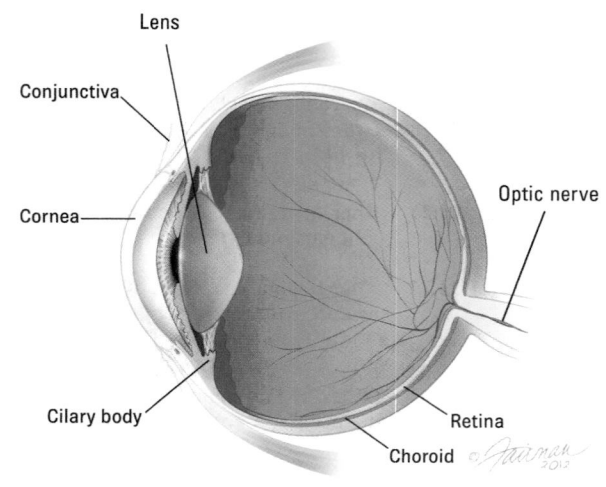

④ **D31** **Benign neoplasm of eye and adnexa**
EXCLUDES 1 benign neoplasm of connective tissue of eyelid (D21.0)
benign neoplasm of optic nerve (D33.3)
benign neoplasm of skin of eyelid (D22.1-, D23.1-)

⑤ **D31.0** Benign neoplasm of conjunctiva

⊟ **IQ** **D31.00** **Benign neoplasm of unspecified conjunctiva**

⊟ **SP** **D31.01** Benign neoplasm of right conjunctiva

⊟ **SP** **D31.02** Benign neoplasm of left conjunctiva

⑤ **D31.1** Benign neoplasm of cornea

⊟ **IQ** **D31.10** **Benign neoplasm of unspecified cornea**

⊟ **SP** **D31.11** Benign neoplasm of right cornea

⊟ **SP** **D31.12** Benign neoplasm of left cornea

⑤ **D31.2** Benign neoplasm of retina
EXCLUDES 1 dark area on retina (D49.81)
hemangioma of retina (D49.81)
neoplasm of unspecified behavior of retina and choroid (D49.81)
retinal freckle (D49.81)

⊟ **IQ** **D31.20** **Benign neoplasm of unspecified retina**

⊟ **SP** **D31.21** Benign neoplasm of right retina

⊟ **SP** **D31.22** Benign neoplasm of left retina

⑤ **D31.3** Benign neoplasm of choroid

⊟ **IQ** **D31.30** **Benign neoplasm of unspecified choroid**

⊟ **SP** **D31.31** Benign neoplasm of right choroid

⊟ **SP** **D31.32** Benign neoplasm of left choroid

⑤ **D31.4** Benign neoplasm of ciliary body

⊟ **IQ** **D31.40** **Benign neoplasm of unspecified ciliary body**

⊟ **SP** **D31.41** Benign neoplasm of right ciliary body

⊟ **SP** **D31.42** Benign neoplasm of left ciliary body

⑤ **D31.5** Benign neoplasm of lacrimal gland and duct
Benign neoplasm of lacrimal sac

④ 4th digit required   ⑤ 5th digit required   ⑥ 6th digit required   ⑦ 7th digit required   ⑦ 7th digit placeholder   ✚ Additional code   ⊟ Laterality

690   *DecisionHealth's* FY 2020 Complete Home Health ICD-10-CM Diagnosis Coding Manual

Benign neoplasm of nasolacrimal duct

☐ IQ D31.50 **Benign neoplasm of unspecified lacrimal gland and duct**

☐ SP D31.51 **Benign neoplasm of right lacrimal gland and duct**

☐ SP D31.52 **Benign neoplasm of left lacrimal gland and duct**

⑤ D31.6 **Benign neoplasm of unspecified site of orbit**

Benign neoplasm of connective tissue of orbit

Benign neoplasm of extraocular muscle

Benign neoplasm of peripheral nerves of orbit

Benign neoplasm of retrobulbar tissue

Benign neoplasm of retro-ocular tissue

EXCLUDES 1 benign neoplasm of orbital bone (D16.4)

☐ IQ D31.60 **Benign neoplasm of unspecified site of unspecified orbit**

☐ SP D31.61 **Benign neoplasm of unspecified site of right orbit**

☐ SP D31.62 **Benign neoplasm of unspecified site of left orbit**

⑤ D31.9 **Benign neoplasm of unspecified part of eye**

Benign neoplasm of eyeball

☐ IQ D31.90 **Benign neoplasm of unspecified part of unspecified eye**

☐ SP D31.91 **Benign neoplasm of unspecified part of right eye**

☐ SP D31.92 **Benign neoplasm of unspecified part of left eye**

④ D32 **Benign neoplasm of meninges**

SP D32.0 **Benign neoplasm of cerebral meninges**

SP D32.1 **Benign neoplasm of spinal meninges**

SP D32.9 **Benign neoplasm of meninges, unspecified**

Meningioma NOS

④ D33 **Benign neoplasm of brain and other parts of central nervous system**

EXCLUDES 1 angioma (D18.0-)
benign neoplasm of meninges (D32.-)
benign neoplasm of peripheral nerves and autonomic nervous system (D36.1-)
hemangioma (D18.0-)
neurofibromatosis (Q85.0-)
retro-ocular benign neoplasm (D31.6-)

CODING TIPS ✓ This code category is used for benign neoplasms of the brain and spinal cord. A personal history of these benign neoplasms is coded to Z86.011.

SP D33.0 **Benign neoplasm of brain, supratentorial**

Benign neoplasm of cerebral ventricle

Benign neoplasm of cerebrum

Benign neoplasm of frontal lobe

Benign neoplasm of occipital lobe

Benign neoplasm of parietal lobe

Benign neoplasm of temporal lobe

EXCLUDES 1 benign neoplasm of fourth ventricle (D33.1)

SP D33.1 **Benign neoplasm of brain, infratentorial**

Benign neoplasm of brain stem

Benign neoplasm of cerebellum

Benign neoplasm of fourth ventricle

SP D33.2 **Benign neoplasm of brain, unspecified**

SP D33.3 **Benign neoplasm of cranial nerves**

Benign neoplasm of olfactory bulb

SP D33.4 **Benign neoplasm of spinal cord**

SP D33.7 **Benign neoplasm of other specified parts of central nervous system**

IQ D33.9 **Benign neoplasm of central nervous system, unspecified**

Benign neoplasm of nervous system (central) NOS

SP + D34 **Benign neoplasm of thyroid gland**

Use additional code to identify any functional activity

+ ④ D35 **Benign neoplasm of other and unspecified endocrine glands**

Use additional code to identify any functional activity

EXCLUDES 1 benign neoplasm of endocrine pancreas (D13.7)
benign neoplasm of ovary (D27.-)
benign neoplasm of testis (D29.2.-)
benign neoplasm of thymus (D15.0)

+ ⑤ D35.0 **Benign neoplasm of adrenal gland**

☐ IQ + D35.00 **Benign neoplasm of unspecified adrenal gland**

☐ SP + D35.01 **Benign neoplasm of right adrenal gland**

☐ SP + D35.02 **Benign neoplasm of left adrenal gland**

SP + D35.1 **Benign neoplasm of parathyroid gland**

SP + D35.2 **Benign neoplasm of pituitary gland**

SP + D35.3 **Benign neoplasm of craniopharyngeal duct**

SP + D35.4 **Benign neoplasm of pineal gland**

SP + D35.5 **Benign neoplasm of carotid body**

SP + D35.6 **Benign neoplasm of aortic body and other paraganglia**

Benign tumor of glomus jugulare

SP + D35.7 **Benign neoplasm of other specified endocrine glands**

IQ + D35.9 **Benign neoplasm of endocrine gland, unspecified**

Benign neoplasm of unspecified endocrine gland

④ D36 **Benign neoplasm of other and unspecified sites**

SP D36.0 **Benign neoplasm of lymph nodes**

EXCLUDES 1 lymphangioma (D18.1)

⑤ D36.1 **Benign neoplasm of peripheral nerves and autonomic nervous system**

EXCLUDES 1 benign neoplasm of peripheral nerves of orbit (D31.6-)
neurofibromatosis (Q85.0-)

SP D36.10 **Benign neoplasm of peripheral nerves and autonomic nervous system, unspecified**

★ New ▲ Revised Px Primary **SP** PDGM Px **SL** Low CoM **SH** High CoM **IQ** Quest. Encounter **Ⓗ** Hospice non-cancer Dx Unspecified **M** *Manifestation*

DecisionHealth's FY 2020 Complete Home Health ICD-10-CM Diagnosis Coding Manual

691

SP D36.11 Benign neoplasm of peripheral nerves and autonomic nervous system of face, head, and neck

SP D36.12 Benign neoplasm of peripheral nerves and autonomic nervous system, upper limb, including shoulder

SP D36.13 Benign neoplasm of peripheral nerves and autonomic nervous system of lower limb, including hip

SP D36.14 Benign neoplasm of peripheral nerves and autonomic nervous system of thorax

SP D36.15 Benign neoplasm of peripheral nerves and autonomic nervous system of abdomen

SP D36.16 Benign neoplasm of peripheral nerves and autonomic nervous system of pelvis

SP D36.17 Benign neoplasm of peripheral nerves and autonomic nervous system of trunk, unspecified

▲ **SP D36.7** Benign neoplasm of other specified sites
Benign neoplasm of back NOS
Benign neoplasm of nose NOS

!Q D36.9 Benign neoplasm, unspecified site

Benign neuroendocrine tumors   (D3A)

✚ **4 D3A** Benign neuroendocrine tumors
Code also:
any associated multiple endocrine neoplasia [MEN] syndromes (E31.2-)
Use additional code to identify any associated endocrine syndrome, such as:
carcinoid syndrome (E34.0)
EXCLUDES 2 benign pancreatic islet cell tumors (D13.7)

✚ **5 D3A.0** Benign carcinoid tumors

!Q ✚ D3A.00 Benign carcinoid tumor of unspecified site

Carcinoid tumor NOS

✚ **6 D3A.01** Benign carcinoid tumors of the small intestine

SP ✚ D3A.010 Benign carcinoid tumor of the duodenum

SP ✚ D3A.011 Benign carcinoid tumor of the jejunum

SP ✚ D3A.012 Benign carcinoid tumor of the ileum

SP ✚ D3A.019 Benign carcinoid tumor of the small intestine, unspecified portion

✚ **6 D3A.02** Benign carcinoid tumors of the appendix, large intestine, and rectum

SP ✚ D3A.020 Benign carcinoid tumor of the appendix

SP ✚ D3A.021 Benign carcinoid tumor of the cecum

SP ✚ D3A.022 Benign carcinoid tumor of the ascending colon

SP ✚ D3A.023 Benign carcinoid tumor of the transverse colon

SP ✚ D3A.024 Benign carcinoid tumor of the descending colon

SP ✚ D3A.025 Benign carcinoid tumor of the sigmoid colon

SP ✚ D3A.026 Benign carcinoid tumor of the rectum

SP ✚ D3A.029 Benign carcinoid tumor of the large intestine, unspecified portion

Benign carcinoid tumor of the colon NOS

✚ **6 D3A.09** Benign carcinoid tumors of other sites

SP ✚ D3A.090 Benign carcinoid tumor of the bronchus and lung

SP ✚ D3A.091 Benign carcinoid tumor of the thymus

SP ✚ D3A.092 Benign carcinoid tumor of the stomach

SP ✚ D3A.093 Benign carcinoid tumor of the kidney

SP ✚ D3A.094 Benign carcinoid tumor of the foregut, unspecified

SP ✚ D3A.095 Benign carcinoid tumor of the midgut, unspecified

SP ✚ D3A.096 Benign carcinoid tumor of the hindgut, unspecified

SP ✚ D3A.098 Benign carcinoid tumors of other sites

SP ✚ D3A.8 Other benign neuroendocrine tumors
Neuroendocrine tumor NOS

Neoplasms of uncertain behavior, polycythemia vera and myelodysplastic syndromes   (D37-D48)

Note:
Categories D37-D44, and D48 classify by site neoplasms of uncertain behavior, i.e., histologic confirmation whether the neoplasm is malignant or benign cannot be made.
EXCLUDES 1 neoplasms of unspecified behavior (D49.-)

CODING TIPS ✓ Codes classifiable to D37-D48 include tumors specifically reported as those of "uncertain behavior." This term is a specific diagnostic statement that must be reported by the physician in order to support assignment of any code from D37-D48, as these tumors include lesions whose behavior cannot be predicted. The status is currently benign, but the tumor could undergo a malignant transformation. These codes are not to be used when a biopsy has not been performed or results are not available.

4 D37 Neoplasm of uncertain behavior of oral cavity and digestive organs
EXCLUDES 1 stromal tumors of uncertain behavior of digestive system (D48.1)

5 D37.0 Neoplasm of uncertain behavior of lip, oral cavity and pharynx
EXCLUDES 1 neoplasm of uncertain behavior of aryepiglottic fold or interarytenoid fold, laryngeal aspect (D38.0)
neoplasm of uncertain behavior of epiglottis NOS (D38.0)
neoplasm of uncertain behavior of skin of lip (D48.5)
neoplasm of uncertain behavior of suprahyoid portion of epiglottis (D38.0)

---

4 4th digit required   **5** 5th digit required   **6** 6th digit required   **7** 7th digit required   **7** 7th digit placeholder   **✚** Additional code   **⬛** Laterality

Chapter 2

C00-D49

SP D37.01 **Neoplasm of uncertain behavior of lip**
Neoplasm of uncertain behavior of vermilion border of lip

SP D37.02 **Neoplasm of uncertain behavior of tongue**

6 D37.03 **Neoplasm of uncertain behavior of the major salivary glands**

SP D37.030 **Neoplasm of uncertain behavior of the parotid salivary glands**

SP D37.031 **Neoplasm of uncertain behavior of the sublingual salivary glands**

SP D37.032 **Neoplasm of uncertain behavior of the submandibular salivary glands**

SP D37.039 **Neoplasm of uncertain behavior of the major salivary glands, unspecified**

SP D37.04 **Neoplasm of uncertain behavior of the minor salivary glands**
Neoplasm of uncertain behavior of submucosal salivary glands of lip
Neoplasm of uncertain behavior of submucosal salivary glands of cheek
Neoplasm of uncertain behavior of submucosal salivary glands of hard palate
Neoplasm of uncertain behavior of submucosal salivary glands of soft palate

SP D37.05 **Neoplasm of uncertain behavior of pharynx**
Neoplasm of uncertain behavior of aryepiglottic fold of pharynx NOS
Neoplasm of uncertain behavior of hypopharyngeal aspect of aryepiglottic fold of pharynx
Neoplasm of uncertain behavior of marginal zone of aryepiglottic fold of pharynx

SP D37.09 **Neoplasm of uncertain behavior of other specified sites of the oral cavity**

SP D37.1 **Neoplasm of uncertain behavior of stomach**

SP D37.2 **Neoplasm of uncertain behavior of small intestine**

SP D37.3 **Neoplasm of uncertain behavior of appendix**

SP D37.4 **Neoplasm of uncertain behavior of colon**

SP D37.5 **Neoplasm of uncertain behavior of rectum**
Neoplasm of uncertain behavior of rectosigmoid junction

SP D37.6 **Neoplasm of uncertain behavior of liver, gallbladder and bile ducts**
Neoplasm of uncertain behavior of ampulla of Vater

SP D37.8 **Neoplasm of uncertain behavior of other specified digestive organs**
Neoplasm of uncertain behavior of anal canal
Neoplasm of uncertain behavior of anal sphincter
Neoplasm of uncertain behavior of anus NOS
Neoplasm of uncertain behavior of esophagus

Neoplasm of uncertain behavior of intestine NOS
Neoplasm of uncertain behavior of pancreas
EXCLUDES 1 neoplasm of uncertain behavior of anal margin (D48.5)
neoplasm of uncertain behavior of anal skin (D48.5)
neoplasm of uncertain behavior of perianal skin (D48.5)

IQ D37.9 **Neoplasm of uncertain behavior of digestive organ, unspecified**

4 D38 **Neoplasm of uncertain behavior of middle ear and respiratory and intrathoracic organs**
EXCLUDES 1 neoplasm of uncertain behavior of heart (D48.7)

SP D38.0 **Neoplasm of uncertain behavior of larynx**
Neoplasm of uncertain behavior of aryepiglottic fold or interarytenoid fold, laryngeal aspect
Neoplasm of uncertain behavior of epiglottis (suprahyoid portion)
EXCLUDES 1 neoplasm of uncertain behavior of aryepiglottic fold or interarytenoid fold NOS (D37.05)
neoplasm of uncertain behavior of hypopharyngeal aspect of aryepiglottic fold (D37.05)
neoplasm of uncertain behavior of marginal zone of aryepiglottic fold (D37.05)

SP D38.1 **Neoplasm of uncertain behavior of trachea, bronchus and lung**

SP D38.2 **Neoplasm of uncertain behavior of pleura**

SP D38.3 **Neoplasm of uncertain behavior of mediastinum**

SP D38.4 **Neoplasm of uncertain behavior of thymus**

SP D38.5 **Neoplasm of uncertain behavior of other respiratory organs**
Neoplasm of uncertain behavior of accessory sinuses
Neoplasm of uncertain behavior of cartilage of nose
Neoplasm of uncertain behavior of middle ear
Neoplasm of uncertain behavior of nasal cavities
EXCLUDES 1 neoplasm of uncertain behavior of ear (external) (skin) (D48.5)
neoplasm of uncertain behavior of nose NOS (D48.7)
neoplasm of uncertain behavior of skin of nose (D48.5)

IQ D38.6 **Neoplasm of uncertain behavior of respiratory organ, unspecified**

★ New ▲ Revised **Px** Primary **SP** PDGM Px **SL** Low CoM **SH** High CoM **IQ** Quest. Encounter **H** Hospice non-cancer Dx   Unspecified   **M** *Manifestation*

4 D39   Neoplasm of uncertain behavior of female genital organs

SP D39.0   Neoplasm of uncertain behavior of uterus

+ 5 D39.1   Neoplasm of uncertain behavior of ovary
Use additional code to identify any functional activity.

⊟ IQ + D39.10   Neoplasm of uncertain behavior of unspecified ovary

⊟ SP + D39.11   Neoplasm of uncertain behavior of right ovary

⊟ SP + D39.12   Neoplasm of uncertain behavior of left ovary

SP D39.2   Neoplasm of uncertain behavior of placenta
Chorioadenoma destruens
Invasive hydatidiform mole
Malignant hydatidiform mole
> **EXCLUDES 1** hydatidiform mole NOS (O01.9)

SP D39.8   Neoplasm of uncertain behavior of other specified female genital organs
Neoplasm of uncertain behavior of skin of female genital organs

IQ D39.9   Neoplasm of uncertain behavior of female genital organ, unspecified

4 D40   Neoplasm of uncertain behavior of male genital organs

SP D40.0   Neoplasm of uncertain behavior of prostate

5 D40.1   Neoplasm of uncertain behavior of testis

⊟ IQ D40.10   Neoplasm of uncertain behavior of unspecified testis

⊟ SP D40.11   Neoplasm of uncertain behavior of right testis

⊟ SP D40.12   Neoplasm of uncertain behavior of left testis

SP D40.8   Neoplasm of uncertain behavior of other specified male genital organs
Neoplasm of uncertain behavior of skin of male genital organs

IQ D40.9   Neoplasm of uncertain behavior of male genital organ, unspecified

4 D41   Neoplasm of uncertain behavior of urinary organs

5 D41.0   Neoplasm of uncertain behavior of kidney
> **EXCLUDES 1** neoplasm of uncertain behavior of renal pelvis (D41.1-)

⊟ IQ D41.00   Neoplasm of uncertain behavior of unspecified kidney

⊟ SP D41.01   Neoplasm of uncertain behavior of right kidney

⊟ SP D41.02   Neoplasm of uncertain behavior of left kidney

5 D41.1   Neoplasm of uncertain behavior of renal pelvis

⊟ IQ D41.10   Neoplasm of uncertain behavior of unspecified renal pelvis

⊟ SP D41.11   Neoplasm of uncertain behavior of right renal pelvis

⊟ SP D41.12   Neoplasm of uncertain behavior of left renal pelvis

5 D41.2   Neoplasm of uncertain behavior of ureter

⊟ IQ D41.20   Neoplasm of uncertain behavior of unspecified ureter

⊟ SP D41.21   Neoplasm of uncertain behavior of right ureter

⊟ SP D41.22   Neoplasm of uncertain behavior of left ureter

SP D41.3   Neoplasm of uncertain behavior of urethra

SP D41.4   Neoplasm of uncertain behavior of bladder

SP D41.8   Neoplasm of uncertain behavior of other specified urinary organs

IQ D41.9   Neoplasm of uncertain behavior of unspecified urinary organ

4 D42   Neoplasm of uncertain behavior of meninges

SP D42.0   Neoplasm of uncertain behavior of cerebral meninges

SP D42.1   Neoplasm of uncertain behavior of spinal meninges

SP D42.9   Neoplasm of uncertain behavior of meninges, unspecified

4 D43   Neoplasm of uncertain behavior of brain and central nervous system
> **EXCLUDES 1** neoplasm of uncertain behavior of peripheral nerves and autonomic nervous system (D48.2)

SP D43.0   Neoplasm of uncertain behavior of brain, supratentorial
Neoplasm of uncertain behavior of cerebral ventricle
Neoplasm of uncertain behavior of cerebrum
Neoplasm of uncertain behavior of frontal lobe
Neoplasm of uncertain behavior of occipital lobe
Neoplasm of uncertain behavior of parietal lobe
Neoplasm of uncertain behavior of temporal lobe
> **EXCLUDES 1** neoplasm of uncertain behavior of fourth ventricle (D43.1)

SP D43.1   Neoplasm of uncertain behavior of brain, infratentorial
Neoplasm of uncertain behavior of brain stem
Neoplasm of uncertain behavior of cerebellum
Neoplasm of uncertain behavior of fourth ventricle

SP D43.2   Neoplasm of uncertain behavior of brain, unspecified

SP D43.3   Neoplasm of uncertain behavior of cranial nerves

SP D43.4   Neoplasm of uncertain behavior of spinal cord

SP D43.8   Neoplasm of uncertain behavior of other specified parts of central nervous system

IQ D43.9   Neoplasm of uncertain behavior of central nervous system, unspecified
Neoplasm of uncertain behavior of nervous system (central) NOS

4 D44   Neoplasm of uncertain behavior of endocrine glands

---

4 4th digit required   5 5th digit required   6 6th digit required   7 7th digit required   7 7th digit placeholder   + Additional code   ⊟ Laterality

EXCLUDES 1 multiple endocrine
adenomatosis (E31.2-)
multiple endocrine neoplasia
(E31.2-)
neoplasm of uncertain behavior
of endocrine pancreas
(D37.8)
neoplasm of uncertain behavior
of ovary (D39.1-)
neoplasm of uncertain behavior
of testis (D40.1-)
neoplasm of uncertain behavior
of thymus (D38.4)

SP D44.0 Neoplasm of uncertain behavior of
thyroid gland

+ 5 D44.1 Neoplasm of uncertain behavior of
adrenal gland
Use additional code to identify any
functional activity.

⊟ IQ + D44.10 Neoplasm of uncertain behavior of
unspecified adrenal gland

⊟ SP + D44.11 Neoplasm of uncertain behavior of
right adrenal gland

⊟ SP + D44.12 Neoplasm of uncertain behavior of
left adrenal gland

SP D44.2 Neoplasm of uncertain behavior of
parathyroid gland

SP + D44.3 Neoplasm of uncertain behavior of
pituitary gland
Use additional code to identify any
functional activity.

SP D44.4 Neoplasm of uncertain behavior of
craniopharyngeal duct

SP D44.5 Neoplasm of uncertain behavior of
pineal gland

SP D44.6 Neoplasm of uncertain behavior of
carotid body

SP D44.7 Neoplasm of uncertain behavior of
aortic body and other paraganglia

IQ D44.9 Neoplasm of uncertain behavior of
unspecified endocrine gland

SP D45 Polycythemia vera
EXCLUDES 1 familial polycythemia (D75.0)
secondary polycythemia
(D75.1)

+ 4 D46 Myelodysplastic syndromes
Use additional code for adverse effect, if
applicable, to identify drug (T36-T50 with
fifth or sixth character 5)
EXCLUDES 2 drug-induced aplastic anemia
(D61.1)

SP + D46.0 Refractory anemia without ring
sideroblasts, so stated
Refractory anemia without sideroblasts,
without excess of blasts

SP + D46.1 Refractory anemia with ring
sideroblasts
RARS

+ 5 D46.2 Refractory anemia with excess of blasts
[RAEB]

SP + D46.20 Refractory anemia with excess of
blasts, unspecified
RAEB NOS

SP + D46.21 Refractory anemia with excess of
blasts 1
RAEB 1

SP + D46.22 Refractory anemia with excess of
blasts 2

RAEB 2

SP + D46.A Refractory cytopenia with multilineage
dysplasia

SP + D46.B Refractory cytopenia with multilineage
dysplasia and ring sideroblasts
RCMD RS

SP + D46.C Myelodysplastic syndrome with isolated
del(5q) chromosomal abnormality
Myelodysplastic syndrome with 5q
deletion
5q minus syndrome NOS

SP + D46.4 Refractory anemia, unspecified

SP + D46.Z Other myelodysplastic syndromes
EXCLUDES 1 chronic myelomonocytic
leukemia (C93.1-)

SP + D46.9 Myelodysplastic syndrome, unspecified
Myelodysplasia NOS

4 D47 Other neoplasms of uncertain behavior of
lymphoid, hematopoietic and related tissue

5 D47.0 Mast cell neoplasms of uncertain
behavior
EXCLUDES 1 congenital cutaneous
mastocytosis (Q82.2)
histiocytic neoplasms of
uncertain behavior
(D47.Z9)
malignant mast cell
neoplasm (C96.2-)

SP D47.01 Cutaneous mastocytosis
Diffuse cutaneous mastocytosis
Maculopapular cutaneous mastocytosis
Solitary mastocytoma
Telangiectasia macularis eruptiva
perstans
Urticaria pigmentosa
EXCLUDES 1 congenital (diffuse)
(maculopapular)
cutaneous mastocytosis
(Q82.2)
congenital urticaria
pigmentosa (Q82.2)
extracutaneous
mastocytoma (D47.09)

SP D47.02 Systemic mastocytosis
Indolent systemic mastocytosis
Isolated bone marrow mastocytosis
Smoldering systemic mastocytosis
Systemic mastocytosis, with an
associated hematological non-mast
cell lineage disease (SM-AHNMD)
Code also, if applicable, any associated
hematological non-mast cell lineage
disease, such as:
acute myeloid leukemia
(C92.6-, C92.A-)
chronic myelomonocytic leukemia
(C93.1-)
essential thrombocytosis (D47.3)
hypereosinophilic syndrome (D72.1)
myelodysplastic syndrome (D46.9)
myeloproliferative syndrome
(D47.1)
non-Hodgkin lymphoma (C82-C85)
plasma cell myeloma (C90.0-)
polycythemia vera (D45)
EXCLUDES 1 aggressive systemic
mastocytosis (C96.21)

★ New ▲ Revised **Px** Primary **SP** PDGM Px **SL** Low CoM **SH** High CoM **IQ** Quest. Encounter **H** Hospice non-cancer Dx Unspecified **M** *Manifestation*

mast cell leukemia
(C94.3-)

SP D47.09 Other mast cell neoplasms of uncertain behavior
Extracutaneous mastocytoma
Mast cell tumor NOS
Mastocytoma NOS
Mastocytosis NOS

SP D47.1 Chronic myeloproliferative disease
Chronic neutrophilic leukemia
Myeloproliferative disease, unspecified
> **EXCLUDES 1** atypical chronic myeloid leukemia BCR/ABL-negative (C92.2-)
> chronic myeloid leukemia BCR/ABL-positive (C92.1-)
> myelofibrosis NOS (D75.81)
> myelophthisic anemia (D61.82)
> myelophthisis (D61.82)
> secondary myelofibrosis NOS (D75.81)

SP D47.2 Monoclonal gammopathy
Monoclonal gammopathy of undetermined significance [MGUS]

SP D47.3 Essential (hemorrhagic) thrombocythemia
Essential thrombocytosis
Idiopathic hemorrhagic thrombocythemia
> **DEFINITION** Rare myeloproliferative disorder characterized by uncontrolled over-production of blood platelet precursor cells, leading to splenomegaly, hemorrhaging from the intestines, gums, or nose, and blood vessel thrombosis.

SP D47.4 Osteomyelofibrosis
Chronic idiopathic myelofibrosis
Myelofibrosis (idiopathic) (with myeloid metaplasia)
Myelosclerosis (megakaryocytic) with myeloid metaplasia
Secondary myelofibrosis in myeloproliferative disease
> **EXCLUDES 1** acute myelofibrosis (C94.4-)

5 D47.Z Other specified neoplasms of uncertain behavior of lymphoid, hematopoietic and related tissue

SP D47.Z1 Post-transplant lymphoproliferative disorder (PTLD)
Code first:
complications of transplanted organs and tissue (T86.-)

SP D47.Z2 Castleman disease
Code also:
if applicable human herpesvirus 8 infection (B10.89)
> **EXCLUDES 2** Kaposi's sarcoma (C46-)

SP D47.Z9 Other specified neoplasms of uncertain behavior of lymphoid, hematopoietic and related tissue
Histiocytic tumors of uncertain behavior

SP D47.9 Neoplasm of uncertain behavior of lymphoid, hematopoietic and related tissue, unspecified
Lymphoproliferative disease NOS

4 D48 Neoplasm of uncertain behavior of other and unspecified sites
> **EXCLUDES 1** neurofibromatosis (nonmalignant) (Q85.0-)

SP D48.0 Neoplasm of uncertain behavior of bone and articular cartilage
> **EXCLUDES 1** neoplasm of uncertain behavior of cartilage of ear (D48.1)
> neoplasm of uncertain behavior of cartilage of larynx (D38.0)
> neoplasm of uncertain behavior of cartilage of nose (D38.5)
> neoplasm of uncertain behavior of connective tissue of eyelid (D48.1)
> neoplasm of uncertain behavior of synovia (D48.1)

SP D48.1 Neoplasm of uncertain behavior of connective and other soft tissue
Neoplasm of uncertain behavior of connective tissue of ear
Neoplasm of uncertain behavior of connective tissue of eyelid
Stromal tumors of uncertain behavior of digestive system
> **EXCLUDES 1** neoplasm of uncertain behavior of articular cartilage (D48.0)
> neoplasm of uncertain behavior of cartilage of larynx (D38.0)
> neoplasm of uncertain behavior of cartilage of nose (D38.5)
> neoplasm of uncertain behavior of connective tissue of breast (D48.6-)

SP D48.2 Neoplasm of uncertain behavior of peripheral nerves and autonomic nervous system
> **EXCLUDES 1** neoplasm of uncertain behavior of peripheral nerves of orbit (D48.7)

SP D48.3 Neoplasm of uncertain behavior of retroperitoneum

SP D48.4 Neoplasm of uncertain behavior of peritoneum

SP D48.5 Neoplasm of uncertain behavior of skin
Neoplasm of uncertain behavior of anal margin
Neoplasm of uncertain behavior of anal skin
Neoplasm of uncertain behavior of perianal skin
Neoplasm of uncertain behavior of skin of breast
> **EXCLUDES 1** neoplasm of uncertain behavior of anus NOS (D37.8)
> neoplasm of uncertain behavior of skin of genital organs (D39.8, D40.8)
> neoplasm of uncertain behavior of vermilion border of lip (D37.0)

---

4 4th digit required   **5** 5th digit required   **6** 6th digit required   **7** 7th digit required   **7** 7th digit placeholder   **+** Additional code   **=** Laterality

696   *DecisionHealth's* FY 2020 Complete Home Health ICD-10-CM Diagnosis Coding Manual

Chapter 2

C00-D49

5 **D48.6 Neoplasm of uncertain behavior of breast**
Neoplasm of uncertain behavior of connective tissue of breast
Cystosarcoma phyllodes
> EXCLUDES 1 neoplasm of uncertain behavior of skin of breast (D48.5)

☐ IQ **D48.60 Neoplasm of uncertain behavior of unspecified breast**

☐ SP **D48.61 Neoplasm of uncertain behavior of right breast**

☐ SP **D48.62 Neoplasm of uncertain behavior of left breast**

SP **D48.7 Neoplasm of uncertain behavior of other specified sites**
Neoplasm of uncertain behavior of eye
Neoplasm of uncertain behavior of heart
Neoplasm of uncertain behavior of peripheral nerves of orbit
> EXCLUDES 1 neoplasm of uncertain behavior of connective tissue (D48.1)
> neoplasm of uncertain behavior of skin of eyelid (D48.5)

IQ **D48.9 Neoplasm of uncertain behavior, unspecified**

Neoplasms of unspecified behavior (D49)

CODING TIPS ✓ Codes classifiable to D49 include tumors that have not been defined as malignant or benign. The term 'mass' should not be interpreted to mean unspecified behavior. The physician should be queried to determine whether neoplasm codes are applicable.

4 **D49 Neoplasms of unspecified behavior**
Note:
Category D49 classifies by site neoplasms of unspecified morphology and behavior. The term 'mass', unless otherwise stated, is not to be regarded as a neoplastic growth.
> INCLUDES 'growth' NOS
> neoplasm NOS
> new growth NOS
> tumor NOS
> EXCLUDES 1 neoplasms of uncertain behavior (D37-D44, D48)

SP **D49.0 Neoplasm of unspecified behavior of digestive system**
> EXCLUDES 1 neoplasm of unspecified behavior of margin of anus (D49.2)
> neoplasm of unspecified behavior of perianal skin (D49.2)
> neoplasm of unspecified behavior of skin of anus (D49.2)

SP **D49.1 Neoplasm of unspecified behavior of respiratory system**

SP **D49.2 Neoplasm of unspecified behavior of bone, soft tissue, and skin**
> EXCLUDES 1 neoplasm of unspecified behavior of anal canal (D49.0)

neoplasm of unspecified behavior of anus NOS (D49.0)
neoplasm of unspecified behavior of bone marrow (D49.89)
neoplasm of unspecified behavior of cartilage of larynx (D49.1)
neoplasm of unspecified behavior of cartilage of nose (D49.1)
neoplasm of unspecified behavior of connective tissue of breast (D49.3)
neoplasm of unspecified behavior of skin of genital organs (D49.59)
neoplasm of unspecified behavior of vermilion border of lip (D49.0)

SP **D49.3 Neoplasm of unspecified behavior of breast**
> EXCLUDES 1 neoplasm of unspecified behavior of skin of breast (D49.2)

SP **D49.4 Neoplasm of unspecified behavior of bladder**

5 **D49.5 Neoplasm of unspecified behavior of other genitourinary organs**

6 **D49.51 Neoplasm of unspecified behavior of kidney**

☐ SP **D49.511 Neoplasm of unspecified behavior of right kidney**

☐ SP **D49.512 Neoplasm of unspecified behavior of left kidney**

☐ IQ **D49.519 Neoplasm of unspecified behavior of unspecified kidney**

SP **D49.59 Neoplasm of unspecified behavior of other genitourinary organ**

SP **D49.6 Neoplasm of unspecified behavior of brain**
> EXCLUDES 1 neoplasm of unspecified behavior of cerebral meninges (D49.7)
> neoplasm of unspecified behavior of cranial nerves (D49.7)

SP **D49.7 Neoplasm of unspecified behavior of endocrine glands and other parts of nervous system**
> EXCLUDES 1 neoplasm of unspecified behavior of peripheral, sympathetic, and parasympathetic nerves and ganglia (D49.2)

5 **D49.8 Neoplasm of unspecified behavior of other specified sites**
> EXCLUDES 1 neoplasm of unspecified behavior of eyelid (skin) (D49.2)
> neoplasm of unspecified behavior of eyelid cartilage (D49.2)
> neoplasm of unspecified behavior of great vessels (D49.2)

★ New ▲ Revised Px Primary SP PDGM Px SL Low CoM SH High CoM IQ Quest. Encounter H Hospice non-cancer Dx Unspecified M Manifestation

DecisionHealth's FY 2020 Complete Home Health ICD-10-CM Diagnosis Coding Manual

697

Chapter 2

C00-D49

> neoplasm of unspecified
> behavior of optic nerve
> (D49.7)

SP D49.81 **Neoplasm of unspecified behavior of retina and choroid**

Dark area on retina
Retinal freckle

SP D49.89 **Neoplasm of unspecified behavior of other specified sites**

IQ D49.9 **Neoplasm of unspecified behavior of unspecified site**

4 4th digit required   **5** 5th digit required   **6** 6th digit required   **7** 7th digit required   **7** 7th digit placeholder   **+** Additional code   **⊟** Laterality

698   *DecisionHealth's* FY 2020 Complete Home Health ICD-10-CM Diagnosis Coding Manual

Chapter 2 Scenarios: Neoplasms (C00-D49)

Lung cancer, dressing changes, drain care

Your patient had a pneumonectomy for cancer of the left lower lobe of the lung. He also has a stage 1 pressure ulcer/injury on the right heel, diabetes and congestive heart failure (CHF). He was referred to home health for aftercare, dressing changes, care of a surgical drain, and teaching of oxygen safety since he is receiving oxygen intermittently at 2 liters/minute. The patient will begin chemotherapy in two weeks.

Description	Code
Primary: Aftercare following surgery for neoplasm	Z48.3
Secondary: Malignant neoplasm of lower lobe, left bronchus of lung	C34.32
Secondary: Pressure ulcer of right heel, Stage 1	L89.611
Secondary: Type 2 diabetes mellitus without complications	E11.9
Secondary: Heart failure, unspecified	I50.9
Secondary: Dependence on supplemental oxygen	Z99.81
Secondary: Acquired absence of lung [part of]	Z90.2

If documentation is present that indicates that the lung cancer is eradicated and requires no further treatment, then the cancer will not be reported as an active diagnosis. However, this patient is still under treatment for his lung cancer, so the cancer is coded. The drain care is included in the aftercare code (Z48.3). There is no indication here that the comorbidities are unstable, so they are coded lower than the active lung cancer and pressure ulcer/injury. Note, Z90.2 includes any part of the lung.

Anemia due to neoplasm

A patient is admitted to home care for management of anemia due to a malignant carcinoid tumor of the stomach.

Description	Code
Primary: Malignant carcinoid tumor of stomach	C7A.092
Secondary: Anemia in neoplastic disease	D63.0

When the admission/encounter is for management of anemia associated with the malignancy and the treatment is only for anemia, the appropriate code for the malignancy is sequenced as the principal or first-listed diagnosis, followed by the appropriate code for the anemia, according to coding guidelines. The coder will see a "code first" note in the Tabular section under the anemia code. Also, note that carcinoid tumors are not listed in the Neoplasm Table. Reference the Index under "Tumor, carcinoid." In the Tabular List, these are not listed in chronological order. They are found after C75.9 as Malignant neuroendocrine tumors (C7A). *[I.C.2.c.1]*

Cancer and hypertension

Your patient has hypertension due to a primary malignant neoplasm of the brain. The focus of care for the patient is the neoplasm.

Description	Code
Primary: Malignant neoplasm of brain, unspecified	C71.9
Secondary: Other secondary hypertension	I15.8

Sequencing is based on the focus of care for the encounter, which is the brain neoplasm in this case. Per official coding guidelines: "If the reason for the encounter is for treatment of a primary malignancy, assign the malignancy as the principal/first-listed diagnosis." *[I.C.2.l.1]*

Dehydration due to neoplasm

A patient who has a primary malignant neoplasm of the lower outer quadrant of her right breast was referred to home care for IV hydration due to severe dehydration that is described as a complication of the neoplasm.

Description	Code
Primary: Dehydration	E86.0
Secondary: Malignant neoplasm of lower-outer quadrant of right female breast	C50.511
Secondary: Encounter for adjustment and management of vascular access device	Z45.2

The dehydration is the focus of care and should, therefore, be coded as the primary diagnosis. Per official coding guidelines: "When the admission/encounter is for management of dehydration due to the malignancy and only the dehydration is being treated (intravenous rehydration), the dehydration is sequenced first, followed by the code(s) for the malignancy." *[I.C.2.c.3]*

Secondary bone cancer and pathological fracture

A patient has a history of prostate cancer that has metastasized to the right femur where it's caused a pathological fracture. He is admitted to home health for nursing and therapy, which will provide routine care of the pathological right femur fracture, which is the focus of care and is healing normally, as well as observation and assessment, strengthening, transfers and pain management. His dosage of morphine, which he has been taking for his neoplasm-related pain, was increased.

Description	Code
Primary: Pathological fracture in neoplastic disease, right femur, subsequent encounter with routine healing	M84.551D
Secondary: Secondary malignant neoplasm, bone	C79.51
Secondary: Neoplasm related pain	G89.3
Secondary: History of prostate cancer	Z85.46
Secondary: Long-term (current) use of opiate analgesic	Z79.891

When an encounter is for a pathological fracture due to a neoplasm and the focus of treatment is the fracture, a code from subcategory M84.5- (Pathological fracture in neoplastic disease) should be sequenced first, followed by the code for the neoplasm, according to coding guidelines. That is the case here and thus M84.551D is assigned in the primary position. Note as well as a seventh character is required to describe the timing of the encounter, such as initial, subsequent or sequela. This is expanded further for fractures to include routine or delayed healing, nonunion or malunion. Routine care for a normally healing fracture is the case here, and thus "D" is the appropriate seventh character. Additional codes are assigned for his neoplasm-related pain, his personal history of prostate cancer and his long-term use of morphine. Do NOT use a code for opioid use from Chapter 5 such as F11.90 in this scenario; these codes should not be assigned without physician documentation of an associated physical, mental or behavioral disorder, according to Q2 2018 Coding Clinic guidance.*[I.C.2.1.6]*

Hodgkin's lymphoma

A 65-year-old man was recently diagnosed with Hodgkin's lymphoma of the lymph nodes of his neck. He is undergoing treatment. He also has hypertension and type 2 diabetes and was admitted to home health for teaching on the disease process and management of new medications.

Description	Code
Primary: Hodgkin lymphoma, unspecified, lymph nodes of head, face, and neck	C81.91
Secondary: Type 2 diabetes mellitus without complications	E11.9
Secondary: Essential (primary) hypertension	I10

As the focus of care, the Hodgkin's lymphoma is coded primary. The lymphoma is affecting the lymph nodes of his neck, so the more specific code C81.91 is assigned. The type 2 diabetes and hypertension are important comorbidities that should be coded even if they're not the focus of care.

HOME HEALTH CODING SCENARIOS

Exacerbated obstructive bronchitis, sessile serrated polyp of the ascending colon

A 78-year-old woman was recently hospitalized for an exacerbation of her chronic obstructive bronchitis. She is admitted to home health to continue her recovery and to teach on and monitor new medications. She also has a sessile serrated polyp of the ascending colon, which her physician wants to monitor but not treat at this time. She also has diabetic polyneuropathy with insulin dependence.

Description	Code
Primary: Chronic obstructive pulmonary disease with (acute) exacerbation	J44.1
Secondary: Benign neoplasm of ascending colon	D12.2
Secondary: Type 2 diabetes mellitus with diabetic polyneuropathy	E11.42
Secondary: Long term (current) use of insulin	Z79.4

The focus of the home health admission is the exacerbated chronic obstructive bronchitis, so that diagnosis is coded primary. The patient also has a sessile serrated polyp of the ascending colon, which is not malignant but can be pre-cancerous and should be coded with D12.2, according to Q2 2018 Coding Clinic guidance. The polyp will require monitoring but isn't the focus of care and thus is coded as a secondary diagnosis. Her diabetic polyneuropathy has the potential to impact her plan of care and is thus also coded. Because she is dependent on insulin but not stated to be a type 1 diabetic, the code for insulin use must be assigned as well.

Aftercare following mastectomy

A 68-year-old female is admitted to home health post-mastectomy of her left breast due to breast cancer of the lower outer quadrant of her left breast. She will begin chemo once the incision is healed. Medical records state she is estrogen receptor positive. The focus of skilled nursing is surgical aftercare and instruction related to the breast cancer.

Description	Code
Primary: Aftercare following surgery for neoplasm	Z48.3
Secondary: Malignant neoplasm of lower-outer quadrant of left female breast	C50.512
Secondary: Estrogen receptor positive status [ER+]	Z17.0
Secondary: Acquired absence of left breast and nipple	Z90.12

The patient is admitted to home health for surgical aftercare following her mastectomy procedure. Her cancer remains under treatment and thus is still coded. Additional Z codes are assigned to capture that she is estrogen receptor positive, which is relevant to her breast cancer diagnosis, and a status code indicating her left breast is now absent following the mastectomy.

Open wounds from lymphoma

A 61-year-old man is admitted to home health following the initial phase of treatment in the hospital for B-cell lymphoma in the lymph nodes of his neck. The lymphoma has caused open wounds on his neck and upper chest, which will require wound care. He also has hypertension and coronary artery disease. The lymphoma and the open wounds are the focus of care.

Description	Code
Primary: Unspecified B-cell lymphoma, lymph nodes of head, face, and neck	C85.11
Secondary: Atherosclerotic heart disease of native coronary artery without angina pectoris	I25.10
Secondary: Essential (primary) hypertension	I10

Since the open wounds were caused by the lymphoma, no additional code is necessary as the lymphoma code covers both conditions. As the focus of care, it is coded primary. Coronary artery disease and hypertension are relevant comorbidities that will require monitoring and so are also coded. Note the ICD-10 classification does not assume a relationship between hypertension and coronary artery disease.

Malignant ascites, lung cancer

A 70-year-old man is admitted to home health for management of malignant ascites caused by cancer in the upper lobe of his right lung. His medical record indicates that he's been a cigarette smoker for the past 30 years and continues to smoke despite his illness.

Description	Code
Primary: Malignant neoplasm of upper lobe, right bronchus or lung	C34.11
Secondary: Malignant ascites	R18.0
Secondary: Nicotine dependence, cigarettes, uncomplicated	F17.210

Though the focus of care is the malignant ascites, there is a "code first" note at R18.0 that says to code the malignancy first. Thus, C34.11 is coded in the primary position. Note that in PDGM, incorrectly coding R18.0 in the ***primary*** position will cause the claim to be sent back to be re-coded. The fact that the patient is a smoker is coded, in accordance with tabular instruction at C34.11. "Smoker" codes to nicotine dependence in the alphabetic index.

Melanoma of eyelid, metastases to brain, liver

An 87-year-old woman comes to home health with a primary diagnosis of metastatic melanoma. The primary site was her left upper eyelid and it has metastasized to her brain and liver. The secondary sites are the focus of care.

Description	Code
Primary: Secondary malignant neoplasm of brain	C79.31
Secondary: Secondary malignant neoplasm of liver and intrahepatic bile duct	C78.7
Secondary: Malignant melanoma of left upper eyelid, including canthus	C43.121

As the focus of care, the secondary neoplasms are coded as the primary diagnosis and the first additional diagnosis. The primary site is coded as an additional secondary diagnosis, in accordance with coding guidelines. *[I.C.2.b]*

HOME HEALTH CODING SCENARIOS

Malignant pericardial effusion, metastatic melanoma

A 79-year-old woman comes to home health for management of malignant pericardial effusion that's causing her symptoms of shortness of breath and fatigue. The cause of the pericardial effusion is documented as metastatic melanoma that began on her forehead and spread to both of her lungs, and her liver and brain.

Description	Code
Primary: Pericardial effusion (noninflammatory)	I31.3
Secondary: Secondary malignant neoplasm of right lung	C78.01
Secondary: Secondary malignant neoplasm of left lung	C78.02
Secondary: Secondary malignant neoplasm of liver and intrahepatic bile duct	C78.7
Secondary: Secondary malignant neoplasm of brain	C79.31
Secondary: Malignant melanoma of other parts of face	C43.39

Malignant pericardial effusion caused by cancer should be captured first with the I31.3, then the codes for the cancer, according to Q1 2019 Coding Clinic guidance. Thus, I31.3 is assigned first, followed by the codes for each of the secondary sites of the metastatic disease, because the metastatic disease is the cause of the pericardial effusion, as well as the primary site. Her symptoms of shortness of breath and fatigue are not separately coded as they are integral to pericardial effusion and are thus included in I31.3.

Chapter 3: Diseases of Blood and Blood-Forming Organs and Certain Disorders Involving the Immune Mechanism (D50 –D89)

This chapter includes five primary categories of conditions, including:

- nutritional, hemolytic and aplastic and other forms of anemia, as well as other bone marrow failure syndromes (D50-D64)

- coagulation defects, purpura and other hemorrhagic conditions (D65- D69)

- Other disorders of blood and blood-forming organs (D70-D77)

- Intraoperative and post-procedural complications of the spleen (D78)

- Certain disorders involving the immune mechanism (D80-D89)

The term "blood-forming organs" refers to the spleen, bone marrow and lymph nodes. Codes from this chapter refer to elements within the blood, such as red blood cells (erythrocytes); white blood cells (leukocytes, lymphocytes, neutrophils, eosinophils, monocytes and basophils); and thrombocytes (platelets or clotting cells).

Sometimes a Chapter 3 code isn't the most appropriate choice. Here are a few situations to watch out for:

- If the documentation indicates a **neoplasm or tumor of a blood-forming organ or of the blood**, coders should look up the term (malignancy, tumor, and adenoma) to find the correct code, most likely a code from Chapter 2.

- If a patient has a **personal or family history of a condition** reported in this chapter, it may be appropriate to select from the Z code section, such as Z85.6 (personal history of leukemia) or Z86.2 (personal history of diseases of the blood and blood-forming organs and certain disorders involving the immune mechanism).

- If a condition reported in this chapter is the **result of injury**, a code from Chapter 19 (Injury, poisoning and certain other consequences of external causes) may be reported, such as a contusion of the spleen (S36.02-), along with a code from this chapter.

- **Symptoms related to blood** are sometimes reported using codes from Chapter 18 (Symptoms, signs and laboratory findings, not elsewhere classified), such as precipitous drop in hematocrit (R71.0) or elevated erythrocyte sedimentation rate (R70.0). Every effort should be made to secure a definitive diagnosis.

- Although rarely coded in home health, if reporting diseases of the blood and blood-forming organs in a **pregnant patient**, when the condition is complicating the pregnancy, report first a code from Chapter 15, such as O99.01- (anemia complicating pregnancy) or O46.00- (antepartum hemorrhage with coagulation defect, unspecified) as the first-listed diagnosis, and a code from this chapter as an additional diagnosis.

Multiple Coding and Sequencing

Codes in this chapter can be either primary or additional diagnoses, depending on the focus of care.

It is important to read the Includes and Excludes notes under codes in this chapter, as well as any other instructions under the code or code category. Here are some examples of multiple coding and sequencing issues for codes in this chapter. Code D57.81- (other sickle-cell disorder with crisis) includes the statement "Use additional code for any associated fever (R50.81)." Therefore, D57.81 is coded first followed by the "fever" code. Another example is code D61.82 (myelophthisis), which includes the statement "Code also the underlying disorder, such a malignant neoplasm of breast (C50-); Tuberculosis (A15-)." Therefore, a code for the neoplasm or tuberculosis is sequenced first, followed by the D61.82 code.

Special Coding Issues

Anemia

Anemia (decrease in either red blood cells or hemoglobin) may be caused by other conditions, such as chronic infections (osteomyelitis, hepatitis, infective endocarditis, tuberculosis, chronic urinary tract infection); inflammatory disorders (rheumatoid disease, burns, systemic lupus erythematosus); and cancer and chronic renal failure. Reporting these conditions requires two codes. For example, anemia in chronic kidney disease (D63.1) has a note to code first underlying chronic kidney disease (N18-).

Anemia may also be related to a malignancy or be the result of treatment for a malignancy. In this situation, there is also a "code first underlying neoplasm" note that applies even when the anemia is the focus of care.

Take note of these three situations and their sequencing rules:

- When the admission/encounter is for management of anemia associated with (or caused by) the malignancy, even if the only treatment is for the anemia, the appropriate code for the malignancy is sequenced as the principal or first-listed diagnosis, followed by the appropriate code for the anemia (such as code D63.0, Anemia in neoplastic disease).

- When the admission/encounter is for management of an anemia associated with an adverse effect of the administration of chemotherapy, immunotherapy or radiation and the only treatment is for the anemia, the anemia code is sequenced first.

Detailed and precise terms are vital to accurately coding any anemia diagnosis. If the home health clinician suspects a specific type of anemia, but the physician documentation is vague, the clinician should check with the physician for verification. For example, anemia due to blood loss from a chronic gastric ulcer would code to D50.0 (iron deficiency anemia secondary to blood loss [chronic]) if the anemia is the focus of care, along with code K25.7 (chronic gastric ulcer without hemorrhage or perforation) as a secondary code to describe the source of the blood loss. Pay attention to the note at K25.- to use an additional code to identify alcohol abuse and dependence (F10-). Most of the time, "hemorrhagic disorder" or "coagulation defects" must be specifically diagnosed and documented by the provider in order to assign codes from category D68 (Other coagulation defects). However, for bleeding symptoms associated with a medication as part of anticoagulation therapy, such as hemoptysis, hematuria, hematemesis and/or hematochezia, assign code D68.32 (Hemorrhagic disorder due to extrinsic circulating anticoagulants), per Q1 2016 Coding Clinic. This is supported by the inclusion term at D68.32 of "Drug-induced hemorrhagic disorder." Sequencing depends on the focus of care.

Note: Assign as many anemia codes as needed to describe the presence of multiple types of anemia.

Neutropenia

Neutropenia is an abnormal decrease of neutrophils in the blood. Neutrophils are the circulating white blood cells essential for phagocytosis and proteolysis that destroy and remove bacteria, cellular debris and other solid particles. Neutrophils can be associated with acute leukemia, infection, rheumatoid arthritis, B12 deficiency and chronic splenomegaly. Symptoms include chills, fever and sores in the throat, stomach or skin.

As with coding from any ICD-10 chapter, the home health agency must determine the principal diagnosis based on the condition that is most relevant to the current plan of care.

The diagnosis may or may not be related to the patient's most recent hospital stay, but must relate to the services the home health agency will be providing.

CHAPTER 3: DISEASES OF THE BLOOD AND BLOOD-FORMING ORGANS AND CERTAIN DISORDERS INVOLVING THE IMMUNE MECHANISM (D50-D89)

EXCLUDES 2   autoimmune disease (systemic) NOS (M35.9)
certain conditions originating in the perinatal period (P00-P96)
complications of pregnancy, childbirth and the puerperium (O00-O9A)
congenital malformations, deformations and chromosomal abnormalities (Q00-Q99)
endocrine, nutritional and metabolic diseases (E00-E88)
human immunodeficiency virus [HIV] disease (B20)
injury, poisoning and certain other consequences of external causes (S00-T88)
neoplasms (C00-D49)
symptoms, signs and abnormal clinical and laboratory findings, not elsewhere classified (R00-R94)

This chapter contains the following blocks:

D50-D53	Nutritional anemias
D55-D59	Hemolytic anemias
D60-D64	Aplastic and other anemias and other bone marrow failure syndromes
D65-D69	Coagulation defects, purpura and other hemorrhagic conditions
D70-D77	Other disorders of blood and blood-forming organs
D78	Intraoperative and postprocedural complications of the spleen
D80-D89	Certain disorders involving the immune mechanism

Nutritional anemias (D50-D53)

4 D50   **Iron deficiency anemia**

     INCLUDES   asiderotic anemia
hypochromic anemia

     ALERT   The assignment of iron deficiency anemia to the home health claim does not provide a supportive diagnosis for medical necessity for the administration of B12 injections by the home health agency under the Medicare part A home health benefit. CMS considers the following conditions reasonable and necessary for the administration of B-12 under the home health benefit: pernicious anemia, megaloblastic anemias, macrocytic anemias, fish tapeworm anemia, gastrectomy, malabsorption syndromes such as sprue and idiopathic steatorrhea, surgical and mechanical disorders such as resection of the small intestine, strictures, anastomosis and blind loop syndrome, and posterolateral sclerosis, other neuropathies associated with pernicious anemia, during the acute phase or acute exacerbation of a neuropathy due to malnutrition and alcoholism.

CODING TIPS ✓   Do not assign codes from category D50 when the record only reports "iron deficiency" but does not specifically state "iron deficiency anemia" or "anemia due to iron deficiency." Iron deficiency (without anemia) should be coded to E61.1.

SP D50.0   **Iron deficiency anemia secondary to blood loss (chronic)**
Posthemorrhagic anemia (chronic)

     EXCLUDES 1   acute posthemorrhagic anemia (D62)
congenital anemia from fetal blood loss (P61.3)

     CODING TIPS ✓   The term "chronic" is a non-essential modifier in the code title for iron deficiency anemia secondary to blood loss (chronic). When the record specifies posthemorrhagic anemia (not specified as acute), D50.0 should be assigned. No time period is specifically required for the condition.

     DEFINITION   Iron depletion from sustained RBC loss in long-term bleeding, often from an ulcerous lesion, causing decreased hemoglobin and insufficient tissue oxygenation.

SP D50.1   **Sideropenic dysphagia**
Kelly-Paterson syndrome
Plummer-Vinson syndrome

SP D50.8   **Other iron deficiency anemias**
Iron deficiency anemia due to inadequate dietary iron intake

     CODING TIPS ✓   Code D50.8 should be used to report anemia due to dietary iron deficiency.

SP D50.9   **Iron deficiency anemia, unspecified**

     CODING TIPS ✓   When the record specifies only "iron deficiency anemia," with no cause provided, report code D50.9.

     DEFINITION   Insufficient stores of iron in the body causing decreased hemoglobin and a reduction in red blood cell oxygen carrying capacity.

4 D51   **Vitamin B12 deficiency anemia**

     EXCLUDES 1   vitamin B12 deficiency (E53.8)

     ALERT   The assignment of B12 deficiency anemia alone to the home health claim does not provide a supportive diagnosis for medical necessity for the administration of B12 injections by the home health agency under the Medicare part A home health benefit. CMS considers the following conditions reasonable and necessary for the administration of B12 under the home health benefit: pernicious anemia, megaloblastic anemias, macrocytic anemias, fish tapeworm anemia, gastrectomy, malabsorption syndromes such as sprue and idiopathic steatorrhea, surgical and mechanical disorders such as resection of the small intestine, strictures, anastomosis and blind loop syndrome, and posterolateral sclerosis, other neuropathies associated with pernicious anemia, during the acute phase or acute exacerbation of a neuropathy due to malnutrition and alcoholism.

Chapter 3

D50-D89

★ New ▲ Revised **Px** Primary   **SP** PDGM Px   **SL** Low CoM   **SH** High CoM   **IQ** Quest. Encounter   **H** Hospice non-cancer Dx   **Unspecified**   **M** *Manifestation*

CODING TIPS ✓   Do not assign codes from category D51 when the record reports "B12 deficiency" but does not specifically state "B12 deficiency anemia" or "anemia due to B12 deficiency." B12 deficiency (without anemia) should be coded to E53.8.

SP D51.0   Vitamin B12 deficiency anemia due to intrinsic factor deficiency
Addison anemia
Biermer anemia
Pernicious (congenital) anemia
Congenital intrinsic factor deficiency
CODING TIPS ✓   When a patient is receiving home health services for the administration of subcutaneous B12 injections, ensure the clinical record contains evidence of an appropriate diagnosis for coverage. Home health coverage for the administration of B12 is limited to specified anemias, such as pernicious, megaloblastic, macrocytic and fish tapeworm (Medicare Benefit Policy Manual, Chapter 7).

CODING TIPS ✓   When a patient is receiving home health services for the administration of subcutaneous B12 injections, the clinical record must contain detailed evidence of why the patient is unable to self administer. For example, a patient with rheumatoid arthritis may have impaired ability to manipulate an injectable medication and self inject. It is not appropriate to use vague terms, such as poor vision or poor manual dexterity. The patient is not expected to self-admiinister IM injections.

DEFINITION   Anemia due to underlying Vitamin B12 malabsorption caused by inadequate production of intrinsic factor in the gastric mucosa.

SP D51.1   Vitamin B12 deficiency anemia due to selective vitamin B12 malabsorption with proteinuria
Imerslund (Gräsbeck) syndrome
Megaloblastic hereditary anemia

SP D51.2   Transcobalamin II deficiency

SP D51.3   Other dietary vitamin B12 deficiency anemia
Vegan anemia
CODING TIPS ✓   Code D51.3 should be used to report anemia due to dietary B12 deficiency. Deficiencies of B Vitamins may result in neuropathies. Look for specific information regarding deficiencies versus anemia.

SP D51.8   Other vitamin B12 deficiency anemias

SP D51.9   Vitamin B12 deficiency anemia, unspecified

4 D52   Folate deficiency anemia
EXCLUDES 1   folate deficiency without anemia (E53.8)

ALERT   The assignment of folate deficiency anemia to the home health claim does not provide a supportive diagnosis for medical necessity for the administration of B12 injections by the home health agency under the Medicare part A home health benefit. CMS considers the following conditions reasonable and necessary for the administration of B-12 under the home health benefit: pernicious anemia, megaloblastic anemias, macrocytic anemias, fish tapeworm anemia, gastrectomy, malabsorption syndromes such as sprue and idiopathic steatorrhea, surgical and mechanical disorders such as resection of the small intestine, strictures, anastomosis and blind loop syndrome, and posterolateral sclerosis, other neuropathies associated with pernicious anemia, during the acute phase or acute exacerbation of a neuropathy due to malnutrition and alcoholism.

DEFINITION   Lack of folic acid causing large, immature, misshapen red blood cells, called megaloblasts, to form in the bone marrow.

SP D52.0   Dietary folate deficiency anemia
Nutritional megaloblastic anemia
CODING TIPS ✓   Code D52.0 should be used to report anemia due to dietary folate deficiency.

SP + D52.1   Drug-induced folate deficiency anemia
Use additional code for adverse effect, if applicable, to identify drug (T36-T50 with fifth or sixth character 5)
CODING TIPS ✓   Code D52.1 indicates folate deficiency anemia due to the effects of a drug. The clinical record should specify the drug and the anemia should be coded as an adverse effect of the drug. A code from T36-T50 should be assigned following D52.1 to identify the drug resulting in anemia.

SP D52.8   Other folate deficiency anemias

SP D52.9   Folate deficiency anemia, unspecified
Folic acid deficiency anemia NOS

4 D53   Other nutritional anemias
INCLUDES   megaloblastic anemia unresponsive to vitamin B12 or folate therapy

SP D53.0   Protein deficiency anemia
Amino-acid deficiency anemia
Orotaciduric anemia
EXCLUDES 1   Lesch-Nyhan syndrome (E79.1)

SP D53.1   Other megaloblastic anemias, not elsewhere classified
Megaloblastic anemia NOS
EXCLUDES 1   Di Guglielmo's disease (C94.0)

SP D53.2   Scorbutic anemia
EXCLUDES 1   scurvy (E54)

SP D53.8   Other specified nutritional anemias
Anemia associated with deficiency of copper
Anemia associated with deficiency of molybdenum
Anemia associated with deficiency of zinc

4 4th digit required   **5** 5th digit required   **6** 6th digit required   **7** 7th digit required   **7** 7th digit placeholder   **+** Additional code   **⊟** Laterality

708   DecisionHealth's FY 2020 Complete Home Health ICD-10-CM Diagnosis Coding Manual

Chapter 3

D50-D89

EXCLUDES 1 nutritional deficiencies without anemia, such as: copper deficiency NOS (E61.0) molybdenum deficiency NOS (E61.5) zinc deficiency NOS (E60)

SP D53.9 Nutritional anemia, unspecified
Simple chronic anemia
EXCLUDES 1 anemia NOS (D64.9)

Hemolytic anemias (D55-D59)

4 D55 Anemia due to enzyme disorders
EXCLUDES 1 drug-induced enzyme deficiency anemia (D59.2)

▲ SP D55.0 Anemia due to glucose-6-phosphate dehydrogenase [G6PD] deficiency
Favism
G6PD deficiency anemia
EXCLUDES 1 glucose-6-phosphate dehydrogenase (G6PD) deficiency without anemia (D75.A)

SP D55.1 Anemia due to other disorders of glutathione metabolism
Anemia (due to) enzyme deficiencies, except G6PD, related to the hexose monophosphate [HMP] shunt pathway
Anemia (due to) hemolytic nonspherocytic (hereditary), type I
DEFINITION Anemia resulting from damage or destruction of RBCs in high numbers due to insufficient glutathione, a tripeptide used by RBCs to protect against oxidative damage.

SP D55.2 Anemia due to disorders of glycolytic enzymes
Hemolytic nonspherocytic (hereditary) anemia, type II
Hexokinase deficiency anemia
Pyruvate kinase [PK] deficiency anemia
Triose-phosphate isomerase deficiency anemia
EXCLUDES 1 disorders of glycolysis not associated with anemia (E74.8)

SP D55.3 Anemia due to disorders of nucleotide metabolism

SP D55.8 Other anemias due to enzyme disorders

SP D55.9 Anemia due to enzyme disorder, unspecified

4 D56 Thalassemia
EXCLUDES 1 sickle-cell thalassemia (D57.4-)

SP + D56.0 Alpha thalassemia
Alpha thalassemia major
Hemoglobin H Constant Spring
Hemoglobin H disease
Hydrops fetalis due to alpha thalassemia
Severe alpha thalassemia
Triple gene defect alpha thalassemia
Use additional code, if applicable, for hydrops fetalis due to alpha thalassemia (P56.99)
EXCLUDES 1 alpha thalassemia trait or minor (D56.3)
asymptomatic alpha thalassemia (D56.3)

hydrops fetalis due to isoimmunization (P56.0)
hydrops fetalis not due to immune hemolysis (P83.2)
DEFINITION Hemoglobinopathy caused by genetic decrease in alpha globin chain formation needed for normal hemoglobin A (2 alpha and 2 beta chains), forming unstable hemoglobin and leading to RBC breakage.

SP D56.1 Beta thalassemia
Beta thalassemia major
Cooley's anemia
Homozygous beta thalassemia
Severe beta thalassemia
Thalassemia intermedia
Thalassemia major
EXCLUDES 1 beta thalassemia minor (D56.3)
beta thalassemia trait (D56.3)
delta-beta thalassemia (D56.2)
hemoglobin E-beta thalassemia (D56.5)
sickle-cell beta thalassemia (D57.4-)
DEFINITION Hemoglobinopathy caused by genetic decrease in beta globin chain formation needed for normal hemoglobin A (2 alpha and 2 beta chains), leaving insoluble alpha chain aggregates that interfere with RBC production, maturation, and membrane function.

SP D56.2 Delta-beta thalassemia
Homozygous delta-beta thalassemia
EXCLUDES 1 delta-beta thalassemia minor (D56.3)
delta-beta thalassemia trait (D56.3)

SP D56.3 Thalassemia minor
Alpha thalassemia minor
Alpha thalassemia silent carrier
Alpha thalassemia trait
Beta thalassemia minor
Beta thalassemia trait
Delta-beta thalassemia minor
Delta-beta thalassemia trait
Thalassemia trait NOS
EXCLUDES 1 alpha thalassemia (D56.0)
beta thalassemia (D56.1)
delta-beta thalassemia (D56.2)
hemoglobin E-beta thalassemia (D56.5)
sickle-cell trait (D57.3)
DEFINITION Alpha, beta, and delta-beta hemoglobinopathies caused by small gene mutations resulting in mild signs and symptoms of anemia, or asymptomatic trait or silent carrier forms.

SP D56.4 Hereditary persistence of fetal hemoglobin [HPFH]

SP D56.5 Hemoglobin E-beta thalassemia
EXCLUDES 1 beta thalassemia (D56.1)
beta thalassemia minor (D56.3)

Chapter 3

D50-D89

★ New ▲Revised Px Primary SP PDGM Px SL Low CoM SH High CoM IQ Quest. Encounter H Hospice non-cancer Dx Unspecified M *Manifestation*

DecisionHealth's FY 2020 Complete Home Health ICD-10-CM Diagnosis Coding Manual

709

beta thalassemia trait
(D56.3)
delta-beta thalassemia
(D56.2)
delta-beta thalassemia trait
(D56.3)
hemoglobin E disease
(D58.2)
other hemoglobinopathies
(D58.2)
sickle-cell beta thalassemia
(D57.4-)

DEFINITION   Hemoglobinopathy caused
by variations in beta globin chain formation,
producing unstable hemoglobin E and
causing microcytic anemia, poor growth,
splenomegaly, and heart failure.

SP D56.8 Other thalassemias
Dominant thalassemia
Hemoglobin C thalassemia
Mixed thalassemia
Thalassemia with other hemoglobinopathy
EXCLUDES 1   hemoglobin C disease
(D58.2)
hemoglobin E disease
(D58.2)
other hemoglobinopathies
(D58.2)
sickle-cell anemia (D57.-)
sickle-cell thalassemia
(D57.4)

SP D56.9   Thalassemia, unspecified
Mediterranean anemia (with other
hemoglobinopathy)
DEFINITION   Inherited blood disease
causing disruption in the normal production
of hemoglobin and a high rate of red blood
cell destruction.

+ 4 D57   Sickle-cell disorders
Use additional code for any associated fever
(R50.81)
EXCLUDES 1   other hemoglobinopathies
(D58.-)

+ 5 D57.0 Hb-SS disease with crisis
Sickle-cell disease NOS with crisis
Hb-SS disease with vasoocclusive pain
CODING TIPS ✓   If vaso-occlusive crisis leads
to a specific identifiable exacerbation, such
as pulmonary infarction, the exacerbation is
also coded.

**SP + D57.00   Hb-SS disease with crisis,
unspecified**
DEFINITION   Hereditary disease in
which RBCs contain abnormal
hemoglobin S, making them elongated
and crescent-shaped. The fragile,
sickled cells become blocked in tiny
blood vessels and break apart, causing
vaso-occlusive pain.

**SP + D57.01   Hb-SS disease with acute chest
syndrome**
DEFINITION   Life-threatening
complication of sickle-cell disease in
which blood clots form in the tiny blood
vessels of the lungs with repeated
episodes of bleeding from the alveoli
and hemosiderin buildup.

**SP + D57.02   Hb-SS disease with splenic
sequestration**
DEFINITION   Life-threatening
complication of sickle-cell disease in
which sickled cells become trapped in
the spleen, causing acute swelling, high
fever, intense abdominal pain, jaundice,
leukocytosis, and tissue infarction.

SP + D57.1 Sickle-cell disease without crisis
Hb-SS disease without crisis
Sickle-cell anemia NOS
Sickle-cell disease NOS
Sickle-cell disorder NOS
DEFINITION   Chronic, hereditary disease
in which red blood cells contain abnormal
hemoglobin S and are stiff and misshapen
like a crescent, inhibiting blood flow through
small blood vessels.

+ 5 D57.2 Sickle-cell/Hb-C disease
Hb-SC disease
Hb-S/Hb-C disease

**SP + D57.20   Sickle-cell/Hb-C disease without
crisis**

+ 6 D57.21   Sickle-cell/Hb-C disease with crisis

**SP + D57.211 Sickle-cell/Hb-C disease with
acute chest syndrome**

**SP + D57.212 Sickle-cell/Hb-C disease with
splenic sequestration**

**SP + D57.219 Sickle-cell/Hb-C disease with
crisis, unspecified**
Sickle-cell/Hb-C disease with crisis
NOS

IQ + D57.3 Sickle-cell trait
Hb-S trait
Heterozygous hemoglobin S
CODING TIPS ✓   When a patient is reported
only to have sickle cell "trait" but no sickle
cell disease is stated, report only D57.3.
DEFINITION   Condition in which a person
carries one gene for normal hemoglobin
and one for abnormal hemoglobin S that
sickles red blood cells, producing only mild
anemia or remaining asymptomatic.

+ 5 D57.4 Sickle-cell thalassemia
Sickle-cell beta thalassemia
Thalassemia Hb-S disease
CODING TIPS ✓   Sickle cell thalassemia
differs from sickle cell disease in that these
patients have a more mild form of sickle cell
disease, with some red blood cells
containing abnormal hemoglobin
(hemoglobin S) and others containing
normal hemoglobin (hemoglobin A).

SP + D57.40   Sickle-cell thalassemia without crisis
Microdrepanocytosis
Sickle-cell thalassemia NOS
DEFINITION   Inherited form of anemia,
occurring mainly among people of
Mediterranean descent, caused by
faulty synthesis of part of the
hemoglobin molecule.

+ 6 D57.41   Sickle-cell thalassemia with crisis
Sickle-cell thalassemia with
vasoocclusive pain

**SP + D57.411 Sickle-cell thalassemia with acute
chest syndrome**

4 4th digit required   **5** 5th digit required   **6** 6th digit required   **7** 7th digit required   **7** 7th digit placeholder   **+** Additional code   **□** Laterality

710   *DecisionHealth's* FY 2020 Complete Home Health ICD-10-CM Diagnosis Coding Manual

Chapter 3

D50-D89

SP **+** **D57.412** Sickle-cell thalassemia with splenic sequestration

SP **+** **D57.419** **Sickle-cell thalassemia with crisis, unspecified**

Sickle-cell thalassemia with crisis NOS

+ **5** **D57.8** **Other sickle-cell disorders**

Hb-SD disease

Hb-SE disease

SP **+** **D57.80** Other sickle-cell disorders without crisis

+ **6** **D57.81** Other sickle-cell disorders with crisis

SP **+** **D57.811** Other sickle-cell disorders with acute chest syndrome

SP **+** **D57.812** Other sickle-cell disorders with splenic sequestration

SP **+** **D57.819** **Other sickle-cell disorders with crisis, unspecified**

Other sickle-cell disorders with crisis NOS

4 **D58** **Other hereditary hemolytic anemias**

EXCLUDES 1 hemolytic anemia of the newborn (P55.-)

SP **D58.0** **Hereditary spherocytosis**

Acholuric (familial) jaundice

Congenital (spherocytic) hemolytic icterus

Minkowski-Chauffard syndrome

DEFINITION Congenital form of spherocytosis with hemolytic anemia, abnormal fragility of erythrocytes, jaundice, and splenomegaly.

SP **D58.1** **Hereditary elliptocytosis**

Elliptocytosis (congenital)

Ovalocytosis (congenital) (hereditary)

SP **D58.2** **Other hemoglobinopathies**

Abnormal hemoglobin NOS

Congenital Heinz body anemia

Hb-C disease

Hb-D disease

Hb-E disease

Hemoglobinopathy NOS

Unstable hemoglobin hemolytic disease

EXCLUDES 1 familial polycythemia (D75.0)

Hb-M disease (D74.0)

hemoglobin E-beta thalassemia (D56.5)

hereditary persistence of fetal hemoglobin [HPFH] (D56.4)

high-altitude polycythemia (D75.1)

methemoglobinemia (D74.-)

other hemoglobinopathies with thalassemia (D56.8)

SP **D58.8** **Other specified hereditary hemolytic anemias**

Stomatocytosis

SP **D58.9** **Hereditary hemolytic anemia, unspecified**

4 **D59** **Acquired hemolytic anemia**

SP **+** **D59.0** **Drug-induced autoimmune hemolytic anemia**

Use additional code for adverse effect, if applicable, to identify drug (T36-T50 with fifth or sixth character 5)

CODING TIPS ✓ Code D59.0 indicates autoimmune hemolytic anemia due to the effects of a drug. The clinical record should specify the drug, and this should be coded as an adverse effect of the drug causing the anemia. A code from T36-T50 should be assigned following D59.0 to identify the drug resulting in anemia.

SP **D59.1** **Other autoimmune hemolytic anemias**

Autoimmune hemolytic disease (cold type) (warm type)

Chronic cold hemagglutinin disease

Cold agglutinin disease

Cold agglutinin hemoglobinuria

Cold type (secondary) (symptomatic) hemolytic anemia

Warm type (secondary) (symptomatic) hemolytic anemia

EXCLUDES 1 Evans syndrome (D69.41)

hemolytic disease of newborn (P55.-)

paroxysmal cold hemoglobinuria (D59.6)

SP **+** **D59.2** **Drug-induced nonautoimmune hemolytic anemia**

Drug-induced enzyme deficiency anemia

Use additional code for adverse effect, if applicable, to identify drug (T36-T50 with fifth or sixth character 5)

CODING TIPS ✓ D59.2 indicates non-autoimmune hemolytic anemia due to the effects of a drug. The clinical record should specify the drug, and this should be coded as an adverse effect of the drug causing the anemia. A code from T36-T50 should be assigned following D59.2 to identify the drug resulting in anemia.

SP **+** **D59.3** **Hemolytic-uremic syndrome**

Use additional code to identify associated:

E. coli infection (B96.2-)

Pneumococcal pneumonia (J13)

Shigella dysenteriae (A03.9)

DEFINITION Condition in which platelets become clogged in narrow renal blood vessels, leading to the destruction of red blood cells and kidney failure. Symptoms include severe abdominal pain, diarrhea, nausea, and vomiting.

SP **D59.4** **Other nonautoimmune hemolytic anemias**

Mechanical hemolytic anemia

Microangiopathic hemolytic anemia

Toxic hemolytic anemia

SP **D59.5** **Paroxysmal nocturnal hemoglobinuria [Marchiafava-Micheli]**

EXCLUDES 1 hemoglobinuria NOS (R82.3)

SP **+** **D59.6** **Hemoglobinuria due to hemolysis from other external causes**

Hemoglobinuria from exertion

March hemoglobinuria

Paroxysmal cold hemoglobinuria

Use additional code (Chapter 20) to identify external cause

EXCLUDES 1 hemoglobinuria NOS (R82.3)

Chapter 3

D50-D89

★ New ▲Revised Px Primary **SP** PDGM Px **SL** Low CoM **SH** High CoM **IQ** Quest. Encounter **H** Hospice non-cancer Dx [Unspecified] **M** *Manifestation*

DecisionHealth's FY 2020 Complete Home Health ICD-10-CM Diagnosis Coding Manual

711

CODING TIPS ✓ Hemoglobinuria is a condition where excess hemoglobin is found in high concentrations in the urine. Code D59.6 only when the hemoglobinuria is stated as due to hemolysis related to a specific other cause (the hemolysis of red blood cells due to another specific cause or condition is resulting in the hemoglobinuria). An external cause code (from Chapter 20) may be assigned to identify the external cause.

SP D59.8 Other acquired hemolytic anemias

SP D59.9 Acquired hemolytic anemia, unspecified
Idiopathic hemolytic anemia, chronic

Aplastic and other anemias and other bone marrow failure syndromes   (D60-D64)

4 D60 Acquired pure red cell aplasia [erythroblastopenia]
INCLUDES red cell aplasia (acquired) (adult) (with thymoma)
EXCLUDES 1 congenital red cell aplasia (D61.01)

SP D60.0 Chronic acquired pure red cell aplasia
DEFINITION Decline of RBC precursor cells in the bone marrow until nearly absent while WBC precursors are present at normal levels; causes normochromic, normoblastic anemia.

SP D60.1 Transient acquired pure red cell aplasia

SP D60.8 Other acquired pure red cell aplasias

SP D60.9 Acquired pure red cell aplasia, unspecified

4 D61 Other aplastic anemias and other bone marrow failure syndromes
EXCLUDES 1 neutropenia (D70.-)

5 D61.0 Constitutional aplastic anemia

SP D61.01 Constitutional (pure) red blood cell aplasia
Blackfan-Diamond syndrome
Congenital (pure) red cell aplasia
Familial hypoplastic anemia
Primary (pure) red cell aplasia
Red cell (pure) aplasia of infants
EXCLUDES 1 acquired red cell aplasia (D60.9)

SP D61.09 Other constitutional aplastic anemia
Fanconi's anemia
Pancytopenia with malformations

SP + D61.1 Drug-induced aplastic anemia
Use additional code for adverse effect, if applicable, to identify drug (T36-T50 with fifth or sixth character 5)

CODING TIPS ✓ When the clinical record specifies aplastic anemia due to antineoplastic chemotherapy, D61.1 should be assigned, followed by the appropriate code to identify the adverse effect of antineoplastic chemotherapy (T36-T50).

SP D61.2 Aplastic anemia due to other external agents
Code first:
, if applicable, toxic effects of substances chiefly nonmedicinal as to source (T51-T65)

SP D61.3 Idiopathic aplastic anemia

5 D61.8 Other specified aplastic anemias and other bone marrow failure syndromes

6 D61.81 Pancytopenia
EXCLUDES 1 pancytopenia (due to) (with) aplastic anemia (D61.9)
pancytopenia (due to) (with) bone marrow infiltration (D61.82)
pancytopenia (due to) (with) congenital (pure) red cell aplasia (D61.01)
pancytopenia (due to) (with) hairy cell leukemia (C91.4-)
pancytopenia (due to) (with) human immunodeficiency virus disease (B20.-)
pancytopenia (due to) (with) leukoerythroblastic anemia (D61.82)
pancytopenia (due to) (with) myeloproliferative disease (D47.1)
EXCLUDES 2 pancytopenia (due to) (with) myelodysplastic syndromes (D46.-)
DEFINITION Decreased count of all elements in the blood: red blood cells, white blood cells, and platelets.

SP D61.810 Antineoplastic chemotherapy induced pancytopenia
EXCLUDES 2 aplastic anemia due to antineoplastic chemotherapy (D61.1)
CODING TIPS ✓ This code is reported when pancytopenia results from antineoplastics. Pancytopenia is a reduction of red and white blood cells, as well as platelets.

SP D61.811 Other drug-induced pancytopenia
EXCLUDES 2 aplastic anemia due to drugs (D61.1)

SP D61.818 Other pancytopenia

SP D61.82 Myelophthisis
Leukoerythroblastic anemia
Myelophthisic anemia
Panmyelophthisis
Code also the underlying disorder, such as:
malignant neoplasm of breast (C50.-)
tuberculosis (A15.-)
EXCLUDES 1 idiopathic myelofibrosis (D47.1)

4 4th digit required   5 5th digit required   6 6th digit required   7 7th digit required   ✓ 7th digit placeholder   + Additional code   ⊟ Laterality

712   DecisionHealth's FY 2020 Complete Home Health ICD-10-CM Diagnosis Coding Manual

Chapter 3

D50-D89

myelofibrosis NOS
(D75.81)
myelofibrosis with
myeloid metaplasia
(D47.4)
primary myelofibrosis
(D47.1)
secondary myelofibrosis
(D75.81)

DEFINITION   Replacement of hemopoietic tissue in the bone marrow by abnormal infiltrates, usually fibrotic tissue or malignant tumors, suppressing bone marrow function.

SP **D61.89   Other specified aplastic anemias and other bone marrow failure syndromes**

SP **D61.9   Aplastic anemia, unspecified**
Hypoplastic anemia NOS
Medullary hypoplasia

SP **D62   Acute posthemorrhagic anemia**
EXCLUDES 1   anemia due to chronic blood loss (D50.0)
blood loss anemia NOS (D50.0)
congenital anemia from fetal blood loss (P61.3)

CODING TIPS ✓   Do not assign D62 when the clinical record documentation specifies only "blood loss," "blood loss anemia" or "chronic blood loss anemia." Code D62 should only be used when posthemorrhagic anemia is specified as acute.

4 **D63   Anemia in chronic diseases classified elsewhere**

IQ **D63.0   Anemia in neoplastic disease**
Code first:
neoplasm (C00-D49)
EXCLUDES 1   aplastic anemia due to antineoplastic chemotherapy (D61.1)
EXCLUDES 2   anemia due to antineoplastic chemotherapy (D64.81)

GUIDELINES   **Section 1.C.2.c.1** When admission/encounter is for management of an anemia associated with the malignancy, and the treatment is only for anemia, the appropriate code for the malignancy is sequenced as the principal or first-listed diagnosis followed by the appropriate code for the anemia (such as code D63.0, Anemia in neoplastic disease).

CODING TIPS ✓   When a patient is admitted for anemia due to neoplastic disease (D63.0), a code for the appropriate neoplasm must be first assigned, regardless of whether the focus of care is the neoplastic disease or the anemia. Anemia is assumed related to the neoplastic disease.

IQ **D63.1   Anemia in chronic kidney disease**
Erythropoietin resistant anemia (EPO resistant anemia)
Code first:
underlying chronic kidney disease (CKD) (N18.-)

ALERT   Watch out for coverage issues with anemia in chronic kidney disease. The treatment is covered under the dialysis benefit. This type of anemia is a related condition if the terminal diagnosis in hospice is ESRD.

M **IQ** **D63.8   *Anemia in other chronic diseases classified elsewhere***
Code first underlying disease, such as:
diphyllobothriasis (B70.0)
hookworm disease (B76.0-B76.9)
hypothyroidism (E00.0-E03.9)
malaria (B50.0-B54)
symptomatic late syphilis (A52.79)
tuberculosis (A18.89)

4 **D64   Other anemias**
EXCLUDES 1   refractory anemia (D46.-)
refractory anemia with excess blasts in transformation [RAEB T] (C92.0-)

SP **D64.0   Hereditary sideroblastic anemia**
Sex-linked hypochromic sideroblastic anemia
DEFINITION   Group of blood disorders in which the bone marrow's ability to produce normal red blood cells is impaired and sideroblasts, or deformed red blood cells, are present in the bloodstream.

IQ **D64.1   Secondary sideroblastic anemia due to disease**
Code first:
underlying disease

SP **+** **D64.2   Secondary sideroblastic anemia due to drugs and toxins**
Code first:
poisoning due to drug or toxin, if applicable (T36-T65 with fifth or sixth character 1-4 or 6)
Use additional code for adverse effect, if applicable, to identify drug (T36-T50 with fifth or sixth character 5)

SP **D64.3   Other sideroblastic anemias**
Sideroblastic anemia NOS
Pyridoxine-responsive sideroblastic anemia NEC

SP **D64.4   Congenital dyserythropoietic anemia**
Dyshematopoietic anemia (congenital)
EXCLUDES 1   Blackfan-Diamond syndrome (D61.01)
Di Guglielmo's disease (C94.0)

CODING TIPS ✓   Congenital dyserythropoietic anemia is defined as a congenital condition resulting in immature red blood cells that are unusually shaped and cannot develop into functional mature cells, leading to a shortage of healthy red blood cells. These patients also frequently have thrombocytopenia, which should be additionally coded if present.

5 **D64.8   Other specified anemias**

SP **D64.81   Anemia due to antineoplastic chemotherapy**
Antineoplastic chemotherapy induced anemia

Chapter 3

D50-D89

★ New ▲ Revised Px Primary **SP** PDGM Px **SL** Low CoM **SH** High CoM **IQ** Quest. Encounter **H** Hospice non-cancer Dx Unspecified **M** *Manifestation*

DecisionHealth's FY 2020 Complete Home Health ICD-10-CM Diagnosis Coding Manual   713

EXCLUDES 1 aplastic anemia due to antineoplastic chemotherapy (D61.1)

EXCLUDES 2 anemia in neoplastic disease (D63.0)

CODING TIPS ✓   Do not assign D64.81 to indicate anemia due to neoplastic disease. Anemia due to neoplastic disease should be coded to D63.0. Anemia is presumed related to neoplasms and to chemotherapy, so both anemias may be coded unless the physician indicates otherwise.

CODING TIPS ✓   Do not assign D64.81 to indicate aplastic anemia due to antineoplastic chemotherapy. If the diagnostic statements specifically report aplastic anemia due to antineoplastic chemotherapy, assign D61.1.

CODING TIPS ✓   Code D64.81 should be followed in the sequencing by the appropriate T code for adverse effect of antineoplastics. When sequencing, follow the guideline on coding adverse effects.

CODING TIPS ✓   Antineoplastic chemotherapy-induced changes usually are short term, and they do not usually reduce the marrow cells to a point of aplasia.

SP D64.89   Other specified anemias
Infantile pseudoleukemia

SP D64.9   Anemia, unspecified

CODING TIPS ✓   There are several conditions presumed related to anemia, such as CKD, neoplastic disease and chemotherapy. Reference the index for anemia and the terms 'with' or 'in' prior to using D64.9.

Coagulation defects, purpura and other hemorrhagic conditions   (D65-D69)

CODING TIPS ✓   The codes in D65-D69 are used for different kinds of hemophilias. If bleeds are related to anticoagulant drugs, see D68.32.

SP D65   Disseminated intravascular coagulation [defibrination syndrome]
Afibrinogenemia, acquired
Consumption coagulopathy
Diffuse or disseminated intravascular coagulation [DIC]
Fibrinolytic hemorrhage, acquired
Fibrinolytic purpura
Purpura fulminans
EXCLUDES 1 disseminated intravascular coagulation (complicating) : abortion or ectopic or molar pregnancy (O00-O07, O08.1) in newborn (P60) pregnancy, childbirth and the puerperium (O45.0, O46.0, O67.0, O72.3)

DEFINITION   Bleeding disorder characterized by an abnormal reduction in the elements involved in blood clotting; marked by profuse hemorrhaging in the late stages.

SP D66   Hereditary factor VIII deficiency
Classical hemophilia
Deficiency factor VIII (with functional defect)
Hemophilia NOS
Hemophilia A
EXCLUDES 1 factor VIII deficiency with vascular defect (D68.0)

DEFINITION   Most common form of hemophilia, referred to as classic hemophilia or hemophilia A; characterized by profuse bleeding from injuries, as well as bleeding from the joints, muscles, digestive tract, and brain.

SP D67   Hereditary factor IX deficiency
Christmas disease
Factor IX deficiency (with functional defect)
Hemophilia B
Plasma thromboplastin component [PTC] deficiency
DEFINITION   A clotting disorder of blood, caused by hereditary deficiency of factor IX.

4 D68   Other coagulation defects
EXCLUDES 1 abnormal coagulation profile (R79.1) coagulation defects complicating abortion or ectopic or molar pregnancy (O00-O07, O08.1) coagulation defects complicating pregnancy, childbirth and the puerperium (O45.0, O46.0, O67.0, O72.3)

SP D68.0   Von Willebrand's disease
Angiohemophilia
Factor VIII deficiency with vascular defect
Vascular hemophilia
EXCLUDES 1 capillary fragility (hereditary) (D69.8) factor VIII deficiency NOS (D66) factor VIII deficiency with functional defect (D66)

SP D68.1   Hereditary factor XI deficiency
Hemophilia C
Plasma thromboplastin antecedent [PTA] deficiency
Rosenthal's disease

SP D68.2   Hereditary deficiency of other clotting factors
AC globulin deficiency
Congenital afibrinogenemia
Deficiency of factor I [fibrinogen]
Deficiency of factor II [prothrombin]
Deficiency of factor V [labile]
Deficiency of factor VII [stable]
Deficiency of factor X [Stuart-Prower]
Deficiency of factor XII [Hageman]
Deficiency of factor XIII [fibrin stabilizing]
Dysfibrinogenemia (congenital)
Hypoproconvertinemia
Owren's disease
Proaccelerin deficiency

5 D68.3   Hemorrhagic disorder due to circulating anticoagulants

6 D68.31   Hemorrhagic disorder due to intrinsic circulating anticoagulants, antibodies, or inhibitors

4 4th digit required   **5** 5th digit required   **6** 6th digit required   **7** 7th digit required   **7** 7th digit placeholder   **+** Additional code   **▤** Laterality

714   *DecisionHealth's* FY 2020 Complete Home Health ICD-10-CM Diagnosis Coding Manual

Chapter 3

D50-D89

SP D68.311 Acquired hemophilia
Autoimmune hemophilia
Autoimmune inhibitors to clotting
factors
Secondary hemophilia

SP D68.312 Antiphospholipid antibody with hemorrhagic disorder
Lupus anticoagulant (LAC) with
hemorrhagic disorder
Systemic lupus erythematosus
[SLE] inhibitor with hemorrhagic
disorder

> **EXCLUDES 1** antiphospholipid
> antibody, finding
> without diagnosis
> (R76.0)
> antiphospholipid
> antibody syndrome
> (D68.61)
> antiphospholipid
> antibody with
> hypercoagulable
> state (D68.61)
> lupus anticoagulant
> (LAC) finding
> without diagnosis
> (R76.0)
> lupus anticoagulant
> (LAC) with
> hypercoagulable
> state (D68.62)
> systemic lupus
> erythematosus
> [SLE] inhibitor
> finding without
> diagnosis (R76.0)
> systemic lupus
> erythematosus
> [SLE] inhibitor with
> hypercoagulable
> state (D68.62)

SP D68.318 Other hemorrhagic disorder due to intrinsic circulating anticoagulants, antibodies, or inhibitors
Antithromboplastinemia
Antithromboplastinogenemia
Hemorrhagic disorder due to
intrinsic increase in antithrombin
Hemorrhagic disorder due to
intrinsic increase in anti-VIIIa
Hemorrhagic disorder due to
intrinsic increase in anti-IXa
Hemorrhagic disorder due to
intrinsic increase in anti-XIa

SP ✚ D68.32 Hemorrhagic disorder due to extrinsic circulating anticoagulants
Drug-induced hemorrhagic disorder
Hemorrhagic disorder due to increase
in anti-IIa
Hemorrhagic disorder due to increase
in anti-Xa
Hyperheparinemia
Use additional code for adverse effect,
if applicable, to identify drug
(T45.515, T45.525)

CODING TIPS ✓ For bleeding such as
hemoptysis, hematuria, hematemesis,
hematochezia, etc., that is associated
with a drug as part of anticoagulation
therapy, assign code D68.32.

CODING TIPS ✓ When a bleed results as
an adverse effect of anticoagulant
therapy, such as a gastric bleed, code
the bleed, D68.32, and then the adverse
effect of the drug or drugs.

SP D68.4 Acquired coagulation factor deficiency
Deficiency of coagulation factor due to
liver disease
Deficiency of coagulation factor due to
vitamin K deficiency

> **EXCLUDES 1** vitamin K deficiency of
> newborn (P53)

5 D68.5 Primary thrombophilia
Primary hypercoagulable states

> **EXCLUDES 1** antiphospholipid syndrome
> (D68.61)
> lupus anticoagulant
> (D68.62)
> secondary activated protein
> C resistance (D68.69)
> secondary antiphospholipid
> antibody syndrome
> (D68.69)
> secondary lupus
> anticoagulant with
> hypercoagulable state
> (D68.69)
> secondary systemic lupus
> erythematosus [SLE]
> inhibitor with
> hypercoagulable state
> (D68.69)
> systemic lupus
> erythematosus [SLE]
> inhibitor finding without
> diagnosis (R76.0)
> systemic lupus
> erythematosus [SLE]
> inhibitor with hemorrhagic
> disorder (D68.312)
> thrombotic
> thrombocytopenic purpura
> (M31.1)

> **DEFINITION** Abnormal development of
> blood clots in arteries or veins.

SP D68.51 Activated protein C resistance
Factor V Leiden mutation

SP D68.52 Prothrombin gene mutation

SP D68.59 Other primary thrombophilia
Antithrombin III deficiency
Hypercoagulable state NOS
Primary hypercoagulable state NEC
Primary thrombophilia NEC
Protein C deficiency
Protein S deficiency
Thrombophilia NOS

5 D68.6 Other thrombophilia
Other hypercoagulable states

> **EXCLUDES 1** diffuse or disseminated
> intravascular coagulation
> [DIC] (D65)

Chapter 3

D50-D89

★ New ▲ Revised Px Primary SP PDGM Px SL Low CoM SH High CoM IQ Quest. Encounter H Hospice non-cancer Dx Unspecified M *Manifestation*

DecisionHealth's FY 2020 Complete Home Health ICD-10-CM Diagnosis Coding Manual

715

heparin induced thrombocytopenia (HIT) (D75.82)

hyperhomocysteinemia (E72.11)

SP D68.61   Antiphospholipid syndrome
Anticardiolipin syndrome
Antiphospholipid antibody syndrome
EXCLUDES 1   anti-phospholipid antibody, finding without diagnosis (R76.0)
anti-phospholipid antibody with hemorrhagic disorder (D68.312)
lupus anticoagulant syndrome (D68.62)

SP D68.62   Lupus anticoagulant syndrome
Lupus anticoagulant
Presence of systemic lupus erythematosus [SLE] inhibitor
EXCLUDES 1   anticardiolipin syndrome (D68.61)
antiphospholipid syndrome (D68.61)
lupus anticoagulant (LAC) finding without diagnosis (R76.0)
lupus anticoagulant (LAC) with hemorrhagic disorder (D68.312)

SP D68.69   Other thrombophilia
Hypercoagulable states NEC
Secondary hypercoagulable state NOS

SP D68.8   Other specified coagulation defects
EXCLUDES 1   hemorrhagic disease of newborn (P53)

SP D68.9   Coagulation defect, unspecified

4 D69   Purpura and other hemorrhagic conditions
EXCLUDES 1   benign hypergammaglobulinemic purpura (D89.0)
cryoglobulinemic purpura (D89.1)
essential (hemorrhagic) thrombocythemia (D47.3)
hemorrhagic thrombocythemia (D47.3)
purpura fulminans (D65)
thrombotic thrombocytopenic purpura (M31.1)
Waldenström hypergammaglobulinemic purpura (D89.0)

SP D69.0   Allergic purpura
Allergic vasculitis
Nonthrombocytopenic hemorrhagic purpura
Nonthrombocytopenic idiopathic purpura
Purpura anaphylactoid
Purpura Henoch(-Schönlein)
Purpura rheumatica
Vascular purpura
EXCLUDES 1   thrombocytopenic hemorrhagic purpura (D69.3)

DEFINITION   Allergic reaction causing hemorrhaging of the skin and mucous membranes; produces purple discolorations on the skin surface.

SP D69.1   Qualitative platelet defects
Bernard-Soulier [giant platelet] syndrome
Glanzmann's disease
Grey platelet syndrome
Thromboasthenia (hemorrhagic) (hereditary)
Thrombocytopathy
EXCLUDES 1   von Willebrand's disease (D68.0)

SP D69.2   Other nonthrombocytopenic purpura
Purpura NOS
Purpura simplex
Senile purpura

SP D69.3   Immune thrombocytopenic purpura
Hemorrhagic (thrombocytopenic) purpura
Idiopathic thrombocytopenic purpura
Tidal platelet dysgenesis

5 D69.4   Other primary thrombocytopenia
EXCLUDES 1   transient neonatal thrombocytopenia (P61.0)
Wiskott-Aldrich syndrome (D82.0)

SP D69.41   Evans syndrome

SP D69.42   Congenital and hereditary thrombocytopenia purpura
Congenital thrombocytopenia
Hereditary thrombocytopenia
Code first congential or hereditary disorder, such as:
thrombocytopenia with absent radius (TAR syndrome) (Q87.2)

SP D69.49   Other primary thrombocytopenia
Megakaryocytic hypoplasia
Primary thrombocytopenia NOS

5 D69.5   Secondary thrombocytopenia
EXCLUDES 1   heparin induced thrombocytopenia (HIT) (D75.82)
transient thrombocytopenia of newborn (P61.0)

DEFINITION   Uncommon but life-threatening adverse reaction in which arterial or venous thrombotic complications develop that can lead to pulmonary embolism, amputation, stroke, or acute myocardial infarction.

SP D69.51   Posttransfusion purpura
Posttransfusion purpura from whole blood (fresh) or blood products
PTP

SP D69.59   Other secondary thrombocytopenia

SP D69.6   Thrombocytopenia, unspecified

SP D69.8   Other specified hemorrhagic conditions
Capillary fragility (hereditary)
Vascular pseudohemophilia

SP D69.9   Hemorrhagic condition, unspecified

Other disorders of blood and blood-forming organs (D70-D77)

+ 4 D70   Neutropenia
INCLUDES   agranulocytosis

4 4th digit required   5 5th digit required   6 6th digit required   7 7th digit required   7 7th digit placeholder   + Additional code   ⊟ Laterality

716   DecisionHealth's FY 2020 Complete Home Health ICD-10-CM Diagnosis Coding Manual

decreased absolute neurophile count (ANC)

Use additional code for any associated:
fever (R50.81)
mucositis (J34.81, K12.3-, K92.81, N76.81)

EXCLUDES 1   neutropenic splenomegaly (D73.81)
transient neonatal neutropenia (P61.5)

SP ✚ D70.0 Congenital agranulocytosis
Congenital neutropenia
Infantile genetic agranulocytosis
Kostmann's disease

SP ✚ D70.1 Agranulocytosis secondary to cancer chemotherapy
Code also:
underlying neoplasm
Use additional code for adverse effect, if applicable, to identify drug (T45.1X5)

SP ✚ D70.2 Other drug-induced agranulocytosis
Use additional code for adverse effect, if applicable, to identify drug (T36-T50 with fifth or sixth character 5)

SP ✚ D70.3 Neutropenia due to infection

SP ✚ D70.4 Cyclic neutropenia
Cyclic hematopoiesis
Periodic neutropenia

SP ✚ D70.8 Other neutropenia

SP ✚ D70.9 Neutropenia, unspecified

SP D71 Functional disorders of polymorphonuclear neutrophils
Cell membrane receptor complex [CR3] defect
Chronic (childhood) granulomatous disease
Congenital dysphagocytosis
Progressive septic granulomatosis

4 D72 Other disorders of white blood cells
EXCLUDES 1   basophilia (D72.824)
immunity disorders (D80-D89)
neutropenia (D70)
preleukemia (syndrome) (D46.9)

SP D72.0 Genetic anomalies of leukocytes
Alder (granulation) (granulocyte) anomaly
Alder syndrome
Hereditary leukocytic hypersegmentation
Hereditary leukocytic hyposegmentation
Hereditary leukomelanopathy
May-Hegglin (granulation) (granulocyte) anomaly
May-Hegglin syndrome
Pelger-Huët (granulation) (granulocyte) anomaly
Pelger-Huët syndrome
EXCLUDES 1   Chédiak (-Steinbrinck) -Higashi syndrome (E70.330)

SP D72.1 Eosinophilia
Allergic eosinophilia
Hereditary eosinophilia
EXCLUDES 1   Löffler's syndrome (J82)
pulmonary eosinophilia (J82)

5 D72.8 Other specified disorders of white blood cells
EXCLUDES 1   leukemia (C91-C95)

6 D72.81 Decreased white blood cell count

EXCLUDES 1   neutropenia (D70.-)

SP D72.810 Lymphocytopenia
Decreased lymphocytes

SP D72.818 Other decreased white blood cell count
Basophilic leukopenia
Eosinophilic leukopenia
Monocytopenia
Other decreased leukocytes
Plasmacytopenia

SP D72.819 Decreased white blood cell count, unspecified
Decreased leukocytes, unspecified
Leukocytopenia, unspecified
Leukopenia
EXCLUDES 1   malignant leukopenia (D70.9)

6 D72.82 Elevated white blood cell count
EXCLUDES 1   eosinophilia (D72.1)

SP D72.820 Lymphocytosis (symptomatic)
Elevated lymphocytes

SP D72.821 Monocytosis (symptomatic)
EXCLUDES 1   infectious mononucleosis (B27.-)

SP D72.822 Plasmacytosis

SP D72.823 Leukemoid reaction
Basophilic leukemoid reaction
Leukemoid reaction NOS
Lymphocytic leukemoid reaction
Monocytic leukemoid reaction
Myelocytic leukemoid reaction
Neutrophilic leukemoid reaction
DEFINITION   A state of circulating blood presenting a clinical picture resembling or indistinguishable from leukemia due to a condition such as infection, bone marrow compromise, liver failure, and inflammatory disorders.

SP D72.824 Basophilia
DEFINITION   Abnormally increased number of basophils in the blood, which release histamine and serotonin upon stimulation.

SP D72.825 Bandemia
Bandemia without diagnosis of specific infection
EXCLUDES 1   confirmed infection - code to infection leukemia (C91.-, C92.-, C93.-, C94.-, C95.-)
DEFINITION   Nonspecific elevated count of immature white blood cells when other white blood cell counts are normal.

SP D72.828 Other elevated white blood cell count

SP D72.829 Elevated white blood cell count, unspecified
Elevated leukocytes, unspecified
Leukocytosis, unspecified

SP D72.89 Other specified disorders of white blood cells
Abnormality of white blood cells NEC

Chapter 3

D50-D89

★ New ▲ Revised Px Primary SP PDGM Px SL Low CoM SH High CoM IQ Quest. Encounter H Hospice non-cancer Dx   Unspecified   M *Manifestation*

DecisionHealth's FY 2020 Complete Home Health ICD-10-CM Diagnosis Coding Manual   717

SP D72.9 Disorder of white blood cells, unspecified

Abnormal leukocyte differential NOS

4 D73 Diseases of spleen

SP D73.0 Hyposplenism

Atrophy of spleen

EXCLUDES 1 asplenia (congenital) (Q89.01)
postsurgical absence of spleen (Z90.81)

SP D73.1 Hypersplenism

EXCLUDES 1 neutropenic splenomegaly (D73.81)
primary splenic neutropenia (D73.81)
splenitis, splenomegaly in late syphilis (A52.79)
splenitis, splenomegaly in tuberculosis (A18.85)
splenomegaly NOS (R16.1)
splenomegaly congenital (Q89.0)

SP D73.2 Chronic congestive splenomegaly

SP D73.3 Abscess of spleen

SP D73.4 Cyst of spleen

SP D73.5 Infarction of spleen

Splenic rupture, nontraumatic
Torsion of spleen

EXCLUDES 1 rupture of spleen due to Plasmodium vivax malaria (B51.0)
traumatic rupture of spleen (S36.03-)

5 D73.8 Other diseases of spleen

SP D73.81 Neutropenic splenomegaly

Werner-Schultz disease

SP D73.89 Other diseases of spleen

Fibrosis of spleen NOS
Perisplenitis
Splenitis NOS

IQ D73.9 Disease of spleen, unspecified

4 D74 Methemoglobinemia

SP D74.0 Congenital methemoglobinemia

Congenital NADH-methemoglobin reductase deficiency
Hemoglobin-M [Hb-M] disease
Methemoglobinemia, hereditary

SP D74.8 Other methemoglobinemias

Acquired methemoglobinemia (with sulfhemoglobinemia)
Toxic methemoglobinemia

SP D74.9 Methemoglobinemia, unspecified

DEFINITION Presence of a higher than normal level of methemoglobin, a form of hemoglobin that does not bind oxygen, in the blood. When its concentration is elevated in red blood cells, anemia and hypoxia may occur.

4 D75 Other and unspecified diseases of blood and blood-forming organs

EXCLUDES 2 acute lymphadenitis (L04.-)
chronic lymphadenitis (I88.1)
enlarged lymph nodes (R59.-)
hypergammaglobulinemia NOS (D89.2)
lymphadenitis NOS (I88.9)
mesenteric lymphadenitis (acute) (chronic) (I88.0)

SP D75.0 Familial erythrocytosis

Benign polycythemia
Familial polycythemia

EXCLUDES 1 hereditary ovalocytosis (D58.1)

SP D75.1 Secondary polycythemia

Acquired polycythemia
Emotional polycythemia
Erythrocytosis NOS
Hypoxemic polycythemia
Nephrogenous polycythemia
Polycythemia due to erythropoietin
Polycythemia due to fall in plasma volume
Polycythemia due to high altitude
Polycythemia due to stress
Polycythemia NOS
Relative polycythemia

EXCLUDES 1 polycythemia neonatorum (P61.1)
polycythemia vera (D45)

5 D75.8 Other specified diseases of blood and blood-forming organs

IQ + D75.81 Myelofibrosis

Myelofibrosis NOS
Secondary myelofibrosis NOS

Code first the underlying disorder, such as:
malignant neoplasm of breast (C50.-)
Use additional code, if applicable, for associated therapy-related myelodysplastic syndrome (D46.-)
Use additional code for adverse effect, if applicable, to identify drug (T45.1X5)

EXCLUDES 1 acute myelofibrosis (C94.4-)
idiopathic myelofibrosis (D47.1)
leukoerythroblastic anemia (D61.82)
myelofibrosis with myeloid metaplasia (D47.4)
myelophthisic anemia (D61.82)
myelophthisis (D61.82)
primary myelofibrosis (D47.1)

SP D75.82 Heparin induced thrombocytopenia (HIT)

SP D75.89 Other specified diseases of blood and blood-forming organs

IQ D75.9 Disease of blood and blood-forming organs, unspecified

★ D75.A Glucose-6-phosphate dehydrogenase (G6PD) deficiency without anemia

EXCLUDES 1 glucose-6-phosphate dehydrogenase (G6PD) deficiency with anemia (D55.0)

4 D76 Other specified diseases with participation of lymphoreticular and reticulohistiocytic tissue

EXCLUDES 1 (Abt-) Letterer-Siwe disease (C96.0)
eosinophilic granuloma (C96.6)

4 4th digit required   5 5th digit required   6 6th digit required   7 7th digit required   7 7th digit placeholder   + Additional code   ⊟ Laterality

718   *DecisionHealth's* FY 2020 Complete Home Health ICD-10-CM Diagnosis Coding Manual

Chapter 3

D50-D89

Hand-Schüller-Christian disease
(C96.5)
histiocytic medullary reticulosis
(C96.9)
histiocytic sarcoma (C96.A)
histiocytosis X, multifocal
(C96.5)
histiocytosis X, unifocal
(C96.6)
Langerhans-cell histiocytosis,
multifocal (C96.5)
Langerhans-cell histiocytosis
NOS (C96.6)
Langerhans-cell histiocytosis,
unifocal (C96.6)
leukemic reticuloendotheliosis
(C91.4-)
lipomelanotic reticulosis
(I89.8)
malignant histiocytosis
(C96.A)
malignant reticulosis (C86.0)
nonlipid reticuloendotheliosis
(C96.0)

SP **D76.1 Hemophagocytic lymphohistiocytosis**
Familial hemophagocytic reticulosis
Histiocytoses of mononuclear phagocytes

SP **+ D76.2 Hemophagocytic syndrome, infection-associated**
Use additional code to identify infectious
agent or disease.

SP **D76.3 Other histiocytosis syndromes**
Reticulohistiocytoma (giant-cell)
Sinus histiocytosis with massive
lymphadenopathy
Xanthogranuloma

M **IQ** **D77** *Other disorders of blood and blood-forming*
organs in diseases classified elsewhere

Code first underlying disease, such as:
amyloidosis (E85.-)
congenital early syphilis (A50.0)
echinococcosis (B67.0-B67.9)
malaria (B50.0-B54)
schistosomiasis [bilharziasis]
(B65.0-B65.9)
vitamin C deficiency (E54)

EXCLUDES 1 rupture of spleen due to
Plasmodium vivax malaria
(B51.0)
splenitis, splenomegaly in late
syphilis (A52.79)
splenitis, splenomegaly in
tuberculosis (A18.85)

Intraoperative and postprocedural complications of the spleen (D78)

CODING TIPS ✓ Conditions classifiable to D78- are classifiable as
intraoperative and postprocedural complications. These
conditions should only be assigned when diagnostic statements
clearly indicate that the condition is a complication of a
procedure.

D78 **Intraoperative and postprocedural**
complications of the spleen

D78.0 Intraoperative hemorrhage and
hematoma of the spleen complicating a
procedure

EXCLUDES 1 intraoperative hemorrhage
and hematoma of the
spleen due to accidental
puncture or laceration
during a procedure
(D78.1-)

SP **D78.01 Intraoperative hemorrhage and**
hematoma of the spleen complicating
a procedure on the spleen

SP **D78.02 Intraoperative hemorrhage and**
hematoma of the spleen complicating
other procedure

D78.1 Accidental puncture and laceration of
the spleen during a procedure

SP **D78.11 Accidental puncture and laceration**
of the spleen during a procedure on
the spleen

SP **D78.12 Accidental puncture and laceration**
of the spleen during other procedure

D78.2 Postprocedural hemorrhage of the
spleen following a procedure

SP **D78.21 Postprocedural hemorrhage of the**
spleen following a procedure on the
spleen

SP **D78.22 Postprocedural hemorrhage of the**
spleen following other procedure

D78.3 Postprocedural hematoma and seroma
of the spleen following a procedure

SP **D78.31 Postprocedural hematoma of the**
spleen following a procedure on the
spleen

SP **D78.32 Postprocedural hematoma of the**
spleen following other procedure

SP **D78.33 Postprocedural seroma of the spleen**
following a procedure on the spleen

SP **D78.34 Postprocedural seroma of the spleen**
following other procedure

+ D78.8 Other intraoperative and
postprocedural complications of the
spleen
Use additional code, if applicable, to
further specify disorder

SP **+ D78.81 Other intraoperative complications**
of the spleen

SP **+ D78.89 Other postprocedural complications**
of the spleen

Certain disorders involving the immune mechanism (D80-D89)

INCLUDES defects in the complement system
immunodeficiency disorders, except human
immunodeficiency virus [HIV] disease
sarcoidosis

EXCLUDES 1 autoimmune disease (systemic) NOS (M35.9)
functional disorders of polymorphonuclear
neutrophils (D71)
human immunodeficiency virus [HIV] disease
(B20)

D80 Immunodeficiency with predominantly
antibody defects

SP **D80.0 Hereditary hypogammaglobulinemia**
Autosomal recessive agammaglobulinemia
(Swiss type)
X-linked agammaglobulinemia [Bruton]
(with growth hormone deficiency)

SP **D80.1 Nonfamilial hypogammaglobulinemia**
Agammaglobulinemia with
immunoglobulin-bearing B-lymphocytes

★ New ▲ Revised **Px** Primary **SP** PDGM Px **SL** Low CoM **SH** High CoM **IQ** Quest. Encounter **H** Hospice non-cancer Dx **Unspecified** **M** *Manifestation*

Common variable agammaglobulinemia
[CVAgamma]

Hypogammaglobulinemia NOS

DEFINITION Loss of the body's ability to respond to infection because of a lack of immunoglobulins (antibodies) in the blood.

SP **D80.2** **Selective deficiency of immunoglobulin A [IgA]**

SP **D80.3** **Selective deficiency of immunoglobulin G [IgG] subclasses**

SP **D80.4** **Selective deficiency of immunoglobulin M [IgM]**

SP **D80.5** **Immunodeficiency with increased immunoglobulin M [IgM]**

SP **D80.6** **Antibody deficiency with near-normal immunoglobulins or with hyperimmunoglobulinemia**

SP **D80.7** **Transient hypogammaglobulinemia of infancy**

SP **D80.8** **Other immunodeficiencies with predominantly antibody defects**
Kappa light chain deficiency

SP **D80.9** **Immunodeficiency with predominantly antibody defects, unspecified**

4 **D81** **Combined immunodeficiencies**
EXCLUDES 1 autosomal recessive agammaglobulinemia (Swiss type) (D80.0)

SP **D81.0** **Severe combined immunodeficiency [SCID] with reticular dysgenesis**

SP **D81.1** **Severe combined immunodeficiency [SCID] with low T- and B-cell numbers**

SP **D81.2** **Severe combined immunodeficiency [SCID] with low or normal B-cell numbers**

▲ **5** **D81.3** **Adenosine deaminase [ADA] deficiency**

★ **D81.30** **Adenosine deaminase deficiency, unspecified**
ADA deficiency NOS

★ **D81.31** **Severe combined immunodeficiency due to adenosine deaminase deficiency**
ADA deficiency with SCID
Adenosine deaminase [ADA] deficiency with severe combined immunodeficiency

DEFINITION Deficiency of Adenosine Deaminase 1 (DADA1) can result in a severe immunodeficiency while any immunodeficiency in deficiency of adenosine deaminase 2 (DADA2) is mild, if present. DADA1 results from a defect of a gene on chromosome 20, whereas DADA2 results from a gene defect on chromosome 22.

★ **D81.32** **Adenosine deaminase 2 deficiency**
ADA2 deficiency
Adenosine deaminase deficiency type 2
Code also, if applicable, any associated manifestations, such as:
polyarteritis nodosa (M30.0)
stroke (I63.-)

DEFINITION Deficiency of Adenosine Deaminase 2 (DADA2), or adenosine deaminase 2 deficiency, is characterized by abnormal inflammation of various tissues, which may be associated with a mottled rash (livedo racemosa), early-onset strokes, other findings of vasculitis (consistent with polyarteritis nodosa), and sometimes immunodeficiency. It is autoinflammatory in nature, and besides the skin and nervous system, may affect the gastrointestinal system or kidneys, and may cause intermittent fevers. It may be associated with hepatosplenomegaly. Onset may be from early childhood to adulthood.

★ **D81.39** **Other adenosine deaminase deficiency**
Adenosine deaminase [ADA] deficiency type 1, NOS
Adenosine deaminase [ADA] deficiency type 1, without SCID
Adenosine deaminase [ADA] deficiency type 1, without severe combined immunodeficiency
Partial ADA deficiency (type 1)
Partial adenosine deaminase deficiency (type 1)

SP **D81.4** **Nezelof's syndrome**

SP **D81.5** **Purine nucleoside phosphorylase [PNP] deficiency**

SP **D81.6** **Major histocompatibility complex class I deficiency**
Bare lymphocyte syndrome

SP **D81.7** **Major histocompatibility complex class II deficiency**

5 **D81.8** **Other combined immunodeficiencies**

6 **D81.81** **Biotin-dependent carboxylase deficiency**
Multiple carboxylase deficiency
EXCLUDES 1 biotin-dependent carboxylase deficiency due to dietary deficiency of biotin (E53.8)

SP **D81.810** **Biotinidase deficiency**

SP **D81.818** **Other biotin-dependent carboxylase deficiency**
Holocarboxylase synthetase deficiency
Other multiple carboxylase deficiency

SP **D81.819** **Biotin-dependent carboxylase deficiency, unspecified**
Multiple carboxylase deficiency, unspecified

SP **D81.89** **Other combined immunodeficiencies**

SP **D81.9** **Combined immunodeficiency, unspecified**
Severe combined immunodeficiency disorder [SCID] NOS

4 **D82** **Immunodeficiency associated with other major defects**
EXCLUDES 1 ataxia telangiectasia [Louis-Bar] (G11.3)

SP **D82.0** **Wiskott-Aldrich syndrome**

44th digit required   **5**5th digit required   **6**6th digit required   **7**7th digit required   **7**7th digit placeholder   **+**Additional code   **⊟**Laterality

720   DecisionHealth's FY 2020 Complete Home Health ICD-10-CM Diagnosis Coding Manual

Chapter 3

D50-D89

Immunodeficiency with thrombocytopenia and eczema

DEFINITION X-linked immunodeficiency syndrome presenting with eczema, thrombocytopenia, and recurrent pyogenic infection.

SP D82.1 Di George's syndrome
Pharyngeal pouch syndrome
Thymic alymphoplasia
Thymic aplasia or hypoplasia with immunodeficiency

DEFINITION Congenital disorder with hypoplasia or aplasia of the thymus and parathyroid glands; associated with congenital heart defects, great vessel anomalies, esophageal atresia, and abnormal facial structure.

SP D82.2 Immunodeficiency with short-limbed stature

SP D82.3 Immunodeficiency following hereditary defective response to Epstein-Barr virus
X-linked lymphoproliferative disease

SP D82.4 Hyperimmunoglobulin E [IgE] syndrome

CODING TIPS ✓ Patients with hyperimmunoglobulin E [IgE] syndrome have a lifelong condition characterized by elevated IgE levels, which may also be referred to as "Job syndrome." These patients are highly prone to problematic skin conditions such as eczema, skin lesions and infections (abscesses), sinus infections, and other respiratory infections, which should be additionally coded when present.

SP D82.8 Immunodeficiency associated with other specified major defects

SP D82.9 Immunodeficiency associated with major defect, unspecified

4 D83 Common variable immunodeficiency

SP D83.0 Common variable immunodeficiency with predominant abnormalities of B-cell numbers and function

SP D83.1 Common variable immunodeficiency with predominant immunoregulatory T-cell disorders

SP D83.2 Common variable immunodeficiency with autoantibodies to B- or T-cells

SP D83.8 Other common variable immunodeficiencies

SP D83.9 Common variable immunodeficiency, unspecified

4 D84 Other immunodeficiencies

SP D84.0 Lymphocyte function antigen-1 [LFA-1] defect

SP D84.1 Defects in the complement system
C1 esterase inhibitor [C1-INH] deficiency

SP D84.8 Other specified immunodeficiencies

SP D84.9 Immunodeficiency, unspecified

4 D86 Sarcoidosis

SP D86.0 Sarcoidosis of lung

SP D86.1 Sarcoidosis of lymph nodes

SP D86.2 Sarcoidosis of lung with sarcoidosis of lymph nodes

SP D86.3 Sarcoidosis of skin

5 D86.8 Sarcoidosis of other sites

SP D86.81 Sarcoid meningitis

SP D86.82 Multiple cranial nerve palsies in sarcoidosis

SP D86.83 Sarcoid iridocyclitis

SP D86.84 Sarcoid pyelonephritis
Tubulo-interstitial nephropathy in sarcoidosis

SP D86.85 Sarcoid myocarditis

SP D86.86 Sarcoid arthropathy
Polyarthritis in sarcoidosis

SP D86.87 Sarcoid myositis

SP D86.89 Sarcoidosis of other sites
Hepatic granuloma
Uveoparotid fever [Heerfordt]

SP D86.9 Sarcoidosis, unspecified

4 D89 Other disorders involving the immune mechanism, not elsewhere classified

EXCLUDES 1 hyperglobulinemia NOS (R77.1)
monoclonal gammopathy (of undetermined significance) (D47.2)

EXCLUDES 2 transplant failure and rejection (T86.-)

SP D89.0 Polyclonal hypergammaglobulinemia
Benign hypergammaglobulinemic purpura
Polyclonal gammopathy NOS

SP D89.1 Cryoglobulinemia
Cryoglobulinemic purpura
Cryoglobulinemic vasculitis
Essential cryoglobulinemia
Idiopathic cryoglobulinemia
Mixed cryoglobulinemia
Primary cryoglobulinemia
Secondary cryoglobulinemia

SP D89.2 Hypergammaglobulinemia, unspecified

SP + D89.3 Immune reconstitution syndrome
Immune reconstitution inflammatory syndrome [IRIS]
Use additional code for adverse effect, if applicable, to identify drug (T36-T50 with fifth or sixth character 5)

5 D89.4 Mast cell activation syndrome and related disorders

EXCLUDES 1 aggressive systemic mastocytosis (C96.21)
congenital cutaneous mastocytosis (Q82.2)
(non-congenital) cutaneous mastocytosis (D47.01)
(indolent) systemic mastocytosis (D47.02)
malignant mast cell neoplasm (C96.2-)
malignant mastocytoma (C96.29)
mast cell leukemia (C94.3-)
mast cell sarcoma (C96.22)
mastocytoma NOS (D47.09)
other mast cell neoplasms of uncertain behavior (D47.09)

Chapter 3

D50-D89

★ New ▲ Revised **Px** Primary **SP** PDGM Px **SL** Low CoM **SH** High CoM **IQ** Quest. Encounter **H** Hospice non-cancer Dx Unspecified **M** *Manifestation*

DecisionHealth's FY 2020 Complete Home Health ICD-10-CM Diagnosis Coding Manual

721

systemic mastocytosis
associated with a clonal
hematologic non-mast cell
lineage disease
(SM-AHNMD) (D47.02)

SP D89.40　Mast cell activation, unspecified

Mast cell activation disorder,
unspecified

Mast cell activation syndrome, NOS

SP D89.41　Monoclonal mast cell activation syndrome

SP D89.42　Idiopathic mast cell activation syndrome

SP D89.43　Secondary mast cell activation

Secondary mast cell activation
syndrome

Code also:
underlying etiology, if known

SP D89.49　Other mast cell activation disorder

Other mast cell activation syndrome

5 D89.8　Other specified disorders involving the immune mechanism, not elsewhere classified

+ 6 D89.81　Graft-versus-host disease

Code first underlying cause, such as:
complications of transplanted organs
and tissue (T86.-)
complications of blood transfusion
(T80.89)

Use additional code to identify
associated manifestations, such as:
desquamative dermatitis (L30.8)
diarrhea (R19.7)
elevated bilirubin (R17)
hair loss (L65.9)

CODING TIPS✓　Code D89.81 may only
be assigned when the provider
specifically indicates this condition.
Development of complicating disease,
such as ESRD or neoplasm in a
transplanted organ, should not be
assumed to indicate graft versus host
disease.

!Q + D89.810　Acute graft-versus-host disease

!Q + D89.811　Chronic graft-versus-host disease

!Q + D89.812　Acute on chronic graft-versus-host disease

!Q + D89.813　Graft-versus-host disease, unspecified

SP D89.82　Autoimmune lymphoproliferative syndrome [ALPS]

SP D89.89　Other specified disorders involving the immune mechanism, not elsewhere classified

EXCLUDES 1　human
immunodeficiency
virus disease (B20)

SP D89.9　Disorder involving the immune mechanism, unspecified

Immune disease NOS

4 4th digit required　　**5** 5th digit required　　**6** 6th digit required　　**7** 7th digit required　　**7v** 7th digit placeholder　　**+** Additional code　　**⊟** Laterality

722　　　　　　　　　　　　　　*DecisionHealth's* FY 2020 Complete Home Health ICD-10-CM Diagnosis Coding Manual

Chapter 3 Scenarios: Diseases of the blood and blood-forming organs and certain disorders involving the immune mechanism (D50-D89)

Anemia due to throat cancer

A 72-year-old male patient is admitted to home health with anemia secondary to a primary malignant neoplasm of his throat. He has a history of tobacco dependence. The anemia will be the focus of care.

Description	Code
Primary: Malignant neoplasm of pharynx, unspecified	C14.0
Secondary: Anemia in neoplastic disease	D63.0
Secondary: Personal history of nicotine dependence	Z87.891

Even though the anemia is the focus of care, official coding guidelines stipulate that the neoplasm causing the anemia must be sequenced first. The patient's history of tobacco dependence is coded, in accordance with the instructional note in the Tabular List for category C14.- to use an additional code to identify the status of tobacco use or exposure, if applicable. *[I.C.2.c.1]*

Antineoplastic chemotherapy induced anemia

An 84-year-old woman was admitted to home health for management of antineoplastic chemotherapy-induced anemia resulting from treatment for primary colon cancer. A physical therapist will also be seeing this patient for strengthening due to weakness.

Description	Code
Primary: Anemia due to antineoplastic chemotherapy	D64.81
Secondary: Malignant neoplasm of colon, unspecified	C18.9
Secondary: Adverse effect of antineoplastic and immunosuppressive drugs, subsequent encounter	T45.1x5D

When the admission is for management of anemia associated with an adverse effect of chemotherapy, and the only treatment is for the anemia, the anemia code is sequenced first followed by the appropriate codes for the neoplasm (C18.9) and the adverse effect of chemotherapy (T45.1x5-), according to coding guidelines. The 7th character of "D" will be commonly used in home care, as it indicates subsequent care. The patient's weakness would be inherent to her condition and would, therefore, not require an additional code. *[I.C.2.c.2]*

Anemia and duodenal ulcer

Home health is seeing a patient for anemia. She has a duodenal ulcer, which her physician suspects may be the cause of her anemia.

Description	Code
Primary: Anemia, unspecified	D64.9
Secondary: Duodenal ulcer, unspecified as acute or chronic, without hemorrhage or perforation	K26.9

Anemia is the focus of care, so it is listed as the primary diagnosis. Since the documentation says that the physician only suspects that the ulcer is the cause of the anemia, it cannot be coded that way; the diagnosis has to be confirmed. Thus, the anemia is coded as unspecified. The duodenal ulcer is also coded as unspecified and without hemorrhage and perforation, since the documentation does not state any additional information.

HOME HEALTH CODING SCENARIOS

Anemia due to chronic gastric ulcer

Your patient has anemia due to blood loss from a chronic gastric ulcer. The focus of care is the medical management of the ulcer.

Description	Code
Primary: Chronic gastric ulcer with hemorrhage	K25.4
Secondary: Iron deficiency anemia secondary to blood loss, chronic	D50.0

Any blood loss specified as due to an ulcer is classified as a hemorrhage even though the blood loss may be slow over time as is frequently seen with chronic gastric ulcers. As the focus of care, the ulcer is coded first and the anemia follows it. Anemia due to blood loss is classified as iron deficiency anemia, according to the alphabetic index.

Chronic graft vs. host disease

A 65-year-old man is admitted to home health with chronic graft versus host disease that is a complication of a stem cell transplant performed a year ago to treat multiple myeloma. The transplant put his multiple myeloma into remission but he continues to experience diarrhea and desquamative dermatitis, which his doctor diagnosed as manifestations of the chronic graft versus host disease. He'll receive skilled nursing for managing new medications, including multiple new immunosuppressive drugs, and physical therapy for muscle strengthening and stamina.

Description	Code
Primary: Complications of stem cell transplant	T86.5
Secondary: Chronic graft-versus-host disease	D89.811
Secondary: Other specified dermatitis	L30.8
Secondary: Diarrhea, unspecified	R19.7
Secondary: Multiple myeloma in remission	C90.01
Secondary: Other long term (current) drug therapy	Z79.899

Since the graft vs. host disease was documented as a complication of his stem cell transplant, T86.5 is coded first, followed by D89.911, in accordance with tabular instruction. Manifestations of chronic graft versus host disease, such as the desquamative dermatitis and diarrhea in this scenario, are assigned as additional diagnoses, in accordance with tabular instructions. His multiple myeloma is in remission but still present so it is coded with C90.01. Finally, Z79.899 is assigned to capture his use of multiple new immunosuppressive drugs.

Non-traumatic compartment syndrome, hemophilia A

A 53-year-old man is admitted to home health for aftercare following surgery for non-traumatic compartment syndrome in his bicep. Medical record documentation indicates that the patient experienced a spontaneous hemorrhage in the muscle due to hemophilia A, which led to the compartment syndrome. It's also indicated that the surgery completely resolved the non-traumatic compartment syndrome.

Description	Code
Primary: Encounter for other orthopedic aftercare	Z47.89
Secondary: Hereditary factor VIII deficiency	D66

The patient requires surgical aftercare following a procedure on the musculoskeletal system. Since there's no specific code for that nor is there a specific code for surgery to treat non-traumatic compartment syndrome, the best code choice is Z47.89. Hemophilia A will impact his recovery from surgery and requires close monitoring by the nurse. This condition is also known as hereditary factor VIII hemophilia. Note as well that Hemophilia A is listed as a clarifying term at D66. Non-traumatic compartment syndrome is not coded because it is completely resolved.

DVTs, Factor V Leiden mutation

A 47-year-old woman was hospitalized for treatment of acute DVTs in the peroneal veins of both her calves. Blood tests in the hospital revealed a Factor V Leiden mutation, which her physician documented is responsible for her DVTs. The focus of the home health admission are the DVTs. She is now on long-term anticoagulant medication and the nurse will be regularly checking PT/INRs.

Description	Code
Primary: Acute embolism and thrombosis of peroneal vein, bilateral	I82.453
Secondary: Activated protein C resistance	D68.51
Secondary: Encounter for therapeutic drug level monitoring	Z51.81
Secondary: Long term (current) use of anticoagulants	Z79.01

As the focus of care, the DVTs are coded in the primary position. Note, in PDGM, if you assign the code for DVTs of *unspecified* distal lower extremity, the claim would be sent back to be recoded. Because the DVTs are specified as affecting the peroneal veins in her calves, I82.452 is appropriately assigned. Her newly diagnosed Factor V Leiden mutation is assigned as the cause of the DVTs, as it is an important condition that will require teaching and monitoring. "Factor V Leiden mutation" is an inclusion term at D68.51. She will be taking long-term anticoagulation therapy and requires blood-level monitoring, thus requiring the assignment of Z51.81 and Z79.01.

Hematochezia due to anticoagulant use

A 67-year-old woman takes anticoagulants prophylactically to treat a chronic deep vein thrombosis (DVT) in the soleal vein of her left calf. Recently she began to pass fresh, red blood in her stools. After being evaluated by her physician, it was determined that the bleeding is related to her long-term use of anticoagulants. The patient's anticoagulant dosage has been adjusted but she continues to take the medication. Management of the DVT is the focus of care.

Description	Code
Primary: Chronic embolism and thrombosis of left calf muscular vein	I82.562
Secondary: Melena	K92.1
Secondary: Hemorrhagic disorder due to extrinsic circulating anticoagulants	D68.32
Secondary: Adverse effect of anticoagulants, subsequent encounter	T45.515D
Secondary: Long term (current) use of anticoagulants	Z79.01

The patient is experiencing bleeding due to her use of anticoagulants, which requires the use of D68.32, according to Q1 2016 Coding Clinic guidance. The condition (bleeding) caused by the drug is coded before the adverse effect code capturing the role of the anticoagulant in causing the bleeding, in accordance with coding guidelines. Since the patient continues to use anticoagulants, Z79.01 also is assigned. The chronic DVT is assigned in the primary position as the focus of care. Be sure that the location of the DVT is specified as non-specific codes are unacceptable primary diagnoses in PDGM. Because the location is specified as the soleal vein of her left calf, I82.562 is coded.

Chapter 4: Endocrine, Nutritional and Metabolic Diseases (E00 – E89)

Chapter 4 addresses a variety of conditions, including endocrine, nutritional and metabolic diseases. Home care clinicians will find themselves flipping to these pages often as this chapter contains the codes for diabetes – a common home care diagnosis. Also, codes in Chapter 4 may be used to identify functional activity associated with any neoplasm code from Chapter 2, or by ectopic endocrine tissue. *Note:* This chapter excludes transitory endocrine and metabolic disorders specific to newborn (codes P70-P74).

Chapter 4 includes codes for a number of different conditions, including:

- Conditions related to the endocrine glands (thyroid, E00-E07); other disorders of glucose regulation and pancreatic internal secretion (E15-E16); disorders of parathyroid, pituitary, hypothalamus, adrenal glands, ovaries, testes, polyglandular disorders; and other endocrine disorders (E20-E35).

- The largest code group for home health is combination codes related to five categories of diabetes codes. These codes include the type of diabetes mellitus, the body system affected and the complications affecting that body system. These categories include:

  - E08, Diabetes mellitus due to underlying conditions

  - E09, Drug or chemically induced diabetes mellitus

  - E10, Type 1 diabetes mellitus

  - E11, Type 2 diabetes mellitus

  - E13, Other specified diabetes mellitus

- Intraoperative complications of endocrine system (E36)

- Conditions related to nutrition, such as malnutrition (E40-E46); other nutritional deficiencies (E50-E64); and overweight, obesity, and other hyperalimentation (E65-E68).

- Metabolic disorders (E70-E88); Conditions related to metabolism as well as cystic fibrosis, volume depletion, dehydration and fluid overload, and hyperkalemia & hypokalemia.

- Post-procedural endocrine and metabolic complications and disorders, not elsewhere classified (E89).

Sometimes a Chapter 4 code isn't the most appropriate choice. See below a few situations to watch out for:

- If the **documentation indicates a neoplasm or tumor of an endocrine organ,** the term (malignancy, tumor, adenoma) that is used in the medical record should be looked up; it is most likely a code from Chapter 2. When a neoplasm affects an endocrine gland, the hormone levels may be unusually high or low and those conditions are used as additional codes to the neoplasm condition. In these situations, an additional code from Chapter 4 may be used to identify any functional activity associated with the neoplasm code from Chapter 2. The neoplasm is coded first and the functional activity is coded as a secondary code.

  Examples are E05.80 (other thyrotoxicosis without crisis) and E31.2 (multiple endocrine neoplasia syndromes)

- If a patient has a **personal or family history** of a condition reported in this chapter, it may be appropriate to select a code from the Z code section, such as Z86.3- (personal history of endocrine, nutritional and metabolic diseases) or Z83.3 (family history of diabetes mellitus). Remember that personal history is far more important than family history in home health coding.

- When reporting endocrine, nutritional and metabolic diseases in a **pregnant patient,** and the condition is complicating the pregnancy, report first a code from Chapter 15, such as O24.41- (diabetes mellitus in pregnancy) or O24.81- (other pre-existing diabetes mellitus in pregnancy). Pay attention to notes to use an additional code from category E11 to further identify any manifestations. Also assign Z79.4 (long-term (current) use of insulin) or Z79.84 (long-term (current) use of oral hypoglycemic drugs) if the diabetes mellitus is being treated with insulin or oral medications. If the patient is treated with both oral medications and insulin, only assign the code for insulin-controlled (Z79.4).

Chapter 4

E00 - E89

Multiple Coding and Sequencing

In this chapter, you will see many instructions to code first and use additional codes as well as instructions to use codes from other chapters. There are many examples of combination codes related to the etiology/manifestations for diabetes. However, there are also "code first" notes related to poisoning due to drugs or toxins and "add an additional code" notes for multiple coding and sequencing issues for codes in this chapter.

If the note to use an additional code references an adverse effect of a drug, refer to the Table of Drugs and Chemicals, as well as codes T36-T50 in Chapter 19 with a 5th or 6th character of '5' to identify the associated drug.

Important: The subterm "with" or "in" within the Index should be interpreted as a link between diabetes and any of those conditions indented under the word "with" or "in", according to coding conventions.

The classification presumes a causal relationship between the two conditions linked by these terms in the Alphabetic Index or Tabular List. These conditions should be coded as related even in the absence of provider documentation explicitly linking them, unless the documentation clearly states the conditions are unrelated or when another guideline exists that specifically requires a documented linkage between two conditions.

Warning: This convention does not apply to 'not elsewhere classified (NEC)' index entries that cover broad categories of conditions. Rather, you must see specific conditions linked by the terms 'with,' 'due to' or 'associated with' in order to assume a connection based on 'with.' Similarly, coronary artery disease cannot be automatically connected to diabetes and coded with E11.59; dementia cannot be automatically connected to diabetes and coded with E11.49; and blindness cannot be automatically connected to diabetes and coded with E11.39; unless explicitly stated as linked by the physician, according to Q4 2017 Coding Clinic guidance.

Special Coding Issues

Diabetes

The most commonly-used and misused diagnosis codes in this chapter are for **diabetes mellitus.**

Again, it's important to note diabetes mellitus codes are combination codes that include the type of diabetes mellitus, the body system affected, and the complications affecting that body system.

Codes E10- and E11- define the condition as Type 1 or Type 2 diabetes. The 4th and 5th characters are used to indicate the complication, such as E11.29 for Type 2 diabetes mellitus with other diabetic kidney complication. Sometimes a 6th character is used to provide further detail. For example, E11.331 for Type 2 diabetes mellitus with moderate nonproliferative diabetic retinopathy with macular edema.

Usually, the term "diabetes" refers to diabetes mellitus (E11-). If the medical record states only "diabetes," assume that it is Type 2 diabetes mellitus.

Although age is not the sole determining factor, most Type 1 diabetics develop the condition before reaching puberty. For this reason Type 1 diabetes mellitus is also referred to as juvenile diabetes. Type 1 diabetic patients must take daily insulin.

If the documentation in the medical record does not indicate the type of diabetes, but does indicate that the patient uses insulin, assign code E11 (Type 2 diabetes) along with Z79.4 (Long-term (current) use of insulin). Code Z79.4 should **not** be assigned if insulin is given temporarily to bring a Type 2 patient's blood sugar under control.

Most Type 2 (formerly called adult onset diabetes or NIDDM) usually is diagnosed in older patients (but not always) and may or may not be treated with insulin. The terms IDDM and NIDDM are archaic and should not be used to determine the type of diabetes.

Take note of the following general rules for coding diabetes mellitus:

- Do not assume that use of terms such as "glycosuria," "glucosuria," "hyperglycemia," or "polyuria" means the patient has diabetes. These are symptoms of diabetes, but may indicate other conditions.

- If the physician documentation indicates that the diabetes is "poorly controlled," "out of control," assign the code for the diabetes mellitus by type with hyperglycemia (EXX.65 code from categories E08-E13). For example, E10.65, Type 1 diabetes mellitus with hyperglycemia; or E11.65, Type 2 diabetes mellitus with hyperglycemia; or any of the other types of diabetes). **But note,** diabetes simply referred to as "uncontrolled" could be either hyperglycemia or hypoglycemia. If documentation isn't clear, query the physician, per Q1 2017 Coding Clinic.

- If the physician states the patient has uncontrolled or "out of control" diabetes plus other complications (manifestations) of diabetes, code them all, including the hyperglycemia. For example, medical record documentation states "uncontrolled Type 2 diabetes with diabetic polyneuropathy." You would code E11.42 and E11.65.

- Do not assume that a young diabetic patient has Type 1.

- Do not assume a patient using insulin has Type 1.

- Do not assume that a patient described as insulin dependent has Type 1.

- If the documentation does not state the type of diabetes, the default code is Type 2. Note that 90% to 95% of patients with diabetes have Type 2.

- If the documentation states Type 1.5, and the physician does not provide more specific information confirming either Type 1 or Type 2, assign a code from E13.-.

Complications due to insulin pump malfunction

Underdose of insulin due to insulin pump failure should be assigned with a specific code from subcategory T85.6 (Mechanical complication of other specified internal and external prosthetic devices, implants and grafts), as the principal or first-listed code. It should be followed by code T38.3x6- (Underdosing of insulin and oral hypoglycemic [antidiabetic] drugs). Additional codes for the type of diabetes mellitus and any associated complications due to the underdosing should also be assigned.

Overdose of insulin due to insulin pump failure: The principal or first-listed code for an encounter due to an insulin pump malfunction resulting in an overdose of insulin should also be T85.6-(Mechanical complication of other specified internal and external prosthetic devices, implants and grafts), followed by code T38.3x1- (Poisoning by insulin and oral hypoglycemic [antidiabetic] drugs, accidental (unintentional).

Include as many codes within a particular category as are necessary to describe all of the complications of the diabetes. They should be sequenced based on the reason for a particular encounter. Assign as many codes from Categories E08 – E13 as needed to identify all of the associated conditions that the patient has.

- For example, for a patient who has Type 2 diabetes mellitus **and** diabetic peripheral angiopathy **and** diabetic gastroparesis, report codes E11.5-(Diabetes with diabetic angiopathy) and E11.43 (Diabetes with diabetic gastroparesis).

- If multiple manifestations apply to a specific body system, then sequence them accordingly. For example, for a patient who has diabetic peripheral angiopathy and gangrene, you would assign E11.52.

- Code Z79.4 (long-term [current] use of insulin) also is reported as an additional diagnosis for patients who have Type 2 diabetes, secondary diabetes, or an unspecified type of diabetes who routinely use insulin. However, code Z79.4 is not reported for patients with Type 1 diabetes. Code Z79.84 (oral antidiabetic/hypoglycemic drugs) is also available to report as an additional diagnosis when applicable.

Secondary diabetes mellitus

Codes under categories E08 (Diabetes mellitus due to underlying condition), E09 (Drug or chemical induced diabetes mellitus) and E13 (Other specified diabetes mellitus) all identify secondary diabetes.

Secondary diabetes is always caused by another condition or event (e.g., cystic fibrosis, malignant neoplasm of the pancreas, pancreatectomy, adverse effect of drug or poisoning). Like primary diabetes mellitus, there are combination codes to identify any complications/manifestations due to secondary diabetes.

Assigning and sequencing secondary diabetes codes and its causes

The sequencing of the secondary diabetes codes in relationship to codes for the cause of the diabetes is based on the Tabular instructions for E08, E09 and E13.

Secondary diabetes due to drugs

Secondary diabetes may be caused by an adverse effect of correctly administered medications, poisoning or sequela of a poisoning.

Secondary diabetes due to pancreatectomy

For post pancreatectomy diabetes mellitus (lack of insulin due to the surgical removal of all or part of the pancreas), assign code E89.1 (Postprocedural hypoinsulinemia), then assign a code from category E13, followed by a code from subcategory Z90.41-(Acquired absence of pancreas).

Coding Diabetes after a Pancreas Transplant

After the transplant, diabetes may no longer be an issue, but lingering manifestations may be. Code as you would any patient with diabetic complications. Assign a code from E11 with the appropriate body system to identify any specific manifestations. The patient still has complications associated with the diabetes because the transplant did not resolve the manifestations of diabetes, even though it did resolve the diabetes.

The manifestations require that diabetes be coded as the etiology even if the patient no longer has diabetes. Also code Z94.83, Organ or tissue replaced by transplant, pancreas.

Diabetic Ulcers

Volume 2 (Alphabetic Index) lists diabetic ulcers as a combination code under each of the diabetes mellitus categories. For example: E08.621, Diabetes mellitus due to underlying condition with foot ulcer; and E08.622, Diabetes mellitus due to underlying condition with other skin ulcer. However there is also a notation to use an additional code to identify site of the foot ulcer (L97.4-, L95.5-), and a notation to an use additional code to identify site of the (other) skin ulcer (L97.1-L97.9, L98.41-L98.49)

Malnutrition (E40-E46)

Malnutrition codes are frequently used with hospice patients to further define their terminal status. The physician must document the actual malnutrition diagnoses but clinicians may and should show an associated Body Mass Index (BMI) code from Z68.- that illustrates the extent of the weight loss.

Overweight, Obesity (E65-E68)

Overweight or obesity is coded only if documented by the physician. Even though the coding of overweight/obesity is limited to physician documentation, the BMI is easily calculated and can be determined by a clinician involved in the care of the patient even in the absence of obesity codes. When coding obesity or overweight, the BMI code Z68.- should also be listed as an additional diagnosis.

Chapter 4

E00 - E89

CHAPTER 4: ENDOCRINE, NUTRITIONAL AND METABOLIC DISEASES (E00-E89)

Note:

All neoplasms, whether functionally active or not, are classified in Chapter 2. Appropriate codes in this chapter (i.e. E05.8, E07.0, E16-E31, E34.-) may be used as additional codes to indicate either functional activity by neoplasms and ectopic endocrine tissue or hyperfunction and hypofunction of endocrine glands associated with neoplasms and other conditions classified elsewhere.

EXCLUDES 1 transitory endocrine and metabolic disorders specific to newborn (P70-P74)

This chapter contains the following blocks:

E00-E07 Disorders of thyroid gland
E08-E13 Diabetes mellitus
E15-E16 Other disorders of glucose regulation and pancreatic internal secretion
E20-E35 Disorders of other endocrine glands
E36 Intraoperative complications of endocrine system
E40-E46 Malnutrition
E50-E64 Other nutritional deficiencies
E65-E68 Overweight, obesity and other hyperalimentation
E70-E88 Metabolic disorders
E89 Postprocedural endocrine and metabolic complications and disorders, not elsewhere classified

Disorders of thyroid gland (E00-E07)

✚ ◢ E00 Congenital iodine-deficiency syndrome
Use additional code (F70-F79) to identify associated intellectual disabilities.

EXCLUDES 1 subclinical iodine-deficiency hypothyroidism (E02)

CODING TIPS ✓ Do not assign a code from E00 to identify any condition that is not reported as "congenital" (present from birth).

DEFINITION Congenital iodine-deficiency syndrome is a congenital disorder often referred to as "cretinism." Congenital iodine-deficiency syndrome results from a thyroid hormone deficiency during fetal development and marked in childhood by dwarfed stature, mental retardation, dystrophy of the bones, and a low basal metabolism.

SP ✚ E00.0 Congenital iodine-deficiency syndrome, neurological type
Endemic cretinism, neurological type
DEFINITION Underactive thyroid gland present at birth with inadequate hormone production and slowed metabolic processes. Untreated, it can cause brain damage, mental retardation, and developmental delays.

SP ✚ E00.1 Congenital iodine-deficiency syndrome, myxedematous type
Endemic hypothyroid cretinism
Endemic cretinism, myxedematous type

SP ✚ E00.2 Congenital iodine-deficiency syndrome, mixed type
Endemic cretinism, mixed type

SP ✚ E00.9 Congenital iodine-deficiency syndrome, unspecified
Congenital iodine-deficiency hypothyroidism NOS

Endemic cretinism NOS

◢ E01 Iodine-deficiency related thyroid disorders and allied conditions
EXCLUDES 1 congenital iodine-deficiency syndrome (E00.-)
subclinical iodine-deficiency hypothyroidism (E02)

SP E01.0 Iodine-deficiency related diffuse (endemic) goiter

SP E01.1 Iodine-deficiency related multinodular (endemic) goiter
Iodine-deficiency related nodular goiter

SP E01.2 Iodine-deficiency related (endemic) goiter, unspecified
Endemic goiter NOS

SP E01.8 Other iodine-deficiency related thyroid disorders and allied conditions
Acquired iodine-deficiency hypothyroidism NOS

SP E02 Subclinical iodine-deficiency hypothyroidism
DEFINITION Early stage of hypothyroidism marked by increased TSH levels and normal free thyroxin T4 levels; occurs when the body requires additional TSH in order to produce enough thyroxin, and developing into overt hypothyroidism in a few years.

◢ E03 Other hypothyroidism
EXCLUDES 1 iodine-deficiency related hypothyroidism (E00-E02)
postprocedural hypothyroidism (E89.0)

CODING TIPS ✓ Report E89.0 for patients with hypothyroidism following a thyroidectomy, not other hypothyroidism (E03).

SP E03.0 Congenital hypothyroidism with diffuse goiter
Congenital parenchymatous goiter (nontoxic)
Congenital goiter (nontoxic) NOS
EXCLUDES 1 transitory congenital goiter with normal function (P72.0)

DEFINITION Abnormal hormone production or blocked TSH receptors in the fetus causing underactive thyroid with diffuse enlargement at birth, tracheal compression, difficulty breathing, and dysphagia.

SP E03.1 Congenital hypothyroidism without goiter
Aplasia of thyroid (with myxedema)
Congenital atrophy of thyroid
Congenital hypothyroidism NOS

IQ ✚ E03.2 Hypothyroidism due to medicaments and other exogenous substances
Code first:
poisoning due to drug or toxin, if applicable
(T36-T65 with fifth or sixth character 1-4 or 6)
Use additional code for adverse effect, if applicable, to identify drug (T36-T50 with fifth or sixth character 5)

Chapter 4

E00-E89

★ New ▲ Revised Px Primary **SP** PDGM Px **SL** Low CoM **SH** High CoM **IQ** Quest. Encounter **H** Hospice non-cancer Dx Unspecified **M** *Manifestation*

DecisionHealth's FY 2020 Complete Home Health ICD-10-CM Diagnosis Coding Manual

731

CODING TIPS ✓ Determine whether the hypothyroidism is due to a poisoning or due to an adverse effect of a medication, such as lithium. Sequencing is determined based on whether the causative factor was a poisoning or an adverse effect. If the physician uses the term "thyroiditis," see E06.4.

SP E03.3 Postinfectious hypothyroidism

DEFINITION Damage to normal thyroid function from a previous infection, resulting in tiredness, weight gain, constipation, cold intolerance, dry skin, slowed mental function, and depression.

SP E03.4 Atrophy of thyroid (acquired)

EXCLUDES 1 congenital atrophy of thyroid (E03.1)

DEFINITION Abnormally small thyroid due to tissue degeneration and wasting; the gland becomes nonviable or severely reduced in function.

SP E03.5 Myxedema coma

DEFINITION Fully symptomatic hypothyroid disease manifesting with coma in a seriously decompensated state, mostly in the elderly, accompanied by hypothermia, hypoventilation with hypoxia, hypercapnia, hyponatremia, and bradycardia.

SP E03.8 Other specified hypothyroidism

SP E03.9 Hypothyroidism, unspecified

Myxedema NOS

DEFINITION Failure of the thyroid gland to produce enough hormone to maintain the body's metabolism, causing fatigue, weight gain, muscle aches and cramps, cold intolerance, memory loss, and depression.

4 E04 Other nontoxic goiter

EXCLUDES 1 congenital goiter (NOS) (diffuse) (parenchymatous) (E03.0)
iodine-deficiency related goiter (E00-E02)

SP E04.0 Nontoxic diffuse goiter

Diffuse (colloid) nontoxic goiter
Simple nontoxic goiter

DEFINITION Generalized, simple, painless thyroid enlargement without impairment of glandular function due to an overload of thyroid-stimulating hormone (TSH) from the pituitary gland.

SP E04.1 Nontoxic single thyroid nodule

Colloid nodule (cystic) (thyroid)
Nontoxic uninodular goiter
Thyroid (cystic) nodule NOS

DEFINITION A simple, painless, cyst-like node or singular goiter on the thyroid that is not impairing the normal glandular function.

SP E04.2 Nontoxic multinodular goiter

Cystic goiter NOS
Multinodular (cystic) goiter NOS

DEFINITION Multiple hard knobs, or cysts, in the thyroid detected by palpation but not impairing function or causing disease.

SP E04.8 Other specified nontoxic goiter

SP E04.9 Nontoxic goiter, unspecified

Goiter NOS
Nodular goiter (nontoxic) NOS

4 E05 Thyrotoxicosis [hyperthyroidism]

EXCLUDES 1 chronic thyroiditis with transient thyrotoxicosis (E06.2)
neonatal thyrotoxicosis (P72.1)

CODING TIPS ✓ Thyrotoxicosis is another term for hyperthyroidism, and these terms may frequently be used interchangeably in clinical records. Unspecified hyperthyroidism should be coded to E05.9-.

CODING TIPS ✓ Codes from category E05 are combination codes that indicate the presence or absence of thyrotoxic crisis or storm. A thyrotoxic crisis (also called "thyroid storm") is a condition that may occur among individuals with hyperthyroidism and is marked by tachycardia, fever, and hypertension, which may or may not result in congestive heart failure and/or shock. Thyrotoxic crisis should only be coded when specified by the physician and cannot be assumed based upon other symptoms alone.

5 E05.0 Thyrotoxicosis with diffuse goiter

Exophthalmic or toxic goiter NOS
Graves' disease
Toxic diffuse goiter

DEFINITION Thyrotropin receptor antibody production that mimics the pituitary's normal regulatory hormone, overriding it and increasing thyroid hormone production, marked by enlarged thyroid and bulging eyes.

SP E05.00 Thyrotoxicosis with diffuse goiter without thyrotoxic crisis or storm

DEFINITION Hyperthyroid conditions with excessive hormone production and speeding up of body functions; increased heart rate and blood pressure, excessive sweating, hand tremors, nervousness and anxiety, insomnia, and weight loss with increased appetite.

SP E05.01 Thyrotoxicosis with diffuse goiter with thyrotoxic crisis or storm

DEFINITION Severe, sudden worsening of hyperthyroid conditions from injury, stress, or gland removal that can lead to coma and death, manifesting with tachycardia, arrhythmia, vomiting, high fever, diarrhea, and dehydration.

5 E05.1 Thyrotoxicosis with toxic single thyroid nodule

Thyrotoxicosis with toxic uninodular goiter

SP E05.10 Thyrotoxicosis with toxic single thyroid nodule without thyrotoxic crisis or storm

SP E05.11 Thyrotoxicosis with toxic single thyroid nodule with thyrotoxic crisis or storm

5 E05.2 Thyrotoxicosis with toxic multinodular goiter

Toxic nodular goiter NOS

---

4 4th digit required   **5** 5th digit required   **6** 6th digit required   **7** 7th digit required   **7** 7th digit placeholder   **+** Additional code   **⊟** Laterality

732   *DecisionHealth's* FY 2020 Complete Home Health ICD-10-CM Diagnosis Coding Manual

Chapter 4

E00-E89

SP E05.20 Thyrotoxicosis with toxic multinodular goiter without thyrotoxic crisis or storm

SP E05.21 Thyrotoxicosis with toxic multinodular goiter with thyrotoxic crisis or storm

5 E05.3 Thyrotoxicosis from ectopic thyroid tissue

SP E05.30 Thyrotoxicosis from ectopic thyroid tissue without thyrotoxic crisis or storm

SP E05.31 Thyrotoxicosis from ectopic thyroid tissue with thyrotoxic crisis or storm

5 E05.4 Thyrotoxicosis factitia

DEFINITION Thyrotoxicosis factitia is a condition of higher than normal thyroid hormones (T3 and T4) resulting from excess ingestion of thyroid hormone (medication). The condition may be iatrogenic (adverse effect resulting from taking prescription correctly) or due to intentional ingestion of excess medication (poisoning). The cause of the condition should be identified and the coder should follow guidelines for coding of adverse effects and poisoning when assigning a code from E05.4-.

SP E05.40 Thyrotoxicosis factitia without thyrotoxic crisis or storm

SP E05.41 Thyrotoxicosis factitia with thyrotoxic crisis or storm

5 E05.8 Other thyrotoxicosis
Overproduction of thyroid-stimulating hormone

SP E05.80 Other thyrotoxicosis without thyrotoxic crisis or storm

SP E05.81 Other thyrotoxicosis with thyrotoxic crisis or storm

5 E05.9 Thyrotoxicosis, unspecified
Hyperthyroidism NOS

SP E05.90 Thyrotoxicosis, unspecified without thyrotoxic crisis or storm

SP E05.91 Thyrotoxicosis, unspecified with thyrotoxic crisis or storm

4 E06 Thyroiditis

EXCLUDES 1 postpartum thyroiditis (O90.5)

DEFINITION Thyroiditis is a condition marked by inflammation of the thyroid (may or may not be infectious in nature), and should not be confused with hyperthyroidism. Various forms of thyroiditis may result in either hyper- or hypothyroidism.

SP + E06.0 Acute thyroiditis
Abscess of thyroid
Pyogenic thyroiditis
Suppurative thyroiditis
Use additional code (B95-B97) to identify infectious agent.

DEFINITION Painful infection of the thyroid gland, often with abscess and pus formation.

SP E06.1 Subacute thyroiditis
de Quervain thyroiditis
Giant-cell thyroiditis
Granulomatous thyroiditis
Nonsuppurative thyroiditis
Viral thyroiditis

EXCLUDES 1 autoimmune thyroiditis (E06.3)

DEFINITION Thyroid inflammation often resulting from another disease, such as mumps or flu, presenting with fever, radiating neck pain, and hyperthyroidism symptoms than can last months.

SP E06.2 Chronic thyroiditis with transient thyrotoxicosis

EXCLUDES 1 autoimmune thyroiditis (E06.3)

SP E06.3 Autoimmune thyroiditis
Hashimoto's thyroiditis
Hashitoxicosis (transient)
Lymphadenoid goiter
Lymphocytic thyroiditis
Struma lymphomatosa

DEFINITION Autoimmune inflammation of the thyroid with lymphocyte infiltration that presents with painless thyroid enlargement and hypothyroid symptoms.

SP + E06.4 Drug-induced thyroiditis
Use additional code for adverse effect, if applicable, to identify drug (T36-T50 with fifth or sixth character 5)

CODING TIPS ✓ Drug-induced thyroiditis should only be coded when clinical record documentation clearly indicates thyroiditis (inflammation of the thyroid), resulting from the administration of a specific drug or chemical. The causative drug or chemical should be identified and the coder should follow guidelines for coding of adverse effects and poisoning when assigning E06.4. If the physician uses the term "hypothyroidism, due to drugs or toxins," see E03.2.

DEFINITION Iatrogenic inflammation of the thyroid due to taking certain medications, such as lithium, or an overdose of iodine.

SP E06.5 Other chronic thyroiditis
Chronic fibrous thyroiditis
Chronic thyroiditis NOS
Ligneous thyroiditis
Riedel thyroiditis

SP E06.9 Thyroiditis, unspecified

DEFINITION Inflammation of the thyroid with noticeable swelling, often on one side, possibly inducing symptoms of hyper- or hypothyroidism, from unspecified causation or acuity.

4 E07 Other disorders of thyroid

SP E07.0 Hypersecretion of calcitonin
C-cell hyperplasia of thyroid
Hypersecretion of thyrocalcitonin

SP E07.1 Dyshormogenetic goiter
Familial dyshormogenetic goiter
Pendred's syndrome

EXCLUDES 1 transitory congenital goiter with normal function (P72.0)

5 E07.8 Other specified disorders of thyroid

SP E07.81 Sick-euthyroid syndrome
Euthyroid sick-syndrome

☆ New ▲ Revised Px Primary SP PDGM Px SL Low CoM SH High CoM IQ Quest. Encounter H Hospice non-cancer Dx Unspecified M Manifestation

DecisionHealth's FY 2020 Complete Home Health ICD-10-CM Diagnosis Coding Manual

733

Chapter 4

E00-E89

DEFINITION   Condition in which thyroid hormone levels are off due to a non-thyroid related problem.

SP E07.89   Other specified disorders of thyroid
Abnormality of thyroid-binding
   globulin
Hemorrhage of thyroid
Infarction of thyroid

IQ E07.9   Disorder of thyroid, unspecified

Diabetes mellitus   (E08-E13)

GUIDELINES   Section I.C.4.a.1)-3)
The diabetes mellitus codes are combination codes that include the type of diabetes mellitus, the body system affected, and the complications affecting that body system. As many codes within a particular category as are necessary to describe all of the complications of the disease may be used. They should be sequenced based on the reason for a particular encounter. Assign as many codes from categories E08 – E13 as needed to identify all of the associated conditions that the patient has.

The age of a patient is not the sole determining factor, though most type 1 diabetics develop the condition before reaching puberty. For this reason type 1 diabetes mellitus is also referred to as juvenile diabetes.

If the type of diabetes mellitus is not documented in the medical record the default is E11.-, Type 2 diabetes mellitus.

If the documentation in a medical record does not indicate the type of diabetes but does indicate that the patient uses insulin, code E11, Type 2 diabetes mellitus, should be assigned. An additional code should be assigned from category Z79 to identify the long-term (current) use of insulin or oral hypoglycemic drugs. If the patient is treated with both oral medications and insulin, only the code for long-term (current) use of insulin should be assigned. Code Z79.4 should not be assigned if insulin is given temporarily to bring a type 2 patient's blood sugar under control during an encounter.

GUIDELINES   Section I.C.4.a.6)
Codes under categories E08, Diabetes mellitus due to underlying condition, E09, Drug or chemical induced diabetes mellitus, and E13, Other specified diabetes mellitus, identify complications/manifestations associated with secondary diabetes mellitus. Secondary diabetes is always caused by another condition or event (e.g., cystic fibrosis, malignant neoplasm of pancreas, pancreatectomy, adverse effect of drug, or poisoning).

CODING TIPS ✓   Codes E08-E13 are combination codes that generally do not require a second code to describe the manifestation unless specified by the code specific convention. Specifically, when coding diabetes with an ulcer, diabetic chronic kidney disease, or speciified manifestations that do not belong in a specific subcategory, a second code is required. A second code to identify gastroparesis (K31.84) may be assigned, optionally, when coding diabetic gastroparesis.

CODING TIPS ✓   Reference the alphabetical index to review conditions that the classification assumes are related to diabetes. All specified manifestations/complications listed under the word 'with' in the index are presumed related unless the physician specified a different cause in documentation, or states they're unrelated. The 'with' convention does not apply to "not elsewhere classified (NEC)" index entries that cover broad categories of conditions. Coding professionals should not assume a causal relationship when the diabetic complication is "NEC."

CODING TIPS ✓   When a patient is receiving home health services for the administration of insulin, the clinical record must contain detailed evidence of the patient's inability to self administer. For example, a patient with rheumatoid arthritis may have impaired ability to manipulate an injectable medication and self inject. It is not appropriate to use vague terms, such as poor vision or poor manual dexterity.

+ 4 E08   Diabetes mellitus due to underlying condition
Code first the underlying condition, such as:
   congenital rubella (P35.0)
   Cushing's syndrome (E24.-)
   cystic fibrosis (E84.-)
   malignant neoplasm (C00-C96)
   malnutrition (E40-E46)
   pancreatitis and other diseases of the
      pancreas (K85-K86.-)
Use additional code to identify control using:
   insulin (Z79.4)
   oral antidiabetic drugs (Z79.84)
   oral hypoglycemic drugs (Z79.84)

EXCLUDES 1   drug or chemical induced
      diabetes mellitus (E09.-)
   gestational diabetes (O24.4-)
   neonatal diabetes mellitus
      (P70.2)
   postpancreatectomy diabetes
      mellitus (E13.-)
   postprocedural diabetes mellitus
      (E13.-)
   secondary diabetes mellitus
      NEC (E13.-)
   type 1 diabetes mellitus (E10.-)
   type 2 diabetes mellitus (E11.-)

CODING TIPS ✓   When coding diabetes mellitus due to an underlying condition, the underlying condition and relationship to diabetes should be specified by the provider.

CODING TIPS ✓   If the patient uses an insulin pump, use Z96.41 as an additional code. If there is a complication involving the insulin pump, use a code from T85.6- or T85.7- instead of the Z code.

CODING TIPS ✓   Use Z79.4 to indicate the use of insulin, OR use Z79.84 to indicate the use of oral anti-glycemics. Use Z79.84 only when the patient does not also take insulin. Do NOT code both.

CODING TIPS ✓   Reference the alphabetical index to review conditions that the classification assumes are related to diabetes. All specified manifestations/complications listed under the word 'with' in the index are presumed related unless the physician specifies a different cause in documentation, or states they're unrelated. The "with" convention does not apply to "not elsewhere classified (NEC)" index entries that cover broad categories of conditions. Specific conditions must be linked by the terms "with," "in," "due to" or "associated with." Coding professionals should not assume a causal relationship when the diabetic complication is "NEC."

---

4 4th digit required   **5** 5th digit required   **6** 6th digit required   **7** 7th digit required   **☑** 7th digit placeholder   **+** Additional code   **☐** Laterality

Chapter 4

E00-E89

CODING TIPS ✓ E08 codes will never be primary. Common conditions causing diabetes due to underlying condition are listed in the "code first" note. If diabetes is related to a malignant neoplasm of the pancreas, query whether the diabetes is caused by the neoplasm itself (E08); the drugs used to treat the neoplasm (E09); or the removal of part or all of the pancreas (E13).

+ ⑤ E08.0 Diabetes mellitus due to underlying condition with hyperosmolarity

IQ + E08.00 Diabetes mellitus due to underlying condition with hyperosmolarity without nonketotic hyperglycemic-hyperosmolar coma (NKHHC)

IQ + E08.01 Diabetes mellitus due to underlying condition with hyperosmolarity with coma

+ ⑤ E08.1 Diabetes mellitus due to underlying condition with ketoacidosis

> **CODING TIPS ✓** Diabetic ketoacidosis is a serious complication of diabetes that occurs when the body produces high levels of blood acids called ketones. This condition is likely resolved before admission to home care, but could be a current diagnosis.

IQ + E08.10 Diabetes mellitus due to underlying condition with ketoacidosis without coma

IQ + E08.11 Diabetes mellitus due to underlying condition with ketoacidosis with coma

+ ⑤ E08.2 Diabetes mellitus due to underlying condition with kidney complications

IQ + E08.21 Diabetes mellitus due to underlying condition with diabetic nephropathy
Diabetes mellitus due to underlying condition with intercapillary glomerulosclerosis
Diabetes mellitus due to underlying condition with intracapillary glomerulonephrosis
Diabetes mellitus due to underlying condition with Kimmelstiel-Wilson disease

IQ + E08.22 Diabetes mellitus due to underlying condition with diabetic chronic kidney disease
Use additional code to identify stage of chronic kidney disease (N18.1-N18.6)

> **CODING TIPS ✓** Assign an additional code from N18- to indicate the stage of CKD. When diabetic nephropathy and CKD are documented, code diabetic CKD, not nephropathy, because CKD is more specific.

CODING TIPS ✓ When diabetes, CKD and hypertension are documented, sequence the appropriate category of diabetes with CKD (E--.22) and the appropriate hypertension code (I12 or I13) prior to N18. The hypertension or the diabetes may be sequenced first depending on the focus of care. Use N18.1-N18.6 or N18.9 to indicate the CKD. The only time that the conditions should be coded differently is if the physician specifically documents that the conditions are not related.

IQ + E08.29 Diabetes mellitus due to underlying condition with other diabetic kidney complication
Renal tubular degeneration in diabetes mellitus due to underlying condition

+ ⑤ E08.3 Diabetes mellitus due to underlying condition with ophthalmic complications

> **CODING TIPS ✓** Diabetic codes indicating specific eye disorders require a 7th character to indicate laterality.

> **CODING TIPS ✓** When a patient has macular edema, the patient also has retinopathy, with the macular edema developing as a complication of the retinopathy. Retinopathy includes three stages: background retinopathy, proliferative retinopathy, and macular edema.

> **CODING TIPS ✓** When coding diabetes with ophthalmic manifestations, review the clinical record and plan of care to ensure that the functional impact of visual impairments is reported. The home health record should clearly report how visual losses impact the function and activities of the patient, including how these conditions impact medication administration, safety, the ability to perform treatments (such as wound care) and other key areas related to the patient's daily living.

+ ⑥ E08.31 Diabetes mellitus due to underlying condition with unspecified diabetic retinopathy

IQ + E08.311 Diabetes mellitus due to underlying condition with unspecified diabetic retinopathy with macular edema

IQ + E08.319 Diabetes mellitus due to underlying condition with unspecified diabetic retinopathy without macular edema

+ ⑥ E08.32 Diabetes mellitus due to underlying condition with mild nonproliferative diabetic retinopathy
Diabetes mellitus due to underlying condition with nonproliferative diabetic retinopathy NOS

Chapter 4

E00-E89

★ New ▲ Revised **Px** Primary **SP** PDGM Px **SL** Low CoM **SH** High CoM **IQ** Quest. Encounter **H** Hospice non-cancer Dx Unspecified **M** *Manifestation*

DecisionHealth's FY 2020 Complete Home Health ICD-10-CM Diagnosis Coding Manual

735

Chapter 4

E00-E89

One of the following 7th characters is to be assigned to codes in subcategory E08.32 to designate laterality of the disease:
1   right eye
2   left eye
3   bilateral
9   unspecified eye

⬒ **IQ** + 7 **E08.321-**   **Diabetes mellitus due to underlying condition with mild nonproliferative diabetic retinopathy with macular edema**

⬒ **IQ** + 7 **E08.329-**   **Diabetes mellitus due to underlying condition with mild nonproliferative diabetic retinopathy without macular edema**

+ 6 **E08.33**   **Diabetes mellitus due to underlying condition with moderate nonproliferative diabetic retinopathy**

One of the following 7th characters is to be assigned to codes in subcategory E08.33 to designate laterality of the disease:
1   right eye
2   left eye
3   bilateral
9   unspecified eye

⬒ **IQ** + 7 **E08.331-**   **Diabetes mellitus due to underlying condition with moderate nonproliferative diabetic retinopathy with macular edema**

⬒ **IQ** + 7 **E08.339-**   **Diabetes mellitus due to underlying condition with moderate nonproliferative diabetic retinopathy without macular edema**

+ 6 **E08.34**   **Diabetes mellitus due to underlying condition with severe nonproliferative diabetic retinopathy**

One of the following 7th characters is to be assigned to codes in subcategory E08.34 to designate laterality of the disease:
1   right eye
2   left eye
3   bilateral
9   unspecified eye

⬒ **IQ** + 7 **E08.341-**   **Diabetes mellitus due to underlying condition with severe nonproliferative diabetic retinopathy with macular edema**

⬒ **IQ** + 7 **E08.349-**   **Diabetes mellitus due to underlying condition with severe nonproliferative diabetic retinopathy without macular edema**

+ 6 **E08.35**   **Diabetes mellitus due to underlying condition with proliferative diabetic retinopathy**

One of the following 7th characters is to be assigned to codes in subcategory E08.35 to designate laterality of the disease:
1   right eye
2   left eye
3   bilateral
9   unspecified eye

⬒ **IQ** + 7 **E08.351-**   **Diabetes mellitus due to underlying condition with proliferative diabetic retinopathy with macular edema**

⬒ **IQ** + 7 **E08.352-**   **Diabetes mellitus due to underlying condition with proliferative diabetic retinopathy with traction retinal detachment involving the macula**

⬒ **IQ** + 7 **E08.353-**   **Diabetes mellitus due to underlying condition with proliferative diabetic retinopathy with traction retinal detachment not involving the macula**

⬒ **IQ** + 7 **E08.354-**   **Diabetes mellitus due to underlying condition with proliferative diabetic retinopathy with combined traction retinal detachment and rhegmatogenous retinal detachment**

⬒ **IQ** + 7 **E08.355-**   **Diabetes mellitus due to underlying condition with stable proliferative diabetic retinopathy**

⬒ **IQ** + 7 **E08.359-**   **Diabetes mellitus due to underlying condition with proliferative diabetic retinopathy without macular edema**

IQ + **E08.36**   **Diabetes mellitus due to underlying condition with diabetic cataract**

CODING TIPS ✓   Cataracts are more common in diabetic patients. The classification assumes a relationship between cataracts and diabetes, when the patient has diabetes. Even cataracts specifically described as "cortical, nuclear and posterior subcapsular" and "nuclear sclerotic" should prompt the assignment of E--.36, along with the code for the specific cataract code (*Q2 2019 Coding Clinic*).

⬒ **IQ** + 7̶ **E08.37X-**   **Diabetes mellitus due to underlying condition with diabetic macular edema, resolved following treatment**

One of the following 7th characters is to be assigned to code E08.37 to designate laterality of the disease:
1   right eye
2   left eye
3   bilateral
9   unspecified eye

---

4 4th digit required   5 5th digit required   6 6th digit required   7 7th digit required   7̶ 7th digit placeholder   **+** Additional code   ⬒ Laterality

CODING TIPS ✓ The macular edema may be resolved, but the retinopathy remains. This code is like a history code for the macular edema.

IQ + E08.39 Diabetes mellitus due to underlying condition with other diabetic ophthalmic complication

Use additional code to identify manifestation, such as: diabetic glaucoma (H40-H42)

CODING TIPS ✓ There is no assumed relationship between diabetes and glaucoma. The coder should seek further clarification regarding the relationship between blindness, glaucoma and diabetes before coding as a diabetic manifestation.

+ ⑤ E08.4 Diabetes mellitus due to underlying condition with neurological complications

CODING TIPS ✓ Diabetes due to an underlying condition with loss of protective sensation or diabetic peripheral neuropathy should be coded to E08.42.

IQ SH SL + E08.40 Diabetes mellitus due to underlying condition with diabetic neuropathy, unspecified

IQ + E08.41 Diabetes mellitus due to underlying condition with diabetic mononeuropathy

IQ SH SL + E08.42 Diabetes mellitus due to underlying condition with diabetic polyneuropathy

Diabetes mellitus due to underlying condition with diabetic neuralgia

CODING TIPS ✓ Diabetic polyneuropathy is the most common type of diabetic neuropathy and causes pain or loss of feeling in the toes, feet, legs, hands and arms.

IQ + E08.43 Diabetes mellitus due to underlying condition with diabetic autonomic (poly)neuropathy

Diabetes mellitus due to underlying condition with diabetic gastroparesis

CODING TIPS ✓ Autonomic neuropathy affects the heart, digestive system and other involuntary functions. This type of neuropathy causes delayed or slowed gastric emptying as well as problems with orthostatic hypotension. This code is not to be used for polyneuropathy of the hands and feet.

CODING TIPS ✓ Gastroparesis (K31.84) may be sequenced after this code as an option.

IQ + E08.44 Diabetes mellitus due to underlying condition with diabetic amyotrophy

CODING TIPS ✓ Diabetic amyotrophy is muscle weakness, characterized by weakness followed by wasting of pelvifemoral muscles, either unilaterally or bilaterally, with associated pain.

IQ + E08.49 Diabetes mellitus due to underlying condition with other diabetic neurological complication

+ ⑤ E08.5 Diabetes mellitus due to underlying condition with circulatory complications

CODING TIPS ✓ Peripheral angiopathy includes arterial, venous and capillary conditions. Peripheral angiopathy may be documented as diabetic PVD. There is an assumed relationship between diabetes and PVD and PAD, including peripheral atherosclerosis and venous insufficiency. Diabetic PVD is coded E--.51. Diabetic arteriosclerosis of the peripheral arteries should be coded E--.51 or E--.52 then the appropriate I70.- code. Diabetic venous insufficiency should be coded E--.51 or E--.52 and I87.2 The presence of diabetes and peripheral arterial disease in the record indicates that both diabetes and PVD should be marked in M1028. Venous disease is not included in M1028.

IQ + E08.51 Diabetes mellitus due to underlying condition with diabetic peripheral angiopathy without gangrene

IQ + E08.52 Diabetes mellitus due to underlying condition with diabetic peripheral angiopathy with gangrene

Diabetes mellitus due to underlying condition with diabetic gangrene

IQ + E08.59 Diabetes mellitus due to underlying condition with other circulatory complications

CODING TIPS ✓ Diabetic circulatory complications other than peripheral angiopathy and gangrene, identified as such by the physician, may be coded to 4th and 5th characters .59. Example: Diabetic CAD or ASHD is documented.

+ ⑤ E08.6 Diabetes mellitus due to underlying condition with other specified complications

+ ⑥ E08.61 Diabetes mellitus due to underlying condition with diabetic arthropathy

IQ + E08.610 Diabetes mellitus due to underlying condition with diabetic neuropathic arthropathy

Diabetes mellitus due to underlying condition with Charcôt's joints

CODING TIPS ✓ Do not add a M14.6 code for Charcot's joint.

IQ + E08.618 Diabetes mellitus due to underlying condition with other diabetic arthropathy

+ ⑥ E08.62 Diabetes mellitus due to underlying condition with skin complications

IQ + E08.620 Diabetes mellitus due to underlying condition with diabetic dermatitis

Diabetes mellitus due to underlying condition with diabetic necrobiosis lipoidica

IQ + E08.621 Diabetes mellitus due to underlying condition with foot ulcer

Use additional code to identify site of ulcer (L97.4-, L97.5-)

★ New ▲ Revised **Px** Primary **SP** PDGM Px **SL** Low CoM **SH** High CoM **IQ** Quest. Encounter **H** Hospice non-cancer Dx   Unspecified   **M** *Manifestation*

CODING TIPS ✓ If the patient has had a diabetic foot ulcer in the past, either healed or amputated, also code Z86.31. Ulceration of the foot is assumed related to diabetes unless another cause is indicated.

IQ ✚ E08.622 Diabetes mellitus due to underlying condition with other skin ulcer

Use additional code to identify site of ulcer (L97.1-L97.9, L98.41-L98.49)

CODING TIPS ✓ Diabetes codes with 4th, 5th and 6th characters .622 are used when an ulcer is located on the lower extremity, beginning at the ankle, and not including the foot. Whereas ulcers located on the foot are assumed related to diabetes, ulcers located elsewhere are not assumed related to diabetes and must be confirmed with the physician.

IQ ✚ E08.628 Diabetes mellitus due to underlying condition with other skin complications

✚ 6 E08.63 Diabetes mellitus due to underlying condition with oral complications

IQ ✚ E08.630 Diabetes mellitus due to underlying condition with periodontal disease

IQ ✚ E08.638 Diabetes mellitus due to underlying condition with other oral complications

✚ 6 E08.64 Diabetes mellitus due to underlying condition with hypoglycemia

IQ ✚ E08.641 Diabetes mellitus due to underlying condition with hypoglycemia with coma

IQ ✚ E08.649 Diabetes mellitus due to underlying condition with hypoglycemia without coma

CODING TIPS ✓ The physician should be queried when the term "uncontrolled" is used to determine whether the patient has hyperglycemia, hypoglycemia or both.

CODING TIPS ✓ If encephalopathy is due to hypoglycemia, use G93.41 as an additional code.

IQ ✚ E08.65 Diabetes mellitus due to underlying condition with hyperglycemia

CODING TIPS ✓ Inadequately controlled, poorly controlled and out of control diabetes are coded with hyperglycemia. The physician should be queried when the term 'uncontrolled' is used to determine whether the patient has hyperglycemia, hypoglycemia, or both. The clinical record should support hyperglycemia. Do not code diabetes with hyperglycemia when ketoacidosis is also documented.

IQ ✚ E08.69 Diabetes mellitus due to underlying condition with other specified complication

Use additional code to identify complication

CODING TIPS ✓ Use this code when the physician specifies a manifestation of diabetes that does not fit in any of the other subcategories. Follow the diabetes code with the code for the specified condition.

CODING TIPS ✓ The classification presumes a cause-and-effect relationship between osteomyelitis and diabetes when no other cause is documented. Osteomyelitis with diabetes is usually associated with ulceration. Use the appropriate code for the osteomyelitis after coding diabetes with other specified manifestation. Although not clear that certain types of diabetes are assumed related to osteomyelitis when referencing diabetes in the index, it is confirmed that osteomyelitis is related to all diabetes types.

IQ ✚ E08.8 Diabetes mellitus due to underlying condition with unspecified complications

CODING TIPS ✓ This code should not be used for unspecified complications. Query the physician for information regarding suspected manifestations that the classification does not presume related.

IQ ✚ E08.9 Diabetes mellitus due to underlying condition without complications

CODING TIPS ✓ This code is acceptable to use for a diabetic without manifestations. Certain specified conditions are assumed related to diabetes by the classification, if listed indented under the word "with" in the alphabetical index, so the use of .9 as a diabetes 4th character should not be common. Query the physician for information regarding suspected manifestations when documentation regarding other potential causes is unclear. This code should be used for a diabetic requiring insulin injections only if teaching is the skill, or other comorbidities, unrelated to diabetes, make it unacceptable for the patient to self-inject. If .9 is used as a 4th character, no other diabetes code may be used.

✚ 4 E09 Drug or chemical induced diabetes mellitus

Code first:
poisoning due to drug or toxin, if applicable (T36-T65 with fifth or sixth character 1-4 or 6)
Use additional code for adverse effect, if applicable, to identify drug (T36-T50 with fifth or sixth character 5)
Use additional code to identify control using:
insulin (Z79.4)
oral antidiabetic drugs (Z79.84)
oral hypoglycemic drugs (Z79.84)

EXCLUDES 1 diabetes mellitus due to underlying condition (E08.-)
gestational diabetes (O24.4-)

4 4th digit required   5 5th digit required   6 6th digit required   7 7th digit required   ✓ 7th digit placeholder   ✚ Additional code   ▤ Laterality

738   *DecisionHealth's* FY 2020 Complete Home Health ICD-10-CM Diagnosis Coding Manual

Chapter 4

E00-E89

neonatal diabetes mellitus (P70.2)

postpancreatectomy diabetes mellitus (E13.-)

postprocedural diabetes mellitus (E13.-)

secondary diabetes mellitus NEC (E13.-)

type 1 diabetes mellitus (E10.-)

type 2 diabetes mellitus (E11.-)

GUIDELINES Section I.C.4.a.6(a)

Codes under categories E08, Diabetes mellitus due to underlying condition, E09, Drug or chemical induced diabetes mellitus, and E13, Other specified diabetes mellitus, identify complications/manifestations associated with secondary diabetes mellitus. Secondary diabetes is always caused by another condition or event (e.g., cystic fibrosis, malignant neoplasm of pancreas, pancreatectomy, adverse effect of drug, or poisoning). For patients with secondary diabetes mellitus who routinely use insulin or oral hypoglycemic drugs, an additional code from category Z79 should be assigned to identify the long-term (current) use of insulin or oral hypoglycemic drugs. If the patient is treated with both oral medications and insulin, only the code for long-term (current) use of insulin should be assigned. Code Z79.4 should not be assigned if insulin is given temporarily to bring a secondary diabetic patient's blood sugar under control during an encounter.

GUIDELINES Section I.C.4.a

The diabetes mellitus codes are combination codes that include the type of diabetes mellitus, the body system affected, and the complications affecting that body system. As many codes within a particular category as are necessary to describe all of the complications of the disease may be used. They should be sequenced based on the reason for a particular encounter. Assign as many codes from categories E08 – E13 as needed to identify all of the associated conditions that the patient has.

CODING TIPS ✓ If the patient uses an insulin pump, use Z96.41 as an additional code. If there is a complication involving the insulin pump, use a code from T85.6- or T85.7- instead of the Z code.

CODING TIPS ✓ Use Z79.4 to indicate the use of insulin, OR use Z79.84 to indicate the use of oral anti-glycemics. Use Z79.84 only when the patient does not also take insulin. Do NOT code both.

CODING TIPS ✓ Reference the alphabetical index to review conditions that the classification assumes are related to diabetes. All specified manifestations/complications listed under the word 'with' in the index are presumed related unless the physician specifies a different cause in documentation, or states they're unrelated. The "with" convention does not apply to "not elsewhere classified (NEC)" index entries that cover broad categories of conditions. Specific conditions must be linked by the terms "with," "in," "due to" or "associated with." Coding professionals should not assume a causal relationship when the diabetic complication is "NEC."

CODING TIPS ✓ If diabetes is related to a malignant neoplasm of the pancreas, query whether the diabetes is caused by the neoplasm itself (E08); the drugs used to treat the neoplasm (E09); or the removal of part or all of the pancreas (E13).

+ 5 E09.0 **Drug or chemical induced diabetes mellitus with hyperosmolarity**

SP + E09.00 **Drug or chemical induced diabetes mellitus with hyperosmolarity without nonketotic hyperglycemic-hyperosmolar coma (NKHHC)**

SP + E09.01 **Drug or chemical induced diabetes mellitus with hyperosmolarity with coma**

+ 5 E09.1 **Drug or chemical induced diabetes mellitus with ketoacidosis**

CODING TIPS ✓ Diabetic ketoacidosis is a serious complication of diabetes that occurs when the body produces high levels of blood acids called ketones. This condition is likely resolved before admission to home care, but could be a current diagnosis.

SP + E09.10 **Drug or chemical induced diabetes mellitus with ketoacidosis without coma**

SP + E09.11 **Drug or chemical induced diabetes mellitus with ketoacidosis with coma**

+ 5 E09.2 **Drug or chemical induced diabetes mellitus with kidney complications**

SP + E09.21 **Drug or chemical induced diabetes mellitus with diabetic nephropathy**

Drug or chemical induced diabetes mellitus with intercapillary glomerulosclerosis

Drug or chemical induced diabetes mellitus with intracapillary glomerulonephrosis

Drug or chemical induced diabetes mellitus with Kimmelstiel-Wilson disease

SP + E09.22 **Drug or chemical induced diabetes mellitus with diabetic chronic kidney disease**

Use additional code to identify stage of chronic kidney disease (N18.1-N18.6)

★ New ▲ Revised **Px** Primary **SP** PDGM Px **SL** Low CoM **SH** High CoM **IQ** Quest. Encounter **H** Hospice non-cancer Dx　Unspecified　**M** *Manifestation*

DecisionHealth's FY 2020 Complete Home Health ICD-10-CM Diagnosis Coding Manual

739

CODING TIPS ✓ Assign an additional code from N18- to indicate the stage of CKD. When diabetic nephropathy and CKD are documented, code diabetic CKD, not nephropathy, because CKD is more specific.

CODING TIPS ✓ When diabetes, CKD and hypertension are documented, sequence the appropriate category of diabetes with CKD (E--.22) and the appropriate hypertension code (I12 or I13) prior to N18. The hypertension or the diabetes may be sequenced first depending on the focus of care. Use N18.1-N18.6 or N18.9 to indicate the CKD. The only time that the conditions should be coded differently is if the physician specifically documents that the conditions are not related.

SP ✚ E09.29 Drug or chemical induced diabetes mellitus with other diabetic kidney complication
Drug or chemical induced diabetes mellitus with renal tubular degeneration

✚ ⑤ E09.3 Drug or chemical induced diabetes mellitus with ophthalmic complications

CODING TIPS ✓ Diabetic codes indicating specific eye disorders require a 7th character to indicate laterality.

CODING TIPS ✓ When coding diabetes with ophthalmic manifestations, review the clinical record and plan of care to ensure that the functional impact of visual impairments is reported. The home health record should clearly report how visual losses impact the function and activities of the patient, including how these conditions impact medication administration, safety, the ability to perform treatments (such as wound care) and other key areas related to the patient's daily living.

CODING TIPS ✓ When a patient has macular edema, the patient also has retinopathy, with the macular edema developing as a complication of the retinopathy. Retinopathy includes three stages: background retinopathy, proliferative retinopathy, and macular edema.

✚ ⑥ E09.31 Drug or chemical induced diabetes mellitus with unspecified diabetic retinopathy

SP ✚ E09.311 Drug or chemical induced diabetes mellitus with unspecified diabetic retinopathy with macular edema

SP ✚ E09.319 Drug or chemical induced diabetes mellitus with unspecified diabetic retinopathy without macular edema

✚ ⑥ E09.32 Drug or chemical induced diabetes mellitus with mild nonproliferative diabetic retinopathy
Drug or chemical induced diabetes mellitus with nonproliferative diabetic retinopathy NOS

One of the following 7th characters is to be assigned to codes in subcategory E09.32 to designate laterality of the disease:
1   right eye
2   left eye
3   bilateral
9   unspecified eye

⊟ SP ✚ ⑦ E09.321- Drug or chemical induced diabetes mellitus with mild nonproliferative diabetic retinopathy with macular edema

⊟ SP ✚ ⑦ E09.329- Drug or chemical induced diabetes mellitus with mild nonproliferative diabetic retinopathy without macular edema

✚ ⑥ E09.33 Drug or chemical induced diabetes mellitus with moderate nonproliferative diabetic retinopathy

One of the following 7th characters is to be assigned to codes in subcategory E09.33 to designate laterality of the disease:
1   right eye
2   left eye
3   bilateral
9   unspecified eye

⊟ SP ✚ ⑦ E09.331- Drug or chemical induced diabetes mellitus with moderate nonproliferative diabetic retinopathy with macular edema

⊟ SP ✚ ⑦ E09.339- Drug or chemical induced diabetes mellitus with moderate nonproliferative diabetic retinopathy without macular edema

✚ ⑥ E09.34 Drug or chemical induced diabetes mellitus with severe nonproliferative diabetic retinopathy

One of the following 7th characters is to be assigned to codes in subcategory E09.34 to designate laterality of the disease:
1   right eye
2   left eye
3   bilateral
9   unspecified eye

⊟ SP ✚ ⑦ E09.341- Drug or chemical induced diabetes mellitus with severe nonproliferative diabetic retinopathy with macular edema

⊟ SP ✚ ⑦ E09.349- Drug or chemical induced diabetes mellitus with severe nonproliferative diabetic retinopathy without macular edema

✚ ⑥ E09.35 Drug or chemical induced diabetes mellitus with proliferative diabetic retinopathy

⑷4th digit required   ⑸5th digit required   ⑹6th digit required   ⑺7th digit required   ⑺7th digit placeholder   ✚Additional code   ⊟Laterality

740   *DecisionHealth's* FY 2020 Complete Home Health ICD-10-CM Diagnosis Coding Manual

Chapter 4

E00-E89

One of the following 7th characters is to be assigned to codes in subcategory E09.35 to designate laterality of the disease:

1   right eye
2   left eye
3   bilateral
9   unspecified eye

⊟ SP + 7 E09.351-   **Drug or chemical induced diabetes mellitus with proliferative diabetic retinopathy with macular edema**

⊟ SP + 7 E09.352-   **Drug or chemical induced diabetes mellitus with proliferative diabetic retinopathy with traction retinal detachment involving the macula**

⊟ SP + 7 E09.353-   **Drug or chemical induced diabetes mellitus with proliferative diabetic retinopathy with traction retinal detachment not involving the macula**

⊟ SP + 7 E09.354-   **Drug or chemical induced diabetes mellitus with proliferative diabetic retinopathy with combined traction retinal detachment and rhegmatogenous retinal detachment**

⊟ SP + 7 E09.355-   **Drug or chemical induced diabetes mellitus with stable proliferative diabetic retinopathy**

⊟ SP + 7 E09.359-   **Drug or chemical induced diabetes mellitus with proliferative diabetic retinopathy without macular edema**

SP + E09.36   **Drug or chemical induced diabetes mellitus with diabetic cataract**

CODING TIPS ✓   Cataracts are more common in diabetic patients. The classification assumes a relationship between cataracts and diabetes, when the patient has diabetes. Even cataracts specifically described as "cortical, nuclear and posterior subcapsular" and "nuclear sclerotic" should prompt the assignment of E--.36, along with the code for the specific cataract code (*Q2 2019 Coding Clinic*).

⊟ SP + 7 E09.37X-   **Drug or chemical induced diabetes mellitus with diabetic macular edema, resolved following treatment**

One of the following 7th characters is to be assigned to code E09.37 to designate laterality of the disease:

1   right eye
2   left eye
3   bilateral
9   unspecified eye

CODING TIPS ✓   The macular edema may be resolved, but the retinopathy remains. This code is like a history code for the macular edema.

SP + E09.39   **Drug or chemical induced diabetes mellitus with other diabetic ophthalmic complication**

Use additional code to identify manifestation, such as:
    diabetic glaucoma (H40-H42)

CODING TIPS ✓   There is no assumed relationship between diabetes and glaucoma. The coder should seek further clarification regarding the relationship between blindness, glaucoma and diabetes before coding as a diabetic manifestation.

+ 5 E09.4   **Drug or chemical induced diabetes mellitus with neurological complications**

CODING TIPS ✓   Drug or chemical-induced diabetes with loss of protective sensation or diabetic peripheral neuropathy should be coded to E09.42.

SP SH SL + E09.40   **Drug or chemical induced diabetes mellitus with neurological complications with diabetic neuropathy, unspecified**

SP + E09.41   **Drug or chemical induced diabetes mellitus with neurological complications with diabetic mononeuropathy**

SP SH SL + E09.42   **Drug or chemical induced diabetes mellitus with neurological complications with diabetic polyneuropathy**

Drug or chemical induced diabetes mellitus with diabetic neuralgia

CODING TIPS ✓   Diabetic polyneuropathy is the most common type of diabetic neuropathy and causes pain or loss of feeling in the toes, feet, legs, hands and arms.

SP + E09.43   **Drug or chemical induced diabetes mellitus with neurological complications with diabetic autonomic (poly)neuropathy**

Drug or chemical induced diabetes mellitus with diabetic gastroparesis

CODING TIPS ✓   Autonomic neuropathy affects the heart, digestive system and other involuntary functions. This type of neuropathy causes delayed or slowed gastric emptying as well as problems with orthostatic hypotension. This code is not to be used for polyneuropathy of the hands and feet.

CODING TIPS ✓   Gastroparesis (K31.84) may be sequenced after this code as an option.

SP + E09.44   **Drug or chemical induced diabetes mellitus with neurological complications with diabetic amyotrophy**

Chapter 4

E00-E89

★ New ▲ Revised Px Primary ⬛SP PDGM Px ⬛SL Low CoM ⬛SH High CoM ⬛IQ Quest. Encounter ⬛H Hospice non-cancer Dx   Unspecified   M *Manifestation*

DecisionHealth's FY 2020 Complete Home Health ICD-10-CM Diagnosis Coding Manual

741

CODING TIPS ✓   Diabetic amyotrophy is muscle weakness, characterized by weakness followed by wasting of pelvifemoral muscles, either unilaterally or bilaterally, with associated pain.

SP ✚ E09.49   Drug or chemical induced diabetes mellitus with neurological complications with other diabetic neurological complication

✚ S E09.5   Drug or chemical induced diabetes mellitus with circulatory complications

CODING TIPS ✓   Peripheral angiopathy includes arterial, venous and capillary conditions. Peripheral angiopathy may be documented as diabetic PVD. There is an assumed relationship between diabetes and PVD and PAD, including peripheral atherosclerosis and venous insufficiency. Diabetic PVD is coded E--.51. Diabetic arteriosclerosis of the peripheral arteries should be coded E--.51 or E--.52 then the appropriate I70.- code. Diabetic venous insufficiency should be coded E--.51 or E--.52 and I87.2 The presence of diabetes and peripheral arterial disease in the record indicates that both diabetes and PVD should be marked in M1028. Venous disease is not included in M1028.

SP ✚ E09.51   Drug or chemical induced diabetes mellitus with diabetic peripheral angiopathy without gangrene

SP ✚ E09.52   Drug or chemical induced diabetes mellitus with diabetic peripheral angiopathy with gangrene
Drug or chemical induced diabetes mellitus with diabetic gangrene

SP ✚ E09.59   Drug or chemical induced diabetes mellitus with other circulatory complications

CODING TIPS ✓   Diabetic circulatory complications other than peripheral angiopathy and gangrene, identified as such by the physician, may be coded to 4th and 5th characters .59. Example: Diabetic CAD or ASHD is documented.

✚ S E09.6   Drug or chemical induced diabetes mellitus with other specified complications

✚ G E09.61   Drug or chemical induced diabetes mellitus with diabetic arthropathy

SP ✚ E09.610   Drug or chemical induced diabetes mellitus with diabetic neuropathic arthropathy
Drug or chemical induced diabetes mellitus with Charcôt's joints

CODING TIPS ✓   Do not add a M14.6 code for Charcot's joint.

SP ✚ E09.618   Drug or chemical induced diabetes mellitus with other diabetic arthropathy

✚ G E09.62   Drug or chemical induced diabetes mellitus with skin complications

SP ✚ E09.620   Drug or chemical induced diabetes mellitus with diabetic dermatitis

Drug or chemical induced diabetes mellitus with diabetic necrobiosis lipoidica

SP ✚ E09.621   Drug or chemical induced diabetes mellitus with foot ulcer
Use additional code to identify site of ulcer (L97.4-, L97.5-)

CODING TIPS ✓   If the patient has had a diabetic foot ulcer in the past, either healed or amputated, also code Z86.31. Ulceration of the foot is assumed related to diabetes unless another cause is indicated.

SP ✚ E09.622   Drug or chemical induced diabetes mellitus with other skin ulcer
Use additional code to identify site of ulcer (L97.1-L97.9, L98.41-L98.49)

CODING TIPS ✓   Diabetes codes with 4th, 5th and 6th characters .622 are used when an ulcer is located on the lower extremity, beginning at the ankle, and not including the foot. Whereas ulcers located on the foot are assumed related to diabetes, ulcers located elsewhere are not assumed related to diabetes and must be confirmed with the physician.

SP ✚ E09.628   Drug or chemical induced diabetes mellitus with other skin complications

✚ G E09.63   Drug or chemical induced diabetes mellitus with oral complications

SP ✚ E09.630   Drug or chemical induced diabetes mellitus with periodontal disease

SP ✚ E09.638   Drug or chemical induced diabetes mellitus with other oral complications

✚ G E09.64   Drug or chemical induced diabetes mellitus with hypoglycemia

SP ✚ E09.641   Drug or chemical induced diabetes mellitus with hypoglycemia with coma

SP ✚ E09.649   Drug or chemical induced diabetes mellitus with hypoglycemia without coma

CODING TIPS ✓   The physician should be queried when the term "uncontrolled" is used to determine whether the patient has hyperglycemia, hypoglycemia or both.

CODING TIPS ✓   If encephalopathy is due to hypoglycemia, use G93.41 as an additional code.

SP ✚ E09.65   Drug or chemical induced diabetes mellitus with hyperglycemia

4 4th digit required   S 5th digit required   G 6th digit required   7 7th digit required   7 7th digit placeholder   ✚ Additional code   S Laterality

742   *DecisionHealth's* FY 2020 Complete Home Health ICD-10-CM Diagnosis Coding Manual

Chapter 4

E00-E89

CODING TIPS ✓ Inadequately controlled, poorly controlled and out of control diabetes are coded with hyperglycemia. The physician should be queried when the term 'uncontrolled' is used to determine whether the patient has hyperglycemia, hypoglycemia, or both. The clinical record should support hyperglycemia. Do not code diabetes with hyperglycemia when ketoacidosis is also documented.

SP ✚ **E09.69 Drug or chemical induced diabetes mellitus with other specified complication**

Use additional code to identify complication

CODING TIPS ✓ Use this code when the physician specifies a manifestation of diabetes that does not fit in any of the other subcategories. Follow the diabetes code with the code for the specified condition.

CODING TIPS ✓ The classification presumes a cause-and-effect relationship between osteomyelitis and diabetes when no other cause is documented. Osteomyelitis with diabetes is usually associated with ulceration. Use the appropriate code for the osteomyelitis after coding diabetes with other specified manifestation. Although not clear that certain types of diabetes are assumed related to osteomyelitis when referencing diabetes in the index, it is confirmed that osteomyelitis is related to all diabetes types.

IQ ✚ **E09.8 Drug or chemical induced diabetes mellitus with unspecified complications**

CODING TIPS ✓ This code should not be used for unspecified complications. Query the physician for information regarding suspected manifestations that the classification does not presume related.

SP ✚ **E09.9 Drug or chemical induced diabetes mellitus without complications**

CODING TIPS ✓ This code is acceptable to use for a diabetic without manifestations. Certain specified conditions are assumed related to diabetes by the classification, if listed indented under the word "with" in the alphabetical index, so the use of .9 as a diabetes 4th character should not be common. Query the physician for information regarding suspected manifestations when documentation regarding other potential causes is unclear. This code should be used for a diabetic requiring insulin injections only if teaching is the skill, or other comorbidities, unrelated to diabetes, make it unacceptable for the patient to self-inject. If .9 is used as a 4th character, no other diabetes code may be used.

4 E10 Type 1 diabetes mellitus

INCLUDES brittle diabetes (mellitus)

diabetes (mellitus) due to autoimmune process
diabetes (mellitus) due to immune mediated pancreatic islet beta-cell destruction
idiopathic diabetes (mellitus)
juvenile onset diabetes (mellitus)
ketosis-prone diabetes (mellitus)

EXCLUDES 1 diabetes mellitus due to underlying condition (E08.-)
drug or chemical induced diabetes mellitus (E09.-)
gestational diabetes (O24.4-)
hyperglycemia NOS (R73.9)
neonatal diabetes mellitus (P70.2)
postpancreatectomy diabetes mellitus (E13.-)
postprocedural diabetes mellitus (E13.-)
secondary diabetes mellitus NEC (E13.-)
type 2 diabetes mellitus (E11.-)

GUIDELINES Section I.C.4.a.1)

The age of a patient is not the sole determining factor, though most type 1 diabetics develop the condition before reaching puberty. For this reason type 1 diabetes mellitus is also referred to as juvenile diabetes.

CODING TIPS ✓ If the patient uses an insulin pump, use Z96.41 as an additional code. If there is a complication involving the insulin pump, use a code from T85.6- or T85.7- instead of the Z code.

CODING TIPS ✓ Reference the alphabetical index to review conditions that the classification assumes are related to diabetes. All specified manifestations/complications listed under the word 'with' in the index are presumed related unless the physician specifies a different cause in documentation, or states they're unrelated. The "with" convention does not apply to "not elsewhere classified (NEC)" index entries that cover broad categories of conditions. Specific conditions must be linked by the terms "with," "in," "due to" or "associated with." Coding professionals should not assume a causal relationship when the diabetic complication is "NEC."

5 E10.1 Type 1 diabetes mellitus with ketoacidosis

CODING TIPS ✓ Diabetic ketoacidosis is a serious complication of diabetes that occurs when the body produces high levels of blood acids called ketones. This condition is likely resolved before admission to home care, but could be a current diagnosis.

DEFINITION Diabetic complication characterized by hyperglycemia, hyperketonemia, and metabolic acidosis; often presents with nausea, vomiting, and abdominal pain; may progress to cerebral edema or lead to coma and/or death.

SP SH E10.10 Type 1 diabetes mellitus with ketoacidosis without coma

---

✶ New ▲ Revised **Px** Primary **SP** PDGM Px **SL** Low CoM **SH** High CoM **IQ** Quest. Encounter **H** Hospice non-cancer Dx   Unspecified   **M** *Manifestation*

DecisionHealth's FY 2020 Complete Home Health ICD-10-CM Diagnosis Coding Manual

743

SP SH E10.11   Type 1 diabetes mellitus with ketoacidosis with coma

5 E10.2   Type 1 diabetes mellitus with kidney complications

SP SH E10.21   Type 1 diabetes mellitus with diabetic nephropathy

Type 1 diabetes mellitus with intercapillary glomerulosclerosis

Type 1 diabetes mellitus with intracapillary glomerulonephrosis

Type 1 diabetes mellitus with Kimmelstiel-Wilson disease

SP SH + E10.22   Type 1 diabetes mellitus with diabetic chronic kidney disease

Use additional code to identify stage of chronic kidney disease (N18.1-N18.6)

CODING TIPS ✓   Assign an additional code from N18- to indicate the stage of CKD. When diabetic nephropathy and CKD are documented, code diabetic CKD, not nephropathy, because CKD is more specific.

CODING TIPS ✓   When diabetes, CKD and hypertension are documented, sequence the appropriate category of diabetes with CKD (E--.22) and the appropriate hypertension code (I12 or I13) prior to N18. The hypertension or the diabetes may be sequenced first depending on the focus of care. Use N18.1-N18.6 or N18.9 to indicate the CKD. The only time that the conditions should be coded differently is if the physician specifically documents that the conditions are not related.

SP SH E10.29   Type 1 diabetes mellitus with other diabetic kidney complication

Type 1 diabetes mellitus with renal tubular degeneration

5 E10.3   Type 1 diabetes mellitus with ophthalmic complications

CODING TIPS ✓   The 7th character codes in this category that are acceptable primary diagnoses in PDGM and contribute to a comorbidity adjustment are those with a 7th character of 1, 2, or 3. Unspecified eye (7th character of 9) is not acceptable as a primary diagnoses in PDGM, nor does it contribute to a comorbidity adjustment.

CODING TIPS ✓   Diabetic codes indicating specific eye disorders require a 7th character to indicate laterality.

CODING TIPS ✓   When a patient has macular edema, the patient also has retinopathy, with the macular edema developing as a complication of the retinopathy. Retinopathy includes three stages: background retinopathy, proliferative retinopathy, and macular edema.

CODING TIPS ✓   When coding diabetes with ophthalmic manifestations, review the clinical record and plan of care to ensure that the functional impact of visual impairments is reported. The home health record should clearly report how visual losses impact the function and activities of the patient, including how these conditions impact medication administration, safety, the ability to perform treatments (such as wound care) and other key areas related to the patient's daily living.

6 E10.31   Type 1 diabetes mellitus with unspecified diabetic retinopathy

SP E10.311   Type 1 diabetes mellitus with unspecified diabetic retinopathy with macular edema

SP SH E10.319   Type 1 diabetes mellitus with unspecified diabetic retinopathy without macular edema

6 E10.32   Type 1 diabetes mellitus with mild nonproliferative diabetic retinopathy

Type 1 diabetes mellitus with nonproliferative diabetic retinopathy NOS

One of the following 7th characters is to be assigned to codes in subcategory E10.32 to designate laterality of the disease:
1   right eye
2   left eye
3   bilateral
9   unspecified eye

⊟ SP 7 E10.321-   Type 1 diabetes mellitus with mild nonproliferative diabetic retinopathy with macular edema

⊟ SP SH 7 E10.329-   Type 1 diabetes mellitus with mild nonproliferative diabetic retinopathy without macular edema

6 E10.33   Type 1 diabetes mellitus with moderate nonproliferative diabetic retinopathy

One of the following 7th characters is to be assigned to codes in subcategory E10.33 to designate laterality of the disease:
1   right eye
2   left eye
3   bilateral
9   unspecified eye

⊟ SP 7 E10.331-   Type 1 diabetes mellitus with moderate nonproliferative diabetic retinopathy with macular edema

⊟ SP SH 7 E10.339-   Type 1 diabetes mellitus with moderate nonproliferative diabetic retinopathy without macular edema

6 E10.34   Type 1 diabetes mellitus with severe nonproliferative diabetic retinopathy

Chapter 4

E00-E89

⬛4th digit required   5 5th digit required   6 6th digit required   7 7th digit required   ☑ 7th digit placeholder   + Additional code   ⊟ Laterality

One of the following 7th characters is to be assigned to codes in subcategory E10.34 to designate laterality of the disease:
1   right eye
2   left eye
3   bilateral
9   unspecified eye

□ SP 7 E10.341- **Type 1 diabetes mellitus with severe nonproliferative diabetic retinopathy with macular edema**

□ SP SH 7 E10.349- **Type 1 diabetes mellitus with severe nonproliferative diabetic retinopathy without macular edema**

6 E10.35 **Type 1 diabetes mellitus with proliferative diabetic retinopathy**

One of the following 7th characters is to be assigned to codes in subcategory E10.35 to designate laterality of the disease:
1   right eye
2   left eye
3   bilateral
9   unspecified eye

□ SP 7 E10.351- **Type 1 diabetes mellitus with proliferative diabetic retinopathy with macular edema**

□ SP SH 7 E10.352- **Type 1 diabetes mellitus with proliferative diabetic retinopathy with traction retinal detachment involving the macula**

□ SP SH 7 E10.353- **Type 1 diabetes mellitus with proliferative diabetic retinopathy with traction retinal detachment not involving the macula**

□ SP SH 7 E10.354- **Type 1 diabetes mellitus with proliferative diabetic retinopathy with combined traction retinal detachment and rhegmatogenous retinal detachment**

□ SP SH 7 E10.355- **Type 1 diabetes mellitus with stable proliferative diabetic retinopathy**

□ SP SH 7 E10.359- **Type 1 diabetes mellitus with proliferative diabetic retinopathy without macular edema**

SP SH E10.36 **Type 1 diabetes mellitus with diabetic cataract**

CODING TIPS ✓ Cataracts are more common in diabetic patients. The classification assumes a relationship between cataracts and diabetes, when the patient has diabetes. Even cataracts specifically described as "cortical, nuclear and posterior subcapsular" and "nuclear sclerotic" should prompt the assignment of E--.36, along with the code for the specific cataract code (*Q2 2019 Coding Clinic*).

□ SP SH 7 E10.37X- **Type 1 diabetes mellitus with diabetic macular edema, resolved following treatment**

One of the following 7th characters is to be assigned to code E10.37 to designate laterality of the disease:
1   right eye
2   left eye
3   bilateral
9   unspecified eye

CODING TIPS ✓ The macular edema may be resolved, but the retinopathy remains. This code is like a history code for the macular edema.

SP SH + E10.39 **Type 1 diabetes mellitus with other diabetic ophthalmic complication**
Use additional code to identify manifestation, such as:
    diabetic glaucoma (H40-H42)
CODING TIPS ✓ There is no assumed relationship between diabetes and glaucoma. The coder should seek further clarification regarding the relationship between blindness, glaucoma and diabetes before coding as a diabetic manifestation.

5 E10.4 **Type 1 diabetes mellitus with neurological complications**
CODING TIPS ✓ Type 1 diabetes with loss of protective sensation or diabetic peripheral neuropathy should be coded to E10.42.

SP SH SL E10.40 **Type 1 diabetes mellitus with diabetic neuropathy, unspecified**

SP SH E10.41 **Type 1 diabetes mellitus with diabetic mononeuropathy**

SP SH SL E10.42 **Type 1 diabetes mellitus with diabetic polyneuropathy**
Type 1 diabetes mellitus with diabetic neuralgia
CODING TIPS ✓ Diabetic polyneuropathy is the most common type of diabetic neuropathy and causes pain or loss of feeling in the toes, feet, legs, hands and arms.

SP SH E10.43 **Type 1 diabetes mellitus with diabetic autonomic (poly)neuropathy**
Type 1 diabetes mellitus with diabetic gastroparesis

Chapter 4

E00-E89

★ New ▲ Revised Px Primary **SP** PDGM Px **SL** Low CoM **SH** High CoM **IQ** Quest. Encounter **H** Hospice non-cancer Dx Unspecified **M** *Manifestation*

DecisionHealth's FY 2020 Complete Home Health ICD-10-CM Diagnosis Coding Manual

745

CODING TIPS ✓ Autonomic neuropathy affects the heart, digestive system and other involuntary functions. This type of neuropathy causes delayed or slowed gastric emptying as well as problems with orthostatic hypotension. This code is not to be used for polyneuropathy of the hands and feet.

CODING TIPS ✓ Gastroparesis (K31.84) may be sequenced after this code as an option.

SP SH E10.44 **Type 1 diabetes mellitus with diabetic amyotrophy**

CODING TIPS ✓ Diabetic amyotrophy is muscle weakness, characterized by weakness followed by wasting of pelvifemoral muscles, either unilaterally or bilaterally, with associated pain.

SP SH E10.49 **Type 1 diabetes mellitus with other diabetic neurological complication**

⑤ E10.5 **Type 1 diabetes mellitus with circulatory complications**

CODING TIPS ✓ Peripheral angiopathy includes arterial, venous and capillary conditions. Peripheral angiopathy may be documented as diabetic PVD. There is an assumed relationship between diabetes and PVD and PAD, including peripheral atherosclerosis and venous insufficiency. Diabetic PVD is coded E--.51. Diabetic arteriosclerosis of the peripheral arteries should be coded E--.51 or E--.52 then the appropriate I70.- code. Diabetic venous insufficiency should be coded E--.51 or E--.52 and I87.2 The presence of diabetes and peripheral arterial disease in the record indicates that both diabetes and PVD should be marked in M1028. Venous disease is not included in M1028.

SP SH E10.51 **Type 1 diabetes mellitus with diabetic peripheral angiopathy without gangrene**

SP SH E10.52 **Type 1 diabetes mellitus with diabetic peripheral angiopathy with gangrene**
Type 1 diabetes mellitus with diabetic gangrene

SP SH E10.59 **Type 1 diabetes mellitus with other circulatory complications**

CODING TIPS ✓ Diabetic circulatory complications other than peripheral angiopathy and gangrene, identified as such by the physician, may be coded to 4th and 5th characters .59. Example: Diabetic CAD or ASHD is documented.

⑤ E10.6 **Type 1 diabetes mellitus with other specified complications**

⑥ E10.61 **Type 1 diabetes mellitus with diabetic arthropathy**

SP SH E10.610 **Type 1 diabetes mellitus with diabetic neuropathic arthropathy**
Type 1 diabetes mellitus with Charcôt's joints

CODING TIPS ✓ Do not add a M14.6 code for Charcot's joint.

SP SH E10.618 **Type 1 diabetes mellitus with other diabetic arthropathy**

⑥ E10.62 **Type 1 diabetes mellitus with skin complications**

SP SH E10.620 **Type 1 diabetes mellitus with diabetic dermatitis**
Type 1 diabetes mellitus with diabetic necrobiosis lipoidica

SP SH ✚ E10.621 **Type 1 diabetes mellitus with foot ulcer**
Use additional code to identify site of ulcer (L97.4-, L97.5-)

CODING TIPS ✓ If the patient has had a diabetic foot ulcer in the past, either healed or amputated, also code Z86.31. Ulceration of the foot is assumed related to diabetes unless another cause is indicated.

SP SH ✚ E10.622 **Type 1 diabetes mellitus with other skin ulcer**
Use additional code to identify site of ulcer (L97.1-L97.9, L98.41-L98.49)

CODING TIPS ✓ Diabetes codes with 4th, 5th and 6th characters .622 are used when an ulcer is located on the lower extremity, beginning at the ankle, and not including the foot. Whereas ulcers located on the foot are assumed related to diabetes, ulcers located elsewhere are not assumed related to diabetes and must be confirmed with the physician.

SP SH E10.628 **Type 1 diabetes mellitus with other skin complications**

⑥ E10.63 **Type 1 diabetes mellitus with oral complications**

SP SH E10.630 **Type 1 diabetes mellitus with periodontal disease**

SP SH E10.638 **Type 1 diabetes mellitus with other oral complications**

⑥ E10.64 **Type 1 diabetes mellitus with hypoglycemia**

SP SH E10.641 **Type 1 diabetes mellitus with hypoglycemia with coma**

SP SH E10.649 **Type 1 diabetes mellitus with hypoglycemia without coma**

CODING TIPS ✓ The physician should be queried when the term "uncontrolled" is used to determine whether the patient has hyperglycemia, hypoglycemia or both.

CODING TIPS ✓ If encephalopathy is due to hypoglycemia, use G93.41 as an additional code.

SP SH E10.65 **Type 1 diabetes mellitus with hyperglycemia**

◰4th digit required ⑤5th digit required ⑥6th digit required ⑦7th digit required ⑦7th digit placeholder ✚Additional code ⊟Laterality

746   *DecisionHealth's* FY 2020 Complete Home Health ICD-10-CM Diagnosis Coding Manual

Chapter 4

E00-E89

CODING TIPS ✓ Inadequately controlled, poorly controlled and out of control diabetes are coded with hyperglycemia. The physician should be queried when the term 'uncontrolled' is used to determine whether the patient has hyperglycemia, hypoglycemia, or both. The clinical record should support hyperglycemia. Do not code diabetes with hyperglycemia when ketoacidosis is also documented.

SP SH ✚ E10.69 Type 1 diabetes mellitus with other specified complication

Use additional code to identify complication

CODING TIPS ✓ Use this code when the physician specifies a manifestation of diabetes that does not fit in any of the other subcategories. Follow the diabetes code with the code for the specified condition.

CODING TIPS ✓ The classification presumes a cause-and-effect relationship between osteomyelitis and diabetes when no other cause is documented. Osteomyelitis with diabetes is usually associated with ulceration. Use the appropriate code for the osteomyelitis after coding diabetes with other specified manifestation. Although not clear that certain types of diabetes are assumed related to osteomyelitis when referencing diabetes in the index, it is confirmed that osteomyelitis is related to all diabetes types.

IQ E10.8 Type 1 diabetes mellitus with unspecified complications

CODING TIPS ✓ This code should not be used for unspecified complications. Query the physician for information regarding suspected manifestations that the classification does not presume related.

SP SH E10.9 Type 1 diabetes mellitus without complications

CODING TIPS ✓ This code is acceptable to use for a diabetic without manifestations. Certain specified conditions are assumed related to diabetes by the classification, if listed indented under the word "with" in the alphabetical index, so the use of .9 as a diabetes 4th character should not be common. Query the physician for information regarding suspected manifestations when documentation regarding other potential causes is unclear. This code should be used for a diabetic requiring insulin injections only if teaching is the skill, or other comorbidities, unrelated to diabetes, make it unacceptable for the patient to self-inject. If .9 is used as a 4th character, no other diabetes code may be used.

✚ 4 E11 Type 2 diabetes mellitus

INCLUDES diabetes (mellitus) due to insulin secretory defect

diabetes NOS
insulin resistant diabetes (mellitus)

Use additional code to identify control using:
insulin (Z79.4)
oral antidiabetic drugs (Z79.84)
oral hypoglycemic drugs (Z79.84)

EXCLUDES 1 diabetes mellitus due to underlying condition (E08.-)
drug or chemical induced diabetes mellitus (E09.-)
gestational diabetes (O24.4-)
neonatal diabetes mellitus (P70.2)
postpancreatectomy diabetes mellitus (E13.-)
postprocedural diabetes mellitus (E13.-)
secondary diabetes mellitus NEC (E13.-)
type 1 diabetes mellitus (E10.-)

GUIDELINES Section I.C.4.a.2)-3)
If the type of diabetes mellitus is not documented in the medical record the default is E11.-, Type 2 diabetes mellitus. If the documentation in a medical record does not indicate the type of diabetes but does indicate that the patient uses insulin, code E11, Type 2 diabetes mellitus, should be assigned. An additional code should be assigned from category Z79 to identify the long-term (current) use of insulin or oral hypoglycemic drugs. If the patient is treated with both oral medications and insulin, only the code for long-term (current) use of insulin should be assigned. Code Z79.4 should not be assigned if insulin is given temporarily to bring a type 2 patient's blood sugar under control during an encounter.

CODING TIPS ✓ If the patient uses an insulin pump, use Z96.41 as an additional code. If there is a complication involving the insulin pump, use a code from T85.6- or T85.7- instead of the Z code.

CODING TIPS ✓ Use Z79.4 to indicate the use of insulin, OR use Z79.84 to indicate the use of oral anti-glycemics. Use Z79.84 only when the patient does not also take insulin. Do NOT code both.

CODING TIPS ✓ Reference the alphabetical index to review conditions that the classification assumes are related to diabetes. All specified manifestations/complications listed under the word 'with' in the index are presumed related unless the physician specifies a different cause in documentation, or states they're unrelated. The "with" convention does not apply to "not elsewhere classified (NEC)" index entries that cover broad categories of conditions. Specific conditions must be linked by the terms "with," "in," "due to" or "associated with." Coding professionals should not assume a causal relationship when the diabetic complication is "NEC."

CODING TIPS ✓ When clinical record diagnostic statements do not indicate a specific type of diabetes, a code from category E11 (Type 2 diabetes) should be assigned.

Chapter 4

E00-E89

★ New ▲ Revised Px Primary SP PDGM Px SL Low CoM SH High CoM IQ Quest. Encounter H Hospice non-cancer Dx   Unspecified   M Manifestation

DecisionHealth's FY 2020 Complete Home Health ICD-10-CM Diagnosis Coding Manual

747

+ ⑤ E11.0 Type 2 diabetes mellitus with hyperosmolarity

DEFINITION   Metabolic diabetic emergency presenting with altered consciousness varying from confusion or disorientation to coma, with extreme dehydration, and high blood concentrations of sugar and sodium.

SP SH + E11.00 Type 2 diabetes mellitus with hyperosmolarity without nonketotic hyperglycemic-hyperosmolar coma (NKHHC)

SP SH + E11.01 Type 2 diabetes mellitus with hyperosmolarity with coma

+ ⑤ E11.1 Type 2 diabetes mellitus with ketoacidosis

SP SH + E11.10 Type 2 diabetes mellitus with ketoacidosis without coma

CODING TIPS ✓   Diabetic ketoacidosis is a serious complication of diabetes that occurs when the body produces high levels of blood acids called ketones. Query the physician to determine if the condition is resolved prior to home care. Diabetic ketoacidosis is rare in type 2 diabetes, so if the documentation states diabetic ketoacidosis, query the physician as to type of diabetes.

SP SH + E11.11 Type 2 diabetes mellitus with ketoacidosis with coma

+ ⑤ E11.2 Type 2 diabetes mellitus with kidney complications

CODING TIPS ✓   Diabetic triopathy refers to the most common types of manifestations of diabetes: nephropathy, retinopathy and neuropathy.

SP SH + E11.21 Type 2 diabetes mellitus with diabetic nephropathy
Type 2 diabetes mellitus with intercapillary glomerulosclerosis
Type 2 diabetes mellitus with intracapillary glomerulonephrosis
Type 2 diabetes mellitus with Kimmelstiel-Wilson disease

SP SH + E11.22 Type 2 diabetes mellitus with diabetic chronic kidney disease
Use additional code to identify stage of chronic kidney disease (N18.1-N18.6)

CODING TIPS ✓   Assign an additional code from N18- to indicate the stage of CKD. When diabetic nephropathy and CKD are documented, code diabetic CKD, not nephropathy, because CKD is more specific.

CODING TIPS ✓   When diabetes, CKD and hypertension are documented, sequence the appropriate category of diabetes with CKD (E--.22) and the appropriate hypertension code (I12 or I13) prior to N18. The hypertension or the diabetes may be sequenced first depending on the focus of care. Use N18.1-N18.6 or N18.9 to indicate the CKD. The only time that the conditions should be coded differently is if the physician specifically documents that the conditions are not related.

SP SH + E11.29 Type 2 diabetes mellitus with other diabetic kidney complication
Type 2 diabetes mellitus with renal tubular degeneration

+ ⑤ E11.3 Type 2 diabetes mellitus with ophthalmic complications

CODING TIPS ✓   The 7th character codes in this category that are acceptable primary diagnoses in PDGM and contribute to a comorbidity adjustment are those with a 7th character of 1, 2, or 3. Unspecified eye (7th character of 9) is not acceptable as a primary diagnoses in PDGM, nor does it contribute to a comorbidity adjustment.

CODING TIPS ✓   Diabetic codes indicating specific eye disorders require a 7th character to indicate laterality.

CODING TIPS ✓   Diabetic triopathy refers to the most common types of manifestations of diabetes: nephropathy, retinopathy and neuropathy.

CODING TIPS ✓   When coding diabetes with ophthalmic manifestations, review the clinical record and plan of care to ensure that the functional impact of visual impairments is reported. The home health record should clearly report how visual losses impact the function and activities of the patient, including how these conditions impact medication administration, safety, the ability to perform treatments (such as wound care) and other key areas related to the patient's daily living.

CODING TIPS ✓   When a patient has macular edema, the patient also has retinopathy, with the macular edema developing as a complication of the retinopathy. Retinopathy includes three stages: background retinopathy, proliferative retinopathy, and macular edema.

+ ⑥ E11.31 Type 2 diabetes mellitus with unspecified diabetic retinopathy

SP + E11.311 Type 2 diabetes mellitus with unspecified diabetic retinopathy with macular edema

SP SH + E11.319 Type 2 diabetes mellitus with unspecified diabetic retinopathy without macular edema

+ ⑥ E11.32 Type 2 diabetes mellitus with mild nonproliferative diabetic retinopathy
Type 2 diabetes mellitus with nonproliferative diabetic retinopathy NOS

---

④ 4th digit required   ⑤ 5th digit required   ⑥ 6th digit required   ⑦ 7th digit required   ⑦ 7th digit placeholder   ✚ Additional code   ⊟ Laterality

Chapter 4

E00-E89

One of the following 7th characters is to be assigned to codes in subcategory E11.32 to designate laterality of the disease:
1 right eye
2 left eye
3 bilateral
9 unspecified eye

目 SP ＋ 7 E11.321- **Type 2 diabetes mellitus with mild nonproliferative diabetic retinopathy with macular edema**

目 SP SH ＋ 7 E11.329- **Type 2 diabetes mellitus with mild nonproliferative diabetic retinopathy without macular edema**

＋ 6 E11.33 **Type 2 diabetes mellitus with moderate nonproliferative diabetic retinopathy**

One of the following 7th characters is to be assigned to codes in subcategory E11.33 to designate laterality of the disease:
1 right eye
2 left eye
3 bilateral
9 unspecified eye

目 SP ＋ 7 E11.331- **Type 2 diabetes mellitus with moderate nonproliferative diabetic retinopathy with macular edema**

目 SP SH ＋ 7 E11.339- **Type 2 diabetes mellitus with moderate nonproliferative diabetic retinopathy without macular edema**

＋ 6 E11.34 **Type 2 diabetes mellitus with severe nonproliferative diabetic retinopathy**

One of the following 7th characters is to be assigned to codes in subcategory E11.34 to designate laterality of the disease:
1 right eye
2 left eye
3 bilateral
9 unspecified eye

目 SP ＋ 7 E11.341- **Type 2 diabetes mellitus with severe nonproliferative diabetic retinopathy with macular edema**

目 SP SH ＋ 7 E11.349- **Type 2 diabetes mellitus with severe nonproliferative diabetic retinopathy without macular edema**

＋ 6 E11.35 **Type 2 diabetes mellitus with proliferative diabetic retinopathy**

One of the following 7th characters is to be assigned to codes in subcategory E11.35 to designate laterality of the disease:
1 right eye
2 left eye
3 bilateral
9 unspecified eye

目 SP ＋ 7 E11.351- **Type 2 diabetes mellitus with proliferative diabetic retinopathy with macular edema**

目 SP SH ＋ 7 E11.352- **Type 2 diabetes mellitus with proliferative diabetic retinopathy with traction retinal detachment involving the macula**

目 SP SH ＋ 7 E11.353- **Type 2 diabetes mellitus with proliferative diabetic retinopathy with traction retinal detachment not involving the macula**

目 SP SH ＋ 7 E11.354- **Type 2 diabetes mellitus with proliferative diabetic retinopathy with combined traction retinal detachment and rhegmatogenous retinal detachment**

目 SP SH ＋ 7 E11.355- **Type 2 diabetes mellitus with stable proliferative diabetic retinopathy**

目 SP SH ＋ 7 E11.359- **Type 2 diabetes mellitus with proliferative diabetic retinopathy without macular edema**

SP SH ＋ E11.36 **Type 2 diabetes mellitus with diabetic cataract**

CODING TIPS ✓ Cataracts are more common in diabetic patients. The classification assumes a relationship between cataracts and diabetes, when the patient has diabetes. Even cataracts specifically described as "cortical, nuclear and posterior subcapsular" and "nuclear sclerotic" should prompt the assignment of E--.36, along with the code for the specific cataract code (*Q2 2019 Coding Clinic*).

目 SP SH ＋ E11.37X- **Type 2 diabetes mellitus with diabetic macular edema, resolved following treatment**
7

One of the following 7th characters is to be assigned to code E11.37 to designate laterality of the disease:
1 right eye
2 left eye
3 bilateral
9 unspecified eye

CODING TIPS ✓ The macular edema may be resolved, but the retinopathy remains. This code is like a history code for the macular edema.

SP SH ＋ E11.39 **Type 2 diabetes mellitus with other diabetic ophthalmic complication**
Use additional code to identify manifestation, such as:
diabetic glaucoma (H40-H42)

CODING TIPS ✓ There is no assumed relationship between diabetes and glaucoma. The coder should seek further clarification regarding the relationship between blindness, glaucoma and diabetes before coding as a diabetic manifestation.

★ New ▲ Revised Px Primary **SP** PDGM Px **SL** Low CoM **SH** High CoM **IQ** Quest. Encounter **H** Hospice non-cancer Dx Unspecified **M** *Manifestation*

DecisionHealth's FY 2020 Complete Home Health ICD-10-CM Diagnosis Coding Manual

749

Chapter 4

E00-E89

+ ⑤ E11.4 Type 2 diabetes mellitus with neurological complications

CODING TIPS✓ Type 2 or unspecified diabetes with loss of protective sensation or diabetic peripheral neuropathy with loss of protective sensation should be coded to E11.42.

CODING TIPS✓ Diabetic triopathy refers to the most common types of manifestations of diabetes: nephropathy, retinopathy and neuropathy.

SP SH SL + E11.40 Type 2 diabetes mellitus with diabetic neuropathy, unspecified

SP SH + E11.41 Type 2 diabetes mellitus with diabetic mononeuropathy

SP SH SL + E11.42 Type 2 diabetes mellitus with diabetic polyneuropathy
Type 2 diabetes mellitus with diabetic neuralgia

CODING TIPS✓ Diabetic polyneuropathy is the most common type of diabetic neuropathy and causes pain or loss of feeling in the toes, feet, legs, hands and arms.

SP SH + E11.43 Type 2 diabetes mellitus with diabetic autonomic (poly)neuropathy
Type 2 diabetes mellitus with diabetic gastroparesis

CODING TIPS✓ Autonomic neuropathy affects the heart, digestive system and other involuntary functions. This type of neuropathy causes delayed or slowed gastric emptying as well as problems with orthostatic hypotension. This code is not to be used for polyneuropathy of the hands and feet.

CODING TIPS✓ Gastroparesis (K31.84) may be sequenced after this code as an option.

SP SH + E11.44 Type 2 diabetes mellitus with diabetic amyotrophy

CODING TIPS✓ Diabetic amyotrophy is muscle weakness, characterized by weakness followed by wasting of pelvifemoral muscles, either unilaterally or bilaterally, with associated pain.

SP SH + E11.49 Type 2 diabetes mellitus with other diabetic neurological complication

+ ⑤ E11.5 Type 2 diabetes mellitus with circulatory complications

CODING TIPS✓ Peripheral angiopathy includes arterial, venous and capillary conditions. Peripheral angiopathy may be documented as diabetic PVD. There is an assumed relationship between diabetes and PVD and PAD, including peripheral atherosclerosis and venous insufficiency. Diabetic PVD is coded E--.51. Diabetic arteriosclerosis of the peripheral arteries should be coded E--.51 or E--.52 then the appropriate I70.- code. Diabetic venous insufficiency should be coded E--.51 or E--.52 and I87.2 The presence of diabetes and peripheral arterial disease in the record indicates that both diabetes and PVD should be marked in M1028. Venous disease is not included in M1028.

SP SH + E11.51 Type 2 diabetes mellitus with diabetic peripheral angiopathy without gangrene

SP SH + E11.52 Type 2 diabetes mellitus with diabetic peripheral angiopathy with gangrene
Type 2 diabetes mellitus with diabetic gangrene

SP SH + E11.59 Type 2 diabetes mellitus with other circulatory complications

CODING TIPS✓ Diabetic circulatory complications other than peripheral angiopathy and gangrene, identified as such by the physician, may be coded to 4th and 5th characters .59. Example: Diabetic CAD or ASHD is documented.

+ ⑤ E11.6 Type 2 diabetes mellitus with other specified complications

+ ⑥ E11.61 Type 2 diabetes mellitus with diabetic arthropathy

SP SH + E11.610 Type 2 diabetes mellitus with diabetic neuropathic arthropathy
Type 2 diabetes mellitus with Charcôt's joints

CODING TIPS✓ Do not add a M14.6 code for Charcot's joint.

SP SH + E11.618 Type 2 diabetes mellitus with other diabetic arthropathy

+ ⑥ E11.62 Type 2 diabetes mellitus with skin complications

SP SH + E11.620 Type 2 diabetes mellitus with diabetic dermatitis
Type 2 diabetes mellitus with diabetic necrobiosis lipoidica

SP SH + E11.621 Type 2 diabetes mellitus with foot ulcer
Use additional code to identify site of ulcer (L97.4-, L97.5-)

CODING TIPS✓ If the patient has had a diabetic foot ulcer in the past, either healed or amputated, also code Z86.31. Ulceration of the foot is assumed related to diabetes unless another cause is indicated.

SP SH + E11.622 Type 2 diabetes mellitus with other skin ulcer
Use additional code to identify site of ulcer (L97.1-L97.9, L98.41-L98.49)

Chapter 4

E00-E89

---

④4th digit required   **⑤**5th digit required   **⑥**6th digit required   **⑦**7th digit required   **⑦**7th digit placeholder   **+**Additional code   **⊟**Laterality

CODING TIPS ✓ Diabetes codes with 4th, 5th and 6th characters .622 are used when an ulcer is located on the lower extremity, beginning at the ankle, and not including the foot. Whereas ulcers located on the foot are assumed related to diabetes, ulcers located elsewhere are not assumed related to diabetes and must be confirmed with the physician.

SP SH + E11.628 Type 2 diabetes mellitus with other skin complications

+ 6 E11.63 Type 2 diabetes mellitus with oral complications

SP SH + E11.630 Type 2 diabetes mellitus with periodontal disease

SP SH + E11.638 Type 2 diabetes mellitus with other oral complications

+ 6 E11.64 Type 2 diabetes mellitus with hypoglycemia

SP SH + E11.641 Type 2 diabetes mellitus with hypoglycemia with coma

SP SH + E11.649 Type 2 diabetes mellitus with hypoglycemia without coma

CODING TIPS ✓ The physician should be queried when the term "uncontrolled" is used to determine whether the patient has hyperglycemia, hypoglycemia or both.

CODING TIPS ✓ If encephalopathy is due to hypoglycemia, use G93.41 as an additional code.

SP SH + E11.65 Type 2 diabetes mellitus with hyperglycemia

CODING TIPS ✓ Inadequately controlled, poorly controlled and out of control diabetes are coded with hyperglycemia. The physician should be queried when the term 'uncontrolled' is used to determine whether the patient has hyperglycemia, hypoglycemia, or both. The clinical record should support hyperglycemia. Do not code diabetes with hyperglycemia when ketoacidosis is also documented.

SP SH + E11.69 Type 2 diabetes mellitus with other specified complication

Use additional code to identify complication

CODING TIPS ✓ Use this code when the physician specifies a manifestation of diabetes that does not fit in any of the other subcategories. Follow the diabetes code with the code for the specified condition.

CODING TIPS ✓ The classification presumes a cause-and-effect relationship between osteomyelitis and diabetes when no other cause is documented. Osteomyelitis with diabetes is usually associated with ulceration. Use the appropriate code for the osteomyelitis after coding diabetes with other specified manifestation. Although not clear that certain types of diabetes are assumed related to osteomyelitis when referencing diabetes in the index, it is confirmed that osteomyelitis is related to all diabetes types.

IQ + E11.8 Type 2 diabetes mellitus with unspecified complications

CODING TIPS ✓ This code should not be used for unspecified complications. Query the physician for information regarding suspected manifestations that the classification does not presume related.

SP SH + E11.9 Type 2 diabetes mellitus without complications

CODING TIPS ✓ This code is acceptable to use for a diabetic without manifestations. Certain specified conditions are assumed related to diabetes by the classification, if listed indented under the word "with" in the alphabetical index, so the use of .9 as a diabetes 4th character should not be common. Query the physician for information regarding suspected manifestations when documentation regarding other potential causes is unclear. This code should be used for a diabetic requiring insulin injections only if teaching is the skill, or other comorbidities, unrelated to diabetes, make it unacceptable for the patient to self-inject. If .9 is used as a 4th character, no other diabetes code may be used.

DEFINITION Underproduction or underutilization of insulin; presents with abnormally high blood sugar (glucose) levels, resulting in impaired carbohydrate and fat metabolism.

+ 4 E13 Other specified diabetes mellitus

INCLUDES diabetes mellitus due to genetic defects of beta-cell function
diabetes mellitus due to genetic defects in insulin action
postpancreatectomy diabetes mellitus
postprocedural diabetes mellitus
secondary diabetes mellitus NEC

Use additional code to identify control using:
insulin (Z79.4)
oral antidiabetic drugs (Z79.84)
oral hypoglycemic drugs (Z79.84)

EXCLUDES 1 diabetes (mellitus) due to autoimmune process (E10.-)
diabetes (mellitus) due to immune mediated pancreatic islet beta-cell destruction (E10.-)

★ New ▲ Revised Px Primary SP PDGM Px SL Low CoM SH High CoM IQ Quest. Encounter H Hospice non-cancer Dx Unspecified M *Manifestation*

DecisionHealth's FY 2020 Complete Home Health ICD-10-CM Diagnosis Coding Manual

751

diabetes mellitus due to
    underlying condition (E08.-)
drug or chemical induced
    diabetes mellitus (E09.-)
gestational diabetes (O24.4-)
neonatal diabetes mellitus
    (P70.2)
type 1 diabetes mellitus (E10.-)

GUIDELINES   Section I.C.4.a.6(a)

Codes under categories E08, Diabetes mellitus due to underlying condition, E09, Drug or chemical induced diabetes mellitus, and E13, Other specified diabetes mellitus, identify complications/manifestations associated with secondary diabetes mellitus. Secondary diabetes is always caused by another condition or event (e.g., cystic fibrosis, malignant neoplasm of pancreas, pancreatectomy, adverse effect of drug, or poisoning).

For patients with secondary diabetes mellitus who routinely use insulin or oral hypoglycemic drugs, an additional code from category Z79 should be assigned to identify the long-term (current) use of insulin or oral hypoglycemic drugs. If the patient is treated with both oral medications and insulin, only the code for long-term (current) use of insulin should be assigned. Code Z79.4 should not be assigned if insulin is given temporarily to bring a secondary diabetic patient's blood sugar under control during an encounter.

GUIDELINES   Section I.C.4.a.6)(b)(i)

For postpancreatectomy diabetes mellitus (lack of insulin due to the surgical removal of all or part of the pancreas), assign code E89.1, Postprocedural hypoinsulinemia. Assign a code from category E13 and a code from subcategory Z90.41-, Acquired absence of pancreas, as additional codes.

CODING TIPS ✓   If the patient uses an insulin pump, use Z96.41 as an additional code. If there is a complication involving the insulin pump, use a code from T85.6- or T85.7- instead of the Z code.

CODING TIPS ✓   Use Z79.4 to indicate the use of insulin, OR use Z79.84 to indicate the use of oral anti-glycemics. Use Z79.84 only when the patient does not also take insulin. Do NOT code both.

CODING TIPS ✓   Reference the alphabetical index to review conditions that the classification assumes are related to diabetes. All specified manifestations/complications listed under the word 'with' in the index are presumed related unless the physician specifies a different cause in documentation, or states they're unrelated. The "with" convention does not apply to "not elsewhere classified (NEC)" index entries that cover broad categories of conditions. Specific conditions must be linked by the terms "with," "in," "due to" or "associated with." Coding professionals should not assume a causal relationship when the diabetic complication is "NEC."

CODING TIPS ✓   If diabetes is related to a malignant neoplasm of the pancreas, query whether the diabetes is caused by the neoplasm itself (E08); the drugs used to treat the neoplasm (E09); or the removal of part or all of the pancreas (E13).

CODING TIPS ✓   When postpancreatectomy or postprocedural diabetes is specified, the coder should first look in the Alphabetic Index and identify the terms "hypoinsulinemia, postprocedural- E89.1." Review of this code in the tabular index will instruct the coder to use an additional code for acquired absence of pancreas (Z90.41-), diabetes mellitus (postpancreatectomy) (postprocedural) (E13.-), and insulin use (Z79.4).

+ 5 E13.0   **Other specified diabetes mellitus with hyperosmolarity**

SP SH + E13.00   **Other specified diabetes mellitus with hyperosmolarity without nonketotic hyperglycemic-hyperosmolar coma (NKHHC)**
    EXCLUDES 2   type 2 diabetes mellitus (E11.-)

SP SH + E13.01   **Other specified diabetes mellitus with hyperosmolarity with coma**

+ 5 E13.1   **Other specified diabetes mellitus with ketoacidosis**
    CODING TIPS ✓   Diabetic ketoacidosis is a serious complication of diabetes that occurs when the body produces high levels of blood acids called ketones. This condition is likely resolved before admission to home care, but could be a current diagnosis.

SP SH + E13.10   **Other specified diabetes mellitus with ketoacidosis without coma**

SP SH + E13.11   **Other specified diabetes mellitus with ketoacidosis with coma**

+ 5 E13.2   **Other specified diabetes mellitus with kidney complications**

SP SH + E13.21   **Other specified diabetes mellitus with diabetic nephropathy**
    Other specified diabetes mellitus with intercapillary glomerulosclerosis
    Other specified diabetes mellitus with intracapillary glomerulonephrosis
    Other specified diabetes mellitus with Kimmelstiel-Wilson disease

SP SH + E13.22   **Other specified diabetes mellitus with diabetic chronic kidney disease**
    Use additional code to identify stage of chronic kidney disease (N18.1-N18.6)
    CODING TIPS ✓   Assign an additional code from N18- to indicate the stage of CKD. When diabetic nephropathy and CKD are documented, code diabetic CKD, not nephropathy, because CKD is more specific.

4 4th digit required   **5** 5th digit required   **6** 6th digit required   **7** 7th digit required   **7** 7th digit placeholder   **+** Additional code   **⊟** Laterality

752   *DecisionHealth's* FY 2020 Complete Home Health ICD-10-CM Diagnosis Coding Manual

CODING TIPS ✓ When diabetes, CKD and hypertension are documented, sequence the appropriate category of diabetes with CKD (E--.22) and the appropriate hypertension code (I12 or I13) prior to N18. The hypertension or the diabetes may be sequenced first depending on the focus of care. Use N18.1-N18.6 or N18.9 to indicate the CKD. The only time that the conditions should be coded differently is if the physician specifically documents that the conditions are not related.

SP SH + E13.29 **Other specified diabetes mellitus with other diabetic kidney complication**
Other specified diabetes mellitus with renal tubular degeneration

+ 5 E13.3 **Other specified diabetes mellitus with ophthalmic complications**

CODING TIPS ✓ The 7th character codes in this category that are acceptable primary diagnoses in PDGM and contribute to a comorbidity adjustment are those with a 7th character of 1, 2, or 3. Unspecified eye (7th character of 9) is not acceptable as a primary diagnoses in PDGM, nor does it contribute to a comorbidity adjustment.

CODING TIPS ✓ Diabetic codes indicating specific eye disorders require a 7th character to indicate laterality.

CODING TIPS ✓ When a patient has macular edema, the patient also has retinopathy, with the macular edema developing as a complication of the retinopathy. Retinopathy includes three stages: background retinopathy, proliferative retinopathy, and macular edema.

CODING TIPS ✓ When coding diabetes with ophthalmic manifestations, review the clinical record and plan of care to ensure that the functional impact of visual impairments is reported. The home health record should clearly report how visual losses impact the function and activities of the patient, including how these conditions impact medication administration, safety, the ability to perform treatments (such as wound care) and other key areas related to the patient's daily living.

+ 6 E13.31 **Other specified diabetes mellitus with unspecified diabetic retinopathy**

SP + E13.311 **Other specified diabetes mellitus with unspecified diabetic retinopathy with macular edema**

SP SH + E13.319 **Other specified diabetes mellitus with unspecified diabetic retinopathy without macular edema**

+ 6 E13.32 **Other specified diabetes mellitus with mild nonproliferative diabetic retinopathy**
Other specified diabetes mellitus with nonproliferative diabetic retinopathy NOS

One of the following 7th characters is to be assigned to codes in subcategory E13.32 to designate laterality of the disease:
1   right eye
2   left eye
3   bilateral
9   unspecified eye

SP + 7 E13.321- **Other specified diabetes mellitus with mild nonproliferative diabetic retinopathy with macular edema**

SP SH + 7 E13.329- **Other specified diabetes mellitus with mild nonproliferative diabetic retinopathy without macular edema**

+ 6 E13.33 **Other specified diabetes mellitus with moderate nonproliferative diabetic retinopathy**

One of the following 7th characters is to be assigned to codes in subcategory E13.33 to designate laterality of the disease:
1   right eye
2   left eye
3   bilateral
9   unspecified eye

SP + 7 E13.331- **Other specified diabetes mellitus with moderate nonproliferative diabetic retinopathy with macular edema**

SP SH + 7 E13.339- **Other specified diabetes mellitus with moderate nonproliferative diabetic retinopathy without macular edema**

+ 6 E13.34 **Other specified diabetes mellitus with severe nonproliferative diabetic retinopathy**

One of the following 7th characters is to be assigned to codes in subcategory E13.34 to designate laterality of the disease:
1   right eye
2   left eye
3   bilateral
9   unspecified eye

SP + 7 E13.341- **Other specified diabetes mellitus with severe nonproliferative diabetic retinopathy with macular edema**

SP SH + 7 E13.349- **Other specified diabetes mellitus with severe nonproliferative diabetic retinopathy without macular edema**

+ 6 E13.35 **Other specified diabetes mellitus with proliferative diabetic retinopathy**

★ New ▲ Revised Px Primary SP PDGM Px SL Low CoM SH High CoM IQ Quest. Encounter H Hospice non-cancer Dx   Unspecified   M *Manifestation*

DecisionHealth's FY 2020 Complete Home Health ICD-10-CM Diagnosis Coding Manual

753

One of the following 7th characters is to be assigned to codes in subcategory E13.35 to designate laterality of the disease:
1   right eye
2   left eye
3   bilateral
9   unspecified eye

⊟ **SP** ✚ **7** **E13.351-**   **Other specified diabetes mellitus with proliferative diabetic retinopathy with macular edema**

⊟ **SP** **SH** ✚ **7** **E13.352-**   **Other specified diabetes mellitus with proliferative diabetic retinopathy with traction retinal detachment involving the macula**

⊟ **SP** **SH** ✚ **7** **E13.353-**   **Other specified diabetes mellitus with proliferative diabetic retinopathy with traction retinal detachment not involving the macula**

⊟ **SP** **SH** ✚ **7** **E13.354-**   **Other specified diabetes mellitus with proliferative diabetic retinopathy with combined traction retinal detachment and rhegmatogenous retinal detachment**

⊟ **SP** **SH** ✚ **7** **E13.355-**   **Other specified diabetes mellitus with stable proliferative diabetic retinopathy**

⊟ **SP** **SH** ✚ **7** **E13.359-**   **Other specified diabetes mellitus with proliferative diabetic retinopathy without macular edema**

SP **SH** ✚ **E13.36**   **Other specified diabetes mellitus with diabetic cataract**

CODING TIPS ✓   Cataracts are more common in diabetic patients. The classification assumes a relationship between cataracts and diabetes, when the patient has diabetes. Even cataracts specifically described as "cortical, nuclear and posterior subcapsular" and "nuclear sclerotic" should prompt the assignment of E--.36, along with the code for the specific cataract code (*Q2 2019 Coding Clinic*).

⊟ **SP** **SH** ✚ **E13.37X-**   **Other specified diabetes mellitus with diabetic macular edema, resolved following treatment**
7

One of the following 7th characters is to be assigned to code E13.37 to designate laterality of the disease:
1   right eye
2   left eye
3   bilateral
9   unspecified eye

CODING TIPS ✓   The macular edema may be resolved, but the retinopathy remains. This code is like a history code for the macular edema.

SP **SH** ✚ **E13.39**   **Other specified diabetes mellitus with other diabetic ophthalmic complication**
Use additional code to identify manifestation, such as:
diabetic glaucoma (H40-H42)

CODING TIPS ✓   There is no assumed relationship between diabetes and glaucoma. The coder should seek further clarification regarding the relationship between blindness, glaucoma and diabetes before coding as a diabetic manifestation.

✚ **5** **E13.4**   **Other specified diabetes mellitus with neurological complications**
CODING TIPS ✓   Other specified diabetes with loss of protective sensation or diabetic peripheral neuropathy should be coded to E13.42.

IQ **SH** **SL** ✚ **E13.40**   **Other specified diabetes mellitus with diabetic neuropathy, unspecified**

SP **SH** ✚ **E13.41**   **Other specified diabetes mellitus with diabetic mononeuropathy**

SP **SH** **SL** ✚ **E13.42**   **Other specified diabetes mellitus with diabetic polyneuropathy**
Other specified diabetes mellitus with diabetic neuralgia

CODING TIPS ✓   Diabetic polyneuropathy is the most common type of diabetic neuropathy and causes pain or loss of feeling in the toes, feet, legs, hands and arms.

SP **SH** ✚ **E13.43**   **Other specified diabetes mellitus with diabetic autonomic (poly)neuropathy**
Other specified diabetes mellitus with diabetic gastroparesis

CODING TIPS ✓   Autonomic neuropathy affects the heart, digestive system and other involuntary functions. This type of neuropathy causes delayed or slowed gastric emptying as well as problems with orthostatic hypotension. This code is not to be used for polyneuropathy of the hands and feet.

CODING TIPS ✓   Gastroparesis (K31.84) may be sequenced after this code as an option.

SP **SH** ✚ **E13.44**   **Other specified diabetes mellitus with diabetic amyotrophy**
CODING TIPS ✓   Diabetic amyotrophy is muscle weakness, characterized by weakness followed by wasting of pelvifemoral muscles, either unilaterally or bilaterally, with associated pain.

SP **SH** ✚ **E13.49**   **Other specified diabetes mellitus with other diabetic neurological complication**

✚ **5** **E13.5**   **Other specified diabetes mellitus with circulatory complications**

4 4th digit required   **5** 5th digit required   **6** 6th digit required   **7** 7th digit required   **7** 7th digit placeholder   ✚ Additional code   ⊟ Laterality

754   *DecisionHealth's* FY 2020 Complete Home Health ICD-10-CM Diagnosis Coding Manual

Chapter 4

E00-E89

CODING TIPS ✓ Peripheral angiopathy includes arterial, venous and capillary conditions. Peripheral angiopathy may be documented as diabetic PVD. There is an assumed relationship between diabetes and PVD and PAD, including peripheral atherosclerosis and venous insufficiency. Diabetic PVD is coded E--.51. Diabetic arteriosclerosis of the peripheral arteries should be coded E--.51 or E--.52 then the appropriate I70.- code. Diabetic venous insufficiency should be coded E--.51 or E--.52 and I87.2 The presence of diabetes and peripheral arterial disease in the record indicates that both diabetes and PVD should be marked in M1028. Venous disease is not included in M1028.

SP **SH** **+** **E13.51** **Other specified diabetes mellitus with diabetic peripheral angiopathy without gangrene**

SP **SH** **+** **E13.52** **Other specified diabetes mellitus with diabetic peripheral angiopathy with gangrene**
Other specified diabetes mellitus with diabetic gangrene

SP **SH** **+** **E13.59** **Other specified diabetes mellitus with other circulatory complications**
CODING TIPS ✓ Diabetic circulatory complications other than peripheral angiopathy and gangrene, identified as such by the physician, may be coded to 4th and 5th characters .59. Example: Diabetic CAD or ASHD is documented.

+ **5** **E13.6** **Other specified diabetes mellitus with other specified complications**

+ **6** **E13.61** **Other specified diabetes mellitus with diabetic arthropathy**

SP **SH** **+** **E13.610** **Other specified diabetes mellitus with diabetic neuropathic arthropathy**
Other specified diabetes mellitus with Charcôt's joints
CODING TIPS ✓ Do not add a M14.6 code for Charcot's joint.

SP **SH** **+** **E13.618** **Other specified diabetes mellitus with other diabetic arthropathy**

+ **6** **E13.62** **Other specified diabetes mellitus with skin complications**

SP **SH** **+** **E13.620** **Other specified diabetes mellitus with diabetic dermatitis**
Other specified diabetes mellitus with diabetic necrobiosis lipoidica

SP **SH** **+** **E13.621** **Other specified diabetes mellitus with foot ulcer**
Use additional code to identify site of ulcer (L97.4-, L97.5-)
CODING TIPS ✓ If the patient has had a diabetic foot ulcer in the past, either healed or amputated, also code Z86.31. Ulceration of the foot is assumed related to diabetes unless another cause is indicated.

SP **SH** **+** **E13.622** **Other specified diabetes mellitus with other skin ulcer**
Use additional code to identify site of ulcer (L97.1-L97.9, L98.41-L98.49)

CODING TIPS ✓ Diabetes codes with 4th, 5th and 6th characters .622 are used when an ulcer is located on the lower extremity, beginning at the ankle, and not including the foot. Whereas ulcers located on the foot are assumed related to diabetes, ulcers located elsewhere are not assumed related to diabetes and must be confirmed with the physician.

SP **SH** **+** **E13.628** **Other specified diabetes mellitus with other skin complications**

+ **6** **E13.63** **Other specified diabetes mellitus with oral complications**

SP **SH** **+** **E13.630** **Other specified diabetes mellitus with periodontal disease**

SP **SH** **+** **E13.638** **Other specified diabetes mellitus with other oral complications**

+ **6** **E13.64** **Other specified diabetes mellitus with hypoglycemia**

SP **SH** **+** **E13.641** **Other specified diabetes mellitus with hypoglycemia with coma**

SP **SH** **+** **E13.649** **Other specified diabetes mellitus with hypoglycemia without coma**
CODING TIPS ✓ The physician should be queried when the term "uncontrolled" is used to determine whether the patient has hyperglycemia, hypoglycemia or both.

CODING TIPS ✓ If encephalopathy is due to hypoglycemia, use G93.41 as an additional code.

SP **SH** **+** **E13.65** **Other specified diabetes mellitus with hyperglycemia**
CODING TIPS ✓ Inadequately controlled, poorly controlled and out of control diabetes are coded with hyperglycemia. The physician should be queried when the term 'uncontrolled' is used to determine whether the patient has hyperglycemia, hypoglycemia, or both. The clinical record should support hyperglycemia. Do not code diabetes with hyperglycemia when ketoacidosis is also documented.

SP **SH** **+** **E13.69** **Other specified diabetes mellitus with other specified complication**
Use additional code to identify complication
CODING TIPS ✓ Use this code when the physician specifies a manifestation of diabetes that does not fit in any of the other subcategories. Follow the diabetes code with the code for the specified condition.

Chapter 4

E00-E89

★ New ▲ Revised Px Primary **SP** PDGM Px **SL** Low CoM **SH** High CoM **IQ** Quest. Encounter **H** Hospice non-cancer Dx Unspecified **M** *Manifestation*

DecisionHealth's FY 2020 Complete Home Health ICD-10-CM Diagnosis Coding Manual

755

CODING TIPS ✓ The classification presumes a cause-and-effect relationship between osteomyelitis and diabetes when no other cause is documented. Osteomyelitis with diabetes is usually associated with ulceration. Use the appropriate code for the osteomyelitis after coding diabetes with other specified manifestation. Although not clear that certain types of diabetes are assumed related to osteomyelitis when referencing diabetes in the index, it is confirmed that osteomyelitis is related to all diabetes types.

IQ ✚ **E13.8   Other specified diabetes mellitus with unspecified complications**

CODING TIPS ✓ This code should not be used for unspecified complications. Query the physician for information regarding suspected manifestations that the classification does not presume related.

SP SH ✚ **E13.9   Other specified diabetes mellitus without complications**

CODING TIPS ✓ This code is acceptable to use for a diabetic without manifestations. Certain specified conditions are assumed related to diabetes by the classification, if listed indented under the word "with" in the alphabetical index, so the use of .9 as a diabetes 4th character should not be common. Query the physician for information regarding suspected manifestations when documentation regarding other potential causes is unclear. This code should be used for a diabetic requiring insulin injections only if teaching is the skill, or other comorbidities, unrelated to diabetes, make it unacceptable for the patient to self-inject. If .9 is used as a 4th character, no other diabetes code may be used.

Other disorders of glucose regulation and pancreatic internal secretion   (E15-E16)

SP E15   Nondiabetic hypoglycemic coma
INCLUDES drug-induced insulin coma in nondiabetic
hyperinsulinism with hypoglycemic coma
hypoglycemic coma NOS

4 E16   Other disorders of pancreatic internal secretion

SP ✚ **E16.0   Drug-induced hypoglycemia without coma**
Use additional code for adverse effect, if applicable, to identify drug (T36-T50 with fifth or sixth character 5)
EXCLUDES 1 diabetes with hypoglycemia without coma (E09.649)
CODING TIPS ✓ Use this code for drug induced hypoglycemia in someone who is not diabetic.

SP E16.1   Other hypoglycemia
Functional hyperinsulinism

Functional nonhyperinsulinemic hypoglycemia
Hyperinsulinism NOS
Hyperplasia of pancreatic islet beta cells NOS
EXCLUDES 1 diabetes with hypoglycemia (E08.649, E10.649, E11.649, E13.649)
hypoglycemia in infant of diabetic mother (P70.1)
neonatal hypoglycemia (P70.4)
CODING TIPS ✓ Do not assign E16.1 to report hypoglycemia in a patient with a known diagnosis of diabetes, including post-procedural hypoinsulinemia.

SP E16.2   Hypoglycemia, unspecified
EXCLUDES 1 diabetes with hypoglycemia (E08.649, E10.649, E11.649, E13.649)
CODING TIPS ✓ Report this code for someone who has hypoglycemia and is not diabetic.
DEFINITION Condition in which blood sugar levels are too low for normal functioning, manifesting as weakness, trembling, hunger, headache, irritability, racing heartbeat, confusion, even convulsions or coma.

SP E16.3   Increased secretion of glucagon
Hyperplasia of pancreatic endocrine cells with glucagon excess

SP E16.4   Increased secretion of gastrin
Hypergastrinemia
Hyperplasia of pancreatic endocrine cells with gastrin excess
Zollinger-Ellison syndrome

SP E16.8   Other specified disorders of pancreatic internal secretion
Increased secretion from endocrine pancreas of growth hormone-releasing hormone
Increased secretion from endocrine pancreas of pancreatic polypeptide
Increased secretion from endocrine pancreas of somatostatin
Increased secretion from endocrine pancreas of vasoactive-intestinal polypeptide
CODING TIPS ✓ Do not use E16.8 for steroid induced diabetes. Use E09 instead.

SP E16.9   Disorder of pancreatic internal secretion, unspecified
Islet-cell hyperplasia NOS
Pancreatic endocrine cell hyperplasia NOS

Disorders of other endocrine glands (E20-E35)

EXCLUDES 1 galactorrhea (N64.3)
gynecomastia (N62)
4 E20   Hypoparathyroidism
EXCLUDES 1 Di George's syndrome (D82.1)
postprocedural hypoparathyroidism (E89.2)
tetany NOS (R29.0)

4 4th digit required   **5** 5th digit required   **6** 6th digit required   **7** 7th digit required   **7** 7th digit placeholder   ✚ Additional code   ⊟ Laterality

756   DecisionHealth's FY 2020 Complete Home Health ICD-10-CM Diagnosis Coding Manual

transitory neonatal
hypoparathyroidism (P71.4)

DEFINITION Reduced production of
parathyroid hormone causing tingling of the
hands, fingers, and mouth, muscle cramps,
and possibly convulsions.

SP **E20.0** **Idiopathic hypoparathyroidism**

SP **E20.1** **Pseudohypoparathyroidism**

CODING TIPS ✓ Patients with
pseudohypoparathyroidism produce
adequate levels of PTH, but are resistant to
its effects due to a genetic abnormality.
These patients typically exhibit low blood
calcium and elevated phosphorus, which
are characteristic of hypoparathyroidism
and should not be separately coded.

DEFINITION Condition of
hypoparathyroidism symptoms manifesting
due to an inadequate response to the
parathyroid hormone, rather than an
insufficient amount of the hormone.

SP **E20.8** **Other hypoparathyroidism**

SP **E20.9** **Hypoparathyroidism, unspecified**
Parathyroid tetany

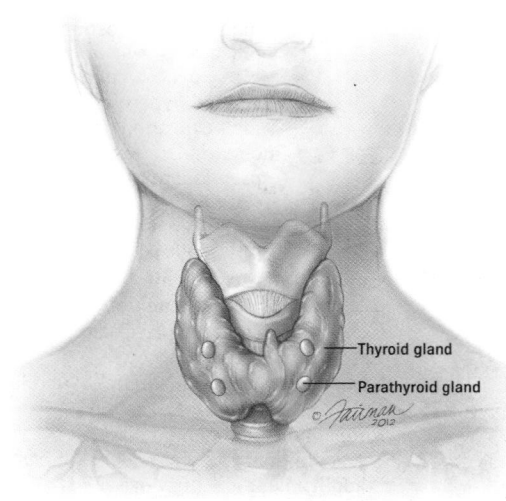

Thyroid gland
Parathyroid gland

4 **E21** **Hyperparathyroidism and other disorders
of parathyroid gland**

EXCLUDES 1 adult osteomalacia (M83.-)
ectopic hyperparathyroidism
(E34.2)
familial hypocalciuric
hypercalcemia (E83.52)
hungry bone syndrome
(E83.81)
infantile and juvenile
osteomalacia (E55.0)

SP **E21.0** **Primary hyperparathyroidism**
Hyperplasia of parathyroid
Osteitis fibrosa cystica generalisata [von
Recklinghausen's disease of bone]

DEFINITION Excessive production of
parathyroid hormone, usually caused by
hyperplasia of the gland itself, causing
decreased calcium levels in bones.

SP **E21.1** **Secondary hyperparathyroidism, not
elsewhere classified**

EXCLUDES 1 secondary
hyperparathyroidism of
renal origin (N25.81)

CODING TIPS ✓ Do not assign E21.1 if the
causative mechanism of the diagnosed
secondary hyperparathyroid disease is of
renal (kidney) origin. E21.1 should only be
assigned when the hyperparathyroidism is
not reported as primary and has a clear
cause reported as not of renal origin.

SP **E21.2** **Other hyperparathyroidism**
Tertiary hyperparathyroidism

EXCLUDES 1 familial hypocalciuric
hypercalcemia (E83.52)

SP **E21.3** **Hyperparathyroidism, unspecified**

SP **E21.4** **Other specified disorders of parathyroid
gland**

IQ **E21.5** **Disorder of parathyroid gland,
unspecified**

4 **E22** **Hyperfunction of pituitary gland**

EXCLUDES 1 Cushing's syndrome (E24.-)
Nelson's syndrome (E24.1)
overproduction of ACTH not
associated with Cushing's
disease (E27.0)
overproduction of pituitary
ACTH (E24.0)
overproduction of thyroid-
stimulating hormone (E05.8-)

SP **E22.0** **Acromegaly and pituitary gigantism**
Overproduction of growth hormone

EXCLUDES 1 constitutional gigantism
(E34.4)
constitutional tall stature
(E34.4)
increased secretion from
endocrine pancreas of
growth hormone-releasing
hormone (E16.8)

DEFINITION Acromegaly: Abnormally
large growth of the hands, feet and facial
features due to the production of too much
growth hormone in adults by the pituitary
gland.

SP **+** **E22.1** **Hyperprolactinemia**
Use additional code for adverse effect, if
applicable, to identify drug (T36-T50
with fifth or sixth character 5)

SP **E22.2** **Syndrome of inappropriate secretion of
antidiuretic hormone**

SP **E22.8** **Other hyperfunction of pituitary gland**
Central precocious puberty

IQ **E22.9** **Hyperfunction of pituitary gland,
unspecified**

4 **E23** **Hypofunction and other disorders of the
pituitary gland**

INCLUDES the listed conditions whether the
disorder is in the pituitary or
the hypothalamus

EXCLUDES 1 postprocedural hypopituitarism
(E89.3)

Chapter 4

E00-E89

★ New ▲ Revised **Px** Primary **SP** PDGM Px **SL** Low CoM **SH** High CoM **IQ** Quest. Encounter **H** Hospice non-cancer Dx **Unspecified** **M** *Manifestation*

DecisionHealth's FY 2020 Complete Home Health ICD-10-CM Diagnosis Coding Manual

757

SP E23.0 Hypopituitarism
Fertile eunuch syndrome
Hypogonadotropic hypogonadism
Idiopathic growth hormone deficiency
Isolated deficiency of gonadotropin
Isolated deficiency of growth hormone
Isolated deficiency of pituitary hormone
Kallmann's syndrome
Lorain-Levi short stature
Necrosis of pituitary gland (postpartum)
Panhypopituitarism
Pituitary cachexia
Pituitary insufficiency NOS
Pituitary short stature
Sheehan's syndrome
Simmonds' disease
DEFINITION   A type of dwarfism with retention of infantile characteristics, due to undersecretion of growth hormone and gonadotropin deficiency.

SP ✚ E23.1 Drug-induced hypopituitarism
Use additional code for adverse effect, if applicable, to identify drug (T36-T50 with fifth or sixth character 5)

IQ E23.2 Diabetes insipidus
EXCLUDES 1   nephrogenic diabetes insipidus (N25.1)
CODING TIPS ✓   E23.2 is one of the less common kinds of diabetes. It is caused by a malfunction of the pituitary gland. Don't confuse with nephrogenic diabetes insipidus, a problem caused by kidneys (N25.2). Diabetes insipidus is not related to diabetes mellitus.
DEFINITION   Insufficient vasopressin production/secretion of antidiuretic hormone (ADH) resulting in intense thirst and excretion of large amounts of urine.

▲ SP E23.3 Hypothalamic dysfunction, not elsewhere classified
EXCLUDES 1   Prader-Willi syndrome (Q87.11)
Russell-Silver syndrome (Q87.19)

SP E23.6 Other disorders of pituitary gland
Abscess of pituitary
Adiposogenital dystrophy

IQ E23.7 Disorder of pituitary gland, unspecified

4 E24 Cushing's syndrome
EXCLUDES 1   congenital adrenal hyperplasia (E25.0)
CODING TIPS ✓   When Cushing's syndrome is stated as the related cause of diabetes (diabetes due to an underlying condition), assign the appropriate code for Cushing's syndrome (classifiable to E24), followed by a code from E08 to indicate diabetes mellitus due to an underlying condition.

SP E24.0 Pituitary-dependent Cushing's disease
Overproduction of pituitary ACTH
Pituitary-dependent hypercorticalism

SP E24.1 Nelson's syndrome

SP ✚ E24.2 Drug-induced Cushing's syndrome
Use additional code for adverse effect, if applicable, to identify drug (T36-T50 with fifth or sixth character 5)

CODING TIPS ✓   Code E24.2 should only be assigned when documentation clearly indicates a relationship between Cushing's syndrome and a drug or chemical as the underlying cause. Assign a code from T36-T50 to indicate the drug and adverse effect.

SP E24.3 Ectopic ACTH syndrome

SP E24.4 Alcohol-induced pseudo-Cushing's syndrome

SP E24.8 Other Cushing's syndrome

SP E24.9 Cushing's syndrome, unspecified
DEFINITION   Disorder caused by prolonged exposure of body tissues to high levels of cortisol, presenting with upper body obesity, thinning arms and legs, brittle bones, severe fatigue, weakness, high blood pressure, and high blood sugar.

4 E25 Adrenogenital disorders
INCLUDES   adrenogenital syndromes, virilizing or feminizing, whether acquired or due to adrenal hyperplasia consequent on inborn enzyme defects in hormone synthesis
Female adrenal pseudohermaphroditism
Female heterosexual precocious pseudopuberty
Male isosexual precocious pseudopuberty
Male macrogenitosomia praecox
Male sexual precocity with adrenal hyperplasia
Male virilization (female)
EXCLUDES 1   indeterminate sex and pseudohermaphroditism (Q56)
chromosomal abnormalities (Q90-Q99)

SP E25.0 Congenital adrenogenital disorders associated with enzyme deficiency
Congenital adrenal hyperplasia
21-Hydroxylase deficiency
Salt-losing congenital adrenal hyperplasia

SP ✚ E25.8 Other adrenogenital disorders
Idiopathic adrenogenital disorder
Use additional code for adverse effect, if applicable, to identify drug (T36-T50 with fifth or sixth character 5)

IQ E25.9 Adrenogenital disorder, unspecified
Adrenogenital syndrome NOS

4 E26 Hyperaldosteronism

5 E26.0 Primary hyperaldosteronism
DEFINITION   Excessive aldosterone production; typically presents with loss of potassium, muscular weakness, and elevated blood pressure.

SP E26.01 Conn's syndrome
Code also:
adrenal adenoma (D35.0-)
DEFINITION   Excess secretion of aldosterone due to an adrenocortical adenoma, causing hypokalemia, alkalosis, muscular weakness, polyuria, polydipsia, and hypertension.

---

4 4th digit required   **5** 5th digit required   **6** 6th digit required   **7** 7th digit required   **☑** 7th digit placeholder   **✚** Additional code   **⊟** Laterality

758   *DecisionHealth's* FY 2020 Complete Home Health ICD-10-CM Diagnosis Coding Manual

SP E26.02 **Glucocorticoid-remediable aldosteronism**
Familial aldosteronism type I

SP E26.09 **Other primary hyperaldosteronism**
Primary aldosteronism due to adrenal hyperplasia (bilateral)

SP E26.1 **Secondary hyperaldosteronism**

5 E26.8 **Other hyperaldosteronism**

SP E26.81 **Bartter's syndrome**
> **DEFINITION** Group of symptoms caused by the kidneys' inability to reabsorb potassium, also known as urinary potassium wasting; causes renal cell enlargement, alkalosis, hyperaldosteronism, cramping, constipation, urinary frequency, and weakness.

SP E26.89 **Other hyperaldosteronism**

!Q E26.9 **Hyperaldosteronism, unspecified**
Aldosteronism NOS
Hyperaldosteronism NOS

4 E27 **Other disorders of adrenal gland**

SP E27.0 **Other adrenocortical overactivity**
Overproduction of ACTH, not associated with Cushing's disease
Premature adrenarche
> **EXCLUDES 1** Cushing's syndrome (E24.-)

SP E27.1 **Primary adrenocortical insufficiency**
Addison's disease
Autoimmune adrenalitis
> **EXCLUDES 1** Addison only phenotype adrenoleukodystrophy (E71.528)
> amyloidosis (E85.-)
> tuberculous Addison's disease (A18.7)
> Waterhouse-Friderichsen syndrome (A39.1)

SP E27.2 **Addisonian crisis**
Adrenal crisis
Adrenocortical crisis
> **CODING TIPS ✓** Do not assign E27.2 to indicate Addison's disease. Code E27.2 indicates Addisonian crisis, a severe and life-threatening condition that may occur in individuals with Addison's disease or other conditions resulting in severely elevated cortisol levels. Addison's disease in the absence of crisis should be coded to E27.1.

> **DEFINITION** Low levels of the glucocorticoid hormone, cortisol, secreted by the adrenal glands and responsible for regulating blood pressure, cardiovascular function, inflammatory response, insulin effects, and metabolism.

SP + E27.3 **Drug-induced adrenocortical insufficiency**
Use additional code for adverse effect, if applicable, to identify drug (T36-T50 with fifth or sixth character 5)

> **CODING TIPS ✓** Code E27.3 should only be assigned when documentation clearly indicates a relationship between adrenocortical insufficiency and a drug or chemical as the underlying cause. Assign a code from T36-T50 following E27.3 to indicate the drug and adverse effect.

5 E27.4 **Other and unspecified adrenocortical insufficiency**
> **EXCLUDES 1** adrenoleukodystrophy [Addison-Schilder] (E71.528)
> Waterhouse-Friderichsen syndrome (A39.1)

!Q E27.40 **Unspecified adrenocortical insufficiency**
Adrenocortical insufficiency NOS
Hypoaldosteronism

!Q E27.49 **Other adrenocortical insufficiency**
Adrenal hemorrhage
Adrenal infarction

SP E27.5 **Adrenomedullary hyperfunction**
Adrenomedullary hyperplasia
Catecholamine hypersecretion
> **DEFINITION** Overproduction of adrenaline hormones by the adrenal medulla, causing heart disease, high blood pressure, and related problems.

SP E27.8 **Other specified disorders of adrenal gland**
Abnormality of cortisol-binding globulin

!Q E27.9 **Disorder of adrenal gland, unspecified**

4 E28 **Ovarian dysfunction**
> **EXCLUDES 1** isolated gonadotropin deficiency (E23.0)
> postprocedural ovarian failure (E89.4-)

SP + E28.0 **Estrogen excess**
Use additional code for adverse effect, if applicable, to identify drug (T36-T50 with fifth or sixth character 5)

SP + E28.1 **Androgen excess**
Hypersecretion of ovarian androgens
Use additional code for adverse effect, if applicable, to identify drug (T36-T50 with fifth or sixth character 5)

SP E28.2 **Polycystic ovarian syndrome**
Sclerocystic ovary syndrome
Stein-Leventhal syndrome
> **CODING TIPS ✓** Polycystic ovarian syndrome (PCOS) is associated with increased risk for a number of other endocrine disorders, including insulin resistance, hypothyroidism and obesity. When present, these other diagnoses should also be reported.

> **DEFINITION** Syndrome in which the ovaries produce too many androgens, causing ovarian cysts and interfering with the menstrual cycle; results in missed, heavy, or irregular periods, infertility, abdominal discomfort, acne, weight gain, and uterine bleeding.

5 E28.3 **Primary ovarian failure**
> **EXCLUDES 1** pure gonadal dysgenesis (Q99.1)
> Turner's syndrome (Q96.-)

★ New ▲ Revised Px Primary **SP** PDGM Px **SL** Low CoM **SH** High CoM **!Q** Quest. Encounter **H** Hospice non-cancer Dx Unspecified M *Manifestation*

6 E28.31   Premature menopause

SP E28.310   Symptomatic premature menopause
Symptoms such as flushing, sleeplessness, headache, lack of concentration, associated with premature menopause

SP E28.319   Asymptomatic premature menopause
Premature menopause NOS

SP E28.39   Other primary ovarian failure
Decreased estrogen
Resistant ovary syndrome

SP E28.8   Other ovarian dysfunction
Ovarian hyperfunction NOS
EXCLUDES 1   postprocedural ovarian failure (E89.4-)

IQ E28.9   Ovarian dysfunction, unspecified

4 E29   Testicular dysfunction
EXCLUDES 1   androgen insensitivity syndrome (E34.5-)
azoospermia or oligospermia NOS (N46.0-N46.1)
isolated gonadotropin deficiency (E23.0)
Klinefelter's syndrome (Q98.0-Q98.1, Q98.4)

SP E29.0   Testicular hyperfunction
Hypersecretion of testicular hormones
DEFINITION   Excessive testosterone production, often due to an active tumor on the testicle. Commonly presents with increased muscle and bone growth in children and increased secondary sex characteristics.

SP + E29.1   Testicular hypofunction
Defective biosynthesis of testicular androgen NOS
5-delta-Reductase deficiency (with male pseudohermaphroditism)
Testicular hypogonadism NOS
Use additional code for adverse effect, if applicable, to identify drug (T36-T50 with fifth or sixth character 5)
EXCLUDES 1   postprocedural testicular hypofunction (E89.5)
DEFINITION   Underdevelopment of all the genital tissues with decreased functional activities of the gonads.

SP E29.8   Other testicular dysfunction

IQ E29.9   Testicular dysfunction, unspecified

4 E30   Disorders of puberty, not elsewhere classified

IQ E30.0   Delayed puberty
Constitutional delay of puberty
Delayed sexual development

IQ E30.1   Precocious puberty
Precocious menstruation
EXCLUDES 1   Albright (-McCune) (-Sternberg) syndrome (Q78.1)
central precocious puberty (E22.8)
congenital adrenal hyperplasia (E25.0)

female heterosexual precocious pseudopuberty (E25.-)
male isosexual precocious pseudopuberty (E25.-)

IQ E30.8   Other disorders of puberty
Premature thelarche

IQ E30.9   Disorder of puberty, unspecified

4 E31   Polyglandular dysfunction
EXCLUDES 1   ataxia telangiectasia [Louis-Bar] (G11.3)
dystrophia myotonica [Steinert] (G71.11)
pseudohypoparathyroidism (E20.1)

SP E31.0   Autoimmune polyglandular failure
Schmidt's syndrome
DEFINITION   Schmidt's syndrome: hypofunction of more than one endocrine gland in different combinations, including the thyroid, adrenals, gonads, parathyroid, and pancreas; occurs primarily in adult females.

SP E31.1   Polyglandular hyperfunction
EXCLUDES 1   multiple endocrine adenomatosis (E31.2-)
multiple endocrine neoplasia (E31.2-)

5 E31.2   Multiple endocrine neoplasia [MEN] syndromes
Multiple endocrine adenomatosis
Code also:
any associated malignancies and other conditions associated with the syndromes
CODING TIPS ✓   MEN syndromes are distinct, inherited autosomal disorders, which may present in conjunction with endocrine tumors.

SP E31.20   Multiple endocrine neoplasia [MEN] syndrome, unspecified
Multiple endocrine adenomatosis NOS
Multiple endocrine neoplasia [MEN] syndrome NOS

SP E31.21   Multiple endocrine neoplasia [MEN] type I
Wermer's syndrome
DEFINITION   Hyperplasia or tumors of the parathyroid, pancreatic islet cells, and pituitary gland; causes oversecretion of hormones, kidney stones, infertility, and severe peptic ulcers.

SP E31.22   Multiple endocrine neoplasia [MEN] type IIA
Sipple's syndrome
DEFINITION   Triad of thyroid medullary carcinoma, adrenal gland tumor, and parathyroid hyperplasia.

SP E31.23   Multiple endocrine neoplasia [MEN] type IIB

SP E31.8   Other polyglandular dysfunction

SP E31.9   Polyglandular dysfunction, unspecified

4 E32   Diseases of thymus

4 4th digit required   5 5th digit required   6 6th digit required   7 7th digit required   ✔ 7th digit placeholder   + Additional code   ⊟ Laterality

760   DecisionHealth's FY 2020 Complete Home Health ICD-10-CM Diagnosis Coding Manual

Chapter 4

E00-E89

EXCLUDES 1 aplasia or hypoplasia of thymus
with immunodeficiency
(D82.1)
myasthenia gravis (G70.0)

IQ E32.0 Persistent hyperplasia of thymus
Hypertrophy of thymus

SP E32.1 Abscess of thymus

SP E32.8 Other diseases of thymus
EXCLUDES 1 aplasia or hypoplasia with
immunodeficiency
(D82.1)
thymoma (D15.0)

IQ E32.9 Disease of thymus, unspecified

4 E34 Other endocrine disorders
EXCLUDES 1 pseudohypoparathyroidism
(E20.1)

SP E34.0 Carcinoid syndrome
Note:
May be used as an additional code to
identify functional activity associated
with a carcinoid tumor.

CODING TIPS ✓ Carcinoid syndrome is a
specific syndrome causing a variety of
symptoms in patients with advanced stage
malignant carcinoid tumors. When coding
carcinoid syndrome, the specific type and
location of the carcinoid tumor should be
identified and additionally coded by
assigning the appropriate code(s) from
category C7A and/or C7B.

DEFINITION Condition in which
cancerous cells secrete hormones into the
bloodstream causing chemical imbalances
in the body with symptoms of periodic
flushing, diarrhea, abdominal pain, and high
blood pressure.

**SP E34.1 Other hypersecretion of intestinal
hormones**

**SP E34.2 Ectopic hormone secretion, not
elsewhere classified**
EXCLUDES 1 ectopic ACTH syndrome
(E24.3)

DEFINITION Condition that occurs when a
glandular tumor metastasizes, moving from
its original location to another area of the
body, and continues to secrete hormones.

▲ SP E34.3 Short stature due to endocrine disorder
Constitutional short stature
Laron-type short stature
EXCLUDES 1 achondroplastic short stature
(Q77.4)
hypochondroplastic short
stature (Q77.4)
nutritional short stature
(E45)
pituitary short stature
(E23.0)
progeria (E34.8)
renal short stature (N25.0)
Russell-Silver syndrome
(Q87.19)
short-limbed stature with
immunodeficiency
(D82.2)

short stature in specific
dysmorphic syndromes -
code to syndrome - see
Alphabetical Index
short stature NOS (R62.52)

SP E34.4 Constitutional tall stature
Constitutional gigantism

5 E34.5 Androgen insensitivity syndrome
DEFINITION Defects in androgen action
causing feminization of external genitalia,
abnormal sexual development, infertility,
and pseudohermaphroditism in males.

**IQ E34.50 Androgen insensitivity syndrome,
unspecified**
Androgen insensitivity NOS

**SP E34.51 Complete androgen insensitivity
syndrome**
Complete androgen insensitivity
de Quervain syndrome
Goldberg-Maxwell syndrome

**SP E34.52 Partial androgen insensitivity
syndrome**
Partial androgen insensitivity
Reifenstein syndrome

SP E34.8 Other specified endocrine disorders
Pineal gland dysfunction
Progeria
EXCLUDES 2 pseudohypoparathyroidism
(E20.1)

IQ E34.9 Endocrine disorder, unspecified
Endocrine disturbance NOS
Hormone disturbance NOS

**M IQ + E35 Disorders of endocrine glands in diseases
classified elsewhere**
Code first underlying disease, such as:
late congenital syphilis of thymus gland
[Dubois disease] (A50.5)
Use additional code, if applicable, to identify:
sequelae of tuberculosis of other organs
(B90.8)
EXCLUDES 1 Echinococcus granulosus
infection of thyroid gland
(B67.3)
meningococcal hemorrhagic
adrenalitis (A39.1)
syphilis of endocrine gland
(A52.79)
tuberculosis of adrenal gland,
except calcification (A18.7)
tuberculosis of endocrine gland
NEC (A18.82)
tuberculosis of thyroid gland
(A18.81)
Waterhouse-Friderichsen
syndrome (A39.1)

Intraoperative complications of endocrine system (E36)

CODING TIPS ✓ Codes classifiable to E36 are complication codes
(intraoperative complications) and should only be coded when
the physician specifically indicates a relationship between the
operative procedure and the specific complication. If no
relationship between the condition suspected to be a
complication and the operative procedure is stated, the provider
may be queried to clarify if the condition is classifiable as a
complication.

★ New ▲ Revised Px Primary SP PDGM Px SL Low CoM SH High CoM IQ Quest. Encounter H Hospice non-cancer Dx   Unspecified   M Manifestation

DecisionHealth's FY 2020 Complete Home Health ICD-10-CM Diagnosis Coding Manual   761

4 E36 Intraoperative complications of endocrine system

> **EXCLUDES 2** postprocedural endocrine and metabolic complications and disorders, not elsewhere classified (E89.-)

5 E36.0 Intraoperative hemorrhage and hematoma of an endocrine system organ or structure complicating a procedure

> **EXCLUDES 1** intraoperative hemorrhage and hematoma of an endocrine system organ or structure due to accidental puncture or laceration during a procedure (E36.1-)

SP E36.01 Intraoperative hemorrhage and hematoma of an endocrine system organ or structure complicating an endocrine system procedure

SP E36.02 Intraoperative hemorrhage and hematoma of an endocrine system organ or structure complicating other procedure

5 E36.1 Accidental puncture and laceration of an endocrine system organ or structure during a procedure

SP E36.11 Accidental puncture and laceration of an endocrine system organ or structure during an endocrine system procedure

SP E36.12 Accidental puncture and laceration of an endocrine system organ or structure during other procedure

SP + E36.8 Other intraoperative complications of endocrine system

> Use additional code, if applicable, to further specify disorder

Malnutrition (E40-E46)

> **EXCLUDES 1** intestinal malabsorption (K90.-)
> sequelae of protein-calorie malnutrition (E64.0)
> **EXCLUDES 2** nutritional anemias (D50-D53)
> starvation (T73.0)

CODING TIPS ✓ Malnutrition is defined as insufficient, excessive or imbalanced nutrient consumption. Not all patients experiencing malnutrition will present with inadequate intake or low body weight/BMI. The specific type of malnutrition (such as severe, moderate, Kwashiorkor, etc.) must be indicated by the patient's provider and cannot be assumed. When documentation only states "malnutrition," assign E46.

SP E40 Kwashiorkor
Severe malnutrition with nutritional edema with dyspigmentation of skin and hair

> **EXCLUDES 1** marasmic kwashiorkor (E42)

> **ALERT** Kwashiorkor is a form of severe protein malnutrition that generally affects children living in tropical and subtropical parts of the world during periods of famine or insufficient food supply. It is typically not found in the United States.

SP E41 Nutritional marasmus
Severe malnutrition with marasmus

> **EXCLUDES 1** marasmic kwashiorkor (E42)

> **CODING TIPS ✓** Assign R64 (Cachexia), not E41 (Nutritional marasmus), for a patient diagnosed with emaciation or described as "emaciated" even though the alphabetic index leads to E41. Using E41 is incorrect because it refers to a type of malnutrition that occurs in infants and young children. Unless that is applicable, do not assign E41, according to Q3 2017 Coding Clinic guidance.

> **DEFINITION** Chronic wasting of body tissues, especially in young children, commonly due to prolonged dietary deficiency of protein and calories.

SP E42 Marasmic kwashiorkor
Intermediate form severe protein-calorie malnutrition
Severe protein-calorie malnutrition with signs of both kwashiorkor and marasmus

SP E43 Unspecified severe protein-calorie malnutrition
Starvation edema

4 E44 Protein-calorie malnutrition of moderate and mild degree

SP E44.0 Moderate protein-calorie malnutrition

SP E44.1 Mild protein-calorie malnutrition

SP E45 Retarded development following protein-calorie malnutrition
Nutritional short stature
Nutritional stunting
Physical retardation due to malnutrition

SP E46 Unspecified protein-calorie malnutrition
Malnutrition NOS
Protein-calorie imbalance NOS

> **EXCLUDES 1** nutritional deficiency NOS (E63.9)

> **ALERT** Hospice claims may be rejected for E46 for non-specificity.

> **CODING TIPS ✓** This code should not be reported as primary in hospice due to its non-specific nature. Query the physician for a more specific code for the malnutrition.

Other nutritional deficiencies (E50-E64)

> **EXCLUDES 2** nutritional anemias (D50-D53)

> **CODING TIPS ✓** Do not use codes from E50-E64 to indicate anemia due to a nutritional deficiency. When a patient has a specific diagnosis of anemia due to a nutritional deficiency, assign the appropriate specified code from Chapter 3.

4 E50 Vitamin A deficiency

> **EXCLUDES 1** sequelae of vitamin A deficiency (E64.1)

SP E50.0 Vitamin A deficiency with conjunctival xerosis

> **DEFINITION** Vitamin A deficiency with dryness of the membrane that lines eyelids and covers the exposed surface of the sclera.

SP E50.1 Vitamin A deficiency with Bitot's spot and conjunctival xerosis
Bitot's spot in the young child

> **DEFINITION** Vitamin A deficiency with superficial spots of keratinized epithelium on the conjunctiva, accompanied by dryness.

4 4th digit required   5 5th digit required   6 6th digit required   7 7th digit required   7 7th digit placeholder   + Additional code   ⊟ Laterality

762   DecisionHealth's FY 2020 Complete Home Health ICD-10-CM Diagnosis Coding Manual

SP E50.2 **Vitamin A deficiency with corneal xerosis**

SP E50.3 **Vitamin A deficiency with corneal ulceration and xerosis**

SP E50.4 **Vitamin A deficiency with keratomalacia**

> **DEFINITION** Vitamin A deficiency with softening of the corneas that may lead to corneal infection or rupture.

SP E50.5 **Vitamin A deficiency with night blindness**

SP E50.6 **Vitamin A deficiency with xerophthalmic scars of cornea**

SP E50.7 **Other ocular manifestations of vitamin A deficiency**
Xerophthalmia NOS

SP E50.8 **Other manifestations of vitamin A deficiency**
Follicular keratosis
Xeroderma

SP E50.9 **Vitamin A deficiency, unspecified**
Hypovitaminosis A NOS

4 E51 **Thiamine deficiency**
> **EXCLUDES 1** sequelae of thiamine deficiency (E64.8)

5 E51.1 **Beriberi**
> **DEFINITION** Severe Vitamin B1 (thiamine) deficiency causing nerve, heart, and/or brain abnormalities.

SP E51.11 **Dry beriberi**
Beriberi NOS
Beriberi with polyneuropathy

SP E51.12 **Wet beriberi**
Beriberi with cardiovascular manifestations
Cardiovascular beriberi
Shoshin disease

SP E51.2 **Wernicke's encephalopathy**

SP E51.8 **Other manifestations of thiamine deficiency**

SP E51.9 **Thiamine deficiency, unspecified**

SP E52 **Niacin deficiency [pellagra]**
Niacin (-tryptophan) deficiency
Nicotinamide deficiency
Pellagra (alcoholic)
> **EXCLUDES 1** sequelae of niacin deficiency (E64.8)

> **DEFINITION** Niacin and amino acid tryptophan deficiency affecting the skin, digestive tract, and brain.

4 E53 **Deficiency of other B group vitamins**
> **EXCLUDES 1** sequelae of vitamin B deficiency (E64.8)

SP E53.0 **Riboflavin deficiency**
Ariboflavinosis
Vitamin B2 deficiency
> **DEFINITION** Riboflavin deficiency causing dry throat and nasal passages, mouth sores, magenta-colored tongue, and overproduction of oil on the skin.

SP E53.1 **Pyridoxine deficiency**
Vitamin B6 deficiency
> **EXCLUDES 1** pyridoxine-responsive sideroblastic anemia (D64.3)

SP E53.8 **Deficiency of other specified B group vitamins**
Biotin deficiency
Cyanocobalamin deficiency
Folate deficiency
Folic acid deficiency
Pantothenic acid deficiency
Vitamin B12 deficiency
> **EXCLUDES 1** folate deficiency anemia (D52.-)
> vitamin B12 deficiency anemia (D51.-)

SP E53.9 **Vitamin B deficiency, unspecified**

SP E54 **Ascorbic acid deficiency**
Deficiency of vitamin C
Scurvy
> **EXCLUDES 1** scorbutic anemia (D53.2)
> sequelae of vitamin C deficiency (E64.2)

> **DEFINITION** Condition known as scurvy caused by deficiency of ascorbic acid (vitamin C) and marked by weakness, anemia, spongy gums, and mucocutaneous hemorrhages.

4 E55 **Vitamin D deficiency**
> **EXCLUDES 1** adult osteomalacia (M83.-)
> osteoporosis (M80.-)
> sequelae of rickets (E64.3)

SP E55.0 **Rickets, active**
Infantile osteomalacia
Juvenile osteomalacia
> **EXCLUDES 1** celiac rickets (K90.0)
> Crohn's rickets (K50.-)
> hereditary vitamin D-dependent rickets (E83.32)
> inactive rickets (E64.3)
> renal rickets (N25.0)
> sequelae of rickets (E64.3)
> vitamin D-resistant rickets (E83.31)

> **DEFINITION** Childhood disease caused by a lack of vitamin D, resulting in soft, spongy bones and bone pain as well as skeletal deformities (e.g., bowlegs, scoliosis), distortion of the rib cage, and oddly-shaped skull.

SP E55.9 **Vitamin D deficiency, unspecified**
Avitaminosis D

4 E56 **Other vitamin deficiencies**
> **EXCLUDES 1** sequelae of other vitamin deficiencies (E64.8)

SP E56.0 **Deficiency of vitamin E**

SP E56.1 **Deficiency of vitamin K**
> **EXCLUDES 1** deficiency of coagulation factor due to vitamin K deficiency (D68.4)
> vitamin K deficiency of newborn (P53)

SP E56.8 **Deficiency of other vitamins**

IQ E56.9 **Vitamin deficiency, unspecified**

SP E58 **Dietary calcium deficiency**
> **EXCLUDES 1** disorders of calcium metabolism (E83.5-)
> sequelae of calcium deficiency (E64.8)

SP E59 **Dietary selenium deficiency**
Keshan disease

★ New ▲ Revised Px Primary **SP** PDGM Px **SL** Low CoM **SH** High CoM **IQ** Quest. Encounter **H** Hospice non-cancer Dx Unspecified **M** *Manifestation*

Chapter 4

E00-E89

EXCLUDES 1 sequelae of selenium deficiency (E64.8)

SP **E60** Dietary zinc deficiency

+ 4 E61 Deficiency of other nutrient elements
Use additional code for adverse effect, if applicable, to identify drug (T36-T50 with fifth or sixth character 5)
EXCLUDES 1 disorders of mineral metabolism (E83.-)
iodine deficiency related thyroid disorders (E00-E02)
sequelae of malnutrition and other nutritional deficiencies (E64.-)

SP + E61.0 Copper deficiency

SP + E61.1 Iron deficiency
EXCLUDES 1 iron deficiency anemia (D50.-)

SP + E61.2 Magnesium deficiency

SP + E61.3 Manganese deficiency

SP + E61.4 Chromium deficiency

SP + E61.5 Molybdenum deficiency

SP + E61.6 Vanadium deficiency

SP + E61.7 Deficiency of multiple nutrient elements

SP + E61.8 Deficiency of other specified nutrient elements

IQ + E61.9 Deficiency of nutrient element, unspecified

4 E63 Other nutritional deficiencies
EXCLUDES 1 dehydration (E86.0)
failure to thrive, adult (R62.7)
failure to thrive, child (R62.51)
feeding problems in newborn (P92.-)
sequelae of malnutrition and other nutritional deficiencies (E64.-)

SP E63.0 Essential fatty acid [EFA] deficiency

SP E63.1 Imbalance of constituents of food intake

SP E63.8 Other specified nutritional deficiencies

IQ E63.9 Nutritional deficiency, unspecified

4 E64 Sequelae of malnutrition and other nutritional deficiencies
Note:
This category is to be used to indicate conditions in categories E43, E44, E46, E50-E63 as the cause of sequelae, which are themselves classified elsewhere. The 'sequelae' include conditions specified as such; they also include the late effects of diseases classifiable to the above categories if the disease itself is no longer present
Code first:
condition resulting from (sequela) of malnutrition and other nutritional deficiencies

SP E64.0 Sequelae of protein-calorie malnutrition
EXCLUDES 2 retarded development following protein-calorie malnutrition (E45)

SP E64.1 Sequelae of vitamin A deficiency

SP E64.2 Sequelae of vitamin C deficiency

SP E64.3 Sequelae of rickets

SP E64.8 Sequelae of other nutritional deficiencies

IQ E64.9 Sequelae of unspecified nutritional deficiency

Overweight, obesity and other hyperalimentation (E65-E68)

SP E65 Localized adiposity
Fat pad

▲ + 4 E66 Overweight and obesity
Code first:
obesity complicating pregnancy, childbirth and the puerperium, if applicable (O99.21-)
Use additional code to identify body mass index (BMI), if known (Z68.-)
EXCLUDES 1 adiposogenital dystrophy (E23.6)
lipomatosis NOS (E88.2)
lipomatosis dolorosa [Dercum] (E88.2)
Prader-Willi syndrome (Q87.11)

GUIDELINES Section I.B.14
For the Body Mass Index (BMI), depth of non-pressure chronic ulcers, pressure ulcer stage, coma scale, and NIH stroke scale (NIHSS) codes, code assignment may be based on medical record documentation from clinicians who are not the patient's provider (i.e., physician or other qualified healthcare practitioner legally accountable for establishing the patient's diagnosis), since this information is typically documented by other clinicians involved in the care of the patient (e.g., a dietitian often documents the BMI, a nurse often documents the pressure ulcer stages, and an emergency medical technician often documents the coma scale). However, the associated diagnosis (such as overweight, obesity, acute stroke, or pressure ulcer) must be documented by the patient's provider.

CODING TIPS ✓ Adult BMI codes are used for people age 20 and over. There are specific BMI codes for ages 2-19 pediatric populations. Code obesity if the physician documents obesity and it is impacting your plan of care.

CODING TIPS ✓ When assigning a code for any overweight, obesity or morbid obesity, physician documentation indicating obesity as a diagnosis is required. If suspected but not present, the coder may query the provider to obtain confirmation of the condition but may not code obesity without confirmation from the provider. BMI may be calculated based upon nursing documentation (height and weight used to calculate); however, the BMI may only be coded if a physician-provided diagnosis, such as overweight, obesity or underweight, is coded.

+ 5 E66.0 Obesity due to excess calories
DEFINITION Increased body weight with excessive accumulation of fat caused by overeating and/or a sedentary lifestyle.

SP + E66.01 Morbid (severe) obesity due to excess calories

---

4 4th digit required   5 5th digit required   6 6th digit required   7 7th digit required   7 7th digit placeholder   + Additional code   B Laterality

764   *DecisionHealth's* FY 2020 Complete Home Health ICD-10-CM Diagnosis Coding Manual

Chapter 4

E00-E89

EXCLUDES 1 morbid (severe) obesity with alveolar hypoventilation (E66.2)

CODING TIPS ✓ Note that the alphabetical index refers to this code for morbid obesity. This code is used when morbid obesity is documented.

SP + E66.09 **Other obesity due to excess calories**

SP + E66.1 **Drug-induced obesity**
Use additional code for adverse effect, if applicable, to identify drug (T36-T50 with fifth or sixth character 5)

CODING TIPS ✓ This code should only be assigned when documentation clearly indicates a relationship between obesity and a drug or chemical as the underlying cause. Assign a code from T36-T50 following E66.1 to indicate the drug and adverse effect.

SP + E66.2 **Morbid (severe) obesity with alveolar hypoventilation**
Obesity hypoventilation syndrome (OHS)
Pickwickian syndrome

SP + E66.3 **Overweight**

SP + E66.8 **Other obesity**

SP + E66.9 **Obesity, unspecified**
Obesity NOS

4 E67 **Other hyperalimentation**
EXCLUDES 1 hyperalimentation NOS (R63.2)
sequelae of hyperalimentation (E68)

SP E67.0 **Hypervitaminosis A**

SP E67.1 **Hypercarotenemia**
DEFINITION Elevated carotene levels in the blood from excessive ingestion of carotenoids or the inability to convert carotenoids to vitamin A; often presents with yellowing of the skin.

SP E67.2 **Megavitamin-B6 syndrome**

SP E67.3 **Hypervitaminosis D**

SP E67.8 **Other specified hyperalimentation**

SP E68 **Sequelae of hyperalimentation**
Code first:
condition resulting from (sequela) of hyperalimentation

Metabolic disorders (E70-E88)

EXCLUDES 1 androgen insensitivity syndrome (E34.5-)
congenital adrenal hyperplasia (E25.0)
Ehlers-Danlos syndrome (Q79.6-)
hemolytic anemias attributable to enzyme disorders (D55.-)
Marfan's syndrome (Q87.4)
5-alpha-reductase deficiency (E29.1)

4 E70 **Disorders of aromatic amino-acid metabolism**

SP E70.0 **Classical phenylketonuria**

DEFINITION Inherited metabolic disorder caused by an enzyme deficiency resulting in accumulation of phenylalanine and its metabolites in the blood with excess excretion in the urine; causes mental retardation, seizures, eczema, and abnormal body odor.

SP E70.1 **Other hyperphenylalaninemias**

5 E70.2 **Disorders of tyrosine metabolism**
EXCLUDES 1 transitory tyrosinemia of newborn (P74.5)

SP E70.20 **Disorder of tyrosine metabolism, unspecified**

SP E70.21 **Tyrosinemia**
Hypertyrosinemia

SP E70.29 **Other disorders of tyrosine metabolism**
Alkaptonuria
Ochronosis

5 E70.3 **Albinism**

SP E70.30 **Albinism, unspecified**

6 E70.31 **Ocular albinism**

SP E70.310 **X-linked ocular albinism**

SP E70.311 **Autosomal recessive ocular albinism**

SP E70.318 **Other ocular albinism**

SP E70.319 **Ocular albinism, unspecified**

6 E70.32 **Oculocutaneous albinism**
EXCLUDES 1 Chediak-Higashi syndrome (E70.330)
Hermansky-Pudlak syndrome (E70.331)

SP E70.320 **Tyrosinase negative oculocutaneous albinism**
Albinism I
Oculocutaneous albinism ty-neg

SP E70.321 **Tyrosinase positive oculocutaneous albinism**
Albinism II
Oculocutaneous albinism ty-pos

SP E70.328 **Other oculocutaneous albinism**
Cross syndrome

SP E70.329 **Oculocutaneous albinism, unspecified**

6 E70.33 **Albinism with hematologic abnormality**

SP E70.330 **Chediak-Higashi syndrome**

SP E70.331 **Hermansky-Pudlak syndrome**

SP E70.338 **Other albinism with hematologic abnormality**

SP E70.339 **Albinism with hematologic abnormality, unspecified**

SP E70.39 **Other specified albinism**
Piebaldism

5 E70.4 **Disorders of histidine metabolism**

SP E70.40 **Disorders of histidine metabolism, unspecified**

SP E70.41 **Histidinemia**

SP E70.49 **Other disorders of histidine metabolism**

SP E70.5 **Disorders of tryptophan metabolism**

SP E70.8 **Other disorders of aromatic amino-acid metabolism**

Chapter 4

E00-E89

★ New ▲ Revised **Px** Primary **SP** PDGM Px **SL** Low CoM **SH** High CoM **IQ** Quest. Encounter **H** Hospice non-cancer Dx Unspecified **M** *Manifestation*

DecisionHealth's FY 2020 Complete Home Health ICD-10-CM Diagnosis Coding Manual

765

SP E70.9 **Disorder of aromatic amino-acid metabolism, unspecified**

4 E71 **Disorders of branched-chain amino-acid metabolism and fatty-acid metabolism**

SP E71.0 **Maple-syrup-urine disease**

5 E71.1 **Other disorders of branched-chain amino-acid metabolism**

6 E71.11 **Branched-chain organic acidurias**

SP E71.110 **Isovaleric acidemia**

SP E71.111 **3-methylglutaconic aciduria**

SP E71.118 **Other branched-chain organic acidurias**

6 E71.12 **Disorders of propionate metabolism**

SP E71.120 **Methylmalonic acidemia**

SP E71.121 **Propionic acidemia**

SP E71.128 **Other disorders of propionate metabolism**

SP E71.19 **Other disorders of branched-chain amino-acid metabolism**
Hyperleucine-isoleucinemia
Hypervalinemia

SP E71.2 **Disorder of branched-chain amino-acid metabolism, unspecified**

5 E71.3 **Disorders of fatty-acid metabolism**
EXCLUDES 1   peroxisomal disorders (E71.5)
Refsum's disease (G60.1)
Schilder's disease (G37.0)
EXCLUDES 2   carnitine deficiency due to inborn error of metabolism (E71.42)

SP E71.30 **Disorder of fatty-acid metabolism, unspecified**

6 E71.31 **Disorders of fatty-acid oxidation**

SP E71.310 **Long chain/very long chain acyl CoA dehydrogenase deficiency**
LCAD
VLCAD

SP E71.311 **Medium chain acyl CoA dehydrogenase deficiency**
MCAD

SP E71.312 **Short chain acyl CoA dehydrogenase deficiency**
SCAD

SP E71.313 **Glutaric aciduria type II**
Glutaric aciduria type II A
Glutaric aciduria type II B
Glutaric aciduria type II C
EXCLUDES 1   glutaric aciduria (type 1) NOS (E72.3)

SP E71.314 **Muscle carnitine palmitoyltransferase deficiency**

SP E71.318 **Other disorders of fatty-acid oxidation**

SP E71.32 **Disorders of ketone metabolism**

SP E71.39 **Other disorders of fatty-acid metabolism**

5 E71.4 **Disorders of carnitine metabolism**
EXCLUDES 1   Muscle carnitine palmitoyltransferase deficiency (E71.314)

SP E71.40 **Disorder of carnitine metabolism, unspecified**

SP E71.41 **Primary carnitine deficiency**

SP E71.42 **Carnitine deficiency due to inborn errors of metabolism**
Code also:
associated inborn error or metabolism

SP E71.43 **Iatrogenic carnitine deficiency**
Carnitine deficiency due to hemodialysis
Carnitine deficiency due to Valproic acid therapy

6 E71.44 **Other secondary carnitine deficiency**

SP E71.440 **Ruvalcaba-Myhre-Smith syndrome**

SP E71.448 **Other secondary carnitine deficiency**

5 E71.5 **Peroxisomal disorders**
EXCLUDES 1   Schilder's disease (G37.0)

SP E71.50 **Peroxisomal disorder, unspecified**

6 E71.51 **Disorders of peroxisome biogenesis**
Group 1 peroxisomal disorders
EXCLUDES 1   Refsum's disease (G60.1)

SP E71.510 **Zellweger syndrome**

SP E71.511 **Neonatal adrenoleukodystrophy**
EXCLUDES 1   X-linked adrenoleukodystrophy (E71.42-)

SP E71.518 **Other disorders of peroxisome biogenesis**

6 E71.52 **X-linked adrenoleukodystrophy**

SP E71.520 **Childhood cerebral X-linked adrenoleukodystrophy**

SP E71.521 **Adolescent X-linked adrenoleukodystrophy**

SP E71.522 **Adrenomyeloneuropathy**

SP E71.528 **Other X-linked adrenoleukodystrophy**
Addison only phenotype adrenoleukodystrophy
Addison-Schilder adrenoleukodystrophy

SP E71.529 **X-linked adrenoleukodystrophy, unspecified type**

SP E71.53 **Other group 2 peroxisomal disorders**

6 E71.54 **Other peroxisomal disorders**

SP E71.540 **Rhizomelic chondrodysplasia punctata**
EXCLUDES 1   chondrodysplasia punctata NOS (Q77.3)

SP E71.541 **Zellweger-like syndrome**

SP E71.542 **Other group 3 peroxisomal disorders**

SP E71.548 **Other peroxisomal disorders**

4 E72 **Other disorders of amino-acid metabolism**
EXCLUDES 1   disorders of:
aromatic amino-acid metabolism (E70.-)
branched-chain amino-acid metabolism (E71.0-E71.2)
fatty-acid metabolism (E71.3)
purine and pyrimidine metabolism (E79.-)
gout (M1A.-, M10.-)

5 E72.0 **Disorders of amino-acid transport**

---

4 4th digit required   5 5th digit required   6 6th digit required   7 7th digit required   ☑ 7th digit placeholder   ✚ Additional code   ⊟ Laterality

766   *DecisionHealth's* FY 2020 Complete Home Health ICD-10-CM Diagnosis Coding Manual

Chapter 4

E00-E89

EXCLUDES 1 disorders of tryptophan metabolism (E70.5)

SP E72.00 Disorders of amino-acid transport, unspecified

SP E72.01 Cystinuria

SP E72.02 Hartnup's disease

SP + E72.03 Lowe's syndrome
Use additional code for associated glaucoma (H42)

SP E72.04 Cystinosis
Fanconi (-de Toni) (-Debré) syndrome with cystinosis
EXCLUDES 1 Fanconi (-de Toni) (-Debré) syndrome without cystinosis (E72.09)

SP E72.09 Other disorders of amino-acid transport
Fanconi (-de Toni) (-Debré) syndrome, unspecified

5 E72.1 Disorders of sulfur-bearing amino-acid metabolism
EXCLUDES 1 cystinosis (E72.04)
cystinuria (E72.01)
transcobalamin II deficiency (D51.2)

SP E72.10 Disorders of sulfur-bearing amino-acid metabolism, unspecified

SP E72.11 Homocystinuria
Cystathionine synthase deficiency

SP E72.12 Methylenetetrahydrofolate reductase deficiency

SP E72.19 Other disorders of sulfur-bearing amino-acid metabolism
Cystathioninuria
Methioninemia
Sulfite oxidase deficiency

5 E72.2 Disorders of urea cycle metabolism
EXCLUDES 1 disorders of ornithine metabolism (E72.4)

SP E72.20 Disorder of urea cycle metabolism, unspecified
Hyperammonemia
EXCLUDES 1 hyperammonemia-hyperornithinemia-homocitrullinemia syndrome E72.4
transient hyperammonemia of newborn (P74.6)

SP E72.21 Argininemia

SP E72.22 Arginosuccinic aciduria

SP E72.23 Citrullinemia

SP E72.29 Other disorders of urea cycle metabolism

SP E72.3 Disorders of lysine and hydroxylysine metabolism
Glutaric aciduria NOS
Glutaric aciduria (type I)
Hydroxylysinemia
Hyperlysinemia
EXCLUDES 1 glutaric aciduria type II (E71.313)
Refsum's disease (G60.1)
Zellweger syndrome (E71.510)

SP E72.4 Disorders of ornithine metabolism

Hyperammonemia-Hyperornithinemia-Homocitrullinemia syndrome
Ornithinemia (types I, II)
Ornithine transcarbamylase deficiency
EXCLUDES 1 hereditary choroidal dystrophy (H31.2-)

5 E72.5 Disorders of glycine metabolism

SP E72.50 Disorder of glycine metabolism, unspecified

SP E72.51 Non-ketotic hyperglycinemia

SP E72.52 Trimethylaminuria

SP E72.53 Primary hyperoxaluria
Oxalosis
Oxaluria

SP E72.59 Other disorders of glycine metabolism
D-glycericacidemia
Hyperhydroxyprolinemia
Hyperprolinemia (types I, II)
Sarcosinemia

5 E72.8 Other specified disorders of amino-acid metabolism

SP E72.81 Disorders of gamma aminobutyric acid metabolism
4-hydroxybutyric aciduria
Disorders of GABA metabolism
GABA metabolic defect
GABA transaminase deficiency
GABA-T deficiency
Gamma-hydroxybutyric aciduria
SSADHD
Succinic semialdehyde dehydrogenase deficiency

SP E72.89 Other specified disorders of amino-acid metabolism
Disorders of beta-amino-acid metabolism
Disorders of gamma-glutamyl cycle

IQ E72.9 Disorder of amino-acid metabolism, unspecified

4 E73 Lactose intolerance

SP E73.0 Congenital lactase deficiency

SP E73.1 Secondary lactase deficiency

SP E73.8 Other lactose intolerance

SP E73.9 Lactose intolerance, unspecified

4 E74 Other disorders of carbohydrate metabolism
EXCLUDES 1 diabetes mellitus (E08-E13)
hypoglycemia NOS (E16.2)
increased secretion of glucagon (E16.3)
mucopolysaccharidosis (E76.0-E76.3)

5 E74.0 Glycogen storage disease

SP E74.00 Glycogen storage disease, unspecified

SP E74.01 von Gierke disease
Type I glycogen storage disease

SP E74.02 Pompe disease
Cardiac glycogenosis
Type II glycogen storage disease

★ New ▲ Revised Px Primary SP PDGM Px SL Low CoM SH High CoM IQ Quest. Encounter H Hospice non-cancer Dx | Unspecified | M *Manifestation*

DEFINITION Pompe disease is also called type II glycogen storage disease and is a congenital disease caused by a metabolic error in which the body deposits an abnormally high amount of glycogen in the kidneys and liver. The disease produces symptoms such as hypoglycemia (low blood sugar) and hyperlipemia (an excess of lipid molecules in the blood, which can lead to problems such as clogged arteries and heart attacks).

SP E74.03 Cori disease
Forbes disease
Type III glycogen storage disease

SP E74.04 McArdle disease
Type V glycogen storage disease

SP E74.09 Other glycogen storage disease
Andersen disease
Hers disease
Tauri disease
Glycogen storage disease, types 0, IV, VI-XI
Liver phosphorylase deficiency
Muscle phosphofructokinase deficiency

5 E74.1 Disorders of fructose metabolism
EXCLUDES 1 muscle phosphofructokinase deficiency (E74.09)

SP E74.10 Disorder of fructose metabolism, unspecified

SP E74.11 Essential fructosuria
Fructokinase deficiency

SP E74.12 Hereditary fructose intolerance
Fructosemia

SP E74.19 Other disorders of fructose metabolism
Fructose-1, 6-diphosphatase deficiency

5 E74.2 Disorders of galactose metabolism

SP E74.20 Disorders of galactose metabolism, unspecified

SP E74.21 Galactosemia

SP E74.29 Other disorders of galactose metabolism
Galactokinase deficiency

5 E74.3 Other disorders of intestinal carbohydrate absorption
EXCLUDES 2 lactose intolerance (E73.-)

SP E74.31 Sucrase-isomaltase deficiency

SP E74.39 Other disorders of intestinal carbohydrate absorption
Disorder of intestinal carbohydrate absorption NOS
Glucose-galactose malabsorption
Sucrase deficiency

SP E74.4 Disorders of pyruvate metabolism and gluconeogenesis
Deficiency of phosphoenolpyruvate carboxykinase
Deficiency of pyruvate carboxylase
Deficiency of pyruvate dehydrogenase
EXCLUDES 1 disorders of pyruvate metabolism and gluconeogenesis with anemia (D55.-)
Leigh's syndrome (G31.82)

SP E74.8 Other specified disorders of carbohydrate metabolism
Essential pentosuria
Renal glycosuria
DEFINITION Excess glucose in the urine with normal levels in the blood, due to renal tubules' inability to reabsorb glucose completely.

!Q E74.9 Disorder of carbohydrate metabolism, unspecified

4 E75 Disorders of sphingolipid metabolism and other lipid storage disorders
EXCLUDES 1 mucolipidosis, types I-III (E77.0-E77.1)
Refsum's disease (G60.1)

5 E75.0 GM2 gangliosidosis

SP E75.00 GM2 gangliosidosis, unspecified

SP E75.01 Sandhoff disease

SP E75.02 Tay-Sachs disease

SP E75.09 Other GM2 gangliosidosis
Adult GM2 gangliosidosis
Juvenile GM2 gangliosidosis

5 E75.1 Other and unspecified gangliosidosis

SP E75.10 Unspecified gangliosidosis
Gangliosidosis NOS

SP E75.11 Mucolipidosis IV

SP E75.19 Other gangliosidosis
GM1 gangliosidosis
GM3 gangliosidosis

5 E75.2 Other sphingolipidosis
EXCLUDES 1 adrenoleukodystrophy [Addison-Schilder] (E71.528)

SP E75.21 Fabry (-Anderson) disease

SP E75.22 Gaucher disease

SP E75.23 Krabbe disease

6 E75.24 Niemann-Pick disease

SP E75.240 Niemann-Pick disease type A

SP E75.241 Niemann-Pick disease type B

SP E75.242 Niemann-Pick disease type C

SP E75.243 Niemann-Pick disease type D

SP E75.248 Other Niemann-Pick disease

SP E75.249 Niemann-Pick disease, unspecified

SP E75.25 Metachromatic leukodystrophy

SP E75.26 Sulfatase deficiency
Multiple sulfatase deficiency (MSD)

SP E75.29 Other sphingolipidosis
Farber's syndrome
Sulfatide lipidosis

SP E75.3 Sphingolipidosis, unspecified

SP E75.4 Neuronal ceroid lipofuscinosis
Batten disease
Bielschowsky-Jansky disease
Kufs disease
Spielmeyer-Vogt disease

SP E75.5 Other lipid storage disorders
Cerebrotendinous cholesterosis [van Bogaert-Scherer-Epstein]
Wolman's disease

SP E75.6 Lipid storage disorder, unspecified

4 E76 Disorders of glycosaminoglycan metabolism

4 4th digit required   **5** 5th digit required   **6** 6th digit required   **7** 7th digit required   **7** 7th digit placeholder   **+** Additional code   **⊟** Laterality

768   *DecisionHealth's* FY 2020 Complete Home Health ICD-10-CM Diagnosis Coding Manual

Chapter 4

E00-E89

⑤ **E76.0 Mucopolysaccharidosis, type I**

SP **E76.01 Hurler's syndrome**

SP **E76.02 Hurler-Scheie syndrome**

SP **E76.03 Scheie's syndrome**

SP **E76.1 Mucopolysaccharidosis, type II**
Hunter's syndrome

⑤ **E76.2 Other mucopolysaccharidoses**

⑥ **E76.21 Morquio mucopolysaccharidoses**

SP **E76.210 Morquio A mucopolysaccharidoses**
Classic Morquio syndrome
Morquio syndrome A
Mucopolysaccharidosis, type IVA

SP **E76.211 Morquio B mucopolysaccharidoses**
Morquio-like mucopolysaccharidoses
Morquio-like syndrome
Morquio syndrome B
Mucopolysaccharidosis, type IVB

SP **E76.219 Morquio mucopolysaccharidoses, unspecified**

Morquio syndrome
Mucopolysaccharidosis, type IV

SP **E76.22 Sanfilippo mucopolysaccharidoses**
Mucopolysaccharidosis, type III (A) (B) (C) (D)
Sanfilippo A syndrome
Sanfilippo B syndrome
Sanfilippo C syndrome
Sanfilippo D syndrome

SP **E76.29 Other mucopolysaccharidoses**
beta-Glucuronidase deficiency
Maroteaux-Lamy (mild) (severe) syndrome
Mucopolysaccharidosis, types VI, VII

SP **E76.3 Mucopolysaccharidosis, unspecified**

SP **E76.8 Other disorders of glucosaminoglycan metabolism**

SP **E76.9 Glucosaminoglycan metabolism disorder, unspecified**

④ **E77 Disorders of glycoprotein metabolism**

SP **E77.0 Defects in post-translational modification of lysosomal enzymes**
Mucolipidosis II [I-cell disease]
Mucolipidosis III [pseudo-Hurler polydystrophy]

SP **E77.1 Defects in glycoprotein degradation**
Aspartylglucosaminuria
Fucosidosis
Mannosidosis
Sialidosis [mucolipidosis I]

SP **E77.8 Other disorders of glycoprotein metabolism**

SP **E77.9 Disorder of glycoprotein metabolism, unspecified**

④ **E78 Disorders of lipoprotein metabolism and other lipidemias**
EXCLUDES 1 sphingolipidosis (E75.0-E75.3)

⑤ **E78.0 Pure hypercholesterolemia**

SP **E78.00 Pure hypercholesterolemia, unspecified**

Fredrickson's hyperlipoproteinemia, type IIa
Hyperbetalipoproteinemia

Low-density-lipoprotein-type [LDL] hyperlipoproteinemia
(Pure) hypercholesterolemia NOS

SP **E78.01 Familial hypercholesterolemia**

SP **E78.1 Pure hyperglyceridemia**
Elevated fasting triglycerides
Endogenous hyperglyceridemia
Fredrickson's hyperlipoproteinemia, type IV
Hyperlipidemia, group B
Hyperprebetalipoproteinemia
Very-low-density-lipoprotein-type [VLDL] hyperlipoproteinemia

SP **E78.2 Mixed hyperlipidemia**
Broad- or floating-betalipoproteinemia
Combined hyperlipidemia NOS
Elevated cholesterol with elevated triglycerides NEC
Fredrickson's hyperlipoproteinemia, type IIb or III
Hyperbetalipoproteinemia with prebetalipoproteinemia
Hypercholesteremia with endogenous hyperglyceridemia
Hyperlipidemia, group C
Tubo-eruptive xanthoma
Xanthoma tuberosum
EXCLUDES 1 cerebrotendinous cholesterosis [van Bogaert-Scherer- Epstein] (E75.5)
familial combined hyperlipidemia (E78.49)

SP **E78.3 Hyperchylomicronemia**
Chylomicron retention disease
Fredrickson's hyperlipoproteinemia, type I or V
Hyperlipidemia, group D
Mixed hyperglyceridemia

⑤ **E78.4 Other hyperlipidemia**

SP **E78.41 Elevated Lipoprotein(a)**
Elevated Lp(a)

SP **E78.49 Other hyperlipidemia**
Familial combined hyperlipidemia

SP **E78.5 Hyperlipidemia, unspecified**

DEFINITION An excess of lipids or fats in the blood.

SP **E78.6 Lipoprotein deficiency**
Abetalipoproteinemia
Depressed HDL cholesterol
High-density lipoprotein deficiency
Hypoalphalipoproteinemia
Hypobetalipoproteinemia (familial)
Lecithin cholesterol acyltransferase deficiency
Tangier disease

⑤ **E78.7 Disorders of bile acid and cholesterol metabolism**
EXCLUDES 1 Niemann-Pick disease type C (E75.242)

SP **E78.70 Disorder of bile acid and cholesterol metabolism, unspecified**

SP **E78.71 Barth syndrome**

SP **E78.72 Smith-Lemli-Opitz syndrome**

SP **E78.79 Other disorders of bile acid and cholesterol metabolism**

⑤ **E78.8 Other disorders of lipoprotein metabolism**

Chapter 4

E00-E89

★ New ▲ Revised Px Primary SP PDGM Px SL Low CoM SH High CoM IQ Quest. Encounter H Hospice non-cancer Dx Unspecified M Manifestation

DecisionHealth's FY 2020 Complete Home Health ICD-10-CM Diagnosis Coding Manual

769

SP E78.81 **Lipoid dermatoarthritis**

SP E78.89 **Other lipoprotein metabolism disorders**

IQ E78.9 **Disorder of lipoprotein metabolism, unspecified**

▲ **4** E79 **Disorders of purine and pyrimidine metabolism**

  EXCLUDES 1 Ataxia-telangiectasia (Q87.19)
  Bloom's syndrome (Q82.8)
  Cockayne's syndrome (Q87.19)
  calculus of kidney (N20.0)
  combined immunodeficiency disorders (D81.-)
  Fanconi's anemia (D61.09)
  gout (M1A.-, M10.-)
  orotaciduric anemia (D53.0)
  progeria (E34.8)
  Werner's syndrome (E34.8)
  xeroderma pigmentosum (Q82.1)

SP E79.0 **Hyperuricemia without signs of inflammatory arthritis and tophaceous disease**
  Asymptomatic hyperuricemia

SP E79.1 **Lesch-Nyhan syndrome**
  HGPRT deficiency

SP E79.2 **Myoadenylate deaminase deficiency**

IQ E79.8 **Other disorders of purine and pyrimidine metabolism**
  Hereditary xanthinuria

SP E79.9 **Disorder of purine and pyrimidine metabolism, unspecified**

4 E80 **Disorders of porphyrin and bilirubin metabolism**
  INCLUDES defects of catalase and peroxidase

SP E80.0 **Hereditary erythropoietic porphyria**
  Congenital erythropoietic porphyria
  Erythropoietic protoporphyria

SP E80.1 **Porphyria cutanea tarda**

5 E80.2 **Other and unspecified porphyria**

SP E80.20 **Unspecified porphyria**
  Porphyria NOS

SP E80.21 **Acute intermittent (hepatic) porphyria**

SP E80.29 **Other porphyria**
  Hereditary coproporphyria

SP E80.3 **Defects of catalase and peroxidase**
  Acatalasia [Takahara]

SP E80.4 **Gilbert syndrome**
  DEFINITION A harmless inborn error of bilirubin metabolism from an abnormal liver enzyme causing a benign elevation of unconjugated bilirubin with no liver damage or hematologic abnormalities.

SP E80.5 **Crigler-Najjar syndrome**

SP E80.6 **Other disorders of bilirubin metabolism**
  Dubin-Johnson syndrome
  Rotor's syndrome

SP E80.7 **Disorder of bilirubin metabolism, unspecified**

4 E83 **Disorders of mineral metabolism**
  EXCLUDES 1 dietary mineral deficiency (E58-E61)
  parathyroid disorders (E20-E21)

vitamin D deficiency (E55.-)

5 E83.0 **Disorders of copper metabolism**

SP E83.00 **Disorder of copper metabolism, unspecified**

SP E83.01 **Wilson's disease**
  Code also:
  associated Kayser Fleischer ring (H18.04-)

SP E83.09 **Other disorders of copper metabolism**
  Menkes' (kinky hair) (steely hair) disease

5 E83.1 **Disorders of iron metabolism**
  EXCLUDES 1 iron deficiency anemia (D50.-)
  sideroblastic anemia (D64.0-D64.3)

SP E83.10 **Disorder of iron metabolism, unspecified**

6 E83.11 **Hemochromatosis**
  EXCLUDES 1 GALD (P78.84)
  Gestational alloimmune liver disease (P78.84)
  Neonatal hemochromatosis (P78.84)

SP E83.110 **Hereditary hemochromatosis**
  Bronzed diabetes
  Pigmentary cirrhosis (of liver)
  Primary (hereditary) hemochromatosis
  DEFINITION A genetic problem causing the body to store too much iron, resulting in liver swelling, skin bronzing, and development of diabetes, arthritis, and organ failure.

SP E83.111 **Hemochromatosis due to repeated red blood cell transfusions**
  Iron overload due to repeated red blood cell transfusions
  Transfusion (red blood cell) associated hemochromatosis

SP E83.118 **Other hemochromatosis**

SP E83.119 **Hemochromatosis, unspecified**

SP ✚ E83.19 **Other disorders of iron metabolism**
  Use additional code, if applicable, for idiopathic pulmonary hemosiderosis (J84.03)

SP E83.2 **Disorders of zinc metabolism**
  Acrodermatitis enteropathica

5 E83.3 **Disorders of phosphorus metabolism and phosphatases**
  EXCLUDES 1 adult osteomalacia (M83.-)
  osteoporosis (M80.-)

SP E83.30 **Disorder of phosphorus metabolism, unspecified**

SP E83.31 **Familial hypophosphatemia**
  Vitamin D-resistant osteomalacia
  Vitamin D-resistant rickets
  EXCLUDES 1 vitamin D-deficiency rickets (E55.0)

SP E83.32 **Hereditary vitamin D-dependent rickets (type 1) (type 2)**
  25-hydroxyvitamin D 1-alpha-hydroxylase deficiency
  Pseudovitamin D deficiency
  Vitamin D receptor defect

4 4th digit required   **5** 5th digit required   **6** 6th digit required   **7** 7th digit required   **7** 7th digit placeholder   ✚ Additional code   **⊟** Laterality

770   DecisionHealth's FY 2020 Complete Home Health ICD-10-CM Diagnosis Coding Manual

Chapter 4

E00-E89

SP E83.39 Other disorders of phosphorus metabolism
Acid phosphatase deficiency
Hypophosphatasia

⑤ E83.4 Disorders of magnesium metabolism

SP E83.40 Disorders of magnesium metabolism, unspecified

SP E83.41 Hypermagnesemia

SP E83.42 Hypomagnesemia

SP E83.49 Other disorders of magnesium metabolism

⑤ E83.5 Disorders of calcium metabolism
EXCLUDES 1   chondrocalcinosis (M11.1-M11.2)
hungry bone syndrome (E83.81)
hyperparathyroidism (E21.0-E21.3)

SP E83.50 Unspecified disorder of calcium metabolism

SP E83.51 Hypocalcemia
DEFINITION   Reduced calcium levels in the blood causing hyperactive deep tendon reflexes, Chvostek's sign, muscle and abdominal cramps, and carpopedal spasm.

SP E83.52 Hypercalcemia
Familial hypocalciuric hypercalcemia
DEFINITION   Excess calcium levels in the blood causing fatigue, muscle weakness, depression, anorexia, nausea, and constipation.

SP E83.59 Other disorders of calcium metabolism

⑤ E83.8 Other disorders of mineral metabolism

SP E83.81 Hungry bone syndrome
DEFINITION   Low levels of calcium due to elevated parathyroid hormone levels or thyrotoxicosis that later return to normal or lower levels after treatment, causing bones to hoard calcium, resulting in increased bone density.

SP E83.89 Other disorders of mineral metabolism

IQ E83.9 Disorder of mineral metabolism, unspecified

④ E84 Cystic fibrosis
INCLUDES   mucoviscidosis
Code also:
exocrine pancreatic insufficiency (K86.81)
CODING TIPS ✓   When reporting a E84 code, do not use an additional code for other disease of the lung. Chronic lung disease with bronchiectasis is an integral part of cystic fibrosis and is not reported separately. However, an infection, such as pneumonia, should be coded separately. A patient with both pulmonary manifestations and gastrointestinal manifestations is coded with E84.0 and E84.1. Other manifestations (E84.8) include diabetes (E08) and right ventricular hypertrophy (I51.7).

SP + E84.0 Cystic fibrosis with pulmonary manifestations
Use additional code to identify any infectious organism present, such as:

Pseudomonas (B96.5)

⑤ E84.1 Cystic fibrosis with intestinal manifestations

SP E84.11 Meconium ileus in cystic fibrosis
EXCLUDES 1   meconium ileus not due to cystic fibrosis (P76.0)

SP E84.19 Cystic fibrosis with other intestinal manifestations
Distal intestinal obstruction syndrome

SP E84.8 Cystic fibrosis with other manifestations

SP E84.9 Cystic fibrosis, unspecified
DEFINITION   Defective gene causing overproduction of mucous that builds up in lung passages, resulting in life-threatening respiratory problems.

④ E85 Amyloidosis
EXCLUDES 2   Alzheimer's disease (G30.0-)

SP E85.0 Non-neuropathic heredofamilial amyloidosis
Hereditary amyloid nephropathy
Code also associated disorders, such as:
autoinflammatory syndromes (M04.-)
EXCLUDES 2   Transthyretin-related (ATTR) familial amyloid cardiomyopathy (E85.4)

SP E85.1 Neuropathic heredofamilial amyloidosis
Amyloid polyneuropathy (Portuguese)
Transthyretin-related (ATTR) familial amyloid polyneuropathy

SP E85.2 Heredofamilial amyloidosis, unspecified

SP E85.3 Secondary systemic amyloidosis
Hemodialysis-associated amyloidosis
DEFINITION   Secondary amyloidosis is also known as reactive systemic amyloidosis, in which the deposited protein fibrils are of the AA type caused by a reaction to a chronic infection or other condition, such as osteomyelitis, rheumatoid arthritis, or a noninfectious disease process such as kidney failure with long term hemodialysis.

SP E85.4 Organ-limited amyloidosis
Localized amyloidosis
Transthyretin-related (ATTR) familial amyloid cardiomyopathy

⑤ E85.8 Other amyloidosis

SP E85.81 Light chain (AL) amyloidosis

SP E85.82 Wild-type transthyretin-related (ATTR) amyloidosis
Senile systemic amyloidosis (SSA)

SP E85.89 Other amyloidosis

SP E85.9 Amyloidosis, unspecified
DEFINITION   Abnormal accumulation of amyloid-like proteins in tissues.

+ ④ E86 Volume depletion
Use additional code(s) for any associated disorders of electrolyte and acid-base balance (E87.-)
EXCLUDES 1   dehydration of newborn (P74.1)
hypovolemic shock NOS (R57.1)
postprocedural hypovolemic shock (T81.19)

Chapter 4

E00-E89

★ New ▲ Revised Px Primary SP PDGM Px SL Low CoM SH High CoM IQ Quest. Encounter H Hospice non-cancer Dx Unspecified M *Manifestation*

DecisionHealth's FY 2020 Complete Home Health ICD-10-CM Diagnosis Coding Manual

771

traumatic hypovolemic shock
(T79.4)

SP ✚ E86.0 Dehydration
> **GUIDELINES** Section I.C.2.c.3)
> When the admission/encounter is for management of dehydration due to the malignancy and only the dehydration is being treated (intravenous rehydration), the dehydration is sequenced first, followed by the code(s) for the malignancy.

SP ✚ E86.1 Hypovolemia
Depletion of volume of plasma
> **DEFINITION** Abnormal decrease in the total volume of circulating blood with a corresponding loss of sodium electrolytes.

SP ✚ E86.9 Volume depletion, unspecified

4️⃣ E87 Other disorders of fluid, electrolyte and acid-base balance
> **EXCLUDES 1** diabetes insipidus (E23.2)
> electrolyte imbalance associated with hyperemesis gravidarum (O21.1)
> electrolyte imbalance following ectopic or molar pregnancy (O08.5)
> familial periodic paralysis (G72.3)

SP E87.0 Hyperosmolality and hypernatremia
Sodium [Na] excess
Sodium [Na] overload

SP E87.1 Hypo-osmolality and hyponatremia
Sodium [Na] deficiency
> **EXCLUDES 1** syndrome of inappropriate secretion of antidiuretic hormone (E22.2)

SP E87.2 Acidosis
Acidosis NOS
Lactic acidosis
Metabolic acidosis
Respiratory acidosis
> **EXCLUDES 1** diabetic acidosis - see categories E08-E10, E13 with ketoacidosis
> **DEFINITION** An abnormal increase in the acidity of body fluids, caused either by accumulation of acids or by depletion of bicarbonates.

SP E87.3 Alkalosis
Alkalosis NOS
Metabolic alkalosis
Respiratory alkalosis

SP E87.4 Mixed disorder of acid-base balance

SP E87.5 Hyperkalemia
Potassium [K] excess
Potassium [K] overload
> **DEFINITION** An abnormally high concentration of potassium ions in the blood.

SP E87.6 Hypokalemia
Potassium [K] deficiency
> **DEFINITION** Low potassium level in the blood causing neuromuscular disorders ranging from weakness to paralysis, electrocardiographic abnormalities, renal disease, and gastrointestinal disorders.

5️⃣ E87.7 Fluid overload

> **EXCLUDES 1** edema NOS (R60.9)
> fluid retention (R60.9)
> **DEFINITION** High infusion rates or transfusion volumes not processed effectively by the recipient, causing circulatory system overload marked by acute respiratory distress.

SP E87.70 Fluid overload, unspecified

SP E87.71 Transfusion associated circulatory overload
Fluid overload due to transfusion (blood) (blood components)
TACO

SP E87.79 Other fluid overload

SP E87.8 Other disorders of electrolyte and fluid balance, not elsewhere classified
Electrolyte imbalance NOS
Hyperchloremia
Hypochloremia

✚ 4️⃣ E88 Other and unspecified metabolic disorders
Use additional codes for associated conditions
> **EXCLUDES 1** histiocytosis X (chronic) (C96.6)

✚ 5️⃣ E88.0 Disorders of plasma-protein metabolism, not elsewhere classified
> **EXCLUDES 1** disorder of lipoprotein metabolism (E78.-)
> monoclonal gammopathy (of undetermined significance) (D47.2)
> polyclonal hypergammaglobulinemia (D89.0)
> Waldenström macroglobulinemia (C88.0)

SP ✚ E88.01 Alpha-1-antitrypsin deficiency
AAT deficiency

▲ SP ✚ E88.02 Plasminogen deficiency
Dysplasminogenemia
Hypoplasminogenemia
Type 1 plasminogen deficiency
Type 2 plasminogen deficiency
Code also:
, if applicable, ligneous conjunctivitis (H10.51)
Use additional code for associated findings, such as:
hydrocephalus (G91.4)
otitis media (H67.-)
respiratory disorder related to plasminogen deficiency (J99)

SP ✚ E88.09 Other disorders of plasma-protein metabolism, not elsewhere classified
Bisalbuminemia

SP ✚ E88.1 Lipodystrophy, not elsewhere classified
Lipodystrophy NOS
> **EXCLUDES 1** Whipple's disease (K90.81)
> **DEFINITION** Defective fat metabolism resulting in abnormal or degenerative subcutaneous fat deposits that appear as lumps or dents under the skin.

SP ✚ E88.2 Lipomatosis, not elsewhere classified
Lipomatosis NOS
Lipomatosis (Check) dolorosa [Dercum]

SP ✚ E88.3 Tumor lysis syndrome
Tumor lysis syndrome (spontaneous)

4️⃣4th digit required   5️⃣5th digit required   6️⃣6th digit required   7️⃣7th digit required   🔽7th digit placeholder   ✚Additional code   ▤Laterality

Tumor lysis syndrome following antineoplastic drug chemotherapy
Use additional code for adverse effect, if applicable, to identify drug (T45.1X5)

+ ⑤ E88.4 Mitochondrial metabolism disorders
> **EXCLUDES 1**   disorders of pyruvate metabolism (E74.4)
> Kearns-Sayre syndrome (H49.81)
> Leber's disease (H47.22)
> Leigh's encephalopathy (G31.82)
> Mitochondrial myopathy, NEC (G71.3)
> Reye's syndrome (G93.7)

SP + E88.40   Mitochondrial metabolism disorder, unspecified

SP + E88.41   MELAS syndrome
Mitochondrial myopathy, encephalopathy, lactic acidosis and stroke-like episodes

SP + E88.42   MERRF syndrome
Myoclonic epilepsy associated with ragged-red fibers
Code also:
> progressive myoclonic epilepsy (G40.3-)

SP + E88.49   Other mitochondrial metabolism disorders

+ ⑤ E88.8   Other specified metabolic disorders

SP + E88.81   Metabolic syndrome
Dysmetabolic syndrome X
Use additional codes for associated manifestations, such as:
> obesity (E66.-)

> **CODING TIPS ✓**   Metabolic syndrome (also called dysmetabolic syndrome X) involves a cluster of symptoms placing individuals at risk for development of a number of disease processes. Manifestations of metabolic syndrome confirmed by the physician, such as obesity (and BMI as calculated by the clinical record documentation), should additionally be coded following E88.81.

SP + E88.89   Other specified metabolic disorders
Launois-Bensaude adenolipomatosis
> **EXCLUDES 1**   adult pulmonary Langerhans cell histiocytosis (J84.82)

IQ + E88.9   Metabolic disorder, unspecified

Postprocedural endocrine and metabolic complications and disorders, not elsewhere classified (E89)

CODING TIPS ✓   Conditions classifiable to E89 are classifiable as postprocedural complications. These conditions should only be assigned when diagnostic statements clearly indicate that the condition is a complication of a procedure.

④ E89   Postprocedural endocrine and metabolic complications and disorders, not elsewhere classified
> **EXCLUDES 2**   intraoperative complications of endocrine system organ or structure (E36.0-, E36.1-, E36.8)

SP E89.0   Postprocedural hypothyroidism
Postirradiation hypothyroidism
Postsurgical hypothyroidism
> **CODING TIPS ✓**   Report E89.0 for patients with hypothyroidism following a thyroidectomy.

> **DEFINITION**   Underactive thyroid gland due to surgery or radiation, causing an inadequate production of thyroid hormone and a slowing of metabolic processes.

SP + E89.1   Postprocedural hypoinsulinemia
Postpancreatectomy hyperglycemia
Postsurgical hypoinsulinemia
Use additional code, if applicable, to identify:
> acquired absence of pancreas (Z90.41-)
> diabetes mellitus (postpancreatectomy) (postprocedural) (E13.-)
> insulin use (Z79.4)
> **EXCLUDES 1**   transient postprocedural hyperglycemia (R73.9)
> transient postprocedural hypoglycemia (E16.2)

> **GUIDELINES**   Section I.C.4.a.6)(b)(i)
> For postpancreatectomy diabetes mellitus (lack of insulin due to the surgical removal of all or part of the pancreas), assign code E89.1, Postprocedural hypoinsulinemia. Assign a code from category E13 and a code from subcategory Z90.41-, Acquired absence of pancreas, as additional codes.

> **CODING TIPS ✓**   Because the pancreas produces insulin, the removal of even a portion of the pancreas can produce diabetic-like symptoms. If manifestations are produced because of the hyperglycemia and lack of insulin, add the codes for manifestations after E89.1 with the appropriate E13 code(s). Also add the acquired absence of pancreas (Z90.41-) and use of insulin (Z79.4).

SP E89.2   Postprocedural hypoparathyroidism
Parathyroprival tetany

SP E89.3   Postprocedural hypopituitarism
Postirradiation hypopituitarism

⑤ E89.4   Postprocedural ovarian failure

SP E89.40   Asymptomatic postprocedural ovarian failure
Postprocedural ovarian failure NOS

SP E89.41   Symptomatic postprocedural ovarian failure
Symptoms such as flushing, sleeplessness, headache, lack of concentration, associated with postprocedural menopause

SP E89.5   Postprocedural testicular hypofunction

SP E89.6   Postprocedural adrenocortical (-medullary) hypofunction

⑤ E89.8   Other postprocedural endocrine and metabolic complications and disorders

⑥ E89.81   Postprocedural hemorrhage of an endocrine system organ or structure following a procedure

SP E89.810   Postprocedural hemorrhage of an endocrine system organ or structure following an endocrine system procedure

---

★ New ▲ Revised **Px** Primary **SP** PDGM Px **SL** Low CoM **SH** High CoM **IQ** Quest. Encounter **H** Hospice non-cancer Dx **Unspecified** **M** *Manifestation*

SP **E89.811** Postprocedural hemorrhage of an
endocrine system organ or
structure following other
procedure

6 **E89.82** Postprocedural hematoma and
seroma of an endocrine system organ
or structure

SP **E89.820** Postprocedural hematoma of an
endocrine system organ or
structure following an endocrine
system procedure

SP **E89.821** Postprocedural hematoma of an
endocrine system organ or
structure following other
procedure

SP **E89.822** Postprocedural seroma of an
endocrine system organ or
structure following an endocrine
system procedure

SP **E89.823** Postprocedural seroma of an
endocrine system organ or
structure following other
procedure

SP **+** **E89.89** Other postprocedural endocrine and
metabolic complications and
disorders
Use additional code, if applicable, to
further specify disorder

4 4th digit required   **5** 5th digit required   **6** 6th digit required   **7** 7th digit required   **7** 7th digit placeholder   **+** Additional code   **⊟** Laterality

774   *DecisionHealth's* FY 2020 Complete Home Health ICD-10-CM Diagnosis Coding Manual

Chapter 4 Scenarios: Endocrine, nutritional and metabolic diseases (E00-E89)

Diabetic macular edema

A 73-year-old man admitted to home care has just been prescribed insulin for his type 2 diabetes. However, the retinopathy and macular edema from his diabetes is severe enough that it has caused legal blindness. Skilled nursing is ordered for teaching and training regarding insulin and use of insulin syringes with magnifiers.

Description	Code
Primary: Type 2 diabetes with unspecified diabetic retinopathy with macular edema	E11.311
Secondary: Legal blindness	H54.8
Secondary: Long-term (current) use of insulin	Z79.4

There's a "code first" note at H54.8 instructing to assign first the reason for the legal blindness - in this case, that would be the one all-inclusive code for diabetic macular edema, E11.311. The long-term (current) use of insulin should be coded, if it is anticipated that the need for insulin will be ongoing. It should not be used for short-term insulin use.

Diabetes with renal manifestation

A patient is admitted to home health for teaching and training about his diabetes with stage 2 chronic kidney disease. He is not currently taking insulin.

Description	Code
Primary: Type 2 diabetes mellitus with diabetic chronic kidney disease	E11.22
Secondary: Chronic kidney disease, stage 2	N18.2

When the type of diabetes is not stated, the default is type 2. There is an assumed relationship in the ICD-10 classification between diabetes and any specific condition listed under "with" in the alphabetic index, and a combination code describes these two conditions: E11.22. Note that E11.22 instructs the coder to use an additional code to identify the stage of chronic kidney disease. Therefore, N18.2 is additionally assigned.

Amyloidosis with arthropathy

Physical therapy is ordered for a patient who has right shoulder arthropathy due to amyloidosis.

Description	Code
Primary: Organ limited amyloidosis (localized)	E85.4
Secondary: Arthropathy in other specified diseases elsewhere, right shoulder	M14.811

Amyloidosis can be limited to one organ; e.g., the musculoskeletal system, the heart or the brain. This is an etiology (amyloidosis) and manifestation (arthropathy) pairing. It is evident when searching the alphabetic index for "arthropathy in (due to) "amyloidosis" and you find "E85.4 *[M14.8-]*." Therefore, the etiology (the amyloidosis) must be immediately followed by the manifestation (the arthropathy).

Type 1 diabetes with neuropathy

A patient is admitted to home care for type 1 diabetes mellitus with neuropathy and with hyperglycemia. She was started on a sliding scale, in addition to her daily insulin, which she is able to administer independently. She also has hypertension, depression and a pressure ulcer/injury of the right buttock (stage 3) that is improving with treatment but still requires dressing changes, which the nurse will be doing twice a week. She also just started taking iron for her anemia. The main reason for admission is diabetic management.

Description	Code
Primary: Type 1 diabetes mellitus with diabetic neuropathy, unspecified	E10.40
Secondary: Type 1 diabetes mellitus with hyperglycemia	E10.65
Secondary: Pressure ulcer of right buttock, stage 3	L89.313
Secondary: Anemia, unspecified	D64.9
Secondary: Essential primary hypertension	I10
Secondary: Depression NOS	F32.9

The patient's diabetes is captured with two separate combination codes, one for the diabetic neuropathy, which is not further specified, and one for diabetes with hyperglycemia. The pressure ulcer/injury code is a combination code, which includes the site, stage and laterality. The other relevant co-morbidities, anemia, hypertension and depression, are additionally coded as they have the potential to impact the patient's plan of care. Though she is taking iron for her anemia, it's not specified as iron deficiency anemia and is thus coded as unspecified.

Secondary diabetes with PVD

Your patient has diabetic peripheral vascular disease (PVD), as a result of prolonged use of prednisone for his asthma. The focus of care is his diabetes. He continues to take prednisone.

Description	Code
Primary: Drug or chemical induced diabetes mellitus with diabetic peripheral angiopathy without gangrene	E09.51
Secondary: Adverse effect of steroids, subsequent encounter	T38.0X5D
Secondary: Asthma NOS	J45.909
Secondary: Long-term (current) use of systemic steroids	Z79.52

Since the patient took the prednisone, as prescribed, and then developed diabetes (which is considered secondary diabetes), this is coded as an adverse effect. Tabular instruction at category E09.- tells you to use an additional code to identify the drug causing the adverse effect, which is found in the Table of Drugs and Chemicals. The reason the drug was taken in the first place, asthma in this case, should be sequenced next. Note, if an existing diagnosis of diabetes worsens due to steroid use, it is not steroid-induced diabetes. Diabetic PVD should be coded as diabetic peripheral angiopathy, according to Q2 2018 Coding Clinic guidance. The patient's continued use of prednisone is captured with Z79.52.

Diabetes, contracture

A patient is referred for home care with worsening type 2 diabetes, now requiring insulin. She has right hand joint contractures after suffering third-degree burns from contact with boiling water three years ago. Orders include nursing for insulin teaching and administration, and occupational therapy to assist with insulin administration strategies.

Description	Code
Primary: Type 2 diabetes without complications	E11.9
Secondary: Contracture, right hand	M24.541
Secondary: Burn of third degree of right hand, unspecified site, sequela	T23.301S
Secondary: Contact with other hot fluids, sequela	X12.XXXS
Secondary: Long term (current) use of insulin	Z79.4

The code for the sequela condition, the contracture, is sequenced immediately before the sequela form of the etiology injury code, the burn, per coding guidelines. When searching the index for sequelae, burn and corrosion, the code provided is for the sequela condition only, indicating this is not a combination code. The code for the sequela condition or residual (the hand contracture) is found by searching the index at contraction, joint, hand joint, and is then sequenced preceding the sequela form of the etiology injury code to fully capture the fact that the now-healed burn left behind the contracture. In the index at sequelae, burn and corrosion, the direction is to code to injury with the seventh character "S." The letter "S" is added to the sequela code to indicate that the code represents a sequela and not an acute burn. An external cause code is assigned to illustrate how the patient sustained the burn that caused the current contracture (contact with boiling water), which is found by searching the Index to External Cause of Injuries. Notice how the external cause code is only three characters long (X12.-) but requires a 7th character, necessitating the use of placeholder "x" for the fourth, fifth and sixth character positions. The external cause code carries the same seventh character as the injury it's describing, in accordance with coding guidelines. Long-term (current) use of insulin, Z79.4, will be coded because the patient uses insulin and is not a type 1 diabetic.

Cystic fibrosis with pseudomonas pneumonia

A 42-year-old man is admitted to home health following a hospitalization where he was treated with IV antibiotics for a pulmonary exacerbation of his cystic fibrosis with pseudomonas pneumonia. The infection is still resolving and he will continue on oral antibiotics for the next six weeks.

Description	Code
Primary: Cystic fibrosis with pulmonary manifestations	E84.0
Secondary: Pneumonia due to Pseudomonas	J15.1
Secondary: Long term (current) use of antibiotics	Z79.2

The pseudomonas pneumonia is coded after the cystic fibrosis in accordance with tabular instructions. The code for antibiotic use is assigned as the patient will continue taking antibiotics for several more weeks.

Diabetic retinopathy secondary to hereditary hemochromatosis

A 68-year-old man comes to home health with a primary diagnosis of diabetic retinopathy in both eyes. He was diagnosed with hereditary hemochromatosis five years ago and developed diabetes two years later as a result. He is insulin-dependent and also has hypertension and will receive skilled nursing visits for teaching on the disease process.

Description	Code
Primary: Hereditary hemochromatosis	E83.110
Secondary: Diabetes mellitus due to underlying condition with unspecified diabetic retinopathy without macular edema	E08.319
Secondary: Essential (primary) hypertension	I10
Secondary: Long term (current) use of insulin	Z79.4

The patient's diabetic retinopathy resulted from hereditary hemochromatosis and is therefore appropriately coded as a manifestation of diabetes due to any underlying condition, with E08.319. Even though the diabetic retinopathy is the focus of care, because it was caused by hemochromatosis, the underlying condition is coded first, according to tabular instruction. Hypertension is an important comorbidity that should be coded whenever it is present. The patient is insulin dependent but not a type 1 diabetic; therefore, the code for insulin use is required.

Diabetes, obesity

A newly diagnosed diabetic on an oral antidiabetic agent is admitted to home health for observation, assessment and teaching on diabetes. The history and physical notes that she is morbidly obese. Her BMI is documented as 56.

Description	Code
Primary: Type 2 diabetes mellitus without complications	E11.9
Secondary: Morbid (severe) obesity due to excess calories	E66.01
Secondary: Body mass index (BMI) 50.0-59.9, adult	z68.43
Secondary: Long term (current) use of oral hypoglycemic drugs	Z79.84

Since the type of diabetes is not stated, the default is type 2. Morbid obesity should always be coded when it's been documented by the physician, according to Q4 2018 Coding Clinic guidance. If not documented or confirmed, the BMI may be calculated, based on the patient's height and weight, by a non-provider, such as a dietitian or nurse, and may be coded without physician verification. Remember to add the code for use of oral hypoglycemic drugs (Z79.84) per the use additional code note at E11.-.

Diabetic osteomyelitis, MRSA

A 69-year-old man with diabetes comes to home health with a primary diagnosis of acute osteomyelitis in the bones of his left big toe. The infecting organism is MRSA. He will receive IV antibiotics for several weeks and is dependent on insulin.

Description	Code
Primary: Type 2 diabetes mellitus with other specified complication	E11.69
Secondary: Other acute osteomyelitis, left ankle and foot	M86.172
Secondary: Methicillin resistant Staphylococcus aureus infection as the cause of diseases classified elsewhere	B95.62
Secondary: Encounter for adjustment and management of vascular access device	Z45.2
Secondary: Long term (current) use of antibiotics	Z79.2
Secondary: Long term (current) use of insulin	Z79.4

The patient's osteomyelitis infection can be assumed to be connected to his diabetes as no other cause was given, according to its listing under the subterm "with" in the alphabetic index. Thus, it is coded as diabetic osteomyelitis. The diabetes is coded as type 2 as the type is not specified and type 2 is the default, according to coding guidelines. The code for osteomyelitis is assigned underneath the diabetes code, in accordance with the etiology-manifestation convention. The infecting organism was specified as MRSA, necessitating the use of B95.62. The administration of IV antibiotics is captured with Z45.2 and Z79.2. As the patient is not specified to be a type 1 diabetes and is dependent on insulin, code Z79.4 is required to capture this. In PDGM, erroneously assigning the code for unspecified osteomyelitis (M86.9) will result in the claim being sent back to be recoded.

Yeast infection, morbid obesity

A 62-year-old woman who is morbidly obese is admitted to home health for medication monitoring, after recently being started on insulin, and physical therapy for a diagnosis of diabetic polyneuropathy. She also requires treatment of a yeast infection in the skin folds of her abdomen. She suffers from severe chafing and irritation from the skin folds constantly rubbing together, which her physician stated led to the yeast infection. Her height is 60 inches and she weighs 502 lbs, which the assessing clinician calculated to 98.

Description	Code
Primary: Type 2 diabetes mellitus with diabetic polyneuropathy	E11.42
Secondary: Erythema intertrigo	L30.4
Secondary: Candidiasis of skin and nail	B37.2
Secondary: Morbid (severe) obesity due to excess calories	E66.01
Secondary: Body mass index (BMI) 70 or greater, adult	Z68.45
Secondary: Long term (current) use of insulin	Z79.4

Diabetic polyneuropathy is captured with the combination code E11.42. As the focus of care, it is coded in the primary position. Codes L30.4 and B37.2 are assigned to capture the irritation in her skin folds from excessive chafing and the resulting yeast infection. Morbid obesity has been diagnosed and must be coded, as it will impact her care and recovery, and because morbid obesity should be coded whenever it has been documented by the physician, according to Q4 2018 Coding Clinic guidance. Her BMI is calculated by the assessing clinician based on her recorded height and weight and coded in accordance with tabular instruction at E66.01. A BMI code can be assigned on the basis of the clinician's documentation, according to coding guidelines. As a type 2 diabetes who uses insulin, an additional code for insulin use, Z79.4, is required.

Sequelae of rickets

A 70-year-old man is admitted to home health for physical therapy due to cervical scoliosis resulting from childhood rickets. He also has advanced degenerative changes in both of his knees.

Description	Code
Primary: Sequelae of rickets	E64.3
Secondary: Spondylopathy in diseases classified elsewhere, cervical region	M49.82
Secondary: Bilateral primary osteoarthritis of knee	M17.0

In this scenario, the sequelae code must be sequenced ahead of the residual (the scoliosis) because the residual code is a manifestation code and must follow its etiology, according to the etiology-manifestation convention. Advanced degenerative changes in the knee joints is coded as osteoarthritis, according to Q2 2018 Coding Clinic guidance. The osteoarthritis will impact his recovery and thus should also be coded. Also, you can code a patient's osteoarthritis as primary osteoarthritis if the type isn't specified, according to Q4 2016 Coding Clinic guidance.

Diabetic hypertension

A 74-year-old man was recently diagnosed with severe hypertension that his physician documented as due to his type 2 diabetes. He also has stage 2 chronic kidney disease, which is also related to the diabetes. The physician confirmed that his additional diagnosis of right heart failure, which predated his diabetes diagnosis, is unrelated to the hypertension. He takes oral hypoglycemic medication. The hypertension is the focus of care.

Description	Code
Primary: Type 2 diabetes mellitus with other circulatory complications	E11.59
Secondary: Hypertension secondary to endocrine disorders	I15.2
Secondary: Type 2 diabetes mellitus with diabetic chronic kidney disease	E11.22
Secondary: Chronic kidney disease, stage 2 (mild)	N18.2
Secondary: Right heart failure, unspecified	I50.810
Secondary: Long term (current) use of oral hypoglycemic drugs	Z79.84

There is no assumed relationship between hypertension and diabetes. However, in this scenario, the physician specifically connected the diagnoses. Thus, it is captured first with E11.59 followed by I15.2. Stage 2 diabetic chronic kidney disease also requires two codes to fully capture the diagnosis: E11.22 and N18.2. While there is normally an assumed relationship between hypertension and heart failure, the physician confirmed the two are unrelated and are thus coded separately, in accordance with coding guidelines.

Chapter 5: Mental, Behavioral and Neurodevelopmental Disorders (F01-F99)

When assigning a diagnosis from this chapter, pay close attention to consistency with OASIS data items related to cognitive and behavioral functioning. **Do not choose a mental disorder as a diagnosis unless that diagnosis is confirmed with the physician.** You'll also want to consider whether your agency will be providing psychiatric nursing when using a code from this chapter as primary, or whether you will be training a caregiver to care for a patient with such a condition. Mental disorders are comorbidities that will impact the care, so ordinarily will be coded as secondary even if psychiatric nursing will not be provided.

Chapter 5 includes codes for a number of different conditions including:

- Psychoses with organic and nonorganic causes such as dementia and schizophrenia.

- Neurotic disorders such as anxiety disorders and phobic disorders.

- Personality disorders such as paranoia and antisocial personality disorder.

- Abuse of alcohol and drugs. In this category, the patient has intense desire to obtain increasing amounts of alcohol or drugs to the exclusion of all other activities, but is not dependent.

- Dependence on alcohol and drugs where the patient has a physical need for the alcohol or drug (addiction) and suffers withdrawal symptoms if it is not available.

- Intellectual disabilities where the patient has an IQ of 70 or less.

- Special symptoms or syndromes, not elsewhere classified, including stuttering and anorexia nervosa.

Some conditions in this chapter use the same or similar terms. It is important to check with the physician if there is any doubt as to which code is correct. For example, obsessive-compulsive disorder may be reported using the appropriate code from category F42.- (Obsessive-compulsive disorder) or F60.5 (Obsessive-compulsive personality disorder). Since there is an Excludes 2 note at both of these codes, they can be coded together as long as both diagnoses are verified by the physician. Another example is major depression unspecified, which may be reported using F32.9 (single episode) or F33.9 (recurrent episodes), F41.8 (mixed anxiety and depressive disorder) or F43.21 (Adjustment disorder with depressed mood).

This chapter also includes some codes that are phobias and disorders not due to substance or known physiological condition, such as shyness disorder of childhood/adolescence (F40.10), adult onset fluency disorder (F98.5), sleep disorders unspecified (F51.9), bedwetting (F98.0). Other disorders coded in this chapter are autism disorder (F84.0) and attention deficit hyperactivity disorder (F90.-).

A few situations to watch out for:

- If a patient has a **personal or family history** of a condition reported in this chapter, it may be appropriate to select from the Z code section, such as Z86.59 (Personal history of other mental and behavioral disorders) or Z81.8 (Family history of other mental and behavioral disorders). **Reminder:** These are vague codes and would not generally be used in home health or hospice.

- If a condition reported in this chapter is the **result of injury or medical treatment**, a code from Chapter 19 may be reported with a code from this chapter.

- **Symptoms** related to mental disorders are sometimes reported using codes from Chapter 18 such as code R41.81 (Age related cognitive decline or senility NOS) or R54 (Age-related physical debility). Every effort should be made to secure a definitive diagnosis. A symptom code from Chapter 18 may be reported as an additional diagnosis when it describes a significant aspect of the condition but is not an integral part of the condition.

- Although not often recorded in home health, if reporting a **mental disorder in a pregnant patient** when the condition is complicating the pregnancy, report first a code from Chapter 15 category O99.3- (Mental disorders and diseases of the nervous system complicating pregnancy, childbirth and the puerperium) with an additional code from Chapter 5 to describe the mental disease or disorder.

Multiple Coding and Sequencing

Includes and Excludes notes should be followed for codes in this chapter, as well as any other instructions under the code or code category. Some examples of multiple coding and sequencing issues for codes in this chapter include:

Disorders that affect the brain

The majority of codes from categories F01-F09 (Mental disorders due to physiological conditions) are reported **following** a code for the underlying physiological condition. For example, a patient with depressed mood disorder due to cerebrovascular disease would be coded I67.9 (cerebrovascular disease, unspecified) followed by F06.31 (Mood disorder due to known physiological condition with depressive features).

Dementia in Alzheimer's disease

Dementia in Alzheimer's disease is reported with code G30.- (Alzheimer's) as the first diagnosis and F02.80 (Dementia in conditions classified elsewhere without behavioral disturbance) or F02.81 (with behavioral disturbance such as physical or verbal aggression) as the additional diagnosis. When coding F02.81, use Z91.83 (Wandering in diseases classified elsewhere) as an additional diagnosis when appropriate. But remember, wandering can only be coded with the F02.81 to indicate behavior problems even though the patient may not have aggressive, violent or combative behavior. There are many neurological conditions in Chapter 6 that are the underlying etiology for F02.8- so be sure to look at the code first note under F02.

Also, an additional code from F02.8- (Dementia in other diseases classified elsewhere) is required for a patient with Lewy body dementia (G31.83). *Note*, dementia is inherent to a diagnosis of Alzheimer's disease and the physician does not have to list it separately in order for it to be coded, the Coding Clinic confirmed in its Q1 2017 update.

Note: F03.- (Unspecified dementia) covers many codes, such as senile and presenile dementia. Vascular dementia is coded from category F01 with a 5th character required to identify with or without behavioral disturbance.

Pain disorders related to psychological factors

Assign code F45.41 for pain that is exclusively related to psychological disorders. As indicated by the Excludes 1 note under category G89 (Pain, not elsewhere classified), a code from category G89 should *not* be assigned with code F45.41.

Code F45.42 (Pain disorders with related psychological factors) should be used with a code from category G89 (Pain not elsewhere classified) if there is documentation of a psychological component for a patient with acute and chronic pain.

Special Coding Issues

Mental and behavioral disorders due to psychoactive substance use

ICD-10-CM has significantly expanded the coding options related to psychoactive substance use. Codes for psychoactive substance use disorders (codes from subcategories F10.9-, F11.9-, F12.9-, F13.9-, F14.9- and F16.9-) should only be assigned based on provider documentation and when they meet the definition of a reportable diagnosis (see Section III, Reporting Additional Diagnoses). The codes are to be used only when the psychoactive substance use is associated

with a physical, mental or behavioral disorder, and such a relationship is documented by the provider, according to coding guidelines.

Selection of codes to indicate "in remission" in categories F10-F19 utilize FXX.11 to indicate abuse in remission, or FXX.21 to indicate dependence in remission. These codes are *assigned only on the basis of physician documentation that the patient is in remission.*

Take note of the following guidelines when coding these diagnoses:

- Capture mild substance abuse disorder in early or sustained remission as substance abuse in remission. Code moderate or severe substance abuse disorder in early or sustained remission as substance dependence in remission.

- When the physician documentation refers to use, abuse and dependence of the same substance (e.g., alcohol, opioid, cannabis, etc.), only one code should be assigned to identify the pattern of use based on the following hierarchy:

  - If both use and abuse are documented, assign only the code for abuse.

  - If both abuse and dependence are documented, assign only the code for dependence.

  - If use, abuse and dependence are all documented, assign only the code for dependence.

  - If both use and dependence are documented, assign only the code for dependence.

- As with all other diagnoses, the codes for psychoactive substance use should only be assigned *based on the physician's documentation and when they meet the definition of a reportable diagnosis.* The definition of other diagnoses is interpreted as additional conditions that affect patient care in terms of requiring:

  - Clinical evaluation, or

  - Therapeutic treatment, or

  - Diagnostic procedures, or extended length of stay, or

  - Increased nursing care and/or monitoring.

The codes are to be used only when the psychoactive substance use is associated with a mental or behavioral disorder, and such a relationship is documented by the physician.

Chapter 5 includes many combination codes that combine the psychoactive substance use with other symptoms such as F10.97 (Alcohol use, unspecified with alcohol-induced persisting dementia) or F10.250 (Alcohol dependence with alcohol induced psychotic disorder with delusions).

CHAPTER 5: MENTAL, BEHAVIORAL AND NEURODEVELOPMENTAL DISORDERS (F01-F99)

INCLUDES disorders of psychological development

EXCLUDES 2 symptoms, signs and abnormal clinical laboratory findings, not elsewhere classified (R00-R99)

CODING TIPS ✓ It is important not to code a patient with dementia or other psychiatric disorder unless documented by the physician. A primary diagnosis of mental disorder may require a psychiatrically trained nurse to provide services. Some services, such as administration of IM medications for treatment of a psychiatric diagnosis, do not require a psychiatrically trained nurse. A mental disorder always impacts the care and should be added as a comorbidity any time the documentation is present.

This chapter contains the following blocks:

F01-F09	Mental disorders due to known physiological conditions
F10-F19	Mental and behavioral disorders due to psychoactive substance use
F20-F29	Schizophrenia, schizotypal, delusional, and other non-mood psychotic disorders
F30-F39	Mood [affective] disorders
F40-F48	Anxiety, dissociative, stress-related, somatoform and other nonpsychotic mental disorders
F50-F59	Behavioral syndromes associated with physiological disturbances and physical factors
F60-F69	Disorders of adult personality and behavior
F70-F79	Intellectual disabilities
F80-F89	Pervasive and specific developmental disorders
F90-F98	Behavioral and emotional disorders with onset usually occurring in childhood and adolescence
F99	Unspecified mental disorder

Mental disorders due to known physiological conditions (F01-F09)

Note:

This block comprises a range of mental disorders grouped together on the basis of their having in common a demonstrable etiology in cerebral disease, brain injury, or other insult leading to cerebral dysfunction. The dysfunction may be primary, as in diseases, injuries, and insults that affect the brain directly and selectively; or secondary, as in systemic diseases and disorders that attack the brain only as one of the multiple organs or systems of the body that are involved.

CODING TIPS ✓ Conditions classifiable here are specifically reportable as due to an underlying cause or condition.

4 F01   Vascular dementia

Vascular dementia as a result of infarction of the brain due to vascular disease, including hypertensive cerebrovascular disease.

INCLUDES arteriosclerotic dementia

Code first:
the underlying physiological condition or sequelae of cerebrovascular disease.

ALERT F01, F02 and F03 will not be accepted as primary codes in hospice.

5 F01.5   Vascular dementia

CODING TIPS ✓ It is inappropriate to code vascular dementia as a sequela of unspecified cerebrovascular disease (I69.918), unless the physician documented the dementia as a sequela of cerebrovascular disease. Vascular dementia can be coded with other types of dementia using the F02.8 subcategory.

CODING TIPS ✓ Vascular dementia may also be reported as "multi-infarct dementia." In this case it should be coded as a sequelae of cerebrovascular accident (stroke). This type of dementia also may be related to other cerebral vascular disorders including vascular hypertension and cerebral atherosclerosis. Major neurocognitive disorder is coded as vascular dementia, if the physician does not specify a cause.

CODING TIPS ✓ F01.5 codes may not be sequenced primary in hospice, and will not qualify as a primary diagnosis in the proposed PDGM. If related to cerebral infarction, home care and hospice coders should use I69.3-. If the patient has not had a stroke, query the physician regarding conditions in I65- I67 as causes of vascular dementia.

IQ F01.50   Vascular dementia without behavioral disturbance

Major neurocognitive disorder without behavioral disturbance

IQ + F01.51   Vascular dementia with behavioral disturbance

Major neurocognitive disorder due to vascular disease, with behavioral disturbance

Major neurocognitive disorder with aggressive behavior

Major neurocognitive disorder with combative behavior

Major neurocognitive disorder with violent behavior

Vascular dementia with aggressive behavior

Vascular dementia with combative behavior

Vascular dementia with violent behavior

Use additional code, if applicable, to identify wandering in vascular dementia (Z91.83)

CODING TIPS ✓ Anxiety is not considered a behavior indicated by a 5th character of 1. Anxiety, when documented by the physician, in addition to dementia, should be coded separately.

CODING TIPS ✓ Use Z91.83 (Wandering in diseases classified elsewhere) as an additional code when appropriate. Wandering can only be coded with the 5th digit indicating behavior problems even though the patient may not have aggressive, violent, combative behavior.

4 F02   Dementia in other diseases classified elsewhere

★ New ▲ Revised **Px** Primary **SP** PDGM Px **SL** Low CoM **SH** High CoM **IQ** Quest. Encounter **H** Hospice non-cancer Dx **Unspecified** **M** *Manifestation*

DecisionHealth's FY 2020 Complete Home Health ICD-10-CM Diagnosis Coding Manual

783

Chapter 5

F01-F99

INCLUDES   Major neurocognitive disorder
in other diseases classified
elsewhere

Code first the underlying physiological
condition, such as:
Alzheimer's (G30.-)
cerebral lipidosis (E75.4)
Creutzfeldt-Jakob disease (A81.0-)
dementia with Lewy bodies (G31.83)
dementia with Parkinsonism (G31.83)
epilepsy and recurrent seizures (G40.-)
frontotemporal dementia (G31.09)
hepatolenticular degeneration (E83.0)
human immunodeficiency virus [HIV]
disease (B20)
Huntington's disease (G10)
hypercalcemia (E83.52)
hypothyroidism, acquired (E00-E03.-)
intoxications (T36-T65)
Jakob-Creutzfeldt disease (A81.0-)
multiple sclerosis (G35)
neurosyphilis (A52.17)
niacin deficiency [pellagra] (E52)
Parkinson's disease (G20)
Pick's disease (G31.01)
polyarteritis nodosa (M30.0)
prion disease (A81.9)
systemic lupus erythematosus (M32.-)
traumatic brain injury (S06.-)
trypanosomiasis (B56.-, B57.-)
vitamin B deficiency (E53.8)

EXCLUDES 2   dementia in alcohol and
psychoactive substance
disorders
(F10-F19, with .17, .27, .97)
vascular dementia (F01.5-)

**⑤ F02.8 Dementia in other diseases classified
elsewhere**

CODING TIPS ✓   Codes F02.80 and F02.81
are manifestation-only codes and should be
used only to report dementia in an
etiology/manifestation pairing. An F02.8-
code should never be used alone and
inappropriate use of these codes may result
in claims edits. Always code the etiology
first, followed by the appropriate F02.8-
code to specify dementia with or without
behavioral disturbance. The physician must
document a diagnosis of dementia and the
presence of behavioral disturbances.

**M IQ SH F02.80   *Dementia in other diseases classified
elsewhere without behavioral
disturbance***

Dementia in other diseases classified
elsewhere NOS
Major neurocognitive disorder in other
diseases classified elsewhere

**M IQ SH ✚ F02.81   *Dementia in other diseases classified
elsewhere with behavioral
disturbance***

Dementia in other diseases classified
elsewhere with aggressive behavior
Dementia in other diseases classified
elsewhere with combative behavior
Dementia in other diseases classified
elsewhere with violent behavior

Major neurocognitive disorder in other
diseases classified elsewhere with
aggressive behavior
Major neurocognitive disorder in other
diseases classified elsewhere with
combative behavior
Major neurocognitive disorder in other
diseases classified elsewhere with
violent behavior

Use additional code, if applicable, to
identify wandering in dementia in
conditions classified elsewhere
(Z91.83)

CODING TIPS ✓   Anxiety is not considered
a behavior indicated by a 5th character
of 1. Anxiety, when documented by the
physician, in addition to dementia,
should be coded separately.

CODING TIPS ✓   Use Z91.83 (Wandering
in diseases classified elsewhere) as an
additional code when appropriate.
Wandering can only be coded with the
5th digit indicating behavior problems
even though the patient may not have
aggressive, violent, combative behavior.

④ F03   Unspecified dementia

Presenile dementia NOS
Presenile psychosis NOS
Primary degenerative dementia NOS
Senile dementia NOS
Senile dementia depressed or paranoid type
Senile psychosis NOS

EXCLUDES 1   senility NOS (R41.81)

EXCLUDES 2   mild memory disturbance due to
known physiological
condition (F06.8)
senile dementia with delirium or
acute confusional state (F05)

DEFINITION   Loss of cognitive and
intellectual functions, such as impaired
memory, judgment, and intellect, without
impaired perception or consciousness.

⑤ F03.9   Unspecified dementia

CODING TIPS ✓   Codes F03.90 and F03.91
are to be used for dementia that is not
specified as due to another condition, and is
reported as unspecified, senile psychosis,
senile dementia (may also state depressed
or paranoid type), primary degenerative
dementia, or presenile dementia/psychosis.
Do not confuse these conditions with
organic brain disease or senility NOS.
Senility NOS should not be coded with an
F03.9- code (see excludes 1 notes) as this
is less specific. When senile dementia is
specified, the appropriate F03.9- code
should be used. If the physician
documentation states major neurocognitive
disorder, do not code as unspecified
dementia.

---

④ 4th digit required   ⑤ 5th digit required   ⑥ 6th digit required   ⑦ 7th digit required   ⑦ 7th digit placeholder   ✚ Additional code   ⊟ Laterality

784   *DecisionHealth's* FY 2020 Complete Home Health ICD-10-CM Diagnosis Coding Manual

CODING TIPS ✓ Hospices should NOT assign a code from F03.9- as primary. When only "dementia" is provided as a diagnostic statement, hospices should query the physician and/or medical director for a more specific diagnosis. Clinical documentation should reflect confirmation of any additional or changed diagnostic statements.

SP SH F03.90 **Unspecified dementia without behavioral disturbance**

Dementia NOS

SP SH + F03.91 **Unspecified dementia with behavioral disturbance**

Unspecified dementia with aggressive behavior

Unspecified dementia with combative behavior

Unspecified dementia with violent behavior

Use additional code, if applicable, to identify wandering in unspecified dementia (Z91.83)

CODING TIPS ✓ Anxiety is not considered a behavior indicated by a 5th character of 1. Anxiety, when documented by the physician, in addition to dementia, should be coded separately.

CODING TIPS ✓ Use Z91.83 (Wandering in diseases classified elsewhere) as an additional code when appropriate. Wandering can only be coded with the 5th digit indicating behavior problems even though the patient may not have aggressive, violent, combative behavior.

IQ SH F04 **Amnestic disorder due to known physiological condition**

Korsakov's psychosis or syndrome, nonalcoholic

Code first:

the underlying physiological condition

EXCLUDES 1 amnesia NOS (R41.3)
anterograde amnesia (R41.1)
dissociative amnesia (F44.0)
retrograde amnesia (R41.2)

EXCLUDES 2 alcohol-induced or unspecified Korsakov's syndrome (F10.26, F10.96)
Korsakov's syndrome induced by other psychoactive substances (F13.26, F13.96, F19.16, F19.26, F19.96)

IQ SH F05 **Delirium due to known physiological condition**

Acute or subacute brain syndrome

Acute or subacute confusional state (nonalcoholic)

Acute or subacute infective psychosis

Acute or subacute organic reaction

Acute or subacute psycho-organic syndrome

Delirium of mixed etiology

Delirium superimposed on dementia

Sundowning

Code first:

the underlying physiological condition

EXCLUDES 1 delirium NOS (R41.0)

EXCLUDES 2 delirium tremens alcohol-induced or unspecified (F10.231, F10.921)

CODING TIPS ✓ Patients with dementia may also have delirium or sundowning. When appropriate, add F05 when dementia is coded.

4 F06 **Other mental disorders due to known physiological condition**

INCLUDES mental disorders due to endocrine disorder
mental disorders due to exogenous hormone
mental disorders due to exogenous toxic substance
mental disorders due to primary cerebral disease
mental disorders due to somatic illness
mental disorders due to systemic disease affecting the brain

Code first:

the underlying physiological condition

EXCLUDES 1 unspecified dementia (F03)

EXCLUDES 2 delirium due to known physiological condition (F05)
dementia as classified in F01-F02
other mental disorders associated with alcohol and other psychoactive substances (F10-F19)

IQ F06.0 **Psychotic disorder with hallucinations due to known physiological condition**

Organic hallucinatory state (nonalcoholic)

EXCLUDES 2 hallucinations and perceptual disturbance induced by alcohol and other psychoactive substances (F10-F19 with .151, .251, .951)
schizophrenia (F20.-)

IQ SH F06.1 **Catatonic disorder due to known physiological condition**

Catatonia associated with another mental disorder

Catatonia NOS

EXCLUDES 1 catatonic stupor (R40.1)
stupor NOS (R40.1)

EXCLUDES 2 catatonic schizophrenia (F20.2)
dissociative stupor (F44.2)

IQ F06.2 **Psychotic disorder with delusions due to known physiological condition**

Paranoid and paranoid-hallucinatory organic states

Schizophrenia-like psychosis in epilepsy

EXCLUDES 2 alcohol and drug-induced psychotic disorder (F10-F19 with .150, .250, .950)
brief psychotic disorder (F23)
delusional disorder (F22)
schizophrenia (F20.-)

5 F06.3 **Mood disorder due to known physiological condition**

★ New ▲ Revised **Px** Primary **SP** PDGM Px **SL** Low CoM **SH** High CoM **IQ** Quest. Encounter **H** Hospice non-cancer Dx Unspecified **M** *Manifestation*

DecisionHealth's FY 2020 Complete Home Health ICD-10-CM Diagnosis Coding Manual

785

Chapter 5

F01-F99

EXCLUDES 2 mood disorders due to alcohol and other psychoactive substances (F10-F19 with .14, .24, .94)

mood disorders, not due to known physiological condition or unspecified (F30-F39)

IQ F06.30 Mood disorder due to known physiological condition, unspecified

IQ F06.31 Mood disorder due to known physiological condition with depressive features
Depressive disorder due to known physiological condition, with depressive features

IQ F06.32 Mood disorder due to known physiological condition with major depressive-like episode
Depressive disorder due to known physiological condition, with major depressive-like episode

IQ F06.33 Mood disorder due to known physiological condition with manic features
Bipolar and related disorder due to a known physiological condition, with manic features
Bipolar and related disorder due to known physiological condition, with manic- or hypomanic-like episodes

IQ F06.34 Mood disorder due to known physiological condition with mixed features
Bipolar and related disorder due to known physiological condition, with mixed features
Depressive disorder due to known physiological condition, with mixed features

IQ F06.4 Anxiety disorder due to known physiological condition
EXCLUDES 2 anxiety disorders due to alcohol and other psychoactive substances (F10-F19 with .180, .280, .980)
anxiety disorders, not due to known physiological condition or unspecified (F40.-, F41.-)

IQ SH F06.8 Other specified mental disorders due to known physiological condition
Epileptic psychosis NOS
Obsessive-compulsive and related disorder due to a known physiological condition
Organic dissociative disorder
Organic emotionally labile [asthenic] disorder

4 F07 Personality and behavioral disorders due to known physiological condition
Code first:
the underlying physiological condition

IQ F07.0 Personality change due to known physiological condition
Frontal lobe syndrome
Limbic epilepsy personality syndrome
Lobotomy syndrome

Organic personality disorder
Organic pseudopsychopathic personality
Organic pseudoretarded personality
Postleucotomy syndrome
Code first:
underlying physiological condition
EXCLUDES 1 mild cognitive impairment (G31.84)
postconcussional syndrome (F07.81)
postencephalitic syndrome (F07.89)
signs and symptoms involving emotional state (R45.-)
EXCLUDES 2 specific personality disorder (F60.-)
DEFINITION Frontal lobe syndrome: Damage to the frontal lobe of the brain, typically manifesting as apathy, a lack of planning, emotional bluntness, the absence of abstract thought and attention, and judgment changes.

5 F07.8 Other personality and behavioral disorders due to known physiological condition

SP + F07.81 Postconcussional syndrome
Postcontusional syndrome (encephalopathy)
Post-traumatic brain syndrome, nonpsychotic
Use additional code to identify associated post-traumatic headache, if applicable (G44.3-)
EXCLUDES 1 current concussion (brain) (S06.0-)
postencephalitic syndrome (F07.89)
CODING TIPS ✓ Code F07.81 should not be used for the patient who has a current concussion (see the Excludes 1 notes).

CODING TIPS ✓ Documentation: Post concussion syndrome is a complex disorder resulting from a mild traumatic brain injury and is not associated with the severity of the initial injury. No documented loss of consciousness with the initial injury is necessary for a diagnosis of post concussion syndrome, but the physician must specify this disorder.

DEFINITION Symptoms such as headache, amnesia, and lack of concentration due to a severe blow to the skull.

SP F07.89 Other personality and behavioral disorders due to known physiological condition
Postencephalitic syndrome
Right hemispheric organic affective disorder

SP F07.9 Unspecified personality and behavioral disorder due to known physiological condition
Organic psychosyndrome

IQ F09 **Unspecified mental disorder due to known physiological condition**

Mental disorder NOS due to known physiological condition
Organic brain syndrome NOS
Organic mental disorder NOS
Organic psychosis NOS
Symptomatic psychosis NOS
Code first:
the underlying physiological condition
EXCLUDES 1 psychosis NOS (F29)

Mental and behavioral disorders due to psychoactive substance use (F10-F19)

GUIDELINES Section I.C.5.b.1)-3)
Selection of codes for "in remission" for categories F10-F19, Mental and behavioral disorders due to psychoactive substance use (categories F10-F19 with -.21), requires the provider's clinical judgment. The appropriate codes for "in remission" are assigned only on the basis of provider documentation (as defined in the Official Guidelines for Coding and Reporting) unless otherwise instructed by the classification.

Mild substance use disorders in early or sustained remission are classified to the appropriate codes for substance abuse in remission, and moderate or severe substance use disorders in early or sustained remission are classified to the appropriate codes for substance dependence in remission.

When the provider documentation refers to use, abuse and dependence of the same substance (e.g. alcohol, opioid, cannabis, etc.), only one code should be assigned to identify the pattern of use based on the following hierarchy:
• If both use and abuse are documented, assign only the code for abuse
• If both abuse and dependence are documented, assign only the code for dependence
• If use, abuse and dependence are all documented, assign only the code for dependence
• If both use and dependence are documented, assign only the code for dependence.

As with all other unspecified diagnoses, the codes for unspecified psychoactive substance use disorders (F10.9-, F11.9-, F12.9-, F13.9-, F14.9-, F15.9-, F16.9-, F18.9-, F19.9-) should only be assigned based on provider documentation and when they meet the definition of a reportable diagnosis (see Section III, Reporting Additional Diagnoses). The codes are to be used only when the psychoactive substance use is associated with a physical, mental or behavioral disorder, and such a relationship is documented by the provider.

CODING TIPS ✓ Codes for psychoactive substance use are to be used only when the psychoactive substance use is associated with a physical, mental or behavioral disorder, and such a relationship is documented by the physician.

+ 4 F10 **Alcohol related disorders**
Use additional code for blood alcohol level, if applicable (Y90.-)
CODING TIPS ✓ There are codes for alcohol use, abuse and dependence. Alcoholism is coded to dependence. Use disorder is coded to abuse or dependence depending on the severity.

CODING TIPS ✓ Alcohol withdrawal is categorized as alcohol dependence, by default.

+ 5 F10.1 **Alcohol abuse**
EXCLUDES 1 alcohol dependence (F10.2-)
alcohol use, unspecified (F10.9-)
SP + F10.10 **Alcohol abuse, uncomplicated**
Alcohol use disorder, mild
IQ + F10.11 **Alcohol abuse, in remission**
Alcohol use disorder, mild, in early remission
Alcohol use disorder, mild, in sustained remission
+ 6 F10.12 **Alcohol abuse with intoxication**
SP + F10.120 **Alcohol abuse with intoxication, uncomplicated**
SP + F10.121 **Alcohol abuse with intoxication delirium**
SP + F10.129 **Alcohol abuse with intoxication, unspecified**
SP + F10.14 **Alcohol abuse with alcohol-induced mood disorder**
Alcohol use disorder, mild, with alcohol-induced bipolar or related disorder
Alcohol use disorder, mild, with alcohol-induced depressive disorder
+ 6 F10.15 **Alcohol abuse with alcohol-induced psychotic disorder**
SP + F10.150 **Alcohol abuse with alcohol-induced psychotic disorder with delusions**
SP + F10.151 **Alcohol abuse with alcohol-induced psychotic disorder with hallucinations**
SP + F10.159 **Alcohol abuse with alcohol-induced psychotic disorder, unspecified**
+ 6 F10.18 **Alcohol abuse with other alcohol-induced disorders**
SP + F10.180 **Alcohol abuse with alcohol-induced anxiety disorder**
SP + F10.181 **Alcohol abuse with alcohol-induced sexual dysfunction**
SP + F10.182 **Alcohol abuse with alcohol-induced sleep disorder**
SP + F10.188 **Alcohol abuse with other alcohol-induced disorder**
SP + F10.19 **Alcohol abuse with unspecified alcohol-induced disorder**
+ 5 F10.2 **Alcohol dependence**
EXCLUDES 1 alcohol abuse (F10.1-)
alcohol use, unspecified (F10.9-)
EXCLUDES 2 toxic effect of alcohol (T51.0-)
CODING TIPS ✓ Alcoholism is coded to alcohol dependence.
SP + F10.20 **Alcohol dependence, uncomplicated**
Alcohol use disorder, moderate
Alcohol use disorder, severe
SP + F10.21 **Alcohol dependence, in remission**
Alcohol use disorder, moderate, in early remission
Alcohol use disorder, moderate, in sustained remission
Alcohol use disorder, severe, in early remission

★ New ▲ Revised **Px** Primary **SP** PDGM Px **SL** Low CoM **SH** High CoM **IQ** Quest. Encounter **H** Hospice non-cancer Dx Unspecified **M** *Manifestation*

DecisionHealth's FY 2020 Complete Home Health ICD-10-CM Diagnosis Coding Manual   787

Chapter 5

F01-F99

Alcohol use disorder, severe, in sustained remission

+ 6 F10.22   Alcohol dependence with intoxication

Acute drunkenness (in alcoholism)

EXCLUDES 2   alcohol dependence with withdrawal (F10.23-)

SP + F10.220   Alcohol dependence with intoxication, uncomplicated

SP + F10.221   Alcohol dependence with intoxication delirium

SP + F10.229   Alcohol dependence with intoxication, unspecified

+ 6 F10.23   Alcohol dependence with withdrawal

EXCLUDES 2   Alcohol dependence with intoxication (F10.22-)

SP + F10.230   Alcohol dependence with withdrawal, uncomplicated

SP + F10.231   Alcohol dependence with withdrawal delirium

DEFINITION   Delirium occurring when an alcoholic is denied alcohol for a significant period of time.

SP + F10.232   Alcohol dependence with withdrawal with perceptual disturbance

SP + F10.239   Alcohol dependence with withdrawal, unspecified

SP + F10.24   Alcohol dependence with alcohol-induced mood disorder

Alcohol use disorder, moderate, with alcohol-induced bipolar or related disorder

Alcohol use disorder, moderate, with alcohol-induced depressive disorder

Alcohol use disorder, severe, with alcohol-induced bipolar or related disorder

Alcohol use disorder, severe, with alcohol-induced depressive disorder

+ 6 F10.25   Alcohol dependence with alcohol-induced psychotic disorder

SP + F10.250   Alcohol dependence with alcohol-induced psychotic disorder with delusions

SP + F10.251   Alcohol dependence with alcohol-induced psychotic disorder with hallucinations

SP + F10.259   Alcohol dependence with alcohol-induced psychotic disorder, unspecified

SP + F10.26   Alcohol dependence with alcohol-induced persisting amnestic disorder

Alcohol use disorder, moderate, with alcohol-induced major neurocognitive disorder, amnestic-confabulatory type

Alcohol use disorder, severe, with alcohol-induced major neurocognitive disorder, amnestic-confabulatory type

SP + F10.27   Alcohol dependence with alcohol-induced persisting dementia

Alcohol use disorder, moderate, with alcohol-induced major neurocognitive disorder, nonamnestic-confabulatory type

Alcohol use disorder, severe, with alcohol-induced major neurocognitive disorder, nonamnestic-confabulatory type

DEFINITION   Lasting state of dementia due to chronic alcoholism.

+ 6 F10.28   Alcohol dependence with other alcohol-induced disorders

SP + F10.280   Alcohol dependence with alcohol-induced anxiety disorder

SP + F10.281   Alcohol dependence with alcohol-induced sexual dysfunction

SP + F10.282   Alcohol dependence with alcohol-induced sleep disorder

SP + F10.288   Alcohol dependence with other alcohol-induced disorder

Alcohol use disorder, moderate, with alcohol-induced mild neurocognitive disorder

Alcohol use disorder, severe, with alcohol-induced mild neurocognitive disorder

CODING TIPS ✓   The physician must link the condition to the alcoholism to use this code.

SP + F10.29   Alcohol dependence with unspecified alcohol-induced disorder

+ 5 F10.9   Alcohol use, unspecified

EXCLUDES 1   alcohol abuse (F10.1-)
alcohol dependence (F10.2-)

CODING TIPS ✓   The use codes are for use of the alcohol associated with a mental, emotional or physical disorder as documented by the physician. The use codes are not to be used for the patient who drinks alcohol occasionally or without the additional physician documentation.

+ 6 F10.92   Alcohol use, unspecified with intoxication

SP + F10.920   Alcohol use, unspecified with intoxication, uncomplicated

SP + F10.921   Alcohol use, unspecified with intoxication delirium

SP + F10.929   Alcohol use, unspecified with intoxication, unspecified

SP + F10.94   Alcohol use, unspecified with alcohol-induced mood disorder

Alcohol induced bipolar or related disorder, without use disorder

Alcohol induced depressive disorder, without use disorder

+ 6 F10.95   Alcohol use, unspecified with alcohol-induced psychotic disorder

SP + F10.950   Alcohol use, unspecified with alcohol-induced psychotic disorder with delusions

SP + F10.951   Alcohol use, unspecified with alcohol-induced psychotic disorder with hallucinations

SP + F10.959   Alcohol use, unspecified with alcohol-induced psychotic disorder, unspecified

Alcohol-induced psychotic disorder without use disorder

---

4 4th digit required   5 5th digit required   6 6th digit required   7 7th digit required   7 7th digit placeholder   **+** Additional code   Laterality

SP + F10.96 Alcohol use, unspecified with alcohol-induced persisting amnestic disorder

Alcohol-induced major neurocognitive disorder, amnestic-confabulatory type, without use disorder

SP + F10.97 Alcohol use, unspecified with alcohol-induced persisting dementia

Alcohol-induced major neurocognitive disorder, nonamnestic-confabulatory type, without use disorder

+ 6 F10.98 Alcohol use, unspecified with other alcohol-induced disorders

SP + F10.980 Alcohol use, unspecified with alcohol-induced anxiety disorder

Alcohol induced anxiety disorder, without use disorder

SP + F10.981 Alcohol use, unspecified with alcohol-induced sexual dysfunction

Alcohol induced sexual dysfunction, without use disorder

SP + F10.982 Alcohol use, unspecified with alcohol-induced sleep disorder

Alcohol induced sleep disorder, without use disorder

DEFINITION Disruption of normal sleep patterns due to the consumption of alcohol.

SP + F10.988 Alcohol use, unspecified with other alcohol-induced disorder

Alcohol induced mild neurocognitive disorder, without use disorder

SP + F10.99 Alcohol use, unspecified with unspecified alcohol-induced disorder

4 F11 Opioid related disorders

CODING TIPS ✓ Do not assign a code for the prescribed opioid use. Without provider documentation of an associated physical, mental or behavioral disorder, "opioid use" is not coded.

5 F11.1 Opioid abuse

EXCLUDES 1 opioid dependence (F11.2-) opioid use, unspecified (F11.9-)

SP F11.10 Opioid abuse, uncomplicated
Opioid use disorder, mild

IQ F11.11 Opioid abuse, in remission
Opioid use disorder, mild, in early remission
Opioid use disorder, mild, in sustained remission

6 F11.12 Opioid abuse with intoxication

SP F11.120 Opioid abuse with intoxication, uncomplicated

SP F11.121 Opioid abuse with intoxication delirium

SP F11.122 Opioid abuse with intoxication with perceptual disturbance

SP F11.129 Opioid abuse with intoxication, unspecified

SP F11.14 Opioid abuse with opioid-induced mood disorder

Opioid use disorder, mild, with opioid-induced depressive disorder

6 F11.15 Opioid abuse with opioid-induced psychotic disorder

SP F11.150 Opioid abuse with opioid-induced psychotic disorder with delusions

SP F11.151 Opioid abuse with opioid-induced psychotic disorder with hallucinations

SP F11.159 Opioid abuse with opioid-induced psychotic disorder, unspecified

6 F11.18 Opioid abuse with other opioid-induced disorder

SP F11.181 Opioid abuse with opioid-induced sexual dysfunction

SP F11.182 Opioid abuse with opioid-induced sleep disorder

SP F11.188 Opioid abuse with other opioid-induced disorder

SP F11.19 Opioid abuse with unspecified opioid-induced disorder

5 F11.2 Opioid dependence

EXCLUDES 1 opioid abuse (F11.1-) opioid use, unspecified (F11.9-)
EXCLUDES 2 opioid poisoning (T40.0-T40.2-)

SP F11.20 Opioid dependence, uncomplicated
Opioid use disorder, moderate
Opioid use disorder, severe

SP F11.21 Opioid dependence, in remission
Opioid use disorder, moderate, in early remission
Opioid use disorder, moderate, in sustained remission
Opioid use disorder, severe, in early remission
Opioid use disorder, severe, in sustained remission

6 F11.22 Opioid dependence with intoxication
EXCLUDES 1 opioid dependence with withdrawal (F11.23)

SP F11.220 Opioid dependence with intoxication, uncomplicated

SP F11.221 Opioid dependence with intoxication delirium

SP F11.222 Opioid dependence with intoxication with perceptual disturbance

SP F11.229 Opioid dependence with intoxication, unspecified

SP F11.23 Opioid dependence with withdrawal
EXCLUDES 1 opioid dependence with intoxication (F11.22-)

SP F11.24 Opioid dependence with opioid-induced mood disorder
Opioid use disorder, moderate, with opioid induced depressive disorder

6 F11.25 Opioid dependence with opioid-induced psychotic disorder

SP F11.250 Opioid dependence with opioid-induced psychotic disorder with delusions

SP F11.251 Opioid dependence with opioid-induced psychotic disorder with hallucinations

---

★ New ▲ Revised Px Primary **SP** PDGM Px **SL** Low CoM **SH** High CoM **IQ** Quest. Encounter **H** Hospice non-cancer Dx Unspecified **M** *Manifestation*

DecisionHealth's FY 2020 Complete Home Health ICD-10-CM Diagnosis Coding Manual

789

Chapter 5

F01-F99

SP F11.259 Opioid dependence with opioid-induced psychotic disorder, unspecified

6 F11.28 Opioid dependence with other opioid-induced disorder

SP F11.281 Opioid dependence with opioid-induced sexual dysfunction

SP F11.282 Opioid dependence with opioid-induced sleep disorder

SP F11.288 Opioid dependence with other opioid-induced disorder

SP F11.29 Opioid dependence with unspecified opioid-induced disorder

5 F11.9 Opioid use, unspecified

> **EXCLUDES 1** opioid abuse (F11.1-)
> opioid dependence (F11.2-)

> **CODING TIPS ✓** The use codes are for use of the opioid associated with (causing) a mental, emotional or physical disorder as documented by the physician. The use codes are not to be used for the patient who uses opioids medicinally or without the additional physician documentation.

> **CODING TIPS ✓** Use disorder is coded to abuse or dependence depending on the severity. Mild is coded to abuse, and moderate and severe are coded to dependence.

SP F11.90 Opioid use, unspecified, uncomplicated

6 F11.92 Opioid use, unspecified with intoxication

> **EXCLUDES 1** opioid use, unspecified with withdrawal (F11.93)

SP F11.920 Opioid use, unspecified with intoxication, uncomplicated

SP F11.921 Opioid use, unspecified with intoxication delirium

Opioid-induced delirium

SP F11.922 Opioid use, unspecified with intoxication with perceptual disturbance

SP F11.929 Opioid use, unspecified with intoxication, unspecified

SP F11.93 Opioid use, unspecified with withdrawal

> **EXCLUDES 1** opioid use, unspecified with intoxication (F11.92-)

SP F11.94 Opioid use, unspecified with opioid-induced mood disorder

Opioid induced depressive disorder, without use disorder

6 F11.95 Opioid use, unspecified with opioid-induced psychotic disorder

SP F11.950 Opioid use, unspecified with opioid-induced psychotic disorder with delusions

SP F11.951 Opioid use, unspecified with opioid-induced psychotic disorder with hallucinations

SP F11.959 Opioid use, unspecified with opioid-induced psychotic disorder, unspecified

6 F11.98 Opioid use, unspecified with other specified opioid-induced disorder

SP F11.981 Opioid use, unspecified with opioid-induced sexual dysfunction

Opioid induced sexual dysfunction, without use disorder

SP F11.982 Opioid use, unspecified with opioid-induced sleep disorder

Opioid induced sleep disorder, without use disorder

SP F11.988 Opioid use, unspecified with other opioid-induced disorder

Opioid induced anxiety disorder, without use disorder

SP F11.99 Opioid use, unspecified with unspecified opioid-induced disorder

4 F12 Cannabis related disorders

> **INCLUDES** marijuana

> **CODING TIPS ✓** Recreational marijuana use or medical use of marijuana should not ordinarily be coded. Do not assign a code for marijuana use, without an associated physical, mental or behavioral disorder documented by the provider.

5 F12.1 Cannabis abuse

> **EXCLUDES 1** cannabis dependence (F12.2-)
> cannabis use, unspecified (F12.9-)

SP F12.10 Cannabis abuse, uncomplicated
Cannabis use disorder, mild

!Q F12.11 Cannabis abuse, in remission
Cannabis use disorder, mild, in early remission
Cannabis use disorder, mild, in sustained remission

6 F12.12 Cannabis abuse with intoxication

SP F12.120 Cannabis abuse with intoxication, uncomplicated

SP F12.121 Cannabis abuse with intoxication delirium

SP F12.122 Cannabis abuse with intoxication with perceptual disturbance

SP F12.129 Cannabis abuse with intoxication, unspecified

6 F12.15 Cannabis abuse with psychotic disorder

SP F12.150 Cannabis abuse with psychotic disorder with delusions

SP F12.151 Cannabis abuse with psychotic disorder with hallucinations

SP F12.159 Cannabis abuse with psychotic disorder, unspecified

6 F12.18 Cannabis abuse with other cannabis-induced disorder

SP F12.180 Cannabis abuse with cannabis-induced anxiety disorder

SP F12.188 Cannabis abuse with other cannabis-induced disorder
Cannabis use disorder, mild, with cannabis-induced sleep disorder

SP F12.19 Cannabis abuse with unspecified cannabis-induced disorder

5 F12.2 Cannabis dependence

> **EXCLUDES 1** cannabis abuse (F12.1-)

---

4 4th digit required   5 5th digit required   6 6th digit required   7 7th digit required   7 7th digit placeholder   ✚ Additional code   ▤ Laterality

790   DecisionHealth's FY 2020 Complete Home Health ICD-10-CM Diagnosis Coding Manual

cannabis use, unspecified (F12.9-)

EXCLUDES 2 cannabis poisoning (T40.7-)

SP **F12.20** **Cannabis dependence, uncomplicated**
Cannabis use disorder, moderate
Cannabis use disorder, severe

SP **F12.21** **Cannabis dependence, in remission**
Cannabis use disorder, moderate, in early remission
Cannabis use disorder, moderate, in sustained remission
Cannabis use disorder, severe, in early remission
Cannabis use disorder, severe, in sustained remission

6 **F12.22** **Cannabis dependence with intoxication**

SP **F12.220** **Cannabis dependence with intoxication, uncomplicated**

SP **F12.221** **Cannabis dependence with intoxication delirium**

SP **F12.222** **Cannabis dependence with intoxication with perceptual disturbance**

SP **F12.229** **Cannabis dependence with intoxication, unspecified**

SP **F12.23** **Cannabis dependence with withdrawal**

6 **F12.25** **Cannabis dependence with psychotic disorder**

SP **F12.250** **Cannabis dependence with psychotic disorder with delusions**

SP **F12.251** **Cannabis dependence with psychotic disorder with hallucinations**

SP **F12.259** **Cannabis dependence with psychotic disorder, unspecified**

6 **F12.28** **Cannabis dependence with other cannabis-induced disorder**

SP **F12.280** **Cannabis dependence with cannabis-induced anxiety disorder**

SP **F12.288** **Cannabis dependence with other cannabis-induced disorder**
Cannabis use disorder, moderate, with cannabis-induced sleep disorder
Cannabis use disorder, severe, with cannabis-induced sleep disorder

SP **F12.29** **Cannabis dependence with unspecified cannabis-induced disorder**

5 **F12.9** **Cannabis use, unspecified**

EXCLUDES 1 cannabis abuse (F12.1-)
cannabis dependence (F12.2-)

CODING TIPS ✓ The use codes are for use of the cannibis associated with (causing) a mental, emotional or physical disorder as documented by the physician. The use codes are not to be used for the patient who uses medical marijuana or uses the marijuana recreationally without the additional physician documentation.

CODING TIPS ✓ Use disorder is coded to abuse or dependence depending on the severity. Mild is coded to abuse, and moderate and severe are coded to dependence.

SP **F12.90** **Cannabis use, unspecified, uncomplicated**

6 **F12.92** **Cannabis use, unspecified with intoxication**

SP **F12.920** **Cannabis use, unspecified with intoxication, uncomplicated**

SP **F12.921** **Cannabis use, unspecified with intoxication delirium**

SP **F12.922** **Cannabis use, unspecified with intoxication with perceptual disturbance**

SP **F12.929** **Cannabis use, unspecified with intoxication, unspecified**

SP **F12.93** **Cannabis use, unspecified with withdrawal**

6 **F12.95** **Cannabis use, unspecified with psychotic disorder**

SP **F12.950** **Cannabis use, unspecified with psychotic disorder with delusions**

SP **F12.951** **Cannabis use, unspecified with psychotic disorder with hallucinations**

SP **F12.959** **Cannabis use, unspecified with psychotic disorder, unspecified**
Cannabis induced psychotic disorder, without use disorder

6 **F12.98** **Cannabis use, unspecified with other cannabis-induced disorder**

SP **F12.980** **Cannabis use, unspecified with anxiety disorder**
Cannabis induced anxiety disorder, without use disorder

SP **F12.988** **Cannabis use, unspecified with other cannabis-induced disorder**
Cannabis induced sleep disorder, without use disorder

SP **F12.99** **Cannabis use, unspecified with unspecified cannabis-induced disorder**

4 **F13** **Sedative, hypnotic, or anxiolytic related disorders**

5 **F13.1** **Sedative, hypnotic or anxiolytic-related abuse**

EXCLUDES 1 sedative, hypnotic or anxiolytic-related dependence (F13.2-)
sedative, hypnotic, or anxiolytic use, unspecified (F13.9-)

SP **F13.10** **Sedative, hypnotic or anxiolytic abuse, uncomplicated**
Sedative, hypnotic, or anxiolytic use disorder, mild

IQ **F13.11** **Sedative, hypnotic or anxiolytic abuse, in remission**
Sedative, hypnotic or anxiolytic use disorder, mild, in early remission
Sedative, hypnotic or anxiolytic use disorder, mild, in sustained remission

---

★ New ▲ Revised **Px** Primary **SP** PDGM Px **SL** Low CoM **SH** High CoM **IQ** Quest. Encounter **H** Hospice non-cancer Dx Unspecified **M** *Manifestation*

Chapter 5

F01-F99

⑥ F13.12 Sedative, hypnotic or anxiolytic abuse with intoxication

SP F13.120 Sedative, hypnotic or anxiolytic abuse with intoxication, uncomplicated

SP F13.121 Sedative, hypnotic or anxiolytic abuse with intoxication delirium

SP F13.129 Sedative, hypnotic or anxiolytic abuse with intoxication, unspecified

SP F13.14 Sedative, hypnotic or anxiolytic abuse with sedative, hypnotic or anxiolytic-induced mood disorder
Sedative, hypnotic, or anxiolytic use disorder, mild, with sedative, hypnotic, or anxiolytic-induced bipolar or related disorder
Sedative, hypnotic, or anxiolytic use disorder, mild, with sedative, hypnotic, or anxiolytic-induced depressive disorder

⑥ F13.15 Sedative, hypnotic or anxiolytic abuse with sedative, hypnotic or anxiolytic-induced psychotic disorder

SP F13.150 Sedative, hypnotic or anxiolytic abuse with sedative, hypnotic or anxiolytic-induced psychotic disorder with delusions

SP F13.151 Sedative, hypnotic or anxiolytic abuse with sedative, hypnotic or anxiolytic-induced psychotic disorder with hallucinations

SP F13.159 Sedative, hypnotic or anxiolytic abuse with sedative, hypnotic or anxiolytic-induced psychotic disorder, unspecified

⑥ F13.18 Sedative, hypnotic or anxiolytic abuse with other sedative, hypnotic or anxiolytic-induced disorders

SP F13.180 Sedative, hypnotic or anxiolytic abuse with sedative, hypnotic or anxiolytic-induced anxiety disorder

SP F13.181 Sedative, hypnotic or anxiolytic abuse with sedative, hypnotic or anxiolytic-induced sexual dysfunction

SP F13.182 Sedative, hypnotic or anxiolytic abuse with sedative, hypnotic or anxiolytic-induced sleep disorder

SP F13.188 Sedative, hypnotic or anxiolytic abuse with other sedative, hypnotic or anxiolytic-induced disorder

SP F13.19 Sedative, hypnotic or anxiolytic abuse with unspecified sedative, hypnotic or anxiolytic-induced disorder

⑤ F13.2 Sedative, hypnotic or anxiolytic-related dependence
| EXCLUDES 1 | sedative, hypnotic or anxiolytic-related abuse (F13.1-)
sedative, hypnotic, or anxiolytic use, unspecified (F13.9-)

| EXCLUDES 2 | sedative, hypnotic, or anxiolytic poisoning (T42.-)

SP F13.20 Sedative, hypnotic or anxiolytic dependence, uncomplicated

SP F13.21 Sedative, hypnotic or anxiolytic dependence, in remission
Sedative, hypnotic or anxiolytic use disorder, moderate, in early remission
Sedative, hypnotic or anxiolytic use disorder, moderate, in sustained remission
Sedative, hypnotic or anxiolytic use disorder, severe, in early remission
Sedative, hypnotic or anxiolytic use disorder, severe, in sustained remission

⑥ F13.22 Sedative, hypnotic or anxiolytic dependence with intoxication
| EXCLUDES 1 | sedative, hypnotic or anxiolytic dependence with withdrawal (F13.23-)

SP F13.220 Sedative, hypnotic or anxiolytic dependence with intoxication, uncomplicated

SP F13.221 Sedative, hypnotic or anxiolytic dependence with intoxication delirium

SP F13.229 Sedative, hypnotic or anxiolytic dependence with intoxication, unspecified

⑥ F13.23 Sedative, hypnotic or anxiolytic dependence with withdrawal
Sedative, hypnotic, or anxiolytic use disorder, moderate
Sedative, hypnotic, or anxiolytic use disorder, severe
| EXCLUDES 1 | sedative, hypnotic or anxiolytic dependence with intoxication (F13.22-)

| DEFINITION | Curtailed drug use, resulting in physical or psychological symptoms lasting hours to weeks, commonly featuring headache, anxiety, depression, chills, sweats, and tremors.

SP F13.230 Sedative, hypnotic or anxiolytic dependence with withdrawal, uncomplicated

SP F13.231 Sedative, hypnotic or anxiolytic dependence with withdrawal delirium

SP F13.232 Sedative, hypnotic or anxiolytic dependence with withdrawal with perceptual disturbance
Sedative, hypnotic, or anxiolytic withdrawal with perceptual disturbances

SP F13.239 Sedative, hypnotic or anxiolytic dependence with withdrawal, unspecified
Sedative, hypnotic, or anxiolytic withdrawal without perceptual disturbances

---

④4th digit required   ⑤5th digit required   ⑥6th digit required   ⑦7th digit required   ☑7th digit placeholder   ➕Additional code   ⊟Laterality

SP F13.24 **Sedative, hypnotic or anxiolytic dependence with sedative, hypnotic or anxiolytic-induced mood disorder**

Sedative, hypnotic, or anxiolytic use disorder, moderate, with sedative, hypnotic, or anxiolytic-induced bipolar or related disorder

Sedative, hypnotic, or anxiolytic use disorder, moderate, with sedative, hypnotic, or anxiolytic-induced depressive disorder

Sedative, hypnotic, or anxiolytic use disorder, severe, with sedative, hypnotic, or anxiolytic-induced bipolar or related disorder

Sedative, hypnotic, or anxiolytic use disorder, severe, with sedative, hypnotic, or anxiolytic-induced depressive disorder

6 F13.25 **Sedative, hypnotic or anxiolytic dependence with sedative, hypnotic or anxiolytic-induced psychotic disorder**

SP F13.250 **Sedative, hypnotic or anxiolytic dependence with sedative, hypnotic or anxiolytic-induced psychotic disorder with delusions**

SP F13.251 **Sedative, hypnotic or anxiolytic dependence with sedative, hypnotic or anxiolytic-induced psychotic disorder with hallucinations**

SP F13.259 **Sedative, hypnotic or anxiolytic dependence with sedative, hypnotic or anxiolytic-induced psychotic disorder, unspecified**

SP F13.26 **Sedative, hypnotic or anxiolytic dependence with sedative, hypnotic or anxiolytic-induced persisting amnestic disorder**

SP F13.27 **Sedative, hypnotic or anxiolytic dependence with sedative, hypnotic or anxiolytic-induced persisting dementia**

Sedative, hypnotic, or anxiolytic use disorder, moderate, with sedative, hypnotic, or anxiolytic-induced major neurocognitive disorder

Sedative, hypnotic, or anxiolytic use disorder, severe, with sedative, hypnotic, or anxiolytic-induced major neurocognitive disorder

6 F13.28 **Sedative, hypnotic or anxiolytic dependence with other sedative, hypnotic or anxiolytic-induced disorders**

SP F13.280 **Sedative, hypnotic or anxiolytic dependence with sedative, hypnotic or anxiolytic-induced anxiety disorder**

SP F13.281 **Sedative, hypnotic or anxiolytic dependence with sedative, hypnotic or anxiolytic-induced sexual dysfunction**

SP F13.282 **Sedative, hypnotic or anxiolytic dependence with sedative, hypnotic or anxiolytic-induced sleep disorder**

SP F13.288 **Sedative, hypnotic or anxiolytic dependence with other sedative, hypnotic or anxiolytic-induced disorder**

Sedative, hypnotic, or anxiolytic use disorder, moderate, with sedative, hypnotic, or anxiolytic-induced mild neurocognitive disorder

Sedative, hypnotic, or anxiolytic use disorder, severe, with sedative, hypnotic, or anxiolytic-induced mild neurocognitive disorder

SP F13.29 **Sedative, hypnotic or anxiolytic dependence with unspecified sedative, hypnotic or anxiolytic-induced disorder**

5 F13.9 **Sedative, hypnotic or anxiolytic-related use, unspecified**

> **EXCLUDES 1** sedative, hypnotic or anxiolytic-related abuse (F13.1-)
> sedative, hypnotic or anxiolytic-related dependence (F13.2-)

> **CODING TIPS ✓** The use codes are for use of sedative, hypnotic or anxiolytic when associated with (causing) a mental, emotional or physical disorder as documented by the physician. The use codes are not to be used for the patient who uses sedatives, hypnotics or anxiolytics without the additional physician documentation.

> **CODING TIPS ✓** Use disorder is coded to abuse or dependence depending on the severity. Mild is coded to abuse, and moderate and severe are coded to dependence.

SP F13.90 **Sedative, hypnotic, or anxiolytic use, unspecified, uncomplicated**

6 F13.92 **Sedative, hypnotic or anxiolytic use, unspecified with intoxication**

> **EXCLUDES 1** sedative, hypnotic or anxiolytic use, unspecified with withdrawal (F13.93-)

SP F13.920 **Sedative, hypnotic or anxiolytic use, unspecified with intoxication, uncomplicated**

SP F13.921 **Sedative, hypnotic or anxiolytic use, unspecified with intoxication delirium**

Sedative, hypnotic, or anxiolytic-induced delirium

SP F13.929 **Sedative, hypnotic or anxiolytic use, unspecified with intoxication, unspecified**

6 F13.93 **Sedative, hypnotic or anxiolytic use, unspecified with withdrawal**

> **EXCLUDES 1** sedative, hypnotic or anxiolytic use, unspecified with intoxication (F13.92-)

SP F13.930 **Sedative, hypnotic or anxiolytic use, unspecified with withdrawal, uncomplicated**

★ New ▲ Revised Px Primary **SP** PDGM Px **SL** Low CoM **SH** High CoM **IQ** Quest. Encounter **H** Hospice non-cancer Dx Unspecified **M** *Manifestation*

Chapter 5

F01-F99

SP F13.931 Sedative, hypnotic or anxiolytic use, unspecified with withdrawal delirium

SP F13.932 Sedative, hypnotic or anxiolytic use, unspecified with withdrawal with perceptual disturbances

SP F13.939 Sedative, hypnotic or anxiolytic use, unspecified with withdrawal, unspecified

SP F13.94 Sedative, hypnotic or anxiolytic use, unspecified with sedative, hypnotic or anxiolytic-induced mood disorder
Sedative, hypnotic, or anxiolytic-induced bipolar or related disorder, without use disorder
Sedative, hypnotic, or anxiolytic-induced depressive disorder, without use disorder

6 F13.95 Sedative, hypnotic or anxiolytic use, unspecified with sedative, hypnotic or anxiolytic-induced psychotic disorder

SP F13.950 Sedative, hypnotic or anxiolytic use, unspecified with sedative, hypnotic or anxiolytic-induced psychotic disorder with delusions

SP F13.951 Sedative, hypnotic or anxiolytic use, unspecified with sedative, hypnotic or anxiolytic-induced psychotic disorder with hallucinations

SP F13.959 Sedative, hypnotic or anxiolytic use, unspecified with sedative, hypnotic or anxiolytic-induced psychotic disorder, unspecified
Sedative, hypnotic, or anxiolytic-induced psychotic disorder, without use disorder

SP F13.96 Sedative, hypnotic or anxiolytic use, unspecified with sedative, hypnotic or anxiolytic-induced persisting amnestic disorder

SP F13.97 Sedative, hypnotic or anxiolytic use, unspecified with sedative, hypnotic or anxiolytic-induced persisting dementia
Sedative, hypnotic, or anxiolytic-induced major neurocognitive disorder, without use disorder

6 F13.98 Sedative, hypnotic or anxiolytic use, unspecified with other sedative, hypnotic or anxiolytic-induced disorders

SP F13.980 Sedative, hypnotic or anxiolytic use, unspecified with sedative, hypnotic or anxiolytic-induced anxiety disorder
Sedative, hypnotic, or anxiolytic-induced anxiety disorder, without use disorder

SP F13.981 Sedative, hypnotic or anxiolytic use, unspecified with sedative, hypnotic or anxiolytic-induced sexual dysfunction

Sedative, hypnotic, or anxiolytic-induced sexual dysfunction disorder, without use disorder

SP F13.982 Sedative, hypnotic or anxiolytic use, unspecified with sedative, hypnotic or anxiolytic-induced sleep disorder
Sedative, hypnotic, or anxiolytic-induced sleep disorder, without use disorder

SP F13.988 Sedative, hypnotic or anxiolytic use, unspecified with other sedative, hypnotic or anxiolytic-induced disorder
Sedative, hypnotic, or anxiolytic-induced mild neurocognitive disorder

SP F13.99 Sedative, hypnotic or anxiolytic use, unspecified with unspecified sedative, hypnotic or anxiolytic-induced disorder

4 F14   Cocaine related disorders
    EXCLUDES 2   other stimulant-related disorders (F15.-)

5 F14.1   Cocaine abuse
    EXCLUDES 1   cocaine dependence (F14.2-)
                cocaine use, unspecified (F14.9-)

SP F14.10   Cocaine abuse, uncomplicated
Cocaine use disorder, mild

!Q F14.11   Cocaine abuse, in remission
Cocaine use disorder, mild, in early remission
Cocaine use disorder, mild, in sustained remission

6 F14.12   Cocaine abuse with intoxication

SP F14.120   Cocaine abuse with intoxication, uncomplicated

SP F14.121   Cocaine abuse with intoxication with delirium

SP F14.122   Cocaine abuse with intoxication with perceptual disturbance

SP F14.129   Cocaine abuse with intoxication, unspecified

SP F14.14   Cocaine abuse with cocaine-induced mood disorder
Cocaine use disorder, mild, with cocaine-induced bipolar or related disorder
Cocaine use disorder, mild, with cocaine-induced depressive disorder

6 F14.15   Cocaine abuse with cocaine-induced psychotic disorder

SP F14.150   Cocaine abuse with cocaine-induced psychotic disorder with delusions

SP F14.151   Cocaine abuse with cocaine-induced psychotic disorder with hallucinations

SP F14.159   Cocaine abuse with cocaine-induced psychotic disorder, unspecified

6 F14.18   Cocaine abuse with other cocaine-induced disorder

SP F14.180   Cocaine abuse with cocaine-induced anxiety disorder

4 4th digit required   5 5th digit required   6 6th digit required   7 7th digit required   7 7th digit placeholder   + Additional code   ⊟ Laterality

794   *DecisionHealth's* FY 2020 Complete Home Health ICD-10-CM Diagnosis Coding Manual

SP F14.181 Cocaine abuse with cocaine-induced sexual dysfunction

SP F14.182 Cocaine abuse with cocaine-induced sleep disorder

SP F14.188 Cocaine abuse with other cocaine-induced disorder
Cocaine use disorder, mild, with cocaine-induced obsessive compulsive or related disorder

SP F14.19 Cocaine abuse with unspecified cocaine-induced disorder

5 F14.2 Cocaine dependence
> **EXCLUDES 1** cocaine abuse (F14.1-)
> cocaine use, unspecified (F14.9-)
> **EXCLUDES 2** cocaine poisoning (T40.5-)

SP F14.20 Cocaine dependence, uncomplicated
Cocaine use disorder, moderate
Cocaine use disorder, severe

SP F14.21 Cocaine dependence, in remission
Cocaine use disorder, moderate, in early remission
Cocaine use disorder, moderate, in sustained remission
Cocaine use disorder, severe, in early remission
Cocaine use disorder, severe, in sustained remission

6 F14.22 Cocaine dependence with intoxication
> **EXCLUDES 1** cocaine dependence with withdrawal (F14.23)

SP F14.220 Cocaine dependence with intoxication, uncomplicated

SP F14.221 Cocaine dependence with intoxication delirium

SP F14.222 Cocaine dependence with intoxication with perceptual disturbance

SP F14.229 Cocaine dependence with intoxication, unspecified

SP F14.23 Cocaine dependence with withdrawal
> **EXCLUDES 1** cocaine dependence with intoxication (F14.22-)

SP F14.24 Cocaine dependence with cocaine-induced mood disorder
Cocaine use disorder, moderate, with cocaine-induced bipolar or related disorder
Cocaine use disorder, moderate, with cocaine-induced depressive disorder
Cocaine use disorder, severe, with cocaine-induced bipolar or related disorder
Cocaine use disorder, severe, with cocaine-induced depressive disorder

6 F14.25 Cocaine dependence with cocaine-induced psychotic disorder

SP F14.250 Cocaine dependence with cocaine-induced psychotic disorder with delusions

SP F14.251 Cocaine dependence with cocaine-induced psychotic disorder with hallucinations

SP F14.259 Cocaine dependence with cocaine-induced psychotic disorder, unspecified

6 F14.28 Cocaine dependence with other cocaine-induced disorder

SP F14.280 Cocaine dependence with cocaine-induced anxiety disorder

SP F14.281 Cocaine dependence with cocaine-induced sexual dysfunction

SP F14.282 Cocaine dependence with cocaine-induced sleep disorder

SP F14.288 Cocaine dependence with other cocaine-induced disorder
Cocaine use disorder, moderate, with cocaine-induced obsessive compulsive or related disorder
Cocaine use disorder, severe, with cocaine-induced obsessive compulsive or related disorder

SP F14.29 Cocaine dependence with unspecified cocaine-induced disorder

5 F14.9 Cocaine use, unspecified
> **EXCLUDES 1** cocaine abuse (F14.1-)
> cocaine dependence (F14.2-)

> **CODING TIPS ✓** The use codes are for use of cocaine when associated with (causing) a mental, emotional or physical disorder as documented by the physician. The use codes are not to be used for the patient who uses cocaine without the additional physician documentation.

> **CODING TIPS ✓** Use disorder is coded to abuse or dependence depending on the severity. Mild is coded to abuse, and moderate and severe are coded to dependence.

SP F14.90 Cocaine use, unspecified, uncomplicated

6 F14.92 Cocaine use, unspecified with intoxication

SP F14.920 Cocaine use, unspecified with intoxication, uncomplicated

SP F14.921 Cocaine use, unspecified with intoxication delirium

SP F14.922 Cocaine use, unspecified with intoxication with perceptual disturbance

SP F14.929 Cocaine use, unspecified with intoxication, unspecified

SP F14.94 Cocaine use, unspecified with cocaine-induced mood disorder
Cocaine induced bipolar or related disorder, without use disorder
Cocaine induced depressive disorder, without use disorder

6 F14.95 Cocaine use, unspecified with cocaine-induced psychotic disorder

SP F14.950 Cocaine use, unspecified with cocaine-induced psychotic disorder with delusions

SP F14.951 Cocaine use, unspecified with cocaine-induced psychotic disorder with hallucinations

SP F14.959 Cocaine use, unspecified with cocaine-induced psychotic disorder, unspecified

★ New ▲ Revised Px Primary **SP** PDGM Px **SL** Low CoM **SH** High CoM **IQ** Quest. Encounter **H** Hospice non-cancer Dx | Unspecified | **M** *Manifestation*

DecisionHealth's FY 2020 Complete Home Health ICD-10-CM Diagnosis Coding Manual | 795

Cocaine induced psychotic disorder, without use disorder

⑥ F14.98 **Cocaine use, unspecified with other specified cocaine-induced disorder**

SP F14.980 **Cocaine use, unspecified with cocaine-induced anxiety disorder**

Cocaine induced anxiety disorder, without use disorder

SP F14.981 **Cocaine use, unspecified with cocaine-induced sexual dysfunction**

Cocaine induced sexual dysfunction, without use disorder

SP F14.982 **Cocaine use, unspecified with cocaine-induced sleep disorder**

Cocaine induced sleep disorder, without use disorder

SP F14.988 **Cocaine use, unspecified with other cocaine-induced disorder**

Cocaine induced obsessive compulsive or related disorder

SP F14.99 **Cocaine use, unspecified with unspecified cocaine-induced disorder**

④ F15 **Other stimulant related disorders**

INCLUDES amphetamine-related disorders
caffeine

EXCLUDES 2 cocaine-related disorders (F14.-)

CODING TIPS ✓ Use this category of codes for methamphetamines and "bath salts" abuse and dependence.

⑤ F15.1 **Other stimulant abuse**

EXCLUDES 1 other stimulant dependence (F15.2-)
other stimulant use, unspecified (F15.9-)

SP F15.10 **Other stimulant abuse, uncomplicated**

Amphetamine type substance use disorder, mild
Other or unspecified stimulant use disorder, mild

IQ F15.11 **Other stimulant abuse, in remission**

Amphetamine type substance use disorder, mild, in early remission
Amphetamine type substance use disorder, mild, in sustained remission
Other or unspecified stimulant use disorder, mild, in early remission
Other or unspecified stimulant use disorder, mild, in sustained remission

⑥ F15.12 **Other stimulant abuse with intoxication**

SP F15.120 **Other stimulant abuse with intoxication, uncomplicated**

SP F15.121 **Other stimulant abuse with intoxication delirium**

SP F15.122 **Other stimulant abuse with intoxication with perceptual disturbance**

Amphetamine or other stimulant use disorder, mild, with amphetamine or other stimulant intoxication, with perceptual disturbances

SP F15.129 **Other stimulant abuse with intoxication, unspecified**

Amphetamine or other stimulant use disorder, mild, with amphetamine or other stimulant intoxication, without perceptual disturbances

SP F15.14 **Other stimulant abuse with stimulant-induced mood disorder**

Amphetamine or other stimulant use disorder, mild, with amphetamine or other stimulant induced bipolar or related disorder
Amphetamine or other stimulant use disorder, mild, with amphetamine or other stimulant induced depressive disorder

⑥ F15.15 **Other stimulant abuse with stimulant-induced psychotic disorder**

SP F15.150 **Other stimulant abuse with stimulant-induced psychotic disorder with delusions**

SP F15.151 **Other stimulant abuse with stimulant-induced psychotic disorder with hallucinations**

SP F15.159 **Other stimulant abuse with stimulant-induced psychotic disorder, unspecified**

⑥ F15.18 **Other stimulant abuse with other stimulant-induced disorder**

SP F15.180 **Other stimulant abuse with stimulant-induced anxiety disorder**

SP F15.181 **Other stimulant abuse with stimulant-induced sexual dysfunction**

SP F15.182 **Other stimulant abuse with stimulant-induced sleep disorder**

SP F15.188 **Other stimulant abuse with other stimulant-induced disorder**

Amphetamine or other stimulant use disorder, mild, with amphetamine or other stimulant induced obsessive-compulsive or related disorder

SP F15.19 **Other stimulant abuse with unspecified stimulant-induced disorder**

⑤ F15.2 **Other stimulant dependence**

EXCLUDES 1 other stimulant abuse (F15.1-)
other stimulant use, unspecified (F15.9-)

SP F15.20 **Other stimulant dependence, uncomplicated**

Amphetamine type substance use disorder, moderate
Amphetamine type substance use disorder, severe
Other or unspecified stimulant use disorder, moderate
Other or unspecified stimulant use disorder, severe

SP F15.21 **Other stimulant dependence, in remission**

Amphetamine type substance use disorder, moderate, in early remission
Amphetamine type substance use disorder, moderate, in sustained remission

---

④4th digit required   ⑤5th digit required   ⑥6th digit required   ⑦7th digit required   ☑7th digit placeholder   ✚Additional code   ▤Laterality

796   *DecisionHealth's* FY 2020 Complete Home Health ICD-10-CM Diagnosis Coding Manual

Amphetamine type substance use disorder, severe, in early remission

Amphetamine type substance use disorder, severe, in sustained remission

Other or unspecified stimulant use disorder, moderate, in early remission

Other or unspecified stimulant use disorder, moderate, in sustained remission

Other or unspecified stimulant use disorder, severe, in early remission

Other or unspecified stimulant use disorder, severe, in sustained remission

⑥ F15.22 Other stimulant dependence with intoxication

> **EXCLUDES 1** other stimulant dependence with withdrawal (F15.23)

SP F15.220 Other stimulant dependence with intoxication, uncomplicated

SP F15.221 Other stimulant dependence with intoxication delirium

SP F15.222 Other stimulant dependence with intoxication with perceptual disturbance

Amphetamine or other stimulant use disorder, moderate, with amphetamine or other stimulant intoxication, with perceptual disturbances

Amphetamine or other stimulant use disorder, severe, with amphetamine or other stimulant intoxication, with perceptual disturbances

SP F15.229 Other stimulant dependence with intoxication, unspecified

Amphetamine or other stimulant use disorder, moderate, with amphetamine or other stimulant intoxication, without perceptual disturbances

Amphetamine or other stimulant use disorder, severe, with amphetamine or other stimulant intoxication, without perceptual disturbances

SP F15.23 Other stimulant dependence with withdrawal

Amphetamine or other stimulant withdrawal

> **EXCLUDES 1** other stimulant dependence with intoxication (F15.22-)

SP F15.24 Other stimulant dependence with stimulant-induced mood disorder

Amphetamine or other stimulant use disorder, moderate, with amphetamine or other stimulant-induced bipolar or related disorder

Amphetamine or other stimulant use disorder, moderate, with amphetamine or other stimulant induced depressive disorder

Amphetamine or other stimulant use disorder, severe, with amphetamine or other stimulant-induced bipolar or related disorder

Amphetamine or other stimulant use disorder, severe, with amphetamine or other stimulant-induced depressive disorder

⑥ F15.25 Other stimulant dependence with stimulant-induced psychotic disorder

SP F15.250 Other stimulant dependence with stimulant-induced psychotic disorder with delusions

SP F15.251 Other stimulant dependence with stimulant-induced psychotic disorder with hallucinations

SP F15.259 Other stimulant dependence with stimulant-induced psychotic disorder, unspecified

⑥ F15.28 Other stimulant dependence with other stimulant-induced disorder

SP F15.280 Other stimulant dependence with stimulant-induced anxiety disorder

SP F15.281 Other stimulant dependence with stimulant-induced sexual dysfunction

SP F15.282 Other stimulant dependence with stimulant-induced sleep disorder

SP F15.288 Other stimulant dependence with other stimulant-induced disorder

Amphetamine or other stimulant use disorder, moderate, with amphetamine or other stimulant induced obsessive compulsive or related disorder

Amphetamine or other stimulant use disorder, severe, with amphetamine or other stimulant induced obsessive compulsive or related disorder

SP F15.29 Other stimulant dependence with unspecified stimulant-induced disorder

⑤ F15.9 Other stimulant use, unspecified

> **EXCLUDES 1** other stimulant abuse (F15.1-)
> other stimulant dependence (F15.2-)

CODING TIPS ✓ The use codes are for use of other stimulants when associated with (causing) a mental, emotional or physical disorder as documented by the physician. The use codes are not to be used for the patient who uses stimulants without the additional physician documentation.

CODING TIPS ✓ Use disorder is coded to abuse or dependence depending on the severity. Mild is coded to abuse, and moderate and severe are coded to dependence.

SP F15.90 Other stimulant use, unspecified, uncomplicated

⑥ F15.92 Other stimulant use, unspecified with intoxication

★ New ▲ Revised Px Primary SP PDGM Px SL Low CoM SH High CoM IQ Quest. Encounter H Hospice non-cancer Dx Unspecified M *Manifestation*

DecisionHealth's FY 2020 Complete Home Health ICD-10-CM Diagnosis Coding Manual

797

Chapter 5

F01-F99

EXCLUDES 1 other stimulant use,
unspecified with
withdrawal (F15.93)

SP **F15.920** **Other stimulant use, unspecified with intoxication, uncomplicated**

SP **F15.921** **Other stimulant use, unspecified with intoxication delirium**

Amphetamine or other stimulant-
induced delirium

SP **F15.922** **Other stimulant use, unspecified with intoxication with perceptual disturbance**

SP **F15.929** **Other stimulant use, unspecified with intoxication, unspecified**

Caffeine intoxication

SP **F15.93** **Other stimulant use, unspecified with withdrawal**

Caffeine withdrawal

EXCLUDES 1 other stimulant use,
unspecified with
intoxication (F15.92-)

SP **F15.94** **Other stimulant use, unspecified with stimulant-induced mood disorder**

Amphetamine or other stimulant-
induced bipolar or related disorder,
without use disorder
Amphetamine or other stimulant-
induced depressive disorder, without
use disorder

6 **F15.95** **Other stimulant use, unspecified with stimulant-induced psychotic disorder**

SP **F15.950** **Other stimulant use, unspecified with stimulant-induced psychotic disorder with delusions**

SP **F15.951** **Other stimulant use, unspecified with stimulant-induced psychotic disorder with hallucinations**

SP **F15.959** **Other stimulant use, unspecified with stimulant-induced psychotic disorder, unspecified**

Amphetamine or other stimulant-
induced psychotic disorder,
without use disorder

6 **F15.98** **Other stimulant use, unspecified with other stimulant-induced disorder**

SP **F15.980** **Other stimulant use, unspecified with stimulant-induced anxiety disorder**

Amphetamine or other stimulant-
induced anxiety disorder, without
use disorder
Caffeine induced anxiety disorder,
without use disorder

SP **F15.981** **Other stimulant use, unspecified with stimulant-induced sexual dysfunction**

Amphetamine or other stimulant-
induced sexual dysfunction,
without use disorder

SP **F15.982** **Other stimulant use, unspecified with stimulant-induced sleep disorder**

Amphetamine or other stimulant-
induced sleep disorder, without
use disorder
Caffeine induced sleep disorder,
without use disorder

SP **F15.988** **Other stimulant use, unspecified with other stimulant-induced disorder**

Amphetamine or other stimulant-
induced obsessive compulsive or
related disorder, without use
disorder

SP **F15.99** **Other stimulant use, unspecified with unspecified stimulant-induced disorder**

4 **F16** **Hallucinogen related disorders**
INCLUDES ecstasy
PCP
phencyclidine

5 **F16.1** **Hallucinogen abuse**
EXCLUDES 1 hallucinogen dependence
(F16.2-)
hallucinogen use,
unspecified (F16.9-)

SP **F16.10** **Hallucinogen abuse, uncomplicated**
Other hallucinogen use disorder, mild
Phencyclidine use disorder, mild

!Q **F16.11** **Hallucinogen abuse, in remission**
Other hallucinogen use disorder, mild,
in early remission
Other hallucinogen use disorder, mild,
in sustained remission
Phencyclidine use disorder, mild, in
early remission
Phencyclidine use disorder, mild, in
sustained remission

6 **F16.12** **Hallucinogen abuse with intoxication**

SP **F16.120** **Hallucinogen abuse with intoxication, uncomplicated**

SP **F16.121** **Hallucinogen abuse with intoxication with delirium**

SP **F16.122** **Hallucinogen abuse with intoxication with perceptual disturbance**

SP **F16.129** **Hallucinogen abuse with intoxication, unspecified**

SP **F16.14** **Hallucinogen abuse with hallucinogen-induced mood disorder**
Other hallucinogen use disorder, mild,
with other hallucinogen induced
bipolar or related disorder
Other hallucinogen use disorder, mild,
with other hallucinogen induced
depressive disorder
Phencyclidine use disorder, mild, with
phencyclidine induced bipolar or
related disorder
Phencyclidine use disorder, mild, with
phencyclidine induced depressive
disorder

6 **F16.15** **Hallucinogen abuse with hallucinogen-induced psychotic disorder**

SP **F16.150** **Hallucinogen abuse with hallucinogen-induced psychotic disorder with delusions**

---

4 4th digit required   **5** 5th digit required   **6** 6th digit required   **7** 7th digit required   **7** 7th digit placeholder   **+** Additional code   **⊟** Laterality

SP **F16.151** Hallucinogen abuse with hallucinogen-induced psychotic disorder with hallucinations

SP **F16.159** Hallucinogen abuse with hallucinogen-induced psychotic disorder, unspecified

6 **F16.18** Hallucinogen abuse with other hallucinogen-induced disorder

SP **F16.180** Hallucinogen abuse with hallucinogen-induced anxiety disorder

SP **F16.183** Hallucinogen abuse with hallucinogen persisting perception disorder (flashbacks)

SP **F16.188** Hallucinogen abuse with other hallucinogen-induced disorder

SP **F16.19** Hallucinogen abuse with unspecified hallucinogen-induced disorder

5 **F16.2** Hallucinogen dependence

> **EXCLUDES 1** hallucinogen abuse (F16.1-)
> hallucinogen use, unspecified (F16.9-)

SP **F16.20** Hallucinogen dependence, uncomplicated

Other hallucinogen use disorder, moderate

Other hallucinogen use disorder, severe

Phencyclidine use disorder, moderate

Phencyclidine use disorder, severe

SP **F16.21** Hallucinogen dependence, in remission

Other hallucinogen use disorder, moderate, in early remission

Other hallucinogen use disorder, moderate, in sustained remission

Other hallucinogen use disorder, severe, in early remission

Other hallucinogen use disorder, severe, in sustained remission

Phencyclidine use disorder, moderate, in early remission

Phencyclidine use disorder, moderate, in sustained remission

Phencyclidine use disorder, severe, in early remission

Phencyclidine use disorder, severe, in sustained remission

6 **F16.22** Hallucinogen dependence with intoxication

SP **F16.220** Hallucinogen dependence with intoxication, uncomplicated

SP **F16.221** Hallucinogen dependence with intoxication with delirium

SP **F16.229** Hallucinogen dependence with intoxication, unspecified

SP **F16.24** Hallucinogen dependence with hallucinogen-induced mood disorder

Other hallucinogen use disorder, moderate, with other hallucinogen induced bipolar or related disorder

Other hallucinogen use disorder, moderate, with other hallucinogen induced depressive disorder

Other hallucinogen use disorder, severe, with other hallucinogen-induced bipolar or related disorder

Other hallucinogen use disorder, severe, with other hallucinogen-induced depressive disorder

Phencyclidine use disorder, moderate, with phencyclidine induced bipolar or related disorder

Phencyclidine use disorder, moderate, with phencyclidine induced depressive disorder

Phencyclidine use disorder, severe, with phencyclidine induced bipolar or related disorder

Phencyclidine use disorder, severe, with phencyclidine-induced depressive disorder

6 **F16.25** Hallucinogen dependence with hallucinogen-induced psychotic disorder

SP **F16.250** Hallucinogen dependence with hallucinogen-induced psychotic disorder with delusions

SP **F16.251** Hallucinogen dependence with hallucinogen-induced psychotic disorder with hallucinations

SP **F16.259** Hallucinogen dependence with hallucinogen-induced psychotic disorder, unspecified

6 **F16.28** Hallucinogen dependence with other hallucinogen-induced disorder

SP **F16.280** Hallucinogen dependence with hallucinogen-induced anxiety disorder

SP **F16.283** Hallucinogen dependence with hallucinogen persisting perception disorder (flashbacks)

SP **F16.288** Hallucinogen dependence with other hallucinogen-induced disorder

SP **F16.29** Hallucinogen dependence with unspecified hallucinogen-induced disorder

5 **F16.9** Hallucinogen use, unspecified

> **EXCLUDES 1** hallucinogen abuse (F16.1-)
> hallucinogen dependence (F16.2-)

CODING TIPS ✓ The use codes are for use of hallucinogens when associated with (causing) a mental, emotional or physical disorder as documented by the physician. The use codes are not to be used for the patient who uses hallucinogens without the additional physician documentation.

CODING TIPS ✓ Use disorder is coded to abuse or dependence depending on the severity. Mild is coded to abuse, and moderate and severe are coded to dependence.

SP **F16.90** Hallucinogen use, unspecified, uncomplicated

6 **F16.92** Hallucinogen use, unspecified with intoxication

SP **F16.920** Hallucinogen use, unspecified with intoxication, uncomplicated

SP **F16.921** Hallucinogen use, unspecified with intoxication with delirium

Other hallucinogen intoxication delirium

★ New ▲ Revised **Px** Primary **SP** PDGM Px **SL** Low CoM **SH** High CoM **IQ** Quest. Encounter **H** Hospice non-cancer Dx Unspecified **M** *Manifestation*

SP F16.929 **Hallucinogen use, unspecified with intoxication, unspecified**

SP F16.94 **Hallucinogen use, unspecified with hallucinogen-induced mood disorder**

Other hallucinogen induced bipolar or related disorder, without use disorder
Other hallucinogen induced depressive disorder, without use disorder
Phencyclidine induced bipolar or related disorder, without use disorder
Phencyclidine induced depressive disorder, without use disorder

6 F16.95 **Hallucinogen use, unspecified with hallucinogen-induced psychotic disorder**

SP F16.950 **Hallucinogen use, unspecified with hallucinogen-induced psychotic disorder with delusions**

SP F16.951 **Hallucinogen use, unspecified with hallucinogen-induced psychotic disorder with hallucinations**

SP F16.959 **Hallucinogen use, unspecified with hallucinogen-induced psychotic disorder, unspecified**

Other hallucinogen induced psychotic disorder, without use disorder
Phencyclidine induced psychotic disorder, without use disorder

6 F16.98 **Hallucinogen use, unspecified with other specified hallucinogen-induced disorder**

SP F16.980 **Hallucinogen use, unspecified with hallucinogen-induced anxiety disorder**

Other hallucinogen-induced anxiety disorder, without use disorder
Phencyclidine induced anxiety disorder, without use disorder

SP F16.983 **Hallucinogen use, unspecified with hallucinogen persisting perception disorder (flashbacks)**

SP F16.988 **Hallucinogen use, unspecified with other hallucinogen-induced disorder**

SP F16.99 **Hallucinogen use, unspecified with unspecified hallucinogen-induced disorder**

4 F17 **Nicotine dependence**

> **EXCLUDES 1** history of tobacco dependence (Z87.891)
> tobacco use NOS (Z72.0)
> **EXCLUDES 2** tobacco use (smoking) during pregnancy, childbirth and the puerperium (O99.33-)
> toxic effect of nicotine (T65.2-)

> **CODING TIPS ✓** Use disorder, regardless of the severity (mild, moderate or severe), is coded to dependence. There is no separate code to indicate abuse.

5 F17.2 **Nicotine dependence**

CODING TIPS ✓ Use the appropriate code to specify nicotine product when known. ICD-10 codes provide for greater specificity, allowing the coder to specify dependence on a specific nicotine product.

6 F17.20 **Nicotine dependence, unspecified**

SP F17.200 **Nicotine dependence, unspecified, uncomplicated**

Tobacco use disorder, mild
Tobacco use disorder, moderate
Tobacco use disorder, severe

SP F17.201 **Nicotine dependence, unspecified, in remission**

Tobacco use disorder, mild, in early remission
Tobacco use disorder, mild, in sustained remission
Tobacco use disorder, moderate, in early remission
Tobacco use disorder, moderate, in sustained remission
Tobacco use disorder, severe, in early remission
Tobacco use disorder, severe, in sustained remission

SP F17.203 **Nicotine dependence unspecified, with withdrawal**

Tobacco withdrawal

SP F17.208 **Nicotine dependence, unspecified, with other nicotine-induced disorders**

SP F17.209 **Nicotine dependence, unspecified, with unspecified nicotine-induced disorders**

6 F17.21 **Nicotine dependence, cigarettes**

CODING TIPS ✓ If the physician documents "smoker" and indicates that it is cigarettes, e.g. 2ppd, use a code from F17.21.

SP F17.210 **Nicotine dependence, cigarettes, uncomplicated**

CODING TIPS ✓ Assign codes F17.210 and F17.290 for a patient who both smokes cigarettes and uses an electronic cigarette. Only assign F17.290 if a person is only using an e-cigarette or "vaping" when nicotine is used.

CODING TIPS ✓ Use this code if the physician documents "smoker" or tobacco/nicotine dependence and indicates cigarettes.

SP F17.211 **Nicotine dependence, cigarettes, in remission**

Tobacco use disorder, cigarettes, mild, in early remission
Tobacco use disorder, cigarettes, mild, in sustained remission
Tobacco use disorder, cigarettes, moderate, in early remission
Tobacco use disorder, cigarettes, moderate, in sustained remission
Tobacco use disorder, cigarettes, severe, in early remission
Tobacco use disorder, cigarettes, severe, in sustained remission

---

4 4th digit required   **5** 5th digit required   **6** 6th digit required   **7** 7th digit required   **7** 7th digit placeholder   **+** Additional code   **⊟** Laterality

CODING TIPS ✓ The use of the code for remission vs. the code for history (Z87.891) is dependent on the physician's documentation. The ICD-10-CM classifies a history of nicotine dependence differently than other types of drug dependence. Reference the term used by the physician in the alphabetical index.

SP F17.213 Nicotine dependence, cigarettes, with withdrawal

SP F17.218 Nicotine dependence, cigarettes, with other nicotine-induced disorders

CODING TIPS ✓ The physician must link the condition to the smoking to use this code.

SP F17.219 Nicotine dependence, cigarettes, with unspecified nicotine-induced disorders

6 F17.22 Nicotine dependence, chewing tobacco

SP F17.220 Nicotine dependence, chewing tobacco, uncomplicated

SP F17.221 Nicotine dependence, chewing tobacco, in remission
Tobacco use disorder, chewing tobacco, mild, in early remission
Tobacco use disorder, chewing tobacco, mild, in sustained remission
Tobacco use disorder, chewing tobacco, moderate, in early remission
Tobacco use disorder, chewing tobacco, moderate, in sustained remission
Tobacco use disorder, chewing tobacco, severe, in early remission
Tobacco use disorder, chewing tobacco, severe, in sustained remission

SP F17.223 Nicotine dependence, chewing tobacco, with withdrawal

SP F17.228 Nicotine dependence, chewing tobacco, with other nicotine-induced disorders

SP F17.229 Nicotine dependence, chewing tobacco, with unspecified nicotine-induced disorders

6 F17.29 Nicotine dependence, other tobacco product

SP F17.290 Nicotine dependence, other tobacco product, uncomplicated

CODING TIPS ✓ Assign codes F17.210 and F17.290 for a patient who both smokes cigarettes and uses an electronic cigarette. Only assign F17.290 if a person is only using an e-cigarette or "vaping" when nicotine is used.

SP F17.291 Nicotine dependence, other tobacco product, in remission
Tobacco use disorder, other tobacco product, mild, in early remission

Tobacco use disorder, other tobacco product, mild, in sustained remission
Tobacco use disorder, other tobacco product, moderate, in early remission
Tobacco use disorder, other tobacco product, moderate, in sustained remission
Tobacco use disorder, other tobacco product, severe, in early remission
Tobacco use disorder, other tobacco product, severe, in sustained remission

SP F17.293 Nicotine dependence, other tobacco product, with withdrawal

SP F17.298 Nicotine dependence, other tobacco product, with other nicotine-induced disorders

SP F17.299 Nicotine dependence, other tobacco product, with unspecified nicotine-induced disorders

4 F18 Inhalant related disorders
INCLUDES volatile solvents

5 F18.1 Inhalant abuse
EXCLUDES 1 inhalant dependence (F18.2-)
inhalant use, unspecified (F18.9-)

SP F18.10 Inhalant abuse, uncomplicated
Inhalant use disorder, mild

IQ F18.11 Inhalant abuse, in remission
Inhalant use disorder, mild, in early remission
Inhalant use disorder, mild, in sustained remission

6 F18.12 Inhalant abuse with intoxication

SP F18.120 Inhalant abuse with intoxication, uncomplicated

SP F18.121 Inhalant abuse with intoxication delirium

SP F18.129 Inhalant abuse with intoxication, unspecified

SP F18.14 Inhalant abuse with inhalant-induced mood disorder
Inhalant use disorder, mild, with inhalant induced depressive disorder

6 F18.15 Inhalant abuse with inhalant-induced psychotic disorder

SP F18.150 Inhalant abuse with inhalant-induced psychotic disorder with delusions

SP F18.151 Inhalant abuse with inhalant-induced psychotic disorder with hallucinations

SP F18.159 Inhalant abuse with inhalant-induced psychotic disorder, unspecified

SP F18.17 Inhalant abuse with inhalant-induced dementia
Inhalant use disorder, mild, with inhalant induced major neurocognitive disorder

6 F18.18 Inhalant abuse with other inhalant-induced disorders

SP F18.180 Inhalant abuse with inhalant-induced anxiety disorder

✦ New ▲ Revised Px Primary **SP** PDGM Px **SL** Low CoM **SH** High CoM **IQ** Quest. Encounter **H** Hospice non-cancer Dx Unspecified **M** *Manifestation*

DecisionHealth's FY 2020 Complete Home Health ICD-10-CM Diagnosis Coding Manual

801

SP F18.188 Inhalant abuse with other inhalant-induced disorder
Inhalant use disorder, mild, with inhalant induced mild neurocognitive disorder

SP F18.19 Inhalant abuse with unspecified inhalant-induced disorder

5 F18.2 Inhalant dependence
EXCLUDES 1   inhalant abuse (F18.1-)
inhalant use, unspecified (F18.9-)

SP F18.20 Inhalant dependence, uncomplicated
Inhalant use disorder, moderate
Inhalant use disorder, severe

SP F18.21 Inhalant dependence, in remission
Inhalant use disorder, moderate, in early remission
Inhalant use disorder, moderate, in sustained remission
Inhalant use disorder, severe, in early remission
Inhalant use disorder, severe, in sustained remission

6 F18.22 Inhalant dependence with intoxication

SP F18.220 Inhalant dependence with intoxication, uncomplicated

SP F18.221 Inhalant dependence with intoxication delirium

SP F18.229 Inhalant dependence with intoxication, unspecified

SP F18.24 Inhalant dependence with inhalant-induced mood disorder
Inhalant use disorder, moderate, with inhalant induced depressive disorder
Inhalant use disorder, severe, with inhalant induced depressive disorder

6 F18.25 Inhalant dependence with inhalant-induced psychotic disorder

SP F18.250 Inhalant dependence with inhalant-induced psychotic disorder with delusions

SP F18.251 Inhalant dependence with inhalant-induced psychotic disorder with hallucinations

SP F18.259 Inhalant dependence with inhalant-induced psychotic disorder, unspecified

SP F18.27 Inhalant dependence with inhalant-induced dementia
Inhalant use disorder, moderate, with inhalant induced major neurocognitive disorder
Inhalant use disorder, severe, with inhalant induced major neurocognitive disorder

6 F18.28 Inhalant dependence with other inhalant-induced disorders

SP F18.280 Inhalant dependence with inhalant-induced anxiety disorder

SP F18.288 Inhalant dependence with other inhalant-induced disorder
Inhalant use disorder, moderate, with inhalant-induced mild neurocognitive disorder
Inhalant use disorder, severe, with inhalant-induced mild neurocognitive disorder

SP F18.29 Inhalant dependence with unspecified inhalant-induced disorder

5 F18.9 Inhalant use, unspecified
EXCLUDES 1   inhalant abuse (F18.1-)
inhalant dependence (F18.2-)

CODING TIPS ✓   The use codes are for use of inhalants when associated with (causing) a mental, emotional or physical disorder as documented by the physician. The use codes are not to be used for the patient who uses inhalants without the additional physician documentation.

CODING TIPS ✓   Use disorder is coded to abuse or dependence depending on the severity. Mild is coded to abuse, and moderate and severe are coded to dependence.

SP F18.90 Inhalant use, unspecified, uncomplicated

6 F18.92 Inhalant use, unspecified with intoxication

SP F18.920 Inhalant use, unspecified with intoxication, uncomplicated

SP F18.921 Inhalant use, unspecified with intoxication with delirium

SP F18.929 Inhalant use, unspecified with intoxication, unspecified

SP F18.94 Inhalant use, unspecified with inhalant-induced mood disorder
Inhalant induced depressive disorder

6 F18.95 Inhalant use, unspecified with inhalant-induced psychotic disorder

SP F18.950 Inhalant use, unspecified with inhalant-induced psychotic disorder with delusions

SP F18.951 Inhalant use, unspecified with inhalant-induced psychotic disorder with hallucinations

SP F18.959 Inhalant use, unspecified with inhalant-induced psychotic disorder, unspecified

SP F18.97 Inhalant use, unspecified with inhalant-induced persisting dementia
Inhalant-induced major neurocognitive disorder

6 F18.98 Inhalant use, unspecified with other inhalant-induced disorders

SP F18.980 Inhalant use, unspecified with inhalant-induced anxiety disorder

SP F18.988 Inhalant use, unspecified with other inhalant-induced disorder
Inhalant-induced mild neurocognitive disorder

SP F18.99 Inhalant use, unspecified with unspecified inhalant-induced disorder

4 F19 Other psychoactive substance related disorders
INCLUDES   polysubstance drug use (indiscriminate drug use)

5 F19.1 Other psychoactive substance abuse

---

4 4th digit required   5 5th digit required   6 6th digit required   7 7th digit required   ☑ 7th digit placeholder   ✚ Additional code   ⊟ Laterality

802   *DecisionHealth's* FY 2020 Complete Home Health ICD-10-CM Diagnosis Coding Manual

EXCLUDES 1 other psychoactive substance dependence (F19.2-)
other psychoactive substance use, unspecified (F19.9-)

SP **F19.10** **Other psychoactive substance abuse, uncomplicated**
Other (or unknown) substance use disorder, mild

IQ **F19.11** **Other psychoactive substance abuse, in remission**
Other (or unknown) substance use disorder, mild, in early remission
Other (or unknown) substance use disorder, mild, in sustained remission

6 **F19.12** **Other psychoactive substance abuse with intoxication**

SP **F19.120** **Other psychoactive substance abuse with intoxication, uncomplicated**

SP **F19.121** **Other psychoactive substance abuse with intoxication delirium**

SP **F19.122** **Other psychoactive substance abuse with intoxication with perceptual disturbances**

SP **F19.129** **Other psychoactive substance abuse with intoxication, unspecified**

SP **F19.14** **Other psychoactive substance abuse with psychoactive substance-induced mood disorder**
Other (or unknown) substance use disorder, mild, with other (or unknown) substance-induced bipolar or related disorder
Other (or unknown) substance use disorder, mild, with other (or unknown) substance-induced depressive disorder

6 **F19.15** **Other psychoactive substance abuse with psychoactive substance-induced psychotic disorder**

SP **F19.150** **Other psychoactive substance abuse with psychoactive substance-induced psychotic disorder with delusions**

SP **F19.151** **Other psychoactive substance abuse with psychoactive substance-induced psychotic disorder with hallucinations**

SP **F19.159** **Other psychoactive substance abuse with psychoactive substance-induced psychotic disorder, unspecified**

SP **F19.16** **Other psychoactive substance abuse with psychoactive substance-induced persisting amnestic disorder**

SP **F19.17** **Other psychoactive substance abuse with psychoactive substance-induced persisting dementia**
Other (or unknown) substance use disorder, mild, with other (or unknown) substance-induced major neurocognitive disorder

6 **F19.18** **Other psychoactive substance abuse with other psychoactive substance-induced disorders**

SP **F19.180** **Other psychoactive substance abuse with psychoactive substance-induced anxiety disorder**

SP **F19.181** **Other psychoactive substance abuse with psychoactive substance-induced sexual dysfunction**

SP **F19.182** **Other psychoactive substance abuse with psychoactive substance-induced sleep disorder**

SP **F19.188** **Other psychoactive substance abuse with other psychoactive substance-induced disorder**
Other (or unknown) substance use disorder, mild, with other (or unknown) substance induced mild neurocognitive disorder
Other (or unknown) substance use disorder, mild, with other (or unknown) substance induced obsessive-compulsive or related disorder

SP **F19.19** **Other psychoactive substance abuse with unspecified psychoactive substance-induced disorder**

5 **F19.2** **Other psychoactive substance dependence**
EXCLUDES 1 other psychoactive substance abuse (F19.1-)
other psychoactive substance use, unspecified (F19.9-)

SP **F19.20** **Other psychoactive substance dependence, uncomplicated**
Other (or unknown) substance use disorder, moderate
Other (or unknown) substance use disorder, severe

SP **F19.21** **Other psychoactive substance dependence, in remission**
Other (or unknown) substance use disorder, moderate, in early remission
Other (or unknown) substance use disorder, moderate, in sustained remission
Other (or unknown) substance use disorder, severe, in early remission
Other (or unknown) substance use disorder, severe, in sustained remission

6 **F19.22** **Other psychoactive substance dependence with intoxication**
EXCLUDES 1 other psychoactive substance dependence with withdrawal (F19.23-)

SP **F19.220** **Other psychoactive substance dependence with intoxication, uncomplicated**

SP **F19.221** **Other psychoactive substance dependence with intoxication delirium**

SP **F19.222** **Other psychoactive substance dependence with intoxication with perceptual disturbance**

SP **F19.229** **Other psychoactive substance dependence with intoxication, unspecified**

★ New ▲ Revised Px Primary **SP** PDGM Px **SL** Low CoM **SH** High CoM **IQ** Quest. Encounter **H** Hospice non-cancer Dx Unspecified **M** *Manifestation*

DecisionHealth's FY 2020 Complete Home Health ICD-10-CM Diagnosis Coding Manual

803

Chapter 5

F01-F99

⑥ **F19.23** **Other psychoactive substance dependence with withdrawal**

　　EXCLUDES 1　other psychoactive substance dependence with intoxication (F19.22-)

SP **F19.230** **Other psychoactive substance dependence with withdrawal, uncomplicated**

SP **F19.231** **Other psychoactive substance dependence with withdrawal delirium**

SP **F19.232** **Other psychoactive substance dependence with withdrawal with perceptual disturbance**

SP **F19.239** **Other psychoactive substance dependence with withdrawal, unspecified**

SP **F19.24** **Other psychoactive substance dependence with psychoactive substance-induced mood disorder**

Other (or unknown) substance use disorder, moderate, with other (or unknown) substance induced bipolar or related disorder

Other (or unknown) substance use disorder, moderate, with other (or unknown) substance induced depressive disorder

Other (or unknown) substance use disorder, severe, with other (or unknown) substance induced bipolar or related disorder

Other (or unknown) substance use disorder, severe, with other (or unknown) substance induced depressive disorder

⑥ **F19.25** **Other psychoactive substance dependence with psychoactive substance-induced psychotic disorder**

SP **F19.250** **Other psychoactive substance dependence with psychoactive substance-induced psychotic disorder with delusions**

SP **F19.251** **Other psychoactive substance dependence with psychoactive substance-induced psychotic disorder with hallucinations**

SP **F19.259** **Other psychoactive substance dependence with psychoactive substance-induced psychotic disorder, unspecified**

SP **F19.26** **Other psychoactive substance dependence with psychoactive substance-induced persisting amnestic disorder**

SP **F19.27** **Other psychoactive substance dependence with psychoactive substance-induced persisting dementia**

Other (or unknown) substance use disorder, moderate, with other (or unknown) substance induced major neurocognitive disorder

Other (or unknown) substance use disorder, severe, with other (or unknown) substance induced major neurocognitive disorder

⑥ **F19.28** **Other psychoactive substance dependence with other psychoactive substance-induced disorders**

SP **F19.280** **Other psychoactive substance dependence with psychoactive substance-induced anxiety disorder**

SP **F19.281** **Other psychoactive substance dependence with psychoactive substance-induced sexual dysfunction**

SP **F19.282** **Other psychoactive substance dependence with psychoactive substance-induced sleep disorder**

SP **F19.288** **Other psychoactive substance dependence with other psychoactive substance-induced disorder**

Other (or unknown) substance use disorder, moderate, with other (or unknown) substance induced mild neurocognitive disorder

Other (or unknown) substance use disorder, severe, with other (or unknown) substance induced mild neurocognitive disorder

Other (or unknown) substance use disorder, moderate, with other (or unknown) substance induced obsessive compulsive or related disorder

Other (or unknown) substance use disorder, severe, with other (or unknown) substance induced obsessive-compulsive or related disorder

SP **F19.29** **Other psychoactive substance dependence with unspecified psychoactive substance-induced disorder**

⑤ **F19.9** **Other psychoactive substance use, unspecified**

　　EXCLUDES 1　other psychoactive substance abuse (F19.1-)
　　　　other psychoactive substance dependence (F19.2-)

　　CODING TIPS ✓　The use codes are for use of psychoactive substances when associated with (causing) a mental, emotional or physical disorder as documented by the physician. The use codes are not to be used for the patient who uses psychoactive substances without the additional physician documentation.

　　CODING TIPS ✓　Use disorder is coded to abuse or dependence depending on the severity. Mild is coded to abuse, and moderate and severe are coded to dependence.

SP **F19.90** **Other psychoactive substance use, unspecified, uncomplicated**

⑥ **F19.92** **Other psychoactive substance use, unspecified with intoxication**

　　EXCLUDES 1　other psychoactive substance use, unspecified with withdrawal (F19.93)

④4th digit required　　⑤5th digit required　　⑥6th digit required　　⑦7th digit required　　☑7th digit placeholder　　✚Additional code　　⊟Laterality

804　　*DecisionHealth's* FY 2020 Complete Home Health ICD-10-CM Diagnosis Coding Manual

SP F19.920 **Other psychoactive substance use, unspecified with intoxication, uncomplicated**

SP F19.921 **Other psychoactive substance use, unspecified with intoxication with delirium**

Other (or unknown) substance-induced delirium

SP F19.922 **Other psychoactive substance use, unspecified with intoxication with perceptual disturbance**

SP F19.929 **Other psychoactive substance use, unspecified with intoxication, unspecified**

6 F19.93 **Other psychoactive substance use, unspecified with withdrawal**

> **EXCLUDES 1** other psychoactive substance use, unspecified with intoxication (F19.92-)

SP F19.930 **Other psychoactive substance use, unspecified with withdrawal, uncomplicated**

SP F19.931 **Other psychoactive substance use, unspecified with withdrawal delirium**

SP F19.932 **Other psychoactive substance use, unspecified with withdrawal with perceptual disturbance**

SP F19.939 **Other psychoactive substance use, unspecified with withdrawal, unspecified**

SP F19.94 **Other psychoactive substance use, unspecified with psychoactive substance-induced mood disorder**

Other (or unknown) substance-induced bipolar or related disorder, without use disorder

Other (or unknown) substance-induced depressive disorder, without use disorder

6 F19.95 **Other psychoactive substance use, unspecified with psychoactive substance-induced psychotic disorder**

SP F19.950 **Other psychoactive substance use, unspecified with psychoactive substance-induced psychotic disorder with delusions**

SP F19.951 **Other psychoactive substance use, unspecified with psychoactive substance-induced psychotic disorder with hallucinations**

SP F19.959 **Other psychoactive substance use, unspecified with psychoactive substance-induced psychotic disorder, unspecified**

Other or unknown substance-induced psychotic disorder, without use disorder

SP F19.96 **Other psychoactive substance use, unspecified with psychoactive substance-induced persisting amnestic disorder**

SP F19.97 **Other psychoactive substance use, unspecified with psychoactive substance-induced persisting dementia**

Other (or unknown) substance-induced major neurocognitive disorder, without use disorder

6 F19.98 **Other psychoactive substance use, unspecified with other psychoactive substance-induced disorders**

SP F19.980 **Other psychoactive substance use, unspecified with psychoactive substance-induced anxiety disorder**

Other (or unknown) substance-induced anxiety disorder, without use disorder

SP F19.981 **Other psychoactive substance use, unspecified with psychoactive substance-induced sexual dysfunction**

Other (or unknown) substance-induced sexual dysfunction, without use disorder

SP F19.982 **Other psychoactive substance use, unspecified with psychoactive substance-induced sleep disorder**

Other (or unknown) substance-induced sleep disorder, without use disorder

SP F19.988 **Other psychoactive substance use, unspecified with other psychoactive substance-induced disorder**

Other (or unknown) substance-induced mild neurocognitive disorder, without use disorder

Other (or unknown) substance-induced obsessive-compulsive or related disorder, without use disorder

SP F19.99 **Other psychoactive substance use, unspecified with unspecified psychoactive substance-induced disorder**

Schizophrenia, schizotypal, delusional, and other non-mood psychotic disorders (F20-F29)

4 F20 **Schizophrenia**
> **EXCLUDES 1** brief psychotic disorder (F23)
> cyclic schizophrenia (F25.0)
> mood [affective] disorders with psychotic symptoms (F30.2, F31.2, F31.5, F31.64, F32.3, F33.3)
> schizoaffective disorder (F25.-)
> schizophrenic reaction NOS (F23)
>
> **EXCLUDES 2** schizophrenic reaction in:
> alcoholism (F10.15-, F10.25-, F10.95-)
> brain disease (F06.2)
> epilepsy (F06.2)
> psychoactive drug use (F11-F19 with .15. .25, .95)

★ New ▲ Revised Px Primary SP PDGM Px SL Low CoM SH High CoM IQ Quest. Encounter H Hospice non-cancer Dx Unspecified M *Manifestation*

DecisionHealth's FY 2020 Complete Home Health ICD-10-CM Diagnosis Coding Manual

805

schizotypal disorder (F21)

CODING TIPS ✓ Schizophrenia will always impact care so it should be coded. Schizophrenia, as a primary diagnosis, usually requires a psychiatric-trained RN.

SP F20.0 Paranoid schizophrenia
Paraphrenic schizophrenia
EXCLUDES 1 involutional paranoid state (F22)
paranoia (F22)
DEFINITION Schizophrenia marked by displays of megalomania, delusions of persecution and/or grandeur, hallucinations, and aggressive behavior.

SP F20.1 Disorganized schizophrenia
Hebephrenic schizophrenia
Hebephrenia

SP F20.2 Catatonic schizophrenia
Schizophrenic catalepsy
Schizophrenic catatonia
Schizophrenic flexibilitas cerea
EXCLUDES 1 catatonic stupor (R40.1)

SP F20.3 Undifferentiated schizophrenia
Atypical schizophrenia
EXCLUDES 1 acute schizophrenia-like psychotic disorder (F23)
EXCLUDES 2 post-schizophrenic depression (F32.89)

SP F20.5 Residual schizophrenia
Restzustand (schizophrenic)
Schizophrenic residual state

5 F20.8 Other schizophrenia
SP F20.81 Schizophreniform disorder
Schizophreniform psychosis NOS
SP F20.89 Other schizophrenia
Cenesthopathic schizophrenia
Simple schizophrenia

SP F20.9 Schizophrenia, unspecified

SP F21 Schizotypal disorder
Borderline schizophrenia
Latent schizophrenia
Latent schizophrenic reaction
Prepsychotic schizophrenia
Prodromal schizophrenia
Pseudoneurotic schizophrenia
Pseudopsychopathic schizophrenia
Schizotypal personality disorder
EXCLUDES 2 Asperger's syndrome (F84.5)
schizoid personality disorder (F60.1)

CODING TIPS ✓ Do not use code F21 when schizophrenia or schizoaffective disorder is specified by the physician. Schizotypal disorder is a personality disorder characterized by behaviors that impact interpersonal relationships, affect appearance and often exacerbate depressive and/or anxious symptoms.

SP F22 Delusional disorders
Delusional dysmorphophobia
Involutional paranoid state
Paranoia
Paranoia querulans
Paranoid psychosis
Paranoid state
Paraphrenia (late)
Sensitiver Beziehungswahn

EXCLUDES 1 mood [affective] disorders with psychotic symptoms (F30.2, F31.2, F31.5, F31.64, F32.3, F33.3)
paranoid schizophrenia (F20.0)
EXCLUDES 2 paranoid personality disorder (F60.0)
paranoid psychosis, psychogenic (F23)
paranoid reaction (F23)
DEFINITION Paranoia: Extreme, irrational distrust of others.

SP F23 Brief psychotic disorder
Paranoid reaction
Psychogenic paranoid psychosis
EXCLUDES 2 mood [affective] disorders with psychotic symptoms (F30.2, F31.2, F31.5, F31.64, F32.3, F33.3)

SP F24 Shared psychotic disorder
Folie à deux
Induced paranoid disorder
Induced psychotic disorder

4 F25 Schizoaffective disorders
EXCLUDES 1 mood [affective] disorders with psychotic symptoms (F30.2, F31.2, F31.5, F31.64, F32.3, F33.3)
schizophrenia (F20.-)

CODING TIPS ✓ Do not use F25.- codes when schizophrenia is specified by the physician. Schizoaffective disorder is diagnosed in patients who do not meet the criteria for either schizophrenia or bipolar disorder but often demonstrate characteristics of both disorders.

SP F25.0 Schizoaffective disorder, bipolar type
Cyclic schizophrenia
Schizoaffective disorder, manic type
Schizoaffective disorder, mixed type
Schizoaffective psychosis, bipolar type
SP F25.1 Schizoaffective disorder, depressive type
Schizoaffective psychosis, depressive type
SP F25.8 Other schizoaffective disorders
SP F25.9 Schizoaffective disorder, unspecified
Schizoaffective psychosis NOS

SP F28 Other psychotic disorder not due to a substance or known physiological condition
Chronic hallucinatory psychosis
Other specified schizophrenia spectrum and other psychotic disorder

SP F29 Unspecified psychosis not due to a substance or known physiological condition
Psychosis NOS
Unspecified schizophrenia spectrum and other psychotic disorder
EXCLUDES 1 mental disorder NOS (F99)
unspecified mental disorder due to known physiological condition (F09)

Mood [affective] disorders (F30-F39)

4 F30 Manic episode
INCLUDES bipolar disorder, single manic episode
mixed affective episode

---

4 4th digit required   **5** 5th digit required   **6** 6th digit required   **7** 7th digit required   **7** 7th digit placeholder   **+** Additional code   **⊟** Laterality

806   *DecisionHealth's* FY 2020 Complete Home Health ICD-10-CM Diagnosis Coding Manual

EXCLUDES 1 bipolar disorder (F31.-)
major depressive disorder,
single episode (F32.-)
major depressive disorder,
recurrent (F33.-)

⑤ F30.1 Manic episode without psychotic symptoms

SP SH F30.10 Manic episode without psychotic symptoms, unspecified

SP SH F30.11 Manic episode without psychotic symptoms, mild

SP SH F30.12 Manic episode without psychotic symptoms, moderate

SP SH F30.13 Manic episode, severe, without psychotic symptoms

SP SH F30.2 Manic episode, severe with psychotic symptoms
Manic stupor
Mania with mood-congruent psychotic symptoms
Mania with mood-incongruent psychotic symptoms

SP SH F30.3 Manic episode in partial remission

SP SH F30.4 Manic episode in full remission

SP SH F30.8 Other manic episodes
Hypomania

SP SH F30.9 Manic episode, unspecified
Mania NOS

④ F31 Bipolar disorder

INCLUDES bipolar I disorder
bipolar type I disorder
manic-depressive illness
manic-depressive psychosis
manic-depressive reaction

EXCLUDES 1 bipolar disorder, single manic
episode (F30.-)
major depressive disorder,
single episode (F32.-)
major depressive disorder,
recurrent (F33.-)

EXCLUDES 2 cyclothymia (F34.0)

CODING TIPS ✓ When assigning a code for bipolar disorder, no additional code for depression or depressive disorder should be assigned if the patient is also reported to have depression and/or depressive symptoms. Individuals with bipolar disorder may have alternating periods of emotional highs and lows reported as cyclothymic features. When cyclothymic features are additionally reported by the physician, cyclothymia (F34.0) should be additionally coded.

SP SH F31.0 Bipolar disorder, current episode hypomanic

⑤ F31.1 Bipolar disorder, current episode manic without psychotic features

SP SH F31.10 Bipolar disorder, current episode manic without psychotic features, unspecified

SP SH F31.11 Bipolar disorder, current episode manic without psychotic features, mild

SP SH F31.12 Bipolar disorder, current episode manic without psychotic features, moderate

SP SH F31.13 Bipolar disorder, current episode manic without psychotic features, severe

SP SH F31.2 Bipolar disorder, current episode manic severe with psychotic features
Bipolar disorder, current episode manic with mood-congruent psychotic symptoms
Bipolar disorder, current episode manic with mood-incongruent psychotic symptoms
Bipolar I disorder, current or most recent episode manic with psychotic features

⑤ F31.3 Bipolar disorder, current episode depressed, mild or moderate severity

SP SH F31.30 Bipolar disorder, current episode depressed, mild or moderate severity, unspecified

SP SH F31.31 Bipolar disorder, current episode depressed, mild

SP SH F31.32 Bipolar disorder, current episode depressed, moderate

SP SH F31.4 Bipolar disorder, current episode depressed, severe, without psychotic features

SP SH F31.5 Bipolar disorder, current episode depressed, severe, with psychotic features
Bipolar disorder, current episode depressed with mood-incongruent psychotic symptoms
Bipolar disorder, current episode depressed with mood-congruent psychotic symptoms
Bipolar I disorder, current or most recent episode depressed, with psychotic features

⑤ F31.6 Bipolar disorder, current episode mixed

SP SH F31.60 Bipolar disorder, current episode mixed, unspecified

SP SH F31.61 Bipolar disorder, current episode mixed, mild

SP SH F31.62 Bipolar disorder, current episode mixed, moderate

SP SH F31.63 Bipolar disorder, current episode mixed, severe, without psychotic features

SP SH F31.64 Bipolar disorder, current episode mixed, severe, with psychotic features
Bipolar disorder, current episode mixed with mood-congruent psychotic symptoms
Bipolar disorder, current episode mixed with mood-incongruent psychotic symptoms

⑤ F31.7 Bipolar disorder, currently in remission

SP SH F31.70 Bipolar disorder, currently in remission, most recent episode unspecified

SP SH F31.71 Bipolar disorder, in partial remission, most recent episode hypomanic

SP SH F31.72 Bipolar disorder, in full remission, most recent episode hypomanic

SP SH F31.73 Bipolar disorder, in partial remission, most recent episode manic

---

★ New ▲ Revised **Px** Primary **SP** PDGM Px **SL** Low CoM **SH** High CoM **IQ** Quest. Encounter **H** Hospice non-cancer Dx [Unspecified] **M** *Manifestation*

SP **F31.74** **Bipolar disorder, in full remission, most recent episode manic**

SP **F31.75** **Bipolar disorder, in partial remission, most recent episode depressed**

SP **F31.76** **Bipolar disorder, in full remission, most recent episode depressed**

SP **SH** **F31.77** **Bipolar disorder, in partial remission, most recent episode mixed**

SP **SH** **F31.78** **Bipolar disorder, in full remission, most recent episode mixed**

5 **F31.8** **Other bipolar disorders**

SP **SH** **F31.81** **Bipolar II disorder**
Bipolar disorder, type 2

SP **SH** **F31.89** **Other bipolar disorder**
Recurrent manic episodes NOS

SP **SH** **F31.9** **Bipolar disorder, unspecified**
Manic depression

4 **F32** **Major depressive disorder, single episode**

> **INCLUDES** single episode of agitated depression
> single episode of depressive reaction
> single episode of major depression
> single episode of psychogenic depression
> single episode of reactive depression
> single episode of vital depression
>
> **EXCLUDES 1** bipolar disorder (F31.-)
> manic episode (F30.-)
> recurrent depressive disorder (F33.-)
>
> **EXCLUDES 2** adjustment disorder (F43.2)

SP **SH** **F32.0** **Major depressive disorder, single episode, mild**

SP **SH** **F32.1** **Major depressive disorder, single episode, moderate**

SP **SH** **F32.2** **Major depressive disorder, single episode, severe without psychotic features**

SP **F32.3** **Major depressive disorder, single episode, severe with psychotic features**
Single episode of major depression with mood-congruent psychotic symptoms
Single episode of major depression with mood-incongruent psychotic symptoms
Single episode of major depression with psychotic symptoms
Single episode of psychogenic depressive psychosis
Single episode of psychotic depression
Single episode of reactive depressive psychosis

SP **SH** **F32.4** **Major depressive disorder, single episode, in partial remission**

SP **F32.5** **Major depressive disorder, single episode, in full remission**

5 **F32.8** **Other depressive episodes**

SP **F32.81** **Premenstrual dysphoric disorder**
> **EXCLUDES 1** premenstrual tension syndrome (N94.3)

> **DEFINITION** Premenstrual dysphoric disorder (PMDD) is a severe form of premenstrual syndrome (PMS). PMDD is characterized by depression, anxiety, tension and irritability that typically begins after release of the ovum.

SP **SH** **F32.89** **Other specified depressive episodes**
Atypical depression
Post-schizophrenic depression
Single episode of 'masked' depression NOS

SP **SH** **F32.9** **Major depressive disorder, single episode, unspecified**
Depression NOS
Depressive disorder NOS
Major depression NOS

> **CODING TIPS ✓** Documentation:
> Unspecified and chronic depression should be coded to F32.9. A physician must provide confirmation of the diagnosis of depression to assign this code, and it should not be assigned based upon the presence of symptoms alone.

4 **F33** **Major depressive disorder, recurrent**

> **INCLUDES** recurrent episodes of depressive reaction
> recurrent episodes of endogenous depression
> recurrent episodes of major depression
> recurrent episodes of psychogenic depression
> recurrent episodes of reactive depression
> recurrent episodes of seasonal depressive disorder
> recurrent episodes of vital depression
>
> **EXCLUDES 1** bipolar disorder (F31.-)
> manic episode (F30.-)

SP **SH** **F33.0** **Major depressive disorder, recurrent, mild**

SP **SH** **F33.1** **Major depressive disorder, recurrent, moderate**

SP **SH** **F33.2** **Major depressive disorder, recurrent severe without psychotic features**

SP **F33.3** **Major depressive disorder, recurrent, severe with psychotic symptoms**
Endogenous depression with psychotic symptoms
Major depressive disorder, recurrent, with psychotic features
Recurrent severe episodes of major depression with mood-congruent psychotic symptoms
Recurrent severe episodes of major depression with mood-incongruent psychotic symptoms
Recurrent severe episodes of major depression with psychotic symptoms
Recurrent severe episodes of psychogenic depressive psychosis
Recurrent severe episodes of psychotic depression
Recurrent severe episodes of reactive depressive psychosis

5 **F33.4** **Major depressive disorder, recurrent, in remission**

---

4 4th digit required   **5** 5th digit required   **6** 6th digit required   **7** 7th digit required   **7** 7th digit placeholder   **+** Additional code   **⊟** Laterality

808   *DecisionHealth's* FY 2020 Complete Home Health ICD-10-CM Diagnosis Coding Manual

SP **SH** **F33.40** Major depressive disorder, recurrent, in remission, unspecified

SP **SH** **F33.41** Major depressive disorder, recurrent, in partial remission

SP **F33.42** Major depressive disorder, recurrent, in full remission

SP **SH** **F33.8** Other recurrent depressive disorders
Recurrent brief depressive episodes

SP **SH** **F33.9** Major depressive disorder, recurrent, unspecified
Monopolar depression NOS

4 **F34** Persistent mood [affective] disorders

SP **F34.0** Cyclothymic disorder
Affective personality disorder
Cycloid personality
Cyclothymia
Cyclothymic personality
DEFINITION Mild mood swings between elevated mood and mild depression.

SP **F34.1** Dysthymic disorder
Depressive neurosis
Depressive personality disorder
Dysthymia
Neurotic depression
Persistent anxiety depression
Persistent depressive disorder
EXCLUDES 2 anxiety depression (mild or not persistent) (F41.8)

5 **F34.8** Other persistent mood [affective] disorders

SP **SH** **F34.81** Disruptive mood dysregulation disorder

SP **SH** **F34.89** Other specified persistent mood disorders

SP **SH** **F34.9** Persistent mood [affective] disorder, unspecified

SP **SH** **F39** Unspecified mood [affective] disorder
Affective psychosis NOS

Anxiety, dissociative, stress-related, somatoform and other nonpsychotic mental disorders (F40-F48)

4 **F40** Phobic anxiety disorders

5 **F40.0** Agoraphobia

SP **F40.00** Agoraphobia, unspecified

SP **F40.01** Agoraphobia with panic disorder
Panic disorder with agoraphobia
EXCLUDES 1 panic disorder without agoraphobia (F41.0)
DEFINITION Fear of open spaces or crowds, traveling, or leaving a safe place, accompanied by panic attacks.

SP **F40.02** Agoraphobia without panic disorder

5 **F40.1** Social phobias
Anthropophobia
Social anxiety disorder
Social anxiety disorder of childhood
Social neurosis
DEFINITION Intense fear of appearing in public, especially in situations where one is the center of attention.

IQ **F40.10** Social phobia, unspecified

SP **F40.11** Social phobia, generalized

5 **F40.2** Specific (isolated) phobias
EXCLUDES 2 dysmorphophobia (nondelusional) (F45.22)
nosophobia (F45.22)

6 **F40.21** Animal type phobia

SP **F40.210** Arachnophobia
Fear of spiders

SP **F40.218** Other animal type phobia

6 **F40.22** Natural environment type phobia

SP **F40.220** Fear of thunderstorms

SP **F40.228** Other natural environment type phobia

6 **F40.23** Blood, injection, injury type phobia

SP **F40.230** Fear of blood

SP **F40.231** Fear of injections and transfusions

SP **F40.232** Fear of other medical care

SP **F40.233** Fear of injury

6 **F40.24** Situational type phobia

SP **F40.240** Claustrophobia

SP **F40.241** Acrophobia

SP **F40.242** Fear of bridges

SP **F40.243** Fear of flying

SP **F40.248** Other situational type phobia

6 **F40.29** Other specified phobia

SP **F40.290** Androphobia
Fear of men

SP **F40.291** Gynephobia
Fear of women

SP **F40.298** Other specified phobia

SP **F40.8** Other phobic anxiety disorders
Phobic anxiety disorder of childhood

IQ **F40.9** Phobic anxiety disorder, unspecified
Phobia NOS
Phobic state NOS

4 **F41** Other anxiety disorders
EXCLUDES 2 anxiety in:
acute stress reaction (F43.0)
transient adjustment reaction (F43.2)
neurasthenia (F48.8)
psychophysiologic disorders (F45.-)
separation anxiety (F93.0)

SP **F41.0** Panic disorder [episodic paroxysmal anxiety]
Panic attack
Panic state
EXCLUDES 1 panic disorder with agoraphobia (F40.01)
DEFINITION Unexplained bouts of intense fear or anxiety, accompanied by physiological symptoms of elevated heart rate, sweating, trembling, dizziness, and dyspnea.

SP **F41.1** Generalized anxiety disorder
Anxiety neurosis
Anxiety reaction
Anxiety state
Overanxious disorder
EXCLUDES 2 neurasthenia (F48.8)

★ New ▲ Revised ℞ Primary **SP** PDGM Px **SL** Low CoM **SH** High CoM **IQ** Quest. Encounter **H** Hospice non-cancer Dx Unspecified **M** *Manifestation*

DecisionHealth's FY 2020 Complete Home Health ICD-10-CM Diagnosis Coding Manual   809

Chapter 5

F01-F99

DEFINITION Persistent, uncontrollable worry about aspects of a person's life; diagnosed when symptoms last longer than six months, with anxiety present on the majority of days in that time.

SP **F41.3** **Other mixed anxiety disorders**

SP **F41.8** **Other specified anxiety disorders**
Anxiety depression (mild or not persistent)
Anxiety hysteria
Mixed anxiety and depressive disorder
CODING TIPS ✓ **Documentation**: Although the classification does *not* assume a relationship, when the physician documentation specifies depression with anxiety, F41.8 should be assigned. The term "with" is considered a relational term and is interpreted to mean "associated with" or "due to."

SP **F41.9** **Anxiety disorder, unspecified**
Anxiety NOS

4 **F42** **Obsessive-compulsive disorder**
EXCLUDES 2 obsessive-compulsive personality (disorder) (F60.5)
obsessive-compulsive symptoms occurring in depression (F32-F33)
obsessive-compulsive symptoms occurring in schizophrenia (F20.-)
DEFINITION Recurrent obsessions of thought or action that are time-consuming or disruptive to daily life and can produce anxiety or distress.

SP **F42.2** **Mixed obsessional thoughts and acts**

SP **F42.3** **Hoarding disorder**
CODING TIPS ✓ Hoarding disorder must be documented by the physician. The personal and public health consequences of hoarding can be substantial, putting people at risk for fire, falling (especially elderly people), poor sanitation and health risks.

SP **F42.4** **Excoriation (skin-picking) disorder**
EXCLUDES 1 factitial dermatitis (L98.1)
other specified behavioral and emotional disorders with onset usually occurring in early childhood and adolescence (F98.8)
CODING TIPS ✓ Skin picking disorder is defined as recurrent skin picking resulting in skin lesions despite repeated attempts to decrease or stop skin picking. Skin picking also leads to clinically significant distress or disability, and patients with skin picking disorder can have important medical sequelae.

SP **F42.8** **Other obsessive-compulsive disorder**
Anancastic neurosis
Obsessive-compulsive neurosis

SP **F42.9** **Obsessive-compulsive disorder, unspecified**

4 **F43** **Reaction to severe stress, and adjustment disorders**

SP **F43.0** **Acute stress reaction**

Acute crisis reaction
Acute reaction to stress
Combat and operational stress reaction
Combat fatigue
Crisis state
Psychic shock

5 **F43.1** **Post-traumatic stress disorder (PTSD)**
Traumatic neurosis
CODING TIPS ✓ Post-traumatic stress disorder is coded with F43.1 and combat fatigue is coded to F43.0. History of combat and operations stress reaction is coded to Z86.51.
DEFINITION Chronic stressful response to traumatic events such as combat, rape, physical assault, and natural disasters with sudden, powerful memories (flashbacks) of the event, anxiety, and panic.

SP **F43.10** **Post-traumatic stress disorder, unspecified**

SP **F43.11** **Post-traumatic stress disorder, acute**

SP **F43.12** **Post-traumatic stress disorder, chronic**

5 **F43.2** **Adjustment disorders**
Culture shock
Grief reaction
Hospitalism in children
EXCLUDES 2 separation anxiety disorder of childhood (F93.0)

SP **F43.20** **Adjustment disorder, unspecified**

SP **F43.21** **Adjustment disorder with depressed mood**
CODING TIPS ✓ Complicated bereavement is coded to F43.21. Bereavement (uncomplicated) is coded Z63.4.
DEFINITION Prolonged depressive state as a reaction to an event or change in the patient's life.

SP **F43.22** **Adjustment disorder with anxiety**

SP **F43.23** **Adjustment disorder with mixed anxiety and depressed mood**

SP **F43.24** **Adjustment disorder with disturbance of conduct**

SP **F43.25** **Adjustment disorder with mixed disturbance of emotions and conduct**

SP **F43.29** **Adjustment disorder with other symptoms**

SP **F43.8** **Other reactions to severe stress**
Other specified trauma and stressor-related disorder

IQ **F43.9** **Reaction to severe stress, unspecified**
Trauma and stressor-related disorder, NOS

4 **F44** **Dissociative and conversion disorders**
INCLUDES conversion hysteria
conversion reaction
hysteria
hysterical psychosis
EXCLUDES 2 malingering [conscious simulation] (Z76.5)

SP **F44.0** **Dissociative amnesia**
EXCLUDES 1 amnesia NOS (R41.3)
anterograde amnesia (R41.1)
dissociative amnesia with dissociative fugue (F44.1)

---

4 4th digit required   **5** 5th digit required   **6** 6th digit required   **7** 7th digit required   **7** 7th digit placeholder   **+** Additional code   **⊟** Laterality

retrograde amnesia (R41.2)

EXCLUDES 2 alcohol-or other
psychoactive substance-
induced amnestic disorder
(F10, F13, F19 with .26,
.96)
amnestic disorder due to
known physiological
condition (F04)
postictal amnesia in epilepsy
(G40.-)

DEFINITION Psychological trauma
causing temporary forgetting of personal
information and inability to perform complex
tasks, like driving or cooking.

SP F44.1 Dissociative fugue
Dissociative amnesia with dissociative
fugue
EXCLUDES 2 postictal fugue in epilepsy
(G40.-)

DEFINITION Disorder occurring in
response to a severe, recent stressor, in
which the patient invents a new personality
and becomes unable to remember his/her
previous identity, lasting days or months.

SP F44.2 Dissociative stupor
EXCLUDES 1 catatonic stupor (R40.1)
stupor NOS (R40.1)
EXCLUDES 2 catatonic disorder due to
known physiological
condition (F06.1)
depressive stupor (F32, F33)
manic stupor (F30, F31)

**SP F44.4 Conversion disorder with motor
symptom or deficit**
Conversion disorder with abnormal
movement
Conversion disorder with speech
symptoms
Conversion disorder with swallowing
symptoms
Conversion disorder with
weakness/paralysis
Dissociative motor disorders
Psychogenic aphonia
Psychogenic dysphonia

**SP F44.5 Conversion disorder with seizures or
convulsions**
Conversion disorder with attacks or
seizures
Dissociative convulsions

**SP F44.6 Conversion disorder with sensory
symptom or deficit**
Conversion disorder with anesthesia or
sensory loss
Conversion disorder with special sensory
symptoms
Dissociative anesthesia and sensory loss
Psychogenic deafness

**SP F44.7 Conversion disorder with mixed
symptom presentation**

**5 F44.8 Other dissociative and conversion
disorders**

SP F44.81 Dissociative identity disorder
Multiple personality disorder

**SP F44.89 Other dissociative and conversion
disorders**
Ganser's syndrome

Psychogenic confusion
Psychogenic twilight state
Trance and possession disorders

**SP F44.9 Dissociative and conversion disorder,
unspecified**
Dissociative disorder NOS

4 F45 Somatoform disorders
EXCLUDES 2 dissociative and conversion
disorders (F44.-)
factitious disorders
(F68.1-, F68.A)
hair-plucking (F63.3)
lalling (F80.0)
lisping (F80.0)
malingering [conscious
simulation] (Z76.5)
nail-biting (F98.8)
psychological or behavioral
factors associated with
disorders or diseases
classified elsewhere (F54)
sexual dysfunction, not due to a
substance or known
physiological condition
(F52.-)
thumb-sucking (F98.8)
tic disorders
(in childhood and
adolescence) (F95.-)
Tourette's syndrome (F95.2)
trichotillomania (F63.3)

SP F45.0 Somatization disorder
Briquet's disorder
Multiple psychosomatic disorder

SP F45.1 Undifferentiated somatoform disorder
Somatic symptom disorder
Undifferentiated psychosomatic disorder

5 F45.2 Hypochondriacal disorders
EXCLUDES 2 delusional dysmorphophobia
(F22)
fixed delusions about bodily
functions or shape (F22)

DEFINITION Chronic worry about
nonexistent illnesses that one believes one
may have.

**SP F45.20 Hypochondriacal disorder,
unspecified**

SP F45.21 Hypochondriasis
Hypochondriacal neurosis
Illness anxiety disorder

SP F45.22 Body dysmorphic disorder
Dysmorphophobia (nondelusional)
Nosophobia

SP F45.29 Other hypochondriacal disorders

**5 F45.4 Pain disorders related to psychological
factors**
EXCLUDES 1 pain NOS (R52)

**SP F45.41 Pain disorder exclusively related to
psychological factors**
Somatoform pain disorder (persistent)
GUIDELINES Section I.C.5.a
Assign code F45.41 for pain that is
exclusively related to psychological
disorders. As indicated by the Excludes
1 note under category G89, a code from
category G89 should not be assigned
with code F45.41.

★ New ▲ Revised **Px** Primary **SP** PDGM Px **SL** Low CoM **SH** High CoM **IQ** Quest. Encounter **H** Hospice non-cancer Dx Unspecified **M** *Manifestation*

DecisionHealth's FY 2020 Complete Home Health ICD-10-CM Diagnosis Coding Manual

811

CODING TIPS ✓   Do not use F45.41 to report somatoform disorder not related to pain, chronic pain syndrome, or psychological factors related to chronic pain disorders (G89.-, F45.42).

SP F45.42   Pain disorder with related psychological factors
Code also:
    associated acute or chronic pain (G89.-)

GUIDELINES   Section I.C.5.a
Code F45.42 should be used with a code from category G89, Pain, not elsewhere classified, if there is documentation of a psychological component for a patient with acute or chronic pain.

CODING TIPS ✓   When the clinical record specifies that the patient has a pain disorder with related psychological factors, this code should be additionally assigned.

SP F45.8   Other somatoform disorders
Psychogenic dysmenorrhea
Psychogenic dysphagia, including 'globus hystericus'
Psychogenic pruritus
Psychogenic torticollis
Somatoform autonomic dysfunction
Teeth grinding
EXCLUDES 1   sleep related teeth grinding (G47.63)

SP F45.9   Somatoform disorder, unspecified
Psychosomatic disorder NOS

4 F48   Other nonpsychotic mental disorders

SP F48.1   Depersonalization-derealization syndrome

SP F48.2   Pseudobulbar affect
Involuntary emotional expression disorder
Code first underlying cause, if known, such as:
    amyotrophic lateral sclerosis (G12.21)
    multiple sclerosis (G35)
    sequelae of cerebrovascular disease (I69.-)
    sequelae of traumatic intracranial injury (S06.-)
CODING TIPS ✓   This is an example of a convention in opposition to a guideline. The guideline says to code the residual condition first followed by the sequela. In this case, the convention states to code first the sequelae of traumatic intracranial injury. The convention is followed.

SP F48.8   Other specified nonpsychotic mental disorders
Dhat syndrome
Neurasthenia
Occupational neurosis, including writer's cramp
Psychasthenia
Psychasthenic neurosis
Psychogenic syncope

SP F48.9   Nonpsychotic mental disorder, unspecified
Neurosis NOS

Behavioral syndromes associated with physiological disturbances and physical factors (F50-F59)

4 F50   Eating disorders
EXCLUDES 1   anorexia NOS (R63.0)
    feeding difficulties (R63.3)
    feeding problems of newborn (P92.-)
    polyphagia (R63.2)
EXCLUDES 2   feeding disorder in infancy or childhood (F98.2-)

5 F50.0   Anorexia nervosa
EXCLUDES 1   loss of appetite (R63.0)
    psychogenic loss of appetite (F50.89)
CODING TIPS ✓   This code can be assigned only if specified as "anorexia nervosa," which is differentiated from simple anorexia (loss of appetite) due to psychological features, including intense fear of weight gain, body image distortions, and a refusal to maintain normal body weight.

SP F50.00   Anorexia nervosa, unspecified

SP F50.01   Anorexia nervosa, restricting type

SP F50.02   Anorexia nervosa, binge eating/purging type
EXCLUDES 1   bulimia nervosa (F50.2)

SP F50.2   Bulimia nervosa
Bulimia NOS
Hyperorexia nervosa
EXCLUDES 1   anorexia nervosa, binge eating/purging type (F50.02)
DEFINITION   Repetitive episodes of binge eating followed by excessive measures to avoid gaining weight, such as self-induced vomiting and extreme exercising.

5 F50.8   Other eating disorders
EXCLUDES 2   pica of infancy and childhood (F98.3)

SP F50.81   Binge eating disorder

SP F50.82   Avoidant/restrictive food intake disorder

SP F50.89   Other specified eating disorder
Pica in adults
Psychogenic loss of appetite
CODING TIPS ✓   Psychogenic loss of appetite may explain the patient's refusal to eat and be used in addition to, or instead of, malnutrition to better explain the patient's loss of weight and further decline.

DEFINITION   This code includes pica in adults. Pica is the urge to eat nonfood substances, such as dirt, paper, paint, and rocks. It also includes the psychogenic loss of appetite characterized by an aversion to food or eating with no pathologic or physiologic explanation.

SP F50.9   Eating disorder, unspecified
Atypical anorexia nervosa
Atypical bulimia nervosa
Feeding or eating disorder, unspecified
Other specified feeding disorder

---

4 4th digit required   **5** 5th digit required   **6** 6th digit required   **7** 7th digit required   **7** 7th digit placeholder   **+** Additional code   **⊟** Laterality

4 F51   Sleep disorders not due to a substance or known physiological condition
    EXCLUDES 2   organic sleep disorders (G47.-)

5 F51.0   Insomnia not due to a substance or known physiological condition
    EXCLUDES 2   alcohol related insomnia
                (F10.182, F10.282,
                F10.982)
            drug-related insomnia
                (F11.182, F11.282,
                F11.982, F13.182,
                F13.282, F13.982,
                F14.182, F14.282,
                F14.982, F15.182,
                F15.282, F15.982,
                F19.182, F19.282,
                F19.982)
            insomnia NOS (G47.0-)
            insomnia due to known
                physiological condition
                (G47.0-)
            organic insomnia (G47.0-)
            sleep deprivation (Z72.820)

SP F51.01   Primary insomnia
    Idiopathic insomnia

SP F51.02   Adjustment insomnia

SP F51.03   Paradoxical insomnia

SP F51.04   Psychophysiologic insomnia

SP F51.05   Insomnia due to other mental disorder
    Code also:
        associated mental disorder

SP F51.09   Other insomnia not due to a substance or known physiological condition

5 F51.1   Hypersomnia not due to a substance or known physiological condition
    EXCLUDES 2   alcohol related hypersomnia
                (F10.182, F10.282,
                F10.982)
            drug-related hypersomnia
                (F11.182, F11.282,
                F11.982, F13.182,
                F13.282, F13.982,
                F14.182, F14.282,
                F14.982, F15.182,
                F15.282, F15.982,
                F19.182, F19.282,
                F19.982)
            hypersomnia NOS (G47.10)
            hypersomnia due to known
                physiological condition
                (G47.10)
            idiopathic hypersomnia
                (G47.11, G47.12)
            narcolepsy (G47.4-)

SP F51.11   Primary hypersomnia

SP F51.12   Insufficient sleep syndrome
    EXCLUDES 1   sleep deprivation
                (Z72.820)

SP F51.13   Hypersomnia due to other mental disorder
    Code also:
        associated mental disorder

SP F51.19   Other hypersomnia not due to a substance or known physiological condition

SP F51.3   Sleepwalking [somnambulism]
    Non-rapid eye movement sleep arousal
        disorders, sleepwalking type

SP F51.4   Sleep terrors [night terrors]
    Non-rapid eye movement sleep arousal
        disorders, sleep terror type

SP F51.5   Nightmare disorder
    Dream anxiety disorder

SP F51.8   Other sleep disorders not due to a substance or known physiological condition

SP F51.9   Sleep disorder not due to a substance or known physiological condition, unspecified
    Emotional sleep disorder NOS

4 F52   Sexual dysfunction not due to a substance or known physiological condition
    EXCLUDES 2   Dhat syndrome (F48.8)

SP F52.0   Hypoactive sexual desire disorder
    Lack or loss of sexual desire
    Male hypoactive sexual desire disorder
    Sexual anhedonia
    EXCLUDES 1   decreased libido (R68.82)
    DEFINITION   Markedly decreased sexual
    desire.

SP F52.1   Sexual aversion disorder
    Sexual aversion and lack of sexual
        enjoyment

5 F52.2   Sexual arousal disorders
    Failure of genital response

SP F52.21   Male erectile disorder
    Erectile disorder
    Psychogenic impotence
    EXCLUDES 1   impotence of organic
                origin (N52.-)
            impotence NOS (N52.-)

SP F52.22   Female sexual arousal disorder
    Female sexual interest/arousal disorder

5 F52.3   Orgasmic disorder
    Inhibited orgasm
    Psychogenic anorgasmy

SP F52.31   Female orgasmic disorder

SP F52.32   Male orgasmic disorder
    Delayed ejaculation

SP F52.4   Premature ejaculation

SP F52.5   Vaginismus not due to a substance or known physiological condition
    Psychogenic vaginismus
    EXCLUDES 2   vaginismus
                (due to a known
                physiological condition)
                (N94.2)

SP F52.6   Dyspareunia not due to a substance or known physiological condition
    Genito-pelvic pain penetration disorder
    Psychogenic dyspareunia
    EXCLUDES 2   dyspareunia
                (due to a known
                physiological condition)
                (N94.1-)

SP F52.8   Other sexual dysfunction not due to a substance or known physiological condition
    Excessive sexual drive
    Nymphomania
    Satyriasis

★ New ▲ Revised Px Primary SP PDGM Px SL Low CoM SH High CoM IQ Quest. Encounter H Hospice non-cancer Dx Unspecified M Manifestation

DecisionHealth's FY 2020 Complete Home Health ICD-10-CM Diagnosis Coding Manual   813

Chapter 5

F01-F99

SP **F52.9** **Unspecified sexual dysfunction not due to a substance or known physiological condition**
Sexual dysfunction NOS

4 **F53** **Mental and behavioral disorders associated with the puerperium, not elsewhere classified**
EXCLUDES 1 mood disorders with psychotic features
(F30.2, F31.2, F31.5, F31.64, F32.3, F33.3)
postpartum dysphoria (O90.6)
psychosis in schizophrenia, schizotypal, delusional, and other psychotic disorders (F20-F29)

SP **F53.0** **Postpartum depression**
Postnatal depression, NOS
Postpartum depression, NOS

SP **F53.1** **Puerperal psychosis**
Postpartum psychosis
Puerperal psychosis, NOS

SP **F54** **Psychological and behavioral factors associated with disorders or diseases classified elsewhere**
Psychological factors affecting physical conditions
Code first the associated physical disorder, such as:
asthma (J45.-)
dermatitis (L23-L25)
gastric ulcer (K25.-)
mucous colitis (K58.-)
ulcerative colitis (K51.-)
urticaria (L50.-)
EXCLUDES 2 tension-type headache (G44.2)

CODING TIPS ✓ Assign code F54 when a psychological condition causes exacerbation of a specific physical condition, such as asthma or ulcers. This code may not be used alone, and documentation should specify that the psychological condition has caused exacerbation of the physical state. Code the physical condition first, followed by F54.

4 **F55** **Abuse of non-psychoactive substances**
EXCLUDES 2 abuse of psychoactive substances (F10-F19)

SP **F55.0** **Abuse of antacids**

SP **F55.1** **Abuse of herbal or folk remedies**

SP **F55.2** **Abuse of laxatives**

SP **F55.3** **Abuse of steroids or hormones**

SP **F55.4** **Abuse of vitamins**

SP **F55.8** **Abuse of other non-psychoactive substances**

SP **F59** **Unspecified behavioral syndromes associated with physiological disturbances and physical factors**
Psychogenic physiological dysfunction NOS
CODING TIPS ✓ Do not use F59 to report psychosomatic disorder. Psychosomatic disorder has a specific code and should be coded to F45.9.

Disorders of adult personality and behavior (F60-F69)

4 **F60** **Specific personality disorders**

SP **F60.0** **Paranoid personality disorder**
Expansive paranoid personality (disorder)
Fanatic personality (disorder)
Querulant personality (disorder)
Paranoid personality (disorder)
Sensitive paranoid personality (disorder)
EXCLUDES 2 paranoia (F22)
paranoia querulans (F22)
paranoid psychosis (F22)
paranoid schizophrenia (F20.0)
paranoid state (F22)

SP **F60.1** **Schizoid personality disorder**
EXCLUDES 2 Asperger's syndrome (F84.5)
delusional disorder (F22)
schizoid disorder of childhood (F84.5)
schizophrenia (F20.-)
schizotypal disorder (F21)

SP **F60.2** **Antisocial personality disorder**
Amoral personality (disorder)
Asocial personality (disorder)
Dissocial personality disorder
Psychopathic personality (disorder)
Sociopathic personality (disorder)
EXCLUDES 1 conduct disorders (F91.-)
EXCLUDES 2 borderline personality disorder (F60.3)

SP **F60.3** **Borderline personality disorder**
Aggressive personality (disorder)
Emotionally unstable personality disorder
Explosive personality (disorder)
EXCLUDES 2 antisocial personality disorder (F60.2)

DEFINITION Disorder in which a person is quick to anger, aggressive, abnormally emotional, and argumentative.

SP **F60.4** **Histrionic personality disorder**
Hysterical personality (disorder)
Psychoinfantile personality (disorder)

SP **F60.5** **Obsessive-compulsive personality disorder**
Anankastic personality (disorder)
Compulsive personality (disorder)
Obsessional personality (disorder)
EXCLUDES 2 obsessive-compulsive disorder (F42-)

SP **F60.6** **Avoidant personality disorder**
Anxious personality disorder

SP **F60.7** **Dependent personality disorder**
Asthenic personality (disorder)
Inadequate personality (disorder)
Passive personality (disorder)

5 **F60.8** **Other specific personality disorders**

SP **F60.81** **Narcissistic personality disorder**

SP **F60.89** **Other specific personality disorders**
Eccentric personality disorder
'Haltlose' type personality disorder
Immature personality disorder
Passive-aggressive personality disorder
Psychoneurotic personality disorder
Self-defeating personality disorder

---

4 4th digit required   **5** 5th digit required   **6** 6th digit required   **7** 7th digit required   **7** 7th digit placeholder   **+** Additional code   **=** Laterality

814   DecisionHealth's FY 2020 Complete Home Health ICD-10-CM Diagnosis Coding Manual

SP F60.9 **Personality disorder, unspecified**
Character disorder NOS
Character neurosis NOS
Pathological personality NOS

4 F63 **Impulse disorders**
> EXCLUDES 2 habitual excessive use of alcohol or psychoactive substances (F10-F19)
> impulse disorders involving sexual behavior (F65.-)

SP F63.0 **Pathological gambling**
Compulsive gambling
Gambling disorder
> EXCLUDES 1 gambling and betting NOS (Z72.6)
> EXCLUDES 2 excessive gambling by manic patients (F30, F31)
> gambling in antisocial personality disorder (F60.2)

SP F63.1 **Pyromania**
Pathological fire-setting
> EXCLUDES 2 fire-setting (by) (in):
> adult with antisocial personality disorder (F60.2)
> alcohol or psychoactive substance intoxication (F10-F19)
> conduct disorders (F91.-)
> mental disorders due to known physiological condition (F01-F09)
> schizophrenia (F20.-)
> DEFINITION Uncontrollable impulse to set fires.

SP F63.2 **Kleptomania**
Pathological stealing
> EXCLUDES 1 shoplifting as the reason for observation for suspected mental disorder (Z03.8)
> EXCLUDES 2 depressive disorder with stealing (F31-F33)
> stealing due to underlying mental condition-code to mental condition
> stealing in mental disorders due to known physiological condition (F01-F09)
> DEFINITION Irresistible impulse to steal.

SP F63.3 **Trichotillomania**
Hair plucking
> EXCLUDES 2 other stereotyped movement disorder (F98.4)

5 F63.8 **Other impulse disorders**

SP F63.81 **Intermittent explosive disorder**

SP F63.89 **Other impulse disorders**

SP F63.9 **Impulse disorder, unspecified**
Impulse control disorder NOS

4 F64 **Gender identity disorders**

SP F64.0 **Transsexualism**
Gender identity disorder in adolescence and adulthood
Gender dysphoria in adolescents and adults

SP + F64.1 **Dual role transvestism**

Use additional code to identify sex reassignment status (Z87.890)
> EXCLUDES 1 gender identity disorder in childhood (F64.2)
> EXCLUDES 2 fetishistic transvestism (F65.1)

SP F64.2 **Gender identity disorder of childhood**
Gender dysphoria in children
> EXCLUDES 1 gender identity disorder in adolescence and adulthood (F64.0)
> EXCLUDES 2 sexual maturation disorder (F66)

SP F64.8 **Other gender identity disorders**
Other specified gender dysphoria

SP F64.9 **Gender identity disorder, unspecified**
Gender dysphoria, unspecified
Gender-role disorder NOS

4 F65 **Paraphilias**

SP F65.0 **Fetishism**
Fetishistic disorder

SP F65.1 **Transvestic fetishism**
Fetishistic transvestism
Transvestic disorder

SP F65.2 **Exhibitionism**
Exhibitionistic disorder
> DEFINITION Compulsion to expose genitals in public.

SP F65.3 **Voyeurism**
Voyeuristic disorder
> DEFINITION Uncontrollable compulsion to covertly observe others who are nude or engaged in sexual activity.

SP F65.4 **Pedophilia**
Pedophilic disorder

5 F65.5 **Sadomasochism**

SP F65.50 **Sadomasochism, unspecified**

SP F65.51 **Sexual masochism**
Sexual masochism disorder
> DEFINITION Psychosexual disorder marked by the need to be humiliated or hurt to achieve sexual gratification.

SP F65.52 **Sexual sadism**
Sexual sadism disorder
> DEFINITION Psychosexual disorder marked by the need to humiliate or injure others to achieve sexual gratification.

5 F65.8 **Other paraphilias**

SP F65.81 **Frotteurism**
Frotteuristic disorder

SP F65.89 **Other paraphilias**
Necrophilia
Other specified paraphilic disorder
> DEFINITION Sexual attraction to corpses.

SP F65.9 **Paraphilia, unspecified**
Paraphilic disorder, unspecified
Sexual deviation NOS

SP F66 **Other sexual disorders**
Sexual maturation disorder
Sexual relationship disorder

4 F68 **Other disorders of adult personality and behavior**

5 F68.1 **Factitious disorder imposed on self**

★ New ▲ Revised **Px** Primary **SP** PDGM Px **SL** Low CoM **SH** High CoM **IQ** Quest. Encounter **H** Hospice non-cancer Dx | Unspecified | **M** *Manifestation*

Compensation neurosis
Elaboration of physical symptoms for
psychological reasons
Hospital hopper syndrome
Münchausen's syndrome
Peregrinating patient
> **EXCLUDES 2** factitial dermatitis (L98.1)
> person feigning illness
> (with obvious motivation)
> (Z76.5)

SP **F68.10** **Factitious disorder imposed on self,
unspecified**

SP **F68.11** **Factitious disorder imposed on self,
with predominantly psychological
signs and symptoms**

SP **F68.12** **Factitious disorder imposed on self,
with predominantly physical signs
and symptoms**

SP **F68.13** **Factitious disorder imposed on self,
with combined psychological and
physical signs and symptoms**

SP **F68.A** **Factitious disorder imposed on another**
Factitious disorder by proxy
Münchausen's by proxy

SP **F68.8** **Other specified disorders of adult
personality and behavior**

IQ **F69** **Unspecified disorder of adult personality
and behavior**

Intellectual Disabilities   (F70-F79)

Code first:
   any associated physical or developmental disorders
> **EXCLUDES 1** borderline intellectual functioning, IQ above 70
> to 84 (R41.83)

CODING TIPS ✓ When IQ is specified, use the appropriate code
from F70-F79 to specify level of intellectual disability based upon
reported IQ. When developmental delays or disorders are
additionally noted in a patient with Intellectual disability, these
should be coded first.

SP **F70** **Mild intellectual disabilities**
IQ level 50-55 to approximately 70
Mild mental subnormality

SP **F71** **Moderate intellectual disabilities**
IQ level 35-40 to 50-55
Moderate mental subnormality

SP **F72** **Severe intellectual disabilities**
IQ 20-25 to 35-40
Severe mental subnormality

SP **F73** **Profound intellectual disabilities**
IQ level below 20-25
Profound mental subnormality

SP **F78** **Other intellectual disabilities**

SP **F79** **Unspecified intellectual disabilities**
Mental deficiency NOS
Mental subnormality NOS

Pervasive and specific developmental
disorders   (F80-F89)

CODING TIPS ✓ Disorders coded to categories F80-F89 should be
specified as related to a developmental origin.

4 **F80** **Specific developmental disorders of speech
and language**

SP **F80.0** **Phonological disorder**
Dyslalia
Functional speech articulation disorder

Lalling
Lisping
Phonological developmental disorder
Speech articulation developmental disorder
Speech-sound disorder
> **EXCLUDES 1** speech articulation
> impairment due to aphasia
> NOS (R47.01)
> speech articulation
> impairment due to apraxia
> (R48.2)
> **EXCLUDES 2** speech articulation
> impairment due to hearing
> loss (F80.4)
> speech articulation
> impairment due to
> intellectual disabilities
> (F70-F79)
> speech articulation
> impairment with
> expressive language
> developmental disorder
> (F80.1)
> speech articulation
> impairment with mixed
> receptive expressive
> language developmental
> disorder (F80.2)

CODING TIPS ✓ Lisping, lalling, dyslalia and
phonological disorder are classified to the
same code, F80.0. Coders should also
carefully note the multiple Excludes 1 and 2
notes for this code to ensure any additional
speech articulation disorders are correctly
coded, when applicable.

SP **F80.1** **Expressive language disorder**
Developmental dysphasia or aphasia,
expressive type
> **EXCLUDES 1** mixed receptive-expressive
> language disorder (F80.2)
> dysphasia and aphasia NOS
> (R47.-)
> **EXCLUDES 2** acquired aphasia with
> epilepsy [Landau-Kleffner]
> (G40.80-)
> selective mutism (F94.0)
> intellectual disabilities
> (F70-F79)
> pervasive developmental
> disorders (F84.-)

CODING TIPS ✓ Language disorders should
not be coded here unless specified as
related to a developmental cause.

SP **F80.2** **Mixed receptive-expressive language
disorder**
Developmental dysphasia or aphasia,
receptive type
Developmental Wernicke's aphasia
> **EXCLUDES 1** central auditory processing
> disorder (H93.25)
> dysphasia or aphasia NOS
> (R47.-)
> expressive language disorder
> (F80.1)
> expressive type dysphasia or
> aphasia (F80.1)
> word deafness (H93.25)

---

4 4th digit required   **5** 5th digit required   **6** 6th digit required   **7** 7th digit required   **7** 7th digit placeholder   **+** Additional code   **⊟** Laterality

EXCLUDES 2 acquired aphasia with epilepsy [Landau-Kleffner] (G40.80-)
pervasive developmental disorders (F84.-)
selective mutism (F94.0)
intellectual disabilities (F70-F79)

DEFINITION Problems comprehending as well as expressing verbal language.

SP F80.4 Speech and language development delay due to hearing loss
Code also:
type of hearing loss (H90.-, H91.-)

5 F80.8 Other developmental disorders of speech and language

SP F80.81 Childhood onset fluency disorder
Cluttering NOS
Stuttering NOS

EXCLUDES 1 adult onset fluency disorder (F98.5)
fluency disorder in conditions classified elsewhere (R47.82)
fluency disorder (stuttering) following cerebrovascular disease (I69. with final characters -23)

CODING TIPS ✓ Presently there are three major recognized forms of stuttering: stuttering with onset in early childhood, stuttering with onset after puberty, and fluency disorder subsequent to brain lesion or disease. F80.81 is the specific code for stuttering with onset in childhood.

SP F80.82 Social pragmatic communication disorder
EXCLUDES 1 Asperger's syndrome (F84.5)
autistic disorder (F84.0)

SP F80.89 Other developmental disorders of speech and language

IQ F80.9 Developmental disorder of speech and language, unspecified
Communication disorder NOS
Language disorder NOS

4 F81 Specific developmental disorders of scholastic skills

IQ F81.0 Specific reading disorder
'Backward reading'
Developmental dyslexia
Specific learning disorder, with impairment in reading
Specific reading retardation
EXCLUDES 1 alexia NOS (R48.0)
dyslexia NOS (R48.0)

IQ F81.2 Mathematics disorder
Developmental acalculia
Developmental arithmetical disorder
Developmental Gerstmann's syndrome
Specific learning disorder, with impairment in mathematics
EXCLUDES 1 acalculia NOS (R48.8)
EXCLUDES 2 arithmetical difficulties associated with a reading disorder (F81.0)

arithmetical difficulties associated with a spelling disorder (F81.81)
arithmetical difficulties due to inadequate teaching (Z55.8)

5 F81.8 Other developmental disorders of scholastic skills

IQ F81.81 Disorder of written expression
Specific learning disorder, with impairment in written expression
Specific spelling disorder

IQ F81.89 Other developmental disorders of scholastic skills

IQ F81.9 Developmental disorder of scholastic skills, unspecified
Knowledge acquisition disability NOS
Learning disability NOS
Learning disorder NOS

SP F82 Specific developmental disorder of motor function
Clumsy child syndrome
Developmental coordination disorder
Developmental dyspraxia
EXCLUDES 1 abnormalities of gait and mobility (R26.-)
lack of coordination (R27.-)
EXCLUDES 2 lack of coordination secondary to intellectual disabilities (F70-F79)

+ 4 F84 Pervasive developmental disorders
Use additional code to identify any associated medical condition and intellectual disabilities.

SP + F84.0 Autistic disorder
Autism spectrum disorder
Infantile autism
Infantile psychosis
Kanner's syndrome
EXCLUDES 1 Asperger's syndrome (F84.5)

DEFINITION Neurological disorder appearing at a young age that impairs social development and communication skills, and resulting in abnormal behavior that varies in degree of severity and ability to function.

SP + F84.2 Rett's syndrome
EXCLUDES 1 Asperger's syndrome (F84.5)
Autistic disorder (F84.0)
Other childhood disintegrative disorder (F84.3)

SP + F84.3 Other childhood disintegrative disorder
Dementia infantilis
Disintegrative psychosis
Heller's syndrome
Symbiotic psychosis
Use additional code to identify any associated neurological condition.
EXCLUDES 1 Asperger's syndrome (F84.5)
Autistic disorder (F84.0)
Rett's syndrome (F84.2)

SP + F84.5 Asperger's syndrome
Asperger's disorder
Autistic psychopathy

★ New ▲ Revised Px Primary **SP** PDGM Px **SL** Low CoM **SH** High CoM **IQ** Quest. Encounter **H** Hospice non-cancer Dx   Unspecified   **M** *Manifestation*

DecisionHealth's FY 2020 Complete Home Health ICD-10-CM Diagnosis Coding Manual

817

Schizoid disorder of childhood

SP ✚ F84.8 Other pervasive developmental disorders
Overactive disorder associated with intellectual disabilities and stereotyped movements

IQ ✚ F84.9 Pervasive developmental disorder, unspecified
Atypical autism

SP F88 Other disorders of psychological development
Developmental agnosia
Global developmental delay
Other specified neurodevelopmental disorder

IQ F89 Unspecified disorder of psychological development
Developmental disorder NOS
Neurodevelopmental disorder NOS

Behavioral and emotional disorders with onset usually occurring in childhood and adolescence (F90-F98)

Note:
Codes within categories F90-F98 may be used regardless of the age of a patient. These disorders generally have onset within the childhood or adolescent years, but may continue throughout life or not be diagnosed until adulthood

CODING TIPS ✓ Disorders classified to categories F90-F98 are frequently diagnosed in childhood and adolescence. However, a diagnosis may be made at any time during an individual's lifetime and may still be reported here when the diagnosis criteria are applicable.

4 F90 Attention-deficit hyperactivity disorders
  INCLUDES attention deficit disorder with hyperactivity
    attention deficit syndrome with hyperactivity
  EXCLUDES 2 anxiety disorders (F40.-, F41.-)
    mood [affective] disorders (F30-F39)
    pervasive developmental disorders (F84.-)
    schizophrenia (F20.-)

SP F90.0 Attention-deficit hyperactivity disorder, predominantly inattentive type
Attention-deficit/hyperactivity disorder, predominantly inattentive presentation

SP F90.1 Attention-deficit hyperactivity disorder, predominantly hyperactive type
Attention-deficit/hyperactivity disorder, predominantly hyperactive impulsive presentation

SP F90.2 Attention-deficit hyperactivity disorder, combined type
Attention-deficit/hyperactivity disorder, combined presentation

SP F90.8 Attention-deficit hyperactivity disorder, other type

SP F90.9 Attention-deficit hyperactivity disorder, unspecified type
Attention-deficit hyperactivity disorder of childhood or adolescence NOS
Attention-deficit hyperactivity disorder NOS

4 F91 Conduct disorders
  EXCLUDES 1 antisocial behavior (Z72.81-)

antisocial personality disorder (F60.2)
  EXCLUDES 2 conduct problems associated with attention-deficit hyperactivity disorder (F90.-)
    mood [affective] disorders (F30-F39)
    pervasive developmental disorders (F84.-)
    schizophrenia (F20.-)

SP F91.0 Conduct disorder confined to family context

SP F91.1 Conduct disorder, childhood-onset type
Unsocialized conduct disorder
Conduct disorder, solitary aggressive type
Unsocialized aggressive disorder

SP F91.2 Conduct disorder, adolescent-onset type
Socialized conduct disorder
Conduct disorder, group type

SP F91.3 Oppositional defiant disorder

SP F91.8 Other conduct disorders
Other specified conduct disorder
Other specified disruptive disorder

IQ F91.9 Conduct disorder, unspecified
Behavioral disorder NOS
Conduct disorder NOS
Disruptive behavior disorder NOS
Disruptive disorder NOS

4 F93 Emotional disorders with onset specific to childhood

SP F93.0 Separation anxiety disorder of childhood
  EXCLUDES 2 mood [affective] disorders (F30-F39)
    nonpsychotic mental disorders (F40-F48)
    phobic anxiety disorder of childhood (F40.8)
    social phobia (F40.1)
  DEFINITION Abnormal anxiety when separated from a parent, guardian, or usual environment.

SP F93.8 Other childhood emotional disorders
Identity disorder
  EXCLUDES 2 gender identity disorder of childhood (F64.2)

IQ F93.9 Childhood emotional disorder, unspecified

4 F94 Disorders of social functioning with onset specific to childhood and adolescence

SP F94.0 Selective mutism
Elective mutism
  EXCLUDES 2 pervasive developmental disorders (F84.-)
    schizophrenia (F20.-)
    specific developmental disorders of speech and language (F80.-)
    transient mutism as part of separation anxiety in young children (F93.0)

SP ✚ F94.1 Reactive attachment disorder of childhood
Use additional code to identify any associated failure to thrive or growth retardation

---

4 4th digit required   5 5th digit required   6 6th digit required   7 7th digit required   7 7th digit placeholder   ✚ Additional code   ▤ Laterality

818   *DecisionHealth's* FY 2020 Complete Home Health ICD-10-CM Diagnosis Coding Manual

EXCLUDES 1 disinhibited attachment disorder of childhood (F94.2)

normal variation in pattern of selective attachment

EXCLUDES 2 Asperger's syndrome (F84.5)

maltreatment syndromes (T74.-)

sexual or physical abuse in childhood, resulting in psychosocial problems (Z62.81-)

SP F94.2 Disinhibited attachment disorder of childhood
Affectionless psychopathy
Institutional syndrome

EXCLUDES 1 reactive attachment disorder of childhood (F94.1)

EXCLUDES 2 Asperger's syndrome (F84.5)

attention-deficit hyperactivity disorders (F90.-)

hospitalism in children (F43.2-)

SP F94.8 Other childhood disorders of social functioning

IQ F94.9 Childhood disorder of social functioning, unspecified

4 F95 Tic disorder

SP F95.0 Transient tic disorder
Provisional tic disorder

SP F95.1 Chronic motor or vocal tic disorder

SP F95.2 Tourette's disorder
Combined vocal and multiple motor tic disorder [de la Tourette]
Tourette's syndrome

SP F95.8 Other tic disorders

IQ F95.9 Tic disorder, unspecified
Tic NOS

4 F98 Other behavioral and emotional disorders with onset usually occurring in childhood and adolescence

EXCLUDES 2 breath-holding spells (R06.89)
gender identity disorder of childhood (F64.2)
Kleine-Levin syndrome (G47.13)
obsessive-compulsive disorder (F42-)
sleep disorders not due to a substance or known physiological condition (F51.-)

SP F98.0 Enuresis not due to a substance or known physiological condition
Enuresis (primary) (secondary) of nonorganic origin
Functional enuresis
Psychogenic enuresis
Urinary incontinence of nonorganic origin

EXCLUDES 1 enuresis NOS (R32)

SP ✚ F98.1 Encopresis not due to a substance or known physiological condition
Functional encopresis
Incontinence of feces of nonorganic origin

Psychogenic encopresis
Use additional code to identify the cause of any coexisting constipation

EXCLUDES 1 encopresis NOS (R15.-)

5 F98.2 Other feeding disorders of infancy and childhood

EXCLUDES 1 feeding difficulties (R63.3)

EXCLUDES 2 anorexia nervosa and other eating disorders (F50.-)
feeding problems of newborn (P92.-)
pica of infancy or childhood (F98.3)

SP F98.21 Rumination disorder of infancy

SP F98.29 Other feeding disorders of infancy and early childhood

SP F98.3 Pica of infancy and childhood
DEFINITION Compulsion to eat inedible substances, such as dirt or rocks.

SP F98.4 Stereotyped movement disorders
Stereotype/habit disorder

EXCLUDES 1 abnormal involuntary movements (R25.-)

EXCLUDES 2 compulsions in obsessive-compulsive disorder (F42-)
hair plucking (F63.3)
movement disorders of organic origin (G20-G25)
nail-biting (F98.8)
nose-picking (F98.8)
stereotypies that are part of a broader psychiatric condition (F01-F95)
thumb-sucking (F98.8)
tic disorders (F95.-)
trichotillomania (F63.3)

SP F98.5 Adult onset fluency disorder

EXCLUDES 1 childhood onset fluency disorder (F80.81)
dysphasia (R47.02)
fluency disorder in conditions classified elsewhere (R47.82)
fluency disorder (stuttering) following cerebrovascular disease (I69. with final characters -23)
tic disorders (F95.-)

CODING TIPS ✓ This code is used for post-childhood onset of stuttering symptoms secondary to emotional stress or trauma. Do not assign F98.5 to report fluency disorder as a sequela of cerebral vascular disease or another cause or to identify dysphasia.

DEFINITION Normal flow of speech disrupted by repeated sounds or pauses.

SP F98.8 Other specified behavioral and emotional disorders with onset usually occurring in childhood and adolescence
Excessive masturbation
Nail-biting
Nose-picking
Thumb-sucking

★ New ▲ Revised **Px** Primary **SP** PDGM Px **SL** Low CoM **SH** High CoM **IQ** Quest. Encounter **H** Hospice non-cancer Dx Unspecified **M** *Manifestation*

DecisionHealth's FY 2020 Complete Home Health ICD-10-CM Diagnosis Coding Manual

819

Chapter 5

F01-F99

IQ F98.9 **Unspecified behavioral and emotional disorders with onset usually occurring in childhood and adolescence**

Unspecified mental disorder (F99)

IQ F99 **Mental disorder, not otherwise specified**
Mental illness NOS

EXCLUDES 1 unspecified mental disorder due to known physiological condition (F09)

CODING TIPS ✓ **Documentation:** Use F99 only when the clinical documentation from the provider reports mental illness but does not specify anything further. Whenever possible, query the provider and obtain information specifying the patient's definitive diagnosis.

◀ 4th digit required　　🅢 5th digit required　　🅖 6th digit required　　🇿 7th digit required　　☑ 7th digit placeholder　　✚ Additional code　　🇪 Laterality

820　　　　　　　　*DecisionHealth's* FY 2020 Complete Home Health ICD-10-CM Diagnosis Coding Manual

Chapter 5 Scenarios: Mental, Behavioral and Neurodevelopmental disorders (F01-F99)

Psychogenic paroxysmal tachycardia

Your patient is diagnosed with psychogenic paroxysmal atrial tachycardia. Home health will monitor this condition and observe for acute exacerbation.

Description	Code
Primary: Paroxysmal atrial tachycardia	I47.1
Secondary: Psychological and behavioral factors associated with disorders or diseases classified elsewhere	F54

F54 is a manifestation code that requires the underlying disease (I47.1) to be coded first.

Unspecified dementia with behavioral disturbance

An 81-year-old woman recently was diagnosed with dementia and prescribed Aricept after being assessed by her primary care physician. Her memory has been poor, she has been forgetting to take her medication and she has started wandering at night. The physician did not indicate a cause for the patient's dementia. Home health skilled nursing is ordered for medication management, assessment of patient's safety at home and instruction of the patient's caregivers regarding management of dementia in the home. She has muscle weakness, which has caused her to fall, so physical therapy has been ordered for strengthening and to develop a home exercise program that the family can administer in the home.

Description	Code
Primary: Dementia, unspecified, with behavioral disturbance	F03.91
Secondary: Wandering in diseases classified elsewhere	Z91.83
Secondary: Muscle weakness (generalized)	M62.81
Secondary: History of falling	Z91.81

F03.9- (Unspecified dementia) codes allow for coding dementia with an unknown etiology with greater specificity and are not "manifestation only" codes. Wandering is considered to be a behavioral disturbance and is not inherent to dementia. Coding muscle weakness requires documentation of measurable muscle weakness. Code Z91.81 (History of falling) is for use when a patient has fallen in the past and is at risk for future falls.

Major depression

A patient is admitted for management of a stage 2 right heel pressure ulcer/injury. He also has a history of anemia, which is not currently a problem and will not be addressed in the plan of care. The caregiver said that the patient cries a lot and says he wishes he would die. He is on Prozac. The assessing nurse called the physician, who confirmed a diagnosis of major depression. He increased the dosage of the anti-depressant and requested that the agency continue to monitor the patient's mental status.

Description	Code
Primary: Pressure ulcer, right heel, stage 2	L89.612
Secondary: Major depressive disorder, single episode, unspecified	F32.9

As the focus of care, the stage 2 right heel pressure ulcer is coded in the primary position. Referencing 'Depression, major' in the Index leads to code F32.9. An inclusion term at F32.9 is "Major depression NOS." Since the anemia is not a current problem and will not be addressed in the plan of care, it is not coded here.

Paranoid schizophrenia

Your patient, who has long-term alcoholism, is admitted to home health with a primary diagnosis of paranoid schizophrenia. The skilled nurse will be administering Haldol injections B.I.D., a new treatment for the schizophrenia, and instructing the caregiver how to administer the medication. The patient also has hypertension and atrial fibrillation for which she takes Coumadin.

Description	Code
Primary: Paranoid schizophrenia	F20.0
Secondary: Alcohol dependence, uncomplicated	F10.20
Secondary: Essential (primary) hypertension	I10
Secondary: Unspecified atrial fibrillation	I48.91
Secondary: Other long term (current) drug therapy	Z79.899
Secondary: Long term (current) use of anticoagulants	Z79.01

The home health focus of care is to administer and teach on the Haldol injections to treat the paranoid schizophrenia. Alcoholism codes to alcohol dependence in the alphabetic index. Alcohol dependence and the other co-morbidities of hypertension and atrial fibrillation are relevant to the current plan of care and should therefore be coded. The Z codes for long-term drug therapy, for the Haldol and Coumadin, are added to provide additional information.

Major recurrent depression

Home health nursing is ordered for a patient with a diagnosis of major recurrent depression for medication teaching and monitoring. He has been on two anti-depressants for years and his physician increased the dosage of each. The history and physical notes that the patient consumes an excessive amount of coffee and soda, and caffeine dependence is documented.

Description	Code
Primary: Major depressive disorder, recurrent, unspecified	F33.9
Secondary: Other stimulant dependence, uncomplicated	F15.20
Secondary: Other long-term drug therapy	Z79.899

Use caution when assigning codes from Chapter 5, Mental, behavioral and neurodevelopmental disorders. Make sure a physician has documented, or confirmed, the diagnosis you are coding. Category F33.- (Major depressive disorder, recurrent) is found in the Alphabetic Index under "Disorder" not "Depression." Search under "disorder, depressive, recurrent." A code for long-term (current) drug use (Z79.899) is added to show the focus on medication monitoring. This code is selected since there is not a code specific for psychiatric drugs. While a psychiatric nurse is often required when a psychiatric diagnosis is the first-listed diagnosis, it does not require a psychiatric nurse to teach or monitor medications. A psychiatric nurse is required if the plan of care involves counseling for the psychiatric condition.

Bipolar disorder, alcoholism

A 68-year-old man was recently diagnosed with bipolar disorder and alcoholism after being hospitalized following a severe alcohol binge. In the hospital he was also found to be in the early stages of alcoholic cirrhosis of the liver. He was admitted to home health to monitor new medications for his bipolar as well as counseling from a certified psych nurse. The bipolar is the focus of care.

Description	Code
Primary: Bipolar disorder, unspecified	F31.9
Secondary: Alcoholic cirrhosis of liver without ascites	K70.30
Secondary: Alcohol dependence with other alcohol-induced disorder	F10.288

The bipolar is the focus of care so it is coded primary. Alcoholism codes to alcohol dependence, according to the alphabetic index. F10.288 is used to indicate that the patient's alcohol dependence has led to alcoholic cirrhosis.

Trichotillomania, hoarding disorder, psych nursing

A 45-year-old woman was recently discharged from an inpatient psych facility where she was diagnosed with severe trichotillomania and hoarding disorder. She will receive counseling and medication management from a certified psych nurse. The nurse will also monitor her hypertension.

Description	Code
Primary: Trichotillomania	F63.3
Secondary: Hoarding disorder	F42.3
Secondary: Essential (primary) hypertension	I10

The patient will receive psych services from a certified psych nurse for her diagnoses of trichotillomania and hoarding disorder. Her hypertension is an important comorbidity that should also be coded.

HOME HEALTH CODING SCENARIOS

Bipolar II, panic disorder, alcoholism

A 55-year-old woman is admitted to home health with primary diagnoses of bipolar II disorder. She also has panic disorder. She's been an alcoholic for the past 10 years. She will receive medication management and visits from the agency's certified psych nurse.

Description	Code
Primary: Bipolar II disorder	F31.81
Secondary: Panic disorder [episodic paroxysmal anxiety]	F41.0
Secondary: Alcohol dependence, uncomplicated	F10.20

The patient's bipolar disorder, which was specified as bipolar II, is the focus of care and thus coded primary. Panic disorder is also coded as it will impact her care. Her alcoholism is a relevant comorbidity that will impact her recovery. Alcoholism codes to alcohol dependence, according to the alphabetic index.

Suicide attempt, anxiety with depression

A 69-year-old man with a years-long history of anxiety with depression attempted to commit suicide by taking all of the remaining contents of a bottle of Tylenol he kept in his cupboard. Following acute care in the hospital, he's admitted to home health for care of symptoms related to the overdose, which are severe abdominal pain and diarrhea, as well as management of new medications.

Description	Code
Primary: Poisoning by 4-Aminophenol derivatives, intentional self-harm, subsequent encounter	T39.1x2D
Secondary: Unspecified abdominal pain	R10.9
Secondary: Diarrhea, unspecified	R19.7
Secondary: Other specified anxiety disorders	F41.8
Secondary: Personal history of self-harm	Z91.5

The patient intentionally took too much Tylenol in a suicide attempt, making it an intentional poisoning. Therefore, it is coded first with a T code for the specific drug. The health issues caused by the poisoning, abdominal pain and diarrhea, are coded next, in accordance with coding guidelines. Be sure to follow proper sequencing instructions for poisoning, which require the T code to be sequenced first. The patient's diagnosis of anxiety with depression is an important comorbidity that will require monitoring and so is also coded. Because it is stated as anxiety with depression, it can be coded with the combination code F41.8. A Z code is included to capture the patient's history of self-harm.

Liver cirrhosis, alcohol dependence, borderline personality disorder

A 46-year-old woman is admitted to home health for management of alcoholic liver cirrhosis. Her medical record indicates long-term alcohol dependence as well as borderline personality disorder. She will also receive psychiatric care from the agency's certified psych nurse.

Description	Code
Primary: Alcoholic cirrhosis of liver without ascites	K70.30
Secondary: Alcohol dependence with other alcohol-induced disorder	F10.288
Secondary: Borderline personality disorder	F60.3

After assigning the primary diagnosis of K70.30 for the alcoholic liver cirrhosis, the code for the patient's alcohol dependence, F10.288, is assigned, in accordance with tabular instruction. The more specific code for alcohol dependence is assigned because it is documented as having caused an alcohol-induced disorder. The patient will receive psychiatric care from the agency, necessitating the capture of her borderline personality disorder. However, psychiatric diagnoses will always affect the plan of care and should always be coded when they've been diagnosed.

Chapter 6: Diseases of the Nervous System (G00- G99)

The nervous system is how the body interprets and acts in response to a stimulus (light, heat, sound, or chemicals within the body). The nervous system consists of two parts: the central nervous system and the peripheral nervous system. Chapter 6 includes:

- Inflammatory diseases of the central nervous system (G00-G09) such as meningitis, encephalitis, myelitis and encephalomyelitis;

- Systemic atrophies primarily affecting the central nervous system (G10-G14)

- Extrapyramidal and movement disorders (G20-G26) such as Parkinson's disease (G20), dystonia (G24.9), and other extrapyramidal and movement disorders (G25.8-)

- Other degenerative diseases of the nervous system such as Alzheimer's disease (G30-) and mild cognitive impairment (G31.84)

- Demyelinating diseases of the central nervous system such as multiple sclerosis (G35), subacute necrotizing myelitis of central nervous system (G37.4)

- Episodic and paroxysmal disorder (G40-G47) such as epilepsy and recurrent seizures; migraine and other headache disorders; TIAs; and sleep disorders.

- Nerve, nerve root and plexus disorders (G50-G59)

- Polyneuropathies and other disorder of the peripheral nervous system (G60-G65)

- Diseases of myoneural junction and muscle (G70-G73) such as muscular dystrophy, myopathies

- Cerebral palsy and other paralytic syndromes (G80-G83), including hemiplegia and hemiparesis, paraplegia (G82.20), and other paralytic syndromes

- Other disorders of the nervous system (G89-G99), including pain not elsewhere classified, disorders of the autonomic nervous system, hydrocephalus, other disorders of the brain and spinal cord as well as intraoperative and postoperative complications and disorders of the nervous system not classified elsewhere

To select the correct code, it is important to understand the differences between the central and peripheral nervous systems.

The central nervous system (CNS) consists of the brain and spinal cord. The CNS receives nerve impulses and interprets them.

The peripheral nervous system (PNS) consists of all nerve fibers outside the CNS. Sensory nerves in the PNS send a nerve impulse to the CNS for interpretation following a stimulus.

Conditions of the PNS include: conditions of cranial nerves (trigeminal and facial nerves); disorders of nerve roots (collections of nerves right outside the spinal cord) and plexuses (large interlacing networks of nerves); and myoneural disorders (conditions involving the place where a nerve meets a muscle).

The somatic nervous system (SNS) includes all nerves controlling the muscular system and external sensory receptors. External sense organs (including skin) are receptors. Muscle fibers and gland cells are effectors. The reflex arc is an automatic, involuntary reaction to stimulus. Examples of reflex arcs include balance, the blinking reflex and the stretch reflex.

Conditions of the eye and associated tissues are in chapter categories H00-H59 in Chapter 7, and conditions of the ear and associated tissues are in categories H60-H95 in chapter 8.

A few situations to watch out for:

- If the documentation indicates **a neoplasm or tumor of an organ in the nervous system**, coders should look up the term (malignancy, tumor, adenoma) used to find the correct code. In most cases, a code from Chapter 2 (C000-D49) may be reported with a code from this chapter.

- **Code Parkinson's disease that's caused dementia** with behavioral disturbance with G20 and F02.81.

- You must **assign an additional code from F02.8- (Dementia in other diseases classified elsewhere) for a patient with Lewy body dementia (G31.83).**

- If a patient has a **personal or family history** of a condition reported in this chapter, it may be appropriate to select from the Z code section, such as Z85.841 (personal history of malignant neoplasm of the brain) or Z86.61(personal history of infection of the central nervous system).

- If a condition reported in this chapter is the **result of injury, poisoning and certain other consequences of external causes**, a code from Chapter 19 (S00-T88) may be reported with a code from this chapter.

- **Symptoms** related to the nervous system and sense organs are sometimes reported using codes from Chapter 18 (Symptoms, signs and abnormal clinical factors). Some examples include categories R43- (disturbances of sensation of smell and taste), R23- (symptoms involving skin) and R29- (other symptoms and signs involving the nervous and musculoskeletal system). Every effort should be made to secure a definitive diagnosis.

- If reporting a **nervous system disease in a pregnant patient** when the condition is complicating the pregnancy, report first a code from Chapter 15 (Pregnancy, childbirth and the puerperium) such as O26.82- (pregnancy related neuritis) or O99.35-(diseases of the nervous system complicating pregnancy, childbirth, and the puerperium), as the first-listed diagnosis, and G40.901 from this chapter as an additional code for epilepsy associated with pregnancy.

Multiple Coding and Sequencing

Many codes in this chapter are related to conditions in other chapters. It is important to read the Includes and Excludes notes under codes in this chapter, as well as any other instructions under the code or code category. Consider this example of multiple coding and sequencing issues for codes in this chapter:

- Meningitis due to listeriosis is reported as A32.11 (listeriosis meningitis) from Chapter 1 as a combination code that includes both the organism and the meningitis. There is an Excludes 1 note under G01 (meningitis in bacterial disease classified elsewhere) that excludes A32.11 from this code.

Special Coding Issues

Dominant/nondominant side

Codes from category G81 (Hemiplegia and hemiparesis) and subcategories G83.1 (Monoplegia of lower limb), G83.2 (Monoplegia of upper limb) and G83.3, (Monoplegia, unspecified) identify whether the dominant or nondominant side is affected. Should the affected side be documented, but not specified as dominant or nondominant, and the classification system does not indicate a default code, code selection is as follows:

- For ambidextrous patients, the default should be dominant.
- If the left side is affected, the default code is nondominant.
- If the right side is affected, the default is dominant.

Coding for Pain

Codes in category G89 (Pain, not elsewhere classified) may be used in conjunction with codes from other categories and chapters to provide more detail about acute and chronic pain and neoplasm-related pain, unless otherwise indicated below.

Take note of the following circumstances:

- If the pain is not specified as acute or chronic, post-thoracotomy, post procedural, or neoplasm related, *do not* assign codes from category G89.
- A code from G89 should *not be assigned* if the underlying (definitive) diagnosis is known, unless the reason for the encounter is pain control/management and **not** management of the underlying condition.
- Category G89 codes are acceptable as the primary, first-listed, code when pain control or pain management is the reason for the admission/ encounter. The underlying cause of the pain (e.g., nerve impingement, severe back pain) should be reported as an additional diagnosis if known.

G89 pain codes may be used in conjunction with site-specific pain codes (including chapter 18 symptom codes) if the category code provides additional information. For example, if the code describes the site of pain, but does not fully describe whether the pain is acute or chronic, then icd codes should be assigned.

The sequencing is dependent on the circumstances of the encounter/admission as follows:

- If the encounter is for pain control or pain management, assign the code from category G89 followed by the code identifying the specific site of pain. For example, encounter for pain management for acute neck pain from trauma is assigned to code G89.11 (Acute pain due to trauma), followed by code M54.2 (Cervicalgia) to identify the site of pain.
- When a patient is admitted for the insertion of a neurostimulator for pain control, assign the appropriate pain code as the principal or first-listed diagnosis.
- When an admission/encounter is for a procedure aimed at treating the underlying condition and a neurostimulator is inserted for pain control during the same admission/encounter, a code for the underlying condition should be assigned as the principal diagnosis and the appropriate pain code should be assigned as a secondary diagnosis.

Postoperative pain is based on the physician documentation. The default code for post-thoracotomy and other postoperative pain not specified as acute or chronic would be the code for the acute form. However, routine or expected pain immediately after surgery should not be coded.

Take note of the following circumstances:

- Postoperative pain not associated with a specific postoperative complication is assigned to the appropriate postoperative pain code in G89.
- Postoperative pain associated with a specific postoperative complication (e.g., painful wire sutures, T81.89) is assigned from chapter 19

(Injury, poisoning, and certain other consequences of external causes). If appropriate, use an additional code from G89.18 (acute pain) or G89.28 (chronic pain).

- For pain due to devices, implants or grafts, report code T85.84- (pain due to internal prosthetic devices, implants and grafts, not elsewhere classified). For complication of a device, implant or graft associated with a specific system, assign a code for the specific system device, such as implant and graft (T84-T88) from Chapter 19 (Injury, poisoning and other consequences of external causes) as the first-listed diagnosis. Also, add a code for the pain if it provides additional information. For example, a subsequent encounter for acute pain due to an infection of a right hip prosthesis is reported as T84.51xD (infection of right hip prosthesis) as the primary diagnosis. Use an additional code to identify the infection, and you may assign G89.18 to indicate that acute post-procedural pain has been documented for this patient by the physician as another additional diagnosis.

There is no time frame defining when pain becomes chronic; the physician's documentation should be used to guide use of these codes.

Neoplasm-related pain (G89.3) is assigned to pain documented as being related, associated or due to cancer, primary or secondary malignancy or tumor, whether the pain is acute or chronic.

- This code may be assigned as first-listed when the stated reason for the admission/encounter is documented as pain control/pain management with the underlying neoplasm reported as an additional diagnosis.

- When the reason for the admission/encounter is management of the neoplasm and the pain associated with the neoplasm is also documented, code G89.3 may be assigned as an additional diagnosis. It is not necessary to assign an additional code for the site of the pain.

- Central pain syndrome (G89.0) and chronic pain syndrome (G89.4) are different than the term "chronic pain" and therefore codes should only be used when the physician has specifically documented this condition.

Epilepsy

One specific nervous system diagnosis that shows up in home health coding is epilepsy (G40-). Epilepsy is a chronic disorder of the brain that is characterized by paroxysmal (sudden and unpredictable) and excessive neuronal discharge of the brain, usually accompanied by an alteration in consciousness.

However, although epilepsy often is diagnosed in those with seizures, not every seizure is epilepsy. For example, stroke, metabolic disorders, tumors and brain injuries are other possible causes of seizure not associated with epilepsy. Those 80 years of age or older have a 3% chance of developing epilepsy and an 11% chance of having at least one seizure.

To find the most precise diagnosis code for epilepsy, it is important to understand the kind of seizure suffered by the patient as ICD-10-CM has greatly expanded the number and detail of available codes for epilepsy and seizures (G40-G47), and the correct code requires specific documentation or confirmation with the physician.

There are two major categories of seizures – general and partial:

Generalized seizures: Those in which the focus or starting point of the neuronal discharge in the brain is not localized. In other words, it seems to be all over the brain. Generalized seizures are further categorized as nonconvulsive and convulsive.

Partial seizures: These begin in a specific brain location and may or may not spread (or generalize) throughout the entire brain. With this in mind, the seizure may or may not affect consciousness. If it does not, it is termed a **simple partial** seizure. If it does impair consciousness, it is termed a **complex partial** seizure.

CHAPTER 6: DISEASES OF THE NERVOUS SYSTEM (G00-G99)

EXCLUDES 2   certain conditions originating in the perinatal period (P04-P96)
certain infectious and parasitic diseases (A00-B99)
complications of pregnancy, childbirth and the puerperium (O00-O9A)
congenital malformations, deformations, and chromosomal abnormalities (Q00-Q99)
endocrine, nutritional and metabolic diseases (E00-E88)
injury, poisoning and certain other consequences of external causes (S00-T88)
neoplasms (C00-D49)
symptoms, signs and abnormal clinical and laboratory findings, not elsewhere classified (R00-R94)

This chapter contains the following blocks:

G00-G09	Inflammatory diseases of the central nervous system
G10-G14	Systemic atrophies primarily affecting the central nervous system
G20-G26	Extrapyramidal and movement disorders
G30-G32	Other degenerative diseases of the nervous system
G35-G37	Demyelinating diseases of the central nervous system
G40-G47	Episodic and paroxysmal disorders
G50-G59	Nerve, nerve root and plexus disorders
G60-G65	Polyneuropathies and other disorders of the peripheral nervous system
G70-G73	Diseases of myoneural junction and muscle
G80-G83	Cerebral palsy and other paralytic syndromes
G89-G99	Other disorders of the nervous system

Inflammatory diseases of the central nervous system   (G00-G09)

CODING TIPS ✓   If the central nervous system infection (CNS) is resolved but has a potential for reoccurence, use Z86.61, personal history of CNS infections. If the CNS infection is resolved, but the patient suffers neurological deficits, code the residual deficit followed by the sequela code G09.

4 G00   Bacterial meningitis, not elsewhere classified
   INCLUDES   bacterial arachnoiditis
   bacterial leptomeningitis
   bacterial meningitis
   bacterial pachymeningitis
   EXCLUDES 1   bacterial meningoencephalitis (G04.2)
   bacterial meningomyelitis (G04.2)

CODING TIPS ✓   Most of these central nervous system infection codes are combination codes and include the bacteria or other organism or are manifestation codes and require that the causative condition be coded first. Follow convention instructions to "code first" or "use additional code."

SP G00.0   Hemophilus meningitis
   Meningitis due to Hemophilus influenzae

DEFINITION   Bacterial infection of the tissues (meninges) surrounding the brain and spinal cord, causing fever, headache, vomiting, malaise, and stiff neck and may progress to confusion, stupor, convulsions, coma, and death.

SP G00.1   Pneumococcal meningitis
   Meningtitis due to Streptococcal pneumoniae

SP + G00.2   Streptococcal meningitis
   Use additional code to further identify organism (B95.0-B95.5)

SP + G00.3   Staphylococcal meningitis
   Use additional code to further identify organism (B95.61-B95.8)

SP + G00.8   Other bacterial meningitis
   Meningitis due to Escherichia coli
   Meningitis due to Friedländer's bacillus
   Meningitis due to Klebsiella
   Use additional code to further identify organism (B96.-)

SP G00.9   Bacterial meningitis, unspecified
   Meningitis due to gram-negative bacteria, unspecified
   Purulent meningitis NOS
   Pyogenic meningitis NOS
   Suppurative meningitis NOS

M IQ G01   *Meningitis in bacterial diseases classified elsewhere*

Code first:
underlying disease
   EXCLUDES 1   meningitis (in) :
   gonococcal (A54.81)
   leptospirosis (A27.81)
   listeriosis (A32.11)
   Lyme disease (A69.21)
   meningococcal (A39.0)
   neurosyphilis (A52.13)
   tuberculosis (A17.0)
   meningoencephalitis and meningomyelitis in bacterial diseases classified elsewhere (G05)

M IQ G02   *Meningitis in other infectious and parasitic diseases classified elsewhere*

Code first underlying disease, such as:
African trypanosomiasis (B56.-)
poliovirus infection (A80.-)
   EXCLUDES 1   candidal meningitis (B37.5)
   coccidioidomycosis meningitis (B38.4)
   cryptococcal meningitis (B45.1)
   herpesviral [herpes simplex] meningitis (B00.3)
   infectious mononucleosis complicated by meningitis (B27.- with fourth character 2)
   measles complicated by meningitis (B05.1)
   meningoencephalitis and meningomyelitis in other infectious and parasitic diseases classified elsewhere (G05)
   mumps meningitis (B26.1)
   rubella meningitis (B06.02)

4 4th digit required   5 5th digit required   6 6th digit required   7 7th digit required   7 7th digit placeholder   +Additional code   ◻Laterality

828   *DecisionHealth's* FY 2020 Complete Home Health ICD-10-CM Diagnosis Coding Manual

varicella [chickenpox]
    meningitis (B01.0)
zoster meningitis (B02.1)

☑ G03   Meningitis due to other and unspecified causes

> INCLUDES   arachnoiditis NOS
> leptomeningitis NOS
> meningitis NOS
> pachymeningitis NOS
> EXCLUDES 1   meningoencephalitis (G04.-)
> meningomyelitis (G04.-)

SP G03.0   Nonpyogenic meningitis
Aseptic meningitis
Nonbacterial meningitis

SP G03.1   Chronic meningitis

SP G03.2   Benign recurrent meningitis [Mollaret]
> CODING TIPS ✓   Do not confuse chronic meningitis with benign recurrent Mollaret's meningitis. Mollaret's meningitis is a rare disorder characterized by a recurrent, mild, and aseptic inflammation of the meninges due to an unknown cause.

IQ G03.8   Meningitis due to other specified causes

IQ G03.9   Meningitis, unspecified
Arachnoiditis (spinal) NOS
> CODING TIPS ✓   Meningitis that is not specified as acute, chronic, or due to a specified cause should be coded to G03.9.

☑ G04   Encephalitis, myelitis and encephalomyelitis

> INCLUDES   acute ascending myelitis
> meningoencephalitis
> meningomyelitis
> EXCLUDES 1   encephalopathy NOS (G93.40)
> EXCLUDES 2   acute transverse myelitis
> (G37.3-)
> alcoholic encephalopathy
> (G31.2)
> benign myalgic
> encephalomyelitis (G93.3)
> multiple sclerosis (G35)
> subacute necrotizing myelitis
> (G37.4)
> toxic encephalitis (G92)
> toxic encephalopathy (G92)

⑤ G04.0   Acute disseminated encephalitis and encephalomyelitis (ADEM)
> EXCLUDES 1   acute necrotizing
> hemorrhagic
> encephalopathy (G04.3-)
> other noninfectious acute
> disseminated
> encephalomyelitis
> (noninfectious ADEM)
> (G04.81)

SP G04.00   Acute disseminated encephalitis and encephalomyelitis, unspecified

SP G04.01   Postinfectious acute disseminated encephalitis and encephalomyelitis (postinfectious ADEM)
> EXCLUDES 1   post chickenpox
> encephalitis (B01.1)
> post measles encephalitis
> (B05.0)
> post measles myelitis
> (B05.1)

SP ✚ G04.02   Postimmunization acute disseminated encephalitis, myelitis and encephalomyelitis
Encephalitis, post immunization
Encephalomyelitis, post immunization
Use additional code to identify the vaccine (T50.A-, T50.B-, T50.Z-)
> CODING TIPS ✓   G04.02 should be assigned for encephalitis, myelitis, and encephalomyelitis that is reported to be caused by the administration of vaccines. Use an additional code from T36-T50 to identify the adverse effect from the vaccine.

SP SH SL G04.1   Tropical spastic paraplegia

SP G04.2   Bacterial meningoencephalitis and meningomyelitis, not elsewhere classified

⑤ G04.3   Acute necrotizing hemorrhagic encephalopathy
> EXCLUDES 1   acute disseminated
> encephalitis and
> encephalomyelitis
> (G04.0-)

SP G04.30   Acute necrotizing hemorrhagic encephalopathy, unspecified

SP G04.31   Postinfectious acute necrotizing hemorrhagic encephalopathy

SP ✚ G04.32   Postimmunization acute necrotizing hemorrhagic encephalopathy
Use additional code to identify the vaccine (T50.A-, T50.B-, T50.Z-)

SP G04.39   Other acute necrotizing hemorrhagic encephalopathy
Code also:
    underlying etiology, if applicable

⑤ G04.8   Other encephalitis, myelitis and encephalomyelitis
Code also:
    any associated seizure (G40.-, R56.9)

SP G04.81   Other encephalitis and encephalomyelitis
Noninfectious acute disseminated encephalomyelitis (noninfectious ADEM)

SP G04.89   Other myelitis

⑤ G04.9   Encephalitis, myelitis and encephalomyelitis, unspecified

SP G04.90   Encephalitis and encephalomyelitis, unspecified
Ventriculitis (cerebral) NOS

SP G04.91   Myelitis, unspecified

☑ G05   Encephalitis, myelitis and encephalomyelitis in diseases classified elsewhere
Code first underlying disease, such as:
    human immunodeficiency virus [HIV]
        disease (B20)
    poliovirus (A80.-)
    suppurative otitis media (H66.01-H66.4)
    trichinellosis (B75)
> EXCLUDES 1   adenoviral encephalitis, myelitis
> and encephalomyelitis
> (A85.1)
> congenital toxoplasmosis
> encephalitis, myelitis and
> encephalomyelitis (P37.1)

Chapter 6

G00-G99

★ New ▲ Revised Px Primary SP PDGM Px SL Low CoM SH High CoM IQ Quest. Encounter H Hospice non-cancer Dx   Unspecified   M *Manifestation*

DecisionHealth's FY 2020 Complete Home Health ICD-10-CM Diagnosis Coding Manual   829

cytomegaloviral encephalitis,
 myelitis and
 encephalomyelitis (B25.8)
encephalitis, myelitis and
 encephalomyelitis (in)
 measles (B05.0)
encephalitis, myelitis and
 encephalomyelitis (in)
 systemic lupus erythematosus
 (M32.19)
enteroviral encephalitis,
 myelitis and
 encephalomyelitis (A85.0)
eosinophilic
 meningoencephalitis (B83.2)
herpesviral [herpes simplex]
 encephalitis, myelitis and
 encephalomyelitis (B00.4)
listerial encephalitis, myelitis
 and encephalomyelitis
 (A32.12)
meningococcal encephalitis,
 myelitis and
 encephalomyelitis (A39.81)
mumps encephalitis, myelitis
 and encephalomyelitis
 (B26.2)
postchickenpox encephalitis,
 myelitis and
 encephalomyelitis (B01.1-)
rubella encephalitis, myelitis
 and encephalomyelitis
 (B06.01)
toxoplasmosis encephalitis,
 myelitis and
 encephalomyelitis (B58.2)
zoster encephalitis, myelitis and
 encephalomyelitis (B02.0)

M IQ G05.3 *Encephalitis and encephalomyelitis in diseases classified elsewhere*
Meningoencephalitis in diseases classified elsewhere

M IQ G05.4 *Myelitis in diseases classified elsewhere*
Meningomyelitis in diseases classified elsewhere

+ 4 G06 **Intracranial and intraspinal abscess and granuloma**
Use additional code (B95-B97) to identify infectious agent.

SP + G06.0 **Intracranial abscess and granuloma**
Brain [any part] abscess (embolic)
Cerebellar abscess (embolic)
Cerebral abscess (embolic)
Intracranial epidural abscess or granuloma
Intracranial extradural abscess or granuloma
Intracranial subdural abscess or granuloma
Otogenic abscess (embolic)
EXCLUDES 1   tuberculous intracranial abscess and granuloma (A17.81)

SP + G06.1 **Intraspinal abscess and granuloma**
Abscess (embolic) of spinal cord [any part]
Intraspinal epidural abscess or granuloma
Intraspinal extradural abscess or granuloma
Intraspinal subdural abscess or granuloma

EXCLUDES 1   tuberculous intraspinal abscess and granuloma (A17.81)

SP + G06.2 **Extradural and subdural abscess, unspecified**

M IQ G07 *Intracranial and intraspinal abscess and granuloma in diseases classified elsewhere*
Code first underlying disease, such as:
schistosomiasis granuloma of brain (B65.-)
EXCLUDES 1   abscess of brain:
amebic (A06.6)
chromomycotic (B43.1)
gonococcal (A54.82)
tuberculous (A17.81)
tuberculoma of meninges (A17.1)

SP G08 **Intracranial and intraspinal phlebitis and thrombophlebitis**
Septic embolism of intracranial or intraspinal venous sinuses and veins
Septic endophlebitis of intracranial or intraspinal venous sinuses and veins
Septic phlebitis of intracranial or intraspinal venous sinuses and veins
Septic thrombophlebitis of intracranial or intraspinal venous sinuses and veins
Septic thrombosis of intracranial or intraspinal venous sinuses and veins
EXCLUDES 1   intracranial phlebitis and thrombophlebitis complicating:
abortion, ectopic or molar pregnancy (O00-O07, O08.7)
pregnancy, childbirth and the puerperium (O22.5, O87.3)
nonpyogenic intracranial phlebitis and thrombophlebitis (I67.6)
EXCLUDES 2   intracranial phlebitis and thrombophlebitis complicating nonpyogenic intraspinal phlebitis and thrombophlebitis (G95.1)

DEFINITION   Inflammation and/or blood clot formation in a large vein or channel for venous blood circulation in the brain or spine.

IQ G09 **Sequelae of inflammatory diseases of central nervous system**
Note:
Category G09 is to be used to indicate conditions whose primary classification is to G00-G08 as the cause of sequelae, themselves classifiable elsewhere. The 'sequelae' include conditions specified as residuals.
Code first:
condition resulting from (sequela) of inflammatory diseases of central nervous system

CODING TIPS ✓   Use G09, not the acute infection, to indicate residual effects or sequelae of meningitis, encephalitis or other CNS inflammatory diseases. If an infectious encephalitis, not coded with codes G00-G08, causes residual conditions, see B94.8. Sequence the residual condition followed by the sequela code unless there is a tabular convention that indicates otherwise.

---

4 4th digit required   5 5th digit required   6 6th digit required   7 7th digit required   7 7th digit placeholder   +Additional code   ⊟ Laterality

830   DecisionHealth's FY 2020 Complete Home Health ICD-10-CM Diagnosis Coding Manual

CODING TIPS ✓ If the central nervous system infection is resolved but has a potential for reoccurrence, use Z86.61, personal history of CNS infections. If the CNS infection is resolved, but the patient suffers neurological deficits, code the neurological deficit and sequela code G09.

Systemic atrophies primarily affecting the central nervous system   (G10-G14)

SP G10   **Huntington's disease**
Huntington's chorea
Huntington's dementia
Code also:
dementia in other diseases classified
elsewhere without behavioral disturbance
(F02.80)

CODING TIPS ✓ Huntington's disease is a progressive neurological disorder that includes mental deterioration and may include dementia as part of its progressive course. When dementia has been diagnosed as related to Huntington's disease, the alpha index instructs to use an additional code (F02-) to identify dementia with or without behavioral disturbance.

DEFINITION A genetic, degenerative disorder of the neurons of the brain, characterized by progressive difficulty with physical and mental tasks until death occurs.

⊿ G11   **Hereditary ataxia**
EXCLUDES 2   cerebral palsy (G80.-)
hereditary and idiopathic
neuropathy (G60.-)
metabolic disorders (E70-E88)

CODING TIPS ✓   **Documentation:** When assigning a code from category G11.-, the coder should review the record in full and assign the most specific code. Coders should not, however, assign codes for early vs. late onset or a hereditary vs. congenital condition unless specifically reported as confirmed by the patient's physician in the record.

SP G11.0   **Congenital nonprogressive ataxia**

SP G11.1   **Early-onset cerebellar ataxia**
Early-onset cerebellar ataxia with essential
tremor
Early-onset cerebellar ataxia with
myoclonus [Hunt's ataxia]
Early-onset cerebellar ataxia with retained
tendon reflexes
Friedreich's ataxia (autosomal recessive)
X-linked recessive spinocerebellar ataxia

SP G11.2   **Late-onset cerebellar ataxia**

▲ SP G11.3   **Cerebellar ataxia with defective DNA
repair**
Ataxia telangiectasia [Louis-Bar]
EXCLUDES 2   Cockayne's syndrome
(Q87.19)
other disorders of purine and
pyrimidine metabolism
(E79.-)
xeroderma pigmentosum
(Q82.1)

SP G11.4   **Hereditary spastic paraplegia**

DEFINITION Hereditary disorder characterized by lower-limb spasticity and near total loss of joint flexibility while the upper limbs remain unaffected.

SP G11.8   **Other hereditary ataxias**

SP G11.9   **Hereditary ataxia, unspecified**
Hereditary cerebellar ataxia NOS
Hereditary cerebellar degeneration
Hereditary cerebellar disease
Hereditary cerebellar syndrome

⊿ G12   **Spinal muscular atrophy and related
syndromes**

SP G12.0   **Infantile spinal muscular atrophy, type I
[Werdnig-Hoffman]**

SP G12.1   **Other inherited spinal muscular atrophy**
Adult form spinal muscular atrophy
Childhood form, type II spinal muscular
atrophy
Distal spinal muscular atrophy
Juvenile form, type III spinal muscular
atrophy [Kugelberg-Welander]
Progressive bulbar palsy of childhood
[Fazio-Londe]
Scapuloperoneal form spinal muscular
atrophy

⑤ G12.2   **Motor neuron disease**

SP G12.20   **Motor neuron disease, unspecified**

H SP G12.21   **Amyotrophic lateral sclerosis**

SP G12.22   **Progressive bulbar palsy**

SP G12.23   **Primary lateral sclerosis**
DEFINITION Primary lateral sclerosis is often mistaken for the more common amyotrophic lateral sclerosis (ALS). However, primary lateral sclerosis progresses more slowly than ALS, and in most cases is not fatal.

SP G12.24   **Familial motor neuron disease**
DEFINITION People with familial MND have the disorder because of a mutation in a gene. Usually at least one other person in the family will have the condition.

SP G12.25   **Progressive spinal muscle atrophy**
DEFINITION Spinal muscular atrophy is a genetic disorder that affects the control of muscle movement. It is caused by a loss of specialized nerve cells, called motor neurons, in the spinal cord and the part of the brain that is connected to the spinal cord (the brainstem).

SP G12.29   **Other motor neuron disease**

SP G12.8   **Other spinal muscular atrophies and
related syndromes**

SP G12.9   **Spinal muscular atrophy, unspecified**

⊿ G13   **Systemic atrophies primarily affecting
central nervous system in diseases
classified elsewhere**

M IQ G13.0   *Paraneoplastic neuromyopathy and
neuropathy*
Carcinomatous neuromyopathy
Sensorial paraneoplastic neuropathy
[Denny Brown]
Code first:
underlying neoplasm (C00-D49)

★ New ▲ Revised **Px** Primary **SP** PDGM Px **SL** Low CoM **SH** High CoM **IQ** Quest. Encounter **H** Hospice non-cancer Dx   Unspecified   **M** *Manifestation*

M IQ G13.1 *Other systemic atrophy primarily affecting central nervous system in neoplastic disease*

Paraneoplastic limbic encephalopathy
Code first:
   underlying neoplasm (C00-D49)

M IQ G13.2 *Systemic atrophy primarily affecting the central nervous system in myxedema*

Code first underlying disease, such as:
   hypothyroidism (E03.-)
   myxedematous congenital iodine
     deficiency (E00.1)

M IQ G13.8 *Systemic atrophy primarily affecting central nervous system in other diseases classified elsewhere*

Code first: ʼ
   underlying disease

SP G14 Postpolio syndrome

   INCLUDES postpolio myelitic syndrome
   EXCLUDES 1 sequelae of poliomyelitis (B91)

   CODING TIPS ✓ The most common symptoms of postpolio syndrome include slowly progressive muscle weakness, fatigue (both generalized and muscular), and a gradual decrease in the size of muscles (muscle atrophy). Pain from joint degeneration and increasing skeletal deformities such as scoliosis (curvature of the spine) is common and may precede the weakness and muscle atrophy.

   CODING TIPS ✓ **Documentation:** G14 should be assigned only when the physician specifically reports "post polio syndrome" in the patient's clinical record. Note that this is differentiated from sequelae of poliomyelitis or residual deficits related to resolved poliomyelitis. When the record only specifies residual deficits related to resolved poliomyelitis, but does not specify post polio syndrome, coders should assign B91, Sequelae of poliomyelitis.

Extrapyramidal and movement disorders (G20-G26)

SP SH SL G20 Parkinson's disease
Hemiparkinsonism
Idiopathic Parkinsonism or Parkinson's
   disease
Paralysis agitans
Parkinsonism or Parkinson's disease NOS
Primary Parkinsonism or Parkinson's disease
   EXCLUDES 1 dementia with Parkinsonism
     (G31.83)

CODING TIPS ✓ Do not confuse a patient who has Parkinson's disease with dementia and a patient who has dementia with Parkinsonism. When a patient is reported to have Parkinson's disease and dementia, assign G20 followed by a code from category F02.8-, Dementia in diseases classified elsewhere. By contrast, dementia with Parkinsonism, which is also known as Lewy body dementia or dementia with Lewy bodies, is coded to G31.83, followed by a code from the F02.8- category. G20 cannot be coded with G31.83. If the physician documents Parkinsons and dementia, but also mentions Parkinsonism or Lewy bodies, the G31.83 code is used instead of G20 along with the code for the dementia (F02.8-).

4 G21 Secondary parkinsonism
   EXCLUDES 1 dementia with Parkinsonism
     (G31.83)
     Huntington's disease (G10)
     Shy-Drager syndrome (G90.3)
     syphilitic Parkinsonism
     (A52.19)

SP + G21.0 Malignant neuroleptic syndrome
Use additional code for adverse effect, if
   applicable, to identify drug (T43.3X5,
   T43.4X5, T43.505, T43.595)
   EXCLUDES 1 neuroleptic induced
     parkinsonism (G21.11)

5 G21.1 Other drug-induced secondary parkinsonism
   CODING TIPS ✓ When coding drug-induced Parkinsonism, be sure to also assign the appropriate code to identify the drug causing the disorder. Drug-induced Parkinsonism is considered an adverse effect of the drug that caused the condition, and the causative relationship must be stated by the physician.

SP SH SL + G21.11 Neuroleptic induced parkinsonism
Use additional code for adverse effect,
   if applicable, to identify drug
   (T43.3X5, T43.4X5, T43.505,
   T43.595)
   EXCLUDES 1 malignant neuroleptic
     syndrome (G21.0)

SP SH SL + G21.19 Other drug induced secondary parkinsonism
Other medication-induced
   parkinsonism
Use additional code for adverse effect,
   if applicable, to identify drug (T36-
   T50 with fifth or sixth character 5)

SP SH SL G21.2 Secondary parkinsonism due to other external agents
Code first:
   (T51-T65) to identify external agent

SP SH SL G21.3 Postencephalitic parkinsonism

SP SH SL G21.4 Vascular parkinsonism

SP SH SL G21.8 Other secondary parkinsonism

SP SH SL G21.9 Secondary parkinsonism, unspecified

4 G23 Other degenerative diseases of basal ganglia
   EXCLUDES 2 multi-system degeneration of
     the autonomic nervous system
     (G90.3)

SP G23.0 Hallervorden-Spatz disease

---

4 4th digit required   5 5th digit required   6 6th digit required   7 7th digit required   7 7th digit placeholder   + Additional code   ⬛ Laterality

832   *DecisionHealth's* FY 2020 Complete Home Health ICD-10-CM Diagnosis Coding Manual

Pigmentary pallidal degeneration

SP **G23.1** **Progressive supranuclear ophthalmoplegia [Steele-Richardson-Olszewski]**
Progressive supranuclear palsy

SP **G23.2** **Striatonigral degeneration**

SP **G23.8** **Other specified degenerative diseases of basal ganglia**
Calcification of basal ganglia

SP **G23.9** **Degenerative disease of basal ganglia, unspecified**

4 **G24** **Dystonia**
> **INCLUDES** dyskinesia
> **EXCLUDES 2** athetoid cerebral palsy (G80.3)
> **CODING TIPS ✓** Dystonias may be specified to congenital or acquired, primary or secondary, and may be anatomically specific. When coding dystonias, the coder should attempt to obtain specific information regarding the origin of the dystonia and the specific type of movement disorder so that the most specific code may be assigned.

+ **5** **G24.0** **Drug induced dystonia**
Use additional code for adverse effect, if applicable, to identify drug (T36-T50 with fifth or sixth character 5)

SP **+** **G24.01** **Drug induced subacute dyskinesia**
Drug induced blepharospasm
Drug induced orofacial dyskinesia
Neuroleptic induced tardive dyskinesia
Tardive dyskinesia
> **CODING TIPS ✓** Tardive dyskinesia due to use of medications, also referred to as lingual-facial-buccal dyskinesia, which presents as uncontrollable movements of the mouth, tongue, jaw, and cheeks, should be coded using G24.01 followed by the appropriate code to identify the drug causing the dyskinesia. This effect is commonly found following the use of neuroleptic medications.
> **DEFINITION** Involuntary repetitive movements of facial, buccal, oral, and cervical muscles, induced by long-term use of antipsychotic agent, sometimes persisting after withdrawal of the agent.

SP **+** **G24.02** **Drug induced acute dystonia**
Acute dystonic reaction to drugs
Neuroleptic induced acute dystonia

SP **+** **G24.09** **Other drug induced dystonia**

SP **G24.1** **Genetic torsion dystonia**
Dystonia deformans progressiva
Dystonia musculorum deformans
Familial torsion dystonia
Idiopathic familial dystonia
Idiopathic (torsion) dystonia NOS
(Schwalbe-) Ziehen-Oppenheim disease

SP **G24.2** **Idiopathic nonfamilial dystonia**

SP **G24.3** **Spasmodic torticollis**
> **EXCLUDES 1** congenital torticollis (Q68.0)
> hysterical torticollis (F44.4)
> ocular torticollis (R29.891)
> psychogenic torticollis (F45.8)
> torticollis NOS (M43.6)

traumatic recurrent torticollis (S13.4)
> **DEFINITION** Contractions of the neck muscles causing contortion, pain, and abnormal head posture.

SP **G24.4** **Idiopathic orofacial dystonia**
Orofacial dyskinesia
> **EXCLUDES 1** drug induced orofacial dyskinesia (G24.01)

SP **G24.5** **Blepharospasm**
> **EXCLUDES 1** drug induced blepharospasm (G24.01)
> **DEFINITION** Spasm of the orbicularis oculi muscle, causing uncontrolled winking or blinking.

SP **G24.8** **Other dystonia**
Acquired torsion dystonia NOS

IQ **G24.9** **Dystonia, unspecified**
Dyskinesia NOS

4 **G25** **Other extrapyramidal and movement disorders**
> **EXCLUDES 2** sleep related movement disorders (G47.6-)

SP **G25.0** **Essential tremor**
Familial tremor
> **EXCLUDES 1** tremor NOS (R25.1)
> **CODING TIPS ✓** Do not assign G25.0 to report unspecified tremors or tremors in a patient with a confirmed diagnosis of Parkinson's disease.

SP **+** **G25.1** **Drug-induced tremor**
Use additional code for adverse effect, if applicable, to identify drug (T36-T50 with fifth or sixth character 5)

SP **G25.2** **Other specified forms of tremor**
Intention tremor

SP **+** **G25.3** **Myoclonus**
Drug-induced myoclonus
Palatal myoclonus
Use additional code for adverse effect, if applicable, to identify drug (T36-T50 with fifth or sixth character 5)
> **EXCLUDES 1** facial myokymia (G51.4)
> myoclonic epilepsy (G40.-)
> **CODING TIPS ✓** Myoclonus is also reported as muscle twitching and is often a symptom of a more specific disease process. When the specific disease process is known, code the underlying disease. If myoclonus is related to the adverse effect of a medication, use an additional code to identify the drug. This code should not be assigned for myoclonic epilepsy or seizures.
> **DEFINITION** Spontaneous contractions of a muscle or group of muscles as a part of a disease process, drug side effect, or abnormal physiological response.

SP **+** **G25.4** **Drug-induced chorea**
Use additional code for adverse effect, if applicable, to identify drug (T36-T50 with fifth or sixth character 5)

SP **G25.5** **Other chorea**
Chorea NOS
> **EXCLUDES 1** chorea NOS with heart involvement (I02.0)

★ New ▲ Revised **Px** Primary **SP** PDGM Px **SL** Low CoM **SH** High CoM **IQ** Quest. Encounter **H** Hospice non-cancer Dx | Unspecified | **M** *Manifestation*

DecisionHealth's FY 2020 Complete Home Health ICD-10-CM Diagnosis Coding Manual

833

Chapter 6

G00-G99

Huntington's chorea (G10)
rheumatic chorea (I02.-)
Sydenham's chorea (I02.-)

⑤ **G25.6 Drug induced tics and other tics of organic origin**

🆂🅿 ✚ **G25.61 Drug induced tics**
Use additional code for adverse effect, if applicable, to identify drug (T36-T50 with fifth or sixth character 5)

🆂🅿 **G25.69 Other tics of organic origin**
EXCLUDES 1 habit spasm (F95.9)
tic NOS (F95.9)
Tourette's syndrome (F95.2)

✚ ⑤ **G25.7 Other and unspecified drug induced movement disorders**
Use additional code for adverse effect, if applicable, to identify drug (T36-T50 with fifth or sixth character 5)

🅸🆀 ✚ **G25.70 Drug induced movement disorder, unspecified**

🆂🅿 ✚ **G25.71 Drug induced akathisia**
Drug induced acathisia
Neuroleptic induced acute akathisia
Tardive akathisia
CODING TIPS ✓ Akathisia is a syndrome characterized by a restless inability to maintain stillness or to "sit still" and is frequently induced by the use of various medications, including antipsychotics. When caused by the effect of a drug, an additional code should be assigned to identify the drug.

🆂🅿 ✚ **G25.79 Other drug induced movement disorders**

⑤ **G25.8 Other specified extrapyramidal and movement disorders**

🆂🅿 **G25.81 Restless legs syndrome**
DEFINITION Irresistible urge to move legs, particularly when sitting or lying down, with leg sensations such as creeping, crawling, itching, tugging, tightening, or pulling alleviated upon movement.

🆂🅿 **G25.82 Stiff-man syndrome**
DEFINITION Progressive fluctuating rigidity of axial and limb muscles in the absence of any signs of cerebral and/or spinal cord disease.

🆂🅿 **G25.83 Benign shuddering attacks**

🆂🅿 **G25.89 Other specified extrapyramidal and movement disorders**

🅸🆀 **G25.9 Extrapyramidal and movement disorder, unspecified**

🆂🅿 **G26 Extrapyramidal and movement disorders in diseases classified elsewhere**
Code first:
underlying disease

Other degenerative diseases of the nervous system (G30-G32)

✚ ④ **G30 Alzheimer's disease**
INCLUDES Alzheimer's dementia senile and presenile forms
Use additional code to identify:
delirium, if applicable (F05)

dementia with behavioral disturbance (F02.81)
dementia without behavioral disturbance (F02.80)
EXCLUDES 1 senile degeneration of brain NEC (G31.1)
senile dementia NOS (F03)
senility NOS (R41.81)
CODING TIPS ✓ **Documentation:** Alzheimer's disease is a particular neurological condition and must be specifically confirmed by a physician. Early onset Alzheimer's is defined as diagnosis prior to the age of 65; however, the designation of early and late onset must be documented by, or confirmed with, the patient's physician and may not be assumed. Query the physician if the information is not readily available and, if unable to make a determination, assign code G30.9 for Alzheimer's disease, unspecified. Alzheimers is a specific type of dementia, so the physician does not have to specifically mention dementia to be able to code it. The Alzheimers is paired with the F02.8- code as a manifestation of Alzheimer's.

DEFINITION Progressive degenerative disease of the brain of unknown cause with diffuse atrophy throughout the cerebral cortex; it initially presents with slight memory disturbance or personality changes that progressively deteriorate to profound memory loss and dementia.

🅷 🆂🅿 ✚ **G30.0 Alzheimer's disease with early onset**
CODING TIPS ✓ Early onset Alzheimer's is very uncommon and is diagnosed prior to the age of 65. Coders may not assume a diagnosis of early onset Alzheimer's disease because of the patient's age, but must have confirmed Early Onset Alzheimers with the patient's physician in order to assign the diagnosis appropriately.

🅷 🆂🅿 ✚ **G30.1 Alzheimer's disease with late onset**
CODING TIPS ✓ Late onset Alzheimer's is the most common type and presents with symptoms after the age of 65. Coders may not assume a diagnosis of late onset Alzheimer's disease but must have confirmed evidence of this from the patient's physician to assign the diagnosis appropriately.

🅷 🆂🅿 ✚ **G30.8 Other Alzheimer's disease**
CODING TIPS ✓ This code is used for the familial type of Alzheimer's, which accounts for less than 1% of cases.

🅷 🆂🅿 ✚ **G30.9 Alzheimer's disease, unspecified**

▲ ✚ ④ **G31 Other degenerative diseases of nervous system, not elsewhere classified**
Use additional For codes G31.0-G31.83, G31.85-G31.9, use additional code to identify:
dementia with behavioral disturbance (F02.81)
dementia without behavioral disturbance (F02.80)
EXCLUDES 2 Reye's syndrome (G93.7)

✚ ⑤ **G31.0 Frontotemporal dementia**

---

④4th digit required   ⑤5th digit required   ⑥6th digit required   ⑦7th digit required   ☑7th digit placeholder   ✚Additional code   ⑤Laterality

H SP + G31.01 Pick's disease
Primary progressive aphasia
Progressive isolated aphasia

DEFINITION Rare, progressive, degenerative disease of the brain, similar to Alzheimer's disease but with cortical atrophy confined to the frontal and temporal lobes.

SP + G31.09 Other frontotemporal dementia
Frontal dementia

H SP + G31.1 Senile degeneration of brain, not elsewhere classified
EXCLUDES 1 Alzheimer's disease (G30.-)
senility NOS (R41.81)

SP + G31.2 Degeneration of nervous system due to alcohol
Alcoholic cerebellar ataxia
Alcoholic cerebellar degeneration
Alcoholic cerebral degeneration
Alcoholic encephalopathy
Dysfunction of the autonomic nervous system due to alcohol
Code also:
associated alcoholism (F10.-)

CODING TIPS ✓ Cerebellar ataxia, encephalopathy, cerebellar degeneration, and autonomic dysfunction/degeneration, when specified as due to alcohol, should be coded to G31.2. Also assign the appropriate F10.- code to identify alcohol dependence/alcoholism, and, when applicable, a code to specify dementia (with or without behavior disturbance) as a manifestation (F02.8-). The dementia in alcohol dependence with alcohol-induced dementia code can be coded with F02.8-.

+ 5 G31.8 Other specified degenerative diseases of nervous system

SP + G31.81 Alpers disease
Grey-matter degeneration

SP + G31.82 Leigh's disease
Subacute necrotizing encephalopathy

SP + G31.83 Dementia with Lewy bodies
Dementia with Parkinsonism
Lewy body dementia
Lewy body disease

CODING TIPS ✓ Parkinsonism dementia, also known as Lewy body dementia (G31.83), has symptoms similar to Parkinson's disease. However, Parkinson's disease is a distinct condition and is coded to G20. For a patient with Lewy body dementia, assign G31.83 followed by a code from category F02.8-, Dementia in diseases classified elsewhere.

SP + G31.84 Mild cognitive impairment, so stated
Mild neurocognitive disorder
EXCLUDES 1 age related cognitive decline (R41.81)
altered mental status (R41.82)
cerebral degeneration (G31.9)
change in mental status (R41.82)

cognitive deficits following (sequelae of) cerebral hemorrhage or infarction (I69.01-, I69.11-, I69.21-, I69.31-, I69.81-, I69.91-)
cognitive impairment due to intracranial or head injury (S06.-)
dementia (F01.-, F02.-, F03)
mild memory disturbance (F06.8)
neurologic neglect syndrome (R41.4)
personality change, nonpsychotic (F68.8)

CODING TIPS ✓ To use this code, the physician must have documented mild cognitive impairment. A patient with mild cognitive impairment does not have dementia. Do not add dementia as an additional code.

DEFINITION Impairment in memory or other specific cognitive function, beyond what is normally seen at a given age, but with function remaining relatively intact in the other cognitive domains.

H SP + G31.85 Corticobasal degeneration

SP + G31.89 Other specified degenerative diseases of nervous system

IQ + G31.9 Degenerative disease of nervous system, unspecified

4 G32 Other degenerative disorders of nervous system in diseases classified elsewhere

M IQ G32.0 Subacute combined degeneration of spinal cord in diseases classified elsewhere
Dana-Putnam syndrome
Sclerosis of spinal cord (combined) (dorsolateral) (posterolateral)
Code first underlying disease, such as:
anemia (D51.9)
dietary (D51.3)
pernicious (D51.0)
vitamin B12 deficiency (E53.8)
EXCLUDES 1 syphilitic combined degeneration of spinal cord (A52.11)

5 G32.8 Other specified degenerative disorders of nervous system in diseases classified elsewhere
Code first underlying disease, such as:
amyloidosis cerebral degeneration (E85.-)
cerebral degeneration (due to) hypothyroidism (E00.0-E03.9)
cerebral degeneration (due to) neoplasm (C00-D49)
cerebral degeneration (due to) vitamin B deficiency, except thiamine (E52-E53.-)
EXCLUDES 1 superior hemorrhagic polioencephalitis [Wernicke's encephalopathy] (E51.2)

★ New ▲ Revised Px Primary SP PDGM Px SL Low CoM SH High CoM IQ Quest. Encounter H Hospice non-cancer Dx Unspecified M Manifestation

DecisionHealth's FY 2020 Complete Home Health ICD-10-CM Diagnosis Coding Manual

835

Chapter 6

G00-G99

M IQ G32.81 *Cerebellar ataxia in diseases classified elsewhere*

Code first underlying disease, such as:
celiac disease (with gluten ataxia) (K90.0)
cerebellar ataxia (in) neoplastic disease (paraneoplastic cerebellar degeneration) (C00-D49)
non-celiac gluten ataxia (M35.9)

EXCLUDES 1 systemic atrophy primarily affecting the central nervous system in alcoholic cerebellar ataxia (G31.2)
systemic atrophy primarily affecting the central nervous system in myxedema (G13.2)

M IQ G32.89 *Other specified degenerative disorders of nervous system in diseases classified elsewhere*

Degenerative encephalopathy in diseases classified elsewhere

Demyelinating diseases of the central nervous system   (G35-G37)

SP SH G35 **Multiple sclerosis**
SL
Disseminated multiple sclerosis
Generalized multiple sclerosis
Multiple sclerosis NOS
Multiple sclerosis of brain stem
Multiple sclerosis of cord

CODING TIPS ✓ Code G35 should be listed primary when the patient is being seen for more than one aspect of the disease. Code associated symptoms of MS from Chapter 18 after code G35 (MS), but only if those symptoms are **not routinely** associated with MS.

4 G36 **Other acute disseminated demyelination**
EXCLUDES 1 postinfectious encephalitis and encephalomyelitis NOS (G04.01)

SP G36.0 **Neuromyelitis optica [Devic]**
Demyelination in optic neuritis
EXCLUDES 1 optic neuritis NOS (H46)

SP G36.1 **Acute and subacute hemorrhagic leukoencephalitis [Hurst]**

SP G36.8 **Other specified acute disseminated demyelination**

SP G36.9 **Acute disseminated demyelination, unspecified**

4 G37 **Other demyelinating diseases of central nervous system**

SP G37.0 **Diffuse sclerosis of central nervous system**
Periaxial encephalitis
Schilder's disease
EXCLUDES 1 X linked adrenoleukodystrophy (E71.52-)

SP G37.1 **Central demyelination of corpus callosum**

SP G37.2 **Central pontine myelinolysis**

SP G37.3 **Acute transverse myelitis in demyelinating disease of central nervous system**
Acute transverse myelitis NOS
Acute transverse myelopathy
EXCLUDES 1 multiple sclerosis (G35)
neuromyelitis optica [Devic] (G36.0)

DEFINITION Spinal cord disorder with inflammatory lesions across the entire width of one level; numbness, back pain, weakness, sensory loss, motor and sphincter deficits, loss of bladder and bowel control appear quickly and progress to paraplegia.

SP G37.4 **Subacute necrotizing myelitis of central nervous system**

SP G37.5 **Concentric sclerosis [Balo] of central nervous system**

SP G37.8 **Other specified demyelinating diseases of central nervous system**

SP G37.9 **Demyelinating disease of central nervous system, unspecified**

Episodic and paroxysmal disorders (G40-G47)

4 G40 **Epilepsy and recurrent seizures**
Note:
the following terms are to be considered equivalent to intractable: pharmacoresistant (pharmacologically resistant), treatment resistant, refractory (medically) and poorly controlled

EXCLUDES 1 conversion disorder with seizures (F44.5)
convulsions NOS (R56.9)
post traumatic seizures (R56.1)
seizure (convulsive) NOS (R56.9)
seizure of newborn (P90)

EXCLUDES 2 hippocampal sclerosis (G93.81)
mesial temporal sclerosis (G93.81)
temporal sclerosis (G93.81)
Todd's paralysis (G83.84)

CODING TIPS ✓ When coding epileptic syndromes, coders should note that seizure(s)/epileptic disorders noted by the physician as treatment- or medication-resistant, refractory, or poorly controlled should be coded to intractable. Coders should not assign R56.9, Unspecified convulsions, for patients experiencing seizure disorders or recurrent seizures. Recurrent seizures and unspecified seizure disorders, when not reported as intractable, should be coded to G40.909.

5 G40.0 **Localization-related (focal) (partial) idiopathic epilepsy and epileptic syndromes with seizures of localized onset**
Benign childhood epilepsy with centrotemporal EEG spikes
Childhood epilepsy with occipital EEG paroxysms

---

4 4th digit required   **5** 5th digit required   **6** 6th digit required   **7** 7th digit required   **7** 7th digit placeholder   **+** Additional code   **=** Laterality

836   *DecisionHealth's* FY 2020 Complete Home Health ICD-10-CM Diagnosis Coding Manual

EXCLUDES 1 adult onset localization-related epilepsy (G40.1-, G40.2-)

⑥ G40.00 Localization-related (focal) (partial) idiopathic epilepsy and epileptic syndromes with seizures of localized onset, not intractable

Localization-related (focal) (partial) idiopathic epilepsy and epileptic syndromes with seizures of localized onset without intractability

SP G40.001 Localization-related (focal) (partial) idiopathic epilepsy and epileptic syndromes with seizures of localized onset, not intractable, with status epilepticus

SP G40.009 Localization-related (focal) (partial) idiopathic epilepsy and epileptic syndromes with seizures of localized onset, not intractable, without status epilepticus

Localization-related (focal) (partial) idiopathic epilepsy and epileptic syndromes with seizures of localized onset NOS

⑥ G40.01 Localization-related (focal) (partial) idiopathic epilepsy and epileptic syndromes with seizures of localized onset, intractable

SP G40.011 Localization-related (focal) (partial) idiopathic epilepsy and epileptic syndromes with seizures of localized onset, intractable, with status epilepticus

SP G40.019 Localization-related (focal) (partial) idiopathic epilepsy and epileptic syndromes with seizures of localized onset, intractable, without status epilepticus

⑤ G40.1 Localization-related (focal) (partial) symptomatic epilepsy and epileptic syndromes with simple partial seizures

Attacks without alteration of consciousness
Epilepsia partialis continua [Kozhevnikof]
Simple partial seizures developing into secondarily generalized seizures

⑥ G40.10 Localization-related (focal) (partial) symptomatic epilepsy and epileptic syndromes with simple partial seizures, not intractable

Localization-related (focal) (partial) symptomatic epilepsy and epileptic syndromes with simple partial seizures without intractability

SP G40.101 Localization-related (focal) (partial) symptomatic epilepsy and epileptic syndromes with simple partial seizures, not intractable, with status epilepticus

SP G40.109 Localization-related (focal) (partial) symptomatic epilepsy and epileptic syndromes with simple partial seizures, not intractable, without status epilepticus

Localization-related (focal) (partial) symptomatic epilepsy and epileptic syndromes with simple partial seizures NOS

⑥ G40.11 Localization-related (focal) (partial) symptomatic epilepsy and epileptic syndromes with simple partial seizures, intractable

SP G40.111 Localization-related (focal) (partial) symptomatic epilepsy and epileptic syndromes with simple partial seizures, intractable, with status epilepticus

SP G40.119 Localization-related (focal) (partial) symptomatic epilepsy and epileptic syndromes with simple partial seizures, intractable, without status epilepticus

⑤ G40.2 Localization-related (focal) (partial) symptomatic epilepsy and epileptic syndromes with complex partial seizures

Attacks with alteration of consciousness, often with automatisms
Complex partial seizures developing into secondarily generalized seizures

⑥ G40.20 Localization-related (focal) (partial) symptomatic epilepsy and epileptic syndromes with complex partial seizures, not intractable

Localization-related (focal) (partial) symptomatic epilepsy and epileptic syndromes with complex partial seizures without intractability

SP G40.201 Localization-related (focal) (partial) symptomatic epilepsy and epileptic syndromes with complex partial seizures, not intractable, with status epilepticus

SP G40.209 Localization-related (focal) (partial) symptomatic epilepsy and epileptic syndromes with complex partial seizures, not intractable, without status epilepticus

Localization-related (focal) (partial) symptomatic epilepsy and epileptic syndromes with complex partial seizures NOS

⑥ G40.21 Localization-related (focal) (partial) symptomatic epilepsy and epileptic syndromes with complex partial seizures, intractable

SP G40.211 Localization-related (focal) (partial) symptomatic epilepsy and epileptic syndromes with complex partial seizures, intractable, with status epilepticus

SP G40.219 Localization-related (focal) (partial) symptomatic epilepsy and epileptic syndromes with complex partial seizures, intractable, without status epilepticus

⑤ G40.3 Generalized idiopathic epilepsy and epileptic syndromes

Code also:
MERRF syndrome, if applicable (E88.42)

⑥ G40.30 Generalized idiopathic epilepsy and epileptic syndromes, not intractable

★ New ▲ Revised Px Primary SP PDGM Px SL Low CoM SH High CoM IQ Quest. Encounter H Hospice non-cancer Dx Unspecified M *Manifestation*

DecisionHealth's FY 2020 Complete Home Health ICD-10-CM Diagnosis Coding Manual

837

Generalized idiopathic epilepsy and epileptic syndromes without intractability

SP **G40.301** **Generalized idiopathic epilepsy and epileptic syndromes, not intractable, with status epilepticus**

SP **G40.309** **Generalized idiopathic epilepsy and epileptic syndromes, not intractable, without status epilepticus**

Generalized idiopathic epilepsy and epileptic syndromes NOS

⑥ **G40.31** **Generalized idiopathic epilepsy and epileptic syndromes, intractable**

SP **G40.311** **Generalized idiopathic epilepsy and epileptic syndromes, intractable, with status epilepticus**

SP **G40.319** **Generalized idiopathic epilepsy and epileptic syndromes, intractable, without status epilepticus**

⑤ **G40.A** **Absence epileptic syndrome**

Childhood absence epilepsy [pyknolepsy]
Juvenile absence epilepsy
Absence epileptic syndrome, NOS

⑥ **G40.A0** **Absence epileptic syndrome, not intractable**

SP **G40.A01** **Absence epileptic syndrome, not intractable, with status epilepticus**

SP **G40.A09** **Absence epileptic syndrome, not intractable, without status epilepticus**

⑥ **G40.A1** **Absence epileptic syndrome, intractable**

SP **G40.A11** **Absence epileptic syndrome, intractable, with status epilepticus**

SP **G40.A19** **Absence epileptic syndrome, intractable, without status epilepticus**

⑤ **G40.B** **Juvenile myoclonic epilepsy [impulsive petit mal]**

⑥ **G40.B0** **Juvenile myoclonic epilepsy, not intractable**

SP **G40.B01** **Juvenile myoclonic epilepsy, not intractable, with status epilepticus**

SP **G40.B09** **Juvenile myoclonic epilepsy, not intractable, without status epilepticus**

⑥ **G40.B1** **Juvenile myoclonic epilepsy, intractable**

SP **G40.B11** **Juvenile myoclonic epilepsy, intractable, with status epilepticus**

SP **G40.B19** **Juvenile myoclonic epilepsy, intractable, without status epilepticus**

⑤ **G40.4** **Other generalized epilepsy and epileptic syndromes**

Epilepsy with grand mal seizures on awakening
Epilepsy with myoclonic absences
Epilepsy with myoclonic-astatic seizures
Grand mal seizure NOS
Nonspecific atonic epileptic seizures
Nonspecific clonic epileptic seizures
Nonspecific myoclonic epileptic seizures
Nonspecific tonic epileptic seizures
Nonspecific tonic-clonic epileptic seizures
Symptomatic early myoclonic encephalopathy

⑥ **G40.40** **Other generalized epilepsy and epileptic syndromes, not intractable**

Other generalized epilepsy and epileptic syndromes without intractability
Other generalized epilepsy and epileptic syndromes NOS

SP **G40.401** **Other generalized epilepsy and epileptic syndromes, not intractable, with status epilepticus**

SP **G40.409** **Other generalized epilepsy and epileptic syndromes, not intractable, without status epilepticus**

⑥ **G40.41** **Other generalized epilepsy and epileptic syndromes, intractable**

SP **G40.411** **Other generalized epilepsy and epileptic syndromes, intractable, with status epilepticus**

SP **G40.419** **Other generalized epilepsy and epileptic syndromes, intractable, without status epilepticus**

✚ **⑤** **G40.5** **Epileptic seizures related to external causes**

Epileptic seizures related to alcohol
Epileptic seizures related to drugs
Epileptic seizures related to hormonal changes
Epileptic seizures related to sleep deprivation
Epileptic seizures related to stress
Code also:
    , if applicable, associated epilepsy and recurrent seizures (G40.-)
Use additional code for adverse effect, if applicable, to identify drug (T36-T50 with fifth or sixth character 5)

✚ **⑥** **G40.50** **Epileptic seizures related to external causes, not intractable**

SP **✚** **G40.501** **Epileptic seizures related to external causes, not intractable, with status epilepticus**

SP **✚** **G40.509** **Epileptic seizures related to external causes, not intractable, without status epilepticus**

Epileptic seizures related to external causes, NOS

⑤ **G40.8** **Other epilepsy and recurrent seizures**

Epilepsies and epileptic syndromes undetermined as to whether they are focal or generalized
Landau-Kleffner syndrome

⑥ **G40.80** **Other epilepsy**

SP **G40.801** **Other epilepsy, not intractable, with status epilepticus**

Other epilepsy without intractability with status epilepticus

SP **G40.802** **Other epilepsy, not intractable, without status epilepticus**

Other epilepsy NOS
Other epilepsy without intractability without status epilepticus

SP **G40.803** **Other epilepsy, intractable, with status epilepticus**

SP **G40.804** **Other epilepsy, intractable, without status epilepticus**

⑥ **G40.81** **Lennox-Gastaut syndrome**

---

④ 4th digit required   **⑤** 5th digit required   **⑥** 6th digit required   **⑦** 7th digit required   **⑦** 7th digit placeholder   **✚** Additional code   **▤** Laterality

SP **G40.811** Lennox-Gastaut syndrome, not intractable, with status epilepticus

SP **G40.812** Lennox-Gastaut syndrome, not intractable, without status epilepticus

SP **G40.813** Lennox-Gastaut syndrome, intractable, with status epilepticus

SP **G40.814** Lennox-Gastaut syndrome, intractable, without status epilepticus

6 **G40.82** Epileptic spasms
Infantile spasms
Salaam attacks
West's syndrome

CODING TIPS ✓ Code G40.82 describes infantile spasms, also known as West's syndrome.

SP **G40.821** Epileptic spasms, not intractable, with status epilepticus

SP **G40.822** Epileptic spasms, not intractable, without status epilepticus

SP **G40.823** Epileptic spasms, intractable, with status epilepticus

SP **G40.824** Epileptic spasms, intractable, without status epilepticus

SP **G40.89** Other seizures

EXCLUDES 1 post traumatic seizures (R56.1)
recurrent seizures NOS (G40.909)
seizure NOS (R56.9)

5 **G40.9** Epilepsy, unspecified

6 **G40.90** Epilepsy, unspecified, not intractable

Epilepsy, unspecified, without intractability

SP **G40.901** Epilepsy, unspecified, not intractable, with status epilepticus

SP **G40.909** Epilepsy, unspecified, not intractable, without status epilepticus

Epilepsy NOS
Epileptic convulsions NOS
Epileptic fits NOS
Epileptic seizures NOS
Recurrent seizures NOS
Seizure disorder NOS

CODING TIPS ✓ Recurrent seizures and unspecified seizure disorders, when not identified as intractable, should be reported using this code. Do not assign R56.9, Unspecified convulsions, to report a diagnosis of recurrent seizures or seizure disorder.

6 **G40.91** Epilepsy, unspecified, intractable
Intractable seizure disorder NOS

SP **G40.911** Epilepsy, unspecified, intractable, with status epilepticus

SP **G40.919** Epilepsy, unspecified, intractable, without status epilepticus

+ **4** **G43** Migraine

Note:
the following terms are to be considered equivalent to intractable: pharmacoresistant (pharmacologically resistant), treatment resistant, refractory (medically) and poorly controlled
Use additional code for adverse effect, if applicable, to identify drug (T36-T50 with fifth or sixth character 5)

EXCLUDES 1 headache NOS (R51)
lower half migraine (G44.00)
EXCLUDES 2 headache syndromes (G44.-)

+ **5** **G43.0** Migraine without aura
Common migraine

EXCLUDES 1 chronic migraine without aura (G43.7-)

+ **6** **G43.00** Migraine without aura, not intractable
Migraine without aura without mention of refractory migraine

SP **+** **G43.001** Migraine without aura, not intractable, with status migrainosus

SP **+** **G43.009** Migraine without aura, not intractable, without status migrainosus
Migraine without aura NOS

+ **6** **G43.01** Migraine without aura, intractable
Migraine without aura with refractory migraine

SP **+** **G43.011** Migraine without aura, intractable, with status migrainosus

SP **+** **G43.019** Migraine without aura, intractable, without status migrainosus

+ **5** **G43.1** Migraine with aura
Basilar migraine
Classical migraine
Migraine equivalents
Migraine preceded or accompanied by transient focal neurological phenomena
Migraine triggered seizures
Migraine with acute-onset aura
Migraine with aura without headache (migraine equivalents)
Migraine with prolonged aura
Migraine with typical aura
Retinal migraine
Code also:
any associated seizure (G40.-, R56.9)

EXCLUDES 1 persistent migraine aura (G43.5-, G43.6-)

+ **6** **G43.10** Migraine with aura, not intractable
Migraine with aura without mention of refractory migraine

SP **+** **G43.101** Migraine with aura, not intractable, with status migrainosus

SP **+** **G43.109** Migraine with aura, not intractable, without status migrainosus
Migraine with aura NOS

+ **6** **G43.11** Migraine with aura, intractable
Migraine with aura with refractory migraine

SP **+** **G43.111** Migraine with aura, intractable, with status migrainosus

★ New ▲ Revised **Px** Primary **SP** PDGM Px **SL** Low CoM **SH** High CoM **IQ** Quest. Encounter **H** Hospice non-cancer Dx ▨ Unspecified **M** *Manifestation*

DecisionHealth's FY 2020 Complete Home Health ICD-10-CM Diagnosis Coding Manual

839

SP **+** **G43.119 Migraine with aura, intractable, without status migrainosus**

+ **5** **G43.4 Hemiplegic migraine**
Familial migraine
Sporadic migraine

+ **6** **G43.40 Hemiplegic migraine, not intractable**
Hemiplegic migraine without refractory migraine

SP **+** **G43.401 Hemiplegic migraine, not intractable, with status migrainosus**

SP **+** **G43.409 Hemiplegic migraine, not intractable, without status migrainosus**
Hemiplegic migraine NOS

+ **6** **G43.41 Hemiplegic migraine, intractable**
Hemiplegic migraine with refractory migraine

SP **+** **G43.411 Hemiplegic migraine, intractable, with status migrainosus**

SP **+** **G43.419 Hemiplegic migraine, intractable, without status migrainosus**

+ **5** **G43.5 Persistent migraine aura without cerebral infarction**

+ **6** **G43.50 Persistent migraine aura without cerebral infarction, not intractable**
Persistent migraine aura without cerebral infarction, without refractory migraine

SP **+** **G43.501 Persistent migraine aura without cerebral infarction, not intractable, with status migrainosus**

SP **+** **G43.509 Persistent migraine aura without cerebral infarction, not intractable, without status migrainosus**
Persistent migraine aura NOS

+ **6** **G43.51 Persistent migraine aura without cerebral infarction, intractable**
Persistent migraine aura without cerebral infarction, with refractory migraine

SP **+** **G43.511 Persistent migraine aura without cerebral infarction, intractable, with status migrainosus**

SP **+** **G43.519 Persistent migraine aura without cerebral infarction, intractable, without status migrainosus**

+ **5** **G43.6 Persistent migraine aura with cerebral infarction**
Code also:
the type of cerebral infarction (I63.-)

+ **6** **G43.60 Persistent migraine aura with cerebral infarction, not intractable**
Persistent migraine aura with cerebral infarction, without refractory migraine

SP **+** **G43.601 Persistent migraine aura with cerebral infarction, not intractable, with status migrainosus**

SP **+** **G43.609 Persistent migraine aura with cerebral infarction, not intractable, without status migrainosus**

+ **6** **G43.61 Persistent migraine aura with cerebral infarction, intractable**

Persistent migraine aura with cerebral infarction, with refractory migraine

SP **+** **G43.611 Persistent migraine aura with cerebral infarction, intractable, with status migrainosus**

SP **+** **G43.619 Persistent migraine aura with cerebral infarction, intractable, without status migrainosus**

+ **5** **G43.7 Chronic migraine without aura**
Transformed migraine
EXCLUDES 1 migraine without aura (G43.0-)

+ **6** **G43.70 Chronic migraine without aura, not intractable**
Chronic migraine without aura, without refractory migraine

SP **+** **G43.701 Chronic migraine without aura, not intractable, with status migrainosus**

SP **+** **G43.709 Chronic migraine without aura, not intractable, without status migrainosus**
Chronic migraine without aura NOS

+ **6** **G43.71 Chronic migraine without aura, intractable**
Chronic migraine without aura, with refractory migraine

SP **+** **G43.711 Chronic migraine without aura, intractable, with status migrainosus**

SP **+** **G43.719 Chronic migraine without aura, intractable, without status migrainosus**

▲ **+** **5** **G43.A Cyclical vomiting**
EXCLUDES 1 cyclical vomiting syndrome unrelated to migraine (R11.15)

▲ **SP** **+** **G43.A0 Cyclical vomiting, in migraine, not intractable**
Cyclical vomiting, without refractory migraine

▲ **SP** **+** **G43.A1 Cyclical vomiting, in migraine, intractable**
Cyclical vomiting, with refractory migraine

+ **5** **G43.B Ophthalmoplegic migraine**

SP **+** **G43.B0 Ophthalmoplegic migraine, not intractable**
Ophthalmoplegic migraine, without refractory migraine

SP **+** **G43.B1 Ophthalmoplegic migraine, intractable**
Ophthalmoplegic migraine, with refractory migraine

+ **5** **G43.C Periodic headache syndromes in child or adult**

SP **+** **G43.C0 Periodic headache syndromes in child or adult, not intractable**
Periodic headache syndromes in child or adult, without refractory migraine

SP **+** **G43.C1 Periodic headache syndromes in child or adult, intractable**
Periodic headache syndromes in child or adult, with refractory migraine

+ **5** **G43.D Abdominal migraine**

SP **+** **G43.D0 Abdominal migraine, not intractable**
Abdominal migraine, without refractory migraine

---

4 4th digit required   **5** 5th digit required   **6** 6th digit required   **7** 7th digit required   **7** 7th digit placeholder   **+** Additional code   **5** Laterality

SP + **G43.D1 Abdominal migraine, intractable**
Abdominal migraine, with refractory migraine

+ 5 **G43.8 Other migraine**

+ 6 **G43.80 Other migraine, not intractable**
Other migraine, without refractory migraine

SP + **G43.801 Other migraine, not intractable, with status migrainosus**

SP + **G43.809 Other migraine, not intractable, without status migrainosus**

+ 6 **G43.81 Other migraine, intractable**
Other migraine, with refractory migraine

SP + **G43.811 Other migraine, intractable, with status migrainosus**

SP + **G43.819 Other migraine, intractable, without status migrainosus**

+ 6 **G43.82 Menstrual migraine, not intractable**
Menstrual headache, not intractable
Menstrual migraine, without refractory migraine
Menstrually related migraine, not intractable
Pre-menstrual headache, not intractable
Pre-menstrual migraine, not intractable
Pure menstrual migraine, not intractable
Code also:
associated premenstrual tension syndrome (N94.3)

SP + **G43.821 Menstrual migraine, not intractable, with status migrainosus**

SP + **G43.829 Menstrual migraine, not intractable, without status migrainosus**
Menstrual migraine NOS

+ 6 **G43.83 Menstrual migraine, intractable**
Menstrual headache, intractable
Menstrual migraine, with refractory migraine
Menstrually related migraine, intractable
Pre-menstrual headache, intractable
Pre-menstrual migraine, intractable
Pure menstrual migraine, intractable
Code also:
associated premenstrual tension syndrome (N94.3)

SP + **G43.831 Menstrual migraine, intractable, with status migrainosus**

SP + **G43.839 Menstrual migraine, intractable, without status migrainosus**

+ 5 **G43.9 Migraine, unspecified**

+ 6 **G43.90 Migraine, unspecified, not intractable**
Migraine, unspecified, without refractory migraine

SP + **G43.901 Migraine, unspecified, not intractable, with status migrainosus**
Status migrainosus NOS

SP + **G43.909 Migraine, unspecified, not intractable, without status migrainosus**
Migraine NOS

+ 6 **G43.91 Migraine, unspecified, intractable**
Migraine, unspecified, with refractory migraine

SP + **G43.911 Migraine, unspecified, intractable, with status migrainosus**

SP + **G43.919 Migraine, unspecified, intractable, without status migrainosus**

4 **G44 Other headache syndromes**

EXCLUDES 1 headache NOS (R51)

EXCLUDES 2 atypical facial pain (G50.1)
headache due to lumbar puncture (G97.1)
migraines (G43.-)
trigeminal neuralgia (G50.0)

5 **G44.0 Cluster headaches and other trigeminal autonomic cephalgias (TAC)**

6 **G44.00 Cluster headache syndrome, unspecified**

Ciliary neuralgia
Cluster headache NOS
Histamine cephalgia
Lower half migraine
Migrainous neuralgia

SP **G44.001 Cluster headache syndrome, unspecified, intractable**

SP **G44.009 Cluster headache syndrome, unspecified, not intractable**
Cluster headache syndrome NOS

6 **G44.01 Episodic cluster headache**

DEFINITION Distinctive headache marked by excruciating, searing pain that develops quickly without warning on one side and occurs in frequent attacks lasting from 15 minutes to 3 hours, in cyclical patterns of up to 12 weeks, followed by remission periods.

SP **G44.011 Episodic cluster headache, intractable**

SP **G44.019 Episodic cluster headache, not intractable**
Episodic cluster headache NOS

6 **G44.02 Chronic cluster headache**

SP **G44.021 Chronic cluster headache, intractable**

SP **G44.029 Chronic cluster headache, not intractable**
Chronic cluster headache NOS

6 **G44.03 Episodic paroxysmal hemicrania**
Paroxysmal hemicrania NOS

DEFINITION Rare headache with severe throbbing or boring pain in the eye or temple on one side and accompanying autonomic responses; occurring in frequent, daily attacks with relatively long headache-free periods.

SP **G44.031 Episodic paroxysmal hemicrania, intractable**

SP **G44.039 Episodic paroxysmal hemicrania, not intractable**
Episodic paroxysmal hemicrania NOS

6 **G44.04 Chronic paroxysmal hemicrania**

SP **G44.041 Chronic paroxysmal hemicrania, intractable**

Chapter 6

G00-G99

★ New ▲ Revised **Px** Primary **SP** PDGM Px **SL** Low CoM **SH** High CoM **IQ** Quest. Encounter **H** Hospice non-cancer Dx Unspecified **M** *Manifestation*

Chapter 6

G00-G99

SP **G44.049** **Chronic paroxysmal hemicrania, not intractable**
Chronic paroxysmal hemicrania NOS

6 **G44.05** **Short lasting unilateral neuralgiform headache with conjunctival injection and tearing (SUNCT)**

SP **G44.051** **Short lasting unilateral neuralgiform headache with conjunctival injection and tearing (SUNCT), intractable**

SP **G44.059** **Short lasting unilateral neuralgiform headache with conjunctival injection and tearing (SUNCT), not intractable**
Short lasting unilateral neuralgiform headache with conjunctival injection and tearing (SUNCT) NOS

6 **G44.09** **Other trigeminal autonomic cephalgias (TAC)**

SP **G44.091** **Other trigeminal autonomic cephalgias (TAC), intractable**

SP **G44.099** **Other trigeminal autonomic cephalgias (TAC), not intractable**

SP **G44.1** **Vascular headache, not elsewhere classified**
EXCLUDES 2   cluster headache (G44.0)
complicated headache syndromes (G44.5-)
drug-induced headache (G44.4-)
migraine (G43.-)
other specified headache syndromes (G44.8-)
post-traumatic headache (G44.3-)
tension-type headache (G44.2-)

5 **G44.2** **Tension-type headache**

6 **G44.20** **Tension-type headache, unspecified**
DEFINITION   Common, muscular contraction headaches, that produce a mild to moderate, dull, achy tightening pain over the forehead and sides like a band encircling the head or pain at the back of the neck or base of the skull.

SP **G44.201** **Tension-type headache, unspecified, intractable**

SP **G44.209** **Tension-type headache, unspecified, not intractable**
Tension headache NOS

6 **G44.21** **Episodic tension-type headache**

SP **G44.211** **Episodic tension-type headache, intractable**

SP **G44.219** **Episodic tension-type headache, not intractable**
Episodic tension-type headache NOS

6 **G44.22** **Chronic tension-type headache**

SP **G44.221** **Chronic tension-type headache, intractable**

SP **G44.229** **Chronic tension-type headache, not intractable**
Chronic tension-type headache NOS

5 **G44.3** **Post-traumatic headache**

6 **G44.30** **Post-traumatic headache, unspecified**
DEFINITION   Headache as a result of head trauma or injury, with frequency and severity diminishing over time; symptoms such as insomnia, concentration problems, personality changes, and dizziness often accompany the headache.

SP **G44.301** **Post-traumatic headache, unspecified, intractable**

SP **G44.309** **Post-traumatic headache, unspecified, not intractable**
Post-traumatic headache NOS

6 **G44.31** **Acute post-traumatic headache**

SP **G44.311** **Acute post-traumatic headache, intractable**

SP **G44.319** **Acute post-traumatic headache, not intractable**
Acute post-traumatic headache NOS

6 **G44.32** **Chronic post-traumatic headache**

SP **G44.321** **Chronic post-traumatic headache, intractable**

SP **G44.329** **Chronic post-traumatic headache, not intractable**
Chronic post-traumatic headache NOS

+ **5** **G44.4** **Drug-induced headache, not elsewhere classified**
Medication overuse headache
Use additional code for adverse effect, if applicable, to identify drug (T36-T50 with fifth or sixth character 5)
DEFINITION   Most common type of chronic daily headache caused by overuse of migraine-abortive ergot alkaloids and analgesic drugs.

SP **+** **G44.40** **Drug-induced headache, not elsewhere classified, not intractable**

SP **+** **G44.41** **Drug-induced headache, not elsewhere classified, intractable**

5 **G44.5** **Complicated headache syndromes**

SP **G44.51** **Hemicrania continua**

SP **G44.52** **New daily persistent headache (NDPH)**

SP **G44.53** **Primary thunderclap headache**
DEFINITION   Dramatic, sudden, severe headache coming without warning, peaking within 60 seconds, then fading over several hours; sometimes signaling a potentially life-threatening condition, such as a ruptured cerebral aneurysm or subarachnoid hemorrhage.

SP **G44.59** **Other complicated headache syndrome**

5 **G44.8** **Other specified headache syndromes**

SP **G44.81** **Hypnic headache**
DEFINITION   Relatively rare headache connected to REM sleep, marked by being awakened with intense throbbing or dull type pain through the head, accompanied by nausea, and lasting about an hour.

4 4th digit required   5 5th digit required   6 6th digit required   7 7th digit required   ☑ 7th digit placeholder   ✚ Additional code   ⊟ Laterality

842   *DecisionHealth's* FY 2020 Complete Home Health ICD-10-CM Diagnosis Coding Manual

SP G44.82 Headache associated with sexual activity
Orgasmic headache
Preorgasmic headache

SP G44.83 Primary cough headache
DEFINITION Headache triggered by bouts of coughing or physically straining movements, such as laughing or sneezing, often described as sharp, stabbing, or splitting on both sides of the head and back of the skull.

SP G44.84 Primary exertional headache

SP G44.85 Primary stabbing headache

SP G44.89 Other headache syndrome

4 G45 Transient cerebral ischemic attacks and related syndromes
EXCLUDES 1 neonatal cerebral ischemia (P91.0)
transient retinal artery occlusion (H34.0-)

SP G45.0 Vertebro-basilar artery syndrome
DEFINITION Obstruction of the vertebral or basilar artery temporarily blocking blood flow to the brain, causing vertigo, diplopia, nystagmus, and muscle weakness.

SP G45.1 Carotid artery syndrome (hemispheric)

SP G45.2 Multiple and bilateral precerebral artery syndromes

SP G45.3 Amaurosis fugax
CODING TIPS ✓ Amaurosis fugax is a sudden loss of vision in one eye related to impaired carotid blood flow and impaired retinal blood supply and is generally temporary. The condition should not be coded on a home health claim as it is classifiable as a type of acute transient ischemic attack. The condition may signal pending stroke and should not be confused with blindness. Coders should not code blindness in a patient with this condition.

SP G45.4 Transient global amnesia
EXCLUDES 1 amnesia NOS (R41.3)

SP G45.8 Other transient cerebral ischemic attacks and related syndromes

SP G45.9 Transient cerebral ischemic attack, unspecified
Spasm of cerebral artery
TIA
Transient cerebral ischemia NOS
CODING TIPS ✓ Note that there is no code in ICD-10 to report sequelae of a TIA, as these are considered to be "transient" and should not cause residual effects. If residual effects are noted, the coder should query the patient's physician to determine if the patient experienced an infarction or stroke. A history of TIA (or CVA) with no residual neurological deficits may be coded to Z86.73, Personal history of transient ischemic attack, and cerebral infarction, without residual deficits.

4 G46 Vascular syndromes of brain in cerebrovascular diseases
Code first:
underlying cerebrovascular disease (I60-I69)

CODING TIPS ✓ Conditions classified to G46.- include conditions specific to syndromes occurring as a result of specific types of cerebral vascular disease (I65-I68) and cerebral vascular accidents (CVA). Home health claims should not include acute CVAs (I60-I63) in any circumstance. When a syndrome classifiable to G46.- occurs as a residual of a CVA, assign the appropriate I69 code to indicate sequelae of cerebrovascular disease. These syndromes may be coded as "other sequelae" of CVAs and should then be coded following the appropriate I69 code with the 5th character '9' and 6th character '8,' for example, I69.398.

SP G46.0 Middle cerebral artery syndrome

SP G46.1 Anterior cerebral artery syndrome

SP G46.2 Posterior cerebral artery syndrome

SP G46.3 Brain stem stroke syndrome
Benedikt syndrome
Claude syndrome
Foville syndrome
Millard-Gubler syndrome
Wallenberg syndrome
Weber syndrome

SP G46.4 Cerebellar stroke syndrome

SP G46.5 Pure motor lacunar syndrome

SP G46.6 Pure sensory lacunar syndrome

SP G46.7 Other lacunar syndromes

SP G46.8 Other vascular syndromes of brain in cerebrovascular diseases

4 G47 Sleep disorders
EXCLUDES 2 nightmares (F51.5)
nonorganic sleep disorders (F51.-)
sleep terrors (F51.4)
sleepwalking (F51.3)

5 G47.0 Insomnia
EXCLUDES 2 alcohol related insomnia (F10.182, F10.282, F10.982)
drug-related insomnia (F11.182, F11.282, F11.982, F13.182, F13.282, F13.982, F14.182, F14.282, F14.982, F15.182, F15.282, F15.982, F19.182, F19.282, F19.982)
idiopathic insomnia (F51.01)
insomnia due to a mental disorder (F51.05)
insomnia not due to a substance or known physiological condition (F51.0-)
nonorganic insomnia (F51.0-)
primary insomnia (F51.01)
sleep apnea (G47.3-)

SP G47.00 Insomnia, unspecified
Insomnia NOS

Chapter 6

G00-G99

★ New ▲ Revised Px Primary SP PDGM Px SL Low CoM SH High CoM IQ Quest. Encounter H Hospice non-cancer Dx Unspecified M Manifestation

DecisionHealth's FY 2020 Complete Home Health ICD-10-CM Diagnosis Coding Manual

843

SP G47.01 **Insomnia due to medical condition**
Code also:
  associated medical condition

SP G47.09 **Other insomnia**

5 G47.1 **Hypersomnia**
  EXCLUDES 2 alcohol-related hypersomnia
              (F10.182, F10.282,
              F10.982)
            drug-related hypersomnia
              (F11.182, F11.282,
              F11.982, F13.182,
              F13.282, F13.982,
              F14.182, F14.282,
              F14.982, F15.182,
              F15.282, F15.982,
              F19.182, F19.282,
              F19.982)
            hypersomnia due to a mental
              disorder (F51.13)
            hypersomnia not due to a
              substance or known
              physiological condition
              (F51.1-)
            primary hypersomnia
              (F51.11)
            sleep apnea (G47.3-)

SP G47.10 **Hypersomnia, unspecified**
Hypersomnia NOS

SP G47.11 **Idiopathic hypersomnia with long sleep time**
Idiopathic hypersomnia NOS

SP G47.12 **Idiopathic hypersomnia without long sleep time**

SP G47.13 **Recurrent hypersomnia**
Kleine-Levin syndrome
Menstrual related hypersomnia

SP G47.14 **Hypersomnia due to medical condition**
Code also:
  associated medical condition

SP G47.19 **Other hypersomnia**

5 G47.2 **Circadian rhythm sleep disorders**
Disorders of the sleep wake schedule
Inversion of nyctohemeral rhythm
Inversion of sleep rhythm

SP G47.20 **Circadian rhythm sleep disorder, unspecified type**
Sleep wake schedule disorder NOS

SP G47.21 **Circadian rhythm sleep disorder, delayed sleep phase type**
Delayed sleep phase syndrome

SP G47.22 **Circadian rhythm sleep disorder, advanced sleep phase type**

SP G47.23 **Circadian rhythm sleep disorder, irregular sleep wake type**
Irregular sleep-wake pattern

SP G47.24 **Circadian rhythm sleep disorder, free running type**
Circadian rhythm sleep disorder, non-24-hour sleep-wake type

SP G47.25 **Circadian rhythm sleep disorder, jet lag type**

SP G47.26 **Circadian rhythm sleep disorder, shift work type**

IQ G47.27 **Circadian rhythm sleep disorder in conditions classified elsewhere**
Code first:
  underlying condition

SP G47.29 **Other circadian rhythm sleep disorder**

5 G47.3 **Sleep apnea**
Code also:
  any associated underlying condition
  EXCLUDES 1 apnea NOS (R06.81)
            Cheyne-Stokes breathing
              (R06.3)
            pickwickian syndrome
              (E66.2)
            sleep apnea of newborn
              (P28.3)

SP G47.30 **Sleep apnea, unspecified**
Sleep apnea NOS

SP G47.31 **Primary central sleep apnea**
Idiopathic central sleep apnea

SP G47.32 **High altitude periodic breathing**

SP G47.33 **Obstructive sleep apnea (adult) (pediatric)**
Obstructive sleep apnea hypopnea
  EXCLUDES 1 obstructive sleep apnea
              of newborn (P28.3)

SP G47.34 **Idiopathic sleep related nonobstructive alveolar hypoventilation**
Sleep related hypoxia

SP G47.35 **Congenital central alveolar hypoventilation syndrome**

IQ G47.36 **Sleep related hypoventilation in conditions classified elsewhere**
Sleep related hypoxemia in conditions
  classified elsewhere
Code first:
  underlying condition

IQ G47.37 **Central sleep apnea in conditions classified elsewhere**
Code first:
  underlying condition

SP G47.39 **Other sleep apnea**

5 G47.4 **Narcolepsy and cataplexy**
  6 G47.41 **Narcolepsy**
    SP G47.411 **Narcolepsy with cataplexy**
    SP G47.419 **Narcolepsy without cataplexy**
             Narcolepsy NOS
  6 G47.42 **Narcolepsy in conditions classified elsewhere**
             Code first:
               underlying condition
    IQ G47.421 **Narcolepsy in conditions classified elsewhere with cataplexy**
    IQ G47.429 **Narcolepsy in conditions classified elsewhere without cataplexy**

5 G47.5 **Parasomnia**
  EXCLUDES 1 alcohol induced parasomnia
              (F10.182, F10.282,
              F10.982)
            drug induced parasomnia
              (F11.182, F11.282,
              F11.982, F13.182,
              F13.282, F13.982,
              F14.182, F14.282,
              F14.982, F15.182,
              F15.282, F15.982,
              F19.182, F19.282,
              F19.982)

◢4th digit required   ⑤5th digit required   ⑥6th digit required   ⑦7th digit required   ⑦7th digit placeholder   ✚Additional code   ▤Laterality

844   *DecisionHealth's* FY 2020 Complete Home Health ICD-10-CM Diagnosis Coding Manual

parasomnia not due to a substance or known physiological condition (F51.8)

SP **G47.50** **Parasomnia, unspecified**
Parasomnia NOS

SP **G47.51** **Confusional arousals**

SP **G47.52** **REM sleep behavior disorder**

SP **G47.53** **Recurrent isolated sleep paralysis**

IQ **G47.54** **Parasomnia in conditions classified elsewhere**
Code first:
underlying condition

SP **G47.59** **Other parasomnia**

5 **G47.6** **Sleep related movement disorders**
EXCLUDES 2 restless legs syndrome (G25.81)

SP **G47.61** **Periodic limb movement disorder**
DEFINITION Involuntary limb movement or jerking during or just before sleep.

SP **G47.62** **Sleep related leg cramps**

SP **G47.63** **Sleep related bruxism**
EXCLUDES 1 psychogenic bruxism (F45.8)
DEFINITION Grinding the teeth during sleep.

SP **G47.69** **Other sleep related movement disorders**

SP **G47.8** **Other sleep disorders**
Other specified sleep-wake disorder

SP **G47.9** **Sleep disorder, unspecified**
Sleep disorder NOS
Unspecified sleep-wake disorder

Nerve, nerve root and plexus disorders (G50-G59)

EXCLUDES 1 current traumatic nerve, nerve root and plexus disorders - see Injury, nerve by body region
neuralgia NOS (M79.2)
neuritis NOS (M79.2)
peripheral neuritis in pregnancy (O26.82-)
radiculitis NOS (M54.1-)

4 **G50** **Disorders of trigeminal nerve**
INCLUDES disorders of 5th cranial nerve

SP **G50.0** **Trigeminal neuralgia**
Syndrome of paroxysmal facial pain
Tic douloureux

SP **G50.1** **Atypical facial pain**

SP **G50.8** **Other disorders of trigeminal nerve**

SP **G50.9** **Disorder of trigeminal nerve, unspecified**

4 **G51** **Facial nerve disorders**
INCLUDES disorders of 7th cranial nerve

SP **G51.0** **Bell's palsy**
Facial palsy
DEFINITION Temporary, unilateral facial muscle weakness or paralysis resulting from damage or trauma to one of the paired facial nerves.

SP **G51.1** **Geniculate ganglionitis**
EXCLUDES 1 postherpetic geniculate ganglionitis (B02.21)
DEFINITION Inflammation of the facial nerve ganglion.

SP **G51.2** **Melkersson's syndrome**
Melkersson-Rosenthal syndrome

5 **G51.3** **Clonic hemifacial spasm**

SP **G51.31** **Clonic hemifacial spasm, right**

SP **G51.32** **Clonic hemifacial spasm, left**

SP **G51.33** **Clonic hemifacial spasm, bilateral**

SP **G51.39** **Clonic hemifacial spasm, unspecified**

SP **G51.4** **Facial myokymia**

SP **G51.8** **Other disorders of facial nerve**

IQ **G51.9** **Disorder of facial nerve, unspecified**

4 **G52** **Disorders of other cranial nerves**
EXCLUDES 2 disorders of acoustic [8th] nerve (H93.3)
disorders of optic [2nd] nerve (H46, H47.0)
paralytic strabismus due to nerve palsy (H49.0-H49.2)

SP **G52.0** **Disorders of olfactory nerve**
Disorders of 1st cranial nerve

SP **G52.1** **Disorders of glossopharyngeal nerve**
Disorder of 9th cranial nerve
Glossopharyngeal neuralgia

SP **G52.2** **Disorders of vagus nerve**
Disorders of pneumogastric [10th] nerve

SP **G52.3** **Disorders of hypoglossal nerve**

Disorders of 12th cranial nerve

SP **G52.7** **Disorders of multiple cranial nerves**
Polyneuritis cranialis

SP **G52.8** **Disorders of other specified cranial nerves**

IQ **G52.9** **Cranial nerve disorder, unspecified**

M IQ **G53** *Cranial nerve disorders in diseases classified elsewhere*

Code first underlying disease, such as:
neoplasm (C00-D49)

EXCLUDES 1 multiple cranial nerve palsy in sarcoidosis (D86.82)
multiple cranial nerve palsy in syphilis (A52.15)
postherpetic geniculate ganglionitis (B02.21)
postherpetic trigeminal neuralgia (B02.22)

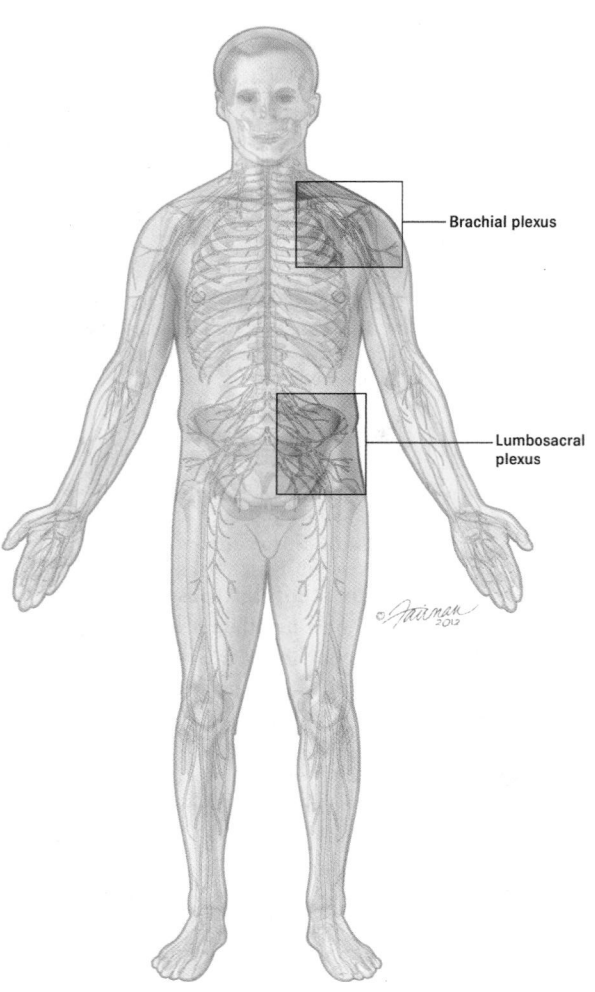
- Brachial plexus
- Lumbosacral plexus

4 G54 **Nerve root and plexus disorders**
EXCLUDES 1 current traumatic nerve root and plexus disorders - see nerve injury by body region
intervertebral disc disorders (M50-M51)
neuralgia or neuritis NOS (M79.2)

neuritis or radiculitis brachial NOS (M54.13)
neuritis or radiculitis lumbar NOS (M54.16)
neuritis or radiculitis lumbosacral NOS (M54.17)
neuritis or radiculitis thoracic NOS (M54.14)
radiculitis NOS (M54.10)
radiculopathy NOS (M54.10)
spondylosis (M47.-)

SP **G54.0** **Brachial plexus disorders**
Thoracic outlet syndrome

SP **G54.1** **Lumbosacral plexus disorders**

SP **G54.2** **Cervical root disorders, not elsewhere classified**

SP **G54.3** **Thoracic root disorders, not elsewhere classified**

SP **G54.4** **Lumbosacral root disorders, not elsewhere classified**

SP **G54.5** **Neuralgic amyotrophy**
Parsonage-Aldren-Turner syndrome
Shoulder-girdle neuritis
EXCLUDES 1 neuralgic amyotrophy in diabetes mellitus (E08-E13 with .44)

CODING TIPS ✓ Do not assign code G54.5 for diabetic amyotrophy. Diabetes with amyotrophy should be coded with the appropriate combination code to specify the type of diabetes and the neuralgic amyotrophy manifestation (E08-E13 with 4th and 5th character .44).

SP **G54.6** **Phantom limb syndrome with pain**

SP **G54.7** **Phantom limb syndrome without pain**
Phantom limb syndrome NOS

SP **G54.8** **Other nerve root and plexus disorders**

IQ **G54.9** **Nerve root and plexus disorder, unspecified**

M IQ **G55** *Nerve root and plexus compressions in diseases classified elsewhere*

Code first underlying disease, such as:
neoplasm (C00-D49)

EXCLUDES 1 nerve root compression (due to) (in) ankylosing spondylitis (M45.-)
nerve root compression (due to) (in) dorsopathies (M53.-, M54.-)
nerve root compression (due to) (in) intervertebral disc disorders (M50.1.-, M51.1.-)
nerve root compression (due to) (in) spondylopathies (M46.-, M48.-)
nerve root compression (due to) (in) spondylosis (M47.0-M47.2.-)

4 G56 **Mononeuropathies of upper limb**
EXCLUDES 1 current traumatic nerve disorder - see nerve injury by body region

4 4th digit required   5 5th digit required   6 6th digit required   7 7th digit required   7 7th digit placeholder   + Additional code   ⊟ Laterality

846   *DecisionHealth's* FY 2020 Complete Home Health ICD-10-CM Diagnosis Coding Manual

CODING TIPS ✓ Complex regional pain syndromes (CRPS Type I or II or unspecified) are no longer classified and coded to causalgias and mononeuropathies. When CRPS Type I, Type II or unspecified is reported, it should be coded to the appropriate G90.5- code.

⑤ **G56.0 Carpal tunnel syndrome**

DEFINITION Pain, burning, tingling and/or numbness in the fingers and hand, often extending to the elbow, due to compression of the median nerve within the carpal tunnel.

☐ **IQ** **G56.00** Carpal tunnel syndrome, unspecified upper limb

☐ **SP** **G56.01** Carpal tunnel syndrome, right upper limb

☐ **SP** **G56.02** Carpal tunnel syndrome, left upper limb

☐ **SP** **G56.03** Carpal tunnel syndrome, bilateral upper limbs

⑤ **G56.1 Other lesions of median nerve**

☐ **IQ** **G56.10** Other lesions of median nerve, unspecified upper limb

☐ **SP** **G56.11** Other lesions of median nerve, right upper limb

☐ **SP** **G56.12** Other lesions of median nerve, left upper limb

☐ **SP** **G56.13** Other lesions of median nerve, bilateral upper limbs

⑤ **G56.2 Lesion of ulnar nerve**
Tardy ulnar nerve palsy

☐ **IQ** **G56.20** Lesion of ulnar nerve, unspecified upper limb

☐ **SP** **G56.21** Lesion of ulnar nerve, right upper limb

☐ **SP** **G56.22** Lesion of ulnar nerve, left upper limb

☐ **SP** **G56.23** Lesion of ulnar nerve, bilateral upper limbs

⑤ **G56.3 Lesion of radial nerve**

☐ **IQ** **G56.30** Lesion of radial nerve, unspecified upper limb

☐ **SP** **G56.31** Lesion of radial nerve, right upper limb

☐ **SP** **G56.32** Lesion of radial nerve, left upper limb

☐ **SP** **G56.33** Lesion of radial nerve, bilateral upper limbs

⑤ **G56.4 Causalgia of upper limb**
Complex regional pain syndrome II of upper limb

EXCLUDES 1 complex regional pain syndrome I of lower limb (G90.52-)
complex regional pain syndrome I of upper limb (G90.51-)
complex regional pain syndrome II of lower limb (G57.7-)
reflex sympathetic dystrophy of lower limb (G90.52-)
reflex sympathetic dystrophy of upper limb (G90.51-)

DEFINITION A burning pain in the arm along the course of a peripheral nerve usually associated with skin changes.

☐ **IQ** **G56.40** Causalgia of unspecified upper limb

☐ **SP** **G56.41** Causalgia of right upper limb

☐ **SP** **G56.42** Causalgia of left upper limb

☐ **SP** **G56.43** Causalgia of bilateral upper limbs

⑤ **G56.8 Other specified mononeuropathies of upper limb**
Interdigital neuroma of upper limb

☐ **IQ** **G56.80** Other specified mononeuropathies of unspecified upper limb

☐ **SP** **G56.81** Other specified mononeuropathies of right upper limb

☐ **SP** **G56.82** Other specified mononeuropathies of left upper limb

☐ **SP** **G56.83** Other specified mononeuropathies of bilateral upper limbs

⑤ **G56.9 Unspecified mononeuropathy of upper limb**

☐ **IQ** **G56.90** Unspecified mononeuropathy of unspecified upper limb

☐ **SP** **G56.91** Unspecified mononeuropathy of right upper limb

☐ **SP** **G56.92** Unspecified mononeuropathy of left upper limb

☐ **SP** **G56.93** Unspecified mononeuropathy of bilateral upper limbs

④ **G57 Mononeuropathies of lower limb**

EXCLUDES 1 current traumatic nerve disorder - see nerve injury by body region

⑤ **G57.0 Lesion of sciatic nerve**

EXCLUDES 1 sciatica NOS (M54.3-)

EXCLUDES 2 sciatica attributed to intervertebral disc disorder (M51.1.-)

CODING TIPS ✓ Report G57.0- for pyriformis (piriformis) syndrome.

☐ **IQ** **G57.00** Lesion of sciatic nerve, unspecified lower limb

☐ **SP** **G57.01** Lesion of sciatic nerve, right lower limb

☐ **SP** **G57.02** Lesion of sciatic nerve, left lower limb

☐ **SP** **G57.03** Lesion of sciatic nerve, bilateral lower limbs

⑤ **G57.1 Meralgia paresthetica**
Lateral cutaneous nerve of thigh syndrome

☐ **IQ** **G57.10** Meralgia paresthetica, unspecified lower limb

☐ **SP** **G57.11** Meralgia paresthetica, right lower limb

☐ **SP** **G57.12** Meralgia paresthetica, left lower limb

☐ **SP** **G57.13** Meralgia paresthetica, bilateral lower limbs

⑤ **G57.2 Lesion of femoral nerve**

☐ **IQ** **G57.20** Lesion of femoral nerve, unspecified lower limb

☐ **SP** **G57.21** Lesion of femoral nerve, right lower limb

☐ **SP** **G57.22** Lesion of femoral nerve, left lower limb

Chapter 6

G00-G99

★ New ▲ Revised **Px** Primary **SP** PDGM Px **SL** Low CoM **SH** High CoM **IQ** Quest. Encounter **H** Hospice non-cancer Dx Unspecified **M** *Manifestation*

DecisionHealth's FY 2020 Complete Home Health ICD-10-CM Diagnosis Coding Manual

847

Chapter 6

G00-G99

☐ **SP** **G57.23** **Lesion of femoral nerve, bilateral lower limbs**

⑤ **G57.3** **Lesion of lateral popliteal nerve**
Peroneal nerve palsy

☐ **IQ** **G57.30** **Lesion of lateral popliteal nerve, unspecified lower limb**

☐ **SP** **G57.31** **Lesion of lateral popliteal nerve, right lower limb**

☐ **SP** **G57.32** **Lesion of lateral popliteal nerve, left lower limb**

☐ **SP** **G57.33** **Lesion of lateral popliteal nerve, bilateral lower limbs**

⑤ **G57.4** **Lesion of medial popliteal nerve**

☐ **IQ** **G57.40** **Lesion of medial popliteal nerve, unspecified lower limb**

☐ **SP** **G57.41** **Lesion of medial popliteal nerve, right lower limb**

☐ **SP** **G57.42** **Lesion of medial popliteal nerve, left lower limb**

☐ **SP** **G57.43** **Lesion of medial popliteal nerve, bilateral lower limbs**

⑤ **G57.5** **Tarsal tunnel syndrome**
> **DEFINITION**   Pain, burning, tingling, and/or numbness of the sole of the foot, often extending to the ankle, due to compression of the posterior tibial nerve or plantar nerves within the tarsal tunnel.

☐ **IQ** **G57.50** **Tarsal tunnel syndrome, unspecified lower limb**

☐ **SP** **G57.51** **Tarsal tunnel syndrome, right lower limb**

☐ **SP** **G57.52** **Tarsal tunnel syndrome, left lower limb**

☐ **SP** **G57.53** **Tarsal tunnel syndrome, bilateral lower limbs**

⑤ **G57.6** **Lesion of plantar nerve**
Morton's metatarsalgia
> **DEFINITION**   Thickening of tissue that surrounds the digital nerve leading to the toes. Most frequently develops between the third and fourth toes, usually in response to irritation, trauma or excessive pressure.

☐ **IQ** **G57.60** **Lesion of plantar nerve, unspecified lower limb**

☐ **SP** **G57.61** **Lesion of plantar nerve, right lower limb**

☐ **SP** **G57.62** **Lesion of plantar nerve, left lower limb**

☐ **SP** **G57.63** **Lesion of plantar nerve, bilateral lower limbs**

⑤ **G57.7** **Causalgia of lower limb**
Complex regional pain syndrome II of lower limb
> **EXCLUDES 1**   complex regional pain syndrome I of lower limb (G90.52-)
> complex regional pain syndrome I of upper limb (G90.51-)
> complex regional pain syndrome II of upper limb (G56.4-)
> reflex sympathetic dystrophy of lower limb (G90.52-)
> reflex sympathetic dystrophy of upper limb (G90.51-)

☐ **IQ** **G57.70** **Causalgia of unspecified lower limb**

☐ **SP** **G57.71** **Causalgia of right lower limb**

☐ **SP** **G57.72** **Causalgia of left lower limb**

☐ **SP** **G57.73** **Causalgia of bilateral lower limbs**

⑤ **G57.8** **Other specified mononeuropathies of lower limb**
Interdigital neuroma of lower limb

☐ **IQ** **G57.80** **Other specified mononeuropathies of unspecified lower limb**

☐ **SP** **G57.81** **Other specified mononeuropathies of right lower limb**

☐ **SP** **G57.82** **Other specified mononeuropathies of left lower limb**

☐ **SP** **G57.83** **Other specified mononeuropathies of bilateral lower limbs**

⑤ **G57.9** **Unspecified mononeuropathy of lower limb**

☐ **IQ** **G57.90** **Unspecified mononeuropathy of unspecified lower limb**

☐ **SP** **G57.91** **Unspecified mononeuropathy of right lower limb**

☐ **SP** **G57.92** **Unspecified mononeuropathy of left lower limb**

☐ **SP** **G57.93** **Unspecified mononeuropathy of bilateral lower limbs**

④ **G58** **Other mononeuropathies**

IQ **G58.0** **Intercostal neuropathy**

SP **G58.7** **Mononeuritis multiplex**

SP **G58.8** **Other specified mononeuropathies**

IQ **G58.9** **Mononeuropathy, unspecified**

IQ **G59** **Mononeuropathy in diseases classified elsewhere**
Code first:
underlying disease
> **EXCLUDES 1**   diabetic mononeuropathy (E08-E13 with .41)
> syphilitic nerve paralysis (A52.19)
> syphilitic neuritis (A52.15)
> tuberculous mononeuropathy (A17.83)

Polyneuropathies and other disorders of the peripheral nervous system   (G60-G65)

> **EXCLUDES 1**   neuralgia NOS (M79.2)
> neuritis NOS (M79.2)
> peripheral neuritis in pregnancy (O26.82-)
> radiculitis NOS (M54.10)

④ **G60** **Hereditary and idiopathic neuropathy**

SP **G60.0** **Hereditary motor and sensory neuropathy**
Charcot-Marie-Tooth disease
Déjérine-Sottas disease
Hereditary motor and sensory neuropathy, types I-IV
Hypertrophic neuropathy of infancy
Peroneal muscular atrophy (axonal type) (hypertrophic type)
Roussy-Levy syndrome

SP **G60.1** **Refsum's disease**
Infantile Refsum disease

SP **G60.2** **Neuropathy in association with hereditary ataxia**

SP **G60.3** **Idiopathic progressive neuropathy**

④4th digit required   ⑤5th digit required   ⑥6th digit required   ⑦7th digit required   ⑦7th digit placeholder   ✚Additional code   ☐Laterality

848   DecisionHealth's FY 2020 Complete Home Health ICD-10-CM Diagnosis Coding Manual

SP G60.8 Other hereditary and idiopathic neuropathies
Dominantly inherited sensory neuropathy
Morvan's disease
Nelaton's syndrome
Recessively inherited sensory neuropathy

SP G60.9 Hereditary and idiopathic neuropathy, unspecified

> **CODING TIPS ✓** The physician should document hereditary and/or idiopathic neuropathy to assign G60.9. If polyneuropathy is documented without a type or cause, assign G62.9.

4 G61 Inflammatory polyneuropathy

> **CODING TIPS ✓** When an inflammatory neuropathy is reported as unresolved, assign the appropriate code from G61.-. If inflammatory neuropathy is documented as resolved but residual neurologic deficits remain as sequelae, assign the appropriate code from category G65.-, Sequelae of inflammatory and toxic polyneuropathies.

SP G61.0 Guillain-Barre syndrome
Acute (post-)infective polyneuritis
Miller Fisher Syndrome

> **CODING TIPS ✓** When Guillain-Barre syndrome is reported as unresolved, assign code G61.0. If a Guillain-Barre syndrome is documented as resolved but residual neurologic deficits remain as sequelae, assign code G65.0, Sequelae of Guillain-Barre syndrome (code first the residual defects when coding G65.0). Acute inflammatory demyelinating polyneuropathy is included in this code.

> **DEFINITION** Disorder that causes the body's immune system to attack the nerves; paralysis begins at the feet and progresses upwards through the legs and torso to the arms and face.

SP + G61.1 Serum neuropathy
Use additional code for adverse effect, if applicable, to identify serum (T50.-)

5 G61.8 Other inflammatory polyneuropathies

SP G61.81 Chronic inflammatory demyelinating polyneuritis

SP G61.82 Multifocal motor neuropathy
MMN

SP G61.89 Other inflammatory polyneuropathies

IQ G61.9 Inflammatory polyneuropathy, unspecified

4 G62 Other and unspecified polyneuropathies

SP + G62.0 Drug-induced polyneuropathy
Use additional code for adverse effect, if applicable, to identify drug (T36-T50 with fifth or sixth character 5)

> **CODING TIPS ✓** Assign G62.0 when the polyneuropathy is specifically reported by the physician as related to the use of a drug. An additional code should be assigned to identify the drug.

SP G62.1 Alcoholic polyneuropathy

> **CODING TIPS ✓** This diagnosis indicates that the alcohol was linked to the disorder, so the use, abuse or dependence of alcohol F10.- code should include 5th and 6th characters .88.

> **CODING TIPS ✓** Assign G62.1 when the physician specifically reports that the polyneuropathy results from alcohol use. The coder should also code any history of, or current use, of alcohol.

> **DEFINITION** Loss of nerve function due to damage from prolonged, excessive alcohol consumption; commonly presents with numbness, weakness, and burning in the feet.

SP G62.2 Polyneuropathy due to other toxic agents
Code first:
(T51-T65) to identify toxic agent

5 G62.8 Other specified polyneuropathies

SP G62.81 Critical illness polyneuropathy
Acute motor neuropathy

SP + G62.82 Radiation-induced polyneuropathy
Use additional external cause code (W88-W90, X39.0-) to identify cause

SP G62.89 Other specified polyneuropathies

IQ G62.9 Polyneuropathy, unspecified
Neuropathy NOS

> **CODING TIPS ✓** The physician should document hereditary and/or idiopathic neuropathy to assign G60.9. If polyneuropathy is documented without a type or cause, assign G62.9.

▲ M IQ G63 *Polyneuropathy in diseases classified elsewhere*
Code first underlying disease, such as:
amyloidosis (E85.-)
endocrine disease, except diabetes (E00-E07, E15-E16, E20-E34)
metabolic diseases (E70-E88)
neoplasm (C00-D49)
nutritional deficiency (E40-E64)

> **EXCLUDES 1** polyneuropathy (in):
diabetes mellitus (E08-E13 with .42)
diphtheria (A36.83)
infectious mononucleosis (B27.0-B27.9 with 1)
Lyme disease (A69.22)
mumps (B26.84)
postherpetic (B02.23)
rheumatoid arthritis (M05.5-)
scleroderma (M34.83)
systemic lupus erythematosus (M32.19)

> **CODING TIPS ✓** Do not assign code G63 for diabetic polyneuropathy. Diabetes with polyneuropathy should be coded with the appropriate combination code to specify the type of diabetes and the polyneuropathy manifestation.

SP G64 Other disorders of peripheral nervous system
Disorder of peripheral nervous system NOS

★ New ▲ Revised Px Primary SP PDGM Px SL Low CoM SH High CoM IQ Quest. Encounter H Hospice non-cancer Dx Unspecified M *Manifestation*

DecisionHealth's FY 2020 Complete Home Health ICD-10-CM Diagnosis Coding Manual

849

⁴ G65 Sequelae of inflammatory and toxic polyneuropathies
Code first:
   condition resulting from (sequela) of
   inflammatory and toxic polyneuropathies

SP G65.0 Sequelae of Guillain-Barré syndrome

SP G65.1 Sequelae of other inflammatory polyneuropathy

SP G65.2 Sequelae of toxic polyneuropathy

Diseases of myoneural junction and muscle   (G70-G73)

⁴ G70 Myasthenia gravis and other myoneural disorders
   EXCLUDES 1 botulism
       (A05.1, A48.51-A48.52)
       transient neonatal myasthenia
       gravis (P94.0)

⁵ G70.0 Myasthenia gravis
   CODING TIPS ✓ When myasthenia gravis is
   not documented as with or without
   exacerbation (no exacerbation is specified),
   assign code G70.00, without (acute)
   exacerbation.

SP G70.00 Myasthenia gravis without (acute) exacerbation
   Myasthenia gravis NOS

SP G70.01 Myasthenia gravis with (acute) exacerbation
   Myasthenia gravis in crisis

SP G70.1 Toxic myoneural disorders
   Code first:
       (T51-T65) to identify toxic agent

SP G70.2 Congenital and developmental myasthenia

⁵ G70.8 Other specified myoneural disorders
   CODING TIPS ✓ Lambert-Eaton myasthenic
   syndrome (LEMS) is an autoimmune
   disorder of the neuromuscular junction, the
   site where nerve cells meet muscle cells
   and help activate the muscles. The
   disruption of electrical impulses is
   associated with antibodies produced as a
   consequence of this autoimmunity.

SP G70.80 Lambert-Eaton syndrome, unspecified
   Lambert-Eaton syndrome NOS

IQ G70.81 Lambert-Eaton syndrome in disease classified elsewhere
   Code first:
       underlying disease
   EXCLUDES 1 Lambert-Eaton syndrome
       in neoplastic disease
       (G73.1)

SP G70.89 Other specified myoneural disorders

IQ G70.9 Myoneural disorder, unspecified

⁴ G71 Primary disorders of muscles
   EXCLUDES 2 arthrogryposis multiplex
       congenita (Q74.3)
       metabolic disorders (E70-E88)
       myositis (M60.-)

⁵ G71.0 Muscular dystrophy

SP G71.00 Muscular dystrophy, unspecified

SP G71.01 Duchenne or Becker muscular dystrophy

Autosomal recessive, childhood type,
   muscular dystrophy resembling
   Duchenne or Becker muscular
   dystrophy
Benign [Becker] muscular dystrophy
Severe [Duchenne] muscular dystrophy

SP G71.02 Facioscapulohumeral muscular dystrophy
Scapulohumeral muscular dystrophy

SP G71.09 Other specified muscular dystrophies
Benign scapuloperoneal muscular
   dystrophy with early contractures
   [Emery-Dreifuss]
Congenital muscular dystrophy NOS
Congenital muscular dystrophy with
   specific morphological abnormalities
   of the muscle fiber
Distal muscular dystrophy
Limb-girdle muscular dystrophy
Ocular muscular dystrophy
Oculopharyngeal muscular dystrophy
Scapuloperoneal muscular dystrophy

⁵ G71.1 Myotonic disorders

SP G71.11 Myotonic muscular dystrophy
Dystrophia myotonica [Steinert]
Myotonia atrophica
Myotonic dystrophy
Proximal myotonic myopathy
   (PROMM)
Steinert disease

SP G71.12 Myotonia congenita
Acetazolamide responsive myotonia
   congenita
Dominant myotonia congenita
   [Thomsen disease]
Myotonia levior
Recessive myotonia congenita [Becker
   disease]

SP G71.13 Myotonic chondrodystrophy
Chondrodystrophic myotonia
Congenital myotonic
   chondrodystrophy
Schwartz-Jampel disease
   DEFINITION Muscle disorder of late
   infancy with distinctive signs: mask-like
   face with small features, short stature or
   dwarfism, limited joint mobility, hip
   dysplasia, and generalized myotonia
   with hypertrophied diaphragmatic
   muscles. Death usually occurs due to
   respiratory compromise.

SP ✚ G71.14 Drug induced myotonia
Use additional code for adverse effect,
   if applicable, to identify drug (T36-
   T50 with fifth or sixth character 5)

SP G71.19 Other specified myotonic disorders
Myotonia fluctuans
Myotonia permanens
Neuromyotonia [Isaacs]
Paramyotonia congenita (of von
   Eulenburg)
Pseudomyotonia
Symptomatic myotonia

SP G71.2 Congenital myopathies
Central core disease
Fiber-type disproportion
Minicore disease

---

⁴4th digit required ⁵5th digit required ⁶6th digit required ⁷7th digit required ⃝7th digit placeholder ✚Additional code ⊟Laterality

850   DecisionHealth's FY 2020 Complete Home Health ICD-10-CM Diagnosis Coding Manual

Multicore disease
Myotubular (centronuclear) myopathy
Nemaline myopathy
> **EXCLUDES 1** arthrogryposis multiplex
> congenita (Q74.3)

SP G71.3 Mitochondrial myopathy, not elsewhere classified
> **EXCLUDES 1** Kearns-Sayre syndrome
> (H49.81)
> Leber's disease (H47.21)
> Leigh's encephalopathy
> (G31.82)
> mitochondrial metabolism
> disorders (E88.4.-)
> Reye's syndrome (G93.7)

SP G71.8 Other primary disorders of muscles

IQ G71.9 Primary disorder of muscle, unspecified
Hereditary myopathy NOS

4 G72 Other and unspecified myopathies
> **EXCLUDES 1** arthrogryposis multiplex
> congenita (Q74.3)
> dermatopolymyositis (M33.-)
> ischemic infarction of muscle
> (M62.2-)
> myositis (M60.-)
> polymyositis (M33.2-)

SP + G72.0 Drug-induced myopathy
Use additional code for adverse effect, if
applicable, to identify drug (T36-T50
with fifth or sixth character 5)

SP + G72.1 Alcoholic myopathy
Use additional code to identify alcoholism
(F10.-)
> **CODING TIPS ✓** This diagnosis indicates that
> the alcohol was linked to the disorder, so
> the use, abuse or dependence of alcohol
> F10.- code should include 5th and 6th
> characters .88.

SP G72.2 Myopathy due to other toxic agents
Code first:
(T51-T65) to identify toxic agent

SP G72.3 Periodic paralysis
Familial periodic paralysis
Hyperkalemic periodic paralysis (familial)
Hypokalemic periodic paralysis (familial)
Myotonic periodic paralysis (familial)
Normokalemic paralysis (familial)
Potassium sensitive periodic paralysis
> **EXCLUDES 1** paramyotonia congenita
> (of von Eulenburg)
> (G71.19)

5 G72.4 Inflammatory and immune myopathies, not elsewhere classified

SP G72.41 Inclusion body myositis [IBM]

SP G72.49 Other inflammatory and immune myopathies, not elsewhere classified
Inflammatory myopathy NOS

5 G72.8 Other specified myopathies

SP G72.81 Critical illness myopathy
Acute necrotizing myopathy
Acute quadriplegic myopathy
Intensive care (ICU) myopathy
Myopathy of critical illness

> **CODING TIPS ✓** Critical illness myopathy
> typically occurs in the ICU among
> patients who have been treated with
> multiple drugs. It commonly occurs in
> sepsis patients and is responsible for
> cachexia and weakness.

> **CODING TIPS ✓** This condition may take
> several weeks to months for a patient to
> fully recover from, and should be coded
> in the home health setting when it
> remains a relevant, current diagnosis for
> the plan of care.

SP G72.89 Other specified myopathies

SP G72.9 Myopathy, unspecified

4 G73 Disorders of myoneural junction and muscle in diseases classified elsewhere

IQ G73.1 Lambert-Eaton syndrome in neoplastic disease
Code first:
underlying neoplasm (C00-D49)
> **EXCLUDES 1** Lambert-Eaton syndrome not
> associated with neoplasm
> (G70.80-G70.81)

> **CODING TIPS ✓** Those with LEMS not
> associated with malignancy have a benign
> overall prognosis. Generally the presence
> of cancer determines the prognosis when
> the LEMS is associated with a neoplasm.

M IQ G73.3 *Myasthenic syndromes in other diseases classified elsewhere*
Code first underlying disease, such as:
neoplasm (C00-D49)
thyrotoxicosis (E05.-)

M IQ G73.7 *Myopathy in diseases classified elsewhere*
Code first underlying disease, such as:
hyperparathyroidism (E21.0, E21.3)
hypoparathyroidism (E20.-)
glycogen storage disease (E74.0)
lipid storage disorders (E75.-)
> **EXCLUDES 1** myopathy in:
> rheumatoid arthritis
> (M05.32)
> sarcoidosis (D86.87)
> scleroderma (M34.82)
> sicca syndrome [Sjögren]
> (M35.03)
> systemic lupus
> erythematosus (M32.19)

Cerebral palsy and other paralytic syndromes (G80-G83)

> **GUIDELINES** Section I.C.6.a
> Codes from category G81, Hemiplegia and hemiparesis, and
> subcategories, G83.1, Monoplegia of lower limb, G83.2,
> Monoplegia of upper limb, and G83.3, Monoplegia, unspecified,
> identify whether the dominant or nondominant side is affected.
> Should the affected side be documented, but not specified as
> dominant or nondominant, and the classification system does not
> indicate a default, code selection is as follows:
> • For ambidextrous patients, the default should be dominant.
> • If the left side is affected, the default is non-dominant.
> • If the right side is affected, the default is dominant.

4 G80 Cerebral palsy
> **EXCLUDES 1** hereditary spastic paraplegia
> (G11.4)

★ New ▲ Revised Px Primary **SP** PDGM Px **SL** Low CoM **SH** High CoM **IQ** Quest. Encounter **H** Hospice non-cancer Dx Unspecified **M** *Manifestation*

DecisionHealth's FY 2020 Complete Home Health ICD-10-CM Diagnosis Coding Manual

851

SP G80.0 Spastic quadriplegic cerebral palsy
Congenital spastic paralysis (cerebral)

DEFINITION   Palsy presenting with spastic paralysis of all four limbs from early brain damage.

SP G80.1 Spastic diplegic cerebral palsy
Spastic cerebral palsy NOS

SP G80.2 Spastic hemiplegic cerebral palsy

DEFINITION   Palsy affecting the limbs on either the left or the right side (e.g., the right arm and right leg).

SP G80.3 Athetoid cerebral palsy
Double athetosis (syndrome)
Dyskinetic cerebral palsy
Dystonic cerebral palsy
Vogt disease

DEFINITION   Permanent, nonprogressive, motor disorder caused by brain damage usually occurring shortly before, during, or after birth and characterized by uncontrolled, writhing movements of the hands, feet, arms, or legs.

SP G80.4 Ataxic cerebral palsy

SP G80.8 Other cerebral palsy
Mixed cerebral palsy syndromes

SP G80.9 Cerebral palsy, unspecified
Cerebral palsy NOS

4 G81 Hemiplegia and hemiparesis
Note:
This category is to be used only when hemiplegia (complete)(incomplete) is reported without further specification, or is stated to be old or longstanding but of unspecified cause. The category is also for use in multiple coding to identify these types of hemiplegia resulting from any cause.

EXCLUDES 1   congenital cerebral palsy
(G80.-)
hemiplegia and hemiparesis due to sequela of cerebrovascular disease
(I69.05-, I69.15-, I69.25-, I69.35-, I69.85-, I69.95-)

CODING TIPS ✓   When coding hemiplegia and monoplegia, the dominance rule stated in the guidelines applies. Coders should note that there is no option to code unspecified side since the classification assumes dominant side.

CODING TIPS ✓   Hemiparesis refers to one-sided weakness and should be coded with G81.-, not M62.81. Hemiplegia with sequela of stroke is included in the combination code, for example I69.351.

CODING TIPS ✓   When paraplegia, hemiplegia, hemiparesis or another paralytic state results from a brain or spinal cord injury, code the paralysis/paresis followed by the code for the brain or spinal injury with the 7th character "S" to report a sequela of the injury.

5 G81.0 Flaccid hemiplegia

CODING TIPS ✓   Words that describe abnormal muscle tonicity as flaccid (hypotonic) or spastic (hypertonic) point to G81.0 and G81.1, respectively. Documentation of complete versus incomplete must come from the physician.

🔲 IQ G81.00 Flaccid hemiplegia affecting unspecified side

🔲 SP SH SL G81.01 Flaccid hemiplegia affecting right dominant side

🔲 SP SH SL G81.02 Flaccid hemiplegia affecting left dominant side

🔲 SP SH SL G81.03 Flaccid hemiplegia affecting right nondominant side

🔲 SP SH SL G81.04 Flaccid hemiplegia affecting left nondominant side

5 G81.1 Spastic hemiplegia

CODING TIPS ✓   Words that describe abnormal muscle tonicity as flaccid (hypotonic) or spastic (hypertonic) point to G81.0 and G81.1, respectively. Documentation of complete versus incomplete must come from the physician.

🔲 IQ G81.10 Spastic hemiplegia affecting unspecified side

🔲 SP SH SL G81.11 Spastic hemiplegia affecting right dominant side

🔲 SP SH SL G81.12 Spastic hemiplegia affecting left dominant side

🔲 SP SH SL G81.13 Spastic hemiplegia affecting right nondominant side

🔲 SP SH SL G81.14 Spastic hemiplegia affecting left nondominant side

5 G81.9 Hemiplegia, unspecified

🔲 IQ G81.90 Hemiplegia, unspecified affecting unspecified side

🔲 SP SH SL G81.91 Hemiplegia, unspecified affecting right dominant side

🔲 SP SH SL G81.92 Hemiplegia, unspecified affecting left dominant side

🔲 SP SH SL G81.93 Hemiplegia, unspecified affecting right nondominant side

🔲 SP SH SL G81.94 Hemiplegia, unspecified affecting left nondominant side

4 G82 Paraplegia (paraparesis) and quadriplegia (quadriparesis)
Note:
This category is to be used only when the listed conditions are reported without further specification, or are stated to be old or longstanding but of unspecified cause. The category is also for use in multiple coding to identify these conditions resulting from any cause

EXCLUDES 1   congenital cerebral palsy
(G80.-)
functional quadriplegia (R53.2)
hysterical paralysis (F44.4)

CODING TIPS ✓   When paraplegia, hemiplegia, hemiparesis or another paralytic state results from a brain or spinal cord injury, code the paralysis/paresis followed by the code for the brain or spinal injury with the 7th character "S" to report a sequela of the injury.

5 G82.2 Paraplegia
Paralysis of both lower limbs NOS

---

4 4th digit required   5 5th digit required   6 6th digit required   7 7th digit required   7 7th digit placeholder   ✚ Additional code   🔲 Laterality

852   DecisionHealth's FY 2020 Complete Home Health ICD-10-CM Diagnosis Coding Manual

Chapter 6

G00-G99

Paraparesis (lower) NOS
Paraplegia (lower) NOS

CODING TIPS ✓ If paraplegia resulted from a spinal cord injury, then code paraplegia followed by the sequela of spinal cord injury code (S14.- with 7th character S for cervical; S24.- with 7th character S for thoracic; S34.- with 7th character S for lumbar). Paraplegia is not likely to result from a CVA. Paraparesis is weakness of both lower limbs without paralysis and is coded with G82.22.

SP SH SL G82.20   Paraplegia, unspecified

ALERT Paraplegia, unspecified, may result in rejected claims in some regions. Query the physician for level of injury and complete/incomplete. "Complete" means that there is complete loss of function below the point of injury. An "incomplete" injury refers to a spinal cord injury in which some feeling or movement is still evident below the point of injury.

SP SH SL G82.21   Paraplegia, complete

SP SH SL G82.22   Paraplegia, incomplete

5 G82.5   Quadriplegia

CODING TIPS ✓ If quadriplegia resulted from a spinal cord injury, then code quadriplegia followed by the sequela of spinal cord injury code (S14.- with 7th character S for cervical; S24.- with 7th character S for thoracic; S34.- with 7th character S for lumbar). If quadriplegia results from a CVA, code the appropriate I69.36- code followed by quadriplegia. Documentation of complete versus incomplete must come from the physician.

SP SH SL G82.50   Quadriplegia, unspecified

ALERT Quadriplegia, unspecified, may result in rejected claims in some regions. Query the physician for level of injury and complete/incomplete. "Complete" means that there is complete loss of function below the point of injury. An "incomplete" injury refers to a spinal cord injury in which some feeling or movement is still evident below the point of injury.

SP SH SL G82.51   Quadriplegia, C1-C4 complete

SP SH SL G82.52   Quadriplegia, C1-C4 incomplete

SP SH SL G82.53   Quadriplegia, C5-C7 complete

SP SH SL G82.54   Quadriplegia, C5-C7 incomplete

4 G83   Other paralytic syndromes

Note:
This category is to be used only when the listed conditions are reported without further specification, or are stated to be old or longstanding but of unspecified cause. The category is also for use in multiple coding to identify these conditions resulting from any cause.

INCLUDES paralysis (complete) (incomplete), except as in G80-G82

CODING TIPS ✓ When coding hemiplegia and monoplegia, the dominance rule stated in the guidelines applies. Coders should note that there is no option to code unspecified side since the classification assumes dominant side.

CODING TIPS ✓ When paraplegia, hemiplegia, hemiparesis or another paralytic state results from a brain or spinal cord injury, code the paralysis/paresis followed by the code for the brain or spinal injury with the 7th character "S" to report a sequela of the injury.

SP G83.0   Diplegia of upper limbs
Diplegia (upper)
Paralysis of both upper limbs

5 G83.1   Monoplegia of lower limb
Paralysis of lower limb

EXCLUDES 1 monoplegia of lower limbs due to sequela of cerebrovascular disease (I69.04-, I69.14-, I69.24-, I69.34-, I69.84-, I69.94-)

CODING TIPS ✓ If monoplegia is the result of an injury, code the monoplegia and then the injury with 7th character S. If monoplegia is the result of a CVA, then code I69.33- and do not assign a code from G83.-. Unlike the G81 codes where hemiparesis is included, monoparesis is not included in the M83 codes. Weakness of a limb wihout mention of muscle weakness is assigned code R29.898, Other symptoms and signs involving the musculoskeletal system. If muscle weakness is documented, assign M62.81.

IQ G83.10   Monoplegia of lower limb affecting unspecified side

ALERT Monoplegia not specifying the limb affected may result in a rejected claim.

SP G83.11   Monoplegia of lower limb affecting right dominant side

SP G83.12   Monoplegia of lower limb affecting left dominant side

SP G83.13   Monoplegia of lower limb affecting right nondominant side

SP G83.14   Monoplegia of lower limb affecting left nondominant side

5 G83.2   Monoplegia of upper limb
Paralysis of upper limb

EXCLUDES 1 monoplegia of upper limbs due to sequela of cerebrovascular disease (I69.03-, I69.13-, I69.23-, I69.33-, I69.83-, I69.93-)

★ New ▲ Revised Px Primary **SP** PDGM Px **SL** Low CoM **SH** High CoM **IQ** Quest. Encounter **H** Hospice non-cancer Dx Unspecified **M** *Manifestation*

DecisionHealth's FY 2020 Complete Home Health ICD-10-CM Diagnosis Coding Manual

853

CODING TIPS ✓ If monoplegia is the result of an injury, code the monoplegia and then the injury with 7th character S. If monoplegia is the result of a CVA, then code I69.33- and do not assign a code from G83.-. Unlike the G81 codes where hemiparesis is included, monoparesis is not included in the M83 codes. Weakness of a limb wihout mention of muscle weakness is assigned code R29.898, Other symptoms and signs involving the musculoskeletal system. If muscle weakness is documented, assign M62.81.

⊟ 🔟 G83.20 Monoplegia of upper limb affecting unspecified side

> **ALERT** Monoplegia not specifying the limb affected may result in a rejected claim.

⊟ SP G83.21 Monoplegia of upper limb affecting right dominant side

⊟ SP G83.22 Monoplegia of upper limb affecting left dominant side

⊟ SP G83.23 Monoplegia of upper limb affecting right nondominant side

⊟ SP G83.24 Monoplegia of upper limb affecting left nondominant side

5 G83.3 Monoplegia, unspecified

> **ALERT** Monoplegia not specifying the limb affected may result in a rejected claim.

⊟ 🔟 G83.30 Monoplegia, unspecified affecting unspecified side

⊟ SP G83.31 Monoplegia, unspecified affecting right dominant side

⊟ SP G83.32 Monoplegia, unspecified affecting left dominant side

⊟ SP G83.33 Monoplegia, unspecified affecting right nondominant side

⊟ SP G83.34 Monoplegia, unspecified affecting left nondominant side

SP G83.4 Cauda equina syndrome
Neurogenic bladder due to cauda equina syndrome

> **EXCLUDES 1** cord bladder NOS (G95.89)
> neurogenic bladder NOS (N31.9)

> **CODING TIPS ✓** Cauda equina syndrome is a rare condition which is commonly denied for lack of documentation to support the diagnosis.

> **CODING TIPS ✓** Assign G83.4 only when the physician specifically reports cauda equina syndrome. This code includes neurogenic bladder, and no additional code for neurogenic bladder should be assigned when present.

> **DEFINITION** Emergent condition due to compression of spinal nerve roots causing dull aching pain in the perineum, bladder, and sacrum with associated paresthesia, bladder dysfunction, and/or paralysis.

SP G83.5 Locked-in state

> **CODING TIPS ✓** If the locked-in state results from a CVA, code the appropriate I69.36- code followed by locked-in state.

5 G83.8 Other specified paralytic syndromes

> **EXCLUDES 1** paralytic syndromes due to current spinal cord injury- code to spinal cord injury (S14, S24, S34)

SP G83.81 Brown-Séquard syndrome

> **CODING TIPS ✓** Brown-Sequard syndrome results when one side of the spinal cord is damaged. There is loss of movement but preserved sensation on one side of the body, while the other side of the body has loss of sensation but preserved movement.

SP G83.82 Anterior cord syndrome

> **CODING TIPS ✓** Anterior cord syndrome is characterized by damage to the front of the spinal cord. This results in impaired movement, touch, pain, and temperature sensations below the point of injury. In most cases of anterior cord syndrome, some movement can later be recovered.

SP G83.83 Posterior cord syndrome

> **CODING TIPS ✓** Posterior cord syndrome is characterized by damage to the back of the spinal cord. Most patients with posterior cord syndrome maintain good muscle power, pain, and temperature sensation, but experience poor coordination.

SP G83.84 Todd's paralysis (postepileptic)

SP G83.89 Other specified paralytic syndromes

🔟 G83.9 Paralytic syndrome, unspecified

> **ALERT** Paralytic syndrome, unspecified may result in a rejected claim. Query the physician for more information.

Other disorders of the nervous system (G89-G99)

4 G89 Pain, not elsewhere classified
Code also:
  related psychological factors associated with pain (F45.42)

> **EXCLUDES 1** generalized pain NOS (R52)
> pain disorders exclusively related to psychological factors (F45.41)
> pain NOS (R52)

> **EXCLUDES 2** atypical face pain (G50.1)
> headache syndromes (G44.-)
> localized pain, unspecified type - code to pain by site, such as:
> abdomen pain (R10.-)
> back pain (M54.9)
> breast pain (N64.4)
> chest pain (R07.1-R07.9)
> ear pain (H92.0-)
> eye pain (H57.1)
> headache (R51)
> joint pain (M25.5-)
> limb pain (M79.6-)
> lumbar region pain (M54.5)
> painful urination (R30.9)
> pelvic and perineal pain (R10.2)
> shoulder pain (M25.51-)

---

4 4th digit required   5 5th digit required   6 6th digit required   7 7th digit required   7 7th digit placeholder   + Additional code   ⊟ Laterality

854   DecisionHealth's FY 2020 Complete Home Health ICD-10-CM Diagnosis Coding Manual

spine pain (M54.-)
throat pain (R07.0)
tongue pain (K14.6)
tooth pain (K08.8)
renal colic (N23)
migraines (G43.-)
myalgia (M79.1-)
pain from prosthetic devices, implants, and grafts (T82.84, T83.84, T84.84, T85.84-)
phantom limb syndrome with pain (G54.6)
vulvar vestibulitis (N94.810)
vulvodynia (N94.81-)

GUIDELINES Section I.C.5.a

Assign code F45.41 for pain that is exclusively related to psychological disorders. As indicated by the Excludes 1 note under category G89, a code from category G89 should not be assigned with code F45.41. Code F45.42, Pain disorders with related psychological factors, should be used with a code from category G89 if there is documentation of a psychological component for a patient with acute or chronic pain.

GUIDELINES Section I.C.6.b.1)

Codes in category G89 may be used in conjunction with codes from other categories and chapters to provide more detail about acute or chronic pain and neoplasm-related pain, unless otherwise indicated below. If the pain is not specified as acute or chronic, postthoracotomy, postprocedural, or neoplasm-related, do not assign codes from category G89. A code from category G89 should not be assigned if the underlying (definitive) diagnosis is known, unless the reason for the encounter is pain control/management and not management of the underlying condition.

When an admission or encounter is for a procedure aimed at treating the underlying condition (e.g., spinal fusion, kyphoplasty), a code for the underlying condition (e.g., vertebral fracture, spinal stenosis) should be assigned as the principal diagnosis. No code from category G89 should be assigned.

CODING TIPS ✓ **Documentation:** Pain disorders should be coded only when specified by the physician and when the plan of care specifically addresses pain with interventions and goals to address the pain as a focus of care.

SP **G89.0** **Central pain syndrome**
Déjérine-Roussy syndrome
Myelopathic pain syndrome
Thalamic pain syndrome (hyperesthetic)
GUIDELINES Section I.C.6.b.6)
Central pain syndrome (G89.0) and chronic pain syndrome (G89.4) are different than the term "chronic pain," and therefore codes should only be used when the provider has specifically documented this condition.

CODING TIPS ✓ Do not code G89.0 unless the physician specifies central pain syndrome. G89.0 may be appropriate if: 1) Traumatic or brain-related damage to the central nervous system (e.g., damage from stroke, MS, tumors, epilepsy, Parkinson's); 2) The character and extent of the pain is partly related to a variety of causes; 3) Treatment includes pain medications. It also might be appropriate for patients on antidepressants and anticonvulsants.

5 **G89.1** **Acute pain, not elsewhere classified**
CODING TIPS ✓ When the clinical record specifies that the patient has a pain disorder with related psychological factors, F45.42 should be additionally assigned.

CODING TIPS ✓ Do not assign codes from the G89.1 and G89.2 subcategories if the underlying/definitive diagnosis is known, unless the addition of the pain code otherwise adds information as to the pain, i.e., acuity and the cause of the pain - post-surgical or post-traumatic. Use these subcategories as primary only if the reason for home care is encounter for pain control/management, and not treatment for an underlying condition.

SP **G89.11** **Acute pain due to trauma**
SP **G89.12** **Acute post-thoracotomy pain**
Post-thoracotomy pain NOS
GUIDELINES Section I.C.6.b.3)(a)-(b)
The provider's documentation should be used to guide the coding of postoperative pain. The default for post-thoracotomy and other postoperative pain not specified as acute or chronic is the code for the acute form. Routine or expected postoperative pain immediately after surgery should not be coded.

(a) Postoperative pain not associated with a specific postoperative complication is assigned to the appropriate postoperative pain code in category G89.

(b) Postoperative pain associated with specific postoperative complication (such as painful wire sutures) is assigned to the appropriate code(s) found in Chapter 19, Injury, poisoning, and certain other consequences of external causes. If appropriate, use additional code(s) from category G89 to identify acute or chronic pain (G89.18 or G89.28).

SP **G89.18** **Other acute postprocedural pain**
Postoperative pain NOS
Postprocedural pain NOS

★ New ▲ Revised **Px** Primary **SP** PDGM Px **SL** Low CoM **SH** High CoM **IQ** Quest. Encounter **H** Hospice non-cancer Dx [Unspecified] **M** *Manifestation*

CODING TIPS ✓ Documentation: Check the clinical record for documentation that the patient is experiencing a level of pain following a procedure that is indicative of a need for specific focus and attention within the plan of care and is being addressed with specific plan of care interventions and goals.

CODING TIPS ✓ G89.18 is the default code for post-operative/post-procedural pain when not specified as acute or chronic. G89.18 should not be coded in all patients who experience pain following a procedure. It is expected that some pain would be experienced following a procedure, and these codes are used for unusual pain.

CODING TIPS ✓ If the post-operative pain is associated with a complication (such as a device left in the body), code the complication and the pain. The exception is if the focus of the care is pain management. In that case, the pain code is sequenced as primary.

⑤ G89.2 Chronic pain, not elsewhere classified

EXCLUDES 1 causalgia, lower limb (G57.7-)
causalgia, upper limb (G56.4-)
central pain syndrome (G89.0)
chronic pain syndrome (G89.4)
complex regional pain syndrome II, lower limb (G57.7-)
complex regional pain syndrome II, upper limb (G56.4-)
neoplasm related chronic pain (G89.3)
reflex sympathetic dystrophy (G90.5-)

GUIDELINES Section I.C.6.b.4)
Chronic pain is classified to subcategory G89.2. There is no time frame defining when pain becomes chronic pain. The provider's documentation should be used to guide use of these codes.

CODING TIPS ✓ When the clinical record specifies that the patient has a pain disorder with related psychological factors, F45.42 should be additionally assigned.

CODING TIPS ✓ No specific time frame is required in order to code pain as chronic. Pain must be specified as chronic by the physician before using these codes. Do not assign codes from the G89.1 and G89.2 subcategories if the underlying/definitive diagnosis is known, unless the addition of the pain code otherwise adds information as to the pain, i.e., acuity and the cause of the pain - post-surgical or post-traumatic. Use these subcategories as primary only if the reason for home care is encounter for pain control/management, and not treatment for an underlying condition.

SP G89.21 Chronic pain due to trauma
SP G89.22 Chronic post-thoracotomy pain
SP G89.28 Other chronic postprocedural pain
Other chronic postoperative pain

CODING TIPS ✓ If chronic pain is associated with a postoperative complication, code the complication and then G89.28.

CODING TIPS ✓ Post-procedural pain that is not specified as acute or chronic should not be coded to G89.28, or to G89.18, Other acute postprocedural pain. Post operative pain should not be coded in all patients who experience pain following a procedure. It is expected that some pain would be experienced following a procedure.

CODING TIPS ✓ Documentation: Check the clinical record for documentation that the patient is experiencing a level of pain following a procedure that is indicative of a need for specific focus and attention within the plan of care and is being addressed with specific plan of care interventions and goals.

SP G89.29 Other chronic pain
SP G89.3 Neoplasm related pain (acute) (chronic)
Cancer associated pain
Pain due to malignancy (primary) (secondary)
Tumor associated pain

GUIDELINES Section I.C.6.b.5)
Code G89.3 is assigned to pain documented as being related, associated or due to cancer, primary or secondary malignancy, or tumor. This code is assigned regardless of whether the pain is acute or chronic. This code may be assigned as the principal or first listed code when the stated reason for the admission/encounter is documented as pain control/pain management. The underlying neoplasm should be reported as an additional diagnosis.

When the reason for the admission/encounter is management of the neoplasm and the pain associated with the neoplasm is also documented, code G89.3 may be assigned as an additional diagnosis. It is not necessary to assign an additional code for the site of the pain.

CODING TIPS ✓ Use G89.3 for chronic or acute pain, when related to a neoplasm, either benign or malignant. Neoplasm related pain may be assigned as primary if the main reason for home care is admission for pain control. Hospices should not report codes from G89 as primary.

SP G89.4 Chronic pain syndrome
Chronic pain associated with significant psychosocial dysfunction

---

⚃4th digit required   ⑤5th digit required   ⑥6th digit required   ⑦7th digit required   ⑦7th digit placeholder   ✚Additional code   ⊟Laterality

856   DecisionHealth's FY 2020 Complete Home Health ICD-10-CM Diagnosis Coding Manual

GUIDELINES Section I.C.6.b.6)
Central pain syndrome (G89.0) and chronic pain syndrome (G89.4) are different than the term "chronic pain," and therefore codes should only be used when the provider has specifically documented this condition.

CODING TIPS ✓ Do not confuse chronic pain syndrome with chronic pain (unspecified). Chronic pain syndrome is a specifically diagnosed condition that must be reported by the patient's physician and includes a cycle of psychological and physical components.

4 G90 Disorders of autonomic nervous system
EXCLUDES 1 dysfunction of the autonomic nervous system due to alcohol (G31.2)

5 G90.0 Idiopathic peripheral autonomic neuropathy

SP G90.01 Carotid sinus syncope
Carotid sinus syndrome

CODING TIPS ✓ Carotid sinus syndrome causes a slow heart rate or decreases the blood pressure without slowing the heart rate. Syncope may result from stimulation of the carotid sinus pressure sensors either internally (high blood pressure) or externally (turning the head). This occurs mostly in elderly men.

DEFINITION Exaggerated response to carotid sinus baroreceptor stimulation causing bradycardia, hypotension, and dizziness.

SP G90.09 Other idiopathic peripheral autonomic neuropathy
Idiopathic peripheral autonomic neuropathy NOS

CODING TIPS ✓ Do not assign G90.09 for polyneuropathy or unspecified peripheral neuropathy. G90.09 is assigned to specify peripheral autonomic neuropathy, a condition that impairs nervous system function between the autonomic nervous system and the brain, resulting in autonomic dysregulation.

SP G90.1 Familial dysautonomia [Riley-Day]

SP G90.2 Horner's syndrome
Bernard(-Horner) syndrome
Cervical sympathetic dystrophy or paralysis

SP G90.3 Multi-system degeneration of the autonomic nervous system
Neurogenic orthostatic hypotension [Shy-Drager]
EXCLUDES 1 orthostatic hypotension NOS (I95.1)

SP ✚ G90.4 Autonomic dysreflexia
Use additional code to identify the cause, such as:
fecal impaction (K56.41)
pressure ulcer (pressure area) (L89.-)
urinary tract infection (N39.0)

5 G90.5 Complex regional pain syndrome I (CRPS I)
Reflex sympathetic dystrophy

EXCLUDES 1 causalgia of lower limb (G57.7-)
causalgia of upper limb (G56.4-)
complex regional pain syndrome II of lower limb (G57.7-)
complex regional pain syndrome II of upper limb (G56.4-)

SP G90.50 Complex regional pain syndrome I, unspecified

6 G90.51 Complex regional pain syndrome I of upper limb

SP G90.511 Complex regional pain syndrome I of right upper limb

SP G90.512 Complex regional pain syndrome I of left upper limb

SP G90.513 Complex regional pain syndrome I of upper limb, bilateral

IQ G90.519 Complex regional pain syndrome I of unspecified upper limb

6 G90.52 Complex regional pain syndrome I of lower limb

SP G90.521 Complex regional pain syndrome I of right lower limb

SP G90.522 Complex regional pain syndrome I of left lower limb

SP G90.523 Complex regional pain syndrome I of lower limb, bilateral

IQ G90.529 Complex regional pain syndrome I of unspecified lower limb

SP G90.59 Complex regional pain syndrome I of other specified site

SP G90.8 Other disorders of autonomic nervous system

IQ G90.9 Disorder of the autonomic nervous system, unspecified

4 G91 Hydrocephalus
INCLUDES acquired hydrocephalus
EXCLUDES 1 Arnold-Chiari syndrome with hydrocephalus (Q07.-)
congenital hydrocephalus (Q03.-)
spina bifida with hydrocephalus (Q05.-)

SP G91.0 Communicating hydrocephalus
Secondary normal pressure hydrocephalus

SP G91.1 Obstructive hydrocephalus

SP G91.2 (Idiopathic) normal pressure hydrocephalus
Normal pressure hydrocephalus NOS
DEFINITION Disruption of normal cerebrospinal fluid circulation and gradual ventricular enlargement without known cause resulting in abnormal gait, cognitive impairment, and urinary incontinence.

SP G91.3 Post-traumatic hydrocephalus, unspecified

M IQ G91.4 *Hydrocephalus in diseases classified elsewhere*
Code first underlying condition, such as:
congenital syphilis (A50.4-)
neoplasm (C00-D49)
plasminogen deficiency (E88.02)

☆ New ▲ Revised Px Primary **SP** PDGM Px **SL** Low CoM **SH** High CoM **IQ** Quest. Encounter **H** Hospice non-cancer Dx Unspecified **M** *Manifestation*

EXCLUDES 1 hydrocephalus due to congenital toxoplasmosis (P37.1)

SP **G91.8** **Other hydrocephalus**

IQ **G91.9** Hydrocephalus, unspecified

SP **G92** **Toxic encephalopathy**
Toxic encephalitis
Toxic metabolic encephalopathy
Code first:
, if applicable, drug induced (T36-T50) (T51-T65) to identify toxic agent

4 **G93** **Other disorders of brain**

SP **G93.0** **Cerebral cysts**
Arachnoid cyst
Porencephalic cyst, acquired
EXCLUDES 1 acquired periventricular cysts of newborn (P91.1)
congenital cerebral cysts (Q04.6)

SP **G93.1** **Anoxic brain damage, not elsewhere classified**
EXCLUDES 1 cerebral anoxia due to anesthesia during labor and delivery (O74.3)
cerebral anoxia due to anesthesia during the puerperium (O89.2)
neonatal anoxia (P84)

CODING TIPS ✓ When the anoxic brain damage is noted as a sequela of an injury and the injury that resulted in the anoxic brain damage is known, a code from Chapter 19, Injury, Poisoning and Certain Other Consequences of External Causes should be additionally assigned (with a 7th character "S").

SP **G93.2** **Benign intracranial hypertension**
EXCLUDES 1 hypertensive encephalopathy (I67.4)

SP **G93.3** **Postviral fatigue syndrome**
Benign myalgic encephalomyelitis
EXCLUDES 1 chronic fatigue syndrome NOS (R53.82)

5 **G93.4** Other and unspecified encephalopathy
EXCLUDES 1 alcoholic encephalopathy (G31.2)
encephalopathy in diseases classified elsewhere (G94)
hypertensive encephalopathy (I67.4)
toxic (metabolic) encephalopathy (G92)

SP **G93.40** Encephalopathy, unspecified

SP **G93.41** **Metabolic encephalopathy**
Septic encephalopathy
CODING TIPS ✓ Assign G93.41 when encephalopathy is documented related to sepsis.

DEFINITION Neuropsychiatric disturbances due to metabolic brain disease, commonly caused by hypoxia, ischemia, hypoglycemia, or diseases of other organs.

SP **G93.49** **Other encephalopathy**
Encephalopathy NEC

CODING TIPS ✓ Assign G93.49 when encephalopathy is documented related to a CVA or stroke.

SP **G93.5** **Compression of brain**
Arnold-Chiari type 1 compression of brain
Compression of brain (stem)
Herniation of brain (stem)
EXCLUDES 1 diffuse traumatic compression of brain (S06.2-)
focal traumatic compression of brain (S06.3-)

SP **G93.6** **Cerebral edema**
EXCLUDES 1 cerebral edema due to birth injury (P11.0)
traumatic cerebral edema (S06.1-)

SP **+ G93.7** **Reye's syndrome**
Code first:
poisoning due to salicylates, if applicable (T39.0-, with sixth character 1-4)
Use additional code for adverse effect due to salicylates, if applicable (T39.0-, with sixth character 5)
DEFINITION Rare, acute, sometimes fatal childhood disease with recurrent vomiting, elevated serum transaminase levels and liver changes, then acute brain swelling, consciousness disturbances and seizures.

5 **G93.8** **Other specified disorders of brain**

SP **G93.81** **Temporal sclerosis**
Hippocampal sclerosis
Mesial temporal sclerosis

IQ **G93.82** **Brain death**

SP **G93.89** **Other specified disorders of brain**
Postradiation encephalopathy

IQ **G93.9** Disorder of brain, unspecified

M IQ **G94** *Other disorders of brain in diseases classified elsewhere*
Code first:
underlying disease
EXCLUDES 1 encephalopathy in congenital syphilis (A50.49)
encephalopathy in influenza (J09.X9, J10.81, J11.81)
encephalopathy in syphilis (A52.19)
hydrocephalus in diseases classified elsewhere (G91.4)

4 **G95** Other and unspecified diseases of spinal cord
EXCLUDES 2 myelitis (G04.-)

SP **G95.0** **Syringomyelia and syringobulbia**
DEFINITION Cyst formation within the spinal cord resulting from trauma, hemorrhage, meningitis, tumor, or Chiari 1 malformation. The growing cyst destroys the cord's center, causing neurologic deficits that progress to greater degrees when not treated surgically.

5 **G95.1** **Vascular myelopathies**
EXCLUDES 2 intraspinal phlebitis and thrombophlebitis, except non-pyogenic (G08)

SP **G95.11** **Acute infarction of spinal cord (embolic) (nonembolic)**

---

4 4th digit required   **5** 5th digit required   **6** 6th digit required   **7** 7th digit required   **☑** 7th digit placeholder   **+** Additional code   **⊟** Laterality

858   *DecisionHealth's* FY 2020 Complete Home Health ICD-10-CM Diagnosis Coding Manual

Anoxia of spinal cord
Arterial thrombosis of spinal cord

SP G95.19 Other vascular myelopathies
Edema of spinal cord
Hematomyelia
Nonpyogenic intraspinal phlebitis and
thrombophlebitis
Subacute necrotic myelopathy

**5 G95.2 Other and unspecified cord
compression**

IQ G95.20 Unspecified cord compression

SP G95.29 Other cord compression

5 G95.8 Other specified diseases of spinal cord
EXCLUDES 1 neurogenic bladder NOS
(N31.9)
neurogenic bladder due to
cauda equina syndrome
(G83.4)
neuromuscular dysfunction
of bladder without spinal
cord lesion (N31.-)

SP G95.81 Conus medullaris syndrome

**SP G95.89 Other specified diseases of spinal
cord**
Cord bladder NOS
Drug-induced myelopathy
Radiation-induced myelopathy
EXCLUDES 1 myelopathy NOS
(G95.9)

IQ G95.9 Disease of spinal cord, unspecified
Myelopathy NOS

4 G96 Other disorders of central nervous system

SP G96.0 Cerebrospinal fluid leak
EXCLUDES 1 cerebrospinal fluid leak from
spinal puncture (G97.0)

**5 G96.1 Disorders of meninges, not elsewhere
classified**

SP G96.11 Dural tear
EXCLUDES 1 accidental puncture or
laceration of dura
during a procedure
(G97.41)

**SP G96.12 Meningeal adhesions (cerebral)
(spinal)**

**SP G96.19 Other disorders of meninges, not
elsewhere classified**

**SP G96.8 Other specified disorders of central
nervous system**

**IQ G96.9 Disorder of central nervous system,
unspecified**

**4 G97 Intraoperative and postprocedural
complications and disorders of nervous
system, not elsewhere classified**
EXCLUDES 2 intraoperative and
postprocedural
cerebrovascular infarction
(I97.81-, I97.82-)

CODING TIPS ✓ **Documentation:** Do not assign
any code for intraoperative and postprocedural
complications and disorders of the nervous
system without specific documentation from
the patient's physician providing a specific
relationship between the complication and the
procedure.

**SP G97.0 Cerebrospinal fluid leak from spinal
puncture**

**SP G97.1 Other reaction to spinal and lumbar
puncture**
Headache due to lumbar puncture

**SP G97.2 Intracranial hypotension following
ventricular shunting**

**5 G97.3 Intraoperative hemorrhage and
hematoma of a nervous system organ or
structure complicating a procedure**
EXCLUDES 1 intraoperative hemorrhage
and hematoma of a
nervous system organ or
structure due to accidental
puncture and laceration
during a procedure
(G97.4-)

**SP G97.31 Intraoperative hemorrhage and
hematoma of a nervous system organ
or structure complicating a nervous
system procedure**

**SP G97.32 Intraoperative hemorrhage and
hematoma of a nervous system organ
or structure complicating other
procedure**

**5 G97.4 Accidental puncture and laceration of a
nervous system organ or structure
during a procedure**

**SP G97.41 Accidental puncture or laceration of
dura during a procedure**
Incidental (inadvertent) durotomy

**SP G97.48 Accidental puncture and laceration
of other nervous system organ or
structure during a nervous system
procedure**

**SP G97.49 Accidental puncture and laceration
of other nervous system organ or
structure during other procedure**

**5 G97.5 Postprocedural hemorrhage of a
nervous system organ or structure
following a procedure**

**SP G97.51 Postprocedural hemorrhage of a
nervous system organ or structure
following a nervous system
procedure**

**SP G97.52 Postprocedural hemorrhage of a
nervous system organ or structure
following other procedure**

**5 G97.6 Postprocedural hematoma and seroma
of a nervous system organ or structure
following a procedure**

**SP G97.61 Postprocedural hematoma of a
nervous system organ or structure
following a nervous system
procedure**

**SP G97.62 Postprocedural hematoma of a
nervous system organ or structure
following other procedure**

**SP G97.63 Postprocedural seroma of a nervous
system organ or structure following
a nervous system procedure**

**SP G97.64 Postprocedural seroma of a nervous
system organ or structure following
other procedure**

**+ 5 G97.8 Other intraoperative and
postprocedural complications and
disorders of nervous system**
Use additional code to further specify
disorder

**SP + G97.81 Other intraoperative complications
of nervous system**

★ New ▲ Revised Px Primary SP PDGM Px SL Low CoM SH High CoM IQ Quest. Encounter H Hospice non-cancer Dx Unspecified M *Manifestation*

DecisionHealth's FY 2020 Complete Home Health ICD-10-CM Diagnosis Coding Manual

859

Chapter 6

G00-G99

SP + G97.82   **Other postprocedural complications and disorders of nervous system**

4 G98   **Other disorders of nervous system not elsewhere classified**

> INCLUDES   nervous system disorder NOS

SP G98.0   **Neurogenic arthritis, not elsewhere classified**

Nonsyphilitic neurogenic arthropathy NEC
Nonsyphilitic neurogenic spondylopathy NEC

> EXCLUDES 1   spondylopathy (in) :
> syringomyelia and
> syringobulbia (G95.0)
> tabes dorsalis (A52.11)

SP G98.8   **Other disorders of nervous system**

Nervous system disorder NOS

4 G99   **Other disorders of nervous system in diseases classified elsewhere**

M IQ G99.0   *Autonomic neuropathy in diseases classified elsewhere*

Code first underlying disease, such as:
  amyloidosis (E85.-)
  gout (M1A.-, M10.-)
  hyperthyroidism (E05.-)

> EXCLUDES 1   diabetic autonomic
> neuropathy
> (E08-E13 with .43)

> CODING TIPS ✓   This neuropathy affects the heart, digestive system and other involuntary functions. This type of neuropathy (G99.0) causes delayed or slowed gastric emptying as well as problems with orthostatic hypotension. This code is not to be used for polyneuropathy of the hands and feet. It is not to be coded as a manifestation of diabetes.

M IQ G99.2   *Myelopathy in diseases classified elsewhere*

Code first underlying disease, such as:
  neoplasm (C00-D49)

> EXCLUDES 1   myelopathy in:
> intervertebral disease
> (M50.0-, M51.0-)
> spondylosis
> (M47.0-, M47.1-)

M IQ G99.8   *Other specified disorders of nervous system in diseases classified elsewhere*

Code first underlying disorder, such as:
  amyloidosis (E85.-)
  avitaminosis (E56.9)

> EXCLUDES 1   nervous system involvement
> in:
> cysticercosis (B69.0)
> rubella (B06.0-)
> syphilis (A52.1-)

Chapter 6

G00-G99

---

4 4th digit required   5 5th digit required   6 6th digit required   7 7th digit required   7 7th digit placeholder   + Additional code   Laterality

Chapter 6 Scenarios: Diseases of the nervous system (G00-G99)

Neoplasm-related pain, breast cancer, liver mets

A 90-year-old woman is admitted to home health to treat severe pain that is reported as related to breast cancer that has spread to her liver.

Description	Code
Primary: Neoplasm-related pain	G89.3
Secondary: Malignant neoplasm of unspecified site of unspecified female breast	C50.919
Secondary: Secondary malignant neoplasm of liver	C78.7

As the focus of care, the neoplasm-related pain is coded in the primary position. The patient's breast cancer and the mets to the liver are coded in the secondary positions as relevant co-morbidities.

Multiple sclerosis

A 48-year-old woman was admitted to the hospital with intractable pain and muscle spasms. The physician diagnosed it as an exacerbation of multiple sclerosis (MS). Upon admission to home care for physical and occupational therapy, she was found to have continued bouts of spasms, muscle weakness, decreased range of motion in her joints, poor functional mobility and an ataxic gait pattern. The referral further stated the patient has hypertension, neurogenic bladder, and a history of urinary tract infections.

Description	Code
Primary: Multiple sclerosis	G35
Secondary: Neurogenic bladder NOS	N31.9
Secondary: Essential (primary) hypertension	I10
Secondary: History of UTI	Z87.440

There are no ICD-10 codes that are specifically for therapy. Rather coding guidelines state to code the reason therapy is seeing the patient, which, in this case, would be the multiple sclerosis. G35 is coded primary as this is the focus of care. No additional codes are required for the weakness, spasms, problems with range of motion, gait or functional mobility as these are all integral symptoms to the multiple sclerosis disease process. As such, they should not be additionally coded. Not all MS patients have neurogenic bladder though. Therefore, it should be coded additionally when present with MS. The additional comorbidities of hypertension and history of UTIs are relevant to the plan of care and thus are coded as well.

PT for Parkinson's with recent falls

A Parkinson's patient requires physical therapy. The referral notes recent falls and requests that the therapist investigate the increase in falls. The therapist's Plan of Care includes instructing the patient on the signs and symptoms of the disease, strategies to address freezing episodes, stretching of anterior muscles, positioning, strengthening of posterior muscles, fall prevention techniques and gait training. The therapist also performs a home-safety evaluation and modifies the patient's environment as needed to reduce the risk of falls.

Description	Code
Primary: Parkinson's disease	G20
Secondary: Repeated Falls	R29.6
Secondary: History of Falling	Z91.81

There are no therapy codes in ICD-10-CM; coding guidelines state to code the primary reason for therapy. In this scenario, the Parkinson's disease is the primary reason for home health and the focus of care for physical therapy, and is therefore coded as primary. The code R29.6, Repeated falls, is assigned when the patient has had recent falls and the plan of care indicates a need to investigate the cause of recent falls. The Excludes 2 note allows the coder to also code Z91.81, history of falling, with R29.6. The code Z91.81 indicates that a patient has previously fallen in the past and continues to be at risk for future falls.

Hemiplegia affecting non-dominant side

A 70-year-old man was in a car accident two years ago and suffered a traumatic brain injury with a subdural hematoma following a loss of consciousness. He was the driver and was involved in a collision with another car. Since the accident the patient has been in a skilled nursing facility. He has recently been sent home and continues to need total care. All home health disciplines have been ordered. He has spastic hemiplegia of the right non-dominant side and dysphagia resulting from the resolved subdural hematoma. He has a PEG tube due to the dysphagia. His family requires teaching on the care of the PEG tube.

Description	Code
Primary: Spastic hemiplegia affecting right non-dominant side	G81.13
Secondary: Dysphagia, unspecified	R13.10
Secondary: Traumatic subdural hemorrhage with loss of consciousness of unspecified duration, sequela	S06.5x9S
Secondary: Encounter for attention to gastrostomy	Z43.1
Secondary: Car driver injured in collision with other type car in traffic accident, sequela	V43.52xS

Sequence first the residual conditions (non-dominant hemiplegia and dysphagia) resulting from the traumatic brain injury, followed by the injury code with the 7th character "S" (sequela), per coding guidelines. Be sure not to code the symptom, dysphagia, as primary as it is considered a questionable encounter code in PDGM. Assign Z43.1 because the agency will be teaching the family to care for the PEG tube. If the patient/family was independent in the care of the PEG tube, Z93.1 would be assigned instead. The external cause code to report the cause of the accident should also be reported with a 7th character "S," in accordance with coding guidelines.

Epilepsy

A patient is admitted for evaluation and control of his intractable seizures. His video EEGs were consistent with epileptiform discharges of the right temporal lobe origin. Family will be instructed in care and management of epilepsy. Dilantin and Phenobarbital must be adjusted and monitored by home health nurses and venipuncture is ordered for therapeutic/toxicity testing. Diagnosis was partial complex epilepsy localized to the right temporal lobe, with impairment of consciousness.

Description	Code
Primary: Localization related symptomatic epilepsy and epileptic syndromes with complex partial seizures, intractable, without status epilepticus	G40.219
Secondary: Encounter for therapeutic drug monitoring	Z51.81
Secondary: Long-term (current) use of other medications	Z79.899

Partial complex epilepsy references G40.219 when intractable. The venipuncture and medication management are captured with Z51.81 and Z79.899.

Early-onset Alzheimer's disease with wandering

A 60-year-old female with early-onset Alzheimer's disease is admitted to home care for safety concerns as to a recent onset of agitation and wandering associated with the Alzheimer's disease. She required a replacement of her gastrostomy tube as she pulled it out, and she has a history of dysphagia. She is visibly agitated during clinical interview and her daughter states this has become worse in past few months.

Description	Code
Primary: Alzheimer's disease with early onset	G30.0
Secondary: Dementia in other disease classified elsewhere with behavioral disturbance	F02.81
Secondary: Wandering in diseases classified elsewhere	Z91.83
Secondary: Dysphagia, unspecified	R13.10
Secondary: Encounter for attention to gastrostomy	Z43.1

The patient has a diagnosis of early-onset Alzheimer's dementia. While early onset Alzheimer's is defined as a diagnosis before the age of 65, you must query the physician to confirm it. Since the diagnosis is confirmed in this case, it is coded with G30.0. The dementia code follows the Alzheimer's code in accordance with the etiology-manifestation convention and in accordance with Q1 2017 Coding Clinic guidance. Because she is experiencing behavioral disturbance, the dementia code F02.81 is assigned to reflect that. Wandering is coded additionally in accordance with tabular instruction.

HOME HEALTH CODING SCENARIOS

Alzheimer's dementia with hypertension

A 72-year-old patient was recently discharged from the hospital where he was treated for uncontrolled hypertension due to inability to take prescribed medications. While there he was diagnosed with late onset Alzheimer's dementia. He is not experiencing behavioral changes, and is now admitted to home care for physical therapy and skilled nursing for safety and medication teaching.

Description	Code
Primary: Alzheimer's disease with late onset	G30.1
Secondary: Dementia in other disease classified elsewhere without behavioral disturbance	F02.80
Secondary: Essential (primary) hypertension	I10
Secondary: Underdosing of other antihypertensive drugs, subsequent encounter	T46.5x6D
Secondary: Patient's unintentional underdosing of medication regimen for other reason	Z91.138

The patient was recently diagnosed with late onset Alzheimer's dementia, so it should be coded with G30.1. An additional code for dementia is also assigned, in accordance with Q1 2017 Coding Clinic guidance. He was treated in the hospital for uncontrolled hypertension, which will require continued monitoring in the home health setting, and thus I10 is assigned to capture that as well. Code T46.5x6D is included to indicate that the patient's uncontrolled hypertension was caused by his inability to take his medication. This code should never be listed primary. Additionally, chapter-specific guidelines instruct the coder to use an additional code to indicate the intent of the patient's non-compliance with his medication regimen and thus Z91.138 is assigned in accordance with this. *[I.C.19.e.5.c]*

Alzheimer's delirium, viral pneumonia

A 56-year-old patient who has had Alzheimer's disease for five years was recently hospitalized with viral pneumonia. She has now been admitted to home care for skilled nursing for continued treatment of the pneumonia. The family says the patient is exhibiting signs of delirium. The nurse queried the physician and confirmed a diagnosis of early onset Alzheimer's with delirium.

Description	Code
Primary: Viral pneumonia, unspecified	J12.9
Secondary: Alzheimer's disease with early onset	G30.0
Secondary: Dementia in other diseases classified elsewhere with behavioral disturbance	F02.81
Secondary: Delirium due to known physiological condition	F05

The patient was diagnosed with Alzheimer's well before the age of 65, and while early onset is defined as a diagnosis before the age of 65, you must query the physician to confirm it, which the nurse did, and thus it is coded with G30.0 As the focus of care, pneumonia is coded primary. The Alzheimer's is coded next because it must be sequenced before the delirium. The dementia code, F02.81, immediately follows the Alzheimer's code as it's part of an etiology/manifestation pairing. Because the patient is experiencing delirium, behavioral disturbance is present and F02.81 is used. The delirium code, F05, follows it.

HOME HEALTH CODING SCENARIOS

ALS with tracheostomy care

A 59-year-old man with amyotrophic lateral sclerosis (ALS) recently had a tracheostomy placed to assist in breathing. His family requires reaching on how to care for it. He is wheelchair bound. The tracheostomy is the focus of care.

Description	Code
Primary: Encounter for attention to tracheostomy	Z43.0
Secondary: Amyotrophic lateral sclerosis	G12.21
Secondary: Dependence on wheelchair	Z99.3

The agency will be providing care to the tracheostomy, so a code from Z43.- (Encounter for attention to artificial openings) is appropriate versus a code from Z93.- (Artificial opening status).

Lewy body dementia

A 77-year-old man is admitted to home health for teaching and medication following a recent diagnosis of Lewy body dementia. He has been experiencing agitation and outbursts. Additional comorbidities include congestive heart failure. The Lewy body dementia with outbursts is the focus of care.

Description	Code
Primary: Dementia with Lewy bodies	G31.83
Secondary: Dementia in other diseases classified elsewhere with behavioral disturbance	F02.81
Secondary: Heart failure, unspecified	I50.9

As the primary diagnosis, Lewy body dementia is coded primary. Because the patient is experiencing behavioral disturbance, F02.81 is assigned immediately after. As a comorbidity that will impact his plan of care, his congestive heart failure is coded.

Alcoholic encephalopathy, alcohol-induced diabetes

A 71-year-old man was admitted to home health with a primary diagnosis of alcoholic encephalopathy, which has led to dementia. He also has type 2 diabetes, which his medical record says is the result of heavy drinking, and hypertension. He's been an alcoholic for 37 years and continues to drink heavily.

Description	Code
Primary: Degeneration of nervous system due to alcohol	G31.2
Secondary: Dementia in other diseases classified elsewhere without behavioral disturbance	F02.80
Secondary: Alcohol dependence with alcohol-induced persisting dementia	F10.27
Secondary: Toxic effect of ethanol, accidental (unintentional), subsequent encounter	T51.0x1D
Secondary: Drug or chemical induced diabetes mellitus without complications	E09.9
Secondary: Essential (primary) hypertension	I10

As the focus of care the alcoholic encephalopathy is coded primary. It has caused dementia, so the necessary dementia manifestation code immediately follows it, in accordance with the etiology-manifestation convention. Code F10.27 is coded to capture his continued alcoholism. Alcoholism codes to dependence in the alphabetic index and the more specific code was chosen to show that the alcoholism ultimately led to dementia. His diabetes is an important comorbidity and since it was caused by alcohol use, it must be coded as drug or chemical-induced diabetes, with the code for the toxic effect of alcohol preceding the diabetes code, in accordance with tabular instruction. Hypertension is coded as a relevant comorbidity.

Neuropathy following Schwannoma removal

A 72-year-old man is admitted to home health with a primary diagnosis of peripheral neuropathy resulting from the removal of Schwannoma tumor on his spinal cord two years ago. The tumor is completely resolved.

Description	Code
Primary: Benign neoplasm of spinal meninges	D32.1
Secondary: Polyneuropathy in diseases classified elsewhere	G63

The patient's neuropathy is the focus of care, but the code for it (G63) is a manifestation code that must be preceded by an etiology code, according to the etiology-manifestation convention. Therefore, the reason for the neuropathy, the Schwannoma tumor, is coded first. Note that even though the Schwannoma is resolved, it must be coded as the cause of the peripheral neuropathy per the instructional note at G63.

Left hip fracture, intractable epilepsy

A 57-year-old woman underwent surgery to repair a fractured left hip sustained during a recent seizure. She has epilepsy that is documented as resistant to treatment. She is admitted to home health to recovery from the fracture and for medication management and occupational therapy.

Description	Code
Primary: Fracture of unspecified part of neck of left femur, subsequent encounter for closed fracture with routine healing	S72.002D
Secondary: Epilepsy, unspecified, intractable, without status epilepticus	G40.919

Though the patient underwent surgery to treat the fracture, a surgical aftercare code is not assigned, in accordance with coding guidelines. Rather, the fracture itself is coded. Since the epilepsy is stated to be resistant to treatment, it is coded as intractable. Be careful to assign the code for the hip fracture that identifies the affected side of the body. Unspecified hip fracture codes are unacceptable primary diagnoses in PDGM.

Chapter 7: Diseases of the Eye and Adnexa (H00-H59)

Chapter 7 includes codes related to conditions of the eye and adnexa, including intraoperative and postprocedural complications and disorders of the eye and adnexa.

Use an external cause code, following the code for the eye condition, if applicable, to identify the cause of the eye condition.

It's important to note that the beginning of this chapter indicates a number of conditions that fall into the Excludes 2 note. In these situations, the conditions are not included in the H00-H59 codes, but may be coded in addition to a code from H00-H59. Refer to the codes in Chapter 7 to determine appropriate sequencing of the codes.

The Excludes 2 note includes the following conditions:

- Certain conditions originating in the perinatal period (P00-P96) located in chapter 16.

- Certain infections and parasitic diseases (A00-B99) located in chapter 1.

- Complications of pregnancy, childbirth and the puerperium (O00–O9A) located in chapter 15.

- Congenital malformations, deformations and chromosomal abnormalities (Q00-Q99) in chapter 17.

- Diabetes mellitus related eye conditions (E09.3-, E10.3-, E11.3-, E13.3-) located in chapter 4.

- Endocrine, nutritional and metabolic diseases (E00-E88) located in chapter 4.

- Injury (trauma) of eye and orbit (S05.-) located in chapter 19.

- Injury, poisoning and certain other consequences of external causes (S00-T88) located in chapter 19.

- Neoplasms (C00-D49) in chapter 2.

- Symptoms, signs and abnormal clinical and laboratory findings (R00-R94) located in chapter 18.

- Syphilis related eye disorders (A50.1, A50.3-, A51.43, A52.71) located in Chapter 1.

Sensory organs

In general, each of the sensory organs has the same basic structure. The sensory organs are composed of sensory receptors, which translate light, mechanical, or chemical stimuli into electrical impulses. Often the tip of the sensory nerve fiber is associated with accessory tissues that amplify the stimulus and increase the sensitivity of the receptor.

Diabetic retinopathy, diabetic glaucoma, and other diabetic vision issues are manifestations of diabetes. In ICD-10-CM, there are combination codes that combine the underlying situation (e.g., diabetes) and the manifestation into one combination code. ***Note:*** Retinopathy due to conditions such as arteriosclerosis and sickle cell disease continue to use the etiology/manifestation convention in coding.

Conjunctivitis of the eye has more than two dozen different ICD-10-CM codes to sift through. When choosing the appropriate ICD-10-CM code for conjunctivitis, it's important to identify the cause of the inflammation.

Blindness can be found under "blindness" in the Alphabetical Index. The key terms 'low' and 'loss' have a "see blindness notation" but also have references for low vision and loss of vision. Blindness and low vision codes in category H54 have a note to code first any associated underlying cause of the blindness.

Code H54.8 (Legal blindness, as defined in USA) includes a table that gives a classification of severity of visual impairment recommended by a 1972 WHO Study Group on the Prevention of Blindness. The term "low vision" in category H54 comprises categories 1 and 2 of the table, the term blindness is in categories 3, 4, and 5, and the term unqualified visual loss is in category 9. Confirm a low vision diagnosis with the physician to support the use of the code.

If "blindness" or "low vision" of both eyes is documented but the visual impairment category is not documented, assign code H54.3, Unqualified visual loss, both eyes. If "blindness" or "low vision" in one eye is documented but the visual impairment category is not documented, assign a code from H54.6-, Unqualified visual loss, one eye, per coding guidelines.

Glaucoma

Assign as many codes from category H40 (Glaucoma) as needed to identify the type of glaucoma, the affected eye and the glaucoma stage.

When a patient has bilateral glaucoma and both eyes are documented as being the same type and stage, and there is a code for bilateral glaucoma, report only the code for the type of glaucoma, bilateral, with the seventh character for the stage.

When a patient has bilateral glaucoma and both eyes are documented as being the same type and stage, and the classification does not provide a code for bilateral glaucoma (i.e., subcategories H40.10, and H40.20) report only one code for the type of glaucoma with the appropriate seventh character for the stage.

When a patient has bilateral glaucoma and each eye is documented as having a different type or stage, and the classification distinguishes laterality, assign the appropriate code for each eye rather than the code for bilateral glaucoma.

When a patient has bilateral glaucoma and each eye is documented as having a different type, and the classification does not distinguish laterality (i.e. H40.10, and H40.20), assign one code for each type of glaucoma with the appropriate seventh character for the stage.

When a patient has bilateral glaucoma and each eye is documented as having the same type, but different stage, and the classification does not distinguish laterality (i.e. subcategories H40.10, and H40.20), assign a code for the type of glaucoma for each eye.

If a patient is admitted with glaucoma and the stage progresses during the admission, assign the code for the highest stage documented.

Assignment of the seventh character "4" for "indeterminate stage" should be based on the clinical documentation. The seventh character "4" is used for glaucoma in which stage cannot be clinically determined. The seventh character "4" should not be confused with the seventh character "0," unspecified, which should be assigned when there is no documentation regarding the stage of the glaucoma.

As with all coding, watch for notes to code first underlying diseases and add additional codes.

CHAPTER 7: DISEASES OF THE EYE AND ADNEXA (H00-H59)

Note:

Use an external cause code following the code for the eye condition, if applicable, to identify the cause of the eye condition

EXCLUDES 2 certain conditions originating in the perinatal period (P04-P96)

certain infectious and parasitic diseases (A00-B99)

complications of pregnancy, childbirth and the puerperium (O00-O9A)

congenital malformations, deformations, and chromosomal abnormalities (Q00-Q99)

diabetes mellitus related eye conditions (E09.3-, E10.3-, E11.3-, E13.3-)

endocrine, nutritional and metabolic diseases (E00-E88)

injury (trauma) of eye and orbit (S05.-)

injury, poisoning and certain other consequences of external causes (S00-T88)

neoplasms (C00-D49)

symptoms, signs and abnormal clinical and laboratory findings, not elsewhere classified (R00-R94)

syphilis related eye disorders (A50.01, A50.3-, A51.43, A52.71)

This chapter contains the following blocks:

H00-H05	Disorders of eyelid, lacrimal system and orbit
H10-H11	Disorders of conjunctiva
H15-H22	Disorders of sclera, cornea, iris and ciliary body
H25-H28	Disorders of lens
H30-H36	Disorders of choroid and retina
H40-H42	Glaucoma
H43-H44	Disorders of vitreous body and globe
H46-H47	Disorders of optic nerve and visual pathways
H49-H52	Disorders of ocular muscles, binocular movement, accommodation and refraction
H53-H54	Visual disturbances and blindness
H55-H57	Other disorders of eye and adnexa
H59	Intraoperative and postprocedural complications and disorders of eye and adnexa, not elsewhere classified

Disorders of eyelid, lacrimal system and orbit (H00-H05)

EXCLUDES 2 open wound of eyelid (S01.1-)
superficial injury of eyelid (S00.1-, S00.2-)

4 H00 Hordeolum and chalazion

5 H00.0 Hordeolum (externum) (internum) of eyelid

6 H00.01 Hordeolum externum
Hordeolum NOS
Stye
DEFINITION Staph infection of an oil gland in an eyelash follicle.

SP H00.011 Hordeolum externum right upper eyelid

SP H00.012 Hordeolum externum right lower eyelid

IQ H00.013 Hordeolum externum right eye, unspecified eyelid

SP H00.014 Hordeolum externum left upper eyelid

SP H00.015 Hordeolum externum left lower eyelid

IQ H00.016 Hordeolum externum left eye, unspecified eyelid

IQ H00.019 Hordeolum externum unspecified eye, unspecified eyelid

6 H00.02 Hordeolum internum
Infection of meibomian gland

SP H00.021 Hordeolum internum right upper eyelid

SP H00.022 Hordeolum internum right lower eyelid

IQ H00.023 Hordeolum internum right eye, unspecified eyelid

SP H00.024 Hordeolum internum left upper eyelid

SP H00.025 Hordeolum internum left lower eyelid

IQ H00.026 Hordeolum internum left eye, unspecified eyelid

IQ H00.029 Hordeolum internum unspecified eye, unspecified eyelid

6 H00.03 Abscess of eyelid
Furuncle of eyelid

SP H00.031 Abscess of right upper eyelid

SP H00.032 Abscess of right lower eyelid

IQ H00.033 Abscess of eyelid right eye, unspecified eyelid

SP H00.034 Abscess of left upper eyelid

SP H00.035 Abscess of left lower eyelid

IQ H00.036 Abscess of eyelid left eye, unspecified eyelid

IQ H00.039 Abscess of eyelid unspecified eye, unspecified eyelid

5 H00.1 Chalazion
Meibomian (gland) cyst
EXCLUDES 2 infected meibomian gland (H00.02-)
DEFINITION Cyst of the tarsal (eyelid) gland.

SP H00.11 Chalazion right upper eyelid

SP H00.12 Chalazion right lower eyelid

IQ H00.13 Chalazion right eye, unspecified eyelid

SP H00.14 Chalazion left upper eyelid

SP H00.15 Chalazion left lower eyelid

IQ H00.16 Chalazion left eye, unspecified eyelid

IQ H00.19 Chalazion unspecified eye, unspecified eyelid

4 H01 Other inflammation of eyelid

5 H01.0 Blepharitis
EXCLUDES 1 blepharoconjunctivitis (H10.5-)

6 H01.00 Unspecified blepharitis
DEFINITION An inflammation of the eyelids or lid margins.

SP H01.001 Unspecified blepharitis right upper eyelid

SP H01.002 Unspecified blepharitis right lower eyelid

IQ H01.003 Unspecified blepharitis right eye, unspecified eyelid

★ New ▲ Revised Px Primary SP PDGM Px SL Low CoM SH High CoM IQ Quest. Encounter H Hospice non-cancer Dx Unspecified M Manifestation

DecisionHealth's FY 2020 Complete Home Health ICD-10-CM Diagnosis Coding Manual

869

Chapter 7

H00-H59

Chapter 7

H00-H59

⊟ SP **H01.004** Unspecified blepharitis left upper eyelid

⊟ SP **H01.005** Unspecified blepharitis left lower eyelid

⊟ IQ **H01.006** Unspecified blepharitis left eye, unspecified eyelid

⊟ IQ **H01.009** Unspecified blepharitis unspecified eye, unspecified eyelid

⊟ SP **H01.00A** Unspecified blepharitis right eye, upper and lower eyelids

⊟ SP **H01.00B** Unspecified blepharitis left eye, upper and lower eyelids

⑥ **H01.01** Ulcerative blepharitis

⊟ SP **H01.011** Ulcerative blepharitis right upper eyelid

⊟ SP **H01.012** Ulcerative blepharitis right lower eyelid

⊟ IQ **H01.013** Ulcerative blepharitis right eye, unspecified eyelid

⊟ SP **H01.014** Ulcerative blepharitis left upper eyelid

⊟ SP **H01.015** Ulcerative blepharitis left lower eyelid

⊟ IQ **H01.016** Ulcerative blepharitis left eye, unspecified eyelid

⊟ IQ **H01.019** Ulcerative blepharitis unspecified eye, unspecified eyelid

⊟ SP **H01.01A** Ulcerative blepharitis right eye, upper and lower eyelids

⊟ SP **H01.01B** Ulcerative blepharitis left eye, upper and lower eyelids

⑥ **H01.02** Squamous blepharitis

⊟ SP **H01.021** Squamous blepharitis right upper eyelid

⊟ SP **H01.022** Squamous blepharitis right lower eyelid

⊟ IQ **H01.023** Squamous blepharitis right eye, unspecified eyelid

⊟ SP **H01.024** Squamous blepharitis left upper eyelid

⊟ SP **H01.025** Squamous blepharitis left lower eyelid

⊟ IQ **H01.026** Squamous blepharitis left eye, unspecified eyelid

⊟ IQ **H01.029** Squamous blepharitis unspecified eye, unspecified eyelid

⊟ SP **H01.02A** Squamous blepharitis right eye, upper and lower eyelids

⊟ SP **H01.02B** Squamous blepharitis left eye, upper and lower eyelids

⑤ **H01.1** Noninfectious dermatoses of eyelid

⑥ **H01.11** Allergic dermatitis of eyelid
Contact dermatitis of eyelid

⊟ SP **H01.111** Allergic dermatitis of right upper eyelid

⊟ SP **H01.112** Allergic dermatitis of right lower eyelid

⊟ IQ **H01.113** Allergic dermatitis of right eye, unspecified eyelid

⊟ SP **H01.114** Allergic dermatitis of left upper eyelid

⊟ SP **H01.115** Allergic dermatitis of left lower eyelid

⊟ IQ **H01.116** Allergic dermatitis of left eye, unspecified eyelid

⊟ IQ **H01.119** Allergic dermatitis of unspecified eye, unspecified eyelid

⑥ **H01.12** Discoid lupus erythematosus of eyelid

⊟ SP **H01.121** Discoid lupus erythematosus of right upper eyelid

⊟ SP **H01.122** Discoid lupus erythematosus of right lower eyelid

⊟ IQ **H01.123** Discoid lupus erythematosus of right eye, unspecified eyelid

⊟ SP **H01.124** Discoid lupus erythematosus of left upper eyelid

⊟ SP **H01.125** Discoid lupus erythematosus of left lower eyelid

⊟ IQ **H01.126** Discoid lupus erythematosus of left eye, unspecified eyelid

⊟ IQ **H01.129** Discoid lupus erythematosus of unspecified eye, unspecified eyelid

⑥ **H01.13** Eczematous dermatitis of eyelid

⊟ SP **H01.131** Eczematous dermatitis of right upper eyelid

⊟ SP **H01.132** Eczematous dermatitis of right lower eyelid

⊟ IQ **H01.133** Eczematous dermatitis of right eye, unspecified eyelid

⊟ SP **H01.134** Eczematous dermatitis of left upper eyelid

⊟ SP **H01.135** Eczematous dermatitis of left lower eyelid

⊟ IQ **H01.136** Eczematous dermatitis of left eye, unspecified eyelid

⊟ IQ **H01.139** Eczematous dermatitis of unspecified eye, unspecified eyelid

⑥ **H01.14** Xeroderma of eyelid

⊟ SP **H01.141** Xeroderma of right upper eyelid

⊟ SP **H01.142** Xeroderma of right lower eyelid

⊟ IQ **H01.143** Xeroderma of right eye, unspecified eyelid

⊟ SP **H01.144** Xeroderma of left upper eyelid

⊟ SP **H01.145** Xeroderma of left lower eyelid

⊟ IQ **H01.146** Xeroderma of left eye, unspecified eyelid

⊟ IQ **H01.149** Xeroderma of unspecified eye, unspecified eyelid

SP **H01.8** Other specified inflammations of eyelid

IQ **H01.9** Unspecified inflammation of eyelid
Inflammation of eyelid NOS

④ **H02** Other disorders of eyelid
EXCLUDES 1 congenital malformations of eyelid (Q10.0-Q10.3)

⑤ **H02.0** Entropion and trichiasis of eyelid

⑥ **H02.00** Unspecified entropion of eyelid
DEFINITION Inward curling of the eyelid margin, usually the bottom, so the lashes irritate the surface of the eyeball.

⊟ SP **H02.001** Unspecified entropion of right upper eyelid

⊟ SP **H02.002** Unspecified entropion of right lower eyelid

---

④4th digit required   ⑤5th digit required   ⑥6th digit required   ⑦7th digit required   ☑7th digit placeholder   ✚Additional code   ⊟Laterality

☰ **IQ** **H02.003** Unspecified entropion of right eye, unspecified eyelid

☰ **SP** **H02.004** Unspecified entropion of left upper eyelid

☰ **SP** **H02.005** Unspecified entropion of left lower eyelid

☰ **IQ** **H02.006** Unspecified entropion of left eye, unspecified eyelid

☰ **IQ** **H02.009** Unspecified entropion of unspecified eye, unspecified eyelid

🄖 **H02.01** Cicatricial entropion of eyelid

☰ **SP** **H02.011** Cicatricial entropion of right upper eyelid

☰ **SP** **H02.012** Cicatricial entropion of right lower eyelid

☰ **IQ** **H02.013** Cicatricial entropion of right eye, unspecified eyelid

☰ **SP** **H02.014** Cicatricial entropion of left upper eyelid

☰ **SP** **H02.015** Cicatricial entropion of left lower eyelid

☰ **IQ** **H02.016** Cicatricial entropion of left eye, unspecified eyelid

☰ **IQ** **H02.019** Cicatricial entropion of unspecified eye, unspecified eyelid

🄖 **H02.02** Mechanical entropion of eyelid

☰ **SP** **H02.021** Mechanical entropion of right upper eyelid

☰ **SP** **H02.022** Mechanical entropion of right lower eyelid

☰ **IQ** **H02.023** Mechanical entropion of right eye, unspecified eyelid

☰ **SP** **H02.024** Mechanical entropion of left upper eyelid

☰ **SP** **H02.025** Mechanical entropion of left lower eyelid

☰ **IQ** **H02.026** Mechanical entropion of left eye, unspecified eyelid

☰ **IQ** **H02.029** Mechanical entropion of unspecified eye, unspecified eyelid

🄖 **H02.03** Senile entropion of eyelid

☰ **SP** **H02.031** Senile entropion of right upper eyelid

☰ **SP** **H02.032** Senile entropion of right lower eyelid

☰ **IQ** **H02.033** Senile entropion of right eye, unspecified eyelid

☰ **SP** **H02.034** Senile entropion of left upper eyelid

☰ **SP** **H02.035** Senile entropion of left lower eyelid

☰ **IQ** **H02.036** Senile entropion of left eye, unspecified eyelid

☰ **IQ** **H02.039** Senile entropion of unspecified eye, unspecified eyelid

🄖 **H02.04** Spastic entropion of eyelid

☰ **SP** **H02.041** Spastic entropion of right upper eyelid

☰ **SP** **H02.042** Spastic entropion of right lower eyelid

☰ **IQ** **H02.043** Spastic entropion of right eye, unspecified eyelid

☰ **SP** **H02.044** Spastic entropion of left upper eyelid

☰ **SP** **H02.045** Spastic entropion of left lower eyelid

☰ **IQ** **H02.046** Spastic entropion of left eye, unspecified eyelid

☰ **IQ** **H02.049** Spastic entropion of unspecified eye, unspecified eyelid

🄖 **H02.05** Trichiasis without entropion

☰ **SP** **H02.051** Trichiasis without entropion right upper eyelid

☰ **SP** **H02.052** Trichiasis without entropion right lower eyelid

☰ **IQ** **H02.053** Trichiasis without entropion right eye, unspecified eyelid

☰ **SP** **H02.054** Trichiasis without entropion left upper eyelid

☰ **SP** **H02.055** Trichiasis without entropion left lower eyelid

☰ **IQ** **H02.056** Trichiasis without entropion left eye, unspecified eyelid

☰ **IQ** **H02.059** Trichiasis without entropion unspecified eye, unspecified eyelid

🄥 **H02.1** Ectropion of eyelid

🄖 **H02.10** Unspecified ectropion of eyelid

DEFINITION Outward curling of the eyelid away from the eye, usually the lower, exposing the inner surface and causing irritation, dryness, pain and possible conjunctivitis and keratitis.

☰ **SP** **H02.101** Unspecified ectropion of right upper eyelid

☰ **SP** **H02.102** Unspecified ectropion of right lower eyelid

☰ **IQ** **H02.103** Unspecified ectropion of right eye, unspecified eyelid

☰ **SP** **H02.104** Unspecified ectropion of left upper eyelid

☰ **IQ** **H02.105** Unspecified ectropion of left lower eyelid

☰ **IQ** **H02.106** Unspecified ectropion of left eye, unspecified eyelid

☰ **IQ** **H02.109** Unspecified ectropion of unspecified eye, unspecified eyelid

🄖 **H02.11** Cicatricial ectropion of eyelid

☰ **SP** **H02.111** Cicatricial ectropion of right upper eyelid

☰ **SP** **H02.112** Cicatricial ectropion of right lower eyelid

☰ **IQ** **H02.113** Cicatricial ectropion of right eye, unspecified eyelid

☰ **SP** **H02.114** Cicatricial ectropion of left upper eyelid

☰ **SP** **H02.115** Cicatricial ectropion of left lower eyelid

☰ **IQ** **H02.116** Cicatricial ectropion of left eye, unspecified eyelid

☰ **IQ** **H02.119** Cicatricial ectropion of unspecified eye, unspecified eyelid

🄖 **H02.12** Mechanical ectropion of eyelid

Chapter 7

H00-H59

★ New ▲ Revised Px Primary **SP** PDGM Px **SL** Low CoM **SH** High CoM **IQ** Quest. Encounter Ⓗ Hospice non-cancer Dx ☐ Unspecified **M** *Manifestation*

DecisionHealth's FY 2020 Complete Home Health ICD-10-CM Diagnosis Coding Manual

871

⊟ SP H02.121 Mechanical ectropion of right upper eyelid

⊟ SP H02.122 Mechanical ectropion of right lower eyelid

⊟ IQ H02.123 Mechanical ectropion of right eye, unspecified eyelid

⊟ SP H02.124 Mechanical ectropion of left upper eyelid

⊟ SP H02.125 Mechanical ectropion of left lower eyelid

⊟ IQ H02.126 Mechanical ectropion of left eye, unspecified eyelid

⊟ IQ H02.129 Mechanical ectropion of unspecified eye, unspecified eyelid

　6 H02.13 Senile ectropion of eyelid

⊟ SP H02.131 Senile ectropion of right upper eyelid

⊟ SP H02.132 Senile ectropion of right lower eyelid

⊟ IQ H02.133 Senile ectropion of right eye, unspecified eyelid

⊟ SP H02.134 Senile ectropion of left upper eyelid

⊟ SP H02.135 Senile ectropion of left lower eyelid

⊟ IQ H02.136 Senile ectropion of left eye, unspecified eyelid

⊟ IQ H02.139 Senile ectropion of unspecified eye, unspecified eyelid

　6 H02.14 Spastic ectropion of eyelid

⊟ SP H02.141 Spastic ectropion of right upper eyelid

⊟ SP H02.142 Spastic ectropion of right lower eyelid

⊟ IQ H02.143 Spastic ectropion of right eye, unspecified eyelid

⊟ SP H02.144 Spastic ectropion of left upper eyelid

⊟ SP H02.145 Spastic ectropion of left lower eyelid

⊟ IQ H02.146 Spastic ectropion of left eye, unspecified eyelid

⊟ IQ H02.149 Spastic ectropion of unspecified eye, unspecified eyelid

　6 H02.15 Paralytic ectropion of eyelid

⊟ SP H02.151 Paralytic ectropion of right upper eyelid

⊟ SP H02.152 Paralytic ectropion of right lower eyelid

⊟ IQ H02.153 Paralytic ectropion of right eye, unspecified eyelid

⊟ SP H02.154 Paralytic ectropion of left upper eyelid

⊟ SP H02.155 Paralytic ectropion of left lower eyelid

⊟ IQ H02.156 Paralytic ectropion of left eye, unspecified eyelid

⊟ IQ H02.159 Paralytic ectropion of unspecified eye, unspecified eyelid

　5 H02.2 Lagophthalmos

　　6 H02.20 Unspecified lagophthalmos

⊟ SP H02.201 Unspecified lagophthalmos right upper eyelid

⊟ SP H02.202 Unspecified lagophthalmos right lower eyelid

⊟ IQ H02.203 Unspecified lagophthalmos right eye, unspecified eyelid

⊟ SP H02.204 Unspecified lagophthalmos left upper eyelid

⊟ SP H02.205 Unspecified lagophthalmos left lower eyelid

⊟ IQ H02.206 Unspecified lagophthalmos left eye, unspecified eyelid

⊟ IQ H02.209 Unspecified lagophthalmos unspecified eye, unspecified eyelid

⊟ SP H02.20A Unspecified lagophthalmos right eye, upper and lower eyelids

⊟ SP H02.20B Unspecified lagophthalmos left eye, upper and lower eyelids

⊟ SP H02.20C Unspecified lagophthalmos, bilateral, upper and lower eyelids

　6 H02.21 Cicatricial lagophthalmos

DEFINITION Inability to completely close the eye due to the presence of scar tissue.

⊟ SP H02.211 Cicatricial lagophthalmos right upper eyelid

⊟ SP H02.212 Cicatricial lagophthalmos right lower eyelid

⊟ IQ H02.213 Cicatricial lagophthalmos right eye, unspecified eyelid

⊟ SP H02.214 Cicatricial lagophthalmos left upper eyelid

⊟ SP H02.215 Cicatricial lagophthalmos left lower eyelid

⊟ IQ H02.216 Cicatricial lagophthalmos left eye, unspecified eyelid

⊟ IQ H02.219 Cicatricial lagophthalmos unspecified eye, unspecified eyelid

⊟ SP H02.21A Cicatricial lagophthalmos right eye, upper and lower eyelids

⊟ SP H02.21B Cicatricial lagophthalmos left eye, upper and lower eyelids

⊟ SP H02.21C Cicatricial lagophthalmos, bilateral, upper and lower eyelids

　6 H02.22 Mechanical lagophthalmos

⊟ SP H02.221 Mechanical lagophthalmos right upper eyelid

⊟ SP H02.222 Mechanical lagophthalmos right lower eyelid

⊟ IQ H02.223 Mechanical lagophthalmos right eye, unspecified eyelid

⊟ SP H02.224 Mechanical lagophthalmos left upper eyelid

⊟ SP H02.225 Mechanical lagophthalmos left lower eyelid

⊟ IQ H02.226 Mechanical lagophthalmos left eye, unspecified eyelid

⊟ IQ H02.229 Mechanical lagophthalmos unspecified eye, unspecified eyelid

⊟ SP H02.22A Mechanical lagophthalmos right eye, upper and lower eyelids

⊟ SP H02.22B Mechanical lagophthalmos left eye, upper and lower eyelids

---

4 4th digit required　　5 5th digit required　　6 6th digit required　　7 7th digit required　　7 7th digit placeholder　　✚ Additional code　　⊟ Laterality

872　　　　　*DecisionHealth's* FY 2020 Complete Home Health ICD-10-CM Diagnosis Coding Manual

Chapter 7

H00-H59

☐ **SP** **H02.22C** Mechanical lagophthalmos, bilateral, upper and lower eyelids

⑥ **H02.23** Paralytic lagophthalmos

☐ **SP** **H02.231** Paralytic lagophthalmos right upper eyelid

☐ **SP** **H02.232** Paralytic lagophthalmos right lower eyelid

☐ **IQ** **H02.233** Paralytic lagophthalmos right eye, unspecified eyelid

☐ **SP** **H02.234** Paralytic lagophthalmos left upper eyelid

☐ **SP** **H02.235** Paralytic lagophthalmos left lower eyelid

☐ **IQ** **H02.236** Paralytic lagophthalmos left eye, unspecified eyelid

☐ **IQ** **H02.239** Paralytic lagophthalmos unspecified eye, unspecified eyelid

☐ **SP** **H02.23A** Paralytic lagophthalmos right eye, upper and lower eyelids

☐ **SP** **H02.23B** Paralytic lagophthalmos left eye, upper and lower eyelids

☐ **SP** **H02.23C** Paralytic lagophthalmos, bilateral, upper and lower eyelids

⑤ **H02.3** Blepharochalasis
Pseudoptosis

DEFINITION Sagging of the skin of the eyelid. In the upper eyelid, the skin sags over the eye obstructing vision; usually due to changes in elastin and collagen, affecting the skin's elasticity.

☐ **IQ** **H02.30** Blepharochalasis unspecified eye, unspecified eyelid

☐ **SP** **H02.31** Blepharochalasis right upper eyelid

☐ **SP** **H02.32** Blepharochalasis right lower eyelid

☐ **IQ** **H02.33** Blepharochalasis right eye, unspecified eyelid

☐ **SP** **H02.34** Blepharochalasis left upper eyelid

☐ **SP** **H02.35** Blepharochalasis left lower eyelid

☐ **IQ** **H02.36** Blepharochalasis left eye, unspecified eyelid

⑤ **H02.4** Ptosis of eyelid

⑥ **H02.40** Unspecified ptosis of eyelid

☐ **SP** **H02.401** Unspecified ptosis of right eyelid

☐ **SP** **H02.402** Unspecified ptosis of left eyelid

☐ **SP** **H02.403** Unspecified ptosis of bilateral eyelids

☐ **IQ** **H02.409** Unspecified ptosis of unspecified eyelid

⑥ **H02.41** Mechanical ptosis of eyelid

☐ **SP** **H02.411** Mechanical ptosis of right eyelid

☐ **SP** **H02.412** Mechanical ptosis of left eyelid

☐ **SP** **H02.413** Mechanical ptosis of bilateral eyelids

☐ **IQ** **H02.419** Mechanical ptosis of unspecified eyelid

⑥ **H02.42** Myogenic ptosis of eyelid

☐ **SP** **H02.421** Myogenic ptosis of right eyelid

☐ **SP** **H02.422** Myogenic ptosis of left eyelid

☐ **SP** **H02.423** Myogenic ptosis of bilateral eyelids

☐ **IQ** **H02.429** Myogenic ptosis of unspecified eyelid

⑥ **H02.43** Paralytic ptosis of eyelid
Neurogenic ptosis of eyelid

☐ **SP** **H02.431** Paralytic ptosis of right eyelid

☐ **SP** **H02.432** Paralytic ptosis of left eyelid

☐ **SP** **H02.433** Paralytic ptosis of bilateral eyelids

☐ **IQ** **H02.439** Paralytic ptosis unspecified eyelid

⑤ **H02.5** Other disorders affecting eyelid function
EXCLUDES 2 blepharospasm (G24.5)
organic tic (G25.69)
psychogenic tic (F95.-)

⑥ **H02.51** Abnormal innervation syndrome

☐ **SP** **H02.511** Abnormal innervation syndrome right upper eyelid

☐ **SP** **H02.512** Abnormal innervation syndrome right lower eyelid

☐ **IQ** **H02.513** Abnormal innervation syndrome right eye, unspecified eyelid

☐ **SP** **H02.514** Abnormal innervation syndrome left upper eyelid

☐ **SP** **H02.515** Abnormal innervation syndrome left lower eyelid

☐ **IQ** **H02.516** Abnormal innervation syndrome left eye, unspecified eyelid

☐ **IQ** **H02.519** Abnormal innervation syndrome unspecified eye, unspecified eyelid

⑥ **H02.52** Blepharophimosis
Ankyloblepharon

DEFINITION Hereditary disorder in which the palpebral fissures (space between the eyelids) is narrowed, giving the appearance of continually squinting.

☐ **SP** **H02.521** Blepharophimosis right upper eyelid

☐ **SP** **H02.522** Blepharophimosis right lower eyelid

☐ **IQ** **H02.523** Blepharophimosis right eye, unspecified eyelid

☐ **SP** **H02.524** Blepharophimosis left upper eyelid

☐ **SP** **H02.525** Blepharophimosis left lower eyelid

☐ **IQ** **H02.526** Blepharophimosis left eye, unspecified eyelid

☐ **IQ** **H02.529** Blepharophimosis unspecified eye, unspecified lid

⑥ **H02.53** Eyelid retraction
Eyelid lag

☐ **SP** **H02.531** Eyelid retraction right upper eyelid

☐ **SP** **H02.532** Eyelid retraction right lower eyelid

☐ **IQ** **H02.533** Eyelid retraction right eye, unspecified eyelid

☐ **SP** **H02.534** Eyelid retraction left upper eyelid

☐ **SP** **H02.535** Eyelid retraction left lower eyelid

☐ **IQ** **H02.536** Eyelid retraction left eye, unspecified eyelid

☐ **IQ** **H02.539** Eyelid retraction unspecified eye, unspecified lid

SP **H02.59** Other disorders affecting eyelid function
Deficient blink reflex
Sensory disorders

★ New ▲ Revised **Px** Primary **SP** PDGM Px **SL** Low CoM **SH** High CoM **IQ** Quest. Encounter ⊞ Hospice non-cancer Dx ▢ Unspecified **M** *Manifestation*

DecisionHealth's FY 2020 Complete Home Health ICD-10-CM Diagnosis Coding Manual

873

⑤ H02.6 Xanthelasma of eyelid

⊟ **!Q** H02.60   Xanthelasma of unspecified eye, unspecified eyelid

⊟ **SP** H02.61   Xanthelasma of right upper eyelid

⊟ **SP** H02.62   Xanthelasma of right lower eyelid

⊟ **!Q** H02.63   Xanthelasma of right eye, unspecified eyelid

⊟ **SP** H02.64   Xanthelasma of left upper eyelid

⊟ **SP** H02.65   Xanthelasma of left lower eyelid

⊟ **!Q** H02.66   Xanthelasma of left eye, unspecified eyelid

⑤ H02.7   Other and unspecified degenerative disorders of eyelid and periocular area

SP H02.70   Unspecified degenerative disorders of eyelid and periocular area

⑥ H02.71   Chloasma of eyelid and periocular area
Dyspigmentation of eyelid
Hyperpigmentation of eyelid

⊟ **SP** H02.711   Chloasma of right upper eyelid and periocular area

⊟ **SP** H02.712   Chloasma of right lower eyelid and periocular area

⊟ **!Q** H02.713   Chloasma of right eye, unspecified eyelid and periocular area

⊟ **SP** H02.714   Chloasma of left upper eyelid and periocular area

⊟ **SP** H02.715   Chloasma of left lower eyelid and periocular area

⊟ **!Q** H02.716   Chloasma of left eye, unspecified eyelid and periocular area

⊟ **!Q** H02.719   Chloasma of unspecified eye, unspecified eyelid and periocular area

⑥ H02.72   Madarosis of eyelid and periocular area
Hypotrichosis of eyelid

⊟ **SP** H02.721   Madarosis of right upper eyelid and periocular area

⊟ **SP** H02.722   Madarosis of right lower eyelid and periocular area

⊟ **!Q** H02.723   Madarosis of right eye, unspecified eyelid and periocular area

⊟ **SP** H02.724   Madarosis of left upper eyelid and periocular area

⊟ **SP** H02.725   Madarosis of left lower eyelid and periocular area

⊟ **!Q** H02.726   Madarosis of left eye, unspecified eyelid and periocular area

⊟ **!Q** H02.729   Madarosis of unspecified eye, unspecified eyelid and periocular area

⑥ H02.73   Vitiligo of eyelid and periocular area
Hypopigmentation of eyelid

⊟ **SP** H02.731   Vitiligo of right upper eyelid and periocular area

⊟ **SP** H02.732   Vitiligo of right lower eyelid and periocular area

⊟ **!Q** H02.733   Vitiligo of right eye, unspecified eyelid and periocular area

⊟ **SP** H02.734   Vitiligo of left upper eyelid and periocular area

⊟ **SP** H02.735   Vitiligo of left lower eyelid and periocular area

⊟ **!Q** H02.736   Vitiligo of left eye, unspecified eyelid and periocular area

⊟ **!Q** H02.739   Vitiligo of unspecified eye, unspecified eyelid and periocular area

SP H02.79   Other degenerative disorders of eyelid and periocular area

⑤ H02.8   Other specified disorders of eyelid

✚ ⑥ H02.81   Retained foreign body in eyelid
Use additional code to identify the type of retained foreign body (Z18.-)

EXCLUDES 1   laceration of eyelid with foreign body (S01.12-)
retained intraocular foreign body (H44.6-, H44.7-)
superficial foreign body of eyelid and periocular area (S00.25-)

⊟ **SP** ✚ H02.811   Retained foreign body in right upper eyelid

⊟ **SP** ✚ H02.812   Retained foreign body in right lower eyelid

⊟ **!Q** ✚ H02.813   Retained foreign body in right eye, unspecified eyelid

⊟ **SP** ✚ H02.814   Retained foreign body in left upper eyelid

⊟ **SP** ✚ H02.815   Retained foreign body in left lower eyelid

⊟ **!Q** ✚ H02.816   Retained foreign body in left eye, unspecified eyelid

⊟ **!Q** ✚ H02.819   Retained foreign body in unspecified eye, unspecified eyelid

⑥ H02.82   Cysts of eyelid
Sebaceous cyst of eyelid

⊟ **SP** H02.821   Cysts of right upper eyelid

⊟ **SP** H02.822   Cysts of right lower eyelid

⊟ **!Q** H02.823   Cysts of right eye, unspecified eyelid

⊟ **SP** H02.824   Cysts of left upper eyelid

⊟ **SP** H02.825   Cysts of left lower eyelid

⊟ **!Q** H02.826   Cysts of left eye, unspecified eyelid

⊟ **!Q** H02.829   Cysts of unspecified eye, unspecified eyelid

⑥ H02.83   Dermatochalasis of eyelid

⊟ **SP** H02.831   Dermatochalasis of right upper eyelid

⊟ **SP** H02.832   Dermatochalasis of right lower eyelid

⊟ **!Q** H02.833   Dermatochalasis of right eye, unspecified eyelid

⊟ **SP** H02.834   Dermatochalasis of left upper eyelid

⊟ **SP** H02.835   Dermatochalasis of left lower eyelid

⊟ **!Q** H02.836   Dermatochalasis of left eye, unspecified eyelid

⊟ **!Q** H02.839   Dermatochalasis of unspecified eye, unspecified eyelid

⑥ H02.84   Edema of eyelid

---

④ 4th digit required   ⑤ 5th digit required   ⑥ 6th digit required   ⑦ 7th digit required   ⑦ 7th digit placeholder   ✚ Additional code   ⊟ Laterality

874   *DecisionHealth's* FY 2020 Complete Home Health ICD-10-CM Diagnosis Coding Manual

Hyperemia of eyelid

▤ **SP** **H02.841** Edema of right upper eyelid

▤ **SP** **H02.842** Edema of right lower eyelid

▤ **IQ** **H02.843** Edema of right eye, unspecified eyelid

▤ **SP** **H02.844** Edema of left upper eyelid

▤ **SP** **H02.845** Edema of left lower eyelid

▤ **IQ** **H02.846** Edema of left eye, unspecified eyelid

▤ **IQ** **H02.849** Edema of unspecified eye, unspecified eyelid

⑥ **H02.85** Elephantiasis of eyelid

▤ **SP** **H02.851** Elephantiasis of right upper eyelid

▤ **SP** **H02.852** Elephantiasis of right lower eyelid

▤ **IQ** **H02.853** Elephantiasis of right eye, unspecified eyelid

▤ **SP** **H02.854** Elephantiasis of left upper eyelid

▤ **SP** **H02.855** Elephantiasis of left lower eyelid

▤ **IQ** **H02.856** Elephantiasis of left eye, unspecified eyelid

▤ **IQ** **H02.859** Elephantiasis of unspecified eye, unspecified eyelid

⑥ **H02.86** Hypertrichosis of eyelid

▤ **SP** **H02.861** Hypertrichosis of right upper eyelid

▤ **SP** **H02.862** Hypertrichosis of right lower eyelid

▤ **IQ** **H02.863** Hypertrichosis of right eye, unspecified eyelid

▤ **SP** **H02.864** Hypertrichosis of left upper eyelid

▤ **SP** **H02.865** Hypertrichosis of left lower eyelid

▤ **IQ** **H02.866** Hypertrichosis of left eye, unspecified eyelid

▤ **IQ** **H02.869** Hypertrichosis of unspecified eye, unspecified eyelid

⑥ **H02.87** Vascular anomalies of eyelid

▤ **SP** **H02.871** Vascular anomalies of right upper eyelid

▤ **SP** **H02.872** Vascular anomalies of right lower eyelid

▤ **IQ** **H02.873** Vascular anomalies of right eye, unspecified eyelid

▤ **SP** **H02.874** Vascular anomalies of left upper eyelid

▤ **SP** **H02.875** Vascular anomalies of left lower eyelid

▤ **IQ** **H02.876** Vascular anomalies of left eye, unspecified eyelid

▤ **IQ** **H02.879** Vascular anomalies of unspecified eye, unspecified eyelid

⑥ **H02.88** Meibomian gland dysfunction of eyelid

▤ **SP** **H02.881** Meibomian gland dysfunction right upper eyelid

▤ **SP** **H02.882** Meibomian gland dysfunction right lower eyelid

▤ **IQ** **H02.883** Meibomian gland dysfunction of right eye, unspecified eyelid

▤ **SP** **H02.884** Meibomian gland dysfunction left upper eyelid

▤ **SP** **H02.885** Meibomian gland dysfunction left lower eyelid

▤ **IQ** **H02.886** Meibomian gland dysfunction of left eye, unspecified eyelid

▤ **IQ** **H02.889** Meibomian gland dysfunction of unspecified eye, unspecified eyelid

▤ **SP** **H02.88A** Meibomian gland dysfunction right eye, upper and lower eyelids

▤ **SP** **H02.88B** Meibomian gland dysfunction left eye, upper and lower eyelids

SP **H02.89** Other specified disorders of eyelid

Hemorrhage of eyelid

IQ **H02.9** Unspecified disorder of eyelid

Disorder of eyelid NOS

④ **H04** Disorders of lacrimal system

EXCLUDES 1 congenital malformations of lacrimal system (Q10.4-Q10.6)

⑤ **H04.0** Dacryoadenitis

⑥ **H04.00** Unspecified dacryoadenitis

DEFINITION Inflammation of the lacrimal gland.

▤ **SP** **H04.001** Unspecified dacryoadenitis, right lacrimal gland

▤ **SP** **H04.002** Unspecified dacryoadenitis, left lacrimal gland

▤ **SP** **H04.003** Unspecified dacryoadenitis, bilateral lacrimal glands

▤ **IQ** **H04.009** Unspecified dacryoadenitis, unspecified lacrimal gland

⑥ **H04.01** Acute dacryoadenitis

▤ **SP** **H04.011** Acute dacryoadenitis, right lacrimal gland

▤ **SP** **H04.012** Acute dacryoadenitis, left lacrimal gland

▤ **SP** **H04.013** Acute dacryoadenitis, bilateral lacrimal glands

▤ **IQ** **H04.019** Acute dacryoadenitis, unspecified lacrimal gland

⑥ **H04.02** Chronic dacryoadenitis

▤ **SP** **H04.021** Chronic dacryoadenitis, right lacrimal gland

▤ **SP** **H04.022** Chronic dacryoadenitis, left lacrimal gland

▤ **SP** **H04.023** Chronic dacryoadenitis, bilateral lacrimal gland

▤ **IQ** **H04.029** Chronic dacryoadenitis, unspecified lacrimal gland

⑥ **H04.03** Chronic enlargement of lacrimal gland

▤ **SP** **H04.031** Chronic enlargement of right lacrimal gland

▤ **SP** **H04.032** Chronic enlargement of left lacrimal gland

▤ **SP** **H04.033** Chronic enlargement of bilateral lacrimal glands

▤ **IQ** **H04.039** Chronic enlargement of unspecified lacrimal gland

⑤ **H04.1** Other disorders of lacrimal gland

⑥ **H04.11** Dacryops

▤ **SP** **H04.111** Dacryops of right lacrimal gland

▤ **SP** **H04.112** Dacryops of left lacrimal gland

▤ **SP** **H04.113** Dacryops of bilateral lacrimal glands

Chapter 7

H00-H59

★ New ▲ Revised **Px** Primary **SP** PDGM Px **SL** Low CoM **SH** High CoM **IQ** Quest. Encounter **H** Hospice non-cancer Dx ⬜ Unspecified **M** *Manifestation*

DecisionHealth's FY 2020 Complete Home Health ICD-10-CM Diagnosis Coding Manual

875

IQ H04.119 Dacryops of unspecified lacrimal gland

6 H04.12 Dry eye syndrome
Tear film insufficiency, NOS

SP H04.121 Dry eye syndrome of right lacrimal gland

SP H04.122 Dry eye syndrome of left lacrimal gland

SP H04.123 Dry eye syndrome of bilateral lacrimal glands

IQ H04.129 Dry eye syndrome of unspecified lacrimal gland

6 H04.13 Lacrimal cyst
Lacrimal cystic degeneration

SP H04.131 Lacrimal cyst, right lacrimal gland

SP H04.132 Lacrimal cyst, left lacrimal gland

SP H04.133 Lacrimal cyst, bilateral lacrimal glands

IQ H04.139 Lacrimal cyst, unspecified lacrimal gland

6 H04.14 Primary lacrimal gland atrophy
DEFINITION Wasting of the lacrimal glands causing severe dryness with decreased tear production.

SP H04.141 Primary lacrimal gland atrophy, right lacrimal gland

SP H04.142 Primary lacrimal gland atrophy, left lacrimal gland

SP H04.143 Primary lacrimal gland atrophy, bilateral lacrimal glands

IQ H04.149 Primary lacrimal gland atrophy, unspecified lacrimal gland

6 H04.15 Secondary lacrimal gland atrophy

SP H04.151 Secondary lacrimal gland atrophy, right lacrimal gland

SP H04.152 Secondary lacrimal gland atrophy, left lacrimal gland

SP H04.153 Secondary lacrimal gland atrophy, bilateral lacrimal glands

IQ H04.159 Secondary lacrimal gland atrophy, unspecified lacrimal gland

6 H04.16 Lacrimal gland dislocation
DEFINITION Lacrimal gland separated from the tear ducts, preventing tears from passing normally to the eye.

SP H04.161 Lacrimal gland dislocation, right lacrimal gland

SP H04.162 Lacrimal gland dislocation, left lacrimal gland

SP H04.163 Lacrimal gland dislocation, bilateral lacrimal glands

IQ H04.169 Lacrimal gland dislocation, unspecified lacrimal gland

SP H04.19 Other specified disorders of lacrimal gland

5 H04.2 Epiphora

6 H04.20 Unspecified epiphora

SP H04.201 Unspecified epiphora, right side

SP H04.202 Unspecified epiphora, left side

SP H04.203 Unspecified epiphora, bilateral

IQ H04.209 Unspecified epiphora, unspecified side

6 H04.21 Epiphora due to excess lacrimation

SP H04.211 Epiphora due to excess lacrimation, right lacrimal gland

SP H04.212 Epiphora due to excess lacrimation, left lacrimal gland

SP H04.213 Epiphora due to excess lacrimation, bilateral lacrimal glands

IQ H04.219 Epiphora due to excess lacrimation, unspecified lacrimal gland

6 H04.22 Epiphora due to insufficient drainage

SP H04.221 Epiphora due to insufficient drainage, right side

SP H04.222 Epiphora due to insufficient drainage, left side

SP H04.223 Epiphora due to insufficient drainage, bilateral

IQ H04.229 Epiphora due to insufficient drainage, unspecified side

5 H04.3 Acute and unspecified inflammation of lacrimal passages
EXCLUDES 1 neonatal dacryocystitis (P39.1)

6 H04.30 Unspecified dacryocystitis
DEFINITION Inflammation of the lacrimal sac in the eye causing obstruction of the tube draining tears into the nose.

SP H04.301 Unspecified dacryocystitis of right lacrimal passage

SP H04.302 Unspecified dacryocystitis of left lacrimal passage

SP H04.303 Unspecified dacryocystitis of bilateral lacrimal passages

IQ H04.309 Unspecified dacryocystitis of unspecified lacrimal passage

6 H04.31 Phlegmonous dacryocystitis

SP H04.311 Phlegmonous dacryocystitis of right lacrimal passage

SP H04.312 Phlegmonous dacryocystitis of left lacrimal passage

SP H04.313 Phlegmonous dacryocystitis of bilateral lacrimal passages

IQ H04.319 Phlegmonous dacryocystitis of unspecified lacrimal passage

6 H04.32 Acute dacryocystitis
Acute dacryopericystitis
DEFINITION Sudden, severe inflammation of the tear sac, usually due to blockage of the tear ducts.

SP H04.321 Acute dacryocystitis of right lacrimal passage

SP H04.322 Acute dacryocystitis of left lacrimal passage

SP H04.323 Acute dacryocystitis of bilateral lacrimal passages

IQ H04.329 Acute dacryocystitis of unspecified lacrimal passage

6 H04.33 Acute lacrimal canaliculitis
DEFINITION Sudden, severe inflammation of the lacrimal passages or tear ducts.

---

4 4th digit required   5 5th digit required   6 6th digit required   7 7th digit required   7 7th digit placeholder   + Additional code   Laterality

876   DecisionHealth's FY 2020 Complete Home Health ICD-10-CM Diagnosis Coding Manual

SP H04.331 Acute lacrimal caniculitis of right lacrimal passage

SP H04.332 Acute lacrimal caniculitis of left lacrimal passage

SP H04.333 Acute lacrimal caniculitis of bilateral lacrimal passages

IQ H04.339 Acute lacrimal caniculitis of unspecified lacrimal passage

5 H04.4 Chronic inflammation of lacrimal passages

6 H04.41 Chronic dacryocystitis

SP H04.411 Chronic dacryocystitis of right lacrimal passage

SP H04.412 Chronic dacryocystitis of left lacrimal passage

SP H04.413 Chronic dacryocystitis of bilateral lacrimal passages

IQ H04.419 Chronic dacryocystitis of unspecified lacrimal passage

6 H04.42 Chronic lacrimal caniculitis

SP H04.421 Chronic lacrimal caniculitis of right lacrimal passage

SP H04.422 Chronic lacrimal caniculitis of left lacrimal passage

SP H04.423 Chronic lacrimal caniculitis of bilateral lacrimal passages

IQ H04.429 Chronic lacrimal caniculitis of unspecified lacrimal passage

6 H04.43 Chronic lacrimal mucocele

> **DEFINITION** Inflammation of the lacrimal system in which the tear ducts, and then the eyes, become filled with mucous.

SP H04.431 Chronic lacrimal mucocele of right lacrimal passage

SP H04.432 Chronic lacrimal mucocele of left lacrimal passage

SP H04.433 Chronic lacrimal mucocele of bilateral lacrimal passages

IQ H04.439 Chronic lacrimal mucocele of unspecified lacrimal passage

5 H04.5 Stenosis and insufficiency of lacrimal passages

6 H04.51 Dacryolith

SP H04.511 Dacryolith of right lacrimal passage

SP H04.512 Dacryolith of left lacrimal passage

SP H04.513 Dacryolith of bilateral lacrimal passages

IQ H04.519 Dacryolith of unspecified lacrimal passage

6 H04.52 Eversion of lacrimal punctum

> **DEFINITION** Tear duct exit turned away from the eye, causing tears to flow directly onto the face instead of moistening the eyeball.

SP H04.521 Eversion of right lacrimal punctum

SP H04.522 Eversion of left lacrimal punctum

SP H04.523 Eversion of bilateral lacrimal punctum

IQ H04.529 Eversion of unspecified lacrimal punctum

6 H04.53 Neonatal obstruction of nasolacrimal duct

EXCLUDES 1 congenital stenosis and stricture of lacrimal duct (Q10.5)

SP H04.531 Neonatal obstruction of right nasolacrimal duct

SP H04.532 Neonatal obstruction of left nasolacrimal duct

SP H04.533 Neonatal obstruction of bilateral nasolacrimal duct

IQ H04.539 Neonatal obstruction of unspecified nasolacrimal duct

6 H04.54 Stenosis of lacrimal canaliculi

SP H04.541 Stenosis of right lacrimal canaliculi

SP H04.542 Stenosis of left lacrimal canaliculi

SP H04.543 Stenosis of bilateral lacrimal canaliculi

IQ H04.549 Stenosis of unspecified lacrimal canaliculi

6 H04.55 Acquired stenosis of nasolacrimal duct

SP H04.551 Acquired stenosis of right nasolacrimal duct

SP H04.552 Acquired stenosis of left nasolacrimal duct

SP H04.553 Acquired stenosis of bilateral nasolacrimal duct

IQ H04.559 Acquired stenosis of unspecified nasolacrimal duct

6 H04.56 Stenosis of lacrimal punctum

SP H04.561 Stenosis of right lacrimal punctum

SP H04.562 Stenosis of left lacrimal punctum

SP H04.563 Stenosis of bilateral lacrimal punctum

IQ H04.569 Stenosis of unspecified lacrimal punctum

6 H04.57 Stenosis of lacrimal sac

SP H04.571 Stenosis of right lacrimal sac

SP H04.572 Stenosis of left lacrimal sac

SP H04.573 Stenosis of bilateral lacrimal sac

IQ H04.579 Stenosis of unspecified lacrimal sac

5 H04.6 Other changes of lacrimal passages

6 H04.61 Lacrimal fistula

SP H04.611 Lacrimal fistula right lacrimal passage

SP H04.612 Lacrimal fistula left lacrimal passage

SP H04.613 Lacrimal fistula bilateral lacrimal passages

IQ H04.619 Lacrimal fistula unspecified lacrimal passage

SP H04.69 Other changes of lacrimal passages

5 H04.8 Other disorders of lacrimal system

6 H04.81 Granuloma of lacrimal passages

SP H04.811 Granuloma of right lacrimal passage

SP H04.812 Granuloma of left lacrimal passage

SP H04.813 Granuloma of bilateral lacrimal passages

IQ H04.819 Granuloma of unspecified lacrimal passage

★ New ▲ Revised **Px** Primary **SP** PDGM Px **SL** Low CoM **SH** High CoM **IQ** Quest. Encounter **H** Hospice non-cancer Dx Unspecified **M** *Manifestation*

SP H04.89 Other disorders of lacrimal system

IQ H04.9 **Disorder of lacrimal system, unspecified**

4 H05 Disorders of orbit

> **EXCLUDES 1** congenital malformation of orbit (Q10.7)

5 H05.0 Acute inflammation of orbit

SP H05.00 **Unspecified acute inflammation of orbit**

6 H05.01 Cellulitis of orbit
Abscess of orbit

SP H05.011 Cellulitis of right orbit

SP H05.012 Cellulitis of left orbit

SP H05.013 Cellulitis of bilateral orbits

IQ H05.019 **Cellulitis of unspecified orbit**

6 H05.02 Osteomyelitis of orbit

SP H05.021 Osteomyelitis of right orbit

SP H05.022 Osteomyelitis of left orbit

SP H05.023 Osteomyelitis of bilateral orbits

IQ H05.029 **Osteomyelitis of unspecified orbit**

6 H05.03 Periostitis of orbit

SP H05.031 Periostitis of right orbit

SP H05.032 Periostitis of left orbit

SP H05.033 Periostitis of bilateral orbits

IQ H05.039 **Periostitis of unspecified orbit**

6 H05.04 Tenonitis of orbit

SP H05.041 Tenonitis of right orbit

SP H05.042 Tenonitis of left orbit

SP H05.043 Tenonitis of bilateral orbits

IQ H05.049 **Tenonitis of unspecified orbit**

5 H05.1 Chronic inflammatory disorders of orbit

SP H05.10 **Unspecified chronic inflammatory disorders of orbit**

6 H05.11 Granuloma of orbit
Pseudotumor (inflammatory) of orbit

SP H05.111 Granuloma of right orbit

SP H05.112 Granuloma of left orbit

SP H05.113 Granuloma of bilateral orbits

IQ H05.119 **Granuloma of unspecified orbit**

6 H05.12 Orbital myositis

> **DEFINITION** Inflammation of one of the muscles that moves the eyeball.

SP H05.121 Orbital myositis, right orbit

SP H05.122 Orbital myositis, left orbit

SP H05.123 Orbital myositis, bilateral

IQ H05.129 **Orbital myositis, unspecified orbit**

5 H05.2 Exophthalmic conditions

SP H05.20 **Unspecified exophthalmos**

6 H05.21 Displacement (lateral) of globe

> **DEFINITION** Condition in which the eyeball is situated towards the side of the head, away from the nose.

SP H05.211 Displacement (lateral) of globe, right eye

SP H05.212 Displacement (lateral) of globe, left eye

SP H05.213 Displacement (lateral) of globe, bilateral

IQ H05.219 **Displacement (lateral) of globe, unspecified eye**

6 H05.22 Edema of orbit
Orbital congestion

SP H05.221 Edema of right orbit

SP H05.222 Edema of left orbit

SP H05.223 Edema of bilateral orbit

IQ H05.229 **Edema of unspecified orbit**

6 H05.23 Hemorrhage of orbit

SP H05.231 Hemorrhage of right orbit

SP H05.232 Hemorrhage of left orbit

SP H05.233 Hemorrhage of bilateral orbit

IQ H05.239 **Hemorrhage of unspecified orbit**

6 H05.24 Constant exophthalmos

SP H05.241 Constant exophthalmos, right eye

SP H05.242 Constant exophthalmos, left eye

SP H05.243 Constant exophthalmos, bilateral

IQ H05.249 **Constant exophthalmos, unspecified eye**

6 H05.25 Intermittent exophthalmos

SP H05.251 Intermittent exophthalmos, right eye

SP H05.252 Intermittent exophthalmos, left eye

SP H05.253 Intermittent exophthalmos, bilateral

IQ H05.259 **Intermittent exophthalmos, unspecified eye**

6 H05.26 Pulsating exophthalmos

SP H05.261 Pulsating exophthalmos, right eye

SP H05.262 Pulsating exophthalmos, left eye

SP H05.263 Pulsating exophthalmos, bilateral

IQ H05.269 **Pulsating exophthalmos, unspecified eye**

5 H05.3 Deformity of orbit

> **EXCLUDES 1** congenital deformity of orbit (Q10.7)
> hypertelorism (Q75.2)

IQ H05.30 **Unspecified deformity of orbit**

6 H05.31 Atrophy of orbit

SP H05.311 Atrophy of right orbit

SP H05.312 Atrophy of left orbit

SP H05.313 Atrophy of bilateral orbit

IQ H05.319 **Atrophy of unspecified orbit**

6 H05.32 Deformity of orbit due to bone disease
Code also:
associated bone disease

SP H05.321 Deformity of right orbit due to bone disease

SP H05.322 Deformity of left orbit due to bone disease

SP H05.323 Deformity of bilateral orbits due to bone disease

IQ H05.329 **Deformity of unspecified orbit due to bone disease**

6 H05.33 Deformity of orbit due to trauma or surgery

SP H05.331 Deformity of right orbit due to trauma or surgery

SP H05.332 Deformity of left orbit due to trauma or surgery

4 4th digit required   **5** 5th digit required   **6** 6th digit required   **7** 7th digit required   **7** 7th digit placeholder   **+** Additional code   **⊟** Laterality

878   *DecisionHealth's* FY 2020 Complete Home Health ICD-10-CM Diagnosis Coding Manual

☐ **SP** **H05.333** Deformity of bilateral orbits due to trauma or surgery

☐ **IQ** **H05.339** Deformity of unspecified orbit due to trauma or surgery

6 **H05.34** Enlargement of orbit

☐ **SP** **H05.341** Enlargement of right orbit

☐ **SP** **H05.342** Enlargement of left orbit

☐ **SP** **H05.343** Enlargement of bilateral orbits

☐ **IQ** **H05.349** Enlargement of unspecified orbit

6 **H05.35** Exostosis of orbit

DEFINITION Abnormal bone growth of the eye socket; can impair vision and prevent the eye from moving properly.

☐ **SP** **H05.351** Exostosis of right orbit

☐ **SP** **H05.352** Exostosis of left orbit

☐ **SP** **H05.353** Exostosis of bilateral orbits

☐ **IQ** **H05.359** Exostosis of unspecified orbit

5 **H05.4** Enophthalmos

6 **H05.40** Unspecified enophthalmos

DEFINITION Condition in which the eye is recessed abnormally deep within the eye socket.

☐ **SP** **H05.401** Unspecified enophthalmos, right eye

☐ **SP** **H05.402** Unspecified enophthalmos, left eye

☐ **SP** **H05.403** Unspecified enophthalmos, bilateral

☐ **IQ** **H05.409** Unspecified enophthalmos, unspecified eye

6 **H05.41** Enophthalmos due to atrophy of orbital tissue

☐ **SP** **H05.411** Enophthalmos due to atrophy of orbital tissue, right eye

☐ **SP** **H05.412** Enophthalmos due to atrophy of orbital tissue, left eye

☐ **SP** **H05.413** Enophthalmos due to atrophy of orbital tissue, bilateral

☐ **IQ** **H05.419** Enophthalmos due to atrophy of orbital tissue, unspecified eye

6 **H05.42** Enophthalmos due to trauma or surgery

☐ **SP** **H05.421** Enophthalmos due to trauma or surgery, right eye

☐ **SP** **H05.422** Enophthalmos due to trauma or surgery, left eye

☐ **SP** **H05.423** Enophthalmos due to trauma or surgery, bilateral

☐ **IQ** **H05.429** Enophthalmos due to trauma or surgery, unspecified eye

+ **5** **H05.5** Retained (old) foreign body following penetrating wound of orbit
Retrobulbar foreign body
Use additional code to identify the type of retained foreign body (Z18.-)

EXCLUDES 1 current penetrating wound of orbit (S05.4-)

EXCLUDES 2 retained foreign body of eyelid (H02.81-)
retained intraocular foreign body (H44.6-, H44.7-)

☐ **IQ** **+** **H05.50** Retained (old) foreign body following penetrating wound of unspecified orbit

☐ **SP** **+** **H05.51** Retained (old) foreign body following penetrating wound of right orbit

☐ **SP** **+** **H05.52** Retained (old) foreign body following penetrating wound of left orbit

☐ **SP** **+** **H05.53** Retained (old) foreign body following penetrating wound of bilateral orbits

5 **H05.8** Other disorders of orbit

6 **H05.81** Cyst of orbit
Encephalocele of orbit

☐ **SP** **H05.811** Cyst of right orbit

☐ **SP** **H05.812** Cyst of left orbit

☐ **SP** **H05.813** Cyst of bilateral orbits

☐ **IQ** **H05.819** Cyst of unspecified orbit

6 **H05.82** Myopathy of extraocular muscles

☐ **SP** **H05.821** Myopathy of extraocular muscles, right orbit

☐ **SP** **H05.822** Myopathy of extraocular muscles, left orbit

☐ **SP** **H05.823** Myopathy of extraocular muscles, bilateral

☐ **IQ** **H05.829** Myopathy of extraocular muscles, unspecified orbit

SP **H05.89** Other disorders of orbit

IQ **H05.9** Unspecified disorder of orbit

Disorders of conjunctiva (H10-H11)

4 **H10** Conjunctivitis

EXCLUDES 1 keratoconjunctivitis (H16.2-)

CODING TIPS ✓ Consider codes from H10 when an infectious organism is not identified and the documentation only supports a clinical picture of conjunctivitis. If a certain bacterial or viral cause is known, a code from the Infectious and parasitic disease chapter may be more appropriate.

5 **H10.0** Mucopurulent conjunctivitis

6 **H10.01** Acute follicular conjunctivitis

☐ **SP** **H10.011** Acute follicular conjunctivitis, right eye

☐ **SP** **H10.012** Acute follicular conjunctivitis, left eye

☐ **SP** **H10.013** Acute follicular conjunctivitis, bilateral

☐ **IQ** **H10.019** Acute follicular conjunctivitis, unspecified eye

6 **H10.02** Other mucopurulent conjunctivitis

CODING TIPS ✓ Subcategory H10.02 is commonly referred to as pink eye.

DEFINITION Inflammation of the conjunctiva with the production of mucous and pus.

☐ **SP** **H10.021** Other mucopurulent conjunctivitis, right eye

☐ **SP** **H10.022** Other mucopurulent conjunctivitis, left eye

☐ **SP** **H10.023** Other mucopurulent conjunctivitis, bilateral

☐ **IQ** **H10.029** Other mucopurulent conjunctivitis, unspecified eye

5 **H10.1** Acute atopic conjunctivitis

★ New ▲ Revised Px Primary **SP** PDGM Px **SL** Low CoM **SH** High CoM **IQ** Quest. Encounter **H** Hospice non-cancer Dx Unspecified **M** *Manifestation*

DecisionHealth's FY 2020 Complete Home Health ICD-10-CM Diagnosis Coding Manual

879

Acute papillary conjunctivitis

> **DEFINITION**   Sudden, severe case of conjunctivitis caused by allergies.

⊟ **!Q** **H10.10**   **Acute atopic conjunctivitis, unspecified eye**

⊟ **SP** **H10.11**   Acute atopic conjunctivitis, right eye

⊟ **SP** **H10.12**   Acute atopic conjunctivitis, left eye

⊟ **SP** **H10.13**   Acute atopic conjunctivitis, bilateral

5 **H10.2**   Other acute conjunctivitis

> **CODING TIPS ✓**   Consider subcategory H10.2 when light or noxious chemicals cause conjunctivitis.

6 **H10.21**   **Acute toxic conjunctivitis**
Acute chemical conjunctivitis
Code first:
  (T51-T65) to identify chemical and intent

> **EXCLUDES 1**   burn and corrosion of eye and adnexa (T26.-)

⊟ **SP** **H10.211**   Acute toxic conjunctivitis, right eye

⊟ **SP** **H10.212**   Acute toxic conjunctivitis, left eye

⊟ **SP** **H10.213**   Acute toxic conjunctivitis, bilateral

⊟ **!Q** **H10.219**   **Acute toxic conjunctivitis, unspecified eye**

6 **H10.22**   **Pseudomembranous conjunctivitis**

⊟ **SP** **H10.221**   Pseudomembranous conjunctivitis, right eye

⊟ **SP** **H10.222**   Pseudomembranous conjunctivitis, left eye

⊟ **SP** **H10.223**   Pseudomembranous conjunctivitis, bilateral

⊟ **SP** **H10.229**   **Pseudomembranous conjunctivitis, unspecified eye**

6 **H10.23**   **Serous conjunctivitis, except viral**
> **EXCLUDES 1**   viral conjunctivitis (B30.-)

⊟ **SP** **H10.231**   Serous conjunctivitis, except viral, right eye

⊟ **SP** **H10.232**   Serous conjunctivitis, except viral, left eye

⊟ **SP** **H10.233**   Serous conjunctivitis, except viral, bilateral

⊟ **!Q** **H10.239**   **Serous conjunctivitis, except viral, unspecified eye**

5 **H10.3**   **Unspecified acute conjunctivitis**
> **EXCLUDES 1**   ophthalmia neonatorum NOS (P39.1)

⊟ **!Q** **H10.30**   **Unspecified acute conjunctivitis, unspecified eye**

⊟ **SP** **H10.31**   **Unspecified acute conjunctivitis, right eye**

⊟ **SP** **H10.32**   **Unspecified acute conjunctivitis, left eye**

⊟ **SP** **H10.33**   **Unspecified acute conjunctivitis, bilateral**

5 **H10.4**   Chronic conjunctivitis

6 **H10.40**   **Unspecified chronic conjunctivitis**

⊟ **SP** **H10.401**   **Unspecified chronic conjunctivitis, right eye**

⊟ **SP** **H10.402**   **Unspecified chronic conjunctivitis, left eye**

⊟ **SP** **H10.403**   **Unspecified chronic conjunctivitis, bilateral**

⊟ **!Q** **H10.409**   **Unspecified chronic conjunctivitis, unspecified eye**

6 **H10.41**   Chronic giant papillary conjunctivitis

⊟ **SP** **H10.411**   Chronic giant papillary conjunctivitis, right eye

⊟ **SP** **H10.412**   Chronic giant papillary conjunctivitis, left eye

⊟ **SP** **H10.413**   Chronic giant papillary conjunctivitis, bilateral

⊟ **!Q** **H10.419**   **Chronic giant papillary conjunctivitis, unspecified eye**

6 **H10.42**   Simple chronic conjunctivitis

⊟ **SP** **H10.421**   Simple chronic conjunctivitis, right eye

⊟ **SP** **H10.422**   Simple chronic conjunctivitis, left eye

⊟ **SP** **H10.423**   Simple chronic conjunctivitis, bilateral

⊟ **!Q** **H10.429**   **Simple chronic conjunctivitis, unspecified eye**

6 **H10.43**   Chronic follicular conjunctivitis

⊟ **SP** **H10.431**   Chronic follicular conjunctivitis, right eye

⊟ **SP** **H10.432**   Chronic follicular conjunctivitis, left eye

⊟ **SP** **H10.433**   Chronic follicular conjunctivitis, bilateral

⊟ **!Q** **H10.439**   **Chronic follicular conjunctivitis, unspecified eye**

SP **H10.44**   Vernal conjunctivitis
> **EXCLUDES 1**   vernal keratoconjunctivitis with limbar and corneal involvement (H16.26-)

> **DEFINITION**   Seasonal inflammation of the conjunctiva due to an allergic reaction to pollen, mold, or another seasonal factor.

SP **H10.45**   Other chronic allergic conjunctivitis

5 **H10.5**   Blepharoconjunctivitis

6 **H10.50**   **Unspecified blepharoconjunctivitis**

⊟ **SP** **H10.501**   **Unspecified blepharoconjunctivitis, right eye**

⊟ **SP** **H10.502**   **Unspecified blepharoconjunctivitis, left eye**

⊟ **SP** **H10.503**   **Unspecified blepharoconjunctivitis, bilateral**

⊟ **!Q** **H10.509**   **Unspecified blepharoconjunctivitis, unspecified eye**

6 **H10.51**   Ligneous conjunctivitis
Code also underlying condition if known, such as:
  plasminogen deficiency (E88.02)

⊟ **SP** **H10.511**   Ligneous conjunctivitis, right eye

⊟ **SP** **H10.512**   Ligneous conjunctivitis, left eye

⊟ **SP** **H10.513**   Ligneous conjunctivitis, bilateral

⊟ **!Q** **H10.519**   **Ligneous conjunctivitis, unspecified eye**

6 **H10.52**   Angular blepharoconjunctivitis

4 4th digit required   **5** 5th digit required   **6** 6th digit required   **7** 7th digit required   **7̄** 7th digit placeholder   **+** Additional code   ⊟ Laterality

880   DecisionHealth's FY 2020 Complete Home Health ICD-10-CM Diagnosis Coding Manual

⊟ **SP** **H10.521** Angular blepharoconjunctivitis, right eye

⊟ **SP** **H10.522** Angular blepharoconjunctivitis, left eye

⊟ **SP** **H10.523** Angular blepharoconjunctivitis, bilateral

⊟ **IQ** **H10.529** Angular blepharoconjunctivitis, unspecified eye

6 **H10.53** Contact blepharoconjunctivitis

⊟ **SP** **H10.531** Contact blepharoconjunctivitis, right eye

⊟ **SP** **H10.532** Contact blepharoconjunctivitis, left eye

⊟ **SP** **H10.533** Contact blepharoconjunctivitis, bilateral

⊟ **IQ** **H10.539** Contact blepharoconjunctivitis, unspecified eye

5 **H10.8** Other conjunctivitis

6 **H10.81** Pingueculitis
   EXCLUDES 1 pinguecula (H11.15-)

   DEFINITION Yellowish, raised areas of limbal conjunctival tissue, usually seen with chronic sun exposure, that become acutely vascularized, irritated, and inflamed.

⊟ **SP** **H10.811** Pingueculitis, right eye

⊟ **SP** **H10.812** Pingueculitis, left eye

⊟ **SP** **H10.813** Pingueculitis, bilateral

⊟ **IQ** **H10.819** Pingueculitis, unspecified eye

6 **H10.82** Rosacea conjunctivitis
   Code first:
      underlying rosacea dermatitis (L71.-)

⊟ **SP** **H10.821** Rosacea conjunctivitis, right eye

⊟ **SP** **H10.822** Rosacea conjunctivitis, left eye

⊟ **SP** **H10.823** Rosacea conjunctivitis, bilateral

⊟ **IQ** **H10.829** Rosacea conjunctivitis, unspecified eye

SP **H10.89** Other conjunctivitis

IQ **H10.9** Unspecified conjunctivitis

4 **H11** Other disorders of conjunctiva
   EXCLUDES 1 keratoconjunctivitis (H16.2-)

5 **H11.0** Pterygium of eye
   EXCLUDES 1 pseudopterygium (H11.81-)

6 **H11.00** Unspecified pterygium of eye

   DEFINITION Raised, wedge-shaped overgrowth of the conjunctiva onto the cornea of the eye.

⊟ **SP** **H11.001** Unspecified pterygium of right eye

⊟ **SP** **H11.002** Unspecified pterygium of left eye

⊟ **SP** **H11.003** Unspecified pterygium of eye, bilateral

⊟ **IQ** **H11.009** Unspecified pterygium of unspecified eye

6 **H11.01** Amyloid pterygium

⊟ **SP** **H11.011** Amyloid pterygium of right eye

⊟ **SP** **H11.012** Amyloid pterygium of left eye

⊟ **SP** **H11.013** Amyloid pterygium of eye, bilateral

⊟ **IQ** **H11.019** Amyloid pterygium of unspecified eye

6 **H11.02** Central pterygium of eye

⊟ **SP** **H11.021** Central pterygium of right eye

⊟ **SP** **H11.022** Central pterygium of left eye

⊟ **SP** **H11.023** Central pterygium of eye, bilateral

⊟ **IQ** **H11.029** Central pterygium of unspecified eye

6 **H11.03** Double pterygium of eye

⊟ **SP** **H11.031** Double pterygium of right eye

⊟ **SP** **H11.032** Double pterygium of left eye

⊟ **SP** **H11.033** Double pterygium of eye, bilateral

⊟ **IQ** **H11.039** Double pterygium of unspecified eye

6 **H11.04** Peripheral pterygium of eye, stationary

⊟ **SP** **H11.041** Peripheral pterygium, stationary, right eye

⊟ **SP** **H11.042** Peripheral pterygium, stationary, left eye

⊟ **SP** **H11.043** Peripheral pterygium, stationary, bilateral

⊟ **IQ** **H11.049** Peripheral pterygium, stationary, unspecified eye

6 **H11.05** Peripheral pterygium of eye, progressive

⊟ **SP** **H11.051** Peripheral pterygium, progressive, right eye

⊟ **SP** **H11.052** Peripheral pterygium, progressive, left eye

⊟ **SP** **H11.053** Peripheral pterygium, progressive, bilateral

⊟ **IQ** **H11.059** Peripheral pterygium, progressive, unspecified eye

6 **H11.06** Recurrent pterygium of eye

⊟ **SP** **H11.061** Recurrent pterygium of right eye

⊟ **SP** **H11.062** Recurrent pterygium of left eye

⊟ **SP** **H11.063** Recurrent pterygium of eye, bilateral

⊟ **IQ** **H11.069** Recurrent pterygium of unspecified eye

5 **H11.1** Conjunctival degenerations and deposits
   EXCLUDES 2 pseudopterygium (H11.81)

IQ **H11.10** Unspecified conjunctival degenerations

6 **H11.11** Conjunctival deposits

⊟ **SP** **H11.111** Conjunctival deposits, right eye

⊟ **SP** **H11.112** Conjunctival deposits, left eye

⊟ **SP** **H11.113** Conjunctival deposits, bilateral

⊟ **IQ** **H11.119** Conjunctival deposits, unspecified eye

6 **H11.12** Conjunctival concretions
   DEFINITION Yellow-white granules or cysts which form just beneath the conjunctiva, wearing it away and causing the sensation of a foreign body in the eye.

⊟ **SP** **H11.121** Conjunctival concretions, right eye

⊟ **SP** **H11.122** Conjunctival concretions, left eye

⊟ **SP** **H11.123** Conjunctival concretions, bilateral

⊟ **IQ** **H11.129** Conjunctival concretions, unspecified eye

Chapter 7

H00-H59

★ New ▲ Revised **Px** Primary **SP** PDGM Px **SL** Low CoM **SH** High CoM **IQ** Quest. Encounter ⊞ Hospice non-cancer Dx Unspecified **M** *Manifestation*

⑥ H11.13 Conjunctival pigmentations
Conjunctival argyrosis [argyria]

☐ SP H11.131 Conjunctival pigmentations, right eye

☐ SP H11.132 Conjunctival pigmentations, left eye

☐ SP H11.133 Conjunctival pigmentations, bilateral

☐ IQ H11.139 Conjunctival pigmentations, unspecified eye

⑥ H11.14 Conjunctival xerosis, unspecified

> **EXCLUDES 1** xerosis of conjunctiva due to vitamin A deficiency (E50.0, E50.1)

☐ SP H11.141 Conjunctival xerosis, unspecified, right eye

☐ SP H11.142 Conjunctival xerosis, unspecified, left eye

☐ SP H11.143 Conjunctival xerosis, unspecified, bilateral

☐ IQ H11.149 Conjunctival xerosis, unspecified, unspecified eye

⑥ H11.15 Pinguecula

> **EXCLUDES 1** pingueculitis (H10.81-)

> **DEFINITION** Small, nonmalignant, yellowish growth on the conjunctiva often asymptomatic and requiring no treatment but may cause irritation.

☐ SP H11.151 Pinguecula, right eye

☐ SP H11.152 Pinguecula, left eye

☐ SP H11.153 Pinguecula, bilateral

☐ IQ H11.159 Pinguecula, unspecified eye

⑤ H11.2 Conjunctival scars

⑥ H11.21 Conjunctival adhesions and strands (localized)

☐ SP H11.211 Conjunctival adhesions and strands (localized), right eye

☐ SP H11.212 Conjunctival adhesions and strands (localized), left eye

☐ SP H11.213 Conjunctival adhesions and strands (localized), bilateral

☐ IQ H11.219 Conjunctival adhesions and strands (localized), unspecified eye

⑥ H11.22 Conjunctival granuloma

☐ SP H11.221 Conjunctival granuloma, right eye

☐ SP H11.222 Conjunctival granuloma, left eye

☐ SP H11.223 Conjunctival granuloma, bilateral

☐ IQ H11.229 Conjunctival granuloma, unspecified

⑥ H11.23 Symblepharon

> **DEFINITION** Conjunctiva of the eyelid that has adhered to the eye, sometimes over the cornea, requiring surgical removal.

☐ SP H11.231 Symblepharon, right eye

☐ SP H11.232 Symblepharon, left eye

☐ SP H11.233 Symblepharon, bilateral

☐ IQ H11.239 Symblepharon, unspecified eye

⑥ H11.24 Scarring of conjunctiva

☐ SP H11.241 Scarring of conjunctiva, right eye

☐ SP H11.242 Scarring of conjunctiva, left eye

☐ SP H11.243 Scarring of conjunctiva, bilateral

☐ IQ H11.249 Scarring of conjunctiva, unspecified eye

⑤ H11.3 Conjunctival hemorrhage
Subconjunctival hemorrhage

☐ IQ H11.30 Conjunctival hemorrhage, unspecified eye

☐ SP H11.31 Conjunctival hemorrhage, right eye

☐ SP H11.32 Conjunctival hemorrhage, left eye

☐ SP H11.33 Conjunctival hemorrhage, bilateral

⑤ H11.4 Other conjunctival vascular disorders and cysts

⑥ H11.41 Vascular abnormalities of conjunctiva
Conjunctival aneurysm

☐ SP H11.411 Vascular abnormalities of conjunctiva, right eye

☐ SP H11.412 Vascular abnormalities of conjunctiva, left eye

☐ SP H11.413 Vascular abnormalities of conjunctiva, bilateral

☐ IQ H11.419 Vascular abnormalities of conjunctiva, unspecified eye

⑥ H11.42 Conjunctival edema

☐ SP H11.421 Conjunctival edema, right eye

☐ SP H11.422 Conjunctival edema, left eye

☐ SP H11.423 Conjunctival edema, bilateral

☐ IQ H11.429 Conjunctival edema, unspecified eye

⑥ H11.43 Conjunctival hyperemia

☐ SP H11.431 Conjunctival hyperemia, right eye

☐ SP H11.432 Conjunctival hyperemia, left eye

☐ SP H11.433 Conjunctival hyperemia, bilateral

☐ IQ H11.439 Conjunctival hyperemia, unspecified eye

⑥ H11.44 Conjunctival cysts

☐ SP H11.441 Conjunctival cysts, right eye

☐ SP H11.442 Conjunctival cysts, left eye

☐ SP H11.443 Conjunctival cysts, bilateral

☐ IQ H11.449 Conjunctival cysts, unspecified eye

⑤ H11.8 Other specified disorders of conjunctiva

⑥ H11.81 Pseudopterygium of conjunctiva

☐ SP H11.811 Pseudopterygium of conjunctiva, right eye

☐ SP H11.812 Pseudopterygium of conjunctiva, left eye

☐ SP H11.813 Pseudopterygium of conjunctiva, bilateral

☐ IQ H11.819 Pseudopterygium of conjunctiva, unspecified eye

⑥ H11.82 Conjunctivochalasis

> **DEFINITION** Loosening of the conjunctiva's attachment to the eye, causing wrinkling, dryness, and a tendency to trap particles in the folds, causing chronic inflammation.

☐ SP H11.821 Conjunctivochalasis, right eye

☐ SP H11.822 Conjunctivochalasis, left eye

☐ SP H11.823 Conjunctivochalasis, bilateral

---

④ 4th digit required   ⑤ 5th digit required   ⑥ 6th digit required   ⑦ 7th digit required   ⑦ 7th digit placeholder   ✚ Additional code   ☐ Laterality

⊟ IQ **H11.829** Conjunctivochalasis, unspecified eye

SP **H11.89** Other specified disorders of conjunctiva

IQ **H11.9** Unspecified disorder of conjunctiva

Disorders of sclera, cornea, iris and ciliary body (H15-H22)

④ **H15** Disorders of sclera

⑤ **H15.0** Scleritis

⑥ **H15.00** Unspecified scleritis

⊟ SP **H15.001** Unspecified scleritis, right eye

⊟ SP **H15.002** Unspecified scleritis, left eye

⊟ SP **H15.003** Unspecified scleritis, bilateral

⊟ IQ **H15.009** Unspecified scleritis, unspecified eye

⑥ **H15.01** Anterior scleritis

⊟ SP **H15.011** Anterior scleritis, right eye

⊟ SP **H15.012** Anterior scleritis, left eye

⊟ SP **H15.013** Anterior scleritis, bilateral

⊟ IQ **H15.019** Anterior scleritis, unspecified eye

⑥ **H15.02** Brawny scleritis

> **DEFINITION** Severe inflammation of the sclera affecting the border between the sclera and the cornea.

⊟ SP **H15.021** Brawny scleritis, right eye

⊟ SP **H15.022** Brawny scleritis, left eye

⊟ SP **H15.023** Brawny scleritis, bilateral

⊟ IQ **H15.029** Brawny scleritis, unspecified eye

⑥ **H15.03** Posterior scleritis
Sclerotenonitis

⊟ SP **H15.031** Posterior scleritis, right eye

⊟ SP **H15.032** Posterior scleritis, left eye

⊟ SP **H15.033** Posterior scleritis, bilateral

⊟ IQ **H15.039** Posterior scleritis, unspecified eye

⑥ **H15.04** Scleritis with corneal involvement

⊟ SP **H15.041** Scleritis with corneal involvement, right eye

⊟ SP **H15.042** Scleritis with corneal involvement, left eye

⊟ SP **H15.043** Scleritis with corneal involvement, bilateral

⊟ IQ **H15.049** Scleritis with corneal involvement, unspecified eye

⑥ **H15.05** Scleromalacia perforans

⊟ SP **H15.051** Scleromalacia perforans, right eye

⊟ SP **H15.052** Scleromalacia perforans, left eye

⊟ SP **H15.053** Scleromalacia perforans, bilateral

⊟ IQ **H15.059** Scleromalacia perforans, unspecified eye

⑥ **H15.09** Other scleritis
Scleral abscess

⊟ SP **H15.091** Other scleritis, right eye

⊟ SP **H15.092** Other scleritis, left eye

⊟ SP **H15.093** Other scleritis, bilateral

⊟ IQ **H15.099** Other scleritis, unspecified eye

⑤ **H15.1** Episcleritis

⑥ **H15.10** Unspecified episcleritis

⊟ SP **H15.101** Unspecified episcleritis, right eye

⊟ SP **H15.102** Unspecified episcleritis, left eye

⊟ SP **H15.103** Unspecified episcleritis, bilateral

⊟ IQ **H15.109** Unspecified episcleritis, unspecified eye

⑥ **H15.11** Episcleritis periodica fugax

> **DEFINITION** Periodic attacks of inflammation of the sclera; typically of rapid onset and short duration.

⊟ SP **H15.111** Episcleritis periodica fugax, right eye

⊟ SP **H15.112** Episcleritis periodica fugax, left eye

⊟ SP **H15.113** Episcleritis periodica fugax, bilateral

⊟ IQ **H15.119** Episcleritis periodica fugax, unspecified eye

⑥ **H15.12** Nodular episcleritis

⊟ SP **H15.121** Nodular episcleritis, right eye

⊟ SP **H15.122** Nodular episcleritis, left eye

⊟ SP **H15.123** Nodular episcleritis, bilateral

⊟ IQ **H15.129** Nodular episcleritis, unspecified eye

⑤ **H15.8** Other disorders of sclera

> **EXCLUDES 2** blue sclera (Q13.5)
> degenerative myopia (H44.2-)

⑥ **H15.81** Equatorial staphyloma

⊟ SP **H15.811** Equatorial staphyloma, right eye

⊟ SP **H15.812** Equatorial staphyloma, left eye

⊟ SP **H15.813** Equatorial staphyloma, bilateral

⊟ IQ **H15.819** Equatorial staphyloma, unspecified eye

⑥ **H15.82** Localized anterior staphyloma

⊟ SP **H15.821** Localized anterior staphyloma, right eye

⊟ SP **H15.822** Localized anterior staphyloma, left eye

⊟ SP **H15.823** Localized anterior staphyloma, bilateral

⊟ IQ **H15.829** Localized anterior staphyloma, unspecified eye

⑥ **H15.83** Staphyloma posticum

⊟ SP **H15.831** Staphyloma posticum, right eye

⊟ SP **H15.832** Staphyloma posticum, left eye

⊟ SP **H15.833** Staphyloma posticum, bilateral

⊟ IQ **H15.839** Staphyloma posticum, unspecified eye

⑥ **H15.84** Scleral ectasia

> **DEFINITION** Contents of the eyeball protrude through an abnormally thin section of the sclera.

⊟ SP **H15.841** Scleral ectasia, right eye

⊟ SP **H15.842** Scleral ectasia, left eye

⊟ SP **H15.843** Scleral ectasia, bilateral

⊟ IQ **H15.849** Scleral ectasia, unspecified eye

⑥ **H15.85** Ring staphyloma

⊟ SP **H15.851** Ring staphyloma, right eye

⊟ SP **H15.852** Ring staphyloma, left eye

⊟ SP **H15.853** Ring staphyloma, bilateral

⊟ IQ **H15.859** Ring staphyloma, unspecified eye

Chapter 7

H00-H59

★ New ▲ Revised Px Primary SP PDGM Px SL Low CoM SH High CoM IQ Quest. Encounter H Hospice non-cancer Dx Unspecified M *Manifestation*

DecisionHealth's FY 2020 Complete Home Health ICD-10-CM Diagnosis Coding Manual

883

SP H15.89 Other disorders of sclera

IQ H15.9 **Unspecified disorder of sclera**

4 H16 Keratitis

5 H16.0 Corneal ulcer

6 H16.00 **Unspecified corneal ulcer**

SP H16.001 **Unspecified corneal ulcer, right eye**

SP H16.002 **Unspecified corneal ulcer, left eye**

SP H16.003 **Unspecified corneal ulcer, bilateral**

IQ H16.009 **Unspecified corneal ulcer, unspecified eye**

6 H16.01 Central corneal ulcer

SP H16.011 Central corneal ulcer, right eye

SP H16.012 Central corneal ulcer, left eye

SP H16.013 Central corneal ulcer, bilateral

IQ H16.019 **Central corneal ulcer, unspecified eye**

6 H16.02 Ring corneal ulcer

> **DEFINITION** Ring of ulceration encircling the entire edge of the cornea.

SP H16.021 Ring corneal ulcer, right eye

SP H16.022 Ring corneal ulcer, left eye

SP H16.023 Ring corneal ulcer, bilateral

IQ H16.029 **Ring corneal ulcer, unspecified eye**

6 H16.03 Corneal ulcer with hypopyon

SP H16.031 Corneal ulcer with hypopyon, right eye

SP H16.032 Corneal ulcer with hypopyon, left eye

SP H16.033 Corneal ulcer with hypopyon, bilateral

IQ H16.039 **Corneal ulcer with hypopyon, unspecified eye**

6 H16.04 Marginal corneal ulcer

SP H16.041 Marginal corneal ulcer, right eye

SP H16.042 Marginal corneal ulcer, left eye

SP H16.043 Marginal corneal ulcer, bilateral

IQ H16.049 **Marginal corneal ulcer, unspecified eye**

6 H16.05 Mooren's corneal ulcer

SP H16.051 Mooren's corneal ulcer, right eye

SP H16.052 Mooren's corneal ulcer, left eye

SP H16.053 Mooren's corneal ulcer, bilateral

IQ H16.059 **Mooren's corneal ulcer, unspecified eye**

6 H16.06 Mycotic corneal ulcer

> **DEFINITION** Corneal ulcer caused by a fungal infection.

SP H16.061 Mycotic corneal ulcer, right eye

SP H16.062 Mycotic corneal ulcer, left eye

SP H16.063 Mycotic corneal ulcer, bilateral

IQ H16.069 **Mycotic corneal ulcer, unspecified eye**

6 H16.07 Perforated corneal ulcer

SP H16.071 Perforated corneal ulcer, right eye

SP H16.072 Perforated corneal ulcer, left eye

SP H16.073 Perforated corneal ulcer, bilateral

IQ H16.079 **Perforated corneal ulcer, unspecified eye**

5 H16.1 **Other and unspecified superficial keratitis without conjunctivitis**

6 H16.10 **Unspecified superficial keratitis**

SP H16.101 **Unspecified superficial keratitis, right eye**

SP H16.102 **Unspecified superficial keratitis, left eye**

SP H16.103 **Unspecified superficial keratitis, bilateral**

IQ H16.109 **Unspecified superficial keratitis, unspecified eye**

6 H16.11 Macular keratitis
Areolar keratitis
Nummular keratitis
Stellate keratitis
Striate keratitis

SP H16.111 Macular keratitis, right eye

SP H16.112 Macular keratitis, left eye

SP H16.113 Macular keratitis, bilateral

IQ H16.119 **Macular keratitis, unspecified eye**

6 H16.12 Filamentary keratitis

> **DEFINITION** Keratitis with twisted filaments of mucoid material on the surface of the cornea.

SP H16.121 Filamentary keratitis, right eye

SP H16.122 Filamentary keratitis, left eye

SP H16.123 Filamentary keratitis, bilateral

IQ H16.129 **Filamentary keratitis, unspecified eye**

6 H16.13 Photokeratitis
Snow blindness
Welders keratitis

> **DEFINITION** Painful, inflamed cornea that develops due to over-exposure to ultraviolet light.

SP H16.131 Photokeratitis, right eye

SP H16.132 Photokeratitis, left eye

SP H16.133 Photokeratitis, bilateral

IQ H16.139 **Photokeratitis, unspecified eye**

6 H16.14 Punctate keratitis

SP H16.141 Punctate keratitis, right eye

SP H16.142 Punctate keratitis, left eye

SP H16.143 Punctate keratitis, bilateral

IQ H16.149 **Punctate keratitis, unspecified eye**

5 H16.2 Keratoconjunctivitis

> **DEFINITION** Inflammation of both the cornea and the conjunctiva; presents with burning, bloodshot, watery eyes sensitive to bright light, blurred vision, and a sensation of something in the eye.

6 H16.20 **Unspecified keratoconjunctivitis**
Superficial keratitis with conjunctivitis NOS

SP H16.201 **Unspecified keratoconjunctivitis, right eye**

SP H16.202 **Unspecified keratoconjunctivitis, left eye**

---

4 4th digit required   5 5th digit required   6 6th digit required   7 7th digit required   7 7th digit placeholder   + Additional code   ⊟ Laterality

884   *DecisionHealth's* FY 2020 Complete Home Health ICD-10-CM Diagnosis Coding Manual

▣ **SP** **H16.203** **Unspecified keratoconjunctivitis, bilateral**

▣ **IQ** **H16.209** **Unspecified keratoconjunctivitis, unspecified eye**

⑥ **H16.21** **Exposure keratoconjunctivitis**
> **DEFINITION** Dryness and inflammation of the cornea and conjunctiva caused by the failure of the eyelid to completely close during sleep and/or blinking.

▣ **SP** **H16.211** **Exposure keratoconjunctivitis, right eye**

▣ **SP** **H16.212** **Exposure keratoconjunctivitis, left eye**

▣ **SP** **H16.213** **Exposure keratoconjunctivitis, bilateral**

▣ **IQ** **H16.219** **Exposure keratoconjunctivitis, unspecified eye**

⑥ **H16.22** **Keratoconjunctivitis sicca, not specified as Sjögren's**
> **EXCLUDES 1** Sjögren's syndrome (M35.01)

▣ **SP** **H16.221** **Keratoconjunctivitis sicca, not specified as Sjögren's, right eye**

▣ **SP** **H16.222** **Keratoconjunctivitis sicca, not specified as Sjögren's, left eye**

▣ **SP** **H16.223** **Keratoconjunctivitis sicca, not specified as Sjögren's, bilateral**

▣ **IQ** **H16.229** **Keratoconjunctivitis sicca, not specified as Sjögren's, unspecified eye**

⑥ **H16.23** **Neurotrophic keratoconjunctivitis**

▣ **SP** **H16.231** **Neurotrophic keratoconjunctivitis, right eye**

▣ **SP** **H16.232** **Neurotrophic keratoconjunctivitis, left eye**

▣ **SP** **H16.233** **Neurotrophic keratoconjunctivitis, bilateral**

▣ **IQ** **H16.239** **Neurotrophic keratoconjunctivitis, unspecified eye**

⑥ **H16.24** **Ophthalmia nodosa**

▣ **SP** **H16.241** **Ophthalmia nodosa, right eye**

▣ **SP** **H16.242** **Ophthalmia nodosa, left eye**

▣ **SP** **H16.243** **Ophthalmia nodosa, bilateral**

▣ **IQ** **H16.249** **Ophthalmia nodosa, unspecified eye**

⑥ **H16.25** **Phlyctenular keratoconjunctivitis**

▣ **SP** **H16.251** **Phlyctenular keratoconjunctivitis, right eye**

▣ **SP** **H16.252** **Phlyctenular keratoconjunctivitis, left eye**

▣ **SP** **H16.253** **Phlyctenular keratoconjunctivitis, bilateral**

▣ **IQ** **H16.259** **Phlyctenular keratoconjunctivitis, unspecified eye**

⑥ **H16.26** **Vernal keratoconjunctivitis, with limbar and corneal involvement**
> **EXCLUDES 1** vernal conjunctivitis without limbar and corneal involvement (H10.44)

▣ **SP** **H16.261** **Vernal keratoconjunctivitis, with limbar and corneal involvement, right eye**

▣ **SP** **H16.262** **Vernal keratoconjunctivitis, with limbar and corneal involvement, left eye**

▣ **SP** **H16.263** **Vernal keratoconjunctivitis, with limbar and corneal involvement, bilateral**

▣ **IQ** **H16.269** **Vernal keratoconjunctivitis, with limbar and corneal involvement, unspecified eye**

⑥ **H16.29** **Other keratoconjunctivitis**

▣ **SP** **H16.291** **Other keratoconjunctivitis, right eye**

▣ **SP** **H16.292** **Other keratoconjunctivitis, left eye**

▣ **SP** **H16.293** **Other keratoconjunctivitis, bilateral**

▣ **IQ** **H16.299** **Other keratoconjunctivitis, unspecified eye**

⑤ **H16.3** **Interstitial and deep keratitis**

⑥ **H16.30** **Unspecified interstitial keratitis**

▣ **SP** **H16.301** **Unspecified interstitial keratitis, right eye**

▣ **SP** **H16.302** **Unspecified interstitial keratitis, left eye**

▣ **SP** **H16.303** **Unspecified interstitial keratitis, bilateral**

▣ **IQ** **H16.309** **Unspecified interstitial keratitis, unspecified eye**

⑥ **H16.31** **Corneal abscess**

▣ **SP** **H16.311** **Corneal abscess, right eye**

▣ **SP** **H16.312** **Corneal abscess, left eye**

▣ **SP** **H16.313** **Corneal abscess, bilateral**

▣ **IQ** **H16.319** **Corneal abscess, unspecified eye**

⑥ **H16.32** **Diffuse interstitial keratitis**
Cogan's syndrome
> **DEFINITION** Rare disorder characterized by recurrent inflammation of the cornea with episodes of dizziness and hearing loss that can lead to blindness and deafness if left untreated.

▣ **SP** **H16.321** **Diffuse interstitial keratitis, right eye**

▣ **SP** **H16.322** **Diffuse interstitial keratitis, left eye**

▣ **SP** **H16.323** **Diffuse interstitial keratitis, bilateral**

▣ **IQ** **H16.329** **Diffuse interstitial keratitis, unspecified eye**

⑥ **H16.33** **Sclerosing keratitis**

▣ **SP** **H16.331** **Sclerosing keratitis, right eye**

▣ **SP** **H16.332** **Sclerosing keratitis, left eye**

▣ **SP** **H16.333** **Sclerosing keratitis, bilateral**

▣ **IQ** **H16.339** **Sclerosing keratitis, unspecified eye**

⑥ **H16.39** **Other interstitial and deep keratitis**

▣ **SP** **H16.391** **Other interstitial and deep keratitis, right eye**

▣ **SP** **H16.392** **Other interstitial and deep keratitis, left eye**

Chapter 7

H00-H59

★ New ▲ Revised **Px** Primary **SP** PDGM Px **SL** Low CoM **SH** High CoM **IQ** Quest. Encounter ⊞ Hospice non-cancer Dx   Unspecified   **M** *Manifestation*

DecisionHealth's FY 2020 Complete Home Health ICD-10-CM Diagnosis Coding Manual

885

☐ SP **H16.393** Other interstitial and deep keratitis, bilateral

☐ IQ **H16.399** Other interstitial and deep keratitis, unspecified eye

5 **H16.4** Corneal neovascularization

6 **H16.40** Unspecified corneal neovascularization

☐ SP **H16.401** Unspecified corneal neovascularization, right eye

☐ SP **H16.402** Unspecified corneal neovascularization, left eye

☐ SP **H16.403** Unspecified corneal neovascularization, bilateral

☐ IQ **H16.409** Unspecified corneal neovascularization, unspecified eye

6 **H16.41** Ghost vessels (corneal)

☐ SP **H16.411** Ghost vessels (corneal), right eye

☐ SP **H16.412** Ghost vessels (corneal), left eye

☐ SP **H16.413** Ghost vessels (corneal), bilateral

☐ IQ **H16.419** Ghost vessels (corneal), unspecified eye

6 **H16.42** Pannus (corneal)

☐ SP **H16.421** Pannus (corneal), right eye

☐ SP **H16.422** Pannus (corneal), left eye

☐ SP **H16.423** Pannus (corneal), bilateral

☐ IQ **H16.429** Pannus (corneal), unspecified eye

6 **H16.43** Localized vascularization of cornea

☐ SP **H16.431** Localized vascularization of cornea, right eye

☐ SP **H16.432** Localized vascularization of cornea, left eye

☐ SP **H16.433** Localized vascularization of cornea, bilateral

☐ IQ **H16.439** Localized vascularization of cornea, unspecified eye

6 **H16.44** Deep vascularization of cornea

☐ SP **H16.441** Deep vascularization of cornea, right eye

☐ SP **H16.442** Deep vascularization of cornea, left eye

☐ SP **H16.443** Deep vascularization of cornea, bilateral

☐ IQ **H16.449** Deep vascularization of cornea, unspecified eye

SP **H16.8** Other keratitis

SP **H16.9** Unspecified keratitis

4 **H17** Corneal scars and opacities

5 **H17.0** Adherent leukoma

☐ IQ **H17.00** Adherent leukoma, unspecified eye

☐ SP **H17.01** Adherent leukoma, right eye

☐ SP **H17.02** Adherent leukoma, left eye

☐ SP **H17.03** Adherent leukoma, bilateral

5 **H17.1** Central corneal opacity

☐ IQ **H17.10** Central corneal opacity, unspecified eye

☐ SP **H17.11** Central corneal opacity, right eye

☐ SP **H17.12** Central corneal opacity, left eye

☐ SP **H17.13** Central corneal opacity, bilateral

5 **H17.8** Other corneal scars and opacities

6 **H17.81** Minor opacity of cornea
Corneal nebula

☐ SP **H17.811** Minor opacity of cornea, right eye

☐ SP **H17.812** Minor opacity of cornea, left eye

☐ SP **H17.813** Minor opacity of cornea, bilateral

☐ IQ **H17.819** Minor opacity of cornea, unspecified eye

6 **H17.82** Peripheral opacity of cornea

☐ SP **H17.821** Peripheral opacity of cornea, right eye

☐ SP **H17.822** Peripheral opacity of cornea, left eye

☐ SP **H17.823** Peripheral opacity of cornea, bilateral

☐ IQ **H17.829** Peripheral opacity of cornea, unspecified eye

SP **H17.89** Other corneal scars and opacities

IQ **H17.9** Unspecified corneal scar and opacity

4 **H18** Other disorders of cornea

5 **H18.0** Corneal pigmentations and deposits

6 **H18.00** Unspecified corneal deposit

☐ SP **H18.001** Unspecified corneal deposit, right eye

☐ SP **H18.002** Unspecified corneal deposit, left eye

☐ SP **H18.003** Unspecified corneal deposit, bilateral

☐ IQ **H18.009** Unspecified corneal deposit, unspecified eye

6 **H18.01** Anterior corneal pigmentations
Staehli's line

☐ SP **H18.011** Anterior corneal pigmentations, right eye

☐ SP **H18.012** Anterior corneal pigmentations, left eye

☐ SP **H18.013** Anterior corneal pigmentations, bilateral

☐ IQ **H18.019** Anterior corneal pigmentations, unspecified eye

6 **H18.02** Argentous corneal deposits

☐ SP **H18.021** Argentous corneal deposits, right eye

☐ SP **H18.022** Argentous corneal deposits, left eye

☐ SP **H18.023** Argentous corneal deposits, bilateral

☐ IQ **H18.029** Argentous corneal deposits, unspecified eye

6 **H18.03** Corneal deposits in metabolic disorders
Code also:
associated metabolic disorder

☐ SP **H18.031** Corneal deposits in metabolic disorders, right eye

☐ SP **H18.032** Corneal deposits in metabolic disorders, left eye

☐ SP **H18.033** Corneal deposits in metabolic disorders, bilateral

☐ IQ **H18.039** Corneal deposits in metabolic disorders, unspecified eye

6 **H18.04** Kayser-Fleischer ring
Code also:
associated Wilson's disease (E83.01)

4 4th digit required   5 5th digit required   6 6th digit required   7 7th digit required   ☑ 7th digit placeholder   ✚ Additional code   ☐ Laterality

886   *DecisionHealth's* FY 2020 Complete Home Health ICD-10-CM Diagnosis Coding Manual

DEFINITION Gray-green or brownish ring of copper deposits on the exterior of the cornea that grow slowly inward; often seen with liver disorders.

▤ SP **H18.041** Kayser-Fleischer ring, right eye

▤ SP **H18.042** Kayser-Fleischer ring, left eye

▤ SP **H18.043** Kayser-Fleischer ring, bilateral

▤ IQ **H18.049** Kayser-Fleischer ring, unspecified eye

6 **H18.05** Posterior corneal pigmentations
Krukenberg's spindle

▤ SP **H18.051** Posterior corneal pigmentations, right eye

▤ SP **H18.052** Posterior corneal pigmentations, left eye

▤ SP **H18.053** Posterior corneal pigmentations, bilateral

▤ IQ **H18.059** Posterior corneal pigmentations, unspecified eye

6 **H18.06** Stromal corneal pigmentations
Hematocornea

▤ SP **H18.061** Stromal corneal pigmentations, right eye

▤ SP **H18.062** Stromal corneal pigmentations, left eye

▤ SP **H18.063** Stromal corneal pigmentations, bilateral

▤ IQ **H18.069** Stromal corneal pigmentations, unspecified eye

5 **H18.1** Bullous keratopathy

▤ IQ **H18.10** Bullous keratopathy, unspecified eye

▤ SP **H18.11** Bullous keratopathy, right eye

▤ SP **H18.12** Bullous keratopathy, left eye

▤ SP **H18.13** Bullous keratopathy, bilateral

5 **H18.2** Other and unspecified corneal edema

SP **H18.20** Unspecified corneal edema

6 **H18.21** Corneal edema secondary to contact lens
EXCLUDES 2 other corneal disorders due to contact lens (H18.82-)

▤ SP **H18.211** Corneal edema secondary to contact lens, right eye

▤ SP **H18.212** Corneal edema secondary to contact lens, left eye

▤ SP **H18.213** Corneal edema secondary to contact lens, bilateral

▤ IQ **H18.219** Corneal edema secondary to contact lens, unspecified eye

6 **H18.22** Idiopathic corneal edema

▤ SP **H18.221** Idiopathic corneal edema, right eye

▤ SP **H18.222** Idiopathic corneal edema, left eye

▤ SP **H18.223** Idiopathic corneal edema, bilateral

▤ IQ **H18.229** Idiopathic corneal edema, unspecified eye

6 **H18.23** Secondary corneal edema

▤ SP **H18.231** Secondary corneal edema, right eye

▤ SP **H18.232** Secondary corneal edema, left eye

▤ SP **H18.233** Secondary corneal edema, bilateral

▤ IQ **H18.239** Secondary corneal edema, unspecified eye

5 **H18.3** Changes of corneal membranes

SP **H18.30** Unspecified corneal membrane change

6 **H18.31** Folds and rupture in Bowman's membrane

▤ SP **H18.311** Folds and rupture in Bowman's membrane, right eye

▤ SP **H18.312** Folds and rupture in Bowman's membrane, left eye

▤ SP **H18.313** Folds and rupture in Bowman's membrane, bilateral

▤ IQ **H18.319** Folds and rupture in Bowman's membrane, unspecified eye

6 **H18.32** Folds in Descemet's membrane
DEFINITION Fold in the membrane between the innermost layer of the cornea and the stroma (strong, supportive layer), affecting vision and preventing the flow of nutrients out of the cornea.

▤ SP **H18.321** Folds in Descemet's membrane, right eye

▤ SP **H18.322** Folds in Descemet's membrane, left eye

▤ SP **H18.323** Folds in Descemet's membrane, bilateral

▤ IQ **H18.329** Folds in Descemet's membrane, unspecified eye

6 **H18.33** Rupture in Descemet's membrane

▤ SP **H18.331** Rupture in Descemet's membrane, right eye

▤ SP **H18.332** Rupture in Descemet's membrane, left eye

▤ SP **H18.333** Rupture in Descemet's membrane, bilateral

▤ IQ **H18.339** Rupture in Descemet's membrane, unspecified eye

5 **H18.4** Corneal degeneration
EXCLUDES 1 Mooren's ulcer (H16.0-)
recurrent erosion of cornea (H18.83-)

SP **H18.40** Unspecified corneal degeneration

6 **H18.41** Arcus senilis
Senile corneal changes

▤ SP **H18.411** Arcus senilis, right eye

▤ SP **H18.412** Arcus senilis, left eye

▤ SP **H18.413** Arcus senilis, bilateral

▤ IQ **H18.419** Arcus senilis, unspecified eye

6 **H18.42** Band keratopathy
DEFINITION Degeneration of the cornea in which calcium deposits are laid in horizontal band-like layers, obscuring the patient's vision.

▤ SP **H18.421** Band keratopathy, right eye

▤ SP **H18.422** Band keratopathy, left eye

▤ SP **H18.423** Band keratopathy, bilateral

▤ IQ **H18.429** Band keratopathy, unspecified eye

SP **H18.43** Other calcerous corneal degeneration

6 **H18.44** Keratomalacia

★ New ▲ Revised Px Primary SP PDGM Px SL Low CoM SH High CoM IQ Quest. Encounter H Hospice non-cancer Dx Unspecified M *Manifestation*

DecisionHealth's FY 2020 Complete Home Health ICD-10-CM Diagnosis Coding Manual

887

EXCLUDES 1 keratomalacia due to vitamin A deficiency (E50.4)

🔵 **SP** **H18.441** **Keratomalacia, right eye**

🔵 **SP** **H18.442** **Keratomalacia, left eye**

🔵 **SP** **H18.443** **Keratomalacia, bilateral**

🔵 **IQ** **H18.449** Keratomalacia, unspecified eye

⑥ **H18.45** **Nodular corneal degeneration**

🔵 **SP** **H18.451** **Nodular corneal degeneration, right eye**

🔵 **SP** **H18.452** **Nodular corneal degeneration, left eye**

🔵 **SP** **H18.453** **Nodular corneal degeneration, bilateral**

🔵 **IQ** **H18.459** Nodular corneal degeneration, unspecified eye

⑥ **H18.46** **Peripheral corneal degeneration**

🔵 **SP** **H18.461** **Peripheral corneal degeneration, right eye**

🔵 **SP** **H18.462** **Peripheral corneal degeneration, left eye**

🔵 **SP** **H18.463** **Peripheral corneal degeneration, bilateral**

🔵 **IQ** **H18.469** Peripheral corneal degeneration, unspecified eye

SP **H18.49** **Other corneal degeneration**

⑤ **H18.5** **Hereditary corneal dystrophies**

IQ **H18.50** Unspecified hereditary corneal dystrophies

SP **H18.51** **Endothelial corneal dystrophy**
Fuchs' dystrophy

SP **H18.52** **Epithelial (juvenile) corneal dystrophy**
DEFINITION Multiple lesions on the outermost layer of the cornea occurring in the early years, which gradually grow together and obscure vision.

SP **H18.53** **Granular corneal dystrophy**

SP **H18.54** **Lattice corneal dystrophy**

SP **H18.55** **Macular corneal dystrophy**

SP **H18.59** **Other hereditary corneal dystrophies**

⑤ **H18.6** **Keratoconus**

⑥ **H18.60** Keratoconus, unspecified

🔵 **SP** **H18.601** Keratoconus, unspecified, right eye

🔵 **SP** **H18.602** Keratoconus, unspecified, left eye

🔵 **SP** **H18.603** Keratoconus, unspecified, bilateral

🔵 **IQ** **H18.609** Keratoconus, unspecified, unspecified eye

⑥ **H18.61** **Keratoconus, stable**

🔵 **SP** **H18.611** **Keratoconus, stable, right eye**

🔵 **SP** **H18.612** **Keratoconus, stable, left eye**

🔵 **SP** **H18.613** **Keratoconus, stable, bilateral**

🔵 **IQ** **H18.619** Keratoconus, stable, unspecified eye

⑥ **H18.62** **Keratoconus, unstable**
Acute hydrops

🔵 **SP** **H18.621** **Keratoconus, unstable, right eye**

🔵 **SP** **H18.622** **Keratoconus, unstable, left eye**

🔵 **SP** **H18.623** **Keratoconus, unstable, bilateral**

🔵 **IQ** **H18.629** Keratoconus, unstable, unspecified eye

⑤ **H18.7** **Other and unspecified corneal deformities**
EXCLUDES 1 congenital malformations of cornea (Q13.3-Q13.4)

IQ **H18.70** Unspecified corneal deformity

⑥ **H18.71** **Corneal ectasia**

🔵 **SP** **H18.711** **Corneal ectasia, right eye**

🔵 **SP** **H18.712** **Corneal ectasia, left eye**

🔵 **SP** **H18.713** **Corneal ectasia, bilateral**

🔵 **IQ** **H18.719** Corneal ectasia, unspecified eye

⑥ **H18.72** **Corneal staphyloma**

🔵 **SP** **H18.721** **Corneal staphyloma, right eye**

🔵 **SP** **H18.722** **Corneal staphyloma, left eye**

🔵 **SP** **H18.723** **Corneal staphyloma, bilateral**

🔵 **IQ** **H18.729** Corneal staphyloma, unspecified eye

⑥ **H18.73** **Descemetocele**

🔵 **SP** **H18.731** **Descemetocele, right eye**

🔵 **SP** **H18.732** **Descemetocele, left eye**

🔵 **SP** **H18.733** **Descemetocele, bilateral**

🔵 **IQ** **H18.739** Descemetocele, unspecified eye

⑥ **H18.79** **Other corneal deformities**

🔵 **SP** **H18.791** **Other corneal deformities, right eye**

🔵 **SP** **H18.792** **Other corneal deformities, left eye**

🔵 **SP** **H18.793** **Other corneal deformities, bilateral**

🔵 **IQ** **H18.799** Other corneal deformities, unspecified eye

⑤ **H18.8** **Other specified disorders of cornea**

⑥ **H18.81** **Anesthesia and hypoesthesia of cornea**
DEFINITION Decreased or complete loss of corneal sensitivity to pain and irritation.

🔵 **SP** **H18.811** **Anesthesia and hypoesthesia of cornea, right eye**

🔵 **SP** **H18.812** **Anesthesia and hypoesthesia of cornea, left eye**

🔵 **SP** **H18.813** **Anesthesia and hypoesthesia of cornea, bilateral**

🔵 **IQ** **H18.819** Anesthesia and hypoesthesia of cornea, unspecified eye

⑥ **H18.82** **Corneal disorder due to contact lens**
EXCLUDES 2 corneal edema due to contact lens (H18.21-)

🔵 **SP** **H18.821** **Corneal disorder due to contact lens, right eye**

🔵 **SP** **H18.822** **Corneal disorder due to contact lens, left eye**

🔵 **SP** **H18.823** **Corneal disorder due to contact lens, bilateral**

🔵 **IQ** **H18.829** Corneal disorder due to contact lens, unspecified eye

⑥ **H18.83** **Recurrent erosion of cornea**

🔵 **SP** **H18.831** **Recurrent erosion of cornea, right eye**

🔵 **SP** **H18.832** **Recurrent erosion of cornea, left eye**

---

④4th digit required ⑤5th digit required ⑥6th digit required ⑦7th digit required ⑦7th digit placeholder ➕Additional code 🔵Laterality

☐ SP **H18.833** Recurrent erosion of cornea, bilateral

☐ IQ **H18.839** Recurrent erosion of cornea, unspecified eye

6 **H18.89** Other specified disorders of cornea

☐ SP **H18.891** Other specified disorders of cornea, right eye

☐ SP **H18.892** Other specified disorders of cornea, left eye

☐ SP **H18.893** Other specified disorders of cornea, bilateral

☐ IQ **H18.899** Other specified disorders of cornea, unspecified eye

IQ **H18.9** Unspecified disorder of cornea

4 **H20** Iridocyclitis

5 **H20.0** Acute and subacute iridocyclitis
Acute anterior uveitis
Acute cyclitis
Acute iritis
Subacute anterior uveitis
Subacute cyclitis
Subacute iritis

EXCLUDES 1 iridocyclitis, iritis, uveitis (due to) (in) diabetes mellitus (E08-E13 with .39)
iridocyclitis, iritis, uveitis (due to) (in) diphtheria (A36.89)
iridocyclitis, iritis, uveitis (due to) (in) gonococcal (A54.32)
iridocyclitis, iritis, uveitis (due to) (in) herpes (simplex) (B00.51)
iridocyclitis, iritis, uveitis (due to) (in) herpes zoster (B02.32)
iridocyclitis, iritis, uveitis (due to) (in) late congenital syphilis (A50.39)
iridocyclitis, iritis, uveitis (due to) (in) late syphilis (A52.71)
iridocyclitis, iritis, uveitis (due to) (in) sarcoidosis (D86.83)
iridocyclitis, iritis, uveitis (due to) (in) syphilis (A51.43)
iridocyclitis, iritis, uveitis (due to) (in) toxoplasmosis (B58.09)
iridocyclitis, iritis, uveitis (due to) (in) tuberculosis (A18.54)

SP **H20.00** Unspecified acute and subacute iridocyclitis

6 **H20.01** Primary iridocyclitis

☐ SP **H20.011** Primary iridocyclitis, right eye

☐ SP **H20.012** Primary iridocyclitis, left eye

☐ SP **H20.013** Primary iridocyclitis, bilateral

☐ IQ **H20.019** Primary iridocyclitis, unspecified eye

6 **H20.02** Recurrent acute iridocyclitis

☐ SP **H20.021** Recurrent acute iridocyclitis, right eye

☐ SP **H20.022** Recurrent acute iridocyclitis, left eye

☐ SP **H20.023** Recurrent acute iridocyclitis, bilateral

☐ IQ **H20.029** Recurrent acute iridocyclitis, unspecified eye

6 **H20.03** Secondary infectious iridocyclitis

☐ SP **H20.031** Secondary infectious iridocyclitis, right eye

☐ SP **H20.032** Secondary infectious iridocyclitis, left eye

☐ SP **H20.033** Secondary infectious iridocyclitis, bilateral

☐ IQ **H20.039** Secondary infectious iridocyclitis, unspecified eye

6 **H20.04** Secondary noninfectious iridocyclitis

☐ SP **H20.041** Secondary noninfectious iridocyclitis, right eye

☐ SP **H20.042** Secondary noninfectious iridocyclitis, left eye

☐ SP **H20.043** Secondary noninfectious iridocyclitis, bilateral

☐ IQ **H20.049** Secondary noninfectious iridocyclitis, unspecified eye

6 **H20.05** Hypopyon

DEFINITION Accumulation of pus in the anterior chamber of the eye between the cornea and the iris and lens.

☐ SP **H20.051** Hypopyon, right eye

☐ SP **H20.052** Hypopyon, left eye

☐ SP **H20.053** Hypopyon, bilateral

☐ IQ **H20.059** Hypopyon, unspecified eye

+ 5 **H20.1** Chronic iridocyclitis
Use additional code for any associated cataract (H26.21-)
EXCLUDES 2 posterior cyclitis (H30.2-)

☐ IQ + **H20.10** Chronic iridocyclitis, unspecified eye

☐ SP + **H20.11** Chronic iridocyclitis, right eye

☐ SP + **H20.12** Chronic iridocyclitis, left eye

☐ SP + **H20.13** Chronic iridocyclitis, bilateral

5 **H20.2** Lens-induced iridocyclitis

☐ IQ **H20.20** Lens-induced iridocyclitis, unspecified eye

☐ SP **H20.21** Lens-induced iridocyclitis, right eye

☐ SP **H20.22** Lens-induced iridocyclitis, left eye

☐ SP **H20.23** Lens-induced iridocyclitis, bilateral

5 **H20.8** Other iridocyclitis

EXCLUDES 2 glaucomatocyclitis crises (H40.4-)
posterior cyclitis (H30.2-)
sympathetic uveitis (H44.13-)

6 **H20.81** Fuchs' heterochromic cyclitis

☐ SP **H20.811** Fuchs' heterochromic cyclitis, right eye

☐ SP **H20.812** Fuchs' heterochromic cyclitis, left eye

☐ SP **H20.813** Fuchs' heterochromic cyclitis, bilateral

★ New ▲ Revised Px Primary SP PDGM Px SL Low CoM SH High CoM IQ Quest. Encounter H Hospice non-cancer Dx Unspecified M *Manifestation*

⊟ !Q **H20.819** Fuchs' heterochromic cyclitis, unspecified eye

⑥ **H20.82** Vogt-Koyanagi syndrome

⊟ SP **H20.821** Vogt-Koyanagi syndrome, right eye

⊟ SP **H20.822** Vogt-Koyanagi syndrome, left eye

⊟ SP **H20.823** Vogt-Koyanagi syndrome, bilateral

⊟ !Q **H20.829** Vogt-Koyanagi syndrome, unspecified eye

SP **H20.9** Unspecified iridocyclitis
Uveitis NOS

④ **H21** Other disorders of iris and ciliary body
EXCLUDES 2 sympathetic uveitis (H44.1-)

⑤ **H21.0** Hyphema
EXCLUDES 1 traumatic hyphema (S05.1-)

DEFINITION Bleeding in the iris that pools in the bottom of the cornea causing vision to be extremely blurred.

⊟ !Q **H21.00** Hyphema, unspecified eye

⊟ SP **H21.01** Hyphema, right eye

⊟ SP **H21.02** Hyphema, left eye

⊟ SP **H21.03** Hyphema, bilateral

⑤ **H21.1** Other vascular disorders of iris and ciliary body
Neovascularization of iris or ciliary body
Rubeosis iridis
Rubeosis of iris

⑥ **H21.1X** Other vascular disorders of iris and ciliary body

⊟ SP **H21.1X1** Other vascular disorders of iris and ciliary body, right eye

⊟ SP **H21.1X2** Other vascular disorders of iris and ciliary body, left eye

⊟ SP **H21.1X3** Other vascular disorders of iris and ciliary body, bilateral

⊟ !Q **H21.1X9** Other vascular disorders of iris and ciliary body, unspecified eye

⑤ **H21.2** Degeneration of iris and ciliary body

⑥ **H21.21** Degeneration of chamber angle

⊟ SP **H21.211** Degeneration of chamber angle, right eye

⊟ SP **H21.212** Degeneration of chamber angle, left eye

⊟ SP **H21.213** Degeneration of chamber angle, bilateral

⊟ !Q **H21.219** Degeneration of chamber angle, unspecified eye

⑥ **H21.22** Degeneration of ciliary body

⊟ SP **H21.221** Degeneration of ciliary body, right eye

⊟ SP **H21.222** Degeneration of ciliary body, left eye

⊟ SP **H21.223** Degeneration of ciliary body, bilateral

⊟ !Q **H21.229** Degeneration of ciliary body, unspecified eye

⑥ **H21.23** Degeneration of iris (pigmentary)
Translucency of iris

DEFINITION Fading of the pigmentation (color) of the iris, allowing light to seep in rather than being blocked; presents with light-sensitivity and blurred vision.

⊟ SP **H21.231** Degeneration of iris (pigmentary), right eye

⊟ SP **H21.232** Degeneration of iris (pigmentary), left eye

⊟ SP **H21.233** Degeneration of iris (pigmentary), bilateral

⊟ !Q **H21.239** Degeneration of iris (pigmentary), unspecified eye

⑥ **H21.24** Degeneration of pupillary margin

⊟ SP **H21.241** Degeneration of pupillary margin, right eye

⊟ SP **H21.242** Degeneration of pupillary margin, left eye

⊟ SP **H21.243** Degeneration of pupillary margin, bilateral

⊟ !Q **H21.249** Degeneration of pupillary margin, unspecified eye

⑥ **H21.25** Iridoschisis

⊟ SP **H21.251** Iridoschisis, right eye

⊟ SP **H21.252** Iridoschisis, left eye

⊟ SP **H21.253** Iridoschisis, bilateral

⊟ !Q **H21.259** Iridoschisis, unspecified eye

⑥ **H21.26** Iris atrophy (essential) (progressive)

⊟ SP **H21.261** Iris atrophy (essential) (progressive), right eye

⊟ SP **H21.262** Iris atrophy (essential) (progressive), left eye

⊟ SP **H21.263** Iris atrophy (essential) (progressive), bilateral

⊟ !Q **H21.269** Iris atrophy (essential) (progressive), unspecified eye

⑥ **H21.27** Miotic pupillary cyst

DEFINITION Fluid-filled pockets in the iris at the pupil's edge, causing the iris to contract and interfering with vision when light is less than optimal.

⊟ SP **H21.271** Miotic pupillary cyst, right eye

⊟ SP **H21.272** Miotic pupillary cyst, left eye

⊟ SP **H21.273** Miotic pupillary cyst, bilateral

⊟ !Q **H21.279** Miotic pupillary cyst, unspecified eye

SP **H21.29** Other iris atrophy

⑤ **H21.3** Cyst of iris, ciliary body and anterior chamber
EXCLUDES 2 miotic pupillary cyst (H21.27-)

⑥ **H21.30** Idiopathic cysts of iris, ciliary body or anterior chamber
Cyst of iris, ciliary body or anterior chamber NOS

⊟ SP **H21.301** Idiopathic cysts of iris, ciliary body or anterior chamber, right eye

⊟ SP **H21.302** Idiopathic cysts of iris, ciliary body or anterior chamber, left eye

⊟ SP **H21.303** Idiopathic cysts of iris, ciliary body or anterior chamber, bilateral

⊟ !Q **H21.309** Idiopathic cysts of iris, ciliary body or anterior chamber, unspecified eye

⑥ **H21.31** Exudative cysts of iris or anterior chamber

---

④ 4th digit required   ⑤ 5th digit required   ⑥ 6th digit required   ⑦ 7th digit required   ⑦ 7th digit placeholder   ✛ Additional code   ⊟ Laterality

▣ **SP** **H21.311** Exudative cysts of iris or anterior chamber, right eye

▣ **SP** **H21.312** Exudative cysts of iris or anterior chamber, left eye

▣ **SP** **H21.313** Exudative cysts of iris or anterior chamber, bilateral

▣ **IQ** **H21.319** Exudative cysts of iris or anterior chamber, unspecified eye

⑥ **H21.32** Implantation cysts of iris, ciliary body or anterior chamber

▣ **SP** **H21.321** Implantation cysts of iris, ciliary body or anterior chamber, right eye

▣ **SP** **H21.322** Implantation cysts of iris, ciliary body or anterior chamber, left eye

▣ **SP** **H21.323** Implantation cysts of iris, ciliary body or anterior chamber, bilateral

▣ **IQ** **H21.329** Implantation cysts of iris, ciliary body or anterior chamber, unspecified eye

⑥ **H21.33** Parasitic cyst of iris, ciliary body or anterior chamber

▣ **SP** **H21.331** Parasitic cyst of iris, ciliary body or anterior chamber, right eye

▣ **SP** **H21.332** Parasitic cyst of iris, ciliary body or anterior chamber, left eye

▣ **SP** **H21.333** Parasitic cyst of iris, ciliary body or anterior chamber, bilateral

▣ **IQ** **H21.339** Parasitic cyst of iris, ciliary body or anterior chamber, unspecified eye

⑥ **H21.34** Primary cyst of pars plana

▣ **SP** **H21.341** Primary cyst of pars plana, right eye

▣ **SP** **H21.342** Primary cyst of pars plana, left eye

▣ **SP** **H21.343** Primary cyst of pars plana, bilateral

▣ **IQ** **H21.349** Primary cyst of pars plana, unspecified eye

⑥ **H21.35** Exudative cyst of pars plana

▣ **SP** **H21.351** Exudative cyst of pars plana, right eye

▣ **SP** **H21.352** Exudative cyst of pars plana, left eye

▣ **SP** **H21.353** Exudative cyst of pars plana, bilateral

▣ **IQ** **H21.359** Exudative cyst of pars plana, unspecified eye

⑤ **H21.4** Pupillary membranes
Iris bombé
Pupillary occlusion
Pupillary seclusion
EXCLUDES 1 congenital pupillary membranes (Q13.8)

▣ **IQ** **H21.40** Pupillary membranes, unspecified eye

▣ **SP** **H21.41** Pupillary membranes, right eye

▣ **SP** **H21.42** Pupillary membranes, left eye

▣ **SP** **H21.43** Pupillary membranes, bilateral

⑤ **H21.5** Other and unspecified adhesions and disruptions of iris and ciliary body
EXCLUDES 1 corectopia (Q13.2)

⑥ **H21.50** Unspecified adhesions of iris

Synechia (iris) NOS

▣ **SP** **H21.501** Unspecified adhesions of iris, right eye

▣ **SP** **H21.502** Unspecified adhesions of iris, left eye

▣ **SP** **H21.503** Unspecified adhesions of iris, bilateral

▣ **IQ** **H21.509** Unspecified adhesions of iris and ciliary body, unspecified eye

⑥ **H21.51** Anterior synechiae (iris)

▣ **SP** **H21.511** Anterior synechiae (iris), right eye

▣ **SP** **H21.512** Anterior synechiae (iris), left eye

▣ **SP** **H21.513** Anterior synechiae (iris), bilateral

▣ **IQ** **H21.519** Anterior synechiae (iris), unspecified eye

⑥ **H21.52** Goniosynechiae
DEFINITION Adhesion of the iris to the posterior surface of the cornea, in the angle of the anterior chamber of the eye.

▣ **SP** **H21.521** Goniosynechiae, right eye

▣ **SP** **H21.522** Goniosynechiae, left eye

▣ **SP** **H21.523** Goniosynechiae, bilateral

▣ **IQ** **H21.529** Goniosynechiae, unspecified eye

⑥ **H21.53** Iridodialysis
DEFINITION Separation or loosening of the iris from its root at the ciliary body, usually from trauma or surgical accident.

▣ **SP** **H21.531** Iridodialysis, right eye

▣ **SP** **H21.532** Iridodialysis, left eye

▣ **SP** **H21.533** Iridodialysis, bilateral

▣ **IQ** **H21.539** Iridodialysis, unspecified eye

⑥ **H21.54** Posterior synechiae (iris)
DEFINITION Adhesion where the lens and the iris grow together, preventing the iris from dilating and contracting properly.

▣ **SP** **H21.541** Posterior synechiae (iris), right eye

▣ **SP** **H21.542** Posterior synechiae (iris), left eye

▣ **SP** **H21.543** Posterior synechiae (iris), bilateral

▣ **IQ** **H21.549** Posterior synechiae (iris), unspecified eye

⑥ **H21.55** Recession of chamber angle

▣ **SP** **H21.551** Recession of chamber angle, right eye

▣ **SP** **H21.552** Recession of chamber angle, left eye

▣ **SP** **H21.553** Recession of chamber angle, bilateral

▣ **IQ** **H21.559** Recession of chamber angle, unspecified eye

⑥ **H21.56** Pupillary abnormalities
Deformed pupil
Ectopic pupil
Rupture of sphincter, pupil
EXCLUDES 1 congenital deformity of pupil (Q13.2-)

▣ **SP** **H21.561** Pupillary abnormality, right eye

▣ **SP** **H21.562** Pupillary abnormality, left eye

▣ **SP** **H21.563** Pupillary abnormality, bilateral

Chapter 7

H00-H59

★ New ▲ Revised Px Primary **SP** PDGM Px **SL** Low CoM **SH** High CoM **IQ** Quest. Encounter **H** Hospice non-cancer Dx Unspecified **M** *Manifestation*

DecisionHealth's FY 2020 Complete Home Health ICD-10-CM Diagnosis Coding Manual

891

■ **IQ** H21.569 **Pupillary abnormality, unspecified eye**

5 H21.8 Other specified disorders of iris and ciliary body

SP ✚ H21.81 **Floppy iris syndrome**
Intraoperative floppy iris syndrome (IFIS)
Use additional code for adverse effect, if applicable, to identify drug (T36-T50 with fifth or sixth character 5)
> **DEFINITION** Syndrome occurring in one who has taken alpha-blockers; a dilated iris does not stay dilated, causing potentially injurious surgical complications.

SP H21.82 **Plateau iris syndrome (post-iridectomy) (postprocedural)**

SP H21.89 **Other specified disorders of iris and ciliary body**

IQ H21.9 **Unspecified disorder of iris and ciliary body**

M **IQ** H22 *Disorders of iris and ciliary body in diseases classified elsewhere*
Code first underlying disease, such as:
gout (M1A.-, M10.-)
leprosy (A30.-)
parasitic disease (B89)

Disorders of lens   (H25-H28)

4 H25 **Age-related cataract**
Senile cataract
> **EXCLUDES 2** capsular glaucoma with pseudoexfoliation of lens (H40.1-)

5 H25.0 Age-related incipient cataract

6 H25.01 Cortical age-related cataract

■ **SP** H25.011 **Cortical age-related cataract, right eye**

■ **SP** H25.012 **Cortical age-related cataract, left eye**

■ **SP** H25.013 **Cortical age-related cataract, bilateral**

■ **IQ** H25.019 **Cortical age-related cataract, unspecified eye**

6 H25.03 Anterior subcapsular polar age-related cataract

■ **SP** H25.031 **Anterior subcapsular polar age-related cataract, right eye**

■ **SP** H25.032 **Anterior subcapsular polar age-related cataract, left eye**

■ **SP** H25.033 **Anterior subcapsular polar age-related cataract, bilateral**

■ **IQ** H25.039 **Anterior subcapsular polar age-related cataract, unspecified eye**

6 H25.04 Posterior subcapsular polar age-related cataract

■ **SP** H25.041 **Posterior subcapsular polar age-related cataract, right eye**

■ **SP** H25.042 **Posterior subcapsular polar age-related cataract, left eye**

■ **SP** H25.043 **Posterior subcapsular polar age-related cataract, bilateral**

■ **IQ** H25.049 **Posterior subcapsular polar age-related cataract, unspecified eye**

6 H25.09 Other age-related incipient cataract
Coronary age-related cataract

Punctate age-related cataract
Water clefts

■ **SP** H25.091 **Other age-related incipient cataract, right eye**

■ **SP** H25.092 **Other age-related incipient cataract, left eye**

■ **SP** H25.093 **Other age-related incipient cataract, bilateral**

■ **IQ** H25.099 **Other age-related incipient cataract, unspecified eye**

5 H25.1 Age-related nuclear cataract
Cataracta brunescens
Nuclear sclerosis cataract

■ **IQ** H25.10 **Age-related nuclear cataract, unspecified eye**

■ **SP** H25.11 **Age-related nuclear cataract, right eye**

■ **SP** H25.12 **Age-related nuclear cataract, left eye**

■ **SP** H25.13 **Age-related nuclear cataract, bilateral**

5 H25.2 Age-related cataract, morgagnian type
Age-related hypermature cataract

■ **IQ** H25.20 **Age-related cataract, morgagnian type, unspecified eye**

■ **SP** H25.21 **Age-related cataract, morgagnian type, right eye**

■ **SP** H25.22 **Age-related cataract, morgagnian type, left eye**

■ **SP** H25.23 **Age-related cataract, morgagnian type, bilateral**

5 H25.8 Other age-related cataract

6 H25.81 Combined forms of age-related cataract

■ **SP** H25.811 **Combined forms of age-related cataract, right eye**

■ **SP** H25.812 **Combined forms of age-related cataract, left eye**

■ **SP** H25.813 **Combined forms of age-related cataract, bilateral**

■ **IQ** H25.819 **Combined forms of age-related cataract, unspecified eye**

SP H25.89 **Other age-related cataract**

SP H25.9 **Unspecified age-related cataract**

| Normal | Anterior subcapsular | Posterior subcapsular | Cortical |

4 H26 **Other cataract**
> **EXCLUDES 1** congenital cataract (Q12.0)
> **DEFINITION** Partial or complete clouding on or in the lens or lens capsule of the eye, obscuring vision.

5 H26.0 Infantile and juvenile cataract

6 H26.00 **Unspecified infantile and juvenile cataract**

---

4 4th digit required   **5** 5th digit required   **6** 6th digit required   **7** 7th digit required   **7** 7th digit placeholder   ✚ Additional code   ■ Laterality

892   *DecisionHealth's* FY 2020 Complete Home Health ICD-10-CM Diagnosis Coding Manual

☰ SP H26.001 Unspecified infantile and juvenile cataract, right eye

☰ SP H26.002 Unspecified infantile and juvenile cataract, left eye

☰ SP H26.003 Unspecified infantile and juvenile cataract, bilateral

☰ IQ H26.009 Unspecified infantile and juvenile cataract, unspecified eye

⑥ H26.01 Infantile and juvenile cortical, lamellar, or zonular cataract

☰ SP H26.011 Infantile and juvenile cortical, lamellar, or zonular cataract, right eye

☰ SP H26.012 Infantile and juvenile cortical, lamellar, or zonular cataract, left eye

☰ SP H26.013 Infantile and juvenile cortical, lamellar, or zonular cataract, bilateral

☰ IQ H26.019 Infantile and juvenile cortical, lamellar, or zonular cataract, unspecified eye

⑥ H26.03 Infantile and juvenile nuclear cataract

☰ SP H26.031 Infantile and juvenile nuclear cataract, right eye

☰ SP H26.032 Infantile and juvenile nuclear cataract, left eye

☰ SP H26.033 Infantile and juvenile nuclear cataract, bilateral

☰ IQ H26.039 Infantile and juvenile nuclear cataract, unspecified eye

⑥ H26.04 Anterior subcapsular polar infantile and juvenile cataract

☰ SP H26.041 Anterior subcapsular polar infantile and juvenile cataract, right eye

☰ SP H26.042 Anterior subcapsular polar infantile and juvenile cataract, left eye

☰ SP H26.043 Anterior subcapsular polar infantile and juvenile cataract, bilateral

☰ IQ H26.049 Anterior subcapsular polar infantile and juvenile cataract, unspecified eye

⑥ H26.05 Posterior subcapsular polar infantile and juvenile cataract

☰ SP H26.051 Posterior subcapsular polar infantile and juvenile cataract, right eye

☰ SP H26.052 Posterior subcapsular polar infantile and juvenile cataract, left eye

☰ SP H26.053 Posterior subcapsular polar infantile and juvenile cataract, bilateral

☰ IQ H26.059 Posterior subcapsular polar infantile and juvenile cataract, unspecified eye

⑥ H26.06 Combined forms of infantile and juvenile cataract

☰ SP H26.061 Combined forms of infantile and juvenile cataract, right eye

☰ SP H26.062 Combined forms of infantile and juvenile cataract, left eye

☰ SP H26.063 Combined forms of infantile and juvenile cataract, bilateral

☰ IQ H26.069 Combined forms of infantile and juvenile cataract, unspecified eye

SP H26.09 Other infantile and juvenile cataract

➕ ⑤ H26.1 Traumatic cataract
Use additional code (Chapter 20) to identify external cause

➕ ⑥ H26.10 Unspecified traumatic cataract

☰ SP ➕ H26.101 Unspecified traumatic cataract, right eye

☰ SP ➕ H26.102 Unspecified traumatic cataract, left eye

☰ SP ➕ H26.103 Unspecified traumatic cataract, bilateral

☰ IQ ➕ H26.109 Unspecified traumatic cataract, unspecified eye

➕ ⑥ H26.11 Localized traumatic opacities

☰ SP ➕ H26.111 Localized traumatic opacities, right eye

☰ SP ➕ H26.112 Localized traumatic opacities, left eye

☰ SP ➕ H26.113 Localized traumatic opacities, bilateral

☰ IQ ➕ H26.119 Localized traumatic opacities, unspecified eye

➕ ⑥ H26.12 Partially resolved traumatic cataract

☰ SP ➕ H26.121 Partially resolved traumatic cataract, right eye

☰ SP ➕ H26.122 Partially resolved traumatic cataract, left eye

☰ SP ➕ H26.123 Partially resolved traumatic cataract, bilateral

☰ IQ ➕ H26.129 Partially resolved traumatic cataract, unspecified eye

➕ ⑥ H26.13 Total traumatic cataract

☰ SP ➕ H26.131 Total traumatic cataract, right eye

☰ SP ➕ H26.132 Total traumatic cataract, left eye

☰ SP ➕ H26.133 Total traumatic cataract, bilateral

☰ IQ ➕ H26.139 Total traumatic cataract, unspecified eye

⑤ H26.2 Complicated cataract

SP H26.20 Unspecified complicated cataract
Cataracta complicata NOS

⑥ H26.21 Cataract with neovascularization
Code also associated condition, such as:
chronic iridocyclitis (H20.1-)

☰ SP H26.211 Cataract with neovascularization, right eye

☰ SP H26.212 Cataract with neovascularization, left eye

☰ SP H26.213 Cataract with neovascularization, bilateral

☰ IQ H26.219 Cataract with neovascularization, unspecified eye

⑥ H26.22 Cataract secondary to ocular disorders (degenerative) (inflammatory)
Code also:
associated ocular disorder

Chapter 7

H00-H59

★ New ▲ Revised Px Primary SP PDGM Px SL Low CoM SH High CoM IQ Quest. Encounter H Hospice non-cancer Dx Unspecified M *Manifestation*

DecisionHealth's FY 2020 Complete Home Health ICD-10-CM Diagnosis Coding Manual

893

⊟ SP **H26.221** **Cataract secondary to ocular disorders (degenerative) (inflammatory), right eye**

⊟ SP **H26.222** **Cataract secondary to ocular disorders (degenerative) (inflammatory), left eye**

⊟ SP **H26.223** **Cataract secondary to ocular disorders (degenerative) (inflammatory), bilateral**

⊟ IQ **H26.229** **Cataract secondary to ocular disorders (degenerative) (inflammatory), unspecified eye**

6 **H26.23** **Glaucomatous flecks (subcapsular)**
Code first:
   underlying glaucoma (H40-H42)

⊟ SP **H26.231** **Glaucomatous flecks (subcapsular), right eye**

⊟ SP **H26.232** **Glaucomatous flecks (subcapsular), left eye**

⊟ SP **H26.233** **Glaucomatous flecks (subcapsular), bilateral**

⊟ IQ **H26.239** **Glaucomatous flecks (subcapsular), unspecified eye**

✚ 5 **H26.3** **Drug-induced cataract**
Toxic cataract
Use additional code for adverse effect, if applicable, to identify drug (T36-T50 with fifth or sixth character 5)
   DEFINITION   Cataract caused by exposure to a drug or other toxic substance, such as a miotic, antimiotic, corticosteroid, metal, nitro compound, or substituted hydrocarbon.

⊟ SP ✚ **H26.30** **Drug-induced cataract, unspecified eye**

⊟ SP ✚ **H26.31** **Drug-induced cataract, right eye**

⊟ SP ✚ **H26.32** **Drug-induced cataract, left eye**

⊟ SP ✚ **H26.33** **Drug-induced cataract, bilateral**

5 **H26.4** **Secondary cataract**

IQ **H26.40** **Unspecified secondary cataract**

6 **H26.41** **Soemmering's ring**
   DEFINITION   Doughnut-shaped remnant of lens behind the pupil, occurring after cataract surgery or secondary to trauma.

⊟ SP **H26.411** **Soemmering's ring, right eye**

⊟ SP **H26.412** **Soemmering's ring, left eye**

⊟ SP **H26.413** **Soemmering's ring, bilateral**

⊟ IQ **H26.419** **Soemmering's ring, unspecified eye**

6 **H26.49** **Other secondary cataract**

⊟ SP **H26.491** **Other secondary cataract, right eye**

⊟ SP **H26.492** **Other secondary cataract, left eye**

⊟ SP **H26.493** **Other secondary cataract, bilateral**

⊟ IQ **H26.499** **Other secondary cataract, unspecified eye**

SP **H26.8** **Other specified cataract**

IQ **H26.9** **Unspecified cataract**

4 **H27** **Other disorders of lens**
   EXCLUDES 1   congenital lens malformations (Q12.-)

mechanical complications of intraocular lens implant (T85.2)
   pseudophakia (Z96.1)

5 **H27.0** **Aphakia**
Acquired absence of lens
Acquired aphakia
Aphakia due to trauma
   EXCLUDES 1   cataract extraction status (Z98.4-)
   congenital absence of lens (Q12.3)
   congenital aphakia (Q12.3)
   DEFINITION   Absence of the crystalline lens of the eye.

⊟ IQ **H27.00** **Aphakia, unspecified eye**

⊟ SP **H27.01** **Aphakia, right eye**

⊟ SP **H27.02** **Aphakia, left eye**

⊟ IQ **H27.03** **Aphakia, bilateral**

5 **H27.1** **Dislocation of lens**

IQ **H27.10** **Unspecified dislocation of lens**

6 **H27.11** **Subluxation of lens**

⊟ SP **H27.111** **Subluxation of lens, right eye**

⊟ SP **H27.112** **Subluxation of lens, left eye**

⊟ SP **H27.113** **Subluxation of lens, bilateral**

⊟ IQ **H27.119** **Subluxation of lens, unspecified eye**

6 **H27.12** **Anterior dislocation of lens**

⊟ SP **H27.121** **Anterior dislocation of lens, right eye**

⊟ SP **H27.122** **Anterior dislocation of lens, left eye**

⊟ SP **H27.123** **Anterior dislocation of lens, bilateral**

⊟ IQ **H27.129** **Anterior dislocation of lens, unspecified eye**

6 **H27.13** **Posterior dislocation of lens**

⊟ SP **H27.131** **Posterior dislocation of lens, right eye**

⊟ SP **H27.132** **Posterior dislocation of lens, left eye**

⊟ SP **H27.133** **Posterior dislocation of lens, bilateral**

⊟ IQ **H27.139** **Posterior dislocation of lens, unspecified eye**

SP **H27.8** **Other specified disorders of lens**

IQ **H27.9** **Unspecified disorder of lens**

M IQ **H28** *Cataract in diseases classified elsewhere*
Code first underlying disease, such as:
   hypoparathyroidism (E20.-)
   myotonia (G71.1-)
   myxedema (E03.-)
   protein-calorie malnutrition (E40-E46)
   EXCLUDES 1   cataract in diabetes mellitus (E08.36, E09.36, E10.36, E11.36, E13.36)

Disorders of choroid and retina   (H30-H36)

4 **H30** **Chorioretinal inflammation**

5 **H30.0** **Focal chorioretinal inflammation**
Focal chorioretinitis
Focal choroiditis
Focal retinitis

---

4 4th digit required   5 5th digit required   6 6th digit required   7 7th digit required   ⊘ 7th digit placeholder   ✚ Additional code   ⊟ Laterality

894   *DecisionHealth's* FY 2020 Complete Home Health ICD-10-CM Diagnosis Coding Manual

Focal retinochoroiditis

6 H30.00 Unspecified focal chorioretinal inflammation

Focal chorioretinitis NOS
Focal choroiditis NOS
Focal retinitis NOS
Focal retinochoroiditis NOS

⊟ SP H30.001 Unspecified focal chorioretinal inflammation, right eye

⊟ SP H30.002 Unspecified focal chorioretinal inflammation, left eye

⊟ SP H30.003 Unspecified focal chorioretinal inflammation, bilateral

⊟ IQ H30.009 Unspecified focal chorioretinal inflammation, unspecified eye

6 H30.01 Focal chorioretinal inflammation, juxtapapillary

⊟ SP H30.011 Focal chorioretinal inflammation, juxtapapillary, right eye

⊟ SP H30.012 Focal chorioretinal inflammation, juxtapapillary, left eye

⊟ SP H30.013 Focal chorioretinal inflammation, juxtapapillary, bilateral

⊟ IQ H30.019 Focal chorioretinal inflammation, juxtapapillary, unspecified eye

6 H30.02 Focal chorioretinal inflammation of posterior pole

⊟ SP H30.021 Focal chorioretinal inflammation of posterior pole, right eye

⊟ SP H30.022 Focal chorioretinal inflammation of posterior pole, left eye

⊟ SP H30.023 Focal chorioretinal inflammation of posterior pole, bilateral

⊟ IQ H30.029 Focal chorioretinal inflammation of posterior pole, unspecified eye

6 H30.03 Focal chorioretinal inflammation, peripheral

⊟ SP H30.031 Focal chorioretinal inflammation, peripheral, right eye

⊟ SP H30.032 Focal chorioretinal inflammation, peripheral, left eye

⊟ SP H30.033 Focal chorioretinal inflammation, peripheral, bilateral

⊟ IQ H30.039 Focal chorioretinal inflammation, peripheral, unspecified eye

6 H30.04 Focal chorioretinal inflammation, macular or paramacular

⊟ SP H30.041 Focal chorioretinal inflammation, macular or paramacular, right eye

⊟ SP H30.042 Focal chorioretinal inflammation, macular or paramacular, left eye

⊟ SP H30.043 Focal chorioretinal inflammation, macular or paramacular, bilateral

⊟ IQ H30.049 Focal chorioretinal inflammation, macular or paramacular, unspecified eye

5 H30.1 Disseminated chorioretinal inflammation

Disseminated chorioretinitis
Disseminated choroiditis
Disseminated retinitis
Disseminated retinochoroiditis

EXCLUDES 2 exudative retinopathy (H35.02-)

6 H30.10 Unspecified disseminated chorioretinal inflammation

Disseminated chorioretinitis NOS
Disseminated choroiditis NOS
Disseminated retinitis NOS
Disseminated retinochoroiditis NOS

⊟ SP H30.101 Unspecified disseminated chorioretinal inflammation, right eye

⊟ SP H30.102 Unspecified disseminated chorioretinal inflammation, left eye

⊟ SP H30.103 Unspecified disseminated chorioretinal inflammation, bilateral

⊟ IQ H30.109 Unspecified disseminated chorioretinal inflammation, unspecified eye

6 H30.11 Disseminated chorioretinal inflammation of posterior pole

⊟ SP H30.111 Disseminated chorioretinal inflammation of posterior pole, right eye

⊟ SP H30.112 Disseminated chorioretinal inflammation of posterior pole, left eye

⊟ SP H30.113 Disseminated chorioretinal inflammation of posterior pole, bilateral

⊟ IQ H30.119 Disseminated chorioretinal inflammation of posterior pole, unspecified eye

6 H30.12 Disseminated chorioretinal inflammation, peripheral

⊟ SP H30.121 Disseminated chorioretinal inflammation, peripheral right eye

⊟ SP H30.122 Disseminated chorioretinal inflammation, peripheral, left eye

⊟ SP H30.123 Disseminated chorioretinal inflammation, peripheral, bilateral

⊟ IQ H30.129 Disseminated chorioretinal inflammation, peripheral, unspecified eye

6 H30.13 Disseminated chorioretinal inflammation, generalized

⊟ SP H30.131 Disseminated chorioretinal inflammation, generalized, right eye

⊟ SP H30.132 Disseminated chorioretinal inflammation, generalized, left eye

⊟ SP H30.133 Disseminated chorioretinal inflammation, generalized, bilateral

⊟ IQ H30.139 Disseminated chorioretinal inflammation, generalized, unspecified eye

6 H30.14 Acute posterior multifocal placoid pigment epitheliopathy

⊟ SP H30.141 Acute posterior multifocal placoid pigment epitheliopathy, right eye

⊟ SP H30.142 Acute posterior multifocal placoid pigment epitheliopathy, left eye

⊟ SP H30.143 Acute posterior multifocal placoid pigment epitheliopathy, bilateral

★ New ▲ Revised Px Primary SP PDGM Px SL Low CoM SH High CoM IQ Quest. Encounter H Hospice non-cancer Dx Unspecified M *Manifestation*

DecisionHealth's FY 2020 Complete Home Health ICD-10-CM Diagnosis Coding Manual

895

☐ IQ H30.149 Acute posterior multifocal placoid pigment epitheliopathy, unspecified eye

⑤ H30.2 Posterior cyclitis
Pars planitis

DEFINITION   Inflammation of the peripheral retina and the ciliary body, the hair-like structures that hold the lens of the eye in place.

☐ IQ H30.20 Posterior cyclitis, unspecified eye

☐ SP **H30.21 Posterior cyclitis, right eye**

☐ SP **H30.22 Posterior cyclitis, left eye**

☐ SP **H30.23 Posterior cyclitis, bilateral**

⑤ H30.8 Other chorioretinal inflammations

⑥ H30.81 Harada's disease

☐ SP **H30.811 Harada's disease, right eye**

☐ SP **H30.812 Harada's disease, left eye**

☐ SP **H30.813 Harada's disease, bilateral**

☐ IQ H30.819 Harada's disease, unspecified eye

⑥ H30.89 Other chorioretinal inflammations

☐ SP **H30.891 Other chorioretinal inflammations, right eye**

☐ SP **H30.892 Other chorioretinal inflammations, left eye**

☐ SP **H30.893 Other chorioretinal inflammations, bilateral**

☐ IQ H30.899 Other chorioretinal inflammations, unspecified eye

⑤ H30.9 Unspecified chorioretinal inflammation
Chorioretinitis NOS
Choroiditis NOS
Neuroretinitis NOS
Retinitis NOS
Retinochoroiditis NOS

☐ IQ H30.90 Unspecified chorioretinal inflammation, unspecified eye

☐ SP H30.91 Unspecified chorioretinal inflammation, right eye

☐ SP H30.92 Unspecified chorioretinal inflammation, left eye

☐ SP H30.93 Unspecified chorioretinal inflammation, bilateral

④ H31 Other disorders of choroid

⑤ H31.0 Chorioretinal scars
EXCLUDES 2   postsurgical chorioretinal scars (H59.81-)

⑥ H31.00 Unspecified chorioretinal scars

☐ SP H31.001 Unspecified chorioretinal scars, right eye

☐ SP H31.002 Unspecified chorioretinal scars, left eye

☐ SP H31.003 Unspecified chorioretinal scars, bilateral

☐ IQ H31.009 Unspecified chorioretinal scars, unspecified eye

⑥ H31.01 Macula scars of posterior pole (postinflammatory) (post-traumatic)
EXCLUDES 1   postprocedural chorioretinal scar (H59.81-)

☐ SP **H31.011 Macula scars of posterior pole (postinflammatory) (post-traumatic), right eye**

☐ SP **H31.012 Macula scars of posterior pole (postinflammatory) (post-traumatic), left eye**

☐ SP **H31.013 Macula scars of posterior pole (postinflammatory) (post-traumatic), bilateral**

☐ IQ H31.019 Macula scars of posterior pole (postinflammatory) (post-traumatic), unspecified eye

⑥ H31.02 Solar retinopathy
DEFINITION   Scar on the retina resulting from solar radiation.

☐ SP **H31.021 Solar retinopathy, right eye**

☐ SP **H31.022 Solar retinopathy, left eye**

☐ SP **H31.023 Solar retinopathy, bilateral**

☐ IQ H31.029 Solar retinopathy, unspecified eye

⑥ H31.09 Other chorioretinal scars

☐ SP **H31.091 Other chorioretinal scars, right eye**

☐ SP **H31.092 Other chorioretinal scars, left eye**

☐ SP **H31.093 Other chorioretinal scars, bilateral**

☐ IQ H31.099 Other chorioretinal scars, unspecified eye

⑤ H31.1 Choroidal degeneration
EXCLUDES 2   angioid streaks of macula (H35.33)

⑥ H31.10 Unspecified choroidal degeneration
Choroidal sclerosis NOS

☐ SP H31.101 Choroidal degeneration, unspecified, right eye

☐ SP H31.102 Choroidal degeneration, unspecified, left eye

☐ SP H31.103 Choroidal degeneration, unspecified, bilateral

☐ IQ H31.109 Choroidal degeneration, unspecified, unspecified eye

⑥ H31.11 Age-related choroidal atrophy

☐ SP **H31.111 Age-related choroidal atrophy, right eye**

☐ SP **H31.112 Age-related choroidal atrophy, left eye**

☐ SP **H31.113 Age-related choroidal atrophy, bilateral**

☐ IQ H31.119 Age-related choroidal atrophy, unspecified eye

⑥ H31.12 Diffuse secondary atrophy of choroid

☐ SP **H31.121 Diffuse secondary atrophy of choroid, right eye**

☐ SP **H31.122 Diffuse secondary atrophy of choroid, left eye**

☐ SP **H31.123 Diffuse secondary atrophy of choroid, bilateral**

☐ IQ H31.129 Diffuse secondary atrophy of choroid, unspecified eye

⑤ H31.2 Hereditary choroidal dystrophy
EXCLUDES 2   hyperornithinemia (E72.4) ornithinemia (E72.4)

SP **H31.20 Hereditary choroidal dystrophy, unspecified**

SP **H31.21 Choroideremia**

SP **H31.22 Choroidal dystrophy (central areolar) (generalized) (peripapillary)**

④ 4th digit required   ⑤ 5th digit required   ⑥ 6th digit required   ⑦ 7th digit required   ⑦ 7th digit placeholder   ✚ Additional code   ☐ Laterality

896   DecisionHealth's FY 2020 Complete Home Health ICD-10-CM Diagnosis Coding Manual

SP H31.23 Gyrate atrophy, choroid

SP H31.29 Other hereditary choroidal dystrophy

5 H31.3 Choroidal hemorrhage and rupture

6 H31.30 Unspecified choroidal hemorrhage

SP H31.301 Unspecified choroidal hemorrhage, right eye

SP H31.302 Unspecified choroidal hemorrhage, left eye

SP H31.303 Unspecified choroidal hemorrhage, bilateral

IQ H31.309 Unspecified choroidal hemorrhage, unspecified eye

6 H31.31 Expulsive choroidal hemorrhage

SP H31.311 Expulsive choroidal hemorrhage, right eye

SP H31.312 Expulsive choroidal hemorrhage, left eye

SP H31.313 Expulsive choroidal hemorrhage, bilateral

IQ H31.319 Expulsive choroidal hemorrhage, unspecified eye

6 H31.32 Choroidal rupture

SP H31.321 Choroidal rupture, right eye

SP H31.322 Choroidal rupture, left eye

SP H31.323 Choroidal rupture, bilateral

IQ H31.329 Choroidal rupture, unspecified eye

5 H31.4 Choroidal detachment

6 H31.40 Unspecified choroidal detachment

SP H31.401 Unspecified choroidal detachment, right eye

SP H31.402 Unspecified choroidal detachment, left eye

SP H31.403 Unspecified choroidal detachment, bilateral

IQ H31.409 Unspecified choroidal detachment, unspecified eye

6 H31.41 Hemorrhagic choroidal detachment

SP H31.411 Hemorrhagic choroidal detachment, right eye

SP H31.412 Hemorrhagic choroidal detachment, left eye

SP H31.413 Hemorrhagic choroidal detachment, bilateral

IQ H31.419 Hemorrhagic choroidal detachment, unspecified eye

6 H31.42 Serous choroidal detachment

SP H31.421 Serous choroidal detachment, right eye

SP H31.422 Serous choroidal detachment, left eye

SP H31.423 Serous choroidal detachment, bilateral

IQ H31.429 Serous choroidal detachment, unspecified eye

SP H31.8 Other specified disorders of choroid

IQ H31.9 Unspecified disorder of choroid

M IQ H32 *Chorioretinal disorders in diseases classified elsewhere*

Code first underlying disease, such as:
congenital toxoplasmosis (P37.1)
histoplasmosis (B39.-)
leprosy (A30.-)

EXCLUDES 1 chorioretinitis (in) :
toxoplasmosis (acquired) (B58.01)
tuberculosis (A18.53)

4 H33 Retinal detachments and breaks

EXCLUDES 1 detachment of retinal pigment epithelium (H35.72-, H35.73-)

DEFINITION Condition in which the retina separates from its underlying layer of cells in the back of the eye, resulting in a decrease in the visual field or blindness.

5 H33.0 Retinal detachment with retinal break
Rhegmatogenous retinal detachment

EXCLUDES 1 serous retinal detachment (without retinal break) (H33.2-)

6 H33.00 Unspecified retinal detachment with retinal break

SP H33.001 Unspecified retinal detachment with retinal break, right eye

SP H33.002 Unspecified retinal detachment with retinal break, left eye

SP H33.003 Unspecified retinal detachment with retinal break, bilateral

IQ H33.009 Unspecified retinal detachment with retinal break, unspecified eye

6 H33.01 Retinal detachment with single break

SP H33.011 Retinal detachment with single break, right eye

SP H33.012 Retinal detachment with single break, left eye

SP H33.013 Retinal detachment with single break, bilateral

IQ H33.019 Retinal detachment with single break, unspecified eye

6 H33.02 Retinal detachment with multiple breaks

SP H33.021 Retinal detachment with multiple breaks, right eye

SP H33.022 Retinal detachment with multiple breaks, left eye

SP H33.023 Retinal detachment with multiple breaks, bilateral

IQ H33.029 Retinal detachment with multiple breaks, unspecified eye

6 H33.03 Retinal detachment with giant retinal tear

SP H33.031 Retinal detachment with giant retinal tear, right eye

SP H33.032 Retinal detachment with giant retinal tear, left eye

SP H33.033 Retinal detachment with giant retinal tear, bilateral

IQ H33.039 Retinal detachment with giant retinal tear, unspecified eye

6 H33.04 Retinal detachment with retinal dialysis

★ New ▲ Revised Px Primary **SP** PDGM Px **SL** Low CoM **SH** High CoM **IQ** Quest. Encounter **H** Hospice non-cancer Dx   Unspecified   **M** *Manifestation*

DecisionHealth's FY 2020 Complete Home Health ICD-10-CM Diagnosis Coding Manual   897

☐ SP **H33.041 Retinal detachment with retinal dialysis, right eye**

☐ SP **H33.042 Retinal detachment with retinal dialysis, left eye**

☐ SP **H33.043 Retinal detachment with retinal dialysis, bilateral**

☐ IQ **H33.049 Retinal detachment with retinal dialysis, unspecified eye**

G **H33.05 Total retinal detachment**

☐ SP **H33.051 Total retinal detachment, right eye**

☐ SP **H33.052 Total retinal detachment, left eye**

☐ SP **H33.053 Total retinal detachment, bilateral**

☐ IQ **H33.059 Total retinal detachment, unspecified eye**

5 **H33.1 Retinoschisis and retinal cysts**
> EXCLUDES 1 congenital retinoschisis (Q14.1)
> microcystoid degeneration of retina (H35.42-)

G **H33.10 Unspecified retinoschisis**

☐ SP **H33.101 Unspecified retinoschisis, right eye**

☐ SP **H33.102 Unspecified retinoschisis, left eye**

☐ SP **H33.103 Unspecified retinoschisis, bilateral**

☐ IQ **H33.109 Unspecified retinoschisis, unspecified eye**

G **H33.11 Cyst of ora serrata**

☐ SP **H33.111 Cyst of ora serrata, right eye**

☐ SP **H33.112 Cyst of ora serrata, left eye**

☐ SP **H33.113 Cyst of ora serrata, bilateral**

☐ IQ **H33.119 Cyst of ora serrata, unspecified eye**

G **H33.12 Parasitic cyst of retina**

☐ SP **H33.121 Parasitic cyst of retina, right eye**

☐ SP **H33.122 Parasitic cyst of retina, left eye**

☐ SP **H33.123 Parasitic cyst of retina, bilateral**

☐ IQ **H33.129 Parasitic cyst of retina, unspecified eye**

G **H33.19 Other retinoschisis and retinal cysts**
Pseudocyst of retina

☐ SP **H33.191 Other retinoschisis and retinal cysts, right eye**

☐ SP **H33.192 Other retinoschisis and retinal cysts, left eye**

☐ SP **H33.193 Other retinoschisis and retinal cysts, bilateral**

☐ IQ **H33.199 Other retinoschisis and retinal cysts, unspecified eye**

5 **H33.2 Serous retinal detachment**
Retinal detachment NOS
Retinal detachment without retinal break
> EXCLUDES 1 central serous chorioretinopathy (H35.71-)

☐ IQ **H33.20 Serous retinal detachment, unspecified eye**

☐ SP **H33.21 Serous retinal detachment, right eye**

☐ SP **H33.22 Serous retinal detachment, left eye**

☐ SP **H33.23 Serous retinal detachment, bilateral**

5 **H33.3 Retinal breaks without detachment**
> EXCLUDES 1 chorioretinal scars after surgery for detachment (H59.81-)
> peripheral retinal degeneration without break (H35.4-)

G **H33.30 Unspecified retinal break**

☐ SP **H33.301 Unspecified retinal break, right eye**

☐ SP **H33.302 Unspecified retinal break, left eye**

☐ SP **H33.303 Unspecified retinal break, bilateral**

☐ IQ **H33.309 Unspecified retinal break, unspecified eye**

G **H33.31 Horseshoe tear of retina without detachment**
Operculum of retina without detachment

☐ SP **H33.311 Horseshoe tear of retina without detachment, right eye**

☐ SP **H33.312 Horseshoe tear of retina without detachment, left eye**

☐ SP **H33.313 Horseshoe tear of retina without detachment, bilateral**

☐ IQ **H33.319 Horseshoe tear of retina without detachment, unspecified eye**

G **H33.32 Round hole of retina without detachment**

☐ SP **H33.321 Round hole, right eye**

☐ SP **H33.322 Round hole, left eye**

☐ SP **H33.323 Round hole, bilateral**

☐ IQ **H33.329 Round hole, unspecified eye**

G **H33.33 Multiple defects of retina without detachment**

☐ SP **H33.331 Multiple defects of retina without detachment, right eye**

☐ SP **H33.332 Multiple defects of retina without detachment, left eye**

☐ SP **H33.333 Multiple defects of retina without detachment, bilateral**

☐ IQ **H33.339 Multiple defects of retina without detachment, unspecified eye**

5 **H33.4 Traction detachment of retina**
Proliferative vitreo-retinopathy with retinal detachment

☐ IQ **H33.40 Traction detachment of retina, unspecified eye**

☐ SP **H33.41 Traction detachment of retina, right eye**

☐ SP **H33.42 Traction detachment of retina, left eye**

☐ SP **H33.43 Traction detachment of retina, bilateral**

SP **H33.8 Other retinal detachments**

4 **H34 Retinal vascular occlusions**
> EXCLUDES 1 amaurosis fugax (G45.3)

5 **H34.0 Transient retinal artery occlusion**

☐ IQ **H34.00 Transient retinal artery occlusion, unspecified eye**

☐ SP **H34.01 Transient retinal artery occlusion, right eye**

☐ SP **H34.02 Transient retinal artery occlusion, left eye**

☐ SP **H34.03 Transient retinal artery occlusion, bilateral**

4 4th digit required   5 5th digit required   G 6th digit required   7 7th digit required   7 7th digit placeholder   + Additional code   ☐ Laterality

898   DecisionHealth's FY 2020 Complete Home Health ICD-10-CM Diagnosis Coding Manual

5 **H34.1 Central retinal artery occlusion**

⊟ IQ **H34.10** Central retinal artery occlusion, unspecified eye

⊟ SP **H34.11** Central retinal artery occlusion, right eye

⊟ SP **H34.12** Central retinal artery occlusion, left eye

⊟ SP **H34.13** Central retinal artery occlusion, bilateral

5 **H34.2 Other retinal artery occlusions**

6 **H34.21** Partial retinal artery occlusion
Hollenhorst's plaque
Retinal microembolism

⊟ SP **H34.211** Partial retinal artery occlusion, right eye

⊟ SP **H34.212** Partial retinal artery occlusion, left eye

⊟ SP **H34.213** Partial retinal artery occlusion, bilateral

⊟ IQ **H34.219** Partial retinal artery occlusion, unspecified eye

6 **H34.23** Retinal artery branch occlusion

⊟ SP **H34.231** Retinal artery branch occlusion, right eye

⊟ SP **H34.232** Retinal artery branch occlusion, left eye

⊟ SP **H34.233** Retinal artery branch occlusion, bilateral

⊟ IQ **H34.239** Retinal artery branch occlusion, unspecified eye

5 **H34.8 Other retinal vascular occlusions**

6 **H34.81** Central retinal vein occlusion

One of the following 7th characters is to be assigned to codes in subcategory H34.81 to designate the severity of the occlusion:
0   with macular edema
1   with retinal neovascularization
2   stable

⊟ SP 7 **H34.811-** Central retinal vein occlusion, right eye

⊟ SP 7 **H34.812-** Central retinal vein occlusion, left eye

⊟ SP 7 **H34.813-** Central retinal vein occlusion, bilateral

⊟ IQ 7 **H34.819-** Central retinal vein occlusion, unspecified eye

6 **H34.82** Venous engorgement
Incipient retinal vein occlusion
Partial retinal vein occlusion

⊟ SP **H34.821** Venous engorgement, right eye

⊟ SP **H34.822** Venous engorgement, left eye

⊟ SP **H34.823** Venous engorgement, bilateral

⊟ IQ **H34.829** Venous engorgement, unspecified eye

6 **H34.83** Tributary (branch) retinal vein occlusion

One of the following 7th characters is to be assigned to codes in subcategory H34.83 to designate the severity of the occlusion:
0   with macular edema
1   with retinal neovascularization
2   stable

⊟ SP 7 **H34.831-** Tributary (branch) retinal vein occlusion, right eye

⊟ SP 7 **H34.832-** Tributary (branch) retinal vein occlusion, left eye

⊟ SP 7 **H34.833-** Tributary (branch) retinal vein occlusion, bilateral

⊟ IQ 7 **H34.839-** Tributary (branch) retinal vein occlusion, unspecified eye

SP **H34.9** Unspecified retinal vascular occlusion

4 **H35 Other retinal disorders**
EXCLUDES 2 diabetic retinal disorders (E08.311-E08.359, E09.311-E09.359, E10.311-E10.359, E11.311-E11.359, E13.311-E13.359)

5 **H35.0 Background retinopathy and retinal vascular changes**
Code also:
any associated hypertension (I10.-)
GUIDELINES   Section I.C.9.a.5)
Subcategory H35.0, Background retinopathy and retinal vascular changes, should be used with a code from category I10-I15, Hypertensive disease to include the systemic hypertension. The sequencing is based on the reason for the encounter.

SP **H35.00** Unspecified background retinopathy

6 **H35.01** Changes in retinal vascular appearance
Retinal vascular sheathing

⊟ SP **H35.011** Changes in retinal vascular appearance, right eye

⊟ SP **H35.012** Changes in retinal vascular appearance, left eye

⊟ SP **H35.013** Changes in retinal vascular appearance, bilateral

⊟ IQ **H35.019** Changes in retinal vascular appearance, unspecified eye

6 **H35.02** Exudative retinopathy
Coats retinopathy

⊟ SP **H35.021** Exudative retinopathy, right eye

⊟ SP **H35.022** Exudative retinopathy, left eye

⊟ SP **H35.023** Exudative retinopathy, bilateral

⊟ IQ **H35.029** Exudative retinopathy, unspecified eye

6 **H35.03** Hypertensive retinopathy

⊟ SP **H35.031** Hypertensive retinopathy, right eye

⊟ SP **H35.032** Hypertensive retinopathy, left eye

⊟ SP **H35.033** Hypertensive retinopathy, bilateral

⊟ IQ **H35.039** Hypertensive retinopathy, unspecified eye

6 **H35.04** Retinal micro-aneurysms, unspecified

⊟ SP **H35.041** Retinal micro-aneurysms, unspecified, right eye

⊟ SP **H35.042** Retinal micro-aneurysms, unspecified, left eye

⊟ SP **H35.043** Retinal micro-aneurysms, unspecified, bilateral

⊟ IQ **H35.049** Retinal micro-aneurysms, unspecified, unspecified eye

Chapter 7

H00-H59

★ New ▲ Revised Px Primary SP PDGM Px SL Low CoM SH High CoM IQ Quest. Encounter H Hospice non-cancer Dx Unspecified M *Manifestation*

DecisionHealth's FY 2020 Complete Home Health ICD-10-CM Diagnosis Coding Manual

899

6 **H35.05** **Retinal neovascularization, unspecified**

SP **H35.051** **Retinal neovascularization, unspecified, right eye**

SP **H35.052** **Retinal neovascularization, unspecified, left eye**

SP **H35.053** **Retinal neovascularization, unspecified, bilateral**

!Q **H35.059** **Retinal neovascularization, unspecified, unspecified eye**

6 **H35.06** **Retinal vasculitis**
Eales disease
Retinal perivasculitis

SP **H35.061** Retinal vasculitis, right eye

SP **H35.062** Retinal vasculitis, left eye

SP **H35.063** Retinal vasculitis, bilateral

!Q **H35.069** **Retinal vasculitis, unspecified eye**

6 **H35.07** Retinal telangiectasis

SP **H35.071** Retinal telangiectasis, right eye

SP **H35.072** Retinal telangiectasis, left eye

SP **H35.073** Retinal telangiectasis, bilateral

!Q **H35.079** **Retinal telangiectasis, unspecified eye**

SP **H35.09** **Other intraretinal microvascular abnormalities**
Retinal varices

5 **H35.1 Retinopathy of prematurity**

6 **H35.10** **Retinopathy of prematurity, unspecified**
Retinopathy of prematurity NOS

SP **H35.101** **Retinopathy of prematurity, unspecified, right eye**

SP **H35.102** **Retinopathy of prematurity, unspecified, left eye**

SP **H35.103** **Retinopathy of prematurity, unspecified, bilateral**

!Q **H35.109** **Retinopathy of prematurity, unspecified, unspecified eye**

6 **H35.11** Retinopathy of prematurity, stage 0

SP **H35.111** Retinopathy of prematurity, stage 0, right eye

SP **H35.112** Retinopathy of prematurity, stage 0, left eye

SP **H35.113** Retinopathy of prematurity, stage 0, bilateral

!Q **H35.119** **Retinopathy of prematurity, stage 0, unspecified eye**

6 **H35.12** Retinopathy of prematurity, stage 1

SP **H35.121** Retinopathy of prematurity, stage 1, right eye

SP **H35.122** Retinopathy of prematurity, stage 1, left eye

SP **H35.123** Retinopathy of prematurity, stage 1, bilateral

!Q **H35.129** **Retinopathy of prematurity, stage 1, unspecified eye**

6 **H35.13** Retinopathy of prematurity, stage 2

SP **H35.131** Retinopathy of prematurity, stage 2, right eye

SP **H35.132** Retinopathy of prematurity, stage 2, left eye

SP **H35.133** Retinopathy of prematurity, stage 2, bilateral

!Q **H35.139** **Retinopathy of prematurity, stage 2, unspecified eye**

6 **H35.14** Retinopathy of prematurity, stage 3

SP **H35.141** Retinopathy of prematurity, stage 3, right eye

SP **H35.142** Retinopathy of prematurity, stage 3, left eye

SP **H35.143** Retinopathy of prematurity, stage 3, bilateral

!Q **H35.149** **Retinopathy of prematurity, stage 3, unspecified eye**

6 **H35.15** Retinopathy of prematurity, stage 4

SP **H35.151** Retinopathy of prematurity, stage 4, right eye

SP **H35.152** Retinopathy of prematurity, stage 4, left eye

SP **H35.153** Retinopathy of prematurity, stage 4, bilateral

!Q **H35.159** **Retinopathy of prematurity, stage 4, unspecified eye**

6 **H35.16** Retinopathy of prematurity, stage 5

SP **H35.161** Retinopathy of prematurity, stage 5, right eye

SP **H35.162** Retinopathy of prematurity, stage 5, left eye

SP **H35.163** Retinopathy of prematurity, stage 5, bilateral

!Q **H35.169** **Retinopathy of prematurity, stage 5, unspecified eye**

6 **H35.17** Retrolental fibroplasia

SP **H35.171** Retrolental fibroplasia, right eye

SP **H35.172** Retrolental fibroplasia, left eye

SP **H35.173** Retrolental fibroplasia, bilateral

!Q **H35.179** **Retrolental fibroplasia, unspecified eye**

5 **H35.2 Other non-diabetic proliferative retinopathy**
Proliferative vitreo-retinopathy
EXCLUDES 1 proliferative vitreo-retinopathy with retinal detachment (H33.4-)

!Q **H35.20** **Other non-diabetic proliferative retinopathy, unspecified eye**

SP **H35.21** Other non-diabetic proliferative retinopathy, right eye

SP **H35.22** Other non-diabetic proliferative retinopathy, left eye

SP **H35.23** Other non-diabetic proliferative retinopathy, bilateral

5 **H35.3 Degeneration of macula and posterior pole**

!Q **H35.30** **Unspecified macular degeneration**
Age-related macular degeneration

6 **H35.31** **Nonexudative age-related macular degeneration**
Atrophic age-related macular degeneration
Dry age-related macular degeneration

4 4th digit required   5 5th digit required   6 6th digit required   7 7th digit required   7 7th digit placeholder   + Additional code   Laterality

900   DecisionHealth's FY 2020 Complete Home Health ICD-10-CM Diagnosis Coding Manual

One of the following 7th characters is to be assigned to codes in subcategory H35.31 to designate the stage of the disease:

0	stage unspecified
1	early dry stage
2	intermediate dry stage
3	advanced atrophic without subfoveal involvement
4	advanced atrophic with subfoveal involvement

▣ **SP** 7 **H35.311-** **Nonexudative age-related macular degeneration, right eye**

▣ **SP** 7 **H35.312-** **Nonexudative age-related macular degeneration, left eye**

▣ **SP** 7 **H35.313-** **Nonexudative age-related macular degeneration, bilateral**

▣ **IQ** 7 **H35.319-** **Nonexudative age-related macular degeneration, unspecified eye**

6 **H35.32 Exudative age-related macular degeneration**
Wet age-related macular degeneration

One of the following 7th characters is to be assigned to codes in subcategory H35.32 to designate the stage of the disease:

0	stage unspecified
1	with active choroidal neovascularization
2	with inactive choroidal neovascularization
3	with inactive scar

▣ **SP** **IQ** 7 **H35.321-** **Exudative age-related macular degeneration, right eye**

▣ **SP** **IQ** 7 **H35.322-** **Exudative age-related macular degeneration, left eye**

▣ **SP** 7 **H35.323-** **Exudative age-related macular degeneration, bilateral**

▣ **IQ** 7 **H35.329-** **Exudative age-related macular degeneration, unspecified eye**

SP **H35.33 Angioid streaks of macula**

6 **H35.34 Macular cyst, hole, or pseudohole**

▣ **SP** **H35.341 Macular cyst, hole, or pseudohole, right eye**

▣ **SP** **H35.342 Macular cyst, hole, or pseudohole, left eye**

▣ **SP** **H35.343 Macular cyst, hole, or pseudohole, bilateral**

▣ **IQ** **H35.349 Macular cyst, hole, or pseudohole, unspecified eye**

6 **H35.35 Cystoid macular degeneration**
　EXCLUDES 1 cystoid macular edema following cataract surgery (H59.03-)

▣ **SP** **H35.351 Cystoid macular degeneration, right eye**

▣ **SP** **H35.352 Cystoid macular degeneration, left eye**

▣ **SP** **H35.353 Cystoid macular degeneration, bilateral**

▣ **IQ** **H35.359 Cystoid macular degeneration, unspecified eye**

6 **H35.36 Drusen (degenerative) of macula**

DEFINITION Small, bright deposits or accumulations of material seen in the retina and/or optic disc that are associated with a variety of eye diseases including macular degeneration, hereditary retinal degeneration, and loss of peripheral vision.

▣ **SP** **H35.361 Drusen (degenerative) of macula, right eye**

▣ **SP** **H35.362 Drusen (degenerative) of macula, left eye**

▣ **SP** **H35.363 Drusen (degenerative) of macula, bilateral**

▣ **IQ** **H35.369 Drusen (degenerative) of macula, unspecified eye**

6 **H35.37 Puckering of macula**

▣ **SP** **H35.371 Puckering of macula, right eye**

▣ **SP** **H35.372 Puckering of macula, left eye**

▣ **SP** **H35.373 Puckering of macula, bilateral**

▣ **IQ** **H35.379 Puckering of macula, unspecified eye**

✚ 6 **H35.38 Toxic maculopathy**
Code first:
　poisoning due to drug or toxin, if applicable
　(T36-T65 with fifth or sixth character 1-4 or 6)
Use additional code for adverse effect, if applicable, to identify drug (T36-T50 with fifth or sixth character 5)

▣ **SP** ✚ **H35.381 Toxic maculopathy, right eye**

▣ **SP** ✚ **H35.382 Toxic maculopathy, left eye**

▣ **SP** ✚ **H35.383 Toxic maculopathy, bilateral**

▣ **IQ** ✚ **H35.389 Toxic maculopathy, unspecified eye**

5 **H35.4 Peripheral retinal degeneration**
　EXCLUDES 1 hereditary retinal degeneration (dystrophy) (H35.5-)
　　peripheral retinal degeneration with retinal break (H33.3-)

IQ **H35.40 Unspecified peripheral retinal degeneration**

6 **H35.41 Lattice degeneration of retina**
Palisade degeneration of retina

▣ **SP** **H35.411 Lattice degeneration of retina, right eye**

▣ **SP** **H35.412 Lattice degeneration of retina, left eye**

▣ **SP** **H35.413 Lattice degeneration of retina, bilateral**

▣ **IQ** **H35.419 Lattice degeneration of retina, unspecified eye**

6 **H35.42 Microcystoid degeneration of retina**

▣ **SP** **H35.421 Microcystoid degeneration of retina, right eye**

▣ **SP** **H35.422 Microcystoid degeneration of retina, left eye**

▣ **SP** **H35.423 Microcystoid degeneration of retina, bilateral**

▣ **IQ** **H35.429 Microcystoid degeneration of retina, unspecified eye**

6 **H35.43 Paving stone degeneration of retina**

Chapter 7

H00-H59

★ New ▲ Revised **Px** Primary **SP** PDGM Px **SL** Low CoM **SH** High CoM **IQ** Quest. Encounter **H** Hospice non-cancer Dx 　Unspecified　 **M** *Manifestation*

⊟ SP H35.431 Paving stone degeneration of retina, right eye

⊟ SP H35.432 Paving stone degeneration of retina, left eye

⊟ SP H35.433 Paving stone degeneration of retina, bilateral

⊟ IQ H35.439 Paving stone degeneration of retina, unspecified eye

⑥ H35.44 Age-related reticular degeneration of retina

⊟ SP H35.441 Age-related reticular degeneration of retina, right eye

⊟ SP H35.442 Age-related reticular degeneration of retina, left eye

⊟ SP H35.443 Age-related reticular degeneration of retina, bilateral

⊟ IQ H35.449 Age-related reticular degeneration of retina, unspecified eye

⑥ H35.45 Secondary pigmentary degeneration

⊟ SP H35.451 Secondary pigmentary degeneration, right eye

⊟ SP H35.452 Secondary pigmentary degeneration, left eye

⊟ SP H35.453 Secondary pigmentary degeneration, bilateral

⊟ IQ H35.459 Secondary pigmentary degeneration, unspecified eye

⑥ H35.46 Secondary vitreoretinal degeneration

⊟ SP H35.461 Secondary vitreoretinal degeneration, right eye

⊟ SP H35.462 Secondary vitreoretinal degeneration, left eye

⊟ SP H35.463 Secondary vitreoretinal degeneration, bilateral

⊟ IQ H35.469 Secondary vitreoretinal degeneration, unspecified eye

⑤ H35.5 Hereditary retinal dystrophy

> **EXCLUDES 1** dystrophies primarily involving Bruch's membrane (H31.1-)

SP H35.50 Unspecified hereditary retinal dystrophy

SP H35.51 Vitreoretinal dystrophy

SP H35.52 Pigmentary retinal dystrophy
Albipunctate retinal dystrophy
Retinitis pigmentosa
Tapetoretinal dystrophy

SP H35.53 Other dystrophies primarily involving the sensory retina
Stargardt's disease

> **DEFINITION** Stargardt's disease: genetic condition causing degeneration of the macula, occurring by age 20, with rapid loss of visual acuity and abnormal pigmentation of the macula.

SP H35.54 Dystrophies primarily involving the retinal pigment epithelium
Vitelliform retinal dystrophy

⑤ H35.6 Retinal hemorrhage

⊟ IQ H35.60 Retinal hemorrhage, unspecified eye

⊟ SP H35.61 Retinal hemorrhage, right eye

⊟ SP H35.62 Retinal hemorrhage, left eye

⊟ SP H35.63 Retinal hemorrhage, bilateral

⑤ H35.7 Separation of retinal layers

> **EXCLUDES 1** retinal detachment (serous) (H33.2-)
> rhegmatogenous retinal detachment (H33.0-)

IQ H35.70 Unspecified separation of retinal layers

⑥ H35.71 Central serous chorioretinopathy

> **DEFINITION** Fluid seepage from the choroid into the retina, causing the retinal layers to fill and separate from each other.

⊟ SP H35.711 Central serous chorioretinopathy, right eye

⊟ SP H35.712 Central serous chorioretinopathy, left eye

⊟ SP H35.713 Central serous chorioretinopathy, bilateral

⊟ IQ H35.719 Central serous chorioretinopathy, unspecified eye

⑥ H35.72 Serous detachment of retinal pigment epithelium

⊟ SP H35.721 Serous detachment of retinal pigment epithelium, right eye

⊟ SP H35.722 Serous detachment of retinal pigment epithelium, left eye

⊟ SP H35.723 Serous detachment of retinal pigment epithelium, bilateral

⊟ IQ H35.729 Serous detachment of retinal pigment epithelium, unspecified eye

⑥ H35.73 Hemorrhagic detachment of retinal pigment epithelium

⊟ SP H35.731 Hemorrhagic detachment of retinal pigment epithelium, right eye

⊟ SP H35.732 Hemorrhagic detachment of retinal pigment epithelium, left eye

⊟ SP H35.733 Hemorrhagic detachment of retinal pigment epithelium, bilateral

⊟ IQ H35.739 Hemorrhagic detachment of retinal pigment epithelium, unspecified eye

⑤ H35.8 Other specified retinal disorders

> **EXCLUDES 2** retinal hemorrhage (H35.6-)

SP H35.81 Retinal edema
Retinal cotton wool spots

SP H35.82 Retinal ischemia

SP H35.89 Other specified retinal disorders

IQ H35.9 Unspecified retinal disorder

M IQ H36 *Retinal disorders in diseases classified elsewhere*

Code first underlying disease, such as:
lipid storage disorders (E75.-)
sickle-cell disorders (D57.-)

> **EXCLUDES 1** arteriosclerotic retinopathy (H35.0-)
> diabetic retinopathy (E08.3-, E09.3-, E10.3-, E11.3-, E13.3-)

Chapter 7 · **H00-H59**

❹ 4th digit required   ❺ 5th digit required   ❻ 6th digit required   ❼ 7th digit required   ⑦ 7th digit placeholder   ✚ Additional code   ⊟ Laterality

902   *DecisionHealth's* FY 2020 Complete Home Health ICD-10-CM Diagnosis Coding Manual

Glaucoma (H40-H42)

Glaucoma

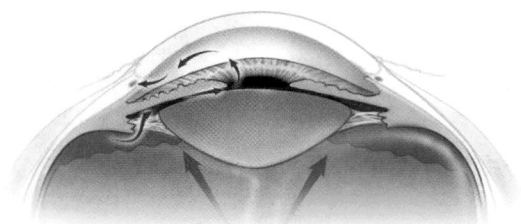

4 H40   Glaucoma

EXCLUDES 1   absolute glaucoma (H44.51-)
congenital glaucoma (Q15.0)
traumatic glaucoma due to birth
injury (P15.3)

GUIDELINES   Section I.C.7.a.1)
Assign as many codes from category H40,
Glaucoma, as needed to identify the type of
glaucoma, the affected eye, and the glaucoma
stage.

GUIDELINES   Section I.C.7.a.2)-3)
When a patient has bilateral glaucoma and
both eyes are documented as being the same
type and stage, and there is a code for bilateral
glaucoma, report only the code for the type of
glaucoma, bilateral, with the seventh character
for the stage.

When a patient has bilateral glaucoma and
each eye is documented as having a different
type or stage, and the classification
distinguishes laterality, assign the appropriate
code for each eye rather than the code for
bilateral glaucoma.

5 H40.0 Glaucoma suspect

DEFINITION   Increase in intraocular
pressure causing pathologic changes in the
optic disk and defects in the field of vision.

6 H40.00   Preglaucoma, unspecified

**SP H40.001   Preglaucoma, unspecified, right
eye**

**SP H40.002   Preglaucoma, unspecified, left
eye**

**SP H40.003   Preglaucoma, unspecified,
bilateral**

**IQ H40.009   Preglaucoma, unspecified,
unspecified eye**

**6 H40.01   Open angle with borderline findings,
low risk**
Open angle, low risk

**SP H40.011   Open angle with borderline
findings, low risk, right eye**

**SP H40.012   Open angle with borderline
findings, low risk, left eye**

**SP H40.013   Open angle with borderline
findings, low risk, bilateral**

**IQ H40.019   Open angle with borderline
findings, low risk, unspecified eye**

**6 H40.02   Open angle with borderline findings,
high risk**
Open angle, high risk

**SP H40.021   Open angle with borderline
findings, high risk, right eye**

**SP H40.022   Open angle with borderline
findings, high risk, left eye**

**SP H40.023   Open angle with borderline
findings, high risk, bilateral**

**IQ H40.029   Open angle with borderline
findings, high risk, unspecified
eye**

6 H40.03   Anatomical narrow angle
Primary angle closure suspect

**SP H40.031   Anatomical narrow angle, right
eye**

SP H40.032   Anatomical narrow angle, left eye

**SP H40.033   Anatomical narrow angle,
bilateral**

**IQ H40.039   Anatomical narrow angle,
unspecified eye**

6 H40.04   Steroid responder

SP H40.041   Steroid responder, right eye

SP H40.042   Steroid responder, left eye

SP H40.043   Steroid responder, bilateral

**IQ H40.049   Steroid responder, unspecified
eye**

6 H40.05   Ocular hypertension

SP H40.051   Ocular hypertension, right eye

SP H40.052   Ocular hypertension, left eye

SP H40.053   Ocular hypertension, bilateral

**IQ H40.059   Ocular hypertension, unspecified
eye**

**6 H40.06   Primary angle closure without
glaucoma damage**

**SP H40.061   Primary angle closure without
glaucoma damage, right eye**

**SP H40.062   Primary angle closure without
glaucoma damage, left eye**

**SP H40.063   Primary angle closure without
glaucoma damage, bilateral**

**IQ H40.069   Primary angle closure without
glaucoma damage, unspecified
eye**

5 H40.1 Open-angle glaucoma

SP 7 H40.10X-   Unspecified open-angle glaucoma

One of the following 7th characters
is to be assigned to code H40.10 to
designate the stage of glaucoma
0   stage unspecified
1   mild stage
2   moderate stage
3   severe stage
4   indeterminate stage

6 H40.11   Primary open-angle glaucoma
Chronic simple glaucoma

★ New ▲ Revised Px Primary SP PDGM Px SL Low CoM SH High CoM IQ Quest. Encounter H Hospice non-cancer Dx   Unspecified   M Manifestation

DecisionHealth's FY 2020 Complete Home Health ICD-10-CM Diagnosis Coding Manual

903

Chapter 7

H00-H59

One of the following 7th characters is to be assigned to each code in subcategory H40.11 to designate the stage of glaucoma
0   stage unspecified
1   mild stage
2   moderate stage
3   severe stage
4   indeterminate stage

☐ **SP** **7** **H40.111-** **Primary open-angle glaucoma, right eye**

☐ **SP** **7** **H40.112-** **Primary open-angle glaucoma, left eye**

☐ **SP** **7** **H40.113-** **Primary open-angle glaucoma, bilateral**

☐ **IQ** **7** **H40.119-** **Primary open-angle glaucoma, unspecified eye**

6 **H40.12** **Low-tension glaucoma**

One of the following 7th characters is to be assigned to each code in subcategory H40.12 to designate the stage of glaucoma
0   stage unspecified
1   mild stage
2   moderate stage
3   severe stage
4   indeterminate stage

☐ **SP** **7** **H40.121-** **Low-tension glaucoma, right eye**

☐ **SP** **7** **H40.122-** **Low-tension glaucoma, left eye**

☐ **SP** **7** **H40.123-** **Low-tension glaucoma, bilateral**

☐ **IQ** **7** **H40.129-** **Low-tension glaucoma, unspecified eye**

6 **H40.13** **Pigmentary glaucoma**

One of the following 7th characters is to be assigned to each code in subcategory H40.13 to designate the stage of glaucoma
0   stage unspecified
1   mild stage
2   moderate stage
3   severe stage
4   indeterminate stage

DEFINITION Granules of pigment coloring the eye break off and block drainage canals, increasing intraocular pressure.

☐ **SP** **7** **H40.131-** **Pigmentary glaucoma, right eye**

☐ **SP** **7** **H40.132-** **Pigmentary glaucoma, left eye**

☐ **SP** **7** **H40.133-** **Pigmentary glaucoma, bilateral**

☐ **IQ** **7** **H40.139-** **Pigmentary glaucoma, unspecified eye**

6 **H40.14** **Capsular glaucoma with pseudoexfoliation of lens**

One of the following 7th characters is to be assigned to each code in subcategory H40.14 to designate the stage of glaucoma
0   stage unspecified
1   mild stage
2   moderate stage
3   severe stage
4   indeterminate stage

☐ **SP** **7** **H40.141-** **Capsular glaucoma with pseudoexfoliation of lens, right eye**

☐ **SP** **7** **H40.142-** **Capsular glaucoma with pseudoexfoliation of lens, left eye**

☐ **SP** **7** **H40.143-** **Capsular glaucoma with pseudoexfoliation of lens, bilateral**

☐ **IQ** **7** **H40.149-** **Capsular glaucoma with pseudoexfoliation of lens, unspecified eye**

6 **H40.15** **Residual stage of open-angle glaucoma**

☐ **SP** **H40.151** **Residual stage of open-angle glaucoma, right eye**

☐ **SP** **H40.152** **Residual stage of open-angle glaucoma, left eye**

☐ **SP** **H40.153** **Residual stage of open-angle glaucoma, bilateral**

☐ **IQ** **H40.159** **Residual stage of open-angle glaucoma, unspecified eye**

5 **H40.2** **Primary angle-closure glaucoma**
 EXCLUDES 1 aqueous misdirection (H40.83-)
 malignant glaucoma (H40.83-)

SP **7** **H40.20X-** **Unspecified primary angle-closure glaucoma**

One of the following 7th characters is to be assigned to code H40.20 to designate the stage of glaucoma
0   stage unspecified
1   mild stage
2   moderate stage
3   severe stage
4   indeterminate stage

6 **H40.21** **Acute angle-closure glaucoma**
Acute angle-closure glaucoma attack
Acute angle-closure glaucoma crisis
 DEFINITION Severe, sudden increase in intraocular pressure due to a blockage of the chamber angle at the junction of the iris and cornea, preventing normal aqueous fluid drainage and causing rapid loss of vision.

☐ **SP** **H40.211** **Acute angle-closure glaucoma, right eye**

☐ **SP** **H40.212** **Acute angle-closure glaucoma, left eye**

☐ **SP** **H40.213** **Acute angle-closure glaucoma, bilateral**

☐ **IQ** **H40.219** **Acute angle-closure glaucoma, unspecified eye**

6 **H40.22** **Chronic angle-closure glaucoma**

4 4th digit required   **5** 5th digit required   **6** 6th digit required   **7** 7th digit required   **7** 7th digit placeholder   **+** Additional code   ☐ Laterality

904   *DecisionHealth's* FY 2020 Complete Home Health ICD-10-CM Diagnosis Coding Manual

Chronic primary angle closure glaucoma

One of the following 7th characters is to be assigned to each code in subcategory H40.22 to designate the stage of glaucoma
0   stage unspecified
1   mild stage
2   moderate stage
3   severe stage
4   indeterminate stage

☰ SP 7 **H40.221-** **Chronic angle-closure glaucoma, right eye**

☰ SP 7 **H40.222-** **Chronic angle-closure glaucoma, left eye**

☰ SP 7 **H40.223-** **Chronic angle-closure glaucoma, bilateral**

☰ IQ 7 **H40.229-** **Chronic angle-closure glaucoma, unspecified eye**

6 **H40.23** **Intermittent angle-closure glaucoma**

☰ SP **H40.231** **Intermittent angle-closure glaucoma, right eye**

☰ SP **H40.232** **Intermittent angle-closure glaucoma, left eye**

☰ SP **H40.233** **Intermittent angle-closure glaucoma, bilateral**

☰ IQ **H40.239** **Intermittent angle-closure glaucoma, unspecified eye**

6 **H40.24** **Residual stage of angle-closure glaucoma**

☰ SP **H40.241** **Residual stage of angle-closure glaucoma, right eye**

☰ SP **H40.242** **Residual stage of angle-closure glaucoma, left eye**

☰ SP **H40.243** **Residual stage of angle-closure glaucoma, bilateral**

☰ IQ **H40.249** **Residual stage of angle-closure glaucoma, unspecified eye**

5 **H40.3** **Glaucoma secondary to eye trauma**
Code also:
    underlying condition

One of the following 7th characters is to be assigned to each code in subcategory H40.3 to designate the stage of glaucoma
0   stage unspecified
1   mild stage
2   moderate stage
3   severe stage
4   indeterminate stage

☰ IQ 7 **H40.30X-** **Glaucoma secondary to eye trauma, unspecified eye**

☰ SP 7 **H40.31X-** **Glaucoma secondary to eye trauma, right eye**

☰ SP 7 **H40.32X-** **Glaucoma secondary to eye trauma, left eye**

☰ SP 7 **H40.33X-** **Glaucoma secondary to eye trauma, bilateral**

5 **H40.4** **Glaucoma secondary to eye inflammation**
Code also:
    underlying condition

One of the following 7th characters is to be assigned to each code in subcategory H40.4 to designate the stage of glaucoma
0   stage unspecified
1   mild stage
2   moderate stage
3   severe stage
4   indeterminate stage

☰ IQ 7 **H40.40X-** **Glaucoma secondary to eye inflammation, unspecified eye**

☰ SP 7 **H40.41X-** **Glaucoma secondary to eye inflammation, right eye**

☰ SP 7 **H40.42X-** **Glaucoma secondary to eye inflammation, left eye**

☰ SP 7 **H40.43X-** **Glaucoma secondary to eye inflammation, bilateral**

5 **H40.5** **Glaucoma secondary to other eye disorders**
Code also:
    underlying eye disorder

One of the following 7th characters is to be assigned to each code in subcategory H40.5 to designate the stage of glaucoma
0   stage unspecified
1   mild stage
2   moderate stage
3   severe stage
4   indeterminate stage

☰ IQ 7 **H40.50X-** **Glaucoma secondary to other eye disorders, unspecified eye**

☰ SP 7 **H40.51X-** **Glaucoma secondary to other eye disorders, right eye**

☰ SP 7 **H40.52X-** **Glaucoma secondary to other eye disorders, left eye**

☰ SP 7 **H40.53X-** **Glaucoma secondary to other eye disorders, bilateral**

✚ 5 **H40.6** **Glaucoma secondary to drugs**
Use additional code for adverse effect, if applicable, to identify drug (T36-T50 with fifth or sixth character 5)

One of the following 7th characters is to be assigned to each code in subcategory H40.6 to designate the stage of glaucoma
0   stage unspecified
1   mild stage
2   moderate stage
3   severe stage
4   indeterminate stage

☰ IQ ✚ 7 **H40.60X-** **Glaucoma secondary to drugs, unspecified eye**

☰ SP ✚ 7 **H40.61X-** **Glaucoma secondary to drugs, right eye**

☰ SP ✚ 7 **H40.62X-** **Glaucoma secondary to drugs, left eye**

☰ SP ✚ 7 **H40.63X-** **Glaucoma secondary to drugs, bilateral**

5 **H40.8** **Other glaucoma**

6 **H40.81** **Glaucoma with increased episcleral venous pressure**
DEFINITION Blood pressure of the veins in the white of the eye increases as the pressure of intraocular fluid increases.

★ New ▲ Revised Px Primary SP PDGM Px SL Low CoM SH High CoM IQ Quest. Encounter H Hospice non-cancer Dx Unspecified M *Manifestation*

DecisionHealth's FY 2020 Complete Home Health ICD-10-CM Diagnosis Coding Manual

905

Chapter 7

H00-H59

Chapter 7

H00-H59

⊟ **SP** **H40.811** Glaucoma with increased episcleral venous pressure, right eye

⊟ **SP** **H40.812** Glaucoma with increased episcleral venous pressure, left eye

⊟ **SP** **H40.813** Glaucoma with increased episcleral venous pressure, bilateral

⊟ **IQ** **H40.819** Glaucoma with increased episcleral venous pressure, unspecified eye

⑥ **H40.82** Hypersecretion glaucoma

> **DEFINITION** Overproduction of ocular fluid rather than insufficient drainage that causes increased intraocular pressure.

⊟ **SP** **H40.821** Hypersecretion glaucoma, right eye

⊟ **SP** **H40.822** Hypersecretion glaucoma, left eye

⊟ **SP** **H40.823** Hypersecretion glaucoma, bilateral

⊟ **IQ** **H40.829** Hypersecretion glaucoma, unspecified eye

⑥ **H40.83** Aqueous misdirection
Malignant glaucoma

⊟ **SP** **H40.831** Aqueous misdirection, right eye

⊟ **SP** **H40.832** Aqueous misdirection, left eye

⊟ **SP** **H40.833** Aqueous misdirection, bilateral

⊟ **IQ** **H40.839** Aqueous misdirection, unspecified eye

SP **H40.89** Other specified glaucoma

SP **H40.9** Unspecified glaucoma

M **IQ** **H42** *Glaucoma in diseases classified elsewhere*

Code first underlying condition, such as:
amyloidosis (E85.-)
aniridia (Q13.1)
glaucoma (in) diabetes mellitus (E08.39, E09.39, E10.39, E11.39, E13.39)
Lowe's syndrome (E72.03)
Reiger's anomaly (Q13.81)
specified metabolic disorder (E70-E88)

> **EXCLUDES 1** glaucoma (in) onchocerciasis (B73.02)
> glaucoma (in) syphilis (A52.71)
> glaucoma (in) tuberculous (A18.59)

Disorders of vitreous body and globe (H43-H44)

④ **H43** Disorders of vitreous body

⑤ **H43.0** Vitreous prolapse

> **EXCLUDES 1** vitreous syndrome following cataract surgery (H59.0-)
> traumatic vitreous prolapse (S05.2-)

⊟ **IQ** **H43.00** Vitreous prolapse, unspecified eye

⊟ **SP** **H43.01** Vitreous prolapse, right eye

⊟ **SP** **H43.02** Vitreous prolapse, left eye

⊟ **SP** **H43.03** Vitreous prolapse, bilateral

⑤ **H43.1** Vitreous hemorrhage

⊟ **IQ** **H43.10** Vitreous hemorrhage, unspecified eye

⊟ **SP** **H43.11** Vitreous hemorrhage, right eye

⊟ **SP** **H43.12** Vitreous hemorrhage, left eye

⊟ **SP** **H43.13** Vitreous hemorrhage, bilateral

⑤ **H43.2** Crystalline deposits in vitreous body

⊟ **IQ** **H43.20** Crystalline deposits in vitreous body, unspecified eye

⊟ **SP** **H43.21** Crystalline deposits in vitreous body, right eye

⊟ **SP** **H43.22** Crystalline deposits in vitreous body, left eye

⊟ **SP** **H43.23** Crystalline deposits in vitreous body, bilateral

⑤ **H43.3** Other vitreous opacities

⑥ **H43.31** Vitreous membranes and strands

⊟ **SP** **H43.311** Vitreous membranes and strands, right eye

⊟ **SP** **H43.312** Vitreous membranes and strands, left eye

⊟ **SP** **H43.313** Vitreous membranes and strands, bilateral

⊟ **IQ** **H43.319** Vitreous membranes and strands, unspecified eye

⑥ **H43.39** Other vitreous opacities
Vitreous floaters

⊟ **SP** **H43.391** Other vitreous opacities, right eye

⊟ **SP** **H43.392** Other vitreous opacities, left eye

⊟ **SP** **H43.393** Other vitreous opacities, bilateral

⊟ **IQ** **H43.399** Other vitreous opacities, unspecified eye

⑤ **H43.8** Other disorders of vitreous body

> **EXCLUDES 1** proliferative vitreo-retinopathy with retinal detachment (H33.4-)
> **EXCLUDES 2** vitreous abscess (H44.02-)

⑥ **H43.81** Vitreous degeneration
Vitreous detachment

⊟ **SP** **H43.811** Vitreous degeneration, right eye

⊟ **SP** **H43.812** Vitreous degeneration, left eye

⊟ **SP** **H43.813** Vitreous degeneration, bilateral

⊟ **IQ** **H43.819** Vitreous degeneration, unspecified eye

⑥ **H43.82** Vitreomacular adhesion
Vitreomacular traction

⊟ **SP** **H43.821** Vitreomacular adhesion, right eye

⊟ **SP** **H43.822** Vitreomacular adhesion, left eye

⊟ **SP** **H43.823** Vitreomacular adhesion, bilateral

⊟ **IQ** **H43.829** Vitreomacular adhesion, unspecified eye

SP **H43.89** Other disorders of vitreous body

IQ **H43.9** Unspecified disorder of vitreous body

---

④4th digit required   ⑤5th digit required   ⑥6th digit required   ⑦7th digit required   ⑦7th digit placeholder   ✚Additional code   ⊟Laterality

906   *DecisionHealth's* FY 2020 Complete Home Health ICD-10-CM Diagnosis Coding Manual

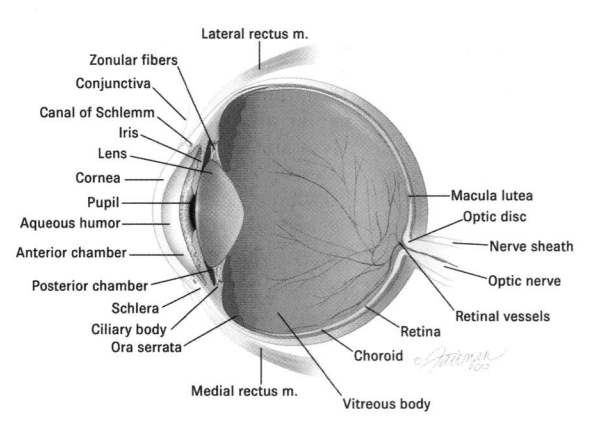

Lateral rectus m.
Zonular fibers
Conjunctiva
Canal of Schlemm
Iris
Lens
Cornea
Pupil
Aqueous humor
Anterior chamber
Posterior chamber
Schlera
Ciliary body
Ora serrata
Medial rectus m.
Vitreous body
Macula lutea
Optic disc
Nerve sheath
Optic nerve
Retinal vessels
Retina
Choroid

4 H44 Disorders of globe

INCLUDES disorders affecting multiple structures of eye

+ 5 H44.0 Purulent endophthalmitis
Use additional code to identify organism

EXCLUDES 1 bleb associated endophthalmitis (H59.4-)

+ 6 H44.00 Unspecified purulent endophthalmitis

▣ **SP + H44.001 Unspecified purulent endophthalmitis, right eye**

▣ **SP + H44.002 Unspecified purulent endophthalmitis, left eye**

▣ **SP + H44.003 Unspecified purulent endophthalmitis, bilateral**

▣ **IQ + H44.009 Unspecified purulent endophthalmitis, unspecified eye**

+ 6 H44.01 Panophthalmitis (acute)

DEFINITION Inflammation affecting all the structures or tissues of the eye.

▣ **SP + H44.011 Panophthalmitis (acute), right eye**

▣ **SP + H44.012 Panophthalmitis (acute), left eye**

▣ **SP + H44.013 Panophthalmitis (acute), bilateral**

▣ **IQ + H44.019 Panophthalmitis (acute), unspecified eye**

+ 6 H44.02 Vitreous abscess (chronic)

▣ **SP + H44.021 Vitreous abscess (chronic), right eye**

▣ **SP + H44.022 Vitreous abscess (chronic), left eye**

▣ **SP + H44.023 Vitreous abscess (chronic), bilateral**

▣ **IQ + H44.029 Vitreous abscess (chronic), unspecified eye**

5 H44.1 Other endophthalmitis

EXCLUDES 1 bleb associated endophthalmitis (H59.4-)

EXCLUDES 2 ophthalmia nodosa (H16.2-)

6 H44.11 Panuveitis

DEFINITION Inflammation of the entire pigmented layer of the eye (uveal tract).

▣ **SP H44.111 Panuveitis, right eye**

▣ **SP H44.112 Panuveitis, left eye**

▣ **SP H44.113 Panuveitis, bilateral**

▣ **IQ H44.119 Panuveitis, unspecified eye**

6 H44.12 Parasitic endophthalmitis, unspecified

▣ **SP H44.121 Parasitic endophthalmitis, unspecified, right eye**

▣ **SP H44.122 Parasitic endophthalmitis, unspecified, left eye**

▣ **SP H44.123 Parasitic endophthalmitis, unspecified, bilateral**

▣ **IQ H44.129 Parasitic endophthalmitis, unspecified, unspecified eye**

6 H44.13 Sympathetic uveitis

▣ **SP H44.131 Sympathetic uveitis, right eye**

▣ **SP H44.132 Sympathetic uveitis, left eye**

▣ **SP H44.133 Sympathetic uveitis, bilateral**

▣ **IQ H44.139 Sympathetic uveitis, unspecified eye**

SP H44.19 Other endophthalmitis

5 H44.2 Degenerative myopia
Malignant myopia

▣ **IQ H44.20 Degenerative myopia, unspecified eye**

▣ **SP H44.21 Degenerative myopia, right eye**

▣ **SP H44.22 Degenerative myopia, left eye**

▣ **SP H44.23 Degenerative myopia, bilateral**

+ 6 H44.2A Degenerative myopia with choroidal neovascularization
Use additional code for any associated choroid disorders (H31.-)

▣ **SP + H44.2A1 Degenerative myopia with choroidal neovascularization, right eye**

▣ **SP + H44.2A2 Degenerative myopia with choroidal neovascularization, left eye**

▣ **SP + H44.2A3 Degenerative myopia with choroidal neovascularization, bilateral eye**

▣ **IQ + H44.2A9 Degenerative myopia with choroidal neovascularization, unspecified eye**

6 H44.2B Degenerative myopia with macular hole

▣ **SP H44.2B1 Degenerative myopia with macular hole, right eye**

▣ **SP H44.2B2 Degenerative myopia with macular hole, left eye**

▣ **SP H44.2B3 Degenerative myopia with macular hole, bilateral eye**

▣ **IQ H44.2B9 Degenerative myopia with macular hole, unspecified eye**

+ 6 H44.2C Degenerative myopia with retinal detachment
Use additional code to identify the retinal detachment (H33.-)

▣ **SP + H44.2C1 Degenerative myopia with retinal detachment, right eye**

▣ **SP + H44.2C2 Degenerative myopia with retinal detachment, left eye**

▣ **SP + H44.2C3 Degenerative myopia with retinal detachment, bilateral eye**

▣ **IQ + H44.2C9 Degenerative myopia with retinal detachment, unspecified eye**

6 H44.2D Degenerative myopia with foveoschisis

Chapter 7

H00-H59

★ New ▲ Revised Px Primary **SP** PDGM Px **SL** Low CoM **SH** High CoM **IQ** Quest. Encounter **H** Hospice non-cancer Dx Unspecified **M** *Manifestation*

DecisionHealth's FY 2020 Complete Home Health ICD-10-CM Diagnosis Coding Manual

907

▣ **SP** **H44.2D1** Degenerative myopia with foveoschisis, right eye

▣ **SP** **H44.2D2** Degenerative myopia with foveoschisis, left eye

▣ **SP** **H44.2D3** Degenerative myopia with foveoschisis, bilateral eye

▣ **IQ** **H44.2D9** Degenerative myopia with foveoschisis, unspecified eye

⑥ **H44.2E** Degenerative myopia with other maculopathy

▣ **SP** **H44.2E1** Degenerative myopia with other maculopathy, right eye

▣ **SP** **H44.2E2** Degenerative myopia with other maculopathy, left eye

▣ **SP** **H44.2E3** Degenerative myopia with other maculopathy, bilateral eye

▣ **IQ** **H44.2E9** Degenerative myopia with other maculopathy, unspecified eye

⑤ **H44.3** Other and unspecified degenerative disorders of globe

IQ **H44.30** Unspecified degenerative disorder of globe

⑥ **H44.31** Chalcosis

▣ **SP** **H44.311** Chalcosis, right eye

▣ **SP** **H44.312** Chalcosis, left eye

▣ **SP** **H44.313** Chalcosis, bilateral

▣ **IQ** **H44.319** Chalcosis, unspecified eye

⑥ **H44.32** Siderosis of eye

▣ **SP** **H44.321** Siderosis of eye, right eye

▣ **SP** **H44.322** Siderosis of eye, left eye.

▣ **SP** **H44.323** Siderosis of eye, bilateral

▣ **IQ** **H44.329** Siderosis of eye, unspecified eye

⑥ **H44.39** Other degenerative disorders of globe

▣ **SP** **H44.391** Other degenerative disorders of globe, right eye

▣ **SP** **H44.392** Other degenerative disorders of globe, left eye

▣ **SP** **H44.393** Other degenerative disorders of globe, bilateral

▣ **IQ** **H44.399** Other degenerative disorders of globe, unspecified eye

⑤ **H44.4** Hypotony of eye

SP **H44.40** Unspecified hypotony of eye

⑥ **H44.41** Flat anterior chamber hypotony of eye

▣ **SP** **H44.411** Flat anterior chamber hypotony of right eye

▣ **SP** **H44.412** Flat anterior chamber hypotony of left eye

▣ **SP** **H44.413** Flat anterior chamber hypotony of eye, bilateral

▣ **IQ** **H44.419** Flat anterior chamber hypotony of unspecified eye

⑥ **H44.42** Hypotony of eye due to ocular fistula

▣ **SP** **H44.421** Hypotony of right eye due to ocular fistula

▣ **SP** **H44.422** Hypotony of left eye due to ocular fistula

▣ **SP** **H44.423** Hypotony of eye due to ocular fistula, bilateral

▣ **IQ** **H44.429** Hypotony of unspecified eye due to ocular fistula

⑥ **H44.43** Hypotony of eye due to other ocular disorders

▣ **SP** **H44.431** Hypotony of eye due to other ocular disorders, right eye

▣ **SP** **H44.432** Hypotony of eye due to other ocular disorders, left eye

▣ **SP** **H44.433** Hypotony of eye due to other ocular disorders, bilateral

▣ **IQ** **H44.439** Hypotony of eye due to other ocular disorders, unspecified eye

⑥ **H44.44** Primary hypotony of eye

▣ **SP** **H44.441** Primary hypotony of right eye

▣ **SP** **H44.442** Primary hypotony of left eye

▣ **SP** **H44.443** Primary hypotony of eye, bilateral

▣ **IQ** **H44.449** Primary hypotony of unspecified eye

⑤ **H44.5** Degenerated conditions of globe

IQ **H44.50** Unspecified degenerated conditions of globe

⑥ **H44.51** Absolute glaucoma

▣ **SP** **H44.511** Absolute glaucoma, right eye

▣ **SP** **H44.512** Absolute glaucoma, left eye

▣ **SP** **H44.513** Absolute glaucoma, bilateral

▣ **IQ** **H44.519** Absolute glaucoma, unspecified eye

⑥ **H44.52** Atrophy of globe
Phthisis bulbi

▣ **SP** **H44.521** Atrophy of globe, right eye

▣ **SP** **H44.522** Atrophy of globe, left eye

▣ **SP** **H44.523** Atrophy of globe, bilateral

▣ **IQ** **H44.529** Atrophy of globe, unspecified eye

⑥ **H44.53** Leucocoria

▣ **SP** **H44.531** Leucocoria, right eye

▣ **SP** **H44.532** Leucocoria, left eye

▣ **SP** **H44.533** Leucocoria, bilateral

▣ **IQ** **H44.539** Leucocoria, unspecified eye

✚ ⑤ **H44.6** Retained (old) intraocular foreign body, magnetic
Use additional code to identify magnetic foreign body (Z18.11)

> **EXCLUDES 1** current intraocular foreign body (S05.-)
> **EXCLUDES 2** retained foreign body in eyelid (H02.81-)
> retained (old) foreign body following penetrating wound of orbit (H05.5-)
> retained (old) intraocular foreign body, nonmagnetic (H44.7-)

✚ ⑥ **H44.60** Unspecified retained (old) intraocular foreign body, magnetic

▣ **SP** ✚ **H44.601** Unspecified retained (old) intraocular foreign body, magnetic, right eye

▣ **SP** ✚ **H44.602** Unspecified retained (old) intraocular foreign body, magnetic, left eye

▣ **SP** ✚ **H44.603** Unspecified retained (old) intraocular foreign body, magnetic, bilateral

④ 4th digit required   ⑤ 5th digit required   ⑥ 6th digit required   ⑦ 7th digit required   ⑦ 7th digit placeholder   ✚ Additional code   ▣ Laterality

908   *DecisionHealth's* FY 2020 Complete Home Health ICD-10-CM Diagnosis Coding Manual

▤ **IQ** ✛ **H44.609** Unspecified retained (old) intraocular foreign body, magnetic, unspecified eye

✛ ⑥ **H44.61** Retained (old) magnetic foreign body in anterior chamber

▤ **SP** ✛ **H44.611** Retained (old) magnetic foreign body in anterior chamber, right eye

▤ **SP** ✛ **H44.612** Retained (old) magnetic foreign body in anterior chamber, left eye

▤ **SP** ✛ **H44.613** Retained (old) magnetic foreign body in anterior chamber, bilateral

▤ **IQ** ✛ **H44.619** Retained (old) magnetic foreign body in anterior chamber, unspecified eye

✛ ⑥ **H44.62** Retained (old) magnetic foreign body in iris or ciliary body

▤ **SP** ✛ **H44.621** Retained (old) magnetic foreign body in iris or ciliary body, right eye

▤ **SP** ✛ **H44.622** Retained (old) magnetic foreign body in iris or ciliary body, left eye

▤ **SP** ✛ **H44.623** Retained (old) magnetic foreign body in iris or ciliary body, bilateral

▤ **IQ** ✛ **H44.629** Retained (old) magnetic foreign body in iris or ciliary body, unspecified eye

✛ ⑥ **H44.63** Retained (old) magnetic foreign body in lens

▤ **SP** ✛ **H44.631** Retained (old) magnetic foreign body in lens, right eye

▤ **SP** ✛ **H44.632** Retained (old) magnetic foreign body in lens, left eye

▤ **SP** ✛ **H44.633** Retained (old) magnetic foreign body in lens, bilateral

▤ **IQ** ✛ **H44.639** Retained (old) magnetic foreign body in lens, unspecified eye

✛ ⑥ **H44.64** Retained (old) magnetic foreign body in posterior wall of globe

▤ **SP** ✛ **H44.641** Retained (old) magnetic foreign body in posterior wall of globe, right eye

▤ **SP** ✛ **H44.642** Retained (old) magnetic foreign body in posterior wall of globe, left eye

▤ **SP** ✛ **H44.643** Retained (old) magnetic foreign body in posterior wall of globe, bilateral

▤ **IQ** ✛ **H44.649** Retained (old) magnetic foreign body in posterior wall of globe, unspecified eye

✛ ⑥ **H44.65** Retained (old) magnetic foreign body in vitreous body

▤ **SP** ✛ **H44.651** Retained (old) magnetic foreign body in vitreous body, right eye

▤ **SP** ✛ **H44.652** Retained (old) magnetic foreign body in vitreous body, left eye

▤ **SP** ✛ **H44.653** Retained (old) magnetic foreign body in vitreous body, bilateral

▤ **IQ** ✛ **H44.659** Retained (old) magnetic foreign body in vitreous body, unspecified eye

✛ ⑥ **H44.69** Retained (old) intraocular foreign body, magnetic, in other or multiple sites

▤ **SP** ✛ **H44.691** Retained (old) intraocular foreign body, magnetic, in other or multiple sites, right eye

▤ **SP** ✛ **H44.692** Retained (old) intraocular foreign body, magnetic, in other or multiple sites, left eye

▤ **SP** ✛ **H44.693** Retained (old) intraocular foreign body, magnetic, in other or multiple sites, bilateral

▤ **IQ** ✛ **H44.699** Retained (old) intraocular foreign body, magnetic, in other or multiple sites, unspecified eye

✛ ⑤ **H44.7** Retained (old) intraocular foreign body, nonmagnetic

Use additional code to identify nonmagnetic foreign body (Z18.01-Z18.10, Z18.12, Z18.2-Z18.9)

EXCLUDES 1 current intraocular foreign body (S05.-)

EXCLUDES 2 retained foreign body in eyelid (H02.81-)
retained (old) foreign body following penetrating wound of orbit (H05.5-)
retained (old) intraocular foreign body, magnetic (H44.6-)

✛ ⑥ **H44.70** Unspecified retained (old) intraocular foreign body, nonmagnetic

▤ **SP** ✛ **H44.701** Unspecified retained (old) intraocular foreign body, nonmagnetic, right eye

▤ **SP** ✛ **H44.702** Unspecified retained (old) intraocular foreign body, nonmagnetic, left eye

▤ **SP** ✛ **H44.703** Unspecified retained (old) intraocular foreign body, nonmagnetic, bilateral

▤ **IQ** ✛ **H44.709** Unspecified retained (old) intraocular foreign body, nonmagnetic, unspecified eye

Retained (old) intraocular foreign body NOS

✛ ⑥ **H44.71** Retained (nonmagnetic) (old) foreign body in anterior chamber

▤ **SP** ✛ **H44.711** Retained (nonmagnetic) (old) foreign body in anterior chamber, right eye

▤ **SP** ✛ **H44.712** Retained (nonmagnetic) (old) foreign body in anterior chamber, left eye

▤ **SP** ✛ **H44.713** Retained (nonmagnetic) (old) foreign body in anterior chamber, bilateral

▤ **IQ** ✛ **H44.719** Retained (nonmagnetic) (old) foreign body in anterior chamber, unspecified eye

✛ ⑥ **H44.72** Retained (nonmagnetic) (old) foreign body in iris or ciliary body

▤ **SP** ✛ **H44.721** Retained (nonmagnetic) (old) foreign body in iris or ciliary body, right eye

Chapter 7

H00-H59

★ New ▲ Revised Px Primary **SP** PDGM Px **SL** Low CoM **SH** High CoM **IQ** Quest. Encounter Ⓗ Hospice non-cancer Dx Unspecified **M** *Manifestation*

DecisionHealth's FY 2020 Complete Home Health ICD-10-CM Diagnosis Coding Manual

909

☐ SP ➕ **H44.722** Retained (nonmagnetic) (old) foreign body in iris or ciliary body, left eye

☐ SP ➕ **H44.723** Retained (nonmagnetic) (old) foreign body in iris or ciliary body, bilateral

☐ SP ➕ **H44.729** Retained (nonmagnetic) (old) foreign body in iris or ciliary body, unspecified eye

➕ 6 **H44.73** Retained (nonmagnetic) (old) foreign body in lens

☐ SP ➕ **H44.731** Retained (nonmagnetic) (old) foreign body in lens, right eye

☐ SP ➕ **H44.732** Retained (nonmagnetic) (old) foreign body in lens, left eye

☐ SP ➕ **H44.733** Retained (nonmagnetic) (old) foreign body in lens, bilateral

☐ IQ ➕ **H44.739** Retained (nonmagnetic) (old) foreign body in lens, unspecified eye

➕ 6 **H44.74** Retained (nonmagnetic) (old) foreign body in posterior wall of globe

☐ SP ➕ **H44.741** Retained (nonmagnetic) (old) foreign body in posterior wall of globe, right eye

☐ SP ➕ **H44.742** Retained (nonmagnetic) (old) foreign body in posterior wall of globe, left eye

☐ SP ➕ **H44.743** Retained (nonmagnetic) (old) foreign body in posterior wall of globe, bilateral

☐ IQ ➕ **H44.749** Retained (nonmagnetic) (old) foreign body in posterior wall of globe, unspecified eye

➕ 6 **H44.75** Retained (nonmagnetic) (old) foreign body in vitreous body

☐ SP ➕ **H44.751** Retained (nonmagnetic) (old) foreign body in vitreous body, right eye

☐ SP ➕ **H44.752** Retained (nonmagnetic) (old) foreign body in vitreous body, left eye

☐ SP ➕ **H44.753** Retained (nonmagnetic) (old) foreign body in vitreous body, bilateral

☐ IQ ➕ **H44.759** Retained (nonmagnetic) (old) foreign body in vitreous body, unspecified eye

➕ 6 **H44.79** Retained (old) intraocular foreign body, nonmagnetic, in other or multiple sites

☐ SP ➕ **H44.791** Retained (old) intraocular foreign body, nonmagnetic, in other or multiple sites, right eye

☐ SP ➕ **H44.792** Retained (old) intraocular foreign body, nonmagnetic, in other or multiple sites, left eye

☐ SP ➕ **H44.793** Retained (old) intraocular foreign body, nonmagnetic, in other or multiple sites, bilateral

☐ IQ ➕ **H44.799** Retained (old) intraocular foreign body, nonmagnetic, in other or multiple sites, unspecified eye

5 **H44.8** Other disorders of globe

6 **H44.81** Hemophthalmos

> **DEFINITION** Accumulation of blood within the eyeball that is not due to a current injury.

☐ SP **H44.811** Hemophthalmos, right eye

☐ SP **H44.812** Hemophthalmos, left eye

☐ SP **H44.813** Hemophthalmos, bilateral

☐ IQ **H44.819** Hemophthalmos, unspecified eye

6 **H44.82** Luxation of globe

☐ SP **H44.821** Luxation of globe, right eye

☐ SP **H44.822** Luxation of globe, left eye

☐ SP **H44.823** Luxation of globe, bilateral

☐ IQ **H44.829** Luxation of globe, unspecified eye

SP **H44.89** Other disorders of globe

IQ **H44.9** Unspecified disorder of globe

Disorders of optic nerve and visual pathways   (H46-H47)

4 **H46** Optic neuritis

> **EXCLUDES 2** ischemic optic neuropathy (H47.01-)
> neuromyelitis optica [Devic] (G36.0)

5 **H46.0** Optic papillitis

> **DEFINITION** Swelling of the optic disc where the optic nerve connects to the retina.

☐ IQ **H46.00** Optic papillitis, unspecified eye

☐ SP **H46.01** Optic papillitis, right eye

☐ SP **H46.02** Optic papillitis, left eye

☐ SP **H46.03** Optic papillitis, bilateral

5 **H46.1** Retrobulbar neuritis
Retrobulbar neuritis NOS

> **EXCLUDES 1** syphilitic retrobulbar neuritis (A52.15)

> **DEFINITION** Inflammation of the optic nerve directly behind the eye.

☐ IQ **H46.10** Retrobulbar neuritis, unspecified eye

☐ SP **H46.11** Retrobulbar neuritis, right eye

☐ SP **H46.12** Retrobulbar neuritis, left eye

☐ SP **H46.13** Retrobulbar neuritis, bilateral

SP **H46.2** Nutritional optic neuropathy

SP **H46.3** Toxic optic neuropathy
Code first:
(T51-T65) to identify cause

SP **H46.8** Other optic neuritis

IQ **H46.9** Unspecified optic neuritis

4 **H47** Other disorders of optic [2nd] nerve and visual pathways

5 **H47.0** Disorders of optic nerve, not elsewhere classified

6 **H47.01** Ischemic optic neuropathy

☐ SP **H47.011** Ischemic optic neuropathy, right eye

☐ SP **H47.012** Ischemic optic neuropathy, left eye

☐ SP **H47.013** Ischemic optic neuropathy, bilateral

☐ IQ **H47.019** Ischemic optic neuropathy, unspecified eye

---

4 4th digit required   5 5th digit required   6 6th digit required   7 7th digit required   7 7th digit placeholder   ➕ Additional code   ☐ Laterality

⑥ H47.02 Hemorrhage in optic nerve sheath

⊟ SP H47.021 Hemorrhage in optic nerve sheath, right eye

⊟ SP H47.022 Hemorrhage in optic nerve sheath, left eye

⊟ SP H47.023 Hemorrhage in optic nerve sheath, bilateral

⊟ IQ H47.029 Hemorrhage in optic nerve sheath, unspecified eye

⑥ H47.03 Optic nerve hypoplasia

⊟ SP H47.031 Optic nerve hypoplasia, right eye

⊟ SP H47.032 Optic nerve hypoplasia, left eye

⊟ SP H47.033 Optic nerve hypoplasia, bilateral

⊟ IQ H47.039 Optic nerve hypoplasia, unspecified eye

⑥ H47.09 Other disorders of optic nerve, not elsewhere classified
Compression of optic nerve

⊟ SP H47.091 Other disorders of optic nerve, not elsewhere classified, right eye

⊟ SP H47.092 Other disorders of optic nerve, not elsewhere classified, left eye

⊟ SP H47.093 Other disorders of optic nerve, not elsewhere classified, bilateral

⊟ IQ H47.099 Other disorders of optic nerve, not elsewhere classified, unspecified eye

⑤ H47.1 Papilledema

SP H47.10 Unspecified papilledema

SP H47.11 Papilledema associated with increased intracranial pressure
DEFINITION Swelling of the optic disk (the part of the retina that connects to the optic nerve) caused by increased intracranial pressure.

SP H47.12 Papilledema associated with decreased ocular pressure

SP H47.13 Papilledema associated with retinal disorder

⑥ H47.14 Foster-Kennedy syndrome
DEFINITION Disease that presents with papilledema in one eye and atrophy of the optic nerve of the other; caused by increased intracranial pressure from a tumor.

⊟ SP H47.141 Foster-Kennedy syndrome, right eye

⊟ SP H47.142 Foster-Kennedy syndrome, left eye

⊟ SP H47.143 Foster-Kennedy syndrome, bilateral

⊟ IQ H47.149 Foster-Kennedy syndrome, unspecified eye

⑤ H47.2 Optic atrophy

SP H47.20 Unspecified optic atrophy

⑥ H47.21 Primary optic atrophy

⊟ SP H47.211 Primary optic atrophy, right eye

⊟ SP H47.212 Primary optic atrophy, left eye

⊟ SP H47.213 Primary optic atrophy, bilateral

⊟ IQ H47.219 Primary optic atrophy, unspecified eye

SP H47.22 Hereditary optic atrophy
Leber's optic atrophy

⑥ H47.23 Glaucomatous optic atrophy

⊟ SP H47.231 Glaucomatous optic atrophy, right eye

⊟ SP H47.232 Glaucomatous optic atrophy, left eye

⊟ SP H47.233 Glaucomatous optic atrophy, bilateral

⊟ IQ H47.239 Glaucomatous optic atrophy, unspecified eye

⑥ H47.29 Other optic atrophy
Temporal pallor of optic disc

⊟ SP H47.291 Other optic atrophy, right eye

⊟ SP H47.292 Other optic atrophy, left eye

⊟ SP H47.293 Other optic atrophy, bilateral

⊟ IQ H47.299 Other optic atrophy, unspecified eye

⑤ H47.3 Other disorders of optic disc

⑥ H47.31 Coloboma of optic disc
DEFINITION Congenital defect of the iris in which there is a gap, hole, or cleft that failed to close; may cause ghost images, blurred or decreased visual activity.

⊟ SP H47.311 Coloboma of optic disc, right eye

⊟ SP H47.312 Coloboma of optic disc, left eye

⊟ SP H47.313 Coloboma of optic disc, bilateral

⊟ IQ H47.319 Coloboma of optic disc, unspecified eye

⑥ H47.32 Drusen of optic disc

⊟ SP H47.321 Drusen of optic disc, right eye

⊟ SP H47.322 Drusen of optic disc, left eye

⊟ SP H47.323 Drusen of optic disc, bilateral

⊟ IQ H47.329 Drusen of optic disc, unspecified eye

⑥ H47.33 Pseudopapilledema of optic disc

⊟ SP H47.331 Pseudopapilledema of optic disc, right eye

⊟ SP H47.332 Pseudopapilledema of optic disc, left eye

⊟ SP H47.333 Pseudopapilledema of optic disc, bilateral

⊟ IQ H47.339 Pseudopapilledema of optic disc, unspecified eye

⑥ H47.39 Other disorders of optic disc

⊟ SP H47.391 Other disorders of optic disc, right eye

⊟ SP H47.392 Other disorders of optic disc, left eye

⊟ SP H47.393 Other disorders of optic disc, bilateral

⊟ IQ H47.399 Other disorders of optic disc, unspecified eye

⑤ H47.4 Disorders of optic chiasm
Code also:
underlying condition

SP H47.41 Disorders of optic chiasm in (due to) inflammatory disorders

SP H47.42 Disorders of optic chiasm in (due to) neoplasm

SP H47.43 Disorders of optic chiasm in (due to) vascular disorders

SP H47.49 Disorders of optic chiasm in (due to) other disorders

⑤ **H47.5 Disorders of other visual pathways**
Disorders of optic tracts, geniculate nuclei and optic radiations
Code also:
  underlying condition

⑥ **H47.51 Disorders of visual pathways in (due to) inflammatory disorders**

⊟ SP **H47.511 Disorders of visual pathways in (due to) inflammatory disorders, right side**

⊟ SP **H47.512 Disorders of visual pathways in (due to) inflammatory disorders, left side**

⊟ IQ **H47.519 Disorders of visual pathways in (due to) inflammatory disorders, unspecified side**

⑥ **H47.52 Disorders of visual pathways in (due to) neoplasm**

⊟ SP **H47.521 Disorders of visual pathways in (due to) neoplasm, right side**

⊟ SP **H47.522 Disorders of visual pathways in (due to) neoplasm, left side**

⊟ IQ **H47.529 Disorders of visual pathways in (due to) neoplasm, unspecified side**

⑥ **H47.53 Disorders of visual pathways in (due to) vascular disorders**

⊟ SP **H47.531 Disorders of visual pathways in (due to) vascular disorders, right side**

⊟ SP **H47.532 Disorders of visual pathways in (due to) vascular disorders, left side**

⊟ IQ **H47.539 Disorders of visual pathways in (due to) vascular disorders, unspecified side**

▲ ⑤ **H47.6 Disorders of visual cortex**
Code also:
  underlying condition
  EXCLUDES 1 injury to visual cortex S04.04-

⑥ **H47.61 Cortical blindness**
  DEFINITION Blindness caused by a defect of the brain and not the eyes.

⊟ SP **H47.611 Cortical blindness, right side of brain**

⊟ SP **H47.612 Cortical blindness, left side of brain**

⊟ IQ **H47.619 Cortical blindness, unspecified side of brain**

⑥ **H47.62 Disorders of visual cortex in (due to) inflammatory disorders**

⊟ SP **H47.621 Disorders of visual cortex in (due to) inflammatory disorders, right side of brain**

⊟ SP **H47.622 Disorders of visual cortex in (due to) inflammatory disorders, left side of brain**

⊟ IQ **H47.629 Disorders of visual cortex in (due to) inflammatory disorders, unspecified side of brain**

⑥ **H47.63 Disorders of visual cortex in (due to) neoplasm**

⊟ SP **H47.631 Disorders of visual cortex in (due to) neoplasm, right side of brain**

⊟ SP **H47.632 Disorders of visual cortex in (due to) neoplasm, left side of brain**

⊟ IQ **H47.639 Disorders of visual cortex in (due to) neoplasm, unspecified side of brain**

⑥ **H47.64 Disorders of visual cortex in (due to) vascular disorders**

⊟ SP **H47.641 Disorders of visual cortex in (due to) vascular disorders, right side of brain**

⊟ SP **H47.642 Disorders of visual cortex in (due to) vascular disorders, left side of brain**

⊟ IQ **H47.649 Disorders of visual cortex in (due to) vascular disorders, unspecified side of brain**

IQ **H47.9 Unspecified disorder of visual pathways**

Disorders of ocular muscles, binocular movement, accommodation and refraction (H49-H52)

EXCLUDES 2 nystagmus and other irregular eye movements (H55)

④ **H49 Paralytic strabismus**
  EXCLUDES 2 internal ophthalmoplegia (H52.51-)
    internuclear ophthalmoplegia (H51.2-)
    progressive supranuclear ophthalmoplegia (G23.1)

⑤ **H49.0 Third [oculomotor] nerve palsy**

⊟ IQ **H49.00 Third [oculomotor] nerve palsy, unspecified eye**

⊟ SP **H49.01 Third [oculomotor] nerve palsy, right eye**

⊟ SP **H49.02 Third [oculomotor] nerve palsy, left eye**

⊟ SP **H49.03 Third [oculomotor] nerve palsy, bilateral**

⑤ **H49.1 Fourth [trochlear] nerve palsy**

⊟ IQ **H49.10 Fourth [trochlear] nerve palsy, unspecified eye**

⊟ SP **H49.11 Fourth [trochlear] nerve palsy, right eye**

⊟ SP **H49.12 Fourth [trochlear] nerve palsy, left eye**

⊟ SP **H49.13 Fourth [trochlear] nerve palsy, bilateral**

⑤ **H49.2 Sixth [abducent] nerve palsy**

⊟ IQ **H49.20 Sixth [abducent] nerve palsy, unspecified eye**

⊟ SP **H49.21 Sixth [abducent] nerve palsy, right eye**

⊟ SP **H49.22 Sixth [abducent] nerve palsy, left eye**

⊟ SP **H49.23 Sixth [abducent] nerve palsy, bilateral**

⑤ **H49.3 Total (external) ophthalmoplegia**
  DEFINITION Paralysis of all of the muscles that move the eye as well as the muscles controlling the diameter of the pupil and shape of the lens.

⊟ IQ **H49.30 Total (external) ophthalmoplegia, unspecified eye**

⊟ SP **H49.31 Total (external) ophthalmoplegia, right eye**

---

④4th digit required   ⑤5th digit required   ⑥6th digit required   ⑦7th digit required   ⑦7th digit placeholder   ✚Additional code   ⊟Laterality

912   *DecisionHealth's* FY 2020 Complete Home Health ICD-10-CM Diagnosis Coding Manual

▤ **SP** **H49.32**   Total (external) ophthalmoplegia, left eye

▤ **SP** **H49.33**   Total (external) ophthalmoplegia, bilateral

▫ **H49.4**   Progressive external ophthalmoplegia

> **EXCLUDES 1**   Kearns-Sayre syndrome (H49.81-)

▤ **IQ** **H49.40**   Progressive external ophthalmoplegia, unspecified eye

▤ **SP** **H49.41**   Progressive external ophthalmoplegia, right eye

▤ **SP** **H49.42**   Progressive external ophthalmoplegia, left eye

▤ **SP** **H49.43**   Progressive external ophthalmoplegia, bilateral

▫ **H49.8**   Other paralytic strabismus

✚ ▫ **H49.81**   Kearns-Sayre syndrome
> Progressive external ophthalmoplegia with pigmentary retinopathy
> Use additional code for other manifestation, such as:
> heart block (I45.9)

▤ **SP** ✚ **H49.811**   Kearns-Sayre syndrome, right eye

▤ **SP** ✚ **H49.812**   Kearns-Sayre syndrome, left eye

▤ **SP** ✚ **H49.813**   Kearns-Sayre syndrome, bilateral

▤ **IQ** ✚ **H49.819**   Kearns-Sayre syndrome, unspecified eye

▫ **H49.88**   Other paralytic strabismus
> External ophthalmoplegia NOS

▤ **SP** **H49.881**   Other paralytic strabismus, right eye

▤ **SP** **H49.882**   Other paralytic strabismus, left eye

▤ **SP** **H49.883**   Other paralytic strabismus, bilateral

▤ **IQ** **H49.889**   Other paralytic strabismus, unspecified eye

SP **H49.9**   Unspecified paralytic strabismus

▣ **H50**   Other strabismus

▫ **H50.0**   Esotropia
> Convergent concomitant strabismus
> **EXCLUDES 1**   intermittent esotropia (H50.31-, H50.32)
> **DEFINITION**   Deviation of the visual axis of one or both eyes inward toward that of the other eye.

SP **H50.00**   Unspecified esotropia

▫ **H50.01**   Monocular esotropia

▤ **SP** **H50.011**   Monocular esotropia, right eye

▤ **SP** **H50.012**   Monocular esotropia, left eye

▫ **H50.02**   Monocular esotropia with A pattern

▤ **SP** **H50.021**   Monocular esotropia with A pattern, right eye

▤ **SP** **H50.022**   Monocular esotropia with A pattern, left eye

▫ **H50.03**   Monocular esotropia with V pattern

▤ **SP** **H50.031**   Monocular esotropia with V pattern, right eye

▤ **SP** **H50.032**   Monocular esotropia with V pattern, left eye

▫ **H50.04**   Monocular esotropia with other noncomitancies

▤ **SP** **H50.041**   Monocular esotropia with other noncomitancies, right eye

▤ **SP** **H50.042**   Monocular esotropia with other noncomitancies, left eye

SP **H50.05**   Alternating esotropia

SP **H50.06**   Alternating esotropia with A pattern

SP **H50.07**   Alternating esotropia with V pattern

SP **H50.08**   Alternating esotropia with other noncomitancies

▫ **H50.1**   Exotropia
> Divergent concomitant strabismus
> **EXCLUDES 1**   intermittent exotropia (H50.33-, H50.34)
> **DEFINITION**   An abnormal alignment of one or both eyes in which one or both eyes deviate outward.

SP **H50.10**   Unspecified exotropia

▫ **H50.11**   Monocular exotropia

▤ **SP** **H50.111**   Monocular exotropia, right eye

▤ **SP** **H50.112**   Monocular exotropia, left eye

▫ **H50.12**   Monocular exotropia with A pattern

▤ **SP** **H50.121**   Monocular exotropia with A pattern, right eye

▤ **SP** **H50.122**   Monocular exotropia with A pattern, left eye

▫ **H50.13**   Monocular exotropia with V pattern

▤ **SP** **H50.131**   Monocular exotropia with V pattern, right eye

▤ **SP** **H50.132**   Monocular exotropia with V pattern, left eye

▫ **H50.14**   Monocular exotropia with other noncomitancies

▤ **SP** **H50.141**   Monocular exotropia with other noncomitancies, right eye

▤ **SP** **H50.142**   Monocular exotropia with other noncomitancies, left eye

SP **H50.15**   Alternating exotropia

SP **H50.16**   Alternating exotropia with A pattern

SP **H50.17**   Alternating exotropia with V pattern

SP **H50.18**   Alternating exotropia with other noncomitancies

▫ **H50.2**   Vertical strabismus
> Hypertropia

▤ **SP** **H50.21**   Vertical strabismus, right eye

▤ **SP** **H50.22**   Vertical strabismus, left eye

▫ **H50.3**   Intermittent heterotropia

SP **H50.30**   Unspecified intermittent heterotropia

▫ **H50.31**   Intermittent monocular esotropia

▤ **SP** **H50.311**   Intermittent monocular esotropia, right eye

▤ **SP** **H50.312**   Intermittent monocular esotropia, left eye

SP **H50.32**   Intermittent alternating esotropia

▫ **H50.33**   Intermittent monocular exotropia

▤ **SP** **H50.331**   Intermittent monocular exotropia, right eye

▤ **SP** **H50.332**   Intermittent monocular exotropia, left eye

SP **H50.34**   Intermittent alternating exotropia

▫ **H50.4**   Other and unspecified heterotropia

SP **H50.40**   Unspecified heterotropia

▫ **H50.41**   Cyclotropia

▤ **SP** **H50.411**   Cyclotropia, right eye

Chapter 7

H00-H59

★ New ▲ Revised **Px** Primary **SP** PDGM Px **SL** Low CoM **SH** High CoM **IQ** Quest. Encounter Ⓗ Hospice non-cancer Dx   Unspecified   **M** *Manifestation*

⊟ SP H50.412 Cyclotropia, left eye

SP H50.42 Monofixation syndrome

SP H50.43 Accommodative component in esotropia

⑤ H50.5 Heterophoria

SP H50.50 Unspecified heterophoria

SP H50.51 Esophoria

SP H50.52 Exophoria

SP H50.53 Vertical heterophoria

SP H50.54 Cyclophoria

SP H50.55 Alternating heterophoria

⑤ H50.6 Mechanical strabismus

SP H50.60 Mechanical strabismus, unspecified

⑥ H50.61 Brown's sheath syndrome

> **DEFINITION** Condition in which the muscle that moves the eye upward and inward is too short, impairing eye movement.

⊟ SP H50.611 Brown's sheath syndrome, right eye

⊟ SP H50.612 Brown's sheath syndrome, left eye

SP H50.69 Other mechanical strabismus
Strabismus due to adhesions
Traumatic limitation of duction of eye muscle

⑤ H50.8 Other specified strabismus

⑥ H50.81 Duane's syndrome

> **DEFINITION** Congenital eye muscle disorder due to cranial nerve dysfunction that inhibits normal rotation of one or both eyes inward and outward, also causing abnormal inward turning with distant viewing and eye retraction when viewing up close.

⊟ SP H50.811 Duane's syndrome, right eye

⊟ SP H50.812 Duane's syndrome, left eye

SP H50.89 Other specified strabismus

SP H50.9 Unspecified strabismus

④ H51 Other disorders of binocular movement

SP H51.0 Palsy (spasm) of conjugate gaze

⑤ H51.1 Convergence insufficiency and excess

SP H51.11 Convergence insufficiency

SP H51.12 Convergence excess

> **DEFINITION** Eyes fail to move in a coordinated fashion when viewing objects up close.

⑤ H51.2 Internuclear ophthalmoplegia

⊟ IQ H51.20 Internuclear ophthalmoplegia, unspecified eye

⊟ SP H51.21 Internuclear ophthalmoplegia, right eye

⊟ SP H51.22 Internuclear ophthalmoplegia, left eye

⊟ SP H51.23 Internuclear ophthalmoplegia, bilateral

SP H51.8 Other specified disorders of binocular movement

IQ H51.9 Unspecified disorder of binocular movement

④ H52 Disorders of refraction and accommodation

⑤ H52.0 Hypermetropia

⊟ IQ H52.00 Hypermetropia, unspecified eye

⊟ SP H52.01 Hypermetropia, right eye

⊟ SP H52.02 Hypermetropia, left eye

⊟ SP H52.03 Hypermetropia, bilateral

⑤ H52.1 Myopia

> **EXCLUDES 1** degenerative myopia (H44.2-)

⊟ IQ H52.10 Myopia, unspecified eye

⊟ SP H52.11 Myopia, right eye

⊟ SP H52.12 Myopia, left eye

⊟ SP H52.13 Myopia, bilateral

⑤ H52.2 Astigmatism

> **DEFINITION** Condition in which the cornea is not shaped perfectly round, causing light to focus on more than one point of the retina and resulting in blurred vision.

⑥ H52.20 Unspecified astigmatism

⊟ SP H52.201 Unspecified astigmatism, right eye

⊟ SP H52.202 Unspecified astigmatism, left eye

⊟ SP H52.203 Unspecified astigmatism, bilateral

⊟ IQ H52.209 Unspecified astigmatism, unspecified eye

⑥ H52.21 Irregular astigmatism

⊟ SP H52.211 Irregular astigmatism, right eye

⊟ SP H52.212 Irregular astigmatism, left eye

⊟ SP H52.213 Irregular astigmatism, bilateral

⊟ IQ H52.219 Irregular astigmatism, unspecified eye

⑥ H52.22 Regular astigmatism

⊟ SP H52.221 Regular astigmatism, right eye

⊟ SP H52.222 Regular astigmatism, left eye

⊟ SP H52.223 Regular astigmatism, bilateral

⊟ IQ H52.229 Regular astigmatism, unspecified eye

⑤ H52.3 Anisometropia and aniseikonia

SP H52.31 Anisometropia

> **DEFINITION** Each eye has a different refractive power.

SP H52.32 Aniseikonia

> **DEFINITION** One eye sees an object differently in size and shape than the way the other eye sees it.

SP H52.4 Presbyopia

> **DEFINITION** Lens of the eye loses its elasticity due to age, making it more difficult to focus on near points.

⑤ H52.5 Disorders of accommodation

⑥ H52.51 Internal ophthalmoplegia (complete) (total)

⊟ SP H52.511 Internal ophthalmoplegia (complete) (total), right eye

⊟ SP H52.512 Internal ophthalmoplegia (complete) (total), left eye

⊟ SP H52.513 Internal ophthalmoplegia (complete) (total), bilateral

⊟ IQ H52.519 Internal ophthalmoplegia (complete) (total), unspecified eye

---

④ 4th digit required   **⑤** 5th digit required   **⑥** 6th digit required   **⑦** 7th digit required   **☑** 7th digit placeholder   **+** Additional code   **⊟** Laterality

914   *DecisionHealth's* FY 2020 Complete Home Health ICD-10-CM Diagnosis Coding Manual

⑥ H52.52 Paresis of accommodation
> **DEFINITION** Paralysis of the ciliary muscles of the eye that results in the loss of visual accommodation.

☐ **SP H52.521 Paresis of accommodation, right eye**

☐ **SP H52.522 Paresis of accommodation, left eye**

☐ **SP H52.523 Paresis of accommodation, bilateral**

☐ **IQ H52.529 Paresis of accommodation, unspecified eye**

⑥ H52.53 Spasm of accommodation
> **DEFINITION** Abnormal, uncontrolled contraction of the ciliary muscle, usually initially presenting as near-sightedness.

☐ **SP H52.531 Spasm of accommodation, right eye**

☐ **SP H52.532 Spasm of accommodation, left eye**

☐ **SP H52.533 Spasm of accommodation, bilateral**

☐ **IQ H52.539 Spasm of accommodation, unspecified eye**

SP H52.6 Other disorders of refraction

IQ H52.7 Unspecified disorder of refraction

Visual disturbances and blindness (H53-H54)

④ H53 Visual disturbances

⑤ H53.0 Amblyopia ex anopsia
> **EXCLUDES 1** amblyopia due to vitamin A deficiency (E50.5)

⑥ H53.00 Unspecified amblyopia

☐ **SP H53.001 Unspecified amblyopia, right eye**

☐ **SP H53.002 Unspecified amblyopia, left eye**

☐ **SP H53.003 Unspecified amblyopia, bilateral**

☐ **IQ H53.009 Unspecified amblyopia, unspecified eye**

⑥ H53.01 Deprivation amblyopia

☐ **SP H53.011 Deprivation amblyopia, right eye**

☐ **SP H53.012 Deprivation amblyopia, left eye**

☐ **SP H53.013 Deprivation amblyopia, bilateral**

☐ **IQ H53.019 Deprivation amblyopia, unspecified eye**

⑥ H53.02 Refractive amblyopia

☐ **SP H53.021 Refractive amblyopia, right eye**

☐ **SP H53.022 Refractive amblyopia, left eye**

☐ **SP H53.023 Refractive amblyopia, bilateral**

☐ **IQ H53.029 Refractive amblyopia, unspecified eye**

⑥ H53.03 Strabismic amblyopia
> **EXCLUDES 1** strabismus (H50.-)

☐ **SP H53.031 Strabismic amblyopia, right eye**

☐ **SP H53.032 Strabismic amblyopia, left eye**

☐ **SP H53.033 Strabismic amblyopia, bilateral**

☐ **IQ H53.039 Strabismic amblyopia, unspecified eye**

⑥ H53.04 Amblyopia suspect

☐ **SP H53.041 Amblyopia suspect, right eye**

☐ **SP H53.042 Amblyopia suspect, left eye**

☐ **SP H53.043 Amblyopia suspect, bilateral**

☐ **IQ H53.049 Amblyopia suspect, unspecified eye**

⑤ H53.1 Subjective visual disturbances
> **EXCLUDES 1** subjective visual disturbances due to vitamin A deficiency (E50.5)
> visual hallucinations (R44.1)

IQ H53.10 Unspecified subjective visual disturbances

SP H53.11 Day blindness
Hemeralopia

⑥ H53.12 Transient visual loss
Scintillating scotoma
> **EXCLUDES 1** amaurosis fugax (G45.3-)
> transient retinal artery occlusion (H34.0-)

☐ **SP H53.121 Transient visual loss, right eye**

☐ **SP H53.122 Transient visual loss, left eye**

☐ **SP H53.123 Transient visual loss, bilateral**

☐ **IQ H53.129 Transient visual loss, unspecified eye**

⑥ H53.13 Sudden visual loss

☐ **SP H53.131 Sudden visual loss, right eye**

☐ **SP H53.132 Sudden visual loss, left eye**

☐ **SP H53.133 Sudden visual loss, bilateral**

☐ **IQ H53.139 Sudden visual loss, unspecified eye**

⑥ H53.14 Visual discomfort
Asthenopia
Photophobia

☐ **SP H53.141 Visual discomfort, right eye**

☐ **SP H53.142 Visual discomfort, left eye**

☐ **SP H53.143 Visual discomfort, bilateral**

☐ **IQ H53.149 Visual discomfort, unspecified**

SP H53.15 Visual distortions of shape and size
Metamorphopsia

SP H53.16 Psychophysical visual disturbances

SP H53.19 Other subjective visual disturbances
Visual halos
> **DEFINITION** Photopsia: sparks or flashes in the field of vision, due to retinal irritation.

SP H53.2 Diplopia
Double vision

⑤ H53.3 Other and unspecified disorders of binocular vision

IQ H53.30 Unspecified disorder of binocular vision

SP H53.31 Abnormal retinal correspondence

SP H53.32 Fusion with defective stereopsis

SP H53.33 Simultaneous visual perception without fusion
> **DEFINITION** Imaging from both eyes reaches the brain and are both processed, but without being merged into a single image; the patient sees two side-by-side images instead of one.

SP H53.34 Suppression of binocular vision

⑤ H53.4 Visual field defects

SP H53.40 Unspecified visual field defects

★ New ▲ Revised Px Primary SP PDGM Px SL Low CoM SH High CoM IQ Quest. Encounter H Hospice non-cancer Dx Unspecified M *Manifestation*

DecisionHealth's FY 2020 Complete Home Health ICD-10-CM Diagnosis Coding Manual

915

H53.41 **Scotoma involving central area**
Central scotoma

H53.411 **Scotoma involving central area, right eye**

H53.412 **Scotoma involving central area, left eye**

H53.413 **Scotoma involving central area, bilateral**

H53.419 **Scotoma involving central area, unspecified eye**

H53.42 **Scotoma of blind spot area**
Enlarged blind spot

DEFINITION Blind spot (scotoma) in the central five degrees of the patient's vision.

H53.421 **Scotoma of blind spot area, right eye**

H53.422 **Scotoma of blind spot area, left eye**

H53.423 **Scotoma of blind spot area, bilateral**

H53.429 **Scotoma of blind spot area, unspecified eye**

H53.43 **Sector or arcuate defects**
Arcuate scotoma
Bjerrum scotoma

H53.431 **Sector or arcuate defects, right eye**

H53.432 **Sector or arcuate defects, left eye**

H53.433 **Sector or arcuate defects, bilateral**

H53.439 **Sector or arcuate defects, unspecified eye**

H53.45 **Other localized visual field defect**
Peripheral visual field defect
Ring scotoma NOS
Scotoma NOS

H53.451 **Other localized visual field defect, right eye**

H53.452 **Other localized visual field defect, left eye**

H53.453 **Other localized visual field defect, bilateral**

H53.459 **Other localized visual field defect, unspecified eye**

H53.46 **Homonymous bilateral field defects**
Homonymous hemianopia
Homonymous hemianopsia
Quadrant anopia
Quadrant anopsia

H53.461 **Homonymous bilateral field defects, right side**

H53.462 **Homonymous bilateral field defects, left side**

H53.469 **Homonymous bilateral field defects, unspecified side**
Homonymous bilateral field defects NOS

H53.47 **Heteronymous bilateral field defects**
Heteronymous hemianop(s)ia

H53.48 **Generalized contraction of visual field**

H53.481 **Generalized contraction of visual field, right eye**

H53.482 **Generalized contraction of visual field, left eye**

H53.483 **Generalized contraction of visual field, bilateral**

H53.489 **Generalized contraction of visual field, unspecified eye**

H53.5 **Color vision deficiencies**
Color blindness

EXCLUDES 2 day blindness (H53.11)

H53.50 **Unspecified color vision deficiencies**
Color blindness NOS

H53.51 **Achromatopsia**
DEFINITION Nonprogressive, hereditary visual disorder and retinal abnormality causing decreased vision, light sensitivity, nystagmus, and complete color blindness.

H53.52 **Acquired color vision deficiency**

H53.53 **Deuteranomaly**
Deuteranopia
DEFINITION A deficiency in color perception primarily affecting red-green hues due to deficient pigment sensitive to green wavelengths, a common form of color blindness.

H53.54 **Protanomaly**
Protanopia

H53.55 **Tritanomaly**
Tritanopia
DEFINITION A deficiency in color perception characterized by an inability to discern blue and yellow due to an absence of blue-sensitive pigment in the retina.

H53.59 **Other color vision deficiencies**

H53.6 **Night blindness**
EXCLUDES 1 night blindness due to vitamin A deficiency (E50.5)

H53.60 **Unspecified night blindness**

H53.61 **Abnormal dark adaptation curve**

H53.62 **Acquired night blindness**

H53.63 **Congenital night blindness**

H53.69 **Other night blindness**

H53.7 **Vision sensitivity deficiencies**

H53.71 **Glare sensitivity**

H53.72 **Impaired contrast sensitivity**

H53.8 **Other visual disturbances**

H53.9 **Unspecified visual disturbance**

H54 **Blindness and low vision**
Note:
For definition of visual impairment categories see table below
Code first:
any associated underlying cause of the blindness
EXCLUDES 1 amaurosis fugax (G45.3)

4 4th digit required **5** 5th digit required **6** 6th digit required **7** 7th digit required **7** 7th digit placeholder **+** Additional code **⊟** Laterality

916   *DecisionHealth's* FY 2020 Complete Home Health ICD-10-CM Diagnosis Coding Manual

GUIDELINES Section I.C.7.b

If "blindness" or "low vision" of both eyes is documented but the visual impairment category is not documented, assign code H54.3, Unqualified visual loss, both eyes. If "blindness" or "low vision" in one eye is documented but the visual impairment category is not documented, assign a code from H54.6-, Unqualified visual loss, one eye. If "blindness" or "visual loss" is documented without any information about whether one or both eyes are affected, assign code H54.7, Unspecified visual loss.

CODING TIPS ✓ Do not use H54 codes for patients with common refractive errors, e.g. farsightedness, nearsightedness, astigmatism, etc. These codes are to indicate the level of vision for those with other eye conditions such as cataracts, retinopathy, glaucoma, hemianopsia, etc. Be careful: OASIS item M1200 options do not equate with these categories of impairment. Blindness should only be coded if documentation supports the code.

⑤ **H54.0 Blindness, both eyes**
Visual impairment categories 3, 4, 5 in both eyes.
CODING TIPS ✓ Do not use H54.0 to indicate blindness in the USA. See H54.3 or H54.8, depending on the physician's documentation.

⑥ **H54.0X Blindness, both eyes, different category levels**
CODING TIPS ✓ The sixth character represents the category of vision in the right eye, and a seventh character represents the category of vision in the left eye.

🔲 **SP** ⑦ **H54.0X3 Blindness right eye, category 3**

🔲 **SP** ⑦ **H54.0X4 Blindness right eye, category 4**

🔲 **SP** ⑦ **H54.0X5 Blindness right eye, category 5**

⑤ **H54.1 Blindness, one eye, low vision other eye**
Visual impairment categories 3, 4, 5 in one eye, with categories 1 or 2 in the other eye.

🔲 **SP** **H54.10** Blindness, one eye, low vision other eye, unspecified eyes

⑥ **H54.11 Blindness, right eye, low vision left eye**
CODING TIPS ✓ The sixth character represents the category of vision in the right eye, and a seventh character represents the category of vision in the left eye.

🔲 **SP** ⑦ **H54.113 Blindness right eye category 3, low vision left eye**

🔲 **SP** ⑦ **H54.114 Blindness right eye category 4, low vision left eye**

🔲 **SP** ⑦ **H54.115 Blindness right eye category 5, low vision left eye**

⑥ **H54.12 Blindness, left eye, low vision right eye**

CODING TIPS ✓ The sixth character represents the category of vision in the right eye, and a seventh character represents the category of vision in the left eye.

🔲 **SP** ⑦ **H54.121 Low vision right eye category 1, blindness left eye**

🔲 **SP** ⑦ **H54.122 Low vision right eye category 2, blindness left eye**

⑤ **H54.2 Low vision, both eyes**
Visual impairment categories 1 or 2 in both eyes.

⑥ **H54.2X Low vision, both eyes, different category levels**
CODING TIPS ✓ The sixth character represents the category of vision in the right eye, and a seventh character represents the category of vision in the left eye.

🔲 **SP** ⑦ **H54.2X1 Low vision, right eye, category 1**

🔲 **SP** ⑦ **H54.2X2 Low vision, right eye, category 2**

SP **H54.3 Unqualified visual loss, both eyes**
Visual impairment category 9 in both eyes.
GUIDELINES Section I.C.7.b
If "blindness" or "low vision" of both eyes is documented but the visual impairment category is not documented, assign code H54.3, Unqualified visual loss, both eyes.

⑤ **H54.4 Blindness, one eye**
Visual impairment categories 3, 4, 5 in one eye [normal vision in other eye]

🔲 **IQ** **H54.40** Blindness, one eye, unspecified eye

⑥ **H54.41 Blindness, right eye, normal vision left eye**
CODING TIPS ✓ The sixth character represents the category of vision in the right eye, and a seventh character represents the category of vision in the left eye.

🔲 **SP** ⑦ **H54.413 Blindness, right eye, category 3**

🔲 **SP** ⑦ **H54.414 Blindness, right eye, category 4**

🔲 **SP** ⑦ **H54.415 Blindness, right eye, category 5**

⑥ **H54.42 Blindness, left eye, normal vision right eye**

🔲 **SP** ⑦ **H54.42A Blindness, left eye, category 3-5**
CODING TIPS ✓ The sixth character represents the category of vision in the right eye, and a seventh character represents the category of vision in the left eye.

⑤ **H54.5 Low vision, one eye**
Visual impairment categories 1 or 2 in one eye [normal vision in other eye].

🔲 **IQ** **H54.50** Low vision, one eye, unspecified eye

⑥ **H54.51 Low vision, right eye, normal vision left eye**
CODING TIPS ✓ The sixth character represents the category of vision in the right eye, and a seventh character represents the category of vision in the left eye.

SP ⑦ **H54.511 Low vision, right eye, category 1-2**

⑥ **H54.52 Low vision, left eye, normal vision right eye**

★ New ▲ Revised **Px** Primary **SP** PDGM Px **SL** Low CoM **SH** High CoM **IQ** Quest. Encounter **H** Hospice non-cancer Dx Unspecified **M** *Manifestation*

SP 7 H54.52A Low vision, left eye, category 1-2
CODING TIPS ✓   The sixth character represents the category of vision in the right eye, and a seventh character represents the category of vision in the left eye.

5 H54.6 Unqualified visual loss, one eye
Visual impairment category 9 in one eye [normal vision in other eye].
GUIDELINES   Section I.C.7.b
If "blindness" or "low vision" in one eye is documented but the visual impairment category is not documented, assign a code from H54.6-, Unqualified visual loss, one eye.

IQ H54.60 Unqualified visual loss, one eye, unspecified

SP H54.61 Unqualified visual loss, right eye, normal vision left eye

SP H54.62 Unqualified visual loss, left eye, normal vision right eye

IQ H54.7 Unspecified visual loss
Visual impairment category 9 NOS
GUIDELINES   Section I.C.7.b
If "blindness" or "visual loss" is documented without any information about whether one or both eyes are affected, assign code H54.7, Unspecified visual loss.

SP H54.8 Legal blindness, as defined in USA
Blindness NOS according to USA definition
Note:
The table below gives a classification of severity of visual impairment recommended by a WHO Study Group on the Prevention of Blindness, Geneva, 6-10 November 1972.
The term 'low vision' in category H54 comprises categories 1 and 2 of the table, the term 'blindness' categories 3, 4 and 5, and the term 'unqualified visual loss' category 9.
If the extent of the visual field is taken into account, patients with a field no greater than 10 but greater than 5 around central fixation should be placed in category 3 and patients with a field no greater than 5 around central fixation should be placed in category 4, even if the central acuity is not impaired.

EXCLUDES 1   legal blindness with specification of impairment level (H54.0-H54.7)

Category of visual impairment	Visual acuity with best possible correction	
	Maximum less than:	**Minimum equal to or better than:**
1	6/18 3/10(0.3) 20/70	6/60 1/10(0.1) 20/200
2	6/60 1/10(0.1) 20/200	3/60 1/20(0.05) 20/400
3	3/60 1/20(0.05) 20/400	1/60(finger counting at one meter) 1/50(0.02) 5/300(20/1200)

CODING TIPS ✓   Use this code when the physician documents blindness without an indication of eyes involved. If "blindness" or "low vision" of both eyes is documented but the visual impairment category is not documented, assign code H54.3, Unqualified visual loss, both eyes.

Other disorders of eye and adnexa (H55-H57)

4 H55 Nystagmus and other irregular eye movements
5 H55.0 Nystagmus
SP H55.00 Unspecified nystagmus
SP H55.01 Congenital nystagmus
SP H55.02 Latent nystagmus
DEFINITION   Involuntary rapid movement of the eyeball occurring only when one eye is covered.
SP H55.03 Visual deprivation nystagmus
SP H55.04 Dissociated nystagmus
DEFINITION   Involuntary rhythmic movements in both eyes that are dissimilar in direction, extent, and frequency of movement.
SP H55.09 Other forms of nystagmus
5 H55.8 Other irregular eye movements
SP H55.81 Saccadic eye movements
DEFINITION   Rapid and involuntary eye movement while changing focus on stationary objects.
SP H55.89 Other irregular eye movements
4 H57 Other disorders of eye and adnexa
5 H57.0 Anomalies of pupillary function
SP H57.00 Unspecified anomaly of pupillary function
SP H57.01 Argyll Robertson pupil, atypical
EXCLUDES 1   syphilitic Argyll Robertson pupil (A52.19)

4 4th digit required   5 5th digit required   6 6th digit required   7 7th digit required   7 7th digit placeholder   + Additional code   = Laterality

918   *DecisionHealth's* FY 2020 Complete Home Health ICD-10-CM Diagnosis Coding Manual

SP H57.02 Anisocoria
> **DEFINITION** Pupils of unequal size.

SP H57.03 Miosis
> **DEFINITION** Constriction of the pupil.

SP H57.04 Mydriasis

6 H57.05 Tonic pupil

SP H57.051 Tonic pupil, right eye

SP H57.052 Tonic pupil, left eye

SP H57.053 Tonic pupil, bilateral

IQ H57.059 Tonic pupil, unspecified eye

SP H57.09 Other anomalies of pupillary function

5 H57.1 Ocular pain

IQ H57.10 Ocular pain, unspecified eye

SP H57.11 Ocular pain, right eye

SP H57.12 Ocular pain, left eye

SP H57.13 Ocular pain, bilateral

5 H57.8 Other specified disorders of eye and adnexa

6 H57.81 Brow ptosis

IQ H57.811 Brow ptosis, right

IQ H57.812 Brow ptosis, left

IQ H57.813 Brow ptosis, bilateral

IQ H57.819 Brow ptosis, unspecified

SP H57.89 Other specified disorders of eye and adnexa

IQ H57.9 Unspecified disorder of eye and adnexa

Intraoperative and postprocedural complications and disorders of eye and adnexa, not elsewhere classified (H59)

4 H59 Intraoperative and postprocedural complications and disorders of eye and adnexa, not elsewhere classified
> **EXCLUDES 1** mechanical complication of intraocular lens (T85.2)
> mechanical complication of other ocular prosthetic devices, implants and grafts (T85.3)
> pseudophakia (Z96.1)
> secondary cataracts (H26.4-)

5 H59.0 Disorders of the eye following cataract surgery

6 H59.01 Keratopathy (bullous aphakic) following cataract surgery
Vitreal corneal syndrome
Vitreous (touch) syndrome

SP H59.011 Keratopathy (bullous aphakic) following cataract surgery, right eye

SP H59.012 Keratopathy (bullous aphakic) following cataract surgery, left eye

SP H59.013 Keratopathy (bullous aphakic) following cataract surgery, bilateral

IQ H59.019 Keratopathy (bullous aphakic) following cataract surgery, unspecified eye

6 H59.02 Cataract (lens) fragments in eye following cataract surgery

SP H59.021 Cataract (lens) fragments in eye following cataract surgery, right eye

SP H59.022 Cataract (lens) fragments in eye following cataract surgery, left eye

SP H59.023 Cataract (lens) fragments in eye following cataract surgery, bilateral

IQ H59.029 Cataract (lens) fragments in eye following cataract surgery, unspecified eye

6 H59.03 Cystoid macular edema following cataract surgery

SP H59.031 Cystoid macular edema following cataract surgery, right eye

SP H59.032 Cystoid macular edema following cataract surgery, left eye

SP H59.033 Cystoid macular edema following cataract surgery, bilateral

IQ H59.039 Cystoid macular edema following cataract surgery, unspecified eye

6 H59.09 Other disorders of the eye following cataract surgery

SP H59.091 Other disorders of the right eye following cataract surgery

SP H59.092 Other disorders of the left eye following cataract surgery

SP H59.093 Other disorders of the eye following cataract surgery, bilateral

IQ H59.099 Other disorders of unspecified eye following cataract surgery

5 H59.1 Intraoperative hemorrhage and hematoma of eye and adnexa complicating a procedure
> **EXCLUDES 1** intraoperative hemorrhage and hematoma of eye and adnexa due to accidental puncture or laceration during a procedure (H59.2-)

6 H59.11 Intraoperative hemorrhage and hematoma of eye and adnexa complicating an ophthalmic procedure

SP H59.111 Intraoperative hemorrhage and hematoma of right eye and adnexa complicating an ophthalmic procedure

SP H59.112 Intraoperative hemorrhage and hematoma of left eye and adnexa complicating an ophthalmic procedure

SP H59.113 Intraoperative hemorrhage and hematoma of eye and adnexa complicating an ophthalmic procedure, bilateral

IQ H59.119 Intraoperative hemorrhage and hematoma of unspecified eye and adnexa complicating an ophthalmic procedure

6 H59.12 Intraoperative hemorrhage and hematoma of eye and adnexa complicating other procedure

SP H59.121 Intraoperative hemorrhage and hematoma of right eye and adnexa complicating other procedure

★ New ▲ Revised Px Primary SP PDGM Px SL Low CoM SH High CoM IQ Quest. Encounter H Hospice non-cancer Dx Unspecified M Manifestation

DecisionHealth's FY 2020 Complete Home Health ICD-10-CM Diagnosis Coding Manual

919

⊟ SP **H59.122** Intraoperative hemorrhage and hematoma of left eye and adnexa complicating other procedure

⊟ SP **H59.123** Intraoperative hemorrhage and hematoma of eye and adnexa complicating other procedure, bilateral

⊟ IQ **H59.129** Intraoperative hemorrhage and hematoma of unspecified eye and adnexa complicating other procedure

⑤ **H59.2** Accidental puncture and laceration of eye and adnexa during a procedure

⑥ **H59.21** Accidental puncture and laceration of eye and adnexa during an ophthalmic procedure

⊟ SP **H59.211** Accidental puncture and laceration of right eye and adnexa during an ophthalmic procedure

⊟ SP **H59.212** Accidental puncture and laceration of left eye and adnexa during an ophthalmic procedure

⊟ SP **H59.213** Accidental puncture and laceration of eye and adnexa during an ophthalmic procedure, bilateral

⊟ IQ **H59.219** Accidental puncture and laceration of unspecified eye and adnexa during an ophthalmic procedure

⑥ **H59.22** Accidental puncture and laceration of eye and adnexa during other procedure

⊟ SP **H59.221** Accidental puncture and laceration of right eye and adnexa during other procedure

⊟ SP **H59.222** Accidental puncture and laceration of left eye and adnexa during other procedure

⊟ SP **H59.223** Accidental puncture and laceration of eye and adnexa during other procedure, bilateral

⊟ IQ **H59.229** Accidental puncture and laceration of unspecified eye and adnexa during other procedure

⑤ **H59.3** Postprocedural hemorrhage, hematoma, and seroma of eye and adnexa following a procedure

⑥ **H59.31** Postprocedural hemorrhage of eye and adnexa following an ophthalmic procedure

⊟ SP **H59.311** Postprocedural hemorrhage of right eye and adnexa following an ophthalmic procedure

⊟ SP **H59.312** Postprocedural hemorrhage of left eye and adnexa following an ophthalmic procedure

⊟ SP **H59.313** Postprocedural hemorrhage of eye and adnexa following an ophthalmic procedure, bilateral

⊟ IQ **H59.319** Postprocedural hemorrhage of unspecified eye and adnexa following an ophthalmic procedure

⑥ **H59.32** Postprocedural hemorrhage of eye and adnexa following other procedure

⊟ SP **H59.321** Postprocedural hemorrhage of right eye and adnexa following other procedure

⊟ SP **H59.322** Postprocedural hemorrhage of left eye and adnexa following other procedure

⊟ SP **H59.323** Postprocedural hemorrhage of eye and adnexa following other procedure, bilateral

⊟ IQ **H59.329** Postprocedural hemorrhage of unspecified eye and adnexa following other procedure

⑥ **H59.33** Postprocedural hematoma of eye and adnexa following an ophthalmic procedure

⊟ SP **H59.331** Postprocedural hematoma of right eye and adnexa following an ophthalmic procedure

⊟ SP **H59.332** Postprocedural hematoma of left eye and adnexa following an ophthalmic procedure

⊟ SP **H59.333** Postprocedural hematoma of eye and adnexa following an ophthalmic procedure, bilateral

⊟ IQ **H59.339** Postprocedural hematoma of unspecified eye and adnexa following an ophthalmic procedure

⑥ **H59.34** Postprocedural hematoma of eye and adnexa following other procedure

⊟ SP **H59.341** Postprocedural hematoma of right eye and adnexa following other procedure

⊟ SP **H59.342** Postprocedural hematoma of left eye and adnexa following other procedure

⊟ SP **H59.343** Postprocedural hematoma of eye and adnexa following other procedure, bilateral

⊟ IQ **H59.349** Postprocedural hematoma of unspecified eye and adnexa following other procedure

⑥ **H59.35** Postprocedural seroma of eye and adnexa following an ophthalmic procedure

⊟ SP **H59.351** Postprocedural seroma of right eye and adnexa following an ophthalmic procedure

⊟ SP **H59.352** Postprocedural seroma of left eye and adnexa following an ophthalmic procedure

⊟ SP **H59.353** Postprocedural seroma of eye and adnexa following an ophthalmic procedure, bilateral

⊟ IQ **H59.359** Postprocedural seroma of unspecified eye and adnexa following an ophthalmic procedure

⑥ **H59.36** Postprocedural seroma of eye and adnexa following other procedure

⊟ SP **H59.361** Postprocedural seroma of right eye and adnexa following other procedure

⊟ SP **H59.362** Postprocedural seroma of left eye and adnexa following other procedure

⑷4th digit required   ⑸5th digit required   ⑹6th digit required   ⑺7th digit required   ⑺7th digit placeholder   +Additional code   ⊟Laterality

920   *DecisionHealth's* FY 2020 Complete Home Health ICD-10-CM Diagnosis Coding Manual

⊟ **SP** **H59.363** Postprocedural seroma of eye and adnexa following other procedure, bilateral

⊟ **IQ** **H59.369** Postprocedural seroma of unspecified eye and adnexa following other procedure

5 **H59.4** Inflammation (infection) of postprocedural bleb
Postprocedural blebitis
EXCLUDES 1 filtering (vitreous) bleb after glaucoma surgery status (Z98.83)

SP **H59.40** Inflammation (infection) of postprocedural bleb, unspecified

SP **H59.41** Inflammation (infection) of postprocedural bleb, stage 1

SP **H59.42** Inflammation (infection) of postprocedural bleb, stage 2

SP **H59.43** Inflammation (infection) of postprocedural bleb, stage 3
Bleb endophthalmitis

5 **H59.8** Other intraoperative and postprocedural complications and disorders of eye and adnexa, not elsewhere classified

6 **H59.81** Chorioretinal scars after surgery for detachment

⊟ **SP** **H59.811** Chorioretinal scars after surgery for detachment, right eye

⊟ **SP** **H59.812** Chorioretinal scars after surgery for detachment, left eye

⊟ **SP** **H59.813** Chorioretinal scars after surgery for detachment, bilateral

⊟ **IQ** **H59.819** Chorioretinal scars after surgery for detachment, unspecified eye

SP **H59.88** Other intraoperative complications of eye and adnexa, not elsewhere classified

SP **H59.89** Other postprocedural complications and disorders of eye and adnexa, not elsewhere classified

Chapter 7

H00-H59

★ New ▲ Revised Px Primary **SP** PDGM Px **SL** Low CoM **SH** High CoM **IQ** Quest. Encounter **H** Hospice non-cancer Dx Unspecified **M** *Manifestation*

DecisionHealth's FY 2020 Complete Home Health ICD-10-CM Diagnosis Coding Manual

921

Chapter 7 Scenarios: Diseases of the eye and adnexa (H00-H59)

Coronary artery bypass graft, glaucoma

An 82-year-old male patient is admitted to home health following surgery for a first-time coronary bypass graft x2 with a history of coronary artery disease. The patient is legally blind due to severe stage open angle glaucoma in both eyes and was recently diagnosed with generalized anxiety disorder. He has a 24-hour caregiver that assists with ADL/IADLs; however, she is not comfortable with managing his surgical site and cardiac status. The physician ordered skilled nursing to assess/monitor the patient's cardiac status and to perform surgical dressing changes.

Description	Code
Primary: Encounter for surgical aftercare following surgery on the circulatory system	Z48.812
Secondary: Atherosclerotic heart disease of native coronary artery without angina pectoris	I25.10
Secondary: Unspecified open-angle glaucoma, severe stage	H40.10x3
Secondary: Legal blindness, as defined in USA	H54.8
Secondary: Generalized anxiety disorder	F41.1
Secondary: Presence of aortocoronary bypass graft	Z95.1

As the focus of care, surgical aftercare is coded primary. The combination code H40.10x3 covers both the type and stage of the patient's glaucoma, which is severe stage unspecified open-angle glaucoma that is occurring in both eyes. "When a patient has bilateral glaucoma and both eyes are documented as being the same type and stage, and the classification does not provide a code for bilateral glaucoma (i.e. subcategories H40.10, and H40.20) report only one code for the type of glaucoma with the appropriate seventh character for the stage," according to coding guidelines. In accordance with tabular instruction, the underlying cause of the blindness (the glaucoma) is coded before the blindness itself. Though coronary artery bypass graft surgery treats the coronary artery disease, it does not resolve it. Therefore, the condition is still coded.

Senile cataracts

An elderly female patient is admitted to home health for teaching and training for a new diagnosis of type 2 diabetes. She does not have any identified manifestations of diabetes and is taking oral medications only. She also has had cortical senile cataracts in both eyes for years but has not had any surgical intervention for them. The cataracts are unrelated to the patient's diabetes. They impact her ability to accurately manage her medications and disease process.

Description	Code
Primary: Type 2 diabetes mellitus without complications	E11.9
Secondary: Cortical age-related cataract, bilateral	H25.013

The patient's cataracts are specified as cortical senile cataracts. In ICD-10 senile cataracts are defined as age-related cataracts. Therefore, H25.013 is the most appropriate code to capture this condition. Though "cataract" appears under the subterm "with" in the alphabetic index "diabetes" listing, they're not related to her diabetes so the "with" convention does not apply and the conditions are coded separately.

Diabetic retinopathy, blindness and low vision

A 73-year-old woman has type 2 diabetes that is out of control and has been started on insulin. She has been found to have proliferative diabetic retinopathy in both eyes. The disease had led to macular edema in her left eye. She is now blind in that eye and has low vision in her right eye. The blindness in her left eye is documented as category 3 and the low vision in her right eye is documented as category 2. She also has hypertension. The focus of the admission is skilled nursing care to teach her how to use insulin to better control her diabetes and for occupational therapy for help completing ADLs/IADLs with her vision deficit.

Description	Code
Primary: Type 2 diabetes mellitus with hyperglycemia	E11.65
Secondary: Type 2 diabetes mellitus with proliferative diabetic retinopathy with macular edema, left eye	E11.3512
Secondary: Type 2 diabetes mellitus with proliferative diabetic retinopathy without macular edema, right eye	E11.3591
Secondary: Low vision right eye category 2, blindness left eye category 3	H54.1223
Secondary: Essential (primary) hypertension	I10
Secondary: Long term (current) use of insulin	Z79.4

Since the focus of care is teaching about insulin use and getting the out of control diabetes under better control, diabetes with hyperglycemia is coded in the primary position. Out of control diabetes codes to diabetes with hyperglycemia, according to the alphabetic index. She also has proliferative diabetic retinopathy in both eyes, and it's caused macular edema in her left eye. Two codes are used to capture the condition's different severity in each eye. Code H54.1223 is assigned to indicate that she's blind in her left eye (documented as category 3) and has low vision in her right (documented as category 2). Hypertension is coded as a relevant comorbidity and her use of insulin, as a non-type 1 diabetic, must be captured with Z79.4.

Diabetic glaucoma

A 63-year-old woman was recently started on an insulin regimen for her type 2 diabetes. She also has diabetic glaucoma, which has left her legally blind.

Description	Code
Primary: Type 2 diabetes mellitus with other diabetic ophthalmic complication	E11.39
Secondary: Glaucoma in diseases classified elsewhere	H42
Secondary: Legal blindness, as defined in USA	H54.8
Secondary: Long term (current) use of insulin	Z79.4

There is no assumed relationship between diabetes and glaucoma. However, a link has been specified in this scenario. The code for glaucoma caused by diabetes, H42, is a manifestation code and cannot be assigned without a preceding etiology. Therefore, E11.39 must be coded immediately before H42. Note the "code first" note at the H54.- category level, instructing the code to first code the underlying cause of the blindness. Since the patient uses insulin but is not a type 2 diabetic, Z79.4 must be assigned.

HOME HEALTH CODING SCENARIOS

Chapter 8: Diseases of the Ear and Mastoid Process (H60-H95)

Chapter 8 includes codes for diseases of the external ear, middle ear and mastoid, internal ear, other disorders of the ear, and intraoperative and postprocedural complications and disorders of the ear and mastoid process, not elsewhere classified.

There is a note at the beginning of this chapter to use an external cause code following the code for the ear condition, if applicable, to identify the cause of the ear condition. Following the note, there is an Excludes 2 note for chapter 8 codes that defines code categories that are not included in the chapter 8 codes, but could be coded in addition to the chapter 8 code if applicable. These include:

- Certain conditions originating in the perinatal period (P00-P96) located in chapter 16.

- Certain infections and parasitic diseases (A00-B99) located in chapter 1.

- Complications of pregnancy, childbirth and the puerperium (O00 –O9A) located in chapter 15.

- Congenital malformations, deformations and chromosomal abnormalities (Q00-Q99) in chapter 17.

- Endocrine, nutritional and metabolic diseases (E00-E88) in chapter 4.

- Injury, poisoning and certain other consequences of external causes (S00-T88) located in chapter 19.

- Neoplasms (C00-D49) in chapter 2.

- Symptoms, signs and abnormal clinical and laboratory findings (R00-R94) located in chapter 18.

To select the appropriate code, it is important to understand the basic anatomy and physiology of the ear and mastoid process. The ear is divided into three sections: the external, middle and inner ear. The outer and middle ear is strictly involved in hearing and sound wave conduction while the inner ear structures function for both hearing and balance, or equilibrium. The external ear canal leads to the structures inside and is surrounded and protected by cranial bones. The opening of the canal, called the external auditory meatus, opens into the middle ear and lies directly above the mastoid process. The mastoid process is the cone-shaped bony prominence that projects from the undersurface of the temporal bone behind the ear. The tissue structure within the mastoid process also aids the hearing function by promoting conductivity of sound between the external and middle ear.

The external ear is made up of the auricle (pinna), which is the visible portion of the ear and the external auditory canal, which is the tube that leads from the outside environment to the middle portion of the ear and the ear drum. Its main function is to act as the conduit into the auditory receptors located within the ear and to amplify incoming sound waves. The second major function of the external ear is self-cleaning and protection of the tympanic membrane and middle and inner ear structures by providing a physical barrier against moisture, microorganisms, foreign bodies and direct injury.

The middle ear is made up of the tympanic cavity within the temporal bone that is filled with air from the nasopharynx through the auditory tube. It contains three tiny bones called ossicles (malleus, incus and the stirrup) that transmit vibration from the tympanic membrane across the middle ear to the inner ear.

The tympanic membrane functions to transmit sound conducted down the ear canal to the ossicles. Perforations of the ear drum are caused by foreign objects stuck in the ear, waves of external pressure from explosions or a slap to the ear, and infections causing internal pressure.

Damage to the middle ear structures affects the ear's ability to conduct sound to the inner ear and results in conductive hearing loss.

The ossicles transmit and amplify sound. Damage to the middle ear also affects the ear's ability to conduct sound towards the inner ear and results in conductive hearing loss.

The Eustachian tube maintains still air in the middle ear to allow the ossicles to function at optimum level and also serves as a drain to carry mucous or bacterial accumulation out of the middle ear to the throat. The shape and size of the Eustachian tube is different in children than adults. The horizontal orientation of the tube in children results in earaches and infections in the middle ear, especially in children under seven years of age. Obstruction of the tube results in hearing impairment, pain and infections.

The middle ear is comprised of a series of bony labyrinths that are lined with periosteum and filled with fluid. The labyrinthine network is made up of the semicircular canals, the vestibule (responsible for balance and equilibrium) and the cochlea which is embedded in the mastoid (responsible for hearing).

Chapter 8

H60 - H95

Common infections

Common infections of the ear and mastoid include: **serous otitis media** (fluid in the inner ear as a result of dysfunction of the Eustachian tube**); suppurative otitis media** (infection of the fluid trapped in the middle ear); **mastoiditis** (infection of the air-filled spaces in the mastoid area and even infects the mastoid bone itself); **otitis externa** (infection of the outer auditory canal); and **myringitis** (infection or inflammation of tympanic membrane).

Neoplasms

There also are several possible neoplasms of the ear and mastoid including:

- **Malignant basal cell or squamous cell tumors** of the external ear most commonly in areas exposed to sun, and most commonly found in the elderly and in fair skinned people.

- Benign tumors: **cholesteatomas**, which are most common in middle ear and external ear canal and can eat into the tiny bones of the ossicular chain or erode the bone separating the middle ear cavity from the mastoid area or brain, and cause deafness, nerve destruction, vertigo and infection risk; **acoustic neuromas** are intracranial tumors on vestibulocochlear branch of 8th cranial nerve near the inner ear where the nerve enters the brain. They are also called schwannomas or glomus tumors, which are highly vascularized masses behind the eardrum that can grow into the mastoid or bony wall or wrap around facial nerves, jugular vein, carotid artery and even invade the brain.

Hearing loss

Hearing loss is coded to category H90 in chapter 8 and includes specific codes for

- conductive and sensorineural hearing loss (largest subcategory of hearing loss codes)

- ototoxic hearing loss

- presbycusis

- sudden idiopathic hearing loss

- other hearing loss

- unspecified hearing loss

Other diseases of ear and mastoid

Other diseases and disorders of ear and mastoid include: **non-infective otitis externa; acquired stenosis; impacted cerumen, tympanosclerosis** (thickening and hardening of tympanic membrane); **adhesive middle ear disease; meniere's disease** (abnormality of inner ear thought to be associated with increased fluid causing swelling and rupture of the membranous labyrinth resulting in unpredictable attacks of vertigo, tinnitus, hearing loss, and/or ear pain/pressure); **vertigo** (many types from severe dizziness/equilibrium dysfunction resulting in a sense that the person or their surroundings are spinning/whirling when there is no motion). *Important note:* Most cases of dizziness are not vertigo and are coded as a symptom, while specific types of vertigo are coded from chapter 8 and not as symptoms.

Otosclerosis is a progressive disease causing abnormal growth of bone of the middle ear that can affect all of the ossicles.

Chapter 8 also includes intraoperative and **postprocedural** codes related to hemorrhage and hematoma; accidental puncture and laceration; stenosis of the ear canal; and other complications and disorders of the ear and mastoid process, not elsewhere classified.

Note: Many of the codes in chapter 8 have laterality designations for greater specificity. As in all coding, the specific codes must be documented or confirmed with the physician.

CHAPTER 8: DISEASES OF THE EAR AND MASTOID PROCESS (H60-H95)

Note:
Use an external cause code following the code for the ear condition, if applicable, to identify the cause of the ear condition

EXCLUDES 2 certain conditions originating in the perinatal period (P04-P96)
certain infectious and parasitic diseases (A00-B99)
complications of pregnancy, childbirth and the puerperium (O00-O9A)
congenital malformations, deformations and chromosomal abnormalities (Q00-Q99)
endocrine, nutritional and metabolic diseases (E00-E88)
injury, poisoning and certain other consequences of external causes (S00-T88)
neoplasms (C00-D49)
symptoms, signs and abnormal clinical and laboratory findings, not elsewhere classified (R00-R94)

This chapter contains the following blocks:
H60-H62   Diseases of external ear
H65-H75   Diseases of middle ear and mastoid
H80-H83   Diseases of inner ear
H90-H94   Other disorders of ear
H95   Intraoperative and postprocedural complications and disorders of ear and mastoid process, not elsewhere classified

Diseases of external ear   (H60-H62)

H60   Otitis externa

H60.0   Abscess of external ear
Boil of external ear
Carbuncle of auricle or external auditory canal
Furuncle of external ear

H60.00   Abscess of external ear, unspecified ear

H60.01   Abscess of right external ear

H60.02   Abscess of left external ear

H60.03   Abscess of external ear, bilateral

H60.1   Cellulitis of external ear
Cellulitis of auricle
Cellulitis of external auditory canal

H60.10   Cellulitis of external ear, unspecified ear

H60.11   Cellulitis of right external ear

H60.12   Cellulitis of left external ear

H60.13   Cellulitis of external ear, bilateral

H60.2   Malignant otitis externa

H60.20   Malignant otitis externa, unspecified ear

H60.21   Malignant otitis externa, right ear

H60.22   Malignant otitis externa, left ear

H60.23   Malignant otitis externa, bilateral

H60.3   Other infective otitis externa

H60.31   Diffuse otitis externa

H60.311   Diffuse otitis externa, right ear

H60.312   Diffuse otitis externa, left ear

H60.313   Diffuse otitis externa, bilateral

H60.319   Diffuse otitis externa, unspecified ear

H60.32   Hemorrhagic otitis externa

H60.321   Hemorrhagic otitis externa, right ear

H60.322   Hemorrhagic otitis externa, left ear

H60.323   Hemorrhagic otitis externa, bilateral

H60.329   Hemorrhagic otitis externa, unspecified ear

H60.33   Swimmer's ear

H60.331   Swimmer's ear, right ear

H60.332   Swimmer's ear, left ear

H60.333   Swimmer's ear, bilateral

H60.339   Swimmer's ear, unspecified ear

H60.39   Other infective otitis externa

H60.391   Other infective otitis externa, right ear

H60.392   Other infective otitis externa, left ear

H60.393   Other infective otitis externa, bilateral

H60.399   Other infective otitis externa, unspecified ear

H60.4   Cholesteatoma of external ear
Keratosis obturans of external ear (canal)
EXCLUDES 2 cholesteatoma of middle ear (H71.-)
recurrent cholesteatoma of postmastoidectomy cavity (H95.0-)

H60.40   Cholesteatoma of external ear, unspecified ear

H60.41   Cholesteatoma of right external ear

H60.42   Cholesteatoma of left external ear

H60.43   Cholesteatoma of external ear, bilateral

H60.5   Acute noninfective otitis externa

H60.50   Unspecified acute noninfective otitis externa
Acute otitis externa NOS

H60.501   Unspecified acute noninfective otitis externa, right ear

H60.502   Unspecified acute noninfective otitis externa, left ear

H60.503   Unspecified acute noninfective otitis externa, bilateral

H60.509   Unspecified acute noninfective otitis externa, unspecified ear

H60.51   Acute actinic otitis externa

H60.511   Acute actinic otitis externa, right ear

H60.512   Acute actinic otitis externa, left ear

H60.513   Acute actinic otitis externa, bilateral

H60.519   Acute actinic otitis externa, unspecified ear

H60.52   Acute chemical otitis externa

H60.521   Acute chemical otitis externa, right ear

H60.522   Acute chemical otitis externa, left ear

★ New ▲ Revised Px Primary **SP** PDGM Px **SL** Low CoM **SH** High CoM **IQ** Quest. Encounter **H** Hospice non-cancer Dx **Unspecified** **M** *Manifestation*

☐ **SP** **H60.523** Acute chemical otitis externa, bilateral

☐ **IQ** **H60.529** Acute chemical otitis externa, unspecified ear

⑥ **H60.53** Acute contact otitis externa

☐ **SP** **H60.531** Acute contact otitis externa, right ear

☐ **SP** **H60.532** Acute contact otitis externa, left ear

☐ **SP** **H60.533** Acute contact otitis externa, bilateral

☐ **IQ** **H60.539** Acute contact otitis externa, unspecified ear

⑥ **H60.54** Acute eczematoid otitis externa

☐ **SP** **H60.541** Acute eczematoid otitis externa, right ear

☐ **SP** **H60.542** Acute eczematoid otitis externa, left ear

☐ **SP** **H60.543** Acute eczematoid otitis externa, bilateral

☐ **IQ** **H60.549** Acute eczematoid otitis externa, unspecified ear

⑥ **H60.55** Acute reactive otitis externa

☐ **SP** **H60.551** Acute reactive otitis externa, right ear

☐ **SP** **H60.552** Acute reactive otitis externa, left ear

☐ **SP** **H60.553** Acute reactive otitis externa, bilateral

☐ **IQ** **H60.559** Acute reactive otitis externa, unspecified ear

⑥ **H60.59** Other noninfective acute otitis externa

☐ **SP** **H60.591** Other noninfective acute otitis externa, right ear

☐ **SP** **H60.592** Other noninfective acute otitis externa, left ear

☐ **SP** **H60.593** Other noninfective acute otitis externa, bilateral

☐ **IQ** **H60.599** Other noninfective acute otitis externa, unspecified ear

⑤ **H60.6** Unspecified chronic otitis externa

☐ **IQ** **H60.60** Unspecified chronic otitis externa, unspecified ear

☐ **SP** **H60.61** Unspecified chronic otitis externa, right ear

☐ **SP** **H60.62** Unspecified chronic otitis externa, left ear

☐ **SP** **H60.63** Unspecified chronic otitis externa, bilateral

⑤ **H60.8** Other otitis externa

⑥ **H60.8X** Other otitis externa

☐ **SP** **H60.8X1** Other otitis externa, right ear

☐ **SP** **H60.8X2** Other otitis externa, left ear

☐ **SP** **H60.8X3** Other otitis externa, bilateral

☐ **IQ** **H60.8X9** Other otitis externa, unspecified ear

⑤ **H60.9** Unspecified otitis externa

☐ **IQ** **H60.90** Unspecified otitis externa, unspecified ear

☐ **SP** **H60.91** Unspecified otitis externa, right ear

☐ **SP** **H60.92** Unspecified otitis externa, left ear

☐ **SP** **H60.93** Unspecified otitis externa, bilateral

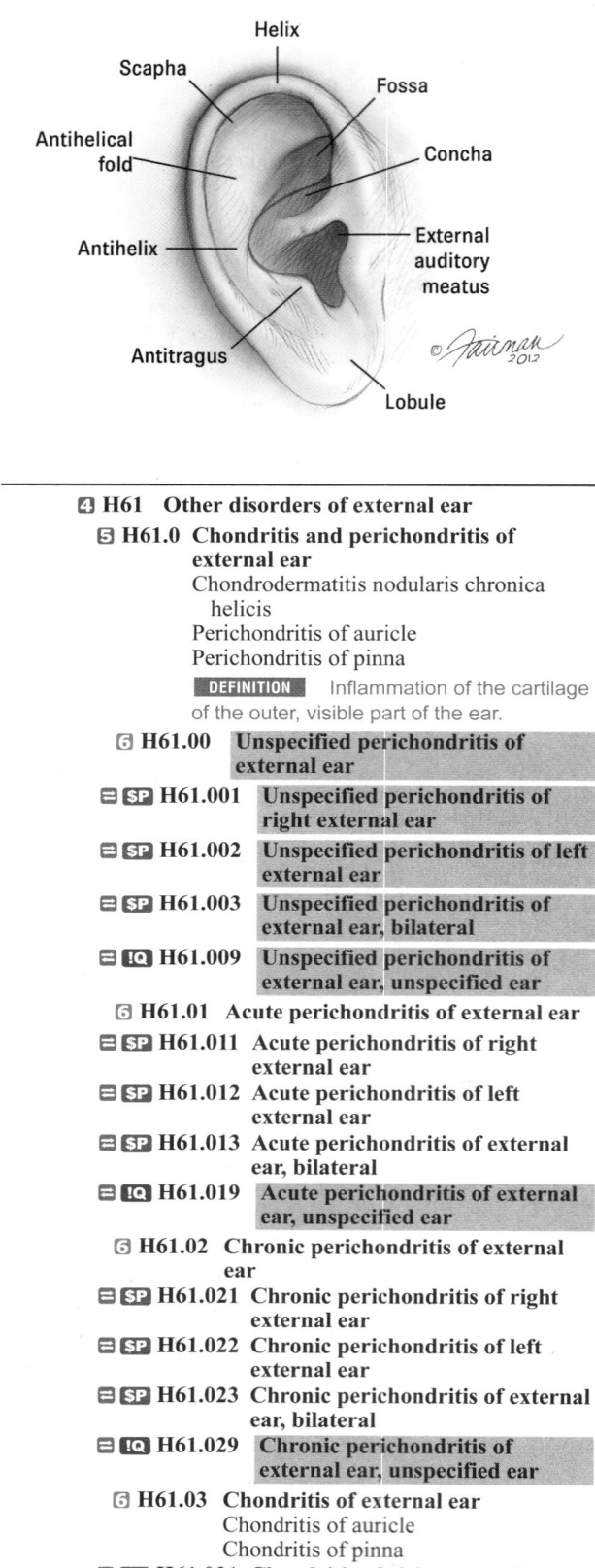

Helix
Scapha
Fossa
Antihelical fold
Concha
Antihelix
External auditory meatus
Antitragus
Lobule

④ **H61** Other disorders of external ear

⑤ **H61.0** Chondritis and perichondritis of external ear
Chondrodermatitis nodularis chronica helicis
Perichondritis of auricle
Perichondritis of pinna
DEFINITION Inflammation of the cartilage of the outer, visible part of the ear.

⑥ **H61.00** Unspecified perichondritis of external ear

☐ **SP** **H61.001** Unspecified perichondritis of right external ear

☐ **SP** **H61.002** Unspecified perichondritis of left external ear

☐ **SP** **H61.003** Unspecified perichondritis of external ear, bilateral

☐ **IQ** **H61.009** Unspecified perichondritis of external ear, unspecified ear

⑥ **H61.01** Acute perichondritis of external ear

☐ **SP** **H61.011** Acute perichondritis of right external ear

☐ **SP** **H61.012** Acute perichondritis of left external ear

☐ **SP** **H61.013** Acute perichondritis of external ear, bilateral

☐ **IQ** **H61.019** Acute perichondritis of external ear, unspecified ear

⑥ **H61.02** Chronic perichondritis of external ear

☐ **SP** **H61.021** Chronic perichondritis of right external ear

☐ **SP** **H61.022** Chronic perichondritis of left external ear

☐ **SP** **H61.023** Chronic perichondritis of external ear, bilateral

☐ **IQ** **H61.029** Chronic perichondritis of external ear, unspecified ear

⑥ **H61.03** Chondritis of external ear
Chondritis of auricle
Chondritis of pinna

☐ **SP** **H61.031** Chondritis of right external ear

☐ **SP** **H61.032** Chondritis of left external ear

Chapter 8

H60-H95

④4th digit required ⑤5th digit required ⑥6th digit required ⑦7th digit required ⑦7th digit placeholder ✛Additional code ☐Laterality

⊟ SP **H61.033** **Chondritis of external ear, bilateral**

⊟ IQ **H61.039** **Chondritis of external ear, unspecified ear**

⑤ **H61.1** **Noninfective disorders of pinna**
  EXCLUDES 2 cauliflower ear (M95.1-)
  gouty tophi of ear (M1A.-)

⑥ **H61.10** **Unspecified noninfective disorders of pinna**
  Disorder of pinna NOS

⊟ SP **H61.101** **Unspecified noninfective disorders of pinna, right ear**

⊟ SP **H61.102** **Unspecified noninfective disorders of pinna, left ear**

⊟ SP **H61.103** **Unspecified noninfective disorders of pinna, bilateral**

⊟ IQ **H61.109** **Unspecified noninfective disorders of pinna, unspecified ear**

⑥ **H61.11** **Acquired deformity of pinna**
  Acquired deformity of auricle
  EXCLUDES 2 cauliflower ear (M95.1-)

⊟ SP **H61.111** **Acquired deformity of pinna, right ear**

⊟ SP **H61.112** **Acquired deformity of pinna, left ear**

⊟ SP **H61.113** **Acquired deformity of pinna, bilateral**

⊟ IQ **H61.119** **Acquired deformity of pinna, unspecified ear**

⑥ **H61.12** **Hematoma of pinna**
  Hematoma of auricle
  DEFINITION Swelling filled with blood on the outer ear.

⊟ SP **H61.121** **Hematoma of pinna, right ear**

⊟ SP **H61.122** **Hematoma of pinna, left ear**

⊟ SP **H61.123** **Hematoma of pinna, bilateral**

⊟ IQ **H61.129** **Hematoma of pinna, unspecified ear**

⑥ **H61.19** **Other noninfective disorders of pinna**

⊟ SP **H61.191** **Noninfective disorders of pinna, right ear**

⊟ SP **H61.192** **Noninfective disorders of pinna, left ear**

⊟ SP **H61.193** **Noninfective disorders of pinna, bilateral**

⊟ IQ **H61.199** **Noninfective disorders of pinna, unspecified ear**

⑤ **H61.2** **Impacted cerumen**
  Wax in ear
  DEFINITION Ear wax blocking the external ear canal.

⊟ IQ **H61.20** **Impacted cerumen, unspecified ear**

⊟ SP **H61.21** **Impacted cerumen, right ear**

⊟ SP **H61.22** **Impacted cerumen, left ear**

⊟ SP **H61.23** **Impacted cerumen, bilateral**

⑤ **H61.3** **Acquired stenosis of external ear canal**
  Collapse of external ear canal
  EXCLUDES 1 postprocedural stenosis of external ear canal (H95.81-)

⑥ **H61.30** **Acquired stenosis of external ear canal, unspecified**

⊟ SP **H61.301** **Acquired stenosis of right external ear canal, unspecified**

⊟ SP **H61.302** **Acquired stenosis of left external ear canal, unspecified**

⊟ SP **H61.303** **Acquired stenosis of external ear canal, unspecified, bilateral**

⊟ IQ **H61.309** **Acquired stenosis of external ear canal, unspecified, unspecified ear**

⑥ **H61.31** **Acquired stenosis of external ear canal secondary to trauma**

⊟ SP **H61.311** **Acquired stenosis of right external ear canal secondary to trauma**

⊟ SP **H61.312** **Acquired stenosis of left external ear canal secondary to trauma**

⊟ SP **H61.313** **Acquired stenosis of external ear canal secondary to trauma, bilateral**

⊟ IQ **H61.319** **Acquired stenosis of external ear canal secondary to trauma, unspecified ear**

⑥ **H61.32** **Acquired stenosis of external ear canal secondary to inflammation and infection**

⊟ SP **H61.321** **Acquired stenosis of right external ear canal secondary to inflammation and infection**

⊟ SP **H61.322** **Acquired stenosis of left external ear canal secondary to inflammation and infection**

⊟ SP **H61.323** **Acquired stenosis of external ear canal secondary to inflammation and infection, bilateral**

⊟ IQ **H61.329** **Acquired stenosis of external ear canal secondary to inflammation and infection, unspecified ear**

⑥ **H61.39** **Other acquired stenosis of external ear canal**

⊟ SP **H61.391** **Other acquired stenosis of right external ear canal**

⊟ SP **H61.392** **Other acquired stenosis of left external ear canal**

⊟ SP **H61.393** **Other acquired stenosis of external ear canal, bilateral**

⊟ IQ **H61.399** **Other acquired stenosis of external ear canal, unspecified ear**

⑤ **H61.8** **Other specified disorders of external ear**

⑥ **H61.81** **Exostosis of external canal**
  DEFINITION A bony growth covered with cartilage on the outer ear.

⊟ SP **H61.811** **Exostosis of right external canal**

⊟ SP **H61.812** **Exostosis of left external canal**

⊟ SP **H61.813** **Exostosis of external canal, bilateral**

⊟ IQ **H61.819** **Exostosis of external canal, unspecified ear**

⑥ **H61.89** **Other specified disorders of external ear**

⊟ SP **H61.891** **Other specified disorders of right external ear**

⊟ SP **H61.892** **Other specified disorders of left external ear**

⊟ SP **H61.893** **Other specified disorders of external ear, bilateral**

Chapter 8

H60-H95

★ New ▲ Revised Px Primary SP PDGM Px SL Low CoM SH High CoM IQ Quest. Encounter H Hospice non-cancer Dx Unspecified M *Manifestation*

DecisionHealth's FY 2020 Complete Home Health ICD-10-CM Diagnosis Coding Manual   929

☐ IQ H61.899 Other specified disorders of external ear, unspecified ear

⑤ H61.9 Disorder of external ear, unspecified

☐ IQ H61.90 Disorder of external ear, unspecified, unspecified ear

☐ IQ H61.91 Disorder of right external ear, unspecified

☐ IQ H61.92 Disorder of left external ear, unspecified

☐ IQ H61.93 Disorder of external ear, unspecified, bilateral

④ H62 Disorders of external ear in diseases classified elsewhere

⑤ H62.4 Otitis externa in other diseases classified elsewhere

Code first underlying disease, such as:
erysipelas (A46)
impetigo (L01.0)
EXCLUDES 1 otitis externa (in):
candidiasis (B37.84)
herpes viral [herpes simplex] (B00.1)
herpes zoster (B02.8)

M ☐ IQ H62.40 *Otitis externa in other diseases classified elsewhere, unspecified ear*

M ☐ IQ H62.41 *Otitis externa in other diseases classified elsewhere, right ear*

M ☐ IQ H62.42 *Otitis externa in other diseases classified elsewhere, left ear*

M ☐ IQ H62.43 *Otitis externa in other diseases classified elsewhere, bilateral*

⑤ H62.8 Other disorders of external ear in diseases classified elsewhere

Code first underlying disease, such as:
gout (M1A.-, M10.-)

⑥ H62.8X Other disorders of external ear in diseases classified elsewhere

☐ IQ H62.8X1 Other disorders of right external ear in diseases classified elsewhere

☐ IQ H62.8X2 Other disorders of left external ear in diseases classified elsewhere

☐ IQ H62.8X3 Other disorders of external ear in diseases classified elsewhere, bilateral

☐ IQ H62.8X9 Other disorders of external ear in diseases classified elsewhere, unspecified ear

---

Diseases of middle ear and mastoid (H65-H75)

▲ + ④ H65 Nonsuppurative otitis media
INCLUDES nonsuppurative otitis media with myringitis
Use additional code for any associated perforated tympanic membrane (H72.-)
Use additional code, if applicable, to identify:
exposure to environmental tobacco smoke (Z77.22)
exposure to tobacco smoke in the perinatal period (P96.81)
history of tobacco dependence (Z87.891)
infectious agent (B95-B97)
occupational exposure to environmental tobacco smoke (Z57.31)
tobacco dependence (F17.-)
tobacco use (Z72.0)

+ ⑤ H65.0 Acute serous otitis media
Acute and subacute secretory otitis

☐ IQ + H65.00 Acute serous otitis media, unspecified ear

☐ SP + H65.01 Acute serous otitis media, right ear

☐ SP + H65.02 Acute serous otitis media, left ear

☐ SP + H65.03 Acute serous otitis media, bilateral

☐ SP + H65.04 Acute serous otitis media, recurrent, right ear

☐ SP + H65.05 Acute serous otitis media, recurrent, left ear

☐ SP + H65.06 Acute serous otitis media, recurrent, bilateral

☐ IQ + H65.07 Acute serous otitis media, recurrent, unspecified ear

+ ⑤ H65.1 Other acute nonsuppurative otitis media
EXCLUDES 1 otitic barotrauma (T70.0)
otitis media (acute) NOS (H66.9)

+ ⑥ H65.11 Acute and subacute allergic otitis media (mucoid) (sanguinous) (serous)

☐ SP + H65.111 Acute and subacute allergic otitis media (mucoid) (sanguinous) (serous), right ear

☐ SP + H65.112 Acute and subacute allergic otitis media (mucoid) (sanguinous) (serous), left ear

☐ SP + H65.113 Acute and subacute allergic otitis media (mucoid) (sanguinous) (serous), bilateral

☐ SP + H65.114 Acute and subacute allergic otitis media (mucoid) (sanguinous) (serous), recurrent, right ear

☐ SP + H65.115 Acute and subacute allergic otitis media (mucoid) (sanguinous) (serous), recurrent, left ear

☐ SP + H65.116 Acute and subacute allergic otitis media (mucoid) (sanguinous) (serous), recurrent, bilateral

☐ IQ + H65.117 Acute and subacute allergic otitis media (mucoid) (sanguinous) (serous), recurrent, unspecified ear

☐ IQ + H65.119 Acute and subacute allergic otitis media (mucoid) (sanguinous) (serous), unspecified ear

+ ⑥ H65.19 Other acute nonsuppurative otitis media
Acute and subacute mucoid otitis media
Acute and subacute nonsuppurative otitis media NOS
Acute and subacute sanguinous otitis media
Acute and subacute seromucinous otitis media

☐ SP + H65.191 Other acute nonsuppurative otitis media, right ear

☐ SP + H65.192 Other acute nonsuppurative otitis media, left ear

☐ SP + H65.193 Other acute nonsuppurative otitis media, bilateral

☐ SP + H65.194 Other acute nonsuppurative otitis media, recurrent, right ear

☐ SP + H65.195 Other acute nonsuppurative otitis media, recurrent, left ear

Chapter 8

H60-H95

---

④4th digit required   ⑤5th digit required   ⑥6th digit required   ⑦7th digit required   ☒7th digit placeholder   +Additional code   ☐Laterality

☐ **SP** ✚ **H65.196** Other acute nonsuppurative otitis media, recurrent, bilateral

☐ **IQ** ✚ **H65.197** Other acute nonsuppurative otitis media recurrent, unspecified ear

☐ **IQ** ✚ **H65.199** Other acute nonsuppurative otitis media, unspecified ear

✚ **5** **H65.2** Chronic serous otitis media
Chronic tubotympanal catarrh

☐ **IQ** ✚ **H65.20** Chronic serous otitis media, unspecified ear

☐ **SP** ✚ **H65.21** Chronic serous otitis media, right ear

☐ **SP** ✚ **H65.22** Chronic serous otitis media, left ear

☐ **SP** ✚ **H65.23** Chronic serous otitis media, bilateral

✚ **5** **H65.3** Chronic mucoid otitis media
Chronic mucinous otitis media
Chronic secretory otitis media
Chronic transudative otitis media
Glue ear

> **EXCLUDES 1** adhesive middle ear disease (H74.1)

> **DEFINITION** Long-term middle ear infection causing mucous to become trapped in the middle ear.

☐ **IQ** ✚ **H65.30** Chronic mucoid otitis media, unspecified ear

☐ **SP** ✚ **H65.31** Chronic mucoid otitis media, right ear

☐ **SP** ✚ **H65.32** Chronic mucoid otitis media, left ear

☐ **SP** ✚ **H65.33** Chronic mucoid otitis media, bilateral

✚ **5** **H65.4** Other chronic nonsuppurative otitis media

✚ **6** **H65.41** Chronic allergic otitis media

☐ **SP** ✚ **H65.411** Chronic allergic otitis media, right ear

☐ **SP** ✚ **H65.412** Chronic allergic otitis media, left ear

☐ **SP** ✚ **H65.413** Chronic allergic otitis media, bilateral

☐ **IQ** ✚ **H65.419** Chronic allergic otitis media, unspecified ear

✚ **6** **H65.49** Other chronic nonsuppurative otitis media
Chronic exudative otitis media
Chronic nonsuppurative otitis media NOS
Chronic otitis media with effusion (nonpurulent)
Chronic seromucinous otitis media

☐ **SP** ✚ **H65.491** Other chronic nonsuppurative otitis media, right ear

☐ **SP** ✚ **H65.492** Other chronic nonsuppurative otitis media, left ear

☐ **SP** ✚ **H65.493** Other chronic nonsuppurative otitis media, bilateral

☐ **IQ** ✚ **H65.499** Other chronic nonsuppurative otitis media, unspecified ear

✚ **5** **H65.9** Unspecified nonsuppurative otitis media
Allergic otitis media NOS
Catarrhal otitis media NOS
Exudative otitis media NOS
Mucoid otitis media NOS
Otitis media with effusion (nonpurulent) NOS

Secretory otitis media NOS
Seromucinous otitis media NOS
Serous otitis media NOS
Transudative otitis media NOS

☐ **IQ** ✚ **H65.90** Unspecified nonsuppurative otitis media, unspecified ear

☐ **SP** ✚ **H65.91** Unspecified nonsuppurative otitis media, right ear

☐ **SP** ✚ **H65.92** Unspecified nonsuppurative otitis media, left ear

☐ **SP** ✚ **H65.93** Unspecified nonsuppurative otitis media, bilateral

✚ **4** **H66** Suppurative and unspecified otitis media

> **INCLUDES** suppurative and unspecified otitis media with myringitis

Use additional code to identify:
exposure to environmental tobacco smoke (Z77.22)
exposure to tobacco smoke in the perinatal period (P96.81)
history of tobacco dependence (Z87.891)
occupational exposure to environmental tobacco smoke (Z57.31)
tobacco dependence (F17.-)
tobacco use (Z72.0)

✚ **5** **H66.0** Acute suppurative otitis media

✚ **6** **H66.00** Acute suppurative otitis media without spontaneous rupture of ear drum

☐ **SP** ✚ **H66.001** Acute suppurative otitis media without spontaneous rupture of ear drum, right ear

☐ **SP** ✚ **H66.002** Acute suppurative otitis media without spontaneous rupture of ear drum, left ear

☐ **SP** ✚ **H66.003** Acute suppurative otitis media without spontaneous rupture of ear drum, bilateral

☐ **SP** ✚ **H66.004** Acute suppurative otitis media without spontaneous rupture of ear drum, recurrent, right ear

☐ **SP** ✚ **H66.005** Acute suppurative otitis media without spontaneous rupture of ear drum, recurrent, left ear

☐ **SP** ✚ **H66.006** Acute suppurative otitis media without spontaneous rupture of ear drum, recurrent, bilateral

☐ **IQ** ✚ **H66.007** Acute suppurative otitis media without spontaneous rupture of ear drum, recurrent, unspecified ear

☐ **IQ** ✚ **H66.009** Acute suppurative otitis media without spontaneous rupture of ear drum, unspecified ear

✚ **6** **H66.01** Acute suppurative otitis media with spontaneous rupture of ear drum

☐ **SP** ✚ **H66.011** Acute suppurative otitis media with spontaneous rupture of ear drum, right ear

☐ **SP** ✚ **H66.012** Acute suppurative otitis media with spontaneous rupture of ear drum, left ear

☐ **SP** ✚ **H66.013** Acute suppurative otitis media with spontaneous rupture of ear drum, bilateral

★ New ▲ Revised Px Primary **SP** PDGM Px **SL** Low CoM **SH** High CoM **IQ** Quest. Encounter **H** Hospice non-cancer Dx   Unspecified   **M** *Manifestation*

DecisionHealth's FY 2020 Complete Home Health ICD-10-CM Diagnosis Coding Manual

931

Chapter 8

H60-H95

⊟ SP ✚ **H66.014** Acute suppurative otitis media with spontaneous rupture of ear drum, recurrent, right ear

⊟ SP ✚ **H66.015** Acute suppurative otitis media with spontaneous rupture of ear drum, recurrent, left ear

⊟ SP ✚ **H66.016** Acute suppurative otitis media with spontaneous rupture of ear drum, recurrent, bilateral

⊟ !Q ✚ **H66.017** Acute suppurative otitis media with spontaneous rupture of ear drum, recurrent, unspecified ear

⊟ !Q ✚ **H66.019** Acute suppurative otitis media with spontaneous rupture of ear drum, unspecified ear

✚ 5 **H66.1** Chronic tubotympanic suppurative otitis media
Benign chronic suppurative otitis media
Chronic tubotympanic disease
Use additional code for any associated perforated tympanic membrane (H72.-)

⊟ !Q ✚ **H66.10** Chronic tubotympanic suppurative otitis media, unspecified

⊟ SP ✚ **H66.11** Chronic tubotympanic suppurative otitis media, right ear

⊟ SP ✚ **H66.12** Chronic tubotympanic suppurative otitis media, left ear

⊟ SP ✚ **H66.13** Chronic tubotympanic suppurative otitis media, bilateral

✚ 5 **H66.2** Chronic atticoantral suppurative otitis media
Chronic atticoantral disease
Use additional code for any associated perforated tympanic membrane (H72.-)

⊟ !Q ✚ **H66.20** Chronic atticoantral suppurative otitis media, unspecified ear

⊟ SP ✚ **H66.21** Chronic atticoantral suppurative otitis media, right ear

⊟ SP ✚ **H66.22** Chronic atticoantral suppurative otitis media, left ear

⊟ SP ✚ **H66.23** Chronic atticoantral suppurative otitis media, bilateral

✚ 5 **H66.3** Other chronic suppurative otitis media
Chronic suppurative otitis media NOS
Use additional code for any associated perforated tympanic membrane (H72.-)
EXCLUDES 1 tuberculous otitis media (A18.6)

✚ 6 **H66.3X** Other chronic suppurative otitis media

⊟ SP ✚ **H66.3X1** Other chronic suppurative otitis media, right ear

⊟ SP ✚ **H66.3X2** Other chronic suppurative otitis media, left ear

⊟ SP ✚ **H66.3X3** Other chronic suppurative otitis media, bilateral

⊟ !Q ✚ **H66.3X9** Other chronic suppurative otitis media, unspecified ear

✚ 5 **H66.4** Suppurative otitis media, unspecified
Purulent otitis media NOS
Use additional code for any associated perforated tympanic membrane (H72.-)

⊟ !Q ✚ **H66.40** Suppurative otitis media, unspecified, unspecified ear

⊟ SP ✚ **H66.41** Suppurative otitis media, unspecified, right ear

⊟ SP ✚ **H66.42** Suppurative otitis media, unspecified, left ear

⊟ SP ✚ **H66.43** Suppurative otitis media, unspecified, bilateral

✚ 5 **H66.9** Otitis media, unspecified
Otitis media NOS
Acute otitis media NOS
Chronic otitis media NOS
Use additional code for any associated perforated tympanic membrane (H72.-)

⊟ !Q ✚ **H66.90** Otitis media, unspecified, unspecified ear

⊟ SP ✚ **H66.91** Otitis media, unspecified, right ear

⊟ SP ✚ **H66.92** Otitis media, unspecified, left ear

⊟ SP ✚ **H66.93** Otitis media, unspecified, bilateral

✚ 4 **H67** Otitis media in diseases classified elsewhere
Code first underlying disease, such as:
plasminogen deficiency (E88.02)
viral disease NEC (B00-B34)
Use additional code for any associated perforated tympanic membrane (H72.-)
EXCLUDES 1 otitis media in:
influenza (J09.X9, J10.83, J11.83)
measles (B05.3)
scarlet fever (A38.0)
tuberculosis (A18.6)

M ⊟ !Q ✚ *H67.1* *Otitis media in diseases classified elsewhere, right ear*

M ⊟ !Q ✚ *H67.2* *Otitis media in diseases classified elsewhere, left ear*

M ⊟ !Q ✚ *H67.3* *Otitis media in diseases classified elsewhere, bilateral*

M ⊟ !Q ✚ *H67.9* *Otitis media in diseases classified elsewhere, unspecified ear*

4 **H68** Eustachian salpingitis and obstruction

5 **H68.0** Eustachian salpingitis

6 **H68.00** Unspecified Eustachian salpingitis

⊟ SP **H68.001** Unspecified Eustachian salpingitis, right ear

⊟ SP **H68.002** Unspecified Eustachian salpingitis, left ear

⊟ SP **H68.003** Unspecified Eustachian salpingitis, bilateral

⊟ !Q **H68.009** Unspecified Eustachian salpingitis, unspecified ear

6 **H68.01** Acute Eustachian salpingitis

⊟ SP **H68.011** Acute Eustachian salpingitis, right ear

⊟ SP **H68.012** Acute Eustachian salpingitis, left ear

⊟ SP **H68.013** Acute Eustachian salpingitis, bilateral

⊟ !Q **H68.019** Acute Eustachian salpingitis, unspecified ear

6 **H68.02** Chronic Eustachian salpingitis

⊟ SP **H68.021** Chronic Eustachian salpingitis, right ear

⊟ SP **H68.022** Chronic Eustachian salpingitis, left ear

⊟ SP **H68.023** Chronic Eustachian salpingitis, bilateral

⊟ !Q **H68.029** Chronic Eustachian salpingitis, unspecified ear

Chapter 8

H60-H95

---

4 4th digit required   5 5th digit required   6 6th digit required   7 7th digit required   ☑ 7th digit placeholder   ✚ Additional code   ⊟ Laterality

5 **H68.1 Obstruction of Eustachian tube**
Stenosis of Eustachian tube
Stricture of Eustachian tube

6 **H68.10   Unspecified obstruction of Eustachian tube**

SP **H68.101   Unspecified obstruction of Eustachian tube, right ear**

SP **H68.102   Unspecified obstruction of Eustachian tube, left ear**

SP **H68.103   Unspecified obstruction of Eustachian tube, bilateral**

IQ **H68.109   Unspecified obstruction of Eustachian tube, unspecified ear**

6 **H68.11   Osseous obstruction of Eustachian tube**

SP **H68.111   Osseous obstruction of Eustachian tube, right ear**

SP **H68.112   Osseous obstruction of Eustachian tube, left ear**

SP **H68.113   Osseous obstruction of Eustachian tube, bilateral**

IQ **H68.119   Osseous obstruction of Eustachian tube, unspecified ear**

6 **H68.12   Intrinsic cartilagenous obstruction of Eustachian tube**

SP **H68.121   Intrinsic cartilagenous obstruction of Eustachian tube, right ear**

SP **H68.122   Intrinsic cartilagenous obstruction of Eustachian tube, left ear**

SP **H68.123   Intrinsic cartilagenous obstruction of Eustachian tube, bilateral**

IQ **H68.129   Intrinsic cartilagenous obstruction of Eustachian tube, unspecified ear**

6 **H68.13   Extrinsic cartilagenous obstruction of Eustachian tube**
Compression of Eustachian tube

SP **H68.131   Extrinsic cartilagenous obstruction of Eustachian tube, right ear**

SP **H68.132   Extrinsic cartilagenous obstruction of Eustachian tube, left ear**

SP **H68.133   Extrinsic cartilagenous obstruction of Eustachian tube, bilateral**

IQ **H68.139   Extrinsic cartilagenous obstruction of Eustachian tube, unspecified ear**

4 **H69   Other and unspecified disorders of Eustachian tube**

5 **H69.0 Patulous Eustachian tube**

IQ **H69.00   Patulous Eustachian tube, unspecified ear**

SP **H69.01   Patulous Eustachian tube, right ear**

SP **H69.02   Patulous Eustachian tube, left ear**

SP **H69.03   Patulous Eustachian tube, bilateral**

5 **H69.8 Other specified disorders of Eustachian tube**

IQ **H69.80   Other specified disorders of Eustachian tube, unspecified ear**

SP **H69.81   Other specified disorders of Eustachian tube, right ear**

SP **H69.82   Other specified disorders of Eustachian tube, left ear**

SP **H69.83   Other specified disorders of Eustachian tube, bilateral**

5 **H69.9   Unspecified Eustachian tube disorder**

IQ **H69.90   Unspecified Eustachian tube disorder, unspecified ear**

SP **H69.91   Unspecified Eustachian tube disorder, right ear**

SP **H69.92   Unspecified Eustachian tube disorder, left ear**

SP **H69.93   Unspecified Eustachian tube disorder, bilateral**

4 **H70   Mastoiditis and related conditions**

5 **H70.0 Acute mastoiditis**
Abscess of mastoid
Empyema of mastoid

6 **H70.00   Acute mastoiditis without complications**

SP **H70.001   Acute mastoiditis without complications, right ear**

SP **H70.002   Acute mastoiditis without complications, left ear**

SP **H70.003   Acute mastoiditis without complications, bilateral**

IQ **H70.009   Acute mastoiditis without complications, unspecified ear**

6 **H70.01   Subperiosteal abscess of mastoid**

SP **H70.011   Subperiosteal abscess of mastoid, right ear**

SP **H70.012   Subperiosteal abscess of mastoid, left ear**

SP **H70.013   Subperiosteal abscess of mastoid, bilateral**

IQ **H70.019   Subperiosteal abscess of mastoid, unspecified ear**

6 **H70.09   Acute mastoiditis with other complications**

SP **H70.091   Acute mastoiditis with other complications, right ear**

SP **H70.092   Acute mastoiditis with other complications, left ear**

SP **H70.093   Acute mastoiditis with other complications, bilateral**

IQ **H70.099   Acute mastoiditis with other complications, unspecified ear**

5 **H70.1 Chronic mastoiditis**
Caries of mastoid
Fistula of mastoid
EXCLUDES 1 tuberculous mastoiditis (A18.03)

IQ **H70.10   Chronic mastoiditis, unspecified ear**

SP **H70.11 Chronic mastoiditis, right ear**

SP **H70.12 Chronic mastoiditis, left ear**

SP **H70.13 Chronic mastoiditis, bilateral**

5 **H70.2 Petrositis**
Inflammation of petrous bone

6 **H70.20   Unspecified petrositis**

DEFINITION Inflammation of the dense, hard bone behind the temple protecting the inner ear.

SP **H70.201   Unspecified petrositis, right ear**

★ New ▲ Revised Px Primary **SP** PDGM Px **SL** Low CoM **SH** High CoM **IQ** Quest. Encounter ⊞ Hospice non-cancer Dx   Unspecified   **M** *Manifestation*

DecisionHealth's FY 2020 Complete Home Health ICD-10-CM Diagnosis Coding Manual

933

⊟ SP **H70.202** **Unspecified petrositis, left ear**

⊟ SP **H70.203** **Unspecified petrositis, bilateral**

⊟ IQ **H70.209** **Unspecified petrositis, unspecified ear**

⑥ **H70.21** Acute petrositis

⊟ SP **H70.211** Acute petrositis, right ear

⊟ SP **H70.212** Acute petrositis, left ear

⊟ SP **H70.213** Acute petrositis, bilateral

⊟ IQ **H70.219** **Acute petrositis, unspecified ear**

⑥ **H70.22** Chronic petrositis

⊟ SP **H70.221** Chronic petrositis, right ear

⊟ SP **H70.222** Chronic petrositis, left ear

⊟ SP **H70.223** Chronic petrositis, bilateral

⊟ IQ **H70.229** **Chronic petrositis, unspecified ear**

⑤ **H70.8** Other mastoiditis and related conditions

> EXCLUDES 1   preauricular sinus and cyst (Q18.1)
> sinus, fistula, and cyst of branchial cleft (Q18.0)

⑥ **H70.81** Postauricular fistula

⊟ SP **H70.811** Postauricular fistula, right ear

⊟ SP **H70.812** Postauricular fistula, left ear

⊟ SP **H70.813** Postauricular fistula, bilateral

⊟ IQ **H70.819** **Postauricular fistula, unspecified ear**

⑥ **H70.89** Other mastoiditis and related conditions

⊟ SP **H70.891** Other mastoiditis and related conditions, right ear

⊟ SP **H70.892** Other mastoiditis and related conditions, left ear

⊟ SP **H70.893** Other mastoiditis and related conditions, bilateral

⊟ IQ **H70.899** **Other mastoiditis and related conditions, unspecified ear**

⑤ **H70.9** **Unspecified mastoiditis**

⊟ IQ **H70.90** **Unspecified mastoiditis, unspecified ear**

⊟ SP **H70.91** **Unspecified mastoiditis, right ear**

⊟ SP **H70.92** **Unspecified mastoiditis, left ear**

⊟ SP **H70.93** **Unspecified mastoiditis, bilateral**

④ **H71** Cholesteatoma of middle ear

> EXCLUDES 2   cholesteatoma of external ear (H60.4-)
> recurrent cholesteatoma of postmastoidectomy cavity (H95.0-)

> DEFINITION   Cyst-like mass filled with cell debris and cholesterol crystals in the middle ear and/or mastoid process that can damage the ossicles, causing deafness, vertigo, and nerve deterioration.

⑤ **H71.0** Cholesteatoma of attic

⊟ IQ **H71.00** **Cholesteatoma of attic, unspecified ear**

⊟ SP **H71.01** Cholesteatoma of attic, right ear

⊟ SP **H71.02** Cholesteatoma of attic, left ear

⊟ SP **H71.03** Cholesteatoma of attic, bilateral

⑤ **H71.1** Cholesteatoma of tympanum

⊟ IQ **H71.10** **Cholesteatoma of tympanum, unspecified ear**

⊟ SP **H71.11** Cholesteatoma of tympanum, right ear

⊟ SP **H71.12** Cholesteatoma of tympanum, left ear

⊟ SP **H71.13** Cholesteatoma of tympanum, bilateral

⑤ **H71.2** Cholesteatoma of mastoid

⊟ IQ **H71.20** **Cholesteatoma of mastoid, unspecified ear**

⊟ SP **H71.21** Cholesteatoma of mastoid, right ear

⊟ SP **H71.22** Cholesteatoma of mastoid, left ear

⊟ SP **H71.23** Cholesteatoma of mastoid, bilateral

⑤ **H71.3** Diffuse cholesteatosis

⊟ IQ **H71.30** **Diffuse cholesteatosis, unspecified ear**

⊟ SP **H71.31** Diffuse cholesteatosis, right ear

⊟ SP **H71.32** Diffuse cholesteatosis, left ear

⊟ SP **H71.33** Diffuse cholesteatosis, bilateral

⑤ **H71.9** **Unspecified cholesteatoma**

⊟ IQ **H71.90** **Unspecified cholesteatoma, unspecified ear**

⊟ SP **H71.91** **Unspecified cholesteatoma, right ear**

⊟ SP **H71.92** **Unspecified cholesteatoma, left ear**

⊟ SP **H71.93** **Unspecified cholesteatoma, bilateral**

④ **H72** Perforation of tympanic membrane

> INCLUDES   persistent post-traumatic perforation of ear drum
> postinflammatory perforation of ear drum

Code first:
  any associated otitis media (H65.-, H66.1-, H66.2-, H66.3-, H66.4-, H66.9-, H67.-)

> EXCLUDES 1   acute suppurative otitis media with rupture of the tympanic membrane (H66.01-)
> traumatic rupture of ear drum (S09.2-)

⑤ **H72.0** Central perforation of tympanic membrane

⊟ IQ **H72.00** **Central perforation of tympanic membrane, unspecified ear**

⊟ SP **H72.01** Central perforation of tympanic membrane, right ear

⊟ SP **H72.02** Central perforation of tympanic membrane, left ear

⊟ SP **H72.03** Central perforation of tympanic membrane, bilateral

⑤ **H72.1** Attic perforation of tympanic membrane
Perforation of pars flaccida

⊟ IQ **H72.10** **Attic perforation of tympanic membrane, unspecified ear**

⊟ SP **H72.11** Attic perforation of tympanic membrane, right ear

⊟ SP **H72.12** Attic perforation of tympanic membrane, left ear

⊟ SP **H72.13** Attic perforation of tympanic membrane, bilateral

⑤ **H72.2** Other marginal perforations of tympanic membrane

Chapter 8

H60-H95

---

④ 4th digit required   ⑤ 5th digit required   ⑥ 6th digit required   ⑦ 7th digit required   ⑦ 7th digit placeholder   ✚ Additional code   ⊟ Laterality

⑥ **H72.2X** **Other marginal perforations of tympanic membrane**

⊟ **SP** **H72.2X1** Other marginal perforations of tympanic membrane, right ear

⊟ **SP** **H72.2X2** Other marginal perforations of tympanic membrane, left ear

⊟ **SP** **H72.2X3** Other marginal perforations of tympanic membrane, bilateral

⊟ **IQ** **H72.2X9** Other marginal perforations of tympanic membrane, unspecified ear

⑤ **H72.8** **Other perforations of tympanic membrane**

⑥ **H72.81** **Multiple perforations of tympanic membrane**

⊟ **SP** **H72.811** Multiple perforations of tympanic membrane, right ear

⊟ **SP** **H72.812** Multiple perforations of tympanic membrane, left ear

⊟ **SP** **H72.813** Multiple perforations of tympanic membrane, bilateral

⊟ **IQ** **H72.819** Multiple perforations of tympanic membrane, unspecified ear

⑥ **H72.82** **Total perforations of tympanic membrane**

⊟ **SP** **H72.821** Total perforations of tympanic membrane, right ear

⊟ **SP** **H72.822** Total perforations of tympanic membrane, left ear

⊟ **SP** **H72.823** Total perforations of tympanic membrane, bilateral

⊟ **IQ** **H72.829** Total perforations of tympanic membrane, unspecified ear

⑤ **H72.9** **Unspecified perforation of tympanic membrane**

⊟ **IQ** **H72.90** Unspecified perforation of tympanic membrane, unspecified ear

⊟ **SP** **H72.91** Unspecified perforation of tympanic membrane, right ear

⊟ **SP** **H72.92** Unspecified perforation of tympanic membrane, left ear

⊟ **SP** **H72.93** Unspecified perforation of tympanic membrane, bilateral

④ **H73** **Other disorders of tympanic membrane**

⑤ **H73.0** **Acute myringitis**

EXCLUDES 1 acute myringitis with otitis media (H65, H66)

⑥ **H73.00** Unspecified acute myringitis
Acute tympanitis NOS

⊟ **SP** **H73.001** Acute myringitis, right ear

⊟ **SP** **H73.002** Acute myringitis, left ear

⊟ **SP** **H73.003** Acute myringitis, bilateral

⊟ **IQ** **H73.009** Acute myringitis, unspecified ear

⑥ **H73.01** **Bullous myringitis**

DEFINITION Inflammation of the eardrum caused by a virus and characterized by blood-filled blisters.

⊟ **SP** **H73.011** Bullous myringitis, right ear

⊟ **SP** **H73.012** Bullous myringitis, left ear

⊟ **SP** **H73.013** Bullous myringitis, bilateral

⊟ **IQ** **H73.019** Bullous myringitis, unspecified ear

⑥ **H73.09** **Other acute myringitis**

⊟ **SP** **H73.091** Other acute myringitis, right ear

⊟ **SP** **H73.092** Other acute myringitis, left ear

⊟ **SP** **H73.093** Other acute myringitis, bilateral

⊟ **IQ** **H73.099** Other acute myringitis, unspecified ear

⑤ **H73.1** **Chronic myringitis**
Chronic tympanitis
EXCLUDES 1 chronic myringitis with otitis media (H65, H66)

⊟ **IQ** **H73.10** Chronic myringitis, unspecified ear

⊟ **SP** **H73.11** Chronic myringitis, right ear

⊟ **SP** **H73.12** Chronic myringitis, left ear

⊟ **SP** **H73.13** Chronic myringitis, bilateral

⑤ **H73.2** **Unspecified myringitis**

⊟ **IQ** **H73.20** Unspecified myringitis, unspecified ear

⊟ **SP** **H73.21** Unspecified myringitis, right ear

⊟ **SP** **H73.22** Unspecified myringitis, left ear

⊟ **SP** **H73.23** Unspecified myringitis, bilateral

⑤ **H73.8** **Other specified disorders of tympanic membrane**

⑥ **H73.81** **Atrophic flaccid tympanic membrane**

DEFINITION Eardrum that has wasted away and lost its tension, resulting in severe hearing loss.

⊟ **SP** **H73.811** Atrophic flaccid tympanic membrane, right ear

⊟ **SP** **H73.812** Atrophic flaccid tympanic membrane, left ear

⊟ **SP** **H73.813** Atrophic flaccid tympanic membrane, bilateral

⊟ **IQ** **H73.819** Atrophic flaccid tympanic membrane, unspecified ear

⑥ **H73.82** **Atrophic nonflaccid tympanic membrane**

⊟ **SP** **H73.821** Atrophic nonflaccid tympanic membrane, right ear

⊟ **SP** **H73.822** Atrophic nonflaccid tympanic membrane, left ear

⊟ **SP** **H73.823** Atrophic nonflaccid tympanic membrane, bilateral

⊟ **IQ** **H73.829** Atrophic nonflaccid tympanic membrane, unspecified ear

⑥ **H73.89** **Other specified disorders of tympanic membrane**

⊟ **SP** **H73.891** Other specified disorders of tympanic membrane, right ear

⊟ **SP** **H73.892** Other specified disorders of tympanic membrane, left ear

⊟ **SP** **H73.893** Other specified disorders of tympanic membrane, bilateral

⊟ **IQ** **H73.899** Other specified disorders of tympanic membrane, unspecified ear

⑤ **H73.9** **Unspecified disorder of tympanic membrane**

⊟ **IQ** **H73.90** Unspecified disorder of tympanic membrane, unspecified ear

⊟ **SP** **H73.91** Unspecified disorder of tympanic membrane, right ear

⊟ **SP** **H73.92** Unspecified disorder of tympanic membrane, left ear

Chapter 8

H60-H95

★ New ▲ Revised **Px** Primary **SP** PDGM Px **SL** Low CoM **SH** High CoM **IQ** Quest. Encounter **H** Hospice non-cancer Dx Unspecified **M** *Manifestation*

DecisionHealth's FY 2020 Complete Home Health ICD-10-CM Diagnosis Coding Manual

935

☰ SP H73.93 **Unspecified disorder of tympanic membrane, bilateral**

4 H74 **Other disorders of middle ear mastoid**
> **EXCLUDES 2** mastoiditis (H70.-)

5 H74.0 Tympanosclerosis
> **DEFINITION** Thickening and hardening of the eardrum, reducing its ability to vibrate and transmit sound.

☰ SP H74.01 Tympanosclerosis, right ear

☰ SP H74.02 Tympanosclerosis, left ear

☰ SP H74.03 Tympanosclerosis, bilateral

☰ IQ H74.09 **Tympanosclerosis, unspecified ear**

5 H74.1 Adhesive middle ear disease
Adhesive otitis
> **EXCLUDES 1** glue ear (H65.3-)

☰ SP H74.11 Adhesive right middle ear disease

☰ SP H74.12 Adhesive left middle ear disease

☰ SP H74.13 Adhesive middle ear disease, bilateral

☰ IQ H74.19 **Adhesive middle ear disease, unspecified ear**

5 H74.2 Discontinuity and dislocation of ear ossicles

☰ IQ H74.20 **Discontinuity and dislocation of ear ossicles, unspecified ear**

☰ SP H74.21 Discontinuity and dislocation of right ear ossicles

☰ SP H74.22 Discontinuity and dislocation of left ear ossicles

☰ SP H74.23 Discontinuity and dislocation of ear ossicles, bilateral

5 H74.3 Other acquired abnormalities of ear ossicles

6 H74.31 Ankylosis of ear ossicles

☰ SP H74.311 Ankylosis of ear ossicles, right ear

☰ SP H74.312 Ankylosis of ear ossicles, left ear

☰ SP H74.313 Ankylosis of ear ossicles, bilateral

☰ IQ H74.319 **Ankylosis of ear ossicles, unspecified ear**

6 H74.32 Partial loss of ear ossicles

☰ SP H74.321 Partial loss of ear ossicles, right ear

☰ SP H74.322 Partial loss of ear ossicles, left ear

☰ SP H74.323 Partial loss of ear ossicles, bilateral

☰ IQ H74.329 **Partial loss of ear ossicles, unspecified ear**

6 H74.39 Other acquired abnormalities of ear ossicles

☰ SP H74.391 Other acquired abnormalities of right ear ossicles

☰ SP H74.392 Other acquired abnormalities of left ear ossicles

☰ SP H74.393 Other acquired abnormalities of ear ossicles, bilateral

☰ IQ H74.399 **Other acquired abnormalities of ear ossicles, unspecified ear**

5 H74.4 Polyp of middle ear

☰ IQ H74.40 **Polyp of middle ear, unspecified ear**

☰ SP H74.41 Polyp of right middle ear

☰ SP H74.42 Polyp of left middle ear

☰ SP H74.43 Polyp of middle ear, bilateral

5 H74.8 Other specified disorders of middle ear and mastoid

6 H74.8X Other specified disorders of middle ear and mastoid

☰ SP H74.8X1 Other specified disorders of right middle ear and mastoid

☰ SP H74.8X2 Other specified disorders of left middle ear and mastoid

☰ SP H74.8X3 Other specified disorders of middle ear and mastoid, bilateral

☰ IQ H74.8X9 **Other specified disorders of middle ear and mastoid, unspecified ear**

5 H74.9 **Unspecified disorder of middle ear and mastoid**

☰ IQ H74.90 **Unspecified disorder of middle ear and mastoid, unspecified ear**

☰ IQ H74.91 **Unspecified disorder of right middle ear and mastoid**

☰ IQ H74.92 **Unspecified disorder of left middle ear and mastoid**

☰ IQ H74.93 **Unspecified disorder of middle ear and mastoid, bilateral**

4 H75 **Other disorders of middle ear and mastoid in diseases classified elsewhere**
Code first:
> underlying disease

5 H75.0 Mastoiditis in infectious and parasitic diseases classified elsewhere
> **EXCLUDES 1** mastoiditis (in):
> syphilis (A52.77)
> tuberculosis (A18.03)

M ☰ IQ H75.00 *Mastoiditis in infectious and parasitic diseases classified elsewhere, unspecified ear*

M ☰ IQ H75.01 *Mastoiditis in infectious and parasitic diseases classified elsewhere, right ear*

M ☰ IQ H75.02 *Mastoiditis in infectious and parasitic diseases classified elsewhere, left ear*

M ☰ IQ H75.03 *Mastoiditis in infectious and parasitic diseases classified elsewhere, bilateral*

5 H75.8 Other specified disorders of middle ear and mastoid in diseases classified elsewhere

☰ IQ H75.80 **Other specified disorders of middle ear and mastoid in diseases classified elsewhere, unspecified ear**

☰ IQ H75.81 Other specified disorders of right middle ear and mastoid in diseases classified elsewhere

☰ IQ H75.82 Other specified disorders of left middle ear and mastoid in diseases classified elsewhere

☰ IQ H75.83 Other specified disorders of middle ear and mastoid in diseases classified elsewhere, bilateral

Diseases of inner ear (H80-H83)

4 H80 **Otosclerosis**
> **INCLUDES** Otospongiosis

5 H80.0 Otosclerosis involving oval window, nonobliterative

Chapter 8

H60-H95

4 4th digit required   5 5th digit required   6 6th digit required   7 7th digit required   7 7th digit placeholder   ✚ Additional code   ☰ Laterality

936   *DecisionHealth's* FY 2020 Complete Home Health ICD-10-CM Diagnosis Coding Manual

⊟ 🔳IQ **H80.00** **Otosclerosis involving oval window, nonobliterative, unspecified ear**

⊟ SP **H80.01** Otosclerosis involving oval window, nonobliterative, right ear

⊟ SP **H80.02** Otosclerosis involving oval window, nonobliterative, left ear

⊟ SP **H80.03** Otosclerosis involving oval window, nonobliterative, bilateral

⑤ **H80.1** Otosclerosis involving oval window, obliterative

⊟ 🔳IQ **H80.10** **Otosclerosis involving oval window, obliterative, unspecified ear**

⊟ SP **H80.11** Otosclerosis involving oval window, obliterative, right ear

⊟ SP **H80.12** Otosclerosis involving oval window, obliterative, left ear

⊟ SP **H80.13** Otosclerosis involving oval window, obliterative, bilateral

⑤ **H80.2** Cochlear otosclerosis
Otosclerosis involving otic capsule
Otosclerosis involving round window

   DEFINITION Formation of bony tissue in the cochlea, causing hearing loss.

⊟ 🔳IQ **H80.20** **Cochlear otosclerosis, unspecified ear**

⊟ SP **H80.21** Cochlear otosclerosis, right ear

⊟ SP **H80.22** Cochlear otosclerosis, left ear

⊟ SP **H80.23** Cochlear otosclerosis, bilateral

⑤ **H80.8** Other otosclerosis

⊟ 🔳IQ **H80.80** **Other otosclerosis, unspecified ear**

⊟ SP **H80.81** Other otosclerosis, right ear

⊟ SP **H80.82** Other otosclerosis, left ear

⊟ SP **H80.83** Other otosclerosis, bilateral

⑤ **H80.9** **Unspecified otosclerosis**

⊟ 🔳IQ **H80.90** **Unspecified otosclerosis, unspecified ear**

⊟ SP **H80.91** **Unspecified otosclerosis, right ear**

⊟ SP **H80.92** **Unspecified otosclerosis, left ear**

⊟ SP **H80.93** **Unspecified otosclerosis, bilateral**

④ **H81** **Disorders of vestibular function**
   EXCLUDES 1 epidemic vertigo (A88.1)
   vertigo NOS (R42)

⑤ **H81.0** Ménière's disease
Labyrinthine hydrops
Ménière's syndrome or vertigo

   DEFINITION Disorder of the inner ear causing attacks of vertigo, tinnitus, and progressive hearing loss involving all tones.

⊟ SP **H81.01** Ménière's disease, right ear

⊟ SP **H81.02** Ménière's disease, left ear

⊟ SP **H81.03** Ménière's disease, bilateral

⊟ 🔳IQ **H81.09** **Ménière's disease, unspecified ear**

⑤ **H81.1** Benign paroxysmal vertigo

⊟ 🔳IQ **H81.10** **Benign paroxysmal vertigo, unspecified ear**

⊟ SP **H81.11** Benign paroxysmal vertigo, right ear

⊟ SP **H81.12** Benign paroxysmal vertigo, left ear

⊟ SP **H81.13** Benign paroxysmal vertigo, bilateral

⑤ **H81.2** Vestibular neuronitis

⊟ 🔳IQ **H81.20** **Vestibular neuronitis, unspecified ear**

⊟ SP **H81.21** Vestibular neuronitis, right ear

⊟ SP **H81.22** Vestibular neuronitis, left ear

⊟ SP **H81.23** Vestibular neuronitis, bilateral

⑤ **H81.3** Other peripheral vertigo

⑥ **H81.31** Aural vertigo

⊟ SP **H81.311** Aural vertigo, right ear

⊟ SP **H81.312** Aural vertigo, left ear

⊟ SP **H81.313** Aural vertigo, bilateral

⊟ 🔳IQ **H81.319** **Aural vertigo, unspecified ear**

⑥ **H81.39** Other peripheral vertigo
Lermoyez' syndrome
Otogenic vertigo
Peripheral vertigo NOS

⊟ SP **H81.391** Other peripheral vertigo, right ear

⊟ SP **H81.392** Other peripheral vertigo, left ear

⊟ SP **H81.393** Other peripheral vertigo, bilateral

⊟ 🔳IQ **H81.399** **Other peripheral vertigo, unspecified ear**

▲ **H81.4** Vertigo of central origin
Central positional nystagmus

⑤ **H81.8** Other disorders of vestibular function

⑥ **H81.8X** Other disorders of vestibular function

⊟ SP **H81.8X1** Other disorders of vestibular function, right ear

⊟ SP **H81.8X2** Other disorders of vestibular function, left ear

⊟ SP **H81.8X3** Other disorders of vestibular function, bilateral

⊟ 🔳IQ **H81.8X9** **Other disorders of vestibular function, unspecified ear**

⑤ **H81.9** **Unspecified disorder of vestibular function**
Vertiginous syndrome NOS

⊟ 🔳IQ **H81.90** **Unspecified disorder of vestibular function, unspecified ear**

⊟ 🔳IQ **H81.91** **Unspecified disorder of vestibular function, right ear**

⊟ 🔳IQ **H81.92** **Unspecified disorder of vestibular function, left ear**

⊟ 🔳IQ **H81.93** **Unspecified disorder of vestibular function, bilateral**

④ **H82** **Vertiginous syndromes in diseases classified elsewhere**
Code first:
   underlying disease
   EXCLUDES 1 epidemic vertigo (A88.1)

⊟ 🔳IQ **H82.1** Vertiginous syndromes in diseases classified elsewhere, right ear

⊟ 🔳IQ **H82.2** Vertiginous syndromes in diseases classified elsewhere, left ear

⊟ 🔳IQ **H82.3** Vertiginous syndromes in diseases classified elsewhere, bilateral

⊟ 🔳IQ **H82.9** **Vertiginous syndromes in diseases classified elsewhere, unspecified ear**

④ **H83** **Other diseases of inner ear**

⑤ **H83.0** Labyrinthitis

⊟ SP **H83.01** Labyrinthitis, right ear

⊟ SP **H83.02** Labyrinthitis, left ear

⊟ SP **H83.03** Labyrinthitis, bilateral

⊟ 🔳IQ **H83.09** **Labyrinthitis, unspecified ear**

★ New ▲ Revised Px Primary SP PDGM Px SL Low CoM SH High CoM IQ Quest. Encounter H Hospice non-cancer Dx | Unspecified | M *Manifestation*

DecisionHealth's FY 2020 Complete Home Health ICD-10-CM Diagnosis Coding Manual

937

Chapter 8

H60-H95

Chapter 8

H60-H95

⑤ H83.1 Labyrinthine fistula

⊟ SP H83.11 Labyrinthine fistula, right ear

⊟ SP H83.12 Labyrinthine fistula, left ear

⊟ SP H83.13 Labyrinthine fistula, bilateral

⊟ IQ H83.19 Labyrinthine fistula, unspecified ear

⑤ H83.2 Labyrinthine dysfunction
Labyrinthine hypersensitivity
Labyrinthine hypofunction
Labyrinthine loss of function

⑥ H83.2X Labyrinthine dysfunction

⊟ SP H83.2X1 Labyrinthine dysfunction, right ear

⊟ SP H83.2X2 Labyrinthine dysfunction, left ear

⊟ SP H83.2X3 Labyrinthine dysfunction, bilateral

⊟ IQ H83.2X9 Labyrinthine dysfunction, unspecified ear

⑤ H83.3 Noise effects on inner ear
Acoustic trauma of inner ear
Noise-induced hearing loss of inner ear

⑥ H83.3X Noise effects on inner ear

⊟ SP H83.3X1 Noise effects on right inner ear

⊟ SP H83.3X2 Noise effects on left inner ear

⊟ SP H83.3X3 Noise effects on inner ear, bilateral

⊟ IQ H83.3X9 Noise effects on inner ear, unspecified ear

⑤ H83.8 Other specified diseases of inner ear

⑥ H83.8X Other specified diseases of inner ear

⊟ SP H83.8X1 Other specified diseases of right inner ear

⊟ SP H83.8X2 Other specified diseases of left inner ear

⊟ SP H83.8X3 Other specified diseases of inner ear, bilateral

⊟ IQ H83.8X9 Other specified diseases of inner ear, unspecified ear

⑤ H83.9 Unspecified disease of inner ear

⊟ IQ H83.90 Unspecified disease of inner ear, unspecified ear

⊟ IQ H83.91 Unspecified disease of right inner ear

⊟ IQ H83.92 Unspecified disease of left inner ear

⊟ IQ H83.93 Unspecified disease of inner ear, bilateral

Other disorders of ear   (H90-H94)

④ H90 Conductive and sensorineural hearing loss
 EXCLUDES 1 deaf nonspeaking NEC (H91.3)
 deafness NOS (H91.9-)
 hearing loss NOS (H91.9-)
 noise-induced hearing loss (H83.3-)
 ototoxic hearing loss (H91.0-)
 sudden (idiopathic) hearing loss (H91.2-)

SP H90.0 Conductive hearing loss, bilateral

⑤ H90.1 Conductive hearing loss, unilateral with unrestricted hearing on the contralateral side

⊟ SP H90.11 Conductive hearing loss, unilateral, right ear, with unrestricted hearing on the contralateral side

⊟ SP H90.12 Conductive hearing loss, unilateral, left ear, with unrestricted hearing on the contralateral side

SP H90.2 Conductive hearing loss, unspecified
Conductive deafness NOS
 DEFINITION Loss of audio acuity caused by transmission interference of sound waves before they can reach the inner ear and the auditory nerve.

SP H90.3 Sensorineural hearing loss, bilateral

⑤ H90.4 Sensorineural hearing loss, unilateral with unrestricted hearing on the contralateral side

⊟ SP H90.41 Sensorineural hearing loss, unilateral, right ear, with unrestricted hearing on the contralateral side

⊟ SP H90.42 Sensorineural hearing loss, unilateral, left ear, with unrestricted hearing on the contralateral side

SP H90.5 Unspecified sensorineural hearing loss
Central hearing loss NOS
Congenital deafness NOS
Neural hearing loss NOS
Perceptive hearing loss NOS
Sensorineural deafness NOS
Sensory hearing loss NOS
 EXCLUDES 1 abnormal auditory perception (H93.2-)
 psychogenic deafness (F44.6)
 DEFINITION Sensory-nerve based hearing loss caused by a disorder affecting the VIII cranial nerve, the inner ear sensory perception, or the central processing area of the brain.

SP H90.6 Mixed conductive and sensorineural hearing loss, bilateral

⑤ H90.7 Mixed conductive and sensorineural hearing loss, unilateral with unrestricted hearing on the contralateral side

⊟ SP H90.71 Mixed conductive and sensorineural hearing loss, unilateral, right ear, with unrestricted hearing on the contralateral side

⊟ SP H90.72 Mixed conductive and sensorineural hearing loss, unilateral, left ear, with unrestricted hearing on the contralateral side

SP H90.8 Mixed conductive and sensorineural hearing loss, unspecified

⑤ H90.A Conductive and sensorineural hearing loss with restricted hearing on the contralateral side

⑥ H90.A1 Conductive hearing loss, unilateral, with restricted hearing on the contralateral side

⊟ SP H90.A11 Conductive hearing loss, unilateral, right ear with restricted hearing on the contralateral side

⊟ SP H90.A12 Conductive hearing loss, unilateral, left ear with restricted hearing on the contralateral side

---

④ 4th digit required   ⑤ 5th digit required   ⑥ 6th digit required   ⑦ 7th digit required   ⑦ 7th digit placeholder   ➕ Additional code   ⊟ Laterality

938   *DecisionHealth's* FY 2020 Complete Home Health ICD-10-CM Diagnosis Coding Manual

⑥ **H90.A2** Sensorineural hearing loss, unilateral, with restricted hearing on the contralateral side

▤ SP **H90.A21** Sensorineural hearing loss, unilateral, right ear, with restricted hearing on the contralateral side

▤ SP **H90.A22** Sensorineural hearing loss, unilateral, left ear, with restricted hearing on the contralateral side

⑥ **H90.A3** Mixed conductive and sensorineural hearing loss, unilateral with restricted hearing on the contralateral side

▤ SP **H90.A31** Mixed conductive and sensorineural hearing loss, unilateral, right ear with restricted hearing on the contralateral side

▤ SP **H90.A32** Mixed conductive and sensorineural hearing loss, unilateral, left ear with restricted hearing on the contralateral side

④ **H91** Other and unspecified hearing loss

> EXCLUDES 1 abnormal auditory perception (H93.2-)
> hearing loss as classified in H90.-
> impacted cerumen (H61.2-)
> noise-induced hearing loss (H83.3-)
> psychogenic deafness (F44.6)
> transient ischemic deafness (H93.01-)

✚ ⑤ **H91.0** Ototoxic hearing loss
> Code first:
> poisoning due to drug or toxin, if applicable (T36-T65 with fifth or sixth character 1-4 or 6)
> Use additional code for adverse effect, if applicable, to identify drug (T36-T50 with fifth or sixth character 5)

▤ SP ✚ **H91.01** Ototoxic hearing loss, right ear

▤ SP ✚ **H91.02** Ototoxic hearing loss, left ear

▤ SP ✚ **H91.03** Ototoxic hearing loss, bilateral

▤ IQ ✚ **H91.09** Ototoxic hearing loss, unspecified ear

⑤ **H91.1** Presbycusis
> Presbyacusia
> DEFINITION Gradual hearing loss that normally occurs with age.

▤ IQ **H91.10** Presbycusis, unspecified ear

▤ SP **H91.11** Presbycusis, right ear

▤ SP **H91.12** Presbycusis, left ear

▤ SP **H91.13** Presbycusis, bilateral

⑤ **H91.2** Sudden idiopathic hearing loss
> Sudden hearing loss NOS

▤ IQ **H91.20** Sudden idiopathic hearing loss, unspecified ear

▤ SP **H91.21** Sudden idiopathic hearing loss, right ear

▤ SP **H91.22** Sudden idiopathic hearing loss, left ear

▤ SP **H91.23** Sudden idiopathic hearing loss, bilateral

SP **H91.3** Deaf nonspeaking, not elsewhere classified

⑤ **H91.8** Other specified hearing loss

⑥ **H91.8X** Other specified hearing loss

▤ SP **H91.8X1** Other specified hearing loss, right ear

▤ SP **H91.8X2** Other specified hearing loss, left ear

▤ SP **H91.8X3** Other specified hearing loss, bilateral

▤ IQ **H91.8X9** Other specified hearing loss, unspecified ear

⑤ **H91.9** Unspecified hearing loss
> Deafness NOS
> High frequency deafness
> Low frequency deafness

▤ IQ **H91.90** Unspecified hearing loss, unspecified ear

▤ SP **H91.91** Unspecified hearing loss, right ear

▤ SP **H91.92** Unspecified hearing loss, left ear

▤ SP **H91.93** Unspecified hearing loss, bilateral

④ **H92** Otalgia and effusion of ear

⑤ **H92.0** Otalgia

▤ SP **H92.01** Otalgia, right ear

▤ SP **H92.02** Otalgia, left ear

▤ SP **H92.03** Otalgia, bilateral

▤ IQ **H92.09** Otalgia, unspecified ear

⑤ **H92.1** Otorrhea
> EXCLUDES 1 leakage of cerebrospinal fluid through ear (G96.0)
> DEFINITION Fluid leaking from the ear.

▤ IQ **H92.10** Otorrhea, unspecified ear

▤ SP **H92.11** Otorrhea, right ear

▤ SP **H92.12** Otorrhea, left ear

▤ SP **H92.13** Otorrhea, bilateral

⑤ **H92.2** Otorrhagia
> EXCLUDES 1 traumatic otorrhagia - code to injury

▤ IQ **H92.20** Otorrhagia, unspecified ear

▤ SP **H92.21** Otorrhagia, right ear

▤ SP **H92.22** Otorrhagia, left ear

▤ SP **H92.23** Otorrhagia, bilateral

④ **H93** Other disorders of ear, not elsewhere classified

⑤ **H93.0** Degenerative and vascular disorders of ear
> EXCLUDES 1 presbycusis (H91.1)

⑥ **H93.01** Transient ischemic deafness
> DEFINITION A passing hearing loss that occurs when blood flow to the auditory organs is decreased due to injury or disease.

▤ SP **H93.011** Transient ischemic deafness, right ear

▤ SP **H93.012** Transient ischemic deafness, left ear

▤ SP **H93.013** Transient ischemic deafness, bilateral

▤ IQ **H93.019** Transient ischemic deafness, unspecified ear

⑥ **H93.09** Unspecified degenerative and vascular disorders of ear

★ New ▲ Revised Px Primary SP PDGM Px SL Low CoM SH High CoM IQ Quest. Encounter H Hospice non-cancer Dx Unspecified M *Manifestation*

DecisionHealth's FY 2020 Complete Home Health ICD-10-CM Diagnosis Coding Manual

939

Chapter 8

H60-H95

⊟ **SP** **H93.091** Unspecified degenerative and vascular disorders of right ear

⊟ **SP** **H93.092** Unspecified degenerative and vascular disorders of left ear

⊟ **SP** **H93.093** Unspecified degenerative and vascular disorders of ear, bilateral

⊟ **!Q** **H93.099** Unspecified degenerative and vascular disorders of unspecified ear

⑤ **H93.1** Tinnitus

> **DEFINITION** Ringing, hissing, roaring or other sound in the ear in the absence of any apparent stimulus.

⊟ **SP** **H93.11** Tinnitus, right ear

⊟ **SP** **H93.12** Tinnitus, left ear

⊟ **SP** **H93.13** Tinnitus, bilateral

⊟ **!Q** **H93.19** Tinnitus, unspecified ear

⑤ **H93.A** Pulsatile tinnitus

⊟ **SP** **H93.A1** Pulsatile tinnitus, right ear

⊟ **SP** **H93.A2** Pulsatile tinnitus, left ear

⊟ **SP** **H93.A3** Pulsatile tinnitus, bilateral

⊟ **!Q** **H93.A9** Pulsatile tinnitus, unspecified ear

⑤ **H93.2** Other abnormal auditory perceptions

> **EXCLUDES 2** auditory hallucinations (R44.0)

⑥ **H93.21** Auditory recruitment

⊟ **SP** **H93.211** Auditory recruitment, right ear

⊟ **SP** **H93.212** Auditory recruitment, left ear

⊟ **SP** **H93.213** Auditory recruitment, bilateral

⊟ **!Q** **H93.219** Auditory recruitment, unspecified ear

⑥ **H93.22** Diplacusis

> **DEFINITION** One sound is heard as two separate sounds at different tones or pitches.

⊟ **SP** **H93.221** Diplacusis, right ear

⊟ **SP** **H93.222** Diplacusis, left ear

⊟ **SP** **H93.223** Diplacusis, bilateral

⊟ **!Q** **H93.229** Diplacusis, unspecified ear

⑥ **H93.23** Hyperacusis

> **DEFINITION** Hearing is abnormally heightened; normal sounds seem amplified, even cause ear pain.

⊟ **SP** **H93.231** Hyperacusis, right ear

⊟ **SP** **H93.232** Hyperacusis, left ear

⊟ **SP** **H93.233** Hyperacusis, bilateral

⊟ **!Q** **H93.239** Hyperacusis, unspecified ear

⑥ **H93.24** Temporary auditory threshold shift

⊟ **SP** **H93.241** Temporary auditory threshold shift, right ear

⊟ **SP** **H93.242** Temporary auditory threshold shift, left ear

⊟ **SP** **H93.243** Temporary auditory threshold shift, bilateral

⊟ **!Q** **H93.249** Temporary auditory threshold shift, unspecified ear

SP **H93.25** Central auditory processing disorder
Congenital auditory imperception
Word deafness

> **EXCLUDES 1** mixed receptive-expressive language disorder (F80.2)

⑥ **H93.29** Other abnormal auditory perceptions

⊟ **SP** **H93.291** Other abnormal auditory perceptions, right ear

⊟ **SP** **H93.292** Other abnormal auditory perceptions, left ear

⊟ **SP** **H93.293** Other abnormal auditory perceptions, bilateral

⊟ **!Q** **H93.299** Other abnormal auditory perceptions, unspecified ear

⑤ **H93.3** Disorders of acoustic nerve
Disorder of 8th cranial nerve

> **EXCLUDES 1** acoustic neuroma (D33.3) syphilitic acoustic neuritis (A52.15)

⑥ **H93.3X** Disorders of acoustic nerve

⊟ **SP** **H93.3X1** Disorders of right acoustic nerve

⊟ **SP** **H93.3X2** Disorders of left acoustic nerve

⊟ **SP** **H93.3X3** Disorders of bilateral acoustic nerves

⊟ **!Q** **H93.3X9** Disorders of unspecified acoustic nerve

⑤ **H93.8** Other specified disorders of ear

⑥ **H93.8X** Other specified disorders of ear

⊟ **SP** **H93.8X1** Other specified disorders of right ear

⊟ **SP** **H93.8X2** Other specified disorders of left ear

⊟ **SP** **H93.8X3** Other specified disorders of ear, bilateral

⊟ **!Q** **H93.8X9** Other specified disorders of ear, unspecified ear

⑤ **H93.9** Unspecified disorder of ear

⊟ **!Q** **H93.90** Unspecified disorder of ear, unspecified ear

⊟ **!Q** **H93.91** Unspecified disorder of right ear

⊟ **!Q** **H93.92** Unspecified disorder of left ear

⊟ **!Q** **H93.93** Unspecified disorder of ear, bilateral

④ **H94** Other disorders of ear in diseases classified elsewhere

⑤ **H94.0** Acoustic neuritis in infectious and parasitic diseases classified elsewhere
Code first underlying disease, such as:
parasitic disease (B65-B89)

> **EXCLUDES 1** acoustic neuritis (in) :
> herpes zoster (B02.29)
> syphilis (A52.15)

M ⊟ **!Q** **H94.00** *Acoustic neuritis in infectious and parasitic diseases classified elsewhere, unspecified ear*

M ⊟ **!Q** **H94.01** *Acoustic neuritis in infectious and parasitic diseases classified elsewhere, right ear*

M ⊟ **!Q** **H94.02** *Acoustic neuritis in infectious and parasitic diseases classified elsewhere, left ear*

M ⊟ **!Q** **H94.03** *Acoustic neuritis in infectious and parasitic diseases classified elsewhere, bilateral*

④ 4th digit required   ⑤ 5th digit required   ⑥ 6th digit required   ⑦ 7th digit required   ☑ 7th digit placeholder   ✚ Additional code   ⊟ Laterality

940   *DecisionHealth's* FY 2020 Complete Home Health ICD-10-CM Diagnosis Coding Manual

⑤ **H94.8 Other specified disorders of ear in diseases classified elsewhere**

Code first underlying disease, such as: congenital syphilis (A50.0)

EXCLUDES 1 aural myiasis (B87.4)
syphilitic labyrinthitis (A52.79)

⊟ **IQ** H94.80 Other specified disorders of ear in diseases classified elsewhere, unspecified ear

⊟ **IQ** H94.81 Other specified disorders of right ear in diseases classified elsewhere

⊟ **IQ** H94.82 Other specified disorders of left ear in diseases classified elsewhere

⊟ **IQ** H94.83 Other specified disorders of ear in diseases classified elsewhere, bilateral

---

Intraoperative and postprocedural complications and disorders of ear and mastoid process, not elsewhere classified (H95)

④ **H95 Intraoperative and postprocedural complications and disorders of ear and mastoid process, not elsewhere classified**

⑤ **H95.0 Recurrent cholesteatoma of postmastoidectomy cavity**

⊟ **IQ** H95.00 Recurrent cholesteatoma of postmastoidectomy cavity, unspecified ear

⊟ **SP** H95.01 Recurrent cholesteatoma of postmastoidectomy cavity, right ear

⊟ **SP** H95.02 Recurrent cholesteatoma of postmastoidectomy cavity, left ear

⊟ **SP** H95.03 Recurrent cholesteatoma of postmastoidectomy cavity, bilateral ears

⑤ **H95.1 Other disorders of ear and mastoid process following mastoidectomy**

⑥ **H95.11 Chronic inflammation of postmastoidectomy cavity**

⊟ **SP** H95.111 Chronic inflammation of postmastoidectomy cavity, right ear

⊟ **SP** H95.112 Chronic inflammation of postmastoidectomy cavity, left ear

⊟ **SP** H95.113 Chronic inflammation of postmastoidectomy cavity, bilateral ears

⊟ **IQ** H95.119 Chronic inflammation of postmastoidectomy cavity, unspecified ear

⑥ **H95.12 Granulation of postmastoidectomy cavity**

⊟ **SP** H95.121 Granulation of postmastoidectomy cavity, right ear

⊟ **SP** H95.122 Granulation of postmastoidectomy cavity, left ear

⊟ **SP** H95.123 Granulation of postmastoidectomy cavity, bilateral ears

⊟ **IQ** H95.129 Granulation of postmastoidectomy cavity, unspecified ear

⑥ **H95.13 Mucosal cyst of postmastoidectomy cavity**

⊟ **SP** H95.131 Mucosal cyst of postmastoidectomy cavity, right ear

⊟ **SP** H95.132 Mucosal cyst of postmastoidectomy cavity, left ear

⊟ **SP** H95.133 Mucosal cyst of postmastoidectomy cavity, bilateral ears

⊟ **IQ** H95.139 Mucosal cyst of postmastoidectomy cavity, unspecified ear

⑥ **H95.19 Other disorders following mastoidectomy**

⊟ **SP** H95.191 Other disorders following mastoidectomy, right ear

⊟ **SP** H95.192 Other disorders following mastoidectomy, left ear

⊟ **SP** H95.193 Other disorders following mastoidectomy, bilateral ears

⊟ **IQ** H95.199 Other disorders following mastoidectomy, unspecified ear

⑤ **H95.2 Intraoperative hemorrhage and hematoma of ear and mastoid process complicating a procedure**

EXCLUDES 1 intraoperative hemorrhage and hematoma of ear and mastoid process due to accidental puncture or laceration during a procedure (H95.3-)

SP H95.21 Intraoperative hemorrhage and hematoma of ear and mastoid process complicating a procedure on the ear and mastoid process

SP H95.22 Intraoperative hemorrhage and hematoma of ear and mastoid process complicating other procedure

⑤ **H95.3 Accidental puncture and laceration of ear and mastoid process during a procedure**

SP H95.31 Accidental puncture and laceration of the ear and mastoid process during a procedure on the ear and mastoid process

SP H95.32 Accidental puncture and laceration of the ear and mastoid process during other procedure

⑤ **H95.4 Postprocedural hemorrhage of ear and mastoid process following a procedure**

SP H95.41 Postprocedural hemorrhage of ear and mastoid process following a procedure on the ear and mastoid process

SP H95.42 Postprocedural hemorrhage of ear and mastoid process following other procedure

⑤ **H95.5 Postprocedural hematoma and seroma of ear and mastoid process following a procedure**

SP H95.51 Postprocedural hematoma of ear and mastoid process following a procedure on the ear and mastoid process

Chapter 8

H60-H95

★ New ▲ Revised **Px** Primary **SP** PDGM Px **SL** Low CoM **SH** High CoM **IQ** Quest. Encounter **H** Hospice non-cancer Dx Unspecified **M** *Manifestation*

DecisionHealth's FY 2020 Complete Home Health ICD-10-CM Diagnosis Coding Manual

941

SP H95.52 Postprocedural hematoma of ear and mastoid process following other procedure

SP H95.53 Postprocedural seroma of ear and mastoid process following a procedure on the ear and mastoid process

SP H95.54 Postprocedural seroma of ear and mastoid process following other procedure

5 H95.8 Other intraoperative and postprocedural complications and disorders of the ear and mastoid process, not elsewhere classified

> **EXCLUDES 2** postprocedural complications and disorders following mastoidectomy (H95.0-, H95.1-)

6 H95.81 Postprocedural stenosis of external ear canal

⊟ SP H95.811 Postprocedural stenosis of right external ear canal

⊟ SP H95.812 Postprocedural stenosis of left external ear canal

⊟ SP H95.813 Postprocedural stenosis of external ear canal, bilateral

⊟ IQ H95.819 Postprocedural stenosis of unspecified external ear canal

SP ✚ H95.88 Other intraoperative complications and disorders of the ear and mastoid process, not elsewhere classified
Use additional code, if applicable, to further specify disorder

SP ✚ H95.89 Other postprocedural complications and disorders of the ear and mastoid process, not elsewhere classified
Use additional code, if applicable, to further specify disorder

Chapter 8

H60-H95

4 4th digit required   5 5th digit required   6 6th digit required   7 7th digit required   ☑ 7th digit placeholder   ✚ Additional code   ⊟ Laterality

942   *DecisionHealth's* FY 2020 Complete Home Health ICD-10-CM Diagnosis Coding Manual

Chapter 8 Scenarios: Diseases of the ear and mastoid process (H60-H95)

Malignant otitis externa, type 1 diabetes

A 68-year-old woman who is a type 1 diabetic comes to home health with a primary diagnosis of malignant otitis externa in bilateral ears. The record indicates the infecting organism is pseudomonas aeruginosa. She will receive IV antibiotics.

Description	Code
Primary: Malignant otitis externa, bilateral	H60.23
Secondary: Pseudomonas (aeruginosa) (mallei) (pseudomallei) as the cause of diseases classified elsewhere	B96.5
Secondary: Type 1 diabetes mellitus without complications	E10.9
Secondary: Encounter for adjustment and management of vascular access device	Z45.2
Secondary: Long term (current) use of antibiotics	Z79.2

The infection is the focus of care and is thus coded primary. The infecting organism immediately follows it. Codes Z45.2 and Z79.2 capture the administration of IV antibiotics. No code for insulin use is assigned because the patient is a type 1 diabetic and insulin dependence is inherent.

Ototoxic hearing loss, ankylosing spondylitis

A 66-year-old man with ankylosing spondylitis is suffering from hearing loss in both ears following the completion of treatment with gentamicin for a severe infection which is now resolved. The physician confirms that the hearing loss is a lingering adverse effect of the gentamicin, which was stopped several weeks ago and is no longer in his system. The focus of care is the hearing loss and the patient will receive occupational therapy.

Description	Code
Primary: Ototoxic hearing loss, bilateral	H91.03
Secondary: Adverse effect of aminoglycosides, sequela	T36.5x5S
Secondary: Ankylosing spondylitis of unspecified sites in spine	M45.9

The focus of care is the hearing loss, which is appropriately coded as ototoxic hearing loss, and placed in the primary position. The adverse effect code for the gentamicin is coded following the code for the problem it caused, in accordance with tabular instruction. The seventh character is "S" because the drug is no longer in his system but has left behind a lingering effect. No code for the infection is assigned as it is now resolved. His ankylosing spondylitis is a relevant comorbidity that will impact his recovery and is thus also coded.

Surgical aftercare, vertigo

A 70-year-old man recently underwent joint replacement surgery on his left hip. He had bilateral osteoarthritis in his hips and will have the other hip replaced later on. While in the hospital, he was diagnosed with severe benign paroxysmal positional vertigo. He is admitted to home health for aftercare, including physical and occupational therapy. The home health physical therapist will help him with exercises designed to ease the vertigo symptoms.

Description	Code
Primary: Aftercare following joint replacement surgery	Z47.1
Secondary: Unilateral primary osteoarthritis, right hip	M16.11
Secondary: Benign paroxysmal vertigo, unspecified ear	H81.10
Secondary: Presence of left artificial hip joint	Z96.642

Surgical aftercare is the focus of care, making Z47.1 the appropriate primary code choice. The patient had bilateral osteoarthritis, but since one hip has been replaced, it is resolved on that side. Thus, unilateral hip osteoarthritis is coded instead, in accordance with coding guidelines. The patient's vertigo is specified as benign paroxysmal positional but the ear was not specified, making the correct diagnosis code H81.10. The status code Z96.642 is assigned to identify the joint that was replaced, in accordance with tabular instruction.

Chapter 9: Diseases of the Circulatory System (I00-I99)

Chapter 9 includes the following blocks:

- I00-I02   Acute rheumatic fever
- I05-I09   Chronic rheumatic heart disease
- I10-I16   Hypertensive diseases
- I20-I25   Ischemic heart disease
- I26-I28   Pulmonary heart disease and diseases of pulmonary circulation
- I30-I52   Other forms of heart disease
- I60-I69   Cerebrovascular diseases
- I70-I79   Diseases of arteries, arterioles, and capillaries
- I80-I89   Diseases of veins, lymphatic vessels and lymph nodes, not elsewhere classified.
- I95-I99   Other and unspecified disorders of the circulatory system

Documentation is critically important in coding for conditions in this chapter. Do not try to decipher the condition from the physician's notes. Rather, ask for additional documentation when necessary. Below are some examples of situations and questions to ask when attempting to obtain additional documentation.

Documentation stating "**atrioventricular block**" (I44 category) means occlusion of the chambers within the heart, but more information is needed, such as is the block first or second degree; does it involve the left or right bundle branches (which transmit electricity throughout the heart), or another type of conduction disorder.

Documentation stating "**heart failure**" (I50 category) means that the heart is not able to pump sufficient blood to the body, but more information is needed, such as is it left-sided failure; is it systolic (contraction phase of heartbeat) failure or diastolic (relaxation phase) failure or both; is it congestive heart failure (the blood backs up into the lungs and the tissues of organs and the legs); is it acute, chronic or acute on chronic failure.

Documentation stating "**atherosclerosis**" (I70 category) means hardening of the arteries, but more information is needed, such as is it a native artery or a graft (autologous, nonautologous, biological, nonbiological, or other type) from a bypass surgery; which artery is affected; what side is affected; is there any intermittent claudication, rest pain, ulceration, or gangrene present. *Note,* the ICD-10 classification assumes a relationship between atherosclerosis of lower extremities and gangrene, ulceration, rest pain and intermittent claudication.

Circulatory organs and functions tie into nearly all other systems so you will find close linkages to other ICD-10-CM chapters. For instance, the respiratory system carries oxygen to the bloodstream and removes excess carbon dioxide from the body (related codes can be found in Chapter 10, diseases of the respiratory system). Other conditions of the lymphatic system are found throughout the book, depending on the location of the lymph node involved and whether it is a site of a tumor (Chapter 2) or infection (Chapter 1).

Conditions related to the blood or blood-forming organs such as anemias, coagulation deficits, neutropenia, disorders of the spleen are reported using codes from Chapter 3 (Diseases of the Blood and Blood-Forming Organs and Certain Disorders Involving the Immune Mechanism).

As is the case with other ICD-10-CM codes, in certain situations you will need to look beyond this chapter to properly code a case. For example:

- If the documentation indicates **a neoplasm or tumor of an organ in the circulatory system,** look up the term (malignancy, tumor, adenoma) to find the correct code, likely a code from Chapter 2 (C00-D49).

- If a patient has **a personal or family history** of a condition reported in this chapter, it may be appropriate to select from the Z code section, such as Z86.7- (Diseases of circulatory system), or Z82.3 (Family history of stroke).

- If a condition reported in this chapter is the **result of injury, poisoning, or certain other consequences of external causes,** a code from Chapter 19 (S00-T88), may be reported with a code from this chapter.

- **Symptoms, signs and abnormal clinical and laboratory findings** related to the circulatory system are sometimes reported using codes from Chapter 18 (R00-R94) such as R09.89 (Symptoms involving cardiovascular system). Every effort should be made to secure a definitive diagnosis. A symptom code from Chapter 18 may be reported as an additional diagnosis when it describes a significant aspect of the condition but is not an integral part of it.

- Although not often coded in home health, if reporting a circulatory disease in a **pregnant patient** when the condition is complicating the pregnancy, report first a code from Chapter 15 (Pregnancy, childbirth and the puerperium), such as O99.411 (Diseases of the circulatory system complicating pregnancy, first trimester).

A code from Chapter 16, Certain conditions originating in the perinatal period (P00-P96), and codes from Chapter 17, Congenital malformations, deformations, and chromosomal abnormalities (Q00-Q99) are not included in codes in this chapter, but may be used as additional codes to describe the patient's situation.

- Additional disorders and conditions that may be present along with a code within this chapter, but are not included in this chapter include endocrine, nutritional and metabolic diseases (E00-E88) in chapter 4; and systemic connective tissue disorders (M30-M36) in chapter 13. Follow the Tabular directions for sequencing these conditions along with a code from chapter 9.

Multiple Coding and Sequencing

It is important to read the Includes and Excludes notes under codes in this chapter, as well as any other instructions under the code or code category. There are many combination codes in chapter 9, which will decrease the need for multiple codes to be assigned.

If heart disease is caused by an infection, be sure to start your search in the Alphabetical Index under the key term 'pericarditis, inflammation of the pericardium,' and confirm the code in the Tabular List after reading all notes. For example, acute pericarditis due to tuberculosis is reported as A18.84 (tuberculosis of the heart), which includes tuberculosis pericarditis as well as several other cardiac conditions. Code I32 (pericarditis in diseases classified elsewhere) is a manifestation code with an Excludes 1 note for tuberculosis pericarditis so the A18.84 code is the only code needed. However, if a patient has staphylococcal pericarditis, the first listed code would be I30.1 (Infective pericarditis) with an additional code of B95.7 (Other staphylococcus as the cause of diseases classified elsewhere) from Chapter 1. However, if the diagnostic statement or confirmation from the physician indicated the pericarditis was due to methicillin susceptible Staphylococcus aureus, code B95.61 (MSSA infection as the cause of diseases classified elsewhere) would be the choice for the additional code.

Category I50 is used to report **heart failure**. There are multiple types of heart failure, such as left sided, systolic, diastolic, combined systolic and diastolic, and right sided failure that can be unspecified, acute, chronic or acute on chronic.

Code I50.1, left-sided heart failure, includes acute pulmonary edema; no additional code needs to be assigned. Never use I50.1 and I50.9 on the same claim.

Code I50.2 indicates systolic heart failure, which is a decrease in the heart's ability to contract. The heart is unable to pump with enough force to push a sufficient amount of blood into the circulation. Systolic heart failure is coded when the documentation indicates HFrEF, which may also be called heart failure with low ejection fraction, or heart failure with reduced systolic function, or other similar terms meaning systolic heart failure. But remember, do not code systolic failure based on ejection fraction numbers without physician interpretation.

Code I50.3 indicates diastolic heart failure, which occurs when the heart has a problem relaxing. Ventricles are not filling during diastole. All codes for heart failure include any associated pulmonary edema. Diastolic heart failure is coded when the documentation indicates HFpEF, which may also be referred to as heart failure with preserved systolic function, and this condition may also be referred to as diastolic heart failure. Do not code diastolic failure based on ejection fraction numbers without physician interpretation.

Diastolic dysfunction or systolic dysfunction is coded to I51.89 if not related to heart failure. If related to heart failure, then diastolic heart failure or systolic heart failure should be coded.

Category I70 is used to report **atherosclerosis**. Within this category, several codes may be appropriate to assign – both from this category and from other chapters. There is a note to use additional codes with I70 to identify: exposure to environmental tobacco smoke (Z77.22), history of tobacco dependence (Z87.891), occupational exposure to environmental tobacco smoke (Z57.31), tobacco dependence (F17.-) and tobacco use (Z72.0).

Take note of the following circumstances:

- Within specific subcategories of atherosclerosis, there are additional code notes. For example, atherosclerosis of native arteries of the extremities (I70.2-) includes a note to add an additional code, if applicable, to identify chronic total occlusion of artery of an extremity (I70.92). Characters 4, 5 and 6 for I70.- codes identify laterality and additional conditions that may be present such as intermittent claudication, rest pain, presence and location of ulceration, and the presence of gangrene. Codes that indicate ulceration also include a note to add an additional code to identify the severity of any ulcer (L98.49-), if applicable.

- Additional codes in category I70.2 to I70.7 utilize expanded subcategories to identify the atherosclerosis of unspecified type of bypass graft(s)(I70.3-); autologous vein bypass graft (I70.4-); nonautologous biological bypass graft(s), (I70.5-); nonbiological bypass graft(s) (I70.6); and other type of bypass graft, (I70.7-) of the extremities.

These are useful terms to know when reviewing documentation related to circulatory disorders:

- Ischemia – decreased blood flow

- Embolism – a clot traveling through the circulatory system

- Infarction – halted blood flow resulting in cellular death

- Occlusion– blockage

- Stenosis – narrowing

- Thrombus – blood clot

- Hemorrhage – heavy or uncontrolled bleeding.

One more pointer: You'll often see the prefixes "epi" and "sub" applied to the anatomical parts. Just remember that "epi" means "upon" and "sub" means "under." Thus, "subarachnoid" means under the arachnoid layer of the meninges.

Special Coding Issues

Hypertension

Hypertensive diseases are organized under one block (I10-I16). Pay attention to the note at the top of the category to use additional codes to identify exposure to environmental tobacco smoke, history of tobacco dependence, occupational exposure to environmental tobacco smoke, tobacco dependence and tobacco use.

The most challenging part of coding for hypertension is establishing its relationship with other conditions. **Remember**, the classification presumes a causal relationship between hypertension and heart involvement and between hypertension and kidney involvement, as the two conditions are linked by the term "with" in the Alphabetic Index. These conditions should be coded as related even in the absence of provider documentation explicitly linking them, unless the documentation clearly states the conditions are unrelated. More specifically:

- **Hypertensive heart disease:** Hypertension with heart conditions classified to I50.-, and I51.4-I51.9, are assigned to a code from category I11 (Hypertensive heart disease) when both conditions are present in the documentation. A cause-and-effect relationship is assumed by the ICD-10 classification system unless the provider states otherwise. If there is uncertainty about the relationship, always query the physician. The hypertensive disease is sequenced first and an additional code is used to identify the specific type(s) of heart disease/failure. If the provider states there is not a relationship between the two conditions, report separate codes for the hypertension and the heart condition in either order based on the impact of each condition on the plan of care.

- **Hypertensive chronic kidney disease:** Report the hypertensive chronic kidney disease (category I12) whether or not a causal relationship is stated in the documentation. Coding Guidelines instruct that you can assume that if both these conditions are present, they are related. You should also report an additional code from category N18 (chronic kidney disease). The classification assumes a relationship between HTN and any condition classifiable to N18 (CKD) and N26. The relationship may be assumed because of the pathology of hypertension, which impacts renal function, often resulting in CKD. However, CKD should not be coded as hypertensive if the physician has specifically documented a different cause. Do not confuse hypertensive chronic kidney disease with renovascular hypertension, a condition in which the kidney dysfunction causes the hypertension. Renovascular hypertension is coded using I15.0.

- **Hypertensive heart and chronic kidney disease (CKD):** Report the hypertensive heart and chronic kidney disease (category I13) when all conditions are present in the documentation. A cause-and-effect relationship is assumed by the ICD-10 classification system unless the provider states otherwise. If there is uncertainty about the relationship, always query the physician. The relationship between the hypertension, heart disease and the chronic kidney disease is presumed by the ICD-10 classification systsem. If heart failure is present, report additional code(s) from category I50 (heart failure) to identify the type(s) of heart failure, and category N18 (chronic kidney disease) to identify the stage of the CKD.

Example: Patient with stage 3 CKD, CHF and hypertension is coded as I13.0, I50.9, N18.3.

- **Hypertensive cerebrovascular disease:** An appropriate code from categories I60-I69 (cerebrovascular disease) is assigned first, followed by the appropriate hypertension code from I10-I16.

- **Hypertensive retinopathy:** Subcategory H35.0 (Background retinopathy and retinal vascular changes) is coded first followed by a code from hypertension category I10 – I16.

- **Hypertension, secondary:** Secondary hypertension is due to an underlying condition. Two codes are required to describe this condition. A code to identify the underlying etiology and a code from category I15, (Secondary hypertension). The actual sequence of the two codes is determined by the reason for admission/encounter.

- **Hypertension transient:** Code R03.0, Elevated blood pressure reading without a diagnosis, is coded unless a patient has an established diagnosis of hypertension.

- **Gestational (pregnancy-induced) hypertension** without significant proteinuria (O13.-), or preeclampsia (O14.-) is coded for transient hypertension associated with pregnancy.

- **Hypertension, controlled** as a diagnosis statement usually refers to an existing state of hypertension under control by therapy. Choose the appropriate code from categories I10-I16 (Hypertensive disease) to describe this situation.

- **Hypertension, uncontrolled** may refer to untreated hypertension or hypertension not responding to current therapeutic regimen. In either case, the appropriate code from categories I10-I16 (Hypertensive disease) is assigned and the terms controlled or uncontrolled do not have any impact on the code assigned. Additional documentation may be included in the medical record to provide this information.

- **Hypertensive Crisis** is assigned with a code from category I16 for documented hypertensive urgency, hypertensive emergency or unspecified hypertensive crisis. Code also any identified hypertensive disease (I10-I15). The sequencing is based on the reason for the encounter.

Atherosclerotic Coronary Artery Disease and Angina

ICD-10-CM has combination codes for atherosclerotic heart disease with angina pectoris: Subcategory I25.11-, Atherosclerotic heart disease of native coronary artery with angina pectoris, and I25.7-, Atherosclerosis of coronary artery bypass graft(s) and coronary artery of transplanted heart with angina pectoris. An additional code for angina pectoris is **not necessary** when using one of these combination codes.

A causal relationship can be assumed in a patient with both atherosclerosis and angina pectoris unless the documentation indicates the angina is due to something other than the atherosclerosis.

If a patient with coronary artery disease is admitted due to an acute myocardial infarction (AMI), the AMI should be sequenced before the coronary artery disease.

CVA

Several conditions, such as a head injury, tumor of the brain or spinal cord, or an infection of the CNS, present with symptoms identical to those found in what a lay person would call "stroke." The symptoms include: weakness, paralysis of facial muscles, clumsiness, paresthesia (numbness), hemiplegia (paralysis in one or both limbs on the same side), loss of sensation, inability to eat or talk, loss of vision or partial vision in one or both eyes, double vision, memory loss, and/or vertigo.

When a physician sees these symptoms, he or she may document the rather generic term "CVA," or "cerebrovascular accident." The acute stage of the condition, reported with codes I60-I63, occurs when brain cells die due to a clot or bleeding in the brain that cuts off the oxygen supply. The acute stage is treated in an inpatient facility, such as with tissue plasminogen activator (t-PA), in order to resolve the clot.

When applicable, use a code from R29.7 to indicate the National Institutes of Health Stroke Scale (NIHSS) score. The NIHSS score can be used as a clinical stroke assessment tool to evaluate and document neurological status in acute stroke patients. The stroke scale is valid for predicting lesion size and can serve as a measure of stroke severity. The NIHSS has been shown to be a predictor of both short and long term outcome of stroke patients.

Sequelae or "late-effects" category I69 includes neurological deficits that persist after the initial onset of conditions classifiable to categories I60-I67. The neurologic deficits caused by cerebrovascular disease may be present from the onset or may arise at any time after the onset of the condition classifiable to I60-I67. You may assign as many of the combination codes in I69 that apply.

Codes from I69 (Sequelae of cerebrovascular disease) that specify hemiplegia, hemiparesis and monoplegia identify whether the dominant or nondominant side is affected. Should the affected side be documented, but not specified as dominant or non-dominant, and the classification system does not indicate a default, code selection is as follows:

- For ambidextrous patients, the default should be dominant.

- If the left side is affected, the default is nondominant.

- If the right side is affected, the default is dominant.

I69 (Sequelae of cerebrovascular disease) codes may be assigned on a health care record **with** codes from I60 – I67, **if** the patient has a current cerebrovascular disease and deficits from an old cerebrovascular disease. However, codes from I69 should not be assigned if the patient does not have neurologic deficits; instead assign Z86.73 (Personal history of TIA and cerebral infarction).

MI

Acute myocardial infarction (AMI) results from a blocked coronary artery that supplies oxygenated blood to a part of the heart's muscle. Interruption of blood and oxygen to the heart muscle causes injury or death of the affected heart muscle tissue. Blockage of a coronary artery that results in a myocardial infarction may be caused by a blood clot due to the rupture of atherosclerotic plaque within arterial walls which causes a blood clot at the site. Other causes of blockage may be mural thrombosis, vegetative endocarditis, or atherosclerotic plaque buildup. A rarer cause of heart attack is spasm of the coronary artery that can prevent blood flow as a result of drug use, such as cocaine.

Types of myocardial infarction:

Transmural infarctions extend through the entire thickness of heart muscle from endocardium to epicardium in the left ventricular wall. These are further classified by site, such as anteriolateral wall or true posterior wall, and are due to complete occlusion of blood supply in the area.

- **STEMI** (ST segment elevation myocardial infarction), the more severe type of MI, occurs when a coronary artery is totally occluded by a blood clot and virtually all the heart muscle dependent on blood supply by that particular artery begins to die. This is a transmural infarction, also known as a Q-wave MI. The ST segment elevation indicates that a large amount of damage to the heart muscle is occurring.

Subendocardial infarctions involve small, multifocal areas of necrosis confined to the inner portion of the wall of the left ventricle, ventricular septum, or papillary muscles and are thought to result from decreased blood supply locally, usually due to narrowing of the vessels.

- **NSTEMI** (non-ST segment elevation myocardial infarction) is a milder form of infarction in which the coronary artery is only partially occluded and only the inner portion of the heart muscle supplied by the coronary artery dies.

The ICD-10-CM codes for type 1 acute myocardial infarction (AMI) identify the site, such as anterolateral wall or true posterior wall. Subcategories I21.0-I21.2 and code I21.3 are used for type 1 ST elevation myocardial infarction (STEMI). Code I21.4, Non-ST elevation (NSTEMI) myocardial infarction, is used for type 1 non ST elevation myocardial infarction (NSTEMI) and nontransmural MIs.

General Guidelines:

- If a type 1 NSTEMI evolves to STEMI, assign the STEMI code.

- If a type 1 STEMI converts to NSTEMI due to thrombolytic therapy, it is still coded as a STEMI.

- If an AMI is documented as nontransmural or subendocardial, but the site is provided, it is still coded as a subendocardial AMI.

- For encounters occurring while the myocardial infarction is equal to, or less than, four weeks old, (including transfers to another acute care setting

or a post-acute setting), and the patient requires continued care for the myocardial infarction, you may continue to report codes from category I21.

- For encounters after the four week time frame and the patient is still receiving care related to the myocardial infarction, the appropriate aftercare code should be assigned rather than a code from category I21. For old or healed MIs, not requiring further care, code I25.2 (Old myocardial infarction) may be assigned.

- Code I21.9 is the default for unspecified acute myocardial infarction or unspecified type. Assign I21.3 if only type 1 STEMI or transmural MI without the site is documented.

Subsequent Acute MI:

Assign a code from category I22 when a patient who has suffered a type 1 or unspecified AMI has a new AMI within the 4 week time frame of the initial AMI. Use a code from category I22 with a code from category I21. The sequencing of the I22 and I21 codes depends on the circumstances of the encounter.

Do not assign I22 for subsequent myocardial infarctions other than type 1 or unspecified. For subsequent type 2 AMI assign only assign I21.A1. For subsequent type 4 or type 5 AMI, assign only I21.A9, per coding guidelines.

Other Types of Myocardial Infarction:

There are options for different types of myocardial infarction. Type 1 myocardial infarctions are assigned to codes I21.0-I21.4. Type 2 myocardial infarction, and myocardial infarction due to demand ischemia or secondary to ischemic balance, is assigned to code I21.A1.

Sequencing of type 2 AMI or the underlying cause should be based on the circumstances of the admission. When a type 2 AMI code is described as NSTEMI or STEMI, only assign code I21.A1. Codes I21.01-I21.4 should only be assigned for type 1 AMIs.

Acute myocardial infarctions type 3, 4a, 4b, 4c and 5 are assigned to code I21.A9, Other myocardial infarction type.

Chapter 9

I00-I99

CHAPTER 9: DISEASES OF THE CIRCULATORY SYSTEM (I00-I99)

EXCLUDES 2 certain conditions originating in the perinatal period (P04-P96)
certain infectious and parasitic diseases (A00-B99)
complications of pregnancy, childbirth and the puerperium (O00-O9A)
congenital malformations, deformations, and chromosomal abnormalities (Q00-Q99)
endocrine, nutritional and metabolic diseases (E00-E88)
injury, poisoning and certain other consequences of external causes (S00-T88)
neoplasms (C00-D49)
symptoms, signs and abnormal clinical and laboratory findings, not elsewhere classified (R00-R94)
systemic connective tissue disorders (M30-M36)
transient cerebral ischemic attacks and related syndromes (G45.-)

This chapter contains the following blocks:

I00-I02   Acute rheumatic fever
I05-I09   Chronic rheumatic heart diseases
I10-I16   Hypertensive diseases
I20-I25   Ischemic heart diseases
I26-I28   Pulmonary heart disease and diseases of pulmonary circulation
I30-I52   Other forms of heart disease
I60-I69   Cerebrovascular diseases
I70-I79   Diseases of arteries, arterioles and capillaries
I80-I89   Diseases of veins, lymphatic vessels and lymph nodes, not elsewhere classified
I95-I99   Other and unspecified disorders of the circulatory system

Acute rheumatic fever   (I00-I02)

SP I00   Rheumatic fever without heart involvement
INCLUDES arthritis, rheumatic, acute or subacute
EXCLUDES 1 rheumatic fever with heart involvement (I01.0 -I01.9)
DEFINITION Delayed, febrile, inflammatory disease resulting about 20 days after streptococcal infection; presents with joint pain, migratory arthritis, skin rash on the trunk and proximal extremities, and nosebleeds; can cause cardiac damage.

4 I01   Rheumatic fever with heart involvement
EXCLUDES 1 chronic diseases of rheumatic origin (I05-I09) unless rheumatic fever is also present or there is evidence of reactivation or activity of the rheumatic process.
CODING TIPS ✓ Pericarditis, endocarditis, and myocarditis are coded with I01-I02 when specified as rheumatic, or associated with rheumatic fever.

SP I01.0   Acute rheumatic pericarditis
Any condition in I00 with pericarditis
Rheumatic pericarditis (acute)
EXCLUDES 1 acute pericarditis not specified as rheumatic (I30.-)

SP I01.1   Acute rheumatic endocarditis

Any condition in I00 with endocarditis or valvulitis
Acute rheumatic valvulitis
SP I01.2   Acute rheumatic myocarditis
Any condition in I00 with myocarditis
SP I01.8   Other acute rheumatic heart disease
Any condition in I00 with other or multiple types of heart involvement
Acute rheumatic pancarditis
SP I01.9   Acute rheumatic heart disease, unspecified
Any condition in I00 with unspecified type of heart involvement
Rheumatic carditis, acute
Rheumatic heart disease, active or acute

4 I02   Rheumatic chorea
INCLUDES Sydenham's chorea
EXCLUDES 1 chorea NOS (G25.5)
Huntington's chorea (G10)
CODING TIPS ✓ Pericarditis, endocarditis, and myocarditis are coded with I01-I02 when specified as rheumatic, or associated with rheumatic fever.
CODING TIPS ✓ Rheumatic chorea may also be referred to as "St. Vitus dance" and is more frequently diagnosed in children and adolescents.

SP I02.0   Rheumatic chorea with heart involvement
Chorea NOS with heart involvement
Rheumatic chorea with heart involvement of any type classifiable under I01.-
SP I02.9   Rheumatic chorea without heart involvement
Rheumatic chorea NOS

Chronic rheumatic heart diseases   (I05-I09)

CODING TIPS ✓ Category I05 -I09 includes disease of the heart valves. Diseases of the mitral and tricuspid heart valves are considered rheumatic, unless specified by the physician as nonrheumatic. Aortic and pulmonary heart valve disease is considered nonrheumatic, unless specified as rheumatic. If multiple valves are involved, ICD-10-CM classifies the disease as rheumatic, unless specified by the physician as non-rheumatic. Pay special attention to includes and excludes 1 notes.

4 I05   Rheumatic mitral valve diseases
INCLUDES conditions classifiable to both I05.0 and I05.2-I05.9, whether specified as rheumatic or not
EXCLUDES 1 mitral valve disease specified as nonrheumatic (I34.-)
mitral valve disease with aortic and/or tricuspid valve involvement (I08.-)
CODING TIPS ✓ Mitral valve disease is assumed to be rheumatic unless specified as nonrheumatic.

SP I05.0   Rheumatic mitral stenosis
Mitral (valve) obstruction (rheumatic)
SP I05.1   Rheumatic mitral insufficiency
Rheumatic mitral incompetence
Rheumatic mitral regurgitation

---

4 4th digit required   **5** 5th digit required   **6** 6th digit required   **7** 7th digit required   **7** 7th digit placeholder   **+** Additional code   **⊟** Laterality

EXCLUDES 1 mitral insufficiency not specified as rheumatic (I34.0)

SP **I05.2** **Rheumatic mitral stenosis with insufficiency**
Rheumatic mitral stenosis with incompetence or regurgitation

SP **I05.8** **Other rheumatic mitral valve diseases**
Rheumatic mitral (valve) failure

SP **I05.9** **Rheumatic mitral valve disease, unspecified**

Rheumatic mitral (valve) disorder (chronic) NOS

4 **I06** **Rheumatic aortic valve diseases**
EXCLUDES 1 aortic valve disease not specified as rheumatic (I35.-)
aortic valve disease with mitral and/or tricuspid valve involvement (I08.-)

CODING TIPS ✓ Aortic valve disease specified as rheumatic is coded to I06. If not specified as rheumatic, see I35.

SP **I06.0** **Rheumatic aortic stenosis**
Rheumatic aortic (valve) obstruction

SP **I06.1** **Rheumatic aortic insufficiency**
Rheumatic aortic incompetence
Rheumatic aortic regurgitation

SP **I06.2** **Rheumatic aortic stenosis with insufficiency**
Rheumatic aortic stenosis with incompetence or regurgitation

SP **I06.8** **Other rheumatic aortic valve diseases**

SP **I06.9** **Rheumatic aortic valve disease, unspecified**

Rheumatic aortic (valve) disease NOS

4 **I07** **Rheumatic tricuspid valve diseases**
INCLUDES rheumatic tricuspid valve diseases specified as rheumatic or unspecified
EXCLUDES 1 tricuspid valve disease specified as nonrheumatic (I36.-)
tricuspid valve disease with aortic and/or mitral valve involvement (I08.-)

CODING TIPS ✓ Tricuspid valve disease is assumed to be rheumatic unless specified as nonrheumatic.

SP **I07.0** **Rheumatic tricuspid stenosis**
Tricuspid (valve) stenosis (rheumatic)

SP **I07.1** **Rheumatic tricuspid insufficiency**
Tricuspid (valve) insufficiency (rheumatic)

SP **I07.2** **Rheumatic tricuspid stenosis and insufficiency**

SP **I07.8** **Other rheumatic tricuspid valve diseases**

SP **I07.9** **Rheumatic tricuspid valve disease, unspecified**

Rheumatic tricuspid valve disorder NOS

4 **I08** **Multiple valve diseases**
INCLUDES multiple valve diseases specified as rheumatic or unspecified
EXCLUDES 1 endocarditis, valve unspecified (I38)

multiple valve disease specified a nonrheumatic (I34.-, I35.-, I36.-, I37.-, I38.-, Q22.-, Q23.-, Q24.8-)
rheumatic valve disease NOS (I09.1)

CODING TIPS ✓ Valve disease involving multiple valves is assumed to be rheumatic unless specified as nonrheumatic. Aortic valve disease, by itself, is considered nonrheumatic, unless specified as rheumatic. When aortic valve disease is combined with other heart valves, it is considered rheumatic.

SP **I08.0** **Rheumatic disorders of both mitral and aortic valves**
Involvement of both mitral and aortic valves specified as rheumatic or unspecified

CODING TIPS ✓ Assign I08.0 for a diagnosis of aortic valve stenosis with mitral valve insufficiency.

SP **I08.1** **Rheumatic disorders of both mitral and tricuspid valves**

SP **I08.2** **Rheumatic disorders of both aortic and tricuspid valves**

SP **I08.3** **Combined rheumatic disorders of mitral, aortic and tricuspid valves**

SP **I08.8** **Other rheumatic multiple valve diseases**
CODING TIPS ✓ When the clinical record reports rheumatic disease of multiple valves but the descriptions in I08.0, .1, .2 or .3 do not apply, e.g., pulmonary valve along with other specified valves, use I08.8.

SP **I08.9** **Rheumatic multiple valve disease, unspecified**

CODING TIPS ✓ When the clinical record reports rheumatic disease of multiple valves, but the affected valves are not specified, assign code I08.9.

4 **I09** **Other rheumatic heart diseases**

SP **I09.0** **Rheumatic myocarditis**
EXCLUDES 1 myocarditis not specified as rheumatic (I51.4)
DEFINITION Chronic inflammation and degeneration of heart muscle due to rheumatic heart disease.

SP **I09.1** **Rheumatic diseases of endocardium, valve unspecified**

Rheumatic endocarditis (chronic)
Rheumatic valvulitis (chronic)
EXCLUDES 1 endocarditis, valve unspecified (I38)

SP **I09.2** **Chronic rheumatic pericarditis**
Adherent pericardium, rheumatic
Chronic rheumatic mediastinopericarditis
Chronic rheumatic myopericarditis
EXCLUDES 1 chronic pericarditis not specified as rheumatic (I31.-)

5 **I09.8** **Other specified rheumatic heart diseases**

SP **SH** **SL** **+** **I09.81** **Rheumatic heart failure**
Use additional code to identify type of heart failure (I50.-)

★ New ▲ Revised **Px** Primary **SP** PDGM Px **SL** Low CoM **SH** High CoM **IQ** Quest. Encounter **H** Hospice non-cancer Dx **Unspecified** **M** *Manifestation*

DecisionHealth's FY 2020 Complete Home Health ICD-10-CM Diagnosis Coding Manual

951

Chapter 9

I00-I99

CODING TIPS ✓ A diagnosis of heart failure in a patient who has rheumatic heart disease, whether specified or presumed, is assigned code I09.81 along with a code from I50 to identify the type of heart failure.

DEFINITION Severe rheumatic damage to heart valves causing heart failure.

SP I09.89 **Other specified rheumatic heart diseases**
Rheumatic disease of pulmonary valve

SP I09.9 **Rheumatic heart disease, unspecified**
Rheumatic carditis
EXCLUDES 1 rheumatoid carditis (M05.31)

Hypertensive diseases   (I10-I16)

Use additional code to identify:
exposure to environmental tobacco smoke (Z77.22)
history of tobacco dependence (Z87.891)
occupational exposure to environmental tobacco smoke (Z57.31)
tobacco dependence (F17.-)
tobacco use (Z72.0)
EXCLUDES 1 neonatal hypertension (P29.2)
primary pulmonary hypertension (I27.0)
EXCLUDES 2 hypertensive disease complicating pregnancy, childbirth and the puerperium (O10-O11, O13-O16)

GUIDELINES Section I.C.9.a.
The classification presumes a causal relationship between hypertension and heart involvement and between hypertension and kidney involvement, as the two conditions are linked by the term "with" in the Alphabetic Index. These conditions should be coded as related even in the absence of provider documentation explicitly linking them, unless the documentation clearly states the conditions are unrelated.
For hypertension and conditions not specifically linked by relational terms such as "with," "associated with" or "due to" in the classification, provider documentation must link the conditions in order to code them as related.

CODING TIPS ✓ Essential hypertension (I10-I13) and pulmonary hypertension (I27) are two different types of hypertension. Essential hypertension, also known as 'high blood pressure' and 'systemic hypertension,' refers to the pressure throughout your body; whereas pulmonary hypertension is high blood pressure that occurs in the arteries in the lungs.

CODING TIPS ✓ Arterial, malignant, benign, and unspecified essential hypertension are included in these codes as nonessential modifiers.

SP I10 **Essential (primary) hypertension**
INCLUDES high blood pressure
hypertension (arterial) (benign) (essential) (malignant) (primary) (systemic)
EXCLUDES 1 hypertensive disease complicating pregnancy, childbirth and the puerperium (O10-O11, O13-O16)
EXCLUDES 2 essential (primary) hypertension involving vessels of brain (I60-I69)

essential (primary) hypertension involving vessels of eye (H35.0-)

CODING TIPS ✓ Essential hypertension is appropriate when no documentation is present indicating the presence of chronic kidney disease (CKD) or heart disease coded as I51.4-I51.7, I51.89, I51.9 and I50.-. If CKD or heart disease coded as I51.4-I51.7, I51.89, I51.9 and I50 are present, I10 is not the correct hypertension code. I10 is only correct in these circumstances if the physician documented that the hypertension **was not related** to CKD or the named heart conditions.

4 I11 **Hypertensive heart disease**
INCLUDES any condition in I50.-, I51.4-I51.9 due to hypertension
GUIDELINES Section I.C.9.a.1)
Hypertension with heart conditions classified to I50.- or I51.4-I51.7, I51.89, I51.9, are assigned to a code from category I11, Hypertensive heart disease. Use additional code(s) from category I50, Heart failure, to identify the type(s) of heart failure in those patients with heart failure.

The same heart conditions (I50.-, I51.4-I51.7, I51.89, I51.9) with hypertension are coded separately if the provider has documented they are unrelated to the hypertension. Sequence according to the circumstances of the admission/encounter.

CODING TIPS ✓ Heart failure (I50.-) and heart conditions included in I51.4-I51.7, I51.89, I51.9 are assumed related to hypertension. The heart conditions in I51.4-I51.7, I51.89, I51.9 are included in I11 and are not coded separately. The code for the heart failure should be added, when heart failure is present. No other heart conditions are assumed related to hypertension. Takotsubo Syndrome (I51.81) is by definition stress related and therefore should not be coded with I11.9, per CC Q2 2018.

SP SH SL I11.0 **Hypertensive heart disease with heart failure**
+
Hypertensive heart failure
Use additional code to identify type of heart failure (I50.-)

SP I11.9 **Hypertensive heart disease without heart failure**
Hypertensive heart disease NOS

4 I12 **Hypertensive chronic kidney disease**
INCLUDES any condition in N18 and N26 - due to hypertension
arteriosclerosis of kidney
arteriosclerotic nephritis (chronic) (interstitial)
hypertensive nephropathy
nephrosclerosis
EXCLUDES 1 hypertension due to kidney disease (I15.0, I15.1)
renovascular hypertension (I15.0)
secondary hypertension (I15.-)
EXCLUDES 2 acute kidney failure (N17.-)

---

4 4th digit required   **5** 5th digit required   **6** 6th digit required   **7** 7th digit required   **7** 7th digit placeholder   **+** Additional code   **⊟** Laterality

GUIDELINES Section I.C.9.a.2)

Assign codes from category I12, Hypertensive chronic kidney disease, when both hypertension and a condition classifiable to category N18, Chronic kidney disease (CKD), are present. CKD should not be coded as hypertensive if the provider indicates the CKD is not related to the hypertension.

The appropriate code from category N18 should be used as a secondary code with a code from category I12 to identify the stage of chronic kidney disease. *See Section I.C.14. Chronic kidney disease.*

If a patient has hypertensive chronic kidney disease and acute renal failure, an additional code for the acute renal failure is required.

CODING TIPS ✓ I12 is coded followed by the appropriate code from N18 to indicate the stage of CKD. If renal sclerosis is documented, use I12.9 and do not code the renal sclerosis as it is considered included in I12.

CODING TIPS ✓ When diabetes, CKD and HTN are documented, sequence the appropriate category of diabetes with CKD (E--.22) and the appropriate hypertension code (I12 or I13) prior to N18. Either the hypertension or the diabetes may be sequenced first. Both diabetes and hypertension are coded as related to the CKD, unless the physician has clearly documented that one condition is not related to the CKD.

CODING TIPS ✓ The I12 classification assumes a relationship between HTN and any condition classifiable to N18 (CKD) and N26. The classification assumes the relationship because of the pathology of hypertension, which impacts renal function, often resulting in CKD. Do not confuse hypertensive chronic kidney disease with renovascular hypertension, a condition in which the kidney dysfunction causes the hypertension. Renovascular hypertension is coded using I15.0.

H SP SH + **I12.0** **Hypertensive chronic kidney disease with stage 5 chronic kidney disease or end stage renal disease**
Use additional code to identify the stage of chronic kidney disease (N18.5, N18.6)

SP SH + **I12.9** **Hypertensive chronic kidney disease with stage 1 through stage 4 chronic kidney disease, or unspecified chronic kidney disease**
Hypertensive chronic kidney disease NOS
Hypertensive renal disease NOS
Use additional code to identify the stage of chronic kidney disease (N18.1-N18.4, N18.9)

4 I13 **Hypertensive heart and chronic kidney disease**
| INCLUDES | any condition in I11.- with any condition in I12.- cardiorenal disease cardiovascular renal disease |

GUIDELINES Section I.C.9.a.3)

Assign codes from combination category I13, Hypertensive heart and chronic kidney disease, when there is hypertension with both heart and kidney involvement. If heart failure is present, assign an additional code from category I50 to identify the type of heart failure.

The appropriate code from category N18, Chronic kidney disease, should be used as a secondary code with a code from category I13 to identify the stage of chronic kidney disease.

The codes in category I13 are combination codes that include hypertension, heart disease and chronic kidney disease. The Includes note at I13 specifies that the conditions included at I11 and I12 are included together in I13. If a patient has hypertension, heart disease and chronic kidney disease, then a code from I13 should be used, not individual codes for hypertension, heart disease and chronic kidney disease, or codes from I11 or I12. For patients with both acute renal failure and chronic kidney disease, an additional code for acute renal failure is required.

CODING TIPS ✓ Heart failure (I50.-) and conditions included in I51.4-I51.7, I51.89, I51.9 are assumed related to hypertension. CKD is assumed related to hypertension. I13 is a combination code that includes the hypertensive heart disease and the hypertensive chronic kidney disease. Do not code I51.4-I51.7, I51.89, I51.9 in addition to I13 as the conditions are already included. The code for the heart failure should be added, if present. The code for the CKD should be added.

CODING TIPS ✓ When diabetes, CKD and HTN are documented, sequence the appropriate category of diabetes with CKD (E--.22) and the appropriate hypertension code (I12 or I13) prior to N18. Either the hypertension or the diabetes may be sequenced first. Both diabetes and hypertension are coded as related to the CKD, unless the physician has clearly documented that one condition is not related to the CKD.

SP SH + **I13.0** **Hypertensive heart and chronic kidney disease with heart failure and stage 1 through stage 4 chronic kidney disease, or unspecified chronic kidney disease**
Use additional code to identify type of heart failure (I50.-)
Use additional code to identify stage of chronic kidney disease (N18.1-N18.4, N18.9)

5 I13.1 **Hypertensive heart and chronic kidney disease without heart failure**

SP SH + **I13.10** **Hypertensive heart and chronic kidney disease without heart failure, with stage 1 through stage 4 chronic kidney disease, or unspecified chronic kidney disease**
Hypertensive heart disease and hypertensive chronic kidney disease NOS

★ New ▲ Revised **Px** Primary **SP** PDGM Px **SL** Low CoM **SH** High CoM **IQ** Quest. Encounter **H** Hospice non-cancer Dx | Unspecified | **M** *Manifestation*

DecisionHealth's FY 2020 Complete Home Health ICD-10-CM Diagnosis Coding Manual

953

Chapter 9

I00-I99

Use additional code to identify the stage of chronic kidney disease (N18.1-N18.4, N18.9)

SP **SH** **+** **I13.11** **Hypertensive heart and chronic kidney disease without heart failure, with stage 5 chronic kidney disease, or end stage renal disease**
Use additional code to identify the stage of chronic kidney disease (N18.5, N18.6)

SP **SH** **+** **I13.2** **Hypertensive heart and chronic kidney disease with heart failure and with stage 5 chronic kidney disease, or end stage renal disease**
Use additional code to identify type of heart failure (I50.-)
Use additional code to identify the stage of chronic kidney disease (N18.5, N18.6)

4 **I15** **Secondary hypertension**
Code also:
underlying condition
EXCLUDES 1 postprocedural hypertension (I97.3)
EXCLUDES 2 secondary hypertension involving vessels of brain (I60-I69)
secondary hypertension involving vessels of eye (H35.0-)

GUIDELINES Section I.C.9.a.6)
Secondary hypertension is due to an underlying condition. Two codes are required: one to identify the underlying etiology and one from category I15 to identify the hypertension. Sequencing of codes is determined by the reason for admission/encounter.

CODING TIPS ✓ It is more common for hypertension to cause the renal dysfunction, however when hypertension is confirmed caused by the kidney (renal) dysfunction, assign a code from I15.-.

SP **I15.0** **Renovascular hypertension**
CODING TIPS ✓ Do not confuse hypertensive chronic kidney disease with renovascular hypertension, a condition in which the kidney dysfunction causes the hypertension. When this is the case, the hypertension is secondary to the renal dysfunction and is coded using I15.0. The two conditions may be coded in either order.

SP **I15.1** **Hypertension secondary to other renal disorders**
SP **I15.2** **Hypertension secondary to endocrine disorders**
CODING TIPS ✓ Assign I15.2 when hypertension is specified as due to Cushing's syndrome, primary aldosteronism, acromegaly, hypo/hyperthyroidism, or another specified endocrine disorder. Do not assign a code from I10-I13.0 when hypertension is specified as secondary to one of these causes.

SP **I15.8** **Other secondary hypertension**
SP **I15.9** **Secondary hypertension, unspecified**

4 **I16** **Hypertensive crisis**
Code also:
any identified hypertensive disease (I10-I15)
GUIDELINES Section I.C.9.a.10)
Assign a code from category I16, Hypertensive crisis, for documented hypertensive urgency, hypertensive emergency or unspecified hypertensive crisis. Code also any identified hypertensive disease (I10-I15). The sequencing is based on the reason for the encounter.

SP **I16.0** **Hypertensive urgency**
CODING TIPS ✓ Code hypertensive urgency when documented by the physician. Hypertensive urgency is a systolic blood pressure greater than 180 or a diastolic pressure greater than 110, without associated progressive organ dysfunction. There may be associated severe headache, shortness of breath, nosebleeds, or severe anxiety.

SP **I16.1** **Hypertensive emergency**
CODING TIPS ✓ Code hypertensive emergency when documented by the physician. Hypertensive emergencies occur when blood pressure reaches levels that lead to impending or progressive organ damage. This usually involves blood pressure levels exceeding 180 systolic or 120 diastolic, but it can occur at even lower levels in patients whose blood pressure had not been previously high. Some potential consequences of uncontrolled blood pressure in this range include stroke, loss of consciousness, memory loss, acute myocardial infarction or angina, aortic dissection, damage to the eyes and kidneys, and pulmonary edema.

SP **I16.9** **Hypertensive crisis, unspecified**
CODING TIPS ✓ Use this code when the physician documents hypertensive crisis. Hypertensive crisis is when a patient has a systolic blood pressure greater than 180 or a diastolic pressure greater than 110, and you do not know yet whether organ damage has occurred.

Ischemic heart diseases (I20-I25)

Use additional code to identify presence of hypertension (I10-I16)

+ **4** **I20** **Angina pectoris**
Use additional code to identify:
exposure to environmental tobacco smoke (Z77.22)
history of tobacco dependence (Z87.891)
occupational exposure to environmental tobacco smoke (Z57.31)
tobacco dependence (F17.-)
tobacco use (Z72.0)
EXCLUDES 1 angina pectoris with atherosclerotic heart disease of native coronary arteries (I25.1-)

4 4th digit required   **5** 5th digit required   **6** 6th digit required   **7** 7th digit required   **7** 7th digit placeholder   **+** Additional code   **=** Laterality

954   *DecisionHealth's* FY 2020 Complete Home Health ICD-10-CM Diagnosis Coding Manual

atherosclerosis of coronary
artery bypass graft (s) and
coronary artery of
transplanted heart with angina
pectoris (I25.7-)
postinfarction angina (I23.7)

GUIDELINES **Section I.C.9.b.** ICD-10-CM has combination codes for atherosclerotic heart disease with angina pectoris. The subcategories for these codes are I25.11, Atherosclerotic heart disease of native coronary artery with angina pectoris and I25.7, Atherosclerosis of coronary artery bypass graft(s) and coronary artery of transplanted heart with angina pectoris.

When using one of these combination codes it is not necessary to use an additional code for angina pectoris. A causal relationship can be assumed in a patient with both atherosclerosis and angina pectoris, unless the documentation indicates the angina is due to something other than the atherosclerosis. If a patient with coronary artery disease is admitted due to an acute myocardial infarction (AMI), the AMI should be sequenced before the coronary artery disease.

CODING TIPS ✓ Do not assign a code from I20.- for a patient who also has coronary artery disease (CAD)/atherosclerotic heart disease (ASHD). Angina in a patient with CAD/ASHD should be coded to the appropriate I25.11- code.

SP SH + **I20.0** **Unstable angina**
Accelerated angina
Crescendo angina
De novo effort angina
Intermediate coronary syndrome
Preinfarction syndrome
Worsening effort angina
CODING TIPS ✓ Unstable angina is also known as angina at rest.

SP SH + **I20.1** **Angina pectoris with documented spasm**
Angiospastic angina
Prinzmetal angina
Spasm-induced angina
Variant angina

SP SH + **I20.8** **Other forms of angina pectoris**
Angina equivalent
Angina of effort
Coronary slow flow syndrome
Stenocardia
Stable angina
Use additional code(s) for symptoms
    associated with angina equivalent

SP SH + **I20.9** **Angina pectoris, unspecified**
Angina NOS
Anginal syndrome
Cardiac angina
Ischemic chest pain

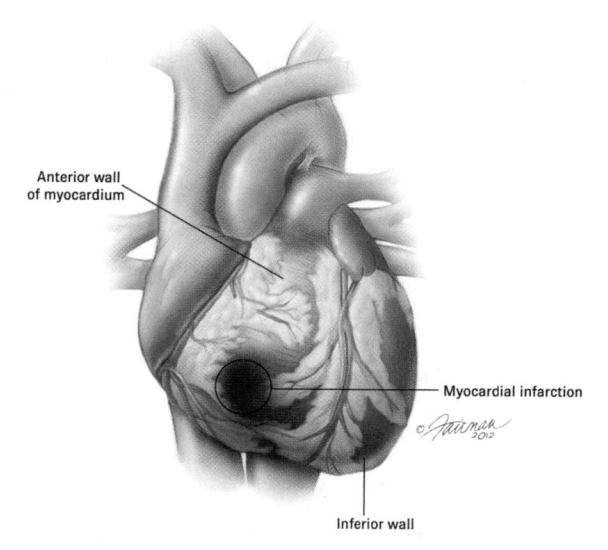

Anterior wall of myocardium

Myocardial infarction

Inferior wall

+ 4 I21 **Acute myocardial infarction**
INCLUDES cardiac infarction
coronary (artery) embolism
coronary (artery) occlusion
coronary (artery) rupture
coronary (artery) thrombosis
infarction of heart,
    myocardium, or ventricle
myocardial infarction specified
    as acute or with a stated
    duration of 4 weeks (28 days)
    or less from onset
Use additional code, if applicable, to identify:
exposure to environmental tobacco smoke
    (Z77.22)
history of tobacco dependence (Z87.891)
occupational exposure to environmental
    tobacco smoke (Z57.31)
status post administration of tPA (rtPA) in a
    different facility within the last 24 hours
    prior to admission to current facility
    (Z92.82)
tobacco dependence (F17.-)
tobacco use (Z72.0)
EXCLUDES 2 old myocardial infarction
    (I25.2)
postmyocardial infarction
    syndrome (I24.1)
subsequent type 1 myocardial
    infarction (I22.-)
GUIDELINES **Section I.C.9.e.4)**
If a subsequent myocardial infarction of one type occurs within 4 weeks of a myocardial infarction of a different type, assign the appropriate codes from category I21 to identify each type. Do not assign a code from I22. Codes from category I22 should only be assigned if both the initial and subsequent myocardial infarctions are type 1 or unspecified.

★ New ▲ Revised Px Primary **SP** PDGM Px **SL** Low CoM **SH** High CoM **IQ** Quest. Encounter ⊞ Hospice non-cancer Dx Unspecified M *Manifestation*

DecisionHealth's FY 2020 Complete Home Health ICD-10-CM Diagnosis Coding Manual

955

GUIDELINES   Section I.C.9.e.1)

The ICD-10-CM codes for type 1 acute myocardial infarction (AMI) identify the site, such as anterolateral wall or true posterior wall. Subcategories I21.0-I21.2 and code I21.3 are used for type 1 ST elevation myocardial infarction (STEMI). Code I21.4, Non-ST elevation (NSTEMI) myocardial infarction, is used for type 1 non ST elevation myocardial infarction (NSTEMI) and nontransmural MIs. If a type 1 NSTEMI evolves to STEMI, assign the STEMI code. If a type 1 STEMI converts to NSTEMI due to thrombolytic therapy, it is still coded as STEMI.

CODING TIPS ✓   When assigning any code from I21.- to report STEMI or NSTEMI, note that ICD-10 coding guidelines only allow assignment of these codes for 4 weeks following the occurrence of the MI. Use I22 codes for any subsequent MI during the same 4 weeks, if both the initial and subsequent MI were Type 1 or unspecified.

CODING TIPS ✓   I21 codes specify STEMI or ST elevation myocardial infarction. If the physician has not documented STEMI, but has documented location, use the specific I21 code for that location. STEMI is more common than NSTEMI, and is the default.

+ 🄂 I21.0   ST elevation (STEMI) myocardial infarction of anterior wall
Type 1 ST elevation myocardial infarction of anterior wall

SP + I21.01   ST elevation (STEMI) myocardial infarction involving left main coronary artery

SP + I21.02   ST elevation (STEMI) myocardial infarction involving left anterior descending coronary artery
ST elevation (STEMI) myocardial infarction involving diagonal coronary artery

SP + I21.09   ST elevation (STEMI) myocardial infarction involving other coronary artery of anterior wall
Acute transmural myocardial infarction of anterior wall
Anteroapical transmural (Q wave) infarction (acute)
Anterolateral transmural (Q wave) infarction (acute)
Anteroseptal transmural (Q wave) infarction (acute)
Transmural (Q wave) infarction (acute) (of) anterior (wall) NOS

+ 🄂 I21.1   ST elevation (STEMI) myocardial infarction of inferior wall
Type 1 ST elevation myocardial infarction of inferior wall

SP + I21.11   ST elevation (STEMI) myocardial infarction involving right coronary artery
Inferoposterior transmural (Q wave) infarction (acute)

SP + I21.19   ST elevation (STEMI) myocardial infarction involving other coronary artery of inferior wall
Acute transmural myocardial infarction of inferior wall

Inferolateral transmural (Q wave) infarction (acute)
Transmural (Q wave) infarction (acute) (of) diaphragmatic wall
Transmural (Q wave) infarction (acute) (of) inferior (wall) NOS
EXCLUDES 2   ST elevation (STEMI) myocardial infarction involving left circumflex coronary artery (I21.21)

+ 🄂 I21.2   ST elevation (STEMI) myocardial infarction of other sites
Type 1 ST elevation myocardial infarction of other sites

SP + I21.21   ST elevation (STEMI) myocardial infarction involving left circumflex coronary artery
ST elevation (STEMI) myocardial infarction involving oblique marginal coronary artery

SP + I21.29   ST elevation (STEMI) myocardial infarction involving other sites
Acute transmural myocardial infarction of other sites
Apical-lateral transmural (Q wave) infarction (acute)
Basal-lateral transmural (Q wave) infarction (acute)
High lateral transmural (Q wave) infarction (acute)
Lateral (wall) NOS transmural (Q wave) infarction (acute)
Posterior (true) transmural (Q wave) infarction (acute)
Posterobasal transmural (Q wave) infarction (acute)
Posterolateral transmural (Q wave) infarction (acute)
Posteroseptal transmural (Q wave) infarction (acute)
Septal transmural (Q wave) infarction (acute) NOS

SP + I21.3   ST elevation (STEMI) myocardial infarction of unspecified site
Acute transmural myocardial infarction of unspecified site
Transmural (Q wave) myocardial infarction NOS
Type 1 ST elevation myocardial infarction of unspecified site
CODING TIPS ✓   This code is used for a documented STEMI, but of unspecified location. Do not use this code for MI, NOS. Do not use this code if the physician has documented Type 2 MI.

SP + I21.4   Non-ST elevation (NSTEMI) myocardial infarction
Acute subendocardial myocardial infarction
Non-Q wave myocardial infarction NOS
Nontransmural myocardial infarction NOS
Type 1 non-ST elevation myocardial infarction

🄂 4th digit required   🄂 5th digit required   🄂 6th digit required   🄂 7th digit required   🄂 7th digit placeholder   ✚ Additional code   🄂 Laterality

GUIDELINES Section I.C.9.e.1)
Code I21.4, Non-ST elevation (NSTEMI) myocardial infarction, is used for type 1 non ST elevation myocardial infarction (NSTEMI) and nontransmural MIs.

GUIDELINES Section I.C.9.e.3)
If an AMI is documented as nontransmural or subendocardial, but the site is provided, it is still coded as a subendocardial AMI.

SP + I21.9 Acute myocardial infarction, unspecified

Myocardial infarction (acute) NOS

GUIDELINES Section I.C.9.e.2)
Code I21.9, Acute myocardial infarction, unspecified, is the default for unspecified acute myocardial infarction or unspecified type. If only type 1 STEMI or transmural MI without the site is documented, assign code I21.3, ST elevation (STEMI) myocardial infarction of unspecified site.

CODING TIPS ✓ This code is used for the initial MI when the physician has not documented the type or location of the infarct.

+ S I21.A Other type of myocardial infarction

CODING TIPS ✓ There is no code for a subsequent MI of types 2, 3, 4, 5. Continue to use I21.A-, remembering that a code can only be used once on a POC/claim.

▲ SP + I21.A1 Myocardial infarction type 2

Myocardial infarction due to demand ischemia

Myocardial infarction secondary to ischemic imbalance

Code first the underlying cause, such as:
anemia (D50.0-D64.9)
chronic obstructive pulmonary disease (J44.-)
paroxysmal tachycardia (I47.0-I47.9)
shock (R57.0-R57.9)

GUIDELINES Section I.C.9.e.5)
The ICD-10-CM provides codes for different types of myocardial infarction. Type 1 myocardial infarctions are assigned to codes I21.0-I21.4, and I21.9.

Type 2 myocardial infarction, and myocardial infarction due to demand ischemia or secondary to ischemic balance, is assigned to code I21.A1, Myocardial infarction type 2 with a code for the underlying cause. Do not assign code I24.8, Other forms of acute ischemic heart disease for the demand ischemia. Sequencing of type 2 AMI or the underlying cause is dependent on the circumstances of admission. When a type 2 AMI code is described as NSTEMI or STEMI, only assign code I21.A1. Codes I21.01-I21.4 should only be assigned for type 1 AMIs.

Acute myocardial infarctions type 3, 4a, 4b, 4c and 5 are assigned to code I21.A9, Other myocardial infarction type. The "Code also" and "Code first" notes should be followed related to complications, and for coding of postprocedural myocardial infarctions during or following cardiac surgery.

CODING TIPS ✓ When the physician documents Type 2 MI, assign I21.A1, even if the physician documents STEMI or NSTEMI. Type 2 MIs are not due to atherosclerotic plaque, but to a problem with supply and demand of oxygen. The documented cause of the problem should be coded first.

▲ IQ + I21.A9 Other myocardial infarction type

Myocardial infarction associated with revascularization procedure
Myocardial infarction type 3
Myocardial infarction type 4a
Myocardial infarction type 4b
Myocardial infarction type 4c
Myocardial infarction type 5

Code first:
, if applicable, postprocedural myocardial infarction following cardiac surgery (I97.190), or postprocedural myocardial infarction during cardiac surgery (I97.790)

Code also complication, if known and applicable, such as:
(acute) stent occlusion (T82.897-)
(acute) stent stenosis (T82.855-)
(acute) stent thrombosis (T82.867-)
cardiac arrest due to underlying cardiac condition (I46.2)
complication of percutaneous coronary intervention (PCI) (I97.89)
occlusion of coronary artery bypass graft (T82.218-)

+ 4 I22 Subsequent ST elevation (STEMI) and non-ST elevation (NSTEMI) myocardial infarction

★ New ▲ Revised Px Primary **SP** PDGM Px **SL** Low CoM **SH** High CoM **IQ** Quest. Encounter **H** Hospice non-cancer Dx Unspecified **M** *Manifestation*

DecisionHealth's FY 2020 Complete Home Health ICD-10-CM Diagnosis Coding Manual

957

Chapter 9

I00-I99

INCLUDES   acute myocardial infarction
occurring within four weeks
(28 days) of a previous acute
myocardial infarction,
regardless of site
cardiac infarction
coronary (artery) embolism
coronary (artery) occlusion
coronary (artery) rupture
coronary (artery) thrombosis
infarction of heart,
myocardium, or ventricle
recurrent myocardial infarction
reinfarction of myocardium
rupture of heart, myocardium,
or ventricle
subsequent type 1 myocardial
infarction

Use additional code, if applicable, to identify:
exposure to environmental tobacco smoke
(Z77.22)
history of tobacco dependence (Z87.891)
occupational exposure to environmental
tobacco smoke (Z57.31)
status post administration of tPA (rtPA) in a
different facility within the last 24 hours
prior to admission to current facility
(Z92.82)
tobacco dependence (F17.-)
tobacco use (Z72.0)

EXCLUDES 1   subsequent myocardial
infarction, type 2 (I21.A1)
subsequent myocardial
infarction of other type
(type 3) (type 4) (type 5)
(I21.A9)

GUIDELINES   Section I.C.9.e.4)
If a subsequent myocardial infarction of one
type occurs within 4 weeks of a myocardial
infarction of a different type, assign the
appropriate codes from category I21 to identify
each type. Do not assign a code from I22.
Codes from category I22 should only be
assigned if both the initial and subsequent
myocardial infarctions are type 1 or
unspecified.

GUIDELINES   Section I.C.9.e.4)
Do not assign code I22 for subsequent
myocardial infarctions other than type 1 or
unspecified. For subsequent type 2 AMI assign
only code I21.A1. For subsequent type 4 or
type 5 AMI, assign only code I21.A9.

CODING TIPS✓   When documentation reports an
acute STEMI or NSTEMI occurring within 4
weeks following a prior acute STEMI or
NSTEMI, a code from I22.- should be
assigned. Codes from I22.- may be assigned
for 4 weeks following the occurrence of the
initial MI. If the time period since the initial MI
(STEMI or NSTEMI) has been less than 4
weeks, then both a code for the initial MI (I21.-)
and subsequent MI (I22.-) should be used. If
the initial MI (STEMI or NSTEMI)
occurred more than 4 weeks ago, then the
initial MI cannot be coded. The subsequent MI
should be assigned with a code from I21.- to
indicate the MI occurring within 4 weeks of
admission to home health or hospice.

CODING TIPS✓   The term "subsequent" refers to
the subsequent MI within the 4 weeks of the
initial MI coded with I21, and not where the
patient has been treated. Code I22 cannot be
coded without an I21.

CODING TIPS✓   I22 codes specify subsequent
myocardial infarction. Even if the physician has
not documented STEMI, but has documented
location, use the specific I22 code for that
location. Do not use I22 codes for Types 2, 3,
4, 5 MIs.

SP + **I22.0   Subsequent ST elevation (STEMI)
myocardial infarction of anterior wall**
Subsequent acute transmural myocardial
infarction of anterior wall
Subsequent transmural (Q wave) infarction
(acute)(of) anterior (wall) NOS
Subsequent anteroapical transmural (Q
wave) infarction (acute)
Subsequent anterolateral transmural (Q
wave) infarction (acute)
Subsequent anteroseptal transmural (Q
wave) infarction (acute)

SP + **I22.1   Subsequent ST elevation (STEMI)
myocardial infarction of inferior wall**
Subsequent acute transmural myocardial
infarction of inferior wall
Subsequent transmural (Q wave) infarction
(acute)(of) diaphragmatic wall
Subsequent transmural (Q wave) infarction
(acute)(of) inferior (wall) NOS
Subsequent inferolateral transmural (Q
wave) infarction (acute)
Subsequent inferoposterior transmural (Q
wave) infarction (acute)

SP + **I22.2   Subsequent non-ST elevation (NSTEMI)
myocardial infarction**
Subsequent acute subendocardial
myocardial infarction
Subsequent non-Q wave myocardial
infarction NOS
Subsequent nontransmural myocardial
infarction NOS

SP + **I22.8   Subsequent ST elevation (STEMI)
myocardial infarction of other sites**
Subsequent acute transmural myocardial
infarction of other sites
Subsequent apical-lateral transmural (Q
wave) myocardial infarction (acute)
Subsequent basal-lateral transmural (Q
wave) myocardial infarction (acute)
Subsequent high lateral transmural (Q
wave) myocardial infarction (acute)
Subsequent transmural (Q wave)
myocardial infarction (acute)(of) lateral
(wall) NOS
Subsequent posterior (true) transmural (Q
wave) myocardial infarction (acute)
Subsequent posterobasal transmural (Q
wave) myocardial infarction (acute)
Subsequent posterolateral transmural (Q
wave) myocardial infarction (acute)
Subsequent posteroseptal transmural (Q
wave) myocardial infarction (acute)
Subsequent septal NOS transmural (Q
wave) myocardial infarction (acute)

---

4 4th digit required   5 5th digit required   6 6th digit required   7 7th digit required   ✓ 7th digit placeholder   + Additional code   ▣ Laterality

SP ✛ I22.9 **Subsequent ST elevation (STEMI) myocardial infarction of unspecified site**

Subsequent acute myocardial infarction of unspecified site

Subsequent myocardial infarction (acute) NOS

CODING TIPS ✓ This code is used for the subsequent MI when the physician has not documented the location of the infarct, regardless of whether it is documented as a STEMI. Do not use I22 codes for types 2, 3, 4, 5 MIs.

⬛ I23 **Certain current complications following ST elevation (STEMI) and non-ST elevation (NSTEMI) myocardial infarction (within the 28 day period)**

CODING TIPS ✓ If a complication occurred after 4 weeks, you can assign a code from I23.-, without a code from I21 or I22. If the complication is post infarction angina and CAD is also present, then code both post infarction angina and CAD with I23.7 and I25.118. If the complication is post infarction angina and it occurs within the 4 weeks, then assign the I23.- code, I21 or I22, I25.118.

SP I23.0 **Hemopericardium as current complication following acute myocardial infarction**

EXCLUDES 1 hemopericardium not specified as current complication following acute myocardial infarction (I31.2)

CODING TIPS ✓ Documentation: Hemopericardium is frequently documented with cardiac wall rupture, including ventricular rupture, following MI, and results in pooling of blood in the pericardial space, leading to tamponade. This life-threatening condition may occur during or shortly after an MI.

SP I23.1 **Atrial septal defect as current complication following acute myocardial infarction**

EXCLUDES 1 acquired atrial septal defect not specified as current complication following acute myocardial infarction (I51.0)

SP I23.2 **Ventricular septal defect as current complication following acute myocardial infarction**

EXCLUDES 1 acquired ventricular septal defect not specified as current complication following acute myocardial infarction (I51.0)

SP I23.3 **Rupture of cardiac wall without hemopericardium as current complication following acute myocardial infarction**

SP I23.4 **Rupture of chordae tendineae as current complication following acute myocardial infarction**

EXCLUDES 1 rupture of chordae tendineae not specified as current complication following acute myocardial infarction (I51.1)

DEFINITION Tear in the fibrous, cord-like tissue connecting the papillary muscles to the valves, holding the valve flaps in place to prevent their eversion.

SP I23.5 **Rupture of papillary muscle as current complication following acute myocardial infarction**

EXCLUDES 1 rupture of papillary muscle not specified as current complication following acute myocardial infarction (I51.2)

SP I23.6 **Thrombosis of atrium, auricular appendage, and ventricle as current complications following acute myocardial infarction**

EXCLUDES 1 thrombosis of atrium, auricular appendage, and ventricle not specified as current complication following acute myocardial infarction (I51.3)

SP I23.7 **Postinfarction angina**

CODING TIPS ✓ If a complication occurred after 4 weeks, you can assign a code from I23.-, without a code from I21 or I22. If the complication is post infarction angina and CAD is also present, then code both post infarction angina and CAD with I23.7 and I25.118. If the complication is post infarction angina and it occurs within the 4 weeks, then assign the I23.- code, I21 or I22, I25.118.

SP I23.8 **Other current complications following acute myocardial infarction**

⬛ I24 **Other acute ischemic heart diseases**

EXCLUDES 1 angina pectoris (I20.-) transient myocardial ischemia in newborn (P29.4)

SP SH I24.0 **Acute coronary thrombosis not resulting in myocardial infarction**

Acute coronary (artery) (vein) embolism not resulting in myocardial infarction

Acute coronary (artery) (vein) occlusion not resulting in myocardial infarction

Acute coronary (artery) (vein) thromboembolism not resulting in myocardial infarction

EXCLUDES 1 atherosclerotic heart disease (I25.1-)

SP SH I24.1 **Dressler's syndrome**

Postmyocardial infarction syndrome

EXCLUDES 1 postinfarction angina (I23.7)

DEFINITION Fever, chest pain, pleuritis, and pericarditis weeks or months after heart injury caused by surgery or myocardial infarction.

SP SH I24.8 **Other forms of acute ischemic heart disease**

EXCLUDES 1 myocardial infarction due to demand ischemia (I21.A1)

★ New ▲ Revised Px Primary **SP** PDGM Px **SL** Low CoM **SH** High CoM **IQ** Quest. Encounter **H** Hospice non-cancer Dx Unspecified **M** *Manifestation*

DecisionHealth's FY 2020 Complete Home Health ICD-10-CM Diagnosis Coding Manual

959

SP **SH** I24.9 **Acute ischemic heart disease, unspecified**

> **EXCLUDES 1** ischemic heart disease (chronic) NOS (I25.9)

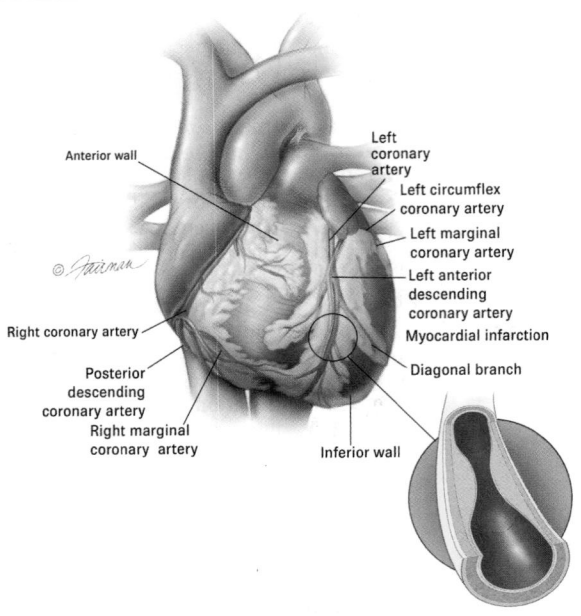

Coronary Artery Disease

+ **4** I25 **Chronic ischemic heart disease**
Use additional code to identify:
chronic total occlusion of coronary artery (I25.82)
exposure to environmental tobacco smoke (Z77.22)
history of tobacco dependence (Z87.891)
occupational exposure to environmental tobacco smoke (Z57.31)
tobacco dependence (F17.-)
tobacco use (Z72.0)

> **GUIDELINES** Section I.C.9.b
> ICD-10-CM has combination codes for atherosclerotic heart disease with angina pectoris. The subcategories for these codes are I25.11, Atherosclerotic heart disease of native coronary artery with angina pectoris, and I25.7, Atherosclerosis of coronary artery bypass graft(s) and coronary artery of transplanted heart with angina pectoris.
>
> When using one of these combination codes it is not necessary to use an additional code for angina pectoris. A causal relationship can be assumed in a patient with both atherosclerosis and angina pectoris, unless the documentation indicates the angina is due to something other than the atherosclerosis.

> **CODING TIPS ✓** When angina occurs with atherosclerotic heart disease, the type of angina is included in the code and is not coded separately with I20 codes.

+ **5** I25.1 **Atherosclerotic heart disease of native coronary artery**
Atherosclerotic cardiovascular disease
Coronary (artery) atheroma
Coronary (artery) atherosclerosis
Coronary (artery) disease
Coronary (artery) sclerosis
Use additional code, if applicable, to identify:
coronary atherosclerosis due to calcified coronary lesion (I25.84)
coronary atherosclerosis due to lipid rich plaque (I25.83)

> **EXCLUDES 2** atheroembolism (I75.-)
> atherosclerosis of coronary artery bypass graft (s) and transplanted heart (I25.7-)

> **CODING TIPS ✓** Atherosclerotic heart disease is coded to the native coronary arteries unless there is physician documentation indicating the ASHD of bypass grafts or transplanted hearts.

SP **SH** **+** I25.10 **Atherosclerotic heart disease of native coronary artery without angina pectoris**
Atherosclerotic heart disease NOS

> **DEFINITION** Clogging of coronary arteries with fatty plaque build-up, restricting blood flow and hardening the arteries.

+ **6** I25.11 **Atherosclerotic heart disease of native coronary artery with angina pectoris**

> **CODING TIPS ✓** When a patient presents with both coronary artery disease (CAD) / atherosclerotic heart disease and angina, a code from I25.11- should be assigned. If the specific type of angina is not specified in the clinical record, assign code I25.119.

SP **+** I25.110 **Atherosclerotic heart disease of native coronary artery with unstable angina pectoris**

> **EXCLUDES 1** unstable angina without atherosclerotic heart disease (I20.0)

> **CODING TIPS ✓** A person with unstable angina is having chest pain at rest and is usually scheduled for an angioplasty or bypass. Unstable angina may be a home health/hospice diagnosis, if the patient is not a surgical candidate.

SP **+** I25.111 **Atherosclerotic heart disease of native coronary artery with angina pectoris with documented spasm**

> **EXCLUDES 1** angina pectoris with documented spasm without atherosclerotic heart disease (I20.1)

SP **+** I25.118 **Atherosclerotic heart disease of native coronary artery with other forms of angina pectoris**

> **EXCLUDES 1** other forms of angina pectoris without atherosclerotic heart disease (I20.8)

4 4th digit required **5** 5th digit required **6** 6th digit required **7** 7th digit required **7** 7th digit placeholder **+** Additional code **⊟** Laterality

960 *DecisionHealth's* FY 2020 Complete Home Health ICD-10-CM Diagnosis Coding Manual

CODING TIPS ✓ If a complication occurred after 4 weeks, you can assign a code from I23.-, without a code from I21 or I22. If the complication is post infarction angina and CAD is also present, then code both post infarction angina and CAD with I23.7 and I25.118. If the complication is post infarction angina and it occurs within the 4 weeks, then assign the I23.- code, I21 or I22, I25.118.

SP + I25.119 **Atherosclerotic heart disease of native coronary artery with unspecified angina pectoris**

Atherosclerotic heart disease with angina NOS

Atherosclerotic heart disease with ischemic chest pain

EXCLUDES 1 unspecified angina pectoris without atherosclerotic heart disease (I20.9)

IQ + I25.2 **Old myocardial infarction**

Healed myocardial infarction

Past myocardial infarction diagnosed by ECG or other investigation, but currently presenting no symptoms

GUIDELINES Section I.C.9.e.1)

For old or healed myocardial infarctions not requiring further care, code I25.2 may be assigned.

CODING TIPS ✓ Assign code I25.2 (old MI) if a myocardial infarction is specified as: old (greater than 4 weeks after acute attack); healed and not currently presenting with symptoms. You can use this code when a patient has no residual effects of a previous MI, even when its presence shows up on the patient's EKG.

SP + I25.3 **Aneurysm of heart**

Mural aneurysm

Ventricular aneurysm

+ 5 I25.4 **Coronary artery aneurysm and dissection**

SP + I25.41 **Coronary artery aneurysm**

Coronary arteriovenous fistula, acquired

EXCLUDES 1 congenital coronary (artery) aneurysm (Q24.5)

SP + I25.42 **Coronary artery dissection**

SP + I25.5 **Ischemic cardiomyopathy**

EXCLUDES 2 coronary atherosclerosis (I25.1-, I25.7-)

SP + I25.6 **Silent myocardial ischemia**

+ 5 I25.7 **Atherosclerosis of coronary artery bypass graft(s) and coronary artery of transplanted heart with angina pectoris**

Use additional code, if applicable, to identify:

coronary atherosclerosis due to calcified coronary lesion (I25.84)

coronary atherosclerosis due to lipid rich plaque (I25.83)

EXCLUDES 1 atherosclerosis of bypass graft (s) of transplanted heart without angina pectoris (I25.812)

atherosclerosis of coronary artery bypass graft (s) without angina pectoris (I25.810)

atherosclerosis of native coronary artery of transplanted heart without angina pectoris (I25.811)

CODING TIPS ✓ Atherosclerotic heart disease (ASHD) involving the bypass graft (as documented by the physician) is coded to I25.7. Do not use this code for ASHD for a patient that has had a bypass in the past unless there is specific documentation of the atherosclerosis being present in the bypass graft.

CODING TIPS ✓ These codes indicate atherosclerotic plaque in the bypass artery or vein grafts. Restenosis of a stent is coded with a complication code.

+ 6 I25.70 **Atherosclerosis of coronary artery bypass graft(s), unspecified, with angina pectoris**

SP + I25.700 **Atherosclerosis of coronary artery bypass graft(s), unspecified, with unstable angina pectoris**

EXCLUDES 1 unstable angina pectoris without atherosclerosis of coronary artery bypass graft (I20.0)

SP + I25.701 **Atherosclerosis of coronary artery bypass graft(s), unspecified, with angina pectoris with documented spasm**

EXCLUDES 1 angina pectoris with documented spasm without atherosclerosis of coronary artery bypass graft (I20.1)

SP + I25.708 **Atherosclerosis of coronary artery bypass graft(s), unspecified, with other forms of angina pectoris**

EXCLUDES 1 other forms of angina pectoris without atherosclerosis of coronary artery bypass graft (I20.8)

SP + I25.709 **Atherosclerosis of coronary artery bypass graft(s), unspecified, with unspecified angina pectoris**

EXCLUDES 1 unspecified angina pectoris without atherosclerosis of coronary artery bypass graft (I20.9)

+ 6 I25.71 **Atherosclerosis of autologous vein coronary artery bypass graft(s) with angina pectoris**

★ New ▲ Revised Px Primary SP PDGM Px SL Low CoM SH High CoM IQ Quest. Encounter H Hospice non-cancer Dx Unspecified M Manifestation

DecisionHealth's FY 2020 Complete Home Health ICD-10-CM Diagnosis Coding Manual

961

SP + I25.710 Atherosclerosis of autologous vein coronary artery bypass graft(s) with unstable angina pectoris

> EXCLUDES 1 unstable angina without atherosclerosis of autologous vein coronary artery bypass graft (s) (I20.0)

> EXCLUDES 2 embolism or thrombus of coronary artery bypass graft (s) (T82.8-)

SP + I25.711 Atherosclerosis of autologous vein coronary artery bypass graft(s) with angina pectoris with documented spasm

> EXCLUDES 1 angina pectoris with documented spasm without atherosclerosis of autologous vein coronary artery bypass graft (s) (I20.1)

SP + I25.718 Atherosclerosis of autologous vein coronary artery bypass graft(s) with other forms of angina pectoris

> EXCLUDES 1 other forms of angina pectoris without atherosclerosis of autologous vein coronary artery bypass graft (s) (I20.8)

SP + I25.719 Atherosclerosis of autologous vein coronary artery bypass graft(s) with unspecified angina pectoris

> EXCLUDES 1 unspecified angina pectoris without atherosclerosis of autologous vein coronary artery bypass graft (s) (I20.9)

+ 6 I25.72 Atherosclerosis of autologous artery coronary artery bypass graft(s) with angina pectoris

Atherosclerosis of internal mammary artery graft with angina pectoris

SP + I25.720 Atherosclerosis of autologous artery coronary artery bypass graft(s) with unstable angina pectoris

> EXCLUDES 1 unstable angina without atherosclerosis of autologous artery coronary artery bypass graft (s) (I20.0)

SP + I25.721 Atherosclerosis of autologous artery coronary artery bypass graft(s) with angina pectoris with documented spasm

> EXCLUDES 1 angina pectoris with documented spasm without atherosclerosis of autologous artery coronary artery bypass graft (s) (I20.1)

SP + I25.728 Atherosclerosis of autologous artery coronary artery bypass graft(s) with other forms of angina pectoris

> EXCLUDES 1 other forms of angina pectoris without atherosclerosis of autologous artery coronary artery bypass graft (s) (I20.8)

SP + I25.729 Atherosclerosis of autologous artery coronary artery bypass graft(s) with unspecified angina pectoris

> EXCLUDES 1 unspecified angina pectoris without atherosclerosis of autologous artery coronary artery bypass graft (s) (I20.9)

+ 6 I25.73 Atherosclerosis of nonautologous biological coronary artery bypass graft(s) with angina pectoris

SP + I25.730 Atherosclerosis of nonautologous biological coronary artery bypass graft(s) with unstable angina pectoris

> EXCLUDES 1 unstable angina without atherosclerosis of nonautologous biological coronary artery bypass graft (s) (I20.0)

SP + I25.731 Atherosclerosis of nonautologous biological coronary artery bypass graft(s) with angina pectoris with documented spasm

> EXCLUDES 1 angina pectoris with documented spasm without atherosclerosis of nonautologous biological coronary artery bypass graft (s) (I20.1)

SP + I25.738 Atherosclerosis of nonautologous biological coronary artery bypass graft(s) with other forms of angina pectoris

> EXCLUDES 1 other forms of angina pectoris without atherosclerosis of nonautologous biological coronary artery bypass graft (s) (I20.8)

4 4th digit required   5 5th digit required   6 6th digit required   7 7th digit required   7 7th digit placeholder   + Additional code   = Laterality

962   DecisionHealth's FY 2020 Complete Home Health ICD-10-CM Diagnosis Coding Manual

SP ✚ **I25.739** Atherosclerosis of nonautologous biological coronary artery bypass graft(s) with unspecified angina pectoris

> **EXCLUDES 1** unspecified angina pectoris without atherosclerosis of nonautologous biological coronary artery bypass graft (s) (I20.9)

✚ Ⓖ **I25.75** Atherosclerosis of native coronary artery of transplanted heart with angina pectoris

> **EXCLUDES 1** atherosclerosis of native coronary artery of transplanted heart without angina pectoris (I25.811)

SP ✚ **I25.750** Atherosclerosis of native coronary artery of transplanted heart with unstable angina

SP ✚ **I25.751** Atherosclerosis of native coronary artery of transplanted heart with angina pectoris with documented spasm

SP ✚ **I25.758** Atherosclerosis of native coronary artery of transplanted heart with other forms of angina pectoris

SP ✚ **I25.759** Atherosclerosis of native coronary artery of transplanted heart with unspecified angina pectoris

✚ Ⓖ **I25.76** Atherosclerosis of bypass graft of coronary artery of transplanted heart with angina pectoris

> **EXCLUDES 1** atherosclerosis of bypass graft of coronary artery of transplanted heart without angina pectoris (I25.812)

SP ✚ **I25.760** Atherosclerosis of bypass graft of coronary artery of transplanted heart with unstable angina

SP ✚ **I25.761** Atherosclerosis of bypass graft of coronary artery of transplanted heart with angina pectoris with documented spasm

SP ✚ **I25.768** Atherosclerosis of bypass graft of coronary artery of transplanted heart with other forms of angina pectoris

SP ✚ **I25.769** Atherosclerosis of bypass graft of coronary artery of transplanted heart with unspecified angina pectoris

✚ Ⓖ **I25.79** Atherosclerosis of other coronary artery bypass graft(s) with angina pectoris

SP ✚ **I25.790** Atherosclerosis of other coronary artery bypass graft(s) with unstable angina pectoris

> **EXCLUDES 1** unstable angina without atherosclerosis of other coronary artery bypass graft (s) (I20.0)

SP ✚ **I25.791** Atherosclerosis of other coronary artery bypass graft(s) with angina pectoris with documented spasm

> **EXCLUDES 1** angina pectoris with documented spasm without atherosclerosis of other coronary artery bypass graft (s) (I20.1)

SP ✚ **I25.798** Atherosclerosis of other coronary artery bypass graft(s) with other forms of angina pectoris

> **EXCLUDES 1** other forms of angina pectoris without atherosclerosis of other coronary artery bypass graft (s) (I20.8)

SP ✚ **I25.799** Atherosclerosis of other coronary artery bypass graft(s) with unspecified angina pectoris

> **EXCLUDES 1** unspecified angina pectoris without atherosclerosis of other coronary artery bypass graft (s) (I20.9)

✚ Ⓢ **I25.8** Other forms of chronic ischemic heart disease

▲ ✚ Ⓖ **I25.81** Atherosclerosis of other coronary vessels without angina pectoris

Use additional code, if applicable, to identify:
coronary atherosclerosis due to calcified coronary lesion (I25.84)
coronary atherosclerosis due to lipid rich plaque (I25.83)

> **EXCLUDES 2** atherosclerotic heart disease of native coronary artery without angina pectoris (I25.10)

SP ✚ **I25.810** Atherosclerosis of coronary artery bypass graft(s) without angina pectoris

Atherosclerosis of coronary artery bypass graft NOS

> **EXCLUDES 1** atherosclerosis of coronary bypass graft (s) with angina pectoris (I25.70-I25.73-, I25.79-)

SP ✚ **I25.811** Atherosclerosis of native coronary artery of transplanted heart without angina pectoris

Atherosclerosis of native coronary artery of transplanted heart NOS

> **EXCLUDES 1** atherosclerosis of native coronary artery of transplanted heart with angina pectoris (I25.75-)

SP ✚ **I25.812** Atherosclerosis of bypass graft of coronary artery of transplanted heart without angina pectoris

★ New ▲ Revised Px Primary **SP** PDGM Px **SL** Low CoM **SH** High CoM **IQ** Quest. Encounter Ⓗ Hospice non-cancer Dx Unspecified **M** Manifestation

DecisionHealth's FY 2020 Complete Home Health ICD-10-CM Diagnosis Coding Manual

963

Atherosclerosis of bypass graft of transplanted heart NOS

EXCLUDES 1 atherosclerosis of bypass graft of transplanted heart with angina pectoris (I25.76)

SP ✚ I25.82 Chronic total occlusion of coronary artery

Complete occlusion of coronary artery
Total occlusion of coronary artery
Code first:
    coronary atherosclerosis
      (I25.1-, I25.7-, I25.81-)

EXCLUDES 1 acute coronary occlusion with myocardial infarction (I21.0-I21.9, I22.-)
acute coronary occlusion without myocardial infarction (I24.0)

SP ✚ I25.83 Coronary atherosclerosis due to lipid rich plaque

Code first:
    coronary atherosclerosis
      (I25.1-, I25.7-, I25.81-)

SP ✚ I25.84 Coronary atherosclerosis due to calcified coronary lesion

Coronary atherosclerosis due to severely calcified coronary lesion
Code first:
    coronary atherosclerosis
      (I25.1-, I25.7-, I25.81-)

CODING TIPS ✓ Calcified lesions are more difficult to treat with angioplasty and stenting because the calcium deposits may block stents from reaching the desired location and may prevent the stent from fully expanding to the optimal size.

SP ✚ I25.89 Other forms of chronic ischemic heart disease

SP ✚ I25.9 Chronic ischemic heart disease, unspecified

Ischemic heart disease (chronic) NOS

Pulmonary heart disease and diseases of pulmonary circulation (I26-I28)

4 I26 Pulmonary embolism

INCLUDES pulmonary (acute) (artery)(vein) infarction
pulmonary (acute) (artery)(vein) thromboembolism
pulmonary (acute) (artery)(vein) thrombosis

EXCLUDES 2 chronic pulmonary embolism (I27.82)
personal history of pulmonary embolism (Z86.711)
pulmonary embolism complicating abortion, ectopic or molar pregnancy (O00-O07, O08.2)

pulmonary embolism complicating pregnancy, childbirth and the puerperium (O88.-)
pulmonary embolism due to trauma (T79.0, T79.1)
pulmonary embolism due to complications of surgical and medical care (T80.0, T81.7-, T82.8-)
septic (non-pulmonary) arterial embolism (I76)

CODING TIPS ✓ Most patients are treated with anticoagulant therapy for an acute embolus for 3-6 months. Do not code chronic pulmonary embolism unless the physician documents chronic pulmonary embolism (I27.82). Assign Z86.711 for history of pulmonary embolism after 3-6 months if the physician has not documented chronic pulmonary embolism. Documentation indicating pulmonary embolism, without further information, is assigned I26.99.

5 I26.0 Pulmonary embolism with acute cor pulmonale

CODING TIPS ✓ Category I26.0- codes should be assigned only when cor pulmonale is reported as occurring and associated with a pulmonary embolus. Cor pulmonale is a right ventricular dysfunction and failure.

SP I26.01 Septic pulmonary embolism with acute cor pulmonale

Code first:
    underlying infection

CODING TIPS ✓ The term septic pulmonary embolism indicates a pulmonary embolus resulting from embolization of infectious particles which enter the lungs in the pulmonary arterial system. This can occur as a result of infectious DVT, periodontal disease, infected venous catheters, endocarditis, or other systemic infections. This code should only be assigned when the embolus is stated as septic and related to an infectious cause. A second code for the underlying/causative infection must be assigned.

SP I26.02 Saddle embolus of pulmonary artery with acute cor pulmonale

SP SL I26.09 Other pulmonary embolism with acute cor pulmonale

Acute cor pulmonale NOS

5 I26.9 Pulmonary embolism without acute cor pulmonale

SP I26.90 Septic pulmonary embolism without acute cor pulmonale

Code first:
    underlying infection

SP I26.92 Saddle embolus of pulmonary artery without acute cor pulmonale

★ I26.93 Single subsegmental pulmonary embolism without acute cor pulmonale

Subsegmental pulmonary embolism NOS

4 4th digit required   5 5th digit required   6 6th digit required   7 7th digit required   ✓ 7th digit placeholder   ✚ Additional code   ▤ Laterality

964   *DecisionHealth's* FY 2020 Complete Home Health ICD-10-CM Diagnosis Coding Manual

DEFINITION Subsegmental PE is defined as PE with no involvement of more proximal pulmonary arteries.

⭐ **I26.94 Multiple subsegmental pulmonary emboli without acute cor pulmonale**
DEFINITION Subsegmental PE is defined as PE with no involvement of more proximal pulmonary arteries.

SP **SL** **I26.99 Other pulmonary embolism without acute cor pulmonale**
Acute pulmonary embolism NOS
Pulmonary embolism NOS
CODING TIPS ✓ Documentation indicating pulmonary embolism, without further information, is assigned I26.99.

4️⃣ I27 Other pulmonary heart diseases
GUIDELINES Section I.C.9.a.11)
Pulmonary hypertension is classified to category I27, Other pulmonary heart diseases. For secondary pulmonary hypertension (I27.1, I27.2-), code also any associated conditions or adverse effects of drugs or toxins. The sequencing is based on the reason for the encounter, except for adverse effects of drugs (See Section I.C.19.e.).

SP **I27.0 Primary pulmonary hypertension**
Heritable pulmonary arterial hypertension
Idiopathic pulmonary arterial hypertension
Primary group 1 pulmonary hypertension
Primary pulmonary arterial hypertension
EXCLUDES 1 persistent pulmonary hypertension of newborn (P29.30)
pulmonary hypertension NOS (I27.20)
secondary pulmonary arterial hypertension (I27.21)
secondary pulmonary hypertension (I27.29)

SP **I27.1 Kyphoscoliotic heart disease**

5️⃣ I27.2 Other secondary pulmonary hypertension
Code also:
associated underlying condition
EXCLUDES 1 Eisenmenger's syndrome (I27.83)

SP **I27.20 Pulmonary hypertension, unspecified**
Pulmonary hypertension NOS

SP **I27.21 Secondary pulmonary arterial hypertension**
(Associated) (drug-induced) (toxin-induced) pulmonary arterial hypertension NOS

(Associated) (drug-induced) (toxin-induced) (secondary) group 1 pulmonary hypertension
Code also associated conditions if applicable, or adverse effects of drugs or toxins, such as:
adverse effect of appetite depressants (T50.5X5)
congenital heart disease (Q20-Q28)
human immunodeficiency virus [HIV] disease (B20)
polymyositis (M33.2-)
portal hypertension (K76.6)
rheumatoid arthritis (M05.-)
schistosomiasis (B65.-)
Sjögren syndrome (M35.0-)
systemic sclerosis (M34.-)

SP **I27.22 Pulmonary hypertension due to left heart disease**
Group 2 pulmonary hypertension
Code also associated left heart disease, if known, such as:
multiple valve disease (I08.-)
rheumatic mitral valve diseases (I05.-)
rheumatic aortic valve diseases (I06.-)

SP **I27.23 Pulmonary hypertension due to lung diseases and hypoxia**
Group 3 pulmonary hypertension
Code also associated lung disease, if known, such as:
bronchiectasis (J47.-)
cystic fibrosis with pulmonary manifestations (E84.0)
interstitial lung disease (J84.-)
pleural effusion (J90)
sleep apnea (G47.3-)

SP **I27.24 Chronic thromboembolic pulmonary hypertension**
Group 4 pulmonary hypertension
Code also:
associated pulmonary embolism, if applicable (I26.-, I27.82)

SP **I27.29 Other secondary pulmonary hypertension**
Group 5 pulmonary hypertension
Pulmonary hypertension with unclear multifactorial mechanisms
Pulmonary hypertension due to hematologic disorders
Pulmonary hypertension due to metabolic disorders
Pulmonary hypertension due to other systemic disorders
Code also other associated disorders, if known, such as:
chronic myeloid leukemia (C92.10- C92.22)
essential thrombocythemia (D47.3)
Gaucher disease (E75.22)
hypertensive chronic kidney disease with end stage renal disease (I12.0, I13.11, I13.2)
hyperthyroidism (E05.-)
hypothyroidism (E00-E03)
polycythemia vera (D45)
sarcoidosis (D86.-)

⭐ New ▲ Revised **Px** Primary **SP** PDGM Px **SL** Low CoM **SH** High CoM **IQ** Quest. Encounter **H** Hospice non-cancer Dx **Unspecified** **M** *Manifestation*

DecisionHealth's FY 2020 Complete Home Health ICD-10-CM Diagnosis Coding Manual

965

5 I27.8   Other specified pulmonary heart diseases

SP I27.81   Cor pulmonale (chronic)
Cor pulmonale NOS
> **EXCLUDES 1**   acute cor pulmonale (I26.0-)

SP ✚ I27.82   Chronic pulmonary embolism
Use additional code, if applicable, for associated long-term (current) use of anticoagulants (Z79.01)
> **EXCLUDES 1**   personal history of pulmonary embolism (Z86.711)

> **CODING TIPS ✓**   Most acute pulmonary emboli do not cause chronic disease. Verify with physician whether chronic disease is being treated or if the patient is being treated prophylactically. Code chronic pulmonary embolism only if the physician has documented the pulmonary embolism as chronic. If treatment persists longer than 3-6 months after the acute pulmonary embolism, query the physician regarding chronicity. If not chronic, code Z86.711 for history of pulmonary embolism.

SP I27.83   Eisenmenger's syndrome
Eisenmenger's complex
(Irreversible) Eisenmenger's disease
Pulmonary hypertension with right to left shunt related to congenital heart disease
Code also underlying heart defect, if known, such as:
atrial septal defect (Q21.1)
Eisenmenger's defect (Q21.8)
patent ductus arteriosus (Q25.0)
ventricular septal defect (Q21.0)

SP I27.89   Other specified pulmonary heart diseases

SP I27.9   Pulmonary heart disease, unspecified
Chronic cardiopulmonary disease

4 I28   Other diseases of pulmonary vessels

SP I28.0   Arteriovenous fistula of pulmonary vessels
> **EXCLUDES 1**   congenital arteriovenous fistula (Q25.72)

> **DEFINITION**   Abnormal passage between the pulmonary arterial and venous systems, which causes unoxygenated blood to enter systemic circulation.

SP I28.1   Aneurysm of pulmonary artery
> **EXCLUDES 1**   congenital aneurysm (Q25.79)
congenital arteriovenous aneurysm (Q25.72)

> **DEFINITION**   Bulging in one portion of the arterial wall that brings blood to the lungs, forming a pouch or sac with the potential for rupture.

SP I28.8   Other diseases of pulmonary vessels
Pulmonary arteritis
Pulmonary endarteritis
Rupture of pulmonary vessels
Stenosis of pulmonary vessels
Stricture of pulmonary vessels

SP I28.9   Disease of pulmonary vessels, unspecified

Other forms of heart disease   (I30-I52)

> **CODING TIPS ✓**   Pericarditis, endocarditis and myocarditis not specified as rheumatic are coded with these codes when a more specific code (such as meningococcal pericarditis) is not appropriate. Heart valve disease of the mitral and tricuspid valves are assumed rheumatic (I05 and I07), unless specified as nonrheumatic. Heart valve disease of the aortic and pulmonary valves are considered nonrheumatic, unless specified as rheumatic. Valve disease affecting multiple valves is considered rheumatic, unless specified by the physician as non-rheumatic. Pay special attention to includes and excludes 1 notes.

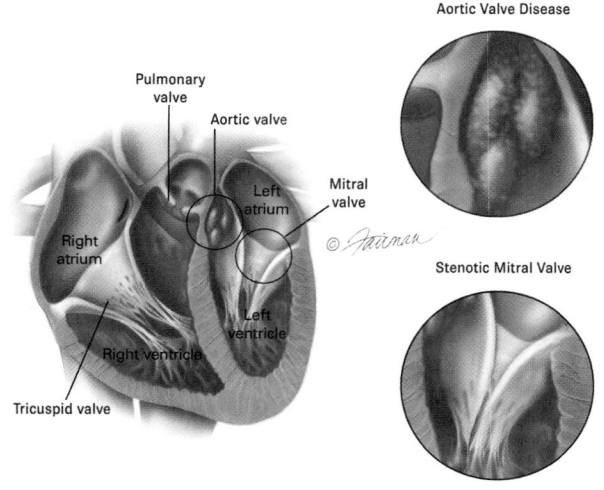

4 I30   Acute pericarditis
> **INCLUDES**   acute mediastinopericarditis
acute myopericarditis
acute pericardial effusion
acute pleuropericarditis
acute pneumopericarditis
> **EXCLUDES 1**   Dressler's syndrome (I24.1)
rheumatic pericarditis (acute) (I01.0)
viral pericarditis due to Coxsakie virus (B33.23)

SP I30.0   Acute nonspecific idiopathic pericarditis

SP ✚ I30.1   Infective pericarditis
Pneumococcal pericarditis
Pneumopyopericardium
Purulent pericarditis
Pyopericarditis
Pyopericardium
Pyopneumopericardium
Staphylococcal pericarditis
Streptococcal pericarditis
Suppurative pericarditis
Viral pericarditis
Use additional code (B95-B97) to identify infectious agent

SP I30.8   Other forms of acute pericarditis

SP I30.9   Acute pericarditis, unspecified

4 I31   Other diseases of pericardium
> **EXCLUDES 1**   diseases of pericardium specified as rheumatic (I09.2)

---

4 4th digit required   5 5th digit required   6 6th digit required   7 7th digit required   ☑ 7th digit placeholder   ✚Additional code   ⊟ Laterality

postcardiotomy syndrome (I97.0)
traumatic injury to pericardium (S26.-)

SP I31.0 **Chronic adhesive pericarditis**
Accretio cordis
Adherent pericardium
Adhesive mediastinopericarditis
DEFINITION Pericardial inflammation with adhesion between the two pericardial layers or between the pericardium and the heart or neighboring structures.

SP I31.1 **Chronic constrictive pericarditis**
Concretio cordis
Pericardial calcification

SP I31.2 **Hemopericardium, not elsewhere classified**
EXCLUDES 1 hemopericardium as current complication following acute myocardial infarction (I23.0)
DEFINITION Bleeding causing the sac around the heart to fill with blood.

SP I31.3 **Pericardial effusion (noninflammatory)**
Chylopericardium
EXCLUDES 1 acute pericardial effusion (I30.9)

SP I31.4 **Cardiac tamponade**
Code first:
underlying cause
DEFINITION Increased pressure on the heart due to fluid in the pericardial sac, impairing ventricular filling action and causing decreased cardiac output.

SP I31.8 **Other specified diseases of pericardium**
Epicardial plaques
Focal pericardial adhesions

SP I31.9 **Disease of pericardium, unspecified**
Pericarditis (chronic) NOS

M SP I32 *Pericarditis in diseases classified elsewhere*
Code first:
underlying disease
EXCLUDES 1 pericarditis (in) :
coxsackie (virus) (B33.23)
gonococcal (A54.83)
meningococcal (A39.53)
rheumatoid (arthritis) (M05.31)
syphilitic (A52.06)
systemic lupus erythematosus (M32.12)
tuberculosis (A18.84)
DEFINITION Inflammation of the membranous sac around the heart occurring with another underlying disease process, causing chest pain, coughing, fatigue, and fever.

4 I33 **Acute and subacute endocarditis**
EXCLUDES 1 acute rheumatic endocarditis (I01.1)
endocarditis NOS (I38)

SP + I33.0 **Acute and subacute infective endocarditis**
Bacterial endocarditis (acute) (subacute)
Infective endocarditis (acute) (subacute) NOS
Endocarditis lenta (acute) (subacute)

Malignant endocarditis (acute) (subacute)
Purulent endocarditis (acute) (subacute)
Septic endocarditis (acute) (subacute)
Ulcerative endocarditis (acute) (subacute)
Vegetative endocarditis (acute) (subacute)
Use additional code (B95-B97) to identify infectious agent

SP I33.9 **Acute and subacute endocarditis, unspecified**
Acute endocarditis NOS
Acute myoendocarditis NOS
Acute periendocarditis NOS
Subacute endocarditis NOS
Subacute myoendocarditis NOS
Subacute periendocarditis NOS

4 I34 **Nonrheumatic mitral valve disorders**
EXCLUDES 1 mitral valve disease (I05.9)
mitral valve failure (I05.8)
mitral valve stenosis (I05.0)
mitral valve disorder of unspecified cause with diseases of aortic and/or tricuspid valve (s) (I08.-)
mitral valve disorder of unspecified cause with mitral stenosis or obstruction (I05.0)
mitral valve disorder specified as congenital (Q23.2, Q23.9)
mitral valve disorder specified as rheumatic (I05.-)
CODING TIPS ✓ Mitral valve disorders are considered rheumatic unless the physician specifies non-rheumatic. See I05.

SP I34.0 **Nonrheumatic mitral (valve) insufficiency**
Nonrheumatic mitral (valve) incompetence NOS
Nonrheumatic mitral (valve) regurgitation NOS

SP I34.1 **Nonrheumatic mitral (valve) prolapse**
Floppy nonrheumatic mitral valve syndrome
EXCLUDES 1 Marfan's syndrome (Q87.4-)

SP I34.2 **Nonrheumatic mitral (valve) stenosis**

SP I34.8 **Other nonrheumatic mitral valve disorders**

SP I34.9 **Nonrheumatic mitral valve disorder, unspecified**

4 I35 **Nonrheumatic aortic valve disorders**
EXCLUDES 1 aortic valve disorder of unspecified cause but with diseases of mitral and/or tricuspid valve (s) (I08.-)
aortic valve disorder specified as congenital (Q23.0, Q23.1)
aortic valve disorder specified as rheumatic (I06.-)
hypertrophic subaortic stenosis (I42.1)
CODING TIPS ✓ Aortic valve disorders are considered nonrheumatic, unless specified as rheumatic. If aortic valve disease exists with other heart valve disease, consider it rheumatic heart disease, unless specified as nonrheumatic multiple valve disease.

SP I35.0 **Nonrheumatic aortic (valve) stenosis**

★ New ▲ Revised Px Primary **SP** PDGM Px **SL** Low CoM **SH** High CoM **IQ** Quest. Encounter **H** Hospice non-cancer Dx Unspecified **M** *Manifestation*

DecisionHealth's FY 2020 Complete Home Health ICD-10-CM Diagnosis Coding Manual

967

Chapter 9

I00-I99

SP I35.1 Nonrheumatic aortic (valve) insufficiency
Nonrheumatic aortic (valve) incompetence NOS
Nonrheumatic aortic (valve) regurgitation NOS

SP I35.2 Nonrheumatic aortic (valve) stenosis with insufficiency

SP I35.8 Other nonrheumatic aortic valve disorders

SP I35.9 Nonrheumatic aortic valve disorder, unspecified

4 I36 Nonrheumatic tricuspid valve disorders
EXCLUDES 1 tricuspid valve disorders of unspecified cause (I07.-)
tricuspid valve disorders specified as congenital (Q22.4, Q22.8, Q22.9)
tricuspid valve disorders specified as rheumatic (I07.-)
tricuspid valve disorders with aortic and/or mitral valve involvement (I08.-)

CODING TIPS ✓ Tricuspid valve disorders are considered rheumatic unless the physician specifies non-rheumatic.

SP I36.0 Nonrheumatic tricuspid (valve) stenosis

SP I36.1 Nonrheumatic tricuspid (valve) insufficiency
Nonrheumatic tricuspid (valve) incompetence
Nonrheumatic tricuspid (valve) regurgitation

SP I36.2 Nonrheumatic tricuspid (valve) stenosis with insufficiency

SP I36.8 Other nonrheumatic tricuspid valve disorders

SP I36.9 Nonrheumatic tricuspid valve disorder, unspecified

4 I37 Nonrheumatic pulmonary valve disorders
EXCLUDES 1 pulmonary valve disorder specified as congenital (Q22.1, Q22.2, Q22.3)
pulmonary valve disorder specified as rheumatic (I09.89)

CODING TIPS ✓ Pulmonary valve disorders are considered nonrheumatic unless the physician specifies rheumatic.

SP I37.0 Nonrheumatic pulmonary valve stenosis

SP I37.1 Nonrheumatic pulmonary valve insufficiency
Nonrheumatic pulmonary valve incompetence
Nonrheumatic pulmonary valve regurgitation

SP I37.2 Nonrheumatic pulmonary valve stenosis with insufficiency

SP I37.8 Other nonrheumatic pulmonary valve disorders

SP I37.9 Nonrheumatic pulmonary valve disorder, unspecified

SP I38 Endocarditis, valve unspecified
INCLUDES endocarditis (chronic) NOS
valvular incompetence NOS
valvular insufficiency NOS
valvular regurgitation NOS
valvular stenosis NOS
valvulitis (chronic) NOS
EXCLUDES 1 congenital insufficiency of cardiac valve NOS (Q24.8)
congenital stenosis of cardiac valve NOS (Q24.8)
endocardial fibroelastosis (I42.4)
endocarditis specified as rheumatic (I09.1)

M IQ I39 Endocarditis and heart valve disorders in diseases classified elsewhere
Code first underlying disease, such as:
Q fever (A78)
EXCLUDES 1 endocardial involvement in:
candidiasis (B37.6)
gonococcal infection (A54.83)
Libman-Sacks disease (M32.11)
listerosis (A32.82)
meningococcal infection (A39.51)
rheumatoid arthritis (M05.31)
syphilis (A52.03)
tuberculosis (A18.84)
typhoid fever (A01.02)

CODING TIPS ✓ I39 is a manifestation code and may be used only in conjunction with a code to report the causative underlying disease process.

CODING TIPS ✓ Documentation: Assign this code only when the clinical record supports a cause and effect relationship between the underlying disease process and the endocarditis/valve disorder.

4 I40 Acute myocarditis
INCLUDES subacute myocarditis
EXCLUDES 1 acute rheumatic myocarditis (I01.2)
DEFINITION Severe inflammation of heart muscle tissue.

SP + I40.0 Infective myocarditis
Septic myocarditis
Use additional code (B95-B97) to identify infectious agent

SP I40.1 Isolated myocarditis
Fiedler's myocarditis
Giant cell myocarditis
Idiopathic myocarditis

SP I40.8 Other acute myocarditis

SP I40.9 Acute myocarditis, unspecified

M IQ I41 Myocarditis in diseases classified elsewhere
Code first underlying disease, such as:
typhus (A75.0-A75.9)
EXCLUDES 1 myocarditis (in) :
Chagas' disease (chronic) (B57.2)
acute (B57.0)
coxsackie (virus) infection (B33.22)
diphtheritic (A36.81)
gonococcal (A54.83)
influenzal (J09.X9, J10.82, J11.82)
meningococcal (A39.52)
mumps (B26.82)
rheumatoid arthritis (M05.31)

---

4 4th digit required   5 5th digit required   6 6th digit required   7 7th digit required   7 7th digit placeholder   + Additional code   B Laterality

968   *DecisionHealth's* FY 2020 Complete Home Health ICD-10-CM Diagnosis Coding Manual

sarcoid (D86.85)
syphilis (A52.06)
toxoplasmosis (B58.81)
tuberculous (A18.84)

CODING TIPS ✓   **Documentation:** Assign this code only when the clinical record supports a cause and effect relationship between the underlying disease process and myocarditis.

CODING TIPS ✓   I41 is a manifestation code and may be used only in conjunction with a code to report the causative underlying disease process.

4 I42   **Cardiomyopathy**

INCLUDES   myocardiopathy

Code first:
  pre-existing cardiomyopathy complicating
    pregnancy and puerperium (O99.4)
EXCLUDES 2   ischemic cardiomyopathy
    (I25.5)
  peripartum cardiomyopathy
    (O90.3)
  ventricular hypertrophy (I51.7)

SP I42.0   **Dilated cardiomyopathy**
Congestive cardiomyopathy

SP I42.1   **Obstructive hypertrophic cardiomyopathy**
Hypertrophic subaortic stenosis
  (idiopathic)

SP I42.2   **Other hypertrophic cardiomyopathy**
Nonobstructive hypertrophic
  cardiomyopathy

SP I42.3   **Endomyocardial (eosinophilic) disease**
Endomyocardial (tropical) fibrosis
Löffler's endocarditis

SP I42.4   **Endocardial fibroelastosis**
Congenital cardiomyopathy
Elastomyofibrosis

SP I42.5   **Other restrictive cardiomyopathy**
Constrictive cardiomyopathy NOS

SP I42.6   **Alcoholic cardiomyopathy**
Code also:
  presence of alcoholism (F10.-)

CODING TIPS ✓   This diagnosis indicates that the alcohol was linked to the disorder, so the use, abuse or dependence of alcohol F10.- code should include 5th and 6th characters .88.

DEFINITION   Dilated disease of the heart muscle due to alcohol abuse.

SP ✚ I42.7   **Cardiomyopathy due to drug and external agent**
Code first:
  poisoning due to drug or toxin, if
    applicable
    (T36-T65 with fifth or sixth character
    1-4 or 6)
  Use additional code for adverse effect, if
    applicable, to identify drug (T36-T50
    with fifth or sixth character 5)

SP I42.8   **Other cardiomyopathies**

SP I42.9   **Cardiomyopathy, unspecified**
Cardiomyopathy (primary) (secondary)
  NOS

M SP I43   **Cardiomyopathy in diseases classified elsewhere**

Code first underlying disease, such as:
  amyloidosis (E85.-)
  glycogen storage disease (E74.0)
  gout (M10.0-)
  thyrotoxicosis (E05.0-E05.9-)
EXCLUDES 1   cardiomyopathy (in) :
  coxsackie (virus) (B33.24)
  diphtheria (A36.81)
  sarcoidosis (D86.85)
  tuberculosis (A18.84)

CODING TIPS ✓   I43 is a manifestation code and may be used only in conjunction with a code to report the causative underlying disease process.

CODING TIPS ✓   **Documentation:** Assign this code only when the clinical record supports a cause and effect relationship between the underlying disease process and cardiomyopathy.

4 I44   **Atrioventricular and left bundle-branch block**

CODING TIPS ✓   When reviewing documentation for heart block, it is important to differentiate heart block degree from heart block type.

SP I44.0   **Atrioventricular block, first degree**

SP I44.1   **Atrioventricular block, second degree**
Atrioventricular block, type I and II
Möbitz block, type I and II
Second degree block, type I and II
Wenckebach's block

SP I44.2   **Atrioventricular block, complete**
Complete heart block NOS
Third degree block

DEFINITION   No conduction of electrical impulses occurs between the atria and ventricles, requiring a pacemaker to maintain rhythm.

5 I44.3   **Other and unspecified atrioventricular block**
Atrioventricular block NOS

⭐ New ▲ Revised **Px** Primary **SP** PDGM Px **SL** Low CoM **SH** High CoM **IQ** Quest. Encounter **H** Hospice non-cancer Dx   Unspecified   **M** *Manifestation*

Chapter 9

I00-I99

SP **I44.30** **Unspecified atrioventricular block**

SP **I44.39** **Other atrioventricular block**

SP **I44.4** **Left anterior fascicular block**

SP **I44.5** **Left posterior fascicular block**

5 **I44.6** **Other and unspecified fascicular block**

SP **I44.60** **Unspecified fascicular block**
Left bundle-branch hemiblock NOS

SP **I44.69** **Other fascicular block**

SP **I44.7** **Left bundle-branch block, unspecified**

4 **I45** **Other conduction disorders**
> **CODING TIPS ✓** When reviewing documentation for heart block, it is important to differentiate heart block degree from heart block type.

SP **I45.0** **Right fascicular block**

5 **I45.1** **Other and unspecified right bundle-branch block**

SP **I45.10** **Unspecified right bundle-branch block**
Right bundle-branch block NOS

SP **I45.19** **Other right bundle-branch block**

SP **I45.2** **Bifascicular block**

SP **I45.3** **Trifascicular block**

SP **I45.4** **Nonspecific intraventricular block**
Bundle-branch block NOS
> **DEFINITION** A condition in which portions of the heart's conduction system are defective and either slow or block the electrical impulses traveling through specialized conduction tissue on the way to the ventricles.

SP **I45.5** **Other specified heart block**
Sinoatrial block
Sinoauricular block
> **EXCLUDES 1** heart block NOS (I45.9)

SP **I45.6** **Pre-excitation syndrome**
Accelerated atrioventricular conduction
Accessory atrioventricular conduction
Anomalous atrioventricular excitation
Lown-Ganong-Levine syndrome
Pre-excitation atrioventricular conduction
Wolff-Parkinson-White syndrome

5 **I45.8** **Other specified conduction disorders**

SP **I45.81** **Long QT syndrome**
> **DEFINITION** Hereditary defect of the heart's electrical conduction system with an abnormally long gap in the time it takes for the ventricles to contract.

SP **I45.89** **Other specified conduction disorders**
Atrioventricular [AV] dissociation
Interference dissociation
Isorhythmic dissociation
Nonparoxysmal AV nodal tachycardia
> **CODING TIPS ✓** This code is used for short QT syndrome.

SP **I45.9** **Conduction disorder, unspecified**
Heart block NOS
Stokes-Adams syndrome

4 **I46** **Cardiac arrest**
> **EXCLUDES 1** cardiogenic shock (R57.0)

> **CODING TIPS ✓** Codes from category I46.- should not be assigned to the home health claim. Use Z86.74 for history of cardiac arrest with successful resuscitation on the home health or hospice claim.

!Q **I46.2** **Cardiac arrest due to underlying cardiac condition**
Code first:
underlying cardiac condition

!Q **I46.8** **Cardiac arrest due to other underlying condition**
Code first:
underlying condition

SP **I46.9** **Cardiac arrest, cause unspecified**

4 **I47** **Paroxysmal tachycardia**
Code first tachycardia complicating:
abortion or ectopic or molar pregnancy (O00-O07, O08.8)
obstetric surgery and procedures (O75.4)
> **EXCLUDES 1** tachycardia NOS (R00.0)
sinoauricular tachycardia NOS (R00.0)
sinus [sinusal] tachycardia NOS (R00.0)

> **CODING TIPS ✓** Do not assign a code from I47.- when only tachycardia is reported in the record and is not specified, or is reported in the record as sinus tachycardia or sinoauricular. When tachycardia is reported as sinus tachycardia or is not specified, report code R00.0 rather than a code from I47.-.

SP **I47.0** **Re-entry ventricular arrhythmia**

SP **I47.1** **Supraventricular tachycardia**
Atrial (paroxysmal) tachycardia
Atrioventricular [AV] (paroxysmal) tachycardia
Atrioventricular re-entrant (nodal) tachycardia [AVNRT] [AVRT]
Junctional (paroxysmal) tachycardia
Nodal (paroxysmal) tachycardia
> **DEFINITION** Abnormally rapid atrial rhythm occurring from time to time, most often in the young.

SP **I47.2** **Ventricular tachycardia**
> **DEFINITION** Potentially lethal rapid heart beat initiating in the ventricles marked by three of more consecutive premature beats.

SP **I47.9** **Paroxysmal tachycardia, unspecified**
Bouveret (-Hoffman) syndrome

4 **I48** **Atrial fibrillation and flutter**
> **CODING TIPS ✓** When assigning a code for atrial fibrillation or flutter, assign the most specific code according to the diagnostic statements given by the patient's physician.
> **DEFINITION** Abnormal heart rhythm that occurs in the atria of the heart.

SP **SH** **SL** **I48.0** **Paroxysmal atrial fibrillation**
> **CODING TIPS ✓** Also known as intermittent atrial fibrillation, paroxysmal atrial fibrillation may spontaneously resolve, only to reappear later.

▲ **5** **I48.1** **Persistent atrial fibrillation**
> **EXCLUDES 1** Permanent atrial fibrillation (I48.21)

---

4 4th digit required   **5** 5th digit required   **6** 6th digit required   **7** 7th digit required   **7** 7th digit placeholder   **+** Additional code   **⊟** Laterality

CODING TIPS ✓ Persistent AF is an abnormal heart rhythm that continues for seven days or longer, or that requires repeat electrical or pharmacological cardioversion. This code may be assigned only with a supportive confirmation diagnosis by the physician. If the provider documents both chronic and persistent AF, assign only a code from category I48.1-, Persistent atrial fibrillation. Persistent AF typically may require repeat pharmacological or electrical cardioversion and does not stop within seven days. Persistent atrial fibrillation that is described as chronic, or just persistent, is coded as I48.19. Pay special attention to the terms the physician uses. Persistent is not to be confused with permanent, which is coded as I48.21.

⭐ **I48.11** **Longstanding persistent atrial fibrillation**

> **DEFINITION** Longstanding persistent atrial fibrillation is persistent and continuous lasting longer than one year.

⭐ **I48.19** **Other persistent atrial fibrillation**
Chronic persistent atrial fibrillation
Persistent atrial fibrillation, NOS

▲ 5️⃣ **I48.2** **Chronic atrial fibrillation**

> **CODING TIPS ✓** Chronic atrial fibrillation is a nonspecific term that could be referring to paroxysmal, persistent, long standing persistent, or permanent atrial fibrillation. If any of these specific terms are used in the diagnostic statement, the specific type should be assigned, and not chronic.

⭐ **I48.20** **Chronic atrial fibrillation, unspecified**

> **EXCLUDES 1** Chronic persistent atrial fibrillation (I48.19)

> **CODING TIPS ✓** **Documentation**: Do not assume a diagnosis of chronic atrial fibrillation in a patient who has a long history of atrial fibrillation or has simply had atrial fibrillation for a long period of time. This code may only be assigned with a supportive confirmation diagnosis by the physician. Without such a diagnostic statement, an unspecified code (I48.91) must be assigned.

⭐ **I48.21** **Permanent atrial fibrillation**

> **CODING TIPS ✓** I48.21 is the correct code when permanent atrial fibrillation is documented. Chronic atrial fibrillation without the use of the word 'permanent' is coded I48.20.

SP **SH** **SL** **I48.3** **Typical atrial flutter**
Type I atrial flutter

SP **SH** **SL** **I48.4** **Atypical atrial flutter**
Type II atrial flutter

5️⃣ **I48.9** **Unspecified atrial fibrillation and atrial flutter**

SP **SH** **SL** **I48.91** **Unspecified atrial fibrillation**

SP **SH** **SL** **I48.92** **Unspecified atrial flutter**

4️⃣ **I49** **Other cardiac arrhythmias**
Code first cardiac arrhythmia complicating:
abortion or ectopic or molar pregnancy (O00-O07, O08.8)
obstetric surgery and procedures (O75.4)

> **EXCLUDES 1** neonatal dysrhythmia (P29.1-)
> sinoatrial bradycardia (R00.1)
> sinus bradycardia (R00.1)
> vagal bradycardia (R00.1)

> **EXCLUDES 2** bradycardia NOS (R00.1)

5️⃣ **I49.0** **Ventricular fibrillation and flutter**

SP **I49.01** **Ventricular fibrillation**

SP **I49.02** **Ventricular flutter**

SP **I49.1** **Atrial premature depolarization**
Atrial premature beats

SP **I49.2** **Junctional premature depolarization**

SP **I49.3** **Ventricular premature depolarization**

5️⃣ **I49.4** **Other and unspecified premature depolarization**

SP **I49.40** **Unspecified premature depolarization**
Premature beats NOS

SP **I49.49** **Other premature depolarization**
Ectopic beats
Extrasystoles
Extrasystolic arrhythmias
Premature contractions

SP **SH** **SL** **I49.5** **Sick sinus syndrome**
Tachycardia-bradycardia syndrome

SP **SH** **SL** **I49.8** **Other specified cardiac arrhythmias**
Brugada syndrome
Coronary sinus rhythm disorder
Ectopic rhythm disorder
Nodal rhythm disorder

SP **SH** **SL** **I49.9** **Cardiac arrhythmia, unspecified**
Arrhythmia (cardiac) NOS

⭐ New ▲ Revised **Px** Primary **SP** PDGM Px **SL** Low CoM **SH** High CoM **IQ** Quest. Encounter **H** Hospice non-cancer Dx Unspecified **M** *Manifestation*

DecisionHealth's FY 2020 Complete Home Health ICD-10-CM Diagnosis Coding Manual

971

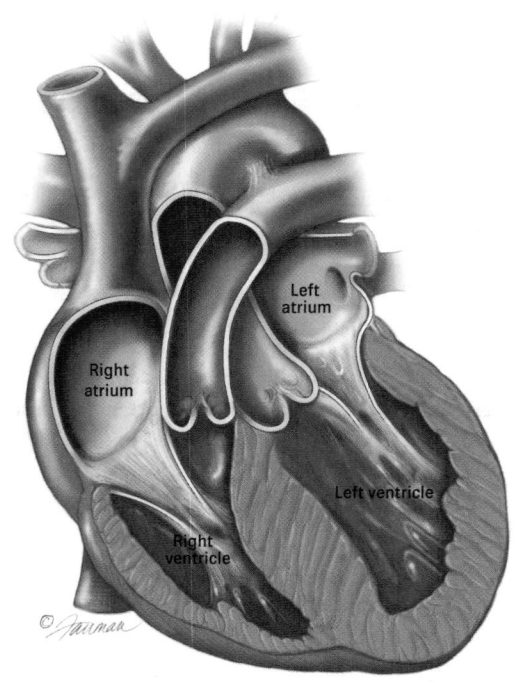

Right atrium

Left atrium

Left ventricle

Right ventricle

© Jarman

H 4 I50   Heart failure
Code first:
 heart failure complicating abortion or
  ectopic or molar pregnancy
  (O00-O07, O08.8)
 heart failure due to hypertension (I11.0)
 heart failure due to hypertension with
  chronic kidney disease (I13.-)
 heart failure following surgery (I97.13-)
 obstetric surgery and procedures (O75.4)
 rheumatic heart failure (I09.81)

EXCLUDES 1 neonatal cardiac failure (P29.0)
EXCLUDES 2 cardiac arrest (I46.-)

GUIDELINES **Section I.C.9.a.1)**
Hypertension with heart conditions classified to
I50.- or I51.4-I51.7, I51.89, I51.9, are assigned
to a code from category I11, Hypertensive
heart disease. Use additional code(s) from
category I50, Heart failure, to identify the
type(s) of heart failure in those patients with
heart failure.

The same heart conditions (I50.-, I51.4-I51.7,
I51.89, I51.9) with hypertension are coded
separately if the provider has documented they
are unrelated to the hypertension. Sequence
according to the circumstances of the
admission/encounter.

CODING TIPS ✓ Stage A of the ABCD
Classification of the American College of
Cardiology (ACC)/American Heart Association
(AHA) is the presence of heart failure risk
factors but no heart disease and no symptoms.
This should not be coded to the regular heart
failure codes, but rather to code Z91.89, Other
specified personal risk factors, not elsewhere
classified. Stage B is where heart disease is
present but there are no symptoms; thus there
are structural changes in the heart before
symptoms occur. Stage C involves structural
heart disease, with symptoms.

CODING TIPS ✓ When both heart failure and a
code from category I11.- will be assigned, the
heart failure (I50.-) code should immediately
follow the code from category I11.-. When both
heart failure and a code from category I13.- will
be assigned, the heart failure code (I50.-) and
the CKD code (N18.-) should immediately
follow the code from I13.- (sequence I50 and
N18 depending on which one has the greatest
impact on the home health plan of care).

CODING TIPS ✓ Decompensated indicates there
has been a flare-up or exacerbation of a
chronic condition.

CODING TIPS ✓ Query the physician on the type
of heart failure (systolic, diastolic, combined
systolic and diastolic HF, end stage, right, or
CHF) to aid in choosing a more specific 4th
character in this category. If the patient has
documented CHF and another type of heart
failure (systolic, diastolic, end stage or
combined) then code just the specific type. If
an acute exacerbation of a chronic failure
occurs, use 5th character 3 for acute on
chronic. An acute heart failure of one type and
chronic of another type should be coded
separately. Do not code the combined type for
these instances.

CODING TIPS ✓ The term "congestive" is a nonessential modifier for heart failure codes. When
coding heart failure, note the non-essential
modifier (congestive) and that no additional
code should be used if a patient has both CHF
and a more specific form of heart failure, such
as diastolic heart failure.

SP SH SL I50.1 Left ventricular failure, unspecified
Cardiac asthma
Edema of lung with heart disease NOS
Edema of lung with heart failure
Left heart failure
Pulmonary edema with heart disease NOS
Pulmonary edema with heart failure

EXCLUDES 1 edema of lung without heart
  disease or heart failure
  (J81.-)
  pulmonary edema without
  heart disease or failure
  (J81.-)

CODING TIPS ✓ Code I50.1, left-sided heart
failure, includes acute pulmonary edema;
no additional code needs to be assigned.
Never use I50.1 and I50.9 on the same
claim.

5 I50.2 Systolic (congestive) heart failure

4 4th digit required **5** 5th digit required **6** 6th digit required **7** 7th digit required **7** 7th digit placeholder **+** Additional code Laterality

972   *DecisionHealth's* FY 2020 Complete Home Health ICD-10-CM Diagnosis Coding Manual

Heart failure with reduced ejection fraction [HFrEF]

Systolic left ventricular heart failure

Code also:
end stage heart failure, if applicable (I50.84)

EXCLUDES 1 combined systolic (congestive) and diastolic (congestive) heart failure (I50.4-)

CODING TIPS ✓ Systolic dysfunction documented as linked to heart failure can be coded as systolic heart failure. If the conditions are not linked by the physician, code them separately with I50.9 and I51.89.

CODING TIPS ✓ Systolic heart failure is coded when the documentation indicates HFrEF, which may also be called heart failure with low ejection fraction, or heart failure with reduced systolic function, or other similar terms meaning systolic heart failure. Do not code systolic failure based on ejection fraction numbers without physician interpretation.

DEFINITION Heart muscle fails to contract with adequate force and not enough oxygen-rich blood is pumped to the body.

SP SH SL I50.20 **Unspecified systolic (congestive) heart failure**

SP SH SL I50.21 **Acute systolic (congestive) heart failure**

SP SH SL I50.22 **Chronic systolic (congestive) heart failure**

SP SH SL I50.23 **Acute on chronic systolic (congestive) heart failure**

CODING TIPS ✓ Decompensated indicates there has been a flare-up or exacerbation of a chronic condition.

5 I50.3 **Diastolic (congestive) heart failure**

Diastolic left ventricular heart failure

Heart failure with normal ejection fraction

Heart failure with preserved ejection fraction [HFpEF]

Code also:
end stage heart failure, if applicable (I50.84)

EXCLUDES 1 combined systolic (congestive) and diastolic (congestive) heart failure (I50.4-)

CODING TIPS ✓ Diastolic dysfunction documented as linked to heart failure can be coded as diastolic heart failure. If the conditions are not linked by the physician, code them separately with I50.9 and I51.89.

CODING TIPS ✓ Diastolic heart failure is coded when the documentation indicates HFpEF, which may also be referred to as heart failure with preserved systolic function, and this condition may also be referred to as diastolic heart failure. Do not code diastolic failure based on ejection fraction numbers without physician interpretation.

CODING TIPS ✓ All codes for heart failure include any associated pulmonary edema.

DEFINITION Heart muscle contracts normally but ventricles fail to relax properly after contraction, resulting in less blood entering the heart.

SP SH SL I50.30 **Unspecified diastolic (congestive) heart failure**

SP SH SL I50.31 **Acute diastolic (congestive) heart failure**

SP SH SL I50.32 **Chronic diastolic (congestive) heart failure**

SP SH SL I50.33 **Acute on chronic diastolic (congestive) heart failure**

CODING TIPS ✓ Decompensated indicates there has been a flare-up or exacerbation of a chronic condition.

5 I50.4 **Combined systolic (congestive) and diastolic (congestive) heart failure**

Combined systolic and diastolic left ventricular heart failure

Heart failure with reduced ejection fraction and diastolic dysfunction

Code also:
end stage heart failure, if applicable (I50.84)

DEFINITION Heart fails both to contract and relax properly, resulting in an insufficient amount of blood moving through the circulatory system.

SP SH SL I50.40 **Unspecified combined systolic (congestive) and diastolic (congestive) heart failure**

SP SH SL I50.41 **Acute combined systolic (congestive) and diastolic (congestive) heart failure**

SP SH SL I50.42 **Chronic combined systolic (congestive) and diastolic (congestive) heart failure**

SP SH SL I50.43 **Acute on chronic combined systolic (congestive) and diastolic (congestive) heart failure**

CODING TIPS ✓ Decompensated indicates there has been a flare-up or exacerbation of a chronic condition.

5 I50.8 **Other heart failure**

6 I50.81 **Right heart failure**

Right ventricular failure

SP SH SL I50.810 **Right heart failure, unspecified**

Right heart failure without mention of left heart failure

Right ventricular failure NOS

SP SH SL I50.811 **Acute right heart failure**

Acute isolated right heart failure

Acute (isolated) right ventricular failure

SP SH SL I50.812 **Chronic right heart failure**

Chronic isolated right heart failure

Chronic (isolated) right ventricular failure

SP SH SL I50.813 **Acute on chronic right heart failure**

Acute on chronic isolated right heart failure

Acute on chronic (isolated) right ventricular failure

Acute decompensation of chronic (isolated) right ventricular failure

---

★ New ▲ Revised Px Primary **SP** PDGM Px **SL** Low CoM **SH** High CoM **IQ** Quest. Encounter **H** Hospice non-cancer Dx Unspecified **M** *Manifestation*

DecisionHealth's FY 2020 Complete Home Health ICD-10-CM Diagnosis Coding Manual

973

Acute exacerbation of chronic (isolated) right ventricular failure

SP SH SL I50.814 **Right heart failure due to left heart failure**
Right ventricular failure secondary to left ventricular failure
Code also:
  the type of left ventricular failure, if known (I50.2-I50.43)
  EXCLUDES 1 Right heart failure with but not due to left heart failure (I50.82)

SP SH SL I50.82 **Biventricular heart failure**
Code also:
  the type of left ventricular failure as systolic, diastolic, or combined, if known (I50.2-I50.43)

SP SH SL I50.83 **High output heart failure**
CODING TIPS ✓ The term "high output heart failure" is a misnomer because the heart in these conditions is normal, capable of generating high cardiac output. The underlying problem in high output failure is a decrease in the systemic vascular resistance that threatens the arterial blood pressure and causes activation of neurohormones, resulting in an increase in salt and water retention by the kidney. Many high output states are curable conditions, and because they are associated with decreased peripheral vascular resistance, the use of vasodilator therapy for treatment of congestion may aggravate the problem.

SP SH SL I50.84 **End stage heart failure**
Stage D heart failure
Code also:
  the type of heart failure as systolic, diastolic, or combined, if known (I50.2-I50.43)
  CODING TIPS ✓ Do not code congestive heart failure with end stage heart failure. Code only specific types of heart failure with end stage heart failure.

DEFINITION Patients with end stage heart failure fall into stage D of the ABCD Classification of the American College of Cardiology (ACC)/American Heart Association (AHA), and are characterized by advanced structural heart disease and pronounced symptoms of heart failure at rest or upon minimal physical exertion, despite maximal medical treatment. They frequently develop intolerance to medical therapy and are developing worsening renal function and diuretic resistance according to current guidelines. This patient population has a 1-year mortality rate of approximately 50%, is at highest risk for re-hospitalization and requires special therapeutic interventions such as ventricular assist devices, artificial hearts and heart transplantation or hospice care.

SP SH SL I50.89 **Other heart failure**

▲ SP SH I50.9 **Heart failure, unspecified**
SL Cardiac, heart or myocardial failure NOS
Congestive heart disease
Congestive heart failure NOS
  EXCLUDES 2 fluid overload unrelated to congestive heart failure (E87.70)

4 I51 **Complications and ill-defined descriptions of heart disease**
  EXCLUDES 1 any condition in I51.4-I51.9 due to hypertension (I11.-)
  any condition in I51.4-I51.9 due to hypertension and chronic kidney disease (I13.-)
  heart disease specified as rheumatic (I00-I09)

SP I51.0 **Cardiac septal defect, acquired**
Acquired septal atrial defect (old)
Acquired septal auricular defect (old)
Acquired septal ventricular defect (old)
  EXCLUDES 1 cardiac septal defect as current complication following acute myocardial infarction (I23.1, I23.2)

SP I51.1 **Rupture of chordae tendineae, not elsewhere classified**
  EXCLUDES 1 rupture of chordae tendineae as current complication following acute myocardial infarction (I23.4)
  DEFINITION Tear in the fibrous, cord-like tissue connecting the papillary muscles to the valves, holding the valve flaps in place to prevent their eversion.

SP I51.2 **Rupture of papillary muscle, not elsewhere classified**
  EXCLUDES 1 rupture of papillary muscle as current complication following acute myocardial infarction (I23.5)

SP SH I51.3 **Intracardiac thrombosis, not elsewhere classified**

4 4th digit required   **5** 5th digit required   **6** 6th digit required   **7** 7th digit required   **7** 7th digit placeholder   **+** Additional code   **□** Laterality

974   *DecisionHealth's* FY 2020 Complete Home Health ICD-10-CM Diagnosis Coding Manual

Apical thrombosis (old)
Atrial thrombosis (old)
Auricular thrombosis (old)
Mural thrombosis (old)
Ventricular thrombosis (old)

> **EXCLUDES 1** intracardiac thrombosis as current complication following acute myocardial infarction (I23.6)

SP I51.4   Myocarditis, unspecified

Chronic (interstitial) myocarditis
Myocardial fibrosis
Myocarditis NOS

> **EXCLUDES 1** acute or subacute myocarditis (I40.-)

> **CODING TIPS ✓** If conditions included in I51.4 -I51.7. I51.89, I51.9 are present with hypertension, then do not code them. These conditions are included in codes I11 and I13.

SP I51.5   Myocardial degeneration

Fatty degeneration of heart or myocardium
Myocardial disease
Senile degeneration of heart or myocardium

> **CODING TIPS ✓** If conditions included in I51.4 -I51.7. I51.89, I51.9 are present with hypertension, then do not code them. These conditions are included in codes I11 and I13.

> **DEFINITION** Wasting away of the heart muscle.

SP I51.7   Cardiomegaly

Cardiac dilatation
Cardiac hypertrophy
Ventricular dilatation

> **CODING TIPS ✓** If conditions included in I51.4 -I51.7. I51.89, I51.9 are present with hypertension, then do not code them. These conditions are included in codes I11 and I13.

S I51.8   Other ill-defined heart diseases

SP I51.81   Takotsubo syndrome

Reversible left ventricular dysfunction following sudden emotional stress
Stress induced cardiomyopathy
Takotsubo cardiomyopathy
Transient left ventricular apical ballooning syndrome

> **CODING TIPS ✓** Takotsubo Syndrome (I51.81) is by definition stress related and therefore should not be coded with I11.9, per CC Q2 2018.

> **DEFINITION** Takutosobu Syndrome presents with chest pain and dypsnea and occurs more frequently in postmenopausal females, with a physical or emotional stressor. They may have ST elevation and a troponin elevation, however cardiac catheterization demonstrates normal coronary arteries in more than 80% of cases.

SP SH I51.89   Other ill-defined heart diseases

Carditis (acute)(chronic)

Pancarditis (acute)(chronic)

> **CODING TIPS ✓** Diastolic dysfunction or systolic dysfunction is coded to I51.89 if not related to heart failure. If related to heart failure, then diastolic heart failure or systolic heart failure should be coded.

> **CODING TIPS ✓** If conditions included in I51.4 -I51.7. I51.89, I51.9 are present with hypertension, then do not code them. These conditions are included in codes I11 and I13.

SP I51.9   Heart disease, unspecified

> **CODING TIPS ✓** This code is assigned for end stage heart disease, but the physician should always be queried for additional information regarding the type of heart disease.

> **CODING TIPS ✓** If conditions included in I51.4 -I51.7. I51.89, I51.9 are present with hypertension, then do not code them. These conditions are included in codes I11 and I13.

M !Q I52   *Other heart disorders in diseases classified elsewhere*

Code first underlying disease, such as:
congenital syphilis (A50.5)
mucopolysaccharidosis (E76.3)
schistosomiasis (B65.0-B65.9)

> **EXCLUDES 1** heart disease (in) : gonococcal infection (A54.83) meningococcal infection (A39.50) rheumatoid arthritis (M05.31) syphilis (A52.06)

Cerebrovascular diseases   (I60-I69)

Use additional code to identify presence of:
alcohol abuse and dependence (F10.-)
exposure to environmental tobacco smoke (Z77.22)
history of tobacco dependence (Z87.891)
hypertension (I10-I16)
occupational exposure to environmental tobacco smoke (Z57.31)
tobacco dependence (F17.-)
tobacco use (Z72.0)

> **EXCLUDES 1** traumatic intracranial hemorrhage (S06.-)

> **CODING TIPS ✓** The hypertensive cerebrovascular disease guideline is based on the instructional note at the I60-I69 block of codes which indicates "use additional code to identify presence of ..." If the physician documents hypertensive cerebrovascular disease, add the code for hypertension.

> **CODING TIPS ✓** A traumatic head injury and a CVA may both be coded if the two conditions are unrelated.

4 I60   Nontraumatic subarachnoid hemorrhage

> **EXCLUDES 1** syphilitic ruptured cerebral aneurysm (A52.05)

> **EXCLUDES 2** sequelae of subarachnoid hemorrhage (I69.0-)

★ New ▲ Revised Px Primary **SP** PDGM Px **SL** Low CoM **SH** High CoM **!Q** Quest. Encounter **H** Hospice non-cancer Dx   Unspecified   **M** *Manifestation*

DecisionHealth's FY 2020 Complete Home Health ICD-10-CM Diagnosis Coding Manual

975

CODING TIPS ✓   Codes from category I60.- should ordinarily not be used on the home health or hospice claim because they indicate a continuing cerebrovascular bleed. If documentation indicates an ongoing bleed, the I60.- codes may continue to be reported in home health and hospice. If there is no indication that the bleed continues, I69.0- is used on home health and hospice claims to indicate residual deficits.

CODING TIPS ✓   Imaging reports may be utilized to provide greater specificity of the anatomic site as documented by the physician. It is appropriate to utilize the imaging report to determine the location of the stroke or infarction, only if the attending or consulting physician has signed or documented otherwise.

CODING TIPS ✓   The use of codes from R29.7 indicate the NIHSS. The NIHSS can be used as a clinical stroke assessment tool to evaluate and document neurological status in acute stroke patients. The stroke scale is valid for predicting lesion size and can serve as a measure of stroke severity. The NIHSS has been shown to be a predictor of both short and long term outcome of stroke patients. The codes are meant for use for acute hospitals only.

🔢 **I60.0**   **Nontraumatic subarachnoid hemorrhage from carotid siphon and bifurcation**

⊟ **SP** **I60.00**   Nontraumatic subarachnoid hemorrhage from unspecified carotid siphon and bifurcation

⊟ **SP** **I60.01**   Nontraumatic subarachnoid hemorrhage from right carotid siphon and bifurcation

⊟ **SP** **I60.02**   Nontraumatic subarachnoid hemorrhage from left carotid siphon and bifurcation

🔢 **I60.1**   **Nontraumatic subarachnoid hemorrhage from middle cerebral artery**

⊟ **SP** **I60.10**   Nontraumatic subarachnoid hemorrhage from unspecified middle cerebral artery

⊟ **SP** **I60.11**   Nontraumatic subarachnoid hemorrhage from right middle cerebral artery

⊟ **SP** **I60.12**   Nontraumatic subarachnoid hemorrhage from left middle cerebral artery

SP **I60.2**   Nontraumatic subarachnoid hemorrhage from anterior communicating artery

🔢 **I60.3**   **Nontraumatic subarachnoid hemorrhage from posterior communicating artery**

⊟ **SP** **I60.30**   Nontraumatic subarachnoid hemorrhage from unspecified posterior communicating artery

⊟ **SP** **I60.31**   Nontraumatic subarachnoid hemorrhage from right posterior communicating artery

⊟ **SP** **I60.32**   Nontraumatic subarachnoid hemorrhage from left posterior communicating artery

SP **I60.4**   Nontraumatic subarachnoid hemorrhage from basilar artery

🔢 **I60.5**   Nontraumatic subarachnoid hemorrhage from vertebral artery

⊟ **SP** **I60.50**   Nontraumatic subarachnoid hemorrhage from unspecified vertebral artery

⊟ **SP** **I60.51**   Nontraumatic subarachnoid hemorrhage from right vertebral artery

⊟ **SP** **I60.52**   Nontraumatic subarachnoid hemorrhage from left vertebral artery

SP **I60.6**   Nontraumatic subarachnoid hemorrhage from other intracranial arteries

SP **I60.7**   Nontraumatic subarachnoid hemorrhage from unspecified intracranial artery

Ruptured (congenital) berry aneurysm
Ruptured (congenital) cerebral aneurysm
Subarachnoid hemorrhage (nontraumatic) from cerebral artery NOS
Subarachnoid hemorrhage (nontraumatic) from communicating artery NOS

EXCLUDES 1   berry aneurysm, nonruptured (I67.1)

SP **I60.8**   Other nontraumatic subarachnoid hemorrhage
Meningeal hemorrhage
Rupture of cerebral arteriovenous malformation

SP **I60.9**   Nontraumatic subarachnoid hemorrhage, unspecified

🔢 **I61**   **Nontraumatic intracerebral hemorrhage**

EXCLUDES 2   sequelae of intracerebral hemorrhage (I69.1-)

CODING TIPS ✓   The use of codes from R29.7 indicate the NIHSS. The NIHSS can be used as a clinical stroke assessment tool to evaluate and document neurological status in acute stroke patients. The stroke scale is valid for predicting lesion size and can serve as a measure of stroke severity. The NIHSS has been shown to be a predictor of both short and long term outcome of stroke patients. The codes are meant for use for acute hospitals only.

CODING TIPS ✓   Imaging reports may be utilized to provide greater specificity of the anatomic site as documented by the physician. It is appropriate to utilize the imaging report to determine the location of the stroke or infarction, only if the attending or consulting physician has signed or documented otherwise.

🔢4th digit required   🔢5th digit required   🔢6th digit required   🔢7th digit required   ☑7th digit placeholder   ➕Additional code   ⊟Laterality

CODING TIPS ✓ Codes from category I61.- should ordinarily not be used on the home health or hospice claim because they indicate a continuing cerebrovascular bleed. If documentation indicates an ongoing bleed, the I61.- codes may continue to be reported in home health and hospice. If there is no indication that the bleed continues, I69.1- is used on home health and hospice claims to indicate residual deficits.

SP I61.0 **Nontraumatic intracerebral hemorrhage in hemisphere, subcortical**
Deep intracerebral hemorrhage (nontraumatic)

SP I61.1 **Nontraumatic intracerebral hemorrhage in hemisphere, cortical**
Cerebral lobe hemorrhage (nontraumatic)
Superficial intracerebral hemorrhage (nontraumatic)

SP I61.2 **Nontraumatic intracerebral hemorrhage in hemisphere, unspecified**

SP I61.3 **Nontraumatic intracerebral hemorrhage in brain stem**

SP I61.4 **Nontraumatic intracerebral hemorrhage in cerebellum**

SP I61.5 **Nontraumatic intracerebral hemorrhage, intraventricular**

SP I61.6 **Nontraumatic intracerebral hemorrhage, multiple localized**

SP I61.8 **Other nontraumatic intracerebral hemorrhage**

SP I61.9 **Nontraumatic intracerebral hemorrhage, unspecified**

4 I62 **Other and unspecified nontraumatic intracranial hemorrhage**
EXCLUDES 2 sequelae of intracranial hemorrhage (I69.2)

CODING TIPS ✓ Codes from category I62.- should ordinarily not be used on the home health or hospice claim because they indicate a continuing cerebrovascular bleed. If documentation indicates an ongoing bleed, the I62.- codes may continue to be reported in home health and hospice. If there is no indication that the bleed continues, I69.2- is used on home health and hospice claims to indicate residual deficits.

CODING TIPS ✓ Imaging reports may be utilized to provide greater specificity of the anatomic site as documented by the physician. It is appropriate to utilize the imaging report to determine the location of the stroke or infarction, only if the attending or consulting physician has signed or documented otherwise.

CODING TIPS ✓ The use of codes from R29.7 indicate the NIHSS. The NIHSS can be used as a clinical stroke assessment tool to evaluate and document neurological status in acute stroke patients. The stroke scale is valid for predicting lesion size and can serve as a measure of stroke severity. The NIHSS has been shown to be a predictor of both short and long term outcome of stroke patients. The codes are meant for use for acute hospitals only.

5 I62.0 **Nontraumatic subdural hemorrhage**

SP I62.00 **Nontraumatic subdural hemorrhage, unspecified**

SP I62.01 **Nontraumatic acute subdural hemorrhage**

SP I62.02 **Nontraumatic subacute subdural hemorrhage**

SP I62.03 **Nontraumatic chronic subdural hemorrhage**

SP I62.1 **Nontraumatic extradural hemorrhage**
Nontraumatic epidural hemorrhage

SP I62.9 **Nontraumatic intracranial hemorrhage, unspecified**

+ 4 I63 **Cerebral infarction**
INCLUDES occlusion and stenosis of cerebral and precerebral arteries, resulting in cerebral infarction
Use additional code, if applicable, to identify status post administration of tPA (rtPA) in a different facility within the last 24 hours prior to admission to current facility (Z92.82)
Use additional code, if known, to indicate National Institutes of Health Stroke Scale (NIHSS) score (R29.7-)
EXCLUDES 2 sequelae of cerebral infarction (I69.3-)

CODING TIPS ✓ The use of codes from R29.7 indicate the NIHSS. The NIHSS can be used as a clinical stroke assessment tool to evaluate and document neurological status in acute stroke patients. The stroke scale is valid for predicting lesion size and can serve as a measure of stroke severity. The NIHSS has been shown to be a predictor of both short and long term outcome of stroke patients. The codes are meant for use for acute hospitals only.

CODING TIPS ✓ Imaging reports may be utilized to provide greater specificity of the anatomic site as documented by the physician. It is appropriate to utilize the imaging report to determine the location of the stroke or infarction, only if the attending or consulting physician has signed or documented otherwise.

CODING TIPS ✓ Codes from category I63.- should ordinarily not be used on the home health or hospice claim because they indicate a continuing cerebrovascular infarction. If documentation indicates an ongoing infarction, the I63.- codes may continue to be reported in home health and hospice. If there is no indication that the infarction continues, I69.3- is used on home health and hospice claims to indicate residual deficits.

+ 5 I63.0 **Cerebral infarction due to thrombosis of precerebral arteries**

SP + I63.00 **Cerebral infarction due to thrombosis of unspecified precerebral artery**

+ 6 I63.01 **Cerebral infarction due to thrombosis of vertebral artery**

⊟ SP + I63.011 **Cerebral infarction due to thrombosis of right vertebral artery**

★ New ▲ Revised Px Primary **SP** PDGM Px **SL** Low CoM **SH** High CoM **IQ** Quest. Encounter ⊟ Hospice non-cancer Dx Unspecified **M** *Manifestation*

DecisionHealth's FY 2020 Complete Home Health ICD-10-CM Diagnosis Coding Manual

977

▤ **SP** ✚ **I63.012**   Cerebral infarction due to thrombosis of left vertebral artery

▤ **SP** ✚ **I63.013**   Cerebral infarction due to thrombosis of bilateral vertebral arteries

▤ **SP** ✚ **I63.019**   Cerebral infarction due to thrombosis of unspecified vertebral artery

SP ✚ **I63.02**   Cerebral infarction due to thrombosis of basilar artery

✚ **6** **I63.03**   Cerebral infarction due to thrombosis of carotid artery

▤ **SP** ✚ **I63.031**   Cerebral infarction due to thrombosis of right carotid artery

▤ **SP** ✚ **I63.032**   Cerebral infarction due to thrombosis of left carotid artery

▤ **SP** ✚ **I63.033**   Cerebral infarction due to thrombosis of bilateral carotid arteries

▤ **SP** ✚ **I63.039**   Cerebral infarction due to thrombosis of unspecified carotid artery

SP ✚ **I63.09**   Cerebral infarction due to thrombosis of other precerebral artery

✚ **5** **I63.1**   Cerebral infarction due to embolism of precerebral arteries

SP ✚ **I63.10**   Cerebral infarction due to embolism of unspecified precerebral artery

✚ **6** **I63.11**   Cerebral infarction due to embolism of vertebral artery

▤ **SP** ✚ **I63.111**   Cerebral infarction due to embolism of right vertebral artery

▤ **SP** ✚ **I63.112**   Cerebral infarction due to embolism of left vertebral artery

▤ **SP** ✚ **I63.113**   Cerebral infarction due to embolism of bilateral vertebral arteries

▤ **SP** ✚ **I63.119**   Cerebral infarction due to embolism of unspecified vertebral artery

SP ✚ **I63.12**   Cerebral infarction due to embolism of basilar artery

✚ **6** **I63.13**   Cerebral infarction due to embolism of carotid artery

▤ **SP** ✚ **I63.131**   Cerebral infarction due to embolism of right carotid artery

▤ **SP** ✚ **I63.132**   Cerebral infarction due to embolism of left carotid artery

▤ **SP** ✚ **I63.133**   Cerebral infarction due to embolism of bilateral carotid arteries

▤ **SP** ✚ **I63.139**   Cerebral infarction due to embolism of unspecified carotid artery

SP ✚ **I63.19**   Cerebral infarction due to embolism of other precerebral artery

✚ **5** **I63.2**   Cerebral infarction due to unspecified occlusion or stenosis of precerebral arteries

SP ✚ **I63.20**   Cerebral infarction due to unspecified occlusion or stenosis of unspecified precerebral arteries

✚ **6** **I63.21**   Cerebral infarction due to unspecified occlusion or stenosis of vertebral arteries

▤ **SP** ✚ **I63.211**   Cerebral infarction due to unspecified occlusion or stenosis of right vertebral artery

▤ **SP** ✚ **I63.212**   Cerebral infarction due to unspecified occlusion or stenosis of left vertebral artery

▤ **SP** ✚ **I63.213**   Cerebral infarction due to unspecified occlusion or stenosis of bilateral vertebral arteries

▤ **SP** ✚ **I63.219**   Cerebral infarction due to unspecified occlusion or stenosis of unspecified vertebral artery

SP ✚ **I63.22**   Cerebral infarction due to unspecified occlusion or stenosis of basilar artery

✚ **6** **I63.23**   Cerebral infarction due to unspecified occlusion or stenosis of carotid arteries

▤ **SP** ✚ **I63.231**   Cerebral infarction due to unspecified occlusion or stenosis of right carotid arteries

▤ **SP** ✚ **I63.232**   Cerebral infarction due to unspecified occlusion or stenosis of left carotid arteries

▤ **SP** ✚ **I63.233**   Cerebral infarction due to unspecified occlusion or stenosis of bilateral carotid arteries

▤ **SP** ✚ **I63.239**   Cerebral infarction due to unspecified occlusion or stenosis of unspecified carotid artery

SP ✚ **I63.29**   Cerebral infarction due to unspecified occlusion or stenosis of other precerebral arteries

✚ **5** **I63.3**   Cerebral infarction due to thrombosis of cerebral arteries

SP ✚ **I63.30**   Cerebral infarction due to thrombosis of unspecified cerebral artery

✚ **6** **I63.31**   Cerebral infarction due to thrombosis of middle cerebral artery

▤ **SP** ✚ **I63.311**   Cerebral infarction due to thrombosis of right middle cerebral artery

▤ **SP** ✚ **I63.312**   Cerebral infarction due to thrombosis of left middle cerebral artery

▤ **SP** ✚ **I63.313**   Cerebral infarction due to thrombosis of bilateral middle cerebral arteries

▤ **SP** ✚ **I63.319**   Cerebral infarction due to thrombosis of unspecified middle cerebral artery

✚ **6** **I63.32**   Cerebral infarction due to thrombosis of anterior cerebral artery

▤ **SP** ✚ **I63.321**   Cerebral infarction due to thrombosis of right anterior cerebral artery

▤ **SP** ✚ **I63.322**   Cerebral infarction due to thrombosis of left anterior cerebral artery

▤ **SP** ✚ **I63.323**   Cerebral infarction due to thrombosis of bilateral anterior cerebral arteries

---

▵ 4th digit required   ▵ 5th digit required   ▵ 6th digit required   ▵ 7th digit required   ▵ 7th digit placeholder   ✚ Additional code   ▤ Laterality

978   *DecisionHealth's* FY 2020 Complete Home Health ICD-10-CM Diagnosis Coding Manual

■ SP + **I63.329** Cerebral infarction due to thrombosis of unspecified anterior cerebral artery

+ 6 **I63.33** Cerebral infarction due to thrombosis of posterior cerebral artery

■ SP + **I63.331** Cerebral infarction due to thrombosis of right posterior cerebral artery

■ SP + **I63.332** Cerebral infarction due to thrombosis of left posterior cerebral artery

■ SP + **I63.333** Cerebral infarction due to thrombosis of bilateral posterior cerebral arteries

■ SP + **I63.339** Cerebral infarction due to thrombosis of unspecified posterior cerebral artery

+ 6 **I63.34** Cerebral infarction due to thrombosis of cerebellar artery

■ SP + **I63.341** Cerebral infarction due to thrombosis of right cerebellar artery

■ SP + **I63.342** Cerebral infarction due to thrombosis of left cerebellar artery

■ SP + **I63.343** Cerebral infarction due to thrombosis of bilateral cerebellar arteries

■ SP + **I63.349** Cerebral infarction due to thrombosis of unspecified cerebellar artery

SP + **I63.39** Cerebral infarction due to thrombosis of other cerebral artery

+ 5 **I63.4** Cerebral infarction due to embolism of cerebral arteries

SP + **I63.40** Cerebral infarction due to embolism of unspecified cerebral artery

+ 6 **I63.41** Cerebral infarction due to embolism of middle cerebral artery

■ SP + **I63.411** Cerebral infarction due to embolism of right middle cerebral artery

■ SP + **I63.412** Cerebral infarction due to embolism of left middle cerebral artery

■ SP + **I63.413** Cerebral infarction due to embolism of bilateral middle cerebral arteries

■ SP + **I63.419** Cerebral infarction due to embolism of unspecified middle cerebral artery

+ 6 **I63.42** Cerebral infarction due to embolism of anterior cerebral artery

■ SP + **I63.421** Cerebral infarction due to embolism of right anterior cerebral artery

■ SP + **I63.422** Cerebral infarction due to embolism of left anterior cerebral artery

■ SP + **I63.423** Cerebral infarction due to embolism of bilateral anterior cerebral arteries

■ SP + **I63.429** Cerebral infarction due to embolism of unspecified anterior cerebral artery

+ 6 **I63.43** Cerebral infarction due to embolism of posterior cerebral artery

■ SP + **I63.431** Cerebral infarction due to embolism of right posterior cerebral artery

■ SP + **I63.432** Cerebral infarction due to embolism of left posterior cerebral artery

■ SP + **I63.433** Cerebral infarction due to embolism of bilateral posterior cerebral arteries

■ SP + **I63.439** Cerebral infarction due to embolism of unspecified posterior cerebral artery

+ 6 **I63.44** Cerebral infarction due to embolism of cerebellar artery

■ SP + **I63.441** Cerebral infarction due to embolism of right cerebellar artery

■ SP + **I63.442** Cerebral infarction due to embolism of left cerebellar artery

■ SP + **I63.443** Cerebral infarction due to embolism of bilateral cerebellar arteries

■ SP + **I63.449** Cerebral infarction due to embolism of unspecified cerebellar artery

SP + **I63.49** Cerebral infarction due to embolism of other cerebral artery

+ 5 **I63.5** Cerebral infarction due to unspecified occlusion or stenosis of cerebral arteries

SP + **I63.50** Cerebral infarction due to unspecified occlusion or stenosis of unspecified cerebral artery

+ 6 **I63.51** Cerebral infarction due to unspecified occlusion or stenosis of middle cerebral artery

■ SP + **I63.511** Cerebral infarction due to unspecified occlusion or stenosis of right middle cerebral artery

■ SP + **I63.512** Cerebral infarction due to unspecified occlusion or stenosis of left middle cerebral artery

■ SP + **I63.513** Cerebral infarction due to unspecified occlusion or stenosis of bilateral middle cerebral arteries

■ SP + **I63.519** Cerebral infarction due to unspecified occlusion or stenosis of unspecified middle cerebral artery

+ 6 **I63.52** Cerebral infarction due to unspecified occlusion or stenosis of anterior cerebral artery

■ SP + **I63.521** Cerebral infarction due to unspecified occlusion or stenosis of right anterior cerebral artery

■ SP + **I63.522** Cerebral infarction due to unspecified occlusion or stenosis of left anterior cerebral artery

■ SP + **I63.523** Cerebral infarction due to unspecified occlusion or stenosis of bilateral anterior cerebral arteries

★ New ▲ Revised Px Primary SP PDGM Px SL Low CoM SH High CoM IQ Quest. Encounter ⊞ Hospice non-cancer Dx Unspecified M *Manifestation*

DecisionHealth's FY 2020 Complete Home Health ICD-10-CM Diagnosis Coding Manual

979

Chapter 9

I00-I99

☐ **SP** + **I63.529**   **Cerebral infarction due to unspecified occlusion or stenosis of unspecified anterior cerebral artery**

+ ⑥ **I63.53**   **Cerebral infarction due to unspecified occlusion or stenosis of posterior cerebral artery**

☐ **SP** + **I63.531**   **Cerebral infarction due to unspecified occlusion or stenosis of right posterior cerebral artery**

☐ **SP** + **I63.532**   **Cerebral infarction due to unspecified occlusion or stenosis of left posterior cerebral artery**

☐ **SP** + **I63.533**   **Cerebral infarction due to unspecified occlusion or stenosis of bilateral posterior cerebral arteries**

☐ **SP** + **I63.539**   **Cerebral infarction due to unspecified occlusion or stenosis of unspecified posterior cerebral artery**

+ ⑥ **I63.54**   **Cerebral infarction due to unspecified occlusion or stenosis of cerebellar artery**

☐ **SP** + **I63.541**   **Cerebral infarction due to unspecified occlusion or stenosis of right cerebellar artery**

☐ **SP** + **I63.542**   **Cerebral infarction due to unspecified occlusion or stenosis of left cerebellar artery**

☐ **SP** + **I63.543**   **Cerebral infarction due to unspecified occlusion or stenosis of bilateral cerebellar arteries**

☐ **SP** + **I63.549**   **Cerebral infarction due to unspecified occlusion or stenosis of unspecified cerebellar artery**

SP + **I63.59**   **Cerebral infarction due to unspecified occlusion or stenosis of other cerebral artery**

SP + **I63.6**   **Cerebral infarction due to cerebral venous thrombosis, nonpyogenic**

+ ⑤ **I63.8**   **Other cerebral infarction**

SP + **I63.81**   **Other cerebral infarction due to occlusion or stenosis of small artery**
Lacunar infarction

SP + **I63.89**   **Other cerebral infarction**

SP + **I63.9**   **Cerebral infarction, unspecified**
Stroke NOS
EXCLUDES 2   transient cerebral ischemic attacks and related syndromes (G45.-)

④ **I65**   **Occlusion and stenosis of precerebral arteries, not resulting in cerebral infarction**
INCLUDES   embolism of precerebral artery
narrowing of precerebral artery
obstruction (complete) (partial) of precerebral artery
thrombosis of precerebral artery
EXCLUDES 1   insufficiency, NOS, of precerebral artery (G45.-)
insufficiency of precerebral arteries causing cerebral infarction (I63.0-I63.2)

CODING TIPS ✓   Codes from categories I65.- and I66.- are used to indicate stenosis and occlusion that do not result in infarction and may be used in the home health setting. Assign the most specific code as appropriate according to diagnostic statements provided by the physician. If the affected artery is not specified, do not assume a code for an affected location, but rather use an unspecified code. If more than one arterial location is affected and a specific code is available for separate locations, separate codes should be assigned.

Imaging reports may be utilized to provide greater specificity of the anatomic site as documented by the physician.

⑤ **I65.0**   **Occlusion and stenosis of vertebral artery**

☐ **SP** **I65.01**   **Occlusion and stenosis of right vertebral artery**

☐ **SP** **I65.02**   **Occlusion and stenosis of left vertebral artery**

☐ **SP** **I65.03**   **Occlusion and stenosis of bilateral vertebral arteries**

☐ **SP** **I65.09**   **Occlusion and stenosis of unspecified vertebral artery**

SP **I65.1**   **Occlusion and stenosis of basilar artery**

⑤ **I65.2**   **Occlusion and stenosis of carotid artery**

☐ **SP** **I65.21**   **Occlusion and stenosis of right carotid artery**

☐ **SP** **I65.22**   **Occlusion and stenosis of left carotid artery**

☐ **SP** **I65.23**   **Occlusion and stenosis of bilateral carotid arteries**

☐ **SP** **I65.29**   **Occlusion and stenosis of unspecified carotid artery**

SP **I65.8**   **Occlusion and stenosis of other precerebral arteries**

SP **I65.9**   **Occlusion and stenosis of unspecified precerebral artery**
Occlusion and stenosis of precerebral artery NOS

④ **I66**   **Occlusion and stenosis of cerebral arteries, not resulting in cerebral infarction**
INCLUDES   embolism of cerebral artery
narrowing of cerebral artery
obstruction (complete) (partial) of cerebral artery
thrombosis of cerebral artery
EXCLUDES 1   Occlusion and stenosis of cerebral artery causing cerebral infarction (I63.3-I63.5)

---

④ 4th digit required   ⑤ 5th digit required   ⑥ 6th digit required   ⑦ 7th digit required   ☑ 7th digit placeholder   + Additional code   ☐ Laterality

980   *DecisionHealth's* FY 2020 Complete Home Health ICD-10-CM Diagnosis Coding Manual

CODING TIPS ✓ Codes from categories I65.- and I66.- are used to indicate stenosis and occlusion that do not result in infarction and may be used in the home health setting. Assign the most specific code as appropriate according to diagnostic statements provided by the physician. If the affected artery is not specified, do not assume a code for an affected location, but rather use an unspecified code. If more than one arterial location is affected and a specific code is available for separate locations, separate codes should be assigned.

Imaging reports may be utilized to provide greater specificity of the anatomic site as documented by the physician.

⑤ I66.0 **Occlusion and stenosis of middle cerebral artery**

⊟ SP I66.01 **Occlusion and stenosis of right middle cerebral artery**

⊟ SP I66.02 **Occlusion and stenosis of left middle cerebral artery**

⊟ SP I66.03 **Occlusion and stenosis of bilateral middle cerebral arteries**

⊟ SP I66.09 **Occlusion and stenosis of unspecified middle cerebral artery**

⑤ I66.1 **Occlusion and stenosis of anterior cerebral artery**

⊟ SP I66.11 **Occlusion and stenosis of right anterior cerebral artery**

⊟ SP I66.12 **Occlusion and stenosis of left anterior cerebral artery**

⊟ SP I66.13 **Occlusion and stenosis of bilateral anterior cerebral arteries**

⊟ SP I66.19 **Occlusion and stenosis of unspecified anterior cerebral artery**

⑤ I66.2 **Occlusion and stenosis of posterior cerebral artery**

⊟ SP I66.21 **Occlusion and stenosis of right posterior cerebral artery**

⊟ SP I66.22 **Occlusion and stenosis of left posterior cerebral artery**

⊟ SP I66.23 **Occlusion and stenosis of bilateral posterior cerebral arteries**

⊟ SP I66.29 **Occlusion and stenosis of unspecified posterior cerebral artery**

SP I66.3 **Occlusion and stenosis of cerebellar arteries**

SP I66.8 **Occlusion and stenosis of other cerebral arteries**
Occlusion and stenosis of perforating arteries

SP I66.9 **Occlusion and stenosis of unspecified cerebral artery**

④ I67 **Other cerebrovascular diseases**
EXCLUDES 2 sequelae of the listed conditions (I69.8)

CODING TIPS ✓ These codes may be used in home health and hospice for various cerebrovascular disease, because the patient has not had a cerebral infarction.

SP I67.0 **Dissection of cerebral arteries, nonruptured**
EXCLUDES 1 ruptured cerebral arteries (I60.7)

SP I67.1 **Cerebral aneurysm, nonruptured**

Cerebral aneurysm NOS
Cerebral arteriovenous fistula, acquired
Internal carotid artery aneurysm, intracranial portion
Internal carotid artery aneurysm, NOS
EXCLUDES 1 congenital cerebral aneurysm, nonruptured (Q28.-)
ruptured cerebral aneurysm (I60.7)

SP SH SL I67.2 **Cerebral atherosclerosis**
Atheroma of cerebral and precerebral arteries

SP I67.3 **Progressive vascular leukoencephalopathy**
Binswanger's disease

SP I67.4 **Hypertensive encephalopathy**
EXCLUDES 2 insufficiency, NOS, of precerebral arteries (G45.2)

SP I67.5 **Moyamoya disease**

SP I67.6 **Nonpyogenic thrombosis of intracranial venous system**
Nonpyogenic thrombosis of cerebral vein
Nonpyogenic thrombosis of intracranial venous sinus
EXCLUDES 1 nonpyogenic thrombosis of intracranial venous system causing infarction (I63.6)

SP I67.7 **Cerebral arteritis, not elsewhere classified**
Granulomatous angiitis of the nervous system
EXCLUDES 1 allergic granulomatous angiitis (M30.1)
DEFINITION Inflammation of an artery in the head.

⑤ I67.8 **Other specified cerebrovascular diseases**

SP SH SL I67.81 **Acute cerebrovascular insufficiency**
Acute cerebrovascular insufficiency unspecified as to location or reversibility

SP SH SL I67.82 **Cerebral ischemia**
Chronic cerebral ischemia

SP I67.83 **Posterior reversible encephalopathy syndrome**
PRES

⑥ I67.84 **Cerebral vasospasm and vasoconstriction**

SP I67.841 **Reversible cerebrovascular vasoconstriction syndrome**
Call-Fleming syndrome
Code first:
underlying condition, if applicable, such as eclampsia (O15.00-O15.9)

SP I67.848 **Other cerebrovascular vasospasm and vasoconstriction**

⑥ I67.85 **Hereditary cerebrovascular diseases**

SP I67.850 **Cerebral autosomal dominant arteriopathy with subcortical infarcts and leukoencephalopathy**
CADASIL
Code also any associated diagnoses, such as:
epilepsy (G40.-)
stroke (I63.-)
vascular dementia (F01.-)

★ New ▲ Revised Px Primary SP PDGM Px SL Low CoM SH High CoM IQ Quest. Encounter H Hospice non-cancer Dx Unspecified M *Manifestation*

DecisionHealth's FY 2020 Complete Home Health ICD-10-CM Diagnosis Coding Manual

981

Chapter 9

I00-I99

SP I67.858 Other hereditary cerebrovascular disease

SP SH SL I67.89 Other cerebrovascular disease

SP I67.9 Cerebrovascular disease, unspecified

> **CODING TIPS ✓** Do not assign I67.9 for sequelae of cerebral vascular accident. Do not assign I67.9 for cerebral atherosclerosis or any other known type of cerebral vascular disorder. If the type of cerebral vascular disease is not specified in the record, query the physician to attempt to obtain a more specific diagnosis.

4 I68 Cerebrovascular disorders in diseases classified elsewhere

> **CODING TIPS ✓** These codes may be used in home health and hospice for various cerebrovascular disease, because the patient has not had a cerebral infarction.

M IQ I68.0 Cerebral amyloid angiopathy

Code first:
  underlying amyloidosis (E85.-)

M IQ I68.2 Cerebral arteritis in other diseases classified elsewhere

Code first:
  underlying disease

> **EXCLUDES 1** cerebral arteritis (in) :
>   listerosis (A32.89)
>   systemic lupus erythematosus (M32.19)
>   syphilis (A52.04)
>   tuberculosis (A18.89)

M IQ I68.8 Other cerebrovascular disorders in diseases classified elsewhere

Code first:
  underlying disease

> **EXCLUDES 1** syphilitic cerebral aneurysm (A52.05)

H 4 I69 Sequelae of cerebrovascular disease

Note:
Category I69 is to be used to indicate conditions in I60-I67 as the cause of sequelae. The 'sequelae' include conditions specified as such or as residuals which may occur at any time after the onset of the causal condition

> **EXCLUDES 1** personal history of cerebral infarction without residual deficit (Z86.73)
>   personal history of prolonged reversible ischemic neurologic deficit (PRIND) (Z86.73)
>   personal history of reversible ischemic neurologcial deficit (RIND) (Z86.73)
>   sequelae of traumatic intracranial injury (S06.-)

GUIDELINES Section I.C.9.d.1)

Category I69 is used to indicate conditions classifiable to categories I60-I67 as the causes of sequela (neurologic deficits), themselves classified elsewhere. These "late effects" include neurologic deficits that persist after initial onset of conditions classifiable to categories I60-I67. The neurologic deficits caused by cerebrovascular disease may be present from the onset or may arise at any time after the onset or may arise at any time after the onset of the condition classifiable to categories I60-I67.

Codes from category I69, Sequelae of cerebrovascular disease, that specify hemiplegia, hemiparesis and monoplegia identify whether the dominant or nondominant side is affected. Should the affected side be documented, but not specified as dominant or nondominant, and the classification system does not indicate a default, code selection is as follows:
• For ambidextrous patients, the default should be dominant.
• If the left side is affected, the default is non-dominant.
• If the right side is affected, the default is dominant.

GUIDELINES Section I.C.9.d.3)

Codes from category I69 should not be assigned if the patient does not have neurologic deficits.

> **CODING TIPS ✓** I69 codes are used to indicate neurologic deficits as sequela of acute CVAs, themselves coded as I60-I63.

5 I69.0 Sequelae of nontraumatic subarachnoid hemorrhage

> **CODING TIPS ✓** Use subcategory I69.0, I69.1 or I69.2 for patients who have had a CVA involving a bleed when residual neurological deficits are apparent. If there are no neurological deficits, use Z86.73 instead. The neurologic deficits caused by cerebrovascular disease may be present from the onset or may arise at any time after the onset of the condition. Some I69.- codes are combination codes that include the residual deficit within the code, e.g., I69.-51. Others are combination codes that require additional information in the form of a secondary code to further specify the deficit, e.g., I69.-91.

> **CODING TIPS ✓** This code is used for residuals from a stroke caused by hemorrhage, not to be confused with a traumatic hemorrhage within or around the brain from an external injury.

IQ I69.00 Unspecified sequelae of nontraumatic subarachnoid hemorrhage

6 I69.01 Cognitive deficits following nontraumatic subarachnoid hemorrhage

SP SH SL I69.010 Attention and concentration deficit following nontraumatic subarachnoid hemorrhage

---

4 4th digit required   **5** 5th digit required   **6** 6th digit required   **7** 7th digit required   **7** 7th digit placeholder   **+** Additional code   **⊟** Laterality

SP SH SL I69.011 Memory deficit following nontraumatic subarachnoid hemorrhage

SP SH SL I69.012 Visuospatial deficit and spatial neglect following nontraumatic subarachnoid hemorrhage

SP SH SL I69.013 Psychomotor deficit following nontraumatic subarachnoid hemorrhage

SP SH SL I69.014 Frontal lobe and executive function deficit following nontraumatic subarachnoid hemorrhage

SP SH SL I69.015 Cognitive social or emotional deficit following nontraumatic subarachnoid hemorrhage

SP SH SL I69.018 Other symptoms and signs involving cognitive functions following nontraumatic subarachnoid hemorrhage

IQ I69.019 Unspecified symptoms and signs involving cognitive functions following nontraumatic subarachnoid hemorrhage

G I69.02 Speech and language deficits following nontraumatic subarachnoid hemorrhage

SP SH SL I69.020 Aphasia following nontraumatic subarachnoid hemorrhage

> **CODING TIPS** ✓ Aphasia is the lack of speech, whereas dysphasia is difficulty speaking.

SP SH SL I69.021 Dysphasia following nontraumatic subarachnoid hemorrhage

> **CODING TIPS** ✓ Aphasia is the lack of speech, whereas dysphasia is difficulty speaking.

> **CODING TIPS** ✓ Distinguish between dysphasia (difficulty speaking) and dysphagia (difficulty swallowing).

SP SH SL I69.022 Dysarthria following nontraumatic subarachnoid hemorrhage

> **CODING TIPS** ✓ Dysarthria is a weakness in the musculature of the mouth and throat causing difficulty with speech.

SP SH SL I69.023 Fluency disorder following nontraumatic subarachnoid hemorrhage

  Stuttering following nontraumatic subarachnoid hemorrhage

SP SH SL I69.028 Other speech and language deficits following nontraumatic subarachnoid hemorrhage

G I69.03 Monoplegia of upper limb following nontraumatic subarachnoid hemorrhage

SP SH SL I69.031 Monoplegia of upper limb following nontraumatic subarachnoid hemorrhage affecting right dominant side

SP SH SL I69.032 Monoplegia of upper limb following nontraumatic subarachnoid hemorrhage affecting left dominant side

SP SH SL I69.033 Monoplegia of upper limb following nontraumatic subarachnoid hemorrhage affecting right non-dominant side

SP SH SL I69.034 Monoplegia of upper limb following nontraumatic subarachnoid hemorrhage affecting left non-dominant side

IQ I69.039 Monoplegia of upper limb following nontraumatic subarachnoid hemorrhage affecting unspecified side

> **ALERT** This code includes unspecified side which may cause the claim to be rejected.

G I69.04 Monoplegia of lower limb following nontraumatic subarachnoid hemorrhage

SP SH SL I69.041 Monoplegia of lower limb following nontraumatic subarachnoid hemorrhage affecting right dominant side

SP SH SL I69.042 Monoplegia of lower limb following nontraumatic subarachnoid hemorrhage affecting left dominant side

SP SH SL I69.043 Monoplegia of lower limb following nontraumatic subarachnoid hemorrhage affecting right non-dominant side

SP SH SL I69.044 Monoplegia of lower limb following nontraumatic subarachnoid hemorrhage affecting left non-dominant side

IQ I69.049 Monoplegia of lower limb following nontraumatic subarachnoid hemorrhage affecting unspecified side

> **ALERT** This code includes unspecified side which may cause the claim to be rejected.

G I69.05 Hemiplegia and hemiparesis following nontraumatic subarachnoid hemorrhage

> **CODING TIPS** ✓ Hemiparesis is weakness of one side of the body due to cerebrovascular disease. This is often documented as "left-sided weakness" or "right-sided weakness." Hemiplegia and hemiparesis are represented by the same code and should be coded when one-sided weakness is described as a result of a stroke. When the side affected is documented, but not dominant or nondominant, the coder may choose dominant if the right side is affected and non-dominant if the left side is affected. Best practice is to obtain information from the clinician regarding dominant side.

SP SH SL I69.051 Hemiplegia and hemiparesis following nontraumatic subarachnoid hemorrhage affecting right dominant side

SP SH SL I69.052 Hemiplegia and hemiparesis following nontraumatic subarachnoid hemorrhage affecting left dominant side

★ New ▲ Revised **Px** Primary **SP** PDGM Px **SL** Low CoM **SH** High CoM **IQ** Quest. Encounter **H** Hospice non-cancer Dx Unspecified **M** *Manifestation*

DecisionHealth's FY 2020 Complete Home Health ICD-10-CM Diagnosis Coding Manual

983

Chapter 9

I00-I99

≡ SP SH SL I69.053 **Hemiplegia and hemiparesis following nontraumatic subarachnoid hemorrhage affecting right non-dominant side**

≡ SP SH SL I69.054 **Hemiplegia and hemiparesis following nontraumatic subarachnoid hemorrhage affecting left non-dominant side**

≡ IQ I69.059 **Hemiplegia and hemiparesis following nontraumatic subarachnoid hemorrhage affecting unspecified side**

> **ALERT** This code includes unspecified side which may cause the claim to be rejected.

+ 6 I69.06 **Other paralytic syndrome following nontraumatic subarachnoid hemorrhage**
Use additional code to identify type of paralytic syndrome, such as:
locked-in state (G83.5)
quadriplegia (G82.5-)

> **EXCLUDES 1** hemiplegia/hemiparesis following nontraumatic subarachnoid hemorrhage (I69.05-)
> monoplegia of lower limb following nontraumatic subarachnoid hemorrhage (I69.04-)
> monoplegia of upper limb following nontraumatic subarachnoid hemorrhage (I69.03-)

≡ SP SH SL + I69.061 **Other paralytic syndrome following nontraumatic subarachnoid hemorrhage affecting right dominant side**

≡ SP SH SL + I69.062 **Other paralytic syndrome following nontraumatic subarachnoid hemorrhage affecting left dominant side**

≡ SP SH SL + I69.063 **Other paralytic syndrome following nontraumatic subarachnoid hemorrhage affecting right non-dominant side**

≡ SP SH SL + I69.064 **Other paralytic syndrome following nontraumatic subarachnoid hemorrhage affecting left non-dominant side**

≡ SP SH SL + I69.065 **Other paralytic syndrome following nontraumatic subarachnoid hemorrhage, bilateral**

≡ IQ + I69.069 **Other paralytic syndrome following nontraumatic subarachnoid hemorrhage affecting unspecified side**

6 I69.09 **Other sequelae of nontraumatic subarachnoid hemorrhage**

SP SH SL I69.090 **Apraxia following nontraumatic subarachnoid hemorrhage**

SP SH SL + I69.091 **Dysphagia following nontraumatic subarachnoid hemorrhage**

Use additional code to identify the type of dysphagia, if known (R13.1-)

> **CODING TIPS ✓** Use an additional code from R13.1 to explain the phase of swallowing affected. Avoid coding unspecified dysphagia. Query the physician regarding phase of dysphagia.

> **CODING TIPS ✓** Distinguish between dysphasia (difficulty speaking) and dysphagia (difficulty swallowing).

SP I69.092 **Facial weakness following nontraumatic subarachnoid hemorrhage**
Facial droop following nontraumatic subarachnoid hemorrhage

SP SH SL I69.093 **Ataxia following nontraumatic subarachnoid hemorrhage**

SP SH SL + I69.098 **Other sequelae following nontraumatic subarachnoid hemorrhage**
Alterations of sensation following nontraumatic subarachnoid hemorrhage
Disturbance of vision following nontraumatic subarachnoid hemorrhage
Use additional code to identify the sequelae

> **CODING TIPS ✓** When generalized muscle weakness, seizures, contractures or other residuals not included in the other sequela codes result from a stroke, assign code I69.398, followed by the code for the specific residual, e.g., M62.81 (muscle weakness), or F48.2 (pseudobulbar affect - also known as involuntary emotional expression disorder).

5 I69.1 **Sequelae of nontraumatic intracerebral hemorrhage**

> **CODING TIPS ✓** Use subcategory I69.0, I69.1 or I69.2 for patients who have had a CVA involving a bleed when residual neurological deficits are apparent. If there are no neurological deficits, use Z86.73 instead. The neurologic deficits caused by cerebrovascular disease may be present from the onset or may arise at any time after the onset of the condition. Some I69.- codes are combination codes that include the residual deficit within the code, e.g., I69.-51. Others are combination codes that require additional information in the form of a secondary code to further specify the deficit, e.g., I69.-91.

> **CODING TIPS ✓** This code is used for residuals from a stroke caused by hemorrhage, not to be confused with a traumatic hemorrhage within or around the brain from an external injury.

SP I69.10 **Unspecified sequelae of nontraumatic intracerebral hemorrhage**

4th digit required   5th digit required   6th digit required   7th digit required   7th digit placeholder   + Additional code   ≡ Laterality

984   *DecisionHealth's* FY 2020 Complete Home Health ICD-10-CM Diagnosis Coding Manual

⑥ I69.11 Cognitive deficits following nontraumatic intracerebral hemorrhage

SP SH SL I69.110 Attention and concentration deficit following nontraumatic intracerebral hemorrhage

SP SH SL I69.111 Memory deficit following nontraumatic intracerebral hemorrhage

SP SH SL I69.112 Visuospatial deficit and spatial neglect following nontraumatic intracerebral hemorrhage

SP SH SL I69.113 Psychomotor deficit following nontraumatic intracerebral hemorrhage

SP SH SL I69.114 Frontal lobe and executive function deficit following nontraumatic intracerebral hemorrhage

SP SH SL I69.115 Cognitive social or emotional deficit following nontraumatic intracerebral hemorrhage

SP SH SL I69.118 Other symptoms and signs involving cognitive functions following nontraumatic intracerebral hemorrhage

IQ I69.119 Unspecified symptoms and signs involving cognitive functions following nontraumatic intracerebral hemorrhage

⑥ I69.12 Speech and language deficits following nontraumatic intracerebral hemorrhage

SP SH SL I69.120 Aphasia following nontraumatic intracerebral hemorrhage

> **CODING TIPS ✓** Aphasia is the lack of speech, whereas dysphasia is difficulty speaking.

SP SH SL I69.121 Dysphasia following nontraumatic intracerebral hemorrhage

> **CODING TIPS ✓** Aphasia is the lack of speech, whereas dysphasia is difficulty speaking.

> **CODING TIPS ✓** Distinguish between dysphasia (difficulty speaking) and dysphagia (difficulty swallowing).

SP SH SL I69.122 Dysarthria following nontraumatic intracerebral hemorrhage

> **CODING TIPS ✓** Dysarthria is a weakness in the musculature of the mouth and throat causing difficulty with speech.

SP SH SL I69.123 Fluency disorder following nontraumatic intracerebral hemorrhage
Stuttering following nontraumatic intracerebral hemorrhage

SP SH SL I69.128 Other speech and language deficits following nontraumatic intracerebral hemorrhage

⑥ I69.13 Monoplegia of upper limb following nontraumatic intracerebral hemorrhage

⊟ SP SH SL I69.131 Monoplegia of upper limb following nontraumatic intracerebral hemorrhage affecting right dominant side

⊟ SP SH SL I69.132 Monoplegia of upper limb following nontraumatic intracerebral hemorrhage affecting left dominant side

⊟ SP SH SL I69.133 Monoplegia of upper limb following nontraumatic intracerebral hemorrhage affecting right non-dominant side

⊟ SP SH SL I69.134 Monoplegia of upper limb following nontraumatic intracerebral hemorrhage affecting left non-dominant side

⊟ IQ I69.139 Monoplegia of upper limb following nontraumatic intracerebral hemorrhage affecting unspecified side

> **ALERT** This code includes unspecified side which may cause the claim to be rejected.

⑥ I69.14 Monoplegia of lower limb following nontraumatic intracerebral hemorrhage

⊟ SP SH SL I69.141 Monoplegia of lower limb following nontraumatic intracerebral hemorrhage affecting right dominant side

⊟ SP SH SL I69.142 Monoplegia of lower limb following nontraumatic intracerebral hemorrhage affecting left dominant side

⊟ SP SH SL I69.143 Monoplegia of lower limb following nontraumatic intracerebral hemorrhage affecting right non-dominant side

⊟ SP SH SL I69.144 Monoplegia of lower limb following nontraumatic intracerebral hemorrhage affecting left non-dominant side

⊟ IQ I69.149 Monoplegia of lower limb following nontraumatic intracerebral hemorrhage affecting unspecified side

> **ALERT** This code includes unspecified side which may cause the claim to be rejected.

⑥ I69.15 Hemiplegia and hemiparesis following nontraumatic intracerebral hemorrhage

> **CODING TIPS ✓** Hemiparesis is weakness of one side of the body due to cerebrovascular disease. This is often documented as "left-sided weakness" or "right-sided weakness." Hemiplegia and hemiparesis are represented by the same code and should be coded when one-sided weakness is described as a result of a stroke. When the side affected is documented, but not dominant or nondominant, the coder may choose dominant if the right side is affected and non-dominant if the left side is affected. Best practice is to obtain information from the clinician regarding dominant side.

★ New ▲ Revised Px Primary **SP** PDGM Px **SL** Low CoM **SH** High CoM **IQ** Quest. Encounter **H** Hospice non-cancer Dx Unspecified **M** *Manifestation*

DecisionHealth's FY 2020 Complete Home Health ICD-10-CM Diagnosis Coding Manual

985

Chapter 9

I00-I99

⊟ SP SH SL **I69.151** **Hemiplegia and hemiparesis following nontraumatic intracerebral hemorrhage affecting right dominant side**

⊟ SP SH SL **I69.152** **Hemiplegia and hemiparesis following nontraumatic intracerebral hemorrhage affecting left dominant side**

⊟ SP SH SL **I69.153** **Hemiplegia and hemiparesis following nontraumatic intracerebral hemorrhage affecting right non-dominant side**

⊟ SP SH SL **I69.154** **Hemiplegia and hemiparesis following nontraumatic intracerebral hemorrhage affecting left non-dominant side**

⊟ IQ **I69.159** **Hemiplegia and hemiparesis following nontraumatic intracerebral hemorrhage affecting unspecified side**

ALERT This code includes unspecified side which may cause the claim to be rejected.

➕ 6 **I69.16** **Other paralytic syndrome following nontraumatic intracerebral hemorrhage**
Use additional code to identify type of paralytic syndrome, such as:
locked-in state (G83.5)
quadriplegia (G82.5-)

EXCLUDES 1 hemiplegia/hemiparesis following nontraumatic intracerebral hemorrhage (I69.15-)
monoplegia of lower limb following nontraumatic intracerebral hemorrhage (I69.14-)
monoplegia of upper limb following nontraumatic intracerebral hemorrhage (I69.13-)

⊟ SP SH SL ➕ **I69.161** **Other paralytic syndrome following nontraumatic intracerebral hemorrhage affecting right dominant side**

⊟ SP SH SL ➕ **I69.162** **Other paralytic syndrome following nontraumatic intracerebral hemorrhage affecting left dominant side**

⊟ SP SH SL ➕ **I69.163** **Other paralytic syndrome following nontraumatic intracerebral hemorrhage affecting right non-dominant side**

⊟ SP SH SL ➕ **I69.164** **Other paralytic syndrome following nontraumatic intracerebral hemorrhage affecting left non-dominant side**

⊟ SP SH SL ➕ **I69.165** **Other paralytic syndrome following nontraumatic intracerebral hemorrhage, bilateral**

⊟ IQ ➕ **I69.169** **Other paralytic syndrome following nontraumatic intracerebral hemorrhage affecting unspecified side**

6 **I69.19** **Other sequelae of nontraumatic intracerebral hemorrhage**

SP SH SL **I69.190** **Apraxia following nontraumatic intracerebral hemorrhage**

SP SH SL ➕ **I69.191** **Dysphagia following nontraumatic intracerebral hemorrhage**
Use additional code to identify the type of dysphagia, if known (R13.1-)

CODING TIPS ✓ Use an additional code from R13.1 to explain the phase of swallowing affected. Avoid coding unspecified dysphagia. Query the physician regarding phase of dysphagia.

CODING TIPS ✓ Distinguish between dysphasia (difficulty speaking) and dysphagia (difficulty swallowing).

SP **I69.192** **Facial weakness following nontraumatic intracerebral hemorrhage**
Facial droop following nontraumatic intracerebral hemorrhage

SP SH SL **I69.193** **Ataxia following nontraumatic intracerebral hemorrhage**

SP SH SL ➕ **I69.198** **Other sequelae of nontraumatic intracerebral hemorrhage**
Alteration of sensations following nontraumatic intracerebral hemorrhage
Disturbance of vision following nontraumatic intracerebral hemorrhage
Use additional code to identify the sequelae

CODING TIPS ✓ When generalized muscle weakness, seizures, contractures or other residuals not included in the other sequela codes result from a stroke, assign code I69.398, followed by the code for the specific residual, e.g., M62.81 (muscle weakness), or F48.2 (pseudobulbar affect - also known as involuntary emotional expression disorder).

5 **I69.2** **Sequelae of other nontraumatic intracranial hemorrhage**

CODING TIPS ✓ Use subcategory I69.0, I69.1 or I69.2 for patients who have had a CVA involving a bleed when residual neurological deficits are apparent. If there are no neurological deficits, use Z86.73 instead. The neurologic deficits caused by cerebrovascular disease may be present from the onset or may arise at any time after the onset of the condition. Some I69.- codes are combination codes that include the residual deficit within the code, e.g., I69.-51. Others are combination codes that require additional information in the form of a secondary code to further specify the deficit, e.g., I69.-91.

---

4 4th digit required   5 5th digit required   6 6th digit required   7 7th digit required   7 7th digit placeholder   ➕ Additional code   ⊟ Laterality

CODING TIPS ✓ This code is used for residuals from a stroke caused by hemorrhage, not to be confused with a traumatic hemorrhage within or around the brain from an external injury.

IQ I69.20 Unspecified sequelae of other nontraumatic intracranial hemorrhage

6 I69.21 Cognitive deficits following other nontraumatic intracranial hemorrhage

SP SH SL I69.210 Attention and concentration deficit following other nontraumatic intracranial hemorrhage

SP SH SL I69.211 Memory deficit following other nontraumatic intracranial hemorrhage

SP SH SL I69.212 Visuospatial deficit and spatial neglect following other nontraumatic intracranial hemorrhage

SP SH SL I69.213 Psychomotor deficit following other nontraumatic intracranial hemorrhage

SP SH SL I69.214 Frontal lobe and executive function deficit following other nontraumatic intracranial hemorrhage

SP SH SL I69.215 Cognitive social or emotional deficit following other nontraumatic intracranial hemorrhage

SP SH SL I69.218 Other symptoms and signs involving cognitive functions following other nontraumatic intracranial hemorrhage

IQ I69.219 Unspecified symptoms and signs involving cognitive functions following other nontraumatic intracranial hemorrhage

6 I69.22 Speech and language deficits following other nontraumatic intracranial hemorrhage

SP SH SL I69.220 Aphasia following other nontraumatic intracranial hemorrhage

CODING TIPS ✓ Aphasia is the lack of speech, whereas dysphasia is difficulty speaking.

SP SH SL I69.221 Dysphasia following other nontraumatic intracranial hemorrhage

CODING TIPS ✓ Aphasia is the lack of speech, whereas dysphasia is difficulty speaking.

CODING TIPS ✓ Distinguish between dysphasia (difficulty speaking) and dysphagia (difficulty swallowing).

SP SH SL I69.222 Dysarthria following other nontraumatic intracranial hemorrhage

CODING TIPS ✓ Dysarthria is a weakness in the musculature of the mouth and throat causing difficulty with speech.

SP SH SL I69.223 Fluency disorder following other nontraumatic intracranial hemorrhage
Stuttering following other nontraumatic intracranial hemorrhage

SP SH SL I69.228 Other speech and language deficits following other nontraumatic intracranial hemorrhage

6 I69.23 Monoplegia of upper limb following other nontraumatic intracranial hemorrhage

⊟ SP SH SL I69.231 Monoplegia of upper limb following other nontraumatic intracranial hemorrhage affecting right dominant side

⊟ SP SH SL I69.232 Monoplegia of upper limb following other nontraumatic intracranial hemorrhage affecting left dominant side

⊟ SP SH SL I69.233 Monoplegia of upper limb following other nontraumatic intracranial hemorrhage affecting right non-dominant side

⊟ SP SH SL I69.234 Monoplegia of upper limb following other nontraumatic intracranial hemorrhage affecting left non-dominant side

⊟ IQ I69.239 Monoplegia of upper limb following other nontraumatic intracranial hemorrhage affecting unspecified side

ALERT This code includes unspecified side which may cause the claim to be rejected.

6 I69.24 Monoplegia of lower limb following other nontraumatic intracranial hemorrhage

⊟ SP SH SL I69.241 Monoplegia of lower limb following other nontraumatic intracranial hemorrhage affecting right dominant side

⊟ SP SH SL I69.242 Monoplegia of lower limb following other nontraumatic intracranial hemorrhage affecting left dominant side

⊟ SP SH SL I69.243 Monoplegia of lower limb following other nontraumatic intracranial hemorrhage affecting right non-dominant side

⊟ SP SH SL I69.244 Monoplegia of lower limb following other nontraumatic intracranial hemorrhage affecting left non-dominant side

⊟ IQ I69.249 Monoplegia of lower limb following other nontraumatic intracranial hemorrhage affecting unspecified side

ALERT This code includes unspecified side which may cause the claim to be rejected.

6 I69.25 Hemiplegia and hemiparesis following other nontraumatic intracranial hemorrhage

★ New ▲ Revised Px Primary SP PDGM Px SL Low CoM SH High CoM IQ Quest. Encounter H Hospice non-cancer Dx Unspecified M Manifestation

DecisionHealth's FY 2020 Complete Home Health ICD-10-CM Diagnosis Coding Manual

987

Chapter 9

I00-I99

CODING TIPS ✓ Hemiparesis is weakness of one side of the body due to cerebrovascular disease. This is often documented as "left-sided weakness" or "right-sided weakness." Hemiplegia and hemiparesis are represented by the same code and should be coded when one-sided weakness is described as a result of a stroke. When the side affected is documented, but not dominant or nondominant, the coder may choose dominant if the right side is affected and non-dominant if the left side is affected. Best practice is to obtain information from the clinician regarding dominant side.

☐ SP SH SL **I69.251** **Hemiplegia and hemiparesis following other nontraumatic intracranial hemorrhage affecting right dominant side**

☐ SP SH SL **I69.252** **Hemiplegia and hemiparesis following other nontraumatic intracranial hemorrhage affecting left dominant side**

☐ SP SH SL **I69.253** **Hemiplegia and hemiparesis following other nontraumatic intracranial hemorrhage affecting right non-dominant side**

☐ SP SH SL **I69.254** **Hemiplegia and hemiparesis following other nontraumatic intracranial hemorrhage affecting left non-dominant side**

☐ IQ **I69.259** **Hemiplegia and hemiparesis following other nontraumatic intracranial hemorrhage affecting unspecified side**

ALERT This code includes unspecified side which may cause the claim to be rejected.

✚ 6 **I69.26** **Other paralytic syndrome following other nontraumatic intracranial hemorrhage**
Use additional code to identify type of paralytic syndrome, such as:
locked-in state (G83.5)
quadriplegia (G82.5-)
EXCLUDES 1 hemiplegia/hemiparesis following other nontraumatic intracranial hemorrhage (I69.25-)
monoplegia of lower limb following other nontraumatic intracranial hemorrhage (I69.24-)
monoplegia of upper limb following other nontraumatic intracranial hemorrhage (I69.23-)

☐ SP SH SL ✚ **I69.261** **Other paralytic syndrome following other nontraumatic intracranial hemorrhage affecting right dominant side**

☐ SP SH SL ✚ **I69.262** **Other paralytic syndrome following other nontraumatic intracranial hemorrhage affecting left dominant side**

☐ SP SH SL ✚ **I69.263** **Other paralytic syndrome following other nontraumatic intracranial hemorrhage affecting right non-dominant side**

☐ SP SH SL ✚ **I69.264** **Other paralytic syndrome following other nontraumatic intracranial hemorrhage affecting left non-dominant side**

☐ SP SH SL ✚ **I69.265** **Other paralytic syndrome following other nontraumatic intracranial hemorrhage, bilateral**

☐ IQ ✚ **I69.269** **Other paralytic syndrome following other nontraumatic intracranial hemorrhage affecting unspecified side**

6 **I69.29** **Other sequelae of other nontraumatic intracranial hemorrhage**

SP SH SL **I69.290** **Apraxia following other nontraumatic intracranial hemorrhage**

SP SH SL ✚ **I69.291** **Dysphagia following other nontraumatic intracranial hemorrhage**
Use additional code to identify the type of dysphagia, if known (R13.1-)
CODING TIPS ✓ Use an additional code from R13.1 to explain the phase of swallowing affected. Avoid coding unspecified dysphagia. Query the physician regarding phase of dysphagia.
CODING TIPS ✓ Distinguish between dysphasia (difficulty speaking) and dysphagia (difficulty swallowing).

SP **I69.292** **Facial weakness following other nontraumatic intracranial hemorrhage**
Facial droop following other nontraumatic intracranial hemorrhage

SP SH SL **I69.293** **Ataxia following other nontraumatic intracranial hemorrhage**

SP SH SL ✚ **I69.298** **Other sequelae of other nontraumatic intracranial hemorrhage**
Alteration of sensation following other nontraumatic intracranial hemorrhage
Disturbance of vision following other nontraumatic intracranial hemorrhage
Use additional code to identify the sequelae

---

4 4th digit required   5 5th digit required   6 6th digit required   7 7th digit required   7 7th digit placeholder   ✚ Additional code   ☐ Laterality

CODING TIPS ✓ When generalized muscle weakness, seizures, contractures or other residuals not included in the other sequela codes result from a stroke, assign code I69.398, followed by the code for the specific residual, e.g., M62.81 (muscle weakness), or F48.2 (pseudobulbar affect - also known as involuntary emotional expression disorder).

5 I69.3 **Sequelae of cerebral infarction**
Sequelae of stroke NOS

CODING TIPS ✓ Use subcategory I69.3 for all stroke patients when residual neurological deficits are apparent. If there are no neurological deficits, use Z86.73 instead. The neurologic deficits caused by cerebrovascular disease may be present from the onset or may arise at any time after the onset of the condition. Some I69.3 codes are combination codes that include the residual deficit within the code, e.g., I69.351. Others are combination codes that require additional information in the form of a secondary code to further specify the deficit, e.g., I69.391.

IQ I69.30 **Unspecified sequelae of cerebral infarction**

6 I69.31 **Cognitive deficits following cerebral infarction**

SP SH SL I69.310 **Attention and concentration deficit following cerebral infarction**

SP SH SL I69.311 **Memory deficit following cerebral infarction**

SP SH SL I69.312 **Visuospatial deficit and spatial neglect following cerebral infarction**

SP SH SL I69.313 **Psychomotor deficit following cerebral infarction**

SP SH SL I69.314 **Frontal lobe and executive function deficit following cerebral infarction**

SP SH SL I69.315 **Cognitive social or emotional deficit following cerebral infarction**

SP SH SL I69.318 **Other symptoms and signs involving cognitive functions following cerebral infarction**

IQ I69.319 **Unspecified symptoms and signs involving cognitive functions following cerebral infarction**

6 I69.32 **Speech and language deficits following cerebral infarction**

SP SH SL I69.320 **Aphasia following cerebral infarction**
CODING TIPS ✓ Aphasia is the lack of speech, whereas dysphasia is difficulty speaking.

SP SH SL I69.321 **Dysphasia following cerebral infarction**
CODING TIPS ✓ Aphasia is the lack of speech, whereas dysphasia is difficulty speaking.

CODING TIPS ✓ Distinguish between dysphasia (difficulty speaking) and dysphagia (difficulty swallowing).

SP SH SL I69.322 **Dysarthria following cerebral infarction**
EXCLUDES 2 transient ischemic attack (TIA) (G45.9)
CODING TIPS ✓ Dysarthria is a weakness in the musculature of the mouth and throat causing difficulty with speech.

SP SH SL I69.323 **Fluency disorder following cerebral infarction**
Stuttering following cerebral infarction

SP SH SL I69.328 **Other speech and language deficits following cerebral infarction**

6 I69.33 **Monoplegia of upper limb following cerebral infarction**
CODING TIPS ✓ Unlike the I69.35 codes where hemiparesis is included, monoparesis is not included in the I69.33 and I69.34 codes. When monoparesis is documented, use I69.398. Weakness of a limb *without mention of muscle weakness* is assigned code R29.898, Other symptoms and signs involving the musculoskeletal system. If muscle weakness is documented, assign M62.81 as an additional code.

SP SH SL I69.331 **Monoplegia of upper limb following cerebral infarction affecting right dominant side**

SP SH SL I69.332 **Monoplegia of upper limb following cerebral infarction affecting left dominant side**

SP SH SL I69.333 **Monoplegia of upper limb following cerebral infarction affecting right non-dominant side**

SP SH SL I69.334 **Monoplegia of upper limb following cerebral infarction affecting left non-dominant side**

IQ I69.339 **Monoplegia of upper limb following cerebral infarction affecting unspecified side**
ALERT This code includes unspecified side which may cause the claim to be rejected.

6 I69.34 **Monoplegia of lower limb following cerebral infarction**
CODING TIPS ✓ Unlike the I69.35 codes where hemiparesis is included, monoparesis is not included in the I69.33 and I69.34 codes. When monoparesis is documented, use I69.398. Weakness of a limb *without mention of muscle weakness* is assigned code R29.898, Other symptoms and signs involving the musculoskeletal system. If muscle weakness is documented, assign M62.81 as an additional code.

★ New ▲ Revised Px Primary SP PDGM Px SL Low CoM SH High CoM IQ Quest. Encounter H Hospice non-cancer Dx Unspecified M *Manifestation*

DecisionHealth's FY 2020 Complete Home Health ICD-10-CM Diagnosis Coding Manual

989

□ SP SH SL I69.341   **Monoplegia of lower limb following cerebral infarction affecting right dominant side**

□ SP SH SL I69.342   **Monoplegia of lower limb following cerebral infarction affecting left dominant side**

□ SP SH SL I69.343   **Monoplegia of lower limb following cerebral infarction affecting right non-dominant side**

□ SP SH SL I69.344   **Monoplegia of lower limb following cerebral infarction affecting left non-dominant side**

□ IQ I69.349   **Monoplegia of lower limb following cerebral infarction affecting unspecified side**

> **ALERT**   This code includes unspecified side which may cause the claim to be rejected.

6 I69.35   **Hemiplegia and hemiparesis following cerebral infarction**

> **CODING TIPS ✓**   Hemiparesis is weakness of one side of the body due to cerebrovascular disease. This is often documented as "left-sided weakness" or "right-sided weakness." Hemiplegia and hemiparesis are represented by the same code and should be coded when one-sided weakness is described as a result of a stroke. When the side affected is documented, but not dominant or nondominant, the coder may choose dominant if the right side is affected and non-dominant if the left side is affected. Best practice is to obtain information from the clinician regarding dominant side.

□ SP SH SL I69.351   **Hemiplegia and hemiparesis following cerebral infarction affecting right dominant side**

> **EXCLUDES 2**   transient ischemic attack (TIA) (G45.9)

□ SP SH SL I69.352   **Hemiplegia and hemiparesis following cerebral infarction affecting left dominant side**

□ SP SH SL I69.353   **Hemiplegia and hemiparesis following cerebral infarction affecting right non-dominant side**

□ SP SH SL I69.354   **Hemiplegia and hemiparesis following cerebral infarction affecting left non-dominant side**

□ IQ I69.359   **Hemiplegia and hemiparesis following cerebral infarction affecting unspecified side**

> **ALERT**   This code includes unspecified side which may cause the claim to be rejected.

+ 6 I69.36   **Other paralytic syndrome following cerebral infarction**
Use additional code to identify type of paralytic syndrome, such as:
locked-in state (G83.5)
quadriplegia (G82.5-)

> **EXCLUDES 1**   hemiplegia/hemiparesis following cerebral infarction (I69.35-)

monoplegia of lower limb following cerebral infarction (I69.34-)
monoplegia of upper limb following cerebral infarction (I69.33-)

□ SP SH SL + I69.361   **Other paralytic syndrome following cerebral infarction affecting right dominant side**

□ SP SH SL + I69.362   **Other paralytic syndrome following cerebral infarction affecting left dominant side**

□ SP SH SL + I69.363   **Other paralytic syndrome following cerebral infarction affecting right non-dominant side**

□ SP SH SL + I69.364   **Other paralytic syndrome following cerebral infarction affecting left non-dominant side**

□ SP SH SL + I69.365   **Other paralytic syndrome following cerebral infarction, bilateral**

□ IQ + I69.369   **Other paralytic syndrome following cerebral infarction affecting unspecified side**

6 I69.39   **Other sequelae of cerebral infarction**

SP SH SL I69.390   **Apraxia following cerebral infarction**

SP SH SL + I69.391   **Dysphagia following cerebral infarction**
Use additional code to identify the type of dysphagia, if known (R13.1-)

> **CODING TIPS ✓**   Use an additional code from R13.1 to explain the phase of swallowing affected. Avoid coding unspecified dysphagia. Query the physician regarding phase of dysphagia.

> **CODING TIPS ✓**   Distinguish between dysphasia (difficulty speaking) and dysphagia (difficulty swallowing).

SP I69.392   **Facial weakness following cerebral infarction**
Facial droop following cerebral infarction

SP SH SL I69.393   **Ataxia following cerebral infarction**

SP SH SL + I69.398   **Other sequelae of cerebral infarction**
Alteration of sensation following cerebral infarction
Disturbance of vision following cerebral infarction
Use additional code to identify the sequelae

> **CODING TIPS ✓**   When generalized muscle weakness, seizures, contractures or other residuals not included in the other sequela codes result from a stroke, assign code I69.398, followed by the code for the specific residual, e.g., M62.81 (muscle weakness), or F48.2 (pseudobulbar affect - also known as involuntary emotional expression disorder).

---

4 4th digit required   **5** 5th digit required   **6** 6th digit required   **7** 7th digit required   **7** 7th digit placeholder   **+** Additional code   **□** Laterality

Chapter 9

I00-I99

5 I69.8 Sequelae of other cerebrovascular diseases

> **EXCLUDES 1** sequelae of traumatic intracranial injury (S06.-)

IQ I69.80 Unspecified sequelae of other cerebrovascular disease

6 I69.81 Cognitive deficits following other cerebrovascular disease

SP SH SL I69.810 Attention and concentration deficit following other cerebrovascular disease

SP SH SL I69.811 Memory deficit following other cerebrovascular disease

SP SH SL I69.812 Visuospatial deficit and spatial neglect following other cerebrovascular disease

SP SH SL I69.813 Psychomotor deficit following other cerebrovascular disease

SP SH SL I69.814 Frontal lobe and executive function deficit following other cerebrovascular disease

SP SH SL I69.815 Cognitive social or emotional deficit following other cerebrovascular disease

SP SH SL I69.818 Other symptoms and signs involving cognitive functions following other cerebrovascular disease

IQ I69.819 Unspecified symptoms and signs involving cognitive functions following other cerebrovascular disease

6 I69.82 Speech and language deficits following other cerebrovascular disease

SP SH SL I69.820 Aphasia following other cerebrovascular disease

SP SH SL I69.821 Dysphasia following other cerebrovascular disease

SP SH SL I69.822 Dysarthria following other cerebrovascular disease

SP SH SL I69.823 Fluency disorder following other cerebrovascular disease
Stuttering following other cerebrovascular disease

SP SH SL I69.828 Other speech and language deficits following other cerebrovascular disease

6 I69.83 Monoplegia of upper limb following other cerebrovascular disease

SP SH SL I69.831 Monoplegia of upper limb following other cerebrovascular disease affecting right dominant side

SP SH SL I69.832 Monoplegia of upper limb following other cerebrovascular disease affecting left dominant side

SP SH SL I69.833 Monoplegia of upper limb following other cerebrovascular disease affecting right non-dominant side

SP SH SL I69.834 Monoplegia of upper limb following other cerebrovascular disease affecting left non-dominant side

IQ I69.839 Monoplegia of upper limb following other cerebrovascular disease affecting unspecified side

> **ALERT** This code includes unspecified side which may cause the claim to be rejected.

6 I69.84 Monoplegia of lower limb following other cerebrovascular disease

SP SH SL I69.841 Monoplegia of lower limb following other cerebrovascular disease affecting right dominant side

SP SH SL I69.842 Monoplegia of lower limb following other cerebrovascular disease affecting left dominant side

SP SH SL I69.843 Monoplegia of lower limb following other cerebrovascular disease affecting right non-dominant side

SP SH SL I69.844 Monoplegia of lower limb following other cerebrovascular disease affecting left non-dominant side

IQ I69.849 Monoplegia of lower limb following other cerebrovascular disease affecting unspecified side

> **ALERT** This code includes unspecified side which may cause the claim to be rejected.

6 I69.85 Hemiplegia and hemiparesis following other cerebrovascular disease

SP SH SL I69.851 Hemiplegia and hemiparesis following other cerebrovascular disease affecting right dominant side

SP SH SL I69.852 Hemiplegia and hemiparesis following other cerebrovascular disease affecting left dominant side

SP SH SL I69.853 Hemiplegia and hemiparesis following other cerebrovascular disease affecting right non-dominant side

SP SH SL I69.854 Hemiplegia and hemiparesis following other cerebrovascular disease affecting left non-dominant side

IQ I69.859 Hemiplegia and hemiparesis following other cerebrovascular disease affecting unspecified side

> **ALERT** This code includes unspecified side which may cause the claim to be rejected.

+ 6 I69.86 Other paralytic syndrome following other cerebrovascular disease
Use additional code to identify type of paralytic syndrome, such as:
locked-in state (G83.5)
quadriplegia (G82.5-)

> **EXCLUDES 1** hemiplegia/hemiparesis following other cerebrovascular disease (I69.85-)

★ New ▲ Revised Px Primary SP PDGM Px SL Low CoM SH High CoM IQ Quest. Encounter H Hospice non-cancer Dx Unspecified M Manifestation

DecisionHealth's FY 2020 Complete Home Health ICD-10-CM Diagnosis Coding Manual

991

Chapter 9

I00-I99

monoplegia of lower limb following other cerebrovascular disease (I69.84-)
monoplegia of upper limb following other cerebrovascular disease (I69.83-)

☐ **SP SH SL** + **I69.861** **Other paralytic syndrome following other cerebrovascular disease affecting right dominant side**

☐ **SP SH SL** + **I69.862** **Other paralytic syndrome following other cerebrovascular disease affecting left dominant side**

☐ **SP SH SL** + **I69.863** **Other paralytic syndrome following other cerebrovascular disease affecting right non-dominant side**

☐ **SP SH SL** + **I69.864** **Other paralytic syndrome following other cerebrovascular disease affecting left non-dominant side**

☐ **SP SH SL** + **I69.865** **Other paralytic syndrome following other cerebrovascular disease, bilateral**

☐ **IQ** + **I69.869** **Other paralytic syndrome following other cerebrovascular disease affecting unspecified side**

6 I69.89 **Other sequelae of other cerebrovascular disease**

SP SH SL I69.890 **Apraxia following other cerebrovascular disease**

SP SH SL + **I69.891** **Dysphagia following other cerebrovascular disease**
Use additional code to identify the type of dysphagia, if known (R13.1-)

SP I69.892 **Facial weakness following other cerebrovascular disease**
Facial droop following other cerebrovascular disease

SP SH SL I69.893 **Ataxia following other cerebrovascular disease**

SP SH SL + **I69.898** **Other sequelae of other cerebrovascular disease**
Alteration of sensation following other cerebrovascular disease
Disturbance of vision following other cerebrovascular disease
Use additional code to identify the sequelae

5 I69.9 **Sequelae of unspecified cerebrovascular diseases**

EXCLUDES 1 sequelae of stroke (I69.3) sequelae of traumatic intracranial injury (S06.-)

CODING TIPS ✓ Do not use this unspecified code for residuals or sequelae of strokes or any other known cerebrovascular diseases. See I69.3-.

IQ I69.90 **Unspecified sequelae of unspecified cerebrovascular disease**

6 I69.91 **Cognitive deficits following unspecified cerebrovascular disease**

SP SH SL I69.910 **Attention and concentration deficit following unspecified cerebrovascular disease**

SP SH SL I69.911 **Memory deficit following unspecified cerebrovascular disease**

SP SH SL I69.912 **Visuospatial deficit and spatial neglect following unspecified cerebrovascular disease**

SP SH SL I69.913 **Psychomotor deficit following unspecified cerebrovascular disease**

SP SH SL I69.914 **Frontal lobe and executive function deficit following unspecified cerebrovascular disease**

SP SH SL I69.915 **Cognitive social or emotional deficit following unspecified cerebrovascular disease**

SP SH SL I69.918 **Other symptoms and signs involving cognitive functions following unspecified cerebrovascular disease**

IQ I69.919 **Unspecified symptoms and signs involving cognitive functions following unspecified cerebrovascular disease**

6 I69.92 **Speech and language deficits following unspecified cerebrovascular disease**

SP SH SL I69.920 **Aphasia following unspecified cerebrovascular disease**

DEFINITION Impaired or complete loss of the ability to communicate with language or symbols resulting from brain damage.

SP SH SL I69.921 **Dysphasia following unspecified cerebrovascular disease**

DEFINITION Impairment in the ability to speak or understand words resulting from brain damage.

SP SH SL I69.922 **Dysarthria following unspecified cerebrovascular disease**

SP SH SL I69.923 **Fluency disorder following unspecified cerebrovascular disease**
Stuttering following unspecified cerebrovascular disease

SP SH SL I69.928 **Other speech and language deficits following unspecified cerebrovascular disease**

6 I69.93 **Monoplegia of upper limb following unspecified cerebrovascular disease**

☐ **SP SH SL I69.931** **Monoplegia of upper limb following unspecified cerebrovascular disease affecting right dominant side**

☐ **SP SH SL I69.932** **Monoplegia of upper limb following unspecified cerebrovascular disease affecting left dominant side**

☐ **SP SH SL I69.933** **Monoplegia of upper limb following unspecified cerebrovascular disease affecting right non-dominant side**

---

4 4th digit required   **5** 5th digit required   **6** 6th digit required   **7** 7th digit required   **7** 7th digit placeholder   **+** Additional code   ☐ Laterality

☰ **SP** **SH** **SL** I69.934 **Monoplegia of upper limb following unspecified cerebrovascular disease affecting left non-dominant side**

☰ **IQ** I69.939 **Monoplegia of upper limb following unspecified cerebrovascular disease affecting unspecified side**

6 I69.94 **Monoplegia of lower limb following unspecified cerebrovascular disease**

☰ **SP** **SH** **SL** I69.941 **Monoplegia of lower limb following unspecified cerebrovascular disease affecting right dominant side**

☰ **SP** **SH** **SL** I69.942 **Monoplegia of lower limb following unspecified cerebrovascular disease affecting left dominant side**

☰ **SP** **SH** **SL** I69.943 **Monoplegia of lower limb following unspecified cerebrovascular disease affecting right non-dominant side**

☰ **SP** **SH** **SL** I69.944 **Monoplegia of lower limb following unspecified cerebrovascular disease affecting left non-dominant side**

☰ **IQ** I69.949 **Monoplegia of lower limb following unspecified cerebrovascular disease affecting unspecified side**

6 I69.95 **Hemiplegia and hemiparesis following unspecified cerebrovascular disease**

DEFINITION Paralysis affecting one side of the body.

☰ **SP** **SH** **SL** I69.951 **Hemiplegia and hemiparesis following unspecified cerebrovascular disease affecting right dominant side**

☰ **SP** **SH** **SL** I69.952 **Hemiplegia and hemiparesis following unspecified cerebrovascular disease affecting left dominant side**

☰ **SP** **SH** **SL** I69.953 **Hemiplegia and hemiparesis following unspecified cerebrovascular disease affecting right non-dominant side**

☰ **SP** **SH** **SL** I69.954 **Hemiplegia and hemiparesis following unspecified cerebrovascular disease affecting left non-dominant side**

☰ **IQ** I69.959 **Hemiplegia and hemiparesis following unspecified cerebrovascular disease affecting unspecified side**

✚ 6 I69.96 **Other paralytic syndrome following unspecified cerebrovascular disease**

Use additional code to identify type of paralytic syndrome, such as:
locked-in state (G83.5)
quadriplegia (G82.5-)

EXCLUDES 1 hemiplegia/hemiparesis following unspecified cerebrovascular disease (I69.95-)

monoplegia of lower limb following unspecified cerebrovascular disease (I69.94-)
monoplegia of upper limb following unspecified cerebrovascular disease (I69.93-)

☰ **SP** **SH** **SL** ✚ I69.961 **Other paralytic syndrome following unspecified cerebrovascular disease affecting right dominant side**

☰ **SP** **SH** **SL** ✚ I69.962 **Other paralytic syndrome following unspecified cerebrovascular disease affecting left dominant side**

☰ **SP** **SH** **SL** ✚ I69.963 **Other paralytic syndrome following unspecified cerebrovascular disease affecting right non-dominant side**

☰ **SP** **SH** **SL** ✚ I69.964 **Other paralytic syndrome following unspecified cerebrovascular disease affecting left non-dominant side**

☰ **IQ** **SH** **SL** ✚ I69.965 **Other paralytic syndrome following unspecified cerebrovascular disease, bilateral**

☰ **IQ** ✚ I69.969 **Other paralytic syndrome following unspecified cerebrovascular disease affecting unspecified side**

6 I69.99 **Other sequelae of unspecified cerebrovascular disease**

SP **SH** **SL** I69.990 **Apraxia following unspecified cerebrovascular disease**

SP **SH** **SL** ✚ I69.991 **Dysphagia following unspecified cerebrovascular disease**

Use additional code to identify the type of dysphagia, if known (R13.1-)

SP I69.992 **Facial weakness following unspecified cerebrovascular disease**

Facial droop following unspecified cerebrovascular disease

SP **SH** **SL** I69.993 **Ataxia following unspecified cerebrovascular disease**

DEFINITION Inability to coordinate muscle movement.

SP **SH** **SL** ✚ I69.998 **Other sequelae following unspecified cerebrovascular disease**

Alteration in sensation following unspecified cerebrovascular disease
Disturbance of vision following unspecified cerebrovascular disease
Use additional code to identify the sequelae

⭐ New ▲ Revised Px Primary **SP** PDGM Px **SL** Low CoM **SH** High CoM **IQ** Quest. Encounter Ⓗ Hospice non-cancer Dx Unspecified **M** *Manifestation*

DecisionHealth's FY 2020 Complete Home Health ICD-10-CM Diagnosis Coding Manual

993

Diseases of arteries, arterioles and capillaries (I70-I79)

+ ☑ I70   Atherosclerosis

| INCLUDES | arteriolosclerosis |

arteriolosclerosis
arterial degeneration
arteriosclerosis
arteriosclerotic vascular disease
arteriovascular degeneration
atheroma
endarteritis deformans or
   obliterans
senile arteritis
senile endarteritis
vascular degeneration

Use additional code to identify:
exposure to environmental tobacco smoke
   (Z77.22)
history of tobacco dependence (Z87.891)
occupational exposure to environmental
   tobacco smoke (Z57.31)
tobacco dependence (F17.-)
tobacco use (Z72.0)

EXCLUDES 2   arteriosclerotic cardiovascular
                   disease (I25.1-)
                 arteriosclerotic heart disease
                   (I25.1-)
                 atheroembolism (I75.-)
                 cerebral atherosclerosis (I67.2)
                 coronary atherosclerosis
                   (I25.1-)
                 mesenteric atherosclerosis
                   (K55.1)
                 precerebral atherosclerosis
                   (I67.2)
                 primary pulmonary
                   atherosclerosis (I27.0)

SP SH + I70.0   Atherosclerosis of aorta

DEFINITION   Fatty plaque deposits in the
aorta that reduce its diameter and elasticity.

SP SH + I70.1   Atherosclerosis of renal artery
Goldblatt's kidney

EXCLUDES 2   atherosclerosis of renal
                   arterioles (I12.-)

CODING TIPS ✓   Atherosclerosis of renal
artery may also be reported as renal artery
stenosis. When renal artery stenosis is
reported as causative of hypertension, an
additional code of I15.0, Renovascular
hypertension, should be reported.

**+ ☑ I70.2   Atherosclerosis of native arteries of the
             extremities**
Mönckeberg's (medial) sclerosis
Use additional code, if applicable, to
   identify chronic total occlusion of artery
   of extremity (I70.92)

EXCLUDES 2   atherosclerosis of bypass
                   graft of extremities
                   (I70.30-I70.79)

CODING TIPS ✓   I70.2 is the correct
subcategory for arteriosclerosis of the
native arteries of the legs. Peripheral
angiopathy may be documented as diabetic
PVD. There is an assumed relationship
between diabetes and PVD and PAD,
including peripheral atherosclerosis.
Diabetic arteriosclerosis of the peripheral
arteries should be coded E--.51 or E--.52
then the appropriate I70.- code. PAD, PVD
on M1028 should be selected.

**+ ☑ I70.20   Unspecified atherosclerosis of native
              arteries of extremities**

**⊟ SP SH + I70.201   Unspecified atherosclerosis of
                     native arteries of extremities,
                     right leg**

**⊟ SP SH + I70.202   Unspecified atherosclerosis of
                     native arteries of extremities, left
                     leg**

**⊟ SP SH + I70.203   Unspecified atherosclerosis of
                     native arteries of extremities,
                     bilateral legs**

**⊟ SP SH + I70.208   Unspecified atherosclerosis of
                     native arteries of extremities,
                     other extremity**

**⊟ IQ + I70.209   Unspecified atherosclerosis of
                  native arteries of extremities,
                  unspecified extremity**

**+ ☑ I70.21   Atherosclerosis of native arteries of
              extremities with intermittent
              claudication**

**⊟ SP SH + I70.211   Atherosclerosis of native arteries
                     of extremities with intermittent
                     claudication, right leg**

**⊟ SP SH + I70.212   Atherosclerosis of native arteries
                     of extremities with intermittent
                     claudication, left leg**

**⊟ SP SH + I70.213   Atherosclerosis of native arteries
                     of extremities with intermittent
                     claudication, bilateral legs**

**⊟ SP SH + I70.218   Atherosclerosis of native arteries
                     of extremities with intermittent
                     claudication, other extremity**

**⊟ IQ + I70.219   Atherosclerosis of native arteries
                  of extremities with intermittent
                  claudication, unspecified
                  extremity**

**+ ☑ I70.22   Atherosclerosis of native arteries of
              extremities with rest pain**

| INCLUDES | any condition classifiable
                 to I70.21-

**⊟ SP SH + I70.221   Atherosclerosis of native arteries
                     of extremities with rest pain, right
                     leg**

**⊟ SP SH + I70.222   Atherosclerosis of native arteries
                     of extremities with rest pain, left
                     leg**

**⊟ SP SH + I70.223   Atherosclerosis of native arteries
                     of extremities with rest pain,
                     bilateral legs**

**⊟ SP SH + I70.228   Atherosclerosis of native arteries
                     of extremities with rest pain, other
                     extremity**

**⊟ IQ + I70.229   Atherosclerosis of native arteries
                  of extremities with rest pain,
                  unspecified extremity**

☑ 4th digit required   ☑ 5th digit required   ☑ 6th digit required   ☑ 7th digit required   ☑ 7th digit placeholder   + Additional code   ⊟ Laterality

994   *DecisionHealth's* FY 2020 Complete Home Health ICD-10-CM Diagnosis Coding Manual

+ ⑥ I70.23 Atherosclerosis of native arteries of right leg with ulceration

> INCLUDES   any condition classifiable to I70.211 and I70.221
> Use additional code to identify severity of ulcer (L97.-)

CODING TIPS ✓ When the physician documents arterial ulcer, query regarding arteriosclerosis.

CODING TIPS ✓ When bilateral ulcers are present or ulcers of multiple specified areas classifiable in a patient with atherosclerosis of the extremities, assign a code for each specific site, taking laterality into account. A second code from category L97.- to specify the severity of the ulcer must be used following each reported site of, atherosclerosis to the extremity with ulceration. The ICD-10 classification assumes a relationship between atherosclerosis of lower extremities and gangrene, ulceration, rest pain and intermittent claudication.

☐ SP SH SL + **I70.231 Atherosclerosis of native arteries of right leg with ulceration of thigh**

☐ SP SH SL + **I70.232 Atherosclerosis of native arteries of right leg with ulceration of calf**

☐ SP SH SL + **I70.233 Atherosclerosis of native arteries of right leg with ulceration of ankle**

☐ SP SH SL + **I70.234 Atherosclerosis of native arteries of right leg with ulceration of heel and midfoot**

> Atherosclerosis of native arteries of right leg with ulceration of plantar surface of midfoot

☐ SP SH SL + **I70.235 Atherosclerosis of native arteries of right leg with ulceration of other part of foot**

> Atherosclerosis of native arteries of right leg extremities with ulceration of toe

▲ ☐ SP SH SL **I70.238 Atherosclerosis of native arteries of right leg with ulceration of other part of lower leg** +

☐ IQ + **I70.239 Atherosclerosis of native arteries of right leg with ulceration of unspecified site**

+ ⑥ I70.24 Atherosclerosis of native arteries of left leg with ulceration

> INCLUDES   any condition classifiable to I70.212 and I70.222
> Use additional code to identify severity of ulcer (L97.-)

CODING TIPS ✓ When the physician documents arterial ulcer, query regarding arteriosclerosis.

CODING TIPS ✓ When bilateral ulcers are present or ulcers of multiple specified areas classifiable in a patient with atherosclerosis of the extremities, assign a code for each specific site, taking laterality into account. A second code from category L97.- to specify the severity of the ulcer must be used following each reported site of atherosclerosis to the extremity with ulceration. The ICD-10 classification assumes a relationship between atherosclerosis of lower extremities and gangrene, ulceration, rest pain and intermittent claudication.

☐ SP SH SL + **I70.241 Atherosclerosis of native arteries of left leg with ulceration of thigh**

☐ SP SH SL + **I70.242 Atherosclerosis of native arteries of left leg with ulceration of calf**

☐ SP SH SL + **I70.243 Atherosclerosis of native arteries of left leg with ulceration of ankle**

☐ SP SH SL + **I70.244 Atherosclerosis of native arteries of left leg with ulceration of heel and midfoot**

> Atherosclerosis of native arteries of left leg with ulceration of plantar surface of midfoot

☐ SP SH SL + **I70.245 Atherosclerosis of native arteries of left leg with ulceration of other part of foot**

> Atherosclerosis of native arteries of left leg extremities with ulceration of toe

▲ ☐ SP SH SL **I70.248 Atherosclerosis of native arteries of left leg with ulceration of other part of lower leg** +

☐ IQ + **I70.249 Atherosclerosis of native arteries of left leg with ulceration of unspecified site**

☐ SP + **I70.25 Atherosclerosis of native arteries of other extremities with ulceration**

> INCLUDES   any condition classifiable to I70.218 and I70.228
> Use additional code to identify the severity of the ulcer (L98.49-)

CODING TIPS ✓ When the physician documents arterial ulcer, query regarding arteriosclerosis.

CODING TIPS ✓ When bilateral ulcers are present or ulcers of multiple specified areas classifiable in a patient with atherosclerosis of the extremities, assign a code for each specific site, taking laterality into account. A second code from category L97.- to specify the severity of the ulcer must be used following each reported site of atherosclerosis to the extremity with ulceration. The ICD-10 classification assumes a relationship between atherosclerosis of lower extremities and gangrene, ulceration, rest pain and intermittent claudication.

+ ⑥ I70.26 Atherosclerosis of native arteries of extremities with gangrene

★ New ▲ Revised Px Primary   SP PDGM Px   SL Low CoM   SH High CoM   IQ Quest. Encounter   H Hospice non-cancer Dx   Unspecified   M *Manifestation*

DecisionHealth's FY 2020 Complete Home Health ICD-10-CM Diagnosis Coding Manual   995

INCLUDES   any condition classifiable
to I70.21-, I70.22-,
I70.23-, I70.24-, and
I70.25-

Use additional code to identify the
severity of any ulcer (L97.-, L98.49-
), if applicable

CODING TIPS ✓   When the clinical record
reports atherosclerosis of the lower
extremities with ulceration and
gangrene, assign a code from
I70.26-. Do not code the gangrene
separately.
An additional code from category L97.-
should be assigned to report the
severity of any ulceration.

☐ SP SH + I70.261 Atherosclerosis of native arteries
of extremities with gangrene, right
leg

☐ SP SH + I70.262 Atherosclerosis of native arteries
of extremities with gangrene, left
leg

☐ SP SH + I70.263 Atherosclerosis of native arteries
of extremities with gangrene,
bilateral legs

☐ SP SH + I70.268 Atherosclerosis of native arteries
of extremities with gangrene,
other extremity

☐ IQ + I70.269 Atherosclerosis of native arteries
of extremities with gangrene,
unspecified extremity

+ ⑥ I70.29 Other atherosclerosis of native
arteries of extremities

☐ SP + I70.291 Other atherosclerosis of native
arteries of extremities, right leg

☐ SP + I70.292 Other atherosclerosis of native
arteries of extremities, left leg

☐ SP + I70.293 Other atherosclerosis of native
arteries of extremities, bilateral
legs

☐ SP + I70.298 Other atherosclerosis of native
arteries of extremities, other
extremity

☐ IQ + I70.299 Other atherosclerosis of native
arteries of extremities,
unspecified extremity

+ ⑤ I70.3 Atherosclerosis of unspecified type of
bypass graft(s) of the extremities

Use additional code, if applicable, to
identify chronic total occlusion of artery
of extremity (I70.92)

EXCLUDES 1   embolism or thrombus of
bypass graft (s) of
extremities (T82.8-)

CODING TIPS ✓   Peripheral angiopathy may
be documented as diabetic PVD. There is
an assumed relationship between diabetes
and PVD and PAD, including peripheral
atherosclerosis. Diabetic arteriosclerosis of
the peripheral arteries should be coded E--
.51 or E--.52 then the appropriate I70.-
code.

+ ⑥ I70.30 Unspecified atherosclerosis of
unspecified type of bypass graft(s)
of the extremities

☐ SP + I70.301 Unspecified atherosclerosis of
unspecified type of bypass
graft(s) of the extremities, right
leg

☐ SP + I70.302 Unspecified atherosclerosis of
unspecified type of bypass
graft(s) of the extremities, left leg

☐ SP + I70.303 Unspecified atherosclerosis of
unspecified type of bypass
graft(s) of the extremities,
bilateral legs

☐ SP + I70.308 Unspecified atherosclerosis of
unspecified type of bypass
graft(s) of the extremities, other
extremity

☐ IQ + I70.309 Unspecified atherosclerosis of
unspecified type of bypass
graft(s) of the extremities,
unspecified extremity

+ ⑥ I70.31 Atherosclerosis of unspecified type
of bypass graft(s) of the extremities
with intermittent claudication

☐ SP + I70.311 Atherosclerosis of unspecified
type of bypass graft(s) of the
extremities with intermittent
claudication, right leg

☐ SP + I70.312 Atherosclerosis of unspecified
type of bypass graft(s) of the
extremities with intermittent
claudication, left leg

☐ SP + I70.313 Atherosclerosis of unspecified
type of bypass graft(s) of the
extremities with intermittent
claudication, bilateral legs

☐ SP + I70.318 Atherosclerosis of unspecified
type of bypass graft(s) of the
extremities with intermittent
claudication, other extremity

☐ IQ + I70.319 Atherosclerosis of unspecified
type of bypass graft(s) of the
extremities with intermittent
claudication, unspecified
extremity

+ ⑥ I70.32 Atherosclerosis of unspecified type
of bypass graft(s) of the extremities
with rest pain

INCLUDES   any condition classifiable
to I70.31-

☐ SP + I70.321 Atherosclerosis of unspecified
type of bypass graft(s) of the
extremities with rest pain, right
leg

☐ SP + I70.322 Atherosclerosis of unspecified
type of bypass graft(s) of the
extremities with rest pain, left leg

☐ SP + I70.323 Atherosclerosis of unspecified
type of bypass graft(s) of the
extremities with rest pain,
bilateral legs

☐ SP + I70.328 Atherosclerosis of unspecified
type of bypass graft(s) of the
extremities with rest pain, other
extremity

④ 4th digit required   ⑤ 5th digit required   ⑥ 6th digit required   ⑦ 7th digit required   ⑦ 7th digit placeholder   ✛ Additional code   ☐ Laterality

996   DecisionHealth's FY 2020 Complete Home Health ICD-10-CM Diagnosis Coding Manual

☰ **IQ** ✛ **I70.329** **Atherosclerosis of unspecified type of bypass graft(s) of the extremities with rest pain, unspecified extremity**

✛ ⑥ **I70.33** **Atherosclerosis of unspecified type of bypass graft(s) of the right leg with ulceration**

> INCLUDES   any condition classifiable to I70.311 and I70.321

Use additional code to identify severity of ulcer (L97.-)

☰ **SP** **SH** **SL** ✛ **I70.331** **Atherosclerosis of unspecified type of bypass graft(s) of the right leg with ulceration of thigh**

☰ **SP** **SH** **SL** ✛ **I70.332** **Atherosclerosis of unspecified type of bypass graft(s) of the right leg with ulceration of calf**

☰ **SP** **SH** **SL** ✛ **I70.333** **Atherosclerosis of unspecified type of bypass graft(s) of the right leg with ulceration of ankle**

☰ **SP** **SH** **SL** ✛ **I70.334** **Atherosclerosis of unspecified type of bypass graft(s) of the right leg with ulceration of heel and midfoot**

Atherosclerosis of unspecified type of bypass graft(s) of right leg with ulceration of plantar surface of midfoot

☰ **SP** **SH** **SL** ✛ **I70.335** **Atherosclerosis of unspecified type of bypass graft(s) of the right leg with ulceration of other part of foot**

Atherosclerosis of unspecified type of bypass graft(s) of the right leg with ulceration of toe

☰ **SP** **SH** **SL** ✛ **I70.338** **Atherosclerosis of unspecified type of bypass graft(s) of the right leg with ulceration of other part of lower leg**

☰ **IQ** **SH** **SL** ✛ **I70.339** **Atherosclerosis of unspecified type of bypass graft(s) of the right leg with ulceration of unspecified site**

✛ ⑥ **I70.34** **Atherosclerosis of unspecified type of bypass graft(s) of the left leg with ulceration**

> INCLUDES   any condition classifiable to I70.312 and I70.322

Use additional code to identify severity of ulcer (L97.-)

☰ **SP** **SH** **SL** ✛ **I70.341** **Atherosclerosis of unspecified type of bypass graft(s) of the left leg with ulceration of thigh**

☰ **SP** **SH** **SL** ✛ **I70.342** **Atherosclerosis of unspecified type of bypass graft(s) of the left leg with ulceration of calf**

☰ **SP** **SH** **SL** ✛ **I70.343** **Atherosclerosis of unspecified type of bypass graft(s) of the left leg with ulceration of ankle**

☰ **SP** **SH** **SL** ✛ **I70.344** **Atherosclerosis of unspecified type of bypass graft(s) of the left leg with ulceration of heel and midfoot**

Atherosclerosis of unspecified type of bypass graft(s) of left leg with ulceration of plantar surface of midfoot

☰ **SP** **SH** **SL** ✛ **I70.345** **Atherosclerosis of unspecified type of bypass graft(s) of the left leg with ulceration of other part of foot**

Atherosclerosis of unspecified type of bypass graft(s) of the left leg with ulceration of toe

☰ **SP** **SH** **SL** ✛ **I70.348** **Atherosclerosis of unspecified type of bypass graft(s) of the left leg with ulceration of other part of lower leg**

☰ **IQ** **SH** **SL** ✛ **I70.349** **Atherosclerosis of unspecified type of bypass graft(s) of the left leg with ulceration of unspecified site**

☰ **SP** ✛ **I70.35** **Atherosclerosis of unspecified type of bypass graft(s) of other extremity with ulceration**

> INCLUDES   any condition classifiable to I70.318 and I70.328

Use additional code to identify severity of ulcer (L98.49-)

✛ ⑥ **I70.36** **Atherosclerosis of unspecified type of bypass graft(s) of the extremities with gangrene**

> INCLUDES   any condition classifiable to I70.31-, I70.32-, I70.33-, I70.34-, I70.35

Use additional code to identify the severity of any ulcer (L97.-, L98.49-), if applicable

☰ **SP** ✛ **I70.361** **Atherosclerosis of unspecified type of bypass graft(s) of the extremities with gangrene, right leg**

☰ **SP** ✛ **I70.362** **Atherosclerosis of unspecified type of bypass graft(s) of the extremities with gangrene, left leg**

☰ **SP** ✛ **I70.363** **Atherosclerosis of unspecified type of bypass graft(s) of the extremities with gangrene, bilateral legs**

☰ **SP** ✛ **I70.368** **Atherosclerosis of unspecified type of bypass graft(s) of the extremities with gangrene, other extremity**

☰ **IQ** ✛ **I70.369** **Atherosclerosis of unspecified type of bypass graft(s) of the extremities with gangrene, unspecified extremity**

✛ ⑥ **I70.39** **Other atherosclerosis of unspecified type of bypass graft(s) of the extremities**

☰ **SP** ✛ **I70.391** **Other atherosclerosis of unspecified type of bypass graft(s) of the extremities, right leg**

☰ **SP** ✛ **I70.392** **Other atherosclerosis of unspecified type of bypass graft(s) of the extremities, left leg**

☰ **SP** ✛ **I70.393** **Other atherosclerosis of unspecified type of bypass graft(s) of the extremities, bilateral legs**

★ New ▲ Revised Px Primary   **SP** PDGM Px   **SL** Low CoM   **SH** High CoM   **IQ** Quest. Encounter   **H** Hospice non-cancer Dx   Unspecified   **M** *Manifestation*

DecisionHealth's FY 2020 Complete Home Health ICD-10-CM Diagnosis Coding Manual

997

Chapter 9

I00-I99

⊟ **SP** ✚ **I70.398**   **Other atherosclerosis of unspecified type of bypass graft(s) of the extremities, other extremity**

⊟ **IQ** ✚ **I70.399**   **Other atherosclerosis of unspecified type of bypass graft(s) of the extremities, unspecified extremity**

✚ **5** **I70.4**   **Atherosclerosis of autologous vein bypass graft(s) of the extremities**
Use additional code, if applicable, to identify chronic total occlusion of artery of extremity (I70.92)

CODING TIPS ✓   Peripheral angiopathy may be documented as diabetic PVD. There is an assumed relationship between diabetes and PVD and PAD, including peripheral atherosclerosis. Diabetic arteriosclerosis of the peripheral arteries should be coded E--.51 or E--.52 then the appropriate I70.- code.

✚ **6** **I70.40**   **Unspecified atherosclerosis of autologous vein bypass graft(s) of the extremities**

⊟ **SP** ✚ **I70.401**   **Unspecified atherosclerosis of autologous vein bypass graft(s) of the extremities, right leg**

⊟ **SP** ✚ **I70.402**   **Unspecified atherosclerosis of autologous vein bypass graft(s) of the extremities, left leg**

⊟ **SP** ✚ **I70.403**   **Unspecified atherosclerosis of autologous vein bypass graft(s) of the extremities, bilateral legs**

⊟ **SP** ✚ **I70.408**   **Unspecified atherosclerosis of autologous vein bypass graft(s) of the extremities, other extremity**

⊟ **IQ** ✚ **I70.409**   **Unspecified atherosclerosis of autologous vein bypass graft(s) of the extremities, unspecified extremity**

✚ **6** **I70.41**   **Atherosclerosis of autologous vein bypass graft(s) of the extremities with intermittent claudication**

⊟ **SP** ✚ **I70.411**   **Atherosclerosis of autologous vein bypass graft(s) of the extremities with intermittent claudication, right leg**

⊟ **SP** ✚ **I70.412**   **Atherosclerosis of autologous vein bypass graft(s) of the extremities with intermittent claudication, left leg**

⊟ **SP** ✚ **I70.413**   **Atherosclerosis of autologous vein bypass graft(s) of the extremities with intermittent claudication, bilateral legs**

⊟ **SP** ✚ **I70.418**   **Atherosclerosis of autologous vein bypass graft(s) of the extremities with intermittent claudication, other extremity**

⊟ **IQ** ✚ **I70.419**   **Atherosclerosis of autologous vein bypass graft(s) of the extremities with intermittent claudication, unspecified extremity**

✚ **6** **I70.42**   **Atherosclerosis of autologous vein bypass graft(s) of the extremities with rest pain**

INCLUDES   any condition classifiable to I70.41-

⊟ **SP** ✚ **I70.421**   **Atherosclerosis of autologous vein bypass graft(s) of the extremities with rest pain, right leg**

⊟ **SP** ✚ **I70.422**   **Atherosclerosis of autologous vein bypass graft(s) of the extremities with rest pain, left leg**

⊟ **SP** ✚ **I70.423**   **Atherosclerosis of autologous vein bypass graft(s) of the extremities with rest pain, bilateral legs**

⊟ **SP** ✚ **I70.428**   **Atherosclerosis of autologous vein bypass graft(s) of the extremities with rest pain, other extremity**

⊟ **IQ** ✚ **I70.429**   **Atherosclerosis of autologous vein bypass graft(s) of the extremities with rest pain, unspecified extremity**

✚ **6** **I70.43**   **Atherosclerosis of autologous vein bypass graft(s) of the right leg with ulceration**

INCLUDES   any condition classifiable to I70.411 and I70.421
Use additional code to identify severity of ulcer (L97.-)

⊟ **SP** **SH** **SL** ✚ **I70.431**   **Atherosclerosis of autologous vein bypass graft(s) of the right leg with ulceration of thigh**

⊟ **SP** **SH** **SL** ✚ **I70.432**   **Atherosclerosis of autologous vein bypass graft(s) of the right leg with ulceration of calf**

⊟ **SP** **SH** **SL** ✚ **I70.433**   **Atherosclerosis of autologous vein bypass graft(s) of the right leg with ulceration of ankle**

⊟ **SP** **SH** **SL** ✚ **I70.434**   **Atherosclerosis of autologous vein bypass graft(s) of the right leg with ulceration of heel and midfoot**
Atherosclerosis of autologous vein bypass graft(s) of right leg with ulceration of plantar surface of midfoot

⊟ **SP** **SH** **SL** ✚ **I70.435**   **Atherosclerosis of autologous vein bypass graft(s) of the right leg with ulceration of other part of foot**
Atherosclerosis of autologous vein bypass graft(s) of right leg with ulceration of toe

⊟ **SP** **SH** **SL** ✚ **I70.438**   **Atherosclerosis of autologous vein bypass graft(s) of the right leg with ulceration of other part of lower leg**

⊟ **IQ** **SH** **SL** ✚ **I70.439**   **Atherosclerosis of autologous vein bypass graft(s) of the right leg with ulceration of unspecified site**

✚ **6** **I70.44**   **Atherosclerosis of autologous vein bypass graft(s) of the left leg with ulceration**

INCLUDES   any condition classifiable to I70.412 and I70.422
Use additional code to identify severity of ulcer (L97.-)

⊟ **SP** **SH** **SL** ✚ **I70.441**   **Atherosclerosis of autologous vein bypass graft(s) of the left leg with ulceration of thigh**

---

4 4th digit required   **5** 5th digit required   **6** 6th digit required   **7** 7th digit required   **7** 7th digit placeholder   ✚ Additional code   ⊟ Laterality

998   *DecisionHealth's* FY 2020 Complete Home Health ICD-10-CM Diagnosis Coding Manual

☐ SP SH SL + **I70.442** **Atherosclerosis of autologous vein bypass graft(s) of the left leg with ulceration of calf**

☐ SP SH SL + **I70.443** **Atherosclerosis of autologous vein bypass graft(s) of the left leg with ulceration of ankle**

☐ SP SH SL + **I70.444** **Atherosclerosis of autologous vein bypass graft(s) of the left leg with ulceration of heel and midfoot**
Atherosclerosis of autologous vein bypass graft(s) of left leg with ulceration of plantar surface of midfoot

☐ SP SH SL + **I70.445** **Atherosclerosis of autologous vein bypass graft(s) of the left leg with ulceration of other part of foot**
Atherosclerosis of autologous vein bypass graft(s) of left leg with ulceration of toe

☐ SP SH SL + **I70.448** **Atherosclerosis of autologous vein bypass graft(s) of the left leg with ulceration of other part of lower leg**

☐ IQ SH SL + **I70.449** **Atherosclerosis of autologous vein bypass graft(s) of the left leg with ulceration of unspecified site**

☐ SP + **I70.45** **Atherosclerosis of autologous vein bypass graft(s) of other extremity with ulceration**
INCLUDES any condition classifiable to I70.418, I70.428, and I70.438
Use additional code to identify severity of ulcer (L98.49)

+ 6 **I70.46** **Atherosclerosis of autologous vein bypass graft(s) of the extremities with gangrene**
INCLUDES any condition classifiable to I70.41-, I70.42-, and I70.43-, I70.44-, I70.45
Use additional code to identify the severity of any ulcer (L97.-, L98.49-), if applicable

☐ SP + **I70.461** **Atherosclerosis of autologous vein bypass graft(s) of the extremities with gangrene, right leg**

☐ SP + **I70.462** **Atherosclerosis of autologous vein bypass graft(s) of the extremities with gangrene, left leg**

☐ SP + **I70.463** **Atherosclerosis of autologous vein bypass graft(s) of the extremities with gangrene, bilateral legs**

☐ SP + **I70.468** **Atherosclerosis of autologous vein bypass graft(s) of the extremities with gangrene, other extremity**

☐ IQ + **I70.469** **Atherosclerosis of autologous vein bypass graft(s) of the extremities with gangrene, unspecified extremity**

+ 6 **I70.49** **Other atherosclerosis of autologous vein bypass graft(s) of the extremities**

☐ SP + **I70.491** **Other atherosclerosis of autologous vein bypass graft(s) of the extremities, right leg**

☐ SP + **I70.492** **Other atherosclerosis of autologous vein bypass graft(s) of the extremities, left leg**

☐ SP + **I70.493** **Other atherosclerosis of autologous vein bypass graft(s) of the extremities, bilateral legs**

☐ SP + **I70.498** **Other atherosclerosis of autologous vein bypass graft(s) of the extremities, other extremity**

☐ IQ + **I70.499** **Other atherosclerosis of autologous vein bypass graft(s) of the extremities, unspecified extremity**

+ 5 **I70.5** **Atherosclerosis of nonautologous biological bypass graft(s) of the extremities**
Use additional code, if applicable, to identify chronic total occlusion of artery of extremity (I70.92)

CODING TIPS ✓ Peripheral angiopathy may be documented as diabetic PVD. There is an assumed relationship between diabetes and PVD and PAD, including peripheral atherosclerosis. Diabetic arteriosclerosis of the peripheral arteries should be coded E--.51 or E--.52 then the appropriate I70.- code.

+ 6 **I70.50** **Unspecified atherosclerosis of nonautologous biological bypass graft(s) of the extremities**

☐ SP + **I70.501** **Unspecified atherosclerosis of nonautologous biological bypass graft(s) of the extremities, right leg**

☐ SP + **I70.502** **Unspecified atherosclerosis of nonautologous biological bypass graft(s) of the extremities, left leg**

☐ SP + **I70.503** **Unspecified atherosclerosis of nonautologous biological bypass graft(s) of the extremities, bilateral legs**

☐ SP + **I70.508** **Unspecified atherosclerosis of nonautologous biological bypass graft(s) of the extremities, other extremity**

☐ IQ + **I70.509** **Unspecified atherosclerosis of nonautologous biological bypass graft(s) of the extremities, unspecified extremity**

+ 6 **I70.51** **Atherosclerosis of nonautologous biological bypass graft(s) of the extremities intermittent claudication**

☐ SP + **I70.511** **Atherosclerosis of nonautologous biological bypass graft(s) of the extremities with intermittent claudication, right leg**

☐ SP + **I70.512** **Atherosclerosis of nonautologous biological bypass graft(s) of the extremities with intermittent claudication, left leg**

☐ SP + **I70.513** **Atherosclerosis of nonautologous biological bypass graft(s) of the extremities with intermittent claudication, bilateral legs**

☐ SP + **I70.518** **Atherosclerosis of nonautologous biological bypass graft(s) of the extremities with intermittent claudication, other extremity**

★ New ▲ Revised Px Primary SP PDGM Px SL Low CoM SH High CoM IQ Quest. Encounter H Hospice non-cancer Dx Unspecified M *Manifestation*

DecisionHealth's FY 2020 Complete Home Health ICD-10-CM Diagnosis Coding Manual 999

⊟ IQ ✛ I70.519 **Atherosclerosis of nonautologous biological bypass graft(s) of the extremities with intermittent claudication, unspecified extremity**

✛ 6 I70.52 **Atherosclerosis of nonautologous biological bypass graft(s) of the extremities with rest pain**
INCLUDES   any condition classifiable to I70.51-

⊟ SP ✛ I70.521 **Atherosclerosis of nonautologous biological bypass graft(s) of the extremities with rest pain, right leg**

⊟ SP ✛ I70.522 **Atherosclerosis of nonautologous biological bypass graft(s) of the extremities with rest pain, left leg**

⊟ SP ✛ I70.523 **Atherosclerosis of nonautologous biological bypass graft(s) of the extremities with rest pain, bilateral legs**

⊟ SP ✛ I70.528 **Atherosclerosis of nonautologous biological bypass graft(s) of the extremities with rest pain, other extremity**

⊟ IQ ✛ I70.529 **Atherosclerosis of nonautologous biological bypass graft(s) of the extremities with rest pain, unspecified extremity**

✛ 6 I70.53 **Atherosclerosis of nonautologous biological bypass graft(s) of the right leg with ulceration**
INCLUDES   any condition classifiable to I70.511 and I70.521
Use additional code to identify severity of ulcer (L97.-)

⊟ SP SH SL ✛ I70.531 **Atherosclerosis of nonautologous biological bypass graft(s) of the right leg with ulceration of thigh**

⊟ SP SH SL ✛ I70.532 **Atherosclerosis of nonautologous biological bypass graft(s) of the right leg with ulceration of calf**

⊟ SP SH SL ✛ I70.533 **Atherosclerosis of nonautologous biological bypass graft(s) of the right leg with ulceration of ankle**

⊟ SP SH SL ✛ I70.534 **Atherosclerosis of nonautologous biological bypass graft(s) of the right leg with ulceration of heel and midfoot**
Atherosclerosis of nonautologous biological bypass graft(s) of right leg with ulceration of plantar surface of midfoot

⊟ SP SH SL ✛ I70.535 **Atherosclerosis of nonautologous biological bypass graft(s) of the right leg with ulceration of other part of foot**
Atherosclerosis of nonautologous biological bypass graft(s) of the right leg with ulceration of toe

⊟ SP SH SL ✛ I70.538 **Atherosclerosis of nonautologous biological bypass graft(s) of the right leg with ulceration of other part of lower leg**

⊟ IQ SH SL ✛ I70.539 **Atherosclerosis of nonautologous biological bypass graft(s) of the right leg with ulceration of unspecified site**

✛ 6 I70.54 **Atherosclerosis of nonautologous biological bypass graft(s) of the left leg with ulceration**
INCLUDES   any condition classifiable to I70.512 and I70.522
Use additional code to identify severity of ulcer (L97.-)

⊟ SP SH SL ✛ I70.541 **Atherosclerosis of nonautologous biological bypass graft(s) of the left leg with ulceration of thigh**

⊟ SP SH SL ✛ I70.542 **Atherosclerosis of nonautologous biological bypass graft(s) of the left leg with ulceration of calf**

⊟ SP SH SL ✛ I70.543 **Atherosclerosis of nonautologous biological bypass graft(s) of the left leg with ulceration of ankle**

⊟ SP SH SL ✛ I70.544 **Atherosclerosis of nonautologous biological bypass graft(s) of the left leg with ulceration of heel and midfoot**
Atherosclerosis of nonautologous biological bypass graft(s) of left leg with ulceration of plantar surface of midfoot

⊟ SP SH SL ✛ I70.545 **Atherosclerosis of nonautologous biological bypass graft(s) of the left leg with ulceration of other part of foot**
Atherosclerosis of nonautologous biological bypass graft(s) of the left leg with ulceration of toe

⊟ SP SH SL ✛ I70.548 **Atherosclerosis of nonautologous biological bypass graft(s) of the left leg with ulceration of other part of lower leg**

⊟ IQ SH SL ✛ I70.549 **Atherosclerosis of nonautologous biological bypass graft(s) of the left leg with ulceration of unspecified site**

⊟ SP ✛ I70.55 **Atherosclerosis of nonautologous biological bypass graft(s) of other extremity with ulceration**
INCLUDES   any condition classifiable to I70.518, I70.528, and I70.538
Use additional code to identify severity of ulcer (L98.49)

✛ 6 I70.56 **Atherosclerosis of nonautologous biological bypass graft(s) of the extremities with gangrene**
INCLUDES   any condition classifiable to I70.51-, I70.52-, and I70.53-, I70.54-, I70.55
Use additional code to identify the severity of any ulcer (L97.-, L98.49-), if applicable

⊟ SP ✛ I70.561 **Atherosclerosis of nonautologous biological bypass graft(s) of the extremities with gangrene, right leg**

⊟ SP ✛ I70.562 **Atherosclerosis of nonautologous biological bypass graft(s) of the extremities with gangrene, left leg**

⊟ SP ✛ I70.563 **Atherosclerosis of nonautologous biological bypass graft(s) of the extremities with gangrene, bilateral legs**

---

4 4th digit required   5 5th digit required   6 6th digit required   7 7th digit required   7 7th digit placeholder   ✛ Additional code   ⊟ Laterality

🔲 SP ➕ I70.568 Atherosclerosis of nonautologous biological bypass graft(s) of the extremities with gangrene, other extremity

🔲 IQ ➕ I70.569 Atherosclerosis of nonautologous biological bypass graft(s) of the extremities with gangrene, unspecified extremity

➕ 6 I70.59 Other atherosclerosis of nonautologous biological bypass graft(s) of the extremities

🔲 SP ➕ I70.591 Other atherosclerosis of nonautologous biological bypass graft(s) of the extremities, right leg

🔲 SP ➕ I70.592 Other atherosclerosis of nonautologous biological bypass graft(s) of the extremities, left leg

🔲 SP ➕ I70.593 Other atherosclerosis of nonautologous biological bypass graft(s) of the extremities, bilateral legs

🔲 SP ➕ I70.598 Other atherosclerosis of nonautologous biological bypass graft(s) of the extremities, other extremity

🔲 IQ ➕ I70.599 Other atherosclerosis of nonautologous biological bypass graft(s) of the extremities, unspecified extremity

➕ 5 I70.6 Atherosclerosis of nonbiological bypass graft(s) of the extremities

Use additional code, if applicable, to identify chronic total occlusion of artery of extremity (I70.92)

CODING TIPS ✓ Peripheral angiopathy may be documented as diabetic PVD. There is an assumed relationship between diabetes and PVD and PAD, including peripheral atherosclerosis. Diabetic arteriosclerosis of the peripheral arteries should be coded E--.51 or E--.52 then the appropriate I70.- code.

➕ 6 I70.60 Unspecified atherosclerosis of nonbiological bypass graft(s) of the extremities

🔲 SP ➕ I70.601 Unspecified atherosclerosis of nonbiological bypass graft(s) of the extremities, right leg

🔲 SP ➕ I70.602 Unspecified atherosclerosis of nonbiological bypass graft(s) of the extremities, left leg

🔲 SP ➕ I70.603 Unspecified atherosclerosis of nonbiological bypass graft(s) of the extremities, bilateral legs

🔲 SP ➕ I70.608 Unspecified atherosclerosis of nonbiological bypass graft(s) of the extremities, other extremity

🔲 IQ ➕ I70.609 Unspecified atherosclerosis of nonbiological bypass graft(s) of the extremities, unspecified extremity

➕ 6 I70.61 Atherosclerosis of nonbiological bypass graft(s) of the extremities with intermittent claudication

🔲 SP ➕ I70.611 Atherosclerosis of nonbiological bypass graft(s) of the extremities with intermittent claudication, right leg

🔲 SP ➕ I70.612 Atherosclerosis of nonbiological bypass graft(s) of the extremities with intermittent claudication, left leg

🔲 SP ➕ I70.613 Atherosclerosis of nonbiological bypass graft(s) of the extremities with intermittent claudication, bilateral legs

🔲 SP ➕ I70.618 Atherosclerosis of nonbiological bypass graft(s) of the extremities with intermittent claudication, other extremity

🔲 IQ ➕ I70.619 Atherosclerosis of nonbiological bypass graft(s) of the extremities with intermittent claudication, unspecified extremity

➕ 6 I70.62 Atherosclerosis of nonbiological bypass graft(s) of the extremities with rest pain
INCLUDES any condition classifiable to I70.61-

🔲 SP ➕ I70.621 Atherosclerosis of nonbiological bypass graft(s) of the extremities with rest pain, right leg

🔲 SP ➕ I70.622 Atherosclerosis of nonbiological bypass graft(s) of the extremities with rest pain, left leg

🔲 SP ➕ I70.623 Atherosclerosis of nonbiological bypass graft(s) of the extremities with rest pain, bilateral legs

🔲 SP ➕ I70.628 Atherosclerosis of nonbiological bypass graft(s) of the extremities with rest pain, other extremity

🔲 IQ ➕ I70.629 Atherosclerosis of nonbiological bypass graft(s) of the extremities with rest pain, unspecified extremity

➕ 6 I70.63 Atherosclerosis of nonbiological bypass graft(s) of the right leg with ulceration
INCLUDES any condition classifiable to I70.611 and I70.621
Use additional code to identify severity of ulcer (L97.-)

🔲 SP SH SL ➕ I70.631 Atherosclerosis of nonbiological bypass graft(s) of the right leg with ulceration of thigh

🔲 SP SH SL ➕ I70.632 Atherosclerosis of nonbiological bypass graft(s) of the right leg with ulceration of calf

🔲 SP SH SL ➕ I70.633 Atherosclerosis of nonbiological bypass graft(s) of the right leg with ulceration of ankle

🔲 SP SH SL ➕ I70.634 Atherosclerosis of nonbiological bypass graft(s) of the right leg with ulceration of heel and midfoot
Atherosclerosis of nonbiological bypass graft(s) of right leg with ulceration of plantar surface of midfoot

🔲 SP SH SL ➕ I70.635 Atherosclerosis of nonbiological bypass graft(s) of the right leg with ulceration of other part of foot

---

★ New ▲ Revised **Px** Primary **SP** PDGM Px **SL** Low CoM **SH** High CoM **IQ** Quest. Encounter **H** Hospice non-cancer Dx | Unspecified | **M** *Manifestation*

Atherosclerosis of nonbiological bypass graft(s) of the right leg with ulceration of toe

☐ **SP** **SH** **SL** ✛ **I70.638**　**Atherosclerosis of nonbiological bypass graft(s) of the right leg with ulceration of other part of lower leg**

☐ **IQ** **SH** **SL** ✛ **I70.639**　**Atherosclerosis of nonbiological bypass graft(s) of the right leg with ulceration of unspecified site**

✛ ⑥ **I70.64**　**Atherosclerosis of nonbiological bypass graft(s) of the left leg with ulceration**

> **INCLUDES**　any condition classifiable to I70.612 and I70.622

Use additional code to identify severity of ulcer (L97.-)

☐ **SP** **SH** **SL** ✛ **I70.641**　**Atherosclerosis of nonbiological bypass graft(s) of the left leg with ulceration of thigh**

☐ **SP** **SH** **SL** ✛ **I70.642**　**Atherosclerosis of nonbiological bypass graft(s) of the left leg with ulceration of calf**

☐ **SP** **SH** **SL** ✛ **I70.643**　**Atherosclerosis of nonbiological bypass graft(s) of the left leg with ulceration of ankle**

☐ **SP** **SH** **SL** ✛ **I70.644**　**Atherosclerosis of nonbiological bypass graft(s) of the left leg with ulceration of heel and midfoot**

Atherosclerosis of nonbiological bypass graft(s) of left leg with ulceration of plantar surface of midfoot

☐ **SP** **SH** **SL** ✛ **I70.645**　**Atherosclerosis of nonbiological bypass graft(s) of the left leg with ulceration of other part of foot**

Atherosclerosis of nonbiological bypass graft(s) of the left leg with ulceration of toe

☐ **SP** **SH** **SL** ✛ **I70.648**　**Atherosclerosis of nonbiological bypass graft(s) of the left leg with ulceration of other part of lower leg**

☐ **IQ** **SH** **SL** ✛ **I70.649**　**Atherosclerosis of nonbiological bypass graft(s) of the left leg with ulceration of unspecified site**

☐ **SP** ✛ **I70.65**　**Atherosclerosis of nonbiological bypass graft(s) of other extremity with ulceration**

> **INCLUDES**　any condition classifiable to I70.618 and I70.628

Use additional code to identify severity of ulcer (L98.49)

✛ ⑥ **I70.66**　**Atherosclerosis of nonbiological bypass graft(s) of the extremities with gangrene**

> **INCLUDES**　any condition classifiable to I70.61-, I70.62-, I70.63-, I70.64-, I70.65

Use additional code to identify the severity of any ulcer (L97.-, L98.49-), if applicable

☐ **SP** ✛ **I70.661**　**Atherosclerosis of nonbiological bypass graft(s) of the extremities with gangrene, right leg**

☐ **SP** ✛ **I70.662**　**Atherosclerosis of nonbiological bypass graft(s) of the extremities with gangrene, left leg**

☐ **SP** ✛ **I70.663**　**Atherosclerosis of nonbiological bypass graft(s) of the extremities with gangrene, bilateral legs**

☐ **SP** ✛ **I70.668**　**Atherosclerosis of nonbiological bypass graft(s) of the extremities with gangrene, other extremity**

☐ **IQ** ✛ **I70.669**　**Atherosclerosis of nonbiological bypass graft(s) of the extremities with gangrene, unspecified extremity**

✛ ⑥ **I70.69**　**Other atherosclerosis of nonbiological bypass graft(s) of the extremities**

☐ **SP** ✛ **I70.691**　**Other atherosclerosis of nonbiological bypass graft(s) of the extremities, right leg**

☐ **SP** ✛ **I70.692**　**Other atherosclerosis of nonbiological bypass graft(s) of the extremities, left leg**

☐ **SP** ✛ **I70.693**　**Other atherosclerosis of nonbiological bypass graft(s) of the extremities, bilateral legs**

☐ **SP** ✛ **I70.698**　**Other atherosclerosis of nonbiological bypass graft(s) of the extremities, other extremity**

☐ **IQ** ✛ **I70.699**　**Other atherosclerosis of nonbiological bypass graft(s) of the extremities, unspecified extremity**

✛ ⑤ **I70.7**　**Atherosclerosis of other type of bypass graft(s) of the extremities**

Use additional code, if applicable, to identify chronic total occlusion of artery of extremity (I70.92)

> **CODING TIPS ✓**　Peripheral angiopathy may be documented as diabetic PVD. There is an assumed relationship between diabetes and PVD and PAD, including peripheral atherosclerosis. Diabetic arteriosclerosis of the peripheral arteries should be coded E--.51 or E--.52 then the appropriate I70.- code.

✛ ⑥ **I70.70**　**Unspecified atherosclerosis of other type of bypass graft(s) of the extremities**

☐ **SP** ✛ **I70.701**　**Unspecified atherosclerosis of other type of bypass graft(s) of the extremities, right leg**

☐ **SP** ✛ **I70.702**　**Unspecified atherosclerosis of other type of bypass graft(s) of the extremities, left leg**

☐ **SP** ✛ **I70.703**　**Unspecified atherosclerosis of other type of bypass graft(s) of the extremities, bilateral legs**

☐ **SP** ✛ **I70.708**　**Unspecified atherosclerosis of other type of bypass graft(s) of the extremities, other extremity**

☐ **IQ** ✛ **I70.709**　**Unspecified atherosclerosis of other type of bypass graft(s) of the extremities, unspecified extremity**

✛ ⑥ **I70.71**　**Atherosclerosis of other type of bypass graft(s) of the extremities with intermittent claudication**

---

④4th digit required　⑤5th digit required　⑥6th digit required　⑦7th digit required　⑦7th digit placeholder　✛Additional code　☐Laterality

1002　　　*DecisionHealth's* FY 2020 Complete Home Health ICD-10-CM Diagnosis Coding Manual

□ SP + **I70.711** **Atherosclerosis of other type of bypass graft(s) of the extremities with intermittent claudication, right leg**

□ SP + **I70.712** **Atherosclerosis of other type of bypass graft(s) of the extremities with intermittent claudication, left leg**

□ SP + **I70.713** **Atherosclerosis of other type of bypass graft(s) of the extremities with intermittent claudication, bilateral legs**

□ SP + **I70.718** **Atherosclerosis of other type of bypass graft(s) of the extremities with intermittent claudication, other extremity**

□ IQ + **I70.719** **Atherosclerosis of other type of bypass graft(s) of the extremities with intermittent claudication, unspecified extremity**

+ 6 **I70.72** **Atherosclerosis of other type of bypass graft(s) of the extremities with rest pain**
> INCLUDES   any condition classifiable to I70.71-

□ SP + **I70.721** **Atherosclerosis of other type of bypass graft(s) of the extremities with rest pain, right leg**

□ SP + **I70.722** **Atherosclerosis of other type of bypass graft(s) of the extremities with rest pain, left leg**

□ SP + **I70.723** **Atherosclerosis of other type of bypass graft(s) of the extremities with rest pain, bilateral legs**

□ SP + **I70.728** **Atherosclerosis of other type of bypass graft(s) of the extremities with rest pain, other extremity**

□ IQ + **I70.729** **Atherosclerosis of other type of bypass graft(s) of the extremities with rest pain, unspecified extremity**

+ 6 **I70.73** **Atherosclerosis of other type of bypass graft(s) of the right leg with ulceration**
> INCLUDES   any condition classifiable to I70.711 and I70.721
> Use additional code to identify severity of ulcer (L97.-)

□ SP SH SL + **I70.731** **Atherosclerosis of other type of bypass graft(s) of the right leg with ulceration of thigh**

□ SP SH SL + **I70.732** **Atherosclerosis of other type of bypass graft(s) of the right leg with ulceration of calf**

□ SP SH SL + **I70.733** **Atherosclerosis of other type of bypass graft(s) of the right leg with ulceration of ankle**

□ SP SH SL + **I70.734** **Atherosclerosis of other type of bypass graft(s) of the right leg with ulceration of heel and midfoot**
Atherosclerosis of other type of bypass graft(s) of right leg with ulceration of plantar surface of midfoot

□ SP SH SL + **I70.735** **Atherosclerosis of other type of bypass graft(s) of the right leg with ulceration of other part of foot**

Atherosclerosis of other type of bypass graft(s) of right leg with ulceration of toe

□ SP SH SL + **I70.738** **Atherosclerosis of other type of bypass graft(s) of the right leg with ulceration of other part of lower leg**

□ IQ SH SL + **I70.739** **Atherosclerosis of other type of bypass graft(s) of the right leg with ulceration of unspecified site**

+ 6 **I70.74** **Atherosclerosis of other type of bypass graft(s) of the left leg with ulceration**
> INCLUDES   any condition classifiable to I70.712 and I70.722
> Use additional code to identify severity of ulcer (L97.-)

□ SP SH SL + **I70.741** **Atherosclerosis of other type of bypass graft(s) of the left leg with ulceration of thigh**

□ SP SH SL + **I70.742** **Atherosclerosis of other type of bypass graft(s) of the left leg with ulceration of calf**

□ SP SH SL + **I70.743** **Atherosclerosis of other type of bypass graft(s) of the left leg with ulceration of ankle**

□ SP SH SL + **I70.744** **Atherosclerosis of other type of bypass graft(s) of the left leg with ulceration of heel and midfoot**
Atherosclerosis of other type of bypass graft(s) of left leg with ulceration of plantar surface of midfoot

□ SP SH SL + **I70.745** **Atherosclerosis of other type of bypass graft(s) of the left leg with ulceration of other part of foot**
Atherosclerosis of other type of bypass graft(s) of left leg with ulceration of toe

□ SP SH SL + **I70.748** **Atherosclerosis of other type of bypass graft(s) of the left leg with ulceration of other part of lower leg**

□ IQ SH SL + **I70.749** **Atherosclerosis of other type of bypass graft(s) of the left leg with ulceration of unspecified site**

□ SP + **I70.75** **Atherosclerosis of other type of bypass graft(s) of other extremity with ulceration**
> INCLUDES   any condition classifiable to I70.718 and I70.728
> Use additional code to identify severity of ulcer (L98.49)

+ 6 **I70.76** **Atherosclerosis of other type of bypass graft(s) of the extremities with gangrene**
> INCLUDES   any condition classifiable to I70.71-, I70.72-, I70.73-, I70.74-, I70.75
> Use additional code to identify the severity of any ulcer (L97.-, L98.49-), if applicable

□ SP + **I70.761** **Atherosclerosis of other type of bypass graft(s) of the extremities with gangrene, right leg**

□ SP + **I70.762** **Atherosclerosis of other type of bypass graft(s) of the extremities with gangrene, left leg**

★ New ▲ Revised Px Primary SP PDGM Px SL Low CoM SH High CoM IQ Quest. Encounter H Hospice non-cancer Dx   Unspecified   M *Manifestation*

DecisionHealth's FY 2020 Complete Home Health ICD-10-CM Diagnosis Coding Manual

1003

Chapter 9

I00-I99

☰ **SP** ✚ **I70.763** Atherosclerosis of other type of bypass graft(s) of the extremities with gangrene, bilateral legs

☰ **SP** ✚ **I70.768** Atherosclerosis of other type of bypass graft(s) of the extremities with gangrene, other extremity

☰ **IQ** ✚ **I70.769** Atherosclerosis of other type of bypass graft(s) of the extremities with gangrene, unspecified extremity

✚ **6** **I70.79** Other atherosclerosis of other type of bypass graft(s) of the extremities

☰ **SP** ✚ **I70.791** Other atherosclerosis of other type of bypass graft(s) of the extremities, right leg

☰ **SP** ✚ **I70.792** Other atherosclerosis of other type of bypass graft(s) of the extremities, left leg

☰ **SP** ✚ **I70.793** Other atherosclerosis of other type of bypass graft(s) of the extremities, bilateral legs

☰ **SP** ✚ **I70.798** Other atherosclerosis of other type of bypass graft(s) of the extremities, other extremity

☰ **IQ** ✚ **I70.799** Other atherosclerosis of other type of bypass graft(s) of the extremities, unspecified extremity

SP ✚ **I70.8** Atherosclerosis of other arteries

CODING TIPS ✓ Peripheral angiopathy may be documented as diabetic PVD. There is an assumed relationship between diabetes and PVD and PAD, including peripheral atherosclerosis. Diabetic arteriosclerosis of the peripheral arteries should be coded E--.51 or E--.52 then the appropriate I70.- code.

✚ **5** **I70.9** Other and unspecified atherosclerosis

SP **SH** ✚ **I70.90** Unspecified atherosclerosis

SP **SH** ✚ **I70.91** Generalized atherosclerosis

SP ✚ **I70.92** Chronic total occlusion of artery of the extremities
Complete occlusion of artery of the extremities
Total occlusion of artery of the extremities
Code first:
atherosclerosis of arteries of the extremities (I70.2-, I70.3-, I70.4-, I70.5-, I70.6-, I70.7-)

4 **I71** Aortic aneurysm and dissection
EXCLUDES 1 aortic ectasia (I77.81-)
syphilitic aortic aneurysm (A52.01)
traumatic aortic aneurysm (S25.09, S35.09)

5 **I71.0** Dissection of aorta

SP **I71.00** Dissection of unspecified site of aorta

SP **I71.01** Dissection of thoracic aorta

SP **I71.02** Dissection of abdominal aorta

SP **I71.03** Dissection of thoracoabdominal aorta

SP **I71.1** Thoracic aortic aneurysm, ruptured

SP **SH** **I71.2** Thoracic aortic aneurysm, without rupture

SP **I71.3** Abdominal aortic aneurysm, ruptured

SP **SH** **I71.4** Abdominal aortic aneurysm, without rupture

SP **I71.5** Thoracoabdominal aortic aneurysm, ruptured

SP **SH** **I71.6** Thoracoabdominal aortic aneurysm, without rupture

IQ **I71.8** Aortic aneurysm of unspecified site, ruptured
Rupture of aorta NOS

IQ **I71.9** Aortic aneurysm of unspecified site, without rupture
Aneurysm of aorta
Dilatation of aorta
Hyaline necrosis of aorta

4 **I72** Other aneurysm
INCLUDES aneurysm (cirsoid) (false) (ruptured)
EXCLUDES 2 acquired aneurysm (I77.0)
aneurysm (of) aorta (I71.-)
aneurysm (of) arteriovenous NOS (Q27.3-)
carotid artery dissection (I77.71)
cerebral (nonruptured) aneurysm (I67.1)
coronary aneurysm (I25.4)
coronary artery dissection (I25.42)
dissection of artery NEC (I77.79)
dissection of precerebral artery, congenital (nonruptured) (Q28.1)
heart aneurysm (I25.3)
iliac artery dissection (I77.72)
precerebral artery, congenital (nonruptured) (Q28.1)
pulmonary artery aneurysm (I28.1)
renal artery dissection (I77.73)
retinal aneurysm (H35.0)
ruptured cerebral aneurysm (I60.7)
varicose aneurysm (I77.0)
vertebral artery dissection (I77.74)

SP **I72.0** Aneurysm of carotid artery
Aneurysm of common carotid artery
Aneurysm of external carotid artery
Aneurysm of internal carotid artery, extracranial portion
EXCLUDES 1 aneurysm of internal carotid artery, intracranial portion (I67.1)
aneurysm of internal carotid artery NOS (I67.1)

SP **I72.1** Aneurysm of artery of upper extremity

SP **I72.2** Aneurysm of renal artery

SP **I72.3** Aneurysm of iliac artery

SP **I72.4** Aneurysm of artery of lower extremity

SP **I72.5** Aneurysm of other precerebral arteries
Aneurysm of basilar artery (trunk)
EXCLUDES 2 aneurysm of carotid artery (I72.0)

---

4 4th digit required   **5** 5th digit required   **6** 6th digit required   **7** 7th digit required   ☑ 7th digit placeholder   ✚ Additional code   ☰ Laterality

aneurysm of vertebral artery
(I72.6)
dissection of carotid artery
(I77.71)
dissection of other
precerebral arteries
(I77.75)
dissection of vertebral artery
(I77.74)

SP I72.6 Aneurysm of vertebral artery
EXCLUDES 2 dissection of vertebral artery
(I77.74)

SP I72.8 Aneurysm of other specified arteries

IQ I72.9 Aneurysm of unspecified site

4 I73 Other peripheral vascular diseases
EXCLUDES 2 chilblains (T69.1)
frostbite (T33-T34)
immersion hand or foot
(T69.0-)
spasm of cerebral artery
(G45.9)

5 I73.0 Raynaud's syndrome
Raynaud's disease
Raynaud's phenomenon (secondary)

SP I73.00 Raynaud's syndrome without gangrene

SP I73.01 Raynaud's syndrome with gangrene
DEFINITION Medium-sized blood
vessels of the hands and feet become
inflamed and blocked by blood clots,
causing gangrene of the extremities.

SP I73.1 Thromboangiitis obliterans [Buerger's disease]

5 I73.8 Other specified peripheral vascular diseases
EXCLUDES 1 diabetic (peripheral)
angiopathy (E08-E13 with
.51-.52)

SP I73.81 Erythromelalgia
DEFINITION Abnormal dilation of
extremity blood vessels, especially in
the feet, causing a painful, burning
sensation, and redness.

SP I73.89 Other specified peripheral vascular diseases
Acrocyanosis
Erythrocyanosis
Simple acroparesthesia [Schultze's
type]
Vasomotor acroparesthesia
[Nothnagel's type]

SP SH I73.9 Peripheral vascular disease, unspecified
Intermittent claudication
Peripheral angiopathy NOS
Spasm of artery
EXCLUDES 1 atherosclerosis of the
extremities (I70.2--I70.7-)

CODING TIPS ✓ Do not assign I73.9
when peripheral atherosclerosis is reported
in the clinical record. Note, atherosclerosis
of the extremities is a more specific
diagnosis and should be coded using a
code from I70.2- through I70.7-. When PVD
is documented in a diabetic, use the
appropriate code for diabetic peripheral
angiopathy instead, and also assign a code
from I70.- if specific information about the
diagnosis if available.

CODING TIPS ✓ I73.9 is used for peripheral
vascular disease and peripheral arterial
disease (angiopathy). If the physician
documents venous disease, I80-I89 should
be referenced.

4 I74 Arterial embolism and thrombosis
INCLUDES embolic infarction
embolic occlusion
thrombotic infarction
thrombotic occlusion
Code first:
embolism and thrombosis complicating
abortion or ectopic or molar pregnancy
(O00-O07, O08.2)
embolism and thrombosis complicating
pregnancy, childbirth and the puerperium
(O88.-)
EXCLUDES 2 atheroembolism (I75.-)
basilar embolism and
thrombosis
(I63.0-I63.2, I65.1)
carotid embolism and
thrombosis
(I63.0-I63.2, I65.2)
cerebral embolism and
thrombosis
(I63.3-I63.5, I66.-)
coronary embolism and
thrombosis (I21-I25)
mesenteric embolism and
thrombosis (K55.0-)
ophthalmic embolism and
thrombosis (H34.-)
precerebral embolism and
thrombosis NOS
(I63.0-I63.2, I65.9)
pulmonary embolism and
thrombosis (I26.-)
renal embolism and thrombosis
(N28.0)
retinal embolism and
thrombosis (H34.-)
septic embolism and thrombosis
(I76)
vertebral embolism and
thrombosis
(I63.0-I63.2, I65.0)

5 I74.0 Embolism and thrombosis of abdominal aorta

SP I74.01 Saddle embolus of abdominal aorta

SP I74.09 Other arterial embolism and thrombosis of abdominal aorta
Aortic bifurcation syndrome
Aortoiliac obstruction
Leriche's syndrome

5 I74.1 Embolism and thrombosis of other and unspecified parts of aorta

---

★ New ▲ Revised Px Primary SP PDGM Px SL Low CoM SH High CoM IQ Quest. Encounter H Hospice non-cancer Dx Unspecified M *Manifestation*

SP I74.10 **Embolism and thrombosis of unspecified parts of aorta**

SP I74.11 **Embolism and thrombosis of thoracic aorta**

SP I74.19 **Embolism and thrombosis of other parts of aorta**

SP I74.2 **Embolism and thrombosis of arteries of the upper extremities**

SP I74.3 **Embolism and thrombosis of arteries of the lower extremities**

!Q I74.4 **Embolism and thrombosis of arteries of extremities, unspecified**
Peripheral arterial embolism NOS

SP I74.5 **Embolism and thrombosis of iliac artery**

SP I74.8 **Embolism and thrombosis of other arteries**

!Q I74.9 **Embolism and thrombosis of unspecified artery**

4 I75 **Atheroembolism**
> INCLUDES   atherothrombotic microembolism
> cholesterol embolism

5 I75.0 **Atheroembolism of extremities**

6 I75.01 **Atheroembolism of upper extremity**

SP I75.011 **Atheroembolism of right upper extremity**

SP I75.012 **Atheroembolism of left upper extremity**

SP I75.013 **Atheroembolism of bilateral upper extremities**

!Q I75.019 **Atheroembolism of unspecified upper extremity**

6 I75.02 **Atheroembolism of lower extremity**

SP I75.021 **Atheroembolism of right lower extremity**

SP I75.022 **Atheroembolism of left lower extremity**

SP I75.023 **Atheroembolism of bilateral lower extremities**

!Q I75.029 **Atheroembolism of unspecified lower extremity**

5 I75.8 **Atheroembolism of other sites**

SP + I75.81 **Atheroembolism of kidney**
Use additional code for any associated acute kidney failure and chronic kidney disease (N17.-, N18.-)

SP I75.89 **Atheroembolism of other site**

SP + I76 **Septic arterial embolism**
Code first underlying infection, such as:
infective endocarditis (I33.0)
lung abscess (J85.-)
Use additional code to identify the site of the embolism (I74.-)
> EXCLUDES 2   septic pulmonary embolism (I26.01, I26.90)

> DEFINITION   Dislodged material from a centralized infection lodged in a small arteriole, causing tissue death due to bacteria and lack of blood supply.

4 I77 **Other disorders of arteries and arterioles**
> EXCLUDES 2   collagen (vascular) diseases (M30-M36)
> hypersensitivity angiitis (M31.0)
> pulmonary artery (I28.-)

SP I77.0 **Arteriovenous fistula, acquired**
Aneurysmal varix
Arteriovenous aneurysm, acquired
> EXCLUDES 1   arteriovenous aneurysm NOS (Q27.3-)
> presence of arteriovenous shunt (fistula) for dialysis (Z99.2)
> traumatic - see injury of blood vessel by body region
> EXCLUDES 2   cerebral (I67.1)
> coronary (I25.4)

SP I77.1 **Stricture of artery**
Narrowing of artery

SP I77.2 **Rupture of artery**
Erosion of artery
Fistula of artery
Ulcer of artery
> EXCLUDES 1   traumatic rupture of artery - see injury of blood vessel by body region

> CODING TIPS ✓   Do not assign code I77.2 for a traumatic rupture of the artery. A fistula, ulcer, or arterial erosion would be coded to I77.2.

SP I77.3 **Arterial fibromuscular dysplasia**
Fibromuscular hyperplasia (of) carotid artery
Fibromuscular hyperplasia (of) renal artery

SP I77.4 **Celiac artery compression syndrome**

SP I77.5 **Necrosis of artery**

SP I77.6 **Arteritis, unspecified**
Aortitis NOS
Endarteritis NOS
> EXCLUDES 1   arteritis or endarteritis:
> aortic arch (M31.4)
> cerebral NEC (I67.7)
> coronary (I25.89)
> deformans (I70.-)
> giant cell (M31.5, M31.6)
> obliterans (I70.-)
> senile (I70.-)

5 I77.7 **Other arterial dissection**
> EXCLUDES 2   dissection of aorta (I71.0-)
> dissection of coronary artery (I25.42)

!Q I77.70 **Dissection of unspecified artery**

SP I77.71 **Dissection of carotid artery**

SP I77.72 **Dissection of iliac artery**

SP I77.73 **Dissection of renal artery**

SP I77.74 **Dissection of vertebral artery**
> EXCLUDES 2   aneurysm of vertebral artery (I72.6)

SP I77.75 **Dissection of other precerebral arteries**
Dissection of basilar artery (trunk)
> EXCLUDES 2   aneurysm of carotid artery (I72.0)
> aneurysm of other precerebral arteries (I72.5)
> aneurysm of vertebral artery (I72.6)
> dissection of carotid artery (I77.71)

---

4 4th digit required   5 5th digit required   6 6th digit required   7 7th digit required   7 7th digit placeholder   + Additional code   E Laterality

1006   DecisionHealth's FY 2020 Complete Home Health ICD-10-CM Diagnosis Coding Manual

dissection of vertebral
artery (I77.74)

SP **I77.76** **Dissection of artery of upper
extremity**

SP **I77.77** **Dissection of artery of lower
extremity**

SP **I77.79** **Dissection of other specified artery**

5 **I77.8** **Other specified disorders of arteries and
arterioles**

6 **I77.81** **Aortic ectasia**
Ectasis aorta
EXCLUDES 1 aortic aneurysm and
dissection (I71.0-)

SP **I77.810** **Thoracic aortic ectasia**

SP **I77.811** **Abdominal aortic ectasia**

SP **I77.812** **Thoracoabdominal aortic ectasia**

SP **I77.819** **Aortic ectasia, unspecified site**

SP **I77.89** **Other specified disorders of arteries
and arterioles**

IQ **I77.9** **Disorder of arteries and arterioles,
unspecified**

4 **I78** **Diseases of capillaries**

SP **I78.0** **Hereditary hemorrhagic telangiectasia**
Rendu-Osler-Weber disease

SP **I78.1** **Nevus, non-neoplastic**
Araneus nevus
Senile nevus
Spider nevus
Stellar nevus
EXCLUDES 1 nevus NOS (D22.-)
vascular NOS (Q82.5)
EXCLUDES 2 blue nevus (D22.-)
flammeus nevus (Q82.5)
hairy nevus (D22.-)
melanocytic nevus (D22.-)
pigmented nevus (D22.-)
portwine nevus (Q82.5)
sanguineous nevus (Q82.5)
strawberry nevus (Q82.5)
verrucous nevus (Q82.5)

SP **I78.8** **Other diseases of capillaries**

IQ **I78.9** **Disease of capillaries, unspecified**

4 **I79** **Disorders of arteries, arterioles and
capillaries in diseases classified elsewhere**
CODING TIPS ✓ Codes from category I79.-
should be coded only when the arterial
disease/dysfunction is specified as due to
another primary disease process. The
causative disease process should be coded
first.

M **IQ** **SH** **I79.0** *Aneurysm of aorta in diseases classified
elsewhere*
Code first:
underlying disease
EXCLUDES 1 syphilitic aneurysm
(A52.01)
CODING TIPS ✓ I79.0 should be coded only
when an aortic aneurysm is specified as
due to another primary disease process.
The causative disease process should be
coded first.

M **IQ** **I79.1** *Aortitis in diseases classified elsewhere*
Code first:
underlying disease
EXCLUDES 1 syphilitic aortitis (A52.02)

M **IQ** **I79.8** *Other disorders of arteries, arterioles
and capillaries in diseases classified
elsewhere*
Code first underlying disease, such as:
amyloidosis (E85.-)
EXCLUDES 1 diabetic (peripheral)
angiopathy (E08-E13 with
.51-.52)
syphilitic endarteritis
(A52.09)
tuberculous endarteritis
(A18.89)

Diseases of veins, lymphatic vessels and lymph nodes, not elsewhere classified (I80-I89)

4 **I80** **Phlebitis and thrombophlebitis**
INCLUDES endophlebitis
inflammation, vein
periphlebitis
suppurative phlebitis
Code first:
phlebitis and thrombophlebitis complicating
abortion, ectopic or molar pregnancy
(O00-O07, O08.7)
phlebitis and thrombophlebitis complicating
pregnancy, childbirth and the puerperium
(O22.-, O87.-)
EXCLUDES 1 venous embolism and
thrombosis of lower
extremities
(I82.4-, I82.5-, I82.81-)

5 **I80.0** **Phlebitis and thrombophlebitis of
superficial vessels of lower extremities**
Phlebitis and thrombophlebitis of
femoropopliteal vein

IQ **I80.00** **Phlebitis and thrombophlebitis of
superficial vessels of unspecified
lower extremity**

SP **I80.01** **Phlebitis and thrombophlebitis of
superficial vessels of right lower
extremity**

SP **I80.02** **Phlebitis and thrombophlebitis of
superficial vessels of left lower
extremity**

SP **I80.03** **Phlebitis and thrombophlebitis of
superficial vessels of lower
extremities, bilateral**

▲ **5** **I80.1** **Phlebitis and thrombophlebitis of
femoral vein**
Phlebitis and thrombophlebitis of common
femoral vein
Phlebitis and thrombophlebitis of deep
femoral vein
CODING TIPS ✓ Deep vein thrombosis in the
proximal deep veins is more significant than
deep vein thrombosis in the distal deep
veins. Veins of the thigh are the iliac and
femoral.

IQ **I80.10** **Phlebitis and thrombophlebitis of
unspecified femoral vein**

SP **I80.11** **Phlebitis and thrombophlebitis of
right femoral vein**

SP **I80.12** **Phlebitis and thrombophlebitis of
left femoral vein**

SP **I80.13** **Phlebitis and thrombophlebitis of
femoral vein, bilateral**

★ New ▲ Revised **Px** Primary **SP** PDGM Px **SL** Low CoM **SH** High CoM **IQ** Quest. Encounter **H** Hospice non-cancer Dx Unspecified **M** *Manifestation*

DecisionHealth's FY 2020 Complete Home Health ICD-10-CM Diagnosis Coding Manual

1007

⑤ I80.2 **Phlebitis and thrombophlebitis of other and unspecified deep vessels of lower extremities**

CODING TIPS ✓ Deep vein thrombosis in the proximal deep veins is more significant than deep vein thrombosis in the distal deep veins. Veins of the calf include the peroneal, gastrocnemial, tibial and soleal. Veins of the thigh are the iliac and femoral.

⑥ I80.20 **Phlebitis and thrombophlebitis of unspecified deep vessels of lower extremities**

🔲 SP I80.201 **Phlebitis and thrombophlebitis of unspecified deep vessels of right lower extremity**

🔲 SP I80.202 **Phlebitis and thrombophlebitis of unspecified deep vessels of left lower extremity**

🔲 SP I80.203 **Phlebitis and thrombophlebitis of unspecified deep vessels of lower extremities, bilateral**

🔲 IQ I80.209 **Phlebitis and thrombophlebitis of unspecified deep vessels of unspecified lower extremity**

▲ ⑥ I80.21 **Phlebitis and thrombophlebitis of iliac vein**
Phlebitis and thrombophlebitis of common iliac vein
Phlebitis and thrombophlebitis of external iliac vein
Phlebitis and thrombophlebitis of internal iliac vein

🔲 SP I80.211 **Phlebitis and thrombophlebitis of right iliac vein**

🔲 SP I80.212 **Phlebitis and thrombophlebitis of left iliac vein**

🔲 SP I80.213 **Phlebitis and thrombophlebitis of iliac vein, bilateral**

🔲 IQ I80.219 **Phlebitis and thrombophlebitis of unspecified iliac vein**

⑥ I80.22 **Phlebitis and thrombophlebitis of popliteal vein**

🔲 SP I80.221 **Phlebitis and thrombophlebitis of right popliteal vein**

🔲 SP I80.222 **Phlebitis and thrombophlebitis of left popliteal vein**

🔲 SP I80.223 **Phlebitis and thrombophlebitis of popliteal vein, bilateral**

🔲 IQ I80.229 **Phlebitis and thrombophlebitis of unspecified popliteal vein**

▲ ⑥ I80.23 **Phlebitis and thrombophlebitis of tibial vein**
Phlebitis and thrombophlebitis of anterior tibial vein
Phlebitis and thrombophlebitis of posterior tibial vein

🔲 SP I80.231 **Phlebitis and thrombophlebitis of right tibial vein**

🔲 SP I80.232 **Phlebitis and thrombophlebitis of left tibial vein**

🔲 SP I80.233 **Phlebitis and thrombophlebitis of tibial vein, bilateral**

🔲 SP I80.239 **Phlebitis and thrombophlebitis of unspecified tibial vein**

★ ⑥ I80.24 **Phlebitis and thrombophlebitis of peroneal vein**

★ 🔲 I80.241 **Phlebitis and thrombophlebitis of right peroneal vein**

★ 🔲 I80.242 **Phlebitis and thrombophlebitis of left peroneal vein**

★ 🔲 I80.243 **Phlebitis and thrombophlebitis of peroneal vein, bilateral**

★ 🔲 I80.249 **Phlebitis and thrombophlebitis of unspecified peroneal vein**

★ ⑥ I80.25 **Phlebitis and thrombophlebitis of calf muscular vein**
Phlebitis and thrombophlebitis of calf muscular vein, NOS
Phlebitis and thrombophlebitis of gastrocnemial vein
Phlebitis and thrombophlebitis of soleal vein

★ 🔲 I80.251 **Phlebitis and thrombophlebitis of right calf muscular vein**

★ 🔲 I80.252 **Phlebitis and thrombophlebitis of left calf muscular vein**

★ 🔲 I80.253 **Phlebitis and thrombophlebitis of calf muscular vein, bilateral**

★ 🔲 I80.259 **Phlebitis and thrombophlebitis of unspecified calf muscular vein**

⑥ I80.29 **Phlebitis and thrombophlebitis of other deep vessels of lower extremities**

🔲 IQ I80.291 **Phlebitis and thrombophlebitis of other deep vessels of right lower extremity**

🔲 SP I80.292 **Phlebitis and thrombophlebitis of other deep vessels of left lower extremity**

🔲 SP I80.293 **Phlebitis and thrombophlebitis of other deep vessels of lower extremity, bilateral**

🔲 IQ I80.299 **Phlebitis and thrombophlebitis of other deep vessels of unspecified lower extremity**

SP I80.3 **Phlebitis and thrombophlebitis of lower extremities, unspecified**

SP I80.8 **Phlebitis and thrombophlebitis of other sites**

IQ I80.9 **Phlebitis and thrombophlebitis of unspecified site**

SP I81 **Portal vein thrombosis**
Portal (vein) obstruction
EXCLUDES 2 hepatic vein thrombosis (I82.0)
phlebitis of portal vein (K75.1)
CODING TIPS ✓ Portal vein thrombosis is a specific clinical condition caused by the occlusion/obstruction of the portal vein but does not include occlusion of the hepatic vein, and is relatively common in cirrhosis patients. It often leads to portal hypertension. When this condition occurs, any comorbid hepatic vein thrombosis and/or portal hypertension should also be coded.

④ I82 **Other venous embolism and thrombosis**
Code first venous embolism and thrombosis complicating:
abortion, ectopic or molar pregnancy (O00-O07, O08.7)
pregnancy, childbirth and the puerperium (O22.-, O87.-)
EXCLUDES 2 venous embolism and thrombosis (of) :

---

④4th digit required   ⑤5th digit required   ⑥6th digit required   ⑦7th digit required   ☑7th digit placeholder   ✚Additional code   🔲Laterality

1008   *DecisionHealth's* FY 2020 Complete Home Health ICD-10-CM Diagnosis Coding Manual

cerebral (I63.6, I67.6)
coronary (I21-I25)
intracranial and intraspinal,
  septic or NOS (G08)
intracranial, nonpyogenic
  (I67.6)
intraspinal, nonpyogenic
  (G95.1)
mesenteric (K55.0-)
portal (I81)
pulmonary (I26.-)

SP SL I82.0 Budd-Chiari syndrome
Hepatic vein thrombosis

> **DEFINITION** Obstruction or occlusion of the hepatic veins, causing an enlarged liver, abdominal pain/tenderness, intractable ascites, mild jaundice, portal hypertension, and liver failure.

SP SL I82.1 Thrombophlebitis migrans

5 I82.2 Embolism and thrombosis of vena cava and other thoracic veins

6 I82.21 Embolism and thrombosis of superior vena cava

SP SL I82.210 Acute embolism and thrombosis of superior vena cava
Embolism and thrombosis of superior vena cava NOS

SP SL I82.211 Chronic embolism and thrombosis of superior vena cava

6 I82.22 Embolism and thrombosis of inferior vena cava

SP SL I82.220 Acute embolism and thrombosis of inferior vena cava
Embolism and thrombosis of inferior vena cava NOS

SP SL I82.221 Chronic embolism and thrombosis of inferior vena cava

6 I82.29 Embolism and thrombosis of other thoracic veins
Embolism and thrombosis of brachiocephalic (innominate) vein

SP SL I82.290 Acute embolism and thrombosis of other thoracic veins

SP SL I82.291 Chronic embolism and thrombosis of other thoracic veins

SP SL I82.3 Embolism and thrombosis of renal vein

5 I82.4 Acute embolism and thrombosis of deep veins of lower extremity

> **CODING TIPS ✓** Acute embolism and thrombosis codes are used unless the physician indicates the condition is chronic.

6 I82.40 Acute embolism and thrombosis of unspecified deep veins of lower extremity
Deep vein thrombosis NOS
DVT NOS

> **EXCLUDES 1** acute embolism and thrombosis of unspecified deep veins of distal lower extremity (I82.4Z-)
> acute embolism and thrombosis of unspecified deep veins of proximal lower extremity (I82.4Y-)

SP SL I82.401 Acute embolism and thrombosis of unspecified deep veins of right lower extremity

SP SL I82.402 Acute embolism and thrombosis of unspecified deep veins of left lower extremity

SP SL I82.403 Acute embolism and thrombosis of unspecified deep veins of lower extremity, bilateral

SP I82.409 Acute embolism and thrombosis of unspecified deep veins of unspecified lower extremity

▲ 6 I82.41 Acute embolism and thrombosis of femoral vein
Acute embolism and thrombosis of common femoral vein
Acute embolism and thrombosis of deep femoral vein

> **CODING TIPS ✓** Deep vein thrombosis in the proximal deep veins is more significant than deep vein thrombosis in the distal deep veins. Veins of the thigh are the iliac and femoral.

SP SL I82.411 Acute embolism and thrombosis of right femoral vein

SP SL I82.412 Acute embolism and thrombosis of left femoral vein

SP SL I82.413 Acute embolism and thrombosis of femoral vein, bilateral

IQ I82.419 Acute embolism and thrombosis of unspecified femoral vein

▲ 6 I82.42 Acute embolism and thrombosis of iliac vein
Acute embolism and thrombosis of common iliac vein
Acute embolism and thrombosis of external iliac vein
Acute embolism and thrombosis of internal iliac vein

> **CODING TIPS ✓** Deep vein thrombosis in the proximal deep veins is more significant than deep vein thrombosis in the distal deep veins. Veins of the thigh are the iliac and femoral.

SP SL I82.421 Acute embolism and thrombosis of right iliac vein

SP SL I82.422 Acute embolism and thrombosis of left iliac vein

SP SL I82.423 Acute embolism and thrombosis of iliac vein, bilateral

IQ I82.429 Acute embolism and thrombosis of unspecified iliac vein

6 I82.43 Acute embolism and thrombosis of popliteal vein

SP SL I82.431 Acute embolism and thrombosis of right popliteal vein

SP SL I82.432 Acute embolism and thrombosis of left popliteal vein

SP SL I82.433 Acute embolism and thrombosis of popliteal vein, bilateral

IQ I82.439 Acute embolism and thrombosis of unspecified popliteal vein

▲ 6 I82.44 Acute embolism and thrombosis of tibial vein
Acute embolism and thrombosis of anterior tibial vein

★ New ▲ Revised Px Primary SP PDGM Px SL Low CoM SH High CoM IQ Quest. Encounter H Hospice non-cancer Dx Unspecified M Manifestation

DecisionHealth's FY 2020 Complete Home Health ICD-10-CM Diagnosis Coding Manual

1009

Chapter 9

I00-I99

Acute embolism and thrombosis of posterior tibial vein

> **CODING TIPS ✓** Deep vein thrombosis in the proximal deep veins is more significant than deep vein thrombosis in the distal deep veins. Veins of the calf include the peroneal, gastrocnemial, tibial and soleal.

⊟ **SP SL I82.441**   **Acute embolism and thrombosis of right tibial vein**

⊟ **SP SL I82.442**   **Acute embolism and thrombosis of left tibial vein**

⊟ **SP SL I82.443**   **Acute embolism and thrombosis of tibial vein, bilateral**

⊟ **IQ I82.449**   **Acute embolism and thrombosis of unspecified tibial vein**

★ 6 **I82.45**   **Acute embolism and thrombosis of peroneal vein**

> **CODING TIPS ✓** Deep vein thrombosis in the proximal deep veins is more significant than deep vein thrombosis in the distal deep veins. Veins of the calf include the peroneal, gastrocnemial, tibial and soleal.

★ ⊟ **I82.451**   **Acute embolism and thrombosis of right peroneal vein**

★ ⊟ **I82.452**   **Acute embolism and thrombosis of left peroneal vein**

★ ⊟ **I82.453**   **Acute embolism and thrombosis of peroneal vein, bilateral**

★ ⊟ **I82.459**   **Acute embolism and thrombosis of unspecified peroneal vein**

★ 6 **I82.46**   **Acute embolism and thrombosis of calf muscular vein**

Acute embolism and thrombosis of calf muscular vein, NOS

Acute embolism and thrombosis of gastrocnemial vein

Acute embolism and thrombosis of soleal vein

> **CODING TIPS ✓** Deep vein thrombosis in the proximal deep veins is more significant than deep vein thrombosis in the distal deep veins. Veins of the calf include the peroneal, gastrocnemial, tibial and soleal.

★ ⊟ **I82.461**   **Acute embolism and thrombosis of right calf muscular vein**

★ ⊟ **I82.462**   **Acute embolism and thrombosis of left calf muscular vein**

★ ⊟ **I82.463**   **Acute embolism and thrombosis of calf muscular vein, bilateral**

★ ⊟ **I82.469**   **Acute embolism and thrombosis of unspecified calf muscular vein**

6 **I82.49**   **Acute embolism and thrombosis of other specified deep vein of lower extremity**

⊟ **SP SL I82.491**   **Acute embolism and thrombosis of other specified deep vein of right lower extremity**

⊟ **SP SL I82.492**   **Acute embolism and thrombosis of other specified deep vein of left lower extremity**

⊟ **SP SL I82.493**   **Acute embolism and thrombosis of other specified deep vein of lower extremity, bilateral**

⊟ **IQ I82.499**   **Acute embolism and thrombosis of other specified deep vein of unspecified lower extremity**

6 **I82.4Y**   **Acute embolism and thrombosis of unspecified deep veins of proximal lower extremity**

Acute embolism and thrombosis of deep vein of thigh NOS

Acute embolism and thrombosis of deep vein of upper leg NOS

⊟ **SP SL I82.4Y1**   **Acute embolism and thrombosis of unspecified deep veins of right proximal lower extremity**

⊟ **SP SL I82.4Y2**   **Acute embolism and thrombosis of unspecified deep veins of left proximal lower extremity**

⊟ **SP SL I82.4Y3**   **Acute embolism and thrombosis of unspecified deep veins of proximal lower extremity, bilateral**

⊟ **IQ I82.4Y9**   **Acute embolism and thrombosis of unspecified deep veins of unspecified proximal lower extremity**

6 **I82.4Z**   **Acute embolism and thrombosis of unspecified deep veins of distal lower extremity**

Acute embolism and thrombosis of deep vein of calf NOS

Acute embolism and thrombosis of deep vein of lower leg NOS

⊟ **SP SL I82.4Z1**   **Acute embolism and thrombosis of unspecified deep veins of right distal lower extremity**

⊟ **SP SL I82.4Z2**   **Acute embolism and thrombosis of unspecified deep veins of left distal lower extremity**

⊟ **SP SL I82.4Z3**   **Acute embolism and thrombosis of unspecified deep veins of distal lower extremity, bilateral**

⊟ **IQ I82.4Z9**   **Acute embolism and thrombosis of unspecified deep veins of unspecified distal lower extremity**

➕ 5 **I82.5**   **Chronic embolism and thrombosis of deep veins of lower extremity**

Use additional code, if applicable, for associated long-term (current) use of anticoagulants (Z79.01)

> **EXCLUDES 1** personal history of venous embolism and thrombosis (Z86.718)

> **CODING TIPS ✓** These conditions are considered acute, unless the physician specifies chronic.

➕ 6 **I82.50**   **Chronic embolism and thrombosis of unspecified deep veins of lower extremity**

> **EXCLUDES 1** chronic embolism and thrombosis of unspecified deep veins of distal lower extremity (I82.5Z-)

4 4th digit required   5 5th digit required   6 6th digit required   7 7th digit required   7 7th digit placeholder   ➕ Additional code   ⊟ Laterality

1010   *DecisionHealth's* FY 2020 Complete Home Health ICD-10-CM Diagnosis Coding Manual

chronic embolism and thrombosis of unspecified deep veins of proximal lower extremity (I82.5Y-)

☐ **SP** **SL** **+** I82.501　Chronic embolism and thrombosis of unspecified deep veins of right lower extremity

☐ **SP** **SL** **+** I82.502　Chronic embolism and thrombosis of unspecified deep veins of left lower extremity

☐ **SP** **SL** **+** I82.503　Chronic embolism and thrombosis of unspecified deep veins of lower extremity, bilateral

☐ **IQ** **+** I82.509　Chronic embolism and thrombosis of unspecified deep veins of unspecified lower extremity

▲ **+** **6** I82.51　Chronic embolism and thrombosis of femoral vein
Chronic embolism and thrombosis of common femoral vein
Chronic embolism and thrombosis of deep femoral vein

CODING TIPS ✓　Deep vein thrombosis in the proximal deep veins is more significant than deep vein thrombosis in the distal deep veins. Veins of the thigh are the iliac and femoral.

☐ **SP** **SL** **+** I82.511　Chronic embolism and thrombosis of right femoral vein

☐ **SP** **SL** **+** I82.512　Chronic embolism and thrombosis of left femoral vein

☐ **SP** **SL** **+** I82.513　Chronic embolism and thrombosis of femoral vein, bilateral

☐ **IQ** **+** I82.519　Chronic embolism and thrombosis of unspecified femoral vein

▲ **+** **6** I82.52　Chronic embolism and thrombosis of iliac vein
Chronic embolism and thrombosis of common iliac vein
Chronic embolism and thrombosis of external iliac vein
Chronic embolism and thrombosis of internal iliac vein

CODING TIPS ✓　Deep vein thrombosis in the proximal deep veins is more significant than deep vein thrombosis in the distal deep veins. Veins of the thigh are the iliac and femoral.

☐ **SP** **SL** **+** I82.521　Chronic embolism and thrombosis of right iliac vein

☐ **SP** **SL** **+** I82.522　Chronic embolism and thrombosis of left iliac vein

☐ **SP** **SL** **+** I82.523　Chronic embolism and thrombosis of iliac vein, bilateral

☐ **IQ** **+** I82.529　Chronic embolism and thrombosis of unspecified iliac vein

+ **6** I82.53　Chronic embolism and thrombosis of popliteal vein

☐ **SP** **SL** **+** I82.531　Chronic embolism and thrombosis of right popliteal vein

☐ **SP** **SL** **+** I82.532　Chronic embolism and thrombosis of left popliteal vein

☐ **SP** **SL** **+** I82.533　Chronic embolism and thrombosis of popliteal vein, bilateral

☐ **IQ** **+** I82.539　Chronic embolism and thrombosis of unspecified popliteal vein

▲ **+** **6** I82.54　Chronic embolism and thrombosis of tibial vein
Chronic embolism and thrombosis of anterior tibial vein
Chronic embolism and thrombosis of posterior tibial vein

CODING TIPS ✓　Deep vein thrombosis in the proximal deep veins is more significant than deep vein thrombosis in the distal deep veins. Veins of the calf include the peroneal, gastrocnemial, tibial and soleal.

☐ **SP** **SL** **+** I82.541　Chronic embolism and thrombosis of right tibial vein

☐ **SP** **SL** **+** I82.542　Chronic embolism and thrombosis of left tibial vein

☐ **SP** **SL** **+** I82.543　Chronic embolism and thrombosis of tibial vein, bilateral

☐ **IQ** **+** I82.549　Chronic embolism and thrombosis of unspecified tibial vein

★ **+** **6** I82.55　Chronic embolism and thrombosis of peroneal vein

CODING TIPS ✓　Deep vein thrombosis in the proximal deep veins is more significant than deep vein thrombosis in the distal deep veins. Veins of the calf include the peroneal, gastrocnemial, tibial and soleal.

★ ☐ **+** I82.551　Chronic embolism and thrombosis of right peroneal vein

★ ☐ **+** I82.552　Chronic embolism and thrombosis of left peroneal vein

★ ☐ **+** I82.553　Chronic embolism and thrombosis of peroneal vein, bilateral

★ ☐ **+** I82.559　Chronic embolism and thrombosis of unspecified peroneal vein

★ **+** **6** I82.56　Chronic embolism and thrombosis of calf muscular vein
Chronic embolism and thrombosis of calf muscular vein NOS
Chronic embolism and thrombosis of gastrocnemial vein
Chronic embolism and thrombosis of soleal vein

CODING TIPS ✓　Deep vein thrombosis in the proximal deep veins is more significant than deep vein thrombosis in the distal deep veins. Veins of the calf include the peroneal, gastrocnemial, tibial and soleal.

★ ☐ **+** I82.561　Chronic embolism and thrombosis of right calf muscular vein

★ ☐ **+** I82.562　Chronic embolism and thrombosis of left calf muscular vein

★ ☐ **+** I82.563　Chronic embolism and thrombosis of calf muscular vein, bilateral

★ ☐ **+** I82.569　Chronic embolism and thrombosis of unspecified calf muscular vein

★ New　▲ Revised　Px Primary　**SP** PDGM Px　**SL** Low CoM　**SH** High CoM　**IQ** Quest. Encounter　**H** Hospice non-cancer Dx　Unspecified　**M** *Manifestation*

DecisionHealth's FY 2020 Complete Home Health ICD-10-CM Diagnosis Coding Manual

1011

✚ ⑥ I82.59 Chronic embolism and thrombosis of other specified deep vein of lower extremity

⊟ SP SL ✚ I82.591 Chronic embolism and thrombosis of other specified deep vein of right lower extremity

⊟ SP SL ✚ I82.592 Chronic embolism and thrombosis of other specified deep vein of left lower extremity

⊟ SP SL ✚ I82.593 Chronic embolism and thrombosis of other specified deep vein of lower extremity, bilateral

⊟ !Q ✚ I82.599 Chronic embolism and thrombosis of other specified deep vein of unspecified lower extremity

✚ ⑥ I82.5Y Chronic embolism and thrombosis of unspecified deep veins of proximal lower extremity

Chronic embolism and thrombosis of deep veins of thigh NOS
Chronic embolism and thrombosis of deep veins of upper leg NOS

⊟ SP SL ✚ I82.5Y1 Chronic embolism and thrombosis of unspecified deep veins of right proximal lower extremity

⊟ SP SL ✚ I82.5Y2 Chronic embolism and thrombosis of unspecified deep veins of left proximal lower extremity

⊟ SP SL ✚ I82.5Y3 Chronic embolism and thrombosis of unspecified deep veins of proximal lower extremity, bilateral

⊟ !Q ✚ I82.5Y9 Chronic embolism and thrombosis of unspecified deep veins of unspecified proximal lower extremity

✚ ⑥ I82.5Z Chronic embolism and thrombosis of unspecified deep veins of distal lower extremity

Chronic embolism and thrombosis of deep veins of calf NOS
Chronic embolism and thrombosis of deep veins of lower leg NOS

⊟ SP SL ✚ I82.5Z1 Chronic embolism and thrombosis of unspecified deep veins of right distal lower extremity

⊟ SP SL ✚ I82.5Z2 Chronic embolism and thrombosis of unspecified deep veins of left distal lower extremity

⊟ SP SL ✚ I82.5Z3 Chronic embolism and thrombosis of unspecified deep veins of distal lower extremity, bilateral

⊟ !Q ✚ I82.5Z9 Chronic embolism and thrombosis of unspecified deep veins of unspecified distal lower extremity

⑤ I82.6 Acute embolism and thrombosis of veins of upper extremity

⑥ I82.60 Acute embolism and thrombosis of unspecified veins of upper extremity

⊟ SP SL I82.601 Acute embolism and thrombosis of unspecified veins of right upper extremity

⊟ SP SL I82.602 Acute embolism and thrombosis of unspecified veins of left upper extremity

⊟ SP SL I82.603 Acute embolism and thrombosis of unspecified veins of upper extremity, bilateral

⊟ !Q I82.609 Acute embolism and thrombosis of unspecified veins of unspecified upper extremity

⑥ I82.61 Acute embolism and thrombosis of superficial veins of upper extremity
Acute embolism and thrombosis of antecubital vein
Acute embolism and thrombosis of basilic vein
Acute embolism and thrombosis of cephalic vein

⊟ SP SL I82.611 Acute embolism and thrombosis of superficial veins of right upper extremity

⊟ SP SL I82.612 Acute embolism and thrombosis of superficial veins of left upper extremity

⊟ SP SL I82.613 Acute embolism and thrombosis of superficial veins of upper extremity, bilateral

⊟ !Q I82.619 Acute embolism and thrombosis of superficial veins of unspecified upper extremity

⑥ I82.62 Acute embolism and thrombosis of deep veins of upper extremity
Acute embolism and thrombosis of brachial vein
Acute embolism and thrombosis of radial vein
Acute embolism and thrombosis of ulnar vein

⊟ SP SL I82.621 Acute embolism and thrombosis of deep veins of right upper extremity

⊟ SP SL I82.622 Acute embolism and thrombosis of deep veins of left upper extremity

⊟ SP SL I82.623 Acute embolism and thrombosis of deep veins of upper extremity, bilateral

⊟ !Q I82.629 Acute embolism and thrombosis of deep veins of unspecified upper extremity

✚ ⑤ I82.7 Chronic embolism and thrombosis of veins of upper extremity
Use additional code, if applicable, for associated long-term (current) use of anticoagulants (Z79.01)
EXCLUDES 1 personal history of venous embolism and thrombosis (Z86.718)
CODING TIPS ✓ These conditions are considered acute, unless the physician specifies chronic.

✚ ⑥ I82.70 Chronic embolism and thrombosis of unspecified veins of upper extremity

---

⬛4th digit required   ⑤5th digit required   ⑥6th digit required   ⬛7th digit required   ☑7th digit placeholder   ✚Additional code   ⊟Laterality

☰ **SP** **SL** ✚ **I82.701** Chronic embolism and thrombosis of unspecified veins of right upper extremity

☰ **SP** **SL** ✚ **I82.702** Chronic embolism and thrombosis of unspecified veins of left upper extremity

☰ **SP** **SL** ✚ **I82.703** Chronic embolism and thrombosis of unspecified veins of upper extremity, bilateral

☰ **IQ** ✚ **I82.709** Chronic embolism and thrombosis of unspecified veins of unspecified upper extremity

✚ ⑥ **I82.71** Chronic embolism and thrombosis of superficial veins of upper extremity
Chronic embolism and thrombosis of antecubital vein
Chronic embolism and thrombosis of basilic vein
Chronic embolism and thrombosis of cephalic vein

☰ **SP** **SL** ✚ **I82.711** Chronic embolism and thrombosis of superficial veins of right upper extremity

☰ **SP** **SL** ✚ **I82.712** Chronic embolism and thrombosis of superficial veins of left upper extremity

☰ **SP** **SL** ✚ **I82.713** Chronic embolism and thrombosis of superficial veins of upper extremity, bilateral

☰ **IQ** ✚ **I82.719** Chronic embolism and thrombosis of superficial veins of unspecified upper extremity

✚ ⑥ **I82.72** Chronic embolism and thrombosis of deep veins of upper extremity
Chronic embolism and thrombosis of brachial vein
Chronic embolism and thrombosis of radial vein
Chronic embolism and thrombosis of ulnar vein

☰ **SP** **SL** ✚ **I82.721** Chronic embolism and thrombosis of deep veins of right upper extremity

☰ **SP** **SL** ✚ **I82.722** Chronic embolism and thrombosis of deep veins of left upper extremity

☰ **SP** **SL** ✚ **I82.723** Chronic embolism and thrombosis of deep veins of upper extremity, bilateral

☰ **IQ** ✚ **I82.729** Chronic embolism and thrombosis of deep veins of unspecified upper extremity

⑤ **I82.A** Embolism and thrombosis of axillary vein

⑥ **I82.A1** Acute embolism and thrombosis of axillary vein

☰ **SP** **SL** **I82.A11** Acute embolism and thrombosis of right axillary vein

☰ **SP** **SL** **I82.A12** Acute embolism and thrombosis of left axillary vein

☰ **SP** **SL** **I82.A13** Acute embolism and thrombosis of axillary vein, bilateral

☰ **IQ** **I82.A19** Acute embolism and thrombosis of unspecified axillary vein

⑥ **I82.A2** Chronic embolism and thrombosis of axillary vein

☰ **SP** **SL** **I82.A21** Chronic embolism and thrombosis of right axillary vein

☰ **SP** **SL** **I82.A22** Chronic embolism and thrombosis of left axillary vein

☰ **SP** **SL** **I82.A23** Chronic embolism and thrombosis of axillary vein, bilateral

☰ **IQ** **I82.A29** Chronic embolism and thrombosis of unspecified axillary vein

⑤ **I82.B** Embolism and thrombosis of subclavian vein

⑥ **I82.B1** Acute embolism and thrombosis of subclavian vein

☰ **SP** **SL** **I82.B11** Acute embolism and thrombosis of right subclavian vein

☰ **SP** **SL** **I82.B12** Acute embolism and thrombosis of left subclavian vein

☰ **SP** **SL** **I82.B13** Acute embolism and thrombosis of subclavian vein, bilateral

☰ **IQ** **I82.B19** Acute embolism and thrombosis of unspecified subclavian vein

⑥ **I82.B2** Chronic embolism and thrombosis of subclavian vein

☰ **SP** **SL** **I82.B21** Chronic embolism and thrombosis of right subclavian vein

☰ **SP** **SL** **I82.B22** Chronic embolism and thrombosis of left subclavian vein

☰ **SP** **SL** **I82.B23** Chronic embolism and thrombosis of subclavian vein, bilateral

☰ **IQ** **I82.B29** Chronic embolism and thrombosis of unspecified subclavian vein

⑤ **I82.C** Embolism and thrombosis of internal jugular vein

⑥ **I82.C1** Acute embolism and thrombosis of internal jugular vein

☰ **SP** **SL** **I82.C11** Acute embolism and thrombosis of right internal jugular vein

☰ **SP** **SL** **I82.C12** Acute embolism and thrombosis of left internal jugular vein

☰ **SP** **SL** **I82.C13** Acute embolism and thrombosis of internal jugular vein, bilateral

☰ **IQ** **I82.C19** Acute embolism and thrombosis of unspecified internal jugular vein

⑥ **I82.C2** Chronic embolism and thrombosis of internal jugular vein

☰ **SP** **SL** **I82.C21** Chronic embolism and thrombosis of right internal jugular vein

☰ **SP** **SL** **I82.C22** Chronic embolism and thrombosis of left internal jugular vein

☰ **SP** **SL** **I82.C23** Chronic embolism and thrombosis of internal jugular vein, bilateral

☰ **IQ** **I82.C29** Chronic embolism and thrombosis of unspecified internal jugular vein

✚ ⑤ **I82.8** Embolism and thrombosis of other specified veins
Use additional code, if applicable, for associated long-term (current) use of anticoagulants (Z79.01)

✚ ⑥ **I82.81** Embolism and thrombosis of superficial veins of lower extremities
Embolism and thrombosis of saphenous vein (greater) (lesser)

★ New ▲ Revised **Px** Primary **SP** PDGM Px **SL** Low CoM **SH** High CoM **IQ** Quest. Encounter **H** Hospice non-cancer Dx ▨ Unspecified **M** *Manifestation*

Chapter 9

I00-I99

☐ **SP** **SL** ✚ **I82.811** **Embolism and thrombosis of superficial veins of right lower extremity**

☐ **SP** **SL** ✚ **I82.812** **Embolism and thrombosis of superficial veins of left lower extremity**

☐ **SP** **SL** ✚ **I82.813** **Embolism and thrombosis of superficial veins of lower extremities, bilateral**

☐ **IQ** ✚ **I82.819** **Embolism and thrombosis of superficial veins of unspecified lower extremity**

✚ **6** **I82.89** **Embolism and thrombosis of other specified veins**

SP **SL** ✚ **I82.890** **Acute embolism and thrombosis of other specified veins**

SP **SL** ✚ **I82.891** **Chronic embolism and thrombosis of other specified veins**

5 **I82.9** **Embolism and thrombosis of unspecified vein**

IQ **I82.90** **Acute embolism and thrombosis of unspecified vein**

Embolism of vein NOS
Thrombosis (vein) NOS

IQ **I82.91** **Chronic embolism and thrombosis of unspecified vein**

4 **I83** **Varicose veins of lower extremities**

EXCLUDES 1 varicose veins complicating pregnancy (O22.0-)
varicose veins complicating the puerperium (O87.4)

CODING TIPS ✓ **Documentation:** When assigning a code from I83.-, coders should assign the most specific code applicable, but cannot assume a specific code. A relationship between a lower extremity wound and varicosity must be stated in the clinical record as a cause and effect relationship by the patient's physician in order to assign a code from I83.2- or I83.0-. Inflammation should not be assumed to be related to varicosities but should be verified by a physician as related before assigning a code from category I83.1-

✚ **5** **I83.0** **Varicose veins of lower extremities with ulcer**

Use additional code to identify severity of ulcer (L97.-)

CODING TIPS ✓ A stasis ulcer associated with varicose vein is coded to I83.0 or I83.2 (varicose veins of lower extremities). An additional code for the ulcer is required to indicate the severity of the ulcer.

✚ **6** **I83.00** **Varicose veins of unspecified lower extremity with ulcer**

IQ ✚ **I83.001** **Varicose veins of unspecified lower extremity with ulcer of thigh**

IQ ✚ **I83.002** **Varicose veins of unspecified lower extremity with ulcer of calf**

IQ ✚ **I83.003** **Varicose veins of unspecified lower extremity with ulcer of ankle**

IQ ✚ **I83.004** **Varicose veins of unspecified lower extremity with ulcer of heel and midfoot**

Varicose veins of unspecified lower extremity with ulcer of plantar surface of midfoot

IQ ✚ **I83.005** **Varicose veins of unspecified lower extremity with ulcer other part of foot**

Varicose veins of unspecified lower extremity with ulcer of toe

IQ ✚ **I83.008** **Varicose veins of unspecified lower extremity with ulcer other part of lower leg**

IQ ✚ **I83.009** **Varicose veins of unspecified lower extremity with ulcer of unspecified site**

✚ **6** **I83.01** **Varicose veins of right lower extremity with ulcer**

☐ **SP** **SL** ✚ **I83.011** **Varicose veins of right lower extremity with ulcer of thigh**

☐ **SP** **SL** ✚ **I83.012** **Varicose veins of right lower extremity with ulcer of calf**

☐ **SP** **SL** ✚ **I83.013** **Varicose veins of right lower extremity with ulcer of ankle**

☐ **SP** **SL** ✚ **I83.014** **Varicose veins of right lower extremity with ulcer of heel and midfoot**

Varicose veins of right lower extremity with ulcer of plantar surface of midfoot

☐ **SP** **SL** ✚ **I83.015** **Varicose veins of right lower extremity with ulcer other part of foot**

Varicose veins of right lower extremity with ulcer of toe

☐ **SP** **SL** ✚ **I83.018** **Varicose veins of right lower extremity with ulcer other part of lower leg**

☐ **IQ** ✚ **I83.019** **Varicose veins of right lower extremity with ulcer of unspecified site**

✚ **6** **I83.02** **Varicose veins of left lower extremity with ulcer**

☐ **SP** **SL** ✚ **I83.021** **Varicose veins of left lower extremity with ulcer of thigh**

☐ **SP** **SL** ✚ **I83.022** **Varicose veins of left lower extremity with ulcer of calf**

☐ **SP** **SL** ✚ **I83.023** **Varicose veins of left lower extremity with ulcer of ankle**

☐ **SP** **SL** ✚ **I83.024** **Varicose veins of left lower extremity with ulcer of heel and midfoot**

Varicose veins of left lower extremity with ulcer of plantar surface of midfoot

☐ **SP** **SL** ✚ **I83.025** **Varicose veins of left lower extremity with ulcer other part of foot**

Varicose veins of left lower extremity with ulcer of toe

☐ **SP** **SL** ✚ **I83.028** **Varicose veins of left lower extremity with ulcer other part of lower leg**

☐ **IQ** ✚ **I83.029** **Varicose veins of left lower extremity with ulcer of unspecified site**

5 **I83.1** **Varicose veins of lower extremities with inflammation**

4 4th digit required   **5** 5th digit required   **6** 6th digit required   **7** 7th digit required   **7** 7th digit placeholder   ✚ Additional code   ☐ Laterality

1014   *DecisionHealth's* FY 2020 Complete Home Health ICD-10-CM Diagnosis Coding Manual

CODING TIPS ✓ Documentation: Do not assume inflammation of the lower extremities to be related to varicosities when present. Inflammation present on assessment should be reported to the patient's physician and a cause and effect relationship confirmed in order to assign a code from category I83.1-.

⊟ **IQ** I83.10 **Varicose veins of unspecified lower extremity with inflammation**

⊟ **SP** **SL** I83.11 **Varicose veins of right lower extremity with inflammation**

⊟ **SP** **SL** I83.12 **Varicose veins of left lower extremity with inflammation**

➕ **5** I83.2 **Varicose veins of lower extremities with both ulcer and inflammation**
Use additional code to identify severity of ulcer (L97.-)

CODING TIPS ✓ If the clinical record reports a confirmed diagnosis of ulcers due to varicosity (condition classifiable to I83.0), as well as inflammation due to varicosity (condition classifiable to I83.1-), then a code from category I83.2- should be reported instead. An additional code is required to indicate the severity of the ulcer.

➕ **6** I83.20 **Varicose veins of unspecified lower extremity with both ulcer and inflammation**

IQ ➕ I83.201 **Varicose veins of unspecified lower extremity with both ulcer of thigh and inflammation**

IQ ➕ I83.202 **Varicose veins of unspecified lower extremity with both ulcer of calf and inflammation**

IQ ➕ I83.203 **Varicose veins of unspecified lower extremity with both ulcer of ankle and inflammation**

IQ ➕ I83.204 **Varicose veins of unspecified lower extremity with both ulcer of heel and midfoot and inflammation**
Varicose veins of unspecified lower extremity with both ulcer of plantar surface of midfoot and inflammation

IQ ➕ I83.205 **Varicose veins of unspecified lower extremity with both ulcer other part of foot and inflammation**
Varicose veins of unspecified lower extremity with both ulcer of toe and inflammation

IQ ➕ I83.208 **Varicose veins of unspecified lower extremity with both ulcer of other part of lower extremity and inflammation**

IQ ➕ I83.209 **Varicose veins of unspecified lower extremity with both ulcer of unspecified site and inflammation**

➕ **6** I83.21 **Varicose veins of right lower extremity with both ulcer and inflammation**

⊟ **SP** **SL** ➕ I83.211 **Varicose veins of right lower extremity with both ulcer of thigh and inflammation**

⊟ **SP** **SL** ➕ I83.212 **Varicose veins of right lower extremity with both ulcer of calf and inflammation**

⊟ **SP** **SL** ➕ I83.213 **Varicose veins of right lower extremity with both ulcer of ankle and inflammation**

⊟ **SP** **SL** ➕ I83.214 **Varicose veins of right lower extremity with both ulcer of heel and midfoot and inflammation**
Varicose veins of right lower extremity with both ulcer of plantar surface of midfoot and inflammation

⊟ **SP** **SL** ➕ I83.215 **Varicose veins of right lower extremity with both ulcer other part of foot and inflammation**
Varicose veins of right lower extremity with both ulcer of toe and inflammation

⊟ **SP** **SL** ➕ I83.218 **Varicose veins of right lower extremity with both ulcer of other part of lower extremity and inflammation**

⊟ **IQ** ➕ I83.219 **Varicose veins of right lower extremity with both ulcer of unspecified site and inflammation**

➕ **6** I83.22 **Varicose veins of left lower extremity with both ulcer and inflammation**

⊟ **SP** **SL** ➕ I83.221 **Varicose veins of left lower extremity with both ulcer of thigh and inflammation**

⊟ **SP** **SL** ➕ I83.222 **Varicose veins of left lower extremity with both ulcer of calf and inflammation**

⊟ **SP** **SL** ➕ I83.223 **Varicose veins of left lower extremity with both ulcer of ankle and inflammation**

⊟ **SP** **SL** ➕ I83.224 **Varicose veins of left lower extremity with both ulcer of heel and midfoot and inflammation**
Varicose veins of left lower extremity with both ulcer of plantar surface of midfoot and inflammation

⊟ **SP** **SL** ➕ I83.225 **Varicose veins of left lower extremity with both ulcer other part of foot and inflammation**
Varicose veins of left lower extremity with both ulcer of toe and inflammation

⊟ **SP** **SL** ➕ I83.228 **Varicose veins of left lower extremity with both ulcer of other part of lower extremity and inflammation**

⊟ **IQ** ➕ I83.229 **Varicose veins of left lower extremity with both ulcer of unspecified site and inflammation**

5 I83.8 **Varicose veins of lower extremities with other complications**

6 I83.81 **Varicose veins of lower extremities with pain**

⊟ **SP** I83.811 **Varicose veins of right lower extremity with pain**

★ New ▲ Revised **Px** Primary **SP** PDGM Px **SL** Low CoM **SH** High CoM **IQ** Quest. Encounter **H** Hospice non-cancer Dx Unspecified **M** *Manifestation*

Chapter 9

I00-I99

☐ SP **I83.812** Varicose veins of left lower extremity with pain

☐ SP **I83.813** Varicose veins of bilateral lower extremities with pain

☐ IQ **I83.819** Varicose veins of unspecified lower extremity with pain

⑥ **I83.89** Varicose veins of lower extremities with other complications
Varicose veins of lower extremities with edema
Varicose veins of lower extremities with swelling

☐ SP **I83.891** Varicose veins of right lower extremity with other complications

☐ SP **I83.892** Varicose veins of left lower extremity with other complications

☐ SP **I83.893** Varicose veins of bilateral lower extremities with other complications

☐ SP **I83.899** Varicose veins of unspecified lower extremity with other complications

⑤ **I83.9** Asymptomatic varicose veins of lower extremities
Phlebectasia of lower extremities
Varicose veins of lower extremities
Varix of lower extremities

CODING TIPS ✓ Before assigning a code from I83.9-, consider if this diagnosis is the correct one, as I83.9- codes indicate asymptomatic varicosities. Also consider the appropriateness of including I83.9- codes on the home health claim, as these codes indicate a stable and asymptomatic condition that should require little to no intervention.

☐ IQ **I83.90** Asymptomatic varicose veins of unspecified lower extremity
Varicose veins NOS

☐ SP **I83.91** Asymptomatic varicose veins of right lower extremity

☐ SP **I83.92** Asymptomatic varicose veins of left lower extremity

☐ SP **I83.93** Asymptomatic varicose veins of bilateral lower extremities

✚ ④ **I85** Esophageal varices
Use additional code to identify:
alcohol abuse and dependence (F10.-)

CODING TIPS ✓ Esophageal varices are coded to vascular disorders, rather than gastrointestinal disorders, due to the nature of their pathophysiology. Bleeding varices can be life-threatening and cause additional complex cardiovascular complications.

✚ ⑤ **I85.0** Esophageal varices
Idiopathic esophageal varices
Primary esophageal varices

SP SL ✚ **I85.00** Esophageal varices without bleeding
Esophageal varices NOS

CODING TIPS ✓ When the clinical record does not specify bleeding or absence of bleeding in a patient with esophageal varices, assign code I85.00, when the varices are not specified as related to any other cause.

SP ✚ **I85.01** Esophageal varices with bleeding

✚ ⑤ **I85.1** Secondary esophageal varices
Esophageal varices secondary to alcoholic liver disease
Esophageal varices secondary to cirrhosis of liver
Esophageal varices secondary to schistosomiasis
Esophageal varices secondary to toxic liver disease
Code first:
underlying disease

CODING TIPS ✓ This diagnosis indicates that the alcohol was linked to the disorder, so the use, abuse or dependence of alcohol F10.- code should include 5th and 6th characters .88.

SP ✚ **I85.10** Secondary esophageal varices without bleeding

SP ✚ **I85.11** Secondary esophageal varices with bleeding

④ **I86** Varicose veins of other sites
EXCLUDES 1 varicose veins of unspecified site (I83.9-)
EXCLUDES 2 retinal varices (H35.0-)

SP **I86.0** Sublingual varices

SP **I86.1** Scrotal varices
Varicocele

SP **I86.2** Pelvic varices

SP **I86.3** Vulval varices
EXCLUDES 1 vulval varices complicating childbirth and the puerperium (O87.8)
vulval varices complicating pregnancy (O22.1-)

SP **I86.4** Gastric varices

SP **I86.8** Varicose veins of other specified sites
Varicose ulcer of nasal septum

④ **I87** Other disorders of veins

⑤ **I87.0** Postthrombotic syndrome
Chronic venous hypertension due to deep vein thrombosis
Postphlebitic syndrome
EXCLUDES 1 chronic venous hypertension without deep vein thrombosis (I87.3-)

⑥ **I87.00** Postthrombotic syndrome without complications
Asymptomatic Postthrombotic syndrome

☐ SP **I87.001** Postthrombotic syndrome without complications of right lower extremity

☐ SP **I87.002** Postthrombotic syndrome without complications of left lower extremity

☐ SP **I87.003** Postthrombotic syndrome without complications of bilateral lower extremity

☐ IQ **I87.009** Postthrombotic syndrome without complications of unspecified extremity
Postthrombotic syndrome NOS

✚ ⑥ **I87.01** Postthrombotic syndrome with ulcer
Use additional code to specify site and severity of ulcer (L97.-)

---

④ 4th digit required   ⑤ 5th digit required   ⑥ 6th digit required   ⑦ 7th digit required   ⑦ 7th digit placeholder   ✚ Additional code   ☐ Laterality

1016   *DecisionHealth's* FY 2020 Complete Home Health ICD-10-CM Diagnosis Coding Manual

CODING TIPS ✓ Postphlebitic or postthrombotic syndrome ulcers require that L97 codes be used to identify the location and laterality of the ulcer.

☐ **SP** ✚ **I87.011** **Postthrombotic syndrome with ulcer of right lower extremity**

☐ **SP** ✚ **I87.012** **Postthrombotic syndrome with ulcer of left lower extremity**

☐ **SP** ✚ **I87.013** **Postthrombotic syndrome with ulcer of bilateral lower extremity**

☐ **IQ** ✚ **I87.019** **Postthrombotic syndrome with ulcer of unspecified lower extremity**

6 **I87.02** **Postthrombotic syndrome with inflammation**

☐ **SP** **I87.021** **Postthrombotic syndrome with inflammation of right lower extremity**

☐ **SP** **I87.022** **Postthrombotic syndrome with inflammation of left lower extremity**

☐ **SP** **I87.023** **Postthrombotic syndrome with inflammation of bilateral lower extremity**

☐ **IQ** **I87.029** **Postthrombotic syndrome with inflammation of unspecified lower extremity**

✚ **6** **I87.03** **Postthrombotic syndrome with ulcer and inflammation**
Use additional code to specify site and severity of ulcer (L97.-)

CODING TIPS ✓ Postphlebitic or postthrombotic syndrome ulcers require that L97 codes be used to identify the location and laterality of the ulcer.

☐ **SP** ✚ **I87.031** **Postthrombotic syndrome with ulcer and inflammation of right lower extremity**

☐ **SP** ✚ **I87.032** **Postthrombotic syndrome with ulcer and inflammation of left lower extremity**

☐ **SP** ✚ **I87.033** **Postthrombotic syndrome with ulcer and inflammation of bilateral lower extremity**

☐ **IQ** ✚ **I87.039** **Postthrombotic syndrome with ulcer and inflammation of unspecified lower extremity**

6 **I87.09** **Postthrombotic syndrome with other complications**

☐ **SP** **I87.091** **Postthrombotic syndrome with other complications of right lower extremity**

☐ **SP** **I87.092** **Postthrombotic syndrome with other complications of left lower extremity**

☐ **SP** **I87.093** **Postthrombotic syndrome with other complications of bilateral lower extremity**

☐ **IQ** **I87.099** **Postthrombotic syndrome with other complications of unspecified lower extremity**

SP **I87.1** **Compression of vein**
Stricture of vein
Vena cava syndrome (inferior) (superior)
EXCLUDES 2 compression of pulmonary vein (I28.8)

SP **I87.2** **Venous insufficiency (chronic) (peripheral)**
Stasis dermatitis
EXCLUDES 1 stasis dermatitis with varicose veins of lower extremities (I83.1-, I83.2-)

CODING TIPS ✓ Chronic venous insufficiency is considered a peripheral angiopathy and is assumed related to diabetes. Use E--.51 prior to coding I87.2 in the diabetic.

CODING TIPS ✓ If the physician documents only "stasis ulcer" then use I87.2 followed by the ulcer code to indicate severity and laterality. Stasis dermatitis, in the absence of varicosities, is included.

5 **I87.3** **Chronic venous hypertension (idiopathic)**
Stasis edema
EXCLUDES 1 chronic venous hypertension due to deep vein thrombosis (I87.0-)
varicose veins of lower extremities (I83.-)

6 **I87.30** **Chronic venous hypertension (idiopathic) without complications**
Asymptomatic chronic venous hypertension (idiopathic)

☐ **SP** **I87.301** **Chronic venous hypertension (idiopathic) without complications of right lower extremity**

☐ **SP** **I87.302** **Chronic venous hypertension (idiopathic) without complications of left lower extremity**

☐ **SP** **I87.303** **Chronic venous hypertension (idiopathic) without complications of bilateral lower extremity**

☐ **IQ** **I87.309** **Chronic venous hypertension (idiopathic) without complications of unspecified lower extremity**
Chronic venous hypertension NOS

✚ **6** **I87.31** **Chronic venous hypertension (idiopathic) with ulcer**
Use additional code to specify site and severity of ulcer (L97.-)

CODING TIPS ✓ To report an ulcer associated with chronic venous hypertension, report first I87.31 or I87.33 and L97 as an additional diagnosis.

☐ **SP** ✚ **I87.311** **Chronic venous hypertension (idiopathic) with ulcer of right lower extremity**

☐ **SP** ✚ **I87.312** **Chronic venous hypertension (idiopathic) with ulcer of left lower extremity**

☐ **SP** ✚ **I87.313** **Chronic venous hypertension (idiopathic) with ulcer of bilateral lower extremity**

☐ **IQ** ✚ **I87.319** **Chronic venous hypertension (idiopathic) with ulcer of unspecified lower extremity**

6 **I87.32** **Chronic venous hypertension (idiopathic) with inflammation**

☐ **SP** **I87.321** **Chronic venous hypertension (idiopathic) with inflammation of right lower extremity**

★ New ▲ Revised **Px** Primary **SP** PDGM Px **SL** Low CoM **SH** High CoM **IQ** Quest. Encounter **H** Hospice non-cancer Dx ☐ Unspecified **M** *Manifestation*

DecisionHealth's FY 2020 Complete Home Health ICD-10-CM Diagnosis Coding Manual

1017

Chapter 9

I00-I99

⊟ **SP** **I87.322** **Chronic venous hypertension (idiopathic) with inflammation of left lower extremity**

⊟ **SP** **I87.323** **Chronic venous hypertension (idiopathic) with inflammation of bilateral lower extremity**

⊟ **IQ** **I87.329** **Chronic venous hypertension (idiopathic) with inflammation of unspecified lower extremity**

✚ **6** **I87.33** **Chronic venous hypertension (idiopathic) with ulcer and inflammation**
Use additional code to specify site and severity of ulcer (L97.-)

CODING TIPS ✓ To report an ulcer associated with chronic venous hypertension, report first I87.31 or I87.33 and L97 as an additional diagnosis.

⊟ **SP** ✚ **I87.331** **Chronic venous hypertension (idiopathic) with ulcer and inflammation of right lower extremity**

⊟ **SP** ✚ **I87.332** **Chronic venous hypertension (idiopathic) with ulcer and inflammation of left lower extremity**

⊟ **SP** ✚ **I87.333** **Chronic venous hypertension (idiopathic) with ulcer and inflammation of bilateral lower extremity**

⊟ **IQ** ✚ **I87.339** **Chronic venous hypertension (idiopathic) with ulcer and inflammation of unspecified lower extremity**

6 **I87.39** **Chronic venous hypertension (idiopathic) with other complications**

⊟ **SP** **I87.391** **Chronic venous hypertension (idiopathic) with other complications of right lower extremity**

⊟ **SP** **I87.392** **Chronic venous hypertension (idiopathic) with other complications of left lower extremity**

⊟ **SP** **I87.393** **Chronic venous hypertension (idiopathic) with other complications of bilateral lower extremity**

⊟ **IQ** **I87.399** **Chronic venous hypertension (idiopathic) with other complications of unspecified lower extremity**

SP **I87.8** **Other specified disorders of veins**
Phlebosclerosis
Venofibrosis

IQ **I87.9** **Disorder of vein, unspecified**

4 **I88** **Nonspecific lymphadenitis**
EXCLUDES 1 acute lymphadenitis, except mesenteric (L04.-)
enlarged lymph nodes NOS (R59.-)
human immunodeficiency virus [HIV] disease resulting in generalized lymphadenopathy (B20)

SP **I88.0** **Nonspecific mesenteric lymphadenitis**
Mesenteric lymphadenitis (acute)(chronic)

SP **I88.1** **Chronic lymphadenitis, except mesenteric**
Adenitis
Lymphadenitis
DEFINITION Chronic enlargement of the lymphatic glands.

SP **I88.8** **Other nonspecific lymphadenitis**

IQ **I88.9** **Nonspecific lymphadenitis, unspecified**
Lymphadenitis NOS

4 **I89** **Other noninfective disorders of lymphatic vessels and lymph nodes**
EXCLUDES 1 chylocele, tunica vaginalis (nonfilarial) NOS (N50.89)
enlarged lymph nodes NOS (R59.-)
filarial chylocele (B74.-)
hereditary lymphedema (Q82.0)

SP **SL** **I89.0** **Lymphedema, not elsewhere classified**
Elephantiasis (nonfilarial) NOS
Lymphangiectasis
Obliteration, lymphatic vessel
Praecox lymphedema
Secondary lymphedema
EXCLUDES 1 postmastectomy lymphedema (I97.2)

CODING TIPS ✓ Lymphedema is not the same as edema associated with other conditions, such as heart failure, and may not be coded without physician confirmation.

SP **I89.1** **Lymphangitis**
Chronic lymphangitis
Lymphangitis NOS
Subacute lymphangitis
EXCLUDES 1 acute lymphangitis (L03.-)

SP **I89.8** **Other specified noninfective disorders of lymphatic vessels and lymph nodes**
Chylocele (nonfilarial)
Chylous ascites
Chylous cyst
Lipomelanotic reticulosis
Lymph node or vessel fistula
Lymph node or vessel infarction
Lymph node or vessel rupture

IQ **I89.9** **Noninfective disorder of lymphatic vessels and lymph nodes, unspecified**
Disease of lymphatic vessels NOS

Other and unspecified disorders of the circulatory system (I95-I99)

4 **I95** **Hypotension**
EXCLUDES 1 cardiovascular collapse (R57.9)
maternal hypotension syndrome (O26.5-)
nonspecific low blood pressure reading NOS (R03.1)

CODING TIPS ✓ A low blood pressure reading in the absence of a diagnosis of hypotension should not be coded to I95.-. A singular low blood pressure reading with no diagnosis of hypotension should be coded to R03.1.

SP **I95.0** **Idiopathic hypotension**

4 4th digit required   **5** 5th digit required   **6** 6th digit required   **7** 7th digit required   ☑ 7th digit placeholder   ✚ Additional code   ⊟ Laterality

1018   *DecisionHealth's* FY 2020 Complete Home Health ICD-10-CM Diagnosis Coding Manual

CODING TIPS ✓ Documentation: Idiopathic hypotension requires a confirmed diagnosis by the patient's physician and may not be assumed. Do not assign I95.0 for a patient with hypotension of uncertain cause, with no physician report of idiopathic etiology, and do not assign for a singular low blood pressure reading.

SP **SH** **I95.1** **Orthostatic hypotension**
Hypotension, postural
> **EXCLUDES 1** neurogenic orthostatic hypotension [Shy-Drager] (G90.3)
> orthostatic hypotension due to drugs (I95.2)

CODING TIPS ✓ Do not assign code I95.1 for orthostasis resulting from medication effects. Hypotension secondary to medication/drug effects is coded to I95.2 and is coded as an adverse effect.

DEFINITION Abnormally low blood pressure that occurs when the patient moves to a standing or upright position.

SP **+** **I95.2** **Hypotension due to drugs**
Orthostatic hypotension due to drugs
Use additional code for adverse effect, if applicable, to identify drug (T36-T50 with fifth or sixth character 5)

CODING TIPS ✓ A patient can have a diagnosis of hypertension and a problem with hypotension at the same time, especially hypotension related to the anti-hypertensive medications. Continue to code the type of hypertension.

CODING TIPS ✓ When hypotension or orthostasis is confirmed and reported in the medical record as resulting from the effects of medications or other drugs, code I95.2 should be assigned. An additional code from category T36-T50 should be assigned to identify the drug.

SP **I95.3** **Hypotension of hemodialysis**
Intra-dialytic hypotension
SL **I95.8** **Other hypotension**
SP **I95.81** **Postprocedural hypotension**
SP **SH** **I95.89** **Other hypotension**
Chronic hypotension
IQ **SH** **I95.9** Hypotension, unspecified

SP **I96** **Gangrene, not elsewhere classified**
Gangrenous cellulitis
> **EXCLUDES 1** gangrene in atherosclerosis of native arteries of the extremities (I70.26)
> gangrene in hernia (K40.1, K40.4, K41.1, K41.4, K42.1, K43.1-, K44.1, K45.1, K46.1)
> gangrene in other peripheral vascular diseases (I73.-)
> gangrene of certain specified sites - see Alphabetical Index
> gas gangrene (A48.0)
> pyoderma gangrenosum (L88)
> **EXCLUDES 2** gangrene in diabetes mellitus (E08-E13 with .52)

CODING TIPS ✓ Gangrene may be documented as gangrenous cellulitis or necrosis, and is also known as dry gangrene.

CODING TIPS ✓ Gangrene associated with a pressure ulcer is coded with I96, then assign the L89.- codes for pressure ulcers. Gangrene associated with pressure ulcers is NOT related to diabetes and is not coded as diabetic gangrene. Note the L89 codes instruct to "code first" any associated gangrene at L89.

CODING TIPS ✓ Do not use I96 to indicate gangrene in diabetes, atherosclerosis or other vascular disease, pyoderma gangrenosum, gas gangrene, or gangrene in a hernia.

DEFINITION Complication of cell death (necrosis), characterized by tissue decay, which becomes black and malodorous, caused by infection or ischemia, resulting from insufficient blood supply.

4 **I97** **Intraoperative and postprocedural complications and disorders of circulatory system, not elsewhere classified**
> **EXCLUDES 2** postprocedural shock (T81.1-)

CODING TIPS ✓ Documentation: Codes in category I97.- are complication codes and require physician documentation and confirmation of a cause and effect relationship between the procedure and the complicated condition. Documentation in the home health clinical record must also support this relationship. They may be described as "post-status" or "post-op".

SP **I97.0** **Postcardiotomy syndrome**
5 **I97.1** **Other postprocedural cardiac functional disturbances**
> **EXCLUDES 2** acute pulmonary insufficiency following thoracic surgery (J95.1)
> intraoperative cardiac functional disturbances (I97.7-)

6 **I97.11** **Postprocedural cardiac insufficiency**
SP **I97.110** **Postprocedural cardiac insufficiency following cardiac surgery**
SP **I97.111** **Postprocedural cardiac insufficiency following other surgery**
6 **I97.12** **Postprocedural cardiac arrest**
SP **I97.120** **Postprocedural cardiac arrest following cardiac surgery**
SP **I97.121** **Postprocedural cardiac arrest following other surgery**
+ **6** **I97.13** **Postprocedural heart failure**
Use additional code to identify the heart failure (I50.-)
SP **+** **I97.130** **Postprocedural heart failure following cardiac surgery**
SP **+** **I97.131** **Postprocedural heart failure following other surgery**
+ **6** **I97.19** **Other postprocedural cardiac functional disturbances**
Use additional code, if applicable, to further specify disorder

★ New ▲ Revised Px Primary **SP** PDGM Px **SL** Low CoM **SH** High CoM **IQ** Quest. Encounter **H** Hospice non-cancer Dx Unspecified **M** *Manifestation*

DecisionHealth's FY 2020 Complete Home Health ICD-10-CM Diagnosis Coding Manual

1019

Chapter 9

I00-I99

SP + I97.190 Other postprocedural cardiac functional disturbances following cardiac surgery
Use additional code, if applicable, for type 4 or type 5 myocardial infarction, to further specify disorder

SP + I97.191 Other postprocedural cardiac functional disturbances following other surgery

SP SL I97.2 Postmastectomy lymphedema syndrome
Elephantiasis due to mastectomy
Obliteration of lymphatic vessels

CODING TIPS ✓   Assign code I97.2 only when lymphedema is specifically reported as related to the effects of a mastectomy.

DEFINITION   Localized edema in the arm following breast and lymph node removal due to lack of lymph circulation through the chest area.

SP I97.3 Postprocedural hypertension

5 I97.4 Intraoperative hemorrhage and hematoma of a circulatory system organ or structure complicating a procedure
EXCLUDES 1   intraoperative hemorrhage and hematoma of a circulatory system organ or structure due to accidental puncture and laceration during a procedure (I97.5-)
EXCLUDES 2   intraoperative cerebrovascular hemorrhage complicating a procedure (G97.3-)

6 I97.41 Intraoperative hemorrhage and hematoma of a circulatory system organ or structure complicating a circulatory system procedure

SP I97.410 Intraoperative hemorrhage and hematoma of a circulatory system organ or structure complicating a cardiac catheterization

SP I97.411 Intraoperative hemorrhage and hematoma of a circulatory system organ or structure complicating a cardiac bypass

SP I97.418 Intraoperative hemorrhage and hematoma of a circulatory system organ or structure complicating other circulatory system procedure

SP I97.42 Intraoperative hemorrhage and hematoma of a circulatory system organ or structure complicating other procedure

5 I97.5 Accidental puncture and laceration of a circulatory system organ or structure during a procedure
EXCLUDES 2   accidental puncture and laceration of brain during a procedure (G97.4-)

SP I97.51 Accidental puncture and laceration of a circulatory system organ or structure during a circulatory system procedure

SP I97.52 Accidental puncture and laceration of a circulatory system organ or structure during other procedure

5 I97.6 Postprocedural hemorrhage, hematoma and seroma of a circulatory system organ or structure following a procedure
EXCLUDES 2   postprocedural cerebrovascular hemorrhage complicating a procedure (G97.5-)

6 I97.61 Postprocedural hemorrhage of a circulatory system organ or structure following a circulatory system procedure

SP I97.610 Postprocedural hemorrhage of a circulatory system organ or structure following a cardiac catheterization

SP I97.611 Postprocedural hemorrhage of a circulatory system organ or structure following cardiac bypass

SP I97.618 Postprocedural hemorrhage of a circulatory system organ or structure following other circulatory system procedure

6 I97.62 Postprocedural hemorrhage, hematoma and seroma of a circulatory system organ or structure following other procedure

SP I97.620 Postprocedural hemorrhage of a circulatory system organ or structure following other procedure

SP I97.621 Postprocedural hematoma of a circulatory system organ or structure following other procedure

SP I97.622 Postprocedural seroma of a circulatory system organ or structure following other procedure

6 I97.63 Postprocedural hematoma of a circulatory system organ or structure following a circulatory system procedure

SP I97.630 Postprocedural hematoma of a circulatory system organ or structure following a cardiac catheterization

SP I97.631 Postprocedural hematoma of a circulatory system organ or structure following cardiac bypass

SP I97.638 Postprocedural hematoma of a circulatory system organ or structure following other circulatory system procedure

6 I97.64 Postprocedural seroma of a circulatory system organ or structure following a circulatory system procedure

SP I97.640 Postprocedural seroma of a circulatory system organ or structure following a cardiac catheterization

SP I97.641 Postprocedural seroma of a circulatory system organ or structure following cardiac bypass

---

4 4th digit required   5 5th digit required   6 6th digit required   7 7th digit required   ☑ 7th digit placeholder   + Additional code   ⊟ Laterality

SP I97.648 Postprocedural seroma of a circulatory system organ or structure following other circulatory system procedure

5 I97.7 Intraoperative cardiac functional disturbances

> EXCLUDES 2 acute pulmonary insufficiency following thoracic surgery (J95.1)
> postprocedural cardiac functional disturbances (I97.1-)

6 I97.71 Intraoperative cardiac arrest

> CODING TIPS ✓ Codes from subcategory I97.71- indicate that the patient experienced cardiac arrest during a surgical procedure. These codes should never be assigned on the home health claim, but history of cardiac arrest with successful resuscitation may be used instead (Z86.74).

SP I97.710 Intraoperative cardiac arrest during cardiac surgery

SP I97.711 Intraoperative cardiac arrest during other surgery

+ 6 I97.79 Other intraoperative cardiac functional disturbances

> Use additional code, if applicable, to further specify disorder

SP + I97.790 Other intraoperative cardiac functional disturbances during cardiac surgery

SP + I97.791 Other intraoperative cardiac functional disturbances during other surgery

+ 5 I97.8 Other intraoperative and postprocedural complications and disorders of the circulatory system, not elsewhere classified

> Use additional code, if applicable, to further specify disorder

+ 6 I97.81 Intraoperative cerebrovascular infarction

> CODING TIPS ✓ Codes from category I97.81- indicate that the patient experienced a cerebral vascular accident *during* a surgical procedure (either a cardiac- I97.810, or non-cardiac- I97.811 procedure). Home health may assign a code from category I69.- (sequelae of cerebral vascular disease) on the home health claim if residual neurological deficits as a result of the cerebral vascular accident remain.

SP + I97.810 Intraoperative cerebrovascular infarction during cardiac surgery

SP + I97.811 Intraoperative cerebrovascular infarction during other surgery

+ 6 I97.82 Postprocedural cerebrovascular infarction

> CODING TIPS ✓ Codes from category I97.82- indicate that the patient experienced a cerebral vascular accident *after* a surgical procedure (either a cardiac- I97.820, or non-cardiac- I97.821 procedure). Home health may assign a code from category I69.- (sequelae of cerebral vascular disease) on the home health claim if residual neurological deficits as a result of the cerebral vascular accident remain.

SP + I97.820 Postprocedural cerebrovascular infarction following cardiac surgery

SP + I97.821 Postprocedural cerebrovascular infarction following other surgery

SP + I97.88 Other intraoperative complications of the circulatory system, not elsewhere classified

SP + I97.89 Other postprocedural complications and disorders of the circulatory system, not elsewhere classified

4 I99 Other and unspecified disorders of circulatory system

SP I99.8 Other disorder of circulatory system

IQ I99.9 Unspecified disorder of circulatory system

★ New ▲ Revised Px Primary SP PDGM Px SL Low CoM SH High CoM IQ Quest. Encounter H Hospice non-cancer Dx Unspecified M *Manifestation*

DecisionHealth's FY 2020 Complete Home Health ICD-10-CM Diagnosis Coding Manual

1021

Chapter 9 Scenarios: Diseases of the circulatory system (I00-I99)

Congestive heart failure

Your agency admitted a 70-year-old woman who was discharged from the hospital with acute exacerbation of her chronic congestive heart failure (CHF) with diastolic heart failure. Her Lasix dose was increased and the physician is requesting daily weights for two weeks and urinary output assessment due to her chronic kidney disease. She also has hypertension and dementia and is described as pleasantly confused without behavioral disturbances.

Description	Code
Primary: Hypertensive heart and chronic kidney disease with heart failure and stage 1 through stage 4 chronic kidney disease, or unspecified chronic kidney disease	I13.0
Secondary: Acute on chronic diastolic (congestive) heart failure	I50.33
Secondary: Chronic kidney disease, unspecified	N18.9
Secondary: Unspecified dementia without behavioral disturbance	F03.90

A cause-and-effect relationship between hypertension, heart failure and chronic kidney disease is assumed by the ICD-10 classification system unless the provider states that the conditions are unrelated. CHF and diastolic (or systolic) heart failure diagnoses are combined into one diagnosis and code. In addition, when an acute exacerbation is reported as superimposed upon a chronic condition, the condition should be coded as "acute on chronic." The appropriate code from N18.- for the stage of chronic kidney disease is also assigned in accordance with tabular instruction. No further information or etiology for the dementia is stated, so only F03.90 can be assigned.

Cerebral vascular accident

A female patient admitted to home health after suffering a CVA with hemiparesis of right side, dysphagia of oral phase and stuttering. Nursing, physical therapy and speech therapy will see the patient. Her co-morbidities of hypertension, diabetes with angiopathy, and well-controlled emphysema are documented. The patient takes insulin and recently has been started on Coumadin. PT/INRs will be monitored. The focus of care is the CVA with hemiparesis.

Description	Code
Primary: Hemiplegia following CVA affecting right dominant side	I69.351
Secondary: Dysphagia following CVA	I69.391
Secondary: Dysphagia oral phase	R13.11
Secondary: Fluency disorder following CVA	I69.323
Secondary: Essential primary hypertension	I10
Secondary: Type 2 diabetes mellitus with angiopathy without gangrene	E11.51
Secondary: Emphysema, unspecified	J43.9
Secondary: Long term (current) use of insulin	Z79.4
Secondary: Encounter for therapeutic drug level monitoring	Z51.81

Even though the documentation does not include whether the right sided CVA is dominant or non-dominant, if the information is not provided, right defaults to dominant, according to official coding guidelines. If the type of diabetes is not specified, it defaults to type 2. Because the patient uses insulin and is not a type 1 diabetic, the code for insulin use is assigned. The patient's emphysema is a relevant comorbidity and is also coded. Code Z79.01 is assigned to capture her Coumadin use. The instructional note on the code for encounter for therapeutic drug monitoring (Z51.81), to also code the condition requiring care, does not include sequencing instructions (code also). The two codes can be in either order. Thus it is sequenced at the bottom of the list.

Exacerbated hypertension, chronic systolic heart failure

A 77-year-old male is admitted to home health with a diagnosis of exacerbated hypertension. He also has chronic systolic heart failure and congestive heart failure (CHF). Hypertension is the focus of care.

Description	Code
Primary: Hypertensive heart disease with heart failure	I11.0
Secondary: Chronic systolic (congestive) heart failure	I50.22

The patient is having an exacerbation of his hypertension, and since it will be the focus of care, it should be listed as the primary diagnosis. A cause-and-effect relationship between hypertension and heart failure is assumed by the ICD-10 classification system unless the provider states they're unrelated. The patient also has two types of heart failure, chronic systolic heart failure and congestive heart failure. Both types of heart failure should be recognized. However, congestive heart failure is included in the code title for chronic systolic heart failure, and therefore only one heart failure code is needed to complete the diagnostic statement in this scenario. Code a patient with chronic systolic heart failure, who does not also have CHF, with I50.22 because "congestive" is a non-essential modifier.

Chronic DVT, wound care, morbid obesity

A 57-year-old patient was referred to home health for wound care to a stage 3 pressure ulcer/injury on her right buttock. She is morbidly obese with a documented BMI of 41. She had a Greenfield filter inserted four years ago after she was diagnosed with a chronic DVT of her deep femoral vein on her right side, following a fem-pop bypass due to severe PVD. As a result of her chronic DVT, she is on chronic anticoagulant therapy and the agency will also be obtaining PT/INR levels.

Description	Code
Primary: Pressure ulcer, stage 3, right buttock	L89.313
Secondary: Peripheral vascular disease, unspecified	I73.9
Secondary: Chronic embolism and thrombosis of right femoral vein	I82.511
Secondary: Morbid (severe) obesity due to excess calories	E66.01
Secondary: Body Mass Index, 40.0-44.9, adult	Z68.41
Secondary: Encounter for therapeutic drug level monitoring	Z51.81
Secondary: Long term (current) use of anticoagulants	Z79.01

The site, stage and laterality of a pressure ulcer/injury are combined into one code. And, as the focus of care, it is coded primary. The chronic DVT should also be coded, since it may be impacted by the peripheral vascular disease and requires long-term anticoagulant therapy. This DVT code (I82.511) also denotes laterality (i.e. the last character 1 = right, indicates laterality). Morbid obesity is a relevant comorbidity and should always be coded when documented, according to Q4 2018 Coding Clinic guidance. It is coded, along with the BMI code, in accordance with tabular instruction. Monitoring of PT/INR levels is captured by Z51.81 and the long-term anticoagulant use is captured with Z79.01.

HOME HEALTH CODING SCENARIOS

Stasis ulcers with MRSA and VRSA

The patient has multiple stasis ulcers on both ankles and both calves that are caused by peripheral venous insufficiency. One on his right ankle includes muscle necrosis; the others are limited to skin. All are infected with MRSA and VRSA. The of focus of care is directed at the ulcers, including wound care and IV administration for antibiotics.

Description	Code
Primary: Peripheral venous insufficiency	I87.2
Secondary: Non-pressure chronic ulcer of right ankle with necrosis of muscle	L97.313
Secondary: Non-pressure chronic ulcer of left ankle limited to breakdown of skin	L97.321
Secondary: Non-pressure chronic ulcer of right calf limited to breakdown of skin	L97.211
Secondary: Non-pressure chronic ulcer of left calf limited to breakdown of skin	L97.221
Secondary: Methicillin resistant Staphylococcus aureus as the cause of diseases classified elsewhere	B95.62
Secondary: Resistance to vancomycin	Z16.21
Secondary: Encounter for adjustment and management of vascular access device	Z45.2
Secondary: Long term (current) use of antibiotics	Z79.2

Non-pressure ulcers are coded after the causal condition, in this case peripheral venous insufficiency. There are codes for the right and left side for most locations. The determination of the 6th character for the level of severity is based on the clinician's documentation. A note at the code level directs the coder to use additional code to report any organism, which is coded following the code for the ulcer. In this case, that code is B95.62 for the MRSA. The resistance to VRSA is also coded, with Z16.21. The administration of IV antibiotics is captured with Z45.2 and Z79.2.

Congestive heart failure, hypertensive chronic kidney disease

The patient has congestive heart failure (CHF) and hypertensive chronic kidney disease (CKD) of unspecified stage. The CHF is focus of care.

Description	Code
Primary: Hypertensive heart and chronic kidney disease with heart failure and stage 1 through stage 4 chronic kidney disease, or unspecified chronic kidney disease	I13.0
Secondary: Heart failure, unspecified	I50.9
Secondary: Chronic kidney disease, unspecified	N18.9

A cause-and-effect relationship between hypertension, heart failure and chronic kidney disease is assumed by the ICD-10 classification system unless the provider states they're unrelated. Additional codes for the type of heart failure and stage of chronic kidney disease are assigned in accordance with tabular instruction.

Hemiplegia after intracerebral hemorrhage, aphasia

The patient is referred for home care after suffering an intracerebral hemorrhage due to uncontrolled hypertension. His deficits include aphasia and left-sided hemiplegia. The patient has a 30-year history of smoking but quit 10 years ago. Nursing, physical therapy, occupational therapy and speech therapy are ordered.

Description	Code
Primary: Hemiplegia following non-traumatic intracerebral hemorrhage affecting left non-dominant side	I69.154
Secondary: Aphasia following non-traumatic intracerebral hemorrhage	I69.120
Secondary: Hypertension	I10
Secondary: Personal history of nicotine dependence	Z87.891

This scenario illustrates how some sequela conditions and the causal illness or injury are combined into one diagnosis code, in this case I69.154 and I69.120. Residual codes are found in the index under the heading "sequelae." Search first for sequelae, hemorrhage, intracerebral, by deficit and then confirm the choice in the tabular. Although the medical record information does not indicate left- or right-hand dominance for the patient, coding guidelines indicate that, when specific information is not available, if the left side of the body is affected, the default code for non-dominant should be used. Tabular instruction at the Hypertensive diseases category level instruct the coder to use an additional code to identify history of tobacco use, which in this case necessitates the addition of Z87.891.

Hypertensive acute systolic heart failure

A 76-year-old woman was admitted to home health with acute systolic heart failure stated in the documentation as secondary to hypertension. She will receive skilled nursing care for management of new medications as well as physical therapy to help increase her stamina in completing ADLs.

Description	Code
Primary: Hypertensive heart disease with heart failure	I11.0
Secondary: Acute systolic (congestive) heart failure	I50.21

The patient's heart failure was caused by her hypertension and is therefore coded as hypertensive heart disease with heart failure. The hypertensive heart disease code is assigned first, in accordance with coding guidelines. An additional code for the specific type of heart failure is also coded, in accordance with tabular instruction.

Secondary hypertension, breast cancer with brain metastasis

A 71-year-old woman comes to home health with uncontrolled hypertension caused by breast cancer in her left breast that has metastasized to her brain. The hypertension is the focus of care.

Description	Code
Primary: Other secondary hypertension	I15.8
Secondary: Secondary malignant neoplasm of brain	C79.31
Secondary: Malignant neoplasm of unspecified site of left female breast	C50.912

The patient's hypertension is caused by the brain neoplasm, so it is coded secondary hypertension. As the focus of care, it is coded first. The brain metastasis is sequenced next as it is causing the hypertension. The original neoplasm is coded as well, as a diagnosis relevant to the plan of care.

HOME HEALTH CODING SCENARIOS

Heart failure with preserved ejection fraction

An 82-year-old woman comes to home health following hospitalization for an exacerbation of the acute heart failure with preserved ejection fraction. The physician wrote the diagnosis as HFpEF.

Description	Code
Primary: Acute diastolic (congestive) heart failure	I50.31

A patient's heart failure documented as HFpEF, which stands for heart failure with preserved ejection fraction, can be coded as diastolic heart failure, according to Q1 2016 Coding Clinic guidance and inclusion terms at the I50.3- subcategory. Because it is described as acute, it is coded with I50.31.

Heart attacks

A 75-year-old man suffered a myocardial infarction. Three weeks and four days later, he suffered another myocardial infarction. After treatment in the hospital, which included the placement of stents via an angioplasty, he was admitted to home health one week later. The focus of care is recovery from the myocardial infarction. He also has a diagnosis of coronary artery disease and a history of resolved prostate cancer.

Description	Code
Primary: Acute myocardial infarction, unspecified	I21.9
Secondary: Old myocardial infarction	I25.2
Secondary: Atherosclerotic heart disease of native coronary artery without angina pectoris	I25.10
Secondary: Presence of coronary angioplasty implant and graft	Z95.5
Secondary: Personal history of malignant neoplasm of prostate	Z85.46

Though the patient has had two recent myocardial infarctions, the first one occurred more than four weeks ago, and is thus no longer an acute condition. Therefore it is coded as an old myocardial infarction with I25.2. The second heart attack is coded as an acute myocardial infarction since it is within the four-week acute timeframe. With no further information available about the type and location of the MI, it is most appropriately captured with I21.9. The patient's coronary artery disease is an important comorbidity and thus is coded, as is the status code (Z95.5) indicating he had a stent placed in the hospital. His personal history of resolved prostate cancer is also important to capture, with Z85.46.

Decompensated chronic obstructive bronchitis, aortic valve disease

A 71-year-old woman is admitted to home health with chronic obstructive bronchitis that is acutely decompensated. She also has aortic valve disease and is awaiting valve replacement surgery once her pulmonary disease is stable.

Description	Code
Primary: Chronic obstructive pulmonary disease with (acute) exacerbation	J44.1
Secondary: Nonrheumatic aortic valve disorder, unspecified	I35.9

The focus of care is acutely decompensated chronic obstructive bronchitis, which codes to the J44.- category. Acutely decompensated chronic obstructive bronchitis can be coded as acutely exacerbated COPD, according to the inclusion terms on J44.1. Her aortic valve disease is an important comorbidity that should also be coded. It codes to I35.9, according to the alphabetic index.

Post-infarction angina

A 67-year-old woman suffered a STEMI 30 days ago, she underwent angioplasty and a stent was placed. She has coronary artery disease and still suffers from post-infarction angina. She also has hypertension and stage 2 kidney disease. The post-infarction angina is the focus of care.

Description	Code
Primary: Postinfarction angina	I23.7
Secondary: Atherosclerotic heart disease of native coronary artery with other forms of angina pectoris	I25.118
Secondary: Hypertensive chronic kidney disease with stage 1 through stage 4 chronic kidney disease, or unspecified chronic kidney disease	I12.9
Secondary: Chronic kidney disease, stage 2 (mild)	N18.2
Secondary: Presence of coronary angioplasty implant and graft	Z95.5

The patient's myocardial infarction is no longer considered an acute condition because it occurred longer than 28 days ago. However, the patient is still experiencing symptoms, which have been specified as post-infarction angina. Even though the 28-day acute period has passed, a post-infarction complication can still be assigned, according to Q2 2017 Coding Clinic guidance. The patient has angina and coronary artery disease, which are assumed to be connected and coded with a combination code, according to coding guidelines. The patient's hypertension and chronic kidney disease are assumed to be connected as well, according to coding guidelines, and are captured with combination codes I12.9 and N18.2. The presence of the stent used to treat the myocardial infarction is captured with Z95.5.

Type 2 myocardial infarction

A 74-year-old man is admitted to home health to continue recovery from a heart attack caused by demand ischemia due to a coronary vasospasm. The vasospasm is now under control and recovery from the heart attack will be the focus of care. He also has chronic obstructive asthma, which is currently stable. The physician's H&P states that he smokes a pack of cigarettes a day.

Description	Code
Primary: Angina pectoris with documented spasm	I20.1
Secondary: Myocardial infarction type 2	I21.A1
Secondary: Chronic obstructive pulmonary disease, unspecified	J44.9
Secondary: Nicotine dependence, cigarettes, uncomplicated	F17.210

A myocardial infarction resulting from demand ischemia due to a coronary vasospasm is a Type 2 heart attack. Because the coronary vasospasm is the underlying cause of the MI, it is coded first, according to the code first note at I21.A1. The patient's chronic obstructive asthma is coded as a relevant comorbidity that could impact his recovery. The patient's tobacco use is captured with F17.210 in accordance with tabular instruction.

HOME HEALTH CODING SCENARIOS

Heart failure with diastolic dysfunction

A 71-year-old man was recently diagnosed with acute congestive heart failure (CHF) with diastolic dysfunction. He is also a type 2 diabetic with additional diagnoses of neuropathy and retinopathy. He uses both insulin and oral antidiabetic medication. The heart failure is the focus of care.

Description	Code
Primary: Acute diastolic (congestive) heart failure	I50.31
Secondary: Type 2 diabetes mellitus with diabetic neuropathy, unspecified	E11.40
Secondary: Type 2 diabetes mellitus with unspecified diabetic retinopathy without macular edema	E11.319
Secondary: Long term (current) use of insulin	Z79.4

A diagnosis of acute congestive heart failure (CHF) with diastolic dysfunction should be coded with I50.31, according to Q1 2017 Coding Clinic guidance. Both the patient's neuropathy and retinopathy can be assumed to be connected to the diagnoses diagnosis, according to the alphabetic index. The patient uses both insulin and oral antidiabetic medication, but only insulin use is coded, in accordance with coding guidelines.

Diabetic ulcer, sick sinus syndrome

A 69-year-old morbidly obese woman with a BMI of 37 comes to home health for wound care to a diabetic foot ulcer on her left heel. The wound has penetrated muscle tissue but there's no mention of necrosis. The documentation also lists a diagnosis of sick sinus syndrome that is controlled with a pacemaker. She is insulin-dependent.

Description	Code
Primary: Type 2 diabetes mellitus with foot ulcer	E11.621
Secondary: Non-pressure chronic ulcer of left heel and midfoot with muscle involvement without evidence of necrosis	L97.425
Secondary: Sick sinus syndrome	I49.5
Secondary: Morbid (severe) obesity due to excess calories	E66.01
Secondary: Presence of cardiac pacemaker	Z95.0
Secondary: Body mass index (BMI) 37.0-37.9, adult	Z68.37
Secondary: Long term (current) use of insulin	Z79.4

Wound care to the diabetic foot ulcer is the focus of care and so it is coded primary. The coding of a diabetic foot ulcer requires two codes – one for the diabetic ulcer and one for the location and severity of the wound. Sick sinus syndrome, even if controlled by a pacemaker, should still be coded, according to Q1 2019 Coding Clinic guidance. Additionally, morbid obesity is always a clinically significant diagnosis and should be coded when it's documented, according to Q4 2018 Coding Clinic guidance. The pacemaker is coded with Z95.0, and an additional status code is assigned to capture the patient's BMI, in accordance with tabular instruction on the obesity code. Finally, since the patient is not a type 1 diabetic, her insulin use must be captured with Z79.4, in accordance with coding guidelines.

Chapter 10: Diseases of the Respiratory System (J00-J99)

The respiratory system includes the airways (nose and nasal passages, pharynx, larynx, trachea, bronchi, alveoli) and lungs. Also included are structures related to these airways such as the vocal cords, tonsils, adenoids, thorax and diaphragm.

The chapter is divided into the following blocks:

J00-J06	Acute upper respiratory infections
J09-J18	Influenza and pneumonia
J20-J22	Other acute lower respiratory infections
J30-J39	Other diseases of the upper respiratory tract
J40-J47	Chronic lower respiratory diseases
J60-J70	Lung diseases due to external agents
J80-J84	Other respiratory diseases principally affecting the interstitium
J85-J86	Suppurative and necrotic conditions of the lower respiratory tract
J90-J94	Other diseases of the pleura
J95	Intraoperative and post procedural complications and disorders of the respiratory system, NEC
J96-J99	Other diseases of the respiratory system

The airways are divided into the upper and lower airways. The upper airways (and upper respiratory tract) include the nasopharynx (nose), oropharynx (mouth), laryngopharynx and larynx. Their purposes are to warm, filter and humidify inhaled air. They also help make sound and send air to the lower airways.

The lower airways begin with the trachea, which then divides into the right and left mainstream bronchial tubes. The bronchial tubes divide into bronchi that are lined with mucus producing ciliated epithelium, which is one of the lung's major defense systems.

The bronchi then divide into secondary bronchi, tertiary bronchi, terminal bronchioles, respiratory bronchioles, alveolar ducts and, finally, into the alveoli, which are the gas exchange units of the lungs.

The right lung is larger and has three lobes: upper, middle and lower. The left lung is smaller and has only an upper and lower lobe. This leaves room for the heart.

Two systems control breathing: an automatic response and a voluntary response. Patients with diagnosed chronic respiratory diseases have a progressive increase in the mechanical work of breathing and limited respiratory reserve capacities. These factors may lead to symptoms of chronic dyspnea on exertion, wheezing, chronic cough and debilitating functional disabilities that limit exercise and

activities of daily living (ADLs). Other respiratory problems that might affect daily life include chronic respiratory inflammation, edema, mucous plugging, hypoxemia, carbon dioxide retention, pulmonary hypertension and pulmonary heart disease.

Codes in this chapter are used to report **pneumonia** (an infection of the lungs). Pneumonia is not a single disease, but refers to many different infections or conditions. Check the documentation for the cause to select the correct code. Pneumonia can be caused by viruses (Category J12.-), bacteria (category J13., J15.-), fungi or organisms called mycoplasma (J15.7), radiation treatment (J70.0), or other causes. Aspiration pneumonia (subcategory J69.0) is caused by the inhalation of substances into the lungs, such as food, vomitus, gastric secretions, milk, oils/essences, etc. Code J18.9 (Pneumonia, organism unspecified) should never be used if the organism or other cause is known.

Some codes are reported for occupational hazards that cause pulmonary problems. Codes in the categories J60-J70 (pneumoconiosis and other lung diseases due to external agents) include conditions involving the aspiration of dust and other substances, such as coal dust (black lung disease at J60) and asbestosis and other mineral fibers (J61), dust containing silica (J62), and other inorganic dusts (J63). Codes from category J67.- (extrinsic allergic alveolitis, pneumonitis due to inhaled organic dust and particles of fungal, actinomycetic or other origin) occur in specific occupations or activities, such as mushroom workers' lung or bird-fanciers' lung.

Other codes found in chapter 10 include: category J98.19 pulmonary collapse (collapsed lung); J98.2, Interstitial emphysema; category J96.-, Respiratory failure (inability of respiratory system to maintain adequate gas exchange); and J95.- Acute pulmonary insufficiency following surgery (problems with the valve between the heart and the artery leading to the lungs).

In certain situations, you'll need to look beyond this chapter to properly code a case. For example:

- If the documentation indicates a **neoplasm or tumor of an organ in the respiratory system,** coders should look up the term (malignancy, tumor, adenoma) to find the correct code in Chapter 2.

- If a patient has a **personal or family history** of a condition reported in this chapter, it may be appropriate to use a code from chapter 21, such as Z87.09 (Diseases of respiratory system); Z85.12 (Personal history of malignant neoplasm of trachea); or Z80.2 (Family history of malignant neoplasm of intrathoracic organs).

- **Symptoms** related to the respiratory system are sometimes reported using codes from Chapter 18 such as code series R09.89 (Symptoms involving respiratory system and other chest symptoms). Every effort should be made to secure a definitive diagnosis. A symptom code from Chapter 18 may be reported as an additional diagnosis when it describes a significant aspect of the condition but is not an integral part of it.

- Although not reported often in home health or hospice, if reporting **a respiratory system disease in a pregnant patient** when the condition is complicating the pregnancy, report a code from Chapter 15 as the first-listed diagnosis and a code from this chapter as an additional diagnosis.

Intraoperative and postprocedural complications and disorders of respiratory system, not elsewhere classified, are coded from category J95. For example, a complication of a tracheostomy is reported using a code from J95.00-J95.09, such as J95.02 (Infection of the tracheostomy stoma) or J95.03 (Mechanical complication of a tracheostomy). Codes such as infection of a tracheostomy state that additional codes should be reported to indicate the type of infection such as cellulitis of the neck (L03.221) or sepsis (A40, A41-).

Multiple Coding and Sequencing

It is important to read the Includes and Excludes 1 and Excludes 2 notes under codes in this chapter, as well as any other instructions under the code or code category. The following are examples of multiple coding and sequencing issues to keep an eye out for in this chapter.

Because of the higher risk of respiratory conditions related to smoking or smoke exposure, there is a note under the heading of the chapter that states to use an additional code, where applicable, to identify:

- exposure to environmental tobacco smoke (Z77.22)

- exposure to tobacco smoke in the prenatal period (P68.81)

- history of tobacco dependence (Z87.891)

- occupational exposure to environmental tobacco smoke (Z57.31)

- tobacco dependence (F17.-)

- tobacco use (Z72.0)

This note is repeated under codes for disorders of the upper respiratory tract, chronic lower respiratory diseases (i.e., asthma, bronchitis) and interstitial pulmonary diseases.

Many of the conditions listed in Chapter 10 involve infections. For example, a note under the acute sinusitis category (J01) states: "Use additional code (B95-B97) to identify infectious agents." With other codes within chapter 10 there are a variety of other notes to code first

or add additional codes for associated conditions and adverse effects.

Some conditions reported with codes in other chapters are reported with manifestations in Chapter 10. For example, cystic fibrosis with pulmonary manifestations (code E84.0 from Chapter 4) is a genetic defect that causes the body to produce abnormally thick, sticky mucus that clogs the airways.

Special Coding Issue

Chronic Obstructive Pulmonary Disease (COPD) and Asthma, emphysema

The codes in categories J44 and J45 distinguish between uncomplicated cases and those in an acute exacerbation. An acute exacerbation is a worsening or a decompensation of a chronic condition. ***An acute exacerbation is not equivalent to an infection superimposed on a chronic condition***, although an exacerbation may be triggered by an infection.

Chronic obstructive pulmonary disease (COPD) (J43-J45) is an irreversible obstruction of the airways. Conditions that fall under the COPD umbrella include chronic obstructive asthma, chronic obstructive bronchitis and emphysema. Code J44.9 is an unspecified code that is reported when a patient has a condition that is classifiable to J44 and there's no information as to whether the condition is exacerbated or occurring with a lower respiratory infection, which would necessitate the coding of J44.1 and J44.0, respectively.

An additional code for the type of asthma should be assigned in a patient with COPD and asthma. For a patient with exacerbated asthma, and a condition classifiable to J44 that's not exacerbated or co-occurring with a lower respiratory infection, you would assign J45.901 along with J44.9. You should not assign an additional code for unspecified asthma in this scenario, but if the asthma is documented as exacerbated, that additional specificity makes the use of an additional asthma code appropriate, according to the Q4 2017 Coding Clinic update.

Assign J43.9 (Emphysema, unspecified) for a patient who has emphysema and acutely exacerbated COPD, according to Q4 2017 Coding Clinic. When it comes to coding COPD, focus on the specificity of the disease, not whether it's exacerbated. If an infection is also present, code it as well and sequence the acute condition first. Conversely, for a diagnosis of exacerbated chronic obstructive bronchitis, the correct code would be J44.1.

Assign a code from J44.0 when a patient has both a condition classifiable to J44 and a diagnosis of a lower respiratory tract infection. An additional code should be assigned to report the infection. If the physician confirms both a diagnosis of a lower respiratory tract infection and exacerbation of chronic obstructive bronchitis, for example, both J44.1, Chronic obstructive pulmonary disease with (acute) exacerbation, and J44.0, Chronic obstructive pulmonary disease with (acute) lower respiratory infection, should be assigned, along with a code for the specific lower respiratory infection. Examples of lower respiratory infections include pneumonia, bronchitis and bronchiolitis. The sequencing of J44.1 and and the lower respiratory infection is discretionary and should be based on the Plan of Care.

Respiratory insufficiency (R06.89) is an integral part of COPD. If the documentation states that the patient has COPD, do not report R06.89 as an additional code.

It is important to locate the diagnosis term in the Alphabetical Index and then review all the notes under the code in the Tabular List to ensure correct code assignment.

Influenza due to certain identified influenza viruses

Code only confirmed cases of influenza due to certain identified influenza viruses (category J09), and due to other identified influenza virus (category J10). In this context, "confirmation" does not require documentation of positive laboratory testing specific for avian or other novel influenza A, or other identified influenza virus. However, coding should be based on the physician's diagnostic statement that the patient has avian influenza, or other novel influenza A, for category J09, or has another particular identified strain influenza, such as H1N1 or H3N2, but not identified as novel or variant, for category J10.

If the physician documents "suspected" or "possible" or "probable" avian influenza, or novel influenza, or other identified influenza, then assign the appropriate influenza code from category J11, Influenza due to unidentified influenza virus. Do not assign a code from category J09, Influenza due to certain identified influenza viruses, or a code from category J10, Influenza due to other identified influenza virus.

Ventilator associated pneumonia

As with all procedural or postprocedural complications, code assignment is based on the physician's documentation of the relationship between the condition and the procedure. Code J95.851, Ventilator associated pneumonia, should be assigned only when the physician has documented ventilator associated pneumonia (VAP). An additional code to identify the organism (e.g., Pseudomonas aeruginosa, code B96.5) should also be assigned. Do not assign an additional code from categories J12-J18 to identify the type of pneumonia.

Code J95.851 should not be assigned in cases where the patient has pneumonia and is on a mechanical ventilator, and the physician has not specifically stated that the pneumonia is ventilator-associated pneumonia. If the documentation is unclear as to whether the patient has pneumonia that is a complication attributable to the mechanical ventilator, query the physician.

If a patient has either aspiration pneumonia or ventilator-associated pneumonia and a condition classifiable to J44, you would not assign J44.0, as neither of the pneumonia diagnoses are considered respiratory infections. For each you'd code J44.9 along with the code for the type of pneumonia, sequenced according to the circumstances of the admission, according to the Q1 2017 Coding Clinic.

CHAPTER 10: DISEASES OF THE RESPIRATORY SYSTEM (J00-J99)

Note:

When a respiratory condition is described as occurring in more than one site and is not specifically indexed, it should be classified to the lower anatomic site (e.g. tracheobronchitis to bronchitis in J40).

Use additional code, where applicable, to identify:

exposure to environmental tobacco smoke (Z77.22)

exposure to tobacco smoke in the perinatal period (P96.81)

history of tobacco dependence (Z87.891)

occupational exposure to environmental tobacco smoke (Z57.31)

tobacco dependence (F17.-)

tobacco use (Z72.0)

EXCLUDES 2 certain conditions originating in the perinatal period (P04-P96)

certain infectious and parasitic diseases (A00-B99)

complications of pregnancy, childbirth and the puerperium (O00-O9A)

congenital malformations, deformations and chromosomal abnormalities (Q00-Q99)

endocrine, nutritional and metabolic diseases (E00-E88)

injury, poisoning and certain other consequences of external causes (S00-T88)

neoplasms (C00-D49)

smoke inhalation (T59.81-)

symptoms, signs and abnormal clinical and laboratory findings, not elsewhere classified (R00-R94)

This chapter contains the following blocks:

J00-J06	Acute upper respiratory infections
J09-J18	Influenza and pneumonia
J20-J22	Other acute lower respiratory infections
J30-J39	Other diseases of upper respiratory tract
J40-J47	Chronic lower respiratory diseases
J60-J70	Lung diseases due to external agents
J80-J84	Other respiratory diseases principally affecting the interstitium
J85-J86	Suppurative and necrotic conditions of the lower respiratory tract
J90-J94	Other diseases of the pleura
J95	Intraoperative and postprocedural complications and disorders of respiratory system, not elsewhere classified
J96-J99	Other diseases of the respiratory system

Acute upper respiratory infections (J00-J06)

EXCLUDES 1 chronic obstructive pulmonary disease with acute lower respiratory infection (J44.0)

influenza virus with other respiratory manifestations (J09.X2, J10.1, J11.1)

CODING TIPS ✓ A patient with an upper respiratory infection (J00-J06), such as laryngitis, pharyngitis, sinus infection, etc., who also has a condition classifiable to J44 would not be coded with J44.0. Code J44.0 is only used when the patient with one of those diagnoses also has a lower respiratory infection, such as bronchitis or pneumonia.

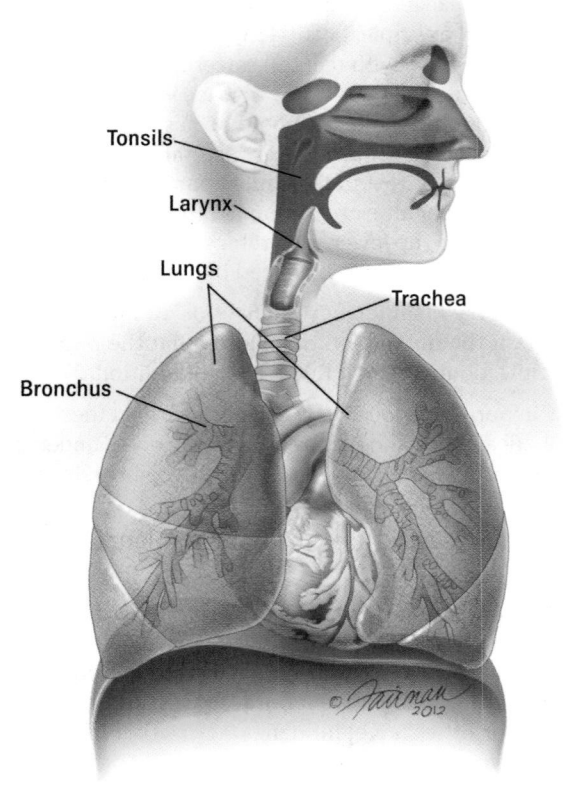

Tonsils

Larynx

Lungs

Trachea

Bronchus

SP J00 **Acute nasopharyngitis [common cold]**

Acute rhinitis

Coryza (acute)

Infective nasopharyngitis NOS

Infective rhinitis

Nasal catarrh, acute

Nasopharyngitis NOS

EXCLUDES 1 acute pharyngitis (J02.-)

acute sore throat NOS (J02.9)

pharyngitis NOS (J02.9)

rhinitis NOS (J31.0)

sore throat NOS (J02.9)

EXCLUDES 2 allergic rhinitis (J30.1-J30.9)

chronic pharyngitis (J31.2)

chronic rhinitis (J31.0)

chronic sore throat (J31.2)

nasopharyngitis, chronic (J31.1)

vasomotor rhinitis (J30.0)

+ 4 J01 **Acute sinusitis**

INCLUDES acute abscess of sinus

acute empyema of sinus

acute infection of sinus

acute inflammation of sinus

acute suppuration of sinus

Use additional code (B95-B97) to identify infectious agent.

EXCLUDES 1 sinusitis NOS (J32.9)

EXCLUDES 2 chronic sinusitis (J32.0-J32.8)

+ 5 J01.0 **Acute maxillary sinusitis**

Acute antritis

---

4 4th digit required   5 5th digit required   6 6th digit required   7 7th digit required   ✓ 7th digit placeholder   + Additional code   ⊟ Laterality

1032   *DecisionHealth's* FY 2020 Complete Home Health ICD-10-CM Diagnosis Coding Manual

SP + J01.00 **Acute maxillary sinusitis, unspecified**

SP + J01.01 **Acute recurrent maxillary sinusitis**

+ S J01.1 **Acute frontal sinusitis**

SP + J01.10 **Acute frontal sinusitis, unspecified**

SP + J01.11 **Acute recurrent frontal sinusitis**

+ S J01.2 **Acute ethmoidal sinusitis**

SP + J01.20 **Acute ethmoidal sinusitis, unspecified**

SP + J01.21 **Acute recurrent ethmoidal sinusitis**

+ S J01.3 **Acute sphenoidal sinusitis**

SP + J01.30 **Acute sphenoidal sinusitis, unspecified**

SP + J01.31 **Acute recurrent sphenoidal sinusitis**

+ S J01.4 **Acute pansinusitis**

SP + J01.40 **Acute pansinusitis, unspecified**

SP + J01.41 **Acute recurrent pansinusitis**

+ S J01.8 **Other acute sinusitis**

SP + J01.80 **Other acute sinusitis**
Acute sinusitis involving more than one sinus but not pansinusitis

SP + J01.81 **Other acute recurrent sinusitis**
Acute recurrent sinusitis involving more than one sinus but not pansinusitis

+ S J01.9 **Acute sinusitis, unspecified**

SP + J01.90 **Acute sinusitis, unspecified**

SP + J01.91 **Acute recurrent sinusitis, unspecified**

4 J02 **Acute pharyngitis**

> INCLUDES | acute sore throat

> EXCLUDES 1 | acute laryngopharyngitis (J06.0)
> peritonsillar abscess (J36)
> pharyngeal abscess (J39.1)
> retropharyngeal abscess (J39.0)

> EXCLUDES 2 | chronic pharyngitis (J31.2)

SP J02.0 **Streptococcal pharyngitis**
Septic pharyngitis
Streptococcal sore throat

> EXCLUDES 2 | scarlet fever (A38.-)

SP + J02.8 **Acute pharyngitis due to other specified organisms**
Use additional code (B95-B97) to identify infectious agent

> EXCLUDES 1 | acute pharyngitis due to coxsackie virus (B08.5)
> acute pharyngitis due to gonococcus (A54.5)
> acute pharyngitis due to herpes [simplex] virus (B00.2)
> acute pharyngitis due to infectious mononucleosis (B27.-)
> enteroviral vesicular pharyngitis (B08.5)

SP J02.9 **Acute pharyngitis, unspecified**
Gangrenous pharyngitis (acute)
Infective pharyngitis (acute) NOS
Pharyngitis (acute) NOS
Sore throat (acute) NOS
Suppurative pharyngitis (acute)
Ulcerative pharyngitis (acute)

4 J03 **Acute tonsillitis**

> EXCLUDES 1 | acute sore throat (J02.-)
> hypertrophy of tonsils (J35.1)
> peritonsillar abscess (J36)
> sore throat NOS (J02.9)
> streptococcal sore throat (J02.0)

> EXCLUDES 2 | chronic tonsillitis (J35.0)

S J03.0 **Streptococcal tonsillitis**

SP J03.00 **Acute streptococcal tonsillitis, unspecified**

SP J03.01 **Acute recurrent streptococcal tonsillitis**

+ S J03.8 **Acute tonsillitis due to other specified organisms**
Use additional code (B95-B97) to identify infectious agent.

> EXCLUDES 1 | diphtheritic tonsillitis (A36.0)
> herpesviral pharyngotonsillitis (B00.2)
> streptococcal tonsillitis (J03.0)
> tuberculous tonsillitis (A15.8)
> Vincent's tonsillitis (A69.1)

SP + J03.80 **Acute tonsillitis due to other specified organisms**

SP + J03.81 **Acute recurrent tonsillitis due to other specified organisms**

S J03.9 **Acute tonsillitis, unspecified**
Follicular tonsillitis (acute)
Gangrenous tonsillitis (acute)
Infective tonsillitis (acute)
Tonsillitis (acute) NOS
Ulcerative tonsillitis (acute)

SP J03.90 **Acute tonsillitis, unspecified**

SP J03.91 **Acute recurrent tonsillitis, unspecified**

+ 4 J04 **Acute laryngitis and tracheitis**
Use additional code (B95-B97) to identify infectious agent.

> EXCLUDES 1 | acute obstructive laryngitis [croup] and epiglottitis (J05.-)

> EXCLUDES 2 | laryngismus (stridulus) (J38.5)

SP + J04.0 **Acute laryngitis**
Edematous laryngitis (acute)
Laryngitis (acute) NOS
Subglottic laryngitis (acute)
Suppurative laryngitis (acute)
Ulcerative laryngitis (acute)

> EXCLUDES 1 | acute obstructive laryngitis (J05.0)

> EXCLUDES 2 | chronic laryngitis (J37.0)

+ S J04.1 **Acute tracheitis**
Acute viral tracheitis
Catarrhal tracheitis (acute)
Tracheitis (acute) NOS

> EXCLUDES 2 | chronic tracheitis (J42)

SP + J04.10 **Acute tracheitis without obstruction**

SP + J04.11 **Acute tracheitis with obstruction**

SP + J04.2 **Acute laryngotracheitis**
Laryngotracheitis NOS
Tracheitis (acute) with laryngitis (acute)

★ New ▲ Revised **Px** Primary **SP** PDGM Px **SL** Low CoM **SH** High CoM **IQ** Quest. Encounter **H** Hospice non-cancer Dx   Unspecified   **M** *Manifestation*

EXCLUDES 1 acute obstructive
laryngotracheitis (J05.0)

EXCLUDES 2 chronic laryngotracheitis
(J37.1)

CODING TIPS ✓ J04.2 is a specific code and should be assigned when the patient is reported as specifically having laryngotracheitis by the physician. This involves inflammation of both the larynx and trachea.

+ ⑤ J04.3   Supraglottitis, unspecified

CODING TIPS ✓ Supraglottitis is a potentially life-threatening inflammation of the supraglottic area of the airway. If airway obstruction is documented, assign J04.31.

SP + J04.30   Supraglottitis, unspecified, without obstruction

SP + J04.31   Supraglottitis, unspecified, with obstruction

+ ④ J05   Acute obstructive laryngitis [croup] and epiglottitis
Use additional code (B95-B97) to identify infectious agent.

SP + J05.0   Acute obstructive laryngitis [croup]
Obstructive laryngitis (acute) NOS
Obstructive laryngotracheitis NOS

+ ⑤ J05.1   Acute epiglottitis
EXCLUDES 2 epiglottitis, chronic (J37.0)

SP + J05.10   Acute epiglottitis without obstruction
Epiglottitis NOS

SP + J05.11   Acute epiglottitis with obstruction

④ J06   Acute upper respiratory infections of multiple and unspecified sites
EXCLUDES 1 acute respiratory infection NOS
(J22)
streptococcal pharyngitis
(J02.0)

SP J06.0   Acute laryngopharyngitis

▲ SP + J06.9   Acute upper respiratory infection, unspecified
Upper respiratory disease, acute
Upper respiratory infection NOS
Use additional code (B95-B97) to identify infectious agent, if known, such as:
respiratory syncytial virus (RSV)
(B97.4)
CODING TIPS ✓ Assign J06.9 for upper respiratory infection NOS only when a more specific diagnosis to identify the type of infection cannot be identified.

Influenza and pneumonia   (J09-J18)

EXCLUDES 2 allergic or eosinophilic pneumonia (J82)
aspiration pneumonia NOS (J69.0)
meconium pneumonia (P24.01)
neonatal aspiration pneumonia (P24.-)
pneumonia due to solids and liquids (J69.-)
congenital pneumonia (P23.9)
lipid pneumonia (J69.1)
rheumatic pneumonia (I00)
ventilator associated pneumonia (J95.851)

CODING TIPS ✓ Assign J43.9 with J18.9 for emphysema, COPD and pneumonia (*Q1 2019 Coding Clinic*).

CODING TIPS ✓ Influenza is not considered a lower respiratory infection for the purposes of coding a condition classifiable to J44 with J44.0. If influenza results in pneumonia, code the condition as J44.0, and the influenza. Sequence according to the focus of care.

CODING TIPS ✓ Pneumonia should be coded to the specific causative organism using a combination code when a specific code is available. Evaluate all available clinical documentation and assign the most specific code for pneumonia. When the causative organism of bacterial pneumonia is known but no combination code exists, assign J15.8.

CODING TIPS ✓ When pneumonia is diagnosed in a patient who also has a condition classifiable to J44, the coder should assign J44.0 and the specific code to indicate the type of pneumonia. Sequence according to the focus of care.

④ J09   Influenza due to certain identified influenza viruses
EXCLUDES 1 influenza A/H1N1 (J10.-)
influenza due to other identified
influenza virus (J10.-)
influenza due to unidentified
influenza virus (J11.-)
seasonal influenza due to other
identified influenza virus
(J10.-)
seasonal influenza due to
unidentified influenza virus
(J11.-)

GUIDELINES Section I.C.10.c
Code only confirmed cases of influenza due to certain identified influenza viruses (category J09), and due to other identified influenza virus (category J10) ... coding should be based on the provider's diagnostic statement that the patient has avian influenza, or other novel influenza A, for category J09, or has another particular identified strain of influenza, such as H1N1 or H3N2, but not identified as novel or variant, for category J10.

If the provider records "suspected" or "possible" or "probable" avian influenza, or novel influenza, or other identified influenza, then the appropriate influenza code from category J11, Influenza due to unidentified influenza virus, should be assigned.

CODING TIPS ✓ J09 is not used for influenza type A. Influenza due to **novel** influenza A is coded to J09 along with manifestations of other respiratory, gastrointestinal and other manifestations. Use additional codes to identify the manifestations.

⑤ J09.X   Influenza due to identified novel influenza A virus
Avian influenza
Bird influenza
Influenza A/H5N1
Influenza of other animal origin, not bird or swine
Swine influenza virus (viruses that normally cause infections in pigs)

SP J09.X1   Influenza due to identified novel influenza A virus with pneumonia
Code also, if applicable, associated:
lung abscess (J85.1)
other specified type of pneumonia

---

④4th digit required   ⑤5th digit required   ⑥6th digit required   ⑦7th digit required   ⑦7th digit placeholder   +Additional code   ⑤Laterality

1034   *DecisionHealth's* FY 2020 Complete Home Health ICD-10-CM Diagnosis Coding Manual

Chapter 10

J00-J99

SP + J09.X2 Influenza due to identified novel influenza A virus with other respiratory manifestations
Influenza due to identified novel influenza A virus NOS
Influenza due to identified novel influenza A virus with laryngitis
Influenza due to identified novel influenza A virus with pharyngitis
Influenza due to identified novel influenza A virus with upper respiratory symptoms
Use additional code, if applicable, for associated:
pleural effusion (J91.8)
sinusitis (J01.-)

SP J09.X3 Influenza due to identified novel influenza A virus with gastrointestinal manifestations
Influenza due to identified novel influenza A virus gastroenteritis
EXCLUDES 1 'intestinal flu' [viral gastroenteritis] (A08.-)

SP + J09.X9 Influenza due to identified novel influenza A virus with other manifestations
Influenza due to identified novel influenza A virus with encephalopathy
Influenza due to identified novel influenza A virus with myocarditis
Influenza due to identified novel influenza A virus with otitis media
Use additional code to identify manifestation

4 J10 Influenza due to other identified influenza virus
EXCLUDES 1 influenza due to avian influenza virus (J09.X-)
influenza due to swine flu (J09.X-)
influenza due to unidentifed influenza virus (J11.-)

GUIDELINES Section I.C.10.c
Code only confirmed cases of influenza due to certain identified influenza viruses (category J09), and due to other identified influenza virus (category J10) ... coding should be based on the provider's diagnostic statement that the patient has avian influenza, or other novel influenza A, for category J09, or has another particular identified strain of influenza, such as H1N1 or H3N2, but not identified as novel or variant, for category J10.

If the provider records "suspected" or "possible" or "probable" avian influenza, or novel influenza, or other identified influenza, then the appropriate influenza code from category J11, Influenza due to unidentified influenza virus, should be assigned.

CODING TIPS ✓ Influenza due to other influenza is coded to J10 along with manifestations of other respiratory, gastrointestinal and other manifestations. Use additional codes to identify the manifestations. If the influenza is identified as influenza A but not documented as novel, use these codes.

5 J10.0 Influenza due to other identified influenza virus with pneumonia
Code also:
associated lung abscess, if applicable (J85.1)

SP J10.00 Influenza due to other identified influenza virus with unspecified type of pneumonia

SP J10.01 Influenza due to other identified influenza virus with the same other identified influenza virus pneumonia

SP J10.08 Influenza due to other identified influenza virus with other specified pneumonia
Code also:
other specified type of pneumonia

SP + J10.1 Influenza due to other identified influenza virus with other respiratory manifestations
Influenza due to other identified influenza virus NOS
Influenza due to other identified influenza virus with laryngitis
Influenza due to other identified influenza virus with pharyngitis
Influenza due to other identified influenza virus with upper respiratory symptoms
Use additional code for associated pleural effusion, if applicable (J91.8)
Use additional code for associated sinusitis, if applicable (J01.-)

SP J10.2 Influenza due to other identified influenza virus with gastrointestinal manifestations
Influenza due to other identified influenza virus gastroenteritis
EXCLUDES 1 'intestinal flu' [viral gastroenteritis] (A08.-)

5 J10.8 Influenza due to other identified influenza virus with other manifestations

SP J10.81 Influenza due to other identified influenza virus with encephalopathy

SP J10.82 Influenza due to other identified influenza virus with myocarditis

SP + J10.83 Influenza due to other identified influenza virus with otitis media
Use additional code for any associated perforated tympanic membrane (H72.-)

SP + J10.89 Influenza due to other identified influenza virus with other manifestations
Use additional codes to identify the manifestations

4 J11 Influenza due to unidentified influenza virus
CODING TIPS ✓ Influenza due to an unspecified influenza virus is coded to J11 along with manifestations of other respiratory, gastrointestinal and other manifestations. Use additional codes to identify the manifestations. Documentation from the physician would indicate "flu" or "influenza" to use J11.

★ New ▲ Revised Px Primary SP PDGM Px SL Low CoM SH High CoM IQ Quest. Encounter H Hospice non-cancer Dx Unspecified M *Manifestation*

DecisionHealth's FY 2020 Complete Home Health ICD-10-CM Diagnosis Coding Manual

1035

Chapter 10

J00-J99

5 J11.0 Influenza due to unidentified influenza virus with pneumonia
Code also:
   associated lung abscess, if applicable (J85.1)

SP J11.00 Influenza due to unidentified influenza virus with unspecified type of pneumonia
Influenza with pneumonia NOS

SP J11.08 Influenza due to unidentified influenza virus with specified pneumonia
Code also:
   other specified type of pneumonia

SP + J11.1 Influenza due to unidentified influenza virus with other respiratory manifestations
Influenza NOS
Influenzal laryngitis NOS
Influenzal pharyngitis NOS
Influenza with upper respiratory symptoms NOS
Use additional code for associated pleural effusion, if applicable (J91.8)
Use additional code for associated sinusitis, if applicable (J01.-)

SP J11.2 Influenza due to unidentified influenza virus with gastrointestinal manifestations
Influenza gastroenteritis NOS
EXCLUDES 1 'intestinal flu' [viral gastroenteritis] (A08.-)

5 J11.8 Influenza due to unidentified influenza virus with other manifestations

SP J11.81 Influenza due to unidentified influenza virus with encephalopathy
Influenzal encephalopathy NOS

SP J11.82 Influenza due to unidentified influenza virus with myocarditis
Influenzal myocarditis NOS

SP + J11.83 Influenza due to unidentified influenza virus with otitis media
Influenzal otitis media NOS
Use additional code for any associated perforated tympanic membrane (H72.-)

SP + J11.89 Influenza due to unidentified influenza virus with other manifestations
Use additional codes to identify the manifestations

4 J12 Viral pneumonia, not elsewhere classified
INCLUDES bronchopneumonia due to viruses other than influenza viruses
Code first:
   associated influenza, if applicable (J09.X1, J10.0-, J11.0-)
Code also:
   associated abscess, if applicable (J85.1)
EXCLUDES 1 aspiration pneumonia due to anesthesia during labor and delivery (O74.0)
   aspiration pneumonia due to anesthesia during pregnancy (O29)
   aspiration pneumonia due to anesthesia during puerperium (O89.0)

aspiration pneumonia due to solids and liquids (J69.-)
aspiration pneumonia NOS (J69.0)
congenital pneumonia (P23.0)
congenital rubella pneumonitis (P35.0)
interstitial pneumonia NOS (J84.9)
lipid pneumonia (J69.1)
neonatal aspiration pneumonia (P24.-)

SP J12.0 Adenoviral pneumonia

▲ SP J12.1 Respiratory syncytial virus pneumonia
RSV pneumonia
CODING TIPS ✓ The description of code J12.1 includes the organism, so no additional code is needed for the organism.

SP J12.2 Parainfluenza virus pneumonia

SP J12.3 Human metapneumovirus pneumonia

5 J12.8 Other viral pneumonia

SP J12.81 Pneumonia due to SARS-associated coronavirus
Severe acute respiratory syndrome NOS

SP J12.89 Other viral pneumonia

SP J12.9 Viral pneumonia, unspecified

SP J13 Pneumonia due to Streptococcus pneumoniae
Bronchopneumonia due to S. pneumoniae
Code first:
   associated influenza, if applicable (J09.X1, J10.0-, J11.0-)
Code also:
   associated abscess, if applicable (J85.1)
EXCLUDES 1 congenital pneumonia due to S. pneumoniae (P23.6)
   lobar pneumonia, unspecified organism (J18.1)
   pneumonia due to other streptococci (J15.3-J15.4)

SP J14 Pneumonia due to Hemophilus influenzae
Bronchopneumonia due to H. influenzae
Code first:
   associated influenza, if applicable (J09.X1, J10.0-, J11.0-)
Code also:
   associated abscess, if applicable (J85.1)
EXCLUDES 1 congenital pneumonia due to H. influenzae (P23.6)

4 J15 Bacterial pneumonia, not elsewhere classified
INCLUDES bronchopneumonia due to bacteria other than S. pneumoniae and H. influenzae
Code first:
   associated influenza, if applicable (J09.X1, J10.0-, J11.0-)
Code also:
   associated abscess, if applicable (J85.1)
EXCLUDES 1 chlamydial pneumonia (J16.0)
   congenital pneumonia (P23.-)
   Legionnaires' disease (A48.1)
   spirochetal pneumonia (A69.8)

---

4 4th digit required   5 5th digit required   6 6th digit required   7 7th digit required   7 7th digit placeholder   + Additional code   5 Laterality

1036   *DecisionHealth's* FY 2020 Complete Home Health ICD-10-CM Diagnosis Coding Manual

CODING TIPS ✓ J15 codes are used for bacterial pneumonia when the bacteria is not Streptococcus pneumoniae (J13) or Hemophilus influenzae (J14).

SP J15.0 **Pneumonia due to Klebsiella pneumoniae**

SP J15.1 **Pneumonia due to Pseudomonas**

5 J15.2 **Pneumonia due to staphylococcus**

SP J15.20 **Pneumonia due to staphylococcus, unspecified**

6 J15.21 **Pneumonia due to staphylococcus aureus**

SP J15.211 **Pneumonia due to Methicillin susceptible Staphylococcus aureus**
MSSA pneumonia
Pneumonia due to Staphylococcus aureus NOS

CODING TIPS ✓ J15.211 is used when the organism causing the pneumonia is identified as MSSA-methicillin susceptible Staph aureus, or Staph aureus without information as to resistance.

SP J15.212 **Pneumonia due to Methicillin resistant Staphylococcus aureus**

GUIDELINES Section I.C.1.e.1)
When a patient is diagnosed with an infection that is due to methicillin resistant Staphylococcus aureus (MRSA), and that infection has a combination code that includes the causal organism (e.g., sepsis, pneumonia) assign the appropriate combination code for the condition (e.g., code A41.02, Sepsis due to Methicillin resistant Staphylococcus aureus or code J15.212, Pneumonia due to Methicillin resistant Staphylococcus aureus). Do not assign code B95.62, Methicillin resistant Staphylococcus aureus infection as the cause of diseases classified elsewhere, as an additional code because the combination code includes the type of infection and the MRSA organism. Do not assign a code from subcategory Z16.11, Resistance to penicillins, as an additional diagnosis.

CODING TIPS ✓ J15.212 is used when the organism causing the pneumonia is methicillin resistant or MRSA. Do not use Z16 codes unless the organism is resistant to a different antibiotic, such as vancomycin - Z16.21.

SP J15.29 **Pneumonia due to other staphylococcus**

CODING TIPS ✓ When pneumonia is identified as "staph" without information as to species, e.g., aureus, use this code.

SP J15.3 **Pneumonia due to streptococcus, group B**

SP J15.4 **Pneumonia due to other streptococci**

EXCLUDES 1 pneumonia due to streptococcus, group B (J15.3)
pneumonia due to Streptococcus pneumoniae (J13)

SP J15.5 **Pneumonia due to Escherichia coli**

SP J15.6 **Pneumonia due to other Gram-negative bacteria**
Pneumonia due to other aerobic Gram-negative bacteria
Pneumonia due to Serratia marcescens

SP J15.7 **Pneumonia due to Mycoplasma pneumoniae**

SP J15.8 **Pneumonia due to other specified bacteria**

CODING TIPS ✓ Do not assign code J15.8 for unspecified pneumonia. J15.8 indicates pneumonia with a specified organism for which no combination code exists.

SP J15.9 **Unspecified bacterial pneumonia**
Pneumonia due to gram-positive bacteria

4 J16 **Pneumonia due to other infectious organisms, not elsewhere classified**
Code first:
associated influenza, if applicable (J09.X1, J10.0-, J11.0-)
Code also:
associated abscess, if applicable (J85.1)
EXCLUDES 1 congenital pneumonia (P23.-)
ornithosis (A70)
pneumocystosis (B59)
pneumonia NOS (J18.9)

SP J16.0 **Chlamydial pneumonia**

SP J16.8 **Pneumonia due to other specified infectious organisms**

M IQ J17 *Pneumonia in diseases classified elsewhere*
Code first underlying disease, such as:
Q fever (A78)
rheumatic fever (I00)
schistosomiasis (B65.0-B65.9)
EXCLUDES 1 candidial pneumonia (B37.1)
chlamydial pneumonia (J16.0)
gonorrheal pneumonia (A54.84)
histoplasmosis pneumonia (B39.0-B39.2)
measles pneumonia (B05.2)
nocardiosis pneumonia (A43.0)
pneumocystosis (B59)
pneumonia due to Pneumocystis carinii (B59)
pneumonia due to Pneumocystis jiroveci (B59)
pneumonia in actinomycosis (A42.0)
pneumonia in anthrax (A22.1)
pneumonia in ascariasis (B77.81)
pneumonia in aspergillosis (B44.0-B44.1)
pneumonia in coccidioidomycosis (B38.0-B38.2)
pneumonia in cytomegalovirus disease (B25.0)
pneumonia in toxoplasmosis (B58.3)

★ New ▲ Revised Px Primary **SP** PDGM Px **SL** Low CoM **SH** High CoM **IQ** Quest. Encounter **H** Hospice non-cancer Dx **Unspecified** **M** *Manifestation*

rubella pneumonia (B06.81)
salmonella pneumonia
(A02.22)
spirochetal infection NEC with
pneumonia (A69.8)
tularemia pneumonia (A21.2)
typhoid fever with pneumonia
(A01.03)
varicella pneumonia (B01.2)
whooping cough with
pneumonia
(A37 with fifth-character 1)

4 J18   Pneumonia, unspecified organism
Code first:
associated influenza, if applicable
(J09.X1, J10.0-, J11.0-)
EXCLUDES 1   abscess of lung with pneumonia
(J85.1)
aspiration pneumonia due to
anesthesia during labor and
delivery (O74.0)
aspiration pneumonia due to
anesthesia during pregnancy
(O29)
aspiration pneumonia due to
anesthesia during puerperium
(O89.0)
aspiration pneumonia due to
solids and liquids (J69.-)
aspiration pneumonia NOS
(J69.0)
congenital pneumonia (P23.0)
drug-induced interstitial lung
disorder (J70.2-J70.4)
interstitial pneumonia NOS
(J84.9)
lipid pneumonia (J69.1)
neonatal aspiration pneumonia
(P24.-)
pneumonitis due to external
agents (J67-J70)
pneumonitis due to fumes and
vapors (J68.0)
usual interstitial pneumonia
(J84.17)
CODING TIPS ✓   Do not use code J18 if the
causative agent is known.

**SP J18.0   Bronchopneumonia, unspecified
organism**
EXCLUDES 1   hypostatic
bronchopneumonia
(J18.2)
lipid pneumonia (J69.1)
EXCLUDES 2   acute bronchiolitis (J21.-)
chronic bronchiolitis (J44.9)
**SP J18.1   Lobar pneumonia, unspecified
organism**
**SP J18.2   Hypostatic pneumonia, unspecified
organism**
Hypostatic bronchopneumonia
Passive pneumonia
**SP J18.8   Other pneumonia, unspecified
organism**
SP J18.9   Pneumonia, unspecified organism
CODING TIPS ✓   Assign J43.9 with J18.9 for
emphysema, COPD and pneumonia (Q1
2019 Coding Clinic).

CODING TIPS ✓   Do not assign J18.9 when
the causative organism or underlying cause
of pneumonia is reported in the clinical
record. If the organism or cause of
pneumonia is known, a combination code
should be assigned. When pneumonia is
diagnosed in a patient who also has COPD,
the coder should assign J44.0 and the type
of pneumonia, and sequence according to
the focus of care.

Other acute lower respiratory infections (J20-J22)

EXCLUDES 2   chronic obstructive pulmonary disease with acute
lower respiratory infection (J44.0)
CODING TIPS ✓   Assign J43.9 and J20.9 for emphysema, COPD
and acute bronchitis when there is no mention of a more specific
type of chronic obstructive lung disease, i.e. chronic obstructive
bronchitis (Q1 2019 Coding Clinic).
CODING TIPS ✓   The presence of conditions in J20-J22 along with
a condition classifiable to J44, require the condition be coded
with J44.0 with the lower respiratory infection code. Sequence
according to the focus of care.
CODING TIPS ✓   **Documentation:** Be cautious to differentiate the
diagnostic differences between bronchitis and bronchiolitis.
These are not interchangeable and are not the same disease
process. Bronchitis is inflammation of the mucous membranes of
the bronchi, while bronchiolitis involves inflammation of the
smaller bronchioles which lead directly to the lungs. Bronchiolitis
is more commonly diagnosed in children.

4 J20   Acute bronchitis
INCLUDES   acute and subacute bronchitis
(with) bronchospasm
acute and subacute bronchitis
(with) tracheitis
acute and subacute bronchitis
(with) tracheobronchitis,
acute
acute and subacute fibrinous
bronchitis
acute and subacute membranous
bronchitis
acute and subacute purulent
bronchitis
acute and subacute septic
bronchitis
EXCLUDES 1   bronchitis NOS (J40)
tracheobronchitis NOS (J40)
EXCLUDES 2   acute bronchitis with
bronchiectasis (J47.0)
acute bronchitis with chronic
obstructive asthma (J44.0)
acute bronchitis with chronic
obstructive pulmonary disease
(J44.0)
allergic bronchitis NOS
(J45.909-)
bronchitis due to chemicals,
fumes and vapors (J68.0)
chronic bronchitis NOS (J42)
chronic mucopurulent
bronchitis (J41.1)
chronic obstructive bronchitis
(J44.-)
chronic obstructive
tracheobronchitis (J44.-)

4 4th digit required   5 5th digit required   6 6th digit required   7 7th digit required   ✓ 7th digit placeholder   + Additional code   ▤ Laterality

1038   DecisionHealth's FY 2020 Complete Home Health ICD-10-CM Diagnosis Coding Manual

chronic simple bronchitis (J41.0)

chronic tracheobronchitis (J42)

CODING TIPS ✓ If the patient also has a condition classifiable to J44, code J44.0 and the appropriate code from J20, and sequence according to the focus of care. You may not assume that a lower respiratory infection is an exacerbation of the COPD. If exacerbation is documented in a condition classifiable to J44, then add J44.1.

SP J20.0 **Acute bronchitis due to Mycoplasma pneumoniae**

SP J20.1 **Acute bronchitis due to Hemophilus influenzae**

SP J20.2 **Acute bronchitis due to streptococcus**

SP J20.3 **Acute bronchitis due to coxsackievirus**

SP J20.4 **Acute bronchitis due to parainfluenza virus**

▲ **SP J20.5** **Acute bronchitis due to respiratory syncytial virus**

Acute bronchitis due to RSV

SP J20.6 **Acute bronchitis due to rhinovirus**

SP J20.7 **Acute bronchitis due to echovirus**

SP J20.8 **Acute bronchitis due to other specified organisms**

SP J20.9 **Acute bronchitis, unspecified**

CODING TIPS ✓ Assign J43.9 and J20.9 for emphysema, COPD and acute bronchitis when there is no mention of a more specific type of chronic obstructive lung disease, i.e. chronic obstructive bronchitis (*Q1 2019 Coding Clinic*).

4 J21 **Acute bronchiolitis**

INCLUDES acute bronchiolitis with bronchospasm

EXCLUDES 2 respiratory bronchiolitis interstitial lung disease (J84.115)

▲ **SP J21.0** **Acute bronchiolitis due to respiratory syncytial virus**

Acute bronchiolitis due to RSV

SP J21.1 **Acute bronchiolitis due to human metapneumovirus**

SP J21.8 **Acute bronchiolitis due to other specified organisms**

SP J21.9 **Acute bronchiolitis, unspecified**

Bronchiolitis (acute)

EXCLUDES 1 chronic bronchiolitis (J44.-)

SP J22 **Unspecified acute lower respiratory infection**

Acute (lower) respiratory (tract) infection NOS

EXCLUDES 1 upper respiratory infection (acute) (J06.9)

Other diseases of upper respiratory tract (J30-J39)

4 J30 **Vasomotor and allergic rhinitis**

INCLUDES spasmodic rhinorrhea

EXCLUDES 1 allergic rhinitis with asthma (bronchial) (J45.909)

rhinitis NOS (J31.0)

SP J30.0 **Vasomotor rhinitis**

SP J30.1 **Allergic rhinitis due to pollen**

Allergy NOS due to pollen

Hay fever

Pollinosis

SP J30.2 **Other seasonal allergic rhinitis**

SP J30.5 **Allergic rhinitis due to food**

5 J30.8 **Other allergic rhinitis**

SP J30.81 **Allergic rhinitis due to animal (cat) (dog) hair and dander**

SP J30.89 **Other allergic rhinitis**

Perennial allergic rhinitis

SP J30.9 **Allergic rhinitis, unspecified**

+ 4 J31 **Chronic rhinitis, nasopharyngitis and pharyngitis**

Use additional code to identify:

exposure to environmental tobacco smoke (Z77.22)

exposure to tobacco smoke in the perinatal period (P96.81)

history of tobacco dependence (Z87.891)

occupational exposure to environmental tobacco smoke (Z57.31)

tobacco dependence (F17.-)

tobacco use (Z72.0)

SP + J31.0 **Chronic rhinitis**

Atrophic rhinitis (chronic)

Granulomatous rhinitis (chronic)

Hypertrophic rhinitis (chronic)

Obstructive rhinitis (chronic)

Ozena

Purulent rhinitis (chronic)

Rhinitis (chronic) NOS

Ulcerative rhinitis (chronic)

EXCLUDES 1 allergic rhinitis (J30.1-J30.9)

vasomotor rhinitis (J30.0)

DEFINITION Long-term inflammation of the nasal mucous membrane, with wasting of the mucous membrane and glands.

SP + J31.1 **Chronic nasopharyngitis**

EXCLUDES 2 acute nasopharyngitis (J00)

DEFINITION Long-term inflammation of the nasal and pharyngeal (throat) mucous membranes.

SP + J31.2 **Chronic pharyngitis**

Chronic sore throat

Atrophic pharyngitis (chronic)

Granular pharyngitis (chronic)

Hypertrophic pharyngitis (chronic)

EXCLUDES 2 acute pharyngitis (J02.9)

+ 4 J32 **Chronic sinusitis**

INCLUDES sinus abscess

sinus empyema

sinus infection

sinus suppuration

Use additional code to identify:

exposure to environmental tobacco smoke (Z77.22)

exposure to tobacco smoke in the perinatal period (P96.81)

history of tobacco dependence (Z87.891)

infectious agent (B95-B97)

occupational exposure to environmental tobacco smoke (Z57.31)

tobacco dependence (F17.-)

tobacco use (Z72.0)

★ New ▲ Revised **Px** Primary **SP** PDGM Px **SL** Low CoM **SH** High CoM **IQ** Quest. Encounter **H** Hospice non-cancer Dx **Unspecified** **M** *Manifestation*

Chapter 10

J00-J99

EXCLUDES 2   acute sinusitis (J01.-)

CODING TIPS ✓   Do not assign a code from J32.- when sinusitis is reported as acute or infectious, unless the patient is reported to have both the chronic and acute form of sinusitis. If both forms are reported as confirmed in the medical record, assign separate and specific codes for each.

SP ➕ **J32.0   Chronic maxillary sinusitis**
Antritis (chronic)
Maxillary sinusitis NOS

SP ➕ **J32.1   Chronic frontal sinusitis**
Frontal sinusitis NOS

SP ➕ **J32.2   Chronic ethmoidal sinusitis**
Ethmoidal sinusitis NOS
EXCLUDES 1   Woakes' ethmoiditis (J33.1)

SP ➕ **J32.3   Chronic sphenoidal sinusitis**
Sphenoidal sinusitis NOS

SP ➕ **J32.4   Chronic pansinusitis**
Pansinusitis NOS

SP ➕ **J32.8   Other chronic sinusitis**
Sinusitis (chronic) involving more than one sinus but not pansinusitis

SP ➕ **J32.9   Chronic sinusitis, unspecified**
Sinusitis (chronic) NOS

➕ **4 J33   Nasal polyp**
Use additional code to identify:
exposure to environmental tobacco smoke (Z77.22)
exposure to tobacco smoke in the perinatal period (P96.81)
history of tobacco dependence (Z87.891)
occupational exposure to environmental tobacco smoke (Z57.31)
tobacco dependence (F17.-)
tobacco use (Z72.0)
EXCLUDES 1   adenomatous polyps (D14.0)

SP ➕ **J33.0   Polyp of nasal cavity**
Choanal polyp
Nasopharyngeal polyp

SP ➕ **J33.1   Polypoid sinus degeneration**
Woakes' syndrome or ethmoiditis

SP ➕ **J33.8   Other polyp of sinus**
Accessory polyp of sinus
Ethmoidal polyp of sinus
Maxillary polyp of sinus
Sphenoidal polyp of sinus

SP ➕ **J33.9   Nasal polyp, unspecified**

4 J34   Other and unspecified disorders of nose and nasal sinuses
EXCLUDES 2   varicose ulcer of nasal septum (I86.8)

SP **J34.0   Abscess, furuncle and carbuncle of nose**
Cellulitis of nose
Necrosis of nose
Ulceration of nose

SP **J34.1   Cyst and mucocele of nose and nasal sinus**

SP **J34.2   Deviated nasal septum**
Deflection or deviation of septum (nasal) (acquired)
EXCLUDES 1   congenital deviated nasal septum (Q67.4)
DEFINITION   Cartilage separating the nostrils is shifted out of position, usually due to an old traumatic injury.

SP **J34.3   Hypertrophy of nasal turbinates**

5 J34.8   Other specified disorders of nose and nasal sinuses

SP **J34.81   Nasal mucositis (ulcerative)**
Code also type of associated therapy, such as:
antineoplastic and immunosuppressive drugs (T45.1X-)
radiological procedure and radiotherapy (Y84.2)
EXCLUDES 2   gastrointestinal mucositis (ulcerative) (K92.81)
mucositis (ulcerative) of vagina and vulva (N76.81)
oral mucositis (ulcerative) (K12.3-)

SP **J34.89   Other specified disorders of nose and nasal sinuses**
Perforation of nasal septum NOS
Rhinolith

IQ **J34.9   Unspecified disorder of nose and nasal sinuses**

➕ **4 J35   Chronic diseases of tonsils and adenoids**
Use additional code to identify:
exposure to environmental tobacco smoke (Z77.22)
exposure to tobacco smoke in the perinatal period (P96.81)
history of tobacco dependence (Z87.891)
occupational exposure to environmental tobacco smoke (Z57.31)
tobacco dependence (F17.-)
tobacco use (Z72.0)

➕ **5 J35.0   Chronic tonsillitis and adenoiditis**
EXCLUDES 2   acute tonsillitis (J03.-)

SP ➕ **J35.01   Chronic tonsillitis**

SP ➕ **J35.02   Chronic adenoiditis**

SP ➕ **J35.03   Chronic tonsillitis and adenoiditis**

SP ➕ **J35.1   Hypertrophy of tonsils**
Enlargement of tonsils
EXCLUDES 1   hypertrophy of tonsils with tonsillitis (J35.0-)

SP ➕ **J35.2   Hypertrophy of adenoids**
Enlargement of adenoids
EXCLUDES 1   hypertrophy of adenoids with adenoiditis (J35.0-)

SP ➕ **J35.3   Hypertrophy of tonsils with hypertrophy of adenoids**
EXCLUDES 1   hypertrophy of tonsils and adenoids with tonsillitis and adenoiditis (J35.03)

SP ➕ **J35.8   Other chronic diseases of tonsils and adenoids**
Adenoid vegetations
Amygdalolith
Calculus, tonsil
Cicatrix of tonsil (and adenoid)
Tonsillar tag
Ulcer of tonsil

IQ ➕ **J35.9   Chronic disease of tonsils and adenoids, unspecified**
Disease (chronic) of tonsils and adenoids NOS

SP ➕ **J36   Peritonsillar abscess**
INCLUDES   abscess of tonsil

---

4 4th digit required   **5** 5th digit required   **6** 6th digit required   **7** 7th digit required   **7** 7th digit placeholder   ➕ Additional code   ⊟ Laterality peritonsillar cellulitis

quinsy

Use additional code (B95-B97) to identify infectious agent.

> **EXCLUDES 1** acute tonsillitis (J03.-)
> chronic tonsillitis (J35.0)
> retropharyngeal abscess (J39.0)
> tonsillitis NOS (J03.9-)

+ 🄴 J37 Chronic laryngitis and laryngotracheitis

Use additional code to identify:

exposure to environmental tobacco smoke (Z77.22)

exposure to tobacco smoke in the perinatal period (P96.81)

history of tobacco dependence (Z87.891)

infectious agent (B95-B97)

occupational exposure to environmental tobacco smoke (Z57.31)

tobacco dependence (F17.-)

tobacco use (Z72.0)

> **CODING TIPS ✓** Assign a code from J37.- only when the physician specifies laryngitis or laryngotracheitis as "chronic."

SP + J37.0 Chronic laryngitis

Catarrhal laryngitis

Hypertrophic laryngitis

Sicca laryngitis

> **EXCLUDES 2** acute laryngitis (J04.0)
> obstructive (acute) laryngitis (J05.0)

SP + J37.1 Chronic laryngotracheitis

Laryngitis, chronic, with tracheitis (chronic)

Tracheitis, chronic, with laryngitis

> **EXCLUDES 1** chronic tracheitis (J42)

> **EXCLUDES 2** acute laryngotracheitis (J04.2)
> acute tracheitis (J04.1)

> **DEFINITION** Long-term inflammation extending past the vocal cords and into the trachea.

+ 🄴 J38 Diseases of vocal cords and larynx, not elsewhere classified

Use additional code to identify:

exposure to environmental tobacco smoke (Z77.22)

exposure to tobacco smoke in the perinatal period (P96.81)

history of tobacco dependence (Z87.891)

occupational exposure to environmental tobacco smoke (Z57.31)

tobacco dependence (F17.-)

tobacco use (Z72.0)

> **EXCLUDES 1** congenital laryngeal stridor (P28.89)
> obstructive laryngitis (acute) (J05.0)
> postprocedural subglottic stenosis (J95.5)
> stridor (R06.1)
> ulcerative laryngitis (J04.0)

+ 🄵 J38.0 Paralysis of vocal cords and larynx

Laryngoplegia

Paralysis of glottis

🅀 + J38.00 Paralysis of vocal cords and larynx, unspecified

SP + J38.01 Paralysis of vocal cords and larynx, unilateral

SP + J38.02 Paralysis of vocal cords and larynx, bilateral

SP + J38.1 Polyp of vocal cord and larynx

> **EXCLUDES 1** adenomatous polyps (D14.1)

SP + J38.2 Nodules of vocal cords

Chorditis (fibrinous)(nodosa)(tuberosa)

Singer's nodes

Teacher's nodes

SP + J38.3 Other diseases of vocal cords

Abscess of vocal cords

Cellulitis of vocal cords

Granuloma of vocal cords

Leukokeratosis of vocal cords

Leukoplakia of vocal cords

SP + J38.4 Edema of larynx

Edema (of) glottis

Subglottic edema

Supraglottic edema

> **EXCLUDES 1** acute obstructive laryngitis [croup] (J05.0)
> edematous laryngitis (J04.0)

SP + J38.5 Laryngeal spasm

Laryngismus (stridulus)

SP + J38.6 Stenosis of larynx

SP + J38.7 Other diseases of larynx

Abscess of larynx

Cellulitis of larynx

Disease of larynx NOS

Necrosis of larynx

Pachyderma of larynx

Perichondritis of larynx

Ulcer of larynx

🄴 J39 Other diseases of upper respiratory tract

> **EXCLUDES 1** acute respiratory infection NOS (J22)
> acute upper respiratory infection (J06.9)
> upper respiratory inflammation due to chemicals, gases, fumes or vapors (J68.2)

SP J39.0 Retropharyngeal and parapharyngeal abscess

Peripharyngeal abscess

> **EXCLUDES 1** peritonsillar abscess (J36)

> **DEFINITION** Pus-filled sore at the back of the throat.

SP J39.1 Other abscess of pharynx

Cellulitis of pharynx

Nasopharyngeal abscess

> **CODING TIPS ✓** Do not assign J39.1 for a diagnosis of pharyngitis. Acute pharyngitis should be coded to J02.-

SP J39.2 Other diseases of pharynx

Cyst of pharynx

Edema of pharynx

> **EXCLUDES 2** chronic pharyngitis (J31.2)
> ulcerative pharyngitis (J02.9)

SP J39.3 Upper respiratory tract hypersensitivity reaction, site unspecified

> **EXCLUDES 1** hypersensitivity reaction of upper respiratory tract, such as:
> extrinsic allergic alveolitis (J67.9)

✱ New ▲ Revised Px Primary **SP** PDGM Px **SL** Low CoM **SH** High CoM **🅀** Quest. Encounter 🄷 Hospice non-cancer Dx Unspecified **M** *Manifestation*

DecisionHealth's FY 2020 Complete Home Health ICD-10-CM Diagnosis Coding Manual

1041

pneumoconiosis (J60-J67.9)

SP J39.8 Other specified diseases of upper respiratory tract

SP J39.9 Disease of upper respiratory tract, unspecified

Chronic lower respiratory diseases (J40-J47)

EXCLUDES 1 bronchitis due to chemicals, gases, fumes and vapors (J68.0)

EXCLUDES 2 cystic fibrosis (E84.-)

Acute Bronchitis

Normal

SP + J40 Bronchitis, not specified as acute or chronic
Bronchitis NOS
Bronchitis with tracheitis NOS
Catarrhal bronchitis
Tracheobronchitis NOS
Use additional code to identify:
    exposure to environmental tobacco smoke (Z77.22)
    exposure to tobacco smoke in the perinatal period (P96.81)
    history of tobacco dependence (Z87.891)
    occupational exposure to environmental tobacco smoke (Z57.31)
    tobacco dependence (F17.-)
    tobacco use (Z72.0)
    EXCLUDES 1 acute bronchitis (J20.-)
        allergic bronchitis NOS (J45.909-)
        asthmatic bronchitis NOS (J45.9-)
        bronchitis due to chemicals, gases, fumes and vapors (J68.0)

CODING TIPS ✓ Do not assign code J40 for chronic, chronic obstructive, or acute bronchitis. J40 should be assigned only when no diagnostic information is available to differentiate the type of bronchitis.

+ 4 J41 Simple and mucopurulent chronic bronchitis
Use additional code to identify:
    exposure to environmental tobacco smoke (Z77.22)
    exposure to tobacco smoke in the perinatal period (P96.81)
    history of tobacco dependence (Z87.891)
    occupational exposure to environmental tobacco smoke (Z57.31)
    tobacco dependence (F17.-)
    tobacco use (Z72.0)
    EXCLUDES 1 chronic bronchitis NOS (J42)
        chronic obstructive bronchitis (J44.-)

CODING TIPS ✓ Chronic bronchitis not specified as "obstructive" should be coded to J41.0-J42. Chronic bronchitis that is specified as obstructive is coded to category J44.-. Chronic indicates cough with mucus most days of the month for at least 3 months out of the year.

SP + J41.0 Simple chronic bronchitis

SP + J41.1 Mucopurulent chronic bronchitis

SP + J41.8 Mixed simple and mucopurulent chronic bronchitis

SP + J42 Unspecified chronic bronchitis
Chronic bronchitis NOS
Chronic tracheitis
Chronic tracheobronchitis
Use additional code to identify:
    exposure to environmental tobacco smoke (Z77.22)
    exposure to tobacco smoke in the perinatal period (P96.81)
    history of tobacco dependence (Z87.891)
    occupational exposure to environmental tobacco smoke (Z57.31)
    tobacco dependence (F17.-)
    tobacco use (Z72.0)
    EXCLUDES 1 chronic asthmatic bronchitis (J44.-)
        chronic bronchitis with airways obstruction (J44.-)
        chronic emphysematous bronchitis (J44.-)
        chronic obstructive pulmonary disease NOS (J44.9)
        simple and mucopurulent chronic bronchitis (J41.-)

CODING TIPS ✓ Chronic bronchitis not specified as "obstructive" should be coded to J41.0-J42. Chronic bronchitis that is specified as obstructive is coded to category J44.-. Chronic indicates cough with mucus most days of the month for at least 3 months out of the year.

+ 4 J43 Emphysema
Use additional code to identify:
    exposure to environmental tobacco smoke (Z77.22)
    history of tobacco dependence (Z87.891)
    occupational exposure to environmental tobacco smoke (Z57.31)
    tobacco dependence (F17.-)
    tobacco use (Z72.0)
    EXCLUDES 1 compensatory emphysema (J98.3)

---

4 4th digit required   5 5th digit required   6 6th digit required   7 7th digit required   7 7th digit placeholder   +Additional code   ⊟ Laterality

emphysema due to inhalation of chemicals, gases, fumes or vapors (J68.4)

emphysema with chronic (obstructive) bronchitis (J44.-)

emphysematous (obstructive) bronchitis (J44.-)

interstitial emphysema (J98.2)

mediastinal emphysema (J98.2)

neonatal interstitial emphysema (P25.0)

surgical (subcutaneous) emphysema (T81.82)

traumatic subcutaneous emphysema (T79.7)

CODING TIPS ✓ Emphysema and COPD (not documented as a specific chronic obstructive bronchitis, chronic obstructive asthma or emphysematous bronchitis) is coded to J43. Emphysema with documented exacerbated COPD is coded to J43, not J44.

CODING TIPS ✓ Do not assign a code from J43.- when the physician documentation reports emphysema with chronic obstructive bronchitis or emphysematous bronchitis. Emphysema with chronic obstructive bronchitis and emphysematous bronchitis should be coded to J44.- and cannot be coded on the same claim as J43.-.

CODING TIPS ✓ Codes in the subclassification J43 include respiratory insufficiency; therefore, do not assign R06.89 as an additional code. However, respiratory failure, if documented, should be coded.

CODING TIPS ✓ When a diagnosis supports coding a more specific code for emphysema, such as interstitial emphysema (J98.2), compensatory emphysema (J98.3), or subcutaneous emphysema due to trauma (T79.7), then do not assign J43.-, but assign the more specific code.

SP + J43.0 Unilateral pulmonary emphysema [MacLeod's syndrome]
Swyer-James syndrome
Unilateral emphysema
Unilateral hyperlucent lung
Unilateral pulmonary artery functional hypoplasia
Unilateral transparency of lung

SP + J43.1 Panlobular emphysema
Panacinar emphysema

SP + J43.2 Centrilobular emphysema

SP + J43.8 Other emphysema

SP + J43.9 Emphysema, unspecified
Bullous emphysema (lung)(pulmonary)
Emphysema (lung)(pulmonary) NOS
Emphysematous bleb
Vesicular emphysema (lung)(pulmonary)

CODING TIPS ✓ Assign J43.9 and J20.9 for emphysema, COPD and acute bronchitis when there's no mention of chronic bronchitis; assign J43.9 with J18.9 for emphysema, COPD and pneumonia; assign J43.9 with a code from J45 for emphysema, COPD and asthma (*Q1 2019 Coding Clinic*)..

DEFINITION Abnormal enlargement of the air sacs in the lungs, which lose their elasticity, making breathing increasingly difficult.

+ ☑ J44 Other chronic obstructive pulmonary disease

INCLUDES asthma with chronic obstructive pulmonary disease
chronic asthmatic (obstructive) bronchitis
chronic bronchitis with airways obstruction
chronic bronchitis with emphysema
chronic emphysematous bronchitis
chronic obstructive asthma
chronic obstructive bronchitis
chronic obstructive tracheobronchitis

Code also:
type of asthma, if applicable (J45.-)
Use additional code to identify:
exposure to environmental tobacco smoke (Z77.22)
history of tobacco dependence (Z87.891)
occupational exposure to environmental tobacco smoke (Z57.31)
tobacco dependence (F17.-)
tobacco use (Z72.0)

EXCLUDES 1 bronchiectasis (J47.-)
chronic bronchitis NOS (J42)
chronic simple and mucopurulent bronchitis (J41.-)
chronic tracheitis (J42)
chronic tracheobronchitis (J42)
emphysema without chronic bronchitis (J43.-)

GUIDELINES Section I.C.10.a
The codes in categories J44 and J45 distinguish between uncomplicated cases and those in acute exacerbation. An acute exacerbation is a worsening or a decompensation of a chronic condition. An acute exacerbation is not equivalent to an infection superimposed on a chronic condition, though an exacerbation may be triggered by an infection.

CODING TIPS ✓ COPD is not the same as chronic bronchitis. COPD is an unspecified term that may encompass multiple components of chronic obstructive pulmonary disease (chronic bronchitis, chronic asthma and emphysema). Code J43.- is used when COPD (unspecified) and emphysema have been documented by the provider.

★ New ▲ Revised Px Primary SP PDGM Px SL Low CoM SH High CoM IQ Quest. Encounter H Hospice non-cancer Dx Unspecified M *Manifestation*

DecisionHealth's FY 2020 Complete Home Health ICD-10-CM Diagnosis Coding Manual

1043

Chapter 10

J00-J99

CODING TIPS ✓ If the type of asthma is specified by the physician, also code the J45 for the type of asthma. If the physician documents that the asthma is exacerbated, but not which type, add J45.901. If the physician has documented asthma, but not specified the type, or exacerbation, do not code the asthma (J45), if the patient has COPD.

▲ **SP** **SH** ✚ **J44.0** **Chronic obstructive pulmonary disease with (acute) lower respiratory infection**
Code also:
  to identify the infection

CODING TIPS ✓ Assign a code from J44.0 when a patient has both a condition classifiable to J44 and a diagnosis of a lower respiratory tract infection. Examples of lower respiratory infections include pneumonia, bronchitis and bronchiolitis. An additional code should be assigned to report the infection, and sequence depending on the focus of care.

CODING TIPS ✓ If the physician confirms both a diagnosis of a lower respiratory tract infection and exacerbation of a condition classifiable to J44, both J44.1 and J44.0 should be assigned, along with a code for the specific lower respiratory infection.

SP **SH** ✚ **J44.1** **Chronic obstructive pulmonary disease with (acute) exacerbation**
Decompensated COPD
Decompensated COPD with (acute) exacerbation
EXCLUDES 2 chronic obstructive pulmonary disease [COPD] with acute bronchitis (J44.0)
  lung diseases due to external agents (J60-J70)

CODING TIPS ✓ **Documentation:** Do not assign this code unless the physician has confirmed that the condition is exacerbated. An exacerbation should be documented by the physician, and changes in treatment and medication regimen do not presume an exacerbation.

CODING TIPS ✓ This code is appropriate when the patient has an acute exacerbation of a condition classifiable to J44, or the disease is decompensating. If the disease is **not** decompensating or exacerbated, use J44.9. If there is a lower respiratory infection, use J44.0, not J44.9.

CODING TIPS ✓ An acute exacerbation is a worsening or decompensation of a chronic condition. Decompensated indicates there has been a flare-up (acute phase) of a chronic condition. It is not equivalent to an infection superimposed on a chronic condition, so do not assume an exacerbation with an infection. The physician must indicate an exacerbation, decompensation or flare-up to use this code.

SP **SH** ✚ **J44.9** **Chronic obstructive pulmonary disease, unspecified**
Chronic obstructive airway disease NOS

Chronic obstructive lung disease NOS
EXCLUDES 2 lung diseases due to external agents (J60-J70)

CODING TIPS ✓ If a condition classifiable to J44 is documented with exacerbation or lower respiratory infection, do not assign J44.9, and use the more specific code(s). If any condition is documented that is included in J44 without an exacerbation or lower respiratory infection, use J44.9. Respiratory insufficiency is an integral part of these diseases; therefore, do not assign additional code R06.89. However, respiratory failure, if indicated, is coded as an additional code.

✚ **4** **J45** **Asthma**
INCLUDES allergic (predominantly) asthma
  allergic bronchitis NOS
  allergic rhinitis with asthma
  atopic asthma
  extrinsic allergic asthma
  hay fever with asthma
  idiosyncratic asthma
  intrinsic nonallergic asthma
  nonallergic asthma
Use additional code to identify:
  exposure to environmental tobacco smoke (Z77.22)
  exposure to tobacco smoke in the perinatal period (P96.81)
  history of tobacco dependence (Z87.891)
  occupational exposure to environmental tobacco smoke (Z57.31)
  tobacco dependence (F17.-)
  tobacco use (Z72.0)
EXCLUDES 1 detergent asthma (J69.8)
  eosinophilic asthma (J82)
  miner's asthma (J60)
  wheezing NOS (R06.2)
  wood asthma (J67.8)
EXCLUDES 2 asthma with chronic obstructive pulmonary disease (J44.9)
  chronic asthmatic (obstructive) bronchitis (J44.9)
  chronic obstructive asthma (J44.9)
GUIDELINES **Section I.C.10.a**
The codes in categories J44 and J45 distinguish between uncomplicated cases and those in acute exacerbation. An acute exacerbation is a worsening or a decompensation of a chronic condition. An acute exacerbation is not equivalent to an infection superimposed on a chronic condition, though an exacerbation may be triggered by an infection.

CODING TIPS ✓ Assign J43.9 with a code from J45 for emphysema, COPD and asthma (*Q1 2019 Coding Clinic*).

CODING TIPS ✓ The patient can have both asthma and other types of COPD, so when documentation indicates a condition classifiable to J44 and any **specified** type of asthma, or exacerbation of asthma, the asthma should also be coded.

---

4 4th digit required   **5** 5th digit required   **6** 6th digit required   **7** 7th digit required   **7** 7th digit placeholder   ✚ Additional code   ⊟ Laterality

CODING TIPS ✓ Status asthmaticus refers to a patient's failure to respond to therapy administered during an asthmatic episode. It is a life-threatening complication that requires emergency care.

CODING TIPS ✓ Patients are classified as having intermittent or persistent (mild, moderate or severe) asthma depending on the degree of impairment and risk. The severity of asthma is determined based on which of the following factors is the worst: daytime or nocturnal symptoms, rescue SABA use, lung function or exacerbation frequency.

DEFINITION Asthma is also known as reactive airway disease. It is an inflammatory process of the lining of the airways of the lungs and is considered reversible. Patients with asthma typically develop wheezing, shortness of breath and cough. Because the inflammation of the lining of the airways is considered reversible, asthma symptoms are intermittent and cover a spectrum from mild-to-severe disease. Several symptoms overlap in patients with COPD and asthma. A history of wheezing strongly suggests a diagnosis of asthma, whereas chronic cough productive of sputum is more indicative of COPD.

+ 5 J45.2 Mild intermittent asthma

SP SH + J45.20 Mild intermittent asthma, uncomplicated
Mild intermittent asthma NOS

SP SH + J45.21 Mild intermittent asthma with (acute) exacerbation

SP SH + J45.22 Mild intermittent asthma with status asthmaticus

+ 5 J45.3 Mild persistent asthma

SP SH + J45.30 Mild persistent asthma, uncomplicated
Mild persistent asthma NOS

SP SH + J45.31 Mild persistent asthma with (acute) exacerbation

SP SH + J45.32 Mild persistent asthma with status asthmaticus

+ 5 J45.4 Moderate persistent asthma

SP SH + J45.40 Moderate persistent asthma, uncomplicated
Moderate persistent asthma NOS

SP SH + J45.41 Moderate persistent asthma with (acute) exacerbation

SP SH + J45.42 Moderate persistent asthma with status asthmaticus

+ 5 J45.5 Severe persistent asthma

SP SH + J45.50 Severe persistent asthma, uncomplicated
Severe persistent asthma NOS

SP SH + J45.51 Severe persistent asthma with (acute) exacerbation

SP SH + J45.52 Severe persistent asthma with status asthmaticus

+ 5 J45.9 Other and unspecified asthma

+ 6 J45.90 Unspecified asthma
Asthmatic bronchitis NOS
Childhood asthma NOS
Late onset asthma

SP SH + J45.901 Unspecified asthma with (acute) exacerbation

SP SH + J45.902 Unspecified asthma with status asthmaticus

SP SH + J45.909 Unspecified asthma, uncomplicated
Asthma NOS
EXCLUDES 2 lung diseases due to external agents (J60-J70)

CODING TIPS ✓ Do not use this code with J44. Asthma is included in the conditions classifiable to J44, and the asthma code should be added only if asthma is specified or exacerbated.

+ 6 J45.99 Other asthma

SP SH + J45.990 Exercise induced bronchospasm

SP SH + J45.991 Cough variant asthma

SP SH + J45.998 Other asthma

+ 4 J47 Bronchiectasis
INCLUDES bronchiolectasis
Use additional code to identify:
    exposure to environmental tobacco smoke (Z77.22)
    exposure to tobacco smoke in the perinatal period (P96.81)
    history of tobacco dependence (Z87.891)
    occupational exposure to environmental tobacco smoke (Z57.31)
    tobacco dependence (F17.-)
    tobacco use (Z72.0)
EXCLUDES 1 congenital bronchiectasis (Q33.4)
    tuberculous bronchiectasis (current disease) (A15.0)

SP SH + J47.0 Bronchiectasis with acute lower respiratory infection
Bronchiectasis with acute bronchitis
Use additional code to identify the infection

SP SH + J47.1 Bronchiectasis with (acute) exacerbation

SP SH + J47.9 Bronchiectasis, uncomplicated
Bronchiectasis NOS
DEFINITION Destruction and widening of the large airways, often due to recurrent, severe infection or inflammation, or following foreign body obstruction.

Lung diseases due to external agents (J60-J70)

EXCLUDES 2 asthma (J45.-)
malignant neoplasm of bronchus and lung (C34.-)

SP J60 Coalworker's pneumoconiosis
Anthracosilicosis
Anthracosis
Black lung disease
Coalworker's lung
EXCLUDES 1 coalworker pneumoconiosis with tuberculosis, any type in A15 (J65)
DEFINITION Silicotic nodules and scar-tissue formation in the lungs due to prolonged inhalation and collection of coal dust particles in the bronchioles.

SP J61 Pneumoconiosis due to asbestos and other mineral fibers

Chapter 10

J00-J99

★ New ▲ Revised **Px** Primary **SP** PDGM Px **SL** Low CoM **SH** High CoM **IQ** Quest. Encounter **H** Hospice non-cancer Dx Unspecified **M** *Manifestation*

DecisionHealth's FY 2020 Complete Home Health ICD-10-CM Diagnosis Coding Manual

1045

Asbestosis

EXCLUDES 1 pleural plaque with asbestosis
(J92.0)
pneumoconiosis with
tuberculosis, any type in A15
(J65)

DEFINITION Chronic lung disease caused by
inhaling asbestos particles over a prolonged
period.

☑ J62 Pneumoconiosis due to dust containing silica

INCLUDES silicotic fibrosis (massive) of
lung

EXCLUDES 1 pneumoconiosis with
tuberculosis, any type in A15

SP J62.0 Pneumoconiosis due to talc dust

**SP J62.8 Pneumoconiosis due to other dust
containing silica**
Silicosis NOS

☑ J63 Pneumoconiosis due to other inorganic dusts

EXCLUDES 1 pneumoconiosis with
tuberculosis, any type in A15
(J65)

SP J63.0 Aluminosis (of lung)

SP J63.1 Bauxite fibrosis (of lung)

SP J63.2 Berylliosis

SP J63.3 Graphite fibrosis (of lung)

SP J63.4 Siderosis

SP J63.5 Stannosis

**SP J63.6 Pneumoconiosis due to other specified
inorganic dusts**

SP J64 Unspecified pneumoconiosis

EXCLUDES 1 pneumonoconiosis with
tuberculosis, any type in A15
(J65)

**SP J65 Pneumoconiosis associated with
tuberculosis**
Any condition in J60-J64 with tuberculosis,
any type in A15
Silicotuberculosis

☑ J66 Airway disease due to specific organic dust

EXCLUDES 2 allergic alveolitis (J67.-)
asbestosis (J61)
bagassosis (J67.1)
farmer's lung (J67.0)
hypersensitivity pneumonitis
due to organic dust (J67.-)
reactive airways dysfunction
syndrome (J68.3)

SP J66.0 Byssinosis
Airway disease due to cotton dust

SP J66.1 Flax-dressers' disease

SP J66.2 Cannabinosis

**SP J66.8 Airway disease due to other specific
organic dusts**

**☑ J67 Hypersensitivity pneumonitis due to
organic dust**

INCLUDES allergic alveolitis and
pneumonitis due to inhaled
organic dust and particles of
fungal, actinomycetic or other
origin

EXCLUDES 1 pneumonitis due to inhalation of
chemicals, gases, fumes or
vapors (J68.0)

SP J67.0 Farmer's lung
Harvester's lung
Haymaker's lung
Moldy hay disease

DEFINITION Inflammation of the small,
inner air sacs in the lungs, due to an allergic
reaction triggered by inhaled organic
substances or microorganisms.

SP J67.1 Bagassosis
Bagasse disease
Bagasse pneumonitis

SP J67.2 Bird fancier's lung
Budgerigar fancier's disease or lung
Pigeon fancier's disease or lung

SP J67.3 Suberosis
Corkhandler's disease or lung
Corkworker's disease or lung

SP J67.4 Maltworker's lung
Alveolitis due to Aspergillus clavatus

SP J67.5 Mushroom-worker's lung

SP J67.6 Maple-bark-stripper's lung
Alveolitis due to Cryptostroma corticale
Cryptostromosis

SP J67.7 Air conditioner and humidifier lung
Allergic alveolitis due to fungal,
thermophilic actinomycetes and other
organisms growing in ventilation [air
conditioning] systems

**SP J67.8 Hypersensitivity pneumonitis due to
other organic dusts**
Cheese-washer's lung
Coffee-worker's lung
Fish-meal worker's lung
Furrier's lung
Sequoiosis

**SP J67.9 Hypersensitivity pneumonitis due to
unspecified organic dust**
Allergic alveolitis (extrinsic) NOS
Hypersensitivity pneumonitis NOS

**+ ☑ J68 Respiratory conditions due to inhalation of
chemicals, gases, fumes and vapors**
Code first:
(T51-T65) to identify cause
Use additional code to identify associated
respiratory conditions, such as:
acute respiratory failure (J96.0-)

**SP + J68.0 Bronchitis and pneumonitis due to
chemicals, gases, fumes and vapors**
Chemical bronchitis (acute)

**SP + J68.1 Pulmonary edema due to chemicals,
gases, fumes and vapors**
Chemical pulmonary edema (acute)
(chronic)

EXCLUDES 1 pulmonary edema (acute)
(chronic) NOS (J81.-)

**SP + J68.2 Upper respiratory inflammation due to
chemicals, gases, fumes and vapors, not
elsewhere classified**

**SP + J68.3 Other acute and subacute respiratory
conditions due to chemicals, gases,
fumes and vapors**
Reactive airways dysfunction syndrome

**SP + J68.4 Chronic respiratory conditions due to
chemicals, gases, fumes and vapors**

☑4th digit required   **☑**5th digit required   **☑**6th digit required   **☑**7th digit required   **☑**7th digit placeholder   **+**Additional code   **☐**Laterality

Emphysema (diffuse) (chronic) due to inhalation of chemicals, gases, fumes and vapors

Obliterative bronchiolitis (chronic) (subacute) due to inhalation of chemicals, gases, fumes and vapors

Pulmonary fibrosis (chronic) due to inhalation of chemicals, gases, fumes and vapors

> **EXCLUDES 1** chronic pulmonary edema due to chemicals, gases, fumes and vapors (J68.1)

SP + J68.8 Other respiratory conditions due to chemicals, gases, fumes and vapors

SP + J68.9 Unspecified respiratory condition due to chemicals, gases, fumes and vapors

4 J69 Pneumonitis due to solids and liquids

> **EXCLUDES 1** neonatal aspiration syndromes (P24.-)
> postprocedural pneumonitis (J95.4)

CODING TIPS ✓ Aspiration pneumonia is not considered an infection (although it can result in an infection). Code J44.0 is NOT to be used with J69, unless a secondary infection is also documented.

SP J69.0 Pneumonitis due to inhalation of food and vomit

Aspiration pneumonia NOS

Aspiration pneumonia (due to) food (regurgitated)

Aspiration pneumonia (due to) gastric secretions

Aspiration pneumonia (due to) milk

Aspiration pneumonia (due to) vomit

Code also:
  any associated foreign body in respiratory tract (T17.-)

> **EXCLUDES 1** chemical pneumonitis due to anesthesia (J95.4)
> obstetric aspiration pneumonitis (O74.0)

CODING TIPS ✓ Code J69.0 for aspiration bronchitis that isn't further specified (Q2 2019 Coding Clinic).

SP J69.1 Pneumonitis due to inhalation of oils and essences

Exogenous lipoid pneumonia

Lipid pneumonia NOS

Code first:
  (T51-T65) to identify substance

> **EXCLUDES 1** endogenous lipoid pneumonia (J84.89)

SP J69.8 Pneumonitis due to inhalation of other solids and liquids

Pneumonitis due to aspiration of blood

Pneumonitis due to aspiration of detergent

Code first:
  (T51-T65) to identify substance

4 J70 Respiratory conditions due to other external agents

SP + J70.0 Acute pulmonary manifestations due to radiation

Radiation pneumonitis

Use additional code (W88-W90, X39.0-) to identify the external cause

SP + J70.1 Chronic and other pulmonary manifestations due to radiation

Fibrosis of lung following radiation

Use additional code (W88-W90, X39.0-) to identify the external cause

SP + J70.2 Acute drug-induced interstitial lung disorders

Use additional code for adverse effect, if applicable, to identify drug (T36-T50 with fifth or sixth character 5)

> **EXCLUDES 1** interstitial pneumonia NOS (J84.9)
> lymphoid interstitial pneumonia (J84.2)

SP + J70.3 Chronic drug-induced interstitial lung disorders

Use additional code for adverse effect, if applicable, to identify drug (T36-T50 with fifth or sixth character 5)

> **EXCLUDES 1** interstitial pneumonia NOS (J84.9)
> lymphoid interstitial pneumonia (J84.2)

SP + J70.4 Drug-induced interstitial lung disorders, unspecified

Use additional code for adverse effect, if applicable, to identify drug (T36-T50 with fifth or sixth character 5)

> **EXCLUDES 1** interstitial pneumonia NOS (J84.9)
> lymphoid interstitial pneumonia (J84.2)

SP J70.5 Respiratory conditions due to smoke inhalation

Smoke inhalation NOS

> **EXCLUDES 1** smoke inhalation due to chemicals, gases, fumes and vapors (J68.9)

SP J70.8 Respiratory conditions due to other specified external agents

Code first:
  (T51-T65) to identify the external agent

SP J70.9 Respiratory conditions due to unspecified external agent

Code first:
  (T51-T65) to identify the external agent

Other respiratory diseases principally affecting the interstitium (J80-J84)

SP J80 Acute respiratory distress syndrome

Acute respiratory distress syndrome in adult or child

Adult hyaline membrane disease

> **EXCLUDES 1** respiratory distress syndrome in newborn (perinatal) (P22.0)

CODING TIPS ✓ Acute respiratory distress syndrome is a life-threatening condition, which requires acute care treatment. J80 should not be assigned as a primary or secondary diagnosis if a current condition.

+ 4 J81 Pulmonary edema

Use additional code to identify:
  exposure to environmental tobacco smoke (Z77.22)
  history of tobacco dependence (Z87.891)
  occupational exposure to environmental tobacco smoke (Z57.31)
  tobacco dependence (F17.-)
  tobacco use (Z72.0)

★ New ▲ Revised Px Primary **SP** PDGM Px **SL** Low CoM **SH** High CoM **IQ** Quest. Encounter **H** Hospice non-cancer Dx Unspecified **M** *Manifestation*

DecisionHealth's FY 2020 Complete Home Health ICD-10-CM Diagnosis Coding Manual

1047

EXCLUDES 1 chemical (acute) pulmonary edema (J68.1)
hypostatic pneumonia (J18.2)
passive pneumonia (J18.2)
pulmonary edema due to external agents (J60-J70)
pulmonary edema with heart disease NOS (I50.1)
pulmonary edema with heart failure (I50.1)

CODING TIPS ✓ Pulmonary congestion is integral to, or routinely associated with, several conditions, such as CHF and pneumonia. Do not use an additional symptom code such as R09.89 when the symptom is routinely associated with the condition.

SP ✚ J81.0   Acute pulmonary edema
Acute edema of lung
DEFINITION Sudden, severe accumulation of fluid in the lungs.

SP ✚ J81.1   Chronic pulmonary edema
Pulmonary congestion (chronic) (passive)
Pulmonary edema NOS

SP J82   Pulmonary eosinophilia, not elsewhere classified
Allergic pneumonia
Eosinophilic asthma
Eosinophilic pneumonia
Löffler's pneumonia
Tropical (pulmonary) eosinophilia NOS
EXCLUDES 1 pulmonary eosinophilia due to aspergillosis (B44.-)
pulmonary eosinophilia due to drugs (J70.2-J70.4)
pulmonary eosinophilia due to specified parasitic infection (B50-B83)
pulmonary eosinophilia due to systemic connective tissue disorders (M30-M36)
pulmonary infiltrate NOS (R91.8)

4️⃣ J84   Other interstitial pulmonary diseases
EXCLUDES 1 drug-induced interstitial lung disorders (J70.2-J70.4)
interstitial emphysema (J98.2)
EXCLUDES 2 lung diseases due to external agents (J60-J70)

5️⃣ J84.0   Alveolar and parieto-alveolar conditions
SP J84.01   Alveolar proteinosis
SP J84.02   Pulmonary alveolar microlithiasis
M IQ J84.03   *Idiopathic pulmonary hemosiderosis*
Essential brown induration of lung
Code first underlying disease, such as:
disorders of iron metabolism (E83.1-)
EXCLUDES 1 acute idiopathic pulmonary hemorrhage in infants [AIPHI] (R04.81)

SP J84.09   Other alveolar and parieto-alveolar conditions
5️⃣ J84.1   Other interstitial pulmonary diseases with fibrosis

EXCLUDES 1 pulmonary fibrosis (chronic) due to inhalation of chemicals, gases, fumes or vapors (J68.4)
pulmonary fibrosis (chronic) following radiation (J70.1)
DEFINITION Formation of fibrous tissue and scarring in the lungs after the lungs have been inflamed for a significant period of time.

SP J84.10   Pulmonary fibrosis, unspecified
Capillary fibrosis of lung
Cirrhosis of lung (chronic) NOS
Fibrosis of lung (atrophic) (chronic) (confluent) (massive) (perialveolar) (peribronchial) NOS
Induration of lung (chronic) NOS
Postinflammatory pulmonary fibrosis

6️⃣ J84.11   Idiopathic interstitial pneumonia
EXCLUDES 1 lymphoid interstitial pneumonia (J84.2)
pneumocystis pneumonia (B59)

SP J84.111   Idiopathic interstitial pneumonia, not otherwise specified
SP J84.112   Idiopathic pulmonary fibrosis
Cryptogenic fibrosing alveolitis
Idiopathic fibrosing alveolitis
SP J84.113   Idiopathic non-specific interstitial pneumonitis
EXCLUDES 1 non-specific interstitial pneumonia NOS, or due to known underlying cause (J84.89)
SP J84.114   Acute interstitial pneumonitis
Hamman-Rich syndrome
EXCLUDES 1 pneumocystis pneumonia (B59)
SP J84.115   Respiratory bronchiolitis interstitial lung disease
SP J84.116   Cryptogenic organizing pneumonia
EXCLUDES 1 organizing pneumonia NOS, or due to known underlying cause (J84.89)
SP J84.117   Desquamative interstitial pneumonia
IQ J84.17   Other interstitial pulmonary diseases with fibrosis in diseases classified elsewhere
Interstitial pneumonia (nonspecific) (usual) due to collagen vascular disease
Interstitial pneumonia (nonspecific) (usual) in diseases classified elsewhere
Organizing pneumonia due to collagen vascular disease

4️⃣ 4th digit required   5️⃣ 5th digit required   6️⃣ 6th digit required   7️⃣ 7th digit required   ☑ 7th digit placeholder   ✚ Additional code   ⊟ Laterality

Organizing pneumonia in diseases
classified elsewhere
Code first underlying disease, such as:
progressive systemic sclerosis
(M34.0)
rheumatoid arthritis
(M05.00-M06.9)
systemic lupus erythematosis
(M32.0-M32.9)

SP **J84.2**   **Lymphoid interstitial pneumonia**
Lymphoid interstitial pneumonitis

5 **J84.8**   **Other specified interstitial pulmonary diseases**

> EXCLUDES 1   exogenous lipoid pneumonia
> (J69.1)
> unspecified lipoid
> pneumonia (J69.1)

SP **J84.81**   **Lymphangioleiomyomatosis**
Lymphangiomyomatosis

SP **J84.82**   **Adult pulmonary Langerhans cell histiocytosis**
Adult PLCH

SP **J84.83**   **Surfactant mutations of the lung**

6 **J84.84**   **Other interstitial lung diseases of childhood**

SP **J84.841**   **Neuroendocrine cell hyperplasia of infancy**

SP **J84.842**   **Pulmonary interstitial glycogenosis**

SP **J84.843**   **Alveolar capillary dysplasia with vein misalignment**

SP **J84.848**   **Other interstitial lung diseases of childhood**

SP **+** **J84.89**   **Other specified interstitial pulmonary diseases**
Endogenous lipoid pneumonia
Interstitial pneumonitis
Non-specific interstitial pneumonitis
NOS
Organizing pneumonia NOS
Code first, if applicable:
poisoning due to drug or toxin
(T51-T65 with fifth or sixth
character to indicate intent) , for
toxic pneumonopathy
underlying cause of pneumonopathy,
if known
Use additional code, for adverse effect,
to identify drug (T36-T50 with fifth
or sixth character 5), if drug-induced

> EXCLUDES 1   cryptogenic organizing
> pneumonia (J84.116)
> idiopathic non-specific
> interstitial pneumonitis
> (J84.113)
> lipoid pneumonia,
> exogenous or
> unspecified (J69.1)
> lymphoid interstitial
> pneumonia (J84.2)

SP **J84.9**   **Interstitial pulmonary disease, unspecified**

Interstitial pneumonia NOS

Suppurative and necrotic conditions of the lower respiratory tract   (J85-J86)

CODING TIPS ✓   When the record specifies the causative organism, use an additional code to report the organism specified, following the instructions to "use an additional code."

+ **4** **J85**   **Abscess of lung and mediastinum**
Use additional code (B95-B97) to identify
infectious agent.

SP **+** **J85.0**   **Gangrene and necrosis of lung**

SP **+** **J85.1**   **Abscess of lung with pneumonia**
Code also:
the type of pneumonia

SP **+** **J85.2**   **Abscess of lung without pneumonia**
Abscess of lung NOS

SP **+** **J85.3**   **Abscess of mediastinum**

+ **4** **J86**   **Pyothorax**
Use additional code (B95-B97) to identify
infectious agent.

> EXCLUDES 1   abscess of lung (J85.-)
> pyothorax due to tuberculosis
> (A15.6)

SP **+** **J86.0**   **Pyothorax with fistula**
Bronchocutaneous fistula
Bronchopleural fistula
Hepatopleural fistula
Mediastinal fistula
Pleural fistula
Thoracic fistula
Any condition classifiable to J86.9 with
fistula

SP **+** **J86.9**   **Pyothorax without fistula**
Abscess of pleura
Abscess of thorax
Empyema (chest) (lung) (pleura)
Fibrinopurulent pleurisy
Purulent pleurisy
Pyopneumothorax
Septic pleurisy
Seropurulent pleurisy
Suppurative pleurisy

Other diseases of the pleura   (J90-J94)

SP **J90**   **Pleural effusion, not elsewhere classified**
Encysted pleurisy
Pleural effusion NOS
Pleurisy with effusion (exudative) (serous)

> EXCLUDES 1   chylous (pleural) effusion
> (J94.0)
> malignant pleural effusion
> (J91.0))
> pleurisy NOS (R09.1)
> tuberculous pleural effusion
> (A15.6)

CODING TIPS ✓   Pleural effusion indicates excess pleural fluid built up and accumulated in the pleural lining causing respiratory distress. While often treated in the inpatient setting, pleural effusion may also be treated in home health with interventions such as a PleurX drainage catheter and other respiratory interventions. Home health should verify the presence or absence of a diagnosed pleural effusion to clarify a need to report the diagnosis as active.

4 **J91**   **Pleural effusion in conditions classified elsewhere**

Chapter 10

J00-J99

★ New ▲ Revised Px Primary **SP** PDGM Px **SL** Low CoM **SH** High CoM **IQ** Quest. Encounter **H** Hospice non-cancer Dx Unspecified **M** *Manifestation*

EXCLUDES 2 pleural effusion in heart failure
(I50.-)
pleural effusion in systemic
lupus erythematosus
(M32.13)

!Q J91.0 Malignant pleural effusion
Code first:
underlying neoplasm

DEFINITION Dangerous fluid
accumulation between the layers of the
membrane lining the chest cavity and lungs,
most often caused by cancers of the breast,
lung, or lymph nodes.

**M !Q J91.8 *Pleural effusion in other conditions
classified elsewhere***
Code first underlying disease, such as:
filariasis (B74.0-B74.9)
influenza (J09.X2, J10.1, J11.1)

CODING TIPS ✓ Pleural effusion (J91.8) may
be used for pleural effusion in systemic
lupus erythematosus and pleural effusion in
heart failure. The code J91.8 is coded after
the condition causing the pleural effusion.
Pleural effusion is ordinarily integral to heart
failure and is not coded separately.
However, if the pleural effusion requires
separate treatment, i.e. chest tube for
drainage, then add the code for pleural
effusion.

4 J92 Pleural plaque
INCLUDES pleural thickening

SP J92.0 Pleural plaque with presence of asbestos

SP J92.9 Pleural plaque without asbestos
Pleural plaque NOS

4 J93 Pneumothorax and air leak
EXCLUDES 1 congenital or perinatal
pneumothorax (P25.1)
postprocedural air leak
(J95.812)
postprocedural pneumothorax
(J95.811)
traumatic pneumothorax
(S27.0)
tuberculous (current disease)
pneumothorax (A15.-)
pyopneumothorax (J86.-)

CODING TIPS ✓ Spontaneous pneumothorax
may be primary or secondary and thus related
to various other conditions. Some causes of
secondary pneumothorax include cystic
fibrosis, spontaneous rupture of the
esophagus, Marfan's syndrome,
lymphangioleiomyomatosis, metastatic cancer,
primary lung cancer, catamenial, pneumocystis
carinii pneumonia, and eosinophilic
pneumonia.

SP J93.0 Spontaneous tension pneumothorax

5 J93.1 Other spontaneous pneumothorax

SP J93.11 Primary spontaneous pneumothorax

**SP J93.12 Secondary spontaneous
pneumothorax**
Code first underlying condition, such
as:
catamenial pneumothorax due to
endometriosis (N80.8)
cystic fibrosis (E84.-)
eosinophilic pneumonia (J82)
lymphangioleiomyomatosis (J84.81)
malignant neoplasm of bronchus and
lung (C34.-)
Marfan's syndrome (Q87.4)
pneumonia due to Pneumocystis
carinii (B59)
secondary malignant neoplasm of
lung (C78.0-)
spontaneous rupture of the esophagus
(K22.3)

5 J93.8 Other pneumothorax and air leak

SP J93.81 Chronic pneumothorax

SP J93.82 Other air leak
Persistent air leak

SP J93.83 Other pneumothorax
Acute pneumothorax
Spontaneous pneumothorax NOS

SP J93.9 Pneumothorax, unspecified
Pneumothorax NOS

4 J94 Other pleural conditions
EXCLUDES 1 pleurisy NOS (R09.1)
traumatic hemopneumothorax
(S27.2)
traumatic hemothorax (S27.1)
tuberculous pleural conditions
(current disease) (A15.-)

SP J94.0 Chylous effusion
Chyliform effusion

SP J94.1 Fibrothorax

SP J94.2 Hemothorax
Hemopneumothorax

SP J94.8 Other specified pleural conditions
Hydropneumothorax
Hydrothorax

!Q J94.9 Pleural condition, unspecified

Intraoperative and postprocedural complications and disorders of respiratory system, not elsewhere classified   (J95)

**4 J95 Intraoperative and postprocedural
complications and disorders of respiratory
system, not elsewhere classified**
EXCLUDES 2 aspiration pneumonia (J69.-)
emphysema (subcutaneous)
resulting from a procedure
(T81.82)
hypostatic pneumonia (J18.2)
pulmonary manifestations due
to radiation (J70.0-J70.1)

CODING TIPS ✓ **Documentation:** Codes in
category J95.- are complication codes and
require physician documentation and
confirmation of a cause and effect relationship
between the procedure and the complicated
condition. Documentation in the home health
clinical record must also support this
relationship. They may be described as "post-
status" or "post-op."

44th digit required **5**5th digit required **6**6th digit required **7**7th digit required **7**7th digit placeholder **+**Additional code **=**Laterality

1050   *DecisionHealth's* FY 2020 Complete Home Health ICD-10-CM Diagnosis Coding Manual

⑤ **J95.0 Tracheostomy complications**

CODING TIPS ✓ Do not use Z93.0 or Z43.0 codes when assigning any code from subcategory J95.0-.

IQ J95.00 Unspecified tracheostomy complication

SP J95.01 Hemorrhage from tracheostomy stoma

SP ✚ J95.02 Infection of tracheostomy stoma
Use additional code to identify type of infection, such as:
cellulitis of neck (L03.221)
sepsis (A40, A41.-)

CODING TIPS ✓ When coding J95.02, use an additional code to indicate the infection, such as cellulitis, sepsis, or the infectious organism, when the specific information is available.

SP J95.03 Malfunction of tracheostomy stoma
Mechanical complication of tracheostomy stoma
Obstruction of tracheostomy airway
Tracheal stenosis due to tracheostomy

SP J95.04 Tracheo-esophageal fistula following tracheostomy

SP J95.09 Other tracheostomy complication

SP J95.1 Acute pulmonary insufficiency following thoracic surgery
EXCLUDES 2 Functional disturbances following cardiac surgery (I97.0, I97.1-)

SP J95.2 Acute pulmonary insufficiency following nonthoracic surgery
EXCLUDES 2 Functional disturbances following cardiac surgery (I97.0, I97.1-)

SP J95.3 Chronic pulmonary insufficiency following surgery
EXCLUDES 2 Functional disturbances following cardiac surgery (I97.0, I97.1-)

SP ✚ J95.4 Chemical pneumonitis due to anesthesia
Mendelson's syndrome
Postprocedural aspiration pneumonia
Use additional code for adverse effect, if applicable, to identify drug (T41.- with fifth or sixth character 5)
EXCLUDES 1 aspiration pneumonitis due to anesthesia complicating labor and delivery (O74.0)
aspiration pneumonitis due to anesthesia complicating pregnancy (O29)
aspiration pneumonitis due to anesthesia complicating the puerperium (O89.01)

SP J95.5 Postprocedural subglottic stenosis

⑤ **J95.6 Intraoperative hemorrhage and hematoma of a respiratory system organ or structure complicating a procedure**
EXCLUDES 1 intraoperative hemorrhage and hematoma of a respiratory system organ or structure due to accidental puncture and laceration during procedure (J95.7-)

SP J95.61 Intraoperative hemorrhage and hematoma of a respiratory system organ or structure complicating a respiratory system procedure

SP J95.62 Intraoperative hemorrhage and hematoma of a respiratory system organ or structure complicating other procedure

⑤ **J95.7 Accidental puncture and laceration of a respiratory system organ or structure during a procedure**
EXCLUDES 2 postprocedural pneumothorax (J95.811)

SP J95.71 Accidental puncture and laceration of a respiratory system organ or structure during a respiratory system procedure

SP J95.72 Accidental puncture and laceration of a respiratory system organ or structure during other procedure

⑤ **J95.8 Other intraoperative and postprocedural complications and disorders of respiratory system, not elsewhere classified**

⑥ **J95.81 Postprocedural pneumothorax and air leak**

SP J95.811 Postprocedural pneumothorax

SP J95.812 Postprocedural air leak

⑥ **J95.82 Postprocedural respiratory failure**
EXCLUDES 1 Respiratory failure in other conditions (J96.-)

SP J95.821 Acute postprocedural respiratory failure
Postprocedural respiratory failure NOS

SP J95.822 Acute and chronic postprocedural respiratory failure

⑥ **J95.83 Postprocedural hemorrhage of a respiratory system organ or structure following a procedure**

SP J95.830 Postprocedural hemorrhage of a respiratory system organ or structure following a respiratory system procedure

SP J95.831 Postprocedural hemorrhage of a respiratory system organ or structure following other procedure

SP J95.84 Transfusion-related acute lung injury (TRALI)

⑥ **J95.85 Complication of respirator [ventilator]**

SP J95.850 Mechanical complication of respirator
EXCLUDES 1 encounter for respirator [ventilator] dependence during power failure (Z99.12)

SP ✚ J95.851 Ventilator associated pneumonia
Ventilator associated pneumonitis
Use additional code to identify the organism, if known (B95.-, B96.-, B97.-)
EXCLUDES 1 ventilator lung in newborn (P27.8)

★ New ▲ Revised Px Primary **SP** PDGM Px **SL** Low CoM **SH** High CoM **IQ** Quest. Encounter **H** Hospice non-cancer Dx Unspecified **M** *Manifestation*

DecisionHealth's FY 2020 Complete Home Health ICD-10-CM Diagnosis Coding Manual

1051

CODING TIPS ✓ VAP is not considered an infection for the purpose of using J44.0.

SP J95.859 Other complication of respirator [ventilator]

6 J95.86 Postprocedural hematoma and seroma of a respiratory system organ or structure following a procedure

SP J95.860 Postprocedural hematoma of a respiratory system organ or structure following a respiratory system procedure

SP J95.861 Postprocedural hematoma of a respiratory system organ or structure following other procedure

SP J95.862 Postprocedural seroma of a respiratory system organ or structure following a respiratory system procedure

SP J95.863 Postprocedural seroma of a respiratory system organ or structure following other procedure

SP J95.88 Other intraoperative complications of respiratory system, not elsewhere classified

SP ✚ J95.89 Other postprocedural complications and disorders of respiratory system, not elsewhere classified

Use additional code to identify disorder, such as:
aspiration pneumonia (J69.-)
bacterial or viral pneumonia (J12-J18)

EXCLUDES 2 acute pulmonary insufficiency following thoracic surgery (J95.1)
postprocedural subglottic stenosis (J95.5)

Other diseases of the respiratory system (J96-J99)

4 J96 Respiratory failure, not elsewhere classified

EXCLUDES 1 acute respiratory distress syndrome (J80)
cardiorespiratory failure (R09.2)
newborn respiratory distress syndrome (P22.0)
postprocedural respiratory failure (J95.82-)
respiratory arrest (R09.2)
respiratory arrest of newborn (P28.81)
respiratory failure of newborn (P28.5)

CODING TIPS ✓ Respiratory failure can be acute (rapid onset) or chronic (ongoing). Acute respiratory failure can develop quickly and may require emergency treatment. Chronic respiratory failure develops more slowly and lasts longer. If the physician documents both acute and chronic respiratory failure, report a code from J96.2.

5 J96.0 Acute respiratory failure

SP J96.00 Acute respiratory failure, unspecified whether with hypoxia or hypercapnia

SP J96.01 Acute respiratory failure with hypoxia

SP J96.02 Acute respiratory failure with hypercapnia

5 J96.1 Chronic respiratory failure

SP J96.10 Chronic respiratory failure, unspecified whether with hypoxia or hypercapnia

SP J96.11 Chronic respiratory failure with hypoxia

SP J96.12 Chronic respiratory failure with hypercapnia

5 J96.2 Acute and chronic respiratory failure
Acute on chronic respiratory failure

SP J96.20 Acute and chronic respiratory failure, unspecified whether with hypoxia or hypercapnia

SP J96.21 Acute and chronic respiratory failure with hypoxia

SP J96.22 Acute and chronic respiratory failure with hypercapnia

5 J96.9 Respiratory failure, unspecified

SP J96.90 Respiratory failure, unspecified, unspecified whether with hypoxia or hypercapnia

SP J96.91 Respiratory failure, unspecified with hypoxia

SP J96.92 Respiratory failure, unspecified with hypercapnia

✚ 4 J98 Other respiratory disorders
Use additional code to identify:
exposure to environmental tobacco smoke (Z77.22)
exposure to tobacco smoke in the perinatal period (P96.81)
history of tobacco dependence (Z87.891)
occupational exposure to environmental tobacco smoke (Z57.31)
tobacco dependence (F17.-)
tobacco use (Z72.0)

EXCLUDES 1 newborn apnea (P28.4)
newborn sleep apnea (P28.3)

EXCLUDES 2 apnea NOS (R06.81)
sleep apnea (G47.3-)

✚ 5 J98.0 Diseases of bronchus, not elsewhere classified

SP ✚ J98.01 Acute bronchospasm

EXCLUDES 1 acute bronchiolitis with bronchospasm (J21.-)
acute bronchitis with bronchospasm (J20.-)
asthma (J45.-)
exercise induced bronchospasm (J45.990)

DEFINITION Constriction or contraction of the smooth muscle in the large air passages, severely limiting airflow.

SP ✚ J98.09 Other diseases of bronchus, not elsewhere classified
Broncholithiasis
Calcification of bronchus
Stenosis of bronchus

4 4th digit required   5 5th digit required   6 6th digit required   7 7th digit required   7 7th digit placeholder   ✚ Additional code   Laterality

1052   *DecisionHealth's* FY 2020 Complete Home Health ICD-10-CM Diagnosis Coding Manual

Tracheobronchial collapse
Tracheobronchial dyskinesia
Ulcer of bronchus

✚ ⑤ J98.1   Pulmonary collapse
> EXCLUDES 1   therapeutic collapse of lung status (Z98.3)

SP ✚ J98.11   Atelectasis
> EXCLUDES 1   newborn atelectasis
> tuberculous atelectasis (current disease) (A15)

SP ✚ J98.19   Other pulmonary collapse

SP ✚ J98.2   Interstitial emphysema
Mediastinal emphysema
> EXCLUDES 1   emphysema NOS (J43.9)
> emphysema in newborn (P25.0)
> surgical emphysema (subcutaneous) (T81.82)
> traumatic subcutaneous emphysema (T79.7)

SP ✚ J98.3   Compensatory emphysema

SP ✚ J98.4   Other disorders of lung
Calcification of lung
Cystic lung disease (acquired)
Lung disease NOS
Pulmolithiasis
> EXCLUDES 1   acute interstitial pneumonitis (J84.114)
> pulmonary insufficiency following surgery (J95.1-J95.2)

✚ ⑤ J98.5   Diseases of mediastinum, not elsewhere classified
> EXCLUDES 2   abscess of mediastinum (J85.3)

SP ✚ J98.51   Mediastinitis
Code first:
> underlying condition, if applicable, such as postoperative mediastinitis (T81.-)

SP ✚ J98.59   Other diseases of mediastinum, not elsewhere classified
Fibrosis of mediastinum
Hernia of mediastinum
Retraction of mediastinum

SP ✚ J98.6   Disorders of diaphragm
Diaphragmatitis
Paralysis of diaphragm
Relaxation of diaphragm
> EXCLUDES 1   congenital malformation of diaphragm NEC (Q79.1)
> congenital diaphragmatic hernia (Q79.0)
> EXCLUDES 2   diaphragmatic hernia (K44.-)

SP ✚ J98.8   Other specified respiratory disorders

IQ ✚ J98.9   Respiratory disorder, unspecified
Respiratory disease (chronic) NOS

M IQ J99   Respiratory disorders in diseases classified elsewhere
Code first underlying disease, such as:
amyloidosis (E85.-)
ankylosing spondylitis (M45)
congenital syphilis (A50.5)
cryoglobulinemia (D89.1)
early congenital syphilis (A50.0)
plasminogen deficiency (E88.02)
schistosomiasis (B65.0-B65.9)
> EXCLUDES 1   respiratory disorders in:
> amebiasis (A06.5)
> blastomycosis (B40.0-B40.2)
> candidiasis (B37.1)
> coccidioidomycosis (B38.0-B38.2)
> cystic fibrosis with pulmonary manifestations (E84.0)
> dermatomyositis (M33.01, M33.11)
> histoplasmosis (B39.0-B39.2)
> late syphilis (A52.72, A52.73)
> polymyositis (M33.21)
> sicca syndrome (M35.02)
> systemic lupus erythematosus (M32.13)
> systemic sclerosis (M34.81)
> Wegener's granulomatosis (M31.30-M31.31)

Chapter 10

J00-J99

★ New ▲ Revised Px Primary SP PDGM Px SL Low CoM SH High CoM IQ Quest. Encounter H Hospice non-cancer Dx Unspecified M *Manifestation*

DecisionHealth's FY 2020 Complete Home Health ICD-10-CM Diagnosis Coding Manual

1053

Chapter 10 Scenarios: Diseases of the respiratory system (J00-J99)

Chronic obstructive bronchitis with chronic obstructive asthma, hypertension

A 75-year-old male patient is admitted to home care with a primary diagnosis of exacerbated chronic obstructive bronchitis with chronic obstructive asthma. He also has hypertension. His history and physical says that he was a cigarette smoker for several decades but quit 12 years ago.

Description	Code
Primary: Chronic obstructive pulmonary disease with acute exacerbation	J44.1
Secondary: Hypertension	I10
Secondary: Personal history of nicotine dependence	Z87.891

The patient's exacerbated chronic obstructive bronchitis and chronic obstructive asthma are appropriately captured with J44.1. The J44.1 code captures both diagnoses. Hypertension is also assigned as a relevant comorbidity. The code for history of tobacco use, required for all codes in Chapter 10 due to chapter-level tabular instruction, is included to capture that the patient is a former smoker.

Emphysema, congestive heart failure, smoker

A 78-year-old female patient is admitted to home health with a primary diagnosis of emphysema. She also has congestive heart failure and the physician documents she is a long-time current cigarette smoker.

Description	Code
Primary: Emphysema, unspecified	J43.9
Secondary: Congestive heart failure, unspecified	I50.9
Secondary: Nicotine dependence, cigarettes, uncomplicated	F17.210

With no other information known about the patient's emphysema, J43.9 is the most appropriate code choice. Congestive heart failure is a relevant comorbidity and is also assigned. Because the patient continues to smoke cigarettes, an additional code is required to report this. The correct code for the cigarette smoking is F17.210, as this is where the alphabetic index leads.

Aftercare of surgery, respiratory issues, GI issues

The patient had gall bladder surgery due to cholecystitis but had an exacerbation of her chronic obstructive bronchitis while in the hospital and additionally developed bacterial pneumonia, which is still being treated with oral antibiotic therapy for 10 days. She also has a gastrostomy that is infected. Her gastrostomy was placed last year because of dysphagia. The focus of care is the exacerbated COPD but she will also receive speech therapy to address the dysphagia.

Description	Code
Primary: Chronic obstructive pulmonary disease with acute exacerbation	J44.1
Secondary: Chronic obstructive pulmonary disease with (acute) lower respiratory infection	J44.0
Secondary: Unspecified bacterial pneumonia	J15.9
Secondary: Gastrostomy infection	K94.22
Secondary: Dysphagia, unspecified	R13.10
Secondary: Encounter for surgical aftercare following surgery on the digestive system	Z48.815

This is a situation in which the patient had surgery, but the aftercare is not the focus of care. Both J44.1 and J44.0 are used as this patient developed an acute lower respiratory tract infection, as well as an exacerbation of her COPD. The Excludes 2 note at J44.1 allows the coder to code both COPD codes. To further specify the lower respiratory tract infection in accordance with tabular instruction, J15.9 (Unspecified bacterial pneumonia) is assigned in this scenario. Code Z43.1 should not be used for the gastrostomy because the gastrostomy is complicated. Dysphagia is coded only if it is a current diagnosis and is addressed by the plan of care, which it is in this case. No code for antibiotic use is assigned because the patient will remain on antibiotics for only 10 days.

Pneumonia, chronic obstructive bronchitis

A patient with chronic obstructive bronchitis is admitted with pneumonia that is still under treatment. The patient's physician confirms that the chronic obstructive bronchitis is acutely exacerbated. The pneumonia is the focus of care.

Description	Code
Primary: Pneumonia, unspecified organism	J18.9
Secondary: Chronic obstructive pulmonary disease with (acute) lower respiratory infection	J44.0
Secondary: Chronic obstructive pulmonary disease with (acute) exacerbation	J44.1

Since the pneumonia is the focus of care, it is coded before both the chronic obstructive bronchitis with lower respiratory infection, and the exacerbated chronic obstructive bronchitis codes. Because the tabular instruction at J44.0 is "code also," either the COPD with lower respiratory infection code, or the code for the infection itself could be sequenced first, depending on the focus of care. The Excludes 2 note at the J44.1 code level directs the coder that chronic obstructive pulmonary disease with a lower respiratory infection is not included in the J44.1 code and, if present, should be coded separately.

HOME HEALTH CODING SCENARIOS

DVT, end-stage COPD

The patient was hospitalized with a DVT of his left gastrocnemial vein. Now discharged home on anticoagulant therapy, home health nursing is ordered for observation and assessment, teaching on the disease process, and weekly lab draws for PT/INR monitoring. His mobility is limited due to severe dyspnea and weakness caused by end-stage/decompensated chronic obstructive bronchitis. He is on continuous oxygen and was a two-pack per day cigarette smoker until three years ago, when he stopped smoking.

Description	Code
Primary: Acute embolism and thrombosis of left calf muscular vein	I82.462
Secondary: Chronic obstructive pulmonary disease with (acute) exacerbation	J44.1
Secondary: Encounter for therapeutic drug level monitoring	Z51.81
Secondary: Long-term (current) use of anticoagulants	Z79.01
Secondary: Dependence on supplemental oxygen	Z99.81
Secondary: Personal history of nicotine dependence	Z87.891

As the focus of care, the DVT is coded in the primary position. Laterality is specified in I82.462 by the last character (2 = left). Ensure that the specific location of the DVT is documented as coding a DVT with an unspecified location in the primary position will result in the claim being sent back to be recoded under PDGM. In this case, since the DVT is documented as occurring in the left gastrocnemial vein, I82.462 is the appropriate code choice, according to inclusion terms at the I82.46- subcategory. There is an instructional note at Z51.81 to code any long-term (current) drug therapy (Z79.-), and at Z79.- to code also any therapeutic drug level monitoring (Z51.81). The status code for supplemental oxygen is included since it adds additional pertinent information. Chronic obstructive bronchitis reported as "decompensated" is coded to J44.1 (Chronic obstructive pulmonary disease with (acute) exacerbation), according to inclusion terms. Category J44.- instructs to use an additional code to identify tobacco use, history of its use or exposure to tobacco smoke. In this case, it is captured with Z87.891.

Influenza with pneumonia, congestive heart failure

A 92-year-old woman was treated in the hospital with influenza that led to a case of pneumonia. Upon release from the hospital, she is admitted to home health, but is still taking Tamiflu and antibiotics, as her influenza and pneumonia have not yet completely resolved. She has a long history of chronic systolic congestive heart failure, which is currently stable, but her physician is concerned about the chronic condition decompensating due to the infection the patient is continuing to fight. Other comorbidities include insulin-dependent diabetes and non-dominant left-sided hemiplegia from an old CVA.

Description	Code
Primary: Influenza due to unidentified influenza virus with unspecified type of pneumonia	J11.00
Secondary: Chronic systolic (congestive) heart failure	I50.22
Secondary: Hemiplegia and hemiparesis following cerebral infarction affecting left non-dominant side	I69.354
Secondary: Type 2 diabetes mellitus without complications	E11.9
Secondary: Long term (current) use of insulin	Z79.4

The patient is still being treated for the influenza with pneumonia and it is the focus of are, so it is coded primary. Her physician is worried that her chronic systolic congestive heart failure may decompensate due to the influenza and pneumonia, and while it is currently stable, it is being closely monitored and thus it is coded directly following the primary diagnosis of influenza with pneumonia. No separate code for congestive heart failure is required as the congestive element of the diagnosis is included in the code for chronic systolic heart failure. With no specific information available about the specific strain of influenza and type of pneumonia, the diagnosis is most appropriately captured with J11.00.

Staph pneumonia

A 71-year-old man was recently hospitalized for treatment of pneumonia, which was specified as caused by staphylococcus aureus bacteria. He improved sufficiently in the hospital and was discharged to home health for continued treatment on a long-term course of oral antibiotic drugs. Three years ago he underwent a kidney transplant and still has stage 2 chronic kidney disease and hypertension.

Description	Code
Primary: Pneumonia due to Methicillin susceptible Staphylococcus aureus	J15.211
Secondary: Hypertensive chronic kidney disease with stage 1 through stage 4 chronic kidney disease, or unspecified chronic kidney disease	I12.9
Secondary: Chronic kidney disease, stage 2 (mild)	N18.2
Secondary: Kidney transplant status	Z94.0
Secondary: Long term (current) use of antibiotics	Z79.2

No separate infecting organism code is required in this scenario because it is included in the pneumonia code. Though the patient underwent a kidney transplant, he still has stage 2 chronic kidney disease. Hypertension and chronic kidney disease are assumed to be connected and are coded as such, as hypertensive chronic kidney disease, in accordance with coding guidelines. The patient is taking oral antibiotics but the course is long-term, making the use of Z79.2 appropriate.

MRSA pneumonia, exacerbated chronic obstructive asthma

A 75-year-old woman is admitted to home health after being hospitalized with MRSA pneumonia, which caused an acute exacerbation of her chronic obstructive asthma. The pneumonia is still resolving and is the focus of care. She will continue taking oral antibiotics for the several weeks.

Description	Code
Primary: Pneumonia due to Methicillin resistant Staphylococcus aureus	J15.212
Secondary: Chronic obstructive pulmonary disease with (acute) lower respiratory infection	J44.0
Secondary: Chronic obstructive pulmonary disease with (acute) exacerbation	J44.1
Secondary: Long term (current) use of antibiotics	Z79.2

As the focus of care, the pneumonia is assigned in the primary position. The code for chronic obstructive asthma with a lower respiratory infection comes next, followed by a code for acutely exacerbated COPD, to show that the pneumonia caused an exacerbation of the chronic condition. An Excludes 2 note on J44.0 allows their assignment of both J44.- codes. Code Z79.2 is assigned to capture continued antibiotics for the next several weeks.

Aspiration pneumonia, Alzheimer's

An 81-year-old woman is admitted to home health with a primary diagnosis of aspiration pneumonia due to the aspiration of food. She suffers from chronic emphysematous bronchitis and Alzheimer's disease.

Description	Code
Primary: Pneumonitis due to inhalation of food and vomit	J69.0
Secondary: Chronic obstructive pulmonary disease, unspecified	J44.9
Secondary: Alzheimer's disease, unspecified	G30.9
Secondary: Dementia in other diseases classified elsewhere without behavioral disturbance	F02.80

The primary diagnosis is aspiration pneumonia due to aspirated food, which codes to J69.0. Code J44.9 is assigned to capture her respiratory condition, and not J44.0, as aspiration pneumonia is not considered a respiratory infection that is included under that code, according to Q1 2017 Coding Clinic guidance. Her Alzheimer's disease is an important comorbidity and is thus coded. Dementia is assigned as a manifestation of Alzheimer's disease. While dementia is not specifically stated, it should be coded along with G30.9, according to Q1 2017 Coding Clinic guidance.

Chemical pneumonia

A 57-year-old man is admitted to home health with a primary diagnosis of chemical pneumonia that his physician diagnosed as caused by inhaling excessive smoke from a campfire. He also has type 2 diabetes and PVD and takes oral hypoglycemic medication.

Description	Code
Primary: Toxic effect of smoke, accidental (unintentional), subsequent encounter	T59.811D
Secondary: Bronchitis and pneumonitis due to chemicals, gases, fumes and vapors	J68.0
Secondary: Type 2 diabetes mellitus with diabetic peripheral angiopathy without gangrene	E11.51
Secondary: Exposure to smoke in controlled fire, not in building or structure, subsequent encounter	X03.1xxD
Secondary: Long term (current) use of oral hypoglycemic drugs	Z79.84

The patient's pneumonia was caused by inhaling excessive smoke during a campfire. Because it is caused by fumes, it is chemical pneumonia. Chemical pneumonia codes to J68.0, according to the alphabetic index. The code for the unintentional poisoning from the smoke is assigned before the pneumonia code, in accordance with tabular instruction. The patient's diabetes and PVD, which can be assumed to be connected via the alphabetic index, are also captured together with the combination code E11.51. An external cause code is used to help show how the patient developed chemical pneumonia, from exposure to smoke. Code Z79.84 is assigned to show that he takes oral hypoglycemic medication for his diabetes.

Exacerbated COPD with emphysema and acute bronchitis

An 87-year-old man was hospitalized with a severe case of acute bronchitis, which caused an exacerbation of his COPD with emphysema. He admitted to home health with still-resolving bronchitis, which is the focus of care, and to help get his emphysema back under control. The patient will be taking oral antibiotics for the next three weeks. He smoked cigarettes as a young man but quit several years ago.

Description	Code
Primary: Acute bronchitis, unspecified	J20.9
Secondary: Emphysema, unspecified	J43.9
Secondary: Long term (current) use of antibiotics	Z79.2
Secondary: Personal history of nicotine dependence	Z87.891

Codes J20.9 and J43.9 are assigned for the patient with his acute bronchitis, and exacerbated COPD with emphysema, according to Q1 2019 Coding Clinic guidance. As the focus of care, the acute bronchitis is coded in the primary position. The patient is taking antibiotics for three weeks, prompting the assignment of Z79.2. Since he has a history of tobacco use and a diagnosis from Chapter 10 (J00-J99), Z87.891 is also assigned. There is a chapter-level tabular instruction covering all of Chapter 10, instructing the coder to assign a code if the patient has been exposed to tobacco, or is a current or former user of tobacco.

Chapter 11: Diseases of the Digestive System (K00- K95)

Chapter 11 includes diseases of the organs of the digestive system: a long, twisting tube stretching from the mouth through the esophagus, stomach, small and large intestines, and ending at the anus. Other areas related to the mouth (teeth, jaws, salivary glands) are also coded in this chapter. Diseases of organs that assist the digestive process (liver, gallbladder, pancreas) are included, as well as diseases of the ducts that carry enzymes and digestive juices from these organs to the intestines (the biliary tract, including the hepatic, cystic and common bile ducts). Finally, this chapter includes conditions affecting the peritoneum (membrane surrounding the organs in the abdominal cavity).

In certain situations you'll need to look beyond this chapter to properly code a case. Here are a few examples of such cases:

- If the documentation indicates a **neoplasm or tumor of an organ in the digestive system**, coders should look up the term (malignancy, tumor, adenoma) to find the correct code, most likely a code from Chapter 2.

- If a patient has a **personal or family history** of a condition reported in this chapter, it may be appropriate to select from chapter 21, the Z code section, such as Z87.11 (Personal history of peptic ulcer disease) or Z87.19 (Personal history of diseases of digestive system), subcategory Z85.0- (Personal history of malignant neoplasm of digestive organs), Z83.79 (Family history of other diseases of digestive system), or Z80.0 (Family history of malignant neoplasm of digestive organs).

- **Symptoms** related to the digestive system are sometimes reported using codes from Chapter 18, such as code series R19.8 (Symptoms involving digestive system and abdomen). Every effort should be made to secure a definitive diagnosis. A symptom code from Chapter 18 may be reported as an additional diagnosis when it describes a significant aspect of the condition but is not an integral part of it.

- Although not coded often in home health, if reporting a **digestive system disease in a pregnant patient** when the condition is complicating the pregnancy, report first a code from Chapter 15, for example O26.61- (Liver and biliary tract disorders in pregnancy), as the first-listed diagnosis and K76.9 (Liver disease unspecified) from this chapter as an additional diagnosis.

Complications of artificial openings of the digestive system are reported using codes from category K94 in this chapter. Each type of ostomy includes specific codes for unspecified complication, hemorrhage, infection (with a note to add an additional code to specify the type of infection), mechanical malfunction and "other" complication. For example, an infection of an esophagostomy is reported using code K94.32 (with an additional code to identify the infection); a mechanical complication of a colostomy is coded as K94.03; a hemorrhage of a gastrostomy is coded as K94.21; and an "other" complication of an enterostomy would be reported as K94.19.

Be aware that if the ostomy is complicated, the complication code is used rather than the Z93.- code for 'status' or the Z43.- code for 'attention to' an artificial opening.

Multiple Coding and Sequencing

Includes and Excludes notes are important to follow, as well as any other instructions under the code or code category. The following are some examples of multiple coding and sequencing issues for codes in this chapter.

- **Peritonitis** is reported using category K65. A note under this code states: use an additional code (B95-B97) if known, to identify infectious agent. Pay close attention to the Excludes 1 note under code K65, since there are many types of peritonitis that are coded using a combination code found in other chapters. Examples include: gonococcal peritonitis (A54.85), neonatal peritonitis (P78.0-P78.1), or aseptic or chemical peritonitis (T81.6-).

- K67 is used as a second diagnosis for disorders of the **peritoneum in infectious diseases** classified elsewhere and includes a note to code first the underlying condition such as helminthiasis (B65.0-B83.9).

- Disorders such as K12.- **(stomatitis and related lesions)** include an extensive note following the category code to use additional codes to identify alcohol abuse and dependence (F10.-) and exposure to tobacco smoke as well as tobacco use, dependence and history of dependence.

- **Oral mucositis** (ulcerative) has notes to add additional codes relative to the cause of the disorder. For example, K12.31 (Mucositis due to antineoplastic therapy) has two instructional notes following the code: use additional code for adverse effect, if applicable, to identify antineoplastic and immunosuppressive drugs (T45.1x5), and use additional code for other neoplastic therapy, such as radiological procedure and radiotherapy (Y84.2).

- Disorders such as **oral thrush (candidiasis)** are not coded in chapter 11. Instead the code is found as a combination code in chapter 1 at B37.0 and provides all of the necessary information with a single code.

- Code K31.84 (**gastroparesis**) includes a note: Code first underlying disease such as anorexia nervosa (F50.0-), scleroderma (M34-) or diabetes mellitus (E08.43, E09.43, E10.43, E11.43, E13.43). However, gastroparesis may be coded alone if the underlying cause is unknown.

- Code K62.81 (**Anal sphincter tear** [healed, old]) includes a note that states: Use additional code for any associated fecal incontinence (R15-).

Special Coding Issues

Ulcers

This chapter includes codes for ulcers (sores or lesions that form in the lining of the stomach or intestinal tract). Code selection depends on the location (stomach, small and large intestine), whether the ulcer is acute, chronic, perforated (lesion extends to entire thickness of organ), hemorrhaging (bleeding), or causing obstruction. Check the physician's documentation carefully in order to report the correct code.

- Category K25.- (stomach ulcer) is used to report a gastric ulcer.

- Category K26.- (duodenal ulcer) is used to report an ulcer involving the duodenum (first section of the small intestine).

- Category K28.- (gastrojejunal ulcer) is used to report an ulcer involving the stomach and jejuneum (second section of the small intestine).

- Category K27.9 (peptic ulcer, site unspecified) is used to report an ulcer in these cases:

  - Ulcer described as gastroduodenal (involving the stomach and duodenum),

  - Ulcer described as a peptic or stress ulcer, or

  - Ulcer is documented as present in digestive tract, but its location is not designated.

Ulcers of the large intestine are reported using codes from either series K51.- (ulcerative colitis), code K63.3 (ulceration of intestine) or code K63.1 (perforation of intestine). If the ulcer is documented as colitis (noninfectious ulcerative colitis), report code K52.9.

Once the location of an ulcer is determined, it's important to recognize the distinguishing factors that most often will lead to the appropriate 4th character. The 4th character denotes whether the ulcer is acute or chronic and whether or not it involves hemorrhage and/or perforation.

Hepatitis

Be careful attaching this diagnosis to your claims. Hepatitis simply means liver inflammation. Do not append a diagnosis of hepatitis because you see elevated liver enzymes on the medical chart because there are two different etiologies for liver inflammation: those due to blockage and those due to infectious or toxic agents.

Hepatitis is due to infectious or toxic agents. Obstructive liver inflammation is not hepatitis. Hepatitis can be caused by alcohol (K70.-), chemical or drug-induced (K71.-), autoimmune (K75.4), or viral (refer to categories B15-B19 in chapter 1), which spans hepatitis A, hepatitis B, hepatitis B with delta and hepatitis C (the most common). Even if an elevated liver enzyme test is present, hepatitis A, B, and C often cannot be differentiated without further lab tests. It is best to use an elevated liver function test diagnosis (code R94.5) until a diagnosis of hepatitis is confirmed. Hepatitis C may be referred to as non-A, non-B or viral.

Once you have a diagnosis, use the patient assessment, coupled with confirmation from the physician, to determine if the hepatitis is: a) chronic or acute, and b) whether it's accompanied by hepatic coma. If newly diagnosed, hepatitis usually is labeled acute since it takes several months to be labeled as chronic. Other diagnosis codes that can be added include those that indicate the mode of transmission, for example, Z20.5 for contact with/exposure to viral hepatitis.

Gastrointestinal Hemorrhage

There are several terms used to describe GI hemorrhage that are linked with the specific area in the GI tract. For example, code K92.2 for GI hemorrhage, unspecified; K29.01 for acute hemorrhagic gastritis; K62.5 for hemorrhage of anus and rectum; K57.- for diverticular disease with hemorrhage; or K25-K28 for peptic ulcer with hemorrhage. The following are some additional terms that describe the presence of GI bleeding:

- Hematemesis, K92.0 (vomiting of blood), indicates acute upper GI hemorrhage;

- Melena, K92.1 (presence of dark-colored blood in the stool), indicates upper or lower GI hemorrhage;

- Occult bleeding (presence of blood in the stool that can be seen only on laboratory exam); and

- Hematochezia/melena (presence of brightly-colored blood in stool), usually indicates blood from the rectum.

Hernias

This chapter also includes codes for hernias in categories K40-K46 (a weakness or defect in the abdominal wall in which the contents of the abdomen protrude into other sites). Check the physician's documentation carefully in order to report the correct code.

Code selection depends first on the location of the hernia: inguinal (into genital area), femoral (into thigh area), umbilical (into area of the navel), hiatal (stomach protruding through the diaphragm), incisional (through an old surgical incision), or ventral (into the front of the abdomen).

Other words describe whether the hernia is obstructing the organs involved. For example, the term "incarcerated" indicates a hernia causing complete obstruction. The term "strangulated" indicates a lack of blood flow to the affected organ due to compression, which can quickly lead to a hernia "with gangrene," in which necrosis or tissue death occurs due to the blocked blood supply and resulting absence of oxygen. You should also know the following terms: unilateral or bilateral (one or both sides, refers to inguinal hernias); recurrent (repaired hernia has reoccurred); reducible, or nonreducible (whether tissue can be put back in its place by manipulation); or sliding (tissue moves into and out of place).

The physician's documentation may include words with the suffix "-cele" or the word "prolapse" (falling, drooping of an organ) to describe hernias. Coders should look up the words used in the documentation to find the correct code since many of the conditions are coded in different body system chapters in ICD-10-CM.

Hernias not related to the digestive system are classified to the system they are associated with. For example, an omphalocele (Q79.2), which is a congenital hernia of the umbilicus, also referred to as an exomphalos, is coded from chapter 17 (Congenital malformations, deformations and chromosomal abnormalities).

Cystocele (herniation of bladder [N81.10]), ureterovaginal prolapse (N81.4), rectocele, prolapse of posterior vaginal wall (N81.6) are other examples of codes found in chapter 14 (Diseases of the genitourinary system) rather than chapter 11.

Constipation

Constipation (Category K59) is the passage of small amounts of hard, dry bowel movements, usually fewer than three times a week. People who are constipated may find it difficult and painful to have a bowel movement. Other symptoms of constipation include feeling bloated, uncomfortable and sluggish.

Constipation codes include:

- Constipation, unspecified (K59.00)
- Slow transit constipation (K59.01)
- Outlet dysfunction constipation (K59.02)
- Drug-induced constipation (K59.03)
- Chronic idiopathic constipation (K59.04)
- Other constipation (K59.09)
- Irritable bowel syndrome with constipation (K58.1)

Diarrhea

Loose, watery stools occurring more than three times in one day is a problem that usually lasts a day or two and resolves on its own. However, prolonged diarrhea can be a sign of other problems and requires use of a more specific code than diarrhea NOS (R19.7), when possible.

Bloody diarrhea is found under Melena (K92.1).

Infectious diarrhea is assigned a code from Chapter 1 when the organism has been identified.

Functional diarrhea is characterized by chronic or recurrent diarrhea not explained by structural or biochemical abnormalities, and is coded with K59.1. This code has an Excludes note: diarrhea, NOS (R19.7); and irritable bowel syndrome with diarrhea (K58.0).

Chapter 11

K00 - K95

CHAPTER 11: DISEASES OF THE DIGESTIVE SYSTEM (K00-K95)

EXCLUDES 2 certain conditions originating in the perinatal period (P04-P96)
certain infectious and parasitic diseases (A00-B99)
complications of pregnancy, childbirth and the puerperium (O00-O9A)
congenital malformations, deformations and chromosomal abnormalities (Q00-Q99)
endocrine, nutritional and metabolic diseases (E00-E88)
injury, poisoning and certain other consequences of external causes (S00-T88)
neoplasms (C00-D49)
symptoms, signs and abnormal clinical and laboratory findings, not elsewhere classified (R00-R94)

This chapter contains the following blocks:
K00-K14   Diseases of oral cavity and salivary glands
K20-K31   Diseases of esophagus, stomach and duodenum
K35-K38   Diseases of appendix
K40-K46   Hernia
K50-K52   Noninfective enteritis and colitis
K55-K64   Other diseases of intestines
K65-K68   Diseases of peritoneum and retroperitoneum
K70-K77   Diseases of liver
K80-K87   Disorders of gallbladder, biliary tract and pancreas
K90-K95   Other diseases of the digestive system

Diseases of oral cavity and salivary glands (K00-K14)

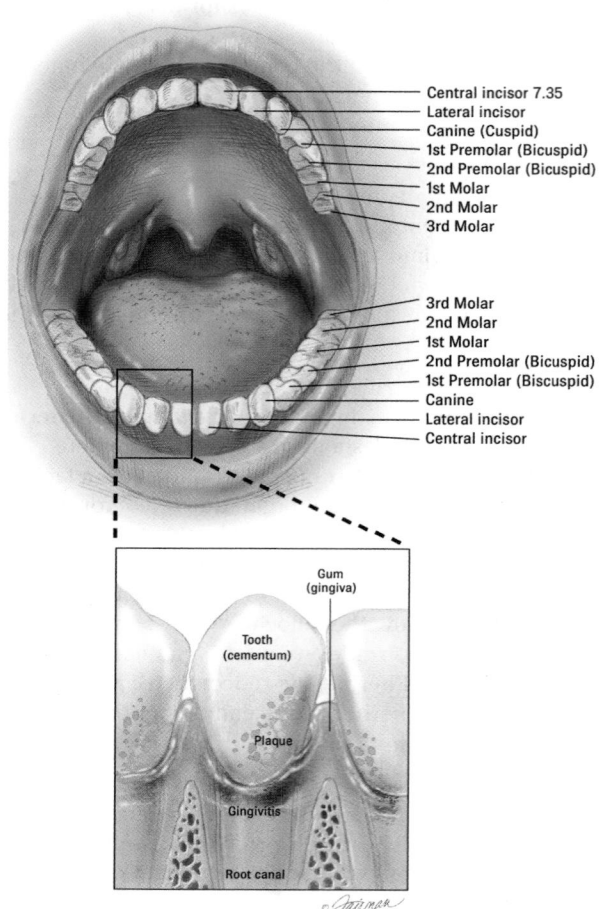

4 K00 Disorders of tooth development and eruption
EXCLUDES 2 embedded and impacted teeth (K01.-)

IQ K00.0 Anodontia
Hypodontia
Oligodontia
EXCLUDES 1 acquired absence of teeth (K08.1-)
DEFINITION Defect in which many or all of the teeth do not develop and are absent from the mouth.

IQ K00.1 Supernumerary teeth
Distomolar
Fourth molar
Mesiodens
Paramolar
Supplementary teeth
EXCLUDES 2 supernumerary roots (K00.2)

IQ K00.2 Abnormalities of size and form of teeth
Concrescence of teeth
Fusion of teeth
Gemination of teeth
Dens evaginatus
Dens in dente
Dens invaginatus

Chapter 11

K00-K95

Enamel pearls
Macrodontia
Microdontia
Peg-shaped [conical] teeth
Supernumerary roots
Taurodontism
Tuberculum paramolare
> **EXCLUDES 1** abnormalities of teeth due to congenital syphilis (A50.5)
> tuberculum Carabelli, which is regarded as a normal variation and should not be coded

!Q K00.3 Mottled teeth
Dental fluorosis
Mottling of enamel
Nonfluoride enamel opacities
> **EXCLUDES 2** deposits [accretions] on teeth (K03.6)

!Q K00.4 Disturbances in tooth formation
Aplasia and hypoplasia of cementum
Dilaceration of tooth
Enamel hypoplasia (neonatal) (postnatal) (prenatal)
Regional odontodysplasia
Turner's tooth
> **EXCLUDES 1** Hutchinson's teeth and mulberry molars in congenital syphilis (A50.5)
> **EXCLUDES 2** mottled teeth (K00.3)

!Q K00.5 Hereditary disturbances in tooth structure, not elsewhere classified
Amelogenesis imperfecta
Dentinogenesis imperfecta
Odontogenesis imperfecta
Dentinal dysplasia
Shell teeth

!Q K00.6 Disturbances in tooth eruption
Dentia praecox
Natal tooth
Neonatal tooth
Premature eruption of tooth
Premature shedding of primary [deciduous] tooth
Prenatal teeth
Retained [persistent] primary tooth
> **EXCLUDES 2** embedded and impacted teeth (K01.-)

!Q K00.7 Teething syndrome

!Q K00.8 Other disorders of tooth development
Color changes during tooth formation
Intrinsic staining of teeth NOS
> **EXCLUDES 2** posteruptive color changes (K03.7)

!Q K00.9 Disorder of tooth development, unspecified
Disorder of odontogenesis NOS

4 K01 Embedded and impacted teeth
> **EXCLUDES 1** abnormal position of fully erupted teeth (M26.3-)

!Q K01.0 Embedded teeth

!Q K01.1 Impacted teeth

4 K02 Dental caries
> **INCLUDES** caries of dentine
> dental cavities
> early childhood caries

pre-eruptive caries
recurrent caries
(dentino enamel junction)
(enamel) (to the pulp)
tooth decay

!Q K02.3 Arrested dental caries
Arrested coronal and root caries

5 K02.5 Dental caries on pit and fissure surface
Dental caries on chewing surface of tooth

!Q K02.51 Dental caries on pit and fissure surface limited to enamel
White spot lesions [initial caries] on pit and fissure surface of tooth

!Q K02.52 Dental caries on pit and fissure surface penetrating into dentin
Primary dental caries, cervical origin

!Q K02.53 Dental caries on pit and fissure surface penetrating into pulp

5 K02.6 Dental caries on smooth surface

!Q K02.61 Dental caries on smooth surface limited to enamel
White spot lesions [initial caries] on smooth surface of tooth

!Q K02.62 Dental caries on smooth surface penetrating into dentin

!Q K02.63 Dental caries on smooth surface penetrating into pulp

!Q K02.7 Dental root caries

!Q K02.9 Dental caries, unspecified

4 K03 Other diseases of hard tissues of teeth
> **EXCLUDES 2** bruxism (F45.8)
> dental caries (K02.-)
> teeth-grinding NOS (F45.8)

!Q K03.0 Excessive attrition of teeth
Approximal wear of teeth
Occlusal wear of teeth
> **DEFINITION** Teeth exhibit excessive wear and tear as a result of tooth-to-tooth contact, often due to grinding the teeth.

!Q K03.1 Abrasion of teeth
Dentifrice abrasion of teeth
Habitual abrasion of teeth
Occupational abrasion of teeth
Ritual abrasion of teeth
Traditional abrasion of teeth
Wedge defect NOS
> **DEFINITION** Teeth exhibit specific wear and tear as a result of tooth contact with another object.

!Q K03.2 Erosion of teeth
Erosion of teeth due to diet
Erosion of teeth due to drugs and medicaments
Erosion of teeth due to persistent vomiting
Erosion of teeth NOS
Idiopathic erosion of teeth
Occupational erosion of teeth

!Q K03.3 Pathological resorption of teeth
Internal granuloma of pulp
Resorption of teeth (external)

!Q K03.4 Hypercementosis
Cementation hyperplasia

!Q K03.5 Ankylosis of teeth
> **DEFINITION** Roots of the teeth grow into and merge with the bone of the jaw; most often occurring during development of baby teeth.

Chapter 11

K00-K95

★ New ▲ Revised Px Primary SP PDGM Px SL Low CoM SH High CoM !Q Quest. Encounter H Hospice non-cancer Dx Unspecified M *Manifestation*

DecisionHealth's FY 2020 Complete Home Health ICD-10-CM Diagnosis Coding Manual 1065

IQ K03.6 Deposits [accretions] on teeth
Betel deposits [accretions] on teeth
Black deposits [accretions] on teeth
Extrinsic staining of teeth NOS
Green deposits [accretions] on teeth
Materia alba deposits [accretions] on teeth
Orange deposits [accretions] on teeth
Staining of teeth NOS
Subgingival dental calculus
Supragingival dental calculus
Tobacco deposits [accretions] on teeth

DEFINITION Calculous deposits or tartar build-up that resists removal by normal brushing and requires professional cleaning.

IQ K03.7 Posteruptive color changes of dental hard tissues
EXCLUDES 2 deposits [accretions] on teeth (K03.6)

5 K03.8 Other specified diseases of hard tissues of teeth

IQ K03.81 Cracked tooth
EXCLUDES 1 asymptomatic craze lines in enamel - omit code broken or fractured tooth due to trauma (S02.5)

IQ K03.89 Other specified diseases of hard tissues of teeth

IQ K03.9 Disease of hard tissues of teeth, unspecified

4 K04 Diseases of pulp and periapical tissues

5 K04.0 Pulpitis
Acute pulpitis
Chronic (hyperplastic) (ulcerative) pulpitis
DEFINITION Painful inflammation of the soft living tissue containing nerves within the center of the tooth.

IQ K04.01 Reversible pulpitis

IQ K04.02 Irreversible pulpitis

IQ K04.1 Necrosis of pulp
Pulpal gangrene

IQ K04.2 Pulp degeneration
Denticles
Pulpal calcifications
Pulpal stones

IQ K04.3 Abnormal hard tissue formation in pulp
Secondary or irregular dentine

IQ K04.4 Acute apical periodontitis of pulpal origin
Acute apical periodontitis NOS
EXCLUDES 1 acute periodontitis (K05.2-)
DEFINITION Severe inflammation of the periodontal ligament connecting the tooth to the jawbone due to infection or necrosis of the soft, living tissue in the center of the tooth.

IQ K04.5 Chronic apical periodontitis
Apical or periapical granuloma
Apical periodontitis NOS
EXCLUDES 1 chronic periodontitis (K05.3-)

IQ K04.6 Periapical abscess with sinus
Dental abscess with sinus
Dentoalveolar abscess with sinus

IQ K04.7 Periapical abscess without sinus
Dental abscess without sinus

Dentoalveolar abscess without sinus

IQ K04.8 Radicular cyst
Apical (periodontal) cyst
Periapical cyst
Residual radicular cyst
EXCLUDES 2 lateral periodontal cyst (K09.0)

5 K04.9 Other and unspecified diseases of pulp and periapical tissues

IQ K04.90 Unspecified diseases of pulp and periapical tissues

IQ K04.99 Other diseases of pulp and periapical tissues

+ 4 K05 Gingivitis and periodontal diseases
Use additional code to identify:
alcohol abuse and dependence (F10.-)
exposure to environmental tobacco smoke (Z77.22)
exposure to tobacco smoke in the perinatal period (P96.81)
history of tobacco dependence (Z87.891)
occupational exposure to environmental tobacco smoke (Z57.31)
tobacco dependence (F17.-)
tobacco use (Z72.0)

+ 5 K05.0 Acute gingivitis
EXCLUDES 1 acute necrotizing ulcerative gingivitis (A69.1)
herpesviral [herpes simplex] gingivostomatitis (B00.2)

IQ + K05.00 Acute gingivitis, plaque induced
Acute gingivitis NOS
Plaque induced gingival disease

IQ + K05.01 Acute gingivitis, non-plaque induced

+ 5 K05.1 Chronic gingivitis
Desquamative gingivitis (chronic)
Gingivitis (chronic) NOS
Hyperplastic gingivitis (chronic)
Pregnancy associated gingivitis
Simple marginal gingivitis (chronic)
Ulcerative gingivitis (chronic)
Code first:
, if applicable, diseases of the digestive system complicating pregnancy (O99.61-)

IQ + K05.10 Chronic gingivitis, plaque induced
Chronic gingivitis NOS
Gingivitis NOS

IQ + K05.11 Chronic gingivitis, non-plaque induced

+ 5 K05.2 Aggressive periodontitis
Acute pericoronitis
EXCLUDES 1 acute apical periodontitis (K04.4)
periapical abscess (K04.7)
periapical abscess with sinus (K04.6)

IQ + K05.20 Aggressive periodontitis, unspecified
DEFINITION Serious and destructive inflammation and infection of the ligaments and bones supporting the teeth, leading to tooth loss.

+ 6 K05.21 Aggressive periodontitis, localized
Periodontal abscess

IQ + K05.211 Aggressive periodontitis, localized, slight

---

4 4th digit required   5 5th digit required   6 6th digit required   7 7th digit required   7 7th digit placeholder   + Additional code   5 Laterality

1066   *DecisionHealth's* FY 2020 Complete Home Health ICD-10-CM Diagnosis Coding Manual

!Q + **K05.212** Aggressive periodontitis, localized, moderate

!Q + **K05.213** Aggressive periodontitis, localized, severe

!Q + **K05.219** Aggressive periodontitis, localized, unspecified severity

+ 6 **K05.22** Aggressive periodontitis, generalized

!Q + **K05.221** Aggressive periodontitis, generalized, slight

!Q + **K05.222** Aggressive periodontitis, generalized, moderate

!Q + **K05.223** Aggressive periodontitis, generalized, severe

!Q + **K05.229** Aggressive periodontitis, generalized, unspecified severity

+ 5 **K05.3** Chronic periodontitis
Chronic pericoronitis
Complex periodontitis
Periodontitis NOS
Simplex periodontitis

> **EXCLUDES 1** chronic apical periodontitis (K04.5)

!Q + **K05.30** Chronic periodontitis, unspecified

+ 6 **K05.31** Chronic periodontitis, localized

!Q + **K05.311** Chronic periodontitis, localized, slight

!Q + **K05.312** Chronic periodontitis, localized, moderate

!Q + **K05.313** Chronic periodontitis, localized, severe

!Q + **K05.319** Chronic periodontitis, localized, unspecified severity

+ 6 **K05.32** Chronic periodontitis, generalized

!Q + **K05.321** Chronic periodontitis, generalized, slight

!Q + **K05.322** Chronic periodontitis, generalized, moderate

!Q + **K05.323** Chronic periodontitis, generalized, severe

!Q + **K05.329** Chronic periodontitis, generalized, unspecified severity

!Q + **K05.4** Periodontosis
Juvenile periodontosis

!Q + **K05.5** Other periodontal diseases
Combined periodontic-endodontic lesion
Narrow gingival width (of periodontal soft tissue)

> **EXCLUDES 2** leukoplakia of gingiva (K13.21)

!Q + **K05.6** Periodontal disease, unspecified

4 **K06** Other disorders of gingiva and edentulous alveolar ridge

> **EXCLUDES 2** acute gingivitis (K05.0)
> atrophy of edentulous alveolar ridge (K08.2)
> chronic gingivitis (K05.1)
> gingivitis NOS (K05.1)

5 **K06.0** Gingival recession
Gingival recession (postinfective) (postprocedural)

> **DEFINITION** Gums that have receded, exposing more tooth.

6 **K06.01** Gingival recession, localized

!Q **K06.010** Localized gingival recession, unspecified
Localized gingival recession, NOS

!Q **K06.011** Localized gingival recession, minimal

!Q **K06.012** Localized gingival recession, moderate

!Q **K06.013** Localized gingival recession, severe

6 **K06.02** Gingival recession, generalized

!Q **K06.020** Generalized gingival recession, unspecified
Generalized gingival recession, NOS

!Q **K06.021** Generalized gingival recession, minimal

!Q **K06.022** Generalized gingival recession, moderate

!Q **K06.023** Generalized gingival recession, severe

!Q **K06.1** Gingival enlargement
Gingival fibromatosis

!Q + **K06.2** Gingival and edentulous alveolar ridge lesions associated with trauma
Irritative hyperplasia of edentulous ridge [denture hyperplasia]
Use additional code (Chapter 20) to identify external cause or denture status (Z97.2)

!Q **K06.3** Horizontal alveolar bone loss

!Q **K06.8** Other specified disorders of gingiva and edentulous alveolar ridge
Fibrous epulis
Flabby alveolar ridge
Giant cell epulis
Peripheral giant cell granuloma of gingiva
Pyogenic granuloma of gingiva
Vertical ridge deficiency

> **EXCLUDES 2** gingival cyst (K09.0)

!Q **K06.9** Disorder of gingiva and edentulous alveolar ridge, unspecified

4 **K08** Other disorders of teeth and supporting structures

> **EXCLUDES 2** dentofacial anomalies [including malocclusion] (M26.-)
> disorders of jaw (M27.-)

!Q **K08.0** Exfoliation of teeth due to systemic causes
Code also:
underlying systemic condition

5 **K08.1** Complete loss of teeth
Acquired loss of teeth, complete

> **EXCLUDES 1** congenital absence of teeth (K00.0)
> exfoliation of teeth due to systemic causes (K08.0)
> partial loss of teeth (K08.4-)

6 **K08.10** Complete loss of teeth, unspecified cause

!Q **K08.101** Complete loss of teeth, unspecified cause, class I

!Q **K08.102** Complete loss of teeth, unspecified cause, class II

!Q **K08.103** Complete loss of teeth, unspecified cause, class III

!Q **K08.104** Complete loss of teeth, unspecified cause, class IV

Chapter 11

K00-K95

★ New ▲ Revised **Px** Primary **SP** PDGM Px **SL** Low CoM **SH** High CoM **!Q** Quest. Encounter **H** Hospice non-cancer Dx   Unspecified   **M** *Manifestation*

DecisionHealth's FY 2020 Complete Home Health ICD-10-CM Diagnosis Coding Manual

1067

IQ K08.109 Complete loss of teeth, unspecified cause, unspecified class

Edentulism NOS

6 K08.11 Complete loss of teeth due to trauma

IQ K08.111 Complete loss of teeth due to trauma, class I

IQ K08.112 Complete loss of teeth due to trauma, class II

IQ K08.113 Complete loss of teeth due to trauma, class III

IQ K08.114 Complete loss of teeth due to trauma, class IV

IQ K08.119 Complete loss of teeth due to trauma, unspecified class

6 K08.12 Complete loss of teeth due to periodontal diseases

IQ K08.121 Complete loss of teeth due to periodontal diseases, class I

IQ K08.122 Complete loss of teeth due to periodontal diseases, class II

IQ K08.123 Complete loss of teeth due to periodontal diseases, class III

IQ K08.124 Complete loss of teeth due to periodontal diseases, class IV

IQ K08.129 Complete loss of teeth due to periodontal diseases, unspecified class

6 K08.13 Complete loss of teeth due to caries

IQ K08.131 Complete loss of teeth due to caries, class I

IQ K08.132 Complete loss of teeth due to caries, class II

IQ K08.133 Complete loss of teeth due to caries, class III

IQ K08.134 Complete loss of teeth due to caries, class IV

IQ K08.139 Complete loss of teeth due to caries, unspecified class

6 K08.19 Complete loss of teeth due to other specified cause

IQ K08.191 Complete loss of teeth due to other specified cause, class I

IQ K08.192 Complete loss of teeth due to other specified cause, class II

IQ K08.193 Complete loss of teeth due to other specified cause, class III

IQ K08.194 Complete loss of teeth due to other specified cause, class IV

IQ K08.199 Complete loss of teeth due to other specified cause, unspecified class

5 K08.2 Atrophy of edentulous alveolar ridge

IQ K08.20 Unspecified atrophy of edentulous alveolar ridge

Atrophy of the mandible NOS
Atrophy of the maxilla NOS

IQ K08.21 Minimal atrophy of the mandible

Minimal atrophy of the edentulous mandible

IQ K08.22 Moderate atrophy of the mandible

Moderate atrophy of the edentulous mandible

IQ K08.23 Severe atrophy of the mandible

Severe atrophy of the edentulous mandible

IQ K08.24 Minimal atrophy of maxilla

Minimal atrophy of the edentulous maxilla

IQ K08.25 Moderate atrophy of the maxilla

Moderate atrophy of the edentulous maxilla

IQ K08.26 Severe atrophy of the maxilla

Severe atrophy of the edentulous maxilla

IQ K08.3 Retained dental root

DEFINITION Part or all of the root structure of a tooth remains in the jaw after the tooth is extracted or otherwise lost.

5 K08.4 Partial loss of teeth

Acquired loss of teeth, partial

EXCLUDES 1 complete loss of teeth (K08.1-)
congenital absence of teeth (K00.0)

EXCLUDES 2 exfoliation of teeth due to systemic causes (K08.0)

6 K08.40 Partial loss of teeth, unspecified cause

IQ K08.401 Partial loss of teeth, unspecified cause, class I

IQ K08.402 Partial loss of teeth, unspecified cause, class II

IQ K08.403 Partial loss of teeth, unspecified cause, class III

IQ K08.404 Partial loss of teeth, unspecified cause, class IV

IQ K08.409 Partial loss of teeth, unspecified cause, unspecified class

Tooth extraction status NOS

6 K08.41 Partial loss of teeth due to trauma

IQ K08.411 Partial loss of teeth due to trauma, class I

IQ K08.412 Partial loss of teeth due to trauma, class II

IQ K08.413 Partial loss of teeth due to trauma, class III

IQ K08.414 Partial loss of teeth due to trauma, class IV

IQ K08.419 Partial loss of teeth due to trauma, unspecified class

6 K08.42 Partial loss of teeth due to periodontal diseases

IQ K08.421 Partial loss of teeth due to periodontal diseases, class I

IQ K08.422 Partial loss of teeth due to periodontal diseases, class II

IQ K08.423 Partial loss of teeth due to periodontal diseases, class III

IQ K08.424 Partial loss of teeth due to periodontal diseases, class IV

IQ K08.429 Partial loss of teeth due to periodontal diseases, unspecified class

6 K08.43 Partial loss of teeth due to caries

IQ K08.431 Partial loss of teeth due to caries, class I

IQ K08.432 Partial loss of teeth due to caries, class II

IQ K08.433 Partial loss of teeth due to caries, class III

---

4 4th digit required   5 5th digit required   6 6th digit required   7 7th digit required   7 7th digit placeholder   +Additional code   Laterality

IQ K08.434 Partial loss of teeth due to caries, class IV

IQ K08.439 Partial loss of teeth due to caries, unspecified class

6 K08.49 Partial loss of teeth due to other specified cause

IQ K08.491 Partial loss of teeth due to other specified cause, class I

IQ K08.492 Partial loss of teeth due to other specified cause, class II

IQ K08.493 Partial loss of teeth due to other specified cause, class III

IQ K08.494 Partial loss of teeth due to other specified cause, class IV

IQ K08.499 Partial loss of teeth due to other specified cause, unspecified class

5 K08.5 Unsatisfactory restoration of tooth
Defective bridge, crown, filling
Defective dental restoration

EXCLUDES 1 dental restoration status (Z98.811)

EXCLUDES 2 endosseous dental implant failure (M27.6-)
unsatisfactory endodontic treatment (M27.5-)

IQ K08.50 Unsatisfactory restoration of tooth, unspecified

Defective dental restoration NOS

IQ K08.51 Open restoration margins of tooth
Dental restoration failure of marginal integrity
Open margin on tooth restoration
Poor gingival margin to tooth restoration

IQ K08.52 Unrepairable overhanging of dental restorative materials
Overhanging of tooth restoration

6 K08.53 Fractured dental restorative material

EXCLUDES 1 cracked tooth (K03.81)
traumatic fracture of tooth (S02.5)

IQ K08.530 Fractured dental restorative material without loss of material

IQ K08.531 Fractured dental restorative material with loss of material

IQ K08.539 Fractured dental restorative material, unspecified

IQ K08.54 Contour of existing restoration of tooth biologically incompatible with oral health
Dental restoration failure of periodontal anatomical integrity
Unacceptable contours of existing restoration of tooth
Unacceptable morphology of existing restoration of tooth

IQ + K08.55 Allergy to existing dental restorative material
Use additional code to identify the specific type of allergy

IQ K08.56 Poor aesthetic of existing restoration of tooth
Dental restoration aesthetically inadequate or displeasing

IQ K08.59 Other unsatisfactory restoration of tooth
Other defective dental restoration

5 K08.8 Other specified disorders of teeth and supporting structures

IQ K08.81 Primary occlusal trauma

IQ K08.82 Secondary occlusal trauma

IQ K08.89 Other specified disorders of teeth and supporting structures
Enlargement of alveolar ridge NOS
Insufficient anatomic crown height
Insufficient clinical crown length
Irregular alveolar process
Toothache NOS

IQ K08.9 Disorder of teeth and supporting structures, unspecified

4 K09 Cysts of oral region, not elsewhere classified

INCLUDES lesions showing histological features both of aneurysmal cyst and of another fibro-osseous lesion

EXCLUDES 2 cysts of jaw (M27.0-, M27.4-)
radicular cyst (K04.8)

IQ K09.0 Developmental odontogenic cysts
Dentigerous cyst
Eruption cyst
Follicular cyst
Gingival cyst
Lateral periodontal cyst
Primordial cyst

EXCLUDES 2 keratocysts (D16.4, D16.5)
odontogenic keratocystic tumors (D16.4, D16.5)

IQ K09.1 Developmental (nonodontogenic) cysts of oral region
Cyst (of) incisive canal
Cyst (of) palatine of papilla
Globulomaxillary cyst
Median palatal cyst
Nasoalveolar cyst
Nasolabial cyst
Nasopalatine duct cyst

IQ K09.8 Other cysts of oral region, not elsewhere classified
Dermoid cyst
Epidermoid cyst
Lymphoepithelial cyst
Epstein's pearl

IQ K09.9 Cyst of oral region, unspecified

+ 4 K11 Diseases of salivary glands
Use additional code to identify:
alcohol abuse and dependence (F10.-)
exposure to environmental tobacco smoke (Z77.22)
exposure to tobacco smoke in the perinatal period (P96.81)
history of tobacco dependence (Z87.891)
occupational exposure to environmental tobacco smoke (Z57.31)
tobacco dependence (F17.-)
tobacco use (Z72.0)

SP + K11.0 Atrophy of salivary gland

DEFINITION Wasting of the saliva glands, resulting in insufficient saliva production.

SP + K11.1 Hypertrophy of salivary gland

+ 5 K11.2 Sialoadenitis
Parotitis

EXCLUDES 1 epidemic parotitis (B26.-)
mumps (B26.-)

Chapter 11

K00-K95

★ New ▲ Revised Px Primary SP PDGM Px SL Low CoM SH High CoM IQ Quest. Encounter H Hospice non-cancer Dx   Unspecified   M *Manifestation*

DecisionHealth's FY 2020 Complete Home Health ICD-10-CM Diagnosis Coding Manual

1069

uveoparotid fever
[Heerfordt] (D86.89)

SP + K11.20 Sialoadenitis, unspecified

SP + K11.21 Acute sialoadenitis
> **EXCLUDES 1** acute recurrent
> sialoadenitis (K11.22)

SP + K11.22 Acute recurrent sialoadenitis

SP + K11.23 Chronic sialoadenitis

SP + K11.3 Abscess of salivary gland

SP + K11.4 Fistula of salivary gland
> **EXCLUDES 1** congenital fistula of salivary
> gland (Q38.4)

SP + K11.5 Sialolithiasis
Calculus of salivary gland or duct
Stone of salivary gland or duct

SP + K11.6 Mucocele of salivary gland
Mucous extravasation cyst of salivary
gland
Mucous retention cyst of salivary gland
Ranula

SP + K11.7 Disturbances of salivary secretion
Hypoptyalism
Ptyalism
Xerostomia
> **EXCLUDES 2** dry mouth NOS (R68.2)

SP + K11.8 Other diseases of salivary glands
Benign lymphoepithelial lesion of salivary
gland
Mikulicz' disease
Necrotizing sialometaplasia
Sialectasia
Stenosis of salivary duct
Stricture of salivary duct
> **EXCLUDES 1** sicca syndrome [Sjögren]
> (M35.0-)

IQ + K11.9 Disease of salivary gland, unspecified
Sialoadenopathy NOS

+ ④ K12 Stomatitis and related lesions
Use additional code to identify:
alcohol abuse and dependence (F10.-)
exposure to environmental tobacco smoke
(Z77.22)
exposure to tobacco smoke in the perinatal
period (P96.81)
history of tobacco dependence (Z87.891)
occupational exposure to environmental
tobacco smoke (Z57.31)
tobacco dependence (F17.-)
tobacco use (Z72.0)
> **EXCLUDES 1** cancrum oris (A69.0)
> cheilitis (K13.0)
> gangrenous stomatitis (A69.0)
> herpesviral [herpes simplex]
> gingivostomatitis (B00.2)
> noma (A69.0)

SP + K12.0 Recurrent oral aphthae
Aphthous stomatitis (major) (minor)
Bednar's aphthae
Periadenitis mucosa necrotica recurrens
Recurrent aphthous ulcer
Stomatitis herpetiformis

SP + K12.1 Other forms of stomatitis
Stomatitis NOS
Denture stomatitis
Ulcerative stomatitis
Vesicular stomatitis

> **EXCLUDES 1** acute necrotizing ulcerative
> stomatitis (A69.1)
> Vincent's stomatitis (A69.1)
> **DEFINITION** Painful inflammation of the
> mucosal soft tissues of the mouth, usually
> from a viral infection that can lead to ulcers
> or vesicular lesions.

SP + K12.2 Cellulitis and abscess of mouth
Cellulitis of mouth (floor)
Submandibular abscess
> **EXCLUDES 2** abscess of salivary gland
> (K11.3)
> abscess of tongue (K14.0)
> periapical abscess
> (K04.6-K04.7)
> periodontal abscess
> (K05.21)
> peritonsillar abscess (J36)

+ ⑤ K12.3 Oral mucositis (ulcerative)
Mucositis (oral) (oropharyneal)
> **EXCLUDES 2** gastrointestinal mucositis
> (ulcerative) (K92.81)
> mucositis (ulcerative) of
> vagina and vulva (N76.81)
> nasal mucositis (ulcerative)
> (J34.81)

SP + K12.30 Oral mucositis (ulcerative),
unspecified

SP + K12.31 Oral mucositis (ulcerative) due to
antineoplastic therapy
Use additional code for adverse effect,
if applicable, to identify
antineoplastic and
immunosuppressive drugs (T45.1X5)
Use additional code for other
antineoplastic therapy, such as:
radiological procedure and
radiotherapy (Y84.2)

SP + K12.32 Oral mucositis (ulcerative) due to
other drugs
Use additional code for adverse effect,
if applicable, to identify drug (T36-
T50 with fifth or sixth character 5)

SP + K12.33 Oral mucositis (ulcerative) due to
radiation
Use additional external cause code
(W88-W90, X39.0-) to identify cause

SP + K12.39 Other oral mucositis (ulcerative)
Viral oral mucositis (ulcerative)

+ ④ K13 Other diseases of lip and oral mucosa
> **INCLUDES** epithelial disturbances of
> tongue
Use additional code to identify:
alcohol abuse and dependence (F10.-)
exposure to environmental tobacco smoke
(Z77.22)
exposure to tobacco smoke in the perinatal
period (P96.81)
history of tobacco dependence (Z87.891)
occupational exposure to environmental
tobacco smoke (Z57.31)
tobacco dependence (F17.-)
tobacco use (Z72.0)
> **EXCLUDES 2** certain disorders of gingiva and
> edentulous alveolar ridge
> (K05-K06)
> cysts of oral region (K09.-)
> diseases of tongue (K14.-)

Chapter 11

K00-K95

④ 4th digit required   ⑤ 5th digit required   ⑥ 6th digit required   ⑦ 7th digit required   ⑦ 7th digit placeholder   ✚ Additional code   ⊟ Laterality

1070   *DecisionHealth's* FY 2020 Complete Home Health ICD-10-CM Diagnosis Coding Manual

stomatitis and related lesions
(K12.-)

SP + K13.0 Diseases of lips
Abscess of lips
Angular cheilitis
Cellulitis of lips
Cheilitis NOS
Cheilodynia
Cheilosis
Exfoliative cheilitis
Fistula of lips
Glandular cheilitis
Hypertrophy of lips
Perlèche NEC

EXCLUDES 1   ariboflavinosis (E53.0)
cheilitis due to radiation-
related disorders
(L55-L59)
congenital fistula of lips
(Q38.0)
congenital hypertrophy of
lips (Q18.6)
Perlèche due to candidiasis
(B37.83)
Perlèche due to riboflavin
deficiency (E53.0)

SP + K13.1 Cheek and lip biting

**+ 5 K13.2 Leukoplakia and other disturbances of
oral epithelium, including tongue**

EXCLUDES 1   carcinoma in situ of oral
epithelium (D00.0-)
hairy leukoplakia (K13.3)

**SP + K13.21 Leukoplakia of oral mucosa,
including tongue**
Leukokeratosis of oral mucosa
Leukoplakia of gingiva, lips, tongue

EXCLUDES 1   hairy leukoplakia
(K13.3)
leukokeratosis nicotina
palati (K13.24)

**SP + K13.22 Minimal keratinized residual ridge
mucosa**
Minimal keratinization of alveolar
ridge mucosa

**SP + K13.23 Excessive keratinized residual ridge
mucosa**
Excessive keratinization of alveolar
ridge mucosa

SP + K13.24 Leukokeratosis nicotina palati
Smoker's palate

**SP + K13.29 Other disturbances of oral
epithelium, including tongue**
Erythroplakia of mouth or tongue
Focal epithelial hyperplasia of mouth
or tongue
Leukoedema of mouth or tongue
Other oral epithelium disturbances

SP + K13.3 Hairy leukoplakia

**SP + K13.4 Granuloma and granuloma-like lesions
of oral mucosa**
Eosinophilic granuloma
Granuloma pyogenicum
Verrucous xanthoma

SP + K13.5 Oral submucous fibrosis
Submucous fibrosis of tongue

DEFINITION   Build-up of fibrous (scar-like)
tissue within the soft tissues of the mouth,
causing rigidity and inability to open the
mouth.

SP + K13.6 Irritative hyperplasia of oral mucosa
EXCLUDES 2   irritative hyperplasia of
edentulous ridge [denture
hyperplasia] (K06.2)

**+ 5 K13.7 Other and unspecified lesions of oral
mucosa**

IQ + K13.70 Unspecified lesions of oral mucosa

SP + K13.79 Other lesions of oral mucosa
Focal oral mucinosis

+ 4 K14 Diseases of tongue
Use additional code to identify:
alcohol abuse and dependence (F10.-)
exposure to environmental tobacco smoke
(Z77.22)
history of tobacco dependence (Z87.891)
occupational exposure to environmental
tobacco smoke (Z57.31)
tobacco dependence (F17.-)
tobacco use (Z72.0)

EXCLUDES 2   erythroplakia (K13.29)
focal epithelial hyperplasia
(K13.29)
leukedema of tongue (K13.29)
leukoplakia of tongue (K13.21)
hairy leukoplakia (K13.3)
macroglossia (congenital)
(Q38.2)
submucous fibrosis of tongue
(K13.5)

SP + K14.0 Glossitis
Abscess of tongue
Ulceration (traumatic) of tongue
EXCLUDES 1   atrophic glossitis (K14.4)

DEFINITION   Changes in the appearance
of the tongue due to inflammation.

SP + K14.1 Geographic tongue
Benign migratory glossitis
Glossitis areata exfoliativa

SP + K14.2 Median rhomboid glossitis

SP + K14.3 Hypertrophy of tongue papillae
Black hairy tongue
Coated tongue
Hypertrophy of foliate papillae
Lingua villosa nigra

SP + K14.4 Atrophy of tongue papillae
Atrophic glossitis

SP + K14.5 Plicated tongue
Fissured tongue
Furrowed tongue
Scrotal tongue
EXCLUDES 1   fissured tongue, congenital
(Q38.3)

SP + K14.6 Glossodynia
Glossopyrosis
Painful tongue
DEFINITION   Pain and/or a burning
sensation in the tongue.

SP + K14.8 Other diseases of tongue
Atrophy of tongue
Crenated tongue
Enlargement of tongue
Glossocele
Glossoptosis

★ New ▲ Revised Px Primary **SP** PDGM Px **SL** Low CoM **SH** High CoM **IQ** Quest. Encounter **H** Hospice non-cancer Dx   Unspecified   **M** *Manifestation*

Hypertrophy of tongue

IQ + K14.9 Disease of tongue, unspecified
Glossopathy NOS

Diseases of esophagus, stomach and duodenum (K20-K31)

EXCLUDES 2 hiatus hernia (K44.-)

+ 4 K20 Esophagitis
Use additional code to identify:
alcohol abuse and dependence (F10.-)
> **EXCLUDES 1** erosion of esophagus (K22.1-)
> esophagitis with gastro-
> esophageal reflux disease
> (K21.0)
> reflux esophagitis (K21.0)
> ulcerative esophagitis (K22.1-)
> **EXCLUDES 2** eosinophilic gastritis or
> gastroenteritis (K52.81)

CODING TIPS ✓ Do not assign a code from
K20.- if gastroesophageal reflux is also
diagnosed. When a patient has confirmed
diagnoses of both gastroesophageal reflux and
esophagitis, code K21.0 should be assigned.

SP + K20.0 Eosinophilic esophagitis

SP + K20.8 Other esophagitis
Abscess of esophagus

SP + K20.9 Esophagitis, unspecified
Esophagitis NOS

4 K21 Gastro-esophageal reflux disease
> **EXCLUDES 1** newborn esophageal reflux
> (P78.83)

SP K21.0 Gastro-esophageal reflux disease with esophagitis
Reflux esophagitis

DEFINITION Esophageal inflammation
due to reflux of gastric acid from the
stomach back up into the esophagus.

SP K21.9 Gastro-esophageal reflux disease without esophagitis
Esophageal reflux NOS

DEFINITION A burning sensation, usually
centered in the middle of the chest near the
breast bone, caused by the reflux of acidic
stomach fluids that enter the lower end of
the esophagus.

4 K22 Other diseases of esophagus
> **EXCLUDES 2** esophageal varices (I85.-)

SP K22.0 Achalasia of cardia
Achalasia NOS
Cardiospasm
> **EXCLUDES 1** congenital cardiospasm
> (Q39.5)

+ 5 K22.1 Ulcer of esophagus
Barrett's ulcer
Erosion of esophagus
Fungal ulcer of esophagus
Peptic ulcer of esophagus
Ulcer of esophagus due to ingestion of
chemicals
Ulcer of esophagus due to ingestion of
drugs and medicaments

Ulcerative esophagitis
Code first:
poisoning due to drug or toxin, if
applicable
(T36-T65 with fifth or sixth character
1-4 or 6)
Use additional code for adverse effect, if
applicable, to identify drug (T36-T50
with fifth or sixth character 5)
> **EXCLUDES 1** Barrett's esophagus (K22.7-)

SP + K22.10 Ulcer of esophagus without bleeding
Ulcer of esophagus NOS

SP + K22.11 Ulcer of esophagus with bleeding
> **EXCLUDES 2** bleeding esophageal
> varices
> (I85.01, I85.11)

SP K22.2 Esophageal obstruction
Compression of esophagus
Constriction of esophagus
Stenosis of esophagus
Stricture of esophagus
> **EXCLUDES 1** congenital stenosis or
> stricture of esophagus
> (Q39.3)

SP K22.3 Perforation of esophagus
Rupture of esophagus
> **EXCLUDES 1** traumatic perforation of
> (thoracic) esophagus
> (S27.8-)

SP K22.4 Dyskinesia of esophagus
Corkscrew esophagus
Diffuse esophageal spasm
Spasm of esophagus
> **EXCLUDES 1** cardiospasm (K22.0)

DEFINITION Weakened, paralyzed, or
uncoordinated movement of esophageal
muscles, causing difficulty swallowing.

SP K22.5 Diverticulum of esophagus, acquired
Esophageal pouch, acquired
> **EXCLUDES 1** diverticulum of esophagus
> (congenital) (Q39.6)

SP K22.6 Gastro-esophageal laceration-hemorrhage syndrome
Mallory-Weiss syndrome

CODING TIPS ✓ Code K22.6 should be
assigned only for patients diagnosed with
Mallory-Weiss syndrome or esophageal
laceration and bleeding due to Mallory-
Weiss tears. When esophageal bleeding is
documented as due to esophageal varices,
assign a code from I85.-.

DEFINITION Esophagus becomes torn
and bleeds near its connection to the
stomach due to prolonged vomiting,
hiccupping, or other spasmodic activity.

5 K22.7 Barrett's esophagus
Barrett's disease
Barrett's syndrome
> **EXCLUDES 1** Barrett's ulcer (K22.1)
> malignant neoplasm of
> esophagus (C15.-)

SP K22.70 Barrett's esophagus without dysplasia
Barrett's esophagus NOS

6 K22.71 Barrett's esophagus with dysplasia

SP K22.710 Barrett's esophagus with low grade dysplasia

4 4th digit required   **5** 5th digit required   **6** 6th digit required   **7** 7th digit required   **7** 7th digit placeholder   **+** Additional code   **B** Laterality

1072   *DecisionHealth's* FY 2020 Complete Home Health ICD-10-CM Diagnosis Coding Manual

SP K22.711 Barrett's esophagus with high grade dysplasia

SP K22.719 Barrett's esophagus with dysplasia, unspecified

SP K22.8 Other specified diseases of esophagus
Hemorrhage of esophagus NOS

EXCLUDES 2 esophageal varices (I85.-)
Paterson-Kelly syndrome (D50.1)

CODING TIPS ✓ Do not assign K22.8 when esophageal hemorrhage is documented as due to Mallory-Weiss syndrome. When Mallory-Weiss syndrome causes laceration and esophageal hemorrhage, assign code K22.6. Also do not assign for esophageal bleeding due to varices. When esophageal bleeding is documented as due to esophageal varices, assign a code from I85.-.

IQ K22.9 Disease of esophagus, unspecified

M IQ K23 Disorders of esophagus in diseases classified elsewhere
Code first underlying disease, such as:
congenital syphilis (A50.5)

EXCLUDES 1 late syphilis (A52.79)
megaesophagus due to Chagas' disease (B57.31)
tuberculosis (A18.83)

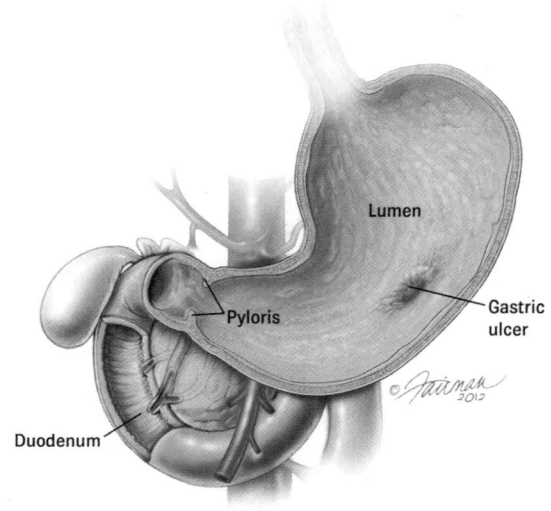

Lumen

Pyloris

Gastric ulcer

Duodenum

+ 4 K25 Gastric ulcer
INCLUDES erosion (acute) of stomach
pylorus ulcer (peptic)
stomach ulcer (peptic)
Use additional code to identify:
alcohol abuse and dependence (F10.-)
EXCLUDES 1 acute gastritis (K29.0-)
peptic ulcer NOS (K27.-)

CODING TIPS ✓ When documentation specifies that any gastric, duodenal or peptic ulcer is related to alcohol abuse or dependence, coders should assign an additional code to specify the abuse/dependence as specified. This is true when assigning code K25, K26 or K27.

CODING TIPS ✓ If the physician documents that the condition is caused or induced by the alcohol, use the appropriate F10 code with 5th and 6th digits .88 to indicate alcohol induced disorder.

CODING TIPS ✓ Gastric ulcers are often documented as stomach ulcers. Carefully read all documentation in order to code ulcers to the proper anatomic location.

SP + K25.0 Acute gastric ulcer with hemorrhage

SP + K25.1 Acute gastric ulcer with perforation

SP + K25.2 Acute gastric ulcer with both hemorrhage and perforation

SP + K25.3 Acute gastric ulcer without hemorrhage or perforation

SP + K25.4 Chronic or unspecified gastric ulcer with hemorrhage

SP + K25.5 Chronic or unspecified gastric ulcer with perforation

SP + K25.6 Chronic or unspecified gastric ulcer with both hemorrhage and perforation

SP + K25.7 Chronic gastric ulcer without hemorrhage or perforation

SP + K25.9 Gastric ulcer, unspecified as acute or chronic, without hemorrhage or perforation

+ 4 K26 Duodenal ulcer
INCLUDES erosion (acute) of duodenum
duodenum ulcer (peptic)
postpyloric ulcer (peptic)
Use additional code to identify:
alcohol abuse and dependence (F10.-)
EXCLUDES 1 peptic ulcer NOS (K27.-)

CODING TIPS ✓ When documentation specifies that any gastric, duodenal or peptic ulcer is related to alcohol abuse or dependence, coders should assign an additional code to specify the abuse/dependence as specified. This is true when assigning code K25, K26 or K27.

CODING TIPS ✓ A peptic ulcer should be coded to K26.- only when specified as duodenal or postpyloric. When documentation reports an ulcer as peptic and does not specify to one of these locations, assign a code from K27.-

SP + K26.0 Acute duodenal ulcer with hemorrhage

SP + K26.1 Acute duodenal ulcer with perforation

SP + K26.2 Acute duodenal ulcer with both hemorrhage and perforation

SP + K26.3 Acute duodenal ulcer without hemorrhage or perforation

SP + K26.4 Chronic or unspecified duodenal ulcer with hemorrhage

SP + K26.5 Chronic or unspecified duodenal ulcer with perforation

SP + K26.6 Chronic or unspecified duodenal ulcer with both hemorrhage and perforation

Chapter 11

K00-K95

★ New ▲ Revised Px Primary **SP** PDGM Px **SL** Low CoM **SH** High CoM **IQ** Quest. Encounter **H** Hospice non-cancer Dx Unspecified **M** *Manifestation*

DecisionHealth's FY 2020 Complete Home Health ICD-10-CM Diagnosis Coding Manual

1073

SP **+** **K26.7**   Chronic duodenal ulcer without hemorrhage or perforation

SP **+** **K26.9**   Duodenal ulcer, unspecified as acute or chronic, without hemorrhage or perforation

+ **4** **K27**   Peptic ulcer, site unspecified

> INCLUDES   gastroduodenal ulcer NOS
> peptic ulcer NOS
> Use additional code to identify:
> alcohol abuse and dependence (F10.-)
> EXCLUDES 1   peptic ulcer of newborn (P78.82)
> CODING TIPS ✓   When documentation specifies that any gastric, duodenal or peptic ulcer is related to alcohol abuse or dependence, coders should assign an additional code to specify the abuse/dependence as specified. This is true when assigning code K25, K26 or K27.

SP **+** **K27.0**   Acute peptic ulcer, site unspecified, with hemorrhage

SP **+** **K27.1**   Acute peptic ulcer, site unspecified, with perforation

SP **+** **K27.2**   Acute peptic ulcer, site unspecified, with both hemorrhage and perforation

SP **+** **K27.3**   Acute peptic ulcer, site unspecified, without hemorrhage or perforation

SP **+** **K27.4**   Chronic or unspecified peptic ulcer, site unspecified, with hemorrhage

SP **+** **K27.5**   Chronic or unspecified peptic ulcer, site unspecified, with perforation

SP **+** **K27.6**   Chronic or unspecified peptic ulcer, site unspecified, with both hemorrhage and perforation

SP **+** **K27.7**   Chronic peptic ulcer, site unspecified, without hemorrhage or perforation

SP **+** **K27.9**   Peptic ulcer, site unspecified, unspecified as acute or chronic, without hemorrhage or perforation

+ **4** **K28**   Gastrojejunal ulcer

> INCLUDES   anastomotic ulcer (peptic) or erosion
> gastrocolic ulcer (peptic) or erosion
> gastrointestinal ulcer (peptic) or erosion
> gastrojejunal ulcer (peptic) or erosion
> jejunal ulcer (peptic) or erosion
> marginal ulcer (peptic) or erosion
> stomal ulcer (peptic) or erosion
> Use additional code to identify:
> alcohol abuse and dependence (F10.-)
> EXCLUDES 1   primary ulcer of small intestine (K63.3)

SP **+** **K28.0**   Acute gastrojejunal ulcer with hemorrhage

SP **+** **K28.1**   Acute gastrojejunal ulcer with perforation

SP **+** **K28.2**   Acute gastrojejunal ulcer with both hemorrhage and perforation

SP **+** **K28.3**   Acute gastrojejunal ulcer without hemorrhage or perforation

SP **+** **K28.4**   Chronic or unspecified gastrojejunal ulcer with hemorrhage

SP **+** **K28.5**   Chronic or unspecified gastrojejunal ulcer with perforation

SP **+** **K28.6**   Chronic or unspecified gastrojejunal ulcer with both hemorrhage and perforation

SP **+** **K28.7**   Chronic gastrojejunal ulcer without hemorrhage or perforation

SP **+** **K28.9**   Gastrojejunal ulcer, unspecified as acute or chronic, without hemorrhage or perforation

4 **K29**   Gastritis and duodenitis

> EXCLUDES 1   eosinophilic gastritis or gastroenteritis (K52.81)
> Zollinger-Ellison syndrome (E16.4)

+ **5** **K29.0**   Acute gastritis

> Use additional code to identify:
> alcohol abuse and dependence (F10.-)
> EXCLUDES 1   erosion (acute) of stomach (K25.-)

SP **+** **K29.00**   Acute gastritis without bleeding

SP **+** **K29.01**   Acute gastritis with bleeding

+ **5** **K29.2**   Alcoholic gastritis

> Use additional code to identify:
> alcohol abuse and dependence (F10.-)

SP **+** **K29.20**   Alcoholic gastritis without bleeding

SP **+** **K29.21**   Alcoholic gastritis with bleeding

5 **K29.3**   Chronic superficial gastritis

SP **K29.30**   Chronic superficial gastritis without bleeding

SP **K29.31**   Chronic superficial gastritis with bleeding

5 **K29.4**   Chronic atrophic gastritis

> Gastric atrophy

SP **K29.40**   Chronic atrophic gastritis without bleeding

SP **K29.41**   Chronic atrophic gastritis with bleeding

5 **K29.5**   Unspecified chronic gastritis

> Chronic antral gastritis
> Chronic fundal gastritis

SP **K29.50**   Unspecified chronic gastritis without bleeding

SP **K29.51**   Unspecified chronic gastritis with bleeding

5 **K29.6**   Other gastritis

> Giant hypertrophic gastritis
> Granulomatous gastritis
> Ménétrier's disease

SP **K29.60**   Other gastritis without bleeding

SP **K29.61**   Other gastritis with bleeding

5 **K29.7**   Gastritis, unspecified

SP **K29.70**   Gastritis, unspecified, without bleeding

SP **K29.71**   Gastritis, unspecified, with bleeding

5 **K29.8**   Duodenitis

SP **K29.80**   Duodenitis without bleeding

SP **K29.81**   Duodenitis with bleeding

5 **K29.9**   Gastroduodenitis, unspecified

SP **K29.90**   Gastroduodenitis, unspecified, without bleeding

---

4 4th digit required   **5** 5th digit required   **6** 6th digit required   **7** 7th digit required   **7** 7th digit placeholder   **+** Additional code   **☐** Laterality

1074   *DecisionHealth's* FY 2020 Complete Home Health ICD-10-CM Diagnosis Coding Manual

SP K29.91 Gastroduodenitis, unspecified, with bleeding

SP K30 Functional dyspepsia
Indigestion
> EXCLUDES 1 dyspepsia NOS (R10.13)
> heartburn (R12)
> nervous dyspepsia (F45.8)
> neurotic dyspepsia (F45.8)
> psychogenic dyspepsia (F45.8)

4 K31 Other diseases of stomach and duodenum
> INCLUDES functional disorders of stomach
> EXCLUDES 2 diabetic gastroparesis
> (E08.43, E09.43, E10.43,
> E11.43, E13.43)
> diverticulum of duodenum
> (K57.00-K57.13)

SP K31.0 Acute dilatation of stomach
Acute distention of stomach
> DEFINITION Distention of the stomach
> due to excessive gas build-up or bowel
> obstruction, preventing passage of food.

SP K31.1 Adult hypertrophic pyloric stenosis
Pyloric stenosis NOS
> EXCLUDES 1 congenital or infantile
> pyloric stenosis (Q40.0)

SP K31.2 Hourglass stricture and stenosis of stomach
> EXCLUDES 1 congenital hourglass
> stomach (Q40.2)
> hourglass contraction of
> stomach (K31.89)

SP K31.3 Pylorospasm, not elsewhere classified
> EXCLUDES 1 congenital or infantile
> pylorospasm (Q40.0)
> neurotic pylorospasm
> (F45.8)
> psychogenic pylorospasm
> (F45.8)

SP K31.4 Gastric diverticulum
> EXCLUDES 1 congenital diverticulum of
> stomach (Q40.2)

SP K31.5 Obstruction of duodenum
Constriction of duodenum
Duodenal ileus (chronic)
Stenosis of duodenum
Stricture of duodenum
Volvulus of duodenum
> EXCLUDES 1 congenital stenosis of
> duodenum (Q41.0)

SP K31.6 Fistula of stomach and duodenum
Gastrocolic fistula
Gastrojejunocolic fistula

SP K31.7 Polyp of stomach and duodenum
> EXCLUDES 1 adenomatous polyp of
> stomach (D13.1)

5 K31.8 Other specified diseases of stomach and duodenum

6 K31.81 Angiodysplasia of stomach and duodenum

SP K31.811 Angiodysplasia of stomach and duodenum with bleeding

SP K31.819 Angiodysplasia of stomach and duodenum without bleeding
Angiodysplasia of stomach and
duodenum NOS

SP K31.82 Dieulafoy lesion (hemorrhagic) of stomach and duodenum

> EXCLUDES 2 Dieulafoy lesion of
> intestine (K63.81)
> DEFINITION Abnormality of arteriole
> within the digestive tract protruding
> through a tiny mucosal defect, usually
> near the gastroesophageal junction, that
> can cause massive gastrointestinal
> bleeding.

SP K31.83 Achlorhydria
> DEFINITION Absence of hydrochloric
> acid in the stomach's gastric secretions,
> most often from antibodies against cells
> producing gastric acid, or a symptom of
> H. pylori infection, atrophic gastritis, or
> cancer.

SP K31.84 Gastroparesis
Gastroparalysis
Code first underlying disease, if
known, such as:
anorexia nervosa (F50.0-)
diabetes mellitus
(E08.43, E09.43, E10.43, E11.43,
E13.43)
scleroderma (M34.-)

SP K31.89 Other diseases of stomach and duodenum

IQ K31.9 Disease of stomach and duodenum, unspecified

Diseases of appendix (K35-K38)

4 K35 Acute appendicitis
> CODING TIPS ✓ With acute appendicitis, the
> single most important distinction is between
> perforation (bacterial contamination of the
> peritoneal space) and no perforation (no
> bacterial contamination), rather than the
> presence or absence of sterile inflammation of
> the peritoneum. The term peritonitis is used by
> different surgeons to mean different things.

> CODING TIPS ✓ When a patient has had an
> appendectomy, usually the condition
> (appendicitis) is resolved. An appendix that is
> ruptured, however, may have caused
> peritonitis that may not be resolved. Acute
> appendicitis progresses from inflammation of
> the appendix, then gangrene, followed by
> perforation. Perforation results in
> contamination of the peritoneal space with
> enteric bacteria, which can result in abscess
> formation or generalized bacterial
> contamination of the peritoneal space
> (generalized peritonitis). Perforation, the
> presence of an abscess, and the presence of
> generalized peritonitis are key characteristics
> of appendicitis that physicians use to describe
> the severity of the disease and determine the
> most appropriate treatment, such as deciding
> whether or not to perform an appendectomy or
> drain abscesses (sometimes percutaneously)
> and determining the duration of antibiotic
> treatment.

5 K35.2 Acute appendicitis with generalized peritonitis
Appendicitis (acute) with generalized
(diffuse) peritonitis following rupture or
perforation of appendix

Chapter 11

K00-K95

★ New ▲ Revised Px Primary SP PDGM Px SL Low CoM SH High CoM IQ Quest. Encounter H Hospice non-cancer Dx   Unspecified   M Manifestation

DecisionHealth's FY 2020 Complete Home Health ICD-10-CM Diagnosis Coding Manual

1075

SP K35.20 Acute appendicitis with generalized peritonitis, without abscess
(Acute) appendicitis with generalized peritonitis NOS

SP K35.21 Acute appendicitis with generalized peritonitis, with abscess

5 K35.3 Acute appendicitis with localized peritonitis

SP K35.30 Acute appendicitis with localized peritonitis, without perforation or gangrene
Acute appendicitis with localized peritonitis NOS

SP K35.31 Acute appendicitis with localized peritonitis and gangrene, without perforation

SP K35.32 Acute appendicitis with perforation and localized peritonitis, without abscess
(Acute) appendicitis with perforation NOS
Perforated appendix NOS
Ruptured appendix (with localized peritonitis) NOS

SP K35.33 Acute appendicitis with perforation and localized peritonitis, with abscess
(Acute) appendicitis with (peritoneal) abscess NOS
Ruptured appendix with localized peritonitis and abscess

5 K35.8 Other and unspecified acute appendicitis

SP K35.80 Unspecified acute appendicitis
Acute appendicitis NOS
Acute appendicitis without (localized) (generalized) peritonitis

6 K35.89 Other acute appendicitis

SP K35.890 Other acute appendicitis without perforation or gangrene

SP K35.891 Other acute appendicitis without perforation, with gangrene
(Acute) appendicitis with gangrene NOS

SP K36 Other appendicitis
Chronic appendicitis
Recurrent appendicitis

SP K37 Unspecified appendicitis
EXCLUDES 1 -unspecified appendicitis with peritonitis (K35.2-, K35.3-)

4 K38 Other diseases of appendix

SP K38.0 Hyperplasia of appendix

SP K38.1 Appendicular concretions
Fecalith of appendix
Stercolith of appendix

SP K38.2 Diverticulum of appendix

SP K38.3 Fistula of appendix

SP K38.8 Other specified diseases of appendix
Intussusception of appendix

!Q K38.9 Disease of appendix, unspecified

Hernia (K40-K46)

Note:
Hernia with both gangrene and obstruction is classified to hernia with gangrene.
INCLUDES acquired hernia

congenital [except diaphragmatic or hiatus] hernia
recurrent hernia

CODING TIPS ✓ **Documentation:** Carefully review all documentation when assigning codes for a hernia. It is important to note the various anatomical positions of each type of hernia, as well as the differences between obstructed and non-obstructed hernias. When a hernia is obstructed, gangrene may occur due to the lack of blood flow related to the obstruction. If the hernia has been repaired, assign the appropriate Z code for aftercare.

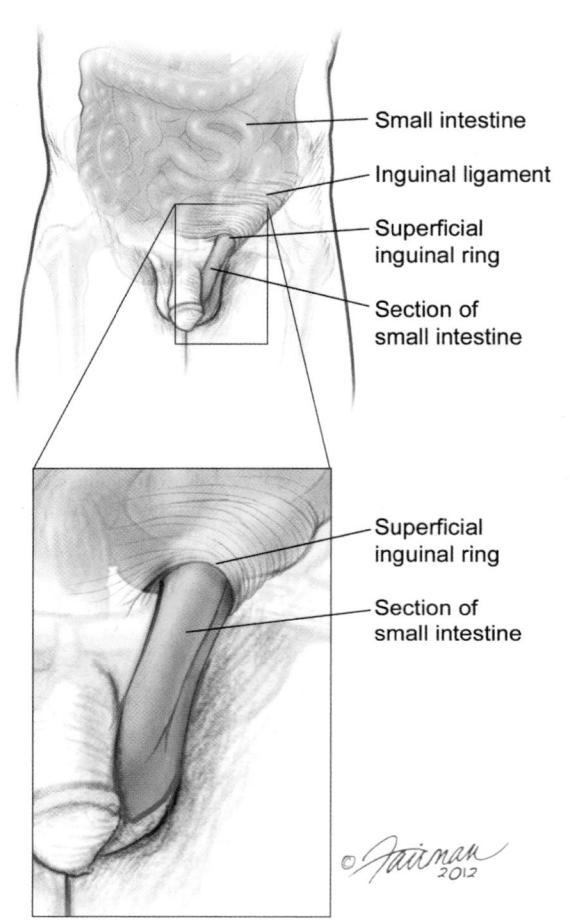

Small intestine
Inguinal ligament
Superficial inguinal ring
Section of small intestine

Superficial inguinal ring
Section of small intestine

4 K40 Inguinal hernia
INCLUDES bubonocele
direct inguinal hernia
double inguinal hernia
indirect inguinal hernia
inguinal hernia NOS
oblique inguinal hernia
scrotal hernia
DEFINITION Weakness in the muscles in the groin area between the abdomen and thigh, allowing part of the intestine to bulge through the muscle wall.

5 K40.0 Bilateral inguinal hernia, with obstruction, without gangrene
Inguinal hernia (bilateral) causing obstruction without gangrene

4 4th digit required   5 5th digit required   6 6th digit required   7 7th digit required   7 7th digit placeholder   ✚ Additional code   ⊟ Laterality

1076   *DecisionHealth's* FY 2020 Complete Home Health ICD-10-CM Diagnosis Coding Manual

Incarcerated inguinal hernia (bilateral)
without gangrene

Irreducible inguinal hernia (bilateral)
without gangrene

Strangulated inguinal hernia (bilateral)
without gangrene

SP **K40.00** **Bilateral inguinal hernia, with obstruction, without gangrene, not specified as recurrent**
Bilateral inguinal hernia, with obstruction, without gangrene NOS

SP **K40.01** **Bilateral inguinal hernia, with obstruction, without gangrene, recurrent**

5 **K40.1** **Bilateral inguinal hernia, with gangrene**

SP **K40.10** **Bilateral inguinal hernia, with gangrene, not specified as recurrent**
Bilateral inguinal hernia, with gangrene NOS

SP **K40.11** **Bilateral inguinal hernia, with gangrene, recurrent**

5 **K40.2** **Bilateral inguinal hernia, without obstruction or gangrene**

SP **K40.20** **Bilateral inguinal hernia, without obstruction or gangrene, not specified as recurrent**
Bilateral inguinal hernia NOS

SP **K40.21** **Bilateral inguinal hernia, without obstruction or gangrene, recurrent**

5 **K40.3** **Unilateral inguinal hernia, with obstruction, without gangrene**
Inguinal hernia (unilateral) causing obstruction without gangrene
Incarcerated inguinal hernia (unilateral) without gangrene
Irreducible inguinal hernia (unilateral) without gangrene
Strangulated inguinal hernia (unilateral) without gangrene

SP **K40.30** **Unilateral inguinal hernia, with obstruction, without gangrene, not specified as recurrent**
Inguinal hernia, with obstruction NOS
Unilateral inguinal hernia, with obstruction, without gangrene NOS

SP **K40.31** **Unilateral inguinal hernia, with obstruction, without gangrene, recurrent**

5 **K40.4** **Unilateral inguinal hernia, with gangrene**

SP **K40.40** **Unilateral inguinal hernia, with gangrene, not specified as recurrent**
Inguinal hernia with gangrene NOS
Unilateral inguinal hernia with gangrene NOS

SP **K40.41** **Unilateral inguinal hernia, with gangrene, recurrent**

5 **K40.9** **Unilateral inguinal hernia, without obstruction or gangrene**

SP **K40.90** **Unilateral inguinal hernia, without obstruction or gangrene, not specified as recurrent**
Inguinal hernia NOS
Unilateral inguinal hernia NOS

SP **K40.91** **Unilateral inguinal hernia, without obstruction or gangrene, recurrent**

4 **K41** **Femoral hernia**

5 **K41.0** **Bilateral femoral hernia, with obstruction, without gangrene**
Femoral hernia (bilateral) causing obstruction, without gangrene
Incarcerated femoral hernia (bilateral), without gangrene
Irreducible femoral hernia (bilateral), without gangrene
Strangulated femoral hernia (bilateral), without gangrene

SP **K41.00** **Bilateral femoral hernia, with obstruction, without gangrene, not specified as recurrent**
Bilateral femoral hernia, with obstruction, without gangrene NOS

SP **K41.01** **Bilateral femoral hernia, with obstruction, without gangrene, recurrent**

5 **K41.1** **Bilateral femoral hernia, with gangrene**

SP **K41.10** **Bilateral femoral hernia, with gangrene, not specified as recurrent**
Bilateral femoral hernia, with gangrene NOS

SP **K41.11** **Bilateral femoral hernia, with gangrene, recurrent**

5 **K41.2** **Bilateral femoral hernia, without obstruction or gangrene**

SP **K41.20** **Bilateral femoral hernia, without obstruction or gangrene, not specified as recurrent**
Bilateral femoral hernia NOS

SP **K41.21** **Bilateral femoral hernia, without obstruction or gangrene, recurrent**

5 **K41.3** **Unilateral femoral hernia, with obstruction, without gangrene**
Femoral hernia (unilateral) causing obstruction, without gangrene
Incarcerated femoral hernia (unilateral), without gangrene
Irreducible femoral hernia (unilateral), without gangrene
Strangulated femoral hernia (unilateral), without gangrene

SP **K41.30** **Unilateral femoral hernia, with obstruction, without gangrene, not specified as recurrent**
Femoral hernia, with obstruction NOS
Unilateral femoral hernia, with obstruction NOS

SP **K41.31** **Unilateral femoral hernia, with obstruction, without gangrene, recurrent**

5 **K41.4** **Unilateral femoral hernia, with gangrene**

SP **K41.40** **Unilateral femoral hernia, with gangrene, not specified as recurrent**
Femoral hernia, with gangrene NOS
Unilateral femoral hernia, with gangrene NOS

SP **K41.41** **Unilateral femoral hernia, with gangrene, recurrent**

5 **K41.9** **Unilateral femoral hernia, without obstruction or gangrene**

SP **K41.90** **Unilateral femoral hernia, without obstruction or gangrene, not specified as recurrent**
Femoral hernia NOS
Unilateral femoral hernia NOS

★ New ▲ Revised Px Primary **SP** PDGM Px **SL** Low CoM **SH** High CoM **IQ** Quest. Encounter **H** Hospice non-cancer Dx Unspecified **M** *Manifestation*

DecisionHealth's FY 2020 Complete Home Health ICD-10-CM Diagnosis Coding Manual

1077

SP K41.91 Unilateral femoral hernia, without obstruction or gangrene, recurrent

4 K42 Umbilical hernia
> INCLUDES   paraumbilical hernia
> EXCLUDES 1   omphalocele (Q79.2)

SP K42.0 Umbilical hernia with obstruction, without gangrene
Umbilical hernia causing obstruction, without gangrene
Incarcerated umbilical hernia, without gangrene
Irreducible umbilical hernia, without gangrene
Strangulated umbilical hernia, without gangrene

SP K42.1 Umbilical hernia with gangrene
Gangrenous umbilical hernia

SP K42.9 Umbilical hernia without obstruction or gangrene
Umbilical hernia NOS

4 K43 Ventral hernia

SP K43.0 Incisional hernia with obstruction, without gangrene
Incisional hernia causing obstruction, without gangrene
Incarcerated incisional hernia, without gangrene
Irreducible incisional hernia, without gangrene
Strangulated incisional hernia, without gangrene

SP K43.1 Incisional hernia with gangrene
Gangrenous incisional hernia

SP K43.2 Incisional hernia without obstruction or gangrene
Incisional hernia NOS

SP K43.3 Parastomal hernia with obstruction, without gangrene
Incarcerated parastomal hernia, without gangrene
Irreducible parastomal hernia, without gangrene
Parastomal hernia causing obstruction, without gangrene
Strangulated parastomal hernia, without gangrene

SP K43.4 Parastomal hernia with gangrene
Gangrenous parastomal hernia

SP K43.5 Parastomal hernia without obstruction or gangrene
Parastomal hernia NOS

SP K43.6 Other and unspecified ventral hernia with obstruction, without gangrene
Epigastric hernia causing obstruction, without gangrene
Hypogastric hernia causing obstruction, without gangrene
Incarcerated epigastric hernia without gangrene
Incarcerated hypogastric hernia without gangrene
Incarcerated midline hernia without gangrene
Incarcerated spigelian hernia without gangrene
Incarcerated subxiphoid hernia without gangrene
Irreducible epigastric hernia without gangrene
Irreducible hypogastric hernia without gangrene
Irreducible midline hernia without gangrene
Irreducible spigelian hernia without gangrene
Irreducible subxiphoid hernia without gangrene
Midline hernia causing obstruction, without gangrene
Spigelian hernia causing obstruction, without gangrene
Strangulated epigastric hernia without gangrene
Strangulated hypogastric hernia without gangrene
Strangulated midline hernia without gangrene
Strangulated spigelian hernia without gangrene
Strangulated subxiphoid hernia without gangrene
Subxiphoid hernia causing obstruction, without gangrene

SP K43.7 Other and unspecified ventral hernia with gangrene
Any condition listed under K43.6 specified as gangrenous

SP K43.9 Ventral hernia without obstruction or gangrene
Epigastric hernia
Ventral hernia NOS

4 K44 Diaphragmatic hernia
> INCLUDES   hiatus hernia (esophageal) (sliding)
> paraesophageal hernia
> EXCLUDES 1   congenital diaphragmatic hernia (Q79.0)
> congenital hiatus hernia (Q40.1)

SP K44.0 Diaphragmatic hernia with obstruction, without gangrene
Diaphragmatic hernia causing obstruction
Incarcerated diaphragmatic hernia
Irreducible diaphragmatic hernia
Strangulated diaphragmatic hernia

SP K44.1 Diaphragmatic hernia with gangrene
Gangrenous diaphragmatic hernia

SP K44.9 Diaphragmatic hernia without obstruction or gangrene
Diaphragmatic hernia NOS

4 K45 Other abdominal hernia
> INCLUDES   abdominal hernia, specified site NEC
> lumbar hernia
> obturator hernia
> pudendal hernia
> retroperitoneal hernia
> sciatic hernia

SP K45.0 Other specified abdominal hernia with obstruction, without gangrene
Other specified abdominal hernia causing obstruction
Other specified incarcerated abdominal hernia
Other specified irreducible abdominal hernia

4 4th digit required   5 5th digit required   6 6th digit required   7 7th digit required   ☑ 7th digit placeholder   + Additional code   ⊟ Laterality

1078   *DecisionHealth's* FY 2020 Complete Home Health ICD-10-CM Diagnosis Coding Manual

Chapter 11

K00-K95

Other specified strangulated abdominal hernia

SP K45.1 **Other specified abdominal hernia with gangrene**
Any condition listed under K45 specified as gangrenous

SP K45.8 **Other specified abdominal hernia without obstruction or gangrene**

4 K46 **Unspecified abdominal hernia**

> **INCLUDES** enterocele
> epiplocele
> hernia NOS
> interstitial hernia
> intestinal hernia
> intra-abdominal hernia
> **EXCLUDES 1** vaginal enterocele (N81.5)

SP K46.0 **Unspecified abdominal hernia with obstruction, without gangrene**
Unspecified abdominal hernia causing obstruction
Unspecified incarcerated abdominal hernia
Unspecified irreducible abdominal hernia
Unspecified strangulated abdominal hernia

IQ K46.1 **Unspecified abdominal hernia with gangrene**
Any condition listed under K46 specified as gangrenous

IQ K46.9 **Unspecified abdominal hernia without obstruction or gangrene**
Abdominal hernia NOS

Noninfective enteritis and colitis (K50-K52)

> **INCLUDES** noninfective inflammatory bowel disease
> **EXCLUDES 1** irritable bowel syndrome (K58.-)
> megacolon (K59.3-)

CODING TIPS ✓ Do not assign a code from K50-K52 when enteritis/colitis is specified as infectious. Infectious colitis requires assignment of a code from Chapter 1, Certain Infectious and Parasitic Diseases.

+ 4 K50 **Crohn's disease [regional enteritis]**
> **INCLUDES** granulomatous enteritis
> Use additional code to identify manifestations, such as:
> pyoderma gangrenosum (L88)
> **EXCLUDES 1** ulcerative colitis (K51.-)

+ 5 K50.0 **Crohn's disease of small intestine**
Crohn's disease [regional enteritis] of duodenum
Crohn's disease [regional enteritis] of ileum
Crohn's disease [regional enteritis] of jejunum
Regional ileitis
Terminal ileitis
> **EXCLUDES 1** Crohn's disease of both small and large intestine (K50.8-)

SP + K50.00 **Crohn's disease of small intestine without complications**

+ 6 K50.01 **Crohn's disease of small intestine with complications**

SP + K50.011 **Crohn's disease of small intestine with rectal bleeding**

SP + K50.012 **Crohn's disease of small intestine with intestinal obstruction**

SP + K50.013 **Crohn's disease of small intestine with fistula**

SP + K50.014 **Crohn's disease of small intestine with abscess**

SP + K50.018 **Crohn's disease of small intestine with other complication**

IQ + K50.019 **Crohn's disease of small intestine with unspecified complications**

+ 5 K50.1 **Crohn's disease of large intestine**
Crohn's disease [regional enteritis] of colon
Crohn's disease [regional enteritis] of large bowel
Crohn's disease [regional enteritis] of rectum
Granulomatous colitis
Regional colitis
> **EXCLUDES 1** Crohn's disease of both small and large intestine (K50.8)

SP + K50.10 **Crohn's disease of large intestine without complications**

+ 6 K50.11 **Crohn's disease of large intestine with complications**

SP + K50.111 **Crohn's disease of large intestine with rectal bleeding**

SP + K50.112 **Crohn's disease of large intestine with intestinal obstruction**

SP + K50.113 **Crohn's disease of large intestine with fistula**

SP + K50.114 **Crohn's disease of large intestine with abscess**

SP + K50.118 **Crohn's disease of large intestine with other complication**

IQ + K50.119 **Crohn's disease of large intestine with unspecified complications**

+ 5 K50.8 **Crohn's disease of both small and large intestine**

SP + K50.80 **Crohn's disease of both small and large intestine without complications**

+ 6 K50.81 **Crohn's disease of both small and large intestine with complications**

SP + K50.811 **Crohn's disease of both small and large intestine with rectal bleeding**

SP + K50.812 **Crohn's disease of both small and large intestine with intestinal obstruction**

SP + K50.813 **Crohn's disease of both small and large intestine with fistula**

SP + K50.814 **Crohn's disease of both small and large intestine with abscess**

SP + K50.818 **Crohn's disease of both small and large intestine with other complication**

IQ + K50.819 **Crohn's disease of both small and large intestine with unspecified complications**

+ 5 K50.9 **Crohn's disease, unspecified**

SP + K50.90 **Crohn's disease, unspecified, without complications**
Crohn's disease NOS
Regional enteritis NOS

+ 6 K50.91 **Crohn's disease, unspecified, with complications**

SP + K50.911 **Crohn's disease, unspecified, with rectal bleeding**

SP + K50.912 **Crohn's disease, unspecified, with intestinal obstruction**

★ New ▲ Revised Px Primary SP PDGM Px SL Low CoM SH High CoM IQ Quest. Encounter H Hospice non-cancer Dx Unspecified M *Manifestation*

DecisionHealth's FY 2020 Complete Home Health ICD-10-CM Diagnosis Coding Manual

1079

SP + **K50.913** **Crohn's disease, unspecified, with fistula**

SP + **K50.914** **Crohn's disease, unspecified, with abscess**

SP + **K50.918** **Crohn's disease, unspecified, with other complication**

IQ + **K50.919** **Crohn's disease, unspecified, with unspecified complications**

+ 4 K51 **Ulcerative colitis**
Use additional code to identify manifestations, such as:
pyoderma gangrenosum (L88)
EXCLUDES 1 Crohn's disease [regional enteritis] (K50.-)

+ 5 K51.0 **Ulcerative (chronic) pancolitis**
Backwash ileitis

SP + **K51.00** **Ulcerative (chronic) pancolitis without complications**
Ulcerative (chronic) pancolitis NOS

+ 6 K51.01 **Ulcerative (chronic) pancolitis with complications**

SP + **K51.011** **Ulcerative (chronic) pancolitis with rectal bleeding**

SP + **K51.012** **Ulcerative (chronic) pancolitis with intestinal obstruction**

SP + **K51.013** **Ulcerative (chronic) pancolitis with fistula**

SP + **K51.014** **Ulcerative (chronic) pancolitis with abscess**

SP + **K51.018** **Ulcerative (chronic) pancolitis with other complication**

IQ + **K51.019** **Ulcerative (chronic) pancolitis with unspecified complications**

+ 5 K51.2 **Ulcerative (chronic) proctitis**

SP + **K51.20** **Ulcerative (chronic) proctitis without complications**
Ulcerative (chronic) proctitis NOS

+ 6 K51.21 **Ulcerative (chronic) proctitis with complications**

SP + **K51.211** **Ulcerative (chronic) proctitis with rectal bleeding**

SP + **K51.212** **Ulcerative (chronic) proctitis with intestinal obstruction**

SP + **K51.213** **Ulcerative (chronic) proctitis with fistula**

SP + **K51.214** **Ulcerative (chronic) proctitis with abscess**

SP + **K51.218** **Ulcerative (chronic) proctitis with other complication**

IQ + **K51.219** **Ulcerative (chronic) proctitis with unspecified complications**

+ 5 K51.3 **Ulcerative (chronic) rectosigmoiditis**

SP + **K51.30** **Ulcerative (chronic) rectosigmoiditis without complications**
Ulcerative (chronic) rectosigmoiditis NOS

+ 6 K51.31 **Ulcerative (chronic) rectosigmoiditis with complications**

SP + **K51.311** **Ulcerative (chronic) rectosigmoiditis with rectal bleeding**

SP + **K51.312** **Ulcerative (chronic) rectosigmoiditis with intestinal obstruction**

SP + **K51.313** **Ulcerative (chronic) rectosigmoiditis with fistula**

SP + **K51.314** **Ulcerative (chronic) rectosigmoiditis with abscess**

SP + **K51.318** **Ulcerative (chronic) rectosigmoiditis with other complication**

IQ + **K51.319** **Ulcerative (chronic) rectosigmoiditis with unspecified complications**

+ 5 K51.4 **Inflammatory polyps of colon**
EXCLUDES 1 adenomatous polyp of colon (D12.6)
polyposis of colon (D12.6)
polyps of colon NOS (K63.5)

SP + **K51.40** **Inflammatory polyps of colon without complications**
Inflammatory polyps of colon NOS

+ 6 K51.41 **Inflammatory polyps of colon with complications**

SP + **K51.411** **Inflammatory polyps of colon with rectal bleeding**

SP + **K51.412** **Inflammatory polyps of colon with intestinal obstruction**

SP + **K51.413** **Inflammatory polyps of colon with fistula**

SP + **K51.414** **Inflammatory polyps of colon with abscess**

SP + **K51.418** **Inflammatory polyps of colon with other complication**

IQ + **K51.419** **Inflammatory polyps of colon with unspecified complications**

+ 5 K51.5 **Left sided colitis**
Left hemicolitis

SP + **K51.50** **Left sided colitis without complications**
Left sided colitis NOS

+ 6 K51.51 **Left sided colitis with complications**

SP + **K51.511** **Left sided colitis with rectal bleeding**

SP + **K51.512** **Left sided colitis with intestinal obstruction**

SP + **K51.513** **Left sided colitis with fistula**

SP + **K51.514** **Left sided colitis with abscess**

SP + **K51.518** **Left sided colitis with other complication**

IQ + **K51.519** **Left sided colitis with unspecified complications**

+ 5 K51.8 **Other ulcerative colitis**

SP + **K51.80** **Other ulcerative colitis without complications**
DEFINITION Inflammation of the intestinal lining with ulcer formation, causing diarrhea as the colon empties frequently.

+ 6 K51.81 **Other ulcerative colitis with complications**

SP + **K51.811** **Other ulcerative colitis with rectal bleeding**

SP + **K51.812** **Other ulcerative colitis with intestinal obstruction**

SP + **K51.813** **Other ulcerative colitis with fistula**

SP + **K51.814** **Other ulcerative colitis with abscess**

SP + **K51.818** **Other ulcerative colitis with other complication**

---

4 4th digit required   **5** 5th digit required   **6** 6th digit required   **7** 7th digit required   **7** 7th digit placeholder   **+** Additional code   **⊟** Laterality

🔲➕ K51.819 Other ulcerative colitis with unspecified complications

➕ ⑤ K51.9 Ulcerative colitis, unspecified

SP ➕ K51.90 Ulcerative colitis, unspecified, without complications

➕ ⑥ K51.91 Ulcerative colitis, unspecified, with complications

SP ➕ K51.911 Ulcerative colitis, unspecified with rectal bleeding

SP ➕ K51.912 Ulcerative colitis, unspecified with intestinal obstruction

SP ➕ K51.913 Ulcerative colitis, unspecified with fistula

SP ➕ K51.914 Ulcerative colitis, unspecified with abscess

SP ➕ K51.918 Ulcerative colitis, unspecified with other complication

🔲➕ K51.919 Ulcerative colitis, unspecified with unspecified complications

④ K52 Other and unspecified noninfective gastroenteritis and colitis

SP K52.0 Gastroenteritis and colitis due to radiation

SP ➕ K52.1 Toxic gastroenteritis and colitis
Drug-induced gastroenteritis and colitis
Code first:
(T51-T65) to identify toxic agent
Use additional code for adverse effect, if applicable, to identify drug (T36-T50 with fifth or sixth character 5)

➕ ⑤ K52.2 Allergic and dietetic gastroenteritis and colitis
Food hypersensitivity gastroenteritis or colitis
Use additional code to identify type of food allergy (Z91.01-, Z91.02-)
> **EXCLUDES 2** allergic eosinophilic colitis (K52.82)
> allergic eosinophilic esophagitis (K20.0)
> allergic eosinophilic gastritis (K52.81)
> allergic eosinophilic gastroenteritis (K52.81)
> food protein-induced proctocolitis (K52.82)

SP ➕ K52.21 Food protein-induced enterocolitis syndrome
FPIES
Use additional code for hypovolemic shock, if present (R57.1)
> **DEFINITION** A nontypical, non-IgE, food allergy affecting infants and young children with serious gastrointestinal effects that result in profound vomiting, severe diarrhea involving both the large and small intestine, and dehydration as well as severe lethargy and dangerous changes in body temperature and blood pressure. Symptoms may not be immediate or show up on standard allergy tests, but will appear after ingesting a food trigger.

SP ➕ K52.22 Food protein-induced enteropathy

> **DEFINITION** A type of food protein intolerance with gastrointestinal manifestations, typically occurring in the pediatric population in the first 6 months of life and most often as intolerance to cow's milk or soy milk protein.

SP ➕ K52.29 Other allergic and dietetic gastroenteritis and colitis
Food hypersensitivity gastroenteritis or colitis
Immediate gastrointestinal hypersensitivity

SP K52.3 Indeterminate colitis
Colonic inflammatory bowel disease unclassified (IBDU)
> **EXCLUDES 1** unspecified colitis (K52.9)

⑤ K52.8 Other specified noninfective gastroenteritis and colitis

SP K52.81 Eosinophilic gastritis or gastroenteritis
Eosinophilic enteritis
> **EXCLUDES 2** eosinophilic esophagitis (K20.0)

SP K52.82 Eosinophilic colitis
Allergic proctocolitis
Food-induced eosinophilic proctocolitis
Food protein-induced proctocolitis
Milk protein-induced proctocolitis

⑥ K52.83 Microscopic colitis

SP K52.831 Collagenous colitis

SP K52.832 Lymphocytic colitis

SP K52.838 Other microscopic colitis

SP K52.839 Microscopic colitis, unspecified

SP K52.89 Other specified noninfective gastroenteritis and colitis

SP K52.9 Noninfective gastroenteritis and colitis, unspecified

Colitis NOS
Enteritis NOS
Gastroenteritis NOS
Ileitis NOS
Jejunitis NOS
Sigmoiditis NOS
> **EXCLUDES 1** diarrhea NOS (R19.7)
> functional diarrhea (K59.1)
> infectious gastroenteritis and colitis NOS (A09)
> neonatal diarrhea (noninfective) (P78.3)
> psychogenic diarrhea (F45.8)

Other diseases of intestines (K55-K64)

④ K55 Vascular disorders of intestine
> **EXCLUDES 1** necrotizing enterocolitis of newborn (P77.-)

⑤ K55.0 Acute vascular disorders of intestine
Infarction of appendices epiploicae
Mesenteric (artery) (vein) embolism
Mesenteric (artery) (vein) infarction
Mesenteric (artery) (vein) thrombosis

⑥ K55.01 Acute (reversible) ischemia of small intestine

★ New ▲ Revised Px Primary SP PDGM Px SL Low CoM SH High CoM 🔲 Quest. Encounter 🗓 Hospice non-cancer Dx Unspecified M *Manifestation*

DecisionHealth's FY 2020 Complete Home Health ICD-10-CM Diagnosis Coding Manual

1081

SP K55.011 Focal (segmental) acute (reversible) ischemia of small intestine

SP K55.012 Diffuse acute (reversible) ischemia of small intestine

SP K55.019 Acute (reversible) ischemia of small intestine, extent unspecified

6 K55.02 Acute infarction of small intestine
Gangrene of small intestine
Necrosis of small intestine

SP K55.021 Focal (segmental) acute infarction of small intestine

SP K55.022 Diffuse acute infarction of small intestine

SP K55.029 Acute infarction of small intestine, extent unspecified

6 K55.03 Acute (reversible) ischemia of large intestine
Acute fulminant ischemic colitis
Subacute ischemic colitis

SP K55.031 Focal (segmental) acute (reversible) ischemia of large intestine

SP K55.032 Diffuse acute (reversible) ischemia of large intestine

SP K55.039 Acute (reversible) ischemia of large intestine, extent unspecified

6 K55.04 Acute infarction of large intestine
Gangrene of large intestine
Necrosis of large intestine

SP K55.041 Focal (segmental) acute infarction of large intestine

SP K55.042 Diffuse acute infarction of large intestine

SP K55.049 Acute infarction of large intestine, extent unspecified

6 K55.05 Acute (reversible) ischemia of intestine, part unspecified

SP K55.051 Focal (segmental) acute (reversible) ischemia of intestine, part unspecified

SP K55.052 Diffuse acute (reversible) ischemia of intestine, part unspecified

SP K55.059 Acute (reversible) ischemia of intestine, part and extent unspecified

6 K55.06 Acute infarction of intestine, part unspecified
Acute intestinal infarction
Gangrene of intestine
Necrosis of intestine

SP K55.061 Focal (segmental) acute infarction of intestine, part unspecified

SP K55.062 Diffuse acute infarction of intestine, part unspecified

SP K55.069 Acute infarction of intestine, part and extent unspecified

SP K55.1 Chronic vascular disorders of intestine
Chronic ischemic colitis
Chronic ischemic enteritis
Chronic ischemic enterocolitis
Ischemic stricture of intestine
Mesenteric atherosclerosis
Mesenteric vascular insufficiency

5 K55.2 Angiodysplasia of colon

SP K55.20 Angiodysplasia of colon without hemorrhage

SP K55.21 Angiodysplasia of colon with hemorrhage

> **DEFINITION** Dilated intestinal blood vessels with corresponding thinning and weakening of vessel walls and bleeding into the intestinal tract.

5 K55.3 Necrotizing enterocolitis

> **EXCLUDES 1** necrotizing enterocolitis of newborn (P77.-)
> **EXCLUDES 2** necrotizing enterocolitis due to Clostridium difficile (A04.7-)

> **CODING TIPS ✓** Necrotizing enterocolitis is characterized by damage to the intestine which can be related to inflammation, infection, or ischemia. This leads to necrosis, which may involve just the intestinal lining, or the full thickness, and can cause perforation, and death. Due to its potential severity, necrotizing enterocolitis is considered a medical emergency.

SP K55.30 Necrotizing enterocolitis, unspecified
Necrotizing enterocolitis, NOS

SP K55.31 Stage 1 necrotizing enterocolitis
Necrotizing enterocolitis without pneumatosis, without perforation

SP K55.32 Stage 2 necrotizing enterocolitis
Necrotizing enterocolitis with pneumatosis, without perforation

SP K55.33 Stage 3 necrotizing enterocolitis
Necrotizing enterocolitis with perforation
Necrotizing enterocolitis with pneumatosis and perforation

SP K55.8 Other vascular disorders of intestine

SP K55.9 Vascular disorder of intestine, unspecified
Ischemic colitis
Ischemic enteritis
Ischemic enterocolitis

4 K56 Paralytic ileus and intestinal obstruction without hernia

> **EXCLUDES 1** congenital stricture or stenosis of intestine (Q41-Q42)
> cystic fibrosis with meconium ileus (E84.11)
> ischemic stricture of intestine (K55.1)
> meconium ileus NOS (P76.0)
> neonatal intestinal obstructions classifiable to P76.-
> obstruction of duodenum (K31.5)
> postprocedural intestinal obstruction (K91.3-)
> stenosis of anus or rectum (K62.4)

SP K56.0 Paralytic ileus
Paralysis of bowel
Paralysis of colon
Paralysis of intestine

> **EXCLUDES 1** gallstone ileus (K56.3)
> ileus NOS (K56.7)

---

4 4th digit required   5 5th digit required   6 6th digit required   7 7th digit required   7 7th digit placeholder   + Additional code   = Laterality

1082   *DecisionHealth's* FY 2020 Complete Home Health ICD-10-CM Diagnosis Coding Manual

obstructive ileus NOS
(K56.69-)

DEFINITION Blockage in the small or large intestine due to nonfunctioning muscle wall; may occur due to fluid imbalance, nerve damage, decreased blood supply, or toxins.

SP K56.1 Intussusception
Intussusception or invagination of bowel
Intussusception or invagination of colon
Intussusception or invagination of intestine
Intussusception or invagination of rectum
EXCLUDES 2 intussusception of appendix (K38.8)

SP K56.2 Volvulus
Strangulation of colon or intestine
Torsion of colon or intestine
Twist of colon or intestine
EXCLUDES 2 volvulus of duodenum (K31.5)

DEFINITION Twisting of the intestine, constricting the passageway and cutting off blood supply to the area; presents with sudden, severe abdominal pain, vomiting, and abdominal distention.

SP K56.3 Gallstone ileus
Obstruction of intestine by gallstone

5 K56.4 Other impaction of intestine

SP K56.41 Fecal impaction
EXCLUDES 1 constipation (K59.0-)
incomplete defecation (R15.0)

SP K56.49 Other impaction of intestine

5 K56.5 Intestinal adhesions [bands] with obstruction (postinfection)
Abdominal hernia due to adhesions with obstruction
Peritoneal adhesions [bands] with intestinal obstruction (postinfection)

CODING TIPS ✓ Intestinal obstruction varies in severity, from partial or intermittent obstruction that resolves without intervention to complete obstruction that requires an operation and may lead to intestinal gangrene and perforation. Physicians frequently describe intestinal obstruction as partial versus complete. These distinctions are relevant because complete obstruction generally requires an operation and partial obstruction usually does not (especially for the small intestine). These descriptors may differentiate between an aftercare code and a condition that may not yet be resolved.

SP K56.50 Intestinal adhesions [bands], unspecified as to partial versus complete obstruction
Intestinal adhesions with obstruction NOS

SP K56.51 Intestinal adhesions [bands], with partial obstruction
Intestinal adhesions with incomplete obstruction

SP K56.52 Intestinal adhesions [bands] with complete obstruction

5 K56.6 Other and unspecified intestinal obstruction

CODING TIPS ✓ Intestinal obstruction varies in severity, from partial or intermittent obstruction that resolves without intervention to complete obstruction that requires an operation and may lead to intestinal gangrene and perforation. Physicians frequently describe intestinal obstruction as partial versus complete. These distinctions are relevant because complete obstruction generally requires an operation and partial obstruction usually does not (especially for the small intestine). These descriptors may differentiate between an aftercare code and a condition that may not yet be resolved.

6 K56.60 Unspecified intestinal obstruction
EXCLUDES 1 intestinal obstruction due to specified condition-code to condition

IQ K56.600 Partial intestinal obstruction, unspecified as to cause
Incomplete intestinal obstruction, NOS

IQ K56.601 Complete intestinal obstruction, unspecified as to cause

IQ K56.609 Unspecified intestinal obstruction, unspecified as to partial versus complete obstruction
Intestinal obstruction NOS

6 K56.69 Other intestinal obstruction
Enterostenosis NOS
Obstructive ileus NOS
Occlusion of colon or intestine NOS
Stenosis of colon or intestine NOS
Stricture of colon or intestine NOS
EXCLUDES 1 intestinal obstruction due to specified condition-code to condition

SP K56.690 Other partial intestinal obstruction
Other incomplete intestinal obstruction

SP K56.691 Other complete intestinal obstruction

SP K56.699 Other intestinal obstruction unspecified as to partial versus complete obstruction
Other intestinal obstruction, NEC

SP K56.7 Ileus, unspecified
EXCLUDES 1 obstructive ileus (K56.69-)
EXCLUDES 2 intestinal obstruction with hernia (K40-K46)

4 K57 Diverticular disease of intestine
Code also:
if applicable peritonitis K65.-
EXCLUDES 1 congenital diverticulum of intestine (Q43.8)
Meckel's diverticulum (Q43.0)
EXCLUDES 2 diverticulum of appendix (K38.2)

CODING TIPS ✓ Do not assign a code from K57.- for diverticular conditions reported as congenital. Congenital diverticulum should be coded to the appropriate Q43.- code.

5 K57.0 Diverticulitis of small intestine with perforation and abscess

Chapter 11

K00-K95

★ New ▲ Revised Px Primary SP PDGM Px SL Low CoM SH High CoM IQ Quest. Encounter H Hospice non-cancer Dx ☐ Unspecified M *Manifestation*

DecisionHealth's FY 2020 Complete Home Health ICD-10-CM Diagnosis Coding Manual

1083

Diverticulitis of small intestine with peritonitis
> **EXCLUDES 1** diverticulitis of both small and large intestine with perforation and abscess (K57.4-)

SP K57.00 **Diverticulitis of small intestine with perforation and abscess without bleeding**

SP K57.01 **Diverticulitis of small intestine with perforation and abscess with bleeding**

5 K57.1 **Diverticular disease of small intestine without perforation or abscess**
> **EXCLUDES 1** diverticular disease of both small and large intestine without perforation or abscess (K57.5-)

SP K57.10 **Diverticulosis of small intestine without perforation or abscess without bleeding**
Diverticular disease of small intestine NOS

SP K57.11 **Diverticulosis of small intestine without perforation or abscess with bleeding**

SP K57.12 **Diverticulitis of small intestine without perforation or abscess without bleeding**

SP K57.13 **Diverticulitis of small intestine without perforation or abscess with bleeding**

5 K57.2 **Diverticulitis of large intestine with perforation and abscess**
Diverticulitis of colon with peritonitis
> **EXCLUDES 1** diverticulitis of both small and large intestine with perforation and abscess (K57.4-)

SP K57.20 **Diverticulitis of large intestine with perforation and abscess without bleeding**

SP K57.21 **Diverticulitis of large intestine with perforation and abscess with bleeding**

5 K57.3 **Diverticular disease of large intestine without perforation or abscess**
> **EXCLUDES 1** diverticular disease of both small and large intestine without perforation or abscess (K57.5-)

SP K57.30 **Diverticulosis of large intestine without perforation or abscess without bleeding**
Diverticular disease of colon NOS

SP K57.31 **Diverticulosis of large intestine without perforation or abscess with bleeding**

SP K57.32 **Diverticulitis of large intestine without perforation or abscess without bleeding**

SP K57.33 **Diverticulitis of large intestine without perforation or abscess with bleeding**

5 K57.4 **Diverticulitis of both small and large intestine with perforation and abscess**
Diverticulitis of both small and large intestine with peritonitis

SP K57.40 **Diverticulitis of both small and large intestine with perforation and abscess without bleeding**

SP K57.41 **Diverticulitis of both small and large intestine with perforation and abscess with bleeding**

5 K57.5 **Diverticular disease of both small and large intestine without perforation or abscess**

SP K57.50 **Diverticulosis of both small and large intestine without perforation or abscess without bleeding**
Diverticular disease of both small and large intestine NOS

SP K57.51 **Diverticulosis of both small and large intestine without perforation or abscess with bleeding**

SP K57.52 **Diverticulitis of both small and large intestine without perforation or abscess without bleeding**

SP K57.53 **Diverticulitis of both small and large intestine without perforation or abscess with bleeding**

5 K57.8 **Diverticulitis of intestine, part unspecified, with perforation and abscess**
Diverticulitis of intestine NOS with peritonitis

SP K57.80 **Diverticulitis of intestine, part unspecified, with perforation and abscess without bleeding**

SP K57.81 **Diverticulitis of intestine, part unspecified, with perforation and abscess with bleeding**

5 K57.9 **Diverticular disease of intestine, part unspecified, without perforation or abscess**

SP K57.90 **Diverticulosis of intestine, part unspecified, without perforation or abscess without bleeding**
Diverticular disease of intestine NOS

SP K57.91 **Diverticulosis of intestine, part unspecified, without perforation or abscess with bleeding**

SP K57.92 **Diverticulitis of intestine, part unspecified, without perforation or abscess without bleeding**

SP K57.93 **Diverticulitis of intestine, part unspecified, without perforation or abscess with bleeding**

4 K58 **Irritable bowel syndrome**
> **INCLUDES** irritable colon
> spastic colon

CODING TIPS ✓ Functional gastrointestinal disorders (FGIDs) can affect any part of the gastrointestinal tract; they are disorders of how the GI tract works, not structural or biochemical abnormalities. Irritable bowel syndrome (IBS) is a chronic functional gastrointestinal disorder characterized by abdominal pain or discomfort associated with altered bowel habits. IBS is classified into subtypes based on the predominant alteration in stool form: IBS with constipation (IBS-C), IBS with diarrhea (IBS-D), both (IBS-M for mixed) or neither (IBS-U for unspecified).

4 4th digit required   5 5th digit required   6 6th digit required   7 7th digit required   7 7th digit placeholder   + Additional code   Laterality

1084   *DecisionHealth's* FY 2020 Complete Home Health ICD-10-CM Diagnosis Coding Manual

Chapter 11

K00-K95

DEFINITION Functional disorder of hypersensitive nerves and muscles in the colon, causing cramping, pain, diarrhea, and/or constipation.

SP K58.0 Irritable bowel syndrome with diarrhea

CODING TIPS✓ Do not assign an additional code for the diarrhea. K58.0 is a combination code and does not require additional coding of the included symptom.

SP K58.1 Irritable bowel syndrome with constipation

SP K58.2 Mixed irritable bowel syndrome

SP K58.8 Other irritable bowel syndrome

SP K58.9 Irritable bowel syndrome without diarrhea
Irritable bowel syndrome NOS

4 K59 Other functional intestinal disorders

EXCLUDES 1 change in bowel habit NOS (R19.4)
intestinal malabsorption (K90.-)
psychogenic intestinal disorders (F45.8)

EXCLUDES 2 functional disorders of stomach (K31.-)

▲ 5 K59.0 Constipation

EXCLUDES 1 fecal impaction (K56.41)
incomplete defecation (R15.0)

SP K59.00 Constipation, unspecified

SP K59.01 Slow transit constipation

DEFINITION Dysfunction of intestinal smooth muscles that move fecal matter, causing slow stool movement.

SP K59.02 Outlet dysfunction constipation

SP ✚ K59.03 Drug induced constipation
Use additional code for adverse effect, if applicable, to identify drug (T36-T50 with fifth or sixth character 5

CODING TIPS✓ Opiate induced constipation is more difficult to manage. Code also the opiate adverse effect.

CODING TIPS✓ Opioids and other medications affect all segments of the stomach and intestine (particularly the colon) altering nerve input to the GI tract which inhibits movement. Constipation from slowed or absent GI motility requires a long-term bowel program and possible colectomy for chronic constipation resistant to treatment.

SP K59.04 Chronic idiopathic constipation
Functional constipation

DEFINITION Chronic idiopathic constipation, also known as functional constipation, is a long-lasting or recurring reduction in stool frequency, usually less than 3 times per week, difficulty passing stools, or both without any underlying illness, medication, or physiological cause, such as hormonal imbalance.

SP K59.09 Other constipation
Chronic constipation

SP K59.1 Functional diarrhea

EXCLUDES 1 diarrhea NOS (R19.7)
irritable bowel syndrome with diarrhea (K58.0)

CODING TIPS✓ K59.1, functional diarrhea, is a condition with no detectable organic cause. When the organism is identified, infectious diarrhea must be assigned from code range A00-A09.

SP K59.2 Neurogenic bowel, not elsewhere classified

DEFINITION Intestinal dysfunction due to spinal cord damage.

5 K59.3 Megacolon, not elsewhere classified
Dilatation of colon
Code first:
, if applicable (T51-T65) to identify toxic agent

EXCLUDES 1 congenital megacolon (aganglionic) (Q43.1)
megacolon (due to) (in) Chagas' disease (B57.32)
megacolon (due to) (in) Clostridium difficile (A04.7-)
megacolon (due to) (in) Hirschsprung's disease (Q43.1)

CODING TIPS✓ Megacolon is an abnormal dilation of the colon, generally accompanied by reduced peristalsis. Do not assign a code from K59.3- if the cause is known to be due to another condition such as *Clostridium difficile* (A04.7), Hirschsprung's disease (Q43.1), or other congenital or known cause. When the cause is known, code the cause of the megacolon.

DEFINITION Enlargement or dilation of the sigmoid colon.

SP K59.31 Toxic megacolon

SP K59.39 Other megacolon
Megacolon NOS

DEFINITION A condition in which the large intestine becomes extremely distended and stretched so that it is much larger than usual. This may be an acute, sudden and severe condition due to infection, or a chronic condition due to abnormal growth. Note: Congenital megacolon and that due to exposure to toxins is classified by other codes.

SP K59.4 Anal spasm
Proctalgia fugax

SP K59.8 Other specified functional intestinal disorders
Atony of colon
Pseudo-obstruction (acute) (chronic) of intestine

SP K59.9 Functional intestinal disorder, unspecified

4 K60 Fissure and fistula of anal and rectal regions

EXCLUDES 1 fissure and fistula of anal and rectal regions with abscess or cellulitis (K61.-)

EXCLUDES 2 anal sphincter tear (healed) (nontraumatic) (old) (K62.81)

Chapter 11

K00-K95

★ New ▲ Revised Px Primary SP PDGM Px SL Low CoM SH High CoM IQ Quest. Encounter H Hospice non-cancer Dx Unspecified M *Manifestation*

DecisionHealth's FY 2020 Complete Home Health ICD-10-CM Diagnosis Coding Manual

1085

SP K60.0 Acute anal fissure

SP K60.1 Chronic anal fissure

SP K60.2 Anal fissure, unspecified

SP K60.3 Anal fistula

> **DEFINITION** An abnormal passage from the anus to the skin.

SP K60.4 Rectal fistula
Fistula of rectum to skin
> **EXCLUDES 1** rectovaginal fistula (N82.3)
> vesicorectal fistual (N32.1)

SP K60.5 Anorectal fistula

4 K61 Abscess of anal and rectal regions
> **INCLUDES** abscess of anal and rectal regions
> cellulitis of anal and rectal regions

SP K61.0 Anal abscess
Perianal abscess
> **EXCLUDES 2** intrasphincteric abscess (K61.4)

SP K61.1 Rectal abscess
Perirectal abscess
> **EXCLUDES 1** ischiorectal abscess (K61.39)

SP K61.2 Anorectal abscess

5 K61.3 Ischiorectal abscess

SP K61.31 Horseshoe abscess

SP K61.39 Other ischiorectal abscess
Abscess of ischiorectal fossa
Ischiorectal abscess, NOS

SP K61.4 Intrasphincteric abscess
Intersphincteric abscess

SP K61.5 Supralevator abscess

4 K62 Other diseases of anus and rectum
> **INCLUDES** anal canal
> **EXCLUDES 2** colostomy and enterostomy malfunction (K94.0-, K94.1-)
> fecal incontinence (R15.-)
> hemorrhoids (K64.-)

SP K62.0 Anal polyp

SP K62.1 Rectal polyp
> **EXCLUDES 1** adenomatous polyp (D12.8)

SP K62.2 Anal prolapse
Prolapse of anal canal

SP K62.3 Rectal prolapse
Prolapse of rectal mucosa
> **DEFINITION** Rectal tissue falls from its usual position, turning itself inside out and protruding from the body in late stages.

SP K62.4 Stenosis of anus and rectum
Stricture of anus (sphincter)

SP K62.5 Hemorrhage of anus and rectum
> **EXCLUDES 1** gastrointestinal bleeding NOS (K92.2)
> melena (K92.1)
> neonatal rectal hemorrhage (P54.2)

SP K62.6 Ulcer of anus and rectum
Solitary ulcer of anus and rectum
Stercoral ulcer of anus and rectum
> **EXCLUDES 1** fissure and fistula of anus and rectum (K60.-)
> ulcerative colitis (K51.-)

> **DEFINITION** Open sore in the rectum and/or anus causing pain that worsens during defecation and blood or mucous in the stool.

SP + K62.7 Radiation proctitis
Use additional code to identify the type of radiation (W90.-)
> **CODING TIPS ✓** Radiation proctitis includes ulceration of the rectal lining due to the adverse effects of radiation. Assign an additional code from W90.- to identify radiation exposure.

5 K62.8 Other specified diseases of anus and rectum
> **EXCLUDES 2** ulcerative proctitis (K51.2)

SP + K62.81 Anal sphincter tear (healed) (nontraumatic) (old)
Tear of anus, nontraumatic
Use additional code for any associated fecal incontinence (R15.-)
> **EXCLUDES 2** anal fissure (K60.-)
> anal sphincter tear (healed) (old) complicating delivery (O34.7-)
> traumatic tear of anal sphincter (S31.831)

SP K62.82 Dysplasia of anus
Anal intraepithelial neoplasia I and II (AIN I and II) (histologically confirmed)
Dysplasia of anus NOS
Mild and moderate dysplasia of anus (histologically confirmed)
> **EXCLUDES 1** abnormal results from anal cytologic examination without histologic confirmation (R85.61-)
> anal intraepithelial neoplasia III (D01.3)
> carcinoma in situ of anus (D01.3)
> HGSIL of anus (R85.613)
> severe dysplasia of anus (D01.3)

SP + K62.89 Other specified diseases of anus and rectum
Proctitis NOS
Use additional code for any associated fecal incontinence (R15.-)

IQ K62.9 Disease of anus and rectum, unspecified

4 K63 Other diseases of intestine

SP K63.0 Abscess of intestine
> **EXCLUDES 1** abscess of intestine with Crohn's disease (K50.014, K50.114, K50.814, K50.914,)
> abscess of intestine with diverticular disease (K57.0, K57.2, K57.4, K57.8)

4 4th digit required   5 5th digit required   6 6th digit required   7 7th digit required   ☑ 7th digit placeholder   + Additional code   ⊟ Laterality

1086 *DecisionHealth's* FY 2020 Complete Home Health ICD-10-CM Diagnosis Coding Manual

abscess of intestine with
ulcerative colitis
(K51.014, K51.214,
K51.314, K51.414,
K51.514, K51.814,
K51.914)

EXCLUDES 2 abscess of anal and rectal
regions (K61.-)
abscess of appendix
(K35.3-)

SP K63.1 Perforation of intestine (nontraumatic)
Perforation (nontraumatic) of rectum

EXCLUDES 1 perforation (nontraumatic)
of duodenum (K26.-)
perforation (nontraumatic)
of intestine with
diverticular disease
(K57.0, K57.2, K57.4,
K57.8)

EXCLUDES 2 perforation (nontraumatic)
of appendix (K35.2-,
K35.3-)

DEFINITION Hole in the intestinal wall
allowing food and/or fecal matter to leak
into the abdominal cavity.

SP K63.2 Fistula of intestine

EXCLUDES 1 fistula of duodenum (K31.6)
fistula of intestine with
Crohn's disease
(K50.013, K50.113,
K50.813, K50.913,)
fistula of intestine with
ulcerative colitis
(K51.013, K51.213,
K51.313, K51.413,
K51.513, K51.813,
K51.913)

EXCLUDES 2 fistula of anal and rectal
regions (K60.-)
fistula of appendix (K38.3)
intestinal-genital fistula,
female (N82.2-N82.4)
vesicointestinal fistula
(N32.1)

DEFINITION Abnormal passageway
between loops of the intestine or the
intestine and another organ or the
abdominal wall.

SP K63.3 Ulcer of intestine
Primary ulcer of small intestine

EXCLUDES 1 duodenal ulcer (K26.-)
gastrointestinal ulcer
(K28.-)
gastrojejunal ulcer (K28.-)
jejunal ulcer (K28.-)
peptic ulcer, site unspecified
(K27.-)
ulcer of intestine with
perforation (K63.1)
ulcer of anus or rectum
(K62.6)
ulcerative colitis (K51.-)

SP K63.4 Enteroptosis

▲ SP K63.5 Polyp of colon

EXCLUDES 1 adenomatous polyp of colon
(D12.-)
inflammatory polyp of colon
(K51.4-)

polyposis of colon (D12.6)

CODING TIPS ✓ Most polyps of the colon are
coded to D12 because they are considered
benign neoplasms. Hyperplastic polyps are
coded to K63.5.

⑤ K63.8 Other specified diseases of intestine

SP K63.81 Dieulafoy lesion of intestine

EXCLUDES 2 Dieulafoy lesion of
stomach and duodenum
(K31.82)

SP K63.89 Other specified diseases of intestine

IQ K63.9 Disease of intestine, unspecified

**④ K64 Hemorrhoids and perianal venous
thrombosis**

INCLUDES piles

EXCLUDES 1 hemorrhoids complicating
childbirth and the puerperium
(O87.2)
hemorrhoids complicating
pregnancy (O22.4)

SP K64.0 First degree hemorrhoids
Grade/stage I hemorrhoids
Hemorrhoids (bleeding) without prolapse
outside of anal canal

SP K64.1 Second degree hemorrhoids
Grade/stage II hemorrhoids
Hemorrhoids (bleeding) that prolapse with
straining, but retract spontaneously

SP K64.2 Third degree hemorrhoids
Grade/stage III hemorrhoids
Hemorrhoids (bleeding) that prolapse with
straining and require manual
replacement back inside anal canal

SP K64.3 Fourth degree hemorrhoids
Grade/stage IV hemorrhoids
Hemorrhoids (bleeding) with prolapsed
tissue that cannot be manually replaced

SP K64.4 Residual hemorrhoidal skin tags
External hemorrhoids, NOS
Skin tags of anus

SP K64.5 Perianal venous thrombosis
External hemorrhoids with thrombosis
Perianal hematoma
Thrombosed hemorrhoids NOS

SP K64.8 Other hemorrhoids
Internal hemorrhoids, without mention of
degree
Prolapsed hemorrhoids, degree not
specified

SP K64.9 Unspecified hemorrhoids
Hemorrhoids (bleeding) NOS
Hemorrhoids (bleeding) without mention
of degree

Chapter 11

K00-K95

★ New ▲ Revised Px Primary SP PDGM Px SL Low CoM SH High CoM IQ Quest. Encounter H Hospice non-cancer Dx Unspecified M *Manifestation*

DecisionHealth's FY 2020 Complete Home Health ICD-10-CM Diagnosis Coding Manual

1087

Diseases of peritoneum and retroperitoneum   (K65-K68)

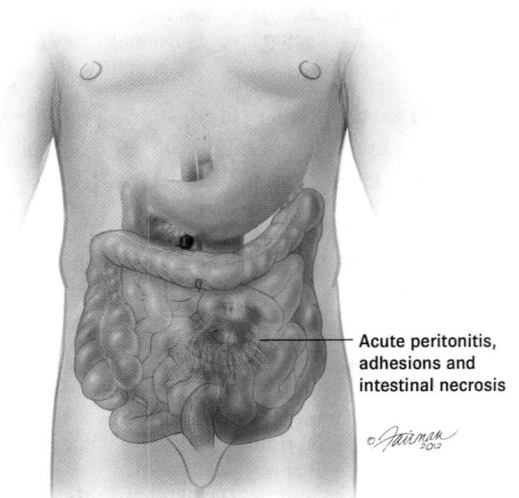

— Acute peritonitis, adhesions and intestinal necrosis

➕ ④ K65   Peritonitis
Code also:
if applicable diverticular disease of intestine (K57.-)
Use additional code (B95-B97), to identify infectious agent, if known

EXCLUDES 1   acute appendicitis with generalized peritonitis (K35.2-)
aseptic peritonitis (T81.6)
benign paroxysmal peritonitis (E85.0)
chemical peritonitis (T81.6)
gonococcal peritonitis (A54.85)
neonatal peritonitis (P78.0-P78.1)
pelvic peritonitis, female (N73.3-N73.5)
periodic familial peritonitis (E85.0)
peritonitis due to talc or other foreign substance (T81.6)
peritonitis in chlamydia (A74.81)
peritonitis in diphtheria (A36.89)
peritonitis in syphilis (late) (A52.74)
peritonitis in tuberculosis (A18.31)
peritonitis with or following abortion or ectopic or molar pregnancy (O00-O07, O08.0)
peritonitis with or following appendicitis (K35.-)
puerperal peritonitis (O85)
retroperitoneal infections (K68.-)

CODING TIPS ✓   When the causative infectious organism is known, always assign an additional code from B95-B97 to identify the infectious agent.

SP ➕ K65.0   Generalized (acute) peritonitis
Pelvic peritonitis (acute), male
Subphrenic peritonitis (acute)
Suppurative peritonitis (acute)

SP ➕ K65.1   Peritoneal abscess
Abdominopelvic abscess
Abscess (of) omentum
Abscess (of) peritoneum
Mesenteric abscess
Retrocecal abscess
Subdiaphragmatic abscess
Subhepatic abscess
Subphrenic abscess

SP ➕ K65.2   Spontaneous bacterial peritonitis
EXCLUDES 1   bacterial peritonitis NOS (K65.9)
CODING TIPS ✓   Do not assign K65.2 unless the physician has specifically provided a diagnosis of "spontaneous" bacterial peritonitis. Bacterial peritonitis not specified as spontaneous is classified to K65.9 (Peritonitis NOS).

SP ➕ K65.3   Choleperitonitis
Peritonitis due to bile

SP ➕ K65.4   Sclerosing mesenteritis
Fat necrosis of peritoneum
(Idiopathic) sclerosing mesenteric fibrosis
Mesenteric lipodystrophy
Mesenteric panniculitis
Retractile mesenteritis
DEFINITION   Rare, idiopathic lesions of fat necrosis, fibrosis, and chronic inflammation causing single or multiple lesions, with diffuse thickening of the mesentery.

SP ➕ K65.8   Other peritonitis
Chronic proliferative peritonitis
Peritonitis due to urine

SP ➕ K65.9   Peritonitis, unspecified
Bacterial peritonitis NOS

④ K66   Other disorders of peritoneum
EXCLUDES 2   ascites (R18.-)
peritoneal effusion (chronic) (R18.8)

SP K66.0   Peritoneal adhesions (postprocedural) (postinfection)
Adhesions (of) abdominal (wall)
Adhesions (of) diaphragm
Adhesions (of) intestine
Adhesions (of) male pelvis
Adhesions (of) omentum
Adhesions (of) stomach
Adhesive bands
Mesenteric adhesions
EXCLUDES 1   female pelvic adhesions [bands] (N73.6)
peritoneal adhesions with intestinal obstruction (K56.5-)

SP K66.1   Hemoperitoneum
EXCLUDES 1   traumatic hemoperitoneum (S36.8-)

SP K66.8   Other specified disorders of peritoneum

!Q K66.9   Disorder of peritoneum, unspecified

---

④4th digit required   ⑤5th digit required   ⑥6th digit required   ⑦7th digit required   ⑦ 7th digit placeholder   ➕Additional code   ⊟Laterality

1088   DecisionHealth's FY 2020 Complete Home Health ICD-10-CM Diagnosis Coding Manual

M IQ K67 *Disorders of peritoneum in infectious diseases classified elsewhere*

Code first underlying disease, such as:
  congenital syphilis (A50.0)
  helminthiasis (B65.0 -B83.9)

    EXCLUDES 1 peritonitis in chlamydia
      (A74.81)
      peritonitis in diphtheria
      (A36.89)
      peritonitis in gonococcal
      (A54.85)
      peritonitis in syphilis (late)
      (A52.74)
      peritonitis in tuberculosis
      (A18.31)

4 K68 **Disorders of retroperitoneum**

5 K68.1 **Retroperitoneal abscess**

SP K68.11 **Postprocedural retroperitoneal abscess**
    EXCLUDES 2 infection following procedure (T81.4-)

SP K68.12 **Psoas muscle abscess**

SP K68.19 **Other retroperitoneal abscess**

SP K68.9 **Other disorders of retroperitoneum**

Diseases of liver (K70-K77)

EXCLUDES 1 jaundice NOS (R17)

EXCLUDES 2 hemochromatosis (E83.11-)
  Reye's syndrome (G93.7)
  viral hepatitis (B15-B19)
  Wilson's disease (E83.0)

+ 4 K70 **Alcoholic liver disease**

Use additional code to identify:
  alcohol abuse and dependence (F10.-)

CODING TIPS ✓ Codes from category K70.- indicate liver disease resulting from alcohol use. An additional code should be assigned to identify alcohol abuse or dependence.

SP + K70.0 **Alcoholic fatty liver**

+ 5 K70.1 **Alcoholic hepatitis**

SP + K70.10 **Alcoholic hepatitis without ascites**

SP + K70.11 **Alcoholic hepatitis with ascites**

H SP + K70.2 **Alcoholic fibrosis and sclerosis of liver**
    DEFINITION Intermediate stage liver disease in which normal, healthy tissue of the liver is replaced by scar tissue due to long-term, excessive alcohol consumption.

+ 5 K70.3 **Alcoholic cirrhosis of liver**
  Alcoholic cirrhosis NOS
    DEFINITION Late stage liver disease characterized by inflammation, debilitating scar tissue, and damaged membranes due to long-term, excessive alcohol consumption.

H SP + K70.30 **Alcoholic cirrhosis of liver without ascites**

H SP + K70.31 **Alcoholic cirrhosis of liver with ascites**

+ 5 K70.4 **Alcoholic hepatic failure**
  Acute alcoholic hepatic failure
  Alcoholic hepatic failure NOS
  Chronic alcoholic hepatic failure
  Subacute alcoholic hepatic failure

SP + K70.40 **Alcoholic hepatic failure without coma**

H SP + K70.41 **Alcoholic hepatic failure with coma**

SP + K70.9 **Alcoholic liver disease, unspecified**

+ 4 K71 **Toxic liver disease**
    INCLUDES drug-induced idiosyncratic (unpredictable) liver disease
      drug-induced toxic (predictable) liver disease

Code first:
  poisoning due to drug or toxin, if applicable (T36-T65 with fifth or sixth character 1-4 or 6)
Use additional code for adverse effect, if applicable, to identify drug (T36-T50 with fifth or sixth character 5)

    EXCLUDES 2 alcoholic liver disease (K70.-)
      Budd-Chiari syndrome (I82.0)

CODING TIPS ✓ Codes from category K71.- indicate liver disease resulting from toxicity or toxic damage to the liver due to chemical exposure, including drugs. When a condition from K71.- is caused by poisoning, code first the appropriate T36-T65 code to indicate poisoning. When the condition is diagnosed as an adverse effect, code the appropriate K71.- code followed by the appropriate code from categories T36-T50 to indicate adverse effect.

H SP + K71.0 **Toxic liver disease with cholestasis**
  Cholestasis with hepatocyte injury
  'Pure' cholestasis

+ 5 K71.1 **Toxic liver disease with hepatic necrosis**
  Hepatic failure (acute) (chronic) due to drugs

H SP + K71.10 **Toxic liver disease with hepatic necrosis, without coma**

H SP + K71.11 **Toxic liver disease with hepatic necrosis, with coma**

H SP + K71.2 **Toxic liver disease with acute hepatitis**

H SP + K71.3 **Toxic liver disease with chronic persistent hepatitis**

H SP + K71.4 **Toxic liver disease with chronic lobular hepatitis**

+ 5 K71.5 **Toxic liver disease with chronic active hepatitis**
  Toxic liver disease with lupoid hepatitis

H SP + K71.50 **Toxic liver disease with chronic active hepatitis without ascites**

H SP + K71.51 **Toxic liver disease with chronic active hepatitis with ascites**

H SP + K71.6 **Toxic liver disease with hepatitis, not elsewhere classified**

H SP + K71.7 **Toxic liver disease with fibrosis and cirrhosis of liver**

H SP + K71.8 **Toxic liver disease with other disorders of liver**
  Toxic liver disease with focal nodular hyperplasia
  Toxic liver disease with hepatic granulomas
  Toxic liver disease with peliosis hepatis
  Toxic liver disease with veno-occlusive disease of liver

H IQ + K71.9 **Toxic liver disease, unspecified**

4 K72 **Hepatic failure, not elsewhere classified**
    INCLUDES fulminant hepatitis NEC, with hepatic failure

Chapter 11

K00-K95

★ New ▲ Revised Px Primary **SP** PDGM Px **SL** Low CoM **SH** High CoM **IQ** Quest. Encounter **H** Hospice non-cancer Dx Unspecified **M** *Manifestation*

DecisionHealth's FY 2020 Complete Home Health ICD-10-CM Diagnosis Coding Manual

1089

hepatic encephalopathy NOS
liver (cell) necrosis with
hepatic failure
malignant hepatitis NEC, with
hepatic failure
yellow liver atrophy or
dystrophy
EXCLUDES 1 alcoholic hepatic failure
(K70.4)
hepatic failure with toxic liver
disease (K71.1-)
icterus of newborn (P55-P59)
postprocedural hepatic failure
(K91.82)
EXCLUDES 2 hepatic failure complicating
abortion or ectopic or molar
pregnancy (O00-O07, O08.8)
hepatic failure complicating
pregnancy, childbirth and the
puerperium (O26.6-)
viral hepatitis with hepatic
coma (B15-B19)

5 K72.0 Acute and subacute hepatic failure
Acute non-viral hepatitis NOS

**SP K72.00 Acute and subacute hepatic failure
without coma**
CODING TIPS ✓ This code is correct for
non-viral acute hepatitis.

**H SP K72.01 Acute and subacute hepatic failure
with coma**

5 K72.1 Chronic hepatic failure

**SP K72.10 Chronic hepatic failure without
coma**

H SP K72.11 Chronic hepatic failure with coma

5 K72.9 Hepatic failure, unspecified

**SP K72.90 Hepatic failure, unspecified without
coma**

**H SP K72.91 Hepatic failure, unspecified with
coma**
Hepatic coma NOS

4 K73 Chronic hepatitis, not elsewhere classified
EXCLUDES 1 alcoholic hepatitis (chronic)
(K70.1-)
drug-induced hepatitis
(chronic) (K71.-)
granulomatous hepatitis
(chronic) NEC (K75.3)
reactive, nonspecific hepatitis
(chronic) (K75.2)
viral hepatitis (chronic) (B15-
B19)

CODING TIPS ✓ Do not assign a code from
category K73.- when hepatitis is specified as
viral or due to a specific cause, such as alcohol
use or toxicity.

**H SP K73.0 Chronic persistent hepatitis, not
elsewhere classified**

**H SP K73.1 Chronic lobular hepatitis, not elsewhere
classified**

**H SP K73.2 Chronic active hepatitis, not elsewhere
classified**

**H SP K73.8 Other chronic hepatitis, not elsewhere
classified**

H SP K73.9 Chronic hepatitis, unspecified

4 K74 Fibrosis and cirrhosis of liver
Code also:
, if applicable, viral hepatitis (acute)
(chronic) (B15-B19)
EXCLUDES 1 alcoholic cirrhosis (of liver)
(K70.3)
alcoholic fibrosis of liver
(K70.2)
cardiac sclerosis of liver
(K76.1)
cirrhosis (of liver) with toxic
liver disease (K71.7)
congenital cirrhosis (of liver)
(P78.81)
pigmentary cirrhosis (of liver)
(E83.110)

CODING TIPS ✓ When viral hepatitis is also
documented as a confirmed diagnosis in a
patient with any diagnosis classifiable to K74.-,
the appropriate code from B15-B19 should
also be assigned. The sequencing of the K74.-
and the viral hepatitis code is according to
focus of care.

H SP K74.0 Hepatic fibrosis

SP K74.1 Hepatic sclerosis

SP K74.2 Hepatic fibrosis with hepatic sclerosis

▲ H SP K74.3 Primary biliary cirrhosis
Chronic nonsuppurative destructive
cholangitis
Primary biliary cholangitis
EXCLUDES 2 primary sclerosing
cholangitis (K83.01)
DEFINITION Scar tissue formation of the
ducts carrying bile from the liver to the small
intestine, resulting in bile build-up and liver
damage leading to cirrhosis.

H SP K74.4 Secondary biliary cirrhosis

H SP K74.5 Biliary cirrhosis, unspecified

5 K74.6 Other and unspecified cirrhosis of liver

H SP K74.60 Unspecified cirrhosis of liver
Cirrhosis (of liver) NOS

H SP K74.69 Other cirrhosis of liver
Cryptogenic cirrhosis (of liver)
Macronodular cirrhosis (of liver)
Micronodular cirrhosis (of liver)
Mixed type cirrhosis (of liver)
Portal cirrhosis (of liver)
Postnecrotic cirrhosis (of liver)

4 K75 Other inflammatory liver diseases
EXCLUDES 2 toxic liver disease (K71.-)

SP K75.0 Abscess of liver
Cholangitic hepatic abscess
Hematogenic hepatic abscess
Hepatic abscess NOS
Lymphogenic hepatic abscess
Pylephlebitic hepatic abscess
EXCLUDES 1 amebic liver abscess
(A06.4)
cholangitis without liver
abscess (K83.09)
pylephlebitis without liver
abscess (K75.1)
EXCLUDES 2 acute or subacute hepatitis
NOS (B17.9)
acute or subacute non-viral
hepatitis (K72.0)

---

4 4th digit required   **5** 5th digit required   **6** 6th digit required   **7** 7th digit required   **7** 7th digit placeholder   **+** Additional code   **⊟** Laterality

1090   DecisionHealth's FY 2020 Complete Home Health ICD-10-CM Diagnosis Coding Manual

chronic hepatitis NEC (K73.8)

SP K75.1 Phlebitis of portal vein
Pylephlebitis
EXCLUDES 1 pylephlebitic liver abscess (K75.0)

H SP K75.2 Nonspecific reactive hepatitis
EXCLUDES 1 acute or subacute hepatitis (K72.0-)
chronic hepatitis NEC (K73.-)
viral hepatitis (B15-B19)

H SP K75.3 Granulomatous hepatitis, not elsewhere classified
EXCLUDES 1 acute or subacute hepatitis (K72.0-)
chronic hepatitis NEC (K73.-)
viral hepatitis (B15-B19)

H SP K75.4 Autoimmune hepatitis
Lupoid hepatitis NEC
DEFINITION Continuous inflammation and necrosis of liver cells that progresses to cirrhosis, in association with autoimmune diseases and not infection, alcohol consumption, or toxic exposure.

S K75.8 Other specified inflammatory liver diseases

H SP K75.81 Nonalcoholic steatohepatitis (NASH)

SP K75.89 Other specified inflammatory liver diseases

SP K75.9 Inflammatory liver disease, unspecified
Hepatitis NOS
EXCLUDES 1 acute or subacute hepatitis (K72.0-)
chronic hepatitis NEC (K73.-)
viral hepatitis (B15-B19)
CODING TIPS ✓ If hepatitis is described as acute and is non-viral, assign code K72.00.
CODING TIPS ✓ Documentation: When documentation confirms only that a patient has hepatitis but does not provide any further detail, assign K75.9 to indicate hepatitis NOS. Do not assign this code if specific cause/type of hepatitis is specified in diagnostic information.

4 K76 Other diseases of liver
EXCLUDES 2 alcoholic liver disease (K70.-)
amyloid degeneration of liver (E85.-)
cystic disease of liver (congenital) (Q44.6)
hepatic vein thrombosis (I82.0)
hepatomegaly NOS (R16.0)
pigmentary cirrhosis (of liver) (E83.110)
portal vein thrombosis (I81)
toxic liver disease (K71.-)

SP K76.0 Fatty (change of) liver, not elsewhere classified
Nonalcoholic fatty liver disease (NAFLD)
EXCLUDES 1 nonalcoholic steatohepatitis (NASH) (K75.81)

SP K76.1 Chronic passive congestion of liver
Cardiac cirrhosis
Cardiac sclerosis

SP K76.2 Central hemorrhagic necrosis of liver
EXCLUDES 1 liver necrosis with hepatic failure (K72.-)

SP K76.3 Infarction of liver

H SP K76.4 Peliosis hepatis
Hepatic angiomatosis

SP K76.5 Hepatic veno-occlusive disease
EXCLUDES 1 Budd-Chiari syndrome (I82.0)

SP + K76.6 Portal hypertension
Use additional code for any associated complications, such as:
portal hypertensive gastropathy (K31.89)
DEFINITION Increase in the pressure within the portal vein which carries blood from the digestive organs to the liver, caused by a blockage of blood flow through the liver.

H SP K76.7 Hepatorenal syndrome
EXCLUDES 1 hepatorenal syndrome following labor and delivery (O90.4)
postprocedural hepatorenal syndrome (K91.83)

S K76.8 Other specified diseases of liver

H SP K76.81 Hepatopulmonary syndrome
Code first underlying liver disease, such as:
alcoholic cirrhosis of liver (K70.3-)
cirrhosis of liver without mention of alcohol (K74.6-)

SP K76.89 Other specified diseases of liver
Cyst (simple) of liver
Focal nodular hyperplasia of liver
Hepatoptosis

IQ K76.9 Liver disease, unspecified

M IQ K77 Liver disorders in diseases classified elsewhere
Code first underlying disease, such as:
amyloidosis (E85.-)
congenital syphilis (A50.0, A50.5)
congenital toxoplasmosis (P37.1)
schistosomiasis (B65.0-B65.9)
EXCLUDES 1 alcoholic hepatitis (K70.1-)
alcoholic liver disease (K70.-)
cytomegaloviral hepatitis (B25.1)
herpesviral [herpes simplex] hepatitis (B00.81)
infectious mononucleosis with liver disease (B27.0-B27.9 with .9)
mumps hepatitis (B26.81)
sarcoidosis with liver disease (D86.89)
secondary syphilis with liver disease (A51.45)
syphilis (late) with liver disease (A52.74)
toxoplasmosis (acquired) hepatitis (B58.1)
tuberculosis with liver disease (A18.83)

★ New ▲ Revised Px Primary **SP** PDGM Px **SL** Low CoM **SH** High CoM **IQ** Quest. Encounter **H** Hospice non-cancer Dx Unspecified **M** *Manifestation*

DecisionHealth's FY 2020 Complete Home Health ICD-10-CM Diagnosis Coding Manual

1091

Disorders of gallbladder, biliary tract and pancreas   (K80-K87)

4 K80   Cholelithiasis

EXCLUDES 1   retained cholelithiasis following cholecystectomy (K91.86)

CODING TIPS ✓   When cholecystitis or cholelithiasis has been diagnosed and treated by surgery, and is resolved by surgery upon home health admission, assign a code for aftercare.

+ 5 K80.0   Calculus of gallbladder with acute cholecystitis
   Any condition listed in K80.2 with acute cholecystitis
   Use additional code if applicable for associated gangrene of gallbladder (K82.A1), or perforation of gallbladder (K82.A2)

SP + K80.00   Calculus of gallbladder with acute cholecystitis without obstruction

SP + K80.01   Calculus of gallbladder with acute cholecystitis with obstruction

+ 5 K80.1   Calculus of gallbladder with other cholecystitis
   Use additional code if applicable for associated gangrene of gallbladder (K82.A1), or perforation of gallbladder (K82.A2)

SP + K80.10   Calculus of gallbladder with chronic cholecystitis without obstruction
   Cholelithiasis with cholecystitis NOS

SP + K80.11   Calculus of gallbladder with chronic cholecystitis with obstruction

SP + K80.12   Calculus of gallbladder with acute and chronic cholecystitis without obstruction

SP + K80.13   Calculus of gallbladder with acute and chronic cholecystitis with obstruction

SP + K80.18   Calculus of gallbladder with other cholecystitis without obstruction

SP + K80.19   Calculus of gallbladder with other cholecystitis with obstruction

5 K80.2   Calculus of gallbladder without cholecystitis
   Cholecystolithiasis without cholecystitis
   Cholelithiasis (without cholecystitis)
   Colic (recurrent) of gallbladder (without cholecystitis)
   Gallstone (impacted) of cystic duct (without cholecystitis)
   Gallstone (impacted) of gallbladder (without cholecystitis)

SP K80.20   Calculus of gallbladder without cholecystitis without obstruction

SP K80.21   Calculus of gallbladder without cholecystitis with obstruction

5 K80.3   Calculus of bile duct with cholangitis
   Any condition listed in K80.5 with cholangitis

SP K80.30   Calculus of bile duct with cholangitis, unspecified, without obstruction

SP K80.31   Calculus of bile duct with cholangitis, unspecified, with obstruction

SP K80.32   Calculus of bile duct with acute cholangitis without obstruction

SP K80.33   Calculus of bile duct with acute cholangitis with obstruction

SP K80.34   Calculus of bile duct with chronic cholangitis without obstruction

SP K80.35   Calculus of bile duct with chronic cholangitis with obstruction

SP K80.36   Calculus of bile duct with acute and chronic cholangitis without obstruction

SP K80.37   Calculus of bile duct with acute and chronic cholangitis with obstruction

+ 5 K80.4   Calculus of bile duct with cholecystitis
   Any condition listed in K80.5 with cholecystitis (with cholangitis)
   Use additional code if applicable for associated gangrene of gallbladder (K82.A1), or perforation of gallbladder (K82.A2)

SP + K80.40   Calculus of bile duct with cholecystitis, unspecified, without obstruction

SP + K80.41   Calculus of bile duct with cholecystitis, unspecified, with obstruction

SP + K80.42   Calculus of bile duct with acute cholecystitis without obstruction

SP + K80.43   Calculus of bile duct with acute cholecystitis with obstruction

SP + K80.44   Calculus of bile duct with chronic cholecystitis without obstruction

SP + K80.45   Calculus of bile duct with chronic cholecystitis with obstruction

SP + K80.46   Calculus of bile duct with acute and chronic cholecystitis without obstruction

SP + K80.47   Calculus of bile duct with acute and chronic cholecystitis with obstruction

5 K80.5   Calculus of bile duct without cholangitis or cholecystitis
   Choledocholithiasis (without cholangitis or cholecystitis)
   Gallstone (impacted) of bile duct NOS (without cholangitis or cholecystitis)
   Gallstone (impacted) of common duct (without cholangitis or cholecystitis)
   Gallstone (impacted) of hepatic duct (without cholangitis or cholecystitis)
   Hepatic cholelithiasis (without cholangitis or cholecystitis)
   Hepatic colic (recurrent) (without cholangitis or cholecystitis)

SP K80.50   Calculus of bile duct without cholangitis or cholecystitis without obstruction

SP K80.51   Calculus of bile duct without cholangitis or cholecystitis with obstruction

+ 5 K80.6   Calculus of gallbladder and bile duct with cholecystitis
   Use additional code if applicable for associated gangrene of gallbladder (K82.A1), or perforation of gallbladder (K82.A2)

SP + K80.60   Calculus of gallbladder and bile duct with cholecystitis, unspecified, without obstruction

---

4 4th digit required   **5** 5th digit required   **6** 6th digit required   **7** 7th digit required   **7** 7th digit placeholder   **+** Additional code   **⊟** Laterality

SP **+** **K80.61** **Calculus of gallbladder and bile duct with cholecystitis, unspecified, with obstruction**

SP **+** **K80.62** Calculus of gallbladder and bile duct with acute cholecystitis without obstruction

SP **+** **K80.63** Calculus of gallbladder and bile duct with acute cholecystitis with obstruction

SP **+** **K80.64** Calculus of gallbladder and bile duct with chronic cholecystitis without obstruction

SP **+** **K80.65** Calculus of gallbladder and bile duct with chronic cholecystitis with obstruction

SP **+** **K80.66** Calculus of gallbladder and bile duct with acute and chronic cholecystitis without obstruction

SP **+** **K80.67** Calculus of gallbladder and bile duct with acute and chronic cholecystitis with obstruction

5 **K80.7** **Calculus of gallbladder and bile duct without cholecystitis**

SP **K80.70** Calculus of gallbladder and bile duct without cholecystitis without obstruction

SP **K80.71** Calculus of gallbladder and bile duct without cholecystitis with obstruction

5 **K80.8** **Other cholelithiasis**

SP **K80.80** Other cholelithiasis without obstruction

SP **K80.81** Other cholelithiasis with obstruction

+ **4** **K81** **Cholecystitis**
Use additional code if applicable for associated gangrene of gallbladder (K82.A1), or perforation of gallbladder (K82.A2)

EXCLUDES 1 cholecystitis with cholelithiasis (K80.-)

CODING TIPS ✓ When cholecystitis or cholelithiasis has been diagnosed and treated by surgery, and is resolved by surgery upon home health admission, assign a code for aftercare.

SP **+** **K81.0** **Acute cholecystitis**
Abscess of gallbladder
Angiocholecystitis
Emphysematous (acute) cholecystitis
Empyema of gallbladder
Gangrene of gallbladder
Gangrenous cholecystitis
Suppurative cholecystitis

SP **+** **K81.1** **Chronic cholecystitis**

SP **+** **K81.2** **Acute cholecystitis with chronic cholecystitis**

SP **+** **K81.9** **Cholecystitis, unspecified**

4 **K82** **Other diseases of gallbladder**
EXCLUDES 1 nonvisualization of gallbladder (R93.2)
postcholecystectomy syndrome (K91.5)

SP **K82.0** **Obstruction of gallbladder**
Occlusion of cystic duct or gallbladder without cholelithiasis
Stenosis of cystic duct or gallbladder without cholelithiasis
Stricture of cystic duct or gallbladder without cholelithiasis
EXCLUDES 1 obstruction of gallbladder with cholelithiasis (K80.-)

SP **K82.1** **Hydrops of gallbladder**
Mucocele of gallbladder
DEFINITION Overly full, distended gallbladder due to accumulation of mucous and watery material rather than stone formation.

SP **K82.2** **Perforation of gallbladder**
Rupture of cystic duct or gallbladder
EXCLUDES 1 Perforation of gallbladder in cholecystitis (K82.A2)

SP **K82.3** **Fistula of gallbladder**
Cholecystocolic fistula
Cholecystoduodenal fistula

SP **K82.4** **Cholesterolosis of gallbladder**
Strawberry gallbladder
EXCLUDES 1 cholesterolosis of gallbladder with cholecystitis (K81.-)
cholesterolosis of gallbladder with cholelithiasis (K80.-)
DEFINITION Build-up of cholesterol deposits on the surface of the gallbladder, giving it a 'strawberry' appearance.

SP **K82.8** **Other specified diseases of gallbladder**
Adhesions of cystic duct or gallbladder
Atrophy of cystic duct or gallbladder
Cyst of cystic duct or gallbladder
Dyskinesia of cystic duct or gallbladder
Hypertrophy of cystic duct or gallbladder
Nonfunctioning of cystic duct or gallbladder
Ulcer of cystic duct or gallbladder

IQ **K82.9** **Disease of gallbladder, unspecified**

5 **K82.A** **Disorders of gallbladder in diseases classified elsewhere**
Code first:
the type of cholecystitis (K81.-), or cholelithiasis with cholecystitis (K80.00-K80.19, K80.40-K80.47, K80.60-K80.67)

M **IQ** **K82.A1** *Gangrene of gallbladder in cholecystitis*

M **IQ** **K82.A2** *Perforation of gallbladder in cholecystitis*

4 **K83** **Other diseases of biliary tract**
EXCLUDES 1 postcholecystectomy syndrome (K91.5)
EXCLUDES 2 conditions involving the gallbladder (K81-K82)
conditions involving the cystic duct (K81-K82)

5 **K83.0** **Cholangitis**
EXCLUDES 1 cholangitic liver abscess (K75.0)
cholangitis with choledocholithiasis (K80.3-, K80.4-)
EXCLUDES 2 chronic nonsuppurative destructive cholangitis (K74.3)
primary biliary cholangitis (K74.3)
primary biliary cirrhosis (K74.3)

★ New ▲ Revised Px Primary **SP** PDGM Px **SL** Low CoM **SH** High CoM **IQ** Quest. Encounter **H** Hospice non-cancer Dx Unspecified **M** *Manifestation*

DecisionHealth's FY 2020 Complete Home Health ICD-10-CM Diagnosis Coding Manual

1093

DEFINITION   Infection of the biliary tract; presents with pain in the upper-right abdomen which may grow worse after a fatty meal, fever, nausea, vomiting, flatulence, pale-colored stool, and yellowing of the eyes and skin.

SP K83.01 **Primary sclerosing cholangitis**

SP K83.09 **Other cholangitis**
Ascending cholangitis
Cholangitis NOS
Primary cholangitis
Recurrent cholangitis
Sclerosing cholangitis
Secondary cholangitis
Stenosing cholangitis
Suppurative cholangitis

SP K83.1 **Obstruction of bile duct**
Occlusion of bile duct without cholelithiasis
Stenosis of bile duct without cholelithiasis
Stricture of bile duct without cholelithiasis
EXCLUDES 1   congenital obstruction of bile duct (Q44.3)
obstruction of bile duct with cholelithiasis (K80.-)

SP K83.2 **Perforation of bile duct**
Rupture of bile duct

SP K83.3 **Fistula of bile duct**
Choledochoduodenal fistula

SP K83.4 **Spasm of sphincter of Oddi**

SP K83.5 **Biliary cyst**

SP K83.8 **Other specified diseases of biliary tract**
Adhesions of biliary tract
Atrophy of biliary tract
Hypertrophy of biliary tract
Ulcer of biliary tract

IQ K83.9 **Disease of biliary tract, unspecified**

4 K85 **Acute pancreatitis**
INCLUDES   acute (recurrent) pancreatitis
subacute pancreatitis

5 K85.0 **Idiopathic acute pancreatitis**

SP K85.00 **Idiopathic acute pancreatitis without necrosis or infection**

SP K85.01 **Idiopathic acute pancreatitis with uninfected necrosis**

SP K85.02 **Idiopathic acute pancreatitis with infected necrosis**

5 K85.1 **Biliary acute pancreatitis**
Gallstone pancreatitis

SP K85.10 **Biliary acute pancreatitis without necrosis or infection**

SP K85.11 **Biliary acute pancreatitis with uninfected necrosis**

SP K85.12 **Biliary acute pancreatitis with infected necrosis**

5 K85.2 **Alcohol induced acute pancreatitis**
EXCLUDES 2   alcohol induced chronic pancreatitis (K86.0)

CODING TIPS ✓   Assign a code from K85.2- only when physician documentation clearly confirms acute pancreatitis due to alcohol use. The appropriate F10 code with 5th and 6th digits .88 should also be added.

SP K85.20 **Alcohol induced acute pancreatitis without necrosis or infection**

SP K85.21 **Alcohol induced acute pancreatitis with uninfected necrosis**

SP K85.22 **Alcohol induced acute pancreatitis with infected necrosis**

+ 5 K85.3 **Drug induced acute pancreatitis**
Use additional code for adverse effect, if applicable, to identify drug (T36-T50 with fifth or sixth character 5)
Use additional code to identify drug abuse and dependence (F11.-F17.-)

SP + K85.30 **Drug induced acute pancreatitis without necrosis or infection**

SP + K85.31 **Drug induced acute pancreatitis with uninfected necrosis**

SP + K85.32 **Drug induced acute pancreatitis with infected necrosis**

5 K85.8 **Other acute pancreatitis**

SP K85.80 **Other acute pancreatitis without necrosis or infection**

SP K85.81 **Other acute pancreatitis with uninfected necrosis**

SP K85.82 **Other acute pancreatitis with infected necrosis**

5 K85.9 **Acute pancreatitis, unspecified**
Pancreatitis NOS

SP K85.90 **Acute pancreatitis without necrosis or infection, unspecified**

SP K85.91 **Acute pancreatitis with uninfected necrosis, unspecified**

SP K85.92 **Acute pancreatitis with infected necrosis, unspecified**

4 K86 **Other diseases of pancreas**
EXCLUDES 2   fibrocystic disease of pancreas (E84.-)
islet cell tumor (of pancreas) (D13.7)
pancreatic steatorrhea (K90.3)

SP + K86.0 **Alcohol-induced chronic pancreatitis**
Code also:
exocrine pancreatic insufficiency (K86.81)
Use additional code to identify:
alcohol abuse and dependence (F10.-)
EXCLUDES 2   alcohol induced acute pancreatitis (K85.2-)

CODING TIPS ✓   Assign code K86.0 only when physician documentation clearly confirms chronic pancreatitis due to alcohol use. The appropriate F10 code with 5th and 6th digits .88 should also be added.

SP K86.1 **Other chronic pancreatitis**
Chronic pancreatitis NOS
Infectious chronic pancreatitis
Recurrent chronic pancreatitis
Relapsing chronic pancreatitis
Code also:
exocrine pancreatic insufficiency (K86.81)

SP K86.2 **Cyst of pancreas**

SP K86.3 **Pseudocyst of pancreas**

5 K86.8 **Other specified diseases of pancreas**

SP K86.81 **Exocrine pancreatic insufficiency**

---

4 4th digit required   **5** 5th digit required   **6** 6th digit required   **7** 7th digit required   **7** 7th digit placeholder   **+** Additional code   **⬒** Laterality

1094   *DecisionHealth's* FY 2020 Complete Home Health ICD-10-CM Diagnosis Coding Manual

DEFINITION Insufficient pancreatic secretory functioning causes malfunctioning digestion and the malabsorption of fats in particular, which leads to malnutrition, and associated diseases of nutritional deficiencies. It is common in cystic fibrosis patients. Symptoms include chronic diarrhea or passing foul-smelling, voluminous stools, bloating, abdominal pain and cramping, weight loss, and steatorrhea.

SP K86.89 Other specified diseases of pancreas
Aseptic pancreatic necrosis, unrelated to acute pancreatitis
Atrophy of pancreas
Calculus of pancreas
Cirrhosis of pancreas
Fibrosis of pancreas
Pancreatic fat necrosis, unrelated to acute pancreatitis
Pancreatic infantilism
Pancreatic necrosis NOS, unrelated to acute pancreatitis

IQ K86.9 Disease of pancreas, unspecified

IQ K87 Disorders of gallbladder, biliary tract and pancreas in diseases classified elsewhere
Code first:
underlying disease
EXCLUDES 1 cytomegaloviral pancreatitis (B25.2)
mumps pancreatitis (B26.3)
syphilitic gallbladder (A52.74)
syphilitic pancreas (A52.74)
tuberculosis of gallbladder (A18.83)
tuberculosis of pancreas (A18.83)

Other diseases of the digestive system (K90-K95)

4 K90 Intestinal malabsorption
EXCLUDES 1 intestinal malabsorption following gastrointestinal surgery (K91.2)
CODING TIPS ✓ Do not assign a code from K90.- when malabsorption is reported as post-surgical or post-procedural. Post-procedural / post-surgical complications affecting the gastrointestinal system are coded to category K91.-

SP + K90.0 Celiac disease
Celiac disease with steatorrhea
Celiac gluten-sensitive enteropathy
Nontropical sprue
Code also:
exocrine pancreatic insufficiency (K86.81)
Use additional code for associated disorders including:
dermatitis herpetiformis (L13.0)
gluten ataxia (G32.81)

DEFINITION Malabsorption syndrome precipitated by ingestion of gluten with loss of villous projections of the intestinal mucosa; manifests with bulky, frothy diarrhea, abdominal distention, flatulence, weight loss, and vitamin and electrolyte depletion.

SP K90.1 Tropical sprue
Sprue NOS
Tropical steatorrhea
DEFINITION A malabsorption syndrome occurring in the tropics and subtropics, marked by inflammation of the mucous tissue of the mouth, diarrhea, and anemia.

SP K90.2 Blind loop syndrome, not elsewhere classified
Blind loop syndrome NOS
EXCLUDES 1 congenital blind loop syndrome (Q43.8)
postsurgical blind loop syndrome (K91.2)

SP K90.3 Pancreatic steatorrhea
DEFINITION Insufficient pancreatic enzyme excretions causing severe malabsorption and nutrient deficiencies with loose stools containing unabsorbed fat.

5 K90.4 Other malabsorption due to intolerance
EXCLUDES 2 celiac gluten-sensitive enteropathy (K90.0)
lactose intolerance (E73.-)

SP K90.41 Non-celiac gluten sensitivity
Gluten sensitivity NOS
Non-celiac gluten sensitive enteropathy

SP K90.49 Malabsorption due to intolerance, not elsewhere classified
Malabsorption due to intolerance to carbohydrate
Malabsorption due to intolerance to fat
Malabsorption due to intolerance to protein
Malabsorption due to intolerance to starch

5 K90.8 Other intestinal malabsorption
SP K90.81 Whipple's disease
SP K90.89 Other intestinal malabsorption
SP K90.9 Intestinal malabsorption, unspecified

4 K91 Intraoperative and postprocedural complications and disorders of digestive system, not elsewhere classified
EXCLUDES 2 complications of artificial opening of digestive system (K94.-)
complications of bariatric procedures (K95.-)
gastrojejunal ulcer (K28.-)
postprocedural (radiation) retroperitoneal abscess (K68.11)
radiation colitis (K52.0)
radiation gastroenteritis (K52.0)
radiation proctitis (K62.7)

Chapter 11

K00-K95

★New ▲Revised Px Primary SP PDGM Px SL Low CoM SH High CoM IQ Quest. Encounter H Hospice non-cancer Dx Unspecified M *Manifestation*

DecisionHealth's FY 2020 Complete Home Health ICD-10-CM Diagnosis Coding Manual

1095

CODING TIPS ✓   Intestinal obstruction varies in severity, from partial or intermittent obstruction that resolves without intervention (usually involving small intestine) to complete obstruction that requires surgical intervention and may lead to intestinal gangrene and perforation. Physicians frequently describe intestinal obstruction as partial versus complete. If the obstruction has been surgically treated without complication, an aftercare code (Z48.815) may be appropriate.

CODING TIPS ✓   **Documentation:** Codes in category K91.- are complication codes and require physician documentation and confirmation of a cause-and-effect relationship between the procedure and the complicated condition. Documentation in the home health clinical record must also support this relationship. Gastrointestinal complications that have been resolved by the time the patient is admitted to home care are coded with aftercare codes, e.g. Z48.815.

SP **K91.0** **Vomiting following gastrointestinal surgery**

SP **K91.1** **Postgastric surgery syndromes**
Dumping syndrome
Postgastrectomy syndrome
Postvagotomy syndrome

SP **K91.2** **Postsurgical malabsorption, not elsewhere classified**
Postsurgical blind loop syndrome
EXCLUDES 1   malabsorption osteomalacia in adults (M83.2)
malabsorption osteoporosis, postsurgical (M80.8-, M81.8)

5 **K91.3** **Postprocedural intestinal obstruction**

SP **K91.30** **Postprocedural intestinal obstruction, unspecified as to partial versus complete**
Postprocedural intestinal obstruction NOS

SP **K91.31** **Postprocedural partial intestinal obstruction**
Postprocedural incomplete intestinal obstruction

SP **K91.32** **Postprocedural complete intestinal obstruction**

SP **K91.5** **Postcholecystectomy syndrome**

5 **K91.6** **Intraoperative hemorrhage and hematoma of a digestive system organ or structure complicating a procedure**
EXCLUDES 1   intraoperative hemorrhage and hematoma of a digestive system organ or structure due to accidental puncture and laceration during a procedure (K91.7-)

SP **K91.61** **Intraoperative hemorrhage and hematoma of a digestive system organ or structure complicating a digestive system procedure**

SP **K91.62** **Intraoperative hemorrhage and hematoma of a digestive system organ or structure complicating other procedure**

5 **K91.7** **Accidental puncture and laceration of a digestive system organ or structure during a procedure**

SP **K91.71** **Accidental puncture and laceration of a digestive system organ or structure during a digestive system procedure**

SP **K91.72** **Accidental puncture and laceration of a digestive system organ or structure during other procedure**

5 **K91.8** **Other intraoperative and postprocedural complications and disorders of digestive system**

SP **K91.81** **Other intraoperative complications of digestive system**

SP **K91.82** **Postprocedural hepatic failure**

SP **K91.83** **Postprocedural hepatorenal syndrome**

6 **K91.84** **Postprocedural hemorrhage of a digestive system organ or structure following a procedure**

SP **K91.840** **Postprocedural hemorrhage of a digestive system organ or structure following a digestive system procedure**

SP **K91.841** **Postprocedural hemorrhage of a digestive system organ or structure following other procedure**

6 **K91.85** **Complications of intestinal pouch**

SP **K91.850** **Pouchitis**
Inflammation of internal ileoanal pouch

SP **K91.858** **Other complications of intestinal pouch**

SP **K91.86** **Retained cholelithiasis following cholecystectomy**

6 **K91.87** **Postprocedural hematoma and seroma of a digestive system organ or structure following a procedure**

SP **K91.870** **Postprocedural hematoma of a digestive system organ or structure following a digestive system procedure**

SP **K91.871** **Postprocedural hematoma of a digestive system organ or structure following other procedure**

SP **K91.872** **Postprocedural seroma of a digestive system organ or structure following a digestive system procedure**

SP **K91.873** **Postprocedural seroma of a digestive system organ or structure following other procedure**

SP **+** **K91.89** **Other postprocedural complications and disorders of digestive system**
Use additional code, if applicable, to further specify disorder
EXCLUDES 2   postprocedural retroperitoneal abscess (K68.11)

4 **K92** **Other diseases of digestive system**
EXCLUDES 1   neonatal gastrointestinal hemorrhage (P54.0-P54.3)

4 4th digit required   **5** 5th digit required   **6** 6th digit required   **7** 7th digit required   **7** 7th digit placeholder   **+** Additional code   **⊟** Laterality

1096   *DecisionHealth's* FY 2020 Complete Home Health ICD-10-CM Diagnosis Coding Manual

CODING TIPS ✓ When gastrointestinal bleeds are related to anti-coagulant or anti-platelet use, also code D68.32 and an additional code to identify the drug.

SP K92.0 **Hematemesis**

SP K92.1 **Melena**

> **EXCLUDES 1** occult blood in feces (R19.5)

SP K92.2 **Gastrointestinal hemorrhage, unspecified**

Gastric hemorrhage NOS
Intestinal hemorrhage NOS

> **EXCLUDES 1** acute hemorrhagic gastritis (K29.01)
> hemorrhage of anus and rectum (K62.5)
> angiodysplasia of stomach with hemorrhage (K31.811)
> diverticular disease with hemorrhage (K57.-)
> gastritis and duodenitis with hemorrhage (K29.-)
> peptic ulcer with hemorrhage (K25-K28)

5 K92.8 **Other specified diseases of the digestive system**

SP K92.81 **Gastrointestinal mucositis (ulcerative)**

Code also type of associated therapy, such as:
antineoplastic and immunosuppressive drugs (T45.1X-)
radiological procedure and radiotherapy (Y84.2)

> **EXCLUDES 2** mucositis (ulcerative) of vagina and vulva (N76.81)
> nasal mucositis (ulcerative) (J34.81)
> oral mucositis (ulcerative) (K12.3-)

SP K92.89 **Other specified diseases of the digestive system**

IQ K92.9 **Disease of digestive system, unspecified**

4 K94 **Complications of artificial openings of the digestive system**

> **CODING TIPS ✓** All colostomy, gastrostomy, enterostomy, and esophagostomy complications are coded to category K94.- . This includes excoriation and denuding of the skin surrounding the ostomy, infection of the ostomy site, hemorrhage of the ostomy site, and other complications. No additional code should be used when coding skin complications unless an infection is present, in which case an additional code should be used to specify the infection. When an ostomy complication is present, do not assign a Z code for the ostomy. Z codes indicate routine ostomy care and are not appropriate in the case of a complicated ostomy.

5 K94.0 **Colostomy complications**

IQ K94.00 **Colostomy complication, unspecified**

SP K94.01 **Colostomy hemorrhage**

SP + K94.02 **Colostomy infection**

Use additional code to specify type of infection, such as:
cellulitis of abdominal wall (L03.311)
sepsis (A40.-, A41.-)

> **CODING TIPS ✓** If the patient has cellulitis at the colostomy site, code the infected colostomy followed by cellulitis.

SP K94.03 **Colostomy malfunction**

Mechanical complication of colostomy

> **CODING TIPS ✓** A mechanical complication may include the denuding of the skin around the stoma due to the appliance not fitting a too-small stoma.

SP K94.09 **Other complications of colostomy**

5 K94.1 **Enterostomy complications**

IQ K94.10 **Enterostomy complication, unspecified**

SP K94.11 **Enterostomy hemorrhage**

SP + K94.12 **Enterostomy infection**

Use additional code to specify type of infection, such as:
cellulitis of abdominal wall (L03.311)
sepsis (A40.-, A41.-)

> **CODING TIPS ✓** If the patient has cellulitis at the enterostomy site, code the infected enterostomy followed by cellulitis.

SP K94.13 **Enterostomy malfunction**

Mechanical complication of enterostomy

SP K94.19 **Other complications of enterostomy**

5 K94.2 **Gastrostomy complications**

> **CODING TIPS ✓** Do not use the Z93.1 (status gastrostomy) or Z43.1 (attention to gastrostomy) codes if the gastrostomy is complicated.

IQ K94.20 **Gastrostomy complication, unspecified**

SP K94.21 **Gastrostomy hemorrhage**

SP + K94.22 **Gastrostomy infection**

Use additional code to specify type of infection, such as:
cellulitis of abdominal wall (L03.311)
sepsis (A40.-, A41.-)

> **CODING TIPS ✓** If the patient has cellulitis at the gastrostomy site, code the infected gastrostomy followed by cellulitis.

SP K94.23 **Gastrostomy malfunction**

Mechanical complication of gastrostomy

SP K94.29 **Other complications of gastrostomy**

5 K94.3 **Esophagostomy complications**

IQ K94.30 **Esophagostomy complications, unspecified**

SP K94.31 **Esophagostomy hemorrhage**

SP + K94.32 **Esophagostomy infection**

Use additional code to identify the infection

★ New ▲ Revised Px Primary **SP** PDGM Px **SL** Low CoM **SH** High CoM **IQ** Quest. Encounter **H** Hospice non-cancer Dx **Unspecified** **M** *Manifestation*

DecisionHealth's FY 2020 Complete Home Health ICD-10-CM Diagnosis Coding Manual

1097

CODING TIPS ✓ If the patient has cellulitis at the esophagostomy site, code the infected esophagostomy followed by cellulitis.

SP K94.33 Esophagostomy malfunction
Mechanical complication of esophagostomy

SP K94.39 Other complications of esophagostomy

4 K95 Complications of bariatric procedures

CODING TIPS ✓ Do not use Z98.84 for bariatric surgery status if there is a complication.

CODING TIPS ✓ Documentation: Codes in category K95.- are complication codes and require physician documentation and confirmation of a cause and effect relationship between the procedure and the complicated condition. Documentation in the home health clinical record must also support this relationship. Gastrointestinal complications that have been resolved by the time the patient is admitted to home care are coded with aftercare codes, e.g. Z48.815.

5 K95.0 Complications of gastric band procedure

SP + K95.01 Infection due to gastric band procedure
Use additional code to specify type of infection or organism, such as:
bacterial and viral infectious agents (B95.-, B96.-)
cellulitis of abdominal wall (L03.311)
sepsis (A40.-, A41.-)

SP + K95.09 Other complications of gastric band procedure
Use additional code, if applicable, to further specify complication

5 K95.8 Complications of other bariatric procedure
EXCLUDES 1 complications of gastric band surgery (K95.0-)

SP + K95.81 Infection due to other bariatric procedure
Use additional code to specify type of infection or organism, such as:
bacterial and viral infectious agents (B95.-, B96.-)
cellulitis of abdominal wall (L03.311)
sepsis (A40.-, A41.-)

SP + K95.89 Other complications of other bariatric procedure
Use additional code, if applicable, to further specify complication

Chapter 11 Scenarios: Diseases of the digestive system (K00-K95)

Infection of gastrostomy

The patient has cellulitis of the abdominal wall extending from an infected gastrostomy site. Documentation confirmed the culture growth of Staphylococcus aureus without mention of MRSA from the gastrostomy site. Home health will focus on the infection. The patient is taking a 3-week course of oral antibiotics.

Description	Code
Primary: Infection of gastrostomy	K94.22
Secondary: Cellulitis of abdominal wall	L03.311
Secondary: Methicillin susceptible Staph aureus infection as the cause of diseases classified elsewhere	B95.61
Secondary: Long term (current) use of antibiotics	Z79.2

Notes at K94.22 instruct coders to use an additional code to identify cellulitis of the abdominal wall (L03.311). The Z code for gastrostomy status should not be used when a complication is present. Because the patient will be taking oral antibiotics for three weeks, Z79.2 is also assigned.

Flare of Crohn's disease

The patient was treated in the hospital for a severe flare of her Crohn's disease of the large intestine, with rectal bleeding. She was placed on new medications for the Crohn's disease in the hospital. Home care is ordered for medical management and education on the new medications.

Description	Code
Primary: Crohn's disease of large intestine with rectal bleeding	K50.111

A flare of her Crohn's disease is the focus of care and since she is currently experiencing rectal bleeding, the code K50.111 is used. No codes are needed for the management of the new medications.

Reflux esophagitis

A patient is admitted to home care for medication management and diet teaching for reflux esophagitis. Patient also has Type 1 diabetes and is on an insulin sliding scale.

Description	Code
Primary: Gastro-esophageal reflux disease with esophagitis	K21.0
Secondary: Type 1 diabetes mellitus without complications	E10.9

This is a case where a disease is coded, not medication management. Medication management itself is not a skilled service and should not be coded primary. Teaching and diet is aimed at the esophagitis so that disease is the code that should be assigned. Within the ICD-10 code set, GERD has separate codes that include the presence or absence of esophagitis. Type 1 diabetes is defined by the E10.- category. There is not an instructional note to list insulin and an additional code for the use of insulin should not be included when coding type 1 diabetes as these diabetics are assumed to require insulin.

Abdominal abscess following surgery

A 70-year-old male is referred to home health for care of a retroperitoneal abscess described as a complication of surgery for sigmoid colon cancer six months prior. After his initial surgery, he developed pain and was diagnosed with a retroperitoneal abscess and an open incision and drainage was performed, with a drain now present to the area. The patient remains on a three month course of IV Vancomycin, which the agency will be administering. The history and physical provided reports that he is also diabetic. The record confirms that the colon cancer is eradicated and the surgical wound is healed.

Description	Code
Primary: Postprocedural retroperitoneal abscess	K68.11
Secondary: Type 2 diabetes mellitus without complications	E11.9
Secondary: Encounter for adjustment and management of vascular device	Z45.2
Secondary: Long term (current) use of antibiotics	Z79.2
Secondary: Personal history of other malignant neoplasm of large intestine	Z85.038

In this scenario, the patient has experienced a GI complication following his surgery to remove the neoplasm. The code for a complication specific to any disease process is located in the chapter specific to diseases of that body system within the ICD-10 code set. For that reason, the code for post-procedural retroperitoneal abscess is found within Chapter 11, Diseases of the digestive system. The history of malignant neoplasm of the large intestine (sigmoid colon) should be included, but is coded using a Z code for personal history, as the cancer has been eliminated/removed and the patient is receiving no further treatment for it.

Barrett's esophagus

A patient is admitted to home health for teaching regarding newly diagnosed Barrett's esophagus with low-grade dysplasia.

Description	Code
Primary: Barrett's esophagus with low grade dysplasia	K22.710

There are three separate codes for Barrett's esophagus with dysplasia in ICD-10, depending on the grade of the dysplasia. In this case, K22.710 is the appropriate code choice.

Alcoholic cirrhosis with ascites

A 77-year-old man comes to home health with a diagnosis of alcoholic cirrhosis with ascites. He also has type 2 diabetes. The liver disease is the focus of care. He has a diagnosis of alcoholism but the medical record says it is in remission and he is not continuing to drink.

Description	Code
Primary: Alcoholic cirrhosis of liver with ascites	K70.31
Secondary: Alcohol dependence, in remission	F10.21
Secondary: Type 2 diabetes mellitus without complications	E11.9

The alcoholic cirrhosis is the focus of care and is therefore coded primary. Because he also has ascites, the combination code indicating the presence of ascites is assigned. His alcoholism is documented was documented as in remission, making F10.21 the appropriate code. Diabetes is an important comorbidity that always must be coded when present.

Chronic pancreatitis, exocrine pancreatic insufficiency

A 69-year-old man is admitted to home health for management of chronic pancreatitis, which has caused exocrine pancreatic insufficiency.

Description	Code
Primary: Other chronic pancreatitis	K86.1
Secondary: Exocrine pancreatic insufficiency	K86.81

As the focus of care, chronic pancreatitis is coded in the primary position. Exocrine pancreatic insufficiency is coded next, in accordance with tabular instruction.

Toxic liver injury

A 67-year-old man is admitted to home health with a primary diagnosis of toxic liver disease caused by an unintentional overdose of prescription ibuprofen that he was taking for back pain. He admitted that he had misread the instructions for dosage and had been taking twice the prescribed amount.

Description	Code
Primary: Poisoning by propionic acid derivatives, accidental (unintentional), subsequent encounter	T39.311D
Secondary: Toxic liver disease, unspecified	K71.9
Secondary: Dorsalgia, unspecified	M54.9

The patient's toxic liver disease was caused by an unintentional overdose of prescription ibuprofen. Because he did not take the drug as prescribed, it is considered a poisoning. The poisoning code must be assigned before the code for the toxic liver disease, according to tabular instruction. The reason the patient was taking the drug causing the poisoning is coded after the toxic liver disease, back pain, is coded immediately after.

Ulcerative colitis with intestinal fistula

A 55-year-old woman is admitted to home health with ulcerative colitis that's caused an intestinal fistula. She also has hypertension and anxiety.

Description	Code
Primary: Ulcerative colitis, unspecified with fistula	K51.913
Secondary: Essential (primary) hypertension	I10
Secondary: Anxiety disorder, unspecified	F41.9

The ulcerative colitis has caused a fistula, necessitating the assignment of K51.913. The patient's hypertension and anxiety are comorbidities that have the potential to impact her care and recovery and thus are coded as secondary diagnoses.

Chapter 12: Diseases of the Skin and Subcutaneous Tissue (L00-L99)

Chapter 12 includes conditions of the skin, sweat glands, hair and nails. Among the most common reasons for home health services are the care of skin lesions, surgical wounds and skin ulcers. The ICD-10-CM codes for skin lesions, including ulcers (except vascular ulcers), are found in this chapter. One of the biggest challenges when selecting a code from Chapter 12 is properly defining the type of wound or skin condition. Some common skin conditions, such as boils (carbuncles), rashes, erythema, abscesses (localized collection of pus), sunburns, baldness (alopecia), hives (urticaria), allergic skin reactions, and blisters (bullae) are reported using these codes. Other conditions, such as bed sores (pressure ulcers), cellulitis (acute spreading infection of skin), and acute lymphadenitis are also reported here.

Sometimes, a Chapter 12 code isn't the most appropriate choice. Here are a few situations to watch out for:

- If the documentation indicates **a neoplasm or tumor of the skin or subcutaneous tissues,** coders should look up the term to find the correct code, most likely a code from Chapter 2 (C00-D49). For example, the Alphabetic Index entry for the term "dermatofibrosarcoma" reads "see Neoplasm, skin, malignant," referring the coder to the Neoplasm Table.

- **Venous (stasis) and arterial ulcers** are coded from Chapter 9, Diseases of the Circulatory system. Atherosclerosis of native arteries of the lower extremities are coded within sub-category I70.23, while ulceration associated with various types of bypass grafts are found at I70.3- to I70.73-. Varicose veins of lower extremity with ulcers are coded from category I83 in Chapter 10.

- **Symptoms** related to skin and subcutaneous tissues are reported using codes from either this chapter or Chapter 18. Chapter 12 includes symptom codes, such as itchiness (pruritis, L29.9). Chapter 18 contains the code series R20-R23 (symptoms involving skin and subcutaneous tissue), which include: disturbances of skin sensations; rash and other nonspecific skin eruption; localized swelling; edema; and other skin changes such as cyanosis, flushing, changes in skin texture, etc.

Every effort should be made to secure a definitive diagnosis. A symptom code from chapters 12 or 18 may be reported as an additional diagnosis when it describes a significant aspect of the condition but is not an integral part of it.

- If a patient has **a personal or family history of a condition of the skin or subcutaneous tissues,** it may be appropriate to select from the V code section, such as Z85.82- (Personal history of malignant neoplasm of skin) or Z87.2 (Personal history of diseases of skin and subcutaneous tissue) or Z84.0 (Family history of skin conditions).

- Although not often found in home care, if reporting a **skin disorder that is complicating pregnancy, childbirth or puerperium**, report a code from Chapter 15, such as O99.71-, as the first-listed diagnosis and a code from this chapter as an additional diagnosis.

- Other code categories that are excluded from chapter 12 include: certain conditions originating in the perinatal period (P00-P96); certain infectious and parasitic diseases (A00-B99); congenital malformations, deformations, and chromosomal abnormalities (Q00-Q99); endocrine, nutritional and metabolic diseases (E00-E88); lipomelanotic reticulosis (I89.8); systemic connective tissue disorders (M30-M36) and viral warts (B07.-).

Multiple Coding and Sequencing

It is very important to read the Includes and Excludes notes under codes in this chapter, as well as any other instructions under the code or code category. Many notes refer to Chapter 1 codes (infections and parasitic conditions). Here are some examples of multiple coding and sequencing issues for codes in this chapter:

A note under classifications L00-L08 (infections of the skin and subcutaneous tissue) states: "Use additional code (B95-B97) to identify infectious agent." The first-listed diagnosis is from chapter 12.

Notes under codes in this chapter may refer to other chapters. For example, a note under the code L97.- non-pressure chronic ulcer of lower limb, not elsewhere classified states: "Code first any associated underlying condition, such as: any associated gangrene (I96). Atherosclerosis of the lower extremities (I70.-), chronic venous hypertension (I87.31-, I87.33-), diabetic ulcers, postphlebitic syndrome (I87.01-, I87.03-), and varicose ulcer (I83.0-, I83.2-)". The code from L97.- is listed following the underlying condition to describe the location and depth of the ulcer.

Important: The L97 "code first" note at means "if present, if applicable." However, if you don't know the underlying etiology you should query the physician, as experts believe auditors will be looking for both codes.

Chapter 12

L00 - L99

Special Coding Issues

Cellulitis (code series L03.-) literally means inflammation of cells. The condition indicates an acute, spreading infection of the dermis and subcutaneous tissues resulting in pain, erythema, edema and warmth. Cellulitis may spread by invading contiguous tissue or through the lymphatic and circulatory systems. If an organism is specified, report the appropriate code from Chapter 1 (B95-B96) as an additional diagnosis. If the cellulitis is associated with a wound or an ostomy, the wound or complicated ostomy is generally coded first.

Cellulitis resulting from a colostomy, enterostomy, gastrostomy and esophagostomy are reported with code K94.- in chapter 11 (Diseases of the digestive system), and cellulitis associated with stomas of the urinary tract are coded with N99.5- codes found in chapter 14 (Diseases of the genitourinary system). A code for the cellulitis from chapter 12 and a code for the organism from chapter 1 are listed as additional diagnoses following the ostomy complication code if cellulitis is present in addition to the ostomy complication. If cellulitis is present and is the focus of care around an ostomy, the cellulitis by location is listed first.

Cellulitis can occur in many areas of the body and therefore, codes from the appropriate chapters should be assigned. For example, cellulitis of the pharynx is reported using code J39.1 from Chapter 10. Cellulitis of the eyelid is reported using code H00.03- from Chapter 7.

Dermatitis and Eczema

Dermatitis is any inflammation of the skin. Eczema is a type of dermatitis with inflammation, erythema (redness), bumps (papules, vesicles, pustules), scales, and/or scabs. All eczema is dermatitis, but not all dermatitis is eczema.

However, in ICD-10, categories L20-L30, the terms dermatitis and eczema are used synonymously and interchangeably. When the cause of the condition is related to contact with the skin, consider categories L24.- to L25.- for contact dermatitis. Allergic contact dermatitis is coded at L23.3 and is used when dermatitis is caused by contact with metals, adhesives, cosmetics, drugs, dyes, food, plants, animal dander and other agents in contact with the skin. Assign an additional code for adverse effects, if applicable, to identify drug (T36-T50 with fifth or sixth character 5) found in the Table of Drugs and Chemicals, to indicate the drug that caused the dermatitis and verify the code in the Tabular List. When the cause of the dermatitis or eczema is unspecified, consider L23.9, allergic contact dermatitis/eczema.

Irritant contact dermatitis is coded at category L24.-, unspecified contact dermatitis is coded at category L25.-. Specific codes for all of the types of irritants are listed in L23.

There are many other conditions "not elsewhere classified" (NEC) that also fall under this category.

For example, intertriginous dermatitis is found between two skin surfaces that rub against each other, such as under the breasts, between the toes, or in the skin folds of the groin. Consider L25.8, Unspecified dermatitis due to other agents.

When dermatitis is known to be the result of an ingested substance, consider category L27.-. When an internally taken drug or medicine causes dermatitis, select a code depending on whether the dermatitis is generalized (L27.0) or localized (L27.1), and remember to add an additional code for adverse effect, if applicable to identify the drug (T36-T50 with fifth or sixth character 5). When the ingested causative agent is food, use L27.2. If another specified substance taken internally is the cause, use L27.8. If the substance is unspecified but known to have been taken internally, use L27.9.

Ulcers

Just as the plan of care and progress notes support nursing interventions, the ICD-10-CM codes support medical necessity for the wound management services provided. If the code is absent or inaccurate, a red flag will be raised when the claim is reviewed and payment may ultimately be delayed.

Codes from the L97.- are often listed as manifestations of other conditions, such as diabetes, atherosclerosis and postphlebitic syndrome. The L97.- codes are not manifestations in the true sense of the word; however, causal conditions should precede the L97.- codes.

More than one L97.- code (non-pressure ulcer of the lower limb) may be used on a claim/record to capture the total number of ulcer locations, but remember that the same code may **not** be used twice in the same diagnosis list. In ICD-10-CM, the L97.- codes are combination codes including the location, laterality (right, left) and the depth of the ulcer. For example, a non-pressure ulcer of the right calf with fat layer exposed is coded L97.212 as an additional code following a code for the underlying condition. If there is no code available for bilateral and the patient has ulcers on both calves, a code for both the right and left calf would be assigned. For example, if there was a chronic skin ulcer of the right calf with fat exposure (L97.212) and another chronic skin ulcer on the left calf with breakdown limited to the skin (L97.221), both would be coded. If there was the same underlying cause for the ulcers, that code would be listed first followed by the two ulcer codes. Necrosis must be evident in the muscle or bone to use an L97.- code with a sixth character of "3" (corresponding to muscle necrosis) or "4" (corresponding to bone necrosis). If you can't see it, you can't code it.

If an ulcer is caused by inadequate venous circulation in the area, then it's most likely a **stasis ulcer**. ICD -10-CM codes designated for non-pressure chronic ulcers of lower limb, not elsewhere classified are found in Category L97. To select a code, you must distinguish between **pressure ulcers** and other kinds of ulcers. Note that **varicose ulcers** are found under "**varix**" in the Alphabetical Index and direct the coder to lower leg with ulcer category I83.- by location on the leg. But **stasis ulcers without varicose veins** are coded with a code from I87.2 (venous insufficiency), or if the statement indicates **venous hypertension** – found under hypertension, venous, idiopathic in the Alphabetical Index and at I87.33- in the Tabular).

If caused by poor arterial circulation, consider it an arterial ulcer. If the etiology is diabetes, the ulcer most likely will be coded as a diabetic ulcer.

Arterial ulcers occur when arterial blood flow is compromised. Atherosclerosis of the right leg with ulceration of the ankle limited to skin breakdown is coded I70.233 followed by L97.311. An arterial ulcer on the toes with gangrene due to atherosclerosis is coded I70.26- (Atherosclerosis of the extremities with gangrene), L98.499 (Non-pressure chronic ulcer of skin of other sites with unspecified severity). In this case, the gangrene is part of the I70.262 combination code and is not coded separately.

Remember that not all arterial ulcers are caused by atherosclerosis. Inflammatory diseases including vasculitis, lupus and scleroderma can cause arterial ulcers, as can an arterial thrombus and other conditions. Always query the physician to determine the etiology of the ulcer. For example, an ulcer due to Raynaud's syndrome would be captured by coding first the Raynaud's I73.00, followed by the ulcer code L97.823 (Ulcer of left lower leg with necrosis of muscle).

Diabetic ulcers are coded with the appropriate code for the type of diabetes from E08.62-, E09.62-, E10.62-, E11.62-, or E13.62- followed by the appropriate code from L97.-. If the physician documents an ulcer as the result of diabetic neuropathy, code the diabetic ulcer as E08.49, E09.49, E10.49, E11.49 or E13.49 followed by L97.- to show the location and depth of ulcer.

Peripheral angiopathy includes arterial, venous and capillary conditions. Peripheral angiopathy may be documented as diabetic PVD. There is an assumed relationship between diabetes and PVD and PAD, including peripheral atherosclerosis and venous insufficiency. Diabetic PVD is coded E--.51. Diabetic arteriosclerosis of the peripheral arteries should be coded E--.51 or E--.52 then the appropriate I70.- code. Diabetic venous insufficiency should be coded E--.51 or E--.52 and I87.2 The presence of diabetes and peripheral arterial disease in the record indicates that both diabetes and PVD should be marked in M1028. Venous disease is not included in M1028.

Always confirm the etiology and type of ulcer with the physician.

A **decubitus ulcer** is a **pressure ulcer,** or what is commonly called a "bed sore." Presentations of pressure ulcers range from a deep red coloration of the skin that does not blanche, to a very deep wound extending to and sometimes into the bone.

Remember, that stage 1 pressure ulcers of patients who are not Caucasian may present as an area of hyperpigmentation (darker coloration of the natural skin tone) that doesn't blanche, and not as an area of non-blanchable redness.

Code a diagnosis of "pressure injury" the same way you would code a "pressure ulcer" by site and stage. The term "pressure injury" represents a change in termination and not a change in definition, per Q3 2016 Coding Clinic guidance.

Home health agencies may adopt the NPUAP guidelines in their clinical practice and documentation. When discrepancies exist between the NPUAP definitions and the OASIS scoring instructions provided in the Guidance Manual and CMS Q&As, providers should rely on the CMS OASIS instructions, according to CMS.

To view the WOCN's most recent guidance, visit *https://cdn.ymaws.com/www.wocn.org/resource/ collection/7406B652-D19C-41C7-906C-0578AABC356B/ OASIS-D_Best_Practice_Document__2019_.pdf.* The NPUAP released new pressure ulcer staging definitions in April 2016. *For the NPUAP new definitions visit http:// tinyurl.com/gnvnhvg. View schematic artwork reflecting the changes in stages for pressure injury at http://bit. ly/1p0NMaE.*

Codes from category L89, pressure ulcer, are combination codes that identify the site of the pressure ulcer as well as the stage of the ulcer. For example, you list only **one code** for a stage 4 pressure ulcer of the right ankle – L89.514.

The ICD-10-CM classifies pressure ulcers based on severity, which is designated by stages 1 - 4, pressure-induced deep tissue damage, unspecified stage, and unstageable. Assign as many codes from category L89 as needed to identify all the pressure ulcers a patient has, if applicable.

Assignment of the code for unstageable pressure ulcer (L89.xx0) should be based on the clinical documentation. These codes are used for pressure ulcers whose stage cannot be clinically determined (e.g., the pressure ulcer is covered by eschar or has been treated with a skin or muscle graft.) This code should not be confused with codes for unspecified stage.

Assignment of the pressure ulcer stage code should be guided by clinical documentation of the stage or documentation of the terms found in the Alphabetical Index. For clinical terms describing the stage that are not found in the Alphabetical Index and when there is no documentation of the stage, you should query the physician.

No code is assigned if the documentation states the pressure ulcer is completely healed. However, pressure ulcers described as "healing" should be assigned the appropriate pressure ulcer stage code

Chapter 12

L00 - L99

based on the documentation in the medical record. If the documentation does not provide information about the stage of the healing pressure ulcer, assign the appropriate code for unspecified stage (L89.899).

If the documentation is unclear about whether the patient has a current pressure ulcer or if the patient is being treated for a healing pressure ulcer, query the physician.

If a patient is admitted with a pressure ulcer at one stage and it progresses to a worse stage, assign the code for the worse stage reported for that site.

CHAPTER 12: DISEASES OF THE SKIN AND SUBCUTANEOUS TISSUE (L00-L99)

EXCLUDES 2 certain conditions originating in the perinatal period (P04-P96)

certain infectious and parasitic diseases (A00-B99)

complications of pregnancy, childbirth and the puerperium (O00-O9A)

congenital malformations, deformations, and chromosomal abnormalities (Q00-Q99)

endocrine, nutritional and metabolic diseases (E00-E88)

lipomelanotic reticulosis (I89.8)

neoplasms (C00-D49)

symptoms, signs and abnormal clinical and laboratory findings, not elsewhere classified (R00-R94)

systemic connective tissue disorders (M30-M36)

viral warts (B07.-)

This chapter contains the following blocks:

L00-L08	Infections of the skin and subcutaneous tissue
L10-L14	Bullous disorders
L20-L30	Dermatitis and eczema
L40-L45	Papulosquamous disorders
L49-L54	Urticaria and erythema
L55-L59	Radiation-related disorders of the skin and subcutaneous tissue
L60-L75	Disorders of skin appendages
L76	Intraoperative and postprocedural complications of skin and subcutaneous tissue
L80-L99	Other disorders of the skin and subcutaneous tissue

Infections of the skin and subcutaneous tissue (L00-L08)

Use additional code (B95-B97) to identify infectious agent.

EXCLUDES 2 hordeolum (H00.0)

infective dermatitis (L30.3)

local infections of skin classified in Chapter 1

lupus panniculitis (L93.2)

panniculitis NOS (M79.3)

panniculitis of neck and back (M54.0-)

Perlèche NOS (K13.0)

Perlèche due to candidiasis (B37.0)

Perlèche due to riboflavin deficiency (E53.0)

pyogenic granuloma (L98.0)

relapsing panniculitis [Weber-Christian] (M35.6)

viral warts (B07.-)

zoster (B02.-)

SP ✚ **L00 Staphylococcal scalded skin syndrome**
Ritter's disease

Use additional code to identify percentage of skin exfoliation (L49.-)

EXCLUDES 1 bullous impetigo (L01.03)
pemphigus neonatorum (L01.03)
toxic epidermal necrolysis [Lyell] (L51.2)

DEFINITION The breakdown of dermal layer cellular structure by staph bacteria causing large sections of skin to slough off and peel away, leaving raw, exposed areas.

4 **L01 Impetigo**
EXCLUDES 1 impetigo herpetiformis (L40.1)

5 **L01.0 Impetigo**
Impetigo contagiosa
Impetigo vulgaris

DEFINITION Bacterial skin infection in children; small pustules form over a reddish rash and burst, leaving an itchy, yellow crust over the affected area.

SP **L01.00 Impetigo, unspecified**
Impetigo NOS

SP **L01.01 Non-bullous impetigo**
DEFINITION Most common type of impetigo due to staph or strep bacteria, in which tiny blisters form (particularly on the face), burst quickly, and leave a small, wet, weeping spot that crusts over and disappears, leaving a red mark that later heals.

SP **L01.02 Bockhart's impetigo**
Impetigo follicularis
Perifolliculitis NOS
Superficial pustular perifolliculitis
DEFINITION Superficial, pustular folliculitis caused by *S. aureus*; characterized by small, painful, tense, yellowish-white domed pustules in crops around follicular orifices that heal in a few days.

SP **L01.03 Bullous impetigo**
Impetigo neonatorum
Pemphigus neonatorum
DEFINITION Impetigo of longer duration (generally due to *S. aureus*), in which large, clear, fluid-filled blisters form on red sores, become cloudy, then burst and ooze, leaving a large, yellowish, crusty scab.

SP **L01.09 Other impetigo**
Ulcerative impetigo
DEFINITION Ulcerative impetigo: A deeper dermis form of impetigo with small, shallow, purulent ulcers that form under a thick, brownish-black crusted surface infection, surrounded by erythema.

SP **L01.1 Impetiginization of other dermatoses**
DEFINITION Impetigo occurring in an area already experiencing a dermatosis; the infected blisters burst, leaving a weeping wet patch that crusts over, worsening the existing condition.

✚ **4** **L02 Cutaneous abscess, furuncle and carbuncle**
Use additional code to identify organism (B95-B96)
EXCLUDES 2 abscess of anus and rectal regions (K61.-)
abscess of female genital organs (external) (N76.4)
abscess of male genital organs (external) (N48.2, N49.-)
CODING TIPS ✓ Abscesses are infected by definition. An aftercare following surgery code is not usually appropriate when an infection is being treated by incision and drainage and/or antibiotics.

Chapter 12

L00-L99

★ New ▲ Revised **Px** Primary **SP** PDGM Px **SL** Low CoM **SH** High CoM **IQ** Quest. Encounter **H** Hospice non-cancer Dx Unspecified **M** *Manifestation*

DecisionHealth's FY 2020 Complete Home Health ICD-10-CM Diagnosis Coding Manual

1107

CODING TIPS ✓ Abscesses, carbuncles and furuncles are coded separately from cellulitis (L03). Furuncles are commonly known as boils. Use an additional code to identify the causative organism.

DEFINITION Furuncle: A bacterial infection of a hair follicle characterized by a painful, red, swollen bump filled with fluid, pus, and cellular debris; also called a boil.

DEFINITION Carbuncle: A group of several infected hair follicles, or furuncles, that join together with more than one opening to drain pus, often extending into deeper tissue.

DEFINITION Abscess: A pocket of pus that collects within an infected area of skin and is generally red and sore.

+ 5 L02.0 Cutaneous abscess, furuncle and carbuncle of face
> **EXCLUDES 2** abscess of ear, external (H60.0)
> abscess of eyelid (H00.0)
> abscess of head [any part, except face] (L02.8)
> abscess of lacrimal gland (H04.0)
> abscess of lacrimal passages (H04.3)
> abscess of mouth (K12.2)
> abscess of nose (J34.0)
> abscess of orbit (H05.0)
> submandibular abscess (K12.2)

SP + L02.01 Cutaneous abscess of face

SP + L02.02 Furuncle of face
> Boil of face
> Folliculitis of face

SP + L02.03 Carbuncle of face

+ 5 L02.1 Cutaneous abscess, furuncle and carbuncle of neck

SP SH SL + L02.11 Cutaneous abscess of neck

SP + L02.12 Furuncle of neck
> Boil of neck
> Folliculitis of neck

SP + L02.13 Carbuncle of neck

+ 5 L02.2 Cutaneous abscess, furuncle and carbuncle of trunk
> **EXCLUDES 1** non-newborn omphalitis (L08.82)
> omphalitis of newborn (P38.-)
> **EXCLUDES 2** abscess of breast (N61.1)
> abscess of buttocks (L02.3)
> abscess of female external genital organs (N76.4)
> abscess of male external genital organs (N48.2, N49.-)
> abscess of hip (L02.4)

+ 6 L02.21 Cutaneous abscess of trunk

SP SH SL + L02.211 Cutaneous abscess of abdominal wall

SP SH SL + L02.212 Cutaneous abscess of back [any part, except buttock]

SP SH SL + L02.213 Cutaneous abscess of chest wall

SP SH SL + L02.214 Cutaneous abscess of groin

SP SH SL + L02.215 Cutaneous abscess of perineum

SP SH SL + L02.216 Cutaneous abscess of umbilicus

SP SH SL + L02.219 Cutaneous abscess of trunk, unspecified

+ 6 L02.22 Furuncle of trunk
> Boil of trunk
> Folliculitis of trunk

SP + L02.221 Furuncle of abdominal wall

SP + L02.222 Furuncle of back [any part, except buttock]

SP + L02.223 Furuncle of chest wall

SP + L02.224 Furuncle of groin

SP + L02.225 Furuncle of perineum

SP + L02.226 Furuncle of umbilicus

SP + L02.229 Furuncle of trunk, unspecified

+ 6 L02.23 Carbuncle of trunk

SP + L02.231 Carbuncle of abdominal wall

SP + L02.232 Carbuncle of back [any part, except buttock]

SP + L02.233 Carbuncle of chest wall

SP + L02.234 Carbuncle of groin

SP + L02.235 Carbuncle of perineum

SP + L02.236 Carbuncle of umbilicus

SP + L02.239 Carbuncle of trunk, unspecified

+ 5 L02.3 Cutaneous abscess, furuncle and carbuncle of buttock
> **EXCLUDES 1** pilonidal cyst with abscess (L05.01)

SP SH SL + L02.31 Cutaneous abscess of buttock
> Cutaneous abscess of gluteal region

SP + L02.32 Furuncle of buttock
> Boil of buttock
> Folliculitis of buttock
> Furuncle of gluteal region

SP + L02.33 Carbuncle of buttock
> Carbuncle of gluteal region

+ 5 L02.4 Cutaneous abscess, furuncle and carbuncle of limb
> **EXCLUDES 2** Cutaneous abscess, furuncle and carbuncle of groin (L02.214, L02.224, L02.234)
> Cutaneous abscess, furuncle and carbuncle of hand (L02.5-)
> Cutaneous abscess, furuncle and carbuncle of foot (L02.6-)

+ 6 L02.41 Cutaneous abscess of limb

⊟ SP SH SL + L02.411 Cutaneous abscess of right axilla

⊟ SP SH SL + L02.412 Cutaneous abscess of left axilla

⊟ SP SH SL + L02.413 Cutaneous abscess of right upper limb

⊟ SP SH SL + L02.414 Cutaneous abscess of left upper limb

⊟ SP SH SL + L02.415 Cutaneous abscess of right lower limb

⊟ SP SH SL + L02.416 Cutaneous abscess of left lower limb

⊟ IQ + L02.419 Cutaneous abscess of limb, unspecified

+ 6 L02.42 Furuncle of limb
> Boil of limb
> Folliculitis of limb

⊟ SP + L02.421 Furuncle of right axilla

4 4th digit required   **5** 5th digit required   **6** 6th digit required   **7** 7th digit required   **7** 7th digit placeholder   **+** Additional code   **⊟** Laterality

1108   *DecisionHealth's* FY 2020 Complete Home Health ICD-10-CM Diagnosis Coding Manual

⊟ SP ✚ **L02.422** Furuncle of left axilla

⊟ SP ✚ **L02.423** Furuncle of right upper limb

⊟ SP ✚ **L02.424** Furuncle of left upper limb

⊟ SP ✚ **L02.425** Furuncle of right lower limb

⊟ SP ✚ **L02.426** Furuncle of left lower limb

⊟ IQ ✚ **L02.429** Furuncle of limb, unspecified

✚ 6 **L02.43** Carbuncle of limb

⊟ SP ✚ **L02.431** Carbuncle of right axilla

⊟ SP ✚ **L02.432** Carbuncle of left axilla

⊟ SP ✚ **L02.433** Carbuncle of right upper limb

⊟ SP ✚ **L02.434** Carbuncle of left upper limb

⊟ SP ✚ **L02.435** Carbuncle of right lower limb

⊟ SP ✚ **L02.436** Carbuncle of left lower limb

⊟ IQ ✚ **L02.439** Carbuncle of limb, unspecified

✚ 5 **L02.5** Cutaneous abscess, furuncle and carbuncle of hand

✚ 6 **L02.51** Cutaneous abscess of hand

⊟ SP SH SL ✚ **L02.511** Cutaneous abscess of right hand

⊟ SP SH SL ✚ **L02.512** Cutaneous abscess of left hand

⊟ IQ ✚ **L02.519** Cutaneous abscess of unspecified hand

✚ 6 **L02.52** Furuncle hand
Boil of hand
Folliculitis of hand

⊟ SP ✚ **L02.521** Furuncle right hand

⊟ SP ✚ **L02.522** Furuncle left hand

⊟ IQ ✚ **L02.529** Furuncle unspecified hand

✚ 6 **L02.53** Carbuncle of hand

⊟ SP ✚ **L02.531** Carbuncle of right hand

⊟ SP ✚ **L02.532** Carbuncle of left hand

⊟ IQ ✚ **L02.539** Carbuncle of unspecified hand

✚ 5 **L02.6** Cutaneous abscess, furuncle and carbuncle of foot

✚ 6 **L02.61** Cutaneous abscess of foot

⊟ SP SH SL ✚ **L02.611** Cutaneous abscess of right foot

⊟ SP SH SL ✚ **L02.612** Cutaneous abscess of left foot

⊟ IQ ✚ **L02.619** Cutaneous abscess of unspecified foot

✚ 6 **L02.62** Furuncle of foot
Boil of foot
Folliculitis of foot

⊟ SP ✚ **L02.621** Furuncle of right foot

⊟ SP ✚ **L02.622** Furuncle of left foot

⊟ IQ ✚ **L02.629** Furuncle of unspecified foot

✚ 6 **L02.63** Carbuncle of foot

⊟ SP ✚ **L02.631** Carbuncle of right foot

⊟ SP ✚ **L02.632** Carbuncle of left foot

⊟ IQ ✚ **L02.639** Carbuncle of unspecified foot

✚ 5 **L02.8** Cutaneous abscess, furuncle and carbuncle of other sites

✚ 6 **L02.81** Cutaneous abscess of other sites

SP SH SL ✚ **L02.811** Cutaneous abscess of head [any part, except face]

SP SH SL ✚ **L02.818** Cutaneous abscess of other sites

✚ 6 **L02.82** Furuncle of other sites
Boil of other sites
Folliculitis of other sites

SP ✚ **L02.821** Furuncle of head [any part, except face]

SP ✚ **L02.828** Furuncle of other sites

✚ 6 **L02.83** Carbuncle of other sites

SP ✚ **L02.831** Carbuncle of head [any part, except face]

SP ✚ **L02.838** Carbuncle of other sites

✚ 5 **L02.9** Cutaneous abscess, furuncle and carbuncle, unspecified

IQ ✚ **L02.91** Cutaneous abscess, unspecified

IQ ✚ **L02.92** Furuncle, unspecified
Boil NOS
Furunculosis NOS

IQ ✚ **L02.93** Carbuncle, unspecified

4 **L03** Cellulitis and acute lymphangitis

EXCLUDES 2 cellulitis of anal and rectal region (K61.-)
cellulitis of external auditory canal (H60.1)
cellulitis of eyelid (H00.0)
cellulitis of female external genital organs (N76.4)
cellulitis of lacrimal apparatus (H04.3)
cellulitis of male external genital organs (N48.2, N49.-)
cellulitis of mouth (K12.2)
cellulitis of nose (J34.0)
eosinophilic cellulitis [Wells] (L98.3)
febrile neutrophilic dermatosis [Sweet] (L98.2)
lymphangitis (chronic) (subacute) (I89.1)

CODING TIPS ✓ L03 includes codes for cellulitis. When diagnostic statements indicate abscess, a code from L02 should be coded.

CODING TIPS ✓ Cellulitis usually presents as an abrupt onset of redness, swelling, pain, or heat in the affected area. Unless a diagnosis of cellulitis is documented by the physician, a code from category L03 should not be assigned. If cellulitis is associated with a wound or ostomy, code the wound or complicated ostomy first, followed by the appropriate L03 code for cellulitis.

DEFINITION Acute lymphangitis: A quickly spreading bacterial infection of the lymph vessels appearing as painful, red streaks visible through the skin surface.

DEFINITION Cellulitis: A spreading bacterial infection of connective soft tissue extending into deep dermal and subcutaneous layers; produces circumscribed swelling, fever, and swollen lymph nodes.

5 **L03.0** Cellulitis and acute lymphangitis of finger and toe
Infection of nail
Onychia
Paronychia
Perionychia

6 **L03.01** Cellulitis of finger
Felon
Whitlow
EXCLUDES 1 herpetic whitlow (B00.89)

⊟ SP **L03.011** Cellulitis of right finger

★ New ▲ Revised Px Primary SP PDGM Px SL Low CoM SH High CoM IQ Quest. Encounter H Hospice non-cancer Dx Unspecified M *Manifestation*

DecisionHealth's FY 2020 Complete Home Health ICD-10-CM Diagnosis Coding Manual

1109

🄴 **SP** L03.012   **Cellulitis of left finger**

🄴 **IQ** L03.019   **Cellulitis of unspecified finger**

🄶 L03.02   **Acute lymphangitis of finger**
Hangnail with lymphangitis of finger

🄴 **SP** L03.021   **Acute lymphangitis of right finger**

🄴 **SP** L03.022   **Acute lymphangitis of left finger**

🄴 **IQ** L03.029   **Acute lymphangitis of unspecified finger**

🄶 L03.03   **Cellulitis of toe**

🄴 **SP** L03.031   **Cellulitis of right toe**

🄴 **SP** L03.032   **Cellulitis of left toe**

🄴 **IQ** L03.039   **Cellulitis of unspecified toe**

🄶 L03.04   **Acute lymphangitis of toe**
Hangnail with lymphangitis of toe

🄴 **SP** L03.041   **Acute lymphangitis of right toe**

🄴 **SP** L03.042   **Acute lymphangitis of left toe**

🄴 **IQ** L03.049   **Acute lymphangitis of unspecified toe**

🄵 L03.1   **Cellulitis and acute lymphangitis of other parts of limb**

🄶 L03.11   **Cellulitis of other parts of limb**
EXCLUDES 2   cellulitis of fingers (L03.01-)
cellulitis of toes (L03.03-)
groin (L03.314)

🄴 **SP SH SL** L03.111   **Cellulitis of right axilla**

🄴 **SP SH SL** L03.112   **Cellulitis of left axilla**

🄴 **SP SH SL** L03.113   **Cellulitis of right upper limb**

🄴 **SP SH SL** L03.114   **Cellulitis of left upper limb**

🄴 **SP SH SL** L03.115   **Cellulitis of right lower limb**

🄴 **SP SH SL** L03.116   **Cellulitis of left lower limb**

🄴 **IQ** L03.119   **Cellulitis of unspecified part of limb**

🄶 L03.12   **Acute lymphangitis of other parts of limb**
EXCLUDES 2   acute lymphangitis of fingers (L03.2-)
acute lymphangitis of toes (L03.04-)
acute lymphangitis of groin (L03.324)

🄴 **SP SH SL** L03.121   **Acute lymphangitis of right axilla**

🄴 **SP SH SL** L03.122   **Acute lymphangitis of left axilla**

🄴 **SP SH SL** L03.123   **Acute lymphangitis of right upper limb**

🄴 **SP SH SL** L03.124   **Acute lymphangitis of left upper limb**

🄴 **SP SH SL** L03.125   **Acute lymphangitis of right lower limb**

🄴 **SP SH SL** L03.126   **Acute lymphangitis of left lower limb**

🄴 **IQ** L03.129   **Acute lymphangitis of unspecified part of limb**

🄵 L03.2   **Cellulitis and acute lymphangitis of face and neck**

🄶 L03.21   **Cellulitis and acute lymphangitis of face**

SP L03.211   **Cellulitis of face**
EXCLUDES 2   abscess of orbit (H05.01-)
cellulitis of ear (H60.1-)

cellulitis of eyelid (H00.0-)
cellulitis of head (L03.81)
cellulitis of lacrimal apparatus (H04.3)
cellulitis of lip (K13.0)
cellulitis of mouth (K12.2)
cellulitis of nose (internal) (J34.0)
cellulitis of orbit (H05.01-)
cellulitis of scalp (L03.81)

SP L03.212   **Acute lymphangitis of face**

SP L03.213   **Periorbital cellulitis**
Preseptal cellulitis

🄶 L03.22   **Cellulitis and acute lymphangitis of neck**

SP SH SL L03.221   **Cellulitis of neck**

SP SH SL L03.222   **Acute lymphangitis of neck**

🄵 L03.3   **Cellulitis and acute lymphangitis of trunk**

🄶 L03.31   **Cellulitis of trunk**
EXCLUDES 2   cellulitis of anal and rectal regions (K61.-)
cellulitis of breast NOS (N61.0)
cellulitis of female external genital organs (N76.4)
cellulitis of male external genital organs (N48.2, N49.-)
omphalitis of newborn (P38.-)
puerperal cellulitis of breast (O91.2)

SP SH SL L03.311   **Cellulitis of abdominal wall**
EXCLUDES 2   cellulitis of umbilicus (L03.316)
cellulitis of groin (L03.314)

SP SH SL L03.312   **Cellulitis of back [any part except buttock]**

SP SH SL L03.313   **Cellulitis of chest wall**

SP SH SL L03.314   **Cellulitis of groin**

SP SH SL L03.315   **Cellulitis of perineum**

SP SH SL L03.316   **Cellulitis of umbilicus**

SP SH SL L03.317   **Cellulitis of buttock**

SP SH SL L03.319   **Cellulitis of trunk, unspecified**

🄶 L03.32   **Acute lymphangitis of trunk**

SP SH SL L03.321   **Acute lymphangitis of abdominal wall**

SP SH SL L03.322   **Acute lymphangitis of back [any part except buttock]**

SP SH SL L03.323   **Acute lymphangitis of chest wall**

SP SH SL L03.324   **Acute lymphangitis of groin**

SP SH SL L03.325   **Acute lymphangitis of perineum**

SP SH SL L03.326   **Acute lymphangitis of umbilicus**

SP SH SL L03.327   **Acute lymphangitis of buttock**

SP SH SL L03.329   **Acute lymphangitis of trunk, unspecified**

🄴4th digit required   🄵5th digit required   🄶6th digit required   🄷7th digit required   🄼7th digit placeholder   ➕Additional code   🄴Laterality

⑤ L03.8 Cellulitis and acute lymphangitis of other sites

⑥ L03.81 Cellulitis of other sites

SP SH SL L03.811 Cellulitis of head [any part, except face]
Cellulitis of scalp
EXCLUDES 2 cellulitis of face (L03.211)

SP SH SL L03.818 Cellulitis of other sites

⑥ L03.89 Acute lymphangitis of other sites

SP SH SL L03.891 Acute lymphangitis of head [any part, except face]

SP SH SL L03.898 Acute lymphangitis of other sites

⑤ L03.9 Cellulitis and acute lymphangitis, unspecified

IQ L03.90 Cellulitis, unspecified

IQ L03.91 Acute lymphangitis, unspecified
EXCLUDES 1 lymphangitis NOS (I89.1)

④ L04 Acute lymphadenitis
INCLUDES abscess (acute) of lymph nodes, except mesenteric
acute lymphadenitis, except mesenteric
EXCLUDES 1 chronic or subacute lymphadenitis, except mesenteric (I88.1)
enlarged lymph nodes (R59.-)
human immunodeficiency virus [HIV] disease resulting in generalized lymphadenopathy (B20)
lymphadenitis NOS (I88.9)
nonspecific mesenteric lymphadenitis (I88.0)

SP L04.0 Acute lymphadenitis of face, head and neck

SP L04.1 Acute lymphadenitis of trunk

SP L04.2 Acute lymphadenitis of upper limb
Acute lymphadenitis of axilla
Acute lymphadenitis of shoulder

SP L04.3 Acute lymphadenitis of lower limb
Acute lymphadenitis of hip
EXCLUDES 2 acute lymphadenitis of groin (L04.1)

SP L04.8 Acute lymphadenitis of other sites

IQ L04.9 Acute lymphadenitis, unspecified

④ L05 Pilonidal cyst and sinus

⑤ L05.0 Pilonidal cyst and sinus with abscess
DEFINITION An abscessed sinus tract draining to the surface and located in the tailbone area, often associated with ingrown hairs.

SP L05.01 Pilonidal cyst with abscess
Pilonidal abscess
Pilonidal dimple with abscess
Postanal dimple with abscess
EXCLUDES 2 congenital sacral dimple (Q82.6)
parasacral dimple (Q82.6)

SP L05.02 Pilonidal sinus with abscess
Coccygeal fistula with abscess
Coccygeal sinus with abscess
Pilonidal fistula with abscess

⑤ L05.9 Pilonidal cyst and sinus without abscess

SP L05.91 Pilonidal cyst without abscess
Pilonidal dimple
Postanal dimple
Pilonidal cyst NOS
EXCLUDES 2 congenital sacral dimple (Q82.6)
parasacral dimple (Q82.6)

SP L05.92 Pilonidal sinus without abscess
Coccygeal fistula
Coccygeal sinus without abscess
Pilonidal fistula

④ L08 Other local infections of skin and subcutaneous tissue

SP L08.0 Pyoderma
Dermatitis gangrenosa
Purulent dermatitis
Septic dermatitis
Suppurative dermatitis
EXCLUDES 1 pyoderma gangrenosum (L88)
pyoderma vegetans (L08.81)
CODING TIPS ✓ Do not assign L08.0 to indicate pyoderma gangrenosum, which is a specific disorder resulting in deep, ulcerative, necrotic ulcers. Pyoderma gangrenosum should be coded to L88 when specified.
DEFINITION A skin condition producing pus.

SP L08.1 Erythrasma
DEFINITION Skin infection caused by Corynebacterium minutissimum in which pink-red patches with fine scales and wrinkling appear in perpetually moist skin folds (intergluteal fold, inframammary fold, armpits, groin) and later turn brown and scaly.

⑤ L08.8 Other specified local infections of the skin and subcutaneous tissue

SP L08.81 Pyoderma vegetans
EXCLUDES 1 pyoderma gangrenosum (L88)
pyoderma NOS (L08.0)

SP L08.82 Omphalitis not of newborn
EXCLUDES 1 omphalitis of newborn (P38.-)

SP L08.89 Other specified local infections of the skin and subcutaneous tissue

SP L08.9 Local infection of the skin and subcutaneous tissue, unspecified

Bullous disorders (L10-L14)

EXCLUDES 1 benign familial pemphigus [Hailey-Hailey] (Q82.8)
staphylococcal scalded skin syndrome (L00)
toxic epidermal necrolysis [Lyell] (L51.2)

④ L10 Pemphigus
EXCLUDES 1 pemphigus neonatorum (L01.03)

SP L10.0 Pemphigus vulgaris

SP L10.1 Pemphigus vegetans

SP L10.2 Pemphigus foliaceous

SP L10.3 Brazilian pemphigus [fogo selvagem]

Chapter 12

L00-L99

★ New ▲ Revised Px Primary SP PDGM Px SL Low CoM SH High CoM IQ Quest. Encounter H Hospice non-cancer Dx ▨ Unspecified M *Manifestation*

DecisionHealth's FY 2020 Complete Home Health ICD-10-CM Diagnosis Coding Manual
1111

SP **L10.4** **Pemphigus erythematosus**
Senear-Usher syndrome

SP + **L10.5** **Drug-induced pemphigus**
Use additional code for adverse effect, if applicable, to identify drug (T36-T50 with fifth or sixth character 5)

CODING TIPS ✓ Code L10.5 should only be assigned when documentation clearly indicates a relationship between pemphigus and a drug or chemical as the underlying cause. Assign a code from T36-T50 following L10.5 to indicate the drug and adverse effect.

5 **L10.8** **Other pemphigus**

SP **L10.81** **Paraneoplastic pemphigus**

SP **L10.89** **Other pemphigus**

SP **L10.9** **Pemphigus, unspecified**

4 **L11** **Other acantholytic disorders**

SP **L11.0** **Acquired keratosis follicularis**
EXCLUDES 1 keratosis follicularis (congenital) [Darier-White] (Q82.8)

SP **L11.1** **Transient acantholytic dermatosis [Grover]**

SP **L11.8** **Other specified acantholytic disorders**

SP **L11.9** **Acantholytic disorder, unspecified**

4 **L12** **Pemphigoid**
EXCLUDES 1 herpes gestationis (O26.4-) impetigo herpetiformis (L40.1)

SP **L12.0** **Bullous pemphigoid**

SP **L12.1** **Cicatricial pemphigoid**
Benign mucous membrane pemphigoid

SP **L12.2** **Chronic bullous disease of childhood**
Juvenile dermatitis herpetiformis

5 **L12.3** **Acquired epidermolysis bullosa**
EXCLUDES 1 epidermolysis bullosa (congenital) (Q81.-)

SP **L12.30** **Acquired epidermolysis bullosa, unspecified**

SP + **L12.31** **Epidermolysis bullosa due to drug**
Use additional code for adverse effect, if applicable, to identify drug (T36-T50 with fifth or sixth character 5)

SP **L12.35** **Other acquired epidermolysis bullosa**

SP **L12.8** **Other pemphigoid**

SP **L12.9** **Pemphigoid, unspecified**

4 **L13** **Other bullous disorders**

SP **L13.0** **Dermatitis herpetiformis**
Duhring's disease
Hydroa herpetiformis
EXCLUDES 1 juvenile dermatitis herpetiformis (L12.2) senile dermatitis herpetiformis (L12.0)

DEFINITION Chronic skin disease that can persist indefinitely, characterized by intensely itchy, symmetrical excoriations on the elbows, knees, lower back, buttocks, and shoulders, often accompanied by burning and stinging hours before an eruption.

SP **L13.1** **Subcorneal pustular dermatitis**
Sneddon-Wilkinson disease

SP **L13.8** **Other specified bullous disorders**

SP **L13.9** **Bullous disorder, unspecified**

IQ **L14** **Bullous disorders in diseases classified elsewhere**
Code first:
underlying disease

Dermatitis and eczema   (L20-L30)

Note:
In this block the terms dermatitis and eczema are used synonymously and interchangeably.
EXCLUDES 2 chronic (childhood) granulomatous disease (D71)
dermatitis gangrenosa (L08.0)
dermatitis herpetiformis (L13.0)
dry skin dermatitis (L85.3)
factitial dermatitis (L98.1)
perioral dermatitis (L71.0)
radiation-related disorders of the skin and subcutaneous tissue (L55-L59)
stasis dermatitis (I87.2)
CODING TIPS ✓ Dermatitis is also referred to as 'rash.'

4 **L20** **Atopic dermatitis**

SP **L20.0** **Besnier's prurigo**

5 **L20.8** **Other atopic dermatitis**
EXCLUDES 2 circumscribed neurodermatitis (L28.0)

SP **L20.81** **Atopic neurodermatitis**
Diffuse neurodermatitis

SP **L20.82** **Flexural eczema**

SP **L20.83** **Infantile (acute) (chronic) eczema**

SP **L20.84** **Intrinsic (allergic) eczema**

SP **L20.89** **Other atopic dermatitis**

SP **L20.9** **Atopic dermatitis, unspecified**

4 **L21** **Seborrheic dermatitis**
EXCLUDES 2 infective dermatitis (L30.3)
seborrheic keratosis (L82.-)

SP **L21.0** **Seborrhea capitis**
Cradle cap
DEFINITION Inflammatory skin rash on the scalp of infants, characterized by flaky or scaly skin with redness.

SP **L21.1** **Seborrheic infantile dermatitis**

SP **L21.8** **Other seborrheic dermatitis**

SP **L21.9** **Seborrheic dermatitis, unspecified**
Seborrhea NOS
DEFINITION Overactivity of the sebaceous (fat) glands, resulting in an inflammatory skin rash.

SP **L22** **Diaper dermatitis**
Diaper erythema
Diaper rash
Psoriasiform diaper rash

4 **L23** **Allergic contact dermatitis**
EXCLUDES 1 allergy NOS (T78.40)
contact dermatitis NOS (L25.9)
dermatitis NOS (L30.9)
EXCLUDES 2 dermatitis due to substances taken internally (L27.-)
dermatitis of eyelid (H01.1-)
diaper dermatitis (L22)
eczema of external ear (H60.5-)
irritant contact dermatitis (L24.-)
perioral dermatitis (L71.0)

4 4th digit required   **5** 5th digit required   **6** 6th digit required   **7** 7th digit required   **7** 7th digit placeholder   **+** Additional code   **=** Laterality

1112   *DecisionHealth's* FY 2020 Complete Home Health ICD-10-CM Diagnosis Coding Manual

radiation-related disorders of the skin and subcutaneous tissue (L55-L59)

CODING TIPS ✓ Do not assign a code from L23 to report a skin reaction or allergy due to drugs or other medications that are ingested (internally). A code from category L27 should be assigned to indicate a skin reaction or allergy due to drugs or other medications ingested internally (with an additional code from T36-T50 assigned to indicate the adverse effect and specific drug).

CODING TIPS ✓ Contact dermatitis indicates that the inflammation of the skin is related to contact with a substance. The specific causative substance that resulted in the condition should be documented and the plan of care should include appropriate interventions for skin care and instruction on prevention of contact with irritants. If the patient had contact with substances and had a non-allergic type reaction, see L24.

DEFINITION Inflammation of the skin upon contact with an allergen, due to hypersensitization.

SP L23.0 Allergic contact dermatitis due to metals
Allergic contact dermatitis due to chromium
Allergic contact dermatitis due to nickel

SP L23.1 Allergic contact dermatitis due to adhesives

SP L23.2 Allergic contact dermatitis due to cosmetics

SP + L23.3 Allergic contact dermatitis due to drugs in contact with skin
Use additional code for adverse effect, if applicable, to identify drug (T36-T50 with fifth or sixth character 5)
EXCLUDES 2 dermatitis due to ingested drugs and medicaments (L27.0-L27.1)

SP L23.4 Allergic contact dermatitis due to dyes

SP L23.5 Allergic contact dermatitis due to other chemical products
Allergic contact dermatitis due to cement
Allergic contact dermatitis due to insecticide
Allergic contact dermatitis due to plastic
Allergic contact dermatitis due to rubber

SP L23.6 Allergic contact dermatitis due to food in contact with the skin
EXCLUDES 2 dermatitis due to ingested food (L27.2)

SP L23.7 Allergic contact dermatitis due to plants, except food
EXCLUDES 2 allergy NOS due to pollen (J30.1)

5 L23.8 Allergic contact dermatitis due to other agents

SP L23.81 Allergic contact dermatitis due to animal (cat) (dog) dander
Allergic contact dermatitis due to animal (cat) (dog) hair

SP L23.89 Allergic contact dermatitis due to other agents

SP L23.9 Allergic contact dermatitis, unspecified cause

Allergic contact eczema NOS

4 L24 Irritant contact dermatitis
EXCLUDES 1 allergy NOS (T78.40)
contact dermatitis NOS (L25.9)
dermatitis NOS (L30.9)
EXCLUDES 2 allergic contact dermatitis (L23.-)
dermatitis due to substances taken internally (L27.-)
dermatitis of eyelid (H01.1-)
diaper dermatitis (L22)
eczema of external ear (H60.5-)
perioral dermatitis (L71.0)
radiation-related disorders of the skin and subcutaneous tissue (L55-L59)

CODING TIPS ✓ Contact dermatitis indicates that the inflammation of the skin is related to contact with a substance. The specific causative substance that resulted in the condition should be documented, and the plan of care should include appropriate interventions for skin care and instruction on prevention of contact with irritants.

SP L24.0 Irritant contact dermatitis due to detergents

SP L24.1 Irritant contact dermatitis due to oils and greases

SP L24.2 Irritant contact dermatitis due to solvents
Irritant contact dermatitis due to chlorocompound
Irritant contact dermatitis due to cyclohexane
Irritant contact dermatitis due to ester
Irritant contact dermatitis due to glycol
Irritant contact dermatitis due to hydrocarbon
Irritant contact dermatitis due to ketone

SP L24.3 Irritant contact dermatitis due to cosmetics

SP + L24.4 Irritant contact dermatitis due to drugs in contact with skin
Use additional code for adverse effect, if applicable, to identify drug (T36-T50 with fifth or sixth character 5)

SP L24.5 Irritant contact dermatitis due to other chemical products
Irritant contact dermatitis due to cement
Irritant contact dermatitis due to insecticide
Irritant contact dermatitis due to plastic
Irritant contact dermatitis due to rubber

SP L24.6 Irritant contact dermatitis due to food in contact with skin
EXCLUDES 2 dermatitis due to ingested food (L27.2)

SP L24.7 Irritant contact dermatitis due to plants, except food
EXCLUDES 2 allergy NOS to pollen (J30.1)

5 L24.8 Irritant contact dermatitis due to other agents

SP L24.81 Irritant contact dermatitis due to metals
Irritant contact dermatitis due to chromium
Irritant contact dermatitis due to nickel

Chapter 12

L00-L99

★ New ▲ Revised Px Primary **SP** PDGM Px **SL** Low CoM **SH** High CoM **IQ** Quest. Encounter **H** Hospice non-cancer Dx Unspecified **M** *Manifestation*

DecisionHealth's FY 2020 Complete Home Health ICD-10-CM Diagnosis Coding Manual

1113

SP L24.89 Irritant contact dermatitis due to other agents
Irritant contact dermatitis due to dyes

SP L24.9 Irritant contact dermatitis, unspecified cause
Irritant contact eczema NOS

4 L25 Unspecified contact dermatitis

EXCLUDES 1 allergic contact dermatitis (L23.-)
allergy NOS (T78.40)
dermatitis NOS (L30.9)
irritant contact dermatitis (L24.-)

EXCLUDES 2 dermatitis due to ingested substances (L27.-)
dermatitis of eyelid (H01.1-)
eczema of external ear (H60.5-)
perioral dermatitis (L71.0)
radiation-related disorders of the skin and subcutaneous tissue (L55-L59)

CODING TIPS ✓ Contact dermatitis indicates that the inflammation of the skin is related to contact with a substance. The specific causative substance that resulted in the condition should be documented, and the plan of care should include appropriate interventions for skin care and instruction on prevention of contact with irritants.

SP L25.0 Unspecified contact dermatitis due to cosmetics

SP + L25.1 Unspecified contact dermatitis due to drugs in contact with skin
Use additional code for adverse effect, if applicable, to identify drug (T36-T50 with fifth or sixth character 5)
EXCLUDES 2 dermatitis due to ingested drugs and medicaments (L27.0-L27.1)

SP L25.2 Unspecified contact dermatitis due to dyes

SP L25.3 Unspecified contact dermatitis due to other chemical products
Unspecified contact dermatitis due to cement
Unspecified contact dermatitis due to insecticide

SP L25.4 Unspecified contact dermatitis due to food in contact with skin
EXCLUDES 2 dermatitis due to ingested food (L27.2)

SP L25.5 Unspecified contact dermatitis due to plants, except food
EXCLUDES 1 nettle rash (L50.9)
EXCLUDES 2 allergy NOS due to pollen (J30.1)

SP L25.8 Unspecified contact dermatitis due to other agents

SP L25.9 Unspecified contact dermatitis, unspecified cause
Contact dermatitis (occupational) NOS
Contact eczema (occupational) NOS

SP L26 Exfoliative dermatitis
Hebra's pityriasis
EXCLUDES 1 Ritter's disease (L00)

4 L27 Dermatitis due to substances taken internally
EXCLUDES 1 allergy NOS (T78.40)
EXCLUDES 2 adverse food reaction, except dermatitis (T78.0-T78.1)
contact dermatitis (L23-L25)
drug photoallergic response (L56.1)
drug phototoxic response (L56.0)
urticaria (L50.-)

SP + L27.0 Generalized skin eruption due to drugs and medicaments taken internally
Use additional code for adverse effect, if applicable, to identify drug (T36-T50 with fifth or sixth character 5)

SP + L27.1 Localized skin eruption due to drugs and medicaments taken internally
Use additional code for adverse effect, if applicable, to identify drug (T36-T50 with fifth or sixth character 5)

SP L27.2 Dermatitis due to ingested food
EXCLUDES 2 dermatitis due to food in contact with skin (L23.6, L24.6, L25.4)

SP L27.8 Dermatitis due to other substances taken internally

SP L27.9 Dermatitis due to unspecified substance taken internally

4 L28 Lichen simplex chronicus and prurigo

SP L28.0 Lichen simplex chronicus
Circumscribed neurodermatitis
Lichen NOS

SP L28.1 Prurigo nodularis

SP L28.2 Other prurigo
Prurigo NOS
Prurigo Hebra
Prurigo mitis
Urticaria papulosa
DEFINITION Chronic inflammatory skin disease featuring blistering papules and severe itching.

4 L29 Pruritus
EXCLUDES 1 neurotic excoriation (L98.1)
psychogenic pruritus (F45.8)
CODING TIPS ✓ Do not confuse pruritis with urticaria. Pruritis refers to "itch" or "itching" while urticaria refers to hives. Urticaria should be coded to L50.

SP L29.0 Pruritus ani
DEFINITION Severe itching of the perianal region.

SP L29.1 Pruritus scroti

SP L29.2 Pruritus vulvae

SP L29.3 Anogenital pruritus, unspecified

SP L29.8 Other pruritus

!Q L29.9 Pruritus, unspecified
Itch NOS

4 L30 Other and unspecified dermatitis
EXCLUDES 2 contact dermatitis (L23-L25)
dry skin dermatitis (L85.3)
small plaque parapsoriasis (L41.3)
stasis dermatitis (I87.2)

SP L30.0 Nummular dermatitis

---

4 4th digit required   5 5th digit required   6 6th digit required   7 7th digit required   7 7th digit placeholder   + Additional code   ⊟ Laterality

1114   DecisionHealth's FY 2020 Complete Home Health ICD-10-CM Diagnosis Coding Manual

Chapter 12

L00-L99

SP L30.1 Dyshidrosis [pompholyx]

SP L30.2 Cutaneous autosensitization
Candidid [levurid]
Dermatophytid
Eczematid

SP L30.3 Infective dermatitis
Infectious eczematoid dermatitis

SP L30.4 Erythema intertrigo

> **CODING TIPS ✓** Consider this code for intertriginous dermatitis for scenarios such as excoriation when two skin surfaces rub together, like between the toes, under the breasts, or between folds of skin.

SP L30.5 Pityriasis alba

SP L30.8 Other specified dermatitis

SP L30.9 Dermatitis, unspecified
Eczema NOS

Papulosquamous disorders (L40-L45)

4 L40 Psoriasis

SP L40.0 Psoriasis vulgaris
Nummular psoriasis
Plaque psoriasis

SP L40.1 Generalized pustular psoriasis
Impetigo herpetiformis
Von Zumbusch's disease

SP L40.2 Acrodermatitis continua

SP L40.3 Pustulosis palmaris et plantaris

SP L40.4 Guttate psoriasis

5 L40.5 Arthropathic psoriasis

SP L40.50 Arthropathic psoriasis, unspecified

SP L40.51 Distal interphalangeal psoriatic arthropathy

SP L40.52 Psoriatic arthritis mutilans

SP L40.53 Psoriatic spondylitis

SP L40.54 Psoriatic juvenile arthropathy

SP L40.59 Other psoriatic arthropathy

SP L40.8 Other psoriasis
Flexural psoriasis

SP L40.9 Psoriasis, unspecified

4 L41 Parapsoriasis
> **EXCLUDES 1** poikiloderma vasculare atrophicans (L94.5)

SP L41.0 Pityriasis lichenoides et varioliformis acuta
Mucha-Habermann disease

SP L41.1 Pityriasis lichenoides chronica

SP L41.3 Small plaque parapsoriasis

SP L41.4 Large plaque parapsoriasis

SP L41.5 Retiform parapsoriasis

SP L41.8 Other parapsoriasis

SP L41.9 Parapsoriasis, unspecified

SP L42 Pityriasis rosea

> **DEFINITION** Skin that is marked with scaling, pink, oval macules, arranged with the long axes parallel to the cleavage lines of the skin.

4 L43 Lichen planus
> **EXCLUDES 1** lichen planopilaris (L66.1)

SP L43.0 Hypertrophic lichen planus

SP L43.1 Bullous lichen planus

SP + L43.2 Lichenoid drug reaction

Use additional code for adverse effect, if applicable, to identify drug (T36-T50 with fifth or sixth character 5)

SP L43.3 Subacute (active) lichen planus
Lichen planus tropicus

SP L43.8 Other lichen planus

SP L43.9 Lichen planus, unspecified

4 L44 Other papulosquamous disorders

SP L44.0 Pityriasis rubra pilaris

> **DEFINITION** Rare skin condition of red-orange, scaly patches spreading over the body, thickened palms and soles, and rough, dry plugs within the rash.

SP L44.1 Lichen nitidus

SP L44.2 Lichen striatus

SP L44.3 Lichen ruber moniliformis

SP L44.4 Infantile papular acrodermatitis [Gianotti-Crosti]

SP L44.8 Other specified papulosquamous disorders

SP L44.9 Papulosquamous disorder, unspecified

IQ L45 Papulosquamous disorders in diseases classified elsewhere
Code first:
underlying disease.

Urticaria and erythema (L49-L54)

> **EXCLUDES 1** Lyme disease (A69.2-)
> rosacea (L71.-)

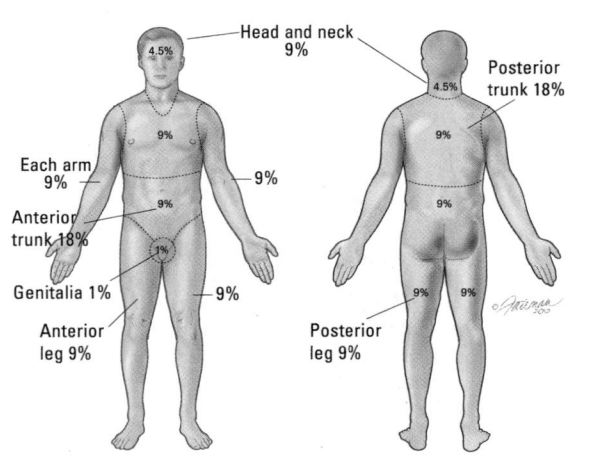

Head and neck 9%
Posterior trunk 18%
Each arm 9%
Anterior trunk 18%
Genitalia 1%
Anterior leg 9%
Posterior leg 9%

4 L49 Exfoliation due to erythematous conditions according to extent of body surface involved
Code first erythematous condition causing exfoliation, such as:
Ritter's disease (L00)
(Staphylococcal) scalded skin syndrome (L00)
Stevens-Johnson syndrome (L51.1)
Stevens-Johnson syndrome-toxic epidermal necrolysis
overlap syndrome (L51.3)
Toxic epidermal necrolysis (L51.2)

> **CODING TIPS ✓** Use the rule of nines to estimate the extent of body surface involved.

Chapter 12

L00-L99

★ New ▲ Revised Px Primary SP PDGM Px SL Low CoM SH High CoM IQ Quest. Encounter H Hospice non-cancer Dx Unspecified M *Manifestation*

DecisionHealth's FY 2020 Complete Home Health ICD-10-CM Diagnosis Coding Manual

1115

!Q L49.0 Exfoliation due to erythematous condition involving less than 10 percent of body surface
Exfoliation due to erythematous condition NOS

!Q L49.1 Exfoliation due to erythematous condition involving 10-19 percent of body surface

!Q L49.2 Exfoliation due to erythematous condition involving 20-29 percent of body surface

!Q L49.3 Exfoliation due to erythematous condition involving 30-39 percent of body surface

!Q L49.4 Exfoliation due to erythematous condition involving 40-49 percent of body surface

!Q L49.5 Exfoliation due to erythematous condition involving 50-59 percent of body surface

!Q L49.6 Exfoliation due to erythematous condition involving 60-69 percent of body surface

!Q L49.7 Exfoliation due to erythematous condition involving 70-79 percent of body surface

!Q L49.8 Exfoliation due to erythematous condition involving 80-89 percent of body surface

!Q L49.9 Exfoliation due to erythematous condition involving 90 or more percent of body surface

▲ 4 L50 Urticaria
   EXCLUDES 1 allergic contact dermatitis (L23.-)
               angioneurotic edema (T78.3)
               giant urticaria (T78.3)
               hereditary angio-edema (D84.1)
               Quincke's edema (T78.3)
               serum urticaria (T80.6-)
               solar urticaria (L56.3)
               urticaria neonatorum (P83.8)
               urticaria papulosa (L28.2)
               urticaria pigmentosa (D47.01)
   CODING TIPS ✓ Do not confuse urticaria with pruritis. Pruritis refers to "itch" or "itching" while urticaria refers to hives. Pruritis should be coded to L29.

SP L50.0 Allergic urticaria
   DEFINITION The most common form of hives in which smooth, raised, pink or white, itchy welts appear on or beneath the skin as a hypersensitivity response of the immune system to an allergic trigger.

SP L50.1 Idiopathic urticaria
   DEFINITION The appearance of hives with no known, apparent cause.

SP L50.2 Urticaria due to cold and heat
   EXCLUDES 2 familial cold urticaria (M04.2)
   DEFINITION The appearance of hives in response to external heat or cold that typically fade after moving to a comfortable temperature.

SP L50.3 Dermatographic urticaria

   DEFINITION The appearance of hives in only one particular area of the body.

SP L50.4 Vibratory urticaria
   DEFINITION Hives brought on by intense, prolonged vibration, such as that which occurs with the use of heavy mechanical equipment.

SP L50.5 Cholinergic urticaria
   DEFINITION Hives that occur in response to a rise in body temperature, such as from exercise, stress, or overheating.

SP L50.6 Contact urticaria

SP L50.8 Other urticaria
   Chronic urticaria
   Recurrent periodic urticaria

SP L50.9 Urticaria, unspecified

＋ 4 L51 Erythema multiforme
   Use additional code for adverse effect, if applicable, to identify drug (T36-T50 with fifth or sixth character 5)
   Use additional code to identify associated manifestations, such as:
      arthropathy associated with dermatological disorders (M14.8-)
      conjunctival edema (H11.42)
      conjunctivitis (H10.22-)
      corneal scars and opacities (H17.-)
      corneal ulcer (H16.0-)
      edema of eyelid (H02.84-)
      inflammation of eyelid (H01.8)
      keratoconjunctivitis sicca (H16.22-)
      mechanical lagophthalmos (H02.22-)
      stomatitis (K12.-)
      symblepharon (H11.23-)
   Use additional code to identify percentage of skin exfoliation (L49.-)
   EXCLUDES 1 staphylococcal scalded skin syndrome (L00)
               Ritter's disease (L00)

SP ＋ L51.0 Nonbullous erythema multiforme

SP ＋ L51.1 Stevens-Johnson syndrome

SP ＋ L51.2 Toxic epidermal necrolysis [Lyell]

SP ＋ L51.3 Stevens-Johnson syndrome-toxic epidermal necrolysis overlap syndrome
   SJS-TEN overlap syndrome

SP ＋ L51.8 Other erythema multiforme

SP ＋ L51.9 Erythema multiforme, unspecified
   Erythema iris
   Erythema multiforme major NOS
   Erythema multiforme minor NOS
   Herpes iris
   DEFINITION Erythema multiforme minor NOS: Acute, localized, self-limiting eruption marked by distinctive, classical target lesions of pink-red blotches with a ring around a pale center.

SP L52 Erythema nodosum
   EXCLUDES 1 tuberculous erythema nodosum (A18.4)
   DEFINITION An inflammatory skin disorder marked by flat, firm, warm, red, tender, or painful nodules about an inch across under the skin that turn purple and fade to brown after several weeks, commonly found on anterior lower legs.

4 4th digit required   5 5th digit required   6 6th digit required   7 7th digit required   7 7th digit placeholder   ＋ Additional code   ⊟ Laterality

1116   *DecisionHealth's* FY 2020 Complete Home Health ICD-10-CM Diagnosis Coding Manual

Chapter 12

L00-L99

▣ L53   Other erythematous conditions
　EXCLUDES 1   erythema ab igne (L59.0)
　　　　　　　erythema due to external agents
　　　　　　　　in contact with skin
　　　　　　　　(L23-L25)
　　　　　　　erythema intertrigo (L30.4)

SP ＋ L53.0   Toxic erythema
　Code first:
　　poisoning due to drug or toxin, if
　　applicable
　　(T36-T65 with fifth or sixth character
　　1-4 or 6)
　Use additional code for adverse effect, if
　　applicable, to identify drug (T36-T50
　　with fifth or sixth character 5)
　　EXCLUDES 1   neonatal erythema toxicum
　　　　　　　(P83.1)

SP L53.1   Erythema annulare centrifugum

SP L53.2   Erythema marginatum

SP L53.3   Other chronic figurate erythema

SP L53.8   Other specified erythematous conditions

IQ L53.9   Erythematous condition, unspecified
　Erythema NOS
　Erythroderma NOS

IQ L54   Erythema in diseases classified elsewhere
　Code first:
　　underlying disease.

Radiation-related disorders of the skin and subcutaneous tissue   (L55-L59)

▣ L55   Sunburn
　CODING TIPS ✓   Sunburns (L55) are
　differentiated by degree. First degree is
　erythema; second degree is blistering; and
　third degree is deep tissue damage.

SP L55.0   Sunburn of first degree

SP L55.1   Sunburn of second degree

SP L55.2   Sunburn of third degree

IQ L55.9   Sunburn, unspecified

＋ ▣ L56   Other acute skin changes due to ultraviolet radiation
　Use additional code to identify the source of
　　the ultraviolet radiation (W89, X32)

SP ＋ L56.0   Drug phototoxic response
　Use additional code for adverse effect, if
　　applicable, to identify drug (T36-T50
　　with fifth or sixth character 5)

SP ＋ L56.1   Drug photoallergic response
　Use additional code for adverse effect, if
　　applicable, to identify drug (T36-T50
　　with fifth or sixth character 5)

SP ＋ L56.2   Photocontact dermatitis [berloque dermatitis]

SP ＋ L56.3   Solar urticaria

SP ＋ L56.4   Polymorphous light eruption

SP ＋ L56.5   Disseminated superficial actinic porokeratosis (DSAP)

SP ＋ L56.8   Other specified acute skin changes due to ultraviolet radiation

SP ＋ L56.9   Acute skin change due to ultraviolet radiation, unspecified

＋ ▣ L57   Skin changes due to chronic exposure to nonionizing radiation

Use additional code to identify the source of
　the ultraviolet radiation (W89)
　CODING TIPS ✓   L57 includes an instruction to
use an additional code to identify the source of
radiation. According to the guidelines, external
cause codes are not required. However, this
instruction is a convention, and conventions
trump guidelines.

SP ＋ L57.0   Actinic keratosis
　Keratosis NOS
　Senile keratosis
　Solar keratosis

SP ＋ L57.1   Actinic reticuloid

SP ＋ L57.2   Cutis rhomboidalis nuchae

SP ＋ L57.3   Poikiloderma of Civatte

SP ＋ L57.4   Cutis laxa senilis
　Elastosis senilis

SP ＋ L57.5   Actinic granuloma

SP ＋ L57.8   Other skin changes due to chronic exposure to nonionizing radiation
　Farmer's skin
　Sailor's skin
　Solar dermatitis
　　DEFINITION   Solar dermatitis: Premature
　aging of the skin and degeneration of the
　elastic tissue of the dermis due to
　prolonged exposure to sunlight.

SP ＋ L57.9   Skin changes due to chronic exposure to nonionizing radiation, unspecified

＋ ▣ L58   Radiodermatitis
　Use additional code to identify the source of
　　the radiation (W88, W90)

SP ＋ L58.0   Acute radiodermatitis

SP ＋ L58.1   Chronic radiodermatitis

SP ＋ L58.9   Radiodermatitis, unspecified

▣ L59   Other disorders of skin and subcutaneous tissue related to radiation

SP L59.0   Erythema ab igne [dermatitis ab igne]

SP L59.8   Other specified disorders of the skin and subcutaneous tissue related to radiation

SP L59.9   Disorder of the skin and subcutaneous tissue related to radiation, unspecified

Disorders of skin appendages   (L60-L75)

EXCLUDES 1   congenital malformations of integument (Q84.-)

▣ L60   Nail disorders
　EXCLUDES 2   clubbing of nails (R68.3)
　　　　　　　onychia and paronychia
　　　　　　　　(L03.0-)

SP L60.0   Ingrowing nail
　CODING TIPS ✓   Care of an ingrown nail
　(regardless of infection) is generally not
　complex. Small and superficial wounds,
　such as caused by an ingrown toenail,
　generally do not require the skills of a
　nurse. Simple wound care is generally not
　covered; however, some conditions can
　increase the complexity. For example, an
　infected ingrown toenail in a diabetic may
　require the skills of a nurse due to the
　potential for complication.

SP L60.1   Onycholysis

SP L60.2   Onychogryphosis

Chapter 12

L00-L99

★ New ▲ Revised Px Primary SP PDGM Px SL Low CoM SH High CoM IQ Quest. Encounter H Hospice non-cancer Dx   Unspecified   M Manifestation

DecisionHealth's FY 2020 Complete Home Health ICD-10-CM Diagnosis Coding Manual   1117

IQ L60.3 Nail dystrophy

IQ L60.4 Beau's lines

IQ L60.5 Yellow nail syndrome

SP L60.8 Other nail disorders

IQ L60.9 Nail disorder, unspecified

M IQ L62 *Nail disorders in diseases classified elsewhere*

Code first underlying disease, such as: pachydermoperiostosis (M89.4-)

4 L63 Alopecia areata

DEFINITION Patchy loss of hair on the head or body.

SP L63.0 Alopecia (capitis) totalis

SP L63.1 Alopecia universalis

SP L63.2 Ophiasis

SP L63.8 Other alopecia areata

SP L63.9 Alopecia areata, unspecified

4 L64 Androgenic alopecia

INCLUDES male-pattern baldness

SP + L64.0 Drug-induced androgenic alopecia

Use additional code for adverse effect, if applicable, to identify drug (T36-T50 with fifth or sixth character 5)

SP L64.8 Other androgenic alopecia

SP L64.9 Androgenic alopecia, unspecified

+ 4 L65 Other nonscarring hair loss

Use additional code for adverse effect, if applicable, to identify drug (T36-T50 with fifth or sixth character 5)

EXCLUDES 1 trichotillomania (F63.3)

SP + L65.0 Telogen effluvium

SP + L65.1 Anagen effluvium

SP + L65.2 Alopecia mucinosa

SP + L65.8 Other specified nonscarring hair loss

IQ + L65.9 Nonscarring hair loss, unspecified

Alopecia NOS

4 L66 Cicatricial alopecia [scarring hair loss]

SP L66.0 Pseudopelade

SP L66.1 Lichen planopilaris

Follicular lichen planus

SP L66.2 Folliculitis decalvans

SP L66.3 Perifolliculitis capitis abscedens

SP L66.4 Folliculitis ulerythematosa reticulata

SP L66.8 Other cicatricial alopecia

SP L66.9 Cicatricial alopecia, unspecified

4 L67 Hair color and hair shaft abnormalities

EXCLUDES 1 monilethrix (Q84.1)
pili annulati (Q84.1)
telogen effluvium (L65.0)

SP L67.0 Trichorrhexis nodosa

IQ L67.1 Variations in hair color

Canities
Greyness, hair (premature)
Heterochromia of hair
Poliosis circumscripta, acquired
Poliosis NOS

IQ L67.8 Other hair color and hair shaft abnormalities

Fragilitas crinium

IQ L67.9 Hair color and hair shaft abnormality, unspecified

4 L68 Hypertrichosis

INCLUDES excess hair

EXCLUDES 1 congenital hypertrichosis (Q84.2)
persistent lanugo (Q84.2)

SP L68.0 Hirsutism

SP L68.1 Acquired hypertrichosis lanuginosa

SP L68.2 Localized hypertrichosis

SP L68.3 Polytrichia

SP L68.8 Other hypertrichosis

SP L68.9 Hypertrichosis, unspecified

4 L70 Acne

EXCLUDES 2 acne keloid (L73.0)

SP L70.0 Acne vulgaris

SP L70.1 Acne conglobata

SP L70.2 Acne varioliformis

Acne necrotica miliaris

SP L70.3 Acne tropica

SP L70.4 Infantile acne

SP L70.5 Acné excoriée

Acné excoriée des jeunes filles
Picker's acne

SP L70.8 Other acne

SP L70.9 Acne, unspecified

+ 4 L71 Rosacea

Use additional code for adverse effect, if applicable, to identify drug (T36-T50 with fifth or sixth character 5)

SP + L71.0 Perioral dermatitis

SP + L71.1 Rhinophyma

SP + L71.8 Other rosacea

SP + L71.9 Rosacea, unspecified

4 L72 Follicular cysts of skin and subcutaneous tissue

SP L72.0 Epidermal cyst

5 L72.1 Pilar and trichodermal cyst

SP L72.11 Pilar cyst

CODING TIPS ✓ Greater than 90% of pilar cysts occur on the scalp. Pilar cysts are the most common cutaneous cyst.

SP L72.12 Trichodermal cyst

Trichilemmal (proliferating) cyst

SP L72.2 Steatocystoma multiplex

SP L72.3 Sebaceous cyst

EXCLUDES 2 pilar cyst (L72.11)
trichilemmal (proliferating) cyst (L72.12)

SP L72.8 Other follicular cysts of the skin and subcutaneous tissue

SP L72.9 Follicular cyst of the skin and subcutaneous tissue, unspecified

4 L73 Other follicular disorders

SP L73.0 Acne keloid

SP L73.1 Pseudofolliculitis barbae

SP L73.2 Hidradenitis suppurativa

SP L73.8 Other specified follicular disorders

Sycosis barbae

IQ L73.9 Follicular disorder, unspecified

4 L74 Eccrine sweat disorders

EXCLUDES 2 generalized hyperhidrosis (R61)

4 4th digit required   5 5th digit required   6 6th digit required   7 7th digit required   7 7th digit placeholder   + Additional code   ⊟ Laterality

1118   *DecisionHealth's* FY 2020 Complete Home Health ICD-10-CM Diagnosis Coding Manual

Chapter 12

L00-L99

SP L74.0 Miliaria rubra

> **DEFINITION** Inflammatory heat rash caused by obstruction of the sweat glands with resultant skin rash of small clusters of red pimples on the skin.

SP L74.1 Miliaria crystallina

SP L74.2 Miliaria profunda
Miliaria tropicalis

SP L74.3 Miliaria, unspecified

SP L74.4 Anhidrosis
Hypohidrosis

5 L74.5 Focal hyperhidrosis

6 L74.51 Primary focal hyperhidrosis

SP L74.510 Primary focal hyperhidrosis, axilla

SP L74.511 Primary focal hyperhidrosis, face

SP L74.512 Primary focal hyperhidrosis, palms

SP L74.513 Primary focal hyperhidrosis, soles

SP L74.519 Primary focal hyperhidrosis, unspecified

SP L74.52 Secondary focal hyperhidrosis
Frey's syndrome

SP L74.8 Other eccrine sweat disorders

SP L74.9 Eccrine sweat disorder, unspecified
Sweat gland disorder NOS

4 L75 Apocrine sweat disorders
> **EXCLUDES 1** dyshidrosis (L30.1)
> hidradenitis suppurativa (L73.2)

SP L75.0 Bromhidrosis

SP L75.1 Chromhidrosis

SP L75.2 Apocrine miliaria
Fox-Fordyce disease

SP L75.8 Other apocrine sweat disorders

SP L75.9 Apocrine sweat disorder, unspecified

Intraoperative and postprocedural complications of skin and subcutaneous tissue (L76)

CODING TIPS ✓ Conditions classifiable to L76 are classifiable as intraoperative and postprocedural complications. These conditions should only be assigned when diagnostic statements clearly indicate that the condition is a complication of a procedure. Complications that are resolved upon admission to home care are coded to Z48.812.

4 L76 Intraoperative and postprocedural complications of skin and subcutaneous tissue

5 L76.0 Intraoperative hemorrhage and hematoma of skin and subcutaneous tissue complicating a procedure
> **EXCLUDES 1** intraoperative hemorrhage and hematoma of skin and subcutaneous tissue due to accidental puncture and laceration during a procedure (L76.1-)

SP L76.01 Intraoperative hemorrhage and hematoma of skin and subcutaneous tissue complicating a dermatologic procedure

SP L76.02 Intraoperative hemorrhage and hematoma of skin and subcutaneous tissue complicating other procedure

5 L76.1 Accidental puncture and laceration of skin and subcutaneous tissue during a procedure

SP L76.11 Accidental puncture and laceration of skin and subcutaneous tissue during a dermatologic procedure

SP L76.12 Accidental puncture and laceration of skin and subcutaneous tissue during other procedure

5 L76.2 Postprocedural hemorrhage of skin and subcutaneous tissue following a procedure

SP L76.21 Postprocedural hemorrhage of skin and subcutaneous tissue following a dermatologic procedure

SP L76.22 Postprocedural hemorrhage of skin and subcutaneous tissue following other procedure

5 L76.3 Postprocedural hematoma and seroma of skin and subcutaneous tissue following a procedure

SP L76.31 Postprocedural hematoma of skin and subcutaneous tissue following a dermatologic procedure

SP L76.32 Postprocedural hematoma of skin and subcutaneous tissue following other procedure

SP L76.33 Postprocedural seroma of skin and subcutaneous tissue following a dermatologic procedure

SP L76.34 Postprocedural seroma of skin and subcutaneous tissue following other procedure

+ 5 L76.8 Other intraoperative and postprocedural complications of skin and subcutaneous tissue
Use additional code, if applicable, to further specify disorder

SP + L76.81 Other intraoperative complications of skin and subcutaneous tissue

SP + L76.82 Other postprocedural complications of skin and subcutaneous tissue

Other disorders of the skin and subcutaneous tissue (L80-L99)

SP L80 Vitiligo
> **EXCLUDES 2** vitiligo of eyelids (H02.73-)
> vitiligo of vulva (N90.89)

> **DEFINITION** White patches devoid of pigmentation appearing on otherwise normal skin.

4 L81 Other disorders of pigmentation
> **EXCLUDES 1** birthmark NOS (Q82.5)
> Peutz-Jeghers syndrome (Q85.8)

> **EXCLUDES 2** nevus - see Alphabetical Index

SP L81.0 Postinflammatory hyperpigmentation

SP L81.1 Chloasma

IQ L81.2 Freckles

IQ L81.3 Café au lait spots

SP L81.4 Other melanin hyperpigmentation
Lentigo

SP L81.5 Leukoderma, not elsewhere classified

★ New ▲ Revised Px Primary **SP** PDGM Px **SL** Low CoM **SH** High CoM **IQ** Quest. Encounter **H** Hospice non-cancer Dx Unspecified **M** *Manifestation*

DecisionHealth's FY 2020 Complete Home Health ICD-10-CM Diagnosis Coding Manual

1119

Chapter 12

L00-L99

SP L81.6 Other disorders of diminished melanin formation

SP L81.7 Pigmented purpuric dermatosis
Angioma serpiginosum

SP L81.8 Other specified disorders of pigmentation
Iron pigmentation
Tattoo pigmentation

IQ L81.9 Disorder of pigmentation, unspecified

4 L82 Seborrheic keratosis
> INCLUDES   basal cell papilloma
> dermatosis papulosa nigra
> Leser-Trélat disease
> EXCLUDES 2 seborrheic dermatitis (L21.-)

SP L82.0 Inflamed seborrheic keratosis
> DEFINITION   Noncancerous, barnacle-like skin lesions appearing in areas of long-term sun exposure in the elderly. Growths are irritated, itchy, inflamed, and may even bleed.

SP L82.1 Other seborrheic keratosis
Seborrheic keratosis NOS
> DEFINITION   Noncancerous skin lesion associated with aging and long periods of sun exposure. Growths appear round or oval, slightly elevated, black, brown, or pale in appearance with a crusty or scaly surface.

SP L83 Acanthosis nigricans
Confluent and reticulated papillomatosis

SP L84 Corns and callosities
Callus
Clavus

4 L85 Other epidermal thickening
> EXCLUDES 2 hypertrophic disorders of the skin (L91.-)

SP L85.0 Acquired ichthyosis
> EXCLUDES 1 congenital ichthyosis (Q80.-)

SP L85.1 Acquired keratosis [keratoderma] palmaris et plantaris
> EXCLUDES 1 inherited keratosis palmaris et plantaris (Q82.8)

SP L85.2 Keratosis punctata (palmaris et plantaris)

SP L85.3 Xerosis cutis
Dry skin dermatitis

SP L85.8 Other specified epidermal thickening
Cutaneous horn

IQ L85.9 Epidermal thickening, unspecified

IQ L86 Keratoderma in diseases classified elsewhere
Code first underlying disease, such as:
Reiter's disease (M02.3-)
> EXCLUDES 1 gonococcal keratoderma (A54.89)
> gonococcal keratosis (A54.89)
> keratoderma due to vitamin A deficiency (E50.8)
> keratosis due to vitamin A deficiency (E50.8)
> xeroderma due to vitamin A deficiency (E50.8)

4 L87 Transepidermal elimination disorders
> EXCLUDES 1 granuloma annulare (perforating) (L92.0)

SP L87.0 Keratosis follicularis et parafollicularis in cutem penetrans
Kyrle disease
Hyperkeratosis follicularis penetrans

SP L87.1 Reactive perforating collagenosis

SP L87.2 Elastosis perforans serpiginosa

SP L87.8 Other transepidermal elimination disorders

IQ L87.9 Transepidermal elimination disorder, unspecified

SP L88 Pyoderma gangrenosum
Phagedenic pyoderma
> EXCLUDES 1 dermatitis gangrenosa (L08.0)

Stage I
Nonblanchable erythema of unbroken skin the sign of lesion of skin ulceration.

Stage II
Limited thickness skin loss concerning dermis, epidermis, or both. Shallow lesion.

Stage III
Total thickness skin loss concerning damage or necrosis of subcutaneous tissue that can expand down to but not underlying fascia. Deep crater-like lesion.

Stage IV
Total thickness skin loss with far-reaching destruction, tissue necrosis.

4 L89 Pressure ulcer
> INCLUDES   bed sore
> decubitus ulcer
> plaster ulcer
> pressure area
> pressure sore

Code first:
any associated gangrene (I96)
> EXCLUDES 2 decubitus (trophic) ulcer of cervix (uteri) (N86)
> diabetic ulcers (E08.621, E08.622, E09.621, E09.622, E10.621, E10.622, E11.621, E11.622, E13.621, E13.622)
> non-pressure chronic ulcer of skin (L97.-)
> skin infections (L00-L08)
> varicose ulcer (I83.0, I83.2)

> GUIDELINES   Section I.C.12.a.1)
Codes from category L89 are combination codes that identify the site of the pressure ulcer as well as the stage of the ulcer. ... Assign as many codes from category L89 as needed to identify all the pressure ulcers the patient has, if applicable.

> GUIDELINES   Section I.C.12.a.4)
No code is assigned if the documentation states that the pressure ulcer is completely healed.

4 4th digit required   5 5th digit required   6 6th digit required   7 7th digit required   ☑ 7th digit placeholder   + Additional code   ⊟ Laterality

1120   DecisionHealth's FY 2020 Complete Home Health ICD-10-CM Diagnosis Coding Manual

Chapter 12

L00-L99

GUIDELINES　Section I.B.14

For the Body Mass Index (BMI), depth of non-pressure chronic ulcers, pressure ulcer stage, coma scale, and NIH stroke scale (NIHSS) codes, code assignment may be based on medical record documentation from clinicians who are not the patient's provider (i.e., physician or other qualified healthcare practitioner legally accountable for establishing the patient's diagnosis), since this information is typically documented by other clinicians involved in the care of the patient (e.g., a dietitian often documents the BMI, a nurse often documents the pressure ulcer stages, and an emergency medical technician often documents the coma scale). However, the associated diagnosis (such as overweight, obesity, acute stroke, or pressure ulcer) must be documented by the patient's provider.

CODING TIPS ✓　Deep Tissue Pressure Injuries (DTPI) presenting with intact skin or partial thickness skin loss should be marked on the **OASIS** as Deep Tissue Injury. DTPI presenting with full thickness loss should be marked on the OASIS as Stage 3 (fatty tissue exposed) or Stage 4 (bone, muscle, ligament, joint capsule). (*4/19 CMS Q&As*)

CODING TIPS ✓　Although not due to pressure, Kennedy ulcers or terminal ulcers are coded to L89. Kennedy ulcers indicate multi-organ failure and are rarely coded in home care, but may be present in hospice patients.

CODING TIPS ✓　Pressure ulcer guidance for the purposes of scoring the OASIS is very different than the guidelines regarding coding pressure ulcers. A pressure ulcer covered with a flap or graft is no longer a pressure ulcer according to OASIS, but is coded as an unstageable pressure ulcer. A pressure ulcer covered with a non-removable dressing is unstageable on the OASIS; however, the stage can be coded based on physician documentation of the stage.

CODING TIPS ✓　Closed stage 3 and 4 pressure ulcers are no longer counted on the OASIS as pressure ulcers even though the closed areas are still at risk for further breakdown. If the physician documents the stage 3 or 4 pressure ulcer as completely healed, do not code the pressure ulcer. Otherwise, the coder should consider whether the pressure ulcer meets the criteria in Section III of the coding guidelines regarding reportable diagnoses.

CODING TIPS ✓　Use category L89 for pressure ulcers/injuries and any ulcer/injury that occurs from pressure or pressure in combination with shear. Note that a pressure ulcer may present as a blister, but not all blisters are pressure ulcers. To code the stage, use descriptions from WOCN and NPUAP.

CODING TIPS ✓　Codes in category L89 are combination codes that include a fifth or sixth character indicating the stage. An assessing clinician may mark the OASIS with pressure ulcer/injury based on the characteristics of the wound utilizing WOCN and NPUAP criteria. The physician must provide confirmation of the diagnosis of pressure ulcer/injury; however, coders may choose the stage based on clinicians' documentation. Home health and hospice coders should never have to use 6th character 9 for unspecified stage.

CODING TIPS ✓　Pressure ulcers/injuries on mucous membranes or where the mucosal membrane meets skin, for example at the urethral meatus, are considered mucosal membrane pressure injuries (MMPI). MMPIs are not considered pressure ulcers/injuries for the purpose of OASIS. They cannot be staged because of the different anatomy.

DEFINITION　**Deep Tissue Pressure Injury (DTPI)** is defined as intact or non-intact skin with localized area of persistent non-blanchable deep red, maroon, purple discoloration or epidermal separation revealing a dark wound bed or blood filled blister. Pain and temperature change often precede skin color changes. Discoloration may appear differently in darkly pigmented skin. This condition results from intense and/or prolonged pressure and shear forces at the bone-muscle interface. The wound may evolve rapidly to reveal the actual extent of tissue injury, or may resolve without tissue loss.

DEFINITION　A pressure-induced ulceration or sore of the skin usually occurring when a patient is confined to bed for long periods of time, due to lack of circulation and oxygenation to the affected tissue.

5 **L89.0**　**Pressure ulcer of elbow**

　6 **L89.00**　**Pressure ulcer of unspecified elbow**

　IQ **L89.000**　**Pressure ulcer of unspecified elbow, unstageable**

　IQ **L89.001**　**Pressure ulcer of unspecified elbow, stage 1**

　　Healing pressure ulcer of unspecified elbow, stage 1

　　Pressure pre-ulcer skin changes limited to persistent focal edema, unspecified elbow

　IQ **L89.002**　**Pressure ulcer of unspecified elbow, stage 2**

　　Healing pressure ulcer of unspecified elbow, stage 2

　　Pressure ulcer with abrasion, blister, partial thickness skin loss involving epidermis and/or dermis, unspecified elbow

　IQ **L89.003**　**Pressure ulcer of unspecified elbow, stage 3**

　　Healing pressure ulcer of unspecified elbow, stage 3

　　Pressure ulcer with full thickness skin loss involving damage or necrosis of subcutaneous tissue, unspecified elbow

Chapter 12

L00-L99

★ New　▲ Revised　**Px** Primary　**SP** PDGM Px　**SL** Low CoM　**SH** High CoM　**IQ** Quest. Encounter　**H** Hospice non-cancer Dx　　Unspecified　**M** *Manifestation*

DecisionHealth's FY 2020 Complete Home Health ICD-10-CM Diagnosis Coding Manual　　　　　1121

IQ L89.004 **Pressure ulcer of unspecified elbow, stage 4**

Healing pressure ulcer of unspecified elbow, stage 4
Pressure ulcer with necrosis of soft tissues through to underlying muscle, tendon, or bone, unspecified elbow

★ **L89.006** **Pressure-induced deep tissue damage of unspecified elbow**

IQ L89.009 **Pressure ulcer of unspecified elbow, unspecified stage**

Healing pressure ulcer of elbow NOS
Healing pressure ulcer of unspecified elbow, unspecified stage

⑥ L89.01 **Pressure ulcer of right elbow**

⊟ SP SH SL L89.010 **Pressure ulcer of right elbow, unstageable**

⊟ SP L89.011 **Pressure ulcer of right elbow, stage 1**

Healing pressure ulcer of right elbow, stage 1
Pressure pre-ulcer skin changes limited to persistent focal edema, right elbow

⊟ SP SH SL L89.012 **Pressure ulcer of right elbow, stage 2**

Healing pressure ulcer of right elbow, stage 2
Pressure ulcer with abrasion, blister, partial thickness skin loss involving epidermis and/or dermis, right elbow

⊟ SP SH SL L89.013 **Pressure ulcer of right elbow, stage 3**

Healing pressure ulcer of right elbow, stage 3
Pressure ulcer with full thickness skin loss involving damage or necrosis of subcutaneous tissue, right elbow

⊟ SP SH SL L89.014 **Pressure ulcer of right elbow, stage 4**

Healing pressure ulcer of right elbow, stage 4
Pressure ulcer with necrosis of soft tissues through to underlying muscle, tendon, or bone, right elbow

★ ⊟ **L89.016** **Pressure-induced deep tissue damage of right elbow**

⊟ IQ L89.019 **Pressure ulcer of right elbow, unspecified stage**

Healing pressure right of elbow NOS
Healing pressure ulcer of right elbow, unspecified stage

⑥ L89.02 **Pressure ulcer of left elbow**

⊟ SP SH SL L89.020 **Pressure ulcer of left elbow, unstageable**

⊟ SP L89.021 **Pressure ulcer of left elbow, stage 1**

Healing pressure ulcer of left elbow, stage 1

Pressure pre-ulcer skin changes limited to persistent focal edema, left elbow

⊟ SP SH SL L89.022 **Pressure ulcer of left elbow, stage 2**

Healing pressure ulcer of left elbow, stage 2
Pressure ulcer with abrasion, blister, partial thickness skin loss involving epidermis and/or dermis, left elbow

⊟ SP SH SL L89.023 **Pressure ulcer of left elbow, stage 3**

Healing pressure ulcer of left elbow, stage 3
Pressure ulcer with full thickness skin loss involving damage or necrosis of subcutaneous tissue, left elbow

⊟ SP SH SL L89.024 **Pressure ulcer of left elbow, stage 4**

Healing pressure ulcer of left elbow, stage 4
Pressure ulcer with necrosis of soft tissues through to underlying muscle, tendon, or bone, left elbow

★ ⊟ **L89.026** **Pressure-induced deep tissue damage of left elbow**

⊟ IQ L89.029 **Pressure ulcer of left elbow, unspecified stage**

Healing pressure ulcer of left of -elbow NOS
Healing pressure ulcer of left elbow, unspecified stage

⑤ L89.1 **Pressure ulcer of back**

⑥ L89.10 **Pressure ulcer of unspecified part of back**

IQ L89.100 **Pressure ulcer of unspecified part of back, unstageable**

IQ L89.101 **Pressure ulcer of unspecified part of back, stage 1**

Healing pressure ulcer of unspecified part of back, stage 1
Pressure pre-ulcer skin changes limited to persistent focal edema, unspecified part of back

IQ SH SL L89.102 **Pressure ulcer of unspecified part of back, stage 2**

Healing pressure ulcer of unspecified part of back, stage 2
Pressure ulcer with abrasion, blister, partial thickness skin loss involving epidermis and/or dermis, unspecified part of back

IQ SH SL L89.103 **Pressure ulcer of unspecified part of back, stage 3**

Healing pressure ulcer of unspecified part of back, stage 3
Pressure ulcer with full thickness skin loss involving damage or necrosis of subcutaneous tissue, unspecified part of back

IQ SH SL L89.104 **Pressure ulcer of unspecified part of back, stage 4**

Healing pressure ulcer of unspecified part of back, stage 4

④4th digit required   **⑤5th digit required**   **⑥6th digit required**   **⑦7th digit required**   **⑦7th digit placeholder**   **✛Additional code**   **⊟Laterality**

1122   *DecisionHealth's* FY 2020 Complete Home Health ICD-10-CM Diagnosis Coding Manual

Chapter 12

L00-L99

Pressure ulcer with necrosis of soft tissues through to underlying muscle, tendon, or bone, unspecified part of back

⭐ **L89.106** **Pressure-induced deep tissue damage of unspecified part of back**

IQ **L89.109** **Pressure ulcer of unspecified part of back, unspecified stage**

Healing pressure ulcer of unspecified part of back NOS

Healing pressure ulcer of unspecified part of back, unspecified stage

6 **L89.11** **Pressure ulcer of right upper back**

Pressure ulcer of right shoulder blade

SP SH SL **L89.110** **Pressure ulcer of right upper back, unstageable**

SP **L89.111** **Pressure ulcer of right upper back, stage 1**

Healing pressure ulcer of right upper back, stage 1

Pressure pre-ulcer skin changes limited to persistent focal edema, right upper back

SP SH SL **L89.112** **Pressure ulcer of right upper back, stage 2**

Healing pressure ulcer of right upper back, stage 2

Pressure ulcer with abrasion, blister, partial thickness skin loss involving epidermis and/or dermis, right upper back

SP SH SL **L89.113** **Pressure ulcer of right upper back, stage 3**

Healing pressure ulcer of right upper back, stage 3

Pressure ulcer with full thickness skin loss involving damage or necrosis of subcutaneous tissue, right upper back

SP SH SL **L89.114** **Pressure ulcer of right upper back, stage 4**

Healing pressure ulcer of right upper back, stage 4

Pressure ulcer with necrosis of soft tissues through to underlying muscle, tendon, or bone, right upper back

⭐ **L89.116** **Pressure-induced deep tissue damage of right upper back**

IQ **L89.119** **Pressure ulcer of right upper back, unspecified stage**

Healing pressure ulcer of right upper back NOS

Healing pressure ulcer of right upper back, unspecified stage

6 **L89.12** **Pressure ulcer of left upper back**

Pressure ulcer of left shoulder blade

SP SH SL **L89.120** **Pressure ulcer of left upper back, unstageable**

SP **L89.121** **Pressure ulcer of left upper back, stage 1**

Healing pressure ulcer of left upper back, stage 1

Pressure pre-ulcer skin changes limited to persistent focal edema, left upper back

SP SH SL **L89.122** **Pressure ulcer of left upper back, stage 2**

Healing pressure ulcer of left upper back, stage 2

Pressure ulcer with abrasion, blister, partial thickness skin loss involving epidermis and/or dermis, left upper back

SP SH SL **L89.123** **Pressure ulcer of left upper back, stage 3**

Healing pressure ulcer of left upper back, stage 3

Pressure ulcer with full thickness skin loss involving damage or necrosis of subcutaneous tissue, left upper back

SP SH SL **L89.124** **Pressure ulcer of left upper back, stage 4**

Healing pressure ulcer of left upper back, stage 4

Pressure ulcer with necrosis of soft tissues through to underlying muscle, tendon, or bone, left upper back

⭐ **L89.126** **Pressure-induced deep tissue damage of left upper back**

IQ **L89.129** **Pressure ulcer of left upper back, unspecified stage**

Healing pressure ulcer of left upper back NOS

Healing pressure ulcer of left upper back, unspecified stage

6 **L89.13** **Pressure ulcer of right lower back**

SP SH SL **L89.130** **Pressure ulcer of right lower back, unstageable**

SP **L89.131** **Pressure ulcer of right lower back, stage 1**

Healing pressure ulcer of right lower back, stage 1

Pressure pre-ulcer skin changes limited to persistent focal edema, right lower back

SP SH SL **L89.132** **Pressure ulcer of right lower back, stage 2**

Healing pressure ulcer of right lower back, stage 2

Pressure ulcer with abrasion, blister, partial thickness skin loss involving epidermis and/or dermis, right lower back

SP SH SL **L89.133** **Pressure ulcer of right lower back, stage 3**

Healing pressure ulcer of right lower back, stage 3

Pressure ulcer with full thickness skin loss involving damage or necrosis of subcutaneous tissue, right lower back

SP SH SL **L89.134** **Pressure ulcer of right lower back, stage 4**

Healing pressure ulcer of right lower back, stage 4

Pressure ulcer with necrosis of soft tissues through to underlying muscle, tendon, or bone, right lower back

⭐ **L89.136** **Pressure-induced deep tissue damage of right lower back**

⭐ New ▲ Revised **Px** Primary **SP** PDGM Px **SL** Low CoM **SH** High CoM **IQ** Quest. Encounter **H** Hospice non-cancer Dx | Unspecified | **M** *Manifestation*

▣ IQ L89.139 Pressure ulcer of right lower back, unspecified stage

Healing pressure ulcer of right lower back NOS

Healing pressure ulcer of right lower back, unspecified stage

⑥ L89.14 Pressure ulcer of left lower back

▣ SP SH SL L89.140 Pressure ulcer of left lower back, unstageable

▣ SP L89.141 Pressure ulcer of left lower back, stage 1

Healing pressure ulcer of left lower back, stage 1

Pressure pre-ulcer skin changes limited to persistent focal edema, left lower back

▣ SP SH SL L89.142 Pressure ulcer of left lower back, stage 2

Healing pressure ulcer of left lower back, stage 2

Pressure ulcer with abrasion, blister, partial thickness skin loss involving epidermis and/or dermis, left lower back

▣ SP SH SL L89.143 Pressure ulcer of left lower back, stage 3

Healing pressure ulcer of left lower back, stage 3

Pressure ulcer with full thickness skin loss involving damage or necrosis of subcutaneous tissue, left lower back

▣ SP SH SL L89.144 Pressure ulcer of left lower back, stage 4

Healing pressure ulcer of left lower back, stage 4

Pressure ulcer with necrosis of soft tissues through to underlying muscle, tendon, or bone, left lower back

★ ▣ L89.146 Pressure-induced deep tissue damage of left lower back

▣ IQ L89.149 Pressure ulcer of left lower back, unspecified stage

Healing pressure ulcer of left lower back NOS

Healing pressure ulcer of left lower back, unspecified stage

⑥ L89.15 Pressure ulcer of sacral region

Pressure ulcer of coccyx

Pressure ulcer of tailbone

SP SH SL L89.150 Pressure ulcer of sacral region, unstageable

SP L89.151 Pressure ulcer of sacral region, stage 1

Healing pressure ulcer of sacral region, stage 1

Pressure pre-ulcer skin changes limited to persistent focal edema, sacral region

SP SH SL L89.152 Pressure ulcer of sacral region, stage 2

Healing pressure ulcer of sacral region, stage 2

Pressure ulcer with abrasion, blister, partial thickness skin loss involving epidermis and/or dermis, sacral region

SP SH SL L89.153 Pressure ulcer of sacral region, stage 3

Healing pressure ulcer of sacral region, stage 3

Pressure ulcer with full thickness skin loss involving damage or necrosis of subcutaneous tissue, sacral region

SP SH SL L89.154 Pressure ulcer of sacral region, stage 4

Healing pressure ulcer of sacral region, stage 4

Pressure ulcer with necrosis of soft tissues through to underlying muscle, tendon, or bone, sacral region

★ L89.156 Pressure-induced deep tissue damage of sacral region

IQ L89.159 Pressure ulcer of sacral region, unspecified stage

Healing pressure ulcer of sacral region NOS

Healing pressure ulcer of sacral region, unspecified stage

⑤ L89.2 Pressure ulcer of hip

⑥ L89.20 Pressure ulcer of unspecified hip

IQ L89.200 Pressure ulcer of unspecified hip, unstageable

IQ L89.201 Pressure ulcer of unspecified hip, stage 1

Healing pressure ulcer of unspecified hip back, stage 1

Pressure pre-ulcer skin changes limited to persistent focal edema, unspecified hip

IQ L89.202 Pressure ulcer of unspecified hip, stage 2

Healing pressure ulcer of unspecified hip, stage 2

Pressure ulcer with abrasion, blister, partial thickness skin loss involving epidermis and/or dermis, unspecified hip

IQ L89.203 Pressure ulcer of unspecified hip, stage 3

Healing pressure ulcer of unspecified hip, stage 3

Pressure ulcer with full thickness skin loss involving damage or necrosis of subcutaneous tissue, unspecified hip

IQ L89.204 Pressure ulcer of unspecified hip, stage 4

Healing pressure ulcer of unspecified hip, stage 4

Pressure ulcer with necrosis of soft tissues through to underlying muscle, tendon, or bone, unspecified hip

★ L89.206 Pressure-induced deep tissue damage of unspecified hip

IQ L89.209 Pressure ulcer of unspecified hip, unspecified stage

Healing pressure ulcer of unspecified hip NOS

Healing pressure ulcer of unspecified hip, unspecified stage

4 4th digit required   **5** 5th digit required   **6** 6th digit required   **7** 7th digit required   **7** 7th digit placeholder   **✚** Additional code   **▣** Laterality

1124   *DecisionHealth's* FY 2020 Complete Home Health ICD-10-CM Diagnosis Coding Manual

⑥ L89.21   Pressure ulcer of right hip

☐ SP SH SL L89.210   Pressure ulcer of right hip, unstageable

☐ SP L89.211   Pressure ulcer of right hip, stage 1
Healing pressure ulcer of right hip back, stage 1
Pressure pre-ulcer skin changes limited to persistent focal edema, right hip

☐ SP SH SL L89.212   Pressure ulcer of right hip, stage 2
Healing pressure ulcer of right hip, stage 2
Pressure ulcer with abrasion, blister, partial thickness skin loss involving epidermis and/or dermis, right hip

☐ SP SH SL L89.213   Pressure ulcer of right hip, stage 3
Healing pressure ulcer of right hip, stage 3
Pressure ulcer with full thickness skin loss involving damage or necrosis of subcutaneous tissue, right hip

☐ SP SH SL L89.214   Pressure ulcer of right hip, stage 4
Healing pressure ulcer of right hip, stage 4
Pressure ulcer with necrosis of soft tissues through to underlying muscle, tendon, or bone, right hip

★ ☐ L89.216   Pressure-induced deep tissue damage of right hip

☐ IQ L89.219   Pressure ulcer of right hip, unspecified stage
Healing pressure ulcer of right hip NOS
Healing pressure ulcer of right hip, unspecified stage

⑥ L89.22   Pressure ulcer of left hip

☐ SP SH SL L89.220   Pressure ulcer of left hip, unstageable

☐ SP L89.221   Pressure ulcer of left hip, stage 1
Healing pressure ulcer of left hip back, stage 1
Pressure pre-ulcer skin changes limited to persistent focal edema, left hip

☐ SP SH SL L89.222   Pressure ulcer of left hip, stage 2
Healing pressure ulcer of left hip, stage 2
Pressure ulcer with abrasion, blister, partial thickness skin loss involving epidermis and/or dermis, left hip

☐ SP SH SL L89.223   Pressure ulcer of left hip, stage 3
Healing pressure ulcer of left hip, stage 3
Pressure ulcer with full thickness skin loss involving damage or necrosis of subcutaneous tissue, left hip

☐ SP SH SL L89.224   Pressure ulcer of left hip, stage 4
Healing pressure ulcer of left hip, stage 4
Pressure ulcer with necrosis of soft tissues through to underlying muscle, tendon, or bone, left hip

★ ☐ L89.226   Pressure-induced deep tissue damage of left hip

☐ IQ L89.229   Pressure ulcer of left hip, unspecified stage
Healing pressure ulcer of left hip NOS
Healing pressure ulcer of left hip, unspecified stage

⑤ L89.3   Pressure ulcer of buttock

CODING TIPS ✓   A pressure ulcer/injury described as being on the ischial tuberosity, is considered to be on the buttock.

⑥ L89.30   Pressure ulcer of unspecified buttock

IQ L89.300   Pressure ulcer of unspecified buttock, unstageable

IQ L89.301   Pressure ulcer of unspecified buttock, stage 1
Healing pressure ulcer of unspecified buttock, stage 1
Pressure pre-ulcer skin changes limited to persistent focal edema, unspecified buttock

IQ L89.302   Pressure ulcer of unspecified buttock, stage 2
Healing pressure ulcer of unspecified buttock, stage 2
Pressure ulcer with abrasion, blister, partial thickness skin loss involving epidermis and/or dermis, unspecified buttock

IQ L89.303   Pressure ulcer of unspecified buttock, stage 3
Healing pressure ulcer of unspecified buttock, stage 3
Pressure ulcer with full thickness skin loss involving damage or necrosis of subcutaneous tissue, unspecified buttock

IQ L89.304   Pressure ulcer of unspecified buttock, stage 4
Healing pressure ulcer of unspecified buttock, stage 4
Pressure ulcer with necrosis of soft tissues through to underlying muscle, tendon, or bone, unspecified buttock

★ L89.306   Pressure-induced deep tissue damage of unspecified buttock

IQ L89.309   Pressure ulcer of unspecified buttock, unspecified stage
Healing pressure ulcer of unspecified buttock NOS
Healing pressure ulcer of unspecified buttock, unspecified stage

⑥ L89.31   Pressure ulcer of right buttock

☐ SP SH SL L89.310   Pressure ulcer of right buttock, unstageable

☐ SP L89.311   Pressure ulcer of right buttock, stage 1
Healing pressure ulcer of right buttock, stage 1
Pressure pre-ulcer skin changes limited to persistent focal edema, right buttock

☐ SP SH SL L89.312   Pressure ulcer of right buttock, stage 2

★ New ▲ Revised Px Primary SP PDGM Px SL Low CoM SH High CoM IQ Quest. Encounter H Hospice non-cancer Dx Unspecified M *Manifestation*

DecisionHealth's FY 2020 Complete Home Health ICD-10-CM Diagnosis Coding Manual

1125

Chapter 12

L00-L99

Healing pressure ulcer of right buttock, stage 2

Pressure ulcer with abrasion, blister, partial thickness skin loss involving epidermis and/or dermis, right buttock

☐ SP SH SL L89.313 Pressure ulcer of right buttock, stage 3

Healing pressure ulcer of right buttock, stage 3

Pressure ulcer with full thickness skin loss involving damage or necrosis of subcutaneous tissue, right buttock

☐ SP SH SL L89.314 Pressure ulcer of right buttock, stage 4

Healing pressure ulcer of right buttock, stage 4

Pressure ulcer with necrosis of soft tissues through to underlying muscle, tendon, or bone, right buttock

★ ☐ L89.316 Pressure-induced deep tissue damage of right buttock

☐ IQ L89.319 Pressure ulcer of right buttock, unspecified stage

Healing pressure ulcer of right buttock NOS

Healing pressure ulcer of right buttock, unspecified stage

6 L89.32 Pressure ulcer of left buttock

☐ SP SH SL L89.320 Pressure ulcer of left buttock, unstageable

☐ SP L89.321 Pressure ulcer of left buttock, stage 1

Healing pressure ulcer of left buttock, stage 1

Pressure pre-ulcer skin changes limited to persistent focal edema, left buttock

☐ SP SH SL L89.322 Pressure ulcer of left buttock, stage 2

Healing pressure ulcer of left buttock, stage 2

Pressure ulcer with abrasion, blister, partial thickness skin loss involving epidermis and/or dermis, left buttock

☐ SP SH SL L89.323 Pressure ulcer of left buttock, stage 3

Healing pressure ulcer of left buttock, stage 3

Pressure ulcer with full thickness skin loss involving damage or necrosis of subcutaneous tissue, left buttock

☐ SP SH SL L89.324 Pressure ulcer of left buttock, stage 4

Healing pressure ulcer of left buttock, stage 4

Pressure ulcer with necrosis of soft tissues through to underlying muscle, tendon, or bone, left buttock

★ ☐ L89.326 Pressure-induced deep tissue damage of left buttock

☐ IQ L89.329 Pressure ulcer of left buttock, unspecified stage

Healing pressure ulcer of left buttock NOS

Healing pressure ulcer of left buttock, unspecified stage

5 L89.4 Pressure ulcer of contiguous site of back, buttock and hip

CODING TIPS ✓ When a patient presents with a pressure ulcer/injury that is contiguous to the surface area of the back, buttock, and/or hip, a code from L89.4- should be assigned. The stage of the ulcer/injury should be assigned as the worst stage identifiable (the area of the ulcer which has deteriorated to its worst stage).

IQ L89.40 Pressure ulcer of contiguous site of back, buttock and hip, unspecified stage

Healing pressure ulcer of contiguous site of back, buttock and hip NOS

Healing pressure ulcer of contiguous site of back, buttock and hip, unspecified stage

SP L89.41 Pressure ulcer of contiguous site of back, buttock and hip, stage 1

Healing pressure ulcer of contiguous site of back, buttock and hip, stage 1

Pressure pre-ulcer skin changes limited to persistent focal edema, contiguous site of back, buttock and hip

SP SH SL L89.42 Pressure ulcer of contiguous site of back, buttock and hip, stage 2

Healing pressure ulcer of contiguous site of back, buttock and hip, stage 2

Pressure ulcer with abrasion, blister, partial thickness skin loss involving epidermis and/or dermis, contiguous site of back, buttock and hip

SP SH SL L89.43 Pressure ulcer of contiguous site of back, buttock and hip, stage 3

Healing pressure ulcer of contiguous site of back, buttock and hip, stage 3

Pressure ulcer with full thickness skin loss involving damage or necrosis of subcutaneous tissue, contiguous site of back, buttock and hip

SP SH SL L89.44 Pressure ulcer of contiguous site of back, buttock and hip, stage 4

Healing pressure ulcer of contiguous site of back, buttock and hip, stage 4

Pressure ulcer with necrosis of soft tissues through to underlying muscle, tendon, or bone, contiguous site of back, buttock and hip

SP SH SL L89.45 Pressure ulcer of contiguous site of back, buttock and hip, unstageable

★ L89.46 Pressure-induced deep tissue damage of contiguous site of back, buttock and hip

5 L89.5 Pressure ulcer of ankle

6 L89.50 Pressure ulcer of unspecified ankle

IQ L89.500 Pressure ulcer of unspecified ankle, unstageable

IQ L89.501 Pressure ulcer of unspecified ankle, stage 1

Healing pressure ulcer of unspecified ankle, stage 1

---

4 4th digit required   5 5th digit required   6 6th digit required   7 7th digit required   7 7th digit placeholder   ✚ Additional code   ☐ Laterality

1126   *DecisionHealth's* FY 2020 Complete Home Health ICD-10-CM Diagnosis Coding Manual

Chapter 12

L00-L99

Pressure pre-ulcer skin changes limited to persistent focal edema, unspecified ankle

IQ **L89.502** **Pressure ulcer of unspecified ankle, stage 2**

Healing pressure ulcer of unspecified ankle, stage 2

Pressure ulcer with abrasion, blister, partial thickness skin loss involving epidermis and/or dermis, unspecified ankle

IQ **L89.503** **Pressure ulcer of unspecified ankle, stage 3**

Healing pressure ulcer of unspecified ankle, stage 3

Pressure ulcer with full thickness skin loss involving damage or necrosis of subcutaneous tissue, unspecified ankle

IQ **L89.504** **Pressure ulcer of unspecified ankle, stage 4**

Healing pressure ulcer of unspecified ankle, stage 4

Pressure ulcer with necrosis of soft tissues through to underlying muscle, tendon, or bone, unspecified ankle

★ **L89.506** **Pressure-induced deep tissue damage of unspecified ankle**

IQ **L89.509** **Pressure ulcer of unspecified ankle, unspecified stage**

Healing pressure ulcer of unspecified ankle NOS

Healing pressure ulcer of unspecified ankle, unspecified stage

6 **L89.51** **Pressure ulcer of right ankle**

⊟ SP SH SL **L89.510** **Pressure ulcer of right ankle, unstageable**

⊟ SP **L89.511** **Pressure ulcer of right ankle, stage 1**

Healing pressure ulcer of right ankle, stage 1

Pressure pre-ulcer skin changes limited to persistent focal edema, right ankle

⊟ SP SH SL **L89.512** **Pressure ulcer of right ankle, stage 2**

Healing pressure ulcer of right ankle, stage 2

Pressure ulcer with abrasion, blister, partial thickness skin loss involving epidermis and/or dermis, right ankle

⊟ SP SH SL **L89.513** **Pressure ulcer of right ankle, stage 3**

Healing pressure ulcer of right ankle, stage 3

Pressure ulcer with full thickness skin loss involving damage or necrosis of subcutaneous tissue, right ankle

⊟ SP SH SL **L89.514** **Pressure ulcer of right ankle, stage 4**

Healing pressure ulcer of right ankle, stage 4

Pressure ulcer with necrosis of soft tissues through to underlying muscle, tendon, or bone, right ankle

★ **⊟ L89.516** **Pressure-induced deep tissue damage of right ankle**

⊟ IQ **L89.519** **Pressure ulcer of right ankle, unspecified stage**

Healing pressure ulcer of right ankle NOS

Healing pressure ulcer of right ankle, unspecified stage

6 **L89.52** **Pressure ulcer of left ankle**

⊟ SP SH SL **L89.520** **Pressure ulcer of left ankle, unstageable**

⊟ SP **L89.521** **Pressure ulcer of left ankle, stage 1**

Healing pressure ulcer of left ankle, stage 1

Pressure pre-ulcer skin changes limited to persistent focal edema, left ankle

⊟ SP SH SL **L89.522** **Pressure ulcer of left ankle, stage 2**

Healing pressure ulcer of left ankle, stage 2

Pressure ulcer with abrasion, blister, partial thickness skin loss involving epidermis and/or dermis, left ankle

⊟ SP SH SL **L89.523** **Pressure ulcer of left ankle, stage 3**

Healing pressure ulcer of left ankle, stage 3

Pressure ulcer with full thickness skin loss involving damage or necrosis of subcutaneous tissue, left ankle

⊟ SP SH SL **L89.524** **Pressure ulcer of left ankle, stage 4**

Healing pressure ulcer of left ankle, stage 4

Pressure ulcer with necrosis of soft tissues through to underlying muscle, tendon, or bone, left ankle

★ **⊟ L89.526** **Pressure-induced deep tissue damage of left ankle**

⊟ IQ **L89.529** **Pressure ulcer of left ankle, unspecified stage**

Healing pressure ulcer of left ankle NOS

Healing pressure ulcer of left ankle, unspecified stage

5 **L89.6** **Pressure ulcer of heel**

6 **L89.60** **Pressure ulcer of unspecified heel**

IQ **L89.600** **Pressure ulcer of unspecified heel, unstageable**

IQ **L89.601** **Pressure ulcer of unspecified heel, stage 1**

Healing pressure ulcer of unspecified heel, stage 1

Pressure pre-ulcer skin changes limited to persistent focal edema, unspecified heel

IQ **L89.602** **Pressure ulcer of unspecified heel, stage 2**

Chapter 12

L00-L99

★ New ▲ Revised **Px** Primary **SP** PDGM Px **SL** Low CoM **SH** High CoM **IQ** Quest. Encounter **H** Hospice non-cancer Dx **Unspecified** **M** *Manifestation*

DecisionHealth's FY 2020 Complete Home Health ICD-10-CM Diagnosis Coding Manual

1127

Healing pressure ulcer of
unspecified heel, stage 2
Pressure ulcer with abrasion, blister,
partial thickness skin loss
involving epidermis and/or
dermis, unspecified heel

IQ L89.603 **Pressure ulcer of unspecified heel, stage 3**

Healing pressure ulcer of
unspecified heel, stage 3
Pressure ulcer with full thickness
skin loss involving damage or
necrosis of subcutaneous tissue,
unspecified heel

IQ L89.604 **Pressure ulcer of unspecified heel, stage 4**

Healing pressure ulcer of
unspecified heel, stage 4
Pressure ulcer with necrosis of soft
tissues through to underlying
muscle, tendon, or bone,
unspecified heel

★ **L89.606** **Pressure-induced deep tissue damage of unspecified heel**

IQ L89.609 **Pressure ulcer of unspecified heel, unspecified stage**

Healing pressure ulcer of
unspecified heel NOS
Healing pressure ulcer of
unspecified heel, unspecified stage

6 L89.61 **Pressure ulcer of right heel**

☐ SP SH SL **L89.610** **Pressure ulcer of right heel, unstageable**

☐ SP **L89.611** **Pressure ulcer of right heel, stage 1**

Healing pressure ulcer of right heel,
stage 1
Pressure pre-ulcer skin changes
limited to persistent focal edema,
right heel

☐ SP SH SL **L89.612** **Pressure ulcer of right heel, stage 2**

Healing pressure ulcer of right heel,
stage 2
Pressure ulcer with abrasion, blister,
partial thickness skin loss
involving epidermis and/or
dermis, right heel

☐ SP SH SL **L89.613** **Pressure ulcer of right heel, stage 3**

Healing pressure ulcer of right heel,
stage 3
Pressure ulcer with full thickness
skin loss involving damage or
necrosis of subcutaneous tissue,
right heel

☐ SP SH SL **L89.614** **Pressure ulcer of right heel, stage 4**

Healing pressure ulcer of right heel,
stage 4
Pressure ulcer with necrosis of soft
tissues through to underlying
muscle, tendon, or bone, right heel

★ ☐ **L89.616** **Pressure-induced deep tissue damage of right heel**

☐ IQ **L89.619** **Pressure ulcer of right heel, unspecified stage**

Healing pressure ulcer of right heel
NOS
Healing pressure ulcer of right heel,
unspecified stage

6 L89.62 **Pressure ulcer of left heel**

☐ SP SH SL **L89.620** **Pressure ulcer of left heel, unstageable**

☐ SP **L89.621** **Pressure ulcer of left heel, stage 1**

Healing pressure ulcer of left heel,
stage 1
Pressure pre-ulcer skin changes
limited to persistent focal edema,
left heel

☐ SP SH SL **L89.622** **Pressure ulcer of left heel, stage 2**

Healing pressure ulcer of left heel,
stage 2
Pressure ulcer with abrasion, blister,
partial thickness skin loss
involving epidermis and/or
dermis, left heel

☐ SP SH SL **L89.623** **Pressure ulcer of left heel, stage 3**

Healing pressure ulcer of left heel,
stage 3
Pressure ulcer with full thickness
skin loss involving damage or
necrosis of subcutaneous tissue,
left heel

☐ SP SH SL **L89.624** **Pressure ulcer of left heel, stage 4**

Healing pressure ulcer of left heel,
stage 4
Pressure ulcer with necrosis of soft
tissues through to underlying
muscle, tendon, or bone, left heel

★ ☐ **L89.626** **Pressure-induced deep tissue damage of left heel**

☐ IQ **L89.629** **Pressure ulcer of left heel, unspecified stage**

Healing pressure ulcer of left heel
NOS
Healing pressure ulcer of left heel,
unspecified stage

5 L89.8 **Pressure ulcer of other site**

CODING TIPS ✓ Use this subcategory for
pressure ulcers/injuries between the knees,
edge of the ear, bridge of the nose and
other areas not covered by the other L89
codes. Do not use L89.9.

6 L89.81 **Pressure ulcer of head**

Pressure ulcer of face

SP SH SL **L89.810** **Pressure ulcer of head, unstageable**

SP **L89.811** **Pressure ulcer of head, stage 1**

Healing pressure ulcer of head,
stage 1
Pressure pre-ulcer skin changes
limited to persistent focal edema,
head

SP SH SL **L89.812** **Pressure ulcer of head, stage 2**

Healing pressure ulcer of head,
stage 2
Pressure ulcer with abrasion, blister,
partial thickness skin loss
involving epidermis and/or
dermis, head

SP SH SL **L89.813** **Pressure ulcer of head, stage 3**

Healing pressure ulcer of head,
stage 3

4 4th digit required   **5** 5th digit required   **6** 6th digit required   **7** 7th digit required   **7** 7th digit placeholder   **+** Additional code   ☐ Laterality

1128   *DecisionHealth's* FY 2020 Complete Home Health ICD-10-CM Diagnosis Coding Manual

Pressure ulcer with full thickness skin loss involving damage or necrosis of subcutaneous tissue, head

SP SH SL L89.814 Pressure ulcer of head, stage 4

Healing pressure ulcer of head, stage 4

Pressure ulcer with necrosis of soft tissues through to underlying muscle, tendon, or bone, head

★ **L89.816 Pressure-induced deep tissue damage of head**

IQ L89.819 Pressure ulcer of head, unspecified stage

Healing pressure ulcer of head NOS

Healing pressure ulcer of head, unspecified stage

6 **L89.89 Pressure ulcer of other site**

SP SH SL L89.890 Pressure ulcer of other site, unstageable

SP L89.891 Pressure ulcer of other site, stage 1

Healing pressure ulcer of other site, stage 1

Pressure pre-ulcer skin changes limited to persistent focal edema, other site

SP SH SL L89.892 Pressure ulcer of other site, stage 2

Healing pressure ulcer of other site, stage 2

Pressure ulcer with abrasion, blister, partial thickness skin loss involving epidermis and/or dermis, other site

SP SH SL L89.893 Pressure ulcer of other site, stage 3

Healing pressure ulcer of other site, stage 3

Pressure ulcer with full thickness skin loss involving damage or necrosis of subcutaneous tissue, other site

SP SH SL L89.894 Pressure ulcer of other site, stage 4

Healing pressure ulcer of other site, stage 4

Pressure ulcer with necrosis of soft tissues through to underlying muscle, tendon, or bone, other site

★ **L89.896 Pressure-induced deep tissue damage of other site**

IQ L89.899 Pressure ulcer of other site, unspecified stage

Healing pressure ulcer of other site NOS

Healing pressure ulcer of other site, unspecified stage

5 **L89.9 Pressure ulcer of unspecified site**

CODING TIPS ✓ Home health and hospice coders should never have to use L89.9- for pressure ulcer of unspecified site.

IQ L89.90 Pressure ulcer of unspecified site, unspecified stage

Healing pressure ulcer of unspecified site NOS

Healing pressure ulcer of unspecified site, unspecified stage

IQ L89.91 Pressure ulcer of unspecified site, stage 1

Healing pressure ulcer of unspecified site, stage 1

Pressure pre-ulcer skin changes limited to persistent focal edema, unspecified site

IQ L89.92 Pressure ulcer of unspecified site, stage 2

Healing pressure ulcer of unspecified site, stage 2

Pressure ulcer with abrasion, blister, partial thickness skin loss involving epidermis and/or dermis, unspecified site

IQ L89.93 Pressure ulcer of unspecified site, stage 3

Healing pressure ulcer of unspecified site, stage 3

Pressure ulcer with full thickness skin loss involving damage or necrosis of subcutaneous tissue, unspecified site

IQ L89.94 Pressure ulcer of unspecified site, stage 4

Healing pressure ulcer of unspecified site, stage 4

Pressure ulcer with necrosis of soft tissues through to underlying muscle, tendon, or bone, unspecified site

IQ L89.95 Pressure ulcer of unspecified site, unstageable

★ **L89.96 Pressure-induced deep tissue damage of unspecified site**

4 **L90 Atrophic disorders of skin**

SP L90.0 Lichen sclerosus et atrophicus

EXCLUDES 2 lichen sclerosus of external female genital organs (N90.4)

lichen sclerosus of external male genital organs (N48.0)

SP L90.1 Anetoderma of Schweninger-Buzzi

SP L90.2 Anetoderma of Jadassohn-Pellizzari

SP L90.3 Atrophoderma of Pasini and Pierini

SP L90.4 Acrodermatitis chronica atrophicans

SP L90.5 Scar conditions and fibrosis of skin

Adherent scar (skin)

Cicatrix

Disfigurement of skin due to scar

Fibrosis of skin NOS

Scar NOS

EXCLUDES 2 hypertrophic scar (L91.0)

keloid scar (L91.0)

SP L90.6 Striae atrophicae

SP L90.8 Other atrophic disorders of skin

IQ L90.9 Atrophic disorder of skin, unspecified

4 **L91 Hypertrophic disorders of skin**

SP L91.0 Hypertrophic scar

Keloid

Keloid scar

EXCLUDES 2 acne keloid (L73.0)

scar NOS (L90.5)

SP L91.8 Other hypertrophic disorders of the skin

Chapter 12

L00-L99

★ New ▲ Revised Px Primary **SP** PDGM Px **SL** Low CoM **SH** High CoM **IQ** Quest. Encounter **H** Hospice non-cancer Dx Unspecified **M** Manifestation

DecisionHealth's FY 2020 Complete Home Health ICD-10-CM Diagnosis Coding Manual

1129

IQ L91.9 Hypertrophic disorder of the skin, unspecified

4 L92 Granulomatous disorders of skin and subcutaneous tissue
> EXCLUDES 2   actinic granuloma (L57.5)

SP L92.0 Granuloma annulare
Perforating granuloma annulare

SP L92.1 Necrobiosis lipoidica, not elsewhere classified
> EXCLUDES 1   necrobiosis lipoidica associated with diabetes mellitus (E08-E13 with .620)

SP L92.2 Granuloma faciale [eosinophilic granuloma of skin]

SP + L92.3 Foreign body granuloma of the skin and subcutaneous tissue
Use additional code to identify the type of retained foreign body (Z18.-)

SP L92.8 Other granulomatous disorders of the skin and subcutaneous tissue

SP L92.9 Granulomatous disorder of the skin and subcutaneous tissue, unspecified
> EXCLUDES 2   umbilical granuloma (P83.81)

+ 4 L93 Lupus erythematosus
Use additional code for adverse effect, if applicable, to identify drug (T36-T50 with fifth or sixth character 5)
> EXCLUDES 1   lupus exedens (A18.4)
> lupus vulgaris (A18.4)
> scleroderma (M34.-)
> systemic lupus erythematosus (M32.-)

SP + L93.0 Discoid lupus erythematosus
Lupus erythematosus NOS

SP + L93.1 Subacute cutaneous lupus erythematosus

SP + L93.2 Other local lupus erythematosus
Lupus erythematosus profundus
Lupus panniculitis

4 L94 Other localized connective tissue disorders
> EXCLUDES 1   systemic connective tissue disorders (M30-M36)

SP L94.0 Localized scleroderma [morphea]
Circumscribed scleroderma

SP L94.1 Linear scleroderma
En coup de sabre lesion

SP L94.2 Calcinosis cutis

SP L94.3 Sclerodactyly

SP L94.4 Gottron's papules

SP L94.5 Poikiloderma vasculare atrophicans

SP L94.6 Ainhum

SP L94.8 Other specified localized connective tissue disorders

IQ L94.9 Localized connective tissue disorder, unspecified

4 L95 Vasculitis limited to skin, not elsewhere classified
> EXCLUDES 1   angioma serpiginosum (L81.7)
> Henoch (-Schönlein) purpura (D69.0)
> hypersensitivity angiitis (M31.0)
> lupus panniculitis (L93.2)
> panniculitis NOS (M79.3)

panniculitis of neck and back (M54.0-)
polyarteritis nodosa (M30.0)
relapsing panniculitis (M35.6)
rheumatoid vasculitis (M05.2)
serum sickness (T80.6-)
urticaria (L50.-)
Wegener's granulomatosis (M31.3-)

SP L95.0 Livedoid vasculitis
Atrophie blanche (en plaque)

SP L95.1 Erythema elevatum diutinum

SP L95.8 Other vasculitis limited to the skin

SP L95.9 Vasculitis limited to the skin, unspecified

4 L97 Non-pressure chronic ulcer of lower limb, not elsewhere classified
> INCLUDES   chronic ulcer of skin of lower limb NOS
> non-healing ulcer of skin
> non-infected sinus of skin
> trophic ulcer NOS
> tropical ulcer NOS
> ulcer of skin of lower limb NOS

Code first any associated underlying condition, such as:
any associated gangrene (I96)
atherosclerosis of the lower extremities (I70.23-, I70.24-, I70.33-, I70.34-, I70.43-, I70.44-, I70.53-, I70.54-, I70.63-, I70.64-, I70.73-, I70.74-)
chronic venous hypertension (I87.31-, I87.33-)
diabetic ulcers (E08.621, E08.622, E09.621, E09.622, E10.621, E10.622, E11.621, E11.622, E13.621, E13.622)
postphlebitic syndrome (I87.01-, I87.03-)
postthrombotic syndrome (I87.01-, I87.03-)
varicose ulcer (I83.0-, I83.2-)
> EXCLUDES 2   pressure ulcer (pressure area) (L89.-)
> skin infections (L00-L08)
> specific infections classified to A00-B99

> GUIDELINES   Section I.B.14
For the Body Mass Index (BMI), depth of non-pressure chronic ulcers, pressure ulcer stage, coma scale, and NIH stroke scale (NIHSS) codes, code assignment may be based on medical record documentation from clinicians who are not the patient's provider (i.e., physician or other qualified healthcare practitioner legally accountable for establishing the patient's diagnosis), since this information is typically documented by other clinicians involved in the care of the patient (e.g., a dietitian often documents the BMI, a nurse often documents the pressure ulcer stages, and an emergency medical technician often documents the coma scale). However, the associated diagnosis (such as overweight, obesity, acute stroke, or pressure ulcer) must be documented by the patient's provider.

---

4 4th digit required   5 5th digit required   6 6th digit required   7 7th digit required   7 7th digit placeholder   + Additional code   ▣ Laterality

CODING TIPS ✓   When coding any non-pressure chronic ulcer classifiable to L97, first code the underlying cause of the ulcer, if known, followed by the appropriate L97 code to identify the ulcer location, site and severity. Gangrene (I96) associated with the ulcer should be coded first prior to sequencing of the L97 code. Skin ulceration on the foot in a diabetic is assumed related to the diabetes, unless otherwise specified by the physician. Skin ulceration on areas other than the foot are not assumed related to diabetes unless documented by the physician. Diabetic neuropathies and peripheral angiopathies are considered co-morbidities and are not coded as causes of diabetic ulcers.

CODING TIPS ✓   If granulation tissue is documented, the 6th character of L97 should at least be a 2. (Ulcers limited to breakdown of skin do not granulate.) Before assigning 6th character 3, there must be evidence of muscle necrosis, not just muscle exposure. Before assigning 6th character 4, there must be evidence of bone necrosis, not just bone exposure. Sixth characters 5 and 6 may be used if muscle or bone, respectively, is involved, but necrosis cannot be determined. Sixth character 8 may be used if documentation of other structures, such as tendon and bone, are documented.

CODING TIPS ✓   L97 codes are specific for location, including laterality and severity (e.g., skin, fat layer exposed, muscle involvement, necrosis of muscle, bone involvement, necrosis of bone, and other specified). The severity of the ulcer may be determined and coded based upon nursing documentation, but the diagnosis of the ulcer must come from the physician.

CODING TIPS ✓   More than one L97 code may be used on a claim/record depending on the number of ulcers, cause of the ulcers, location on the lower limb, and severity of the ulcers. The same code may only be used once. Watch out for laterality. Do not choose an unspecified side code. There are no codes for bilateral, so if the condition is bilateral, a code for the right and a code for the left must be used. Two ulcers at the same location, but of different severity, may both be coded.

�5 **L97.1   Non-pressure chronic ulcer of thigh**

�6 **L97.10   Non-pressure chronic ulcer of unspecified thigh**

!Q L97.101   Non-pressure chronic ulcer of unspecified thigh limited to breakdown of skin

!Q L97.102   Non-pressure chronic ulcer of unspecified thigh with fat layer exposed

!Q L97.103   Non-pressure chronic ulcer of unspecified thigh with necrosis of muscle

!Q L97.104   Non-pressure chronic ulcer of unspecified thigh with necrosis of bone

!Q L97.105   Non-pressure chronic ulcer of unspecified thigh with muscle involvement without evidence of necrosis

!Q L97.106   Non-pressure chronic ulcer of unspecified thigh with bone involvement without evidence of necrosis

!Q L97.108   Non-pressure chronic ulcer of unspecified thigh with other specified severity

!Q L97.109   Non-pressure chronic ulcer of unspecified thigh with unspecified severity

�6 **L97.11   Non-pressure chronic ulcer of right thigh**

⇄ **SP SH SL L97.111   Non-pressure chronic ulcer of right thigh limited to breakdown of skin**

⇄ **SP SH SL L97.112   Non-pressure chronic ulcer of right thigh with fat layer exposed**

⇄ **SP SH SL L97.113   Non-pressure chronic ulcer of right thigh with necrosis of muscle**

⇄ **SP SH SL L97.114   Non-pressure chronic ulcer of right thigh with necrosis of bone**

⇄ **SP SH SL L97.115   Non-pressure chronic ulcer of right thigh with muscle involvement without evidence of necrosis**

⇄ **SP SH SL L97.116   Non-pressure chronic ulcer of right thigh with bone involvement without evidence of necrosis**

⇄ **SP SH SL L97.118   Non-pressure chronic ulcer of right thigh with other specified severity**

⇄ **SP SH SL L97.119   Non-pressure chronic ulcer of right thigh with unspecified severity**

�6 **L97.12   Non-pressure chronic ulcer of left thigh**

⇄ **SP SH SL L97.121   Non-pressure chronic ulcer of left thigh limited to breakdown of skin**

⇄ **SP SH SL L97.122   Non-pressure chronic ulcer of left thigh with fat layer exposed**

⇄ **SP SH SL L97.123   Non-pressure chronic ulcer of left thigh with necrosis of muscle**

⇄ **SP SH SL L97.124   Non-pressure chronic ulcer of left thigh with necrosis of bone**

⇄ **SP SH SL L97.125   Non-pressure chronic ulcer of left thigh with muscle involvement without evidence of necrosis**

⇄ **SP SH SL L97.126   Non-pressure chronic ulcer of left thigh with bone involvement without evidence of necrosis**

⇄ **SP SH SL L97.128   Non-pressure chronic ulcer of left thigh with other specified severity**

⇄ **SP SH SL L97.129   Non-pressure chronic ulcer of left thigh with unspecified severity**

�5 **L97.2   Non-pressure chronic ulcer of calf**

�6 **L97.20   Non-pressure chronic ulcer of unspecified calf**

!Q L97.201   Non-pressure chronic ulcer of unspecified calf limited to breakdown of skin

!Q L97.202   Non-pressure chronic ulcer of unspecified calf with fat layer exposed

★ New ▲ Revised Px Primary SP PDGM Px SL Low CoM SH High CoM !Q Quest. Encounter H Hospice non-cancer Dx   Unspecified   M *Manifestation*

DecisionHealth's FY 2020 Complete Home Health ICD-10-CM Diagnosis Coding Manual

1131

Chapter 12

L00-L99

!Q L97.203 Non-pressure chronic ulcer of unspecified calf with necrosis of muscle

!Q L97.204 Non-pressure chronic ulcer of unspecified calf with necrosis of bone

!Q L97.205 Non-pressure chronic ulcer of unspecified calf with muscle involvement without evidence of necrosis

!Q L97.206 Non-pressure chronic ulcer of unspecified calf with bone involvement without evidence of necrosis

!Q L97.208 Non-pressure chronic ulcer of unspecified calf with other specified severity

!Q L97.209 Non-pressure chronic ulcer of unspecified calf with unspecified severity

6 L97.21 Non-pressure chronic ulcer of right calf

SP SH SL L97.211 Non-pressure chronic ulcer of right calf limited to breakdown of skin

SP SH SL L97.212 Non-pressure chronic ulcer of right calf with fat layer exposed

SP SH SL L97.213 Non-pressure chronic ulcer of right calf with necrosis of muscle

SP SH SL L97.214 Non-pressure chronic ulcer of right calf with necrosis of bone

SP SH SL L97.215 Non-pressure chronic ulcer of right calf with muscle involvement without evidence of necrosis

SP SH SL L97.216 Non-pressure chronic ulcer of right calf with bone involvement without evidence of necrosis

SP SH SL L97.218 Non-pressure chronic ulcer of right calf with other specified severity

SP SH SL L97.219 Non-pressure chronic ulcer of right calf with unspecified severity

6 L97.22 Non-pressure chronic ulcer of left calf

SP SH SL L97.221 Non-pressure chronic ulcer of left calf limited to breakdown of skin

SP SH SL L97.222 Non-pressure chronic ulcer of left calf with fat layer exposed

SP SH SL L97.223 Non-pressure chronic ulcer of left calf with necrosis of muscle

SP SH SL L97.224 Non-pressure chronic ulcer of left calf with necrosis of bone

SP SH SL L97.225 Non-pressure chronic ulcer of left calf with muscle involvement without evidence of necrosis

SP SH SL L97.226 Non-pressure chronic ulcer of left calf with bone involvement without evidence of necrosis

SP SH SL L97.228 Non-pressure chronic ulcer of left calf with other specified severity

SP SH SL L97.229 Non-pressure chronic ulcer of left calf with unspecified severity

5 L97.3 Non-pressure chronic ulcer of ankle

6 L97.30 Non-pressure chronic ulcer of unspecified ankle

SP L97.301 Non-pressure chronic ulcer of unspecified ankle limited to breakdown of skin

!Q L97.302 Non-pressure chronic ulcer of unspecified ankle with fat layer exposed

!Q L97.303 Non-pressure chronic ulcer of unspecified ankle with necrosis of muscle

!Q L97.304 Non-pressure chronic ulcer of unspecified ankle with necrosis of bone

!Q L97.305 Non-pressure chronic ulcer of unspecified ankle with muscle involvement without evidence of necrosis

!Q L97.306 Non-pressure chronic ulcer of unspecified ankle with bone involvement without evidence of necrosis

!Q L97.308 Non-pressure chronic ulcer of unspecified ankle with other specified severity

!Q L97.309 Non-pressure chronic ulcer of unspecified ankle with unspecified severity

6 L97.31 Non-pressure chronic ulcer of right ankle

SP SH SL L97.311 Non-pressure chronic ulcer of right ankle limited to breakdown of skin

SP SH SL L97.312 Non-pressure chronic ulcer of right ankle with fat layer exposed

SP SH SL L97.313 Non-pressure chronic ulcer of right ankle with necrosis of muscle

SP SH SL L97.314 Non-pressure chronic ulcer of right ankle with necrosis of bone

SP SH SL L97.315 Non-pressure chronic ulcer of right ankle with muscle involvement without evidence of necrosis

SP SH SL L97.316 Non-pressure chronic ulcer of right ankle with bone involvement without evidence of necrosis

SP SH SL L97.318 Non-pressure chronic ulcer of right ankle with other specified severity

SP SH SL L97.319 Non-pressure chronic ulcer of right ankle with unspecified severity

6 L97.32 Non-pressure chronic ulcer of left ankle

SP SH SL L97.321 Non-pressure chronic ulcer of left ankle limited to breakdown of skin

SP SH SL L97.322 Non-pressure chronic ulcer of left ankle with fat layer exposed

SP SH SL L97.323 Non-pressure chronic ulcer of left ankle with necrosis of muscle

SP SH SL L97.324 Non-pressure chronic ulcer of left ankle with necrosis of bone

SP SH SL L97.325 Non-pressure chronic ulcer of left ankle with muscle involvement without evidence of necrosis

Chapter 12

L00-L99

---

4 4th digit required   5 5th digit required   6 6th digit required   7 7th digit required   7 7th digit placeholder   **+** Additional code   Laterality

⊟ SP SH SL **L97.326** Non-pressure chronic ulcer of left ankle with bone involvement without evidence of necrosis

⊟ SP SH SL **L97.328** Non-pressure chronic ulcer of left ankle with other specified severity

⊟ SP SH SL **L97.329** Non-pressure chronic ulcer of left ankle with unspecified severity

⑤ **L97.4** Non-pressure chronic ulcer of heel and midfoot
Non-pressure chronic ulcer of plantar surface of midfoot

⑥ **L97.40** Non-pressure chronic ulcer of unspecified heel and midfoot

IQ **L97.401** Non-pressure chronic ulcer of unspecified heel and midfoot limited to breakdown of skin

IQ **L97.402** Non-pressure chronic ulcer of unspecified heel and midfoot with fat layer exposed

IQ **L97.403** Non-pressure chronic ulcer of unspecified heel and midfoot with necrosis of muscle

IQ **L97.404** Non-pressure chronic ulcer of unspecified heel and midfoot with necrosis of bone

IQ **L97.405** Non-pressure chronic ulcer of unspecified heel and midfoot with muscle involvement without evidence of necrosis

IQ **L97.406** Non-pressure chronic ulcer of unspecified heel and midfoot with bone involvement without evidence of necrosis

IQ **L97.408** Non-pressure chronic ulcer of unspecified heel and midfoot with other specified severity

IQ **L97.409** Non-pressure chronic ulcer of unspecified heel and midfoot with unspecified severity

⑥ **L97.41** Non-pressure chronic ulcer of right heel and midfoot

⊟ SP SH SL **L97.411** Non-pressure chronic ulcer of right heel and midfoot limited to breakdown of skin

⊟ SP SH SL **L97.412** Non-pressure chronic ulcer of right heel and midfoot with fat layer exposed

⊟ SP SH SL **L97.413** Non-pressure chronic ulcer of right heel and midfoot with necrosis of muscle

⊟ SP SH SL **L97.414** Non-pressure chronic ulcer of right heel and midfoot with necrosis of bone

⊟ SP SH SL **L97.415** Non-pressure chronic ulcer of right heel and midfoot with muscle involvement without evidence of necrosis

⊟ SP SH SL **L97.416** Non-pressure chronic ulcer of right heel and midfoot with bone involvement without evidence of necrosis

⊟ SP SH SL **L97.418** Non-pressure chronic ulcer of right heel and midfoot with other specified severity

⊟ SP SH SL **L97.419** Non-pressure chronic ulcer of right heel and midfoot with unspecified severity

⑥ **L97.42** Non-pressure chronic ulcer of left heel and midfoot

⊟ SP SH SL **L97.421** Non-pressure chronic ulcer of left heel and midfoot limited to breakdown of skin

⊟ SP SH SL **L97.422** Non-pressure chronic ulcer of left heel and midfoot with fat layer exposed

⊟ SP SH SL **L97.423** Non-pressure chronic ulcer of left heel and midfoot with necrosis of muscle

⊟ SP SH SL **L97.424** Non-pressure chronic ulcer of left heel and midfoot with necrosis of bone

⊟ SP SH SL **L97.425** Non-pressure chronic ulcer of left heel and midfoot with muscle involvement without evidence of necrosis

⊟ SP SH SL **L97.426** Non-pressure chronic ulcer of left heel and midfoot with bone involvement without evidence of necrosis

⊟ SP SH SL **L97.428** Non-pressure chronic ulcer of left heel and midfoot with other specified severity

⊟ SP SH SL **L97.429** Non-pressure chronic ulcer of left heel and midfoot with unspecified severity

⑤ **L97.5** Non-pressure chronic ulcer of other part of foot
Non-pressure chronic ulcer of toe

⑥ **L97.50** Non-pressure chronic ulcer of other part of unspecified foot

IQ **L97.501** Non-pressure chronic ulcer of other part of unspecified foot limited to breakdown of skin

IQ **L97.502** Non-pressure chronic ulcer of other part of unspecified foot with fat layer exposed

IQ **L97.503** Non-pressure chronic ulcer of other part of unspecified foot with necrosis of muscle

IQ **L97.504** Non-pressure chronic ulcer of other part of unspecified foot with necrosis of bone

IQ **L97.505** Non-pressure chronic ulcer of other part of unspecified foot with muscle involvement without evidence of necrosis

IQ **L97.506** Non-pressure chronic ulcer of other part of unspecified foot with bone involvement without evidence of necrosis

IQ **L97.508** Non-pressure chronic ulcer of other part of unspecified foot with other specified severity

IQ **L97.509** Non-pressure chronic ulcer of other part of unspecified foot with unspecified severity

⑥ **L97.51** Non-pressure chronic ulcer of other part of right foot

⊟ SP SH SL **L97.511** Non-pressure chronic ulcer of other part of right foot limited to breakdown of skin

⊟ SP SH SL **L97.512** Non-pressure chronic ulcer of other part of right foot with fat layer exposed

Chapter 12

L00-L99

★ New ▲ Revised Px Primary **SP** PDGM Px **SL** Low CoM **SH** High CoM **IQ** Quest. Encounter ⊞ Hospice non-cancer Dx Unspecified **M** *Manifestation*

DecisionHealth's FY 2020 Complete Home Health ICD-10-CM Diagnosis Coding Manual

1133

🔲 SP SH SL **L97.513** Non-pressure chronic ulcer of other part of right foot with necrosis of muscle

🔲 SP SH SL **L97.514** Non-pressure chronic ulcer of other part of right foot with necrosis of bone

🔲 SP SH SL **L97.515** Non-pressure chronic ulcer of other part of right foot with muscle involvement without evidence of necrosis

🔲 SP SH SL **L97.516** Non-pressure chronic ulcer of other part of right foot with bone involvement without evidence of necrosis

🔲 SP SH SL **L97.518** Non-pressure chronic ulcer of other part of right foot with other specified severity

🔲 SP SH SL **L97.519** **Non-pressure chronic ulcer of other part of right foot with unspecified severity**

6️⃣ **L97.52** Non-pressure chronic ulcer of other part of left foot

🔲 SP SH SL **L97.521** Non-pressure chronic ulcer of other part of left foot limited to breakdown of skin

🔲 SP SH SL **L97.522** Non-pressure chronic ulcer of other part of left foot with fat layer exposed

🔲 SP SH SL **L97.523** Non-pressure chronic ulcer of other part of left foot with necrosis of muscle

🔲 SP SH SL **L97.524** Non-pressure chronic ulcer of other part of left foot with necrosis of bone

🔲 SP SH SL **L97.525** Non-pressure chronic ulcer of other part of left foot with muscle involvement without evidence of necrosis

🔲 SP SH SL **L97.526** Non-pressure chronic ulcer of other part of left foot with bone involvement without evidence of necrosis

🔲 SP SH SL **L97.528** Non-pressure chronic ulcer of other part of left foot with other specified severity

🔲 SP SH SL **L97.529** **Non-pressure chronic ulcer of left foot with unspecified severity**

5️⃣ **L97.8** Non-pressure chronic ulcer of other part of lower leg

6️⃣ **L97.80** **Non-pressure chronic ulcer of other part of unspecified lower leg**

IQ **L97.801** **Non-pressure chronic ulcer of other part of unspecified lower leg limited to breakdown of skin**

IQ **L97.802** **Non-pressure chronic ulcer of other part of unspecified lower leg with fat layer exposed**

IQ **L97.803** **Non-pressure chronic ulcer of other part of unspecified lower leg with necrosis of muscle**

IQ **L97.804** **Non-pressure chronic ulcer of other part of unspecified lower leg with necrosis of bone**

IQ **L97.805** **Non-pressure chronic ulcer of other part of unspecified lower leg with muscle involvement without evidence of necrosis**

IQ **L97.806** **Non-pressure chronic ulcer of other part of unspecified lower leg with bone involvement without evidence of necrosis**

IQ **L97.808** **Non-pressure chronic ulcer of other part of unspecified lower leg with other specified severity**

IQ **L97.809** **Non-pressure chronic ulcer of other part of unspecified lower leg with unspecified severity**

6️⃣ **L97.81** Non-pressure chronic ulcer of other part of right lower leg

🔲 SP SH SL **L97.811** Non-pressure chronic ulcer of other part of right lower leg limited to breakdown of skin

🔲 SP SH SL **L97.812** Non-pressure chronic ulcer of other part of right lower leg with fat layer exposed

🔲 SP SH SL **L97.813** Non-pressure chronic ulcer of other part of right lower leg with necrosis of muscle

🔲 SP SH SL **L97.814** Non-pressure chronic ulcer of other part of right lower leg with necrosis of bone

🔲 SP SH SL **L97.815** Non-pressure chronic ulcer of other part of right lower leg with muscle involvement without evidence of necrosis

🔲 SP SH SL **L97.816** Non-pressure chronic ulcer of other part of right lower leg with bone involvement without evidence of necrosis

🔲 SP SH SL **L97.818** Non-pressure chronic ulcer of other part of right lower leg with other specified severity

🔲 SP SH SL **L97.819** **Non-pressure chronic ulcer of other part of right lower leg with unspecified severity**

6️⃣ **L97.82** Non-pressure chronic ulcer of other part of left lower leg

🔲 SP SH SL **L97.821** Non-pressure chronic ulcer of other part of left lower leg limited to breakdown of skin

🔲 SP SH SL **L97.822** Non-pressure chronic ulcer of other part of left lower leg with fat layer exposed

🔲 SP SH SL **L97.823** Non-pressure chronic ulcer of other part of left lower leg with necrosis of muscle

🔲 SP SH SL **L97.824** Non-pressure chronic ulcer of other part of left lower leg with necrosis of bone

🔲 SP SH SL **L97.825** Non-pressure chronic ulcer of other part of left lower leg with muscle involvement without evidence of necrosis

🔲 SP SH SL **L97.826** Non-pressure chronic ulcer of other part of left lower leg with bone involvement without evidence of necrosis

🔲 SP SH SL **L97.828** Non-pressure chronic ulcer of other part of left lower leg with other specified severity

4️⃣ 4th digit required   5️⃣ 5th digit required   6️⃣ 6th digit required   7️⃣ 7th digit required   7️⃣ 7th digit placeholder   ✚ Additional code   🔲 Laterality

1134   *DecisionHealth's* FY 2020 Complete Home Health ICD-10-CM Diagnosis Coding Manual

Chapter 12

L00-L99

☐ SP SH SL **L97.829** Non-pressure chronic ulcer of other part of left lower leg with unspecified severity

5 **L97.9** Non-pressure chronic ulcer of unspecified part of lower leg

CODING TIPS ✓ Coders should not have to use L97.9 as the location of the ulcer should be documented.

6 **L97.90** Non-pressure chronic ulcer of unspecified part of unspecified lower leg

IQ **L97.901** Non-pressure chronic ulcer of unspecified part of unspecified lower leg limited to breakdown of skin

IQ **L97.902** Non-pressure chronic ulcer of unspecified part of unspecified lower leg with fat layer exposed

IQ **L97.903** Non-pressure chronic ulcer of unspecified part of unspecified lower leg with necrosis of muscle

IQ **L97.904** Non-pressure chronic ulcer of unspecified part of unspecified lower leg with necrosis of bone

IQ **L97.905** Non-pressure chronic ulcer of unspecified part of unspecified lower leg with muscle involvement without evidence of necrosis

IQ **L97.906** Non-pressure chronic ulcer of unspecified part of unspecified lower leg with bone involvement without evidence of necrosis

IQ **L97.908** Non-pressure chronic ulcer of unspecified part of unspecified lower leg with other specified severity

IQ **L97.909** Non-pressure chronic ulcer of unspecified part of unspecified lower leg with unspecified severity

6 **L97.91** Non-pressure chronic ulcer of unspecified part of right lower leg

☐ SP SH SL **L97.911** Non-pressure chronic ulcer of unspecified part of right lower leg limited to breakdown of skin

☐ SP SH SL **L97.912** Non-pressure chronic ulcer of unspecified part of right lower leg with fat layer exposed

☐ SP SH SL **L97.913** Non-pressure chronic ulcer of unspecified part of right lower leg with necrosis of muscle

☐ SP SH SL **L97.914** Non-pressure chronic ulcer of unspecified part of right lower leg with necrosis of bone

☐ SP SH SL **L97.915** Non-pressure chronic ulcer of unspecified part of right lower leg with muscle involvement without evidence of necrosis

☐ SP SH SL **L97.916** Non-pressure chronic ulcer of unspecified part of right lower leg with bone involvement without evidence of necrosis

☐ SP SH SL **L97.918** Non-pressure chronic ulcer of unspecified part of right lower leg with other specified severity

☐ SP SH SL **L97.919** Non-pressure chronic ulcer of unspecified part of right lower leg with unspecified severity

6 **L97.92** Non-pressure chronic ulcer of unspecified part of left lower leg

☐ SP SH SL **L97.921** Non-pressure chronic ulcer of unspecified part of left lower leg limited to breakdown of skin

☐ SP SH SL **L97.922** Non-pressure chronic ulcer of unspecified part of left lower leg with fat layer exposed

☐ SP SH SL **L97.923** Non-pressure chronic ulcer of unspecified part of left lower leg with necrosis of muscle

☐ SP SH SL **L97.924** Non-pressure chronic ulcer of unspecified part of left lower leg with necrosis of bone

☐ SP SH SL **L97.925** Non-pressure chronic ulcer of unspecified part of left lower leg with muscle involvement without evidence of necrosis

☐ SP SH SL **L97.926** Non-pressure chronic ulcer of unspecified part of left lower leg with bone involvement without evidence of necrosis

☐ SP SH SL **L97.928** Non-pressure chronic ulcer of unspecified part of left lower leg with other specified severity

☐ SP SH SL **L97.929** Non-pressure chronic ulcer of unspecified part of left lower leg with unspecified severity

4 **L98** Other disorders of skin and subcutaneous tissue, not elsewhere classified

SP **L98.0** Pyogenic granuloma

EXCLUDES 2 pyogenic granuloma of gingiva (K06.8)
pyogenic granuloma of maxillary alveolar ridge (K04.5)
pyogenic granuloma of oral mucosa (K13.4)

SP **L98.1** Factitial dermatitis
Neurotic excoriation

EXCLUDES 1 Excoriation (skin-picking) disorder (F42.4)

CODING TIPS ✓ Factitial dermatitis, L98.1, may also be referred to as neurotic excoriation or dermatitis artefacta and is characterized by deliberate, self-inflicted skin lesions produced as a result of underlying psychological conditions. When specified, any underlying or additional psychological conditions should also be coded. An example of a psychological condition is skin-picking disorder (F42.4).

SP **L98.2** Febrile neutrophilic dermatosis [Sweet]

SP SH SL **L98.3** Eosinophilic cellulitis [Wells]

5 **L98.4** Non-pressure chronic ulcer of skin, not elsewhere classified
Chronic ulcer of skin NOS
Tropical ulcer NOS
Ulcer of skin NOS

★ New ▲ Revised Px Primary ☐SP PDGM Px ☐SL Low CoM ☐SH High CoM ☐IQ Quest. Encounter ☐H Hospice non-cancer Dx ☐ Unspecified M *Manifestation*

DecisionHealth's FY 2020 Complete Home Health ICD-10-CM Diagnosis Coding Manual

1135

EXCLUDES 2   pressure ulcer
(pressure area) (L89.-)
gangrene (I96)
skin infections (L00-L08)
specific infections classified
to A00-B99
ulcer of lower limb NEC
(L97.-)
varicose ulcer (I83.0-I82.2)

CODING TIPS ✓   Do not use L98 to indicate a pressure ulcer/injury. All pressure ulcers/injuries are coded to the L89 category. L98.4 is used for ulcers that are not pressure ulcers/injuries and are not on lower extremities.

6 L98.41   Non-pressure chronic ulcer of buttock

SP L98.411   Non-pressure chronic ulcer of buttock limited to breakdown of skin

SP L98.412   Non-pressure chronic ulcer of buttock with fat layer exposed

SP L98.413   Non-pressure chronic ulcer of buttock with necrosis of muscle

SP L98.414   Non-pressure chronic ulcer of buttock with necrosis of bone

SP L98.415   Non-pressure chronic ulcer of buttock with muscle involvement without evidence of necrosis

SP L98.416   Non-pressure chronic ulcer of buttock with bone involvement without evidence of necrosis

SP L98.418   Non-pressure chronic ulcer of buttock with other specified severity

SP L98.419   Non-pressure chronic ulcer of buttock with unspecified severity

6 L98.42   Non-pressure chronic ulcer of back

SP L98.421   Non-pressure chronic ulcer of back limited to breakdown of skin

SP L98.422   Non-pressure chronic ulcer of back with fat layer exposed

SP L98.423   Non-pressure chronic ulcer of back with necrosis of muscle

SP L98.424   Non-pressure chronic ulcer of back with necrosis of bone

SP L98.425   Non-pressure chronic ulcer of back with muscle involvement without evidence of necrosis

SP L98.426   Non-pressure chronic ulcer of back with bone involvement without evidence of necrosis

SP L98.428   Non-pressure chronic ulcer of back with other specified severity

SP L98.429   Non-pressure chronic ulcer of back with unspecified severity

6 L98.49   Non-pressure chronic ulcer of skin of other sites
Non-pressure chronic ulcer of skin NOS

CODING TIPS ✓   Locally advanced, metastatic or recurrent cancer may infiltrate the skin, disrupt its integrity, and cause chronic, poorly healing, and fungating wounds. When an ulcer/wound is the result of cancer, code only the cancer. Query the physician for metastasis to the skin, e.g. C79.2. Do not use L98.49.

SP L98.491   Non-pressure chronic ulcer of skin of other sites limited to breakdown of skin

SP L98.492   Non-pressure chronic ulcer of skin of other sites with fat layer exposed

SP L98.493   Non-pressure chronic ulcer of skin of other sites with necrosis of muscle

SP L98.494   Non-pressure chronic ulcer of skin of other sites with necrosis of bone

SP L98.495   Non-pressure chronic ulcer of skin of other sites with muscle involvement without evidence of necrosis

SP L98.496   Non-pressure chronic ulcer of skin of other sites with bone involvement without evidence of necrosis

SP L98.498   Non-pressure chronic ulcer of skin of other sites with other specified severity

SP L98.499   Non-pressure chronic ulcer of skin of other sites with unspecified severity

SP L98.5   Mucinosis of the skin
Focal mucinosis
Lichen myxedematosus
Reticular erythematous mucinosis
EXCLUDES 1   focal oral mucinosis (K13.79)
myxedema (E03.9)

SP L98.6   Other infiltrative disorders of the skin and subcutaneous tissue
EXCLUDES 1   hyalinosis cutis et mucosae (E78.89)

SP L98.7   Excessive and redundant skin and subcutaneous tissue
Loose or sagging skin following bariatric surgery weight loss
Loose or sagging skin following dietary weight loss
Loose or sagging skin, NOS
EXCLUDES 2   acquired excess or redundant skin of eyelid (H02.3-)
congenital excess or redundant skin of eyelid (Q10.3)
skin changes due to chronic exposure to nonionizing radiation (L57.-)

SP L98.8   Other specified disorders of the skin and subcutaneous tissue

IQ L98.9   Disorder of the skin and subcutaneous tissue, unspecified

M IQ L99   *Other disorders of skin and subcutaneous tissue in diseases classified elsewhere*
Code first underlying disease, such as:
amyloidosis (E85.-)

☐4 4th digit required   ☐5 5th digit required   ☐6 6th digit required   ☐7 7th digit required   ☑ 7th digit placeholder   + Additional code   ☐ Laterality

1136   *DecisionHealth's* FY 2020 Complete Home Health ICD-10-CM Diagnosis Coding Manual

EXCLUDES 1	skin disorders in diabetes (E08-E13 with .62)
	skin disorders in gonorrhea (A54.89)
	skin disorders in syphilis (A51.31, A52.79)

★ New ▲ Revised Px Primary **SP** PDGM Px **SL** Low CoM **SH** High CoM **IQ** Quest. Encounter **H** Hospice non-cancer Dx   Unspecified   **M** *Manifestation*

DecisionHealth's FY 2020 Complete Home Health ICD-10-CM Diagnosis Coding Manual

1137

Chapter 12 Scenarios: Diseases of the skin and subcutaneous tissue (L00-L99)

Pressure ulcers/injuries, old spinal stroke

Your new 66-year-old patient was referred for care of a stage 3 pressure ulcer/injury on her right buttock and a stage 2 pressure ulcer/injury on her right hip. Skilled nursing has been ordered for wound care. She also has hypertension and is a paraplegic due to an old spinal stroke

Description	Code
Primary: Pressure ulcer right buttock, stage 3	L89.313
Secondary: Pressure ulcer right hip, stage 2	L89.212
Secondary: Paraplegia	G82.20
Secondary: Essential (primary) hypertension	I10
Secondary: Dependence on wheelchair	Z99.3

ICD-10 provides a great deal of specificity with regard to the pressure ulcers/injuries. For example, take L89.313 and break it down: the L89.3.- root code indicates the buttock, the 5th digit "1" indicates the right side, and the 6th digit "3" indicates the stage of the pressure ulcer/injury. In this scenario, the paraplegia is also reported as due to an old spinal stroke. Only the code for the paraplegia is assigned as there is currently no code for sequela of a spinal stroke, according to Q3 2017 Coding Clinic guidance.

Bilateral pressure ulcers/injuries

A 72-year-old male patient has stage 2 pressure ulcers/injuries on both elbows, for which he will be receiving wound care.

Description	Code
Primary: Pressure ulcer of right elbow, stage 2	L89.012
Secondary: Pressure ulcer of left elbow, stage 2	L89.022

There is no single code to indicate a bilateral pressure ulcer/injury in ICD-10. Thus, both ulcers/injuries are captured by their unique body site codes. No separate code is required for the stage, because the ICD-10 combination code includes the stage.

Venous insufficiency, non-healing stasis ulcer

A 72-year-old man is admitted to home care with diagnoses of venous insufficiency and hypertension. He has skin breakdown on his left heel, diagnosed by the physician as a stasis ulcer and the ulcer is considered non-healing. Wound care is ordered as well as medication management for his hypertension.

Description	Code
Primary: Venous insufficiency (chronic) (peripheral)	I87.2
Secondary: Non-pressure chronic ulcer of left heel and mid-foot limited to breakdown of skin	L97.421
Secondary: Essential (primary) hypertension	I10

The L97.- codes allow you to identify not only the location, but the severity of the ulcer. In this case, the documentation states the severity is limited to the breakdown of the skin so a 6th character of "1" is appropriate. The L97.421 code includes that the ulcer is non-healing. Hypertension is coded as a relevant comorbidity.

Varicose veins, infected non-healing stasis ulcer

A 79-year-old woman is admitted to home care for wound care of an infected, non-healing stasis ulcer on her right ankle that has exposed the fat layer. The stasis ulcer is a result of varicose veins and is infected with Methicillin resistant staphylococcus aureus (MRSA). She will require IV antibiotics.

Description	Code
Primary: Varicose veins of right lower extremity with ulcer of ankle	I83.013
Secondary: Non-pressure chronic ulcer of right ankle with fat layer exposed	L97.312
Secondary: Methicillin resistant Staphylococcus aureus infection as the cause of diseases classified elsewhere	B95.62
Secondary: Encounter for adjustment and management of vascular access device	Z45.2
Secondary: Long term (current) use of antibiotics	Z79.2

Tabular instruction under I83.0- tells coders to "use additional code to identify severity of ulcer (L97.-)." In this case, the documentation states the severity includes exposure of the fat layer so L97.312 should be used. The fact that the ulcer is non-healing is captured in the L97.312 code. Because it's infected with MRSA, an additional code (B95.62) is assigned to capture that. Codes Z45.2 and Z79.2 are assigned to capture the administration of IV antibiotics.

Arterial ulcer

A 75-year-old woman comes to home health after developing an ulcer on her calf, which her physician diagnosed as caused by atherosclerosis. The clinician documents that the ulcer is on her right calf, measures two millimeters in depth and four millimeters in diameter, and that it has gone beyond the skin layers into the patient's fatty tissue. The patient also has hypertension. The nurse also documents that while the patient has never smoked, her husband has been a smoker for 35 years, and continues to smoke. Home health will provide wound care.

Description	Code
Primary: Atherosclerosis of native arteries of right leg, with ulceration of calf	I70.232
Secondary: Non-pressure chronic ulcer of right calf with fat layer exposed	L97.212
Secondary: Essential (primary) hypertension	I10
Secondary: Exposure to environmental tobacco smoke	Z77.22

Diagnosed as an arterial ulcer caused by atherosclerosis, the wound is coded as such. Descriptions of laterality and severity are required in ICD-10, and thus the wound is specified as being on the patient's right calf and extending into the fatty layer of tissue. Hypertension is also coded as a relevant comorbidity. ICD-10 atherosclerosis codes include an instructional note to include, if applicable, whether the patient has any dependence on tobacco. In this case, the patient isn't dependent on tobacco, but is exposed to it, and that should be documented and coded.

Cellulitis

A patient initially sustained a minor laceration injury to her right index finger from the sharp edge of a tin can lid. This injury caused cellulitis and the patient requires treatment with IV antibiotics, as several rounds of oral antibiotics were not successful. The initial wound is still healing but does not require treatment from the agency. The focus of the admission is on the cellulitis.

Description	Code
Primary: Cellulitis of right (index) finger	L03.011
Secondary: Laceration without foreign body right index finger (without damage to nail) subsequent encounter	S61.210D
Secondary: Encounter for adjustment and management of vascular device	Z45.2
Secondary: Long term (current) use of antibiotics	Z79.2
Secondary: Contact with other sharp object(s), not elsewhere classified, subsequent encounter	W26.8XXD

The wound typically is coded before the cellulitis, except when the wound does not require care or is no longer present. Tabular instructions at S61.- state, "code also any associated wound infection." Note that this instruction is different from a "code first" instruction and does not provide any sequencing direction. If the wound is now closed, then it would not be coded. Because the wound is not receiving active treatment from the agency, the 7th character "D" for subsequent encounter is appropriate. The external cause code is added to help explain how the patient sustained the wound that led to the cellulitis. It carries the same 7th character ("D") as the code it is explaining (S61.210D), in accordance with official coding guidelines. Codes Z45.2 and Z79.2 capture the administration of IV antibiotics.

Adverse effect of Lovenox, hives

An 82-year-old man recently was diagnosed with paroxysmal atrial fibrillation and was given injections of Lovenox. The drug was given as directed, but the patient suffered an allergic reaction that caused him to break out in hives. His physician has prescribed new medication and the patient has been admitted to home health for medication management and monitoring.

Description	Code
Primary: Allergic urticaria	L50.0
Secondary: Adverse effect of anticoagulants, subsequent encounter	T45.515D
Secondary: Paroxysmal atrial fibrillation	I48.0

The drug was given correctly but the patient experienced a problem anyway. Therefore, the scenario is an adverse effect. The adverse effect of the drug, the hives, is coded first, in accordance with coding guidelines. The code for an adverse effect caused by Lovenox is T45.515-, according to the table of drugs and chemicals. A seventh character of "D" is assigned to indicate the subsequent nature of the encounter. The reason the drug was given is coded after the adverse effect code.

Scar from burn

A 68-year-old female developed an extensive scar on her left forearm after a second degree burn healed. The burn occurred when she accidentally dropped a hot iron. The scar causes her severe pain and difficulty with mobility and completing ADLs/IADLs. She was admitted to home health for nursing care and occupational therapy. She also has peripheral vascular disease and chronic atrial fibrillation, for which she is on long-term anticoagulant therapy.

Description	Code
Primary: Scar conditions and fibrosis of skin	L90.5
Secondary: Burn of second degree of left forearm, sequela	T22.212S
Secondary: Peripheral vascular disease, unspecified	I73.9
Secondary: Chronic atrial fibrillation	I48.2
Secondary: Long term (current) use of anticoagulants	Z79.01
Secondary: Contact with other hot household appliances, sequela	X15.8xxS

The burn, though healed, left behind a scar that is causing the patient significant distress. Therefore, the burn is coded with a seventh character "S" to indicate that it is healed but has caused a residual condition, or sequela. The residual condition, the scar, is coded prior to the injury that caused it, in accordance with coding guidelines. As comorbidities that will impact her ability to heal, her peripheral vascular disease and chronic atrial fibrillation are coded as well. Her use of anticoagulant medication carries certain risks and thus should be coded with Z79.01. An external cause code is used to describe how the patient sustained the burn.

Diaper dermatitis

A 98-year-old woman is bedbound and debilitated. She is incontinent of urine and feces and was recently found to have excoriation of the skin around genital and buttocks areas caused by contact with urine and feces in her diaper. The dermatitis is the focus of care.

Description	Code
Primary: Diaper dermatitis	L22
Secondary: Unspecified urinary incontinence	R32
Secondary: Full incontinence of feces	R15.9
Secondary: Other malaise	R53.81
Secondary: Bed confinement status	Z74.01

Excoriation of the skin from contact with urine and feces is diaper dermatitis. As the focus of care, it is coded in the primary position. Her fecal and urine incontinence are coded with R32 and R15.9 and her debility and bedbound status are coded with R53.81 and Z74.01.

Ulcer due to PVD, GERD

An 82-year-old male patient is admitted to home health for wound care to an ulcer of his right lateral plantar foot; the wound is showing bone involvement but there's no evidence of necrosis. The ulcer was caused by PVD. He also has GERD and was recently prescribed new medication for it. The patient complains of pain in his legs with ambulation.

Description	Code
Primary: Peripheral vascular disease, unspecified	I73.9
Secondary: Non-pressure chronic ulcer of other part of right foot with bone involvement without evidence of necrosis	L97.516
Secondary: Gastro-esophageal reflux disease without esophagitis	K21.9

The patient's ulcer has been said to be caused by PVD but there's no mention of atherosclerosis. Thus, I73.9 must be assigned to capture the etiology of the ulcer. The L97.516 code, which specifies that the ulcer is on his right foot and that there is bone involvement but no necrosis, is assigned immediately following. GERD is coded as a relevant comorbidity.

Stasis ulcer

A 76-year-old woman was referred to home health for wound care for an ulcer on her left ankle caused by chronic venous hypertension. Muscle tissue is evident in the wound on her ankle but there's no necrosis.

Description	Code
Primary: Chronic venous hypertension (idiopathic) with ulcer of left lower extremity	I87.312
Secondary: Non-pressure chronic ulcer of left ankle with muscle involvement without evidence of necrosis	L97.325

The wound is the result of chronic venous hypertension and it thus captured first with the combination code I87.312. The L97.325, which specifies that the ulcer is on her left ankle and that muscle tissue is visible but there's no necrosis, is assigned following the code for chronic venous hypertension with ulcer.

Gangrenous pressure ulcer, diabetic neuropathy

A 71-year-old woman is admitted to home health for wound care to a gangrenous stage 3 pressure ulcer to her right heel that's documented as associated with diabetic neuropathy. The diabetes is documented as Type 1.5. She uses both insulin and oral hypoglycemic medication.

Description	Code
Primary: Gangrene, not elsewhere classified	I96
Secondary: Pressure ulcer of right heel, stage 3	L89.613
Secondary: Other specified diabetes mellitus with diabetic polyneuropathy	E13.42
Secondary: Long term (current) use of insulin	Z79.4

A gangrenous pressure ulcer on the heel is not a diabetic ulcer and should not be coded as a diabetic manifestation, according to Q3 2018 Coding Clinic guidance. It is coded as gangrenous pressure ulcer, first with I96 followed by L89.612, in accordance with tabular instruction. The gangrene code must be assigned before the pressure ulcer code, according to a "code first" note at the L89.- category level. Since the diabetes is documented as type 1.5, a diabetes code from the E13.- category is assigned, according to Q3 2018 Coding Clinic guidance. The patient uses both insulin and oral hypoglycemic medication; only the code for insulin use is assigned, in accordance with coding guidelines.

HOME HEALTH CODING SCENARIOS

Chapter 13: Diseases of Musculoskeletal System and Connective Tissue (M00-M99)

Note that traumatic fracture codes and pathological fractures codes are **not** grouped together in ICD-10. Traumatic fracture codes are found in Chapter 19 (Injury, poisoning and certain other consequences of external causes), while codes for pathological fractures are found in Chapter 13 (Diseases of the Musculoskeletal System and Connective Tissue). This isn't a change from ICD-9, but it is a common mistake for coders to assume that all fractures are found in the same chapter.

"Connective tissue" is material that helps give tissue form and strength, including the structures around joints (cartilage, bursae, and synovial cavity). Chapter 13 includes conditions affecting bones, joints, muscles, ligaments, tendons and connective tissues. The conditions found in this chapter include inflammation, displacement, degeneration, and rupture of these structures.

Pathologic fractures (in which the bone is weakened by a disease, such as cancer or osteoporosis) are reported using codes in this chapter. Traumatic fractures (in which bone is broken by external force or violence), injuries to muscles and tendons, as well as dislocations, are reported using codes from Chapter 19 (Injury, poisoning, and certain other consequences of external causes).

Chapter 13 is divided into 18 blocks of similar conditions, which include:

- M00-M02 **Infectious arthropathies** are arthropathies due to microbiological agents that may result in direct infection of the joint or indirect infection which may be reactive or postinfective arthropathy.

- M04 **Autoinflammatory syndromes**

- M05-M14 **Inflammatory polyarthropathies** include conditions such as: **rheumatoid arthritis**, an autoimmune disorder that causes chronic inflammation of the joints, particularly those in the hands and feet. It differs from other types of arthritis in that it affects the joint lining causing painful swelling that can eventually result in joint deformity; **enteropathic arthropathies**, which are diseases of the joints associated or linked to gastrointestinal tract inflammation causing the joints to become inflamed and tender; and **gout,** which is a form of inflammatory polyarthropathy and includes acute idiopathic gout or chronic gout (category M1A). Gouty arthritis or crystal arthropathy is a form of arthritis caused by deposits of urate crystals around one or more joints; and villonodular synovitis, a condition that affects joints lined with synovial tissue.

- M15-M19 **Osteoarthritis**

- M20-M25 **Other joint disorders** includes acquired deformities of joints, recurrent dislocations, contractures, pain, stiffness and other joint disorders of upper and lower extremities.

- M26-M27 **Dentofacial anomalies** including malocclusion and other disorders of the jaw.

- M30-M36 **Systemic connective tissue disorders**, which include polyarteritis nodosa, necrotizing vasculopathies, systemic lupus erythematosis, scleroderma and manifestations of diseases classified elswhere

- M40-M43 **Deforming dorsopathies,** such as kyphosis, lordosis, scoliosis, osteochondrosis of spine.

- M45-M49 **Spondylopathies**, which is a degenerative or developmental anomaly of vertebrae, enthesopathy (disorders of ligamentous or muscular attachments of the spine), spondylosis (degenerative arthritis of spine), fatigue fracture of vertebra, collapsed vertebrae, and other disorders of spine.

- M50-M54 **Other dorsopathies**, include spinal disc disorders, radiculopathy, sciatica, lumbago, etc.

- M60-M63 **Disorders of muscles** such as myositis; paralytic calcification and ossification of muscles; non-traumatic separation, rupture and ischemic infarction of muscles; contracture of muscle; muscle wasting & atrophy; rhabdomyolysis, disintegration or destruction of muscle); and disorders of muscles in diseases classified elsewhere.

- M65-M67 **Disorders of synovium and tendon** such as synovitis/tenosynovitis; abscess of tendon sheath; calcific tendinitis; and spontaneous rupture of synovium & tendons;

- M70-M79 **Other soft tissue disorders**, including conditions related to use, overuse & pressure such as bursitis; calcium deposits; fibroblastic disorders; necrotizing fasciitis; non-traumatic rotator cuff tears; bone spurs; rheumatism; myalgia; pain in limbs; and nontraumatic compartment syndrome.

- M80-M85 **Disorders of bone density and structure** such as osteoporosis, pathological fractures, stress fractures; fibrous dysplasia; & bone cysts.

- M86-M90 **Other osteopathies** such as osteomyelitis; osteonecrosis; osteitis deformans (Paget's disease); algoneurodystrophy; disorders of bone development; osteolysis and osteopathy; major osseous defect, and osteonecrosis in diseases classified elsewhere.

- M91-M94 **Chondropathies** (diseases of the cartilage)

- M95 **Other disorders of the musculoskeletal system and connective tissue**

- M96 **Intraoperative and post procedural complications and disorders** of the musculoskeletal system, not elsewhere classified

- M97 **Periprosthetic fracture around internal prosthetic joint**

- M99 **Biomechanical lesions, not elsewhere classified** such as segmental and somatic dysfunction; subluxation complex (vertebral); and stenosis of neural canal.

As noted by the contents in the blocks, the terminology is considerably different in ICD-10 than ICD-9 so a current medical dictionary will be a useful tool in determining the correct diagnosis. Refer to the term used in the physician's documentation in order to select the correct code. If the documentation is unclear, query the physician.

Sometimes a Chapter 13 code is not the most appropriate choice. The following chapters are all referenced in an Excludes 2 note at the start of the chapter.

- If the documentation indicates a **neoplasm or tumor of the bone, joint or connective tissue**, look up the term (malignancy, tumor, adenoma, or specific name) in the Alphabetical index and verify the correct code in the Tabular List, most likely a code from Chapter 2. The Alpha Index will direct the coder to the neoplasm table and the correct column to use.

- This chapter includes some general **symptom codes**, such as pain in joint (category M25.-), low back pain (M54.5), and pain in limb (subcategory M79.6-). Symptoms may be reported using codes from Chapter 18, such as difficulty walking (R26.2), symptoms involving nervous and musculoskeletal systems (R29.9-); abnormality of gait (R26.9) and lack of coordination (R27.9). Every effort should be made to secure a definitive diagnosis. A symptom code may be reported as an additional diagnosis when it indicates a significant aspect of the condition, but is not an integral part of it. If the documentation is unclear, query the physician.

- If a patient has a **personal or family history** of a condition reported in this chapter, it may be appropriate to select from the Z code section, such as Z85.830 (Personal history of malignant neoplasm, bone), Z87.311 (Personal history of pathologic fracture), Z87.312 (Personal history of stress fracture), Z82.61 (Family history of arthritis),

or Z82.62 (Family history of osteoporosis).

There is an Excludes 2 note at the beginning of chapter 13 that indicates the following situations are not included in Chapter 13 codes, but may be coded in addition, if applicable to the situation. Code selection and sequencing will be determined by finding the code in the Alphabetical Index and verifying it in the Tabular as well as following all instructional notes. Take note of the following conditions **not** included in Chapter 13:

- arthropathic psoriasis (L40.5-)

- certain conditions originating in the perinatal period (P00-P96)

- certain infections and parasitic diseases (A00-B99)

- compartment syndrome (traumatic) (T79.A-)

- complications of pregnancy, childbirth and the puerperium (O00-O9A)

- congenital malformations, deformations, and chromosomal abnormalities (Q00-Q99)

- endocrine, nutritional and metabolic diseases (E00-E88)

- injury, poisoning and certain other consequences of external causes (S00-T88)

- neoplasms (C00-D49)

- symptoms, signs and abnormal clinical and laboratory findings, not elsewhere classified (R00-R94)

General Guidance

Site and laterality

Most of the codes within this chapter have site and laterality designations. The site represents the bone, joint or muscle involved. For some conditions, when more than one bone, joint or muscle is usually involved, such as osteoarthritis, there is a "multiple sites" code available, for example, M15.3, Secondary multiple arthritis. There also are codes to indicate bilateral presence of the condition, such as M16.0, bilateral primary osteoarthritis of hip.

For categories where no multiple site code is provided and more than one bone, joint or muscle is involved, multiple codes should be used to indicate the different sites involved. For example, code both M62.251 and M62.261 for nontraumatic ischemic infarction of muscle right thigh and right lower leg.

Bone versus joint

For certain conditions, the bone may be affected at the upper or lower end (e.g., avascular necrosis of the bone (M87), and osteoporosis (M80, M81). Though the portion of the bone affected may be at the joint, the site designation will be the bone, not the joint. Examples include M87.022, idiopathic avascular necrosis of left humerus; or M80.061D, Subsequent encounter for age related osteoporosis with routine healing of current pathological fracture, right lower leg.

Acute traumatic versus chronic or recurrent musculoskeletal conditions

Many musculoskeletal conditions are a result of previous injury or trauma to a site, or are recurrent conditions. Bone, joint or muscle conditions that are a result of a healed injury or a recurrent condition are usually found in Chapter 13. However, any current acute injury should be coded to the appropriate injury code from Chapter 19. If it is difficult to determine from the documentation in the record which code is best to describe a condition, query the provider.

Coding pathological fractures

Pathological fracture codes are combination codes that include a 7th character to indicate whether the care encounter is initial, subsequent or sequela. The 7th character A is used as long as the patient is receiving active treatment for the fracture. Examples of active treatment are: surgical treatment, emergency department encounter, evaluation and treatment by a new physician. The 7th character D is used for encounters for routine healing after the patient has completed active treatment. The remaining 7th characters, listed under each subcategory in the Tabular List, are to be used for subsequent encounters for treatment of problems associated with the healing, such as delayed healing, malunions, nonunions, and sequelae.

Care for complications of surgical treatment for fracture repairs during the healing or recovery phase should be coded as appropriate complication codes.

Multiple Coding and Sequencing

It is important to read the Includes and Excludes notes under codes in this chapter, as well as any other instructions under the code or code category.

Note, there is an instructional note at the beginning of Chapter 13 that states: use an external cause code following the code for the musculoskeletal condition, if applicable, to identify the cause of the musculoskeletal condition.

Here are some examples of multiple coding and sequencing issues for codes in this chapter:

- **Infectious arthropathies** include pyogenic arthritis (category M00) that include codes for arthritis caused by microbiological organisms of specific joints. Several of the subcategories have an instructional note to add an additional code to identify the bacterial agent. For example, Staphylococcal arthritis, right hip, requires two

codes, M00.051 as the first-listed code followed by a code from B95.61-B95.8 to identify the type of staphylococcus involved.

- Codes from category M01, **direct infections of joints** due to infectious and parasitic diseases classified elsewhere, and category M02, postinfective and reactive arthropathies, have a code first note to code the underlying disease that refers to infection codes in chapter 1. The code from chapter 1 is reported as the first-listed code followed by the code from chapter 13.

- Some codes require you to code also any associated conditions, For example, codes from category M07 (**enteropathic arthopathies**) require you to code also any associated enteropathy, such as regional enteritis (Crohn's disease K50- or ulcerative colitis K51-). Also category M08 (juvenile arthritis) instructs to code also any associated underlying conditions as an additional code.

- Code category M63 (**disorders of muscles in diseases classified elsewhere**) requires a code first for the underlying disease from chapter 1.

Throughout Chapter 13, there are many categories that include notes to code first or use an additional code for adverse effect, if applicable, to identify the drug (T36-T50 with fifth or sixth character 5). An example is M81.8 (Drug-induced osteoporosis without current pathological fracture).

Special Coding Issues

Fractures

Spontaneous chronic or pathological fractures are reported using codes from this chapter (subcategory M84.4-), while pathological fractures in neoplastic disease are coded at subcategory M84.5- with a note to code also the underlying neoplasm. Stress fractures are coded to subcategory M84.3, while fatigue fractures of the vertebrae are coded to subcategory M48.4- and collapsed fractures of the vertebra are coded to M48.5-.

All of the pathological, stress, fatigue, and collapsed fractures require the appropriate 7th character to indicate whether the encounter is initial, subsequent or a sequela. There are specific 7th character designations for subsequent encounter for fractures with routine healing, delayed healing, and with nonunion or malunion. **Aftercare codes for healing pathological fractures are not used in ICD-10-CM**.

Traumatic fractures are assigned the appropriate code by site and type of fracture from Chapter 19 (Injury, poisoning and certain other consequences of external causes (S00-S99)).

Report a code from M97 for fractures around a prosthesis that are not complications of the prosthesis, but the result of the same conditions as other fractures, that is, trauma or pathological conditions. Periprosthetic fractures can occur around any prosthesis, but the most common would be the hip, knee, ankle, shoulder, or elbow.

Code T84 includes all of the complications of orthopedic prostheses, implants and grafts. Periprosthetic fractures are not considered complications and can be found in M97. Subcategory T84.0 includes complications of internal prosthetic joints. Most include the joint affected, so there is no need to add Z96.6 for the joint unless the complication code does not indicate the joint. A code from M96.6- or M97.- may provide additional information.

Joint replacements

Continue to assign the injury code for patient who underwent a joint replacement to treat a hip fracture. The aftercare code Z47.1 (Aftercare following joint replacement surgery) is ***not** appropriate* in these types of scenarios, according to the Coding Clinic Q3 2016 guidance.

Osteoporosis

Osteoporosis is a systemic condition, meaning that all bones of the musculoskeletal system are affected. Therefore site is not a component of the codes under M81, Osteoporosis without current pathological fracture. The site codes under category M80, Osteoporosis with current pathological fracture, identify the site of the fracture, not the osteoporosis.

Osteoporosis without current pathological fracture, Category M81, is used for patients with osteoporosis who do not currently have a pathological fracture due to osteoporosis, even if they had one in the past. For patients with a history of osteoporosis fractures, status code Z87.310 (Personal history of (healed) osteoporosis fracture) should follow the code from M81.

Category 80, Osteoporosis with current pathological fracture, is for patients who have a current pathological fracture at the time of the encounter. The codes under M80 identify the site of the fracture. A code from M80, not a traumatic fracture code, should be used for any patient with known osteoporosis who suffers a fracture, even if the patient had a minor fall or trauma, if that fall or trauma would not usually break a normal, healthy bone.

Arthropathies (M00-M25)

It is incorrect to code an arthropathy and pain in joint separately because pain is integral to the disease.

ICD-10-CM has greatly expanded the codes for arthropathies addressing them in multiple blocks and including many instructional notes within the code categories. Specific sites and laterality are included in the combination codes.

Osteoarthritis

Osteoarthritis also is referred to as degenerative arthritis or degenerative joint disease. It is the most common form of inflammatory joint disease, caused by deterioration of the cartilage that covers the ends of the bones and typically occurs slowly over a long period of time. As the cartilage deteriorates, it becomes rough and causes irritation of the joint. As deterioration continues, the bone itself becomes exposed and eventually joint movement results in bone rubbing against bone, causing pain and damage to the bone itself. When coding osteoarthritis, differentiate between primary and secondary.

Primary osteoarthritis is without a specific known cause other than the progressive wearing down of the cartilage in the joints and is also referred to as idiopathic osteoarthopathy. Codes by specific site are found at categories M15-M19. Primary arthritis NOS or unspecified osteoarthritis, unspecified site, is coded as M19.90.

Secondary osteoarthritis refers to degenerative disease of the synovial joints that results from some predisposing condition, such as trauma/injury, or the result of congenital or other disease that has adversely altered the articular cartilage and/or subchondral bone of the affected joints. Secondary osteoarthritis codes are found in ICD-10-CM at M19.2- (Secondary osteoarthritis of other joints), or M89.4- in the Tabular defined as Other hypertrophic osteoarthropathy by site.

Code osteoarthritis in a patient's joint as primary osteoarthritis if the type of OA, such as primary, secondary or generalized, is not specified. "When the type of osteoarthritis is not specified, "primary" is the default." For example, you should assign M16.0 (Bilateral primary osteoarthritis of hip) for a patient documented has having bilateral osteoarthritis of the hips, according to Q4 2016 Coding Clinic guidance.

When coding arthritis conditions, you must:

- specify the type of arthritis (rheumatoid, infective/pyogenic, reactive/Reiter's disease, osteoarthritis,/degenerative, etc); ***and***

- specify the site – do not use multiple sites code; code each affected site separately. M12.9 is arthropathy unspecified, so it is the best choice if information about the specific type of arthritis is unknown. Traumatic arthropathy (subcategory M12.5-) is an example of a residual effect that occurred because of an injury in the past, but excludes a current injury. Consider this example: The patient fractured her right ankle three years ago and now has arthritis in that ankle (M12.571).

In its early stages, Charcot's arthropathy (M14.60-), also known as neuropathic arthropathy, often is confused with osteoarthritis (OA). Some pain, a prominent and often hemorrhagic effusion, and subluxation and instability of the joint are usually present. Acute joint dislocation sometimes occurs at this stage. Neurogenic arthropathy progresses more rapidly than OA. Arthropathy may not develop until long after onset of the neuropathic condition, but can progress rapidly and lead to complete joint disorganization in a few months.

If the patient has Charcot's joints arthropathy due to diabetes type 2, the correct code would be a combination code E11.610 from chapter 4.

CHAPTER 13: DISEASES OF THE MUSCULOSKELETAL SYSTEM AND CONNECTIVE TISSUE (M00-M99)

Note:
Use an external cause code following the code for the musculoskeletal condition, if applicable, to identify the cause of the musculoskeletal condition

EXCLUDES 2 arthropathic psoriasis (L40.5-)
certain conditions originating in the perinatal period (P04-P96)
certain infectious and parasitic diseases (A00-B99)
compartment syndrome (traumatic) (T79.A-)
complications of pregnancy, childbirth and the puerperium (O00-O9A)
congenital malformations, deformations, and chromosomal abnormalities (Q00-Q99)
endocrine, nutritional and metabolic diseases (E00-E88)
injury, poisoning and certain other consequences of external causes (S00-T88)
neoplasms (C00-D49)
symptoms, signs and abnormal clinical and laboratory findings, not elsewhere classified (R00-R94)

GUIDELINES Section I.C.13.a
Most of the codes within Chapter 13 have site and laterality designations. The site represents the bone, joint or the muscle involved. For some conditions where more than one bone, joint or muscle is usually involved, such as osteoarthritis, there is a "multiple sites" code available. For categories where no multiple site code is provided and more than one bone, joint or muscle is involved, multiple codes should be used to indicate the different sites involved.

GUIDELINES Section I.C.13.a.1)
For certain conditions, the bone may be affected at the upper or lower end, (e.g., avascular necrosis of bone, M87, Osteoporosis, M80, M81). Though the portion of the bone affected may be at the joint, the site designation will be the bone, not the joint.

GUIDELINES Section I.C.13.b
Many musculoskeletal conditions are a result of previous injury or trauma to a site, or are recurrent conditions. Bone, joint or muscle conditions that are the result of a healed injury are usually found in chapter 13. Recurrent bone, joint or muscle conditions are also usually found in chapter 13. Any current, acute injury should be coded to the appropriate injury code from chapter 19. Chronic or recurrent conditions should generally be coded with a code from chapter 13. If it is difficult to determine from the documentation in the record which code is best to describe a condition, query the provider.

This chapter contains the following blocks:

M00-M02	Infectious arthropathies
M04	Autoinflammatory syndromes
M05-M14	Inflammatory polyarthropathies
M15-M19	Osteoarthritis
M20-M25	Other joint disorders
M26-M27	Dentofacial anomalies [including malocclusion] and other disorders of jaw
M30-M36	Systemic connective tissue disorders
M40-M43	Deforming dorsopathies
M45-M49	Spondylopathies
M50-M54	Other dorsopathies
M60-M63	Disorders of muscles
M65-M67	Disorders of synovium and tendon
M70-M79	Other soft tissue disorders
M80-M85	Disorders of bone density and structure
M86-M90	Other osteopathies
M91-M94	Chondropathies
M95	Other disorders of the musculoskeletal system and connective tissue
M96	Intraoperative and postprocedural complications and disorders of musculoskeletal system, not elsewhere classified
M97	Periprosthetic fracture around internal prosthetic joint
M99	Biomechanical lesions, not elsewhere classified

Arthropathies (M00-M25)

INCLUDES Disorders affecting predominantly peripheral (limb) joints

Infectious arthropathies (M00-M02)

Note:
This block comprises arthropathies due to microbiological agents. Distinction is made between the following types of etiological relationship:
a) direct infection of joint, where organisms invade synovial tissue and microbial antigen is present in the joint;
b) indirect infection, which may be of two types: a reactive arthropathy, where microbial infection of the body is established but neither organisms nor antigens can be identified in the joint, and a postinfective arthropathy, where microbial antigen is present but recovery of an organism is inconstant and evidence of local multiplication is lacking.

4 M00 Pyogenic arthritis
CODING TIPS✓ Also known as septic joint or septic arthritis, M00.- may be coded in addition to the infection/inflammation of a joint prosthesis.

+ 5 M00.0 Staphylococcal arthritis and polyarthritis
Use additional code (B95.61-B95.8) to identify bacterial agent
EXCLUDES 2 infection and inflammatory reaction due to internal joint prosthesis (T84.5-)

IQ + M00.00 Staphylococcal arthritis, unspecified joint

+ 6 M00.01 Staphylococcal arthritis, shoulder
⊟ SP + M00.011 Staphylococcal arthritis, right shoulder
⊟ SP + M00.012 Staphylococcal arthritis, left shoulder
⊟ IQ + M00.019 Staphylococcal arthritis, unspecified shoulder

+ 6 M00.02 Staphylococcal arthritis, elbow
⊟ SP + M00.021 Staphylococcal arthritis, right elbow
⊟ SP + M00.022 Staphylococcal arthritis, left elbow
⊟ IQ + M00.029 Staphylococcal arthritis, unspecified elbow

+ 6 M00.03 Staphylococcal arthritis, wrist
Staphylococcal arthritis of carpal bones
⊟ SP + M00.031 Staphylococcal arthritis, right wrist
⊟ SP + M00.032 Staphylococcal arthritis, left wrist
⊟ IQ + M00.039 Staphylococcal arthritis, unspecified wrist

+ 6 M00.04 Staphylococcal arthritis, hand

⬛4th digit required   ⬛5th digit required   ⬛6th digit required   ⬛7th digit required   ⬛7th digit placeholder   ✚Additional code   ⊟Laterality

1150   DecisionHealth's FY 2020 Complete Home Health ICD-10-CM Diagnosis Coding Manual

Staphylococcal arthritis of metacarpus and phalanges

▣ SP ✚ **M00.041** Staphylococcal arthritis, right hand

▣ SP ✚ **M00.042** Staphylococcal arthritis, left hand

▣ IQ ✚ **M00.049** Staphylococcal arthritis, unspecified hand

✚ ⑥ **M00.05** Staphylococcal arthritis, hip

▣ SP ✚ **M00.051** Staphylococcal arthritis, right hip

▣ SP ✚ **M00.052** Staphylococcal arthritis, left hip

▣ IQ ✚ **M00.059** Staphylococcal arthritis, unspecified hip

✚ ⑥ **M00.06** Staphylococcal arthritis, knee

▣ SP ✚ **M00.061** Staphylococcal arthritis, right knee

▣ SP ✚ **M00.062** Staphylococcal arthritis, left knee

▣ IQ ✚ **M00.069** Staphylococcal arthritis, unspecified knee

✚ ⑥ **M00.07** Staphylococcal arthritis, ankle and foot
Staphylococcal arthritis, tarsus, metatarsus and phalanges

▣ SP ✚ **M00.071** Staphylococcal arthritis, right ankle and foot

▣ SP ✚ **M00.072** Staphylococcal arthritis, left ankle and foot

▣ IQ ✚ **M00.079** Staphylococcal arthritis, unspecified ankle and foot

SP ✚ **M00.08** Staphylococcal arthritis, vertebrae

SP ✚ **M00.09** Staphylococcal polyarthritis

⑤ **M00.1** Pneumococcal arthritis and polyarthritis

IQ **M00.10** Pneumococcal arthritis, unspecified joint

⑥ **M00.11** Pneumococcal arthritis, shoulder

▣ SP **M00.111** Pneumococcal arthritis, right shoulder

▣ SP **M00.112** Pneumococcal arthritis, left shoulder

▣ IQ **M00.119** Pneumococcal arthritis, unspecified shoulder

⑥ **M00.12** Pneumococcal arthritis, elbow

▣ SP **M00.121** Pneumococcal arthritis, right elbow

▣ SP **M00.122** Pneumococcal arthritis, left elbow

▣ IQ **M00.129** Pneumococcal arthritis, unspecified elbow

⑥ **M00.13** Pneumococcal arthritis, wrist
Pneumococcal arthritis of carpal bones

▣ SP **M00.131** Pneumococcal arthritis, right wrist

▣ SP **M00.132** Pneumococcal arthritis, left wrist

▣ IQ **M00.139** Pneumococcal arthritis, unspecified wrist

⑥ **M00.14** Pneumococcal arthritis, hand
Pneumococcal arthritis of metacarpus and phalanges

▣ SP **M00.141** Pneumococcal arthritis, right hand

▣ SP **M00.142** Pneumococcal arthritis, left hand

▣ IQ **M00.149** Pneumococcal arthritis, unspecified hand

⑥ **M00.15** Pneumococcal arthritis, hip

▣ SP **M00.151** Pneumococcal arthritis, right hip

▣ SP **M00.152** Pneumococcal arthritis, left hip

▣ IQ **M00.159** Pneumococcal arthritis, unspecified hip

⑥ **M00.16** Pneumococcal arthritis, knee

▣ SP **M00.161** Pneumococcal arthritis, right knee

▣ SP **M00.162** Pneumococcal arthritis, left knee

▣ IQ **M00.169** Pneumococcal arthritis, unspecified knee

⑥ **M00.17** Pneumococcal arthritis, ankle and foot
Pneumococcal arthritis, tarsus, metatarsus and phalanges

▣ SP **M00.171** Pneumococcal arthritis, right ankle and foot

▣ SP **M00.172** Pneumococcal arthritis, left ankle and foot

▣ IQ **M00.179** Pneumococcal arthritis, unspecified ankle and foot

SP **M00.18** Pneumococcal arthritis, vertebrae

SP **M00.19** Pneumococcal polyarthritis

✚ ⑤ **M00.2** Other streptococcal arthritis and polyarthritis
Use additional code (B95.0-B95.2, B95.4-B95.5) to identify bacterial agent

IQ ✚ **M00.20** Other streptococcal arthritis, unspecified joint

✚ ⑥ **M00.21** Other streptococcal arthritis, shoulder

▣ SP ✚ **M00.211** Other streptococcal arthritis, right shoulder

▣ SP ✚ **M00.212** Other streptococcal arthritis, left shoulder

▣ IQ ✚ **M00.219** Other streptococcal arthritis, unspecified shoulder

✚ ⑥ **M00.22** Other streptococcal arthritis, elbow

▣ SP ✚ **M00.221** Other streptococcal arthritis, right elbow

▣ SP ✚ **M00.222** Other streptococcal arthritis, left elbow

▣ IQ ✚ **M00.229** Other streptococcal arthritis, unspecified elbow

✚ ⑥ **M00.23** Other streptococcal arthritis, wrist
Other streptococcal arthritis of carpal bones

▣ SP ✚ **M00.231** Other streptococcal arthritis, right wrist

▣ SP ✚ **M00.232** Other streptococcal arthritis, left wrist

▣ IQ ✚ **M00.239** Other streptococcal arthritis, unspecified wrist

✚ ⑥ **M00.24** Other streptococcal arthritis, hand
Other streptococcal arthritis metacarpus and phalanges

▣ SP ✚ **M00.241** Other streptococcal arthritis, right hand

▣ SP ✚ **M00.242** Other streptococcal arthritis, left hand

▣ IQ ✚ **M00.249** Other streptococcal arthritis, unspecified hand

✚ ⑥ **M00.25** Other streptococcal arthritis, hip

▣ SP ✚ **M00.251** Other streptococcal arthritis, right hip

★ New　▲ Revised　Px Primary　SP PDGM Px　SL Low CoM　SH High CoM　IQ Quest. Encounter　H Hospice non-cancer Dx　Unspecified　M *Manifestation*

Chapter 13

M00-M99

☐ 🆂🅿 ➕ **M00.252 Other streptococcal arthritis, left hip**

☐ 🅸🆀 ➕ **M00.259 Other streptococcal arthritis, unspecified hip**

➕ �６ **M00.26 Other streptococcal arthritis, knee**

☐ 🆂🅿 ➕ **M00.261 Other streptococcal arthritis, right knee**

☐ 🆂🅿 ➕ **M00.262 Other streptococcal arthritis, left knee**

☐ 🅸🆀 ➕ **M00.269 Other streptococcal arthritis, unspecified knee**

➕ �６ **M00.27 Other streptococcal arthritis, ankle and foot**
Other streptococcal arthritis, tarsus, metatarsus and phalanges

☐ 🆂🅿 ➕ **M00.271 Other streptococcal arthritis, right ankle and foot**

☐ 🆂🅿 ➕ **M00.272 Other streptococcal arthritis, left ankle and foot**

☐ 🅸🆀 ➕ **M00.279 Other streptococcal arthritis, unspecified ankle and foot**

🆂🅿 ➕ **M00.28 Other streptococcal arthritis, vertebrae**

🆂🅿 ➕ **M00.29 Other streptococcal polyarthritis**

➕ �５ **M00.8 Arthritis and polyarthritis due to other bacteria**
Use additional code (B96) to identify bacteria

🅸🆀 ➕ **M00.80 Arthritis due to other bacteria, unspecified joint**

➕ �６ **M00.81 Arthritis due to other bacteria, shoulder**

☐ 🆂🅿 ➕ **M00.811 Arthritis due to other bacteria, right shoulder**

☐ 🆂🅿 ➕ **M00.812 Arthritis due to other bacteria, left shoulder**

☐ 🅸🆀 ➕ **M00.819 Arthritis due to other bacteria, unspecified shoulder**

➕ �６ **M00.82 Arthritis due to other bacteria, elbow**

☐ 🆂🅿 ➕ **M00.821 Arthritis due to other bacteria, right elbow**

☐ 🆂🅿 ➕ **M00.822 Arthritis due to other bacteria, left elbow**

☐ 🅸🆀 ➕ **M00.829 Arthritis due to other bacteria, unspecified elbow**

➕ �６ **M00.83 Arthritis due to other bacteria, wrist**
Arthritis due to other bacteria, carpal bones

☐ 🆂🅿 ➕ **M00.831 Arthritis due to other bacteria, right wrist**

☐ 🆂🅿 ➕ **M00.832 Arthritis due to other bacteria, left wrist**

☐ 🅸🆀 ➕ **M00.839 Arthritis due to other bacteria, unspecified wrist**

➕ �６ **M00.84 Arthritis due to other bacteria, hand**
Arthritis due to other bacteria, metacarpus and phalanges

☐ 🆂🅿 ➕ **M00.841 Arthritis due to other bacteria, right hand**

☐ 🆂🅿 ➕ **M00.842 Arthritis due to other bacteria, left hand**

☐ 🅸🆀 ➕ **M00.849 Arthritis due to other bacteria, unspecified hand**

➕ �６ **M00.85 Arthritis due to other bacteria, hip**

☐ 🆂🅿 ➕ **M00.851 Arthritis due to other bacteria, right hip**

☐ 🆂🅿 ➕ **M00.852 Arthritis due to other bacteria, left hip**

☐ 🅸🆀 ➕ **M00.859 Arthritis due to other bacteria, unspecified hip**

➕ �６ **M00.86 Arthritis due to other bacteria, knee**

☐ 🆂🅿 ➕ **M00.861 Arthritis due to other bacteria, right knee**

☐ 🆂🅿 ➕ **M00.862 Arthritis due to other bacteria, left knee**

☐ 🅸🆀 ➕ **M00.869 Arthritis due to other bacteria, unspecified knee**

➕ �６ **M00.87 Arthritis due to other bacteria, ankle and foot**
Arthritis due to other bacteria, tarsus, metatarsus, and phalanges

☐ 🆂🅿 ➕ **M00.871 Arthritis due to other bacteria, right ankle and foot**

☐ 🆂🅿 ➕ **M00.872 Arthritis due to other bacteria, left ankle and foot**

☐ 🅸🆀 ➕ **M00.879 Arthritis due to other bacteria, unspecified ankle and foot**

🆂🅿 ➕ **M00.88 Arthritis due to other bacteria, vertebrae**

🆂🅿 ➕ **M00.89 Polyarthritis due to other bacteria**

🆂🅿 **M00.9 Pyogenic arthritis, unspecified**
Infective arthritis NOS

🄴 **M01 Direct infections of joint in infectious and parasitic diseases classified elsewhere**
Code first underlying disease, such as:
leprosy [Hansen's disease] (A30.-)
mycoses (B35-B49)
O'nyong-nyong fever (A92.1)
paratyphoid fever (A01.1-A01.4)

EXCLUDES 1 arthropathy in Lyme disease (A69.23)
gonococcal arthritis (A54.42)
meningococcal arthritis (A39.83)
mumps arthritis (B26.85)
postinfective arthropathy (M02.-)
postmeningococcal arthritis (A39.84)
reactive arthritis (M02.3)
rubella arthritis (B06.82)
sarcoidosis arthritis (D86.86)
typhoid fever arthritis (A01.04)
tuberculosis arthritis (A18.01-A18.02)

🄵 **M01.X Direct infection of joint in infectious and parasitic diseases classified elsewhere**

🅼 🅸🆀 **M01.X0 *Direct infection of unspecified joint in infectious and parasitic diseases classified elsewhere***

🄶 **M01.X1 Direct infection of shoulder joint in infectious and parasitic diseases classified elsewhere**

🅼 ☐ 🅸🆀 **M01.X11 *Direct infection of right shoulder in infectious and parasitic diseases classified elsewhere***

🅼 ☐ 🅸🆀 **M01.X12 *Direct infection of left shoulder in infectious and parasitic diseases classified elsewhere***

🄴 4th digit required   🄵 5th digit required   🄶 6th digit required   🄷 7th digit required   🅦 7th digit placeholder   ➕ Additional code   ☐ Laterality

1152   *DecisionHealth's* FY 2020 Complete Home Health ICD-10-CM Diagnosis Coding Manual

M ⊟ **IQ** M01.X19 *Direct infection of unspecified shoulder in infectious and parasitic diseases classified elsewhere*

⑥ M01.X2 Direct infection of elbow in infectious and parasitic diseases classified elsewhere

M ⊟ **IQ** M01.X21 *Direct infection of right elbow in infectious and parasitic diseases classified elsewhere*

M ⊟ **IQ** M01.X22 *Direct infection of left elbow in infectious and parasitic diseases classified elsewhere*

M ⊟ **IQ** M01.X29 *Direct infection of unspecified elbow in infectious and parasitic diseases classified elsewhere*

⑥ M01.X3 Direct infection of wrist in infectious and parasitic diseases classified elsewhere
Direct infection of carpal bones in infectious and parasitic diseases classified elsewhere

M ⊟ **IQ** M01.X31 *Direct infection of right wrist in infectious and parasitic diseases classified elsewhere*

M ⊟ **IQ** M01.X32 *Direct infection of left wrist in infectious and parasitic diseases classified elsewhere*

M ⊟ **IQ** M01.X39 *Direct infection of unspecified wrist in infectious and parasitic diseases classified elsewhere*

⑥ M01.X4 Direct infection of hand in infectious and parasitic diseases classified elsewhere
Direct infection of metacarpus and phalanges in infectious and parasitic diseases classified elsewhere

M ⊟ **IQ** M01.X41 *Direct infection of right hand in infectious and parasitic diseases classified elsewhere*

M ⊟ **IQ** M01.X42 *Direct infection of left hand in infectious and parasitic diseases classified elsewhere*

M ⊟ **IQ** M01.X49 *Direct infection of unspecified hand in infectious and parasitic diseases classified elsewhere*

⑥ M01.X5 Direct infection of hip in infectious and parasitic diseases classified elsewhere

M ⊟ **IQ** M01.X51 *Direct infection of right hip in infectious and parasitic diseases classified elsewhere*

M ⊟ **IQ** M01.X52 *Direct infection of left hip in infectious and parasitic diseases classified elsewhere*

M ⊟ **IQ** M01.X59 *Direct infection of unspecified hip in infectious and parasitic diseases classified elsewhere*

⑥ M01.X6 Direct infection of knee in infectious and parasitic diseases classified elsewhere

M ⊟ **IQ** M01.X61 *Direct infection of right knee in infectious and parasitic diseases classified elsewhere*

M ⊟ **IQ** M01.X62 *Direct infection of left knee in infectious and parasitic diseases classified elsewhere*

M ⊟ **IQ** M01.X69 *Direct infection of unspecified knee in infectious and parasitic diseases classified elsewhere*

⑥ M01.X7 Direct infection of ankle and foot in infectious and parasitic diseases classified elsewhere
Direct infection of tarsus, metatarsus and phalanges in infectious and parasitic diseases classified elsewhere

M ⊟ **IQ** M01.X71 *Direct infection of right ankle and foot in infectious and parasitic diseases classified elsewhere*

M ⊟ **IQ** M01.X72 *Direct infection of left ankle and foot in infectious and parasitic diseases classified elsewhere*

M ⊟ **IQ** M01.X79 *Direct infection of unspecified ankle and foot in infectious and parasitic diseases classified elsewhere*

M **IQ** M01.X8 *Direct infection of vertebrae in infectious and parasitic diseases classified elsewhere*

M **IQ** M01.X9 *Direct infection of multiple joints in infectious and parasitic diseases classified elsewhere*

④ M02 **Postinfective and reactive arthropathies**
Code first underlying disease, such as:
congenital syphilis [Clutton's joints] (A50.5)
enteritis due to Yersinia enterocolitica (A04.6)
infective endocarditis (I33.0)
viral hepatitis (B15-B19)

EXCLUDES 1 Behçet's disease (M35.2)
direct infections of joint in infectious and parasitic diseases classified elsewhere (M01.-)
postmeningococcal arthritis (A39.84)
mumps arthritis (B26.85)
rubella arthritis (B06.82)
syphilis arthritis (late) (A52.77)
rheumatic fever (I00)
tabetic arthropathy [Charcôt's] (A52.16)

CODING TIPS ✓ M02.- codes indicate arthropathy due to another cause. The identified underlying cause should be coded first.

⑤ M02.0 **Arthropathy following intestinal bypass**

IQ M02.00 **Arthropathy following intestinal bypass, unspecified site**

⑥ M02.01 **Arthropathy following intestinal bypass, shoulder**

⊟ **SP** M02.011 Arthropathy following intestinal bypass, right shoulder

⊟ **SP** M02.012 Arthropathy following intestinal bypass, left shoulder

⊟ **IQ** M02.019 **Arthropathy following intestinal bypass, unspecified shoulder**

★ New ▲ Revised **Px** Primary **SP** PDGM Px **SL** Low CoM **SH** High CoM **IQ** Quest. Encounter ⊞ Hospice non-cancer Dx ⬛ Unspecified **M** *Manifestation*

DecisionHealth's FY 2020 Complete Home Health ICD-10-CM Diagnosis Coding Manual

1153

⑥ **M02.02** Arthropathy following intestinal bypass, elbow

☐ SP **M02.021** Arthropathy following intestinal bypass, right elbow

☐ SP **M02.022** Arthropathy following intestinal bypass, left elbow

☐ IQ **M02.029** Arthropathy following intestinal bypass, unspecified elbow

⑥ **M02.03** Arthropathy following intestinal bypass, wrist
Arthropathy following intestinal bypass, carpal bones

☐ SP **M02.031** Arthropathy following intestinal bypass, right wrist

☐ SP **M02.032** Arthropathy following intestinal bypass, left wrist

☐ IQ **M02.039** Arthropathy following intestinal bypass, unspecified wrist

⑥ **M02.04** Arthropathy following intestinal bypass, hand
Arthropathy following intestinal bypass, metacarpals and phalanges

☐ SP **M02.041** Arthropathy following intestinal bypass, right hand

☐ SP **M02.042** Arthropathy following intestinal bypass, left hand

☐ IQ **M02.049** Arthropathy following intestinal bypass, unspecified hand

⑥ **M02.05** Arthropathy following intestinal bypass, hip

☐ SP **M02.051** Arthropathy following intestinal bypass, right hip

☐ SP **M02.052** Arthropathy following intestinal bypass, left hip

☐ IQ **M02.059** Arthropathy following intestinal bypass, unspecified hip

⑥ **M02.06** Arthropathy following intestinal bypass, knee

☐ SP **M02.061** Arthropathy following intestinal bypass, right knee

☐ SP **M02.062** Arthropathy following intestinal bypass, left knee

☐ IQ **M02.069** Arthropathy following intestinal bypass, unspecified knee

⑥ **M02.07** Arthropathy following intestinal bypass, ankle and foot
Arthropathy following intestinal bypass, tarsus, metatarsus and phalanges

☐ SP **M02.071** Arthropathy following intestinal bypass, right ankle and foot

☐ SP **M02.072** Arthropathy following intestinal bypass, left ankle and foot

☐ IQ **M02.079** Arthropathy following intestinal bypass, unspecified ankle and foot

SP **M02.08** Arthropathy following intestinal bypass, vertebrae

SP **M02.09** Arthropathy following intestinal bypass, multiple sites

⑤ **M02.1** Postdysenteric arthropathy

IQ **M02.10** Postdysenteric arthropathy, unspecified site

⑥ **M02.11** Postdysenteric arthropathy, shoulder

☐ SP **M02.111** Postdysenteric arthropathy, right shoulder

☐ SP **M02.112** Postdysenteric arthropathy, left shoulder

☐ IQ **M02.119** Postdysenteric arthropathy, unspecified shoulder

⑥ **M02.12** Postdysenteric arthropathy, elbow

☐ SP **M02.121** Postdysenteric arthropathy, right elbow

☐ SP **M02.122** Postdysenteric arthropathy, left elbow

☐ IQ **M02.129** Postdysenteric arthropathy, unspecified elbow

⑥ **M02.13** Postdysenteric arthropathy, wrist
Postdysenteric arthropathy, carpal bones

☐ SP **M02.131** Postdysenteric arthropathy, right wrist

☐ SP **M02.132** Postdysenteric arthropathy, left wrist

☐ IQ **M02.139** Postdysenteric arthropathy, unspecified wrist

⑥ **M02.14** Postdysenteric arthropathy, hand
Postdysenteric arthropathy, metacarpus and phalanges

☐ SP **M02.141** Postdysenteric arthropathy, right hand

☐ SP **M02.142** Postdysenteric arthropathy, left hand

☐ IQ **M02.149** Postdysenteric arthropathy, unspecified hand

⑥ **M02.15** Postdysenteric arthropathy, hip

☐ SP **M02.151** Postdysenteric arthropathy, right hip

☐ SP **M02.152** Postdysenteric arthropathy, left hip

☐ IQ **M02.159** Postdysenteric arthropathy, unspecified hip

⑥ **M02.16** Postdysenteric arthropathy, knee

☐ SP **M02.161** Postdysenteric arthropathy, right knee

☐ SP **M02.162** Postdysenteric arthropathy, left knee

☐ IQ **M02.169** Postdysenteric arthropathy, unspecified knee

⑥ **M02.17** Postdysenteric arthropathy, ankle and foot
Postdysenteric arthropathy, tarsus, metatarsus and phalanges

☐ SP **M02.171** Postdysenteric arthropathy, right ankle and foot

☐ SP **M02.172** Postdysenteric arthropathy, left ankle and foot

☐ IQ **M02.179** Postdysenteric arthropathy, unspecified ankle and foot

SP **M02.18** Postdysenteric arthropathy, vertebrae

SP **M02.19** Postdysenteric arthropathy, multiple sites

⑤ **M02.2** Postimmunization arthropathy

IQ **M02.20** Postimmunization arthropathy, unspecified site

⑥ **M02.21** Postimmunization arthropathy, shoulder

☐ SP **M02.211** Postimmunization arthropathy, right shoulder

☐ SP **M02.212** Postimmunization arthropathy, left shoulder

---

④ 4th digit required   ⑤ 5th digit required   ⑥ 6th digit required   ⑦ 7th digit required   ⑦ 7th digit placeholder   ✚ Additional code   ☐ Laterality

1154   *DecisionHealth's* FY 2020 Complete Home Health ICD-10-CM Diagnosis Coding Manual

🟦 **IQ** **M02.219 Postimmunization arthropathy, unspecified shoulder**

⑥ **M02.22 Postimmunization arthropathy, elbow**

🟦 **SP** M02.221 Postimmunization arthropathy, right elbow

🟦 **SP** M02.222 Postimmunization arthropathy, left elbow

🟦 **IQ** **M02.229 Postimmunization arthropathy, unspecified elbow**

⑥ **M02.23 Postimmunization arthropathy, wrist**
Postimmunization arthropathy, carpal bones

🟦 **SP** M02.231 Postimmunization arthropathy, right wrist

🟦 **SP** M02.232 Postimmunization arthropathy, left wrist

🟦 **IQ** **M02.239 Postimmunization arthropathy, unspecified wrist**

⑥ **M02.24 Postimmunization arthropathy, hand**
Postimmunization arthropathy, metacarpus and phalanges

🟦 **SP** M02.241 Postimmunization arthropathy, right hand

🟦 **SP** M02.242 Postimmunization arthropathy, left hand

🟦 **IQ** **M02.249 Postimmunization arthropathy, unspecified hand**

⑥ **M02.25 Postimmunization arthropathy, hip**

🟦 **SP** M02.251 Postimmunization arthropathy, right hip

🟦 **SP** M02.252 Postimmunization arthropathy, left hip

🟦 **IQ** **M02.259 Postimmunization arthropathy, unspecified hip**

⑥ **M02.26 Postimmunization arthropathy, knee**

🟦 **SP** M02.261 Postimmunization arthropathy, right knee

🟦 **SP** M02.262 Postimmunization arthropathy, left knee

🟦 **IQ** **M02.269 Postimmunization arthropathy, unspecified knee**

⑥ **M02.27 Postimmunization arthropathy, ankle and foot**
Postimmunization arthropathy, tarsus, metatarsus and phalanges

🟦 **SP** M02.271 Postimmunization arthropathy, right ankle and foot

🟦 **SP** M02.272 Postimmunization arthropathy, left ankle and foot

🟦 **IQ** **M02.279 Postimmunization arthropathy, unspecified ankle and foot**

SP M02.28 Postimmunization arthropathy, vertebrae

SP M02.29 Postimmunization arthropathy, multiple sites

⑤ **M02.3 Reiter's disease**
Reactive arthritis

IQ **M02.30 Reiter's disease, unspecified site**

⑥ **M02.31 Reiter's disease, shoulder**

🟦 **SP** M02.311 Reiter's disease, right shoulder

🟦 **SP** M02.312 Reiter's disease, left shoulder

🟦 **IQ** **M02.319 Reiter's disease, unspecified shoulder**

⑥ **M02.32 Reiter's disease, elbow**

🟦 **SP** M02.321 Reiter's disease, right elbow

🟦 **SP** M02.322 Reiter's disease, left elbow

🟦 **IQ** **M02.329 Reiter's disease, unspecified elbow**

⑥ **M02.33 Reiter's disease, wrist**
Reiter's disease, carpal bones

🟦 **SP** M02.331 Reiter's disease, right wrist

🟦 **SP** M02.332 Reiter's disease, left wrist

🟦 **IQ** **M02.339 Reiter's disease, unspecified wrist**

⑥ **M02.34 Reiter's disease, hand**
Reiter's disease, metacarpus and phalanges

🟦 **SP** M02.341 Reiter's disease, right hand

🟦 **SP** M02.342 Reiter's disease, left hand

🟦 **IQ** **M02.349 Reiter's disease, unspecified hand**

⑥ **M02.35 Reiter's disease, hip**

🟦 **SP** M02.351 Reiter's disease, right hip

🟦 **SP** M02.352 Reiter's disease, left hip

🟦 **IQ** **M02.359 Reiter's disease, unspecified hip**

⑥ **M02.36 Reiter's disease, knee**

🟦 **SP** M02.361 Reiter's disease, right knee

🟦 **SP** M02.362 Reiter's disease, left knee

🟦 **IQ** **M02.369 Reiter's disease, unspecified knee**

⑥ **M02.37 Reiter's disease, ankle and foot**
Reiter's disease, tarsus, metatarsus and phalanges

🟦 **SP** M02.371 Reiter's disease, right ankle and foot

🟦 **SP** M02.372 Reiter's disease, left ankle and foot

🟦 **IQ** **M02.379 Reiter's disease, unspecified ankle and foot**

SP M02.38 Reiter's disease, vertebrae

SP M02.39 Reiter's disease, multiple sites

⑤ **M02.8 Other reactive arthropathies**

IQ **M02.80 Other reactive arthropathies, unspecified site**

⑥ **M02.81 Other reactive arthropathies, shoulder**

🟦 **IQ** M02.811 Other reactive arthropathies, right shoulder

🟦 **IQ** M02.812 Other reactive arthropathies, left shoulder

🟦 **IQ** **M02.819 Other reactive arthropathies, unspecified shoulder**

⑥ **M02.82 Other reactive arthropathies, elbow**

🟦 **IQ** M02.821 Other reactive arthropathies, right elbow

🟦 **IQ** M02.822 Other reactive arthropathies, left elbow

🟦 **IQ** **M02.829 Other reactive arthropathies, unspecified elbow**

⑥ **M02.83 Other reactive arthropathies, wrist**
Other reactive arthropathies, carpal bones

🟦 **IQ** M02.831 Other reactive arthropathies, right wrist

🟦 **IQ** M02.832 Other reactive arthropathies, left wrist

🟦 **IQ** **M02.839 Other reactive arthropathies, unspecified wrist**

⑥ **M02.84 Other reactive arthropathies, hand**

★ New ▲ Revised Px Primary **SP** PDGM Px **SL** Low CoM **SH** High CoM **IQ** Quest. Encounter ⊞ Hospice non-cancer Dx   Unspecified   **M** *Manifestation*

DecisionHealth's FY 2020 Complete Home Health ICD-10-CM Diagnosis Coding Manual   1155

Other reactive arthropathies, metacarpus and phalanges

☐ **🔲 M02.841 Other reactive arthropathies, right hand**

☐ **🔲 M02.842 Other reactive arthropathies, left hand**

☐ **🔲 M02.849 Other reactive arthropathies, unspecified hand**

⑥ M02.85 Other reactive arthropathies, hip

☐ **🔲 M02.851 Other reactive arthropathies, right hip**

☐ **🔲 M02.852 Other reactive arthropathies, left hip**

☐ **🔲 M02.859 Other reactive arthropathies, unspecified hip**

⑥ M02.86 Other reactive arthropathies, knee

☐ **🔲 M02.861 Other reactive arthropathies, right knee**

☐ **🔲 M02.862 Other reactive arthropathies, left knee**

☐ **🔲 M02.869 Other reactive arthropathies, unspecified knee**

⑥ M02.87 Other reactive arthropathies, ankle and foot
Other reactive arthropathies, tarsus, metatarsus and phalanges

☐ **🔲 M02.871 Other reactive arthropathies, right ankle and foot**

☐ **🔲 M02.872 Other reactive arthropathies, left ankle and foot**

☐ **🔲 M02.879 Other reactive arthropathies, unspecified ankle and foot**

🔲 M02.88 Other reactive arthropathies, vertebrae

🔲 M02.89 Other reactive arthropathies, multiple sites

🔲 M02.9 Reactive arthropathy, unspecified

Autoinflammatory syndromes (M04)

④ M04 Autoinflammatory syndromes
EXCLUDES 2 Crohn's disease (K50.-)

SP M04.1 Periodic fever syndromes
Familial Mediterranean fever
Hyperimmunoglobin D syndrome
Mevalonate kinase deficiency
Tumor necrosis factor receptor associated periodic syndrome [TRAPS]
DEFINITION The disease is characterized by recurrent attacks of fever; intense inflammatory response pain in the abdomen, joints, and chest; and red, swollen skin lesions; it often leads to kidney failure.

SP M04.2 Cryopyrin-associated periodic syndromes
Chronic infantile neurological, cutaneous and articular syndrome [CINCA]
Familial cold autoinflammatory syndrome
Familial cold urticaria
Muckle-Wells syndrome
Neonatal onset multisystemic inflammatory disorder [NOMID]

SP M04.8 Other autoinflammatory syndromes
Blau syndrome
Deficiency of interleukin 1 receptor antagonist [DIRA]

Majeed syndrome
Periodic fever, aphthous stomatitis, pharyngitis, and adenopathy syndrome [PFAPA]
Pyogenic arthritis, pyoderma gangrenosum, and acne syndrome [PAPA]

🔲 M04.9 Autoinflammatory syndrome, unspecified

Inflammatory polyarthropathies (M05-M14)

④ M05 Rheumatoid arthritis with rheumatoid factor
EXCLUDES 1 rheumatic fever (I00)
juvenile rheumatoid arthritis (M08.-)
rheumatoid arthritis of spine (M45.-)
CODING TIPS ✓ Rheumatoid arthritis classified here includes rheumatoid arthritis and associated conditions (see combination codes) that have an identified rheumatoid factor present. Do not assume the presence of rheumatoid factor when a diagnosis of rheumatoid arthritis is noted in the clinical record. Rheumatoid arthritis that is not specified with rheumatoid factor is coded to M06.-. There are many associated conditions that the classification assumes are related to rheumatoid arthritis. Consult the alphabetic index "arthritis, rheumatoid, with."

⑤ M05.0 Felty's syndrome
Rheumatoid arthritis with splenoadenomegaly and leukopenia
DEFINITION Atypical form of rheumatoid arthritis presenting with fever, enlarged spleen, recurring infections, and decreased white cell count.

🔲 M05.00 Felty's syndrome, unspecified site

⑥ M05.01 Felty's syndrome, shoulder

☐ **SP M05.011 Felty's syndrome, right shoulder**

☐ **SP M05.012 Felty's syndrome, left shoulder**

☐ **🔲 M05.019 Felty's syndrome, unspecified shoulder**

⑥ M05.02 Felty's syndrome, elbow

☐ **SP M05.021 Felty's syndrome, right elbow**

☐ **SP M05.022 Felty's syndrome, left elbow**

☐ **🔲 M05.029 Felty's syndrome, unspecified elbow**

⑥ M05.03 Felty's syndrome, wrist
Felty's syndrome, carpal bones

☐ **SP M05.031 Felty's syndrome, right wrist**

☐ **SP M05.032 Felty's syndrome, left wrist**

☐ **🔲 M05.039 Felty's syndrome, unspecified wrist**

⑥ M05.04 Felty's syndrome, hand
Felty's syndrome, metacarpus and phalanges

☐ **SP M05.041 Felty's syndrome, right hand**

☐ **SP M05.042 Felty's syndrome, left hand**

☐ **🔲 M05.049 Felty's syndrome, unspecified hand**

⑥ M05.05 Felty's syndrome, hip

---

④4th digit required   ⑤5th digit required   ⑥6th digit required   ⑦7th digit required   ⑦7th digit placeholder   ✚Additional code   ☐Laterality

☐ **SP** M05.051 Felty's syndrome, right hip

☐ **SP** M05.052 Felty's syndrome, left hip

☐ **IQ** M05.059 Felty's syndrome, unspecified hip

⑥ M05.06 Felty's syndrome, knee

☐ **SP** M05.061 Felty's syndrome, right knee

☐ **SP** M05.062 Felty's syndrome, left knee

☐ **IQ** M05.069 Felty's syndrome, unspecified knee

⑥ M05.07 Felty's syndrome, ankle and foot
Felty's syndrome, tarsus, metatarsus and phalanges

☐ **SP** M05.071 Felty's syndrome, right ankle and foot

☐ **SP** M05.072 Felty's syndrome, left ankle and foot

☐ **IQ** M05.079 Felty's syndrome, unspecified ankle and foot

SP M05.09 Felty's syndrome, multiple sites

⑤ M05.1 Rheumatoid lung disease with rheumatoid arthritis

IQ M05.10 Rheumatoid lung disease with rheumatoid arthritis of unspecified site

⑥ M05.11 Rheumatoid lung disease with rheumatoid arthritis of shoulder

☐ **SP** M05.111 Rheumatoid lung disease with rheumatoid arthritis of right shoulder

☐ **SP** M05.112 Rheumatoid lung disease with rheumatoid arthritis of left shoulder

☐ **IQ** M05.119 Rheumatoid lung disease with rheumatoid arthritis of unspecified shoulder

⑥ M05.12 Rheumatoid lung disease with rheumatoid arthritis of elbow

☐ **SP** M05.121 Rheumatoid lung disease with rheumatoid arthritis of right elbow

☐ **SP** M05.122 Rheumatoid lung disease with rheumatoid arthritis of left elbow

☐ **IQ** M05.129 Rheumatoid lung disease with rheumatoid arthritis of unspecified elbow

⑥ M05.13 Rheumatoid lung disease with rheumatoid arthritis of wrist
Rheumatoid lung disease with rheumatoid arthritis, carpal bones

☐ **SP** M05.131 Rheumatoid lung disease with rheumatoid arthritis of right wrist

☐ **SP** M05.132 Rheumatoid lung disease with rheumatoid arthritis of left wrist

☐ **IQ** M05.139 Rheumatoid lung disease with rheumatoid arthritis of unspecified wrist

⑥ M05.14 Rheumatoid lung disease with rheumatoid arthritis of hand
Rheumatoid lung disease with rheumatoid arthritis, metacarpus and phalanges

☐ **SP** M05.141 Rheumatoid lung disease with rheumatoid arthritis of right hand

☐ **SP** M05.142 Rheumatoid lung disease with rheumatoid arthritis of left hand

☐ **IQ** M05.149 Rheumatoid lung disease with rheumatoid arthritis of unspecified hand

⑥ M05.15 Rheumatoid lung disease with rheumatoid arthritis of hip

☐ **SP** M05.151 Rheumatoid lung disease with rheumatoid arthritis of right hip

☐ **SP** M05.152 Rheumatoid lung disease with rheumatoid arthritis of left hip

☐ **IQ** M05.159 Rheumatoid lung disease with rheumatoid arthritis of unspecified hip

⑥ M05.16 Rheumatoid lung disease with rheumatoid arthritis of knee

☐ **SP** M05.161 Rheumatoid lung disease with rheumatoid arthritis of right knee

☐ **SP** M05.162 Rheumatoid lung disease with rheumatoid arthritis of left knee

☐ **IQ** M05.169 Rheumatoid lung disease with rheumatoid arthritis of unspecified knee

⑥ M05.17 Rheumatoid lung disease with rheumatoid arthritis of ankle and foot
Rheumatoid lung disease with rheumatoid arthritis, tarsus, metatarsus and phalanges

☐ **SP** M05.171 Rheumatoid lung disease with rheumatoid arthritis of right ankle and foot

☐ **SP** M05.172 Rheumatoid lung disease with rheumatoid arthritis of left ankle and foot

☐ **IQ** M05.179 Rheumatoid lung disease with rheumatoid arthritis of unspecified ankle and foot

SP M05.19 Rheumatoid lung disease with rheumatoid arthritis of multiple sites

⑤ M05.2 Rheumatoid vasculitis with rheumatoid arthritis

IQ M05.20 Rheumatoid vasculitis with rheumatoid arthritis of unspecified site

⑥ M05.21 Rheumatoid vasculitis with rheumatoid arthritis of shoulder

☐ **SP** M05.211 Rheumatoid vasculitis with rheumatoid arthritis of right shoulder

☐ **SP** M05.212 Rheumatoid vasculitis with rheumatoid arthritis of left shoulder

☐ **IQ** M05.219 Rheumatoid vasculitis with rheumatoid arthritis of unspecified shoulder

⑥ M05.22 Rheumatoid vasculitis with rheumatoid arthritis of elbow

☐ **SP** M05.221 Rheumatoid vasculitis with rheumatoid arthritis of right elbow

☐ **SP** M05.222 Rheumatoid vasculitis with rheumatoid arthritis of left elbow

☐ **IQ** M05.229 Rheumatoid vasculitis with rheumatoid arthritis of unspecified elbow

⑥ M05.23 Rheumatoid vasculitis with rheumatoid arthritis of wrist

★ New ▲ Revised **Px** Primary **SP** PDGM Px **SL** Low CoM **SH** High CoM **IQ** Quest. Encounter Ⓗ Hospice non-cancer Dx Unspecified **M** *Manifestation*

DecisionHealth's FY 2020 Complete Home Health ICD-10-CM Diagnosis Coding Manual

1157

Rheumatoid vasculitis with rheumatoid arthritis, carpal bones

SP M05.231 **Rheumatoid vasculitis with rheumatoid arthritis of right wrist**

SP M05.232 **Rheumatoid vasculitis with rheumatoid arthritis of left wrist**

IQ M05.239 **Rheumatoid vasculitis with rheumatoid arthritis of unspecified wrist**

6 M05.24 **Rheumatoid vasculitis with rheumatoid arthritis of hand**
Rheumatoid vasculitis with rheumatoid arthritis, metacarpus and phalanges

SP M05.241 **Rheumatoid vasculitis with rheumatoid arthritis of right hand**

SP M05.242 **Rheumatoid vasculitis with rheumatoid arthritis of left hand**

IQ M05.249 **Rheumatoid vasculitis with rheumatoid arthritis of unspecified hand**

6 M05.25 **Rheumatoid vasculitis with rheumatoid arthritis of hip**

SP M05.251 **Rheumatoid vasculitis with rheumatoid arthritis of right hip**

SP M05.252 **Rheumatoid vasculitis with rheumatoid arthritis of left hip**

IQ M05.259 **Rheumatoid vasculitis with rheumatoid arthritis of unspecified hip**

6 M05.26 **Rheumatoid vasculitis with rheumatoid arthritis of knee**

SP M05.261 **Rheumatoid vasculitis with rheumatoid arthritis of right knee**

SP M05.262 **Rheumatoid vasculitis with rheumatoid arthritis of left knee**

IQ M05.269 **Rheumatoid vasculitis with rheumatoid arthritis of unspecified knee**

6 M05.27 **Rheumatoid vasculitis with rheumatoid arthritis of ankle and foot**
Rheumatoid vasculitis with rheumatoid arthritis, tarsus, metatarsus and phalanges

SP M05.271 **Rheumatoid vasculitis with rheumatoid arthritis of right ankle and foot**

SP M05.272 **Rheumatoid vasculitis with rheumatoid arthritis of left ankle and foot**

IQ M05.279 **Rheumatoid vasculitis with rheumatoid arthritis of unspecified ankle and foot**

SP M05.29 **Rheumatoid vasculitis with rheumatoid arthritis of multiple sites**

5 M05.3 **Rheumatoid heart disease with rheumatoid arthritis**
Rheumatoid carditis
Rheumatoid endocarditis
Rheumatoid myocarditis
Rheumatoid pericarditis

IQ M05.30 **Rheumatoid heart disease with rheumatoid arthritis of unspecified site**

6 M05.31 **Rheumatoid heart disease with rheumatoid arthritis of shoulder**

SP M05.311 **Rheumatoid heart disease with rheumatoid arthritis of right shoulder**

SP M05.312 **Rheumatoid heart disease with rheumatoid arthritis of left shoulder**

IQ M05.319 **Rheumatoid heart disease with rheumatoid arthritis of unspecified shoulder**

6 M05.32 **Rheumatoid heart disease with rheumatoid arthritis of elbow**

SP M05.321 **Rheumatoid heart disease with rheumatoid arthritis of right elbow**

SP M05.322 **Rheumatoid heart disease with rheumatoid arthritis of left elbow**

IQ M05.329 **Rheumatoid heart disease with rheumatoid arthritis of unspecified elbow**

6 M05.33 **Rheumatoid heart disease with rheumatoid arthritis of wrist**
Rheumatoid heart disease with rheumatoid arthritis, carpal bones

SP M05.331 **Rheumatoid heart disease with rheumatoid arthritis of right wrist**

SP M05.332 **Rheumatoid heart disease with rheumatoid arthritis of left wrist**

IQ M05.339 **Rheumatoid heart disease with rheumatoid arthritis of unspecified wrist**

6 M05.34 **Rheumatoid heart disease with rheumatoid arthritis of hand**
Rheumatoid heart disease with rheumatoid arthritis, metacarpus and phalanges

SP M05.341 **Rheumatoid heart disease with rheumatoid arthritis of right hand**

SP M05.342 **Rheumatoid heart disease with rheumatoid arthritis of left hand**

IQ M05.349 **Rheumatoid heart disease with rheumatoid arthritis of unspecified hand**

6 M05.35 **Rheumatoid heart disease with rheumatoid arthritis of hip**

SP M05.351 **Rheumatoid heart disease with rheumatoid arthritis of right hip**

SP M05.352 **Rheumatoid heart disease with rheumatoid arthritis of left hip**

IQ M05.359 **Rheumatoid heart disease with rheumatoid arthritis of unspecified hip**

6 M05.36 **Rheumatoid heart disease with rheumatoid arthritis of knee**

SP M05.361 **Rheumatoid heart disease with rheumatoid arthritis of right knee**

SP M05.362 **Rheumatoid heart disease with rheumatoid arthritis of left knee**

IQ M05.369 **Rheumatoid heart disease with rheumatoid arthritis of unspecified knee**

6 M05.37 **Rheumatoid heart disease with rheumatoid arthritis of ankle and foot**
Rheumatoid heart disease with rheumatoid arthritis, tarsus, metatarsus and phalanges

---

4 4th digit required　　**5** 5th digit required　　**6** 6th digit required　　**7** 7th digit required　　**7** 7th digit placeholder　　**+** Additional code　　Laterality

1158　　*DecisionHealth's* FY 2020 Complete Home Health ICD-10-CM Diagnosis Coding Manual

☐ SP **M05.371** Rheumatoid heart disease with rheumatoid arthritis of right ankle and foot

☐ SP **M05.372** Rheumatoid heart disease with rheumatoid arthritis of left ankle and foot

☐ IQ **M05.379** Rheumatoid heart disease with rheumatoid arthritis of unspecified ankle and foot

SP **M05.39** Rheumatoid heart disease with rheumatoid arthritis of multiple sites

5 **M05.4** Rheumatoid myopathy with rheumatoid arthritis

IQ **M05.40** Rheumatoid myopathy with rheumatoid arthritis of unspecified site

6 **M05.41** Rheumatoid myopathy with rheumatoid arthritis of shoulder

☐ SP **M05.411** Rheumatoid myopathy with rheumatoid arthritis of right shoulder

☐ SP **M05.412** Rheumatoid myopathy with rheumatoid arthritis of left shoulder

☐ IQ **M05.419** Rheumatoid myopathy with rheumatoid arthritis of unspecified shoulder

6 **M05.42** Rheumatoid myopathy with rheumatoid arthritis of elbow

☐ SP **M05.421** Rheumatoid myopathy with rheumatoid arthritis of right elbow

☐ SP **M05.422** Rheumatoid myopathy with rheumatoid arthritis of left elbow

☐ IQ **M05.429** Rheumatoid myopathy with rheumatoid arthritis of unspecified elbow

6 **M05.43** Rheumatoid myopathy with rheumatoid arthritis of wrist
Rheumatoid myopathy with rheumatoid arthritis, carpal bones

☐ SP **M05.431** Rheumatoid myopathy with rheumatoid arthritis of right wrist

☐ SP **M05.432** Rheumatoid myopathy with rheumatoid arthritis of left wrist

☐ IQ **M05.439** Rheumatoid myopathy with rheumatoid arthritis of unspecified wrist

6 **M05.44** Rheumatoid myopathy with rheumatoid arthritis of hand
Rheumatoid myopathy with rheumatoid arthritis, metacarpus and phalanges

☐ SP **M05.441** Rheumatoid myopathy with rheumatoid arthritis of right hand

☐ SP **M05.442** Rheumatoid myopathy with rheumatoid arthritis of left hand

☐ IQ **M05.449** Rheumatoid myopathy with rheumatoid arthritis of unspecified hand

6 **M05.45** Rheumatoid myopathy with rheumatoid arthritis of hip

☐ SP **M05.451** Rheumatoid myopathy with rheumatoid arthritis of right hip

☐ SP **M05.452** Rheumatoid myopathy with rheumatoid arthritis of left hip

☐ IQ **M05.459** Rheumatoid myopathy with rheumatoid arthritis of unspecified hip

6 **M05.46** Rheumatoid myopathy with rheumatoid arthritis of knee

☐ SP **M05.461** Rheumatoid myopathy with rheumatoid arthritis of right knee

☐ SP **M05.462** Rheumatoid myopathy with rheumatoid arthritis of left knee

☐ IQ **M05.469** Rheumatoid myopathy with rheumatoid arthritis of unspecified knee

6 **M05.47** Rheumatoid myopathy with rheumatoid arthritis of ankle and foot
Rheumatoid myopathy with rheumatoid arthritis, tarsus, metatarsus and phalanges

☐ SP **M05.471** Rheumatoid myopathy with rheumatoid arthritis of right ankle and foot

☐ SP **M05.472** Rheumatoid myopathy with rheumatoid arthritis of left ankle and foot

☐ IQ **M05.479** Rheumatoid myopathy with rheumatoid arthritis of unspecified ankle and foot

SP **M05.49** Rheumatoid myopathy with rheumatoid arthritis of multiple sites

5 **M05.5** Rheumatoid polyneuropathy with rheumatoid arthritis

IQ **M05.50** Rheumatoid polyneuropathy with rheumatoid arthritis of unspecified site

6 **M05.51** Rheumatoid polyneuropathy with rheumatoid arthritis of shoulder

☐ SP **M05.511** Rheumatoid polyneuropathy with rheumatoid arthritis of right shoulder

☐ SP **M05.512** Rheumatoid polyneuropathy with rheumatoid arthritis of left shoulder

☐ IQ **M05.519** Rheumatoid polyneuropathy with rheumatoid arthritis of unspecified shoulder

6 **M05.52** Rheumatoid polyneuropathy with rheumatoid arthritis of elbow

☐ SP **M05.521** Rheumatoid polyneuropathy with rheumatoid arthritis of right elbow

☐ SP **M05.522** Rheumatoid polyneuropathy with rheumatoid arthritis of left elbow

☐ IQ **M05.529** Rheumatoid polyneuropathy with rheumatoid arthritis of unspecified elbow

6 **M05.53** Rheumatoid polyneuropathy with rheumatoid arthritis of wrist
Rheumatoid polyneuropathy with rheumatoid arthritis, carpal bones

☐ SP **M05.531** Rheumatoid polyneuropathy with rheumatoid arthritis of right wrist

☐ SP **M05.532** Rheumatoid polyneuropathy with rheumatoid arthritis of left wrist

☐ IQ **M05.539** Rheumatoid polyneuropathy with rheumatoid arthritis of unspecified wrist

---

★ New ▲ Revised Px Primary SP PDGM Px SL Low CoM SH High CoM IQ Quest. Encounter H Hospice non-cancer Dx Unspecified M *Manifestation*

DecisionHealth's FY 2020 Complete Home Health ICD-10-CM Diagnosis Coding Manual

1159

6 **M05.54** **Rheumatoid polyneuropathy with rheumatoid arthritis of hand**
Rheumatoid polyneuropathy with rheumatoid arthritis, metacarpus and phalanges

SP **M05.541** **Rheumatoid polyneuropathy with rheumatoid arthritis of right hand**

SP **M05.542** **Rheumatoid polyneuropathy with rheumatoid arthritis of left hand**

IQ **M05.549** **Rheumatoid polyneuropathy with rheumatoid arthritis of unspecified hand**

6 **M05.55** **Rheumatoid polyneuropathy with rheumatoid arthritis of hip**

SP **M05.551** **Rheumatoid polyneuropathy with rheumatoid arthritis of right hip**

SP **M05.552** **Rheumatoid polyneuropathy with rheumatoid arthritis of left hip**

IQ **M05.559** **Rheumatoid polyneuropathy with rheumatoid arthritis of unspecified hip**

6 **M05.56** **Rheumatoid polyneuropathy with rheumatoid arthritis of knee**

SP **M05.561** **Rheumatoid polyneuropathy with rheumatoid arthritis of right knee**

SP **M05.562** **Rheumatoid polyneuropathy with rheumatoid arthritis of left knee**

IQ **M05.569** **Rheumatoid polyneuropathy with rheumatoid arthritis of unspecified knee**

6 **M05.57** **Rheumatoid polyneuropathy with rheumatoid arthritis of ankle and foot**
Rheumatoid polyneuropathy with rheumatoid arthritis, tarsus, metatarsus and phalanges

SP **M05.571** **Rheumatoid polyneuropathy with rheumatoid arthritis of right ankle and foot**

SP **M05.572** **Rheumatoid polyneuropathy with rheumatoid arthritis of left ankle and foot**

IQ **M05.579** **Rheumatoid polyneuropathy with rheumatoid arthritis of unspecified ankle and foot**

SP **M05.59** **Rheumatoid polyneuropathy with rheumatoid arthritis of multiple sites**

5 **M05.6** **Rheumatoid arthritis with involvement of other organs and systems**

SP **M05.60** **Rheumatoid arthritis of unspecified site with involvement of other organs and systems**

6 **M05.61** **Rheumatoid arthritis of shoulder with involvement of other organs and systems**

SP **M05.611** **Rheumatoid arthritis of right shoulder with involvement of other organs and systems**

SP **M05.612** **Rheumatoid arthritis of left shoulder with involvement of other organs and systems**

IQ **M05.619** **Rheumatoid arthritis of unspecified shoulder with involvement of other organs and systems**

6 **M05.62** **Rheumatoid arthritis of elbow with involvement of other organs and systems**

SP **M05.621** **Rheumatoid arthritis of right elbow with involvement of other organs and systems**

SP **M05.622** **Rheumatoid arthritis of left elbow with involvement of other organs and systems**

IQ **M05.629** **Rheumatoid arthritis of unspecified elbow with involvement of other organs and systems**

6 **M05.63** **Rheumatoid arthritis of wrist with involvement of other organs and systems**
Rheumatoid arthritis of carpal bones with involvement of other organs and systems

SP **M05.631** **Rheumatoid arthritis of right wrist with involvement of other organs and systems**

SP **M05.632** **Rheumatoid arthritis of left wrist with involvement of other organs and systems**

IQ **M05.639** **Rheumatoid arthritis of unspecified wrist with involvement of other organs and systems**

6 **M05.64** **Rheumatoid arthritis of hand with involvement of other organs and systems**
Rheumatoid arthritis of metacarpus and phalanges with involvement of other organs and systems

SP **M05.641** **Rheumatoid arthritis of right hand with involvement of other organs and systems**

SP **M05.642** **Rheumatoid arthritis of left hand with involvement of other organs and systems**

IQ **M05.649** **Rheumatoid arthritis of unspecified hand with involvement of other organs and systems**

6 **M05.65** **Rheumatoid arthritis of hip with involvement of other organs and systems**

SP **M05.651** **Rheumatoid arthritis of right hip with involvement of other organs and systems**

SP **M05.652** **Rheumatoid arthritis of left hip with involvement of other organs and systems**

IQ **M05.659** **Rheumatoid arthritis of unspecified hip with involvement of other organs and systems**

6 **M05.66** **Rheumatoid arthritis of knee with involvement of other organs and systems**

SP **M05.661** **Rheumatoid arthritis of right knee with involvement of other organs and systems**

SP **M05.662** **Rheumatoid arthritis of left knee with involvement of other organs and systems**

IQ **M05.669** **Rheumatoid arthritis of unspecified knee with involvement of other organs and systems**

4 4th digit required   5 5th digit required   6 6th digit required   7 7th digit required   7 7th digit placeholder   + Additional code   Laterality

1160   *DecisionHealth's* FY 2020 Complete Home Health ICD-10-CM Diagnosis Coding Manual

⑥ **M05.67 Rheumatoid arthritis of ankle and foot with involvement of other organs and systems**
Rheumatoid arthritis of tarsus, metatarsus and phalanges with involvement of other organs and systems

⊟ SP **M05.671 Rheumatoid arthritis of right ankle and foot with involvement of other organs and systems**

⊟ SP **M05.672 Rheumatoid arthritis of left ankle and foot with involvement of other organs and systems**

⊟ IQ **M05.679 Rheumatoid arthritis of unspecified ankle and foot with involvement of other organs and systems**

SP **M05.69 Rheumatoid arthritis of multiple sites with involvement of other organs and systems**

⑤ **M05.7 Rheumatoid arthritis with rheumatoid factor without organ or systems involvement**

SP **M05.70 Rheumatoid arthritis with rheumatoid factor of unspecified site without organ or systems involvement**

⑥ **M05.71 Rheumatoid arthritis with rheumatoid factor of shoulder without organ or systems involvement**

⊟ IQ **M05.711 Rheumatoid arthritis with rheumatoid factor of right shoulder without organ or systems involvement**

⊟ SP **M05.712 Rheumatoid arthritis with rheumatoid factor of left shoulder without organ or systems involvement**

⊟ IQ **M05.719 Rheumatoid arthritis with rheumatoid factor of unspecified shoulder without organ or systems involvement**

⑥ **M05.72 Rheumatoid arthritis with rheumatoid factor of elbow without organ or systems involvement**

⊟ SP **M05.721 Rheumatoid arthritis with rheumatoid factor of right elbow without organ or systems involvement**

⊟ SP **M05.722 Rheumatoid arthritis with rheumatoid factor of left elbow without organ or systems involvement**

⊟ IQ **M05.729 Rheumatoid arthritis with rheumatoid factor of unspecified elbow without organ or systems involvement**

⑥ **M05.73 Rheumatoid arthritis with rheumatoid factor of wrist without organ or systems involvement**

⊟ SP **M05.731 Rheumatoid arthritis with rheumatoid factor of right wrist without organ or systems involvement**

⊟ SP **M05.732 Rheumatoid arthritis with rheumatoid factor of left wrist without organ or systems involvement**

⊟ IQ **M05.739 Rheumatoid arthritis with rheumatoid factor of unspecified wrist without organ or systems involvement**

⑥ **M05.74 Rheumatoid arthritis with rheumatoid factor of hand without organ or systems involvement**

⊟ SP **M05.741 Rheumatoid arthritis with rheumatoid factor of right hand without organ or systems involvement**

⊟ SP **M05.742 Rheumatoid arthritis with rheumatoid factor of left hand without organ or systems involvement**

⊟ IQ **M05.749 Rheumatoid arthritis with rheumatoid factor of unspecified hand without organ or systems involvement**

⑥ **M05.75 Rheumatoid arthritis with rheumatoid factor of hip without organ or systems involvement**

⊟ SP **M05.751 Rheumatoid arthritis with rheumatoid factor of right hip without organ or systems involvement**

⊟ SP **M05.752 Rheumatoid arthritis with rheumatoid factor of left hip without organ or systems involvement**

⊟ IQ **M05.759 Rheumatoid arthritis with rheumatoid factor of unspecified hip without organ or systems involvement**

⑥ **M05.76 Rheumatoid arthritis with rheumatoid factor of knee without organ or systems involvement**

⊟ SP **M05.761 Rheumatoid arthritis with rheumatoid factor of right knee without organ or systems involvement**

⊟ SP **M05.762 Rheumatoid arthritis with rheumatoid factor of left knee without organ or systems involvement**

⊟ IQ **M05.769 Rheumatoid arthritis with rheumatoid factor of unspecified knee without organ or systems involvement**

⑥ **M05.77 Rheumatoid arthritis with rheumatoid factor of ankle and foot without organ or systems involvement**

⊟ SP **M05.771 Rheumatoid arthritis with rheumatoid factor of right ankle and foot without organ or systems involvement**

⊟ SP **M05.772 Rheumatoid arthritis with rheumatoid factor of left ankle and foot without organ or systems involvement**

★ New ▲ Revised Px Primary SP PDGM Px SL Low CoM SH High CoM IQ Quest. Encounter H Hospice non-cancer Dx Unspecified M *Manifestation*

DecisionHealth's FY 2020 Complete Home Health ICD-10-CM Diagnosis Coding Manual

1161

M05.779 Rheumatoid arthritis with rheumatoid factor of unspecified ankle and foot without organ or systems involvement

M05.79 Rheumatoid arthritis with rheumatoid factor of multiple sites without organ or systems involvement

M05.8 Other rheumatoid arthritis with rheumatoid factor

M05.80 Other rheumatoid arthritis with rheumatoid factor of unspecified site

M05.81 Other rheumatoid arthritis with rheumatoid factor of shoulder

M05.811 Other rheumatoid arthritis with rheumatoid factor of right shoulder

M05.812 Other rheumatoid arthritis with rheumatoid factor of left shoulder

M05.819 Other rheumatoid arthritis with rheumatoid factor of unspecified shoulder

M05.82 Other rheumatoid arthritis with rheumatoid factor of elbow

M05.821 Other rheumatoid arthritis with rheumatoid factor of right elbow

M05.822 Other rheumatoid arthritis with rheumatoid factor of left elbow

M05.829 Other rheumatoid arthritis with rheumatoid factor of unspecified elbow

M05.83 Other rheumatoid arthritis with rheumatoid factor of wrist

M05.831 Other rheumatoid arthritis with rheumatoid factor of right wrist

M05.832 Other rheumatoid arthritis with rheumatoid factor of left wrist

M05.839 Other rheumatoid arthritis with rheumatoid factor of unspecified wrist

M05.84 Other rheumatoid arthritis with rheumatoid factor of hand

M05.841 Other rheumatoid arthritis with rheumatoid factor of right hand

M05.842 Other rheumatoid arthritis with rheumatoid factor of left hand

M05.849 Other rheumatoid arthritis with rheumatoid factor of unspecified hand

M05.85 Other rheumatoid arthritis with rheumatoid factor of hip

M05.851 Other rheumatoid arthritis with rheumatoid factor of right hip

M05.852 Other rheumatoid arthritis with rheumatoid factor of left hip

M05.859 Other rheumatoid arthritis with rheumatoid factor of unspecified hip

M05.86 Other rheumatoid arthritis with rheumatoid factor of knee

M05.861 Other rheumatoid arthritis with rheumatoid factor of right knee

M05.862 Other rheumatoid arthritis with rheumatoid factor of left knee

M05.869 Other rheumatoid arthritis with rheumatoid factor of unspecified knee

M05.87 Other rheumatoid arthritis with rheumatoid factor of ankle and foot

M05.871 Other rheumatoid arthritis with rheumatoid factor of right ankle and foot

M05.872 Other rheumatoid arthritis with rheumatoid factor of left ankle and foot

M05.879 Other rheumatoid arthritis with rheumatoid factor of unspecified ankle and foot

M05.89 Other rheumatoid arthritis with rheumatoid factor of multiple sites

M05.9 Rheumatoid arthritis with rheumatoid factor, unspecified

M06 Other rheumatoid arthritis

M06.0 Rheumatoid arthritis without rheumatoid factor

M06.00 Rheumatoid arthritis without rheumatoid factor, unspecified site

M06.01 Rheumatoid arthritis without rheumatoid factor, shoulder

M06.011 Rheumatoid arthritis without rheumatoid factor, right shoulder

M06.012 Rheumatoid arthritis without rheumatoid factor, left shoulder

M06.019 Rheumatoid arthritis without rheumatoid factor, unspecified shoulder

M06.02 Rheumatoid arthritis without rheumatoid factor, elbow

M06.021 Rheumatoid arthritis without rheumatoid factor, right elbow

M06.022 Rheumatoid arthritis without rheumatoid factor, left elbow

M06.029 Rheumatoid arthritis without rheumatoid factor, unspecified elbow

M06.03 Rheumatoid arthritis without rheumatoid factor, wrist

M06.031 Rheumatoid arthritis without rheumatoid factor, right wrist

M06.032 Rheumatoid arthritis without rheumatoid factor, left wrist

M06.039 Rheumatoid arthritis without rheumatoid factor, unspecified wrist

M06.04 Rheumatoid arthritis without rheumatoid factor, hand

M06.041 Rheumatoid arthritis without rheumatoid factor, right hand

M06.042 Rheumatoid arthritis without rheumatoid factor, left hand

M06.049 Rheumatoid arthritis without rheumatoid factor, unspecified hand

M06.05 Rheumatoid arthritis without rheumatoid factor, hip

M06.051 Rheumatoid arthritis without rheumatoid factor, right hip

M06.052 Rheumatoid arthritis without rheumatoid factor, left hip

4 4th digit required   5 5th digit required   6 6th digit required   7 7th digit required   7 7th digit placeholder   + Additional code   ⊟ Laterality

1162   *DecisionHealth's* FY 2020 Complete Home Health ICD-10-CM Diagnosis Coding Manual

M06.059 Rheumatoid arthritis without rheumatoid factor, unspecified hip

M06.06 Rheumatoid arthritis without rheumatoid factor, knee

M06.061 Rheumatoid arthritis without rheumatoid factor, right knee

M06.062 Rheumatoid arthritis without rheumatoid factor, left knee

M06.069 Rheumatoid arthritis without rheumatoid factor, unspecified knee

M06.07 Rheumatoid arthritis without rheumatoid factor, ankle and foot

M06.071 Rheumatoid arthritis without rheumatoid factor, right ankle and foot

M06.072 Rheumatoid arthritis without rheumatoid factor, left ankle and foot

M06.079 Rheumatoid arthritis without rheumatoid factor, unspecified ankle and foot

M06.08 Rheumatoid arthritis without rheumatoid factor, vertebrae

M06.09 Rheumatoid arthritis without rheumatoid factor, multiple sites

M06.1 Adult-onset Still's disease
> **EXCLUDES 1** Still's disease NOS (M08.2-)

M06.2 Rheumatoid bursitis

M06.20 Rheumatoid bursitis, unspecified site

M06.21 Rheumatoid bursitis, shoulder

M06.211 Rheumatoid bursitis, right shoulder

M06.212 Rheumatoid bursitis, left shoulder

M06.219 Rheumatoid bursitis, unspecified shoulder

M06.22 Rheumatoid bursitis, elbow

M06.221 Rheumatoid bursitis, right elbow

M06.222 Rheumatoid bursitis, left elbow

M06.229 Rheumatoid bursitis, unspecified elbow

M06.23 Rheumatoid bursitis, wrist

M06.231 Rheumatoid bursitis, right wrist

M06.232 Rheumatoid bursitis, left wrist

M06.239 Rheumatoid bursitis, unspecified wrist

M06.24 Rheumatoid bursitis, hand

M06.241 Rheumatoid bursitis, right hand

M06.242 Rheumatoid bursitis, left hand

M06.249 Rheumatoid bursitis, unspecified hand

M06.25 Rheumatoid bursitis, hip

M06.251 Rheumatoid bursitis, right hip

M06.252 Rheumatoid bursitis, left hip

M06.259 Rheumatoid bursitis, unspecified hip

M06.26 Rheumatoid bursitis, knee

M06.261 Rheumatoid bursitis, right knee

M06.262 Rheumatoid bursitis, left knee

M06.269 Rheumatoid bursitis, unspecified knee

M06.27 Rheumatoid bursitis, ankle and foot

M06.271 Rheumatoid bursitis, right ankle and foot

M06.272 Rheumatoid bursitis, left ankle and foot

M06.279 Rheumatoid bursitis, unspecified ankle and foot

M06.28 Rheumatoid bursitis, vertebrae

M06.29 Rheumatoid bursitis, multiple sites

M06.3 Rheumatoid nodule

M06.30 Rheumatoid nodule, unspecified site

M06.31 Rheumatoid nodule, shoulder

M06.311 Rheumatoid nodule, right shoulder

M06.312 Rheumatoid nodule, left shoulder

M06.319 Rheumatoid nodule, unspecified shoulder

M06.32 Rheumatoid nodule, elbow

M06.321 Rheumatoid nodule, right elbow

M06.322 Rheumatoid nodule, left elbow

M06.329 Rheumatoid nodule, unspecified elbow

M06.33 Rheumatoid nodule, wrist

M06.331 Rheumatoid nodule, right wrist

M06.332 Rheumatoid nodule, left wrist

M06.339 Rheumatoid nodule, unspecified wrist

M06.34 Rheumatoid nodule, hand

M06.341 Rheumatoid nodule, right hand

M06.342 Rheumatoid nodule, left hand

M06.349 Rheumatoid nodule, unspecified hand

M06.35 Rheumatoid nodule, hip

M06.351 Rheumatoid nodule, right hip

M06.352 Rheumatoid nodule, left hip

M06.359 Rheumatoid nodule, unspecified hip

M06.36 Rheumatoid nodule, knee

M06.361 Rheumatoid nodule, right knee

M06.362 Rheumatoid nodule, left knee

M06.369 Rheumatoid nodule, unspecified knee

M06.37 Rheumatoid nodule, ankle and foot

M06.371 Rheumatoid nodule, right ankle and foot

M06.372 Rheumatoid nodule, left ankle and foot

M06.379 Rheumatoid nodule, unspecified ankle and foot

M06.38 Rheumatoid nodule, vertebrae

M06.39 Rheumatoid nodule, multiple sites

M06.4 Inflammatory polyarthropathy
> **EXCLUDES 1** polyarthritis NOS (M13.0)

M06.8 Other specified rheumatoid arthritis

M06.80 Other specified rheumatoid arthritis, unspecified site

M06.81 Other specified rheumatoid arthritis, shoulder

★ New ▲ Revised Px Primary **SP** PDGM Px **SL** Low CoM **SH** High CoM **IQ** Quest. Encounter **H** Hospice non-cancer Dx Unspecified **M** *Manifestation*

⊟ SP **M06.811** Other specified rheumatoid arthritis, right shoulder

⊟ SP **M06.812** Other specified rheumatoid arthritis, left shoulder

⊟ IQ **M06.819** Other specified rheumatoid arthritis, unspecified shoulder

⑥ **M06.82** Other specified rheumatoid arthritis, elbow

⊟ SP **M06.821** Other specified rheumatoid arthritis, right elbow

⊟ SP **M06.822** Other specified rheumatoid arthritis, left elbow

⊟ IQ **M06.829** Other specified rheumatoid arthritis, unspecified elbow

⑥ **M06.83** Other specified rheumatoid arthritis, wrist

⊟ SP **M06.831** Other specified rheumatoid arthritis, right wrist

⊟ SP **M06.832** Other specified rheumatoid arthritis, left wrist

⊟ IQ **M06.839** Other specified rheumatoid arthritis, unspecified wrist

⑥ **M06.84** Other specified rheumatoid arthritis, hand

⊟ SP **M06.841** Other specified rheumatoid arthritis, right hand

⊟ SP **M06.842** Other specified rheumatoid arthritis, left hand

⊟ IQ **M06.849** Other specified rheumatoid arthritis, unspecified hand

⑥ **M06.85** Other specified rheumatoid arthritis, hip

⊟ SP **M06.851** Other specified rheumatoid arthritis, right hip

⊟ SP **M06.852** Other specified rheumatoid arthritis, left hip

⊟ IQ **M06.859** Other specified rheumatoid arthritis, unspecified hip

⑥ **M06.86** Other specified rheumatoid arthritis, knee

⊟ SP **M06.861** Other specified rheumatoid arthritis, right knee

⊟ SP **M06.862** Other specified rheumatoid arthritis, left knee

⊟ IQ **M06.869** Other specified rheumatoid arthritis, unspecified knee

⑥ **M06.87** Other specified rheumatoid arthritis, ankle and foot

⊟ SP **M06.871** Other specified rheumatoid arthritis, right ankle and foot

⊟ SP **M06.872** Other specified rheumatoid arthritis, left ankle and foot

⊟ IQ **M06.879** Other specified rheumatoid arthritis, unspecified ankle and foot

SP **M06.88** Other specified rheumatoid arthritis, vertebrae

SP **M06.89** Other specified rheumatoid arthritis, multiple sites

IQ **M06.9** Rheumatoid arthritis, unspecified

④ **M07** Enteropathic arthropathies
  Code also associated enteropathy, such as:
  regional enteritis [Crohn's disease] (K50.-)
  ulcerative colitis (K51.-)
  EXCLUDES 1 psoriatic arthropathies (L40.5-)

⑤ **M07.6** Enteropathic arthropathies

IQ **M07.60** Enteropathic arthropathies, unspecified site

⑥ **M07.61** Enteropathic arthropathies, shoulder

⊟ SP **M07.611** Enteropathic arthropathies, right shoulder

⊟ SP **M07.612** Enteropathic arthropathies, left shoulder

⊟ IQ **M07.619** Enteropathic arthropathies, unspecified shoulder

⑥ **M07.62** Enteropathic arthropathies, elbow

⊟ SP **M07.621** Enteropathic arthropathies, right elbow

⊟ SP **M07.622** Enteropathic arthropathies, left elbow

⊟ IQ **M07.629** Enteropathic arthropathies, unspecified elbow

⑥ **M07.63** Enteropathic arthropathies, wrist

⊟ SP **M07.631** Enteropathic arthropathies, right wrist

⊟ SP **M07.632** Enteropathic arthropathies, left wrist

⊟ IQ **M07.639** Enteropathic arthropathies, unspecified wrist

⑥ **M07.64** Enteropathic arthropathies, hand

⊟ SP **M07.641** Enteropathic arthropathies, right hand

⊟ SP **M07.642** Enteropathic arthropathies, left hand

⊟ IQ **M07.649** Enteropathic arthropathies, unspecified hand

⑥ **M07.65** Enteropathic arthropathies, hip

⊟ SP **M07.651** Enteropathic arthropathies, right hip

⊟ SP **M07.652** Enteropathic arthropathies, left hip

⊟ IQ **M07.659** Enteropathic arthropathies, unspecified hip

⑥ **M07.66** Enteropathic arthropathies, knee

⊟ SP **M07.661** Enteropathic arthropathies, right knee

⊟ SP **M07.662** Enteropathic arthropathies, left knee

⊟ IQ **M07.669** Enteropathic arthropathies, unspecified knee

⑥ **M07.67** Enteropathic arthropathies, ankle and foot

⊟ SP **M07.671** Enteropathic arthropathies, right ankle and foot

⊟ SP **M07.672** Enteropathic arthropathies, left ankle and foot

⊟ IQ **M07.679** Enteropathic arthropathies, unspecified ankle and foot

SP **M07.68** Enteropathic arthropathies, vertebrae

SP **M07.69** Enteropathic arthropathies, multiple sites

④ **M08** Juvenile arthritis
  Code also any associated underlying condition, such as:
  regional enteritis [Crohn's disease] (K50.-)
  ulcerative colitis (K51.-)
  EXCLUDES 1 arthropathy in Whipple's disease (M14.8)
  Felty's syndrome (M05.0)

---

④4th digit required   ⑤5th digit required   ⑥6th digit required   ⑦7th digit required   ⑦7th digit placeholder   ✚Additional code   ⊟Laterality

juvenile dermatomyositis
(M33.0-)
psoriatic juvenile arthropathy
(L40.54)

CODING TIPS ✓ Juvenile arthritis generally
indicates arthritic conditions that have
developed in individuals under 16 years of age.
Autoimmune disorders are often the cause of
these conditions, and all available records
should be carefully reviewed to assign the
most specific diagnosis and identify any
underlying conditions.

⑤ M08.0 **Unspecified juvenile rheumatoid arthritis**

Juvenile rheumatoid arthritis with or
without rheumatoid factor

🄠 M08.00 **Unspecified juvenile rheumatoid arthritis of unspecified site**

⑥ M08.01 **Unspecified juvenile rheumatoid arthritis, shoulder**

▤ SP M08.011 **Unspecified juvenile rheumatoid arthritis, right shoulder**

▤ SP M08.012 **Unspecified juvenile rheumatoid arthritis, left shoulder**

▤ 🄠 M08.019 **Unspecified juvenile rheumatoid arthritis, unspecified shoulder**

⑥ M08.02 **Unspecified juvenile rheumatoid arthritis of elbow**

▤ SP M08.021 **Unspecified juvenile rheumatoid arthritis, right elbow**

▤ SP M08.022 **Unspecified juvenile rheumatoid arthritis, left elbow**

▤ 🄠 M08.029 **Unspecified juvenile rheumatoid arthritis, unspecified elbow**

⑥ M08.03 **Unspecified juvenile rheumatoid arthritis, wrist**

▤ SP M08.031 **Unspecified juvenile rheumatoid arthritis, right wrist**

▤ SP M08.032 **Unspecified juvenile rheumatoid arthritis, left wrist**

▤ 🄠 M08.039 **Unspecified juvenile rheumatoid arthritis, unspecified wrist**

⑥ M08.04 **Unspecified juvenile rheumatoid arthritis, hand**

▤ SP M08.041 **Unspecified juvenile rheumatoid arthritis, right hand**

▤ SP M08.042 **Unspecified juvenile rheumatoid arthritis, left hand**

▤ 🄠 M08.049 **Unspecified juvenile rheumatoid arthritis, unspecified hand**

⑥ M08.05 **Unspecified juvenile rheumatoid arthritis, hip**

▤ SP M08.051 **Unspecified juvenile rheumatoid arthritis, right hip**

▤ SP M08.052 **Unspecified juvenile rheumatoid arthritis, left hip**

▤ 🄠 M08.059 **Unspecified juvenile rheumatoid arthritis, unspecified hip**

⑥ M08.06 **Unspecified juvenile rheumatoid arthritis, knee**

▤ SP M08.061 **Unspecified juvenile rheumatoid arthritis, right knee**

▤ SP M08.062 **Unspecified juvenile rheumatoid arthritis, left knee**

▤ 🄠 M08.069 **Unspecified juvenile rheumatoid arthritis, unspecified knee**

⑥ M08.07 **Unspecified juvenile rheumatoid arthritis, ankle and foot**

▤ SP M08.071 **Unspecified juvenile rheumatoid arthritis, right ankle and foot**

▤ SP M08.072 **Unspecified juvenile rheumatoid arthritis, left ankle and foot**

▤ 🄠 M08.079 **Unspecified juvenile rheumatoid arthritis, unspecified ankle and foot**

SP M08.08 **Unspecified juvenile rheumatoid arthritis, vertebrae**

SP M08.09 **Unspecified juvenile rheumatoid arthritis, multiple sites**

SP M08.1 Juvenile ankylosing spondylitis
EXCLUDES 1 ankylosing spondylitis in
adults (M45.0-)

⑤ M08.2 Juvenile rheumatoid arthritis with systemic onset
Still's disease NOS
EXCLUDES 1 adult-onset Still's disease
(M06.1-)

🄠 M08.20 **Juvenile rheumatoid arthritis with systemic onset, unspecified site**

⑥ M08.21 **Juvenile rheumatoid arthritis with systemic onset, shoulder**

▤ SP M08.211 Juvenile rheumatoid arthritis with systemic onset, right shoulder

▤ SP M08.212 Juvenile rheumatoid arthritis with systemic onset, left shoulder

▤ 🄠 M08.219 **Juvenile rheumatoid arthritis with systemic onset, unspecified shoulder**

⑥ M08.22 Juvenile rheumatoid arthritis with systemic onset, elbow

▤ SP M08.221 Juvenile rheumatoid arthritis with systemic onset, right elbow

▤ SP M08.222 Juvenile rheumatoid arthritis with systemic onset, left elbow

▤ 🄠 M08.229 **Juvenile rheumatoid arthritis with systemic onset, unspecified elbow**

⑥ M08.23 Juvenile rheumatoid arthritis with systemic onset, wrist

▤ SP M08.231 Juvenile rheumatoid arthritis with systemic onset, right wrist

▤ SP M08.232 Juvenile rheumatoid arthritis with systemic onset, left wrist

▤ 🄠 M08.239 **Juvenile rheumatoid arthritis with systemic onset, unspecified wrist**

⑥ M08.24 Juvenile rheumatoid arthritis with systemic onset, hand

▤ SP M08.241 Juvenile rheumatoid arthritis with systemic onset, right hand

▤ SP M08.242 Juvenile rheumatoid arthritis with systemic onset, left hand

▤ 🄠 M08.249 **Juvenile rheumatoid arthritis with systemic onset, unspecified hand**

⑥ M08.25 Juvenile rheumatoid arthritis with systemic onset, hip

★ New ▲ Revised Px Primary SP PDGM Px SL Low CoM SH High CoM 🄠 Quest. Encounter 🄷 Hospice non-cancer Dx Unspecified M *Manifestation*

DecisionHealth's FY 2020 Complete Home Health ICD-10-CM Diagnosis Coding Manual 1165

☐ SP **M08.251** Juvenile rheumatoid arthritis with systemic onset, right hip

☐ SP **M08.252** Juvenile rheumatoid arthritis with systemic onset, left hip

☐ IQ **M08.259** Juvenile rheumatoid arthritis with systemic onset, unspecified hip

⑥ **M08.26** Juvenile rheumatoid arthritis with systemic onset, knee

☐ SP **M08.261** Juvenile rheumatoid arthritis with systemic onset, right knee

☐ SP **M08.262** Juvenile rheumatoid arthritis with systemic onset, left knee

☐ IQ **M08.269** Juvenile rheumatoid arthritis with systemic onset, unspecified knee

⑥ **M08.27** Juvenile rheumatoid arthritis with systemic onset, ankle and foot

☐ SP **M08.271** Juvenile rheumatoid arthritis with systemic onset, right ankle and foot

☐ SP **M08.272** Juvenile rheumatoid arthritis with systemic onset, left ankle and foot

☐ IQ **M08.279** Juvenile rheumatoid arthritis with systemic onset, unspecified ankle and foot

SP **M08.28** Juvenile rheumatoid arthritis with systemic onset, vertebrae

SP **M08.29** Juvenile rheumatoid arthritis with systemic onset, multiple sites

SP **M08.3** Juvenile rheumatoid polyarthritis (seronegative)

⑤ **M08.4** Pauciarticular juvenile rheumatoid arthritis

IQ **M08.40** Pauciarticular juvenile rheumatoid arthritis, unspecified site

⑥ **M08.41** Pauciarticular juvenile rheumatoid arthritis, shoulder

☐ SP **M08.411** Pauciarticular juvenile rheumatoid arthritis, right shoulder

☐ SP **M08.412** Pauciarticular juvenile rheumatoid arthritis, left shoulder

☐ IQ **M08.419** Pauciarticular juvenile rheumatoid arthritis, unspecified shoulder

⑥ **M08.42** Pauciarticular juvenile rheumatoid arthritis, elbow

☐ SP **M08.421** Pauciarticular juvenile rheumatoid arthritis, right elbow

☐ SP **M08.422** Pauciarticular juvenile rheumatoid arthritis, left elbow

☐ IQ **M08.429** Pauciarticular juvenile rheumatoid arthritis, unspecified elbow

⑥ **M08.43** Pauciarticular juvenile rheumatoid arthritis, wrist

☐ SP **M08.431** Pauciarticular juvenile rheumatoid arthritis, right wrist

☐ SP **M08.432** Pauciarticular juvenile rheumatoid arthritis, left wrist

☐ IQ **M08.439** Pauciarticular juvenile rheumatoid arthritis, unspecified wrist

⑥ **M08.44** Pauciarticular juvenile rheumatoid arthritis, hand

☐ SP **M08.441** Pauciarticular juvenile rheumatoid arthritis, right hand

☐ SP **M08.442** Pauciarticular juvenile rheumatoid arthritis, left hand

☐ IQ **M08.449** Pauciarticular juvenile rheumatoid arthritis, unspecified hand

⑥ **M08.45** Pauciarticular juvenile rheumatoid arthritis, hip

☐ SP **M08.451** Pauciarticular juvenile rheumatoid arthritis, right hip

☐ SP **M08.452** Pauciarticular juvenile rheumatoid arthritis, left hip

☐ IQ **M08.459** Pauciarticular juvenile rheumatoid arthritis, unspecified hip

⑥ **M08.46** Pauciarticular juvenile rheumatoid arthritis, knee

☐ SP **M08.461** Pauciarticular juvenile rheumatoid arthritis, right knee

☐ SP **M08.462** Pauciarticular juvenile rheumatoid arthritis, left knee

☐ IQ **M08.469** Pauciarticular juvenile rheumatoid arthritis, unspecified knee

⑥ **M08.47** Pauciarticular juvenile rheumatoid arthritis, ankle and foot

☐ SP **M08.471** Pauciarticular juvenile rheumatoid arthritis, right ankle and foot

☐ SP **M08.472** Pauciarticular juvenile rheumatoid arthritis, left ankle and foot

☐ IQ **M08.479** Pauciarticular juvenile rheumatoid arthritis, unspecified ankle and foot

SP **M08.48** Pauciarticular juvenile rheumatoid arthritis, vertebrae

⑤ **M08.8** Other juvenile arthritis

IQ **M08.80** Other juvenile arthritis, unspecified site

⑥ **M08.81** Other juvenile arthritis, shoulder

☐ SP **M08.811** Other juvenile arthritis, right shoulder

☐ SP **M08.812** Other juvenile arthritis, left shoulder

☐ IQ **M08.819** Other juvenile arthritis, unspecified shoulder

⑥ **M08.82** Other juvenile arthritis, elbow

☐ SP **M08.821** Other juvenile arthritis, right elbow

☐ SP **M08.822** Other juvenile arthritis, left elbow

☐ IQ **M08.829** Other juvenile arthritis, unspecified elbow

⑥ **M08.83** Other juvenile arthritis, wrist

☐ SP **M08.831** Other juvenile arthritis, right wrist

☐ SP **M08.832** Other juvenile arthritis, left wrist

☐ IQ **M08.839** Other juvenile arthritis, unspecified wrist

⑥ **M08.84** Other juvenile arthritis, hand

☐ SP **M08.841** Other juvenile arthritis, right hand

☐ SP **M08.842** Other juvenile arthritis, left hand

---

④ 4th digit required   ⑤ 5th digit required   ⑥ 6th digit required   ⑦ 7th digit required   ⑦ 7th digit placeholder   ✛ Additional code   ☐ Laterality

Chapter 13

M00-M99

IQ M08.849 Other juvenile arthritis, unspecified hand

6 **M08.85 Other juvenile arthritis, hip**

SP **M08.851 Other juvenile arthritis, right hip**

SP **M08.852 Other juvenile arthritis, left hip**

IQ M08.859 Other juvenile arthritis, unspecified hip

6 **M08.86 Other juvenile arthritis, knee**

SP **M08.861 Other juvenile arthritis, right knee**

SP **M08.862 Other juvenile arthritis, left knee**

IQ M08.869 Other juvenile arthritis, unspecified knee

6 **M08.87 Other juvenile arthritis, ankle and foot**

SP **M08.871 Other juvenile arthritis, right ankle and foot**

SP **M08.872 Other juvenile arthritis, left ankle and foot**

IQ M08.879 Other juvenile arthritis, unspecified ankle and foot

SP **M08.88 Other juvenile arthritis, other specified site**
Other juvenile arthritis, vertebrae

SP **M08.89 Other juvenile arthritis, multiple sites**

5 **M08.9 Juvenile arthritis, unspecified**

> EXCLUDES 1 juvenile rheumatoid arthritis, unspecified (M08.0-)

IQ M08.90 Juvenile arthritis, unspecified, unspecified site

6 **M08.91 Juvenile arthritis, unspecified, shoulder**

SP **M08.911 Juvenile arthritis, unspecified, right shoulder**

SP **M08.912 Juvenile arthritis, unspecified, left shoulder**

IQ M08.919 Juvenile arthritis, unspecified, unspecified shoulder

6 **M08.92 Juvenile arthritis, unspecified, elbow**

SP **M08.921 Juvenile arthritis, unspecified, right elbow**

SP **M08.922 Juvenile arthritis, unspecified, left elbow**

IQ M08.929 Juvenile arthritis, unspecified, unspecified elbow

6 **M08.93 Juvenile arthritis, unspecified, wrist**

SP **M08.931 Juvenile arthritis, unspecified, right wrist**

SP **M08.932 Juvenile arthritis, unspecified, left wrist**

IQ M08.939 Juvenile arthritis, unspecified, unspecified wrist

6 **M08.94 Juvenile arthritis, unspecified, hand**

SP **M08.941 Juvenile arthritis, unspecified, right hand**

SP **M08.942 Juvenile arthritis, unspecified, left hand**

IQ M08.949 Juvenile arthritis, unspecified, unspecified hand

6 **M08.95 Juvenile arthritis, unspecified, hip**

SP **M08.951 Juvenile arthritis, unspecified, right hip**

SP **M08.952 Juvenile arthritis, unspecified, left hip**

IQ M08.959 Juvenile arthritis, unspecified, unspecified hip

6 **M08.96 Juvenile arthritis, unspecified, knee**

SP **M08.961 Juvenile arthritis, unspecified, right knee**

SP **M08.962 Juvenile arthritis, unspecified, left knee**

IQ M08.969 Juvenile arthritis, unspecified, unspecified knee

6 **M08.97 Juvenile arthritis, unspecified, ankle and foot**

SP **M08.971 Juvenile arthritis, unspecified, right ankle and foot**

SP **M08.972 Juvenile arthritis, unspecified, left ankle and foot**

IQ M08.979 Juvenile arthritis, unspecified, unspecified ankle and foot

SP **M08.98 Juvenile arthritis, unspecified, vertebrae**

SP **M08.99 Juvenile arthritis, unspecified, multiple sites**

+ 4 **M1A Chronic gout**
Use additional code to identify:
Autonomic neuropathy in diseases classified elsewhere (G99.0)
Calculus of urinary tract in diseases classified elsewhere (N22)
Cardiomyopathy in diseases classified elsewhere (I43)
Disorders of external ear in diseases classified elsewhere (H61.1-, H62.8-)
Disorders of iris and ciliary body in diseases classified elsewhere (H22)
Glomerular disorders in diseases classified elsewhere (N08)

> EXCLUDES 1 gout NOS (M10.-)

> EXCLUDES 2 acute gout (M10.-)

The appropriate 7th character is to be added to each code from category M1A
0   without tophus (tophi)
1   with tophus (tophi)

CODING TIPS ✓ Do not assign a code from category M1A.- unless the physician has specifically provided a diagnosis of "chronic" gout.

+ 5 **M1A.0 Idiopathic chronic gout**
Chronic gouty bursitis
Primary chronic gout

IQ + 7 M1A.00X- Idiopathic chronic gout, unspecified site

+ 6 **M1A.01 Idiopathic chronic gout, shoulder**

SP + 7 **M1A.011- Idiopathic chronic gout, right shoulder**

SP + 7 **M1A.012- Idiopathic chronic gout, left shoulder**

IQ + 7 M1A.019- Idiopathic chronic gout, unspecified shoulder

+ 6 **M1A.02 Idiopathic chronic gout, elbow**

★ New ▲ Revised Px Primary SP PDGM Px SL Low CoM SH High CoM IQ Quest. Encounter H Hospice non-cancer Dx | Unspecified | M Manifestation

DecisionHealth's FY 2020 Complete Home Health ICD-10-CM Diagnosis Coding Manual | 1167

☰ **SP** ✛ 7 **M1A.021-** Idiopathic chronic gout, right elbow

☰ **SP** ✛ 7 **M1A.022-** Idiopathic chronic gout, left elbow

☰ **IQ** ✛ 7 **M1A.029-** Idiopathic chronic gout, unspecified elbow

✛ 6 **M1A.03** Idiopathic chronic gout, wrist

☰ **SP** ✛ 7 **M1A.031-** Idiopathic chronic gout, right wrist

☰ **SP** ✛ 7 **M1A.032-** Idiopathic chronic gout, left wrist

☰ **IQ** ✛ 7 **M1A.039-** Idiopathic chronic gout, unspecified wrist

✛ 6 **M1A.04** Idiopathic chronic gout, hand

☰ **SP** ✛ 7 **M1A.041-** Idiopathic chronic gout, right hand

☰ **SP** ✛ 7 **M1A.042-** Idiopathic chronic gout, left hand

☰ **IQ** ✛ 7 **M1A.049-** Idiopathic chronic gout, unspecified hand

✛ 6 **M1A.05** Idiopathic chronic gout, hip

☰ **SP** ✛ 7 **M1A.051-** Idiopathic chronic gout, right hip

☰ **SP** ✛ 7 **M1A.052-** Idiopathic chronic gout, left hip

☰ **IQ** ✛ 7 **M1A.059-** Idiopathic chronic gout, unspecified hip

✛ 6 **M1A.06** Idiopathic chronic gout, knee

☰ **SP** ✛ 7 **M1A.061-** Idiopathic chronic gout, right knee

☰ **SP** ✛ 7 **M1A.062-** Idiopathic chronic gout, left knee

☰ **IQ** ✛ 7 **M1A.069-** Idiopathic chronic gout, unspecified knee

✛ 6 **M1A.07** Idiopathic chronic gout, ankle and foot

☰ **SP** ✛ 7 **M1A.071-** Idiopathic chronic gout, right ankle and foot

☰ **SP** ✛ 7 **M1A.072-** Idiopathic chronic gout, left ankle and foot

☰ **IQ** ✛ 7 **M1A.079-** Idiopathic chronic gout, unspecified ankle and foot

SP ✛ ☑ **M1A.08X-** Idiopathic chronic gout, vertebrae

SP ✛ ☑ **M1A.09X-** Idiopathic chronic gout, multiple sites

✛ 5 **M1A.1** Lead-induced chronic gout
  Code first:
    toxic effects of lead and its compounds (T56.0-)

IQ ✛ ☑ **M1A.10X-** Lead-induced chronic gout, unspecified site

✛ 6 **M1A.11** Lead-induced chronic gout, shoulder

☰ **SP** ✛ 7 **M1A.111-** Lead-induced chronic gout, right shoulder

☰ **SP** ✛ 7 **M1A.112-** Lead-induced chronic gout, left shoulder

☰ **IQ** ✛ 7 **M1A.119-** Lead-induced chronic gout, unspecified shoulder

✛ 6 **M1A.12** Lead-induced chronic gout, elbow

☰ **SP** ✛ 7 **M1A.121-** Lead-induced chronic gout, right elbow

☰ **SP** ✛ 7 **M1A.122-** Lead-induced chronic gout, left elbow

☰ **IQ** ✛ 7 **M1A.129-** Lead-induced chronic gout, unspecified elbow

✛ 6 **M1A.13** Lead-induced chronic gout, wrist

☰ **SP** ✛ 7 **M1A.131-** Lead-induced chronic gout, right wrist

☰ **SP** ✛ 7 **M1A.132-** Lead-induced chronic gout, left wrist

☰ **IQ** ✛ 7 **M1A.139-** Lead-induced chronic gout, unspecified wrist

✛ 6 **M1A.14** Lead-induced chronic gout, hand

☰ **SP** ✛ 7 **M1A.141-** Lead-induced chronic gout, right hand

☰ **SP** ✛ 7 **M1A.142-** Lead-induced chronic gout, left hand

☰ **IQ** ✛ 7 **M1A.149-** Lead-induced chronic gout, unspecified hand

✛ 6 **M1A.15** Lead-induced chronic gout, hip

☰ **SP** ✛ 7 **M1A.151-** Lead-induced chronic gout, right hip

☰ **SP** ✛ 7 **M1A.152-** Lead-induced chronic gout, left hip

☰ **IQ** ✛ 7 **M1A.159-** Lead-induced chronic gout, unspecified hip

✛ 6 **M1A.16** Lead-induced chronic gout, knee

☰ **SP** ✛ 7 **M1A.161-** Lead-induced chronic gout, right knee

☰ **SP** ✛ 7 **M1A.162-** Lead-induced chronic gout, left knee

☰ **IQ** ✛ 7 **M1A.169-** Lead-induced chronic gout, unspecified knee

✛ 6 **M1A.17** Lead-induced chronic gout, ankle and foot

☰ **SP** ✛ 7 **M1A.171-** Lead-induced chronic gout, right ankle and foot

☰ **SP** ✛ 7 **M1A.172-** Lead-induced chronic gout, left ankle and foot

☰ **IQ** ✛ 7 **M1A.179-** Lead-induced chronic gout, unspecified ankle and foot

SP ✛ ☑ **M1A.18X-** Lead-induced chronic gout, vertebrae

SP ✛ ☑ **M1A.19X-** Lead-induced chronic gout, multiple sites

✛ 5 **M1A.2** Drug-induced chronic gout
  Use additional code for adverse effect, if applicable, to identify drug (T36-T50 with fifth or sixth character 5)

IQ ✛ ☑ **M1A.20X-** Drug-induced chronic gout, unspecified site

✛ 6 **M1A.21** Drug-induced chronic gout, shoulder

☰ **SP** ✛ 7 **M1A.211-** Drug-induced chronic gout, right shoulder

☰ **SP** ✛ 7 **M1A.212-** Drug-induced chronic gout, left shoulder

☰ **IQ** ✛ 7 **M1A.219-** Drug-induced chronic gout, unspecified shoulder

✛ 6 **M1A.22** Drug-induced chronic gout, elbow

☰ **SP** ✛ 7 **M1A.221-** Drug-induced chronic gout, right elbow

☰ **SP** ✛ 7 **M1A.222-** Drug-induced chronic gout, left elbow

☰ **IQ** ✛ 7 **M1A.229-** Drug-induced chronic gout, unspecified elbow

✛ 6 **M1A.23** Drug-induced chronic gout, wrist

☰ **SP** ✛ 7 **M1A.231-** Drug-induced chronic gout, right wrist

☰ **SP** ✛ 7 **M1A.232-** Drug-induced chronic gout, left wrist

---

4 4th digit required   5 5th digit required   6 6th digit required   7 7th digit required   ☑ 7th digit placeholder   ✛ Additional code   ☰ Laterality

🔲 **IQ** ✚ 7 **M1A.239-** Drug-induced chronic gout, unspecified wrist

✚ 6 **M1A.24** Drug-induced chronic gout, hand

🔲 **SP** ✚ 7 **M1A.241-** Drug-induced chronic gout, right hand

🔲 **SP** ✚ 7 **M1A.242-** Drug-induced chronic gout, left hand

🔲 **IQ** ✚ 7 **M1A.249-** Drug-induced chronic gout, unspecified hand

✚ 6 **M1A.25** Drug-induced chronic gout, hip

🔲 **SP** ✚ 7 **M1A.251-** Drug-induced chronic gout, right hip

🔲 **SP** ✚ 7 **M1A.252-** Drug-induced chronic gout, left hip

🔲 **IQ** ✚ 7 **M1A.259-** Drug-induced chronic gout, unspecified hip

✚ 6 **M1A.26** Drug-induced chronic gout, knee

🔲 **SP** ✚ 7 **M1A.261-** Drug-induced chronic gout, right knee

🔲 **SP** ✚ 7 **M1A.262-** Drug-induced chronic gout, left knee

🔲 **IQ** ✚ 7 **M1A.269-** Drug-induced chronic gout, unspecified knee

✚ 6 **M1A.27** Drug-induced chronic gout, ankle and foot

🔲 **SP** ✚ 7 **M1A.271-** Drug-induced chronic gout, right ankle and foot

🔲 **SP** ✚ 7 **M1A.272-** Drug-induced chronic gout, left ankle and foot

🔲 **IQ** ✚ 7 **M1A.279-** Drug-induced chronic gout, unspecified ankle and foot

SP ✚ 7 **M1A.28X-** Drug-induced chronic gout, vertebrae

SP ✚ 7 **M1A.29X-** Drug-induced chronic gout, multiple sites

✚ 5 **M1A.3** Chronic gout due to renal impairment
Code first:
    associated renal disease

IQ ✚ 7 **M1A.30X-** Chronic gout due to renal impairment, unspecified site

✚ 6 **M1A.31** Chronic gout due to renal impairment, shoulder

🔲 **SP** ✚ 7 **M1A.311-** Chronic gout due to renal impairment, right shoulder

🔲 **SP** ✚ 7 **M1A.312-** Chronic gout due to renal impairment, left shoulder

🔲 **IQ** ✚ 7 **M1A.319-** Chronic gout due to renal impairment, unspecified shoulder

✚ 6 **M1A.32** Chronic gout due to renal impairment, elbow

🔲 **SP** ✚ 7 **M1A.321-** Chronic gout due to renal impairment, right elbow

🔲 **SP** ✚ 7 **M1A.322-** Chronic gout due to renal impairment, left elbow

🔲 **IQ** ✚ 7 **M1A.329-** Chronic gout due to renal impairment, unspecified elbow

✚ 6 **M1A.33** Chronic gout due to renal impairment, wrist

🔲 **SP** ✚ 7 **M1A.331-** Chronic gout due to renal impairment, right wrist

🔲 **SP** ✚ 7 **M1A.332-** Chronic gout due to renal impairment, left wrist

🔲 **IQ** ✚ 7 **M1A.339-** Chronic gout due to renal impairment, unspecified wrist

✚ 6 **M1A.34** Chronic gout due to renal impairment, hand

🔲 **SP** ✚ 7 **M1A.341-** Chronic gout due to renal impairment, right hand

🔲 **SP** ✚ 7 **M1A.342-** Chronic gout due to renal impairment, left hand

🔲 **IQ** ✚ 7 **M1A.349-** Chronic gout due to renal impairment, unspecified hand

✚ 6 **M1A.35** Chronic gout due to renal impairment, hip

🔲 **SP** ✚ 7 **M1A.351-** Chronic gout due to renal impairment, right hip

🔲 **SP** ✚ 7 **M1A.352-** Chronic gout due to renal impairment, left hip

🔲 **IQ** ✚ 7 **M1A.359-** Chronic gout due to renal impairment, unspecified hip

✚ 6 **M1A.36** Chronic gout due to renal impairment, knee

🔲 **SP** ✚ 7 **M1A.361-** Chronic gout due to renal impairment, right knee

🔲 **SP** ✚ 7 **M1A.362-** Chronic gout due to renal impairment, left knee

🔲 **IQ** ✚ 7 **M1A.369-** Chronic gout due to renal impairment, unspecified knee

✚ 6 **M1A.37** Chronic gout due to renal impairment, ankle and foot

🔲 **SP** ✚ 7 **M1A.371-** Chronic gout due to renal impairment, right ankle and foot

🔲 **SP** ✚ 7 **M1A.372-** Chronic gout due to renal impairment, left ankle and foot

🔲 **IQ** ✚ 7 **M1A.379-** Chronic gout due to renal impairment, unspecified ankle and foot

SP ✚ 7 **M1A.38X-** Chronic gout due to renal impairment, vertebrae

SP ✚ 7 **M1A.39X-** Chronic gout due to renal impairment, multiple sites

✚ 5 **M1A.4** Other secondary chronic gout
Code first:
    associated condition

IQ ✚ 7 **M1A.40X-** Other secondary chronic gout, unspecified site

✚ 6 **M1A.41** Other secondary chronic gout, shoulder

🔲 **SP** ✚ 7 **M1A.411-** Other secondary chronic gout, right shoulder

🔲 **SP** ✚ 7 **M1A.412-** Other secondary chronic gout, left shoulder

🔲 **IQ** ✚ 7 **M1A.419-** Other secondary chronic gout, unspecified shoulder

✚ 6 **M1A.42** Other secondary chronic gout, elbow

🔲 **SP** ✚ 7 **M1A.421-** Other secondary chronic gout, right elbow

🔲 **SP** ✚ 7 **M1A.422-** Other secondary chronic gout, left elbow

🔲 **IQ** ✚ 7 **M1A.429-** Other secondary chronic gout, unspecified elbow

✚ 6 **M1A.43** Other secondary chronic gout, wrist

🔲 **SP** ✚ 7 **M1A.431-** Other secondary chronic gout, right wrist

🔲 **SP** ✚ 7 **M1A.432-** Other secondary chronic gout, left wrist

🔲 **IQ** ✚ 7 **M1A.439-** Other secondary chronic gout, unspecified wrist

✚ 6 **M1A.44** Other secondary chronic gout, hand

★ New ▲ Revised **Px** Primary **SP** PDGM Px **SL** Low CoM **SH** High CoM **IQ** Quest. Encounter Ⓗ Hospice non-cancer Dx Unspecified **M** *Manifestation*

⊟ SP + 7 M1A.441- Other secondary chronic gout, right hand

⊟ SP + 7 M1A.442- Other secondary chronic gout, left hand

⊟ IQ + 7 M1A.449- Other secondary chronic gout, unspecified hand

+ 6 M1A.45 Other secondary chronic gout, hip

⊟ SP + 7 M1A.451- Other secondary chronic gout, right hip

⊟ SP + 7 M1A.452- Other secondary chronic gout, left hip

⊟ IQ + 7 M1A.459- Other secondary chronic gout, unspecified hip

+ 6 M1A.46 Other secondary chronic gout, knee

⊟ SP + 7 M1A.461- Other secondary chronic gout, right knee

⊟ SP + 7 M1A.462- Other secondary chronic gout, left knee

⊟ IQ + 7 M1A.469- Other secondary chronic gout, unspecified knee

+ 6 M1A.47 Other secondary chronic gout, ankle and foot

⊟ SP + 7 M1A.471- Other secondary chronic gout, right ankle and foot

⊟ SP + 7 M1A.472- Other secondary chronic gout, left ankle and foot

⊟ IQ + 7 M1A.479- Other secondary chronic gout, unspecified ankle and foot

SP + 7 M1A.48X- Other secondary chronic gout, vertebrae

SP + 7 M1A.49X- Other secondary chronic gout, multiple sites

SP + 7 M1A.9XX- Chronic gout, unspecified

+ 4 M10 Gout
    Acute gout
    Gout attack
    Gout flare
    Podagra
    Use additional code to identify:
      Autonomic neuropathy in diseases classified elsewhere (G99.0)
      Calculus of urinary tract in diseases classified elsewhere (N22)
      Cardiomyopathy in diseases classified elsewhere (I43)
      Disorders of external ear in diseases classified elsewhere (H61.1-, H62.8-)
      Disorders of iris and ciliary body in diseases classified elsewhere (H22)
      Glomerular disorders in diseases classified elsewhere (N08)
    EXCLUDES 2 chronic gout (M1A.-)

+ 5 M10.0 Idiopathic gout
    Gouty bursitis
    Primary gout

IQ + M10.00 Idiopathic gout, unspecified site

+ 6 M10.01 Idiopathic gout, shoulder

⊟ SP + M10.011 Idiopathic gout, right shoulder

⊟ SP + M10.012 Idiopathic gout, left shoulder

⊟ IQ + M10.019 Idiopathic gout, unspecified shoulder

+ 6 M10.02 Idiopathic gout, elbow

⊟ SP + M10.021 Idiopathic gout, right elbow

⊟ SP + M10.022 Idiopathic gout, left elbow

⊟ IQ + M10.029 Idiopathic gout, unspecified elbow

+ 6 M10.03 Idiopathic gout, wrist

⊟ SP + M10.031 Idiopathic gout, right wrist

⊟ SP + M10.032 Idiopathic gout, left wrist

⊟ IQ + M10.039 Idiopathic gout, unspecified wrist

+ 6 M10.04 Idiopathic gout, hand

⊟ SP + M10.041 Idiopathic gout, right hand

⊟ SP + M10.042 Idiopathic gout, left hand

⊟ IQ + M10.049 Idiopathic gout, unspecified hand

+ 6 M10.05 Idiopathic gout, hip

⊟ SP + M10.051 Idiopathic gout, right hip

⊟ SP + M10.052 Idiopathic gout, left hip

⊟ IQ + M10.059 Idiopathic gout, unspecified hip

+ 6 M10.06 Idiopathic gout, knee

⊟ SP + M10.061 Idiopathic gout, right knee

⊟ SP + M10.062 Idiopathic gout, left knee

⊟ IQ + M10.069 Idiopathic gout, unspecified knee

+ 6 M10.07 Idiopathic gout, ankle and foot

⊟ SP + M10.071 Idiopathic gout, right ankle and foot

⊟ SP + M10.072 Idiopathic gout, left ankle and foot

⊟ IQ + M10.079 Idiopathic gout, unspecified ankle and foot

SP + M10.08 Idiopathic gout, vertebrae

SP + M10.09 Idiopathic gout, multiple sites

+ 5 M10.1 Lead-induced gout
    Code first:
      toxic effects of lead and its compounds (T56.0-)

IQ + M10.10 Lead-induced gout, unspecified site

+ 6 M10.11 Lead-induced gout, shoulder

⊟ SP + M10.111 Lead-induced gout, right shoulder

⊟ SP + M10.112 Lead-induced gout, left shoulder

⊟ IQ + M10.119 Lead-induced gout, unspecified shoulder

+ 6 M10.12 Lead-induced gout, elbow

⊟ SP + M10.121 Lead-induced gout, right elbow

⊟ SP + M10.122 Lead-induced gout, left elbow

⊟ IQ + M10.129 Lead-induced gout, unspecified elbow

+ 6 M10.13 Lead-induced gout, wrist

⊟ SP + M10.131 Lead-induced gout, right wrist

⊟ SP + M10.132 Lead-induced gout, left wrist

⊟ IQ + M10.139 Lead-induced gout, unspecified wrist

+ 6 M10.14 Lead-induced gout, hand

⊟ SP + M10.141 Lead-induced gout, right hand

⊟ SP + M10.142 Lead-induced gout, left hand

⊟ IQ + M10.149 Lead-induced gout, unspecified hand

+ 6 M10.15 Lead-induced gout, hip

⊟ SP + M10.151 Lead-induced gout, right hip

⊟ SP + M10.152 Lead-induced gout, left hip

⊟ IQ + M10.159 Lead-induced gout, unspecified hip

+ 6 M10.16 Lead-induced gout, knee

---

4 4th digit required   5 5th digit required   6 6th digit required   7 7th digit required   7 7th digit placeholder   + Additional code   ⊟ Laterality

☰ **SP** ✚ **M10.161** Lead-induced gout, right knee

☰ **SP** ✚ **M10.162** Lead-induced gout, left knee

☰ **IQ** ✚ **M10.169** Lead-induced gout, unspecified knee

✚ ⑥ **M10.17** Lead-induced gout, ankle and foot

☰ **SP** ✚ **M10.171** Lead-induced gout, right ankle and foot

☰ **SP** ✚ **M10.172** Lead-induced gout, left ankle and foot

☰ **IQ** ✚ **M10.179** Lead-induced gout, unspecified ankle and foot

SP ✚ **M10.18** Lead-induced gout, vertebrae

SP ✚ **M10.19** Lead-induced gout, multiple sites

✚ ⑤ **M10.2 Drug-induced gout**

Use additional code for adverse effect, if applicable, to identify drug (T36-T50 with fifth or sixth character 5)

IQ ✚ **M10.20** Drug-induced gout, unspecified site

✚ ⑥ **M10.21** Drug-induced gout, shoulder

☰ **SP** ✚ **M10.211** Drug-induced gout, right shoulder

☰ **SP** ✚ **M10.212** Drug-induced gout, left shoulder

☰ **IQ** ✚ **M10.219** Drug-induced gout, unspecified shoulder

✚ ⑥ **M10.22** Drug-induced gout, elbow

☰ **SP** ✚ **M10.221** Drug-induced gout, right elbow

☰ **SP** ✚ **M10.222** Drug-induced gout, left elbow

☰ **IQ** ✚ **M10.229** Drug-induced gout, unspecified elbow

✚ ⑥ **M10.23** Drug-induced gout, wrist

☰ **SP** ✚ **M10.231** Drug-induced gout, right wrist

☰ **SP** ✚ **M10.232** Drug-induced gout, left wrist

☰ **IQ** ✚ **M10.239** Drug-induced gout, unspecified wrist

✚ ⑥ **M10.24** Drug-induced gout, hand

☰ **SP** ✚ **M10.241** Drug-induced gout, right hand

☰ **SP** ✚ **M10.242** Drug-induced gout, left hand

☰ **IQ** ✚ **M10.249** Drug-induced gout, unspecified hand

✚ ⑥ **M10.25** Drug-induced gout, hip

☰ **SP** ✚ **M10.251** Drug-induced gout, right hip

☰ **SP** ✚ **M10.252** Drug-induced gout, left hip

☰ **IQ** ✚ **M10.259** Drug-induced gout, unspecified hip

✚ ⑥ **M10.26** Drug-induced gout, knee

☰ **SP** ✚ **M10.261** Drug-induced gout, right knee

☰ **SP** ✚ **M10.262** Drug-induced gout, left knee

☰ **IQ** ✚ **M10.269** Drug-induced gout, unspecified knee

✚ ⑥ **M10.27** Drug-induced gout, ankle and foot

☰ **SP** ✚ **M10.271** Drug-induced gout, right ankle and foot

☰ **SP** ✚ **M10.272** Drug-induced gout, left ankle and foot

☰ **IQ** ✚ **M10.279** Drug-induced gout, unspecified ankle and foot

SP ✚ **M10.28** Drug-induced gout, vertebrae

SP ✚ **M10.29** Drug-induced gout, multiple sites

✚ ⑤ **M10.3 Gout due to renal impairment**

Code first:
  associated renal disease

IQ ✚ **M10.30** Gout due to renal impairment, unspecified site

✚ ⑥ **M10.31** Gout due to renal impairment, shoulder

☰ **SP** ✚ **M10.311** Gout due to renal impairment, right shoulder

☰ **SP** ✚ **M10.312** Gout due to renal impairment, left shoulder

☰ **IQ** ✚ **M10.319** Gout due to renal impairment, unspecified shoulder

✚ ⑥ **M10.32** Gout due to renal impairment, elbow

☰ **SP** ✚ **M10.321** Gout due to renal impairment, right elbow

☰ **SP** ✚ **M10.322** Gout due to renal impairment, left elbow

☰ **IQ** ✚ **M10.329** Gout due to renal impairment, unspecified elbow

✚ ⑥ **M10.33** Gout due to renal impairment, wrist

☰ **SP** ✚ **M10.331** Gout due to renal impairment, right wrist

☰ **SP** ✚ **M10.332** Gout due to renal impairment, left wrist

☰ **IQ** ✚ **M10.339** Gout due to renal impairment, unspecified wrist

✚ ⑥ **M10.34** Gout due to renal impairment, hand

☰ **SP** ✚ **M10.341** Gout due to renal impairment, right hand

☰ **SP** ✚ **M10.342** Gout due to renal impairment, left hand

☰ **IQ** ✚ **M10.349** Gout due to renal impairment, unspecified hand

✚ ⑥ **M10.35** Gout due to renal impairment, hip

☰ **SP** ✚ **M10.351** Gout due to renal impairment, right hip

☰ **SP** ✚ **M10.352** Gout due to renal impairment, left hip

☰ **IQ** ✚ **M10.359** Gout due to renal impairment, unspecified hip

✚ ⑥ **M10.36** Gout due to renal impairment, knee

☰ **SP** ✚ **M10.361** Gout due to renal impairment, right knee

☰ **SP** ✚ **M10.362** Gout due to renal impairment, left knee

☰ **IQ** ✚ **M10.369** Gout due to renal impairment, unspecified knee

✚ ⑥ **M10.37** Gout due to renal impairment, ankle and foot

☰ **SP** ✚ **M10.371** Gout due to renal impairment, right ankle and foot

☰ **SP** ✚ **M10.372** Gout due to renal impairment, left ankle and foot

☰ **IQ** ✚ **M10.379** Gout due to renal impairment, unspecified ankle and foot

SP ✚ **M10.38** Gout due to renal impairment, vertebrae

SP ✚ **M10.39** Gout due to renal impairment, multiple sites

✚ ⑤ **M10.4 Other secondary gout**

Code first:
  associated condition

IQ ✚ **M10.40** Other secondary gout, unspecified site

✚ ⑥ **M10.41** Other secondary gout, shoulder

☰ **SP** ✚ **M10.411** Other secondary gout, right shoulder

★ New ▲ Revised Px Primary **SP** PDGM Px **SL** Low CoM **SH** High CoM **IQ** Quest. Encounter **H** Hospice non-cancer Dx   Unspecified   **M** *Manifestation*

DecisionHealth's FY 2020 Complete Home Health ICD-10-CM Diagnosis Coding Manual

1171

Chapter 13

M00-M99

⊟ SP ✚ **M10.412** Other secondary gout, left shoulder

⊟ IQ ✚ **M10.419** Other secondary gout, unspecified shoulder

✚ 6 **M10.42** Other secondary gout, elbow

⊟ SP ✚ **M10.421** Other secondary gout, right elbow

⊟ SP ✚ **M10.422** Other secondary gout, left elbow

⊟ IQ ✚ **M10.429** Other secondary gout, unspecified elbow

✚ 6 **M10.43** Other secondary gout, wrist

⊟ SP ✚ **M10.431** Other secondary gout, right wrist

⊟ SP ✚ **M10.432** Other secondary gout, left wrist

⊟ IQ ✚ **M10.439** Other secondary gout, unspecified wrist

✚ 6 **M10.44** Other secondary gout, hand

⊟ SP ✚ **M10.441** Other secondary gout, right hand

⊟ SP ✚ **M10.442** Other secondary gout, left hand

⊟ IQ ✚ **M10.449** Other secondary gout, unspecified hand

✚ 6 **M10.45** Other secondary gout, hip

⊟ SP ✚ **M10.451** Other secondary gout, right hip

⊟ SP ✚ **M10.452** Other secondary gout, left hip

⊟ IQ ✚ **M10.459** Other secondary gout, unspecified hip

✚ 6 **M10.46** Other secondary gout, knee

⊟ SP ✚ **M10.461** Other secondary gout, right knee

⊟ SP ✚ **M10.462** Other secondary gout, left knee

⊟ IQ ✚ **M10.469** Other secondary gout, unspecified knee

✚ 6 **M10.47** Other secondary gout, ankle and foot

⊟ SP ✚ **M10.471** Other secondary gout, right ankle and foot

⊟ SP ✚ **M10.472** Other secondary gout, left ankle and foot

⊟ IQ ✚ **M10.479** Other secondary gout, unspecified ankle and foot

SP ✚ **M10.48** Other secondary gout, vertebrae

SP ✚ **M10.49** Other secondary gout, multiple sites

SP ✚ **M10.9** Gout, unspecified

Gout NOS

4 **M11** Other crystal arthropathies

5 **M11.0** Hydroxyapatite deposition disease

IQ **M11.00** Hydroxyapatite deposition disease, unspecified site

6 **M11.01** Hydroxyapatite deposition disease, shoulder

⊟ SP **M11.011** Hydroxyapatite deposition disease, right shoulder

⊟ SP **M11.012** Hydroxyapatite deposition disease, left shoulder

⊟ IQ **M11.019** Hydroxyapatite deposition disease, unspecified shoulder

6 **M11.02** Hydroxyapatite deposition disease, elbow

⊟ SP **M11.021** Hydroxyapatite deposition disease, right elbow

⊟ SP **M11.022** Hydroxyapatite deposition disease, left elbow

⊟ IQ **M11.029** Hydroxyapatite deposition disease, unspecified elbow

6 **M11.03** Hydroxyapatite deposition disease, wrist

⊟ SP **M11.031** Hydroxyapatite deposition disease, right wrist

⊟ SP **M11.032** Hydroxyapatite deposition disease, left wrist

⊟ IQ **M11.039** Hydroxyapatite deposition disease, unspecified wrist

6 **M11.04** Hydroxyapatite deposition disease, hand

⊟ SP **M11.041** Hydroxyapatite deposition disease, right hand

⊟ SP **M11.042** Hydroxyapatite deposition disease, left hand

⊟ IQ **M11.049** Hydroxyapatite deposition disease, unspecified hand

6 **M11.05** Hydroxyapatite deposition disease, hip

⊟ SP **M11.051** Hydroxyapatite deposition disease, right hip

⊟ SP **M11.052** Hydroxyapatite deposition disease, left hip

⊟ IQ **M11.059** Hydroxyapatite deposition disease, unspecified hip

6 **M11.06** Hydroxyapatite deposition disease, knee

⊟ SP **M11.061** Hydroxyapatite deposition disease, right knee

⊟ SP **M11.062** Hydroxyapatite deposition disease, left knee

⊟ IQ **M11.069** Hydroxyapatite deposition disease, unspecified knee

6 **M11.07** Hydroxyapatite deposition disease, ankle and foot

⊟ SP **M11.071** Hydroxyapatite deposition disease, right ankle and foot

⊟ SP **M11.072** Hydroxyapatite deposition disease, left ankle and foot

⊟ IQ **M11.079** Hydroxyapatite deposition disease, unspecified ankle and foot

SP **M11.08** Hydroxyapatite deposition disease, vertebrae

SP **M11.09** Hydroxyapatite deposition disease, multiple sites

5 **M11.1** Familial chondrocalcinosis

IQ **M11.10** Familial chondrocalcinosis, unspecified site

6 **M11.11** Familial chondrocalcinosis, shoulder

⊟ SP **M11.111** Familial chondrocalcinosis, right shoulder

⊟ SP **M11.112** Familial chondrocalcinosis, left shoulder

⊟ IQ **M11.119** Familial chondrocalcinosis, unspecified shoulder

6 **M11.12** Familial chondrocalcinosis, elbow

⊟ IQ **M11.121** Familial chondrocalcinosis, right elbow

⊟ SP **M11.122** Familial chondrocalcinosis, left elbow

⊟ IQ **M11.129** Familial chondrocalcinosis, unspecified elbow

6 **M11.13** Familial chondrocalcinosis, wrist

⊟ SP **M11.131** Familial chondrocalcinosis, right wrist

---

4 4th digit required   5 5th digit required   6 6th digit required   7 7th digit required   ✓ 7th digit placeholder   ✚ Additional code   ⊟ Laterality

☰ SP M11.132 Familial chondrocalcinosis, left wrist

☰ IQ M11.139 Familial chondrocalcinosis, unspecified wrist

⑥ M11.14 Familial chondrocalcinosis, hand

☰ SP M11.141 Familial chondrocalcinosis, right hand

☰ SP M11.142 Familial chondrocalcinosis, left hand

☰ IQ M11.149 Familial chondrocalcinosis, unspecified hand

⑥ M11.15 Familial chondrocalcinosis, hip

☰ SP M11.151 Familial chondrocalcinosis, right hip

☰ SP M11.152 Familial chondrocalcinosis, left hip

☰ IQ M11.159 Familial chondrocalcinosis, unspecified hip

⑥ M11.16 Familial chondrocalcinosis, knee

☰ SP M11.161 Familial chondrocalcinosis, right knee

☰ SP M11.162 Familial chondrocalcinosis, left knee

☰ IQ M11.169 Familial chondrocalcinosis, unspecified knee

⑥ M11.17 Familial chondrocalcinosis, ankle and foot

☰ SP M11.171 Familial chondrocalcinosis, right ankle and foot

☰ SP M11.172 Familial chondrocalcinosis, left ankle and foot

☰ IQ M11.179 Familial chondrocalcinosis, unspecified ankle and foot

SP M11.18 Familial chondrocalcinosis, vertebrae

SP M11.19 Familial chondrocalcinosis, multiple sites

⑤ M11.2 Other chondrocalcinosis
Chondrocalcinosis NOS

IQ M11.20 Other chondrocalcinosis, unspecified site

⑥ M11.21 Other chondrocalcinosis, shoulder

☰ SP M11.211 Other chondrocalcinosis, right shoulder

☰ SP M11.212 Other chondrocalcinosis, left shoulder

☰ IQ M11.219 Other chondrocalcinosis, unspecified shoulder

⑥ M11.22 Other chondrocalcinosis, elbow

☰ SP M11.221 Other chondrocalcinosis, right elbow

☰ SP M11.222 Other chondrocalcinosis, left elbow

☰ IQ M11.229 Other chondrocalcinosis, unspecified elbow

⑥ M11.23 Other chondrocalcinosis, wrist

☰ SP M11.231 Other chondrocalcinosis, right wrist

☰ SP M11.232 Other chondrocalcinosis, left wrist

☰ IQ M11.239 Other chondrocalcinosis, unspecified wrist

⑥ M11.24 Other chondrocalcinosis, hand

☰ SP M11.241 Other chondrocalcinosis, right hand

☰ SP M11.242 Other chondrocalcinosis, left hand

☰ IQ M11.249 Other chondrocalcinosis, unspecified hand

⑥ M11.25 Other chondrocalcinosis, hip

☰ SP M11.251 Other chondrocalcinosis, right hip

☰ SP M11.252 Other chondrocalcinosis, left hip

☰ IQ M11.259 Other chondrocalcinosis, unspecified hip

⑥ M11.26 Other chondrocalcinosis, knee

☰ SP M11.261 Other chondrocalcinosis, right knee

☰ SP M11.262 Other chondrocalcinosis, left knee

☰ IQ M11.269 Other chondrocalcinosis, unspecified knee

⑥ M11.27 Other chondrocalcinosis, ankle and foot

☰ SP M11.271 Other chondrocalcinosis, right ankle and foot

☰ SP M11.272 Other chondrocalcinosis, left ankle and foot

☰ IQ M11.279 Other chondrocalcinosis, unspecified ankle and foot

SP M11.28 Other chondrocalcinosis, vertebrae

SP M11.29 Other chondrocalcinosis, multiple sites

⑤ M11.8 Other specified crystal arthropathies

IQ M11.80 Other specified crystal arthropathies, unspecified site

⑥ M11.81 Other specified crystal arthropathies, shoulder

☰ SP M11.811 Other specified crystal arthropathies, right shoulder

☰ SP M11.812 Other specified crystal arthropathies, left shoulder

☰ IQ M11.819 Other specified crystal arthropathies, unspecified shoulder

⑥ M11.82 Other specified crystal arthropathies, elbow

☰ SP M11.821 Other specified crystal arthropathies, right elbow

☰ SP M11.822 Other specified crystal arthropathies, left elbow

☰ IQ M11.829 Other specified crystal arthropathies, unspecified elbow

⑥ M11.83 Other specified crystal arthropathies, wrist

☰ SP M11.831 Other specified crystal arthropathies, right wrist

☰ SP M11.832 Other specified crystal arthropathies, left wrist

☰ IQ M11.839 Other specified crystal arthropathies, unspecified wrist

⑥ M11.84 Other specified crystal arthropathies, hand

☰ SP M11.841 Other specified crystal arthropathies, right hand

☰ SP M11.842 Other specified crystal arthropathies, left hand

☰ IQ M11.849 Other specified crystal arthropathies, unspecified hand

⑥ M11.85 Other specified crystal arthropathies, hip

☰ SP M11.851 Other specified crystal arthropathies, right hip

★ New ▲ Revised Px Primary SP PDGM Px SL Low CoM SH High CoM IQ Quest. Encounter H Hospice non-cancer Dx Unspecified M Manifestation

DecisionHealth's FY 2020 Complete Home Health ICD-10-CM Diagnosis Coding Manual

1173

☰ **SP** **M11.852** Other specified crystal arthropathies, left hip

☰ **IQ** **M11.859** Other specified crystal arthropathies, unspecified hip

⑥ **M11.86** Other specified crystal arthropathies, knee

☰ **SP** **M11.861** Other specified crystal arthropathies, right knee

☰ **SP** **M11.862** Other specified crystal arthropathies, left knee

☰ **IQ** **M11.869** Other specified crystal arthropathies, unspecified knee

⑥ **M11.87** Other specified crystal arthropathies, ankle and foot

☰ **SP** **M11.871** Other specified crystal arthropathies, right ankle and foot

☰ **SP** **M11.872** Other specified crystal arthropathies, left ankle and foot

☰ **IQ** **M11.879** Other specified crystal arthropathies, unspecified ankle and foot

SP **M11.88** Other specified crystal arthropathies, vertebrae

SP **M11.89** Other specified crystal arthropathies, multiple sites

IQ **M11.9** Crystal arthropathy, unspecified

④ **M12** Other and unspecified arthropathy

> **EXCLUDES 1** arthrosis (M15-M19)
> cricoarytenoid arthropathy (J38.7)

⑤ **M12.0** Chronic postrheumatic arthropathy [Jaccoud]

IQ **M12.00** Chronic postrheumatic arthropathy [Jaccoud], unspecified site

⑥ **M12.01** Chronic postrheumatic arthropathy [Jaccoud], shoulder

☰ **SP** **M12.011** Chronic postrheumatic arthropathy [Jaccoud], right shoulder

☰ **SP** **M12.012** Chronic postrheumatic arthropathy [Jaccoud], left shoulder

☰ **IQ** **M12.019** Chronic postrheumatic arthropathy [Jaccoud], unspecified shoulder

⑥ **M12.02** Chronic postrheumatic arthropathy [Jaccoud], elbow

☰ **SP** **M12.021** Chronic postrheumatic arthropathy [Jaccoud], right elbow

☰ **SP** **M12.022** Chronic postrheumatic arthropathy [Jaccoud], left elbow

☰ **IQ** **M12.029** Chronic postrheumatic arthropathy [Jaccoud], unspecified elbow

⑥ **M12.03** Chronic postrheumatic arthropathy [Jaccoud], wrist

☰ **SP** **M12.031** Chronic postrheumatic arthropathy [Jaccoud], right wrist

☰ **SP** **M12.032** Chronic postrheumatic arthropathy [Jaccoud], left wrist

☰ **IQ** **M12.039** Chronic postrheumatic arthropathy [Jaccoud], unspecified wrist

⑥ **M12.04** Chronic postrheumatic arthropathy [Jaccoud], hand

☰ **SP** **M12.041** Chronic postrheumatic arthropathy [Jaccoud], right hand

☰ **SP** **M12.042** Chronic postrheumatic arthropathy [Jaccoud], left hand

☰ **IQ** **M12.049** Chronic postrheumatic arthropathy [Jaccoud], unspecified hand

⑥ **M12.05** Chronic postrheumatic arthropathy [Jaccoud], hip

☰ **SP** **M12.051** Chronic postrheumatic arthropathy [Jaccoud], right hip

☰ **SP** **M12.052** Chronic postrheumatic arthropathy [Jaccoud], left hip

☰ **IQ** **M12.059** Chronic postrheumatic arthropathy [Jaccoud], unspecified hip

⑥ **M12.06** Chronic postrheumatic arthropathy [Jaccoud], knee

☰ **SP** **M12.061** Chronic postrheumatic arthropathy [Jaccoud], right knee

☰ **SP** **M12.062** Chronic postrheumatic arthropathy [Jaccoud], left knee

☰ **IQ** **M12.069** Chronic postrheumatic arthropathy [Jaccoud], unspecified knee

⑥ **M12.07** Chronic postrheumatic arthropathy [Jaccoud], ankle and foot

☰ **SP** **M12.071** Chronic postrheumatic arthropathy [Jaccoud], right ankle and foot

☰ **SP** **M12.072** Chronic postrheumatic arthropathy [Jaccoud], left ankle and foot

☰ **IQ** **M12.079** Chronic postrheumatic arthropathy [Jaccoud], unspecified ankle and foot

SP **M12.08** Chronic postrheumatic arthropathy [Jaccoud], other specified site
Chronic postrheumatic arthropathy [Jaccoud], vertebrae

SP **M12.09** Chronic postrheumatic arthropathy [Jaccoud], multiple sites

⑤ **M12.1** Kaschin-Beck disease
Osteochondroarthrosis deformans endemica

IQ **M12.10** Kaschin-Beck disease, unspecified site

⑥ **M12.11** Kaschin-Beck disease, shoulder

☰ **SP** **M12.111** Kaschin-Beck disease, right shoulder

☰ **SP** **M12.112** Kaschin-Beck disease, left shoulder

☰ **IQ** **M12.119** Kaschin-Beck disease, unspecified shoulder

⑥ **M12.12** Kaschin-Beck disease, elbow

☰ **SP** **M12.121** Kaschin-Beck disease, right elbow

☰ **SP** **M12.122** Kaschin-Beck disease, left elbow

☰ **IQ** **M12.129** Kaschin-Beck disease, unspecified elbow

⑥ **M12.13** Kaschin-Beck disease, wrist

☰ **SP** **M12.131** Kaschin-Beck disease, right wrist

☰ **SP** **M12.132** Kaschin-Beck disease, left wrist

☰ **IQ** **M12.139** Kaschin-Beck disease, unspecified wrist

⑥ **M12.14** Kaschin-Beck disease, hand

---

④4th digit required   ⑤5th digit required   ⑥6th digit required   ⑦7th digit required   ☑7th digit placeholder   ✚Additional code   ☰Laterality

1174   *DecisionHealth's* FY 2020 Complete Home Health ICD-10-CM Diagnosis Coding Manual

☐ SP M12.141 Kaschin-Beck disease, right hand
☐ SP M12.142 Kaschin-Beck disease, left hand
☐ IQ M12.149 Kaschin-Beck disease, unspecified hand
⑥ M12.15 Kaschin-Beck disease, hip
☐ SP M12.151 Kaschin-Beck disease, right hip
☐ SP M12.152 Kaschin-Beck disease, left hip
☐ IQ M12.159 Kaschin-Beck disease, unspecified hip
⑥ M12.16 Kaschin-Beck disease, knee
☐ SP M12.161 Kaschin-Beck disease, right knee
☐ SP M12.162 Kaschin-Beck disease, left knee
☐ IQ M12.169 Kaschin-Beck disease, unspecified knee
⑥ M12.17 Kaschin-Beck disease, ankle and foot
☐ SP M12.171 Kaschin-Beck disease, right ankle and foot
☐ SP M12.172 Kaschin-Beck disease, left ankle and foot
☐ IQ M12.179 Kaschin-Beck disease, unspecified ankle and foot
SP M12.18 Kaschin-Beck disease, vertebrae
SP M12.19 Kaschin-Beck disease, multiple sites
⑤ M12.2 Villonodular synovitis (pigmented)
IQ M12.20 Villonodular synovitis (pigmented), unspecified site
⑥ M12.21 Villonodular synovitis (pigmented), shoulder
☐ SP M12.211 Villonodular synovitis (pigmented), right shoulder
☐ SP M12.212 Villonodular synovitis (pigmented), left shoulder
☐ IQ M12.219 Villonodular synovitis (pigmented), unspecified shoulder
⑥ M12.22 Villonodular synovitis (pigmented), elbow
☐ SP M12.221 Villonodular synovitis (pigmented), right elbow
☐ SP M12.222 Villonodular synovitis (pigmented), left elbow
☐ IQ M12.229 Villonodular synovitis (pigmented), unspecified elbow
⑥ M12.23 Villonodular synovitis (pigmented), wrist
☐ SP M12.231 Villonodular synovitis (pigmented), right wrist
☐ SP M12.232 Villonodular synovitis (pigmented), left wrist
☐ IQ M12.239 Villonodular synovitis (pigmented), unspecified wrist
⑥ M12.24 Villonodular synovitis (pigmented), hand
☐ SP M12.241 Villonodular synovitis (pigmented), right hand
☐ SP M12.242 Villonodular synovitis (pigmented), left hand
☐ IQ M12.249 Villonodular synovitis (pigmented), unspecified hand
⑥ M12.25 Villonodular synovitis (pigmented), hip
☐ SP M12.251 Villonodular synovitis (pigmented), right hip

☐ SP M12.252 Villonodular synovitis (pigmented), left hip
☐ IQ M12.259 Villonodular synovitis (pigmented), unspecified hip
⑥ M12.26 Villonodular synovitis (pigmented), knee
☐ SP M12.261 Villonodular synovitis (pigmented), right knee
☐ SP M12.262 Villonodular synovitis (pigmented), left knee
☐ IQ M12.269 Villonodular synovitis (pigmented), unspecified knee
⑥ M12.27 Villonodular synovitis (pigmented), ankle and foot
☐ SP M12.271 Villonodular synovitis (pigmented), right ankle and foot
☐ SP M12.272 Villonodular synovitis (pigmented), left ankle and foot
☐ IQ M12.279 Villonodular synovitis (pigmented), unspecified ankle and foot
SP M12.28 Villonodular synovitis (pigmented), other specified site
Villonodular synovitis (pigmented), vertebrae
SP M12.29 Villonodular synovitis (pigmented), multiple sites
⑤ M12.3 Palindromic rheumatism
IQ M12.30 Palindromic rheumatism, unspecified site
⑥ M12.31 Palindromic rheumatism, shoulder
☐ SP M12.311 Palindromic rheumatism, right shoulder
☐ SP M12.312 Palindromic rheumatism, left shoulder
☐ IQ M12.319 Palindromic rheumatism, unspecified shoulder
⑥ M12.32 Palindromic rheumatism, elbow
☐ SP M12.321 Palindromic rheumatism, right elbow
☐ SP M12.322 Palindromic rheumatism, left elbow
☐ IQ M12.329 Palindromic rheumatism, unspecified elbow
⑥ M12.33 Palindromic rheumatism, wrist
☐ SP M12.331 Palindromic rheumatism, right wrist
☐ SP M12.332 Palindromic rheumatism, left wrist
☐ IQ M12.339 Palindromic rheumatism, unspecified wrist
⑥ M12.34 Palindromic rheumatism, hand
☐ SP M12.341 Palindromic rheumatism, right hand
☐ SP M12.342 Palindromic rheumatism, left hand
☐ IQ M12.349 Palindromic rheumatism, unspecified hand
⑥ M12.35 Palindromic rheumatism, hip
☐ SP M12.351 Palindromic rheumatism, right hip
☐ SP M12.352 Palindromic rheumatism, left hip
☐ IQ M12.359 Palindromic rheumatism, unspecified hip
⑥ M12.36 Palindromic rheumatism, knee

★ New ▲ Revised Px Primary SP PDGM Px SL Low CoM SH High CoM IQ Quest. Encounter Ⓗ Hospice non-cancer Dx Unspecified M *Manifestation*

DecisionHealth's FY 2020 Complete Home Health ICD-10-CM Diagnosis Coding Manual

1175

⊟ SP **M12.361 Palindromic rheumatism, right knee**

⊟ SP **M12.362 Palindromic rheumatism, left knee**

⊟ IQ **M12.369 Palindromic rheumatism, unspecified knee**

⑥ **M12.37 Palindromic rheumatism, ankle and foot**

⊟ SP **M12.371 Palindromic rheumatism, right ankle and foot**

⊟ SP **M12.372 Palindromic rheumatism, left ankle and foot**

⊟ IQ **M12.379 Palindromic rheumatism, unspecified ankle and foot**

SP **M12.38 Palindromic rheumatism, other specified site**
　　Palindromic rheumatism, vertebrae

SP **M12.39 Palindromic rheumatism, multiple sites**

⑤ **M12.4 Intermittent hydrarthrosis**

IQ **M12.40 Intermittent hydrarthrosis, unspecified site**

⑥ **M12.41 Intermittent hydrarthrosis, shoulder**

⊟ SP **M12.411 Intermittent hydrarthrosis, right shoulder**

⊟ SP **M12.412 Intermittent hydrarthrosis, left shoulder**

⊟ IQ **M12.419 Intermittent hydrarthrosis, unspecified shoulder**

⑥ **M12.42 Intermittent hydrarthrosis, elbow**

⊟ SP **M12.421 Intermittent hydrarthrosis, right elbow**

⊟ SP **M12.422 Intermittent hydrarthrosis, left elbow**

⊟ IQ **M12.429 Intermittent hydrarthrosis, unspecified elbow**

⑥ **M12.43 Intermittent hydrarthrosis, wrist**

⊟ SP **M12.431 Intermittent hydrarthrosis, right wrist**

⊟ SP **M12.432 Intermittent hydrarthrosis, left wrist**

⊟ IQ **M12.439 Intermittent hydrarthrosis, unspecified wrist**

⑥ **M12.44 Intermittent hydrarthrosis, hand**

⊟ SP **M12.441 Intermittent hydrarthrosis, right hand**

⊟ SP **M12.442 Intermittent hydrarthrosis, left hand**

⊟ IQ **M12.449 Intermittent hydrarthrosis, unspecified hand**

⑥ **M12.45 Intermittent hydrarthrosis, hip**

⊟ SP **M12.451 Intermittent hydrarthrosis, right hip**

⊟ SP **M12.452 Intermittent hydrarthrosis, left hip**

⊟ IQ **M12.459 Intermittent hydrarthrosis, unspecified hip**

⑥ **M12.46 Intermittent hydrarthrosis, knee**

⊟ SP **M12.461 Intermittent hydrarthrosis, right knee**

⊟ SP **M12.462 Intermittent hydrarthrosis, left knee**

⊟ IQ **M12.469 Intermittent hydrarthrosis, unspecified knee**

⑥ **M12.47 Intermittent hydrarthrosis, ankle and foot**

⊟ SP **M12.471 Intermittent hydrarthrosis, right ankle and foot**

⊟ SP **M12.472 Intermittent hydrarthrosis, left ankle and foot**

⊟ IQ **M12.479 Intermittent hydrarthrosis, unspecified ankle and foot**

SP **M12.48 Intermittent hydrarthrosis, other site**

SP **M12.49 Intermittent hydrarthrosis, multiple sites**

⑤ **M12.5 Traumatic arthropathy**
　　EXCLUDES 1 　current injury-see Alphabetic Index
　　　　post-traumatic osteoarthritis of first carpometacarpal joint (M18.2-M18.3)
　　　　post-traumatic osteoarthritis of hip (M16.4-M16.5)
　　　　post-traumatic osteoarthritis of knee (M17.2-M17.3)
　　　　post-traumatic osteoarthritis NOS (M19.1-)
　　　　post-traumatic osteoarthritis of other single joints (M19.1-)

　　CODING TIPS ✓　Report the injury that caused the traumatic arthropathy using a code from Chapter 19 (Injury, Poisoning and Certain Other Consequences of External Causes). If the injury requires a 7th character, use "S" for sequela.

IQ **M12.50 Traumatic arthropathy, unspecified site**

⑥ **M12.51 Traumatic arthropathy, shoulder**

⊟ SP **M12.511 Traumatic arthropathy, right shoulder**

⊟ SP **M12.512 Traumatic arthropathy, left shoulder**

⊟ IQ **M12.519 Traumatic arthropathy, unspecified shoulder**

⑥ **M12.52 Traumatic arthropathy, elbow**

⊟ SP **M12.521 Traumatic arthropathy, right elbow**

⊟ SP **M12.522 Traumatic arthropathy, left elbow**

⊟ IQ **M12.529 Traumatic arthropathy, unspecified elbow**

⑥ **M12.53 Traumatic arthropathy, wrist**

⊟ SP **M12.531 Traumatic arthropathy, right wrist**

⊟ SP **M12.532 Traumatic arthropathy, left wrist**

⊟ IQ **M12.539 Traumatic arthropathy, unspecified wrist**

⑥ **M12.54 Traumatic arthropathy, hand**

⊟ SP **M12.541 Traumatic arthropathy, right hand**

⊟ SP **M12.542 Traumatic arthropathy, left hand**

⊟ IQ **M12.549 Traumatic arthropathy, unspecified hand**

⑥ **M12.55 Traumatic arthropathy, hip**

⊟ SP **M12.551 Traumatic arthropathy, right hip**

⊟ SP **M12.552 Traumatic arthropathy, left hip**

⊟ IQ **M12.559 Traumatic arthropathy, unspecified hip**

---

❹4th digit required　❺5th digit required　❻6th digit required　❼7th digit required　❼7th digit placeholder　✚Additional code　⊟Laterality

1176　　*DecisionHealth's* FY 2020 Complete Home Health ICD-10-CM Diagnosis Coding Manual

⑥ **M12.56** Traumatic arthropathy, knee

⊟ 🅢🅟 **M12.561** Traumatic arthropathy, right knee

⊟ 🅢🅟 **M12.562** Traumatic arthropathy, left knee

⊟ 🅘🅠 **M12.569** Traumatic arthropathy, unspecified knee

⑥ **M12.57** Traumatic arthropathy, ankle and foot

⊟ 🅢🅟 **M12.571** Traumatic arthropathy, right ankle and foot

⊟ 🅢🅟 **M12.572** Traumatic arthropathy, left ankle and foot

⊟ 🅘🅠 **M12.579** Traumatic arthropathy, unspecified ankle and foot

🅢🅟 **M12.58** Traumatic arthropathy, other specified site
Traumatic arthropathy, vertebrae

🅢🅟 **M12.59** Traumatic arthropathy, multiple sites

⑤ **M12.8** Other specific arthropathies, not elsewhere classified
Transient arthropathy

🅘🅠 **M12.80** Other specific arthropathies, not elsewhere classified, unspecified site

⑥ **M12.81** Other specific arthropathies, not elsewhere classified, shoulder

⊟ 🅢🅟 **M12.811** Other specific arthropathies, not elsewhere classified, right shoulder

⊟ 🅢🅟 **M12.812** Other specific arthropathies, not elsewhere classified, left shoulder

⊟ 🅘🅠 **M12.819** Other specific arthropathies, not elsewhere classified, unspecified shoulder

⑥ **M12.82** Other specific arthropathies, not elsewhere classified, elbow

⊟ 🅢🅟 **M12.821** Other specific arthropathies, not elsewhere classified, right elbow

⊟ 🅢🅟 **M12.822** Other specific arthropathies, not elsewhere classified, left elbow

⊟ 🅘🅠 **M12.829** Other specific arthropathies, not elsewhere classified, unspecified elbow

⑥ **M12.83** Other specific arthropathies, not elsewhere classified, wrist

⊟ 🅢🅟 **M12.831** Other specific arthropathies, not elsewhere classified, right wrist

⊟ 🅢🅟 **M12.832** Other specific arthropathies, not elsewhere classified, left wrist

⊟ 🅘🅠 **M12.839** Other specific arthropathies, not elsewhere classified, unspecified wrist

⑥ **M12.84** Other specific arthropathies, not elsewhere classified, hand

⊟ 🅢🅟 **M12.841** Other specific arthropathies, not elsewhere classified, right hand

⊟ 🅢🅟 **M12.842** Other specific arthropathies, not elsewhere classified, left hand

⊟ 🅘🅠 **M12.849** Other specific arthropathies, not elsewhere classified, unspecified hand

⑥ **M12.85** Other specific arthropathies, not elsewhere classified, hip

⊟ 🅢🅟 **M12.851** Other specific arthropathies, not elsewhere classified, right hip

⊟ 🅢🅟 **M12.852** Other specific arthropathies, not elsewhere classified, left hip

⊟ 🅘🅠 **M12.859** Other specific arthropathies, not elsewhere classified, unspecified hip

⑥ **M12.86** Other specific arthropathies, not elsewhere classified, knee

⊟ 🅢🅟 **M12.861** Other specific arthropathies, not elsewhere classified, right knee

⊟ 🅢🅟 **M12.862** Other specific arthropathies, not elsewhere classified, left knee

⊟ 🅘🅠 **M12.869** Other specific arthropathies, not elsewhere classified, unspecified knee

⑥ **M12.87** Other specific arthropathies, not elsewhere classified, ankle and foot

⊟ 🅢🅟 **M12.871** Other specific arthropathies, not elsewhere classified, right ankle and foot

⊟ 🅢🅟 **M12.872** Other specific arthropathies, not elsewhere classified, left ankle and foot

⊟ 🅘🅠 **M12.879** Other specific arthropathies, not elsewhere classified, unspecified ankle and foot

🅢🅟 **M12.88** Other specific arthropathies, not elsewhere classified, other specified site
Other specific arthropathies, not elsewhere classified, vertebrae

🅢🅟 **M12.89** Other specific arthropathies, not elsewhere classified, multiple sites

🅢🅟 **M12.9** Arthropathy, unspecified

CODING TIPS ✓ This code should **not** be used in home care, unless the physician specifically documents arthropathy. Arthritis should be coded to osteoarthritis, unless the physician has specifically stated another type.

④ **M13** Other arthritis
EXCLUDES 1 arthrosis (M15-M19)
osteoarthritis (M15-M19)

🅢🅟 **M13.0** Polyarthritis, unspecified

⑤ **M13.1** Monoarthritis, not elsewhere classified

🅘🅠 **M13.10** Monoarthritis, not elsewhere classified, unspecified site

⑥ **M13.11** Monoarthritis, not elsewhere classified, shoulder

⊟ 🅢🅟 **M13.111** Monoarthritis, not elsewhere classified, right shoulder

⊟ 🅢🅟 **M13.112** Monoarthritis, not elsewhere classified, left shoulder

⊟ 🅘🅠 **M13.119** Monoarthritis, not elsewhere classified, unspecified shoulder

⑥ **M13.12** Monoarthritis, not elsewhere classified, elbow

⊟ 🅢🅟 **M13.121** Monoarthritis, not elsewhere classified, right elbow

⊟ 🅢🅟 **M13.122** Monoarthritis, not elsewhere classified, left elbow

⊟ 🅘🅠 **M13.129** Monoarthritis, not elsewhere classified, unspecified elbow

⑥ **M13.13** Monoarthritis, not elsewhere classified, wrist

⊟ 🅢🅟 **M13.131** Monoarthritis, not elsewhere classified, right wrist

⊟ 🅢🅟 **M13.132** Monoarthritis, not elsewhere classified, left wrist

★ New ▲ Revised Px Primary 🅢🅟 PDGM Px 🅢🅛 Low CoM 🅢🅗 High CoM 🅘🅠 Quest. Encounter 🄷 Hospice non-cancer Dx   Unspecified   ᴍ *Manifestation*

DecisionHealth's FY 2020 Complete Home Health ICD-10-CM Diagnosis Coding Manual

1177

☐ **IQ** **M13.139** Monoarthritis, not elsewhere classified, unspecified wrist

⑥ **M13.14** Monoarthritis, not elsewhere classified, hand

☐ **SP** **M13.141** Monoarthritis, not elsewhere classified, right hand

☐ **SP** **M13.142** Monoarthritis, not elsewhere classified, left hand

☐ **IQ** **M13.149** Monoarthritis, not elsewhere classified, unspecified hand

⑥ **M13.15** Monoarthritis, not elsewhere classified, hip

☐ **SP** **M13.151** Monoarthritis, not elsewhere classified, right hip

☐ **SP** **M13.152** Monoarthritis, not elsewhere classified, left hip

☐ **IQ** **M13.159** Monoarthritis, not elsewhere classified, unspecified hip

⑥ **M13.16** Monoarthritis, not elsewhere classified, knee

☐ **SP** **M13.161** Monoarthritis, not elsewhere classified, right knee

☐ **SP** **M13.162** Monoarthritis, not elsewhere classified, left knee

☐ **IQ** **M13.169** Monoarthritis, not elsewhere classified, unspecified knee

⑥ **M13.17** Monoarthritis, not elsewhere classified, ankle and foot

☐ **SP** **M13.171** Monoarthritis, not elsewhere classified, right ankle and foot

☐ **SP** **M13.172** Monoarthritis, not elsewhere classified, left ankle and foot

☐ **IQ** **M13.179** Monoarthritis, not elsewhere classified, unspecified ankle and foot

⑤ **M13.8** Other specified arthritis
Allergic arthritis
EXCLUDES 1 osteoarthritis (M15-M19)

SP **M13.80** Other specified arthritis, unspecified site

⑥ **M13.81** Other specified arthritis, shoulder

☐ **SP** **M13.811** Other specified arthritis, right shoulder

☐ **SP** **M13.812** Other specified arthritis, left shoulder

☐ **SP** **M13.819** Other specified arthritis, unspecified shoulder

⑥ **M13.82** Other specified arthritis, elbow

☐ **SP** **M13.821** Other specified arthritis, right elbow

☐ **SP** **M13.822** Other specified arthritis, left elbow

☐ **IQ** **M13.829** Other specified arthritis, unspecified elbow

⑥ **M13.83** Other specified arthritis, wrist

☐ **SP** **M13.831** Other specified arthritis, right wrist

☐ **SP** **M13.832** Other specified arthritis, left wrist

☐ **IQ** **M13.839** Other specified arthritis, unspecified wrist

⑥ **M13.84** Other specified arthritis, hand

☐ **SP** **M13.841** Other specified arthritis, right hand

☐ **SP** **M13.842** Other specified arthritis, left hand

☐ **IQ** **M13.849** Other specified arthritis, unspecified hand

⑥ **M13.85** Other specified arthritis, hip

☐ **SP** **M13.851** Other specified arthritis, right hip

☐ **SP** **M13.852** Other specified arthritis, left hip

☐ **IQ** **M13.859** Other specified arthritis, unspecified hip

⑥ **M13.86** Other specified arthritis, knee

☐ **SP** **M13.861** Other specified arthritis, right knee

☐ **SP** **M13.862** Other specified arthritis, left knee

☐ **IQ** **M13.869** Other specified arthritis, unspecified knee

⑥ **M13.87** Other specified arthritis, ankle and foot

☐ **SP** **M13.871** Other specified arthritis, right ankle and foot

☐ **SP** **M13.872** Other specified arthritis, left ankle and foot

☐ **IQ** **M13.879** Other specified arthritis, unspecified ankle and foot

SP **M13.88** Other specified arthritis, other site

SP **M13.89** Other specified arthritis, multiple sites

④ **M14** Arthropathies in other diseases classified elsewhere
EXCLUDES 1 arthropathy in:
diabetes mellitus (E08-E13 with .61-)
hematological disorders (M36.2-M36.3)
hypersensitivity reactions (M36.4)
neoplastic disease (M36.1)
neurosyphillis (A52.16)
sarcoidosis (D86.86)
enteropathic arthropathies (M07.-)
juvenile psoriatic arthropathy (L40.54)
lipoid dermatoarthritis (E78.81)

⑤ **M14.6** Charcôt's joint
Neuropathic arthropathy
EXCLUDES 1 Charcôt's joint in diabetes mellitus (E08-E13 with .610)
Charcôt's joint in tabes dorsalis (A52.16)

CODING TIPS ✓ Do not assign a code from M14.6- to report Charcot arthropathy in diabetes or syphilis. Charcot's joint in diabetes mellitus should be coded to the appropriate combination code from E08-E13 indicating the manifestation.

IQ **M14.60** Charcôt's joint, unspecified site

⑥ **M14.61** Charcôt's joint, shoulder

☐ **SP** **M14.611** Charcôt's joint, right shoulder

☐ **SP** **M14.612** Charcôt's joint, left shoulder

☐ **IQ** **M14.619** Charcôt's joint, unspecified shoulder

⑥ **M14.62** Charcôt's joint, elbow

☐ **SP** **M14.621** Charcôt's joint, right elbow

☐ **SP** **M14.622** Charcôt's joint, left elbow

④4th digit required   ⑤5th digit required   ⑥6th digit required   ⑦7th digit required   ⑦7th digit placeholder   ✚Additional code   ☐Laterality

1178   *DecisionHealth's* FY 2020 Complete Home Health ICD-10-CM Diagnosis Coding Manual

☰ IQ M14.629 Charcôt's joint, unspecified elbow

G M14.63 Charcôt's joint, wrist

☰ SP M14.631 Charcôt's joint, right wrist

☰ SP M14.632 Charcôt's joint, left wrist

☰ IQ M14.639 Charcôt's joint, unspecified wrist

G M14.64 Charcôt's joint, hand

☰ SP M14.641 Charcôt's joint, right hand

☰ SP M14.642 Charcôt's joint, left hand

☰ IQ M14.649 Charcôt's joint, unspecified hand

G M14.65 Charcôt's joint, hip

☰ SP M14.651 Charcôt's joint, right hip

☰ SP M14.652 Charcôt's joint, left hip

☰ IQ M14.659 Charcôt's joint, unspecified hip

G M14.66 Charcôt's joint, knee

☰ SP M14.661 Charcôt's joint, right knee

☰ SP M14.662 Charcôt's joint, left knee

☰ IQ M14.669 Charcôt's joint, unspecified knee

G M14.67 Charcôt's joint, ankle and foot

☰ SP M14.671 Charcôt's joint, right ankle and foot

☰ SP M14.672 Charcôt's joint, left ankle and foot

☰ IQ M14.679 Charcôt's joint, unspecified ankle and foot

SP M14.68 Charcôt's joint, vertebrae

SP M14.69 Charcôt's joint, multiple sites

5 M14.8 Arthropathies in other specified diseases classified elsewhere

Code first underlying disease, such as:
amyloidosis (E85.-)
erythema multiforme (L51.-)
erythema nodosum (L52)
hemochromatosis (E83.11-)
hyperparathyroidism (E21.-)
hypothyroidism (E00-E03)
sickle-cell disorders (D57.-)
thyrotoxicosis [hyperthyroidism] (E05.-)
Whipple's disease (K90.81)

M IQ M14.80 *Arthropathies in other specified diseases classified elsewhere, unspecified site*

G M14.81 Arthropathies in other specified diseases classified elsewhere, shoulder

M ☰ IQ M14.811 *Arthropathies in other specified diseases classified elsewhere, right shoulder*

M ☰ IQ M14.812 *Arthropathies in other specified diseases classified elsewhere, left shoulder*

M ☰ IQ M14.819 *Arthropathies in other specified diseases classified elsewhere, unspecified shoulder*

G M14.82 Arthropathies in other specified diseases classified elsewhere, elbow

M ☰ IQ M14.821 *Arthropathies in other specified diseases classified elsewhere, right elbow*

M ☰ IQ M14.822 *Arthropathies in other specified diseases classified elsewhere, left elbow*

M ☰ IQ M14.829 *Arthropathies in other specified diseases classified elsewhere, unspecified elbow*

G M14.83 Arthropathies in other specified diseases classified elsewhere, wrist

M ☰ IQ M14.831 *Arthropathies in other specified diseases classified elsewhere, right wrist*

M ☰ IQ M14.832 *Arthropathies in other specified diseases classified elsewhere, left wrist*

M ☰ IQ M14.839 *Arthropathies in other specified diseases classified elsewhere, unspecified wrist*

G M14.84 Arthropathies in other specified diseases classified elsewhere, hand

M ☰ IQ M14.841 *Arthropathies in other specified diseases classified elsewhere, right hand*

M ☰ IQ M14.842 *Arthropathies in other specified diseases classified elsewhere, left hand*

M ☰ IQ M14.849 *Arthropathies in other specified diseases classified elsewhere, unspecified hand*

G M14.85 Arthropathies in other specified diseases classified elsewhere, hip

M ☰ IQ M14.851 *Arthropathies in other specified diseases classified elsewhere, right hip*

M ☰ IQ M14.852 *Arthropathies in other specified diseases classified elsewhere, left hip*

M ☰ IQ M14.859 *Arthropathies in other specified diseases classified elsewhere, unspecified hip*

G M14.86 Arthropathies in other specified diseases classified elsewhere, knee

M ☰ IQ M14.861 *Arthropathies in other specified diseases classified elsewhere, right knee*

M ☰ IQ M14.862 *Arthropathies in other specified diseases classified elsewhere, left knee*

M ☰ IQ M14.869 *Arthropathies in other specified diseases classified elsewhere, unspecified knee*

G M14.87 Arthropathies in other specified diseases classified elsewhere, ankle and foot

M ☰ IQ M14.871 *Arthropathies in other specified diseases classified elsewhere, right ankle and foot*

M ☰ IQ M14.872 *Arthropathies in other specified diseases classified elsewhere, left ankle and foot*

M ☰ IQ M14.879 *Arthropathies in other specified diseases classified elsewhere, unspecified ankle and foot*

M IQ M14.88 *Arthropathies in other specified diseases classified elsewhere, vertebrae*

M IQ M14.89 *Arthropathies in other specified diseases classified elsewhere, multiple sites*

★ New ▲ Revised Px Primary **SP** PDGM Px **SL** Low CoM **SH** High CoM **IQ** Quest. Encounter **H** Hospice non-cancer Dx Unspecified **M** *Manifestation*

Osteoarthritis　(M15-M19)

EXCLUDES 2　osteoarthritis of spine　(M47.-)

ALERT　　Laterality is important. Most of the osteoarthritis codes may be subject to review if laterality is not coded. Query for additional information to avoid assigning a last digit of 9.

CODING TIPS ✓　　Osteoarthritis/degenerative joint disease (Categories M15-M19) is the most common type of arthritis in the elderly, and is the default if the physician documents arthritis. If the arthritis is in the spine, refer to Category M47. When coding osteoarthritis, review the medical records to determine whether the OA is localized or generalized; primary or secondary. Bilateral osteoarthritis of the same site is considered localized. Osteoarthritis, when the joint is known, is considered primary by default. If the joints affected are unknown, primary is not assumed.　Generalized OA affects multiple joints (M15). Primary osteoarthritis is caused by aging. Secondary OA is caused by other conditions such as obesity.

CODING TIPS ✓　　Documented arthritis defaults to osteoarthritis, and osteoarthritis defaults to primary, when the joints are known, and when otherwise not noted to be secondary or due to some other cause.

☲ M15　Polyosteoarthritis
    INCLUDES　arthritis of multiple sites
    EXCLUDES 1　bilateral involvement of single
           joint　(M16-M19)

SP M15.0　Primary generalized (osteo)arthritis

SP M15.1　Heberden's nodes (with arthropathy)
    Interphalangeal distal osteoarthritis

SP M15.2　Bouchard's nodes (with arthropathy)
    Juxtaphalangeal distal osteoarthritis

SP M15.3　Secondary multiple arthritis
    Post-traumatic polyosteoarthritis

SP M15.4　Erosive (osteo)arthritis

SP M15.8　Other polyosteoarthritis

SP M15.9　Polyosteoarthritis, unspecified
    Generalized osteoarthritis NOS

☲ M16　Osteoarthritis of hip

SP M16.0　Bilateral primary osteoarthritis of hip

  ☴ M16.1　Unilateral primary osteoarthritis of hip
    Primary osteoarthritis of hip NOS

⊟ IQ M16.10　Unilateral primary osteoarthritis, unspecified hip

⊟ SP M16.11　Unilateral primary osteoarthritis, right hip

⊟ SP M16.12　Unilateral primary osteoarthritis, left hip

SP M16.2　Bilateral osteoarthritis resulting from hip dysplasia

  ☴ M16.3　Unilateral osteoarthritis resulting from hip dysplasia
    Dysplastic osteoarthritis of hip NOS

⊟ IQ M16.30　Unilateral osteoarthritis resulting from hip dysplasia, unspecified hip

⊟ SP M16.31　Unilateral osteoarthritis resulting from hip dysplasia, right hip

⊟ SP M16.32　Unilateral osteoarthritis resulting from hip dysplasia, left hip

SP M16.4　Bilateral post-traumatic osteoarthritis of hip

  ☴ M16.5　Unilateral post-traumatic osteoarthritis of hip
    Post-traumatic osteoarthritis of hip NOS

⊟ IQ M16.50　Unilateral post-traumatic osteoarthritis, unspecified hip

⊟ SP M16.51　Unilateral post-traumatic osteoarthritis, right hip

⊟ SP M16.52　Unilateral post-traumatic osteoarthritis, left hip

SP M16.6　Other bilateral secondary osteoarthritis of hip

SP M16.7　Other unilateral secondary osteoarthritis of hip
    Secondary osteoarthritis of hip NOS

IQ M16.9　Osteoarthritis of hip, unspecified

☲ M17　Osteoarthritis of knee

SP M17.0　Bilateral primary osteoarthritis of knee

  ☴ M17.1　Unilateral primary osteoarthritis of knee
    Primary osteoarthritis of knee NOS

⊟ IQ M17.10　Unilateral primary osteoarthritis, unspecified knee

⊟ SP M17.11　Unilateral primary osteoarthritis, right knee

⊟ SP M17.12　Unilateral primary osteoarthritis, left knee

SP M17.2　Bilateral post-traumatic osteoarthritis of knee

  ☴ M17.3　Unilateral post-traumatic osteoarthritis of knee
    Post-traumatic osteoarthritis of knee NOS

⊟ IQ M17.30　Unilateral post-traumatic osteoarthritis, unspecified knee

⊟ SP M17.31　Unilateral post-traumatic osteoarthritis, right knee

⊟ SP M17.32　Unilateral post-traumatic osteoarthritis, left knee

SP M17.4　Other bilateral secondary osteoarthritis of knee

SP M17.5　Other unilateral secondary osteoarthritis of knee
    Secondary osteoarthritis of knee NOS

IQ M17.9　Osteoarthritis of knee, unspecified

☲ M18　Osteoarthritis of first carpometacarpal joint

SP M18.0　Bilateral primary osteoarthritis of first carpometacarpal joints

  ☴ M18.1　Unilateral primary osteoarthritis of first carpometacarpal joint
    Primary osteoarthritis of first carpometacarpal joint NOS

⊟ IQ M18.10　Unilateral primary osteoarthritis of first carpometacarpal joint, unspecified hand

⊟ SP M18.11　Unilateral primary osteoarthritis of first carpometacarpal joint, right hand

⊟ SP M18.12　Unilateral primary osteoarthritis of first carpometacarpal joint, left hand

SP M18.2　Bilateral post-traumatic osteoarthritis of first carpometacarpal joints

  ☴ M18.3　Unilateral post-traumatic osteoarthritis of first carpometacarpal joint
    Post-traumatic osteoarthritis of first carpometacarpal joint NOS

⊟ IQ M18.30　Unilateral post-traumatic osteoarthritis of first carpometacarpal joint, unspecified hand

⊟ SP M18.31　Unilateral post-traumatic osteoarthritis of first carpometacarpal joint, right hand

---

☲4th digit required　　**☴**5th digit required　　**☵**6th digit required　　**☷**7th digit required　　**☑** 7th digit placeholder　　**✛** Additional code　　**⊟** Laterality

⊟ **SP** **M18.32** Unilateral post-traumatic osteoarthritis of first carpometacarpal joint, left hand

SP **M18.4** Other bilateral secondary osteoarthritis of first carpometacarpal joints

⑤ **M18.5** Other unilateral secondary osteoarthritis of first carpometacarpal joint

Secondary osteoarthritis of first carpometacarpal joint NOS

⊟ **IQ** **M18.50** Other unilateral secondary osteoarthritis of first carpometacarpal joint, unspecified hand

⊟ **SP** **M18.51** Other unilateral secondary osteoarthritis of first carpometacarpal joint, right hand

⊟ **SP** **M18.52** Other unilateral secondary osteoarthritis of first carpometacarpal joint, left hand

IQ **M18.9** Osteoarthritis of first carpometacarpal joint, unspecified

④ **M19** Other and unspecified osteoarthritis

EXCLUDES 1	polyarthritis (M15.-)
EXCLUDES 2	arthrosis of spine (M47.-)
	hallux rigidus (M20.2)
	osteoarthritis of spine (M47.-)

⑤ **M19.0** Primary osteoarthritis of other joints

ALERT Laterality is important. Osteoarthritis not specifying the joint affected may result in medical claim rejection. Query for additional information to avoid assigning a last digit 9.

⑥ **M19.01** Primary osteoarthritis, shoulder

⊟ **SP** **M19.011** Primary osteoarthritis, right shoulder

⊟ **SP** **M19.012** Primary osteoarthritis, left shoulder

⊟ **IQ** **M19.019** Primary osteoarthritis, unspecified shoulder

⑥ **M19.02** Primary osteoarthritis, elbow

⊟ **SP** **M19.021** Primary osteoarthritis, right elbow

⊟ **SP** **M19.022** Primary osteoarthritis, left elbow

⊟ **IQ** **M19.029** Primary osteoarthritis, unspecified elbow

⑥ **M19.03** Primary osteoarthritis, wrist

⊟ **SP** **M19.031** Primary osteoarthritis, right wrist

⊟ **SP** **M19.032** Primary osteoarthritis, left wrist

⊟ **IQ** **M19.039** Primary osteoarthritis, unspecified wrist

⑥ **M19.04** Primary osteoarthritis, hand

EXCLUDES 2	primary osteoarthritis of first carpometacarpal joint (M18.0-, M18.1-)

⊟ **SP** **M19.041** Primary osteoarthritis, right hand

⊟ **SP** **M19.042** Primary osteoarthritis, left hand

⊟ **IQ** **M19.049** Primary osteoarthritis, unspecified hand

⑥ **M19.07** Primary osteoarthritis ankle and foot

⊟ **SP** **M19.071** Primary osteoarthritis, right ankle and foot

⊟ **SP** **M19.072** Primary osteoarthritis, left ankle and foot

⊟ **IQ** **M19.079** Primary osteoarthritis, unspecified ankle and foot

⑤ **M19.1** Post-traumatic osteoarthritis of other joints

⑥ **M19.11** Post-traumatic osteoarthritis, shoulder

⊟ **SP** **M19.111** Post-traumatic osteoarthritis, right shoulder

⊟ **SP** **M19.112** Post-traumatic osteoarthritis, left shoulder

⊟ **IQ** **M19.119** Post-traumatic osteoarthritis, unspecified shoulder

⑥ **M19.12** Post-traumatic osteoarthritis, elbow

⊟ **SP** **M19.121** Post-traumatic osteoarthritis, right elbow

⊟ **SP** **M19.122** Post-traumatic osteoarthritis, left elbow

⊟ **IQ** **M19.129** Post-traumatic osteoarthritis, unspecified elbow

⑥ **M19.13** Post-traumatic osteoarthritis, wrist

⊟ **SP** **M19.131** Post-traumatic osteoarthritis, right wrist

⊟ **SP** **M19.132** Post-traumatic osteoarthritis, left wrist

⊟ **IQ** **M19.139** Post-traumatic osteoarthritis, unspecified wrist

⑥ **M19.14** Post-traumatic osteoarthritis, hand

EXCLUDES 2	post-traumatic osteoarthritis of first carpometacarpal joint (M18.2-, M18.3-)

⊟ **SP** **M19.141** Post-traumatic osteoarthritis, right hand

⊟ **SP** **M19.142** Post-traumatic osteoarthritis, left hand

⊟ **IQ** **M19.149** Post-traumatic osteoarthritis, unspecified hand

⑥ **M19.17** Post-traumatic osteoarthritis, ankle and foot

⊟ **SP** **M19.171** Post-traumatic osteoarthritis, right ankle and foot

⊟ **SP** **M19.172** Post-traumatic osteoarthritis, left ankle and foot

⊟ **IQ** **M19.179** Post-traumatic osteoarthritis, unspecified ankle and foot

⑤ **M19.2** Secondary osteoarthritis of other joints

⑥ **M19.21** Secondary osteoarthritis, shoulder

⊟ **SP** **M19.211** Secondary osteoarthritis, right shoulder

⊟ **SP** **M19.212** Secondary osteoarthritis, left shoulder

⊟ **IQ** **M19.219** Secondary osteoarthritis, unspecified shoulder

⑥ **M19.22** Secondary osteoarthritis, elbow

⊟ **SP** **M19.221** Secondary osteoarthritis, right elbow

⊟ **SP** **M19.222** Secondary osteoarthritis, left elbow

⊟ **IQ** **M19.229** Secondary osteoarthritis, unspecified elbow

⑥ **M19.23** Secondary osteoarthritis, wrist

⊟ **SP** **M19.231** Secondary osteoarthritis, right wrist

⊟ **SP** **M19.232** Secondary osteoarthritis, left wrist

★ New ▲ Revised Px Primary **SP** PDGM Px **SL** Low CoM **SH** High CoM **IQ** Quest. Encounter ⊞ Hospice non-cancer Dx Unspecified **M** *Manifestation*

DecisionHealth's FY 2020 Complete Home Health ICD-10-CM Diagnosis Coding Manual

1181

🔲 !Q **M19.239　Secondary osteoarthritis, unspecified wrist**

⑥ **M19.24　Secondary osteoarthritis, hand**

🔲 SP **M19.241　Secondary osteoarthritis, right hand**

🔲 SP **M19.242　Secondary osteoarthritis, left hand**

🔲 !Q **M19.249　Secondary osteoarthritis, unspecified hand**

⑥ **M19.27　Secondary osteoarthritis, ankle and foot**

🔲 SP **M19.271　Secondary osteoarthritis, right ankle and foot**

🔲 SP **M19.272　Secondary osteoarthritis, left ankle and foot**

🔲 !Q **M19.279　Secondary osteoarthritis, unspecified ankle and foot**

⑤ **M19.9　Osteoarthritis, unspecified site**

> **ALERT**　Osteoarthritis not specifying the joint affected may result in a medical claim rejection. Query for additional information to avoid assigning a last digit 9.

> **CODING TIPS ✓**　If the site is known, do not use M19.9- codes. Code to site. The default is primary.

!Q **M19.90　Unspecified osteoarthritis, unspecified site**

Arthrosis NOS
Arthritis NOS
Osteoarthritis NOS

> **CODING TIPS ✓**　Avoid using M19.90. M19.90 is assigned when no information is available regarding the osteoarthritis.

!Q **M19.91　Primary osteoarthritis, unspecified site**

Primary osteoarthritis NOS

> **CODING TIPS ✓**　Avoid using M19.91. This code is appropriate only when the physician documents "primary osteoarthritis" without naming joints affected.

!Q **M19.92　Post-traumatic osteoarthritis, unspecified site**

Post-traumatic osteoarthritis NOS

!Q **M19.93　Secondary osteoarthritis, unspecified site**

Secondary osteoarthritis NOS

Other joint disorders　(M20-M25)

EXCLUDES 2　joints of the spine　(M40-M54)

④ **M20　Acquired deformities of fingers and toes**

> **EXCLUDES 1**　acquired absence of fingers and toes　(Z89.-)
> congenital absence of fingers and toes　(Q71.3-, Q72.3-)
> congenital deformities and malformations of fingers and toes　(Q66.-, Q68-Q70, Q74.-)

> **CODING TIPS ✓**　Acquired deformities are different than congenital deformities. If the deformity was present at birth or considered congenital, refer to the Q codes.

⑤ **M20.0　Deformity of finger(s)**

> **EXCLUDES 1**　clubbing of fingers　(R68.3)

palmar fascial fibromatosis [Dupuytren]　(M72.0)
trigger finger　(M65.3)

⑥ **M20.00　Unspecified deformity of finger(s)**

🔲 !Q **M20.001　Unspecified deformity of right finger(s)**

🔲 !Q **M20.002　Unspecified deformity of left finger(s)**

🔲 !Q **M20.009　Unspecified deformity of unspecified finger(s)**

⑥ **M20.01　Mallet finger**

🔲 SP **M20.011　Mallet finger of right finger(s)**

🔲 SP **M20.012　Mallet finger of left finger(s)**

🔲 !Q **M20.019　Mallet finger of unspecified finger(s)**

⑥ **M20.02　Boutonnière deformity**

🔲 SP **M20.021　Boutonnière deformity of right finger(s)**

🔲 SP **M20.022　Boutonnière deformity of left finger(s)**

🔲 !Q **M20.029　Boutonnière deformity of unspecified finger(s)**

⑥ **M20.03　Swan-neck deformity**

🔲 SP **M20.031　Swan-neck deformity of right finger(s)**

🔲 SP **M20.032　Swan-neck deformity of left finger(s)**

🔲 !Q **M20.039　Swan-neck deformity of unspecified finger(s)**

⑥ **M20.09　Other deformity of finger(s)**

🔲 SP **M20.091　Other deformity of right finger(s)**

🔲 SP **M20.092　Other deformity of left finger(s)**

🔲 !Q **M20.099　Other deformity of finger(s), unspecified finger(s)**

⑤ **M20.1　Hallux valgus (acquired)**

> **EXCLUDES 2**　bunion　(M21.6-)

🔲 !Q **M20.10　Hallux valgus (acquired), unspecified foot**

🔲 SP **M20.11　Hallux valgus (acquired), right foot**

🔲 SP **M20.12　Hallux valgus (acquired), left foot**

⑤ **M20.2　Hallux rigidus**

> **DEFINITION**　Inflexible, stiff great toe, with limited motion at the metatarsophalangeal joint.

🔲 !Q **M20.20　Hallux rigidus, unspecified foot**

🔲 SP **M20.21　Hallux rigidus, right foot**

🔲 SP **M20.22　Hallux rigidus, left foot**

⑤ **M20.3　Hallux varus (acquired)**

> **DEFINITION**　Displaced joint of the big toe which is pointed away from the rest of the toes.

🔲 !Q **M20.30　Hallux varus (acquired), unspecified foot**

🔲 SP **M20.31　Hallux varus (acquired), right foot**

🔲 SP **M20.32　Hallux varus (acquired), left foot**

⑤ **M20.4　Other hammer toe(s) (acquired)**

🔲 !Q **M20.40　Other hammer toe(s) (acquired), unspecified foot**

🔲 SP **M20.41　Other hammer toe(s) (acquired), right foot**

---

④ 4th digit required　　⑤ 5th digit required　　⑥ 6th digit required　　⑦ 7th digit required　　⑦ 7th digit placeholder　　✚ Additional code　　🔲 Laterality

☐ 🆂🅿 **M20.42 Other hammer toe(s) (acquired), left foot**

🗏 **M20.5 Other deformities of toe(s) (acquired)**

　⑥ **M20.5X Other deformities of toe(s) (acquired)**

☐ 🆂🅿 **M20.5X1 Other deformities of toe(s) (acquired), right foot**

☐ 🆂🅿 **M20.5X2 Other deformities of toe(s) (acquired), left foot**

☐ 🅸🆀 **M20.5X9 Other deformities of toe(s) (acquired), unspecified foot**

　🗏 **M20.6 Acquired deformities of toe(s), unspecified**

☐ 🅸🆀 **M20.60 Acquired deformities of toe(s), unspecified, unspecified foot**

☐ 🅸🆀 **M20.61 Acquired deformities of toe(s), unspecified, right foot**

☐ 🅸🆀 **M20.62 Acquired deformities of toe(s), unspecified, left foot**

🄸 **M21 Other acquired deformities of limbs**

　　EXCLUDES 1　acquired absence of limb (Z89.-)
　　　　　congenital absence of limbs (Q71-Q73)
　　　　　congenital deformities and malformations of limbs (Q65-Q66, Q68-Q74)
　　EXCLUDES 2　acquired deformities of fingers or toes (M20.-)
　　　　　coxa plana (M91.2)

▲ 🗏 **M21.0 Valgus deformity, not elsewhere classified**

　　EXCLUDES 1　metatarsus valgus (Q66.6)
　　　　　talipes calcaneovalgus (Q66.4-)

🅸🆀 **M21.00 Valgus deformity, not elsewhere classified, unspecified site**

　⑥ **M21.02 Valgus deformity, not elsewhere classified, elbow**
　　Cubitus valgus

☐ 🆂🅿 **M21.021 Valgus deformity, not elsewhere classified, right elbow**

☐ 🆂🅿 **M21.022 Valgus deformity, not elsewhere classified, left elbow**

☐ 🅸🆀 **M21.029 Valgus deformity, not elsewhere classified, unspecified elbow**

　⑥ **M21.05 Valgus deformity, not elsewhere classified, hip**

☐ 🆂🅿 **M21.051 Valgus deformity, not elsewhere classified, right hip**

☐ 🆂🅿 **M21.052 Valgus deformity, not elsewhere classified, left hip**

☐ 🅸🆀 **M21.059 Valgus deformity, not elsewhere classified, unspecified hip**

　⑥ **M21.06 Valgus deformity, not elsewhere classified, knee**
　　Genu valgum
　　Knock knee

　　DEFINITION　Deformity in which the knees are angled abnormally close together with the ankles apart when standing erect with the legs straightened.

☐ 🆂🅿 **M21.061 Valgus deformity, not elsewhere classified, right knee**

☐ 🆂🅿 **M21.062 Valgus deformity, not elsewhere classified, left knee**

☐ 🅸🆀 **M21.069 Valgus deformity, not elsewhere classified, unspecified knee**

　⑥ **M21.07 Valgus deformity, not elsewhere classified, ankle**

☐ 🆂🅿 **M21.071 Valgus deformity, not elsewhere classified, right ankle**

☐ 🆂🅿 **M21.072 Valgus deformity, not elsewhere classified, left ankle**

☐ 🅸🆀 **M21.079 Valgus deformity, not elsewhere classified, unspecified ankle**

▲ 🗏 **M21.1 Varus deformity, not elsewhere classified**

　　EXCLUDES 1　metatarsus varus (Q66.22-)
　　　　　tibia vara (M92.5)

🅸🆀 **M21.10 Varus deformity, not elsewhere classified, unspecified site**

　⑥ **M21.12 Varus deformity, not elsewhere classified, elbow**
　　Cubitus varus, elbow

☐ 🆂🅿 **M21.121 Varus deformity, not elsewhere classified, right elbow**

☐ 🆂🅿 **M21.122 Varus deformity, not elsewhere classified, left elbow**

☐ 🅸🆀 **M21.129 Varus deformity, not elsewhere classified, unspecified elbow**

　⑥ **M21.15 Varus deformity, not elsewhere classified, hip**

☐ 🆂🅿 **M21.151 Varus deformity, not elsewhere classified, right hip**

☐ 🆂🅿 **M21.152 Varus deformity, not elsewhere classified, left hip**

☐ 🅸🆀 **M21.159 Varus deformity, not elsewhere classified, unspecified**

　⑥ **M21.16 Varus deformity, not elsewhere classified, knee**
　　Bow leg
　　Genu varum

☐ 🆂🅿 **M21.161 Varus deformity, not elsewhere classified, right knee**

☐ 🆂🅿 **M21.162 Varus deformity, not elsewhere classified, left knee**

☐ 🅸🆀 **M21.169 Varus deformity, not elsewhere classified, unspecified knee**

　⑥ **M21.17 Varus deformity, not elsewhere classified, ankle**

　　DEFINITION　Inward angulation of the tibia and fibula on the talus generally due to trauma or overpull by the tibialis posterior and anterior tendons.

☐ 🆂🅿 **M21.171 Varus deformity, not elsewhere classified, right ankle**

☐ 🆂🅿 **M21.172 Varus deformity, not elsewhere classified, left ankle**

☐ 🅸🆀 **M21.179 Varus deformity, not elsewhere classified, unspecified ankle**

🗏 **M21.2 Flexion deformity**

🅸🆀 **M21.20 Flexion deformity, unspecified site**

　⑥ **M21.21 Flexion deformity, shoulder**

☐ 🆂🅿 **M21.211 Flexion deformity, right shoulder**

☐ 🆂🅿 **M21.212 Flexion deformity, left shoulder**

☐ 🅸🆀 **M21.219 Flexion deformity, unspecified shoulder**

　⑥ **M21.22 Flexion deformity, elbow**

☐ 🆂🅿 **M21.221 Flexion deformity, right elbow**

★ New　▲ Revised　Px Primary　🆂🅿 PDGM Px　🆂🅻 Low CoM　🆂🅷 High CoM　🅸🆀 Quest. Encounter　🅷 Hospice non-cancer Dx　Unspecified　🅼 *Manifestation*

DecisionHealth's FY 2020 Complete Home Health ICD-10-CM Diagnosis Coding Manual

1183

☐ **SP** **M21.222** Flexion deformity, left elbow

☐ **IQ** **M21.229** Flexion deformity, unspecified elbow

　6 **M21.23** Flexion deformity, wrist

☐ **SP** **M21.231** Flexion deformity, right wrist

☐ **SP** **M21.232** Flexion deformity, left wrist

☐ **IQ** **M21.239** Flexion deformity, unspecified wrist

　6 **M21.24** Flexion deformity, finger joints

☐ **SP** **M21.241** Flexion deformity, right finger joints

☐ **SP** **M21.242** Flexion deformity, left finger joints

☐ **IQ** **M21.249** Flexion deformity, unspecified finger joints

　6 **M21.25** Flexion deformity, hip

☐ **SP** **M21.251** Flexion deformity, right hip

☐ **SP** **M21.252** Flexion deformity, left hip

☐ **IQ** **M21.259** Flexion deformity, unspecified hip

　6 **M21.26** Flexion deformity, knee

☐ **SP** **M21.261** Flexion deformity, right knee

☐ **SP** **M21.262** Flexion deformity, left knee

☐ **IQ** **M21.269** Flexion deformity, unspecified knee

　6 **M21.27** Flexion deformity, ankle and toes

☐ **SP** **M21.271** Flexion deformity, right ankle and toes

☐ **SP** **M21.272** Flexion deformity, left ankle and toes

☐ **IQ** **M21.279** Flexion deformity, unspecified ankle and toes

　5 **M21.3** Wrist or foot drop (acquired)

　6 **M21.33** Wrist drop (acquired)

☐ **SP** **M21.331** Wrist drop, right wrist

☐ **SP** **M21.332** Wrist drop, left wrist

☐ **IQ** **M21.339** Wrist drop, unspecified wrist

　6 **M21.37** Foot drop (acquired)

☐ **SP** **M21.371** Foot drop, right foot

☐ **SP** **M21.372** Foot drop, left foot

☐ **IQ** **M21.379** Foot drop, unspecified foot

　5 **M21.4** Flat foot [pes planus] (acquired)
　　　EXCLUDES 1　congenital pes planus (Q66.5-)

☐ **IQ** **M21.40** Flat foot [pes planus] (acquired), unspecified foot

☐ **SP** **M21.41** Flat foot [pes planus] (acquired), right foot

☐ **SP** **M21.42** Flat foot [pes planus] (acquired), left foot

　5 **M21.5** Acquired clawhand, clubhand, clawfoot and clubfoot
　　　EXCLUDES 1　clubfoot, not specified as acquired (Q66.89)

　6 **M21.51** Acquired clawhand

☐ **SP** **M21.511** Acquired clawhand, right hand

☐ **SP** **M21.512** Acquired clawhand, left hand

☐ **IQ** **M21.519** Acquired clawhand, unspecified hand

　6 **M21.52** Acquired clubhand

☐ **SP** **M21.521** Acquired clubhand, right hand

☐ **SP** **M21.522** Acquired clubhand, left hand

☐ **IQ** **M21.529** Acquired clubhand, unspecified hand

　6 **M21.53** Acquired clawfoot

☐ **SP** **M21.531** Acquired clawfoot, right foot

☐ **SP** **M21.532** Acquired clawfoot, left foot

☐ **IQ** **M21.539** Acquired clawfoot, unspecified foot

　6 **M21.54** Acquired clubfoot

☐ **SP** **M21.541** Acquired clubfoot, right foot

☐ **SP** **M21.542** Acquired clubfoot, left foot

☐ **IQ** **M21.549** Acquired clubfoot, unspecified foot

　5 **M21.6** Other acquired deformities of foot
　　　EXCLUDES 2　deformities of toe (acquired) (M20.1-M20.6-)

　6 **M21.61** Bunion

☐ **SP** **M21.611** Bunion of right foot

☐ **SP** **M21.612** Bunion of left foot

☐ **IQ** **M21.619** Bunion of unspecified foot

　6 **M21.62** Bunionette

☐ **SP** **M21.621** Bunionette of right foot

☐ **SP** **M21.622** Bunionette of left foot

☐ **IQ** **M21.629** Bunionette of unspecified foot

　6 **M21.6X** Other acquired deformities of foot

☐ **SP** **M21.6X1** Other acquired deformities of right foot

☐ **SP** **M21.6X2** Other acquired deformities of left foot

☐ **IQ** **M21.6X9** Other acquired deformities of unspecified foot

　5 **M21.7** Unequal limb length (acquired)
　　　Note:
　　　The site used should correspond to the shorter limb
　　　CODING TIPS ✓　Acquired unequal limb length is usually due to an injury. Consider adding the injury with 7th character S.

☐ **IQ** **M21.70** Unequal limb length (acquired), unspecified site

　6 **M21.72** Unequal limb length (acquired), humerus

☐ **SP** **M21.721** Unequal limb length (acquired), right humerus

☐ **SP** **M21.722** Unequal limb length (acquired), left humerus

☐ **IQ** **M21.729** Unequal limb length (acquired), unspecified humerus

　6 **M21.73** Unequal limb length (acquired), ulna and radius

☐ **SP** **M21.731** Unequal limb length (acquired), right ulna

☐ **SP** **M21.732** Unequal limb length (acquired), left ulna

☐ **SP** **M21.733** Unequal limb length (acquired), right radius

☐ **SP** **M21.734** Unequal limb length (acquired), left radius

☐ **IQ** **M21.739** Unequal limb length (acquired), unspecified ulna and radius

　6 **M21.75** Unequal limb length (acquired), femur

4 4th digit required　　**5** 5th digit required　　**6** 6th digit required　　**7** 7th digit required　　**7** 7th digit placeholder　　**+** Additional code　　☐ Laterality

1184　　　*DecisionHealth's* FY 2020 Complete Home Health ICD-10-CM Diagnosis Coding Manual

⊟ SP **M21.751** Unequal limb length (acquired), right femur

⊟ SP **M21.752** Unequal limb length (acquired), left femur

⊟ IQ **M21.759** Unequal limb length (acquired), unspecified femur

6 **M21.76** Unequal limb length (acquired), tibia and fibula

⊟ SP **M21.761** Unequal limb length (acquired), right tibia

⊟ SP **M21.762** Unequal limb length (acquired), left tibia

⊟ SP **M21.763** Unequal limb length (acquired), right fibula

⊟ SP **M21.764** Unequal limb length (acquired), left fibula

⊟ IQ **M21.769** Unequal limb length (acquired), unspecified tibia and fibula

5 **M21.8** Other specified acquired deformities of limbs

> **EXCLUDES 2**   coxa plana (M91.2)

IQ **M21.80** Other specified acquired deformities of unspecified limb

6 **M21.82** Other specified acquired deformities of upper arm

⊟ SP **M21.821** Other specified acquired deformities of right upper arm

⊟ SP **M21.822** Other specified acquired deformities of left upper arm

⊟ IQ **M21.829** Other specified acquired deformities of unspecified upper arm

6 **M21.83** Other specified acquired deformities of forearm

⊟ SP **M21.831** Other specified acquired deformities of right forearm

⊟ SP **M21.832** Other specified acquired deformities of left forearm

⊟ IQ **M21.839** Other specified acquired deformities of unspecified forearm

6 **M21.85** Other specified acquired deformities of thigh

⊟ SP **M21.851** Other specified acquired deformities of right thigh

⊟ SP **M21.852** Other specified acquired deformities of left thigh

⊟ IQ **M21.859** Other specified acquired deformities of unspecified thigh

6 **M21.86** Other specified acquired deformities of lower leg

⊟ SP **M21.861** Other specified acquired deformities of right lower leg

⊟ SP **M21.862** Other specified acquired deformities of left lower leg

⊟ IQ **M21.869** Other specified acquired deformities of unspecified lower leg

5 **M21.9** Unspecified acquired deformity of limb and hand

IQ **M21.90** Unspecified acquired deformity of unspecified limb

6 **M21.92** Unspecified acquired deformity of upper arm

⊟ SP **M21.921** Unspecified acquired deformity of right upper arm

⊟ SP **M21.922** Unspecified acquired deformity of left upper arm

⊟ IQ **M21.929** Unspecified acquired deformity of unspecified upper arm

6 **M21.93** Unspecified acquired deformity of forearm

⊟ SP **M21.931** Unspecified acquired deformity of right forearm

⊟ SP **M21.932** Unspecified acquired deformity of left forearm

⊟ IQ **M21.939** Unspecified acquired deformity of unspecified forearm

6 **M21.94** Unspecified acquired deformity of hand

⊟ SP **M21.941** Unspecified acquired deformity of hand, right hand

⊟ SP **M21.942** Unspecified acquired deformity of hand, left hand

⊟ IQ **M21.949** Unspecified acquired deformity of hand, unspecified hand

6 **M21.95** Unspecified acquired deformity of thigh

⊟ SP **M21.951** Unspecified acquired deformity of right thigh

⊟ SP **M21.952** Unspecified acquired deformity of left thigh

⊟ IQ **M21.959** Unspecified acquired deformity of unspecified thigh

6 **M21.96** Unspecified acquired deformity of lower leg

⊟ SP **M21.961** Unspecified acquired deformity of right lower leg

⊟ SP **M21.962** Unspecified acquired deformity of left lower leg

⊟ IQ **M21.969** Unspecified acquired deformity of unspecified lower leg

4 **M22** Disorder of patella

> **EXCLUDES 1**   traumatic dislocation of patella (S83.0-)

5 **M22.0** Recurrent dislocation of patella

⊟ IQ **M22.00** Recurrent dislocation of patella, unspecified knee

⊟ SP **M22.01** Recurrent dislocation of patella, right knee

⊟ SP **M22.02** Recurrent dislocation of patella, left knee

5 **M22.1** Recurrent subluxation of patella
Incomplete dislocation of patella

⊟ IQ **M22.10** Recurrent subluxation of patella, unspecified knee

⊟ SP **M22.11** Recurrent subluxation of patella, right knee

⊟ SP **M22.12** Recurrent subluxation of patella, left knee

5 **M22.2** Patellofemoral disorders

6 **M22.2X** Patellofemoral disorders

⊟ SP **M22.2X1** Patellofemoral disorders, right knee

⊟ SP **M22.2X2** Patellofemoral disorders, left knee

⊟ IQ **M22.2X9** Patellofemoral disorders, unspecified knee

5 **M22.3** Other derangements of patella

6 **M22.3X** Other derangements of patella

★ New ▲ Revised Px Primary SP PDGM Px SL Low CoM SH High CoM IQ Quest. Encounter H Hospice non-cancer Dx   Unspecified   M *Manifestation*

DecisionHealth's FY 2020 Complete Home Health ICD-10-CM Diagnosis Coding Manual

1185

Chapter 13

M00-M99

⊟ **SP** **M22.3X1** Other derangements of patella, right knee

⊟ **SP** **M22.3X2** Other derangements of patella, left knee

⊟ **IQ** **M22.3X9** Other derangements of patella, unspecified knee

⑤ **M22.4** Chondromalacia patellae

> **CODING TIPS** ✓   Chondromalacia patellae (CMP) is also referred to as "runner's knee."

⊟ **IQ** **M22.40** Chondromalacia patellae, unspecified knee

⊟ **SP** **M22.41** Chondromalacia patellae, right knee

⊟ **SP** **M22.42** Chondromalacia patellae, left knee

⑤ **M22.8** Other disorders of patella

⑥ **M22.8X** Other disorders of patella

⊟ **SP** **M22.8X1** Other disorders of patella, right knee

⊟ **SP** **M22.8X2** Other disorders of patella, left knee

⊟ **IQ** **M22.8X9** Other disorders of patella, unspecified knee

⑤ **M22.9** Unspecified disorder of patella

⊟ **IQ** **M22.90** Unspecified disorder of patella, unspecified knee

⊟ **SP** **M22.91** Unspecified disorder of patella, right knee

⊟ **SP** **M22.92** Unspecified disorder of patella, left knee

④ **M23** Internal derangement of knee

> **EXCLUDES 1**   ankylosis (M24.66)
> current injury - see injury of knee and lower leg (S80-S89)
> deformity of knee (M21.-)
> osteochondritis dissecans (M93.2)
> recurrent dislocation or subluxation of joints (M24.4)
> recurrent dislocation or subluxation of patella (M22.0-M22.1)

> **CODING TIPS** ✓   Categories M23 and M24 are used for patients who have old injuries. New injuries are coded with codes from Chapter 19.

⑤ **M23.0** Cystic meniscus

⑥ **M23.00** Cystic meniscus, unspecified meniscus

> Cystic meniscus, unspecified lateral meniscus
> Cystic meniscus, unspecified medial meniscus

⊟ **SP** **M23.000** Cystic meniscus, unspecified lateral meniscus, right knee

⊟ **SP** **M23.001** Cystic meniscus, unspecified lateral meniscus, left knee

⊟ **IQ** **M23.002** Cystic meniscus, unspecified lateral meniscus, unspecified knee

⊟ **SP** **M23.003** Cystic meniscus, unspecified medial meniscus, right knee

⊟ **SP** **M23.004** Cystic meniscus, unspecified medial meniscus, left knee

⊟ **IQ** **M23.005** Cystic meniscus, unspecified medial meniscus, unspecified knee

⊟ **SP** **M23.006** Cystic meniscus, unspecified meniscus, right knee

⊟ **SP** **M23.007** Cystic meniscus, unspecified meniscus, left knee

⊟ **IQ** **M23.009** Cystic meniscus, unspecified meniscus, unspecified knee

⑥ **M23.01** Cystic meniscus, anterior horn of medial meniscus

⊟ **SP** **M23.011** Cystic meniscus, anterior horn of medial meniscus, right knee

⊟ **SP** **M23.012** Cystic meniscus, anterior horn of medial meniscus, left knee

⊟ **IQ** **M23.019** Cystic meniscus, anterior horn of medial meniscus, unspecified knee

⑥ **M23.02** Cystic meniscus, posterior horn of medial meniscus

⊟ **SP** **M23.021** Cystic meniscus, posterior horn of medial meniscus, right knee

⊟ **SP** **M23.022** Cystic meniscus, posterior horn of medial meniscus, left knee

⊟ **IQ** **M23.029** Cystic meniscus, posterior horn of medial meniscus, unspecified knee

⑥ **M23.03** Cystic meniscus, other medial meniscus

⊟ **SP** **M23.031** Cystic meniscus, other medial meniscus, right knee

⊟ **SP** **M23.032** Cystic meniscus, other medial meniscus, left knee

⊟ **IQ** **M23.039** Cystic meniscus, other medial meniscus, unspecified knee

⑥ **M23.04** Cystic meniscus, anterior horn of lateral meniscus

⊟ **SP** **M23.041** Cystic meniscus, anterior horn of lateral meniscus, right knee

⊟ **SP** **M23.042** Cystic meniscus, anterior horn of lateral meniscus, left knee

⊟ **IQ** **M23.049** Cystic meniscus, anterior horn of lateral meniscus, unspecified knee

⑥ **M23.05** Cystic meniscus, posterior horn of lateral meniscus

⊟ **SP** **M23.051** Cystic meniscus, posterior horn of lateral meniscus, right knee

⊟ **SP** **M23.052** Cystic meniscus, posterior horn of lateral meniscus, left knee

⊟ **IQ** **M23.059** Cystic meniscus, posterior horn of lateral meniscus, unspecified knee

⑥ **M23.06** Cystic meniscus, other lateral meniscus

⊟ **SP** **M23.061** Cystic meniscus, other lateral meniscus, right knee

⊟ **SP** **M23.062** Cystic meniscus, other lateral meniscus, left knee

⊟ **IQ** **M23.069** Cystic meniscus, other lateral meniscus, unspecified knee

⑤ **M23.2** Derangement of meniscus due to old tear or injury

> Old bucket-handle tear

⑥ **M23.20** Derangement of unspecified meniscus due to old tear or injury

> Derangement of unspecified lateral meniscus due to old tear or injury

---

④ 4th digit required   ⑤ 5th digit required   ⑥ 6th digit required   ⑦ 7th digit required   ⑦ 7th digit placeholder   ✚ Additional code   ⊟ Laterality

1186   *DecisionHealth's* FY 2020 Complete Home Health ICD-10-CM Diagnosis Coding Manual

Derangement of unspecified medial meniscus due to old tear or injury

☰ SP **M23.200** **Derangement of unspecified lateral meniscus due to old tear or injury, right knee**

☰ SP **M23.201** **Derangement of unspecified lateral meniscus due to old tear or injury, left knee**

☰ IQ **M23.202** **Derangement of unspecified lateral meniscus due to old tear or injury, unspecified knee**

☰ SP **M23.203** **Derangement of unspecified medial meniscus due to old tear or injury, right knee**

☰ SP **M23.204** **Derangement of unspecified medial meniscus due to old tear or injury, left knee**

☰ IQ **M23.205** **Derangement of unspecified medial meniscus due to old tear or injury, unspecified knee**

☰ SP **M23.206** **Derangement of unspecified meniscus due to old tear or injury, right knee**

☰ SP **M23.207** **Derangement of unspecified meniscus due to old tear or injury, left knee**

☰ IQ **M23.209** **Derangement of unspecified meniscus due to old tear or injury, unspecified knee**

⑥ **M23.21** Derangement of anterior horn of medial meniscus due to old tear or injury

☰ SP **M23.211** Derangement of anterior horn of medial meniscus due to old tear or injury, right knee

☰ SP **M23.212** Derangement of anterior horn of medial meniscus due to old tear or injury, left knee

☰ IQ **M23.219** **Derangement of anterior horn of medial meniscus due to old tear or injury, unspecified knee**

⑥ **M23.22** Derangement of posterior horn of medial meniscus due to old tear or injury

☰ SP **M23.221** Derangement of posterior horn of medial meniscus due to old tear or injury, right knee

☰ SP **M23.222** Derangement of posterior horn of medial meniscus due to old tear or injury, left knee

☰ IQ **M23.229** **Derangement of posterior horn of medial meniscus due to old tear or injury, unspecified knee**

⑥ **M23.23** Derangement of other medial meniscus due to old tear or injury

☰ SP **M23.231** Derangement of other medial meniscus due to old tear or injury, right knee

☰ SP **M23.232** Derangement of other medial meniscus due to old tear or injury, left knee

☰ IQ **M23.239** **Derangement of other medial meniscus due to old tear or injury, unspecified knee**

⑥ **M23.24** Derangement of anterior horn of lateral meniscus due to old tear or injury

☰ SP **M23.241** Derangement of anterior horn of lateral meniscus due to old tear or injury, right knee

☰ SP **M23.242** Derangement of anterior horn of lateral meniscus due to old tear or injury, left knee

☰ IQ **M23.249** **Derangement of anterior horn of lateral meniscus due to old tear or injury, unspecified knee**

⑥ **M23.25** Derangement of posterior horn of lateral meniscus due to old tear or injury

☰ SP **M23.251** Derangement of posterior horn of lateral meniscus due to old tear or injury, right knee

☰ SP **M23.252** Derangement of posterior horn of lateral meniscus due to old tear or injury, left knee

☰ IQ **M23.259** **Derangement of posterior horn of lateral meniscus due to old tear or injury, unspecified knee**

⑥ **M23.26** Derangement of other lateral meniscus due to old tear or injury

☰ SP **M23.261** Derangement of other lateral meniscus due to old tear or injury, right knee

☰ SP **M23.262** Derangement of other lateral meniscus due to old tear or injury, left knee

☰ IQ **M23.269** **Derangement of other lateral meniscus due to old tear or injury, unspecified knee**

⑤ **M23.3** Other meniscus derangements
Degenerate meniscus
Detached meniscus
Retained meniscus

⑥ **M23.30** **Other meniscus derangements, unspecified meniscus**

Other meniscus derangements, unspecified lateral meniscus
Other meniscus derangements, unspecified medial meniscus

☰ SP **M23.300** **Other meniscus derangements, unspecified lateral meniscus, right knee**

☰ SP **M23.301** **Other meniscus derangements, unspecified lateral meniscus, left knee**

☰ IQ **M23.302** **Other meniscus derangements, unspecified lateral meniscus, unspecified knee**

☰ SP **M23.303** **Other meniscus derangements, unspecified medial meniscus, right knee**

☰ SP **M23.304** **Other meniscus derangements, unspecified medial meniscus, left knee**

☰ IQ **M23.305** **Other meniscus derangements, unspecified medial meniscus, unspecified knee**

☰ SP **M23.306** **Other meniscus derangements, unspecified meniscus, right knee**

☰ SP **M23.307** **Other meniscus derangements, unspecified meniscus, left knee**

★ New ▲ Revised Px Primary SP PDGM Px SL Low CoM SH High CoM IQ Quest. Encounter H Hospice non-cancer Dx ▣ Unspecified M *Manifestation*

DecisionHealth's FY 2020 Complete Home Health ICD-10-CM Diagnosis Coding Manual

1187

Chapter 13

M00-M99

☐ **IQ** M23.309 **Other meniscus derangements, unspecified meniscus, unspecified knee**

⑥ M23.31 Other meniscus derangements, anterior horn of medial meniscus
☐ **SP** M23.311 Other meniscus derangements, anterior horn of medial meniscus, right knee
☐ **SP** M23.312 Other meniscus derangements, anterior horn of medial meniscus, left knee
☐ **IQ** M23.319 **Other meniscus derangements, anterior horn of medial meniscus, unspecified knee**

⑥ M23.32 Other meniscus derangements, posterior horn of medial meniscus
☐ **SP** M23.321 Other meniscus derangements, posterior horn of medial meniscus, right knee
☐ **SP** M23.322 Other meniscus derangements, posterior horn of medial meniscus, left knee
☐ **IQ** M23.329 **Other meniscus derangements, posterior horn of medial meniscus, unspecified knee**

⑥ M23.33 Other meniscus derangements, other medial meniscus
☐ **SP** M23.331 Other meniscus derangements, other medial meniscus, right knee
☐ **SP** M23.332 Other meniscus derangements, other medial meniscus, left knee
☐ **IQ** M23.339 **Other meniscus derangements, other medial meniscus, unspecified knee**

⑥ M23.34 Other meniscus derangements, anterior horn of lateral meniscus
☐ **SP** M23.341 Other meniscus derangements, anterior horn of lateral meniscus, right knee
☐ **SP** M23.342 Other meniscus derangements, anterior horn of lateral meniscus, left knee
☐ **IQ** M23.349 **Other meniscus derangements, anterior horn of lateral meniscus, unspecified knee**

⑥ M23.35 Other meniscus derangements, posterior horn of lateral meniscus
☐ **SP** M23.351 Other meniscus derangements, posterior horn of lateral meniscus, right knee
☐ **SP** M23.352 Other meniscus derangements, posterior horn of lateral meniscus, left knee
☐ **IQ** M23.359 **Other meniscus derangements, posterior horn of lateral meniscus, unspecified knee**

⑥ M23.36 Other meniscus derangements, other lateral meniscus
☐ **SP** M23.361 Other meniscus derangements, other lateral meniscus, right knee
☐ **SP** M23.362 Other meniscus derangements, other lateral meniscus, left knee
☐ **IQ** M23.369 **Other meniscus derangements, other lateral meniscus, unspecified knee**

⑤ M23.4 Loose body in knee

☐ **IQ** M23.40 **Loose body in knee, unspecified knee**
☐ **SP** M23.41 Loose body in knee, right knee
☐ **SP** M23.42 Loose body in knee, left knee
⑤ M23.5 Chronic instability of knee
☐ **IQ** M23.50 **Chronic instability of knee, unspecified knee**
☐ **SP** M23.51 Chronic instability of knee, right knee
☐ **SP** M23.52 Chronic instability of knee, left knee
⑤ M23.6 Other spontaneous disruption of ligament(s) of knee
⑥ M23.60 **Other spontaneous disruption of unspecified ligament of knee**
☐ **SP** M23.601 **Other spontaneous disruption of unspecified ligament of right knee**
☐ **SP** M23.602 **Other spontaneous disruption of unspecified ligament of left knee**
☐ **IQ** M23.609 **Other spontaneous disruption of unspecified ligament of unspecified knee**

⑥ M23.61 Other spontaneous disruption of anterior cruciate ligament of knee
☐ **SP** M23.611 Other spontaneous disruption of anterior cruciate ligament of right knee
☐ **SP** M23.612 Other spontaneous disruption of anterior cruciate ligament of left knee
☐ **IQ** M23.619 **Other spontaneous disruption of anterior cruciate ligament of unspecified knee**

⑥ M23.62 Other spontaneous disruption of posterior cruciate ligament of knee
☐ **SP** M23.621 Other spontaneous disruption of posterior cruciate ligament of right knee
☐ **SP** M23.622 Other spontaneous disruption of posterior cruciate ligament of left knee
☐ **IQ** M23.629 **Other spontaneous disruption of posterior cruciate ligament of unspecified knee**

⑥ M23.63 Other spontaneous disruption of medial collateral ligament of knee
☐ **SP** M23.631 Other spontaneous disruption of medial collateral ligament of right knee
☐ **SP** M23.632 Other spontaneous disruption of medial collateral ligament of left knee
☐ **IQ** M23.639 **Other spontaneous disruption of medial collateral ligament of unspecified knee**

⑥ M23.64 Other spontaneous disruption of lateral collateral ligament of knee
☐ **SP** M23.641 Other spontaneous disruption of lateral collateral ligament of right knee
☐ **SP** M23.642 Other spontaneous disruption of lateral collateral ligament of left knee
☐ **IQ** M23.649 **Other spontaneous disruption of lateral collateral ligament of unspecified knee**

---

④ 4th digit required   ⑤ 5th digit required   ⑥ 6th digit required   ⑦ 7th digit required   ⑦ 7th digit placeholder   ✚ Additional code   ☐ Laterality

⑥ M23.67 Other spontaneous disruption of capsular ligament of knee

☐ SP M23.671 Other spontaneous disruption of capsular ligament of right knee

☐ SP M23.672 Other spontaneous disruption of capsular ligament of left knee

☐ IQ M23.679 Other spontaneous disruption of capsular ligament of unspecified knee

⑤ M23.8 Other internal derangements of knee
　　Laxity of ligament of knee
　　Snapping knee

⑥ M23.8X Other internal derangements of knee

☐ SP M23.8X1 Other internal derangements of right knee

☐ SP M23.8X2 Other internal derangements of left knee

☐ IQ M23.8X9 Other internal derangements of unspecified knee

⑤ M23.9 Unspecified internal derangement of knee

☐ IQ M23.90 Unspecified internal derangement of unspecified knee

☐ IQ M23.91 Unspecified internal derangement of right knee

☐ IQ M23.92 Unspecified internal derangement of left knee

④ M24 Other specific joint derangements

EXCLUDES 1　current injury - see injury of joint by body region

EXCLUDES 2　ganglion (M67.4)
　　snapping knee (M23.8-)
　　temporomandibular joint disorders (M26.6-)

CODING TIPS ✓　Categories M23 and M24 are used for patients who have old injuries. New injuries are coded with codes from Chapter 19.

⑤ M24.0 Loose body in joint

EXCLUDES 2　loose body in knee (M23.4)

IQ M24.00 Loose body in unspecified joint

⑥ M24.01 Loose body in shoulder

☐ SP M24.011 Loose body in right shoulder

☐ SP M24.012 Loose body in left shoulder

☐ IQ M24.019 Loose body in unspecified shoulder

⑥ M24.02 Loose body in elbow

☐ SP M24.021 Loose body in right elbow

☐ SP M24.022 Loose body in left elbow

☐ IQ M24.029 Loose body in unspecified elbow

⑥ M24.03 Loose body in wrist

☐ SP M24.031 Loose body in right wrist

☐ SP M24.032 Loose body in left wrist

☐ IQ M24.039 Loose body in unspecified wrist

⑥ M24.04 Loose body in finger joints

☐ SP M24.041 Loose body in right finger joint(s)

☐ SP M24.042 Loose body in left finger joint(s)

☐ IQ M24.049 Loose body in unspecified finger joint(s)

⑥ M24.05 Loose body in hip

☐ SP M24.051 Loose body in right hip

☐ SP M24.052 Loose body in left hip

☐ IQ M24.059 Loose body in unspecified hip

⑥ M24.07 Loose body in ankle and toe joints

☐ SP M24.071 Loose body in right ankle

☐ SP M24.072 Loose body in left ankle

☐ IQ M24.073 Loose body in unspecified ankle

☐ SP M24.074 Loose body in right toe joint(s)

☐ SP M24.075 Loose body in left toe joint(s)

☐ IQ M24.076 Loose body in unspecified toe joints

SP M24.08 Loose body, other site

⑤ M24.1 Other articular cartilage disorders

EXCLUDES 2　chondrocalcinosis (M11.1, M11.2-)
　　internal derangement of knee (M23.-)
　　metastatic calcification (E83.5)
　　ochronosis (E70.2)

IQ M24.10 Other articular cartilage disorders, unspecified site

⑥ M24.11 Other articular cartilage disorders, shoulder

☐ SP M24.111 Other articular cartilage disorders, right shoulder

☐ SP M24.112 Other articular cartilage disorders, left shoulder

☐ IQ M24.119 Other articular cartilage disorders, unspecified shoulder

⑥ M24.12 Other articular cartilage disorders, elbow

☐ SP M24.121 Other articular cartilage disorders, right elbow

☐ SP M24.122 Other articular cartilage disorders, left elbow

☐ IQ M24.129 Other articular cartilage disorders, unspecified elbow

⑥ M24.13 Other articular cartilage disorders, wrist

☐ SP M24.131 Other articular cartilage disorders, right wrist

☐ SP M24.132 Other articular cartilage disorders, left wrist

☐ IQ M24.139 Other articular cartilage disorders, unspecified wrist

⑥ M24.14 Other articular cartilage disorders, hand

☐ SP M24.141 Other articular cartilage disorders, right hand

☐ SP M24.142 Other articular cartilage disorders, left hand

☐ IQ M24.149 Other articular cartilage disorders, unspecified hand

⑥ M24.15 Other articular cartilage disorders, hip

☐ SP M24.151 Other articular cartilage disorders, right hip

☐ SP M24.152 Other articular cartilage disorders, left hip

☐ IQ M24.159 Other articular cartilage disorders, unspecified hip

⑥ M24.17 Other articular cartilage disorders, ankle and foot

☐ SP M24.171 Other articular cartilage disorders, right ankle

☐ SP M24.172 Other articular cartilage disorders, left ankle

★ New ▲ Revised Px Primary SP PDGM Px SL Low CoM SH High CoM IQ Quest. Encounter H Hospice non-cancer Dx　Unspecified　M Manifestation

DecisionHealth's FY 2020 Complete Home Health ICD-10-CM Diagnosis Coding Manual

1189

☐ **IQ** **M24.173** Other articular cartilage disorders, unspecified ankle

☐ **SP** **M24.174** Other articular cartilage disorders, right foot

☐ **SP** **M24.175** Other articular cartilage disorders, left foot

☐ **IQ** **M24.176** Other articular cartilage disorders, unspecified foot

▲ **5** **M24.2** **Disorder of ligament**
    Instability secondary to old ligament injury
    Ligamentous laxity NOS
    EXCLUDES 1 familial ligamentous laxity (M35.7)
    EXCLUDES 2 internal derangement of knee (M23.5-M23.8X9)

IQ **M24.20** Disorder of ligament, unspecified site

6 **M24.21** Disorder of ligament, shoulder

☐ **SP** **M24.211** Disorder of ligament, right shoulder

☐ **SP** **M24.212** Disorder of ligament, left shoulder

☐ **IQ** **M24.219** Disorder of ligament, unspecified shoulder

6 **M24.22** Disorder of ligament, elbow

☐ **SP** **M24.221** Disorder of ligament, right elbow

☐ **SP** **M24.222** Disorder of ligament, left elbow

☐ **IQ** **M24.229** Disorder of ligament, unspecified elbow

6 **M24.23** Disorder of ligament, wrist

☐ **SP** **M24.231** Disorder of ligament, right wrist

☐ **SP** **M24.232** Disorder of ligament, left wrist

☐ **IQ** **M24.239** Disorder of ligament, unspecified wrist

6 **M24.24** Disorder of ligament, hand

☐ **SP** **M24.241** Disorder of ligament, right hand

☐ **SP** **M24.242** Disorder of ligament, left hand

☐ **IQ** **M24.249** Disorder of ligament, unspecified hand

6 **M24.25** Disorder of ligament, hip

☐ **SP** **M24.251** Disorder of ligament, right hip

☐ **SP** **M24.252** Disorder of ligament, left hip

☐ **IQ** **M24.259** Disorder of ligament, unspecified hip

6 **M24.27** Disorder of ligament, ankle and foot

☐ **SP** **M24.271** Disorder of ligament, right ankle

☐ **SP** **M24.272** Disorder of ligament, left ankle

☐ **IQ** **M24.273** Disorder of ligament, unspecified ankle

☐ **SP** **M24.274** Disorder of ligament, right foot

☐ **SP** **M24.275** Disorder of ligament, left foot

☐ **IQ** **M24.276** Disorder of ligament, unspecified foot

SP **M24.28** Disorder of ligament, vertebrae

5 **M24.3** Pathological dislocation of joint, not elsewhere classified
    EXCLUDES 1 congenital dislocation or displacement of joint- see congenital malformations and deformations of the musculoskeletal system (Q65-Q79)

current injury - see injury of joints and ligaments by body region
recurrent dislocation of joint (M24.4-)

IQ **M24.30** Pathological dislocation of unspecified joint, not elsewhere classified

6 **M24.31** Pathological dislocation of shoulder, not elsewhere classified

☐ **SP** **M24.311** Pathological dislocation of right shoulder, not elsewhere classified

☐ **SP** **M24.312** Pathological dislocation of left shoulder, not elsewhere classified

☐ **IQ** **M24.319** Pathological dislocation of unspecified shoulder, not elsewhere classified

6 **M24.32** Pathological dislocation of elbow, not elsewhere classified

☐ **SP** **M24.321** Pathological dislocation of right elbow, not elsewhere classified

☐ **SP** **M24.322** Pathological dislocation of left elbow, not elsewhere classified

☐ **IQ** **M24.329** Pathological dislocation of unspecified elbow, not elsewhere classified

6 **M24.33** Pathological dislocation of wrist, not elsewhere classified

☐ **SP** **M24.331** Pathological dislocation of right wrist, not elsewhere classified

☐ **SP** **M24.332** Pathological dislocation of left wrist, not elsewhere classified

☐ **IQ** **M24.339** Pathological dislocation of unspecified wrist, not elsewhere classified

6 **M24.34** Pathological dislocation of hand, not elsewhere classified

☐ **SP** **M24.341** Pathological dislocation of right hand, not elsewhere classified

☐ **SP** **M24.342** Pathological dislocation of left hand, not elsewhere classified

☐ **IQ** **M24.349** Pathological dislocation of unspecified hand, not elsewhere classified

6 **M24.35** Pathological dislocation of hip, not elsewhere classified

☐ **SP** **M24.351** Pathological dislocation of right hip, not elsewhere classified

☐ **SP** **M24.352** Pathological dislocation of left hip, not elsewhere classified

☐ **IQ** **M24.359** Pathological dislocation of unspecified hip, not elsewhere classified

6 **M24.36** Pathological dislocation of knee, not elsewhere classified

☐ **SP** **M24.361** Pathological dislocation of right knee, not elsewhere classified

☐ **SP** **M24.362** Pathological dislocation of left knee, not elsewhere classified

☐ **IQ** **M24.369** Pathological dislocation of unspecified knee, not elsewhere classified

6 **M24.37** Pathological dislocation of ankle and foot, not elsewhere classified

☐ **SP** **M24.371** Pathological dislocation of right ankle, not elsewhere classified

4 4th digit required   **5** 5th digit required   **6** 6th digit required   **7** 7th digit required   **7** 7th digit placeholder   **+** Additional code   ☐ Laterality

1190   *DecisionHealth's* FY 2020 Complete Home Health ICD-10-CM Diagnosis Coding Manual

☐ 𝖲𝖯 **M24.372** Pathological dislocation of left ankle, not elsewhere classified

☐ 𝗜𝗤 **M24.373** Pathological dislocation of unspecified ankle, not elsewhere classified

☐ 𝖲𝖯 **M24.374** Pathological dislocation of right foot, not elsewhere classified

☐ 𝖲𝖯 **M24.375** Pathological dislocation of left foot, not elsewhere classified

☐ 𝗜𝗤 **M24.376** Pathological dislocation of unspecified foot, not elsewhere classified

⑤ **M24.4 Recurrent dislocation of joint**
Recurrent subluxation of joint
EXCLUDES 2 recurrent dislocation of patella (M22.0-M22.1)
recurrent vertebral dislocation (M43.3-, M43.4, M43.5-)

𝗜𝗤 **M24.40** Recurrent dislocation, unspecified joint

⑥ **M24.41** Recurrent dislocation, shoulder

☐ 𝖲𝖯 **M24.411** Recurrent dislocation, right shoulder

☐ 𝖲𝖯 **M24.412** Recurrent dislocation, left shoulder

☐ 𝗜𝗤 **M24.419** Recurrent dislocation, unspecified shoulder

⑥ **M24.42** Recurrent dislocation, elbow

☐ 𝖲𝖯 **M24.421** Recurrent dislocation, right elbow

☐ 𝖲𝖯 **M24.422** Recurrent dislocation, left elbow

☐ 𝗜𝗤 **M24.429** Recurrent dislocation, unspecified elbow

⑥ **M24.43** Recurrent dislocation, wrist

☐ 𝖲𝖯 **M24.431** Recurrent dislocation, right wrist

☐ 𝖲𝖯 **M24.432** Recurrent dislocation, left wrist

☐ 𝗜𝗤 **M24.439** Recurrent dislocation, unspecified wrist

⑥ **M24.44** Recurrent dislocation, hand and finger(s)

☐ 𝖲𝖯 **M24.441** Recurrent dislocation, right hand

☐ 𝖲𝖯 **M24.442** Recurrent dislocation, left hand

☐ 𝗜𝗤 **M24.443** Recurrent dislocation, unspecified hand

☐ 𝖲𝖯 **M24.444** Recurrent dislocation, right finger

☐ 𝖲𝖯 **M24.445** Recurrent dislocation, left finger

☐ 𝗜𝗤 **M24.446** Recurrent dislocation, unspecified finger

⑥ **M24.45** Recurrent dislocation, hip

☐ 𝖲𝖯 **M24.451** Recurrent dislocation, right hip

☐ 𝖲𝖯 **M24.452** Recurrent dislocation, left hip

☐ 𝗜𝗤 **M24.459** Recurrent dislocation, unspecified hip

⑥ **M24.46** Recurrent dislocation, knee

☐ 𝖲𝖯 **M24.461** Recurrent dislocation, right knee

☐ 𝖲𝖯 **M24.462** Recurrent dislocation, left knee

☐ 𝗜𝗤 **M24.469** Recurrent dislocation, unspecified knee

⑥ **M24.47** Recurrent dislocation, ankle, foot and toes

☐ 𝖲𝖯 **M24.471** Recurrent dislocation, right ankle

☐ 𝖲𝖯 **M24.472** Recurrent dislocation, left ankle

☐ 𝗜𝗤 **M24.473** Recurrent dislocation, unspecified ankle

☐ 𝖲𝖯 **M24.474** Recurrent dislocation, right foot

☐ 𝖲𝖯 **M24.475** Recurrent dislocation, left foot

☐ 𝗜𝗤 **M24.476** Recurrent dislocation, unspecified foot

☐ 𝖲𝖯 **M24.477** Recurrent dislocation, right toe(s)

☐ 𝖲𝖯 **M24.478** Recurrent dislocation, left toe(s)

☐ 𝗜𝗤 **M24.479** Recurrent dislocation, unspecified toe(s)

⑤ **M24.5 Contracture of joint**
EXCLUDES 1 contracture of muscle without contracture of joint (M62.4-)
contracture of tendon (sheath) without contracture of joint (M62.4-)
Dupuytren's contracture (M72.0)
EXCLUDES 2 acquired deformities of limbs (M20-M21)

𝗜𝗤 **M24.50** Contracture, unspecified joint

⑥ **M24.51** Contracture, shoulder

☐ 𝖲𝖯 **M24.511** Contracture, right shoulder

☐ 𝖲𝖯 **M24.512** Contracture, left shoulder

☐ 𝗜𝗤 **M24.519** Contracture, unspecified shoulder

⑥ **M24.52** Contracture, elbow

☐ 𝖲𝖯 **M24.521** Contracture, right elbow

☐ 𝖲𝖯 **M24.522** Contracture, left elbow

☐ 𝗜𝗤 **M24.529** Contracture, unspecified elbow

⑥ **M24.53** Contracture, wrist

☐ 𝖲𝖯 **M24.531** Contracture, right wrist

☐ 𝖲𝖯 **M24.532** Contracture, left wrist

☐ 𝗜𝗤 **M24.539** Contracture, unspecified wrist

⑥ **M24.54** Contracture, hand

☐ 𝖲𝖯 **M24.541** Contracture, right hand

☐ 𝖲𝖯 **M24.542** Contracture, left hand

☐ 𝗜𝗤 **M24.549** Contracture, unspecified hand

⑥ **M24.55** Contracture, hip

☐ 𝖲𝖯 **M24.551** Contracture, right hip

☐ 𝖲𝖯 **M24.552** Contracture, left hip

☐ 𝗜𝗤 **M24.559** Contracture, unspecified hip

⑥ **M24.56** Contracture, knee

☐ 𝖲𝖯 **M24.561** Contracture, right knee

☐ 𝖲𝖯 **M24.562** Contracture, left knee

☐ 𝗜𝗤 **M24.569** Contracture, unspecified knee

⑥ **M24.57** Contracture, ankle and foot

☐ 𝖲𝖯 **M24.571** Contracture, right ankle

☐ 𝖲𝖯 **M24.572** Contracture, left ankle

☐ 𝗜𝗤 **M24.573** Contracture, unspecified ankle

☐ 𝖲𝖯 **M24.574** Contracture, right foot

☐ 𝖲𝖯 **M24.575** Contracture, left foot

☐ 𝗜𝗤 **M24.576** Contracture, unspecified foot

⑤ **M24.6 Ankylosis of joint**
EXCLUDES 1 stiffness of joint without ankylosis (M25.6-)
EXCLUDES 2 spine (M43.2-)

★ New ▲ Revised Px Primary 𝖲𝖯 PDGM Px 𝖲𝖫 Low CoM 𝖲𝖧 High CoM 𝗜𝗤 Quest. Encounter 𝗛 Hospice non-cancer Dx Unspecified **M** *Manifestation*

DecisionHealth's FY 2020 Complete Home Health ICD-10-CM Diagnosis Coding Manual

1191

IQ M24.60   Ankylosis, unspecified joint

   6 M24.61   Ankylosis, shoulder

SP M24.611   Ankylosis, right shoulder

SP M24.612   Ankylosis, left shoulder

IQ M24.619   Ankylosis, unspecified shoulder

   6 M24.62   Ankylosis, elbow

SP M24.621   Ankylosis, right elbow

SP M24.622   Ankylosis, left elbow

IQ M24.629   Ankylosis, unspecified elbow

   6 M24.63   Ankylosis, wrist

SP M24.631   Ankylosis, right wrist

SP M24.632   Ankylosis, left wrist

IQ M24.639   Ankylosis, unspecified wrist

   6 M24.64   Ankylosis, hand

SP M24.641   Ankylosis, right hand

SP M24.642   Ankylosis, left hand

IQ M24.649   Ankylosis, unspecified hand

   6 M24.65   Ankylosis, hip

SP M24.651   Ankylosis, right hip

SP M24.652   Ankylosis, left hip

IQ M24.659   Ankylosis, unspecified hip

   6 M24.66   Ankylosis, knee

SP M24.661   Ankylosis, right knee

SP M24.662   Ankylosis, left knee

IQ M24.669   Ankylosis, unspecified knee

   6 M24.67   Ankylosis, ankle and foot

SP M24.671   Ankylosis, right ankle

SP M24.672   Ankylosis, left ankle

IQ M24.673   Ankylosis, unspecified ankle

SP M24.674   Ankylosis, right foot

SP M24.675   Ankylosis, left foot

IQ M24.676   Ankylosis, unspecified foot

SP M24.7   Protrusio acetabuli

5 M24.8   Other specific joint derangements, not elsewhere classified

    EXCLUDES 2   iliotibial band syndrome (M76.3)

IQ M24.80   Other specific joint derangements of unspecified joint, not elsewhere classified

   6 M24.81   Other specific joint derangements of shoulder, not elsewhere classified

SP M24.811   Other specific joint derangements of right shoulder, not elsewhere classified

SP M24.812   Other specific joint derangements of left shoulder, not elsewhere classified

IQ M24.819   Other specific joint derangements of unspecified shoulder, not elsewhere classified

   6 M24.82   Other specific joint derangements of elbow, not elsewhere classified

SP M24.821   Other specific joint derangements of right elbow, not elsewhere classified

SP M24.822   Other specific joint derangements of left elbow, not elsewhere classified

IQ M24.829   Other specific joint derangements of unspecified elbow, not elsewhere classified

   6 M24.83   Other specific joint derangements of wrist, not elsewhere classified

SP M24.831   Other specific joint derangements of right wrist, not elsewhere classified

SP M24.832   Other specific joint derangements of left wrist, not elsewhere classified

IQ M24.839   Other specific joint derangements of unspecified wrist, not elsewhere classified

   6 M24.84   Other specific joint derangements of hand, not elsewhere classified

SP M24.841   Other specific joint derangements of right hand, not elsewhere classified

SP M24.842   Other specific joint derangements of left hand, not elsewhere classified

IQ M24.849   Other specific joint derangements of unspecified hand, not elsewhere classified

   6 M24.85   Other specific joint derangements of hip, not elsewhere classified
     Irritable hip

SP M24.851   Other specific joint derangements of right hip, not elsewhere classified

SP M24.852   Other specific joint derangements of left hip, not elsewhere classified

IQ M24.859   Other specific joint derangements of unspecified hip, not elsewhere classified

   6 M24.87   Other specific joint derangements of ankle and foot, not elsewhere classified

SP M24.871   Other specific joint derangements of right ankle, not elsewhere classified

SP M24.872   Other specific joint derangements of left ankle, not elsewhere classified

IQ M24.873   Other specific joint derangements of unspecified ankle, not elsewhere classified

SP M24.874   Other specific joint derangements of right foot, not elsewhere classified

SP M24.875   Other specific joint derangements left foot, not elsewhere classified

IQ M24.876   Other specific joint derangements of unspecified foot, not elsewhere classified

IQ M24.9   Joint derangement, unspecified

4 M25   Other joint disorder, not elsewhere classified

    EXCLUDES 2   abnormality of gait and mobility (R26.-)
      acquired deformities of limb (M20-M21)
      calcification of bursa (M71.4-)
      calcification of shoulder (joint) (M75.3)

4 4th digit required   **5** 5th digit required   **6** 6th digit required   **7** 7th digit required   **7** 7th digit placeholder   **+** Additional code   **⊟** Laterality

1192   *DecisionHealth's* FY 2020 Complete Home Health ICD-10-CM Diagnosis Coding Manual

calcification of tendon
(M65.2-)
difficulty in walking (R26.2)
temporomandibular joint
disorder (M26.6-)

⑤ M25.0 Hemarthrosis

> EXCLUDES 1   current injury - see injury of
> joint by body region
> hemophilic arthropathy
> (M36.2)

IQ M25.00   Hemarthrosis, unspecified joint

⑥ M25.01 Hemarthrosis, shoulder

⊟ SP M25.011 Hemarthrosis, right shoulder

⊟ SP M25.012 Hemarthrosis, left shoulder

**⊟ IQ M25.019   Hemarthrosis, unspecified
shoulder**

⑥ M25.02 Hemarthrosis, elbow

⊟ SP M25.021 Hemarthrosis, right elbow

⊟ SP M25.022 Hemarthrosis, left elbow

⊟ IQ M25.029   Hemarthrosis, unspecified elbow

⑥ M25.03 Hemarthrosis, wrist

⊟ SP M25.031 Hemarthrosis, right wrist

⊟ SP M25.032 Hemarthrosis, left wrist

⊟ IQ M25.039   Hemarthrosis, unspecified wrist

⑥ M25.04 Hemarthrosis, hand

⊟ SP M25.041 Hemarthrosis, right hand

⊟ SP M25.042 Hemarthrosis, left hand

⊟ IQ M25.049   Hemarthrosis, unspecified hand

⑥ M25.05 Hemarthrosis, hip

⊟ SP M25.051 Hemarthrosis, right hip

⊟ SP M25.052 Hemarthrosis, left hip

⊟ IQ M25.059   Hemarthrosis, unspecified hip

⑥ M25.06 Hemarthrosis, knee

⊟ SP M25.061 Hemarthrosis, right knee

⊟ SP M25.062 Hemarthrosis, left knee

⊟ IQ M25.069   Hemarthrosis, unspecified knee

⑥ M25.07 Hemarthrosis, ankle and foot

⊟ SP M25.071 Hemarthrosis, right ankle

⊟ SP M25.072 Hemarthrosis, left ankle

⊟ IQ M25.073   Hemarthrosis, unspecified ankle

⊟ SP M25.074 Hemarthrosis, right foot

⊟ SP M25.075 Hemarthrosis, left foot

⊟ IQ M25.076   Hemarthrosis, unspecified foot

SP M25.08 Hemarthrosis, other specified site
Hemarthrosis, vertebrae

⑤ M25.1 Fistula of joint

IQ M25.10   Fistula, unspecified joint

⑥ M25.11 Fistula, shoulder

⊟ SP M25.111 Fistula, right shoulder

⊟ SP M25.112 Fistula, left shoulder

⊟ IQ M25.119   Fistula, unspecified shoulder

⑥ M25.12 Fistula, elbow

⊟ SP M25.121 Fistula, right elbow

⊟ SP M25.122 Fistula, left elbow

⊟ IQ M25.129   Fistula, unspecified elbow

⑥ M25.13 Fistula, wrist

⊟ SP M25.131 Fistula, right wrist

⊟ SP M25.132 Fistula, left wrist

⊟ IQ M25.139   Fistula, unspecified wrist

⑥ M25.14 Fistula, hand

⊟ SP M25.141 Fistula, right hand

⊟ SP M25.142 Fistula, left hand

⊟ IQ M25.149   Fistula, unspecified hand

⑥ M25.15 Fistula, hip

⊟ SP M25.151 Fistula, right hip

⊟ SP M25.152 Fistula, left hip

⊟ IQ M25.159   Fistula, unspecified hip

⑥ M25.16 Fistula, knee

⊟ SP M25.161 Fistula, right knee

⊟ SP M25.162 Fistula, left knee

⊟ IQ M25.169   Fistula, unspecified knee

⑥ M25.17 Fistula, ankle and foot

⊟ SP M25.171 Fistula, right ankle

⊟ SP M25.172 Fistula, left ankle

⊟ IQ M25.173   Fistula, unspecified ankle

⊟ SP M25.174 Fistula, right foot

⊟ SP M25.175 Fistula, left foot

⊟ IQ M25.176   Fistula, unspecified foot

SP M25.18 Fistula, other specified site
Fistula, vertebrae

⑤ M25.2 Flail joint

IQ M25.20   Flail joint, unspecified joint

⑥ M25.21 Flail joint, shoulder

⊟ SP M25.211 Flail joint, right shoulder

⊟ SP M25.212 Flail joint, left shoulder

⊟ IQ M25.219   Flail joint, unspecified shoulder

⑥ M25.22 Flail joint, elbow

⊟ SP M25.221 Flail joint, right elbow

⊟ SP M25.222 Flail joint, left elbow

⊟ IQ M25.229   Flail joint, unspecified elbow

⑥ M25.23 Flail joint, wrist

⊟ SP M25.231 Flail joint, right wrist

⊟ SP M25.232 Flail joint, left wrist

⊟ IQ M25.239   Flail joint, unspecified wrist

⑥ M25.24 Flail joint, hand

⊟ SP M25.241 Flail joint, right hand

⊟ SP M25.242 Flail joint, left hand

⊟ IQ M25.249   Flail joint, unspecified hand

⑥ M25.25 Flail joint, hip

⊟ SP M25.251 Flail joint, right hip

⊟ SP M25.252 Flail joint, left hip

⊟ IQ M25.259   Flail joint, unspecified hip

⑥ M25.26 Flail joint, knee

⊟ SP M25.261 Flail joint, right knee

⊟ SP M25.262 Flail joint, left knee

⊟ IQ M25.269   Flail joint, unspecified knee

⑥ M25.27 Flail joint, ankle and foot

⊟ SP M25.271 Flail joint, right ankle and foot

⊟ SP M25.272 Flail joint, left ankle and foot

**⊟ IQ M25.279   Flail joint, unspecified ankle and
foot**

SP M25.28 Flail joint, other site

⑤ M25.3 Other instability of joint

★ New ▲ Revised Px Primary SP PDGM Px SL Low CoM SH High CoM IQ Quest. Encounter H Hospice non-cancer Dx   Unspecified   M *Manifestation*

DecisionHealth's FY 2020 Complete Home Health ICD-10-CM Diagnosis Coding Manual   1193

EXCLUDES 1 instability of joint secondary to old ligament injury (M24.2-)
instability of joint secondary to removal of joint prosthesis (M96.8-)

EXCLUDES 2 spinal instabilities (M53.2-)

IQ M25.30 Other instability, unspecified joint

6 M25.31 Other instability, shoulder

SP M25.311 Other instability, right shoulder

SP M25.312 Other instability, left shoulder

IQ M25.319 Other instability, unspecified shoulder

6 M25.32 Other instability, elbow

SP M25.321 Other instability, right elbow

SP M25.322 Other instability, left elbow

IQ M25.329 Other instability, unspecified elbow

6 M25.33 Other instability, wrist

SP M25.331 Other instability, right wrist

SP M25.332 Other instability, left wrist

IQ M25.339 Other instability, unspecified wrist

6 M25.34 Other instability, hand

SP M25.341 Other instability, right hand

SP M25.342 Other instability, left hand

IQ M25.349 Other instability, unspecified hand

6 M25.35 Other instability, hip

SP M25.351 Other instability, right hip

SP M25.352 Other instability, left hip

IQ M25.359 Other instability, unspecified hip

6 M25.36 Other instability, knee

SP M25.361 Other instability, right knee

SP M25.362 Other instability, left knee

IQ M25.369 Other instability, unspecified knee

6 M25.37 Other instability, ankle and foot

SP M25.371 Other instability, right ankle

SP M25.372 Other instability, left ankle

IQ M25.373 Other instability, unspecified ankle

SP M25.374 Other instability, right foot

SP M25.375 Other instability, left foot

IQ M25.376 Other instability, unspecified foot

5 M25.4 Effusion of joint

EXCLUDES 1 hydrarthrosis in yaws (A66.6)
intermittent hydrarthrosis (M12.4-)
other infective (teno) synovitis (M65.1-)

IQ M25.40 Effusion, unspecified joint

6 M25.41 Effusion, shoulder

SP M25.411 Effusion, right shoulder

SP M25.412 Effusion, left shoulder

IQ M25.419 Effusion, unspecified shoulder

6 M25.42 Effusion, elbow

SP M25.421 Effusion, right elbow

SP M25.422 Effusion, left elbow

IQ M25.429 Effusion, unspecified elbow

6 M25.43 Effusion, wrist

SP M25.431 Effusion, right wrist

SP M25.432 Effusion, left wrist

IQ M25.439 Effusion, unspecified wrist

6 M25.44 Effusion, hand

SP M25.441 Effusion, right hand

SP M25.442 Effusion, left hand

IQ M25.449 Effusion, unspecified hand

6 M25.45 Effusion, hip

SP M25.451 Effusion, right hip

SP M25.452 Effusion, left hip

IQ M25.459 Effusion, unspecified hip

6 M25.46 Effusion, knee

SP M25.461 Effusion, right knee

SP M25.462 Effusion, left knee

IQ M25.469 Effusion, unspecified knee

6 M25.47 Effusion, ankle and foot

SP M25.471 Effusion, right ankle

SP M25.472 Effusion, left ankle

IQ M25.473 Effusion, unspecified ankle

SP M25.474 Effusion, right foot

SP M25.475 Effusion, left foot

IQ M25.476 Effusion, unspecified foot

SP M25.48 Effusion, other site

5 M25.5 Pain in joint

EXCLUDES 2 pain in hand (M79.64-)
pain in fingers (M79.64-)
pain in foot (M79.67-)
pain in limb (M79.6-)
pain in toes (M79.67-)

CODING TIPS ✓ These codes should be used when 1) the cause of the pain is unknown; 2) the pain is a sequela of an injury; or 3) in conjunction with a G89 code. Do not use these codes with conditions like arthritis.

IQ M25.50 Pain in unspecified joint

6 M25.51 Pain in shoulder

IQ M25.511 Pain in right shoulder

IQ M25.512 Pain in left shoulder

IQ M25.519 Pain in unspecified shoulder

6 M25.52 Pain in elbow

IQ M25.521 Pain in right elbow

IQ M25.522 Pain in left elbow

IQ M25.529 Pain in unspecified elbow

6 M25.53 Pain in wrist

IQ M25.531 Pain in right wrist

IQ M25.532 Pain in left wrist

IQ M25.539 Pain in unspecified wrist

6 M25.54 Pain in joints of hand

IQ M25.541 Pain in joints of right hand

IQ M25.542 Pain in joints of left hand

IQ M25.549 Pain in joints of unspecified hand
Pain in joints of hand NOS

6 M25.55 Pain in hip

IQ M25.551 Pain in right hip

---

4 4th digit required   5 5th digit required   6 6th digit required   7 7th digit required   7 7th digit placeholder   + Additional code   Laterality

1194   *DecisionHealth's* FY 2020 Complete Home Health ICD-10-CM Diagnosis Coding Manual

☐ **IQ** M25.552 Pain in left hip

☐ **IQ** M25.559 Pain in unspecified hip

⑥ M25.56 Pain in knee

☐ **IQ** M25.561 Pain in right knee

☐ **IQ** M25.562 Pain in left knee

☐ **IQ** M25.569 Pain in unspecified knee

⑥ M25.57 Pain in ankle and joints of foot

☐ **IQ** M25.571 Pain in right ankle and joints of right foot

☐ **IQ** M25.572 Pain in left ankle and joints of left foot

☐ **IQ** M25.579 Pain in unspecified ankle and joints of unspecified foot

⑤ M25.6 Stiffness of joint, not elsewhere classified

> **EXCLUDES 1** ankylosis of joint (M24.6-)
> contracture of joint (M24.5-)
>
> **CODING TIPS ✓** These codes should be used when 1) the cause of the stiffness is unknown; 2) the stiffness is a sequela of an injury. Do not use these codes with conditions like arthritis.

IQ M25.60 Stiffness of unspecified joint, not elsewhere classified

⑥ M25.61 Stiffness of shoulder, not elsewhere classified

☐ **IQ** M25.611 Stiffness of right shoulder, not elsewhere classified

☐ **IQ** M25.612 Stiffness of left shoulder, not elsewhere classified

☐ **IQ** M25.619 Stiffness of unspecified shoulder, not elsewhere classified

⑥ M25.62 Stiffness of elbow, not elsewhere classified

☐ **IQ** M25.621 Stiffness of right elbow, not elsewhere classified

☐ **IQ** M25.622 Stiffness of left elbow, not elsewhere classified

☐ **IQ** M25.629 Stiffness of unspecified elbow, not elsewhere classified

⑥ M25.63 Stiffness of wrist, not elsewhere classified

☐ **IQ** M25.631 Stiffness of right wrist, not elsewhere classified

☐ **IQ** M25.632 Stiffness of left wrist, not elsewhere classified

☐ **IQ** M25.639 Stiffness of unspecified wrist, not elsewhere classified

⑥ M25.64 Stiffness of hand, not elsewhere classified

☐ **IQ** M25.641 Stiffness of right hand, not elsewhere classified

☐ **IQ** M25.642 Stiffness of left hand, not elsewhere classified

☐ **IQ** M25.649 Stiffness of unspecified hand, not elsewhere classified

⑥ M25.65 Stiffness of hip, not elsewhere classified

☐ **IQ** M25.651 Stiffness of right hip, not elsewhere classified

☐ **IQ** M25.652 Stiffness of left hip, not elsewhere classified

☐ **IQ** M25.659 Stiffness of unspecified hip, not elsewhere classified

⑥ M25.66 Stiffness of knee, not elsewhere classified

☐ **IQ** M25.661 Stiffness of right knee, not elsewhere classified

☐ **IQ** M25.662 Stiffness of left knee, not elsewhere classified

☐ **IQ** M25.669 Stiffness of unspecified knee, not elsewhere classified

⑥ M25.67 Stiffness of ankle and foot, not elsewhere classified

☐ **IQ** M25.671 Stiffness of right ankle, not elsewhere classified

☐ **IQ** M25.672 Stiffness of left ankle, not elsewhere classified

☐ **IQ** M25.673 Stiffness of unspecified ankle, not elsewhere classified

☐ **IQ** M25.674 Stiffness of right foot, not elsewhere classified

☐ **IQ** M25.675 Stiffness of left foot, not elsewhere classified

☐ **IQ** M25.676 Stiffness of unspecified foot, not elsewhere classified

⑤ M25.7 Osteophyte

IQ M25.70 Osteophyte, unspecified joint

⑥ M25.71 Osteophyte, shoulder

☐ **SP** M25.711 Osteophyte, right shoulder

☐ **SP** M25.712 Osteophyte, left shoulder

☐ **IQ** M25.719 Osteophyte, unspecified shoulder

⑥ M25.72 Osteophyte, elbow

☐ **SP** M25.721 Osteophyte, right elbow

☐ **SP** M25.722 Osteophyte, left elbow

☐ **IQ** M25.729 Osteophyte, unspecified elbow

⑥ M25.73 Osteophyte, wrist

☐ **SP** M25.731 Osteophyte, right wrist

☐ **SP** M25.732 Osteophyte, left wrist

☐ **IQ** M25.739 Osteophyte, unspecified wrist

⑥ M25.74 Osteophyte, hand

☐ **SP** M25.741 Osteophyte, right hand

☐ **SP** M25.742 Osteophyte, left hand

☐ **IQ** M25.749 Osteophyte, unspecified hand

⑥ M25.75 Osteophyte, hip

☐ **SP** M25.751 Osteophyte, right hip

☐ **SP** M25.752 Osteophyte, left hip

☐ **IQ** M25.759 Osteophyte, unspecified hip

⑥ M25.76 Osteophyte, knee

☐ **SP** M25.761 Osteophyte, right knee

☐ **SP** M25.762 Osteophyte, left knee

☐ **IQ** M25.769 Osteophyte, unspecified knee

⑥ M25.77 Osteophyte, ankle and foot

☐ **SP** M25.771 Osteophyte, right ankle

☐ **SP** M25.772 Osteophyte, left ankle

☐ **IQ** M25.773 Osteophyte, unspecified ankle

☐ **SP** M25.774 Osteophyte, right foot

☐ **SP** M25.775 Osteophyte, left foot

☐ **IQ** M25.776 Osteophyte, unspecified foot

SP M25.78 Osteophyte, vertebrae

⑤ M25.8 Other specified joint disorders

IQ M25.80 Other specified joint disorders, unspecified joint

★ New ▲ Revised Px Primary **SP** PDGM Px **SL** Low CoM **SH** High CoM **IQ** Quest. Encounter **H** Hospice non-cancer Dx Unspecified **M** *Manifestation*

DecisionHealth's FY 2020 Complete Home Health ICD-10-CM Diagnosis Coding Manual

1195

Chapter 13

M00-M99

6 **M25.81** Other specified joint disorders, shoulder

SP **M25.811** Other specified joint disorders, right shoulder

SP **M25.812** Other specified joint disorders, left shoulder

IQ **M25.819** Other specified joint disorders, unspecified shoulder

6 **M25.82** Other specified joint disorders, elbow

SP **M25.821** Other specified joint disorders, right elbow

SP **M25.822** Other specified joint disorders, left elbow

IQ **M25.829** Other specified joint disorders, unspecified elbow

6 **M25.83** Other specified joint disorders, wrist

SP **M25.831** Other specified joint disorders, right wrist

SP **M25.832** Other specified joint disorders, left wrist

IQ **M25.839** Other specified joint disorders, unspecified wrist

6 **M25.84** Other specified joint disorders, hand

SP **M25.841** Other specified joint disorders, right hand

SP **M25.842** Other specified joint disorders, left hand

IQ **M25.849** Other specified joint disorders, unspecified hand

6 **M25.85** Other specified joint disorders, hip

SP **M25.851** Other specified joint disorders, right hip

SP **M25.852** Other specified joint disorders, left hip

IQ **M25.859** Other specified joint disorders, unspecified hip

6 **M25.86** Other specified joint disorders, knee

SP **M25.861** Other specified joint disorders, right knee

SP **M25.862** Other specified joint disorders, left knee

IQ **M25.869** Other specified joint disorders, unspecified knee

6 **M25.87** Other specified joint disorders, ankle and foot

SP **M25.871** Other specified joint disorders, right ankle and foot

SP **M25.872** Other specified joint disorders, left ankle and foot

IQ **M25.879** Other specified joint disorders, unspecified ankle and foot

IQ **M25.9** Joint disorder, unspecified

Dentofacial anomalies [including malocclusion] and other disorders of jaw (M26-M27)

EXCLUDES 1　hemifacial atrophy or hypertrophy (Q67.4) unilateral condylar hyperplasia or hypoplasia (M27.8)

4 **M26** Dentofacial anomalies [including malocclusion]

5 **M26.0** Major anomalies of jaw size

EXCLUDES 1　acromegaly (E22.0)

Robin's syndrome (Q87.0)

IQ **M26.00** Unspecified anomaly of jaw size

IQ **M26.01** Maxillary hyperplasia

IQ **M26.02** Maxillary hypoplasia

IQ **M26.03** Mandibular hyperplasia

IQ **M26.04** Mandibular hypoplasia

IQ **M26.05** Macrogenia

DEFINITION　　Abnormally large chin.

IQ **M26.06** Microgenia

IQ **M26.07** Excessive tuberosity of jaw
Entire maxillary tuberosity

IQ **M26.09** Other specified anomalies of jaw size

5 **M26.1** Anomalies of jaw-cranial base relationship

IQ **M26.10** Unspecified anomaly of jaw-cranial base relationship

IQ **M26.11** Maxillary asymmetry

IQ **M26.12** Other jaw asymmetry

IQ **M26.19** Other specified anomalies of jaw-cranial base relationship

5 **M26.2** Anomalies of dental arch relationship

IQ **M26.20** Unspecified anomaly of dental arch relationship

6 **M26.21** Malocclusion, Angle's class

IQ **M26.211** Malocclusion, Angle's class I
Neutro-occlusion

IQ **M26.212** Malocclusion, Angle's class II
Disto-occlusion Division I
Disto-occlusion Division II

IQ **M26.213** Malocclusion, Angle's class III
Mesio-occlusion

IQ **M26.219** Malocclusion, Angle's class, unspecified

6 **M26.22** Open occlusal relationship

IQ **M26.220** Open anterior occlusal relationship
Anterior open bite

IQ **M26.221** Open posterior occlusal relationship
Posterior open bite

IQ **M26.23** Excessive horizontal overlap
Excessive horizontal overjet

IQ **M26.24** Reverse articulation
Crossbite (anterior) (posterior)

IQ **M26.25** Anomalies of interarch distance

IQ **M26.29** Other anomalies of dental arch relationship
Midline deviation of dental arch
Overbite (excessive) deep
Overbite (excessive) horizontal
Overbite (excessive) vertical
Posterior lingual occlusion of mandibular teeth

5 **M26.3** Anomalies of tooth position of fully erupted tooth or teeth

EXCLUDES 2　embedded and impacted teeth (K01.-)

IQ **M26.30** Unspecified anomaly of tooth position of fully erupted tooth or teeth
Abnormal spacing of fully erupted tooth or teeth NOS
Displacement of fully erupted tooth or teeth NOS

---

4 4th digit required　　5 5th digit required　　6 6th digit required　　7 7th digit required　　7 7th digit placeholder　　+ Additional code　　Laterality

1196　　　　　*DecisionHealth's* FY 2020 Complete Home Health ICD-10-CM Diagnosis Coding Manual

Transposition of fully erupted tooth or teeth NOS

[IQ] M26.31 Crowding of fully erupted teeth

[IQ] M26.32 Excessive spacing of fully erupted teeth
Diastema of fully erupted tooth or teeth NOS

[IQ] M26.33 Horizontal displacement of fully erupted tooth or teeth
Tipped tooth or teeth
Tipping of fully erupted tooth

[IQ] M26.34 Vertical displacement of fully erupted tooth or teeth
Extruded tooth
Infraeruption of tooth or teeth
Supraeruption of tooth or teeth

[IQ] M26.35 Rotation of fully erupted tooth or teeth

[IQ] M26.36 Insufficient interocclusal distance of fully erupted teeth (ridge)
Lack of adequate intermaxillary vertical dimension of fully erupted teeth

[IQ] M26.37 Excessive interocclusal distance of fully erupted teeth
Excessive intermaxillary vertical dimension of fully erupted teeth
Loss of occlusal vertical dimension of fully erupted teeth

[IQ] M26.39 Other anomalies of tooth position of fully erupted tooth or teeth

[IQ] M26.4 Malocclusion, unspecified

[5] M26.5 Dentofacial functional abnormalities
EXCLUDES 1   bruxism (F45.8)
teeth-grinding NOS (F45.8)

[IQ] M26.50 Dentofacial functional abnormalities, unspecified

[IQ] M26.51 Abnormal jaw closure

[IQ] M26.52 Limited mandibular range of motion

[IQ] M26.53 Deviation in opening and closing of the mandible

[IQ] M26.54 Insufficient anterior guidance
Insufficient anterior occlusal guidance

[IQ] M26.55 Centric occlusion maximum intercuspation discrepancy
EXCLUDES 1   centric occlusion NOS (M26.59)

[IQ] M26.56 Non-working side interference
Balancing side interference

[IQ] M26.57 Lack of posterior occlusal support

[IQ] M26.59 Other dentofacial functional abnormalities
Centric occlusion (of teeth) NOS
Malocclusion due to abnormal swallowing
Malocclusion due to mouth breathing
Malocclusion due to tongue, lip or finger habits

[5] M26.6 Temporomandibular joint disorders
EXCLUDES 2   current temporomandibular joint dislocation (S03.0)
current temporomandibular joint sprain (S03.4)

[6] M26.60 Temporomandibular joint disorder, unspecified

[IQ] M26.601 Right temporomandibular joint disorder, unspecified

[IQ] M26.602 Left temporomandibular joint disorder, unspecified

[IQ] M26.603 Bilateral temporomandibular joint disorder, unspecified

[IQ] M26.609 Unspecified temporomandibular joint disorder, unspecified side
Temporomandibular joint disorder NOS

[6] M26.61 Adhesions and ankylosis of temporomandibular joint

[IQ] M26.611 Adhesions and ankylosis of right temporomandibular joint

[IQ] M26.612 Adhesions and ankylosis of left temporomandibular joint

[IQ] M26.613 Adhesions and ankylosis of bilateral temporomandibular joint

[IQ] M26.619 Adhesions and ankylosis of temporomandibular joint, unspecified side

[6] M26.62 Arthralgia of temporomandibular joint

[IQ] M26.621 Arthralgia of right temporomandibular joint

[IQ] M26.622 Arthralgia of left temporomandibular joint

[IQ] M26.623 Arthralgia of bilateral temporomandibular joint

[IQ] M26.629 Arthralgia of temporomandibular joint, unspecified side

[6] M26.63 Articular disc disorder of temporomandibular joint

[IQ] M26.631 Articular disc disorder of right temporomandibular joint

[IQ] M26.632 Articular disc disorder of left temporomandibular joint

[IQ] M26.633 Articular disc disorder of bilateral temporomandibular joint

[IQ] M26.639 Articular disc disorder of temporomandibular joint, unspecified side

[IQ] M26.69 Other specified disorders of temporomandibular joint

[5] M26.7 Dental alveolar anomalies

[IQ] M26.70 Unspecified alveolar anomaly

[IQ] M26.71 Alveolar maxillary hyperplasia

[IQ] M26.72 Alveolar mandibular hyperplasia

[IQ] M26.73 Alveolar maxillary hypoplasia

[IQ] M26.74 Alveolar mandibular hypoplasia

[IQ] M26.79 Other specified alveolar anomalies

[5] M26.8 Other dentofacial anomalies

[IQ] M26.81 Anterior soft tissue impingement
Anterior soft tissue impingement on teeth

[IQ] M26.82 Posterior soft tissue impingement
Posterior soft tissue impingement on teeth

[IQ] M26.89 Other dentofacial anomalies

[IQ] M26.9 Dentofacial anomaly, unspecified

[4] M27 Other diseases of jaws

[IQ] M27.0 Developmental disorders of jaws
Latent bone cyst of jaw
Stafne's cyst
Torus mandibularis
Torus palatinus

★ New ▲ Revised Px Primary SP PDGM Px SL Low CoM SH High CoM IQ Quest. Encounter H Hospice non-cancer Dx   Unspecified   M *Manifestation*

DecisionHealth's FY 2020 Complete Home Health ICD-10-CM Diagnosis Coding Manual

1197

IQ M27.1 Giant cell granuloma, central
Giant cell granuloma NOS
> **EXCLUDES 1** peripheral giant cell
> granuloma (K06.8)

SP ➕ M27.2 Inflammatory conditions of jaws
Osteitis of jaw(s)
Osteomyelitis (neonatal) jaw(s)
Osteoradionecrosis jaw(s)
Periostitis jaw(s)
Sequestrum of jaw bone
Use additional code (W88-W90, X39.0) to
identify radiation, if radiation-induced
> **EXCLUDES 2** osteonecrosis of jaw due to
> drug (M87.180)

IQ M27.3 Alveolitis of jaws
Alveolar osteitis
Dry socket
> **DEFINITION** Inflammation of the tooth
sockets.

5 M27.4 Other and unspecified cysts of jaw
> **EXCLUDES 1** cysts of oral region (K09.-)
> latent bone cyst of jaw
> (M27.0)
> Stafne's cyst (M27.0)

IQ M27.40 Unspecified cyst of jaw
Cyst of jaw NOS

IQ M27.49 Other cysts of jaw
Aneurysmal cyst of jaw
Hemorrhagic cyst of jaw
Traumatic cyst of jaw

**5 M27.5 Periradicular pathology associated with
previous endodontic treatment**

**IQ M27.51 Perforation of root canal space due
to endodontic treatment**

IQ M27.52 Endodontic overfill

IQ M27.53 Endodontic underfill

**IQ M27.59 Other periradicular pathology
associated with previous endodontic
treatment**

5 M27.6 Endosseous dental implant failure

**IQ M27.61 Osseointegration failure of dental
implant**
Hemorrhagic complications of dental
implant placement
Iatrogenic osseointegration failure of
dental implant
Osseointegration failure of dental
implant due to complications of
systemic disease
Osseointegration failure of dental
implant due to poor bone quality
Pre-integration failure of dental
implant NOS
Pre-osseointegration failure of dental
implant

**IQ M27.62 Post-osseointegration biological
failure of dental implant**
Failure of dental implant due to lack of
attached gingiva
Failure of dental implant due to
occlusal trauma (caused by poor
prosthetic design)
Failure of dental implant due to
parafunctional habits
Failure of dental implant due to
periodontal infection (peri-
implantitis)

Failure of dental implant due to poor
oral hygiene
Iatrogenic post-osseointegration failure
of dental implant
Post-osseointegration failure of dental
implant due to complications of
systemic disease

**IQ M27.63 Post-osseointegration mechanical
failure of dental implant**
Failure of dental prosthesis causing
loss of dental implant
Fracture of dental implant
> **EXCLUDES 2** cracked tooth (K03.81)
> fractured dental
> restorative material
> with loss of material
> (K08.531)
> fractured dental
> restorative material
> without loss of material
> (K08.530)
> fractured tooth (S02.5)

**IQ M27.69 Other endosseous dental implant
failure**
Dental implant failure NOS

IQ M27.8 Other specified diseases of jaws
Cherubism
Exostosis
Fibrous dysplasia
Unilateral condylar hyperplasia
Unilateral condylar hypoplasia
> **EXCLUDES 1** jaw pain (R68.84)

IQ M27.9 Disease of jaws, unspecified

Systemic connective tissue disorders (M30-M36)

> **INCLUDES** autoimmune disease NOS
> collagen (vascular) disease NOS
> systemic autoimmune disease
> systemic collagen (vascular) disease
> **EXCLUDES 1** autoimmune disease, single organ or single cell-
> type -code to relevant condition category

---

4 4th digit required   **5** 5th digit required   **6** 6th digit required   **7** 7th digit required   **7** 7th digit placeholder   **➕** Additional code   **⊟** Laterality

Muscle

Medullary bone

Effusion
Osteoarthritis

M30 Polyarteritis nodosa and related conditions
> **EXCLUDES 1** microscopic polyarteritis (M31.7)

SP M30.0 Polyarteritis nodosa
> **DEFINITION** The body's immune system mistakenly attacks small and medium-sized blood vessels, resulting in tissue death.

SP M30.1 Polyarteritis with lung involvement [Churg-Strauss]
Allergic granulomatous angiitis

SP M30.2 Juvenile polyarteritis

SP M30.3 Mucocutaneous lymph node syndrome [Kawasaki]

SP M30.8 Other conditions related to polyarteritis nodosa
Polyangiitis overlap syndrome

M31 Other necrotizing vasculopathies

SP M31.0 Hypersensitivity angiitis
Goodpasture's syndrome

SP M31.1 Thrombotic microangiopathy
Thrombotic thrombocytopenic purpura

SP M31.2 Lethal midline granuloma
> **DEFINITION** Tumor associated with infection that appears in the nose or sinuses that may be fatal if not diagnosed and treated in time.

M31.3 Wegener's granulomatosis
Necrotizing respiratory granulomatosis

SP M31.30 Wegener's granulomatosis without renal involvement
Wegener's granulomatosis NOS

SP M31.31 Wegener's granulomatosis with renal involvement

SP M31.4 Aortic arch syndrome [Takayasu]

SP M31.5 Giant cell arteritis with polymyalgia rheumatica

SP M31.6 Other giant cell arteritis

SP M31.7 Microscopic polyangiitis
Microscopic polyarteritis
> **EXCLUDES 1** polyarteritis nodosa (M30.0)

SP M31.8 Other specified necrotizing vasculopathies
Hypocomplementemic vasculitis
Septic vasculitis

SP M31.9 Necrotizing vasculopathy, unspecified

M32 Systemic lupus erythematosus (SLE)
> **EXCLUDES 1** lupus erythematosus (discoid) (NOS) (L93.0)
> **CODING TIPS ✓** Do not assign a code from category M32.- unless lupus is specified as systemic.

SP ✛ M32.0 Drug-induced systemic lupus erythematosus
Use additional code for adverse effect, if applicable, to identify drug (T36-T50 with fifth or sixth character 5)
> **CODING TIPS ✓** Assign code M32.0 only when documentation clearly confirms that the systemic lupus diagnosis is secondary to the effects of a drug. An additional code from categories T36-T50 should be used to identify the drug.

M32.1 Systemic lupus erythematosus with organ or system involvement

SP M32.10 Systemic lupus erythematosus, organ or system involvement unspecified

SP M32.11 Endocarditis in systemic lupus erythematosus
Libman-Sacks disease

SP M32.12 Pericarditis in systemic lupus erythematosus
Lupus pericarditis

SP M32.13 Lung involvement in systemic lupus erythematosus
Pleural effusion due to systemic lupus erythematosus

SP M32.14 Glomerular disease in systemic lupus erythematosus
Lupus renal disease NOS

SP M32.15 Tubulo-interstitial nephropathy in systemic lupus erythematosus

SP M32.19 Other organ or system involvement in systemic lupus erythematosus

SP M32.8 Other forms of systemic lupus erythematosus

SP M32.9 Systemic lupus erythematosus, unspecified
SLE NOS
Systemic lupus erythematosus NOS
Systemic lupus erythematosus without organ involvement

M33 Dermatopolymyositis

M33.0 Juvenile dermatomyositis

SP M33.00 Juvenile dermatomyositis, organ involvement unspecified

SP M33.01 Juvenile dermatomyositis with respiratory involvement

SP M33.02 Juvenile dermatomyositis with myopathy

SP M33.03 Juvenile dermatomyositis without myopathy

SP M33.09 Juvenile dermatomyositis with other organ involvement

M33.1 Other dermatomyositis
Adult dermatomyositis

★ New ▲ Revised **Px** Primary **SP** PDGM Px **SL** Low CoM **SH** High CoM **IQ** Quest. Encounter **H** Hospice non-cancer Dx | Unspecified | **M** *Manifestation*

DecisionHealth's FY 2020 Complete Home Health ICD-10-CM Diagnosis Coding Manual

1199

SP M33.10 Other dermatomyositis, organ involvement unspecified

SP M33.11 Other dermatomyositis with respiratory involvement

SP M33.12 Other dermatomyositis with myopathy

SP M33.13 Other dermatomyositis without myopathy
Dermatomyositis NOS

SP M33.19 Other dermatomyositis with other organ involvement

5 M33.2 Polymyositis

SP M33.20 Polymyositis, organ involvement unspecified

SP M33.21 Polymyositis with respiratory involvement

SP M33.22 Polymyositis with myopathy

SP M33.29 Polymyositis with other organ involvement

5 M33.9 Dermatopolymyositis, unspecified

SP M33.90 Dermatopolymyositis, unspecified, organ involvement unspecified

SP M33.91 Dermatopolymyositis, unspecified with respiratory involvement

SP M33.92 Dermatopolymyositis, unspecified with myopathy

SP M33.93 Dermatopolymyositis, unspecified without myopathy

SP M33.99 Dermatopolymyositis, unspecified with other organ involvement

▲ 4 M34 Systemic sclerosis [scleroderma]
EXCLUDES 1   circumscribed scleroderma (L94.0)
neonatal scleroderma (P83.88)

SP M34.0 Progressive systemic sclerosis

SP M34.1 CR(E)ST syndrome
Combination of calcinosis, Raynaud's phenomenon, esophageal dysfunction, sclerodactyly, telangiectasia

SP ✚ M34.2 Systemic sclerosis induced by drug and chemical
Code first:
poisoning due to drug or toxin, if applicable (T36-T65 with fifth or sixth character 1-4 or 6)
Use additional code for adverse effect, if applicable, to identify drug (T36-T50 with fifth or sixth character 5)

5 M34.8 Other forms of systemic sclerosis

SP M34.81 Systemic sclerosis with lung involvement

SP M34.82 Systemic sclerosis with myopathy

SP M34.83 Systemic sclerosis with polyneuropathy

SP M34.89 Other systemic sclerosis

SP M34.9 Systemic sclerosis, unspecified

4 M35 Other systemic involvement of connective tissue
EXCLUDES 1   reactive perforating collagenosis (L87.1)

5 M35.0 Sicca syndrome [Sjögren]

SP M35.00 Sicca syndrome, unspecified

SP M35.01 Sicca syndrome with keratoconjunctivitis

SP M35.02 Sicca syndrome with lung involvement

SP M35.03 Sicca syndrome with myopathy

SP M35.04 Sicca syndrome with tubulo-interstitial nephropathy
Renal tubular acidosis in sicca syndrome

SP M35.09 Sicca syndrome with other organ involvement

SP M35.1 Other overlap syndromes
Mixed connective tissue disease
EXCLUDES 1   polyangiitis overlap syndrome (M30.8)

SP M35.2 Behçet's disease
DEFINITION   Relapsing inflammatory disorder with recurring painful sores of the mouth, skin, and genitals, swollen joints, severe uveitis, retinal vasculitis, optic atrophy, and digestive system involvement.

SP M35.3 Polymyalgia rheumatica
EXCLUDES 1   polymyalgia rheumatica with giant cell arteritis (M31.5)

SP M35.4 Diffuse (eosinophilic) fasciitis

SP M35.5 Multifocal fibrosclerosis

SP M35.6 Relapsing panniculitis [Weber-Christian]
EXCLUDES 1   lupus panniculitis (L93.2) panniculitis NOS (M79.3-)

▲ SP M35.7 Hypermobility syndrome
Familial ligamentous laxity
EXCLUDES 1   Ehlers-Danlos syndrome (Q79.6-)
ligamentous laxity, NOS (M24.2-)

SP M35.8 Other specified systemic involvement of connective tissue

!Q M35.9 Systemic involvement of connective tissue, unspecified
Autoimmune disease (systemic) NOS
Collagen (vascular) disease NOS

4 M36 Systemic disorders of connective tissue in diseases classified elsewhere
EXCLUDES 2   arthropathies in diseases classified elsewhere (M14.-)

M !Q M36.0 *Dermato(poly)myositis in neoplastic disease*
Code first:
underlying neoplasm (C00-D49)

M !Q M36.1 *Arthropathy in neoplastic disease*
Code first underlying neoplasm, such as:
leukemia (C91-C95)
malignant histiocytosis (C96.A)
multiple myeloma (C90.0)

M !Q M36.2 *Hemophilic arthropathy*
Hemarthrosis in hemophilic arthropathy
Code first underlying disease, such as:
factor VIII deficiency (D66)
with vascular defect (D68.0)
factor IX deficiency (D67)
hemophilia (classical) (D66)
hemophilia B (D67)
hemophilia C (D68.1)

M !Q M36.3 *Arthropathy in other blood disorders*

---

4 4th digit required   **5** 5th digit required   **6** 6th digit required   **7** 7th digit required   **7** 7th digit placeholder   ✚ Additional code   ⊟ Laterality

M **IQ** **M36.4** *Arthropathy in hypersensitivity reactions classified elsewhere*

Code first underlying disease, such as:
Henoch (-Schönlein) purpura (D69.0)
serum sickness (T80.6-)

M **IQ** **M36.8** *Systemic disorders of connective tissue in other diseases classified elsewhere*

Code first underlying disease, such as:
alkaptonuria (E70.2)
hypogammaglobulinemia (D80.-)
ochronosis (E70.2)

Dorsopathies (M40-M54)

Deforming dorsopathies (M40-M43)

4 **M40 Kyphosis and lordosis**

> EXCLUDES 1   congenital kyphosis and lordosis (Q76.4)
> kyphoscoliosis (M41.-)
> postprocedural kyphosis and lordosis (M96.-)

5 **M40.0 Postural kyphosis**

> EXCLUDES 1   osteochondrosis of spine (M42.-)

IQ **M40.00** Postural kyphosis, site unspecified

SP **M40.03** Postural kyphosis, cervicothoracic region

SP **M40.04** Postural kyphosis, thoracic region

SP **M40.05** Postural kyphosis, thoracolumbar region

5 **M40.1 Other secondary kyphosis**

IQ **M40.10** Other secondary kyphosis, site unspecified

SP **M40.12** Other secondary kyphosis, cervical region

SP **M40.13** Other secondary kyphosis, cervicothoracic region

SP **M40.14** Other secondary kyphosis, thoracic region

SP **M40.15** Other secondary kyphosis, thoracolumbar region

5 **M40.2 Other and unspecified kyphosis**

6 **M40.20** Unspecified kyphosis

SP **M40.202** Unspecified kyphosis, cervical region

SP **M40.203** Unspecified kyphosis, cervicothoracic region

SP **M40.204** Unspecified kyphosis, thoracic region

SP **M40.205** Unspecified kyphosis, thoracolumbar region

IQ **M40.209** Unspecified kyphosis, site unspecified

6 **M40.29** Other kyphosis

SP **M40.292** Other kyphosis, cervical region

SP **M40.293** Other kyphosis, cervicothoracic region

SP **M40.294** Other kyphosis, thoracic region

SP **M40.295** Other kyphosis, thoracolumbar region

IQ **M40.299** Other kyphosis, site unspecified

5 **M40.3 Flatback syndrome**

IQ **M40.30** Flatback syndrome, site unspecified

SP **M40.35** Flatback syndrome, thoracolumbar region

SP **M40.36** Flatback syndrome, lumbar region

SP **M40.37** Flatback syndrome, lumbosacral region

5 **M40.4 Postural lordosis**
Acquired lordosis

IQ **M40.40** Postural lordosis, site unspecified

SP **M40.45** Postural lordosis, thoracolumbar region

SP **M40.46** Postural lordosis, lumbar region

SP **M40.47** Postural lordosis, lumbosacral region

5 **M40.5 Lordosis, unspecified**

IQ **M40.50** Lordosis, unspecified, site unspecified

SP **M40.55** Lordosis, unspecified, thoracolumbar region

SP **M40.56** Lordosis, unspecified, lumbar region

SP **M40.57** Lordosis, unspecified, lumbosacral region

4 **M41 Scoliosis**

> INCLUDES   kyphoscoliosis

> EXCLUDES 1   congenital scoliosis NOS (Q67.5)
> congenital scoliosis due to bony malformation (Q76.3)
> postural congenital scoliosis (Q67.5)
> kyphoscoliotic heart disease (I27.1)
> postprocedural scoliosis (M96.-)

> CODING TIPS ✓   The correct aftercare code to use for surgeries for treatment of scoliosis is Z47.82.

5 **M41.0 Infantile idiopathic scoliosis**

IQ **M41.00** Infantile idiopathic scoliosis, site unspecified

SP **M41.02** Infantile idiopathic scoliosis, cervical region

SP **M41.03** Infantile idiopathic scoliosis, cervicothoracic region

SP **M41.04** Infantile idiopathic scoliosis, thoracic region

SP **M41.05** Infantile idiopathic scoliosis, thoracolumbar region

SP **M41.06** Infantile idiopathic scoliosis, lumbar region

SP **M41.07** Infantile idiopathic scoliosis, lumbosacral region

SP **M41.08** Infantile idiopathic scoliosis, sacral and sacrococcygeal region

5 **M41.1 Juvenile and adolescent idiopathic scoliosis**

6 **M41.11** Juvenile idiopathic scoliosis

SP **M41.112** Juvenile idiopathic scoliosis, cervical region

SP **M41.113** Juvenile idiopathic scoliosis, cervicothoracic region

SP **M41.114** Juvenile idiopathic scoliosis, thoracic region

SP **M41.115** Juvenile idiopathic scoliosis, thoracolumbar region

★ New ▲ Revised Px Primary SP PDGM Px SL Low CoM SH High CoM IQ Quest. Encounter H Hospice non-cancer Dx   Unspecified   M *Manifestation*

DecisionHealth's FY 2020 Complete Home Health ICD-10-CM Diagnosis Coding Manual

1201

SP M41.116 Juvenile idiopathic scoliosis, lumbar region

SP M41.117 Juvenile idiopathic scoliosis, lumbosacral region

IQ M41.119 Juvenile idiopathic scoliosis, site unspecified

6 M41.12 Adolescent scoliosis

SP M41.122 Adolescent idiopathic scoliosis, cervical region

SP M41.123 Adolescent idiopathic scoliosis, cervicothoracic region

SP M41.124 Adolescent idiopathic scoliosis, thoracic region

SP M41.125 Adolescent idiopathic scoliosis, thoracolumbar region

SP M41.126 Adolescent idiopathic scoliosis, lumbar region

SP M41.127 Adolescent idiopathic scoliosis, lumbosacral region

IQ M41.129 Adolescent idiopathic scoliosis, site unspecified

5 M41.2 Other idiopathic scoliosis

SP M41.20 Other idiopathic scoliosis, site unspecified

SP M41.22 Other idiopathic scoliosis, cervical region

SP M41.23 Other idiopathic scoliosis, cervicothoracic region

SP M41.24 Other idiopathic scoliosis, thoracic region

SP M41.25 Other idiopathic scoliosis, thoracolumbar region

SP M41.26 Other idiopathic scoliosis, lumbar region

SP M41.27 Other idiopathic scoliosis, lumbosacral region

5 M41.3 Thoracogenic scoliosis

IQ M41.30 Thoracogenic scoliosis, site unspecified

SP M41.34 Thoracogenic scoliosis, thoracic region

SP M41.35 Thoracogenic scoliosis, thoracolumbar region

5 M41.4 Neuromuscular scoliosis
Scoliosis secondary to cerebral palsy, Friedreich's ataxia, poliomyelitis and other neuromuscular disorders
Code also:
underlying condition

IQ M41.40 Neuromuscular scoliosis, site unspecified

SP M41.41 Neuromuscular scoliosis, occipito-atlanto-axial region

SP M41.42 Neuromuscular scoliosis, cervical region

SP M41.43 Neuromuscular scoliosis, cervicothoracic region

SP M41.44 Neuromuscular scoliosis, thoracic region

SP M41.45 Neuromuscular scoliosis, thoracolumbar region

SP M41.46 Neuromuscular scoliosis, lumbar region

SP M41.47 Neuromuscular scoliosis, lumbosacral region

5 M41.5 Other secondary scoliosis

IQ M41.50 Other secondary scoliosis, site unspecified

SP M41.52 Other secondary scoliosis, cervical region

SP M41.53 Other secondary scoliosis, cervicothoracic region

SP M41.54 Other secondary scoliosis, thoracic region

SP M41.55 Other secondary scoliosis, thoracolumbar region

SP M41.56 Other secondary scoliosis, lumbar region

SP M41.57 Other secondary scoliosis, lumbosacral region

5 M41.8 Other forms of scoliosis

IQ M41.80 Other forms of scoliosis, site unspecified

SP M41.82 Other forms of scoliosis, cervical region

SP M41.83 Other forms of scoliosis, cervicothoracic region

SP M41.84 Other forms of scoliosis, thoracic region

SP M41.85 Other forms of scoliosis, thoracolumbar region

SP M41.86 Other forms of scoliosis, lumbar region

SP M41.87 Other forms of scoliosis, lumbosacral region

SP M41.9 Scoliosis, unspecified

4 M42 Spinal osteochondrosis

5 M42.0 Juvenile osteochondrosis of spine
Calvé's disease
Scheuermann's disease
EXCLUDES 1 postural kyphosis (M40.0)

IQ M42.00 Juvenile osteochondrosis of spine, site unspecified

SP M42.01 Juvenile osteochondrosis of spine, occipito-atlanto-axial region

SP M42.02 Juvenile osteochondrosis of spine, cervical region

SP M42.03 Juvenile osteochondrosis of spine, cervicothoracic region

SP M42.04 Juvenile osteochondrosis of spine, thoracic region

SP M42.05 Juvenile osteochondrosis of spine, thoracolumbar region

SP M42.06 Juvenile osteochondrosis of spine, lumbar region

SP M42.07 Juvenile osteochondrosis of spine, lumbosacral region

SP M42.08 Juvenile osteochondrosis of spine, sacral and sacrococcygeal region

SP M42.09 Juvenile osteochondrosis of spine, multiple sites in spine

5 M42.1 Adult osteochondrosis of spine

IQ M42.10 Adult osteochondrosis of spine, site unspecified

SP M42.11 Adult osteochondrosis of spine, occipito-atlanto-axial region

SP M42.12 Adult osteochondrosis of spine, cervical region

SP M42.13 Adult osteochondrosis of spine, cervicothoracic region

SP M42.14 Adult osteochondrosis of spine, thoracic region

4 4th digit required   **5** 5th digit required   **6** 6th digit required   **7** 7th digit required   **7** 7th digit placeholder   **+** Additional code   **⊟** Laterality

1202   *DecisionHealth's* FY 2020 Complete Home Health ICD-10-CM Diagnosis Coding Manual

SP M42.15 Adult osteochondrosis of spine, thoracolumbar region

SP M42.16 Adult osteochondrosis of spine, lumbar region

SP M42.17 Adult osteochondrosis of spine, lumbosacral region

SP M42.18 Adult osteochondrosis of spine, sacral and sacrococcygeal region

SP M42.19 Adult osteochondrosis of spine, multiple sites in spine

SP M42.9 Spinal osteochondrosis, unspecified

4 M43 Other deforming dorsopathies

> **EXCLUDES 1** congenital spondylolysis and spondylolisthesis (Q76.2)
> hemivertebra (Q76.3-Q76.4)
> Klippel-Feil syndrome (Q76.1)
> lumbarization and sacralization (Q76.4)
> platyspondylisis (Q76.4)
> spina bifida occulta (Q76.0)
> spinal curvature in osteoporosis (M80.-)
> spinal curvature in Paget's disease of bone [osteitis deformans] (M88.-)

5 M43.0 Spondylolysis

> **EXCLUDES 1** congenital spondylolysis (Q76.2)
> spondylolisthesis (M43.1)

> **DEFINITION** A defect of the pars interarticularis segment of vertebral bone that connects the facet joints, causing stress fracture and predisposing to slippage; occurs most commonly in the lumbar region (specifically L5) during adolescence.

IQ M43.00 Spondylolysis, site unspecified

SP M43.01 Spondylolysis, occipito-atlanto-axial region

SP M43.02 Spondylolysis, cervical region

SP M43.03 Spondylolysis, cervicothoracic region

SP M43.04 Spondylolysis, thoracic region

SP M43.05 Spondylolysis, thoracolumbar region

SP M43.06 Spondylolysis, lumbar region

SP M43.07 Spondylolysis, lumbosacral region

SP M43.08 Spondylolysis, sacral and sacrococcygeal region

SP M43.09 Spondylolysis, multiple sites in spine

5 M43.1 Spondylolisthesis

> **EXCLUDES 1** acute traumatic of lumbosacral region (S33.1)
> acute traumatic of sites other than lumbosacral- code to Fracture, vertebra, by region
> congenital spondylolisthesis (Q76.2)

> **DEFINITION** An acquired condition in which one vertebra slips forward over the one below it, often from degenerative aging or a small fracture in the piece of bone (pars interarticularis) connecting the facet joint above to the one below.

IQ M43.10 Spondylolisthesis, site unspecified

SP M43.11 Spondylolisthesis, occipito-atlanto-axial region

SP M43.12 Spondylolisthesis, cervical region

SP M43.13 Spondylolisthesis, cervicothoracic region

SP M43.14 Spondylolisthesis, thoracic region

SP M43.15 Spondylolisthesis, thoracolumbar region

SP M43.16 Spondylolisthesis, lumbar region

SP M43.17 Spondylolisthesis, lumbosacral region

SP M43.18 Spondylolisthesis, sacral and sacrococcygeal region

SP M43.19 Spondylolisthesis, multiple sites in spine

5 M43.2 Fusion of spine

> Ankylosis of spinal joint
> **EXCLUDES 1** ankylosing spondylitis (M45.0-)
> congenital fusion of spine (Q76.4)
> **EXCLUDES 2** arthrodesis status (Z98.1)
> pseudoarthrosis after fusion or arthrodesis (M96.0)

> **CODING TIPS ✓** Ankylosis of the joint is caused by arthritis, traumatic injury or infection. The joint will assume the least painful position and become permanently fixed. A surgical fusion is coded Z98.1.

IQ M43.20 Fusion of spine, site unspecified

SP M43.21 Fusion of spine, occipito-atlanto-axial region

SP M43.22 Fusion of spine, cervical region

SP M43.23 Fusion of spine, cervicothoracic region

SP M43.24 Fusion of spine, thoracic region

SP M43.25 Fusion of spine, thoracolumbar region

SP M43.26 Fusion of spine, lumbar region

SP M43.27 Fusion of spine, lumbosacral region

SP M43.28 Fusion of spine, sacral and sacrococcygeal region

SP M43.3 Recurrent atlantoaxial dislocation with myelopathy

SP M43.4 Other recurrent atlantoaxial dislocation

5 M43.5 Other recurrent vertebral dislocation

> **EXCLUDES 1** biomechanical lesions NEC (M99.-)

6 M43.5X Other recurrent vertebral dislocation

SP M43.5X2 Other recurrent vertebral dislocation, cervical region

SP M43.5X3 Other recurrent vertebral dislocation, cervicothoracic region

SP M43.5X4 Other recurrent vertebral dislocation, thoracic region

SP M43.5X5 Other recurrent vertebral dislocation, thoracolumbar region

SP M43.5X6 Other recurrent vertebral dislocation, lumbar region

SP M43.5X7 Other recurrent vertebral dislocation, lumbosacral region

SP M43.5X8 Other recurrent vertebral dislocation, sacral and sacrococcygeal region

---

★ New ▲ Revised **Px** Primary **SP** PDGM Px **SL** Low CoM **SH** High CoM **IQ** Quest. Encounter **H** Hospice non-cancer Dx ☐ Unspecified **M** *Manifestation*

Chapter 13

M00-M99

!Q M43.5X9 Other recurrent vertebral dislocation, site unspecified

SP M43.6 Torticollis

> EXCLUDES 1　congenital (sternomastoid) torticollis (Q68.0)
> current injury - see Injury, of spine, by body region
> ocular torticollis (R29.891)
> psychogenic torticollis (F45.8)
> spasmodic torticollis (G24.3)
> torticollis due to birth injury (P15.2)

> DEFINITION　Contraction of the neck muscles causing limited neck motion and head positioned to one side.

⑤ M43.8 Other specified deforming dorsopathies

> EXCLUDES 2　kyphosis and lordosis (M40.-)
> scoliosis (M41.-)

⑥ M43.8X Other specified deforming dorsopathies

SP M43.8X1 Other specified deforming dorsopathies, occipito-atlanto-axial region

SP M43.8X2 Other specified deforming dorsopathies, cervical region

SP M43.8X3 Other specified deforming dorsopathies, cervicothoracic region

SP M43.8X4 Other specified deforming dorsopathies, thoracic region

SP M43.8X5 Other specified deforming dorsopathies, thoracolumbar region

SP M43.8X6 Other specified deforming dorsopathies, lumbar region

SP M43.8X7 Other specified deforming dorsopathies, lumbosacral region

SP M43.8X8 Other specified deforming dorsopathies, sacral and sacrococcygeal region

!Q M43.8X9 Other specified deforming dorsopathies, site unspecified

!Q M43.9 Deforming dorsopathy, unspecified
> Curvature of spine NOS

Spondylopathies (M45-M49)

④ M45 Ankylosing spondylitis
> Rheumatoid arthritis of spine

> EXCLUDES 1　arthropathy in Reiter's disease (M02.3-)
> juvenile (ankylosing) spondylitis (M08.1)

> EXCLUDES 2　Behçet's disease (M35.2)

> DEFINITION　Autoimmune arthritis causing chronic inflammation of the spine and sacroiliac joints, eventually leading to spinal fusion from calcification of ligaments and discs that progresses up the spine, possibly affecting other organs.

SP M45.0 Ankylosing spondylitis of multiple sites in spine

SP M45.1 Ankylosing spondylitis of occipito-atlanto-axial region

SP M45.2 Ankylosing spondylitis of cervical region

SP M45.3 Ankylosing spondylitis of cervicothoracic region

SP M45.4 Ankylosing spondylitis of thoracic region

SP M45.5 Ankylosing spondylitis of thoracolumbar region

SP M45.6 Ankylosing spondylitis lumbar region

SP M45.7 Ankylosing spondylitis of lumbosacral region

SP M45.8 Ankylosing spondylitis sacral and sacrococcygeal region

!Q M45.9 Ankylosing spondylitis of unspecified sites in spine

④ M46 Other inflammatory spondylopathies

⑤ M46.0 Spinal enthesopathy
> Disorder of ligamentous or muscular attachments of spine

!Q M46.00 Spinal enthesopathy, site unspecified

SP M46.01 Spinal enthesopathy, occipito-atlanto-axial region

SP M46.02 Spinal enthesopathy, cervical region

SP M46.03 Spinal enthesopathy, cervicothoracic region

SP M46.04 Spinal enthesopathy, thoracic region

SP M46.05 Spinal enthesopathy, thoracolumbar region

SP M46.06 Spinal enthesopathy, lumbar region

SP M46.07 Spinal enthesopathy, lumbosacral region

SP M46.08 Spinal enthesopathy, sacral and sacrococcygeal region

SP M46.09 Spinal enthesopathy, multiple sites in spine

SP M46.1 Sacroiliitis, not elsewhere classified

⑤ M46.2 Osteomyelitis of vertebra

!Q M46.20 Osteomyelitis of vertebra, site unspecified

SP M46.21 Osteomyelitis of vertebra, occipito-atlanto-axial region

SP M46.22 Osteomyelitis of vertebra, cervical region

SP M46.23 Osteomyelitis of vertebra, cervicothoracic region

SP M46.24 Osteomyelitis of vertebra, thoracic region

SP M46.25 Osteomyelitis of vertebra, thoracolumbar region

SP M46.26 Osteomyelitis of vertebra, lumbar region

SP M46.27 Osteomyelitis of vertebra, lumbosacral region

SP M46.28 Osteomyelitis of vertebra, sacral and sacrococcygeal region

✚ ⑤ M46.3 Infection of intervertebral disc (pyogenic)
> Use additional code (B95-B97) to identify infectious agent.

!Q ✚ M46.30 Infection of intervertebral disc (pyogenic), site unspecified

SP ✚ M46.31 Infection of intervertebral disc (pyogenic), occipito-atlanto-axial region

SP ✚ M46.32 Infection of intervertebral disc (pyogenic), cervical region

---

④ 4th digit required　　⑤ 5th digit required　　⑥ 6th digit required　　⑦ 7th digit required　　⑦ 7th digit placeholder　　✚ Additional code　　⊟ Laterality

SP ✚ **M46.33** Infection of intervertebral disc (pyogenic), cervicothoracic region

SP ✚ **M46.34** Infection of intervertebral disc (pyogenic), thoracic region

SP ✚ **M46.35** Infection of intervertebral disc (pyogenic), thoracolumbar region

SP ✚ **M46.36** Infection of intervertebral disc (pyogenic), lumbar region

SP ✚ **M46.37** Infection of intervertebral disc (pyogenic), lumbosacral region

SP ✚ **M46.38** Infection of intervertebral disc (pyogenic), sacral and sacrococcygeal region

SP ✚ **M46.39** Infection of intervertebral disc (pyogenic), multiple sites in spine

5 **M46.4** Discitis, unspecified

IQ **M46.40** Discitis, unspecified, site unspecified

SP **M46.41** Discitis, unspecified, occipito-atlanto-axial region

SP **M46.42** Discitis, unspecified, cervical region

SP **M46.43** Discitis, unspecified, cervicothoracic region

SP **M46.44** Discitis, unspecified, thoracic region

SP **M46.45** Discitis, unspecified, thoracolumbar region

SP **M46.46** Discitis, unspecified, lumbar region

SP **M46.47** Discitis, unspecified, lumbosacral region

SP **M46.48** Discitis, unspecified, sacral and sacrococcygeal region

SP **M46.49** Discitis, unspecified, multiple sites in spine

5 **M46.5** Other infective spondylopathies

IQ **M46.50** Other infective spondylopathies, site unspecified

SP **M46.51** Other infective spondylopathies, occipito-atlanto-axial region

SP **M46.52** Other infective spondylopathies, cervical region

SP **M46.53** Other infective spondylopathies, cervicothoracic region

SP **M46.54** Other infective spondylopathies, thoracic region

SP **M46.55** Other infective spondylopathies, thoracolumbar region

SP **M46.56** Other infective spondylopathies, lumbar region

SP **M46.57** Other infective spondylopathies, lumbosacral region

SP **M46.58** Other infective spondylopathies, sacral and sacrococcygeal region

SP **M46.59** Other infective spondylopathies, multiple sites in spine

5 **M46.8** Other specified inflammatory spondylopathies

IQ **M46.80** Other specified inflammatory spondylopathies, site unspecified

SP **M46.81** Other specified inflammatory spondylopathies, occipito-atlanto-axial region

SP **M46.82** Other specified inflammatory spondylopathies, cervical region

SP **M46.83** Other specified inflammatory spondylopathies, cervicothoracic region

SP **M46.84** Other specified inflammatory spondylopathies, thoracic region

SP **M46.85** Other specified inflammatory spondylopathies, thoracolumbar region

SP **M46.86** Other specified inflammatory spondylopathies, lumbar region

SP **M46.87** Other specified inflammatory spondylopathies, lumbosacral region

SP **M46.88** Other specified inflammatory spondylopathies, sacral and sacrococcygeal region

SP **M46.89** Other specified inflammatory spondylopathies, multiple sites in spine

5 **M46.9** Unspecified inflammatory spondylopathy

IQ **M46.90** Unspecified inflammatory spondylopathy, site unspecified

SP **M46.91** Unspecified inflammatory spondylopathy, occipito-atlanto-axial region

SP **M46.92** Unspecified inflammatory spondylopathy, cervical region

SP **M46.93** Unspecified inflammatory spondylopathy, cervicothoracic region

SP **M46.94** Unspecified inflammatory spondylopathy, thoracic region

SP **M46.95** Unspecified inflammatory spondylopathy, thoracolumbar region

SP **M46.96** Unspecified inflammatory spondylopathy, lumbar region

SP **M46.97** Unspecified inflammatory spondylopathy, lumbosacral region

SP **M46.98** Unspecified inflammatory spondylopathy, sacral and sacrococcygeal region

SP **M46.99** Unspecified inflammatory spondylopathy, multiple sites in spine

4 **M47** Spondylosis

> **INCLUDES** arthrosis or osteoarthritis of spine
> degeneration of facet joints

> **CODING TIPS** ✓ OA of spine is coded M47.-. OA of the spine causing weakness, spasticity, clumsiness, altered tonus, but generally no pain, should be coded M47.1-. OA of the spine causing pain, numbness and weakness is coded as M47.2. Query the physician for more specificity when clinical documentation includes those symptoms.

5 **M47.0** Anterior spinal and vertebral artery compression syndromes

6 **M47.01** Anterior spinal artery compression syndromes

SP **M47.011** Anterior spinal artery compression syndromes, occipito-atlanto-axial region

SP **M47.012** Anterior spinal artery compression syndromes, cervical region

★ New ▲ Revised Px Primary **SP** PDGM Px **SL** Low CoM **SH** High CoM **IQ** Quest. Encounter ⊞ Hospice non-cancer Dx Unspecified **M** *Manifestation*

DecisionHealth's FY 2020 Complete Home Health ICD-10-CM Diagnosis Coding Manual 1205

SP M47.013 Anterior spinal artery compression syndromes, cervicothoracic region

SP M47.014 Anterior spinal artery compression syndromes, thoracic region

SP M47.015 Anterior spinal artery compression syndromes, thoracolumbar region

SP M47.016 Anterior spinal artery compression syndromes, lumbar region

IQ M47.019 Anterior spinal artery compression syndromes, site unspecified

6 M47.02 Vertebral artery compression syndromes

SP M47.021 Vertebral artery compression syndromes, occipito-atlanto-axial region

SP M47.022 Vertebral artery compression syndromes, cervical region

IQ M47.029 Vertebral artery compression syndromes, site unspecified

▲ **5 M47.1** Other spondylosis with myelopathy
Spondylogenic compression of spinal cord
EXCLUDES 1 vertebral subluxation (M43.3-M43.5X9)
CODING TIPS ✓ Myelopathy refers to weakness, spasticity, clumsiness, altered tonus, hyperreflexia and pathological reflexes, but generally no pain.

IQ M47.10 Other spondylosis with myelopathy, site unspecified

SP M47.11 Other spondylosis with myelopathy, occipito-atlanto-axial region

SP M47.12 Other spondylosis with myelopathy, cervical region

SP M47.13 Other spondylosis with myelopathy, cervicothoracic region

SP M47.14 Other spondylosis with myelopathy, thoracic region

SP M47.15 Other spondylosis with myelopathy, thoracolumbar region

SP M47.16 Other spondylosis with myelopathy, lumbar region

5 M47.2 Other spondylosis with radiculopathy
CODING TIPS ✓ Radiculopathy refers to symptoms of pain, numbness and weakness in a pattern consistent with the distribution of a particular nerve root.

IQ M47.20 Other spondylosis with radiculopathy, site unspecified

SP M47.21 Other spondylosis with radiculopathy, occipito-atlanto-axial region

SP M47.22 Other spondylosis with radiculopathy, cervical region

SP M47.23 Other spondylosis with radiculopathy, cervicothoracic region

SP M47.24 Other spondylosis with radiculopathy, thoracic region

SP M47.25 Other spondylosis with radiculopathy, thoracolumbar region

SP M47.26 Other spondylosis with radiculopathy, lumbar region

SP M47.27 Other spondylosis with radiculopathy, lumbosacral region

SP M47.28 Other spondylosis with radiculopathy, sacral and sacrococcygeal region

5 M47.8 Other spondylosis

6 M47.81 Spondylosis without myelopathy or radiculopathy

SP M47.811 Spondylosis without myelopathy or radiculopathy, occipito-atlanto-axial region

SP M47.812 Spondylosis without myelopathy or radiculopathy, cervical region

SP M47.813 Spondylosis without myelopathy or radiculopathy, cervicothoracic region

SP M47.814 Spondylosis without myelopathy or radiculopathy, thoracic region

SP M47.815 Spondylosis without myelopathy or radiculopathy, thoracolumbar region

SP M47.816 Spondylosis without myelopathy or radiculopathy, lumbar region

SP M47.817 Spondylosis without myelopathy or radiculopathy, lumbosacral region

SP M47.818 Spondylosis without myelopathy or radiculopathy, sacral and sacrococcygeal region

IQ M47.819 Spondylosis without myelopathy or radiculopathy, site unspecified

6 M47.89 Other spondylosis

SP M47.891 Other spondylosis, occipito-atlanto-axial region

SP M47.892 Other spondylosis, cervical region

SP M47.893 Other spondylosis, cervicothoracic region

SP M47.894 Other spondylosis, thoracic region

SP M47.895 Other spondylosis, thoracolumbar region

SP M47.896 Other spondylosis, lumbar region

SP M47.897 Other spondylosis, lumbosacral region

SP M47.898 Other spondylosis, sacral and sacrococcygeal region

IQ M47.899 Other spondylosis, site unspecified

IQ M47.9 Spondylosis, unspecified

4 M48 Other spondylopathies

5 M48.0 Spinal stenosis
Caudal stenosis
CODING TIPS ✓ To determine if spinal stenosis has been resolved by surgery, look for physician documentation regarding decompression or release.

IQ M48.00 Spinal stenosis, site unspecified

SP M48.01 Spinal stenosis, occipito-atlanto-axial region

SP M48.02 Spinal stenosis, cervical region

SP M48.03 Spinal stenosis, cervicothoracic region

SP M48.04 Spinal stenosis, thoracic region

SP M48.05 Spinal stenosis, thoracolumbar region

6 M48.06 Spinal stenosis, lumbar region

4 4th digit required   **5** 5th digit required   **6** 6th digit required   **7** 7th digit required   **7** 7th digit placeholder   **+** Additional code   **⊟** Laterality

1206   *DecisionHealth's* FY 2020 Complete Home Health ICD-10-CM Diagnosis Coding Manual

DEFINITION   Neurogenic claudication may present in one or both legs and usually presents as some combination of discomfort, pain, numbness and weakness in the calves, buttocks, and/or thighs.

SP M48.061 Spinal stenosis, lumbar region without neurogenic claudication
Spinal stenosis, lumbar region NOS

SP M48.062 Spinal stenosis, lumbar region with neurogenic claudication

SP M48.07 Spinal stenosis, lumbosacral region

SP M48.08 Spinal stenosis, sacral and sacrococcygeal region

5 M48.1 Ankylosing hyperostosis [Forestier]
Diffuse idiopathic skeletal hyperostosis [DISH]

SP M48.10 Ankylosing hyperostosis [Forestier], site unspecified

SP M48.11 Ankylosing hyperostosis [Forestier], occipito-atlanto-axial region

SP M48.12 Ankylosing hyperostosis [Forestier], cervical region

SP M48.13 Ankylosing hyperostosis [Forestier], cervicothoracic region

SP M48.14 Ankylosing hyperostosis [Forestier], thoracic region

SP M48.15 Ankylosing hyperostosis [Forestier], thoracolumbar region

SP M48.16 Ankylosing hyperostosis [Forestier], lumbar region

SP M48.17 Ankylosing hyperostosis [Forestier], lumbosacral region

SP M48.18 Ankylosing hyperostosis [Forestier], sacral and sacrococcygeal region

SP M48.19 Ankylosing hyperostosis [Forestier], multiple sites in spine

5 M48.2 Kissing spine

IQ M48.20 Kissing spine, site unspecified

SP M48.21 Kissing spine, occipito-atlanto-axial region

SP M48.22 Kissing spine, cervical region

SP M48.23 Kissing spine, cervicothoracic region

SP M48.24 Kissing spine, thoracic region

SP M48.25 Kissing spine, thoracolumbar region

SP M48.26 Kissing spine, lumbar region

SP M48.27 Kissing spine, lumbosacral region

5 M48.3 Traumatic spondylopathy

IQ M48.30 Traumatic spondylopathy, site unspecified

SP M48.31 Traumatic spondylopathy, occipito-atlanto-axial region

SP M48.32 Traumatic spondylopathy, cervical region

SP M48.33 Traumatic spondylopathy, cervicothoracic region

SP M48.34 Traumatic spondylopathy, thoracic region

SP M48.35 Traumatic spondylopathy, thoracolumbar region

SP M48.36 Traumatic spondylopathy, lumbar region

SP M48.37 Traumatic spondylopathy, lumbosacral region

SP M48.38 Traumatic spondylopathy, sacral and sacrococcygeal region

5 M48.4 Fatigue fracture of vertebra
Stress fracture of vertebra
EXCLUDES 1   pathological fracture NOS (M84.4-)
pathological fracture of vertebra due to neoplasm (M84.58)
pathological fracture of vertebra due to other diagnosis (M84.68)
pathological fracture of vertebra due to osteoporosis (M80.-)
traumatic fracture of vertebrae (S12.0-S12.3-, S22.0-, S32.0-)

The appropriate 7th character is to be added to each code from subcategory M48.4:
A   initial encounter for fracture
D   subsequent encounter for fracture with routine healing
G   subsequent encounter for fracture with delayed healing
S   sequela of fracture

CODING TIPS ✓   Fractures repaired by joint replacements are NOT coded with Z47.1. Fractures repaired by any other orthopedic surgery are NOT coded with Z47.89. Z codes are not appropriate for fractures of any kind. Code the fracture with 7th character D for fractures undergoing surgical repair.

IQ ☑ M48.40X- Fatigue fracture of vertebra, site unspecified

SP ☑ M48.41X- Fatigue fracture of vertebra, occipito-atlanto-axial region

SP ☑ M48.42X- Fatigue fracture of vertebra, cervical region

SP ☑ M48.43X- Fatigue fracture of vertebra, cervicothoracic region

SP ☑ M48.44X- Fatigue fracture of vertebra, thoracic region

SP ☑ M48.45X- Fatigue fracture of vertebra, thoracolumbar region

SP ☑ M48.46X- Fatigue fracture of vertebra, lumbar region

SP ☑ M48.47X- Fatigue fracture of vertebra, lumbosacral region

SP ☑ M48.48X- Fatigue fracture of vertebra, sacral and sacrococcygeal region

5 M48.5 Collapsed vertebra, not elsewhere classified
Collapsed vertebra NOS
Compression fracture of vertebra NOS
Wedging of vertebra NOS
EXCLUDES 1   current injury - see Injury of spine, by body region
fatigue fracture of vertebra (M48.4)
pathological fracture of vertebra due to neoplasm (M84.58)

★ New ▲ Revised Px Primary **SP** PDGM Px **SL** Low CoM **SH** High CoM **IQ** Quest. Encounter **H** Hospice non-cancer Dx   Unspecified   **M** *Manifestation*

pathological fracture of vertebra due to other diagnosis (M84.68)
pathological fracture of vertebra due to osteoporosis (M80.-)
pathological fracture NOS (M84.4-)
stress fracture of vertebra (M48.4-)
traumatic fracture of vertebra (S12.-, S22.-, S32.-)

The appropriate 7th character is to be added to each code from subcategory M48.5:
A   initial encounter for fracture
D   subsequent encounter for fracture with routine healing
G   subsequent encounter for fracture with delayed healing
S   sequela of fracture

CODING TIPS ✓ Fractures repaired by joint replacements are NOT coded with Z47.1. Fractures repaired by any other orthopedic surgery are NOT coded with Z47.89. Z codes are not appropriate for fractures of any kind. Code the fracture with 7th character D for fractures undergoing surgical repair.

IQ ☑ M48.50X- **Collapsed vertebra, not elsewhere classified, site unspecified**

SP ☑ M48.51X- Collapsed vertebra, not elsewhere classified, occipito-atlanto-axial region

SP ☑ M48.52X- Collapsed vertebra, not elsewhere classified, cervical region

SP ☑ M48.53X- Collapsed vertebra, not elsewhere classified, cervicothoracic region

SP ☑ M48.54X- Collapsed vertebra, not elsewhere classified, thoracic region

SP ☑ M48.55X- Collapsed vertebra, not elsewhere classified, thoracolumbar region

SP ☑ M48.56X- Collapsed vertebra, not elsewhere classified, lumbar region

SP ☑ M48.57X- Collapsed vertebra, not elsewhere classified, lumbosacral region

SP ☑ M48.58X- Collapsed vertebra, not elsewhere classified, sacral and sacrococcygeal region

⑤ M48.8 Other specified spondylopathies
Ossification of posterior longitudinal ligament

⑥ M48.8X Other specified spondylopathies

SP M48.8X1 Other specified spondylopathies, occipito-atlanto-axial region

SP M48.8X2 Other specified spondylopathies, cervical region

SP M48.8X3 Other specified spondylopathies, cervicothoracic region

SP M48.8X4 Other specified spondylopathies, thoracic region

SP M48.8X5 Other specified spondylopathies, thoracolumbar region

SP M48.8X6 Other specified spondylopathies, lumbar region

SP M48.8X7 Other specified spondylopathies, lumbosacral region

SP M48.8X8 Other specified spondylopathies, sacral and sacrococcygeal region

IQ M48.8X9 **Other specified spondylopathies, site unspecified**

SP M48.9 **Spondylopathy, unspecified**

④ M49 Spondylopathies in diseases classified elsewhere

INCLUDES curvature of spine in diseases classified elsewhere
deformity of spine in diseases classified elsewhere
kyphosis in diseases classified elsewhere
scoliosis in diseases classified elsewhere
spondylopathy in diseases classified elsewhere

Code first underlying disease, such as:
brucellosis (A23.-)
Charcot-Marie-Tooth disease (G60.0)
enterobacterial infections (A01-A04)
osteitis fibrosa cystica (E21.0)

EXCLUDES 1 curvature of spine in tuberculosis [Pott's] (A18.01)
enteropathic arthropathies (M07.-)
gonococcal spondylitis (A54.41)
neuropathic [tabes dorsalis] spondylitis (A52.11)
neuropathic spondylopathy in syringomyelia (G95.0)
neuropathic spondylopathy in tabes dorsalis (A52.11)
nonsyphilitic neuropathic spondylopathy NEC (G98.0)
spondylitis in syphilis (acquired) (A52.77)
tuberculous spondylitis (A18.01)
typhoid fever spondylitis (A01.05)

⑤ M49.8 Spondylopathy in diseases classified elsewhere

CODING TIPS ✓ M49.8- codes indicate spondylopathy due to an underlying condition. The underlying condition should be identified and coded first.

M IQ M49.80 *Spondylopathy in diseases classified elsewhere, site unspecified*

M IQ M49.81 *Spondylopathy in diseases classified elsewhere, occipito-atlanto-axial region*

M IQ M49.82 *Spondylopathy in diseases classified elsewhere, cervical region*

M IQ M49.83 *Spondylopathy in diseases classified elsewhere, cervicothoracic region*

M IQ M49.84 *Spondylopathy in diseases classified elsewhere, thoracic region*

M IQ M49.85 *Spondylopathy in diseases classified elsewhere, thoracolumbar region*

M IQ M49.86 *Spondylopathy in diseases classified elsewhere, lumbar region*

M IQ M49.87 *Spondylopathy in diseases classified elsewhere, lumbosacral region*

---

④ 4th digit required   ⑤ 5th digit required   ⑥ 6th digit required   ☑ 7th digit required   ☑ 7th digit placeholder   **+** Additional code   ⊟ Laterality

M IQ M49.88 *Spondylopathy in diseases classified elsewhere, sacral and sacrococcygeal region*

M IQ M49.89 *Spondylopathy in diseases classified elsewhere, multiple sites in spine*

Other dorsopathies (M50-M54)

EXCLUDES 1   current injury - see injury of spine by body region
discitis NOS (M46.4-)

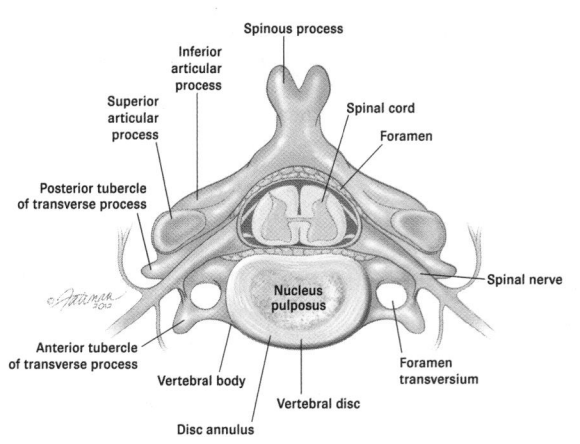

4 M50   Cervical disc disorders
Note:
code to the most superior level of disorder
INCLUDES   cervicothoracic disc disorders
with cervicalgia
cervicothoracic disc disorders
CODING TIPS ✓   If the patient has a disc disorder at more than one region, code to the highest level of each region. Note the excludes 2 note at M51.

5 M50.0 Cervical disc disorder with myelopathy
CODING TIPS ✓   Myelopathy refers to weakness, spasticity, clumsiness, altered tonus, hyperreflexia and pathological reflexes, but generally no pain.

SP M50.00   Cervical disc disorder with myelopathy, unspecified cervical region

SP M50.01   Cervical disc disorder with myelopathy, high cervical region
C2-C3 disc disorder with myelopathy
C3-C4 disc disorder with myelopathy

6 M50.02   Cervical disc disorder with myelopathy, mid-cervical region
IQ M50.020   Cervical disc disorder with myelopathy, mid-cervical region, unspecified level

SP M50.021 Cervical disc disorder at C4-C5 level with myelopathy
C4-C5 disc disorder with myelopathy

SP M50.022 Cervical disc disorder at C5-C6 level with myelopathy
C5-C6 disc disorder with myelopathy

SP M50.023 Cervical disc disorder at C6-C7 level with myelopathy
C6-C7 disc disorder with myelopathy

SP M50.03   Cervical disc disorder with myelopathy, cervicothoracic region
C7-T1 disc disorder with myelopathy

5 M50.1 Cervical disc disorder with radiculopathy
EXCLUDES 2   brachial radiculitis NOS (M54.13)
CODING TIPS ✓   Radiculopathy refers to symptoms of pain, numbness and weakness in a pattern consistent with the distribution of a particular nerve root.

IQ M50.10   Cervical disc disorder with radiculopathy, unspecified cervical region

SP M50.11   Cervical disc disorder with radiculopathy, high cervical region
C2-C3 disc disorder with radiculopathy
C3 radiculopathy due to disc disorder
C3-C4 disc disorder with radiculopathy
C4 radiculopathy due to disc disorder

6 M50.12   Cervical disc disorder with radiculopathy, mid-cervical region
▲ IQ M50.120   Mid-cervical disc disorder, unspecified level

SP M50.121 Cervical disc disorder at C4-C5 level with radiculopathy
C4-C5 disc disorder with radiculopathy
C5 radiculopathy due to disc disorder

SP M50.122 Cervical disc disorder at C5-C6 level with radiculopathy
C5-C6 disc disorder with radiculopathy
C6 radiculopathy due to disc disorder

SP M50.123 Cervical disc disorder at C6-C7 level with radiculopathy
C6-C7 disc disorder with radiculopathy
C7 radiculopathy due to disc disorder

SP M50.13   Cervical disc disorder with radiculopathy, cervicothoracic region
C7-T1 disc disorder with radiculopathy
C8 radiculopathy due to disc disorder

5 M50.2 Other cervical disc displacement
IQ M50.20   Other cervical disc displacement, unspecified cervical region

SP M50.21   Other cervical disc displacement, high cervical region
Other C2-C3 cervical disc displacement
Other C3-C4 cervical disc displacement

6 M50.22   Other cervical disc displacement, mid-cervical region
IQ M50.220   Other cervical disc displacement, mid-cervical region, unspecified level

SP M50.221 Other cervical disc displacement at C4-C5 level

★ New ▲ Revised Px Primary SP PDGM Px SL Low CoM SH High CoM IQ Quest. Encounter H Hospice non-cancer Dx   Unspecified   M *Manifestation*

DecisionHealth's FY 2020 Complete Home Health ICD-10-CM Diagnosis Coding Manual   1209

Other C4-C5 cervical disc
displacement

SP M50.222 Other cervical disc displacement at C5-C6 level
Other C5-C6 cervical disc
displacement

SP M50.223 Other cervical disc displacement at C6-C7 level
Other C6-C7 cervical disc
displacement

SP M50.23 Other cervical disc displacement, cervicothoracic region
Other C7-T1 cervical disc
displacement

5 M50.3 Other cervical disc degeneration

!Q M50.30 Other cervical disc degeneration, unspecified cervical region

SP M50.31 Other cervical disc degeneration, high cervical region
Other C2-C3 cervical disc degeneration
Other C3-C4 cervical disc degeneration

6 M50.32 Other cervical disc degeneration, mid-cervical region

!Q M50.320 Other cervical disc degeneration, mid-cervical region, unspecified level

SP M50.321 Other cervical disc degeneration at C4-C5 level
Other C4-C5 cervical disc
degeneration

SP M50.322 Other cervical disc degeneration at C5-C6 level
Other C5-C6 cervical disc
degeneration

SP M50.323 Other cervical disc degeneration at C6-C7 level
Other C6-C7 cervical disc
degeneration

SP M50.33 Other cervical disc degeneration, cervicothoracic region
Other C7-T1 cervical disc degeneration

5 M50.8 Other cervical disc disorders

!Q M50.80 Other cervical disc disorders, unspecified cervical region

SP M50.81 Other cervical disc disorders, high cervical region
Other C2-C3 cervical disc disorders
Other C3-C4 cervical disc disorders

6 M50.82 Other cervical disc disorders, mid-cervical region

!Q M50.820 Other cervical disc disorders, mid-cervical region, unspecified level

SP M50.821 Other cervical disc disorders at C4-C5 level
Other C4-C5 cervical disc disorders

SP M50.822 Other cervical disc disorders at C5-C6 level
Other C5-C6 cervical disc disorders

SP M50.823 Other cervical disc disorders at C6-C7 level
Other C6-C7 cervical disc disorders

SP M50.83 Other cervical disc disorders, cervicothoracic region
Other C7-T1 cervical disc disorders

5 M50.9 Cervical disc disorder, unspecified

!Q M50.90 Cervical disc disorder, unspecified, unspecified cervical region

SP M50.91 Cervical disc disorder, unspecified, high cervical region
C2-C3 cervical disc disorder,
unspecified
C3-C4 cervical disc disorder,
unspecified

6 M50.92 Cervical disc disorder, unspecified, mid-cervical region

!Q M50.920 Unspecified cervical disc disorder, mid-cervical region, unspecified level

SP M50.921 Unspecified cervical disc disorder at C4-C5 level
Unspecified C4-C5 cervical disc
disorder

SP M50.922 Unspecified cervical disc disorder at C5-C6 level
Unspecified C5-C6 cervical disc
disorder

SP M50.923 Unspecified cervical disc disorder at C6-C7 level
Unspecified C6-C7 cervical disc
disorder

SP M50.93 Cervical disc disorder, unspecified, cervicothoracic region
C7-T1 cervical disc disorder,
unspecified

4 M51 Thoracic, thoracolumbar, and lumbosacral intervertebral disc disorders
> **EXCLUDES 2** cervical and cervicothoracic disc disorders (M50.-)
> sacral and sacrococcygeal disorders (M53.3)

> **CODING TIPS ✓** If the patient has a disc disorder at more than one region, code to the highest level of each region. Note the excludes 2 note at M51.

5 M51.0 Thoracic, thoracolumbar and lumbosacral intervertebral disc disorders with myelopathy
> **CODING TIPS ✓** Myelopathy refers to weakness, spasticity, clumsiness, altered tonus, hyperreflexia and pathological reflexes, but generally no pain.

SP M51.04 Intervertebral disc disorders with myelopathy, thoracic region

SP M51.05 Intervertebral disc disorders with myelopathy, thoracolumbar region

SP M51.06 Intervertebral disc disorders with myelopathy, lumbar region

5 M51.1 Thoracic, thoracolumbar and lumbosacral intervertebral disc disorders with radiculopathy
Sciatica due to intervertebral disc disorder
> **EXCLUDES 1** lumbar radiculitis NOS (M54.16)
> sciatica NOS (M54.3)

> **CODING TIPS ✓** Radiculopathy refers to symptoms of pain, numbness and weakness in a pattern consistent with the distribution of a particular nerve root.

SP M51.14 Intervertebral disc disorders with radiculopathy, thoracic region

---

4 4th digit required   5 5th digit required   6 6th digit required   7 7th digit required   7⃣ 7th digit placeholder   + Additional code   ⊟ Laterality

1210   *DecisionHealth's* FY 2020 Complete Home Health ICD-10-CM Diagnosis Coding Manual

SP M51.15 Intervertebral disc disorders with radiculopathy, thoracolumbar region

SP M51.16 Intervertebral disc disorders with radiculopathy, lumbar region

SP M51.17 Intervertebral disc disorders with radiculopathy, lumbosacral region

5 M51.2 Other thoracic, thoracolumbar and lumbosacral intervertebral disc displacement
Lumbago due to displacement of intervertebral disc

SP M51.24 Other intervertebral disc displacement, thoracic region

SP M51.25 Other intervertebral disc displacement, thoracolumbar region

SP M51.26 Other intervertebral disc displacement, lumbar region

SP M51.27 Other intervertebral disc displacement, lumbosacral region

5 M51.3 Other thoracic, thoracolumbar and lumbosacral intervertebral disc degeneration

SP M51.34 Other intervertebral disc degeneration, thoracic region

SP M51.35 Other intervertebral disc degeneration, thoracolumbar region

SP M51.36 Other intervertebral disc degeneration, lumbar region

SP M51.37 Other intervertebral disc degeneration, lumbosacral region

5 M51.4 Schmorl's nodes

SP M51.44 Schmorl's nodes, thoracic region

SP M51.45 Schmorl's nodes, thoracolumbar region

SP M51.46 Schmorl's nodes, lumbar region

SP M51.47 Schmorl's nodes, lumbosacral region

5 M51.8 Other thoracic, thoracolumbar and lumbosacral intervertebral disc disorders

SP M51.84 Other intervertebral disc disorders, thoracic region

SP M51.85 Other intervertebral disc disorders, thoracolumbar region

SP M51.86 Other intervertebral disc disorders, lumbar region

SP M51.87 Other intervertebral disc disorders, lumbosacral region

SP M51.9 Unspecified thoracic, thoracolumbar and lumbosacral intervertebral disc disorder

4 M53 Other and unspecified dorsopathies, not elsewhere classified

SP M53.0 Cervicocranial syndrome
Posterior cervical sympathetic syndrome

SP M53.1 Cervicobrachial syndrome
EXCLUDES 2 cervical disc disorder (M50.-)
thoracic outlet syndrome (G54.0)

5 M53.2 Spinal instabilities

6 M53.2X Spinal instabilities

SP M53.2X1 Spinal instabilities, occipito-atlanto-axial region

SP M53.2X2 Spinal instabilities, cervical region

SP M53.2X3 Spinal instabilities, cervicothoracic region

SP M53.2X4 Spinal instabilities, thoracic region

SP M53.2X5 Spinal instabilities, thoracolumbar region

SP M53.2X6 Spinal instabilities, lumbar region

SP M53.2X7 Spinal instabilities, lumbosacral region

SP M53.2X8 Spinal instabilities, sacral and sacrococcygeal region

IQ M53.2X9 Spinal instabilities, site unspecified

SP M53.3 Sacrococcygeal disorders, not elsewhere classified
Coccygodynia

5 M53.8 Other specified dorsopathies

IQ M53.80 Other specified dorsopathies, site unspecified

SP M53.81 Other specified dorsopathies, occipito-atlanto-axial region

SP M53.82 Other specified dorsopathies, cervical region

SP M53.83 Other specified dorsopathies, cervicothoracic region

SP M53.84 Other specified dorsopathies, thoracic region

SP M53.85 Other specified dorsopathies, thoracolumbar region

SP M53.86 Other specified dorsopathies, lumbar region

SP M53.87 Other specified dorsopathies, lumbosacral region

SP M53.88 Other specified dorsopathies, sacral and sacrococcygeal region

IQ M53.9 Dorsopathy, unspecified

4 M54 Dorsalgia
EXCLUDES 1 psychogenic dorsalgia (F45.41)

5 M54.0 Panniculitis affecting regions of neck and back
EXCLUDES 1 lupus panniculitis (L93.2)
panniculitis NOS (M79.3)
relapsing [Weber-Christian] panniculitis (M35.6)

IQ M54.00 Panniculitis affecting regions of neck and back, site unspecified

SP M54.01 Panniculitis affecting regions of neck and back, occipito-atlanto-axial region

SP M54.02 Panniculitis affecting regions of neck and back, cervical region

SP M54.03 Panniculitis affecting regions of neck and back, cervicothoracic region

SP M54.04 Panniculitis affecting regions of neck and back, thoracic region

SP M54.05 Panniculitis affecting regions of neck and back, thoracolumbar region

SP M54.06 Panniculitis affecting regions of neck and back, lumbar region

SP M54.07 Panniculitis affecting regions of neck and back, lumbosacral region

SP M54.08 Panniculitis affecting regions of neck and back, sacral and sacrococcygeal region

SP M54.09 Panniculitis affecting regions, neck and back, multiple sites in spine

5 M54.1 Radiculopathy
Brachial neuritis or radiculitis NOS
Lumbar neuritis or radiculitis NOS

★ New ▲ Revised Px Primary **SP** PDGM Px **SL** Low CoM **SH** High CoM **IQ** Quest. Encounter **H** Hospice non-cancer Dx   Unspecified   **M** *Manifestation*

Lumbosacral neuritis or radiculitis NOS
Thoracic neuritis or radiculitis NOS
Radiculitis NOS

EXCLUDES 1 neuralgia and neuritis NOS (M79.2)
radiculopathy with cervical disc disorder (M50.1)
radiculopathy with lumbar and other intervertebral disc disorder (M51.1-)
radiculopathy with spondylosis (M47.2-)

CODING TIPS ✓ Radiculopathy associated with a certain disc disorder should not be coded to M54.1. Note the excludes 1 note.

IQ M54.10 Radiculopathy, site unspecified

SP M54.11 Radiculopathy, occipito-atlanto-axial region

SP M54.12 Radiculopathy, cervical region

SP M54.13 Radiculopathy, cervicothoracic region

SP M54.14 Radiculopathy, thoracic region

SP M54.15 Radiculopathy, thoracolumbar region

SP M54.16 Radiculopathy, lumbar region

SP M54.17 Radiculopathy, lumbosacral region

SP M54.18 Radiculopathy, sacral and sacrococcygeal region

SP M54.2 Cervicalgia

EXCLUDES 1 cervicalgia due to intervertebral cervical disc disorder (M50.-)

CODING TIPS ✓ Cervicalgia associated with a certain disc disorder should not be coded to M54.2. Note the excludes 1 note.

5 M54.3 Sciatica

EXCLUDES 1 lesion of sciatic nerve (G57.0)
sciatica due to intervertebral disc disorder (M51.1-)
sciatica with lumbago (M54.4-)

CODING TIPS ✓ Sciatica associated with a certain disc disorder should not be coded to M54.3. Note the excludes 1 note.

DEFINITION Severe pain in the sciatic nerve running down the lower back through the leg; usually resulting from nerve compression or pinching.

▤ IQ M54.30 Sciatica, unspecified side

▤ SP M54.31 Sciatica, right side

▤ SP M54.32 Sciatica, left side

5 M54.4 Lumbago with sciatica

EXCLUDES 1 lumbago with sciatica due to intervertebral disc disorder (M51.1-)

CODING TIPS ✓ Lumbago associated with a certain disc disorder should not be coded with this code. Note the excludes 1 note.

▤ IQ M54.40 Lumbago with sciatica, unspecified side

▤ SP M54.41 Lumbago with sciatica, right side

▤ SP M54.42 Lumbago with sciatica, left side

IQ M54.5 Low back pain

Loin pain
Lumbago NOS

EXCLUDES 1 low back strain (S39.012)
lumbago due to intervertebral disc displacement (M51.2-)
lumbago with sciatica (M54.4-)

CODING TIPS ✓ Lumbago associated with a certain disc disorder should not be coded with this code. Note the excludes 1 note.

IQ M54.6 Pain in thoracic spine

EXCLUDES 1 pain in thoracic spine due to intervertebral disc disorder (M51.-)

5 M54.8 Other dorsalgia

EXCLUDES 1 dorsalgia in thoracic region (M54.6)
low back pain (M54.5)

SP M54.81 Occipital neuralgia

SP M54.89 Other dorsalgia

IQ M54.9 Dorsalgia, unspecified

Backache NOS
Back pain NOS

Soft tissue disorders   (M60-M79)

Disorders of muscles   (M60-M63)

EXCLUDES 1 dermatopolymyositis (M33.-)
muscular dystrophies and myopathies (G71-G72)
myopathy in amyloidosis (E85.-)
myopathy in polyarteritis nodosa (M30.0)
myopathy in rheumatoid arthritis (M05.32)
myopathy in scleroderma (M34.-)
myopathy in Sjögren's syndrome (M35.03)
myopathy in systemic lupus erythematosus (M32.-)

4 M60   Myositis

EXCLUDES 2 inclusion body myositis [IBM] (G72.41)

CODING TIPS ✓ **Documentation:** Myositis indicates inflammation of the muscles. This may be caused by inflammatory disorders/autoimmune conditions, infection, or injury. Review all clinical documentation carefully to identify any cause and assign the most specific code for the condition.

CODING TIPS ✓ Category M60.- does not include inflammatory myositis specified as inclusion body myositis (IBM), a chronic progressive neurologic condition leading to inflammation and weakness of the muscle. IBM should be coded to G72.41.

+ 5 M60.0 Infective myositis

Tropical pyomyositis
Use additional code (B95-B97) to identify infectious agent

+ 6 M60.00   Infective myositis, unspecified site

▤ SP + M60.000   Infective myositis, unspecified right arm

Infective myositis, right upper limb NOS

▤ SP + M60.001   Infective myositis, unspecified left arm

---

4 4th digit required   **5** 5th digit required   **6** 6th digit required   **7** 7th digit required   **7** 7th digit placeholder   **+** Additional code   **▤** Laterality

Infective myositis, left upper limb NOS

☰ **IQ** ✚ **M60.002 Infective myositis, unspecified arm**

Infective myositis, upper limb NOS

☰ **SP** ✚ **M60.003 Infective myositis, unspecified right leg**

Infective myositis, right lower limb NOS

☰ **SP** ✚ **M60.004 Infective myositis, unspecified left leg**

Infective myositis, left lower limb NOS

☰ **IQ** ✚ **M60.005 Infective myositis, unspecified leg**

Infective myositis, lower limb NOS

☰ **IQ** ✚ **M60.009 Infective myositis, unspecified site**

✚ **⑥ M60.01 Infective myositis, shoulder**

☰ **SP** ✚ M60.011 Infective myositis, right shoulder

☰ **SP** ✚ M60.012 Infective myositis, left shoulder

☰ **IQ** ✚ **M60.019 Infective myositis, unspecified shoulder**

✚ **⑥ M60.02 Infective myositis, upper arm**

☰ **SP** ✚ M60.021 Infective myositis, right upper arm

☰ **SP** ✚ M60.022 Infective myositis, left upper arm

☰ **IQ** ✚ **M60.029 Infective myositis, unspecified upper arm**

✚ **⑥ M60.03 Infective myositis, forearm**

☰ **SP** ✚ M60.031 Infective myositis, right forearm

☰ **SP** ✚ M60.032 Infective myositis, left forearm

☰ **IQ** ✚ **M60.039 Infective myositis, unspecified forearm**

✚ **⑥ M60.04 Infective myositis, hand and fingers**

☰ **SP** ✚ M60.041 Infective myositis, right hand

☰ **SP** ✚ M60.042 Infective myositis, left hand

☰ **IQ** ✚ **M60.043 Infective myositis, unspecified hand**

☰ **IQ** ✚ M60.044 Infective myositis, right finger(s)

☰ **IQ** ✚ M60.045 Infective myositis, left finger(s)

☰ **IQ** ✚ **M60.046 Infective myositis, unspecified finger(s)**

✚ **⑥ M60.05 Infective myositis, thigh**

☰ **SP** ✚ M60.051 Infective myositis, right thigh

☰ **SP** ✚ M60.052 Infective myositis, left thigh

☰ **IQ** ✚ **M60.059 Infective myositis, unspecified thigh**

✚ **⑥ M60.06 Infective myositis, lower leg**

☰ **SP** ✚ M60.061 Infective myositis, right lower leg

☰ **SP** ✚ M60.062 Infective myositis, left lower leg

☰ **IQ** ✚ **M60.069 Infective myositis, unspecified lower leg**

✚ **⑥ M60.07 Infective myositis, ankle, foot and toes**

☰ **SP** ✚ M60.070 Infective myositis, right ankle

☰ **SP** ✚ M60.071 Infective myositis, left ankle

☰ **IQ** ✚ **M60.072 Infective myositis, unspecified ankle**

☰ **SP** ✚ M60.073 Infective myositis, right foot

☰ **SP** ✚ M60.074 Infective myositis, left foot

☰ **IQ** ✚ **M60.075 Infective myositis, unspecified foot**

☰ **SP** ✚ M60.076 Infective myositis, right toe(s)

☰ **SP** ✚ M60.077 Infective myositis, left toe(s)

☰ **IQ** ✚ **M60.078 Infective myositis, unspecified toe(s)**

SP ✚ M60.08 Infective myositis, other site

SP ✚ M60.09 Infective myositis, multiple sites

⑤ M60.1 Interstitial myositis

IQ **M60.10 Interstitial myositis of unspecified site**

⑥ M60.11 Interstitial myositis, shoulder

☰ **SP** M60.111 Interstitial myositis, right shoulder

☰ **SP** M60.112 Interstitial myositis, left shoulder

☰ **IQ** **M60.119 Interstitial myositis, unspecified shoulder**

⑥ M60.12 Interstitial myositis, upper arm

☰ **SP** M60.121 Interstitial myositis, right upper arm

☰ **SP** M60.122 Interstitial myositis, left upper arm

☰ **IQ** **M60.129 Interstitial myositis, unspecified upper arm**

⑥ M60.13 Interstitial myositis, forearm

☰ **SP** M60.131 Interstitial myositis, right forearm

☰ **IQ** M60.132 Interstitial myositis, left forearm

☰ **IQ** **M60.139 Interstitial myositis, unspecified forearm**

⑥ M60.14 Interstitial myositis, hand

☰ **SP** M60.141 Interstitial myositis, right hand

☰ **SP** M60.142 Interstitial myositis, left hand

☰ **IQ** **M60.149 Interstitial myositis, unspecified hand**

⑥ M60.15 Interstitial myositis, thigh

☰ **SP** M60.151 Interstitial myositis, right thigh

☰ **SP** M60.152 Interstitial myositis, left thigh

☰ **IQ** **M60.159 Interstitial myositis, unspecified thigh**

⑥ M60.16 Interstitial myositis, lower leg

☰ **SP** M60.161 Interstitial myositis, right lower leg

☰ **SP** M60.162 Interstitial myositis, left lower leg

☰ **IQ** **M60.169 Interstitial myositis, unspecified lower leg**

⑥ M60.17 Interstitial myositis, ankle and foot

☰ **SP** M60.171 Interstitial myositis, right ankle and foot

☰ **SP** M60.172 Interstitial myositis, left ankle and foot

☰ **IQ** **M60.179 Interstitial myositis, unspecified ankle and foot**

SP M60.18 Interstitial myositis, other site

SP M60.19 Interstitial myositis, multiple sites

✚ ⑤ **M60.2 Foreign body granuloma of soft tissue, not elsewhere classified**

Use additional code to identify the type of retained foreign body (Z18.-)

EXCLUDES 1 foreign body granuloma of skin and subcutaneous tissue (L92.3)

★ New ▲ Revised **Px** Primary **SP** PDGM Px **SL** Low CoM **SH** High CoM **IQ** Quest. Encounter Ⓗ Hospice non-cancer Dx Unspecified **M** *Manifestation*

DecisionHealth's FY 2020 Complete Home Health ICD-10-CM Diagnosis Coding Manual

1213

IQ **+** **M60.20** Foreign body granuloma of soft tissue, not elsewhere classified, unspecified site

+ **6** **M60.21** Foreign body granuloma of soft tissue, not elsewhere classified, shoulder

SP **+** **M60.211** Foreign body granuloma of soft tissue, not elsewhere classified, right shoulder

SP **+** **M60.212** Foreign body granuloma of soft tissue, not elsewhere classified, left shoulder

IQ **+** **M60.219** Foreign body granuloma of soft tissue, not elsewhere classified, unspecified shoulder

+ **6** **M60.22** Foreign body granuloma of soft tissue, not elsewhere classified, upper arm

SP **+** **M60.221** Foreign body granuloma of soft tissue, not elsewhere classified, right upper arm

SP **+** **M60.222** Foreign body granuloma of soft tissue, not elsewhere classified, left upper arm

IQ **+** **M60.229** Foreign body granuloma of soft tissue, not elsewhere classified, unspecified upper arm

+ **6** **M60.23** Foreign body granuloma of soft tissue, not elsewhere classified, forearm

SP **+** **M60.231** Foreign body granuloma of soft tissue, not elsewhere classified, right forearm

SP **+** **M60.232** Foreign body granuloma of soft tissue, not elsewhere classified, left forearm

IQ **+** **M60.239** Foreign body granuloma of soft tissue, not elsewhere classified, unspecified forearm

+ **6** **M60.24** Foreign body granuloma of soft tissue, not elsewhere classified, hand

SP **+** **M60.241** Foreign body granuloma of soft tissue, not elsewhere classified, right hand

SP **+** **M60.242** Foreign body granuloma of soft tissue, not elsewhere classified, left hand

IQ **+** **M60.249** Foreign body granuloma of soft tissue, not elsewhere classified, unspecified hand

+ **6** **M60.25** Foreign body granuloma of soft tissue, not elsewhere classified, thigh

SP **+** **M60.251** Foreign body granuloma of soft tissue, not elsewhere classified, right thigh

SP **+** **M60.252** Foreign body granuloma of soft tissue, not elsewhere classified, left thigh

IQ **+** **M60.259** Foreign body granuloma of soft tissue, not elsewhere classified, unspecified thigh

+ **6** **M60.26** Foreign body granuloma of soft tissue, not elsewhere classified, lower leg

SP **+** **M60.261** Foreign body granuloma of soft tissue, not elsewhere classified, right lower leg

SP **+** **M60.262** Foreign body granuloma of soft tissue, not elsewhere classified, left lower leg

IQ **+** **M60.269** Foreign body granuloma of soft tissue, not elsewhere classified, unspecified lower leg

+ **6** **M60.27** Foreign body granuloma of soft tissue, not elsewhere classified, ankle and foot

SP **+** **M60.271** Foreign body granuloma of soft tissue, not elsewhere classified, right ankle and foot

SP **+** **M60.272** Foreign body granuloma of soft tissue, not elsewhere classified, left ankle and foot

IQ **+** **M60.279** Foreign body granuloma of soft tissue, not elsewhere classified, unspecified ankle and foot

SP **+** **M60.28** Foreign body granuloma of soft tissue, not elsewhere classified, other site

5 **M60.8** Other myositis

IQ **M60.80** Other myositis, unspecified site

6 **M60.81** Other myositis shoulder

SP **M60.811** Other myositis, right shoulder

SP **M60.812** Other myositis, left shoulder

IQ **M60.819** Other myositis, unspecified shoulder

6 **M60.82** Other myositis, upper arm

SP **M60.821** Other myositis, right upper arm

SP **M60.822** Other myositis, left upper arm

IQ **M60.829** Other myositis, unspecified upper arm

6 **M60.83** Other myositis, forearm

SP **M60.831** Other myositis, right forearm

SP **M60.832** Other myositis, left forearm

IQ **M60.839** Other myositis, unspecified forearm

6 **M60.84** Other myositis, hand

SP **M60.841** Other myositis, right hand

SP **M60.842** Other myositis, left hand

IQ **M60.849** Other myositis, unspecified hand

6 **M60.85** Other myositis, thigh

SP **M60.851** Other myositis, right thigh

SP **M60.852** Other myositis, left thigh

IQ **M60.859** Other myositis, unspecified thigh

6 **M60.86** Other myositis, lower leg

SP **M60.861** Other myositis, right lower leg

SP **M60.862** Other myositis, left lower leg

IQ **M60.869** Other myositis, unspecified lower leg

6 **M60.87** Other myositis, ankle and foot

SP **M60.871** Other myositis, right ankle and foot

SP **M60.872** Other myositis, left ankle and foot

IQ **M60.879** Other myositis, unspecified ankle and foot

SP **M60.88** Other myositis, other site

SP **M60.89** Other myositis, multiple sites

IQ **M60.9** Myositis, unspecified

4 **M61** Calcification and ossification of muscle

4 4th digit required   **5** 5th digit required   **6** 6th digit required   **7** 7th digit required   **7** 7th digit placeholder   **+** Additional code   **⊟** Laterality

1214   *DecisionHealth's* FY 2020 Complete Home Health ICD-10-CM Diagnosis Coding Manual

⑤ **M61.0 Myositis ossificans traumatica**

🔢 **M61.00 Myositis ossificans traumatica, unspecified site**

⑥ **M61.01 Myositis ossificans traumatica, shoulder**

▱ 🆂🅿 **M61.011 Myositis ossificans traumatica, right shoulder**

▱ 🆂🅿 **M61.012 Myositis ossificans traumatica, left shoulder**

▱ 🔢 **M61.019 Myositis ossificans traumatica, unspecified shoulder**

⑥ **M61.02 Myositis ossificans traumatica, upper arm**

▱ 🆂🅿 **M61.021 Myositis ossificans traumatica, right upper arm**

▱ 🆂🅿 **M61.022 Myositis ossificans traumatica, left upper arm**

▱ 🔢 **M61.029 Myositis ossificans traumatica, unspecified upper arm**

⑥ **M61.03 Myositis ossificans traumatica, forearm**

▱ 🆂🅿 **M61.031 Myositis ossificans traumatica, right forearm**

▱ 🆂🅿 **M61.032 Myositis ossificans traumatica, left forearm**

▱ 🔢 **M61.039 Myositis ossificans traumatica, unspecified forearm**

⑥ **M61.04 Myositis ossificans traumatica, hand**

▱ 🆂🅿 **M61.041 Myositis ossificans traumatica, right hand**

▱ 🆂🅿 **M61.042 Myositis ossificans traumatica, left hand**

▱ 🔢 **M61.049 Myositis ossificans traumatica, unspecified hand**

⑥ **M61.05 Myositis ossificans traumatica, thigh**

▱ 🆂🅿 **M61.051 Myositis ossificans traumatica, right thigh**

▱ 🆂🅿 **M61.052 Myositis ossificans traumatica, left thigh**

▱ 🔢 **M61.059 Myositis ossificans traumatica, unspecified thigh**

⑥ **M61.06 Myositis ossificans traumatica, lower leg**

▱ 🆂🅿 **M61.061 Myositis ossificans traumatica, right lower leg**

▱ 🆂🅿 **M61.062 Myositis ossificans traumatica, left lower leg**

▱ 🔢 **M61.069 Myositis ossificans traumatica, unspecified lower leg**

⑥ **M61.07 Myositis ossificans traumatica, ankle and foot**

▱ 🆂🅿 **M61.071 Myositis ossificans traumatica, right ankle and foot**

▱ 🆂🅿 **M61.072 Myositis ossificans traumatica, left ankle and foot**

▱ 🔢 **M61.079 Myositis ossificans traumatica, unspecified ankle and foot**

🆂🅿 **M61.08 Myositis ossificans traumatica, other site**

🆂🅿 **M61.09 Myositis ossificans traumatica, multiple sites**

⑤ **M61.1 Myositis ossificans progressiva**
Fibrodysplasia ossificans progressiva

🔢 **M61.10 Myositis ossificans progressiva, unspecified site**

⑥ **M61.11 Myositis ossificans progressiva, shoulder**

▱ 🆂🅿 **M61.111 Myositis ossificans progressiva, right shoulder**

▱ 🆂🅿 **M61.112 Myositis ossificans progressiva, left shoulder**

▱ 🔢 **M61.119 Myositis ossificans progressiva, unspecified shoulder**

⑥ **M61.12 Myositis ossificans progressiva, upper arm**

▱ 🆂🅿 **M61.121 Myositis ossificans progressiva, right upper arm**

▱ 🆂🅿 **M61.122 Myositis ossificans progressiva, left upper arm**

▱ 🔢 **M61.129 Myositis ossificans progressiva, unspecified arm**

⑥ **M61.13 Myositis ossificans progressiva, forearm**

▱ 🆂🅿 **M61.131 Myositis ossificans progressiva, right forearm**

▱ 🆂🅿 **M61.132 Myositis ossificans progressiva, left forearm**

▱ 🔢 **M61.139 Myositis ossificans progressiva, unspecified forearm**

⑥ **M61.14 Myositis ossificans progressiva, hand and finger(s)**

▱ 🆂🅿 **M61.141 Myositis ossificans progressiva, right hand**

▱ 🆂🅿 **M61.142 Myositis ossificans progressiva, left hand**

▱ 🔢 **M61.143 Myositis ossificans progressiva, unspecified hand**

▱ 🆂🅿 **M61.144 Myositis ossificans progressiva, right finger(s)**

▱ 🆂🅿 **M61.145 Myositis ossificans progressiva, left finger(s)**

▱ 🔢 **M61.146 Myositis ossificans progressiva, unspecified finger(s)**

⑥ **M61.15 Myositis ossificans progressiva, thigh**

▱ 🆂🅿 **M61.151 Myositis ossificans progressiva, right thigh**

▱ 🆂🅿 **M61.152 Myositis ossificans progressiva, left thigh**

▱ 🔢 **M61.159 Myositis ossificans progressiva, unspecified thigh**

⑥ **M61.16 Myositis ossificans progressiva, lower leg**

▱ 🆂🅿 **M61.161 Myositis ossificans progressiva, right lower leg**

▱ 🆂🅿 **M61.162 Myositis ossificans progressiva, left lower leg**

▱ 🔢 **M61.169 Myositis ossificans progressiva, unspecified lower leg**

⑥ **M61.17 Myositis ossificans progressiva, ankle, foot and toe(s)**

▱ 🆂🅿 **M61.171 Myositis ossificans progressiva, right ankle**

▱ 🆂🅿 **M61.172 Myositis ossificans progressiva, left ankle**

▱ 🔢 **M61.173 Myositis ossificans progressiva, unspecified ankle**

▱ 🆂🅿 **M61.174 Myositis ossificans progressiva, right foot**

▱ 🆂🅿 **M61.175 Myositis ossificans progressiva, left foot**

★ New ▲ Revised Px Primary 🆂🅿 PDGM Px 🆂🅛 Low CoM 🆂🅗 High CoM 🔢 Quest. Encounter Ⓗ Hospice non-cancer Dx Unspecified Ⓜ *Manifestation*

DecisionHealth's FY 2020 Complete Home Health ICD-10-CM Diagnosis Coding Manual

1215

Chapter 13

M00-M99

☱ **IQ** **M61.176** Myositis ossificans progressiva, unspecified foot

☱ **SP** **M61.177** Myositis ossificans progressiva, right toe(s)

☱ **SP** **M61.178** Myositis ossificans progressiva, left toe(s)

☱ **IQ** **M61.179** Myositis ossificans progressiva, unspecified toe(s)

SP **M61.18** Myositis ossificans progressiva, other site

SP **M61.19** Myositis ossificans progressiva, multiple sites

5 **M61.2** Paralytic calcification and ossification of muscle
    Myositis ossificans associated with quadriplegia or paraplegia

IQ **M61.20** Paralytic calcification and ossification of muscle, unspecified site

6 **M61.21** Paralytic calcification and ossification of muscle, shoulder

☱ **SP** **M61.211** Paralytic calcification and ossification of muscle, right shoulder

☱ **SP** **M61.212** Paralytic calcification and ossification of muscle, left shoulder

☱ **IQ** **M61.219** Paralytic calcification and ossification of muscle, unspecified shoulder

6 **M61.22** Paralytic calcification and ossification of muscle, upper arm

☱ **SP** **M61.221** Paralytic calcification and ossification of muscle, right upper arm

☱ **SP** **M61.222** Paralytic calcification and ossification of muscle, left upper arm

☱ **IQ** **M61.229** Paralytic calcification and ossification of muscle, unspecified upper arm

6 **M61.23** Paralytic calcification and ossification of muscle, forearm

☱ **SP** **M61.231** Paralytic calcification and ossification of muscle, right forearm

☱ **SP** **M61.232** Paralytic calcification and ossification of muscle, left forearm

☱ **IQ** **M61.239** Paralytic calcification and ossification of muscle, unspecified forearm

6 **M61.24** Paralytic calcification and ossification of muscle, hand

☱ **SP** **M61.241** Paralytic calcification and ossification of muscle, right hand

☱ **SP** **M61.242** Paralytic calcification and ossification of muscle, left hand

☱ **IQ** **M61.249** Paralytic calcification and ossification of muscle, unspecified hand

6 **M61.25** Paralytic calcification and ossification of muscle, thigh

☱ **SP** **M61.251** Paralytic calcification and ossification of muscle, right thigh

☱ **SP** **M61.252** Paralytic calcification and ossification of muscle, left thigh

☱ **IQ** **M61.259** Paralytic calcification and ossification of muscle, unspecified thigh

6 **M61.26** Paralytic calcification and ossification of muscle, lower leg

☱ **SP** **M61.261** Paralytic calcification and ossification of muscle, right lower leg

☱ **SP** **M61.262** Paralytic calcification and ossification of muscle, left lower leg

☱ **IQ** **M61.269** Paralytic calcification and ossification of muscle, unspecified lower leg

6 **M61.27** Paralytic calcification and ossification of muscle, ankle and foot

☱ **SP** **M61.271** Paralytic calcification and ossification of muscle, right ankle and foot

☱ **SP** **M61.272** Paralytic calcification and ossification of muscle, left ankle and foot

☱ **IQ** **M61.279** Paralytic calcification and ossification of muscle, unspecified ankle and foot

SP **M61.28** Paralytic calcification and ossification of muscle, other site

SP **M61.29** Paralytic calcification and ossification of muscle, multiple sites

5 **M61.3** Calcification and ossification of muscles associated with burns
    Myositis ossificans associated with burns

IQ **M61.30** Calcification and ossification of muscles associated with burns, unspecified site

6 **M61.31** Calcification and ossification of muscles associated with burns, shoulder

☱ **SP** **M61.311** Calcification and ossification of muscles associated with burns, right shoulder

☱ **SP** **M61.312** Calcification and ossification of muscles associated with burns, left shoulder

☱ **IQ** **M61.319** Calcification and ossification of muscles associated with burns, unspecified shoulder

6 **M61.32** Calcification and ossification of muscles associated with burns, upper arm

☱ **SP** **M61.321** Calcification and ossification of muscles associated with burns, right upper arm

☱ **SP** **M61.322** Calcification and ossification of muscles associated with burns, left upper arm

☱ **IQ** **M61.329** Calcification and ossification of muscles associated with burns, unspecified upper arm

6 **M61.33** Calcification and ossification of muscles associated with burns, forearm

☱ **SP** **M61.331** Calcification and ossification of muscles associated with burns, right forearm

☱ **SP** **M61.332** Calcification and ossification of muscles associated with burns, left forearm

---

4 4th digit required   **5** 5th digit required   **6** 6th digit required   **7** 7th digit required   **7** 7th digit placeholder   **+** Additional code   ☱ Laterality

☐ **IQ** **M61.339** Calcification and ossification of muscles associated with burns, unspecified forearm

☐ **M61.34** Calcification and ossification of muscles associated with burns, hand

☐ **SP** **M61.341** Calcification and ossification of muscles associated with burns, right hand

☐ **SP** **M61.342** Calcification and ossification of muscles associated with burns, left hand

☐ **IQ** **M61.349** Calcification and ossification of muscles associated with burns, unspecified hand

☐ **M61.35** Calcification and ossification of muscles associated with burns, thigh

☐ **SP** **M61.351** Calcification and ossification of muscles associated with burns, right thigh

☐ **SP** **M61.352** Calcification and ossification of muscles associated with burns, left thigh

☐ **IQ** **M61.359** Calcification and ossification of muscles associated with burns, unspecified thigh

☐ **M61.36** Calcification and ossification of muscles associated with burns, lower leg

☐ **SP** **M61.361** Calcification and ossification of muscles associated with burns, right lower leg

☐ **SP** **M61.362** Calcification and ossification of muscles associated with burns, left lower leg

☐ **IQ** **M61.369** Calcification and ossification of muscles associated with burns, unspecified lower leg

☐ **M61.37** Calcification and ossification of muscles associated with burns, ankle and foot

☐ **SP** **M61.371** Calcification and ossification of muscles associated with burns, right ankle and foot

☐ **SP** **M61.372** Calcification and ossification of muscles associated with burns, left ankle and foot

☐ **IQ** **M61.379** Calcification and ossification of muscles associated with burns, unspecified ankle and foot

SP **M61.38** Calcification and ossification of muscles associated with burns, other site

SP **M61.39** Calcification and ossification of muscles associated with burns, multiple sites

☐ **M61.4** Other calcification of muscle

> **EXCLUDES 1** calcific tendinitis NOS (M65.2-)
> calcific tendinitis of shoulder (M75.3)

IQ **M61.40** Other calcification of muscle, unspecified site

☐ **M61.41** Other calcification of muscle, shoulder

☐ **SP** **M61.411** Other calcification of muscle, right shoulder

☐ **SP** **M61.412** Other calcification of muscle, left shoulder

☐ **IQ** **M61.419** Other calcification of muscle, unspecified shoulder

☐ **M61.42** Other calcification of muscle, upper arm

☐ **SP** **M61.421** Other calcification of muscle, right upper arm

☐ **SP** **M61.422** Other calcification of muscle, left upper arm

☐ **IQ** **M61.429** Other calcification of muscle, unspecified upper arm

☐ **M61.43** Other calcification of muscle, forearm

☐ **SP** **M61.431** Other calcification of muscle, right forearm

☐ **SP** **M61.432** Other calcification of muscle, left forearm

☐ **IQ** **M61.439** Other calcification of muscle, unspecified forearm

☐ **M61.44** Other calcification of muscle, hand

☐ **SP** **M61.441** Other calcification of muscle, right hand

☐ **SP** **M61.442** Other calcification of muscle, left hand

☐ **IQ** **M61.449** Other calcification of muscle, unspecified hand

☐ **M61.45** Other calcification of muscle, thigh

☐ **SP** **M61.451** Other calcification of muscle, right thigh

☐ **SP** **M61.452** Other calcification of muscle, left thigh

☐ **IQ** **M61.459** Other calcification of muscle, unspecified thigh

☐ **M61.46** Other calcification of muscle, lower leg

☐ **SP** **M61.461** Other calcification of muscle, right lower leg

☐ **SP** **M61.462** Other calcification of muscle, left lower leg

☐ **IQ** **M61.469** Other calcification of muscle, unspecified lower leg

☐ **M61.47** Other calcification of muscle, ankle and foot

☐ **SP** **M61.471** Other calcification of muscle, right ankle and foot

☐ **SP** **M61.472** Other calcification of muscle, left ankle and foot

☐ **IQ** **M61.479** Other calcification of muscle, unspecified ankle and foot

SP **M61.48** Other calcification of muscle, other site

SP **M61.49** Other calcification of muscle, multiple sites

☐ **M61.5** Other ossification of muscle

IQ **M61.50** Other ossification of muscle, unspecified site

☐ **M61.51** Other ossification of muscle, shoulder

☐ **SP** **M61.511** Other ossification of muscle, right shoulder

☐ **SP** **M61.512** Other ossification of muscle, left shoulder

☐ **IQ** **M61.519** Other ossification of muscle, unspecified shoulder

☐ **M61.52** Other ossification of muscle, upper arm

★ New ▲ Revised **Px** Primary **SP** PDGM Px **SL** Low CoM **SH** High CoM **IQ** Quest. Encounter **H** Hospice non-cancer Dx Unspecified **M** *Manifestation*

☐ SP **M61.521** Other ossification of muscle, right upper arm

☐ SP **M61.522** Other ossification of muscle, left upper arm

☐ IQ **M61.529** Other ossification of muscle, unspecified upper arm

⑥ **M61.53** Other ossification of muscle, forearm

☐ SP **M61.531** Other ossification of muscle, right forearm

☐ SP **M61.532** Other ossification of muscle, left forearm

☐ IQ **M61.539** Other ossification of muscle, unspecified forearm

⑥ **M61.54** Other ossification of muscle, hand

☐ SP **M61.541** Other ossification of muscle, right hand

☐ SP **M61.542** Other ossification of muscle, left hand

☐ IQ **M61.549** Other ossification of muscle, unspecified hand

⑥ **M61.55** Other ossification of muscle, thigh

☐ SP **M61.551** Other ossification of muscle, right thigh

☐ SP **M61.552** Other ossification of muscle, left thigh

☐ IQ **M61.559** Other ossification of muscle, unspecified thigh

⑥ **M61.56** Other ossification of muscle, lower leg

☐ SP **M61.561** Other ossification of muscle, right lower leg

☐ SP **M61.562** Other ossification of muscle, left lower leg

☐ IQ **M61.569** Other ossification of muscle, unspecified lower leg

⑥ **M61.57** Other ossification of muscle, ankle and foot

☐ SP **M61.571** Other ossification of muscle, right ankle and foot

☐ SP **M61.572** Other ossification of muscle, left ankle and foot

☐ IQ **M61.579** Other ossification of muscle, unspecified ankle and foot

SP **M61.58** Other ossification of muscle, other site

SP **M61.59** Other ossification of muscle, multiple sites

IQ **M61.9** Calcification and ossification of muscle, unspecified

④ **M62** Other disorders of muscle

> **EXCLUDES 1** alcoholic myopathy (G72.1)
> cramp and spasm (R25.2)
> drug-induced myopathy (G72.0)
> myalgia (M79.1-)
> stiff-man syndrome (G25.82)
>
> **EXCLUDES 2** nontraumatic hematoma of muscle (M79.81)

⑤ **M62.0** Separation of muscle (nontraumatic)
> Diastasis of muscle
>
> **EXCLUDES 1** diastasis recti complicating pregnancy, labor and delivery (O71.8)
> traumatic separation of muscle- see strain of muscle by body region

CODING TIPS ✓ Codes classified in M62.0- through M62.28 indicate muscle separation, rupture and ischemia of a non-traumatic origin. When a traumatic muscle injury is reported, do not assign a code from M62.0- through M62.28, but instead assign a code from Chapter 19, Injury, Poisoning and Certain Other Consequences of External Causes.

IQ **M62.00** Separation of muscle (nontraumatic), unspecified site

⑥ **M62.01** Separation of muscle (nontraumatic), shoulder

☐ SP **M62.011** Separation of muscle (nontraumatic), right shoulder

☐ SP **M62.012** Separation of muscle (nontraumatic), left shoulder

☐ IQ **M62.019** Separation of muscle (nontraumatic), unspecified shoulder

⑥ **M62.02** Separation of muscle (nontraumatic), upper arm

☐ SP **M62.021** Separation of muscle (nontraumatic), right upper arm

☐ SP **M62.022** Separation of muscle (nontraumatic), left upper arm

☐ IQ **M62.029** Separation of muscle (nontraumatic), unspecified upper arm

⑥ **M62.03** Separation of muscle (nontraumatic), forearm

☐ SP **M62.031** Separation of muscle (nontraumatic), right forearm

☐ SP **M62.032** Separation of muscle (nontraumatic), left forearm

☐ IQ **M62.039** Separation of muscle (nontraumatic), unspecified forearm

⑥ **M62.04** Separation of muscle (nontraumatic), hand

☐ SP **M62.041** Separation of muscle (nontraumatic), right hand

☐ SP **M62.042** Separation of muscle (nontraumatic), left hand

☐ IQ **M62.049** Separation of muscle (nontraumatic), unspecified hand

⑥ **M62.05** Separation of muscle (nontraumatic), thigh

☐ SP **M62.051** Separation of muscle (nontraumatic), right thigh

☐ SP **M62.052** Separation of muscle (nontraumatic), left thigh

☐ IQ **M62.059** Separation of muscle (nontraumatic), unspecified thigh

⑥ **M62.06** Separation of muscle (nontraumatic), lower leg

☐ SP **M62.061** Separation of muscle (nontraumatic), right lower leg

☐ SP **M62.062** Separation of muscle (nontraumatic), left lower leg

☐ IQ **M62.069** Separation of muscle (nontraumatic), unspecified lower leg

⑥ **M62.07** Separation of muscle (nontraumatic), ankle and foot

---

④4th digit required   ⑤5th digit required   ⑥6th digit required   ⑦7th digit required   ⑦7th digit placeholder   ➕Additional code   ☐Laterality

1218   *DecisionHealth's* FY 2020 Complete Home Health ICD-10-CM Diagnosis Coding Manual

⊟ **SP** **M62.071** Separation of muscle (nontraumatic), right ankle and foot

⊟ **SP** **M62.072** Separation of muscle (nontraumatic), left ankle and foot

⊟ **IQ** **M62.079** Separation of muscle (nontraumatic), unspecified ankle and foot

SP **M62.08** Separation of muscle (nontraumatic), other site

⑤ **M62.1** Other rupture of muscle (nontraumatic)

> **EXCLUDES 1** traumatic rupture of muscle - see strain of muscle by body region
>
> **EXCLUDES 2** rupture of tendon (M66.-)
>
> **CODING TIPS ✓** Codes classified in M62.0- through M62.28 indicate muscle separation, rupture and ischemia of a non-traumatic origin. When a traumatic muscle injury is reported, do not assign a code from M62.0- through M62.28, but instead assign a code from Chapter 19, Injury, Poisoning and Certain Other Consequences of External Causes.

IQ **M62.10** Other rupture of muscle (nontraumatic), unspecified site

⑥ **M62.11** Other rupture of muscle (nontraumatic), shoulder

⊟ **SP** **M62.111** Other rupture of muscle (nontraumatic), right shoulder

⊟ **SP** **M62.112** Other rupture of muscle (nontraumatic), left shoulder

⊟ **IQ** **M62.119** Other rupture of muscle (nontraumatic), unspecified shoulder

⑥ **M62.12** Other rupture of muscle (nontraumatic), upper arm

⊟ **SP** **M62.121** Other rupture of muscle (nontraumatic), right upper arm

⊟ **SP** **M62.122** Other rupture of muscle (nontraumatic), left upper arm

⊟ **IQ** **M62.129** Other rupture of muscle (nontraumatic), unspecified upper arm

⑥ **M62.13** Other rupture of muscle (nontraumatic), forearm

⊟ **SP** **M62.131** Other rupture of muscle (nontraumatic), right forearm

⊟ **SP** **M62.132** Other rupture of muscle (nontraumatic), left forearm

⊟ **IQ** **M62.139** Other rupture of muscle (nontraumatic), unspecified forearm

⑥ **M62.14** Other rupture of muscle (nontraumatic), hand

⊟ **SP** **M62.141** Other rupture of muscle (nontraumatic), right hand

⊟ **SP** **M62.142** Other rupture of muscle (nontraumatic), left hand

⊟ **IQ** **M62.149** Other rupture of muscle (nontraumatic), unspecified hand

⑥ **M62.15** Other rupture of muscle (nontraumatic), thigh

⊟ **SP** **M62.151** Other rupture of muscle (nontraumatic), right thigh

⊟ **SP** **M62.152** Other rupture of muscle (nontraumatic), left thigh

⊟ **IQ** **M62.159** Other rupture of muscle (nontraumatic), unspecified thigh

⑥ **M62.16** Other rupture of muscle (nontraumatic), lower leg

⊟ **SP** **M62.161** Other rupture of muscle (nontraumatic), right lower leg

⊟ **SP** **M62.162** Other rupture of muscle (nontraumatic), left lower leg

⊟ **IQ** **M62.169** Other rupture of muscle (nontraumatic), unspecified lower leg

⑥ **M62.17** Other rupture of muscle (nontraumatic), ankle and foot

⊟ **SP** **M62.171** Other rupture of muscle (nontraumatic), right ankle and foot

⊟ **SP** **M62.172** Other rupture of muscle (nontraumatic), left ankle and foot

⊟ **IQ** **M62.179** Other rupture of muscle (nontraumatic), unspecified ankle and foot

SP **M62.18** Other rupture of muscle (nontraumatic), other site

⑤ **M62.2** Nontraumatic ischemic infarction of muscle

> **EXCLUDES 1** compartment syndrome (traumatic) (T79.A-) nontraumatic compartment syndrome (M79.A-) traumatic ischemia of muscle (T79.6) rhabdomyolysis (M62.82) Volkmann's ischemic contracture (T79.6)
>
> **CODING TIPS ✓** Codes classified in M62.0- through M62.28 indicate muscle separation, rupture and ischemia of a non-traumatic origin. When a traumatic muscle injury is reported, do not assign a code from M62.0- through M62.28, but instead assign a code from Chapter 19, Injury, Poisoning and Certain Other Consequences of External Causes.

IQ **M62.20** Nontraumatic ischemic infarction of muscle, unspecified site

⑥ **M62.21** Nontraumatic ischemic infarction of muscle, shoulder

⊟ **SP** **M62.211** Nontraumatic ischemic infarction of muscle, right shoulder

⊟ **SP** **M62.212** Nontraumatic ischemic infarction of muscle, left shoulder

⊟ **IQ** **M62.219** Nontraumatic ischemic infarction of muscle, unspecified shoulder

⑥ **M62.22** Nontraumatic ischemic infarction of muscle, upper arm

⊟ **SP** **M62.221** Nontraumatic ischemic infarction of muscle, right upper arm

⊟ **SP** **M62.222** Nontraumatic ischemic infarction of muscle, left upper arm

⊟ **IQ** **M62.229** Nontraumatic ischemic infarction of muscle, unspecified upper arm

⑥ **M62.23** Nontraumatic ischemic infarction of muscle, forearm

⊟ **SP** **M62.231** Nontraumatic ischemic infarction of muscle, right forearm

---

★ New ▲ Revised Px Primary **SP** PDGM Px **SL** Low CoM **SH** High CoM **IQ** Quest. Encounter **H** Hospice non-cancer Dx Unspecified **M** *Manifestation*

DecisionHealth's FY 2020 Complete Home Health ICD-10-CM Diagnosis Coding Manual

1219

SP M62.232 Nontraumatic ischemic infarction of muscle, left forearm

IQ M62.239 Nontraumatic ischemic infarction of muscle, unspecified forearm

M62.24 Nontraumatic ischemic infarction of muscle, hand

SP M62.241 Nontraumatic ischemic infarction of muscle, right hand

SP M62.242 Nontraumatic ischemic infarction of muscle, left hand

IQ M62.249 Nontraumatic ischemic infarction of muscle, unspecified hand

M62.25 Nontraumatic ischemic infarction of muscle, thigh

SP M62.251 Nontraumatic ischemic infarction of muscle, right thigh

SP M62.252 Nontraumatic ischemic infarction of muscle, left thigh

IQ M62.259 Nontraumatic ischemic infarction of muscle, unspecified thigh

M62.26 Nontraumatic ischemic infarction of muscle, lower leg

SP M62.261 Nontraumatic ischemic infarction of muscle, right lower leg

SP M62.262 Nontraumatic ischemic infarction of muscle, left lower leg

IQ M62.269 Nontraumatic ischemic infarction of muscle, unspecified lower leg

M62.27 Nontraumatic ischemic infarction of muscle, ankle and foot

SP M62.271 Nontraumatic ischemic infarction of muscle, right ankle and foot

SP M62.272 Nontraumatic ischemic infarction of muscle, left ankle and foot

IQ M62.279 Nontraumatic ischemic infarction of muscle, unspecified ankle and foot

SP M62.28 Nontraumatic ischemic infarction of muscle, other site

SP M62.3 Immobility syndrome (paraplegic)

> **CODING TIPS ✓**   Do not assign M62.3 for paraplegia that is due to a neurologic condition or injury. M62.3 indicates paraplegia of a non-neurologic origin. Do not use this code when the condition is due to an injury or other neurologic condition.

M62.4 Contracture of muscle
   Contracture of tendon (sheath)
   > **EXCLUDES 1**   contracture of joint (M24.5-)

IQ M62.40 Contracture of muscle, unspecified site

M62.41 Contracture of muscle, shoulder

IQ M62.411 Contracture of muscle, right shoulder

IQ M62.412 Contracture of muscle, left shoulder

IQ M62.419 Contracture of muscle, unspecified shoulder

M62.42 Contracture of muscle, upper arm

IQ M62.421 Contracture of muscle, right upper arm

IQ M62.422 Contracture of muscle, left upper arm

IQ M62.429 Contracture of muscle, unspecified upper arm

M62.43 Contracture of muscle, forearm

IQ M62.431 Contracture of muscle, right forearm

IQ M62.432 Contracture of muscle, left forearm

IQ M62.439 Contracture of muscle, unspecified forearm

M62.44 Contracture of muscle, hand

IQ M62.441 Contracture of muscle, right hand

IQ M62.442 Contracture of muscle, left hand

IQ M62.449 Contracture of muscle, unspecified hand

M62.45 Contracture of muscle, thigh

IQ M62.451 Contracture of muscle, right thigh

IQ M62.452 Contracture of muscle, left thigh

IQ M62.459 Contracture of muscle, unspecified thigh

M62.46 Contracture of muscle, lower leg

IQ M62.461 Contracture of muscle, right lower leg

IQ M62.462 Contracture of muscle, left lower leg

IQ M62.469 Contracture of muscle, unspecified lower leg

M62.47 Contracture of muscle, ankle and foot

IQ M62.471 Contracture of muscle, right ankle and foot

IQ M62.472 Contracture of muscle, left ankle and foot

IQ M62.479 Contracture of muscle, unspecified ankle and foot

IQ M62.48 Contracture of muscle, other site

IQ M62.49 Contracture of muscle, multiple sites

M62.5 Muscle wasting and atrophy, not elsewhere classified
   Disuse atrophy NEC
   > **EXCLUDES 1**   neuralgic amyotrophy (G54.5)
   > progressive muscular atrophy (G12.21)
   > sarcopenia (M62.84)
   > **EXCLUDES 2**   pelvic muscle wasting (N81.84)

IQ M62.50 Muscle wasting and atrophy, not elsewhere classified, unspecified site

M62.51 Muscle wasting and atrophy, not elsewhere classified, shoulder

SP M62.511 Muscle wasting and atrophy, not elsewhere classified, right shoulder

SP M62.512 Muscle wasting and atrophy, not elsewhere classified, left shoulder

IQ M62.519 Muscle wasting and atrophy, not elsewhere classified, unspecified shoulder

M62.52 Muscle wasting and atrophy, not elsewhere classified, upper arm

SP M62.521 Muscle wasting and atrophy, not elsewhere classified, right upper arm

---

◆4th digit required   ⑤5th digit required   ⑥6th digit required   ⑦7th digit required   ⑦7th digit placeholder   ✚Additional code   ⊟Laterality

1220   *DecisionHealth's* FY 2020 Complete Home Health ICD-10-CM Diagnosis Coding Manual

☐ SP **M62.522 Muscle wasting and atrophy, not elsewhere classified, left upper arm**

☐ IQ **M62.529 Muscle wasting and atrophy, not elsewhere classified, unspecified upper arm**

6 **M62.53 Muscle wasting and atrophy, not elsewhere classified, forearm**

☐ SP **M62.531 Muscle wasting and atrophy, not elsewhere classified, right forearm**

☐ SP **M62.532 Muscle wasting and atrophy, not elsewhere classified, left forearm**

☐ IQ **M62.539 Muscle wasting and atrophy, not elsewhere classified, unspecified forearm**

6 **M62.54 Muscle wasting and atrophy, not elsewhere classified, hand**

☐ SP **M62.541 Muscle wasting and atrophy, not elsewhere classified, right hand**

☐ SP **M62.542 Muscle wasting and atrophy, not elsewhere classified, left hand**

☐ IQ **M62.549 Muscle wasting and atrophy, not elsewhere classified, unspecified hand**

6 **M62.55 Muscle wasting and atrophy, not elsewhere classified, thigh**

☐ SP **M62.551 Muscle wasting and atrophy, not elsewhere classified, right thigh**

☐ SP **M62.552 Muscle wasting and atrophy, not elsewhere classified, left thigh**

☐ IQ **M62.559 Muscle wasting and atrophy, not elsewhere classified, unspecified thigh**

6 **M62.56 Muscle wasting and atrophy, not elsewhere classified, lower leg**

☐ SP **M62.561 Muscle wasting and atrophy, not elsewhere classified, right lower leg**

☐ SP **M62.562 Muscle wasting and atrophy, not elsewhere classified, left lower leg**

☐ IQ **M62.569 Muscle wasting and atrophy, not elsewhere classified, unspecified lower leg**

6 **M62.57 Muscle wasting and atrophy, not elsewhere classified, ankle and foot**

☐ SP **M62.571 Muscle wasting and atrophy, not elsewhere classified, right ankle and foot**

☐ SP **M62.572 Muscle wasting and atrophy, not elsewhere classified, left ankle and foot**

☐ IQ **M62.579 Muscle wasting and atrophy, not elsewhere classified, unspecified ankle and foot**

SP **M62.58 Muscle wasting and atrophy, not elsewhere classified, other site**

SP **M62.59 Muscle wasting and atrophy, not elsewhere classified, multiple sites**

5 **M62.8 Other specified disorders of muscle**

> **EXCLUDES 2** nontraumatic hematoma of muscle (M79.81)

IQ **M62.81 Muscle weakness (generalized)**

> **EXCLUDES 1** muscle weakness in sarcopenia (M62.84)

CODING TIPS ✓ Use M62.81 for true muscle weakness. Muscle weakness may be the result of musculoskeletal disorders, neuromuscular disease or degenerative disease otherwise unidentified. If muscle weakness is part of a condition, do not use the code. Unilateral weakness associated with stroke, brain disorders or injury is coded to hemiplegia/hemiparesis, not M62.81. Muscle group measurements are not required, but measurable muscle weakness must be documented.

SP **M62.82 Rhabdomyolysis**

> **EXCLUDES 1** traumatic rhabdomyolysis (T79.6)

6 **M62.83 Muscle spasm**

SP **M62.830 Muscle spasm of back**

IQ **M62.831 Muscle spasm of calf**
Charley-horse

IQ **M62.838 Other muscle spasm**

SP **M62.84 Sarcopenia**
Age-related sarcopenia
Code first underlying disease, if applicable, such as:
> disorders of myoneural junction and muscle disease in diseases classified elsewhere (G73.-)
> other and unspecified myopathies (G72.-)
> primary disorders of muscles (G71.-)

CODING TIPS ✓ Patients with sarcopenia typically experience mobility limitations and other functional issues such as an inability to carry out activities of daily living. Low grip strength and slow gait speed are strongly correlated with decreased ability to recover from serious injury, falls, disability, hospital and nursing home admissions, and increased mortality. Conditions which may be associated with sarcopenia include hip fracture, bed rest with immobilization, chronic obstructive pulmonary disease, diabetes mellitus Type 2, stroke, Parkinson's disease and congestive heart failure. While all people lose muscle mass and strength as they age, some older adults may have accelerated loss of muscle and may develop sarcopenia without having any of these conditions.

SP **M62.89 Other specified disorders of muscle**
Muscle (sheath) hernia

IQ **M62.9 Disorder of muscle, unspecified**

4 **M63 Disorders of muscle in diseases classified elsewhere**
Code first underlying disease, such as:
> leprosy (A30.-)
> neoplasm (C49.-, C79.89, D21.-, D48.1)
> schistosomiasis (B65.-)
> trichinellosis (B75)
> **EXCLUDES 1** myopathy in cysticercosis (B69.81)
> myopathy in endocrine diseases (G73.7)

★ New ▲ Revised Px Primary SP PDGM Px SL Low CoM SH High CoM IQ Quest. Encounter H Hospice non-cancer Dx Unspecified M *Manifestation*

Chapter 13

M00-M99

myopathy in metabolic diseases
(G73.7)
myopathy in sarcoidosis
(D86.87)
myopathy in secondary syphilis
(A51.49)
myopathy in syphilis (late)
(A52.78)
myopathy in toxoplasmosis
(B58.82)
myopathy in tuberculosis
(A18.09)

⑤ **M63.8 Disorders of muscle in diseases classified elsewhere**

Ⓜ Ⓘ🅀 **M63.80** *Disorders of muscle in diseases classified elsewhere, unspecified site*

⑥ **M63.81 Disorders of muscle in diseases classified elsewhere, shoulder**

Ⓜ ☰ Ⓘ🅀 **M63.811** *Disorders of muscle in diseases classified elsewhere, right shoulder*

Ⓜ ☰ Ⓘ🅀 **M63.812** *Disorders of muscle in diseases classified elsewhere, left shoulder*

Ⓜ ☰ Ⓘ🅀 **M63.819** *Disorders of muscle in diseases classified elsewhere, unspecified shoulder*

⑥ **M63.82 Disorders of muscle in diseases classified elsewhere, upper arm**

Ⓜ ☰ Ⓘ🅀 **M63.821** *Disorders of muscle in diseases classified elsewhere, right upper arm*

Ⓜ ☰ Ⓘ🅀 **M63.822** *Disorders of muscle in diseases classified elsewhere, left upper arm*

Ⓜ ☰ Ⓘ🅀 **M63.829** *Disorders of muscle in diseases classified elsewhere, unspecified upper arm*

⑥ **M63.83 Disorders of muscle in diseases classified elsewhere, forearm**

Ⓜ ☰ Ⓘ🅀 **M63.831** *Disorders of muscle in diseases classified elsewhere, right forearm*

Ⓜ ☰ Ⓘ🅀 **M63.832** *Disorders of muscle in diseases classified elsewhere, left forearm*

Ⓜ ☰ Ⓘ🅀 **M63.839** *Disorders of muscle in diseases classified elsewhere, unspecified forearm*

⑥ **M63.84 Disorders of muscle in diseases classified elsewhere, hand**

Ⓜ ☰ Ⓘ🅀 **M63.841** *Disorders of muscle in diseases classified elsewhere, right hand*

Ⓜ ☰ Ⓘ🅀 **M63.842** *Disorders of muscle in diseases classified elsewhere, left hand*

Ⓜ ☰ Ⓘ🅀 **M63.849** *Disorders of muscle in diseases classified elsewhere, unspecified hand*

⑥ **M63.85 Disorders of muscle in diseases classified elsewhere, thigh**

Ⓜ ☰ Ⓘ🅀 **M63.851** *Disorders of muscle in diseases classified elsewhere, right thigh*

Ⓜ ☰ Ⓘ🅀 **M63.852** *Disorders of muscle in diseases classified elsewhere, left thigh*

Ⓜ ☰ Ⓘ🅀 **M63.859** *Disorders of muscle in diseases classified elsewhere, unspecified thigh*

⑥ **M63.86 Disorders of muscle in diseases classified elsewhere, lower leg**

Ⓜ ☰ Ⓘ🅀 **M63.861** *Disorders of muscle in diseases classified elsewhere, right lower leg*

Ⓜ ☰ Ⓘ🅀 **M63.862** *Disorders of muscle in diseases classified elsewhere, left lower leg*

Ⓜ ☰ Ⓘ🅀 **M63.869** *Disorders of muscle in diseases classified elsewhere, unspecified lower leg*

⑥ **M63.87 Disorders of muscle in diseases classified elsewhere, ankle and foot**

Ⓜ ☰ Ⓘ🅀 **M63.871** *Disorders of muscle in diseases classified elsewhere, right ankle and foot*

Ⓜ ☰ Ⓘ🅀 **M63.872** *Disorders of muscle in diseases classified elsewhere, left ankle and foot*

Ⓜ ☰ Ⓘ🅀 **M63.879** *Disorders of muscle in diseases classified elsewhere, unspecified ankle and foot*

Ⓜ Ⓘ🅀 **M63.88** *Disorders of muscle in diseases classified elsewhere, other site*

Ⓜ Ⓘ🅀 **M63.89** *Disorders of muscle in diseases classified elsewhere, multiple sites*

Disorders of synovium and tendon (M65-M67)

④ **M65   Synovitis and tenosynovitis**

> **EXCLUDES 1**   chronic crepitant synovitis of hand and wrist (M70.0-)
> current injury - see injury of ligament or tendon by body region
> soft tissue disorders related to use, overuse and pressure (M70.-)

✚ ⑤ **M65.0 Abscess of tendon sheath**
Use additional code (B95-B96) to identify bacterial agent.

Ⓘ🅀 ✚ **M65.00** Abscess of tendon sheath, unspecified site

✚ ⑥ **M65.01 Abscess of tendon sheath, shoulder**

☰ 🆂🅿 ✚ **M65.011** Abscess of tendon sheath, right shoulder

☰ 🆂🅿 ✚ **M65.012** Abscess of tendon sheath, left shoulder

☰ Ⓘ🅀 ✚ **M65.019** Abscess of tendon sheath, unspecified shoulder

✚ ⑥ **M65.02 Abscess of tendon sheath, upper arm**

☰ 🆂🅿 ✚ **M65.021** Abscess of tendon sheath, right upper arm

☰ 🆂🅿 ✚ **M65.022** Abscess of tendon sheath, left upper arm

☰ Ⓘ🅀 ✚ **M65.029** Abscess of tendon sheath, unspecified upper arm

✚ ⑥ **M65.03 Abscess of tendon sheath, forearm**

☰ 🆂🅿 ✚ **M65.031** Abscess of tendon sheath, right forearm

☰ 🆂🅿 ✚ **M65.032** Abscess of tendon sheath, left forearm

☰ Ⓘ🅀 ✚ **M65.039** Abscess of tendon sheath, unspecified forearm

✚ ⑥ **M65.04 Abscess of tendon sheath, hand**

☰ 🆂🅿 ✚ **M65.041** Abscess of tendon sheath, right hand

④4th digit required   ⑤5th digit required   ⑥6th digit required   ⑦7th digit required   ⑦7th digit placeholder   ✚Additional code   ☰Laterality

1222   *DecisionHealth's* FY 2020 Complete Home Health ICD-10-CM Diagnosis Coding Manual

☰ SP ✚ M65.042 Abscess of tendon sheath, left hand

☰ IQ ✚ M65.049 Abscess of tendon sheath, unspecified hand

✚ ⑥ M65.05 Abscess of tendon sheath, thigh

☰ SP ✚ M65.051 Abscess of tendon sheath, right thigh

☰ SP ✚ M65.052 Abscess of tendon sheath, left thigh

☰ IQ ✚ M65.059 Abscess of tendon sheath, unspecified thigh

✚ ⑥ M65.06 Abscess of tendon sheath, lower leg

☰ SP ✚ M65.061 Abscess of tendon sheath, right lower leg

☰ SP ✚ M65.062 Abscess of tendon sheath, left lower leg

☰ IQ ✚ M65.069 Abscess of tendon sheath, unspecified lower leg

✚ ⑥ M65.07 Abscess of tendon sheath, ankle and foot

☰ SP ✚ M65.071 Abscess of tendon sheath, right ankle and foot

☰ SP ✚ M65.072 Abscess of tendon sheath, left ankle and foot

☰ IQ ✚ M65.079 Abscess of tendon sheath, unspecified ankle and foot

SP ✚ M65.08 Abscess of tendon sheath, other site

⑤ M65.1 Other infective (teno)synovitis

IQ M65.10 Other infective (teno)synovitis, unspecified site

⑥ M65.11 Other infective (teno)synovitis, shoulder

☰ SP M65.111 Other infective (teno)synovitis, right shoulder

☰ SP M65.112 Other infective (teno)synovitis, left shoulder

☰ IQ M65.119 Other infective (teno)synovitis, unspecified shoulder

⑥ M65.12 Other infective (teno)synovitis, elbow

☰ SP M65.121 Other infective (teno)synovitis, right elbow

☰ SP M65.122 Other infective (teno)synovitis, left elbow

☰ IQ M65.129 Other infective (teno)synovitis, unspecified elbow

⑥ M65.13 Other infective (teno)synovitis, wrist

☰ SP M65.131 Other infective (teno)synovitis, right wrist

☰ SP M65.132 Other infective (teno)synovitis, left wrist

☰ IQ M65.139 Other infective (teno)synovitis, unspecified wrist

⑥ M65.14 Other infective (teno)synovitis, hand

☰ SP M65.141 Other infective (teno)synovitis, right hand

☰ SP M65.142 Other infective (teno)synovitis, left hand

☰ IQ M65.149 Other infective (teno)synovitis, unspecified hand

⑥ M65.15 Other infective (teno)synovitis, hip

☰ SP M65.151 Other infective (teno)synovitis, right hip

☰ SP M65.152 Other infective (teno)synovitis, left hip

☰ IQ M65.159 Other infective (teno)synovitis, unspecified hip

⑥ M65.16 Other infective (teno)synovitis, knee

☰ SP M65.161 Other infective (teno)synovitis, right knee

☰ SP M65.162 Other infective (teno)synovitis, left knee

☰ IQ M65.169 Other infective (teno)synovitis, unspecified knee

⑥ M65.17 Other infective (teno)synovitis, ankle and foot

☰ SP M65.171 Other infective (teno)synovitis, right ankle and foot

☰ SP M65.172 Other infective (teno)synovitis, left ankle and foot

☰ IQ M65.179 Other infective (teno)synovitis, unspecified ankle and foot

SP M65.18 Other infective (teno)synovitis, other site

SP M65.19 Other infective (teno)synovitis, multiple sites

⑤ M65.2 Calcific tendinitis

EXCLUDES 1 tendinitis as classified in M75-M77
calcified tendinitis of shoulder (M75.3)

IQ M65.20 Calcific tendinitis, unspecified site

⑥ M65.22 Calcific tendinitis, upper arm

☰ SP M65.221 Calcific tendinitis, right upper arm

☰ SP M65.222 Calcific tendinitis, left upper arm

☰ IQ M65.229 Calcific tendinitis, unspecified upper arm

⑥ M65.23 Calcific tendinitis, forearm

☰ SP M65.231 Calcific tendinitis, right forearm

☰ SP M65.232 Calcific tendinitis, left forearm

☰ IQ M65.239 Calcific tendinitis, unspecified forearm

⑥ M65.24 Calcific tendinitis, hand

☰ SP M65.241 Calcific tendinitis, right hand

☰ SP M65.242 Calcific tendinitis, left hand

☰ IQ M65.249 Calcific tendinitis, unspecified hand

⑥ M65.25 Calcific tendinitis, thigh

☰ SP M65.251 Calcific tendinitis, right thigh

☰ SP M65.252 Calcific tendinitis, left thigh

☰ IQ M65.259 Calcific tendinitis, unspecified thigh

⑥ M65.26 Calcific tendinitis, lower leg

☰ SP M65.261 Calcific tendinitis, right lower leg

☰ SP M65.262 Calcific tendinitis, left lower leg

☰ IQ M65.269 Calcific tendinitis, unspecified lower leg

⑥ M65.27 Calcific tendinitis, ankle and foot

☰ SP M65.271 Calcific tendinitis, right ankle and foot

☰ SP M65.272 Calcific tendinitis, left ankle and foot

☰ IQ M65.279 Calcific tendinitis, unspecified ankle and foot

SP M65.28 Calcific tendinitis, other site

SP M65.29 Calcific tendinitis, multiple sites

★ New ▲ Revised Px Primary SP PDGM Px SL Low CoM SH High CoM IQ Quest. Encounter H Hospice non-cancer Dx Unspecified M *Manifestation*

⑤ **M65.3 Trigger finger**
Nodular tendinous disease

IQ M65.30 Trigger finger, unspecified finger

⑥ **M65.31** Trigger thumb

⊟ **SP M65.311** Trigger thumb, right thumb

⊟ **SP M65.312** Trigger thumb, left thumb

⊟ **IQ M65.319** Trigger thumb, unspecified thumb

⑥ **M65.32** Trigger finger, index finger

⊟ **SP M65.321** Trigger finger, right index finger

⊟ **SP M65.322** Trigger finger, left index finger

⊟ **IQ M65.329** Trigger finger, unspecified index finger

⑥ **M65.33** Trigger finger, middle finger

⊟ **SP M65.331** Trigger finger, right middle finger

⊟ **SP M65.332** Trigger finger, left middle finger

⊟ **IQ M65.339** Trigger finger, unspecified middle finger

⑥ **M65.34** Trigger finger, ring finger

⊟ **SP M65.341** Trigger finger, right ring finger

⊟ **SP M65.342** Trigger finger, left ring finger

⊟ **IQ M65.349** Trigger finger, unspecified ring finger

⑥ **M65.35** Trigger finger, little finger

⊟ **SP M65.351** Trigger finger, right little finger

⊟ **SP M65.352** Trigger finger, left little finger

⊟ **IQ M65.359** Trigger finger, unspecified little finger

SP M65.4 Radial styloid tenosynovitis [de Quervain]

⑤ **M65.8 Other synovitis and tenosynovitis**

IQ M65.80 Other synovitis and tenosynovitis, unspecified site

⑥ **M65.81** Other synovitis and tenosynovitis, shoulder

⊟ **SP M65.811** Other synovitis and tenosynovitis, right shoulder

⊟ **SP M65.812** Other synovitis and tenosynovitis, left shoulder

⊟ **IQ M65.819** Other synovitis and tenosynovitis, unspecified shoulder

⑥ **M65.82** Other synovitis and tenosynovitis, upper arm

⊟ **SP M65.821** Other synovitis and tenosynovitis, right upper arm

⊟ **SP M65.822** Other synovitis and tenosynovitis, left upper arm

⊟ **IQ M65.829** Other synovitis and tenosynovitis, unspecified upper arm

⑥ **M65.83** Other synovitis and tenosynovitis, forearm

⊟ **SP M65.831** Other synovitis and tenosynovitis, right forearm

⊟ **SP M65.832** Other synovitis and tenosynovitis, left forearm

⊟ **IQ M65.839** Other synovitis and tenosynovitis, unspecified forearm

⑥ **M65.84** Other synovitis and tenosynovitis, hand

⊟ **SP M65.841** Other synovitis and tenosynovitis, right hand

⊟ **SP M65.842** Other synovitis and tenosynovitis, left hand

⊟ **IQ M65.849** Other synovitis and tenosynovitis, unspecified hand

⑥ **M65.85** Other synovitis and tenosynovitis, thigh

⊟ **SP M65.851** Other synovitis and tenosynovitis, right thigh

⊟ **SP M65.852** Other synovitis and tenosynovitis, left thigh

⊟ **IQ M65.859** Other synovitis and tenosynovitis, unspecified thigh

⑥ **M65.86** Other synovitis and tenosynovitis, lower leg

⊟ **SP M65.861** Other synovitis and tenosynovitis, right lower leg

⊟ **SP M65.862** Other synovitis and tenosynovitis, left lower leg

⊟ **IQ M65.869** Other synovitis and tenosynovitis, unspecified lower leg

⑥ **M65.87** Other synovitis and tenosynovitis, ankle and foot

⊟ **SP M65.871** Other synovitis and tenosynovitis, right ankle and foot

⊟ **SP M65.872** Other synovitis and tenosynovitis, left ankle and foot

⊟ **IQ M65.879** Other synovitis and tenosynovitis, unspecified ankle and foot

SP M65.88 Other synovitis and tenosynovitis, other site

SP M65.89 Other synovitis and tenosynovitis, multiple sites

IQ M65.9 Synovitis and tenosynovitis, unspecified

④ **M66 Spontaneous rupture of synovium and tendon**

| INCLUDES | rupture that occurs when a normal force is applied to tissues that are inferred to have less than normal strength |
| EXCLUDES 2 | rotator cuff syndrome (M75.1-) rupture where an abnormal force is applied to normal tissue - see injury of tendon by body region |

SP M66.0 Rupture of popliteal cyst

⑤ **M66.1 Rupture of synovium**
Rupture of synovial cyst

| EXCLUDES 2 | rupture of popliteal cyst (M66.0) |

IQ M66.10 Rupture of synovium, unspecified joint

⑥ **M66.11** Rupture of synovium, shoulder

⊟ **SP M66.111** Rupture of synovium, right shoulder

⊟ **SP M66.112** Rupture of synovium, left shoulder

⊟ **IQ M66.119** Rupture of synovium, unspecified shoulder

⑥ **M66.12** Rupture of synovium, elbow

⊟ **SP M66.121** Rupture of synovium, right elbow

⊟ **SP M66.122** Rupture of synovium, left elbow

---

④4th digit required   ⑤5th digit required   ⑥6th digit required   ⑦7th digit required   ⑦7th digit placeholder   ✚Additional code   ⊟Laterality

1224   *DecisionHealth's* FY 2020 Complete Home Health ICD-10-CM Diagnosis Coding Manual

☐ **IQ** **M66.129** Rupture of synovium, unspecified elbow

⑥ **M66.13** Rupture of synovium, wrist

☐ **SP** **M66.131** Rupture of synovium, right wrist

☐ **SP** **M66.132** Rupture of synovium, left wrist

☐ **IQ** **M66.139** Rupture of synovium, unspecified wrist

⑥ **M66.14** Rupture of synovium, hand and fingers

☐ **SP** **M66.141** Rupture of synovium, right hand

☐ **SP** **M66.142** Rupture of synovium, left hand

☐ **IQ** **M66.143** Rupture of synovium, unspecified hand

☐ **SP** **M66.144** Rupture of synovium, right finger(s)

☐ **SP** **M66.145** Rupture of synovium, left finger(s)

☐ **IQ** **M66.146** Rupture of synovium, unspecified finger(s)

⑥ **M66.15** Rupture of synovium, hip

☐ **SP** **M66.151** Rupture of synovium, right hip

☐ **SP** **M66.152** Rupture of synovium, left hip

☐ **IQ** **M66.159** Rupture of synovium, unspecified hip

⑥ **M66.17** Rupture of synovium, ankle, foot and toes

☐ **SP** **M66.171** Rupture of synovium, right ankle

☐ **SP** **M66.172** Rupture of synovium, left ankle

☐ **IQ** **M66.173** Rupture of synovium, unspecified ankle

☐ **SP** **M66.174** Rupture of synovium, right foot

☐ **SP** **M66.175** Rupture of synovium, left foot

☐ **IQ** **M66.176** Rupture of synovium, unspecified foot

☐ **SP** **M66.177** Rupture of synovium, right toe(s)

☐ **SP** **M66.178** Rupture of synovium, left toe(s)

☐ **IQ** **M66.179** Rupture of synovium, unspecified toe(s)

SP **M66.18** Rupture of synovium, other site

⑤ **M66.2** Spontaneous rupture of extensor tendons

IQ **M66.20** Spontaneous rupture of extensor tendons, unspecified site

⑥ **M66.21** Spontaneous rupture of extensor tendons, shoulder

☐ **SP** **M66.211** Spontaneous rupture of extensor tendons, right shoulder

☐ **SP** **M66.212** Spontaneous rupture of extensor tendons, left shoulder

☐ **IQ** **M66.219** Spontaneous rupture of extensor tendons, unspecified shoulder

⑥ **M66.22** Spontaneous rupture of extensor tendons, upper arm

☐ **SP** **M66.221** Spontaneous rupture of extensor tendons, right upper arm

☐ **SP** **M66.222** Spontaneous rupture of extensor tendons, left upper arm

☐ **IQ** **M66.229** Spontaneous rupture of extensor tendons, unspecified upper arm

⑥ **M66.23** Spontaneous rupture of extensor tendons, forearm

☐ **SP** **M66.231** Spontaneous rupture of extensor tendons, right forearm

☐ **SP** **M66.232** Spontaneous rupture of extensor tendons, left forearm

☐ **IQ** **M66.239** Spontaneous rupture of extensor tendons, unspecified forearm

⑥ **M66.24** Spontaneous rupture of extensor tendons, hand

☐ **SP** **M66.241** Spontaneous rupture of extensor tendons, right hand

☐ **SP** **M66.242** Spontaneous rupture of extensor tendons, left hand

☐ **IQ** **M66.249** Spontaneous rupture of extensor tendons, unspecified hand

⑥ **M66.25** Spontaneous rupture of extensor tendons, thigh

☐ **SP** **M66.251** Spontaneous rupture of extensor tendons, right thigh

☐ **SP** **M66.252** Spontaneous rupture of extensor tendons, left thigh

☐ **IQ** **M66.259** Spontaneous rupture of extensor tendons, unspecified thigh

⑥ **M66.26** Spontaneous rupture of extensor tendons, lower leg

☐ **SP** **M66.261** Spontaneous rupture of extensor tendons, right lower leg

☐ **SP** **M66.262** Spontaneous rupture of extensor tendons, left lower leg

☐ **IQ** **M66.269** Spontaneous rupture of extensor tendons, unspecified lower leg

⑥ **M66.27** Spontaneous rupture of extensor tendons, ankle and foot

☐ **SP** **M66.271** Spontaneous rupture of extensor tendons, right ankle and foot

☐ **SP** **M66.272** Spontaneous rupture of extensor tendons, left ankle and foot

☐ **IQ** **M66.279** Spontaneous rupture of extensor tendons, unspecified ankle and foot

SP **M66.28** Spontaneous rupture of extensor tendons, other site

SP **M66.29** Spontaneous rupture of extensor tendons, multiple sites

⑤ **M66.3** Spontaneous rupture of flexor tendons

IQ **M66.30** Spontaneous rupture of flexor tendons, unspecified site

⑥ **M66.31** Spontaneous rupture of flexor tendons, shoulder

☐ **SP** **M66.311** Spontaneous rupture of flexor tendons, right shoulder

☐ **SP** **M66.312** Spontaneous rupture of flexor tendons, left shoulder

☐ **IQ** **M66.319** Spontaneous rupture of flexor tendons, unspecified shoulder

⑥ **M66.32** Spontaneous rupture of flexor tendons, upper arm

☐ **SP** **M66.321** Spontaneous rupture of flexor tendons, right upper arm

☐ **SP** **M66.322** Spontaneous rupture of flexor tendons, left upper arm

☐ **IQ** **M66.329** Spontaneous rupture of flexor tendons, unspecified upper arm

⑥ **M66.33** Spontaneous rupture of flexor tendons, forearm

☐ **SP** **M66.331** Spontaneous rupture of flexor tendons, right forearm

☐ **SP** **M66.332** Spontaneous rupture of flexor tendons, left forearm

★ New ▲ Revised **Px** Primary **SP** PDGM Px **SL** Low CoM **SH** High CoM **IQ** Quest. Encounter **H** Hospice non-cancer Dx | Unspecified | **M** *Manifestation*

DecisionHealth's FY 2020 Complete Home Health ICD-10-CM Diagnosis Coding Manual

1225

Chapter 13

M00-M99

⊟ **!Q** **M66.339** Spontaneous rupture of flexor tendons, unspecified forearm

6 **M66.34** Spontaneous rupture of flexor tendons, hand

⊟ **SP** **M66.341** Spontaneous rupture of flexor tendons, right hand

⊟ **SP** **M66.342** Spontaneous rupture of flexor tendons, left hand

⊟ **!Q** **M66.349** Spontaneous rupture of flexor tendons, unspecified hand

6 **M66.35** Spontaneous rupture of flexor tendons, thigh

⊟ **SP** **M66.351** Spontaneous rupture of flexor tendons, right thigh

⊟ **SP** **M66.352** Spontaneous rupture of flexor tendons, left thigh

⊟ **!Q** **M66.359** Spontaneous rupture of flexor tendons, unspecified thigh

6 **M66.36** Spontaneous rupture of flexor tendons, lower leg

⊟ **SP** **M66.361** Spontaneous rupture of flexor tendons, right lower leg

⊟ **SP** **M66.362** Spontaneous rupture of flexor tendons, left lower leg

⊟ **!Q** **M66.369** Spontaneous rupture of flexor tendons, unspecified lower leg

6 **M66.37** Spontaneous rupture of flexor tendons, ankle and foot

⊟ **SP** **M66.371** Spontaneous rupture of flexor tendons, right ankle and foot

⊟ **SP** **M66.372** Spontaneous rupture of flexor tendons, left ankle and foot

⊟ **!Q** **M66.379** Spontaneous rupture of flexor tendons, unspecified ankle and foot

SP **M66.38** Spontaneous rupture of flexor tendons, other site

SP **M66.39** Spontaneous rupture of flexor tendons, multiple sites

5 **M66.8** Spontaneous rupture of other tendons

!Q **M66.80** Spontaneous rupture of other tendons, unspecified site

6 **M66.81** Spontaneous rupture of other tendons, shoulder

⊟ **SP** **M66.811** Spontaneous rupture of other tendons, right shoulder

⊟ **SP** **M66.812** Spontaneous rupture of other tendons, left shoulder

⊟ **!Q** **M66.819** Spontaneous rupture of other tendons, unspecified shoulder

6 **M66.82** Spontaneous rupture of other tendons, upper arm

⊟ **SP** **M66.821** Spontaneous rupture of other tendons, right upper arm

⊟ **SP** **M66.822** Spontaneous rupture of other tendons, left upper arm

⊟ **!Q** **M66.829** Spontaneous rupture of other tendons, unspecified upper arm

6 **M66.83** Spontaneous rupture of other tendons, forearm

⊟ **SP** **M66.831** Spontaneous rupture of other tendons, right forearm

⊟ **SP** **M66.832** Spontaneous rupture of other tendons, left forearm

⊟ **!Q** **M66.839** Spontaneous rupture of other tendons, unspecified forearm

6 **M66.84** Spontaneous rupture of other tendons, hand

⊟ **SP** **M66.841** Spontaneous rupture of other tendons, right hand

⊟ **SP** **M66.842** Spontaneous rupture of other tendons, left hand

⊟ **!Q** **M66.849** Spontaneous rupture of other tendons, unspecified hand

6 **M66.85** Spontaneous rupture of other tendons, thigh

⊟ **SP** **M66.851** Spontaneous rupture of other tendons, right thigh

⊟ **SP** **M66.852** Spontaneous rupture of other tendons, left thigh

⊟ **!Q** **M66.859** Spontaneous rupture of other tendons, unspecified thigh

6 **M66.86** Spontaneous rupture of other tendons, lower leg

⊟ **SP** **M66.861** Spontaneous rupture of other tendons, right lower leg

⊟ **SP** **M66.862** Spontaneous rupture of other tendons, left lower leg

⊟ **!Q** **M66.869** Spontaneous rupture of other tendons, unspecified lower leg

6 **M66.87** Spontaneous rupture of other tendons, ankle and foot

⊟ **SP** **M66.871** Spontaneous rupture of other tendons, right ankle and foot

⊟ **SP** **M66.872** Spontaneous rupture of other tendons, left ankle and foot

⊟ **!Q** **M66.879** Spontaneous rupture of other tendons, unspecified ankle and foot

▲ **SP** **M66.88** Spontaneous rupture of other tendons, other sites

SP **M66.89** Spontaneous rupture of other tendons, multiple sites

!Q **M66.9** Spontaneous rupture of unspecified tendon

     Rupture at musculotendinous junction, nontraumatic

4 **M67** **Other disorders of synovium and tendon**

     EXCLUDES 1 palmar fascial fibromatosis [Dupuytren] (M72.0)
           tendinitis NOS (M77.9-)
           xanthomatosis localized to tendons (E78.2)

5 **M67.0** Short Achilles tendon (acquired)

⊟ **!Q** **M67.00** Short Achilles tendon (acquired), unspecified ankle

⊟ **SP** **M67.01** Short Achilles tendon (acquired), right ankle

⊟ **SP** **M67.02** Short Achilles tendon (acquired), left ankle

5 **M67.2** Synovial hypertrophy, not elsewhere classified

     EXCLUDES 1 villonodular synovitis (pigmented) (M12.2-)

!Q **M67.20** Synovial hypertrophy, not elsewhere classified, unspecified site

6 **M67.21** Synovial hypertrophy, not elsewhere classified, shoulder

⊟ **SP** **M67.211** Synovial hypertrophy, not elsewhere classified, right shoulder

⊟ **SP** **M67.212** Synovial hypertrophy, not elsewhere classified, left shoulder

---

4 4th digit required   **5** 5th digit required   **6** 6th digit required   **7** 7th digit required   **7** 7th digit placeholder   **+** Additional code   ⊟ Laterality

☰ **IQ** **M67.219** Synovial hypertrophy, not elsewhere classified, unspecified shoulder

⑥ **M67.22** Synovial hypertrophy, not elsewhere classified, upper arm

☰ **SP** **M67.221** Synovial hypertrophy, not elsewhere classified, right upper arm

☰ **SP** **M67.222** Synovial hypertrophy, not elsewhere classified, left upper arm

☰ **IQ** **M67.229** Synovial hypertrophy, not elsewhere classified, unspecified upper arm

⑥ **M67.23** Synovial hypertrophy, not elsewhere classified, forearm

☰ **SP** **M67.231** Synovial hypertrophy, not elsewhere classified, right forearm

☰ **SP** **M67.232** Synovial hypertrophy, not elsewhere classified, left forearm

☰ **IQ** **M67.239** Synovial hypertrophy, not elsewhere classified, unspecified forearm

⑥ **M67.24** Synovial hypertrophy, not elsewhere classified, hand

☰ **SP** **M67.241** Synovial hypertrophy, not elsewhere classified, right hand

☰ **SP** **M67.242** Synovial hypertrophy, not elsewhere classified, left hand

☰ **IQ** **M67.249** Synovial hypertrophy, not elsewhere classified, unspecified hand

⑥ **M67.25** Synovial hypertrophy, not elsewhere classified, thigh

☰ **SP** **M67.251** Synovial hypertrophy, not elsewhere classified, right thigh

☰ **SP** **M67.252** Synovial hypertrophy, not elsewhere classified, left thigh

☰ **IQ** **M67.259** Synovial hypertrophy, not elsewhere classified, unspecified thigh

⑥ **M67.26** Synovial hypertrophy, not elsewhere classified, lower leg

☰ **SP** **M67.261** Synovial hypertrophy, not elsewhere classified, right lower leg

☰ **SP** **M67.262** Synovial hypertrophy, not elsewhere classified, left lower leg

☰ **IQ** **M67.269** Synovial hypertrophy, not elsewhere classified, unspecified lower leg

⑥ **M67.27** Synovial hypertrophy, not elsewhere classified, ankle and foot

☰ **SP** **M67.271** Synovial hypertrophy, not elsewhere classified, right ankle and foot

☰ **SP** **M67.272** Synovial hypertrophy, not elsewhere classified, left ankle and foot

☰ **IQ** **M67.279** Synovial hypertrophy, not elsewhere classified, unspecified ankle and foot

SP **M67.28** Synovial hypertrophy, not elsewhere classified, other site

SP **M67.29** Synovial hypertrophy, not elsewhere classified, multiple sites

⑤ **M67.3** Transient synovitis

Toxic synovitis

> **EXCLUDES 1** palindromic rheumatism (M12.3-)

IQ **M67.30** Transient synovitis, unspecified site

⑥ **M67.31** Transient synovitis, shoulder

☰ **SP** **M67.311** Transient synovitis, right shoulder

☰ **SP** **M67.312** Transient synovitis, left shoulder

☰ **IQ** **M67.319** Transient synovitis, unspecified shoulder

⑥ **M67.32** Transient synovitis, elbow

☰ **SP** **M67.321** Transient synovitis, right elbow

☰ **SP** **M67.322** Transient synovitis, left elbow

☰ **IQ** **M67.329** Transient synovitis, unspecified elbow

⑥ **M67.33** Transient synovitis, wrist

☰ **SP** **M67.331** Transient synovitis, right wrist

☰ **SP** **M67.332** Transient synovitis, left wrist

☰ **IQ** **M67.339** Transient synovitis, unspecified wrist

⑥ **M67.34** Transient synovitis, hand

☰ **SP** **M67.341** Transient synovitis, right hand

☰ **SP** **M67.342** Transient synovitis, left hand

☰ **IQ** **M67.349** Transient synovitis, unspecified hand

⑥ **M67.35** Transient synovitis, hip

☰ **SP** **M67.351** Transient synovitis, right hip

☰ **SP** **M67.352** Transient synovitis, left hip

☰ **IQ** **M67.359** Transient synovitis, unspecified hip

⑥ **M67.36** Transient synovitis, knee

☰ **SP** **M67.361** Transient synovitis, right knee

☰ **SP** **M67.362** Transient synovitis, left knee

☰ **IQ** **M67.369** Transient synovitis, unspecified knee

⑥ **M67.37** Transient synovitis, ankle and foot

☰ **SP** **M67.371** Transient synovitis, right ankle and foot

☰ **SP** **M67.372** Transient synovitis, left ankle and foot

☰ **IQ** **M67.379** Transient synovitis, unspecified ankle and foot

SP **M67.38** Transient synovitis, other site

SP **M67.39** Transient synovitis, multiple sites

⑤ **M67.4** Ganglion

Ganglion of joint or tendon (sheath)

> **EXCLUDES 1** ganglion in yaws (A66.6)
>
> **EXCLUDES 2** cyst of bursa (M71.2-M71.3)
> cyst of synovium (M71.2-M71.3)

IQ **M67.40** Ganglion, unspecified site

⑥ **M67.41** Ganglion, shoulder

☰ **SP** **M67.411** Ganglion, right shoulder

☰ **SP** **M67.412** Ganglion, left shoulder

☰ **IQ** **M67.419** Ganglion, unspecified shoulder

⑥ **M67.42** Ganglion, elbow

☰ **SP** **M67.421** Ganglion, right elbow

☰ **SP** **M67.422** Ganglion, left elbow

☰ **IQ** **M67.429** Ganglion, unspecified elbow

★ New ▲ Revised Px Primary **SP** PDGM Px **SL** Low CoM **SH** High CoM **IQ** Quest. Encounter **H** Hospice non-cancer Dx Unspecified **M** *Manifestation*

DecisionHealth's FY 2020 Complete Home Health ICD-10-CM Diagnosis Coding Manual

1227

⑥ **M67.43** Ganglion, wrist
⊟ SP **M67.431** Ganglion, right wrist
⊟ SP **M67.432** Ganglion, left wrist
⊟ IQ **M67.439** Ganglion, unspecified wrist
　⑥ **M67.44** Ganglion, hand
⊟ SP **M67.441** Ganglion, right hand
⊟ SP **M67.442** Ganglion, left hand
⊟ IQ **M67.449** Ganglion, unspecified hand
　⑥ **M67.45** Ganglion, hip
⊟ SP **M67.451** Ganglion, right hip
⊟ SP **M67.452** Ganglion, left hip
⊟ IQ **M67.459** Ganglion, unspecified hip
　⑥ **M67.46** Ganglion, knee
⊟ SP **M67.461** Ganglion, right knee
⊟ SP **M67.462** Ganglion, left knee
⊟ IQ **M67.469** Ganglion, unspecified knee
　⑥ **M67.47** Ganglion, ankle and foot
⊟ SP **M67.471** Ganglion, right ankle and foot
⊟ SP **M67.472** Ganglion, left ankle and foot
⊟ IQ **M67.479** Ganglion, unspecified ankle and foot
　SP **M67.48** Ganglion, other site
　SP **M67.49** Ganglion, multiple sites
⑤ **M67.5** Plica syndrome
　　Plica knee
⊟ IQ **M67.50** Plica syndrome, unspecified knee
⊟ SP **M67.51** Plica syndrome, right knee
⊟ SP **M67.52** Plica syndrome, left knee
⑤ **M67.8** Other specified disorders of synovium and tendon
　IQ **M67.80** Other specified disorders of synovium and tendon, unspecified site
　⑥ **M67.81** Other specified disorders of synovium and tendon, shoulder
⊟ SP **M67.811** Other specified disorders of synovium, right shoulder
⊟ SP **M67.812** Other specified disorders of synovium, left shoulder
⊟ SP **M67.813** Other specified disorders of tendon, right shoulder
⊟ SP **M67.814** Other specified disorders of tendon, left shoulder
⊟ IQ **M67.819** Other specified disorders of synovium and tendon, unspecified shoulder
　⑥ **M67.82** Other specified disorders of synovium and tendon, elbow
⊟ SP **M67.821** Other specified disorders of synovium, right elbow
⊟ SP **M67.822** Other specified disorders of synovium, left elbow
⊟ SP **M67.823** Other specified disorders of tendon, right elbow
⊟ SP **M67.824** Other specified disorders of tendon, left elbow
⊟ IQ **M67.829** Other specified disorders of synovium and tendon, unspecified elbow
　⑥ **M67.83** Other specified disorders of synovium and tendon, wrist

⊟ SP **M67.831** Other specified disorders of synovium, right wrist
⊟ SP **M67.832** Other specified disorders of synovium, left wrist
⊟ SP **M67.833** Other specified disorders of tendon, right wrist
⊟ SP **M67.834** Other specified disorders of tendon, left wrist
▲⊟ IQ **M67.839** Other specified disorders of synovium and tendon, unspecified wrist
　⑥ **M67.84** Other specified disorders of synovium and tendon, hand
⊟ SP **M67.841** Other specified disorders of synovium, right hand
⊟ SP **M67.842** Other specified disorders of synovium, left hand
⊟ SP **M67.843** Other specified disorders of tendon, right hand
⊟ SP **M67.844** Other specified disorders of tendon, left hand
⊟ IQ **M67.849** Other specified disorders of synovium and tendon, unspecified hand
　⑥ **M67.85** Other specified disorders of synovium and tendon, hip
⊟ SP **M67.851** Other specified disorders of synovium, right hip
⊟ SP **M67.852** Other specified disorders of synovium, left hip
⊟ SP **M67.853** Other specified disorders of tendon, right hip
⊟ SP **M67.854** Other specified disorders of tendon, left hip
⊟ IQ **M67.859** Other specified disorders of synovium and tendon, unspecified hip
　⑥ **M67.86** Other specified disorders of synovium and tendon, knee
⊟ SP **M67.861** Other specified disorders of synovium, right knee
⊟ SP **M67.862** Other specified disorders of synovium, left knee
⊟ SP **M67.863** Other specified disorders of tendon, right knee
⊟ SP **M67.864** Other specified disorders of tendon, left knee
⊟ IQ **M67.869** Other specified disorders of synovium and tendon, unspecified knee
　⑥ **M67.87** Other specified disorders of synovium and tendon, ankle and foot
⊟ SP **M67.871** Other specified disorders of synovium, right ankle and foot
⊟ SP **M67.872** Other specified disorders of synovium, left ankle and foot
⊟ SP **M67.873** Other specified disorders of tendon, right ankle and foot
⊟ SP **M67.874** Other specified disorders of tendon, left ankle and foot
⊟ IQ **M67.879** Other specified disorders of synovium and tendon, unspecified ankle and foot
　SP **M67.88** Other specified disorders of synovium and tendon, other site
　SP **M67.89** Other specified disorders of synovium and tendon, multiple sites

---

④ 4th digit required　⑤ 5th digit required　⑥ 6th digit required　⑦ 7th digit required　⑦ 7th digit placeholder　✚ Additional code　⊟ Laterality

1228　　　*DecisionHealth's* FY 2020 Complete Home Health ICD-10-CM Diagnosis Coding Manual

5 M67.9 Unspecified disorder of synovium and tendon

!Q M67.90 Unspecified disorder of synovium and tendon, unspecified site

6 M67.91 Unspecified disorder of synovium and tendon, shoulder

⊟ SP M67.911 Unspecified disorder of synovium and tendon, right shoulder

⊟ SP M67.912 Unspecified disorder of synovium and tendon, left shoulder

⊟ !Q M67.919 Unspecified disorder of synovium and tendon, unspecified shoulder

6 M67.92 Unspecified disorder of synovium and tendon, upper arm

⊟ SP M67.921 Unspecified disorder of synovium and tendon, right upper arm

⊟ SP M67.922 Unspecified disorder of synovium and tendon, left upper arm

⊟ !Q M67.929 Unspecified disorder of synovium and tendon, unspecified upper arm

6 M67.93 Unspecified disorder of synovium and tendon, forearm

⊟ SP M67.931 Unspecified disorder of synovium and tendon, right forearm

⊟ SP M67.932 Unspecified disorder of synovium and tendon, left forearm

⊟ !Q M67.939 Unspecified disorder of synovium and tendon, unspecified forearm

6 M67.94 Unspecified disorder of synovium and tendon, hand

⊟ SP M67.941 Unspecified disorder of synovium and tendon, right hand

⊟ SP M67.942 Unspecified disorder of synovium and tendon, left hand

⊟ !Q M67.949 Unspecified disorder of synovium and tendon, unspecified hand

6 M67.95 Unspecified disorder of synovium and tendon, thigh

⊟ SP M67.951 Unspecified disorder of synovium and tendon, right thigh

⊟ SP M67.952 Unspecified disorder of synovium and tendon, left thigh

⊟ !Q M67.959 Unspecified disorder of synovium and tendon, unspecified thigh

6 M67.96 Unspecified disorder of synovium and tendon, lower leg

⊟ SP M67.961 Unspecified disorder of synovium and tendon, right lower leg

⊟ SP M67.962 Unspecified disorder of synovium and tendon, left lower leg

⊟ !Q M67.969 Unspecified disorder of synovium and tendon, unspecified lower leg

6 M67.97 Unspecified disorder of synovium and tendon, ankle and foot

⊟ SP M67.971 Unspecified disorder of synovium and tendon, right ankle and foot

⊟ SP M67.972 Unspecified disorder of synovium and tendon, left ankle and foot

⊟ !Q M67.979 Unspecified disorder of synovium and tendon, unspecified ankle and foot

SP M67.98 Unspecified disorder of synovium and tendon, other site

SP M67.99 Unspecified disorder of synovium and tendon, multiple sites

Other soft tissue disorders (M70-M79)

+ 4 M70 Soft tissue disorders related to use, overuse and pressure

> **INCLUDES** soft tissue disorders of occupational origin
>
> Use additional external cause code to identify activity causing disorder (Y93.-)
>
> **EXCLUDES 1** bursitis NOS (M71.9-)
>
> **EXCLUDES 2** bursitis of shoulder (M75.5) enthesopathies (M76-M77) pressure ulcer (pressure area) (L89.-)

+ 5 M70.0 Crepitant synovitis (acute) (chronic) of hand and wrist

+ 6 M70.03 Crepitant synovitis (acute) (chronic), wrist

⊟ SP + M70.031 Crepitant synovitis (acute) (chronic), right wrist

⊟ SP + M70.032 Crepitant synovitis (acute) (chronic), left wrist

⊟ !Q + M70.039 Crepitant synovitis (acute) (chronic), unspecified wrist

+ 6 M70.04 Crepitant synovitis (acute) (chronic), hand

⊟ SP + M70.041 Crepitant synovitis (acute) (chronic), right hand

⊟ SP + M70.042 Crepitant synovitis (acute) (chronic), left hand

⊟ !Q + M70.049 Crepitant synovitis (acute) (chronic), unspecified hand

+ 5 M70.1 Bursitis of hand

⊟ !Q + M70.10 Bursitis, unspecified hand

⊟ SP + M70.11 Bursitis, right hand

⊟ SP + M70.12 Bursitis, left hand

+ 5 M70.2 Olecranon bursitis

⊟ !Q + M70.20 Olecranon bursitis, unspecified elbow

⊟ SP + M70.21 Olecranon bursitis, right elbow

⊟ SP + M70.22 Olecranon bursitis, left elbow

+ 5 M70.3 Other bursitis of elbow

⊟ !Q + M70.30 Other bursitis of elbow, unspecified elbow

⊟ SP + M70.31 Other bursitis of elbow, right elbow

⊟ SP + M70.32 Other bursitis of elbow, left elbow

+ 5 M70.4 Prepatellar bursitis

⊟ !Q + M70.40 Prepatellar bursitis, unspecified knee

⊟ SP + M70.41 Prepatellar bursitis, right knee

⊟ SP + M70.42 Prepatellar bursitis, left knee

+ 5 M70.5 Other bursitis of knee

⊟ !Q + M70.50 Other bursitis of knee, unspecified knee

⊟ SP + M70.51 Other bursitis of knee, right knee

⊟ SP + M70.52 Other bursitis of knee, left knee

+ 5 M70.6 Trochanteric bursitis
Trochanteric tendinitis

★ New ▲ Revised Px Primary SP PDGM Px SL Low CoM SH High CoM !Q Quest. Encounter H Hospice non-cancer Dx Unspecified M Manifestation

DecisionHealth's FY 2020 Complete Home Health ICD-10-CM Diagnosis Coding Manual

1229

Chapter 13

M00-M99

▣ **!Q** ✚ **M70.60 Trochanteric bursitis, unspecified hip**

▣ **SP** ✚ M70.61 Trochanteric bursitis, right hip

▣ **SP** ✚ M70.62 Trochanteric bursitis, left hip

✚ **5** **M70.7 Other bursitis of hip**
  Ischial bursitis

▣ **!Q** ✚ **M70.70 Other bursitis of hip, unspecified hip**

▣ **SP** ✚ M70.71 Other bursitis of hip, right hip

▣ **SP** ✚ M70.72 Other bursitis of hip, left hip

✚ **5** **M70.8 Other soft tissue disorders related to use, overuse and pressure**

!Q ✚ **M70.80 Other soft tissue disorders related to use, overuse and pressure of unspecified site**

✚ **6** **M70.81 Other soft tissue disorders related to use, overuse and pressure of shoulder**

▣ **SP** ✚ M70.811 Other soft tissue disorders related to use, overuse and pressure, right shoulder

▣ **SP** ✚ M70.812 Other soft tissue disorders related to use, overuse and pressure, left shoulder

▣ **!Q** ✚ **M70.819 Other soft tissue disorders related to use, overuse and pressure, unspecified shoulder**

✚ **6** **M70.82 Other soft tissue disorders related to use, overuse and pressure of upper arm**

▣ **SP** ✚ M70.821 Other soft tissue disorders related to use, overuse and pressure, right upper arm

▣ **SP** ✚ M70.822 Other soft tissue disorders related to use, overuse and pressure, left upper arm

▣ **!Q** ✚ **M70.829 Other soft tissue disorders related to use, overuse and pressure, unspecified upper arms**

✚ **6** **M70.83 Other soft tissue disorders related to use, overuse and pressure of forearm**

▣ **SP** ✚ M70.831 Other soft tissue disorders related to use, overuse and pressure, right forearm

▣ **SP** ✚ M70.832 Other soft tissue disorders related to use, overuse and pressure, left forearm

▣ **!Q** ✚ **M70.839 Other soft tissue disorders related to use, overuse and pressure, unspecified forearm**

✚ **6** **M70.84 Other soft tissue disorders related to use, overuse and pressure of hand**

▣ **SP** ✚ M70.841 Other soft tissue disorders related to use, overuse and pressure, right hand

▣ **SP** ✚ M70.842 Other soft tissue disorders related to use, overuse and pressure, left hand

▣ **!Q** ✚ **M70.849 Other soft tissue disorders related to use, overuse and pressure, unspecified hand**

✚ **6** **M70.85 Other soft tissue disorders related to use, overuse and pressure of thigh**

▣ **SP** ✚ M70.851 Other soft tissue disorders related to use, overuse and pressure, right thigh

▣ **SP** ✚ M70.852 Other soft tissue disorders related to use, overuse and pressure, left thigh

▣ **!Q** ✚ **M70.859 Other soft tissue disorders related to use, overuse and pressure, unspecified thigh**

✚ **6** **M70.86 Other soft tissue disorders related to use, overuse and pressure lower leg**

▣ **SP** ✚ M70.861 Other soft tissue disorders related to use, overuse and pressure, right lower leg

▣ **SP** ✚ M70.862 Other soft tissue disorders related to use, overuse and pressure, left lower leg

▣ **!Q** ✚ **M70.869 Other soft tissue disorders related to use, overuse and pressure, unspecified leg**

✚ **6** **M70.87 Other soft tissue disorders related to use, overuse and pressure of ankle and foot**

▣ **SP** ✚ M70.871 Other soft tissue disorders related to use, overuse and pressure, right ankle and foot

▣ **SP** ✚ M70.872 Other soft tissue disorders related to use, overuse and pressure, left ankle and foot

▣ **!Q** ✚ **M70.879 Other soft tissue disorders related to use, overuse and pressure, unspecified ankle and foot**

SP ✚ M70.88 Other soft tissue disorders related to use, overuse and pressure other site

SP ✚ M70.89 Other soft tissue disorders related to use, overuse and pressure multiple sites

✚ **5** **M70.9 Unspecified soft tissue disorder related to use, overuse and pressure**

!Q ✚ **M70.90 Unspecified soft tissue disorder related to use, overuse and pressure of unspecified site**

✚ **6** **M70.91 Unspecified soft tissue disorder related to use, overuse and pressure of shoulder**

▣ **!Q** ✚ **M70.911 Unspecified soft tissue disorder related to use, overuse and pressure, right shoulder**

▣ **!Q** ✚ **M70.912 Unspecified soft tissue disorder related to use, overuse and pressure, left shoulder**

▣ **!Q** ✚ **M70.919 Unspecified soft tissue disorder related to use, overuse and pressure, unspecified shoulder**

✚ **6** **M70.92 Unspecified soft tissue disorder related to use, overuse and pressure of upper arm**

▣ **SP** ✚ **M70.921 Unspecified soft tissue disorder related to use, overuse and pressure, right upper arm**

▣ **SP** ✚ **M70.922 Unspecified soft tissue disorder related to use, overuse and pressure, left upper arm**

▣ **!Q** ✚ **M70.929 Unspecified soft tissue disorder related to use, overuse and pressure, unspecified upper arm**

---

4 4th digit required **5** 5th digit required **6** 6th digit required **7** 7th digit required **7** 7th digit placeholder ✚ Additional code ▣ Laterality

1230 *DecisionHealth's* FY 2020 Complete Home Health ICD-10-CM Diagnosis Coding Manual

+ 6 M70.93 Unspecified soft tissue disorder related to use, overuse and pressure of forearm

⊟ SP + M70.931 Unspecified soft tissue disorder related to use, overuse and pressure, right forearm

⊟ SP + M70.932 Unspecified soft tissue disorder related to use, overuse and pressure, left forearm

⊟ IQ + M70.939 Unspecified soft tissue disorder related to use, overuse and pressure, unspecified forearm

+ 6 M70.94 Unspecified soft tissue disorder related to use, overuse and pressure of hand

⊟ SP + M70.941 Unspecified soft tissue disorder related to use, overuse and pressure, right hand

⊟ SP + M70.942 Unspecified soft tissue disorder related to use, overuse and pressure, left hand

⊟ IQ + M70.949 Unspecified soft tissue disorder related to use, overuse and pressure, unspecified hand

+ 6 M70.95 Unspecified soft tissue disorder related to use, overuse and pressure of thigh

⊟ SP + M70.951 Unspecified soft tissue disorder related to use, overuse and pressure, right thigh

⊟ SP + M70.952 Unspecified soft tissue disorder related to use, overuse and pressure, left thigh

⊟ IQ + M70.959 Unspecified soft tissue disorder related to use, overuse and pressure, unspecified thigh

+ 6 M70.96 Unspecified soft tissue disorder related to use, overuse and pressure lower leg

⊟ SP + M70.961 Unspecified soft tissue disorder related to use, overuse and pressure, right lower leg

⊟ SP + M70.962 Unspecified soft tissue disorder related to use, overuse and pressure, left lower leg

⊟ IQ + M70.969 Unspecified soft tissue disorder related to use, overuse and pressure, unspecified lower leg

+ 6 M70.97 Unspecified soft tissue disorder related to use, overuse and pressure of ankle and foot

⊟ SP + M70.971 Unspecified soft tissue disorder related to use, overuse and pressure, right ankle and foot

⊟ SP + M70.972 Unspecified soft tissue disorder related to use, overuse and pressure, left ankle and foot

⊟ IQ + M70.979 Unspecified soft tissue disorder related to use, overuse and pressure, unspecified ankle and foot

SP + M70.98 Unspecified soft tissue disorder related to use, overuse and pressure other

SP + M70.99 Unspecified soft tissue disorder related to use, overuse and pressure multiple sites

4 M71 Other bursopathies

> **EXCLUDES 1** bunion (M20.1)
> bursitis related to use, overuse or pressure (M70.-)
> enthesopathies (M76-M77)

+ 5 M71.0 Abscess of bursa

> Use additional code (B95.-, B96.-) to identify causative organism

IQ + M71.00 Abscess of bursa, unspecified site

+ 6 M71.01 Abscess of bursa, shoulder

⊟ SP + M71.011 Abscess of bursa, right shoulder

⊟ SP + M71.012 Abscess of bursa, left shoulder

⊟ IQ + M71.019 Abscess of bursa, unspecified shoulder

+ 6 M71.02 Abscess of bursa, elbow

⊟ SP + M71.021 Abscess of bursa, right elbow

⊟ SP + M71.022 Abscess of bursa, left elbow

⊟ IQ + M71.029 Abscess of bursa, unspecified elbow

+ 6 M71.03 Abscess of bursa, wrist

⊟ SP + M71.031 Abscess of bursa, right wrist

⊟ SP + M71.032 Abscess of bursa, left wrist

⊟ IQ + M71.039 Abscess of bursa, unspecified wrist

+ 6 M71.04 Abscess of bursa, hand

⊟ SP + M71.041 Abscess of bursa, right hand

⊟ SP + M71.042 Abscess of bursa, left hand

⊟ IQ + M71.049 Abscess of bursa, unspecified hand

+ 6 M71.05 Abscess of bursa, hip

⊟ SP + M71.051 Abscess of bursa, right hip

⊟ SP + M71.052 Abscess of bursa, left hip

⊟ IQ + M71.059 Abscess of bursa, unspecified hip

+ 6 M71.06 Abscess of bursa, knee

⊟ SP + M71.061 Abscess of bursa, right knee

⊟ SP + M71.062 Abscess of bursa, left knee

⊟ IQ + M71.069 Abscess of bursa, unspecified knee

+ 6 M71.07 Abscess of bursa, ankle and foot

⊟ SP + M71.071 Abscess of bursa, right ankle and foot

⊟ SP + M71.072 Abscess of bursa, left ankle and foot

⊟ IQ + M71.079 Abscess of bursa, unspecified ankle and foot

SP + M71.08 Abscess of bursa, other site

SP + M71.09 Abscess of bursa, multiple sites

+ 5 M71.1 Other infective bursitis

> Use additional code (B95.-, B96.-) to identify causative organism

IQ + M71.10 Other infective bursitis, unspecified site

+ 6 M71.11 Other infective bursitis, shoulder

⊟ SP + M71.111 Other infective bursitis, right shoulder

⊟ SP + M71.112 Other infective bursitis, left shoulder

★ New ▲ Revised Px Primary SP PDGM Px SL Low CoM SH High CoM IQ Quest. Encounter H Hospice non-cancer Dx Unspecified M *Manifestation*

Chapter 13

M00-M99

☐ 🔲 ✚ **M71.119** Other infective bursitis, unspecified shoulder

✚ 6️⃣ **M71.12** Other infective bursitis, elbow

☐ SP ✚ **M71.121** Other infective bursitis, right elbow

☐ SP ✚ **M71.122** Other infective bursitis, left elbow

☐ 🔲 ✚ **M71.129** Other infective bursitis, unspecified elbow

✚ 6️⃣ **M71.13** Other infective bursitis, wrist

☐ SP ✚ **M71.131** Other infective bursitis, right wrist

☐ SP ✚ **M71.132** Other infective bursitis, left wrist

☐ 🔲 ✚ **M71.139** Other infective bursitis, unspecified wrist

✚ 6️⃣ **M71.14** Other infective bursitis, hand

☐ SP ✚ **M71.141** Other infective bursitis, right hand

☐ SP ✚ **M71.142** Other infective bursitis, left hand

☐ 🔲 ✚ **M71.149** Other infective bursitis, unspecified hand

✚ 6️⃣ **M71.15** Other infective bursitis, hip

☐ SP ✚ **M71.151** Other infective bursitis, right hip

☐ SP ✚ **M71.152** Other infective bursitis, left hip

☐ 🔲 ✚ **M71.159** Other infective bursitis, unspecified hip

✚ 6️⃣ **M71.16** Other infective bursitis, knee

☐ SP ✚ **M71.161** Other infective bursitis, right knee

☐ SP ✚ **M71.162** Other infective bursitis, left knee

☐ 🔲 ✚ **M71.169** Other infective bursitis, unspecified knee

✚ 6️⃣ **M71.17** Other infective bursitis, ankle and foot

☐ SP ✚ **M71.171** Other infective bursitis, right ankle and foot

☐ SP ✚ **M71.172** Other infective bursitis, left ankle and foot

☐ 🔲 ✚ **M71.179** Other infective bursitis, unspecified ankle and foot

SP ✚ **M71.18** Other infective bursitis, other site

SP ✚ **M71.19** Other infective bursitis, multiple sites

5️⃣ **M71.2** Synovial cyst of popliteal space [Baker]

EXCLUDES 1   synovial cyst of popliteal space with rupture (M66.0)

DEFINITION   Collection of synovial fluid that has escaped from the knee joint or bursa and has formed a synovial-lined sac behind the knee.

☐ 🔲 **M71.20** Synovial cyst of popliteal space [Baker], unspecified knee

☐ SP **M71.21** Synovial cyst of popliteal space [Baker], right knee

☐ SP **M71.22** Synovial cyst of popliteal space [Baker], left knee

5️⃣ **M71.3** Other bursal cyst

Synovial cyst NOS

EXCLUDES 1   synovial cyst with rupture (M66.1-)

🔲 **M71.30** Other bursal cyst, unspecified site

6️⃣ **M71.31** Other bursal cyst, shoulder

☐ SP **M71.311** Other bursal cyst, right shoulder

☐ SP **M71.312** Other bursal cyst, left shoulder

☐ 🔲 **M71.319** Other bursal cyst, unspecified shoulder

6️⃣ **M71.32** Other bursal cyst, elbow

☐ SP **M71.321** Other bursal cyst, right elbow

☐ SP **M71.322** Other bursal cyst, left elbow

☐ 🔲 **M71.329** Other bursal cyst, unspecified elbow

6️⃣ **M71.33** Other bursal cyst, wrist

☐ SP **M71.331** Other bursal cyst, right wrist

☐ SP **M71.332** Other bursal cyst, left wrist

☐ 🔲 **M71.339** Other bursal cyst, unspecified wrist

6️⃣ **M71.34** Other bursal cyst, hand

☐ SP **M71.341** Other bursal cyst, right hand

☐ SP **M71.342** Other bursal cyst, left hand

☐ 🔲 **M71.349** Other bursal cyst, unspecified hand

6️⃣ **M71.35** Other bursal cyst, hip

☐ SP **M71.351** Other bursal cyst, right hip

☐ SP **M71.352** Other bursal cyst, left hip

☐ 🔲 **M71.359** Other bursal cyst, unspecified hip

6️⃣ **M71.37** Other bursal cyst, ankle and foot

☐ SP **M71.371** Other bursal cyst, right ankle and foot

☐ SP **M71.372** Other bursal cyst, left ankle and foot

☐ 🔲 **M71.379** Other bursal cyst, unspecified ankle and foot

SP **M71.38** Other bursal cyst, other site

SP **M71.39** Other bursal cyst, multiple sites

5️⃣ **M71.4** Calcium deposit in bursa

EXCLUDES 2   calcium deposit in bursa of shoulder (M75.3)

🔲 **M71.40** Calcium deposit in bursa, unspecified site

6️⃣ **M71.42** Calcium deposit in bursa, elbow

☐ SP **M71.421** Calcium deposit in bursa, right elbow

☐ SP **M71.422** Calcium deposit in bursa, left elbow

☐ 🔲 **M71.429** Calcium deposit in bursa, unspecified elbow

6️⃣ **M71.43** Calcium deposit in bursa, wrist

☐ SP **M71.431** Calcium deposit in bursa, right wrist

☐ SP **M71.432** Calcium deposit in bursa, left wrist

☐ 🔲 **M71.439** Calcium deposit in bursa, unspecified wrist

6️⃣ **M71.44** Calcium deposit in bursa, hand

☐ SP **M71.441** Calcium deposit in bursa, right hand

☐ SP **M71.442** Calcium deposit in bursa, left hand

☐ 🔲 **M71.449** Calcium deposit in bursa, unspecified hand

6️⃣ **M71.45** Calcium deposit in bursa, hip

☐ SP **M71.451** Calcium deposit in bursa, right hip

4️⃣ 4th digit required   5️⃣ 5th digit required   6️⃣ 6th digit required   7️⃣ 7th digit required   ✔️ 7th digit placeholder   ✚ Additional code   ☐ Laterality

1232   *DecisionHealth's* FY 2020 Complete Home Health ICD-10-CM Diagnosis Coding Manual

◨ **SP** **M71.452** Calcium deposit in bursa, left hip

◨ **IQ** **M71.459** Calcium deposit in bursa, unspecified hip

⑥ **M71.46** Calcium deposit in bursa, knee

◨ **SP** **M71.461** Calcium deposit in bursa, right knee

◨ **SP** **M71.462** Calcium deposit in bursa, left knee

◨ **IQ** **M71.469** Calcium deposit in bursa, unspecified knee

⑥ **M71.47** Calcium deposit in bursa, ankle and foot

◨ **SP** **M71.471** Calcium deposit in bursa, right ankle and foot

◨ **SP** **M71.472** Calcium deposit in bursa, left ankle and foot

◨ **IQ** **M71.479** Calcium deposit in bursa, unspecified ankle and foot

SP **M71.48** Calcium deposit in bursa, other site

SP **M71.49** Calcium deposit in bursa, multiple sites

⑤ **M71.5** Other bursitis, not elsewhere classified

> **EXCLUDES 1** bursitis NOS (M71.9-)
>
> **EXCLUDES 2** bursitis of shoulder (M75.5)
> bursitis of tibial collateral [Pellegrini-Stieda] (M76.4-)

IQ **M71.50** Other bursitis, not elsewhere classified, unspecified site

⑥ **M71.52** Other bursitis, not elsewhere classified, elbow

◨ **SP** **M71.521** Other bursitis, not elsewhere classified, right elbow

◨ **SP** **M71.522** Other bursitis, not elsewhere classified, left elbow

◨ **IQ** **M71.529** Other bursitis, not elsewhere classified, unspecified elbow

⑥ **M71.53** Other bursitis, not elsewhere classified, wrist

◨ **SP** **M71.531** Other bursitis, not elsewhere classified, right wrist

◨ **SP** **M71.532** Other bursitis, not elsewhere classified, left wrist

◨ **IQ** **M71.539** Other bursitis, not elsewhere classified, unspecified wrist

⑥ **M71.54** Other bursitis, not elsewhere classified, hand

◨ **SP** **M71.541** Other bursitis, not elsewhere classified, right hand

◨ **SP** **M71.542** Other bursitis, not elsewhere classified, left hand

◨ **IQ** **M71.549** Other bursitis, not elsewhere classified, unspecified hand

⑥ **M71.55** Other bursitis, not elsewhere classified, hip

◨ **SP** **M71.551** Other bursitis, not elsewhere classified, right hip

◨ **SP** **M71.552** Other bursitis, not elsewhere classified, left hip

◨ **IQ** **M71.559** Other bursitis, not elsewhere classified, unspecified hip

⑥ **M71.56** Other bursitis, not elsewhere classified, knee

◨ **SP** **M71.561** Other bursitis, not elsewhere classified, right knee

◨ **SP** **M71.562** Other bursitis, not elsewhere classified, left knee

◨ **IQ** **M71.569** Other bursitis, not elsewhere classified, unspecified knee

⑥ **M71.57** Other bursitis, not elsewhere classified, ankle and foot

◨ **SP** **M71.571** Other bursitis, not elsewhere classified, right ankle and foot

◨ **SP** **M71.572** Other bursitis, not elsewhere classified, left ankle and foot

◨ **IQ** **M71.579** Other bursitis, not elsewhere classified, unspecified ankle and foot

SP **M71.58** Other bursitis, not elsewhere classified, other site

⑤ **M71.8** Other specified bursopathies

IQ **M71.80** Other specified bursopathies, unspecified site

⑥ **M71.81** Other specified bursopathies, shoulder

◨ **SP** **M71.811** Other specified bursopathies, right shoulder

◨ **SP** **M71.812** Other specified bursopathies, left shoulder

◨ **IQ** **M71.819** Other specified bursopathies, unspecified shoulder

⑥ **M71.82** Other specified bursopathies, elbow

◨ **SP** **M71.821** Other specified bursopathies, right elbow

◨ **SP** **M71.822** Other specified bursopathies, left elbow

◨ **IQ** **M71.829** Other specified bursopathies, unspecified elbow

⑥ **M71.83** Other specified bursopathies, wrist

◨ **SP** **M71.831** Other specified bursopathies, right wrist

◨ **SP** **M71.832** Other specified bursopathies, left wrist

◨ **IQ** **M71.839** Other specified bursopathies, unspecified wrist

⑥ **M71.84** Other specified bursopathies, hand

◨ **SP** **M71.841** Other specified bursopathies, right hand

◨ **SP** **M71.842** Other specified bursopathies, left hand

◨ **IQ** **M71.849** Other specified bursopathies, unspecified hand

⑥ **M71.85** Other specified bursopathies, hip

◨ **SP** **M71.851** Other specified bursopathies, right hip

◨ **SP** **M71.852** Other specified bursopathies, left hip

◨ **IQ** **M71.859** Other specified bursopathies, unspecified hip

⑥ **M71.86** Other specified bursopathies, knee

◨ **SP** **M71.861** Other specified bursopathies, right knee

◨ **SP** **M71.862** Other specified bursopathies, left knee

◨ **IQ** **M71.869** Other specified bursopathies, unspecified knee

⑥ **M71.87** Other specified bursopathies, ankle and foot

◨ **SP** **M71.871** Other specified bursopathies, right ankle and foot

★ New ▲ Revised Px Primary **SP** PDGM Px **SL** Low CoM **SH** High CoM **IQ** Quest. Encounter Ⓗ Hospice non-cancer Dx Unspecified **M** *Manifestation*

DecisionHealth's FY 2020 Complete Home Health ICD-10-CM Diagnosis Coding Manual

1233

⊟ SP M71.872 Other specified bursopathies, left ankle and foot

⊟ IQ M71.879 Other specified bursopathies, unspecified ankle and foot

SP M71.88 Other specified bursopathies, other site

SP M71.89 Other specified bursopathies, multiple sites

IQ M71.9 Bursopathy, unspecified
Bursitis NOS

4 M72 Fibroblastic disorders
　EXCLUDES 2　retroperitoneal fibromatosis (D48.3)

SP M72.0 Palmar fascial fibromatosis [Dupuytren]

SP M72.1 Knuckle pads

SP M72.2 Plantar fascial fibromatosis
Plantar fasciitis

SP M72.4 Pseudosarcomatous fibromatosis
Nodular fasciitis

SP + M72.6 Necrotizing fasciitis
Use additional code (B95.-, B96.-) to identify causative organism

SP + M72.8 Other fibroblastic disorders
Abscess of fascia
Fasciitis NEC
Other infective fasciitis
Use additional code to (B95.-, B96.-) identify causative organism
　EXCLUDES 1　diffuse (eosinophilic) fasciitis (M35.4)
　　necrotizing fasciitis (M72.6)
　　nodular fasciitis (M72.4)
　　perirenal fasciitis NOS (N13.5)
　　perirenal fasciitis with infection (N13.6)
　　plantar fasciitis (M72.2)

IQ M72.9 Fibroblastic disorder, unspecified
Fasciitis NOS
Fibromatosis NOS

4 M75 Shoulder lesions
　EXCLUDES 2　shoulder-hand syndrome (M89.0-)

5 M75.0 Adhesive capsulitis of shoulder
Frozen shoulder
Periarthritis of shoulder

⊟ IQ M75.00 Adhesive capsulitis of unspecified shoulder

⊟ SP M75.01 Adhesive capsulitis of right shoulder

⊟ SP M75.02 Adhesive capsulitis of left shoulder

5 M75.1 Rotator cuff tear or rupture, not specified as traumatic
Rotator cuff syndrome
Supraspinatus tear or rupture, not specified as traumatic
Supraspinatus syndrome
　EXCLUDES 1　tear of rotator cuff, traumatic (S46.01-)

6 M75.10 Unspecified rotator cuff tear or rupture, not specified as traumatic

⊟ IQ M75.100 Unspecified rotator cuff tear or rupture of unspecified shoulder, not specified as traumatic

⊟ SP M75.101 Unspecified rotator cuff tear or rupture of right shoulder, not specified as traumatic

⊟ SP M75.102 Unspecified rotator cuff tear or rupture of left shoulder, not specified as traumatic

6 M75.11 Incomplete rotator cuff tear or rupture not specified as traumatic
CODING TIPS ✓　A partial tear of the rotator cuff is an area of damage to the rotator cuff tendons, where the tear does not go all the way through the tendons. Note that a complete tear is coded to M75.12. A traumatic tear is coded to S46.01-.

⊟ IQ M75.110 Incomplete rotator cuff tear or rupture of unspecified shoulder, not specified as traumatic

⊟ SP M75.111 Incomplete rotator cuff tear or rupture of right shoulder, not specified as traumatic

⊟ SP M75.112 Incomplete rotator cuff tear or rupture of left shoulder, not specified as traumatic

6 M75.12 Complete rotator cuff tear or rupture not specified as traumatic

⊟ IQ M75.120 Complete rotator cuff tear or rupture of unspecified shoulder, not specified as traumatic

⊟ SP M75.121 Complete rotator cuff tear or rupture of right shoulder, not specified as traumatic

⊟ SP M75.122 Complete rotator cuff tear or rupture of left shoulder, not specified as traumatic

5 M75.2 Bicipital tendinitis

⊟ IQ M75.20 Bicipital tendinitis, unspecified shoulder

⊟ SP M75.21 Bicipital tendinitis, right shoulder

⊟ SP M75.22 Bicipital tendinitis, left shoulder

5 M75.3 Calcific tendinitis of shoulder
Calcified bursa of shoulder

⊟ IQ M75.30 Calcific tendinitis of unspecified shoulder

⊟ SP M75.31 Calcific tendinitis of right shoulder

⊟ SP M75.32 Calcific tendinitis of left shoulder

5 M75.4 Impingement syndrome of shoulder

⊟ IQ M75.40 Impingement syndrome of unspecified shoulder

⊟ SP M75.41 Impingement syndrome of right shoulder

⊟ SP M75.42 Impingement syndrome of left shoulder

5 M75.5 Bursitis of shoulder

⊟ IQ M75.50 Bursitis of unspecified shoulder

⊟ SP M75.51 Bursitis of right shoulder

⊟ SP M75.52 Bursitis of left shoulder

5 M75.8 Other shoulder lesions

⊟ IQ M75.80 Other shoulder lesions, unspecified shoulder

⊟ SP M75.81 Other shoulder lesions, right shoulder

⊟ SP M75.82 Other shoulder lesions, left shoulder

5 M75.9 Shoulder lesion, unspecified

⊟ IQ M75.90 Shoulder lesion, unspecified, unspecified shoulder

---

4 4th digit required　　5 5th digit required　　6 6th digit required　　7 7th digit required　　7 7th digit placeholder　　+ Additional code　　⊟ Laterality

⊟ SP **M75.91** Shoulder lesion, unspecified, right shoulder

⊟ SP **M75.92** Shoulder lesion, unspecified, left shoulder

④ **M76** Enthesopathies, lower limb, excluding foot
　EXCLUDES 2　bursitis due to use, overuse and pressure (M70.-)
　　enthesopathies of ankle and foot (M77.5-)

　⑤ **M76.0** Gluteal tendinitis

⊟ IQ **M76.00** Gluteal tendinitis, unspecified hip

⊟ SP **M76.01** Gluteal tendinitis, right hip

⊟ SP **M76.02** Gluteal tendinitis, left hip

　⑤ **M76.1** Psoas tendinitis

⊟ IQ **M76.10** Psoas tendinitis, unspecified hip

⊟ SP **M76.11** Psoas tendinitis, right hip

⊟ SP **M76.12** Psoas tendinitis, left hip

　⑤ **M76.2** Iliac crest spur

⊟ IQ **M76.20** Iliac crest spur, unspecified hip

⊟ SP **M76.21** Iliac crest spur, right hip

⊟ SP **M76.22** Iliac crest spur, left hip

　⑤ **M76.3** Iliotibial band syndrome

⊟ IQ **M76.30** Iliotibial band syndrome, unspecified leg

⊟ SP **M76.31** Iliotibial band syndrome, right leg

⊟ SP **M76.32** Iliotibial band syndrome, left leg

　⑤ **M76.4** Tibial collateral bursitis [Pellegrini-Stieda]

⊟ IQ **M76.40** Tibial collateral bursitis [Pellegrini-Stieda], unspecified leg

⊟ SP **M76.41** Tibial collateral bursitis [Pellegrini-Stieda], right leg

⊟ SP **M76.42** Tibial collateral bursitis [Pellegrini-Stieda], left leg

　⑤ **M76.5** Patellar tendinitis

⊟ IQ **M76.50** Patellar tendinitis, unspecified knee

⊟ SP **M76.51** Patellar tendinitis, right knee

⊟ SP **M76.52** Patellar tendinitis, left knee

　⑤ **M76.6** Achilles tendinitis
　　Achilles bursitis

⊟ IQ **M76.60** Achilles tendinitis, unspecified leg

⊟ SP **M76.61** Achilles tendinitis, right leg

⊟ SP **M76.62** Achilles tendinitis, left leg

　⑤ **M76.7** Peroneal tendinitis

⊟ IQ **M76.70** Peroneal tendinitis, unspecified leg

⊟ SP **M76.71** Peroneal tendinitis, right leg

⊟ SP **M76.72** Peroneal tendinitis, left leg

　⑤ **M76.8** Other specified enthesopathies of lower limb, excluding foot

　　⑥ **M76.81** Anterior tibial syndrome

⊟ SP **M76.811** Anterior tibial syndrome, right leg

⊟ SP **M76.812** Anterior tibial syndrome, left leg

⊟ IQ **M76.819** Anterior tibial syndrome, unspecified leg

　　⑥ **M76.82** Posterior tibial tendinitis

⊟ SP **M76.821** Posterior tibial tendinitis, right leg

⊟ SP **M76.822** Posterior tibial tendinitis, left leg

⊟ IQ **M76.829** Posterior tibial tendinitis, unspecified leg

⑥ **M76.89** Other specified enthesopathies of lower limb, excluding foot

⊟ SP **M76.891** Other specified enthesopathies of right lower limb, excluding foot

⊟ SP **M76.892** Other specified enthesopathies of left lower limb, excluding foot

⊟ IQ **M76.899** Other specified enthesopathies of unspecified lower limb, excluding foot

SP **M76.9** Unspecified enthesopathy, lower limb, excluding foot

④ **M77** Other enthesopathies
　EXCLUDES 1　bursitis NOS (M71.9-)
　EXCLUDES 2　bursitis due to use, overuse and pressure (M70.-)
　　osteophyte (M25.7)
　　spinal enthesopathy (M46.0-)

　⑤ **M77.0** Medial epicondylitis

⊟ IQ **M77.00** Medial epicondylitis, unspecified elbow

⊟ SP **M77.01** Medial epicondylitis, right elbow

⊟ SP **M77.02** Medial epicondylitis, left elbow

　⑤ **M77.1** Lateral epicondylitis
　　Tennis elbow
　　DEFINITION　A painful inflammation of the tendons that anchor the extensor carpi radialis brevis muscle to the outer aspect of the humerus at the elbow.

⊟ IQ **M77.10** Lateral epicondylitis, unspecified elbow

⊟ SP **M77.11** Lateral epicondylitis, right elbow

⊟ SP **M77.12** Lateral epicondylitis, left elbow

　⑤ **M77.2** Periarthritis of wrist

⊟ IQ **M77.20** Periarthritis, unspecified wrist

⊟ SP **M77.21** Periarthritis, right wrist

⊟ SP **M77.22** Periarthritis, left wrist

　⑤ **M77.3** Calcaneal spur

⊟ IQ **M77.30** Calcaneal spur, unspecified foot

⊟ SP **M77.31** Calcaneal spur, right foot

⊟ SP **M77.32** Calcaneal spur, left foot

　⑤ **M77.4** Metatarsalgia
　　EXCLUDES 1　Morton's metatarsalgia (G57.6)

⊟ IQ **M77.40** Metatarsalgia, unspecified foot

⊟ SP **M77.41** Metatarsalgia, right foot

⊟ SP **M77.42** Metatarsalgia, left foot

▲ ⑤ **M77.5** Other enthesopathy of foot and ankle

▲ ⊟ IQ **M77.50** Other enthesopathy of unspecified foot and ankle

▲ ⊟ SP **M77.51** Other enthesopathy of right foot and ankle

▲ ⊟ SP **M77.52** Other enthesopathy of left foot and ankle

SP **M77.8** Other enthesopathies, not elsewhere classified

IQ **M77.9** Enthesopathy, unspecified
　　Bone spur NOS
　　Capsulitis NOS
　　Periarthritis NOS
　　Tendinitis NOS

④ **M79** Other and unspecified soft tissue disorders, not elsewhere classified

★ New ▲ Revised Px Primary SP PDGM Px SL Low CoM SH High CoM IQ Quest. Encounter H Hospice non-cancer Dx Unspecified M *Manifestation*

DecisionHealth's FY 2020 Complete Home Health ICD-10-CM Diagnosis Coding Manual

1235

EXCLUDES 1   psychogenic rheumatism
(F45.8)
soft tissue pain, psychogenic
(F45.41)

SP M79.0 **Rheumatism, unspecified**
EXCLUDES 1   fibromyalgia (M79.7)
palindromic rheumatism
(M12.3-)

5 M79.1 Myalgia
Myofascial pain syndrome
EXCLUDES 1   fibromyalgia (M79.7)
myositis (M60.-)

SP M79.10   **Myalgia, unspecified site**

SP M79.11   **Myalgia of mastication muscle**

SP M79.12   **Myalgia of auxiliary muscles, head and neck**

SP M79.18   **Myalgia, other site**

SP M79.2   **Neuralgia and neuritis, unspecified**
EXCLUDES 1   brachial radiculitis NOS
(M54.1)
lumbosacral radiculitis NOS
(M54.1)
mononeuropathies
(G56-G58)
radiculitis NOS (M54.1)
sciatica (M54.3-M54.4)

SP M79.3   **Panniculitis, unspecified**
EXCLUDES 1   lupus panniculitis (L93.2)
neck and back panniculitis
(M54.0-)
relapsing [Weber-Christian]
panniculitis (M35.6)

SP M79.4 Hypertrophy of (infrapatellar) fat pad

SP M79.5 Residual foreign body in soft tissue
EXCLUDES 1   foreign body granuloma of
skin and subcutaneous
tissue (L92.3)
foreign body granuloma of
soft tissue (M60.2-)

5 M79.6 Pain in limb, hand, foot, fingers and toes
EXCLUDES 2   pain in joint (M25.5-)

CODING TIPS ✓   These codes should be used
when 1) the cause of the pain is
unknown; 2) the pain is a sequela of an
injury; or 3) in conjunction with a G89 code.
Do not use these codes with conditions
where this type is integral.

6 M79.60   **Pain in limb, unspecified**

▣ IQ M79.601 Pain in right arm
Pain in right upper limb NOS

▣ IQ M79.602 Pain in left arm
Pain in left upper limb NOS

▣ IQ M79.603   Pain in arm, unspecified
Pain in upper limb NOS

▣ IQ M79.604 Pain in right leg
Pain in right lower limb NOS

▣ IQ M79.605 Pain in left leg
Pain in left lower limb NOS

▣ IQ M79.606   Pain in leg, unspecified
Pain in lower limb NOS

▣ IQ M79.609   Pain in unspecified limb
Pain in limb NOS

6 M79.62 Pain in upper arm
Pain in axillary region

▣ IQ M79.621 Pain in right upper arm

▣ IQ M79.622 Pain in left upper arm

▣ IQ M79.629   Pain in unspecified upper arm

6 M79.63 Pain in forearm

▣ IQ M79.631 Pain in right forearm

▣ IQ M79.632 Pain in left forearm

▣ IQ M79.639   Pain in unspecified forearm

6 M79.64 Pain in hand and fingers

▣ IQ M79.641 Pain in right hand

▣ IQ M79.642 Pain in left hand

▣ IQ M79.643   Pain in unspecified hand

▣ IQ M79.644 Pain in right finger(s)

▣ IQ M79.645 Pain in left finger(s)

▣ IQ M79.646   Pain in unspecified finger(s)

6 M79.65 Pain in thigh

▣ IQ M79.651 Pain in right thigh

▣ IQ M79.652 Pain in left thigh

▣ IQ M79.659   Pain in unspecified thigh

6 M79.66 Pain in lower leg

▣ IQ M79.661 Pain in right lower leg

▣ IQ M79.662 Pain in left lower leg

▣ IQ M79.669   Pain in unspecified lower leg

6 M79.67 Pain in foot and toes

▣ IQ M79.671 Pain in right foot

▣ IQ M79.672 Pain in left foot

▣ IQ M79.673   Pain in unspecified foot

▣ IQ M79.674 Pain in right toe(s)

▣ IQ M79.675 Pain in left toe(s)

▣ IQ M79.676   Pain in unspecified toe(s)

SP M79.7 Fibromyalgia
Fibromyositis
Fibrositis
Myofibrositis

5 M79.A Nontraumatic compartment syndrome
Code first:
, if applicable, associated postprocedural
complication
EXCLUDES 1   compartment syndrome NOS
(T79.A-)
fibromyalgia (M79.7)
nontraumatic ischemic
infarction of muscle
(M62.2-)
traumatic compartment
syndrome (T79.A-)

**6 M79.A1 Nontraumatic compartment
syndrome of upper extremity**
Nontraumatic compartment syndrome
of shoulder, arm, forearm, wrist,
hand, and fingers

**▣ SP M79.A11 Nontraumatic compartment
syndrome of right upper
extremity**

**▣ SP M79.A12 Nontraumatic compartment
syndrome of left upper extremity**

**▣ IQ M79.A19   Nontraumatic compartment
syndrome of unspecified upper
extremity**

**6 M79.A2 Nontraumatic compartment
syndrome of lower extremity**
Nontraumatic compartment syndrome
of hip, buttock, thigh, leg, foot, and
toes

---

4 4th digit required   **5** 5th digit required   **6** 6th digit required   **7** 7th digit required   **7** 7th digit placeholder   **+** Additional code   **▣** Laterality

⊟ 𝗦𝗣 **M79.A21** Nontraumatic compartment syndrome of right lower extremity

⊟ 𝗦𝗣 **M79.A22** Nontraumatic compartment syndrome of left lower extremity

⊟ 𝗜𝗤 **M79.A29** Nontraumatic compartment syndrome of unspecified lower extremity

𝗦𝗣 **M79.A3** Nontraumatic compartment syndrome of abdomen

𝗦𝗣 **M79.A9** Nontraumatic compartment syndrome of other sites

𝟱 **M79.8** Other specified soft tissue disorders

𝗦𝗣 **M79.81** Nontraumatic hematoma of soft tissue
Nontraumatic hematoma of muscle
Nontraumatic seroma of muscle and soft tissue

DEFINITION A spontaneous, nontraumatic localized collection of partially clotted blood within a soft tissue such as muscle.

𝗦𝗣 **M79.89** Other specified soft tissue disorders
Polyalgia

𝗜𝗤 **M79.9** Soft tissue disorder, unspecified

Osteopathies and chondropathies (M80-M94)

Disorders of bone density and structure (M80-M85)

+ ◢ **M80** Osteoporosis with current pathological fracture

INCLUDES osteoporosis with current fragility fracture

Use additional code to identify major osseous defect, if applicable (M89.7-)

EXCLUDES 1 collapsed vertebra NOS (M48.5)
pathological fracture NOS (M84.4)
wedging of vertebra NOS (M48.5)

EXCLUDES 2 personal history of (healed) osteoporosis fracture (Z87.310)

The appropriate 7th character is to be added to each code from category M80:
A   initial encounter for fracture
D   subsequent encounter for fracture with routine healing
G   subsequent encounter for fracture with delayed healing
K   subsequent encounter for fracture with nonunion
P   subsequent encounter for fracture with malunion
S   sequela

GUIDELINES Section I.C.13.c
Coding of Pathologic Fractures: 7th character D is to be used for encounters after the patient has completed active treatment for the fracture and is receiving routine care for the fracture during the healing or recovery phase. The other 7th characters, listed under each subcategory in the Tabular List, are to be used for subsequent encounters for treatment of problems associated with the healing, such as malunions, nonunions, and sequelae.
Care for complications of surgical treatment for fracture repairs during the healing or recovery phase should be coded with the appropriate complication codes.

GUIDELINES Section I.C.13.d.2)
Category M80, Osteoporosis with current pathological fracture, is for patients who have a current pathologic fracture at the time of an encounter. The codes under M80 identify the site of the fracture. A code from category M80, not a traumatic fracture code, should be used for any patient with known osteoporosis who suffers a fracture, even if the patient had a minor fall or trauma, if that fall or trauma would not usually break a normal, healthy bone.

GUIDELINES Section I.C.13.a.1)
For certain conditions, the bone may be affected at the upper or lower end, (e.g., avascular necrosis of bone, M87, Osteoporosis, M80, M81). Though the portion of the bone affected may be at the joint, the site designation will be the bone, not the joint.

CODING TIPS ✓ Fractures repaired by joint replacements are NOT coded with Z47.1. Fractures repaired by any other orthopedic surgery are NOT coded with Z47.89. Z codes are not appropriate for fractures of any kind. Code the fracture with 7th character D for fractures undergoing surgical repair.

CODING TIPS ✓ When a patient with osteoporosis is noted to have an active fracture, use the osteoporosis fracture codes, unless the physician has identified the fracture as a trauma fracture. Age-related osteoporosis includes post-menopausal and senile osteoporosis, as well as unspecified. Age-related osteoporosis is the default if the type of osteoporosis is not identified. Code Z87.310 is assigned for an osteoporosis fracture that has healed.

+ 𝟱 **M80.0** Age-related osteoporosis with current pathological fracture
Involutional osteoporosis with current pathological fracture
Osteoporosis NOS with current pathological fracture
Postmenopausal osteoporosis with current pathological fracture
Senile osteoporosis with current pathological fracture

𝗜𝗤 **+** ☑ **M80.00X-** Age-related osteoporosis with current pathological fracture, unspecified site

★ New ▲ Revised 𝗣𝘅 Primary 𝗦𝗣 PDGM Px 𝗦𝗟 Low CoM 𝗦𝗛 High CoM 𝗜𝗤 Quest. Encounter 𝗛 Hospice non-cancer Dx Unspecified 𝗠 *Manifestation*

DecisionHealth's FY 2020 Complete Home Health ICD-10-CM Diagnosis Coding Manual

1237

CODING TIPS ✓   Use this code for osteoporosis fractures of the rib and pelvis. It is the best choice until the classification can be updated.

+ ⑥ **M80.01** Age-related osteoporosis with current pathological fracture, shoulder

⊟ **SP** **+** ⑦ **M80.011-** Age-related osteoporosis with current pathological fracture, right shoulder

⊟ **SP** **+** ⑦ **M80.012-** Age-related osteoporosis with current pathological fracture, left shoulder

⊟ **!Q** **+** ⑦ **M80.019-** Age-related osteoporosis with current pathological fracture, unspecified shoulder

+ ⑥ **M80.02** Age-related osteoporosis with current pathological fracture, humerus

⊟ **SP** **+** ⑦ **M80.021-** Age-related osteoporosis with current pathological fracture, right humerus

⊟ **SP** **+** ⑦ **M80.022-** Age-related osteoporosis with current pathological fracture, left humerus

⊟ **!Q** **+** ⑦ **M80.029-** Age-related osteoporosis with current pathological fracture, unspecified humerus

+ ⑥ **M80.03** Age-related osteoporosis with current pathological fracture, forearm
Age-related osteoporosis with current pathological fracture of wrist

⊟ **SP** **+** ⑦ **M80.031-** Age-related osteoporosis with current pathological fracture, right forearm

⊟ **SP** **+** ⑦ **M80.032-** Age-related osteoporosis with current pathological fracture, left forearm

⊟ **!Q** **+** ⑦ **M80.039-** Age-related osteoporosis with current pathological fracture, unspecified forearm

+ ⑥ **M80.04** Age-related osteoporosis with current pathological fracture, hand

⊟ **SP** **+** ⑦ **M80.041-** Age-related osteoporosis with current pathological fracture, right hand

⊟ **SP** **+** ⑦ **M80.042-** Age-related osteoporosis with current pathological fracture, left hand

⊟ **!Q** **+** ⑦ **M80.049-** Age-related osteoporosis with current pathological fracture, unspecified hand

+ ⑥ **M80.05** Age-related osteoporosis with current pathological fracture, femur
Age-related osteoporosis with current pathological fracture of hip

⊟ **SP** **+** ⑦ **M80.051-** Age-related osteoporosis with current pathological fracture, right femur

⊟ **SP** **+** ⑦ **M80.052-** Age-related osteoporosis with current pathological fracture, left femur

⊟ **!Q** **+** ⑦ **M80.059-** Age-related osteoporosis with current pathological fracture, unspecified femur

+ ⑥ **M80.06** Age-related osteoporosis with current pathological fracture, lower leg

⊟ **SP** **+** ⑦ **M80.061-** Age-related osteoporosis with current pathological fracture, right lower leg

⊟ **SP** **+** ⑦ **M80.062-** Age-related osteoporosis with current pathological fracture, left lower leg

⊟ **!Q** **+** ⑦ **M80.069-** Age-related osteoporosis with current pathological fracture, unspecified lower leg

+ ⑥ **M80.07** Age-related osteoporosis with current pathological fracture, ankle and foot

⊟ **SP** **+** ⑦ **M80.071-** Age-related osteoporosis with current pathological fracture, right ankle and foot

⊟ **SP** **+** ⑦ **M80.072-** Age-related osteoporosis with current pathological fracture, left ankle and foot

⊟ **!Q** **+** ⑦ **M80.079-** Age-related osteoporosis with current pathological fracture, unspecified ankle and foot

SP **+** ☑ **M80.08X-** Age-related osteoporosis with current pathological fracture, vertebra(e)

+ ⑤ **M80.8** Other osteoporosis with current pathological fracture
Drug-induced osteoporosis with current pathological fracture
Idiopathic osteoporosis with current pathological fracture
Osteoporosis of disuse with current pathological fracture
Postoophorectomy osteoporosis with current pathological fracture
Postsurgical malabsorption osteoporosis with current pathological fracture
Post-traumatic osteoporosis with current pathological fracture
Use additional code for adverse effect, if applicable, to identify drug (T36-T50 with fifth or sixth character 5)

!Q **+** ☑ **M80.80X-** Other osteoporosis with current pathological fracture, unspecified site

+ ⑥ **M80.81** Other osteoporosis with pathological fracture, shoulder

⊟ **SP** **+** ☑ **M80.811-** Other osteoporosis with current pathological fracture, right shoulder

⊟ **SP** **+** ☑ **M80.812-** Other osteoporosis with current pathological fracture, left shoulder

⊟ **!Q** **+** ☑ **M80.819-** Other osteoporosis with current pathological fracture, unspecified shoulder

+ ⑥ **M80.82** Other osteoporosis with current pathological fracture, humerus

⊟ **SP** **+** ☑ **M80.821-** Other osteoporosis with current pathological fracture, right humerus

⊟ **SP** **+** ☑ **M80.822-** Other osteoporosis with current pathological fracture, left humerus

---

④ 4th digit required   ⑤ 5th digit required   ⑥ 6th digit required   ⑦ 7th digit required   ☑ 7th digit placeholder   **+** Additional code   ⊟ Laterality

1238   *DecisionHealth's* FY 2020 Complete Home Health ICD-10-CM Diagnosis Coding Manual

☐ **IQ** ✛ 🔟 **M80.829-** Other osteoporosis with current pathological fracture, unspecified humerus

✛ 🔞 **M80.83** Other osteoporosis with current pathological fracture, forearm
Other osteoporosis with current pathological fracture of wrist

☐ **SP** ✛ 🔟 **M80.831-** Other osteoporosis with current pathological fracture, right forearm

☐ **SP** ✛ 🔟 **M80.832-** Other osteoporosis with current pathological fracture, left forearm

☐ **IQ** ✛ 🔟 **M80.839-** Other osteoporosis with current pathological fracture, unspecified forearm

✛ 🔞 **M80.84** Other osteoporosis with current pathological fracture, hand

☐ **SP** ✛ 🔟 **M80.841-** Other osteoporosis with current pathological fracture, right hand

☐ **SP** ✛ 🔟 **M80.842-** Other osteoporosis with current pathological fracture, left hand

☐ **IQ** ✛ 🔟 **M80.849-** Other osteoporosis with current pathological fracture, unspecified hand

✛ 🔞 **M80.85** Other osteoporosis with current pathological fracture, femur
Other osteoporosis with current pathological fracture of hip

☐ **SP** ✛ 🔟 **M80.851-** Other osteoporosis with current pathological fracture, right femur

☐ **SP** ✛ 🔟 **M80.852-** Other osteoporosis with current pathological fracture, left femur

☐ **IQ** ✛ 🔟 **M80.859-** Other osteoporosis with current pathological fracture, unspecified femur

✛ 🔞 **M80.86** Other osteoporosis with current pathological fracture, lower leg

☐ **SP** ✛ 🔟 **M80.861-** Other osteoporosis with current pathological fracture, right lower leg

☐ **SP** ✛ 🔟 **M80.862-** Other osteoporosis with current pathological fracture, left lower leg

☐ **IQ** ✛ 🔟 **M80.869-** Other osteoporosis with current pathological fracture, unspecified lower leg

✛ 🔞 **M80.87** Other osteoporosis with current pathological fracture, ankle and foot

☐ **SP** ✛ 🔟 **M80.871-** Other osteoporosis with current pathological fracture, right ankle and foot

☐ **SP** ✛ 🔟 **M80.872-** Other osteoporosis with current pathological fracture, left ankle and foot

☐ **IQ** ✛ 🔟 **M80.879-** Other osteoporosis with current pathological fracture, unspecified ankle and foot

SP ✛ 🔽 **M80.88X-** Other osteoporosis with current pathological fracture, vertebra(e)

✛ 🔠 **M81** Osteoporosis without current pathological fracture
Use additional code to identify:
major osseous defect, if applicable (M89.7-)
personal history of (healed) osteoporosis fracture, if applicable (Z87.310)

EXCLUDES 1 osteoporosis with current pathological fracture (M80.-)
Sudeck's atrophy (M89.0)

GUIDELINES Section I.C.13.a.1)
For certain conditions, the bone may be affected at the upper or lower end, (e.g., avascular necrosis of bone, M87, Osteoporosis, M80, M81). Though the portion of the bone affected may be at the joint, the site designation will be the bone, not the joint.

GUIDELINES Section I.C.13.d.1)
Category M81, Osteoporosis without current pathological fracture, is for use for patients with osteoporosis who do not currently have a pathologic fracture due to the osteoporosis, even if they have had a fracture in the past. For patients with a history of osteoporosis fractures, status code Z87.310, Personal history of (healed) osteoporosis fracture, should follow the code from M81.

CODING TIPS ✓ M81 is coded for patients with osteoporosis with no current fracture. Osteoporosis is not site-specific since it's considered a systemic condition.

SP ✛ **M81.0** Age-related osteoporosis without current pathological fracture
Involutional osteoporosis without current pathological fracture
Osteoporosis NOS
Postmenopausal osteoporosis without current pathological fracture
Senile osteoporosis without current pathological fracture

SP ✛ **M81.6** Localized osteoporosis [Lequesne]
EXCLUDES 1 Sudeck's atrophy (M89.0)

SP ✛ **M81.8** Other osteoporosis without current pathological fracture
Drug-induced osteoporosis without current pathological fracture
Idiopathic osteoporosis without current pathological fracture
Osteoporosis of disuse without current pathological fracture
Postoophorectomy osteoporosis without current pathological fracture
Postsurgical malabsorption osteoporosis without current pathological fracture
Post-traumatic osteoporosis without current pathological fracture
Use additional code for adverse effect, if applicable, to identify drug (T36-T50 with fifth or sixth character 5)

🔠 **M83** Adult osteomalacia
EXCLUDES 1 infantile and juvenile osteomalacia (E55.0)
renal osteodystrophy (N25.0)
rickets (active) (E55.0)
rickets (active) sequelae (E64.3)
vitamin D-resistant osteomalacia (E83.3)
vitamin D-resistant rickets (active) (E83.3)

DEFINITION Deficient levels of calcium in the bone, resulting in bone softening.

SP **M83.0** Puerperal osteomalacia

SP **M83.1** Senile osteomalacia

★ New ▲ Revised **Px** Primary **SP** PDGM Px **SL** Low CoM **SH** High CoM **IQ** Quest. Encounter **H** Hospice non-cancer Dx Unspecified **M** *Manifestation*

DecisionHealth's FY 2020 Complete Home Health ICD-10-CM Diagnosis Coding Manual

1239

Chapter 13

M00-M99

SP **M83.2** **Adult osteomalacia due to malabsorption**
Postsurgical malabsorption osteomalacia in adults

SP **M83.3** **Adult osteomalacia due to malnutrition**

SP **M83.4** **Aluminum bone disease**

SP **+** **M83.5** **Other drug-induced osteomalacia in adults**
Use additional code for adverse effect, if applicable, to identify drug (T36-T50 with fifth or sixth character 5)

SP **M83.8** **Other adult osteomalacia**

SP **M83.9** Adult osteomalacia, unspecified

4 **M84** **Disorder of continuity of bone**

EXCLUDES 2   traumatic fracture of bone-see fracture, by site

GUIDELINES   Section I.C.13.c
Coding of Pathologic Fractures: 7th character D is to be used for encounters after the patient has completed active treatment for the fracture and is receiving routine care for the fracture during the healing or recovery phase. The other 7th characters, listed under each subcategory in the Tabular List, are to be used for subsequent encounters for treatment of problems associated with the healing, such as malunions, nonunions, and sequelae.
Care for complications of surgical treatment for fracture repairs during the healing or recovery phase should be coded with the appropriate complication codes.

+ **5** **M84.3** **Stress fracture**
Fatigue fracture
March fracture
Stress fracture NOS
Stress reaction
Use additional external cause code(s) to identify the cause of the stress fracture

EXCLUDES 1   pathological fracture NOS (M84.4.-)
pathological fracture due to osteoporosis (M80.-)
traumatic fracture (S12.-, S22.-, S32.-, S42.-, S52.-, S62.-, S72.-, S82.-, S92.-)

EXCLUDES 2   personal history of (healed) stress (fatigue) fracture (Z87.312)
stress fracture of vertebra (M48.4-)

The appropriate 7th character is to be added to each code from subcategory M84.3:
A   initial encounter for fracture
D   subsequent encounter for fracture with routine healing
G   subsequent encounter for fracture with delayed healing
K   subsequent encounter for fracture with nonunion
P   subsequent encounter for fracture with malunion
S   sequela

CODING TIPS ✓   Fractures repaired by joint replacements are NOT coded with Z47.1. Fractures repaired by any other orthopedic surgery are NOT coded with Z47.89. Z codes are not appropriate for fractures of any kind. Code the fracture with 7th character D for fractures undergoing surgical repair.

CODING TIPS ✓   Stress fractures are coded with M84.3. History of healed stress fracture is coded to Z87.312.

DEFINITION   Small, hairline crack(s) in the surface of a bone due to overuse or activity that applies a repetitive force to a particular area, most commonly occurring in the lower legs and feet.

IQ **+** **7** **M84.30X-**   Stress fracture, unspecified site

+ **6** **M84.31** **Stress fracture, shoulder**

SP **+** **7** **M84.311-** **Stress fracture, right shoulder**

SP **+** **7** **M84.312-** **Stress fracture, left shoulder**

IQ **+** **7** **M84.319-**   Stress fracture, unspecified shoulder

+ **6** **M84.32** **Stress fracture, humerus**

SP **+** **7** **M84.321-** **Stress fracture, right humerus**

SP **+** **7** **M84.322-** **Stress fracture, left humerus**

IQ **+** **7** **M84.329-**   Stress fracture, unspecified humerus

+ **6** **M84.33** **Stress fracture, ulna and radius**

SP **+** **7** **M84.331-** **Stress fracture, right ulna**

SP **+** **7** **M84.332-** **Stress fracture, left ulna**

SP **+** **7** **M84.333-** **Stress fracture, right radius**

SP **+** **7** **M84.334-** **Stress fracture, left radius**

IQ **+** **7** **M84.339-**   Stress fracture, unspecified ulna and radius

+ **6** **M84.34** **Stress fracture, hand and fingers**

SP **+** **7** **M84.341-** **Stress fracture, right hand**

SP **+** **7** **M84.342-** **Stress fracture, left hand**

IQ **+** **7** **M84.343-**   Stress fracture, unspecified hand

SP **+** **7** **M84.344-** **Stress fracture, right finger(s)**

SP **+** **7** **M84.345-** **Stress fracture, left finger(s)**

IQ **+** **7** **M84.346-**   Stress fracture, unspecified finger(s)

+ **6** **M84.35** **Stress fracture, pelvis and femur**
Stress fracture, hip

SP **+** **7** **M84.350-** **Stress fracture, pelvis**

SP **+** **7** **M84.351-** **Stress fracture, right femur**

SP **+** **7** **M84.352-** **Stress fracture, left femur**

IQ **+** **7** **M84.353-**   Stress fracture, unspecified femur

IQ **+** **7** **M84.359-**   Stress fracture, hip, unspecified

+ **6** **M84.36** **Stress fracture, tibia and fibula**

SP **+** **7** **M84.361-** **Stress fracture, right tibia**

SP **+** **7** **M84.362-** **Stress fracture, left tibia**

SP **+** **7** **M84.363-** **Stress fracture, right fibula**

SP **+** **7** **M84.364-** **Stress fracture, left fibula**

IQ **+** **7** **M84.369-**   Stress fracture, unspecified tibia and fibula

+ **6** **M84.37** **Stress fracture, ankle, foot and toes**

---

4 4th digit required   **5** 5th digit required   **6** 6th digit required   **7** 7th digit required   **7** 7th digit placeholder   **+** Additional code   **⊟** Laterality

⊟ SP ✚ 7 M84.371- Stress fracture, right ankle

⊟ SP ✚ 7 M84.372- Stress fracture, left ankle

⊟ IQ ✚ 7 M84.373- **Stress fracture, unspecified ankle**

⊟ SP ✚ 7 M84.374- Stress fracture, right foot

⊟ SP ✚ 7 M84.375- Stress fracture, left foot

⊟ IQ ✚ 7 M84.376- **Stress fracture, unspecified foot**

⊟ SP ✚ 7 M84.377- Stress fracture, right toe(s)

⊟ SP ✚ 7 M84.378- Stress fracture, left toe(s)

⊟ IQ ✚ 7 M84.379- **Stress fracture, unspecified toe(s)**

SP ✚ 7 M84.38X- Stress fracture, other site

> EXCLUDES 2   stress fracture of vertebra (M48.4-)

5 **M84.4 Pathological fracture, not elsewhere classified**
Chronic fracture
Pathological fracture NOS

> EXCLUDES 1   collapsed vertebra NEC (M48.5)
> pathological fracture in neoplastic disease (M84.5-)
> pathological fracture in osteoporosis (M80.-)
> pathological fracture in other disease (M84.6-)
> stress fracture (M84.3-)
> traumatic fracture (S12.-, S22.-, S32.-, S42.-, S52.-, S62.-, S72.-, S82.-, S92.-)

> EXCLUDES 2   personal history of (healed) pathological fracture (Z87.311)

The appropriate 7th character is to be added to each code from subcategory M84.4:

A   initial encounter for fracture
D   subsequent encounter for fracture with routine healing
G   subsequent encounter for fracture with delayed healing
K   subsequent encounter for fracture with nonunion
P   subsequent encounter for fracture with malunion
S   sequela

CODING TIPS ✓   Fractures repaired by joint replacements are NOT coded with Z47.1. Fractures repaired by any other orthopedic surgery are NOT coded with Z47.89. Z codes are not appropriate for fractures of any kind. Code the fracture with 7th character D for fractures undergoing surgical repair.

CODING TIPS ✓   Spontaneous fractures occur without external blunt trauma and are almost always considered pathologic. Compression fractures are considered pathologic fractures. If the patient falls and has a compression fracture or unusual fracture, ask the physician whether it is considered trauma or pathologic. Pathologic fractures due to osteoporosis (M80) and due to neoplasm (M84.5) are not coded here. Pathologic fractures may be coded with 7th character D or S. Aftercare codes are not used in ICD-10 for fractures.

CODING TIPS ✓   Watch out for laterality. Do not choose unspecified. Use Z87.311 for history of healed pathological fracture. Collapsed vertebra or compression fracture of the vertebra is coded to M48.5 when no other cause is identified.

DEFINITION   A break resulting from widespread lesions or disease process that destroys normal bone mass, causing the weakened bone to break spontaneously without obvious external force.

IQ 7 M84.40X- **Pathological fracture, unspecified site**

6 **M84.41 Pathological fracture, shoulder**

⊟ SP 7 M84.411- Pathological fracture, right shoulder

⊟ SP 7 M84.412- Pathological fracture, left shoulder

⊟ IQ 7 M84.419- **Pathological fracture, unspecified shoulder**

6 **M84.42 Pathological fracture, humerus**

⊟ SP 7 M84.421- Pathological fracture, right humerus

⊟ SP 7 M84.422- Pathological fracture, left humerus

⊟ IQ 7 M84.429- **Pathological fracture, unspecified humerus**

6 **M84.43 Pathological fracture, ulna and radius**

⊟ SP 7 M84.431- Pathological fracture, right ulna

⊟ SP 7 M84.432- Pathological fracture, left ulna

⊟ SP 7 M84.433- Pathological fracture, right radius

⊟ SP 7 M84.434- Pathological fracture, left radius

⊟ IQ 7 M84.439- **Pathological fracture, unspecified ulna and radius**

6 **M84.44 Pathological fracture, hand and fingers**

⊟ SP 7 M84.441- Pathological fracture, right hand

⊟ SP 7 M84.442- Pathological fracture, left hand

⊟ IQ 7 M84.443- **Pathological fracture, unspecified hand**

⊟ SP 7 M84.444- Pathological fracture, right finger(s)

⊟ SP 7 M84.445- Pathological fracture, left finger(s)

⊟ IQ 7 M84.446- **Pathological fracture, unspecified finger(s)**

6 **M84.45 Pathological fracture, femur and pelvis**

★ New ▲ Revised Px Primary   SP PDGM Px   SL Low CoM   SH High CoM   IQ Quest. Encounter   H Hospice non-cancer Dx   Unspecified   M *Manifestation*

DecisionHealth's FY 2020 Complete Home Health ICD-10-CM Diagnosis Coding Manual   1241

☐ **SP** **7** **M84.451-** Pathological fracture, right femur

☐ **SP** **7** **M84.452-** Pathological fracture, left femur

☐ **IQ** **7** **M84.453-** Pathological fracture, unspecified femur

☐ **SP** **7** **M84.454-** Pathological fracture, pelvis

☐ **IQ** **7** **M84.459-** Pathological fracture, hip, unspecified

　6 **M84.46** Pathological fracture, tibia and fibula

☐ **SP** **7** **M84.461-** Pathological fracture, right tibia

☐ **SP** **7** **M84.462-** Pathological fracture, left tibia

☐ **SP** **7** **M84.463-** Pathological fracture, right fibula

☐ **SP** **7** **M84.464-** Pathological fracture, left fibula

☐ **IQ** **7** **M84.469-** Pathological fracture, unspecified tibia and fibula

　6 **M84.47** Pathological fracture, ankle, foot and toes

☐ **SP** **7** **M84.471-** Pathological fracture, right ankle

☐ **SP** **7** **M84.472-** Pathological fracture, left ankle

☐ **IQ** **7** **M84.473-** Pathological fracture, unspecified ankle

☐ **SP** **7** **M84.474-** Pathological fracture, right foot

☐ **SP** **7** **M84.475-** Pathological fracture, left foot

☐ **IQ** **7** **M84.476-** Pathological fracture, unspecified foot

☐ **SP** **7** **M84.477-** Pathological fracture, right toe(s)

☐ **SP** **7** **M84.478-** Pathological fracture, left toe(s)

☐ **IQ** **7** **M84.479-** Pathological fracture, unspecified toe(s)

SP **7** **M84.48X-** Pathological fracture, other site

　5 **M84.5** Pathological fracture in neoplastic disease
　Code also:
　　underlying neoplasm

The appropriate 7th character is to be added to each code from subcategory M84.5:

A	initial encounter for fracture
D	subsequent encounter for fracture with routine healing
G	subsequent encounter for fracture with delayed healing
K	subsequent encounter for fracture with nonunion
P	subsequent encounter for fracture with malunion
S	sequela

GUIDELINES　Section I.C.2.I.6)
When an encounter is for a pathological fracture due to a neoplasm, and the focus of treatment is the fracture, a code from subcategory M84.5, Pathological fracture in neoplastic disease, should be sequenced first, followed by the code for the neoplasm. If the focus of treatment is the neoplasm with an associated pathological fracture, the neoplasm code should be sequenced first, followed by a code from M84.5 for the pathological fracture.

CODING TIPS ✓　Fractures repaired by joint replacements are NOT coded with Z47.1. Fractures repaired by any other orthopedic surgery are NOT coded with Z47.89. Z codes are not appropriate for fractures of any kind. Code the fracture with 7th character D for fractures undergoing surgical repair.

CODING TIPS ✓　M84.5 indicates pathological fractures related to a neoplasm, most likely a primary or secondary neoplasm to the bone. The neoplasm is also coded and sequenced depending on the focus of care.

DEFINITION　A break resulting from metastatic invasion or tumor growth that destroys normal bone mass, resulting in fracture without obvious trauma to the bone.

IQ **7** **M84.50X-** Pathological fracture in neoplastic disease, unspecified site

　6 **M84.51** Pathological fracture in neoplastic disease, shoulder

☐ **SP** **7** **M84.511-** Pathological fracture in neoplastic disease, right shoulder

☐ **SP** **7** **M84.512-** Pathological fracture in neoplastic disease, left shoulder

☐ **IQ** **7** **M84.519-** Pathological fracture in neoplastic disease, unspecified shoulder

　6 **M84.52** Pathological fracture in neoplastic disease, humerus

☐ **SP** **7** **M84.521-** Pathological fracture in neoplastic disease, right humerus

☐ **SP** **7** **M84.522-** Pathological fracture in neoplastic disease, left humerus

☐ **IQ** **7** **M84.529-** Pathological fracture in neoplastic disease, unspecified humerus

　6 **M84.53** Pathological fracture in neoplastic disease, ulna and radius

☐ **SP** **7** **M84.531-** Pathological fracture in neoplastic disease, right ulna

☐ **SP** **7** **M84.532-** Pathological fracture in neoplastic disease, left ulna

☐ **SP** **7** **M84.533-** Pathological fracture in neoplastic disease, right radius

☐ **SP** **7** **M84.534-** Pathological fracture in neoplastic disease, left radius

☐ **IQ** **7** **M84.539-** Pathological fracture in neoplastic disease, unspecified ulna and radius

　6 **M84.54** Pathological fracture in neoplastic disease, hand

☐ **SP** **7** **M84.541-** Pathological fracture in neoplastic disease, right hand

☐ **SP** **7** **M84.542-** Pathological fracture in neoplastic disease, left hand

☐ **IQ** **7** **M84.549-** Pathological fracture in neoplastic disease, unspecified hand

　6 **M84.55** Pathological fracture in neoplastic disease, pelvis and femur

☐ **SP** **7** **M84.550-** Pathological fracture in neoplastic disease, pelvis

☐ **SP** **7** **M84.551-** Pathological fracture in neoplastic disease, right femur

---

4 4th digit required　　**5** 5th digit required　　**6** 6th digit required　　**7** 7th digit required　　**7** 7th digit placeholder　　**+** Additional code　　☐ Laterality

1242　　　　*DecisionHealth's* FY 2020 Complete Home Health ICD-10-CM Diagnosis Coding Manual

⊟ **SP** **7** **M84.552-** Pathological fracture in neoplastic disease, left femur

⊟ **IQ** **7** **M84.553-** Pathological fracture in neoplastic disease, unspecified femur

⊟ **IQ** **7** **M84.559-** Pathological fracture in neoplastic disease, hip, unspecified

6 **M84.56** Pathological fracture in neoplastic disease, tibia and fibula

⊟ **SP** **7** **M84.561-** Pathological fracture in neoplastic disease, right tibia

⊟ **SP** **7** **M84.562-** Pathological fracture in neoplastic disease, left tibia

⊟ **SP** **7** **M84.563-** Pathological fracture in neoplastic disease, right fibula

⊟ **SP** **7** **M84.564-** Pathological fracture in neoplastic disease, left fibula

⊟ **IQ** **7** **M84.569-** Pathological fracture in neoplastic disease, unspecified tibia and fibula

6 **M84.57** Pathological fracture in neoplastic disease, ankle and foot

⊟ **SP** **7** **M84.571-** Pathological fracture in neoplastic disease, right ankle

⊟ **SP** **7** **M84.572-** Pathological fracture in neoplastic disease, left ankle

⊟ **IQ** **7** **M84.573-** Pathological fracture in neoplastic disease, unspecified ankle

⊟ **SP** **7** **M84.574-** Pathological fracture in neoplastic disease, right foot

⊟ **SP** **7** **M84.575-** Pathological fracture in neoplastic disease, left foot

⊟ **IQ** **7** **M84.576-** Pathological fracture in neoplastic disease, unspecified foot

SP **7** **M84.58X-** Pathological fracture in neoplastic disease, other specified site
Pathological fracture in neoplastic disease, vertebrae

5 **M84.6** Pathological fracture in other disease
Code also:
underlying condition
EXCLUDES 1 pathological fracture in osteoporosis (M80.-)

The appropriate 7th character is to be added to each code from subcategory M84.6:
A	initial encounter for fracture
D	subsequent encounter for fracture with routine healing
G	subsequent encounter for fracture with delayed healing
K	subsequent encounter for fracture with nonunion
P	subsequent encounter for fracture with malunion
S	sequela

CODING TIPS ✓ Fractures repaired by joint replacements are NOT coded with Z47.1. Fractures repaired by any other orthopedic surgery are NOT coded with Z47.89. Z codes are not appropriate for fractures of any kind. Code the fracture with 7th character D for fractures undergoing surgical repair.

IQ **7** **M84.60X-** Pathological fracture in other disease, unspecified site

6 **M84.61** Pathological fracture in other disease, shoulder

⊟ **SP** **7** **M84.611-** Pathological fracture in other disease, right shoulder

⊟ **SP** **7** **M84.612-** Pathological fracture in other disease, left shoulder

⊟ **IQ** **7** **M84.619-** Pathological fracture in other disease, unspecified shoulder

6 **M84.62** Pathological fracture in other disease, humerus

⊟ **SP** **7** **M84.621-** Pathological fracture in other disease, right humerus

⊟ **SP** **7** **M84.622-** Pathological fracture in other disease, left humerus

⊟ **IQ** **7** **M84.629-** Pathological fracture in other disease, unspecified humerus

6 **M84.63** Pathological fracture in other disease, ulna and radius

⊟ **SP** **7** **M84.631-** Pathological fracture in other disease, right ulna

⊟ **SP** **7** **M84.632-** Pathological fracture in other disease, left ulna

⊟ **SP** **7** **M84.633-** Pathological fracture in other disease, right radius

⊟ **SP** **7** **M84.634-** Pathological fracture in other disease, left radius

⊟ **IQ** **7** **M84.639-** Pathological fracture in other disease, unspecified ulna and radius

6 **M84.64** Pathological fracture in other disease, hand

⊟ **SP** **7** **M84.641-** Pathological fracture in other disease, right hand

⊟ **SP** **7** **M84.642-** Pathological fracture in other disease, left hand

⊟ **IQ** **7** **M84.649-** Pathological fracture in other disease, unspecified hand

6 **M84.65** Pathological fracture in other disease, pelvis and femur

⊟ **SP** **7** **M84.650-** Pathological fracture in other disease, pelvis

⊟ **SP** **7** **M84.651-** Pathological fracture in other disease, right femur

⊟ **SP** **7** **M84.652-** Pathological fracture in other disease, left femur

⊟ **IQ** **7** **M84.653-** Pathological fracture in other disease, unspecified femur

⊟ **IQ** **7** **M84.659-** Pathological fracture in other disease, hip, unspecified

6 **M84.66** Pathological fracture in other disease, tibia and fibula

⊟ **SP** **7** **M84.661-** Pathological fracture in other disease, right tibia

⊟ **SP** **7** **M84.662-** Pathological fracture in other disease, left tibia

---

★ New ▲ Revised **Px** Primary **SP** PDGM Px **SL** Low CoM **SH** High CoM **IQ** Quest. Encounter **H** Hospice non-cancer Dx Unspecified **M** *Manifestation*

≡ SP 7 M84.663- Pathological fracture in other disease, right fibula

≡ SP 7 M84.664- Pathological fracture in other disease, left fibula

≡ !Q 7 M84.669- Pathological fracture in other disease, unspecified tibia and fibula

6 M84.67 Pathological fracture in other disease, ankle and foot

≡ SP 7 M84.671- Pathological fracture in other disease, right ankle

≡ SP 7 M84.672- Pathological fracture in other disease, left ankle

≡ !Q 7 M84.673- Pathological fracture in other disease, unspecified ankle

≡ SP 7 M84.674- Pathological fracture in other disease, right foot

≡ SP 7 M84.675- Pathological fracture in other disease, left foot

≡ !Q 7 M84.676- Pathological fracture in other disease, unspecified foot

SP 7 M84.68X- Pathological fracture in other disease, other site

5 M84.7 Nontraumatic fracture, not elsewhere classified

> **CODING TIPS ✓** Fractures repaired by joint replacements are NOT coded with Z47.1. Fractures repaired by any other orthopedic surgery are NOT coded with Z47.89. Z codes are not appropriate for fractures of any kind. Code the fracture with 7th character D for fractures undergoing surgical repair.

6 M84.75 Atypical femoral fracture

> The appropriate 7th character is to be added to each code from M84.75:
> | | |
> |---|---|
> | A | initial encounter for fracture |
> | D | subsequent encounter for fracture with routine healing |
> | G | subsequent encounter for fracture with delayed healing |
> | K | subsequent encounter for fracture with nonunion |
> | P | subsequent encounter for fracture with malunion |
> | S | sequela |

!Q 7 M84.750- Atypical femoral fracture, unspecified

≡ SP 7 M84.751- Incomplete atypical femoral fracture, right leg

≡ SP 7 M84.752- Incomplete atypical femoral fracture, left leg

≡ !Q 7 M84.753- Incomplete atypical femoral fracture, unspecified leg

≡ SP 7 M84.754- Complete transverse atypical femoral fracture, right leg

≡ SP 7 M84.755- Complete transverse atypical femoral fracture, left leg

≡ !Q 7 M84.756- Complete transverse atypical femoral fracture, unspecified leg

≡ SP 7 M84.757- Complete oblique atypical femoral fracture, right leg

≡ SP 7 M84.758- Complete oblique atypical femoral fracture, left leg

≡ !Q 7 M84.759- Complete oblique atypical femoral fracture, unspecified leg

5 M84.8 Other disorders of continuity of bone

!Q M84.80 Other disorders of continuity of bone, unspecified site

6 M84.81 Other disorders of continuity of bone, shoulder

≡ SP M84.811 Other disorders of continuity of bone, right shoulder

≡ SP M84.812 Other disorders of continuity of bone, left shoulder

≡ !Q M84.819 Other disorders of continuity of bone, unspecified shoulder

6 M84.82 Other disorders of continuity of bone, humerus

≡ SP M84.821 Other disorders of continuity of bone, right humerus

≡ SP M84.822 Other disorders of continuity of bone, left humerus

≡ !Q M84.829 Other disorders of continuity of bone, unspecified humerus

6 M84.83 Other disorders of continuity of bone, ulna and radius

≡ SP M84.831 Other disorders of continuity of bone, right ulna

≡ SP M84.832 Other disorders of continuity of bone, left ulna

≡ SP M84.833 Other disorders of continuity of bone, right radius

≡ SP M84.834 Other disorders of continuity of bone, left radius

≡ !Q M84.839 Other disorders of continuity of bone, unspecified ulna and radius

6 M84.84 Other disorders of continuity of bone, hand

≡ SP M84.841 Other disorders of continuity of bone, right hand

≡ SP M84.842 Other disorders of continuity of bone, left hand

≡ !Q M84.849 Other disorders of continuity of bone, unspecified hand

6 M84.85 Other disorders of continuity of bone, pelvic region and thigh

≡ SP M84.851 Other disorders of continuity of bone, right pelvic region and thigh

≡ SP M84.852 Other disorders of continuity of bone, left pelvic region and thigh

≡ !Q M84.859 Other disorders of continuity of bone, unspecified pelvic region and thigh

6 M84.86 Other disorders of continuity of bone, tibia and fibula

≡ SP M84.861 Other disorders of continuity of bone, right tibia

≡ SP M84.862 Other disorders of continuity of bone, left tibia

≡ SP M84.863 Other disorders of continuity of bone, right fibula

≡ SP M84.864 Other disorders of continuity of bone, left fibula

≡ !Q M84.869 Other disorders of continuity of bone, unspecified tibia and fibula

6 M84.87 Other disorders of continuity of bone, ankle and foot

≡ SP M84.871 Other disorders of continuity of bone, right ankle and foot

≡ SP M84.872 Other disorders of continuity of bone, left ankle and foot

---

4 4th digit required **5** 5th digit required **6** 6th digit required **7** 7th digit required **7** 7th digit placeholder **+** Additional code **≡** Laterality

☐ **IQ** **M84.879** Other disorders of continuity of bone, unspecified ankle and foot

SP **M84.88** Other disorders of continuity of bone, other site

IQ **M84.9** Disorder of continuity of bone, unspecified

④ **M85** Other disorders of bone density and structure

> **EXCLUDES 1** osteogenesis imperfecta (Q78.0)
> osteopetrosis (Q78.2)
> osteopoikilosis (Q78.8)
> polyostotic fibrous dysplasia (Q78.1)

⑤ **M85.0** Fibrous dysplasia (monostotic)

> **EXCLUDES 2** fibrous dysplasia of jaw (M27.8)

IQ **M85.00** Fibrous dysplasia (monostotic), unspecified site

⑥ **M85.01** Fibrous dysplasia (monostotic), shoulder

☐ **SP** **M85.011** Fibrous dysplasia (monostotic), right shoulder

☐ **SP** **M85.012** Fibrous dysplasia (monostotic), left shoulder

☐ **IQ** **M85.019** Fibrous dysplasia (monostotic), unspecified shoulder

⑥ **M85.02** Fibrous dysplasia (monostotic), upper arm

☐ **SP** **M85.021** Fibrous dysplasia (monostotic), right upper arm

☐ **SP** **M85.022** Fibrous dysplasia (monostotic), left upper arm

☐ **IQ** **M85.029** Fibrous dysplasia (monostotic), unspecified upper arm

⑥ **M85.03** Fibrous dysplasia (monostotic), forearm

☐ **SP** **M85.031** Fibrous dysplasia (monostotic), right forearm

☐ **SP** **M85.032** Fibrous dysplasia (monostotic), left forearm

☐ **IQ** **M85.039** Fibrous dysplasia (monostotic), unspecified forearm

⑥ **M85.04** Fibrous dysplasia (monostotic), hand

☐ **SP** **M85.041** Fibrous dysplasia (monostotic), right hand

☐ **SP** **M85.042** Fibrous dysplasia (monostotic), left hand

☐ **IQ** **M85.049** Fibrous dysplasia (monostotic), unspecified hand

⑥ **M85.05** Fibrous dysplasia (monostotic), thigh

☐ **SP** **M85.051** Fibrous dysplasia (monostotic), right thigh

☐ **SP** **M85.052** Fibrous dysplasia (monostotic), left thigh

☐ **IQ** **M85.059** Fibrous dysplasia (monostotic), unspecified thigh

⑥ **M85.06** Fibrous dysplasia (monostotic), lower leg

☐ **SP** **M85.061** Fibrous dysplasia (monostotic), right lower leg

☐ **SP** **M85.062** Fibrous dysplasia (monostotic), left lower leg

☐ **IQ** **M85.069** Fibrous dysplasia (monostotic), unspecified lower leg

⑥ **M85.07** Fibrous dysplasia (monostotic), ankle and foot

☐ **SP** **M85.071** Fibrous dysplasia (monostotic), right ankle and foot

☐ **SP** **M85.072** Fibrous dysplasia (monostotic), left ankle and foot

☐ **IQ** **M85.079** Fibrous dysplasia (monostotic), unspecified ankle and foot

SP **M85.08** Fibrous dysplasia (monostotic), other site

SP **M85.09** Fibrous dysplasia (monostotic), multiple sites

⑤ **M85.1** Skeletal fluorosis

IQ **M85.10** Skeletal fluorosis, unspecified site

⑥ **M85.11** Skeletal fluorosis, shoulder

☐ **SP** **M85.111** Skeletal fluorosis, right shoulder

☐ **SP** **M85.112** Skeletal fluorosis, left shoulder

☐ **IQ** **M85.119** Skeletal fluorosis, unspecified shoulder

⑥ **M85.12** Skeletal fluorosis, upper arm

☐ **SP** **M85.121** Skeletal fluorosis, right upper arm

☐ **SP** **M85.122** Skeletal fluorosis, left upper arm

☐ **IQ** **M85.129** Skeletal fluorosis, unspecified upper arm

⑥ **M85.13** Skeletal fluorosis, forearm

☐ **SP** **M85.131** Skeletal fluorosis, right forearm

☐ **SP** **M85.132** Skeletal fluorosis, left forearm

☐ **IQ** **M85.139** Skeletal fluorosis, unspecified forearm

⑥ **M85.14** Skeletal fluorosis, hand

☐ **SP** **M85.141** Skeletal fluorosis, right hand

☐ **SP** **M85.142** Skeletal fluorosis, left hand

☐ **IQ** **M85.149** Skeletal fluorosis, unspecified hand

⑥ **M85.15** Skeletal fluorosis, thigh

☐ **SP** **M85.151** Skeletal fluorosis, right thigh

☐ **SP** **M85.152** Skeletal fluorosis, left thigh

☐ **IQ** **M85.159** Skeletal fluorosis, unspecified thigh

⑥ **M85.16** Skeletal fluorosis, lower leg

☐ **SP** **M85.161** Skeletal fluorosis, right lower leg

☐ **SP** **M85.162** Skeletal fluorosis, left lower leg

☐ **IQ** **M85.169** Skeletal fluorosis, unspecified lower leg

⑥ **M85.17** Skeletal fluorosis, ankle and foot

☐ **SP** **M85.171** Skeletal fluorosis, right ankle and foot

☐ **SP** **M85.172** Skeletal fluorosis, left ankle and foot

☐ **IQ** **M85.179** Skeletal fluorosis, unspecified ankle and foot

SP **M85.18** Skeletal fluorosis, other site

SP **M85.19** Skeletal fluorosis, multiple sites

IQ **M85.2** Hyperostosis of skull

⑤ **M85.3** Osteitis condensans

IQ **M85.30** Osteitis condensans, unspecified site

⑥ **M85.31** Osteitis condensans, shoulder

☐ **SP** **M85.311** Osteitis condensans, right shoulder

☐ **SP** **M85.312** Osteitis condensans, left shoulder

★ New ▲ Revised **Px** Primary **SP** PDGM Px **SL** Low CoM **SH** High CoM **IQ** Quest. Encounter ⊞ Hospice non-cancer Dx │ Unspecified │ **M** *Manifestation*

⊟ **IQ** **M85.319** Osteitis condensans, unspecified shoulder

⑥ **M85.32** Osteitis condensans, upper arm

⊟ **SP** **M85.321** Osteitis condensans, right upper arm

⊟ **SP** **M85.322** Osteitis condensans, left upper arm

⊟ **IQ** **M85.329** Osteitis condensans, unspecified upper arm

⑥ **M85.33** Osteitis condensans, forearm

⊟ **SP** **M85.331** Osteitis condensans, right forearm

⊟ **SP** **M85.332** Osteitis condensans, left forearm

⊟ **IQ** **M85.339** Osteitis condensans, unspecified forearm

⑥ **M85.34** Osteitis condensans, hand

⊟ **SP** **M85.341** Osteitis condensans, right hand

⊟ **SP** **M85.342** Osteitis condensans, left hand

⊟ **IQ** **M85.349** Osteitis condensans, unspecified hand

⑥ **M85.35** Osteitis condensans, thigh

⊟ **SP** **M85.351** Osteitis condensans, right thigh

⊟ **SP** **M85.352** Osteitis condensans, left thigh

⊟ **IQ** **M85.359** Osteitis condensans, unspecified thigh

⑥ **M85.36** Osteitis condensans, lower leg

⊟ **SP** **M85.361** Osteitis condensans, right lower leg

⊟ **SP** **M85.362** Osteitis condensans, left lower leg

⊟ **IQ** **M85.369** Osteitis condensans, unspecified lower leg

⑥ **M85.37** Osteitis condensans, ankle and foot

⊟ **SP** **M85.371** Osteitis condensans, right ankle and foot

⊟ **SP** **M85.372** Osteitis condensans, left ankle and foot

⊟ **IQ** **M85.379** Osteitis condensans, unspecified ankle and foot

SP **M85.38** Osteitis condensans, other site

SP **M85.39** Osteitis condensans, multiple sites

⑤ **M85.4** Solitary bone cyst

    EXCLUDES 2   solitary cyst of jaw (M27.4)

IQ **M85.40** Solitary bone cyst, unspecified site

⑥ **M85.41** Solitary bone cyst, shoulder

⊟ **SP** **M85.411** Solitary bone cyst, right shoulder

⊟ **SP** **M85.412** Solitary bone cyst, left shoulder

⊟ **IQ** **M85.419** Solitary bone cyst, unspecified shoulder

⑥ **M85.42** Solitary bone cyst, humerus

⊟ **SP** **M85.421** Solitary bone cyst, right humerus

⊟ **SP** **M85.422** Solitary bone cyst, left humerus

⊟ **IQ** **M85.429** Solitary bone cyst, unspecified humerus

⑥ **M85.43** Solitary bone cyst, ulna and radius

⊟ **SP** **M85.431** Solitary bone cyst, right ulna and radius

⊟ **SP** **M85.432** Solitary bone cyst, left ulna and radius

⊟ **IQ** **M85.439** Solitary bone cyst, unspecified ulna and radius

⑥ **M85.44** Solitary bone cyst, hand

⊟ **SP** **M85.441** Solitary bone cyst, right hand

⊟ **SP** **M85.442** Solitary bone cyst, left hand

⊟ **IQ** **M85.449** Solitary bone cyst, unspecified hand

⑥ **M85.45** Solitary bone cyst, pelvis

⊟ **SP** **M85.451** Solitary bone cyst, right pelvis

⊟ **SP** **M85.452** Solitary bone cyst, left pelvis

⊟ **IQ** **M85.459** Solitary bone cyst, unspecified pelvis

⑥ **M85.46** Solitary bone cyst, tibia and fibula

⊟ **SP** **M85.461** Solitary bone cyst, right tibia and fibula

⊟ **SP** **M85.462** Solitary bone cyst, left tibia and fibula

⊟ **IQ** **M85.469** Solitary bone cyst, unspecified tibia and fibula

⑥ **M85.47** Solitary bone cyst, ankle and foot

⊟ **SP** **M85.471** Solitary bone cyst, right ankle and foot

⊟ **SP** **M85.472** Solitary bone cyst, left ankle and foot

⊟ **IQ** **M85.479** Solitary bone cyst, unspecified ankle and foot

SP **M85.48** Solitary bone cyst, other site

⑤ **M85.5** Aneurysmal bone cyst

    EXCLUDES 2   aneurysmal cyst of jaw (M27.4)

IQ **M85.50** Aneurysmal bone cyst, unspecified site

⑥ **M85.51** Aneurysmal bone cyst, shoulder

⊟ **SP** **M85.511** Aneurysmal bone cyst, right shoulder

⊟ **SP** **M85.512** Aneurysmal bone cyst, left shoulder

⊟ **IQ** **M85.519** Aneurysmal bone cyst, unspecified shoulder

⑥ **M85.52** Aneurysmal bone cyst, upper arm

⊟ **SP** **M85.521** Aneurysmal bone cyst, right upper arm

⊟ **SP** **M85.522** Aneurysmal bone cyst, left upper arm

⊟ **IQ** **M85.529** Aneurysmal bone cyst, unspecified upper arm

⑥ **M85.53** Aneurysmal bone cyst, forearm

⊟ **SP** **M85.531** Aneurysmal bone cyst, right forearm

⊟ **SP** **M85.532** Aneurysmal bone cyst, left forearm

⊟ **IQ** **M85.539** Aneurysmal bone cyst, unspecified forearm

⑥ **M85.54** Aneurysmal bone cyst, hand

⊟ **SP** **M85.541** Aneurysmal bone cyst, right hand

⊟ **SP** **M85.542** Aneurysmal bone cyst, left hand

⊟ **IQ** **M85.549** Aneurysmal bone cyst, unspecified hand

⑥ **M85.55** Aneurysmal bone cyst, thigh

⊟ **SP** **M85.551** Aneurysmal bone cyst, right thigh

⊟ **SP** **M85.552** Aneurysmal bone cyst, left thigh

⊟ **IQ** **M85.559** Aneurysmal bone cyst, unspecified thigh

⑥ **M85.56** Aneurysmal bone cyst, lower leg

---

④ 4th digit required   ⑤ 5th digit required   ⑥ 6th digit required   ⑦ 7th digit required   ⑦ 7th digit placeholder   ✚ Additional code   ⊟ Laterality

1246   *DecisionHealth's* FY 2020 Complete Home Health ICD-10-CM Diagnosis Coding Manual

☰ **SP** **M85.561** Aneurysmal bone cyst, right lower leg

☰ **SP** **M85.562** Aneurysmal bone cyst, left lower leg

☰ **IQ** **M85.569** Aneurysmal bone cyst, unspecified lower leg

⑥ **M85.57** Aneurysmal bone cyst, ankle and foot

☰ **SP** **M85.571** Aneurysmal bone cyst, right ankle and foot

☰ **SP** **M85.572** Aneurysmal bone cyst, left ankle and foot

☰ **IQ** **M85.579** Aneurysmal bone cyst, unspecified ankle and foot

SP **M85.58** Aneurysmal bone cyst, other site

SP **M85.59** Aneurysmal bone cyst, multiple sites

⑤ **M85.6** Other cyst of bone

> **EXCLUDES 1** cyst of jaw NEC (M27.4)
> osteitis fibrosa cystica
> generalisata [von
> Recklinghausen's disease
> of bone] (E21.0)

IQ **M85.60** Other cyst of bone, unspecified site

⑥ **M85.61** Other cyst of bone, shoulder

☰ **SP** **M85.611** Other cyst of bone, right shoulder

☰ **SP** **M85.612** Other cyst of bone, left shoulder

☰ **IQ** **M85.619** Other cyst of bone, unspecified shoulder

⑥ **M85.62** Other cyst of bone, upper arm

☰ **SP** **M85.621** Other cyst of bone, right upper arm

☰ **SP** **M85.622** Other cyst of bone, left upper arm

☰ **IQ** **M85.629** Other cyst of bone, unspecified upper arm

⑥ **M85.63** Other cyst of bone, forearm

☰ **SP** **M85.631** Other cyst of bone, right forearm

☰ **SP** **M85.632** Other cyst of bone, left forearm

☰ **IQ** **M85.639** Other cyst of bone, unspecified forearm

⑥ **M85.64** Other cyst of bone, hand

☰ **SP** **M85.641** Other cyst of bone, right hand

☰ **SP** **M85.642** Other cyst of bone, left hand

☰ **IQ** **M85.649** Other cyst of bone, unspecified hand

⑥ **M85.65** Other cyst of bone, thigh

☰ **SP** **M85.651** Other cyst of bone, right thigh

☰ **SP** **M85.652** Other cyst of bone, left thigh

☰ **IQ** **M85.659** Other cyst of bone, unspecified thigh

⑥ **M85.66** Other cyst of bone, lower leg

☰ **SP** **M85.661** Other cyst of bone, right lower leg

☰ **SP** **M85.662** Other cyst of bone, left lower leg

☰ **IQ** **M85.669** Other cyst of bone, unspecified lower leg

⑥ **M85.67** Other cyst of bone, ankle and foot

☰ **SP** **M85.671** Other cyst of bone, right ankle and foot

☰ **SP** **M85.672** Other cyst of bone, left ankle and foot

☰ **IQ** **M85.679** Other cyst of bone, unspecified ankle and foot

SP **M85.68** Other cyst of bone, other site

SP **M85.69** Other cyst of bone, multiple sites

⑤ **M85.8** Other specified disorders of bone density and structure

> Hyperostosis of bones, except skull
> Osteosclerosis, acquired
>
> **EXCLUDES 1** diffuse idiopathic skeletal
> hyperostosis [DISH]
> (M48.1)
> osteosclerosis congenita
> (Q77.4)
> osteosclerosis fragilitas
> (generalista) (Q78.2)
> osteosclerosis myelofibrosis
> (D75.81)

IQ **M85.80** Other specified disorders of bone density and structure, unspecified site

⑥ **M85.81** Other specified disorders of bone density and structure, shoulder

☰ **SP** **M85.811** Other specified disorders of bone density and structure, right shoulder

☰ **SP** **M85.812** Other specified disorders of bone density and structure, left shoulder

☰ **IQ** **M85.819** Other specified disorders of bone density and structure, unspecified shoulder

⑥ **M85.82** Other specified disorders of bone density and structure, upper arm

☰ **SP** **M85.821** Other specified disorders of bone density and structure, right upper arm

☰ **SP** **M85.822** Other specified disorders of bone density and structure, left upper arm

☰ **IQ** **M85.829** Other specified disorders of bone density and structure, unspecified upper arm

⑥ **M85.83** Other specified disorders of bone density and structure, forearm

☰ **SP** **M85.831** Other specified disorders of bone density and structure, right forearm

☰ **SP** **M85.832** Other specified disorders of bone density and structure, left forearm

☰ **IQ** **M85.839** Other specified disorders of bone density and structure, unspecified forearm

⑥ **M85.84** Other specified disorders of bone density and structure, hand

☰ **SP** **M85.841** Other specified disorders of bone density and structure, right hand

☰ **SP** **M85.842** Other specified disorders of bone density and structure, left hand

☰ **IQ** **M85.849** Other specified disorders of bone density and structure, unspecified hand

⑥ **M85.85** Other specified disorders of bone density and structure, thigh

☰ **SP** **M85.851** Other specified disorders of bone density and structure, right thigh

☰ **SP** **M85.852** Other specified disorders of bone density and structure, left thigh

---

★ New ▲ Revised **Px** Primary **SP** PDGM Px **SL** Low CoM **SH** High CoM **IQ** Quest. Encounter **H** Hospice non-cancer Dx   Unspecified   **M** *Manifestation*

DecisionHealth's FY 2020 Complete Home Health ICD-10-CM Diagnosis Coding Manual

1247

☐ **IQ** **M85.859** Other specified disorders of bone density and structure, unspecified thigh

G **M85.86** Other specified disorders of bone density and structure, lower leg

☐ **SP** **M85.861** Other specified disorders of bone density and structure, right lower leg

☐ **SP** **M85.862** Other specified disorders of bone density and structure, left lower leg

☐ **IQ** **M85.869** Other specified disorders of bone density and structure, unspecified lower leg

G **M85.87** Other specified disorders of bone density and structure, ankle and foot

☐ **SP** **M85.871** Other specified disorders of bone density and structure, right ankle and foot

☐ **SP** **M85.872** Other specified disorders of bone density and structure, left ankle and foot

☐ **IQ** **M85.879** Other specified disorders of bone density and structure, unspecified ankle and foot

SP **M85.88** Other specified disorders of bone density and structure, other site

SP **M85.89** Other specified disorders of bone density and structure, multiple sites

IQ **M85.9** Disorder of bone density and structure, unspecified

Other osteopathies   (M86-M90)

EXCLUDES 1 postprocedural osteopathies (M96.-)

+ **4** **M86** **Osteomyelitis**
Use additional code (B95-B97) to identify infectious agent
Use additional code to identify major osseous defect, if applicable (M89.7-)

EXCLUDES 1 osteomyelitis due to:
echinococcus (B67.2)
gonococcus (A54.43)
salmonella (A02.24)

EXCLUDES 2 ostemyelitis of:
orbit (H05.0-)
petrous bone (H70.2-)
vertebra (M46.2-)

CODING TIPS✓ Osteomyelitis commonly occurs in diabetic patients. When osteomyelitis occurs in a diabetic patient and the physician has not clearly stated they are unrelated, the appropriate code from E08-E13 should be assigned with 4th and 5th characters of .69 followed by the appropriate code for osteomyelitis. When the osteomyelitis does not involve the lower extremity, look carefully for a different cause other than diabetes.

CODING TIPS✓ Codes classified to M86.- do not include osteomyelitis of the orbit, petrous bone, or vertebrae. Look for other causes of the osteomyelitis in the record, besides diabetes.

+ **5** **M86.0** Acute hematogenous osteomyelitis

IQ + **M86.00** Acute hematogenous osteomyelitis, unspecified site

+ **G** **M86.01** Acute hematogenous osteomyelitis, shoulder

☐ **SP** + **M86.011** Acute hematogenous osteomyelitis, right shoulder

☐ **SP** + **M86.012** Acute hematogenous osteomyelitis, left shoulder

☐ **IQ** + **M86.019** Acute hematogenous osteomyelitis, unspecified shoulder

+ **G** **M86.02** Acute hematogenous osteomyelitis, humerus

☐ **SP** + **M86.021** Acute hematogenous osteomyelitis, right humerus

☐ **SP** + **M86.022** Acute hematogenous osteomyelitis, left humerus

☐ **IQ** + **M86.029** Acute hematogenous osteomyelitis, unspecified humerus

+ **G** **M86.03** Acute hematogenous osteomyelitis, radius and ulna

☐ **SP** + **M86.031** Acute hematogenous osteomyelitis, right radius and ulna

☐ **SP** + **M86.032** Acute hematogenous osteomyelitis, left radius and ulna

☐ **IQ** + **M86.039** Acute hematogenous osteomyelitis, unspecified radius and ulna

+ **G** **M86.04** Acute hematogenous osteomyelitis, hand

☐ **SP** + **M86.041** Acute hematogenous osteomyelitis, right hand

☐ **SP** + **M86.042** Acute hematogenous osteomyelitis, left hand

☐ **IQ** + **M86.049** Acute hematogenous osteomyelitis, unspecified hand

+ **G** **M86.05** Acute hematogenous osteomyelitis, femur

☐ **SP** + **M86.051** Acute hematogenous osteomyelitis, right femur

☐ **SP** + **M86.052** Acute hematogenous osteomyelitis, left femur

☐ **IQ** + **M86.059** Acute hematogenous osteomyelitis, unspecified femur

+ **G** **M86.06** Acute hematogenous osteomyelitis, tibia and fibula

☐ **SP** + **M86.061** Acute hematogenous osteomyelitis, right tibia and fibula

☐ **SP** + **M86.062** Acute hematogenous osteomyelitis, left tibia and fibula

☐ **IQ** + **M86.069** Acute hematogenous osteomyelitis, unspecified tibia and fibula

+ **G** **M86.07** Acute hematogenous osteomyelitis, ankle and foot

☐ **SP** + **M86.071** Acute hematogenous osteomyelitis, right ankle and foot

☐ **SP** + **M86.072** Acute hematogenous osteomyelitis, left ankle and foot

☐ **IQ** + **M86.079** Acute hematogenous osteomyelitis, unspecified ankle and foot

SP + **M86.08** Acute hematogenous osteomyelitis, other sites

SP + **M86.09** Acute hematogenous osteomyelitis, multiple sites

+ **5** **M86.1** Other acute osteomyelitis

4 4th digit required   **5** 5th digit required   **G** 6th digit required   **7** 7th digit required   **7** 7th digit placeholder   + Additional code   ☐ Laterality

1248   *DecisionHealth's* FY 2020 Complete Home Health ICD-10-CM Diagnosis Coding Manual

IQ + M86.10 Other acute osteomyelitis, unspecified site

+ 6 M86.11 Other acute osteomyelitis, shoulder

SP + M86.111 Other acute osteomyelitis, right shoulder

SP + M86.112 Other acute osteomyelitis, left shoulder

IQ + M86.119 Other acute osteomyelitis, unspecified shoulder

+ 6 M86.12 Other acute osteomyelitis, humerus

SP + M86.121 Other acute osteomyelitis, right humerus

SP + M86.122 Other acute osteomyelitis, left humerus

IQ + M86.129 Other acute osteomyelitis, unspecified humerus

+ 6 M86.13 Other acute osteomyelitis, radius and ulna

SP + M86.131 Other acute osteomyelitis, right radius and ulna

SP + M86.132 Other acute osteomyelitis, left radius and ulna

IQ + M86.139 Other acute osteomyelitis, unspecified radius and ulna

+ 6 M86.14 Other acute osteomyelitis, hand

SP + M86.141 Other acute osteomyelitis, right hand

SP + M86.142 Other acute osteomyelitis, left hand

IQ + M86.149 Other acute osteomyelitis, unspecified hand

+ 6 M86.15 Other acute osteomyelitis, femur

SP + M86.151 Other acute osteomyelitis, right femur

SP + M86.152 Other acute osteomyelitis, left femur

IQ + M86.159 Other acute osteomyelitis, unspecified femur

+ 6 M86.16 Other acute osteomyelitis, tibia and fibula

SP + M86.161 Other acute osteomyelitis, right tibia and fibula

SP + M86.162 Other acute osteomyelitis, left tibia and fibula

IQ + M86.169 Other acute osteomyelitis, unspecified tibia and fibula

+ 6 M86.17 Other acute osteomyelitis, ankle and foot

SP + M86.171 Other acute osteomyelitis, right ankle and foot

SP + M86.172 Other acute osteomyelitis, left ankle and foot

IQ + M86.179 Other acute osteomyelitis, unspecified ankle and foot

SP + M86.18 Other acute osteomyelitis, other site

SP + M86.19 Other acute osteomyelitis, multiple sites

+ 5 M86.2 Subacute osteomyelitis

IQ + M86.20 Subacute osteomyelitis, unspecified site

+ 6 M86.21 Subacute osteomyelitis, shoulder

SP + M86.211 Subacute osteomyelitis, right shoulder

SP + M86.212 Subacute osteomyelitis, left shoulder

IQ + M86.219 Subacute osteomyelitis, unspecified shoulder

+ 6 M86.22 Subacute osteomyelitis, humerus

SP + M86.221 Subacute osteomyelitis, right humerus

SP + M86.222 Subacute osteomyelitis, left humerus

IQ + M86.229 Subacute osteomyelitis, unspecified humerus

+ 6 M86.23 Subacute osteomyelitis, radius and ulna

SP + M86.231 Subacute osteomyelitis, right radius and ulna

SP + M86.232 Subacute osteomyelitis, left radius and ulna

IQ + M86.239 Subacute osteomyelitis, unspecified radius and ulna

+ 6 M86.24 Subacute osteomyelitis, hand

SP + M86.241 Subacute osteomyelitis, right hand

SP + M86.242 Subacute osteomyelitis, left hand

IQ + M86.249 Subacute osteomyelitis, unspecified hand

+ 6 M86.25 Subacute osteomyelitis, femur

SP + M86.251 Subacute osteomyelitis, right femur

SP + M86.252 Subacute osteomyelitis, left femur

IQ + M86.259 Subacute osteomyelitis, unspecified femur

+ 6 M86.26 Subacute osteomyelitis, tibia and fibula

SP + M86.261 Subacute osteomyelitis, right tibia and fibula

SP + M86.262 Subacute osteomyelitis, left tibia and fibula

IQ + M86.269 Subacute osteomyelitis, unspecified tibia and fibula

+ 6 M86.27 Subacute osteomyelitis, ankle and foot

SP + M86.271 Subacute osteomyelitis, right ankle and foot

SP + M86.272 Subacute osteomyelitis, left ankle and foot

IQ + M86.279 Subacute osteomyelitis, unspecified ankle and foot

SP + M86.28 Subacute osteomyelitis, other site

SP + M86.29 Subacute osteomyelitis, multiple sites

+ 5 M86.3 Chronic multifocal osteomyelitis

IQ + M86.30 Chronic multifocal osteomyelitis, unspecified site

+ 6 M86.31 Chronic multifocal osteomyelitis, shoulder

SP + M86.311 Chronic multifocal osteomyelitis, right shoulder

SP + M86.312 Chronic multifocal osteomyelitis, left shoulder

IQ + M86.319 Chronic multifocal osteomyelitis, unspecified shoulder

+ 6 M86.32 Chronic multifocal osteomyelitis, humerus

SP + M86.321 Chronic multifocal osteomyelitis, right humerus

SP + M86.322 Chronic multifocal osteomyelitis, left humerus

★ New ▲ Revised **Px** Primary **SP** PDGM Px **SL** Low CoM **SH** High CoM **IQ** Quest. Encounter **H** Hospice non-cancer Dx ⬚ Unspecified **M** *Manifestation*

Chapter 13

M00-M99

☐ **IQ** ✛ **M86.329** Chronic multifocal osteomyelitis, unspecified humerus

✛ ⑥ **M86.33** Chronic multifocal osteomyelitis, radius and ulna

☐ **SP** ✛ **M86.331** Chronic multifocal osteomyelitis, right radius and ulna

☐ **SP** ✛ **M86.332** Chronic multifocal osteomyelitis, left radius and ulna

☐ **IQ** ✛ **M86.339** Chronic multifocal osteomyelitis, unspecified radius and ulna

✛ ⑥ **M86.34** Chronic multifocal osteomyelitis, hand

☐ **SP** ✛ **M86.341** Chronic multifocal osteomyelitis, right hand

☐ **SP** ✛ **M86.342** Chronic multifocal osteomyelitis, left hand

☐ **IQ** ✛ **M86.349** Chronic multifocal osteomyelitis, unspecified hand

✛ ⑥ **M86.35** Chronic multifocal osteomyelitis, femur

☐ **SP** ✛ **M86.351** Chronic multifocal osteomyelitis, right femur

☐ **SP** ✛ **M86.352** Chronic multifocal osteomyelitis, left femur

☐ **IQ** ✛ **M86.359** Chronic multifocal osteomyelitis, unspecified femur

✛ ⑥ **M86.36** Chronic multifocal osteomyelitis, tibia and fibula

☐ **SP** ✛ **M86.361** Chronic multifocal osteomyelitis, right tibia and fibula

☐ **SP** ✛ **M86.362** Chronic multifocal osteomyelitis, left tibia and fibula

☐ **IQ** ✛ **M86.369** Chronic multifocal osteomyelitis, unspecified tibia and fibula

✛ ⑥ **M86.37** Chronic multifocal osteomyelitis, ankle and foot

☐ **SP** ✛ **M86.371** Chronic multifocal osteomyelitis, right ankle and foot

☐ **SP** ✛ **M86.372** Chronic multifocal osteomyelitis, left ankle and foot

☐ **IQ** ✛ **M86.379** Chronic multifocal osteomyelitis, unspecified ankle and foot

SP ✛ **M86.38** Chronic multifocal osteomyelitis, other site

SP ✛ **M86.39** Chronic multifocal osteomyelitis, multiple sites

✛ ⑤ **M86.4** Chronic osteomyelitis with draining sinus

IQ ✛ **M86.40** Chronic osteomyelitis with draining sinus, unspecified site

✛ ⑥ **M86.41** Chronic osteomyelitis with draining sinus, shoulder

☐ **SP** ✛ **M86.411** Chronic osteomyelitis with draining sinus, right shoulder

☐ **SP** ✛ **M86.412** Chronic osteomyelitis with draining sinus, left shoulder

☐ **IQ** ✛ **M86.419** Chronic osteomyelitis with draining sinus, unspecified shoulder

✛ ⑥ **M86.42** Chronic osteomyelitis with draining sinus, humerus

☐ **SP** ✛ **M86.421** Chronic osteomyelitis with draining sinus, right humerus

☐ **SP** ✛ **M86.422** Chronic osteomyelitis with draining sinus, left humerus

☐ **IQ** ✛ **M86.429** Chronic osteomyelitis with draining sinus, unspecified humerus

✛ ⑥ **M86.43** Chronic osteomyelitis with draining sinus, radius and ulna

☐ **SP** ✛ **M86.431** Chronic osteomyelitis with draining sinus, right radius and ulna

☐ **SP** ✛ **M86.432** Chronic osteomyelitis with draining sinus, left radius and ulna

☐ **IQ** ✛ **M86.439** Chronic osteomyelitis with draining sinus, unspecified radius and ulna

✛ ⑥ **M86.44** Chronic osteomyelitis with draining sinus, hand

☐ **SP** ✛ **M86.441** Chronic osteomyelitis with draining sinus, right hand

☐ **SP** ✛ **M86.442** Chronic osteomyelitis with draining sinus, left hand

☐ **IQ** ✛ **M86.449** Chronic osteomyelitis with draining sinus, unspecified hand

✛ ⑥ **M86.45** Chronic osteomyelitis with draining sinus, femur

☐ **SP** ✛ **M86.451** Chronic osteomyelitis with draining sinus, right femur

☐ **SP** ✛ **M86.452** Chronic osteomyelitis with draining sinus, left femur

☐ **IQ** ✛ **M86.459** Chronic osteomyelitis with draining sinus, unspecified femur

✛ ⑥ **M86.46** Chronic osteomyelitis with draining sinus, tibia and fibula

☐ **SP** ✛ **M86.461** Chronic osteomyelitis with draining sinus, right tibia and fibula

☐ **SP** ✛ **M86.462** Chronic osteomyelitis with draining sinus, left tibia and fibula

☐ **IQ** ✛ **M86.469** Chronic osteomyelitis with draining sinus, unspecified tibia and fibula

✛ ⑥ **M86.47** Chronic osteomyelitis with draining sinus, ankle and foot

☐ **SP** ✛ **M86.471** Chronic osteomyelitis with draining sinus, right ankle and foot

☐ **SP** ✛ **M86.472** Chronic osteomyelitis with draining sinus, left ankle and foot

☐ **IQ** ✛ **M86.479** Chronic osteomyelitis with draining sinus, unspecified ankle and foot

SP ✛ **M86.48** Chronic osteomyelitis with draining sinus, other site

SP ✛ **M86.49** Chronic osteomyelitis with draining sinus, multiple sites

✛ ⑤ **M86.5** Other chronic hematogenous osteomyelitis

IQ ✛ **M86.50** Other chronic hematogenous osteomyelitis, unspecified site

✛ ⑥ **M86.51** Other chronic hematogenous osteomyelitis, shoulder

☐ **SP** ✛ **M86.511** Other chronic hematogenous osteomyelitis, right shoulder

☐ **SP** ✛ **M86.512** Other chronic hematogenous osteomyelitis, left shoulder

④ 4th digit required　　⑤ 5th digit required　　⑥ 6th digit required　　⑦ 7th digit required　　⑦ 7th digit placeholder　　✛ Additional code　　☐ Laterality

1250　　　　　*DecisionHealth's* FY 2020 Complete Home Health ICD-10-CM Diagnosis Coding Manual

☐ IQ ✚ **M86.519** Other chronic hematogenous osteomyelitis, unspecified shoulder

✚ 6 **M86.52** Other chronic hematogenous osteomyelitis, humerus

☐ SP ✚ **M86.521** Other chronic hematogenous osteomyelitis, right humerus

☐ SP ✚ **M86.522** Other chronic hematogenous osteomyelitis, left humerus

☐ IQ ✚ **M86.529** Other chronic hematogenous osteomyelitis, unspecified humerus

✚ 6 **M86.53** Other chronic hematogenous osteomyelitis, radius and ulna

☐ SP ✚ **M86.531** Other chronic hematogenous osteomyelitis, right radius and ulna

☐ SP ✚ **M86.532** Other chronic hematogenous osteomyelitis, left radius and ulna

☐ IQ ✚ **M86.539** Other chronic hematogenous osteomyelitis, unspecified radius and ulna

✚ 6 **M86.54** Other chronic hematogenous osteomyelitis, hand

☐ SP ✚ **M86.541** Other chronic hematogenous osteomyelitis, right hand

☐ SP ✚ **M86.542** Other chronic hematogenous osteomyelitis, left hand

☐ IQ ✚ **M86.549** Other chronic hematogenous osteomyelitis, unspecified hand

✚ 6 **M86.55** Other chronic hematogenous osteomyelitis, femur

☐ SP ✚ **M86.551** Other chronic hematogenous osteomyelitis, right femur

☐ SP ✚ **M86.552** Other chronic hematogenous osteomyelitis, left femur

☐ IQ ✚ **M86.559** Other chronic hematogenous osteomyelitis, unspecified femur

✚ 6 **M86.56** Other chronic hematogenous osteomyelitis, tibia and fibula

☐ SP ✚ **M86.561** Other chronic hematogenous osteomyelitis, right tibia and fibula

☐ SP ✚ **M86.562** Other chronic hematogenous osteomyelitis, left tibia and fibula

☐ IQ ✚ **M86.569** Other chronic hematogenous osteomyelitis, unspecified tibia and fibula

✚ 6 **M86.57** Other chronic hematogenous osteomyelitis, ankle and foot

☐ SP ✚ **M86.571** Other chronic hematogenous osteomyelitis, right ankle and foot

☐ SP ✚ **M86.572** Other chronic hematogenous osteomyelitis, left ankle and foot

☐ IQ ✚ **M86.579** Other chronic hematogenous osteomyelitis, unspecified ankle and foot

SP ✚ **M86.58** Other chronic hematogenous osteomyelitis, other site

SP ✚ **M86.59** Other chronic hematogenous osteomyelitis, multiple sites

✚ 5 **M86.6** Other chronic osteomyelitis

IQ ✚ **M86.60** Other chronic osteomyelitis, unspecified site

✚ 6 **M86.61** Other chronic osteomyelitis, shoulder

☐ SP ✚ **M86.611** Other chronic osteomyelitis, right shoulder

☐ SP ✚ **M86.612** Other chronic osteomyelitis, left shoulder

☐ IQ ✚ **M86.619** Other chronic osteomyelitis, unspecified shoulder

✚ 6 **M86.62** Other chronic osteomyelitis, humerus

☐ SP ✚ **M86.621** Other chronic osteomyelitis, right humerus

☐ SP ✚ **M86.622** Other chronic osteomyelitis, left humerus

☐ IQ ✚ **M86.629** Other chronic osteomyelitis, unspecified humerus

✚ 6 **M86.63** Other chronic osteomyelitis, radius and ulna

☐ SP ✚ **M86.631** Other chronic osteomyelitis, right radius and ulna

☐ SP ✚ **M86.632** Other chronic osteomyelitis, left radius and ulna

☐ IQ ✚ **M86.639** Other chronic osteomyelitis, unspecified radius and ulna

✚ 6 **M86.64** Other chronic osteomyelitis, hand

☐ SP ✚ **M86.641** Other chronic osteomyelitis, right hand

☐ SP ✚ **M86.642** Other chronic osteomyelitis, left hand

☐ IQ ✚ **M86.649** Other chronic osteomyelitis, unspecified hand

✚ 6 **M86.65** Other chronic osteomyelitis, thigh

☐ SP ✚ **M86.651** Other chronic osteomyelitis, right thigh

☐ SP ✚ **M86.652** Other chronic osteomyelitis, left thigh

☐ IQ ✚ **M86.659** Other chronic osteomyelitis, unspecified thigh

✚ 6 **M86.66** Other chronic osteomyelitis, tibia and fibula

☐ SP ✚ **M86.661** Other chronic osteomyelitis, right tibia and fibula

☐ SP ✚ **M86.662** Other chronic osteomyelitis, left tibia and fibula

☐ IQ ✚ **M86.669** Other chronic osteomyelitis, unspecified tibia and fibula

✚ 6 **M86.67** Other chronic osteomyelitis, ankle and foot

☐ SP ✚ **M86.671** Other chronic osteomyelitis, right ankle and foot

☐ SP ✚ **M86.672** Other chronic osteomyelitis, left ankle and foot

☐ IQ ✚ **M86.679** Other chronic osteomyelitis, unspecified ankle and foot

SP ✚ **M86.68** Other chronic osteomyelitis, other site

SP ✚ **M86.69** Other chronic osteomyelitis, multiple sites

✚ 5 **M86.8** Other osteomyelitis
  Brodie's abscess

✚ 6 **M86.8X** Other osteomyelitis

SP ✚ **M86.8X0** Other osteomyelitis, multiple sites

SP ✚ **M86.8X1** Other osteomyelitis, shoulder

SP ✚ **M86.8X2** Other osteomyelitis, upper arm

SP ✚ **M86.8X3** Other osteomyelitis, forearm

SP ✚ **M86.8X4** Other osteomyelitis, hand

SP ✚ **M86.8X5** Other osteomyelitis, thigh

☆ New ▲ Revised **Px** Primary **SP** PDGM Px **SL** Low CoM **SH** High CoM **IQ** Quest. Encounter **H** Hospice non-cancer Dx | Unspecified | **M** *Manifestation*

SP **+** **M86.8X6** Other osteomyelitis, lower leg

SP **+** **M86.8X7** Other osteomyelitis, ankle and foot

SP **+** **M86.8X8** Other osteomyelitis, other site

SP **+** **M86.8X9** Other osteomyelitis, unspecified sites

!Q **+** **M86.9** Osteomyelitis, unspecified
Infection of bone NOS
Periostitis without osteomyelitis

+ **④** **M87** Osteonecrosis
INCLUDES   avascular necrosis of bone
Use additional code to identify major osseous defect, if applicable (M89.7-)
EXCLUDES 1   juvenile osteonecrosis (M91-M92)
osteochondropathies (M90-M93)

GUIDELINES   Section I.C.13.a.1)
For certain conditions, the bone may be affected at the upper or lower end, (e.g., avascular necrosis of bone, M87, Osteoporosis, M80, M81). Though the portion of the bone affected may be at the joint, the site designation will be the bone, not the joint.

CODING TIPS ✓   **Documentation:** Osteonecrosis also may be termed avascular necrosis or aseptic necrosis of the bone. The condition indicates a necrosis of bone due to impaired blood supply and may be related to trauma, use of drugs or another cause. Review documentation carefully to determine if a causative condition is known.

DEFINITION   The death of bone tissue from an interruption of its blood supply.

+ **⑤** **M87.0** Idiopathic aseptic necrosis of bone
DEFINITION   The death of bone tissue from ischemia of unknown cause.

!Q **+** **M87.00** Idiopathic aseptic necrosis of unspecified bone

+ **⑥** **M87.01** Idiopathic aseptic necrosis of shoulder
Idiopathic aseptic necrosis of clavicle and scapula

⊟ **!Q** **+** **M87.011** Idiopathic aseptic necrosis of right shoulder

⊟ **!Q** **+** **M87.012** Idiopathic aseptic necrosis of left shoulder

⊟ **!Q** **+** **M87.019** Idiopathic aseptic necrosis of unspecified shoulder

+ **⑥** **M87.02** Idiopathic aseptic necrosis of humerus

⊟ **SP** **+** **M87.021** Idiopathic aseptic necrosis of right humerus

⊟ **SP** **+** **M87.022** Idiopathic aseptic necrosis of left humerus

⊟ **!Q** **+** **M87.029** Idiopathic aseptic necrosis of unspecified humerus

+ **⑥** **M87.03** Idiopathic aseptic necrosis of radius, ulna and carpus

⊟ **SP** **+** **M87.031** Idiopathic aseptic necrosis of right radius

⊟ **SP** **+** **M87.032** Idiopathic aseptic necrosis of left radius

⊟ **!Q** **+** **M87.033** Idiopathic aseptic necrosis of unspecified radius

⊟ **SP** **+** **M87.034** Idiopathic aseptic necrosis of right ulna

⊟ **SP** **+** **M87.035** Idiopathic aseptic necrosis of left ulna

⊟ **!Q** **+** **M87.036** Idiopathic aseptic necrosis of unspecified ulna

⊟ **SP** **+** **M87.037** Idiopathic aseptic necrosis of right carpus

⊟ **SP** **+** **M87.038** Idiopathic aseptic necrosis of left carpus

⊟ **!Q** **+** **M87.039** Idiopathic aseptic necrosis of unspecified carpus

+ **⑥** **M87.04** Idiopathic aseptic necrosis of hand and fingers
Idiopathic aseptic necrosis of metacarpals and phalanges of hands

⊟ **SP** **+** **M87.041** Idiopathic aseptic necrosis of right hand

⊟ **SP** **+** **M87.042** Idiopathic aseptic necrosis of left hand

⊟ **!Q** **+** **M87.043** Idiopathic aseptic necrosis of unspecified hand

⊟ **SP** **+** **M87.044** Idiopathic aseptic necrosis of right finger(s)

⊟ **SP** **+** **M87.045** Idiopathic aseptic necrosis of left finger(s)

⊟ **!Q** **+** **M87.046** Idiopathic aseptic necrosis of unspecified finger(s)

+ **⑥** **M87.05** Idiopathic aseptic necrosis of pelvis and femur

⊟ **SP** **+** **M87.050** Idiopathic aseptic necrosis of pelvis

⊟ **SP** **+** **M87.051** Idiopathic aseptic necrosis of right femur

⊟ **SP** **+** **M87.052** Idiopathic aseptic necrosis of left femur

⊟ **!Q** **+** **M87.059** Idiopathic aseptic necrosis of unspecified femur
Idiopathic aseptic necrosis of hip NOS

+ **⑥** **M87.06** Idiopathic aseptic necrosis of tibia and fibula

⊟ **SP** **+** **M87.061** Idiopathic aseptic necrosis of right tibia

⊟ **SP** **+** **M87.062** Idiopathic aseptic necrosis of left tibia

⊟ **!Q** **+** **M87.063** Idiopathic aseptic necrosis of unspecified tibia

⊟ **SP** **+** **M87.064** Idiopathic aseptic necrosis of right fibula

⊟ **SP** **+** **M87.065** Idiopathic aseptic necrosis of left fibula

⊟ **!Q** **+** **M87.066** Idiopathic aseptic necrosis of unspecified fibula

+ **⑥** **M87.07** Idiopathic aseptic necrosis of ankle, foot and toes
Idiopathic aseptic necrosis of metatarsus, tarsus, and phalanges of toes

⊟ **SP** **+** **M87.071** Idiopathic aseptic necrosis of right ankle

⊟ **SP** **+** **M87.072** Idiopathic aseptic necrosis of left ankle

⊟ **!Q** **+** **M87.073** Idiopathic aseptic necrosis of unspecified ankle

⊟ **SP** **+** **M87.074** Idiopathic aseptic necrosis of right foot

---

④4th digit required   **⑤**5th digit required   **⑥**6th digit required   **⑦**7th digit required   **⑦**7th digit placeholder   **+**Additional code   **⊟**Laterality

1252   *DecisionHealth's* FY 2020 Complete Home Health ICD-10-CM Diagnosis Coding Manual

🖩 SP ✚ **M87.075** Idiopathic aseptic necrosis of left foot

🖩 IQ ✚ **M87.076** Idiopathic aseptic necrosis of unspecified foot

🖩 SP ✚ **M87.077** Idiopathic aseptic necrosis of right toe(s)

🖩 SP ✚ **M87.078** Idiopathic aseptic necrosis of left toe(s)

🖩 IQ ✚ **M87.079** Idiopathic aseptic necrosis of unspecified toe(s)

SP ✚ **M87.08** Idiopathic aseptic necrosis of bone, other site

SP ✚ **M87.09** Idiopathic aseptic necrosis of bone, multiple sites

✚ 5 **M87.1** Osteonecrosis due to drugs
    Use additional code for adverse effect, if applicable, to identify drug (T36-T50 with fifth or sixth character 5)

IQ ✚ **M87.10** Osteonecrosis due to drugs, unspecified bone

✚ 6 **M87.11** Osteonecrosis due to drugs, shoulder

🖩 SP ✚ **M87.111** Osteonecrosis due to drugs, right shoulder

🖩 SP ✚ **M87.112** Osteonecrosis due to drugs, left shoulder

🖩 IQ ✚ **M87.119** Osteonecrosis due to drugs, unspecified shoulder

✚ 6 **M87.12** Osteonecrosis due to drugs, humerus

🖩 SP ✚ **M87.121** Osteonecrosis due to drugs, right humerus

🖩 SP ✚ **M87.122** Osteonecrosis due to drugs, left humerus

🖩 IQ ✚ **M87.129** Osteonecrosis due to drugs, unspecified humerus

✚ 6 **M87.13** Osteonecrosis due to drugs of radius, ulna and carpus

🖩 SP ✚ **M87.131** Osteonecrosis due to drugs of right radius

🖩 SP ✚ **M87.132** Osteonecrosis due to drugs of left radius

🖩 IQ ✚ **M87.133** Osteonecrosis due to drugs of unspecified radius

🖩 SP ✚ **M87.134** Osteonecrosis due to drugs of right ulna

🖩 SP ✚ **M87.135** Osteonecrosis due to drugs of left ulna

🖩 IQ ✚ **M87.136** Osteonecrosis due to drugs of unspecified ulna

🖩 SP ✚ **M87.137** Osteonecrosis due to drugs of right carpus

🖩 SP ✚ **M87.138** Osteonecrosis due to drugs of left carpus

🖩 IQ ✚ **M87.139** Osteonecrosis due to drugs of unspecified carpus

✚ 6 **M87.14** Osteonecrosis due to drugs, hand and fingers

🖩 SP ✚ **M87.141** Osteonecrosis due to drugs, right hand

🖩 SP ✚ **M87.142** Osteonecrosis due to drugs, left hand

🖩 IQ ✚ **M87.143** Osteonecrosis due to drugs, unspecified hand

🖩 SP ✚ **M87.144** Osteonecrosis due to drugs, right finger(s)

🖩 SP ✚ **M87.145** Osteonecrosis due to drugs, left finger(s)

🖩 IQ ✚ **M87.146** Osteonecrosis due to drugs, unspecified finger(s)

✚ 6 **M87.15** Osteonecrosis due to drugs, pelvis and femur

🖩 SP ✚ **M87.150** Osteonecrosis due to drugs, pelvis

🖩 SP ✚ **M87.151** Osteonecrosis due to drugs, right femur

🖩 SP ✚ **M87.152** Osteonecrosis due to drugs, left femur

🖩 IQ ✚ **M87.159** Osteonecrosis due to drugs, unspecified femur

✚ 6 **M87.16** Osteonecrosis due to drugs, tibia and fibula

🖩 SP ✚ **M87.161** Osteonecrosis due to drugs, right tibia

🖩 SP ✚ **M87.162** Osteonecrosis due to drugs, left tibia

🖩 IQ ✚ **M87.163** Osteonecrosis due to drugs, unspecified tibia

🖩 SP ✚ **M87.164** Osteonecrosis due to drugs, right fibula

🖩 SP ✚ **M87.165** Osteonecrosis due to drugs, left fibula

🖩 IQ ✚ **M87.166** Osteonecrosis due to drugs, unspecified fibula

✚ 6 **M87.17** Osteonecrosis due to drugs, ankle, foot and toes

🖩 SP ✚ **M87.171** Osteonecrosis due to drugs, right ankle

🖩 SP ✚ **M87.172** Osteonecrosis due to drugs, left ankle

🖩 IQ ✚ **M87.173** Osteonecrosis due to drugs, unspecified ankle

🖩 SP ✚ **M87.174** Osteonecrosis due to drugs, right foot

🖩 SP ✚ **M87.175** Osteonecrosis due to drugs, left foot

🖩 IQ ✚ **M87.176** Osteonecrosis due to drugs, unspecified foot

🖩 SP ✚ **M87.177** Osteonecrosis due to drugs, right toe(s)

🖩 SP ✚ **M87.178** Osteonecrosis due to drugs, left toe(s)

🖩 IQ ✚ **M87.179** Osteonecrosis due to drugs, unspecified toe(s)

✚ 6 **M87.18** Osteonecrosis due to drugs, other site

SP ✚ **M87.180** Osteonecrosis due to drugs, jaw

SP ✚ **M87.188** Osteonecrosis due to drugs, other site

SP ✚ **M87.19** Osteonecrosis due to drugs, multiple sites

✚ 5 **M87.2** Osteonecrosis due to previous trauma

IQ ✚ **M87.20** Osteonecrosis due to previous trauma, unspecified bone

✚ 6 **M87.21** Osteonecrosis due to previous trauma, shoulder

🖩 SP ✚ **M87.211** Osteonecrosis due to previous trauma, right shoulder

🖩 SP ✚ **M87.212** Osteonecrosis due to previous trauma, left shoulder

🖩 IQ ✚ **M87.219** Osteonecrosis due to previous trauma, unspecified shoulder

✚ 6 **M87.22** Osteonecrosis due to previous trauma, humerus

★ New ▲ Revised Px Primary SP PDGM Px SL Low CoM SH High CoM IQ Quest. Encounter H Hospice non-cancer Dx   Unspecified   M *Manifestation*

DecisionHealth's FY 2020 Complete Home Health ICD-10-CM Diagnosis Coding Manual   1253

☐ SP ✚ **M87.221** Osteonecrosis due to previous trauma, right humerus

☐ SP ✚ **M87.222** Osteonecrosis due to previous trauma, left humerus

☐ IQ ✚ **M87.229** Osteonecrosis due to previous trauma, unspecified humerus

✚ 6 **M87.23** Osteonecrosis due to previous trauma of radius, ulna and carpus

☐ SP ✚ **M87.231** Osteonecrosis due to previous trauma of right radius

☐ SP ✚ **M87.232** Osteonecrosis due to previous trauma of left radius

☐ IQ ✚ **M87.233** Osteonecrosis due to previous trauma of unspecified radius

☐ SP ✚ **M87.234** Osteonecrosis due to previous trauma of right ulna

☐ SP ✚ **M87.235** Osteonecrosis due to previous trauma of left ulna

☐ IQ ✚ **M87.236** Osteonecrosis due to previous trauma of unspecified ulna

☐ SP ✚ **M87.237** Osteonecrosis due to previous trauma of right carpus

☐ SP ✚ **M87.238** Osteonecrosis due to previous trauma of left carpus

☐ IQ ✚ **M87.239** Osteonecrosis due to previous trauma of unspecified carpus

✚ 6 **M87.24** Osteonecrosis due to previous trauma, hand and fingers

☐ SP ✚ **M87.241** Osteonecrosis due to previous trauma, right hand

☐ SP ✚ **M87.242** Osteonecrosis due to previous trauma, left hand

☐ IQ ✚ **M87.243** Osteonecrosis due to previous trauma, unspecified hand

☐ SP ✚ **M87.244** Osteonecrosis due to previous trauma, right finger(s)

☐ SP ✚ **M87.245** Osteonecrosis due to previous trauma, left finger(s)

☐ IQ ✚ **M87.246** Osteonecrosis due to previous trauma, unspecified finger(s)

✚ 6 **M87.25** Osteonecrosis due to previous trauma, pelvis and femur

☐ SP ✚ **M87.250** Osteonecrosis due to previous trauma, pelvis

☐ SP ✚ **M87.251** Osteonecrosis due to previous trauma, right femur

☐ SP ✚ **M87.252** Osteonecrosis due to previous trauma, left femur

☐ IQ ✚ **M87.256** Osteonecrosis due to previous trauma, unspecified femur

✚ 6 **M87.26** Osteonecrosis due to previous trauma, tibia and fibula

☐ SP ✚ **M87.261** Osteonecrosis due to previous trauma, right tibia

☐ SP ✚ **M87.262** Osteonecrosis due to previous trauma, left tibia

☐ IQ ✚ **M87.263** Osteonecrosis due to previous trauma, unspecified tibia

☐ SP ✚ **M87.264** Osteonecrosis due to previous trauma, right fibula

☐ SP ✚ **M87.265** Osteonecrosis due to previous trauma, left fibula

☐ IQ ✚ **M87.266** Osteonecrosis due to previous trauma, unspecified fibula

✚ 6 **M87.27** Osteonecrosis due to previous trauma, ankle, foot and toes

☐ SP ✚ **M87.271** Osteonecrosis due to previous trauma, right ankle

☐ SP ✚ **M87.272** Osteonecrosis due to previous trauma, left ankle

☐ IQ ✚ **M87.273** Osteonecrosis due to previous trauma, unspecified ankle

☐ SP ✚ **M87.274** Osteonecrosis due to previous trauma, right foot

☐ SP ✚ **M87.275** Osteonecrosis due to previous trauma, left foot

☐ IQ ✚ **M87.276** Osteonecrosis due to previous trauma, unspecified foot

☐ SP ✚ **M87.277** Osteonecrosis due to previous trauma, right toe(s)

☐ SP ✚ **M87.278** Osteonecrosis due to previous trauma, left toe(s)

☐ IQ ✚ **M87.279** Osteonecrosis due to previous trauma, unspecified toe(s)

SP ✚ **M87.28** Osteonecrosis due to previous trauma, other site

SP ✚ **M87.29** Osteonecrosis due to previous trauma, multiple sites

✚ 5 **M87.3** Other secondary osteonecrosis

IQ ✚ **M87.30** Other secondary osteonecrosis, unspecified bone

✚ 6 **M87.31** Other secondary osteonecrosis, shoulder

☐ SP ✚ **M87.311** Other secondary osteonecrosis, right shoulder

☐ SP ✚ **M87.312** Other secondary osteonecrosis, left shoulder

☐ IQ ✚ **M87.319** Other secondary osteonecrosis, unspecified shoulder

✚ 6 **M87.32** Other secondary osteonecrosis, humerus

☐ SP ✚ **M87.321** Other secondary osteonecrosis, right humerus

☐ SP ✚ **M87.322** Other secondary osteonecrosis, left humerus

☐ IQ ✚ **M87.329** Other secondary osteonecrosis, unspecified humerus

✚ 6 **M87.33** Other secondary osteonecrosis of radius, ulna and carpus

☐ SP ✚ **M87.331** Other secondary osteonecrosis of right radius

☐ SP ✚ **M87.332** Other secondary osteonecrosis of left radius

☐ IQ ✚ **M87.333** Other secondary osteonecrosis of unspecified radius

☐ SP ✚ **M87.334** Other secondary osteonecrosis of right ulna

☐ SP ✚ **M87.335** Other secondary osteonecrosis of left ulna

☐ IQ ✚ **M87.336** Other secondary osteonecrosis of unspecified ulna

☐ SP ✚ **M87.337** Other secondary osteonecrosis of right carpus

☐ SP ✚ **M87.338** Other secondary osteonecrosis of left carpus

☐ IQ ✚ **M87.339** Other secondary osteonecrosis of unspecified carpus

✚ 6 **M87.34** Other secondary osteonecrosis, hand and fingers

☐ SP ✚ **M87.341** Other secondary osteonecrosis, right hand

---

4 4th digit required   5 5th digit required   6 6th digit required   7 7th digit required   7 7th digit placeholder   ✚ Additional code   ☐ Laterality

1254   *DecisionHealth's* FY 2020 Complete Home Health ICD-10-CM Diagnosis Coding Manual

☐ SP ✚ M87.342 Other secondary osteonecrosis, left hand

☐ IQ ✚ M87.343 Other secondary osteonecrosis, unspecified hand

☐ SP ✚ M87.344 Other secondary osteonecrosis, right finger(s)

☐ SP ✚ M87.345 Other secondary osteonecrosis, left finger(s)

☐ IQ ✚ M87.346 Other secondary osteonecrosis, unspecified finger(s)

✚ ⑥ M87.35 Other secondary osteonecrosis, pelvis and femur

☐ SP ✚ M87.350 Other secondary osteonecrosis, pelvis

☐ SP ✚ M87.351 Other secondary osteonecrosis, right femur

☐ SP ✚ M87.352 Other secondary osteonecrosis, left femur

☐ IQ ✚ M87.353 Other secondary osteonecrosis, unspecified femur

✚ ⑥ M87.36 Other secondary osteonecrosis, tibia and fibula

☐ SP ✚ M87.361 Other secondary osteonecrosis, right tibia

☐ SP ✚ M87.362 Other secondary osteonecrosis, left tibia

☐ IQ ✚ M87.363 Other secondary osteonecrosis, unspecified tibia

☐ SP ✚ M87.364 Other secondary osteonecrosis, right fibula

☐ SP ✚ M87.365 Other secondary osteonecrosis, left fibula

☐ IQ ✚ M87.366 Other secondary osteonecrosis, unspecified fibula

✚ ⑥ M87.37 Other secondary osteonecrosis, ankle and foot

☐ SP ✚ M87.371 Other secondary osteonecrosis, right ankle

☐ SP ✚ M87.372 Other secondary osteonecrosis, left ankle

☐ IQ ✚ M87.373 Other secondary osteonecrosis, unspecified ankle

☐ SP ✚ M87.374 Other secondary osteonecrosis, right foot

☐ SP ✚ M87.375 Other secondary osteonecrosis, left foot

☐ IQ ✚ M87.376 Other secondary osteonecrosis, unspecified foot

☐ SP ✚ M87.377 Other secondary osteonecrosis, right toe(s)

☐ SP ✚ M87.378 Other secondary osteonecrosis, left toe(s)

☐ IQ ✚ M87.379 Other secondary osteonecrosis, unspecified toe(s)

SP ✚ M87.38 Other secondary osteonecrosis, other site

SP ✚ M87.39 Other secondary osteonecrosis, multiple sites

✚ ⑤ M87.8 Other osteonecrosis

IQ ✚ M87.80 Other osteonecrosis, unspecified bone

✚ ⑥ M87.81 Other osteonecrosis, shoulder

☐ SP ✚ M87.811 Other osteonecrosis, right shoulder

☐ SP ✚ M87.812 Other osteonecrosis, left shoulder

☐ IQ ✚ M87.819 Other osteonecrosis, unspecified shoulder

✚ ⑥ M87.82 Other osteonecrosis, humerus

☐ SP ✚ M87.821 Other osteonecrosis, right humerus

☐ SP ✚ M87.822 Other osteonecrosis, left humerus

☐ IQ ✚ M87.829 Other osteonecrosis, unspecified humerus

✚ ⑥ M87.83 Other osteonecrosis of radius, ulna and carpus

☐ SP ✚ M87.831 Other osteonecrosis of right radius

☐ SP ✚ M87.832 Other osteonecrosis of left radius

☐ IQ ✚ M87.833 Other osteonecrosis of unspecified radius

☐ SP ✚ M87.834 Other osteonecrosis of right ulna

☐ SP ✚ M87.835 Other osteonecrosis of left ulna

☐ IQ ✚ M87.836 Other osteonecrosis of unspecified ulna

☐ SP ✚ M87.837 Other osteonecrosis of right carpus

☐ SP ✚ M87.838 Other osteonecrosis of left carpus

☐ IQ ✚ M87.839 Other osteonecrosis of unspecified carpus

✚ ⑥ M87.84 Other osteonecrosis, hand and fingers

☐ SP ✚ M87.841 Other osteonecrosis, right hand

☐ SP ✚ M87.842 Other osteonecrosis, left hand

☐ IQ ✚ M87.843 Other osteonecrosis, unspecified hand

☐ SP ✚ M87.844 Other osteonecrosis, right finger(s)

☐ SP ✚ M87.845 Other osteonecrosis, left finger(s)

☐ IQ ✚ M87.849 Other osteonecrosis, unspecified finger(s)

✚ ⑥ M87.85 Other osteonecrosis, pelvis and femur

☐ SP ✚ M87.850 Other osteonecrosis, pelvis

☐ SP ✚ M87.851 Other osteonecrosis, right femur

☐ SP ✚ M87.852 Other osteonecrosis, left femur

☐ IQ ✚ M87.859 Other osteonecrosis, unspecified femur

✚ ⑥ M87.86 Other osteonecrosis, tibia and fibula

☐ SP ✚ M87.861 Other osteonecrosis, right tibia

☐ SP ✚ M87.862 Other osteonecrosis, left tibia

☐ IQ ✚ M87.863 Other osteonecrosis, unspecified tibia

☐ SP ✚ M87.864 Other osteonecrosis, right fibula

☐ SP ✚ M87.865 Other osteonecrosis, left fibula

☐ IQ ✚ M87.869 Other osteonecrosis, unspecified fibula

✚ ⑥ M87.87 Other osteonecrosis, ankle, foot and toes

☐ SP ✚ M87.871 Other osteonecrosis, right ankle

☐ SP ✚ M87.872 Other osteonecrosis, left ankle

☐ IQ ✚ M87.873 Other osteonecrosis, unspecified ankle

☐ SP ✚ M87.874 Other osteonecrosis, right foot

☐ SP ✚ M87.875 Other osteonecrosis, left foot

☐ IQ ✚ M87.876 Other osteonecrosis, unspecified foot

★ New ▲ Revised Px Primary SP PDGM Px SL Low CoM SH High CoM IQ Quest. Encounter H Hospice non-cancer Dx Unspecified M Manifestation

DecisionHealth's FY 2020 Complete Home Health ICD-10-CM Diagnosis Coding Manual

1255

Chapter 13

M00-M99

⊟ **SP** ✚ **M87.877** Other osteonecrosis, right toe(s)

⊟ **SP** ✚ **M87.878** Other osteonecrosis, left toe(s)

⊟ **IQ** ✚ **M87.879** Other osteonecrosis, unspecified toe(s)

SP ✚ **M87.88** Other osteonecrosis, other site

SP ✚ **M87.89** Other osteonecrosis, multiple sites

IQ ✚ **M87.9** Osteonecrosis, unspecified

    Necrosis of bone NOS

4 **M88** Osteitis deformans [Paget's disease of bone]

> **EXCLUDES 1**   osteitis deformans in neoplastic disease (M90.6)

> **DEFINITION**   A bone disorder characterized by cycles of bone loss followed by excessive attempts at repair; results in painful, deformed, enlarged bones of porous tissue prone to fractures and arthritic affected joints.

SP **M88.0** Osteitis deformans of skull

> **DEFINITION**   Excessive breakdown and rebuilding of bone tissue in the skull, resulting in an enlarged head with abnormally remodeled skull bones that may press on nerves causing headache, vertigo, tinnitus, or hearing loss.

SP **M88.1** Osteitis deformans of vertebrae

> **DEFINITION**   Excessive breakdown and rebuilding of the vertebrae with bone material that is less dense, resulting in an abnormally remodeled, thickened spine prone to fracture that may compress nerve roots causing pain, numbness, and tingling in arms or legs.

5 **M88.8** Osteitis deformans of other bones

6 **M88.81** Osteitis deformans of shoulder

⊟ **SP** **M88.811** Osteitis deformans of right shoulder

⊟ **SP** **M88.812** Osteitis deformans of left shoulder

⊟ **IQ** **M88.819** Osteitis deformans of unspecified shoulder

6 **M88.82** Osteitis deformans of upper arm

⊟ **SP** **M88.821** Osteitis deformans of right upper arm

⊟ **SP** **M88.822** Osteitis deformans of left upper arm

⊟ **IQ** **M88.829** Osteitis deformans of unspecified upper arm

6 **M88.83** Osteitis deformans of forearm

⊟ **SP** **M88.831** Osteitis deformans of right forearm

⊟ **SP** **M88.832** Osteitis deformans of left forearm

⊟ **IQ** **M88.839** Osteitis deformans of unspecified forearm

6 **M88.84** Osteitis deformans of hand

⊟ **SP** **M88.841** Osteitis deformans of right hand

⊟ **SP** **M88.842** Osteitis deformans of left hand

⊟ **IQ** **M88.849** Osteitis deformans of unspecified hand

6 **M88.85** Osteitis deformans of thigh

⊟ **SP** **M88.851** Osteitis deformans of right thigh

⊟ **SP** **M88.852** Osteitis deformans of left thigh

⊟ **IQ** **M88.859** Osteitis deformans of unspecified thigh

6 **M88.86** Osteitis deformans of lower leg

⊟ **SP** **M88.861** Osteitis deformans of right lower leg

⊟ **SP** **M88.862** Osteitis deformans of left lower leg

⊟ **IQ** **M88.869** Osteitis deformans of unspecified lower leg

6 **M88.87** Osteitis deformans of ankle and foot

⊟ **SP** **M88.871** Osteitis deformans of right ankle and foot

⊟ **SP** **M88.872** Osteitis deformans of left ankle and foot

⊟ **IQ** **M88.879** Osteitis deformans of unspecified ankle and foot

SP **M88.88** Osteitis deformans of other bones

> **EXCLUDES 2**   osteitis deformans of skull (M88.0)
> osteitis deformans of vertebrae (M88.1)

SP **M88.89** Osteitis deformans of multiple sites

IQ **M88.9** Osteitis deformans of unspecified bone

4 **M89** Other disorders of bone

5 **M89.0** Algoneurodystrophy

    Shoulder-hand syndrome

    Sudeck's atrophy

> **EXCLUDES 1**   causalgia, lower limb (G57.7-)
> causalgia, upper limb (G56.4-)
> complex regional pain syndrome II, lower limb (G57.7-)
> complex regional pain syndrome II, upper limb (G56.4-)
> reflex sympathetic dystrophy (G90.5-)

> **DEFINITION**   Acute wasting away of bone(s) following relatively minor injury; presents with severe burning pain in the affected extremity, trophic changes in bone, and vasomotor disturbances without specific nerve injury.

IQ **M89.00** Algoneurodystrophy, unspecified site

6 **M89.01** Algoneurodystrophy, shoulder

⊟ **SP** **M89.011** Algoneurodystrophy, right shoulder

⊟ **SP** **M89.012** Algoneurodystrophy, left shoulder

⊟ **IQ** **M89.019** Algoneurodystrophy, unspecified shoulder

6 **M89.02** Algoneurodystrophy, upper arm

⊟ **SP** **M89.021** Algoneurodystrophy, right upper arm

⊟ **SP** **M89.022** Algoneurodystrophy, left upper arm

⊟ **IQ** **M89.029** Algoneurodystrophy, unspecified upper arm

6 **M89.03** Algoneurodystrophy, forearm

⊟ **SP** **M89.031** Algoneurodystrophy, right forearm

⊟ **SP** **M89.032** Algoneurodystrophy, left forearm

⊟ **IQ** **M89.039** Algoneurodystrophy, unspecified forearm

---

4 4th digit required   **5** 5th digit required   **6** 6th digit required   **7** 7th digit required   ☑ 7th digit placeholder   ✚ Additional code   ⊟ Laterality

⑥ **M89.04** Algoneurodystrophy, hand

⊟ **SP** **M89.041** Algoneurodystrophy, right hand

⊟ **SP** **M89.042** Algoneurodystrophy, left hand

⊟ **IQ** **M89.049** Algoneurodystrophy, unspecified hand

⑥ **M89.05** Algoneurodystrophy, thigh

⊟ **SP** **M89.051** Algoneurodystrophy, right thigh

⊟ **SP** **M89.052** Algoneurodystrophy, left thigh

⊟ **IQ** **M89.059** Algoneurodystrophy, unspecified thigh

⑥ **M89.06** Algoneurodystrophy, lower leg

⊟ **SP** **M89.061** Algoneurodystrophy, right lower leg

⊟ **SP** **M89.062** Algoneurodystrophy, left lower leg

⊟ **IQ** **M89.069** Algoneurodystrophy, unspecified lower leg

⑥ **M89.07** Algoneurodystrophy, ankle and foot

⊟ **SP** **M89.071** Algoneurodystrophy, right ankle and foot

⊟ **SP** **M89.072** Algoneurodystrophy, left ankle and foot

⊟ **IQ** **M89.079** Algoneurodystrophy, unspecified ankle and foot

SP **M89.08** Algoneurodystrophy, other site

SP **M89.09** Algoneurodystrophy, multiple sites

⑤ **M89.1** Physeal arrest
Arrest of growth plate
Epiphyseal arrest
Growth plate arrest

⑥ **M89.12** Physeal arrest, humerus

⊟ **SP** **M89.121** Complete physeal arrest, right proximal humerus

⊟ **SP** **M89.122** Complete physeal arrest, left proximal humerus

⊟ **SP** **M89.123** Partial physeal arrest, right proximal humerus

⊟ **SP** **M89.124** Partial physeal arrest, left proximal humerus

⊟ **SP** **M89.125** Complete physeal arrest, right distal humerus

⊟ **SP** **M89.126** Complete physeal arrest, left distal humerus

⊟ **SP** **M89.127** Partial physeal arrest, right distal humerus

⊟ **SP** **M89.128** Partial physeal arrest, left distal humerus

⊟ **IQ** **M89.129** Physeal arrest, humerus, unspecified

⑥ **M89.13** Physeal arrest, forearm

⊟ **SP** **M89.131** Complete physeal arrest, right distal radius

⊟ **SP** **M89.132** Complete physeal arrest, left distal radius

⊟ **SP** **M89.133** Partial physeal arrest, right distal radius

⊟ **SP** **M89.134** Partial physeal arrest, left distal radius

⊟ **SP** **M89.138** Other physeal arrest of forearm

⊟ **IQ** **M89.139** Physeal arrest, forearm, unspecified

⑥ **M89.15** Physeal arrest, femur

⊟ **SP** **M89.151** Complete physeal arrest, right proximal femur

⊟ **SP** **M89.152** Complete physeal arrest, left proximal femur

⊟ **SP** **M89.153** Partial physeal arrest, right proximal femur

⊟ **SP** **M89.154** Partial physeal arrest, left proximal femur

⊟ **SP** **M89.155** Complete physeal arrest, right distal femur

⊟ **SP** **M89.156** Complete physeal arrest, left distal femur

⊟ **SP** **M89.157** Partial physeal arrest, right distal femur

⊟ **SP** **M89.158** Partial physeal arrest, left distal femur

⊟ **IQ** **M89.159** Physeal arrest, femur, unspecified

⑥ **M89.16** Physeal arrest, lower leg

⊟ **SP** **M89.160** Complete physeal arrest, right proximal tibia

⊟ **SP** **M89.161** Complete physeal arrest, left proximal tibia

⊟ **SP** **M89.162** Partial physeal arrest, right proximal tibia

⊟ **SP** **M89.163** Partial physeal arrest, left proximal tibia

⊟ **SP** **M89.164** Complete physeal arrest, right distal tibia

⊟ **SP** **M89.165** Complete physeal arrest, left distal tibia

⊟ **SP** **M89.166** Partial physeal arrest, right distal tibia

⊟ **SP** **M89.167** Partial physeal arrest, left distal tibia

⊟ **SP** **M89.168** Other physeal arrest of lower leg

⊟ **IQ** **M89.169** Physeal arrest, lower leg, unspecified

SP **M89.18** Physeal arrest, other site

⑤ **M89.2** Other disorders of bone development and growth

IQ **M89.20** Other disorders of bone development and growth, unspecified site

⑥ **M89.21** Other disorders of bone development and growth, shoulder

⊟ **SP** **M89.211** Other disorders of bone development and growth, right shoulder

⊟ **SP** **M89.212** Other disorders of bone development and growth, left shoulder

⊟ **IQ** **M89.219** Other disorders of bone development and growth, unspecified shoulder

⑥ **M89.22** Other disorders of bone development and growth, humerus

⊟ **SP** **M89.221** Other disorders of bone development and growth, right humerus

⊟ **SP** **M89.222** Other disorders of bone development and growth, left humerus

⊟ **IQ** **M89.229** Other disorders of bone development and growth, unspecified humerus

⑥ **M89.23** Other disorders of bone development and growth, ulna and radius

★ New ▲ Revised Px Primary **SP** PDGM Px **SL** Low CoM **SH** High CoM **IQ** Quest. Encounter Ⓗ Hospice non-cancer Dx ⬚ Unspecified **M** *Manifestation*

DecisionHealth's FY 2020 Complete Home Health ICD-10-CM Diagnosis Coding Manual

1257

⊟ SP **M89.231** Other disorders of bone development and growth, right ulna

⊟ SP **M89.232** Other disorders of bone development and growth, left ulna

⊟ SP **M89.233** Other disorders of bone development and growth, right radius

⊟ SP **M89.234** Other disorders of bone development and growth, left radius

⊟ IQ **M89.239** Other disorders of bone development and growth, unspecified ulna and radius

⑥ **M89.24** Other disorders of bone development and growth, hand

⊟ SP **M89.241** Other disorders of bone development and growth, right hand

⊟ SP **M89.242** Other disorders of bone development and growth, left hand

⊟ IQ **M89.249** Other disorders of bone development and growth, unspecified hand

⑥ **M89.25** Other disorders of bone development and growth, femur

⊟ SP **M89.251** Other disorders of bone development and growth, right femur

⊟ SP **M89.252** Other disorders of bone development and growth, left femur

⊟ IQ **M89.259** Other disorders of bone development and growth, unspecified femur

⑥ **M89.26** Other disorders of bone development and growth, tibia and fibula

⊟ SP **M89.261** Other disorders of bone development and growth, right tibia

⊟ SP **M89.262** Other disorders of bone development and growth, left tibia

⊟ SP **M89.263** Other disorders of bone development and growth, right fibula

⊟ SP **M89.264** Other disorders of bone development and growth, left fibula

⊟ IQ **M89.269** Other disorders of bone development and growth, unspecified lower leg

⑥ **M89.27** Other disorders of bone development and growth, ankle and foot

⊟ SP **M89.271** Other disorders of bone development and growth, right ankle and foot

⊟ SP **M89.272** Other disorders of bone development and growth, left ankle and foot

⊟ IQ **M89.279** Other disorders of bone development and growth, unspecified ankle and foot

SP **M89.28** Other disorders of bone development and growth, other site

SP **M89.29** Other disorders of bone development and growth, multiple sites

⑤ **M89.3 Hypertrophy of bone**

IQ **M89.30** Hypertrophy of bone, unspecified site

⑥ **M89.31** Hypertrophy of bone, shoulder

⊟ SP **M89.311** Hypertrophy of bone, right shoulder

⊟ SP **M89.312** Hypertrophy of bone, left shoulder

⊟ IQ **M89.319** Hypertrophy of bone, unspecified shoulder

⑥ **M89.32** Hypertrophy of bone, humerus

⊟ SP **M89.321** Hypertrophy of bone, right humerus

⊟ SP **M89.322** Hypertrophy of bone, left humerus

⊟ IQ **M89.329** Hypertrophy of bone, unspecified humerus

⑥ **M89.33** Hypertrophy of bone, ulna and radius

⊟ SP **M89.331** Hypertrophy of bone, right ulna

⊟ SP **M89.332** Hypertrophy of bone, left ulna

⊟ SP **M89.333** Hypertrophy of bone, right radius

⊟ SP **M89.334** Hypertrophy of bone, left radius

⊟ IQ **M89.339** Hypertrophy of bone, unspecified ulna and radius

⑥ **M89.34** Hypertrophy of bone, hand

⊟ SP **M89.341** Hypertrophy of bone, right hand

⊟ SP **M89.342** Hypertrophy of bone, left hand

⊟ IQ **M89.349** Hypertrophy of bone, unspecified hand

⑥ **M89.35** Hypertrophy of bone, femur

⊟ SP **M89.351** Hypertrophy of bone, right femur

⊟ SP **M89.352** Hypertrophy of bone, left femur

⊟ IQ **M89.359** Hypertrophy of bone, unspecified femur

⑥ **M89.36** Hypertrophy of bone, tibia and fibula

⊟ SP **M89.361** Hypertrophy of bone, right tibia

⊟ SP **M89.362** Hypertrophy of bone, left tibia

⊟ SP **M89.363** Hypertrophy of bone, right fibula

⊟ SP **M89.364** Hypertrophy of bone, left fibula

⊟ IQ **M89.369** Hypertrophy of bone, unspecified tibia and fibula

⑥ **M89.37** Hypertrophy of bone, ankle and foot

⊟ SP **M89.371** Hypertrophy of bone, right ankle and foot

⊟ SP **M89.372** Hypertrophy of bone, left ankle and foot

⊟ IQ **M89.379** Hypertrophy of bone, unspecified ankle and foot

SP **M89.38** Hypertrophy of bone, other site

SP **M89.39** Hypertrophy of bone, multiple sites

⑤ **M89.4 Other hypertrophic osteoarthropathy**
Marie-Bamberger disease
Pachydermoperiostosis

IQ **M89.40** Other hypertrophic osteoarthropathy, unspecified site

⑥ **M89.41** Other hypertrophic osteoarthropathy, shoulder

⊟ SP **M89.411** Other hypertrophic osteoarthropathy, right shoulder

◢4th digit required   ⑤5th digit required   ⑥6th digit required   ⑦7th digit required   ⑦7th digit placeholder   ✚Additional code   ⊟Laterality

1258   *DecisionHealth's* FY 2020 Complete Home Health ICD-10-CM Diagnosis Coding Manual

⊟ SP M89.412 Other hypertrophic osteoarthropathy, left shoulder

⊟ IQ M89.419 Other hypertrophic osteoarthropathy, unspecified shoulder

⑥ M89.42 Other hypertrophic osteoarthropathy, upper arm

⊟ SP M89.421 Other hypertrophic osteoarthropathy, right upper arm

⊟ SP M89.422 Other hypertrophic osteoarthropathy, left upper arm

⊟ IQ M89.429 Other hypertrophic osteoarthropathy, unspecified upper arm

⑥ M89.43 Other hypertrophic osteoarthropathy, forearm

⊟ SP M89.431 Other hypertrophic osteoarthropathy, right forearm

⊟ SP M89.432 Other hypertrophic osteoarthropathy, left forearm

⊟ IQ M89.439 Other hypertrophic osteoarthropathy, unspecified forearm

⑥ M89.44 Other hypertrophic osteoarthropathy, hand

⊟ SP M89.441 Other hypertrophic osteoarthropathy, right hand

⊟ SP M89.442 Other hypertrophic osteoarthropathy, left hand

⊟ IQ M89.449 Other hypertrophic osteoarthropathy, unspecified hand

⑥ M89.45 Other hypertrophic osteoarthropathy, thigh

⊟ SP M89.451 Other hypertrophic osteoarthropathy, right thigh

⊟ SP M89.452 Other hypertrophic osteoarthropathy, left thigh

⊟ IQ M89.459 Other hypertrophic osteoarthropathy, unspecified thigh

⑥ M89.46 Other hypertrophic osteoarthropathy, lower leg

⊟ SP M89.461 Other hypertrophic osteoarthropathy, right lower leg

⊟ SP M89.462 Other hypertrophic osteoarthropathy, left lower leg

⊟ IQ M89.469 Other hypertrophic osteoarthropathy, unspecified lower leg

⑥ M89.47 Other hypertrophic osteoarthropathy, ankle and foot

⊟ SP M89.471 Other hypertrophic osteoarthropathy, right ankle and foot

⊟ SP M89.472 Other hypertrophic osteoarthropathy, left ankle and foot

⊟ IQ M89.479 Other hypertrophic osteoarthropathy, unspecified ankle and foot

SP M89.48 Other hypertrophic osteoarthropathy, other site

SP M89.49 Other hypertrophic osteoarthropathy, multiple sites

➕ ⑤ M89.5 Osteolysis

Use additional code to identify major osseous defect, if applicable (M89.7-)

EXCLUDES 2 periprosthetic osteolysis of internal prosthetic joint (T84.05-)

IQ ➕ M89.50 Osteolysis, unspecified site

➕ ⑥ M89.51 Osteolysis, shoulder

⊟ SP ➕ M89.511 Osteolysis, right shoulder

⊟ SP ➕ M89.512 Osteolysis, left shoulder

⊟ IQ ➕ M89.519 Osteolysis, unspecified shoulder

➕ ⑥ M89.52 Osteolysis, upper arm

⊟ SP ➕ M89.521 Osteolysis, right upper arm

⊟ SP ➕ M89.522 Osteolysis, left upper arm

⊟ IQ ➕ M89.529 Osteolysis, unspecified upper arm

➕ ⑥ M89.53 Osteolysis, forearm

⊟ SP ➕ M89.531 Osteolysis, right forearm

⊟ SP ➕ M89.532 Osteolysis, left forearm

⊟ IQ ➕ M89.539 Osteolysis, unspecified forearm

➕ ⑥ M89.54 Osteolysis, hand

⊟ SP ➕ M89.541 Osteolysis, right hand

⊟ SP ➕ M89.542 Osteolysis, left hand

⊟ IQ ➕ M89.549 Osteolysis, unspecified hand

➕ ⑥ M89.55 Osteolysis, thigh

⊟ SP ➕ M89.551 Osteolysis, right thigh

⊟ SP ➕ M89.552 Osteolysis, left thigh

⊟ IQ ➕ M89.559 Osteolysis, unspecified thigh

➕ ⑥ M89.56 Osteolysis, lower leg

⊟ SP ➕ M89.561 Osteolysis, right lower leg

⊟ SP ➕ M89.562 Osteolysis, left lower leg

⊟ IQ ➕ M89.569 Osteolysis, unspecified lower leg

➕ ⑥ M89.57 Osteolysis, ankle and foot

⊟ SP ➕ M89.571 Osteolysis, right ankle and foot

⊟ SP ➕ M89.572 Osteolysis, left ankle and foot

⊟ IQ ➕ M89.579 Osteolysis, unspecified ankle and foot

SP ➕ M89.58 Osteolysis, other site

SP ➕ M89.59 Osteolysis, multiple sites

➕ ⑤ M89.6 Osteopathy after poliomyelitis

Use additional code (B91) to identify previous poliomyelitis

EXCLUDES 1 postpolio syndrome (G14)

IQ ➕ M89.60 Osteopathy after poliomyelitis, unspecified site

CODING TIPS ✓ Osteopathy caused by polio will be coded as a sequela of polio with code B91 as an additional code.

➕ ⑥ M89.61 Osteopathy after poliomyelitis, shoulder

⊟ SP ➕ M89.611 Osteopathy after poliomyelitis, right shoulder

⊟ SP ➕ M89.612 Osteopathy after poliomyelitis, left shoulder

⊟ IQ ➕ M89.619 Osteopathy after poliomyelitis, unspecified shoulder

➕ ⑥ M89.62 Osteopathy after poliomyelitis, upper arm

⊟ SP ➕ M89.621 Osteopathy after poliomyelitis, right upper arm

★ New ▲ Revised Px Primary SP PDGM Px SL Low CoM SH High CoM IQ Quest. Encounter H Hospice non-cancer Dx   Unspecified   M *Manifestation*

DecisionHealth's FY 2020 Complete Home Health ICD-10-CM Diagnosis Coding Manual   1259

⊟ **SP** ✚ **M89.622** Osteopathy after poliomyelitis, left upper arm

⊟ **IQ** ✚ **M89.629** Osteopathy after poliomyelitis, unspecified upper arm

✚ **⑥ M89.63** Osteopathy after poliomyelitis, forearm

⊟ **SP** ✚ **M89.631** Osteopathy after poliomyelitis, right forearm

⊟ **SP** ✚ **M89.632** Osteopathy after poliomyelitis, left forearm

⊟ **IQ** ✚ **M89.639** Osteopathy after poliomyelitis, unspecified forearm

✚ **⑥ M89.64** Osteopathy after poliomyelitis, hand

⊟ **SP** ✚ **M89.641** Osteopathy after poliomyelitis, right hand

⊟ **SP** ✚ **M89.642** Osteopathy after poliomyelitis, left hand

⊟ **IQ** ✚ **M89.649** Osteopathy after poliomyelitis, unspecified hand

✚ **⑥ M89.65** Osteopathy after poliomyelitis, thigh

⊟ **SP** ✚ **M89.651** Osteopathy after poliomyelitis, right thigh

⊟ **SP** ✚ **M89.652** Osteopathy after poliomyelitis, left thigh

⊟ **IQ** ✚ **M89.659** Osteopathy after poliomyelitis, unspecified thigh

✚ **⑥ M89.66** Osteopathy after poliomyelitis, lower leg

⊟ **SP** ✚ **M89.661** Osteopathy after poliomyelitis, right lower leg

⊟ **SP** ✚ **M89.662** Osteopathy after poliomyelitis, left lower leg

⊟ **IQ** ✚ **M89.669** Osteopathy after poliomyelitis, unspecified lower leg

✚ **⑥ M89.67** Osteopathy after poliomyelitis, ankle and foot

⊟ **SP** ✚ **M89.671** Osteopathy after poliomyelitis, right ankle and foot

⊟ **SP** ✚ **M89.672** Osteopathy after poliomyelitis, left ankle and foot

⊟ **IQ** ✚ **M89.679** Osteopathy after poliomyelitis, unspecified ankle and foot

SP ✚ **M89.68** Osteopathy after poliomyelitis, other site

SP ✚ **M89.69** Osteopathy after poliomyelitis, multiple sites

⑤ M89.7 Major osseous defect
> Code first underlying disease, if known, such as:
> aseptic necrosis of bone (M87.-)
> malignant neoplasm of bone (C40.-)
> osteolysis (M89.5)
> osteomyelitis (M86.-)
> osteonecrosis (M87.-)
> osteoporosis (M80.-, M81.-)
> periprosthetic osteolysis (T84.05-)

IQ **M89.70** Major osseous defect, unspecified site

⑥ M89.71 Major osseous defect, shoulder region
> Major osseous defect clavicle or scapula

⊟ **SP** **M89.711** Major osseous defect, right shoulder region

⊟ **SP** **M89.712** Major osseous defect, left shoulder region

⊟ **IQ** **M89.719** Major osseous defect, unspecified shoulder region

⑥ M89.72 Major osseous defect, humerus

⊟ **SP** **M89.721** Major osseous defect, right humerus

⊟ **SP** **M89.722** Major osseous defect, left humerus

⊟ **IQ** **M89.729** Major osseous defect, unspecified humerus

⑥ M89.73 Major osseous defect, forearm
> Major osseous defect of radius and ulna

⊟ **SP** **M89.731** Major osseous defect, right forearm

⊟ **SP** **M89.732** Major osseous defect, left forearm

⊟ **IQ** **M89.739** Major osseous defect, unspecified forearm

⑥ M89.74 Major osseous defect, hand
> Major osseous defect of carpus, fingers, metacarpus

⊟ **SP** **M89.741** Major osseous defect, right hand

⊟ **SP** **M89.742** Major osseous defect, left hand

⊟ **IQ** **M89.749** Major osseous defect, unspecified hand

⑥ M89.75 Major osseous defect, pelvic region and thigh
> Major osseous defect of femur and pelvis

⊟ **SP** **M89.751** Major osseous defect, right pelvic region and thigh

⊟ **SP** **M89.752** Major osseous defect, left pelvic region and thigh

⊟ **IQ** **M89.759** Major osseous defect, unspecified pelvic region and thigh

⑥ M89.76 Major osseous defect, lower leg
> Major osseous defect of fibula and tibia

⊟ **SP** **M89.761** Major osseous defect, right lower leg

⊟ **SP** **M89.762** Major osseous defect, left lower leg

⊟ **IQ** **M89.769** Major osseous defect, unspecified lower leg

⑥ M89.77 Major osseous defect, ankle and foot
> Major osseous defect of metatarsus, tarsus, toes

⊟ **SP** **M89.771** Major osseous defect, right ankle and foot

⊟ **SP** **M89.772** Major osseous defect, left ankle and foot

⊟ **IQ** **M89.779** Major osseous defect, unspecified ankle and foot

SP **M89.78** Major osseous defect, other site

SP **M89.79** Major osseous defect, multiple sites

⑤ M89.8 Other specified disorders of bone
> Infantile cortical hyperostoses
> Post-traumatic subperiosteal ossification

⑥ M89.8X Other specified disorders of bone

SP **M89.8X0** Other specified disorders of bone, multiple sites

SP **M89.8X1** Other specified disorders of bone, shoulder

SP **M89.8X2** Other specified disorders of bone, upper arm

SP **M89.8X3** Other specified disorders of bone, forearm

44th digit required   **5**5th digit required   **6**6th digit required   **7**7th digit required   **⑦**7th digit placeholder   ✚Additional code   ⊟Laterality

1260   *DecisionHealth's* FY 2020 Complete Home Health ICD-10-CM Diagnosis Coding Manual

SP M89.8X4 Other specified disorders of bone, hand

SP M89.8X5 Other specified disorders of bone, thigh

SP M89.8X6 Other specified disorders of bone, lower leg

SP M89.8X7 Other specified disorders of bone, ankle and foot

SP M89.8X8 Other specified disorders of bone, other site

IQ M89.8X9 Other specified disorders of bone, unspecified site

IQ M89.9 Disorder of bone, unspecified

4 M90 Osteopathies in diseases classified elsewhere

> EXCLUDES 1 osteochondritis, osteomyelitis, and osteopathy (in) :
> cryptococcosis (B45.3)
> diabetes mellitus (E08-E13 with .69-)
> gonococcal (A54.43)
> neurogenic syphilis (A52.11)
> renal osteodystrophy (N25.0)
> salmonellosis (A02.24)
> secondary syphilis (A51.46)
> syphilis (late) (A52.77)

5 M90.5 Osteonecrosis in diseases classified elsewhere

> Code first underlying disease, such as:
> caisson disease (T70.3)
> hemoglobinopathy (D50-D64)

M IQ M90.50 *Osteonecrosis in diseases classified elsewhere, unspecified site*

6 M90.51 Osteonecrosis in diseases classified elsewhere, shoulder

M ⊟ IQ M90.511 *Osteonecrosis in diseases classified elsewhere, right shoulder*

M ⊟ IQ M90.512 *Osteonecrosis in diseases classified elsewhere, left shoulder*

M ⊟ IQ M90.519 *Osteonecrosis in diseases classified elsewhere, unspecified shoulder*

6 M90.52 Osteonecrosis in diseases classified elsewhere, upper arm

M ⊟ IQ M90.521 *Osteonecrosis in diseases classified elsewhere, right upper arm*

M ⊟ IQ M90.522 *Osteonecrosis in diseases classified elsewhere, left upper arm*

M ⊟ IQ M90.529 *Osteonecrosis in diseases classified elsewhere, unspecified upper arm*

6 M90.53 Osteonecrosis in diseases classified elsewhere, forearm

M ⊟ IQ M90.531 *Osteonecrosis in diseases classified elsewhere, right forearm*

M ⊟ IQ M90.532 *Osteonecrosis in diseases classified elsewhere, left forearm*

M ⊟ IQ M90.539 *Osteonecrosis in diseases classified elsewhere, unspecified forearm*

6 M90.54 Osteonecrosis in diseases classified elsewhere, hand

M ⊟ IQ M90.541 *Osteonecrosis in diseases classified elsewhere, right hand*

M ⊟ IQ M90.542 *Osteonecrosis in diseases classified elsewhere, left hand*

M ⊟ IQ M90.549 *Osteonecrosis in diseases classified elsewhere, unspecified hand*

6 M90.55 Osteonecrosis in diseases classified elsewhere, thigh

M ⊟ IQ M90.551 *Osteonecrosis in diseases classified elsewhere, right thigh*

M ⊟ IQ M90.552 *Osteonecrosis in diseases classified elsewhere, left thigh*

M ⊟ IQ M90.559 *Osteonecrosis in diseases classified elsewhere, unspecified thigh*

6 M90.56 Osteonecrosis in diseases classified elsewhere, lower leg

M ⊟ IQ M90.561 *Osteonecrosis in diseases classified elsewhere, right lower leg*

M ⊟ IQ M90.562 *Osteonecrosis in diseases classified elsewhere, left lower leg*

M ⊟ IQ M90.569 *Osteonecrosis in diseases classified elsewhere, unspecified lower leg*

6 M90.57 Osteonecrosis in diseases classified elsewhere, ankle and foot

M ⊟ IQ M90.571 *Osteonecrosis in diseases classified elsewhere, right ankle and foot*

M ⊟ IQ M90.572 *Osteonecrosis in diseases classified elsewhere, left ankle and foot*

M ⊟ IQ M90.579 *Osteonecrosis in diseases classified elsewhere, unspecified ankle and foot*

M IQ M90.58 *Osteonecrosis in diseases classified elsewhere, other site*

M IQ M90.59 *Osteonecrosis in diseases classified elsewhere, multiple sites*

5 M90.6 Osteitis deformans in neoplastic diseases
Osteitis deformans in malignant neoplasm of bone

> Code first:
> the neoplasm (C40.-, C41.-)
> EXCLUDES 1 osteitis deformans [Paget's disease of bone] (M88.-)
> DEFINITION Excessive breakdown with abnormal reformation of bone tissue in the presence of a malignant neoplasm of the bone; results in painful, deformed bones prone to pathological fractures.

M IQ M90.60 *Osteitis deformans in neoplastic diseases, unspecified site*

6 M90.61 Osteitis deformans in neoplastic diseases, shoulder

M ⊟ IQ M90.611 *Osteitis deformans in neoplastic diseases, right shoulder*

M ⊟ IQ M90.612 *Osteitis deformans in neoplastic diseases, left shoulder*

M ⊟ IQ M90.619 *Osteitis deformans in neoplastic diseases, unspecified shoulder*

6 M90.62 Osteitis deformans in neoplastic diseases, upper arm

★ New ▲ Revised Px Primary SP PDGM Px SL Low CoM SH High CoM IQ Quest. Encounter H Hospice non-cancer Dx Unspecified M *Manifestation*

DecisionHealth's FY 2020 Complete Home Health ICD-10-CM Diagnosis Coding Manual

1261

M ⊟ IQ **M90.621** *Osteitis deformans in neoplastic diseases, right upper arm*

M ⊟ IQ **M90.622** *Osteitis deformans in neoplastic diseases, left upper arm*

M ⊟ IQ **M90.629** *Osteitis deformans in neoplastic diseases, unspecified upper arm*

⑥ **M90.63** Osteitis deformans in neoplastic diseases, forearm

M ⊟ IQ **M90.631** *Osteitis deformans in neoplastic diseases, right forearm*

M ⊟ IQ **M90.632** *Osteitis deformans in neoplastic diseases, left forearm*

M ⊟ IQ **M90.639** *Osteitis deformans in neoplastic diseases, unspecified forearm*

⑥ **M90.64** Osteitis deformans in neoplastic diseases, hand

M ⊟ IQ **M90.641** *Osteitis deformans in neoplastic diseases, right hand*

M ⊟ IQ **M90.642** *Osteitis deformans in neoplastic diseases, left hand*

M ⊟ IQ **M90.649** *Osteitis deformans in neoplastic diseases, unspecified hand*

⑥ **M90.65** Osteitis deformans in neoplastic diseases, thigh

M ⊟ IQ **M90.651** *Osteitis deformans in neoplastic diseases, right thigh*

M ⊟ IQ **M90.652** *Osteitis deformans in neoplastic diseases, left thigh*

M ⊟ IQ **M90.659** *Osteitis deformans in neoplastic diseases, unspecified thigh*

⑥ **M90.66** Osteitis deformans in neoplastic diseases, lower leg

M ⊟ IQ **M90.661** *Osteitis deformans in neoplastic diseases, right lower leg*

M ⊟ IQ **M90.662** *Osteitis deformans in neoplastic diseases, left lower leg*

M ⊟ IQ **M90.669** *Osteitis deformans in neoplastic diseases, unspecified lower leg*

⑥ **M90.67** Osteitis deformans in neoplastic diseases, ankle and foot

M ⊟ IQ **M90.671** *Osteitis deformans in neoplastic diseases, right ankle and foot*

M ⊟ IQ **M90.672** *Osteitis deformans in neoplastic diseases, left ankle and foot*

M ⊟ IQ **M90.679** *Osteitis deformans in neoplastic diseases, unspecified ankle and foot*

M IQ **M90.68** *Osteitis deformans in neoplastic diseases, other site*

M IQ **M90.69** *Osteitis deformans in neoplastic diseases, multiple sites*

⑤ **M90.8** Osteopathy in diseases classified elsewhere

Code first underlying disease, such as:
  rickets (E55.0)
  vitamin-D-resistant rickets (E83.3)

CODING TIPS ✓   The addition of this code is not necessary for diabetic osteomyelitis. If diabetic osteomyelitis is confirmed, use the appropriate diabetes category (E08-E13) with 4th and 5th digits .69 followed by the osteomyelitis. Query the physician if acute or chronic is not documented.

M IQ **M90.80** *Osteopathy in diseases classified elsewhere, unspecified site*

⑥ **M90.81** Osteopathy in diseases classified elsewhere, shoulder

M ⊟ IQ **M90.811** *Osteopathy in diseases classified elsewhere, right shoulder*

M ⊟ IQ **M90.812** *Osteopathy in diseases classified elsewhere, left shoulder*

M ⊟ IQ **M90.819** *Osteopathy in diseases classified elsewhere, unspecified shoulder*

⑥ **M90.82** Osteopathy in diseases classified elsewhere, upper arm

M ⊟ IQ **M90.821** *Osteopathy in diseases classified elsewhere, right upper arm*

M ⊟ IQ **M90.822** *Osteopathy in diseases classified elsewhere, left upper arm*

M ⊟ IQ **M90.829** *Osteopathy in diseases classified elsewhere, unspecified upper arm*

⑥ **M90.83** Osteopathy in diseases classified elsewhere, forearm

M ⊟ IQ **M90.831** *Osteopathy in diseases classified elsewhere, right forearm*

M ⊟ IQ **M90.832** *Osteopathy in diseases classified elsewhere, left forearm*

M ⊟ IQ **M90.839** *Osteopathy in diseases classified elsewhere, unspecified forearm*

⑥ **M90.84** Osteopathy in diseases classified elsewhere, hand

M ⊟ IQ **M90.841** *Osteopathy in diseases classified elsewhere, right hand*

M ⊟ IQ **M90.842** *Osteopathy in diseases classified elsewhere, left hand*

M ⊟ IQ **M90.849** *Osteopathy in diseases classified elsewhere, unspecified hand*

⑥ **M90.85** Osteopathy in diseases classified elsewhere, thigh

M ⊟ IQ **M90.851** *Osteopathy in diseases classified elsewhere, right thigh*

M ⊟ IQ **M90.852** *Osteopathy in diseases classified elsewhere, left thigh*

M ⊟ IQ **M90.859** *Osteopathy in diseases classified elsewhere, unspecified thigh*

⑥ **M90.86** Osteopathy in diseases classified elsewhere, lower leg

M ⊟ IQ **M90.861** *Osteopathy in diseases classified elsewhere, right lower leg*

M ⊟ IQ **M90.862** *Osteopathy in diseases classified elsewhere, left lower leg*

M ⊟ IQ **M90.869** *Osteopathy in diseases classified elsewhere, unspecified lower leg*

⑥ **M90.87** Osteopathy in diseases classified elsewhere, ankle and foot

M ⊟ IQ **M90.871** *Osteopathy in diseases classified elsewhere, right ankle and foot*

M ⊟ IQ **M90.872** *Osteopathy in diseases classified elsewhere, left ankle and foot*

M ⊟ IQ **M90.879** *Osteopathy in diseases classified elsewhere, unspecified ankle and foot*

M IQ **M90.88** *Osteopathy in diseases classified elsewhere, other site*

M IQ **M90.89** *Osteopathy in diseases classified elsewhere, multiple sites*

---

④4th digit required   ⑤5th digit required   ⑥6th digit required   ⑦7th digit required   ⑦7th digit placeholder   ✚Additional code   ⊟Laterality

Chondropathies (M91-M94)

EXCLUDES 1 postprocedural chondropathies (M96.-)

4 M91 Juvenile osteochondrosis of hip and pelvis

   EXCLUDES 1 slipped upper femoral epiphysis (nontraumatic) (M93.0)

SP M91.0 Juvenile osteochondrosis of pelvis
Osteochondrosis (juvenile) of acetabulum
Osteochondrosis (juvenile) of iliac crest [Buchanan]
Osteochondrosis (juvenile) of ischiopubic synchondrosis [van Neck]
Osteochondrosis (juvenile) of symphysis pubis [Pierson]

5 M91.1 Juvenile osteochondrosis of head of femur [Legg-Calvé-Perthes]

   DEFINITION Disruption of blood supply to the femoral head epiphysis in children, resulting in death of bone; occurs most commonly in boys age 4-8.

IQ M91.10 Juvenile osteochondrosis of head of femur [Legg-Calvé-Perthes], unspecified leg

SP M91.11 Juvenile osteochondrosis of head of femur [Legg-Calvé-Perthes], right leg

SP M91.12 Juvenile osteochondrosis of head of femur [Legg-Calvé-Perthes], left leg

5 M91.2 Coxa plana
Hip deformity due to previous juvenile osteochondrosis

   DEFINITION Residual effect of Legg-Calve-Perthes in which the necrotic bone of the normally rounded femoral head is flattened due to gradual bone replacement; secondary deformity of the acetabulum occurs with growth.

IQ M91.20 Coxa plana, unspecified hip

SP M91.21 Coxa plana, right hip

SP M91.22 Coxa plana, left hip

5 M91.3 Pseudocoxalgia

IQ M91.30 Pseudocoxalgia, unspecified hip

SP M91.31 Pseudocoxalgia, right hip

SP M91.32 Pseudocoxalgia, left hip

5 M91.4 Coxa magna

   DEFINITION Residual effect of Legg-Calve-Perthes in which the femoral head is enlarged, becoming broad and overgrown due to the gradual bone replacement process.

IQ M91.40 Coxa magna, unspecified hip

SP M91.41 Coxa magna, right hip

SP M91.42 Coxa magna, left hip

5 M91.8 Other juvenile osteochondrosis of hip and pelvis
Juvenile osteochondrosis after reduction of congenital dislocation of hip

IQ M91.80 Other juvenile osteochondrosis of hip and pelvis, unspecified leg

SP M91.81 Other juvenile osteochondrosis of hip and pelvis, right leg

SP M91.82 Other juvenile osteochondrosis of hip and pelvis, left leg

5 M91.9 Juvenile osteochondrosis of hip and pelvis, unspecified

IQ M91.90 Juvenile osteochondrosis of hip and pelvis, unspecified, unspecified leg

SP M91.91 Juvenile osteochondrosis of hip and pelvis, unspecified, right leg

SP M91.92 Juvenile osteochondrosis of hip and pelvis, unspecified, left leg

4 M92 Other juvenile osteochondrosis

   DEFINITION Condition of unknown etiology affecting the developing growth plate and ossification centers in children where increased stress occurs; genetics, repeated trauma, mechanical factors, hormone imbalances, and vascular abnormalities may be a factor.

5 M92.0 Juvenile osteochondrosis of humerus
Osteochondrosis (juvenile) of capitulum of humerus [Panner]
Osteochondrosis (juvenile) of head of humerus [Haas]

IQ M92.00 Juvenile osteochondrosis of humerus, unspecified arm

SP M92.01 Juvenile osteochondrosis of humerus, right arm

SP M92.02 Juvenile osteochondrosis of humerus, left arm

5 M92.1 Juvenile osteochondrosis of radius and ulna
Osteochondrosis (juvenile) of lower ulna [Burns]
Osteochondrosis (juvenile) of radial head [Brailsford]

IQ M92.10 Juvenile osteochondrosis of radius and ulna, unspecified arm

SP M92.11 Juvenile osteochondrosis of radius and ulna, right arm

SP M92.12 Juvenile osteochondrosis of radius and ulna, left arm

5 M92.2 Juvenile osteochondrosis, hand

6 M92.20 Unspecified juvenile osteochondrosis, hand

SP M92.201 Unspecified juvenile osteochondrosis, right hand

SP M92.202 Unspecified juvenile osteochondrosis, left hand

IQ M92.209 Unspecified juvenile osteochondrosis, unspecified hand

6 M92.21 Osteochondrosis (juvenile) of carpal lunate [Kienböck]

SP M92.211 Osteochondrosis (juvenile) of carpal lunate [Kienböck], right hand

SP M92.212 Osteochondrosis (juvenile) of carpal lunate [Kienböck], left hand

IQ M92.219 Osteochondrosis (juvenile) of carpal lunate [Kienböck], unspecified hand

6 M92.22 Osteochondrosis (juvenile) of metacarpal heads [Mauclaire]

SP M92.221 Osteochondrosis (juvenile) of metacarpal heads [Mauclaire], right hand

---

★ New ▲ Revised Px Primary SP PDGM Px SL Low CoM SH High CoM IQ Quest. Encounter H Hospice non-cancer Dx Unspecified M *Manifestation*

DecisionHealth's FY 2020 Complete Home Health ICD-10-CM Diagnosis Coding Manual   1263

⊟ **SP** **M92.222** Osteochondrosis (juvenile) of metacarpal heads [Mauclaire], left hand

⊟ **IQ** **M92.229** Osteochondrosis (juvenile) of metacarpal heads [Mauclaire], unspecified hand

⑥ **M92.29** Other juvenile osteochondrosis, hand

⊟ **SP** **M92.291** Other juvenile osteochondrosis, right hand

⊟ **SP** **M92.292** Other juvenile osteochondrosis, left hand

⊟ **IQ** **M92.299** Other juvenile osteochondrosis, unspecified hand

⑤ **M92.3** Other juvenile osteochondrosis, upper limb

⊟ **IQ** **M92.30** Other juvenile osteochondrosis, unspecified upper limb

⊟ **SP** **M92.31** Other juvenile osteochondrosis, right upper limb

⊟ **SP** **M92.32** Other juvenile osteochondrosis, left upper limb

⑤ **M92.4** Juvenile osteochondrosis of patella
Osteochondrosis (juvenile) of primary patellar center [Köhler]
Osteochondrosis (juvenile) of secondary patellar centre [Sinding Larsen]

⊟ **IQ** **M92.40** Juvenile osteochondrosis of patella, unspecified knee

⊟ **SP** **M92.41** Juvenile osteochondrosis of patella, right knee

⊟ **SP** **M92.42** Juvenile osteochondrosis of patella, left knee

⑤ **M92.5** Juvenile osteochondrosis of tibia and fibula
Osteochondrosis (juvenile) of proximal tibia [Blount]
Osteochondrosis (juvenile) of tibial tubercle [Osgood-Schlatter]
Tibia vara

⊟ **IQ** **M92.50** Juvenile osteochondrosis of tibia and fibula, unspecified leg

⊟ **SP** **M92.51** Juvenile osteochondrosis of tibia and fibula, right leg

⊟ **SP** **M92.52** Juvenile osteochondrosis of tibia and fibula, left leg

⑤ **M92.6** Juvenile osteochondrosis of tarsus
Osteochondrosis (juvenile) of calcaneum [Sever]
Osteochondrosis (juvenile) of os tibiale externum [Haglund]
Osteochondrosis (juvenile) of talus [Diaz]
Osteochondrosis (juvenile) of tarsal navicular [Köhler]

⊟ **IQ** **M92.60** Juvenile osteochondrosis of tarsus, unspecified ankle

⊟ **SP** **M92.61** Juvenile osteochondrosis of tarsus, right ankle

⊟ **SP** **M92.62** Juvenile osteochondrosis of tarsus, left ankle

⑤ **M92.7** Juvenile osteochondrosis of metatarsus
Osteochondrosis (juvenile) of fifth metatarsus [Iselin]
Osteochondrosis (juvenile) of second metatarsus [Freiberg]

⊟ **IQ** **M92.70** Juvenile osteochondrosis of metatarsus, unspecified foot

⊟ **SP** **M92.71** Juvenile osteochondrosis of metatarsus, right foot

⊟ **SP** **M92.72** Juvenile osteochondrosis of metatarsus, left foot

SP **M92.8** Other specified juvenile osteochondrosis
Calcaneal apophysitis

IQ **M92.9** Juvenile osteochondrosis, unspecified
Juvenile apophysitis NOS
Juvenile epiphysitis NOS
Juvenile osteochondritis NOS
Juvenile osteochondrosis NOS

④ **M93** Other osteochondropathies
EXCLUDES 2   osteochondrosis of spine (M42.-)

➕ ⑤ **M93.0** Slipped upper femoral epiphysis (nontraumatic)
Use additional code for associated chondrolysis (M94.3)
DEFINITION   Nontraumatic slippage of the femoral head of the epiphysis occurring in adolescence.

➕ ⑥ **M93.00** Unspecified slipped upper femoral epiphysis (nontraumatic)

⊟ **SP** ➕ **M93.001** Unspecified slipped upper femoral epiphysis (nontraumatic), right hip

⊟ **SP** ➕ **M93.002** Unspecified slipped upper femoral epiphysis (nontraumatic), left hip

⊟ **IQ** ➕ **M93.003** Unspecified slipped upper femoral epiphysis (nontraumatic), unspecified hip

➕ ⑥ **M93.01** Acute slipped upper femoral epiphysis (nontraumatic)

⊟ **SP** ➕ **M93.011** Acute slipped upper femoral epiphysis (nontraumatic), right hip

⊟ **SP** ➕ **M93.012** Acute slipped upper femoral epiphysis (nontraumatic), left hip

⊟ **IQ** ➕ **M93.013** Acute slipped upper femoral epiphysis (nontraumatic), unspecified hip

➕ ⑥ **M93.02** Chronic slipped upper femoral epiphysis (nontraumatic)

⊟ **SP** ➕ **M93.021** Chronic slipped upper femoral epiphysis (nontraumatic), right hip

⊟ **SP** ➕ **M93.022** Chronic slipped upper femoral epiphysis (nontraumatic), left hip

⊟ **IQ** ➕ **M93.023** Chronic slipped upper femoral epiphysis (nontraumatic), unspecified hip

➕ ⑥ **M93.03** Acute on chronic slipped upper femoral epiphysis (nontraumatic)

⊟ **SP** ➕ **M93.031** Acute on chronic slipped upper femoral epiphysis (nontraumatic), right hip

⊟ **SP** ➕ **M93.032** Acute on chronic slipped upper femoral epiphysis (nontraumatic), left hip

⊟ **IQ** ➕ **M93.033** Acute on chronic slipped upper femoral epiphysis (nontraumatic), unspecified hip

SP **M93.1** Kienböck's disease of adults
Adult osteochondrosis of carpal lunates

---

④4th digit required   ⑤5th digit required   ⑥6th digit required   ⑦7th digit required   ⑦7th digit placeholder   ➕Additional code   ⊟Laterality

1264   *DecisionHealth's* FY 2020 Complete Home Health ICD-10-CM Diagnosis Coding Manual

DEFINITION Idiopathic disruption of blood supply to the carpal lunate bone in adults, resulting in death of the bone tissue.

⑤ **M93.2 Osteochondritis dissecans**

DEFINITION Joint condition in which a piece of cartilage and thin, underlying bone detaches from the bone's end; occurs most often in boys age 10-20 after a joint injury, and commonly affecting the knee.

IQ M93.20 Osteochondritis dissecans of unspecified site

⑥ M93.21 Osteochondritis dissecans of shoulder

SP M93.211 Osteochondritis dissecans, right shoulder

SP M93.212 Osteochondritis dissecans, left shoulder

IQ M93.219 Osteochondritis dissecans, unspecified shoulder

⑥ M93.22 Osteochondritis dissecans of elbow

SP M93.221 Osteochondritis dissecans, right elbow

SP M93.222 Osteochondritis dissecans, left elbow

IQ M93.229 Osteochondritis dissecans, unspecified elbow

⑥ M93.23 Osteochondritis dissecans of wrist

SP M93.231 Osteochondritis dissecans, right wrist

SP M93.232 Osteochondritis dissecans, left wrist

IQ M93.239 Osteochondritis dissecans, unspecified wrist

⑥ M93.24 Osteochondritis dissecans of joints of hand

SP M93.241 Osteochondritis dissecans, joints of right hand

SP M93.242 Osteochondritis dissecans, joints of left hand

IQ M93.249 Osteochondritis dissecans, joints of unspecified hand

⑥ M93.25 Osteochondritis dissecans of hip

SP M93.251 Osteochondritis dissecans, right hip

SP M93.252 Osteochondritis dissecans, left hip

IQ M93.259 Osteochondritis dissecans, unspecified hip

⑥ M93.26 Osteochondritis dissecans knee

SP M93.261 Osteochondritis dissecans, right knee

SP M93.262 Osteochondritis dissecans, left knee

IQ M93.269 Osteochondritis dissecans, unspecified knee

⑥ M93.27 Osteochondritis dissecans of ankle and joints of foot

SP M93.271 Osteochondritis dissecans, right ankle and joints of right foot

SP M93.272 Osteochondritis dissecans, left ankle and joints of left foot

IQ M93.279 Osteochondritis dissecans, unspecified ankle and joints of foot

SP M93.28 Osteochondritis dissecans other site

SP M93.29 Osteochondritis dissecans multiple sites

⑤ **M93.8 Other specified osteochondropathies**

DEFINITION Other conditions affecting bone and cartilage at any age, noted by abnormal endochondral ossification.

IQ M93.80 Other specified osteochondropathies of unspecified site

⑥ M93.81 Other specified osteochondropathies of shoulder

SP M93.811 Other specified osteochondropathies, right shoulder

SP M93.812 Other specified osteochondropathies, left shoulder

IQ M93.819 Other specified osteochondropathies, unspecified shoulder

⑥ M93.82 Other specified osteochondropathies of upper arm

SP M93.821 Other specified osteochondropathies, right upper arm

SP M93.822 Other specified osteochondropathies, left upper arm

IQ M93.829 Other specified osteochondropathies, unspecified upper arm

⑥ M93.83 Other specified osteochondropathies of forearm

SP M93.831 Other specified osteochondropathies, right forearm

SP M93.832 Other specified osteochondropathies, left forearm

IQ M93.839 Other specified osteochondropathies, unspecified forearm

⑥ M93.84 Other specified osteochondropathies of hand

SP M93.841 Other specified osteochondropathies, right hand

SP M93.842 Other specified osteochondropathies, left hand

IQ M93.849 Other specified osteochondropathies, unspecified hand

⑥ M93.85 Other specified osteochondropathies of thigh

SP M93.851 Other specified osteochondropathies, right thigh

SP M93.852 Other specified osteochondropathies, left thigh

IQ M93.859 Other specified osteochondropathies, unspecified thigh

⑥ M93.86 Other specified osteochondropathies lower leg

SP M93.861 Other specified osteochondropathies, right lower leg

SP M93.862 Other specified osteochondropathies, left lower leg

---

★ New ▲ Revised Px Primary **SP** PDGM Px **SL** Low CoM **SH** High CoM **IQ** Quest. Encounter ⊞ Hospice non-cancer Dx Unspecified **M** *Manifestation*

DecisionHealth's FY 2020 Complete Home Health ICD-10-CM Diagnosis Coding Manual

1265

Chapter 13

M00-M99

⊟ !Q M93.869 **Other specified osteochondropathies, unspecified lower leg**

6 M93.87 **Other specified osteochondropathies of ankle and foot**

⊟ SP M93.871 **Other specified osteochondropathies, right ankle and foot**

⊟ SP M93.872 **Other specified osteochondropathies, left ankle and foot**

⊟ !Q M93.879 **Other specified osteochondropathies, unspecified ankle and foot**

SP M93.88 **Other specified osteochondropathies other**

SP M93.89 **Other specified osteochondropathies multiple sites**

5 M93.9 **Osteochondropathy, unspecified**
    Apophysitis NOS
    Epiphysitis NOS
    Osteochondritis NOS
    Osteochondrosis NOS

!Q M93.90 **Osteochondropathy, unspecified of unspecified site**

6 M93.91 **Osteochondropathy, unspecified of shoulder**

⊟ SP M93.911 **Osteochondropathy, unspecified, right shoulder**

⊟ SP M93.912 **Osteochondropathy, unspecified, left shoulder**

⊟ !Q M93.919 **Osteochondropathy, unspecified, unspecified shoulder**

6 M93.92 **Osteochondropathy, unspecified of upper arm**

⊟ SP M93.921 **Osteochondropathy, unspecified, right upper arm**

⊟ SP M93.922 **Osteochondropathy, unspecified, left upper arm**

⊟ !Q M93.929 **Osteochondropathy, unspecified, unspecified upper arm**

6 M93.93 **Osteochondropathy, unspecified of forearm**

⊟ SP M93.931 **Osteochondropathy, unspecified, right forearm**

⊟ SP M93.932 **Osteochondropathy, unspecified, left forearm**

⊟ !Q M93.939 **Osteochondropathy, unspecified, unspecified forearm**

6 M93.94 **Osteochondropathy, unspecified of hand**

⊟ SP M93.941 **Osteochondropathy, unspecified, right hand**

⊟ SP M93.942 **Osteochondropathy, unspecified, left hand**

⊟ !Q M93.949 **Osteochondropathy, unspecified, unspecified hand**

6 M93.95 **Osteochondropathy, unspecified of thigh**

⊟ SP M93.951 **Osteochondropathy, unspecified, right thigh**

⊟ SP M93.952 **Osteochondropathy, unspecified, left thigh**

⊟ !Q M93.959 **Osteochondropathy, unspecified, unspecified thigh**

6 M93.96 **Osteochondropathy, unspecified lower leg**

⊟ SP M93.961 **Osteochondropathy, unspecified, right lower leg**

⊟ SP M93.962 **Osteochondropathy, unspecified, left lower leg**

⊟ !Q M93.969 **Osteochondropathy, unspecified, unspecified lower leg**

6 M93.97 **Osteochondropathy, unspecified of ankle and foot**

⊟ SP M93.971 **Osteochondropathy, unspecified, right ankle and foot**

⊟ SP M93.972 **Osteochondropathy, unspecified, left ankle and foot**

⊟ !Q M93.979 **Osteochondropathy, unspecified, unspecified ankle and foot**

!Q M93.98 **Osteochondropathy, unspecified other**

SP M93.99 **Osteochondropathy, unspecified multiple sites**

4 **M94 Other disorders of cartilage**

SP **M94.0 Chondrocostal junction syndrome [Tietze]**
    Costochondritis

SP **M94.1 Relapsing polychondritis**

5 **M94.2 Chondromalacia**
    EXCLUDES 1   chondromalacia patellae (M22.4)
    DEFINITION   Joint cartilage softens and degenerates, causing tenderness, pain, and a grinding sensation.

!Q **M94.20 Chondromalacia, unspecified site**

6 **M94.21 Chondromalacia, shoulder**

⊟ SP **M94.211 Chondromalacia, right shoulder**

⊟ SP **M94.212 Chondromalacia, left shoulder**

⊟ !Q **M94.219 Chondromalacia, unspecified shoulder**

6 **M94.22 Chondromalacia, elbow**

⊟ SP **M94.221 Chondromalacia, right elbow**

⊟ SP **M94.222 Chondromalacia, left elbow**

⊟ !Q **M94.229 Chondromalacia, unspecified elbow**

6 **M94.23 Chondromalacia, wrist**

⊟ SP **M94.231 Chondromalacia, right wrist**

⊟ SP **M94.232 Chondromalacia, left wrist**

⊟ !Q **M94.239 Chondromalacia, unspecified wrist**

6 **M94.24 Chondromalacia, joints of hand**

⊟ SP **M94.241 Chondromalacia, joints of right hand**

⊟ SP **M94.242 Chondromalacia, joints of left hand**

⊟ !Q **M94.249 Chondromalacia, joints of unspecified hand**

6 **M94.25 Chondromalacia, hip**

⊟ SP **M94.251 Chondromalacia, right hip**

⊟ SP **M94.252 Chondromalacia, left hip**

⊟ !Q **M94.259 Chondromalacia, unspecified hip**

6 **M94.26 Chondromalacia, knee**

---

4 4th digit required   5 5th digit required   6 6th digit required   7 7th digit required   7 7th digit placeholder   + Additional code   ⊟ Laterality

CODING TIPS ✓ Do not assign M94.26-
for chondromalacia patellae (also called
"runner's knee" or CMP).
Chondromalacia patellae is an
inflammation of the underside of the
patella and is coded to M22.4.

⊟ **SP** M94.261 Chondromalacia, right knee

⊟ **SP** M94.262 Chondromalacia, left knee

⊟ **IQ** M94.269 Chondromalacia, unspecified
knee

⑥ M94.27 Chondromalacia, ankle and joints of
foot

⊟ **SP** M94.271 Chondromalacia, right ankle and
joints of right foot

⊟ **SP** M94.272 Chondromalacia, left ankle and
joints of left foot

⊟ **IQ** M94.279 Chondromalacia, unspecified
ankle and joints of foot

SP M94.28 Chondromalacia, other site

SP M94.29 Chondromalacia, multiple sites

⑤ M94.3 Chondrolysis

Code first:
any associated slipped upper femoral
epiphysis (nontraumatic) (M93.0-)

DEFINITION Sudden, severe damage to
joint cartilage causing rapid death of normal
cartilage cells and abrupt loss of the joint's
cartilage layer.

⑥ M94.35 Chondrolysis, hip

⊟ **SP** M94.351 Chondrolysis, right hip

⊟ **SP** M94.352 Chondrolysis, left hip

⊟ **IQ** M94.359 Chondrolysis, unspecified hip

⑤ M94.8 Other specified disorders of cartilage

⑥ M94.8X Other specified disorders of cartilage

SP M94.8X0 Other specified disorders of
cartilage, multiple sites

SP M94.8X1 Other specified disorders of
cartilage, shoulder

SP M94.8X2 Other specified disorders of
cartilage, upper arm

SP M94.8X3 Other specified disorders of
cartilage, forearm

SP M94.8X4 Other specified disorders of
cartilage, hand

SP M94.8X5 Other specified disorders of
cartilage, thigh

SP M94.8X6 Other specified disorders of
cartilage, lower leg

SP M94.8X7 Other specified disorders of
cartilage, ankle and foot

SP M94.8X8 Other specified disorders of
cartilage, other site

IQ M94.8X9 Other specified disorders of
cartilage, unspecified sites

IQ M94.9 Disorder of cartilage, unspecified

Other disorders of the musculoskeletal system and connective tissue (M95)

④ M95 Other acquired deformities of
musculoskeletal system and connective
tissue

EXCLUDES 2 acquired absence of limbs and
organs (Z89-Z90)

acquired deformities of limbs
(M20-M21)
congenital malformations and
deformations of the
musculoskeletal system
(Q65-Q79)
deforming dorsopathies
(M40-M43)
dentofacial anomalies
[including malocclusion]
(M26.-)
postprocedural musculoskeletal
disorders (M96.-)

IQ M95.0 Acquired deformity of nose

EXCLUDES 2 deviated nasal septum
(J34.2)

⑤ M95.1 Cauliflower ear

EXCLUDES 2 other acquired deformities of
ear (H61.1)

⊟ **IQ** M95.10 Cauliflower ear, unspecified ear

⊟ **SP** M95.11 Cauliflower ear, right ear

⊟ **SP** M95.12 Cauliflower ear, left ear

SP M95.2 Other acquired deformity of head

SP M95.3 Acquired deformity of neck

SP M95.4 Acquired deformity of chest and rib

SP M95.5 Acquired deformity of pelvis

EXCLUDES 1 maternal care for known or
suspected disproportion
(O33.-)

SP M95.8 Other specified acquired deformities of
musculoskeletal system

IQ M95.9 Acquired deformity of musculoskeletal
system, unspecified

Intraoperative and postprocedural complications and disorders of musculoskeletal system, not elsewhere classified (M96)

④ M96 Intraoperative and postprocedural
complications and disorders of
musculoskeletal system, not elsewhere
classified

EXCLUDES 2 arthropathy following intestinal
bypass (M02.0-)
complications of internal
orthopedic prosthetic devices,
implants and grafts (T84.-)
disorders associated with
osteoporosis (M80)
periprosthetic fracture around
internal prosthetic joint
(M97.-)
presence of functional implants
and other devices (Z96-Z97)

CODING TIPS ✓ These conditions may be used
in addition to complication codes found in the T
chapter.

CODING TIPS ✓ **Documentation:** Codes in
category M96.- are complication codes and
require physician documentation and
confirmation of a cause and effect relationship
between the procedure and the complicated
condition. Documentation in the home health
clinical record must also support this
relationship.

★ New ▲ Revised Px Primary **SP** PDGM Px **SL** Low CoM **SH** High CoM **IQ** Quest. Encounter **H** Hospice non-cancer Dx Unspecified **M** *Manifestation*

DecisionHealth's FY 2020 Complete Home Health ICD-10-CM Diagnosis Coding Manual

1267

SP M96.0 Pseudarthrosis after fusion or arthrodesis

SP M96.1 Postlaminectomy syndrome, not elsewhere classified

SP M96.2 Postradiation kyphosis

SP M96.3 Postlaminectomy kyphosis

SP M96.4 Postsurgical lordosis

SP M96.5 Postradiation scoliosis

5 M96.6 Fracture of bone following insertion of orthopedic implant, joint prosthesis, or bone plate
Intraoperative fracture of bone during insertion of orthopedic implant, joint prosthesis, or bone plate
> EXCLUDES 2 complication of internal orthopedic devices, implants or grafts (T84.-)

6 M96.62 Fracture of humerus following insertion of orthopedic implant, joint prosthesis, or bone plate

SP M96.621 Fracture of humerus following insertion of orthopedic implant, joint prosthesis, or bone plate, right arm

SP M96.622 Fracture of humerus following insertion of orthopedic implant, joint prosthesis, or bone plate, left arm

IQ M96.629 Fracture of humerus following insertion of orthopedic implant, joint prosthesis, or bone plate, unspecified arm

6 M96.63 Fracture of radius or ulna following insertion of orthopedic implant, joint prosthesis, or bone plate

SP M96.631 Fracture of radius or ulna following insertion of orthopedic implant, joint prosthesis, or bone plate, right arm

SP M96.632 Fracture of radius or ulna following insertion of orthopedic implant, joint prosthesis, or bone plate, left arm

IQ M96.639 Fracture of radius or ulna following insertion of orthopedic implant, joint prosthesis, or bone plate, unspecified arm

SP M96.65 Fracture of pelvis following insertion of orthopedic implant, joint prosthesis, or bone plate

6 M96.66 Fracture of femur following insertion of orthopedic implant, joint prosthesis, or bone plate

SP M96.661 Fracture of femur following insertion of orthopedic implant, joint prosthesis, or bone plate, right leg

SP M96.662 Fracture of femur following insertion of orthopedic implant, joint prosthesis, or bone plate, left leg

IQ M96.669 Fracture of femur following insertion of orthopedic implant, joint prosthesis, or bone plate, unspecified leg

6 M96.67 Fracture of tibia or fibula following insertion of orthopedic implant, joint prosthesis, or bone plate

SP M96.671 Fracture of tibia or fibula following insertion of orthopedic implant, joint prosthesis, or bone plate, right leg

SP M96.672 Fracture of tibia or fibula following insertion of orthopedic implant, joint prosthesis, or bone plate, left leg

IQ M96.679 Fracture of tibia or fibula following insertion of orthopedic implant, joint prosthesis, or bone plate, unspecified leg

SP M96.69 Fracture of other bone following insertion of orthopedic implant, joint prosthesis, or bone plate

5 M96.8 Other intraoperative and postprocedural complications and disorders of musculoskeletal system, not elsewhere classified

6 M96.81 Intraoperative hemorrhage and hematoma of a musculoskeletal structure complicating a procedure
> EXCLUDES 1 intraoperative hemorrhage and hematoma of a musculoskeletal structure due to accidental puncture and laceration during a procedure (M96.82-)

SP M96.810 Intraoperative hemorrhage and hematoma of a musculoskeletal structure complicating a musculoskeletal system procedure

SP M96.811 Intraoperative hemorrhage and hematoma of a musculoskeletal structure complicating other procedure

6 M96.82 Accidental puncture and laceration of a musculoskeletal structure during a procedure

SP M96.820 Accidental puncture and laceration of a musculoskeletal structure during a musculoskeletal system procedure

SP M96.821 Accidental puncture and laceration of a musculoskeletal structure during other procedure

6 M96.83 Postprocedural hemorrhage of a musculoskeletal structure following a procedure

SP M96.830 Postprocedural hemorrhage of a musculoskeletal structure following a musculoskeletal system procedure

SP M96.831 Postprocedural hemorrhage of a musculoskeletal structure following other procedure

6 M96.84 Postprocedural hematoma and seroma of a musculoskeletal structure following a procedure

SP M96.840 Postprocedural hematoma of a musculoskeletal structure following a musculoskeletal system procedure

SP M96.841 Postprocedural hematoma of a musculoskeletal structure following other procedure

---

4 4th digit required   **5** 5th digit required   **6** 6th digit required   **7** 7th digit required   **7** 7th digit placeholder   **+** Additional code   **⊟** Laterality

SP **M96.842** Postprocedural seroma of a musculoskeletal structure following a musculoskeletal system procedure

SP **M96.843** Postprocedural seroma of a musculoskeletal structure following other procedure

SP **+** **M96.89** Other intraoperative and postprocedural complications and disorders of the musculoskeletal system

Instability of joint secondary to removal of joint prosthesis

Use additional code, if applicable, to further specify disorder

Periprosthetic fracture around internal prosthetic joint   (M97)

4 **M97** Periprosthetic fracture around internal prosthetic joint

> **EXCLUDES 2** fracture of bone following insertion of orthopedic implant, joint prosthesis or bone plate (M96.6-)
> breakage (fracture) of prosthetic joint (T84.01-)

> The appropriate 7th character is to be added to each code from category M97
> A   initial encounter
> D   subsequent encounter
> S   sequela

> **CODING TIPS ✓**   Fractures around a prosthesis are not complications of the prosthesis, but the result of the same conditions as other fractures, that is, trauma or pathological conditions. Periprosthetic fractures can occur around any prosthesis, but the most common is the hip, knee, ankle, shoulder, or elbow. Sequence the traumatic or pathologic fracture first and then follow it with the periprosthetic fracture code.

5 **M97.0** Periprosthetic fracture around internal prosthetic hip joint

SP **M97.01X-** Periprosthetic fracture around internal prosthetic right hip joint

SP **M97.02X-** Periprosthetic fracture around internal prosthetic left hip joint

5 **M97.1** Periprosthetic fracture around internal prosthetic knee joint

SP **M97.11X-** Periprosthetic fracture around internal prosthetic right knee joint

SP **M97.12X-** Periprosthetic fracture around internal prosthetic left knee joint

5 **M97.2** Periprosthetic fracture around internal prosthetic ankle joint

SP **M97.21X-** Periprosthetic fracture around internal prosthetic right ankle joint

SP **M97.22X-** Periprosthetic fracture around internal prosthetic left ankle joint

5 **M97.3** Periprosthetic fracture around internal prosthetic shoulder joint

SP **M97.31X-** Periprosthetic fracture around internal prosthetic right shoulder joint

SP **M97.32X-** Periprosthetic fracture around internal prosthetic left shoulder joint

5 **M97.4** Periprosthetic fracture around internal prosthetic elbow joint

SP **M97.41X-** Periprosthetic fracture around internal prosthetic right elbow joint

SP **M97.42X-** Periprosthetic fracture around internal prosthetic left elbow joint

SP **+** **M97.8XX-** Periprosthetic fracture around other internal prosthetic joint

Periprosthetic fracture around internal prosthetic finger joint
Periprosthetic fracture around internal prosthetic spinal joint
Periprosthetic fracture around internal prosthetic toe joint
Periprosthetic fracture around internal prosthetic wrist joint

Use additional code to identify the joint (Z96.6-)

IQ **M97.9XX-** Periprosthetic fracture around unspecified internal prosthetic joint

Biomechanical lesions, not elsewhere classified   (M99)

4 **M99** Biomechanical lesions, not elsewhere classified

Note:
This category should not be used if the condition can be classified elsewhere.

5 **M99.0** Segmental and somatic dysfunction

SP **M99.00** Segmental and somatic dysfunction of head region

SP **M99.01** Segmental and somatic dysfunction of cervical region

SP **M99.02** Segmental and somatic dysfunction of thoracic region

SP **M99.03** Segmental and somatic dysfunction of lumbar region

SP **M99.04** Segmental and somatic dysfunction of sacral region

SP **M99.05** Segmental and somatic dysfunction of pelvic region

SP **M99.06** Segmental and somatic dysfunction of lower extremity

SP **M99.07** Segmental and somatic dysfunction of upper extremity

SP **M99.08** Segmental and somatic dysfunction of rib cage

SP **M99.09** Segmental and somatic dysfunction of abdomen and other regions

5 **M99.1** Subluxation complex (vertebral)

SP **M99.10** Subluxation complex (vertebral) of head region

SP **M99.11** Subluxation complex (vertebral) of cervical region

SP **M99.12** Subluxation complex (vertebral) of thoracic region

SP **M99.13** Subluxation complex (vertebral) of lumbar region

SP **M99.14** Subluxation complex (vertebral) of sacral region

SP **M99.15** Subluxation complex (vertebral) of pelvic region

---

✱ New ▲ Revised Px Primary **SP** PDGM Px **SL** Low CoM **SH** High CoM **IQ** Quest. Encounter **H** Hospice non-cancer Dx   Unspecified   **M** *Manifestation*

SP M99.16 Subluxation complex (vertebral) of lower extremity

SP M99.17 Subluxation complex (vertebral) of upper extremity

SP M99.18 Subluxation complex (vertebral) of rib cage

SP M99.19 Subluxation complex (vertebral) of abdomen and other regions

5 M99.2 Subluxation stenosis of neural canal

SP M99.20 Subluxation stenosis of neural canal of head region

SP M99.21 Subluxation stenosis of neural canal of cervical region

SP M99.22 Subluxation stenosis of neural canal of thoracic region

SP M99.23 Subluxation stenosis of neural canal of lumbar region

SP M99.24 Subluxation stenosis of neural canal of sacral region

SP M99.25 Subluxation stenosis of neural canal of pelvic region

SP M99.26 Subluxation stenosis of neural canal of lower extremity

SP M99.27 Subluxation stenosis of neural canal of upper extremity

SP M99.28 Subluxation stenosis of neural canal of rib cage

SP M99.29 Subluxation stenosis of neural canal of abdomen and other regions

5 M99.3 Osseous stenosis of neural canal

SP M99.30 Osseous stenosis of neural canal of head region

SP M99.31 Osseous stenosis of neural canal of cervical region

SP M99.32 Osseous stenosis of neural canal of thoracic region

SP M99.33 Osseous stenosis of neural canal of lumbar region

SP M99.34 Osseous stenosis of neural canal of sacral region

SP M99.35 Osseous stenosis of neural canal of pelvic region

SP M99.36 Osseous stenosis of neural canal of lower extremity

SP M99.37 Osseous stenosis of neural canal of upper extremity

SP M99.38 Osseous stenosis of neural canal of rib cage

SP M99.39 Osseous stenosis of neural canal of abdomen and other regions

5 M99.4 Connective tissue stenosis of neural canal

SP M99.40 Connective tissue stenosis of neural canal of head region

SP M99.41 Connective tissue stenosis of neural canal of cervical region

SP M99.42 Connective tissue stenosis of neural canal of thoracic region

SP M99.43 Connective tissue stenosis of neural canal of lumbar region

SP M99.44 Connective tissue stenosis of neural canal of sacral region

SP M99.45 Connective tissue stenosis of neural canal of pelvic region

SP M99.46 Connective tissue stenosis of neural canal of lower extremity

SP M99.47 Connective tissue stenosis of neural canal of upper extremity

SP M99.48 Connective tissue stenosis of neural canal of rib cage

SP M99.49 Connective tissue stenosis of neural canal of abdomen and other regions

5 M99.5 Intervertebral disc stenosis of neural canal

SP M99.50 Intervertebral disc stenosis of neural canal of head region

SP M99.51 Intervertebral disc stenosis of neural canal of cervical region

SP M99.52 Intervertebral disc stenosis of neural canal of thoracic region

SP M99.53 Intervertebral disc stenosis of neural canal of lumbar region

SP M99.54 Intervertebral disc stenosis of neural canal of sacral region

SP M99.55 Intervertebral disc stenosis of neural canal of pelvic region

SP M99.56 Intervertebral disc stenosis of neural canal of lower extremity

SP M99.57 Intervertebral disc stenosis of neural canal of upper extremity

SP M99.58 Intervertebral disc stenosis of neural canal of rib cage

SP M99.59 Intervertebral disc stenosis of neural canal of abdomen and other regions

5 M99.6 Osseous and subluxation stenosis of intervertebral foramina

SP M99.60 Osseous and subluxation stenosis of intervertebral foramina of head region

SP M99.61 Osseous and subluxation stenosis of intervertebral foramina of cervical region

SP M99.62 Osseous and subluxation stenosis of intervertebral foramina of thoracic region

SP M99.63 Osseous and subluxation stenosis of intervertebral foramina of lumbar region

SP M99.64 Osseous and subluxation stenosis of intervertebral foramina of sacral region

SP M99.65 Osseous and subluxation stenosis of intervertebral foramina of pelvic region

SP M99.66 Osseous and subluxation stenosis of intervertebral foramina of lower extremity

SP M99.67 Osseous and subluxation stenosis of intervertebral foramina of upper extremity

SP M99.68 Osseous and subluxation stenosis of intervertebral foramina of rib cage

SP M99.69 Osseous and subluxation stenosis of intervertebral foramina of abdomen and other regions

5 M99.7 Connective tissue and disc stenosis of intervertebral foramina

SP M99.70 Connective tissue and disc stenosis of intervertebral foramina of head region

SP M99.71 Connective tissue and disc stenosis of intervertebral foramina of cervical region

SP M99.72 Connective tissue and disc stenosis of intervertebral foramina of thoracic region

4 4th digit required　　5 5th digit required　　6 6th digit required　　7 7th digit required　　7 7th digit placeholder　　+ Additional code　　Laterality

1270　　　*DecisionHealth's* FY 2020 Complete Home Health ICD-10-CM Diagnosis Coding Manual

SP M99.73 Connective tissue and disc stenosis of intervertebral foramina of lumbar region

SP M99.74 Connective tissue and disc stenosis of intervertebral foramina of sacral region

SP M99.75 Connective tissue and disc stenosis of intervertebral foramina of pelvic region

SP M99.76 Connective tissue and disc stenosis of intervertebral foramina of lower extremity

SP M99.77 Connective tissue and disc stenosis of intervertebral foramina of upper extremity

SP M99.78 Connective tissue and disc stenosis of intervertebral foramina of rib cage

SP M99.79 Connective tissue and disc stenosis of intervertebral foramina of abdomen and other regions

5 M99.8 Other biomechanical lesions

SP M99.80 Other biomechanical lesions of head region

SP M99.81 Other biomechanical lesions of cervical region

SP M99.82 Other biomechanical lesions of thoracic region

SP M99.83 Other biomechanical lesions of lumbar region

SP M99.84 Other biomechanical lesions of sacral region

SP M99.85 Other biomechanical lesions of pelvic region

SP M99.86 Other biomechanical lesions of lower extremity

SP M99.87 Other biomechanical lesions of upper extremity

SP M99.88 Other biomechanical lesions of rib cage

SP M99.89 Other biomechanical lesions of abdomen and other regions

IQ M99.9 Biomechanical lesion, unspecified

★ New ▲ Revised Px Primary **SP** PDGM Px **SL** Low CoM **SH** High CoM **IQ** Quest. Encounter **H** Hospice non-cancer Dx   Unspecified   **M** *Manifestation*

DecisionHealth's FY 2020 Complete Home Health ICD-10-CM Diagnosis Coding Manual   1271

Chapter 13 Scenarios: Diseases of the musculoskeletal system and connective tissue (M00-M99)

Osteoporosis and pathologic fracture

An elderly gentleman is admitted for home care after undergoing surgery for a pathological fracture of the left femur. Physical therapy is ordered for muscle strengthening and gait training. Skilled nursing is ordered for surgical wound assessment. Medical documentation includes hypertension, seizure disorder and osteoporosis.

Description	Code
Primary: Age-related osteoporosis with current pathological fracture, left femur	M80.052D
Secondary: HTN, unspecified	I10
Secondary: Seizure disorder NOS	G40.909

A code from category M80.-, not a traumatic fracture code, should be used for any patient with known osteoporosis who suffers a fracture, even if the patient had a minor fall or trauma, if that fall or trauma would not usually break a normal, healthy bone, according to coding guidelines. The M80.0- subcategory indicates age-related osteoporosis with current pathologic fracture. The fifth digit "5" indicates femur, the sixth digit "2" indicates the left side and the seventh character "D" indicates subsequent care. Osteoporosis that is not otherwise specified codes to age-related osteoporosis within the ICD-10 classification system.

Pathologic fracture, bone cancer

A 75-year-old male patient has brain cancer that has metastasized to his bones. As a result, he has suffered a pathologic fracture to his right femur, which was treated surgically in the hospital. The focus of the home health admission is the fracture aftercare, which is routine.

Description	Code
Primary: Pathologic fracture in neoplastic disease, right femur, subsequent encounter with routine healing	M84.551D
Secondary: Secondary malignant neoplasm of bone	C79.51
Secondary: Malignant neoplasm of brain, unspecified	C71.9

As the focus of care, the pathological fracture caused by the bone metastasis is coded in the primary position. When an encounter is for a pathological fracture due to a neoplasm, and the focus of treatment is the fracture, a code from subcategory M84.5- (Pathological fracture in neoplastic disease) should be sequenced first followed by the code for the neoplasm, according to coding guidelines. As the reason for the pathological fracture, the secondary malignant neoplasm in the bones is coded before the primary malignant neoplasm in the brain. The care is routine, so the appropriate seventh character is D, which specifies that the case is a subsequent encounter for fracture with routine healing. The underlying neoplasms also are coded, as required by the note in the tabular.

Multiple therapies and fracture

Your patient sustained a pathological fracture of her left femur when rolling over in bed. She has a diagnosis of senile osteoporosis. Skilled nursing and physical and occupational therapy are ordered. She had a vertebral pathologic fracture one year ago.

Description	Code
Primary: Age-related osteoporosis with current pathologic fracture of left femur, subsequent encounter with routine healing	M80.052D
Secondary: Personal history of (healed) osteoporosis fracture	Z87.310

The combination code M80.052D covers both the patient's osteoporosis and pathological fracture of her left femur. The seventh character "D" identifies the subsequent nature of the encounter. Her personal history of a healed pathological fracture is relevant to this case and is thus coded. Senile osteoporosis is coded as age-related osteoporosis, according to the alphabetic index.

Spinal stenosis

The home health agency received a referral for a home care assessment for a patient recently discharged from the hospital after a myocardial infarction (MI) and sudden cardiac arrest within the last two weeks. The patient has acute back pain in the lumbar area, diagnosed as spinal stenosis of the lumbar region with neurogenic claudication, and is deficient in vitamin B. The focus for home care is the spinal stenosis/back pain. The nursing staff is to assess her response to pain medications and new cardiac medications, and perform venipuncture for Digoxin levels. Physical therapy will provide therapeutic exercises and training, and occupational therapy will provide ADL training, adaptive equipment, and motor/sensory treatment.

Description	Code
Primary: Spinal stenosis, lumbar region with neurogenic claudication	M48.062
Secondary: Acute myocardial infarction, unspecified	I21.9
Secondary: Vitamin B deficiency, unspecified	E53.9
Secondary: Encounter for therapeutic drug level monitoring	Z51.81
Secondary: Other long term (current) drug therapy	Z79.899
Secondary: Personal history of sudden cardiac arrest	Z86.74

The combination code M48.062 covers both the spinal stenosis of the lumbar region and the neurogenic claudication. It is not acceptable to code spinal stenosis of an **unspecified** location as primary under PDGM. Back pain is integral to spinal stenosis and thus no additional code is required to capture it. An "acute" MI is acute for four weeks post-heart attack and with no further detail given about the MI, I21.9 is the appropriate code choice. The Z code for history of sudden cardiac arrest is used when there has been a cardiac arrest with successful resuscitation. Venipuncture and monitoring for Digoxin levels are captured with Z51.81 and Z79.899.

Ankle arthritis

A 73-year-old man was admitted for physical therapy for difficulty in ambulating. Per the medical record, the patient sustained a left ankle fracture four years ago, and now has arthritis in the joint as a result. Due to the pain, the patient has fallen several times in recent weeks.

Description	Code
Primary: Traumatic arthropathy, left ankle and foot	M12.572
Secondary: Other fracture of left lower leg, sequela	S82.892S
Secondary: Repeated falls	R29.6
Secondary: History of falling	Z91.81

Traumatic arthropathy is coded as it is a residual effect that occurred because of an injury in the past. The now-resolved ankle fracture, which is the reason for the traumatic arthritis, is coded immediately following the arthritis code, in accordance with coding guidelines. It includes the seventh character "S" to indicate that it is not an active condition but rather has left behind a residual, or sequela. The repeated falls code (R29.6) is used when a patient has recently fallen and the reason for the fall is being investigated. The history of falling code (Z91.81) is used when a patient has fallen in the past and is at risk for future falls.

Rheumatoid arthritis, monthly infusions

A 67-year-old man receives home health care for monthly infusions of Actemra to treat his severe rheumatoid arthritis (RA) of both hands. He is positive for rheumatoid factor. He is frequently monitored for potential side effects and complications from the long-term use of Actemra.

Description	Code
Primary: Rheumatoid arthritis with rheumatoid factor of right hand without organ or systems involvement	M05.741
Secondary: Rheumatoid arthritis with rheumatoid factor of left hand without organ or systems involvement	M05.742
Secondary: Encounter for adjustment and management of vascular access device	Z45.2
Secondary: Other long term (current) drug therapy	Z79.899

Two codes are assigned to capture the rheumatoid arthritis being present in both hands, since a bilateral code is not available. Code Z45.2 is assigned to capture the care of the vascular access device used to deliver the infusion. Additionally, Z79.899 is assigned to capture the patient's long-term use of Actemra; in the absence of a more specific code from Z79.-, Z79.899 is the most appropriate in this case. Note that it is not acceptable to code unspecified rheumatoid arthritis as the primary reason for home health in PDGM. A more specific code, which requires knowing which joints are affected and which type of the disease (i.e. seropositive, seronegative, etc.) is present, must be assigned in order to be used as the primary diagnosis.

Traumatic arthritis, stroke sequela

A 67-year-old woman suffered a stroke last year, in which she lost consciousness, fell and broke her left wrist. After the stroke, she continues to suffer from right dominant side hemiplegia, aphasia and dysphagia. Additionally, she has traumatic arthritis in her left wrist as a result of the now-healed fracture. She has orders for physical, occupational and speech therapy to continue her recovery from the stroke sequela. The hemiplegia is the focus of care.

Description	Code
Primary: Hemiplegia and hemiparesis following cerebral infarction affecting right dominant side	I69.351
Secondary: Aphasia following cerebral infarction	I69.320
Secondary: Dysphagia following cerebral infarction	I69.391
Secondary: Dysphagia, unspecified	R13.10
Secondary: Traumatic arthropathy, left wrist	M12.532
Secondary: Fracture of unspecified carpal bone, left wrist, sequela	S62.102S

Though it is a therapy-only case, there is no need to assign a rehab code in ICD-10. The conditions requiring therapy will suffice. As the focus of care, the right dominant side hemiplegia is coded primary. An additional code for dysphagia is assigned, in accordance with tabular instructions at I69.391. The patient's arthritis has been specified as traumatic arthritis, resulting from an old healed wrist fracture. Though the fracture is healed, it left the patient with arthritis. Therefore, the code for the fracture is assigned immediately following the residual it caused (the traumatic arthritis) with the seventh character "S" to indicate that it's no longer an active condition but a sequela.

Nephritis due to lupus

A 60-year-old woman comes to home health for nephritis secondary to systemic lupus erythematosus. She will receive skilled nursing for management of medications, including an increased dosage of systemic steroids, which she has taken for the last year. The nephritis is the focus of care.

Description	Code
Primary: Glomerular disease in systemic lupus erythematosus	M32.14
Secondary: Long term (current) use of systemic steroids	Z79.52

The patient's nephritis is documented as being caused by systemic lupus erythematosus. Thus it is appropriate to code it with the combination code M32.14. As the focus of care, it is coded in the primary position. Since the combination code covers both conditions, an additional code for the lupus is not necessary. The patient has taken systemic steroids over a long period of time, which carries certain risks and thus must be captured with Z79.52.

Chronic idiopathic gout

A 67-year-old man is admitted to home health for skilled nursing, managing new medications, and physical and occupational therapy to address trouble with ADLs/IADLs due to a primary diagnosis of chronic idiopathic gout that affects both of his elbows. He also has a diagnosis of hypertension for which he was recently prescribed new medication.

Description	Code
Primary: Idiopathic chronic gout, right elbow, without tophus (tophi)	M1A.0210
Secondary: Idiopathic chronic gout, left elbow, without tophus (tophi)	M1A.0220
Secondary: Essential (primary) hypertension	I10

The patient's gout is specified as chronic idiopathic gout of both elbows. Because no bilateral code is available, two codes (one for the right and one for the left) are used. It's imperative to know the specific joint affected by the gout, as codes for gout in an unspecified location and laterality are not acceptable as primary diagnoses in PDGM. His hypertension will require monitoring and thus should also be coded.

Pseudogout

A 70-year-old man is experiencing a severe flare of pseudogout in bilateral ankles. He was admitted to home health for management of medications, including prednisone, and physical therapy.

Description	Code
Primary: Other chondrocalcinosis, right ankle and foot	M11.271
Secondary: Other chondrocalcinosis, left ankle and foot	M11.272
Secondary: Long term (current) use of systemic steroids	Z79.52

Pseudogout is classified under chondrocalcinosis. Because there is not a code that captures chondrocalcinosis in both ankles, two codes are used for the right and left ankles. The specific joint and side of the body must be documented in order to code pseudogout as a primary diagnosis in home health. Note, codes for pseudogout in an unspecified location or that don't specify the left or right side of the body are not acceptable as primary diagnoses in PDGM. Taking the systemic steroid drug prednisone comes with certain risks, so it should be captured with Z79.52.

Pathological periprosthetic fracture

An 84-year-old woman with a left knee prosthesis was walking in her home when she felt a sharp pain in her left lower leg and heard a snap sound. She was admitted to the hospital where a fracture of the tibia, around the left knee prosthesis, was discovered. The hospitalist diagnosed the fracture as a pathological periprosthetic fracture and ordered home health for skilled nursing, physical and occupational therapy with a focus on care to and recovery from the fracture. She also has diagnoses of hypertension and depression.

Description	Code
Primary: Pathological fracture, left tibia, subsequent encounter for fracture with routine healing	M84.462D
Secondary: Periprosthetic fracture around internal prosthetic left knee joint, subsequent encounter	M97.12xD
Secondary: Essential (primary) hypertension	I10
Secondary: Major depressive disorder, single episode, unspecified	F32.9

The fracture was diagnosed as a pathological periprosthetic fracture around the left knee prosthesis. Therefore, the pathologic fracture is sequenced first, followed by the periprosthetic fracture code, in accordance with Q4 2016 Coding Clinic guidance. The patient's hypertension and depression are important comorbidities that will impact her ability to recover and are thus coded as secondary diagnoses.

Pseudogout, alcoholism

A 67-year-old man with long-term alcoholism is admitted to home health for physical and occupation therapy for pseudogout affecting both knees.

Description	Code
Primary: Other chondrocalcinosis, right knee	M11.261
Secondary: Other chondrocalcinosis, left knee	M11.262
Secondary: Alcohol dependence, uncomplicated	F10.20

Note that there is no listing for "pseudogout" in the alphabetic index. Codes for pseudogout are found in the index by searching under "chondrocalcinosis." Because the diagnosis is affecting both knees and there is no bilateral code, two codes are assigned – one for each knee, in accordance with coding guidelines. Alcoholism codes to alcohol dependence, according to the alphabetic index. Be sure to specify the laterality of the affected joint.

Chapter 14: Diseases of the Genitourinary System (N00-N99)

Chapter 14 includes codes arranged in the following blocks:

- Glomerular diseases such as nephritic syndrome, hematuria and hereditary nephropathy (N00-N08);

- Renal tubulo-interstitial diseases and disorders such as hereditary nephritis and chronic pylonephritis, hydronephrosis, and vesicoureteral-reflux nephropathy (N10-N16);

- Acute kidney failure and chronic kidney disease (N17-N19);

- Urolithiasis (N20-N23);

- Other disorders of kidney and ureter including nephrogenic diabetes insipidus, secondary hyperparathyroidism of renal origin, contracted (small) kidney, ischemia and infarction of kidney, and acquired cyst of kidney (N25-N29);

- Other disorders of urinary system including cystitis, neuromuscular dysfunction of the bladder, overactive bladder, uretheral stricture, UTI and urinary incontinence (N30-N39);

- Diseases of male genital organs including enlarged prostate, inflammatory diseases of prostate, hydrocele & spermatocele, noninflammatory disorders of testes, orchitis & epididymitis, male infertility, inflammatory disorders of penis, priaprism, inflammatory disorders of male genitalia, and erectile dysfunction (N40-N53);

- Disorders of breast including benign mammary dysplasia, cystic mastopathy, fibroadenosis of breast & mammary ducts, other inflammatory disorders of breast – hypertrophy & hypoplasia, fat necrosis of breast, other signs and symptoms in breast, and deformity & disproportion of reconstructed breast (N60-N65);

- Inflammatory diseases of female pelvic organs including salpingitis & oophoritis, inflammatory disease of uterus and cervix, pelvic inflammatory diseases and other inflammation of vagina and vulva (N70-N77);

- Noninflammatory disorders of female genital tract including endometriosis, female genital prolapses, urethrocele, cystocele, and rectocele, genital prolapsed, fistulas involving female genital tract, atrophy & polyps genital organs, cervical and vaginal disorders, female genital mutilation status, abnormal uterine & vaginal bleeding, menopausal and perimenopausal disorders and female infertility (N80-N98); and

- Intraoperative and postprocedural complications and disorders of genitourinary system such as uretheral strictures, adhesions, complications of urinary tract stomas, hemorrhage, and accidental puncture and lacerations (N99).

This chapter also includes a number of codes for symptoms, such as N95 for those related to menopausal and perimenopausal disorders and N64.4 for mastodynia (breast pain). Codes in category N92 for conditions related to menstrual periods (unusually heavy [menorrhagia], unusually light [oligomenorrhea], painful [dysmenorrhea], or no periods at all [amenorrhea]). Every effort should be made to secure a definitive diagnosis.

Home health and hospice coding will deal mostly with these areas of Chapter 14:

- Chronic kidney failure (N18.-)

- Urinary incontinence (N39.3, N39.4-)

- Cystitis (N30.-) and Urinary tract infection (N39.0)

- Problems with prostate (N40.- , N41.-, N42.-)

Symptoms related to the genitourinary system are sometimes reported using codes from Chapter 18, symptoms, signs and abnormal clinical and laboratory findings, not elsewhere classified. More specifically, using codes in subcategory R39.- (symptoms involving urinary system) and R82.-(nonspecific findings on examination of urine). Every effort should be made to secure a definitive diagnosis. A symptom code from Chapter 18 may be reported as an additional diagnosis when it describes a significant aspect of the condition but is not an integral part of it.

Other situations when codes outside of Chapter 14 are needed include:

- If the documentation indicates a **neoplasm or tumor of an organ in the genitourinary system**, look up the term (malignancy, tumor, adenoma) to find the correct code, most likely a code from C00 – D49 in Chapter 2.

- If a patient has a **personal or family history** of a condition reported in this chapter, it may be more appropriate to select from the Z code section, such as Z87.448 (Personal history disorder of urinary system), Z85.40 and Z85.45 (Personal history of malignant neoplasm of female and male genital organs), or Z80.4 (Family history of malignant neoplasm of genital organs).

- If a condition reported in this chapter is the result of **injury, poisoning and certain other consequences** of external causes, a code from

Chapter 14

N00 - N99

Chapter 19 may be reported with or instead of a code from this chapter.

- Additional codes in the following categories may be coded in addition to or instead of codes from chapter 14. Refer to the Alphabetical List for the code and follow the notes, if applicable, at the appropriate code. They are:
  - Certain conditions originating in the perinatal period (P00-P96)
  - Complications of pregnancy, childbirth or the puerperium (O00-O9A)
  - Congenital malformations, deformations and chromosomal abnormalities (Q00-O99)
  - Certain infectious and parasitic diseases (A00-B99)
  - Endocrine, nutritional and metabolic diseases (E00-E88)

Multiple Coding and Sequencing

It is important to read the Includes and Excludes notes under codes in this chapter, as well as any other instructions under the code or code category. Below are some examples of multiple coding and sequencing issues for codes in this chapter.

Codes N40.1 (Benign prostatic hyperplasia with lower urinary tract symptoms) and N40.3 (Nodular prostate with lower urinary tract symptoms) include a note that states: "Use additional code(s) for associated symptoms when specified." The note lists symptoms such as incomplete bladder emptying, nocturia, straining on urination, urinary frequency, hesitancy, incontinence, obstruction, retention, urgency and weak urinary stream from Chapter 18, including signs and symptoms involving the genitourinary system (R30-R39), as well as codes N13.8 and N39.4- from this chapter.

Special Coding Issues

There are many more specific combination codes in ICD-10 CM that reduce the need for multiple codes related to genitourinary conditions. Therefore, all codes must be referenced in the Alphabetical Index and then verified in the Tabular list to ensure the correct code is selected.

The Kidneys

The kidneys are responsible for removing waste from the body, regulating electrolyte balance and blood pressure, and stimulating red blood cell production. Although inflammation, scarring, or a decrease in membrane surface area lowers the rate of glomerular filtration, the kidney so effectively compensates that

people rarely know they have lost kidney function until only 10% to 20% remains. High blood pressure and anemia may develop with increasing frequency after loss of 30% to 50% kidney function, but these signs develop so gradually they often produce no symptoms.

Because of their intimate relationship with such a large portion of the circulating blood, up to 25% of diseases of the kidney, or any disturbance in the kidney's delicate mechanism, can adversely influence blood pressure, and in turn, may alter kidney function.

Chronic Kidney Disease (CKD)

There are two notes found at N18, Chronic kidney disease. First is a code first note to assign any associated disease, such as:

- diabetic chronic kidney disease (E08.22. E09.22, E10.22, E11.22, E13.22)
- hypertensive chronic kidney disease (I12.-, I13.-)

There is also a note to use an additional code to identify kidney transplant status, such as Z94.0, if applicable.

Stages of chronic kidney disease (CKD)

Chronic kidney disease is classified according to severity. The severity of CKD is designated by stages 1 – 5. Stage 2, code N18.2, equates to mild CKD; stage 3, code N18.3, equates to moderate CKD; stage 4, N18.4, equates to severe CKD. Code N18.6, End stage renal disease (ESRD), is assigned when the provider has documented end-stage-renal disease (ESRD) or chronic kidney disease requiring long-term dialysis. If both a stage of CKD and ESRD are documented, assign code N18.6 only.

When both hypertension and a condition classifiable to category N18, Chronic kidney disease (CKD), are present, assign codes from category I12, Hypertensive chronic kidney disease. CKD should not be coded as hypertensive if the physician has specifically documented a different cause. The appropriate code from category N18 should be used as a secondary code with a code from category I12 to identify the stage of chronic kidney disease.

Abnormal lab findings are not coded and reported unless the provider indicates clinical significance. Therefore, it would be inappropriate to assign a stage for CKD based solely on glomerular filtration rate (GFR). If that information is not available, the coder may select N18.9 for unspecified CKD, or N18.6, if the patient is undergoing dialysis.

If CKD, hypertension and heart disease are all present, it may be appropriate to report a code from Category I13.- (**hypertensive heart and chronic kidney disease**). A code from N18.- (CKD) is reported as an additional code. The classification assumes a relationship between HTN and any condition classifiable to N18 (CKD) and N26. The relationship may be assumed because of the pathology of hypertension, which impacts renal function, often resulting in CKD. Do not confuse hypertensive chronic kidney disease with renovascular hypertension, a condition in which the kidney dysfunction causes the hypertension. Renovascular hypertension is coded using I15.0.

Chronic kidney disease and kidney transplant status

Patients who have undergone a kidney transplant may still have some form of CKD because the kidney transplant may not fully restore kidney function. Therefore, the presence of CKD alone does not constitute a transplant complication. Assign the appropriate N18 code for the patient's stage of CKD and code Z94.0, kidney transplant status. If a transplant complication, such as failure or rejection or other transplant complication is documented, refer to section I.C.19.g of the Official Coding Guidelines for information on coding complications of a kidney transplant. If the documentation is unclear as to whether the patient has a complication of the transplant, query the physician.

Chronic kidney disease with other complications

Patients with CKD may also suffer from other serious conditions, most commonly diabetes mellitus and hypertension. The sequencing of the CKD code in relationship to codes for other contributing conditions is based on conventions in the Tabular List.

Kidney failure is the inability of the kidneys to excrete waste products and occurs for various reasons. It may be acute (N17.-) or chronic (N18.9) in nature. Causes include surgery or trauma, pregnancy, various medical conditions, nephrotoxins, and irreversible conditions that diminish nephron function.

Acute kidney failure (N17.-) most often is due to reduced blood volume or perfusion of the kidney. Causes include infections, severe dehydration, vascular disease, and damage to renal tissues. Factors outside the kidney, such as obstruction, stones, prostatic hypertrophy and tumors also may cause acute kidney failure. Depending on the cause, severity, and medical treatment, 30% to 60% of acute kidney failure patients will recover.

Note: Code N08 (Glomerular disorders in diseases classified elsewhere) is a manifestation code that is assigned when there is not specific information about the kidney disease provided. The code first note at N08 lists the most common causes of glomerulonephritis, nephritis and nephropathy.

Diabetic nephropathy is coded using a code from the most appropriate diabetes category (E08-E13) with a 4th and 5th character of XXX.21. One of the diabetic category codes with 4th and 5th characters, XXX.22 is used when the diagnosis is diabetic

chronic kidney disease and requires a second additional code from N18 to identify the stage of the chronic kidney disease (stage 1, 2, 3, 4, 5, or ESRD). ESRD is not technically a stage but used for any patient with CKD who requires chronic dialysis. If both a specific stage of CKD and dialysis are documented for a patient, only N18.6 is assigned.

Acquired renal cysts are classified to N28.1, while a congenital cyst of the kidney is coded Q61.- from chapter 17.

Infections

E. coli is the most common disease-causing organism for urinary system infections, but other organisms including Staphylococcus may be the culprit. When the organism is known, an additional code from B95-B97, infection in diseases classified elsewhere, is added to identify the infectious agent.

Cystitis

Category N30.-, or inflammation of the bladder, usually resulting from a urinary tract infection may also involve other associated organs, such as the kidney, prostate or urethra. Cystitis is more common in women than men. Nonetheless, the diagnosis must be documented by the physician before being coded. Sexual intercourse, trauma or poor hygiene allows bacteria to enter the bladder — typically a sterile vesicle. Urinary frequency, urgency, difficulty and pain just above the pubic area are all symptoms of urinary tract infections. There are a number of combination codes within the N30.- category to describe cystitis as acute, chronic, interstitial, with or without hematuria or other conditions present for greater specificity.

Pyelonephritis, an inflammation of the kidney and renal pelvis, is a more severe condition, which occurs when the invading organisms reach the renal pelvis and kidney tissue. When coded to N12, this condition is also referred to as tubule-interstitial nephritis, not specified as acute or chronic. If the documentation states acute tubulo-interstitial nephritis or acute pyelonephritis, the appropriate code is N10. If the documentation states chronic pyelonephritis or chronic tubule-interstitial nephritis, the appropriate code is N11.-. An additional code is added from B95-B97 to identify the infectious agent, when known, in each of these situations.

Urinary tract infection

Category N39.0, Urinary tract infection site not specified, also has a note to use an additional code (B95-B97) to identify the infectious agent.

A urinary tract infection occurring in a patient with a urinary catheter is **not assumed** to be a complication of the catheter. Therefore, code N39.0 and code Z46.6 (fitting and adjustment of urinary device) can be assigned unless the physician documentation supports the infection was caused by the catheter.

If the infection is caused by the catheter, assign a code from T83.51- (infection and inflammatory reaction due to urinary catheter). When T83.51- is used, do not use the Z46.6 code for catheter care. Follow the T83.51- code with an additional code for the specified infection, such as UTI (N39.0 plus an additional code from B95-B97).

Other Issues

The urethra differs in men and women. The female urethra is about 9.5 cm long and the male urethra is about 20 cm long. In men, it serves the dual purpose of conveying sperm and discharging urine from the bladder. The female urethra performs only the latter function.

Neurogenic bladder or neuromuscular dysfunction of bladder, unspecified normally is coded N31.9. There is a note at the N31 category to use an additional code to identify any associated urinary incontinence (N39.3-, N39.4-). Another code for neurogenic bladder, G83.4 (Neurogenic bladder due to cauda equina syndrome) is from Chapter 6, Diseases of the nervous system, but it should not be used unless it is documented or verified with the physician. Improper use of neurogenic bladder codes is a red flag and typically leads to denials. Rarely will a neurogenic bladder be accurately coded at G83.4.

Hyperplasia (benign) of the prostate is coded to N40.- in ICD-10. Prostate growth involves hormones, occurs in different types of tissue (e.g., muscular, glandular), and affects men differently. As a result of these differences, treatment varies in each case. There is no cure for BPH and once prostate growth starts, it often continues unless medical therapy is started.

The prostate can grow in two different ways. In one type of growth, cells multiply around the urethra and squeeze it, much like squeezing a straw. The second type of growth is middle-lobe prostate growth in which cells grow into the urethra and the bladder outlet area. This type of growth typically requires surgery. Hyperplasia, or enlarged prostate, causes a number of symptoms, such as hematuria from straining, a weak urine stream and dribbling. When an enlarged prostate has associated lower urinary tract symptoms, assign code N40.1 first followed by codes to identify the lower urinary tract symptoms (LUTS).

CHAPTER 14: DISEASES OF THE GENITOURINARY SYSTEM (N00-N99)

EXCLUDES 2 certain conditions originating in the perinatal period (P04-P96)

certain infectious and parasitic diseases (A00-B99)

complications of pregnancy, childbirth and the puerperium (O00-O9A)

congenital malformations, deformations and chromosomal abnormalities (Q00-Q99)

endocrine, nutritional and metabolic diseases (E00-E88)

injury, poisoning and certain other consequences of external causes (S00-T88)

neoplasms (C00-D49)

symptoms, signs and abnormal clinical and laboratory findings, not elsewhere classified (R00-R94)

This chapter contains the following blocks:

N00-N08	Glomerular diseases
N10-N16	Renal tubulo-interstitial diseases
N17-N19	Acute kidney failure and chronic kidney disease
N20-N23	Urolithiasis
N25-N29	Other disorders of kidney and ureter
N30-N39	Other diseases of the urinary system
N40-N53	Diseases of male genital organs
N60-N65	Disorders of breast
N70-N77	Inflammatory diseases of female pelvic organs
N80-N98	Noninflammatory disorders of female genital tract
N99	Intraoperative and postprocedural complications and disorders of genitourinary system, not elsewhere classified

Glomerular diseases   (N00-N08)

Code also:

any associated kidney failure (N17-N19) .

EXCLUDES 1 hypertensive chronic kidney disease (I12.-)

4 N00   Acute nephritic syndrome

INCLUDES acute glomerular disease
acute glomerulonephritis
acute nephritis

EXCLUDES 1 acute tubulo-interstitial nephritis (N10)
nephritic syndrome NOS (N05.-)

SP N00.0 Acute nephritic syndrome with minor glomerular abnormality
Acute nephritic syndrome with minimal change lesion

SP N00.1 Acute nephritic syndrome with focal and segmental glomerular lesions
Acute nephritic syndrome with focal and segmental hyalinosis
Acute nephritic syndrome with focal and segmental sclerosis
Acute nephritic syndrome with focal glomerulonephritis

SP N00.2 Acute nephritic syndrome with diffuse membranous glomerulonephritis

SP N00.3 Acute nephritic syndrome with diffuse mesangial proliferative glomerulonephritis

SP N00.4 Acute nephritic syndrome with diffuse endocapillary proliferative glomerulonephritis

SP N00.5 Acute nephritic syndrome with diffuse mesangiocapillary glomerulonephritis
Acute nephritic syndrome with membranoproliferative glomerulonephritis, types 1 and 3, or NOS

SP N00.6 Acute nephritic syndrome with dense deposit disease
Acute nephritic syndrome with membranoproliferative glomerulonephritis, type 2

SP N00.7 Acute nephritic syndrome with diffuse crescentic glomerulonephritis
Acute nephritic syndrome with extracapillary glomerulonephritis

SP N00.8 Acute nephritic syndrome with other morphologic changes
Acute nephritic syndrome with proliferative glomerulonephritis NOS

IQ N00.9 Acute nephritic syndrome with unspecified morphologic changes

4 N01   Rapidly progressive nephritic syndrome

INCLUDES rapidly progressive glomerular disease
rapidly progressive glomerulonephritis
rapidly progressive nephritis

EXCLUDES 1 nephritic syndrome NOS (N05.-)

SP N01.0 Rapidly progressive nephritic syndrome with minor glomerular abnormality
Rapidly progressive nephritic syndrome with minimal change lesion

SP N01.1 Rapidly progressive nephritic syndrome with focal and segmental glomerular lesions
Rapidly progressive nephritic syndrome with focal and segmental hyalinosis
Rapidly progressive nephritic syndrome with focal and segmental sclerosis
Rapidly progressive nephritic syndrome with focal glomerulonephritis

SP N01.2 Rapidly progressive nephritic syndrome with diffuse membranous glomerulonephritis

SP N01.3 Rapidly progressive nephritic syndrome with diffuse mesangial proliferative glomerulonephritis

SP N01.4 Rapidly progressive nephritic syndrome with diffuse endocapillary proliferative glomerulonephritis

SP N01.5 Rapidly progressive nephritic syndrome with diffuse mesangiocapillary glomerulonephritis
Rapidly progressive nephritic syndrome with membranoproliferative glomerulonephritis, types 1 and 3, or NOS

SP N01.6 Rapidly progressive nephritic syndrome with dense deposit disease
Rapidly progressive nephritic syndrome with membranoproliferative glomerulonephritis, type 2

SP N01.7 Rapidly progressive nephritic syndrome with diffuse crescentic glomerulonephritis
Rapidly progressive nephritic syndrome with extracapillary glomerulonephritis

Chapter 14

N00-N99

★ New ▲ Revised **Px** Primary **SP** PDGM Px **SL** Low CoM **SH** High CoM **IQ** Quest. Encounter **H** Hospice non-cancer Dx   Unspecified   **M** *Manifestation*

DecisionHealth's FY 2020 Complete Home Health ICD-10-CM Diagnosis Coding Manual

1281

SP **N01.8** **Rapidly progressive nephritic syndrome with other morphologic changes**
Rapidly progressive nephritic syndrome with proliferative glomerulonephritis NOS

IQ **N01.9** **Rapidly progressive nephritic syndrome with unspecified morphologic changes**

4 **N02** **Recurrent and persistent hematuria**
EXCLUDES 1 acute cystitis with hematuria (N30.01)
hematuria NOS (R31.9)
hematuria not associated with specified morphologic lesions (R31.-)

SP **N02.0** **Recurrent and persistent hematuria with minor glomerular abnormality**
Recurrent and persistent hematuria with minimal change lesion

SP **N02.1** **Recurrent and persistent hematuria with focal and segmental glomerular lesions**
Recurrent and persistent hematuria with focal and segmental hyalinosis
Recurrent and persistent hematuria with focal and segmental sclerosis
Recurrent and persistent hematuria with focal glomerulonephritis

SP **N02.2** **Recurrent and persistent hematuria with diffuse membranous glomerulonephritis**

SP **N02.3** **Recurrent and persistent hematuria with diffuse mesangial proliferative glomerulonephritis**

SP **N02.4** **Recurrent and persistent hematuria with diffuse endocapillary proliferative glomerulonephritis**

SP **N02.5** **Recurrent and persistent hematuria with diffuse mesangiocapillary glomerulonephritis**
Recurrent and persistent hematuria with membranoproliferative glomerulonephritis, types 1 and 3, or NOS

SP **N02.6** **Recurrent and persistent hematuria with dense deposit disease**
Recurrent and persistent hematuria with membranoproliferative glomerulonephritis, type 2

SP **N02.7** **Recurrent and persistent hematuria with diffuse crescentic glomerulonephritis**
Recurrent and persistent hematuria with extracapillary glomerulonephritis

SP **N02.8** **Recurrent and persistent hematuria with other morphologic changes**
Recurrent and persistent hematuria with proliferative glomerulonephritis NOS

IQ **N02.9** **Recurrent and persistent hematuria with unspecified morphologic changes**

4 **N03** **Chronic nephritic syndrome**
INCLUDES chronic glomerular disease
chronic glomerulonephritis
chronic nephritis
EXCLUDES 1 chronic tubulo-interstitial nephritis (N11.-)
diffuse sclerosing glomerulonephritis (N05.8-)

nephritic syndrome NOS (N05.-)

SP **N03.0** **Chronic nephritic syndrome with minor glomerular abnormality**
Chronic nephritic syndrome with minimal change lesion

SP **N03.1** **Chronic nephritic syndrome with focal and segmental glomerular lesions**
Chronic nephritic syndrome with focal and segmental hyalinosis
Chronic nephritic syndrome with focal and segmental sclerosis
Chronic nephritic syndrome with focal glomerulonephritis

SP **N03.2** **Chronic nephritic syndrome with diffuse membranous glomerulonephritis**

SP **N03.3** **Chronic nephritic syndrome with diffuse mesangial proliferative glomerulonephritis**

SP **N03.4** **Chronic nephritic syndrome with diffuse endocapillary proliferative glomerulonephritis**

SP **N03.5** **Chronic nephritic syndrome with diffuse mesangiocapillary glomerulonephritis**
Chronic nephritic syndrome with membranoproliferative glomerulonephritis, types 1 and 3, or NOS

SP **N03.6** **Chronic nephritic syndrome with dense deposit disease**
Chronic nephritic syndrome with membranoproliferative glomerulonephritis, type 2

SP **N03.7** **Chronic nephritic syndrome with diffuse crescentic glomerulonephritis**
Chronic nephritic syndrome with extracapillary glomerulonephritis

SP **N03.8** **Chronic nephritic syndrome with other morphologic changes**
Chronic nephritic syndrome with proliferative glomerulonephritis NOS

IQ **N03.9** **Chronic nephritic syndrome with unspecified morphologic changes**

4 **N04** **Nephrotic syndrome**
INCLUDES congenital nephrotic syndrome
lipoid nephrosis

SP **N04.0** **Nephrotic syndrome with minor glomerular abnormality**
Nephrotic syndrome with minimal change lesion

SP **N04.1** **Nephrotic syndrome with focal and segmental glomerular lesions**
Nephrotic syndrome with focal and segmental hyalinosis
Nephrotic syndrome with focal and segmental sclerosis
Nephrotic syndrome with focal glomerulonephritis

SP **N04.2** **Nephrotic syndrome with diffuse membranous glomerulonephritis**

SP **N04.3** **Nephrotic syndrome with diffuse mesangial proliferative glomerulonephritis**

SP **N04.4** **Nephrotic syndrome with diffuse endocapillary proliferative glomerulonephritis**

SP **N04.5** **Nephrotic syndrome with diffuse mesangiocapillary glomerulonephritis**

Chapter 14

N00-N99

Nephrotic syndrome with membranoproliferative glomerulonephritis, types 1 and 3, or NOS

SP N04.6 Nephrotic syndrome with dense deposit disease

Nephrotic syndrome with membranoproliferative glomerulonephritis, type 2

SP N04.7 Nephrotic syndrome with diffuse crescentic glomerulonephritis

Nephrotic syndrome with extracapillary glomerulonephritis

SP N04.8 Nephrotic syndrome with other morphologic changes

Nephrotic syndrome with proliferative glomerulonephritis NOS

IQ N04.9 Nephrotic syndrome with unspecified morphologic changes

4 N05 Unspecified nephritic syndrome

> INCLUDES
> glomerular disease NOS
> glomerulonephritis NOS
> nephritis NOS
> nephropathy NOS and renal disease NOS with morphological lesion specified in .0-.8
>
> EXCLUDES 1
> nephropathy NOS with no stated morphological lesion (N28.9)
> renal disease NOS with no stated morphological lesion (N28.9)
> tubulo-interstitial nephritis NOS (N12)

SP N05.0 Unspecified nephritic syndrome with minor glomerular abnormality

Unspecified nephritic syndrome with minimal change lesion

SP N05.1 Unspecified nephritic syndrome with focal and segmental glomerular lesions

Unspecified nephritic syndrome with focal and segmental hyalinosis
Unspecified nephritic syndrome with focal and segmental sclerosis
Unspecified nephritic syndrome with focal glomerulonephritis

SP N05.2 Unspecified nephritic syndrome with diffuse membranous glomerulonephritis

SP N05.3 Unspecified nephritic syndrome with diffuse mesangial proliferative glomerulonephritis

SP N05.4 Unspecified nephritic syndrome with diffuse endocapillary proliferative glomerulonephritis

SP N05.5 Unspecified nephritic syndrome with diffuse mesangiocapillary glomerulonephritis

Unspecified nephritic syndrome with membranoproliferative glomerulonephritis, types 1 and 3, or NOS

SP N05.6 Unspecified nephritic syndrome with dense deposit disease

Unspecified nephritic syndrome with membranoproliferative glomerulonephritis, type 2

SP N05.7 Unspecified nephritic syndrome with diffuse crescentic glomerulonephritis

Unspecified nephritic syndrome with extracapillary glomerulonephritis

SP N05.8 Unspecified nephritic syndrome with other morphologic changes

Unspecified nephritic syndrome with proliferative glomerulonephritis NOS

IQ N05.9 Unspecified nephritic syndrome with unspecified morphologic changes

4 N06 Isolated proteinuria with specified morphological lesion

> EXCLUDES 1
> Proteinuria not associated with specific morphologic lesions (R80.0)

SP N06.0 Isolated proteinuria with minor glomerular abnormality

Isolated proteinuria with minimal change lesion

SP N06.1 Isolated proteinuria with focal and segmental glomerular lesions

Isolated proteinuria with focal and segmental hyalinosis
Isolated proteinuria with focal and segmental sclerosis
Isolated proteinuria with focal glomerulonephritis

SP N06.2 Isolated proteinuria with diffuse membranous glomerulonephritis

SP N06.3 Isolated proteinuria with diffuse mesangial proliferative glomerulonephritis

SP N06.4 Isolated proteinuria with diffuse endocapillary proliferative glomerulonephritis

SP N06.5 Isolated proteinuria with diffuse mesangiocapillary glomerulonephritis

Isolated proteinuria with membranoproliferative glomerulonephritis, types 1 and 3, or NOS

SP N06.6 Isolated proteinuria with dense deposit disease

Isolated proteinuria with membranoproliferative glomerulonephritis, type 2

SP N06.7 Isolated proteinuria with diffuse crescentic glomerulonephritis

Isolated proteinuria with extracapillary glomerulonephritis

SP N06.8 Isolated proteinuria with other morphologic lesion

Isolated proteinuria with proliferative glomerulonephritis NOS

IQ N06.9 Isolated proteinuria with unspecified morphologic lesion

4 N07 Hereditary nephropathy, not elsewhere classified

> EXCLUDES 2
> Alport's syndrome (Q87.81-)
> hereditary amyloid nephropathy (E85.-)
> nail patella syndrome (Q87.2)
> non-neuropathic heredofamilial amyloidosis (E85.-)

★ New ▲ Revised Px Primary SP PDGM Px SL Low CoM SH High CoM IQ Quest. Encounter H Hospice non-cancer Dx Unspecified M *Manifestation*

DecisionHealth's FY 2020 Complete Home Health ICD-10-CM Diagnosis Coding Manual

1283

Chapter 14

N00-N99

SP N07.0 Hereditary nephropathy, not elsewhere classified with minor glomerular abnormality
Hereditary nephropathy, not elsewhere classified with minimal change lesion

SP N07.1 Hereditary nephropathy, not elsewhere classified with focal and segmental glomerular lesions
Hereditary nephropathy, not elsewhere classified with focal and segmental hyalinosis
Hereditary nephropathy, not elsewhere classified with focal and segmental sclerosis
Hereditary nephropathy, not elsewhere classified with focal glomerulonephritis

SP N07.2 Hereditary nephropathy, not elsewhere classified with diffuse membranous glomerulonephritis

SP N07.3 Hereditary nephropathy, not elsewhere classified with diffuse mesangial proliferative glomerulonephritis

SP N07.4 Hereditary nephropathy, not elsewhere classified with diffuse endocapillary proliferative glomerulonephritis

SP N07.5 Hereditary nephropathy, not elsewhere classified with diffuse mesangiocapillary glomerulonephritis
Hereditary nephropathy, not elsewhere classified with membranoproliferative glomerulonephritis, types 1 and 3, or NOS

SP N07.6 Hereditary nephropathy, not elsewhere classified with dense deposit disease
Hereditary nephropathy, not elsewhere classified with membranoproliferative glomerulonephritis, type 2

SP N07.7 Hereditary nephropathy, not elsewhere classified with diffuse crescentic glomerulonephritis
Hereditary nephropathy, not elsewhere classified with extracapillary glomerulonephritis

SP N07.8 Hereditary nephropathy, not elsewhere classified with other morphologic lesions
Hereditary nephropathy, not elsewhere classified with proliferative glomerulonephritis NOS

IQ N07.9 Hereditary nephropathy, not elsewhere classified with unspecified morphologic lesions

M IQ N08 *Glomerular disorders in diseases classified elsewhere*
Glomerulonephritis
Nephritis
Nephropathy
Code first underlying disease, such as:
amyloidosis (E85.-)
congenital syphilis (A50.5)
cryoglobulinemia (D89.1)
disseminated intravascular coagulation (D65)
gout (M1A.-, M10.-)
microscopic polyangiitis (M31.7)
multiple myeloma (C90.0-)
sepsis (A40.0-A41.9)
sickle-cell disease (D57.0-D57.8)
EXCLUDES 1 glomerulonephritis, nephritis and nephropathy (in) :

antiglomerular basement membrane disease (M31.0)
diabetes (E08-E13 with .21)
gonococcal (A54.21)
Goodpasture's syndrome (M31.0)
hemolytic-uremic syndrome (D59.3)
lupus (M32.14)
mumps (B26.83)
syphilis (A52.75)
systemic lupus erythematosus (M32.14)
Wegener's granulomatosis (M31.31)
pyelonephritis in diseases classified elsewhere (N16)
renal tubulo-interstitial disorders classified elsewhere (N16)

CODING TIPS ✓ Do not assign code N08 for a patient diagnosed with diabetic nephropathy. For a patient diagnosed with diabetic nephropathy, choose and assign the appropriate combination code to specify the manifestation from categories E08-E13 with 4th and 5th characters .21.

Renal tubulo-interstitial diseases (N10-N16)

INCLUDES pyelonephritis
EXCLUDES 1 pyeloureteritis cystica (N28.85)
CODING TIPS ✓ If the urinary tract infection is resolved, or if the patient has recurrent infections, consider the use of Z87.440.

SP + N10 Acute pyelonephritis
Acute infectious interstitial nephritis
Acute pyelitis
Acute tubulo-interstitial nephritis
Hemoglobin nephrosis
Myoglobin nephrosis
Use additional code (B95-B97), to identify infectious agent.

+ 4 N11 Chronic tubulo-interstitial nephritis
INCLUDES chronic infectious interstitial nephritis
chronic pyelitis
chronic pyelonephritis
Use additional code (B95-B97), to identify infectious agent.

SP SH + N11.0 Nonobstructive reflux-associated chronic pyelonephritis
Pyelonephritis (chronic) associated with (vesicoureteral) reflux
EXCLUDES 1 vesicoureteral reflux NOS (N13.70)

SP SH + N11.1 Chronic obstructive pyelonephritis
Pyelonephritis (chronic) associated with anomaly of pelviureteric junction
Pyelonephritis (chronic) associated with anomaly of pyeloureteric junction
Pyelonephritis (chronic) associated with crossing of vessel
Pyelonephritis (chronic) associated with kinking of ureter
Pyelonephritis (chronic) associated with obstruction of ureter

4 4th digit required   5 5th digit required   6 6th digit required   7 7th digit required   ☑ 7th digit placeholder   ✚ Additional code   ▤ Laterality

1284   *DecisionHealth's* FY 2020 Complete Home Health ICD-10-CM Diagnosis Coding Manual

Pyelonephritis (chronic) associated with
stricture of pelviureteric junction
Pyelonephritis (chronic) associated with
stricture of ureter

> **EXCLUDES 1** calculous pyelonephritis
> (N20.9)
> obstructive uropathy (N13.-)

SP **SH** **+** **N11.8** **Other chronic tubulo-interstitial
nephritis**
Nonobstructive chronic pyelonephritis
NOS

SP **+** **N11.9** **Chronic tubulo-interstitial nephritis,
unspecified**

Chronic interstitial nephritis NOS
Chronic pyelitis NOS
Chronic pyelonephritis NOS

SP **N12** **Tubulo-interstitial nephritis, not specified
as acute or chronic**
Interstitial nephritis NOS
Pyelitis NOS
Pyelonephritis NOS

> **EXCLUDES 1** calculous pyelonephritis
> (N20.9)

> **CODING TIPS ✓** A patient with unspecified
> pyelonephritis and urinary calculus unspecified
> is coded as N12 and N20 in either order.

4 **N13** **Obstructive and reflux uropathy**

> **EXCLUDES 2** calculus of kidney and ureter
> without hydronephrosis
> (N20.-)
> congenital obstructive defects
> of renal pelvis and ureter
> (Q62.0-Q62.3)
> hydronephrosis with
> ureteropelvic junction
> obstruction (Q62.11)
> obstructive pyelonephritis
> (N11.1)

SP **N13.0** **Hydronephrosis with ureteropelvic
junction obstruction**
Hydronephrosis due to acquired occlusion
of ureteropelvic junction

> **EXCLUDES 2** Hydronephrosis with
> ureteropelvic junction
> obstruction due to calculus
> (N13.2)

SP **N13.1** **Hydronephrosis with ureteral stricture,
not elsewhere classified**

> **EXCLUDES 1** Hydronephrosis with ureteral
> stricture with infection
> (N13.6)

SP **SH** **N13.2** **Hydronephrosis with renal and ureteral
calculous obstruction**

> **EXCLUDES 1** Hydronephrosis with renal
> and ureteral calculous
> obstruction with infection
> (N13.6)

5 **N13.3** **Other and unspecified hydronephrosis**

> **EXCLUDES 1** hydronephrosis with
> infection (N13.6)

SP **N13.30** **Unspecified hydronephrosis**

SP **N13.39** **Other hydronephrosis**

SP **N13.4** **Hydroureter**

> **EXCLUDES 1** congenital hydroureter
> (Q62.3-)
> hydroureter with infection
> (N13.6)

vesicoureteral-reflux with
hydroureter (N13.73-)

SP **N13.5** **Crossing vessel and stricture of ureter
without hydronephrosis**
Kinking and stricture of ureter without
hydronephrosis

> **EXCLUDES 1** Crossing vessel and stricture
> of ureter without
> hydronephrosis with
> infection (N13.6)

SP **+** **N13.6** **Pyonephrosis**
Conditions in N13.0-N13.5 with infection
Obstructive uropathy with infection
Use additional code (B95-B97), to identify
infectious agent.

5 **N13.7** **Vesicoureteral-reflux**

> **EXCLUDES 1** reflux-associated
> pyelonephritis (N11.0)

SP **N13.70** **Vesicoureteral-reflux, unspecified**
Vesicoureteral-reflux NOS

> **DEFINITION** Abnormal retrograde flow
> of urine from bladder back into the
> ureter and kidney; may cause
> progressive, long-term damage.

SP **N13.71** **Vesicoureteral-reflux without reflux
nephropathy**

6 **N13.72** **Vesicoureteral-reflux with reflux
nephropathy without hydroureter**

SP **N13.721** **Vesicoureteral-reflux with reflux
nephropathy without hydroureter,
unilateral**

SP **N13.722** **Vesicoureteral-reflux with reflux
nephropathy without hydroureter,
bilateral**

IQ **N13.729** **Vesicoureteral-reflux with reflux
nephropathy without
hydroureter, unspecified**

6 **N13.73** **Vesicoureteral-reflux with reflux
nephropathy with hydroureter**

SP **N13.731** **Vesicoureteral-reflux with reflux
nephropathy with hydroureter,
unilateral**

SP **N13.732** **Vesicoureteral-reflux with reflux
nephropathy with hydroureter,
bilateral**

IQ **N13.739** **Vesicoureteral-reflux with reflux
nephropathy with hydroureter,
unspecified**

SP **N13.8** **Other obstructive and reflux uropathy**
Urinary tract obstruction due to specified
cause
Code first, if applicable, any causal
condition, such as:
enlarged prostate (N40.1)

SP **N13.9** **Obstructive and reflux uropathy,
unspecified**
Urinary tract obstruction NOS

+ **4** **N14** **Drug- and heavy-metal-induced tubulo-
interstitial and tubular conditions**
Code first:
poisoning due to drug or toxin, if applicable
(T36-T65 with fifth or sixth character 1-4
or 6)
Use additional code for adverse effect, if
applicable, to identify drug (T36-T50 with
fifth or sixth character 5)

★ New ▲ Revised Px Primary **SP** PDGM Px **SL** Low CoM **SH** High CoM **IQ** Quest. Encounter **H** Hospice non-cancer Dx | Unspecified | **M** *Manifestation*

DecisionHealth's FY 2020 Complete Home Health ICD-10-CM Diagnosis Coding Manual

1285

CODING TIPS ✓ Conditions classified to N14.- indicate nephropathy due to drugs, metals, or other toxic exposure. When one of these conditions has been specifically reported, first assign the appropriate code from T36-T65 when the condition is due to a poisoning. Or, to indicate adverse effect, assign a second code from T36-T50 following the appropriate N14.-code.

SP + N14.0 **Analgesic nephropathy**

SP + N14.1 **Nephropathy induced by other drugs, medicaments and biological substances**

SP + N14.2 **Nephropathy induced by unspecified drug, medicament or biological substance**

SP + N14.3 **Nephropathy induced by heavy metals**

SP + N14.4 **Toxic nephropathy, not elsewhere classified**

④ N15 **Other renal tubulo-interstitial diseases**

SP N15.0 **Balkan nephropathy**
Balkan endemic nephropathy

SP N15.1 **Renal and perinephric abscess**

SP N15.8 **Other specified renal tubulo-interstitial diseases**

SP N15.9 **Renal tubulo-interstitial disease, unspecified**

Infection of kidney NOS
EXCLUDES 1 urinary tract infection NOS (N39.0)

M IQ N16 *Renal tubulo-interstitial disorders in diseases classified elsewhere*

Pyelonephritis
Tubulo-interstitial nephritis
Code first underlying disease, such as:
brucellosis (A23.0-A23.9)
cryoglobulinemia (D89.1)
glycogen storage disease (E74.0)
leukemia (C91-C95)
lymphoma (C81.0-C85.9, C96.0-C96.9)
multiple myeloma (C90.0-)
sepsis (A40.0-A41.9)
Wilson's disease (E83.0)
EXCLUDES 1 diphtheritic pyelonephritis and tubulo-interstitial nephritis (A36.84)
pyelonephritis and tubulo-interstitial nephritis in candidiasis (B37.49)
pyelonephritis and tubulo-interstitial nephritis in cystinosis (E72.04)
pyelonephritis and tubulo-interstitial nephritis in salmonella infection (A02.25)
pyelonephritis and tubulo-interstitial nephritis in sarcoidosis (D86.84)
pyelonephritis and tubulo-interstitial nephritis in sicca syndrome [Sjogren's] (M35.04)
pyelonephritis and tubulo-interstitial nephritis in systemic lupus erythematosus (M32.15)

pyelonephritis and tubulo-interstitial nephritis in toxoplasmosis (B58.83)
renal tubular degeneration in diabetes (E08-E13 with .29)
syphilitic pyelonephritis and tubulo-interstitial nephritis (A52.75)

Acute kidney failure and chronic kidney disease   (N17-N19)

EXCLUDES 2 congenital renal failure (P96.0)
drug- and heavy-metal-induced tubulo-interstitial and tubular conditions (N14.-)
extrarenal uremia (R39.2)
hemolytic-uremic syndrome (D59.3)
hepatorenal syndrome (K76.7)
postpartum hepatorenal syndrome (O90.4)
posttraumatic renal failure (T79.5)
prerenal uremia (R39.2)
renal failure complicating abortion or ectopic or molar pregnancy (O00-O07, O08.4)
renal failure following labor and delivery (O90.4)
renal failure postprocedural (N99.0)

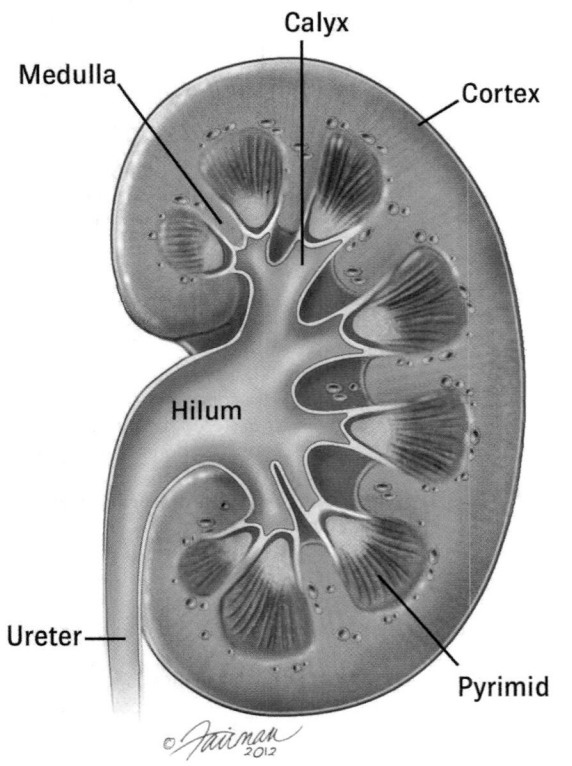

④ N17 **Acute kidney failure**
Code also:
associated underlying condition
EXCLUDES 1 posttraumatic renal failure (T79.5)

---

④4th digit required   **⑤**5th digit required   **⑥**6th digit required   **⑦**7th digit required   **⑦**7th digit placeholder   **+**Additional code   **⊟**Laterality

1286   *DecisionHealth's* FY 2020 Complete Home Health ICD-10-CM Diagnosis Coding Manual

GUIDELINES Section I.C.9.a.2)
If a patient has hypertensive chronic kidney disease and acute renal failure, an additional code for the acute renal failure [category N17] is required.

CODING TIPS✓ When both acute kidney failure and chronic kidney disease (CKD) are present, both conditions should be coded. It should be verified with the physician to identify if acute kidney failure is resolved when a patient returns to home health. Home health may continue to treat acute kidney failure in the home until it is completely resolved, if it had not resolved prior to the patient's discharge home.

H SP N17.0 Acute kidney failure with tubular necrosis
Acute tubular necrosis
Renal tubular necrosis
Tubular necrosis NOS

H SP N17.1 Acute kidney failure with acute cortical necrosis
Acute cortical necrosis
Cortical necrosis NOS
Renal cortical necrosis

H SP N17.2 Acute kidney failure with medullary necrosis
Medullary [papillary] necrosis NOS
Acute medullary [papillary] necrosis
Renal medullary [papillary] necrosis

H SP N17.8 Other acute kidney failure

H SP N17.9 Acute kidney failure, unspecified
Acute kidney injury (nontraumatic)
EXCLUDES 2 traumatic kidney injury (S37.0-)

+ 4 N18 Chronic kidney disease (CKD)
Code first any associated:
diabetic chronic kidney disease (E08.22, E09.22, E10.22, E11.22, E13.22)
hypertensive chronic kidney disease (I12.-, I13.-)
Use additional code to identify kidney transplant status, if applicable, (Z94.0)

GUIDELINES Section I.C.14.a.1)
The ICD-10-CM classifies CKD based on severity. The severity of CKD is designated by stages 1-5. Stage 2, code N18.2, equates to mild CKD; stage 3, code N18.3, equates to moderate CKD; and stage 4, code N18.4, equates to severe CKD. Code N18.6, End stage renal disease (ESRD), is assigned when the provider has documented end-stage-renal disease (ESRD). If both a stage of CKD and ESRD are documented, assign code N18.6 only.

GUIDELINES Section I.C.14.a.3)
Patients with CKD may also suffer from other serious conditions, most commonly diabetes mellitus and hypertension. The sequencing of the CKD code in relationship to codes for other contributing conditions is based on the conventions in the Tabular List.

CODING TIPS✓ The stage of CKD may not be coded based on lab data such as glomerular filtration rates (GFR).

CODING TIPS✓ Chronic kidney disease (CKD) is assumed related to hypertension and diabetes. Hypertension (I12 or I13) is sequenced prior to chronic kidney disease (CKD) if both are present. Any associated diabetes also must be sequenced prior to the CKD. Diabetic CKD and hypertension is coded either E11.22, I12.9, N18.9 or I12.9, E11.22, N18.9. If documentation indicates hypertensive heart and kidney disease, the hypertension code will be from the I13 category.

CODING TIPS✓ The presence of CKD alone after a kidney transplant doesn't necessarily mean the transplant is complicated. Patients who have undergone a kidney transplant may still have some form of CKD because the kidney transplant may not fully restore kidney function. Assign the appropriate N18 code (chronic kidney disease) to indicate the stage of CKD, and code Z94.0 (kidney organ or tissue replaced by transplant), if a transplant complication is not documented.

SP SH + N18.1 Chronic kidney disease, stage 1

SP SH + N18.2 Chronic kidney disease, stage 2 (mild)

SP SH + N18.3 Chronic kidney disease, stage 3 (moderate)

SP SH + N18.4 Chronic kidney disease, stage 4 (severe)

IQ SH + N18.5 Chronic kidney disease, stage 5
EXCLUDES 1 chronic kidney disease, stage 5 requiring chronic dialysis (N18.6)

H IQ SH + N18.6 End stage renal disease
Chronic kidney disease requiring chronic dialysis
Use additional code to identify dialysis status (Z99.2)

ALERT ESRD is not appropriate for assignment to the primary diagnosis in home care. ESRD and related care to the dialysis catheter is the responsibility of the dialysis center.

CODING TIPS✓ If ESRD is documented along with another stage of CKD, code only N18.6.

CODING TIPS✓ All CKD patients requiring dialysis are coded as N18.6, even if the physician documents a different stage. Do not code ESRD as primary in home health. Add the appropriate Z99.2 or Z91.15 if on dialysis. If the patient with ESRD is not on dialysis, then the code for palliative care may be appropriate (Z51.5).

IQ + N18.9 Chronic kidney disease, unspecified
Chronic renal disease
Chronic renal failure NOS
Chronic renal insufficiency
Chronic uremia NOS
Diffuse sclerosing glomerulonephritis NOS

H IQ N19 Unspecified kidney failure
Uremia NOS
EXCLUDES 1 acute kidney failure (N17.-)
chronic kidney disease (N18.-)
chronic uremia (N18.9)
extrarenal uremia (R39.2)
prerenal uremia (R39.2)

★ New ▲ Revised Px Primary **SP** PDGM Px **SL** Low CoM **SH** High CoM **IQ** Quest. Encounter **H** Hospice non-cancer Dx Unspecified **M** *Manifestation*

renal insufficiency (acute)
(N28.9)
uremia of newborn (P96.0)

Urolithiasis (N20-N23)

4 N20   Calculus of kidney and ureter
Calculous pyelonephritis
EXCLUDES 1 nephrocalcinosis (E83.5)
that with hydronephrosis
(N13.2)

CODING TIPS ✓ If the renal calculi is resolved, or
if the patient has recurrent kidney stones,
consider the use of Z87.442.

CODING TIPS ✓ A patient with unspecified
pyelonephritis and urinary calculus unspecified
is coded as N12 and N20 in either order.

SP SH N20.0 Calculus of kidney
Nephrolithiasis NOS
Renal calculus
Renal stone
Staghorn calculus
Stone in kidney

SP N20.1 Calculus of ureter
Ureteric stone

**SP SH N20.2 Calculus of kidney with calculus of
ureter**

IQ N20.9   Urinary calculus, unspecified

4 N21   Calculus of lower urinary tract
INCLUDES calculus of lower urinary tract
with cystitis and urethritis

SP N21.0 Calculus in bladder
Calculus in diverticulum of bladder
Urinary bladder stone
EXCLUDES 2 staghorn calculus (N20.0)

DEFINITION An abnormal concretion of
mineral salts, occurring in the bladder.

SP N21.1 Calculus in urethra
EXCLUDES 2 calculus of prostate (N42.0)

SP N21.8 Other lower urinary tract calculus

**IQ N21.9   Calculus of lower urinary tract,
unspecified**
EXCLUDES 1 calculus of urinary tract NOS
(N20.9)

**M IQ N22   *Calculus of urinary tract in diseases
classified elsewhere***
Code first underlying disease, such as:
gout (M1A.-, M10.-)
schistosomiasis (B65.0-B65.9)

SP N23   Unspecified renal colic

Other disorders of kidney and ureter (N25-N29)

EXCLUDES 2 disorders of kidney and ureter with urolithiasis
(N20-N23)

**4 N25   Disorders resulting from impaired renal
tubular function**

SP N25.0 Renal osteodystrophy
Azotemic osteodystrophy
Phosphate-losing tubular disorders
Renal rickets
Renal short stature
EXCLUDES 2 metabolic disorders
classifiable to E70-E88

SP SH N25.1 Nephrogenic diabetes insipidus

EXCLUDES 1 diabetes insipidus NOS
(E23.2)

**5 N25.8 Other disorders resulting from impaired
renal tubular function**

**SP N25.81 Secondary hyperparathyroidism of
renal origin**
EXCLUDES 1 secondary
hyperparathyroidism,
non-renal (E21.1)
EXCLUDES 2 metabolic disorders
classifiable to E70-E88

**SP N25.89 Other disorders resulting from
impaired renal tubular function**
Hypokalemic nephropathy
Lightwood-Albright syndrome
Renal tubular acidosis NOS

**IQ N25.9   Disorder resulting from impaired renal
tubular function, unspecified**

4 N26   Unspecified contracted kidney
EXCLUDES 1 contracted kidney due to
hypertension (I12.-)
diffuse sclerosing
glomerulonephritis (N05.8.-)
hypertensive nephrosclerosis
(arteriolar) (arteriosclerotic)
(I12.-)
small kidney of unknown cause
(N27.-)

CODING TIPS ✓ When a condition classifiable to
N26.-is present with a diagnosis of
hypertension, I12.9 should be assigned, unless
the physician documents secondary
hypertension. N26 is included in I12.

SP N26.1 Atrophy of kidney (terminal)

SP N26.2 Page kidney

IQ N26.9   Renal sclerosis, unspecified

4 N27   Small kidney of unknown cause
INCLUDES oligonephronia

SP N27.0 Small kidney, unilateral

SP N27.1 Small kidney, bilateral

IQ N27.9   Small kidney, unspecified

**4 N28   Other disorders of kidney and ureter, not
elsewhere classified**

SP N28.0 Ischemia and infarction of kidney
Renal artery embolism
Renal artery obstruction
Renal artery occlusion
Renal artery thrombosis
Renal infarct
EXCLUDES 1 atherosclerosis of renal
artery (extrarenal part)
(I70.1)
congenital stenosis of renal
artery (Q27.1)
Goldblatt's kidney (I70.1)

SP N28.1 Cyst of kidney, acquired
Cyst (multiple) (solitary) of kidney
(acquired)
EXCLUDES 1 cystic kidney disease
(congenital) (Q61.-)

4 4th digit required   **5** 5th digit required   **6** 6th digit required   **7** 7th digit required   **7** 7th digit placeholder   **+** Additional code   **⊟** Laterality

1288   *DecisionHealth's* FY 2020 Complete Home Health ICD-10-CM Diagnosis Coding Manual

CODING TIPS ✓ N28.1 is coded only for acquired renal cysts. If the medical record does not indicate acquired or congenital, ICD-10 assumes the cyst is congenital (Q61). Carefully review documentation provided to ensure the cysts are in the kidney when assigning this code. Cysts noted to be present in the ureters are not classified here.

⑤ N28.8   Other specified disorders of kidney and ureter

> **EXCLUDES 1** hydroureter (N13.4)
> ureteric stricture with hydronephrosis (N13.1)
> ureteric stricture without hydronephrosis (N13.5)

SP N28.81   Hypertrophy of kidney

SP N28.82   Megaloureter

SP N28.83   Nephroptosis

SP N28.84   Pyelitis cystica

SP N28.85   Pyeloureteritis cystica

> **DEFINITION** Infection of the renal pelvis and ureter with development of small cysts in the kidney and ureter.

SP N28.86   Ureteritis cystica

SP N28.89   Other specified disorders of kidney and ureter

IQ N28.9   Disorder of kidney and ureter, unspecified

> Nephropathy NOS
> Renal disease (acute) NOS
> Renal insufficiency (acute)
> **EXCLUDES 1** chronic renal insufficiency (N18.9)
> unspecified nephritic syndrome (N05.-)

M IQ SH N29   *Other disorders of kidney and ureter in diseases classified elsewhere*

> Code first underlying disease, such as:
> amyloidosis (E85.-)
> nephrocalcinosis (E83.5)
> schistosomiasis (B65.0-B65.9)
> **EXCLUDES 1** disorders of kidney and ureter in:
> cystinosis (E72.0)
> gonorrhea (A54.21)
> syphilis (A52.75)
> tuberculosis (A18.11)

Other diseases of the urinary system (N30-N39)

> **EXCLUDES 1** urinary infection (complicating) :
> abortion or ectopic or molar pregnancy (O00-O07, O08.8)
> pregnancy, childbirth and the puerperium (O23.-, O75.3, O86.2-)

+ ④ N30   Cystitis

> Use additional code to identify infectious agent (B95-B97)
> **EXCLUDES 1** prostatocystitis (N41.3)

> **CODING TIPS ✓** If the urinary tract infection is resolved, or if the patient has recurrent infections, consider the use of Z87.440.

CODING TIPS ✓ Gross hematuria means that the blood in the urine can be seen with the naked eye. If hematuria is related to anticoagulant/antiplatelets, also code D68.32 and the T code for the drug.

CODING TIPS ✓ Cystitis indicates inflammation and/or infection localized to the bladder. When a urinary tract infection is specified as cystitis, assign the appropriate N30.- code. Also assign a code for the causative organism, when known. An unspecified urinary tract infection should be coded to N39.0.

+ ⑤ N30.0   Acute cystitis

> **EXCLUDES 1** irradiation cystitis (N30.4-)
> trigonitis (N30.3-)

SP + N30.00   Acute cystitis without hematuria

SP + N30.01   Acute cystitis with hematuria

+ ⑤ N30.1   Interstitial cystitis (chronic)

SP + N30.10   Interstitial cystitis (chronic) without hematuria

SP + N30.11   Interstitial cystitis (chronic) with hematuria

+ ⑤ N30.2   Other chronic cystitis

SP + N30.20   Other chronic cystitis without hematuria

SP + N30.21   Other chronic cystitis with hematuria

+ ⑤ N30.3   Trigonitis

> Urethrotrigonitis
> **DEFINITION** Inflammation of the mouth of the bladder where it drains into the urethra.

SP + N30.30   Trigonitis without hematuria

SP + N30.31   Trigonitis with hematuria

+ ⑤ N30.4   Irradiation cystitis

SP + N30.40   Irradiation cystitis without hematuria

SP + N30.41   Irradiation cystitis with hematuria

+ ⑤ N30.8   Other cystitis

> Abscess of bladder

SP + N30.80   Other cystitis without hematuria

SP + N30.81   Other cystitis with hematuria

> **DEFINITION** Bullous (cystic) cystitis: Inflammation of the bladder with formation of cysts on the interior bladder wall.

+ ⑤ N30.9   Cystitis, unspecified

SP + N30.90   Cystitis, unspecified without hematuria

SP + N30.91   Cystitis, unspecified with hematuria

+ ④ N31   Neuromuscular dysfunction of bladder, not elsewhere classified

> Use additional code to identify any associated urinary incontinence (N39.3-N39.4-)
> **EXCLUDES 1** cord bladder NOS (G95.89)
> neurogenic bladder due to cauda equina syndrome (G83.4)
> neuromuscular dysfunction due to spinal cord lesion (G95.89)

SP SH + N31.0   Uninhibited neuropathic bladder, not elsewhere classified

SP SH + N31.1   Reflex neuropathic bladder, not elsewhere classified

---

★ New ▲ Revised **Px** Primary **SP** PDGM Px **SL** Low CoM **SH** High CoM **IQ** Quest. Encounter **H** Hospice non-cancer Dx Unspecified **M** *Manifestation*

SP ✚ **N31.2 Flaccid neuropathic bladder, not elsewhere classified**
Atonic (motor) (sensory) neuropathic bladder
Autonomous neuropathic bladder
Nonreflex neuropathic bladder

SP ✚ **N31.8 Other neuromuscular dysfunction of bladder**

SP **SH** ✚ **N31.9 Neuromuscular dysfunction of bladder, unspecified**
Neurogenic bladder dysfunction NOS

4 N32 Other disorders of bladder
> EXCLUDES 2   calculus of bladder (N21.0)
> cystocele (N81.1-)
> hernia or prolapse of bladder, female (N81.1-)

SP N32.0 Bladder-neck obstruction
Bladder-neck stenosis (acquired)
> EXCLUDES 1   congenital bladder-neck obstruction (Q64.3-)
> DEFINITION   Blockage in the opening between the bladder and the urethra, causing bladder distention and decreased urine output.

SP N32.1 Vesicointestinal fistula
Vesicorectal fistula
> DEFINITION   Abnormal passage between the bladder and the intestines.

SP N32.2 Vesical fistula, not elsewhere classified
> EXCLUDES 1   fistula between bladder and female genital tract (N82.0-N82.1)

SP N32.3 Diverticulum of bladder
> EXCLUDES 1   congenital diverticulum of bladder (Q64.6)
> diverticulitis of bladder (N30.8-)

5 N32.8 Other specified disorders of bladder

SP N32.81 Overactive bladder
Detrusor muscle hyperactivity
> EXCLUDES 1   frequent urination due to specified bladder condition- code to condition

SP N32.89 Other specified disorders of bladder
Bladder hemorrhage
Bladder hypertrophy
Calcified bladder
Contracted bladder

IQ N32.9 Bladder disorder, unspecified

M IQ N33 Bladder disorders in diseases classified elsewhere
Code first underlying disease, such as:
schistosomiasis (B65.0-B65.9)
> EXCLUDES 1   bladder disorder in syphilis (A52.76)
> bladder disorder in tuberculosis (A18.12)
> candidal cystitis (B37.41)
> chlamydial cystitis (A56.01)
> cystitis in gonorrhea (A54.01)
> cystitis in neurogenic bladder (N31.-)
> diphtheritic cystitis (A36.85)
> syphilitic cystitis (A52.76)
> trichomonal cystitis (A59.03)

✚ **4 N34 Urethritis and urethral syndrome**

Use additional code (B95-B97), to identify infectious agent.
> EXCLUDES 2   Reiter's disease (M02.3-)
> urethritis in diseases with a predominantly sexual mode of transmission (A50-A64)
> urethrotrigonitis (N30.3-)

SP ✚ **N34.0 Urethral abscess**
Abscess (of) Cowper's gland
Abscess (of) Littré's gland
Abscess (of) urethral (gland)
Periurethral abscess
> EXCLUDES 1   urethral caruncle (N36.2)

SP ✚ **N34.1 Nonspecific urethritis**
Nongonococcal urethritis
Nonvenereal urethritis

SP ✚ **N34.2 Other urethritis**
Meatitis, urethral
Postmenopausal urethritis
Ulcer of urethra (meatus)
Urethritis NOS

SP ✚ **N34.3 Urethral syndrome, unspecified**

4 N35 Urethral stricture
> EXCLUDES 1   congenital urethral stricture (Q64.3-)
> postprocedural urethral stricture (N99.1-)

5 N35.0 Post-traumatic urethral stricture
Urethral stricture due to injury
> EXCLUDES 1   postprocedural urethral stricture (N99.1-)

6 N35.01 Post-traumatic urethral stricture, male

SP N35.010 Post-traumatic urethral stricture, male, meatal

SP N35.011 Post-traumatic bulbous urethral stricture

SP N35.012 Post-traumatic membranous urethral stricture

SP N35.013 Post-traumatic anterior urethral stricture

SP N35.014 Post-traumatic urethral stricture, male, unspecified

SP N35.016 Post-traumatic urethral stricture, male, overlapping sites

6 N35.02 Post-traumatic urethral stricture, female

SP N35.021 Urethral stricture due to childbirth

SP N35.028 Other post-traumatic urethral stricture, female

5 N35.1 Postinfective urethral stricture, not elsewhere classified
> EXCLUDES 1   urethral stricture associated with schistosomiasis (B65.-, N29)
> gonococcal urethral stricture (A54.01)
> syphilitic urethral stricture (A52.76)

6 N35.11 Postinfective urethral stricture, not elsewhere classified, male

SP N35.111 Postinfective urethral stricture, not elsewhere classified, male, meatal

SP N35.112 Postinfective bulbous urethral stricture, not elsewhere classified, male

---

4 4th digit required   5 5th digit required   6 6th digit required   7 7th digit required   7 7th digit placeholder   ✚ Additional code   ⬡ Laterality

1290   DecisionHealth's FY 2020 Complete Home Health ICD-10-CM Diagnosis Coding Manual

SP N35.113 Postinfective membranous urethral stricture, not elsewhere classified, male

SP N35.114 Postinfective anterior urethral stricture, not elsewhere classified, male

SP N35.116 Postinfective urethral stricture, not elsewhere classified, male, overlapping sites

SP N35.119 Postinfective urethral stricture, not elsewhere classified, male, unspecified

SP N35.12 Postinfective urethral stricture, not elsewhere classified, female

⑤ N35.8 Other urethral stricture

> **EXCLUDES 1** postprocedural urethral stricture (N99.1-)

⑥ N35.81 Other urethral stricture, male

SP N35.811 Other urethral stricture, male, meatal

SP N35.812 Other urethral bulbous stricture, male

SP N35.813 Other membranous urethral stricture, male

▲ SP N35.814 Other anterior urethral stricture, male

SP N35.816 Other urethral stricture, male, overlapping sites

SP N35.819 Other urethral stricture, male, unspecified site

SP N35.82 Other urethral stricture, female

⑤ N35.9 Urethral stricture, unspecified

⑥ N35.91 Urethral stricture, unspecified, male

SP N35.911 Unspecified urethral stricture, male, meatal

SP N35.912 Unspecified bulbous urethral stricture, male

SP N35.913 Unspecified membranous urethral stricture, male

SP N35.914 Unspecified anterior urethral stricture, male

SP N35.916 Unspecified urethral stricture, male, overlapping sites

SP N35.919 Unspecified urethral stricture, male, unspecified site

> Pinhole meatus NOS
> Urethral stricture NOS

SP N35.92 Unspecified urethral stricture, female

④ N36 Other disorders of urethra

SP N36.0 Urethral fistula

> Urethroperineal fistula
> Urethrorectal fistula
> Urinary fistula NOS

> **EXCLUDES 1** urethroscrotal fistula (N50.89)
> urethrovaginal fistula (N82.1)
> urethrovesicovaginal fistula (N82.1)

> **DEFINITION** An abnormal passage communicating with the urethra.

SP N36.1 Urethral diverticulum

> **DEFINITION** Sac-like out-pouching of the urethral wall.

SP N36.2 Urethral caruncle

> **DEFINITION** A fleshy outgrowth in the urethra that may be normal or abnormal, often growing from mucous membranes.

➕ ⑤ N36.4 Urethral functional and muscular disorders

> Use additional code to identify associated urinary stress incontinence (N39.3)

SP ➕ N36.41 Hypermobility of urethra

SP ➕ N36.42 Intrinsic sphincter deficiency (ISD)

SP ➕ N36.43 Combined hypermobility of urethra and intrinsic sphincter deficiency

SP ➕ N36.44 Muscular disorders of urethra

> Bladder sphincter dyssynergy

SP N36.5 Urethral false passage

SP N36.8 Other specified disorders of urethra

> **EXCLUDES 1** congenital urethrocele (Q64.7)
> female urethrocele (N81.0)

IQ N36.9 Urethral disorder, unspecified

M IQ N37 *Urethral disorders in diseases classified elsewhere*

> Code first:
> underlying disease

> **EXCLUDES 1** urethritis (in) :
> candidal infection (B37.41)
> chlamydial (A56.01)
> gonorrhea (A54.01)
> syphilis (A52.76)
> trichomonal infection (A59.03)
> tuberculosis (A18.13)

④ N39 Other disorders of urinary system

> **EXCLUDES 2** hematuria NOS (R31.-)
> recurrent or persistent hematuria (N02.-)
> recurrent or persistent hematuria with specified morphological lesion (N02.-)
> proteinuria NOS (R80.-)

▲ SP SH ➕ N39.0 Urinary tract infection, site not specified

> Use additional code (B95-B97), to identify infectious agent.

> **EXCLUDES 1** candidiasis of urinary tract (B37.4-)
> neonatal urinary tract infection (P39.3)
> pyuria (R82.81)
> urinary tract infection of specified site, such as:
> cystitis (N30.-)
> urethritis (N34.-)

> **CODING TIPS ✓** Bacteriuria is a condition where there are bacteria present in a microscopic examination of the urine. Do not code bacteriuria as a UTI. See R82.7.

> **CODING TIPS ✓** The urinary tract includes the kidneys, ureters, bladder and urethra. Infection involving the bladder is coded with category N30. Infection of the kidney should be coded N15.9 (unless specific information is available). Urethritis is coded with category N34. Infection involving the ureter(s) should be coded with N28.86. Query for specific information.

★ New ▲ Revised Px Primary SP PDGM Px SL Low CoM SH High CoM IQ Quest. Encounter H Hospice non-cancer Dx [Unspecified] M *Manifestation*

DecisionHealth's FY 2020 Complete Home Health ICD-10-CM Diagnosis Coding Manual 1291

CODING TIPS ✓ If UTI is not a confirmed diagnosis, report a symptom code (e.g., codes in R30-R39 series) instead of this code.

CODING TIPS ✓ Code N39.0 is appropriate only when the site of the UTI is unspecified. Remember to use additional code (B95-B97) to identify infectious agent. If the urinary tract infection is resolved, or if the patient has recurrent infections, consider the use of Z87.440.

SP N39.3 Stress incontinence (female) (male)
Code also:
   any associated overactive bladder (N32.81)
   EXCLUDES 1 mixed incontinence (N39.46)
   DEFINITION Involuntary loss of bladder control during physical movements, such as coughing, sneezing, or other strenuous activity.

5 N39.4 Other specified urinary incontinence
Code also:
   any associated overactive bladder (N32.81)
   EXCLUDES 1 enuresis NOS (R32)
     functional urinary incontinence (R39.81)
     urinary incontinence associated with cognitive impairment (R39.81)
     urinary incontinence NOS (R32)
     urinary incontinence of nonorganic origin (F98.0)

SP N39.41 Urge incontinence
   EXCLUDES 1 mixed incontinence (N39.46)
   DEFINITION Inability to control urination after the urge to urinate.

SP N39.42 Incontinence without sensory awareness
Insensible (urinary) incontinence

!Q N39.43 Post-void dribbling

!Q N39.44 Nocturnal enuresis

!Q N39.45 Continuous leakage

SP N39.46 Mixed incontinence
Urge and stress incontinence

6 N39.49 Other specified urinary incontinence

SP N39.490 Overflow incontinence
   DEFINITION Urinary incontinence due to pressure of retained urine in the bladder, after the bladder has contracted to its limits, with dribbling urine.

SP N39.491 Coital incontinence

SP N39.492 Postural (urinary) incontinence

SP N39.498 Other specified urinary incontinence
Reflex incontinence
Total incontinence

SP N39.8 Other specified disorders of urinary system

!Q N39.9 Disorder of urinary system, unspecified

Diseases of male genital organs (N40-N53)

4 N40 Benign prostatic hyperplasia
   INCLUDES adenofibromatous hypertrophy of prostate
     benign hypertrophy of the prostate
     benign prostatic hypertrophy
     BPH
     enlarged prostate
     nodular prostate
     polyp of prostate
   EXCLUDES 1 benign neoplasms of prostate (adenoma, benign) (fibroadenoma) (fibroma) (myoma) (D29.1)
   EXCLUDES 2 malignant neoplasm of prostate (C61)

CODING TIPS ✓ Enlarged prostate disorders no longer include the benign neoplasms of the prostate. Benign tumors of the prostate are coded to D29.1, not N40.

CODING TIPS ✓ Although hyperplasia (increase in number of cells) and hypertrophy (increase in size of cells) are not synonymous, benign prostatic hyperplasia and benign prostatic hypertrophy are classified to the same code. When a patient diagnosed with a condition classifiable to N40.- also has lower urinary tract symptoms present – such as obstruction, incontinence, hesitancy, frequency, urgency or other included conditions – assign code N40.1 and the associated symptoms.

SP N40.0 Benign prostatic hyperplasia without lower urinary tract symptoms
Enlarged prostate without LUTS
Enlarged prostate NOS

SP SH + N40.1 Benign prostatic hyperplasia with lower urinary tract symptoms
Enlarged prostate with LUTS
Use additional code for associated symptoms, when specified:
   incomplete bladder emptying (R39.14)
   nocturia (R35.1)
   straining on urination (R39.16)
   urinary frequency (R35.0)
   urinary hesitancy (R39.11)
   urinary incontinence (N39.4-)
   urinary obstruction (N13.8)
   urinary retention (R33.8)
   urinary urgency (R39.15)
   weak urinary stream (R39.12)

SP N40.2 Nodular prostate without lower urinary tract symptoms
Nodular prostate without LUTS

SP + N40.3 Nodular prostate with lower urinary tract symptoms
Use additional code for associated symptoms, when specified:
   incomplete bladder emptying (R39.14)
   nocturia (R35.1)
   straining on urination (R39.16)
   urinary frequency (R35.0)
   urinary hesitancy (R39.11)
   urinary incontinence (N39.4-)
   urinary obstruction (N13.8)
   urinary retention (R33.8)
   urinary urgency (R39.15)

4 4th digit required   **5** 5th digit required   **6** 6th digit required   **7** 7th digit required   **7** 7th digit placeholder   **+** Additional code   **⊟** Laterality

1292   *DecisionHealth's* FY 2020 Complete Home Health ICD-10-CM Diagnosis Coding Manual

weak urinary stream (R39.12)

+ 4 N41 Inflammatory diseases of prostate
Use additional code (B95-B97), to identify infectious agent.

SP + N41.0 Acute prostatitis

SP + N41.1 Chronic prostatitis

SP + N41.2 Abscess of prostate

SP + N41.3 Prostatocystitis

SP + N41.4 Granulomatous prostatitis

SP + N41.8 Other inflammatory diseases of prostate

IQ + N41.9 Inflammatory disease of prostate, unspecified
Prostatitis NOS

4 N42 Other and unspecified disorders of prostate

SP N42.0 Calculus of prostate
Prostatic stone

SP N42.1 Congestion and hemorrhage of prostate
> EXCLUDES 1 enlarged prostate (N40.-)
> hematuria (R31.-)
> hyperplasia of prostate (N40.-)
> inflammatory diseases of prostate (N41.-)

5 N42.3 Dysplasia of prostate

SP N42.30 Unspecified dysplasia of prostate

SP N42.31 Prostatic intraepithelial neoplasia
PIN
Prostatic intraepithelial neoplasia I (PIN I)
Prostatic intraepithelial neoplasia II (PIN II)
> EXCLUDES 1 prostatic intraepithelial neoplasia III (PIN III) (D07.5)

SP N42.32 Atypical small acinar proliferation of prostate

SP N42.39 Other dysplasia of prostate

5 N42.8 Other specified disorders of prostate

SP N42.81 Prostatodynia syndrome
Painful prostate syndrome

SP N42.82 Prostatosis syndrome

SP N42.83 Cyst of prostate

SP N42.89 Other specified disorders of prostate

IQ N42.9 Disorder of prostate, unspecified

4 N43 Hydrocele and spermatocele
> INCLUDES hydrocele of spermatic cord, testis or tunica vaginalis ·
> EXCLUDES 1 congenital hydrocele (P83.5)

CODING TIPS ✓ Conditions classifiable to N43.- indicate cysts of fluid that develop near the head of the epididymis (spermatocele), or surrounding the testicle (hydrocele). They are often painless but may cause discomfort due to pressure on surrounding areas. When a hydrocele is reported as infected, assign N43.1 with an additional code for the causative organism, if known.

SP N43.0 Encysted hydrocele

SP + N43.1 Infected hydrocele
Use additional code (B95-B97), to identify infectious agent

SP N43.2 Other hydrocele

IQ N43.3 Hydrocele, unspecified
DEFINITION Collection of serous fluid on the tunica vaginalis, spermatic cord, or testicle from acute local injury, infection, radiotherapy, or gradual fluid accumulation.

5 N43.4 Spermatocele of epididymis
Spermatic cyst
DEFINITION Cyst on the epididymis containing sperm.

IQ N43.40 Spermatocele of epididymis, unspecified

SP N43.41 Spermatocele of epididymis, single

SP N43.42 Spermatocele of epididymis, multiple

4 N44 Noninflammatory disorders of testis

5 N44.0 Torsion of testis

SP N44.00 Torsion of testis, unspecified
DEFINITION Testicle becomes twisted inside the scrotum, cutting off the blood supply.

SP N44.01 Extravaginal torsion of spermatic cord

SP N44.02 Intravaginal torsion of spermatic cord
Torsion of spermatic cord NOS

SP N44.03 Torsion of appendix testis

SP N44.04 Torsion of appendix epididymis

SP N44.1 Cyst of tunica albuginea testis

SP N44.2 Benign cyst of testis

SP N44.8 Other noninflammatory disorders of the testis

+ 4 N45 Orchitis and epididymitis
Use additional code (B95-B97), to identify infectious agent.

CODING TIPS ✓ When coding conditions classifiable to N45.-, review documentation to identify the causative organism(s) if known, and assign an additional code.

SP + N45.1 Epididymitis

SP + N45.2 Orchitis

SP + N45.3 Epididymo-orchitis

SP + N45.4 Abscess of epididymis or testis

4 N46 Male infertility
> EXCLUDES 1 vasectomy status (Z98.52)

5 N46.0 Azoospermia
Absolute male infertility
Male infertility due to germinal (cell) aplasia
Male infertility due to spermatogenic arrest (complete)

IQ N46.01 Organic azoospermia
Azoospermia NOS

6 N46.02 Azoospermia due to extratesticular causes
Code also:
associated cause

IQ N46.021 Azoospermia due to drug therapy

IQ N46.022 Azoospermia due to infection

IQ N46.023 Azoospermia due to obstruction of efferent ducts

IQ N46.024 Azoospermia due to radiation

IQ N46.025 Azoospermia due to systemic disease

★ New ▲ Revised Px Primary SP PDGM Px SL Low CoM SH High CoM IQ Quest. Encounter H Hospice non-cancer Dx Unspecified M *Manifestation*

Chapter 14

N00-N99

IQ N46.029 Azoospermia due to other extratesticular causes

5 N46.1 Oligospermia
Male infertility due to germinal cell desquamation
Male infertility due to hypospermatogenesis
Male infertility due to incomplete spermatogenic arrest
DEFINITION Insufficient spermatozoa in the semen.

IQ N46.11 Organic oligospermia
Oligospermia NOS

6 N46.12 Oligospermia due to extratesticular causes
Code also:
associated cause

IQ N46.121 Oligospermia due to drug therapy

IQ N46.122 Oligospermia due to infection

IQ N46.123 Oligospermia due to obstruction of efferent ducts

IQ N46.124 Oligospermia due to radiation

IQ N46.125 Oligospermia due to systemic disease

IQ N46.129 Oligospermia due to other extratesticular causes

IQ N46.8 Other male infertility

IQ N46.9 Male infertility, unspecified

4 N47 Disorders of prepuce

SP N47.0 Adherent prepuce, newborn

SP N47.1 Phimosis

SP N47.2 Paraphimosis

SP N47.3 Deficient foreskin

SP N47.4 Benign cyst of prepuce

SP N47.5 Adhesions of prepuce and glans penis

SP + N47.6 Balanoposthitis
Use additional code (B95-B97), to identify infectious agent.
EXCLUDES 1 balanitis (N48.1)
DEFINITION Inflammation of the head of the penis and foreskin.

SP + N47.7 Other inflammatory diseases of prepuce
Use additional code (B95-B97), to identify infectious agent.

SP N47.8 Other disorders of prepuce

4 N48 Other disorders of penis

SP N48.0 Leukoplakia of penis
Balanitis xerotica obliterans
Kraurosis of penis
Lichen sclerosus of external male genital organs
EXCLUDES 1 carcinoma in situ of penis (D07.4)
DEFINITION Chronic skin condition of the penis causing atrophic, white, patches on the foreskin and glans with hardened, indurated tissue near the meatus.

SP + N48.1 Balanitis
Use additional code (B95-B97), to identify infectious agent
EXCLUDES 1 amebic balanitis (A06.8)
balanitis xerotica obliterans (N48.0)
candidal balanitis (B37.42)

gonococcal balanitis (A54.23)
herpesviral [herpes simplex] balanitis (A60.01)
DEFINITION Inflammation of the glans penis (the head of the penis).

+ 5 N48.2 Other inflammatory disorders of penis
Use additional code (B95-B97), to identify infectious agent.
EXCLUDES 1 balanitis (N48.1)
balanitis xerotica obliterans (N48.0)
balanoposthitis (N47.6)

SP + N48.21 Abscess of corpus cavernosum and penis

SP + N48.22 Cellulitis of corpus cavernosum and penis

SP + N48.29 Other inflammatory disorders of penis

5 N48.3 Priapism
Painful erection
Code first:
underlying cause

SP N48.30 Priapism, unspecified

SP N48.31 Priapism due to trauma

IQ N48.32 Priapism due to disease classified elsewhere

SP N48.33 Priapism, drug-induced

SP N48.39 Other priapism

SP N48.5 Ulcer of penis

SP N48.6 Induration penis plastica
Peyronie's disease
Plastic induration of penis

5 N48.8 Other specified disorders of penis

SP N48.81 Thrombosis of superficial vein of penis

SP N48.82 Acquired torsion of penis
Acquired torsion of penis NOS
EXCLUDES 1 congenital torsion of penis (Q55.63)

SP N48.83 Acquired buried penis
EXCLUDES 1 congenital hidden penis (Q55.64)

SP N48.89 Other specified disorders of penis

IQ N48.9 Disorder of penis, unspecified

+ 4 N49 Inflammatory disorders of male genital organs, not elsewhere classified
Use additional code (B95-B97), to identify infectious agent
EXCLUDES 1 inflammation of penis (N48.1, N48.2-)
orchitis and epididymitis (N45.-)

SP + N49.0 Inflammatory disorders of seminal vesicle
Vesiculitis NOS

SP + N49.1 Inflammatory disorders of spermatic cord, tunica vaginalis and vas deferens
Vasitis

SP + N49.2 Inflammatory disorders of scrotum

SP + N49.3 Fournier gangrene

| 4 4th digit required | 5 5th digit required | 6 6th digit required | 7 7th digit required | 7 7th digit placeholder | + Additional code | ⊟ Laterality |

CODING TIPS ✓ Fournier gangrene is a specific condition typically occurring in males, which includes a necrotizing or gangrenous infection of the perineal region often including a mix of aerobic and anaerobic bacteria. An additional code should be assigned to identify causative organism(s).

DEFINITION Necrosis affecting the perineal, genital, or perianal regions, characterized by black and malodorous tissue decay caused by infection or ischemia.

SP + N49.8 Inflammatory disorders of other specified male genital organs
Inflammation of multiple sites in male genital organs

IQ + N49.9 Inflammatory disorder of unspecified male genital organ
Abscess of unspecified male genital organ
Boil of unspecified male genital organ
Carbuncle of unspecified male genital organ
Cellulitis of unspecified male genital organ

4 N50 Other and unspecified disorders of male genital organs
EXCLUDES 2 torsion of testis (N44.0-)

SP N50.0 Atrophy of testis

SP N50.1 Vascular disorders of male genital organs
Hematocele, NOS, of male genital organs
Hemorrhage of male genital organs
Thrombosis of male genital organs

SP N50.3 Cyst of epididymis

5 N50.8 Other specified disorders of male genital organs
DEFINITION Chylocele: A cyst-like lesion resulting from the escape of chyle (milky fluid consisting of lymph and emulsified fat) into the tunica vaginalis of the testes.

6 N50.81 Testicular pain

⊟ SP N50.811 Right testicular pain

⊟ SP N50.812 Left testicular pain

⊟ IQ N50.819 Testicular pain, unspecified

SP N50.82 Scrotal pain

SP N50.89 Other specified disorders of the male genital organs
Atrophy of scrotum, seminal vesicle, spermatic cord, tunica vaginalis and vas deferens
Chylocele, tunica vaginalis (nonfilarial) NOS
Edema of scrotum, seminal vesicle, spermatic cord, tunica vaginalis and vas deferens
Hypertrophy of scrotum, seminal vesicle, spermatic cord, tunica vaginalis and vas deferens
Stricture of spermatic cord, tunica vaginalis, and vas deferens
Ulcer of scrotum, seminal vesicle, spermatic cord, testis, tunica vaginalis and vas deferens
Urethroscrotal fistula

IQ N50.9 Disorder of male genital organs, unspecified

M IQ N51 Disorders of male genital organs in diseases classified elsewhere
Code first underlying disease, such as:
filariasis (B74.0-B74.9)
EXCLUDES 1 amebic balanitis (A06.8)
candidal balanitis (B37.42)
gonococcal balanitis (A54.23)
gonococcal prostatitis (A54.22)
herpesviral [herpes simplex] balanitis (A60.01)
trichomonal prostatitis (A59.02)
tuberculous prostatitis (A18.14)

4 N52 Male erectile dysfunction
EXCLUDES 1 psychogenic impotence (F52.21)

5 N52.0 Vasculogenic erectile dysfunction

SP N52.01 Erectile dysfunction due to arterial insufficiency

SP N52.02 Corporo-venous occlusive erectile dysfunction

SP N52.03 Combined arterial insufficiency and corporo-venous occlusive erectile dysfunction

IQ N52.1 Erectile dysfunction due to diseases classified elsewhere
Code first:
underlying disease

SP N52.2 Drug-induced erectile dysfunction

5 N52.3 Postprocedural erectile dysfunction

SP N52.31 Erectile dysfunction following radical prostatectomy

SP N52.32 Erectile dysfunction following radical cystectomy

SP N52.33 Erectile dysfunction following urethral surgery

SP N52.34 Erectile dysfunction following simple prostatectomy

SP N52.35 Erectile dysfunction following radiation therapy

SP N52.36 Erectile dysfunction following interstitial seed therapy

SP N52.37 Erectile dysfunction following prostate ablative therapy
Erectile dysfunction following cryotherapy
Erectile dysfunction following other prostate ablative therapies
Erectile dysfunction following ultrasound ablative therapies

SP N52.39 Other and unspecified postprocedural erectile dysfunction

SP N52.8 Other male erectile dysfunction

SP N52.9 Male erectile dysfunction, unspecified
Impotence NOS

4 N53 Other male sexual dysfunction
EXCLUDES 1 psychogenic sexual dysfunction (F52.-)

5 N53.1 Ejaculatory dysfunction
EXCLUDES 1 premature ejaculation (F52.4)

SP N53.11 Retarded ejaculation

SP N53.12 Painful ejaculation

SP N53.13 Anejaculatory orgasm

★ New ▲ Revised Px Primary **SP** PDGM Px **SL** Low CoM **SH** High CoM **IQ** Quest. Encounter ⊞ Hospice non-cancer Dx Unspecified **M** *Manifestation*

SP N53.14 Retrograde ejaculation

SP N53.19 Other ejaculatory dysfunction
Ejaculatory dysfunction NOS

SP N53.8 Other male sexual dysfunction

IQ N53.9 Unspecified male sexual dysfunction

Disorders of breast   (N60-N65)

EXCLUDES 1   disorders of breast associated with childbirth (O91-O92)

CODING TIPS ✓   Code malignancies of the breast to Category C50.

4 N60 Benign mammary dysplasia
INCLUDES   fibrocystic mastopathy

5 N60.0 Solitary cyst of breast
Cyst of breast

SP N60.01 Solitary cyst of right breast

SP N60.02 Solitary cyst of left breast

IQ N60.09 Solitary cyst of unspecified breast

5 N60.1 Diffuse cystic mastopathy
Cystic breast
Fibrocystic disease of breast
EXCLUDES 1   diffuse cystic mastopathy with epithelial proliferation (N60.3-)

SP N60.11 Diffuse cystic mastopathy of right breast

SP N60.12 Diffuse cystic mastopathy of left breast

IQ N60.19 Diffuse cystic mastopathy of unspecified breast

5 N60.2 Fibroadenosis of breast
Adenofibrosis of breast
EXCLUDES 2   fibroadenoma of breast (D24.-)

SP N60.21 Fibroadenosis of right breast

SP N60.22 Fibroadenosis of left breast

IQ N60.29 Fibroadenosis of unspecified breast

5 N60.3 Fibrosclerosis of breast
Cystic mastopathy with epithelial proliferation

SP N60.31 Fibrosclerosis of right breast

SP N60.32 Fibrosclerosis of left breast

IQ N60.39 Fibrosclerosis of unspecified breast

5 N60.4 Mammary duct ectasia
DEFINITION   Dilated milk duct filled with fluid; becomes inflamed and clogged with a thick, sticky substance, causing discharge and tenderness.

SP N60.41 Mammary duct ectasia of right breast

SP N60.42 Mammary duct ectasia of left breast

IQ N60.49 Mammary duct ectasia of unspecified breast

5 N60.8 Other benign mammary dysplasias

SP N60.81 Other benign mammary dysplasias of right breast

SP N60.82 Other benign mammary dysplasias of left breast

IQ N60.89 Other benign mammary dysplasias of unspecified breast

5 N60.9 Unspecified benign mammary dysplasia

SP N60.91 Unspecified benign mammary dysplasia of right breast

SP N60.92 Unspecified benign mammary dysplasia of left breast

IQ N60.99 Unspecified benign mammary dysplasia of unspecified breast

4 N61 Inflammatory disorders of breast
EXCLUDES 1   inflammatory carcinoma of breast (C50.9)
inflammatory disorder of breast associated with childbirth (O91.-)
neonatal infective mastitis (P39.0)
thrombophlebitis of breast [Mondor's disease] (I80.8)
CODING TIPS ✓   Do not assign a code from N61.- for patients who also have breast cancer.

SP N61.0 Mastitis without abscess
Infective mastitis (acute) (nonpuerperal) (subacute)
Mastitis (acute) (nonpuerperal) (subacute) NOS
Cellulitis (acute) (nonpuerperal) (subacute) of breast NOS
Cellulitis (acute) (nonpuerperal) (subacute) of nipple NOS

SP N61.1 Abscess of the breast and nipple
Abscess (acute) (chronic) (nonpuerperal) of areola
Abscess (acute) (chronic) (nonpuerperal) of breast
Carbuncle of breast
Mastitis with abscess

SP N62 Hypertrophy of breast
Gynecomastia
Hypertrophy of breast NOS
Massive pubertal hypertrophy of breast
EXCLUDES 1   breast engorgement of newborn (P83.4)
disproportion of reconstructed breast (N65.1)
DEFINITION   Abnormal largeness of the breast.

4 N63 Unspecified lump in breast
Nodule(s) NOS in breast
CODING TIPS ✓   These codes are for abnormal nodules or lumps in the breast that are not identified as a neoplasm or tumor.

IQ N63.0 Unspecified lump in unspecified breast

5 N63.1 Unspecified lump in the right breast

SP N63.10 Unspecified lump in the right breast, unspecified quadrant

SP N63.11 Unspecified lump in the right breast, upper outer quadrant

SP N63.12 Unspecified lump in the right breast, upper inner quadrant

SP N63.13 Unspecified lump in the right breast, lower outer quadrant

SP N63.14 Unspecified lump in the right breast, lower inner quadrant

★ N63.15 Unspecified lump in the right breast, overlapping quadrants

5 N63.2 Unspecified lump in the left breast

---

4 4th digit required   5 5th digit required   6 6th digit required   7 7th digit required   7 7th digit placeholder   + Additional code   Laterality

1296   DecisionHealth's FY 2020 Complete Home Health ICD-10-CM Diagnosis Coding Manual

⊟ SP **N63.20** Unspecified lump in the left breast, unspecified quadrant

⊟ SP **N63.21** Unspecified lump in the left breast, upper outer quadrant

⊟ SP **N63.22** Unspecified lump in the left breast, upper inner quadrant

⊟ SP **N63.23** Unspecified lump in the left breast, lower outer quadrant

⊟ SP **N63.24** Unspecified lump in the left breast, lower inner quadrant

★ ⊟ **N63.25** Unspecified lump in the left breast, overlapping quadrants

⑤ **N63.3** Unspecified lump in axillary tail

⊟ SP **N63.31** Unspecified lump in axillary tail of the right breast

⊟ SP **N63.32** Unspecified lump in axillary tail of the left breast

⑤ **N63.4** Unspecified lump in breast, subareolar

⊟ SP **N63.41** Unspecified lump in right breast, subareolar

⊟ SP **N63.42** Unspecified lump in left breast, subareolar

④ **N64** Other disorders of breast

> **EXCLUDES 2** mechanical complication of breast prosthesis and implant (T85.4-)

SP **N64.0** Fissure and fistula of nipple

SP **N64.1** Fat necrosis of breast
Fat necrosis (segmental) of breast
Code first:
> breast necrosis due to breast graft (T85.898)

SP **N64.2** Atrophy of breast

SP **N64.3** Galactorrhea not associated with childbirth

> **DEFINITION** Inappropriate discharge of milk from the breast.

SP **N64.4** Mastodynia

⑤ **N64.5** Other signs and symptoms in breast

> **EXCLUDES 2** abnormal findings on diagnostic imaging of breast (R92.-)

SP **N64.51** Induration of breast

SP **N64.52** Nipple discharge

> **EXCLUDES 1** abnormal findings in nipple discharge (R89.-)

SP **N64.53** Retraction of nipple

SP **N64.59** Other signs and symptoms in breast

⑤ **N64.8** Other specified disorders of breast

SP **N64.81** Ptosis of breast

> **EXCLUDES 1** ptosis of native breast in relation to reconstructed breast (N65.1)

> **DEFINITION** Falling, drooping, or sagging of the breast tissue which can occur naturally, or following pregnancy or weight gain and loss.

SP **N64.82** Hypoplasia of breast
Micromastia

> **EXCLUDES 1** congenital absence of breast (Q83.0)

hypoplasia of native breast in relation to reconstructed breast (N65.1)

SP **N64.89** Other specified disorders of breast
Galactocele
Subinvolution of breast (postlactational)

IQ **N64.9** Disorder of breast, unspecified

④ **N65** Deformity and disproportion of reconstructed breast

SP **N65.0** Deformity of reconstructed breast
Contour irregularity in reconstructed breast
Excess tissue in reconstructed breast
Misshapen reconstructed breast

SP **N65.1** Disproportion of reconstructed breast
Breast asymmetry between native breast and reconstructed breast
Disproportion between native breast and reconstructed breast

Inflammatory diseases of female pelvic organs (N70-N77)

> **EXCLUDES 1** inflammatory diseases of female pelvic organs complicating:
> abortion or ectopic or molar pregnancy (O00-O07, O08.0)
> pregnancy, childbirth and the puerperium (O23.-, O75.3, O85, O86.-)

✚ ④ **N70** Salpingitis and oophoritis

> **INCLUDES** abscess (of) fallopian tube
> abscess (of) ovary
> pyosalpinx
> salpingo-oophoritis
> tubo-ovarian abscess
> tubo-ovarian inflammatory disease

Use additional code (B95-B97), to identify infectious agent

> **EXCLUDES 1** gonococcal infection (A54.24)
> tuberculous infection (A18.17)

> **CODING TIPS ✓** When coding a condition classifiable to N70.-, review documentation to identify the causative organism(s) if known, and assign an additional code.

✚ ⑤ **N70.0** Acute salpingitis and oophoritis

SP ✚ **N70.01** Acute salpingitis

SP ✚ **N70.02** Acute oophoritis

SP ✚ **N70.03** Acute salpingitis and oophoritis

✚ ⑤ **N70.1** Chronic salpingitis and oophoritis
Hydrosalpinx

SP ✚ **N70.11** Chronic salpingitis

SP ✚ **N70.12** Chronic oophoritis

SP ✚ **N70.13** Chronic salpingitis and oophoritis

✚ ⑤ **N70.9** Salpingitis and oophoritis, unspecified

> **DEFINITION** Inflammation of appendages of the uterus (adnexa uteri).

SP ✚ **N70.91** Salpingitis, unspecified

SP ✚ **N70.92** Oophoritis, unspecified

SP ✚ **N70.93** Salpingitis and oophoritis, unspecified

✚ ④ **N71** Inflammatory disease of uterus, except cervix

> **INCLUDES** endo (myo) metritis

★ New ▲ Revised Px Primary SP PDGM Px SL Low CoM SH High CoM IQ Quest. Encounter H Hospice non-cancer Dx Unspecified M *Manifestation*

metritis
myometritis
pyometra
uterine abscess
Use additional code (B95-B97), to identify
infectious agent
EXCLUDES 1   hyperplastic endometritis
(N85.0-)
infection of uterus following
delivery (O85, O86.-)

SP + **N71.0 Acute inflammatory disease of uterus**

SP + **N71.1 Chronic inflammatory disease of uterus**

IQ + **N71.9 Inflammatory disease of uterus,
unspecified**

SP + **N72   Inflammatory disease of cervix uteri**
INCLUDES   cervicitis
(with or without erosion or
ectropion)
endocervicitis
(with or without erosion or
ectropion)
exocervicitis
(with or without erosion or
ectropion)
Use additional code (B95-B97), to identify
infectious agent
EXCLUDES 1   erosion and ectropion of cervix
without cervicitis (N86)

+ **4** **N73   Other female pelvic inflammatory diseases**
Use additional code (B95-B97), to identify
infectious agent.

SP + **N73.0 Acute parametritis and pelvic cellulitis**
Abscess of broad ligament
Abscess of parametrium
Pelvic cellulitis, female

SP + **N73.1 Chronic parametritis and pelvic
cellulitis**
Any condition in N73.0 specified as
chronic
EXCLUDES 1   tuberculous parametritis and
pelvic cellultis (A18.17)

SP + **N73.2 Unspecified parametritis and pelvic
cellulitis**
Any condition in N73.0 unspecified
whether acute or chronic

SP + **N73.3 Female acute pelvic peritonitis**

SP + **N73.4 Female chronic pelvic peritonitis**
EXCLUDES 1   tuberculous pelvic (female)
peritonitis (A18.17)

SP + **N73.5 Female pelvic peritonitis, unspecified**

SP + **N73.6 Female pelvic peritoneal adhesions
(postinfective)**
EXCLUDES 2   postprocedural pelvic
peritoneal adhesions
(N99.4)

SP + **N73.8 Other specified female pelvic
inflammatory diseases**

IQ + **N73.9 Female pelvic inflammatory disease,
unspecified**
Female pelvic infection or inflammation
NOS

IQ **N74   Female pelvic inflammatory disorders in
diseases classified elsewhere**
Code first:
underlying disease
EXCLUDES 1   chlamydial cervicitis (A56.02)

chlamydial pelvic inflammatory
disease (A56.11)
gonococcal cervicitis (A54.03)
gonococcal pelvic inflammatory
disease (A54.24)
herpesviral [herpes simplex]
cervicitis (A60.03)
herpesviral [herpes simplex]
pelvic inflammatory disease
(A60.09)
syphilitic cervicitis (A52.76)
syphilitic pelvic inflammatory
disease (A52.76)
trichomonal cervicitis (A59.09)
tuberculous cervicitis (A18.16)
tuberculous pelvic
inflammatory disease
(A18.17)

4 **N75   Diseases of Bartholin's gland**

SP **N75.0 Cyst of Bartholin's gland**

SP **N75.1 Abscess of Bartholin's gland**

SP **N75.8 Other diseases of Bartholin's gland**
Bartholinitis

IQ **N75.9 Disease of Bartholin's gland,
unspecified**

+ **4** **N76   Other inflammation of vagina and vulva**
Use additional code (B95-B97), to identify
infectious agent
EXCLUDES 2   senile (atrophic) vaginitis
(N95.2)
vulvar vestibulitis (N94.810)

SP + **N76.0 Acute vaginitis**
Acute vulvovaginitis
Vaginitis NOS
Vulvovaginitis NOS

SP + **N76.1 Subacute and chronic vaginitis**
Chronic vulvovaginitis
Subacute vulvovaginitis

SP + **N76.2 Acute vulvitis**
Vulvitis NOS

SP + **N76.3 Subacute and chronic vulvitis**

SP + **N76.4 Abscess of vulva**
Furuncle of vulva

SP + **N76.5 Ulceration of vagina**

SP + **N76.6 Ulceration of vulva**

+ **5** **N76.8 Other specified inflammation of vagina
and vulva**

SP + **N76.81 Mucositis (ulcerative) of vagina and
vulva**
Code also type of associated therapy,
such as:
antineoplastic and
immunosuppressive drugs
(T45.1X-)
radiological procedure and
radiotherapy (Y84.2)
EXCLUDES 2   gastrointestinal mucositis
(ulcerative) (K92.81)
nasal mucositis
(ulcerative) (J34.81)
oral mucositis
(ulcerative) (K12.3-)

SP + **N76.89 Other specified inflammation of
vagina and vulva**

4 **N77   Vulvovaginal ulceration and inflammation
in diseases classified elsewhere**

44th digit required   **5**5th digit required   **6**6th digit required   **7**7th digit required   **☑**7th digit placeholder   **+**Additional code   **▣**Laterality

M **IQ** **N77.0** *Ulceration of vulva in diseases classified elsewhere*

Code first underlying disease, such as: Behçet's disease (M35.2)

> **EXCLUDES 1** ulceration of vulva in gonococcal infection (A54.02)
> ulceration of vulva in herpesviral [herpes simplex] infection (A60.04)
> ulceration of vulva in syphilis (A51.0)
> ulceration of vulva in tuberculosis (A18.18)

M **IQ** **N77.1** *Vaginitis, vulvitis and vulvovaginitis in diseases classified elsewhere*

Code first underlying disease, such as: pinworm (B80)

> **EXCLUDES 1** candidal vulvovaginitis (B37.3)
> chlamydial vulvovaginitis (A56.02)
> gonococcal vulvovaginitis (A54.02)
> herpesviral [herpes simplex] vulvovaginitis (A60.04)
> trichomonal vulvovaginitis (A59.01)
> tuberculous vulvovaginitis (A18.18)
> vulvovaginitis in early syphilis (A51.0)
> vulvovaginitis in late syphilis (A52.76)

Noninflammatory disorders of female genital tract (N80-N98)

4 **N80** Endometriosis

> **DEFINITION** Tissue that lines the uterus growing outside the uterus in the pelvis, abdomen, and on other organs; causes pain and infertility.

SP **N80.0** Endometriosis of uterus
Adenomyosis

> **EXCLUDES 1** stromal endometriosis (D39.0)

SP **N80.1** Endometriosis of ovary

SP **N80.2** Endometriosis of fallopian tube

SP **N80.3** Endometriosis of pelvic peritoneum

SP **N80.4** Endometriosis of rectovaginal septum and vagina

SP **N80.5** Endometriosis of intestine

SP **N80.6** Endometriosis in cutaneous scar

SP **N80.8** Other endometriosis
Endometriosis of thorax

SP **N80.9** Endometriosis, unspecified

4 **N81** Female genital prolapse

> **EXCLUDES 1** genital prolapse complicating pregnancy, labor or delivery (O34.5-)
> prolapse and hernia of ovary and fallopian tube (N83.4-)
> prolapse of vaginal vault after hysterectomy (N99.3)

SP **N81.0** Urethrocele

> **EXCLUDES 1** urethrocele with cystocele (N81.1-)
> urethrocele with prolapse of uterus (N81.2-N81.4)

5 **N81.1** Cystocele
Cystocele with urethrocele
Cystourethrocele

> **EXCLUDES 1** cystocele with prolapse of uterus (N81.2-N81.4)

SP **N81.10** Cystocele, unspecified
Prolapse of (anterior) vaginal wall NOS

SP **N81.11** Cystocele, midline

SP **N81.12** Cystocele, lateral
Paravaginal cystocele

> **DEFINITION** Bladder bulges through the side wall of the vagina.

SP **N81.2** Incomplete uterovaginal prolapse
First degree uterine prolapse
Prolapse of cervix NOS
Second degree uterine prolapse

> **EXCLUDES 1** cervical stump prolapse (N81.85)

SP **N81.3** Complete uterovaginal prolapse
Procidentia (uteri) NOS
Third degree uterine prolapse

SP **N81.4** Uterovaginal prolapse, unspecified
Prolapse of uterus NOS

SP **N81.5** Vaginal enterocele

> **EXCLUDES 1** enterocele with prolapse of uterus (N81.2-N81.4)

SP **+** **N81.6** Rectocele
Prolapse of posterior vaginal wall
Use additional code for any associated fecal incontinence, if applicable (R15.-)

> **EXCLUDES 2** perineocele (N81.81)
> rectal prolapse (K62.3)
> rectocele with prolapse of uterus (N81.2-N81.4)

5 **N81.8** Other female genital prolapse

SP **N81.81** Perineocele

SP **N81.82** Incompetence or weakening of pubocervical tissue

SP **N81.83** Incompetence or weakening of rectovaginal tissue

SP **N81.84** Pelvic muscle wasting
Disuse atrophy of pelvic muscles and anal sphincter

SP **N81.85** Cervical stump prolapse

> **CODING TIPS** ✓ A cervical stump prolapse, N81.85, occurs when the cervix falls into the vaginal vault following a supracervical hysterectomy.

SP **N81.89** Other female genital prolapse
Deficient perineum
Old laceration of muscles of pelvic floor

SP **N81.9** Female genital prolapse, unspecified

4 **N82** Fistulae involving female genital tract

> **EXCLUDES 1** vesicointestinal fistulae (N32.1)

SP **N82.0** Vesicovaginal fistula

SP **N82.1** Other female urinary-genital tract fistulae
Cervicovesical fistula

★ New ▲ Revised Px Primary **SP** PDGM Px **SL** Low CoM **SH** High CoM **IQ** Quest. Encounter **H** Hospice non-cancer Dx **Unspecified** **M** *Manifestation*

DecisionHealth's FY 2020 Complete Home Health ICD-10-CM Diagnosis Coding Manual

1299

Chapter 14

N00-N99

Ureterovaginal fistula
Urethrovaginal fistula
Uteroureteric fistula
Uterovesical fistula

SP N82.2 Fistula of vagina to small intestine

SP N82.3 Fistula of vagina to large intestine
Rectovaginal fistula

SP N82.4 Other female intestinal-genital tract fistulae
Intestinouterine fistula

SP N82.5 Female genital tract-skin fistulae
Uterus to abdominal wall fistula
Vaginoperineal fistula

SP N82.8 Other female genital tract fistulae

IQ N82.9 Female genital tract fistula, unspecified

4 N83 Noninflammatory disorders of ovary, fallopian tube and broad ligament
　　EXCLUDES 2 hydrosalpinx (N70.1-)

5 N83.0 Follicular cyst of ovary
Cyst of graafian follicle
Hemorrhagic follicular cyst (of ovary)
　　DEFINITION Fluid-filled sac on the ovary caused by larger than normal growth of a follicle that does not rupture to release the egg.

☐ IQ N83.00 Follicular cyst of ovary, unspecified side

☐ SP N83.01 Follicular cyst of right ovary

☐ SP N83.02 Follicular cyst of left ovary

5 N83.1 Corpus luteum cyst
Hemorrhagic corpus luteum cyst

☐ IQ N83.10 Corpus luteum cyst of ovary, unspecified side

☐ SP N83.11 Corpus luteum cyst of right ovary

☐ SP N83.12 Corpus luteum cyst of left ovary

5 N83.2 Other and unspecified ovarian cysts
　　EXCLUDES 1 developmental ovarian cyst (Q50.1)
neoplastic ovarian cyst (D27.-)
polycystic ovarian syndrome (E28.2)
Stein-Leventhal syndrome (E28.2)

6 N83.20 Unspecified ovarian cysts

☐ SP N83.201 Unspecified ovarian cyst, right side

☐ SP N83.202 Unspecified ovarian cyst, left side

☐ IQ N83.209 Unspecified ovarian cyst, unspecified side
Ovarian cyst, NOS

6 N83.29 Other ovarian cysts
Retention cyst of ovary
Simple cyst of ovary

☐ SP N83.291 Other ovarian cyst, right side

☐ SP N83.292 Other ovarian cyst, left side

☐ IQ N83.299 Other ovarian cyst, unspecified side

5 N83.3 Acquired atrophy of ovary and fallopian tube

6 N83.31 Acquired atrophy of ovary

☐ SP N83.311 Acquired atrophy of right ovary

☐ SP N83.312 Acquired atrophy of left ovary

☐ IQ N83.319 Acquired atrophy of ovary, unspecified side
Acquired atrophy of ovary, NOS

6 N83.32 Acquired atrophy of fallopian tube

☐ SP N83.321 Acquired atrophy of right fallopian tube

☐ SP N83.322 Acquired atrophy of left fallopian tube

☐ IQ N83.329 Acquired atrophy of fallopian tube, unspecified side
Acquired atrophy of fallopian tube, NOS

6 N83.33 Acquired atrophy of ovary and fallopian tube

☐ SP N83.331 Acquired atrophy of right ovary and fallopian tube

☐ SP N83.332 Acquired atrophy of left ovary and fallopian tube

☐ IQ N83.339 Acquired atrophy of ovary and fallopian tube, unspecified side
Acquired atrophy of ovary and fallopian tube, NOS

5 N83.4 Prolapse and hernia of ovary and fallopian tube

☐ IQ N83.40 Prolapse and hernia of ovary and fallopian tube, unspecified side
Prolapse and hernia of ovary and fallopian tube, NOS

☐ SP N83.41 Prolapse and hernia of right ovary and fallopian tube

☐ SP N83.42 Prolapse and hernia of left ovary and fallopian tube

5 N83.5 Torsion of ovary, ovarian pedicle and fallopian tube
Torsion of accessory tube

6 N83.51 Torsion of ovary and ovarian pedicle

☐ SP N83.511 Torsion of right ovary and ovarian pedicle

☐ SP N83.512 Torsion of left ovary and ovarian pedicle

☐ IQ N83.519 Torsion of ovary and ovarian pedicle, unspecified side
Torsion of ovary and ovarian pedicle, NOS

6 N83.52 Torsion of fallopian tube
Torsion of hydatid of Morgagni

☐ SP N83.521 Torsion of right fallopian tube

☐ SP N83.522 Torsion of left fallopian tube

☐ IQ N83.529 Torsion of fallopian tube, unspecified side
Torsion of fallopian tube, NOS

SP N83.53 Torsion of ovary, ovarian pedicle and fallopian tube

SP N83.6 Hematosalpinx
　　EXCLUDES 1 hematosalpinx (with) (in):
hematocolpos (N89.7)
hematometra (N85.7)
tubal pregnancy (O00.1-)

SP N83.7 Hematoma of broad ligament

SP N83.8 Other noninflammatory disorders of ovary, fallopian tube and broad ligament
Broad ligament laceration syndrome [Allen-Masters]

---

4 4th digit required　　5 5th digit required　　6 6th digit required　　7 7th digit required　　7 7th digit placeholder　　+Additional code　　☐ Laterality

1300　　　　　　　　*DecisionHealth's* FY 2020 Complete Home Health ICD-10-CM Diagnosis Coding Manual

IQ N83.9 **Noninflammatory disorder of ovary, fallopian tube and broad ligament, unspecified**

4 N84 **Polyp of female genital tract**
> EXCLUDES 1 adenomatous polyp (D28.-)
> placental polyp (O90.89)

SP N84.0 **Polyp of corpus uteri**
Polyp of endometrium
Polyp of uterus NOS
> EXCLUDES 1 polypoid endometrial hyperplasia (N85.0-)

SP N84.1 **Polyp of cervix uteri**
Mucous polyp of cervix

SP N84.2 **Polyp of vagina**

SP N84.3 **Polyp of vulva**
Polyp of labia

SP N84.8 **Polyp of other parts of female genital tract**

IQ N84.9 **Polyp of female genital tract, unspecified**

4 N85 **Other noninflammatory disorders of uterus, except cervix**
> EXCLUDES 1 endometriosis (N80.-)
> inflammatory diseases of uterus (N71.-)
> noninflammatory disorders of cervix, except malposition (N86-N88)
> polyp of corpus uteri (N84.0)
> uterine prolapse (N81.-)

5 N85.0 **Endometrial hyperplasia**
> DEFINITION Overgrowth of cells lining the uterus.

SP N85.00 **Endometrial hyperplasia, unspecified**
Hyperplasia (adenomatous) (cystic) (glandular) of endometrium
Hyperplastic endometritis

SP N85.01 **Benign endometrial hyperplasia**
Endometrial hyperplasia (complex) (simple) without atypia

SP N85.02 **Endometrial intraepithelial neoplasia [EIN]**
Endometrial hyperplasia with atypia
> EXCLUDES 1 malignant neoplasm of endometrium (with endometrial intraepithelial neoplasia [EIN]) (C54.1)

SP N85.2 **Hypertrophy of uterus**
Bulky or enlarged uterus
> EXCLUDES 1 puerperal hypertrophy of uterus (O90.89)

SP N85.3 **Subinvolution of uterus**
> EXCLUDES 1 puerperal subinvolution of uterus (O90.89)

SP N85.4 **Malposition of uterus**
Anteversion of uterus
Retroflexion of uterus
Retroversion of uterus
> EXCLUDES 1 malposition of uterus complicating pregnancy, labor or delivery (O34.5-, O65.5)

SP N85.5 **Inversion of uterus**

> EXCLUDES 1 current obstetric trauma (O71.2)
> postpartum inversion of uterus (O71.2)

SP N85.6 **Intrauterine synechiae**

SP N85.7 **Hematometra**
Hematosalpinx with hematometra
> EXCLUDES 1 hematometra with hematocolpos (N89.7)
> DEFINITION Blood accumulated in the uterus.

SP N85.8 **Other specified noninflammatory disorders of uterus**
Atrophy of uterus, acquired
Fibrosis of uterus NOS

IQ N85.9 **Noninflammatory disorder of uterus, unspecified**
Disorder of uterus NOS

SP N86 **Erosion and ectropion of cervix uteri**
Decubitus (trophic) ulcer of cervix
Eversion of cervix
> EXCLUDES 1 erosion and ectropion of cervix with cervicitis (N72)

4 N87 **Dysplasia of cervix uteri**
> EXCLUDES 1 abnormal results from cervical cytologic examination without histologic confirmation (R87.61-)
> carcinoma in situ of cervix uteri (D06.-)
> cervical intraepithelial neoplasia III [CIN III] (D06.-)
> HGSIL of cervix (R87.613)
> severe dysplasia of cervix uteri (D06.-)

> CODING TIPS ✓ Mild and moderate dysplasia of the cervix is coded to this category. Class III is coded to D06.

SP N87.0 **Mild cervical dysplasia**
Cervical intraepithelial neoplasia I [CIN I]

SP N87.1 **Moderate cervical dysplasia**
Cervical intraepithelial neoplasia II [CIN II]

SP N87.9 **Dysplasia of cervix uteri, unspecified**
Anaplasia of cervix
Cervical atypism
Cervical dysplasia NOS

4 N88 **Other noninflammatory disorders of cervix uteri**
> EXCLUDES 2 inflammatory disease of cervix (N72)
> polyp of cervix (N84.1)

SP N88.0 **Leukoplakia of cervix uteri**

SP N88.1 **Old laceration of cervix uteri**
Adhesions of cervix
> EXCLUDES 1 current obstetric trauma (O71.3)

SP N88.2 **Stricture and stenosis of cervix uteri**
> EXCLUDES 1 stricture and stenosis of cervix uteri complicating labor (O65.5)

SP N88.3 **Incompetence of cervix uteri**
Investigation and management of (suspected) cervical incompetence in a nonpregnant woman

Chapter 14

N00-N99

★ New ▲ Revised Px Primary SP PDGM Px SL Low CoM SH High CoM IQ Quest. Encounter H Hospice non-cancer Dx Unspecified M Manifestation

DecisionHealth's FY 2020 Complete Home Health ICD-10-CM Diagnosis Coding Manual

1301

Chapter 14

N00-N99

EXCLUDES 1 cervical incompetence complicating pregnancy (O34.3-)

SP N88.4 Hypertrophic elongation of cervix uteri

SP N88.8 Other specified noninflammatory disorders of cervix uteri
EXCLUDES 1 current obstetric trauma (O71.3)

!Q N88.9 Noninflammatory disorder of cervix uteri, unspecified

4 N89 Other noninflammatory disorders of vagina
EXCLUDES 1 abnormal results from vaginal cytologic examination without histologic confirmation (R87.62-)
carcinoma in situ of vagina (D07.2)
HGSIL of vagina (R87.623)
inflammation of vagina (N76.-)
senile (atrophic) vaginitis (N95.2)
severe dysplasia of vagina (D07.2)
trichomonal leukorrhea (A59.00)
vaginal intraepithelial neoplasia [VAIN], grade III (D07.2)

SP N89.0 Mild vaginal dysplasia
Vaginal intraepithelial neoplasia [VAIN], grade I

SP N89.1 Moderate vaginal dysplasia
Vaginal intraepithelial neoplasia [VAIN], grade II

SP N89.3 Dysplasia of vagina, unspecified

SP N89.4 Leukoplakia of vagina
DEFINITION White plaque on the mucosal surface of the vagina that develops into thickened, rough-textured grayish white lesions.

SP N89.5 Stricture and atresia of vagina
Vaginal adhesions
Vaginal stenosis
EXCLUDES 1 congenital atresia or stricture (Q52.4)
postprocedural adhesions of vagina (N99.2)

SP N89.6 Tight hymenal ring
Rigid hymen
Tight introitus
EXCLUDES 1 imperforate hymen (Q52.3)

SP N89.7 Hematocolpos
Hematocolpos with hematometra or hematosalpinx

SP N89.8 Other specified noninflammatory disorders of vagina
Leukorrhea NOS
Old vaginal laceration
Pessary ulcer of vagina
EXCLUDES 1 current obstetric trauma (O70.-, O71.4, O71.7-O71.8)
old laceration involving muscles of pelvic floor (N81.8)

!Q N89.9 Noninflammatory disorder of vagina, unspecified

4 N90 Other noninflammatory disorders of vulva and perineum
EXCLUDES 1 anogenital (venereal) warts (A63.0)
carcinoma in situ of vulva (D07.1)
condyloma acuminatum (A63.0)
current obstetric trauma (O70.-, O71.7-O71.8)
inflammation of vulva (N76.-)
severe dysplasia of vulva (D07.1)
vulvar intraepithelial neoplasm III [VIN III] (D07.1)

SP N90.0 Mild vulvar dysplasia
Vulvar intraepithelial neoplasia [VIN], grade I

SP N90.1 Moderate vulvar dysplasia
Vulvar intraepithelial neoplasia [VIN], grade II

SP N90.3 Dysplasia of vulva, unspecified

SP N90.4 Leukoplakia of vulva
Dystrophy of vulva
Kraurosis of vulva
Lichen sclerosus of external female genital organs

SP N90.5 Atrophy of vulva
Stenosis of vulva

5 N90.6 Hypertrophy of vulva

SP N90.60 Unspecified hypertrophy of vulva
Unspecified hypertrophy of labia

SP N90.61 Childhood asymmetric labium majus enlargement
CALME

SP N90.69 Other specified hypertrophy of vulva
Other specified hypertrophy of labia

SP N90.7 Vulvar cyst

5 N90.8 Other specified noninflammatory disorders of vulva and perineum

6 N90.81 Female genital mutilation status
Female genital cutting status

SP N90.810 Female genital mutilation status, unspecified
Female genital cutting status, unspecified
Female genital mutilation status NOS

SP N90.811 Female genital mutilation Type I status
Clitorectomy status
Female genital cutting Type I status

SP N90.812 Female genital mutilation Type II status
Clitorectomy with excision of labia minora status
Female genital cutting Type II status

SP N90.813 Female genital mutilation Type III status
Female genital cutting Type III status
Infibulation status

SP N90.818 Other female genital mutilation status
Female genital cutting Type IV status

---

4 4th digit required **5** 5th digit required **6** 6th digit required **7** 7th digit required **7** 7th digit placeholder **+** Additional code **⊟** Laterality

1302 *DecisionHealth's* FY 2020 Complete Home Health ICD-10-CM Diagnosis Coding Manual

Female genital mutilation Type IV status

Other female genital cutting status

SP N90.89 **Other specified noninflammatory disorders of vulva and perineum**

Adhesions of vulva

Hypertrophy of clitoris

IQ N90.9 **Noninflammatory disorder of vulva and perineum, unspecified**

N91 **Absent, scanty and rare menstruation**

EXCLUDES 1 ovarian dysfunction (E28.-)

SP N91.0 **Primary amenorrhea**

SP N91.1 **Secondary amenorrhea**

IQ N91.2 **Amenorrhea, unspecified**

SP N91.3 **Primary oligomenorrhea**

SP N91.4 **Secondary oligomenorrhea**

IQ N91.5 **Oligomenorrhea, unspecified**

Hypomenorrhea NOS

N92 **Excessive, frequent and irregular menstruation**

EXCLUDES 1 postmenopausal bleeding (N95.0)

precocious puberty (menstruation) (E30.1)

IQ N92.0 **Excessive and frequent menstruation with regular cycle**

Heavy periods NOS

Menorrhagia NOS

Polymenorrhea

IQ N92.1 **Excessive and frequent menstruation with irregular cycle**

Irregular intermenstrual bleeding

Irregular, shortened intervals between menstrual bleeding

Menometrorrhagia

Metrorrhagia

IQ N92.2 **Excessive menstruation at puberty**

Excessive bleeding associated with onset of menstrual periods

Pubertal menorrhagia

Puberty bleeding

IQ N92.3 **Ovulation bleeding**

Regular intermenstrual bleeding

▲ SP N92.4 **Excessive bleeding in the premenopausal period**

Climacteric menorrhagia or metrorrhagia

Menopausal menorrhagia or metrorrhagia

Perimenopausal bleeding

Perimenopausal menorrhagia or metrorrhagia

Preclimacteric menorrhagia or metrorrhagia

Premenopausal menorrhagia or metrorrhagia

SP N92.5 **Other specified irregular menstruation**

IQ N92.6 **Irregular menstruation, unspecified**

Irregular bleeding NOS

Irregular periods NOS

EXCLUDES 1 irregular menstruation with:

lengthened intervals or scanty bleeding (N91.3-N91.5)

shortened intervals or excessive bleeding (N92.1)

N93 **Other abnormal uterine and vaginal bleeding**

EXCLUDES 1 neonatal vaginal hemorrhage (P54.6)

precocious puberty (menstruation) (E30.1)

pseudomenses (P54.6)

SP N93.0 **Postcoital and contact bleeding**

DEFINITION Bleeding after sexual intercourse.

SP N93.1 **Pre-pubertal vaginal bleeding**

SP N93.8 **Other specified abnormal uterine and vaginal bleeding**

Dysfunctional or functional uterine or vaginal bleeding NOS

IQ N93.9 **Abnormal uterine and vaginal bleeding, unspecified**

N94 **Pain and other conditions associated with female genital organs and menstrual cycle**

SP N94.0 **Mittelschmerz**

DEFINITION Pain accompanying ovulation, usually occurring midway between menstruation periods.

N94.1 **Dyspareunia**

EXCLUDES 1 psychogenic dyspareunia (F52.6)

DEFINITION Pain during sexual intercourse.

SP N94.10 **Unspecified dyspareunia**

SP N94.11 **Superficial (introital) dyspareunia**

SP N94.12 **Deep dyspareunia**

SP N94.19 **Other specified dyspareunia**

SP N94.2 **Vaginismus**

EXCLUDES 1 psychogenic vaginismus (F52.5)

DEFINITION Severe, painful spasms of the vaginal muscles that prevent sexual intercourse.

SP N94.3 **Premenstrual tension syndrome**

Code also:

associated menstrual migraine (G43.82-, G43.83-)

EXCLUDES 1 Premenstrual dysphoric disorder (F32.81)

SP N94.4 **Primary dysmenorrhea**

SP N94.5 **Secondary dysmenorrhea**

SP N94.6 **Dysmenorrhea, unspecified**

EXCLUDES 1 psychogenic dysmenorrhea (F45.8)

N94.8 **Other specified conditions associated with female genital organs and menstrual cycle**

N94.81 **Vulvodynia**

SP N94.810 **Vulvar vestibulitis**

DEFINITION Pain, tenderness, and redness in the vestibule area of the female external genitalia of unknown cause.

SP N94.818 **Other vulvodynia**

SP N94.819 **Vulvodynia, unspecified**

Vulvodynia NOS

SP N94.89 **Other specified conditions associated with female genital organs and menstrual cycle**

★ New ▲ Revised Px Primary **SP** PDGM Px **SL** Low CoM **SH** High CoM **IQ** Quest. Encounter **H** Hospice non-cancer Dx Unspecified **M** *Manifestation*

Chapter 14

N00-N99

IQ N94.9 **Unspecified condition associated with female genital organs and menstrual cycle**

4 N95 **Menopausal and other perimenopausal disorders**
Menopausal and other perimenopausal disorders due to naturally occurring (age-related) menopause and perimenopause

> EXCLUDES 1   excessive bleeding in the premenopausal period (N92.4)
> menopausal and perimenopausal disorders due to artificial or premature menopause (E89.4-, E28.31-)
> premature menopause (E28.31-)
>
> EXCLUDES 2   postmenopausal osteoporosis (M81.0-)
> postmenopausal osteoporosis with current pathological fracture (M80.0-)
> postmenopausal urethritis (N34.2)

SP N95.0 **Postmenopausal bleeding**

SP + N95.1 **Menopausal and female climacteric states**
Symptoms such as flushing, sleeplessness, headache, lack of concentration, associated with natural (age-related) menopause
Use additional code for associated symptoms

> EXCLUDES 1   asymptomatic menopausal state (Z78.0)
> symptoms associated with artificial menopause (E89.41)
> symptoms associated with premature menopause (E28.310)

SP N95.2 **Postmenopausal atrophic vaginitis**
Senile (atrophic) vaginitis

> DEFINITION   Thinning of vaginal epithelium due to decreased estrogen levels.

SP N95.8 **Other specified menopausal and perimenopausal disorders**

IQ N95.9 **Unspecified menopausal and perimenopausal disorder**

SP N96 **Recurrent pregnancy loss**
Investigation or care in a nonpregnant woman with history of recurrent pregnancy loss

> EXCLUDES 1   recurrent pregancy loss with current pregnancy (O26.2-)

4 N97 **Female infertility**

> INCLUDES   inability to achieve a pregnancy sterility, female NOS
>
> EXCLUDES 1   female infertility associated with:
> hypopituitarism (E23.0)
> Stein-Leventhal syndrome (E28.2)
>
> EXCLUDES 2   incompetence of cervix uteri (N88.3)

SP N97.0 **Female infertility associated with anovulation**

SP N97.1 **Female infertility of tubal origin**
Female infertility associated with congenital anomaly of tube
Female infertility due to tubal block
Female infertility due to tubal occlusion
Female infertility due to tubal stenosis

SP N97.2 **Female infertility of uterine origin**
Female infertility associated with congenital anomaly of uterus
Female infertility due to nonimplantation of ovum

SP N97.8 **Female infertility of other origin**

IQ N97.9 **Female infertility, unspecified**

4 N98 **Complications associated with artificial fertilization**

SP N98.0 **Infection associated with artificial insemination**

SP N98.1 **Hyperstimulation of ovaries**
Hyperstimulation of ovaries NOS
Hyperstimulation of ovaries associated with induced ovulation

SP N98.2 **Complications of attempted introduction of fertilized ovum following in vitro fertilization**

SP N98.3 **Complications of attempted introduction of embryo in embryo transfer**

SP N98.8 **Other complications associated with artificial fertilization**

IQ N98.9 **Complication associated with artificial fertilization, unspecified**

Intraoperative and postprocedural complications and disorders of genitourinary system, not elsewhere classified   (N99)

4 N99 **Intraoperative and postprocedural complications and disorders of genitourinary system, not elsewhere classified**

> EXCLUDES 2   irradiation cystitis (N30.4-)
> postoophorectomy osteoporosis with current pathological fracture (M80.8-)
> postoophorectomy osteoporosis without current pathological fracture (M81.8)

> CODING TIPS ✓   **Documentation:** Codes in category N99.- are complication codes and require physician documentation and confirmation of a cause and effect relationship between any specified procedure and the complicated condition. Documentation in the home health clinical record must also support this relationship. If the complication has been resolved, the aftercare code may be appropriate (Z48.816).

SP + N99.0 **Postprocedural (acute) (chronic) kidney failure**
Use additional code to type of kidney disease

5 N99.1 **Postprocedural urethral stricture**
Postcatheterization urethral stricture

6 N99.11 **Postprocedural urethral stricture, male**

SP N99.110 **Postprocedural urethral stricture, male, meatal**

---

4 4th digit required   5 5th digit required   6 6th digit required   7 7th digit required   7 7th digit placeholder   + Additional code   Laterality

1304   *DecisionHealth's* FY 2020 Complete Home Health ICD-10-CM Diagnosis Coding Manual

SP **N99.111** Postprocedural bulbous urethral stricture, male

SP **N99.112** Postprocedural membranous urethral stricture, male

SP **N99.113** Postprocedural anterior bulbous urethral stricture, male

SP **N99.114** Postprocedural urethral stricture, male, unspecified

SP **N99.115** Postprocedural fossa navicularis urethral stricture

SP **N99.116** Postprocedural urethral stricture, male, overlapping sites

SP **N99.12** Postprocedural urethral stricture, female

SP **N99.2** Postprocedural adhesions of vagina

SP **N99.3** Prolapse of vaginal vault after hysterectomy

SP **N99.4** Postprocedural pelvic peritoneal adhesions

> **EXCLUDES 2** pelvic peritoneal adhesions NOS (N73.6)
> postinfective pelvic peritoneal adhesions (N73.6)

5 **N99.5** Complications of stoma of urinary tract

> **EXCLUDES 2** mechanical complication of urinary catheter (T83.0-)

> **CODING TIPS ✓** All cystostomy and other urinary stoma complications (including ileoconduit, urostomy and nephrostomy) are coded to N99.51-N99.53. This includes excoriation and denuding of the skin surrounding the ostomy, infection of the ostomy site, hemorrhage of the ostomy site and other complications. No additional code should be used when coding skin complications unless an infection is present, in which case an additional code should be used to specify the infection. When an ostomy complication is present, do not assign a Z code for the ostomy. Z codes indicate routine ostomy care, which is not appropriate in the case of a complicated ostomy.

6 **N99.51** Complication of cystostomy

SP **N99.510** Cystostomy hemorrhage

SP **N99.511** Cystostomy infection

> **CODING TIPS ✓** Code the cystostomy infection first, followed by cellulitis (if documented), followed by the bacteria causing the infection, if known.

SP **N99.512** Cystostomy malfunction

SP **N99.518** Other cystostomy complication

6 **N99.52** Complication of incontinent external stoma of urinary tract

SP **N99.520** Hemorrhage of incontinent external stoma of urinary tract

SP **N99.521** Infection of incontinent external stoma of urinary tract

SP **N99.522** Malfunction of incontinent external stoma of urinary tract

SP **N99.523** Herniation of incontinent stoma of urinary tract

SP **N99.524** Stenosis of incontinent stoma of urinary tract

SP **N99.528** Other complication of incontinent external stoma of urinary tract

6 **N99.53** Complication of continent stoma of urinary tract

SP **N99.530** Hemorrhage of continent stoma of urinary tract

SP **N99.531** Infection of continent stoma of urinary tract

SP **N99.532** Malfunction of continent stoma of urinary tract

SP **N99.533** Herniation of continent stoma of urinary tract

SP **N99.534** Stenosis of continent stoma of urinary tract

SP **N99.538** Other complication of continent stoma of urinary tract

5 **N99.6** Intraoperative hemorrhage and hematoma of a genitourinary system organ or structure complicating a procedure

> **EXCLUDES 1** intraoperative hemorrhage and hematoma of a genitourinary system organ or structure due to accidental puncture or laceration during a procedure (N99.7-)

SP **N99.61** Intraoperative hemorrhage and hematoma of a genitourinary system organ or structure complicating a genitourinary system procedure

SP **N99.62** Intraoperative hemorrhage and hematoma of a genitourinary system organ or structure complicating other procedure

5 **N99.7** Accidental puncture and laceration of a genitourinary system organ or structure during a procedure

SP **N99.71** Accidental puncture and laceration of a genitourinary system organ or structure during a genitourinary system procedure

SP **N99.72** Accidental puncture and laceration of a genitourinary system organ or structure during other procedure

5 **N99.8** Other intraoperative and postprocedural complications and disorders of genitourinary system

SP **N99.81** Other intraoperative complications of genitourinary system

6 **N99.82** Postprocedural hemorrhage of a genitourinary system organ or structure following a procedure

SP **N99.820** Postprocedural hemorrhage of a genitourinary system organ or structure following a genitourinary system procedure

SP **N99.821** Postprocedural hemorrhage of a genitourinary system organ or structure following other procedure

SP **N99.83** Residual ovary syndrome

6 **N99.84** Postprocedural hematoma and seroma of a genitourinary system organ or structure following a procedure

Chapter 14

N00-N99

★ New ▲ Revised Px Primary **SP** PDGM Px **SL** Low CoM **SH** High CoM **IQ** Quest. Encounter **H** Hospice non-cancer Dx Unspecified **M** *Manifestation*

DecisionHealth's FY 2020 Complete Home Health ICD-10-CM Diagnosis Coding Manual

1305

SP N99.840 Postprocedural hematoma of a genitourinary system organ or structure following a genitourinary system procedure

SP N99.841 Postprocedural hematoma of a genitourinary system organ or structure following other procedure

SP N99.842 Postprocedural seroma of a genitourinary system organ or structure following a genitourinary system procedure

SP N99.843 Postprocedural seroma of a genitourinary system organ or structure following other procedure

⭐ **N99.85** Post endometrial ablation syndrome

SP N99.89 Other postprocedural complications and disorders of genitourinary system

🔢4th digit required   🔢5th digit required   🔢6th digit required   🔢7th digit required   🔢7th digit placeholder   ✚Additional code   ⊟Laterality

1306   *DecisionHealth's* FY 2020 Complete Home Health ICD-10-CM Diagnosis Coding Manual

Chapter 14 Scenarios: Diseases of the genitourinary system (N00-N99)

UTI, catheter care, functional incontinence

A 72-year-old woman who is incontinent of urine is referred to home health with a urinary tract infection (UTI). She had a suprapubic catheter placed while she was in the hospital in hopes that it would be less likely than a Foley to cause UTIs. The patient also had a stroke four years ago that left her with residual conditions of left-sided hemiplegia (left side dominant) and aphasia. There is no indication that the stroke is the cause of her incontinence, except that she cannot get to the toilet in time due to her decreased mobility. Documentation in the chart offers no indication that the UTI is secondary to the indwelling catheter, and calls to the physician's office seeking clarification were not returned. The plan of care will focus on treatment of the UTI, as well as teaching care of the new suprapubic catheter.

Description	Code
Primary: Urinary tract infection, site not specified	N39.0
Secondary: Encounter for attention to cystostomy	Z43.5
Secondary: Functional urinary incontinence	R39.81
Secondary: Hemiplegia and hemiparesis following cerebral infarction affecting left dominant side	I69.352
Secondary: Aphasia following cerebral infarction	I69.320

N39.0 has a "Use additional code" note for the infectious agent to be included if known. No organism is listed here so none can be coded. The UTI cannot be assumed to be a complication of the catheter unless the physician has said that it is. Since that is not the case, it is not coded as a complication. Functional urinary incontinence, R39.81, is used to clarify the cause of the incontinence, distinguishing it from a medical condition. Code Z43.5 (Encounter for attention to cystostomy) is used for the catheter care because the agency is changing and caring for a patient's suprapubic catheter and the code captures "attention to" which communicates the provision of more comprehensive care such as assessing, cleaning and teaching, versus simply changing the catheter.

Multiple sclerosis, neurogenic bladder, history of UTI

A 50-year-old woman, diagnosed with multiple sclerosis for the past 20 years, has decreased visual acuity and some impaired mobility, balance and fine motor control, all of which have been relatively stable for six months. She requires home care for the management of her neurogenic bladder, which is causing urinary retention and incontinence without awareness and is managed with a chronic Foley catheter. She has had several UTIs. A nurse visits every four weeks to change the catheter, perform other care associated with the Foley catheter, monitor for signs of urinary tract infection and perform management of the neurogenic bladder.

Description	Code
Primary: Neurogenic bladder NOS	N31.9
Secondary: Multiple sclerosis	G35
Secondary: Incontinence without sensory awareness	N39.42
Secondary: Fitting and adjustment of urinary devices	Z46.6
Secondary: Personal history of urinary (tract) infection	Z87.440

Code N31.9 (neurogenic bladder) is the principal diagnosis code because it represents the most acute condition, which requires the most intensive services. Instruction at N31.- states to use an additional code for urinary incontinence. Assign G35, multiple sclerosis, if the patient is being seen for more than one aspect of this chronic condition. In this case, the neurogenic bladder is the focus of care. History of UTIs (Z87.440) is also assigned.

Diabetic kidney disease

A 67-year-old female patient is admitted to home health with a new diagnosis of chronic kidney disease stage 2 due to diabetes. The patient also has restless leg syndrome and lives alone. The focus of care is the newly diagnosed kidney disease.

Description	Code
Primary: Type 2 diabetes mellitus with diabetic chronic kidney disease	E11.22
Secondary: Chronic kidney disease stage 2	N18.2
Secondary: Restless leg syndrome	G25.81
Secondary: Problems related to living alone	Z60.2

Even though the kidney disease is the main reason for admission, manifestation sequencing rules take precedence, so the underlying etiology must be listed primary. Many ICD-10 diabetes codes are combination codes and do not require an additional code. However, diabetes with kidney disease has an instruction in the Tabular to "use additional code" to identify the stage of kidney disease. Restless leg syndrome is a pertinent comorbidity and should be addressed in the plan of care. However, the physician should be queried to determine if this syndrome is attributed to the diabetes, relating to a more direct condition of neuropathy, etc. A Z code should be added describing that the patient lives alone to further paint the picture for this patient. Codes in categories Z55-Z65 can be reported based on information in other clinicians' assessments, not just the physician's, according to Q1 2018 Coding Clinic guidance.

Congestive heart failure, hypertension, chronic kidney disease

A patient is admitted to home health after being hospitalized for congestive heart failure with shortness of breath, chest pain and acute renal failure. The patient's comorbidities include hypertension and stage 3 chronic kidney disease (CKD). The patient continues to have edema, but other acute symptoms, as well as the acute renal failure, are resolved upon admission to home care. Skilled nursing is ordered to teach on the disease process and monitor symptoms.

Description	Code
Primary: Hypertensive heart and chronic kidney disease with heart failure and stage 1 through stage 4 chronic kidney disease, or unspecified chronic kidney disease	I13.0
Secondary: Heart failure, unspecified	I50.9
Secondary: Chronic kidney disease, stage 3 (moderate)	N18.3

A cause-and-effect relationship between hypertension, heart failure and chronic kidney disease is assumed by the ICD-10 classification system unless the provider states otherwise. The heart failure is not specified as systolic or diastolic, and therefore would be unspecified. An additional code from N18.- is assigned for the stage of chronic kidney disease in accordance with tabular instruction. The edema is not coded as it is a symptom of the congestive heart failure.

Stage 3 CKD with kidney transplant

A patient was admitted to home health for skilled nursing care following a successful kidney transplant. He still has stage 3 chronic kidney disease (CKD).

Description	Code
Primary: Aftercare following kidney transplant	Z48.22
Secondary: Chronic kidney disease, stage 3 (moderate)	N18.3

Patients who have undergone a kidney transplant may still have some form of CKD because the kidney transplant may not fully restore kidney function. Therefore, the presence of CKD alone does not constitute a transplant complication, and would not be coded as such, according to coding guidelines. Assign the appropriate N18.- code for the patient's stage of CKD. Code Z94.0 (Kidney transplant status) is not required here because the aftercare code already identifies the patient's transplanted organ. *[I.C.14.a.2]*

Benign prostatic hyperplasia

An 85-year-old man is admitted to home health with benign prostatic hyperplasia (BPH) to address debilitating symptoms of urinary overflow incontinence and nocturia. He will receive skilled nursing and occupational therapy. He also has hypertension.

Description	Code
Primary: Benign prostatic hyperplasia with lower urinary tract symptoms	N40.1
Secondary: Overflow incontinence	N39.490
Secondary: Nocturia	R35.1
Secondary: Essential (primary) hypertension	I10

Even though incontinence and nocturia are symptoms of an enlarged prostate, or benign prostatic hyperplasia (BPH), and would not normally be additionally coded, they are in this scenario because tabular instructions call for it. Be sure to follow tabular instructions that state to assign the symptom codes after the BPH code. R35.1 Hypertension is coded as a relevant comorbidity.

Cellulitis around cystostomy site

A 71-year-old woman has a cystostomy in place due to paraplegia. Recently the site around the opening became irritated and her physician diagnosed cellulitis due to group B streptococcus bacteria. She was prescribed a 10-day course of antibiotics and will receive skilled nursing visits to monitor the infection until it resolves. She is wheelchair bound.

Description	Code
Primary: Cystostomy infection	N99.511
Secondary: Cellulitis of groin	L03.314
Secondary: Streptococcus, group B, as the cause of diseases classified elsewhere	B95.1
Secondary: Paraplegia, unspecified	G82.20
Secondary: Dependence on wheelchair	Z99.3

The infection is affecting the skin around the stoma and should thus be coded as a complication of the stoma, with N99.511. Codes for the cellulitis and the group B streptococcus bacteria are added to further describe the infection, in accordance with tabular instruction. The patient's paraplegia and wheelchair dependence are coded as relevant comorbidity factors that will impact the patient's recovery. Long-term antibiotic use is not coded as she is only taking antibiotics for 10 days.

Urethral stricture of overlapping sites

A 75-year-old man comes to home health with a primary diagnosis of a urethral stricture affecting the membranous and bulbous areas. He requires Foley care and teaching. There is no documented cause stated for the urethral stricture in the medical record. He also has diabetic PVD and hypertension. He takes oral hypoglycemic medication for his diabetes.

Description	Code
Primary: Unspecified urethral stricture, male, overlapping sites	N35.916
Secondary: Encounter for fitting and adjustment of urinary device	Z46.6
Secondary: Type 2 diabetes mellitus with diabetic peripheral angiopathy without gangrene	E11.51
Secondary: Essential (primary) hypertension	I10
Secondary: Long term (current) use of oral hypoglycemic drugs	Z79.84

The patient has a primary diagnosis of a urethral stricture affecting overlapping sites that has no documented etiology, which is appropriately coded with N35.916. The care and teaching for the Foley catheter is coded with Z46.6. The patient's diabetic PVD and hypertension have the potential to impact his care and recovery and are thus coded as secondary diagnoses as well. His use of oral hypoglycemic medication is captured with Z79.84.

Sickle cell nephropathy

A 51-year-old woman is admitted to home health with a primary diagnosis of sickle cell nephropathy.

Description	Code
Primary: Other sickle-cell disorders without crisis	D57.80
Secondary: Glomerular disorders in diseases classified elsewhere	N08

Sickle cell nephropathy is coded first with a code from the D57.- category (Other sickle-cell disorders without crisis) followed immediately by N08, according to the alphabetic index. Note that the way the codes are listed in the index specifies that they are an unbreakable etiology-manifestation pair, meaning that the N08 code must always immediately follow the D57.- code, according to coding guidelines.

Chapter 15: Pregnancy, Childbirth and the Puerperium (O00-O9A)

Codes from Chapter 15 are reported for ectopic pregnancies (the implantation of a fertilized egg outside the uterus) and molar pregnancies (abnormal products of conception), abortions (including miscarriages), and pregnancy complications. Complications of pregnancy may occur during the antepartum period (before delivery), intrapartum period (during labor and delivery), or puerperium (postpartum period of six weeks following delivery).

The pregnancy codes found here include problems and symptoms related to both the mother and the fetus. The conditions in the mother may have been present before she became pregnant, or developed during the pregnancy or postpartum period. Complication codes in this chapter are reported when the maternal or fetal conditions are affecting management of the pregnancy, or are requiring diagnostic tests, additional observation, special care, or termination of the pregnancy. If it is unclear whether the condition is affecting the management, query the physician.

Codes from this chapter are used only on the mother's medical record, never on the newborn's record. To report complications for a newborn or a fetus during delivery, see Chapter 16 (perinatal period) and Chapter 17 (congenital anomalies).

The principal diagnosis code assignment should correspond to the complication of pregnancy that was the reason for the patient encounter. Conditions usually classified in other chapters of ICD-10-CM are reclassified in Chapter 15 when they are related to or are aggravated by the pregnancy, childbirth, or by the puerperium.

Hypertension, for example, is classified in category O10.- during pregnancy, delivery, and the puerperium.

The majority of codes in Chapter 15 have a final character indicating the trimester of pregnancy. The timeframe for trimesters are:

- 1st trimester – less than 14 weeks 0 days

- 2nd trimester – 14 weeks 0 days to less than 28 weeks 0 days

- 3rd trimester – 28 weeks 0 days until delivery

If the trimester is not a component of a code, it is because the condition always occurs in a specific trimester, or the concept of trimester of pregnancy is not applicable. Certain codes have characters for only certain trimesters because the condition does not occur in all trimesters, but it may occur in more than one.

Assignment of the final character for trimester should be based on the provider's (physician's) documentation of the trimester (or number of weeks) for the current admission/encounter. This applies to the assignment of trimester for pre-existing conditions as well as those that develop during or are due to pregnancy. The provider's documentation of the number of weeks may be used to assign the appropriate code identifying the trimester.

Whenever delivery occurs during the current admission, and there is an "in childbirth" option for the obstetric complication being coded, the "in childbirth" code should be assigned.

Each category that includes codes for trimester has a code for "unspecified trimester." The "unspecified trimester" code should rarely be used, such as when the documentation in the record is insufficient to determine the trimester and it is not possible to obtain clarification.

Chapter 15 codes have sequencing priority over codes from other chapters. An additional code from category Z3A, weeks of gestation, is used with codes from this chapter to identify specific weeks of pregnancy following any complications of pregnancy, childbirth and the puerperium. An outcome of delivery code, Z37.0-Z37.9, should be included on every maternal record when a delivery has occurred.

Maternity and postpartum care is a specialty in home care. OASIS is not involved with these patients if the care is provided for maternity reasons. Should the pregnancy be incidental to the home care encounter, then code Z33.1, Pregnant state incidental, should be used in place of any Chapter 15 codes. It is the physician's responsibility to state that the condition being treated is not affecting the pregnancy.

The circumstances of the encounter govern the selection of the principal diagnosis.

In episodes when no delivery occurs, the principal diagnosis should correspond to the principal complication of the pregnancy that necessitated the encounter. When more than one complication is being treated or monitored, any of the complication codes may be sequenced first.

Codes from category O35 (Maternal care for known or suspected fetal abnormality and damage), and category O36 (Maternal care for other fetal problems), are assigned only when the fetal condition is actually responsible for modifying the management of the mother, i.e., by requiring diagnostic studies, additional observation, special care, or termination of pregnancy. The fact that the fetal condition exists does not justify assigning a code from this series to the mother's record.

In cases when surgery is performed on the fetus, a diagnosis code from category O35, Maternal care for known or suspected fetal abnormality and damage, should be assigned to identify the fetal condition.

No code from Chapter 16, the perinatal codes, should be used on the mother's record to identify fetal conditions. Surgery performed in utero on a fetus is still to be coded as an obstetric encounter.

The postpartum period begins immediately after delivery and continues for six weeks following delivery. The peripartum period is defined as the last month of pregnancy to five months postpartum. A postpartum complication is any complication occurring within the six-week period. (NOTE: Chapter 15 codes also may be used to describe pregnancy-related complications of the mother after the six-week period, should the physician document that a condition is pregnancy related). It is acceptable to use codes specifically for the puerperium with codes complicating pregnancy and childbirth if a condition arises postpartum during the delivery encounter.

Code O94, Sequelae of complication of pregnancy, childbirth, and the puerperium, is used when an initial complication of a pregnancy develops a sequelae requiring treatment at a future date. This code may be used at any time after the initial postpartum period. This code, like all sequela codes, is to be sequenced following the code describing the sequelae of the complication.

Sometimes a Chapter 15 code is not the most appropriate choice. Here are a few situations to watch out for:

- If the documentation indicates **a neoplasm or tumor of an organ**, coders should look up the term (malignancy, tumor, adenoma) used in the medical record to find the correct code, most likely a code from Chapter 2. A code from Chapter 15 is reported (such as subcategory O9A.1- Malignant neoplasm complicating pregnancy, childbirth and the puerperium) as the first- listed diagnosis with an additional code (C00-C96) to identify the neoplasm.

- If a patient has a **personal history of a condition that may complicate the pregnancy in the future but is not currently a complication,** use a code from the Z code section. Examples are Z22.330 (Carrier or suspected carrier of Group B streptococcus), or Z87.51 (Personal history of pre-term labor. However, use code O09.21- (Supervision of pregnancy with history of pre-term labor) if the patient is currently pregnant. If a code from Chapter 15 also is being reported, the Z code is reported as an additional diagnosis.

General Rules for OB Cases

7th Character for Fetus Identification

Where applicable, a 7th character is to be assigned for certain categories (such as O31, O32, O33.3- O33.7, O35, O40, O41, O60.1, O60.2, O64, and O69) to identify the fetus for which the complication code applies. In some of these code categories, there are specific codes for each option. In other code subcategories, coders will need to refer to the 7th character boxes for the definition of the 7th character options.

Assign 7th character "0":

- For single gestations

- When the documentation in the record is insufficient to determine the fetus affected and it is not possible to obtain clarification.

- When it is not possible to clinically determine which fetus is affected.

Selection of OB Principal or First-Listed Diagnosis

For **routine outpatient prenatal visits** when no complications are present, a code from category Z34, Encounter for supervision of normal pregnancy, should be used as a first-listed diagnosis. These codes should not be used in conjunction with Chapter 15 codes, according to the coding guidelines.

For routine prenatal outpatient visits for patients with high-risk pregnancies, a code from category O09 (Supervision of high risk pregnancy) should be used as the first-listed diagnosis. Secondary Chapter 15 codes may be used in conjunction with these codes, if appropriate.

In episodes when no delivery occurs, the principal diagnosis should correspond to the principal complication of the pregnancy which necessitated the encounter. Should more than one complication exist, all of which are treated or monitored, any of the complications codes may be sequenced first.

When an obstetric patient is admitted and delivers during that admission, the condition that prompted the admission should be sequenced as the principal diagnosis. If multiple conditions prompted the admission, sequence the one most related to the delivery as the principal diagnosis. A code for any complication of the delivery should be assigned as an additional diagnosis. In cases of cesarean delivery, the selection of the principal diagnosis should be the condition established after study that was responsible for the patient's admission. If the patient was admitted with a condition that resulted in the performance of the cesarean procedure, then that condition should be selected as the principal diagnosis. If the reason for the admission/encounter was unrelated to the condition resulting in the cesarean delivery, the condition related to the reason for the admission/encounter should be selected as the principal diagnosis.

A code from category Z37, Outcome of delivery, should be included on every maternal record when a delivery has occurred. These codes are not to be used on subsequent records or on the newborn record.

Pre-existing Conditions versus Conditions due to pregnancy

Certain categories in Chapter 15 distinguish between conditions of the mother that existed prior to the pregnancy (pre-existing) and those that are a direct result of pregnancy. When assigning codes from Chapter 15, it is important to assess if a condition was pre-existing prior to pregnancy or developed during or due to pregnancy in order to assign the correct code.

Categories that do not distinguish between pre-existing and pregnancy-related conditions may be used for either.

Pre-existing hypertension in pregnancy

Category O10 (pre-existing hypertension complicating pregnancy, childbirth and the puerperium) includes codes for hypertensive heart and hypertensive chronic kidney disease. When assigning one of the O10 codes that includes hypertensive heart disease or hypertensive chronic kidney disease, it is necessary to add a secondary code from the appropriate hypertension category to specify the type of heart failure or chronic kidney disease.

Multiple Coding and Sequencing

Codes from this chapter almost always are reported as the first-listed diagnosis. Exceptions are category O94 (Sequelae of pregnancy, childbirth and the puerperium), which requires coding first the condition resulting from (sequel) of complication of pregnancy, childbirth and the puerperium, and some Z codes designated as primary only in the Tabular List.

Most complication codes include notes instructing the coder to report an additional code to provide more information as to the nature of the complication. The following are some examples of coding for complications during pregnancy, delivery and the postpartum periods:

- During pregnancy, childbirth or the puerperium, a patient admitted because of an **HIV-related illness** should receive a principal diagnosis from subcategory O98.7-, Human immunodeficiency [HIV] disease complicating pregnancy, childbirth and the puerperium, followed by the code(s)

for the HIV-related illness(es). Patients with asymptomatic HIV infection status admitted during pregnancy, childbirth and the puerperium should be assigned codes O98.7- and Z21, Asymptomatic human immunodeficiency virus [HIV] infection status.

- **Diabetes mellitus** is a significant complicating factor in pregnancy. Pregnant women who are diabetic should be assigned a code from category O24, Diabetes mellitus in pregnancy, childbirth and the puerperium, first, followed by the appropriate code(s) (E08-E13) from chapter 4. Code Z79.4, Long-term (current) use of insulin, or code Z79.84, Long-term (current) use of oral hypoglycemic drugs, should also be assigned if the diabetes mellitus is being treated with insulin or oral medications. If the patient is treated with both oral medications and insulin, only the code for insulin-controlled should be assigned, per the FY2017 Chapter 15 coding guidelines. Remember, these are chapter specific guidelines and therefore only apply to Chapter 15 codes.

- **Gestational (pregnancy induced) diabetes** can occur during the second and third trimester of pregnancy in women who were not diabetic prior to pregnancy. Gestational diabetes can cause complications in the pregnancy similar to those of pre-existing diabetes mellitus. It also puts the woman at greater risk of developing diabetes after the pregnancy. Codes for gestational diabetes are in subcategory O24.4, Gestational diabetes mellitus. No other code from category O24, Diabetes mellitus in pregnancy, childbirth, and the puerperium should be used with a code from O24.4.

The codes under subcategory O24.4 include diet controlled, insulin controlled, and controlled by oral hypoglycemic drugs. If a patient with gestational diabetes is treated with both diet and insulin, only assign the code for insulin-controlled. If a patient with gestational diabetes is treated with both diet and oral hypoglycemic medications, only assign the code for "controlled by oral hypoglycemic drugs." Code Z79.4 or code Z79.84 should not be assigned with codes from subcategory O24.4.

An abnormal glucose tolerance in pregnancy is assigned a code from subcategory O99.81, Abnormal glucose complicating pregnancy, childbirth and the puerperium.

Sepsis and septic shock complicating abortion, pregnancy, childbirth and the puerperium

When assigning a chapter 15 code for sepsis complicating abortion, pregnancy, childbirth, and the puerperium, a code for the specific type of infection should be assigned as an additional diagnosis. If severe sepsis is present, a code from subcategory R65.2, Severe sepsis, and code(s) for associated organ dysfunction(s) should also be assigned as additional diagnoses.

Code O85, Puerperal sepsis, should be assigned with a secondary code to identify the causal organism (e.g., for a bacterial infection, assign a code from category B95-B96, bacterial infections in conditions classified elsewhere). A code from category A40, streptococcal sepsis, or A41, other sepsis, should not be used for puerperal sepsis. If applicable, use additional codes to identify severe sepsis (R65.2-) and any associated acute organ dysfunction.

Pregnancy-related Cardiomyopathy

Pregnancy associated cardiomyopathy, code O90.3, is unique in that it may be diagnosed in the third trimester of pregnancy but may continue to progress months after the delivery. For this reason, it is referred to as peripartum cardiomyopathy. Code O90.3 is only for use when the cardiomyopathy develops as a result of pregnancy in a woman who did not have pre-existing heart disease.

Alcohol and tobacco use during pregnancy, childbirth and the puerperium

Codes under subcategory O99.31, Alcohol use complicating pregnancy, childbirth and the puerperium, should be assigned for any pregnancy case when a mother uses alcohol during the pregnancy or postpartum. A secondary code from category F10, alcohol related disorders, should also be assigned to identify manifestations of alcohol use.

Codes under subcategory O99.33, Tobacco use disorder complicating pregnancy, childbirth, and the puerperium, should be assigned for any pregnancy case when a mother used any type of tobacco product during the pregnancy or postpartum. A secondary code from F17, nicotine dependence, should also be assigned to identify the type of nicotine dependence.

Poisoning, toxic effects, adverse effects and underdosing in a pregnant patient

A code from subcategory O9A.2, Injury, poisoning and certain other consequences of external causes complicating pregnancy, childbirth, and the puerperium, should be sequenced first, followed by the appropriate injury, poisoning, toxic effect, adverse effect, or underdosing code, and then the additional code(s) that specifies the condition caused by the poisoning, toxic effect, adverse effect or underdosing.

Abuse in a Pregnant Patient

For suspected or confirmed cases of abuse of a pregnant patient, a code(s) from subcategories O9A.3, Physical abuse complicating pregnancy, childbirth, and the puerperium, O9A.4, Sexual abuse complicating pregnancy, childbirth, and the puerperium, and O9A.5, Psychological abuse complicating pregnancy, childbirth, and the puerperium, should be sequenced first, followed by the appropriate codes (if applicable) to identify any associated current injury due to physical abuse, sexual abuse, and the perpetrator of abuse. Refer to chapter 19 for codes related to current injuries and Y07- for codes to describe the perpetrator of abuse.

CHAPTER 15: PREGNANCY, CHILDBIRTH AND THE PUERPERIUM (O00-O9A)

Note:

CODES FROM THIS CHAPTER ARE FOR USE ONLY ON MATERNAL RECORDS, NEVER ON NEWBORN RECORDS

Codes from this chapter are for use for conditions related to or aggravated by the pregnancy, childbirth, or by the puerperium (maternal causes or obstetric causes)

Trimesters are counted from the first day of the last menstrual period. They are defined as follows:

1st trimester- less than 14 weeks 0 days
2nd trimester- 14 weeks 0 days to less than 28 weeks 0 days
3rd trimester- 28 weeks 0 days until delivery

Use additional code from category Z3A, Weeks of gestation, to identify the specific week of the pregnancy, if known.

EXCLUDES 1   supervision of normal pregnancy (Z34.-)

EXCLUDES 2   mental and behavioral disorders associated with the puerperium (F53.-)
obstetrical tetanus (A34)
postpartum necrosis of pituitary gland (E23.0)
puerperal osteomalacia (M83.0)

GUIDELINES   Section I.C.15.a.1)

Obstetric cases require codes from chapter 15, codes in the range O00-O9A, Pregnancy, Childbirth, and the Puerperium. Chapter 15 codes have sequencing priority over codes from other chapters. Additional codes from other chapters may be used in conjunction with chapter 15 codes to further specify conditions. Should the provider document that the pregnancy is incidental to the encounter, then code Z33.1, Pregnant state, incidental, should be used in place of any chapter 15 codes. It is the provider's responsibility to state that the condition being treated is not affecting the pregnancy.

GUIDELINES   Section I.C.15.a.2)

Chapter 15 codes are to be used only on the maternal record, never on the record of the newborn.

GUIDELINES   Section I.C.15.c

When assigning codes from Chapter 15, it is important to assess if a condition was pre-existing prior to pregnancy or developed during or due to the pregnancy in order to assign the correct code. Categories that do not distinguish between pre-existing and pregnancy related conditions may be used for either. It is acceptable to use codes specifically for the puerperium with codes complicating pregnancy and childbirth if a condition arises postpartum during the delivery encounter.

This chapter contains the following blocks:

O00-O08   Pregnancy with abortive outcome
O09   Supervision of high risk pregnancy
O10-O16   Edema, proteinuria and hypertensive disorders in pregnancy, childbirth and the puerperium
O20-O29   Other maternal disorders predominantly related to pregnancy
O30-O48   Maternal care related to the fetus and amniotic cavity and possible delivery problems
O60-O77   Complications of labor and delivery
O80-O82   Encounter for delivery
O85-O92   Complications predominantly related to the puerperium
O94-O9A   Other obstetric conditions, not elsewhere classified

Pregnancy with abortive outcome (O00-O08)

EXCLUDES 1   continuing pregnancy in multiple gestation after abortion of one fetus or more (O31.1-, O31.3-)

+ ④ O00   **Ectopic pregnancy**
   INCLUDES   ruptured ectopic pregnancy
   Use additional code from category O08 to identify any associated complication

+ ⑤ O00.0   **Abdominal pregnancy**
   EXCLUDES 1   maternal care for viable fetus in abdominal pregnancy (O36.7-)

SP + O00.00   **Abdominal pregnancy without intrauterine pregnancy**
   Abdominal pregnancy NOS

SP + O00.01   **Abdominal pregnancy with intrauterine pregnancy**

+ ⑤ O00.1   **Tubal pregnancy**
   Fallopian pregnancy
   Rupture of (fallopian) tube due to pregnancy
   Tubal abortion
   DEFINITION   Fertilized egg implants itself within the fallopian tube where the embryo grows and may rupture the tube.

+ ⑥ O00.10   **Tubal pregnancy without intrauterine pregnancy**
   Tubal pregnancy NOS

☰ SP + O00.101   **Right tubal pregnancy without intrauterine pregnancy**

☰ SP + O00.102   **Left tubal pregnancy without intrauterine pregnancy**

☰ SP + O00.109   **Unspecified tubal pregnancy without intrauterine pregnancy**

+ ⑥ O00.11   **Tubal pregnancy with intrauterine pregnancy**

☰ SP + O00.111   **Right tubal pregnancy with intrauterine pregnancy**

☰ SP + O00.112   **Left tubal pregnancy with intrauterine pregnancy**

☰ SP + O00.119   **Unspecified tubal pregnancy with intrauterine pregnancy**

+ ⑤ O00.2   **Ovarian pregnancy**

+ ⑥ O00.20   **Ovarian pregnancy without intrauterine pregnancy**
   Ovarian pregnancy NOS

☰ SP + O00.201   **Right ovarian pregnancy without intrauterine pregnancy**

☰ SP + O00.202   **Left ovarian pregnancy without intrauterine pregnancy**

☰ SP + O00.209   **Unspecified ovarian pregnancy without intrauterine pregnancy**

+ ⑥ O00.21   **Ovarian pregnancy with intrauterine pregnancy**

☰ SP + O00.211   **Right ovarian pregnancy with intrauterine pregnancy**

☰ SP + O00.212   **Left ovarian pregnancy with intrauterine pregnancy**

☰ SP + O00.219   **Unspecified ovarian pregnancy with intrauterine pregnancy**

+ ⑤ O00.8   **Other ectopic pregnancy**
   Cervical pregnancy
   Cornual pregnancy
   Intraligamentous pregnancy
   Mural pregnancy

SP + O00.80   **Other ectopic pregnancy without intrauterine pregnancy**
   Other ectopic pregnancy NOS

SP + O00.81   **Other ectopic pregnancy with intrauterine pregnancy**

★ New   ▲ Revised   **Px** Primary   **SP** PDGM Px   **SL** Low CoM   **SH** High CoM   **IQ** Quest. Encounter   **H** Hospice non-cancer Dx   Unspecified   **M** *Manifestation*

+ 5 O00.9 **Ectopic pregnancy, unspecified**

SP + O00.90 **Unspecified ectopic pregnancy without intrauterine pregnancy**

Ectopic pregnancy NOS

SP + O00.91 **Unspecified ectopic pregnancy with intrauterine pregnancy**

+ 4 O01 **Hydatidiform mole**
Use additional code from category O08 to identify any associated complication.
> EXCLUDES 1   chorioadenoma (destruens) (D39.2)
> malignant hydatidiform mole (D39.2)

SP + O01.0 **Classical hydatidiform mole**
Complete hydatidiform mole

SP + O01.1 **Incomplete and partial hydatidiform mole**

SP + O01.9 **Hydatidiform mole, unspecified**
Trophoblastic disease NOS
Vesicular mole NOS

+ 4 O02 **Other abnormal products of conception**
Use additional code from category O08 to identify any associated complication.
> EXCLUDES 1   papyraceous fetus (O31.0-)

SP + O02.0 **Blighted ovum and nonhydatidiform mole**
Carneous mole
Fleshy mole
Intrauterine mole NOS
Molar pregnancy NEC
Pathological ovum

SP + O02.1 **Missed abortion**
Early fetal death, before completion of 20 weeks of gestation, with retention of dead fetus
> EXCLUDES 1   failed induced abortion (O07.-)
> fetal death (intrauterine) (late) (O36.4)
> missed abortion with blighted ovum (O02.0)
> missed abortion with hydatidiform mole (O01.-)
> missed abortion with nonhydatidiform (O02.0)
> missed abortion with other abnormal products of conception (O02.8-)
> missed delivery (O36.4)
> stillbirth (P95)

+ 5 O02.8 **Other specified abnormal products of conception**
> EXCLUDES 1   abnormal products of conception with blighted ovum (O02.0)
> abnormal products of conception with hydatidiform mole (O01.-)
> abnormal products of conception with nonhydatidiform mole (O02.0)

SP + O02.81 **Inappropriate change in quantitative human chorionic gonadotropin (hCG) in early pregnancy**
Biochemical pregnancy
Chemical pregnancy

Inappropriate level of quantitative human chorionic gonadotropin (hCG) for gestational age in early pregnancy

SP + O02.89 **Other abnormal products of conception**

SP + O02.9 **Abnormal product of conception, unspecified**

4 O03 **Spontaneous abortion**
Note:
Incomplete abortion includes retained products of conception following spontaneous abortion
> INCLUDES   miscarriage

SP O03.0 **Genital tract and pelvic infection following incomplete spontaneous abortion**
Endometritis following incomplete spontaneous abortion
Oophoritis following incomplete spontaneous abortion
Parametritis following incomplete spontaneous abortion
Pelvic peritonitis following incomplete spontaneous abortion
Salpingitis following incomplete spontaneous abortion
Salpingo-oophoritis following incomplete spontaneous abortion
> EXCLUDES 1   sepsis following incomplete spontaneous abortion (O03.37)
> urinary tract infection following incomplete spontaneous abortion (O03.38)

SP O03.1 **Delayed or excessive hemorrhage following incomplete spontaneous abortion**
Afibrinogenemia following incomplete spontaneous abortion
Defibrination syndrome following incomplete spontaneous abortion
Hemolysis following incomplete spontaneous abortion
Intravascular coagulation following incomplete spontaneous abortion

SP O03.2 **Embolism following incomplete spontaneous abortion**
Air embolism following incomplete spontaneous abortion
Amniotic fluid embolism following incomplete spontaneous abortion
Blood-clot embolism following incomplete spontaneous abortion
Embolism NOS following incomplete spontaneous abortion
Fat embolism following incomplete spontaneous abortion
Pulmonary embolism following incomplete spontaneous abortion
Pyemic embolism following incomplete spontaneous abortion
Septic or septicopyemic embolism following incomplete spontaneous abortion
Soap embolism following incomplete spontaneous abortion

---

4 4th digit required   5 5th digit required   6 6th digit required   7 7th digit required   7 7th digit placeholder   + Additional code   5 Laterality

5 O03.3 **Other and unspecified complications following incomplete spontaneous abortion**

SP O03.30 **Unspecified complication following incomplete spontaneous abortion**

SP O03.31 **Shock following incomplete spontaneous abortion**
Circulatory collapse following incomplete spontaneous abortion
Shock (postprocedural) following incomplete spontaneous abortion
> **EXCLUDES 1** shock due to infection following incomplete spontaneous abortion (O03.37)

SP O03.32 **Renal failure following incomplete spontaneous abortion**
Kidney failure (acute) following incomplete spontaneous abortion
Oliguria following incomplete spontaneous abortion
Renal shutdown following incomplete spontaneous abortion
Renal tubular necrosis following incomplete spontaneous abortion
Uremia following incomplete spontaneous abortion

SP O03.33 **Metabolic disorder following incomplete spontaneous abortion**

SP O03.34 **Damage to pelvic organs following incomplete spontaneous abortion**
Laceration, perforation, tear or chemical damage of bladder following incomplete spontaneous abortion
Laceration, perforation, tear or chemical damage of bowel following incomplete spontaneous abortion
Laceration, perforation, tear or chemical damage of broad ligament following incomplete spontaneous abortion
Laceration, perforation, tear or chemical damage of cervix following incomplete spontaneous abortion
Laceration, perforation, tear or chemical damage of periurethral tissue following incomplete spontaneous abortion
Laceration, perforation, tear or chemical damage of uterus following incomplete spontaneous abortion
Laceration, perforation, tear or chemical damage of vagina following incomplete spontaneous abortion

SP O03.35 **Other venous complications following incomplete spontaneous abortion**

SP O03.36 **Cardiac arrest following incomplete spontaneous abortion**

SP ✚ O03.37 **Sepsis following incomplete spontaneous abortion**
Use additional code to identify infectious agent (B95-B97)
Use additional code to identify severe sepsis, if applicable (R65.2-)

> **EXCLUDES 1** septic or septicopyemic embolism following incomplete spontaneous abortion (O03.2)

SP O03.38 **Urinary tract infection following incomplete spontaneous abortion**
Cystitis following incomplete spontaneous abortion

SP O03.39 **Incomplete spontaneous abortion with other complications**

SP O03.4 **Incomplete spontaneous abortion without complication**

SP O03.5 **Genital tract and pelvic infection following complete or unspecified spontaneous abortion**
Endometritis following complete or unspecified spontaneous abortion
Oophoritis following complete or unspecified spontaneous abortion
Parametritis following complete or unspecified spontaneous abortion
Pelvic peritonitis following complete or unspecified spontaneous abortion
Salpingitis following complete or unspecified spontaneous abortion
Salpingo-oophoritis following complete or unspecified spontaneous abortion
> **EXCLUDES 1** sepsis following complete or unspecified spontaneous abortion (O03.87)
> urinary tract infection following complete or unspecified spontaneous abortion (O03.88)

SP O03.6 **Delayed or excessive hemorrhage following complete or unspecified spontaneous abortion**
Afibrinogenemia following complete or unspecified spontaneous abortion
Defibrination syndrome following complete or unspecified spontaneous abortion
Hemolysis following complete or unspecified spontaneous abortion
Intravascular coagulation following complete or unspecified spontaneous abortion

SP O03.7 **Embolism following complete or unspecified spontaneous abortion**
Air embolism following complete or unspecified spontaneous abortion
Amniotic fluid embolism following complete or unspecified spontaneous abortion
Blood-clot embolism following complete or unspecified spontaneous abortion
Embolism NOS following complete or unspecified spontaneous abortion
Fat embolism following complete or unspecified spontaneous abortion
Pulmonary embolism following complete or unspecified spontaneous abortion
Pyemic embolism following complete or unspecified spontaneous abortion
Septic or septicopyemic embolism following complete or unspecified spontaneous abortion

Chapter 15

O00-O9A

★ New ▲ Revised **Px** Primary **SP** PDGM Px **SL** Low CoM **SH** High CoM **IQ** Quest. Encounter **H** Hospice non-cancer Dx Unspecified **M** *Manifestation*

Soap embolism following complete or unspecified spontaneous abortion

⑤ O03.8 **Other and unspecified complications following complete or unspecified spontaneous abortion**

SP O03.80 **Unspecified complication following complete or unspecified spontaneous abortion**

SP O03.81 **Shock following complete or unspecified spontaneous abortion**

Circulatory collapse following complete or unspecified spontaneous abortion

Shock (postprocedural) following complete or unspecified spontaneous abortion

> **EXCLUDES 1** shock due to infection following complete or unspecified spontaneous abortion (O03.87)

SP O03.82 **Renal failure following complete or unspecified spontaneous abortion**

Kidney failure (acute) following complete or unspecified spontaneous abortion

Oliguria following complete or unspecified spontaneous abortion

Renal shutdown following complete or unspecified spontaneous abortion

Renal tubular necrosis following complete or unspecified spontaneous abortion

Uremia following complete or unspecified spontaneous abortion

SP O03.83 **Metabolic disorder following complete or unspecified spontaneous abortion**

SP O03.84 **Damage to pelvic organs following complete or unspecified spontaneous abortion**

Laceration, perforation, tear or chemical damage of bladder following complete or unspecified spontaneous abortion

Laceration, perforation, tear or chemical damage of bowel following complete or unspecified spontaneous abortion

Laceration, perforation, tear or chemical damage of broad ligament following complete or unspecified spontaneous abortion

Laceration, perforation, tear or chemical damage of cervix following complete or unspecified spontaneous abortion

Laceration, perforation, tear or chemical damage of periurethral tissue following complete or unspecified spontaneous abortion

Laceration, perforation, tear or chemical damage of uterus following complete or unspecified spontaneous abortion

Laceration, perforation, tear or chemical damage of vagina following complete or unspecified spontaneous abortion

SP O03.85 **Other venous complications following complete or unspecified spontaneous abortion**

SP O03.86 **Cardiac arrest following complete or unspecified spontaneous abortion**

SP ✚ O03.87 **Sepsis following complete or unspecified spontaneous abortion**

Use additional code to identify infectious agent (B95-B97)

Use additional code to identify severe sepsis, if applicable (R65.2-)

> **EXCLUDES 1** septic or septicopyemic embolism following complete or unspecified spontaneous abortion (O03.7)

SP O03.88 **Urinary tract infection following complete or unspecified spontaneous abortion**

Cystitis following complete or unspecified spontaneous abortion

SP O03.89 **Complete or unspecified spontaneous abortion with other complications**

SP O03.9 **Complete or unspecified spontaneous abortion without complication**

Miscarriage NOS

Spontaneous abortion NOS

④ O04 **Complications following (induced) termination of pregnancy**

> **INCLUDES** complications following (induced) termination of pregnancy

> **EXCLUDES 1** encounter for elective termination of pregnancy, uncomplicated (Z33.2)
> failed attempted termination of pregnancy (O07.-)

SP O04.5 **Genital tract and pelvic infection following (induced) termination of pregnancy**

Endometritis following (induced) termination of pregnancy

Oophoritis following (induced) termination of pregnancy

Parametritis following (induced) termination of pregnancy

Pelvic peritonitis following (induced) termination of pregnancy

Salpingitis following (induced) termination of pregnancy

Salpingo-oophoritis following (induced) termination of pregnancy

> **EXCLUDES 1** sepsis following (induced) termination of pregnancy (O04.87)
> urinary tract infection following (induced) termination of pregnancy (O04.88)

SP O04.6 **Delayed or excessive hemorrhage following (induced) termination of pregnancy**

---

④ 4th digit required   ⑤ 5th digit required   ⑥ 6th digit required   ⑦ 7th digit required   ⑦ 7th digit placeholder   ✚ Additional code   ⊟ Laterality

1318   *DecisionHealth's* FY 2020 Complete Home Health ICD-10-CM Diagnosis Coding Manual

Afibrinogenemia following (induced) termination of pregnancy

Defibrination syndrome following (induced) termination of pregnancy

Hemolysis following (induced) termination of pregnancy

Intravascular coagulation following (induced) termination of pregnancy

SP O04.7 Embolism following (induced) termination of pregnancy

Air embolism following (induced) termination of pregnancy

Amniotic fluid embolism following (induced) termination of pregnancy

Blood-clot embolism following (induced) termination of pregnancy

Embolism NOS following (induced) termination of pregnancy

Fat embolism following (induced) termination of pregnancy

Pulmonary embolism following (induced) termination of pregnancy

Pyemic embolism following (induced) termination of pregnancy

Septic or septicopyemic embolism following (induced) termination of pregnancy

Soap embolism following (induced) termination of pregnancy

5 O04.8 (Induced) termination of pregnancy with other and unspecified complications

SP O04.80 (Induced) termination of pregnancy with unspecified complications

SP O04.81 Shock following (induced) termination of pregnancy

Circulatory collapse following (induced) termination of pregnancy

Shock (postprocedural) following (induced) termination of pregnancy

EXCLUDES 1 shock due to infection following (induced) termination of pregnancy (O04.87)

SP O04.82 Renal failure following (induced) termination of pregnancy

Kidney failure (acute) following (induced) termination of pregnancy

Oliguria following (induced) termination of pregnancy

Renal shutdown following (induced) termination of pregnancy

Renal tubular necrosis following (induced) termination of pregnancy

Uremia following (induced) termination of pregnancy

SP O04.83 Metabolic disorder following (induced) termination of pregnancy

SP O04.84 Damage to pelvic organs following (induced) termination of pregnancy

Laceration, perforation, tear or chemical damage of bladder following (induced) termination of pregnancy

Laceration, perforation, tear or chemical damage of bowel following (induced) termination of pregnancy

Laceration, perforation, tear or chemical damage of broad ligament following (induced) termination of pregnancy

Laceration, perforation, tear or chemical damage of cervix following (induced) termination of pregnancy

Laceration, perforation, tear or chemical damage of periurethral tissue following (induced) termination of pregnancy

Laceration, perforation, tear or chemical damage of uterus following (induced) termination of pregnancy

Laceration, perforation, tear or chemical damage of vagina following (induced) termination of pregnancy

SP O04.85 Other venous complications following (induced) termination of pregnancy

SP O04.86 Cardiac arrest following (induced) termination of pregnancy

SP + O04.87 Sepsis following (induced) termination of pregnancy

Use additional code to identify infectious agent (B95-B97)

Use additional code to identify severe sepsis, if applicable (R65.2-)

EXCLUDES 1 septic or septicopyemic embolism following (induced) termination of pregnancy (O04.7)

SP O04.88 Urinary tract infection following (induced) termination of pregnancy

Cystitis following (induced) termination of pregnancy

SP O04.89 (Induced) termination of pregnancy with other complications

4 O07 Failed attempted termination of pregnancy

INCLUDES failure of attempted induction of termination of pregnancy incomplete elective abortion

EXCLUDES 1 incomplete spontaneous abortion (O03.0-)

SP O07.0 Genital tract and pelvic infection following failed attempted termination of pregnancy

Endometritis following failed attempted termination of pregnancy

Oophoritis following failed attempted termination of pregnancy

Parametritis following failed attempted termination of pregnancy

Pelvic peritonitis following failed attempted termination of pregnancy

Salpingitis following failed attempted termination of pregnancy

Salpingo-oophoritis following failed attempted termination of pregnancy

EXCLUDES 1 sepsis following failed attempted termination of pregnancy (O07.37)

urinary tract infection following failed attempted termination of pregnancy (O07.38)

SP O07.1 Delayed or excessive hemorrhage following failed attempted termination of pregnancy

Chapter 15

O00-O9A

★ New ▲ Revised Px Primary SP PDGM Px SL Low CoM SH High CoM IQ Quest. Encounter H Hospice non-cancer Dx Unspecified M *Manifestation*

DecisionHealth's FY 2020 Complete Home Health ICD-10-CM Diagnosis Coding Manual

1319

Afibrinogenemia following failed attempted termination of pregnancy

Defibrination syndrome following failed attempted termination of pregnancy

Hemolysis following failed attempted termination of pregnancy

Intravascular coagulation following failed attempted termination of pregnancy

SP O07.2 **Embolism following failed attempted termination of pregnancy**

Air embolism following failed attempted termination of pregnancy

Amniotic fluid embolism following failed attempted termination of pregnancy

Blood-clot embolism following failed attempted termination of pregnancy

Embolism NOS following failed attempted termination of pregnancy

Fat embolism following failed attempted termination of pregnancy

Pulmonary embolism following failed attempted termination of pregnancy

Pyemic embolism following failed attempted termination of pregnancy

Septic or septicopyemic embolism following failed attempted termination of pregnancy

Soap embolism following failed attempted termination of pregnancy

5 O07.3 **Failed attempted termination of pregnancy with other and unspecified complications**

SP O07.30 **Failed attempted termination of pregnancy with unspecified complications**

SP O07.31 **Shock following failed attempted termination of pregnancy**

Circulatory collapse following failed attempted termination of pregnancy

Shock (postprocedural) following failed attempted termination of pregnancy

EXCLUDES 1 shock due to infection following failed attempted termination of pregnancy (O07.37)

SP O07.32 **Renal failure following failed attempted termination of pregnancy**

Kidney failure (acute) following failed attempted termination of pregnancy

Oliguria following failed attempted termination of pregnancy

Renal shutdown following failed attempted termination of pregnancy

Renal tubular necrosis following failed attempted termination of pregnancy

Uremia following failed attempted termination of pregnancy

SP O07.33 **Metabolic disorder following failed attempted termination of pregnancy**

SP O07.34 **Damage to pelvic organs following failed attempted termination of pregnancy**

Laceration, perforation, tear or chemical damage of bladder following failed attempted termination of pregnancy

Laceration, perforation, tear or chemical damage of bowel following failed attempted termination of pregnancy

Laceration, perforation, tear or chemical damage of broad ligament following failed attempted termination of pregnancy

Laceration, perforation, tear or chemical damage of cervix following failed attempted termination of pregnancy

Laceration, perforation, tear or chemical damage of periurethral tissue following failed attempted termination of pregnancy

Laceration, perforation, tear or chemical damage of uterus following failed attempted termination of pregnancy

Laceration, perforation, tear or chemical damage of vagina following failed attempted termination of pregnancy

SP O07.35 **Other venous complications following failed attempted termination of pregnancy**

SP O07.36 **Cardiac arrest following failed attempted termination of pregnancy**

SP + O07.37 **Sepsis following failed attempted termination of pregnancy**

Use additional code (B95-B97), to identify infectious agent

Use additional code (R65.2-) to identify severe sepsis, if applicable

EXCLUDES 1 septic or septicopyemic embolism following failed attempted termination of pregnancy (O07.2)

SP O07.38 **Urinary tract infection following failed attempted termination of pregnancy**

Cystitis following failed attempted termination of pregnancy

SP O07.39 **Failed attempted termination of pregnancy with other complications**

SP O07.4 **Failed attempted termination of pregnancy without complication**

4 O08 **Complications following ectopic and molar pregnancy**

This category is for use with categories O00-O02 to identify any associated complications

SP O08.0 **Genital tract and pelvic infection following ectopic and molar pregnancy**

Endometritis following ectopic and molar pregnancy

Oophoritis following ectopic and molar pregnancy

Parametritis following ectopic and molar pregnancy

Pelvic peritonitis following ectopic and molar pregnancy

Salpingitis following ectopic and molar pregnancy

Salpingo-oophoritis following ectopic and molar pregnancy

4 4th digit required   5 5th digit required   6 6th digit required   7 7th digit required   7 7th digit placeholder   + Additional code   ⊟ Laterality

1320   DecisionHealth's FY 2020 Complete Home Health ICD-10-CM Diagnosis Coding Manual

EXCLUDES 1   sepsis following ectopic and molar pregnancy (O08.82)
urinary tract infection (O08.83)

SP O08.1 Delayed or excessive hemorrhage following ectopic and molar pregnancy

Afibrinogenemia following ectopic and molar pregnancy

Defibrination syndrome following ectopic and molar pregnancy

Hemolysis following ectopic and molar pregnancy

Intravascular coagulation following ectopic and molar pregnancy

EXCLUDES 1   delayed or excessive hemorrhage due to incomplete abortion (O03.1)

SP O08.2 Embolism following ectopic and molar pregnancy

Air embolism following ectopic and molar pregnancy

Amniotic fluid embolism following ectopic and molar pregnancy

Blood-clot embolism following ectopic and molar pregnancy

Embolism NOS following ectopic and molar pregnancy

Fat embolism following ectopic and molar pregnancy

Pulmonary embolism following ectopic and molar pregnancy

Pyemic embolism following ectopic and molar pregnancy

Septic or septicopyemic embolism following ectopic and molar pregnancy

Soap embolism following ectopic and molar pregnancy

SP O08.3 Shock following ectopic and molar pregnancy

Circulatory collapse following ectopic and molar pregnancy

Shock (postprocedural) following ectopic and molar pregnancy

EXCLUDES 1   shock due to infection following ectopic and molar pregnancy (O08.82)

SP O08.4 Renal failure following ectopic and molar pregnancy

Kidney failure (acute) following ectopic and molar pregnancy

Oliguria following ectopic and molar pregnancy

Renal shutdown following ectopic and molar pregnancy

Renal tubular necrosis following ectopic and molar pregnancy

Uremia following ectopic and molar pregnancy

SP O08.5 Metabolic disorders following an ectopic and molar pregnancy

SP O08.6 Damage to pelvic organs and tissues following an ectopic and molar pregnancy

Laceration, perforation, tear or chemical damage of bladder following an ectopic and molar pregnancy

Laceration, perforation, tear or chemical damage of bowel following an ectopic and molar pregnancy

Laceration, perforation, tear or chemical damage of broad ligament following an ectopic and molar pregnancy

Laceration, perforation, tear or chemical damage of cervix following an ectopic and molar pregnancy

Laceration, perforation, tear or chemical damage of periurethral tissue following an ectopic and molar pregnancy

Laceration, perforation, tear or chemical damage of uterus following an ectopic and molar pregnancy

Laceration, perforation, tear or chemical damage of vagina following an ectopic and molar pregnancy

SP O08.7 Other venous complications following an ectopic and molar pregnancy

5 O08.8 Other complications following an ectopic and molar pregnancy

SP O08.81 Cardiac arrest following an ectopic and molar pregnancy

SP + O08.82 Sepsis following ectopic and molar pregnancy

Use additional code (B95-B97), to identify infectious agent

Use additional code (R65.2-) to identify severe sepsis, if applicable

EXCLUDES 1   septic or septicopyemic embolism following ectopic and molar pregnancy (O08.2)

SP O08.83 Urinary tract infection following an ectopic and molar pregnancy

Cystitis following an ectopic and molar pregnancy

SP O08.89 Other complications following an ectopic and molar pregnancy

SP O08.9 Unspecified complication following an ectopic and molar pregnancy

Supervision of high risk pregnancy   (O09)

4 O09 Supervision of high risk pregnancy

5 O09.0 Supervision of pregnancy with history of infertility

IQ O09.00 Supervision of pregnancy with history of infertility, unspecified trimester

SP O09.01 Supervision of pregnancy with history of infertility, first trimester

SP O09.02 Supervision of pregnancy with history of infertility, second trimester

SP O09.03 Supervision of pregnancy with history of infertility, third trimester

5 O09.1 Supervision of pregnancy with history of ectopic pregnancy

IQ O09.10 Supervision of pregnancy with history of ectopic pregnancy, unspecified trimester

SP O09.11 Supervision of pregnancy with history of ectopic pregnancy, first trimester

SP O09.12 Supervision of pregnancy with history of ectopic pregnancy, second trimester

Chapter 15

O00-O9A

★ New ▲ Revised Px Primary SP PDGM Px SL Low CoM SH High CoM IQ Quest. Encounter H Hospice non-cancer Dx   Unspecified   M Manifestation

DecisionHealth's FY 2020 Complete Home Health ICD-10-CM Diagnosis Coding Manual

1321

SP O09.13 Supervision of pregnancy with history of ectopic pregnancy, third trimester

⑤ O09.A Supervision of pregnancy with history of molar pregnancy

> **DEFINITION** An abnormal product of conception that occurs when the cells proliferate out of control, creating a growth or mass of cell clusters that causes the body to continue producing hormones as if in pregnancy, even though there is no fetus developing. This gives a false positive pregnancy result. Molar pregnancies have the potential of developing into a cancerous growth, called choriocarinoma if left untreated.

!Q O09.A0 Supervision of pregnancy with history of molar pregnancy, unspecified trimester

SP O09.A1 Supervision of pregnancy with history of molar pregnancy, first trimester

SP O09.A2 Supervision of pregnancy with history of molar pregnancy, second trimester

SP O09.A3 Supervision of pregnancy with history of molar pregnancy, third trimester

⑤ O09.2 Supervision of pregnancy with other poor reproductive or obstetric history

> **EXCLUDES 2** pregnancy care for patient with history of recurrent pregnancy loss (O26.2-)

⑥ O09.21 Supervision of pregnancy with history of pre-term labor

SP O09.211 Supervision of pregnancy with history of pre-term labor, first trimester

SP O09.212 Supervision of pregnancy with history of pre-term labor, second trimester

SP O09.213 Supervision of pregnancy with history of pre-term labor, third trimester

!Q O09.219 Supervision of pregnancy with history of pre-term labor, unspecified trimester

⑥ O09.29 Supervision of pregnancy with other poor reproductive or obstetric history

> Supervision of pregnancy with history of neonatal death
> Supervision of pregnancy with history of stillbirth

SP O09.291 Supervision of pregnancy with other poor reproductive or obstetric history, first trimester

SP O09.292 Supervision of pregnancy with other poor reproductive or obstetric history, second trimester

SP O09.293 Supervision of pregnancy with other poor reproductive or obstetric history, third trimester

!Q O09.299 Supervision of pregnancy with other poor reproductive or obstetric history, unspecified trimester

⑤ O09.3 Supervision of pregnancy with insufficient antenatal care

> Supervision of concealed pregnancy
> Supervision of hidden pregnancy

!Q O09.30 Supervision of pregnancy with insufficient antenatal care, unspecified trimester

SP O09.31 Supervision of pregnancy with insufficient antenatal care, first trimester

SP O09.32 Supervision of pregnancy with insufficient antenatal care, second trimester

SP O09.33 Supervision of pregnancy with insufficient antenatal care, third trimester

⑤ O09.4 Supervision of pregnancy with grand multiparity

!Q O09.40 Supervision of pregnancy with grand multiparity, unspecified trimester

SP O09.41 Supervision of pregnancy with grand multiparity, first trimester

SP O09.42 Supervision of pregnancy with grand multiparity, second trimester

SP O09.43 Supervision of pregnancy with grand multiparity, third trimester

⑤ O09.5 Supervision of elderly primigravida and multigravida

> Pregnancy for a female 35 years and older at expected date of delivery

⑥ O09.51 Supervision of elderly primigravida

SP O09.511 Supervision of elderly primigravida, first trimester

SP O09.512 Supervision of elderly primigravida, second trimester

SP O09.513 Supervision of elderly primigravida, third trimester

!Q O09.519 Supervision of elderly primigravida, unspecified trimester

⑥ O09.52 Supervision of elderly multigravida

SP O09.521 Supervision of elderly multigravida, first trimester

SP O09.522 Supervision of elderly multigravida, second trimester

SP O09.523 Supervision of elderly multigravida, third trimester

!Q O09.529 Supervision of elderly multigravida, unspecified trimester

⑤ O09.6 Supervision of young primigravida and multigravida

> Supervision of pregnancy for a female less than 16 years old at expected date of delivery

⑥ O09.61 Supervision of young primigravida

SP O09.611 Supervision of young primigravida, first trimester

SP O09.612 Supervision of young primigravida, second trimester

SP O09.613 Supervision of young primigravida, third trimester

!Q O09.619 Supervision of young primigravida, unspecified trimester

⑥ O09.62 Supervision of young multigravida

⬛4 4th digit required   ⬛5 5th digit required   ⬛6 6th digit required   ⬛7 7th digit required   ⬛x 7th digit placeholder   ✚ Additional code   ⬛ Laterality

SP O09.621 Supervision of young multigravida, first trimester

SP O09.622 Supervision of young multigravida, second trimester

SP O09.623 Supervision of young multigravida, third trimester

IQ O09.629 Supervision of young multigravida, unspecified trimester

5 O09.7 Supervision of high risk pregnancy due to social problems

IQ O09.70 Supervision of high risk pregnancy due to social problems, unspecified trimester

IQ O09.71 Supervision of high risk pregnancy due to social problems, first trimester

IQ O09.72 Supervision of high risk pregnancy due to social problems, second trimester

IQ O09.73 Supervision of high risk pregnancy due to social problems, third trimester

5 O09.8 Supervision of other high risk pregnancies

6 O09.81 Supervision of pregnancy resulting from assisted reproductive technology
　　Supervision of pregnancy resulting from in-vitro fertilization
　　EXCLUDES 2 gestational carrier status (Z33.3)

SP O09.811 Supervision of pregnancy resulting from assisted reproductive technology, first trimester

SP O09.812 Supervision of pregnancy resulting from assisted reproductive technology, second trimester

SP O09.813 Supervision of pregnancy resulting from assisted reproductive technology, third trimester

IQ O09.819 Supervision of pregnancy resulting from assisted reproductive technology, unspecified trimester

6 O09.82 Supervision of pregnancy with history of in utero procedure during previous pregnancy

SP O09.821 Supervision of pregnancy with history of in utero procedure during previous pregnancy, first trimester

SP O09.822 Supervision of pregnancy with history of in utero procedure during previous pregnancy, second trimester

SP O09.823 Supervision of pregnancy with history of in utero procedure during previous pregnancy, third trimester

IQ O09.829 Supervision of pregnancy with history of in utero procedure during previous pregnancy, unspecified trimester

EXCLUDES 1 supervision of pregnancy affected by in utero procedure during current pregnancy (O35.7)

6 O09.89 Supervision of other high risk pregnancies

SP O09.891 Supervision of other high risk pregnancies, first trimester

SP O09.892 Supervision of other high risk pregnancies, second trimester

SP O09.893 Supervision of other high risk pregnancies, third trimester

IQ O09.899 Supervision of other high risk pregnancies, unspecified trimester

5 O09.9 Supervision of high risk pregnancy, unspecified

IQ O09.90 Supervision of high risk pregnancy, unspecified, unspecified trimester

SP O09.91 Supervision of high risk pregnancy, unspecified, first trimester

SP O09.92 Supervision of high risk pregnancy, unspecified, second trimester

SP O09.93 Supervision of high risk pregnancy, unspecified, third trimester

Edema, proteinuria and hypertensive disorders in pregnancy, childbirth and the puerperium (O10-O16)

4 O10 Pre-existing hypertension complicating pregnancy, childbirth and the puerperium
　　INCLUDES pre-existing hypertension with pre-existing proteinuria complicating pregnancy, childbirth and the puerperium
　　EXCLUDES 2 pre-existing hypertension with superimposed pre-eclampsia complicating pregnancy, childbirth and the puerperium (O11.-)
　　GUIDELINES Section I.C.15.d
　　Category O10 includes codes for hypertensive heart and hypertensive chronic kidney disease. When assigning one of the O10 codes that includes hypertensive heart disease or hypertensive chronic kidney disease, it is necessary to add a secondary code from the appropriate hypertension category to specify the type of heart failure or chronic kidney disease.

5 O10.0 Pre-existing essential hypertension complicating pregnancy, childbirth and the puerperium
　　Any condition in I10 specified as a reason for obstetric care during pregnancy, childbirth or the puerperium

6 O10.01 Pre-existing essential hypertension complicating pregnancy,

SP O10.011 Pre-existing essential hypertension complicating pregnancy, first trimester

SP O10.012 Pre-existing essential hypertension complicating pregnancy, second trimester

★ New ▲ Revised **Px** Primary **SP** PDGM Px **SL** Low CoM **SH** High CoM **IQ** Quest. Encounter **H** Hospice non-cancer Dx **Unspecified** **M** *Manifestation*

DecisionHealth's FY 2020 Complete Home Health ICD-10-CM Diagnosis Coding Manual

1323

SP O10.013 Pre-existing essential hypertension complicating pregnancy, third trimester

IQ O10.019 Pre-existing essential hypertension complicating pregnancy, unspecified trimester

SP O10.02 Pre-existing essential hypertension complicating childbirth

SP O10.03 Pre-existing essential hypertension complicating the puerperium

+ 5 O10.1 Pre-existing hypertensive heart disease complicating pregnancy, childbirth and the puerperium

Any condition in I11 specified as a reason for obstetric care during pregnancy, childbirth or the puerperium

Use additional code from I11 to identify the type of hypertensive heart disease

+ 6 O10.11 Pre-existing hypertensive heart disease complicating pregnancy

SP + O10.111 Pre-existing hypertensive heart disease complicating pregnancy, first trimester

SP + O10.112 Pre-existing hypertensive heart disease complicating pregnancy, second trimester

SP + O10.113 Pre-existing hypertensive heart disease complicating pregnancy, third trimester

IQ + O10.119 Pre-existing hypertensive heart disease complicating pregnancy, unspecified trimester

SP + O10.12 Pre-existing hypertensive heart disease complicating childbirth

SP + O10.13 Pre-existing hypertensive heart disease complicating the puerperium

+ 5 O10.2 Pre-existing hypertensive chronic kidney disease complicating pregnancy, childbirth and the puerperium

Any condition in I12 specified as a reason for obstetric care during pregnancy, childbirth or the puerperium

Use additional code from I12 to identify the type of hypertensive chronic kidney disease

+ 6 O10.21 Pre-existing hypertensive chronic kidney disease complicating pregnancy

SP + O10.211 Pre-existing hypertensive chronic kidney disease complicating pregnancy, first trimester

SP + O10.212 Pre-existing hypertensive chronic kidney disease complicating pregnancy, second trimester

SP + O10.213 Pre-existing hypertensive chronic kidney disease complicating pregnancy, third trimester

IQ + O10.219 Pre-existing hypertensive chronic kidney disease complicating pregnancy, unspecified trimester

SP + O10.22 Pre-existing hypertensive chronic kidney disease complicating childbirth

SP + O10.23 Pre-existing hypertensive chronic kidney disease complicating the puerperium

+ 5 O10.3 Pre-existing hypertensive heart and chronic kidney disease complicating pregnancy, childbirth and the puerperium

Any condition in I13 specified as a reason for obstetric care during pregnancy, childbirth or the puerperium

Use additional code from I13 to identify the type of hypertensive heart and chronic kidney disease

+ 6 O10.31 Pre-existing hypertensive heart and chronic kidney disease complicating pregnancy

SP + O10.311 Pre-existing hypertensive heart and chronic kidney disease complicating pregnancy, first trimester

SP + O10.312 Pre-existing hypertensive heart and chronic kidney disease complicating pregnancy, second trimester

SP + O10.313 Pre-existing hypertensive heart and chronic kidney disease complicating pregnancy, third trimester

IQ + O10.319 Pre-existing hypertensive heart and chronic kidney disease complicating pregnancy, unspecified trimester

SP + O10.32 Pre-existing hypertensive heart and chronic kidney disease complicating childbirth

SP + O10.33 Pre-existing hypertensive heart and chronic kidney disease complicating the puerperium

+ 5 O10.4 Pre-existing secondary hypertension complicating pregnancy, childbirth and the puerperium

Any condition in I15 specified as a reason for obstetric care during pregnancy, childbirth or the puerperium

Use additional code from I15 to identify the type of secondary hypertension

+ 6 O10.41 Pre-existing secondary hypertension complicating pregnancy

SP + O10.411 Pre-existing secondary hypertension complicating pregnancy, first trimester

SP + O10.412 Pre-existing secondary hypertension complicating pregnancy, second trimester

SP + O10.413 Pre-existing secondary hypertension complicating pregnancy, third trimester

IQ + O10.419 Pre-existing secondary hypertension complicating pregnancy, unspecified trimester

SP + O10.42 Pre-existing secondary hypertension complicating childbirth

SP + O10.43 Pre-existing secondary hypertension complicating the puerperium

5 O10.9 Unspecified pre-existing hypertension complicating pregnancy, childbirth and the puerperium

6 O10.91 Unspecified pre-existing hypertension complicating pregnancy

☐4 4th digit required   ☐5 5th digit required   ☐6 6th digit required   ☐7 7th digit required   ☑ 7th digit placeholder   **+**Additional code   ⊟ Laterality

1324   *DecisionHealth's* FY 2020 Complete Home Health ICD-10-CM Diagnosis Coding Manual

SP O10.911 Unspecified pre-existing hypertension complicating pregnancy, first trimester

SP O10.912 Unspecified pre-existing hypertension complicating pregnancy, second trimester

SP O10.913 Unspecified pre-existing hypertension complicating pregnancy, third trimester

IQ O10.919 Unspecified pre-existing hypertension complicating pregnancy, unspecified trimester

SP O10.92 Unspecified pre-existing hypertension complicating childbirth

SP O10.93 Unspecified pre-existing hypertension complicating the puerperium

+ ◢ O11 Pre-existing hypertension with pre-eclampsia

INCLUDES conditions in Ol0 complicated by pre-eclampsia
pre-eclampsia superimposed pre-existing hypertension

Use additional code from O10 to identify the type of hypertension

SP + O11.1 Pre-existing hypertension with pre-eclampsia, first trimester

SP + O11.2 Pre-existing hypertension with pre-eclampsia, second trimester

SP + O11.3 Pre-existing hypertension with pre-eclampsia, third trimester

SP + O11.4 Pre-existing hypertension with pre-eclampsia, complicating childbirth

SP + O11.5 Pre-existing hypertension with pre-eclampsia, complicating the puerperium

IQ + O11.9 Pre-existing hypertension with pre-eclampsia, unspecified trimester

◢ O12 Gestational [pregnancy-induced] edema and proteinuria without hypertension

⑤ O12.0 Gestational edema

IQ O12.00 Gestational edema, unspecified trimester

SP O12.01 Gestational edema, first trimester

SP O12.02 Gestational edema, second trimester

SP O12.03 Gestational edema, third trimester

SP O12.04 Gestational edema, complicating childbirth

SP O12.05 Gestational edema, complicating the puerperium

⑤ O12.1 Gestational proteinuria

IQ O12.10 Gestational proteinuria, unspecified trimester

SP O12.11 Gestational proteinuria, first trimester

SP O12.12 Gestational proteinuria, second trimester

SP O12.13 Gestational proteinuria, third trimester

SP O12.14 Gestational proteinuria, complicating childbirth

SP O12.15 Gestational proteinuria, complicating the puerperium

⑤ O12.2 Gestational edema with proteinuria

IQ O12.20 Gestational edema with proteinuria, unspecified trimester

SP O12.21 Gestational edema with proteinuria, first trimester

SP O12.22 Gestational edema with proteinuria, second trimester

SP O12.23 Gestational edema with proteinuria, third trimester

SP O12.24 Gestational edema with proteinuria, complicating childbirth

SP O12.25 Gestational edema with proteinuria, complicating the puerperium

◢ O13 Gestational [pregnancy-induced] hypertension without significant proteinuria

INCLUDES gestational hypertension NOS
transient hypertension of pregnancy

GUIDELINES Section I.9.a.7)
Unless patient has an established diagnosis of hypertension, assign code O13.-, Gestational [pregnancy-induced] hypertension without significant proteinuria, or O14.-, Pre-eclampsia, for transient hypertension of pregnancy.

SP O13.1 Gestational [pregnancy-induced] hypertension without significant proteinuria, first trimester

SP O13.2 Gestational [pregnancy-induced] hypertension without significant proteinuria, second trimester

SP O13.3 Gestational [pregnancy-induced] hypertension without significant proteinuria, third trimester

SP O13.4 Gestational [pregnancy-induced] hypertension without significant proteinuria, complicating childbirth

SP O13.5 Gestational [pregnancy-induced] hypertension without significant proteinuria, complicating the puerperium

IQ O13.9 Gestational [pregnancy-induced] hypertension without significant proteinuria, unspecified trimester

◢ O14 Pre-eclampsia

EXCLUDES 1 pre-existing hypertension with pre-eclampsia (O11)

GUIDELINES Section I.9.a.7)
Unless patient has an established diagnosis of hypertension, assign code O13.-, Gestational [pregnancy-induced] hypertension without significant proteinuria, or O14.-, Pre-eclampsia, for transient hypertension of pregnancy.

⑤ O14.0 Mild to moderate pre-eclampsia

DEFINITION Hypertension (BP >140/90 mmHg) after the 20th week of gestation and up to 6 weeks postpartum, with proteinuria.

IQ O14.00 Mild to moderate pre-eclampsia, unspecified trimester

SP O14.02 Mild to moderate pre-eclampsia, second trimester

SP O14.03 Mild to moderate pre-eclampsia, third trimester

SP O14.04 Mild to moderate pre-eclampsia, complicating childbirth

SP O14.05 Mild to moderate pre-eclampsia, complicating the puerperium

⑤ O14.1 Severe pre-eclampsia

Chapter 15

O00-O9A

★ New ▲ Revised Px Primary SP PDGM Px SL Low CoM SH High CoM IQ Quest. Encounter H Hospice non-cancer Dx Unspecified M Manifestation

DecisionHealth's FY 2020 Complete Home Health ICD-10-CM Diagnosis Coding Manual

1325

EXCLUDES 1 HELLP syndrome (O14.2-)

DEFINITION Severe hypertension (BP >160/110 mmHg) after the 20th week of gestation and up to 6 weeks postpartum, with proteinuria, and additional symptoms such as pulmonary edema, upper abdominal pain, severe headaches, and blurred vision.

SP **O14.10** Severe pre-eclampsia, unspecified trimester

SP **O14.12** Severe pre-eclampsia, second trimester

SP **O14.13** Severe pre-eclampsia, third trimester

SP **O14.14** Severe pre-eclampsia complicating childbirth

SP **O14.15** Severe pre-eclampsia, complicating the puerperium

5 **O14.2** HELLP syndrome
Severe pre-eclampsia with hemolysis, elevated liver enzymes and low platelet count (HELLP)

DEFINITION Severe pre-eclampsia with hemolysis, elevated liver enzymes and low platelet count (HELLP).

IQ **O14.20** HELLP syndrome (HELLP), unspecified trimester

SP **O14.22** HELLP syndrome (HELLP), second trimester

SP **O14.23** HELLP syndrome (HELLP), third trimester

SP **O14.24** HELLP syndrome, complicating childbirth

SP **O14.25** HELLP syndrome, complicating the puerperium

5 **O14.9** Unspecified pre-eclampsia

IQ **O14.90** Unspecified pre-eclampsia, unspecified trimester

SP **O14.92** Unspecified pre-eclampsia, second trimester

SP **O14.93** Unspecified pre-eclampsia, third trimester

SP **O14.94** Unspecified pre-eclampsia, complicating childbirth

SP **O14.95** Unspecified pre-eclampsia, complicating the puerperium

4 **O15** Eclampsia
INCLUDES convulsions following conditions in O10-O14 and O16

5 **O15.0** Eclampsia complicating pregnancy

SP **O15.00** Eclampsia complicating pregnancy, unspecified trimester

SP **O15.02** Eclampsia complicating pregnancy, second trimester

SP **O15.03** Eclampsia complicating pregnancy, third trimester

SP **O15.1** Eclampsia complicating labor

SP **O15.2** Eclampsia complicating the puerperium

IQ **O15.9** Eclampsia, unspecified as to time period
Eclampsia NOS

4 **O16** Unspecified maternal hypertension

SP **O16.1** Unspecified maternal hypertension, first trimester

SP **O16.2** Unspecified maternal hypertension, second trimester

SP **O16.3** Unspecified maternal hypertension, third trimester

SP **O16.4** Unspecified maternal hypertension, complicating childbirth

SP **O16.5** Unspecified maternal hypertension, complicating the puerperium

IQ **O16.9** Unspecified maternal hypertension, unspecified trimester

Other maternal disorders predominantly related to pregnancy (O20-O29)

EXCLUDES 2 maternal care related to the fetus and amniotic cavity and possible delivery problems (O30-O48)
maternal diseases classifiable elsewhere but complicating pregnancy, labor and delivery, and the puerperium (O98-O99)

4 **O20** Hemorrhage in early pregnancy
INCLUDES hemorrhage before completion of 20 weeks gestation
EXCLUDES 1 pregnancy with abortive outcome (O00-O08)

SP **O20.0** Threatened abortion
Hemorrhage specified as due to threatened abortion

SP **O20.8** Other hemorrhage in early pregnancy

SP **O20.9** Hemorrhage in early pregnancy, unspecified

4 **O21** Excessive vomiting in pregnancy

SP **O21.0** Mild hyperemesis gravidarum
Hyperemesis gravidarum, mild or unspecified, starting before the end of the 20th week of gestation

SP **O21.1** Hyperemesis gravidarum with metabolic disturbance
Hyperemesis gravidarum, starting before the end of the 20th week of gestation, with metabolic disturbance such as carbohydrate depletion
Hyperemesis gravidarum, starting before the end of the 20th week of gestation, with metabolic disturbance such as dehydration
Hyperemesis gravidarum, starting before the end of the 20th week of gestation, with metabolic disturbance such as electrolyte imbalance

SP **O21.2** Late vomiting of pregnancy
Excessive vomiting starting after 20 completed weeks of gestation

SP ✚ **O21.8** Other vomiting complicating pregnancy
Vomiting due to diseases classified elsewhere, complicating pregnancy
Use additional code, to identify cause.

SP **O21.9** Vomiting of pregnancy, unspecified

4 **O22** Venous complications and hemorrhoids in pregnancy
EXCLUDES 1 venous complications of:
abortion NOS (O03.9)
ectopic or molar pregnancy (O08.7)
failed attempted abortion (O07.35)
induced abortion (O04.85)

4 4th digit required   **5** 5th digit required   **6** 6th digit required   **7** 7th digit required   **7** 7th digit placeholder   **✚** Additional code   **⊟** Laterality

1326   DecisionHealth's FY 2020 Complete Home Health ICD-10-CM Diagnosis Coding Manual

Chapter 15

O00-O9A

spontaneous abortion (O03.89)

EXCLUDES 2 obstetric pulmonary embolism (O88.-)

venous complications and hemorrhoids of childbirth and the puerperium (O87.-)

⑤ O22.0 Varicose veins of lower extremity in pregnancy
Varicose veins NOS in pregnancy

IQ O22.00 Varicose veins of lower extremity in pregnancy, unspecified trimester

SP O22.01 Varicose veins of lower extremity in pregnancy, first trimester

SP O22.02 Varicose veins of lower extremity in pregnancy, second trimester

SP O22.03 Varicose veins of lower extremity in pregnancy, third trimester

⑤ O22.1 Genital varices in pregnancy
Perineal varices in pregnancy
Vaginal varices in pregnancy
Vulval varices in pregnancy

IQ O22.10 Genital varices in pregnancy, unspecified trimester

SP O22.11 Genital varices in pregnancy, first trimester

SP O22.12 Genital varices in pregnancy, second trimester

SP O22.13 Genital varices in pregnancy, third trimester

✛ ⑤ O22.2 Superficial thrombophlebitis in pregnancy
Phlebitis in pregnancy NOS
Thrombophlebitis of legs in pregnancy
Thrombosis in pregnancy NOS
Use additional code to identify the superficial thrombophlebitis (I80.0-)

IQ ✛ O22.20 Superficial thrombophlebitis in pregnancy, unspecified trimester

SP ✛ O22.21 Superficial thrombophlebitis in pregnancy, first trimester

SP ✛ O22.22 Superficial thrombophlebitis in pregnancy, second trimester

SP ✛ O22.23 Superficial thrombophlebitis in pregnancy, third trimester

✛ ⑤ O22.3 Deep phlebothrombosis in pregnancy
Deep vein thrombosis, antepartum
Use additional code to identify the deep vein thrombosis (I82.4-, I82.5-, I82.62-, I82.72-)
Use additional code, if applicable, for associated long-term (current) use of anticoagulants (Z79.01)

IQ ✛ O22.30 Deep phlebothrombosis in pregnancy, unspecified trimester

SP ✛ O22.31 Deep phlebothrombosis in pregnancy, first trimester

SP ✛ O22.32 Deep phlebothrombosis in pregnancy, second trimester

SP ✛ O22.33 Deep phlebothrombosis in pregnancy, third trimester

⑤ O22.4 Hemorrhoids in pregnancy

IQ O22.40 Hemorrhoids in pregnancy, unspecified trimester

SP O22.41 Hemorrhoids in pregnancy, first trimester

SP O22.42 Hemorrhoids in pregnancy, second trimester

SP O22.43 Hemorrhoids in pregnancy, third trimester

⑤ O22.5 Cerebral venous thrombosis in pregnancy
Cerebrovenous sinus thrombosis in pregnancy

IQ O22.50 Cerebral venous thrombosis in pregnancy, unspecified trimester

SP O22.51 Cerebral venous thrombosis in pregnancy, first trimester

SP O22.52 Cerebral venous thrombosis in pregnancy, second trimester

SP O22.53 Cerebral venous thrombosis in pregnancy, third trimester

⑤ O22.8 Other venous complications in pregnancy

⑥ O22.8X Other venous complications in pregnancy

SP O22.8X1 Other venous complications in pregnancy, first trimester

SP O22.8X2 Other venous complications in pregnancy, second trimester

SP O22.8X3 Other venous complications in pregnancy, third trimester

IQ O22.8X9 Other venous complications in pregnancy, unspecified trimester

⑤ O22.9 Venous complication in pregnancy, unspecified
Gestational phlebitis NOS
Gestational phlebopathy NOS
Gestational thrombosis NOS

IQ O22.90 Venous complication in pregnancy, unspecified, unspecified trimester

SP O22.91 Venous complication in pregnancy, unspecified, first trimester

SP O22.92 Venous complication in pregnancy, unspecified, second trimester

SP O22.93 Venous complication in pregnancy, unspecified, third trimester

✛ ④ O23 Infections of genitourinary tract in pregnancy
Use additional code to identify organism (B95.-, B96.-)

EXCLUDES 2 gonococcal infections complicating pregnancy, childbirth and the puerperium (O98.2)

infections with a predominantly sexual mode of transmission NOS complicating pregnancy, childbirth and the puerperium (O98.3)

syphilis complicating pregnancy, childbirth and the puerperium (O98.1)

tuberculosis of genitourinary system complicating pregnancy, childbirth and the puerperium (O98.0)

venereal disease NOS complicating pregnancy, childbirth and the puerperium (O98.3)

✛ ⑤ O23.0 Infections of kidney in pregnancy
Pyelonephritis in pregnancy

IQ ✛ O23.00 Infections of kidney in pregnancy, unspecified trimester

★ New ▲ Revised **Px** Primary **SP** PDGM Px **SL** Low CoM **SH** High CoM **IQ** Quest. Encounter **H** Hospice non-cancer Dx Unspecified **M** *Manifestation*

DecisionHealth's FY 2020 Complete Home Health ICD-10-CM Diagnosis Coding Manual

1327

SP + O23.01 Infections of kidney in pregnancy, first trimester

SP + O23.02 Infections of kidney in pregnancy, second trimester

SP + O23.03 Infections of kidney in pregnancy, third trimester

+ 5 O23.1 Infections of bladder in pregnancy

IQ + O23.10 Infections of bladder in pregnancy, unspecified trimester

SP + O23.11 Infections of bladder in pregnancy, first trimester

SP + O23.12 Infections of bladder in pregnancy, second trimester

SP + O23.13 Infections of bladder in pregnancy, third trimester

+ 5 O23.2 Infections of urethra in pregnancy

IQ + O23.20 Infections of urethra in pregnancy, unspecified trimester

SP + O23.21 Infections of urethra in pregnancy, first trimester

SP + O23.22 Infections of urethra in pregnancy, second trimester

SP + O23.23 Infections of urethra in pregnancy, third trimester

+ 5 O23.3 Infections of other parts of urinary tract in pregnancy

IQ + O23.30 Infections of other parts of urinary tract in pregnancy, unspecified trimester

SP + O23.31 Infections of other parts of urinary tract in pregnancy, first trimester

SP + O23.32 Infections of other parts of urinary tract in pregnancy, second trimester

SP + O23.33 Infections of other parts of urinary tract in pregnancy, third trimester

+ 5 O23.4 Unspecified infection of urinary tract in pregnancy

IQ + O23.40 Unspecified infection of urinary tract in pregnancy, unspecified trimester

SP + O23.41 Unspecified infection of urinary tract in pregnancy, first trimester

SP + O23.42 Unspecified infection of urinary tract in pregnancy, second trimester

SP + O23.43 Unspecified infection of urinary tract in pregnancy, third trimester

+ 5 O23.5 Infections of the genital tract in pregnancy

+ 6 O23.51 Infection of cervix in pregnancy

SP + O23.511 Infections of cervix in pregnancy, first trimester

SP + O23.512 Infections of cervix in pregnancy, second trimester

SP + O23.513 Infections of cervix in pregnancy, third trimester

IQ + O23.519 Infections of cervix in pregnancy, unspecified trimester

· + 6 O23.52 Salpingo-oophoritis in pregnancy
Oophoritis in pregnancy
Salpingitis in pregnancy

SP + O23.521 Salpingo-oophoritis in pregnancy, first trimester

SP + O23.522 Salpingo-oophoritis in pregnancy, second trimester

SP + O23.523 Salpingo-oophoritis in pregnancy, third trimester

IQ + O23.529 Salpingo-oophoritis in pregnancy, unspecified trimester

+ 6 O23.59 Infection of other part of genital tract in pregnancy

SP + O23.591 Infection of other part of genital tract in pregnancy, first trimester

SP + O23.592 Infection of other part of genital tract in pregnancy, second trimester

SP + O23.593 Infection of other part of genital tract in pregnancy, third trimester

IQ + O23.599 Infection of other part of genital tract in pregnancy, unspecified trimester

+ 5 O23.9 Unspecified genitourinary tract infection in pregnancy
Genitourinary tract infection in pregnancy NOS

IQ + O23.90 Unspecified genitourinary tract infection in pregnancy, unspecified trimester

SP + O23.91 Unspecified genitourinary tract infection in pregnancy, first trimester

SP + O23.92 Unspecified genitourinary tract infection in pregnancy, second trimester

SP + O23.93 Unspecified genitourinary tract infection in pregnancy, third trimester

4 O24 Diabetes mellitus in pregnancy, childbirth, and the puerperium

GUIDELINES Section I.C.15.g-h

Diabetes mellitus is a significant complicating factor in pregnancy. Pregnant women who are diabetic should be assigned a code from category O24, Diabetes mellitus in pregnancy, childbirth, and the puerperium, first, followed by the appropriate diabetes code(s) (E08-E13) from Chapter 4.

An additional code should be assigned from category Z79 to identify the long-term (current) use of insulin or oral hypoglycemic drugs. If the patient is treated with both oral medications and insulin, only the code for long-term (current) use of insulin should be assigned. Code Z79.4 should not be assigned if insulin is given temporarily to bring a type 2 patient's blood sugar under control during an encounter.

+ 5 O24.0 Pre-existing type 1 diabetes mellitus, in pregnancy, childbirth and the puerperium
Juvenile onset diabetes mellitus, in pregnancy, childbirth and the puerperium
Ketosis-prone diabetes mellitus in pregnancy, childbirth and the puerperium
Use additional code from category E10 to further identify any manifestations

+ 6 O24.01 Pre-existing type 1 diabetes mellitus, in pregnancy

SP + O24.011 Pre-existing type 1 diabetes mellitus, in pregnancy, first trimester

SP + O24.012 Pre-existing type 1 diabetes mellitus, in pregnancy, second trimester

---

4 4th digit required   5 5th digit required   6 6th digit required   7 7th digit required   7 7th digit placeholder   + Additional code   ⊟ Laterality

Chapter 15

O00-O9A

SP ✚ **O24.013 Pre-existing type 1 diabetes mellitus, in pregnancy, third trimester**

IQ ✚ **O24.019 Pre-existing type 1 diabetes mellitus, in pregnancy, unspecified trimester**

SP ✚ **O24.02 Pre-existing type 1 diabetes mellitus, in childbirth**

SP ✚ **O24.03 Pre-existing type 1 diabetes mellitus, in the puerperium**

✚ **5 O24.1 Pre-existing type 2 diabetes mellitus, in pregnancy, childbirth and the puerperium**

Insulin-resistant diabetes mellitus in pregnancy, childbirth and the puerperium

Use additional code (for):
from category E11 to further identify any manifestations
long-term (current) use of insulin (Z79.4)

✚ **6 O24.11 Pre-existing type 2 diabetes mellitus, in pregnancy**

SP ✚ **O24.111 Pre-existing type 2 diabetes mellitus, in pregnancy, first trimester**

SP ✚ **O24.112 Pre-existing type 2 diabetes mellitus, in pregnancy, second trimester**

SP ✚ **O24.113 Pre-existing type 2 diabetes mellitus, in pregnancy, third trimester**

IQ ✚ **O24.119 Pre-existing type 2 diabetes mellitus, in pregnancy, unspecified trimester**

SP ✚ **O24.12 Pre-existing type 2 diabetes mellitus, in childbirth**

SP ✚ **O24.13 Pre-existing type 2 diabetes mellitus, in the puerperium**

✚ **5 O24.3 Unspecified pre-existing diabetes mellitus in pregnancy, childbirth and the puerperium**

Use additional code (for):
from category E11 to further identify any manifestation
long-term (current) use of insulin (Z79.4)

✚ **6 O24.31 Unspecified pre-existing diabetes mellitus in pregnancy**

SP ✚ **O24.311 Unspecified pre-existing diabetes mellitus in pregnancy, first trimester**

SP ✚ **O24.312 Unspecified pre-existing diabetes mellitus in pregnancy, second trimester**

SP ✚ **O24.313 Unspecified pre-existing diabetes mellitus in pregnancy, third trimester**

IQ ✚ **O24.319 Unspecified pre-existing diabetes mellitus in pregnancy, unspecified trimester**

SP ✚ **O24.32 Unspecified pre-existing diabetes mellitus in childbirth**

SP ✚ **O24.33 Unspecified pre-existing diabetes mellitus in the puerperium**

5 O24.4 Gestational diabetes mellitus
Diabetes mellitus arising in pregnancy
Gestational diabetes mellitus NOS

GUIDELINES Section I.C.15.i

Gestational (pregnancy induced) diabetes can occur during the second and third trimester of pregnancy in women who were not diabetic prior to pregnancy. Gestational diabetes can cause complications in the pregnancy similar to those of pre-existing diabetes mellitus. It also puts the woman at greater risk of developing diabetes after the pregnancy. Codes for gestational diabetes are in subcategory O24.4, Gestational diabetes mellitus. No other code from category O24, Diabetes mellitus in pregnancy, childbirth, and the puerperium, should be used with a code from O24.4. The codes under subcategory O24.4 include diet controlled, insulin controlled, and controlled by oral hypoglycemic drugs. If a patient with gestational diabetes is treated with both diet and insulin, only the code for insulin-controlled is required. If a patient with gestational diabetes is treated with both diet and oral hypoglycemic medications, only the code for "controlled by oral hypoglycemic drugs" is required. An abnormal glucose tolerance in pregnancy is assigned a code from subcategory O99.81, Abnormal glucose complicating pregnancy, childbirth, and the puerperium.

CODING TIPS ✓ Do not use O24.4 if diabetes persists after pregnancy. Use E08 -E13 code.

6 O24.41 Gestational diabetes mellitus in pregnancy

SP O24.410 Gestational diabetes mellitus in pregnancy, diet controlled

SP O24.414 Gestational diabetes mellitus in pregnancy, insulin controlled

SP O24.415 Gestational diabetes mellitus in pregnancy, controlled by oral hypoglycemic drugs
Gestational diabetes mellitus in pregnancy, controlled by oral antidiabetic drugs

SP O24.419 Gestational diabetes mellitus in pregnancy, unspecified control

6 O24.42 Gestational diabetes mellitus in childbirth

SP O24.420 Gestational diabetes mellitus in childbirth, diet controlled

SP O24.424 Gestational diabetes mellitus in childbirth, insulin controlled

SP O24.425 Gestational diabetes mellitus in childbirth, controlled by oral hypoglycemic drugs
Gestational diabetes mellitus in childbirth, controlled by oral antidiabetic drugs

SP O24.429 Gestational diabetes mellitus in childbirth, unspecified control

6 O24.43 Gestational diabetes mellitus in the puerperium

SP O24.430 Gestational diabetes mellitus in the puerperium, diet controlled

SP O24.434 Gestational diabetes mellitus in the puerperium, insulin controlled

Chapter 15

O00-O9A

★ New ▲ Revised Px Primary **SP** PDGM Px **SL** Low CoM **SH** High CoM **IQ** Quest. Encounter **H** Hospice non-cancer Dx Unspecified **M** *Manifestation*

DecisionHealth's FY 2020 Complete Home Health ICD-10-CM Diagnosis Coding Manual

1329

Chapter 15

O00-O9A

SP O24.435 Gestational diabetes mellitus in puerperium, controlled by oral hypoglycemic drugs
Gestational diabetes mellitus in puerperium, controlled by oral antidiabetic drugs

SP O24.439 Gestational diabetes mellitus in the puerperium, unspecified control

+ 5 O24.8 Other pre-existing diabetes mellitus in pregnancy, childbirth, and the puerperium
Use additional code (for):
from categories E08, E09 and E13 to further identify any manifestation
long-term (current) use of insulin (Z79.4)

CODING TIPS ✓ Use this code for the obstetric patient who had pre-existing diabetes before pregnancy. Use an additional code for the type of diabetes, E08-E13.

+ 6 O24.81 Other pre-existing diabetes mellitus in pregnancy

SP + O24.811 Other pre-existing diabetes mellitus in pregnancy, first trimester

SP + O24.812 Other pre-existing diabetes mellitus in pregnancy, second trimester

SP + O24.813 Other pre-existing diabetes mellitus in pregnancy, third trimester

!Q + O24.819 Other pre-existing diabetes mellitus in pregnancy, unspecified trimester

SP + O24.82 Other pre-existing diabetes mellitus in childbirth

SP + O24.83 Other pre-existing diabetes mellitus in the puerperium

+ 5 O24.9 Unspecified diabetes mellitus in pregnancy, childbirth and the puerperium
Use additional code for long-term (current) use of insulin (Z79.4)

+ 6 O24.91 Unspecified diabetes mellitus in pregnancy

SP + O24.911 Unspecified diabetes mellitus in pregnancy, first trimester

SP + O24.912 Unspecified diabetes mellitus in pregnancy, second trimester

SP + O24.913 Unspecified diabetes mellitus in pregnancy, third trimester

!Q + O24.919 Unspecified diabetes mellitus in pregnancy, unspecified trimester

SP + O24.92 Unspecified diabetes mellitus in childbirth

SP + O24.93 Unspecified diabetes mellitus in the puerperium

4 O25 Malnutrition in pregnancy, childbirth and the puerperium

5 O25.1 Malnutrition in pregnancy

!Q O25.10 Malnutrition in pregnancy, unspecified trimester

SP O25.11 Malnutrition in pregnancy, first trimester

SP O25.12 Malnutrition in pregnancy, second trimester

SP O25.13 Malnutrition in pregnancy, third trimester

SP O25.2 Malnutrition in childbirth

SP O25.3 Malnutrition in the puerperium

4 O26 Maternal care for other conditions predominantly related to pregnancy

5 O26.0 Excessive weight gain in pregnancy
EXCLUDES 2 gestational edema (O12.0, O12.2)

!Q O26.00 Excessive weight gain in pregnancy, unspecified trimester

SP O26.01 Excessive weight gain in pregnancy, first trimester

SP O26.02 Excessive weight gain in pregnancy, second trimester

SP O26.03 Excessive weight gain in pregnancy, third trimester

5 O26.1 Low weight gain in pregnancy

!Q O26.10 Low weight gain in pregnancy, unspecified trimester

SP O26.11 Low weight gain in pregnancy, first trimester

SP O26.12 Low weight gain in pregnancy, second trimester

SP O26.13 Low weight gain in pregnancy, third trimester

5 O26.2 Pregnancy care for patient with recurrent pregnancy loss

!Q O26.20 Pregnancy care for patient with recurrent pregnancy loss, unspecified trimester

SP O26.21 Pregnancy care for patient with recurrent pregnancy loss, first trimester

SP O26.22 Pregnancy care for patient with recurrent pregnancy loss, second trimester

SP O26.23 Pregnancy care for patient with recurrent pregnancy loss, third trimester

5 O26.3 Retained intrauterine contraceptive device in pregnancy

!Q O26.30 Retained intrauterine contraceptive device in pregnancy, unspecified trimester

SP O26.31 Retained intrauterine contraceptive device in pregnancy, first trimester

SP O26.32 Retained intrauterine contraceptive device in pregnancy, second trimester

SP O26.33 Retained intrauterine contraceptive device in pregnancy, third trimester

5 O26.4 Herpes gestationis

!Q O26.40 Herpes gestationis, unspecified trimester

SP O26.41 Herpes gestationis, first trimester

SP O26.42 Herpes gestationis, second trimester

SP O26.43 Herpes gestationis, third trimester

5 O26.5 Maternal hypotension syndrome
Supine hypotensive syndrome

!Q O26.50 Maternal hypotension syndrome, unspecified trimester

SP O26.51 Maternal hypotension syndrome, first trimester

---

4 4th digit required   5 5th digit required   6 6th digit required   7 7th digit required   7 7th digit placeholder   + Additional code   ▣ Laterality

SP O26.52 Maternal hypotension syndrome, second trimester

SP O26.53 Maternal hypotension syndrome, third trimester

+ 5 O26.6 Liver and biliary tract disorders in pregnancy, childbirth and the puerperium

Use additional code to identify the specific disorder

> **EXCLUDES 2** hepatorenal syndrome following labor and delivery (O90.4)

+ 6 O26.61 Liver and biliary tract disorders in pregnancy

SP + O26.611 Liver and biliary tract disorders in pregnancy, first trimester

IQ + O26.612 Liver and biliary tract disorders in pregnancy, second trimester

SP + O26.613 Liver and biliary tract disorders in pregnancy, third trimester

IQ + O26.619 Liver and biliary tract disorders in pregnancy, unspecified trimester

SP + O26.62 Liver and biliary tract disorders in childbirth

SP + O26.63 Liver and biliary tract disorders in the puerperium

5 O26.7 Subluxation of symphysis (pubis) in pregnancy, childbirth and the puerperium

> **EXCLUDES 1** traumatic separation of symphysis (pubis) during childbirth (O71.6)

6 O26.71 Subluxation of symphysis (pubis) in pregnancy

SP O26.711 Subluxation of symphysis (pubis) in pregnancy, first trimester

SP O26.712 Subluxation of symphysis (pubis) in pregnancy, second trimester

SP O26.713 Subluxation of symphysis (pubis) in pregnancy, third trimester

IQ O26.719 Subluxation of symphysis (pubis) in pregnancy, unspecified trimester

SP O26.72 Subluxation of symphysis (pubis) in childbirth

SP O26.73 Subluxation of symphysis (pubis) in the puerperium

5 O26.8 Other specified pregnancy related conditions

6 O26.81 Pregnancy related exhaustion and fatigue

SP O26.811 Pregnancy related exhaustion and fatigue, first trimester

SP O26.812 Pregnancy related exhaustion and fatigue, second trimester

SP O26.813 Pregnancy related exhaustion and fatigue, third trimester

IQ O26.819 Pregnancy related exhaustion and fatigue, unspecified trimester

6 O26.82 Pregnancy related peripheral neuritis

SP O26.821 Pregnancy related peripheral neuritis, first trimester

SP O26.822 Pregnancy related peripheral neuritis, second trimester

SP O26.823 Pregnancy related peripheral neuritis, third trimester

IQ O26.829 Pregnancy related peripheral neuritis, unspecified trimester

+ 6 O26.83 Pregnancy related renal disease

Use additional code to identify the specific disorder

SP + O26.831 Pregnancy related renal disease, first trimester

SP + O26.832 Pregnancy related renal disease, second trimester

SP + O26.833 Pregnancy related renal disease, third trimester

IQ + O26.839 Pregnancy related renal disease, unspecified trimester

6 O26.84 Uterine size-date discrepancy complicating pregnancy

> **EXCLUDES 1** encounter for suspected problem with fetal growth ruled out (Z03.74)

SP O26.841 Uterine size-date discrepancy, first trimester

SP O26.842 Uterine size-date discrepancy, second trimester

SP O26.843 Uterine size-date discrepancy, third trimester

IQ O26.849 Uterine size-date discrepancy, unspecified trimester

6 O26.85 Spotting complicating pregnancy

SP O26.851 Spotting complicating pregnancy, first trimester

SP O26.852 Spotting complicating pregnancy, second trimester

SP O26.853 Spotting complicating pregnancy, third trimester

IQ O26.859 Spotting complicating pregnancy, unspecified trimester

SP O26.86 Pruritic urticarial papules and plaques of pregnancy (PUPPP)

Polymorphic eruption of pregnancy

6 O26.87 Cervical shortening

> **EXCLUDES 1** encounter for suspected cervical shortening ruled out (Z03.75)

SP O26.872 Cervical shortening, second trimester

> **DEFINITION** Sonographic evidence of a cervix shortened to 2.5 cm or less in the second trimester; a warning of impending premature birth in women with a prior history of early delivery.

SP O26.873 Cervical shortening, third trimester

IQ O26.879 Cervical shortening, unspecified trimester

6 O26.89 Other specified pregnancy related conditions

SP O26.891 Other specified pregnancy related conditions, first trimester

SP O26.892 Other specified pregnancy related conditions, second trimester

SP O26.893 Other specified pregnancy related conditions, third trimester

IQ O26.899 Other specified pregnancy related conditions, unspecified trimester

★ New ▲ Revised **Px** Primary **SP** PDGM Px **SL** Low CoM **SH** High CoM **IQ** Quest. Encounter **H** Hospice non-cancer Dx | Unspecified | **M** *Manifestation*

DecisionHealth's FY 2020 Complete Home Health ICD-10-CM Diagnosis Coding Manual

1331

5 O26.9 **Pregnancy related conditions, unspecified**

IQ O26.90 **Pregnancy related conditions, unspecified, unspecified trimester**

IQ O26.91 **Pregnancy related conditions, unspecified, first trimester**

IQ O26.92 **Pregnancy related conditions, unspecified, second trimester**

IQ O26.93 **Pregnancy related conditions, unspecified, third trimester**

4 O28 **Abnormal findings on antenatal screening of mother**

> EXCLUDES 1　diagnostic findings classified elsewhere - see Alphabetical Index

IQ O28.0 **Abnormal hematological finding on antenatal screening of mother**

IQ O28.1 **Abnormal biochemical finding on antenatal screening of mother**

IQ O28.2 **Abnormal cytological finding on antenatal screening of mother**

IQ O28.3 **Abnormal ultrasonic finding on antenatal screening of mother**

IQ O28.4 **Abnormal radiological finding on antenatal screening of mother**

IQ O28.5 **Abnormal chromosomal and genetic finding on antenatal screening of mother**

IQ O28.8 **Other abnormal findings on antenatal screening of mother**

IQ O28.9 **Unspecified abnormal findings on antenatal screening of mother**

+ 4 O29 **Complications of anesthesia during pregnancy**

> INCLUDES　maternal complications arising from the administration of a general, regional or local anesthetic, analgesic or other sedation during pregnancy

Use additional code, if necessary, to identify the complication

> EXCLUDES 2　complications of anesthesia during labor and delivery (O74.-)
> complications of anesthesia during the puerperium (O89.-)

+ 5 O29.0 **Pulmonary complications of anesthesia during pregnancy**

+ 6 O29.01 **Aspiration pneumonitis due to anesthesia during pregnancy**

Inhalation of stomach contents or secretions NOS due to anesthesia during pregnancy

Mendelson's syndrome due to anesthesia during pregnancy

SP + O29.011 **Aspiration pneumonitis due to anesthesia during pregnancy, first trimester**

SP + O29.012 **Aspiration pneumonitis due to anesthesia during pregnancy, second trimester**

SP + O29.013 **Aspiration pneumonitis due to anesthesia during pregnancy, third trimester**

IQ + O29.019 **Aspiration pneumonitis due to anesthesia during pregnancy, unspecified trimester**

+ 6 O29.02 **Pressure collapse of lung due to anesthesia during pregnancy**

SP + O29.021 **Pressure collapse of lung due to anesthesia during pregnancy, first trimester**

SP + O29.022 **Pressure collapse of lung due to anesthesia during pregnancy, second trimester**

SP + O29.023 **Pressure collapse of lung due to anesthesia during pregnancy, third trimester**

IQ + O29.029 **Pressure collapse of lung due to anesthesia during pregnancy, unspecified trimester**

+ 6 O29.09 **Other pulmonary complications of anesthesia during pregnancy**

SP + O29.091 **Other pulmonary complications of anesthesia during pregnancy, first trimester**

SP + O29.092 **Other pulmonary complications of anesthesia during pregnancy, second trimester**

SP + O29.093 **Other pulmonary complications of anesthesia during pregnancy, third trimester**

IQ + O29.099 **Other pulmonary complications of anesthesia during pregnancy, unspecified trimester**

+ 5 O29.1 Cardiac complications of anesthesia during pregnancy

+ 6 O29.11 **Cardiac arrest due to anesthesia during pregnancy**

SP + O29.111 **Cardiac arrest due to anesthesia during pregnancy, first trimester**

SP + O29.112 **Cardiac arrest due to anesthesia during pregnancy, second trimester**

SP + O29.113 **Cardiac arrest due to anesthesia during pregnancy, third trimester**

IQ + O29.119 **Cardiac arrest due to anesthesia during pregnancy, unspecified trimester**

+ 6 O29.12 **Cardiac failure due to anesthesia during pregnancy**

SP + O29.121 **Cardiac failure due to anesthesia during pregnancy, first trimester**

SP + O29.122 **Cardiac failure due to anesthesia during pregnancy, second trimester**

SP + O29.123 **Cardiac failure due to anesthesia during pregnancy, third trimester**

IQ + O29.129 **Cardiac failure due to anesthesia during pregnancy, unspecified trimester**

+ 6 O29.19 **Other cardiac complications of anesthesia during pregnancy**

SP + O29.191 **Other cardiac complications of anesthesia during pregnancy, first trimester**

SP + O29.192 **Other cardiac complications of anesthesia during pregnancy, second trimester**

SP + O29.193 **Other cardiac complications of anesthesia during pregnancy, third trimester**

IQ + O29.199 **Other cardiac complications of anesthesia during pregnancy, unspecified trimester**

4 4th digit required　5 5th digit required　6 6th digit required　7 7th digit required　7 7th digit placeholder　+ Additional code　= Laterality

1332　　DecisionHealth's FY 2020 Complete Home Health ICD-10-CM Diagnosis Coding Manual

+ 5 O29.2 Central nervous system complications of anesthesia during pregnancy

 + 6 O29.21 Cerebral anoxia due to anesthesia during pregnancy

  SP **+ O29.211 Cerebral anoxia due to anesthesia during pregnancy, first trimester**

  SP **+ O29.212 Cerebral anoxia due to anesthesia during pregnancy, second trimester**

  SP **+ O29.213 Cerebral anoxia due to anesthesia during pregnancy, third trimester**

  IQ **+ O29.219 Cerebral anoxia due to anesthesia during pregnancy, unspecified trimester**

 + 6 O29.29 Other central nervous system complications of anesthesia during pregnancy

  SP **+ O29.291 Other central nervous system complications of anesthesia during pregnancy, first trimester**

  SP **+ O29.292 Other central nervous system complications of anesthesia during pregnancy, second trimester**

  SP **+ O29.293 Other central nervous system complications of anesthesia during pregnancy, third trimester**

  IQ **+ O29.299 Other central nervous system complications of anesthesia during pregnancy, unspecified trimester**

+ 5 O29.3 Toxic reaction to local anesthesia during pregnancy

 + 6 O29.3X Toxic reaction to local anesthesia during pregnancy

  SP **+ O29.3X1 Toxic reaction to local anesthesia during pregnancy, first trimester**

  SP **+ O29.3X2 Toxic reaction to local anesthesia during pregnancy, second trimester**

  SP **+ O29.3X3 Toxic reaction to local anesthesia during pregnancy, third trimester**

  IQ **+ O29.3X9 Toxic reaction to local anesthesia during pregnancy, unspecified trimester**

+ 5 O29.4 Spinal and epidural anesthesia induced headache during pregnancy

 IQ **+ O29.40 Spinal and epidural anesthesia induced headache during pregnancy, unspecified trimester**

 SP **+ O29.41 Spinal and epidural anesthesia induced headache during pregnancy, first trimester**

 SP **+ O29.42 Spinal and epidural anesthesia induced headache during pregnancy, second trimester**

 SP **+ O29.43 Spinal and epidural anesthesia induced headache during pregnancy, third trimester**

+ 5 O29.5 Other complications of spinal and epidural anesthesia during pregnancy

 + 6 O29.5X Other complications of spinal and epidural anesthesia during pregnancy

  SP **+ O29.5X1 Other complications of spinal and epidural anesthesia during pregnancy, first trimester**

  SP **+ O29.5X2 Other complications of spinal and epidural anesthesia during pregnancy, second trimester**

  SP **+ O29.5X3 Other complications of spinal and epidural anesthesia during pregnancy, third trimester**

  IQ **+ O29.5X9 Other complications of spinal and epidural anesthesia during pregnancy, unspecified trimester**

+ 5 O29.6 Failed or difficult intubation for anesthesia during pregnancy

 IQ **+ O29.60 Failed or difficult intubation for anesthesia during pregnancy, unspecified trimester**

 SP **+ O29.61 Failed or difficult intubation for anesthesia during pregnancy, first trimester**

 SP **+ O29.62 Failed or difficult intubation for anesthesia during pregnancy, second trimester**

 SP **+ O29.63 Failed or difficult intubation for anesthesia during pregnancy, third trimester**

+ 5 O29.8 Other complications of anesthesia during pregnancy

 + 6 O29.8X Other complications of anesthesia during pregnancy

  SP **+ O29.8X1 Other complications of anesthesia during pregnancy, first trimester**

  SP **+ O29.8X2 Other complications of anesthesia during pregnancy, second trimester**

  SP **+ O29.8X3 Other complications of anesthesia during pregnancy, third trimester**

  IQ **+ O29.8X9 Other complications of anesthesia during pregnancy, unspecified trimester**

+ 5 O29.9 Unspecified complication of anesthesia during pregnancy

 IQ **+ O29.90 Unspecified complication of anesthesia during pregnancy, unspecified trimester**

 IQ **+ O29.91 Unspecified complication of anesthesia during pregnancy, first trimester**

 IQ **+ O29.92 Unspecified complication of anesthesia during pregnancy, second trimester**

 IQ **+ O29.93 Unspecified complication of anesthesia during pregnancy, third trimester**

Maternal care related to the fetus and amniotic cavity and possible delivery problems (O30-O48)

4 O30 Multiple gestation
 Code also:
  any complications specific to multiple gestation

5 O30.0 Twin pregnancy

 6 O30.00 Twin pregnancy, unspecified number of placenta and unspecified number of amniotic sacs

★ New ▲ Revised Px Primary SP PDGM Px SL Low CoM SH High CoM IQ Quest. Encounter H Hospice non-cancer Dx Unspecified M Manifestation

DecisionHealth's FY 2020 Complete Home Health ICD-10-CM Diagnosis Coding Manual

1333

!Q O30.001 **Twin pregnancy, unspecified number of placenta and unspecified number of amniotic sacs, first trimester**

!Q O30.002 **Twin pregnancy, unspecified number of placenta and unspecified number of amniotic sacs, second trimester**

!Q O30.003 **Twin pregnancy, unspecified number of placenta and unspecified number of amniotic sacs, third trimester**

!Q O30.009 **Twin pregnancy, unspecified number of placenta and unspecified number of amniotic sacs, unspecified trimester**

6 O30.01 Twin pregnancy, monochorionic/monoamniotic
Twin pregnancy, one placenta, one amniotic sac
EXCLUDES 1 conjoined twins (O30.02-)

!Q O30.011 Twin pregnancy, monochorionic/monoamniotic, first trimester

!Q O30.012 Twin pregnancy, monochorionic/monoamniotic, second trimester

!Q O30.013 Twin pregnancy, monochorionic/monoamniotic, third trimester

!Q O30.019 **Twin pregnancy, monochorionic/monoamniotic, unspecified trimester**

6 O30.02 Conjoined twin pregnancy

SP O30.021 Conjoined twin pregnancy, first trimester

SP O30.022 Conjoined twin pregnancy, second trimester

SP O30.023 Conjoined twin pregnancy, third trimester

!Q O30.029 **Conjoined twin pregnancy, unspecified trimester**

6 O30.03 Twin pregnancy, monochorionic/diamniotic
Twin pregnancy, one placenta, two amniotic sacs

!Q O30.031 Twin pregnancy, monochorionic/diamniotic, first trimester

!Q O30.032 Twin pregnancy, monochorionic/diamniotic, second trimester

!Q O30.033 Twin pregnancy, monochorionic/diamniotic, third trimester

!Q O30.039 **Twin pregnancy, monochorionic/diamniotic, unspecified trimester**

6 O30.04 Twin pregnancy, dichorionic/diamniotic
Twin pregnancy, two placentae, two amniotic sacs

!Q O30.041 Twin pregnancy, dichorionic/diamniotic, first trimester

!Q O30.042 Twin pregnancy, dichorionic/diamniotic, second trimester

!Q O30.043 Twin pregnancy, dichorionic/diamniotic, third trimester

!Q O30.049 **Twin pregnancy, dichorionic/diamniotic, unspecified trimester**

6 O30.09 Twin pregnancy, unable to determine number of placenta and number of amniotic sacs

!Q O30.091 Twin pregnancy, unable to determine number of placenta and number of amniotic sacs, first trimester

!Q O30.092 Twin pregnancy, unable to determine number of placenta and number of amniotic sacs, second trimester

!Q O30.093 Twin pregnancy, unable to determine number of placenta and number of amniotic sacs, third trimester

!Q O30.099 **Twin pregnancy, unable to determine number of placenta and number of amniotic sacs, unspecified trimester**

5 O30.1 Triplet pregnancy

6 O30.10 **Triplet pregnancy, unspecified number of placenta and unspecified number of amniotic sacs**

!Q O30.101 **Triplet pregnancy, unspecified number of placenta and unspecified number of amniotic sacs, first trimester**

!Q O30.102 **Triplet pregnancy, unspecified number of placenta and unspecified number of amniotic sacs, second trimester**

!Q O30.103 **Triplet pregnancy, unspecified number of placenta and unspecified number of amniotic sacs, third trimester**

!Q O30.109 **Triplet pregnancy, unspecified number of placenta and unspecified number of amniotic sacs, unspecified trimester**

6 O30.11 Triplet pregnancy with two or more monochorionic fetuses

!Q O30.111 Triplet pregnancy with two or more monochorionic fetuses, first trimester

!Q O30.112 Triplet pregnancy with two or more monochorionic fetuses, second trimester

!Q O30.113 Triplet pregnancy with two or more monochorionic fetuses, third trimester

!Q O30.119 **Triplet pregnancy with two or more monochorionic fetuses, unspecified trimester**

6 O30.12 Triplet pregnancy with two or more monoamniotic fetuses

!Q O30.121 Triplet pregnancy with two or more monoamniotic fetuses, first trimester

4 4th digit required   **5** 5th digit required   **6** 6th digit required   **7** 7th digit required   **7** 7th digit placeholder   **+** Additional code   **⊟** Laterality

1334   *DecisionHealth's* FY 2020 Complete Home Health ICD-10-CM Diagnosis Coding Manual

IQ O30.122 Triplet pregnancy with two or more monoamniotic fetuses, second trimester

IQ O30.123 Triplet pregnancy with two or more monoamniotic fetuses, third trimester

IQ O30.129 Triplet pregnancy with two or more monoamniotic fetuses, unspecified trimester

6 O30.13 Triplet pregnancy, trichorionic/triamniotic

IQ O30.131 Triplet pregnancy, trichorionic/triamniotic, first trimester

IQ O30.132 Triplet pregnancy, trichorionic/triamniotic, second trimester

IQ O30.133 Triplet pregnancy, trichorionic/triamniotic, third trimester

IQ O30.139 Triplet pregnancy, trichorionic/triamniotic, unspecified trimester

6 O30.19 Triplet pregnancy, unable to determine number of placenta and number of amniotic sacs

IQ O30.191 Triplet pregnancy, unable to determine number of placenta and number of amniotic sacs, first trimester

IQ O30.192 Triplet pregnancy, unable to determine number of placenta and number of amniotic sacs, second trimester

IQ O30.193 Triplet pregnancy, unable to determine number of placenta and number of amniotic sacs, third trimester

IQ O30.199 Triplet pregnancy, unable to determine number of placenta and number of amniotic sacs, unspecified trimester

5 O30.2 Quadruplet pregnancy

6 O30.20 Quadruplet pregnancy, unspecified number of placenta and unspecified number of amniotic sacs

IQ O30.201 Quadruplet pregnancy, unspecified number of placenta and unspecified number of amniotic sacs, first trimester

IQ O30.202 Quadruplet pregnancy, unspecified number of placenta and unspecified number of amniotic sacs, second trimester

IQ O30.203 Quadruplet pregnancy, unspecified number of placenta and unspecified number of amniotic sacs, third trimester

IQ O30.209 Quadruplet pregnancy, unspecified number of placenta and unspecified number of amniotic sacs, unspecified trimester

6 O30.21 Quadruplet pregnancy with two or more monochorionic fetuses

IQ O30.211 Quadruplet pregnancy with two or more monochorionic fetuses, first trimester

IQ O30.212 Quadruplet pregnancy with two or more monochorionic fetuses, second trimester

IQ O30.213 Quadruplet pregnancy with two or more monochorionic fetuses, third trimester

IQ O30.219 Quadruplet pregnancy with two or more monochorionic fetuses, unspecified trimester

6 O30.22 Quadruplet pregnancy with two or more monoamniotic fetuses

IQ O30.221 Quadruplet pregnancy with two or more monoamniotic fetuses, first trimester

IQ O30.222 Quadruplet pregnancy with two or more monoamniotic fetuses, second trimester

IQ O30.223 Quadruplet pregnancy with two or more monoamniotic fetuses, third trimester

IQ O30.229 Quadruplet pregnancy with two or more monoamniotic fetuses, unspecified trimester

6 O30.23 Quadruplet pregnancy, quadrachorionic/quadra-amniotic

IQ O30.231 Quadruplet pregnancy, quadrachorionic/quadra-amniotic, first trimester

IQ O30.232 Quadruplet pregnancy, quadrachorionic/quadra-amniotic, second trimester

IQ O30.233 Quadruplet pregnancy, quadrachorionic/quadra-amniotic, third trimester

IQ O30.239 Quadruplet pregnancy, quadrachorionic/quadra-amniotic, unspecified trimester

6 O30.29 Quadruplet pregnancy, unable to determine number of placenta and number of amniotic sacs

IQ O30.291 Quadruplet pregnancy, unable to determine number of placenta and number of amniotic sacs, first trimester

IQ O30.292 Quadruplet pregnancy, unable to determine number of placenta and number of amniotic sacs, second trimester

IQ O30.293 Quadruplet pregnancy, unable to determine number of placenta and number of amniotic sacs, third trimester

IQ O30.299 Quadruplet pregnancy, unable to determine number of placenta and number of amniotic sacs, unspecified trimester

5 O30.8 Other specified multiple gestation
Multiple gestation pregnancy greater then quadruplets

6 O30.80 Other specified multiple gestation, unspecified number of placenta and unspecified number of amniotic sacs

★ New ▲ Revised Px Primary SP PDGM Px SL Low CoM SH High CoM IQ Quest. Encounter H Hospice non-cancer Dx   Unspecified   M Manifestation

DecisionHealth's FY 2020 Complete Home Health ICD-10-CM Diagnosis Coding Manual

1335

Chapter 15

O00-O9A

!Q O30.801 Other specified multiple gestation, unspecified number of placenta and unspecified number of amniotic sacs, first trimester

!Q O30.802 Other specified multiple gestation, unspecified number of placenta and unspecified number of amniotic sacs, second trimester

!Q O30.803 Other specified multiple gestation, unspecified number of placenta and unspecified number of amniotic sacs, third trimester

!Q O30.809 Other specified multiple gestation, unspecified number of placenta and unspecified number of amniotic sacs, unspecified trimester

6 O30.81 Other specified multiple gestation with two or more monochorionic fetuses

!Q O30.811 Other specified multiple gestation with two or more monochorionic fetuses, first trimester

!Q O30.812 Other specified multiple gestation with two or more monochorionic fetuses, second trimester

!Q O30.813 Other specified multiple gestation with two or more monochorionic fetuses, third trimester

!Q O30.819 Other specified multiple gestation with two or more monochorionic fetuses, unspecified trimester

6 O30.82 Other specified multiple gestation with two or more monoamniotic fetuses

!Q O30.821 Other specified multiple gestation with two or more monoamniotic fetuses, first trimester

!Q O30.822 Other specified multiple gestation with two or more monoamniotic fetuses, second trimester

!Q O30.823 Other specified multiple gestation with two or more monoamniotic fetuses, third trimester

!Q O30.829 Other specified multiple gestation with two or more monoamniotic fetuses, unspecified trimester

6 O30.83 Other specified multiple gestation, number of chorions and amnions are both equal to the number of fetuses
    Pentachorionic, penta-amniotic pregnancy (quintuplets)
    Hexachorionic, hexa-amniotic pregnancy (sextuplets)
    Heptachorionic, hepta-amniotic pregnancy (septuplets)

!Q O30.831 Other specified multiple gestation, number of chorions and amnions are both equal to the number of fetuses, first trimester

!Q O30.832 Other specified multiple gestation, number of chorions and amnions are both equal to the number of fetuses, second trimester

!Q O30.833 Other specified multiple gestation, number of chorions and amnions are both equal to the number of fetuses, third trimester

!Q O30.839 Other specified multiple gestation, number of chorions and amnions are both equal to the number of fetuses, unspecified trimester

6 O30.89 Other specified multiple gestation, unable to determine number of placenta and number of amniotic sacs

!Q O30.891 Other specified multiple gestation, unable to determine number of placenta and number of amniotic sacs, first trimester

!Q O30.892 Other specified multiple gestation, unable to determine number of placenta and number of amniotic sacs, second trimester

!Q O30.893 Other specified multiple gestation, unable to determine number of placenta and number of amniotic sacs, third trimester

!Q O30.899 Other specified multiple gestation, unable to determine number of placenta and number of amniotic sacs, unspecified trimester

5 O30.9 Multiple gestation, unspecified
    Multiple pregnancy NOS

!Q O30.90 Multiple gestation, unspecified, unspecified trimester

!Q O30.91 Multiple gestation, unspecified, first trimester

!Q O30.92 Multiple gestation, unspecified, second trimester

!Q O30.93 Multiple gestation, unspecified, third trimester

4 O31 Complications specific to multiple gestation
    EXCLUDES 2 delayed delivery of second twin, triplet, etc. (O63.2)
    malpresentation of one fetus or more (O32.9)
    placental transfusion syndromes (O43.0-)

One of the following 7th characters is to be assigned to each code under category O31. 7th character 0 is for single gestations and multiple gestations where the fetus is unspecified. 7th characters 1 through 9 are for cases of multiple gestations to identify the fetus for which the code applies. The appropriate code from category O30, Multiple gestation, must also be assigned when assigning a code from category O31 that has a 7th character of 1 through 9.

0	not applicable or unspecified
1	fetus 1
2	fetus 2
3	fetus 3
4	fetus 4
5	fetus 5
9	other fetus

5 O31.0 Papyraceous fetus

---

4 4th digit required **5** 5th digit required **6** 6th digit required **7** 7th digit required **7** 7th digit placeholder **+** Additional code **⊟** Laterality

Fetus compressus

IQ **7** **O31.00X-** **Papyraceous fetus, unspecified trimester**

IQ **7** **O31.01X-** **Papyraceous fetus, first trimester**

IQ **7** **O31.02X-** **Papyraceous fetus, second trimester**

IQ **7** **O31.03X-** **Papyraceous fetus, third trimester**

5 **O31.1** **Continuing pregnancy after spontaneous abortion of one fetus or more**

IQ **7** **O31.10X-** **Continuing pregnancy after spontaneous abortion of one fetus or more, unspecified trimester**

IQ **7** **O31.11X-** **Continuing pregnancy after spontaneous abortion of one fetus or more, first trimester**

IQ **7** **O31.12X-** **Continuing pregnancy after spontaneous abortion of one fetus or more, second trimester**

IQ **7** **O31.13X-** **Continuing pregnancy after spontaneous abortion of one fetus or more, third trimester**

5 **O31.2** **Continuing pregnancy after intrauterine death of one fetus or more**

IQ **7** **O31.20X-** **Continuing pregnancy after intrauterine death of one fetus or more, unspecified trimester**

IQ **7** **O31.21X-** **Continuing pregnancy after intrauterine death of one fetus or more, first trimester**

IQ **7** **O31.22X-** **Continuing pregnancy after intrauterine death of one fetus or more, second trimester**

IQ **7** **O31.23X-** **Continuing pregnancy after intrauterine death of one fetus or more, third trimester**

5 **O31.3** **Continuing pregnancy after elective fetal reduction of one fetus or more**
Continuing pregnancy after selective termination of one fetus or more

IQ **7** **O31.30X-** **Continuing pregnancy after elective fetal reduction of one fetus or more, unspecified trimester**

IQ **7** **O31.31X-** **Continuing pregnancy after elective fetal reduction of one fetus or more, first trimester**

IQ **7** **O31.32X-** **Continuing pregnancy after elective fetal reduction of one fetus or more, second trimester**

IQ **7** **O31.33X-** **Continuing pregnancy after elective fetal reduction of one fetus or more, third trimester**

5 **O31.8** **Other complications specific to multiple gestation**

6 **O31.8X** **Other complications specific to multiple gestation**

IQ **7** **O31.8X1-** **Other complications specific to multiple gestation, first trimester**

IQ **7** **O31.8X2-** **Other complications specific to multiple gestation, second trimester**

IQ **7** **O31.8X3-** **Other complications specific to multiple gestation, third trimester**

IQ **7** **O31.8X9-** **Other complications specific to multiple gestation, unspecified trimester**

4 **O32** **Maternal care for malpresentation of fetus**

> **INCLUDES** the listed conditions as a reason for observation, hospitalization or other obstetric care of the mother, or for cesarean delivery before onset of labor
>
> **EXCLUDES 1** malpresentation of fetus with obstructed labor (O64.-)

One of the following 7th characters is to be assigned to each code under category O32. 7th character 0 is for single gestations and multiple gestations where the fetus is unspecified. 7th characters 1 through 9 are for cases of multiple gestations to identify the fetus for which the code applies. The appropriate code from category O30, Multiple gestation, must also be assigned when assigning a code from category O32 that has a 7th character of 1 through 9.

0	not applicable or unspecified
1	fetus 1
2	fetus 2
3	fetus 3
4	fetus 4
5	fetus 5
9	other fetus

IQ **7** **O32.0XX-** **Maternal care for unstable lie**

IQ **7** **O32.1XX-** **Maternal care for breech presentation**

Maternal care for buttocks presentation
Maternal care for complete breech
Maternal care for frank breech
> **EXCLUDES 1** footling presentation (O32.8)
> incomplete breech (O32.8)

IQ **7** **O32.2XX-** **Maternal care for transverse and oblique lie**

Maternal care for oblique presentation
Maternal care for transverse presentation

IQ **7** **O32.3XX-** **Maternal care for face, brow and chin presentation**

IQ **7** **O32.4XX-** **Maternal care for high head at term**

Maternal care for failure of head to enter pelvic brim

IQ **7** **O32.6XX-** **Maternal care for compound presentation**

IQ **7** **O32.8XX-** **Maternal care for other malpresentation of fetus**

Maternal care for footling presentation
Maternal care for incomplete breech

IQ **7** **O32.9XX-** **Maternal care for malpresentation of fetus, unspecified**

4 **O33** **Maternal care for disproportion**

★ New ▲ Revised **Px** Primary **SP** PDGM Px **SL** Low CoM **SH** High CoM **IQ** Quest. Encounter **H** Hospice non-cancer Dx | Unspecified | **M** *Manifestation*

DecisionHealth's FY 2020 Complete Home Health ICD-10-CM Diagnosis Coding Manual 1337

Chapter 15

O00-O9A

| INCLUDES | the listed conditions as a reason for observation, hospitalization or other obstetric care of the mother, or for cesarean delivery before onset of labor |
| EXCLUDES 1 | disproportion with obstructed labor (O65-O66) |

!Q O33.0 Maternal care for disproportion due to deformity of maternal pelvic bones

Maternal care for disproportion due to pelvic deformity causing disproportion NOS

!Q O33.1 Maternal care for disproportion due to generally contracted pelvis

Maternal care for disproportion due to contracted pelvis NOS causing disproportion

!Q O33.2 Maternal care for disproportion due to inlet contraction of pelvis

Maternal care for disproportion due to inlet contraction (pelvis) causing disproportion

!Q ☑ O33.3XX-   Maternal care for disproportion due to outlet contraction of pelvis

Maternal care for disproportion due to mid-cavity contraction (pelvis)

Maternal care for disproportion due to outlet contraction (pelvis)

One of the following 7th characters is to be assigned to code O33.3. 7th character 0 is for single gestations and multiple gestations where the fetus is unspecified. 7th characters 1 through 9 are for cases of multiple gestations to identify the fetus for which the code applies. The appropriate code from category O30, Multiple gestation, must also be assigned when assigning code O33.3 with a 7th character of 1 through 9.

0	not applicable or unspecified
1	fetus 1
2	fetus 2
3	fetus 3
4	fetus 4
5	fetus 5
9	other fetus

!Q ☑ O33.4XX-   Maternal care for disproportion of mixed maternal and fetal origin

One of the following 7th characters is to be assigned to code O33.4. 7th character 0 is for single gestations and multiple gestations where the fetus is unspecified. 7th characters 1 through 9 are for cases of multiple gestations to identify the fetus for which the code applies. The appropriate code from category O30, Multiple gestation, must also be assigned when assigning code O33.4 with a 7th character of 1 through 9.

0	not applicable or unspecified
1	fetus 1
2	fetus 2
3	fetus 3
4	fetus 4
5	fetus 5
9	other fetus

!Q ☑ O33.5XX-   Maternal care for disproportion due to unusually large fetus

Maternal care for disproportion due to disproportion of fetal origin with normally formed fetus

Maternal care for disproportion due to fetal disproportion NOS

One of the following 7th characters is to be assigned to code O33.5. 7th character 0 is for single gestations and multiple gestations where the fetus is unspecified. 7th characters 1 through 9 are for cases of multiple gestations to identify the fetus for which the code applies. The appropriate code from category O30, Multiple gestation, must also be assigned when assigning code O33.5 with a 7th character of 1 through 9.

0	not applicable or unspecified
1	fetus 1
2	fetus 2
3	fetus 3
4	fetus 4
5	fetus 5
9	other fetus

!Q ☑ O33.6XX-   Maternal care for disproportion due to hydrocephalic fetus

▲4th digit required   ⑤5th digit required   ⑥6th digit required   ⑦7th digit required   ☑7th digit placeholder   ✚Additional code   ⊟Laterality

1338   *DecisionHealth's* FY 2020 Complete Home Health ICD-10-CM Diagnosis Coding Manual

One of the following 7th characters is to be assigned to code O33.6. 7th character 0 is for single gestations and multiple gestations where the fetus is unspecified. 7th characters 1 through 9 are for cases of multiple gestations to identify the fetus for which the code applies. The appropriate code from category O30, Multiple gestation, must also be assigned when assigning code O33.6 with a 7th character of 1 through 9.

0	not applicable or unspecified
1	fetus 1
2	fetus 2
3	fetus 3
4	fetus 4
5	fetus 5
9	other fetus

!Q ☑7 O33.7XX- **Maternal care for disproportion due to other fetal deformities**

Maternal care for disproportion due to fetal ascites

Maternal care for disproportion due to fetal hydrops

Maternal care for disproportion due to fetal meningomyelocele

Maternal care for disproportion due to fetal sacral teratoma

Maternal care for disproportion due to fetal tumor

EXCLUDES 1 obstructed labor due to other fetal deformities (O66.3)

One of the following 7th characters is to be assigned to code O33.7. 7th character 0 is for single gestations and multiple gestations where the fetus is unspecified. 7th characters 1 through 9 are for cases of multiple gestations to identify the fetus for which the code applies. The appropriate code from category O30, Multiple gestation, must also be assigned when assigning code O33.7 with a 7th character of 1 through 9.

0	not applicable or unspecified
1	fetus 1
2	fetus 2
3	fetus 3
4	fetus 4
5	fetus 5
9	other fetus

!Q O33.8 **Maternal care for disproportion of other origin**

!Q O33.9 **Maternal care for disproportion, unspecified**

Maternal care for disproportion due to cephalopelvic disproportion NOS

Maternal care for disproportion due to fetopelvic disproportion NOS

+ ☑4 O34 **Maternal care for abnormality of pelvic organs**

INCLUDES the listed conditions as a reason for hospitalization or other obstetric care of the mother, or for cesarean delivery before onset of labor

Code first:
any associated obstructed labor (O65.5)
Use additional code for specific condition

+ ☑5 O34.0 **Maternal care for congenital malformation of uterus**

Maternal care for double uterus
Maternal care for uterus bicornis

!Q + O34.00 **Maternal care for unspecified congenital malformation of uterus, unspecified trimester**

!Q + O34.01 **Maternal care for unspecified congenital malformation of uterus, first trimester**

!Q + O34.02 **Maternal care for unspecified congenital malformation of uterus, second trimester**

!Q + O34.03 **Maternal care for unspecified congenital malformation of uterus, third trimester**

+ ☑5 O34.1 **Maternal care for benign tumor of corpus uteri**

EXCLUDES 2 maternal care for benign tumor of cervix (O34.4-)
maternal care for malignant neoplasm of uterus (O9A.1-)

!Q + O34.10 **Maternal care for benign tumor of corpus uteri, unspecified trimester**

!Q + O34.11 **Maternal care for benign tumor of corpus uteri, first trimester**

!Q + O34.12 **Maternal care for benign tumor of corpus uteri, second trimester**

!Q + O34.13 **Maternal care for benign tumor of corpus uteri, third trimester**

+ ☑5 O34.2 **Maternal care due to uterine scar from previous surgery**

+ ☑6 O34.21 **Maternal care for scar from previous cesarean delivery**

!Q + O34.211 **Maternal care for low transverse scar from previous cesarean delivery**

!Q + O34.212 **Maternal care for vertical scar from previous cesarean delivery**

Maternal care for classical scar from previous cesarean delivery

!Q + O34.219 **Maternal care for unspecified type scar from previous cesarean delivery**

!Q + O34.29 **Maternal care due to uterine scar from other previous surgery**

Maternal care due to uterine scar from other transmural uterine incision

+ ☑5 O34.3 **Maternal care for cervical incompetence**

Maternal care for cerclage with or without cervical incompetence

Maternal care for Shirodkar suture with or without cervical incompetence

!Q + O34.30 **Maternal care for cervical incompetence, unspecified trimester**

!Q + O34.31 **Maternal care for cervical incompetence, first trimester**

★ New ▲ Revised Px Primary SP PDGM Px SL Low CoM SH High CoM !Q Quest. Encounter H Hospice non-cancer Dx ☐ Unspecified M *Manifestation*

DecisionHealth's FY 2020 Complete Home Health ICD-10-CM Diagnosis Coding Manual

1339

!Q **+** **O34.32** Maternal care for cervical incompetence, second trimester

!Q **+** **O34.33** Maternal care for cervical incompetence, third trimester

+ **⑤** **O34.4** Maternal care for other abnormalities of cervix

!Q **+** **O34.40** Maternal care for other abnormalities of cervix, unspecified trimester

!Q **+** **O34.41** Maternal care for other abnormalities of cervix, first trimester

!Q **+** **O34.42** Maternal care for other abnormalities of cervix, second trimester

!Q **+** **O34.43** Maternal care for other abnormalities of cervix, third trimester

+ **⑤** **O34.5** Maternal care for other abnormalities of gravid uterus

+ **⑥** **O34.51** Maternal care for incarceration of gravid uterus

!Q **+** **O34.511** Maternal care for incarceration of gravid uterus, first trimester

!Q **+** **O34.512** Maternal care for incarceration of gravid uterus, second trimester

!Q **+** **O34.513** Maternal care for incarceration of gravid uterus, third trimester

!Q **+** **O34.519** Maternal care for incarceration of gravid uterus, unspecified trimester

+ **⑥** **O34.52** Maternal care for prolapse of gravid uterus

!Q **+** **O34.521** Maternal care for prolapse of gravid uterus, first trimester

!Q **+** **O34.522** Maternal care for prolapse of gravid uterus, second trimester

!Q **+** **O34.523** Maternal care for prolapse of gravid uterus, third trimester

!Q **+** **O34.529** Maternal care for prolapse of gravid uterus, unspecified trimester

+ **⑥** **O34.53** Maternal care for retroversion of gravid uterus

!Q **+** **O34.531** Maternal care for retroversion of gravid uterus, first trimester

!Q **+** **O34.532** Maternal care for retroversion of gravid uterus, second trimester

!Q **+** **O34.533** Maternal care for retroversion of gravid uterus, third trimester

!Q **+** **O34.539** Maternal care for retroversion of gravid uterus, unspecified trimester

+ **⑥** **O34.59** Maternal care for other abnormalities of gravid uterus

!Q **+** **O34.591** Maternal care for other abnormalities of gravid uterus, first trimester

!Q **+** **O34.592** Maternal care for other abnormalities of gravid uterus, second trimester

!Q **+** **O34.593** Maternal care for other abnormalities of gravid uterus, third trimester

!Q **+** **O34.599** Maternal care for other abnormalities of gravid uterus, unspecified trimester

+ **⑤** **O34.6** Maternal care for abnormality of vagina

> **EXCLUDES 2** maternal care for vaginal varices in pregnancy (O22.1-)

!Q **+** **O34.60** Maternal care for abnormality of vagina, unspecified trimester

!Q **+** **O34.61** Maternal care for abnormality of vagina, first trimester

!Q **+** **O34.62** Maternal care for abnormality of vagina, second trimester

!Q **+** **O34.63** Maternal care for abnormality of vagina, third trimester

+ **⑤** **O34.7** Maternal care for abnormality of vulva and perineum

> **EXCLUDES 2** maternal care for perineal and vulval varices in pregnancy (O22.1-)

!Q **+** **O34.70** Maternal care for abnormality of vulva and perineum, unspecified trimester

!Q **+** **O34.71** Maternal care for abnormality of vulva and perineum, first trimester

!Q **+** **O34.72** Maternal care for abnormality of vulva and perineum, second trimester

!Q **+** **O34.73** Maternal care for abnormality of vulva and perineum, third trimester

+ **⑤** **O34.8** Maternal care for other abnormalities of pelvic organs

!Q **+** **O34.80** Maternal care for other abnormalities of pelvic organs, unspecified trimester

!Q **+** **O34.81** Maternal care for other abnormalities of pelvic organs, first trimester

!Q **+** **O34.82** Maternal care for other abnormalities of pelvic organs, second trimester

!Q **+** **O34.83** Maternal care for other abnormalities of pelvic organs, third trimester

+ **⑤** **O34.9** Maternal care for abnormality of pelvic organ, unspecified

!Q **+** **O34.90** Maternal care for abnormality of pelvic organ, unspecified, unspecified trimester

!Q **+** **O34.91** Maternal care for abnormality of pelvic organ, unspecified, first trimester

!Q **+** **O34.92** Maternal care for abnormality of pelvic organ, unspecified, second trimester

!Q **+** **O34.93** Maternal care for abnormality of pelvic organ, unspecified, third trimester

④ **O35** Maternal care for known or suspected fetal abnormality and damage

> **INCLUDES** the listed conditions in the fetus as a reason for hospitalization or other obstetric care to the mother, or for termination of pregnancy

Code also:
any associated maternal condition

> **EXCLUDES 1** encounter for suspected maternal and fetal conditions ruled out (Z03.7-)

④ 4th digit required   **⑤** 5th digit required   **⑥** 6th digit required   **⑦** 7th digit required   **⑦** 7th digit placeholder   **+** Additional code   **⊟** Laterality

1340   *DecisionHealth's* FY 2020 Complete Home Health ICD-10-CM Diagnosis Coding Manual

One of the following 7th characters is to be assigned to each code under category O35. 7th character 0 is for single gestations and multiple gestations where the fetus is unspecified. 7th characters 1 through 9 are for cases of multiple gestations to identify the fetus for which the code applies. The appropriate code from category O30, Multiple gestation, must also be assigned when assigning a code from category O35 that has a 7th character of 1 through 9.

0	not applicable or unspecified
1	fetus 1
2	fetus 2
3	fetus 3
4	fetus 4
5	fetus 5
9	other fetus

!Q ✓ O35.0XX- **Maternal care for (suspected) central nervous system malformation in fetus**

Maternal care for fetal anencephaly
Maternal care for fetal hydrocephalus
Maternal care for fetal spina bifida

EXCLUDES 2 chromosomal abnormality in fetus (O35.1)

!Q ✓ O35.1XX- **Maternal care for (suspected) chromosomal abnormality in fetus**

!Q ✓ O35.2XX- **Maternal care for (suspected) hereditary disease in fetus**

EXCLUDES 2 chromosomal abnormality in fetus (O35.1)

!Q ✓ O35.3XX- **Maternal care for (suspected) damage to fetus from viral disease in mother**

Maternal care for damage to fetus from maternal cytomegalovirus infection
Maternal care for damage to fetus from maternal rubella

!Q ✓ O35.4XX- **Maternal care for (suspected) damage to fetus from alcohol**

!Q ✓ O35.5XX- **Maternal care for (suspected) damage to fetus by drugs**

Maternal care for damage to fetus from drug addiction

!Q ✓ O35.6XX- **Maternal care for (suspected) damage to fetus by radiation**

!Q ✓ O35.7XX- **Maternal care for (suspected) damage to fetus by other medical procedures**

Maternal care for damage to fetus by amniocentesis
Maternal care for damage to fetus by biopsy procedures
Maternal care for damage to fetus by hematological investigation
Maternal care for damage to fetus by intrauterine contraceptive device
Maternal care for damage to fetus by intrauterine surgery

!Q ✓ O35.8XX- **Maternal care for other (suspected) fetal abnormality and damage**

Maternal care for damage to fetus from maternal listeriosis
Maternal care for damage to fetus from maternal toxoplasmosis

!Q ✓ O35.9XX- **Maternal care for (suspected) fetal abnormality and damage, unspecified**

4 O36 **Maternal care for other fetal problems**

INCLUDES the listed conditions in the fetus as a reason for hospitalization or other obstetric care of the mother, or for termination of pregnancy

EXCLUDES 1 encounter for suspected maternal and fetal conditions ruled out (Z03.7-)
placental transfusion syndromes (O43.0-)

EXCLUDES 2 labor and delivery complicated by fetal stress (O77.-)

One of the following 7th characters is to be assigned to each code under category O36. 7th character 0 is for single gestations and multiple gestations where the fetus is unspecified. 7th characters 1 through 9 are for cases of multiple gestations to identify the fetus for which the code applies. The appropriate code from category O30, Multiple gestation, must also be assigned when assigning a code from category O36 that has a 7th character of 1 through 9.

0	not applicable or unspecified
1	fetus 1
2	fetus 2
3	fetus 3
4	fetus 4
5	fetus 5
9	other fetus

CODING TIPS ✓ It is common to have abnormalities of the fetal heart rate or rhythm during the antepartum period, including fetal tachycardia, fetal bradycardia, decelerations of the fetal heart rate and loss of variability. Abnormalities during antenatal tests such as non-stress tests (NSTs) and contraction stress tests (CSTs) are also reported.

5 O36.0 **Maternal care for rhesus isoimmunization**

Maternal care for Rh incompatibility (with hydrops fetalis)

6 O36.01 **Maternal care for anti-D [Rh] antibodies**

!Q 7 O36.011- **Maternal care for anti-D [Rh] antibodies, first trimester**

!Q 7 O36.012- **Maternal care for anti-D [Rh] antibodies, second trimester**

!Q 7 O36.013- **Maternal care for anti-D [Rh] antibodies, third trimester**

!Q 7 O36.019- **Maternal care for anti-D [Rh] antibodies, unspecified trimester**

6 O36.09 **Maternal care for other rhesus isoimmunization**

!Q 7 O36.091- **Maternal care for other rhesus isoimmunization, first trimester**

★ New ▲ Revised **Px** Primary **SP** PDGM Px **SL** Low CoM **SH** High CoM **!Q** Quest. Encounter **H** Hospice non-cancer Dx   Unspecified   **M** *Manifestation*

Chapter 15

O00-O9A

IQ 7 O36.092- Maternal care for other rhesus isoimmunization, second trimester

IQ 7 O36.093- Maternal care for other rhesus isoimmunization, third trimester

IQ 7 O36.099- Maternal care for other rhesus isoimmunization, unspecified trimester

5 O36.1 Maternal care for other isoimmunization
Maternal care for ABO isoimmunization

6 O36.11 Maternal care for Anti-A sensitization
Maternal care for isoimmunization NOS (with hydrops fetalis)

IQ 7 O36.111- Maternal care for Anti-A sensitization, first trimester

IQ 7 O36.112- Maternal care for Anti-A sensitization, second trimester

IQ 7 O36.113- Maternal care for Anti-A sensitization, third trimester

IQ 7 O36.119- Maternal care for Anti-A sensitization, unspecified trimester

6 O36.19 Maternal care for other isoimmunization
Maternal care for Anti-B sensitization

IQ 7 O36.191- Maternal care for other isoimmunization, first trimester

IQ 7 O36.192- Maternal care for other isoimmunization, second trimester

IQ 7 O36.193- Maternal care for other isoimmunization, third trimester

IQ 7 O36.199- Maternal care for other isoimmunization, unspecified trimester

5 O36.2 Maternal care for hydrops fetalis
Maternal care for hydrops fetalis NOS
Maternal care for hydrops fetalis not associated with isoimmunization
EXCLUDES 1 hydrops fetalis associated with ABO isoimmunization (O36.1-)
hydrops fetalis associated with rhesus isoimmunization (O36.0-)

IQ 7 O36.20X- Maternal care for hydrops fetalis, unspecified trimester

IQ 7 O36.21X- Maternal care for hydrops fetalis, first trimester

IQ 7 O36.22X- Maternal care for hydrops fetalis, second trimester

IQ 7 O36.23X- Maternal care for hydrops fetalis, third trimester

IQ 7 O36.4XX- Maternal care for intrauterine death
Maternal care for intrauterine fetal death NOS
Maternal care for intrauterine fetal death after completion of 20 weeks of gestation
Maternal care for late fetal death
Maternal care for missed delivery

EXCLUDES 1 missed abortion (O02.1)
stillbirth (P95)

5 O36.5 Maternal care for known or suspected poor fetal growth

6 O36.51 Maternal care for known or suspected placental insufficiency

IQ 7 O36.511- Maternal care for known or suspected placental insufficiency, first trimester

IQ 7 O36.512- Maternal care for known or suspected placental insufficiency, second trimester

IQ 7 O36.513- Maternal care for known or suspected placental insufficiency, third trimester

IQ 7 O36.519- Maternal care for known or suspected placental insufficiency, unspecified trimester

6 O36.59 Maternal care for other known or suspected poor fetal growth
Maternal care for known or suspected light-for-dates NOS
Maternal care for known or suspected small-for-dates NOS

IQ 7 O36.591- Maternal care for other known or suspected poor fetal growth, first trimester

IQ 7 O36.592- Maternal care for other known or suspected poor fetal growth, second trimester

IQ 7 O36.593- Maternal care for other known or suspected poor fetal growth, third trimester

IQ 7 O36.599- Maternal care for other known or suspected poor fetal growth, unspecified trimester

5 O36.6 Maternal care for excessive fetal growth
Maternal care for known or suspected large-for-dates

IQ 7 O36.60X- Maternal care for excessive fetal growth, unspecified trimester

IQ 7 O36.61X- Maternal care for excessive fetal growth, first trimester

IQ 7 O36.62X- Maternal care for excessive fetal growth, second trimester

IQ 7 O36.63X- Maternal care for excessive fetal growth, third trimester

5 O36.7 Maternal care for viable fetus in abdominal pregnancy

IQ 7 O36.70X- Maternal care for viable fetus in abdominal pregnancy, unspecified trimester

IQ 7 O36.71X- Maternal care for viable fetus in abdominal pregnancy, first trimester

IQ 7 O36.72X- Maternal care for viable fetus in abdominal pregnancy, second trimester

IQ 7 O36.73X- Maternal care for viable fetus in abdominal pregnancy, third trimester

5 O36.8 Maternal care for other specified fetal problems

---

4 4th digit required   5 5th digit required   6 6th digit required   7 7th digit required   7 7th digit placeholder   + Additional code   Laterality

IQ ☑ O36.80X- **Pregnancy with inconclusive fetal viability**
Encounter to determine fetal viability of pregnancy

⑥ O36.81 Decreased fetal movements

IQ ⑦ O36.812- **Decreased fetal movements, second trimester**

IQ ⑦ O36.813- **Decreased fetal movements, third trimester**

IQ ⑦ O36.819- **Decreased fetal movements, unspecified trimester**

⑥ O36.82 Fetal anemia and thrombocytopenia

IQ ⑦ O36.821- **Fetal anemia and thrombocytopenia, first trimester**

IQ ⑦ O36.822- **Fetal anemia and thrombocytopenia, second trimester**

IQ ⑦ O36.823- **Fetal anemia and thrombocytopenia, third trimester**

IQ ⑦ O36.829- **Fetal anemia and thrombocytopenia, unspecified trimester**

▲ ⑥ O36.83 Maternal care for abnormalities of the fetal heart rate or rhythm
Maternal care for depressed fetal heart rate tones
Maternal care for fetal bradycardia
Maternal care for fetal heart rate abnormal variability
Maternal care for fetal heart rate decelerations
Maternal care for fetal heart rate irregularity
Maternal care for fetal tachycardia
Maternal care for non-reassuring fetal heart rate or rhythm

IQ ⑦ O36.831- **Maternal care for abnormalities of the fetal heart rate or rhythm, first trimester**

IQ ⑦ O36.832- **Maternal care for abnormalities of the fetal heart rate or rhythm, second trimester**

IQ ⑦ O36.833- **Maternal care for abnormalities of the fetal heart rate or rhythm, third trimester**

IQ ⑦ O36.839- **Maternal care for abnormalities of the fetal heart rate or rhythm, unspecified trimester**

⑥ O36.89 Maternal care for other specified fetal problems

IQ ⑦ O36.891- **Maternal care for other specified fetal problems, first trimester**

IQ ⑦ O36.892- **Maternal care for other specified fetal problems, second trimester**

IQ ⑦ O36.893- **Maternal care for other specified fetal problems, third trimester**

IQ ⑦ O36.899- **Maternal care for other specified fetal problems, unspecified trimester**

⑤ O36.9 **Maternal care for fetal problem, unspecified**

IQ ☑ O36.90X- **Maternal care for fetal problem, unspecified, unspecified trimester**

IQ ☑ O36.91X- **Maternal care for fetal problem, unspecified, first trimester**

IQ ☑ O36.92X- **Maternal care for fetal problem, unspecified, second trimester**

IQ ☑ O36.93X- **Maternal care for fetal problem, unspecified, third trimester**

④ O40 Polyhydramnios
INCLUDES hydramnios
EXCLUDES 1 encounter for suspected maternal and fetal conditions ruled out (Z03.7-)

One of the following 7th characters is to be assigned to each code under category O40. 7th character 0 is for single gestations and multiple gestations where the fetus is unspecified. 7th characters 1 through 9 are for cases of multiple gestations to identify the fetus for which the code applies. The appropriate code from category O30, Multiple gestation, must also be assigned when assigning a code from category O40 that has a 7th character of 1 through 9.
0   not applicable or unspecified
1   fetus 1
2   fetus 2
3   fetus 3
4   fetus 4
5   fetus 5
9   other fetus

SP IQ ☑ O40.1XX- **Polyhydramnios, first trimester**

SP ☑ O40.2XX- **Polyhydramnios, second trimester**

SP ☑ O40.3XX- **Polyhydramnios, third trimester**

IQ ☑ O40.9XX- **Polyhydramnios, unspecified trimester**

④ O41 Other disorders of amniotic fluid and membranes
EXCLUDES 1 encounter for suspected maternal and fetal conditions ruled out (Z03.7-)

One of the following 7th characters is to be assigned to each code under category O41. 7th character 0 is for single gestations and multiple gestations where the fetus is unspecified. 7th characters 1 through 9 are for cases of multiple gestations to identify the fetus for which the code applies. The appropriate code from category O30, Multiple gestation, must also be assigned when assigning a code from category O41 that has a 7th character of 1 through 9.
0   not applicable or unspecified
1   fetus 1
2   fetus 2
3   fetus 3
4   fetus 4
5   fetus 5
9   other fetus

⑤ O41.0 Oligohydramnios
Oligohydramnios without rupture of membranes

Chapter 15

O00-O9A

★ New ▲ Revised Px Primary SP PDGM Px SL Low CoM SH High CoM IQ Quest. Encounter H Hospice non-cancer Dx   Unspecified   M *Manifestation*

DecisionHealth's FY 2020 Complete Home Health ICD-10-CM Diagnosis Coding Manual

1343

IQ 7 O41.00X- Oligohydramnios, unspecified trimester

SP 7 O41.01X- Oligohydramnios, first trimester

SP 7 O41.02X- Oligohydramnios, second trimester

SP 7 O41.03X- Oligohydramnios, third trimester

5 O41.1 Infection of amniotic sac and membranes

6 O41.10 Infection of amniotic sac and membranes, unspecified

IQ 7 O41.101- Infection of amniotic sac and membranes, unspecified, first trimester

IQ 7 O41.102- Infection of amniotic sac and membranes, unspecified, second trimester

IQ 7 O41.103- Infection of amniotic sac and membranes, unspecified, third trimester

IQ 7 O41.109- Infection of amniotic sac and membranes, unspecified, unspecified trimester

6 O41.12 Chorioamnionitis

SP 7 O41.121- Chorioamnionitis, first trimester

SP 7 O41.122- Chorioamnionitis, second trimester

SP 7 O41.123- Chorioamnionitis, third trimester

IQ 7 O41.129- Chorioamnionitis, unspecified trimester

6 O41.14 Placentitis

SP 7 O41.141- Placentitis, first trimester

SP 7 O41.142- Placentitis, second trimester

SP 7 O41.143- Placentitis, third trimester

IQ 7 O41.149- Placentitis, unspecified trimester

5 O41.8 Other specified disorders of amniotic fluid and membranes

6 O41.8X Other specified disorders of amniotic fluid and membranes

SP 7 O41.8X1- Other specified disorders of amniotic fluid and membranes, first trimester

SP 7 O41.8X2- Other specified disorders of amniotic fluid and membranes, second trimester

SP 7 O41.8X3- Other specified disorders of amniotic fluid and membranes, third trimester

IQ 7 O41.8X9- Other specified disorders of amniotic fluid and membranes, unspecified trimester

5 O41.9 Disorder of amniotic fluid and membranes, unspecified

IQ 7 O41.90X- Disorder of amniotic fluid and membranes, unspecified, unspecified trimester

IQ 7 O41.91X- Disorder of amniotic fluid and membranes, unspecified, first trimester

IQ 7 O41.92X- Disorder of amniotic fluid and membranes, unspecified, second trimester

IQ 7 O41.93X- Disorder of amniotic fluid and membranes, unspecified, third trimester

4 O42 Premature rupture of membranes

5 O42.0 Premature rupture of membranes, onset of labor within 24 hours of rupture

IQ O42.00 Premature rupture of membranes, onset of labor within 24 hours of rupture, unspecified weeks of gestation

6 O42.01 Preterm premature rupture of membranes, onset of labor within 24 hours of rupture
Premature rupture of membranes before 37 completed weeks of gestation

SP O42.011 Preterm premature rupture of membranes, onset of labor within 24 hours of rupture, first trimester

SP O42.012 Preterm premature rupture of membranes, onset of labor within 24 hours of rupture, second trimester

SP O42.013 Preterm premature rupture of membranes, onset of labor within 24 hours of rupture, third trimester

IQ O42.019 Preterm premature rupture of membranes, onset of labor within 24 hours of rupture, unspecified trimester

SP O42.02 Full-term premature rupture of membranes, onset of labor within 24 hours of rupture
Premature rupture of membranes at or after 37 completed weeks of gestation, onset of labor within 24 hours of rupture

5 O42.1 Premature rupture of membranes, onset of labor more than 24 hours following rupture

IQ O42.10 Premature rupture of membranes, onset of labor more than 24 hours following rupture, unspecified weeks of gestation

6 O42.11 Preterm premature rupture of membranes, onset of labor more than 24 hours following rupture
Premature rupture of membranes before 37 completed weeks of gestation

SP O42.111 Preterm premature rupture of membranes, onset of labor more than 24 hours following rupture, first trimester

SP O42.112 Preterm premature rupture of membranes, onset of labor more than 24 hours following rupture, second trimester

SP O42.113 Preterm premature rupture of membranes, onset of labor more than 24 hours following rupture, third trimester

---

4 4th digit required   5 5th digit required   6 6th digit required   7 7th digit required   7 7th digit placeholder   ✚ Additional code   ⊟ Laterality

IQ O42.119 Preterm premature rupture of membranes, onset of labor more than 24 hours following rupture, unspecified trimester

SP O42.12 Full-term premature rupture of membranes, onset of labor more than 24 hours following rupture
Premature rupture of membranes at or after 37 completed weeks of gestation, onset of labor more than 24 hours following rupture

5 O42.9 Premature rupture of membranes, unspecified as to length of time between rupture and onset of labor

IQ O42.90 Premature rupture of membranes, unspecified as to length of time between rupture and onset of labor, unspecified weeks of gestation

6 O42.91 Preterm premature rupture of membranes, unspecified as to length of time between rupture and onset of labor
Premature rupture of membranes before 37 completed weeks of gestation

SP O42.911 Preterm premature rupture of membranes, unspecified as to length of time between rupture and onset of labor, first trimester

SP O42.912 Preterm premature rupture of membranes, unspecified as to length of time between rupture and onset of labor, second trimester

SP O42.913 Preterm premature rupture of membranes, unspecified as to length of time between rupture and onset of labor, third trimester

IQ O42.919 Preterm premature rupture of membranes, unspecified as to length of time between rupture and onset of labor, unspecified trimester

SP O42.92 Full-term premature rupture of membranes, unspecified as to length of time between rupture and onset of labor
Premature rupture of membranes at or after 37 completed weeks of gestation, unspecified as to length of time between rupture and onset of labor

4 O43 Placental disorders
> EXCLUDES 2   maternal care for poor fetal growth due to placental insufficiency (O36.5-)
> placenta previa (O44.-)
> placental polyp (O90.89)
> placentitis (O41.14-)
> premature separation of placenta [abruptio placentae] (O45.-)

5 O43.0 Placental transfusion syndromes

6 O43.01 Fetomaternal placental transfusion syndrome

Maternofetal placental transfusion syndrome

SP O43.011 Fetomaternal placental transfusion syndrome, first trimester

SP O43.012 Fetomaternal placental transfusion syndrome, second trimester

SP O43.013 Fetomaternal placental transfusion syndrome, third trimester

IQ O43.019 Fetomaternal placental transfusion syndrome, unspecified trimester

6 O43.02 Fetus-to-fetus placental transfusion syndrome

SP O43.021 Fetus-to-fetus placental transfusion syndrome, first trimester

SP O43.022 Fetus-to-fetus placental transfusion syndrome, second trimester

SP O43.023 Fetus-to-fetus placental transfusion syndrome, third trimester

IQ O43.029 Fetus-to-fetus placental transfusion syndrome, unspecified trimester

5 O43.1 Malformation of placenta

6 O43.10 Malformation of placenta, unspecified

Abnormal placenta NOS

IQ O43.101 Malformation of placenta, unspecified, first trimester

IQ O43.102 Malformation of placenta, unspecified, second trimester

IQ O43.103 Malformation of placenta, unspecified, third trimester

IQ O43.109 Malformation of placenta, unspecified, unspecified trimester

6 O43.11 Circumvallate placenta

SP O43.111 Circumvallate placenta, first trimester

SP O43.112 Circumvallate placenta, second trimester

SP O43.113 Circumvallate placenta, third trimester

IQ O43.119 Circumvallate placenta, unspecified trimester

6 O43.12 Velamentous insertion of umbilical cord

SP O43.121 Velamentous insertion of umbilical cord, first trimester

SP O43.122 Velamentous insertion of umbilical cord, second trimester

SP O43.123 Velamentous insertion of umbilical cord, third trimester

IQ O43.129 Velamentous insertion of umbilical cord, unspecified trimester

6 O43.19 Other malformation of placenta

SP O43.191 Other malformation of placenta, first trimester

SP O43.192 Other malformation of placenta, second trimester

★ New ▲ Revised **Px** Primary **SP** PDGM Px **SL** Low CoM **SH** High CoM **IQ** Quest. Encounter **H** Hospice non-cancer Dx   Unspecified   **M** *Manifestation*

DecisionHealth's FY 2020 Complete Home Health ICD-10-CM Diagnosis Coding Manual   1345

SP **O43.193** Other malformation of placenta, third trimester

!Q **O43.199** Other malformation of placenta, unspecified trimester

5 **O43.2** Morbidly adherent placenta
Code also:
associated third stage postpartum hemorrhage, if applicable (O72.0)
EXCLUDES 1 retained placenta (O73.-)

6 **O43.21** Placenta accreta

SP **O43.211** Placenta accreta, first trimester

SP **O43.212** Placenta accreta, second trimester

SP **O43.213** Placenta accreta, third trimester

!Q **O43.219** Placenta accreta, unspecified trimester

6 **O43.22** Placenta increta

SP **O43.221** Placenta increta, first trimester

SP **O43.222** Placenta increta, second trimester

SP **O43.223** Placenta increta, third trimester

!Q **O43.229** Placenta increta, unspecified trimester

6 **O43.23** Placenta percreta

SP **O43.231** Placenta percreta, first trimester

SP **O43.232** Placenta percreta, second trimester

SP **O43.233** Placenta percreta, third trimester

!Q **O43.239** Placenta percreta, unspecified trimester

5 **O43.8** Other placental disorders

6 **O43.81** Placental infarction

SP **O43.811** Placental infarction, first trimester

SP **O43.812** Placental infarction, second trimester

SP **O43.813** Placental infarction, third trimester

!Q **O43.819** Placental infarction, unspecified trimester

6 **O43.89** Other placental disorders
Placental dysfunction

SP **O43.891** Other placental disorders, first trimester

SP **O43.892** Other placental disorders, second trimester

SP **O43.893** Other placental disorders, third trimester

!Q **O43.899** Other placental disorders, unspecified trimester

5 **O43.9** Unspecified placental disorder

!Q **O43.90** Unspecified placental disorder, unspecified trimester

!Q **O43.91** Unspecified placental disorder, first trimester

!Q **O43.92** Unspecified placental disorder, second trimester

!Q **O43.93** Unspecified placental disorder, third trimester

4 **O44** Placenta previa

5 **O44.0** Complete placenta previa NOS or without hemorrhage
Placenta previa NOS

!Q **O44.00** Complete placenta previa NOS or without hemorrhage, unspecified trimester

SP **O44.01** Complete placenta previa NOS or without hemorrhage, first trimester

SP **O44.02** Complete placenta previa NOS or without hemorrhage, second trimester

SP **O44.03** Complete placenta previa NOS or without hemorrhage, third trimester

5 **O44.1** Complete placenta previa with hemorrhage
EXCLUDES 1 labor and delivery complicated by hemorrhage from vasa previa (O69.4)

!Q **O44.10** Complete placenta previa with hemorrhage, unspecified trimester

SP **O44.11** Complete placenta previa with hemorrhage, first trimester

SP **O44.12** Complete placenta previa with hemorrhage, second trimester

SP **O44.13** Complete placenta previa with hemorrhage, third trimester

5 **O44.2** Partial placenta previa without hemorrhage
Marginal placenta previa, NOS or without hemorrhage

!Q **O44.20** Partial placenta previa NOS or without hemorrhage, unspecified trimester

SP **O44.21** Partial placenta previa NOS or without hemorrhage, first trimester

SP **O44.22** Partial placenta previa NOS or without hemorrhage, second trimester

SP **O44.23** Partial placenta previa NOS or without hemorrhage, third trimester

5 **O44.3** Partial placenta previa with hemorrhage
Marginal placenta previa with hemorrhage

!Q **O44.30** Partial placenta previa with hemorrhage, unspecified trimester

SP **O44.31** Partial placenta previa with hemorrhage, first trimester

SP **O44.32** Partial placenta previa with hemorrhage, second trimester

SP **O44.33** Partial placenta previa with hemorrhage, third trimester

5 **O44.4** Low lying placenta NOS or without hemorrhage
Low implantation of placenta NOS or without hemorrhage

!Q **O44.40** Low lying placenta NOS or without hemorrhage, unspecified trimester

SP **O44.41** Low lying placenta NOS or without hemorrhage, first trimester

SP **O44.42** Low lying placenta NOS or without hemorrhage, second trimester

SP **O44.43** Low lying placenta NOS or without hemorrhage, third trimester

5 **O44.5** Low lying placenta with hemorrhage
Low implantation of placenta with hemorrhage

!Q **O44.50** Low lying placenta with hemorrhage, unspecified trimester

SP **O44.51** Low lying placenta with hemorrhage, first trimester

4 4th digit required   **5** 5th digit required   **6** 6th digit required   **7** 7th digit required   **7** 7th digit placeholder   **+** Additional code   **5** Laterality

1346   *DecisionHealth's* FY 2020 Complete Home Health ICD-10-CM Diagnosis Coding Manual

SP O44.52 Low lying placenta with hemorrhage, second trimester

SP O44.53 Low lying placenta with hemorrhage, third trimester

4 O45 Premature separation of placenta [abruptio placentae]

5 O45.0 Premature separation of placenta with coagulation defect

6 O45.00 Premature separation of placenta with coagulation defect, unspecified

IQ O45.001 Premature separation of placenta with coagulation defect, unspecified, first trimester

SP O45.002 Premature separation of placenta with coagulation defect, unspecified, second trimester

SP O45.003 Premature separation of placenta with coagulation defect, unspecified, third trimester

IQ O45.009 Premature separation of placenta with coagulation defect, unspecified, unspecified trimester

6 O45.01 Premature separation of placenta with afibrinogenemia
Premature separation of placenta with hypofibrinogenemia

SP O45.011 Premature separation of placenta with afibrinogenemia, first trimester

SP O45.012 Premature separation of placenta with afibrinogenemia, second trimester

SP O45.013 Premature separation of placenta with afibrinogenemia, third trimester

IQ O45.019 Premature separation of placenta with afibrinogenemia, unspecified trimester

6 O45.02 Premature separation of placenta with disseminated intravascular coagulation

SP O45.021 Premature separation of placenta with disseminated intravascular coagulation, first trimester

SP O45.022 Premature separation of placenta with disseminated intravascular coagulation, second trimester

SP O45.023 Premature separation of placenta with disseminated intravascular coagulation, third trimester

IQ O45.029 Premature separation of placenta with disseminated intravascular coagulation, unspecified trimester

6 O45.09 Premature separation of placenta with other coagulation defect

SP O45.091 Premature separation of placenta with other coagulation defect, first trimester

SP O45.092 Premature separation of placenta with other coagulation defect, second trimester

SP O45.093 Premature separation of placenta with other coagulation defect, third trimester

IQ O45.099 Premature separation of placenta with other coagulation defect, unspecified trimester

5 O45.8 Other premature separation of placenta

6 O45.8X Other premature separation of placenta

SP O45.8X1 Other premature separation of placenta, first trimester

SP O45.8X2 Other premature separation of placenta, second trimester

SP O45.8X3 Other premature separation of placenta, third trimester

IQ O45.8X9 Other premature separation of placenta, unspecified trimester

5 O45.9 Premature separation of placenta, unspecified
Abruptio placentae NOS

IQ O45.90 Premature separation of placenta, unspecified, unspecified trimester

SP O45.91 Premature separation of placenta, unspecified, first trimester

SP O45.92 Premature separation of placenta, unspecified, second trimester

SP O45.93 Premature separation of placenta, unspecified, third trimester

4 O46 Antepartum hemorrhage, not elsewhere classified

EXCLUDES 1 hemorrhage in early pregnancy (O20.-)
intrapartum hemorrhage NEC (O67.-)
placenta previa (O44.-)
premature separation of placenta [abruptio placentae] (O45.-)

5 O46.0 Antepartum hemorrhage with coagulation defect

6 O46.00 Antepartum hemorrhage with coagulation defect, unspecified

SP O46.001 Antepartum hemorrhage with coagulation defect, unspecified, first trimester

SP O46.002 Antepartum hemorrhage with coagulation defect, unspecified, second trimester

SP O46.003 Antepartum hemorrhage with coagulation defect, unspecified, third trimester

IQ O46.009 Antepartum hemorrhage with coagulation defect, unspecified, unspecified trimester

6 O46.01 Antepartum hemorrhage with afibrinogenemia
Antepartum hemorrhage with hypofibrinogenemia

SP O46.011 Antepartum hemorrhage with afibrinogenemia, first trimester

SP O46.012 Antepartum hemorrhage with afibrinogenemia, second trimester

SP O46.013 Antepartum hemorrhage with afibrinogenemia, third trimester

IQ O46.019 Antepartum hemorrhage with afibrinogenemia, unspecified trimester

---

★ New ▲ Revised Px Primary **SP** PDGM Px **SL** Low CoM **SH** High CoM **IQ** Quest. Encounter **H** Hospice non-cancer Dx | Unspecified | **M** *Manifestation*

6 O46.02   Antepartum hemorrhage with disseminated intravascular coagulation

SP O46.021   Antepartum hemorrhage with disseminated intravascular coagulation, first trimester

SP O46.022   Antepartum hemorrhage with disseminated intravascular coagulation, second trimester

SP O46.023   Antepartum hemorrhage with disseminated intravascular coagulation, third trimester

IQ O46.029   Antepartum hemorrhage with disseminated intravascular coagulation, unspecified trimester

6 O46.09   Antepartum hemorrhage with other coagulation defect

SP O46.091   Antepartum hemorrhage with other coagulation defect, first trimester

SP O46.092   Antepartum hemorrhage with other coagulation defect, second trimester

SP O46.093   Antepartum hemorrhage with other coagulation defect, third trimester

IQ O46.099   Antepartum hemorrhage with other coagulation defect, unspecified trimester

5 O46.8   Other antepartum hemorrhage

6 O46.8X   Other antepartum hemorrhage

SP O46.8X1   Other antepartum hemorrhage, first trimester

SP O46.8X2   Other antepartum hemorrhage, second trimester

SP O46.8X3   Other antepartum hemorrhage, third trimester

IQ O46.8X9   Other antepartum hemorrhage, unspecified trimester

5 O46.9   Antepartum hemorrhage, unspecified

IQ O46.90   Antepartum hemorrhage, unspecified, unspecified trimester

SP O46.91   Antepartum hemorrhage, unspecified, first trimester

SP O46.92   Antepartum hemorrhage, unspecified, second trimester

SP O46.93   Antepartum hemorrhage, unspecified, third trimester

4 O47   False labor
INCLUDES   Braxton Hicks contractions
threatened labor
EXCLUDES 1   preterm labor (O60.-)

5 O47.0   False labor before 37 completed weeks of gestation

IQ O47.00   False labor before 37 completed weeks of gestation, unspecified trimester

SP O47.02   False labor before 37 completed weeks of gestation, second trimester

SP O47.03   False labor before 37 completed weeks of gestation, third trimester

SP O47.1   False labor at or after 37 completed weeks of gestation

IQ O47.9   False labor, unspecified

4 O48   Late pregnancy

SP O48.0   Post-term pregnancy
Pregnancy over 40 completed weeks to 42 completed weeks gestation

SP O48.1   Prolonged pregnancy
Pregnancy which has advanced beyond 42 completed weeks gestation

Complications of labor and delivery (O60-O77)

4 O60   Preterm labor
INCLUDES   onset (spontaneous) of labor before 37 completed weeks of gestation
EXCLUDES 1   false labor (O47.0-)
threatened labor NOS (O47.0-)

5 O60.0   Preterm labor without delivery

IQ O60.00   Preterm labor without delivery, unspecified trimester

SP O60.02   Preterm labor without delivery, second trimester

SP O60.03   Preterm labor without delivery, third trimester

5 O60.1   Preterm labor with preterm delivery

One of the following 7th characters is to be assigned to each code under subcategory O60.1. 7th character 0 is for single gestations and multiple gestations where the fetus is unspecified. 7th characters 1 through 9 are for cases of multiple gestations to identify the fetus for which the code applies. The appropriate code from category O30, Multiple gestation, must also be assigned when assigning a code from subcategory O60.1 that has a 7th character of 1 through 9.
0   not applicable or unspecified
1   fetus 1
2   fetus 2
3   fetus 3
4   fetus 4
5   fetus 5
9   other fetus

IQ ☑ O60.10X-   Preterm labor with preterm delivery, unspecified trimester
Preterm labor with delivery NOS

SP ☑ O60.12X-   Preterm labor second trimester with preterm delivery second trimester

SP ☑ O60.13X-   Preterm labor second trimester with preterm delivery third trimester

SP ☑ O60.14X-   Preterm labor third trimester with preterm delivery third trimester

5 O60.2   Term delivery with preterm labor

---

4 4th digit required   5 5th digit required   6 6th digit required   7 7th digit required   ☑ 7th digit placeholder   ✚ Additional code   ▤ Laterality

1348   DecisionHealth's FY 2020 Complete Home Health ICD-10-CM Diagnosis Coding Manual

One of the following 7th characters is to be assigned to each code under subcategory O60.2. 7th character 0 is for single gestations and multiple gestations where the fetus is unspecified. 7th characters 1 through 9 are for cases of multiple gestations to identify the fetus for which the code applies. The appropriate code from category O30, Multiple gestation, must also be assigned when assigning a code from subcategory O60.2 that has a 7th character of 1 through 9.

0	not applicable or unspecified
1	fetus 1
2	fetus 2
3	fetus 3
4	fetus 4
5	fetus 5
9	other fetus

[IQ] [☑] O60.20X- **Term delivery with preterm labor, unspecified trimester**

[SP] [☑] O60.22X- **Term delivery with preterm labor, second trimester**

[SP] [☑] O60.23X- **Term delivery with preterm labor, third trimester**

[4] O61 **Failed induction of labor**

[IQ] O61.0 **Failed medical induction of labor**
Failed induction (of labor) by oxytocin
Failed induction (of labor) by prostaglandins

[IQ] O61.1 **Failed instrumental induction of labor**
Failed mechanical induction (of labor)
Failed surgical induction (of labor)

[IQ] O61.8 **Other failed induction of labor**

[IQ] O61.9 **Failed induction of labor, unspecified**

[4] O62 **Abnormalities of forces of labor**

[IQ] O62.0 **Primary inadequate contractions**
Failure of cervical dilatation
Primary hypotonic uterine dysfunction
Uterine inertia during latent phase of labor

[IQ] O62.1 **Secondary uterine inertia**
Arrested active phase of labor
Secondary hypotonic uterine dysfunction

[IQ] O62.2 **Other uterine inertia**
Atony of uterus without hemorrhage
Atony of uterus NOS
Desultory labor
Hypotonic uterine dysfunction NOS
Irregular labor
Poor contractions
Slow slope active phase of labor
Uterine inertia NOS
EXCLUDES 1 atony of uterus with hemorrhage (postpartum) (O72.1)
postpartum atony of uterus without hemorrhage (O75.89)

[IQ] O62.3 **Precipitate labor**
DEFINITION Labor occurring quickly, with rapid expulsion of the fetus.

[IQ] O62.4 **Hypertonic, incoordinate, and prolonged uterine contractions**
Cervical spasm
Contraction ring dystocia
Dyscoordinate labor

Hour-glass contraction of uterus
Hypertonic uterine dysfunction
Incoordinate uterine action
Tetanic contractions
Uterine dystocia NOS
Uterine spasm
EXCLUDES 1 dystocia (fetal) (maternal) NOS (O66.9)

[IQ] O62.8 **Other abnormalities of forces of labor**

[IQ] O62.9 **Abnormality of forces of labor, unspecified**

[4] O63 **Long labor**

[IQ] O63.0 **Prolonged first stage (of labor)**

[IQ] O63.1 **Prolonged second stage (of labor)**

[IQ] O63.2 **Delayed delivery of second twin, triplet, etc.**

[IQ] O63.9 **Long labor, unspecified**
Prolonged labor NOS

[4] O64 **Obstructed labor due to malposition and malpresentation of fetus**

One of the following 7th characters is to be assigned to each code under category O64. 7th character 0 is for single gestations and multiple gestations where the fetus is unspecified. 7th characters 1 through 9 are for cases of multiple gestations to identify the fetus for which the code applies. The appropriate code from category O30, Multiple gestation, must also be assigned when assigning a code from category O64 that has a 7th character of 1 through 9.

0	not applicable or unspecified
1	fetus 1
2	fetus 2
3	fetus 3
4	fetus 4
5	fetus 5
9	other fetus

[IQ] [☑] O64.0XX- **Obstructed labor due to incomplete rotation of fetal head**
Deep transverse arrest
Obstructed labor due to persistent occipitoiliac (position)
Obstructed labor due to persistent occipitoposterior (position)
Obstructed labor due to persistent occipitosacral (position)
Obstructed labor due to persistent occipitotransverse (position)

[IQ] [☑] O64.1XX- **Obstructed labor due to breech presentation**
Obstructed labor due to buttocks presentation
Obstructed labor due to complete breech presentation
Obstructed labor due to frank breech presentation

[IQ] [☑] O64.2XX- **Obstructed labor due to face presentation**
Obstructed labor due to chin presentation

[IQ] [☑] O64.3XX- **Obstructed labor due to brow presentation**

[IQ] [☑] O64.4XX- **Obstructed labor due to shoulder presentation**

★ New ▲ Revised Px Primary **SP** PDGM Px **SL** Low CoM **SH** High CoM **IQ** Quest. Encounter **H** Hospice non-cancer Dx Unspecified **M** *Manifestation*

DecisionHealth's FY 2020 Complete Home Health ICD-10-CM Diagnosis Coding Manual

1349

Chapter 15

O00-O9A

Prolapsed arm
EXCLUDES 1 impacted shoulders
(O66.0)
shoulder dystocia
(O66.0)

IQ ☑ **O64.5XX- Obstructed labor due to compound presentation**

IQ ☑ **O64.8XX- Obstructed labor due to other malposition and malpresentation**
Obstructed labor due to footling presentation
Obstructed labor due to incomplete breech presentation

IQ ☑ **O64.9XX- Obstructed labor due to malposition and malpresentation, unspecified**

4 O65 Obstructed labor due to maternal pelvic abnormality

IQ O65.0 Obstructed labor due to deformed pelvis

IQ O65.1 Obstructed labor due to generally contracted pelvis

IQ O65.2 Obstructed labor due to pelvic inlet contraction

IQ O65.3 Obstructed labor due to pelvic outlet and mid-cavity contraction

IQ O65.4 Obstructed labor due to fetopelvic disproportion, unspecified
EXCLUDES 1 dystocia due to abnormality of fetus (O66.2-O66.3)

IQ + O65.5 Obstructed labor due to abnormality of maternal pelvic organs
Obstructed labor due to conditions listed in O34.-
Use additional code to identify abnormality of pelvic organs O34.-

IQ O65.8 Obstructed labor due to other maternal pelvic abnormalities

IQ O65.9 Obstructed labor due to maternal pelvic abnormality, unspecified

4 O66 Other obstructed labor

IQ O66.0 Obstructed labor due to shoulder dystocia
Impacted shoulders
DEFINITION Shoulders of the fetus become caught in the pelvis during delivery.

IQ O66.1 Obstructed labor due to locked twins

IQ O66.2 Obstructed labor due to unusually large fetus

IQ + O66.3 Obstructed labor due to other abnormalities of fetus
Dystocia due to fetal ascites
Dystocia due to fetal hydrops
Dystocia due to fetal meningomyelocele
Dystocia due to fetal sacral teratoma
Dystocia due to fetal tumor
Dystocia due to hydrocephalic fetus
Use additional code to identify cause of obstruction

5 O66.4 Failed trial of labor

IQ O66.40 Failed trial of labor, unspecified

IQ O66.41 Failed attempted vaginal birth after previous cesarean delivery
Code first:
rupture of uterus, if applicable (O71.0-, O71.1)

IQ O66.5 Attempted application of vacuum extractor and forceps
Attempted application of vacuum or forceps, with subsequent delivery by forceps or cesarean delivery

IQ O66.6 Obstructed labor due to other multiple fetuses

IQ + O66.8 Other specified obstructed labor
Use additional code to identify cause of obstruction

IQ O66.9 Obstructed labor, unspecified
Dystocia NOS
Fetal dystocia NOS
Maternal dystocia NOS

4 O67 Labor and delivery complicated by intrapartum hemorrhage, not elsewhere classified
EXCLUDES 1 antepartum hemorrhage NEC (O46.-)
placenta previa (O44.-)
premature separation of placenta [abruptio placentae] (O45.-)
EXCLUDES 2 postpartum hemorrhage (O72.-)

SP O67.0 Intrapartum hemorrhage with coagulation defect
Intrapartum hemorrhage (excessive) associated with afibrinogenemia
Intrapartum hemorrhage (excessive) associated with disseminated intravascular coagulation
Intrapartum hemorrhage (excessive) associated with hyperfibrinolysis
Intrapartum hemorrhage (excessive) associated with hypofibrinogenemia

SP O67.8 Other intrapartum hemorrhage
Excessive intrapartum hemorrhage

SP O67.9 Intrapartum hemorrhage, unspecified

SP O68 Labor and delivery complicated by abnormality of fetal acid-base balance
Fetal acidemia complicating labor and delivery
Fetal acidosis complicating labor and delivery
Fetal alkalosis complicating labor and delivery
Fetal metabolic acidemia complicating labor and delivery
EXCLUDES 1 fetal stress NOS (O77.9)
labor and delivery complicated by electrocardiographic evidence of fetal stress (O77.8)
labor and delivery complicated by ultrasonic evidence of fetal stress (O77.8)
EXCLUDES 2 abnormality in fetal heart rate or rhythm (O76)
labor and delivery complicated by meconium in amniotic fluid (O77.0)

4 O69 Labor and delivery complicated by umbilical cord complications

---

4 4th digit required   **5** 5th digit required   **6** 6th digit required   **7** 7th digit required   ☑ 7th digit placeholder   **+** Additional code   **⊟** Laterality

Chapter 15

O00-O9A

One of the following 7th characters is to be assigned to each code under category O69. 7th character 0 is for single gestations and multiple gestations where the fetus is unspecified. 7th characters 1 through 9 are for cases of multiple gestations to identify the fetus for which the code applies. The appropriate code from category O30, Multiple gestation, must also be assigned when assigning a code from category O69 that has a 7th character of 1 through 9.

0	not applicable or unspecified
1	fetus 1
2	fetus 2
3	fetus 3
4	fetus 4
5	fetus 5
9	other fetus

!Q ☑ O69.0XX- **Labor and delivery complicated by prolapse of cord**

!Q ☑ O69.1XX- **Labor and delivery complicated by cord around neck, with compression**

> **EXCLUDES 1** labor and delivery complicated by cord around neck, without compression (O69.81)

!Q ☑ O69.2XX- **Labor and delivery complicated by other cord entanglement, with compression**

Labor and delivery complicated by compression of cord NOS
Labor and delivery complicated by entanglement of cords of twins in monoamniotic sac
Labor and delivery complicated by knot in cord

> **EXCLUDES 1** labor and delivery complicated by other cord entanglement, without compression (O69.82)

!Q ☑ O69.3XX- **Labor and delivery complicated by short cord**

!Q ☑ O69.4XX- **Labor and delivery complicated by vasa previa**

Labor and delivery complicated by hemorrhage from vasa previa

!Q ☑ O69.5XX- **Labor and delivery complicated by vascular lesion of cord**

Labor and delivery complicated by cord bruising
Labor and delivery complicated by cord hematoma
Labor and delivery complicated by thrombosis of umbilical vessels

⑤ O69.8 Labor and delivery complicated by other cord complications

!Q ☑ O69.81X- **Labor and delivery complicated by cord around neck, without compression**

!Q ☑ O69.82X- **Labor and delivery complicated by other cord entanglement, without compression**

!Q ☑ O69.89X- **Labor and delivery complicated by other cord complications**

!Q ☑ O69.9XX- **Labor and delivery complicated by cord complication, unspecified**

④ O70 Perineal laceration during delivery

> **INCLUDES** episiotomy extended by laceration

> **EXCLUDES 1** obstetric high vaginal laceration alone (O71.4)

SP O70.0 First degree perineal laceration during delivery

Perineal laceration, rupture or tear involving fourchette during delivery
Perineal laceration, rupture or tear involving labia during delivery
Perineal laceration, rupture or tear involving skin during delivery
Perineal laceration, rupture or tear involving vagina during delivery
Perineal laceration, rupture or tear involving vulva during delivery
Slight perineal laceration, rupture or tear during delivery

SP O70.1 Second degree perineal laceration during delivery

Perineal laceration, rupture or tear during delivery as in O70.0, also involving pelvic floor
Perineal laceration, rupture or tear during delivery as in O70.0, also involving perineal muscles
Perineal laceration, rupture or tear during delivery as in O70.0, also involving vaginal muscles

> **EXCLUDES 1** perineal laceration involving anal sphincter (O70.2)

⑤ O70.2 Third degree perineal laceration during delivery

Perineal laceration, rupture or tear during delivery as in O70.1, also involving anal sphincter
Perineal laceration, rupture or tear during delivery as in O70.1, also involving rectovaginal septum
Perineal laceration, rupture or tear during delivery as in O70.1, also involving sphincter NOS

> **EXCLUDES 1** anal sphincter tear during delivery without third degree perineal laceration (O70.4)
> perineal laceration involving anal or rectal mucosa (O70.3)

SP O70.20 **Third degree perineal laceration during delivery, unspecified**

SP O70.21 Third degree perineal laceration during delivery, IIIa

Third degree perineal laceration during delivery with less than 50% of external anal sphincter (EAS) thickness torn

SP O70.22 Third degree perineal laceration during delivery, IIIb

Third degree perineal laceration during delivery with more than 50% external anal sphincter (EAS) thickness torn

---

★ New ▲ Revised **Px** Primary **SP** PDGM Px **SL** Low CoM **SH** High CoM **!Q** Quest. Encounter **H** Hospice non-cancer Dx Unspecified **M** *Manifestation*

SP O70.23 Third degree perineal laceration during delivery, IIIc
Third degree perineal laceration during delivery with both external anal sphincter (EAS) and internal anal sphincter (IAS) torn

SP O70.3 Fourth degree perineal laceration during delivery
Perineal laceration, rupture or tear during delivery as in O70.2, also involving anal mucosa
Perineal laceration, rupture or tear during delivery as in O70.2, also involving rectal mucosa

SP O70.4 Anal sphincter tear complicating delivery, not associated with third degree laceration
EXCLUDES 1 anal sphincter tear with third degree perineal laceration (O70.2)

SP O70.9 Perineal laceration during delivery, unspecified

4 O71 Other obstetric trauma
INCLUDES obstetric damage from instruments

5 O71.0 Rupture of uterus (spontaneous) before onset of labor
EXCLUDES 1 disruption of (current) cesarean delivery wound (O90.0)
laceration of uterus, NEC (O71.81)

IQ O71.00 Rupture of uterus before onset of labor, unspecified trimester

SP O71.02 Rupture of uterus before onset of labor, second trimester

SP O71.03 Rupture of uterus before onset of labor, third trimester

SP O71.1 Rupture of uterus during labor
Rupture of uterus not stated as occurring before onset of labor
EXCLUDES 1 disruption of cesarean delivery wound (O90.0)
laceration of uterus, NEC (O71.81)

SP O71.2 Postpartum inversion of uterus

SP O71.3 Obstetric laceration of cervix
Annular detachment of cervix

SP O71.4 Obstetric high vaginal laceration alone
Laceration of vaginal wall without perineal laceration
EXCLUDES 1 obstetric high vaginal laceration with perineal laceration (O70.-)

SP O71.5 Other obstetric injury to pelvic organs
Obstetric injury to bladder
Obstetric injury to urethra
EXCLUDES 2 obstetric periurethral trauma (O71.82)

SP O71.6 Obstetric damage to pelvic joints and ligaments
Obstetric avulsion of inner symphyseal cartilage
Obstetric damage to coccyx
Obstetric traumatic separation of symphysis (pubis)

SP O71.7 Obstetric hematoma of pelvis
Obstetric hematoma of perineum

Obstetric hematoma of vagina
Obstetric hematoma of vulva

5 O71.8 Other specified obstetric trauma

SP O71.81 Laceration of uterus, not elsewhere classified

SP O71.82 Other specified trauma to perineum and vulva
Obstetric periurethral trauma

SP O71.89 Other specified obstetric trauma

IQ O71.9 Obstetric trauma, unspecified

4 O72 Postpartum hemorrhage
INCLUDES hemorrhage after delivery of fetus or infant

SP O72.0 Third-stage hemorrhage
Hemorrhage associated with retained, trapped or adherent placenta
Retained placenta NOS
Code also:
type of adherent placenta (O43.2-)

SP O72.1 Other immediate postpartum hemorrhage
Hemorrhage following delivery of placenta
Postpartum hemorrhage (atonic) NOS
Uterine atony with hemorrhage
EXCLUDES 1 uterine atony NOS (O62.2)
uterine atony without hemorrhage (O62.2)
postpartum atony of uterus without hemorrhage (O75.89)

SP O72.2 Delayed and secondary postpartum hemorrhage
Hemorrhage associated with retained portions of placenta or membranes after the first 24 hours following delivery of placenta
Retained products of conception NOS, following delivery

SP O72.3 Postpartum coagulation defects
Postpartum afibrinogenemia
Postpartum fibrinolysis

4 O73 Retained placenta and membranes, without hemorrhage
EXCLUDES 1 placenta accreta (O43.21-)
placenta increta (O43.22-)
placenta percreta (O43.23-)

SP O73.0 Retained placenta without hemorrhage
Adherent placenta, without hemorrhage
Trapped placenta without hemorrhage

SP O73.1 Retained portions of placenta and membranes, without hemorrhage
Retained products of conception following delivery, without hemorrhage

+ 4 O74 Complications of anesthesia during labor and delivery
INCLUDES maternal complications arising from the administration of a general, regional or local anesthetic, analgesic or other sedation during labor and delivery
Use additional code, if applicable, to identify specific complication

SP + O74.0 Aspiration pneumonitis due to anesthesia during labor and delivery
Inhalation of stomach contents or secretions NOS due to anesthesia during labor and delivery

4 4th digit required   5 5th digit required   6 6th digit required   7 7th digit required   7 7th digit placeholder   + Additional code   ☰ Laterality

1352   DecisionHealth's FY 2020 Complete Home Health ICD-10-CM Diagnosis Coding Manual

Chapter 15

O00-O9A

Mendelson's syndrome due to anesthesia during labor and delivery

SP ✚ O74.1 **Other pulmonary complications of anesthesia during labor and delivery**

SP ✚ O74.2 **Cardiac complications of anesthesia during labor and delivery**

SP ✚ O74.3 **Central nervous system complications of anesthesia during labor and delivery**

SP ✚ O74.4 **Toxic reaction to local anesthesia during labor and delivery**

SP ✚ O74.5 **Spinal and epidural anesthesia-induced headache during labor and delivery**

SP ✚ O74.6 **Other complications of spinal and epidural anesthesia during labor and delivery**

SP ✚ O74.7 **Failed or difficult intubation for anesthesia during labor and delivery**

SP ✚ O74.8 **Other complications of anesthesia during labor and delivery**

IQ ✚ O74.9 **Complication of anesthesia during labor and delivery, unspecified**

◢ O75 **Other complications of labor and delivery, not elsewhere classified**

> EXCLUDES 2 puerperal (postpartum) infection (O86.-)
> puerperal (postpartum) sepsis (O85)

SP O75.0 **Maternal distress during labor and delivery**

SP O75.1 **Shock during or following labor and delivery**

Obstetric shock following labor and delivery

SP O75.2 **Pyrexia during labor, not elsewhere classified**

SP ✚ O75.3 **Other infection during labor**

Sepsis during labor

Use additional code (B95-B97), to identify infectious agent

SP ✚ O75.4 **Other complications of obstetric surgery and procedures**

Cardiac arrest following obstetric surgery or procedures

Cardiac failure following obstetric surgery or procedures

Cerebral anoxia following obstetric surgery or procedures

Pulmonary edema following obstetric surgery or procedures

Use additional code to identify specific complication

> EXCLUDES 2 complications of anesthesia during labor and delivery (O74.-)
> disruption of obstetrical (surgical) wound (O90.0-O90.1)
> hematoma of obstetrical (surgical) wound (O90.2)
> infection of obstetrical (surgical) wound (O86.0-)

SP O75.5 **Delayed delivery after artificial rupture of membranes**

⑤ O75.8 **Other specified complications of labor and delivery**

SP O75.81 **Maternal exhaustion complicating labor and delivery**

IQ O75.82 **Onset (spontaneous) of labor after 37 completed weeks of gestation but before 39 completed weeks gestation, with delivery by (planned) cesarean section**

Delivery by (planned) cesarean section occurring after 37 completed weeks of gestation but before 39 completed weeks gestation due to (spontaneous) onset of labor

Code first to specify reason for planned cesarean section such as:
cephalopelvic disproportion (normally formed fetus) (O33.9)
previous cesarean delivery (O34.21)

SP O75.89 **Other specified complications of labor and delivery**

IQ O75.9 **Complication of labor and delivery, unspecified**

SP O76 **Abnormality in fetal heart rate and rhythm complicating labor and delivery**

Depressed fetal heart rate tones complicating labor and delivery

Fetal bradycardia complicating labor and delivery

Fetal heart rate decelerations complicating labor and delivery

Fetal heart rate irregularity complicating labor and delivery

Fetal heart rate abnormal variability complicating labor and delivery

Fetal tachycardia complicating labor and delivery

Non-reassuring fetal heart rate or rhythm complicating labor and delivery

> EXCLUDES 1 fetal stress NOS (O77.9)
> labor and delivery complicated by electrocardiographic evidence of fetal stress (O77.8)
> labor and delivery complicated by ultrasonic evidence of fetal stress (O77.8)

> EXCLUDES 2 fetal metabolic acidemia (O68)
> other fetal stress (O77.0-O77.1)

◢ O77 **Other fetal stress complicating labor and delivery**

SP O77.0 **Labor and delivery complicated by meconium in amniotic fluid**

SP O77.1 **Fetal stress in labor or delivery due to drug administration**

SP O77.8 **Labor and delivery complicated by other evidence of fetal stress**

Labor and delivery complicated by electrocardiographic evidence of fetal stress

Labor and delivery complicated by ultrasonic evidence of fetal stress

> EXCLUDES 1 abnormality of fetal acid-base balance (O68)
> abnormality in fetal heart rate or rhythm (O76)
> fetal metabolic acidemia (O68)

IQ O77.9 **Labor and delivery complicated by fetal stress, unspecified**

> EXCLUDES 1 abnormality of fetal acid-base balance (O68)

★ New ▲ Revised Px Primary **SP** PDGM Px **SL** Low CoM **SH** High CoM **IQ** Quest. Encounter **H** Hospice non-cancer Dx Unspecified **M** *Manifestation*

DecisionHealth's FY 2020 Complete Home Health ICD-10-CM Diagnosis Coding Manual

1353

Chapter 15

O00-O9A

abnormality in fetal heart
rate or rhythm (O76)
fetal metabolic acidemia
(O68)

Encounter for delivery   (O80-O82)

IQ + O80   **Encounter for full-term uncomplicated delivery**
Delivery requiring minimal or no assistance, with or without episiotomy, without fetal manipulation [e.g., rotation version] or instrumentation [forceps] of a spontaneous, cephalic, vaginal, full-term, single, live-born infant. This code is for use as a single diagnosis code and is not to be used with any other code from chapter 15.
Use additional code to indicate outcome of delivery (Z37.0)

IQ + O82   **Encounter for cesarean delivery without indication**
Use additional code to indicate outcome of delivery (Z37.0)

Complications predominantly related to the puerperium   (O85-O92)

EXCLUDES 2   mental and behavioral disorders associated with the puerperium (F53.-)
obstetrical tetanus (A34)
puerperal osteomalacia (M83.0)

GUIDELINES   **Section I.C.15.a.2)**
Chapter 15 codes are to be used only on the maternal record, never on the record of the newborn.

SP + O85   **Puerperal sepsis**
Postpartum sepsis
Puerperal peritonitis
Puerperal pyemia
Use additional code (B95-B97), to identify infectious agent
Use additional code (R65.2-) to identify severe sepsis, if applicable
EXCLUDES 1   fever of unknown origin following delivery (O86.4)
genital tract infection following delivery (O86.1-)
obstetric pyemic and septic embolism (O88.3-)
puerperal septic thrombophlebitis (O86.81)
urinary tract infection following delivery (O86.2-)
EXCLUDES 2   sepsis during labor (O75.3)

+ 4 O86   **Other puerperal infections**
Use additional code (B95-B97), to identify infectious agent
EXCLUDES 2   infection during labor (O75.3)
obstetrical tetanus (A34)

GUIDELINES   Section I.C.1.d.5)(b-c)
For infections following a procedure, a code from T81.40, to T81.43 Infection following a procedure, or a code from O86.00 to O86.03, Infection of obstetric surgical wound, that identifies the site of the infection should be coded first, if known. Assign an additional code for sepsis following a procedure (T81.44) or sepsis following an obstetrical procedure (O86.04). Use an additional code to identify the infectious agent. If the patient has severe sepsis, the appropriate code from subcategory R65.2 should also be assigned with the additional code(s) for any acute organ dysfunction.

If a postprocedural infection has resulted in postprocedural septic shock, assign the codes indicated above for sepsis due to a postprocedural infection, followed by code T81.12-, Postprocedural septic shock. Do not assign code R65.21, Severe sepsis with septic shock. Additional code(s) should be assigned for any acute organ dysfunction.

+ 5 O86.0   **Infection of obstetric surgical wound**
Infected cesarean delivery wound following delivery
Infected perineal repair following delivery
EXCLUDES 1   complications of procedures, not elsewhere classified (T81.4-)
postprocedural fever NOS (R50.82)
postprocedural retroperitoneal abscess (K68.11)

SP + O86.00   **Infection of obstetric surgical wound, unspecified**

SP + O86.01   **Infection of obstetric surgical wound, superficial incisional site**
Subcutaneous abscess following an obstetrical procedure
Stitch abscess following an obstetrical procedure

▲ SP + O86.02   **Infection of obstetric surgical wound, deep incisional site**
Intramuscular abscess following an obstetrical procedure
Sub-fascial abscess following an obstetrical procedure

SP + O86.03   **Infection of obstetric surgical wound, organ and space site**
Intraabdominal abscess following an obstetrical procedure
Subphrenic abscess following an obstetrical procedure

SP + O86.04   **Sepsis following an obstetrical procedure**
Use additional code to identify the sepsis

SP + O86.09   **Infection of obstetric surgical wound, other surgical site**

+ 5 O86.1   **Other infection of genital tract following delivery**

SP + O86.11   **Cervicitis following delivery**

SP + O86.12   **Endometritis following delivery**

SP + O86.13   **Vaginitis following delivery**

---

4 4th digit required   5 5th digit required   6 6th digit required   7 7th digit required   7 7th digit placeholder   +Additional code   ⬛ Laterality

1354   *DecisionHealth's* FY 2020 Complete Home Health ICD-10-CM Diagnosis Coding Manual

Chapter 15

O00-O9A

SP + O86.19 Other infection of genital tract following delivery

+ 5 O86.2 Urinary tract infection following delivery

SP + O86.20 Urinary tract infection following delivery, unspecified
Puerperal urinary tract infection NOS

SP + O86.21 Infection of kidney following delivery

SP + O86.22 Infection of bladder following delivery
Infection of urethra following delivery

SP + O86.29 Other urinary tract infection following delivery

SP + O86.4 Pyrexia of unknown origin following delivery
Puerperal infection NOS following delivery
Puerperal pyrexia NOS following delivery
EXCLUDES 2 pyrexia during labor (O75.2)

+ 5 O86.8 Other specified puerperal infections

SP + O86.81 Puerperal septic thrombophlebitis

SP + O86.89 Other specified puerperal infections

4 O87 Venous complications and hemorrhoids in the puerperium
INCLUDES venous complications in labor, delivery and the puerperium
EXCLUDES 2 obstetric embolism (O88.-)
puerperal septic thrombophlebitis (O86.81)
venous complications in pregnancy (O22.-)

SP O87.0 Superficial thrombophlebitis in the puerperium
Puerperal phlebitis NOS
Puerperal thrombosis NOS

SP + O87.1 Deep phlebothrombosis in the puerperium
Deep vein thrombosis, postpartum
Pelvic thrombophlebitis, postpartum
Use additional code to identify the deep vein thrombosis (I82.4-, I82.5-, I82.62-. I82.72-)
Use additional code, if applicable, for associated long-term (current) use of anticoagulants (Z79.01)

SP O87.2 Hemorrhoids in the puerperium

SP O87.3 Cerebral venous thrombosis in the puerperium
Cerebrovenous sinus thrombosis in the puerperium

SP O87.4 Varicose veins of lower extremity in the puerperium

SP O87.8 Other venous complications in the puerperium
Genital varices in the puerperium

SP O87.9 Venous complication in the puerperium, unspecified
Puerperal phlebopathy NOS

4 O88 Obstetric embolism
EXCLUDES 1 embolism complicating abortion NOS (O03.2)
embolism complicating ectopic or molar pregnancy (O08.2)
embolism complicating failed attempted abortion (O07.2)

embolism complicating induced abortion (O04.7)
embolism complicating spontaneous abortion (O03.2, O03.7)

5 O88.0 Obstetric air embolism

6 O88.01 Obstetric air embolism in pregnancy

SP O88.011 Air embolism in pregnancy, first trimester

SP O88.012 Air embolism in pregnancy, second trimester

SP O88.013 Air embolism in pregnancy, third trimester

SP O88.019 Air embolism in pregnancy, unspecified trimester

SP O88.02 Air embolism in childbirth

SP O88.03 Air embolism in the puerperium

5 O88.1 Amniotic fluid embolism
Anaphylactoid syndrome in pregnancy

6 O88.11 Amniotic fluid embolism in pregnancy

SP O88.111 Amniotic fluid embolism in pregnancy, first trimester

SP O88.112 Amniotic fluid embolism in pregnancy, second trimester

SP O88.113 Amniotic fluid embolism in pregnancy, third trimester

SP O88.119 Amniotic fluid embolism in pregnancy, unspecified trimester

SP O88.12 Amniotic fluid embolism in childbirth

SP O88.13 Amniotic fluid embolism in the puerperium

5 O88.2 Obstetric thromboembolism

6 O88.21 Thromboembolism in pregnancy
Obstetric (pulmonary) embolism NOS

SP O88.211 Thromboembolism in pregnancy, first trimester

SP O88.212 Thromboembolism in pregnancy, second trimester

SP O88.213 Thromboembolism in pregnancy, third trimester

SP O88.219 Thromboembolism in pregnancy, unspecified trimester

SP O88.22 Thromboembolism in childbirth

SP O88.23 Thromboembolism in the puerperium
Puerperal (pulmonary) embolism NOS

5 O88.3 Obstetric pyemic and septic embolism

6 O88.31 Pyemic and septic embolism in pregnancy

SP O88.311 Pyemic and septic embolism in pregnancy, first trimester

SP O88.312 Pyemic and septic embolism in pregnancy, second trimester

SP O88.313 Pyemic and septic embolism in pregnancy, third trimester

SP O88.319 Pyemic and septic embolism in pregnancy, unspecified trimester

SP O88.32 Pyemic and septic embolism in childbirth

SP O88.33 Pyemic and septic embolism in the puerperium

5 O88.8 Other obstetric embolism
Obstetric fat embolism

Chapter 15

O00-O9A

★ New ▲ Revised Px Primary **SP** PDGM Px **SL** Low CoM **SH** High CoM **IQ** Quest. Encounter **H** Hospice non-cancer Dx Unspecified **M** *Manifestation*

⑥ O88.81 Other embolism in pregnancy

SP O88.811 Other embolism in pregnancy, first trimester

SP O88.812 Other embolism in pregnancy, second trimester

SP O88.813 Other embolism in pregnancy, third trimester

SP O88.819 Other embolism in pregnancy, unspecified trimester

SP O88.82 Other embolism in childbirth

SP O88.83 Other embolism in the puerperium

➕ ④ O89 Complications of anesthesia during the puerperium
> **INCLUDES** maternal complications arising from the administration of a general, regional or local anesthetic, analgesic or other sedation during the puerperium

Use additional code, if applicable, to identify specific complication

➕ ⑤ O89.0 Pulmonary complications of anesthesia during the puerperium

SP ➕ O89.01 Aspiration pneumonitis due to anesthesia during the puerperium
Inhalation of stomach contents or secretions NOS due to anesthesia during the puerperium
Mendelson's syndrome due to anesthesia during the puerperium

SP ➕ O89.09 Other pulmonary complications of anesthesia during the puerperium

SP ➕ O89.1 Cardiac complications of anesthesia during the puerperium

SP ➕ O89.2 Central nervous system complications of anesthesia during the puerperium

SP ➕ O89.3 Toxic reaction to local anesthesia during the puerperium

SP ➕ O89.4 Spinal and epidural anesthesia-induced headache during the puerperium

SP ➕ O89.5 Other complications of spinal and epidural anesthesia during the puerperium

SP ➕ O89.6 Failed or difficult intubation for anesthesia during the puerperium

SP ➕ O89.8 Other complications of anesthesia during the puerperium

SP ➕ O89.9 Complication of anesthesia during the puerperium, unspecified

④ O90 Complications of the puerperium, not elsewhere classified

SP O90.0 Disruption of cesarean delivery wound
Dehiscence of cesarean delivery wound
> **EXCLUDES 1** rupture of uterus (spontaneous) before onset of labor (O71.0-)
> rupture of uterus during labor (O71.1)

SP O90.1 Disruption of perineal obstetric wound
Disruption of wound of episiotomy
Disruption of wound of perineal laceration
Secondary perineal tear

SP O90.2 Hematoma of obstetric wound

SP O90.3 Peripartum cardiomyopathy
Conditions in I42.- arising during pregnancy and the puerperium

> **EXCLUDES 1** pre-existing heart disease complicating pregnancy and the puerperium (O99.4-)

> **GUIDELINES** Section I.C.15.o.5)
Pregnancy associated cardiomyopathy, code O90.3, is unique in that it may be diagnosed in the third trimester of pregnancy but may continue to progress months after delivery. For this reason, it is referred to as peripartum cardiomyopathy. Code O90.3 is only for use when the cardiomyopathy develops as a result of pregnancy in a woman who did not have pre-existing heart disease.

SP O90.4 Postpartum acute kidney failure
Hepatorenal syndrome following labor and delivery

SP O90.5 Postpartum thyroiditis

SP O90.6 Postpartum mood disturbance
Postpartum blues
Postpartum dysphoria
Postpartum sadness
> **EXCLUDES 1** postpartum depression (F53.0)
> puerperal psychosis (F53.1)

⑤ O90.8 Other complications of the puerperium, not elsewhere classified

SP O90.81 Anemia of the puerperium
Postpartum anemia NOS
> **EXCLUDES 1** pre-existing anemia complicating the puerperium (O99.03)

> **CODING TIPS ✓** Use O90.81 for diagnosed anemia complicating the postpartum period. Use O99.01 for anemia complicating pregnancy. Use O99.03 for pre-existing anemia complicating the puerperium.

SP O90.89 Other complications of the puerperium, not elsewhere classified
Placental polyp

SP O90.9 Complication of the puerperium, unspecified

➕ ④ O91 Infections of breast associated with pregnancy, the puerperium and lactation
Use additional code to identify infection

➕ ⑤ O91.0 Infection of nipple associated with pregnancy, the puerperium and lactation

➕ ⑥ O91.01 Infection of nipple associated with pregnancy
Gestational abscess of nipple

SP ➕ O91.011 Infection of nipple associated with pregnancy, first trimester

SP ➕ O91.012 Infection of nipple associated with pregnancy, second trimester

SP ➕ O91.013 Infection of nipple associated with pregnancy, third trimester

SP ➕ O91.019 Infection of nipple associated with pregnancy, unspecified trimester

SP ➕ O91.02 Infection of nipple associated with the puerperium
Puerperal abscess of nipple

SP ➕ O91.03 Infection of nipple associated with lactation

---

④4th digit required   ⑤5th digit required   ⑥6th digit required   ⑦7th digit required   ☑7th digit placeholder   ➕Additional code   ⊟Laterality

Abscess of nipple associated with lactation

+ ⑤ O91.1 Abscess of breast associated with pregnancy, the puerperium and lactation

+ ⑥ O91.11 Abscess of breast associated with pregnancy
Gestational mammary abscess
Gestational purulent mastitis
Gestational subareolar abscess

⑤ᴾ + O91.111 Abscess of breast associated with pregnancy, first trimester

⑤ᴾ + O91.112 Abscess of breast associated with pregnancy, second trimester

⑤ᴾ + O91.113 Abscess of breast associated with pregnancy, third trimester

⑤ᴾ + O91.119 Abscess of breast associated with pregnancy, unspecified trimester

⑤ᴾ + O91.12 Abscess of breast associated with the puerperium
Puerperal mammary abscess
Puerperal purulent mastitis
Puerperal subareolar abscess

⑤ᴾ + O91.13 Abscess of breast associated with lactation
Mammary abscess associated with lactation
Purulent mastitis associated with lactation
Subareolar abscess associated with lactation

+ ⑤ O91.2 Nonpurulent mastitis associated with pregnancy, the puerperium and lactation

+ ⑥ O91.21 Nonpurulent mastitis associated with pregnancy
Gestational interstitial mastitis
Gestational lymphangitis of breast
Gestational mastitis NOS
Gestational parenchymatous mastitis

⑤ᴾ + O91.211 Nonpurulent mastitis associated with pregnancy, first trimester

⑤ᴾ + O91.212 Nonpurulent mastitis associated with pregnancy, second trimester

⑤ᴾ + O91.213 Nonpurulent mastitis associated with pregnancy, third trimester

!ᴑ + O91.219 Nonpurulent mastitis associated with pregnancy, unspecified trimester

⑤ᴾ + O91.22 Nonpurulent mastitis associated with the puerperium
Puerperal interstitial mastitis
Puerperal lymphangitis of breast
Puerperal mastitis NOS
Puerperal parenchymatous mastitis

⑤ᴾ + O91.23 Nonpurulent mastitis associated with lactation
Interstitial mastitis associated with lactation
Lymphangitis of breast associated with lactation
Mastitis NOS associated with lactation
Parenchymatous mastitis associated with lactation

④ O92 Other disorders of breast and disorders of lactation associated with pregnancy and the puerperium

⑤ O92.0 Retracted nipple associated with pregnancy, the puerperium, and lactation

⑥ O92.01 Retracted nipple associated with pregnancy

⑤ᴾ O92.011 Retracted nipple associated with pregnancy, first trimester

⑤ᴾ O92.012 Retracted nipple associated with pregnancy, second trimester

⑤ᴾ O92.013 Retracted nipple associated with pregnancy, third trimester

!ᴑ O92.019 Retracted nipple associated with pregnancy, unspecified trimester

⑤ᴾ O92.02 Retracted nipple associated with the puerperium

⑤ᴾ O92.03 Retracted nipple associated with lactation

⑤ O92.1 Cracked nipple associated with pregnancy, the puerperium, and lactation
Fissure of nipple, gestational or puerperal

⑥ O92.11 Cracked nipple associated with pregnancy

⑤ᴾ O92.111 Cracked nipple associated with pregnancy, first trimester

⑤ᴾ O92.112 Cracked nipple associated with pregnancy, second trimester

⑤ᴾ O92.113 Cracked nipple associated with pregnancy, third trimester

!ᴑ O92.119 Cracked nipple associated with pregnancy, unspecified trimester

⑤ᴾ O92.12 Cracked nipple associated with the puerperium

⑤ᴾ O92.13 Cracked nipple associated with lactation

⑤ O92.2 Other and unspecified disorders of breast associated with pregnancy and the puerperium

!ᴑ O92.20 Unspecified disorder of breast associated with pregnancy and the puerperium

⑤ᴾ O92.29 Other disorders of breast associated with pregnancy and the puerperium

⑤ᴾ O92.3 Agalactia
Primary agalactia
> **EXCLUDES 1** Elective agalactia (O92.5)
> Secondary agalactia (O92.5)
> Therapeutic agalactia (O92.5)

⑤ᴾ O92.4 Hypogalactia

⑤ᴾ O92.5 Suppressed lactation
Elective agalactia
Secondary agalactia
Therapeutic agalactia
> **EXCLUDES 1** primary agalactia (O92.3)

⑤ᴾ O92.6 Galactorrhea

⑤ O92.7 Other and unspecified disorders of lactation

!ᴑ O92.70 Unspecified disorders of lactation

⑤ᴾ O92.79 Other disorders of lactation
Puerperal galactocele

★ New ▲ Revised Px Primary ⑤ᴾ PDGM Px ⑤ᴸ Low CoM ⑤ᴴ High CoM !ᴑ Quest. Encounter Ⓗ Hospice non-cancer Dx Unspecified M *Manifestation*

DecisionHealth's FY 2020 Complete Home Health ICD-10-CM Diagnosis Coding Manual

1357

Chapter 15

O00-O9A

Other obstetric conditions, not elsewhere classified (O94-O9A)

SP O94 Sequelae of complication of pregnancy, childbirth, and the puerperium
Note:
This category is to be used to indicate conditions in O00-O77.-, O85-O94 and O98-O9A.- as the cause of late effects. The sequelae include conditions specified as such, or as late effects, which may occur at any time after the puerperium
Code first:
condition resulting from (sequela) of complication of pregnancy, childbirth, and the puerperium

GUIDELINES Section I.C.15.p.1)-3)
Code O94 is for use in those cases when an initial complication of a pregnancy develops a sequelae requiring care or treatment at a future date. This code may be used at any time after the initial postpartum period. This code, like all sequela codes, is to be sequenced following the code describing the sequelae of the complication.

+ 4 O98 Maternal infectious and parasitic diseases classifiable elsewhere but complicating pregnancy, childbirth and the puerperium
INCLUDES the listed conditions when complicating the pregnant state, when aggravated by the pregnancy, or as a reason for obstetric care
Use additional code (Chapter 1), to identify specific infectious or parasitic disease
EXCLUDES 2 herpes gestationis (O26.4-)
infectious carrier state (O99.82-, O99.83-)
obstetrical tetanus (A34)
puerperal infection (O86.-)
puerperal sepsis (O85)
when the reason for maternal care is that the disease is known or suspected to have affected the fetus (O35-O36)

+ 5 O98.0 Tuberculosis complicating pregnancy, childbirth and the puerperium
Conditions in A15-A19
+ 6 O98.01 Tuberculosis complicating pregnancy
SP + O98.011 Tuberculosis complicating pregnancy, first trimester
SP + O98.012 Tuberculosis complicating pregnancy, second trimester
SP + O98.013 Tuberculosis complicating pregnancy, third trimester
IQ + O98.019 Tuberculosis complicating pregnancy, unspecified trimester
SP + O98.02 Tuberculosis complicating childbirth
SP + O98.03 Tuberculosis complicating the puerperium
+ 5 O98.1 Syphilis complicating pregnancy, childbirth and the puerperium
Conditions in A50-A53
+ 6 O98.11 Syphilis complicating pregnancy
SP + O98.111 Syphilis complicating pregnancy, first trimester

SP + O98.112 Syphilis complicating pregnancy, second trimester
SP + O98.113 Syphilis complicating pregnancy, third trimester
IQ + O98.119 Syphilis complicating pregnancy, unspecified trimester
SP + O98.12 Syphilis complicating childbirth
SP + O98.13 Syphilis complicating the puerperium
+ 5 O98.2 Gonorrhea complicating pregnancy, childbirth and the puerperium
Conditions in A54.-
+ 6 O98.21 Gonorrhea complicating pregnancy
SP + O98.211 Gonorrhea complicating pregnancy, first trimester
SP + O98.212 Gonorrhea complicating pregnancy, second trimester
SP + O98.213 Gonorrhea complicating pregnancy, third trimester
IQ + O98.219 Gonorrhea complicating pregnancy, unspecified trimester
SP + O98.22 Gonorrhea complicating childbirth
SP + O98.23 Gonorrhea complicating the puerperium
+ 5 O98.3 Other infections with a predominantly sexual mode of transmission complicating pregnancy, childbirth and the puerperium
Conditions in A55-A64
+ 6 O98.31 Other infections with a predominantly sexual mode of transmission complicating pregnancy
SP + O98.311 Other infections with a predominantly sexual mode of transmission complicating pregnancy, first trimester
SP + O98.312 Other infections with a predominantly sexual mode of transmission complicating pregnancy, second trimester
SP + O98.313 Other infections with a predominantly sexual mode of transmission complicating pregnancy, third trimester
IQ + O98.319 Other infections with a predominantly sexual mode of transmission complicating pregnancy, unspecified trimester
SP + O98.32 Other infections with a predominantly sexual mode of transmission complicating childbirth
SP + O98.33 Other infections with a predominantly sexual mode of transmission complicating the puerperium
+ 5 O98.4 Viral hepatitis complicating pregnancy, childbirth and the puerperium
Conditions in B15-B19
+ 6 O98.41 Viral hepatitis complicating pregnancy
SP + O98.411 Viral hepatitis complicating pregnancy, first trimester
SP + O98.412 Viral hepatitis complicating pregnancy, second trimester
SP + O98.413 Viral hepatitis complicating pregnancy, third trimester

---

4 4th digit required   5 5th digit required   6 6th digit required   7 7th digit required   7 7th digit placeholder   + Additional code   ⊟ Laterality

IQ ✚ **O98.419** Viral hepatitis complicating pregnancy, unspecified trimester

SP ✚ **O98.42** Viral hepatitis complicating childbirth

SP ✚ **O98.43** Viral hepatitis complicating the puerperium

✚ 5 **O98.5** Other viral diseases complicating pregnancy, childbirth and the puerperium

Conditions in A80-B09, B25-B34, R87.81-, R87.82-

> **EXCLUDES 1** human immunodeficiency virus [HIV] disease complicating pregnancy, childbirth and the puerperium (O98.7-)

✚ 6 **O98.51** Other viral diseases complicating pregnancy

SP ✚ **O98.511** Other viral diseases complicating pregnancy, first trimester

SP ✚ **O98.512** Other viral diseases complicating pregnancy, second trimester

SP ✚ **O98.513** Other viral diseases complicating pregnancy, third trimester

IQ ✚ **O98.519** Other viral diseases complicating pregnancy, unspecified trimester

SP ✚ **O98.52** Other viral diseases complicating childbirth

SP ✚ **O98.53** Other viral diseases complicating the puerperium

✚ 5 **O98.6** Protozoal diseases complicating pregnancy, childbirth and the puerperium

Conditions in B50-B64

✚ 6 **O98.61** Protozoal diseases complicating pregnancy

SP ✚ **O98.611** Protozoal diseases complicating pregnancy, first trimester

SP ✚ **O98.612** Protozoal diseases complicating pregnancy, second trimester

SP ✚ **O98.613** Protozoal diseases complicating pregnancy, third trimester

IQ ✚ **O98.619** Protozoal diseases complicating pregnancy, unspecified trimester

SP ✚ **O98.62** Protozoal diseases complicating childbirth

SP ✚ **O98.63** Protozoal diseases complicating the puerperium

✚ 5 **O98.7** Human immunodeficiency virus [HIV] disease complicating pregnancy, childbirth and the puerperium

Use additional code to identify the type of HIV disease:
Acquired immune deficiency syndrome (AIDS) (B20)
Asymptomatic HIV status (Z21)
HIV positive NOS (Z21)
Symptomatic HIV disease (B20)

> **GUIDELINES** Section I.C.1.a.2)(g)
> During pregnancy, childbirth or the puerperium, a patient admitted (or presenting for a health care encounter) because of an HIV-related illness should receive a principal diagnosis code of O98.7-, followed by B20 and the code(s) for the HIV-related illness(es). Codes from Chapter 15 always take sequencing priority.
>
> Patients with asymptomatic HIV infection status admitted (or presenting for a health care encounter) during pregnancy, childbirth, or the puerperium should receive codes of O98.7- and Z21.

✚ 6 **O98.71** Human immunodeficiency virus [HIV] disease complicating pregnancy

SP ✚ **O98.711** Human immunodeficiency virus [HIV] disease complicating pregnancy, first trimester

SP ✚ **O98.712** Human immunodeficiency virus [HIV] disease complicating pregnancy, second trimester

SP ✚ **O98.713** Human immunodeficiency virus [HIV] disease complicating pregnancy, third trimester

IQ ✚ **O98.719** Human immunodeficiency virus [HIV] disease complicating pregnancy, unspecified trimester

SP ✚ **O98.72** Human immunodeficiency virus [HIV] disease complicating childbirth

SP ✚ **O98.73** Human immunodeficiency virus [HIV] disease complicating the puerperium

✚ 5 **O98.8** Other maternal infectious and parasitic diseases complicating pregnancy, childbirth and the puerperium

✚ 6 **O98.81** Other maternal infectious and parasitic diseases complicating pregnancy

SP ✚ **O98.811** Other maternal infectious and parasitic diseases complicating pregnancy, first trimester

SP ✚ **O98.812** Other maternal infectious and parasitic diseases complicating pregnancy, second trimester

SP ✚ **O98.813** Other maternal infectious and parasitic diseases complicating pregnancy, third trimester

IQ ✚ **O98.819** Other maternal infectious and parasitic diseases complicating pregnancy, unspecified trimester

SP ✚ **O98.82** Other maternal infectious and parasitic diseases complicating childbirth

SP ✚ **O98.83** Other maternal infectious and parasitic diseases complicating the puerperium

✚ 5 **O98.9** Unspecified maternal infectious and parasitic disease complicating pregnancy, childbirth and the puerperium

✚ 6 **O98.91** Unspecified maternal infectious and parasitic disease complicating pregnancy

Chapter 15

O00-O9A

✶ New ▲ Revised **Px** Primary **SP** PDGM Px **SL** Low CoM **SH** High CoM **IQ** Quest. Encounter **H** Hospice non-cancer Dx Unspecified **M** *Manifestation*

IQ + O98.911 Unspecified maternal infectious and parasitic disease complicating pregnancy, first trimester

IQ + O98.912 Unspecified maternal infectious and parasitic disease complicating pregnancy, second trimester

IQ + O98.913 Unspecified maternal infectious and parasitic disease complicating pregnancy, third trimester

IQ + O98.919 Unspecified maternal infectious and parasitic disease complicating pregnancy, unspecified trimester

IQ + O98.92 Unspecified maternal infectious and parasitic disease complicating childbirth

IQ + O98.93 Unspecified maternal infectious and parasitic disease complicating the puerperium

+ 4 O99 Other maternal diseases classifiable elsewhere but complicating pregnancy, childbirth and the puerperium

INCLUDES   conditions which complicate the pregnant state, are aggravated by the pregnancy or are a main reason for obstetric care

Use additional code to identify specific condition

EXCLUDES 2   when the reason for maternal care is that the condition is known or suspected to have affected the fetus (O35-O36)

+ 5 O99.0 Anemia complicating pregnancy, childbirth and the puerperium

Conditions in D50-D64

EXCLUDES 1   anemia arising in the puerperium (O90.81) postpartum anemia NOS (O90.81)

+ 6 O99.01 Anemia complicating pregnancy

CODING TIPS ✓   Use O90.81 for diagnosed anemia complicating the postpartum period. Use O99.01 for anemia complicating pregnancy. Use O99.03 for pre-existing anemia complicating the puerperium.

SP + O99.011 Anemia complicating pregnancy, first trimester

SP + O99.012 Anemia complicating pregnancy, second trimester

SP + O99.013 Anemia complicating pregnancy, third trimester

IQ + O99.019 Anemia complicating pregnancy, unspecified trimester

SP + O99.02 Anemia complicating childbirth

SP + O99.03 Anemia complicating the puerperium

EXCLUDES 1   postpartum anemia not pre-existing prior to delivery (O90.81)

CODING TIPS ✓   Use O90.81 for diagnosed anemia complicating the postpartum period. Use O99.01 for anemia complicating pregnancy. Use O99.03 for pre-existing anemia complicating the puerperium.

+ 5 O99.1 Other diseases of the blood and blood-forming organs and certain disorders involving the immune mechanism complicating pregnancy, childbirth and the puerperium

Conditions in D65-D89

EXCLUDES 1   hemorrhage with coagulation defects (O45.-, O46.0-, O67.0, O72.3)

+ 6 O99.11 Other diseases of the blood and blood-forming organs and certain disorders involving the immune mechanism complicating pregnancy

SP + O99.111 Other diseases of the blood and blood-forming organs and certain disorders involving the immune mechanism complicating pregnancy, first trimester

SP + O99.112 Other diseases of the blood and blood-forming organs and certain disorders involving the immune mechanism complicating pregnancy, second trimester

SP + O99.113 Other diseases of the blood and blood-forming organs and certain disorders involving the immune mechanism complicating pregnancy, third trimester

IQ + O99.119 Other diseases of the blood and blood-forming organs and certain disorders involving the immune mechanism complicating pregnancy, unspecified trimester

SP + O99.12 Other diseases of the blood and blood-forming organs and certain disorders involving the immune mechanism complicating childbirth

SP + O99.13 Other diseases of the blood and blood-forming organs and certain disorders involving the immune mechanism complicating the puerperium

+ 5 O99.2 Endocrine, nutritional and metabolic diseases complicating pregnancy, childbirth and the puerperium

Conditions in E00-E88

EXCLUDES 2   diabetes mellitus (O24.-) malnutrition (O25.-) postpartum thyroiditis (O90.5)

+ 6 O99.21 Obesity complicating pregnancy, childbirth, and the puerperium

Use additional code to identify the type of obesity (E66.-)

IQ + O99.210 Obesity complicating pregnancy, unspecified trimester

SP + O99.211 Obesity complicating pregnancy, first trimester

SP + O99.212 Obesity complicating pregnancy, second trimester

4 4th digit required   5 5th digit required   6 6th digit required   7 7th digit required   7 7th digit placeholder   + Additional code   ⊟ Laterality

1360   DecisionHealth's FY 2020 Complete Home Health ICD-10-CM Diagnosis Coding Manual

SP **+** **O99.213** **Obesity complicating pregnancy, third trimester**

SP **+** **O99.214** **Obesity complicating childbirth**

SP **+** **O99.215** **Obesity complicating the puerperium**

+ **6** **O99.28** **Other endocrine, nutritional and metabolic diseases complicating pregnancy, childbirth and the puerperium**

IQ **+** **O99.280** Endocrine, nutritional and metabolic diseases complicating pregnancy, unspecified trimester

SP **+** **O99.281** **Endocrine, nutritional and metabolic diseases complicating pregnancy, first trimester**

SP **+** **O99.282** **Endocrine, nutritional and metabolic diseases complicating pregnancy, second trimester**

SP **+** **O99.283** **Endocrine, nutritional and metabolic diseases complicating pregnancy, third trimester**

SP **+** **O99.284** **Endocrine, nutritional and metabolic diseases complicating childbirth**

SP **+** **O99.285** **Endocrine, nutritional and metabolic diseases complicating the puerperium**

+ **5** **O99.3** **Mental disorders and diseases of the nervous system complicating pregnancy, childbirth and the puerperium**

+ **6** **O99.31** **Alcohol use complicating pregnancy, childbirth, and the puerperium**
Use additional code(s) from F10 to identify manifestations of the alcohol use

IQ **+** **O99.310** Alcohol use complicating pregnancy, unspecified trimester

SP **+** **O99.311** **Alcohol use complicating pregnancy, first trimester**

SP **+** **O99.312** **Alcohol use complicating pregnancy, second trimester**

SP **+** **O99.313** **Alcohol use complicating pregnancy, third trimester**

SP **+** **O99.314** **Alcohol use complicating childbirth**

SP **+** **O99.315** **Alcohol use complicating the puerperium**

+ **6** **O99.32** **Drug use complicating pregnancy, childbirth, and the puerperium**
Use additional code(s) from F11-F16 and F18-F19 to identify manifestations of the drug use

IQ **+** **O99.320** Drug use complicating pregnancy, unspecified trimester

SP **+** **O99.321** **Drug use complicating pregnancy, first trimester**

SP **+** **O99.322** **Drug use complicating pregnancy, second trimester**

SP **+** **O99.323** **Drug use complicating pregnancy, third trimester**

SP **+** **O99.324** **Drug use complicating childbirth**

SP **+** **O99.325** **Drug use complicating the puerperium**

+ **6** **O99.33** **Tobacco use disorder complicating pregnancy, childbirth, and the puerperium**
Smoking complicating pregnancy, childbirth, and the puerperium

Use additional code from category F17 to identify type of tobacco nicotine dependence

IQ **+** **O99.330** Smoking (tobacco) complicating pregnancy, unspecified trimester

SP **+** **O99.331** **Smoking (tobacco) complicating pregnancy, first trimester**

SP **+** **O99.332** **Smoking (tobacco) complicating pregnancy, second trimester**

SP **+** **O99.333** **Smoking (tobacco) complicating pregnancy, third trimester**

SP **+** **O99.334** **Smoking (tobacco) complicating childbirth**

SP **+** **O99.335** **Smoking (tobacco) complicating the puerperium**

▲ **+** **6** **O99.34** **Other mental disorders complicating pregnancy, childbirth, and the puerperium**
Conditions in F01-F09, F20-F99 and F54-F99
> **EXCLUDES 2** postpartum mood disturbance (O90.6)
> postnatal psychosis (F53.1)
> puerperal psychosis (F53.1)

IQ **+** **O99.340** Other mental disorders complicating pregnancy, unspecified trimester

SP **+** **O99.341** **Other mental disorders complicating pregnancy, first trimester**

SP **+** **O99.342** **Other mental disorders complicating pregnancy, second trimester**

SP **+** **O99.343** **Other mental disorders complicating pregnancy, third trimester**

SP **+** **O99.344** **Other mental disorders complicating childbirth**

SP **+** **O99.345** **Other mental disorders complicating the puerperium**

+ **6** **O99.35** **Diseases of the nervous system complicating pregnancy, childbirth, and the puerperium**
Conditions in G00-G99
> **EXCLUDES 2** pregnancy related peripheral neuritis (O26.8-)

IQ **+** **O99.350** Diseases of the nervous system complicating pregnancy, unspecified trimester

SP **+** **O99.351** **Diseases of the nervous system complicating pregnancy, first trimester**

SP **+** **O99.352** **Diseases of the nervous system complicating pregnancy, second trimester**

SP **+** **O99.353** **Diseases of the nervous system complicating pregnancy, third trimester**

SP **+** **O99.354** **Diseases of the nervous system complicating childbirth**

SP **+** **O99.355** **Diseases of the nervous system complicating the puerperium**

+ **5** **O99.4** **Diseases of the circulatory system complicating pregnancy, childbirth and the puerperium**

Chapter 15

O00-O9A

★ New ▲ Revised Px Primary **SP** PDGM Px **SL** Low CoM **SH** High CoM **IQ** Quest. Encounter **H** Hospice non-cancer Dx ▊ Unspecified **M** *Manifestation*

DecisionHealth's FY 2020 Complete Home Health ICD-10-CM Diagnosis Coding Manual

1361

Conditions in I00-I99

EXCLUDES 1 peripartum cardiomyopathy (O90.3)

EXCLUDES 2 hypertensive disorders (O10-O16)
obstetric embolism (O88.-)
venous complications and cerebrovenous sinus thrombosis in labor, childbirth and the puerperium (O87.-)
venous complications and cerebrovenous sinus thrombosis in pregnancy (O22.-)

+ ⑥ O99.41 Diseases of the circulatory system complicating pregnancy

SP + O99.411 Diseases of the circulatory system complicating pregnancy, first trimester

SP + O99.412 Diseases of the circulatory system complicating pregnancy, second trimester

SP + O99.413 Diseases of the circulatory system complicating pregnancy, third trimester

IQ + O99.419 Diseases of the circulatory system complicating pregnancy, unspecified trimester

SP + O99.42 Diseases of the circulatory system complicating childbirth

SP + O99.43 Diseases of the circulatory system complicating the puerperium

+ ⑤ O99.5 Diseases of the respiratory system complicating pregnancy, childbirth and the puerperium
Conditions in J00-J99

+ ⑥ O99.51 Diseases of the respiratory system complicating pregnancy

SP + O99.511 Diseases of the respiratory system complicating pregnancy, first trimester

SP + O99.512 Diseases of the respiratory system complicating pregnancy, second trimester

SP + O99.513 Diseases of the respiratory system complicating pregnancy, third trimester

IQ + O99.519 Diseases of the respiratory system complicating pregnancy, unspecified trimester

SP + O99.52 Diseases of the respiratory system complicating childbirth

SP + O99.53 Diseases of the respiratory system complicating the puerperium

+ ⑤ O99.6 Diseases of the digestive system complicating pregnancy, childbirth and the puerperium
Conditions in K00-K93

EXCLUDES 2 hemorrhoids in pregnancy (O22.4-)
liver and biliary tract disorders in pregnancy, childbirth and the puerperium (O26.6-)

+ ⑥ O99.61 Diseases of the digestive system complicating pregnancy

SP + O99.611 Diseases of the digestive system complicating pregnancy, first trimester

SP + O99.612 Diseases of the digestive system complicating pregnancy, second trimester

SP + O99.613 Diseases of the digestive system complicating pregnancy, third trimester

IQ + O99.619 Diseases of the digestive system complicating pregnancy, unspecified trimester

SP + O99.62 Diseases of the digestive system complicating childbirth

SP + O99.63 Diseases of the digestive system complicating the puerperium

+ ⑤ O99.7 Diseases of the skin and subcutaneous tissue complicating pregnancy, childbirth and the puerperium
Conditions in L00-L99

EXCLUDES 2 herpes gestationis (O26.4)
pruritic urticarial papules and plaques of pregnancy (PUPPP) (O26.86)

+ ⑥ O99.71 Diseases of the skin and subcutaneous tissue complicating pregnancy

SP + O99.711 Diseases of the skin and subcutaneous tissue complicating pregnancy, first trimester

SP + O99.712 Diseases of the skin and subcutaneous tissue complicating pregnancy, second trimester

SP + O99.713 Diseases of the skin and subcutaneous tissue complicating pregnancy, third trimester

IQ + O99.719 Diseases of the skin and subcutaneous tissue complicating pregnancy, unspecified trimester

SP + O99.72 Diseases of the skin and subcutaneous tissue complicating childbirth

SP + O99.73 Diseases of the skin and subcutaneous tissue complicating the puerperium

▲ + ⑤ O99.8 Other specified diseases and conditions complicating pregnancy, childbirth and the puerperium
Conditions in D00-D48, H00-H95, M00-N99, and Q00-Q99
Use additional code to identify condition

EXCLUDES 2 genitourinary infections in pregnancy (O23.-)
infection of genitourinary tract following delivery (O86.1-O86.4)
malignant neoplasm complicating pregnancy, childbirth and the puerperium (O9A.1-)
maternal care for known or suspected abnormality of maternal pelvic organs (O34.-)
postpartum acute kidney failure (O90.4)
traumatic injuries in pregnancy (O9A.2-)

---

④ 4th digit required   **⑤** 5th digit required   **⑥** 6th digit required   **⑦** 7th digit required   **☑** 7th digit placeholder   **+** Additional code   **▤** Laterality

+ ⑥ O99.81 Abnormal glucose complicating pregnancy, childbirth and the puerperium
> EXCLUDES 1 gestational diabetes (O24.4-)

SP + O99.810 Abnormal glucose complicating pregnancy

SP + O99.814 Abnormal glucose complicating childbirth

SP + O99.815 Abnormal glucose complicating the puerperium

+ ⑥ O99.82 Streptococcus B carrier state complicating pregnancy, childbirth and the puerperium
> EXCLUDES 1 Carrier of streptococcus group B (GBS) in a nonpregnant woman (Z22.330)

SP + O99.820 Streptococcus B carrier state complicating pregnancy

SP + O99.824 Streptococcus B carrier state complicating childbirth

SP + O99.825 Streptococcus B carrier state complicating the puerperium

+ ⑥ O99.83 Other infection carrier state complicating pregnancy, childbirth and the puerperium
> Use additional code to identify the carrier state (Z22.-)

SP + O99.830 Other infection carrier state complicating pregnancy

SP + O99.834 Other infection carrier state complicating childbirth

SP + O99.835 Other infection carrier state complicating the puerperium

+ ⑥ O99.84 Bariatric surgery status complicating pregnancy, childbirth and the puerperium
> Gastric banding status complicating pregnancy, childbirth and the puerperium
> Gastric bypass status for obesity complicating pregnancy, childbirth and the puerperium
> Obesity surgery status complicating pregnancy, childbirth and the puerperium

IQ + O99.840 Bariatric surgery status complicating pregnancy, unspecified trimester

SP + O99.841 Bariatric surgery status complicating pregnancy, first trimester

SP + O99.842 Bariatric surgery status complicating pregnancy, second trimester

SP + O99.843 Bariatric surgery status complicating pregnancy, third trimester

SP + O99.844 Bariatric surgery status complicating childbirth

SP + O99.845 Bariatric surgery status complicating the puerperium

SP + O99.89 Other specified diseases and conditions complicating pregnancy, childbirth and the puerperium

④ O9A Maternal malignant neoplasms, traumatic injuries and abuse classifiable elsewhere but complicating pregnancy, childbirth and the puerperium

+ ⑤ O9A.1 Malignant neoplasm complicating pregnancy, childbirth and the puerperium
> Conditions in C00-C96
> Use additional code to identify neoplasm
> EXCLUDES 2 maternal care for benign tumor of corpus uteri (O34.1-)
> maternal care for benign tumor of cervix (O34.4-)

+ ⑥ O9A.11 Malignant neoplasm complicating pregnancy

SP + O9A.111 Malignant neoplasm complicating pregnancy, first trimester

SP + O9A.112 Malignant neoplasm complicating pregnancy, second trimester

SP + O9A.113 Malignant neoplasm complicating pregnancy, third trimester

IQ + O9A.119 Malignant neoplasm complicating pregnancy, unspecified trimester

SP + O9A.12 Malignant neoplasm complicating childbirth

SP + O9A.13 Malignant neoplasm complicating the puerperium

+ ⑤ O9A.2 Injury, poisoning and certain other consequences of external causes complicating pregnancy, childbirth and the puerperium
> Conditions in S00-T88, except T74 and T76
> Use additional code(s) to identify the injury or poisoning
> EXCLUDES 2 physical, sexual and psychological abuse complicating pregnancy, childbirth and the puerperium (O9A.3-, O9A.4-, O9A.5-)

+ ⑥ O9A.21 Injury, poisoning and certain other consequences of external causes complicating pregnancy

SP + O9A.211 Injury, poisoning and certain other consequences of external causes complicating pregnancy, first trimester

SP + O9A.212 Injury, poisoning and certain other consequences of external causes complicating pregnancy, second trimester

SP + O9A.213 Injury, poisoning and certain other consequences of external causes complicating pregnancy, third trimester

IQ + O9A.219 Injury, poisoning and certain other consequences of external causes complicating pregnancy, unspecified trimester

SP + O9A.22 Injury, poisoning and certain other consequences of external causes complicating childbirth

SP + O9A.23 Injury, poisoning and certain other consequences of external causes complicating the puerperium

Chapter 15

O00-O9A

★ New ▲ Revised Px Primary SP PDGM Px SL Low CoM SH High CoM IQ Quest. Encounter H Hospice non-cancer Dx   Unspecified   M *Manifestation*

+ 5 O9A.3 Physical abuse complicating pregnancy, childbirth and the puerperium
Conditions in T74.11 or T76.11
Use additional code (if applicable):
to identify any associated current injury due to physical abuse
to identify the perpetrator of abuse (Y07.-)

EXCLUDES 2 sexual abuse complicating pregnancy, childbirth and the puerperium (O9A.4)

GUIDELINES Section I.C.15.r
For suspected or confirmed cases of abuse of a pregnant patient, a code(s) from subcategories O9A.3, O9A.4, and O9A.5, should be sequenced first, followed by the appropriate codes (if applicable) to identify any associated current injury due to physical abuse, sexual abuse, and the perpetrator of abuse.

+ 6 O9A.31 Physical abuse complicating pregnancy

SP + O9A.311 Physical abuse complicating pregnancy, first trimester

SP + O9A.312 Physical abuse complicating pregnancy, second trimester

SP + O9A.313 Physical abuse complicating pregnancy, third trimester

IQ + O9A.319 Physical abuse complicating pregnancy, unspecified trimester

SP + O9A.32 Physical abuse complicating childbirth

SP + O9A.33 Physical abuse complicating the puerperium

+ 5 O9A.4 Sexual abuse complicating pregnancy, childbirth and the puerperium
Conditions in T74.21 or T76.21
Use additional code (if applicable):
to identify any associated current injury due to sexual abuse
to identify the perpetrator of abuse (Y07.-)

+ 6 O9A.41 Sexual abuse complicating pregnancy

SP + O9A.411 Sexual abuse complicating pregnancy, first trimester

SP + O9A.412 Sexual abuse complicating pregnancy, second trimester

SP + O9A.413 Sexual abuse complicating pregnancy, third trimester

IQ + O9A.419 Sexual abuse complicating pregnancy, unspecified trimester

SP + O9A.42 Sexual abuse complicating childbirth

SP + O9A.43 Sexual abuse complicating the puerperium

+ 5 O9A.5 Psychological abuse complicating pregnancy, childbirth and the puerperium
Conditions in T74.31 or T76.31
Use additional code to identify the perpetrator of abuse (Y07.-)

+ 6 O9A.51 Psychological abuse complicating pregnancy

SP + O9A.511 Psychological abuse complicating pregnancy, first trimester

SP + O9A.512 Psychological abuse complicating pregnancy, second trimester

SP + O9A.513 Psychological abuse complicating pregnancy, third trimester

IQ + O9A.519 Psychological abuse complicating pregnancy, unspecified trimester

SP + O9A.52 Psychological abuse complicating childbirth

SP + O9A.53 Psychological abuse complicating the puerperium

Chapter 15

O00-O9A

---

4 4th digit required   5 5th digit required   6 6th digit required   7 7th digit required   7 7th digit placeholder   + Additional code   ⊟ Laterality

Chapter 16: Certain Conditions Originating in the Perinatal Period (P00-P96)

The codes in this chapter are for conditions that have their origin in the fetal or perinatal period (before birth and through the first 28 days after birth) even if morbidity occurs later. If a condition originates in the perinatal period and continues throughout life, the perinatal code should continue to be used, regardless of the age of the patient.

Codes from this chapter **_are used on newborn records only, never on maternal records_**. Codes from chapter 15, the obstetric chapter, are never permitted on the newborn record.

When coding the birth episode in a newborn record, assign a code from category Z38, Liveborn infants according to place of birth and type of delivery, as the principal diagnosis. A code from category Z38 is assigned only once, to a newborn at the time of birth. If a newborn is transferred to another institution, a code from category Z38 should not be used at the receiving hospital.

All clinically significant conditions noted during the routine newborn examination should be coded. A condition is clinically significant if it requires any of the following: clinical evaluation; therapeutic treatment; diagnostic procedures; extended length of hospital stay, increased nursing care and/or monitoring; or if the condition has implications for future health care needs. Codes should be assigned for conditions that have been specified by the provider as having implications for future health care needs.

Codes from other chapters may be used with codes from Chapter 16 if the codes from the other chapters provide more detail. If the reason for the encounter is a perinatal condition, the code from chapter 16 should be sequenced first.

If a newborn has **a condition that may be either due to the birth process or community-acquired** and the documentation does not indicate whether it is congenital or community-acquired, the default code choice is due to the birth process, and the code from Chapter 16 should be used.

If the condition is community-acquired, a code from Chapter 16 should not be assigned. For example, a newborn may have an injured shoulder. Unless otherwise specified, assume that the condition is related to the delivery and report a code P03.1, (Newborn affected by other malpresentation, malposition and disproportion during labor and delivery) as the first-listed diagnosis.

Special Coding Issues

Newborn affected by maternal factors and by complications of pregnancy, labor, and delivery

Codes P00-P04 are used when the listed maternal conditions are specified as the cause of confirmed morbidity or potential morbidity which have their origin in the perinatal period. Several of these codes have a note to code first any current condition in the newborn.

Just because the mother had a medical condition or experienced some complication of pregnancy, labor or delivery does not mean the mother's condition affected the newborn. For example, the mother may have had hypertension (category O10-O11, O13-O16) listed on her chart. If the condition affected the newborn, then code P00.0 (Newborn affected by maternal hypertensive disorders) should be reported on the newborn's chart. If the mother's condition did not affect the fetus, code P00.0 is not reported.

Expanded codes reference specific types of complications. Read the notes under each code carefully to determine the specific code to use.

Prematurity and Fetal Growth Retardation

Providers utilize different criteria in determining prematurity. A code for prematurity should not be assigned unless it is documented. Assignment of codes in categories P05, Disorders of newborn related to slow fetal growth and fetal malnutrition, and P07, Disorders of newborn related to short gestation and low birth weight, not elsewhere classified, should be based on the recorded birth weight and estimated gestational age. Codes from category P05 should not be assigned with codes from subcategory P07.0 or P07.1.

When both birth weight and gestational age are available, two codes from category P07 should be assigned, with the code for birth weight sequenced before the code for gestational age.

Codes from category P07, Disorders of newborn related to short gestation and low birth weight, not elsewhere classified, are for use for a child or adult who was premature or had a low birth weight as a newborn and this is affecting the patient's current health status.

Bacterial Sepsis of Newborn

Category P36, Bacterial sepsis of newborn, includes congenital sepsis. If a perinate is documented as having sepsis without documentation of congenital or community acquired, the default is congenital and a code from category P36 should be assigned. If the P36 code includes the causal organism, an additional code from category B95, Streptococcus, Staphylococcus, and Enterococcus as the cause of diseases classified elsewhere, or B96, Other bacterial agents as the cause of disease classified elsewhere, should not be assigned. If the P36 code does not include the causal organism, assign an additional code from category B96. If applicable, use additional codes to identify severe sepsis (R65.2-) and any associated acute organ dysfunction.

Chapter 16

P00 - P96

CHAPTER 16: CERTAIN CONDITIONS ORIGINATING IN THE PERINATAL PERIOD (P00-P96)

Note:

Codes from this chapter are for use on newborn records only, never on maternal records

| INCLUDES | conditions that have their origin in the fetal or perinatal period (before birth through the first 28 days after birth) even if morbidity occurs later

| EXCLUDES 2 | congenital malformations, deformations and chromosomal abnormalities (Q00-Q99)

endocrine, nutritional and metabolic diseases (E00-E88)

injury, poisoning and certain other consequences of external causes (S00-T88)

neoplasms (C00-D49)

tetanus neonatorum (A33)

| ALERT | Sometimes payer policy conflicts with official guidelines, rules and conventions, and other official guidance. When a payer refuses to pay based on code(s) used in compliance with that guidance, take the following steps: 1) Determine whether the denial or rejection is truly a coding dispute and not a different coverage or payment issue; 2) Remind the payer that following official guidelines and conventions is required by HIPAA code set standards and provide the official guidance in question. If a payer does have a policy that clearly conflicts with official coding rules or guidelines, every effort should be made to resolve the issue with the payer; 3) If the payer refuses to change its policy, obtain the payer requirements in writing. If the payer refuses to provide their policy in writing, document all discussions, including dates and names of individuals involved; 4) Conform to the payer's policy if the payer continues to deny or reject the claim; 5) Keep a permanent file of the documentation obtained regarding payer coding policies. It may be come in handy in the event of an audit.

This chapter contains the following blocks:

P00-P04	Newborn affected by maternal factors and by complications of pregnancy, labor, and delivery
P05-P08	Disorders of newborn related to length of gestation and fetal growth
P09	Abnormal findings on neonatal screening
P10-P15	Birth trauma
P19-P29	Respiratory and cardiovascular disorders specific to the perinatal period
P35-P39	Infections specific to the perinatal period
P50-P61	Hemorrhagic and hematological disorders of newborn
P70-P74	Transitory endocrine and metabolic disorders specific to newborn
P76-P78	Digestive system disorders of newborn
P80-P83	Conditions involving the integument and temperature regulation of newborn
P84	Other problems with newborn
P90-P96	Other disorders originating in the perinatal period

Newborn affected by maternal factors and by complications of pregnancy, labor, and delivery (P00-P04)

Note:

These codes are for use when the listed maternal conditions are specified as the cause of confirmed morbidity or potential morbidity which have their origin in the perinatal period (before birth through the first 28 days after birth).

⁴ P00 Newborn affected by maternal conditions that may be unrelated to present pregnancy

Code first:

any current condition in newborn

| EXCLUDES 2 | encounter for observation of newborn for suspected diseases and conditions ruled out (Z05.-)

newborn affected by maternal complications of pregnancy (P01.-)

newborn affected by maternal endocrine and metabolic disorders (P70-P74)

newborn affected by noxious substances transmitted via placenta or breast milk (P04.-)

SP P00.0 Newborn affected by maternal hypertensive disorders

Newborn affected by maternal conditions classifiable to O10-O11, O13-O16

SP P00.1 Newborn affected by maternal renal and urinary tract diseases

Newborn affected by maternal conditions classifiable to N00-N39

SP P00.2 Newborn affected by maternal infectious and parasitic diseases

Newborn affected by maternal infectious disease classifiable to A00-B99, J09 and J10

| EXCLUDES 1 | maternal genital tract or other localized infections (P00.8)

| EXCLUDES 2 | infections specific to the perinatal period (P35-P39)

SP P00.3 Newborn affected by other maternal circulatory and respiratory diseases

Newborn affected by maternal conditions classifiable to I00-I99, J00-J99, Q20-Q34 and not included in P00.0, P00.2

SP P00.4 Newborn affected by maternal nutritional disorders

Newborn affected by maternal disorders classifiable to E40-E64

Maternal malnutrition NOS

SP P00.5 Newborn affected by maternal injury

Newborn affected by maternal conditions classifiable to O9A.2-

SP P00.6 Newborn affected by surgical procedure on mother

Newborn affected by amniocentesis

| EXCLUDES 1 | Cesarean delivery for present delivery (P03.4)

damage to placenta from amniocentesis, Cesarean delivery or surgical induction (P02.1)

previous surgery to uterus or pelvic organs (P03.89)

| EXCLUDES 2 | newborn affected by complication of (fetal) intrauterine procedure (P96.5)

SP P00.7 Newborn affected by other medical procedures on mother, not elsewhere classified

Newborn affected by radiation to mother

★ New ▲ Revised Px Primary | SP | PDGM Px | SL | Low CoM | SH | High CoM | IQ | Quest. Encounter | H | Hospice non-cancer Dx | Unspecified | M | Manifestation

DecisionHealth's FY 2020 Complete Home Health ICD-10-CM Diagnosis Coding Manual

1367

EXCLUDES 1 damage to placenta from amniocentesis, cesarean delivery or surgical induction (P02.1)
newborn affected by other complications of labor and delivery (P03.-)

5 P00.8 Newborn affected by other maternal conditions

SP P00.81 Newborn affected by periodontal disease in mother

SP P00.89 Newborn affected by other maternal conditions
Newborn affected by conditions classifiable to T80-T88
Newborn affected by maternal genital tract or other localized infections
Newborn affected by maternal systemic lupus erythematosus

IQ P00.9 Newborn affected by unspecified maternal condition

4 P01 Newborn affected by maternal complications of pregnancy
Code first:
any current condition in newborn
EXCLUDES 2 encounter for observation of newborn for suspected diseases and conditions ruled out (Z05.-)

SP P01.0 Newborn affected by incompetent cervix

SP P01.1 Newborn affected by premature rupture of membranes

SP P01.2 Newborn affected by oligohydramnios
EXCLUDES 1 oligohydramnios due to premature rupture of membranes (P01.1)
DEFINITION Inadequate amount of amniotic fluid in the womb affecting the fetus.

SP P01.3 Newborn affected by polyhydramnios
Newborn affected by hydramnios
DEFINITION Excessive amount of amniotic fluid in the womb affecting the fetus.

SP P01.4 Newborn affected by ectopic pregnancy
Newborn affected by abdominal pregnancy

SP P01.5 Newborn affected by multiple pregnancy
Newborn affected by triplet (pregnancy)
Newborn affected by twin (pregnancy)

SP P01.6 Newborn affected by maternal death

SP P01.7 Newborn affected by malpresentation before labor
Newborn affected by breech presentation before labor
Newborn affected by external version before labor
Newborn affected by face presentation before labor
Newborn affected by transverse lie before labor
Newborn affected by unstable lie before labor

SP P01.8 Newborn affected by other maternal complications of pregnancy

SP P01.9 Newborn affected by maternal complication of pregnancy, unspecified

4 P02 Newborn affected by complications of placenta, cord and membranes
Code first:
any current condition in newborn
EXCLUDES 2 encounter for observation of newborn for suspected diseases and conditions ruled out (Z05.-)

SP P02.0 Newborn affected by placenta previa

SP P02.1 Newborn affected by other forms of placental separation and hemorrhage
Newborn affected by abruptio placenta
Newborn affected by accidental hemorrhage
Newborn affected by antepartum hemorrhage
Newborn affected by damage to placenta from amniocentesis, cesarean delivery or surgical induction
Newborn affected by maternal blood loss
Newborn affected by premature separation of placenta

5 P02.2 Newborn affected by other and unspecified morphological and functional abnormalities of placenta

SP P02.20 Newborn affected by unspecified morphological and functional abnormalities of placenta

SP P02.29 Newborn affected by other morphological and functional abnormalities of placenta
Newborn affected by placental dysfunction
Newborn affected by placental infarction
Newborn affected by placental insufficiency

SP P02.3 Newborn affected by placental transfusion syndromes
Newborn affected by placental and cord abnormalities resulting in twin-to-twin or other transplacental transfusion

SP P02.4 Newborn affected by prolapsed cord

SP P02.5 Newborn affected by other compression of umbilical cord
Newborn affected by umbilical cord (tightly) around neck
Newborn affected by entanglement of umbilical cord
Newborn affected by knot in umbilical cord

5 P02.6 Newborn affected by other and unspecified conditions of umbilical cord

SP P02.60 Newborn affected by unspecified conditions of umbilical cord

SP P02.69 Newborn affected by other conditions of umbilical cord
Newborn affected by short umbilical cord
Newborn affected by vasa previa
EXCLUDES 1 newborn affected by single umbilical artery (Q27.0)

5 P02.7 Newborn affected by chorioamnionitis

SP P02.70 Newborn affected by fetal inflammatory response syndrome

Chapter 16

P00-P96

Newborn affected by FIRS

SP P02.78 Newborn affected by other conditions from chorioamnionitis
Newborn affected by amnionitis
Newborn affected by membranitis
Newborn affected by placentitis

SP P02.8 Newborn affected by other abnormalities of membranes

SP P02.9 Newborn affected by abnormality of membranes, unspecified

4 P03 Newborn affected by other complications of labor and delivery
Code first:
any current condition in newborn
> **EXCLUDES 2** encounter for observation of newborn for suspected diseases and conditions ruled out (Z05.-)

SP P03.0 Newborn affected by breech delivery and extraction

SP P03.1 Newborn affected by other malpresentation, malposition and disproportion during labor and delivery
Newborn affected by contracted pelvis
Newborn affected by conditions classifiable to O64-O66
Newborn affected by persistent occipitoposterior
Newborn affected by transverse lie

SP P03.2 Newborn affected by forceps delivery

SP P03.3 Newborn affected by delivery by vacuum extractor [ventouse]

SP P03.4 Newborn affected by Cesarean delivery

SP P03.5 Newborn affected by precipitate delivery
Newborn affected by rapid second stage
> **DEFINITION** Fetus affected by labor occurring quickly, with rapid expulsion.

SP P03.6 Newborn affected by abnormal uterine contractions
Newborn affected by conditions classifiable to O62.-, except O62.3
Newborn affected by hypertonic labor
Newborn affected by uterine inertia

5 P03.8 Newborn affected by other specified complications of labor and delivery

6 P03.81 Newborn affected by abnormality in fetal (intrauterine) heart rate or rhythm
> **EXCLUDES 1** neonatal cardiac dysrhythmia (P29.1-)

SP P03.810 Newborn affected by abnormality in fetal (intrauterine) heart rate or rhythm before the onset of labor

SP P03.811 Newborn affected by abnormality in fetal (intrauterine) heart rate or rhythm during labor

SP P03.819 Newborn affected by abnormality in fetal (intrauterine) heart rate or rhythm, unspecified as to time of onset

SP P03.82 Meconium passage during delivery
> **EXCLUDES 1** meconium aspiration (P24.00, P24.01)
> meconium staining (P96.83)

SP P03.89 Newborn affected by other specified complications of labor and delivery
Newborn affected by abnormality of maternal soft tissues
Newborn affected by conditions classifiable to O60-O75 and by procedures used in labor and delivery not included in P02.- and P03.0-P03.6
Newborn affected by induction of labor

IQ P03.9 Newborn affected by complication of labor and delivery, unspecified

4 P04 Newborn affected by noxious substances transmitted via placenta or breast milk
> **INCLUDES** nonteratogenic effects of substances transmitted via placenta
> **EXCLUDES 2** congenital malformations (Q00-Q99)
> encounter for observation of newborn for suspected diseases and conditions ruled out (Z05.-)
> neonatal jaundice from excessive hemolysis due to drugs or toxins transmitted from mother (P58.4)
> newborn in contact with and (suspected) exposures hazardous to health not transmitted via placenta or breast milk (Z77.-)

SP P04.0 Newborn affected by maternal anesthesia and analgesia in pregnancy, labor and delivery
Newborn affected by reactions and intoxications from maternal opiates and tranquilizers administered for procedures during pregnancy or labor and delivery
> **EXCLUDES 2** newborn affected by other maternal medication (P04.1-)

5 P04.1 Newborn affected by other maternal medication
Code first:
withdrawal symptoms from maternal use of drugs of addiction, if applicable (P96.1)
> **EXCLUDES 1** dysmorphism due to warfarin (Q86.2)
> fetal hydantoin syndrome (Q86.1)
> **EXCLUDES 2** maternal anesthesia and analgesia in pregnancy, labor and delivery (P04.0)
> maternal use of drugs of addiction (P04.4-)

SP P04.11 Newborn affected by maternal antineoplastic chemotherapy

SP P04.12 Newborn affected by maternal cytotoxic drugs

SP P04.13 Newborn affected by maternal use of anticonvulsants

SP P04.14 Newborn affected by maternal use of opiates

SP P04.15 Newborn affected by maternal use of antidepressants

SP P04.16 Newborn affected by maternal use of amphetamines

Chapter 16

P00-P96

★ New ▲ Revised Px Primary **SP** PDGM Px **SL** Low CoM **SH** High CoM **IQ** Quest. Encounter **H** Hospice non-cancer Dx   Unspecified   **M** *Manifestation*

DecisionHealth's FY 2020 Complete Home Health ICD-10-CM Diagnosis Coding Manual

1369

SP P04.17 Newborn affected by maternal use of sedative-hypnotics

SP P04.1A Newborn affected by maternal use of anxiolytics

SP P04.18 Newborn affected by other maternal medication

SP P04.19 Newborn affected by maternal use of unspecified medication

SP P04.2 Newborn affected by maternal use of tobacco
Newborn affected by exposure in utero to tobacco smoke
> **EXCLUDES 2** newborn exposure to environmental tobacco smoke (P96.81)

SP P04.3 Newborn affected by maternal use of alcohol
> **EXCLUDES 1** fetal alcohol syndrome (Q86.0)

5 P04.4 Newborn affected by maternal use of drugs of addiction

SP P04.40 Newborn affected by maternal use of unspecified drugs of addiction

▲ **SP P04.41** Newborn affected by maternal use of cocaine

SP P04.42 Newborn affected by maternal use of hallucinogens
> **EXCLUDES 2** newborn affected by other maternal medication (P04.1-)

SP P04.49 Newborn affected by maternal use of other drugs of addiction
> **EXCLUDES 2** newborn affected by maternal anesthesia and analgesia (P04.0)
> withdrawal symptoms from maternal use of drugs of addiction (P96.1)

SP P04.5 Newborn affected by maternal use of nutritional chemical substances

SP P04.6 Newborn affected by maternal exposure to environmental chemical substances

5 P04.8 Newborn affected by other maternal noxious substances

SP P04.81 Newborn affected by maternal use of cannabis

SP P04.89 Newborn affected by other maternal noxious substances

IQ P04.9 Newborn affected by maternal noxious substance, unspecified

Disorders of newborn related to length of gestation and fetal growth   (P05-P08)

4 P05 Disorders of newborn related to slow fetal growth and fetal malnutrition

5 P05.0 Newborn light for gestational age
Newborn light-for-dates
Weight below but length above 10th percentile for gestational age

IQ P05.00 Newborn light for gestational age, unspecified weight

SP P05.01 Newborn light for gestational age, less than 500 grams

SP P05.02 Newborn light for gestational age, 500-749 grams

SP P05.03 Newborn light for gestational age, 750-999 grams

SP P05.04 Newborn light for gestational age, 1000-1249 grams

SP P05.05 Newborn light for gestational age, 1250-1499 grams

SP P05.06 Newborn light for gestational age, 1500-1749 grams

SP P05.07 Newborn light for gestational age, 1750-1999 grams

SP P05.08 Newborn light for gestational age, 2000-2499 grams

SP P05.09 Newborn light for gestational age, 2500 grams and over
Newborn light for gestational age, other

5 P05.1 Newborn small for gestational age
Newborn small-and-light-for-dates
Newborn small-for-dates
Weight and length below 10th percentile for gestational age

IQ P05.10 Newborn small for gestational age, unspecified weight

SP P05.11 Newborn small for gestational age, less than 500 grams

SP P05.12 Newborn small for gestational age, 500-749 grams

SP P05.13 Newborn small for gestational age, 750-999 grams

SP P05.14 Newborn small for gestational age, 1000-1249 grams

SP P05.15 Newborn small for gestational age, 1250-1499 grams

SP P05.16 Newborn small for gestational age, 1500-1749 grams

SP P05.17 Newborn small for gestational age, 1750-1999 grams

SP P05.18 Newborn small for gestational age, 2000-2499 grams

SP P05.19 Newborn small for gestational age, other
Newborn small for gestational age, 2500 grams and over

SP P05.2 Newborn affected by fetal (intrauterine) malnutrition not light or small for gestational age
Infant, not light or small for gestational age, showing signs of fetal malnutrition, such as dry, peeling skin and loss of subcutaneous tissue
> **EXCLUDES 1** newborn affected by fetal malnutrition with light for gestational age (P05.0-)
> newborn affected by fetal malnutrition with small for gestational age (P05.1-)

SP P05.9 Newborn affected by slow intrauterine growth, unspecified
Newborn affected by fetal growth retardation NOS

4 P07 Disorders of newborn related to short gestation and low birth weight, not elsewhere classified
Note:
When both birth weight and gestational age of the newborn are available, both should be coded with birth weight sequenced before gestational age

---

4 4th digit required   **5** 5th digit required   **6** 6th digit required   **7** 7th digit required   **7** 7th digit placeholder   **+** Additional code   **⊟** Laterality

1370   *DecisionHealth's* FY 2020 Complete Home Health ICD-10-CM Diagnosis Coding Manual

Chapter 16

P00-P96

INCLUDES the listed conditions, without
further specification, as the
cause of morbidity or
additional care, in newborn

5 **P07.0** **Extremely low birth weight newborn**
Newborn birth weight 999 g. or less
EXCLUDES 1 low birth weight due to slow
fetal growth and fetal
malnutrition (P05.-)

IQ **P07.00** **Extremely low birth weight**
newborn, unspecified weight

SP **P07.01** **Extremely low birth weight**
newborn, less than 500 grams

SP **P07.02** **Extremely low birth weight**
newborn, 500-749 grams

SP **P07.03** **Extremely low birth weight**
newborn, 750-999 grams

5 **P07.1** **Other low birth weight newborn**
Newborn birth weight 1000-2499 g.
EXCLUDES 1 low birth weight due to slow
fetal growth and fetal
malnutrition (P05.-)

IQ **P07.10** **Other low birth weight newborn,**
unspecified weight

SP **P07.14** **Other low birth weight newborn,**
1000-1249 grams

SP **P07.15** **Other low birth weight newborn,**
1250-1499 grams

SP **P07.16** **Other low birth weight newborn,**
1500-1749 grams

SP **P07.17** **Other low birth weight newborn,**
1750-1999 grams

SP **P07.18** **Other low birth weight newborn,**
2000-2499 grams

5 **P07.2** **Extreme immaturity of newborn**
Less than 28 completed weeks (less than
196 completed days) of gestation.

IQ **P07.20** **Extreme immaturity of newborn,**
unspecified weeks of gestation
Gestational age less than 28 completed
weeks NOS

SP **P07.21** **Extreme immaturity of newborn,**
gestational age less than 23
completed weeks
Extreme immaturity of newborn,
gestational age less than 23 weeks, 0
days

SP **P07.22** **Extreme immaturity of newborn,**
gestational age 23 completed weeks
Extreme immaturity of newborn,
gestational age 23 weeks, 0 days
through 23 weeks, 6 days

SP **P07.23** **Extreme immaturity of newborn,**
gestational age 24 completed weeks
Extreme immaturity of newborn,
gestational age 24 weeks, 0 days
through 24 weeks, 6 days

SP **P07.24** **Extreme immaturity of newborn,**
gestational age 25 completed weeks
Extreme immaturity of newborn,
gestational age 25 weeks, 0 days
through 25 weeks, 6 days

SP **P07.25** **Extreme immaturity of newborn,**
gestational age 26 completed weeks
Extreme immaturity of newborn,
gestational age 26 weeks, 0 days
through 26 weeks, 6 days

SP **P07.26** **Extreme immaturity of newborn,**
gestational age 27 completed weeks
Extreme immaturity of newborn,
gestational age 27 weeks, 0 days
through 27 weeks, 6 days

5 **P07.3** **Preterm [premature] newborn [other]**
28 completed weeks or more but less than
37 completed weeks (196 completed
days but less than 259 completed days)
of gestation.
Prematurity NOS

IQ **P07.30** **Preterm newborn, unspecified**
weeks of gestation

SP **P07.31** **Preterm newborn, gestational age 28**
completed weeks
Preterm newborn, gestational age 28
weeks, 0 days through 28 weeks, 6
days

SP **P07.32** **Preterm newborn, gestational age 29**
completed weeks
Preterm newborn, gestational age 29
weeks, 0 days through 29 weeks, 6
days

SP **P07.33** **Preterm newborn, gestational age 30**
completed weeks
Preterm newborn, gestational age 30
weeks, 0 days through 30 weeks, 6
days

SP **P07.34** **Preterm newborn, gestational age 31**
completed weeks
Preterm newborn, gestational age 31
weeks, 0 days through 31 weeks, 6
days

SP **P07.35** **Preterm newborn, gestational age 32**
completed weeks
Preterm newborn, gestational age 32
weeks, 0 days through 32 weeks, 6
days

SP **P07.36** **Preterm newborn, gestational age 33**
completed weeks
Preterm newborn, gestational age 33
weeks, 0 days through 33 weeks, 6
days

SP **P07.37** **Preterm newborn, gestational age 34**
completed weeks
Preterm newborn, gestational age 34
weeks, 0 days through 34 weeks, 6
days

SP **P07.38** **Preterm newborn, gestational age 35**
completed weeks
Preterm newborn, gestational age 35
weeks, 0 days through 35 weeks, 6
days

SP **P07.39** **Preterm newborn, gestational age 36**
completed weeks
Preterm newborn, gestational age 36
weeks, 0 days through 36 weeks, 6
days

4 **P08** **Disorders of newborn related to long**
gestation and high birth weight
Note:
When both birth weight and gestational age of
the newborn are available, priority of
assignment should be given to birth weight
INCLUDES the listed conditions, without
further specification, as
causes of morbidity or
additional care, in newborn

★ New ▲ Revised Px Primary SP PDGM Px SL Low CoM SH High CoM IQ Quest. Encounter H Hospice non-cancer Dx Unspecified M *Manifestation*

DecisionHealth's FY 2020 Complete Home Health ICD-10-CM Diagnosis Coding Manual

1371

SP P08.0   Exceptionally large newborn baby
Usually implies a birth weight of 4500 g.
or more
> **EXCLUDES 1**   syndrome of infant of
> diabetic mother (P70.1)
> syndrome of infant of mother
> with gestational diabetes
> (P70.0)

**SP P08.1   Other heavy for gestational age
newborn**
Other newborn heavy- or large-for-dates
regardless of period of gestation
Usually implies a birth weight of 4000 g.
to 4499 g.
> **EXCLUDES 1**   newborn with a birth weight
> of 4500 or more (P08.0)
> syndrome of infant of
> diabetic mother (P70.1)
> syndrome of infant of mother
> with gestational diabetes
> (P70.0) .

**5 P08.2   Late newborn, not heavy for gestational
age**

SP P08.21   Post-term newborn
Newborn with gestation period over 40
completed weeks to 42 completed
weeks

SP P08.22   Prolonged gestation of newborn
Newborn with gestation period over 42
completed weeks (294 days or more),
not heavy- or large-for-dates.
Postmaturity NOS

Abnormal findings on neonatal screening (P09)

SP ✚ P09   Abnormal findings on neonatal screening
Use additional code to identify signs,
symptoms and conditions associated with
the screening
> **EXCLUDES 2**   nonspecific serologic evidence
> of human immunodeficiency
> virus [HIV] (R75)

Birth trauma   (P10-P15)

**4 P10   Intracranial laceration and hemorrhage
due to birth injury**
> **EXCLUDES 1**   intracranial hemorrhage of
> newborn NOS (P52.9)
> intracranial hemorrhage of
> newborn due to anoxia or
> hypoxia (P52.-)
> nontraumatic intracranial
> hemorrhage of newborn
> (P52.-)

**SP P10.0   Subdural hemorrhage due to birth
injury**
Subdural hematoma (localized) due to
birth injury
> **EXCLUDES 1**   subdural hemorrhage
> accompanying tentorial
> tear (P10.4)

**SP P10.1   Cerebral hemorrhage due to birth
injury**

**SP P10.2   Intraventricular hemorrhage due to
birth injury**

**SP P10.3   Subarachnoid hemorrhage due to birth
injury**

SP P10.4   Tentorial tear due to birth injury

**SP P10.8   Other intracranial lacerations and
hemorrhages due to birth injury**

**!Q P10.9   Unspecified intracranial laceration and
hemorrhage due to birth injury**

**4 P11   Other birth injuries to central nervous
system**

SP P11.0   Cerebral edema due to birth injury

**SP P11.1   Other specified brain damage due to
birth injury**

**!Q P11.2   Unspecified brain damage due to birth
injury**

SP P11.3   Birth injury to facial nerve
Facial palsy due to birth injury
> **DEFINITION**   Facial muscle weakness or
> paralysis resulting from damage or trauma
> to one of the paired facial nerves.

SP P11.4   Birth injury to other cranial nerves

SP P11.5   Birth injury to spine and spinal cord
Fracture of spine due to birth injury

**!Q P11.9   Birth injury to central nervous system,
unspecified**

4 P12   Birth injury to scalp

SP P12.0   Cephalhematoma due to birth injury

**SP P12.1   Chignon (from vacuum extraction) due
to birth injury**

**SP P12.2   Epicranial subaponeurotic hemorrhage
due to birth injury**
Subgaleal hemorrhage

SP P12.3   Bruising of scalp due to birth injury

**SP P12.4   Injury of scalp of newborn due to
monitoring equipment**
Sampling incision of scalp of newborn
Scalp clip (electrode) injury of newborn

5 P12.8   Other birth injuries to scalp

SP P12.81   Caput succedaneum

SP P12.89   Other birth injuries to scalp

!Q P12.9   Birth injury to scalp, unspecified

4 P13   Birth injury to skeleton
> **EXCLUDES 2**   birth injury to spine (P11.5)

SP P13.0   Fracture of skull due to birth injury

SP P13.1   Other birth injuries to skull
> **EXCLUDES 1**   cephalhematoma (P12.0)

SP P13.2   Birth injury to femur

SP P13.3   Birth injury to other long bones

SP P13.4   Fracture of clavicle due to birth injury

SP P13.8   Birth injuries to other parts of skeleton

!Q P13.9   Birth injury to skeleton, unspecified

4 P14   Birth injury to peripheral nervous system

SP P14.0   Erb's paralysis due to birth injury

SP P14.1   Klumpke's paralysis due to birth injury

**SP P14.2   Phrenic nerve paralysis due to birth
injury**

SP P14.3   Other brachial plexus birth injuries

**SP P14.8   Birth injuries to other parts of
peripheral nervous system**

**!Q P14.9   Birth injury to peripheral nervous
system, unspecified**

4 P15   Other birth injuries

SP P15.0   Birth injury to liver
Rupture of liver due to birth injury

---

4 4th digit required   5 5th digit required   6 6th digit required   7 7th digit required   7 7th digit placeholder   ✚ Additional code   Laterality

SP P15.1 Birth injury to spleen
Rupture of spleen due to birth injury

SP P15.2 Sternomastoid injury due to birth injury

SP P15.3 Birth injury to eye
Subconjunctival hemorrhage due to birth injury
Traumatic glaucoma due to birth injury

SP P15.4 Birth injury to face
Facial congestion due to birth injury

SP P15.5 Birth injury to external genitalia

SP P15.6 Subcutaneous fat necrosis due to birth injury

SP P15.8 Other specified birth injuries

IQ P15.9 Birth injury, unspecified

Respiratory and cardiovascular disorders specific to the perinatal period (P19-P29)

4 P19 Metabolic acidemia in newborn
INCLUDES metabolic acidemia in newborn

SP P19.0 Metabolic acidemia in newborn first noted before onset of labor

SP P19.1 Metabolic acidemia in newborn first noted during labor

SP P19.2 Metabolic acidemia noted at birth

SP P19.9 Metabolic acidemia, unspecified

▲ 4 P22 Respiratory distress of newborn

▲ SP P22.0 Respiratory distress syndrome of newborn
Cardiorespiratory distress syndrome of newborn
Hyaline membrane disease
Idiopathic respiratory distress syndrome [IRDS or RDS] of newborn
Pulmonary hypoperfusion syndrome
Respiratory distress syndrome, type I
EXCLUDES 2 respiratory arrest of newborn (P28.81)
respiratory failure of newborn NOS (P28.5)

SP P22.1 Transient tachypnea of newborn
Idiopathic tachypnea of newborn
Respiratory distress syndrome, type II
Wet lung syndrome
DEFINITION Rapid breathing of a newborn.

▲ SP P22.8 Other respiratory distress of newborn
EXCLUDES 1 respiratory arrest of newborn (P28.81)
respiratory failure of newborn NOS (P28.5)

▲ SP P22.9 Respiratory distress of newborn, unspecified
EXCLUDES 1 respiratory arrest of newborn (P28.81)
respiratory failure of newborn NOS (P28.5)

4 P23 Congenital pneumonia
INCLUDES infective pneumonia acquired in utero or during birth
EXCLUDES 1 neonatal pneumonia resulting from aspiration (P24.-)

SP + P23.0 Congenital pneumonia due to viral agent
Use additional code (B97) to identify organism

EXCLUDES 1 congenital rubella pneumonitis (P35.0)

SP P23.1 Congenital pneumonia due to Chlamydia

SP P23.2 Congenital pneumonia due to staphylococcus

SP P23.3 Congenital pneumonia due to streptococcus, group B

SP P23.4 Congenital pneumonia due to Escherichia coli

SP P23.5 Congenital pneumonia due to Pseudomonas

SP + P23.6 Congenital pneumonia due to other bacterial agents
Congenital pneumonia due to Hemophilus influenzae
Congenital pneumonia due to Klebsiella pneumoniae
Congenital pneumonia due to Mycoplasma
Congenital pneumonia due to Streptococcus, except group B
Use additional code (B95-B96) to identify organism

SP P23.8 Congenital pneumonia due to other organisms

IQ P23.9 Congenital pneumonia, unspecified

4 P24 Neonatal aspiration
INCLUDES aspiration in utero and during delivery

5 P24.0 Meconium aspiration
EXCLUDES 1 meconium passage (without aspiration) during delivery (P03.82)
meconium staining (P96.83)

SP P24.00 Meconium aspiration without respiratory symptoms
Meconium aspiration NOS

SP + P24.01 Meconium aspiration with respiratory symptoms
Meconium aspiration pneumonia
Meconium aspiration pneumonitis
Meconium aspiration syndrome NOS
Use additional code to identify any secondary pulmonary hypertension, if applicable (I27.2-)

5 P24.1 Neonatal aspiration of (clear) amniotic fluid and mucus
Neonatal aspiration of liquor (amnii)

SP P24.10 Neonatal aspiration of (clear) amniotic fluid and mucus without respiratory symptoms
Neonatal aspiration of amniotic fluid and mucus NOS

SP + P24.11 Neonatal aspiration of (clear) amniotic fluid and mucus with respiratory symptoms
Neonatal aspiration of amniotic fluid and mucus with pneumonia
Neonatal aspiration of amniotic fluid and mucus with pneumonitis
Use additional code to identify any secondary pulmonary hypertension, if applicable (I27.2-)

5 P24.2 Neonatal aspiration of blood

SP P24.20 Neonatal aspiration of blood without respiratory symptoms
Neonatal aspiration of blood NOS

Chapter 16

P00-P96

★ New ▲ Revised Px Primary SP PDGM Px SL Low CoM SH High CoM IQ Quest. Encounter H Hospice non-cancer Dx Unspecified M *Manifestation*

DecisionHealth's FY 2020 Complete Home Health ICD-10-CM Diagnosis Coding Manual

1373

SP + P24.21 Neonatal aspiration of blood with respiratory symptoms
Neonatal aspiration of blood with pneumonia
Neonatal aspiration of blood with pneumonitis
Use additional code to identify any secondary pulmonary hypertension, if applicable (I27.2-)

5 P24.3 Neonatal aspiration of milk and regurgitated food
Neonatal aspiration of stomach contents

SP P24.30 Neonatal aspiration of milk and regurgitated food without respiratory symptoms
Neonatal aspiration of milk and regurgitated food NOS

SP + P24.31 Neonatal aspiration of milk and regurgitated food with respiratory symptoms
Neonatal aspiration of milk and regurgitated food with pneumonia
Neonatal aspiration of milk and regurgitated food with pneumonitis
Use additional code to identify any secondary pulmonary hypertension, if applicable (I27.2-)

5 P24.8 Other neonatal aspiration

SP P24.80 Other neonatal aspiration without respiratory symptoms
Neonatal aspiration NEC

SP + P24.81 Other neonatal aspiration with respiratory symptoms
Neonatal aspiration pneumonia NEC
Neonatal aspiration with pneumonitis NEC
Neonatal aspiration with pneumonia NOS
Neonatal aspiration with pneumonitis NOS
Use additional code to identify any secondary pulmonary hypertension, if applicable (I27.2-)

SP P24.9 Neonatal aspiration, unspecified

4 P25 Interstitial emphysema and related conditions originating in the perinatal period

SP P25.0 Interstitial emphysema originating in the perinatal period

SP P25.1 Pneumothorax originating in the perinatal period

SP P25.2 Pneumomediastinum originating in the perinatal period

SP P25.3 Pneumopericardium originating in the perinatal period

SP P25.8 Other conditions related to interstitial emphysema originating in the perinatal period

4 P26 Pulmonary hemorrhage originating in the perinatal period
EXCLUDES 1 acute idiopathic hemorrhage in infants over 28 days old (R04.81)

SP P26.0 Tracheobronchial hemorrhage originating in the perinatal period

SP P26.1 Massive pulmonary hemorrhage originating in the perinatal period

SP P26.8 Other pulmonary hemorrhages originating in the perinatal period

SP P26.9 Unspecified pulmonary hemorrhage originating in the perinatal period

4 P27 Chronic respiratory disease originating in the perinatal period
EXCLUDES 2 respiratory distress of newborn (P22.0-P22.9)

SP P27.0 Wilson-Mikity syndrome
Pulmonary dysmaturity

SP P27.1 Bronchopulmonary dysplasia originating in the perinatal period

SP P27.8 Other chronic respiratory diseases originating in the perinatal period
Congenital pulmonary fibrosis
Ventilator lung in newborn

!Q P27.9 Unspecified chronic respiratory disease originating in the perinatal period

4 P28 Other respiratory conditions originating in the perinatal period
EXCLUDES 1 congenital malformations of the respiratory system (Q30-Q34)

SP P28.0 Primary atelectasis of newborn
Primary failure to expand terminal respiratory units
Pulmonary hypoplasia associated with short gestation
Pulmonary immaturity NOS

5 P28.1 Other and unspecified atelectasis of newborn

SP P28.10 Unspecified atelectasis of newborn
Atelectasis of newborn NOS

SP P28.11 Resorption atelectasis without respiratory distress syndrome
EXCLUDES 1 resorption atelectasis with respiratory distress syndrome (P22.0)

SP P28.19 Other atelectasis of newborn
Partial atelectasis of newborn
Secondary atelectasis of newborn

SP P28.2 Cyanotic attacks of newborn
EXCLUDES 1 apnea of newborn (P28.3-P28.4)
DEFINITION A newborn with normal skin tone suddenly turns blue due to a lack of oxygen for a certain period of time before returning to normal color.

SP P28.3 Primary sleep apnea of newborn
Central sleep apnea of newborn
Obstructive sleep apnea of newborn
Sleep apnea of newborn NOS

SP P28.4 Other apnea of newborn
Apnea of prematurity
Obstructive apnea of newborn
EXCLUDES 1 obstructive sleep apnea of newborn (P28.3)

SP P28.5 Respiratory failure of newborn
EXCLUDES 1 respiratory arrest of newborn (P28.81)
respiratory distress of newborn (P22.0-)

5 P28.8 Other specified respiratory conditions of newborn

SP P28.81 Respiratory arrest of newborn

---

4 4th digit required   5 5th digit required   6 6th digit required   7 7th digit required   7 7th digit placeholder   + Additional code   Laterality

1374   *DecisionHealth's* FY 2020 Complete Home Health ICD-10-CM Diagnosis Coding Manual

SP P28.89 **Other specified respiratory conditions of newborn**
Congenital laryngeal stridor
Sniffles in newborn
Snuffles in newborn
> **EXCLUDES 1** early congenital syphilitic rhinitis (A50.05)

IQ P28.9 **Respiratory condition of newborn, unspecified**
Respiratory depression in newborn

4 P29 **Cardiovascular disorders originating in the perinatal period**
> **EXCLUDES 1** congenital malformations of the circulatory system (Q20-Q28)

SP P29.0 **Neonatal cardiac failure**

5 P29.1 **Neonatal cardiac dysrhythmia**

SP P29.11 **Neonatal tachycardia**

SP P29.12 **Neonatal bradycardia**
> **DEFINITION** Abnormally slow newborn heartbeat.

SP P29.2 **Neonatal hypertension**

5 P29.3 **Persistent fetal circulation**

IQ P29.30 **Pulmonary hypertension of newborn**
Persistent pulmonary hypertension of newborn

IQ P29.38 **Other persistent fetal circulation**
Delayed closure of ductus arteriosus

SP P29.4 **Transient myocardial ischemia in newborn**

5 P29.8 **Other cardiovascular disorders originating in the perinatal period**

SP P29.81 **Cardiac arrest of newborn**

SP P29.89 **Other cardiovascular disorders originating in the perinatal period**

IQ P29.9 **Cardiovascular disorder originating in the perinatal period, unspecified**

Infections specific to the perinatal period (P35-P39)

Infections acquired in utero, during birth via the umbilicus, or during the first 28 days after birth
> **EXCLUDES 2** asymptomatic human immunodeficiency virus [HIV] infection status (Z21)
> congenital gonococcal infection (A54.-)
> congenital pneumonia (P23.-)
> congenital syphilis (A50.-)
> human immunodeficiency virus [HIV] disease (B20)
> infant botulism (A48.51)
> infectious diseases not specific to the perinatal period (A00-B99, J09, J10.-)
> intestinal infectious disease (A00-A09)
> laboratory evidence of human immunodeficiency virus [HIV] (R75)
> tetanus neonatorum (A33)

4 P35 **Congenital viral diseases**
> **INCLUDES** infections acquired in utero or during birth

SP P35.0 **Congenital rubella syndrome**
Congenital rubella pneumonitis

SP P35.1 **Congenital cytomegalovirus infection**

SP P35.2 **Congenital herpesviral [herpes simplex] infection**

SP P35.3 **Congenital viral hepatitis**

SP + P35.4 **Congenital Zika virus disease**
Use additional code to identify manifestations of congenital Zika virus disease

SP P35.8 **Other congenital viral diseases**
Congenital varicella [chickenpox]

IQ P35.9 **Congenital viral disease, unspecified**

+ 4 P36 **Bacterial sepsis of newborn**
> **INCLUDES** congenital sepsis
Use additional code(s), if applicable, to identify severe sepsis (R65.2-) and associated acute organ dysfunction(s)

SP + P36.0 **Sepsis of newborn due to streptococcus, group B**

+ 5 P36.1 **Sepsis of newborn due to other and unspecified streptococci**

SP + P36.10 **Sepsis of newborn due to unspecified streptococci**

SP + P36.19 **Sepsis of newborn due to other streptococci**

SP + P36.2 **Sepsis of newborn due to Staphylococcus aureus**

+ 5 P36.3 **Sepsis of newborn due to other and unspecified staphylococci**

SP + P36.30 **Sepsis of newborn due to unspecified staphylococci**

SP + P36.39 **Sepsis of newborn due to other staphylococci**

SP + P36.4 **Sepsis of newborn due to Escherichia coli**

SP + P36.5 **Sepsis of newborn due to anaerobes**

SP + P36.8 **Other bacterial sepsis of newborn**
Use additional code from category B96 to identify organism

SP + P36.9 **Bacterial sepsis of newborn, unspecified**

4 P37 **Other congenital infectious and parasitic diseases**
> **EXCLUDES 2** congenital syphilis (A50.-)
> infectious neonatal diarrhea (A00-A09)
> necrotizing enterocolitis in newborn (P77.-)
> noninfectious neonatal diarrhea (P78.3)
> ophthalmia neonatorum due to gonococcus (A54.31)
> tetanus neonatorum (A33)

SP P37.0 **Congenital tuberculosis**

SP P37.1 **Congenital toxoplasmosis**
Hydrocephalus due to congenital toxoplasmosis

SP P37.2 **Neonatal (disseminated) listeriosis**

SP P37.3 **Congenital falciparum malaria**

SP P37.4 **Other congenital malaria**

SP P37.5 **Neonatal candidiasis**

SP P37.8 **Other specified congenital infectious and parasitic diseases**

IQ P37.9 **Congenital infectious or parasitic disease, unspecified**

4 P38 **Omphalitis of newborn**
> **EXCLUDES 1** omphalitis not of newborn (L08.82)
> tetanus omphalitis (A33)

Chapter 16

P00-P96

★ New ▲ Revised Px Primary **SP** PDGM Px **SL** Low CoM **SH** High CoM **IQ** Quest. Encounter **H** Hospice non-cancer Dx Unspecified **M** *Manifestation*

DecisionHealth's FY 2020 Complete Home Health ICD-10-CM Diagnosis Coding Manual

1375

umbilical hemorrhage of newborn (P51.-)

SP **P38.1** **Omphalitis with mild hemorrhage**

SP **P38.9** **Omphalitis without hemorrhage**
Omphalitis of newborn NOS

+ **☑ P39** **Other infections specific to the perinatal period**
Use additional code to identify organism or specific infection

SP + **P39.0** **Neonatal infective mastitis**
EXCLUDES 1 breast engorgement of newborn (P83.4)
noninfective mastitis of newborn (P83.4)
DEFINITION Inflammation of the breast in a newborn.

SP + **P39.1** **Neonatal conjunctivitis and dacryocystitis**
Neonatal chlamydial conjunctivitis
Ophthalmia neonatorum NOS
EXCLUDES 1 gonococcal conjunctivitis (A54.31)

SP + **P39.2** **Intra-amniotic infection affecting newborn, not elsewhere classified**

SP + **P39.3** **Neonatal urinary tract infection**

SP + **P39.4** **Neonatal skin infection**
Neonatal pyoderma
EXCLUDES 1 pemphigus neonatorum (L00)
staphylococcal scalded skin syndrome (L00)

SP + **P39.8** **Other specified infections specific to the perinatal period**

!Q + **P39.9** **Infection specific to the perinatal period, unspecified**

Hemorrhagic and hematological disorders of newborn   (P50-P61)

EXCLUDES 1 congenital stenosis and stricture of bile ducts (Q44.3)
Crigler-Najjar syndrome (E80.5)
Dubin-Johnson syndrome (E80.6)
Gilbert syndrome (E80.4)
hereditary hemolytic anemias (D55-D58)

☑ P50 **Newborn affected by intrauterine (fetal) blood loss**
EXCLUDES 1 congenital anemia from intrauterine (fetal) blood loss (P61.3)

SP **P50.0** **Newborn affected by intrauterine (fetal) blood loss from vasa previa**

SP **P50.1** **Newborn affected by intrauterine (fetal) blood loss from ruptured cord**

SP **P50.2** **Newborn affected by intrauterine (fetal) blood loss from placenta**

SP **P50.3** **Newborn affected by hemorrhage into co-twin**

SP **P50.4** **Newborn affected by hemorrhage into maternal circulation**

SP **P50.5** **Newborn affected by intrauterine (fetal) blood loss from cut end of co-twin's cord**

SP **P50.8** **Newborn affected by other intrauterine (fetal) blood loss**

SP **P50.9** **Newborn affected by intrauterine (fetal) blood loss, unspecified**

Newborn affected by fetal hemorrhage NOS

☑ P51 **Umbilical hemorrhage of newborn**
EXCLUDES 1 omphalitis with mild hemorrhage (P38.1)
umbilical hemorrhage from cut end of co-twins cord (P50.5)

SP **P51.0** **Massive umbilical hemorrhage of newborn**

SP **P51.8** **Other umbilical hemorrhages of newborn**
Slipped umbilical ligature NOS

SP **P51.9** **Umbilical hemorrhage of newborn, unspecified**

☑ P52 **Intracranial nontraumatic hemorrhage of newborn**
INCLUDES intracranial hemorrhage due to anoxia or hypoxia
EXCLUDES 1 intracranial hemorrhage due to birth injury (P10.-)
intracranial hemorrhage due to other injury (S06.-)

SP **P52.0** **Intraventricular (nontraumatic) hemorrhage, grade 1, of newborn**
Subependymal hemorrhage (without intraventricular extension)
Bleeding into germinal matrix

SP **P52.1** **Intraventricular (nontraumatic) hemorrhage, grade 2, of newborn**
Subependymal hemorrhage with intraventricular extension
Bleeding into ventricle

☑ P52.2 **Intraventricular (nontraumatic) hemorrhage, grade 3 and grade 4, of newborn**

SP **P52.21** **Intraventricular (nontraumatic) hemorrhage, grade 3, of newborn**
Subependymal hemorrhage with intraventricular extension with enlargement of ventricle

SP **P52.22** **Intraventricular (nontraumatic) hemorrhage, grade 4, of newborn**
Bleeding into cerebral cortex
Subependymal hemorrhage with intracerebral extension

!Q **P52.3** **Unspecified intraventricular (nontraumatic) hemorrhage of newborn**

SP **P52.4** **Intracerebral (nontraumatic) hemorrhage of newborn**

SP **P52.5** **Subarachnoid (nontraumatic) hemorrhage of newborn**

SP **P52.6** **Cerebellar (nontraumatic) and posterior fossa hemorrhage of newborn**

SP **P52.8** **Other intracranial (nontraumatic) hemorrhages of newborn**

!Q **P52.9** **Intracranial (nontraumatic) hemorrhage of newborn, unspecified**

SP **P53** **Hemorrhagic disease of newborn**
Vitamin K deficiency of newborn

☑ P54 **Other neonatal hemorrhages**
EXCLUDES 1 newborn affected by (intrauterine) blood loss (P50.-)
pulmonary hemorrhage originating in the perinatal period (P26.-)

SP **P54.0** **Neonatal hematemesis**

☑ 4th digit required   ☑ 5th digit required   ☑ 6th digit required   ☑ 7th digit required   ☑ 7th digit placeholder   + Additional code   ▣ Laterality

1376   DecisionHealth's FY 2020 Complete Home Health ICD-10-CM Diagnosis Coding Manual

EXCLUDES 1 neonatal hematemesis due to swallowed maternal blood (P78.2)

SP **P54.1** **Neonatal melena**
    EXCLUDES 1 neonatal melena due to swallowed maternal blood (P78.2)

SP **P54.2** **Neonatal rectal hemorrhage**

SP **P54.3** **Other neonatal gastrointestinal hemorrhage**

SP **P54.4** **Neonatal adrenal hemorrhage**

SP **P54.5** **Neonatal cutaneous hemorrhage**
Neonatal bruising
Neonatal ecchymoses
Neonatal petechiae
Neonatal superficial hematomata
    EXCLUDES 2 bruising of scalp due to birth injury (P12.3)
        cephalhematoma due to birth injury (P12.0)
    DEFINITION Minute red spots on the surface of the skin, due to escape of a small amount of blood from the vessels.

SP **P54.6** **Neonatal vaginal hemorrhage**
Neonatal pseudomenses

SP **P54.8** **Other specified neonatal hemorrhages**

IQ **P54.9** **Neonatal hemorrhage, unspecified**

4 **P55** **Hemolytic disease of newborn**

SP **P55.0** **Rh isoimmunization of newborn**

SP **P55.1** **ABO isoimmunization of newborn**

SP **P55.8** **Other hemolytic diseases of newborn**

IQ **P55.9** **Hemolytic disease of newborn, unspecified**

4 **P56** **Hydrops fetalis due to hemolytic disease**
    EXCLUDES 1 hydrops fetalis NOS (P83.2)

SP **P56.0** **Hydrops fetalis due to isoimmunization**

5 **P56.9** **Hydrops fetalis due to other and unspecified hemolytic disease**

IQ **P56.90** **Hydrops fetalis due to unspecified hemolytic disease**

SP **P56.99** **Hydrops fetalis due to other hemolytic disease**

4 **P57** **Kernicterus**

SP **P57.0** **Kernicterus due to isoimmunization**
    DEFINITION Encephalopathy due to severe jaundice caused by destruction of the infant's red blood cells by the mother's immune system. Excess bilirubin crosses the blood-brain barrier and accumulates toxically in the brain.

SP **P57.8** **Other specified kernicterus**
    EXCLUDES 1 Crigler-Najjar syndrome (E80.5)

SP **P57.9** **Kernicterus, unspecified**

4 **P58** **Neonatal jaundice due to other excessive hemolysis**
    EXCLUDES 1 jaundice due to isoimmunization (P55-P57)

SP **P58.0** **Neonatal jaundice due to bruising**

SP **P58.1** **Neonatal jaundice due to bleeding**

SP **P58.2** **Neonatal jaundice due to infection**

SP **P58.3** **Neonatal jaundice due to polycythemia**

+ **5** **P58.4** **Neonatal jaundice due to drugs or toxins transmitted from mother or given to newborn**
Code first:
  poisoning due to drug or toxin, if applicable
    (T36-T65 with fifth or sixth character 1-4 or 6)
Use additional code for adverse effect, if applicable, to identify drug (T36-T50 with fifth or sixth character 5)

SP **+** **P58.41** **Neonatal jaundice due to drugs or toxins transmitted from mother**

SP **+** **P58.42** **Neonatal jaundice due to drugs or toxins given to newborn**

SP **P58.5** **Neonatal jaundice due to swallowed maternal blood**

SP **P58.8** **Neonatal jaundice due to other specified excessive hemolysis**

SP **P58.9** **Neonatal jaundice due to excessive hemolysis, unspecified**

4 **P59** **Neonatal jaundice from other and unspecified causes**
    EXCLUDES 1 jaundice due to inborn errors of metabolism (E70-E88)
        kernicterus (P57.-)

SP **P59.0** **Neonatal jaundice associated with preterm delivery**
Hyperbilirubinemia of prematurity
Jaundice due to delayed conjugation associated with preterm delivery

SP **P59.1** **Inspissated bile syndrome**

5 **P59.2** **Neonatal jaundice from other and unspecified hepatocellular damage**
    EXCLUDES 1 congenital viral hepatitis (P35.3)

SP **P59.20** **Neonatal jaundice from unspecified hepatocellular damage**

SP **P59.29** **Neonatal jaundice from other hepatocellular damage**
Neonatal giant cell hepatitis
Neonatal (idiopathic) hepatitis

SP **P59.3** **Neonatal jaundice from breast milk inhibitor**

SP **P59.8** **Neonatal jaundice from other specified causes**

SP **P59.9** **Neonatal jaundice, unspecified**
Neonatal physiological jaundice (intense)(prolonged) NOS

SP **P60** **Disseminated intravascular coagulation of newborn**
Defibrination syndrome of newborn

4 **P61** **Other perinatal hematological disorders**
    EXCLUDES 1 transient hypogammaglobulinemia of infancy (D80.7)

SP **P61.0** **Transient neonatal thrombocytopenia**
Neonatal thrombocytopenia due to exchange transfusion
Neonatal thrombocytopenia due to idiopathic maternal thrombocytopenia
Neonatal thrombocytopenia due to isoimmunization

SP **P61.1** **Polycythemia neonatorum**
    DEFINITION Abnormally increased number of red blood cells in the neonate's bloodstream.

Chapter 16

P00-P96

★ New ▲ Revised **Px** Primary **SP** PDGM Px **SL** Low CoM **SH** High CoM **IQ** Quest. Encounter **H** Hospice non-cancer Dx Unspecified **M** *Manifestation*

DecisionHealth's FY 2020 Complete Home Health ICD-10-CM Diagnosis Coding Manual

1377

SP **P61.2** **Anemia of prematurity**

SP **P61.3** **Congenital anemia from fetal blood loss**

SP **P61.4** **Other congenital anemias, not elsewhere classified**
Congenital anemia NOS

SP **P61.5** **Transient neonatal neutropenia**
EXCLUDES 1 congenital neutropenia (nontransient) (D70.0)

SP **P61.6** **Other transient neonatal disorders of coagulation**

SP **P61.8** **Other specified perinatal hematological disorders**

IQ **P61.9** **Perinatal hematological disorder, unspecified**

Transitory endocrine and metabolic disorders specific to newborn (P70-P74)

INCLUDES transitory endocrine and metabolic disturbances caused by the infant's response to maternal endocrine and metabolic factors, or its adjustment to extrauterine environment

4 **P70** **Transitory disorders of carbohydrate metabolism specific to newborn**

SP **P70.0** **Syndrome of infant of mother with gestational diabetes**
Newborn (with hypoglycemia) affected by maternal gestational diabetes
EXCLUDES 1 newborn (with hypoglycemia) affected by maternal (pre-existing) diabetes mellitus (P70.1)
syndrome of infant of a diabetic mother (P70.1)

SP **P70.1** **Syndrome of infant of a diabetic mother**
Newborn (with hypoglycemia) affected by maternal (pre-existing) diabetes mellitus
EXCLUDES 1 newborn (with hypoglycemia) affected by maternal gestational diabetes (P70.0)
syndrome of infant of mother with gestational diabetes (P70.0)

SP **P70.2** **Neonatal diabetes mellitus**

SP **P70.3** **Iatrogenic neonatal hypoglycemia**

SP **P70.4** **Other neonatal hypoglycemia**
Transitory neonatal hypoglycemia

SP **P70.8** **Other transitory disorders of carbohydrate metabolism of newborn**

SP **P70.9** **Transitory disorder of carbohydrate metabolism of newborn, unspecified**

4 **P71** **Transitory neonatal disorders of calcium and magnesium metabolism**

SP **P71.0** **Cow's milk hypocalcemia in newborn**

SP **P71.1** **Other neonatal hypocalcemia**
EXCLUDES 1 neonatal hypoparathyroidism (P71.4)

SP **P71.2** **Neonatal hypomagnesemia**

SP **P71.3** **Neonatal tetany without calcium or magnesium deficiency**
Neonatal tetany NOS

SP **P71.4** **Transitory neonatal hypoparathyroidism**

SP **P71.8** **Other transitory neonatal disorders of calcium and magnesium metabolism**

SP **P71.9** **Transitory neonatal disorder of calcium and magnesium metabolism, unspecified**

4 **P72** **Other transitory neonatal endocrine disorders**
EXCLUDES 1 congenital hypothyroidism with or without goiter (E03.0-E03.1)
dyshormogenetic goiter (E07.1)
Pendred's syndrome (E07.1)

SP **P72.0** **Neonatal goiter, not elsewhere classified**
Transitory congenital goiter with normal functioning

SP **P72.1** **Transitory neonatal hyperthyroidism**
Neonatal thyrotoxicosis
DEFINITION Abnormally high levels of thyroid hormone in the neonate.

SP **P72.2** **Other transitory neonatal disorders of thyroid function, not elsewhere classified**
Transitory neonatal hypothyroidism

SP **P72.8** **Other specified transitory neonatal endocrine disorders**

IQ **P72.9** **Transitory neonatal endocrine disorder, unspecified**

4 **P74** **Other transitory neonatal electrolyte and metabolic disturbances**

SP **P74.0** **Late metabolic acidosis of newborn**
EXCLUDES 1 (fetal) metabolic acidosis of newborn (P19)
DEFINITION Imbalance in the acid to alkaline ratio in the blood, most often affecting premature infants in the 2nd and 3rd week of life.

SP **P74.1** **Dehydration of newborn**

5 **P74.2** **Disturbances of sodium balance of newborn**

SP **P74.21** **Hypernatremia of newborn**

SP **P74.22** **Hyponatremia of newborn**

5 **P74.3** **Disturbances of potassium balance of newborn**

SP **P74.31** **Hyperkalemia of newborn**

SP **P74.32** **Hypokalemia of newborn**

5 **P74.4** **Other transitory electrolyte disturbances of newborn**

SP **P74.41** **Alkalosis of newborn**
Hyperbicarbonatemia

6 **P74.42** **Disturbances of chlorine balance of newborn**

▲ **SP** **P74.421** **Hyperchloremia of newborn**
Hyperchloremic metabolic acidosis
EXCLUDES 2 late metabolic acidosis of the newborn (P74.0)

SP **P74.422** **Hypochloremia of newborn**

SP **P74.49** **Other transitory electrolyte disturbance of newborn**

SP **P74.5** **Transitory tyrosinemia of newborn**

SP **P74.6** **Transitory hyperammonemia of newborn**

SP **P74.8** **Other transitory metabolic disturbances of newborn**
Amino-acid metabolic disorders described as transitory

4 4th digit required **5** 5th digit required **6** 6th digit required **7** 7th digit required **☑** 7th digit placeholder **+** Additional code **⊟** Laterality

1378   *DecisionHealth's* FY 2020 Complete Home Health ICD-10-CM Diagnosis Coding Manual

Chapter 16

P00-P96

IQ P74.9 Transitory metabolic disturbance of newborn, unspecified

Digestive system disorders of newborn (P76-P78)

4 P76 Other intestinal obstruction of newborn

SP P76.0 Meconium plug syndrome
Meconium ileus NOS

> **EXCLUDES 1** meconium ileus in cystic fibrosis (E84.11)

> **DEFINITION** Dark green feces that normally comprises a newborn's first bowel movement does not pass through the bowel, causing blockage of the intestine.

SP P76.1 Transitory ileus of newborn

> **EXCLUDES 1** Hirschsprung's disease (Q43.1)

SP P76.2 Intestinal obstruction due to inspissated milk

SP P76.8 Other specified intestinal obstruction of newborn

> **EXCLUDES 1** intestinal obstruction classifiable to K56.-

IQ P76.9 Intestinal obstruction of newborn, unspecified

4 P77 Necrotizing enterocolitis of newborn

SP P77.1 Stage 1 necrotizing enterocolitis in newborn
Necrotizing enterocolitis without pneumatosis, without perforation

SP P77.2 Stage 2 necrotizing enterocolitis in newborn
Necrotizing enterocolitis with pneumatosis, without perforation

SP P77.3 Stage 3 necrotizing enterocolitis in newborn
Necrotizing enterocolitis with perforation
Necrotizing enterocolitis with pneumatosis and perforation

IQ P77.9 Necrotizing enterocolitis in newborn, unspecified
Necrotizing enterocolitis in newborn, NOS

4 P78 Other perinatal digestive system disorders

> **EXCLUDES 1** cystic fibrosis (E84.0-E84.9)
> neonatal gastrointestinal hemorrhages (P54.0-P54.3)

SP P78.0 Perinatal intestinal perforation
Meconium peritonitis

SP P78.1 Other neonatal peritonitis
Neonatal peritonitis NOS

SP P78.2 Neonatal hematemesis and melena due to swallowed maternal blood

SP P78.3 Noninfective neonatal diarrhea
Neonatal diarrhea NOS

5 P78.8 Other specified perinatal digestive system disorders

SP P78.81 Congenital cirrhosis (of liver)

SP P78.82 Peptic ulcer of newborn

SP P78.83 Newborn esophageal reflux
Neonatal esophageal reflux

SP P78.84 Gestational alloimmune liver disease
GALD
Neonatal hemochromatosis

> **EXCLUDES 1** hemochromatosis (E83.11-)

SP P78.89 Other specified perinatal digestive system disorders

SP P78.9 Perinatal digestive system disorder, unspecified

Conditions involving the integument and temperature regulation of newborn (P80-P83)

4 P80 Hypothermia of newborn

SP P80.0 Cold injury syndrome
Severe and usually chronic hypothermia associated with a pink flushed appearance, edema and neurological and biochemical abnormalities.

> **EXCLUDES 1** mild hypothermia of newborn (P80.8)

SP P80.8 Other hypothermia of newborn
Mild hypothermia of newborn

SP P80.9 Hypothermia of newborn, unspecified

4 P81 Other disturbances of temperature regulation of newborn

SP P81.0 Environmental hyperthermia of newborn

SP P81.8 Other specified disturbances of temperature regulation of newborn

SP P81.9 Disturbance of temperature regulation of newborn, unspecified
Fever of newborn NOS

4 P83 Other conditions of integument specific to newborn

> **EXCLUDES 1** congenital malformations of skin and integument (Q80-Q84)
> hydrops fetalis due to hemolytic disease (P56.-)
> neonatal skin infection (P39.4)
> staphylococcal scalded skin syndrome (L00)

> **EXCLUDES 2** cradle cap (L21.0)
> diaper [napkin] dermatitis (L22)

SP P83.0 Sclerema neonatorum

SP P83.1 Neonatal erythema toxicum

SP P83.2 Hydrops fetalis not due to hemolytic disease
Hydrops fetalis NOS

5 P83.3 Other and unspecified edema specific to newborn

SP P83.30 Unspecified edema specific to newborn

SP P83.39 Other edema specific to newborn

SP P83.4 Breast engorgement of newborn
Noninfective mastitis of newborn

SP P83.5 Congenital hydrocele

SP P83.6 Umbilical polyp of newborn

5 P83.8 Other specified conditions of integument specific to newborn

SP P83.81 Umbilical granuloma

> **EXCLUDES 2** Granulomatous disorder of the skin and subcutaneous tissue, unspecified (L92.9)

SP P83.88 Other specified conditions of integument specific to newborn
Bronze baby syndrome

★ New ▲ Revised Px Primary SP PDGM Px SL Low CoM SH High CoM IQ Quest. Encounter H Hospice non-cancer Dx Unspecified M Manifestation

DecisionHealth's FY 2020 Complete Home Health ICD-10-CM Diagnosis Coding Manual

1379

Neonatal scleroderma

Urticaria neonatorum

IQ P83.9   Condition of the integument specific to newborn, unspecified

Other problems with newborn (P84)

SP P84   Other problems with newborn

Acidemia of newborn

Acidosis of newborn

Anoxia of newborn NOS

Asphyxia of newborn NOS

Hypercapnia of newborn

Hypoxemia of newborn

Hypoxia of newborn NOS

Mixed metabolic and respiratory acidosis of newborn

> **EXCLUDES 1**   intracranial hemorrhage due to anoxia or hypoxia (P52.-)
> hypoxic ischemic encephalopathy [HIE] (P91.6-)
> late metabolic acidosis of newborn (P74.0)

Other disorders originating in the perinatal period (P90-P96)

SP P90   Convulsions of newborn

> **EXCLUDES 1**   benign myoclonic epilepsy in infancy (G40.3-)
> benign neonatal convulsions (familial) (G40.3-)

4 P91   Other disturbances of cerebral status of newborn

SP P91.0   Neonatal cerebral ischemia

SP P91.1   Acquired periventricular cysts of newborn

SP P91.2   Neonatal cerebral leukomalacia

Periventricular leukomalacia

SP P91.3   Neonatal cerebral irritability

SP P91.4   Neonatal cerebral depression

SP P91.5   Neonatal coma

5 P91.6   Hypoxic ischemic encephalopathy [HIE]

> **EXCLUDES 1**   Neonatal cerebral depression (P91.4)
> Neonatal cerebral irritability (P91.3)
> Neonatal coma (P91.5)

SP P91.60   Hypoxic ischemic encephalopathy [HIE], unspecified

SP P91.61   Mild hypoxic ischemic encephalopathy [HIE]

SP P91.62   Moderate hypoxic ischemic encephalopathy [HIE]

SP P91.63   Severe hypoxic ischemic encephalopathy [HIE]

5 P91.8   Other specified disturbances of cerebral status of newborn

6 P91.81   Neonatal encephalopathy

IQ P91.811   Neonatal encephalopathy in diseases classified elsewhere

Code first underlying condition, if known, such as:

congenital cirrhosis (of liver) (P78.81)

intracranial nontraumatic hemorrhage of newborn (P52.-)

kernicterus (P57.-)

SP P91.819   Neonatal encephalopathy, unspecified

SP P91.88   Other specified disturbances of cerebral status of newborn

IQ P91.9   Disturbance of cerebral status of newborn, unspecified

4 P92   Feeding problems of newborn

> **EXCLUDES 1**   eating disorders (F50.-)
> feeding problems in child over 28 days old (R63.3)

5 P92.0   Vomiting of newborn

> **EXCLUDES 1**   vomiting of child over 28 days old (R11.-)

SP P92.01   Bilious vomiting of newborn

> **EXCLUDES 1**   bilious vomiting in child over 28 days old (R11.14)

SP P92.09   Other vomiting of newborn

> **EXCLUDES 1**   regurgitation of food in newborn (P92.1)

SP P92.1   Regurgitation and rumination of newborn

SP P92.2   Slow feeding of newborn

SP P92.3   Underfeeding of newborn

SP P92.4   Overfeeding of newborn

SP P92.5   Neonatal difficulty in feeding at breast

SP P92.6   Failure to thrive in newborn

> **EXCLUDES 1**   failure to thrive in child over 28 days old (R62.51)

SP P92.8   Other feeding problems of newborn

IQ P92.9   Feeding problem of newborn, unspecified

4 P93   Reactions and intoxications due to drugs administered to newborn

> **INCLUDES**   reactions and intoxications due to drugs administered to fetus affecting newborn

> **EXCLUDES 1**   jaundice due to drugs or toxins transmitted from mother or given to newborn (P58.4-)
> reactions and intoxications from maternal opiates, tranquilizers and other medication (P04.0-P04.1, P04.4-)
> withdrawal symptoms from maternal use of drugs of addiction (P96.1)
> withdrawal symptoms from therapeutic use of drugs in newborn (P96.2)

SP P93.0   Grey baby syndrome

Grey syndrome from chloramphenicol administration in newborn

SP + P93.8   Other reactions and intoxications due to drugs administered to newborn

Use additional code for adverse effect, if applicable, to identify drug (T36-T50 with fifth or sixth character 5)

Chapter 16

P00-P96

---

4 4th digit required   **5** 5th digit required   **6** 6th digit required   **7** 7th digit required   **7** 7th digit placeholder   **+** Additional code   **▱** Laterality

4 P94 **Disorders of muscle tone of newborn**

SP P94.0 **Transient neonatal myasthenia gravis**
>> **EXCLUDES 1** myasthenia gravis (G70.0)

SP P94.1 **Congenital hypertonia**

SP P94.2 **Congenital hypotonia**
Floppy baby syndrome, unspecified

SP P94.8 **Other disorders of muscle tone of newborn**

IQ P94.9 **Disorder of muscle tone of newborn, unspecified**

IQ P95 **Stillbirth**
Deadborn fetus NOS
Fetal death of unspecified cause
Stillbirth NOS
>> **EXCLUDES 1** maternal care for intrauterine death (O36.4)
>> missed abortion (O02.1)
>> outcome of delivery, stillbirth (Z37.1, Z37.3, Z37.4, Z37.7)

4 P96 **Other conditions originating in the perinatal period**

SP P96.0 **Congenital renal failure**
Uremia of newborn

SP P96.1 **Neonatal withdrawal symptoms from maternal use of drugs of addiction**
Drug withdrawal syndrome in infant of dependent mother
Neonatal abstinence syndrome
>> **EXCLUDES 1** reactions and intoxications from maternal opiates and tranquilizers administered during labor and delivery (P04.0)

SP P96.2 **Withdrawal symptoms from therapeutic use of drugs in newborn**

SP P96.3 **Wide cranial sutures of newborn**
Neonatal craniotabes

SP P96.5 **Complication to newborn due to (fetal) intrauterine procedure**
>> **EXCLUDES 2** newborn affected by amniocentesis (P00.6)

5 P96.8 **Other specified conditions originating in the perinatal period**

SP P96.81 **Exposure to (parental) (environmental) tobacco smoke in the perinatal period**
>> **EXCLUDES 2** newborn affected by in utero exposure to tobacco (P04.2)
>> exposure to environmental tobacco smoke after the perinatal period (Z77.22)

SP P96.82 **Delayed separation of umbilical cord**

IQ P96.83 **Meconium staining**
>> **EXCLUDES 1** meconium aspiration (P24.00, P24.01)
>> meconium passage during delivery (P03.82)

SP + P96.89 **Other specified conditions originating in the perinatal period**
Use additional code to specify condition

IQ P96.9 **Condition originating in the perinatal period, unspecified**

Congenital debility NOS

★ New ▲ Revised Px Primary SP PDGM Px SL Low CoM SH High CoM IQ Quest. Encounter H Hospice non-cancer Dx Unspecified M *Manifestation*

DecisionHealth's FY 2020 Complete Home Health ICD-10-CM Diagnosis Coding Manual

1381

Chapter 16

P00-P96

Chapter 17: Congenital Malformations, Deformations and Chromosomal Abnormalities (Q00-Q99)

"Congenital" indicates a condition that is present at birth. A congenital anomaly may be caused by an inherited abnormality (such as webbed fingers or syndactyly), or due to environmental factors (such as fetal alcohol syndrome). Chapter 17 includes codes for congenital conditions related to problems inherited from parents as well as environmental causes. Chapter 16 includes congenital conditions related to environmental problems or injuries occurring during birth.

Codes for these conditions are located in the Alphabetic Index under the terms "anomaly", malformations, deformity/deformations or abnormal chromosomal.

Assign appropriate codes from this chapter when a malformation/deformation or chromosomal abnormality is documented. The diagnosis may be principal/first-listed or a secondary diagnosis.

Codes in this chapter most often are reported for pediatric patients, but may be listed throughout the patient's life. Some anomalies are present at birth but do not become apparent until later in life, e.g., arteriovenous malformations in the brain. Whenever the condition is diagnosed during the patient's lifetime, it is appropriate to assign a code from code range Q00-Q99.

If a congenital malformation or deformity has been corrected, a personal history code should be used to **identify the history of the malformation or deformity. Note,** codes from this chapter are not for use on maternal records.

Multiple Coding and Sequencing

It is important to read the Includes and Excludes notes under codes in this chapter, as well as any other instructions under the code or code category. The following are examples of multiple coding and sequencing issues for codes in this chapter:

- When a congenital anomaly does not have a unique code assignment, assign additional codes for any manifestation that may be present. An example is the use of code Q79.1 (Other congenital malformations of diaphragm) for a patient with congenital absence of diaphragm. Report the associated respiratory conditions as additional diagnoses to provide more information.

- When the code assignment specifically identifies the malformation, deformity or chromosomal abnormality, manifestations that are an inherent component of the anomaly should not be coded separately. An example is code Q21.3 (Tetralogy of Fallot). The individual cardiac conditions associated with this anomaly such as ventricular septal defect with pulmonary stenosis

or atresia, dextroposition of aorta, and hypertrophy of right ventricle, are not reported separately. However, additional codes should be assigned for manifestations that are not an inherent component of the condition.

When a malformation, deformation or chromosomal abnormality does not have a unique code assignment, assign additional codes for any manifestations that may be present,

- For the birth admission, the appropriate code from category Z38, Liveborn infants, according to place of birth and type of delivery, should be sequenced as the principal diagnosis, followed by any congenital anomaly codes (Q00-Q99) as additional diagnoses.

Special Coding Issues – Congenital or Acquired

Coders should be cautious when selecting codes from this chapter. Some conditions can be either congenital or acquired (developed after birth). The Alphabetical Index in ICD-10 shows acquired and congenital as subentries under the main term.

Defect
      Circulation I99.9
            congenital Q28.9

A congenital circulation defect is reported using code Q28.9; an acquired defect is reported using code I99.9. If not specified as acquired or congenital, query the physician or report as acquired.

The Alphabetic Index sometimes indicates an acquired condition using parentheses as a nonessential modifier. For example, the index for cyst of kidney reads:

Cyst
      Kidney (acquired) N28.1
            congenital Q61.00

Congenital cysts are reported using code Q61.00; acquired cysts are reported using code N28.1. If not specified as acquired or congenital, query the physician or report as acquired.

Coders often make mistakes when referencing the Alphabetic Index for the status codes for absent body parts, such as amputation status codes. Many entries under the term "absence" include two choices – one for the congenital absence of the body part and one for the acquired absence. Acquired absence is usually the result of surgical removal. Reference: 'Absence, lung.' The first code listed is Q33.3 for the congenital absence of the lung. The second code listed is Z90.2 for the acquired absence of lung, i.e., surgical removal.

Chapter 17

Q00-Q99

CHAPTER 17: CONGENITAL MALFORMATIONS, DEFORMATIONS AND CHROMOSOMAL ABNORMALITIES (Q00-Q99)

Note:

Codes from this chapter are not for use on maternal records

EXCLUDES 2 inborn errors of metabolism (E70-E88)

ALERT Sometimes payer policy conflicts with official guidelines, rules and conventions, and other official guidance. When a payer refuses to pay based on code(s) used in compliance with that guidance, take the following steps: 1) Determine whether the denial or rejection is truly a coding dispute and not a different coverage or payment issue; 2) Remind the payer that following official guidelines and conventions is required by HIPAA code set standards and provide the official guidance in question. If a payer does have a policy that clearly conflicts with official coding rules or guidelines, every effort should be made to resolve the issue with the payer; 3) If the payer refuses to change its policy, obtain the payer requirements in writing. If the payer refuses to provide their policy in writing, document all discussions, including dates and names of individuals involved; 4) Conform to the payer's policy if the payer continues to deny or reject the claim; 5) Keep a permanent file of the documentation obtained regarding payer coding policies. It may be come in handy in the event of an audit.

GUIDELINES Section I.C.17

Codes from Chapter 17 may be used throughout the life of the patient. If a congenital malformation or deformity has been corrected, a personal history code should be used to identify the history of the malformation or deformity. Although present at birth, malformation/deformation/or chromosomal abnormality may not be identified until later in life. Whenever the condition is diagnosed by the physician, it is appropriate to assign a code from codes Q00-Q99. For the birth admission, the appropriate code from category Z38, Liveborn infants, according to place of birth and type of delivery, should be sequenced as the principal diagnosis, followed by any congenital anomaly codes, Q00- Q99.

This chapter contains the following blocks:

Q00-Q07	Congenital malformations of the nervous system
Q10-Q18	Congenital malformations of eye, ear, face and neck
Q20-Q28	Congenital malformations of the circulatory system
Q30-Q34	Congenital malformations of the respiratory system
Q35-Q37	Cleft lip and cleft palate
Q38-Q45	Other congenital malformations of the digestive system
Q50-Q56	Congenital malformations of genital organs
Q60-Q64	Congenital malformations of the urinary system
Q65-Q79	Congenital malformations and deformations of the musculoskeletal system
Q80-Q89	Other congenital malformations
Q90-Q99	Chromosomal abnormalities, not elsewhere classified

Congenital malformations of the nervous system (Q00-Q07)

4 Q00 Anencephaly and similar malformations

IQ Q00.0 Anencephaly
Acephaly
Acrania
Amyelencephaly
Hemianencephaly

Hemicephaly

IQ Q00.1 Craniorachischisis

IQ Q00.2 Iniencephaly

DEFINITION Neural tube birth defect in which the fetal head is severely bent backwards, the neck is usually absent, and other severe birth defects are present.

4 Q01 Encephalocele

INCLUDES Arnold-Chiari syndrome, type III
encephalocystocele
encephalomyelocele
hydroencephalocele
hydromeningocele, cranial
meningocele, cerebral
meningoencephalocele

EXCLUDES 1 Meckel-Gruber syndrome (Q61.9)

IQ Q01.0 Frontal encephalocele

IQ Q01.1 Nasofrontal encephalocele

IQ Q01.2 Occipital encephalocele

IQ Q01.8 Encephalocele of other sites

IQ Q01.9 Encephalocele, unspecified

▲ **IQ Q02** Microcephaly

INCLUDES hydromicrocephaly
micrencephalon

Code first:
, if applicable, congenital Zika virus disease

EXCLUDES 1 Meckel-Gruber syndrome (Q61.9)

DEFINITION Abnormal smallness of the head.

4 Q03 Congenital hydrocephalus

INCLUDES hydrocephalus in newborn

EXCLUDES 1 Arnold-Chiari syndrome, type II (Q07.0-)
acquired hydrocephalus (G91.-)
hydrocephalus due to congenital toxoplasmosis (P37.1)
hydrocephalus with spina bifida (Q05.0-Q05.4)

CODING TIPS ✓ Use Z98.2 as a secondary code to indicate a cerebrospinal fluid drainage shunt.

IQ Q03.0 Malformations of aqueduct of Sylvius
Anomaly of aqueduct of Sylvius
Obstruction of aqueduct of Sylvius, congenital
Stenosis of aqueduct of Sylvius

IQ Q03.1 Atresia of foramina of Magendie and Luschka
Dandy-Walker syndrome

IQ Q03.8 Other congenital hydrocephalus

IQ Q03.9 Congenital hydrocephalus, unspecified

4 Q04 Other congenital malformations of brain

EXCLUDES 1 cyclopia (Q87.0)
macrocephaly (Q75.3)

IQ Q04.0 Congenital malformations of corpus callosum
Agenesis of corpus callosum

IQ Q04.1 Arhinencephaly

IQ Q04.2 Holoprosencephaly

IQ Q04.3 Other reduction deformities of brain
Absence of part of brain
Agenesis of part of brain

---

4 4th digit required   **5** 5th digit required   **6** 6th digit required   **7** 7th digit required   **7** 7th digit placeholder   **+** Additional code   **⬚** Laterality

1384   *DecisionHealth's* FY 2020 Complete Home Health ICD-10-CM Diagnosis Coding Manual

Agyria
Aplasia of part of brain
Hydranencephaly
Hypoplasia of part of brain
Lissencephaly
Microgyria
Pachygyria

EXCLUDES 1   congenital malformations of corpus callosum (Q04.0)

IQ **Q04.4 Septo-optic dysplasia of brain**

IQ **Q04.5 Megalencephaly**

IQ **Q04.6 Congenital cerebral cysts**
Porencephaly
Schizencephaly

EXCLUDES 1   acquired porencephalic cyst (G93.0)

IQ **Q04.8 Other specified congenital malformations of brain**
Arnold-Chiari syndrome, type IV
Macrogyria

IQ **Q04.9 Congenital malformation of brain, unspecified**
Congenital anomaly NOS of brain
Congenital deformity NOS of brain
Congenital disease or lesion NOS of brain
Multiple anomalies NOS of brain, congenital

+ 4 Q05   Spina bifida
INCLUDES   hydromeningocele (spinal)
meningocele (spinal)
meningomyelocele
myelocele
myelomeningocele
rachischisis
spina bifida (aperta) (cystica)
syringomyelocele

Use additional code for any associated paraplegia (paraparesis) (G82.2-)

EXCLUDES 1   Arnold-Chiari syndrome, type II (Q07.0-)
spina bifida occulta (Q76.0)

CODING TIPS ✓   Use Z98.2 as a secondary code to indicate a cerebrospinal fluid drainage shunt.

SP + Q05.0   Cervical spina bifida with hydrocephalus

SP + Q05.1   Thoracic spina bifida with hydrocephalus
Dorsal spina bifida with hydrocephalus
Thoracolumbar spina bifida with hydrocephalus

SP + Q05.2   Lumbar spina bifida with hydrocephalus
Lumbosacral spina bifida with hydrocephalus

SP + Q05.3   Sacral spina bifida with hydrocephalus

SP + Q05.4   Unspecified spina bifida with hydrocephalus

SP + Q05.5   Cervical spina bifida without hydrocephalus

SP + Q05.6   Thoracic spina bifida without hydrocephalus
Dorsal spina bifida NOS
Thoracolumbar spina bifida NOS

SP + Q05.7   Lumbar spina bifida without hydrocephalus
Lumbosacral spina bifida NOS

SP + Q05.8   Sacral spina bifida without hydrocephalus

SP + Q05.9   Spina bifida, unspecified

4 Q06   Other congenital malformations of spinal cord

IQ **Q06.0 Amyelia**

IQ **Q06.1 Hypoplasia and dysplasia of spinal cord**
Atelomyelia
Myelatelia
Myelodysplasia of spinal cord

IQ **Q06.2 Diastematomyelia**

IQ **Q06.3 Other congenital cauda equina malformations**

IQ **Q06.4 Hydromyelia**
Hydrorachis

IQ **Q06.8 Other specified congenital malformations of spinal cord**

IQ **Q06.9 Congenital malformation of spinal cord, unspecified**
Congenital anomaly NOS of spinal cord
Congenital deformity NOS of spinal cord
Congenital disease or lesion NOS of spinal cord

4 Q07   Other congenital malformations of nervous system
EXCLUDES 2   congenital central alveolar hypoventilation syndrome (G47.35)
familial dysautonomia [Riley-Day] (G90.1)
neurofibromatosis (nonmalignant) (Q85.0-)

CODING TIPS ✓   Chiari malformation, also referred to as Arnold-Chiari malformation, is an anomaly where cerebellar tissue extends into the spinal canal. The most common form, type IV, includes spina bifida and hydrocephalus. Type IV is an anomaly where cerebellar hypoplasia is present.

5 Q07.0   Arnold-Chiari syndrome
Arnold-Chiari syndrome, type II
EXCLUDES 1   Arnold-Chiari syndrome, type III (Q01.-)
Arnold-Chiari syndrome, type IV (Q04.8)

SP Q07.00   Arnold-Chiari syndrome without spina bifida or hydrocephalus

SP Q07.01   Arnold-Chiari syndrome with spina bifida

SP Q07.02   Arnold-Chiari syndrome with hydrocephalus

SP Q07.03   Arnold-Chiari syndrome with spina bifida and hydrocephalus

SP Q07.8   Other specified congenital malformations of nervous system
Agenesis of nerve
Displacement of brachial plexus
Jaw-winking syndrome
Marcus Gunn's syndrome

IQ **Q07.9 Congenital malformation of nervous system, unspecified**
Congenital anomaly NOS of nervous system
Congenital deformity NOS of nervous system
Congenital disease or lesion NOS of nervous system

★ New ▲ Revised   **Px** Primary   **SP** PDGM Px   **SL** Low CoM   **SH** High CoM   **IQ** Quest. Encounter   **H** Hospice non-cancer Dx   Unspecified   **M** *Manifestation*

DecisionHealth's FY 2020 Complete Home Health ICD-10-CM Diagnosis Coding Manual   1385

Chapter 17

Q00-Q99

Congenital malformations of eye, ear, face and neck (Q10-Q18)

EXCLUDES 2   cleft lip and cleft palate (Q35-Q37)
congenital malformation of cervical spine (Q05.0, Q05.5, Q67.5, Q76.0-Q76.4)
congenital malformation of larynx (Q31.-)
congenital malformation of lip NEC (Q38.0)
congenital malformation of nose (Q30.-)
congenital malformation of parathyroid gland (Q89.2)
congenital malformation of thyroid gland (Q89.2)

4 Q10   Congenital malformations of eyelid, lacrimal apparatus and orbit
> **EXCLUDES 1**   cryptophthalmos NOS (Q11.2)
> cryptophthalmos syndrome (Q87.0)

IQ Q10.0   Congenital ptosis
> **DEFINITION**   Congenital drooping of the upper eyelid.

IQ Q10.1   Congenital ectropion

IQ Q10.2   Congenital entropion

IQ Q10.3   Other congenital malformations of eyelid
Ablepharon
Blepharophimosis, congenital
Coloboma of eyelid
Congenital absence or agenesis of cilia
Congenital absence or agenesis of eyelid
Congenital accessory eyelid
Congenital accessory eye muscle
Congenital malformation of eyelid NOS

IQ Q10.4   Absence and agenesis of lacrimal apparatus
Congenital absence of punctum lacrimale

IQ Q10.5   Congenital stenosis and stricture of lacrimal duct

IQ Q10.6   Other congenital malformations of lacrimal apparatus
Congenital malformation of lacrimal apparatus NOS

IQ Q10.7   Congenital malformation of orbit

4 Q11   Anophthalmos, microphthalmos and macrophthalmos

IQ Q11.0   Cystic eyeball

IQ Q11.1   Other anophthalmos
Anophthalmos NOS
Agenesis of eye
Aplasia of eye

IQ Q11.2   Microphthalmos
Cryptophthalmos NOS
Dysplasia of eye
Hypoplasia of eye
Rudimentary eye
> **EXCLUDES 1**   cryptophthalmos syndrome (Q87.0)
> **DEFINITION**   Abnormal smallness in all dimensions of one or both eyes.

IQ Q11.3   Macrophthalmos
> **EXCLUDES 1**   macrophthalmos in congenital glaucoma (Q15.0)

4 Q12   Congenital lens malformations

IQ Q12.0   Congenital cataract

IQ Q12.1   Congenital displaced lens

IQ Q12.2   Coloboma of lens

IQ Q12.3   Congenital aphakia

IQ Q12.4   Spherophakia

IQ Q12.8   Other congenital lens malformations
Microphakia

IQ Q12.9   Congenital lens malformation, unspecified

4 Q13   Congenital malformations of anterior segment of eye

IQ Q13.0   Coloboma of iris
Coloboma NOS

IQ + Q13.1   Absence of iris
Aniridia
Use additional code for associated glaucoma (H42)

IQ Q13.2   Other congenital malformations of iris
Anisocoria, congenital
Atresia of pupil
Congenital malformation of iris NOS
Corectopia

IQ Q13.3   Congenital corneal opacity

IQ Q13.4   Other congenital corneal malformations
Congenital malformation of cornea NOS
Microcornea
Peter's anomaly

IQ Q13.5   Blue sclera

5 Q13.8   Other congenital malformations of anterior segment of eye

IQ + Q13.81   Rieger's anomaly
> Use additional code for associated glaucoma (H42)

IQ Q13.89   Other congenital malformations of anterior segment of eye

IQ Q13.9   Congenital malformation of anterior segment of eye, unspecified

4 Q14   Congenital malformations of posterior segment of eye
> **EXCLUDES 2**   optic nerve hypoplasia (H47.03-)

IQ Q14.0   Congenital malformation of vitreous humor
Congenital vitreous opacity

IQ Q14.1   Congenital malformation of retina
Congenital retinal aneurysm

IQ Q14.2   Congenital malformation of optic disc
Coloboma of optic disc

IQ Q14.3   Congenital malformation of choroid

IQ Q14.8   Other congenital malformations of posterior segment of eye
Coloboma of the fundus

IQ Q14.9   Congenital malformation of posterior segment of eye, unspecified

4 Q15   Other congenital malformations of eye
> **EXCLUDES 1**   congenital nystagmus (H55.01)
> ocular albinism (E70.31-)
> optic nerve hypoplasia (H47.03-)
> retinitis pigmentosa (H35.52)

IQ Q15.0   Congenital glaucoma
Axenfeld's anomaly
Buphthalmos
Glaucoma of childhood
Glaucoma of newborn
Hydrophthalmos
Keratoglobus, congenital, with glaucoma
Macrocornea with glaucoma

---

4 4th digit required   5 5th digit required   6 6th digit required   7 7th digit required   7 7th digit placeholder   + Additional code   Laterality

Macrophthalmos in congenital glaucoma
Megalocornea with glaucoma

DEFINITION   Disease of infancy, marked by an increase of intraocular fluid, elevated eye pressure, and enlargement of the eyeball.

!Q Q15.8 Other specified congenital malformations of eye

!Q Q15.9 Congenital malformation of eye, unspecified

Congenital anomaly of eye
Congenital deformity of eye

4 Q16 Congenital malformations of ear causing impairment of hearing

EXCLUDES 1   congenital deafness (H90.-)

!Q Q16.0 Congenital absence of (ear) auricle

!Q Q16.1 Congenital absence, atresia and stricture of auditory canal (external)

Congenital atresia or stricture of osseous meatus

!Q Q16.2 Absence of eustachian tube

!Q Q16.3 Congenital malformation of ear ossicles

Congenital fusion of ear ossicles

!Q Q16.4 Other congenital malformations of middle ear

Congenital malformation of middle ear NOS

!Q Q16.5 Congenital malformation of inner ear

Congenital anomaly of membranous labyrinth
Congenital anomaly of organ of Corti

!Q Q16.9 Congenital malformation of ear causing impairment of hearing, unspecified

Congenital absence of ear NOS

4 Q17 Other congenital malformations of ear

EXCLUDES 1   congenital malformations of ear with impairment of hearing (Q16.0-Q16.9)
preauricular sinus (Q18.1)

!Q Q17.0 Accessory auricle

Accessory tragus
Polyotia
Preauricular appendage or tag
Supernumerary ear
Supernumerary lobule

!Q Q17.1 Macrotia

DEFINITION   Excessive enlargement of the auricle (outer portion of ear).

!Q Q17.2 Microtia

!Q Q17.3 Other misshapen ear

Pointed ear

!Q Q17.4 Misplaced ear

Low-set ears

EXCLUDES 1   cervical auricle (Q18.2)

!Q Q17.5 Prominent ear

Bat ear

!Q Q17.8 Other specified congenital malformations of ear

Congenital absence of lobe of ear

!Q Q17.9 Congenital malformation of ear, unspecified

Congenital anomaly of ear NOS

4 Q18 Other congenital malformations of face and neck

EXCLUDES 1   cleft lip and cleft palate (Q35-Q37)
conditions classified to Q67.0-Q67.4
congenital malformations of skull and face bones (Q75.-)
cyclopia (Q87.0)
dentofacial anomalies [including malocclusion] (M26.-)
malformation syndromes affecting facial appearance (Q87.0)
persistent thyroglossal duct (Q89.2)

!Q Q18.0 Sinus, fistula and cyst of branchial cleft

Branchial vestige

!Q Q18.1 Preauricular sinus and cyst

Fistula of auricle, congenital
Cervicoaural fistula

!Q Q18.2 Other branchial cleft malformations

Branchial cleft malformation NOS
Cervical auricle
Otocephaly

!Q Q18.3 Webbing of neck

Pterygium colli

DEFINITION   A thick flap of skin extending from the side of the neck to the shoulder, often in concert with other birth defects.

!Q Q18.4 Macrostomia

DEFINITION   Abnormally large mouth.

!Q Q18.5 Microstomia

DEFINITION   Abnormally small mouth.

!Q Q18.6 Macrocheilia

Hypertrophy of lip, congenital

DEFINITION   Abnormally large lips.

!Q Q18.7 Microcheilia

!Q Q18.8 Other specified congenital malformations of face and neck

Medial cyst of face and neck
Medial fistula of face and neck
Medial sinus of face and neck

!Q Q18.9 Congenital malformation of face and neck, unspecified

Congenital anomaly NOS of face and neck

★ New ▲ Revised Px Primary   SP PDGM Px   SL Low CoM   SH High CoM   !Q Quest. Encounter   H Hospice non-cancer Dx   Unspecified   M *Manifestation*

DecisionHealth's FY 2020 Complete Home Health ICD-10-CM Diagnosis Coding Manual   1387

Chapter 17

Q00-Q99

Congenital malformations of the circulatory system   (Q20-Q28)

Normal Heart   Double Outlet Right Ventricle   Double Inlet Ventricle
           Double Outlet Left Ventricle   Tetrology of Fallot

Discordant Ventricularerial   Discordant Atrioventricular Connection
Connection   Malformation of Cardiac Chambers

4️⃣ Q20   Congenital malformations of cardiac chambers and connections
> **EXCLUDES 1**   dextrocardia with situs inversus (Q89.3)
> mirror-image atrial arrangement with situs inversus (Q89.3)

SP Q20.0   Common arterial trunk
Persistent truncus arteriosus
> **EXCLUDES 1**   aortic septal defect (Q21.4)

> **DEFINITION**   Congenital anomaly in which there is abnormal communication between the ascending aorta and pulmonary artery, near the semilunar valve.

SP Q20.1   Double outlet right ventricle
Taussig-Bing syndrome

SP Q20.2   Double outlet left ventricle

SP Q20.3   Discordant ventriculoarterial connection
Dextrotransposition of aorta
Transposition of great vessels (complete)

SP Q20.4   Double inlet ventricle
Common ventricle
Cor triloculare biatriatum
Single ventricle
> **DEFINITION**   No septum or membrane is present dividing the right ventricle from the left ventricle.

SP Q20.5   Discordant atrioventricular connection
Corrected transposition
Levotransposition
Ventricular inversion

SP Q20.6   Isomerism of atrial appendages
Isomerism of atrial appendages with asplenia or polysplenia

SP Q20.8   Other congenital malformations of cardiac chambers and connections
Cor binoculare

IQ Q20.9   Congenital malformation of cardiac chambers and connections, unspecified

4️⃣ Q21   Congenital malformations of cardiac septa
> **EXCLUDES 1**   acquired cardiac septal defect (I51.0)

SP Q21.0   Ventricular septal defect
Roger's disease

SP Q21.1   Atrial septal defect
Coronary sinus defect
Patent or persistent foramen ovale
Patent or persistent ostium secundum defect (type II)
Patent or persistent sinus venosus defect

SP Q21.2   Atrioventricular septal defect
Common atrioventricular canal
Endocardial cushion defect
Ostium primum atrial septal defect (type I)

SP Q21.3   Tetralogy of Fallot
Ventricular septal defect with pulmonary stenosis or atresia, dextroposition of aorta and hypertrophy of right ventricle.

SP Q21.4   Aortopulmonary septal defect
Aortic septal defect
Aortopulmonary window

SP Q21.8   Other congenital malformations of cardiac septa
Eisenmenger's defect
Pentalogy of Fallot
Code also if applicable:
   Eisenmenger's complex (I27.83)
   Eisenmenger's syndrome (I27.83)

IQ Q21.9   Congenital malformation of cardiac septum, unspecified
Septal (heart) defect NOS

4️⃣ Q22   Congenital malformations of pulmonary and tricuspid valves

SP Q22.0   Pulmonary valve atresia
> **DEFINITION**   Congenital absence of a normal valvular opening into the pulmonary artery.

SP Q22.1   Congenital pulmonary valve stenosis

SP Q22.2   Congenital pulmonary valve insufficiency
Congenital pulmonary valve regurgitation

SP Q22.3   Other congenital malformations of pulmonary valve
Congenital malformation of pulmonary valve NOS
Supernumerary cusps of pulmonary valve

SP Q22.4   Congenital tricuspid stenosis
Congenital tricuspid atresia
> **DEFINITION**   Abnormal narrowing of the valve that prevents blood from flowing back into the right atrium from the right ventricle.

SP Q22.5   Ebstein's anomaly

SP Q22.6   Hypoplastic right heart syndrome

SP Q22.8   Other congenital malformations of tricuspid valve

SP Q22.9   Congenital malformation of tricuspid valve, unspecified

4️⃣ Q23   Congenital malformations of aortic and mitral valves

SP Q23.0   Congenital stenosis of aortic valve
Congenital aortic atresia
Congenital aortic stenosis NOS
> **EXCLUDES 1**   congenital stenosis of aortic valve in hypoplastic left heart syndrome (Q23.4)
> congenital subaortic stenosis (Q24.4)
> supravalvular aortic stenosis (congenital) (Q25.3)

4️⃣ 4th digit required   5️⃣ 5th digit required   6️⃣ 6th digit required   7️⃣ 7th digit required   7️⃣ 7th digit placeholder   ➕ Additional code   ⊟ Laterality

SP Q23.1 Congenital insufficiency of aortic valve
Bicuspid aortic valve
Congenital aortic insufficiency

SP Q23.2 Congenital mitral stenosis
Congenital mitral atresia

SP Q23.3 Congenital mitral insufficiency

SP Q23.4 Hypoplastic left heart syndrome

SP Q23.8 Other congenital malformations of aortic and mitral valves

IQ Q23.9 Congenital malformation of aortic and mitral valves, unspecified

4 Q24 Other congenital malformations of heart
EXCLUDES 1 endocardial fibroelastosis (I42.4)

SP Q24.0 Dextrocardia
EXCLUDES 1 dextrocardia with situs inversus (Q89.3)
isomerism of atrial appendages (with asplenia or polysplenia) (Q20.6)
mirror-image atrial arrangement with situs inversus (Q89.3)

SP Q24.1 Levocardia

SP Q24.2 Cor triatriatum
DEFINITION The heart has three atrial chambers with the left atrium divided into two segments.

SP Q24.3 Pulmonary infundibular stenosis
Subvalvular pulmonic stenosis

SP Q24.4 Congenital subaortic stenosis

SP Q24.5 Malformation of coronary vessels
Congenital coronary (artery) aneurysm

SP Q24.6 Congenital heart block

SP Q24.8 Other specified congenital malformations of heart
Congenital diverticulum of left ventricle
Congenital malformation of myocardium
Congenital malformation of pericardium
Malposition of heart
Uhl's disease

IQ Q24.9 Congenital malformation of heart, unspecified
Congenital anomaly of heart
Congenital disease of heart

4 Q25 Congenital malformations of great arteries
CODING TIPS ✓ If the condition has been corrected or is no longer a problem, then code Z87.74, Personal history of (corrected) congenital malformations of heart and circulatory system.

SP Q25.0 Patent ductus arteriosus
Patent ductus Botallo
Persistent ductus arteriosus

SP Q25.1 Coarctation of aorta
Coarctation of aorta (preductal) (postductal)
Stenosis of aorta

5 Q25.2 Atresia of aorta

SP Q25.21 Interruption of aortic arch
Atresia of aortic arch

SP Q25.29 Other atresia of aorta
Atresia of aorta

SP Q25.3 Supravalvular aortic stenosis

EXCLUDES 1 congenital aortic stenosis NOS (Q23.0)
congenital stenosis of aortic valve (Q23.0)

5 Q25.4 Other congenital malformations of aorta
EXCLUDES 1 hypoplasia of aorta in hypoplastic left heart syndrome (Q23.4)

IQ Q25.40 Congenital malformation of aorta unspecified

SP Q25.41 Absence and aplasia of aorta

SP Q25.42 Hypoplasia of aorta

SP Q25.43 Congenital aneurysm of aorta
Congenital aneurysm of aortic root
Congenital aneurysm of aortic sinus

SP Q25.44 Congenital dilation of aorta

SP Q25.45 Double aortic arch
Vascular ring of aorta

SP Q25.46 Tortuous aortic arch
Persistent convolutions of aortic arch

SP Q25.47 Right aortic arch
Persistent right aortic arch

SP Q25.48 Anomalous origin of subclavian artery

SP Q25.49 Other congenital malformations of aorta
Aortic arch
Bovine arch

SP Q25.5 Atresia of pulmonary artery

SP Q25.6 Stenosis of pulmonary artery
Supravalvular pulmonary stenosis

5 Q25.7 Other congenital malformations of pulmonary artery

SP Q25.71 Coarctation of pulmonary artery

SP Q25.72 Congenital pulmonary arteriovenous malformation
Congenital pulmonary arteriovenous aneurysm

SP Q25.79 Other congenital malformations of pulmonary artery
Aberrant pulmonary artery
Agenesis of pulmonary artery
Congenital aneurysm of pulmonary artery
Congenital anomaly of pulmonary artery
Hypoplasia of pulmonary artery

SP Q25.8 Other congenital malformations of other great arteries

IQ Q25.9 Congenital malformation of great arteries, unspecified

4 Q26 Congenital malformations of great veins

SP Q26.0 Congenital stenosis of vena cava
Congenital stenosis of vena cava (inferior)(superior)

SP Q26.1 Persistent left superior vena cava

SP Q26.2 Total anomalous pulmonary venous connection
Total anomalous pulmonary venous return [TAPVR], subdiaphragmatic
Total anomalous pulmonary venous return [TAPVR], supradiaphragmatic

SP Q26.3 Partial anomalous pulmonary venous connection
Partial anomalous pulmonary venous return

★ New ▲ Revised Px Primary **SP** PDGM Px **SL** Low CoM **SH** High CoM **IQ** Quest. Encounter **H** Hospice non-cancer Dx Unspecified **M** *Manifestation*

DecisionHealth's FY 2020 Complete Home Health ICD-10-CM Diagnosis Coding Manual 1389

Chapter 17

Q00-Q99

SP Q26.4 Anomalous pulmonary venous connection, unspecified

SP Q26.5 Anomalous portal venous connection

SP Q26.6 Portal vein-hepatic artery fistula

SP Q26.8 Other congenital malformations of great veins
Absence of vena cava (inferior) (superior)
Azygos continuation of inferior vena cava
Persistent left posterior cardinal vein
Scimitar syndrome

SP Q26.9 Congenital malformation of great vein, unspecified
Congenital anomaly of vena cava (inferior) (superior) NOS

4 Q27 Other congenital malformations of peripheral vascular system
EXCLUDES 2   anomalies of cerebral and
precerebral vessels
(Q28.0-Q28.3)
anomalies of coronary vessels
(Q24.5)
anomalies of pulmonary artery
(Q25.5-Q25.7)
congenital retinal aneurysm
(Q14.1)
hemangioma and
lymphangioma (D18.-)

SP Q27.0 Congenital absence and hypoplasia of umbilical artery
Single umbilical artery

SP Q27.1 Congenital renal artery stenosis

SP Q27.2 Other congenital malformations of renal artery
Congenital malformation of renal artery
NOS
Multiple renal arteries

5 Q27.3 Arteriovenous malformation (peripheral)
Arteriovenous aneurysm
EXCLUDES 1   acquired arteriovenous
aneurysm (I77.0)
EXCLUDES 2   arteriovenous malformation
of cerebral vessels
(Q28.2)
arteriovenous malformation
of precerebral vessels
(Q28.0)

IQ Q27.30 Arteriovenous malformation, site unspecified

SP Q27.31 Arteriovenous malformation of vessel of upper limb

SP Q27.32 Arteriovenous malformation of vessel of lower limb

SP Q27.33 Arteriovenous malformation of digestive system vessel

SP Q27.34 Arteriovenous malformation of renal vessel

SP Q27.39 Arteriovenous malformation, other site

SP Q27.4 Congenital phlebectasia

SP Q27.8 Other specified congenital malformations of peripheral vascular system
Absence of peripheral vascular system
Atresia of peripheral vascular system
Congenital aneurysm (peripheral)
Congenital stricture, artery

Congenital varix
EXCLUDES 1   arteriovenous malformation
(Q27.3-)

IQ Q27.9 Congenital malformation of peripheral vascular system, unspecified
Anomaly of artery or vein NOS

4 Q28 Other congenital malformations of circulatory system
EXCLUDES 1   congenital aneurysm NOS
(Q27.8)
congenital coronary aneurysm
(Q24.5)
ruptured cerebral arteriovenous
malformation (I60.8)
ruptured malformation of
precerebral vessels (I72.0)
EXCLUDES 2   congenital peripheral aneurysm
(Q27.8)
congenital pulmonary aneurysm
(Q25.79)
congenital retinal aneurysm
(Q14.1)

SP Q28.0 Arteriovenous malformation of precerebral vessels
Congenital arteriovenous precerebral
aneurysm (nonruptured)

SP Q28.1 Other malformations of precerebral vessels
Congenital malformation of precerebral
vessels NOS
Congenital precerebral aneurysm
(nonruptured)

SP Q28.2 Arteriovenous malformation of cerebral vessels
Arteriovenous malformation of brain NOS
Congenital arteriovenous cerebral
aneurysm (nonruptured)

SP Q28.3 Other malformations of cerebral vessels
Congenital cerebral aneurysm
(nonruptured)
Congenital malformation of cerebral
vessels NOS
Developmental venous anomaly

SP Q28.8 Other specified congenital malformations of circulatory system
Congenital aneurysm, specified site NEC
Spinal vessel anomaly

IQ Q28.9 Congenital malformation of circulatory system, unspecified

Congenital malformations of the respiratory system (Q30-Q34)

4 Q30 Congenital malformations of nose
EXCLUDES 1   congenital deviation of nasal
septum (Q67.4)

SP Q30.0 Choanal atresia
Atresia of nares (anterior) (posterior)
Congenital stenosis of nares (anterior)
(posterior)
DEFINITION   Fetal nasal airways are
obstructed by membranous or bony tissue;
infant is unable to breathe and nurse
simultaneously.

SP Q30.1 Agenesis and underdevelopment of nose
Congenital absent of nose

SP Q30.2 Fissured, notched and cleft nose

SP Q30.3 Congenital perforated nasal septum

---

4 4th digit required   5 5th digit required   6 6th digit required   7 7th digit required   7 7th digit placeholder   ✚ Additional code   ⊟ Laterality

SP Q30.8 Other congenital malformations of nose
Accessory nose
Congenital anomaly of nasal sinus wall

IQ Q30.9 Congenital malformation of nose, unspecified

4 Q31 Congenital malformations of larynx
> **EXCLUDES 1** congenital laryngeal stridor NOS (P28.89)

SP Q31.0 Web of larynx
Glottic web of larynx
Subglottic web of larynx
Web of larynx NOS

SP Q31.1 Congenital subglottic stenosis

SP Q31.2 Laryngeal hypoplasia

SP Q31.3 Laryngocele

SP Q31.5 Congenital laryngomalacia

SP Q31.8 Other congenital malformations of larynx
Absence of larynx
Agenesis of larynx
Atresia of larynx
Congenital cleft thyroid cartilage
Congenital fissure of epiglottis
Congenital stenosis of larynx NEC
Posterior cleft of cricoid cartilage

IQ Q31.9 Congenital malformation of larynx, unspecified

4 Q32 Congenital malformations of trachea and bronchus
> **EXCLUDES 1** congenital bronchiectasis (Q33.4)

SP Q32.0 Congenital tracheomalacia

SP Q32.1 Other congenital malformations of trachea
Atresia of trachea
Congenital anomaly of tracheal cartilage
Congenital dilatation of trachea
Congenital malformation of trachea
Congenital stenosis of trachea
Congenital tracheocele

SP Q32.2 Congenital bronchomalacia

SP Q32.3 Congenital stenosis of bronchus

SP Q32.4 Other congenital malformations of bronchus
Absence of bronchus
Agenesis of bronchus
Atresia of bronchus
Congenital diverticulum of bronchus
Congenital malformation of bronchus NOS

4 Q33 Congenital malformations of lung

SP Q33.0 Congenital cystic lung
Congenital cystic lung disease
Congenital honeycomb lung
Congenital polycystic lung disease
> **EXCLUDES 1** cystic fibrosis (E84.0)
> cystic lung disease, acquired or unspecified (J98.4)

SP Q33.1 Accessory lobe of lung
Azygos lobe (fissured), lung

SP Q33.2 Sequestration of lung

SP Q33.3 Agenesis of lung
Congenital absence of lung (lobe)

SP Q33.4 Congenital bronchiectasis

SP Q33.5 Ectopic tissue in lung

SP Q33.6 Congenital hypoplasia and dysplasia of lung

> **EXCLUDES 1** pulmonary hypoplasia associated with short gestation (P28.0)

SP Q33.8 Other congenital malformations of lung

IQ Q33.9 Congenital malformation of lung, unspecified

4 Q34 Other congenital malformations of respiratory system
> **EXCLUDES 2** congenital central alveolar hypoventilation syndrome (G47.35)

SP Q34.0 Anomaly of pleura

SP Q34.1 Congenital cyst of mediastinum

SP Q34.8 Other specified congenital malformations of respiratory system
Atresia of nasopharynx

IQ Q34.9 Congenital malformation of respiratory system, unspecified
Congenital absence of respiratory system
Congenital anomaly of respiratory system NOS

Cleft lip and cleft palate (Q35-Q37)

Use additional code to identify associated malformation of the nose (Q30.2)
> **EXCLUDES 1** Robin's syndrome (Q87.0)

4 Q35 Cleft palate
> **INCLUDES** fissure of palate
> palatoschisis
> **EXCLUDES 1** cleft palate with cleft lip (Q37.-)

IQ Q35.1 Cleft hard palate

IQ Q35.3 Cleft soft palate

IQ Q35.5 Cleft hard palate with cleft soft palate

IQ Q35.7 Cleft uvula

IQ Q35.9 Cleft palate, unspecified
Cleft palate NOS
> **DEFINITION** A congenital fissure in the roof of the mouth, resulting from incomplete fusion of the palate during embryonic development.

4 Q36 Cleft lip
> **INCLUDES** cheiloschisis
> congenital fissure of lip
> harelip
> labium leporinum
> **EXCLUDES 1** cleft lip with cleft palate (Q37.-)
> **CODING TIPS ✓** If the cleft palate/cleft lip has been corrected, use Z87.730, Personal history of (corrected) congenital malformations of cleft lip and palate.

SP Q36.0 Cleft lip, bilateral

SP Q36.1 Cleft lip, median

IQ Q36.9 Cleft lip, unilateral
Cleft lip NOS

4 Q37 Cleft palate with cleft lip
> **INCLUDES** cheilopalatoschisis
> **CODING TIPS ✓** If the cleft palate/cleft lip has been corrected, use Z87.730, Personal history of (corrected) congenital malformations of cleft lip and palate.

SP Q37.0 Cleft hard palate with bilateral cleft lip

★ New ▲ Revised Px Primary **SP** PDGM Px **SL** Low CoM **SH** High CoM **IQ** Quest. Encounter **H** Hospice non-cancer Dx Unspecified M *Manifestation*

SP Q37.1 Cleft hard palate with unilateral cleft lip
Cleft hard palate with cleft lip NOS

SP Q37.2 Cleft soft palate with bilateral cleft lip

SP Q37.3 Cleft soft palate with unilateral cleft lip
Cleft soft palate with cleft lip NOS

SP Q37.4 Cleft hard and soft palate with bilateral cleft lip

SP Q37.5 Cleft hard and soft palate with unilateral cleft lip
Cleft hard and soft palate with cleft lip NOS

SP Q37.8 Unspecified cleft palate with bilateral cleft lip

IQ Q37.9 Unspecified cleft palate with unilateral cleft lip
Cleft palate with cleft lip NOS

Other congenital malformations of the digestive system   (Q38-Q45)

4 Q38 Other congenital malformations of tongue, mouth and pharynx
EXCLUDES 1   dentofacial anomalies (M26.-)
macrostomia (Q18.4)
microstomia (Q18.5)

SP Q38.0 Congenital malformations of lips, not elsewhere classified
Congenital fistula of lip
Congenital malformation of lip NOS
Van der Woude's syndrome
EXCLUDES 1   cleft lip (Q36.-)
cleft lip with cleft palate (Q37.-)
macrocheilia (Q18.6)
microcheilia (Q18.7)

SP Q38.1 Ankyloglossia
Tongue tie

SP Q38.2 Macroglossia
Congenital hypertrophy of tongue
DEFINITION   Congenital enlargement of the tongue.

SP Q38.3 Other congenital malformations of tongue
Aglossia
Bifid tongue
Congenital adhesion of tongue
Congenital fissure of tongue
Congenital malformation of tongue NOS
Double tongue
Hypoglossia
Hypoplasia of tongue
Microglossia

SP Q38.4 Congenital malformations of salivary glands and ducts
Atresia of salivary glands and ducts
Congenital absence of salivary glands and ducts
Congenital accessory salivary glands and ducts
Congenital fistula of salivary gland
DEFINITION   Congenital salivary gland fistula: Abnormal passage communicating with a salivary gland and present at birth.

SP Q38.5 Congenital malformations of palate, not elsewhere classified
Congenital absence of uvula
Congenital malformation of palate NOS
Congenital high arched palate
EXCLUDES 1   cleft palate (Q35.-)
cleft palate with cleft lip (Q37.-)

SP Q38.6 Other congenital malformations of mouth
Congenital malformation of mouth NOS

SP Q38.7 Congenital pharyngeal pouch
Congenital diverticulum of pharynx
EXCLUDES 1   pharyngeal pouch syndrome (D82.1)

SP Q38.8 Other congenital malformations of pharynx
Congenital malformation of pharynx NOS
Imperforate pharynx

4 Q39 Congenital malformations of esophagus

SP Q39.0 Atresia of esophagus without fistula
Atresia of esophagus NOS

SP Q39.1 Atresia of esophagus with tracheo-esophageal fistula
Atresia of esophagus with broncho-esophageal fistula
CODING TIPS ✓   Code Q39.1 is used for a congenital tracheoesophageal fistula (TE fistula). A fistula as a complication of a tracheostomy is coded J95.04.

SP Q39.2 Congenital tracheo-esophageal fistula without atresia
Congenital tracheo-esophageal fistula NOS

SP Q39.3 Congenital stenosis and stricture of esophagus

SP Q39.4 Esophageal web

SP Q39.5 Congenital dilatation of esophagus
Congenital cardiospasm

SP Q39.6 Congenital diverticulum of esophagus
Congenital esophageal pouch

SP Q39.8 Other congenital malformations of esophagus
Congenital absence of esophagus
Congenital displacement of esophagus
Congenital duplication of esophagus

IQ Q39.9 Congenital malformation of esophagus, unspecified

4 Q40 Other congenital malformations of upper alimentary tract

SP Q40.0 Congenital hypertrophic pyloric stenosis
Congenital or infantile constriction
Congenital or infantile hypertrophy
Congenital or infantile spasm
Congenital or infantile stenosis
Congenital or infantile stricture
DEFINITION   Congenital narrowing and partial obstruction of the gastric outlet due to muscular hypertrophy and mucosal edema of the ring-like muscle at the lower end of the stomach (pyloric orifice) in newborns.

SP Q40.1 Congenital hiatus hernia
Congenital displacement of cardia through esophageal hiatus
EXCLUDES 1   congenital diaphragmatic hernia (Q79.0)

SP Q40.2 Other specified congenital malformations of stomach
Congenital displacement of stomach
Congenital diverticulum of stomach
Congenital hourglass stomach

---

4 4th digit required   5 5th digit required   6 6th digit required   7 7th digit required   ☑ 7th digit placeholder   ✚ Additional code   ⊟ Laterality

Congenital duplication of stomach
Megalogastria
Microgastria

IQ Q40.3 **Congenital malformation of stomach, unspecified**

SP Q40.8 **Other specified congenital malformations of upper alimentary tract**

IQ Q40.9 **Congenital malformation of upper alimentary tract, unspecified**

Congenital anomaly of upper alimentary tract
Congenital deformity of upper alimentary tract

4 Q41 **Congenital absence, atresia and stenosis of small intestine**

INCLUDES congenital obstruction, occlusion or stricture of small intestine or intestine NOS

EXCLUDES 1 cystic fibrosis with intestinal manifestation (E84.11)
meconium ileus NOS (without cystic fibrosis) (P76.0)

SP Q41.0 **Congenital absence, atresia and stenosis of duodenum**

SP Q41.1 **Congenital absence, atresia and stenosis of jejunum**
Apple peel syndrome
Imperforate jejunum

SP Q41.2 **Congenital absence, atresia and stenosis of ileum**

SP Q41.8 **Congenital absence, atresia and stenosis of other specified parts of small intestine**

SP Q41.9 **Congenital absence, atresia and stenosis of small intestine, part unspecified**

Congenital absence, atresia and stenosis of intestine NOS

4 Q42 **Congenital absence, atresia and stenosis of large intestine**

INCLUDES congenital obstruction, occlusion and stricture of large intestine

SP Q42.0 **Congenital absence, atresia and stenosis of rectum with fistula**

SP Q42.1 **Congenital absence, atresia and stenosis of rectum without fistula**
Imperforate rectum

SP Q42.2 **Congenital absence, atresia and stenosis of anus with fistula**

SP Q42.3 **Congenital absence, atresia and stenosis of anus without fistula**
Imperforate anus

SP Q42.8 **Congenital absence, atresia and stenosis of other parts of large intestine**

SP Q42.9 **Congenital absence, atresia and stenosis of large intestine, part unspecified**

4 Q43 **Other congenital malformations of intestine**

SP Q43.0 **Meckel's diverticulum (displaced) (hypertrophic)**
Persistent omphalomesenteric duct
Persistent vitelline duct

SP Q43.1 **Hirschsprung's disease**
Aganglionosis
Congenital (aganglionic) megacolon

SP Q43.2 **Other congenital functional disorders of colon**
Congenital dilatation of colon

SP Q43.3 **Congenital malformations of intestinal fixation**
Congenital omental, anomalous adhesions [bands]
Congenital peritoneal adhesions [bands]
Incomplete rotation of cecum and colon
Insufficient rotation of cecum and colon
Jackson's membrane
Malrotation of colon
Rotation failure of cecum and colon
Universal mesentery

SP Q43.4 **Duplication of intestine**

SP Q43.5 **Ectopic anus**

SP Q43.6 **Congenital fistula of rectum and anus**

EXCLUDES 1 congenital fistula of anus with absence, atresia and stenosis (Q42.2)
congenital fistula of rectum with absence, atresia and stenosis (Q42.0)
congenital rectovaginal fistula (Q52.2)
congenital urethrorectal fistula (Q64.73)
pilonidal fistula or sinus (L05.-)

SP Q43.7 **Persistent cloaca**
Cloaca NOS

SP Q43.8 **Other specified congenital malformations of intestine**
Congenital blind loop syndrome
Congenital diverticulitis, colon
Congenital diverticulum, intestine
Dolichocolon
Megaloappendix
Megaloduodenum
Microcolon
Transposition of appendix
Transposition of colon
Transposition of intestine

IQ Q43.9 **Congenital malformation of intestine, unspecified**

4 Q44 **Congenital malformations of gallbladder, bile ducts and liver**

SP Q44.0 **Agenesis, aplasia and hypoplasia of gallbladder**
Congenital absence of gallbladder

SP Q44.1 **Other congenital malformations of gallbladder**
Congenital malformation of gallbladder NOS
Intrahepatic gallbladder

SP Q44.2 **Atresia of bile ducts**

SP Q44.3 **Congenital stenosis and stricture of bile ducts**

SP Q44.4 **Choledochal cyst**

SP Q44.5 **Other congenital malformations of bile ducts**
Accessory hepatic duct
Biliary duct duplication
Congenital malformation of bile duct NOS
Cystic duct duplication

SP Q44.6 **Cystic disease of liver**
Fibrocystic disease of liver

★ New ▲ Revised Px Primary **SP** PDGM Px **SL** Low CoM **SH** High CoM **IQ** Quest. Encounter 🄷 Hospice non-cancer Dx Unspecified **M** *Manifestation*

DecisionHealth's FY 2020 Complete Home Health ICD-10-CM Diagnosis Coding Manual

1393

SP Q44.7 Other congenital malformations of liver
Accessory liver
Alagille's syndrome
Congenital absence of liver
Congenital hepatomegaly
Congenital malformation of liver NOS

4 Q45 Other congenital malformations of digestive system
EXCLUDES 2   congenital diaphragmatic hernia
(Q79.0)
congenital hiatus hernia
(Q40.1)

SP Q45.0 Agenesis, aplasia and hypoplasia of pancreas
Congenital absence of pancreas

SP Q45.1 Annular pancreas

SP Q45.2 Congenital pancreatic cyst

SP Q45.3 Other congenital malformations of pancreas and pancreatic duct
Accessory pancreas
Congenital malformation of pancreas or pancreatic duct NOS
EXCLUDES 1   congenital diabetes mellitus
(E10.-)
cystic fibrosis
(E84.0-E84.9)
fibrocystic disease of pancreas (E84.-)
neonatal diabetes mellitus
(P70.2)

SP Q45.8 Other specified congenital malformations of digestive system
Absence (complete) (partial) of alimentary tract NOS
Duplication of digestive system
Malposition, congenital of digestive system

IQ Q45.9 Congenital malformation of digestive system, unspecified
Congenital anomaly of digestive system
Congenital deformity of digestive system

Congenital malformations of genital organs (Q50-Q56)

EXCLUDES 1   androgen insensitivity syndrome (E34.5-)
syndromes associated with anomalies in the number and form of chromosomes (Q90-Q99)

4 Q50 Congenital malformations of ovaries, fallopian tubes and broad ligaments

5 Q50.0 Congenital absence of ovary
EXCLUDES 1   Turner's syndrome (Q96.-)

SP Q50.01 Congenital absence of ovary, unilateral

SP Q50.02 Congenital absence of ovary, bilateral

SP Q50.1 Developmental ovarian cyst

SP Q50.2 Congenital torsion of ovary

5 Q50.3 Other congenital malformations of ovary

SP Q50.31 Accessory ovary

SP Q50.32 Ovarian streak
46, XX with streak gonads

SP Q50.39 Other congenital malformation of ovary
Congenital malformation of ovary NOS

SP Q50.4 Embryonic cyst of fallopian tube
Fimbrial cyst

SP Q50.5 Embryonic cyst of broad ligament
Epoophoron cyst
Parovarian cyst

SP Q50.6 Other congenital malformations of fallopian tube and broad ligament
Absence of fallopian tube and broad ligament
Accessory fallopian tube and broad ligament
Atresia of fallopian tube and broad ligament
Congenital malformation of fallopian tube or broad ligament NOS

4 Q51 Congenital malformations of uterus and cervix

SP Q51.0 Agenesis and aplasia of uterus
Congenital absence of uterus

5 Q51.1 Doubling of uterus with doubling of cervix and vagina

SP Q51.10 Doubling of uterus with doubling of cervix and vagina without obstruction
Doubling of uterus with doubling of cervix and vagina NOS

SP Q51.11 Doubling of uterus with doubling of cervix and vagina with obstruction

5 Q51.2 Other doubling of uterus
Doubling of uterus NOS
Septate uterus

SP Q51.20 Other doubling of uterus, unspecified
Septate uterus, unspecified

SP Q51.21 Other complete doubling of uterus
Complete septate uterus

SP Q51.22 Other partial doubling of uterus
Partial septate uterus

SP Q51.28 Other doubling of uterus, other specified
Septate uterus, other specified

SP Q51.3 Bicornate uterus
Bicornate uterus, complete or partial

SP Q51.4 Unicornate uterus
Unicornate uterus with or without a separate uterine horn
Uterus with only one functioning horn

SP Q51.5 Agenesis and aplasia of cervix
Congenital absence of cervix

SP Q51.6 Embryonic cyst of cervix

SP Q51.7 Congenital fistulae between uterus and digestive and urinary tracts

5 Q51.8 Other congenital malformations of uterus and cervix

6 Q51.81 Other congenital malformations of uterus

SP Q51.810 Arcuate uterus
Arcuatus uterus

SP Q51.811 Hypoplasia of uterus

SP Q51.818 Other congenital malformations of uterus
Müllerian anomaly of uterus NEC

6 Q51.82 Other congenital malformations of cervix

SP Q51.820 Cervical duplication

SP Q51.821 Hypoplasia of cervix

---

4 4th digit required   5 5th digit required   6 6th digit required   7 7th digit required   7 7th digit placeholder   + Additional code   ⊟ Laterality

SP Q51.828 Other congenital malformations of cervix

IQ Q51.9 Congenital malformation of uterus and cervix, unspecified

4 Q52 Other congenital malformations of female genitalia

SP Q52.0 Congenital absence of vagina
Vaginal agenesis, total or partial

5 Q52.1 Doubling of vagina
> **EXCLUDES 1** doubling of vagina with doubling of uterus and cervix (Q51.1-)

SP Q52.10 Doubling of vagina, unspecified
Septate vagina NOS

SP Q52.11 Transverse vaginal septum

6 Q52.12 Longitudinal vaginal septum

SP Q52.120 Longitudinal vaginal septum, nonobstructing

SP Q52.121 Longitudinal vaginal septum, obstructing, right side

SP Q52.122 Longitudinal vaginal septum, obstructing, left side

SP Q52.123 Longitudinal vaginal septum, microperforate, right side

SP Q52.124 Longitudinal vaginal septum, microperforate, left side

SP Q52.129 Other and unspecified longitudinal vaginal septum

SP Q52.2 Congenital rectovaginal fistula
> **EXCLUDES 1** cloaca (Q43.7)

SP Q52.3 Imperforate hymen

SP Q52.4 Other congenital malformations of vagina
Canal of Nuck cyst, congenital
Congenital malformation of vagina NOS
Embryonic vaginal cyst
Gartner's duct cyst

SP Q52.5 Fusion of labia

SP Q52.6 Congenital malformation of clitoris

5 Q52.7 Other and unspecified congenital malformations of vulva

IQ Q52.70 Unspecified congenital malformations of vulva
Congenital malformation of vulva NOS

SP Q52.71 Congenital absence of vulva

SP Q52.79 Other congenital malformations of vulva
Congenital cyst of vulva

SP Q52.8 Other specified congenital malformations of female genitalia

IQ Q52.9 Congenital malformation of female genitalia, unspecified

4 Q53 Undescended and ectopic testicle

5 Q53.0 Ectopic testis

IQ Q53.00 Ectopic testis, unspecified

SP Q53.01 Ectopic testis, unilateral

SP Q53.02 Ectopic testes, bilateral

5 Q53.1 Undescended testicle, unilateral

IQ Q53.10 Unspecified undescended testicle, unilateral

6 Q53.11 Abdominal testis, unilateral

SP Q53.111 Unilateral intraabdominal testis

SP Q53.112 Unilateral inguinal testis

SP Q53.12 Ectopic perineal testis, unilateral

SP Q53.13 Unilateral high scrotal testis

5 Q53.2 Undescended testicle, bilateral

SP Q53.20 Undescended testicle, unspecified, bilateral

6 Q53.21 Abdominal testis, bilateral

SP Q53.211 Bilateral intraabdominal testes

SP Q53.212 Bilateral inguinal testes

SP Q53.22 Ectopic perineal testis, bilateral

SP Q53.23 Bilateral high scrotal testes

IQ Q53.9 Undescended testicle, unspecified
Cryptorchism NOS

4 Q54 Hypospadias
> **EXCLUDES 1** epispadias (Q64.0)

> **CODING TIPS ✓** Use category Q54 when hypospadias is still present. If the condition has been corrected, then code Z87.710, Personal history of hypospadias.

SP Q54.0 Hypospadias, balanic
Hypospadias, coronal
Hypospadias, glandular

SP Q54.1 Hypospadias, penile

SP Q54.2 Hypospadias, penoscrotal

SP Q54.3 Hypospadias, perineal

SP Q54.4 Congenital chordee
Chordee without hypospadias
> **DEFINITION** Abnormal downward or upward bowing of the penis, due to a congenital anomaly.

SP Q54.8 Other hypospadias
Hypospadias with intersex state

SP Q54.9 Hypospadias, unspecified

4 Q55 Other congenital malformations of male genital organs
> **EXCLUDES 1** congenital hydrocele (P83.5)
> hypospadias (Q54.-)

SP Q55.0 Absence and aplasia of testis
Monorchism

SP Q55.1 Hypoplasia of testis and scrotum
Fusion of testes

5 Q55.2 Other and unspecified congenital malformations of testis and scrotum

IQ Q55.20 Unspecified congenital malformations of testis and scrotum
Congenital malformation of testis or scrotum NOS

SP Q55.21 Polyorchism

SP Q55.22 Retractile testis

SP Q55.23 Scrotal transposition

SP Q55.29 Other congenital malformations of testis and scrotum

SP Q55.3 Atresia of vas deferens
Code first:
any associated cystic fibrosis (E84.-)

SP Q55.4 Other congenital malformations of vas deferens, epididymis, seminal vesicles and prostate
Absence or aplasia of prostate
Absence or aplasia of spermatic cord
Congenital malformation of vas deferens, epididymis, seminal vesicles or prostate NOS

SP Q55.5 Congenital absence and aplasia of penis

★ New ▲ Revised Px Primary SP PDGM Px SL Low CoM SH High CoM IQ Quest. Encounter H Hospice non-cancer Dx Unspecified M Manifestation

DecisionHealth's FY 2020 Complete Home Health ICD-10-CM Diagnosis Coding Manual

1395

5 Q55.6 Other congenital malformations of penis

SP Q55.61 Curvature of penis (lateral)

SP Q55.62 Hypoplasia of penis
Micropenis

SP Q55.63 Congenital torsion of penis
EXCLUDES 1   acquired torsion of penis (N48.82)

SP Q55.64 Hidden penis
Buried penis
Concealed penis
EXCLUDES 1   acquired buried penis (N48.83)

SP Q55.69 Other congenital malformation of penis
Congenital malformation of penis NOS

SP Q55.7 Congenital vasocutaneous fistula

SP Q55.8 Other specified congenital malformations of male genital organs

!Q Q55.9 Congenital malformation of male genital organ, unspecified
Congenital anomaly of male genital organ
Congenital deformity of male genital organ

4 Q56 Indeterminate sex and pseudohermaphroditism
EXCLUDES 1   46,XX true hermaphrodite (Q99.1)
androgen insensitivity syndrome (E34.5-)
chimera 46,XX/46,XY true hermaphrodite (Q99.0)
female pseudohermaphroditism with adrenocortical disorder (E25.-)
pseudohermaphroditism with specified chromosomal anomaly (Q96-Q99)
pure gonadal dysgenesis (Q99.1)

SP Q56.0 Hermaphroditism, not elsewhere classified
Ovotestis

SP Q56.1 Male pseudohermaphroditism, not elsewhere classified
46, XY with streak gonads
Male pseudohermaphroditism NOS

SP Q56.2 Female pseudohermaphroditism, not elsewhere classified
Female pseudohermaphroditism NOS

SP Q56.3 Pseudohermaphroditism, unspecified

SP Q56.4 Indeterminate sex, unspecified
Ambiguous genitalia

Congenital malformations of the urinary system (Q60-Q64)

4 Q60 Renal agenesis and other reduction defects of kidney
INCLUDES   congenital absence of kidney
congenital atrophy of kidney
infantile atrophy of kidney

SP Q60.0 Renal agenesis, unilateral

SP Q60.1 Renal agenesis, bilateral

!Q Q60.2 Renal agenesis, unspecified

SP Q60.3 Renal hypoplasia, unilateral

SP Q60.4 Renal hypoplasia, bilateral

!Q Q60.5 Renal hypoplasia, unspecified

SP Q60.6 Potter's syndrome

4 Q61 Cystic kidney disease
EXCLUDES 1   acquired cyst of kidney (N28.1)
Potter's syndrome (Q60.6)

5 Q61.0 Congenital renal cyst

SP Q61.00 Congenital renal cyst, unspecified
Cyst of kidney NOS (congenital)

SP Q61.01 Congenital single renal cyst

SP Q61.02 Congenital multiple renal cysts

5 Q61.1 Polycystic kidney, infantile type
Polycystic kidney, autosomal recessive

SP Q61.11 Cystic dilatation of collecting ducts

SP Q61.19 Other polycystic kidney, infantile type

SP Q61.2 Polycystic kidney, adult type
Polycystic kidney, autosomal dominant

SP Q61.3 Polycystic kidney, unspecified

SP Q61.4 Renal dysplasia
Multicystic dysplastic kidney
Multicystic kidney (development)
Multicystic kidney disease
Multicystic renal dysplasia
EXCLUDES 1   polycystic kidney disease (Q61.11-Q61.3)

SP Q61.5 Medullary cystic kidney
Nephronopthisis
Sponge kidney NOS

SP Q61.8 Other cystic kidney diseases
Fibrocystic kidney
Fibrocystic renal degeneration or disease

!Q Q61.9 Cystic kidney disease, unspecified
Meckel-Gruber syndrome

4 Q62 Congenital obstructive defects of renal pelvis and congenital malformations of ureter

SP Q62.0 Congenital hydronephrosis

5 Q62.1 Congenital occlusion of ureter
Atresia and stenosis of ureter

SP Q62.10 Congenital occlusion of ureter, unspecified

SP Q62.11 Congenital occlusion of ureteropelvic junction

SP Q62.12 Congenital occlusion of ureterovesical orifice

SP Q62.2 Congenital megaureter
Congenital dilatation of ureter

5 Q62.3 Other obstructive defects of renal pelvis and ureter

SP Q62.31 Congenital ureterocele, orthotopic

SP Q62.32 Cecoureterocele
Ectopic ureterocele

SP Q62.39 Other obstructive defects of renal pelvis and ureter
Ureteropelvic junction obstruction NOS

SP Q62.4 Agenesis of ureter
Congenital absence ureter

SP Q62.5 Duplication of ureter
Accessory ureter
Double ureter

5 Q62.6 Malposition of ureter

SP Q62.60 Malposition of ureter, unspecified

SP Q62.61 Deviation of ureter

SP Q62.62 Displacement of ureter

SP Q62.63 Anomalous implantation of ureter

---

4 4th digit required   5 5th digit required   6 6th digit required   7 7th digit required   ✓ 7th digit placeholder   ✚ Additional code   ⊟ Laterality

Ectopia of ureter

Ectopic ureter

SP Q62.69 Other malposition of ureter

SP Q62.7 Congenital vesico-uretero-renal reflux

SP Q62.8 Other congenital malformations of ureter

Anomaly of ureter NOS

▣ Q63 Other congenital malformations of kidney

EXCLUDES 1 congenital nephrotic syndrome (N04.-)

SP Q63.0 Accessory kidney

SP Q63.1 Lobulated, fused and horseshoe kidney

SP Q63.2 Ectopic kidney

Congenital displaced kidney

Malrotation of kidney

SP Q63.3 Hyperplastic and giant kidney

Compensatory hypertrophy of kidney

SP Q63.8 Other specified congenital malformations of kidney

Congenital renal calculi

IQ Q63.9 Congenital malformation of kidney, unspecified

▣ Q64 Other congenital malformations of urinary system

SP Q64.0 Epispadias

EXCLUDES 1 hypospadias (Q54.-)

DEFINITION A rare, congenital defect in which the urethra typically opens on the upper penile surface in boys, although, the urethral opening may also be positioned in the abdomen.

⑤ Q64.1 Exstrophy of urinary bladder

SP Q64.10 Exstrophy of urinary bladder, unspecified

Ectopia vesicae

SP Q64.11 Supravesical fissure of urinary bladder

SP Q64.12 Cloacal exstrophy of urinary bladder

SP Q64.19 Other exstrophy of urinary bladder

Extroversion of bladder

SP Q64.2 Congenital posterior urethral valves

⑤ Q64.3 Other atresia and stenosis of urethra and bladder neck

SP Q64.31 Congenital bladder neck obstruction

Congenital obstruction of vesicourethral orifice

SP Q64.32 Congenital stricture of urethra

SP Q64.33 Congenital stricture of urinary meatus

SP Q64.39 Other atresia and stenosis of urethra and bladder neck

Atresia and stenosis of urethra and bladder neck NOS

SP Q64.4 Malformation of urachus

Cyst of urachus

Patent urachus

Prolapse of urachus

SP Q64.5 Congenital absence of bladder and urethra

SP Q64.6 Congenital diverticulum of bladder

⑤ Q64.7 Other and unspecified congenital malformations of bladder and urethra

EXCLUDES 1 congenital prolapse of bladder (mucosa) (Q79.4)

IQ Q64.70 Unspecified congenital malformation of bladder and urethra

Malformation of bladder or urethra NOS

SP Q64.71 Congenital prolapse of urethra

SP Q64.72 Congenital prolapse of urinary meatus

SP Q64.73 Congenital urethrorectal fistula

SP Q64.74 Double urethra

SP Q64.75 Double urinary meatus

SP Q64.79 Other congenital malformations of bladder and urethra

SP Q64.8 Other specified congenital malformations of urinary system

IQ Q64.9 Congenital malformation of urinary system, unspecified

Congenital anomaly NOS of urinary system

Congenital deformity NOS of urinary system

Congenital malformations and deformations of the musculoskeletal system (Q65-Q79)

▣ Q65 Congenital deformities of hip

EXCLUDES 1 clicking hip (R29.4)

⑤ Q65.0 Congenital dislocation of hip, unilateral

⊟ IQ Q65.00 Congenital dislocation of unspecified hip, unilateral

⊟ SP Q65.01 Congenital dislocation of right hip, unilateral

⊟ SP Q65.02 Congenital dislocation of left hip, unilateral

SP Q65.1 Congenital dislocation of hip, bilateral

IQ Q65.2 Congenital dislocation of hip, unspecified

⑤ Q65.3 Congenital partial dislocation of hip, unilateral

⊟ IQ Q65.30 Congenital partial dislocation of unspecified hip, unilateral

⊟ SP Q65.31 Congenital partial dislocation of right hip, unilateral

⊟ SP Q65.32 Congenital partial dislocation of left hip, unilateral

SP Q65.4 Congenital partial dislocation of hip, bilateral

IQ Q65.5 Congenital partial dislocation of hip, unspecified

SP Q65.6 Congenital unstable hip

Congenital dislocatable hip

⑤ Q65.8 Other congenital deformities of hip

SP Q65.81 Congenital coxa valga

SP Q65.82 Congenital coxa vara

SP Q65.89 Other specified congenital deformities of hip

Anteversion of femoral neck

Congenital acetabular dysplasia

IQ Q65.9 Congenital deformity of hip, unspecified

▣ Q66 Congenital deformities of feet

EXCLUDES 1 reduction defects of feet (Q72.-)

★ New ▲ Revised Px Primary SP PDGM Px SL Low CoM SH High CoM IQ Quest. Encounter ⊞ Hospice non-cancer Dx Unspecified M *Manifestation*

DecisionHealth's FY 2020 Complete Home Health ICD-10-CM Diagnosis Coding Manual

1397

valgus deformities (acquired)
(M21.0-)
varus deformities (acquired)
(M21.1-)

▲ �5 **Q66.0** Congenital talipes equinovarus

☆ 🖻 **Q66.00** Congenital talipes equinovarus, unspecified foot

☆ 🖻 **Q66.01** Congenital talipes equinovarus, right foot

☆ 🖻 **Q66.02** Congenital talipes equinovarus, left foot

▲ �5 **Q66.1** Congenital talipes calcaneovarus

☆ 🖻 **Q66.10** Congenital talipes calcaneovarus, unspecified foot

☆ 🖻 **Q66.11** Congenital talipes calcaneovarus, right foot

☆ 🖻 **Q66.12** Congenital talipes calcaneovarus, left foot

�5 **Q66.2** Congenital metatarsus (primus) varus

▲ 🄖 **Q66.21** Congenital metatarsus primus varus

☆ 🖻 **Q66.211** Congenital metatarsus primus varus, right foot

☆ 🖻 **Q66.212** Congenital metatarsus primus varus, left foot

☆ 🖻 **Q66.219** Congenital metatarsus primus varus, unspecified foot

▲ 🄖 **Q66.22** Congenital metatarsus adductus
Congenital metatarsus varus

☆ 🖻 **Q66.221** Congenital metatarsus adductus, right foot

☆ 🖻 **Q66.222** Congenital metatarsus adductus, left foot

☆ 🖻 **Q66.229** Congenital metatarsus adductus, unspecified foot

▲ �5 **Q66.3** Other congenital varus deformities of feet
Hallux varus, congenital

☆ 🖻 **Q66.30** Other congenital varus deformities of feet, unspecified foot

☆ 🖻 **Q66.31** Other congenital varus deformities of feet, right foot

☆ 🖻 **Q66.32** Other congenital varus deformities of feet, left foot

▲ �5 **Q66.4** Congenital talipes calcaneovalgus

☆ 🖻 **Q66.40** Congenital talipes calcaneovalgus, unspecified foot

☆ 🖻 **Q66.41** Congenital talipes calcaneovalgus, right foot

☆ 🖻 **Q66.42** Congenital talipes calcaneovalgus, left foot

�5 **Q66.5** Congenital pes planus
Congenital flat foot
Congenital rigid flat foot
Congenital spastic (everted) flat foot
EXCLUDES 1 pes planus, acquired (M21.4)

🖻 🄎 **Q66.50** Congenital pes planus, unspecified foot

🖻 🆂🅿 **Q66.51** Congenital pes planus, right foot

🖻 🆂🅿 **Q66.52** Congenital pes planus, left foot

🆂🅿 **Q66.6** Other congenital valgus deformities of feet
Congenital metatarsus valgus

▲ �5 **Q66.7** Congenital pes cavus

★ 🖻 **Q66.70** Congenital pes cavus, unspecified foot

★ 🖻 **Q66.71** Congenital pes cavus, right foot

★ 🖻 **Q66.72** Congenital pes cavus, left foot

�5 **Q66.8** Other congenital deformities of feet

🖻 🄎 **Q66.80** Congenital vertical talus deformity, unspecified foot

🖻 🆂🅿 **Q66.81** Congenital vertical talus deformity, right foot

🖻 🆂🅿 **Q66.82** Congenital vertical talus deformity, left foot

🖻 🆂🅿 **Q66.89** Other specified congenital deformities of feet
Congenital asymmetric talipes
Congenital clubfoot NOS
Congenital talipes NOS
Congenital tarsal coalition
Hammer toe, congenital

▲ �5 **Q66.9** Congenital deformity of feet, unspecified

★ 🖻 **Q66.90** Congenital deformity of feet, unspecified, unspecified foot

★ 🖻 **Q66.91** Congenital deformity of feet, unspecified, right foot

★ 🖻 **Q66.92** Congenital deformity of feet, unspecified, left foot

🄘 **Q67** Congenital musculoskeletal deformities of head, face, spine and chest
EXCLUDES 1 congenital malformation syndromes classified to Q87.-
Potter's syndrome (Q60.6)

🆂🅿 **Q67.0** Congenital facial asymmetry

🆂🅿 **Q67.1** Congenital compression facies

🆂🅿 **Q67.2** Dolichocephaly

🆂🅿 **Q67.3** Plagiocephaly

🆂🅿 **Q67.4** Other congenital deformities of skull, face and jaw
Congenital depressions in skull
Congenital hemifacial atrophy or hypertrophy
Deviation of nasal septum, congenital
Squashed or bent nose, congenital
EXCLUDES 1 dentofacial anomalies [including malocclusion] (M26.-)
syphilitic saddle nose (A50.5)

🆂🅿 **Q67.5** Congenital deformity of spine
Congenital postural scoliosis
Congenital scoliosis NOS
EXCLUDES 1 infantile idiopathic scoliosis (M41.0)
scoliosis due to congenital bony malformation (Q76.3)

🆂🅿 **Q67.6** Pectus excavatum
Congenital funnel chest

🆂🅿 **Q67.7** Pectus carinatum
Congenital pigeon chest
DEFINITION A protrusion deformity of the chest wall in which the sternum and ribs are prominent, due to obstruction of infantile respiration or to rickets.

🆂🅿 **Q67.8** Other congenital deformities of chest
Congenital deformity of chest wall NOS

🄠 4th digit required   �5 5th digit required   🄖 6th digit required   �7 7th digit required   🅥 7th digit placeholder   ➕ Additional code   🖻 Laterality

Q68 **Other congenital musculoskeletal deformities**

> EXCLUDES 1   reduction defects of limb (s) (Q71-Q73)
>
> EXCLUDES 2   congenital myotonic chondrodystrophy (G71.13)

SP Q68.0 **Congenital deformity of sternocleidomastoid muscle**

Congenital contracture of sternocleidomastoid (muscle)

Congenital (sternomastoid) torticollis

Sternomastoid tumor (congenital)

SP Q68.1 **Congenital deformity of finger(s) and hand**

Congenital clubfinger

Spade-like hand (congenital)

SP Q68.2 **Congenital deformity of knee**

Congenital dislocation of knee

Congenital genu recurvatum

SP Q68.3 **Congenital bowing of femur**

> EXCLUDES 1   anteversion of femur (neck) (Q65.89)

SP Q68.4 **Congenital bowing of tibia and fibula**

IQ Q68.5 **Congenital bowing of long bones of leg, unspecified**

SP Q68.6 **Discoid meniscus**

SP Q68.8 **Other specified congenital musculoskeletal deformities**

Congenital deformity of clavicle

Congenital deformity of elbow

Congenital deformity of forearm

Congenital deformity of scapula

Congenital deformity of wrist

Congenital dislocation of elbow

Congenital dislocation of shoulder

Congenital dislocation of wrist

Q69 **Polydactyly**

SP Q69.0 **Accessory finger(s)**

SP Q69.1 **Accessory thumb(s)**

SP Q69.2 **Accessory toe(s)**

Accessory hallux

IQ Q69.9 **Polydactyly, unspecified**

Supernumerary digit(s) NOS

> DEFINITION   An extra number of digits on a hand or foot.

Q70 **Syndactyly**

Q70.0 **Fused fingers**

Complex syndactyly of fingers with synostosis

IQ Q70.00 **Fused fingers, unspecified hand**

SP Q70.01 **Fused fingers, right hand**

SP Q70.02 **Fused fingers, left hand**

SP Q70.03 **Fused fingers, bilateral**

Q70.1 **Webbed fingers**

Simple syndactyly of fingers without synostosis

IQ Q70.10 **Webbed fingers, unspecified hand**

SP Q70.11 **Webbed fingers, right hand**

SP Q70.12 **Webbed fingers, left hand**

SP Q70.13 **Webbed fingers, bilateral**

Q70.2 **Fused toes**

Complex syndactyly of toes with synostosis

IQ Q70.20 **Fused toes, unspecified foot**

SP Q70.21 **Fused toes, right foot**

SP Q70.22 **Fused toes, left foot**

SP Q70.23 **Fused toes, bilateral**

Q70.3 **Webbed toes**

Simple syndactyly of toes without synostosis

IQ Q70.30 **Webbed toes, unspecified foot**

IQ Q70.31 **Webbed toes, right foot**

SP Q70.32 **Webbed toes, left foot**

SP Q70.33 **Webbed toes, bilateral**

SP Q70.4 **Polysyndactyly, unspecified**

> EXCLUDES 1   specified syndactyly of hand and feet - code to specified conditions (Q70.0- -Q70.3-)

SP Q70.9 **Syndactyly, unspecified**

Symphalangy NOS

> DEFINITION   Partial or total webbing connecting two or more fingers or toes; may involve skin/soft tissue only or include fusion of bone.

Q71 **Reduction defects of upper limb**

Q71.0 **Congenital complete absence of upper limb**

IQ Q71.00 **Congenital complete absence of unspecified upper limb**

SP Q71.01 **Congenital complete absence of right upper limb**

SP Q71.02 **Congenital complete absence of left upper limb**

SP Q71.03 **Congenital complete absence of upper limb, bilateral**

Q71.1 **Congenital absence of upper arm and forearm with hand present**

IQ Q71.10 **Congenital absence of unspecified upper arm and forearm with hand present**

SP Q71.11 **Congenital absence of right upper arm and forearm with hand present**

SP Q71.12 **Congenital absence of left upper arm and forearm with hand present**

SP Q71.13 **Congenital absence of upper arm and forearm with hand present, bilateral**

Q71.2 **Congenital absence of both forearm and hand**

IQ Q71.20 **Congenital absence of both forearm and hand, unspecified upper limb**

SP Q71.21 **Congenital absence of both forearm and hand, right upper limb**

SP Q71.22 **Congenital absence of both forearm and hand, left upper limb**

SP Q71.23 **Congenital absence of both forearm and hand, bilateral**

Q71.3 **Congenital absence of hand and finger**

IQ Q71.30 **Congenital absence of unspecified hand and finger**

SP Q71.31 **Congenital absence of right hand and finger**

SP Q71.32 **Congenital absence of left hand and finger**

SP Q71.33 **Congenital absence of hand and finger, bilateral**

Q71.4 **Longitudinal reduction defect of radius**

Clubhand (congenital)

★ New   ▲ Revised   Px Primary   **SP** PDGM Px   **SL** Low CoM   **SH** High CoM   **IQ** Quest. Encounter   **H** Hospice non-cancer Dx   Unspecified   **M** *Manifestation*

Radial clubhand

☐ **IQ** Q71.40 **Longitudinal reduction defect of unspecified radius**

☐ **SP** Q71.41 **Longitudinal reduction defect of right radius**

☐ **SP** Q71.42 **Longitudinal reduction defect of left radius**

☐ **SP** Q71.43 **Longitudinal reduction defect of radius, bilateral**

5 Q71.5 **Longitudinal reduction defect of ulna**

☐ **IQ** Q71.50 **Longitudinal reduction defect of unspecified ulna**

☐ **SP** Q71.51 **Longitudinal reduction defect of right ulna**

☐ **SP** Q71.52 **Longitudinal reduction defect of left ulna**

☐ **SP** Q71.53 **Longitudinal reduction defect of ulna, bilateral**

5 Q71.6 **Lobster-claw hand**

☐ **IQ** Q71.60 **Lobster-claw hand, unspecified hand**

☐ **SP** Q71.61 **Lobster-claw right hand**

☐ **SP** Q71.62 **Lobster-claw left hand**

☐ **SP** Q71.63 **Lobster-claw hand, bilateral**

5 Q71.8 **Other reduction defects of upper limb**

6 Q71.81 **Congenital shortening of upper limb**

☐ **SP** Q71.811 **Congenital shortening of right upper limb**

☐ **SP** Q71.812 **Congenital shortening of left upper limb**

☐ **SP** Q71.813 **Congenital shortening of upper limb, bilateral**

☐ **IQ** Q71.819 **Congenital shortening of unspecified upper limb**

6 Q71.89 **Other reduction defects of upper limb**

☐ **SP** Q71.891 **Other reduction defects of right upper limb**

☐ **SP** Q71.892 **Other reduction defects of left upper limb**

☐ **SP** Q71.893 **Other reduction defects of upper limb, bilateral**

☐ **IQ** Q71.899 **Other reduction defects of unspecified upper limb**

5 Q71.9 **Unspecified reduction defect of upper limb**

☐ **SP** Q71.90 **Unspecified reduction defect of unspecified upper limb**

☐ **SP** Q71.91 **Unspecified reduction defect of right upper limb**

☐ **SP** Q71.92 **Unspecified reduction defect of left upper limb**

☐ **SP** Q71.93 **Unspecified reduction defect of upper limb, bilateral**

4 Q72 **Reduction defects of lower limb**

5 Q72.0 **Congenital complete absence of lower limb**

☐ **SP** Q72.00 **Congenital complete absence of unspecified lower limb**

☐ **SP** Q72.01 **Congenital complete absence of right lower limb**

☐ **SP** Q72.02 **Congenital complete absence of left lower limb**

☐ **SP** Q72.03 **Congenital complete absence of lower limb, bilateral**

5 Q72.1 **Congenital absence of thigh and lower leg with foot present**

☐ **IQ** Q72.10 **Congenital absence of unspecified thigh and lower leg with foot present**

☐ **SP** Q72.11 **Congenital absence of right thigh and lower leg with foot present**

☐ **SP** Q72.12 **Congenital absence of left thigh and lower leg with foot present**

☐ **SP** Q72.13 **Congenital absence of thigh and lower leg with foot present, bilateral**

5 Q72.2 **Congenital absence of both lower leg and foot**

☐ **IQ** Q72.20 **Congenital absence of both lower leg and foot, unspecified lower limb**

☐ **SP** Q72.21 **Congenital absence of both lower leg and foot, right lower limb**

☐ **SP** Q72.22 **Congenital absence of both lower leg and foot, left lower limb**

☐ **SP** Q72.23 **Congenital absence of both lower leg and foot, bilateral**

5 Q72.3 **Congenital absence of foot and toe(s)**

☐ **IQ** Q72.30 **Congenital absence of unspecified foot and toe(s)**

☐ **SP** Q72.31 **Congenital absence of right foot and toe(s)**

☐ **SP** Q72.32 **Congenital absence of left foot and toe(s)**

☐ **SP** Q72.33 **Congenital absence of foot and toe(s), bilateral**

5 Q72.4 **Longitudinal reduction defect of femur**

Proximal femoral focal deficiency

☐ **IQ** Q72.40 **Longitudinal reduction defect of unspecified femur**

☐ **SP** Q72.41 **Longitudinal reduction defect of right femur**

☐ **SP** Q72.42 **Longitudinal reduction defect of left femur**

☐ **SP** Q72.43 **Longitudinal reduction defect of femur, bilateral**

5 Q72.5 **Longitudinal reduction defect of tibia**

☐ **IQ** Q72.50 **Longitudinal reduction defect of unspecified tibia**

☐ **SP** Q72.51 **Longitudinal reduction defect of right tibia**

☐ **SP** Q72.52 **Longitudinal reduction defect of left tibia**

☐ **SP** Q72.53 **Longitudinal reduction defect of tibia, bilateral**

5 Q72.6 **Longitudinal reduction defect of fibula**

☐ **IQ** Q72.60 **Longitudinal reduction defect of unspecified fibula**

☐ **SP** Q72.61 **Longitudinal reduction defect of right fibula**

☐ **SP** Q72.62 **Longitudinal reduction defect of left fibula**

☐ **SP** Q72.63 **Longitudinal reduction defect of fibula, bilateral**

5 Q72.7 **Split foot**

☐ **IQ** Q72.70 **Split foot, unspecified lower limb**

☐ **SP** Q72.71 **Split foot, right lower limb**

☐ **SP** Q72.72 **Split foot, left lower limb**

☐ **SP** Q72.73 **Split foot, bilateral**

---

4 4th digit required   **5** 5th digit required   **6** 6th digit required   **7** 7th digit required   **7** 7th digit placeholder   **+** Additional code   ☐ Laterality

⑤ **Q72.8 Other reduction defects of lower limb**

  ⑥ **Q72.81 Congenital shortening of lower limb**

⊟ SP **Q72.811 Congenital shortening of right lower limb**

⊟ SP **Q72.812 Congenital shortening of left lower limb**

⊟ SP **Q72.813 Congenital shortening of lower limb, bilateral**

⊟ IQ **Q72.819 Congenital shortening of unspecified lower limb**

  ⑥ **Q72.89 Other reduction defects of lower limb**

⊟ SP **Q72.891 Other reduction defects of right lower limb**

⊟ SP **Q72.892 Other reduction defects of left lower limb**

⊟ SP **Q72.893 Other reduction defects of lower limb, bilateral**

⊟ IQ **Q72.899 Other reduction defects of unspecified lower limb**

⑤ **Q72.9 Unspecified reduction defect of lower limb**

⊟ IQ **Q72.90 Unspecified reduction defect of unspecified lower limb**

⊟ SP **Q72.91 Unspecified reduction defect of right lower limb**

⊟ SP **Q72.92 Unspecified reduction defect of left lower limb**

⊟ SP **Q72.93 Unspecified reduction defect of lower limb, bilateral**

④ **Q73 Reduction defects of unspecified limb**

IQ **Q73.0 Congenital absence of unspecified limb(s)**
Amelia NOS

IQ **Q73.1 Phocomelia, unspecified limb(s)**
Phocomelia NOS

IQ **Q73.8 Other reduction defects of unspecified limb(s)**
Longitudinal reduction deformity of unspecified limb(s)
Ectromelia of limb NOS
Hemimelia of limb NOS
Reduction defect of limb NOS

④ **Q74 Other congenital malformations of limb(s)**
EXCLUDES 1   polydactyly (Q69.-)
reduction defect of limb (Q71-Q73)
syndactyly (Q70.-)

SP **Q74.0 Other congenital malformations of upper limb(s), including shoulder girdle**
Accessory carpal bones
Cleidocranial dysostosis
Congenital pseudarthrosis of clavicle
Macrodactylia (fingers)
Madelung's deformity
Radioulnar synostosis
Sprengel's deformity
Triphalangeal thumb

SP **Q74.1 Congenital malformation of knee**
Congenital absence of patella
Congenital dislocation of patella
Congenital genu valgum
Congenital genu varum
Rudimentary patella
EXCLUDES 1   congenital dislocation of knee (Q68.2)

congenital genu recurvatum (Q68.2)
nail patella syndrome (Q87.2)

SP **Q74.2 Other congenital malformations of lower limb(s), including pelvic girdle**
Congenital fusion of sacroiliac joint
Congenital malformation of ankle joint
Congenital malformation of sacroiliac joint
EXCLUDES 1   anteversion of femur (neck) (Q65.89)

SP **Q74.3 Arthrogryposis multiplex congenita**

SP **Q74.8 Other specified congenital malformations of limb(s)**

IQ **Q74.9 Unspecified congenital malformation of limb(s)**
Congenital anomaly of limb(s) NOS

④ **Q75 Other congenital malformations of skull and face bones**
EXCLUDES 1   congenital malformation of face NOS (Q18.-)
congenital malformation syndromes classified to Q87.-
dentofacial anomalies [including malocclusion] (M26.-)
musculoskeletal deformities of head and face (Q67.0-Q67.4)
skull defects associated with congenital anomalies of brain such as:
anencephaly (Q00.0)
encephalocele (Q01.-)
hydrocephalus (Q03.-)
microcephaly (Q02)

SP **Q75.0 Craniosynostosis**
Acrocephaly
Imperfect fusion of skull
Oxycephaly
Trigonocephaly

SP **Q75.1 Craniofacial dysostosis**
Crouzon's disease

SP **Q75.2 Hypertelorism**

SP **Q75.3 Macrocephaly**

SP **Q75.4 Mandibulofacial dysostosis**
Franceschetti syndrome
Treacher Collins syndrome

SP **Q75.5 Oculomandibular dysostosis**

SP **Q75.8 Other specified congenital malformations of skull and face bones**
Absence of skull bone, congenital
Congenital deformity of forehead
Platybasia

IQ **Q75.9 Congenital malformation of skull and face bones, unspecified**
Congenital anomaly of face bones NOS
Congenital anomaly of skull NOS

④ **Q76 Congenital malformations of spine and bony thorax**
EXCLUDES 1   congenital musculoskeletal deformities of spine and chest (Q67.5-Q67.8)

SP **Q76.0 Spina bifida occulta**
EXCLUDES 1   meningocele (spinal) (Q05.-)
spina bifida (aperta) (cystica) (Q05.-)

★ New ▲ Revised Px Primary SP PDGM Px SL Low CoM SH High CoM IQ Quest. Encounter H Hospice non-cancer Dx Unspecified M *Manifestation*

DecisionHealth's FY 2020 Complete Home Health ICD-10-CM Diagnosis Coding Manual   1401

SP Q76.1 Klippel-Feil syndrome
Cervical fusion syndrome

SP Q76.2 Congenital spondylolisthesis
Congenital spondylolysis
EXCLUDES 1 spondylolisthesis (acquired) (M43.1-)
spondylolysis (acquired) (M43.0-)

SP Q76.3 Congenital scoliosis due to congenital bony malformation
Hemivertebra fusion or failure of segmentation with scoliosis

5 Q76.4 Other congenital malformations of spine, not associated with scoliosis

6 Q76.41 Congenital kyphosis

SP Q76.411 Congenital kyphosis, occipito-atlanto-axial region

SP Q76.412 Congenital kyphosis, cervical region

SP Q76.413 Congenital kyphosis, cervicothoracic region

SP Q76.414 Congenital kyphosis, thoracic region

SP Q76.415 Congenital kyphosis, thoracolumbar region

IQ Q76.419 Congenital kyphosis, unspecified region

6 Q76.42 Congenital lordosis

SP Q76.425 Congenital lordosis, thoracolumbar region

SP Q76.426 Congenital lordosis, lumbar region

SP Q76.427 Congenital lordosis, lumbosacral region

SP Q76.428 Congenital lordosis, sacral and sacrococcygeal region

IQ Q76.429 Congenital lordosis, unspecified region

SP Q76.49 Other congenital malformations of spine, not associated with scoliosis
Congenital absence of vertebra NOS
Congenital fusion of spine NOS
Congenital malformation of lumbosacral (joint) (region) NOS
Congenital malformation of spine NOS
Hemivertebra NOS
Malformation of spine NOS
Platyspondylisis NOS
Supernumerary vertebra NOS

SP Q76.5 Cervical rib
Supernumerary rib in cervical region

SP Q76.6 Other congenital malformations of ribs
Accessory rib
Congenital absence of rib
Congenital fusion of ribs
Congenital malformation of ribs NOS
EXCLUDES 1 short rib syndrome (Q77.2)

SP Q76.7 Congenital malformation of sternum
Congenital absence of sternum
Sternum bifidum

SP Q76.8 Other congenital malformations of bony thorax

IQ Q76.9 Congenital malformation of bony thorax, unspecified

4 Q77 Osteochondrodysplasia with defects of growth of tubular bones and spine

EXCLUDES 1 mucopolysaccharidosis (E76.0-E76.3)
EXCLUDES 2 congenital myotonic chondrodystrophy (G71.13)

SP Q77.0 Achondrogenesis
Hypochondrogenesis

SP Q77.1 Thanatophoric short stature

SP Q77.2 Short rib syndrome
Asphyxiating thoracic dysplasia [Jeune]

SP Q77.3 Chondrodysplasia punctata
EXCLUDES 1 Rhizomelic chondrodysplasia punctata (E71.43)

SP Q77.4 Achondroplasia
Hypochondroplasia
Osteosclerosis congenita

SP Q77.5 Diastrophic dysplasia

SP Q77.6 Chondroectodermal dysplasia
Ellis-van Creveld syndrome

SP Q77.7 Spondyloepiphyseal dysplasia

SP Q77.8 Other osteochondrodysplasia with defects of growth of tubular bones and spine

SP Q77.9 Osteochondrodysplasia with defects of growth of tubular bones and spine, unspecified

4 Q78 Other osteochondrodysplasias
EXCLUDES 2 congenital myotonic chondrodystrophy (G71.13)

SP Q78.0 Osteogenesis imperfecta
Fragilitas ossium
Osteopsathyrosis

SP Q78.1 Polyostotic fibrous dysplasia
Albright(-McCune)(-Sternberg) syndrome
DEFINITION Genetic bone disorder causing multiple areas of normal bone to be replaced by bands of abnormal fibrous tissue, causing pain, fractures, and deformity.

SP Q78.2 Osteopetrosis
Albers-Schönberg syndrome
Osteosclerosis NOS

SP Q78.3 Progressive diaphyseal dysplasia
Camurati-Engelmann syndrome

SP Q78.4 Enchondromatosis
Maffucci's syndrome
Ollier's disease

SP Q78.5 Metaphyseal dysplasia
Pyle's syndrome

SP Q78.6 Multiple congenital exostoses
Diaphyseal aclasis

SP Q78.8 Other specified osteochondrodysplasias
Osteopoikilosis

IQ Q78.9 Osteochondrodysplasia, unspecified
Chondrodystrophy NOS
Osteodystrophy NOS

4 Q79 Congenital malformations of musculoskeletal system, not elsewhere classified
EXCLUDES 2 congenital (sternomastoid) torticollis (Q68.0)

SP Q79.0 Congenital diaphragmatic hernia
EXCLUDES 1 congenital hiatus hernia (Q40.1)

SP Q79.1 Other congenital malformations of diaphragm
Absence of diaphragm

---

4 4th digit required   5 5th digit required   6 6th digit required   7 7th digit required   7 7th digit placeholder   + Additional code   ⊟ Laterality

1402   DecisionHealth's FY 2020 Complete Home Health ICD-10-CM Diagnosis Coding Manual

Congenital malformation of diaphragm NOS

Eventration of diaphragm

SP **Q79.2** **Exomphalos**

Omphalocele

EXCLUDES 1 umbilical hernia (K42.-)

SP **Q79.3** **Gastroschisis**

SP **Q79.4** **Prune belly syndrome**

Congenital prolapse of bladder mucosa

Eagle-Barrett syndrome

5 **Q79.5** **Other congenital malformations of abdominal wall**

EXCLUDES 1 umbilical hernia (K42.-)

SP **Q79.51** **Congenital hernia of bladder**

SP **Q79.59** **Other congenital malformations of abdominal wall**

▲ **5** **Q79.6** **Ehlers-Danlos syndromes**

DEFINITION Ehlers-Danlos syndromes are a clinically and genetically heterogeneous group of heritable connective tissue disorders characterized by articular hypermobility, skin hyperextensibility or laxity, and tissue fragility affecting virtually every organ system: skin, ligaments, joints, bone, muscle, blood vessels and various organs.

⭐ **Q79.60** **Ehlers-Danlos syndrome, unspecified**

⭐ **Q79.61** **Classical Ehlers-Danlos syndrome**

Classical EDS (cEDS)

⭐ **Q79.62** **Hypermobile Ehlers-Danlos syndrome**

Hypermobile EDS (hEDS)

⭐ **Q79.63** **Vascular Ehlers-Danlos syndrome**

Vascular EDS (vEDS)

⭐ **Q79.69** **Other Ehlers-Danlos syndromes**

SP **Q79.8** **Other congenital malformations of musculoskeletal system**

Absence of muscle

Absence of tendon

Accessory muscle

Amyotrophia congenita

Congenital constricting bands

Congenital shortening of tendon

Poland syndrome

IQ **Q79.9** **Congenital malformation of musculoskeletal system, unspecified**

Congenital anomaly of musculoskeletal system NOS

Congenital deformity of musculoskeletal system NOS

Other congenital malformations (Q80-Q89)

4 **Q80** **Congenital ichthyosis**

EXCLUDES 1 Refsum's disease (G60.1)

IQ **Q80.0** **Ichthyosis vulgaris**

IQ **Q80.1** **X-linked ichthyosis**

IQ **Q80.2** **Lamellar ichthyosis**

Collodion baby

IQ **Q80.3** **Congenital bullous ichthyosiform erythroderma**

IQ **Q80.4** **Harlequin fetus**

IQ **Q80.8** **Other congenital ichthyosis**

IQ **Q80.9** **Congenital ichthyosis, unspecified**

4 **Q81** **Epidermolysis bullosa**

▲ **SP** **Q81.0** **Epidermolysis bullosa simplex**

EXCLUDES 1 Cockayne's syndrome (Q87.19)

SP **Q81.1** **Epidermolysis bullosa letalis**

Herlitz' syndrome

SP **Q81.2** **Epidermolysis bullosa dystrophica**

SP **Q81.8** **Other epidermolysis bullosa**

IQ **Q81.9** **Epidermolysis bullosa, unspecified**

4 **Q82** **Other congenital malformations of skin**

EXCLUDES 1 acrodermatitis enteropathica (E83.2)

congenital erythropoietic porphyria (E80.0)

pilonidal cyst or sinus (L05.-)

Sturge-Weber (-Dimitri) syndrome (Q85.8)

SP **Q82.0** **Hereditary lymphedema**

SP **Q82.1** **Xeroderma pigmentosum**

SP **Q82.2** **Congenital cutaneous mastocytosis**

Congenital diffuse cutaneous mastocytosis

Congenital maculopapular cutaneous mastocytosis

Congenital urticaria pigmentosa

EXCLUDES 1 cutaneous mastocytosis NOS (D47.01)

diffuse cutaneous mastocytosis (with onset after newborn period) (D47.01)

malignant mastocytosis (C96.2-)

systemic mastocytosis (D47.02)

urticaria pigmentosa (non-congenital) (with onset after newborn period) (D47.01)

SP **Q82.3** **Incontinentia pigmenti**

SP **Q82.4** **Ectodermal dysplasia (anhidrotic)**

EXCLUDES 1 Ellis-van Creveld syndrome (Q77.6)

SP **Q82.5** **Congenital non-neoplastic nevus**

Birthmark NOS

Flammeus Nevus

Portwine Nevus

Sanguineous Nevus

Strawberry Nevus

Vascular Nevus NOS

Verrucous Nevus

EXCLUDES 2 Café au lait spots (L81.3)

lentigo (L81.4)

nevus NOS (D22.-)

araneus nevus (I78.1)

melanocytic nevus (D22.-)

pigmented nevus (D22.-)

spider nevus (I78.1)

stellar nevus (I78.1)

SP **Q82.6** **Congenital sacral dimple**

Parasacral dimple

EXCLUDES 2 pilonidal cyst with abscess (L05.01)

pilonidal cyst without abscess (L05.91)

▲ **SP** **Q82.8** **Other specified congenital malformations of skin**

Abnormal palmar creases

⭐ New ▲ Revised Px Primary **SP** PDGM Px **SL** Low CoM **SH** High CoM **IQ** Quest. Encounter ⊞ Hospice non-cancer Dx **Unspecified** **M** *Manifestation*

Accessory skin tags
Benign familial pemphigus [Hailey-
  Hailey]
Congenital poikiloderma
Cutis laxa (hyperelastica)
Dermatoglyphic anomalies
Inherited keratosis palmaris et plantaris
Keratosis follicularis [Darier-White]
EXCLUDES 1   Ehlers-Danlos syndrome
  (Q79.6-)

IQ Q82.9 **Congenital malformation of skin, unspecified**

4 Q83 **Congenital malformations of breast**
EXCLUDES 2   absence of pectoral muscle
  (Q79.8)
  hypoplasia of breast (N64.82)
  micromastia (N64.82)

SP Q83.0 **Congenital absence of breast with absent nipple**

SP Q83.1 **Accessory breast**
Supernumerary breast

SP Q83.2 **Absent nipple**

SP Q83.3 **Accessory nipple**
Supernumerary nipple

SP Q83.8 **Other congenital malformations of breast**

IQ Q83.9 **Congenital malformation of breast, unspecified**

4 Q84 **Other congenital malformations of integument**

SP Q84.0 **Congenital alopecia**
Congenital atrichosis

IQ Q84.1 **Congenital morphological disturbances of hair, not elsewhere classified**
Beaded hair
Monilethrix
Pili annulati
EXCLUDES 1   Menkes' kinky hair
  syndrome (E83.0)

IQ Q84.2 **Other congenital malformations of hair**
Congenital hypertrichosis
Congenital malformation of hair NOS
Persistent lanugo

IQ Q84.3 **Anonychia**
EXCLUDES 1   nail patella syndrome
  (Q87.2)

IQ Q84.4 **Congenital leukonychia**

IQ Q84.5 **Enlarged and hypertrophic nails**
Congenital onychauxis
Pachyonychia

IQ Q84.6 **Other congenital malformations of nails**
Congenital clubnail
Congenital koilonychia
Congenital malformation of nail NOS

SP Q84.8 **Other specified congenital malformations of integument**
Aplasia cutis congenita

IQ Q84.9 **Congenital malformation of integument, unspecified**
Congenital anomaly of integument NOS
Congenital deformity of integument NOS

4 Q85 **Phakomatoses, not elsewhere classified**
EXCLUDES 1   ataxia telangiectasia [Louis-
  Bar] (G11.3)
  familial dysautonomia [Riley-
  Day] (G90.1)

5 Q85.0 **Neurofibromatosis (nonmalignant)**

SP Q85.00 **Neurofibromatosis, unspecified**

SP Q85.01 **Neurofibromatosis, type 1**
Von Recklinghausen disease

SP Q85.02 **Neurofibromatosis, type 2**
Acoustic neurofibromatosis

SP Q85.03 **Schwannomatosis**
DEFINITION   A rare type of
neurofibromatosis causing tumors on
nerve sheaths of spinal, peripheral, and
cranial nerves - except the eighth
(vestibular) cranial nerve.

SP Q85.09 **Other neurofibromatosis**

SP Q85.1 **Tuberous sclerosis**
Bourneville's disease
Epiloia

SP Q85.8 **Other phakomatoses, not elsewhere classified**
Peutz-Jeghers Syndrome
Sturge-Weber(-Dimitri) syndrome
von Hippel-Lindau syndrome
EXCLUDES 1   Meckel-Gruber syndrome
  (Q61.9)

SP Q85.9 **Phakomatosis, unspecified**
Hamartosis NOS

4 Q86 **Congenital malformation syndromes due to known exogenous causes, not elsewhere classified**
EXCLUDES 2   iodine-deficiency-related
  hypothyroidism (E00-E02)
  nonteratogenic effects of
  substances transmitted via
  placenta or breast milk
  (P04.-)

SP Q86.0 **Fetal alcohol syndrome (dysmorphic)**

SP Q86.1 **Fetal hydantoin syndrome**
Meadow's syndrome

SP Q86.2 **Dysmorphism due to warfarin**

SP Q86.8 **Other congenital malformation syndromes due to known exogenous causes**

+ 4 Q87 **Other specified congenital malformation syndromes affecting multiple systems**
Use additional code(s) to identify all
associated manifestations

SP + Q87.0 **Congenital malformation syndromes predominantly affecting facial appearance**
Acrocephalopolysyndactyly
Acrocephalosyndactyly [Apert]
Cryptophthalmos syndrome
Cyclopia
Goldenhar syndrome
Moebius syndrome
Oro-facial-digital syndrome
Robin syndrome
Whistling face

▲ + 5 Q87.1 **Congenital malformation syndromes predominantly associated with short stature**
EXCLUDES 1   Ellis-van Creveld syndrome
  (Q77.6)
  Smith-Lemli-Opitz
  syndrome (E78.72)

★ + Q87.11 **Prader-Willi syndrome**

★ + Q87.19 **Other congenital malformation syndromes predominantly associated with short stature**

---

4 4th digit required **5** 5th digit required **6** 6th digit required **7** 7th digit required **7** 7th digit placeholder **+** Additional code **⊟** Laterality

1404   *DecisionHealth's* FY 2020 Complete Home Health ICD-10-CM Diagnosis Coding Manual

Aarskog syndrome
Cockayne syndrome
De Lange syndrome
Dubowitz syndrome
Noonan syndrome
Robinow-Silverman-Smith syndrome
Russell-Silver syndrome
Seckel syndrome

SP + Q87.2 Congenital malformation syndromes predominantly involving limbs
Holt-Oram syndrome
Klippel-Trenaunay-Weber syndrome
Nail patella syndrome
Rubinstein-Taybi syndrome
Sirenomelia syndrome
Thrombocytopenia with absent radius [TAR] syndrome
VATER syndrome

SP + Q87.3 Congenital malformation syndromes involving early overgrowth
Beckwith-Wiedemann syndrome
Sotos syndrome
Weaver syndrome

+ 5 Q87.4 Marfan's syndrome

SP + Q87.40 Marfan's syndrome, unspecified

+ 6 Q87.41 Marfan's syndrome with cardiovascular manifestations

SP + Q87.410 Marfan's syndrome with aortic dilation

SP + Q87.418 Marfan's syndrome with other cardiovascular manifestations

SP + Q87.42 Marfan's syndrome with ocular manifestations

SP + Q87.43 Marfan's syndrome with skeletal manifestation

SP + Q87.5 Other congenital malformation syndromes with other skeletal changes

+ 5 Q87.8 Other specified congenital malformation syndromes, not elsewhere classified
EXCLUDES 1 Zellweger syndrome (E71.510)

SP + Q87.81 Alport syndrome
Use additional code to identify stage of chronic kidney disease (N18.1-N18.6)

SP + Q87.82 Arterial tortuosity syndrome

SP + Q87.89 Other specified congenital malformation syndromes, not elsewhere classified
Laurence-Moon (-Bardet)-Biedl syndrome

4 Q89 Other congenital malformations, not elsewhere classified

5 Q89.0 Congenital absence and malformations of spleen
EXCLUDES 1 isomerism of atrial appendages (with asplenia or polysplenia) (Q20.6)

SP Q89.01 Asplenia (congenital)

SP Q89.09 Congenital malformations of spleen
Congenital splenomegaly

SP Q89.1 Congenital malformations of adrenal gland
EXCLUDES 1 adrenogenital disorders (E25.-)
congenital adrenal hyperplasia (E25.0)

SP Q89.2 Congenital malformations of other endocrine glands
Congenital malformation of parathyroid or thyroid gland
Persistent thyroglossal duct
Thyroglossal cyst
EXCLUDES 1 congenital goiter (E03.0)
congenital hypothyroidism (E03.1)

SP Q89.3 Situs inversus
Dextrocardia with situs inversus
Mirror-image atrial arrangement with situs inversus
Situs inversus or transversus abdominalis
Situs inversus or transversus thoracis
Transposition of abdominal viscera
Transposition of thoracic viscera
EXCLUDES 1 dextrocardia NOS (Q24.0)

DEFINITION Congenital disorder in which the position of all major organs in the chest and abdomen are reversed horizontally.

SP Q89.4 Conjoined twins
Craniopagus
Dicephaly
Pygopagus
Thoracopagus

SP Q89.7 Multiple congenital malformations, not elsewhere classified
Multiple congenital anomalies NOS
Multiple congenital deformities NOS
EXCLUDES 1 congenital malformation syndromes affecting multiple systems (Q87.-)

SP + Q89.8 Other specified congenital malformations
Use additional code(s) to identify all associated manifestations

IQ Q89.9 Congenital malformation, unspecified
Congenital anomaly NOS
Congenital deformity NOS

Chromosomal abnormalities, not elsewhere classified (Q90-Q99)

EXCLUDES 2 mitochondrial metabolic disorders (E88.4-)

+ 4 Q90 Down syndrome
Use additional code(s) to identify any associated physical conditions and degree of intellectual disabilities (F70-F79)

SP + Q90.0 Trisomy 21, nonmosaicism (meiotic nondisjunction)

SP + Q90.1 Trisomy 21, mosaicism (mitotic nondisjunction)

SP + Q90.2 Trisomy 21, translocation

SP + Q90.9 Down syndrome, unspecified
Trisomy 21 NOS

4 Q91 Trisomy 18 and Trisomy 13

SP Q91.0 Trisomy 18, nonmosaicism (meiotic nondisjunction)

SP Q91.1 Trisomy 18, mosaicism (mitotic nondisjunction)

SP Q91.2 Trisomy 18, translocation

SP Q91.3 Trisomy 18, unspecified

SP Q91.4 Trisomy 13, nonmosaicism (meiotic nondisjunction)

★ New ▲ Revised Px Primary SP PDGM Px SL Low CoM SH High CoM IQ Quest. Encounter H Hospice non-cancer Dx Unspecified M Manifestation

DecisionHealth's FY 2020 Complete Home Health ICD-10-CM Diagnosis Coding Manual

1405

SP Q91.5 Trisomy 13, mosaicism (mitotic nondisjunction)

SP Q91.6 Trisomy 13, translocation

SP Q91.7 Trisomy 13, unspecified

4 Q92 Other trisomies and partial trisomies of the autosomes, not elsewhere classified
INCLUDES unbalanced translocations and insertions
EXCLUDES 1 trisomies of chromosomes 13, 18, 21 (Q90-Q91)

SP Q92.0 Whole chromosome trisomy, nonmosaicism (meiotic nondisjunction)

SP Q92.1 Whole chromosome trisomy, mosaicism (mitotic nondisjunction)

SP Q92.2 Partial trisomy
Less than whole arm duplicated
Whole arm or more duplicated
EXCLUDES 1 partial trisomy due to unbalanced translocation (Q92.5)

SP Q92.5 Duplications with other complex rearrangements
Partial trisomy due to unbalanced translocations
Code also:
  any associated deletions due to unbalanced translocations, inversions and insertions (Q93.7)

5 Q92.6 Marker chromosomes
Trisomies due to dicentrics
Trisomies due to extra rings
Trisomies due to isochromosomes
Individual with marker heterochromatin

SP Q92.61 Marker chromosomes in normal individual

SP Q92.62 Marker chromosomes in abnormal individual

SP Q92.7 Triploidy and polyploidy

SP Q92.8 Other specified trisomies and partial trisomies of autosomes
Duplications identified by fluorescence in situ hybridization (FISH)
Duplications identified by in situ hybridization (ISH)
Duplications seen only at prometaphase

IQ Q92.9 Trisomy and partial trisomy of autosomes, unspecified

4 Q93 Monosomies and deletions from the autosomes, not elsewhere classified

SP Q93.0 Whole chromosome monosomy, nonmosaicism (meiotic nondisjunction)

SP Q93.1 Whole chromosome monosomy, mosaicism (mitotic nondisjunction)

SP Q93.2 Chromosome replaced with ring, dicentric or isochromosome

SP Q93.3 Deletion of short arm of chromosome 4
Wolff-Hirschorn syndrome

SP Q93.4 Deletion of short arm of chromosome 5
Cri-du-chat syndrome

5 Q93.5 Other deletions of part of a chromosome

SP Q93.51 Angelman syndrome

SP Q93.59 Other deletions of part of a chromosome

SP Q93.7 Deletions with other complex rearrangements

Deletions due to unbalanced translocations, inversions and insertions
Code also:
  any associated duplications due to unbalanced translocations, inversions and insertions (Q92.5)

5 Q93.8 Other deletions from the autosomes

SP Q93.81 Velo-cardio-facial syndrome
Deletion 22q11.2

SP Q93.82 Williams syndrome

SP Q93.88 Other microdeletions
Miller-Dieker syndrome
Smith-Magenis syndrome

SP Q93.89 Other deletions from the autosomes
Deletions identified by fluorescence in situ hybridization (FISH)
Deletions identified by in situ hybridization (ISH)
Deletions seen only at prometaphase

IQ Q93.9 Deletion from autosomes, unspecified

4 Q95 Balanced rearrangements and structural markers, not elsewhere classified
INCLUDES Robertsonian and balanced reciprocal translocations and insertions

SP Q95.0 Balanced translocation and insertion in normal individual

SP Q95.1 Chromosome inversion in normal individual

SP Q95.2 Balanced autosomal rearrangement in abnormal individual

SP Q95.3 Balanced sex/autosomal rearrangement in abnormal individual

SP Q95.5 Individual with autosomal fragile site

SP Q95.8 Other balanced rearrangements and structural markers

SP Q95.9 Balanced rearrangement and structural marker, unspecified

▲ 4 Q96 Turner's syndrome
EXCLUDES 1 Noonan syndrome (Q87.19)

SP Q96.0 Karyotype 45, X

SP Q96.1 Karyotype 46, X iso (Xq)
Karyotype 46, isochromosome Xq

SP Q96.2 Karyotype 46, X with abnormal sex chromosome, except iso (Xq)
Karyotype 46, X with abnormal sex chromosome, except isochromosome Xq

SP Q96.3 Mosaicism, 45, X/46, XX or XY

SP Q96.4 Mosaicism, 45, X/other cell line(s) with abnormal sex chromosome

SP Q96.8 Other variants of Turner's syndrome

SP Q96.9 Turner's syndrome, unspecified

4 Q97 Other sex chromosome abnormalities, female phenotype, not elsewhere classified
EXCLUDES 1 Turner's syndrome (Q96.-)

SP Q97.0 Karyotype 47, XXX

SP Q97.1 Female with more than three X chromosomes

SP Q97.2 Mosaicism, lines with various numbers of X chromosomes

SP Q97.3 Female with 46, XY karyotype

SP Q97.8 Other specified sex chromosome abnormalities, female phenotype

SP Q97.9 Sex chromosome abnormality, female phenotype, unspecified

---

4 4th digit required   5 5th digit required   6 6th digit required   7 7th digit required   7 7th digit placeholder   + Additional code   ▤ Laterality

4 Q98 Other sex chromosome abnormalities, male phenotype, not elsewhere classified

SP Q98.0 Klinefelter syndrome karyotype 47, XXY

SP Q98.1 Klinefelter syndrome, male with more than two X chromosomes

SP Q98.3 Other male with 46, XX karyotype

SP Q98.4 Klinefelter syndrome, unspecified

SP Q98.5 Karyotype 47, XYY

SP Q98.6 Male with structurally abnormal sex chromosome

SP Q98.7 Male with sex chromosome mosaicism

SP Q98.8 Other specified sex chromosome abnormalities, male phenotype

SP Q98.9 Sex chromosome abnormality, male phenotype, unspecified

4 Q99 Other chromosome abnormalities, not elsewhere classified

SP Q99.0 Chimera 46, XX/46, XY
    Chimera 46, XX/46, XY true hermaphrodite

SP Q99.1 46, XX true hermaphrodite
    46, XX with streak gonads
    46, XY with streak gonads
    Pure gonadal dysgenesis

SP Q99.2 Fragile X chromosome
    Fragile X syndrome

SP Q99.8 Other specified chromosome abnormalities

IQ Q99.9 Chromosomal abnormality, unspecified

★ New ▲ Revised Px Primary SP PDGM Px SL Low CoM SH High CoM IQ Quest. Encounter H Hospice non-cancer Dx | Unspecified | M *Manifestation*

DecisionHealth's FY 2020 Complete Home Health ICD-10-CM Diagnosis Coding Manual

1407

Chapter 17 Scenarios: Congenital malformations, deformations and chromosomal abnormalities (Q00-Q99)

Pressure ulcers/injuries, spina bifida

A 21-year-old woman who was born with spina bifida is admitted to home health for wound care to a stage 3 pressure ulcer/injury on her right buttock and a stage 2 pressure ulcer/injury on her sacrum. She is confined to a wheelchair.

Description	Code
Primary: Pressure ulcer of right buttock, stage 3	L89.313
Secondary: Pressure ulcer of sacral region, stage 2	L89.152
Secondary: Spina bifida, unspecified	Q05.9
Secondary: Dependence on wheelchair	Z99.3

As the focus of care, the pressure ulcers/injuries are coded primary. Her spina bifida and wheelchair dependence are also coded as it will impact her care.

Tetralogy of Fallot

A 28-year-old man is admitted for aftercare following surgery to replace his pulmonary valve with a prosthetic one. He was diagnosed with Tetralogy of Fallot as a baby, which necessitated the valve replacement. He has had numerous heart surgeries over the years. He also has a history of melanoma, requiring the removal of several moles and is frequently monitored for recurrence.

Description	Code
Primary: Encounter for surgical aftercare following surgery on the circulatory system	Z48.812
Secondary: Tetralogy of Fallot	Q21.3
Secondary: Presence of prosthetic heart valve	Z95.2
Secondary: Personal history of malignant melanoma of skin	Z85.820

Surgical aftercare is the focus of care, making Z48.812 the appropriate primary diagnosis code. The surgical procedure treats an aspect of the heart condition, Tetralogy of Fallot, but does not cure it. Thus, it is still coded. Tetralogy of Fallot is a congenital condition and as such may be assigned throughout the life of the patient, according to coding guidelines. Code Z95.2 is assigned to indicate the presence of a prosthetic heart valve. An additional code is assigned to capture his history of malignant melanoma and need for frequent monitoring.

Down syndrome, E. coli pneumonia

A 52-year-old man is admitted to home health to continue recovery from E. coli pneumonia. He continues to take oral antibiotics and will for several weeks. He has Down syndrome with severe intellectual disabilities.

Description	Code
Primary: Pneumonia due to Escherichia coli	J15.5
Secondary: Down syndrome, unspecified	Q90.9
Secondary: Severe intellectual disabilities	F72
Secondary: Long term (current) use of antibiotics	Z79.2

As the focus of care, the E. coli pneumonia is coded primary. His Down syndrome will impact his plan of care and is thus coded. His severe intellectual disabilities are also coded, following the Down syndrome code, in accordance with tabular instruction. Since he will be taking antibiotics for several more weeks, the code for long-term antibiotic use is assigned.

Open heart surgery, Marfan syndrome

A 65-year-old man underwent open heart surgery to replace his aortic root as well as his aortic valve. The surgery resolved aortic dilation associated with Marfan syndrome. He was admitted to home health for routine surgical aftercare.

Description	Code
Primary: Encounter for surgical aftercare following surgery on the circulatory system	Z48.812
Secondary: Marfan's syndrome, unspecified	Q87.40

Routine surgical aftercare following cardiac surgery is coded with Z48.812. Note that aftercare codes should only be used routine care. The open heart surgery resolved the aortic dilation but did not resolve the Marfan syndrome, which is a congenital condition that can cause a variety of manifestations. Thus, Q87.40 is assigned to capture it.

HOME HEALTH CODING SCENARIOS

Chapter 18: Symptoms, Signs and Abnormal Clinical and Laboratory Findings, not Elsewhere Classified (R00-R99)

Chapter 18 includes symptoms, signs, abnormal results of clinical or other investigative procedures, and ill-defined conditions where no diagnosis classifiable elsewhere is recorded. Signs and symptoms that point rather definitively to a given diagnosis have been assigned to a category in other chapters within ICD-10-CM. In general, categories in this chapter include the less well-defined conditions and symptoms that, without the necessary study of the case to establish a final diagnosis, point perhaps equally to two or more diseases or to two or more systems of the body. Practically all categories in the chapter should be designated "not otherwise specified," "unknown etiology" or "transient." The Alphabetical Index should be consulted to determine which signs and symptoms are to be allocated here and which to other chapters. The residual subcategories numbered .8 are generally provided for other relevant symptoms that cannot be allocated elsewhere in the classification.

Note, in the new home health payment system, the Patient-Driven Groupings Model (PDGM), which is set to take effect Jan. 1, 2020, many common home health symptom codes carry a questionable encounter designation.

Using a questionable encounter code as a primary diagnosis could result in claims getting kicked back, payment delays and potential red flags for auditors.

CMS states that "the majority of the R codes (codes that describe signs and symptoms, as opposed to diagnoses) are not appropriate as principal diagnosis codes for grouping home health periods into clinical groups" under PDGM.

To avoid these issues, take steps to identify which symptom codes your agency uses and work to gather more detailed information that will lead to more specific, acceptable codes instead.

The conditions and signs or symptoms included in categories R00-R99 of this chapter consist of:

- cases for which no more specific diagnosis can be made even after all the facts bearing on the case have been investigated;

- signs or symptoms existing at the time of initial encounter that proved to be transient and whose causes could not be determined;

- provisional diagnosis in a patient who failed to return for further investigation or care;

- cases referred elsewhere for investigation or treatment before the diagnosis was made;

- cases in which a more precise diagnosis was not available for any other reason;

- certain symptoms, for which supplementary information is provided, that represent important problems in medical care in their own right.

There is an Excludes 2 note at the beginning of this chapter for conditions, signs or symptoms that may be coded in addition to a code from Chapter 18, but are not included as part of the codes that are available in this chapter such as abnormal findings on antenatal screening of the mother (O28.-), certain conditions originating in the perinatal period (P00-P96), signs and symptoms classified in the body system chapters, and signs and symptoms of the breast (N63, N64.5).

The chapter is organized into blocks that correspond to signs and symptoms involving specific body systems such as circulatory, digestive, skin and subcutaneous tissue, nervous and musculoskeletal, genitourinary, cognitive perception/emotional state/behavior, and speech and voice; general signs and symptoms; abnormal findings on examination of blood, urine, other body fluids, substances and tissues; abnormal findings on diagnostic imaging and in functional studies; abnormal tumor markers; and ill-defined and unknown cause of mortality.

A "symptom" is any subjective evidence of disease, or a patient's condition, as reported by the patient. A "sign" is an indication of a problem that is observed by the physician or the clinician. For example, a patient may report a **symptom** by stating that he/she is feeling dizzy. A physician may report a **sign**, such as fever or irregular heartbeat.

More thorough examination may be needed to determine the cause of the symptom or sign (a definitive diagnosis). Coders should not assume a condition is present based on documentation of symptoms. If the documentation lists symptoms but no definitive diagnosis, query the doctor for a definitive diagnosis.

Many codes have an Excludes 1 note that lists more definitive diagnoses. If any of these conditions are documented, do not report the symptom code. For example, category R22, (Localized superficial swelling, mass or lump of skin) includes this note: "Excludes 1: abnormal findings on diagnostic imaging (R90-R93), edema (R60.-), enlarged lymph nodes (R59.-), localized adiposity (E65), and swelling of joint (M25.4-).

Sometimes, a Chapter 18 code is not the most appropriate choice. **Symptom codes also are found in other chapters.** Here are a few situations to watch out for:

• A breast mass or lump is reported using code N63 (lump or mass in breast) from Chapter 14.

• An itch is reported using code Subcategory L29.9 (pruritus and related conditions) from Chapter 12.

• Pain in the eye is reported using code H57.1- (pain in or around the eye) from Chapter 7.

Multiple Coding and Sequencing

It is important to read the Includes and Excludes notes under codes in this chapter, as well as any other instructions under the code or code category. Below are some examples of multiple coding and sequencing issues for codes in this chapter.

A symptom code is not reported if the symptom is an integral part of the condition. For example, congestive heart failure and edema would be reported using only a code from the I50.- category (heart failure) because the edema is an integral part of the heart failure.

A symptom code is reported as an additional diagnosis when it describes a significant aspect of the condition but is not an integral part of it. Code N40.1 Benign prostatic hyperplasia with lower urinary tract symptoms has a note that reads: "Use additional codes to identify symptoms," and lists subcategory N39.4- (Urinary incontinence), code N13.8 (Urinary obstruction) plus several codes from subcategories R33.-, R35.- or R39.- to report the urinary symptoms present.

Category R50 (Fever of other and unknown origin) includes R50.81, fever in conditions classified elsewhere, with a note stating to code first the underlying condition when fever is present – such as with leukemia, neutropenia and sickle-cell disease. Fever is not an integral part of these conditions; therefore, it is reported as an additional diagnosis when present. There are many symptom codes for fever in certain situations: R50.2 (drug induced); R50.82 (postprocedural); R50.83 postvaccination; R50.84 (Febrile nonhemolytic transfusion reaction); and R50.9, (unspecified). However, there are dozens of codes, especially in Chapter 1, for specific diseases in which fever is an integral symptom and a code from category R50 is not used.

Special Coding Issues

Symptoms as reasons for receiving home care

Neither coding nor OASIS instructions prevent an agency from reporting a symptom when a related definitive diagnosis has not been established (confirmed by the provider). However, every effort should be made to establish/confirm a definitive diagnosis. As previously noted, "the majority of the R codes (codes that describe signs and symptoms, as opposed to diagnoses) are not appropriate as **principal** diagnosis codes for grouping home health periods into clinical groups" under PDGM, according to CMS. Codes for signs and symptoms may be reported in addition to a related definitive diagnosis when the sign or symptom is not routinely associated with that diagnosis, such as the various signs and symptoms associated with complex syndromes. The definitive diagnosis should be sequenced before the symptom code.

Signs or symptoms that are associated routinely with a disease process should not be assigned as additional codes, unless otherwise instructed by the classification.

Gait training

For patients needing gait training, the correct principal diagnosis code usually is the illness, especially if there is a disease code indicating gait problem as part of the illness. For example, **abnormality of gait and mobility** (R26.-) is integral to a patient with hemiplegia due to a CVA, lower back pain, or when using aftercare following joint replacement (Z47.1) of the lower extremity. If the therapist or physician documents "abnormal gait" or "unsteady gait," attempt to obtain the definitive diagnosis or a more specific description of the abnormal gait problem, such as R26.0 (Ataxic gait), R26.1 (Paralytic gait), R26.81 (Unsteadiness on feet gait), R26.89 (Other abnormalities of gait and mobility) or R26.9 (Unspecified abnormalities of gait and mobility).

Clinicians should investigate the cause of the gait abnormality. If the gait abnormality is integral to the condition causing the abnormal gait, then code the condition and not the abnormal gait.

Repeated falls (R29.6) is for use for encounters when a patient has recently fallen or has a tendency to fall and the reason for the fall is being investigated. There is an Excludes 2 note at this code to indicate at risk of or history of falling (Z91.81) is not included in this code, but may be coded as either a first-listed or additional code with R29.6.

Combination codes – ICD-10-CM contains a number of combination codes that identify both the definitive diagnosis and common symptoms of that diagnosis. When using one of these combination codes, an additional code should not be assigned for the symptom. The physician must identify a cause-and-effect relationship, if one exists. For example, in some elderly patients with incontinence, the incontinence may be attributed to one of several diseases or conditions.

Gangrene is a complication of necrosis (i.e., cell death) characterized by the decay of body tissues, which become black and malodorous. It is usually the result of critically insufficient blood supply (e.g., peripheral vascular disease) and often is associated with diabetes and long-term smoking. In ICD-10-CM, gangrene is included in multiple combination codes when it is present with another diagnosis or condition. A separate code for gangrene has been reassigned to I96 in Chapter 9, Diseases of the circulatory system and is no longer within the Symptoms chapter. Refer to the Alphabetical Index for the correct combination code based on the diagnostic statement.

Coma scale codes (R40.2-) can be used in conjunction with traumatic brain injury codes, acute cerebrovascular disease or sequelae of cerebrovascular disease codes. These codes are primarily for use by trauma registries, but they may be used in any setting where this information is collected. The coma scale codes should be sequenced after the diagnosis code(s).

These codes, one from each subcategory, are needed to complete the scale. The 7th character indicates when the scale was recorded and should match on all three codes. At a minimum, report the initial score documented on presentation at your facility. This may be a score from the emergency medical technician (EMT) or in the emergency department. If desired, a facility may choose to capture multiple coma scale scores.

Functional quadriplegia (R53.2) is the lack of ability to use one's limbs or ambulate due to extreme debility. It is not associated with neurologic deficit or injury, and code R53.2 should not be used for cases of neurologic quadriplegia. It should be assigned only if functional quadriplegia is specifically documented in the medical record.

SIRS due to non-infectious process – The systemic inflammatory response syndrome (SIRS) can develop as a result of certain non-infectious disease processes, such as trauma, malignant neoplasm or pancreatitis. When SIRS is documented with a noninfectious condition, and no subsequent infection is documented, the code for the underlying condition, such as an injury, should be assigned followed by code R65.10, Systemic inflammatory response syndrome (SIRS) of non-infectious origin without acute organ dysfunction, or code R65.11, Systemic inflammatory response syndrome (SIRS) of non-infectious origin with acute organ dysfunction. If an associated acute organ dysfunction is documented, the appropriate code(s) for the specific type of organ dysfunction(s) should be assigned in addition to code R65.11. If acute organ dysfunction is documented, but it cannot be determined if the acute organ dysfunction is associated with SIRS or due to another condition (e.g., directly due to the trauma), the provider should be queried.

Death NOS – Code R99, Ill-defined and unknown cause of mortality, is only for use in the very limited circumstance when a patient who has already died is brought into an emergency department or other health care facility and is pronounced dead upon arrival. It does not represent the discharge disposition of death.

A patient's **National Institutes of Health Stroke Scale** (NIHSS) score can be reported with the new **R29.7-** codes. The NIHSS score can be used as a clinical stroke assessment tool to evaluate and document neurological status in acute stroke patients. The stroke scale is valid for predicting lesion size and can serve as a measure of stroke severity.

The NIHSS has been shown to be a predictor of both short and long term outcome of stroke patients. Additionally, the stroke scale serves as a data collection tool for planning patient care and provides a common language for information exchanges among healthcare providers. The scale is designed to be a simple, valid and reliable tool that can be administered at the bedside consistently by physicians, nurses or therapists.

The NIH stroke scale (NIHSS) codes (R29.7- -) can be used in conjunction with acute stroke codes (I63) to identify the patient's neurological status and the severity of the stroke. The stroke scale codes should be sequenced after the acute stroke diagnosis code(s). At a minimum, report the initial score documented. If desired, a facility may choose to capture multiple stroke scale scores, per coding guidelines.

For coma scale and NIHSS codes, code assignment may be based on medical record documentation from clinicians who are not the patient's provider such as an emergency medical technician. However, the associated diagnosis (such as acute stroke) must be documented by patient's provider.

CHAPTER 18: SYMPTOMS, SIGNS AND ABNORMAL CLINICAL AND LABORATORY FINDINGS, NOT ELSEWHERE CLASSIFIED (R00-R99)

Note:

This chapter includes symptoms, signs, abnormal results of clinical or other investigative procedures, and ill-defined conditions regarding which no diagnosis classifiable elsewhere is recorded.

Signs and symptoms that point rather definitely to a given diagnosis have been assigned to a category in other chapters of the classification. In general, categories in this chapter include the less well-defined conditions and symptoms that, without the necessary study of the case to establish a final diagnosis, point perhaps equally to two or more diseases or to two or more systems of the body. Practically all categories in the chapter could be designated 'not otherwise specified', 'unknown etiology' or 'transient'. The Alphabetical Index should be consulted to determine which symptoms and signs are to be allocated here and which to other chapters. The residual subcategories, numbered .8, are generally provided for other relevant symptoms that cannot be allocated elsewhere in the classification.

The conditions and signs or symptoms included in categories R00-R94 consist of:

(a) cases for which no more specific diagnosis can be made even after all the facts bearing on the case have been investigated;

(b) signs or symptoms existing at the time of initial encounter that proved to be transient and whose causes could not be determined;

(c) provisional diagnosis in a patient who failed to return for further investigation or care;

(d) cases referred elsewhere for investigation or treatment before the diagnosis was made;

(e) cases in which a more precise diagnosis was not available for any other reason;

(f) certain symptoms, for which supplementary information is provided, that represent important problems in medical care in their own right.

EXCLUDES 2 abnormal findings on antenatal screening of mother (O28.-)
certain conditions originating in the perinatal period (P04-P96)
signs and symptoms classified in the body system chapters
signs and symptoms of breast (N63, N64.5)

GUIDELINES Section I.C.18.a-c

Codes that describe symptoms and signs are acceptable for reporting purposes when a related definitive diagnosis has not been established (confirmed) by the provider.

Codes for signs and symptoms may be reported in addition to a related definitive diagnosis when the sign or symptom is not routinely associated with that diagnosis, such as the various signs and symptoms associated with complex syndromes. The definitive diagnosis code should be sequenced before the symptom code. Signs or symptoms that are associated routinely with a disease process should not be assigned as additional codes, unless otherwise instructed by the classification.

ICD-10-CM contains a number of combination codes that identify both the definitive diagnosis and common symptoms of that diagnosis. When using one of these combination codes, an additional code should not be assigned for the symptom.

CODING TIPS ✓ R codes are not allowed as primary under the proposed PDGM. They are allowed as secondary codes when not routinely associated with the definitive diagnosis. Symptom/sign diagnoses should be coded if there is no definitive diagnosis or the symptom/sign is not routinely associated with the definitive diagnosis, e.g. hemoptysis with pneumonia.

This chapter contains the following blocks:

R00-R09 Symptoms and signs involving the circulatory and respiratory systems
R10-R19 Symptoms and signs involving the digestive system and abdomen
R20-R23 Symptoms and signs involving the skin and subcutaneous tissue
R25-R29 Symptoms and signs involving the nervous and musculoskeletal systems
R30-R39 Symptoms and signs involving the genitourinary system
R40-R46 Symptoms and signs involving cognition, perception, emotional state and behavior
R47-R49 Symptoms and signs involving speech and voice
R50-R69 General symptoms and signs
R70-R79 Abnormal findings on examination of blood, without diagnosis
R80-R82 Abnormal findings on examination of urine, without diagnosis
R83-R89 Abnormal findings on examination of other body fluids, substances and tissues, without diagnosis
R90-R94 Abnormal findings on diagnostic imaging and in function studies, without diagnosis
R97 Abnormal tumor markers
R99 Ill-defined and unknown cause of mortality

Symptoms and signs involving the circulatory and respiratory systems (R00-R09)

4 R00   Abnormalities of heart beat
   EXCLUDES 1 abnormalities originating in the perinatal period (P29.1-)
   EXCLUDES 2 specified arrhythmias (I47-I49)

IQ R00.0   Tachycardia, unspecified
   Rapid heart beat
   Sinoauricular tachycardia NOS
   Sinus [sinusal] tachycardia NOS
   EXCLUDES 1 neonatal tachycardia (P29.11)
   paroxysmal tachycardia (I47.-)

   CODING TIPS ✓ Tachycardia that is not specified as due to a specific arrhythmia or any particular cause is coded here. When the record reports "sinus tachycardia," assign code R00.0. Sinus tachycardia indicates a high heart rate with an impulse that continues to originate from the SA node.

IQ SH SL R00.1   Bradycardia, unspecified
   +
   Sinoatrial bradycardia
   Sinus bradycardia
   Slow heart beat
   Vagal bradycardia
   Use additional code for adverse effect, if applicable, to identify drug (T36-T50 with fifth or sixth character 5)
   EXCLUDES 1 neonatal bradycardia (P29.12)

IQ R00.2   Palpitations

---

4 4th digit required   5 5th digit required   6 6th digit required   7 7th digit required   7 7th digit placeholder   + Additional code   ▤ Laterality

1414   DecisionHealth's FY 2020 Complete Home Health ICD-10-CM Diagnosis Coding Manual

Awareness of heart beat

DEFINITION   Sensation of feeling the heart beat.

!Q R00.8   Other abnormalities of heart beat

!Q R00.9   Unspecified abnormalities of heart beat

4 R01   Cardiac murmurs and other cardiac sounds

EXCLUDES 1   cardiac murmurs and sounds originating in the perinatal period (P29.8)

!Q R01.0   Benign and innocent cardiac murmurs
Functional cardiac murmur

!Q R01.1   Cardiac murmur, unspecified
Cardiac bruit NOS
Heart murmur NOS
Systolic murmur NOS

!Q R01.2   Other cardiac sounds
Cardiac dullness, increased or decreased
Precordial friction

4 R03   Abnormal blood-pressure reading, without diagnosis

!Q R03.0   Elevated blood-pressure reading, without diagnosis of hypertension
Note:
This category is to be used to record an episode of elevated blood pressure in a patient in whom no formal diagnosis of hypertension has been made, or as an isolated incidental finding.

GUIDELINES   Section I.C.9.a.7)
Assign code R03.0, Elevated blood pressure reading without diagnosis of hypertension, unless patient has an established diagnosis of hypertension. Assign code O13.-, Gestational [pregnancy-induced] hypertension without significant proteinuria, or O14.-, Pre-eclampsia, for transient hypertension of pregnancy.

CODING TIPS ✓   Do not assign this code for a patient with a diagnosis of hypertension (I10-I13).

!Q R03.1   Nonspecific low blood-pressure reading

EXCLUDES 1   hypotension (I95.-)
maternal hypotension syndrome (O26.5-)
neurogenic orthostatic hypotension (G90.3)

CODING TIPS ✓   Assign code R03.1 when a patient has a low blood pressure reading but has not been diagnosed with hypotension or orthostasis.

4 R04   Hemorrhage from respiratory passages

CODING TIPS ✓   If these bleeds are the result of an adverse effect of anticoagulant, add D68.32 and the T code for anticoagulant from the Table of Drugs and Chemicals.

!Q R04.0   Epistaxis
Hemorrhage from nose
Nosebleed

!Q R04.1   Hemorrhage from throat

EXCLUDES 2   hemoptysis (R04.2)

!Q R04.2   Hemoptysis
Blood-stained sputum
Cough with hemorrhage

DEFINITION   Coughing up blood or bloody mucous.

5 R04.8   Hemorrhage from other sites in respiratory passages

!Q R04.81   Acute idiopathic pulmonary hemorrhage in infants
AIPHI
Acute idiopathic hemorrhage in infants over 28 days old

EXCLUDES 1   perinatal pulmonary hemorrhage (P26.-)
von Willebrand's disease (D68.0)

!Q R04.89   Hemorrhage from other sites in respiratory passages
Pulmonary hemorrhage NOS

!Q R04.9   Hemorrhage from respiratory passages, unspecified

!Q R05   Cough

EXCLUDES 1   cough with hemorrhage (R04.2)
smoker's cough (J41.0)

CODING TIPS ✓   Do not assign R05 as an additional code when the cough is an integral symptom of another disease process also coded, such as COPD, bronchitis, asthma, or another pulmonary condition known to be the cause of the cough.

4 R06   Abnormalities of breathing

EXCLUDES 1   acute respiratory distress syndrome (J80)
respiratory arrest (R09.2)
respiratory arrest of newborn (P28.81)
respiratory distress syndrome of newborn (P22.-)
respiratory failure (J96.-)
respiratory failure of newborn (P28.5)

CODING TIPS ✓   Do not assign a code from R06.- as an additional code when the respiratory symptom is routinely associated with another disease process also coded, such as COPD, bronchitis, asthma, or another condition known to be the cause of the presenting symptom. The more specific condition should be coded.

5 R06.0   Dyspnea

EXCLUDES 1   tachypnea NOS (R06.82)
transient tachypnea of newborn (P22.1)

!Q R06.00   Dyspnea, unspecified

!Q R06.01   Orthopnea

DEFINITION   Difficulty breathing while lying down, necessitating sleeping propped up or in a chair.

!Q R06.02   Shortness of breath

!Q R06.03   Acute respiratory distress

!Q R06.09   Other forms of dyspnea

!Q R06.1   Stridor

EXCLUDES 1   congenital laryngeal stridor (P28.89)
laryngismus (stridulus) (J38.5)

DEFINITION   A whistling sound when breathing, usually heard on inspiration, indicating obstruction of the trachea or larynx.

★ New ▲ Revised Px Primary SP PDGM Px SL Low CoM SH High CoM !Q Quest. Encounter H Hospice non-cancer Dx   Unspecified   M *Manifestation*

DecisionHealth's FY 2020 Complete Home Health ICD-10-CM Diagnosis Coding Manual   1415

Chapter 18

R00-R99

IQ R06.2 Wheezing
> **EXCLUDES 1** Asthma (J45.-)

IQ R06.3 Periodic breathing
Cheyne-Stokes breathing

IQ R06.4 Hyperventilation
> **EXCLUDES 1** psychogenic hyperventilation (F45.8)

IQ R06.5 Mouth breathing
> **EXCLUDES 2** dry mouth NOS (R68.2)

IQ R06.6 Hiccough
> **EXCLUDES 1** psychogenic hiccough (F45.8)

> **DEFINITION** Sharp sound of inhalation, with spasm of the glottis and diaphragm.

IQ R06.7 Sneezing

5 R06.8 Other abnormalities of breathing

IQ R06.81 Apnea, not elsewhere classified
Apnea NOS
> **EXCLUDES 1** apnea (of) newborn (P28.4)
> sleep apnea (G47.3-)
> sleep apnea of newborn (primary) (P28.3)

> **DEFINITION** Temporary cessation of breathing.

IQ R06.82 Tachypnea, not elsewhere classified
Tachypnea NOS
> **EXCLUDES 1** transitory tachypnea of newborn (P22.1)

> **DEFINITION** Rapid breathing.

IQ R06.83 Snoring

IQ R06.89 Other abnormalities of breathing
Breath-holding (spells)
Sighing
> **CODING TIPS ✓** Respiratory **insufficiency** is part of COPD and therefore is not coded separately. Respiratory **failure** is coded in addition to COPD when documented. Respiratory failure is often confused with respiratory arrest. Respiratory failure means not enough oxygen is getting into the blood and there is a carbon dioxide buildup.

IQ R06.9 Unspecified abnormalities of breathing

4 R07 Pain in throat and chest
> **EXCLUDES 1** epidemic myalgia (B33.0)
> **EXCLUDES 2** jaw pain R68.84
> pain in breast (N64.4)

> **CODING TIPS ✓** Do not assign a code from R07.- for a patient with angina. Chest pain due to angina should be coded to the appropriate I20.- or I25.- code

IQ R07.0 Pain in throat
> **EXCLUDES 1** chronic sore throat (J31.2)
> sore throat (acute) NOS (J02.9)
> **EXCLUDES 2** dysphagia (R13.1-)
> pain in neck (M54.2)

IQ R07.1 Chest pain on breathing
Painful respiration

IQ R07.2 Precordial pain

5 R07.8 Other chest pain

IQ R07.81 Pleurodynia
Pleurodynia NOS

> **EXCLUDES 1** epidemic pleurodynia (B33.0)

IQ R07.82 Intercostal pain

IQ R07.89 Other chest pain
Anterior chest-wall pain NOS

IQ R07.9 Chest pain, unspecified

4 R09 Other symptoms and signs involving the circulatory and respiratory system
> **EXCLUDES 1** acute respiratory distress syndrome (J80)
> respiratory arrest of newborn (P28.81)
> respiratory distress syndrome of newborn (P22.0)
> respiratory failure (J96.-)
> respiratory failure of newborn (P28.5)

5 R09.0 Asphyxia and hypoxemia
> **EXCLUDES 1** asphyxia due to carbon monoxide (T58.-)
> asphyxia due to foreign body in respiratory tract (T17.-)
> birth (intrauterine) asphyxia (P84)
> hyperventilation (R06.4)
> traumatic asphyxia (T71.-)
> **EXCLUDES 2** hypercapnia (R06.89)

IQ R09.01 Asphyxia
> **DEFINITION** Extreme decrease in the amount of oxygen in the body, accompanied by an increase of carbon dioxide, leading to loss of consciousness or death.

IQ R09.02 Hypoxemia
> **DEFINITION** Abnormally low levels of oxygen in arterial blood.

IQ R09.1 Pleurisy
> **EXCLUDES 1** pleurisy with effusion (J90)

IQ R09.2 Respiratory arrest
Cardiorespiratory failure
> **EXCLUDES 1** cardiac arrest (I46.-)
> respiratory arrest of newborn (P28.81)
> respiratory distress of newborn (P22.0)
> respiratory failure (J96.-)
> respiratory failure of newborn (P28.5)
> respiratory insufficiency (R06.89)
> respiratory insufficiency of newborn (P28.5)

IQ R09.3 Abnormal sputum
Abnormal amount of sputum
Abnormal color of sputum
Abnormal odor of sputum
Excessive sputum
> **EXCLUDES 1** blood-stained sputum (R04.2)

5 R09.8 Other specified symptoms and signs involving the circulatory and respiratory systems

IQ R09.81 Nasal congestion

IQ R09.82 Postnasal drip

IQ R09.89 Other specified symptoms and signs involving the circulatory and respiratory systems

---

4 4th digit required 5 5th digit required 6 6th digit required 7 7th digit required 7 7th digit placeholder + Additional code ▭ Laterality

1416   *DecisionHealth's* FY 2020 Complete Home Health ICD-10-CM Diagnosis Coding Manual

Bruit (arterial)
Abnormal chest percussion
Feeling of foreign body in throat
Friction sounds in chest
Chest tympany
Choking sensation
Rales
Weak pulse

EXCLUDES 2   foreign body in throat
(T17.2-)
wheezing (R06.2)

CODING TIPS ✓   Pulmonary congestion is integral to, or routinely associated with, several conditions, such as CHF and pneumonia. Do not use an additional symptom code such as R09.89 when the symptom is routinely associated with the condition.

Symptoms and signs involving the digestive system and abdomen   (R10-R19)

EXCLUDES 2   congenital or infantile pylorospasm (Q40.0)
gastrointestinal hemorrhage (K92.0-K92.2)
intestinal obstruction (K56.-)
newborn gastrointestinal hemorrhage (P54.0-P54.3)
newborn intestinal obstruction (P76.-)
pylorospasm (K31.3)
signs and symptoms involving the urinary system (R30-R39)
symptoms referable to female genital organs (N94.-)
symptoms referable to male genital organs (N48-N50)

4 R10   Abdominal and pelvic pain

EXCLUDES 1   renal colic (N23)

EXCLUDES 2   dorsalgia (M54.-)
flatulence and related conditions (R14.-)

IQ R10.0   Acute abdomen
Severe abdominal pain (generalized) (with abdominal rigidity)
EXCLUDES 1   abdominal rigidity NOS (R19.3)
generalized abdominal pain NOS (R10.84)
localized abdominal pain (R10.1-R10.3-)

5 R10.1   Pain localized to upper abdomen

IQ R10.10   Upper abdominal pain, unspecified

IQ R10.11   Right upper quadrant pain

IQ R10.12   Left upper quadrant pain

IQ R10.13   Epigastric pain
Dyspepsia
EXCLUDES 1   functional dyspepsia (K30)

IQ R10.2   Pelvic and perineal pain
EXCLUDES 1   vulvodynia (N94.81)

5 R10.3   Pain localized to other parts of lower abdomen

IQ R10.30   Lower abdominal pain, unspecified

IQ R10.31   Right lower quadrant pain

IQ R10.32   Left lower quadrant pain

IQ R10.33   Periumbilical pain

5 R10.8   Other abdominal pain

6 R10.81   Abdominal tenderness
Abdominal tenderness NOS

IQ R10.811   Right upper quadrant abdominal tenderness

IQ R10.812   Left upper quadrant abdominal tenderness

IQ R10.813   Right lower quadrant abdominal tenderness

IQ R10.814   Left lower quadrant abdominal tenderness

IQ R10.815   Periumbilic abdominal tenderness

IQ R10.816   Epigastric abdominal tenderness

IQ R10.817   Generalized abdominal tenderness

IQ R10.819   Abdominal tenderness, unspecified site

6 R10.82   Rebound abdominal tenderness

IQ R10.821   Right upper quadrant rebound abdominal tenderness

IQ R10.822   Left upper quadrant rebound abdominal tenderness

IQ R10.823   Right lower quadrant rebound abdominal tenderness

IQ R10.824   Left lower quadrant rebound abdominal tenderness

IQ R10.825   Periumbilic rebound abdominal tenderness

IQ R10.826   Epigastric rebound abdominal tenderness

IQ R10.827   Generalized rebound abdominal tenderness

IQ R10.829   Rebound abdominal tenderness, unspecified site

IQ R10.83   Colic
Colic NOS
Infantile colic
EXCLUDES 1   colic in adult and child over 12 months old (R10.84)

IQ R10.84   Generalized abdominal pain
EXCLUDES 1   generalized abdominal pain associated with acute abdomen (R10.0)

IQ R10.9   Unspecified abdominal pain

4 R11   Nausea and vomiting
EXCLUDES 1   cyclical vomiting associated with migraine (G43.A-)
excessive vomiting in pregnancy (O21.-)
hematemesis (K92.0)
neonatal hematemesis (P54.0)
newborn vomiting (P92.0-)
psychogenic vomiting (F50.89)
vomiting associated with bulimia nervosa (F50.2)
vomiting following gastrointestinal surgery (K91.0)

IQ R11.0   Nausea
Nausea NOS
Nausea without vomiting

5 R11.1   Vomiting

IQ R11.10   Vomiting, unspecified
Vomiting NOS

IQ R11.11   Vomiting without nausea

★ New ▲ Revised Px Primary **SP** PDGM Px **SL** Low CoM **SH** High CoM **IQ** Quest. Encounter 🖫 Hospice non-cancer Dx   Unspecified   **M** *Manifestation*

IQ R11.12 **Projectile vomiting**

IQ R11.13 **Vomiting of fecal matter**

IQ R11.14 **Bilious vomiting**
Bilious emesis

★ **R11.15** **Cyclical vomiting syndrome unrelated to migraine**
Cyclic vomiting syndrome NOS
Persistent vomiting
> EXCLUDES 1   cyclical vomiting in migraine (G43.A-)
> EXCLUDES 2   bulimia nervosa (F50.2)
> diabetes mellitus due to underlying condition (E08.-)

IQ R11.2   **Nausea with vomiting, unspecified**
Persistent nausea with vomiting NOS

IQ R12 **Heartburn**
> EXCLUDES 1   dyspepsia NOS (R10.13)
> functional dyspepsia (K30)

4 R13 **Aphagia and dysphagia**

IQ R13.0 **Aphagia**
Inability to swallow
> EXCLUDES 1   psychogenic aphagia (F50.9)

5 R13.1 **Dysphagia**
Code first:
, if applicable, dysphagia following cerebrovascular disease (I69. with final characters -91)
> EXCLUDES 1   psychogenic dysphagia (F45.8)

> CODING TIPS ✓   The results from tests such as the video fluoroscopic swallowing study, video endoscopic swallowing study, barium-contrast esophagogram or an upper endoscopy or manometry may identify the swallowing stage affected.

> CODING TIPS ✓   Assign a code from R13.1- following a code from I69.- when dysphagia is reported as a sequela of cerebral vascular disease to report the specified level of dysphagia.

> DEFINITION   Difficulty in swallowing.

IQ R13.10   **Dysphagia, unspecified**
Difficulty in swallowing NOS

IQ R13.11 **Dysphagia, oral phase**

IQ R13.12 **Dysphagia, oropharyngeal phase**

IQ R13.13 **Dysphagia, pharyngeal phase**

IQ R13.14 **Dysphagia, pharyngoesophageal phase**

IQ R13.19 **Other dysphagia**
Cervical dysphagia
Neurogenic dysphagia

4 R14 **Flatulence and related conditions**
> EXCLUDES 1   psychogenic aerophagy (F45.8)

IQ R14.0 **Abdominal distension (gaseous)**
Bloating
Tympanites (abdominal) (intestinal)

IQ R14.1 **Gas pain**

IQ R14.2 **Eructation**

IQ R14.3 **Flatulence**

4 R15 **Fecal incontinence**
> INCLUDES   encopresis NOS

> EXCLUDES 1   fecal incontinence of nonorganic origin (F98.1)

IQ R15.0 **Incomplete defecation**
> EXCLUDES 1   constipation (K59.0-)
> fecal impaction (K56.41)

IQ R15.1 **Fecal smearing**
Fecal soiling

IQ R15.2 **Fecal urgency**

IQ R15.9 **Full incontinence of feces**
Fecal incontinence NOS

4 R16 **Hepatomegaly and splenomegaly, not elsewhere classified**

IQ R16.0 **Hepatomegaly, not elsewhere classified**
Hepatomegaly NOS

IQ R16.1 **Splenomegaly, not elsewhere classified**
Splenomegaly NOS

IQ R16.2 **Hepatomegaly with splenomegaly, not elsewhere classified**
Hepatosplenomegaly NOS

IQ R17   **Unspecified jaundice**
> EXCLUDES 1   neonatal jaundice (P55, P57-P59)

4 R18 **Ascites**
> INCLUDES   fluid in peritoneal cavity
> EXCLUDES 1   ascites in alcoholic cirrhosis (K70.31)
> ascites in alcoholic hepatitis (K70.11)
> ascites in toxic liver disease with chronic active hepatitis (K71.51)

IQ R18.0 **Malignant ascites**
Code first malignancy, such as:
malignant neoplasm of ovary (C56.-)
secondary malignant neoplasm of retroperitoneum and peritoneum (C78.6)
> DEFINITION   Abnormal accumulation of fluid containing cancer cells in the peritoneal cavity, usually from metastatic spread of a malignancy.

IQ R18.8 **Other ascites**
Ascites NOS
Peritoneal effusion (chronic)

4 R19 **Other symptoms and signs involving the digestive system and abdomen**
> EXCLUDES 1   acute abdomen (R10.0)

5 R19.0 **Intra-abdominal and pelvic swelling, mass and lump**
> EXCLUDES 1   abdominal distension (gaseous) (R14.-)
> ascites (R18.-)

> CODING TIPS ✓   A mass should not be coded for an area that has been clearly identified as a neoplasm. If a mass has been biopsied and reported as a neoplasm, code the appropriate neoplasm code.

IQ R19.00   **Intra-abdominal and pelvic swelling, mass and lump, unspecified site**

≡ IQ R19.01 **Right upper quadrant abdominal swelling, mass and lump**

≡ IQ R19.02 **Left upper quadrant abdominal swelling, mass and lump**

≡ IQ R19.03 **Right lower quadrant abdominal swelling, mass and lump**

---

4 4th digit required   **5** 5th digit required   **6** 6th digit required   **7** 7th digit required   **7** 7th digit placeholder   **✚** Additional code   **≡** Laterality

☐ IQ R19.04 Left lower quadrant abdominal swelling, mass and lump

IQ R19.05 Periumbilic swelling, mass or lump
Diffuse or generalized umbilical swelling or mass

IQ R19.06 Epigastric swelling, mass or lump

IQ R19.07 Generalized intra-abdominal and pelvic swelling, mass and lump
Diffuse or generalized intra-abdominal swelling or mass NOS
Diffuse or generalized pelvic swelling or mass NOS

IQ R19.09 Other intra-abdominal and pelvic swelling, mass and lump

5 R19.1 Abnormal bowel sounds

IQ R19.11 Absent bowel sounds

IQ R19.12 Hyperactive bowel sounds

IQ R19.15 Other abnormal bowel sounds
Abnormal bowel sounds NOS

IQ R19.2 Visible peristalsis
Hyperperistalsis

5 R19.3 Abdominal rigidity
EXCLUDES 1 abdominal rigidity with severe abdominal pain (R10.0)

IQ R19.30 Abdominal rigidity, unspecified site

☐ IQ R19.31 Right upper quadrant abdominal rigidity

☐ IQ R19.32 Left upper quadrant abdominal rigidity

☐ IQ R19.33 Right lower quadrant abdominal rigidity

☐ IQ R19.34 Left lower quadrant abdominal rigidity

IQ R19.35 Periumbilic abdominal rigidity

IQ R19.36 Epigastric abdominal rigidity

IQ R19.37 Generalized abdominal rigidity

IQ R19.4 Change in bowel habit
EXCLUDES 1 constipation (K59.0-)
functional diarrhea (K59.1)

IQ R19.5 Other fecal abnormalities
Abnormal stool color
Bulky stools
Mucus in stools
Occult blood in feces
Occult blood in stools
EXCLUDES 1 melena (K92.1)
neonatal melena (P54.1)

IQ R19.6 Halitosis

IQ R19.7 Diarrhea, unspecified
Diarrhea NOS
EXCLUDES 1 functional diarrhea (K59.1)
neonatal diarrhea (P78.3)
psychogenic diarrhea (F45.8)

IQ R19.8 Other specified symptoms and signs involving the digestive system and abdomen

Symptoms and signs involving the skin and subcutaneous tissue   (R20-R23)

EXCLUDES 2 symptoms relating to breast (N64.4-N64.5)

4 R20 Disturbances of skin sensation
EXCLUDES 1 dissociative anesthesia and sensory loss (F44.6)

psychogenic disturbances (F45.8)

IQ R20.0 Anesthesia of skin

IQ R20.1 Hypoesthesia of skin

IQ R20.2 Paresthesia of skin
Formication
Pins and needles
Tingling skin
EXCLUDES 1 acroparesthesia (I73.8)

IQ R20.3 Hyperesthesia

IQ R20.8 Other disturbances of skin sensation

IQ R20.9 Unspecified disturbances of skin sensation

IQ R21 Rash and other nonspecific skin eruption
INCLUDES rash NOS
EXCLUDES 1 specified type of rash- code to condition
vesicular eruption (R23.8)

4 R22 Localized swelling, mass and lump of skin and subcutaneous tissue
INCLUDES subcutaneous nodules (localized) (superficial)
EXCLUDES 1 abnormal findings on diagnostic imaging (R90-R93)
edema (R60.-)
enlarged lymph nodes (R59.-)
localized adiposity (E65)
swelling of joint (M25.4-)

IQ R22.0 Localized swelling, mass and lump, head

IQ R22.1 Localized swelling, mass and lump, neck

IQ R22.2 Localized swelling, mass and lump, trunk
EXCLUDES 1 intra-abdominal or pelvic mass and lump (R19.0-)
intra-abdominal or pelvic swelling (R19.0-)
EXCLUDES 2 breast mass and lump (N63)

5 R22.3 Localized swelling, mass and lump, upper limb

☐ IQ R22.30 Localized swelling, mass and lump, unspecified upper limb

☐ IQ R22.31 Localized swelling, mass and lump, right upper limb

☐ IQ R22.32 Localized swelling, mass and lump, left upper limb

☐ IQ R22.33 Localized swelling, mass and lump, upper limb, bilateral

5 R22.4 Localized swelling, mass and lump, lower limb

☐ IQ R22.40 Localized swelling, mass and lump, unspecified lower limb

☐ IQ R22.41 Localized swelling, mass and lump, right lower limb

☐ IQ R22.42 Localized swelling, mass and lump, left lower limb

☐ IQ R22.43 Localized swelling, mass and lump, lower limb, bilateral

IQ R22.9 Localized swelling, mass and lump, unspecified

4 R23 Other skin changes

IQ R23.0 Cyanosis
EXCLUDES 1 acrocyanosis (I73.8)
cyanotic attacks of newborn (P28.2)

★ New ▲ Revised Px Primary SP PDGM Px SL Low CoM SH High CoM IQ Quest. Encounter H Hospice non-cancer Dx Unspecified M *Manifestation*

DEFINITION Bluish tint of the skin from lack of oxygen.

!Q R23.1 Pallor
Clammy skin
DEFINITION Excessive paleness of the skin, especially the face.

!Q R23.2 Flushing
Excessive blushing
Code first:
, if applicable, menopausal and female climacteric states (N95.1)

!Q R23.3 Spontaneous ecchymoses
Petechiae
EXCLUDES 1 ecchymoses of newborn (P54.5)
purpura (D69.-)
DEFINITION Minute red spots on the skin, due to escape of a small amount of blood from the vessels.

!Q R23.4 Changes in skin texture
Desquamation of skin
Induration of skin
Scaling of skin
EXCLUDES 1 epidermal thickening NOS (L85.9)

!Q R23.8 Other skin changes
CODING TIPS ✓ When vesicular ulcerations (weeping ulcers) occur to the lower extremities as a result of edema (such as due to CHF or other edema producing conditions), assign R23.8 to indicate the resulting open vesicular (blister) ulceration. Do not assign this code to indicate other ulcerations such as due to friction or unspecified ulcers.

CODING TIPS ✓ Because this code may be assigned to report blistering due to edema, it is important that clear assessment of the patient's patterns of edema are present in the clinical record. The plan of care should include interventions to address the patient's edema, as well as the resulting ulcers.

!Q R23.9 Unspecified skin changes

Symptoms and signs involving the nervous and musculoskeletal systems   (R25-R29)

4 R25 Abnormal involuntary movements
EXCLUDES 1 specific movement disorders (G20-G26)
stereotyped movement disorders (F98.4)
tic disorders (F95.-)

!Q R25.0 Abnormal head movements

!Q R25.1 Tremor, unspecified
EXCLUDES 1 chorea NOS (G25.5)
essential tremor (G25.0)
hysterical tremor (F44.4)
intention tremor (G25.2)

!Q R25.2 Cramp and spasm
EXCLUDES 2 carpopedal spasm (R29.0)
charley-horse (M62.831)
infantile spasms (G40.4-)
muscle spasm of back (M62.830)

muscle spasm of calf (M62.831)

!Q R25.3 Fasciculation
Twitching NOS

!Q R25.8 Other abnormal involuntary movements

!Q R25.9 Unspecified abnormal involuntary movements

4 R26 Abnormalities of gait and mobility
EXCLUDES 1 ataxia NOS (R27.0)
hereditary ataxia (G11.-)
locomotor (syphilitic) ataxia (A52.11)
immobility syndrome (paraplegic) (M62.3)

CODING TIPS ✓ Code gait issues based on physician documentation, not therapy documentation. Even if documented by the physician, symptom codes should not be used when the symptom is routinely associated with the condition. For example, do not code difficulty walking (R26.2) for a diagnosis of arthritis. If the gait issue is the result of Parkinsons, then use Parkinsons, not abnormality of gait. The rules specifiying the restricted use of symptom coding apply to therapy "codes." Report the code for the type of gait that is documented by the physician when the symptom is not routinely associated with the condition.

Clinicians should investigate the cause of the gait abnormality when documented by the physician. Note the exclusions under R26. Consider M62.81 or M23 when the focus is on progressive muscle strengthening or limitations of motion (respectively) for affecting activities of daily living. Use R27, lack of coordination, if equilibrium or nonequilibrium tests show considerable muscle weakness, limitations of movement (LOMs) and balance problems.

!Q R26.0 Ataxic gait
Staggering gait
CODING TIPS ✓ Ataxia involves all four limbs and is coded to R27.

!Q R26.1 Paralytic gait
Spastic gait

!Q R26.2 Difficulty in walking, not elsewhere classified
EXCLUDES 1 falling (R29.6)
unsteadiness on feet (R26.81)

5 R26.8 Other abnormalities of gait and mobility

!Q R26.81 Unsteadiness on feet

!Q R26.89 Other abnormalities of gait and mobility

!Q R26.9 Unspecified abnormalities of gait and mobility
CODING TIPS ✓ Keep in mind when assigning R26.9 that if the cause of the gait abnormality is known, the code for the underlying cause of the gait abnormality should be assigned. It is not appropriate to assign the code for a symptom when a more specific condition has been identified.

4 R27 Other lack of coordination
EXCLUDES 1 ataxic gait (R26.0)

---

4 4th digit required   **5** 5th digit required   **6** 6th digit required   **7** 7th digit required   **7** 7th digit placeholder   **+** Additional code   **=** Laterality

hereditary ataxia (G11.-)
vertigo NOS (R42)

CODING TIPS ✓   Category R27 includes problems related to equilibrium (vestibular/balance coordination) and nonequilibrium (nonvestibular coordination) issues. This results from neurological conditions or can indirectly result from orthopedic corrective treatment.

!Q R27.0   Ataxia, unspecified

EXCLUDES 1   ataxia following cerebrovascular disease (I69. with final characters -93)

DEFINITION   Distortion or impairment of voluntary movement.

!Q R27.8   Other lack of coordination

!Q R27.9   Unspecified lack of coordination

4 R29   Other symptoms and signs involving the nervous and musculoskeletal systems.

!Q R29.0   Tetany
Carpopedal spasm

EXCLUDES 1   hysterical tetany (F44.5)
neonatal tetany (P71.3)
parathyroid tetany (E20.9)
post-thyroidectomy tetany (E89.2)

!Q R29.1   Meningismus

!Q R29.2   Abnormal reflex

EXCLUDES 2   abnormal pupillary reflex (H57.0)
hyperactive gag reflex (J39.2)
vasovagal reaction or syncope (R55)

!Q R29.3   Abnormal posture

!Q R29.4   Clicking hip

EXCLUDES 1   congenital deformities of hip (Q65.-)

!Q R29.5   Transient paralysis
Code first:
any associated spinal cord injury (S14.0, S14.1-, S24.0, S24.1-, S34.0-, S34.1-)

EXCLUDES 1   transient ischemic attack (G45.9)

!Q R29.6   Repeated falls
Falling
Tendency to fall

EXCLUDES 2   at risk for falling (Z91.81)
history of falling (Z91.81)

GUIDELINES   Section I.C.18.d
Code R29.6, Repeated falls, is for use for encounters when a patient has recently fallen and the reason for the fall is being investigated. Code Z91.81, History of falling, is for use when a patient has fallen in the past and is at risk for future falls. When appropriate, both codes R29.6 and Z91.81 may be assigned together.

CODING TIPS ✓   Code R29.6 indicates that a patient has been experiencing recent falls. When home health will be assessing the patient's pattern of falls and home safety, as well as addressing methods to reduce the falls, this code may be assigned to provide additional information.

5 R29.7   National Institutes of Health Stroke Scale (NIHSS) score
Code first:
the type of cerebral infarction (I63-)

CODING TIPS ✓   The NIHSS is used as a clinical stroke assessment tool to evaluate and document neurological status in acute stroke patients and is used for inpatient admissions only. The stroke scale is valid for predicting lesion size and can serve as a measure of stroke severity. The NIHSS has been shown to be a predictor of both short and long term outcome of stroke patients. The stroke scale also serves as a data collection tool for planning patient care and provides a common language for information exchanges among healthcare providers. The scale is designed to be a simple, valid, and reliable tool that can be administered at the bedside consistently by physicians, nurses or therapists.

6 R29.70   NIHSS score 0-9

!Q R29.700   NIHSS score 0

!Q R29.701   NIHSS score 1

!Q R29.702   NIHSS score 2

!Q R29.703   NIHSS score 3

!Q R29.704   NIHSS score 4

!Q R29.705   NIHSS score 5

!Q R29.706   NIHSS score 6

!Q R29.707   NIHSS score 7

!Q R29.708   NIHSS score 8

!Q R29.709   NIHSS score 9

6 R29.71   NIHSS score 10-19

!Q R29.710   NIHSS score 10

!Q R29.711   NIHSS score 11

!Q R29.712   NIHSS score 12

!Q R29.713   NIHSS score 13

!Q R29.714   NIHSS score 14

!Q R29.715   NIHSS score 15

!Q R29.716   NIHSS score 16

!Q R29.717   NIHSS score 17

!Q R29.718   NIHSS score 18

!Q R29.719   NIHSS score 19

6 R29.72   NIHSS score 20-29

!Q R29.720   NIHSS score 20

!Q R29.721   NIHSS score 21

!Q R29.722   NIHSS score 22

!Q R29.723   NIHSS score 23

!Q R29.724   NIHSS score 24

!Q R29.725   NIHSS score 25

!Q R29.726   NIHSS score 26

!Q R29.727   NIHSS score 27

!Q R29.728   NIHSS score 28

Chapter 18

R00-R99

★ New ▲ Revised Px Primary **SP** PDGM Px **SL** Low CoM **SH** High CoM **!Q** Quest. Encounter **H** Hospice non-cancer Dx   Unspecified   **M** *Manifestation*

DecisionHealth's FY 2020 Complete Home Health ICD-10-CM Diagnosis Coding Manual   1421

IQ R29.729 NIHSS score 29
6 R29.73 NIHSS score 30-39
IQ R29.730 NIHSS score 30
IQ R29.731 NIHSS score 31
IQ R29.732 NIHSS score 32
IQ R29.733 NIHSS score 33
IQ R29.734 NIHSS score 34
IQ R29.735 NIHSS score 35
IQ R29.736 NIHSS score 36
IQ R29.737 NIHSS score 37
IQ R29.738 NIHSS score 38
IQ R29.739 NIHSS score 39
6 R29.74 NIHSS score 40-42
IQ R29.740 NIHSS score 40
IQ R29.741 NIHSS score 41
IQ R29.742 NIHSS score 42

5 R29.8 Other symptoms and signs involving the nervous and musculoskeletal systems
6 R29.81 Other symptoms and signs involving the nervous system
IQ R29.810 Facial weakness
Facial droop

> **EXCLUDES 1** Bell's palsy (G51.0)
> facial weakness following cerebrovascular disease (I69. with final characters -92)

IQ R29.818 Other symptoms and signs involving the nervous system

> **CODING TIPS ✓** R29.818 is a nonspecific code, so be sure that documentation supports its use.

6 R29.89 Other symptoms and signs involving the musculoskeletal system

> **EXCLUDES 2** pain in limb (M79.6-)

IQ R29.890 Loss of height

> **EXCLUDES 1** osteoporosis (M80-M81)

IQ R29.891 Ocular torticollis

> **EXCLUDES 1** congenital (sternomastoid) torticollis Q68.0
> psychogenic torticollis (F45.8)
> spasmodic torticollis (G24.3)
> torticollis due to birth injury (P15.8)
> torticollis NOS M43.6

IQ R29.898 Other symptoms and signs involving the musculoskeletal system

5 R29.9 Unspecified symptoms and signs involving the nervous and musculoskeletal systems
IQ R29.90 Unspecified symptoms and signs involving the nervous system
IQ R29.91 Unspecified symptoms and signs involving the musculoskeletal system

Symptoms and signs involving the genitourinary system (R30-R39)

4 R30 Pain associated with micturition

> **EXCLUDES 1** psychogenic pain associated with micturition (F45.8)

IQ R30.0 Dysuria
Strangury
IQ R30.1 Vesical tenesmus
IQ R30.9 Painful micturition, unspecified
Painful urination NOS

4 R31 Hematuria

> **EXCLUDES 1** hematuria included with underlying conditions, such as:
> acute cystitis with hematuria (N30.01)
> recurrent and persistent hematuria in glomerular diseases (N02.-)

IQ R31.0 Gross hematuria

> **CODING TIPS ✓** Gross hematuria means that the blood in the urine can be seen with the naked eye. If hematuria is related to anticoagulant/antiplatelets, also code D68.32 and the T code for the drug.

IQ R31.1 Benign essential microscopic hematuria
5 R31.2 Other microscopic hematuria
IQ R31.21 Asymptomatic microscopic hematuria
AMH
IQ R31.29 Other microscopic hematuria
IQ R31.9 Hematuria, unspecified

> **DEFINITION** Presence of blood in the urine.

IQ R32 Unspecified urinary incontinence
Enuresis NOS

> **EXCLUDES 1** functional urinary incontinence (R39.81)
> nonorganic enuresis (F98.0)
> stress incontinence and other specified urinary incontinence (N39.3-N39.4-)
> urinary incontinence associated with cognitive impairment (R39.81)

4 R33 Retention of urine

> **EXCLUDES 1** psychogenic retention of urine (F45.8)

IQ ✛ R33.0 Drug induced retention of urine
Use additional code for adverse effect, if applicable, to identify drug (T36-T50 with fifth or sixth character 5)

IQ R33.8 Other retention of urine
Code first, if applicable, any causal condition, such as:
enlarged prostate (N40.1)

IQ R33.9 Retention of urine, unspecified

IQ R34 Anuria and oliguria

> **EXCLUDES 1** anuria and oliguria complicating abortion or ectopic or molar pregnancy (O00-O07, O08.4)
> anuria and oliguria complicating pregnancy (O26.83-)

---

4 4th digit required   5 5th digit required   6 6th digit required   7 7th digit required   7 7th digit placeholder   ✛ Additional code   ▱ Laterality

anuria and oliguria
    complicating the puerperium
    (O90.4)

4 R35   Polyuria
    Code first, if applicable, any causal condition,
        such as:
    enlarged prostate (N40.1)
    EXCLUDES 1   psychogenic polyuria (F45.8)

IQ R35.0 Frequency of micturition

IQ R35.1 Nocturia

IQ R35.8 Other polyuria
    Polyuria NOS

4 R36   Urethral discharge

IQ R36.0 Urethral discharge without blood

IQ R36.1 Hematospermia

IQ R36.9 Urethral discharge, unspecified
    Penile discharge NOS
    Urethrorrhea

IQ R37   Sexual dysfunction, unspecified

**4 R39   Other and unspecified symptoms and
    signs involving the genitourinary system**

IQ R39.0 Extravasation of urine

5 R39.1 Other difficulties with micturition
    Code first, if applicable, any causal
        condition, such as:
    enlarged prostate (N40.1)

IQ R39.11 Hesitancy of micturition
    DEFINITION   Difficulty starting
    urination.

IQ R39.12 Poor urinary stream
    Weak urinary steam

IQ R39.13 Splitting of urinary stream

**IQ R39.14 Feeling of incomplete bladder
    emptying**

IQ R39.15 Urgency of urination
    EXCLUDES 1   urge incontinence
        (N39.41, N39.46)

IQ R39.16 Straining to void

6 R39.19 Other difficulties with micturition

IQ R39.191 Need to immediately re-void

IQ R39.192 Position dependent micturition
    CODING TIPS ✓   Having to take
    specific positions to be able to
    micturate spontaneously or to
    improve bladder emptying (for
    example, leaning forwards or
    backwards on the toilet seat or
    voiding in the semi-standing position)
    is called position-dependent
    micturition.

IQ R39.198 Other difficulties with micturition

IQ R39.2 Extrarenal uremia
    Prerenal uremia
    EXCLUDES 1   uremia NOS (N19)

**5 R39.8 Other symptoms and signs involving the
    genitourinary system**

IQ R39.81 Functional urinary incontinence
    Urinary incontinence due to cognitive
        impairment, or severe physical
        disability or immobility
    EXCLUDES 1   stress incontinence and
        other specified urinary
        incontinence
        (N39.3-N39.4-)

urinary incontinence
    NOS (R32)
    DEFINITION   Leaking urine due to
cognitive impairment or physical
disability leading to the inability for
volitional control over bladder function.

IQ R39.82 Chronic bladder pain

IQ R39.83 Unilateral non-palpable testicle

IQ R39.84 Bilateral non-palpable testicles

**IQ R39.89 Other symptoms and signs involving
    the genitourinary system**

**IQ R39.9 Unspecified symptoms and signs
    involving the genitourinary system**

Symptoms and signs involving cognition, perception, emotional state and behavior (R40-R46)

EXCLUDES 2   symptoms and signs constituting part of a pattern
    of mental disorder (F01-F99)

4 R40   Somnolence, stupor and coma
    EXCLUDES 1   neonatal coma (P91.5)
        somnolence, stupor and coma in
            diabetes (E08-E13)
        somnolence, stupor and coma in
            hepatic failure (K72.-)
        somnolence, stupor and coma in
            hypoglycemia (nondiabetic)
            (E15)

IQ R40.0 Somnolence
    Drowsiness
    EXCLUDES 1   coma (R40.2-)

IQ R40.1 Stupor
    Catatonic stupor
    Semicoma
    EXCLUDES 1   catatonic schizophrenia
        (F20.2)
        coma (R40.2-)
        depressive stupor (F31-F33)
        dissociative stupor (F44.2)
        manic stupor (F30.2)

H 5 R40.2 Coma
    Note:
    One code from each subcategory, R40.21-
        R40.23, is required to complete the coma
        scale
    Code first any associated:
        fracture of skull (S02.-)
        intracranial injury (S06.-)

Chapter 18

R00-R99

✻ New ▲ Revised Px Primary **SP** PDGM Px **SL** Low CoM **SH** High CoM **IQ** Quest. Encounter **H** Hospice non-cancer Dx   Unspecified   **M** *Manifestation*

DecisionHealth's FY 2020 Complete Home Health ICD-10-CM Diagnosis Coding Manual   1423

Chapter 18

R00-R99

GUIDELINES Section I.B.14

For the Body Mass Index (BMI), depth of non-pressure chronic ulcers, pressure ulcer stage, coma scale, and NIH stroke scale (NIHSS) codes, code assignment may be based on medical record documentation from clinicians who are not the patient's provider (i.e., physician or other qualified healthcare practitioner legally accountable for establishing the patient's diagnosis), since this information is typically documented by other clinicians involved in the care of the patient (e.g., a dietitian often documents the BMI, a nurse often documents the pressure ulcer stages, and an emergency medical technician often documents the coma scale). However, the associated diagnosis (such as overweight, obesity, acute stroke, or pressure ulcer) must be documented by the patient's provider.

CODING TIPS ✓ If the provider's documentation clearly shows that the ratings are specific scores or numeric values for the Glasgow scale, rather than description, i.e., eyes open to pain, it would be appropriate to report codes from R40.21, R40.22 and R40.23.

CODING TIPS ✓ Non-physician documentation is appropriate for coding of the Glasgow Coma Scale. It would be appropriate to use the pre-hospital report containing the EMT's documentation and other non-physician documentation to determine the Glasgow coma score.

CODING TIPS ✓ Coma takes at least 3 codes unless the Glasgow Coma Scale total score is available. A 7th character is needed to indicate when the scale was performed.

!Q R40.20   Unspecified coma
Coma NOS
Unconsciousness NOS

6 R40.21   Coma scale, eyes open

The following appropriate 7th character is to be added to subcategory R40.21-:
0	unspecified time
1	in the field [EMT or ambulance]
2	at arrival to emergency department
3	at hospital admission
4	24 hours or more after hospital admission

!Q 7 R40.211-   Coma scale, eyes open, never
Coma scale eye opening score of 1

!Q 7 R40.212-   Coma scale, eyes open, to pain
Coma scale eye opening score of 2

!Q 7 R40.213-   Coma scale, eyes open, to sound
Coma scale eye opening score of 3

!Q 7 R40.214-   Coma scale, eyes open, spontaneous
Coma scale eye opening score of 4

6 R40.22   Coma scale, best verbal response

The following appropriate 7th character is to be added to subcategory R40.22-:
0	unspecified time
1	in the field [EMT or ambulance]
2	at arrival to emergency department
3	at hospital admission
4	24 hours or more after hospital admission

!Q 7 R40.221-   Coma scale, best verbal response, none
Coma scale verbal score of 1

!Q 7 R40.222-   Coma scale, best verbal response, incomprehensible words
Coma scale verbal score of 2
Incomprehensible sounds (2-5 years of age)
Moans/grunts to pain; restless (<2 years old)

!Q 7 R40.223-   Coma scale, best verbal response, inappropriate words
Coma scale verbal score of 3
Inappropriate crying or screaming (< 2 years of age)
Screaming (2-5 years of age)

!Q 7 R40.224-   Coma scale, best verbal response, confused conversation
Coma scale verbal score of 4
Inappropriate words (2-5 years of age)
Irritable cries (< 2 years of age)

!Q 7 R40.225-   Coma scale, best verbal response, oriented
Coma scale verbal score of 5
Cooing or babbling or crying appropriately (< 2 years of age)
Uses appropriate words (2- 5 years of age)

6 R40.23   Coma scale, best motor response

The following appropriate 7th character is to be added to subcategory R40.23-:
0	unspecified time
1	in the field [EMT or ambulance]
2	at arrival to emergency department
3	at hospital admission
4	24 hours or more after hospital admission

!Q 7 R40.231-   Coma scale, best motor response, none
Coma scale motor score of 1

!Q 7 R40.232-   Coma scale, best motor response, extension
Abnormal extensor posturing to pain or noxious stimuli (< 2 years of age)
Coma scale motor score of 2
Extensor posturing to pain or noxious stimuli (2-5 years of age)

4 4th digit required   5 5th digit required   6 6th digit required   7 7th digit required   7 7th digit placeholder   + Additional code   ☐ Laterality

1424   *DecisionHealth's* FY 2020 Complete Home Health ICD-10-CM Diagnosis Coding Manual

IQ 7 R40.233- **Coma scale, best motor response, abnormal flexion**

Abnormal flexure posturing to pain or noxious stimuli (2-5 years of age)

Coma scale motor score of 3

Flexion/decorticate posturing (< 2 years of age)

IQ 7 R40.234- **Coma scale, best motor response, flexion withdrawal**

Coma scale motor score of 4

Withdraws from pain or noxious stimuli (2-5 years of age)

IQ 7 R40.235- **Coma scale, best motor response, localizes pain**

Coma scale motor score of 5

Localizes pain (2-5 years of age)

Withdraws to touch (< 2 years of age)

IQ 7 R40.236- **Coma scale, best motor response, obeys commands**

Coma scale motor score of 6

Normal or spontaneous movement (< 2 years of age)

Obeys commands (2-5 years of age)

6 R40.24 **Glasgow coma scale, total score**

Note:

Assign a code from subcategory R40.24, when only the total coma score is documented

The following appropriate 7th character is to be added to subcategory R40.24-:
0	unspecified time
1	in the field [EMT or ambulance]
2	at arrival to emergency department
3	at hospital admission
4	24 hours or more after hospital admission

CODING TIPS ✓ If the total score is documented, do not code the individual scores for the Glasgow Coma Scale.

IQ 7 R40.241- **Glasgow coma scale score 13-15**

IQ 7 R40.242- **Glasgow coma scale score 9-12**

IQ 7 R40.243- **Glasgow coma scale score 3-8**

IQ 7 R40.244- **Other coma, without documented Glasgow coma scale score, or with partial score reported**

IQ R40.3 **Persistent vegetative state**

CODING TIPS ✓ Assign code R40.3 only when the physician has specifically confirmed persistent vegetative state (PVS). Also note that PVS differs from coma.

IQ R40.4 **Transient alteration of awareness**

CODING TIPS ✓ Code R40.4 for transient alteration of awareness that is not associated with delirium or with another identified condition. It may be prevalent for those at the end of life.

4 R41 **Other symptoms and signs involving cognitive functions and awareness**

EXCLUDES 1 dissociative [conversion] disorders (F44.-)
mild cognitive impairment, so stated (G31.84)

IQ R41.0 **Disorientation, unspecified**

Confusion NOS

Delirium NOS

IQ R41.1 **Anterograde amnesia**

IQ R41.2 **Retrograde amnesia**

IQ R41.3 **Other amnesia**

Amnesia NOS

Memory loss NOS

EXCLUDES 1 amnestic disorder due to known physiologic condition (F04)
amnestic syndrome due to psychoactive substance use (F10-F19 with 5th character .6)
mild memory disturbance due to known physiological condition (F06.8)
transient global amnesia (G45.4)

IQ R41.4 **Neurologic neglect syndrome**

Asomatognosia

Hemi-akinesia

Hemi-inattention

Hemispatial neglect

Left-sided neglect

Sensory neglect

Visuospatial neglect

EXCLUDES 1 visuospatial deficit (R41.842)

CODING TIPS ✓ If neurologic neglect syndrome is related to a stroke, use the sequela code for the visuospatial neglect, for example I69.312.

5 R41.8 **Other symptoms and signs involving cognitive functions and awareness**

IQ R41.81 **Age-related cognitive decline**

Senility NOS

IQ R41.82 **Altered mental status, unspecified**

Change in mental status NOS

EXCLUDES 1 altered level of consciousness (R40.-)
altered mental status due to known condition - code to condition
delirium NOS (R41.0)

CODING TIPS ✓ Code R41.82 is used for an altered mental status such as an acute onset of confusion with unknown cause. If altered mental status is due to another condition, code that condition instead.

IQ R41.83 **Borderline intellectual functioning**

IQ level 71 to 84

EXCLUDES 1 intellectual disabilities (F70-F79)

CODING TIPS ✓ Do not assign R41.83 when intellectual disability is specified. Intellectual disabilities are coded to categories F70-F79.

6 R41.84 **Other specified cognitive deficit**

★ New ▲ Revised Px Primary SP PDGM Px SL Low CoM SH High CoM IQ Quest. Encounter H Hospice non-cancer Dx Unspecified M Manifestation

DecisionHealth's FY 2020 Complete Home Health ICD-10-CM Diagnosis Coding Manual 1425

Chapter 18

R00-R99

EXCLUDES 1   cognitive deficits as sequelae of cerebrovascular disease (I69.01-, I69.11-, I69.21-, I69.31-, I69.81-, I69.91-)

CODING TIPS ✓   The R41.84 codes were created to identify cognitive deficits related to a traumatic brain injury (TBI) and other neurological conditions. They describe cognitive impairments such as problems with memory, concentration, attention, communication and executive function. They are intended to be used as supplementary codes when the cause of the deficit is known as well as before a more specific diagnosis is made. R41.84 codes are not to be used for sequelae of cerebral infarction/strokes. For sequelae of strokes, reference I69.-1 for specific codes, for example I69.311 (Memory deficit following cerebral infarction).

IQ R41.840   Attention and concentration deficit
    EXCLUDES 1   attention-deficit hyperactivity disorders (F90.-)

IQ R41.841   Cognitive communication deficit

IQ R41.842   Visuospatial deficit

IQ R41.843   Psychomotor deficit

IQ R41.844   Frontal lobe and executive function deficit

IQ R41.89   Other symptoms and signs involving cognitive functions and awareness
    Anosognosia

IQ R41.9   Unspecified symptoms and signs involving cognitive functions and awareness
    Unspecified neurocognitive disorder

IQ R42   Dizziness and giddiness
    Light-headedness
    Vertigo NOS
    EXCLUDES 1   vertiginous syndromes (H81.-)
        vertigo from infrasound (T75.23)

4 R43   Disturbances of smell and taste

IQ R43.0   Anosmia

IQ R43.1   Parosmia

IQ R43.2   Parageusia

IQ R43.8   Other disturbances of smell and taste
    Mixed disturbance of smell and taste

IQ R43.9   Unspecified disturbances of smell and taste

4 R44   Other symptoms and signs involving general sensations and perceptions
    EXCLUDES 1   alcoholic hallucinations (F1.5)
        hallucinations in drug psychosis (F11-F19 with .5)
        hallucinations in mood disorders with psychotic symptoms (F30.2, F31.5, F32.3, F33.3)
        hallucinations in schizophrenia, schizotypal and delusional disorders (F20-F29)

    EXCLUDES 2   disturbances of skin sensation (R20.-)

IQ R44.0   Auditory hallucinations

IQ R44.1   Visual hallucinations

IQ R44.2   Other hallucinations

IQ R44.3   Hallucinations, unspecified

IQ R44.8   Other symptoms and signs involving general sensations and perceptions

IQ R44.9   Unspecified symptoms and signs involving general sensations and perceptions

4 R45   Symptoms and signs involving emotional state

IQ R45.0   Nervousness
    Nervous tension

IQ R45.1   Restlessness and agitation

IQ R45.2   Unhappiness

IQ R45.3   Demoralization and apathy
    EXCLUDES 1   anhedonia (R45.84)

IQ R45.4   Irritability and anger

IQ R45.5   Hostility

IQ R45.6   Violent behavior

IQ R45.7   State of emotional shock and stress, unspecified

5 R45.8   Other symptoms and signs involving emotional state

IQ R45.81   Low self-esteem

IQ R45.82   Worries

IQ R45.83   Excessive crying of child, adolescent or adult
    EXCLUDES 1   excessive crying of infant (baby) R68.11

IQ R45.84   Anhedonia
    CODING TIPS ✓   R45.84 is a nonspecific code used to describe a decreased desire to engage in activities, often with decreased motivation. Anhedonia is frequently identified as a symptom of psychiatric conditions such as depression. Report a more specific code when the cause of anhedonia is known.

6 R45.85   Homicidal and suicidal ideations
    EXCLUDES 1   suicide attempt (T14.91)

IQ R45.850   Homicidal ideations

IQ R45.851   Suicidal ideations

IQ R45.86   Emotional lability

IQ R45.87   Impulsiveness

IQ R45.89   Other symptoms and signs involving emotional state

4 R46   Symptoms and signs involving appearance and behavior
    EXCLUDES 1   appearance and behavior in schizophrenia, schizotypal and delusional disorders (F20-F29)
        mental and behavioral disorders (F01-F99)

IQ R46.0   Very low level of personal hygiene

IQ R46.1   Bizarre personal appearance

IQ R46.2   Strange and inexplicable behavior

IQ R46.3   Overactivity

IQ R46.4   Slowness and poor responsiveness

---

4 4th digit required   5 5th digit required   6 6th digit required   7 7th digit required   7 7th digit placeholder   ➕Additional code   ⊟ Laterality

1426   *DecisionHealth's* FY 2020 Complete Home Health ICD-10-CM Diagnosis Coding Manual

EXCLUDES 1 stupor (R40.1)

IQ R46.5 Suspiciousness and marked evasiveness

IQ R46.6 Undue concern and preoccupation with stressful events

IQ R46.7 Verbosity and circumstantial detail obscuring reason for contact

5 R46.8 Other symptoms and signs involving appearance and behavior

IQ R46.81 Obsessive-compulsive behavior

EXCLUDES 1 obsessive-compulsive disorder (F42-)

IQ R46.89 Other symptoms and signs involving appearance and behavior

Symptoms and signs involving speech and voice (R47-R49)

4 R47 Speech disturbances, not elsewhere classified

EXCLUDES 1 autism (F84.0)
cluttering (F80.81)
specific developmental disorders of speech and language (F80.-)
stuttering (F80.81)

5 R47.0 Dysphasia and aphasia

CODING TIPS ✓ Do not use R47.0 codes for sequela of cerebral infarctions or stroke. Use, for example, I69.32 instead for these sequelae. Do not confuse dysphasia with dysphagia (difficulty in swallowing), which is another possible sequela of a stroke.

IQ R47.01 Aphasia

EXCLUDES 1 aphasia following cerebrovascular disease (I69. with final characters -20)
progressive isolated aphasia (G31.01)

DEFINITION The inability to speak, write, or understand spoken or written language.

IQ R47.02 Dysphasia

EXCLUDES 1 dysphasia following cerebrovascular disease (I69. with final characters -21)

IQ R47.1 Dysarthria and anarthria

EXCLUDES 1 dysarthria following cerebrovascular disease (I69. with final characters -22)

5 R47.8 Other speech disturbances

EXCLUDES 1 dysarthria following cerebrovascular disease (I69. with final characters -28)

IQ R47.81 Slurred speech

IQ R47.82 Fluency disorder in conditions classified elsewhere
Stuttering in conditions classified elsewhere
Code first underlying disease or condition, such as:
Parkinson's disease (G20)

EXCLUDES 1 adult onset fluency disorder (F98.5)
childhood onset fluency disorder (F80.81)
fluency disorder (stuttering) following cerebrovascular disease (I69. with final characters -23)

IQ R47.89 Other speech disturbances

IQ R47.9 Unspecified speech disturbances

4 R48 Dyslexia and other symbolic dysfunctions, not elsewhere classified

EXCLUDES 1 specific developmental disorders of scholastic skills (F81.-)

IQ R48.0 Dyslexia and alexia

IQ R48.1 Agnosia
Astereognosia (astereognosis)
Autotopagnosia

EXCLUDES 1 visual object agnosia (R48.3)

IQ R48.2 Apraxia

EXCLUDES 1 apraxia following cerebrovascular disease (I69. with final characters -90)

IQ R48.3 Visual agnosia
Prosopagnosia
Simultanagnosia (asimultagnosia)

IQ R48.8 Other symbolic dysfunctions
Acalculia
Agraphia

IQ R48.9 Unspecified symbolic dysfunctions

4 R49 Voice and resonance disorders

EXCLUDES 1 psychogenic voice and resonance disorders (F44.4)

CODING TIPS ✓ Do not use R49 codes for sequelae of cerebral infarctions or stroke. Use, for example, I69.32 instead for these sequelae.

IQ R49.0 Dysphonia
Hoarseness

IQ R49.1 Aphonia
Loss of voice

DEFINITION Inability to produce vocal sounds.

5 R49.2 Hypernasality and hyponasality

IQ R49.21 Hypernasality

IQ R49.22 Hyponasality

IQ R49.8 Other voice and resonance disorders

IQ R49.9 Unspecified voice and resonance disorder
Change in voice NOS
Resonance disorder NOS

General symptoms and signs (R50-R69)

4 R50 Fever of other and unknown origin

EXCLUDES 1 chills without fever (R68.83)
febrile convulsions (R56.0-)
fever of unknown origin during labor (O75.2)
fever of unknown origin in newborn (P81.9)
hypothermia due to illness (R68.0)
malignant hyperthermia due to anesthesia (T88.3)

Chapter 18

R00-R99

★ New ▲ Revised Px Primary **SP** PDGM Px **SL** Low CoM **SH** High CoM **IQ** Quest. Encounter **H** Hospice non-cancer Dx | Unspecified | **M** *Manifestation*

DecisionHealth's FY 2020 Complete Home Health ICD-10-CM Diagnosis Coding Manual | 1427

puerperal pyrexia NOS (O86.4)

IQ + R50.2   **Drug induced fever**
Use additional code for adverse effect, if applicable, to identify drug (T36-T50 with fifth or sixth character 5)
> **EXCLUDES 1**   postvaccination (postimmunization) fever (R50.83)

5 R50.8   **Other specified fever**

IQ R50.81   **Fever presenting with conditions classified elsewhere**
Code first underlying condition when associated fever is present, such as with:
leukemia (C91-C95)
neutropenia (D70.-)
sickle-cell disease (D57.-)

IQ R50.82   **Postprocedural fever**
> **EXCLUDES 1**   postprocedural infection (T81.4-)
> posttransfusion fever (R50.84)
> postvaccination (postimmunization) fever (R50.83)

IQ R50.83   **Postvaccination fever**
Postimmunization fever

IQ R50.84   **Febrile nonhemolytic transfusion reaction**
FNHTR
Posttransfusion fever

IQ R50.9   **Fever, unspecified**
Fever NOS
Fever of unknown origin [FUO]
Fever with chills
Fever with rigors
Hyperpyrexia NOS
Persistent fever
Pyrexia NOS
> **CODING TIPS ✓**   When an infection causing a fever has been diagnosed, do not assign R50.9, but instead code the causative infectious disease specifically.

IQ R51   **Headache**
Facial pain NOS
> **EXCLUDES 1**   atypical face pain (G50.1)
> migraine and other headache syndromes (G43-G44)
> trigeminal neuralgia (G50.0)

IQ R52   **Pain, unspecified**
Acute pain NOS
Generalized pain NOS
Pain NOS
> **EXCLUDES 1**   acute and chronic pain, not elsewhere classified (G89.-)
> localized pain, unspecified type - code to pain by site, such as:
> abdomen pain (R10.-)
> back pain (M54.9)
> breast pain (N64.4)
> chest pain (R07.1-R07.9)
> ear pain (H92.0-)
> eye pain (H57.1)
> headache (R51)
> joint pain (M25.5-)
> limb pain (M79.6-)
> lumbar region pain (M54.5)

pelvic and perineal pain (R10.2)
shoulder pain (M25.51-)
spine pain (M54.-)
throat pain (R07.0)
tongue pain (K14.6)
tooth pain (K08.8)
renal colic (N23)
pain disorders exclusively related to psychological factors (F45.41)
> **CODING TIPS ✓**   R52 should not be coded to identify pain when the underlying cause of pain is known. Code the specific cause of the pain when a diagnosis is present for the cause, such as osteoarthritis. Pay special attention to the Excludes 1 note.

4 R53   **Malaise and fatigue**

IQ R53.0   **Neoplastic (malignant) related fatigue**
Code first:
associated neoplasm

IQ R53.1   **Weakness**
Asthenia NOS
> **EXCLUDES 1**   age-related weakness (R54)
> muscle weakness (M62.8-)
> sarcopenia (M62.84)
> senile asthenia (R54)
> **CODING TIPS ✓**   Also known as general weakness. If code R53.1 is used to support therapy, documentation should establish medical necessity. The condition may include excessive tiredness, lacking energy, listlessness, and/or sleepiness. Excludes generalized muscle weakness. Generally used for patients with cardiorespiratory diseases. May be part of many different illnesses, including the flu, pneumonia, congestive heart failure (CHF) and arteriosclerotic heart disease (ASHD).
> **CODING TIPS ✓**   Do not assign R53.1 to indicate muscle weakness or weakness resulting as a sequela of a cerebral vascular accident. Muscle weakness is coded to M62.8-.

IQ R53.2   **Functional quadriplegia**
Complete immobility due to severe physical disability or frailty
> **EXCLUDES 1**   frailty NOS (R54)
> hysterical paralysis (F44.4)
> immobility syndrome (M62.3)
> neurologic quadriplegia (G82.5-)
> quadriplegia (G82.50)
> **CODING TIPS ✓**   Functional quadriplegia refers to the inability to move due to another condition (such as severe contractures or arthritis), resulting in the patient being quadriplegia-like. Do not use code R53.2 for quadriplegia or in addition to quadriplegia. Code only if documented by the physician.
> **DEFINITION**   Inability to move due to non-neurological condition, such as severe spasticity, arthritis, or severe muscle contracture.

5 R53.8   **Other malaise and fatigue**

---

4 4th digit required   **5** 5th digit required   **6** 6th digit required   **7** 7th digit required   **✓** 7th digit placeholder   **+** Additional code   **□** Laterality

1428   *DecisionHealth's* FY 2020 Complete Home Health ICD-10-CM Diagnosis Coding Manual

EXCLUDES 1 combat exhaustion and
  fatigue (F43.0)
  congenital debility (P96.9)
  exhaustion and fatigue due to
  excessive exertion (T73.3)
  exhaustion and fatigue due to
  exposure (T73.2)
  exhaustion and fatigue due to
  heat (T67.-)
  exhaustion and fatigue due to
  pregnancy (O26.8-)
  exhaustion and fatigue due to
  recurrent depressive
  episode (F33)
  exhaustion and fatigue due to
  senile debility (R54)

IQ R53.81 Other malaise
Chronic debility
Debility NOS
General physical deterioration
Malaise NOS
Nervous debility

> **EXCLUDES 1** age-related physical
> debility (R54)

> **ALERT** This diagnosis is
> prohibited from use as a terminal
> diagnosis in hospice.

> **CODING TIPS ✓** Note that debility is a
> non-specific condition characterized by
> weight loss, functional decline,
> malnutrition and multiple chronic
> conditions. Coding a non-specific
> diagnosis such as this should be
> avoided if possible. If the diagnosis
> causing the debility is known, code that
> condition.

IQ R53.82 Chronic fatigue, unspecified
Chronic fatigue syndrome NOS
> **EXCLUDES 1** postviral fatigue
> syndrome (G93.3)

IQ R53.83 Other fatigue
Fatigue NOS
Lack of energy
Lethargy
Tiredness
> **EXCLUDES 2** exhaustion and fatigue
> due to depressive
> episode (F32.-)

IQ R54 Age-related physical debility
Frailty
Old age
Senescence
Senile asthenia
Senile debility
> **EXCLUDES 1** age-related cognitive decline
> (R41.81)
> sarcopenia (M62.84)
> senile psychosis (F03)
> senility NOS (R41.81)

> **CODING TIPS ✓** Note that debility is a non-
> specific condition characterized by weight loss,
> functional decline, malnutrition and multiple
> chronic conditions. Coding a non-specific
> diagnosis such as this should be avoided if
> possible. If the diagnosis causing the debility is
> known, code that condition.

IQ R55 Syncope and collapse
Blackout

Fainting
Vasovagal attack
> **EXCLUDES 1** cardiogenic shock (R57.0)
> carotid sinus syncope (G90.01)
> heat syncope (T67.1)
> neurocirculatory asthenia
> (F45.8)
> neurogenic orthostatic
> hypotension (G90.3)
> orthostatic hypotension (I95.1)
> postprocedural shock (T81.1-)
> psychogenic syncope (F48.8)
> shock NOS (R57.9)
> shock complicating or
> following abortion or ectopic
> or molar pregnancy
> (O00-O07, O08.3)
> shock complicating or
> following labor and delivery
> (O75.1)
> Stokes-Adams attack (I45.9)
> unconsciousness NOS (R40.2-)

> **DEFINITION** Fainting and collapse due to a
> lack of blood flow to the brain.

4 R56 Convulsions, not elsewhere classified
> **EXCLUDES 1** dissociative convulsions and
> seizures (F44.5)
> epileptic convulsions and
> seizures (G40.-)
> newborn convulsions and
> seizures (P90)

5 R56.0 Febrile convulsions
> **DEFINITION** A convulsion accompanying
> high fever, characterized by loss of
> consciousness with stiffness and jerking of
> the limbs. The skin may become pale or
> turn blue. Once the jerking subsides, the
> child goes limp and then normal color and
> consciousness return.

IQ R56.00 Simple febrile convulsions
Febrile convulsion NOS
Febrile seizure NOS
> **CODING TIPS ✓** Febrile seizures, code
> R56.00, affect 3%-5% of all children.
> Fever triggers these seizures.

IQ R56.01 Complex febrile convulsions
Atypical febrile seizure
Complex febrile seizure
Complicated febrile seizure
> **EXCLUDES 1** status epilepticus
> (G40.901)

IQ R56.1 Post traumatic seizures
> **EXCLUDES 1** post traumatic epilepsy
> (G40.-)

IQ R56.9 Unspecified convulsions
Convulsion disorder
Fit NOS
Recurrent convulsions
Seizure(s) (convulsive) NOS
> **CODING TIPS ✓** Do not assign R56.9 when a
> patient has had recurrent seizures or a
> seizure disorder. When recurrent seizures
> or seizure disorder are present, report the
> appropriate code from category G40.-.

4 R57 Shock, not elsewhere classified
> **EXCLUDES 1** anaphylactic shock NOS
> (T78.2)

Chapter 18

R00-R99

★ New ▲ Revised Px Primary **SP** PDGM Px **SL** Low CoM **SH** High CoM **IQ** Quest. Encounter **H** Hospice non-cancer Dx Unspecified **M** *Manifestation*

Chapter 18

R00-R99

anaphylactic reaction or shock
   due to adverse food reaction
   (T78.0-)
anaphylactic shock due to
   adverse effect of correct drug
   or medicament properly
   administered (T88.6)
anaphylactic shock due to
   serum (T80.5-)
anesthetic shock (T88.3)
electric shock (T75.4)
obstetric shock (O75.1)
postprocedural shock (T81.1-)
psychic shock (F43.0)
shock complicating or
   following ectopic or molar
   pregnancy (O00-O07, O08.3)
shock due to lightning (T75.01)
traumatic shock (T79.4)
toxic shock syndrome (A48.3)

R57.0 Cardiogenic shock
   EXCLUDES 2   septic shock (R65.21)

R57.1 Hypovolemic shock

R57.8 Other shock

R57.9 Shock, unspecified
   Failure of peripheral circulation NOS

R58 Hemorrhage, not elsewhere classified
   Hemorrhage NOS
   EXCLUDES 1   hemorrhage included with
      underlying conditions, such
      as:
   acute duodenal ulcer with
      hemorrhage (K26.0)
   acute gastritis with bleeding
      (K29.01)
   ulcerative enterocolitis with
      rectal bleeding (K51.01)

R59 Enlarged lymph nodes
   INCLUDES   swollen glands
   EXCLUDES 1   lymphadenitis NOS (I88.9)
      acute lymphadenitis (L04.-)
      chronic lymphadenitis (I88.1)
      mesenteric (acute) (chronic)
         lymphadenitis (I88.0)

R59.0 Localized enlarged lymph nodes

R59.1 Generalized enlarged lymph nodes
   Lymphadenopathy NOS

R59.9 Enlarged lymph nodes, unspecified

R60 Edema, not elsewhere classified
   EXCLUDES 1   angioneurotic edema (T78.3)
      ascites (R18.-)
      cerebral edema (G93.6)
      cerebral edema due to birth
         injury (P11.0)
      edema of larynx (J38.4)
      edema of nasopharynx (J39.2)
      edema of pharynx (J39.2)
      gestational edema (O12.0-)
      hereditary edema (Q82.0)
      hydrops fetalis NOS (P83.2)
      hydrothorax (J94.8)
      hydrops fetalis NOS (P83.2)
      newborn edema (P83.3)
      pulmonary edema (J81.-)

CODING TIPS ✓   Report R60 only when the
cause of the edema is unknown, as it is usually
integral to another condition where you would
not report this symptom code. Never code
edema in addition to CHF.

R60.0 Localized edema
   CODING TIPS ✓   Do not report R60.0 in a
   patient with heart failure or any other known
   cause for the edema.

R60.1 Generalized edema
   EXCLUDES 2   nutritional edema (E40-E46)

R60.9 Edema, unspecified
   Fluid retention NOS

R61 Generalized hyperhidrosis
   Excessive sweating
   Night sweats
   Secondary hyperhidrosis
   Code first:
      , if applicable, menopausal and female
         climacteric states (N95.1)
   EXCLUDES 1   focal (primary) (secondary)
         hyperhidrosis (L74.5-)
      Frey's syndrome (L74.52)
      localized (primary)
         (secondary) hyperhidrosis
         (L74.5-)

**R62 Lack of expected normal physiological
development in childhood and adults**
   EXCLUDES 1   delayed puberty (E30.0)
      gonadal dysgenesis (Q99.1)
      hypopituitarism (E23.0)

R62.0 Delayed milestone in childhood
   Delayed attainment of expected
      physiological developmental stage
   Late talker
   Late walker

**R62.5 Other and unspecified lack of expected
normal physiological development in
childhood**
   EXCLUDES 1   HIV disease resulting in
         failure to thrive (B20)
      physical retardation due to
         malnutrition (E45)

**R62.50 Unspecified lack of expected normal
physiological development in
childhood**
   Infantilism NOS

R62.51 Failure to thrive (child)
   Failure to gain weight
   EXCLUDES 1   failure to thrive in child
         under 28 days old
         (P92.6)

R62.52 Short stature (child)
   Lack of growth
   Physical retardation
   Short stature NOS
   EXCLUDES 1   short stature due to
         endocrine disorder
         (E34.3)

**R62.59 Other lack of expected normal
physiological development in
childhood**

R62.7 Adult failure to thrive
   ALERT   This diagnosis is prohibited
   from use as a primary terminal diagnosis.

4️⃣4th digit required   5️⃣5th digit required   6️⃣6th digit required   7️⃣7th digit required   ☑️7th digit placeholder   ➕Additional code   ▣Laterality

1430   DecisionHealth's FY 2020 Complete Home Health ICD-10-CM Diagnosis Coding Manual

CODING TIPS ✓ When coding failure to thrive, identify the conditions leading to the patient's failure to thrive and code these underlying conditions first.

▲ **◿ R63   Symptoms and signs concerning food and fluid intake**

EXCLUDES 1 bulimia NOS (F50.2)

!Q R63.0   Anorexia

Loss of appetite

EXCLUDES 1 anorexia nervosa (F50.0-)
loss of appetite of
nonorganic origin
(F50.89)

CODING TIPS ✓ Anorexia indicates a loss of appetite or intake resulting from appetite loss. Note that anorexia nervosa, which is coded to F50.0-, differs from anorexia coded to R63.0 in that anorexia nervosa includes a psychological component of body image disturbance.

!Q R63.1   Polydipsia

Excessive thirst

!Q R63.2   Polyphagia

Excessive eating
Hyperalimentation NOS

!Q R63.3   Feeding difficulties

Feeding problem (elderly) (infant) NOS
Picky eater

EXCLUDES 1 eating disorders (F50.-)
feeding problems of
newborn (P92.-)
infant feeding disorder of
nonorganic origin (F98.2-)

!Q R63.4   Abnormal weight loss

CODING TIPS ✓ Code also for BMI (Z68) with code R63.4. The Z68 codes are for adults 20 years of age and older.

!Q R63.5   Abnormal weight gain

EXCLUDES 1 excessive weight gain in
pregnancy (O26.0-)
obesity (E66.-)

!Q ✚ R63.6   Underweight

Use additional code to identify body mass index (BMI), if known (Z68.-)

EXCLUDES 1 abnormal weight loss
(R63.4)
anorexia nervosa (F50.0-)
malnutrition (E40-E46)

!Q R63.8   Other symptoms and signs concerning food and fluid intake

!Q R64   Cachexia

Wasting syndrome

Code first:
underlying condition, if known

EXCLUDES 1 abnormal weight loss (R63.4)
nutritional marasmus (E41)

CODING TIPS ✓ Assign R64 (Cachexia), not E41 (Nutritional marasmus), for a patient diagnosed with emaciation or described as "emaciated" even though the alphabetic index leads to E41. Using E41 is incorrect because it refers to a type of malnutrition that occurs in infants and young children. Unless that is applicable, do not assign E41, according to Q3 2017 Coding Clinic guidance.

◿ R65   Symptoms and signs specifically associated with systemic inflammation and infection

GUIDELINES Section I.C.1.d.6)
Only one code from category R65, Symptoms and signs specifically associated with systemic inflammation and infection, should be assigned. Therefore, when a non-infectious condition leads to an infection resulting in severe sepsis, assign the appropriate code from subcategory R65.2, Severe sepsis. Do not additionally assign a code from subcategory R65.1, Systemic inflammatory response syndrome (SIRS) of noninfectious origin.

▲ **⑤ R65.1   Systemic inflammatory response syndrome (SIRS) of non-infectious origin**

Code first underlying condition, such as:
heatstroke (T67.0-)
injury and trauma (S00-T88)

EXCLUDES 1 sepsis- code to infection
severe sepsis (R65.2)

CODING TIPS ✓ R65.1 codes are used for systemic inflammatory response syndrome (SIRS) of non-infectious origin. Some physicians will document "sepsis," but not indicate an infectious process, for example, "due to a pulmonary embolism." Sepsis implies an infection, so the physician should be queried. SIRS is an overreaction to the inflammatory process that triggers changes throughout the body.

!Q R65.10   Systemic inflammatory response syndrome (SIRS) of non-infectious origin without acute organ dysfunction

Systemic inflammatory response syndrome (SIRS) NOS

!Q ✚ R65.11   Systemic inflammatory response syndrome (SIRS) of non-infectious origin with acute organ dysfunction

Use additional code to identify specific acute organ dysfunction, such as:
acute kidney failure (N17.-)
acute respiratory failure (J96.0-)
critical illness myopathy (G72.81)
critical illness polyneuropathy (G62.81)
disseminated intravascular coagulopathy [DIC] (D65)
encephalopathy (metabolic) (septic) (G93.41)
hepatic failure (K72.0-)

★ New ▲ Revised **Px** Primary **SP** PDGM Px **SL** Low CoM **SH** High CoM **!Q** Quest. Encounter **H** Hospice non-cancer Dx   Unspecified   **M** *Manifestation*

DecisionHealth's FY 2020 Complete Home Health ICD-10-CM Diagnosis Coding Manual   1431

GUIDELINES Section I.C.18.g

The systemic inflammatory response syndrome (SIRS) can develop as a result of certain non-infectious disease processes, such as trauma, malignant neoplasm, or pancreatitis. When SIRS is documented with a noninfectious condition, and no subsequent infection is documented, the code for the underlying condition, such as an injury, should be assigned, followed by code R65.10, Systemic inflammatory response syndrome (SIRS) of non-infectious origin without acute organ dysfunction, or code R65.11, Systemic inflammatory response syndrome (SIRS) of non-infectious origin with acute organ dysfunction. If an associated acute organ dysfunction is documented, the appropriate code(s) for the specific type of organ dysfunction(s) should be assigned in addition to code R65.11. If acute organ dysfunction is documented, but it cannot be determined if the acute organ dysfunction is associated with SIRS or due to another condition (e.g., directly due to the trauma), the provider should be queried.

+ ⑤ R65.2 Severe sepsis
   Infection with associated acute organ dysfunction
   Sepsis with acute organ dysfunction
   Sepsis with multiple organ dysfunction
   Systemic inflammatory response syndrome due to infectious process with acute organ dysfunction
   Code first underlying infection, such as:
     infection following a procedure (T81.4-)
     infections following infusion, transfusion and therapeutic injection (T80.2-)
     puerperal sepsis (O85)
     sepsis following complete or unspecified spontaneous abortion (O03.87)
     sepsis following ectopic and molar pregnancy (O08.82)
     sepsis following incomplete spontaneous abortion (O03.37)
     sepsis following (induced) termination of pregnancy (O04.87)
     sepsis NOS (A41.9)
   Use additional code to identify specific acute organ dysfunction, such as:
     acute kidney failure (N17.-)
     acute respiratory failure (J96.0-)
     critical illness myopathy (G72.81)
     critical illness polyneuropathy (G62.81)
     disseminated intravascular coagulopathy [DIC] (D65)
     encephalopathy (metabolic) (septic) (G93.41)
     hepatic failure (K72.0-)

GUIDELINES Section I.C.1.d.4)

If the reason for admission is both sepsis or severe sepsis and a localized infection, such as pneumonia or cellulitis, a code(s) for the underlying systemic infection should be assigned first and the code for the localized infection should be assigned as a secondary diagnosis. If the patient has severe sepsis, a code from subcategory R65.2 should also be assigned as a secondary diagnosis. If the patient is admitted with a localized infection, such as pneumonia, and sepsis/severe sepsis doesn't develop until after admission, the localized infection should be assigned first, followed by the appropriate sepsis/severe sepsis codes.

GUIDELINES Section I.C.1.d.1)(a)(iv)

If a patient has sepsis and an acute organ dysfunction, but the medical record documentation indicates that the acute organ dysfunction is related to a medical condition other than the sepsis, do not assign a code from subcategory R65.2, Severe sepsis. An acute organ dysfunction must be associated with the sepsis in order to assign the severe sepsis code. If the documentation is not clear as to whether an acute organ dysfunction is related to the sepsis or another medical condition, query the provider.

GUIDELINES Section I.C.1.d.1)(b)

The coding of severe sepsis requires a minimum of two codes: first a code for the underlying systemic infection, followed by a code from subcategory R65.2, Severe sepsis. If the causal organism is not documented, assign code A41.9, Sepsis, unspecified organism, for the infection. Additional code(s) for the associated acute organ dysfunction are also required. Due to the complex nature of severe sepsis, some cases may require querying the provider prior to assignment of the codes.

CODING TIPS ✓ When severe sepsis is present in a patient (sepsis with the additional presence of organ dysfunction, hypotension, or hypoperfusion), a code from R65.2- must be assigned in addition to the code identifying the underlying infection. An additional code(s) also should be assigned to identify all organ dysfunction present.

IQ + R65.20 Severe sepsis without septic shock
   Severe sepsis NOS

□ 4th digit required   ⑤ 5th digit required   ⑥ 6th digit required   ⑦ 7th digit required   ⑦ 7th digit placeholder   + Additional code   ⊟ Laterality

1432   DecisionHealth's FY 2020 Complete Home Health ICD-10-CM Diagnosis Coding Manual

GUIDELINES   Section I.C.1.d.5)(b-c)

For infections following a procedure, a code from T81.40, to T81.43 Infection following a procedure, or a code from O86.00 to O86.03, Infection of obstetric surgical wound, that identifies the site of the infection should be coded first, if known. Assign an additional code for sepsis following a procedure (T81.44) or sepsis following an obstetrical procedure (O86.04). Use an additional code to identify the infectious agent. If the patient has severe sepsis, the appropriate code from subcategory R65.2 should also be assigned with the additional code(s) for any acute organ dysfunction.

If a postprocedural infection has resulted in postprocedural septic shock, assign the codes indicated above for sepsis due to a postprocedural infection, followed by code T81.12-, Postprocedural septic shock. Do not assign code R65.21, Severe sepsis with septic shock. Additional code(s) should be assigned for any acute organ dysfunction.

!Q ✚ R65.21   Severe sepsis with septic shock

GUIDELINES   Section I.C.1.d.2)(a)

Septic shock generally refers to circulatory failure associated with severe sepsis, and therefore, it represents a type of acute organ dysfunction. For cases of septic shock, the code for the systemic infection should be sequenced first, followed by code R65.21, Severe sepsis with septic shock or code T81.12, Postprocedural septic shock. Any additional codes for the other acute organ dysfunctions should also be assigned. As noted in the sequencing instructions in the Tabular List, the code for septic shock cannot be assigned as a principal diagnosis.

4 R68   Other general symptoms and signs

!Q R68.0   Hypothermia, not associated with low environmental temperature

EXCLUDES 1   hypothermia NOS (accidental) (T68)
hypothermia due to anesthesia (T88.51)
hypothermia due to low environmental temperature (T68)
newborn hypothermia (P80.-)

5 R68.1   Nonspecific symptoms peculiar to infancy

EXCLUDES 1   colic, infantile (R10.83)
neonatal cerebral irritability (P91.3)
teething syndrome (K00.7)

!Q R68.11   Excessive crying of infant (baby)

EXCLUDES 1   excessive crying of child, adolescent, or adult (R45.83)

!Q R68.12   Fussy infant (baby)
Irritable infant

!Q ✚ R68.13   Apparent life threatening event in infant (ALTE)
Apparent life threatening event in newborn
Brief resolved unexplained event (BRUE)
Code first:
confirmed diagnosis, if known
Use additional code(s) for associated signs and symptoms if no confirmed diagnosis established, or if signs and symptoms are not associated routinely with confirmed diagnosis, or provide additional information for cause of ALTE

!Q R68.19   Other nonspecific symptoms peculiar to infancy

!Q R68.2   Dry mouth, unspecified

EXCLUDES 1   dry mouth due to dehydration (E86.0)
dry mouth due to sicca syndrome [Sjögren] (M35.0-)
salivary gland hyposecretion (K11.7)

!Q R68.3   Clubbing of fingers
Clubbing of nails
EXCLUDES 1   congenital clubfinger (Q68.1)

5 R68.8   Other general symptoms and signs

!Q R68.81   Early satiety

!Q R68.82   Decreased libido
Decreased sexual desire

!Q R68.83   Chills (without fever)
Chills NOS
EXCLUDES 1   chills with fever (R50.9)

!Q R68.84   Jaw pain
Mandibular pain
Maxilla pain
EXCLUDES 1   temporomandibular joint arthralgia (M26.62-)

CODING TIPS ✓   Jaw pain may be a symptom of myocardial infarction. If the condition causing the pain is known, such as a jaw disorder, then, for example, use a M26.62 code instead.

!Q R68.89   Other general symptoms and signs

!Q R69   Illness, unspecified
Unknown and unspecified cases of morbidity
CODING TIPS ✓   R69 indicates unknown illness of unknown origin and should not be assigned on a home health claim.

Abnormal findings on examination of blood, without diagnosis   (R70-R79)

EXCLUDES 2   abnormal findings on antenatal screening of mother (O28.-)
abnormalities of lipids (E78.-)
abnormalities of platelets and thrombocytes (D69.-)

★ New ▲ Revised Px Primary SP PDGM Px SL Low CoM SH High CoM !Q Quest. Encounter H Hospice non-cancer Dx   Unspecified   M *Manifestation*

DecisionHealth's FY 2020 Complete Home Health ICD-10-CM Diagnosis Coding Manual   1433

Chapter 18

R00-R99

abnormalities of white blood cells classified elsewhere (D70-D72)

coagulation hemorrhagic disorders (D65-D68)

diagnostic abnormal findings classified elsewhere - see Alphabetical Index

hemorrhagic and hematological disorders of newborn (P50-P61)

⁴ R70   Elevated erythrocyte sedimentation rate and abnormality of plasma viscosity

IQ R70.0 Elevated erythrocyte sedimentation rate

IQ R70.1 Abnormal plasma viscosity

⁴ R71   Abnormality of red blood cells

> **EXCLUDES 1**   anemias (D50-D64)
> anemia of premature infant (P61.2)
> benign (familial) polycythemia (D75.0)
> congenital anemias (P61.2-P61.4)
> newborn anemia due to isoimmunization (P55.-)
> polycythemia neonatorum (P61.1)
> polycythemia NOS (D75.1)
> polycythemia vera (D45)
> secondary polycythemia (D75.1)

IQ R71.0 Precipitous drop in hematocrit
Drop (precipitous) in hemoglobin
Drop in hematocrit

IQ R71.8 Other abnormality of red blood cells
Abnormal red-cell morphology NOS
Abnormal red-cell volume NOS
Anisocytosis
Poikilocytosis

⁴ R73   Elevated blood glucose level

> **EXCLUDES 1**   diabetes mellitus (E08-E13)
> diabetes mellitus in pregnancy, childbirth and the puerperium (O24.-)
> neonatal disorders (P70.0-P70.2)
> postsurgical hypoinsulinemia (E89.1)

⁵ R73.0 Abnormal glucose

> **EXCLUDES 1**   abnormal glucose in pregnancy (O99.81-)
> diabetes mellitus (E08-E13)
> dysmetabolic syndrome X (E88.81)
> gestational diabetes (O24.4-)
> glycosuria (R81)
> hypoglycemia (E16.2)

IQ R73.01 Impaired fasting glucose
Elevated fasting glucose

IQ R73.02 Impaired glucose tolerance (oral)
Elevated glucose tolerance

IQ R73.03 Prediabetes
Latent diabetes

> **CODING TIPS✓**   Prediabetes is defined as having an impaired fasting glucose (IFG): fasting blood glucose of 100-125 mg/dL, impaired glucose tolerance (IGT): blood glucose of 140-199 mg/dL 2 hours after a 75 g oral glucose tolerance test (OGTT) or a hemoglobin A1c value of 5.7%-6.4%.

> **DEFINITION**   An elevated blood sugar level that is higher than normal, but not high enough to be diagnosed as type 2 diabetes. When left untreated, prediabetes progresses to type 2 diabetes in less than 10 years. For many people, prediabetes has no signs or symptoms.

IQ R73.09 Other abnormal glucose
Abnormal glucose NOS
Abnormal non-fasting glucose tolerance

IQ R73.9   Hyperglycemia, unspecified

> **CODING TIPS✓**   Hyperglycemia should be coded to R73.9 only when not associated with diabetes mellitus or any form of post-procedural hyperinsulinemia. R73.9 indicates hyperglycemia that is of an unspecified origin.

⁴ R74   Abnormal serum enzyme levels

IQ R74.0 Nonspecific elevation of levels of transaminase and lactic acid dehydrogenase [LDH]

IQ R74.8 Abnormal levels of other serum enzymes
Abnormal level of acid phosphatase
Abnormal level of alkaline phosphatase
Abnormal level of amylase
Abnormal level of lipase [triacylglycerol lipase]

IQ R74.9   Abnormal serum enzyme level, unspecified

IQ R75   Inconclusive laboratory evidence of human immunodeficiency virus [HIV]
Nonconclusive HIV-test finding in infants

> **EXCLUDES 1**   asymptomatic human immunodeficiency virus [HIV] infection status (Z21)
> human immunodeficiency virus [HIV] disease (B20)

> **GUIDELINES**   Section I.C.1.a.2)(f)
> Patients with any known prior diagnosis of an HIV-related illness should be coded to B20. Once a patient has developed an HIV-related illness, the patient should always be assigned code B20 on every subsequent admission/ encounter. Patients previously diagnosed with any HIV illness (B20) should never be assigned to R75 or Z21, Asymptomatic human immunodeficiency virus [HIV] infection status.

> **GUIDELINES**   Section I.C.1.a.2)(e)
> Patients with inconclusive HIV serology, but no definitive diagnosis or manifestations of the illness, may be assigned code R75, Inconclusive laboratory evidence of human immunodeficiency virus [HIV].

⁴ R76   Other abnormal immunological findings in serum

IQ R76.0 Raised antibody titer

> **EXCLUDES 1**   isoimmunization in pregnancy (O36.0-O36.1)
> isoimmunization affecting newborn (P55.-)

⁵ R76.1 Nonspecific reaction to test for tuberculosis

IQ R76.11 Nonspecific reaction to tuberculin skin test without active tuberculosis
Abnormal result of Mantoux test

---

⁴4th digit required   ⁵5th digit required   ⁶6th digit required   ⁷7th digit required   ⑦7th digit placeholder   ✚Additional code   ▤Laterality

PPD positive
Tuberculin (skin test) positive
Tuberculin (skin test) reactor

> **EXCLUDES 1** nonspecific reaction to cell mediated immunity measurement of gamma interferon antigen response without active tuberculosis (R76.12)

IQ R76.12 Nonspecific reaction to cell mediated immunity measurement of gamma interferon antigen response without active tuberculosis
Nonspecific reaction to QuantiFERON-TB test (QFT) without active tuberculosis

> **EXCLUDES 1** nonspecific reaction to tuberculin skin test without active tuberculosis (R76.11)
> positive tuberculin skin test (R76.11)

IQ R76.8 Other specified abnormal immunological findings in serum
Raised level of immunoglobulins NOS

IQ R76.9 Abnormal immunological finding in serum, unspecified

4 R77 Other abnormalities of plasma proteins

> **EXCLUDES 1** disorders of plasma-protein metabolism (E88.0-)

IQ R77.0 Abnormality of albumin

IQ R77.1 Abnormality of globulin
Hyperglobulinemia NOS

IQ R77.2 Abnormality of alphafetoprotein

IQ R77.8 Other specified abnormalities of plasma proteins

IQ R77.9 Abnormality of plasma protein, unspecified

+ 4 R78 Findings of drugs and other substances, not normally found in blood
Use additional code to identify the any retained foreign body, if applicable (Z18.-)

> **EXCLUDES 1** mental or behavioral disorders due to psychoactive substance use (F10-F19)

IQ + R78.0 Finding of alcohol in blood
Use additional external cause code (Y90.-), for detail regarding alcohol level.

IQ + R78.1 Finding of opiate drug in blood

IQ + R78.2 Finding of cocaine in blood

IQ + R78.3 Finding of hallucinogen in blood

IQ + R78.4 Finding of other drugs of addictive potential in blood

IQ + R78.5 Finding of other psychotropic drug in blood

IQ + R78.6 Finding of steroid agent in blood

+ 5 R78.7 Finding of abnormal level of heavy metals in blood

IQ + R78.71 Abnormal lead level in blood

> **EXCLUDES 1** lead poisoning (T56.0-)

IQ + R78.79 Finding of abnormal level of heavy metals in blood

+ 5 R78.8 Finding of other specified substances, not normally found in blood

IQ + R78.81 Bacteremia

> **EXCLUDES 1** sepsis-code to specified infection

> **CODING TIPS ✓** Do not assign code R78.81 to indicate the presence of sepsis. Bacteremia only indicates the presence of bacteria identified in the bloodstream, not the infectious process. Do not assign R78.81 with any code identifying sepsis. Sepsis should be coded to the appropriate code identifying the specific type of sepsis present.

> **DEFINITION** The presence of small numbers of bacteria in the bloodstream, usually as a temporary condition, and without causing symptoms.

IQ + R78.89 Finding of other specified substances, not normally found in blood
Finding of abnormal level of lithium in blood

> **CODING TIPS ✓** Code R78.89 indicates that the patient has elevated non-therapeutic levels of a drug found in the blood on testing, but has no adverse effects of the drug. If the clinical record indicates poisoning or adverse effect, reference the Table of Drugs and Chemicals for the correct code, including drug and intent.

IQ + R78.9 Finding of unspecified substance, not normally found in blood

+ 4 R79 Other abnormal findings of blood chemistry
Use additional code to identify any retained foreign body, if applicable (Z18.-)

> **EXCLUDES 1** asymptomatic hyperuricemia (E79.0)
> hyperglycemia NOS (R73.9)
> hypoglycemia NOS (E16.2)
> neonatal hypoglycemia (P70.3-P70.4)
> specific findings indicating disorder of amino-acid metabolism (E70-E72)
> specific findings indicating disorder of carbohydrate metabolism (E73-E74)
> specific findings indicating disorder of lipid metabolism (E75.-)

IQ + R79.0 Abnormal level of blood mineral
Abnormal blood level of cobalt
Abnormal blood level of copper
Abnormal blood level of iron
Abnormal blood level of magnesium
Abnormal blood level of mineral NEC
Abnormal blood level of zinc

> **EXCLUDES 1** abnormal level of lithium (R78.89)
> disorders of mineral metabolism (E83.-)
> neonatal hypomagnesemia (P71.2)
> nutritional mineral deficiency (E58-E61)

IQ + R79.1 Abnormal coagulation profile
Abnormal or prolonged bleeding time

★ New ▲ Revised Px Primary SP PDGM Px SL Low CoM SH High CoM IQ Quest. Encounter H Hospice non-cancer Dx   Unspecified   M Manifestation

DecisionHealth's FY 2020 Complete Home Health ICD-10-CM Diagnosis Coding Manual   1435

Chapter 18

R00-R99

Abnormal or prolonged coagulation time
Abnormal or prolonged partial thromboplastin time [PTT]
Abnormal or prolonged prothrombin time [PT]

EXCLUDES 1   coagulation defects (D68.-)

EXCLUDES 2   abnormality of fluid, electrolyte or acid-base balance (E86-E87)

CODING TIPS ✓   This code is not for those on Coumadin or other blood thinners for prophylactic purposes. Use Z51.81 and Z79.01 instead. If a bleed has occurred because of anticoagulants/antiplatelets, code the bleed and D68.32 and the T code for the drug.

＋ 5 R79.8   Other specified abnormal findings of blood chemistry

!Q ＋ R79.81   Abnormal blood-gas level

DEFINITION   Abnormal oxygen or carbon dioxide level in the blood.

!Q ＋ R79.82   Elevated C-reactive protein (CRP)

!Q ＋ R79.89   Other specified abnormal findings of blood chemistry

!Q ＋ R79.9   Abnormal finding of blood chemistry, unspecified

Abnormal findings on examination of urine, without diagnosis   (R80-R82)

EXCLUDES 1   abnormal findings on antenatal screening of mother (O28.-)
diagnostic abnormal findings classified elsewhere - see Alphabetical Index
specific findings indicating disorder of amino-acid metabolism (E70-E72)
specific findings indicating disorder of carbohydrate metabolism (E73-E74)

4 R80   Proteinuria

EXCLUDES 1   gestational proteinuria (O12.1-)

!Q R80.0   Isolated proteinuria
Idiopathic proteinuria

EXCLUDES 1   isolated proteinuria with specific morphological lesion (N06.-)

!Q R80.1   Persistent proteinuria, unspecified

!Q R80.2   Orthostatic proteinuria, unspecified
Postural proteinuria

!Q R80.3   Bence Jones proteinuria

!Q R80.8   Other proteinuria

!Q R80.9   Proteinuria, unspecified
Albuminuria NOS

!Q R81   Glycosuria

EXCLUDES 1   renal glycosuria (E74.8)

＋ 4 R82   Other and unspecified abnormal findings in urine

INCLUDES   chromoabnormalities in urine

Use additional code to identify any retained foreign body, if applicable (Z18.-)

EXCLUDES 2   hematuria (R31.-)

!Q ＋ R82.0   Chyluria

EXCLUDES 1   filarial chyluria (B74.-)

!Q ＋ R82.1   Myoglobinuria

!Q ＋ R82.2   Biliuria

!Q ＋ R82.3   Hemoglobinuria

EXCLUDES 1   hemoglobinuria due to hemolysis from external causes NEC (D59.6)
hemoglobinuria due to paroxysmal nocturnal [Marchiafava-Micheli] (D59.5)

!Q ＋ R82.4   Acetonuria
Ketonuria

!Q ＋ R82.5   Elevated urine levels of drugs, medicaments and biological substances
Elevated urine levels of catecholamines
Elevated urine levels of indoleacetic acid
Elevated urine levels of 17-ketosteroids
Elevated urine levels of steroids

!Q ＋ R82.6   Abnormal urine levels of substances chiefly nonmedicinal as to source
Abnormal urine level of heavy metals

＋ 5 R82.7   Abnormal findings on microbiological examination of urine

EXCLUDES 1   colonization status (Z22.-)

CODING TIPS ✓   Bacteriuria is a condition where there are bacteria present in a microscopic examination of the urine. It is not definitive evidence of a UTI.

!Q ＋ R82.71   Bacteriuria

DEFINITION   The presence of bacteria identified in the urine. It affects more women than men and commonly occurs asymptomatically.

!Q ＋ R82.79   Other abnormal findings on microbiological examination of urine
Positive culture findings of urine

▲ ＋ 5 R82.8   Abnormal findings on cytological and histological examination of urine

★ ＋ R82.81   Pyuria
Sterile pyuria

★ ＋ R82.89   Other abnormal findings on cytological and histological examination of urine

＋ 5 R82.9   Other and unspecified abnormal findings in urine

!Q ＋ R82.90   Unspecified abnormal findings in urine

!Q ＋ R82.91   Other chromoabnormalities of urine
Chromoconversion (dipstick)
Idiopathic dipstick converts positive for blood with no cellular forms in sediment

EXCLUDES 1   hemoglobinuria (R82.3)
myoglobinuria (R82.1)

＋ 6 R82.99   Other abnormal findings in urine

!Q ＋ R82.991   Hypocitraturia

!Q ＋ R82.992   Hyperoxaluria

EXCLUDES 1   Primary hyperoxaluria (E72.53)

▲ !Q ＋ R82.993   Hyperuricosuria

!Q ＋ R82.994   Hypercalciuria
Idiopathic hypercalciuria

!Q ＋ R82.998   Other abnormal findings in urine
Cells and casts in urine
Crystalluria
Melanuria

---

4 4th digit required   **5** 5th digit required   **6** 6th digit required   **7** 7th digit required   **7** 7th digit placeholder   **＋** Additional code   **⊟** Laterality

Abnormal findings on examination of other body fluids, substances and tissues, without diagnosis   (R83-R89)

EXCLUDES 1 abnormal findings on antenatal screening of mother (O28.-)

diagnostic abnormal findings classified elsewhere - see Alphabetical Index

EXCLUDES 2 abnormal findings on examination of blood, without diagnosis (R70-R79)

abnormal findings on examination of urine, without diagnosis (R80-R82)

abnormal tumor markers (R97.-)

4 R83   Abnormal findings in cerebrospinal fluid

IQ R83.0   Abnormal level of enzymes in cerebrospinal fluid

IQ R83.1   Abnormal level of hormones in cerebrospinal fluid

IQ R83.2   Abnormal level of other drugs, medicaments and biological substances in cerebrospinal fluid

IQ R83.3   Abnormal level of substances chiefly nonmedicinal as to source in cerebrospinal fluid

IQ R83.4   Abnormal immunological findings in cerebrospinal fluid

IQ R83.5   Abnormal microbiological findings in cerebrospinal fluid

Positive culture findings in cerebrospinal fluid

EXCLUDES 1 colonization status (Z22.-)

IQ R83.6   Abnormal cytological findings in cerebrospinal fluid

IQ R83.8   Other abnormal findings in cerebrospinal fluid

Abnormal chromosomal findings in cerebrospinal fluid

IQ R83.9   Unspecified abnormal finding in cerebrospinal fluid

4 R84   Abnormal findings in specimens from respiratory organs and thorax

INCLUDES abnormal findings in bronchial washings

abnormal findings in nasal secretions

abnormal findings in pleural fluid

abnormal findings in sputum

abnormal findings in throat scrapings

EXCLUDES 1 blood-stained sputum (R04.2)

IQ R84.0   Abnormal level of enzymes in specimens from respiratory organs and thorax

IQ R84.1   Abnormal level of hormones in specimens from respiratory organs and thorax

IQ R84.2   Abnormal level of other drugs, medicaments and biological substances in specimens from respiratory organs and thorax

IQ R84.3   Abnormal level of substances chiefly nonmedicinal as to source in specimens from respiratory organs and thorax

IQ R84.4   Abnormal immunological findings in specimens from respiratory organs and thorax

IQ R84.5   Abnormal microbiological findings in specimens from respiratory organs and thorax

Positive culture findings in specimens from respiratory organs and thorax

EXCLUDES 1 colonization status (Z22.-)

IQ R84.6   Abnormal cytological findings in specimens from respiratory organs and thorax

IQ R84.7   Abnormal histological findings in specimens from respiratory organs and thorax

IQ R84.8   Other abnormal findings in specimens from respiratory organs and thorax

Abnormal chromosomal findings in specimens from respiratory organs and thorax

IQ R84.9   Unspecified abnormal finding in specimens from respiratory organs and thorax

4 R85   Abnormal findings in specimens from digestive organs and abdominal cavity

INCLUDES abnormal findings in peritoneal fluid

abnormal findings in saliva

EXCLUDES 1 cloudy peritoneal dialysis effluent (R88.0)

fecal abnormalities (R19.5)

IQ R85.0   Abnormal level of enzymes in specimens from digestive organs and abdominal cavity

IQ R85.1   Abnormal level of hormones in specimens from digestive organs and abdominal cavity

IQ R85.2   Abnormal level of other drugs, medicaments and biological substances in specimens from digestive organs and abdominal cavity

IQ R85.3   Abnormal level of substances chiefly nonmedicinal as to source in specimens from digestive organs and abdominal cavity

IQ R85.4   Abnormal immunological findings in specimens from digestive organs and abdominal cavity

IQ R85.5   Abnormal microbiological findings in specimens from digestive organs and abdominal cavity

Positive culture findings in specimens from digestive organs and abdominal cavity

EXCLUDES 1 colonization status (Z22.-)

5 R85.6   Abnormal cytological findings in specimens from digestive organs and abdominal cavity

6 R85.61   Abnormal cytologic smear of anus

EXCLUDES 1 abnormal cytological findings in specimens from other digestive organs and abdominal cavity (R85.69)

carcinoma in situ of anus (histologically confirmed) (D01.3)

anal intraepithelial neoplasia I [AIN I] (K62.82)

★ New ▲ Revised Px Primary SP PDGM Px SL Low CoM SH High CoM IQ Quest. Encounter H Hospice non-cancer Dx   Unspecified   M Manifestation

DecisionHealth's FY 2020 Complete Home Health ICD-10-CM Diagnosis Coding Manual   1437

anal intraepithelial
neoplasia II [AIN II]
(K62.82)
anal intraepithelial
neoplasia III [AIN III]
(D01.3)
dysplasia (mild)
(moderate) of anus
(histologically
confirmed) (K62.82)
severe dysplasia of anus
(histologically
confirmed) (D01.3)

EXCLUDES 2 anal high risk human
papillomavirus (HPV)
DNA test positive
(R85.81)
anal low risk human
papillomavirus (HPV)
DNA test positive
(R85.82)

IQ **R85.610 Atypical squamous cells of
undetermined significance on
cytologic smear of anus (ASC-US)**

IQ **R85.611 Atypical squamous cells cannot
exclude high grade squamous
intraepithelial lesion on cytologic
smear of anus (ASC-H)**

IQ **R85.612 Low grade squamous
intraepithelial lesion on cytologic
smear of anus (LGSIL)**

IQ **R85.613 High grade squamous
intraepithelial lesion on cytologic
smear of anus (HGSIL)**

IQ **R85.614 Cytologic evidence of malignancy
on smear of anus**

IQ **R85.615 Unsatisfactory cytologic smear of
anus**
Inadequate sample of cytologic
smear of anus

IQ **R85.616 Satisfactory anal smear but
lacking transformation zone**

IQ **R85.618 Other abnormal cytological
findings on specimens from anus**

IQ **R85.619 Unspecified abnormal cytological
findings in specimens from anus**
Abnormal anal cytology NOS
Atypical glandular cells of anus
NOS

IQ **R85.69 Abnormal cytological findings in
specimens from other digestive
organs and abdominal cavity**

IQ **R85.7 Abnormal histological findings in
specimens from digestive organs and
abdominal cavity**

5 **R85.8 Other abnormal findings in specimens
from digestive organs and abdominal
cavity**

IQ **R85.81 Anal high risk human
papillomavirus (HPV) DNA test
positive**
EXCLUDES 1 anogenital warts due to
human papillomavirus
(HPV) (A63.0)
condyloma acuminatum
(A63.0)

IQ + **R85.82 Anal low risk human papillomavirus
(HPV) DNA test positive**

Use additional code for associated
human papillomavirus (B97.7)

IQ **R85.89 Other abnormal findings in
specimens from digestive organs and
abdominal cavity**
Abnormal chromosomal findings in
specimens from digestive organs and
abdominal cavity

IQ **R85.9 Unspecified abnormal finding in
specimens from digestive organs and
abdominal cavity**

4 **R86 Abnormal findings in specimens from male
genital organs**
INCLUDES abnormal findings in prostatic
secretions
abnormal findings in semen,
seminal fluid
abnormal spermatozoa
EXCLUDES 1 azoospermia (N46.0-)
oligospermia (N46.1-)

IQ **R86.0 Abnormal level of enzymes in specimens
from male genital organs**

IQ **R86.1 Abnormal level of hormones in
specimens from male genital organs**

IQ **R86.2 Abnormal level of other drugs,
medicaments and biological substances
in specimens from male genital organs**

IQ **R86.3 Abnormal level of substances chiefly
nonmedicinal as to source in specimens
from male genital organs**

IQ **R86.4 Abnormal immunological findings in
specimens from male genital organs**

IQ **R86.5 Abnormal microbiological findings in
specimens from male genital organs**
Positive culture findings in specimens
from male genital organs
EXCLUDES 1 colonization status (Z22.-)

IQ **R86.6 Abnormal cytological findings in
specimens from male genital organs**

IQ **R86.7 Abnormal histological findings in
specimens from male genital organs**

IQ **R86.8 Other abnormal findings in specimens
from male genital organs**
Abnormal chromosomal findings in
specimens from male genital organs

IQ **R86.9 Unspecified abnormal finding in
specimens from male genital organs**

4 **R87 Abnormal findings in specimens from
female genital organs**
INCLUDES abnormal findings in secretion
and smears from cervix uteri
abnormal findings in secretion
and smears from vagina
abnormal findings in secretion
and smears from vulva

IQ **R87.0 Abnormal level of enzymes in specimens
from female genital organs**

IQ **R87.1 Abnormal level of hormones in
specimens from female genital organs**

IQ **R87.2 Abnormal level of other drugs,
medicaments and biological substances
in specimens from female genital organs**

IQ **R87.3 Abnormal level of substances chiefly
nonmedicinal as to source in specimens
from female genital organs**

IQ **R87.4 Abnormal immunological findings in
specimens from female genital organs**

---

4 4th digit required   5 5th digit required   6 6th digit required   7 7th digit required   7 7th digit placeholder   + Additional code   = Laterality

1438   DecisionHealth's FY 2020 Complete Home Health ICD-10-CM Diagnosis Coding Manual

IQ R87.5 Abnormal microbiological findings in specimens from female genital organs
Positive culture findings in specimens from female genital organs
EXCLUDES 1 colonization status (Z22.-)

⑤ R87.6 Abnormal cytological findings in specimens from female genital organs

⑥ R87.61 Abnormal cytological findings in specimens from cervix uteri
EXCLUDES 1 abnormal cytological findings in specimens from other female genital organs (R87.69)
abnormal cytological findings in specimens from vagina (R87.62-)
carcinoma in situ of cervix uteri (histologically confirmed) (D06.-)
cervical intraepithelial neoplasia I [CIN I] (N87.0)
cervical intraepithelial neoplasia II [CIN II] (N87.1)
cervical intraepithelial neoplasia III [CIN III] (D06.-)
dysplasia (mild) (moderate) of cervix uteri (histologically confirmed) (N87.-)
severe dysplasia of cervix uteri (histologically confirmed) (D06.-)
EXCLUDES 2 cervical high risk human papillomavirus (HPV) DNA test positive (R87.810)
cervical low risk human papillomavirus (HPV) DNA test positive (R87.820)

IQ R87.610 Atypical squamous cells of undetermined significance on cytologic smear of cervix (ASC-US)

IQ R87.611 Atypical squamous cells cannot exclude high grade squamous intraepithelial lesion on cytologic smear of cervix (ASC-H)

IQ R87.612 Low grade squamous intraepithelial lesion on cytologic smear of cervix (LGSIL)

IQ R87.613 High grade squamous intraepithelial lesion on cytologic smear of cervix (HGSIL)

IQ R87.614 Cytologic evidence of malignancy on smear of cervix

IQ R87.615 Unsatisfactory cytologic smear of cervix
Inadequate sample of cytologic smear of cervix

IQ R87.616 Satisfactory cervical smear but lacking transformation zone

IQ R87.618 Other abnormal cytological findings on specimens from cervix uteri

IQ R87.619 Unspecified abnormal cytological findings in specimens from cervix uteri
Abnormal cervical cytology NOS
Abnormal Papanicolaou smear of cervix NOS
Abnormal thin preparation smear of cervix NOS
Atypical endocervial cells of cervix NOS
Atypical endometrial cells of cervix NOS
Atypical glandular cells of cervix NOS

+ ⑥ R87.62 Abnormal cytological findings in specimens from vagina
Use additional code to identify acquired absence of uterus and cervix, if applicable (Z90.71-)
EXCLUDES 1 abnormal cytological findings in specimens from cervix uteri (R87.61-)
abnormal cytological findings in specimens from other female genital organs (R87.69)
carcinoma in situ of vagina (histologically confirmed) (D07.2)
vaginal intraepithelial neoplasia I [VAIN I] (N89.0)
vaginal intraepithelial neoplasia II [VAIN II] (N89.1)
vaginal intraepithelial neoplasia III [VAIN III] (D07.2)
dysplasia (mild) (moderate) of vagina (histologically confirmed) (N89.-)
severe dysplasia of vagina (histologically confirmed) (D07.2)
EXCLUDES 2 vaginal high risk human papillomavirus (HPV) DNA test positive (R87.811)
vaginal low risk human papillomavirus (HPV) DNA test positive (R87.821)

IQ + R87.620 Atypical squamous cells of undetermined significance on cytologic smear of vagina (ASC-US)

IQ + R87.621 Atypical squamous cells cannot exclude high grade squamous intraepithelial lesion on cytologic smear of vagina (ASC-H)

★ New ▲ Revised Px Primary SP PDGM Px SL Low CoM SH High CoM IQ Quest. Encounter H Hospice non-cancer Dx   Unspecified   M *Manifestation*

DecisionHealth's FY 2020 Complete Home Health ICD-10-CM Diagnosis Coding Manual   1439

[IQ] + R87.622   **Low grade squamous intraepithelial lesion on cytologic smear of vagina (LGSIL)**

[IQ] + R87.623   **High grade squamous intraepithelial lesion on cytologic smear of vagina (HGSIL)**

[IQ] + R87.624   **Cytologic evidence of malignancy on smear of vagina**

[IQ] + R87.625   **Unsatisfactory cytologic smear of vagina**
Inadequate sample of cytologic smear of vagina

[IQ] + R87.628   **Other abnormal cytological findings on specimens from vagina**

[IQ] + R87.629   **Unspecified abnormal cytological findings in specimens from vagina**
Abnormal Papanicolaou smear of vagina NOS
Abnormal thin preparation smear of vagina NOS
Abnormal vaginal cytology NOS
Atypical endocervical cells of vagina NOS
Atypical endometrial cells of vagina NOS
Atypical glandular cells of vagina NOS

[IQ] R87.69   **Abnormal cytological findings in specimens from other female genital organs**
Abnormal cytological findings in specimens from female genital organs NOS
> **EXCLUDES 1**   dysplasia of vulva (histologically confirmed) (N90.0-N90.3)

[IQ] R87.7   **Abnormal histological findings in specimens from female genital organs**
> **EXCLUDES 1**   carcinoma in situ (histologically confirmed) of female genital organs (D06-D07.3)
> cervical intraepithelial neoplasia I [CIN I] (N87.0)
> cervical intraepithelial neoplasia II [CIN II] (N87.1)
> cervical intraepithelial neoplasia III [CIN III] (D06.-)
> dysplasia (mild) (moderate) of cervix uteri (histologically confirmed) (N87.-)
> dysplasia (mild) (moderate) of vagina (histologically confirmed) (N89.-)
> vaginal intraepithelial neoplasia I [VAIN I] (N89.0)
> vaginal intraepithelial neoplasia II [VAIN II] (N89.1)

> vaginal intraepithelial neoplasia III [VAIN III] (D07.2)
> severe dysplasia of cervix uteri (histologically confirmed) (D06.-)
> severe dysplasia of vagina (histologically confirmed) (D07.2)

[5] R87.8   **Other abnormal findings in specimens from female genital organs**

[6] R87.81   **High risk human papillomavirus (HPV) DNA test positive from female genital organs**
> **EXCLUDES 1**   anogenital warts due to human papillomavirus (HPV) (A63.0)
> condyloma acuminatum (A63.0)

[IQ] R87.810   **Cervical high risk human papillomavirus (HPV) DNA test positive**

[IQ] R87.811   **Vaginal high risk human papillomavirus (HPV) DNA test positive**

+ [6] R87.82   **Low risk human papillomavirus (HPV) DNA test positive from female genital organs**
Use additional code for associated human papillomavirus (B97.7)

[IQ] + R87.820   **Cervical low risk human papillomavirus (HPV) DNA test positive**

[IQ] + R87.821   **Vaginal low risk human papillomavirus (HPV) DNA test positive**

[IQ] R87.89   **Other abnormal findings in specimens from female genital organs**
Abnormal chromosomal findings in specimens from female genital organs

[IQ] R87.9   **Unspecified abnormal finding in specimens from female genital organs**

[4] R88   **Abnormal findings in other body fluids and substances**

[IQ] R88.0   **Cloudy (hemodialysis) (peritoneal) dialysis effluent**

[IQ] R88.8   **Abnormal findings in other body fluids and substances**

[4] R89   **Abnormal findings in specimens from other organs, systems and tissues**
> **INCLUDES**   abnormal findings in nipple discharge
> abnormal findings in synovial fluid
> abnormal findings in wound secretions

[IQ] R89.0   **Abnormal level of enzymes in specimens from other organs, systems and tissues**

[IQ] R89.1   **Abnormal level of hormones in specimens from other organs, systems and tissues**

[IQ] R89.2   **Abnormal level of other drugs, medicaments and biological substances in specimens from other organs, systems and tissues**

---

[4] 4th digit required   **[5]** 5th digit required   **[6]** 6th digit required   **[7]** 7th digit required   **[7]** 7th digit placeholder   **+** Additional code   **[=]** Laterality

!Q R89.3 **Abnormal level of substances chiefly nonmedicinal as to source in specimens from other organs, systems and tissues**

!Q R89.4 **Abnormal immunological findings in specimens from other organs, systems and tissues**

!Q R89.5 **Abnormal microbiological findings in specimens from other organs, systems and tissues**

Positive culture findings in specimens from other organs, systems and tissues

EXCLUDES 1 colonization status (Z22.-)

!Q R89.6 **Abnormal cytological findings in specimens from other organs, systems and tissues**

!Q R89.7 **Abnormal histological findings in specimens from other organs, systems and tissues**

!Q R89.8 **Other abnormal findings in specimens from other organs, systems and tissues**

Abnormal chromosomal findings in specimens from other organs, systems and tissues

!Q R89.9 **Unspecified abnormal finding in specimens from other organs, systems and tissues**

Abnormal findings on diagnostic imaging and in function studies, without diagnosis (R90-R94)

INCLUDES nonspecific abnormal findings on diagnostic imaging by computerized axial tomography [CAT scan]

nonspecific abnormal findings on diagnostic imaging by magnetic resonance imaging [MRI][NMR]

nonspecific abnormal findings on diagnostic imaging by positron emission tomography [PET scan]

nonspecific abnormal findings on diagnostic imaging by thermography

nonspecific abnormal findings on diagnostic imaging by ultrasound [echogram]

nonspecific abnormal findings on diagnostic imaging by X-ray examination

EXCLUDES 1 abnormal findings on antenatal screening of mother (O28.-)

diagnostic abnormal findings classified elsewhere - see Alphabetical Index

4 R90 **Abnormal findings on diagnostic imaging of central nervous system**

!Q R90.0 **Intracranial space-occupying lesion found on diagnostic imaging of central nervous system**

5 R90.8 **Other abnormal findings on diagnostic imaging of central nervous system**

!Q R90.81 **Abnormal echoencephalogram**

!Q R90.82 **White matter disease, unspecified**

!Q R90.89 **Other abnormal findings on diagnostic imaging of central nervous system**

Other cerebrovascular abnormality found on diagnostic imaging of central nervous system

4 R91 **Abnormal findings on diagnostic imaging of lung**

!Q R91.1 **Solitary pulmonary nodule**

Coin lesion lung

Solitary pulmonary nodule, subsegmental branch of the bronchial tree

!Q R91.8 **Other nonspecific abnormal finding of lung field**

Lung mass NOS found on diagnostic imaging of lung

Pulmonary infiltrate NOS

Shadow, lung

4 R92 **Abnormal and inconclusive findings on diagnostic imaging of breast**

!Q R92.0 **Mammographic microcalcification found on diagnostic imaging of breast**

EXCLUDES 2 mammographic calcification (calculus) found on diagnostic imaging of breast (R92.1)

!Q R92.1 **Mammographic calcification found on diagnostic imaging of breast**

Mammographic calculus found on diagnostic imaging of breast

!Q R92.2 **Inconclusive mammogram**

Dense breasts NOS

Inconclusive mammogram NEC

Inconclusive mammography due to dense breasts

Inconclusive mammography NEC

!Q R92.8 **Other abnormal and inconclusive findings on diagnostic imaging of breast**

4 R93 **Abnormal findings on diagnostic imaging of other body structures**

!Q R93.0 **Abnormal findings on diagnostic imaging of skull and head, not elsewhere classified**

EXCLUDES 1 intracranial space-occupying lesion found on diagnostic imaging (R90.0)

!Q R93.1 **Abnormal findings on diagnostic imaging of heart and coronary circulation**

Abnormal echocardiogram NOS

Abnormal heart shadow

!Q R93.2 **Abnormal findings on diagnostic imaging of liver and biliary tract**

Nonvisualization of gallbladder

!Q R93.3 **Abnormal findings on diagnostic imaging of other parts of digestive tract**

5 R93.4 **Abnormal findings on diagnostic imaging of urinary organs**

EXCLUDES 2 hypertrophy of kidney (N28.81)

!Q R93.41 **Abnormal radiologic findings on diagnostic imaging of renal pelvis, ureter, or bladder**

Filling defect of bladder found on diagnostic imaging

Filling defect of renal pelvis found on diagnostic imaging

Filling defect of ureter found on diagnostic imaging

6 R93.42 **Abnormal radiologic findings on diagnostic imaging of kidney**

⊟ !Q R93.421 **Abnormal radiologic findings on diagnostic imaging of right kidney**

⊟ !Q R93.422 **Abnormal radiologic findings on diagnostic imaging of left kidney**

Chapter 18

R00-R99

★ New ▲ Revised Px Primary SP PDGM Px SL Low CoM SH High CoM !Q Quest. Encounter H Hospice non-cancer Dx Unspecified M Manifestation

DecisionHealth's FY 2020 Complete Home Health ICD-10-CM Diagnosis Coding Manual   1441

Chapter 18

R00-R99

⊟ IQ R93.429 Abnormal radiologic findings on diagnostic imaging of unspecified kidney

IQ R93.49 Abnormal radiologic findings on diagnostic imaging of other urinary organs

IQ R93.5 Abnormal findings on diagnostic imaging of other abdominal regions, including retroperitoneum

IQ R93.6 Abnormal findings on diagnostic imaging of limbs

> EXCLUDES 2   abnormal finding in skin and subcutaneous tissue (R93.8-)

IQ R93.7 Abnormal findings on diagnostic imaging of other parts of musculoskeletal system

> EXCLUDES 2   abnormal findings on diagnostic imaging of skull (R93.0)

⑤ R93.8 Abnormal findings on diagnostic imaging of other specified body structures

⑥ R93.81 Abnormal radiologic findings on diagnostic imaging of testis

⊟ IQ R93.811 Abnormal radiologic findings on diagnostic imaging of right testicle

⊟ IQ R93.812 Abnormal radiologic findings on diagnostic imaging of left testicle

⊟ IQ R93.813 Abnormal radiologic findings on diagnostic imaging of testicles, bilateral

⊟ IQ R93.819 Abnormal radiologic findings on diagnostic imaging of unspecified testicle

IQ R93.89 Abnormal findings on diagnostic imaging of other specified body structures

Abnormal finding by radioisotope localization of placenta

Abnormal radiological finding in skin and subcutaneous tissue

Mediastinal shift

IQ R93.9 Diagnostic imaging inconclusive due to excess body fat of patient

④ R94 Abnormal results of function studies

> INCLUDES   abnormal results of radionuclide [radioisotope] uptake studies abnormal results of scintigraphy

⑤ R94.0 Abnormal results of function studies of central nervous system

IQ R94.01 Abnormal electroencephalogram [EEG]

IQ R94.02 Abnormal brain scan

IQ R94.09 Abnormal results of other function studies of central nervous system

⑤ R94.1 Abnormal results of function studies of peripheral nervous system and special senses

⑥ R94.11 Abnormal results of function studies of eye

IQ R94.110 Abnormal electro-oculogram [EOG]

IQ R94.111 Abnormal electroretinogram [ERG]

Abnormal retinal function study

IQ R94.112 Abnormal visually evoked potential [VEP]

IQ R94.113 Abnormal oculomotor study

IQ R94.118 Abnormal results of other function studies of eye

⑥ R94.12 Abnormal results of function studies of ear and other special senses

IQ R94.120 Abnormal auditory function study

IQ R94.121 Abnormal vestibular function study

IQ R94.128 Abnormal results of other function studies of ear and other special senses

⑥ R94.13 Abnormal results of function studies of peripheral nervous system

IQ R94.130 Abnormal response to nerve stimulation, unspecified

IQ R94.131 Abnormal electromyogram [EMG]

> EXCLUDES 1   electromyogram of eye (R94.113)

IQ R94.138 Abnormal results of other function studies of peripheral nervous system

IQ R94.2 Abnormal results of pulmonary function studies

Reduced ventilatory capacity

Reduced vital capacity

⑤ R94.3 Abnormal results of cardiovascular function studies

IQ R94.30 Abnormal result of cardiovascular function study, unspecified

IQ R94.31 Abnormal electrocardiogram [ECG] [EKG]

> EXCLUDES 1   long QT syndrome (I45.81)

IQ R94.39 Abnormal result of other cardiovascular function study

Abnormal electrophysiological intracardiac studies

Abnormal phonocardiogram

Abnormal vectorcardiogram

IQ R94.4 Abnormal results of kidney function studies

Abnormal renal function test

IQ R94.5 Abnormal results of liver function studies

IQ R94.6 Abnormal results of thyroid function studies

IQ R94.7 Abnormal results of other endocrine function studies

> EXCLUDES 2   abnormal glucose (R73.0-)

IQ R94.8 Abnormal results of function studies of other organs and systems

Abnormal basal metabolic rate [BMR]

Abnormal bladder function test

Abnormal splenic function test

Abnormal tumor markers   (R97)

④ R97 Abnormal tumor markers

Elevated tumor associated antigens [TAA]

Elevated tumor specific antigens [TSA]

IQ R97.0 Elevated carcinoembryonic antigen [CEA]

IQ R97.1 Elevated cancer antigen 125 [CA 125]

⑤ R97.2 Elevated prostate specific antigen [PSA]

IQ R97.20 Elevated prostate specific antigen [PSA]

④4th digit required   ⑤5th digit required   ⑥6th digit required   ⑦7th digit required   ☑7th digit placeholder   ✚Additional code   ⊟Laterality

1442   DecisionHealth's FY 2020 Complete Home Health ICD-10-CM Diagnosis Coding Manual

DEFINITION Elevated levels of prostate specific antigen (PSA) in the bloodstream can indicate prostate cancer, or precursor conditions that can develop into prostate cancer.

IQ R97.21 Rising PSA following treatment for malignant neoplasm of prostate

IQ R97.8 Other abnormal tumor markers

Ill-defined and unknown cause of mortality (R99)

H IQ R99 Ill-defined and unknown cause of mortality
Death (unexplained) NOS
Unspecified cause of mortality

CODING TIPS ✓ Code R99 indicates that a patient has expired. This code should never be assigned on a home health claim.

Chapter 18

R00-R99

★ New ▲ Revised Px Primary SP PDGM Px SL Low CoM SH High CoM IQ Quest. Encounter H Hospice non-cancer Dx   Unspecified   M *Manifestation*

DecisionHealth's FY 2020 Complete Home Health ICD-10-CM Diagnosis Coding Manual
1443

Chapter 18 Scenarios: Symptoms, signs and abnormal clinical and laboratory findings, not elsewhere classified (R00-R99)

Gait abnormality, orthostatic hypotension

A patient is admitted for gait abnormality documented by the physician as unsteadiness on feet. The patient has experienced repeated falls. It was determined that the unsteadiness is due to the patient's severe orthostatic hypotension. The patient will receive physical and occupational therapy to address the gait as well as safety concerns in the home.

Description	Code
Primary: Orthostatic hypotension	I95.1
Secondary: Unsteadiness on feet	R26.81
Secondary: History of falling	Z91.81

It is imperative to determine the underlying diagnosis behind a patient's symptoms as most symptom codes are not acceptable as primary diagnoses in the PDGM system. In this case, because orthostatic hypotension was determined to be the underlying diagnosis and the focus of the admission, it is assigned first. You may code symptoms when a more definitive diagnosis is known but the symptom is not integral to the condition and provides important additional information. The history of falling code (Z91.81) is used when a patient has fallen in the past and is at risk for future falls.

Gastrostomy care, Alzheimer's

An elderly male patient with severe late-onset Alzheimer's with dementia and a seizure disorder had a bout of aspiration pneumonia, resulting from dysphagia, that required hospitalization. The patient is debilitated, and has been for years, is nonverbal, and needs 24-hour care. Before his admission to home health, the pneumonia resolved but the patient has a gastrostomy tube with continuous tube feedings due to the dysphagia. The home health nurse will visit three times a week to educate his wife on tube feedings, make sure his nutritional needs are met, and assess for risks of further aspiration. The focus of care is the care and teaching of the g-tube.

Description	Code
Primary: Encounter for attention to gastrostomy	Z43.1
Secondary: Dysphagia, unspecified	R13.10
Secondary: Alzheimer's disease with late onset	G30.1
Secondary: Dementia in other diseases classified elsewhere without behavioral disturbance	F02.80
Secondary: Epilepsy, unspecified, not intractable, without status epilepticus	G40.909
Secondary: Other malaise	R53.81
Secondary: Personal history of pneumonia (recurrent)	Z87.01

Do not assign a symptom code, such as R13.10, in the primary position, as it does not support the primary reason for a home health admission. In this case, since the focus of care is the g-tube, Z43.1 is assigned primary. The Alzheimer's disease has been specified as late-onset and is thus coded that way. The code for dementia follows the Alzheimer's code in accordance with the etiology-manifestation convention and the Q1 2017 Coding Clinic guidance. Debility is sequenced after the conditions causing the debility. Though the pneumonia is resolved, the patient is at risk for future aspiration, thus Z87.01 is assigned.

Dysphagia, stroke sequelae

A patient is referred to home care for skilled nursing and speech-language therapy for treatment of dysphagia, dysarthria and dysphonia, all of which resulted from a stroke. Nursing is teaching on medications and diet. The patient also has a history of MRSA.

Description	Code
Primary: Dysphagia following cerebral infarction	I69.391
Secondary: Dysphagia, unspecified	R13.10
Secondary: Dysarthria following cerebral infarction	I69.322
Secondary: Other speech and language deficits following cerebral infarction	I69.328
Secondary: Dysphonia	R49.0
Secondary: Personal history of Methicillin resistant Staphylococcus aureus infection	Z86.14

The patient's dysphagia, dysarthria and dysphonia are all stroke sequela. While the combination code I69.322 covers both the dysarthria and the fact that it's stroke-related, two codes are required for the other two sequelae. In the case of the dysphagia, tabular instruction requires the assignment of R13.10 after I69.391. For the dysphonia, there is no unique code for it as a sequela, so the code for other speech-related deficits is assigned with an additional symptom code to specify that it's dysphonia. Be aware that most coding symptom codes are unacceptable in the PDGM payment system when assigned as primary. Coders must make every effort to determine the underlying cause of the symptoms. The MRSA, while not an active diagnosis, can have an effect on a patient's health and should be coded as a personal history code.

Chronic Afib, unspecified nausea, atypical chest pain

A 94-year-old female patient is admitted to home health for teaching on new medications prescribed for chronic atrial fibrillation and hypertension. Lately, she's also been experiencing nausea without vomiting, atypical chest pain, and epigastric pain. Radiology suggests possible gastric outlet obstruction or gastric volvulus.

Description	Code
Primary: Chronic atrial fibrillation, unspecified	I48.20
Secondary: Essential (primary) hypertension	I10
Secondary: Nausea without vomiting	R11.0
Secondary: Anterior chest-wall pain NOS	R07.89
Secondary: Epigastric pain	R10.13

The patient is admitted for teaching on new medications for chronic Afib and hypertension; thus they are assigned as primary and first secondary diagnosis. Her additional symptoms of nausea, chest pain and epigastric pain are not associated by the physician with her definitive diagnoses, and so they are coded separately. The physician's differential diagnoses may not be used until confirmed. Remember, most symptom codes are not acceptable as primary diagnosese in PDGM.

Exacerbated CAD with angina, fall with hip pain

A 93-year-old female is admitted to home health with exacerbated coronary artery disease with angina. She's also complaining of left hip pain after tripping over a root in her yard and landing on her left side. The physician documents a possible subtle fracture and sends her home with an order for a home health skilled nursing and physical therapy. Her history includes chronic obstructive tracheobronchitis, resolved breast cancer and a past right hip replacement. Her left hip x-ray was inconclusive.

Description	Code
Primary: Atherosclerotic heart disease of native coronary artery with unspecified angina pectoris	I25.119
Secondary: Pain in left hip	M25.552
Secondary: Chronic obstructive pulmonary disease, unspecified	J44.9
Secondary: Personal history of malignant neoplasm of breast	Z85.3
Secondary: Presence of right artificial hip joint	Z96.641
Secondary: Fall on same level from slipping, tripping and stumbling without subsequent striking against object, subsequent encounter	W01.0xxD

As the focus of care, CAD with angina is coded in the primary position. Although the physician suspects a hip fracture, testing so far is inconclusive and, therefore, only her symptoms can be coded. Note that most symptom codes are not acceptable primary diagnoses in the PDGM system.

Generalized anxiety disorder, syncope

A 93-year-old woman was hospitalized after fainting during a bingo game at the senior center. While in the hospital she was diagnosed with generalized anxiety disorder and was later admitted to home health for teaching on the condition, new medications prescribed to manage her symptoms and to monitor her for continued fainting episodes. She has mild hypertension but it is well-controlled with medication.

Description	Code
Primary: Generalized anxiety disorder	F41.1
Secondary: Syncope and collapse	R55
Secondary: Essential (primary) hypertension	I10

Generalized anxiety disorder is the focus of care and is thus coded primary. Since her syncope symptoms will be monitored, the symptom code is also assigned. Hypertension should always be coded when present. Remember, most symptom codes are unacceptable as primary diagnoses in PDGM.

Crohn's, seizures

A 70-year-old man suffered three seizures in two days and was hospitalized for investigate the cause. There is no diagnosis of epilepsy or any other reason given for the seizures. While in the hospital, he also suffered a flare of his Crohn's disease. He is admitted to home health with new medication for the Crohn's flare and to manage the seizure symptoms, for which no cause has been found.

Description	Code
Primary: Crohn's disease, unspecified, without complications	K50.90
Secondary: Unspecified convulsions	R56.9

As the focus of care, Crohn's is coded primary. Without an underlying diagnosis for the seizures, you must assign a symptom code. Remember, most symptom codes are unacceptable as primary diagnoses in PDGM.

Heart failure exacerbation, epistaxis from anticoagulant

A 70-year-old man is experiencing an acute exacerbation of chronic systolic heart failure. He also takes Coumadin for paroxysmal atrial fibrillation and began experiencing nosebleeds as an adverse effect from long-term use of the anticoagulant. He is still taking Coumadin.

Description	Code
Primary: Acute on chronic systolic (congestive) heart failure	I50.23
Secondary: Epistaxis	R04.0
Secondary: Adverse effect of anticoagulants, subsequent encounter	T45.515D
Secondary: Paroxysmal atrial fibrillation	I48.0
Secondary: Long term (current) use of anticoagulants	Z79.01

The acute heart failure exacerbation is the focus of care and is thus coded primary. Epistaxis, being caused by anticoagulant medication, is coded before the adverse effect of the drug code, in accordance with coding guidelines. The reason for the drug that caused the adverse effect, the paroxysmal atrial fibrillation, is assigned next. The patient's continued use of Coumadin is captured with Z79.01. Remember that most symptom codes cannot be a coded as the primary reason for home health under PDGM.

Nausea and vomiting from ibuprofen, rheumatoid arthritis

A 71-year-old woman is admitted to home health after being hospitalized for severe nausea and vomiting. It was determined that she took several 800-mg tablets of ibuprofen to manage joint pain caused by rheumatoid arthritis. The ibuprofen tablets had originally been prescribed for her daughter, with whom she lives. The patient thought they were the same as the over-the-counter Advil, which are 200-mg, she normally takes. She also suffers from mild hypertension.

Description	Code
Primary: Poisoning by propionic acid derivatives, accidental (unintentional), subsequent encounter	T39.311D
Secondary: Nausea with vomiting, unspecified	R11.2
Secondary: Rheumatoid arthritis, unspecified	M06.9
Secondary: Essential (primary) hypertension	I10

The patient took a medication that was prescribed for someone else and believed she was taking a smaller dose than what she actually was. Therefore, this scenario is a poisoning and the T code for the drug is coded before what it caused, the nausea and vomiting. The reason the patient was taking the ibuprofen, rheumatoid arthritis, is also coded. Since no further detail is provided, the unspecified code M06.9, must be used. Note that without more detail about which joints are affected and whether the diagnosis is seropositive, etc., a more specific rheumatoid arthritis code cannot be assigned. Her hypertension will require monitoring and thus it is coded.

Cancer surgery, elevated blood pressure

A 70-year-old woman recently underwent surgery for Kupffer cell sarcoma and is admitted to home health for aftercare. Her hospital record indicates that she's had elevated blood pressure following the surgery and anti-hypertensive medication has been prescribed. However, no diagnosis of hypertension was documented, and the physician did not respond to a query.

Description	Code
Primary: Aftercare following surgery for neoplasm	Z48.3
Secondary: Angiosarcoma of liver	C22.3
Secondary: Elevated blood-pressure reading, without diagnosis of hypertension	R03.0

Surgery was done for cancer, which necessitates the use of the Z48.3 aftercare code. The cancer is not stated as resolved and is thus coded as an active diagnosis. Kupffer cell sarcoma codes to angiosarcoma of liver, according to the alphabetic index. While the patient has elevated blood pressure and has been prescribed anti-hypertension medication, not hypertension diagnosis has been documented nor has been confirmed. Thus, only the symptom code, R03.0, can be assigned.

Chapter 19: Injury, Poisoning and Certain Other Consequences of External Causes (S00-T88)

Chapter 19 includes injuries, organized by body part or site beginning with the head and concluding with the ankle and foot, rather than by categories of injury. Other blocks within this chapter include effects of foreign body entering through natural orifice; burns and corrosions; frostbite; poisoning by, adverse effect of and under-dosing of drugs, medicaments and biological substances; toxic effects of substances chiefly non-medicinal as to source; other and unspecified effects of external causes; certain early complications of trauma; and complications of surgical and medical care, not elsewhere classified.

This chapter is the largest in the ICD-10-CM manual and encompasses the S and T alpha characters. The S-section is used for coding different types of injuries related to single body regions and the T-section covers injuries to unspecified body regions as well as poisoning and certain other consequences of external causes.

Secondary code(s) from Chapter 20, External causes of morbidity, are used to indicate the cause of injury. Codes within the T section that include the external cause do not require an additional external cause code.

A note at the beginning of the chapter indicates an additional code should be used to identify any retained foreign body, if applicable (Z18.-)

Chapter 19 has an Excludes 1 note indicating that this chapter specifically excludes birth trauma, found in Chapter 16 (P10-P15) and obstetrical trauma found in Chapter 15 (O70-O71).

Application of 7th Characters

Most categories in Chapter 19 have a 7th character requirement for each applicable code. With the exception of fractures, most categories have one of three 7th character values: A for initial encounter; D for subsequent encounter; and S for sequela. Categories for traumatic fractures have additional 7th character values. In general, focus on whether the patient is *still receiving active treatment* for the condition described by the code title when you choose a seventh character that corresponds to either an "initial" or "subsequent" encounter, according to the Coding Clinic. Note, the physician must determine whether the patient is receiving active treatment or ongoing care for the condition.

More specifically:

- 7th character "A", initial encounter, is used while the patient is receiving active treatment for the condition. Examples of active treatment

are: surgical treatment, emergency department encounter, and evaluation and treatment by a new physician. It doesn't matter if your agency isn't the first provider to see the patient for the condition, as long as your agency is providing active treatment for it, the seventh character "A" is what you should assign.

Specifically, antibiotic therapy for infected post-operative wounds as well as wound vac treatment for trauma wounds or dehisced wounds are both examples of active treatment that should be coded with an "A," regardless of setting.

- 7th character "D", subsequent encounter, is used for encounters after the patient has received active treatment of the condition and is receiving routine care for the condition during the healing or recovery phase. Examples of subsequent care are: cast change or removal, removal of external or internal fixation device, medication adjustment, routine aftercare and fracture care with the exception of when the patient delays seeking treatment and it results in a malunion or nonunion, and follow up visits following treatment of the injury or condition. *The aftercare Z codes should not be used for aftercare for conditions such as injuries or poisonings, where the 7th characters are provided to identify subsequent care.* For example, for aftercare of an injury, assign the original injury code with the 7th character "D" (subsequent encounter). **Also note**, you will continue to assign the injury code for patient who underwent a joint replacement to treat a hip fracture. The aftercare code Z47.1 (Aftercare following joint replacement surgery) is *not appropriate* in these types of scenarios, according to Coding Clinic Q3 2016 guidance.

- 7th character "S", sequela, is used for complications or conditions that arise as a direct result of an injury, such as scar formation and skin contractures after a burn, traumatic arthritis and quadriplegia after a spinal cord injury. The scars are sequelae of the burn, traumatic arthritis and quadriplegia after a spinal cord injury. When using a 7th character "S", it is necessary to use both the injury code that precipitated the sequela and the code for the sequela itself. The "S" is added only to the injury code, not the sequela code. The 7th character "S" identifies the injury responsible for the sequela. The specific type of sequela (e.g., scar) is sequenced first, followed by the injury code.

Note: 7th characters D and S do not apply to codes in category S06 with 6th character 7 - death due to brain injury prior to regaining consciousness, or 8 - death due to other cause prior to regaining consciousness.

In general, scenarios involving complications in which the agency is providing continuing treatment, such as for infected and dehisced wounds, are the most appropriate for considering the assignment of an initial encounter seventh character.

Situations that aren't truly complicated, like routine fracture healing, routine aftercare or when a patient experiences a complication in the hospital that resolves prior to the home health admission, don't meet these criteria and shouldn't be coded as initial encounters.

Nevertheless, be aware that every code choice must be supportable and defensible.

Coding of Injuries

Codes for traumatic wounds are classified in different ways, which may overlap. Consider:

- Wounds may be open (e.g., lacerations, punctures, animal bites, fractures), superficial (e.g., insect bites, splinters, abrasions, skin tears), or open/internal (e.g., intracranial hematoma, organ rupture, fractures).

- Wounds may be described as with or without an opening into a cavity. Example: S31.604D, Subsequent encounter for care of an unspecified open wound of abdominal wall, left lower quadrant with penetration into peritoneal cavity.

- Wounds may be described as complicated or without mention of complication. A wound is considered complicated if there is delayed healing, presence of a foreign body in the wound, or an infection.

A common error made by new coders is reporting a code for an open wound (trauma) injury for surgical wound complications or other wounds, including ulcers, because the referral information referred to **"an open wound"** of a particular location rather than the type of wound.

Almost all amputations are the result of other medical conditions rather than accidents and are not coded with codes from Chapter 19 unless there are complications of the post-surgical amputation stump, such as dehiscence (T87.81), infection (T87.4-), necrosis (T85.5-) or neuroma (T87.3-).

When coding injuries, assign separate codes for each injury unless a combination code is provided, in which case the combination code is assigned. Code T07, unspecified multiple injuries, should **not** be used in the inpatient setting unless information for a more specific code is not available. Traumatic injury codes (S00-T14.9) are **not** to be used for normal, healing surgical wounds or to identify complications of surgical wounds. The

code for the most serious injury, as determined by the provider and the focus of treatment, is sequenced first.

- Superficial injuries, such as abrasions or contusions, are not coded when associated with more severe injuries of the same site.

- When a primary injury results in damage to peripheral nerves or blood vessels, the primary injury is sequenced first with additional code(s) for injuries to the nerves and spinal cord (such as category S04), and/or injury to blood vessels (such as category S15). When the primary injury is to the blood vessels or nerves, that injury should be sequenced first.

Coding of Traumatic Fractures

The principles of multiple coding of injuries should be followed in coding fractures. Fractures of specific sites are coded individually by site in accordance with both the provisions within categories S02, S12, S22, S32, S42, S49, S52, S59, S62, S72, S79, S82, S89, S92 and the level of detail furnished by the medical record content. Multiple fractures are sequenced in accordance with the severity of the fracture.

Fracture codes require a great amount of specificity in order to code them accurately. Information that may be found in fracture codes includes the type of fracture (open or closed), specific anatomical site, whether the fracture is displaced or not, laterality, and healing status (i.e., routine healing versus delayed healing, nonunion or malunion). Laterality and identification of encounter type (initial, subsequent or sequela) are significant components of the code expansion.

A fracture not indicated as open or closed should be coded as closed. A fracture not indicated as displaced or not displaced should be coded as displaced.

More specific guidelines for traumatic fractures include:

- Traumatic fractures are coded using the appropriate 7th character for initial encounter (i.e., A, B, C) while receiving active treatment for the fracture. Examples of active treatment for the fracture are: surgical treatment, emergency department encounter, and evaluation and treatment by a new physician. The appropriate 7th character for initial encounter should also be assigned for a patient who delayed seeking treatment for the fracture or non-union. **Home health and hospice never use the 7th characters A, B or C when coding fractures**.

- In home health and hospice, fractures are coded using the appropriate 7th character for subsequent care for encounters after the patient has completed active treatment of the fracture and is receiving routine care for the fracture during the healing or recovery phase. Examples of fracture aftercare are: cast change or removal, removal of external or internal fixation device, medication adjustment, and follow-up visits following fracture treatment.

- Care for complications of surgical treatment for fracture repairs during the healing or recovery phase should be coded with the appropriate complication codes.

- Care of complications of fractures, such as malunion and nonunion, should be reported with the appropriate 7th character for subsequent care with nonunion (i.e., K, M, N) or subsequent care with malunion (i.e., P, Q, R).

- Some fracture categories provide for 7th character extensions to designate the type of open fracture based on the Gustilo open fracture classification. Refer to the shaded box of 7th character extension definitions at the top of category S52, (fracture of upper end of ulna) for a listing of all 7th character extension codes as an example. ***Coders must pay special attention to the list of appropriate 7th character codes at the top of each category of fracture in Chapter 19 to select the most appropriate code.***

Some situations related to fractures are coded from chapters other than chapter 19 such as the following:

- A code from category M80 should be used for any patient with known osteoporosis who suffers a fracture, even if the patient had a minor fall or trauma, if that fall or trauma would not usually break a normal, healthy bone. (Refer to M80, Osteoporosis with current pathological fracture in Chapter 13, Diseases of Musculoskeletal System.)

- Refer to Chapter 13, Diseases of the Musculoskeletal System and Connective Tissue for codes related to stress fractures (M84.3-), pathological fractures (M84.5-) or collapsed vertebrae (M48.5-).

- The aftercare Z codes should **not** be used for aftercare for traumatic fractures. For aftercare of a traumatic fracture, assign the original (acute) fracture code with the appropriate 7th character.

Coding of Burns and Corrosions

ICD-10-CM makes a distinction between burns and corrosions. The burn codes are for thermal burns, except sunburns, that come from a heat source, such as a fire or hot appliance. The burn codes are also for burns resulting from electricity and radiation. Corrosions are burns due to chemicals. The guidelines are the same for burns and corrosions.

Current burns (T20-T25) are classified by depth, extent and by agent (X code). Burns are classified as first degree (erythema), second degree (blistering), and third degree (full-thickness involvement). Burns of the

eye and internal organs (T26-T28) are classified by site, but not by degree.

Sequencing of burn and related condition codes

- Sequence first the code that reflects the highest degree of burn when more than one burn is present.

- When the reason for the admission or encounter is for treatment of multiple external burns, sequence first the code that reflects the burn of the highest degree.

- When the patient has both internal and external burns, the circumstances of admission govern the selection of the principal or first-listed diagnosis.

- When a patient is admitted for burn injuries and other related conditions, such as smoke inhalation and/or respiratory failure, the circumstances of admission govern the selection of the principal or first-listed diagnosis.

- Classify **burns of the same local site** (three character category level, T20-T28) but of different degrees to the subcategory identifying the highest degree recorded in the diagnosis.

- **Non-healing burns** are coded as acute burns.

- **Necrosis of burned skin** should be coded as a non-healing burn.

- For any documented **infected burn site**, use an additional code for the infection.

- Burns treated with **skin grafts** should be coded with the trauma codes for burns; and when applicable you can also code aftercare for transplant if you're also caring for the donor site (Z48.298).

Burns and corrosions Classified According to Extent of Body Surface Involved

Assign codes from category T31, Burns classified according to the extent of body surface involved, or T32, Corrosions classified to the extent of body surface involved, when the site of the burn is not specified or when there is a need for additional data. It is advisable to use category T31 as additional coding, when needed, to provide data for evaluating burn mortality, such as that needed by burn units. It also is advisable to use category T31 as an additional code for reporting purposes when there is mention of a third-degree burn involving 20% or more of the body surface.

Categories T31 and T32 are based on the classic "rule of nines" in estimating body surface: head and neck are assigned 9%, each arm 9%, each leg 18%, the anterior and posterior trunk 18% each, and genitalia 1%. Providers may change these percentage assignments where necessary to accommodate infants and children who have proportionately larger heads than adults, and adults who have large buttocks, thighs or abdomen that involve burns.

Coding sequela of burns

Encounters **for treatment of sequela** (late effects) of burns (i.e., scars or joint contractures) should be coded with the 7th character "S".

When appropriate, **both a code for a current burn or corrosion** with a 7th character of "D" and a burn or corrosion code with a 7th character "S" may be assigned on the same record (when both a current burn and a sequel of an old burn exist). Burns and corrosions do not heal at the same rate and a current healing wound may still exist with sequela of a healed burn or corrosion.

An **external cause code** should be used with burns and corrosions to identify the source and intent of the burn, as well as the place where it occurred.

Adverse Effects, Poisoning, Underdosing and Toxic Effects

Codes in categories T36-T65 are combination codes that include the substance that was taken as well as the intent. No additional external cause code is required for poisoning, toxic effects, adverse effects and underdosing codes.

- Do not code directly from the Table of Drugs and Chemicals. Always refer back to the Tabular List to confirm the correct code.

- Use as many codes as necessary to describe completely all drugs, medicinal or biological substances.

- If the same code would describe the causative agent for more than one adverse reaction, poisoning, toxic effect or underdosing, assign the code only once.

- If two or more drugs, medicinal or biological substances are reported, code each individually unless a combination code is listed in the Table of Drugs and Chemicals.

The occurrence of drug toxicity is classified in ICD-10-CM as follows:

Adverse Effect

When coding an adverse effect (hypersensitivity, reaction) of a drug that has been correctly prescribed and properly administered, assign the appropriate code for the nature of the adverse effect followed by the appropriate code for the adverse effect of the drug (T36-T50). The code for the drug should have a 5th or 6th character "5" (e.g., T36.0X5-). Examples of the nature of an adverse effect are tachycardia, delirium, gastrointestinal hemorrhaging, vomiting, hypokalemia, hepatitis, renal failure or respiratory failure.

Poisoning

When coding a poisoning or reaction to the improper use of a medication (e.g., overdose, wrong substance given or taken in error, wrong route of administration), first assign the appropriate code from categories T36-T50, followed by additional code(s) for all manifestations of the poisoning. The poisoning codes have an associated intent as their 5th or 6th character (accidental, intentional self-harm, assault, and undetermined). When no intent of poisoning is indicated, code to accidental. Undetermined intent is only used when there is specific documentation in the record that the intent of the poisoning cannot be determined.

If there is also a diagnosis of abuse or dependence of the substance, the abuse or dependence is assigned as an additional code.

Examples of poisoning include:

- **Error** was made in drug prescription or in the administration of the drug by provider, nurse, patient or other person.

- If an **overdose of a drug** was intentionally taken or administered and resulted in drug toxicity, it would be coded as a poisoning.

- **Nonprescription drug or medicinal agent taken in combination with a correctly prescribed** and properly administered drug, any drug toxicity or other reaction resulting from the interaction of the two drugs would be classified as a poisoning.

- When a reaction results from the **interaction of drug(s) and alcohol,** this would be classified as a poisoning.

Underdosing

Underdosing refers to taking less of a medication than is prescribed by the provider or as instructed by the manufacturer whether inadvertently or deliberately. For underdosing, a code from categories T36-T50 with a fifth or sixth character of "6" is used.

Use an additional code for underdosing intent such as patient's non-compliance with medical treatment and regimen (Z91.12-, Z91.13- or Z91.14) or failure in dosage during surgical and medical care (Y63.6-Y63.9). Reminder, the physician needs to confirm this occurrence.

Codes for underdosing should never be assigned as principal or first-listed codes. If a patient has a relapse or exacerbation of the medical condition for which the drug is prescribed because of the reduction in dose, then the medical condition itself should be coded.

Toxic Effects

A toxic effect is classified when a harmful substance is ingested or comes in contact with a person. Codes for the toxic effect of substances that are chiefly nonmedicinal as a source (T51-T65) include a 7th character to indicate the intention.

There are multiple notes at the top of this block of codes. One states to use an additional code for all associated manifestations of toxic effect, such as respiratory conditions due to external agents (J60-J70), personal history of foreign body fully removed (Z87.821) and to identify any retained foreign body, if applicable (Z18.-). The second instructional note states: when no intent is indicated, code to accidental. Undetermined intent is only for use when there is specific documentation in the record that the intent of the toxic effect cannot be determined.

Adult and child abuse, neglect and other maltreatment

Sequence first the appropriate code from categories T74.- (Adult and child abuse, neglect and other maltreatment, confirmed) or T76.- (Adult and child abuse, neglect and other maltreatment, unspecified) for any abuse, neglect and other maltreatment, followed by any accompanying mental health or injury code(s).

If the documentation in the medical record states abuse or neglect, it is coded as confirmed (T74.-). An external cause code from the assault section (X92-Y08) for the cause of any physical injuries and a perpetrator code (Y07) also should be added if the perpetrator of the abuse is known for cases of confirmed abuse or neglect.

If **suspected abuse and neglect** is documented in the medical record, the abuse or neglect is coded as suspected (T76.-) without an external cause or perpetrator code reported.

Complications of care

Code assignment for complications of care is *based on the provider's documentation of the relationship between the condition and the care or procedure.* This guideline applies to any complication of care, regardless of the chapter the code is located in. There must be a cause-and-effect relationship between the care provided and the condition, and an indication in the documentation that it is a complication. *Reminder: Not all conditions that occur during or following medical care or surgery are classified as complications.*

Pain due to medical devices

Pain associated with devices, implants or grafts left in a surgical site is assigned to the appropriate code(s) found in Chapter 19. Specific codes for pain due to medical devices are found in the T code section of ICD-10-CM, according to type of device.

Use additional code(s) from category G89 to identify acute or chronic pain due to the presence of a device, implant or graft (G89.18 or G89.28). Example: a subsequent encounter for a painful hip prosthesis is coded T84.84xD. Additional pain codes are located in multiple body system chapters.

Transplant complications

Codes under category T86, Complications of transplanted organs and tissues, are used for both complications and rejection of transplanted organs. A transplant complication code is only assigned if the complication affects the function of the transplanted organ. Two codes are required to fully describe a transplant complication: the appropriate code from category T86 and a secondary code that identifies the complication.

Pre-existing conditions or conditions that develop after the transplant are not coded as complications unless they affect the function of the transplanted organs.

Patients who have undergone kidney transplant may still have some form of chronic kidney disease (CKD) because the kidney transplant may not fully restore kidney function. A code from T86.1- should be assigned for documented complications of a kidney transplant, such as a transplant failure or rejection or other transplant complication. A code from T86.1- should <u>not</u> be assigned for post kidney transplant patients who have chronic kidney disease (CKD) unless a transplant complication such as transplant failure or rejection is documented. If the documentation is unclear as to whether the patient has a complication of the transplant, query the provider.

Conditions that affect the function of the transplanted kidney, other than CKD, should be assigned a code from T86.1-, Complications of kidney transplant, and a secondary code that identifies the complication. For patients with CKD following a kidney transplant, but who do not have complications such as failure or rejection, refer to codes in category N18 for CKD stages.

Complication codes that include external cause

As with certain other T codes, some of the complications of care codes have the external cause included in the code. These combination codes include the nature of the complication as well as the type of procedure that caused the complication. No external cause code indicating the type of procedure is necessary for these codes.

Complications of care codes within body system chapters

Intraoperative and postprocedural complication codes are found within body system chapters with codes specific to the organs and structures to that body system. These codes should be sequenced first, followed by a code(s) for the specific complication, if applicable.

Codes for personal or family history of conditions that have been resolved related to injuries such as traumatic fractures, and other consequences are found in chapter 21, Factors influencing health status and contact with health services, rather than in Chapter 19. Some examples include: Z87.81, Personal history of healed traumatic fracture; and Personal history of abuse or neglect (childhood Z62.81- or adult Z91.41-).

Codes for complications of surgical and medical care not elsewhere classified include:

- Complications following infusion, transfusion and therapeutic injection (e.g., T80.212-, Local infection due to central venous catheter)

- ABO, Rh and non-ABO incompatibility reactions due to transfusions of blood and blood products. Anaphylactic reaction due to serum, administration of blood and blood products, vaccine, and other serum (T80.3-T80.89).

- Complications of procedures, not elsewhere classified such as postprocedural shock (T81.1-T81.19); disruption of wound (T81.30-T81.33); infection following a procedure (T81.4-), with an additional code to identify infection and an additional code from R65.2- to identify severe sepsis, if applicable; and complications of foreign body accidentally left in the body (T81.5-, T81.6-)

- Complications of cardiac and vascular prosthetic devices, implants and grafts (T82.-)

- Complications of genitourinary prosthetic devices, implants and grafts (T83.-), which includes complications of urinary catheters, cystostomy catheters, other urinary devices and implants, and complications related to prosthetic devices, implants and grafts of the genitourinary tract.

- Complications of internal orthopedic prosthetic devices, implants and grafts. (T84.-).

- Complications of other internal prosthetic devices, implants and grafts. (T85.-)

- Complications of transplanted organs and tissues (T86.-).

- Complications peculiar to reattachment and amputation (T87.-)

- Other complications of surgical and medical care, not elsewhere classified (T88.-).

Complications involving stoma may be reported elsewhere. For example, a tracheostomy complication is reported using a code from J95.0- in Chapter 10. A complication of an esophagostomy, colostomy or enterostomy is reported using a code from K94.- from Chapter 11.

Special Coding Issues

Wounds

Many wounds in the Medicare home care population are the intentional result of medical treatment. Coding surgical wounds and medical amputations using Chapter 19 open wound codes is a mistake because those codes are reserved for injuries (from accidents or violence). Medically-caused wounds should not be coded from Chapter 19, unless they are complicated. Even then, they should never be coded as open wounds. If there is a complication of a surgery, a code from Chapter 19 will be used instead of the Z code for aftercare. The term "complication" should be referenced in the Volume 2 Alphabetic Index. Once the term "complication" is found, reference the type of complication, such as infection or mechanical, to find the correct code.

Superficial injuries

Skin tears or partial thickness wounds are typically superficial injuries and are coded as such. Reference "injury, superficial" in the Alphabetic Index. Care for skin tears is typically not covered by Medicare because the wound care is simple. If the skin tear is complicated in some way – the tear no longer has a flap and is infected or there is an underlying condition that is complicating the wound's healing – then you may consider coding the skin tear as a trauma wound. For the trauma wound to be coded as primary, documentation must support the skilled care needed and the underlying condition. Consult your specific MAC's instructions for coding skin tears that require skilled care.

Infection/complication coding

Occasionally, a post-surgical infection or other surgical complication code may be appropriate. OASIS requires that home care clinicians use the WOCN guidelines to indicate the status of the surgical wound. "Not healing" includes signs and symptoms of infection and delayed healing. If there are signs and symptoms of infection, do not use the aftercare code for that surgery. The aftercare code is indicated only for routine, uncomplicated care. Subcategory T81.4- codes are commonly used for a post-surgical infection; however, some post-operative infections have more specific codes, such as infected amputation, which is coded with T87.4-. Reference the Alphabetic Index to find the most specific code.

The T81.4- subcategory allows coders to report the depth of the infection. There are codes to specify whether the surgical wound infection is affecting the superficial incision surgical site (T81.41-), the deep incisional surgical site (T81.42-) or the organ and space surgical site (T81.43-). Other surgical site and unspecified options are also available (T81.49- and T81.40-). Each of these codes requires a seventh character: "A," "D" or "S." Also, make note of the inclusion terms at each code, such as "subcutaneous abscess following a procedure," to help guide the appropriate code choice.

When a patient is admitted to home care primarily for **surgical wound assessment and treatment**, the presence of a surgical drain is not a complication; it is a normal part of care for some surgical wounds. Care of surgical drains is included in the aftercare code for routine surgical care. If care includes removal or changing of the surgical drain, use Z48.03.

What counts as a wound?

A **lesion** is a broad term used to describe an area of pathologically altered tissue. Sores, ulcers, rashes, crusts, edema, trauma wounds, etc. are all considered lesions.

The **port-a-cath or mediport site** is considered a surgical wound as long as it is present, even if healed over. Implanted infusion devices or venous access devices are considered surgical wounds, and it does not matter whether the device is accessed with any particular frequency. Only **central venous catheters** are considered surgical wounds. Care of the uncomplicated venous or arterial line is coded Z45.2, Adjustment and management of a vascular catheter. Subsequent encounter to care for a bloodstream infection due to central venous catheter is coded T80.211D. Local infection at the exit or insertion site due to central venous catheter is coded with T80.212D, but central line associated infections (including PICC lines) are coded to T80.218D.

Extravasation or infiltration of a vesicant agent into surrounding tissue is a more serious complication of IV therapy and is coded to T80.810 if related to the administration of vesicant antineoplastic chemotherapy or T80.818 if there is extravasation of another vesicant agent.

Chapter 19

S00 - T88

CHAPTER 19: INJURY, POISONING AND CERTAIN OTHER CONSEQUENCES OF EXTERNAL CAUSES (S00-T88)

Note:

Use secondary code(s) from Chapter 20, External causes of morbidity, to indicate cause of injury. Codes within the T section that include the external cause do not require an additional external cause code

The chapter uses the S-section for coding different types of injuries related to single body regions and the T-section to cover injuries to unspecified body regions as well as poisoning and certain other consequences of external causes.

Use additional code to identify any retained foreign body, if applicable (Z18.-)

EXCLUDES 1   birth trauma (P10-P15)
obstetric trauma (O70-O71)

GUIDELINES   Section I.C.19.a

Most categories in chapter 19 have a 7th character requirement for each applicable code ... While the patient may be seen by a new or different provider over the course of treatment for an injury, assignment of the 7th character is based on whether the patient is undergoing active treatment and not whether the provider is seeing the patient for the first time ... 7th character "D" subsequent encounter is used for encounters after the patient has completed active treatment of the condition and is receiving routine care for the condition during the healing or recovery phase.

The aftercare Z codes should not be used for aftercare for conditions such as injuries or poisonings, where 7th characters are provided to identify subsequent care. For example, for aftercare of an injury, assign the acute injury code with the 7th character "D" (subsequent encounter).

7th character "S", sequela, is for use for complications or conditions that arise as a direct result of a condition, such as scar formation after a burn. The scars are sequelae of the burn. When using 7th character "S", it is necessary to use both the injury code that precipitated the sequela and the code for the sequela itself. The "S" is added only to the injury code, not the sequela code. The 7th character "S" identifies the injury responsible for the sequela. The specific type of sequela (e.g. scar) is sequenced first, followed by the injury code.

CODING TIPS ✓   7th character A is acceptable in home health and hospice when active treatment is provided, such as antibiotics for an infected wound or a wound vac for a dehisced wound. D is used when the complication or injury is now healing. Think of D as aftercare. S is used for sequela of the injury or complication. Sequela is a residual deficit or condition produced as a result of the injury or complication after the original injury or complication has healed.

This chapter contains the following blocks:

S00-S09	Injuries to the head
S10-S19	Injuries to the neck
S20-S29	Injuries to the thorax
S30-S39	Injuries to the abdomen, lower back, lumbar spine, pelvis and external genitals
S40-S49	Injuries to the shoulder and upper arm
S50-S59	Injuries to the elbow and forearm
S60-S69	Injuries to the wrist, hand and fingers
S70-S79	Injuries to the hip and thigh
S80-S89	Injuries to the knee and lower leg
S90-S99	Injuries to the ankle and foot
T07	Injuries involving multiple body regions

T14	Injury of unspecified body region
T15-T19	Effects of foreign body entering through natural orifice
T20-T25	Burns and corrosions of external body surface, specified by site
T26-T28	Burns and corrosions confined to eye and internal organs
T30-T32	Burns and corrosions of multiple and unspecified body regions
T33-T34	Frostbite
T36-T50	Poisoning by, adverse effect of and underdosing of drugs, medicaments and biological substances
T51-T65	Toxic effects of substances chiefly nonmedicinal as to source
T66-T78	Other and unspecified effects of external causes
T79	Certain early complications of trauma
T80-T88	Complications of surgical and medical care, not elsewhere classified

Injuries to the head   (S00-S09)

INCLUDES   injuries of ear
injuries of eye
injuries of face [any part]
injuries of gum
injuries of jaw
injuries of oral cavity
injuries of palate
injuries of periocular area
injuries of scalp
injuries of temporomandibular joint area
injuries of tongue
injuries of tooth

Code also:
for any associated infection

EXCLUDES 2   burns and corrosions (T20-T32)
effects of foreign body in ear (T16)
effects of foreign body in larynx (T17.3)
effects of foreign body in mouth NOS (T18.0)
effects of foreign body in nose (T17.0-T17.1)
effects of foreign body in pharynx (T17.2)
effects of foreign body on external eye (T15.-)
frostbite (T33-T34)
insect bite or sting, venomous (T63.4)

GUIDELINES   Section I.C.19.c.2)

Multiple fractures are sequenced in accordance with the severity of the fracture.

GUIDELINES   Section I.C.19.b.1)-2)

When coding injuries, assign separate codes for each injury unless a combination code is provided, in which case the combination code is assigned ... Traumatic injury codes (S00-T14.9) are not to be used for normal, healing surgical wounds or to identify complications of surgical wounds. The code for the most serious injury, as determined by the provider and the focus of treatment, is sequenced first.

1) Superficial injuries such as abrasions or contusions are not coded when associated with more severe injuries of the same site.

2) When a primary injury results in minor damage to peripheral nerves or blood vessels, the primary injury is sequenced first with additional code(s) for injuries to nerves and spinal cord (such as category S04), and/or injury to blood vessels (such as category S15). When the primary injury is to the blood vessels or nerves, that injury should be sequenced first.

4 4th digit required   **5** 5th digit required   **6** 6th digit required   **7** 7th digit required   **✓** 7th digit placeholder   **+** Additional code   **⊟** Laterality

1456   *DecisionHealth's* FY 2020 Complete Home Health ICD-10-CM Diagnosis Coding Manual

Chapter 19

S00-T88

GUIDELINES Section I.C.19.c
Coding of Traumatic Fractures: The principles of multiple coding of injuries should be followed in coding fractures. Fractures of specified sites are coded individually by site in accordance with both the provisions within categories S02, S12, S22, S32, S42, S49, S52, S59, S62, S72, S79, S82, S89, S92 and the level of detail furnished by medical record content. A fracture not indicated as open or closed should be coded to closed. A fracture not indicated whether displaced or not displaced should be coded to displaced.

CODING TIPS ✓ 7th character A is acceptable in home health and hospice when active treatment is provided, such as antibiotics for an infected wound or a wound vac for a dehisced wound. D is used when the complication or injury is now healing. Think of D as aftercare. S is used for sequela of the injury or complication. Sequela is a residual deficit or condition produced as a result of the injury or complication after the original injury or complication has healed.

4 S00 Superficial injury of head
> **EXCLUDES 1** diffuse cerebral contusion
> (S06.2-)
> focal cerebral contusion
> (S06.3-)
> injury of eye and orbit (S05.-)
> open wound of head (S01.-)

> The appropriate 7th character is to be added to each code from category S00
> A   initial encounter
> D   subsequent encounter
> S   sequela

5 S00.0 Superficial injury of scalp

!Q 7 S00.00X- Unspecified superficial injury of scalp

!Q 7 S00.01X- Abrasion of scalp

!Q 7 S00.02X- Blister (nonthermal) of scalp

!Q 7 S00.03X- Contusion of scalp
Bruise of scalp
Hematoma of scalp

!Q 7 S00.04X- External constriction of part of scalp

!Q 7 S00.05X- Superficial foreign body of scalp
Splinter in the scalp

!Q 7 S00.06X- Insect bite (nonvenomous) of scalp

!Q 7 S00.07X- Other superficial bite of scalp
> **EXCLUDES 1** open bite of scalp
> (S01.05)

5 S00.1 Contusion of eyelid and periocular area
Black eye
> **EXCLUDES 2** contusion of eyeball and
> orbital tissues (S05.1)

!Q 7 S00.10X- Contusion of unspecified eyelid and periocular area

!Q 7 S00.11X- Contusion of right eyelid and periocular area

!Q 7 S00.12X- Contusion of left eyelid and periocular area

5 S00.2 Other and unspecified superficial injuries of eyelid and periocular area
> **EXCLUDES 2** superficial injury of
> conjunctiva and cornea
> (S05.0-)

6 S00.20 Unspecified superficial injury of eyelid and periocular area

!Q 7 S00.201- Unspecified superficial injury of right eyelid and periocular area

!Q 7 S00.202- Unspecified superficial injury of left eyelid and periocular area

!Q 7 S00.209- Unspecified superficial injury of unspecified eyelid and periocular area

6 S00.21 Abrasion of eyelid and periocular area

!Q 7 S00.211- Abrasion of right eyelid and periocular area

!Q 7 S00.212- Abrasion of left eyelid and periocular area

!Q 7 S00.219- Abrasion of unspecified eyelid and periocular area

6 S00.22 Blister (nonthermal) of eyelid and periocular area

!Q 7 S00.221- Blister (nonthermal) of right eyelid and periocular area

!Q 7 S00.222- Blister (nonthermal) of left eyelid and periocular area

!Q 7 S00.229- Blister (nonthermal) of unspecified eyelid and periocular area

6 S00.24 External constriction of eyelid and periocular area

!Q 7 S00.241- External constriction of right eyelid and periocular area

!Q 7 S00.242- External constriction of left eyelid and periocular area

!Q 7 S00.249- External constriction of unspecified eyelid and periocular area

6 S00.25 Superficial foreign body of eyelid and periocular area
Splinter of eyelid and periocular area
> **EXCLUDES 2** retained foreign body in
> eyelid (H02.81-)

!Q 7 S00.251- Superficial foreign body of right eyelid and periocular area

!Q 7 S00.252- Superficial foreign body of left eyelid and periocular area

!Q 7 S00.259- Superficial foreign body of unspecified eyelid and periocular area

6 S00.26 Insect bite (nonvenomous) of eyelid and periocular area

!Q 7 S00.261- Insect bite (nonvenomous) of right eyelid and periocular area

!Q 7 S00.262- Insect bite (nonvenomous) of left eyelid and periocular area

!Q 7 S00.269- Insect bite (nonvenomous) of unspecified eyelid and periocular area

6 S00.27 Other superficial bite of eyelid and periocular area
> **EXCLUDES 1** open bite of eyelid and
> periocular area
> (S01.15)

!Q 7 S00.271- Other superficial bite of right eyelid and periocular area

!Q 7 S00.272- Other superficial bite of left eyelid and periocular area

!Q 7 S00.279- Other superficial bite of unspecified eyelid and periocular area

★ New ▲ Revised **Px** Primary **SP** PDGM Px **SL** Low CoM **SH** High CoM **!Q** Quest. Encounter **H** Hospice non-cancer Dx   Unspecified   **M** *Manifestation*

DecisionHealth's FY 2020 Complete Home Health ICD-10-CM Diagnosis Coding Manual

1457

⑤ S00.3   **Superficial injury of nose**

!Q 7⃣ S00.30X-   Unspecified superficial injury of nose

!Q 7⃣ S00.31X-   Abrasion of nose

!Q 7⃣ S00.32X-   Blister (nonthermal) of nose

!Q 7⃣ S00.33X-   Contusion of nose
Bruise of nose
Hematoma of nose

!Q 7⃣ S00.34X-   External constriction of nose

!Q 7⃣ S00.35X-   Superficial foreign body of nose
Splinter in the nose

!Q 7⃣ S00.36X-   Insect bite (nonvenomous) of nose

!Q 7⃣ S00.37X-   Other superficial bite of nose
EXCLUDES 1   open bite of nose (S01.25)

⑤ S00.4   **Superficial injury of ear**

⑥ S00.40   Unspecified superficial injury of ear

⊟ !Q 7⃣ S00.401-   Unspecified superficial injury of right ear

⊟ !Q 7⃣ S00.402-   Unspecified superficial injury of left ear

⊟ !Q 7⃣ S00.409-   Unspecified superficial injury of unspecified ear

⑥ S00.41   Abrasion of ear

⊟ !Q 7⃣ S00.411-   Abrasion of right ear

⊟ !Q 7⃣ S00.412-   Abrasion of left ear

⊟ !Q 7⃣ S00.419-   Abrasion of unspecified ear

⑥ S00.42   Blister (nonthermal) of ear

⊟ !Q 7⃣ S00.421-   Blister (nonthermal) of right ear

⊟ !Q 7⃣ S00.422-   Blister (nonthermal) of left ear

⊟ !Q 7⃣ S00.429-   Blister (nonthermal) of unspecified ear

⑥ S00.43   Contusion of ear
Bruise of ear
Hematoma of ear

⊟ !Q 7⃣ S00.431-   Contusion of right ear

⊟ !Q 7⃣ S00.432-   Contusion of left ear

⊟ !Q 7⃣ S00.439-   Contusion of unspecified ear

⑥ S00.44   External constriction of ear

⊟ !Q 7⃣ S00.441-   External constriction of right ear

⊟ !Q 7⃣ S00.442-   External constriction of left ear

⊟ !Q 7⃣ S00.449-   External constriction of unspecified ear

⑥ S00.45   Superficial foreign body of ear
Splinter in the ear

⊟ !Q 7⃣ S00.451-   Superficial foreign body of right ear

⊟ !Q 7⃣ S00.452-   Superficial foreign body of left ear

⊟ !Q 7⃣ S00.459-   Superficial foreign body of unspecified ear

⑥ S00.46   Insect bite (nonvenomous) of ear

⊟ !Q 7⃣ S00.461-   Insect bite (nonvenomous) of right ear

⊟ !Q 7⃣ S00.462-   Insect bite (nonvenomous) of left ear

⊟ !Q 7⃣ S00.469-   Insect bite (nonvenomous) of unspecified ear

⑥ S00.47   Other superficial bite of ear
EXCLUDES 1   open bite of ear (S01.35)

⊟ !Q 7⃣ S00.471-   Other superficial bite of right ear

⊟ !Q 7⃣ S00.472-   Other superficial bite of left ear

⊟ !Q 7⃣ S00.479-   Other superficial bite of unspecified ear

⑤ S00.5   **Superficial injury of lip and oral cavity**

⑥ S00.50   Unspecified superficial injury of lip and oral cavity

!Q 7⃣ S00.501-   Unspecified superficial injury of lip

!Q 7⃣ S00.502-   Unspecified superficial injury of oral cavity

⑥ S00.51   Abrasion of lip and oral cavity

!Q 7⃣ S00.511-   Abrasion of lip

!Q 7⃣ S00.512-   Abrasion of oral cavity

⑥ S00.52   Blister (nonthermal) of lip and oral cavity

!Q 7⃣ S00.521-   Blister (nonthermal) of lip

!Q 7⃣ S00.522-   Blister (nonthermal) of oral cavity

⑥ S00.53   Contusion of lip and oral cavity

!Q 7⃣ S00.531-   Contusion of lip
Bruise of lip
Hematoma of lip

!Q 7⃣ S00.532-   Contusion of oral cavity
Bruise of oral cavity
Hematoma of oral cavity

⑥ S00.54   External constriction of lip and oral cavity

!Q 7⃣ S00.541-   External constriction of lip

!Q 7⃣ S00.542-   External constriction of oral cavity

⑥ S00.55   Superficial foreign body of lip and oral cavity

!Q 7⃣ S00.551-   Superficial foreign body of lip
Splinter of lip and oral cavity

!Q 7⃣ S00.552-   Superficial foreign body of oral cavity
Splinter of lip and oral cavity

⑥ S00.56   Insect bite (nonvenomous) of lip and oral cavity

!Q 7⃣ S00.561-   Insect bite (nonvenomous) of lip

!Q 7⃣ S00.562-   Insect bite (nonvenomous) of oral cavity

⑥ S00.57   Other superficial bite of lip and oral cavity

!Q 7⃣ S00.571-   Other superficial bite of lip
EXCLUDES 1   open bite of lip (S01.551)

!Q 7⃣ S00.572-   Other superficial bite of oral cavity
EXCLUDES 1   open bite of oral cavity (S01.552)

⑤ S00.8   **Superficial injury of other parts of head**
Superficial injuries of face [any part]

!Q 7⃣ S00.80X-   Unspecified superficial injury of other part of head

!Q 7⃣ S00.81X-   Abrasion of other part of head

!Q 7⃣ S00.82X-   Blister (nonthermal) of other part of head

!Q 7⃣ S00.83X-   Contusion of other part of head
Bruise of other part of head
Hematoma of other part of head

!Q 7⃣ S00.84X-   External constriction of other part of head

!Q 7⃣ S00.85X-   Superficial foreign body of other part of head

---

4⃣ 4th digit required   ⑤ 5th digit required   ⑥ 6th digit required   7⃣ 7th digit required   7⃣ 7th digit placeholder   ✚ Additional code   ⊟ Laterality

1458   *DecisionHealth's* FY 2020 Complete Home Health ICD-10-CM Diagnosis Coding Manual

Splinter in other part of head

!Q ☑ S00.86X- **Insect bite (nonvenomous) of other part of head**

!Q ☑ S00.87X- **Other superficial bite of other part of head**

EXCLUDES 1 open bite of other part of head (S01.85)

⑤ S00.9 **Superficial injury of unspecified part of head**

!Q ☑ S00.90X- **Unspecified superficial injury of unspecified part of head**

!Q ☑ S00.91X- **Abrasion of unspecified part of head**

!Q ☑ S00.92X- **Blister (nonthermal) of unspecified part of head**

!Q ☑ S00.93X- **Contusion of unspecified part of head**

Bruise of head
Hematoma of head

!Q ☑ S00.94X- **External constriction of unspecified part of head**

!Q ☑ S00.95X- **Superficial foreign body of unspecified part of head**

Splinter of head

!Q ☑ S00.96X- **Insect bite (nonvenomous) of unspecified part of head**

!Q ☑ S00.97X- **Other superficial bite of unspecified part of head**

EXCLUDES 1 open bite of head (S01.95)

④ S01 **Open wound of head**

Code also any associated:
injury of cranial nerve (S04.-)
injury of muscle and tendon of head (S09.1-)
intracranial injury (S06.-)
wound infection

EXCLUDES 1 open skull fracture (S02.- with 7th character B)

EXCLUDES 2 injury of eye and orbit (S05.-)
traumatic amputation of part of head (S08.-)

The appropriate 7th character is to be added to each code from category S01
A   initial encounter
D   subsequent encounter
S   sequela

CODING TIPS ✓ Open wound codes are used for wounds caused by trauma. Do not assign a code for "open wound" unless the etiology of the wound is related to trauma. Do not use Z codes for any aspect of care of a trauma wound, e.g. no Z code for dressing changes, drain care, or suture removal.

CODING TIPS ✓ No aftercare code applies. The 7th character "D" is the default for home care and hospice when providing aftercare for a healing or resolving condition; "A" is used for active treatment such as antibiotics or more than routine wound care; "S" may be used to indicate a residual condition after the original injury has healed.

⑤ S01.0 **Open wound of scalp**
EXCLUDES 1 avulsion of scalp (S08.0)

SP ☑ S01.00X- **Unspecified open wound of scalp**

SP ☑ S01.01X- **Laceration without foreign body of scalp**

SP ☑ S01.02X- **Laceration with foreign body of scalp**

SP ☑ S01.03X- **Puncture wound without foreign body of scalp**

SP ☑ S01.04X- **Puncture wound with foreign body of scalp**

SP ☑ S01.05X- **Open bite of scalp**
Bite of scalp NOS
EXCLUDES 1 superficial bite of scalp (S00.06, S00.07-)

⑤ S01.1 **Open wound of eyelid and periocular area**
Open wound of eyelid and periocular area with or without involvement of lacrimal passages

⑥ S01.10 **Unspecified open wound of eyelid and periocular area**

⊟ SP 7 S01.101- **Unspecified open wound of right eyelid and periocular area**

⊟ SP 7 S01.102- **Unspecified open wound of left eyelid and periocular area**

⊟ !Q 7 S01.109- **Unspecified open wound of unspecified eyelid and periocular area**

⑥ S01.11 **Laceration without foreign body of eyelid and periocular area**

⊟ SP 7 S01.111- **Laceration without foreign body of right eyelid and periocular area**

⊟ SP 7 S01.112- **Laceration without foreign body of left eyelid and periocular area**

⊟ !Q 7 S01.119- **Laceration without foreign body of unspecified eyelid and periocular area**

⑥ S01.12 **Laceration with foreign body of eyelid and periocular area**

⊟ SP 7 S01.121- **Laceration with foreign body of right eyelid and periocular area**

⊟ SP 7 S01.122- **Laceration with foreign body of left eyelid and periocular area**

⊟ !Q 7 S01.129- **Laceration with foreign body of unspecified eyelid and periocular area**

⑥ S01.13 **Puncture wound without foreign body of eyelid and periocular area**

⊟ SP 7 S01.131- **Puncture wound without foreign body of right eyelid and periocular area**

⊟ SP 7 S01.132- **Puncture wound without foreign body of left eyelid and periocular area**

⊟ !Q 7 S01.139- **Puncture wound without foreign body of unspecified eyelid and periocular area**

⑥ S01.14 **Puncture wound with foreign body of eyelid and periocular area**

⊟ SP 7 S01.141- **Puncture wound with foreign body of right eyelid and periocular area**

⊟ SP 7 S01.142- **Puncture wound with foreign body of left eyelid and periocular area**

★ New ▲ Revised Px Primary SP PDGM Px SL Low CoM SH High CoM !Q Quest. Encounter Ⓗ Hospice non-cancer Dx Unspecified M Manifestation

DecisionHealth's FY 2020 Complete Home Health ICD-10-CM Diagnosis Coding Manual

1459

Chapter 19

S00-T88

☐ **IQ** 7 **S01.149-** Puncture wound with foreign body of unspecified eyelid and periocular area

6 **S01.15** Open bite of eyelid and periocular area
Bite of eyelid and periocular area NOS
EXCLUDES 1 superficial bite of eyelid and periocular area (S00.26, S00.27)

☐ **SP** 7 **S01.151-** Open bite of right eyelid and periocular area

☐ **SP** 7 **S01.152-** Open bite of left eyelid and periocular area

☐ **IQ** 7 **S01.159-** Open bite of unspecified eyelid and periocular area

5 **S01.2** Open wound of nose

SP ☑ **S01.20X-** Unspecified open wound of nose

SP ☑ **S01.21X-** Laceration without foreign body of nose

SP ☑ **S01.22X-** Laceration with foreign body of nose

SP ☑ **S01.23X-** Puncture wound without foreign body of nose

SP ☑ **S01.24X-** Puncture wound with foreign body of nose

SP ☑ **S01.25X-** Open bite of nose
Bite of nose NOS
EXCLUDES 1 superficial bite of nose (S00.36, S00.37)

5 **S01.3** Open wound of ear

6 **S01.30** Unspecified open wound of ear

☐ **SP** 7 **S01.301-** Unspecified open wound of right ear

☐ **SP** 7 **S01.302-** Unspecified open wound of left ear

☐ **IQ** 7 **S01.309-** Unspecified open wound of unspecified ear

6 **S01.31** Laceration without foreign body of ear

☐ **SP** 7 **S01.311-** Laceration without foreign body of right ear

☐ **SP** 7 **S01.312-** Laceration without foreign body of left ear

☐ **IQ** 7 **S01.319-** Laceration without foreign body of unspecified ear

6 **S01.32** Laceration with foreign body of ear

☐ **SP** 7 **S01.321-** Laceration with foreign body of right ear

☐ **SP** 7 **S01.322-** Laceration with foreign body of left ear

☐ **IQ** 7 **S01.329-** Laceration with foreign body of unspecified ear

6 **S01.33** Puncture wound without foreign body of ear

☐ **SP** 7 **S01.331-** Puncture wound without foreign body of right ear

☐ **SP** 7 **S01.332-** Puncture wound without foreign body of left ear

☐ **IQ** 7 **S01.339-** Puncture wound without foreign body of unspecified ear

6 **S01.34** Puncture wound with foreign body of ear

☐ **SP** 7 **S01.341-** Puncture wound with foreign body of right ear

☐ **SP** 7 **S01.342-** Puncture wound with foreign body of left ear

☐ **IQ** 7 **S01.349-** Puncture wound with foreign body of unspecified ear

6 **S01.35** Open bite of ear
Bite of ear NOS
EXCLUDES 1 superficial bite of ear (S00.46, S00.47)

☐ **SP** 7 **S01.351-** Open bite of right ear

☐ **SP** 7 **S01.352-** Open bite of left ear

☐ **IQ** 7 **S01.359-** Open bite of unspecified ear

5 **S01.4** Open wound of cheek and temporomandibular area

6 **S01.40** Unspecified open wound of cheek and temporomandibular area

☐ **SP** 7 **S01.401-** Unspecified open wound of right cheek and temporomandibular area

☐ **SP** 7 **S01.402-** Unspecified open wound of left cheek and temporomandibular area

☐ **IQ** 7 **S01.409-** Unspecified open wound of unspecified cheek and temporomandibular area

6 **S01.41** Laceration without foreign body of cheek and temporomandibular area

☐ **SP** 7 **S01.411-** Laceration without foreign body of right cheek and temporomandibular area

☐ **SP** 7 **S01.412-** Laceration without foreign body of left cheek and temporomandibular area

☐ **IQ** 7 **S01.419-** Laceration without foreign body of unspecified cheek and temporomandibular area

6 **S01.42** Laceration with foreign body of cheek and temporomandibular area

☐ **SP** 7 **S01.421-** Laceration with foreign body of right cheek and temporomandibular area

☐ **SP** 7 **S01.422-** Laceration with foreign body of left cheek and temporomandibular area

☐ **IQ** 7 **S01.429-** Laceration with foreign body of unspecified cheek and temporomandibular area

6 **S01.43** Puncture wound without foreign body of cheek and temporomandibular area

☐ **SP** 7 **S01.431-** Puncture wound without foreign body of right cheek and temporomandibular area

☐ **SP** 7 **S01.432-** Puncture wound without foreign body of left cheek and temporomandibular area

☐ **IQ** 7 **S01.439-** Puncture wound without foreign body of unspecified cheek and temporomandibular area

6 **S01.44** Puncture wound with foreign body of cheek and temporomandibular area

☐ **SP** 7 **S01.441-** Puncture wound with foreign body of right cheek and temporomandibular area

☐ **SP** 7 **S01.442-** Puncture wound with foreign body of left cheek and temporomandibular area

4 4th digit required   5 5th digit required   6 6th digit required   7 7th digit required   ☑ 7th digit placeholder   + Additional code   ☐ Laterality

1460   DecisionHealth's FY 2020 Complete Home Health ICD-10-CM Diagnosis Coding Manual

☐ **IQ** **7** **S01.449-** **Puncture wound with foreign body of unspecified cheek and temporomandibular area**

6 **S01.45** **Open bite of cheek and temporomandibular area**
Bite of cheek and temporomandibular area NOS
> **EXCLUDES 2** superficial bite of cheek and temporomandibular area (S00.86, S00.87)

☐ **SP** **7** **S01.451-** **Open bite of right cheek and temporomandibular area**

☐ **SP** **7** **S01.452-** **Open bite of left cheek and temporomandibular area**

☐ **IQ** **7** **S01.459-** **Open bite of unspecified cheek and temporomandibular area**

5 **S01.5** **Open wound of lip and oral cavity**
> **EXCLUDES 2** tooth dislocation (S03.2)
> tooth fracture (S02.5)

6 **S01.50** **Unspecified open wound of lip and oral cavity**

SP **7** **S01.501-** **Unspecified open wound of lip**

SP **7** **S01.502-** **Unspecified open wound of oral cavity**

6 **S01.51** **Laceration of lip and oral cavity without foreign body**

SP **7** **S01.511-** **Laceration without foreign body of lip**

SP **7** **S01.512-** **Laceration without foreign body of oral cavity**

6 **S01.52** **Laceration of lip and oral cavity with foreign body**

SP **7** **S01.521-** **Laceration with foreign body of lip**

SP **7** **S01.522-** **Laceration with foreign body of oral cavity**

6 **S01.53** **Puncture wound of lip and oral cavity without foreign body**

SP **7** **S01.531-** **Puncture wound without foreign body of lip**

SP **7** **S01.532-** **Puncture wound without foreign body of oral cavity**

6 **S01.54** **Puncture wound of lip and oral cavity with foreign body**

SP **7** **S01.541-** **Puncture wound with foreign body of lip**

SP **7** **S01.542-** **Puncture wound with foreign body of oral cavity**

6 **S01.55** **Open bite of lip and oral cavity**

SP **7** **S01.551-** **Open bite of lip**
Bite of lip NOS
> **EXCLUDES 1** superficial bite of lip (S00.571)

SP **7** **S01.552-** **Open bite of oral cavity**
Bite of oral cavity NOS
> **EXCLUDES 1** superficial bite of oral cavity (S00.572)

5 **S01.8** **Open wound of other parts of head**

SP **7** **S01.80X-** **Unspecified open wound of other part of head**

SP **7** **S01.81X-** **Laceration without foreign body of other part of head**

SP **7** **S01.82X-** **Laceration with foreign body of other part of head**

SP **7** **S01.83X-** **Puncture wound without foreign body of other part of head**

SP **7** **S01.84X-** **Puncture wound with foreign body of other part of head**

SP **7** **S01.85X-** **Open bite of other part of head**
Bite of other part of head NOS
> **EXCLUDES 1** superficial bite of other part of head (S00.87)

5 **S01.9** **Open wound of unspecified part of head**

IQ **7** **S01.90X-** **Unspecified open wound of unspecified part of head**

IQ **7** **S01.91X-** **Laceration without foreign body of unspecified part of head**

IQ **7** **S01.92X-** **Laceration with foreign body of unspecified part of head**

IQ **7** **S01.93X-** **Puncture wound without foreign body of unspecified part of head**

IQ **7** **S01.94X-** **Puncture wound with foreign body of unspecified part of head**

IQ **7** **S01.95X-** **Open bite of unspecified part of head**
Bite of head NOS
> **EXCLUDES 1** superficial bite of head NOS (S00.97)

4 **S02** **Fracture of skull and facial bones**
Note:
A fracture not indicated as open or closed should be coded to closed
Code also:
any associated intracranial injury (S06.-)

> The appropriate 7th character is to be added to each code from category S02
> A   initial encounter for closed fracture
> B   initial encounter for open fracture
> D   subsequent encounter for fracture with routine healing
> G   subsequent encounter for fracture with delayed healing
> K   subsequent encounter for fracture with nonunion
> S   sequela

CODING TIPS ✓ Fractures are not coded with aftercare codes. Displaced and closed are default choices when documentation is absent. "D" is the 7th character for home care and hospice unless the physician has documented delayed healing, nonunion or malunion. A sequela is a condition left after the fracture has healed.

Chapter 19
S00-T88

★ New ▲ Revised Px Primary **SP** PDGM Px **SL** Low CoM **SH** High CoM **IQ** Quest. Encounter ⊞ Hospice non-cancer Dx Unspecified **M** *Manifestation*

DecisionHealth's FY 2020 Complete Home Health ICD-10-CM Diagnosis Coding Manual 1461

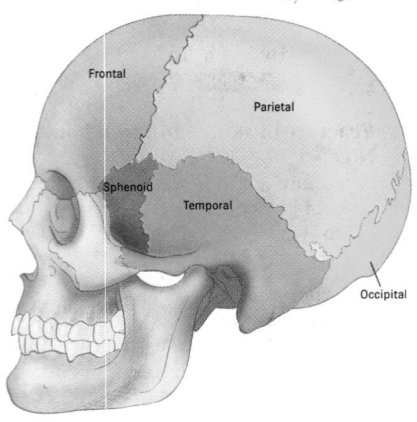

SP 7 S02.0XX- Fracture of vault of skull
 Fracture of frontal bone
 Fracture of parietal bone

▲ **5 S02.1** Fracture of base of skull
 EXCLUDES 2 lateral orbital wall (S02.84-)
 medial orbital wall
  (S02.83-)
 orbital floor (S02.3-)

 6 S02.10 Unspecified fracture of base of skull

SP 7 S02.101- Fracture of base of skull, right side

SP 7 S02.102- Fracture of base of skull, left side

IQ 7 S02.109- Fracture of base of skull, unspecified side

 6 S02.11 Fracture of occiput

IQ 7 S02.110- Type I occipital condyle fracture, unspecified side

IQ 7 S02.111- Type II occipital condyle fracture, unspecified side

IQ 7 S02.112- Type III occipital condyle fracture, unspecified side

SP 7 S02.113- Unspecified occipital condyle fracture

IQ 7 S02.118- Other fracture of occiput, unspecified side

SP 7 S02.119- Unspecified fracture of occiput

SP 7 S02.11A- Type I occipital condyle fracture, right side

SP 7 S02.11B- Type I occipital condyle fracture, left side

SP 7 S02.11C- Type II occipital condyle fracture, right side

SP 7 S02.11D- Type II occipital condyle fracture, left side

SP 7 S02.11E- Type III occipital condyle fracture, right side

SP 7 S02.11F- Type III occipital condyle fracture, left side

SP 7 S02.11G- Other fracture of occiput, right side

SP 7 S02.11H- Other fracture of occiput, left side

★ **6 S02.12** Fracture of orbital roof
 CODING TIPS ✓ Orbital fractures may be defined in terms of anatomic location, including isolated fractures of the orbital floor, medial wall, temporal wall, and roof. These fractures are commonly seen with midfacial trauma.

★ **7 S02.121-** Fracture of orbital roof, right side

★ **7 S02.122-** Fracture of orbital roof, left side

★ **7 S02.129-** Fracture of orbital roof, unspecified side

▲ **SP 7 S02.19X-** Other fracture of base of skull
 Fracture of anterior fossa of base of skull
 Fracture of ethmoid sinus
 Fracture of frontal sinus
 Fracture of middle fossa of base of skull
 Fracture of posterior fossa of base of skull
 Fracture of sphenoid
 Fracture of temporal bone

SP 7 S02.2XX- Fracture of nasal bones

▲ **5 S02.3** Fracture of orbital floor
 Fracture of inferior orbital wall
 EXCLUDES 1 orbit NOS (S02.85)
 EXCLUDES 2 lateral orbital wall (S02.84-)
  medial orbital wall
   (S02.83-)
  orbital roof (S02.1-)

IQ 7 S02.30X- Fracture of orbital floor, unspecified side

SP 7 S02.31X- Fracture of orbital floor, right side

SP 7 S02.32X- Fracture of orbital floor, left side

 5 S02.4 Fracture of malar, maxillary and zygoma bones
 Fracture of superior maxilla
 Fracture of upper jaw (bone)
 Fracture of zygomatic process of temporal bone

 6 S02.40 Fracture of malar, maxillary and zygoma bones, unspecified

IQ 7 S02.400- Malar fracture, unspecified side

IQ 7 S02.401- Maxillary fracture, unspecified side

IQ 7 S02.402- Zygomatic fracture, unspecified side

4 4th digit required **5** 5th digit required **6** 6th digit required **7** 7th digit required **7** 7th digit placeholder **+** Additional code **⊟** Laterality

1462   DecisionHealth's FY 2020 Complete Home Health ICD-10-CM Diagnosis Coding Manual

☰ SP 7 **S02.40A-** Malar fracture, right side

☰ SP 7 **S02.40B-** Malar fracture, left side

☰ SP 7 **S02.40C-** Maxillary fracture, right side

☰ SP 7 **S02.40D-** Maxillary fracture, left side

☰ SP 7 **S02.40E-** Zygomatic fracture, right side

☰ SP 7 **S02.40F-** Zygomatic fracture, left side

6 **S02.41** LeFort fracture

SP 7 **S02.411-** LeFort I fracture

SP 7 **S02.412-** LeFort II fracture

SP 7 **S02.413-** LeFort III fracture

SP 7 **S02.42X-** Fracture of alveolus of maxilla

IQ 7 **S02.5XX-** Fracture of tooth (traumatic)
Broken tooth
EXCLUDES 1 cracked tooth
(nontraumatic)
(K03.81)

5 **S02.6** Fracture of mandible
Fracture of lower jaw (bone)

6 **S02.60** Fracture of mandible, unspecified

☰ IQ 7 **S02.600-** Fracture of unspecified part of body of mandible, unspecified side

☰ SP 7 **S02.601-** Fracture of unspecified part of body of right mandible

☰ SP 7 **S02.602-** Fracture of unspecified part of body of left mandible

SP 7 **S02.609-** Fracture of mandible, unspecified

6 **S02.61** Fracture of condylar process of mandible

☰ IQ 7 **S02.610-** Fracture of condylar process of mandible, unspecified side

☰ SP 7 **S02.611-** Fracture of condylar process of right mandible

☰ SP 7 **S02.612-** Fracture of condylar process of left mandible

6 **S02.62** Fracture of subcondylar process of mandible

☰ IQ 7 **S02.620-** Fracture of subcondylar process of mandible, unspecified side

☰ SP 7 **S02.621-** Fracture of subcondylar process of right mandible

☰ SP 7 **S02.622-** Fracture of subcondylar process of left mandible

6 **S02.63** Fracture of coronoid process of mandible

☰ IQ 7 **S02.630-** Fracture of coronoid process of mandible, unspecified side

☰ SP 7 **S02.631-** Fracture of coronoid process of right mandible

☰ SP 7 **S02.632-** Fracture of coronoid process of left mandible

6 **S02.64** Fracture of ramus of mandible

☰ IQ 7 **S02.640-** Fracture of ramus of mandible, unspecified side

☰ SP 7 **S02.641-** Fracture of ramus of right mandible

☰ SP 7 **S02.642-** Fracture of ramus of left mandible

6 **S02.65** Fracture of angle of mandible

☰ IQ 7 **S02.650-** Fracture of angle of mandible, unspecified side

☰ SP 7 **S02.651-** Fracture of angle of right mandible

☰ SP 7 **S02.652-** Fracture of angle of left mandible

SP 7 **S02.66X-** Fracture of symphysis of mandible

6 **S02.67** Fracture of alveolus of mandible

☰ IQ 7 **S02.670-** Fracture of alveolus of mandible, unspecified side

☰ SP 7 **S02.671-** Fracture of alveolus of right mandible

☰ SP 7 **S02.672-** Fracture of alveolus of left mandible

SP 7 **S02.69X-** Fracture of mandible of other specified site

▲ 5 **S02.8** Fractures of other specified skull and facial bones
Fracture of palate
EXCLUDES 2 fracture of orbital floor (S02.3-)
fracture of orbital roof (S02.12-)

☰ IQ 7 **S02.80X-** Fracture of other specified skull and facial bones, unspecified side

☰ SP 7 **S02.81X-** Fracture of other specified skull and facial bones, right side

☰ SP 7 **S02.82X-** Fracture of other specified skull and facial bones, left side

★ 6 **S02.83** Fracture of medial orbital wall
EXCLUDES 2 orbital floor (S02.3-)
orbital roof (S02.12-)
CODING TIPS ✓ Orbital fractures may be defined in terms of anatomic location, including isolated fractures of the orbital floor, medial wall, temporal wall, and roof. These fractures are commonly seen with midfacial trauma.

★ ☰ 7 **S02.831-** Fracture of medial orbital wall, right side

★ ☰ 7 **S02.832-** Fracture of medial orbital wall, left side

★ ☰ 7 **S02.839-** Fracture of medial orbital wall, unspecified side

★ 6 **S02.84** Fracture of lateral orbital wall
EXCLUDES 2 orbital floor (S02.3-)
orbital roof (S02.12-)
CODING TIPS ✓ Orbital fractures may be defined in terms of anatomic location, including isolated fractures of the orbital floor, medial wall, temporal wall, and roof. These fractures are commonly seen with midfacial trauma.

★ ☰ 7 **S02.841-** Fracture of lateral orbital wall, right side

★ ☰ 7 **S02.842-** Fracture of lateral orbital wall, left side

★ ☰ 7 **S02.849-** Fracture of lateral orbital wall, unspecified side

★ 7 **S02.85X-** Fracture of orbit, unspecified
Fracture of orbit NOS
Fracture of orbit wall NOS
EXCLUDES 1 lateral orbital wall (S02.84-)
medial orbital wall (S02.83-)
orbital floor (S02.3-)
orbital roof (S02.12-)

★ New ▲ Revised Px Primary SP PDGM Px SL Low CoM SH High CoM IQ Quest. Encounter H Hospice non-cancer Dx Unspecified M *Manifestation*

DecisionHealth's FY 2020 Complete Home Health ICD-10-CM Diagnosis Coding Manual

1463

Chapter 19

S00-T88

Chapter 19

S00-T88

CODING TIPS ✓ Orbital fractures may be defined in terms of anatomic location, including isolated fractures of the orbital floor, medial wall, temporal wall, and roof. These fractures are commonly seen with midfacial trauma.

⑤ **S02.9**   **Fracture of unspecified skull and facial bones**

SP ☑ **S02.91X-**   **Unspecified fracture of skull**

SP ☑ **S02.92X-**   **Unspecified fracture of facial bones**

④ **S03**   **Dislocation and sprain of joints and ligaments of head**

     INCLUDES   avulsion of joint (capsule) or ligament of head
            laceration of cartilage, joint (capsule) or ligament of head
            sprain of cartilage, joint (capsule) or ligament of head
            traumatic hemarthrosis of joint or ligament of head
            traumatic rupture of joint or ligament of head
            traumatic subluxation of joint or ligament of head
            traumatic tear of joint or ligament of head

Code also:
   any associated open wound
     EXCLUDES 2   Strain of muscle or tendon of head (S09.1)

The appropriate 7th character is to be added to each code from category S03
A   initial encounter
D   subsequent encounter
S   sequela

⑤ **S03.0**   **Dislocation of jaw**
Dislocation of jaw (cartilage) (meniscus)
Dislocation of mandible
Dislocation of temporomandibular (joint)

⊟ **IQ** ☑ **S03.00X-**   **Dislocation of jaw, unspecified side**

⊟ **SP** ☑ **S03.01X-**   **Dislocation of jaw, right side**

⊟ **SP** ☑ **S03.02X-**   **Dislocation of jaw, left side**

⊟ **SP** ☑ **S03.03X-**   **Dislocation of jaw, bilateral**

SP ☑ **S03.1XX-**   **Dislocation of septal cartilage of nose**

IQ ☑ **S03.2XX-**   **Dislocation of tooth**

⑤ **S03.4**   **Sprain of jaw**
Sprain of temporomandibular (joint) (ligament)

⊟ **IQ** ☑ **S03.40X-**   **Sprain of jaw, unspecified side**

⊟ **SP** ☑ **S03.41X-**   **Sprain of jaw, right side**

⊟ **SP** ☑ **S03.42X-**   **Sprain of jaw, left side**

⊟ **SP** ☑ **S03.43X-**   **Sprain of jaw, bilateral**

SP ☑ **S03.8XX-**   **Sprain of joints and ligaments of other parts of head**

SP ☑ **S03.9XX-**   **Sprain of joints and ligaments of unspecified parts of head**

④ **S04**   **Injury of cranial nerve**

The selection of side should be based on the side of the body being affected
Code first:
   any associated intracranial injury (S06.-)
Code also any associated:
   open wound of head (S01.-)
   skull fracture (S02.-)

The appropriate 7th character is to be added to each code from category S04
A   initial encounter
D   subsequent encounter
S   sequela

✚ ⑤ **S04.0**   **Injury of optic nerve and pathways**
Use additional code to identify any visual field defect or blindness (H53.4-, H54.-)

✚ ⑥ **S04.01**   **Injury of optic nerve**
Injury of 2nd cranial nerve

⊟ **SP** ✚ ⑦ **S04.011-**   **Injury of optic nerve, right eye**

⊟ **SP** ✚ ⑦ **S04.012-**   **Injury of optic nerve, left eye**

⊟ **IQ** ✚ ⑦ **S04.019-**   **Injury of optic nerve, unspecified eye**
Injury of optic nerve NOS

SP ✚ ☑ **S04.02X-**   **Injury of optic chiasm**

✚ ⑥ **S04.03**   **Injury of optic tract and pathways**
Injury of optic radiation

⊟ **SP** ✚ ⑦ **S04.031-**   **Injury of optic tract and pathways, right side**

⊟ **SP** ✚ ⑦ **S04.032-**   **Injury of optic tract and pathways, left side**

⊟ **IQ** ✚ ⑦ **S04.039-**   **Injury of optic tract and pathways, unspecified side**
Injury of optic tract and pathways NOS

✚ ⑥ **S04.04**   **Injury of visual cortex**

⊟ **SP** ✚ ⑦ **S04.041-**   **Injury of visual cortex, right side**

⊟ **SP** ✚ ⑦ **S04.042-**   **Injury of visual cortex, left side**

⊟ **IQ** ✚ ⑦ **S04.049-**   **Injury of visual cortex, unspecified side**
Injury of visual cortex NOS

⑤ **S04.1**   **Injury of oculomotor nerve**
Injury of 3rd cranial nerve

⊟ **IQ** ☑ **S04.10X-**   **Injury of oculomotor nerve, unspecified side**

⊟ **SP** ☑ **S04.11X-**   **Injury of oculomotor nerve, right side**

⊟ **SP** ☑ **S04.12X-**   **Injury of oculomotor nerve, left side**

⑤ **S04.2**   **Injury of trochlear nerve**
Injury of 4th cranial nerve

⊟ **IQ** ☑ **S04.20X-**   **Injury of trochlear nerve, unspecified side**

⊟ **SP** ☑ **S04.21X-**   **Injury of trochlear nerve, right side**

⊟ **SP** ☑ **S04.22X-**   **Injury of trochlear nerve, left side**

⑤ **S04.3**   **Injury of trigeminal nerve**
Injury of 5th cranial nerve

⊟ **IQ** ☑ **S04.30X-**   **Injury of trigeminal nerve, unspecified side**

⊟ **SP** ☑ **S04.31X-**   **Injury of trigeminal nerve, right side**

⊟ **SP** ☑ **S04.32X-**   **Injury of trigeminal nerve, left side**

⑤ **S04.4**   **Injury of abducent nerve**
Injury of 6th cranial nerve

---

④4th digit required   ⑤5th digit required   ⑥6th digit required   ⑦7th digit required   ☑7th digit placeholder   ✚Additional code   ⊟Laterality

☐ **IQ** ☑ **S04.40X-** **Injury of abducent nerve, unspecified side**

☐ **SP** ☑ **S04.41X-** Injury of abducent nerve, right side

☐ **SP** ☑ **S04.42X-** Injury of abducent nerve, left side

⑤ **S04.5** **Injury of facial nerve**
Injury of 7th cranial nerve

☐ **IQ** ☑ **S04.50X-** **Injury of facial nerve, unspecified side**

☐ **SP** ☑ **S04.51X-** Injury of facial nerve, right side

☐ **SP** ☑ **S04.52X-** Injury of facial nerve, left side

⑤ **S04.6** **Injury of acoustic nerve**
Injury of auditory nerve
Injury of 8th cranial nerve

☐ **IQ** ☑ **S04.60X-** **Injury of acoustic nerve, unspecified side**

☐ **SP** ☑ **S04.61X-** Injury of acoustic nerve, right side

☐ **SP** ☑ **S04.62X-** Injury of acoustic nerve, left side

⑤ **S04.7** **Injury of accessory nerve**
Injury of 11th cranial nerve

☐ **IQ** ☑ **S04.70X-** **Injury of accessory nerve, unspecified side**

☐ **SP** ☑ **S04.71X-** Injury of accessory nerve, right side

☐ **SP** ☑ **S04.72X-** Injury of accessory nerve, left side

⑤ **S04.8** **Injury of other cranial nerves**

⑥ **S04.81** **Injury of olfactory [1st] nerve**

☐ **SP** 7 **S04.811-** Injury of olfactory [1st] nerve, right side

☐ **SP** 7 **S04.812-** Injury of olfactory [1st] nerve, left side

☐ **IQ** 7 **S04.819-** **Injury of olfactory [1st] nerve, unspecified side**

⑥ **S04.89** **Injury of other cranial nerves**
Injury of vagus [10th] nerve

☐ **SP** 7 **S04.891-** Injury of other cranial nerves, right side

☐ **SP** 7 **S04.892-** Injury of other cranial nerves, left side

☐ **IQ** 7 **S04.899-** **Injury of other cranial nerves, unspecified side**

IQ ☑ **S04.9XX-** **Injury of unspecified cranial nerve**

④ **S05** **Injury of eye and orbit**
INCLUDES	open wound of eye and orbit
EXCLUDES 2	2nd cranial [optic] nerve injury (S04.0-)
	3rd cranial [oculomotor] nerve injury (S04.1-)
	open wound of eyelid and periocular area (S01.1-)
	orbital bone fracture (S02.1-, S02.3-, S02.8-)
	superficial injury of eyelid (S00.1-S00.2)

The appropriate 7th character is to be added to each code from category S05
A   initial encounter
D   subsequent encounter
S   sequela

⑤ **S05.0** **Injury of conjunctiva and corneal abrasion without foreign body**
| EXCLUDES 1 | foreign body in conjunctival sac (T15.1) |

foreign body in cornea (T15.0)

☐ **IQ** ☑ **S05.00X-** **Injury of conjunctiva and corneal abrasion without foreign body, unspecified eye**

☐ **IQ** ☑ **S05.01X-** Injury of conjunctiva and corneal abrasion without foreign body, right eye

☐ **IQ** ☑ **S05.02X-** Injury of conjunctiva and corneal abrasion without foreign body, left eye

⑤ **S05.1** **Contusion of eyeball and orbital tissues**
Traumatic hyphema
| EXCLUDES 2 | black eye NOS (S00.1) |
| | contusion of eyelid and periocular area (S00.1) |

☐ **IQ** ☑ **S05.10X-** **Contusion of eyeball and orbital tissues, unspecified eye**

☐ **IQ** ☑ **S05.11X-** Contusion of eyeball and orbital tissues, right eye

☐ **IQ** ☑ **S05.12X-** Contusion of eyeball and orbital tissues, left eye

⑤ **S05.2** **Ocular laceration and rupture with prolapse or loss of intraocular tissue**

☐ **IQ** ☑ **S05.20X-** **Ocular laceration and rupture with prolapse or loss of intraocular tissue, unspecified eye**

☐ **SP** ☑ **S05.21X-** Ocular laceration and rupture with prolapse or loss of intraocular tissue, right eye

☐ **SP** ☑ **S05.22X-** Ocular laceration and rupture with prolapse or loss of intraocular tissue, left eye

⑤ **S05.3** **Ocular laceration without prolapse or loss of intraocular tissue**
Laceration of eye NOS

☐ **IQ** ☑ **S05.30X-** **Ocular laceration without prolapse or loss of intraocular tissue, unspecified eye**

☐ **SP** ☑ **S05.31X-** Ocular laceration without prolapse or loss of intraocular tissue, right eye

☐ **SP** ☑ **S05.32X-** Ocular laceration without prolapse or loss of intraocular tissue, left eye

⑤ **S05.4** **Penetrating wound of orbit with or without foreign body**
| EXCLUDES 2 | retained (old) foreign body following penetrating wound in orbit (H05.5-) |

☐ **IQ** ☑ **S05.40X-** **Penetrating wound of orbit with or without foreign body, unspecified eye**

☐ **SP** ☑ **S05.41X-** Penetrating wound of orbit with or without foreign body, right eye

☐ **SP** ☑ **S05.42X-** Penetrating wound of orbit with or without foreign body, left eye

⑤ **S05.5** **Penetrating wound with foreign body of eyeball**
| EXCLUDES 2 | retained (old) intraocular foreign body (H44.6-, H44.7) |

☐ **IQ** ☑ **S05.50X-** **Penetrating wound with foreign body of unspecified eyeball**

☐ **SP** ☑ **S05.51X-** Penetrating wound with foreign body of right eyeball

★ New ▲ Revised Px Primary **SP** PDGM Px **SL** Low CoM **SH** High CoM **IQ** Quest. Encounter **H** Hospice non-cancer Dx   Unspecified   **M** *Manifestation*

DecisionHealth's FY 2020 Complete Home Health ICD-10-CM Diagnosis Coding Manual

1465

Chapter 19

S00-T88

☐ **SP** ☑ **S05.52X-**   **Penetrating wound with foreign body of left eyeball**

☐ **S05.6**   **Penetrating wound without foreign body of eyeball**
Ocular penetration NOS

☐ **IQ** ☑ **S05.60X-**   **Penetrating wound without foreign body of unspecified eyeball**

☐ **SP** ☑ **S05.61X-**   **Penetrating wound without foreign body of right eyeball**

☐ **SP** ☑ **S05.62X-**   **Penetrating wound without foreign body of left eyeball**

☐ **S05.7**   **Avulsion of eye**
Traumatic enucleation

☐ **IQ** ☑ **S05.70X-**   **Avulsion of unspecified eye**

☐ **SP** ☑ **S05.71X-**   **Avulsion of right eye**

☐ **SP** ☑ **S05.72X-**   **Avulsion of left eye**

☐ **S05.8**   **Other injuries of eye and orbit**
Lacrimal duct injury

☐ **S05.8X**   **Other injuries of eye and orbit**

☐ **SP** ☑ **S05.8X1-**   **Other injuries of right eye and orbit**

☐ **SP** ☑ **S05.8X2-**   **Other injuries of left eye and orbit**

☐ **IQ** ☑ **S05.8X9-**   **Other injuries of unspecified eye and orbit**

☐ **S05.9**   **Unspecified injury of eye and orbit**
Injury of eye NOS

☐ **IQ** ☑ **S05.90X-**   **Unspecified injury of unspecified eye and orbit**

☐ **IQ** ☑ **S05.91X-**   **Unspecified injury of right eye and orbit**

☐ **IQ** ☑ **S05.92X-**   **Unspecified injury of left eye and orbit**

☐ **S06**   **Intracranial injury**
Note:
7th characters D and S do not apply to codes in category S06 with 6th character 7 - death due to brain injury prior to regaining consciousness, or 8 - death due to other cause prior to regaining consciousness.

  INCLUDES   traumatic brain injury

Code also any associated:
open wound of head (S01.-)
skull fracture (S02.-)

  EXCLUDES 1   head injury NOS (S09.90)

The appropriate 7th character is to be added to each code from category S06
A   initial encounter
D   subsequent encounter
S   sequela

CODING TIPS ✓   Intracranial injuries are caused by trauma, not strokes. To determine whether the intracranial injury with 7th character "D" or "S" should be used, look at the plan of care (POC) and the length of time since the head injury. Is the POC directed at the head injury or the residuals of the head injury?

CODING TIPS ✓   When coding sequelae of a traumatic brain injury, the guideline indicates to first list the residual condition(s), followed by the specific traumatic brain injury diagnosed, using the appropriate code from category S06 with the seventh character "S" to indicate sequelae. In some cases with traumatic brain injury, there is a tabular convention that indicates to code the intracranial injury first and then the residual, e.g. R40.2-. A convention always overrules a conflicting guideline.

☐ **S06.0**   **Concussion**
Commotio cerebri

  EXCLUDES 1   concussion with other intracranial injuries classified in subcategories S06.1- to S06.6- , S06.81- and S06.82- code to specified intracranial injury

CODING TIPS ✓   Loss of consciousness (LOC) of more than 30 minutes should not be classified as a concussion or mild traumatic brain injury. Query the physician if documentation indicates longer than 30 minutes LOC.

☐ **S06.0X**   **Concussion**

SP ☑ **S06.0X0-**   **Concussion without loss of consciousness**

SP ☑ **S06.0X1-**   **Concussion with loss of consciousness of 30 minutes or less**

SP ☑ **S06.0X9-**   **Concussion with loss of consciousness of unspecified duration**
Concussion NOS

☐ **S06.1**   **Traumatic cerebral edema**
Diffuse traumatic cerebral edema
Focal traumatic cerebral edema

☐ **S06.1X**   **Traumatic cerebral edema**

SP ☑ **S06.1X0-**   **Traumatic cerebral edema without loss of consciousness**

SP ☑ **S06.1X1-**   **Traumatic cerebral edema with loss of consciousness of 30 minutes or less**

SP ☑ **S06.1X2-**   **Traumatic cerebral edema with loss of consciousness of 31 minutes to 59 minutes**

SP ☑ **S06.1X3-**   **Traumatic cerebral edema with loss of consciousness of 1 hour to 5 hours 59 minutes**

SP ☑ **S06.1X4-**   **Traumatic cerebral edema with loss of consciousness of 6 hours to 24 hours**

SP ☑ **S06.1X5-**   **Traumatic cerebral edema with loss of consciousness greater than 24 hours with return to pre-existing conscious level**

SP ☑ **S06.1X6-**   **Traumatic cerebral edema with loss of consciousness greater than 24 hours without return to pre-existing conscious level with patient surviving**

☐ 4th digit required   ☐ 5th digit required   ☐ 6th digit required   ☑ 7th digit required   ☑ 7th digit placeholder   ✚ Additional code   ☐ Laterality

1466   *DecisionHealth's* FY 2020 Complete Home Health ICD-10-CM Diagnosis Coding Manual

IQ **7** **S06.1X7-** Traumatic cerebral edema with loss of consciousness of any duration with death due to brain injury prior to regaining consciousness

IQ **7** **S06.1X8-** Traumatic cerebral edema with loss of consciousness of any duration with death due to other cause prior to regaining consciousness

SP **7** **S06.1X9-** Traumatic cerebral edema with loss of consciousness of unspecified duration
Traumatic cerebral edema NOS

5 **S06.2** **Diffuse traumatic brain injury**
Diffuse axonal brain injury
EXCLUDES 1 traumatic diffuse cerebral edema (S06.1X-)

6 **S06.2X** **Diffuse traumatic brain injury**

SP **7** **S06.2X0-** Diffuse traumatic brain injury without loss of consciousness

SP **7** **S06.2X1-** Diffuse traumatic brain injury with loss of consciousness of 30 minutes or less

SP **7** **S06.2X2-** Diffuse traumatic brain injury with loss of consciousness of 31 minutes to 59 minutes

SP **7** **S06.2X3-** Diffuse traumatic brain injury with loss of consciousness of 1 hour to 5 hours 59 minutes

SP **7** **S06.2X4-** Diffuse traumatic brain injury with loss of consciousness of 6 hours to 24 hours

SP **7** **S06.2X5-** Diffuse traumatic brain injury with loss of consciousness greater than 24 hours with return to pre-existing conscious levels

SP **7** **S06.2X6-** Diffuse traumatic brain injury with loss of consciousness greater than 24 hours without return to pre-existing conscious level with patient surviving

IQ **7** **S06.2X7-** Diffuse traumatic brain injury with loss of consciousness of any duration with death due to brain injury prior to regaining consciousness

IQ **7** **S06.2X8-** Diffuse traumatic brain injury with loss of consciousness of any duration with death due to other cause prior to regaining consciousness

SP **7** **S06.2X9-** Diffuse traumatic brain injury with loss of consciousness of unspecified duration
Diffuse traumatic brain injury NOS

5 **S06.3** **Focal traumatic brain injury**
EXCLUDES 1 any condition classifiable to S06.4-S06.6
focal cerebral edema (S06.1)

6 **S06.30** **Unspecified focal traumatic brain injury**

SP **7** **S06.300-** Unspecified focal traumatic brain injury without loss of consciousness

SP **7** **S06.301-** Unspecified focal traumatic brain injury with loss of consciousness of 30 minutes or less

SP **7** **S06.302-** Unspecified focal traumatic brain injury with loss of consciousness of 31 minutes to 59 minutes

SP **7** **S06.303-** Unspecified focal traumatic brain injury with loss of consciousness of 1 hour to 5 hours 59 minutes

SP **7** **S06.304-** Unspecified focal traumatic brain injury with loss of consciousness of 6 hours to 24 hours

SP **7** **S06.305-** Unspecified focal traumatic brain injury with loss of consciousness greater than 24 hours with return to pre-existing conscious level

SP **7** **S06.306-** Unspecified focal traumatic brain injury with loss of consciousness greater than 24 hours without return to pre-existing conscious level with patient surviving

IQ **7** **S06.307-** Unspecified focal traumatic brain injury with loss of consciousness of any duration with death due to brain injury prior to regaining consciousness

IQ **7** **S06.308-** Unspecified focal traumatic brain injury with loss of consciousness of any duration with death due to other cause prior to regaining consciousness

SP **7** **S06.309-** Unspecified focal traumatic brain injury with loss of consciousness of unspecified duration
Unspecified focal traumatic brain injury NOS

6 **S06.31** **Contusion and laceration of right cerebrum**

SP **7** **S06.310-** Contusion and laceration of right cerebrum without loss of consciousness

SP **7** **S06.311-** Contusion and laceration of right cerebrum with loss of consciousness of 30 minutes or less

SP **7** **S06.312-** Contusion and laceration of right cerebrum with loss of consciousness of 31 minutes to 59 minutes

SP **7** **S06.313-** Contusion and laceration of right cerebrum with loss of consciousness of 1 hour to 5 hours 59 minutes

SP **7** **S06.314-** Contusion and laceration of right cerebrum with loss of consciousness of 6 hours to 24 hours

Chapter 19

S00-T88

★ New ▲ Revised Px Primary **SP** PDGM Px **SL** Low CoM **SH** High CoM **IQ** Quest. Encounter **H** Hospice non-cancer Dx Unspecified **M** *Manifestation*

DecisionHealth's FY 2020 Complete Home Health ICD-10-CM Diagnosis Coding Manual

1467

SP 7 S06.315- **Contusion and laceration of right cerebrum with loss of consciousness greater than 24 hours with return to pre-existing conscious level**

SP 7 S06.316- **Contusion and laceration of right cerebrum with loss of consciousness greater than 24 hours without return to pre-existing conscious level with patient surviving**

IQ 7 S06.317- **Contusion and laceration of right cerebrum with loss of consciousness of any duration with death due to brain injury prior to regaining consciousness**

IQ 7 S06.318- **Contusion and laceration of right cerebrum with loss of consciousness of any duration with death due to other cause prior to regaining consciousness**

SP 7 S06.319- **Contusion and laceration of right cerebrum with loss of consciousness of unspecified duration**
Contusion and laceration of right cerebrum NOS

6 S06.32 **Contusion and laceration of left cerebrum**

SP 7 S06.320- **Contusion and laceration of left cerebrum without loss of consciousness**

SP 7 S06.321- **Contusion and laceration of left cerebrum with loss of consciousness of 30 minutes or less**

SP 7 S06.322- **Contusion and laceration of left cerebrum with loss of consciousness of 31 minutes to 59 minutes**

SP 7 S06.323- **Contusion and laceration of left cerebrum with loss of consciousness of 1 hour to 5 hours 59 minutes**

SP 7 S06.324- **Contusion and laceration of left cerebrum with loss of consciousness of 6 hours to 24 hours**

SP 7 S06.325- **Contusion and laceration of left cerebrum with loss of consciousness greater than 24 hours with return to pre-existing conscious level**

SP 7 S06.326- **Contusion and laceration of left cerebrum with loss of consciousness greater than 24 hours without return to pre-existing conscious level with patient surviving**

IQ 7 S06.327- **Contusion and laceration of left cerebrum with loss of consciousness of any duration with death due to brain injury prior to regaining consciousness**

IQ 7 S06.328- **Contusion and laceration of left cerebrum with loss of consciousness of any duration with death due to other cause prior to regaining consciousness**

SP 7 S06.329- **Contusion and laceration of left cerebrum with loss of consciousness of unspecified duration**
Contusion and laceration of left cerebrum NOS

6 S06.33 **Contusion and laceration of cerebrum, unspecified**

SP 7 S06.330- **Contusion and laceration of cerebrum, unspecified, without loss of consciousness**

SP 7 S06.331- **Contusion and laceration of cerebrum, unspecified, with loss of consciousness of 30 minutes or less**

SP 7 S06.332- **Contusion and laceration of cerebrum, unspecified, with loss of consciousness of 31 minutes to 59 minutes**

SP 7 S06.333- **Contusion and laceration of cerebrum, unspecified, with loss of consciousness of 1 hour to 5 hours 59 minutes**

SP 7 S06.334- **Contusion and laceration of cerebrum, unspecified, with loss of consciousness of 6 hours to 24 hours**

SP 7 S06.335- **Contusion and laceration of cerebrum, unspecified, with loss of consciousness greater than 24 hours with return to pre-existing conscious level**

SP 7 S06.336- **Contusion and laceration of cerebrum, unspecified, with loss of consciousness greater than 24 hours without return to pre-existing conscious level with patient surviving**

IQ 7 S06.337- **Contusion and laceration of cerebrum, unspecified, with loss of consciousness of any duration with death due to brain injury prior to regaining consciousness**

IQ 7 S06.338- **Contusion and laceration of cerebrum, unspecified, with loss of consciousness of any duration with death due to other cause prior to regaining consciousness**

SP 7 S06.339- **Contusion and laceration of cerebrum, unspecified, with loss of consciousness of unspecified duration**
Contusion and laceration of cerebrum NOS

6 S06.34 **Traumatic hemorrhage of right cerebrum**
Traumatic intracerebral hemorrhage and hematoma of right cerebrum

SP 7 S06.340- **Traumatic hemorrhage of right cerebrum without loss of consciousness**

SP 7 S06.341- **Traumatic hemorrhage of right cerebrum with loss of consciousness of 30 minutes or less**

4 4th digit required   5 5th digit required   6 6th digit required   7 7th digit required   7 7th digit placeholder   + Additional code   Laterality

1468   DecisionHealth's FY 2020 Complete Home Health ICD-10-CM Diagnosis Coding Manual

Chapter 19

S00-T88

⊟ **SP** 7 **S06.342-** Traumatic hemorrhage of right cerebrum with loss of consciousness of 31 minutes to 59 minutes

⊟ **SP** 7 **S06.343-** Traumatic hemorrhage of right cerebrum with loss of consciousness of 1 hours to 5 hours 59 minutes

⊟ **SP** 7 **S06.344-** Traumatic hemorrhage of right cerebrum with loss of consciousness of 6 hours to 24 hours

⊟ **SP** 7 **S06.345-** Traumatic hemorrhage of right cerebrum with loss of consciousness greater than 24 hours with return to pre-existing conscious level

⊟ **SP** **IQ** 7 **S06.346-** Traumatic hemorrhage of right cerebrum with loss of consciousness greater than 24 hours without return to pre-existing conscious level with patient surviving

⊟ **IQ** 7 **S06.347-** Traumatic hemorrhage of right cerebrum with loss of consciousness of any duration with death due to brain injury prior to regaining consciousness

⊟ **IQ** 7 **S06.348-** Traumatic hemorrhage of right cerebrum with loss of consciousness of any duration with death due to other cause prior to regaining consciousness

⊟ **SP** 7 **S06.349-** Traumatic hemorrhage of right cerebrum with loss of consciousness of unspecified duration

Traumatic hemorrhage of right cerebrum NOS

6 **S06.35** Traumatic hemorrhage of left cerebrum

Traumatic intracerebral hemorrhage and hematoma of left cerebrum

⊟ **SP** 7 **S06.350-** Traumatic hemorrhage of left cerebrum without loss of consciousness

⊟ **SP** 7 **S06.351-** Traumatic hemorrhage of left cerebrum with loss of consciousness of 30 minutes or less

⊟ **SP** 7 **S06.352-** Traumatic hemorrhage of left cerebrum with loss of consciousness of 31 minutes to 59 minutes

⊟ **SP** 7 **S06.353-** Traumatic hemorrhage of left cerebrum with loss of consciousness of 1 hours to 5 hours 59 minutes

⊟ **SP** 7 **S06.354-** Traumatic hemorrhage of left cerebrum with loss of consciousness of 6 hours to 24 hours

⊟ **SP** 7 **S06.355-** Traumatic hemorrhage of left cerebrum with loss of consciousness greater than 24 hours with return to pre-existing conscious level

⊟ **SP** 7 **S06.356-** Traumatic hemorrhage of left cerebrum with loss of consciousness greater than 24 hours without return to pre-existing conscious level with patient surviving

⊟ **IQ** 7 **S06.357-** Traumatic hemorrhage of left cerebrum with loss of consciousness of any duration with death due to brain injury prior to regaining consciousness

⊟ **IQ** 7 **S06.358-** Traumatic hemorrhage of left cerebrum with loss of consciousness of any duration with death due to other cause prior to regaining consciousness

⊟ **SP** 7 **S06.359-** Traumatic hemorrhage of left cerebrum with loss of consciousness of unspecified duration

Traumatic hemorrhage of left cerebrum NOS

6 **S06.36** Traumatic hemorrhage of cerebrum, unspecified

Traumatic intracerebral hemorrhage and hematoma, unspecified

SP 7 **S06.360-** Traumatic hemorrhage of cerebrum, unspecified, without loss of consciousness

SP 7 **S06.361-** Traumatic hemorrhage of cerebrum, unspecified, with loss of consciousness of 30 minutes or less

SP 7 **S06.362-** Traumatic hemorrhage of cerebrum, unspecified, with loss of consciousness of 31 minutes to 59 minutes

SP 7 **S06.363-** Traumatic hemorrhage of cerebrum, unspecified, with loss of consciousness of 1 hours to 5 hours 59 minutes

SP 7 **S06.364-** Traumatic hemorrhage of cerebrum, unspecified, with loss of consciousness of 6 hours to 24 hours

SP 7 **S06.365-** Traumatic hemorrhage of cerebrum, unspecified, with loss of consciousness greater than 24 hours with return to pre-existing conscious level

SP 7 **S06.366-** Traumatic hemorrhage of cerebrum, unspecified, with loss of consciousness greater than 24 hours without return to pre-existing conscious level with patient surviving

IQ 7 **S06.367-** Traumatic hemorrhage of cerebrum, unspecified, with loss of consciousness of any duration with death due to brain injury prior to regaining consciousness

IQ 7 **S06.368-** Traumatic hemorrhage of cerebrum, unspecified, with loss of consciousness of any duration with death due to other cause prior to regaining consciousness

✦ New ▲ Revised Px Primary **SP** PDGM Px **SL** Low CoM **SH** High CoM **IQ** Quest. Encounter ⊞ Hospice non-cancer Dx │ Unspecified │ **M** *Manifestation*

DecisionHealth's FY 2020 Complete Home Health ICD-10-CM Diagnosis Coding Manual

1469

SP 7 S06.369- Traumatic hemorrhage of cerebrum, unspecified, with loss of consciousness of unspecified duration

Traumatic hemorrhage of cerebrum NOS

6 S06.37 Contusion, laceration, and hemorrhage of cerebellum

SP 7 S06.370- Contusion, laceration, and hemorrhage of cerebellum without loss of consciousness

SP 7 S06.371- Contusion, laceration, and hemorrhage of cerebellum with loss of consciousness of 30 minutes or less

SP 7 S06.372- Contusion, laceration, and hemorrhage of cerebellum with loss of consciousness of 31 minutes to 59 minutes

SP 7 S06.373- Contusion, laceration, and hemorrhage of cerebellum with loss of consciousness of 1 hour to 5 hours 59 minutes

SP 7 S06.374- Contusion, laceration, and hemorrhage of cerebellum with loss of consciousness of 6 hours to 24 hours

SP 7 S06.375- Contusion, laceration, and hemorrhage of cerebellum with loss of consciousness greater than 24 hours with return to pre-existing conscious level

SP 7 S06.376- Contusion, laceration, and hemorrhage of cerebellum with loss of consciousness greater than 24 hours without return to pre-existing conscious level with patient surviving

IQ 7 S06.377- Contusion, laceration, and hemorrhage of cerebellum with loss of consciousness of any duration with death due to brain injury prior to regaining consciousness

IQ 7 S06.378- Contusion, laceration, and hemorrhage of cerebellum with loss of consciousness of any duration with death due to other cause prior to regaining consciousness

SP 7 S06.379- Contusion, laceration, and hemorrhage of cerebellum with loss of consciousness of unspecified duration

Contusion, laceration, and hemorrhage of cerebellum NOS

6 S06.38 Contusion, laceration, and hemorrhage of brainstem

SP 7 S06.380- Contusion, laceration, and hemorrhage of brainstem without loss of consciousness

SP 7 S06.381- Contusion, laceration, and hemorrhage of brainstem with loss of consciousness of 30 minutes or less

SP 7 S06.382- Contusion, laceration, and hemorrhage of brainstem with loss of consciousness of 31 minutes to 59 minutes

SP 7 S06.383- Contusion, laceration, and hemorrhage of brainstem with loss of consciousness of 1 hour to 5 hours 59 minutes

SP 7 S06.384- Contusion, laceration, and hemorrhage of brainstem with loss of consciousness of 6 hours to 24 hours

SP 7 S06.385- Contusion, laceration, and hemorrhage of brainstem with loss of consciousness greater than 24 hours with return to pre-existing conscious level

SP 7 S06.386- Contusion, laceration, and hemorrhage of brainstem with loss of consciousness greater than 24 hours without return to pre-existing conscious level with patient surviving

IQ 7 S06.387- Contusion, laceration, and hemorrhage of brainstem with loss of consciousness of any duration with death due to brain injury prior to regaining consciousness

IQ 7 S06.388- Contusion, laceration, and hemorrhage of brainstem with loss of consciousness of any duration with death due to other cause prior to regaining consciousness

SP 7 S06.389- Contusion, laceration, and hemorrhage of brainstem with loss of consciousness of unspecified duration

Contusion, laceration, and hemorrhage of brainstem NOS

5 S06.4 Epidural hemorrhage

Extradural hemorrhage NOS

Extradural hemorrhage (traumatic)

6 S06.4X Epidural hemorrhage

SP 7 S06.4X0- Epidural hemorrhage without loss of consciousness

SP 7 S06.4X1- Epidural hemorrhage with loss of consciousness of 30 minutes or less

SP 7 S06.4X2- Epidural hemorrhage with loss of consciousness of 31 minutes to 59 minutes

SP 7 S06.4X3- Epidural hemorrhage with loss of consciousness of 1 hour to 5 hours 59 minutes

SP 7 S06.4X4- Epidural hemorrhage with loss of consciousness of 6 hours to 24 hours

SP 7 S06.4X5- Epidural hemorrhage with loss of consciousness greater than 24 hours with return to pre-existing conscious level

SP 7 S06.4X6- Epidural hemorrhage with loss of consciousness greater than 24 hours without return to pre-existing conscious level with patient surviving

IQ 7 S06.4X7- Epidural hemorrhage with loss of consciousness of any duration with death due to brain injury prior to regaining consciousness

---

4 4th digit required   5 5th digit required   6 6th digit required   7 7th digit required   7 7th digit placeholder   + Additional code   ▱ Laterality

1470   *DecisionHealth's* FY 2020 Complete Home Health ICD-10-CM Diagnosis Coding Manual

IQ 7 S06.4X8- Epidural hemorrhage with loss of consciousness of any duration with death due to other causes prior to regaining consciousness

SP 7 S06.4X9- Epidural hemorrhage with loss of consciousness of unspecified duration

Epidural hemorrhage NOS

5 S06.5 Traumatic subdural hemorrhage

6 S06.5X Traumatic subdural hemorrhage

SP 7 S06.5X0- Traumatic subdural hemorrhage without loss of consciousness

SP 7 S06.5X1- Traumatic subdural hemorrhage with loss of consciousness of 30 minutes or less

SP 7 S06.5X2- Traumatic subdural hemorrhage with loss of consciousness of 31 minutes to 59 minutes

SP 7 S06.5X3- Traumatic subdural hemorrhage with loss of consciousness of 1 hour to 5 hours 59 minutes

SP 7 S06.5X4- Traumatic subdural hemorrhage with loss of consciousness of 6 hours to 24 hours

SP 7 S06.5X5- Traumatic subdural hemorrhage with loss of consciousness greater than 24 hours with return to pre-existing conscious level

SP 7 S06.5X6- Traumatic subdural hemorrhage with loss of consciousness greater than 24 hours without return to pre-existing conscious level with patient surviving

IQ 7 S06.5X7- Traumatic subdural hemorrhage with loss of consciousness of any duration with death due to brain injury before regaining consciousness

IQ 7 S06.5X8- Traumatic subdural hemorrhage with loss of consciousness of any duration with death due to other cause before regaining consciousness

SP 7 S06.5X9- Traumatic subdural hemorrhage with loss of consciousness of unspecified duration

Traumatic subdural hemorrhage NOS

5 S06.6 Traumatic subarachnoid hemorrhage

6 S06.6X Traumatic subarachnoid hemorrhage

SP 7 S06.6X0- Traumatic subarachnoid hemorrhage without loss of consciousness

SP 7 S06.6X1- Traumatic subarachnoid hemorrhage with loss of consciousness of 30 minutes or less

SP 7 S06.6X2- Traumatic subarachnoid hemorrhage with loss of consciousness of 31 minutes to 59 minutes

SP 7 S06.6X3- Traumatic subarachnoid hemorrhage with loss of consciousness of 1 hour to 5 hours 59 minutes

SP 7 S06.6X4- Traumatic subarachnoid hemorrhage with loss of consciousness of 6 hours to 24 hours

SP 7 S06.6X5- Traumatic subarachnoid hemorrhage with loss of consciousness greater than 24 hours with return to pre-existing conscious level

SP 7 S06.6X6- Traumatic subarachnoid hemorrhage with loss of consciousness greater than 24 hours without return to pre-existing conscious level with patient surviving

IQ 7 S06.6X7- Traumatic subarachnoid hemorrhage with loss of consciousness of any duration with death due to brain injury prior to regaining consciousness

IQ 7 S06.6X8- Traumatic subarachnoid hemorrhage with loss of consciousness of any duration with death due to other cause prior to regaining consciousness

SP 7 S06.6X9- Traumatic subarachnoid hemorrhage with loss of consciousness of unspecified duration

Traumatic subarachnoid hemorrhage NOS

5 S06.8 Other specified intracranial injuries

6 S06.81 Injury of right internal carotid artery, intracranial portion, not elsewhere classified

SP 7 S06.810- Injury of right internal carotid artery, intracranial portion, not elsewhere classified without loss of consciousness

SP 7 S06.811- Injury of right internal carotid artery, intracranial portion, not elsewhere classified with loss of consciousness of 30 minutes or less

SP 7 S06.812- Injury of right internal carotid artery, intracranial portion, not elsewhere classified with loss of consciousness of 31 minutes to 59 minutes

SP 7 S06.813- Injury of right internal carotid artery, intracranial portion, not elsewhere classified with loss of consciousness of 1 hour to 5 hours 59 minutes

SP 7 S06.814- Injury of right internal carotid artery, intracranial portion, not elsewhere classified with loss of consciousness of 6 hours to 24 hours

SP 7 S06.815- Injury of right internal carotid artery, intracranial portion, not elsewhere classified with loss of consciousness greater than 24 hours with return to pre-existing conscious level

Chapter 19

S00-T88

★ New ▲ Revised Px Primary SP PDGM Px SL Low CoM SH High CoM IQ Quest. Encounter H Hospice non-cancer Dx   Unspecified   M Manifestation

DecisionHealth's FY 2020 Complete Home Health ICD-10-CM Diagnosis Coding Manual

1471

⊟ SP 7 S06.816-   Injury of right internal carotid artery, intracranial portion, not elsewhere classified with loss of consciousness greater than 24 hours without return to pre-existing conscious level with patient surviving

⊟ IQ 7 S06.817-   Injury of right internal carotid artery, intracranial portion, not elsewhere classified with loss of consciousness of any duration with death due to brain injury prior to regaining consciousness

⊟ IQ 7 S06.818-   Injury of right internal carotid artery, intracranial portion, not elsewhere classified with loss of consciousness of any duration with death due to other cause prior to regaining consciousness

⊟ SP 7 S06.819-   Injury of right internal carotid artery, intracranial portion, not elsewhere classified with loss of consciousness of unspecified duration

     Injury of right internal carotid artery, intracranial portion, not elsewhere classified NOS

6 S06.82   Injury of left internal carotid artery, intracranial portion, not elsewhere classified

⊟ SP 7 S06.820-   Injury of left internal carotid artery, intracranial portion, not elsewhere classified without loss of consciousness

⊟ SP 7 S06.821-   Injury of left internal carotid artery, intracranial portion, not elsewhere classified with loss of consciousness of 30 minutes or less

⊟ SP 7 S06.822-   Injury of left internal carotid artery, intracranial portion, not elsewhere classified with loss of consciousness of 31 minutes to 59 minutes

⊟ SP 7 S06.823-   Injury of left internal carotid artery, intracranial portion, not elsewhere classified with loss of consciousness of 1 hour to 5 hours 59 minutes

⊟ SP 7 S06.824-   Injury of left internal carotid artery, intracranial portion, not elsewhere classified with loss of consciousness of 6 hours to 24 hours

⊟ SP 7 S06.825-   Injury of left internal carotid artery, intracranial portion, not elsewhere classified with loss of consciousness greater than 24 hours with return to pre-existing conscious level

⊟ SP 7 S06.826-   Injury of left internal carotid artery, intracranial portion, not elsewhere classified with loss of consciousness greater than 24 hours without return to pre-existing conscious level with patient surviving

⊟ IQ 7 S06.827-   Injury of left internal carotid artery, intracranial portion, not elsewhere classified with loss of consciousness of any duration with death due to brain injury prior to regaining consciousness

⊟ IQ 7 S06.828-   Injury of left internal carotid artery, intracranial portion, not elsewhere classified with loss of consciousness of any duration with death due to other cause prior to regaining consciousness

⊟ SP 7 S06.829-   Injury of left internal carotid artery, intracranial portion, not elsewhere classified with loss of consciousness of unspecified duration

     Injury of left internal carotid artery, intracranial portion, not elsewhere classified NOS

6 S06.89   Other specified intracranial injury

     EXCLUDES 1   concussion (S06.0X-)

SP 7 S06.890-   Other specified intracranial injury without loss of consciousness

SP 7 S06.891-   Other specified intracranial injury with loss of consciousness of 30 minutes or less

SP 7 S06.892-   Other specified intracranial injury with loss of consciousness of 31 minutes to 59 minutes

SP 7 S06.893-   Other specified intracranial injury with loss of consciousness of 1 hour to 5 hours 59 minutes

SP 7 S06.894-   Other specified intracranial injury with loss of consciousness of 6 hours to 24 hours

SP 7 S06.895-   Other specified intracranial injury with loss of consciousness greater than 24 hours with return to pre-existing conscious level

SP 7 S06.896-   Other specified intracranial injury with loss of consciousness greater than 24 hours without return to pre-existing conscious level with patient surviving

SP 7 S06.897-   Other specified intracranial injury with loss of consciousness of any duration with death due to brain injury prior to regaining consciousness

IQ 7 S06.898-   Other specified intracranial injury with loss of consciousness of any duration with death due to other cause prior to regaining consciousness

SP 7 S06.899-   Other specified intracranial injury with loss of consciousness of unspecified duration

5 S06.9   Unspecified intracranial injury

     Brain injury NOS
     Head injury NOS with loss of consciousness
     Traumatic brain injury NOS

4 4th digit required   **5** 5th digit required   **6** 6th digit required   **7** 7th digit required   **7** 7th digit placeholder   **+** Additional code   ⊟ Laterality

1472   *DecisionHealth's* FY 2020 Complete Home Health ICD-10-CM Diagnosis Coding Manual

EXCLUDES 1 conditions classifiable to S06.0- to S06.8-code to specified intracranial injury
head injury NOS (S09.90)

6 S06.9X   Unspecified intracranial injury

!Q 7 S06.9X0-   Unspecified intracranial injury without loss of consciousness

!Q 7 S06.9X1-   Unspecified intracranial injury with loss of consciousness of 30 minutes or less

!Q 7 S06.9X2-   Unspecified intracranial injury with loss of consciousness of 31 minutes to 59 minutes

!Q 7 S06.9X3-   Unspecified intracranial injury with loss of consciousness of 1 hour to 5 hours 59 minutes

!Q 7 S06.9X4-   Unspecified intracranial injury with loss of consciousness of 6 hours to 24 hours

!Q 7 S06.9X5-   Unspecified intracranial injury with loss of consciousness greater than 24 hours with return to pre-existing conscious level

!Q 7 S06.9X6-   Unspecified intracranial injury with loss of consciousness greater than 24 hours without return to pre-existing conscious level with patient surviving

!Q 7 S06.9X7-   Unspecified intracranial injury with loss of consciousness of any duration with death due to brain injury prior to regaining consciousness

!Q 7 S06.9X8-   Unspecified intracranial injury with loss of consciousness of any duration with death due to other cause prior to regaining consciousness

!Q 7 S06.9X9-   Unspecified intracranial injury with loss of consciousness of unspecified duration

+ 4 S07   Crushing injury of head
Use additional code for all associated injuries, such as:
intracranial injuries (S06.-)
skull fractures (S02.-)

The appropriate 7th character is to be added to each code from category S07
A   initial encounter
D   subsequent encounter
S   sequela

SP + 7 S07.0XX-   Crushing injury of face
SP + 7 S07.1XX-   Crushing injury of skull
SP + 7 S07.8XX-   Crushing injury of other parts of head
SP + 7 S07.9XX-   Crushing injury of head, part unspecified

4 S08   Avulsion and traumatic amputation of part of head
An amputation not identified as partial or complete should be coded to complete

The appropriate 7th character is to be added to each code from category S08
A   initial encounter
D   subsequent encounter
S   sequela

SP 7 S08.0XX-   Avulsion of scalp

5 S08.1   Traumatic amputation of ear

6 S08.11   Complete traumatic amputation of ear

= SP 7 S08.111-   Complete traumatic amputation of right ear

= SP 7 S08.112-   Complete traumatic amputation of left ear

= !Q 7 S08.119-   Complete traumatic amputation of unspecified ear

6 S08.12   Partial traumatic amputation of ear

= SP 7 S08.121-   Partial traumatic amputation of right ear

= SP 7 S08.122-   Partial traumatic amputation of left ear

= !Q 7 S08.129-   Partial traumatic amputation of unspecified ear

5 S08.8   Traumatic amputation of other parts of head

6 S08.81   Traumatic amputation of nose

SP 7 S08.811-   Complete traumatic amputation of nose

SP 7 S08.812-   Partial traumatic amputation of nose

SP 7 S08.89X-   Traumatic amputation of other parts of head

4 S09   Other and unspecified injuries of head

The appropriate 7th character is to be added to each code from category S09
A   initial encounter
D   subsequent encounter
S   sequela

SP 7 S09.0XX-   Injury of blood vessels of head, not elsewhere classified
EXCLUDES 1 injury of cerebral blood vessels (S06.-)
injury of precerebral blood vessels (S15.-)

5 S09.1   Injury of muscle and tendon of head
Code also:
any associated open wound (S01.-)
EXCLUDES 2 sprain to joints and ligament of head (S03.9)

!Q 7 S09.10X-   Unspecified injury of muscle and tendon of head
Injury of muscle and tendon of head NOS

!Q 7 S09.11X-   Strain of muscle and tendon of head

SP 7 S09.12X-   Laceration of muscle and tendon of head

!Q 7 S09.19X-   Other specified injury of muscle and tendon of head

5 S09.2   Traumatic rupture of ear drum
EXCLUDES 1 traumatic rupture of ear drum due to blast injury (S09.31-)

= !Q 7 S09.20X-   Traumatic rupture of unspecified ear drum

★ New ▲ Revised Px Primary SP PDGM Px SL Low CoM SH High CoM !Q Quest. Encounter H Hospice non-cancer Dx Unspecified M Manifestation

DecisionHealth's FY 2020 Complete Home Health ICD-10-CM Diagnosis Coding Manual   1473

☐ SP ⑦ **S09.21X-** **Traumatic rupture of right ear drum**

☐ SP ⑦ **S09.22X-** **Traumatic rupture of left ear drum**

⑤ **S09.3** **Other specified and unspecified injury of middle and inner ear**

> EXCLUDES 1 injury to ear NOS (S09.91-)
>
> EXCLUDES 2 injury to external ear (S00.4-, S01.3-, S08.1-)

⑥ **S09.30** **Unspecified injury of middle and inner ear**

☐ !Q ⑦ **S09.301-** **Unspecified injury of right middle and inner ear**

☐ !Q ⑦ **S09.302-** **Unspecified injury of left middle and inner ear**

☐ !Q ⑦ **S09.309-** **Unspecified injury of unspecified middle and inner ear**

⑥ **S09.31** **Primary blast injury of ear**
Blast injury of ear NOS

☐ SP ⑦ **S09.311-** **Primary blast injury of right ear**

☐ SP ⑦ **S09.312-** **Primary blast injury of left ear**

☐ SP ⑦ **S09.313-** **Primary blast injury of ear, bilateral**

☐ !Q ⑦ **S09.319-** **Primary blast injury of unspecified ear**

⑥ **S09.39** **Other specified injury of middle and inner ear**
Secondary blast injury to ear

☐ SP ⑦ **S09.391-** **Other specified injury of right middle and inner ear**

☐ SP ⑦ **S09.392-** **Other specified injury of left middle and inner ear**

☐ !Q ⑦ **S09.399-** **Other specified injury of unspecified middle and inner ear**

SP ⑦ **S09.8XX-** **Other specified injuries of head**

⑤ **S09.9** **Unspecified injury of face and head**

!Q ⑦ **S09.90X-** **Unspecified injury of head**
Head injury NOS

> EXCLUDES 1 brain injury NOS (S06.9-)
> head injury NOS with loss of consciousness (S06.9-)
> intracranial injury NOS (S06.9-)

!Q ⑦ **S09.91X-** **Unspecified injury of ear**
Injury of ear NOS

!Q ⑦ **S09.92X-** **Unspecified injury of nose**
Injury of nose NOS

!Q ⑦ **S09.93X-** **Unspecified injury of face**
Injury of face NOS

Injuries to the neck (S10-S19)

> INCLUDES injuries of nape
> injuries of supraclavicular region
> injuries of throat
>
> EXCLUDES 2 burns and corrosions (T20-T32)
> effects of foreign body in esophagus (T18.1)
> effects of foreign body in larynx (T17.3)
> effects of foreign body in pharynx (T17.2)
> effects of foreign body in trachea (T17.4)
> frostbite (T33-T34)

insect bite or sting, venomous (T63.4)

GUIDELINES Section I.C.19.c.2)
Multiple fractures are sequenced in accordance with the severity of the fracture.

GUIDELINES Section I.C.19.b.1)-2)
When coding injuries, assign separate codes for each injury unless a combination code is provided, in which case the combination code is assigned ... Traumatic injury codes (S00-T14.9) are not to be used for normal, healing surgical wounds or to identify complications of surgical wounds. The code for the most serious injury, as determined by the provider and the focus of treatment, is sequenced first.

1) Superficial injuries such as abrasions or contusions are not coded when associated with more severe injuries of the same site.

2) When a primary injury results in minor damage to peripheral nerves or blood vessels, the primary injury is sequenced first with additional code(s) for injuries to nerves and spinal cord (such as category S04), and/or injury to blood vessels (such as category S15). When the primary injury is to the blood vessels or nerves, that injury should be sequenced first.

GUIDELINES Section I.C.19.c
Coding of Traumatic Fractures: The principles of multiple coding of injuries should be followed in coding fractures. Fractures of specified sites are coded individually by site in accordance with both the provisions within categories S02, S12, S22, S32, S42, S49, S52, S59, S62, S72, S79, S82, S89, S92 and the level of detail furnished by medical record content. A fracture not indicated as open or closed should be coded to closed. A fracture not indicated whether displaced or not displaced should be coded to displaced.

CODING TIPS ✓ 7th character A is acceptable in home health and hospice when active treatment is provided, such as antibiotics for an infected wound or a wound vac for a dehisced wound. D is used when the complication or injury is now healing. Think of D as aftercare. S is used for sequela of the injury or complication. Sequela is a residual deficit or condition produced as a result of the injury or complication after the original injury or complication has healed.

④ **S10** **Superficial injury of neck**

> The appropriate 7th character is to be added to each code from category S10
> A initial encounter
> D subsequent encounter
> S sequela

!Q ⑦ **S10.0XX-** **Contusion of throat**
Contusion of cervical esophagus
Contusion of larynx
Contusion of pharynx
Contusion of trachea

⑤ **S10.1** **Other and unspecified superficial injuries of throat**

!Q ⑦ **S10.10X-** **Unspecified superficial injuries of throat**

!Q ⑦ **S10.11X-** **Abrasion of throat**

!Q ⑦ **S10.12X-** **Blister (nonthermal) of throat**

!Q ⑦ **S10.14X-** **External constriction of part of throat**

!Q ⑦ **S10.15X-** **Superficial foreign body of throat**
Splinter in the throat

---

④ 4th digit required   ⑤ 5th digit required   ⑥ 6th digit required   ⑦ 7th digit required   ⑦ 7th digit placeholder   ➕ Additional code   ☐ Laterality

IQ ☑ S10.16X- Insect bite (nonvenomous) of throat

IQ ☑ S10.17X- Other superficial bite of throat
> **EXCLUDES 1** open bite of throat (S11.85)

⑤ S10.8 Superficial injury of other specified parts of neck

IQ ☑ S10.80X- Unspecified superficial injury of other specified part of neck

IQ ☑ S10.81X- Abrasion of other specified part of neck

IQ ☑ S10.82X- Blister (nonthermal) of other specified part of neck

IQ ☑ S10.83X- Contusion of other specified part of neck

IQ ☑ S10.84X- External constriction of other specified part of neck

IQ ☑ S10.85X- Superficial foreign body of other specified part of neck
Splinter in other specified part of neck

IQ ☑ S10.86X- Insect bite of other specified part of neck

IQ ☑ S10.87X- Other superficial bite of other specified part of neck
> **EXCLUDES 1** open bite of other specified parts of neck (S11.85)

⑤ S10.9 Superficial injury of unspecified part of neck

IQ ☑ S10.90X- Unspecified superficial injury of unspecified part of neck

IQ ☑ S10.91X- Abrasion of unspecified part of neck

IQ ☑ S10.92X- Blister (nonthermal) of unspecified part of neck

IQ ☑ S10.93X- Contusion of unspecified part of neck

IQ ☑ S10.94X- External constriction of unspecified part of neck

IQ ☑ S10.95X- Superficial foreign body of unspecified part of neck

IQ ☑ S10.96X- Insect bite of unspecified part of neck

IQ ☑ S10.97X- Other superficial bite of unspecified part of neck

④ S11 Open wound of neck
Code also any associated:
spinal cord injury (S14.0, S14.1-)
wound infection
> **EXCLUDES 2** open fracture of vertebra (S12.- with 7th character B)

The appropriate 7th character is to be added to each code from category S11
A   initial encounter
D   subsequent encounter
S   sequela

CODING TIPS ✓ Open wound codes are used for wounds caused by trauma. Do not assign a code for "open wound" unless the etiology of the wound is related to trauma. Do not use Z codes for any aspect of care of a trauma wound, e.g. no Z code for dressing changes, drain care, or suture removal.

CODING TIPS ✓ No aftercare code applies. The 7th character "D" is the default for home care and hospice when providing aftercare for a healing or resolving condition; "A" is used for active treatment such as antibiotics or more than routine wound care; "S" may be used to indicate a residual condition after the original injury has healed.

⑤ S11.0 Open wound of larynx and trachea

⑥ S11.01 Open wound of larynx
> **EXCLUDES 2** open wound of vocal cord (S11.03)

SP ⑦ S11.011- Laceration without foreign body of larynx

SP ⑦ S11.012- Laceration with foreign body of larynx

SP ⑦ S11.013- Puncture wound without foreign body of larynx

SP ⑦ S11.014- Puncture wound with foreign body of larynx

SP ⑦ S11.015- Open bite of larynx
Bite of larynx NOS

SP ⑦ S11.019- Unspecified open wound of larynx

⑥ S11.02 Open wound of trachea
Open wound of cervical trachea
Open wound of trachea NOS
> **EXCLUDES 2** open wound of thoracic trachea (S27.5-)

SP ⑦ S11.021- Laceration without foreign body of trachea

SP ⑦ S11.022- Laceration with foreign body of trachea

SP ⑦ S11.023- Puncture wound without foreign body of trachea

SP ⑦ S11.024- Puncture wound with foreign body of trachea

SP ⑦ S11.025- Open bite of trachea
Bite of trachea NOS

SP ⑦ S11.029- Unspecified open wound of trachea

⑥ S11.03 Open wound of vocal cord

SP ⑦ S11.031- Laceration without foreign body of vocal cord

SP ⑦ S11.032- Laceration with foreign body of vocal cord

SP ⑦ S11.033- Puncture wound without foreign body of vocal cord

SP ⑦ S11.034- Puncture wound with foreign body of vocal cord

SP ⑦ S11.035- Open bite of vocal cord
Bite of vocal cord NOS

SP ⑦ S11.039- Unspecified open wound of vocal cord

⑤ S11.1 Open wound of thyroid gland

SP ☑ S11.10X- Unspecified open wound of thyroid gland

SP ☑ S11.11X- Laceration without foreign body of thyroid gland

SP ☑ S11.12X- Laceration with foreign body of thyroid gland

SP ☑ S11.13X- Puncture wound without foreign body of thyroid gland

SP ☑ S11.14X- Puncture wound with foreign body of thyroid gland

SP ☑ S11.15X- Open bite of thyroid gland

★ New ▲ Revised Px Primary SP PDGM Px SL Low CoM SH High CoM IQ Quest. Encounter H Hospice non-cancer Dx Unspecified M Manifestation

DecisionHealth's FY 2020 Complete Home Health ICD-10-CM Diagnosis Coding Manual

1475

Chapter 19

S00-T88

Bite of thyroid gland NOS

⑤ S11.2 Open wound of pharynx and cervical esophagus

> **EXCLUDES 1** open wound of esophagus NOS (S27.8-)

SP ☑ S11.20X- **Unspecified open wound of pharynx and cervical esophagus**

SP ☑ S11.21X- Laceration without foreign body of pharynx and cervical esophagus

SP ☑ S11.22X- Laceration with foreign body of pharynx and cervical esophagus

SP ☑ S11.23X- Puncture wound without foreign body of pharynx and cervical esophagus

SP ☑ S11.24X- Puncture wound with foreign body of pharynx and cervical esophagus

SP ☑ S11.25X- Open bite of pharynx and cervical esophagus

Bite of pharynx and cervical esophagus NOS

⑤ S11.8 Open wound of other specified parts of neck

SP ☑ S11.80X- **Unspecified open wound of other specified part of neck**

SP ☑ S11.81X- Laceration without foreign body of other specified part of neck

SP ☑ S11.82X- Laceration with foreign body of other specified part of neck

SP ☑ S11.83X- Puncture wound without foreign body of other specified part of neck

SP ☑ S11.84X- Puncture wound with foreign body of other specified part of neck

SP ☑ S11.85X- Open bite of other specified part of neck

Bite of other specified part of neck NOS

> **EXCLUDES 1** superficial bite of other specified part of neck (S10.87)

SP ☑ S11.89X- Other open wound of other specified part of neck

⑤ S11.9 Open wound of unspecified part of neck

SP ☑ S11.90X- **Unspecified open wound of unspecified part of neck**

SP ☑ S11.91X- **Laceration without foreign body of unspecified part of neck**

SP ☑ S11.92X- **Laceration with foreign body of unspecified part of neck**

IQ ☑ S11.93X- **Puncture wound without foreign body of unspecified part of neck**

IQ ☑ S11.94X- **Puncture wound with foreign body of unspecified part of neck**

IQ ☑ S11.95X- **Open bite of unspecified part of neck**

Bite of neck NOS

> **EXCLUDES 1** superficial bite of neck (S10.97)

④ S12 Fracture of cervical vertebra and other parts of neck

Note:

A fracture not indicated as displaced or nondisplaced should be coded to displaced

A fracture not indicated as open or closed should be coded to closed

INCLUDES fracture of cervical neural arch
fracture of cervical spine
fracture of cervical spinous process
fracture of cervical transverse process
fracture of cervical vertebral arch
fracture of neck

Code first:
any associated cervical spinal cord injury (S14.0, S14.1-)

The appropriate 7th character is to be added to all codes from subcategories S12.0-S12.6

A	initial encounter for closed fracture
B	initial encounter for open fracture
D	subsequent encounter for fracture with routine healing
G	subsequent encounter for fracture with delayed healing
K	subsequent encounter for fracture with nonunion
S	sequela

CODING TIPS ✓ Fractures repaired by joint replacements are NOT coded with Z47.1. Fractures repaired by any other orthopedic surgery are NOT coded with Z47.89. Z codes are not appropriate for fractures of any kind. Code the fracture with 7th character D for fractures undergoing surgical repair.

CODING TIPS ✓ A fracture not indicated as displaced or nondisplaced should be coded to displaced. A fracture not indicated as open or closed should be coded to closed.

CODING TIPS ✓ 'D' is the 7th character for home care and hospice unless the physician has documented delayed healing, nonunion or malunion. A sequela is a condition left after the fracture has healed. The Gustilo open fracture classification must be used for open fractures. The default 7th character for open fractures is E.

⑤ S12.0 Fracture of first cervical vertebra
Atlas

⑥ S12.00 **Unspecified fracture of first cervical vertebra**

SP ⑦ S12.000- **Unspecified displaced fracture of first cervical vertebra**

SP ⑦ S12.001- **Unspecified nondisplaced fracture of first cervical vertebra**

SP ☑ S12.01X- Stable burst fracture of first cervical vertebra

SP ☑ S12.02X- Unstable burst fracture of first cervical vertebra

⑥ S12.03 Posterior arch fracture of first cervical vertebra

SP ⑦ S12.030- Displaced posterior arch fracture of first cervical vertebra

SP ⑦ S12.031- Nondisplaced posterior arch fracture of first cervical vertebra

⑥ S12.04 Lateral mass fracture of first cervical vertebra

SP ⑦ S12.040- Displaced lateral mass fracture of first cervical vertebra

---

④4th digit required ⑤5th digit required ⑥6th digit required ⑦7th digit required ☑7th digit placeholder ✚Additional code ▣Laterality

1476   *DecisionHealth's* FY 2020 Complete Home Health ICD-10-CM Diagnosis Coding Manual

SP 7 S12.041- Nondisplaced lateral mass fracture of first cervical vertebra

6 S12.09 Other fracture of first cervical vertebra

SP 7 S12.090- Other displaced fracture of first cervical vertebra

SP 7 S12.091- Other nondisplaced fracture of first cervical vertebra

5 S12.1 Fracture of second cervical vertebra
Axis

6 S12.10 Unspecified fracture of second cervical vertebra

SP 7 S12.100- Unspecified displaced fracture of second cervical vertebra

SP 7 S12.101- Unspecified nondisplaced fracture of second cervical vertebra

6 S12.11 Type II dens fracture

SP 7 S12.110- Anterior displaced Type II dens fracture

SP 7 S12.111- Posterior displaced Type II dens fracture

SP 7 S12.112- Nondisplaced Type II dens fracture

6 S12.12 Other dens fracture

SP 7 S12.120- Other displaced dens fracture

SP 7 S12.121- Other nondisplaced dens fracture

6 S12.13 Unspecified traumatic spondylolisthesis of second cervical vertebra

SP 7 S12.130- Unspecified traumatic displaced spondylolisthesis of second cervical vertebra

SP 7 S12.131- Unspecified traumatic nondisplaced spondylolisthesis of second cervical vertebra

SP 7 S12.14X- Type III traumatic spondylolisthesis of second cervical vertebra

6 S12.15 Other traumatic spondylolisthesis of second cervical vertebra

SP 7 S12.150- Other traumatic displaced spondylolisthesis of second cervical vertebra

SP 7 S12.151- Other traumatic nondisplaced spondylolisthesis of second cervical vertebra

6 S12.19 Other fracture of second cervical vertebra

SP 7 S12.190- Other displaced fracture of second cervical vertebra

SP 7 S12.191- Other nondisplaced fracture of second cervical vertebra

5 S12.2 Fracture of third cervical vertebra

6 S12.20 Unspecified fracture of third cervical vertebra

SP 7 S12.200- Unspecified displaced fracture of third cervical vertebra

SP 7 S12.201- Unspecified nondisplaced fracture of third cervical vertebra

6 S12.23 Unspecified traumatic spondylolisthesis of third cervical vertebra

SP 7 S12.230- Unspecified traumatic displaced spondylolisthesis of third cervical vertebra

SP 7 S12.231- Unspecified traumatic nondisplaced spondylolisthesis of third cervical vertebra

SP 7 S12.24X- Type III traumatic spondylolisthesis of third cervical vertebra

6 S12.25 Other traumatic spondylolisthesis of third cervical vertebra

SP 7 S12.250- Other traumatic displaced spondylolisthesis of third cervical vertebra

SP 7 S12.251- Other traumatic nondisplaced spondylolisthesis of third cervical vertebra

6 S12.29 Other fracture of third cervical vertebra

SP 7 S12.290- Other displaced fracture of third cervical vertebra

SP 7 S12.291- Other nondisplaced fracture of third cervical vertebra

5 S12.3 Fracture of fourth cervical vertebra

6 S12.30 Unspecified fracture of fourth cervical vertebra

SP 7 S12.300- Unspecified displaced fracture of fourth cervical vertebra

SP 7 S12.301- Unspecified nondisplaced fracture of fourth cervical vertebra

6 S12.33 Unspecified traumatic spondylolisthesis of fourth cervical vertebra

SP 7 S12.330- Unspecified traumatic displaced spondylolisthesis of fourth cervical vertebra

SP 7 S12.331- Unspecified traumatic nondisplaced spondylolisthesis of fourth cervical vertebra

SP 7 S12.34X- Type III traumatic spondylolisthesis of fourth cervical vertebra

6 S12.35 Other traumatic spondylolisthesis of fourth cervical vertebra

SP 7 S12.350- Other traumatic displaced spondylolisthesis of fourth cervical vertebra

SP 7 S12.351- Other traumatic nondisplaced spondylolisthesis of fourth cervical vertebra

6 S12.39 Other fracture of fourth cervical vertebra

SP 7 S12.390- Other displaced fracture of fourth cervical vertebra

SP 7 S12.391- Other nondisplaced fracture of fourth cervical vertebra

5 S12.4 Fracture of fifth cervical vertebra

6 S12.40 Unspecified fracture of fifth cervical vertebra

SP 7 S12.400- Unspecified displaced fracture of fifth cervical vertebra

SP 7 S12.401- Unspecified nondisplaced fracture of fifth cervical vertebra

Chapter 19

S00-T88

★ New ▲ Revised Px Primary **SP** PDGM Px **SL** Low CoM **SH** High CoM **IQ** Quest. Encounter H Hospice non-cancer Dx Unspecified M *Manifestation*

DecisionHealth's FY 2020 Complete Home Health ICD-10-CM Diagnosis Coding Manual

1477

⑥ **S12.43** **Unspecified traumatic spondylolisthesis of fifth cervical vertebra**

SP ⑦ **S12.430-** **Unspecified traumatic displaced spondylolisthesis of fifth cervical vertebra**

SP ⑦ **S12.431-** **Unspecified traumatic nondisplaced spondylolisthesis of fifth cervical vertebra**

SP ⑦ **S12.44X-** Type III traumatic spondylolisthesis of fifth cervical vertebra

⑥ **S12.45** Other traumatic spondylolisthesis of fifth cervical vertebra

SP ⑦ **S12.450-** Other traumatic displaced spondylolisthesis of fifth cervical vertebra

SP ⑦ **S12.451-** Other traumatic nondisplaced spondylolisthesis of fifth cervical vertebra

⑥ **S12.49** Other fracture of fifth cervical vertebra

SP ⑦ **S12.490-** Other displaced fracture of fifth cervical vertebra

SP ⑦ **S12.491-** Other nondisplaced fracture of fifth cervical vertebra

⑤ **S12.5** Fracture of sixth cervical vertebra

⑥ **S12.50** **Unspecified fracture of sixth cervical vertebra**

SP ⑦ **S12.500-** **Unspecified displaced fracture of sixth cervical vertebra**

SP ⑦ **S12.501-** **Unspecified nondisplaced fracture of sixth cervical vertebra**

⑥ **S12.53** **Unspecified traumatic spondylolisthesis of sixth cervical vertebra**

SP ⑦ **S12.530-** **Unspecified traumatic displaced spondylolisthesis of sixth cervical vertebra**

SP ⑦ **S12.531-** **Unspecified traumatic nondisplaced spondylolisthesis of sixth cervical vertebra**

SP ⑦ **S12.54X-** Type III traumatic spondylolisthesis of sixth cervical vertebra

⑥ **S12.55** Other traumatic spondylolisthesis of sixth cervical vertebra

SP ⑦ **S12.550-** Other traumatic displaced spondylolisthesis of sixth cervical vertebra

SP ⑦ **S12.551-** Other traumatic nondisplaced spondylolisthesis of sixth cervical vertebra

⑥ **S12.59** Other fracture of sixth cervical vertebra

SP ⑦ **S12.590-** Other displaced fracture of sixth cervical vertebra

SP ⑦ **S12.591-** Other nondisplaced fracture of sixth cervical vertebra

⑤ **S12.6** Fracture of seventh cervical vertebra

⑥ **S12.60** **Unspecified fracture of seventh cervical vertebra**

SP ⑦ **S12.600-** **Unspecified displaced fracture of seventh cervical vertebra**

SP ⑦ **S12.601-** **Unspecified nondisplaced fracture of seventh cervical vertebra**

⑥ **S12.63** **Unspecified traumatic spondylolisthesis of seventh cervical vertebra**

SP ⑦ **S12.630-** **Unspecified traumatic displaced spondylolisthesis of seventh cervical vertebra**

SP ⑦ **S12.631-** **Unspecified traumatic nondisplaced spondylolisthesis of seventh cervical vertebra**

SP ⑦ **S12.64X-** Type III traumatic spondylolisthesis of seventh cervical vertebra

⑥ **S12.65** Other traumatic spondylolisthesis of seventh cervical vertebra

SP ⑦ **S12.650-** Other traumatic displaced spondylolisthesis of seventh cervical vertebra

SP ⑦ **S12.651-** Other traumatic nondisplaced spondylolisthesis of seventh cervical vertebra

⑥ **S12.69** Other fracture of seventh cervical vertebra

SP ⑦ **S12.690-** Other displaced fracture of seventh cervical vertebra

SP ⑦ **S12.691-** Other nondisplaced fracture of seventh cervical vertebra

SP ⑦ **S12.8XX-** **Fracture of other parts of neck**
Hyoid bone
Larynx
Thyroid cartilage
Trachea

The appropriate 7th character is to be added to code S12.8
A   initial encounter
D   subsequent encounter
S   sequela

SP ⑦ **S12.9XX-** **Fracture of neck, unspecified**

Fracture of neck NOS
Fracture of cervical spine NOS
Fracture of cervical vertebra NOS

The appropriate 7th character is to be added to code S12.9
A   initial encounter
D   subsequent encounter
S   sequela

④ **S13** **Dislocation and sprain of joints and ligaments at neck level**

INCLUDES   avulsion of joint or ligament at neck level
laceration of cartilage, joint or ligament at neck level
sprain of cartilage, joint or ligament at neck level
traumatic hemarthrosis of joint or ligament at neck level
traumatic rupture of joint or ligament at neck level
traumatic subluxation of joint or ligament at neck level
traumatic tear of joint or ligament at neck level

Code also:
any associated open wound

④ 4th digit required   ⑤ 5th digit required   ⑥ 6th digit required   ⑦ 7th digit required   ⑦ 7th digit placeholder   ✚ Additional code   ⊟ Laterality

1478   DecisionHealth's FY 2020 Complete Home Health ICD-10-CM Diagnosis Coding Manual

EXCLUDES 2 strain of muscle or tendon at neck level (S16.1)

The appropriate 7th character is to be added to each code from category S13
A   initial encounter
D   subsequent encounter
S   sequela

SP 7 S13.0XX- **Traumatic rupture of cervical intervertebral disc**
    EXCLUDES 1 rupture or displacement (nontraumatic) of cervical intervertebral disc NOS (M50.-)

5 S13.1 **Subluxation and dislocation of cervical vertebrae**
Code also any associated:
   open wound of neck (S11.-)
   spinal cord injury (S14.1-)
    EXCLUDES 2 fracture of cervical vertebrae (S12.0-S12.3-)

6 S13.10 **Subluxation and dislocation of unspecified cervical vertebrae**

SP 7 S13.100- **Subluxation of unspecified cervical vertebrae**

SP 7 S13.101- **Dislocation of unspecified cervical vertebrae**

6 S13.11 **Subluxation and dislocation of C0/C1 cervical vertebrae**
Subluxation and dislocation of atlantooccipital joint
Subluxation and dislocation of atloidooccipital joint
Subluxation and dislocation of occipitoatloid joint

SP 7 S13.110- Subluxation of C0/C1 cervical vertebrae

SP 7 S13.111- Dislocation of C0/C1 cervical vertebrae

6 S13.12 **Subluxation and dislocation of C1/C2 cervical vertebrae**
Subluxation and dislocation of atlantoaxial joint

SP 7 S13.120- Subluxation of C1/C2 cervical vertebrae

SP 7 S13.121- Dislocation of C1/C2 cervical vertebrae

6 S13.13 **Subluxation and dislocation of C2/C3 cervical vertebrae**

SP 7 S13.130- Subluxation of C2/C3 cervical vertebrae

SP 7 S13.131- Dislocation of C2/C3 cervical vertebrae

6 S13.14 **Subluxation and dislocation of C3/C4 cervical vertebrae**

SP 7 S13.140- Subluxation of C3/C4 cervical vertebrae

SP 7 S13.141- Dislocation of C3/C4 cervical vertebrae

6 S13.15 **Subluxation and dislocation of C4/C5 cervical vertebrae**

SP 7 S13.150- Subluxation of C4/C5 cervical vertebrae

SP 7 S13.151- Dislocation of C4/C5 cervical vertebrae

6 S13.16 **Subluxation and dislocation of C5/C6 cervical vertebrae**

SP 7 S13.160- Subluxation of C5/C6 cervical vertebrae

SP 7 S13.161- Dislocation of C5/C6 cervical vertebrae

6 S13.17 **Subluxation and dislocation of C6/C7 cervical vertebrae**

SP 7 S13.170- Subluxation of C6/C7 cervical vertebrae

SP 7 S13.171- Dislocation of C6/C7 cervical vertebrae

6 S13.18 **Subluxation and dislocation of C7/T1 cervical vertebrae**

SP 7 S13.180- Subluxation of C7/T1 cervical vertebrae

SP 7 S13.181- Dislocation of C7/T1 cervical vertebrae

5 S13.2 **Dislocation of other and unspecified parts of neck**

SP 7 S13.20X- **Dislocation of unspecified parts of neck**

SP 7 S13.29X- **Dislocation of other parts of neck**

SP 7 S13.4XX- **Sprain of ligaments of cervical spine**
Sprain of anterior longitudinal (ligament), cervical
Sprain of atlanto-axial (joints)
Sprain of atlanto-occipital (joints)
Whiplash injury of cervical spine

SP 7 S13.5XX- **Sprain of thyroid region**
Sprain of cricoarytenoid (joint) (ligament)
Sprain of cricothyroid (joint) (ligament)
Sprain of thyroid cartilage

SP 7 S13.8XX- **Sprain of joints and ligaments of other parts of neck**

SP 7 S13.9XX- **Sprain of joints and ligaments of unspecified parts of neck**

Chapter 19

S00-T88

★ New ▲ Revised **Px** Primary **SP** PDGM Px **SL** Low CoM **SH** High CoM **IQ** Quest. Encounter **H** Hospice non-cancer Dx   Unspecified   **M** *Manifestation*

DecisionHealth's FY 2020 Complete Home Health ICD-10-CM Diagnosis Coding Manual

1479

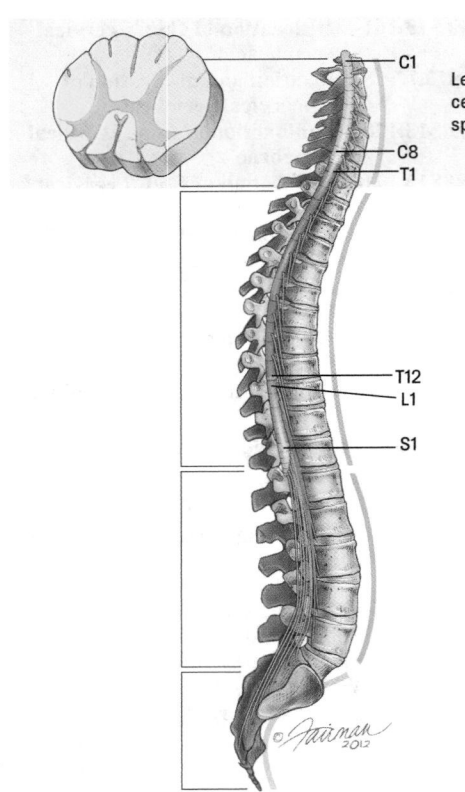

C1
Level of
cervical
spinal cord
C8
T1
T12
L1
S1

Chapter 19

S00-T88

4 S14   Injury of nerves and spinal cord at neck level

Note:
Code to highest level of cervical cord injury
Code also any associated:
  fracture of cervical vertebra
    (S12.0--S12.6.-)
  open wound of neck (S11.-)
  transient paralysis (R29.5)

The appropriate 7th character is to be added to each code from category S14
A   initial encounter
D   subsequent encounter
S   sequela

CODING TIPS ✓   When coding sequelae of a cervical spinal cord injury, first list the residual condition(s), followed by the specific spinal cord injury diagnosed using the appropriate code from this category with the seventh character "S" to indicate sequelae. If there are multiple levels of injury, code only the highest injury in each section of the spine (cervical, thoracic, and lumbar).

SP 7 S14.0XX-   Concussion and edema of cervical spinal cord

5 S14.1   Other and unspecified injuries of cervical spinal cord

6 S14.10   Unspecified injury of cervical spinal cord

!Q 7 S14.101-   Unspecified injury at C1 level of cervical spinal cord

!Q 7 S14.102-   Unspecified injury at C2 level of cervical spinal cord

!Q 7 S14.103-   Unspecified injury at C3 level of cervical spinal cord

!Q 7 S14.104-   Unspecified injury at C4 level of cervical spinal cord

!Q 7 S14.105-   Unspecified injury at C5 level of cervical spinal cord

!Q 7 S14.106-   Unspecified injury at C6 level of cervical spinal cord

!Q 7 S14.107-   Unspecified injury at C7 level of cervical spinal cord

!Q 7 S14.108-   Unspecified injury at C8 level of cervical spinal cord

!Q 7 S14.109-   Unspecified injury at unspecified level of cervical spinal cord

Injury of cervical spinal cord NOS

6 S14.11   Complete lesion of cervical spinal cord

SP 7 S14.111-   Complete lesion at C1 level of cervical spinal cord

SP 7 S14.112-   Complete lesion at C2 level of cervical spinal cord

SP 7 S14.113-   Complete lesion at C3 level of cervical spinal cord

SP 7 S14.114-   Complete lesion at C4 level of cervical spinal cord

SP 7 S14.115-   Complete lesion at C5 level of cervical spinal cord

SP 7 S14.116-   Complete lesion at C6 level of cervical spinal cord

SP 7 S14.117-   Complete lesion at C7 level of cervical spinal cord

SP 7 S14.118-   Complete lesion at C8 level of cervical spinal cord

!Q 7 S14.119-   Complete lesion at unspecified level of cervical spinal cord

6 S14.12   Central cord syndrome of cervical spinal cord

SP 7 S14.121-   Central cord syndrome at C1 level of cervical spinal cord

SP 7 S14.122-   Central cord syndrome at C2 level of cervical spinal cord

SP 7 S14.123-   Central cord syndrome at C3 level of cervical spinal cord

SP 7 S14.124-   Central cord syndrome at C4 level of cervical spinal cord

SP 7 S14.125-   Central cord syndrome at C5 level of cervical spinal cord

SP 7 S14.126-   Central cord syndrome at C6 level of cervical spinal cord

SP 7 S14.127-   Central cord syndrome at C7 level of cervical spinal cord

SP 7 S14.128-   Central cord syndrome at C8 level of cervical spinal cord

!Q 7 S14.129-   Central cord syndrome at unspecified level of cervical spinal cord

6 S14.13   Anterior cord syndrome of cervical spinal cord

SP 7 S14.131-   Anterior cord syndrome at C1 level of cervical spinal cord

SP 7 S14.132-   Anterior cord syndrome at C2 level of cervical spinal cord

4 4th digit required   5 5th digit required   6 6th digit required   7 7th digit required   7 7th digit placeholder   ✚ Additional code   ⊟ Laterality

1480   *DecisionHealth's* FY 2020 Complete Home Health ICD-10-CM Diagnosis Coding Manual

SP **7** **S14.133-** Anterior cord syndrome at C3 level of cervical spinal cord

SP **7** **S14.134-** Anterior cord syndrome at C4 level of cervical spinal cord

SP **7** **S14.135-** Anterior cord syndrome at C5 level of cervical spinal cord

SP **7** **S14.136-** Anterior cord syndrome at C6 level of cervical spinal cord

SP **7** **S14.137-** Anterior cord syndrome at C7 level of cervical spinal cord

SP **7** **S14.138-** Anterior cord syndrome at C8 level of cervical spinal cord

!Q **7** **S14.139-** Anterior cord syndrome at unspecified level of cervical spinal cord

6 **S14.14** Brown-Séquard syndrome of cervical spinal cord

SP **7** **S14.141-** Brown-Séquard syndrome at C1 level of cervical spinal cord

SP **7** **S14.142-** Brown-Séquard syndrome at C2 level of cervical spinal cord

SP **7** **S14.143-** Brown-Séquard syndrome at C3 level of cervical spinal cord

SP **7** **S14.144-** Brown-Séquard syndrome at C4 level of cervical spinal cord

SP **7** **S14.145-** Brown-Séquard syndrome at C5 level of cervical spinal cord

SP **7** **S14.146-** Brown-Séquard syndrome at C6 level of cervical spinal cord

SP **7** **S14.147-** Brown-Séquard syndrome at C7 level of cervical spinal cord

SP **7** **S14.148-** Brown-Séquard syndrome at C8 level of cervical spinal cord

!Q **7** **S14.149-** Brown-Séquard syndrome at unspecified level of cervical spinal cord

6 **S14.15** Other incomplete lesions of cervical spinal cord
Incomplete lesion of cervical spinal cord NOS
Posterior cord syndrome of cervical spinal cord

SP **7** **S14.151-** Other incomplete lesion at C1 level of cervical spinal cord

SP **7** **S14.152-** Other incomplete lesion at C2 level of cervical spinal cord

SP **7** **S14.153-** Other incomplete lesion at C3 level of cervical spinal cord

SP **7** **S14.154-** Other incomplete lesion at C4 level of cervical spinal cord

SP **7** **S14.155-** Other incomplete lesion at C5 level of cervical spinal cord

SP **7** **S14.156-** Other incomplete lesion at C6 level of cervical spinal cord

SP **7** **S14.157-** Other incomplete lesion at C7 level of cervical spinal cord

SP **7** **S14.158-** Other incomplete lesion at C8 level of cervical spinal cord

!Q **7** **S14.159-** Other incomplete lesion at unspecified level of cervical spinal cord

SP **☑** **S14.2XX-** Injury of nerve root of cervical spine

SP **☑** **S14.3XX-** Injury of brachial plexus

SP **☑** **S14.4XX-** Injury of peripheral nerves of neck

SP **☑** **S14.5XX-** Injury of cervical sympathetic nerves

SP **☑** **S14.8XX-** Injury of other specified nerves of neck

!Q **☑** **S14.9XX-** Injury of unspecified nerves of neck

4 **S15** Injury of blood vessels at neck level
Code also:
  any associated open wound (S11.-)

> The appropriate 7th character is to be added to each code from category S15
> A   initial encounter
> D   subsequent encounter
> S   sequela

5 **S15.0** Injury of carotid artery of neck
Injury of carotid artery (common) (external) (internal, extracranial portion)
Injury of carotid artery NOS
  EXCLUDES 1 injury of internal carotid artery, intracranial portion (S06.8)

6 **S15.00** Unspecified injury of carotid artery

⊟ **!Q** **7** **S15.001-** Unspecified injury of right carotid artery

⊟ **!Q** **7** **S15.002-** Unspecified injury of left carotid artery

⊟ **!Q** **7** **S15.009-** Unspecified injury of unspecified carotid artery

6 **S15.01** Minor laceration of carotid artery
Incomplete transection of carotid artery
Laceration of carotid artery NOS
Superficial laceration of carotid artery

⊟ **SP** **7** **S15.011-** Minor laceration of right carotid artery

⊟ **SP** **7** **S15.012-** Minor laceration of left carotid artery

⊟ **SP** **!Q** **7** **S15.019-** Minor laceration of unspecified carotid artery

6 **S15.02** Major laceration of carotid artery
Complete transection of carotid artery
Traumatic rupture of carotid artery

⊟ **SP** **7** **S15.021-** Major laceration of right carotid artery

⊟ **SP** **7** **S15.022-** Major laceration of left carotid artery

⊟ **SP** **!Q** **7** **S15.029-** Major laceration of unspecified carotid artery

6 **S15.09** Other specified injury of carotid artery

⊟ **SP** **7** **S15.091-** Other specified injury of right carotid artery

⊟ **SP** **7** **S15.092-** Other specified injury of left carotid artery

⊟ **!Q** **7** **S15.099-** Other specified injury of unspecified carotid artery

5 **S15.1** Injury of vertebral artery

6 **S15.10** Unspecified injury of vertebral artery

⊟ **!Q** **7** **S15.101-** Unspecified injury of right vertebral artery

⊟ **!Q** **7** **S15.102-** Unspecified injury of left vertebral artery

⊟ **!Q** **7** **S15.109-** Unspecified injury of unspecified vertebral artery

6 **S15.11** Minor laceration of vertebral artery
Incomplete transection of vertebral artery

★ New ▲ Revised Px Primary **SP** PDGM Px **SL** Low CoM **SH** High CoM **!Q** Quest. Encounter **H** Hospice non-cancer Dx   Unspecified   **M** *Manifestation*

DecisionHealth's FY 2020 Complete Home Health ICD-10-CM Diagnosis Coding Manual

1481

Chapter 19

S00-T88

Laceration of vertebral artery NOS
Superficial laceration of vertebral artery

🔲 SP 7 **S15.111-** **Minor laceration of right vertebral artery**

🔲 SP 7 **S15.112-** **Minor laceration of left vertebral artery**

🔲 SP IQ 7 **S15.119-** **Minor laceration of unspecified vertebral artery**

6 **S15.12** **Major laceration of vertebral artery**
Complete transection of vertebral artery
Traumatic rupture of vertebral artery

🔲 SP 7 **S15.121-** **Major laceration of right vertebral artery**

🔲 SP 7 **S15.122-** **Major laceration of left vertebral artery**

🔲 SP IQ 7 **S15.129-** **Major laceration of unspecified vertebral artery**

6 **S15.19** **Other specified injury of vertebral artery**

🔲 SP 7 **S15.191-** **Other specified injury of right vertebral artery**

🔲 SP 7 **S15.192-** **Other specified injury of left vertebral artery**

🔲 IQ 7 **S15.199-** **Other specified injury of unspecified vertebral artery**

5 **S15.2** **Injury of external jugular vein**

6 **S15.20** **Unspecified injury of external jugular vein**

🔲 IQ 7 **S15.201-** **Unspecified injury of right external jugular vein**

🔲 IQ 7 **S15.202-** **Unspecified injury of left external jugular vein**

🔲 IQ 7 **S15.209-** **Unspecified injury of unspecified external jugular vein**

6 **S15.21** **Minor laceration of external jugular vein**
Incomplete transection of external jugular vein
Laceration of external jugular vein NOS
Superficial laceration of external jugular vein

🔲 SP 7 **S15.211-** **Minor laceration of right external jugular vein**

🔲 SP 7 **S15.212-** **Minor laceration of left external jugular vein**

🔲 IQ 7 **S15.219-** **Minor laceration of unspecified external jugular vein**

6 **S15.22** **Major laceration of external jugular vein**
Complete transection of external jugular vein
Traumatic rupture of external jugular vein

🔲 SP 7 **S15.221-** **Major laceration of right external jugular vein**

🔲 SP 7 **S15.222-** **Major laceration of left external jugular vein**

🔲 IQ 7 **S15.229-** **Major laceration of unspecified external jugular vein**

6 **S15.29** **Other specified injury of external jugular vein**

🔲 SP 7 **S15.291-** **Other specified injury of right external jugular vein**

🔲 SP 7 **S15.292-** **Other specified injury of left external jugular vein**

🔲 IQ 7 **S15.299-** **Other specified injury of unspecified external jugular vein**

5 **S15.3** **Injury of internal jugular vein**

6 **S15.30** **Unspecified injury of internal jugular vein**

🔲 IQ 7 **S15.301-** **Unspecified injury of right internal jugular vein**

🔲 IQ 7 **S15.302-** **Unspecified injury of left internal jugular vein**

🔲 IQ 7 **S15.309-** **Unspecified injury of unspecified internal jugular vein**

6 **S15.31** **Minor laceration of internal jugular vein**
Incomplete transection of internal jugular vein
Laceration of internal jugular vein NOS
Superficial laceration of internal jugular vein

🔲 SP 7 **S15.311-** **Minor laceration of right internal jugular vein**

🔲 SP 7 **S15.312-** **Minor laceration of left internal jugular vein**

🔲 IQ 7 **S15.319-** **Minor laceration of unspecified internal jugular vein**

6 **S15.32** **Major laceration of internal jugular vein**
Complete transection of internal jugular vein
Traumatic rupture of internal jugular vein

🔲 SP 7 **S15.321-** **Major laceration of right internal jugular vein**

🔲 SP 7 **S15.322-** **Major laceration of left internal jugular vein**

🔲 IQ 7 **S15.329-** **Major laceration of unspecified internal jugular vein**

6 **S15.39** **Other specified injury of internal jugular vein**

🔲 SP 7 **S15.391-** **Other specified injury of right internal jugular vein**

🔲 SP 7 **S15.392-** **Other specified injury of left internal jugular vein**

🔲 IQ 7 **S15.399-** **Other specified injury of unspecified internal jugular vein**

SP 7 **S15.8XX-** **Injury of other specified blood vessels at neck level**

IQ 7 **S15.9XX-** **Injury of unspecified blood vessel at neck level**

4 **S16** **Injury of muscle, fascia and tendon at neck level**
Code also:
any associated open wound (S11.-)
EXCLUDES 2 sprain of joint or ligament at neck level (S13.9)

---

4 4th digit required   5 5th digit required   6 6th digit required   7 7th digit required   7 7th digit placeholder   ✚ Additional code   🔲 Laterality

1482   *DecisionHealth's* FY 2020 Complete Home Health ICD-10-CM Diagnosis Coding Manual

The appropriate 7th character is to be added to each code from category S16
A   initial encounter
D   subsequent encounter
S   sequela

SP ☑ **S16.1XX-**   **Strain of muscle, fascia and tendon at neck level**

SP ☑ **S16.2XX-**   **Laceration of muscle, fascia and tendon at neck level**

IQ ☑ **S16.8XX-**   **Other specified injury of muscle, fascia and tendon at neck level**

IQ ☑ **S16.9XX-**   **Unspecified injury of muscle, fascia and tendon at neck level**

+ **4** **S17**   **Crushing injury of neck**
Use additional code for all associated injuries, such as:
injury of blood vessels (S15.-)
open wound of neck (S11.-)
spinal cord injury (S14.0, S14.1-)
vertebral fracture (S12.0--S12.3-)

The appropriate 7th character is to be added to each code from category S17
A   initial encounter
D   subsequent encounter
S   sequela

SP **+** ☑ **S17.0XX-**   **Crushing injury of larynx and trachea**

SP **+** ☑ **S17.8XX-**   **Crushing injury of other specified parts of neck**

IQ **+** ☑ **S17.9XX-**   **Crushing injury of neck, part unspecified**

4 **S19**   **Other specified and unspecified injuries of neck**

The appropriate 7th character is to be added to each code from category S19
A   initial encounter
D   subsequent encounter
S   sequela

5 **S19.8**   **Other specified injuries of neck**

SP ☑ **S19.80X-**   **Other specified injuries of unspecified part of neck**

SP ☑ **S19.81X-**   **Other specified injuries of larynx**

SP ☑ **S19.82X-**   **Other specified injuries of cervical trachea**
     EXCLUDES 2   other specified injury of thoracic trachea (S27.5-)

SP ☑ **S19.83X-**   **Other specified injuries of vocal cord**

SP ☑ **S19.84X-**   **Other specified injuries of thyroid gland**

SP ☑ **S19.85X-**   **Other specified injuries of pharynx and cervical esophagus**

SP ☑ **S19.89X-**   **Other specified injuries of other specified part of neck**

IQ ☑ **S19.9XX-**   **Unspecified injury of neck**

Injuries to the thorax   (S20-S29)

INCLUDES   injuries of breast
injuries of chest (wall)
injuries of interscapular area
EXCLUDES 2   burns and corrosions (T20-T32)
effects of foreign body in bronchus (T17.5)
effects of foreign body in esophagus (T18.1)

effects of foreign body in lung (T17.8)
effects of foreign body in trachea (T17.4)
frostbite (T33-T34)
injuries of axilla
injuries of clavicle
injuries of scapular region
injuries of shoulder
insect bite or sting, venomous (T63.4)

GUIDELINES   Section I.C.19.c.2)
Multiple fractures are sequenced in accordance with the severity of the fracture.

GUIDELINES   Section I.C.19.b.1)-2)
When coding injuries, assign separate codes for each injury unless a combination code is provided, in which case the combination code is assigned ... Traumatic injury codes (S00-T14.9) are not to be used for normal, healing surgical wounds or to identify complications of surgical wounds. The code for the most serious injury, as determined by the provider and the focus of treatment, is sequenced first.

1) Superficial injuries such as abrasions or contusions are not coded when associated with more severe injuries of the same site.

2) When a primary injury results in minor damage to peripheral nerves or blood vessels, the primary injury is sequenced first with additional code(s) for injuries to nerves and spinal cord (such as category S04), and/or injury to blood vessels (such as category S15). When the primary injury is to the blood vessels or nerves, that injury should be sequenced first.

GUIDELINES   Section I.C.19.c
Coding of Traumatic Fractures: The principles of multiple coding of injuries should be followed in coding fractures. Fractures of specified sites are coded individually by site in accordance with both the provisions within categories S02, S12, S22, S32, S42, S49, S52, S59, S62, S72, S79, S82, S89, S92 and the level of detail furnished by medical record content. A fracture not indicated as open or closed should be coded to closed. A fracture not indicated whether displaced or not displaced should be coded to displaced.

CODING TIPS ✓   7th character A is acceptable in home health and hospice when active treatment is provided, such as antibiotics for an infected wound or a wound vac for a dehisced wound. D is used when the complication or injury is now healing. Think of D as aftercare. S is used for sequela of the injury or complication. Sequela is a residual deficit or condition produced as a result of the injury or complication after the original injury or complication has healed.

4 **S20**   **Superficial injury of thorax**

The appropriate 7th character is to be added to each code from category S20
A   initial encounter
D   subsequent encounter
S   sequela

5 **S20.0**   **Contusion of breast**

⊟ **IQ** ☑ **S20.00X-**   **Contusion of breast, unspecified breast**

⊟ **IQ** ☑ **S20.01X-**   **Contusion of right breast**

⊟ **IQ** ☑ **S20.02X-**   **Contusion of left breast**

5 **S20.1**   **Other and unspecified superficial injuries of breast**

Chapter 19

S00-T88

★New ▲Revised Px Primary **SP** PDGM Px **SL** Low CoM **SH** High CoM **IQ** Quest. Encounter ⊞Hospice non-cancer Dx   Unspecified   **M** *Manifestation*

DecisionHealth's FY 2020 Complete Home Health ICD-10-CM Diagnosis Coding Manual   1483

⑥ **S20.10** **Unspecified superficial injuries of breast**

▤ !Q ⑦ **S20.101-** **Unspecified superficial injuries of breast, right breast**

▤ !Q ⑦ **S20.102-** **Unspecified superficial injuries of breast, left breast**

▤ !Q ⑦ **S20.109-** **Unspecified superficial injuries of breast, unspecified breast**

⑥ **S20.11** Abrasion of breast

▤ !Q ⑦ **S20.111-** Abrasion of breast, right breast

▤ !Q ⑦ **S20.112-** Abrasion of breast, left breast

▤ !Q ⑦ **S20.119-** **Abrasion of breast, unspecified breast**

⑥ **S20.12** Blister (nonthermal) of breast

▤ !Q ⑦ **S20.121-** Blister (nonthermal) of breast, right breast

▤ !Q ⑦ **S20.122-** Blister (nonthermal) of breast, left breast

▤ !Q ⑦ **S20.129-** **Blister (nonthermal) of breast, unspecified breast**

⑥ **S20.14** External constriction of part of breast

▤ !Q ⑦ **S20.141-** External constriction of part of breast, right breast

▤ !Q ⑦ **S20.142-** External constriction of part of breast, left breast

▤ !Q ⑦ **S20.149-** **External constriction of part of breast, unspecified breast**

⑥ **S20.15** Superficial foreign body of breast
Splinter in the breast

▤ !Q ⑦ **S20.151-** Superficial foreign body of breast, right breast

▤ !Q ⑦ **S20.152-** Superficial foreign body of breast, left breast

▤ !Q ⑦ **S20.159-** **Superficial foreign body of breast, unspecified breast**

⑥ **S20.16** Insect bite (nonvenomous) of breast

▤ !Q ⑦ **S20.161-** Insect bite (nonvenomous) of breast, right breast

▤ !Q ⑦ **S20.162-** Insect bite (nonvenomous) of breast, left breast

▤ !Q ⑦ **S20.169-** **Insect bite (nonvenomous) of breast, unspecified breast**

⑥ **S20.17** Other superficial bite of breast
EXCLUDES 1 open bite of breast (S21.05-)

▤ !Q ⑦ **S20.171-** Other superficial bite of breast, right breast

▤ !Q ⑦ **S20.172-** Other superficial bite of breast, left breast

▤ !Q ⑦ **S20.179-** **Other superficial bite of breast, unspecified breast**

⑤ **S20.2** Contusion of thorax

!Q ⑦ **S20.20X-** **Contusion of thorax, unspecified**

⑥ **S20.21** Contusion of front wall of thorax

▤ SP ⑦ **S20.211-** Contusion of right front wall of thorax

▤ SP ⑦ **S20.212-** Contusion of left front wall of thorax

▤ !Q ⑦ **S20.219-** **Contusion of unspecified front wall of thorax**

⑥ **S20.22** Contusion of back wall of thorax

▤ SP ⑦ **S20.221-** Contusion of right back wall of thorax

▤ SP ⑦ **S20.222-** Contusion of left back wall of thorax

▤ !Q ⑦ **S20.229-** **Contusion of unspecified back wall of thorax**

⑤ **S20.3** **Other and unspecified superficial injuries of front wall of thorax**

⑥ **S20.30** **Unspecified superficial injuries of front wall of thorax**

▤ !Q ⑦ **S20.301-** **Unspecified superficial injuries of right front wall of thorax**

▤ !Q ⑦ **S20.302-** **Unspecified superficial injuries of left front wall of thorax**

▤ !Q ⑦ **S20.309-** **Unspecified superficial injuries of unspecified front wall of thorax**

⑥ **S20.31** Abrasion of front wall of thorax

▤ !Q ⑦ **S20.311-** Abrasion of right front wall of thorax

▤ !Q ⑦ **S20.312-** Abrasion of left front wall of thorax

▤ !Q ⑦ **S20.319-** **Abrasion of unspecified front wall of thorax**

⑥ **S20.32** Blister (nonthermal) of front wall of thorax

▤ !Q ⑦ **S20.321-** Blister (nonthermal) of right front wall of thorax

▤ !Q ⑦ **S20.322-** Blister (nonthermal) of left front wall of thorax

▤ !Q ⑦ **S20.329-** **Blister (nonthermal) of unspecified front wall of thorax**

⑥ **S20.34** External constriction of front wall of thorax

▤ !Q ⑦ **S20.341-** External constriction of right front wall of thorax

▤ !Q ⑦ **S20.342-** External constriction of left front wall of thorax

▤ !Q ⑦ **S20.349-** **External constriction of unspecified front wall of thorax**

⑥ **S20.35** Superficial foreign body of front wall of thorax
Splinter in front wall of thorax

▤ !Q ⑦ **S20.351-** Superficial foreign body of right front wall of thorax

▤ !Q ⑦ **S20.352-** Superficial foreign body of left front wall of thorax

▤ !Q ⑦ **S20.359-** **Superficial foreign body of unspecified front wall of thorax**

⑥ **S20.36** Insect bite (nonvenomous) of front wall of thorax

▤ !Q ⑦ **S20.361-** Insect bite (nonvenomous) of right front wall of thorax

▤ !Q ⑦ **S20.362-** Insect bite (nonvenomous) of left front wall of thorax

▤ !Q ⑦ **S20.369-** **Insect bite (nonvenomous) of unspecified front wall of thorax**

⑥ **S20.37** Other superficial bite of front wall of thorax
EXCLUDES 1 open bite of front wall of thorax (S21.14)

▤ !Q ⑦ **S20.371-** Other superficial bite of right front wall of thorax

▤ !Q ⑦ **S20.372-** Other superficial bite of left front wall of thorax

▤ !Q ⑦ **S20.379-** **Other superficial bite of unspecified front wall of thorax**

④ 4th digit required ⑤ 5th digit required ⑥ 6th digit required ⑦ 7th digit required ⑦ 7th digit placeholder ✚ Additional code ▤ Laterality

1484 *DecisionHealth's* FY 2020 Complete Home Health ICD-10-CM Diagnosis Coding Manual

5 S20.4 Other and unspecified superficial injuries of back wall of thorax

6 S20.40 Unspecified superficial injuries of back wall of thorax

☰ !Q 7 **S20.401- Unspecified superficial injuries of right back wall of thorax**

☰ !Q 7 **S20.402- Unspecified superficial injuries of left back wall of thorax**

☰ !Q 7 **S20.409- Unspecified superficial injuries of unspecified back wall of thorax**

6 S20.41 Abrasion of back wall of thorax

☰ !Q 7 **S20.411- Abrasion of right back wall of thorax**

☰ !Q 7 **S20.412- Abrasion of left back wall of thorax**

☰ !Q 7 **S20.419- Abrasion of unspecified back wall of thorax**

6 S20.42 Blister (nonthermal) of back wall of thorax

☰ !Q 7 **S20.421- Blister (nonthermal) of right back wall of thorax**

☰ !Q 7 **S20.422- Blister (nonthermal) of left back wall of thorax**

☰ !Q 7 **S20.429- Blister (nonthermal) of unspecified back wall of thorax**

6 S20.44 External constriction of back wall of thorax

☰ !Q 7 **S20.441- External constriction of right back wall of thorax**

☰ !Q 7 **S20.442- External constriction of left back wall of thorax**

☰ !Q 7 **S20.449- External constriction of unspecified back wall of thorax**

6 S20.45 Superficial foreign body of back wall of thorax
Splinter of back wall of thorax

☰ !Q 7 **S20.451- Superficial foreign body of right back wall of thorax**

☰ !Q 7 **S20.452- Superficial foreign body of left back wall of thorax**

☰ !Q 7 **S20.459- Superficial foreign body of unspecified back wall of thorax**

6 S20.46 Insect bite (nonvenomous) of back wall of thorax

☰ !Q 7 **S20.461- Insect bite (nonvenomous) of right back wall of thorax**

☰ !Q 7 **S20.462- Insect bite (nonvenomous) of left back wall of thorax**

☰ !Q 7 **S20.469- Insect bite (nonvenomous) of unspecified back wall of thorax**

6 S20.47 Other superficial bite of back wall of thorax
EXCLUDES 1 open bite of back wall of thorax (S21.24)

☰ !Q 7 **S20.471- Other superficial bite of right back wall of thorax**

☰ !Q 7 **S20.472- Other superficial bite of left back wall of thorax**

☰ !Q 7 **S20.479- Other superficial bite of unspecified back wall of thorax**

5 S20.9 Superficial injury of unspecified parts of thorax
EXCLUDES 1 contusion of thorax NOS (S20.20)

!Q 7 **S20.90X- Unspecified superficial injury of unspecified parts of thorax**
Superficial injury of thoracic wall NOS

!Q 7 **S20.91X- Abrasion of unspecified parts of thorax**

!Q 7 **S20.92X- Blister (nonthermal) of unspecified parts of thorax**

!Q 7 **S20.94X- External constriction of unspecified parts of thorax**

!Q 7 **S20.95X- Superficial foreign body of unspecified parts of thorax**
Splinter in thorax NOS

!Q 7 **S20.96X- Insect bite (nonvenomous) of unspecified parts of thorax**

!Q 7 **S20.97X- Other superficial bite of unspecified parts of thorax**
EXCLUDES 1 open bite of thorax NOS (S21.95)

4 S21 Open wound of thorax
Code also any associated injury, such as:
  injury of heart (S26.-)
  injury of intrathoracic organs (S27.-)
  rib fracture (S22.3-, S22.4-)
  spinal cord injury (S24.0-, S24.1-)
  traumatic hemopneumothorax (S27.3)
  traumatic hemothorax (S27.1)
  traumatic pneumothorax (S27.0)
  wound infection
EXCLUDES 1 traumatic amputation (partial) of thorax (S28.1)

The appropriate 7th character is to be added to each code from category S21
A   initial encounter
D   subsequent encounter
S   sequela

CODING TIPS ✓   Open wound codes are used for wounds caused by trauma. Do not assign a code for "open wound" unless the etiology of the wound is related to trauma. Do not use Z codes for any aspect of care of a trauma wound, e.g. no Z code for dressing changes, drain care, or suture removal.

CODING TIPS ✓   No aftercare code applies. The 7th character "D" is the default for home care and hospice when providing aftercare for a healing or resolving condition; "A" is used for active treatment such as antibiotics or more than routine wound care; "S" may be used to indicate a residual condition after the original injury has healed.

5 S21.0 Open wound of breast

6 S21.00 Unspecified open wound of breast

☰ SP 7 **S21.001- Unspecified open wound of right breast**

☰ SP 7 **S21.002- Unspecified open wound of left breast**

☰ !Q 7 **S21.009- Unspecified open wound of unspecified breast**

6 S21.01 Laceration without foreign body of breast

☰ SP 7 **S21.011- Laceration without foreign body of right breast**

☰ SP 7 **S21.012- Laceration without foreign body of left breast**

★ New ▲ Revised Px Primary SP PDGM Px SL Low CoM SH High CoM !Q Quest. Encounter H Hospice non-cancer Dx Unspecified M *Manifestation*

DecisionHealth's FY 2020 Complete Home Health ICD-10-CM Diagnosis Coding Manual   1485

Chapter 19

S00-T88

⊟ **IQ** **7** S21.019- **Laceration without foreign body of unspecified breast**

6 S21.02 **Laceration with foreign body of breast**

⊟ **SP** **7** S21.021- **Laceration with foreign body of right breast**

⊟ **SP** **7** S21.022- **Laceration with foreign body of left breast**

⊟ **IQ** **7** S21.029- **Laceration with foreign body of unspecified breast**

6 S21.03 **Puncture wound without foreign body of breast**

⊟ **SP** **7** S21.031- **Puncture wound without foreign body of right breast**

⊟ **SP** **7** S21.032- **Puncture wound without foreign body of left breast**

⊟ **IQ** **7** S21.039- **Puncture wound without foreign body of unspecified breast**

6 S21.04 **Puncture wound with foreign body of breast**

⊟ **SP** **7** S21.041- **Puncture wound with foreign body of right breast**

⊟ **SP** **7** S21.042- **Puncture wound with foreign body of left breast**

⊟ **IQ** **7** S21.049- **Puncture wound with foreign body of unspecified breast**

6 S21.05 **Open bite of breast**
Bite of breast NOS
> **EXCLUDES 1** superficial bite of breast (S20.17)

⊟ **SP** **7** S21.051- **Open bite of right breast**

⊟ **SP** **7** S21.052- **Open bite of left breast**

⊟ **IQ** **7** S21.059- **Open bite of unspecified breast**

5 S21.1 **Open wound of front wall of thorax without penetration into thoracic cavity**
Open wound of chest without penetration into thoracic cavity

6 S21.10 **Unspecified open wound of front wall of thorax without penetration into thoracic cavity**

⊟ **SP** **7** S21.101- **Unspecified open wound of right front wall of thorax without penetration into thoracic cavity**

⊟ **SP** **7** S21.102- **Unspecified open wound of left front wall of thorax without penetration into thoracic cavity**

⊟ **SP** **7** S21.109- **Unspecified open wound of unspecified front wall of thorax without penetration into thoracic cavity**

6 S21.11 **Laceration without foreign body of front wall of thorax without penetration into thoracic cavity**

⊟ **SP** **7** S21.111- **Laceration without foreign body of right front wall of thorax without penetration into thoracic cavity**

⊟ **SP** **7** S21.112- **Laceration without foreign body of left front wall of thorax without penetration into thoracic cavity**

⊟ **SP** **7** S21.119- **Laceration without foreign body of unspecified front wall of thorax without penetration into thoracic cavity**

6 S21.12 **Laceration with foreign body of front wall of thorax without penetration into thoracic cavity**

⊟ **SP** **7** S21.121- **Laceration with foreign body of right front wall of thorax without penetration into thoracic cavity**

⊟ **SP** **7** S21.122- **Laceration with foreign body of left front wall of thorax without penetration into thoracic cavity**

⊟ **SP** **7** S21.129- **Laceration with foreign body of unspecified front wall of thorax without penetration into thoracic cavity**

6 S21.13 **Puncture wound without foreign body of front wall of thorax without penetration into thoracic cavity**

⊟ **SP** **7** S21.131- **Puncture wound without foreign body of right front wall of thorax without penetration into thoracic cavity**

⊟ **SP** **7** S21.132- **Puncture wound without foreign body of left front wall of thorax without penetration into thoracic cavity**

⊟ **IQ** **7** S21.139- **Puncture wound without foreign body of unspecified front wall of thorax without penetration into thoracic cavity**

6 S21.14 **Puncture wound with foreign body of front wall of thorax without penetration into thoracic cavity**

⊟ **SP** **7** S21.141- **Puncture wound with foreign body of right front wall of thorax without penetration into thoracic cavity**

⊟ **SP** **7** S21.142- **Puncture wound with foreign body of left front wall of thorax without penetration into thoracic cavity**

⊟ **IQ** **7** S21.149- **Puncture wound with foreign body of unspecified front wall of thorax without penetration into thoracic cavity**

6 S21.15 **Open bite of front wall of thorax without penetration into thoracic cavity**
Bite of front wall of thorax NOS
> **EXCLUDES 1** superficial bite of front wall of thorax (S20.37)

⊟ **SP** **7** S21.151- **Open bite of right front wall of thorax without penetration into thoracic cavity**

⊟ **SP** **7** S21.152- **Open bite of left front wall of thorax without penetration into thoracic cavity**

⊟ **IQ** **7** S21.159- **Open bite of unspecified front wall of thorax without penetration into thoracic cavity**

5 S21.2 **Open wound of back wall of thorax without penetration into thoracic cavity**

6 S21.20 **Unspecified open wound of back wall of thorax without penetration into thoracic cavity**

---

4 4th digit required   **5** 5th digit required   **6** 6th digit required   **7** 7th digit required   **7** 7th digit placeholder   **+** Additional code   ⊟ Laterality

☐ **SP** ⑦ **S21.201-** Unspecified open wound of right back wall of thorax without penetration into thoracic cavity

☐ **SP** ⑦ **S21.202-** Unspecified open wound of left back wall of thorax without penetration into thoracic cavity

☐ **SP** ⑦ **S21.209-** Unspecified open wound of unspecified back wall of thorax without penetration into thoracic cavity

⑥ **S21.21** Laceration without foreign body of back wall of thorax without penetration into thoracic cavity

☐ **SP** ⑦ **S21.211-** Laceration without foreign body of right back wall of thorax without penetration into thoracic cavity

☐ **SP** ⑦ **S21.212-** Laceration without foreign body of left back wall of thorax without penetration into thoracic cavity

☐ **SP** ⑦ **S21.219-** Laceration without foreign body of unspecified back wall of thorax without penetration into thoracic cavity

⑥ **S21.22** Laceration with foreign body of back wall of thorax without penetration into thoracic cavity

☐ **SP** ⑦ **S21.221-** Laceration with foreign body of right back wall of thorax without penetration into thoracic cavity

☐ **SP** ⑦ **S21.222-** Laceration with foreign body of left back wall of thorax without penetration into thoracic cavity

☐ **SP** ⑦ **S21.229-** Laceration with foreign body of unspecified back wall of thorax without penetration into thoracic cavity

⑥ **S21.23** Puncture wound without foreign body of back wall of thorax without penetration into thoracic cavity

☐ **SP** ⑦ **S21.231-** Puncture wound without foreign body of right back wall of thorax without penetration into thoracic cavity

☐ **SP** ⑦ **S21.232-** Puncture wound without foreign body of left back wall of thorax without penetration into thoracic cavity

☐ **IQ** ⑦ **S21.239-** Puncture wound without foreign body of unspecified back wall of thorax without penetration into thoracic cavity

⑥ **S21.24** Puncture wound with foreign body of back wall of thorax without penetration into thoracic cavity

☐ **SP** ⑦ **S21.241-** Puncture wound with foreign body of right back wall of thorax without penetration into thoracic cavity

☐ **SP** ⑦ **S21.242-** Puncture wound with foreign body of left back wall of thorax without penetration into thoracic cavity

☐ **IQ** ⑦ **S21.249-** Puncture wound with foreign body of unspecified back wall of thorax without penetration into thoracic cavity

⑥ **S21.25** Open bite of back wall of thorax without penetration into thoracic cavity
Bite of back wall of thorax NOS
EXCLUDES 1 superficial bite of back wall of thorax (S20.47)

☐ **SP** ⑦ **S21.251-** Open bite of right back wall of thorax without penetration into thoracic cavity

☐ **SP** ⑦ **S21.252-** Open bite of left back wall of thorax without penetration into thoracic cavity

☐ **IQ** ⑦ **S21.259-** Open bite of unspecified back wall of thorax without penetration into thoracic cavity

⑤ **S21.3** Open wound of front wall of thorax with penetration into thoracic cavity
Open wound of chest with penetration into thoracic cavity

⑥ **S21.30** Unspecified open wound of front wall of thorax with penetration into thoracic cavity

☐ **SP** ⑦ **S21.301-** Unspecified open wound of right front wall of thorax with penetration into thoracic cavity

☐ **SP** ⑦ **S21.302-** Unspecified open wound of left front wall of thorax with penetration into thoracic cavity

☐ **SP** ⑦ **S21.309-** Unspecified open wound of unspecified front wall of thorax with penetration into thoracic cavity

⑥ **S21.31** Laceration without foreign body of front wall of thorax with penetration into thoracic cavity

☐ **SP** ⑦ **S21.311-** Laceration without foreign body of right front wall of thorax with penetration into thoracic cavity

☐ **SP** ⑦ **S21.312-** Laceration without foreign body of left front wall of thorax with penetration into thoracic cavity

☐ **SP** ⑦ **S21.319-** Laceration without foreign body of unspecified front wall of thorax with penetration into thoracic cavity

⑥ **S21.32** Laceration with foreign body of front wall of thorax with penetration into thoracic cavity

☐ **SP** ⑦ **S21.321-** Laceration with foreign body of right front wall of thorax with penetration into thoracic cavity

☐ **SP** ⑦ **S21.322-** Laceration with foreign body of left front wall of thorax with penetration into thoracic cavity

☐ **SP** ⑦ **S21.329-** Laceration with foreign body of unspecified front wall of thorax with penetration into thoracic cavity

⑥ **S21.33** Puncture wound without foreign body of front wall of thorax with penetration into thoracic cavity

Chapter 19

S00-T88

★ New ▲ Revised **Px** Primary **SP** PDGM Px **SL** Low CoM **SH** High CoM **IQ** Quest. Encounter ☐ Hospice non-cancer Dx Unspecified **M** *Manifestation*

DecisionHealth's FY 2020 Complete Home Health ICD-10-CM Diagnosis Coding Manual

1487

Chapter 19

S00-T88

⊟ SP 7 **S21.331-** Puncture wound without foreign body of right front wall of thorax with penetration into thoracic cavity

⊟ SP 7 **S21.332-** Puncture wound without foreign body of left front wall of thorax with penetration into thoracic cavity

⊟ !Q 7 **S21.339-** Puncture wound without foreign body of unspecified front wall of thorax with penetration into thoracic cavity

6 **S21.34** Puncture wound with foreign body of front wall of thorax with penetration into thoracic cavity

⊟ SP 7 **S21.341-** Puncture wound with foreign body of right front wall of thorax with penetration into thoracic cavity

⊟ SP 7 **S21.342-** Puncture wound with foreign body of left front wall of thorax with penetration into thoracic cavity

⊟ !Q 7 **S21.349-** Puncture wound with foreign body of unspecified front wall of thorax with penetration into thoracic cavity

6 **S21.35** Open bite of front wall of thorax with penetration into thoracic cavity
EXCLUDES 1 superficial bite of front wall of thorax (S20.37)

⊟ SP 7 **S21.351-** Open bite of right front wall of thorax with penetration into thoracic cavity

⊟ SP 7 **S21.352-** Open bite of left front wall of thorax with penetration into thoracic cavity

⊟ !Q 7 **S21.359-** Open bite of unspecified front wall of thorax with penetration into thoracic cavity

5 **S21.4** Open wound of back wall of thorax with penetration into thoracic cavity

6 **S21.40** Unspecified open wound of back wall of thorax with penetration into thoracic cavity

⊟ SP 7 **S21.401-** Unspecified open wound of right back wall of thorax with penetration into thoracic cavity

⊟ SP 7 **S21.402-** Unspecified open wound of left back wall of thorax with penetration into thoracic cavity

⊟ SP 7 **S21.409-** Unspecified open wound of unspecified back wall of thorax with penetration into thoracic cavity

6 **S21.41** Laceration without foreign body of back wall of thorax with penetration into thoracic cavity

⊟ SP 7 **S21.411-** Laceration without foreign body of right back wall of thorax with penetration into thoracic cavity

⊟ SP 7 **S21.412-** Laceration without foreign body of left back wall of thorax with penetration into thoracic cavity

⊟ SP 7 **S21.419-** Laceration without foreign body of unspecified back wall of thorax with penetration into thoracic cavity

6 **S21.42** Laceration with foreign body of back wall of thorax with penetration into thoracic cavity

⊟ SP 7 **S21.421-** Laceration with foreign body of right back wall of thorax with penetration into thoracic cavity

⊟ SP 7 **S21.422-** Laceration with foreign body of left back wall of thorax with penetration into thoracic cavity

⊟ SP 7 **S21.429-** Laceration with foreign body of unspecified back wall of thorax with penetration into thoracic cavity

6 **S21.43** Puncture wound without foreign body of back wall of thorax with penetration into thoracic cavity

⊟ SP 7 **S21.431-** Puncture wound without foreign body of right back wall of thorax with penetration into thoracic cavity

⊟ SP 7 **S21.432-** Puncture wound without foreign body of left back wall of thorax with penetration into thoracic cavity

⊟ !Q 7 **S21.439-** Puncture wound without foreign body of unspecified back wall of thorax with penetration into thoracic cavity

6 **S21.44** Puncture wound with foreign body of back wall of thorax with penetration into thoracic cavity

⊟ SP 7 **S21.441-** Puncture wound with foreign body of right back wall of thorax with penetration into thoracic cavity

⊟ SP 7 **S21.442-** Puncture wound with foreign body of left back wall of thorax with penetration into thoracic cavity

⊟ !Q 7 **S21.449-** Puncture wound with foreign body of unspecified back wall of thorax with penetration into thoracic cavity

6 **S21.45** Open bite of back wall of thorax with penetration into thoracic cavity
Bite of back wall of thorax NOS
EXCLUDES 1 superficial bite of back wall of thorax (S20.47)

⊟ SP 7 **S21.451-** Open bite of right back wall of thorax with penetration into thoracic cavity

⊟ SP 7 **S21.452-** Open bite of left back wall of thorax with penetration into thoracic cavity

⊟ !Q 7 **S21.459-** Open bite of unspecified back wall of thorax with penetration into thoracic cavity

5 **S21.9** Open wound of unspecified part of thorax
Open wound of thoracic wall NOS

SP 7 **S21.90X-** Unspecified open wound of unspecified part of thorax

---

4 4th digit required   5 5th digit required   6 6th digit required   7 7th digit required   7 7th digit placeholder   ✚ Additional code   ⊟ Laterality

SP ☑ S21.91X- **Laceration without foreign body of unspecified part of thorax**

SP ☑ S21.92X- **Laceration with foreign body of unspecified part of thorax**

IQ ☑ S21.93X- **Puncture wound without foreign body of unspecified part of thorax**

IQ ☑ S21.94X- **Puncture wound with foreign body of unspecified part of thorax**

IQ ☑ S21.95X- **Open bite of unspecified part of thorax**

> **EXCLUDES 1** superficial bite of thorax (S20.97)

④ S22 **Fracture of rib(s), sternum and thoracic spine**

Note:

A fracture not indicated as displaced or nondisplaced should be coded to displaced

A fracture not indicated as open or closed should be coded to closed

> **INCLUDES** fracture of thoracic neural arch
> fracture of thoracic spinous process
> fracture of thoracic transverse process
> fracture of thoracic vertebra
> fracture of thoracic vertebral arch

Code first any associated:
injury of intrathoracic organ (S27.-)
spinal cord injury (S24.0-, S24.1-)

> **EXCLUDES 1** transection of thorax (S28.1)
> **EXCLUDES 2** fracture of clavicle (S42.0-)
> fracture of scapula (S42.1-)

The appropriate 7th character is to be added to each code from category S22

A	initial encounter for closed fracture
B	initial encounter for open fracture
D	subsequent encounter for fracture with routine healing
G	subsequent encounter for fracture with delayed healing
K	subsequent encounter for fracture with nonunion
S	sequela

CODING TIPS ✓ Fractures repaired by joint replacements are NOT coded with Z47.1. Fractures repaired by any other orthopedic surgery are NOT coded with Z47.89. Z codes are not appropriate for fractures of any kind. Code the fracture with 7th character D for fractures undergoing surgical repair.

CODING TIPS ✓ A fracture not indicated as displaced or nondisplaced should be coded to displaced. A fracture not indicated as open or closed should be coded to closed.

CODING TIPS ✓ 'D' is the 7th character for home care and hospice unless the physician has documented delayed healing, nonunion or malunion. A sequela is a condition left after the fracture has healed. The Gustilo open fracture classification must be used for open fractures. The default 7th character for open fractures is E.

⑤ S22.0 **Fracture of thoracic vertebra**

⑥ S22.00 **Fracture of unspecified thoracic vertebra**

SP ⑦ S22.000- **Wedge compression fracture of unspecified thoracic vertebra**

SP ⑦ S22.001- **Stable burst fracture of unspecified thoracic vertebra**

SP ⑦ S22.002- **Unstable burst fracture of unspecified thoracic vertebra**

SP ⑦ S22.008- **Other fracture of unspecified thoracic vertebra**

SP ⑦ S22.009- **Unspecified fracture of unspecified thoracic vertebra**

⑥ S22.01 **Fracture of first thoracic vertebra**

SP ⑦ S22.010- **Wedge compression fracture of first thoracic vertebra**

SP ⑦ S22.011- **Stable burst fracture of first thoracic vertebra**

SP ⑦ S22.012- **Unstable burst fracture of first thoracic vertebra**

SP ⑦ S22.018- **Other fracture of first thoracic vertebra**

SP ⑦ S22.019- **Unspecified fracture of first thoracic vertebra**

⑥ S22.02 **Fracture of second thoracic vertebra**

SP ⑦ S22.020- **Wedge compression fracture of second thoracic vertebra**

SP ⑦ S22.021- **Stable burst fracture of second thoracic vertebra**

SP ⑦ S22.022- **Unstable burst fracture of second thoracic vertebra**

SP ⑦ S22.028- **Other fracture of second thoracic vertebra**

SP ⑦ S22.029- **Unspecified fracture of second thoracic vertebra**

⑥ S22.03 **Fracture of third thoracic vertebra**

SP ⑦ S22.030- **Wedge compression fracture of third thoracic vertebra**

SP ⑦ S22.031- **Stable burst fracture of third thoracic vertebra**

SP ⑦ S22.032- **Unstable burst fracture of third thoracic vertebra**

SP ⑦ S22.038- **Other fracture of third thoracic vertebra**

SP ⑦ S22.039- **Unspecified fracture of third thoracic vertebra**

⑥ S22.04 **Fracture of fourth thoracic vertebra**

SP ⑦ S22.040- **Wedge compression fracture of fourth thoracic vertebra**

SP ⑦ S22.041- **Stable burst fracture of fourth thoracic vertebra**

SP ⑦ S22.042- **Unstable burst fracture of fourth thoracic vertebra**

SP ⑦ S22.048- **Other fracture of fourth thoracic vertebra**

SP ⑦ S22.049- **Unspecified fracture of fourth thoracic vertebra**

⑥ S22.05 **Fracture of T5-T6 vertebra**

SP ⑦ S22.050- **Wedge compression fracture of T5-T6 vertebra**

SP ⑦ S22.051- **Stable burst fracture of T5-T6 vertebra**

SP ⑦ S22.052- **Unstable burst fracture of T5-T6 vertebra**

SP ⑦ S22.058- **Other fracture of T5-T6 vertebra**

Chapter 19

S00-T88

★ New ▲ Revised Px Primary SP PDGM Px SL Low CoM SH High CoM IQ Quest. Encounter H Hospice non-cancer Dx | Unspecified | M *Manifestation*

DecisionHealth's FY 2020 Complete Home Health ICD-10-CM Diagnosis Coding Manual | 1489

SP 7 S22.059- Unspecified fracture of T5-T6 vertebra

6 S22.06 Fracture of T7-T8 vertebra

SP 7 S22.060- Wedge compression fracture of T7-T8 vertebra

SP 7 S22.061- Stable burst fracture of T7-T8 vertebra

SP 7 S22.062- Unstable burst fracture of T7-T8 vertebra

SP 7 S22.068- Other fracture of T7-T8 thoracic vertebra

SP 7 S22.069- Unspecified fracture of T7-T8 vertebra

6 S22.07 Fracture of T9-T10 vertebra

SP 7 S22.070- Wedge compression fracture of T9-T10 vertebra

SP 7 S22.071- Stable burst fracture of T9-T10 vertebra

SP 7 S22.072- Unstable burst fracture of T9-T10 vertebra

SP 7 S22.078- Other fracture of T9-T10 vertebra

SP 7 S22.079- Unspecified fracture of T9-T10 vertebra

6 S22.08 Fracture of T11-T12 vertebra

SP 7 S22.080- Wedge compression fracture of T11-T12 vertebra

SP 7 S22.081- Stable burst fracture of T11-T12 vertebra

SP 7 S22.082- Unstable burst fracture of T11-T12 vertebra

SP 7 S22.088- Other fracture of T11-T12 vertebra

SP 7 S22.089- Unspecified fracture of T11-T12 vertebra

5 S22.2 Fracture of sternum

SP 7 S22.20X- Unspecified fracture of sternum

SP 7 S22.21X- Fracture of manubrium

SP 7 S22.22X- Fracture of body of sternum

SP 7 S22.23X- Sternal manubrial dissociation

SP 7 S22.24X- Fracture of xiphoid process

5 S22.3 Fracture of one rib

⊟ SP 7 S22.31X- Fracture of one rib, right side

⊟ SP 7 S22.32X- Fracture of one rib, left side

⊟ !Q 7 S22.39X- Fracture of one rib, unspecified side

5 S22.4 Multiple fractures of ribs
Fractures of two or more ribs
EXCLUDES 1 flail chest (S22.5-)

⊟ SP 7 S22.41X- Multiple fractures of ribs, right side

⊟ SP 7 S22.42X- Multiple fractures of ribs, left side

⊟ SP 7 S22.43X- Multiple fractures of ribs, bilateral

⊟ !Q 7 S22.49X- Multiple fractures of ribs, unspecified side

SP 7 S22.5XX- Flail chest

SP 7 S22.9XX- Fracture of bony thorax, part unspecified

4 S23 Dislocation and sprain of joints and ligaments of thorax
INCLUDES avulsion of joint or ligament of thorax

laceration of cartilage, joint or ligament of thorax
sprain of cartilage, joint or ligament of thorax
traumatic hemarthrosis of joint or ligament of thorax
traumatic rupture of joint or ligament of thorax
traumatic subluxation of joint or ligament of thorax
traumatic tear of joint or ligament of thorax
Code also:
any associated open wound
EXCLUDES 2 dislocation, sprain of sternoclavicular joint (S43.2, S43.6)
strain of muscle or tendon of thorax (S29.01-)

The appropriate 7th character is to be added to each code from category S23
A   initial encounter
D   subsequent encounter
S   sequela

SP 7 S23.0XX- Traumatic rupture of thoracic intervertebral disc
EXCLUDES 1 rupture or displacement (nontraumatic) of thoracic intervertebral disc NOS (M51.- with fifth character 4)

5 S23.1 Subluxation and dislocation of thoracic vertebra
Code also:
any associated
open wound of thorax (S21.-)
spinal cord injury (S24.0-, S24.1-)
EXCLUDES 2 fracture of thoracic vertebrae (S22.0-)

6 S23.10 Subluxation and dislocation of unspecified thoracic vertebra

!Q 7 S23.100- Subluxation of unspecified thoracic vertebra

!Q 7 S23.101- Dislocation of unspecified thoracic vertebra

6 S23.11 Subluxation and dislocation of T1/T2 thoracic vertebra

SP 7 S23.110- Subluxation of T1/T2 thoracic vertebra

SP 7 S23.111- Dislocation of T1/T2 thoracic vertebra

6 S23.12 Subluxation and dislocation of T2/T3-T3/T4 thoracic vertebra

SP 7 S23.120- Subluxation of T2/T3 thoracic vertebra

SP 7 S23.121- Dislocation of T2/T3 thoracic vertebra

SP 7 S23.122- Subluxation of T3/T4 thoracic vertebra

SP 7 S23.123- Dislocation of T3/T4 thoracic vertebra

6 S23.13 Subluxation and dislocation of T4/T5-T5/T6 thoracic vertebra

SP 7 S23.130- Subluxation of T4/T5 thoracic vertebra

SP 7 S23.131- Dislocation of T4/T5 thoracic vertebra

4 4th digit required   5 5th digit required   6 6th digit required   7 7th digit required   7 7th digit placeholder   + Additional code   ⊟ Laterality

1490   DecisionHealth's FY 2020 Complete Home Health ICD-10-CM Diagnosis Coding Manual

SP 7 S23.132- Subluxation of T5/T6 thoracic vertebra

SP 7 S23.133- Dislocation of T5/T6 thoracic vertebra

6 S23.14 Subluxation and dislocation of T6/T7-T7/T8 thoracic vertebra

SP 7 S23.140- Subluxation of T6/T7 thoracic vertebra

SP 7 S23.141- Dislocation of T6/T7 thoracic vertebra

SP 7 S23.142- Subluxation of T7/T8 thoracic vertebra

SP 7 S23.143- Dislocation of T7/T8 thoracic vertebra

6 S23.15 Subluxation and dislocation of T8/T9-T9/T10 thoracic vertebra

SP 7 S23.150- Subluxation of T8/T9 thoracic vertebra

SP 7 S23.151- Dislocation of T8/T9 thoracic vertebra

SP 7 S23.152- Subluxation of T9/T10 thoracic vertebra

SP 7 S23.153- Dislocation of T9/T10 thoracic vertebra

6 S23.16 Subluxation and dislocation of T10/T11-T11/T12 thoracic vertebra

SP 7 S23.160- Subluxation of T10/T11 thoracic vertebra

SP 7 S23.161- Dislocation of T10/T11 thoracic vertebra

SP 7 S23.162- Subluxation of T11/T12 thoracic vertebra

SP 7 S23.163- Dislocation of T11/T12 thoracic vertebra

6 S23.17 Subluxation and dislocation of T12/L1 thoracic vertebra

SP 7 S23.170- Subluxation of T12/L1 thoracic vertebra

SP 7 S23.171- Dislocation of T12/L1 thoracic vertebra

5 S23.2 Dislocation of other and unspecified parts of thorax

IQ 7 S23.20X- Dislocation of unspecified part of thorax

IQ 7 S23.29X- Dislocation of other parts of thorax

SP 7 S23.3XX- Sprain of ligaments of thoracic spine

5 S23.4 Sprain of ribs and sternum

SP 7 S23.41X- Sprain of ribs

6 S23.42 Sprain of sternum

SP 7 S23.420- Sprain of sternoclavicular (joint) (ligament)

SP 7 S23.421- Sprain of chondrosternal joint

SP 7 S23.428- Other sprain of sternum

SP 7 S23.429- Unspecified sprain of sternum

SP 7 S23.8XX- Sprain of other specified parts of thorax

SP 7 S23.9XX- Sprain of unspecified parts of thorax

4 S24 Injury of nerves and spinal cord at thorax level
Note:
Code to highest level of thoracic spinal cord injury

Injuries to the spinal cord (S24.0 and S24.1) refer to the cord level and not bone level injury, and can affect nerve roots at and below the level given.
Code also any associated:
fracture of thoracic vertebra (S22.0-)
open wound of thorax (S21.-)
transient paralysis (R29.5)
EXCLUDES 2 injury of brachial plexus (S14.3)

The appropriate 7th character is to be added to each code from category S24
A   initial encounter
D   subsequent encounter
S   sequela

CODING TIPS ✓ When coding sequelae of a cervical spinal cord injury, first list the residual condition(s), followed by the specific spinal cord injury diagnosed using the appropriate code from this category with the seventh character "S" to indicate sequelae. If there are multiple levels of injury, code only the highest injury in each section of the spine (cervical, thoracic, and lumbar).

SP 7 S24.0XX- Concussion and edema of thoracic spinal cord

5 S24.1 Other and unspecified injuries of thoracic spinal cord

6 S24.10 Unspecified injury of thoracic spinal cord

IQ 7 S24.101- Unspecified injury at T1 level of thoracic spinal cord

IQ 7 S24.102- Unspecified injury at T2-T6 level of thoracic spinal cord

IQ 7 S24.103- Unspecified injury at T7-T10 level of thoracic spinal cord

IQ 7 S24.104- Unspecified injury at T11-T12 level of thoracic spinal cord

IQ 7 S24.109- Unspecified injury at unspecified level of thoracic spinal cord
Injury of thoracic spinal cord NOS

6 S24.11 Complete lesion of thoracic spinal cord

SP 7 S24.111- Complete lesion at T1 level of thoracic spinal cord

SP 7 S24.112- Complete lesion at T2-T6 level of thoracic spinal cord

SP 7 S24.113- Complete lesion at T7-T10 level of thoracic spinal cord

SP 7 S24.114- Complete lesion at T11-T12 level of thoracic spinal cord

IQ 7 S24.119- Complete lesion at unspecified level of thoracic spinal cord

6 S24.13 Anterior cord syndrome of thoracic spinal cord

SP 7 S24.131- Anterior cord syndrome at T1 level of thoracic spinal cord

SP 7 S24.132- Anterior cord syndrome at T2-T6 level of thoracic spinal cord

SP 7 S24.133- Anterior cord syndrome at T7-T10 level of thoracic spinal cord

SP 7 S24.134- Anterior cord syndrome at T11-T12 level of thoracic spinal cord

Chapter 19

S00-T88

✷ New ▲ Revised Px Primary **SP** PDGM Px **SL** Low CoM **SH** High CoM **IQ** Quest. Encounter ⊞ Hospice non-cancer Dx   Unspecified   **M** *Manifestation*

DecisionHealth's FY 2020 Complete Home Health ICD-10-CM Diagnosis Coding Manual

1491

!Q 7 S24.139- **Anterior cord syndrome at unspecified level of thoracic spinal cord**

6 S24.14 **Brown-Séquard syndrome of thoracic spinal cord**

SP 7 S24.141- **Brown-Séquard syndrome at T1 level of thoracic spinal cord**

SP 7 S24.142- **Brown-Séquard syndrome at T2-T6 level of thoracic spinal cord**

SP 7 S24.143- **Brown-Séquard syndrome at T7-T10 level of thoracic spinal cord**

SP 7 S24.144- **Brown-Séquard syndrome at T11-T12 level of thoracic spinal cord**

!Q 7 S24.149- **Brown-Séquard syndrome at unspecified level of thoracic spinal cord**

6 S24.15 **Other incomplete lesions of thoracic spinal cord**
Incomplete lesion of thoracic spinal cord NOS
Posterior cord syndrome of thoracic spinal cord

SP 7 S24.151- **Other incomplete lesion at T1 level of thoracic spinal cord**

SP 7 S24.152- **Other incomplete lesion at T2-T6 level of thoracic spinal cord**

SP 7 S24.153- **Other incomplete lesion at T7-T10 level of thoracic spinal cord**

SP 7 S24.154- **Other incomplete lesion at T11-T12 level of thoracic spinal cord**

!Q 7 S24.159- **Other incomplete lesion at unspecified level of thoracic spinal cord**

SP 7 S24.2XX- **Injury of nerve root of thoracic spine**

SP 7 S24.3XX- **Injury of peripheral nerves of thorax**

SP 7 S24.4XX- **Injury of thoracic sympathetic nervous system**
Injury of cardiac plexus
Injury of esophageal plexus
Injury of pulmonary plexus
Injury of stellate ganglion
Injury of thoracic sympathetic ganglion

SP 7 S24.8XX- **Injury of other specified nerves of thorax**

!Q 7 S24.9XX- **Injury of unspecified nerve of thorax**

4 S25 **Injury of blood vessels of thorax**
Code also:
any associated open wound (S21.-)

The appropriate 7th character is to be added to each code from category S25
A   initial encounter
D   subsequent encounter
S   sequela

5 S25.0 **Injury of thoracic aorta**
Injury of aorta NOS

!Q 7 S25.00X- **Unspecified injury of thoracic aorta**

SP 7 S25.01X- **Minor laceration of thoracic aorta**
Incomplete transection of thoracic aorta
Laceration of thoracic aorta NOS
Superficial laceration of thoracic aorta

SP 7 S25.02X- **Major laceration of thoracic aorta**
Complete transection of thoracic aorta
Traumatic rupture of thoracic aorta

SP 7 S25.09X- **Other specified injury of thoracic aorta**

5 S25.1 **Injury of innominate or subclavian artery**

6 S25.10 **Unspecified injury of innominate or subclavian artery**

⊟ !Q 7 S25.101- **Unspecified injury of right innominate or subclavian artery**

⊟ !Q 7 S25.102- **Unspecified injury of left innominate or subclavian artery**

⊟ !Q 7 S25.109- **Unspecified injury of unspecified innominate or subclavian artery**

6 S25.11 **Minor laceration of innominate or subclavian artery**
Incomplete transection of innominate or subclavian artery
Laceration of innominate or subclavian artery NOS
Superficial laceration of innominate or subclavian artery

⊟ SP 7 S25.111- **Minor laceration of right innominate or subclavian artery**

⊟ SP 7 S25.112- **Minor laceration of left innominate or subclavian artery**

⊟ !Q 7 S25.119- **Minor laceration of unspecified innominate or subclavian artery**

6 S25.12 **Major laceration of innominate or subclavian artery**
Complete transection of innominate or subclavian artery
Traumatic rupture of innominate or subclavian artery

⊟ SP 7 S25.121- **Major laceration of right innominate or subclavian artery**

⊟ SP 7 S25.122- **Major laceration of left innominate or subclavian artery**

⊟ !Q 7 S25.129- **Major laceration of unspecified innominate or subclavian artery**

6 S25.19 **Other specified injury of innominate or subclavian artery**

⊟ SP 7 S25.191- **Other specified injury of right innominate or subclavian artery**

⊟ SP 7 S25.192- **Other specified injury of left innominate or subclavian artery**

⊟ !Q 7 S25.199- **Other specified injury of unspecified innominate or subclavian artery**

5 S25.2 **Injury of superior vena cava**
Injury of vena cava NOS

!Q 7 S25.20X- **Unspecified injury of superior vena cava**

SP 7 S25.21X- **Minor laceration of superior vena cava**
Incomplete transection of superior vena cava
Laceration of superior vena cava NOS
Superficial laceration of superior vena cava

---

4 4th digit required   5 5th digit required   6 6th digit required   7 7th digit required   7 7th digit placeholder   + Additional code   ⊟ Laterality

1492   *DecisionHealth's* FY 2020 Complete Home Health ICD-10-CM Diagnosis Coding Manual

SP 7 S25.22X- Major laceration of superior vena cava
Complete transection of superior vena cava
Traumatic rupture of superior vena cava

SP 7 S25.29X- Other specified injury of superior vena cava

5 S25.3 Injury of innominate or subclavian vein

6 S25.30 Unspecified injury of innominate or subclavian vein

IQ 7 S25.301- Unspecified injury of right innominate or subclavian vein

IQ 7 S25.302- Unspecified injury of left innominate or subclavian vein

IQ 7 S25.309- Unspecified injury of unspecified innominate or subclavian vein

6 S25.31 Minor laceration of innominate or subclavian vein
Incomplete transection of innominate or subclavian vein
Laceration of innominate or subclavian vein NOS
Superficial laceration of innominate or subclavian vein

SP 7 S25.311- Minor laceration of right innominate or subclavian vein

SP 7 S25.312- Minor laceration of left innominate or subclavian vein

IQ 7 S25.319- Minor laceration of unspecified innominate or subclavian vein

6 S25.32 Major laceration of innominate or subclavian vein
Complete transection of innominate or subclavian vein
Traumatic rupture of innominate or subclavian vein

SP 7 S25.321- Major laceration of right innominate or subclavian vein

SP 7 S25.322- Major laceration of left innominate or subclavian vein

IQ 7 S25.329- Major laceration of unspecified innominate or subclavian vein

6 S25.39 Other specified injury of innominate or subclavian vein

SP 7 S25.391- Other specified injury of right innominate or subclavian vein

SP 7 S25.392- Other specified injury of left innominate or subclavian vein

IQ 7 S25.399- Other specified injury of unspecified innominate or subclavian vein

5 S25.4 Injury of pulmonary blood vessels

6 S25.40 Unspecified injury of pulmonary blood vessels

IQ 7 S25.401- Unspecified injury of right pulmonary blood vessels

IQ 7 S25.402- Unspecified injury of left pulmonary blood vessels

IQ 7 S25.409- Unspecified injury of unspecified pulmonary blood vessels

6 S25.41 Minor laceration of pulmonary blood vessels
Incomplete transection of pulmonary blood vessels
Laceration of pulmonary blood vessels NOS
Superficial laceration of pulmonary blood vessels

SP 7 S25.411- Minor laceration of right pulmonary blood vessels

SP 7 S25.412- Minor laceration of left pulmonary blood vessels

IQ 7 S25.419- Minor laceration of unspecified pulmonary blood vessels

6 S25.42 Major laceration of pulmonary blood vessels
Complete transection of pulmonary blood vessels
Traumatic rupture of pulmonary blood vessels

SP 7 S25.421- Major laceration of right pulmonary blood vessels

SP 7 S25.422- Major laceration of left pulmonary blood vessels

IQ 7 S25.429- Major laceration of unspecified pulmonary blood vessels

6 S25.49 Other specified injury of pulmonary blood vessels

SP 7 S25.491- Other specified injury of right pulmonary blood vessels

SP 7 S25.492- Other specified injury of left pulmonary blood vessels

IQ 7 S25.499- Other specified injury of unspecified pulmonary blood vessels

5 S25.5 Injury of intercostal blood vessels

6 S25.50 Unspecified injury of intercostal blood vessels

IQ 7 S25.501- Unspecified injury of intercostal blood vessels, right side

IQ 7 S25.502- Unspecified injury of intercostal blood vessels, left side

IQ 7 S25.509- Unspecified injury of intercostal blood vessels, unspecified side

6 S25.51 Laceration of intercostal blood vessels

SP 7 S25.511- Laceration of intercostal blood vessels, right side

SP 7 S25.512- Laceration of intercostal blood vessels, left side

SP IQ 7 S25.519- Laceration of intercostal blood vessels, unspecified side

6 S25.59 Other specified injury of intercostal blood vessels

SP 7 S25.591- Other specified injury of intercostal blood vessels, right side

SP 7 S25.592- Other specified injury of intercostal blood vessels, left side

IQ 7 S25.599- Other specified injury of intercostal blood vessels, unspecified side

5 S25.8 Injury of other blood vessels of thorax
Injury of azygos vein
Injury of mammary artery or vein

6 S25.80 Unspecified injury of other blood vessels of thorax

★New ▲Revised **Px** Primary **SP** PDGM Px **SL** Low CoM **SH** High CoM **IQ** Quest. Encounter **H** Hospice non-cancer Dx Unspecified **M** *Manifestation*

DecisionHealth's FY 2020 Complete Home Health ICD-10-CM Diagnosis Coding Manual

1493

☰ !Q 7 **S25.801-** **Unspecified injury of other blood vessels of thorax, right side**

☰ !Q 7 **S25.802-** **Unspecified injury of other blood vessels of thorax, left side**

☰ !Q 7 **S25.809-** **Unspecified injury of other blood vessels of thorax, unspecified side**

6 **S25.81** **Laceration of other blood vessels of thorax**

☰ SP 7 **S25.811-** **Laceration of other blood vessels of thorax, right side**

☰ SP 7 **S25.812-** **Laceration of other blood vessels of thorax, left side**

☰ !Q 7 **S25.819-** **Laceration of other blood vessels of thorax, unspecified side**

6 **S25.89** **Other specified injury of other blood vessels of thorax**

☰ SP 7 **S25.891-** **Other specified injury of other blood vessels of thorax, right side**

☰ SP 7 **S25.892-** **Other specified injury of other blood vessels of thorax, left side**

☰ !Q 7 **S25.899-** **Other specified injury of other blood vessels of thorax, unspecified side**

5 **S25.9** **Injury of unspecified blood vessel of thorax**

!Q ☑ **S25.90X-** **Unspecified injury of unspecified blood vessel of thorax**

!Q ☑ **S25.91X-** **Laceration of unspecified blood vessel of thorax**

!Q ☑ **S25.99X-** **Other specified injury of unspecified blood vessel of thorax**

4 **S26** **Injury of heart**
Code also any associated:
  open wound of thorax (S21.-)
  traumatic hemopneumothorax (S27.2)
  traumatic hemothorax (S27.1)
  traumatic pneumothorax (S27.0)

The appropriate 7th character is to be added to each code from category S26
A   initial encounter
D   subsequent encounter
S   sequela

5 **S26.0** **Injury of heart with hemopericardium**

!Q ☑ **S26.00X-** **Unspecified injury of heart with hemopericardium**

SP ☑ **S26.01X-** **Contusion of heart with hemopericardium**

6 **S26.02** **Laceration of heart with hemopericardium**

SP 7 **S26.020-** **Mild laceration of heart with hemopericardium**
Laceration of heart without penetration of heart chamber

SP 7 **S26.021-** **Moderate laceration of heart with hemopericardium**
Laceration of heart with penetration of heart chamber

SP 7 **S26.022-** **Major laceration of heart with hemopericardium**
Laceration of heart with penetration of multiple heart chambers

SP ☑ **S26.09X-** **Other injury of heart with hemopericardium**

5 **S26.1** **Injury of heart without hemopericardium**

!Q ☑ **S26.10X-** **Unspecified injury of heart without hemopericardium**

SP ☑ **S26.11X-** **Contusion of heart without hemopericardium**

SP ☑ **S26.12X-** **Laceration of heart without hemopericardium**

SP ☑ **S26.19X-** **Other injury of heart without hemopericardium**

5 **S26.9** **Injury of heart, unspecified with or without hemopericardium**

!Q ☑ **S26.90X-** **Unspecified injury of heart, unspecified with or without hemopericardium**

SP ☑ **S26.91X-** **Contusion of heart, unspecified with or without hemopericardium**

SP ☑ **S26.92X-** **Laceration of heart, unspecified with or without hemopericardium**
Laceration of heart NOS

SP ☑ **S26.99X-** **Other injury of heart, unspecified with or without hemopericardium**

4 **S27** **Injury of other and unspecified intrathoracic organs**
Code also:
  any associated open wound of thorax (S21.-)
  EXCLUDES 2 injury of cervical esophagus (S10-S19)
    injury of trachea (cervical) (S10-S19)

The appropriate 7th character is to be added to each code from category S27
A   initial encounter
D   subsequent encounter
S   sequela

SP ☑ **S27.0XX-** **Traumatic pneumothorax**
  EXCLUDES 1 spontaneous pneumothorax (J93.-)
  CODING TIPS ✓ Do not assign S27.0- to indicate a pneumothorax that is not specifically identified as due to trauma. Chapter 19 codes are for those diagnoses due to injury and trauma. S27.0- indicates pneumothorax resulting from traumatic origin. Nontraumatic (spontaneous or unspecified pneumothorax) should be coded to J93.-.

SP ☑ **S27.1XX-** **Traumatic hemothorax**

SP ☑ **S27.2XX-** **Traumatic hemopneumothorax**

5 **S27.3** **Other and unspecified injuries of lung**

6 **S27.30** **Unspecified injury of lung**

!Q 7 **S27.301-** **Unspecified injury of lung, unilateral**

!Q 7 **S27.302-** **Unspecified injury of lung, bilateral**

!Q 7 **S27.309-** **Unspecified injury of lung, unspecified**

6 **S27.31** **Primary blast injury of lung**
Blast injury of lung NOS

4 4th digit required   5 5th digit required   6 6th digit required   7 7th digit required   ☑ 7th digit placeholder   + Additional code   ☰ Laterality

1494   *DecisionHealth's* FY 2020 Complete Home Health ICD-10-CM Diagnosis Coding Manual

SP **7** S27.311- Primary blast injury of lung, unilateral

SP **7** S27.312- Primary blast injury of lung, bilateral

SP **7** S27.319- Primary blast injury of lung, unspecified

6 S27.32 Contusion of lung

SP **7** S27.321- Contusion of lung, unilateral

SP **7** S27.322- Contusion of lung, bilateral

SP **7** S27.329- Contusion of lung, unspecified

6 S27.33 Laceration of lung

SP **7** S27.331- Laceration of lung, unilateral

SP **7** S27.332- Laceration of lung, bilateral

IQ **7** S27.339- Laceration of lung, unspecified

6 S27.39 Other injuries of lung
Secondary blast injury of lung

SP **7** S27.391- Other injuries of lung, unilateral

SP **7** S27.392- Other injuries of lung, bilateral

IQ **7** S27.399- Other injuries of lung, unspecified

5 S27.4 Injury of bronchus

6 S27.40 Unspecified injury of bronchus

IQ **7** S27.401- Unspecified injury of bronchus, unilateral

IQ **7** S27.402- Unspecified injury of bronchus, bilateral

IQ **7** S27.409- Unspecified injury of bronchus, unspecified

6 S27.41 Primary blast injury of bronchus
Blast injury of bronchus NOS

SP **7** S27.411- Primary blast injury of bronchus, unilateral

SP **7** S27.412- Primary blast injury of bronchus, bilateral

IQ **7** S27.419- Primary blast injury of bronchus, unspecified

6 S27.42 Contusion of bronchus

SP **7** S27.421- Contusion of bronchus, unilateral

SP **7** S27.422- Contusion of bronchus, bilateral

IQ **7** S27.429- Contusion of bronchus, unspecified

6 S27.43 Laceration of bronchus

SP **7** S27.431- Laceration of bronchus, unilateral

SP **7** S27.432- Laceration of bronchus, bilateral

IQ **7** S27.439- Laceration of bronchus, unspecified

6 S27.49 Other injury of bronchus
Secondary blast injury of bronchus

SP **7** S27.491- Other injury of bronchus, unilateral

SP **7** S27.492- Other injury of bronchus, bilateral

IQ **7** S27.499- Other injury of bronchus, unspecified

5 S27.5 Injury of thoracic trachea

IQ **7** S27.50X- Unspecified injury of thoracic trachea

SP **7** S27.51X- Primary blast injury of thoracic trachea
Blast injury of thoracic trachea NOS

SP **7** S27.52X- Contusion of thoracic trachea

SP **7** S27.53X- Laceration of thoracic trachea

SP **7** S27.59X- Other injury of thoracic trachea
Secondary blast injury of thoracic trachea

5 S27.6 Injury of pleura

IQ **7** S27.60X- Unspecified injury of pleura

SP **7** S27.63X- Laceration of pleura

SP **7** S27.69X- Other injury of pleura

5 S27.8 Injury of other specified intrathoracic organs

6 S27.80 Injury of diaphragm

SP **7** S27.802- Contusion of diaphragm

SP **7** S27.803- Laceration of diaphragm

SP **7** S27.808- Other injury of diaphragm

IQ **7** S27.809- Unspecified injury of diaphragm

6 S27.81 Injury of esophagus (thoracic part)

SP **7** S27.812- Contusion of esophagus (thoracic part)

SP **7** S27.813- Laceration of esophagus (thoracic part)

SP **7** S27.818- Other injury of esophagus (thoracic part)

IQ **7** S27.819- Unspecified injury of esophagus (thoracic part)

6 S27.89 Injury of other specified intrathoracic organs
Injury of lymphatic thoracic duct
Injury of thymus gland

SP **7** S27.892- Contusion of other specified intrathoracic organs

SP **7** S27.893- Laceration of other specified intrathoracic organs

SP **7** S27.898- Other injury of other specified intrathoracic organs

IQ **7** S27.899- Unspecified injury of other specified intrathoracic organs

IQ **7** S27.9XX- Injury of unspecified intrathoracic organ

4 S28 Crushing injury of thorax, and traumatic amputation of part of thorax

The appropriate 7th character is to be added to each code from category S28
A   initial encounter
D   subsequent encounter
S   sequela

SP **+** **7** S28.0XX- Crushed chest
Use additional code for all associated injuries
EXCLUDES 1 flail chest (S22.5)

SP **7** S28.1XX- Traumatic amputation (partial) of part of thorax, except breast

5 S28.2 Traumatic amputation of breast

6 S28.21 Complete traumatic amputation of breast
Traumatic amputation of breast NOS

= **SP** **7** S28.211- Complete traumatic amputation of right breast

= **SP** **7** S28.212- Complete traumatic amputation of left breast

= **IQ** **7** S28.219- Complete traumatic amputation of unspecified breast

---

★ New ▲ Revised Px Primary **SP** PDGM Px **SL** Low CoM **SH** High CoM **IQ** Quest. Encounter **H** Hospice non-cancer Dx Unspecified **M** *Manifestation*

Chapter 19

S00-T88

⑥ **S28.22   Partial traumatic amputation of breast**

⊟ SP ⑦ **S28.221-   Partial traumatic amputation of right breast**

⊟ SP ⑦ **S28.222-   Partial traumatic amputation of left breast**

⊟ !Q ⑦ **S28.229-   Partial traumatic amputation of unspecified breast**

④ S29   **Other and unspecified injuries of thorax**

Code also:
   any associated open wound (S21.-)

The appropriate 7th character is to be added to each code from category S29
A   initial encounter
D   subsequent encounter
S   sequela

⑤ **S29.0   Injury of muscle and tendon at thorax level**

⑥ **S29.00   Unspecified injury of muscle and tendon of thorax**

!Q ⑦ **S29.001-   Unspecified injury of muscle and tendon of front wall of thorax**

!Q ⑦ **S29.002-   Unspecified injury of muscle and tendon of back wall of thorax**

!Q ⑦ **S29.009-   Unspecified injury of muscle and tendon of unspecified wall of thorax**

⑥ **S29.01   Strain of muscle and tendon of thorax**

SP ⑦ **S29.011-   Strain of muscle and tendon of front wall of thorax**

SP ⑦ **S29.012-   Strain of muscle and tendon of back wall of thorax**

SP ⑦ **S29.019-   Strain of muscle and tendon of unspecified wall of thorax**

⑥ **S29.02   Laceration of muscle and tendon of thorax**

SP ⑦ **S29.021-   Laceration of muscle and tendon of front wall of thorax**

SP ⑦ **S29.022-   Laceration of muscle and tendon of back wall of thorax**

!Q ⑦ **S29.029-   Laceration of muscle and tendon of unspecified wall of thorax**

⑥ **S29.09   Other injury of muscle and tendon of thorax**

SP ⑦ **S29.091-   Other injury of muscle and tendon of front wall of thorax**

SP ⑦ **S29.092-   Other injury of muscle and tendon of back wall of thorax**

!Q ⑦ **S29.099-   Other injury of muscle and tendon of unspecified wall of thorax**

SP ⑦ **S29.8XX-   Other specified injuries of thorax**

!Q ⑦ **S29.9XX-   Unspecified injury of thorax**

Injuries to the abdomen, lower back, lumbar spine, pelvis and external genitals (S30-S39)

INCLUDES   injuries to the abdominal wall
injuries to the anus
injuries to the buttock
injuries to the external genitalia
injuries to the flank
injuries to the groin

EXCLUDES 2   burns and corrosions (T20-T32)
effects of foreign body in anus and rectum (T18.5)
effects of foreign body in genitourinary tract (T19.-)
effects of foreign body in stomach, small intestine and colon (T18.2-T18.4)
frostbite (T33-T34)
insect bite or sting, venomous (T63.4)

GUIDELINES   Section I.C.19.c.2)
Multiple fractures are sequenced in accordance with the severity of the fracture.

GUIDELINES   Section I.C.19.b.1)-2)
When coding injuries, assign separate codes for each injury unless a combination code is provided, in which case the combination code is assigned ... Traumatic injury codes (S00-T14.9) are not to be used for normal, healing surgical wounds or to identify complications of surgical wounds. The code for the most serious injury, as determined by the provider and the focus of treatment, is sequenced first.

1) Superficial injuries such as abrasions or contusions are not coded when associated with more severe injuries of the same site.

2) When a primary injury results in minor damage to peripheral nerves or blood vessels, the primary injury is sequenced first with additional code(s) for injuries to nerves and spinal cord (such as category S04), and/or injury to blood vessels (such as category S15). When the primary injury is to the blood vessels or nerves, that injury should be sequenced first.

GUIDELINES   Section I.C.19.c
Coding of Traumatic Fractures: The principles of multiple coding of injuries should be followed in coding fractures. Fractures of specified sites are coded individually by site in accordance with both the provisions within categories S02, S12, S22, S32, S42, S49, S52, S59, S62, S72, S79, S82, S89, S92 and the level of detail furnished by medical record content. A fracture not indicated as open or closed should be coded to closed. A fracture not indicated whether displaced or not displaced should be coded to displaced.

CODING TIPS ✓   7th character A is acceptable in home health and hospice when active treatment is provided, such as antibiotics for an infected wound or a wound vac for a dehisced wound. D is used when the complication or injury is now healing. Think of D as aftercare. S is used for sequela of the injury or complication. Sequela is a residual deficit or condition produced as a result of the injury or complication after the original injury or complication has healed.

④ S30   **Superficial injury of abdomen, lower back, pelvis and external genitals**

EXCLUDES 2   superficial injury of hip (S70.-)

The appropriate 7th character is to be added to each code from category S30
A   initial encounter
D   subsequent encounter
S   sequela

SP ⑦ **S30.0XX-   Contusion of lower back and pelvis**
Contusion of buttock

SP ⑦ **S30.1XX-   Contusion of abdominal wall**

---

④4th digit required   ⑤5th digit required   ⑥6th digit required   ⑦7th digit required   ⑦ 7th digit placeholder   +Additional code   ⊟Laterality

1496   *DecisionHealth's* FY 2020 Complete Home Health ICD-10-CM Diagnosis Coding Manual

Contusion of flank
Contusion of groin

5 **S30.2** **Contusion of external genital organs**

6 **S30.20** **Contusion of unspecified external genital organ**

SP 7 **S30.201-** **Contusion of unspecified external genital organ, male**

SP IQ 7 **S30.202-** **Contusion of unspecified external genital organ, female**

SP 7 **S30.21X-** Contusion of penis

SP 7 **S30.22X-** Contusion of scrotum and testes

SP 7 **S30.23X-** Contusion of vagina and vulva

SP 7 **S30.3XX-** Contusion of anus

5 **S30.8** **Other superficial injuries of abdomen, lower back, pelvis and external genitals**

6 **S30.81** **Abrasion of abdomen, lower back, pelvis and external genitals**

IQ 7 **S30.810-** Abrasion of lower back and pelvis

IQ 7 **S30.811-** Abrasion of abdominal wall

IQ 7 **S30.812-** Abrasion of penis

IQ 7 **S30.813-** Abrasion of scrotum and testes

IQ 7 **S30.814-** Abrasion of vagina and vulva

IQ 7 **S30.815-** **Abrasion of unspecified external genital organs, male**

IQ 7 **S30.816-** **Abrasion of unspecified external genital organs, female**

IQ 7 **S30.817-** Abrasion of anus

6 **S30.82** **Blister (nonthermal) of abdomen, lower back, pelvis and external genitals**

IQ 7 **S30.820-** Blister (nonthermal) of lower back and pelvis

IQ 7 **S30.821-** Blister (nonthermal) of abdominal wall

IQ 7 **S30.822-** Blister (nonthermal) of penis

IQ 7 **S30.823-** Blister (nonthermal) of scrotum and testes

IQ 7 **S30.824-** Blister (nonthermal) of vagina and vulva

IQ 7 **S30.825-** **Blister (nonthermal) of unspecified external genital organs, male**

IQ 7 **S30.826-** **Blister (nonthermal) of unspecified external genital organs, female**

IQ 7 **S30.827-** Blister (nonthermal) of anus

6 **S30.84** **External constriction of abdomen, lower back, pelvis and external genitals**

IQ 7 **S30.840-** External constriction of lower back and pelvis

IQ 7 **S30.841-** External constriction of abdominal wall

IQ + 7 **S30.842-** External constriction of penis
Hair tourniquet syndrome of penis
Use additional cause code to identify the constricting item (W49.0-)

IQ 7 **S30.843-** External constriction of scrotum and testes

IQ 7 **S30.844-** External constriction of vagina and vulva

IQ 7 **S30.845-** **External constriction of unspecified external genital organs, male**

IQ 7 **S30.846-** **External constriction of unspecified external genital organs, female**

6 **S30.85** Superficial foreign body of abdomen, lower back, pelvis and external genitals
Splinter in the abdomen, lower back, pelvis and external genitals

IQ 7 **S30.850-** Superficial foreign body of lower back and pelvis

IQ 7 **S30.851-** Superficial foreign body of abdominal wall

IQ 7 **S30.852-** Superficial foreign body of penis

IQ 7 **S30.853-** Superficial foreign body of scrotum and testes

IQ 7 **S30.854-** Superficial foreign body of vagina and vulva

IQ 7 **S30.855-** **Superficial foreign body of unspecified external genital organs, male**

IQ 7 **S30.856-** **Superficial foreign body of unspecified external genital organs, female**

IQ 7 **S30.857-** Superficial foreign body of anus

6 **S30.86** Insect bite (nonvenomous) of abdomen, lower back, pelvis and external genitals

IQ 7 **S30.860-** Insect bite (nonvenomous) of lower back and pelvis

IQ 7 **S30.861-** Insect bite (nonvenomous) of abdominal wall

IQ 7 **S30.862-** Insect bite (nonvenomous) of penis

IQ 7 **S30.863-** Insect bite (nonvenomous) of scrotum and testes

IQ 7 **S30.864-** Insect bite (nonvenomous) of vagina and vulva

IQ 7 **S30.865-** **Insect bite (nonvenomous) of unspecified external genital organs, male**

IQ 7 **S30.866-** **Insect bite (nonvenomous) of unspecified external genital organs, female**

IQ 7 **S30.867-** Insect bite (nonvenomous) of anus

6 **S30.87** Other superficial bite of abdomen, lower back, pelvis and external genitals
EXCLUDES 1 open bite of abdomen, lower back, pelvis and external genitals (S31.05, S31.15, S31.25, S31.35, S31.45, S31.55)

IQ 7 **S30.870-** Other superficial bite of lower back and pelvis

IQ 7 **S30.871-** Other superficial bite of abdominal wall

IQ 7 **S30.872-** Other superficial bite of penis

IQ 7 **S30.873-** Other superficial bite of scrotum and testes

IQ 7 **S30.874-** Other superficial bite of vagina and vulva

Chapter 19

S00-T88

★ New ▲ Revised Px Primary SP PDGM Px SL Low CoM SH High CoM IQ Quest. Encounter H Hospice non-cancer Dx Unspecified M *Manifestation*

IQ 7 S30.875- Other superficial bite of unspecified external genital organs, male

IQ 7 S30.876- Other superficial bite of unspecified external genital organs, female

IQ 7 S30.877- Other superficial bite of anus

5 S30.9 Unspecified superficial injury of abdomen, lower back, pelvis and external genitals

IQ 7 S30.91X- Unspecified superficial injury of lower back and pelvis

IQ 7 S30.92X- Unspecified superficial injury of abdominal wall

IQ 7 S30.93X- Unspecified superficial injury of penis

IQ 7 S30.94X- Unspecified superficial injury of scrotum and testes

IQ 7 S30.95X- Unspecified superficial injury of vagina and vulva

IQ 7 S30.96X- Unspecified superficial injury of unspecified external genital organs, male

IQ 7 S30.97X- Unspecified superficial injury of unspecified external genital organs, female

IQ 7 S30.98X- Unspecified superficial injury of anus

4 S31 Open wound of abdomen, lower back, pelvis and external genitals
Code also any associated:
spinal cord injury
(S24.0, S24.1-, S34.0-, S34.1-)
wound infection
> **EXCLUDES 1** traumatic amputation of part of abdomen, lower back and pelvis (S38.2-, S38.3)
> **EXCLUDES 2** open wound of hip (S71.00-S71.02)
> open fracture of pelvis (S32.1--S32.9 with 7th character B)

The appropriate 7th character is to be added to each code from category S31
A   initial encounter
D   subsequent encounter
S   sequela

CODING TIPS ✓ Open wound codes are used for wounds caused by trauma. Do not assign a code for "open wound" unless the etiology of the wound is related to trauma. Do not use Z codes for any aspect of care of a trauma wound, e.g. no Z code for dressing changes, drain care, or suture removal.

CODING TIPS ✓ No aftercare code applies, including those indicating dressing changes, drain care, or suture removal. 7th character 'D' is the default for home care and hospice when providing aftercare for a healing or resolving condition; 'A' is used for active treatment such as antibiotics or more than routine wound care; 'S' may be used to indicate a residual condition after the original injury has healed.

5 S31.0 Open wound of lower back and pelvis

6 S31.00 Unspecified open wound of lower back and pelvis

SP 7 S31.000- Unspecified open wound of lower back and pelvis without penetration into retroperitoneum
Unspecified open wound of lower back and pelvis NOS

SP 7 S31.001- Unspecified open wound of lower back and pelvis with penetration into retroperitoneum

6 S31.01 Laceration without foreign body of lower back and pelvis

SP 7 S31.010- Laceration without foreign body of lower back and pelvis without penetration into retroperitoneum
Laceration without foreign body of lower back and pelvis NOS

SP 7 S31.011- Laceration without foreign body of lower back and pelvis with penetration into retroperitoneum

6 S31.02 Laceration with foreign body of lower back and pelvis

SP 7 S31.020- Laceration with foreign body of lower back and pelvis without penetration into retroperitoneum
Laceration with foreign body of lower back and pelvis NOS

SP 7 S31.021- Laceration with foreign body of lower back and pelvis with penetration into retroperitoneum

6 S31.03 Puncture wound without foreign body of lower back and pelvis

SP 7 S31.030- Puncture wound without foreign body of lower back and pelvis without penetration into retroperitoneum
Puncture wound without foreign body of lower back and pelvis NOS

SP 7 S31.031- Puncture wound without foreign body of lower back and pelvis with penetration into retroperitoneum

6 S31.04 Puncture wound with foreign body of lower back and pelvis

SP 7 S31.040- Puncture wound with foreign body of lower back and pelvis without penetration into retroperitoneum
Puncture wound with foreign body of lower back and pelvis NOS

SP 7 S31.041- Puncture wound with foreign body of lower back and pelvis with penetration into retroperitoneum

6 S31.05 Open bite of lower back and pelvis
Bite of lower back and pelvis NOS
> **EXCLUDES 1** superficial bite of lower back and pelvis (S30.860, S30.870)

SP 7 S31.050- Open bite of lower back and pelvis without penetration into retroperitoneum
Open bite of lower back and pelvis NOS

---

4 4th digit required   5 5th digit required   6 6th digit required   7 7th digit required   7 7th digit placeholder   + Additional code   ▣ Laterality

1498   DecisionHealth's FY 2020 Complete Home Health ICD-10-CM Diagnosis Coding Manual

SP 7 S31.051- Open bite of lower back and pelvis with penetration into retroperitoneum

5 S31.1 Open wound of abdominal wall without penetration into peritoneal cavity

Open wound of abdominal wall NOS

EXCLUDES 2 open wound of abdominal wall with penetration into peritoneal cavity (S31.6-)

6 S31.10 Unspecified open wound of abdominal wall without penetration into peritoneal cavity

SP 7 S31.100- Unspecified open wound of abdominal wall, right upper quadrant without penetration into peritoneal cavity

SP 7 S31.101- Unspecified open wound of abdominal wall, left upper quadrant without penetration into peritoneal cavity

SP 7 S31.102- Unspecified open wound of abdominal wall, epigastric region without penetration into peritoneal cavity

SP 7 S31.103- Unspecified open wound of abdominal wall, right lower quadrant without penetration into peritoneal cavity

SP 7 S31.104- Unspecified open wound of abdominal wall, left lower quadrant without penetration into peritoneal cavity

SP 7 S31.105- Unspecified open wound of abdominal wall, periumbilic region without penetration into peritoneal cavity

SP 7 S31.109- Unspecified open wound of abdominal wall, unspecified quadrant without penetration into peritoneal cavity

Unspecified open wound of abdominal wall NOS

6 S31.11 Laceration without foreign body of abdominal wall without penetration into peritoneal cavity

SP 7 S31.110- Laceration without foreign body of abdominal wall, right upper quadrant without penetration into peritoneal cavity

SP 7 S31.111- Laceration without foreign body of abdominal wall, left upper quadrant without penetration into peritoneal cavity

SP 7 S31.112- Laceration without foreign body of abdominal wall, epigastric region without penetration into peritoneal cavity

SP 7 S31.113- Laceration without foreign body of abdominal wall, right lower quadrant without penetration into peritoneal cavity

SP 7 S31.114- Laceration without foreign body of abdominal wall, left lower quadrant without penetration into peritoneal cavity

SP 7 S31.115- Laceration without foreign body of abdominal wall, periumbilic region without penetration into peritoneal cavity

SP 7 S31.119- Laceration without foreign body of abdominal wall, unspecified quadrant without penetration into peritoneal cavity

6 S31.12 Laceration with foreign body of abdominal wall without penetration into peritoneal cavity

SP 7 S31.120- Laceration of abdominal wall with foreign body, right upper quadrant without penetration into peritoneal cavity

SP 7 S31.121- Laceration of abdominal wall with foreign body, left upper quadrant without penetration into peritoneal cavity

SP 7 S31.122- Laceration of abdominal wall with foreign body, epigastric region without penetration into peritoneal cavity

SP 7 S31.123- Laceration of abdominal wall with foreign body, right lower quadrant without penetration into peritoneal cavity

SP 7 S31.124- Laceration of abdominal wall with foreign body, left lower quadrant without penetration into peritoneal cavity

SP 7 S31.125- Laceration of abdominal wall with foreign body, periumbilic region without penetration into peritoneal cavity

SP 7 S31.129- Laceration of abdominal wall with foreign body, unspecified quadrant without penetration into peritoneal cavity

6 S31.13 Puncture wound of abdominal wall without foreign body without penetration into peritoneal cavity

SP 7 S31.130- Puncture wound of abdominal wall without foreign body, right upper quadrant without penetration into peritoneal cavity

SP 7 S31.131- Puncture wound of abdominal wall without foreign body, left upper quadrant without penetration into peritoneal cavity

SP 7 S31.132- Puncture wound of abdominal wall without foreign body, epigastric region without penetration into peritoneal cavity

SP 7 S31.133- Puncture wound of abdominal wall without foreign body, right lower quadrant without penetration into peritoneal cavity

SP 7 S31.134- Puncture wound of abdominal wall without foreign body, left lower quadrant without penetration into peritoneal cavity

SP 7 S31.135- Puncture wound of abdominal wall without foreign body, periumbilic region without penetration into peritoneal cavity

Chapter 19

S00-T88

★ New ▲ Revised Px Primary SP PDGM Px SL Low CoM SH High CoM IQ Quest. Encounter H Hospice non-cancer Dx   Unspecified   M *Manifestation*

DecisionHealth's FY 2020 Complete Home Health ICD-10-CM Diagnosis Coding Manual

1499

Chapter 19

S00-T88

▣ **IQ** ⑦ **S31.139-** Puncture wound of abdominal wall without foreign body, unspecified quadrant without penetration into peritoneal cavity

⑥ **S31.14** Puncture wound of abdominal wall with foreign body without penetration into peritoneal cavity

▣ **SP** ⑦ **S31.140-** Puncture wound of abdominal wall with foreign body, right upper quadrant without penetration into peritoneal cavity

▣ **SP** ⑦ **S31.141-** Puncture wound of abdominal wall with foreign body, left upper quadrant without penetration into peritoneal cavity

▣ **SP** ⑦ **S31.142-** Puncture wound of abdominal wall with foreign body, epigastric region without penetration into peritoneal cavity

▣ **SP** ⑦ **S31.143-** Puncture wound of abdominal wall with foreign body, right lower quadrant without penetration into peritoneal cavity

▣ **SP** ⑦ **S31.144-** Puncture wound of abdominal wall with foreign body, left lower quadrant without penetration into peritoneal cavity

▣ **SP** ⑦ **S31.145-** Puncture wound of abdominal wall with foreign body, periumbilic region without penetration into peritoneal cavity

▣ **IQ** ⑦ **S31.149-** Puncture wound of abdominal wall with foreign body, unspecified quadrant without penetration into peritoneal cavity

⑥ **S31.15** Open bite of abdominal wall without penetration into peritoneal cavity
Bite of abdominal wall NOS
EXCLUDES 1 superficial bite of abdominal wall (S30.871)

▣ **SP** ⑦ **S31.150-** Open bite of abdominal wall, right upper quadrant without penetration into peritoneal cavity

▣ **SP** ⑦ **S31.151-** Open bite of abdominal wall, left upper quadrant without penetration into peritoneal cavity

▣ **SP** ⑦ **S31.152-** Open bite of abdominal wall, epigastric region without penetration into peritoneal cavity

▣ **SP** ⑦ **S31.153-** Open bite of abdominal wall, right lower quadrant without penetration into peritoneal cavity

▣ **SP** ⑦ **S31.154-** Open bite of abdominal wall, left lower quadrant without penetration into peritoneal cavity

▣ **SP** ⑦ **S31.155-** Open bite of abdominal wall, periumbilic region without penetration into peritoneal cavity

▣ **IQ** ⑦ **S31.159-** Open bite of abdominal wall, unspecified quadrant without penetration into peritoneal cavity

⑤ **S31.2** Open wound of penis

SP ⑰ **S31.20X-** Unspecified open wound of penis

SP ⑰ **S31.21X-** Laceration without foreign body of penis

SP ⑰ **S31.22X-** Laceration with foreign body of penis

SP ⑰ **S31.23X-** Puncture wound without foreign body of penis

SP ⑰ **S31.24X-** Puncture wound with foreign body of penis

SP ⑰ **S31.25X-** Open bite of penis
Bite of penis NOS
EXCLUDES 1 superficial bite of penis (S30.862, S30.872)

⑤ **S31.3** Open wound of scrotum and testes

SP ⑰ **S31.30X-** Unspecified open wound of scrotum and testes

SP ⑰ **S31.31X-** Laceration without foreign body of scrotum and testes

SP ⑰ **S31.32X-** Laceration with foreign body of scrotum and testes

SP ⑰ **S31.33X-** Puncture wound without foreign body of scrotum and testes

SP ⑰ **S31.34X-** Puncture wound with foreign body of scrotum and testes

SP ⑰ **S31.35X-** Open bite of scrotum and testes
Bite of scrotum and testes NOS
EXCLUDES 1 superficial bite of scrotum and testes (S30.863, S30.873)

⑤ **S31.4** Open wound of vagina and vulva
EXCLUDES 1 injury to vagina and vulva during delivery (O70.-, O71.4)

SP ⑰ **S31.40X-** Unspecified open wound of vagina and vulva

SP ⑰ **S31.41X-** Laceration without foreign body of vagina and vulva

SP ⑰ **S31.42X-** Laceration with foreign body of vagina and vulva

SP ⑰ **S31.43X-** Puncture wound without foreign body of vagina and vulva

SP ⑰ **S31.44X-** Puncture wound with foreign body of vagina and vulva

SP ⑰ **S31.45X-** Open bite of vagina and vulva
Bite of vagina and vulva NOS
EXCLUDES 1 superficial bite of vagina and vulva (S30.864, S30.874)

⑤ **S31.5** Open wound of unspecified external genital organs
EXCLUDES 1 traumatic amputation of external genital organs (S38.21, S38.22)

⑥ **S31.50** Unspecified open wound of unspecified external genital organs

IQ ⑦ **S31.501-** Unspecified open wound of unspecified external genital organs, male

IQ ⑦ **S31.502-** Unspecified open wound of unspecified external genital organs, female

⑥ **S31.51** Laceration without foreign body of unspecified external genital organs

IQ ⑦ **S31.511-** Laceration without foreign body of unspecified external genital organs, male

---

❹ 4th digit required ⑤ 5th digit required ⑥ 6th digit required ⑦ 7th digit required ⑰ 7th digit placeholder ✚ Additional code ▣ Laterality

1500 *DecisionHealth's* FY 2020 Complete Home Health ICD-10-CM Diagnosis Coding Manual

!Q 7 S31.512- Laceration without foreign body of unspecified external genital organs, female

6 S31.52 Laceration with foreign body of unspecified external genital organs

!Q 7 S31.521- Laceration with foreign body of unspecified external genital organs, male

!Q 7 S31.522- Laceration with foreign body of unspecified external genital organs, female

6 S31.53 Puncture wound without foreign body of unspecified external genital organs

!Q 7 S31.531- Puncture wound without foreign body of unspecified external genital organs, male

!Q 7 S31.532- Puncture wound without foreign body of unspecified external genital organs, female

6 S31.54 Puncture wound with foreign body of unspecified external genital organs

!Q 7 S31.541- Puncture wound with foreign body of unspecified external genital organs, male

!Q 7 S31.542- Puncture wound with foreign body of unspecified external genital organs, female

6 S31.55 Open bite of unspecified external genital organs

Bite of unspecified external genital organs NOS

> **EXCLUDES 1** superficial bite of unspecified external genital organs (S30.865, S30.866, S30.875, S30.876)

!Q 7 S31.551- Open bite of unspecified external genital organs, male

!Q 7 S31.552- Open bite of unspecified external genital organs, female

5 S31.6 Open wound of abdominal wall with penetration into peritoneal cavity

6 S31.60 Unspecified open wound of abdominal wall with penetration into peritoneal cavity

SP 7 S31.600- Unspecified open wound of abdominal wall, right upper quadrant with penetration into peritoneal cavity

SP 7 S31.601- Unspecified open wound of abdominal wall, left upper quadrant with penetration into peritoneal cavity

SP 7 S31.602- Unspecified open wound of abdominal wall, epigastric region with penetration into peritoneal cavity

SP 7 S31.603- Unspecified open wound of abdominal wall, right lower quadrant with penetration into peritoneal cavity

SP 7 S31.604- Unspecified open wound of abdominal wall, left lower quadrant with penetration into peritoneal cavity

SP 7 S31.605- Unspecified open wound of abdominal wall, periumbilic region with penetration into peritoneal cavity

SP 7 S31.609- Unspecified open wound of abdominal wall, unspecified quadrant with penetration into peritoneal cavity

6 S31.61 Laceration without foreign body of abdominal wall with penetration into peritoneal cavity

SP 7 S31.610- Laceration without foreign body of abdominal wall, right upper quadrant with penetration into peritoneal cavity

SP 7 S31.611- Laceration without foreign body of abdominal wall, left upper quadrant with penetration into peritoneal cavity

SP 7 S31.612- Laceration without foreign body of abdominal wall, epigastric region with penetration into peritoneal cavity

SP 7 S31.613- Laceration without foreign body of abdominal wall, right lower quadrant with penetration into peritoneal cavity

SP 7 S31.614- Laceration without foreign body of abdominal wall, left lower quadrant with penetration into peritoneal cavity

SP 7 S31.615- Laceration without foreign body of abdominal wall, periumbilic region with penetration into peritoneal cavity

SP 7 S31.619- Laceration without foreign body of abdominal wall, unspecified quadrant with penetration into peritoneal cavity

6 S31.62 Laceration with foreign body of abdominal wall with penetration into peritoneal cavity

SP 7 S31.620- Laceration with foreign body of abdominal wall, right upper quadrant with penetration into peritoneal cavity

SP 7 S31.621- Laceration with foreign body of abdominal wall, left upper quadrant with penetration into peritoneal cavity

SP 7 S31.622- Laceration with foreign body of abdominal wall, epigastric region with penetration into peritoneal cavity

SP 7 S31.623- Laceration with foreign body of abdominal wall, right lower quadrant with penetration into peritoneal cavity

SP 7 S31.624- Laceration with foreign body of abdominal wall, left lower quadrant with penetration into peritoneal cavity

★ New ▲ Revised Px Primary SP PDGM Px SL Low CoM SH High CoM !Q Quest. Encounter H Hospice non-cancer Dx Unspecified M *Manifestation*

DecisionHealth's FY 2020 Complete Home Health ICD-10-CM Diagnosis Coding Manual

1501

Chapter 19

S00-T88

⊟ SP 7 **S31.625-** Laceration with foreign body of abdominal wall, periumbilic region with penetration into peritoneal cavity

⊟ SP 7 **S31.629-** Laceration with foreign body of abdominal wall, unspecified quadrant with penetration into peritoneal cavity

6 **S31.63** Puncture wound without foreign body of abdominal wall with penetration into peritoneal cavity

⊟ SP 7 **S31.630-** Puncture wound without foreign body of abdominal wall, right upper quadrant with penetration into peritoneal cavity

⊟ SP 7 **S31.631-** Puncture wound without foreign body of abdominal wall, left upper quadrant with penetration into peritoneal cavity

⊟ SP 7 **S31.632-** Puncture wound without foreign body of abdominal wall, epigastric region with penetration into peritoneal cavity

⊟ SP 7 **S31.633-** Puncture wound without foreign body of abdominal wall, right lower quadrant with penetration into peritoneal cavity

⊟ SP 7 **S31.634-** Puncture wound without foreign body of abdominal wall, left lower quadrant with penetration into peritoneal cavity

⊟ SP 7 **S31.635-** Puncture wound without foreign body of abdominal wall, periumbilic region with penetration into peritoneal cavity

⊟ !Q 7 **S31.639-** Puncture wound without foreign body of abdominal wall, unspecified quadrant with penetration into peritoneal cavity

6 **S31.64** Puncture wound with foreign body of abdominal wall with penetration into peritoneal cavity

⊟ SP 7 **S31.640-** Puncture wound with foreign body of abdominal wall, right upper quadrant with penetration into peritoneal cavity

⊟ SP 7 **S31.641-** Puncture wound with foreign body of abdominal wall, left upper quadrant with penetration into peritoneal cavity

⊟ SP 7 **S31.642-** Puncture wound with foreign body of abdominal wall, epigastric region with penetration into peritoneal cavity

⊟ SP 7 **S31.643-** Puncture wound with foreign body of abdominal wall, right lower quadrant with penetration into peritoneal cavity

⊟ SP 7 **S31.644-** Puncture wound with foreign body of abdominal wall, left lower quadrant with penetration into peritoneal cavity

⊟ SP 7 **S31.645-** Puncture wound with foreign body of abdominal wall, periumbilic region with penetration into peritoneal cavity

⊟ !Q 7 **S31.649-** Puncture wound with foreign body of abdominal wall, unspecified quadrant with penetration into peritoneal cavity

6 **S31.65** Open bite of abdominal wall with penetration into peritoneal cavity
EXCLUDES 1 superficial bite of abdominal wall (S30.861, S30.871)

⊟ SP 7 **S31.650-** Open bite of abdominal wall, right upper quadrant with penetration into peritoneal cavity

⊟ SP 7 **S31.651-** Open bite of abdominal wall, left upper quadrant with penetration into peritoneal cavity

⊟ SP 7 **S31.652-** Open bite of abdominal wall, epigastric region with penetration into peritoneal cavity

⊟ SP 7 **S31.653-** Open bite of abdominal wall, right lower quadrant with penetration into peritoneal cavity

⊟ SP 7 **S31.654-** Open bite of abdominal wall, left lower quadrant with penetration into peritoneal cavity

⊟ SP 7 **S31.655-** Open bite of abdominal wall, periumbilic region with penetration into peritoneal cavity

⊟ !Q 7 **S31.659-** Open bite of abdominal wall, unspecified quadrant with penetration into peritoneal cavity

5 **S31.8** Open wound of other parts of abdomen, lower back and pelvis

6 **S31.80** Open wound of unspecified buttock

!Q 7 **S31.801-** Laceration without foreign body of unspecified buttock

!Q 7 **S31.802-** Laceration with foreign body of unspecified buttock

!Q 7 **S31.803-** Puncture wound without foreign body of unspecified buttock

!Q 7 **S31.804-** Puncture wound with foreign body of unspecified buttock

!Q 7 **S31.805-** Open bite of unspecified buttock
Bite of buttock NOS
EXCLUDES 1 superficial bite of buttock (S30.870)

!Q 7 **S31.809-** Unspecified open wound of unspecified buttock

6 **S31.81** Open wound of right buttock

⊟ SP 7 **S31.811-** Laceration without foreign body of right buttock

⊟ SP 7 **S31.812-** Laceration with foreign body of right buttock

⊟ SP 7 **S31.813-** Puncture wound without foreign body of right buttock

⊟ SP 7 **S31.814-** Puncture wound with foreign body of right buttock

⊟ SP 7 **S31.815-** Open bite of right buttock
Bite of right buttock NOS
EXCLUDES 1 superficial bite of buttock (S30.870)

⊟ SP 7 **S31.819-** Unspecified open wound of right buttock

4 4th digit required   5 5th digit required   6 6th digit required   7 7th digit required   7 7th digit placeholder   + Additional code   ⊟ Laterality

1502   DecisionHealth's FY 2020 Complete Home Health ICD-10-CM Diagnosis Coding Manual

◧ **S31.82   Open wound of left buttock**

⊟ **SP** 7 **S31.821-   Laceration without foreign body of left buttock**

⊟ **SP** 7 **S31.822-   Laceration with foreign body of left buttock**

⊟ **SP** 7 **S31.823-   Puncture wound without foreign body of left buttock**

⊟ **SP** 7 **S31.824-   Puncture wound with foreign body of left buttock**

⊟ **SP** 7 **S31.825-   Open bite of left buttock**
Bite of left buttock NOS
> **EXCLUDES 1**   superficial bite of buttock (S30.870)

⊟ **SP** 7 **S31.829-   Unspecified open wound of left buttock**

◧ **S31.83   Open wound of anus**

SP 7 **S31.831-   Laceration without foreign body of anus**

SP 7 **S31.832-   Laceration with foreign body of anus**

SP 7 **S31.833-   Puncture wound without foreign body of anus**

SP 7 **S31.834-   Puncture wound with foreign body of anus**

SP 7 **S31.835-   Open bite of anus**
Bite of anus NOS
> **EXCLUDES 1**   superficial bite of anus (S30.877)

SP 7 **S31.839-   Unspecified open wound of anus**

▣ **S32   Fracture of lumbar spine and pelvis**
Note:
A fracture not indicated as displaced or nondisplaced should be coded to displaced
A fracture not indicated as opened or closed should be coded to closed
> **INCLUDES**   fracture of lumbosacral neural arch
> fracture of lumbosacral spinous process
> fracture of lumbosacral transverse process
> fracture of lumbosacral vertebra
> fracture of lumbosacral vertebral arch

Code first:
any associated spinal cord and spinal nerve injury (S34.-)
> **EXCLUDES 1**   transection of abdomen (S38.3)
> **EXCLUDES 2**   fracture of hip NOS (S72.0-)

The appropriate 7th character is to be added to each code from category S32
A   initial encounter for closed fracture
B   initial encounter for open fracture
D   subsequent encounter for fracture with routine healing
G   subsequent encounter for fracture with delayed healing
K   subsequent encounter for fracture with nonunion
S   sequela

CODING TIPS ✓   Fractures repaired by joint replacements are NOT coded with Z47.1. Fractures repaired by any other orthopedic surgery are NOT coded with Z47.89. Z codes are not appropriate for fractures of any kind. Code the fracture with 7th character D for fractures undergoing surgical repair.

CODING TIPS ✓   'D' is the 7th character for home care and hospice unless the physician has documented delayed healing, nonunion or malunion. A sequela is a condition left after the fracture has healed. The Gustilo open fracture classification must be used for open fractures. The default 7th character for open fractures is E.

CODING TIPS ✓   A fracture not indicated as displaced or nondisplaced should be coded to displaced. A fracture not indicated as open or closed should be coded to closed.

▤ **S32.0   Fracture of lumbar vertebra**
Fracture of lumbar spine NOS

◧ **S32.00   Fracture of unspecified lumbar vertebra**

SP 7 **S32.000-   Wedge compression fracture of unspecified lumbar vertebra**

SP 7 **S32.001-   Stable burst fracture of unspecified lumbar vertebra**

SP 7 **S32.002-   Unstable burst fracture of unspecified lumbar vertebra**

SP 7 **S32.008-   Other fracture of unspecified lumbar vertebra**

SP 7 **S32.009-   Unspecified fracture of unspecified lumbar vertebra**

◧ **S32.01   Fracture of first lumbar vertebra**

SP 7 **S32.010-   Wedge compression fracture of first lumbar vertebra**

SP 7 **S32.011-   Stable burst fracture of first lumbar vertebra**

SP 7 **S32.012-   Unstable burst fracture of first lumbar vertebra**

SP 7 **S32.018-   Other fracture of first lumbar vertebra**

SP 7 **S32.019-   Unspecified fracture of first lumbar vertebra**

◧ **S32.02   Fracture of second lumbar vertebra**

SP 7 **S32.020-   Wedge compression fracture of second lumbar vertebra**

SP 7 **S32.021-   Stable burst fracture of second lumbar vertebra**

SP 7 **S32.022-   Unstable burst fracture of second lumbar vertebra**

SP 7 **S32.028-   Other fracture of second lumbar vertebra**

SP 7 **S32.029-   Unspecified fracture of second lumbar vertebra**

◧ **S32.03   Fracture of third lumbar vertebra**

SP 7 **S32.030-   Wedge compression fracture of third lumbar vertebra**

SP 7 **S32.031-   Stable burst fracture of third lumbar vertebra**

SP 7 **S32.032-   Unstable burst fracture of third lumbar vertebra**

SP 7 **S32.038-   Other fracture of third lumbar vertebra**

Chapter 19

S00-T88

★ New ▲ Revised **Px** Primary **SP** PDGM Px **SL** Low CoM **SH** High CoM **IQ** Quest. Encounter H Hospice non-cancer Dx   Unspecified   **M** *Manifestation*

DecisionHealth's FY 2020 Complete Home Health ICD-10-CM Diagnosis Coding Manual   1503

SP 7 S32.039-   Unspecified fracture of third lumbar vertebra

6 S32.04   Fracture of fourth lumbar vertebra

SP 7 S32.040-   Wedge compression fracture of fourth lumbar vertebra

SP 7 S32.041-   Stable burst fracture of fourth lumbar vertebra

SP 7 S32.042-   Unstable burst fracture of fourth lumbar vertebra

SP 7 S32.048-   Other fracture of fourth lumbar vertebra

SP 7 S32.049-   Unspecified fracture of fourth lumbar vertebra

6 S32.05   Fracture of fifth lumbar vertebra

SP 7 S32.050-   Wedge compression fracture of fifth lumbar vertebra

SP 7 S32.051-   Stable burst fracture of fifth lumbar vertebra

SP 7 S32.052-   Unstable burst fracture of fifth lumbar vertebra

SP 7 S32.058-   Other fracture of fifth lumbar vertebra

SP 7 S32.059-   Unspecified fracture of fifth lumbar vertebra

5 S32.1   Fracture of sacrum
> For vertical fractures, code to most medial fracture extension
> Use two codes if both a vertical and transverse fracture are present
> Code also:
> > any associated fracture of pelvic ring (S32.8-)

SP 7 S32.10X-   Unspecified fracture of sacrum

6 S32.11   Zone I fracture of sacrum
> Vertical sacral ala fracture of sacrum

SP 7 S32.110-   Nondisplaced Zone I fracture of sacrum

SP 7 S32.111-   Minimally displaced Zone I fracture of sacrum

SP 7 S32.112-   Severely displaced Zone I fracture of sacrum

SP 7 S32.119-   Unspecified Zone I fracture of sacrum

6 S32.12   Zone II fracture of sacrum
> Vertical foraminal region fracture of sacrum

SP 7 S32.120-   Nondisplaced Zone II fracture of sacrum

SP 7 S32.121-   Minimally displaced Zone II fracture of sacrum

SP 7 S32.122-   Severely displaced Zone II fracture of sacrum

SP 7 S32.129-   Unspecified Zone II fracture of sacrum

6 S32.13   Zone III fracture of sacrum
> Vertical fracture into spinal canal region of sacrum

SP 7 S32.130-   Nondisplaced Zone III fracture of sacrum

SP 7 S32.131-   Minimally displaced Zone III fracture of sacrum

SP 7 S32.132-   Severely displaced Zone III fracture of sacrum

SP 7 S32.139-   Unspecified Zone III fracture of sacrum

SP 7 S32.14X-   Type 1 fracture of sacrum

Transverse flexion fracture of sacrum without displacement

SP 7 S32.15X-   Type 2 fracture of sacrum
Transverse flexion fracture of sacrum with posterior displacement

SP 7 S32.16X-   Type 3 fracture of sacrum
Transverse extension fracture of sacrum with anterior displacement

SP 7 S32.17X-   Type 4 fracture of sacrum
Transverse segmental comminution of upper sacrum

SP 7 S32.19X-   Other fracture of sacrum

SP 7 S32.2XX-   Fracture of coccyx

5 S32.3   Fracture of ilium
> **EXCLUDES 1**   fracture of ilium with associated disruption of pelvic ring (S32.8-)

6 S32.30   Unspecified fracture of ilium

⊟ SP 7 S32.301-   Unspecified fracture of right ilium

⊟ SP 7 S32.302-   Unspecified fracture of left ilium

⊟ IQ 7 S32.309-   Unspecified fracture of unspecified ilium

6 S32.31   Avulsion fracture of ilium

⊟ SP 7 S32.311-   Displaced avulsion fracture of right ilium

⊟ SP 7 S32.312-   Displaced avulsion fracture of left ilium

⊟ IQ 7 S32.313-   Displaced avulsion fracture of unspecified ilium

⊟ SP 7 S32.314-   Nondisplaced avulsion fracture of right ilium

⊟ SP 7 S32.315-   Nondisplaced avulsion fracture of left ilium

⊟ IQ 7 S32.316-   Nondisplaced avulsion fracture of unspecified ilium

6 S32.39   Other fracture of ilium

⊟ SP 7 S32.391-   Other fracture of right ilium

⊟ SP 7 S32.392-   Other fracture of left ilium

⊟ IQ 7 S32.399-   Other fracture of unspecified ilium

5 S32.4   Fracture of acetabulum
> Code also:
> > any associated fracture of pelvic ring (S32.8-)

6 S32.40   Unspecified fracture of acetabulum

⊟ SP 7 S32.401-   Unspecified fracture of right acetabulum

⊟ SP 7 S32.402-   Unspecified fracture of left acetabulum

⊟ IQ 7 S32.409-   Unspecified fracture of unspecified acetabulum

6 S32.41   Fracture of anterior wall of acetabulum

⊟ SP 7 S32.411-   Displaced fracture of anterior wall of right acetabulum

⊟ SP 7 S32.412-   Displaced fracture of anterior wall of left acetabulum

⊟ IQ 7 S32.413-   Displaced fracture of anterior wall of unspecified acetabulum

⊟ SP 7 S32.414-   Nondisplaced fracture of anterior wall of right acetabulum

---

⬛4 4th digit required   ⬛5 5th digit required   ⬛6 6th digit required   ⬛7 7th digit required   ⑦ 7th digit placeholder   ✚Additional code   ⊟Laterality

▣ **SP** 7 **S32.415-** Nondisplaced fracture of anterior wall of left acetabulum

▣ **SP** **IQ** 7 **S32.416-** Nondisplaced fracture of anterior wall of unspecified acetabulum

6 **S32.42** Fracture of posterior wall of acetabulum

▣ **SP** 7 **S32.421-** Displaced fracture of posterior wall of right acetabulum

▣ **SP** 7 **S32.422-** Displaced fracture of posterior wall of left acetabulum

▣ **IQ** 7 **S32.423-** Displaced fracture of posterior wall of unspecified acetabulum

▣ **SP** 7 **S32.424-** Nondisplaced fracture of posterior wall of right acetabulum

▣ **SP** 7 **S32.425-** Nondisplaced fracture of posterior wall of left acetabulum

▣ **IQ** 7 **S32.426-** Nondisplaced fracture of posterior wall of unspecified acetabulum

6 **S32.43** Fracture of anterior column [iliopubic] of acetabulum

▣ **SP** 7 **S32.431-** Displaced fracture of anterior column [iliopubic] of right acetabulum

▣ **SP** 7 **S32.432-** Displaced fracture of anterior column [iliopubic] of left acetabulum

▣ **IQ** 7 **S32.433-** Displaced fracture of anterior column [iliopubic] of unspecified acetabulum

▣ **SP** 7 **S32.434-** Nondisplaced fracture of anterior column [iliopubic] of right acetabulum

▣ **SP** 7 **S32.435-** Nondisplaced fracture of anterior column [iliopubic] of left acetabulum

▣ **IQ** 7 **S32.436-** Nondisplaced fracture of anterior column [iliopubic] of unspecified acetabulum

6 **S32.44** Fracture of posterior column [ilioischial] of acetabulum

▣ **SP** 7 **S32.441-** Displaced fracture of posterior column [ilioischial] of right acetabulum

▣ **SP** 7 **S32.442-** Displaced fracture of posterior column [ilioischial] of left acetabulum

▣ **IQ** 7 **S32.443-** Displaced fracture of posterior column [ilioischial] of unspecified acetabulum

▣ **SP** 7 **S32.444-** Nondisplaced fracture of posterior column [ilioischial] of right acetabulum

▣ **SP** 7 **S32.445-** Nondisplaced fracture of posterior column [ilioischial] of left acetabulum

▣ **IQ** 7 **S32.446-** Nondisplaced fracture of posterior column [ilioischial] of unspecified acetabulum

6 **S32.45** Transverse fracture of acetabulum

▣ **SP** 7 **S32.451-** Displaced transverse fracture of right acetabulum

▣ **SP** 7 **S32.452-** Displaced transverse fracture of left acetabulum

▣ **IQ** 7 **S32.453-** Displaced transverse fracture of unspecified acetabulum

▣ **SP** 7 **S32.454-** Nondisplaced transverse fracture of right acetabulum

▣ **SP** 7 **S32.455-** Nondisplaced transverse fracture of left acetabulum

▣ **IQ** 7 **S32.456-** Nondisplaced transverse fracture of unspecified acetabulum

6 **S32.46** Associated transverse-posterior fracture of acetabulum

▣ **SP** 7 **S32.461-** Displaced associated transverse-posterior fracture of right acetabulum

▣ **SP** 7 **S32.462-** Displaced associated transverse-posterior fracture of left acetabulum

▣ **IQ** 7 **S32.463-** Displaced associated transverse-posterior fracture of unspecified acetabulum

▣ **SP** 7 **S32.464-** Nondisplaced associated transverse-posterior fracture of right acetabulum

▣ **SP** 7 **S32.465-** Nondisplaced associated transverse-posterior fracture of left acetabulum

▣ **IQ** 7 **S32.466-** Nondisplaced associated transverse-posterior fracture of unspecified acetabulum

6 **S32.47** Fracture of medial wall of acetabulum

▣ **SP** 7 **S32.471-** Displaced fracture of medial wall of right acetabulum

▣ **SP** 7 **S32.472-** Displaced fracture of medial wall of left acetabulum

▣ **IQ** 7 **S32.473-** Displaced fracture of medial wall of unspecified acetabulum

▣ **SP** 7 **S32.474-** Nondisplaced fracture of medial wall of right acetabulum

▣ **SP** 7 **S32.475-** Nondisplaced fracture of medial wall of left acetabulum

▣ **IQ** 7 **S32.476-** Nondisplaced fracture of medial wall of unspecified acetabulum

6 **S32.48** Dome fracture of acetabulum

▣ **SP** 7 **S32.481-** Displaced dome fracture of right acetabulum

▣ **SP** 7 **S32.482-** Displaced dome fracture of left acetabulum

▣ **IQ** 7 **S32.483-** Displaced dome fracture of unspecified acetabulum

▣ **SP** 7 **S32.484-** Nondisplaced dome fracture of right acetabulum

▣ **SP** 7 **S32.485-** Nondisplaced dome fracture of left acetabulum

▣ **IQ** 7 **S32.486-** Nondisplaced dome fracture of unspecified acetabulum

6 **S32.49** Other specified fracture of acetabulum

▣ **SP** 7 **S32.491-** Other specified fracture of right acetabulum

▣ **SP** 7 **S32.492-** Other specified fracture of left acetabulum

▣ **IQ** 7 **S32.499-** Other specified fracture of unspecified acetabulum

5 **S32.5** Fracture of pubis

★ New ▲ Revised **Px** Primary **SP** PDGM Px **SL** Low CoM **SH** High CoM **IQ** Quest. Encounter **H** Hospice non-cancer Dx Unspecified **M** *Manifestation*

DecisionHealth's FY 2020 Complete Home Health ICD-10-CM Diagnosis Coding Manual

1505

Chapter 19

S00-T88

EXCLUDES 1 fracture of pubis with
associated disruption of
pelvic ring (S32.8-)

6 **S32.50   Unspecified fracture of pubis**

☐ SP 7 **S32.501-   Unspecified fracture of right
pubis**

☐ SP 7 **S32.502-   Unspecified fracture of left
pubis**

☐ SP IQ 7 **S32.509-   Unspecified fracture of
unspecified pubis**

6 **S32.51   Fracture of superior rim of pubis**

☐ SP 7 **S32.511-   Fracture of superior rim of right
pubis**

☐ SP 7 **S32.512-   Fracture of superior rim of left
pubis**

☐ IQ 7 **S32.519-   Fracture of superior rim of
unspecified pubis**

6 **S32.59   Other specified fracture of pubis**

☐ SP 7 **S32.591-   Other specified fracture of right
pubis**

☐ SP 7 **S32.592-   Other specified fracture of left
pubis**

☐ IQ 7 **S32.599-   Other specified fracture of
unspecified pubis**

5 **S32.6   Fracture of ischium**

EXCLUDES 1 fracture of ischium with
associated disruption of
pelvic ring (S32.8-)

6 **S32.60   Unspecified fracture of ischium**

☐ SP 7 **S32.601-   Unspecified fracture of right
ischium**

☐ SP 7 **S32.602-   Unspecified fracture of left
ischium**

☐ IQ 7 **S32.609-   Unspecified fracture of
unspecified ischium**

6 **S32.61   Avulsion fracture of ischium**

☐ SP 7 **S32.611-   Displaced avulsion fracture of
right ischium**

☐ SP 7 **S32.612-   Displaced avulsion fracture of
left ischium**

☐ IQ 7 **S32.613-   Displaced avulsion fracture of
unspecified ischium**

☐ SP 7 **S32.614-   Nondisplaced avulsion fracture
of right ischium**

☐ SP 7 **S32.615-   Nondisplaced avulsion fracture
of left ischium**

☐ IQ 7 **S32.616-   Nondisplaced avulsion fracture
of unspecified ischium**

6 **S32.69   Other specified fracture of ischium**

☐ SP 7 **S32.691-   Other specified fracture of right
ischium**

☐ SP 7 **S32.692-   Other specified fracture of left
ischium**

☐ IQ 7 **S32.699-   Other specified fracture of
unspecified ischium**

5 **S32.8   Fracture of other parts of pelvis**
Code also any associated:
   fracture of acetabulum (S32.4-)
   sacral fracture (S32.1-)

6 **S32.81   Multiple fractures of pelvis with
disruption of pelvic ring**
Multiple pelvic fractures with
disruption of pelvic circle

SP 7 **S32.810-   Multiple fractures of pelvis with
stable disruption of pelvic ring**

SP 7 **S32.811-   Multiple fractures of pelvis with
unstable disruption of pelvic ring**

SP ☑ **S32.82X-   Multiple fractures of pelvis
without disruption of pelvic ring**
Multiple pelvic fractures without
disruption of pelvic circle

SP ☑ **S32.89X-   Fracture of other parts of pelvis**

IQ ☑ **S32.9XX-   Fracture of unspecified parts of
lumbosacral spine and pelvis**
Fracture of lumbosacral spine NOS
Fracture of pelvis NOS

4 **S33   Dislocation and sprain of joints and
ligaments of lumbar spine and pelvis**

INCLUDES avulsion of joint or ligament of
lumbar spine and pelvis
laceration of cartilage, joint or
ligament of lumbar spine and
pelvis
sprain of cartilage, joint or
ligament of lumbar spine and
pelvis
traumatic hemarthrosis of joint
or ligament of lumbar spine
and pelvis
traumatic rupture of joint or
ligament of lumbar spine and
pelvis
traumatic subluxation of joint or
ligament of lumbar spine and
pelvis
traumatic tear of joint or
ligament of lumbar spine and
pelvis

Code also:
any associated open wound

EXCLUDES 1 nontraumatic rupture or
displacement of lumbar
intervertebral disc NOS
(M51.-)
obstetric damage to pelvic joints
and ligaments (O71.6)

EXCLUDES 2 dislocation and sprain of joints
and ligaments of hip (S73.-)
strain of muscle of lower back
and pelvis (S39.01-)

The appropriate 7th character is to be added to
each code from category S33
A   initial encounter
D   subsequent encounter
S   sequela

SP ☑ **S33.0XX-   Traumatic rupture of lumbar
intervertebral disc**

EXCLUDES 1 rupture or displacement
(nontraumatic) of
lumbar intervertebral
disc NOS (M51.- with
fifth character 6)

5 **S33.1   Subluxation and dislocation of lumbar
vertebra**
Code also any associated:
   open wound of abdomen, lower back and
   pelvis (S31)
   spinal cord injury
   (S24.0, S24.1-, S34.0-, S34.1-)

EXCLUDES 2 fracture of lumbar vertebrae
(S32.0-)

4 4th digit required   5 5th digit required   6 6th digit required   7 7th digit required   ☑ 7th digit placeholder   ✚ Additional code   ☐ Laterality

1506   *DecisionHealth's* FY 2020 Complete Home Health ICD-10-CM Diagnosis Coding Manual

🔢 S33.10　**Subluxation and dislocation of unspecified lumbar vertebra**

!Q 7️⃣ S33.100-　**Subluxation of unspecified lumbar vertebra**

!Q 7️⃣ S33.101-　**Dislocation of unspecified lumbar vertebra**

🔢 S33.11　Subluxation and dislocation of L1/L2 lumbar vertebra

SP 7️⃣ S33.110-　Subluxation of L1/L2 lumbar vertebra

SP 7️⃣ S33.111-　Dislocation of L1/L2 lumbar vertebra

🔢 S33.12　Subluxation and dislocation of L2/L3 lumbar vertebra

SP 7️⃣ S33.120-　Subluxation of L2/L3 lumbar vertebra

SP 7️⃣ S33.121-　Dislocation of L2/L3 lumbar vertebra

🔢 S33.13　Subluxation and dislocation of L3/L4 lumbar vertebra

SP 7️⃣ S33.130-　Subluxation of L3/L4 lumbar vertebra

SP 7️⃣ S33.131-　Dislocation of L3/L4 lumbar vertebra

🔢 S33.14　Subluxation and dislocation of L4/L5 lumbar vertebra

SP 7️⃣ S33.140-　Subluxation of L4/L5 lumbar vertebra

SP 7️⃣ S33.141-　Dislocation of L4/L5 lumbar vertebra

SP 7️⃣ S33.2XX-　Dislocation of sacroiliac and sacrococcygeal joint

5️⃣ S33.3　**Dislocation of other and unspecified parts of lumbar spine and pelvis**

!Q 7️⃣ S33.30X-　**Dislocation of unspecified parts of lumbar spine and pelvis**

SP 7️⃣ S33.39X-　Dislocation of other parts of lumbar spine and pelvis

SP 7️⃣ S33.4XX-　Traumatic rupture of symphysis pubis

SP 7️⃣ S33.5XX-　Sprain of ligaments of lumbar spine

SP 7️⃣ S33.6XX-　Sprain of sacroiliac joint

SP 7️⃣ S33.8XX-　Sprain of other parts of lumbar spine and pelvis

SP 7️⃣ S33.9XX-　**Sprain of unspecified parts of lumbar spine and pelvis**

4️⃣ S34　**Injury of lumbar and sacral spinal cord and nerves at abdomen, lower back and pelvis level**
Note:
Code to highest level of lumbar cord injury
Injuries to the spinal cord (S34.0 and S34.1) refer to the cord level and not bone level injury, and can affect nerve roots at and below the level given.
Code also any associated:
　fracture of vertebra　(S22.0-, S32.0-)
　open wound of abdomen, lower back and pelvis (S31.-)
　transient paralysis　(R29.5)

The appropriate 7th character is to be added to each code from category S34
A　　initial encounter
D　　subsequent encounter
S　　sequela

CODING TIPS ✓　　When coding sequelae of a cervical spinal cord injury, first list the residual condition(s), followed by the specific spinal cord injury diagnosed using the appropriate code from this category with the seventh character "S" to indicate sequelae. If there are multiple levels of injury, code only the highest injury in each section of the spine (cervical, thoracic, and lumbar).

5️⃣ S34.0　Concussion and edema of lumbar and sacral spinal cord

SP ☑️ S34.01X-　Concussion and edema of lumbar spinal cord

SP ☑️ S34.02X-　Concussion and edema of sacral spinal cord
Concussion and edema of conus medullaris

5️⃣ S34.1　**Other and unspecified injury of lumbar and sacral spinal cord**

🔢 S34.10　**Unspecified injury to lumbar spinal cord**

!Q 7️⃣ S34.101-　**Unspecified injury to L1 level of lumbar spinal cord**
Unspecified injury to lumbar spinal cord level 1

!Q 7️⃣ S34.102-　**Unspecified injury to L2 level of lumbar spinal cord**
Unspecified injury to lumbar spinal cord level 2

!Q 7️⃣ S34.103-　**Unspecified injury to L3 level of lumbar spinal cord**
Unspecified injury to lumbar spinal cord level 3

!Q 7️⃣ S34.104-　**Unspecified injury to L4 level of lumbar spinal cord**
Unspecified injury to lumbar spinal cord level 4

!Q 7️⃣ S34.105-　**Unspecified injury to L5 level of lumbar spinal cord**
Unspecified injury to lumbar spinal cord level 5

!Q 7️⃣ S34.109-　**Unspecified injury to unspecified level of lumbar spinal cord**

🔢 S34.11　Complete lesion of lumbar spinal cord

SP 7️⃣ S34.111-　Complete lesion of L1 level of lumbar spinal cord
Complete lesion of lumbar spinal cord level 1

SP 7️⃣ S34.112-　Complete lesion of L2 level of lumbar spinal cord
Complete lesion of lumbar spinal cord level 2

SP 7️⃣ S34.113-　Complete lesion of L3 level of lumbar spinal cord
Complete lesion of lumbar spinal cord level 3

SP 7️⃣ S34.114-　Complete lesion of L4 level of lumbar spinal cord
Complete lesion of lumbar spinal cord level 4

SP 7️⃣ S34.115-　Complete lesion of L5 level of lumbar spinal cord
Complete lesion of lumbar spinal cord level 5

Chapter 19

S00-T88

★ New ▲ Revised Px Primary SP PDGM Px SL Low CoM SH High CoM !Q Quest. Encounter H Hospice non-cancer Dx　Unspecified　M Manifestation

DecisionHealth's FY 2020 Complete Home Health ICD-10-CM Diagnosis Coding Manual

1507

Chapter 19

S00-T88

!Q 7 S34.119-   **Complete lesion of unspecified level of lumbar spinal cord**

6 S34.12   **Incomplete lesion of lumbar spinal cord**

SP 7 S34.121-   **Incomplete lesion of L1 level of lumbar spinal cord**
Incomplete lesion of lumbar spinal cord level 1

SP 7 S34.122-   **Incomplete lesion of L2 level of lumbar spinal cord**
Incomplete lesion of lumbar spinal cord level 2

SP 7 S34.123-   **Incomplete lesion of L3 level of lumbar spinal cord**
Incomplete lesion of lumbar spinal cord level 3

SP 7 S34.124-   **Incomplete lesion of L4 level of lumbar spinal cord**
Incomplete lesion of lumbar spinal cord level 4

SP 7 S34.125-   **Incomplete lesion of L5 level of lumbar spinal cord**
Incomplete lesion of lumbar spinal cord level 5

!Q 7 S34.129-   **Incomplete lesion of unspecified level of lumbar spinal cord**

6 S34.13   **Other and unspecified injury to sacral spinal cord**
Other injury to conus medullaris

SP 7 S34.131-   **Complete lesion of sacral spinal cord**
Complete lesion of conus medullaris

SP 7 S34.132-   **Incomplete lesion of sacral spinal cord**
Incomplete lesion of conus medullaris

!Q 7 S34.139-   **Unspecified injury to sacral spinal cord**
Unspecified injury of conus medullaris

5 S34.2   **Injury of nerve root of lumbar and sacral spine**

SP ☑ S34.21X-   **Injury of nerve root of lumbar spine**

SP ☑ S34.22X-   **Injury of nerve root of sacral spine**

SP ☑ S34.3XX-   **Injury of cauda equina**

SP ☑ S34.4XX-   **Injury of lumbosacral plexus**

SP ☑ S34.5XX-   **Injury of lumbar, sacral and pelvic sympathetic nerves**
Injury of celiac ganglion or plexus
Injury of hypogastric plexus
Injury of mesenteric plexus (inferior) (superior)
Injury of splanchnic nerve

SP ☑ S34.6XX-   **Injury of peripheral nerve(s) at abdomen, lower back and pelvis level**

SP ☑ S34.8XX-   **Injury of other nerves at abdomen, lower back and pelvis level**

!Q ☑ S34.9XX-   **Injury of unspecified nerves at abdomen, lower back and pelvis level**

4 S35   **Injury of blood vessels at abdomen, lower back and pelvis level**
Code also:
any associated open wound (S31.-)

The appropriate 7th character is to be added to each code from category S35
A   initial encounter
D   subsequent encounter
S   sequela

5 S35.0   **Injury of abdominal aorta**
EXCLUDES 1   injury of aorta NOS (S25.0)

!Q ☑ S35.00X-   **Unspecified injury of abdominal aorta**

SP ☑ S35.01X-   **Minor laceration of abdominal aorta**
Incomplete transection of abdominal aorta
Laceration of abdominal aorta NOS
Superficial laceration of abdominal aorta

SP ☑ S35.02X-   **Major laceration of abdominal aorta**
Complete transection of abdominal aorta
Traumatic rupture of abdominal aorta

SP ☑ S35.09X-   **Other injury of abdominal aorta**

5 S35.1   **Injury of inferior vena cava**
Injury of hepatic vein
EXCLUDES 1   injury of vena cava NOS (S25.2)

!Q ☑ S35.10X-   **Unspecified injury of inferior vena cava**

SP ☑ S35.11X-   **Minor laceration of inferior vena cava**
Incomplete transection of inferior vena cava
Laceration of inferior vena cava NOS
Superficial laceration of inferior vena cava

SP ☑ S35.12X-   **Major laceration of inferior vena cava**
Complete transection of inferior vena cava
Traumatic rupture of inferior vena cava

SP ☑ S35.19X-   **Other injury of inferior vena cava**

5 S35.2   **Injury of celiac or mesenteric artery and branches**

6 S35.21   **Injury of celiac artery**

SP 7 S35.211-   **Minor laceration of celiac artery**
Incomplete transection of celiac artery
Laceration of celiac artery NOS
Superficial laceration of celiac artery

SP 7 S35.212-   **Major laceration of celiac artery**
Complete transection of celiac artery
Traumatic rupture of celiac artery

SP 7 S35.218-   **Other injury of celiac artery**

!Q 7 S35.219-   **Unspecified injury of celiac artery**

6 S35.22   **Injury of superior mesenteric artery**

SP 7 S35.221-   **Minor laceration of superior mesenteric artery**
Incomplete transection of superior mesenteric artery

■4th digit required   ■5th digit required   ■6th digit required   ■7th digit required   ☑7th digit placeholder   ✚Additional code   ⊟Laterality

1508   *DecisionHealth's* FY 2020 Complete Home Health ICD-10-CM Diagnosis Coding Manual

Laceration of superior mesenteric artery NOS
Superficial laceration of superior mesenteric artery

SP **7** S35.222-   **Major laceration of superior mesenteric artery**
Complete transection of superior mesenteric artery
Traumatic rupture of superior mesenteric artery

SP **7** S35.228-   **Other injury of superior mesenteric artery**

IQ **7** S35.229-   Unspecified injury of superior mesenteric artery

6 S35.23   **Injury of inferior mesenteric artery**

SP **7** S35.231-   **Minor laceration of inferior mesenteric artery**
Incomplete transection of inferior mesenteric artery
Laceration of inferior mesenteric artery NOS
Superficial laceration of inferior mesenteric artery

SP **7** S35.232-   **Major laceration of inferior mesenteric artery**
Complete transection of inferior mesenteric artery
Traumatic rupture of inferior mesenteric artery

SP **7** S35.238-   **Other injury of inferior mesenteric artery**

IQ **7** S35.239-   Unspecified injury of inferior mesenteric artery

6 S35.29   **Injury of branches of celiac and mesenteric artery**
Injury of gastric artery
Injury of gastroduodenal artery
Injury of hepatic artery
Injury of splenic artery

SP **7** S35.291-   **Minor laceration of branches of celiac and mesenteric artery**
Incomplete transection of branches of celiac and mesenteric artery
Laceration of branches of celiac and mesenteric artery NOS
Superficial laceration of branches of celiac and mesenteric artery

SP **7** S35.292-   **Major laceration of branches of celiac and mesenteric artery**
Complete transection of branches of celiac and mesenteric artery
Traumatic rupture of branches of celiac and mesenteric artery

SP **7** S35.298-   **Other injury of branches of celiac and mesenteric artery**

IQ **7** S35.299-   Unspecified injury of branches of celiac and mesenteric artery

5 S35.3   **Injury of portal or splenic vein and branches**

6 S35.31   **Injury of portal vein**

SP **7** S35.311-   **Laceration of portal vein**

SP **7** S35.318-   **Other specified injury of portal vein**

IQ **7** S35.319-   Unspecified injury of portal vein

6 S35.32   **Injury of splenic vein**

SP **7** S35.321-   **Laceration of splenic vein**

SP **7** S35.328-   **Other specified injury of splenic vein**

IQ **7** S35.329-   Unspecified injury of splenic vein

6 S35.33   **Injury of superior mesenteric vein**

SP **7** S35.331-   **Laceration of superior mesenteric vein**

SP **7** S35.338-   **Other specified injury of superior mesenteric vein**

IQ **7** S35.339-   Unspecified injury of superior mesenteric vein

6 S35.34   **Injury of inferior mesenteric vein**

SP **7** S35.341-   **Laceration of inferior mesenteric vein**

SP **7** S35.348-   **Other specified injury of inferior mesenteric vein**

IQ **7** S35.349-   Unspecified injury of inferior mesenteric vein

5 S35.4   **Injury of renal blood vessels**

6 S35.40   Unspecified injury of renal blood vessel

IQ **7** S35.401-   Unspecified injury of right renal artery

IQ **7** S35.402-   Unspecified injury of left renal artery

IQ **7** S35.403-   Unspecified injury of unspecified renal artery

IQ **7** S35.404-   Unspecified injury of right renal vein

IQ **7** S35.405-   Unspecified injury of left renal vein

IQ **7** S35.406-   Unspecified injury of unspecified renal vein

6 S35.41   **Laceration of renal blood vessel**

SP **7** S35.411-   **Laceration of right renal artery**

SP **7** S35.412-   **Laceration of left renal artery**

IQ **7** S35.413-   Laceration of unspecified renal artery

SP **7** S35.414-   **Laceration of right renal vein**

SP **7** S35.415-   **Laceration of left renal vein**

IQ **7** S35.416-   Laceration of unspecified renal vein

6 S35.49   **Other specified injury of renal blood vessel**

SP **7** S35.491-   **Other specified injury of right renal artery**

SP **7** S35.492-   **Other specified injury of left renal artery**

IQ **7** S35.493-   Other specified injury of unspecified renal artery

SP **7** S35.494-   **Other specified injury of right renal vein**

SP **7** S35.495-   **Other specified injury of left renal vein**

IQ **7** S35.496-   Other specified injury of unspecified renal vein

5 S35.5   **Injury of iliac blood vessels**

IQ **7** S35.50X-   Injury of unspecified iliac blood vessel(s)

6 S35.51   **Injury of iliac artery or vein**
Injury of hypogastric artery or vein

SP **7** S35.511-   **Injury of right iliac artery**

SP **7** S35.512-   **Injury of left iliac artery**

★ New ▲ Revised Px Primary **SP** PDGM Px **SL** Low CoM **SH** High CoM **IQ** Quest. Encounter **H** Hospice non-cancer Dx ▢ Unspecified **M** *Manifestation*

DecisionHealth's FY 2020 Complete Home Health ICD-10-CM Diagnosis Coding Manual   1509

Chapter 19

S00-T88

Chapter 19

S00-T88

☐ !Q 7 **S35.513-** **Injury of unspecified iliac artery**

☐ SP 7 **S35.514-** Injury of right iliac vein

☐ SP 7 **S35.515-** Injury of left iliac vein

☐ !Q 7 **S35.516-** **Injury of unspecified iliac vein**

6 **S35.53** Injury of uterine artery or vein

☐ SP 7 **S35.531-** Injury of right uterine artery

☐ SP 7 **S35.532-** Injury of left uterine artery

☐ !Q 7 **S35.533-** **Injury of unspecified uterine artery**

☐ SP 7 **S35.534-** Injury of right uterine vein

☐ SP 7 **S35.535-** Injury of left uterine vein

☐ !Q 7 **S35.536-** **Injury of unspecified uterine vein**

SP ☑ **S35.59X-** Injury of other iliac blood vessels

5 **S35.8** **Injury of other blood vessels at abdomen, lower back and pelvis level**
Injury of ovarian artery or vein

6 **S35.8X** Injury of other blood vessels at abdomen, lower back and pelvis level

SP 7 **S35.8X1-** Laceration of other blood vessels at abdomen, lower back and pelvis level

SP 7 **S35.8X8-** Other specified injury of other blood vessels at abdomen, lower back and pelvis level

!Q 7 **S35.8X9-** **Unspecified injury of other blood vessels at abdomen, lower back and pelvis level**

5 **S35.9** **Injury of unspecified blood vessel at abdomen, lower back and pelvis level**

!Q ☑ **S35.90X-** **Unspecified injury of unspecified blood vessel at abdomen, lower back and pelvis level**

!Q ☑ **S35.91X-** **Laceration of unspecified blood vessel at abdomen, lower back and pelvis level**

!Q ☑ **S35.99X-** **Other specified injury of unspecified blood vessel at abdomen, lower back and pelvis level**

4 **S36** **Injury of intra-abdominal organs**
Code also:
any associated open wound (S31.-)

The appropriate 7th character is to be added to each code from category S36
A   initial encounter
D   subsequent encounter
S   sequela

CODING TIPS ✓ Codes from category S36 do not include injury to intra-abdominal organs resulting from intraoperative complications. When intraoperative complications occur, the appropriate complication code from the disease-specific chapter should be assigned (intraoperative and post-procedural complications), as well as any T codes indicating further information on the complication.

5 **S36.0** Injury of spleen

!Q ☑ **S36.00X-** **Unspecified injury of spleen**

6 **S36.02** Contusion of spleen

SP 7 **S36.020-** Minor contusion of spleen

Contusion of spleen less than 2 cm

SP 7 **S36.021-** Major contusion of spleen
Contusion of spleen greater than 2 cm

!Q 7 **S36.029-** **Unspecified contusion of spleen**

6 **S36.03** Laceration of spleen

SP 7 **S36.030-** Superficial (capsular) laceration of spleen
Laceration of spleen less than 1 cm
Minor laceration of spleen

SP 7 **S36.031-** Moderate laceration of spleen
Laceration of spleen 1 to 3 cm

SP 7 **S36.032-** Major laceration of spleen
Avulsion of spleen
Laceration of spleen greater than 3 cm
Massive laceration of spleen
Multiple moderate lacerations of spleen
Stellate laceration of spleen

!Q 7 **S36.039-** **Unspecified laceration of spleen**

SP ☑ **S36.09X-** Other injury of spleen

5 **S36.1** Injury of liver and gallbladder and bile duct

6 **S36.11** Injury of liver

SP 7 **S36.112-** Contusion of liver

SP 7 **S36.113-** **Laceration of liver, unspecified degree**

SP 7 **S36.114-** Minor laceration of liver
Laceration involving capsule only, or, without significant involvement of hepatic parenchyma [i.e., less than 1 cm deep]

SP 7 **S36.115-** Moderate laceration of liver
Laceration involving parenchyma but without major disruption of parenchyma [i.e., less than 10 cm long and less than 3 cm deep]

SP 7 **S36.116-** Major laceration of liver
Laceration with significant disruption of hepatic parenchyma [i.e., greater than 10 cm long and 3 cm deep]
Multiple moderate lacerations, with or without hematoma
Stellate laceration of liver

SP 7 **S36.118-** Other injury of liver

!Q 7 **S36.119-** **Unspecified injury of liver**

6 **S36.12** Injury of gallbladder

SP 7 **S36.122-** Contusion of gallbladder

SP 7 **S36.123-** Laceration of gallbladder

SP 7 **S36.128-** Other injury of gallbladder

!Q 7 **S36.129-** **Unspecified injury of gallbladder**

SP ☑ **S36.13X-** Injury of bile duct

5 **S36.2** Injury of pancreas

6 **S36.20** **Unspecified injury of pancreas**

!Q 7 **S36.200-** **Unspecified injury of head of pancreas**

!Q 7 **S36.201-** **Unspecified injury of body of pancreas**

!Q 7 **S36.202-** **Unspecified injury of tail of pancreas**

4 4th digit required   5 5th digit required   6 6th digit required   7 7th digit required   ☑ 7th digit placeholder   ＋Additional code   ☐ Laterality

1510   *DecisionHealth's* FY 2020 Complete Home Health ICD-10-CM Diagnosis Coding Manual

!Q 7 S36.209-   Unspecified injury of unspecified part of pancreas

6 S36.22   Contusion of pancreas

SP 7 S36.220-   Contusion of head of pancreas

SP 7 S36.221-   Contusion of body of pancreas

SP 7 S36.222-   Contusion of tail of pancreas

!Q 7 S36.229-   Contusion of unspecified part of pancreas

6 S36.23   Laceration of pancreas, unspecified degree

SP 7 S36.230-   Laceration of head of pancreas, unspecified degree

SP 7 S36.231-   Laceration of body of pancreas, unspecified degree

SP 7 S36.232-   Laceration of tail of pancreas, unspecified degree

!Q 7 S36.239-   Laceration of unspecified part of pancreas, unspecified degree

6 S36.24   Minor laceration of pancreas

SP 7 S36.240-   Minor laceration of head of pancreas

SP 7 S36.241-   Minor laceration of body of pancreas

SP 7 S36.242-   Minor laceration of tail of pancreas

!Q 7 S36.249-   Minor laceration of unspecified part of pancreas

6 S36.25   Moderate laceration of pancreas

SP 7 S36.250-   Moderate laceration of head of pancreas

SP 7 S36.251-   Moderate laceration of body of pancreas

SP 7 S36.252-   Moderate laceration of tail of pancreas

!Q 7 S36.259-   Moderate laceration of unspecified part of pancreas

6 S36.26   Major laceration of pancreas

SP 7 S36.260-   Major laceration of head of pancreas

SP 7 S36.261-   Major laceration of body of pancreas

SP 7 S36.262-   Major laceration of tail of pancreas

!Q 7 S36.269-   Major laceration of unspecified part of pancreas

6 S36.29   Other injury of pancreas

SP 7 S36.290-   Other injury of head of pancreas

SP 7 S36.291-   Other injury of body of pancreas

SP 7 S36.292-   Other injury of tail of pancreas

SP !Q 7 S36.299-   Other injury of unspecified part of pancreas

5 S36.3   Injury of stomach

!Q 7 S36.30X-   Unspecified injury of stomach

SP 7 S36.32X-   Contusion of stomach

SP 7 S36.33X-   Laceration of stomach

SP 7 S36.39X-   Other injury of stomach

5 S36.4   Injury of small intestine

6 S36.40   Unspecified injury of small intestine

!Q 7 S36.400-   Unspecified injury of duodenum

!Q 7 S36.408-   Unspecified injury of other part of small intestine

!Q 7 S36.409-   Unspecified injury of unspecified part of small intestine

6 S36.41   Primary blast injury of small intestine
Blast injury of small intestine NOS

SP 7 S36.410-   Primary blast injury of duodenum

SP 7 S36.418-   Primary blast injury of other part of small intestine

!Q 7 S36.419-   Primary blast injury of unspecified part of small intestine

6 S36.42   Contusion of small intestine

SP 7 S36.420-   Contusion of duodenum

SP 7 S36.428-   Contusion of other part of small intestine

!Q 7 S36.429-   Contusion of unspecified part of small intestine

6 S36.43   Laceration of small intestine

SP 7 S36.430-   Laceration of duodenum

SP 7 S36.438-   Laceration of other part of small intestine

!Q 7 S36.439-   Laceration of unspecified part of small intestine

6 S36.49   Other injury of small intestine

SP 7 S36.490-   Other injury of duodenum

SP 7 S36.498-   Other injury of other part of small intestine

!Q 7 S36.499-   Other injury of unspecified part of small intestine

5 S36.5   Injury of colon
> **EXCLUDES 2**   injury of rectum (S36.6-)

6 S36.50   Unspecified injury of colon

!Q 7 S36.500-   Unspecified injury of ascending [right] colon

!Q 7 S36.501-   Unspecified injury of transverse colon

!Q 7 S36.502-   Unspecified injury of descending [left] colon

!Q 7 S36.503-   Unspecified injury of sigmoid colon

!Q 7 S36.508-   Unspecified injury of other part of colon

!Q 7 S36.509-   Unspecified injury of unspecified part of colon

6 S36.51   Primary blast injury of colon
Blast injury of colon NOS

SP 7 S36.510-   Primary blast injury of ascending [right] colon

SP 7 S36.511-   Primary blast injury of transverse colon

SP 7 S36.512-   Primary blast injury of descending [left] colon

SP 7 S36.513-   Primary blast injury of sigmoid colon

SP 7 S36.518-   Primary blast injury of other part of colon

!Q 7 S36.519-   Primary blast injury of unspecified part of colon

6 S36.52   Contusion of colon

SP 7 S36.520-   Contusion of ascending [right] colon

SP 7 S36.521-   Contusion of transverse colon

★ New ▲ Revised **Px** Primary **SP** PDGM Px **SL** Low CoM **SH** High CoM **!Q** Quest. Encounter **H** Hospice non-cancer Dx   Unspecified   **M** *Manifestation*

SP **7** **S36.522-** Contusion of descending [left] colon

SP **7** **S36.523-** Contusion of sigmoid colon

SP **7** **S36.528-** Contusion of other part of colon

IQ **7** **S36.529-** Contusion of unspecified part of colon

6 **S36.53** Laceration of colon

SP **7** **S36.530-** Laceration of ascending [right] colon

SP **7** **S36.531-** Laceration of transverse colon

SP **7** **S36.532-** Laceration of descending [left] colon

SP **7** **S36.533-** Laceration of sigmoid colon

SP **7** **S36.538-** Laceration of other part of colon

IQ **7** **S36.539-** Laceration of unspecified part of colon

6 **S36.59** Other injury of colon
Secondary blast injury of colon

SP **7** **S36.590-** Other injury of ascending [right] colon

SP **7** **S36.591-** Other injury of transverse colon

SP **7** **S36.592-** Other injury of descending [left] colon

SP **7** **S36.593-** Other injury of sigmoid colon

SP **7** **S36.598-** Other injury of other part of colon

IQ **7** **S36.599-** Other injury of unspecified part of colon

5 **S36.6** Injury of rectum

IQ **7** **S36.60X-** Unspecified injury of rectum

SP **7** **S36.61X-** Primary blast injury of rectum
Blast injury of rectum NOS

SP **7** **S36.62X-** Contusion of rectum

SP **7** **S36.63X-** Laceration of rectum

SP **7** **S36.69X-** Other injury of rectum
Secondary blast injury of rectum

5 **S36.8** Injury of other intra-abdominal organs

SP **7** **S36.81X-** Injury of peritoneum

6 **S36.89** Injury of other intra-abdominal organs
Injury of retroperitoneum

SP **7** **S36.892-** Contusion of other intra-abdominal organs

SP **7** **S36.893-** Laceration of other intra-abdominal organs

SP **7** **S36.898-** Other injury of other intra-abdominal organs

IQ **7** **S36.899-** Unspecified injury of other intra-abdominal organs

5 **S36.9** Injury of unspecified intra-abdominal organ

IQ **7** **S36.90X-** Unspecified injury of unspecified intra-abdominal organ

IQ **7** **S36.92X-** Contusion of unspecified intra-abdominal organ

IQ **7** **S36.93X-** Laceration of unspecified intra-abdominal organ

IQ **7** **S36.99X-** Other injury of unspecified intra-abdominal organ

4 **S37** Injury of urinary and pelvic organs
Code also:
any associated open wound (S31.-)

EXCLUDES 1 obstetric trauma to pelvic organs (O71.-)
EXCLUDES 2 injury of peritoneum (S36.81)
injury of retroperitoneum (S36.89-)

The appropriate 7th character is to be added to each code from category S37
A   initial encounter
D   subsequent encounter
S   sequela

CODING TIPS ✓ Codes from category S37 do not include injury to urinary and pelvic organs resulting from intraoperative complications. When intraoperative complications occur, the appropriate complication code from the disease-specific chapter should be assigned (intraoperative and post-procedural complications), as well as any T codes indicating further information on the complication.

5 **S37.0** Injury of kidney
EXCLUDES 2 acute kidney injury (nontraumatic) (N17.9)

6 **S37.00** Unspecified injury of kidney

IQ **7** **S37.001-** Unspecified injury of right kidney

IQ **7** **S37.002-** Unspecified injury of left kidney

IQ **7** **S37.009-** Unspecified injury of unspecified kidney

6 **S37.01** Minor contusion of kidney
Contusion of kidney less than 2 cm
Contusion of kidney NOS

SP **7** **S37.011-** Minor contusion of right kidney

SP **7** **S37.012-** Minor contusion of left kidney

SP **7** **S37.019-** Minor contusion of unspecified kidney

6 **S37.02** Major contusion of kidney
Contusion of kidney greater than 2 cm

SP **7** **S37.021-** Major contusion of right kidney

SP **7** **S37.022-** Major contusion of left kidney

IQ **7** **S37.029-** Major contusion of unspecified kidney

6 **S37.03** Laceration of kidney, unspecified degree

SP **7** **S37.031-** Laceration of right kidney, unspecified degree

SP **7** **S37.032-** Laceration of left kidney, unspecified degree

IQ **7** **S37.039-** Laceration of unspecified kidney, unspecified degree

6 **S37.04** Minor laceration of kidney
Laceration of kidney less than 1 cm

SP **7** **S37.041-** Minor laceration of right kidney

SP **7** **S37.042-** Minor laceration of left kidney

IQ **7** **S37.049-** Minor laceration of unspecified kidney

6 **S37.05** Moderate laceration of kidney
Laceration of kidney 1 to 3 cm

SP **7** **S37.051-** Moderate laceration of right kidney

SP **7** **S37.052-** Moderate laceration of left kidney

---

4 4th digit required   **5** 5th digit required   **6** 6th digit required   **7** 7th digit required   **7** 7th digit placeholder   **+** Additional code   **Ⓔ** Laterality

1512   *DecisionHealth's* FY 2020 Complete Home Health ICD-10-CM Diagnosis Coding Manual

▣ **IQ** **7** **S37.059-** Moderate laceration of unspecified kidney

6 **S37.06** **Major laceration of kidney**
Avulsion of kidney
Laceration of kidney greater than 3 cm
Massive laceration of kidney
Multiple moderate lacerations of kidney
Stellate laceration of kidney

▣ **SP** **7** **S37.061-** Major laceration of right kidney

▣ **SP** **7** **S37.062-** Major laceration of left kidney

▣ **SP** **7** **S37.069-** Major laceration of unspecified kidney

6 **S37.09** **Other injury of kidney**

▣ **SP** **7** **S37.091-** Other injury of right kidney

▣ **SP** **7** **S37.092-** Other injury of left kidney

▣ **IQ** **7** **S37.099-** Other injury of unspecified kidney

5 **S37.1** **Injury of ureter**

IQ **7** **S37.10X-** Unspecified injury of ureter

SP **7** **S37.12X-** Contusion of ureter

SP **7** **S37.13X-** Laceration of ureter

SP **7** **S37.19X-** Other injury of ureter

5 **S37.2** **Injury of bladder**

IQ **7** **S37.20X-** Unspecified injury of bladder

SP **7** **S37.22X-** Contusion of bladder

SP **7** **S37.23X-** Laceration of bladder

SP **7** **S37.29X-** Other injury of bladder

5 **S37.3** **Injury of urethra**

IQ **7** **S37.30X-** Unspecified injury of urethra

SP **7** **S37.32X-** Contusion of urethra

SP **7** **S37.33X-** Laceration of urethra

SP **7** **S37.39X-** Other injury of urethra

5 **S37.4** **Injury of ovary**

6 **S37.40** Unspecified injury of ovary

IQ **7** **S37.401-** Unspecified injury of ovary, unilateral

IQ **7** **S37.402-** Unspecified injury of ovary, bilateral

IQ **7** **S37.409-** Unspecified injury of ovary, unspecified

6 **S37.42** **Contusion of ovary**

SP **7** **S37.421-** Contusion of ovary, unilateral

SP **7** **S37.422-** Contusion of ovary, bilateral

IQ **7** **S37.429-** Contusion of ovary, unspecified

6 **S37.43** **Laceration of ovary**

SP **7** **S37.431-** Laceration of ovary, unilateral

SP **7** **S37.432-** Laceration of ovary, bilateral

IQ **7** **S37.439-** Laceration of ovary, unspecified

6 **S37.49** **Other injury of ovary**

SP **7** **S37.491-** Other injury of ovary, unilateral

SP **7** **S37.492-** Other injury of ovary, bilateral

IQ **7** **S37.499-** Other injury of ovary, unspecified

5 **S37.5** **Injury of fallopian tube**

6 **S37.50** Unspecified injury of fallopian tube

IQ **7** **S37.501-** Unspecified injury of fallopian tube, unilateral

IQ **7** **S37.502-** Unspecified injury of fallopian tube, bilateral

IQ **7** **S37.509-** Unspecified injury of fallopian tube, unspecified

6 **S37.51** **Primary blast injury of fallopian tube**
Blast injury of fallopian tube NOS

SP **7** **S37.511-** Primary blast injury of fallopian tube, unilateral

SP **7** **S37.512-** Primary blast injury of fallopian tube, bilateral

IQ **7** **S37.519-** Primary blast injury of fallopian tube, unspecified

6 **S37.52** **Contusion of fallopian tube**

SP **7** **S37.521-** Contusion of fallopian tube, unilateral

SP **7** **S37.522-** Contusion of fallopian tube, bilateral

IQ **7** **S37.529-** Contusion of fallopian tube, unspecified

6 **S37.53** **Laceration of fallopian tube**

SP **7** **S37.531-** Laceration of fallopian tube, unilateral

SP **7** **S37.532-** Laceration of fallopian tube, bilateral

IQ **7** **S37.539-** Laceration of fallopian tube, unspecified

6 **S37.59** **Other injury of fallopian tube**
Secondary blast injury of fallopian tube

SP **7** **S37.591-** Other injury of fallopian tube, unilateral

SP **7** **S37.592-** Other injury of fallopian tube, bilateral

IQ **7** **S37.599-** Other injury of fallopian tube, unspecified

5 **S37.6** **Injury of uterus**
EXCLUDES 1 injury to gravid uterus (O9A.2-)
injury to uterus during delivery (O71.-)

IQ **7** **S37.60X-** Unspecified injury of uterus

SP **7** **S37.62X-** Contusion of uterus

SP **7** **S37.63X-** Laceration of uterus

SP **7** **S37.69X-** Other injury of uterus

5 **S37.8** **Injury of other urinary and pelvic organs**

6 **S37.81** **Injury of adrenal gland**

SP **7** **S37.812-** Contusion of adrenal gland

SP **7** **S37.813-** Laceration of adrenal gland

SP **7** **S37.818-** Other injury of adrenal gland

IQ **7** **S37.819-** Unspecified injury of adrenal gland

6 **S37.82** **Injury of prostate**

SP **7** **S37.822-** Contusion of prostate

SP **7** **S37.823-** Laceration of prostate

SP **7** **S37.828-** Other injury of prostate

IQ **7** **S37.829-** Unspecified injury of prostate

6 **S37.89** **Injury of other urinary and pelvic organ**

SP **7** **S37.892-** Contusion of other urinary and pelvic organ

SP **7** **S37.893-** Laceration of other urinary and pelvic organ

★ New ▲ Revised **Px** Primary **SP** PDGM Px **SL** Low CoM **SH** High CoM **IQ** Quest. Encounter Ⓗ Hospice non-cancer Dx Unspecified **M** *Manifestation*

DecisionHealth's FY 2020 Complete Home Health ICD-10-CM Diagnosis Coding Manual

1513

Chapter 19

S00-T88

SP 7 S37.898- Other injury of other urinary and pelvic organ

IQ 7 S37.899- Unspecified injury of other urinary and pelvic organ

5 S37.9 Injury of unspecified urinary and pelvic organ

IQ 7 S37.90X- Unspecified injury of unspecified urinary and pelvic organ

IQ 7 S37.92X- Contusion of unspecified urinary and pelvic organ

IQ 7 S37.93X- Laceration of unspecified urinary and pelvic organ

IQ 7 S37.99X- Other injury of unspecified urinary and pelvic organ

4 S38 Crushing injury and traumatic amputation of abdomen, lower back, pelvis and external genitals

An amputation not identified as partial or complete should be coded to complete

The appropriate 7th character is to be added to each code from category S38
A   initial encounter
D   subsequent encounter
S   sequela

CODING TIPS ✓   Use these codes only when the amputation was due to trauma. There is no need for adding Z89 with traumatic amputations. See Z47.81 for care of amputations not due to trauma.

+ 5 S38.0 Crushing injury of external genital organs
Use additional code for any associated injuries

+ 6 S38.00 Crushing injury of unspecified external genital organs

IQ + 7 S38.001- Crushing injury of unspecified external genital organs, male

IQ + 7 S38.002- Crushing injury of unspecified external genital organs, female

SP + 7 S38.01X- Crushing injury of penis

SP + 7 S38.02X- Crushing injury of scrotum and testis

SP + 7 S38.03X- Crushing injury of vulva

SP + 7 S38.1XX- Crushing injury of abdomen, lower back, and pelvis
Use additional code for all associated injuries, such as:
fracture of thoracic or lumbar spine and pelvis (S22.0-, S32.-)
injury to intra-abdominal organs (S36.-)
injury to urinary and pelvic organs (S37.-)
open wound of abdominal wall (S31.-)
spinal cord injury (S34.0, S34.1-)
EXCLUDES 2 crushing injury of external genital organs (S38.0-)

5 S38.2 Traumatic amputation of external genital organs

6 S38.21 Traumatic amputation of female external genital organs
Traumatic amputation of clitoris

Traumatic amputation of labium (majus) (minus)
Traumatic amputation of vulva

SP 7 S38.211- Complete traumatic amputation of female external genital organs

SP 7 S38.212- Partial traumatic amputation of female external genital organs

6 S38.22 Traumatic amputation of penis

SP 7 S38.221- Complete traumatic amputation of penis

SP 7 S38.222- Partial traumatic amputation of penis

6 S38.23 Traumatic amputation of scrotum and testis

SP 7 S38.231- Complete traumatic amputation of scrotum and testis

SP 7 S38.232- Partial traumatic amputation of scrotum and testis

SP 7 S38.3XX- Transection (partial) of abdomen

4 S39 Other and unspecified injuries of abdomen, lower back, pelvis and external genitals

Code also:
any associated open wound (S31.-)
EXCLUDES 2 sprain of joints and ligaments of lumbar spine and pelvis (S33.-)

The appropriate 7th character is to be added to each code from category S39
A   initial encounter
D   subsequent encounter
S   sequela

5 S39.0 Injury of muscle, fascia and tendon of abdomen, lower back and pelvis

6 S39.00 Unspecified injury of muscle, fascia and tendon of abdomen, lower back and pelvis

IQ 7 S39.001- Unspecified injury of muscle, fascia and tendon of abdomen

IQ 7 S39.002- Unspecified injury of muscle, fascia and tendon of lower back

IQ 7 S39.003- Unspecified injury of muscle, fascia and tendon of pelvis

6 S39.01 Strain of muscle, fascia and tendon of abdomen, lower back and pelvis

SP 7 S39.011- Strain of muscle, fascia and tendon of abdomen

SP 7 S39.012- Strain of muscle, fascia and tendon of lower back

SP 7 S39.013- Strain of muscle, fascia and tendon of pelvis

6 S39.02 Laceration of muscle, fascia and tendon of abdomen, lower back and pelvis

SP 7 S39.021- Laceration of muscle, fascia and tendon of abdomen

SP 7 S39.022- Laceration of muscle, fascia and tendon of lower back

SP 7 S39.023- Laceration of muscle, fascia and tendon of pelvis

6 S39.09 Other injury of muscle, fascia and tendon of abdomen, lower back and pelvis

SP 7 S39.091- Other injury of muscle, fascia and tendon of abdomen

---

4 4th digit required   **5** 5th digit required   **6** 6th digit required   **7** 7th digit required   **7** 7th digit placeholder   **+** Additional code   **☐** Laterality

1514   *DecisionHealth's* FY 2020 Complete Home Health ICD-10-CM Diagnosis Coding Manual

SP 7 **S39.092-** Other injury of muscle, fascia and tendon of lower back

SP 7 **S39.093-** Other injury of muscle, fascia and tendon of pelvis

5 **S39.8** Other specified injuries of abdomen, lower back, pelvis and external genitals

SP ☑ **S39.81X-** Other specified injuries of abdomen

SP ☑ **S39.82X-** Other specified injuries of lower back

SP ☑ **S39.83X-** Other specified injuries of pelvis

6 **S39.84** Other specified injuries of external genitals

SP 7 **S39.840-** Fracture of corpus cavernosum penis

SP 7 **S39.848-** Other specified injuries of external genitals

5 **S39.9** Unspecified injury of abdomen, lower back, pelvis and external genitals

IQ ☑ **S39.91X-** Unspecified injury of abdomen

IQ ☑ **S39.92X-** Unspecified injury of lower back

IQ ☑ **S39.93X-** Unspecified injury of pelvis

IQ ☑ **S39.94X-** Unspecified injury of external genitals

Injuries to the shoulder and upper arm (S40-S49)

INCLUDES	injuries of axilla
	injuries of scapular region
EXCLUDES 2	burns and corrosions (T20-T32)
	frostbite (T33-T34)
	injuries of elbow (S50-S59)
	insect bite or sting, venomous (T63.4)

GUIDELINES Section I.C.19.c.2)

Multiple fractures are sequenced in accordance with the severity of the fracture.

GUIDELINES Section I.C.19.b.1)-2)

When coding injuries, assign separate codes for each injury unless a combination code is provided, in which case the combination code is assigned ... Traumatic injury codes (S00-T14.9) are not to be used for normal, healing surgical wounds or to identify complications of surgical wounds. The code for the most serious injury, as determined by the provider and the focus of treatment, is sequenced first.

1) Superficial injuries such as abrasions or contusions are not coded when associated with more severe injuries of the same site.

2) When a primary injury results in minor damage to peripheral nerves or blood vessels, the primary injury is sequenced first with additional code(s) for injuries to nerves and spinal cord (such as category S04), and/or injury to blood vessels (such as category S15). When the primary injury is to the blood vessels or nerves, that injury should be sequenced first.

GUIDELINES Section I.C.19.c

Coding of Traumatic Fractures: The principles of multiple coding of injuries should be followed in coding fractures. Fractures of specified sites are coded individually by site in accordance with both the provisions within categories S02, S12, S22, S32, S42, S49, S52, S59, S62, S72, S79, S82, S89, S92 and the level of detail furnished by medical record content. A fracture not indicated as open or closed should be coded to closed. A fracture not indicated whether displaced or not displaced should be coded to displaced.

CODING TIPS ✓ 7th character A is acceptable in home health and hospice when active treatment is provided, such as antibiotics for an infected wound or a wound vac for a dehisced wound. D is used when the complication or injury is now healing. Think of D as aftercare. S is used for sequela of the injury or complication. Sequela is a residual deficit or condition produced as a result of the injury or complication after the original injury or complication has healed.

4 **S40** Superficial injury of shoulder and upper arm

The appropriate 7th character is to be added to each code from category S40
A   initial encounter
D   subsequent encounter
S   sequela

5 **S40.0** Contusion of shoulder and upper arm

6 **S40.01** Contusion of shoulder

⊟ **IQ** 7 **S40.011-** Contusion of right shoulder

⊟ **IQ** 7 **S40.012-** Contusion of left shoulder

⊟ **IQ** 7 **S40.019-** Contusion of unspecified shoulder

6 **S40.02** Contusion of upper arm

⊟ **IQ** 7 **S40.021-** Contusion of right upper arm

⊟ **IQ** 7 **S40.022-** Contusion of left upper arm

⊟ **IQ** 7 **S40.029-** Contusion of unspecified upper arm

5 **S40.2** Other superficial injuries of shoulder

6 **S40.21** Abrasion of shoulder

⊟ **IQ** 7 **S40.211-** Abrasion of right shoulder

⊟ **IQ** 7 **S40.212-** Abrasion of left shoulder

⊟ **IQ** 7 **S40.219-** Abrasion of unspecified shoulder

6 **S40.22** Blister (nonthermal) of shoulder

⊟ **IQ** 7 **S40.221-** Blister (nonthermal) of right shoulder

⊟ **IQ** 7 **S40.222-** Blister (nonthermal) of left shoulder

⊟ **IQ** 7 **S40.229-** Blister (nonthermal) of unspecified shoulder

6 **S40.24** External constriction of shoulder

⊟ **IQ** 7 **S40.241-** External constriction of right shoulder

⊟ **IQ** 7 **S40.242-** External constriction of left shoulder

⊟ **IQ** 7 **S40.249-** External constriction of unspecified shoulder

6 **S40.25** Superficial foreign body of shoulder
Splinter in the shoulder

⊟ **IQ** 7 **S40.251-** Superficial foreign body of right shoulder

⊟ **IQ** 7 **S40.252-** Superficial foreign body of left shoulder

Chapter 19

S00-T88

★ New ▲ Revised Px Primary **SP** PDGM Px **SL** Low CoM **SH** High CoM **IQ** Quest. Encounter **H** Hospice non-cancer Dx Unspecified **M** *Manifestation*

DecisionHealth's FY 2020 Complete Home Health ICD-10-CM Diagnosis Coding Manual

1515

Chapter 19

S00-T88

☐ !Q 7 **S40.259-** Superficial foreign body of unspecified shoulder

6 **S40.26** Insect bite (nonvenomous) of shoulder

☐ !Q 7 **S40.261-** Insect bite (nonvenomous) of right shoulder

☐ !Q 7 **S40.262-** Insect bite (nonvenomous) of left shoulder

☐ !Q 7 **S40.269-** Insect bite (nonvenomous) of unspecified shoulder

6 **S40.27** Other superficial bite of shoulder
EXCLUDES 1 open bite of shoulder (S41.05)

☐ !Q 7 **S40.271-** Other superficial bite of right shoulder

☐ !Q 7 **S40.272-** Other superficial bite of left shoulder

☐ !Q 7 **S40.279-** Other superficial bite of unspecified shoulder

5 **S40.8** Other superficial injuries of upper arm

6 **S40.81** Abrasion of upper arm

☐ !Q 7 **S40.811-** Abrasion of right upper arm

☐ !Q 7 **S40.812-** Abrasion of left upper arm

☐ !Q 7 **S40.819-** Abrasion of unspecified upper arm

6 **S40.82** Blister (nonthermal) of upper arm

☐ !Q 7 **S40.821-** Blister (nonthermal) of right upper arm

☐ !Q 7 **S40.822-** Blister (nonthermal) of left upper arm

☐ !Q 7 **S40.829-** Blister (nonthermal) of unspecified upper arm

6 **S40.84** External constriction of upper arm

☐ !Q 7 **S40.841-** External constriction of right upper arm

☐ !Q 7 **S40.842-** External constriction of left upper arm

☐ !Q 7 **S40.849-** External constriction of unspecified upper arm

6 **S40.85** Superficial foreign body of upper arm
Splinter in the upper arm

☐ !Q 7 **S40.851-** Superficial foreign body of right upper arm

☐ !Q 7 **S40.852-** Superficial foreign body of left upper arm

☐ !Q 7 **S40.859-** Superficial foreign body of unspecified upper arm

6 **S40.86** Insect bite (nonvenomous) of upper arm

☐ !Q 7 **S40.861-** Insect bite (nonvenomous) of right upper arm

☐ !Q 7 **S40.862-** Insect bite (nonvenomous) of left upper arm

☐ !Q 7 **S40.869-** Insect bite (nonvenomous) of unspecified upper arm

6 **S40.87** Other superficial bite of upper arm
EXCLUDES 1 open bite of upper arm (S41.14)
EXCLUDES 2 other superficial bite of shoulder (S40.27-)

☐ !Q 7 **S40.871-** Other superficial bite of right upper arm

☐ !Q 7 **S40.872-** Other superficial bite of left upper arm

☐ !Q 7 **S40.879-** Other superficial bite of unspecified upper arm

5 **S40.9** Unspecified superficial injury of shoulder and upper arm

6 **S40.91** Unspecified superficial injury of shoulder

☐ !Q 7 **S40.911-** Unspecified superficial injury of right shoulder

☐ !Q 7 **S40.912-** Unspecified superficial injury of left shoulder

☐ !Q 7 **S40.919-** Unspecified superficial injury of unspecified shoulder

6 **S40.92** Unspecified superficial injury of upper arm

☐ !Q 7 **S40.921-** Unspecified superficial injury of right upper arm

☐ !Q 7 **S40.922-** Unspecified superficial injury of left upper arm

☐ !Q 7 **S40.929-** Unspecified superficial injury of unspecified upper arm

4 **S41** Open wound of shoulder and upper arm
Code also:
any associated wound infection
EXCLUDES 1 traumatic amputation of shoulder and upper arm (S48.-)
EXCLUDES 2 open fracture of shoulder and upper arm (S42.- with 7th character B or C)

The appropriate 7th character is to be added to each code from category S41
A initial encounter
D subsequent encounter
S sequela

CODING TIPS ✓ Open wound codes indicate a wound resulting from a traumatic origin. Do not assign a code for "open wound" unless the etiology of the wound is related to trauma.

CODING TIPS ✓ No aftercare code applies, including those indicating dressing changes, drain care, or suture removal. 7th character 'D' is the default for home care and hospice when providing aftercare for a healing or resolving condition; 'A' is used for active treatment such as antibiotics or more than routine wound care; 'S' may be used to indicate a residual condition after the original injury has healed.

5 **S41.0** Open wound of shoulder

6 **S41.00** Unspecified open wound of shoulder

☐ SP 7 **S41.001-** Unspecified open wound of right shoulder

☐ SP 7 **S41.002-** Unspecified open wound of left shoulder

☐ !Q 7 **S41.009-** Unspecified open wound of unspecified shoulder

6 **S41.01** Laceration without foreign body of shoulder

☐ SP 7 **S41.011-** Laceration without foreign body of right shoulder

☐ SP 7 **S41.012-** Laceration without foreign body of left shoulder

☐ !Q 7 **S41.019-** Laceration without foreign body of unspecified shoulder

---

4 4th digit required   5 5th digit required   6 6th digit required   7 7th digit required   7 7th digit placeholder   + Additional code   ☐ Laterality

1516   DecisionHealth's FY 2020 Complete Home Health ICD-10-CM Diagnosis Coding Manual

6 **S41.02** Laceration with foreign body of shoulder

☐ SP 7 **S41.021-** Laceration with foreign body of right shoulder

☐ SP 7 **S41.022-** Laceration with foreign body of left shoulder

☐ !Q 7 **S41.029-** Laceration with foreign body of unspecified shoulder

6 **S41.03** Puncture wound without foreign body of shoulder

☐ SP 7 **S41.031-** Puncture wound without foreign body of right shoulder

☐ SP 7 **S41.032-** Puncture wound without foreign body of left shoulder

☐ !Q 7 **S41.039-** Puncture wound without foreign body of unspecified shoulder

6 **S41.04** Puncture wound with foreign body of shoulder

☐ SP 7 **S41.041-** Puncture wound with foreign body of right shoulder

☐ SP 7 **S41.042-** Puncture wound with foreign body of left shoulder

☐ !Q 7 **S41.049-** Puncture wound with foreign body of unspecified shoulder

6 **S41.05** Open bite of shoulder
Bite of shoulder NOS
EXCLUDES 1 superficial bite of shoulder (S40.27)

☐ SP 7 **S41.051-** Open bite of right shoulder

☐ SP 7 **S41.052-** Open bite of left shoulder

☐ !Q 7 **S41.059-** Open bite of unspecified shoulder

5 **S41.1** Open wound of upper arm

6 **S41.10** Unspecified open wound of upper arm

☐ SP 7 **S41.101-** Unspecified open wound of right upper arm

☐ SP 7 **S41.102-** Unspecified open wound of left upper arm

☐ !Q 7 **S41.109-** Unspecified open wound of unspecified upper arm

6 **S41.11** Laceration without foreign body of upper arm

☐ SP 7 **S41.111-** Laceration without foreign body of right upper arm

☐ SP 7 **S41.112-** Laceration without foreign body of left upper arm

☐ !Q 7 **S41.119-** Laceration without foreign body of unspecified upper arm

6 **S41.12** Laceration with foreign body of upper arm

☐ SP 7 **S41.121-** Laceration with foreign body of right upper arm

☐ SP 7 **S41.122-** Laceration with foreign body of left upper arm

☐ !Q 7 **S41.129-** Laceration with foreign body of unspecified upper arm

6 **S41.13** Puncture wound without foreign body of upper arm

☐ SP 7 **S41.131-** Puncture wound without foreign body of right upper arm

☐ SP 7 **S41.132-** Puncture wound without foreign body of left upper arm

☐ !Q 7 **S41.139-** Puncture wound without foreign body of unspecified upper arm

6 **S41.14** Puncture wound with foreign body of upper arm

☐ SP 7 **S41.141-** Puncture wound with foreign body of right upper arm

☐ SP 7 **S41.142-** Puncture wound with foreign body of left upper arm

☐ !Q 7 **S41.149-** Puncture wound with foreign body of unspecified upper arm

6 **S41.15** Open bite of upper arm
Bite of upper arm NOS
EXCLUDES 1 superficial bite of upper arm (S40.87)

☐ SP 7 **S41.151-** Open bite of right upper arm

☐ SP 7 **S41.152-** Open bite of left upper arm

☐ !Q 7 **S41.159-** Open bite of unspecified upper arm

4 **S42** Fracture of shoulder and upper arm
Note:
A fracture not indicated as displaced or nondisplaced should be coded to displaced
A fracture not indicated as open or closed should be coded to closed
EXCLUDES 1 traumatic amputation of shoulder and upper arm (S48.-)

The appropriate 7th character is to be added to all codes from category S42
A initial encounter for closed fracture
B initial encounter for open fracture
D subsequent encounter for fracture with routine healing
G subsequent encounter for fracture with delayed healing
K subsequent encounter for fracture with nonunion
P subsequent encounter for fracture with malunion
S sequela

CODING TIPS ✓ Fractures repaired by joint replacements are NOT coded with Z47.1. Fractures repaired by any other orthopedic surgery are NOT coded with Z47.89. Z codes are not appropriate for fractures of any kind. Code the fracture with 7th character D for fractures undergoing surgical repair.

CODING TIPS ✓ 'D' is the 7th character for home care and hospice unless the physician has documented delayed healing, nonunion or malunion. A sequela is a condition left after the fracture has healed. The Gustilo open fracture classification must be used for open fractures. The default 7th character for open fractures is E.

CODING TIPS ✓ A fracture not indicated as displaced or nondisplaced should be coded to displaced. A fracture not indicated as open or closed should be coded to closed.

5 **S42.0** Fracture of clavicle

6 **S42.00** Fracture of unspecified part of clavicle

☐ SP 7 **S42.001-** Fracture of unspecified part of right clavicle

Chapter 19

S00-T88

☰ SP 7 **S42.002-**   **Fracture of unspecified part of left clavicle**

☰ !Q 7 **S42.009-**   **Fracture of unspecified part of unspecified clavicle**

⑥ **S42.01**   Fracture of sternal end of clavicle

☰ SP 7 **S42.011-**   Anterior displaced fracture of sternal end of right clavicle

☰ SP 7 **S42.012-**   Anterior displaced fracture of sternal end of left clavicle

☰ !Q 7 **S42.013-**   **Anterior displaced fracture of sternal end of unspecified clavicle**

     Displaced fracture of sternal end of clavicle NOS

☰ SP 7 **S42.014-**   Posterior displaced fracture of sternal end of right clavicle

☰ SP 7 **S42.015-**   Posterior displaced fracture of sternal end of left clavicle

☰ !Q 7 **S42.016-**   **Posterior displaced fracture of sternal end of unspecified clavicle**

☰ SP 7 **S42.017-**   Nondisplaced fracture of sternal end of right clavicle

☰ SP 7 **S42.018-**   Nondisplaced fracture of sternal end of left clavicle

☰ !Q 7 **S42.019-**   **Nondisplaced fracture of sternal end of unspecified clavicle**

⑥ **S42.02**   Fracture of shaft of clavicle

☰ SP 7 **S42.021-**   Displaced fracture of shaft of right clavicle

☰ SP 7 **S42.022-**   Displaced fracture of shaft of left clavicle

☰ SP !Q 7 **S42.023-**   **Displaced fracture of shaft of unspecified clavicle**

☰ SP 7 **S42.024-**   Nondisplaced fracture of shaft of right clavicle

☰ SP 7 **S42.025-**   Nondisplaced fracture of shaft of left clavicle

☰ !Q 7 **S42.026-**   **Nondisplaced fracture of shaft of unspecified clavicle**

⑥ **S42.03**   Fracture of lateral end of clavicle
     Fracture of acromial end of clavicle

☰ SP 7 **S42.031-**   Displaced fracture of lateral end of right clavicle

☰ SP 7 **S42.032-**   Displaced fracture of lateral end of left clavicle

☰ !Q 7 **S42.033-**   **Displaced fracture of lateral end of unspecified clavicle**

☰ SP 7 **S42.034-**   Nondisplaced fracture of lateral end of right clavicle

☰ SP 7 **S42.035-**   Nondisplaced fracture of lateral end of left clavicle

☰ !Q 7 **S42.036-**   **Nondisplaced fracture of lateral end of unspecified clavicle**

⑤ **S42.1**   Fracture of scapula

⑥ **S42.10**   **Fracture of unspecified part of scapula**

☰ SP 7 **S42.101-**   **Fracture of unspecified part of scapula, right shoulder**

☰ SP 7 **S42.102-**   **Fracture of unspecified part of scapula, left shoulder**

☰ !Q 7 **S42.109-**   **Fracture of unspecified part of scapula, unspecified shoulder**

⑥ **S42.11**   Fracture of body of scapula

☰ SP 7 **S42.111-**   Displaced fracture of body of scapula, right shoulder

☰ SP 7 **S42.112-**   Displaced fracture of body of scapula, left shoulder

☰ !Q 7 **S42.113-**   **Displaced fracture of body of scapula, unspecified shoulder**

☰ SP 7 **S42.114-**   Nondisplaced fracture of body of scapula, right shoulder

☰ SP 7 **S42.115-**   Nondisplaced fracture of body of scapula, left shoulder

☰ !Q 7 **S42.116-**   **Nondisplaced fracture of body of scapula, unspecified shoulder**

⑥ **S42.12**   Fracture of acromial process

☰ SP 7 **S42.121-**   Displaced fracture of acromial process, right shoulder

☰ SP 7 **S42.122-**   Displaced fracture of acromial process, left shoulder

☰ !Q 7 **S42.123-**   **Displaced fracture of acromial process, unspecified shoulder**

☰ SP 7 **S42.124-**   Nondisplaced fracture of acromial process, right shoulder

☰ SP 7 **S42.125-**   Nondisplaced fracture of acromial process, left shoulder

☰ !Q 7 **S42.126-**   **Nondisplaced fracture of acromial process, unspecified shoulder**

⑥ **S42.13**   Fracture of coracoid process

☰ SP 7 **S42.131-**   Displaced fracture of coracoid process, right shoulder

☰ SP 7 **S42.132-**   Displaced fracture of coracoid process, left shoulder

☰ !Q 7 **S42.133-**   **Displaced fracture of coracoid process, unspecified shoulder**

☰ SP 7 **S42.134-**   Nondisplaced fracture of coracoid process, right shoulder

☰ SP 7 **S42.135-**   Nondisplaced fracture of coracoid process, left shoulder

☰ !Q 7 **S42.136-**   **Nondisplaced fracture of coracoid process, unspecified shoulder**

⑥ **S42.14**   Fracture of glenoid cavity of scapula

☰ SP 7 **S42.141-**   Displaced fracture of glenoid cavity of scapula, right shoulder

☰ SP 7 **S42.142-**   Displaced fracture of glenoid cavity of scapula, left shoulder

☰ !Q 7 **S42.143-**   **Displaced fracture of glenoid cavity of scapula, unspecified shoulder**

☰ SP 7 **S42.144-**   Nondisplaced fracture of glenoid cavity of scapula, right shoulder

☰ SP 7 **S42.145-**   Nondisplaced fracture of glenoid cavity of scapula, left shoulder

☰ !Q 7 **S42.146-**   **Nondisplaced fracture of glenoid cavity of scapula, unspecified shoulder**

⑥ **S42.15**   Fracture of neck of scapula

☰ SP 7 **S42.151-**   Displaced fracture of neck of scapula, right shoulder

☰ SP 7 **S42.152-**   Displaced fracture of neck of scapula, left shoulder

☰ !Q 7 **S42.153-**   **Displaced fracture of neck of scapula, unspecified shoulder**

☰ SP 7 **S42.154-**   Nondisplaced fracture of neck of scapula, right shoulder

☰ SP 7 **S42.155-**   Nondisplaced fracture of neck of scapula, left shoulder

Chapter 19

S00-T88

4️⃣4th digit required   5️⃣5th digit required   6️⃣6th digit required   7️⃣7th digit required   7️⃣7th digit placeholder   ✚Additional code   ☰Laterality

☰ 🔘 7 **S42.156-** Nondisplaced fracture of neck of scapula, unspecified shoulder

6 S42.19 Fracture of other part of scapula

☰ SP 7 **S42.191-** Fracture of other part of scapula, right shoulder

☰ SP 7 **S42.192-** Fracture of other part of scapula, left shoulder

☰ 🔘 7 **S42.199-** Fracture of other part of scapula, unspecified shoulder

5 S42.2 Fracture of upper end of humerus
Fracture of proximal end of humerus
EXCLUDES 2 fracture of shaft of humerus (S42.3-)
physeal fracture of upper end of humerus (S49.0-)

6 S42.20 Unspecified fracture of upper end of humerus

☰ SP 7 **S42.201-** Unspecified fracture of upper end of right humerus

☰ SP 7 **S42.202-** Unspecified fracture of upper end of left humerus

☰ 🔘 7 **S42.209-** Unspecified fracture of upper end of unspecified humerus

6 S42.21 Unspecified fracture of surgical neck of humerus
Fracture of neck of humerus NOS

☰ SP 7 **S42.211-** Unspecified displaced fracture of surgical neck of right humerus

☰ SP 7 **S42.212-** Unspecified displaced fracture of surgical neck of left humerus

☰ 🔘 7 **S42.213-** Unspecified displaced fracture of surgical neck of unspecified humerus

☰ SP 7 **S42.214-** Unspecified nondisplaced fracture of surgical neck of right humerus

☰ SP 7 **S42.215-** Unspecified nondisplaced fracture of surgical neck of left humerus

☰ 🔘 7 **S42.216-** Unspecified nondisplaced fracture of surgical neck of unspecified humerus

6 S42.22 2-part fracture of surgical neck of humerus

☰ SP 7 **S42.221-** 2-part displaced fracture of surgical neck of right humerus

☰ SP 7 **S42.222-** 2-part displaced fracture of surgical neck of left humerus

☰ 🔘 7 **S42.223-** 2-part displaced fracture of surgical neck of unspecified humerus

☰ SP 7 **S42.224-** 2-part nondisplaced fracture of surgical neck of right humerus

☰ SP 7 **S42.225-** 2-part nondisplaced fracture of surgical neck of left humerus

☰ 🔘 7 **S42.226-** 2-part nondisplaced fracture of surgical neck of unspecified humerus

6 S42.23 3-part fracture of surgical neck of humerus

☰ SP 7 **S42.231-** 3-part fracture of surgical neck of right humerus

☰ SP 7 **S42.232-** 3-part fracture of surgical neck of left humerus

☰ 🔘 7 **S42.239-** 3-part fracture of surgical neck of unspecified humerus

6 S42.24 4-part fracture of surgical neck of humerus

☰ SP 7 **S42.241-** 4-part fracture of surgical neck of right humerus

☰ SP 7 **S42.242-** 4-part fracture of surgical neck of left humerus

☰ 🔘 7 **S42.249-** 4-part fracture of surgical neck of unspecified humerus

6 S42.25 Fracture of greater tuberosity of humerus

☰ SP 7 **S42.251-** Displaced fracture of greater tuberosity of right humerus

☰ SP 7 **S42.252-** Displaced fracture of greater tuberosity of left humerus

☰ 🔘 7 **S42.253-** Displaced fracture of greater tuberosity of unspecified humerus

☰ SP 7 **S42.254-** Nondisplaced fracture of greater tuberosity of right humerus

☰ SP 7 **S42.255-** Nondisplaced fracture of greater tuberosity of left humerus

☰ 🔘 7 **S42.256-** Nondisplaced fracture of greater tuberosity of unspecified humerus

6 S42.26 Fracture of lesser tuberosity of humerus

☰ SP 7 **S42.261-** Displaced fracture of lesser tuberosity of right humerus

☰ SP 7 **S42.262-** Displaced fracture of lesser tuberosity of left humerus

☰ 🔘 7 **S42.263-** Displaced fracture of lesser tuberosity of unspecified humerus

☰ SP 7 **S42.264-** Nondisplaced fracture of lesser tuberosity of right humerus

☰ SP 7 **S42.265-** Nondisplaced fracture of lesser tuberosity of left humerus

☰ 🔘 7 **S42.266-** Nondisplaced fracture of lesser tuberosity of unspecified humerus

6 S42.27 Torus fracture of upper end of humerus

The appropriate 7th character is to be added to all codes in subcategory S42.27
A	initial encounter for closed fracture
D	subsequent encounter for fracture with routine healing
G	subsequent encounter for fracture with delayed healing
K	subsequent encounter for fracture with nonunion
P	subsequent encounter for fracture with malunion
S	sequela

☰ SP 7 **S42.271-** Torus fracture of upper end of right humerus

☰ SP 7 **S42.272-** Torus fracture of upper end of left humerus

☰ 🔘 7 **S42.279-** Torus fracture of upper end of unspecified humerus

6 S42.29 Other fracture of upper end of humerus

★ New ▲ Revised Px Primary SP PDGM Px SL Low CoM SH High CoM IQ Quest. Encounter H Hospice non-cancer Dx Unspecified M Manifestation

DecisionHealth's FY 2020 Complete Home Health ICD-10-CM Diagnosis Coding Manual

1519

Fracture of anatomical neck of humerus

Fracture of articular head of humerus

⊟ **SP** 7 S42.291-   **Other displaced fracture of upper end of right humerus**

⊟ **SP** 7 S42.292-   **Other displaced fracture of upper end of left humerus**

⊟ **IQ** 7 S42.293-   **Other displaced fracture of upper end of unspecified humerus**

⊟ **SP** 7 S42.294-   **Other nondisplaced fracture of upper end of right humerus**

⊟ **SP** 7 S42.295-   **Other nondisplaced fracture of upper end of left humerus**

⊟ **IQ** 7 S42.296-   **Other nondisplaced fracture of upper end of unspecified humerus**

5 **S42.3   Fracture of shaft of humerus**

Fracture of humerus NOS

Fracture of upper arm NOS

> **EXCLUDES 2**   physeal fractures of upper end of humerus (S49.0-)
>
> physeal fractures of lower end of humerus (S49.1-)

6 **S42.30   Unspecified fracture of shaft of humerus**

⊟ **SP** 7 S42.301-   **Unspecified fracture of shaft of humerus, right arm**

⊟ **SP** 7 S42.302-   **Unspecified fracture of shaft of humerus, left arm**

⊟ **IQ** 7 S42.309-   **Unspecified fracture of shaft of humerus, unspecified arm**

6 **S42.31   Greenstick fracture of shaft of humerus**

The appropriate 7th character is to be added to all codes in subcategory S42.31

A   initial encounter for closed fracture

D   subsequent encounter for fracture with routine healing

G   subsequent encounter for fracture with delayed healing

K   subsequent encounter for fracture with nonunion

P   subsequent encounter for fracture with malunion

S   sequela

⊟ **SP** 7 S42.311-   **Greenstick fracture of shaft of humerus, right arm**

⊟ **SP** 7 S42.312-   **Greenstick fracture of shaft of humerus, left arm**

⊟ **IQ** 7 S42.319-   **Greenstick fracture of shaft of humerus, unspecified arm**

6 **S42.32   Transverse fracture of shaft of humerus**

⊟ **SP** 7 S42.321-   **Displaced transverse fracture of shaft of humerus, right arm**

⊟ **SP** 7 S42.322-   **Displaced transverse fracture of shaft of humerus, left arm**

⊟ **IQ** 7 S42.323-   **Displaced transverse fracture of shaft of humerus, unspecified arm**

⊟ **SP** 7 S42.324-   **Nondisplaced transverse fracture of shaft of humerus, right arm**

⊟ **SP** 7 S42.325-   **Nondisplaced transverse fracture of shaft of humerus, left arm**

⊟ **IQ** 7 S42.326-   **Nondisplaced transverse fracture of shaft of humerus, unspecified arm**

6 **S42.33   Oblique fracture of shaft of humerus**

⊟ **SP** 7 S42.331-   **Displaced oblique fracture of shaft of humerus, right arm**

⊟ **SP** 7 S42.332-   **Displaced oblique fracture of shaft of humerus, left arm**

⊟ **IQ** 7 S42.333-   **Displaced oblique fracture of shaft of humerus, unspecified arm**

⊟ **SP** 7 S42.334-   **Nondisplaced oblique fracture of shaft of humerus, right arm**

⊟ **SP** 7 S42.335-   **Nondisplaced oblique fracture of shaft of humerus, left arm**

⊟ **IQ** 7 S42.336-   **Nondisplaced oblique fracture of shaft of humerus, unspecified arm**

6 **S42.34   Spiral fracture of shaft of humerus**

⊟ **SP** 7 S42.341-   **Displaced spiral fracture of shaft of humerus, right arm**

⊟ **SP** 7 S42.342-   **Displaced spiral fracture of shaft of humerus, left arm**

⊟ **IQ** 7 S42.343-   **Displaced spiral fracture of shaft of humerus, unspecified arm**

⊟ **SP** 7 S42.344-   **Nondisplaced spiral fracture of shaft of humerus, right arm**

⊟ **SP** 7 S42.345-   **Nondisplaced spiral fracture of shaft of humerus, left arm**

⊟ **IQ** 7 S42.346-   **Nondisplaced spiral fracture of shaft of humerus, unspecified arm**

6 **S42.35   Comminuted fracture of shaft of humerus**

⊟ **SP** 7 S42.351-   **Displaced comminuted fracture of shaft of humerus, right arm**

⊟ **SP** 7 S42.352-   **Displaced comminuted fracture of shaft of humerus, left arm**

⊟ **IQ** 7 S42.353-   **Displaced comminuted fracture of shaft of humerus, unspecified arm**

⊟ **SP** 7 S42.354-   **Nondisplaced comminuted fracture of shaft of humerus, right arm**

⊟ **SP** 7 S42.355-   **Nondisplaced comminuted fracture of shaft of humerus, left arm**

⊟ **IQ** 7 S42.356-   **Nondisplaced comminuted fracture of shaft of humerus, unspecified arm**

6 **S42.36   Segmental fracture of shaft of humerus**

⊟ **SP** 7 S42.361-   **Displaced segmental fracture of shaft of humerus, right arm**

⊟ **SP** 7 S42.362-   **Displaced segmental fracture of shaft of humerus, left arm**

⊟ **IQ** 7 S42.363-   **Displaced segmental fracture of shaft of humerus, unspecified arm**

⊟ **SP** 7 S42.364-   **Nondisplaced segmental fracture of shaft of humerus, right arm**

⊟ **SP** 7 S42.365-   **Nondisplaced segmental fracture of shaft of humerus, left arm**

4 4th digit required   5 5th digit required   6 6th digit required   7 7th digit required   7 7th digit placeholder   + Additional code   ⊟ Laterality

1520   *DecisionHealth's* FY 2020 Complete Home Health ICD-10-CM Diagnosis Coding Manual

⊟ **IQ** 7 S42.366- **Nondisplaced segmental fracture of shaft of humerus, unspecified arm**

⑥ S42.39 **Other fracture of shaft of humerus**

⊟ **SP** 7 S42.391- **Other fracture of shaft of right humerus**

⊟ **SP** 7 S42.392- **Other fracture of shaft of left humerus**

⊟ **IQ** 7 S42.399- **Other fracture of shaft of unspecified humerus**

⑤ S42.4 **Fracture of lower end of humerus**
Fracture of distal end of humerus
EXCLUDES 2 fracture of shaft of humerus (S42.3-)
physeal fracture of lower end of humerus (S49.1-)

⑥ S42.40 **Unspecified fracture of lower end of humerus**
Fracture of elbow NOS

⊟ **SP** 7 S42.401- **Unspecified fracture of lower end of right humerus**

⊟ **SP** 7 S42.402- **Unspecified fracture of lower end of left humerus**

⊟ **IQ** 7 S42.409- **Unspecified fracture of lower end of unspecified humerus**

⑥ S42.41 **Simple supracondylar fracture without intercondylar fracture of humerus**

⊟ **SP** 7 S42.411- **Displaced simple supracondylar fracture without intercondylar fracture of right humerus**

⊟ **SP** 7 S42.412- **Displaced simple supracondylar fracture without intercondylar fracture of left humerus**

⊟ **IQ** 7 S42.413- **Displaced simple supracondylar fracture without intercondylar fracture of unspecified humerus**

⊟ **SP** 7 S42.414- **Nondisplaced simple supracondylar fracture without intercondylar fracture of right humerus**

⊟ **SP** 7 S42.415- **Nondisplaced simple supracondylar fracture without intercondylar fracture of left humerus**

⊟ **IQ** 7 S42.416- **Nondisplaced simple supracondylar fracture without intercondylar fracture of unspecified humerus**

⑥ S42.42 **Comminuted supracondylar fracture without intercondylar fracture of humerus**

⊟ **SP** 7 S42.421- **Displaced comminuted supracondylar fracture without intercondylar fracture of right humerus**

⊟ **SP** 7 S42.422- **Displaced comminuted supracondylar fracture without intercondylar fracture of left humerus**

⊟ **IQ** 7 S42.423- **Displaced comminuted supracondylar fracture without intercondylar fracture of unspecified humerus**

⊟ **SP** 7 S42.424- **Nondisplaced comminuted supracondylar fracture without intercondylar fracture of right humerus**

⊟ **SP** 7 S42.425- **Nondisplaced comminuted supracondylar fracture without intercondylar fracture of left humerus**

⊟ **IQ** 7 S42.426- **Nondisplaced comminuted supracondylar fracture without intercondylar fracture of unspecified humerus**

⑥ S42.43 **Fracture (avulsion) of lateral epicondyle of humerus**

⊟ **SP** 7 S42.431- **Displaced fracture (avulsion) of lateral epicondyle of right humerus**

⊟ **SP** 7 S42.432- **Displaced fracture (avulsion) of lateral epicondyle of left humerus**

⊟ **IQ** 7 S42.433- **Displaced fracture (avulsion) of lateral epicondyle of unspecified humerus**

⊟ **SP** 7 S42.434- **Nondisplaced fracture (avulsion) of lateral epicondyle of right humerus**

⊟ **SP** 7 S42.435- **Nondisplaced fracture (avulsion) of lateral epicondyle of left humerus**

⊟ **IQ** 7 S42.436- **Nondisplaced fracture (avulsion) of lateral epicondyle of unspecified humerus**

⑥ S42.44 **Fracture (avulsion) of medial epicondyle of humerus**

⊟ **SP** 7 S42.441- **Displaced fracture (avulsion) of medial epicondyle of right humerus**

⊟ **SP** 7 S42.442- **Displaced fracture (avulsion) of medial epicondyle of left humerus**

⊟ **IQ** 7 S42.443- **Displaced fracture (avulsion) of medial epicondyle of unspecified humerus**

⊟ **SP** 7 S42.444- **Nondisplaced fracture (avulsion) of medial epicondyle of right humerus**

⊟ **SP** 7 S42.445- **Nondisplaced fracture (avulsion) of medial epicondyle of left humerus**

⊟ **IQ** 7 S42.446- **Nondisplaced fracture (avulsion) of medial epicondyle of unspecified humerus**

⊟ **SP** 7 S42.447- **Incarcerated fracture (avulsion) of medial epicondyle of right humerus**

⊟ **SP** 7 S42.448- **Incarcerated fracture (avulsion) of medial epicondyle of left humerus**

⊟ **IQ** 7 S42.449- **Incarcerated fracture (avulsion) of medial epicondyle of unspecified humerus**

⑥ S42.45 **Fracture of lateral condyle of humerus**
Fracture of capitellum of humerus

⊟ **SP** 7 S42.451- **Displaced fracture of lateral condyle of right humerus**

⊟ **SP** 7 S42.452- **Displaced fracture of lateral condyle of left humerus**

★ New ▲ Revised Px Primary **SP** PDGM Px **SL** Low CoM **SH** High CoM **IQ** Quest. Encounter ⊞ Hospice non-cancer Dx Unspecified **M** Manifestation

DecisionHealth's FY 2020 Complete Home Health ICD-10-CM Diagnosis Coding Manual

1521

Chapter 19

S00-T88

☰ 🔳 7 **S42.453-** **Displaced fracture of lateral condyle of unspecified humerus**

☰ SP 7 **S42.454-** Nondisplaced fracture of lateral condyle of right humerus

☰ SP 7 **S42.455-** Nondisplaced fracture of lateral condyle of left humerus

☰ 🔳 7 **S42.456-** **Nondisplaced fracture of lateral condyle of unspecified humerus**

6 **S42.46** **Fracture of medial condyle of humerus**
Trochlea fracture of humerus

☰ SP 7 **S42.461-** Displaced fracture of medial condyle of right humerus

☰ SP 7 **S42.462-** Displaced fracture of medial condyle of left humerus

☰ 🔳 7 **S42.463-** **Displaced fracture of medial condyle of unspecified humerus**

☰ SP 7 **S42.464-** Nondisplaced fracture of medial condyle of right humerus

☰ SP 7 **S42.465-** Nondisplaced fracture of medial condyle of left humerus

☰ 🔳 7 **S42.466-** **Nondisplaced fracture of medial condyle of unspecified humerus**

6 **S42.47** **Transcondylar fracture of humerus**

☰ SP 7 **S42.471-** Displaced transcondylar fracture of right humerus

☰ SP 7 **S42.472-** Displaced transcondylar fracture of left humerus

☰ 🔳 7 **S42.473-** **Displaced transcondylar fracture of unspecified humerus**

☰ SP 7 **S42.474-** Nondisplaced transcondylar fracture of right humerus

☰ SP 7 **S42.475-** Nondisplaced transcondylar fracture of left humerus

☰ 🔳 7 **S42.476-** **Nondisplaced transcondylar fracture of unspecified humerus**

6 **S42.48** **Torus fracture of lower end of humerus**

The appropriate 7th character is to be added to all codes in subcategory S42.48
A   initial encounter for closed fracture
D   subsequent encounter for fracture with routine healing
G   subsequent encounter for fracture with delayed healing
K   subsequent encounter for fracture with nonunion
P   subsequent encounter for fracture with malunion
S   sequela

☰ SP 7 **S42.481-** Torus fracture of lower end of right humerus

☰ SP 7 **S42.482-** Torus fracture of lower end of left humerus

☰ 🔳 7 **S42.489-** **Torus fracture of lower end of unspecified humerus**

6 **S42.49** **Other fracture of lower end of humerus**

☰ SP 7 **S42.491-** Other displaced fracture of lower end of right humerus

☰ SP 7 **S42.492-** Other displaced fracture of lower end of left humerus

☰ 🔳 7 **S42.493-** **Other displaced fracture of lower end of unspecified humerus**

☰ SP 7 **S42.494-** Other nondisplaced fracture of lower end of right humerus

☰ SP 7 **S42.495-** Other nondisplaced fracture of lower end of left humerus

☰ 🔳 7 **S42.496-** **Other nondisplaced fracture of lower end of unspecified humerus**

5 **S42.9** **Fracture of shoulder girdle, part unspecified**
Fracture of shoulder NOS

☰ 🔳 7 **S42.90X-** **Fracture of unspecified shoulder girdle, part unspecified**

☰ SP 7 **S42.91X-** **Fracture of right shoulder girdle, part unspecified**

☰ SP 7 **S42.92X-** **Fracture of left shoulder girdle, part unspecified**

4 **S43** **Dislocation and sprain of joints and ligaments of shoulder girdle**

INCLUDES   avulsion of joint or ligament of shoulder girdle
laceration of cartilage, joint or ligament of shoulder girdle
sprain of cartilage, joint or ligament of shoulder girdle
traumatic hemarthrosis of joint or ligament of shoulder girdle
traumatic rupture of joint or ligament of shoulder girdle
traumatic subluxation of joint or ligament of shoulder girdle
traumatic tear of joint or ligament of shoulder girdle

Code also:
any associated open wound

EXCLUDES 2   strain of muscle, fascia and tendon of shoulder and upper arm (S46.-)

The appropriate 7th character is to be added to each code from category S43
A   initial encounter
D   subsequent encounter
S   sequela

5 **S43.0** **Subluxation and dislocation of shoulder joint**
Dislocation of glenohumeral joint
Subluxation of glenohumeral joint

6 **S43.00** **Unspecified subluxation and dislocation of shoulder joint**
Dislocation of humerus NOS
Subluxation of humerus NOS

☰ SP 7 **S43.001-** **Unspecified subluxation of right shoulder joint**

☰ SP 7 **S43.002-** **Unspecified subluxation of left shoulder joint**

☰ 🔳 7 **S43.003-** **Unspecified subluxation of unspecified shoulder joint**

☰ SP 7 **S43.004-** **Unspecified dislocation of right shoulder joint**

☰ SP 7 **S43.005-** **Unspecified dislocation of left shoulder joint**

☰ 🔳 7 **S43.006-** **Unspecified dislocation of unspecified shoulder joint**

---

4 4th digit required   5 5th digit required   6 6th digit required   7 7th digit required   ☑ 7th digit placeholder   ✚ Additional code   ☰ Laterality

6 **S43.01** Anterior subluxation and dislocation of humerus

☐ SP 7 **S43.011-** Anterior subluxation of right humerus

☐ SP 7 **S43.012-** Anterior subluxation of left humerus

☐ IQ 7 **S43.013-** Anterior subluxation of unspecified humerus

☐ SP 7 **S43.014-** Anterior dislocation of right humerus

☐ SP 7 **S43.015-** Anterior dislocation of left humerus

☐ IQ 7 **S43.016-** Anterior dislocation of unspecified humerus

6 **S43.02** Posterior subluxation and dislocation of humerus

☐ SP 7 **S43.021-** Posterior subluxation of right humerus

☐ SP 7 **S43.022-** Posterior subluxation of left humerus

☐ IQ 7 **S43.023-** Posterior subluxation of unspecified humerus

☐ SP 7 **S43.024-** Posterior dislocation of right humerus

☐ SP 7 **S43.025-** Posterior dislocation of left humerus

☐ IQ 7 **S43.026-** Posterior dislocation of unspecified humerus

6 **S43.03** Inferior subluxation and dislocation of humerus

☐ SP 7 **S43.031-** Inferior subluxation of right humerus

☐ SP 7 **S43.032-** Inferior subluxation of left humerus

☐ IQ 7 **S43.033-** Inferior subluxation of unspecified humerus

☐ SP 7 **S43.034-** Inferior dislocation of right humerus

☐ SP 7 **S43.035-** Inferior dislocation of left humerus

☐ IQ 7 **S43.036-** Inferior dislocation of unspecified humerus

6 **S43.08** Other subluxation and dislocation of shoulder joint

☐ SP 7 **S43.081-** Other subluxation of right shoulder joint

☐ SP 7 **S43.082-** Other subluxation of left shoulder joint

☐ IQ 7 **S43.083-** Other subluxation of unspecified shoulder joint

☐ SP 7 **S43.084-** Other dislocation of right shoulder joint

☐ SP 7 **S43.085-** Other dislocation of left shoulder joint

☐ IQ 7 **S43.086-** Other dislocation of unspecified shoulder joint

5 **S43.1** Subluxation and dislocation of acromioclavicular joint

6 **S43.10** Unspecified dislocation of acromioclavicular joint

☐ SP 7 **S43.101-** Unspecified dislocation of right acromioclavicular joint

☐ SP 7 **S43.102-** Unspecified dislocation of left acromioclavicular joint

☐ IQ 7 **S43.109-** Unspecified dislocation of unspecified acromioclavicular joint

6 **S43.11** Subluxation of acromioclavicular joint

☐ SP 7 **S43.111-** Subluxation of right acromioclavicular joint

☐ SP 7 **S43.112-** Subluxation of left acromioclavicular joint

☐ IQ 7 **S43.119-** Subluxation of unspecified acromioclavicular joint

6 **S43.12** Dislocation of acromioclavicular joint, 100%-200% displacement

☐ SP 7 **S43.121-** Dislocation of right acromioclavicular joint, 100%-200% displacement

☐ SP 7 **S43.122-** Dislocation of left acromioclavicular joint, 100%-200% displacement

☐ IQ 7 **S43.129-** Dislocation of unspecified acromioclavicular joint, 100%-200% displacement

6 **S43.13** Dislocation of acromioclavicular joint, greater than 200% displacement

☐ SP 7 **S43.131-** Dislocation of right acromioclavicular joint, greater than 200% displacement

☐ SP 7 **S43.132-** Dislocation of left acromioclavicular joint, greater than 200% displacement

☐ IQ 7 **S43.139-** Dislocation of unspecified acromioclavicular joint, greater than 200% displacement

6 **S43.14** Inferior dislocation of acromioclavicular joint

☐ SP 7 **S43.141-** Inferior dislocation of right acromioclavicular joint

☐ SP 7 **S43.142-** Inferior dislocation of left acromioclavicular joint

☐ IQ 7 **S43.149-** Inferior dislocation of unspecified acromioclavicular joint

6 **S43.15** Posterior dislocation of acromioclavicular joint

☐ SP 7 **S43.151-** Posterior dislocation of right acromioclavicular joint

☐ SP 7 **S43.152-** Posterior dislocation of left acromioclavicular joint

☐ IQ 7 **S43.159-** Posterior dislocation of unspecified acromioclavicular joint

5 **S43.2** Subluxation and dislocation of sternoclavicular joint

6 **S43.20** Unspecified subluxation and dislocation of sternoclavicular joint

☐ SP 7 **S43.201-** Unspecified subluxation of right sternoclavicular joint

☐ SP 7 **S43.202-** Unspecified subluxation of left sternoclavicular joint

☐ IQ 7 **S43.203-** Unspecified subluxation of unspecified sternoclavicular joint

☐ SP 7 **S43.204-** Unspecified dislocation of right sternoclavicular joint

Chapter 19

S00-T88

★ New ▲ Revised Px Primary SP PDGM Px SL Low CoM SH High CoM IQ Quest. Encounter H Hospice non-cancer Dx Unspecified M *Manifestation*

DecisionHealth's FY 2020 Complete Home Health ICD-10-CM Diagnosis Coding Manual

1523

☐ **SP** 7 **S43.205-** **Unspecified dislocation of left sternoclavicular joint**

☐ **!Q** 7 **S43.206-** **Unspecified dislocation of unspecified sternoclavicular joint**

6 **S43.21** **Anterior subluxation and dislocation of sternoclavicular joint**

☐ **SP** 7 **S43.211-** **Anterior subluxation of right sternoclavicular joint**

☐ **SP** 7 **S43.212-** **Anterior subluxation of left sternoclavicular joint**

☐ **!Q** 7 **S43.213-** **Anterior subluxation of unspecified sternoclavicular joint**

☐ **SP** 7 **S43.214-** **Anterior dislocation of right sternoclavicular joint**

☐ **SP** 7 **S43.215-** **Anterior dislocation of left sternoclavicular joint**

☐ **!Q** 7 **S43.216-** **Anterior dislocation of unspecified sternoclavicular joint**

6 **S43.22** **Posterior subluxation and dislocation of sternoclavicular joint**

☐ **SP** 7 **S43.221-** **Posterior subluxation of right sternoclavicular joint**

☐ **SP** 7 **S43.222-** **Posterior subluxation of left sternoclavicular joint**

☐ **!Q** 7 **S43.223-** **Posterior subluxation of unspecified sternoclavicular joint**

☐ **SP** 7 **S43.224-** **Posterior dislocation of right sternoclavicular joint**

☐ **SP** 7 **S43.225-** **Posterior dislocation of left sternoclavicular joint**

☐ **!Q** 7 **S43.226-** **Posterior dislocation of unspecified sternoclavicular joint**

5 **S43.3** **Subluxation and dislocation of other and unspecified parts of shoulder girdle**

6 **S43.30** **Subluxation and dislocation of unspecified parts of shoulder girdle**
Dislocation of shoulder girdle NOS
Subluxation of shoulder girdle NOS

☐ **SP** 7 **S43.301-** **Subluxation of unspecified parts of right shoulder girdle**

☐ **SP** 7 **S43.302-** **Subluxation of unspecified parts of left shoulder girdle**

☐ **!Q** 7 **S43.303-** **Subluxation of unspecified parts of unspecified shoulder girdle**

☐ **SP** 7 **S43.304-** **Dislocation of unspecified parts of right shoulder girdle**

☐ **SP** 7 **S43.305-** **Dislocation of unspecified parts of left shoulder girdle**

☐ **!Q** 7 **S43.306-** **Dislocation of unspecified parts of unspecified shoulder girdle**

6 **S43.31** **Subluxation and dislocation of scapula**

☐ **SP** 7 **S43.311-** **Subluxation of right scapula**

☐ **SP** 7 **S43.312-** **Subluxation of left scapula**

☐ **!Q** 7 **S43.313-** **Subluxation of unspecified scapula**

☐ **SP** 7 **S43.314-** **Dislocation of right scapula**

☐ **SP** 7 **S43.315-** **Dislocation of left scapula**

☐ **!Q** 7 **S43.316-** **Dislocation of unspecified scapula**

6 **S43.39** **Subluxation and dislocation of other parts of shoulder girdle**

☐ **SP** 7 **S43.391-** **Subluxation of other parts of right shoulder girdle**

☐ **SP** 7 **S43.392-** **Subluxation of other parts of left shoulder girdle**

☐ **SP** 7 **S43.393-** **Subluxation of other parts of unspecified shoulder girdle**

☐ **SP** 7 **S43.394-** **Dislocation of other parts of right shoulder girdle**

☐ **SP** 7 **S43.395-** **Dislocation of other parts of left shoulder girdle**

☐ **!Q** 7 **S43.396-** **Dislocation of other parts of unspecified shoulder girdle**

5 **S43.4** **Sprain of shoulder joint**

6 **S43.40** **Unspecified sprain of shoulder joint**

☐ **SP** 7 **S43.401-** **Unspecified sprain of right shoulder joint**

☐ **SP** 7 **S43.402-** **Unspecified sprain of left shoulder joint**

☐ **!Q** 7 **S43.409-** **Unspecified sprain of unspecified shoulder joint**

6 **S43.41** **Sprain of coracohumeral (ligament)**

☐ **SP** 7 **S43.411-** **Sprain of right coracohumeral (ligament)**

☐ **SP** 7 **S43.412-** **Sprain of left coracohumeral (ligament)**

☐ **!Q** 7 **S43.419-** **Sprain of unspecified coracohumeral (ligament)**

6 **S43.42** **Sprain of rotator cuff capsule**
EXCLUDES 1 rotator cuff syndrome (complete) (incomplete), not specified as traumatic (M75.1-)
EXCLUDES 2 injury of tendon of rotator cuff (S46.0-)

☐ **SP** 7 **S43.421-** **Sprain of right rotator cuff capsule**

☐ **SP** 7 **S43.422-** **Sprain of left rotator cuff capsule**

☐ **!Q** 7 **S43.429-** **Sprain of unspecified rotator cuff capsule**

6 **S43.43** **Superior glenoid labrum lesion**
SLAP lesion

☐ **SP** 7 **S43.431-** **Superior glenoid labrum lesion of right shoulder**

☐ **SP** 7 **S43.432-** **Superior glenoid labrum lesion of left shoulder**

☐ **!Q** 7 **S43.439-** **Superior glenoid labrum lesion of unspecified shoulder**

6 **S43.49** **Other sprain of shoulder joint**

☐ **SP** 7 **S43.491-** **Other sprain of right shoulder joint**

☐ **SP** 7 **S43.492-** **Other sprain of left shoulder joint**

☐ **!Q** 7 **S43.499-** **Other sprain of unspecified shoulder joint**

5 **S43.5** **Sprain of acromioclavicular joint**
Sprain of acromioclavicular ligament

☐ **!Q** 7 **S43.50X-** **Sprain of unspecified acromioclavicular joint**

☐ **SP** 7 **S43.51X-** **Sprain of right acromioclavicular joint**

---

4 4th digit required   5 5th digit required   6 6th digit required   7 7th digit required   7 7th digit placeholder   + Additional code   ☐ Laterality

Chapter 19

S00-T88

⊟ **SP** ✅ **S43.52X-** Sprain of left acromioclavicular joint

⑤ **S43.6** Sprain of sternoclavicular joint

⊟ **IQ** ✅ **S43.60X-** Sprain of unspecified sternoclavicular joint

⊟ **SP** ✅ **S43.61X-** Sprain of right sternoclavicular joint

⊟ **SP** ✅ **S43.62X-** Sprain of left sternoclavicular joint

⑤ **S43.8** Sprain of other specified parts of shoulder girdle

⊟ **IQ** ✅ **S43.80X-** Sprain of other specified parts of unspecified shoulder girdle

⊟ **SP** ✅ **S43.81X-** Sprain of other specified parts of right shoulder girdle

⊟ **SP** ✅ **S43.82X-** Sprain of other specified parts of left shoulder girdle

⑤ **S43.9** Sprain of unspecified parts of shoulder girdle

⊟ **IQ** ✅ **S43.90X-** Sprain of unspecified parts of unspecified shoulder girdle

Sprain of shoulder girdle NOS

⊟ **SP** ✅ **S43.91X-** Sprain of unspecified parts of right shoulder girdle

⊟ **SP** ✅ **S43.92X-** Sprain of unspecified parts of left shoulder girdle

④ **S44** Injury of nerves at shoulder and upper arm level
Code also:
any associated open wound (S41.-)
EXCLUDES 2 injury of brachial plexus (S14.3-)

The appropriate 7th character is to be added to each code from category S44
A initial encounter
D subsequent encounter
S sequela

⑤ **S44.0** Injury of ulnar nerve at upper arm level
EXCLUDES 1 ulnar nerve NOS (S54.0)

⊟ **IQ** ✅ **S44.00X-** Injury of ulnar nerve at upper arm level, unspecified arm

⊟ **SP** ✅ **S44.01X-** Injury of ulnar nerve at upper arm level, right arm

⊟ **SP** ✅ **S44.02X-** Injury of ulnar nerve at upper arm level, left arm

⑤ **S44.1** Injury of median nerve at upper arm level
EXCLUDES 1 median nerve NOS (S54.1)

⊟ **IQ** ✅ **S44.10X-** Injury of median nerve at upper arm level, unspecified arm

⊟ **SP** ✅ **S44.11X-** Injury of median nerve at upper arm level, right arm

⊟ **SP** ✅ **S44.12X-** Injury of median nerve at upper arm level, left arm

⑤ **S44.2** Injury of radial nerve at upper arm level
EXCLUDES 1 radial nerve NOS (S54.2)

⊟ **IQ** ✅ **S44.20X-** Injury of radial nerve at upper arm level, unspecified arm

⊟ **SP** ✅ **S44.21X-** Injury of radial nerve at upper arm level, right arm

⊟ **SP** ✅ **S44.22X-** Injury of radial nerve at upper arm level, left arm

⑤ **S44.3** Injury of axillary nerve

⊟ **IQ** ✅ **S44.30X-** Injury of axillary nerve, unspecified arm

⊟ **SP** ✅ **S44.31X-** Injury of axillary nerve, right arm

⊟ **SP** ✅ **S44.32X-** Injury of axillary nerve, left arm

⑤ **S44.4** Injury of musculocutaneous nerve

⊟ **IQ** ✅ **S44.40X-** Injury of musculocutaneous nerve, unspecified arm

⊟ **SP** ✅ **S44.41X-** Injury of musculocutaneous nerve, right arm

⊟ **SP** ✅ **S44.42X-** Injury of musculocutaneous nerve, left arm

⑤ **S44.5** Injury of cutaneous sensory nerve at shoulder and upper arm level

⊟ **IQ** ✅ **S44.50X-** Injury of cutaneous sensory nerve at shoulder and upper arm level, unspecified arm

⊟ **SP** ✅ **S44.51X-** Injury of cutaneous sensory nerve at shoulder and upper arm level, right arm

⊟ **SP** ✅ **S44.52X-** Injury of cutaneous sensory nerve at shoulder and upper arm level, left arm

⑤ **S44.8** Injury of other nerves at shoulder and upper arm level

⑥ **S44.8X** Injury of other nerves at shoulder and upper arm level

⊟ **SP** ✅ **S44.8X1-** Injury of other nerves at shoulder and upper arm level, right arm

⊟ **SP** ✅ **S44.8X2-** Injury of other nerves at shoulder and upper arm level, left arm

⊟ **IQ** ✅ **S44.8X9-** Injury of other nerves at shoulder and upper arm level, unspecified arm

⑤ **S44.9** Injury of unspecified nerve at shoulder and upper arm level

⊟ **IQ** ✅ **S44.90X-** Injury of unspecified nerve at shoulder and upper arm level, unspecified arm

⊟ **IQ** ✅ **S44.91X-** Injury of unspecified nerve at shoulder and upper arm level, right arm

⊟ **IQ** ✅ **S44.92X-** Injury of unspecified nerve at shoulder and upper arm level, left arm

④ **S45** Injury of blood vessels at shoulder and upper arm level
Code also:
any associated open wound (S41.-)
EXCLUDES 2 injury of subclavian artery (S25.1)
injury of subclavian vein (S25.3)

The appropriate 7th character is to be added to each code from category S45
A initial encounter
D subsequent encounter
S sequela

⑤ **S45.0** Injury of axillary artery

⑥ **S45.00** Unspecified injury of axillary artery

⊟ **IQ** ✅ **S45.001-** Unspecified injury of axillary artery, right side

⊟ **IQ** ✅ **S45.002-** Unspecified injury of axillary artery, left side

---

★ New ▲ Revised Px Primary **SP** PDGM Px **SL** Low CoM **SH** High CoM **IQ** Quest. Encounter ⊞ Hospice non-cancer Dx Unspecified **M** *Manifestation*

Chapter 19

S00-T88

🔲 **!Q** 7️⃣ S45.009-   Unspecified injury of axillary artery, unspecified side

6️⃣ S45.01   Laceration of axillary artery

🔲 **SP** 7️⃣ S45.011-   Laceration of axillary artery, right side

🔲 **SP** 7️⃣ S45.012-   Laceration of axillary artery, left side

🔲 **!Q** 7️⃣ S45.019-   Laceration of axillary artery, unspecified side

6️⃣ S45.09   Other specified injury of axillary artery

🔲 **SP** 7️⃣ S45.091-   Other specified injury of axillary artery, right side

🔲 **SP** 7️⃣ S45.092-   Other specified injury of axillary artery, left side

🔲 **!Q** 7️⃣ S45.099-   Other specified injury of axillary artery, unspecified side

5️⃣ S45.1   Injury of brachial artery

6️⃣ S45.10   Unspecified injury of brachial artery

🔲 **!Q** 7️⃣ S45.101-   Unspecified injury of brachial artery, right side

🔲 **!Q** 7️⃣ S45.102-   Unspecified injury of brachial artery, left side

🔲 **!Q** 7️⃣ S45.109-   Unspecified injury of brachial artery, unspecified side

6️⃣ S45.11   Laceration of brachial artery

🔲 **SP** 7️⃣ S45.111-   Laceration of brachial artery, right side

🔲 **SP** 7️⃣ S45.112-   Laceration of brachial artery, left side

🔲 **!Q** 7️⃣ S45.119-   Laceration of brachial artery, unspecified side

6️⃣ S45.19   Other specified injury of brachial artery

🔲 **SP** 7️⃣ S45.191-   Other specified injury of brachial artery, right side

🔲 **SP** 7️⃣ S45.192-   Other specified injury of brachial artery, left side

🔲 **!Q** 7️⃣ S45.199-   Other specified injury of brachial artery, unspecified side

5️⃣ S45.2   Injury of axillary or brachial vein

6️⃣ S45.20   Unspecified injury of axillary or brachial vein

🔲 **!Q** 7️⃣ S45.201-   Unspecified injury of axillary or brachial vein, right side

🔲 **!Q** 7️⃣ S45.202-   Unspecified injury of axillary or brachial vein, left side

🔲 **!Q** 7️⃣ S45.209-   Unspecified injury of axillary or brachial vein, unspecified side

6️⃣ S45.21   Laceration of axillary or brachial vein

🔲 **SP** 7️⃣ S45.211-   Laceration of axillary or brachial vein, right side

🔲 **SP** 7️⃣ S45.212-   Laceration of axillary or brachial vein, left side

🔲 **!Q** 7️⃣ S45.219-   Laceration of axillary or brachial vein, unspecified side

6️⃣ S45.29   Other specified injury of axillary or brachial vein

🔲 **SP** 7️⃣ S45.291-   Other specified injury of axillary or brachial vein, right side

🔲 **SP** 7️⃣ S45.292-   Other specified injury of axillary or brachial vein, left side

🔲 **!Q** 7️⃣ S45.299-   Other specified injury of axillary or brachial vein, unspecified side

5️⃣ S45.3   Injury of superficial vein at shoulder and upper arm level

6️⃣ S45.30   Unspecified injury of superficial vein at shoulder and upper arm level

🔲 **!Q** 7️⃣ S45.301-   Unspecified injury of superficial vein at shoulder and upper arm level, right arm

🔲 **!Q** 7️⃣ S45.302-   Unspecified injury of superficial vein at shoulder and upper arm level, left arm

🔲 **!Q** 7️⃣ S45.309-   Unspecified injury of superficial vein at shoulder and upper arm level, unspecified arm

6️⃣ S45.31   Laceration of superficial vein at shoulder and upper arm level

🔲 **SP** 7️⃣ S45.311-   Laceration of superficial vein at shoulder and upper arm level, right arm

🔲 **SP** 7️⃣ S45.312-   Laceration of superficial vein at shoulder and upper arm level, left arm

🔲 **!Q** 7️⃣ S45.319-   Laceration of superficial vein at shoulder and upper arm level, unspecified arm

6️⃣ S45.39   Other specified injury of superficial vein at shoulder and upper arm level

🔲 **SP** 7️⃣ S45.391-   Other specified injury of superficial vein at shoulder and upper arm level, right arm

🔲 **SP** 7️⃣ S45.392-   Other specified injury of superficial vein at shoulder and upper arm level, left arm

🔲 **!Q** 7️⃣ S45.399-   Other specified injury of superficial vein at shoulder and upper arm level, unspecified arm

5️⃣ S45.8   Injury of other specified blood vessels at shoulder and upper arm level

6️⃣ S45.80   Unspecified injury of other specified blood vessels at shoulder and upper arm level

🔲 **!Q** 7️⃣ S45.801-   Unspecified injury of other specified blood vessels at shoulder and upper arm level, right arm

🔲 **!Q** 7️⃣ S45.802-   Unspecified injury of other specified blood vessels at shoulder and upper arm level, left arm

🔲 **!Q** 7️⃣ S45.809-   Unspecified injury of other specified blood vessels at shoulder and upper arm level, unspecified arm

6️⃣ S45.81   Laceration of other specified blood vessels at shoulder and upper arm level

🔲 **SP** 7️⃣ S45.811-   Laceration of other specified blood vessels at shoulder and upper arm level, right arm

🔲 **SP** 7️⃣ S45.812-   Laceration of other specified blood vessels at shoulder and upper arm level, left arm

---

4️⃣ 4th digit required   5️⃣ 5th digit required   6️⃣ 6th digit required   7️⃣ 7th digit required   7️⃣ 7th digit placeholder   ✚ Additional code   🔲 Laterality

1526   *DecisionHealth's* FY 2020 Complete Home Health ICD-10-CM Diagnosis Coding Manual

🔲 **IQ** ⑦ **S45.819-** Laceration of other specified blood vessels at shoulder and upper arm level, unspecified arm

⑥ **S45.89** Other specified injury of other specified blood vessels at shoulder and upper arm level

🔲 **SP** ⑦ **S45.891-** Other specified injury of other specified blood vessels at shoulder and upper arm level, right arm

🔲 **SP** ⑦ **S45.892-** Other specified injury of other specified blood vessels at shoulder and upper arm level, left arm

🔲 **IQ** ⑦ **S45.899-** Other specified injury of other specified blood vessels at shoulder and upper arm level, unspecified arm

⑤ **S45.9** Injury of unspecified blood vessel at shoulder and upper arm level

⑥ **S45.90** Unspecified injury of unspecified blood vessel at shoulder and upper arm level

🔲 **IQ** ⑦ **S45.901-** Unspecified injury of unspecified blood vessel at shoulder and upper arm level, right arm

🔲 **IQ** ⑦ **S45.902-** Unspecified injury of unspecified blood vessel at shoulder and upper arm level, left arm

🔲 **IQ** ⑦ **S45.909-** Unspecified injury of unspecified blood vessel at shoulder and upper arm level, unspecified arm

⑥ **S45.91** Laceration of unspecified blood vessel at shoulder and upper arm level

🔲 **IQ** ⑦ **S45.911-** Laceration of unspecified blood vessel at shoulder and upper arm level, right arm

🔲 **IQ** ⑦ **S45.912-** Laceration of unspecified blood vessel at shoulder and upper arm level, left arm

🔲 **IQ** ⑦ **S45.919-** Laceration of unspecified blood vessel at shoulder and upper arm level, unspecified arm

⑥ **S45.99** Other specified injury of unspecified blood vessel at shoulder and upper arm level

🔲 **IQ** ⑦ **S45.991-** Other specified injury of unspecified blood vessel at shoulder and upper arm level, right arm

🔲 **IQ** ⑦ **S45.992-** Other specified injury of unspecified blood vessel at shoulder and upper arm level, left arm

🔲 **IQ** ⑦ **S45.999-** Other specified injury of unspecified blood vessel at shoulder and upper arm level, unspecified arm

④ **S46** Injury of muscle, fascia and tendon at shoulder and upper arm level
Code also:
  any associated open wound (S41.-)
  EXCLUDES 2 injury of muscle, fascia and tendon at elbow (S56.-)
  sprain of joints and ligaments of shoulder girdle (S43.9)

The appropriate 7th character is to be added to each code from category S46
A   initial encounter
D   subsequent encounter
S   sequela

⑤ **S46.0** Injury of muscle(s) and tendon(s) of the rotator cuff of shoulder

⑥ **S46.00** Unspecified injury of muscle(s) and tendon(s) of the rotator cuff of shoulder

🔲 **IQ** ⑦ **S46.001-** Unspecified injury of muscle(s) and tendon(s) of the rotator cuff of right shoulder

🔲 **IQ** ⑦ **S46.002-** Unspecified injury of muscle(s) and tendon(s) of the rotator cuff of left shoulder

🔲 **IQ** ⑦ **S46.009-** Unspecified injury of muscle(s) and tendon(s) of the rotator cuff of unspecified shoulder

⑥ **S46.01** Strain of muscle(s) and tendon(s) of the rotator cuff of shoulder

🔲 **SP** ⑦ **S46.011-** Strain of muscle(s) and tendon(s) of the rotator cuff of right shoulder

🔲 **SP** ⑦ **S46.012-** Strain of muscle(s) and tendon(s) of the rotator cuff of left shoulder

🔲 **IQ** ⑦ **S46.019-** Strain of muscle(s) and tendon(s) of the rotator cuff of unspecified shoulder

⑥ **S46.02** Laceration of muscle(s) and tendon(s) of the rotator cuff of shoulder

🔲 **SP** ⑦ **S46.021-** Laceration of muscle(s) and tendon(s) of the rotator cuff of right shoulder

🔲 **SP** ⑦ **S46.022-** Laceration of muscle(s) and tendon(s) of the rotator cuff of left shoulder

🔲 **IQ** ⑦ **S46.029-** Laceration of muscle(s) and tendon(s) of the rotator cuff of unspecified shoulder

⑥ **S46.09** Other injury of muscle(s) and tendon(s) of the rotator cuff of shoulder

🔲 **SP** ⑦ **S46.091-** Other injury of muscle(s) and tendon(s) of the rotator cuff of right shoulder

🔲 **SP** ⑦ **S46.092-** Other injury of muscle(s) and tendon(s) of the rotator cuff of left shoulder

🔲 **IQ** ⑦ **S46.099-** Other injury of muscle(s) and tendon(s) of the rotator cuff of unspecified shoulder

⑤ **S46.1** Injury of muscle, fascia and tendon of long head of biceps

⑥ **S46.10** Unspecified injury of muscle, fascia and tendon of long head of biceps

Chapter 19

S00-T88

★ New ▲ Revised Px Primary **SP** PDGM Px **SL** Low CoM **SH** High CoM **IQ** Quest. Encounter **H** Hospice non-cancer Dx   Unspecified   **M** *Manifestation*

DecisionHealth's FY 2020 Complete Home Health ICD-10-CM Diagnosis Coding Manual   1527

Chapter 19

S00-T88

☐ IQ 7 **S46.101-** **Unspecified injury of muscle, fascia and tendon of long head of biceps, right arm**

☐ IQ 7 **S46.102-** **Unspecified injury of muscle, fascia and tendon of long head of biceps, left arm**

☐ IQ 7 **S46.109-** **Unspecified injury of muscle, fascia and tendon of long head of biceps, unspecified arm**

6 **S46.11** Strain of muscle, fascia and tendon of long head of biceps

☐ SP 7 **S46.111-** Strain of muscle, fascia and tendon of long head of biceps, right arm

☐ SP 7 **S46.112-** Strain of muscle, fascia and tendon of long head of biceps, left arm

☐ IQ 7 **S46.119-** **Strain of muscle, fascia and tendon of long head of biceps, unspecified arm**

6 **S46.12** Laceration of muscle, fascia and tendon of long head of biceps

☐ SP 7 **S46.121-** Laceration of muscle, fascia and tendon of long head of biceps, right arm

☐ SP 7 **S46.122-** Laceration of muscle, fascia and tendon of long head of biceps, left arm

☐ IQ 7 **S46.129-** **Laceration of muscle, fascia and tendon of long head of biceps, unspecified arm**

6 **S46.19** Other injury of muscle, fascia and tendon of long head of biceps

☐ SP 7 **S46.191-** Other injury of muscle, fascia and tendon of long head of biceps, right arm

☐ SP 7 **S46.192-** Other injury of muscle, fascia and tendon of long head of biceps, left arm

☐ IQ 7 **S46.199-** **Other injury of muscle, fascia and tendon of long head of biceps, unspecified arm**

5 **S46.2** Injury of muscle, fascia and tendon of other parts of biceps

6 **S46.20** **Unspecified injury of muscle, fascia and tendon of other parts of biceps**

☐ IQ 7 **S46.201-** **Unspecified injury of muscle, fascia and tendon of other parts of biceps, right arm**

☐ IQ 7 **S46.202-** **Unspecified injury of muscle, fascia and tendon of other parts of biceps, left arm**

☐ IQ 7 **S46.209-** **Unspecified injury of muscle, fascia and tendon of other parts of biceps, unspecified arm**

6 **S46.21** Strain of muscle, fascia and tendon of other parts of biceps

☐ SP 7 **S46.211-** Strain of muscle, fascia and tendon of other parts of biceps, right arm

☐ SP 7 **S46.212-** Strain of muscle, fascia and tendon of other parts of biceps, left arm

☐ IQ 7 **S46.219-** **Strain of muscle, fascia and tendon of other parts of biceps, unspecified arm**

6 **S46.22** Laceration of muscle, fascia and tendon of other parts of biceps

☐ SP 7 **S46.221-** Laceration of muscle, fascia and tendon of other parts of biceps, right arm

☐ SP 7 **S46.222-** Laceration of muscle, fascia and tendon of other parts of biceps, left arm

☐ IQ 7 **S46.229-** **Laceration of muscle, fascia and tendon of other parts of biceps, unspecified arm**

6 **S46.29** Other injury of muscle, fascia and tendon of other parts of biceps

☐ SP 7 **S46.291-** Other injury of muscle, fascia and tendon of other parts of biceps, right arm

☐ SP 7 **S46.292-** Other injury of muscle, fascia and tendon of other parts of biceps, left arm

☐ IQ 7 **S46.299-** **Other injury of muscle, fascia and tendon of other parts of biceps, unspecified arm**

5 **S46.3** Injury of muscle, fascia and tendon of triceps

6 **S46.30** **Unspecified injury of muscle, fascia and tendon of triceps**

☐ IQ 7 **S46.301-** **Unspecified injury of muscle, fascia and tendon of triceps, right arm**

☐ IQ 7 **S46.302-** **Unspecified injury of muscle, fascia and tendon of triceps, left arm**

☐ IQ 7 **S46.309-** **Unspecified injury of muscle, fascia and tendon of triceps, unspecified arm**

6 **S46.31** Strain of muscle, fascia and tendon of triceps

☐ SP 7 **S46.311-** Strain of muscle, fascia and tendon of triceps, right arm

☐ SP 7 **S46.312-** Strain of muscle, fascia and tendon of triceps, left arm

☐ IQ 7 **S46.319-** **Strain of muscle, fascia and tendon of triceps, unspecified arm**

6 **S46.32** Laceration of muscle, fascia and tendon of triceps

☐ SP 7 **S46.321-** Laceration of muscle, fascia and tendon of triceps, right arm

☐ SP 7 **S46.322-** Laceration of muscle, fascia and tendon of triceps, left arm

☐ IQ 7 **S46.329-** **Laceration of muscle, fascia and tendon of triceps, unspecified arm**

6 **S46.39** Other injury of muscle, fascia and tendon of triceps

☐ SP 7 **S46.391-** Other injury of muscle, fascia and tendon of triceps, right arm

☐ SP 7 **S46.392-** Other injury of muscle, fascia and tendon of triceps, left arm

☐ IQ 7 **S46.399-** **Other injury of muscle, fascia and tendon of triceps, unspecified arm**

5 **S46.8** Injury of other muscles, fascia and tendons at shoulder and upper arm level

6 **S46.80** **Unspecified injury of other muscles, fascia and tendons at shoulder and upper arm level**

---

4 4th digit required   5 5th digit required   6 6th digit required   7 7th digit required   7 7th digit placeholder   ✚ Additional code   ☐ Laterality

☐ **IQ** **7** **S46.801-** Unspecified injury of other muscles, fascia and tendons at shoulder and upper arm level, right arm

☐ **IQ** **7** **S46.802-** Unspecified injury of other muscles, fascia and tendons at shoulder and upper arm level, left arm

☐ **IQ** **7** **S46.809-** Unspecified injury of other muscles, fascia and tendons at shoulder and upper arm level, unspecified arm

6 **S46.81** Strain of other muscles, fascia and tendons at shoulder and upper arm level

☐ **SP** **7** **S46.811-** Strain of other muscles, fascia and tendons at shoulder and upper arm level, right arm

☐ **SP** **7** **S46.812-** Strain of other muscles, fascia and tendons at shoulder and upper arm level, left arm

☐ **IQ** **7** **S46.819-** Strain of other muscles, fascia and tendons at shoulder and upper arm level, unspecified arm

6 **S46.82** Laceration of other muscles, fascia and tendons at shoulder and upper arm level

☐ **SP** **7** **S46.821-** Laceration of other muscles, fascia and tendons at shoulder and upper arm level, right arm

☐ **SP** **7** **S46.822-** Laceration of other muscles, fascia and tendons at shoulder and upper arm level, left arm

☐ **SP** **7** **S46.829-** Laceration of other muscles, fascia and tendons at shoulder and upper arm level, unspecified arm

6 **S46.89** Other injury of other muscles, fascia and tendons at shoulder and upper arm level

☐ **SP** **7** **S46.891-** Other injury of other muscles, fascia and tendons at shoulder and upper arm level, right arm

☐ **SP** **7** **S46.892-** Other injury of other muscles, fascia and tendons at shoulder and upper arm level, left arm

☐ **IQ** **7** **S46.899-** Other injury of other muscles, fascia and tendons at shoulder and upper arm level, unspecified arm

5 **S46.9** Injury of unspecified muscle, fascia and tendon at shoulder and upper arm level

6 **S46.90** Unspecified injury of unspecified muscle, fascia and tendon at shoulder and upper arm level

☐ **IQ** **7** **S46.901-** Unspecified injury of unspecified muscle, fascia and tendon at shoulder and upper arm level, right arm

☐ **IQ** **7** **S46.902-** Unspecified injury of unspecified muscle, fascia and tendon at shoulder and upper arm level, left arm

☐ **IQ** **7** **S46.909-** Unspecified injury of unspecified muscle, fascia and tendon at shoulder and upper arm level, unspecified arm

6 **S46.91** Strain of unspecified muscle, fascia and tendon at shoulder and upper arm level

☐ **SP** **7** **S46.911-** Strain of unspecified muscle, fascia and tendon at shoulder and upper arm level, right arm

☐ **SP** **7** **S46.912-** Strain of unspecified muscle, fascia and tendon at shoulder and upper arm level, left arm

☐ **IQ** **7** **S46.919-** Strain of unspecified muscle, fascia and tendon at shoulder and upper arm level, unspecified arm

6 **S46.92** Laceration of unspecified muscle, fascia and tendon at shoulder and upper arm level

☐ **SP** **7** **S46.921-** Laceration of unspecified muscle, fascia and tendon at shoulder and upper arm level, right arm

☐ **SP** **7** **S46.922-** Laceration of unspecified muscle, fascia and tendon at shoulder and upper arm level, left arm

☐ **IQ** **7** **S46.929-** Laceration of unspecified muscle, fascia and tendon at shoulder and upper arm level, unspecified arm

6 **S46.99** Other injury of unspecified muscle, fascia and tendon at shoulder and upper arm level

☐ **SP** **7** **S46.991-** Other injury of unspecified muscle, fascia and tendon at shoulder and upper arm level, right arm

☐ **SP** **7** **S46.992-** Other injury of unspecified muscle, fascia and tendon at shoulder and upper arm level, left arm

☐ **IQ** **7** **S46.999-** Other injury of unspecified muscle, fascia and tendon at shoulder and upper arm level, unspecified arm

+ **4** **S47** Crushing injury of shoulder and upper arm
Use additional code for all associated injuries
EXCLUDES 2 crushing injury of elbow (S57.0-)

The appropriate 7th character is to be added to each code from category S47
A   initial encounter
D   subsequent encounter
S   sequela

☐ **SP** **+** **7** **S47.1XX-** Crushing injury of right shoulder and upper arm

☐ **SP** **+** **7** **S47.2XX-** Crushing injury of left shoulder and upper arm

☐ **IQ** **+** **7** **S47.9XX-** Crushing injury of shoulder and upper arm, unspecified arm

4 **S48** Traumatic amputation of shoulder and upper arm

★ New ▲ Revised Px Primary **SP** PDGM Px **SL** Low CoM **SH** High CoM **IQ** Quest. Encounter **H** Hospice non-cancer Dx   Unspecified   **M** *Manifestation*

DecisionHealth's FY 2020 Complete Home Health ICD-10-CM Diagnosis Coding Manual

1529

An amputation not identified as partial or complete should be coded to complete traumatic amputation at elbow
EXCLUDES 1 level (S58.0)

The appropriate 7th character is to be added to each code from category S48
A   initial encounter
D   subsequent encounter
S   sequela

CODING TIPS ✓ Use these codes only when the amputation was due to trauma. There is no need for adding Z89 with traumatic amputations. See Z47.81 for care of amputations not due to trauma.

⑤ **S48.0**   **Traumatic amputation at shoulder joint**

   ⑥ **S48.01**   **Complete traumatic amputation at shoulder joint**

☰ **SP** ⑦ **S48.011-**   **Complete traumatic amputation at right shoulder joint**

☰ **SP** ⑦ **S48.012-**   **Complete traumatic amputation at left shoulder joint**

☰ **IQ** ⑦ **S48.019-**   **Complete traumatic amputation at unspecified shoulder joint**

   ⑥ **S48.02**   **Partial traumatic amputation at shoulder joint**

☰ **SP** ⑦ **S48.021-**   **Partial traumatic amputation at right shoulder joint**

☰ **SP** ⑦ **S48.022-**   **Partial traumatic amputation at left shoulder joint**

☰ **IQ** ⑦ **S48.029-**   **Partial traumatic amputation at unspecified shoulder joint**

⑤ **S48.1**   **Traumatic amputation at level between shoulder and elbow**

   ⑥ **S48.11**   **Complete traumatic amputation at level between shoulder and elbow**

☰ **SP** ⑦ **S48.111-**   **Complete traumatic amputation at level between right shoulder and elbow**

☰ **SP** ⑦ **S48.112-**   **Complete traumatic amputation at level between left shoulder and elbow**

☰ **IQ** ⑦ **S48.119-**   **Complete traumatic amputation at level between unspecified shoulder and elbow**

   ⑥ **S48.12**   **Partial traumatic amputation at level between shoulder and elbow**

☰ **SP** ⑦ **S48.121-**   **Partial traumatic amputation at level between right shoulder and elbow**

☰ **SP** ⑦ **S48.122-**   **Partial traumatic amputation at level between left shoulder and elbow**

☰ **IQ** ⑦ **S48.129-**   **Partial traumatic amputation at level between unspecified shoulder and elbow**

⑤ **S48.9**   **Traumatic amputation of shoulder and upper arm, level unspecified**

   ⑥ **S48.91**   **Complete traumatic amputation of shoulder and upper arm, level unspecified**

☰ **IQ** ⑦ **S48.911-**   **Complete traumatic amputation of right shoulder and upper arm, level unspecified**

☰ **IQ** ⑦ **S48.912-**   **Complete traumatic amputation of left shoulder and upper arm, level unspecified**

☰ **IQ** ⑦ **S48.919-**   **Complete traumatic amputation of unspecified shoulder and upper arm, level unspecified**

   ⑥ **S48.92**   **Partial traumatic amputation of shoulder and upper arm, level unspecified**

☰ **IQ** ⑦ **S48.921-**   **Partial traumatic amputation of right shoulder and upper arm, level unspecified**

☰ **IQ** ⑦ **S48.922-**   **Partial traumatic amputation of left shoulder and upper arm, level unspecified**

☰ **IQ** ⑦ **S48.929-**   **Partial traumatic amputation of unspecified shoulder and upper arm, level unspecified**

④ **S49**   **Other and unspecified injuries of shoulder and upper arm**

The appropriate 7th character is to be added to each code from subcategories S49.0 and S49.1
A   initial encounter for closed fracture
D   subsequent encounter for fracture with routine healing
G   subsequent encounter for fracture with delayed healing
K   subsequent encounter for fracture with nonunion
P   subsequent encounter for fracture with malunion
S   sequela

⑤ **S49.0**   **Physeal fracture of upper end of humerus**

   ⑥ **S49.00**   **Unspecified physeal fracture of upper end of humerus**

☰ **SP** ⑦ **S49.001-**   **Unspecified physeal fracture of upper end of humerus, right arm**

☰ **SP** ⑦ **S49.002-**   **Unspecified physeal fracture of upper end of humerus, left arm**

☰ **IQ** ⑦ **S49.009-**   **Unspecified physeal fracture of upper end of humerus, unspecified arm**

   ⑥ **S49.01**   **Salter-Harris Type I physeal fracture of upper end of humerus**

☰ **SP** ⑦ **S49.011-**   **Salter-Harris Type I physeal fracture of upper end of humerus, right arm**

☰ **SP** ⑦ **S49.012-**   **Salter-Harris Type I physeal fracture of upper end of humerus, left arm**

☰ **IQ** ⑦ **S49.019-**   **Salter-Harris Type I physeal fracture of upper end of humerus, unspecified arm**

   ⑥ **S49.02**   **Salter-Harris Type II physeal fracture of upper end of humerus**

☰ **SP** ⑦ **S49.021-**   **Salter-Harris Type II physeal fracture of upper end of humerus, right arm**

☰ **SP** ⑦ **S49.022-**   **Salter-Harris Type II physeal fracture of upper end of humerus, left arm**

☰ **IQ** ⑦ **S49.029-**   **Salter-Harris Type II physeal fracture of upper end of humerus, unspecified arm**

④4th digit required   ⑤5th digit required   ⑥6th digit required   ⑦7th digit required   ⑦7th digit placeholder   ✚Additional code   ☰Laterality

1530   *DecisionHealth's* FY 2020 Complete Home Health ICD-10-CM Diagnosis Coding Manual

🄖 **S49.03** Salter-Harris Type III physeal fracture of upper end of humerus

🄳 🆂🅿 �7 **S49.031-** Salter-Harris Type III physeal fracture of upper end of humerus, right arm

🄳 🆂🅿 �7 **S49.032-** Salter-Harris Type III physeal fracture of upper end of humerus, left arm

🄳 🄸🅀 �7 **S49.039-** Salter-Harris Type III physeal fracture of upper end of humerus, unspecified arm

🄖 **S49.04** Salter-Harris Type IV physeal fracture of upper end of humerus

🄳 🆂🅿 �7 **S49.041-** Salter-Harris Type IV physeal fracture of upper end of humerus, right arm

🄳 🆂🅿 �7 **S49.042-** Salter-Harris Type IV physeal fracture of upper end of humerus, left arm

🄳 🄸🅀 �7 **S49.049-** Salter-Harris Type IV physeal fracture of upper end of humerus, unspecified arm

🄖 **S49.09** Other physeal fracture of upper end of humerus

🄳 🆂🅿 �7 **S49.091-** Other physeal fracture of upper end of humerus, right arm

🄳 🆂🅿 �7 **S49.092-** Other physeal fracture of upper end of humerus, left arm

🄳 🄸🅀 �7 **S49.099-** Other physeal fracture of upper end of humerus, unspecified arm

🄢 **S49.1** Physeal fracture of lower end of humerus

🄖 **S49.10** Unspecified physeal fracture of lower end of humerus

🄳 🆂🅿 �7 **S49.101-** Unspecified physeal fracture of lower end of humerus, right arm

🄳 🆂🅿 �7 **S49.102-** Unspecified physeal fracture of lower end of humerus, left arm

🄳 🄸🅀 �7 **S49.109-** Unspecified physeal fracture of lower end of humerus, unspecified arm

🄖 **S49.11** Salter-Harris Type I physeal fracture of lower end of humerus

🄳 🆂🅿 �7 **S49.111-** Salter-Harris Type I physeal fracture of lower end of humerus, right arm

🄳 🆂🅿 �7 **S49.112-** Salter-Harris Type I physeal fracture of lower end of humerus, left arm

🄳 🄸🅀 �7 **S49.119-** Salter-Harris Type I physeal fracture of lower end of humerus, unspecified arm

🄖 **S49.12** Salter-Harris Type II physeal fracture of lower end of humerus

🄳 🆂🅿 �7 **S49.121-** Salter-Harris Type II physeal fracture of lower end of humerus, right arm

🄳 🆂🅿 �7 **S49.122-** Salter-Harris Type II physeal fracture of lower end of humerus, left arm

🄳 🄸🅀 �7 **S49.129-** Salter-Harris Type II physeal fracture of lower end of humerus, unspecified arm

🄖 **S49.13** Salter-Harris Type III physeal fracture of lower end of humerus

🄳 🆂🅿 �7 **S49.131-** Salter-Harris Type III physeal fracture of lower end of humerus, right arm

🄳 🆂🅿 �7 **S49.132-** Salter-Harris Type III physeal fracture of lower end of humerus, left arm

🄳 🄸🅀 �7 **S49.139-** Salter-Harris Type III physeal fracture of lower end of humerus, unspecified arm

🄖 **S49.14** Salter-Harris Type IV physeal fracture of lower end of humerus

🄳 🆂🅿 �7 **S49.141-** Salter-Harris Type IV physeal fracture of lower end of humerus, right arm

🄳 🆂🅿 �7 **S49.142-** Salter-Harris Type IV physeal fracture of lower end of humerus, left arm

🄳 🆂🅿 🄸🅀 �7 **S49.149-** Salter-Harris Type IV physeal fracture of lower end of humerus, unspecified arm

🄖 **S49.19** Other physeal fracture of lower end of humerus

🄳 🆂🅿 �7 **S49.191-** Other physeal fracture of lower end of humerus, right arm

🄳 🆂🅿 �7 **S49.192-** Other physeal fracture of lower end of humerus, left arm

🄳 🄸🅀 �7 **S49.199-** Other physeal fracture of lower end of humerus, unspecified arm

🄢 **S49.8** Other specified injuries of shoulder and upper arm

The appropriate 7th character is to be added to each code in subcategory S49.8
A   initial encounter
D   subsequent encounter
S   sequela

🄳 🄸🅀 �7 **S49.80X-** Other specified injuries of shoulder and upper arm, unspecified arm

🄳 🆂🅿 �7 **S49.81X-** Other specified injuries of right shoulder and upper arm

🄳 🆂🅿 �7 **S49.82X-** Other specified injuries of left shoulder and upper arm

🄢 **S49.9** Unspecified injury of shoulder and upper arm

The appropriate 7th character is to be added to each code in subcategory S49.9
A   initial encounter
D   subsequent encounter
S   sequela

🄳 🄸🅀 �7 **S49.90X-** Unspecified injury of shoulder and upper arm, unspecified arm

🄳 🄸🅀 �7 **S49.91X-** Unspecified injury of right shoulder and upper arm

🄳 🄸🅀 �7 **S49.92X-** Unspecified injury of left shoulder and upper arm

Injuries to the elbow and forearm (S50-S59)

EXCLUDES 2 burns and corrosions (T20-T32)
frostbite (T33-T34)
injuries of wrist and hand (S60-S69)
insect bite or sting, venomous (T63.4)

Chapter 19

S00-T88

★ New ▲ Revised Px Primary 🆂🅿 PDGM Px 🆂🄻 Low CoM 🆂🄷 High CoM 🄸🅀 Quest. Encounter 🄷 Hospice non-cancer Dx   Unspecified   M *Manifestation*

DecisionHealth's FY 2020 Complete Home Health ICD-10-CM Diagnosis Coding Manual   1531

GUIDELINES Section I.C.19.c.2)

Multiple fractures are sequenced in accordance with the severity of the fracture.

GUIDELINES Section I.C.19.b.1)-2)

When coding injuries, assign separate codes for each injury unless a combination code is provided, in which case the combination code is assigned ... Traumatic injury codes (S00-T14.9) are not to be used for normal, healing surgical wounds or to identify complications of surgical wounds. The code for the most serious injury, as determined by the provider and the focus of treatment, is sequenced first.

1) Superficial injuries such as abrasions or contusions are not coded when associated with more severe injuries of the same site.

2) When a primary injury results in minor damage to peripheral nerves or blood vessels, the primary injury is sequenced first with additional code(s) for injuries to nerves and spinal cord (such as category S04), and/or injury to blood vessels (such as category S15). When the primary injury is to the blood vessels or nerves, that injury should be sequenced first.

GUIDELINES Section I.C.19.c

Coding of Traumatic Fractures: The principles of multiple coding of injuries should be followed in coding fractures. Fractures of specified sites are coded individually by site in accordance with both the provisions within categories S02, S12, S22, S32, S42, S49, S52, S59, S62, S72, S79, S82, S89, S92 and the level of detail furnished by medical record content. A fracture not indicated as open or closed should be coded to closed. A fracture not indicated whether displaced or not displaced should be coded to displaced.

CODING TIPS ✓ 7th character A is acceptable in home health and hospice when active treatment is provided, such as antibiotics for an infected wound or a wound vac for a dehisced wound. D is used when the complication or injury is now healing. Think of D as aftercare. S is used for sequela of the injury or complication. Sequela is a residual deficit or condition produced as a result of the injury or complication after the original injury or complication has healed.

4 S50 Superficial injury of elbow and forearm
    EXCLUDES 2 superficial injury of wrist and hand (S60.-)

The appropriate 7th character is to be added to each code from category S50
A   initial encounter
D   subsequent encounter
S   sequela

5 S50.0 Contusion of elbow
S50.00X- Contusion of unspecified elbow
S50.01X- Contusion of right elbow
S50.02X- Contusion of left elbow
5 S50.1 Contusion of forearm
S50.10X- Contusion of unspecified forearm
S50.11X- Contusion of right forearm
S50.12X- Contusion of left forearm
5 S50.3 Other superficial injuries of elbow
6 S50.31 Abrasion of elbow
S50.311- Abrasion of right elbow
S50.312- Abrasion of left elbow

S50.319- Abrasion of unspecified elbow
6 S50.32 Blister (nonthermal) of elbow
S50.321- Blister (nonthermal) of right elbow
S50.322- Blister (nonthermal) of left elbow
S50.329- Blister (nonthermal) of unspecified elbow
6 S50.34 External constriction of elbow
S50.341- External constriction of right elbow
S50.342- External constriction of left elbow
S50.349- External constriction of unspecified elbow
6 S50.35 Superficial foreign body of elbow
    Splinter in the elbow
S50.351- Superficial foreign body of right elbow
S50.352- Superficial foreign body of left elbow
S50.359- Superficial foreign body of unspecified elbow
6 S50.36 Insect bite (nonvenomous) of elbow
S50.361- Insect bite (nonvenomous) of right elbow
S50.362- Insect bite (nonvenomous) of left elbow
S50.369- Insect bite (nonvenomous) of unspecified elbow
6 S50.37 Other superficial bite of elbow
    EXCLUDES 1 open bite of elbow (S51.04)
S50.371- Other superficial bite of right elbow
S50.372- Other superficial bite of left elbow
S50.379- Other superficial bite of unspecified elbow
5 S50.8 Other superficial injuries of forearm
6 S50.81 Abrasion of forearm
S50.811- Abrasion of right forearm
S50.812- Abrasion of left forearm
S50.819- Abrasion of unspecified forearm
6 S50.82 Blister (nonthermal) of forearm
S50.821- Blister (nonthermal) of right forearm
S50.822- Blister (nonthermal) of left forearm
S50.829- Blister (nonthermal) of unspecified forearm
6 S50.84 External constriction of forearm
S50.841- External constriction of right forearm
S50.842- External constriction of left forearm
S50.849- External constriction of unspecified forearm
6 S50.85 Superficial foreign body of forearm
    Splinter in the forearm
S50.851- Superficial foreign body of right forearm
S50.852- Superficial foreign body of left forearm

4 4th digit required   **5** 5th digit required   **6** 6th digit required   **7** 7th digit required   **7** 7th digit placeholder   **+** Additional code   **⊟** Laterality

1532   *DecisionHealth's* FY 2020 Complete Home Health ICD-10-CM Diagnosis Coding Manual

Chapter 19

S00-T88

☐ **!Q** 7 **S50.859-** **Superficial foreign body of unspecified forearm**

6 **S50.86** **Insect bite (nonvenomous) of forearm**

☐ **!Q** 7 **S50.861-** **Insect bite (nonvenomous) of right forearm**

☐ **!Q** 7 **S50.862-** **Insect bite (nonvenomous) of left forearm**

☐ **!Q** 7 **S50.869-** **Insect bite (nonvenomous) of unspecified forearm**

6 **S50.87** **Other superficial bite of forearm**
 EXCLUDES 1 open bite of forearm (S51.84)

☐ **!Q** 7 **S50.871-** **Other superficial bite of right forearm**

☐ **!Q** 7 **S50.872-** **Other superficial bite of left forearm**

☐ **!Q** 7 **S50.879-** **Other superficial bite of unspecified forearm**

5 **S50.9** **Unspecified superficial injury of elbow and forearm**

6 **S50.90** **Unspecified superficial injury of elbow**

☐ **!Q** 7 **S50.901-** **Unspecified superficial injury of right elbow**

☐ **!Q** 7 **S50.902-** **Unspecified superficial injury of left elbow**

☐ **!Q** 7 **S50.909-** **Unspecified superficial injury of unspecified elbow**

6 **S50.91** **Unspecified superficial injury of forearm**

☐ **!Q** 7 **S50.911-** **Unspecified superficial injury of right forearm**

☐ **!Q** 7 **S50.912-** **Unspecified superficial injury of left forearm**

☐ **!Q** 7 **S50.919-** **Unspecified superficial injury of unspecified forearm**

4 **S51** **Open wound of elbow and forearm**
 Code also:
  any associated wound infection
 EXCLUDES 1 open fracture of elbow and forearm (S52.- with open fracture 7th character)
  traumatic amputation of elbow and forearm (S58.-)
 EXCLUDES 2 open wound of wrist and hand (S61.-)

 The appropriate 7th character is to be added to each code from category S51
 A initial encounter
 D subsequent encounter
 S sequela

 CODING TIPS ✓ Open wound codes indicate a wound resulting from a traumatic origin. Do not assign a code for "open wound" unless the etiology of the wound is related to trauma.

 CODING TIPS ✓ No aftercare code applies, including those indicating dressing changes, drain care, or suture removal. 7th character 'D' is the default for home care and hospice when providing aftercare for a healing or resolving condition; 'A' is used for active treatment such as antibiotics or more than routine wound care; 'S' may be used to indicate a residual condition after the original injury has healed.

5 **S51.0** **Open wound of elbow**

6 **S51.00** **Unspecified open wound of elbow**

☐ **SP** 7 **S51.001-** **Unspecified open wound of right elbow**

☐ **SP** 7 **S51.002-** **Unspecified open wound of left elbow**

☐ **!Q** 7 **S51.009-** **Unspecified open wound of unspecified elbow**
 Open wound of elbow NOS

6 **S51.01** **Laceration without foreign body of elbow**

☐ **SP** 7 **S51.011-** **Laceration without foreign body of right elbow**

☐ **SP** 7 **S51.012-** **Laceration without foreign body of left elbow**

☐ **!Q** 7 **S51.019-** **Laceration without foreign body of unspecified elbow**

6 **S51.02** **Laceration with foreign body of elbow**

☐ **SP** 7 **S51.021-** **Laceration with foreign body of right elbow**

☐ **SP** 7 **S51.022-** **Laceration with foreign body of left elbow**

☐ **!Q** 7 **S51.029-** **Laceration with foreign body of unspecified elbow**

6 **S51.03** **Puncture wound without foreign body of elbow**

☐ **SP** 7 **S51.031-** **Puncture wound without foreign body of right elbow**

☐ **SP** 7 **S51.032-** **Puncture wound without foreign body of left elbow**

☐ **!Q** 7 **S51.039-** **Puncture wound without foreign body of unspecified elbow**

6 **S51.04** **Puncture wound with foreign body of elbow**

☐ **SP** 7 **S51.041-** **Puncture wound with foreign body of right elbow**

☐ **SP** 7 **S51.042-** **Puncture wound with foreign body of left elbow**

☐ **!Q** 7 **S51.049-** **Puncture wound with foreign body of unspecified elbow**

6 **S51.05** **Open bite of elbow**
 Bite of elbow NOS
 EXCLUDES 1 superficial bite of elbow (S50.36, S50.37)

☐ **SP** 7 **S51.051-** **Open bite, right elbow**

☐ **SP** 7 **S51.052-** **Open bite, left elbow**

☐ **!Q** 7 **S51.059-** **Open bite, unspecified elbow**

5 **S51.8** **Open wound of forearm**
 EXCLUDES 2 open wound of elbow (S51.0-)

6 **S51.80** **Unspecified open wound of forearm**

☐ **SP** 7 **S51.801-** **Unspecified open wound of right forearm**

★ New ▲ Revised **Px** Primary **SP** PDGM Px **SL** Low CoM **SH** High CoM **!Q** Quest. Encounter **H** Hospice non-cancer Dx   Unspecified   **M** *Manifestation*

DecisionHealth's FY 2020 Complete Home Health ICD-10-CM Diagnosis Coding Manual   1533

☐ SP 7 **S51.802-** **Unspecified open wound of left forearm**

☐ IQ 7 **S51.809-** **Unspecified open wound of unspecified forearm**

Open wound of forearm NOS

6 **S51.81** **Laceration without foreign body of forearm**

☐ SP 7 **S51.811-** **Laceration without foreign body of right forearm**

☐ SP 7 **S51.812-** **Laceration without foreign body of left forearm**

☐ IQ 7 **S51.819-** **Laceration without foreign body of unspecified forearm**

6 **S51.82** **Laceration with foreign body of forearm**

☐ SP 7 **S51.821-** **Laceration with foreign body of right forearm**

☐ SP 7 **S51.822-** **Laceration with foreign body of left forearm**

☐ IQ 7 **S51.829-** **Laceration with foreign body of unspecified forearm**

6 **S51.83** **Puncture wound without foreign body of forearm**

☐ SP 7 **S51.831-** **Puncture wound without foreign body of right forearm**

☐ SP 7 **S51.832-** **Puncture wound without foreign body of left forearm**

☐ IQ 7 **S51.839-** **Puncture wound without foreign body of unspecified forearm**

6 **S51.84** **Puncture wound with foreign body of forearm**

☐ SP 7 **S51.841-** **Puncture wound with foreign body of right forearm**

☐ SP 7 **S51.842-** **Puncture wound with foreign body of left forearm**

☐ IQ 7 **S51.849-** **Puncture wound with foreign body of unspecified forearm**

6 **S51.85** **Open bite of forearm**

Bite of forearm NOS

EXCLUDES 1 superficial bite of forearm (S50.86, S50.87)

☐ SP 7 **S51.851-** **Open bite of right forearm**

☐ SP 7 **S51.852-** **Open bite of left forearm**

☐ IQ 7 **S51.859-** **Open bite of unspecified forearm**

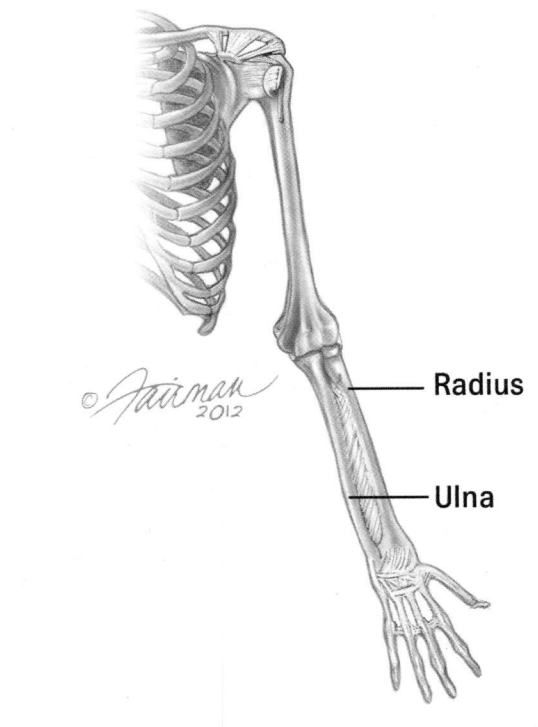

Radius

Ulna

4 **S52** **Fracture of forearm**

Note:

A fracture not indicated as displaced or nondisplaced should be coded to displaced

A fracture not indicated as open or closed should be coded to closed

The open fracture designations are based on the Gustilo open fracture classification

EXCLUDES 1 traumatic amputation of forearm (S58.-)

EXCLUDES 2 fracture at wrist and hand level (S62.-)

4 4th digit required　　5 5th digit required　　6 6th digit required　　7 7th digit required　　7 7th digit placeholder　　+ Additional code　　☐ Laterality

1534　　　　*DecisionHealth's* FY 2020 Complete Home Health ICD-10-CM Diagnosis Coding Manual

Chapter 19

S00-T88

The appropriate 7th character is to be added to all codes from category S52

A   initial encounter for closed fracture

B   initial encounter for open fracture type I or II

C   initial encounter for open fracture type IIIA, IIIB, or IIIC

D   subsequent encounter for closed fracture with routine healing

E   subsequent encounter for open fracture type I or II with routine healing

F   subsequent encounter for open fracture type IIIA, IIIB, or IIIC with routine healing

G   subsequent encounter for closed fracture with delayed healing

H   subsequent encounter for open fracture type I or II with delayed healing

J   subsequent encounter for open fracture type IIIA, IIIB, or IIIC with delayed healing

K   subsequent encounter for closed fracture with nonunion

M   subsequent encounter for open fracture type I or II with nonunion

N   subsequent encounter for open fracture type IIIA, IIIB, or IIIC with nonunion

P   subsequent encounter for closed fracture with malunion

Q   subsequent encounter for open fracture type I or II with malunion

R   subsequent encounter for open fracture type IIIA, IIIB, or IIIC with malunion

S   sequela

CODING TIPS ✓ Fractures repaired by joint replacements are NOT coded with Z47.1. Fractures repaired by any other orthopedic surgery are NOT coded with Z47.89. Z codes are not appropriate for fractures of any kind. Code the fracture with 7th character D for fractures undergoing surgical repair.

CODING TIPS ✓ A fracture not indicated as displaced or nondisplaced should be coded to displaced. A fracture not indicated as open or closed should be coded to closed. The open fracture designations are based on the Gustilo open fracture classification. The 7th characters E, H, M and Q are the default for the Gustilo classification when no information is available. Always query the physician.

CODING TIPS ✓ "D" is the 7th character for home care and hospice unless the physician has documented delayed healing, nonunion or malunion. A sequela is a condition left after the fracture has healed.

5 S52.0 **Fracture of upper end of ulna**
Fracture of proximal end of ulna
EXCLUDES 2 fracture of elbow NOS (S42.40-)
fractures of shaft of ulna (S52.2-)

6 S52.00 **Unspecified fracture of upper end of ulna**

⊟ SP 7 S52.001- Unspecified fracture of upper end of right ulna

⊟ SP 7 S52.002- Unspecified fracture of upper end of left ulna

⊟ !Q 7 S52.009- Unspecified fracture of upper end of unspecified ulna

6 S52.01 **Torus fracture of upper end of ulna**

The appropriate 7th character is to be added to all codes in subcategory S52.01

A   initial encounter for closed fracture

D   subsequent encounter for fracture with routine healing

G   subsequent encounter for fracture with delayed healing

K   subsequent encounter for fracture with nonunion

P   subsequent encounter for fracture with malunion

S   sequela

CODING TIPS ✓ Open fractures do not occur with torus fractures and greenstick fractures, therefore the 7th characters for open fractures are not available.

⊟ SP 7 S52.011- Torus fracture of upper end of right ulna

⊟ SP 7 S52.012- Torus fracture of upper end of left ulna

⊟ !Q 7 S52.019- Torus fracture of upper end of unspecified ulna

6 S52.02 **Fracture of olecranon process without intraarticular extension of ulna**

⊟ SP 7 S52.021- Displaced fracture of olecranon process without intraarticular extension of right ulna

⊟ SP 7 S52.022- Displaced fracture of olecranon process without intraarticular extension of left ulna

⊟ !Q 7 S52.023- Displaced fracture of olecranon process without intraarticular extension of unspecified ulna

⊟ SP 7 S52.024- Nondisplaced fracture of olecranon process without intraarticular extension of right ulna

⊟ SP 7 S52.025- Nondisplaced fracture of olecranon process without intraarticular extension of left ulna

⊟ !Q 7 S52.026- Nondisplaced fracture of olecranon process without intraarticular extension of unspecified ulna

6 S52.03 **Fracture of olecranon process with intraarticular extension of ulna**

⊟ SP 7 S52.031- Displaced fracture of olecranon process with intraarticular extension of right ulna

⊟ SP 7 S52.032- Displaced fracture of olecranon process with intraarticular extension of left ulna

★ New ▲ Revised **Px** Primary **SP** PDGM Px **SL** Low CoM **SH** High CoM **!Q** Quest. Encounter **H** Hospice non-cancer Dx Unspecified **M** *Manifestation*

DecisionHealth's FY 2020 Complete Home Health ICD-10-CM Diagnosis Coding Manual   1535

☐ !Q 7 **S52.033-** **Displaced fracture of olecranon process with intraarticular extension of unspecified ulna**

☐ SP 7 **S52.034-** Nondisplaced fracture of olecranon process with intraarticular extension of right ulna

☐ SP 7 **S52.035-** Nondisplaced fracture of olecranon process with intraarticular extension of left ulna

☐ !Q 7 **S52.036-** **Nondisplaced fracture of olecranon process with intraarticular extension of unspecified ulna**

6 **S52.04** Fracture of coronoid process of ulna

☐ SP 7 **S52.041-** Displaced fracture of coronoid process of right ulna

☐ SP 7 **S52.042-** Displaced fracture of coronoid process of left ulna

☐ !Q 7 **S52.043-** **Displaced fracture of coronoid process of unspecified ulna**

☐ SP 7 **S52.044-** Nondisplaced fracture of coronoid process of right ulna

☐ SP 7 **S52.045-** Nondisplaced fracture of coronoid process of left ulna

☐ !Q 7 **S52.046-** **Nondisplaced fracture of coronoid process of unspecified ulna**

6 **S52.09** Other fracture of upper end of ulna

☐ SP 7 **S52.091-** Other fracture of upper end of right ulna

☐ SP 7 **S52.092-** Other fracture of upper end of left ulna

☐ !Q 7 **S52.099-** **Other fracture of upper end of unspecified ulna**

5 **S52.1** Fracture of upper end of radius
Fracture of proximal end of radius
EXCLUDES 2 physeal fractures of upper end of radius (S59.2-)
fracture of shaft of radius (S52.3-)

6 **S52.10** **Unspecified fracture of upper end of radius**

☐ SP 7 **S52.101-** **Unspecified fracture of upper end of right radius**

☐ SP 7 **S52.102-** **Unspecified fracture of upper end of left radius**

☐ !Q 7 **S52.109-** **Unspecified fracture of upper end of unspecified radius**

6 **S52.11** Torus fracture of upper end of radius

The appropriate 7th character is to be added to all codes in subcategory S52.11
A   initial encounter for closed fracture
D   subsequent encounter for fracture with routine healing
G   subsequent encounter for fracture with delayed healing
K   subsequent encounter for fracture with nonunion
P   subsequent encounter for fracture with malunion
S   sequela

CODING TIPS ✓ Open fractures do not occur with torus fractures and greenstick fractures, therefore the 7th characters for open fractures are not available.

☐ SP 7 **S52.111-** Torus fracture of upper end of right radius

☐ SP 7 **S52.112-** Torus fracture of upper end of left radius

☐ !Q 7 **S52.119-** **Torus fracture of upper end of unspecified radius**

6 **S52.12** Fracture of head of radius

☐ SP 7 **S52.121-** Displaced fracture of head of right radius

☐ SP 7 **S52.122-** Displaced fracture of head of left radius

☐ !Q 7 **S52.123-** **Displaced fracture of head of unspecified radius**

☐ SP 7 **S52.124-** Nondisplaced fracture of head of right radius

☐ SP 7 **S52.125-** Nondisplaced fracture of head of left radius

☐ !Q 7 **S52.126-** **Nondisplaced fracture of head of unspecified radius**

6 **S52.13** Fracture of neck of radius

☐ SP 7 **S52.131-** Displaced fracture of neck of right radius

☐ SP 7 **S52.132-** Displaced fracture of neck of left radius

☐ !Q 7 **S52.133-** **Displaced fracture of neck of unspecified radius**

☐ SP 7 **S52.134-** Nondisplaced fracture of neck of right radius

☐ SP 7 **S52.135-** Nondisplaced fracture of neck of left radius

☐ !Q 7 **S52.136-** **Nondisplaced fracture of neck of unspecified radius**

6 **S52.18** Other fracture of upper end of radius

☐ SP 7 **S52.181-** Other fracture of upper end of right radius

☐ SP 7 **S52.182-** Other fracture of upper end of left radius

☐ !Q 7 **S52.189-** **Other fracture of upper end of unspecified radius**

5 **S52.2** Fracture of shaft of ulna

6 **S52.20** **Unspecified fracture of shaft of ulna**
Fracture of ulna NOS

☐ SP 7 **S52.201-** **Unspecified fracture of shaft of right ulna**

⁴ 4th digit required   ⁵ 5th digit required   ⁶ 6th digit required   ⁷ 7th digit required   ⑦ 7th digit placeholder   ✚ Additional code   ☐ Laterality

1536   DecisionHealth's FY 2020 Complete Home Health ICD-10-CM Diagnosis Coding Manual

🔲 **SP** 7 **S52.202-** Unspecified fracture of shaft of left ulna

🔲 **IQ** 7 **S52.209-** Unspecified fracture of shaft of unspecified ulna

   6 **S52.21** Greenstick fracture of shaft of ulna

> The appropriate 7th character is to be added to all codes in subcategory S52.21
>
> A   initial encounter for closed fracture
> D   subsequent encounter for fracture with routine healing
> G   subsequent encounter for fracture with delayed healing
> K   subsequent encounter for fracture with nonunion
> P   subsequent encounter for fracture with malunion
> S   sequela

CODING TIPS ✓ Open fractures do not occur with torus fractures and greenstick fractures, therefore the 7th characters for open fractures are not available.

🔲 **SP** 7 **S52.211-** Greenstick fracture of shaft of right ulna

🔲 **SP** 7 **S52.212-** Greenstick fracture of shaft of left ulna

🔲 **IQ** 7 **S52.219-** Greenstick fracture of shaft of unspecified ulna

   6 **S52.22** Transverse fracture of shaft of ulna

🔲 **SP** 7 **S52.221-** Displaced transverse fracture of shaft of right ulna

🔲 **SP** 7 **S52.222-** Displaced transverse fracture of shaft of left ulna

🔲 **IQ** 7 **S52.223-** Displaced transverse fracture of shaft of unspecified ulna

🔲 **SP** 7 **S52.224-** Nondisplaced transverse fracture of shaft of right ulna

🔲 **SP** 7 **S52.225-** Nondisplaced transverse fracture of shaft of left ulna

🔲 **IQ** 7 **S52.226-** Nondisplaced transverse fracture of shaft of unspecified ulna

   6 **S52.23** Oblique fracture of shaft of ulna

🔲 **SP** 7 **S52.231-** Displaced oblique fracture of shaft of right ulna

🔲 **SP** 7 **S52.232-** Displaced oblique fracture of shaft of left ulna

🔲 **IQ** 7 **S52.233-** Displaced oblique fracture of shaft of unspecified ulna

🔲 **SP** 7 **S52.234-** Nondisplaced oblique fracture of shaft of right ulna

🔲 **SP** 7 **S52.235-** Nondisplaced oblique fracture of shaft of left ulna

🔲 **IQ** 7 **S52.236-** Nondisplaced oblique fracture of shaft of unspecified ulna

   6 **S52.24** Spiral fracture of shaft of ulna

🔲 **SP IQ** 7 **S52.241-** Displaced spiral fracture of shaft of ulna, right arm

🔲 **SP** 7 **S52.242-** Displaced spiral fracture of shaft of ulna, left arm

🔲 **IQ** 7 **S52.243-** Displaced spiral fracture of shaft of ulna, unspecified arm

🔲 **SP** 7 **S52.244-** Nondisplaced spiral fracture of shaft of ulna, right arm

🔲 **SP** 7 **S52.245-** Nondisplaced spiral fracture of shaft of ulna, left arm

🔲 **IQ** 7 **S52.246-** Nondisplaced spiral fracture of shaft of ulna, unspecified arm

   6 **S52.25** Comminuted fracture of shaft of ulna

🔲 **SP** 7 **S52.251-** Displaced comminuted fracture of shaft of ulna, right arm

🔲 **SP** 7 **S52.252-** Displaced comminuted fracture of shaft of ulna, left arm

🔲 **IQ** 7 **S52.253-** Displaced comminuted fracture of shaft of ulna, unspecified arm

🔲 **SP** 7 **S52.254-** Nondisplaced comminuted fracture of shaft of ulna, right arm

🔲 **SP** 7 **S52.255-** Nondisplaced comminuted fracture of shaft of ulna, left arm

🔲 **IQ** 7 **S52.256-** Nondisplaced comminuted fracture of shaft of ulna, unspecified arm

   6 **S52.26** Segmental fracture of shaft of ulna

🔲 **SP** 7 **S52.261-** Displaced segmental fracture of shaft of ulna, right arm

🔲 **SP** 7 **S52.262-** Displaced segmental fracture of shaft of ulna, left arm

🔲 **IQ** 7 **S52.263-** Displaced segmental fracture of shaft of ulna, unspecified arm

🔲 **SP** 7 **S52.264-** Nondisplaced segmental fracture of shaft of ulna, right arm

🔲 **SP** 7 **S52.265-** Nondisplaced segmental fracture of shaft of ulna, left arm

🔲 **IQ** 7 **S52.266-** Nondisplaced segmental fracture of shaft of ulna, unspecified arm

   6 **S52.27** Monteggia's fracture of ulna
      Fracture of upper shaft of ulna with dislocation of radial head

🔲 **SP** 7 **S52.271-** Monteggia's fracture of right ulna

🔲 **SP** 7 **S52.272-** Monteggia's fracture of left ulna

🔲 **IQ** 7 **S52.279-** Monteggia's fracture of unspecified ulna

   6 **S52.28** Bent bone of ulna

🔲 **SP** 7 **S52.281-** Bent bone of right ulna

🔲 **SP** 7 **S52.282-** Bent bone of left ulna

🔲 **IQ** 7 **S52.283-** Bent bone of unspecified ulna

   6 **S52.29** Other fracture of shaft of ulna

🔲 **SP** 7 **S52.291-** Other fracture of shaft of right ulna

🔲 **SP** 7 **S52.292-** Other fracture of shaft of left ulna

🔲 **IQ** 7 **S52.299-** Other fracture of shaft of unspecified ulna

  5 **S52.3** Fracture of shaft of radius

   6 **S52.30** Unspecified fracture of shaft of radius

🔲 **SP** 7 **S52.301-** Unspecified fracture of shaft of right radius

🔲 **SP** 7 **S52.302-** Unspecified fracture of shaft of left radius

🔲 **IQ** 7 **S52.309-** Unspecified fracture of shaft of unspecified radius

★ New ▲ Revised **Px** Primary **SP** PDGM Px **SL** Low CoM **SH** High CoM **IQ** Quest. Encounter 🔲 Hospice non-cancer Dx   Unspecified   **M** *Manifestation*

DecisionHealth's FY 2020 Complete Home Health ICD-10-CM Diagnosis Coding Manual

1537

Chapter 19

S00-T88

⑥ **S52.31**   Greenstick fracture of shaft of radius

> The appropriate 7th character is to be added to all codes in subcategory S52.31
> A   initial encounter for closed fracture
> D   subsequent encounter for fracture with routine healing
> G   subsequent encounter for fracture with delayed healing
> K   subsequent encounter for fracture with nonunion
> P   subsequent encounter for fracture with malunion
> S   sequela

CODING TIPS ✓   Open fractures do not occur with torus fractures and greenstick fractures, therefore the 7th characters for open fractures are not available.

☐ SP 7 **S52.311-**   Greenstick fracture of shaft of radius, right arm

☐ SP 7 **S52.312-**   Greenstick fracture of shaft of radius, left arm

☐ IQ 7 **S52.319-**   Greenstick fracture of shaft of radius, unspecified arm

⑥ **S52.32**   Transverse fracture of shaft of radius

☐ SP 7 **S52.321-**   Displaced transverse fracture of shaft of right radius

☐ SP 7 **S52.322-**   Displaced transverse fracture of shaft of left radius

☐ IQ 7 **S52.323-**   Displaced transverse fracture of shaft of unspecified radius

☐ SP 7 **S52.324-**   Nondisplaced transverse fracture of shaft of right radius

☐ SP 7 **S52.325-**   Nondisplaced transverse fracture of shaft of left radius

☐ IQ 7 **S52.326-**   Nondisplaced transverse fracture of shaft of unspecified radius

⑥ **S52.33**   Oblique fracture of shaft of radius

☐ SP 7 **S52.331-**   Displaced oblique fracture of shaft of right radius

☐ SP 7 **S52.332-**   Displaced oblique fracture of shaft of left radius

☐ IQ 7 **S52.333-**   Displaced oblique fracture of shaft of unspecified radius

☐ SP 7 **S52.334-**   Nondisplaced oblique fracture of shaft of right radius

☐ SP 7 **S52.335-**   Nondisplaced oblique fracture of shaft of left radius

☐ IQ 7 **S52.336-**   Nondisplaced oblique fracture of shaft of unspecified radius

⑥ **S52.34**   Spiral fracture of shaft of radius

☐ SP 7 **S52.341-**   Displaced spiral fracture of shaft of radius, right arm

☐ SP 7 **S52.342-**   Displaced spiral fracture of shaft of radius, left arm

☐ IQ 7 **S52.343-**   Displaced spiral fracture of shaft of radius, unspecified arm

☐ SP 7 **S52.344-**   Nondisplaced spiral fracture of shaft of radius, right arm

☐ SP 7 **S52.345-**   Nondisplaced spiral fracture of shaft of radius, left arm

☐ IQ 7 **S52.346-**   Nondisplaced spiral fracture of shaft of radius, unspecified arm

⑥ **S52.35**   Comminuted fracture of shaft of radius

☐ SP 7 **S52.351-**   Displaced comminuted fracture of shaft of radius, right arm

☐ SP 7 **S52.352-**   Displaced comminuted fracture of shaft of radius, left arm

☐ IQ 7 **S52.353-**   Displaced comminuted fracture of shaft of radius, unspecified arm

☐ SP 7 **S52.354-**   Nondisplaced comminuted fracture of shaft of radius, right arm

☐ SP 7 **S52.355-**   Nondisplaced comminuted fracture of shaft of radius, left arm

☐ IQ 7 **S52.356-**   Nondisplaced comminuted fracture of shaft of radius, unspecified arm

⑥ **S52.36**   Segmental fracture of shaft of radius

☐ SP 7 **S52.361-**   Displaced segmental fracture of shaft of radius, right arm

☐ SP 7 **S52.362-**   Displaced segmental fracture of shaft of radius, left arm

☐ IQ 7 **S52.363-**   Displaced segmental fracture of shaft of radius, unspecified arm

☐ SP 7 **S52.364-**   Nondisplaced segmental fracture of shaft of radius, right arm

☐ SP 7 **S52.365-**   Nondisplaced segmental fracture of shaft of radius, left arm

☐ IQ 7 **S52.366-**   Nondisplaced segmental fracture of shaft of radius, unspecified arm

⑥ **S52.37**   Galeazzi's fracture
    Fracture of lower shaft of radius with radioulnar joint dislocation

☐ SP 7 **S52.371-**   Galeazzi's fracture of right radius

☐ SP 7 **S52.372-**   Galeazzi's fracture of left radius

☐ IQ 7 **S52.379-**   Galeazzi's fracture of unspecified radius

⑥ **S52.38**   Bent bone of radius

☐ SP 7 **S52.381-**   Bent bone of right radius

☐ SP 7 **S52.382-**   Bent bone of left radius

☐ SP IQ 7 **S52.389-**   Bent bone of unspecified radius

⑥ **S52.39**   Other fracture of shaft of radius

☐ SP 7 **S52.391-**   Other fracture of shaft of radius, right arm

☐ SP 7 **S52.392-**   Other fracture of shaft of radius, left arm

☐ IQ 7 **S52.399-**   Other fracture of shaft of radius, unspecified arm

⑤ **S52.5**   Fracture of lower end of radius
    Fracture of distal end of radius
    EXCLUDES 2   physeal fractures of lower end of radius (S59.2-)

⑥ **S52.50**   Unspecified fracture of the lower end of radius

☐ SP 7 **S52.501-**   Unspecified fracture of the lower end of right radius

☐ SP 7 **S52.502-**   Unspecified fracture of the lower end of left radius

☐ IQ 7 **S52.509-**   Unspecified fracture of the lower end of unspecified radius

---

④ 4th digit required   ⑤ 5th digit required   ⑥ 6th digit required   ⑦ 7th digit required   ⑦ 7th digit placeholder   ✚ Additional code   ☐ Laterality

1538   *DecisionHealth's* FY 2020 Complete Home Health ICD-10-CM Diagnosis Coding Manual

⑥ **S52.51** Fracture of radial styloid process

⊟ **SP** 7 **S52.511-** Displaced fracture of right radial styloid process

⊟ **SP** 7 **S52.512-** Displaced fracture of left radial styloid process

⊟ **!Q** 7 **S52.513-** Displaced fracture of unspecified radial styloid process

⊟ **SP** 7 **S52.514-** Nondisplaced fracture of right radial styloid process

⊟ **SP** 7 **S52.515-** Nondisplaced fracture of left radial styloid process

⊟ **!Q** 7 **S52.516-** Nondisplaced fracture of unspecified radial styloid process

⑥ **S52.52** Torus fracture of lower end of radius

The appropriate 7th character is to be added to all codes in subcategory S52.52

A initial encounter for closed fracture

D subsequent encounter for fracture with routine healing

G subsequent encounter for fracture with delayed healing

K subsequent encounter for fracture with nonunion

P subsequent encounter for fracture with malunion

S sequela

CODING TIPS ✓ Open fractures do not occur with torus fractures and greenstick fractures, therefore the 7th characters for open fractures are not available.

⊟ **SP** 7 **S52.521-** Torus fracture of lower end of right radius

⊟ **SP** 7 **S52.522-** Torus fracture of lower end of left radius

⊟ **!Q** 7 **S52.529-** Torus fracture of lower end of unspecified radius

⑥ **S52.53** Colles' fracture

DEFINITION Break in the lower end of the radius with posterior displacement of the wrist, often caused by breaking a fall with an extended, outstretched hand.

⊟ **SP** 7 **S52.531-** Colles' fracture of right radius

⊟ **SP** 7 **S52.532-** Colles' fracture of left radius

⊟ **!Q** 7 **S52.539-** Colles' fracture of unspecified radius

⑥ **S52.54** Smith's fracture

DEFINITION Break in the lower end of the radius with palmar displacement of the wrist; a reverse Colles' fracture.

⊟ **SP** 7 **S52.541-** Smith's fracture of right radius

⊟ **SP** 7 **S52.542-** Smith's fracture of left radius

⊟ **!Q** 7 **S52.549-** Smith's fracture of unspecified radius

⑥ **S52.55** Other extraarticular fracture of lower end of radius

⊟ **SP** 7 **S52.551-** Other extraarticular fracture of lower end of right radius

⊟ **SP** 7 **S52.552-** Other extraarticular fracture of lower end of left radius

⊟ **!Q** 7 **S52.559-** Other extraarticular fracture of lower end of unspecified radius

⑥ **S52.56** Barton's fracture

⊟ **SP** 7 **S52.561-** Barton's fracture of right radius

⊟ **SP** 7 **S52.562-** Barton's fracture of left radius

⊟ **!Q** 7 **S52.569-** Barton's fracture of unspecified radius

⑥ **S52.57** Other intraarticular fracture of lower end of radius

⊟ **SP** 7 **S52.571-** Other intraarticular fracture of lower end of right radius

⊟ **SP** 7 **S52.572-** Other intraarticular fracture of lower end of left radius

⊟ **!Q** 7 **S52.579-** Other intraarticular fracture of lower end of unspecified radius

⑥ **S52.59** Other fractures of lower end of radius

⊟ **SP** 7 **S52.591-** Other fractures of lower end of right radius

⊟ **SP** 7 **S52.592-** Other fractures of lower end of left radius

⊟ **!Q** 7 **S52.599-** Other fractures of lower end of unspecified radius

⑤ **S52.6** Fracture of lower end of ulna

⑥ **S52.60** Unspecified fracture of lower end of ulna

⊟ **SP** 7 **S52.601-** Unspecified fracture of lower end of right ulna

⊟ **SP** 7 **S52.602-** Unspecified fracture of lower end of left ulna

⊟ **!Q** 7 **S52.609-** Unspecified fracture of lower end of unspecified ulna

⑥ **S52.61** Fracture of ulna styloid process

⊟ **SP** 7 **S52.611-** Displaced fracture of right ulna styloid process

⊟ **SP** 7 **S52.612-** Displaced fracture of left ulna styloid process

⊟ **!Q** 7 **S52.613-** Displaced fracture of unspecified ulna styloid process

⊟ **SP** 7 **S52.614-** Nondisplaced fracture of right ulna styloid process

⊟ **SP** 7 **S52.615-** Nondisplaced fracture of left ulna styloid process

⊟ **SP** **!Q** 7 **S52.616-** Nondisplaced fracture of unspecified ulna styloid process

⑥ **S52.62** Torus fracture of lower end of ulna

The appropriate 7th character is to be added to all codes in subcategory S52.62

A initial encounter for closed fracture

D subsequent encounter for fracture with routine healing

G subsequent encounter for fracture with delayed healing

K subsequent encounter for fracture with nonunion

P subsequent encounter for fracture with malunion

S sequela

⊟ **SP** 7 **S52.621-** Torus fracture of lower end of right ulna

⊟ **SP** 7 **S52.622-** Torus fracture of lower end of left ulna

Chapter 19

S00-T88

★ New ▲ Revised Px Primary **SP** PDGM Px **SL** Low CoM **SH** High CoM **!Q** Quest. Encounter ⊞ Hospice non-cancer Dx Unspecified **M** Manifestation

DecisionHealth's FY 2020 Complete Home Health ICD-10-CM Diagnosis Coding Manual 1539

☐ IQ 7 **S52.629-** **Torus fracture of lower end of unspecified ulna**

6 **S52.69** Other fracture of lower end of ulna

☐ SP 7 **S52.691-** Other fracture of lower end of right ulna

☐ SP 7 **S52.692-** Other fracture of lower end of left ulna

☐ SP IQ 7 **S52.699-** **Other fracture of lower end of unspecified ulna**

5 **S52.9** **Unspecified fracture of forearm**

☐ IQ 7 **S52.90X-** **Unspecified fracture of unspecified forearm**

☐ SP 7 **S52.91X-** **Unspecified fracture of right forearm**

☐ SP 7 **S52.92X-** **Unspecified fracture of left forearm**

4 **S53** **Dislocation and sprain of joints and ligaments of elbow**

| INCLUDES | avulsion of joint or ligament of elbow |

laceration of cartilage, joint or ligament of elbow

sprain of cartilage, joint or ligament of elbow

traumatic hemarthrosis of joint or ligament of elbow

traumatic rupture of joint or ligament of elbow

traumatic subluxation of joint or ligament of elbow

traumatic tear of joint or ligament of elbow

Code also:
any associated open wound

| EXCLUDES 2 | strain of muscle, fascia and tendon at forearm level (S56.-) |

The appropriate 7th character is to be added to each code from category S53
A   initial encounter
D   subsequent encounter
S   sequela

5 **S53.0** **Subluxation and dislocation of radial head**
Dislocation of radiohumeral joint
Subluxation of radiohumeral joint

| EXCLUDES 1 | Monteggia's fracture-dislocation (S52.27-) |

6 **S53.00** **Unspecified subluxation and dislocation of radial head**

☐ SP 7 **S53.001-** **Unspecified subluxation of right radial head**

☐ SP 7 **S53.002-** **Unspecified subluxation of left radial head**

☐ IQ 7 **S53.003-** **Unspecified subluxation of unspecified radial head**

☐ SP IQ 7 **S53.004-** **Unspecified dislocation of right radial head**

☐ SP 7 **S53.005-** **Unspecified dislocation of left radial head**

☐ IQ 7 **S53.006-** **Unspecified dislocation of unspecified radial head**

6 **S53.01** **Anterior subluxation and dislocation of radial head**

Anteriomedial subluxation and dislocation of radial head

☐ SP 7 **S53.011-** **Anterior subluxation of right radial head**

☐ SP 7 **S53.012-** **Anterior subluxation of left radial head**

☐ IQ 7 **S53.013-** **Anterior subluxation of unspecified radial head**

☐ SP 7 **S53.014-** **Anterior dislocation of right radial head**

☐ SP 7 **S53.015-** **Anterior dislocation of left radial head**

☐ IQ 7 **S53.016-** **Anterior dislocation of unspecified radial head**

6 **S53.02** **Posterior subluxation and dislocation of radial head**
Posteriolateral subluxation and dislocation of radial head

☐ SP 7 **S53.021-** **Posterior subluxation of right radial head**

☐ SP 7 **S53.022-** **Posterior subluxation of left radial head**

☐ IQ 7 **S53.023-** **Posterior subluxation of unspecified radial head**

☐ SP 7 **S53.024-** **Posterior dislocation of right radial head**

☐ SP 7 **S53.025-** **Posterior dislocation of left radial head**

☐ !Q 7 **S53.026-** **Posterior dislocation of unspecified radial head**

6 **S53.03** **Nursemaid's elbow**

☐ SP 7 **S53.031-** **Nursemaid's elbow, right elbow**

☐ SP 7 **S53.032-** **Nursemaid's elbow, left elbow**

☐ IQ 7 **S53.033-** **Nursemaid's elbow, unspecified elbow**

6 **S53.09** **Other subluxation and dislocation of radial head**

☐ SP 7 **S53.091-** **Other subluxation of right radial head**

☐ SP 7 **S53.092-** **Other subluxation of left radial head**

☐ !Q 7 **S53.093-** **Other subluxation of unspecified radial head**

☐ SP 7 **S53.094-** **Other dislocation of right radial head**

☐ SP 7 **S53.095-** **Other dislocation of left radial head**

☐ IQ 7 **S53.096-** **Other dislocation of unspecified radial head**

5 **S53.1** **Subluxation and dislocation of ulnohumeral joint**
Subluxation and dislocation of elbow NOS

| EXCLUDES 1 | dislocation of radial head alone (S53.0-) |

6 **S53.10** **Unspecified subluxation and dislocation of ulnohumeral joint**

☐ SP 7 **S53.101-** **Unspecified subluxation of right ulnohumeral joint**

☐ SP 7 **S53.102-** **Unspecified subluxation of left ulnohumeral joint**

☐ !Q 7 **S53.103-** **Unspecified subluxation of unspecified ulnohumeral joint**

☐ SP 7 **S53.104-** **Unspecified dislocation of right ulnohumeral joint**

4 4th digit required   5 5th digit required   6 6th digit required   7 7th digit required   7 7th digit placeholder   + Additional code   ☐ Laterality

1540   DecisionHealth's FY 2020 Complete Home Health ICD-10-CM Diagnosis Coding Manual

Chapter 19

S00-T88

▤ **SP** 7 S53.105- **Unspecified dislocation of left ulnohumeral joint**

▤ **!Q** 7 S53.106- **Unspecified dislocation of unspecified ulnohumeral joint**

6 S53.11 Anterior subluxation and dislocation of ulnohumeral joint

▤ **SP** 7 S53.111- Anterior subluxation of right ulnohumeral joint

▤ **SP** 7 S53.112- Anterior subluxation of left ulnohumeral joint

▤ **!Q** 7 S53.113- **Anterior subluxation of unspecified ulnohumeral joint**

▤ **SP** 7 S53.114- Anterior dislocation of right ulnohumeral joint

▤ **SP** 7 S53.115- Anterior dislocation of left ulnohumeral joint

▤ **!Q** 7 S53.116- **Anterior dislocation of unspecified ulnohumeral joint**

6 S53.12 Posterior subluxation and dislocation of ulnohumeral joint

▤ **SP** 7 S53.121- Posterior subluxation of right ulnohumeral joint

▤ **SP** 7 S53.122- Posterior subluxation of left ulnohumeral joint

▤ **!Q** 7 S53.123- **Posterior subluxation of unspecified ulnohumeral joint**

▤ **SP** 7 S53.124- Posterior dislocation of right ulnohumeral joint

▤ **SP** 7 S53.125- Posterior dislocation of left ulnohumeral joint

▤ **!Q** 7 S53.126- **Posterior dislocation of unspecified ulnohumeral joint**

6 S53.13 Medial subluxation and dislocation of ulnohumeral joint

▤ **SP** 7 S53.131- Medial subluxation of right ulnohumeral joint

▤ **SP** 7 S53.132- Medial subluxation of left ulnohumeral joint

▤ **!Q** 7 S53.133- **Medial subluxation of unspecified ulnohumeral joint**

▤ **SP** 7 S53.134- Medial dislocation of right ulnohumeral joint

▤ **SP** 7 S53.135- Medial dislocation of left ulnohumeral joint

▤ **!Q** 7 S53.136- **Medial dislocation of unspecified ulnohumeral joint**

6 S53.14 Lateral subluxation and dislocation of ulnohumeral joint

▤ **SP** 7 S53.141- Lateral subluxation of right ulnohumeral joint

▤ **SP** 7 S53.142- Lateral subluxation of left ulnohumeral joint

▤ **!Q** 7 S53.143- **Lateral subluxation of unspecified ulnohumeral joint**

▤ **SP** 7 S53.144- Lateral dislocation of right ulnohumeral joint

▤ **SP** 7 S53.145- Lateral dislocation of left ulnohumeral joint

▤ **!Q** 7 S53.146- **Lateral dislocation of unspecified ulnohumeral joint**

6 S53.19 Other subluxation and dislocation of ulnohumeral joint

▤ **SP** 7 S53.191- Other subluxation of right ulnohumeral joint

▤ **SP** 7 S53.192- Other subluxation of left ulnohumeral joint

▤ **!Q** 7 S53.193- **Other subluxation of unspecified ulnohumeral joint**

▤ **SP** 7 S53.194- Other dislocation of right ulnohumeral joint

▤ **SP** 7 S53.195- Other dislocation of left ulnohumeral joint

▤ **!Q** 7 S53.196- **Other dislocation of unspecified ulnohumeral joint**

5 S53.2 Traumatic rupture of radial collateral ligament
> **EXCLUDES 1** sprain of radial collateral ligament NOS (S53.43-)

▤ **!Q** 7 S53.20X- **Traumatic rupture of unspecified radial collateral ligament**

▤ **SP** 7 S53.21X- Traumatic rupture of right radial collateral ligament

▤ **SP** 7 S53.22X- Traumatic rupture of left radial collateral ligament

5 S53.3 Traumatic rupture of ulnar collateral ligament
> **EXCLUDES 1** sprain of ulnar collateral ligament (S53.44-)

▤ **!Q** 7 S53.30X- **Traumatic rupture of unspecified ulnar collateral ligament**

▤ **SP** 7 S53.31X- Traumatic rupture of right ulnar collateral ligament

▤ **SP** 7 S53.32X- Traumatic rupture of left ulnar collateral ligament

5 S53.4 Sprain of elbow
> **EXCLUDES 2** traumatic rupture of radial collateral ligament (S53.2-)
> traumatic rupture of ulnar collateral ligament (S53.3-)

6 S53.40 **Unspecified sprain of elbow**

▤ **SP** 7 S53.401- **Unspecified sprain of right elbow**

▤ **SP** 7 S53.402- **Unspecified sprain of left elbow**

▤ **!Q** 7 S53.409- **Unspecified sprain of unspecified elbow**
Sprain of elbow NOS

6 S53.41 Radiohumeral (joint) sprain

▤ **SP** 7 S53.411- Radiohumeral (joint) sprain of right elbow

▤ **SP** 7 S53.412- Radiohumeral (joint) sprain of left elbow

▤ **!Q** 7 S53.419- **Radiohumeral (joint) sprain of unspecified elbow**

6 S53.42 Ulnohumeral (joint) sprain

▤ **SP** 7 S53.421- Ulnohumeral (joint) sprain of right elbow

▤ **SP** 7 S53.422- Ulnohumeral (joint) sprain of left elbow

▤ **!Q** 7 S53.429- **Ulnohumeral (joint) sprain of unspecified elbow**

6 S53.43 Radial collateral ligament sprain

▤ **SP** 7 S53.431- Radial collateral ligament sprain of right elbow

▤ **SP** 7 S53.432- Radial collateral ligament sprain of left elbow

▤ **!Q** 7 S53.439- **Radial collateral ligament sprain of unspecified elbow**

6 S53.44 Ulnar collateral ligament sprain

★ New ▲ Revised Px Primary **SP** PDGM Px **SL** Low CoM **SH** High CoM **!Q** Quest. Encounter ⊞ Hospice non-cancer Dx Unspecified M *Manifestation*

DecisionHealth's FY 2020 Complete Home Health ICD-10-CM Diagnosis Coding Manual

1541

Chapter 19

S00-T88

⊟ SP 7 **S53.441-** Ulnar collateral ligament sprain of right elbow

⊟ SP 7 **S53.442-** Ulnar collateral ligament sprain of left elbow

⊟ IQ 7 **S53.449-** Ulnar collateral ligament sprain of unspecified elbow

6 **S53.49** Other sprain of elbow

⊟ SP 7 **S53.491-** Other sprain of right elbow

⊟ SP 7 **S53.492-** Other sprain of left elbow

⊟ IQ 7 **S53.499-** Other sprain of unspecified elbow

4 **S54** **Injury of nerves at forearm level**
Code also:
  any associated open wound (S51.-)
  EXCLUDES 2 injury of nerves at wrist and hand level (S64.-)

The appropriate 7th character is to be added to each code from category S54
A   initial encounter
D   subsequent encounter
S   sequela

5 **S54.0** **Injury of ulnar nerve at forearm level**
Injury of ulnar nerve NOS

⊟ IQ 7 **S54.00X-** Injury of ulnar nerve at forearm level, unspecified arm

⊟ SP 7 **S54.01X-** Injury of ulnar nerve at forearm level, right arm

⊟ SP 7 **S54.02X-** Injury of ulnar nerve at forearm level, left arm

5 **S54.1** **Injury of median nerve at forearm level**
Injury of median nerve NOS

⊟ IQ 7 **S54.10X-** Injury of median nerve at forearm level, unspecified arm

⊟ SP 7 **S54.11X-** Injury of median nerve at forearm level, right arm

⊟ SP 7 **S54.12X-** Injury of median nerve at forearm level, left arm

5 **S54.2** **Injury of radial nerve at forearm level**
Injury of radial nerve NOS

⊟ IQ 7 **S54.20X-** Injury of radial nerve at forearm level, unspecified arm

⊟ SP 7 **S54.21X-** Injury of radial nerve at forearm level, right arm

⊟ SP 7 **S54.22X-** Injury of radial nerve at forearm level, left arm

5 **S54.3** **Injury of cutaneous sensory nerve at forearm level**

⊟ IQ 7 **S54.30X-** Injury of cutaneous sensory nerve at forearm level, unspecified arm

⊟ SP 7 **S54.31X-** Injury of cutaneous sensory nerve at forearm level, right arm

⊟ SP 7 **S54.32X-** Injury of cutaneous sensory nerve at forearm level, left arm

5 **S54.8** **Injury of other nerves at forearm level**

6 **S54.8X** Injury of other nerves at forearm level

⊟ SP 7 **S54.8X1-** Injury of other nerves at forearm level, right arm

⊟ SP 7 **S54.8X2-** Injury of other nerves at forearm level, left arm

⊟ IQ 7 **S54.8X9-** Injury of other nerves at forearm level, unspecified arm

5 **S54.9** **Injury of unspecified nerve at forearm level**

⊟ IQ 7 **S54.90X-** Injury of unspecified nerve at forearm level, unspecified arm

⊟ IQ 7 **S54.91X-** Injury of unspecified nerve at forearm level, right arm

⊟ IQ 7 **S54.92X-** Injury of unspecified nerve at forearm level, left arm

4 **S55** **Injury of blood vessels at forearm level**
Code also:
  any associated open wound (S51.-)
  EXCLUDES 2 injury of blood vessels at wrist and hand level (S65.-)
  injury of brachial vessels (S45.1-S45.2)

The appropriate 7th character is to be added to each code from category S55
A   initial encounter
D   subsequent encounter
S   sequela

5 **S55.0** **Injury of ulnar artery at forearm level**

6 **S55.00** Unspecified injury of ulnar artery at forearm level

⊟ IQ 7 **S55.001-** Unspecified injury of ulnar artery at forearm level, right arm

⊟ IQ 7 **S55.002-** Unspecified injury of ulnar artery at forearm level, left arm

⊟ IQ 7 **S55.009-** Unspecified injury of ulnar artery at forearm level, unspecified arm

6 **S55.01** Laceration of ulnar artery at forearm level

⊟ SP 7 **S55.011-** Laceration of ulnar artery at forearm level, right arm

⊟ SP 7 **S55.012-** Laceration of ulnar artery at forearm level, left arm

⊟ IQ 7 **S55.019-** Laceration of ulnar artery at forearm level, unspecified arm

6 **S55.09** Other specified injury of ulnar artery at forearm level

⊟ SP 7 **S55.091-** Other specified injury of ulnar artery at forearm level, right arm

⊟ SP 7 **S55.092-** Other specified injury of ulnar artery at forearm level, left arm

⊟ IQ 7 **S55.099-** Other specified injury of ulnar artery at forearm level, unspecified arm

5 **S55.1** **Injury of radial artery at forearm level**

6 **S55.10** Unspecified injury of radial artery at forearm level

⊟ IQ 7 **S55.101-** Unspecified injury of radial artery at forearm level, right arm

⊟ IQ 7 **S55.102-** Unspecified injury of radial artery at forearm level, left arm

⊟ IQ 7 **S55.109-** Unspecified injury of radial artery at forearm level, unspecified arm

6 **S55.11** Laceration of radial artery at forearm level

⊟ SP 7 **S55.111-** Laceration of radial artery at forearm level, right arm

⊟ SP 7 **S55.112-** Laceration of radial artery at forearm level, left arm

---

4 4th digit required   5 5th digit required   6 6th digit required   7 7th digit required   ☑ 7th digit placeholder   +Additional code   ⊟ Laterality

☰ !Q 7 **S55.119-** **Laceration of radial artery at forearm level, unspecified arm**

6 S55.19 Other specified injury of radial artery at forearm level

☰ SP 7 S55.191- Other specified injury of radial artery at forearm level, right arm

☰ SP 7 S55.192- Other specified injury of radial artery at forearm level, left arm

☰ !Q 7 **S55.199-** **Other specified injury of radial artery at forearm level, unspecified arm**

5 S55.2 Injury of vein at forearm level

6 S55.20 **Unspecified injury of vein at forearm level**

☰ !Q 7 **S55.201-** **Unspecified injury of vein at forearm level, right arm**

☰ !Q 7 **S55.202-** **Unspecified injury of vein at forearm level, left arm**

☰ !Q 7 **S55.209-** **Unspecified injury of vein at forearm level, unspecified arm**

6 S55.21 Laceration of vein at forearm level

☰ SP 7 S55.211- Laceration of vein at forearm level, right arm

☰ SP 7 S55.212- Laceration of vein at forearm level, left arm

☰ !Q 7 **S55.219-** **Laceration of vein at forearm level, unspecified arm**

6 S55.29 Other specified injury of vein at forearm level

☰ SP 7 S55.291- Other specified injury of vein at forearm level, right arm

☰ SP 7 S55.292- Other specified injury of vein at forearm level, left arm

☰ !Q 7 **S55.299-** **Other specified injury of vein at forearm level, unspecified arm**

5 S55.8 Injury of other blood vessels at forearm level

6 S55.80 **Unspecified injury of other blood vessels at forearm level**

☰ !Q 7 **S55.801-** **Unspecified injury of other blood vessels at forearm level, right arm**

☰ !Q 7 **S55.802-** **Unspecified injury of other blood vessels at forearm level, left arm**

☰ !Q 7 **S55.809-** **Unspecified injury of other blood vessels at forearm level, unspecified arm**

6 S55.81 Laceration of other blood vessels at forearm level

☰ SP 7 S55.811- Laceration of other blood vessels at forearm level, right arm

☰ SP 7 S55.812- Laceration of other blood vessels at forearm level, left arm

☰ !Q 7 **S55.819-** **Laceration of other blood vessels at forearm level, unspecified arm**

6 S55.89 Other specified injury of other blood vessels at forearm level

☰ SP 7 S55.891- Other specified injury of other blood vessels at forearm level, right arm

☰ SP 7 S55.892- Other specified injury of other blood vessels at forearm level, left arm

☰ !Q 7 **S55.899-** **Other specified injury of other blood vessels at forearm level, unspecified arm**

5 S55.9 Injury of unspecified blood vessel at forearm level

6 S55.90 **Unspecified injury of unspecified blood vessel at forearm level**

☰ !Q 7 **S55.901-** **Unspecified injury of unspecified blood vessel at forearm level, right arm**

☰ !Q 7 **S55.902-** **Unspecified injury of unspecified blood vessel at forearm level, left arm**

☰ !Q 7 **S55.909-** **Unspecified injury of unspecified blood vessel at forearm level, unspecified arm**

6 S55.91 **Laceration of unspecified blood vessel at forearm level**

☰ SP 7 **S55.911-** **Laceration of unspecified blood vessel at forearm level, right arm**

☰ SP 7 **S55.912-** **Laceration of unspecified blood vessel at forearm level, left arm**

☰ !Q 7 **S55.919-** **Laceration of unspecified blood vessel at forearm level, unspecified arm**

6 S55.99 **Other specified injury of unspecified blood vessel at forearm level**

☰ SP 7 **S55.991-** **Other specified injury of unspecified blood vessel at forearm level, right arm**

☰ SP 7 **S55.992-** **Other specified injury of unspecified blood vessel at forearm level, left arm**

☰ !Q 7 **S55.999-** **Other specified injury of unspecified blood vessel at forearm level, unspecified arm**

4 S56 **Injury of muscle, fascia and tendon at forearm level**
Code also:
any associated open wound (S51.-)
EXCLUDES 2 injury of muscle, fascia and tendon at or below wrist (S66.-)
sprain of joints and ligaments of elbow (S53.4-)

The appropriate 7th character is to be added to each code from category S56
A   initial encounter
D   subsequent encounter
S   sequela

5 S56.0 **Injury of flexor muscle, fascia and tendon of thumb at forearm level**

6 S56.00 **Unspecified injury of flexor muscle, fascia and tendon of thumb at forearm level**

☰ !Q 7 **S56.001-** **Unspecified injury of flexor muscle, fascia and tendon of right thumb at forearm level**

★ New ▲ Revised Px Primary SP PDGM Px SL Low CoM SH High CoM !Q Quest. Encounter H Hospice non-cancer Dx   Unspecified   M *Manifestation*

DecisionHealth's FY 2020 Complete Home Health ICD-10-CM Diagnosis Coding Manual   1543

Chapter 19

S00-T88

Chapter 19

S00-T88

▣ **!Q** 7 S56.002- Unspecified injury of flexor muscle, fascia and tendon of left thumb at forearm level

▣ **!Q** 7 S56.009- Unspecified injury of flexor muscle, fascia and tendon of unspecified thumb at forearm level

6 S56.01 Strain of flexor muscle, fascia and tendon of thumb at forearm level

▣ **SP** 7 S56.011- Strain of flexor muscle, fascia and tendon of right thumb at forearm level

▣ **SP** 7 S56.012- Strain of flexor muscle, fascia and tendon of left thumb at forearm level

▣ **SP** 7 S56.019- Strain of flexor muscle, fascia and tendon of unspecified thumb at forearm level

6 S56.02 Laceration of flexor muscle, fascia and tendon of thumb at forearm level

▣ **SP** 7 S56.021- Laceration of flexor muscle, fascia and tendon of right thumb at forearm level

▣ **SP** 7 S56.022- Laceration of flexor muscle, fascia and tendon of left thumb at forearm level

▣ **!Q** 7 S56.029- Laceration of flexor muscle, fascia and tendon of unspecified thumb at forearm level

6 S56.09 Other injury of flexor muscle, fascia and tendon of thumb at forearm level

▣ **SP** 7 S56.091- Other injury of flexor muscle, fascia and tendon of right thumb at forearm level

▣ **SP** 7 S56.092- Other injury of flexor muscle, fascia and tendon of left thumb at forearm level

▣ **!Q** 7 S56.099- Other injury of flexor muscle, fascia and tendon of unspecified thumb at forearm level

5 S56.1 Injury of flexor muscle, fascia and tendon of other and unspecified finger at forearm level

6 S56.10 Unspecified injury of flexor muscle, fascia and tendon of other and unspecified finger at forearm level

▣ **!Q** 7 S56.101- Unspecified injury of flexor muscle, fascia and tendon of right index finger at forearm level

▣ **!Q** 7 S56.102- Unspecified injury of flexor muscle, fascia and tendon of left index finger at forearm level

▣ **!Q** 7 S56.103- Unspecified injury of flexor muscle, fascia and tendon of right middle finger at forearm level

▣ **!Q** 7 S56.104- Unspecified injury of flexor muscle, fascia and tendon of left middle finger at forearm level

▣ **!Q** 7 S56.105- Unspecified injury of flexor muscle, fascia and tendon of right ring finger at forearm level

▣ **!Q** 7 S56.106- Unspecified injury of flexor muscle, fascia and tendon of left ring finger at forearm level

▣ **!Q** 7 S56.107- Unspecified injury of flexor muscle, fascia and tendon of right little finger at forearm level

▣ **!Q** 7 S56.108- Unspecified injury of flexor muscle, fascia and tendon of left little finger at forearm level

▣ **!Q** 7 S56.109- Unspecified injury of flexor muscle, fascia and tendon of unspecified finger at forearm level

6 S56.11 Strain of flexor muscle, fascia and tendon of other and unspecified finger at forearm level

▣ **SP** 7 S56.111- Strain of flexor muscle, fascia and tendon of right index finger at forearm level

▣ **SP** 7 S56.112- Strain of flexor muscle, fascia and tendon of left index finger at forearm level

▣ **SP** 7 S56.113- Strain of flexor muscle, fascia and tendon of right middle finger at forearm level

▣ **SP** 7 S56.114- Strain of flexor muscle, fascia and tendon of left middle finger at forearm level

▣ **SP** 7 S56.115- Strain of flexor muscle, fascia and tendon of right ring finger at forearm level

▣ **SP** 7 S56.116- Strain of flexor muscle, fascia and tendon of left ring finger at forearm level

▣ **SP** 7 S56.117- Strain of flexor muscle, fascia and tendon of right little finger at forearm level

▣ **SP** 7 S56.118- Strain of flexor muscle, fascia and tendon of left little finger at forearm level

▣ **!Q** 7 S56.119- Strain of flexor muscle, fascia and tendon of finger of unspecified finger at forearm level

6 S56.12 Laceration of flexor muscle, fascia and tendon of other and unspecified finger at forearm level

▣ **SP** 7 S56.121- Laceration of flexor muscle, fascia and tendon of right index finger at forearm level

▣ **SP** 7 S56.122- Laceration of flexor muscle, fascia and tendon of left index finger at forearm level

▣ **SP** 7 S56.123- Laceration of flexor muscle, fascia and tendon of right middle finger at forearm level

▣ **SP** 7 S56.124- Laceration of flexor muscle, fascia and tendon of left middle finger at forearm level

▣ **SP** 7 S56.125- Laceration of flexor muscle, fascia and tendon of right ring finger at forearm level

▣ **SP** 7 S56.126- Laceration of flexor muscle, fascia and tendon of left ring finger at forearm level

---

4 4th digit required   5 5th digit required   6 6th digit required   7 7th digit required   ⁊ 7th digit placeholder   + Additional code   ▣ Laterality

1544   *DecisionHealth's* FY 2020 Complete Home Health ICD-10-CM Diagnosis Coding Manual

SP 7 S56.127- Laceration of flexor muscle, fascia and tendon of right little finger at forearm level

SP 7 S56.128- Laceration of flexor muscle, fascia and tendon of left little finger at forearm level

IQ 7 S56.129- Laceration of flexor muscle, fascia and tendon of unspecified finger at forearm level

6 S56.19 Other injury of flexor muscle, fascia and tendon of other and unspecified finger at forearm level

SP 7 S56.191- Other injury of flexor muscle, fascia and tendon of right index finger at forearm level

SP 7 S56.192- Other injury of flexor muscle, fascia and tendon of left index finger at forearm level

SP 7 S56.193- Other injury of flexor muscle, fascia and tendon of right middle finger at forearm level

SP 7 S56.194- Other injury of flexor muscle, fascia and tendon of left middle finger at forearm level

SP 7 S56.195- Other injury of flexor muscle, fascia and tendon of right ring finger at forearm level

SP 7 S56.196- Other injury of flexor muscle, fascia and tendon of left ring finger at forearm level

SP 7 S56.197- Other injury of flexor muscle, fascia and tendon of right little finger at forearm level

SP 7 S56.198- Other injury of flexor muscle, fascia and tendon of left little finger at forearm level

IQ 7 S56.199- Other injury of flexor muscle, fascia and tendon of unspecified finger at forearm level

5 S56.2 Injury of other flexor muscle, fascia and tendon at forearm level

6 S56.20 Unspecified injury of other flexor muscle, fascia and tendon at forearm level

IQ 7 S56.201- Unspecified injury of other flexor muscle, fascia and tendon at forearm level, right arm

IQ 7 S56.202- Unspecified injury of other flexor muscle, fascia and tendon at forearm level, left arm

IQ 7 S56.209- Unspecified injury of other flexor muscle, fascia and tendon at forearm level, unspecified arm

6 S56.21 Strain of other flexor muscle, fascia and tendon at forearm level

SP 7 S56.211- Strain of other flexor muscle, fascia and tendon at forearm level, right arm

SP 7 S56.212- Strain of other flexor muscle, fascia and tendon at forearm level, left arm

IQ 7 S56.219- Strain of other flexor muscle, fascia and tendon at forearm level, unspecified arm

6 S56.22 Laceration of other flexor muscle, fascia and tendon at forearm level

SP 7 S56.221- Laceration of other flexor muscle, fascia and tendon at forearm level, right arm

SP 7 S56.222- Laceration of other flexor muscle, fascia and tendon at forearm level, left arm

IQ 7 S56.229- Laceration of other flexor muscle, fascia and tendon at forearm level, unspecified arm

6 S56.29 Other injury of other flexor muscle, fascia and tendon at forearm level

SP 7 S56.291- Other injury of other flexor muscle, fascia and tendon at forearm level, right arm

SP 7 S56.292- Other injury of other flexor muscle, fascia and tendon at forearm level, left arm

IQ 7 S56.299- Other injury of other flexor muscle, fascia and tendon at forearm level, unspecified arm

5 S56.3 Injury of extensor or abductor muscles, fascia and tendons of thumb at forearm level

6 S56.30 Unspecified injury of extensor or abductor muscles, fascia and tendons of thumb at forearm level

IQ 7 S56.301- Unspecified injury of extensor or abductor muscles, fascia and tendons of right thumb at forearm level

IQ 7 S56.302- Unspecified injury of extensor or abductor muscles, fascia and tendons of left thumb at forearm level

IQ 7 S56.309- Unspecified injury of extensor or abductor muscles, fascia and tendons of unspecified thumb at forearm level

6 S56.31 Strain of extensor or abductor muscles, fascia and tendons of thumb at forearm level

SP 7 S56.311- Strain of extensor or abductor muscles, fascia and tendons of right thumb at forearm level

SP 7 S56.312- Strain of extensor or abductor muscles, fascia and tendons of left thumb at forearm level

IQ 7 S56.319- Strain of extensor or abductor muscles, fascia and tendons of unspecified thumb at forearm level

6 S56.32 Laceration of extensor or abductor muscles, fascia and tendons of thumb at forearm level

SP 7 S56.321- Laceration of extensor or abductor muscles, fascia and tendons of right thumb at forearm level

SP 7 S56.322- Laceration of extensor or abductor muscles, fascia and tendons of left thumb at forearm level

SP IQ 7 S56.329- Laceration of extensor or abductor muscles, fascia and tendons of unspecified thumb at forearm level

★ New ▲ Revised Px Primary **SP** PDGM Px **SL** Low CoM **SH** High CoM **IQ** Quest. Encounter **H** Hospice non-cancer Dx Unspecified **M** *Manifestation*

DecisionHealth's FY 2020 Complete Home Health ICD-10-CM Diagnosis Coding Manual

1545

⑥ S56.39 Other injury of extensor or abductor muscles, fascia and tendons of thumb at forearm level

☐ **SP** ⑦ **S56.391-** Other injury of extensor or abductor muscles, fascia and tendons of right thumb at forearm level

☐ **SP** ⑦ **S56.392-** Other injury of extensor or abductor muscles, fascia and tendons of left thumb at forearm level

☐ **IQ** ⑦ **S56.399-** Other injury of extensor or abductor muscles, fascia and tendons of unspecified thumb at forearm level

⑤ S56.4 Injury of extensor muscle, fascia and tendon of other and unspecified finger at forearm level

⑥ S56.40 Unspecified injury of extensor muscle, fascia and tendon of other and unspecified finger at forearm level

☐ **IQ** ⑦ **S56.401-** Unspecified injury of extensor muscle, fascia and tendon of right index finger at forearm level

☐ **IQ** ⑦ **S56.402-** Unspecified injury of extensor muscle, fascia and tendon of left index finger at forearm level

☐ **IQ** ⑦ **S56.403-** Unspecified injury of extensor muscle, fascia and tendon of right middle finger at forearm level

☐ **IQ** ⑦ **S56.404-** Unspecified injury of extensor muscle, fascia and tendon of left middle finger at forearm level

☐ **IQ** ⑦ **S56.405-** Unspecified injury of extensor muscle, fascia and tendon of right ring finger at forearm level

☐ **IQ** ⑦ **S56.406-** Unspecified injury of extensor muscle, fascia and tendon of left ring finger at forearm level

☐ **IQ** ⑦ **S56.407-** Unspecified injury of extensor muscle, fascia and tendon of right little finger at forearm level

☐ **IQ** ⑦ **S56.408-** Unspecified injury of extensor muscle, fascia and tendon of left little finger at forearm level

☐ **IQ** ⑦ **S56.409-** Unspecified injury of extensor muscle, fascia and tendon of unspecified finger at forearm level

⑥ S56.41 Strain of extensor muscle, fascia and tendon of other and unspecified finger at forearm level

☐ **SP** ⑦ **S56.411-** Strain of extensor muscle, fascia and tendon of right index finger at forearm level

☐ **SP** ⑦ **S56.412-** Strain of extensor muscle, fascia and tendon of left index finger at forearm level

☐ **SP** ⑦ **S56.413-** Strain of extensor muscle, fascia and tendon of right middle finger at forearm level

☐ **SP** ⑦ **S56.414-** Strain of extensor muscle, fascia and tendon of left middle finger at forearm level

☐ **SP** ⑦ **S56.415-** Strain of extensor muscle, fascia and tendon of right ring finger at forearm level

☐ **SP** ⑦ **S56.416-** Strain of extensor muscle, fascia and tendon of left ring finger at forearm level

☐ **SP** ⑦ **S56.417-** Strain of extensor muscle, fascia and tendon of right little finger at forearm level

☐ **SP** ⑦ **S56.418-** Strain of extensor muscle, fascia and tendon of left little finger at forearm level

☐ **IQ** ⑦ **S56.419-** Strain of extensor muscle, fascia and tendon of finger, unspecified finger at forearm level

⑥ S56.42 Laceration of extensor muscle, fascia and tendon of other and unspecified finger at forearm level

☐ **SP** ⑦ **S56.421-** Laceration of extensor muscle, fascia and tendon of right index finger at forearm level

☐ **SP** ⑦ **S56.422-** Laceration of extensor muscle, fascia and tendon of left index finger at forearm level

☐ **SP** ⑦ **S56.423-** Laceration of extensor muscle, fascia and tendon of right middle finger at forearm level

☐ **SP** ⑦ **S56.424-** Laceration of extensor muscle, fascia and tendon of left middle finger at forearm level

☐ **SP** ⑦ **S56.425-** Laceration of extensor muscle, fascia and tendon of right ring finger at forearm level

☐ **SP** ⑦ **S56.426-** Laceration of extensor muscle, fascia and tendon of left ring finger at forearm level

☐ **SP** ⑦ **S56.427-** Laceration of extensor muscle, fascia and tendon of right little finger at forearm level

☐ **SP** ⑦ **S56.428-** Laceration of extensor muscle, fascia and tendon of left little finger at forearm level

☐ **IQ** ⑦ **S56.429-** Laceration of extensor muscle, fascia and tendon of unspecified finger at forearm level

⑥ S56.49 Other injury of extensor muscle, fascia and tendon of other and unspecified finger at forearm level

☐ **SP** ⑦ **S56.491-** Other injury of extensor muscle, fascia and tendon of right index finger at forearm level

☐ **SP** ⑦ **S56.492-** Other injury of extensor muscle, fascia and tendon of left index finger at forearm level

☐ **SP** ⑦ **S56.493-** Other injury of extensor muscle, fascia and tendon of right middle finger at forearm level

☐ **SP** ⑦ **S56.494-** Other injury of extensor muscle, fascia and tendon of left middle finger at forearm level

☐ **SP** ⑦ **S56.495-** Other injury of extensor muscle, fascia and tendon of right ring finger at forearm level

④4th digit required   ⑤5th digit required   ⑥6th digit required   ⑦7th digit required   ⑦7th digit placeholder   ➕Additional code   ☐Laterality

1546   *DecisionHealth's* FY 2020 Complete Home Health ICD-10-CM Diagnosis Coding Manual

☐ SP 7 S56.496- Other injury of extensor muscle, fascia and tendon of left ring finger at forearm level

☐ SP 7 S56.497- Other injury of extensor muscle, fascia and tendon of right little finger at forearm level

☐ SP 7 S56.498- Other injury of extensor muscle, fascia and tendon of left little finger at forearm level

☐ IQ 7 S56.499- Other injury of extensor muscle, fascia and tendon of unspecified finger at forearm level

5 S56.5 Injury of other extensor muscle, fascia and tendon at forearm level

6 S56.50 Unspecified injury of other extensor muscle, fascia and tendon at forearm level

☐ IQ 7 S56.501- Unspecified injury of other extensor muscle, fascia and tendon at forearm level, right arm

☐ IQ 7 S56.502- Unspecified injury of other extensor muscle, fascia and tendon at forearm level, left arm

☐ IQ 7 S56.509- Unspecified injury of other extensor muscle, fascia and tendon at forearm level, unspecified arm

6 S56.51 Strain of other extensor muscle, fascia and tendon at forearm level

☐ SP 7 S56.511- Strain of other extensor muscle, fascia and tendon at forearm level, right arm

☐ SP 7 S56.512- Strain of other extensor muscle, fascia and tendon at forearm level, left arm

☐ IQ 7 S56.519- Strain of other extensor muscle, fascia and tendon at forearm level, unspecified arm

6 S56.52 Laceration of other extensor muscle, fascia and tendon at forearm level

☐ SP 7 S56.521- Laceration of other extensor muscle, fascia and tendon at forearm level, right arm

☐ SP 7 S56.522- Laceration of other extensor muscle, fascia and tendon at forearm level, left arm

☐ IQ 7 S56.529- Laceration of other extensor muscle, fascia and tendon at forearm level, unspecified arm

6 S56.59 Other injury of other extensor muscle, fascia and tendon at forearm level

☐ SP 7 S56.591- Other injury of other extensor muscle, fascia and tendon at forearm level, right arm

☐ SP 7 S56.592- Other injury of other extensor muscle, fascia and tendon at forearm level, left arm

☐ IQ 7 S56.599- Other injury of other extensor muscle, fascia and tendon at forearm level, unspecified arm

5 S56.8 Injury of other muscles, fascia and tendons at forearm level

6 S56.80 Unspecified injury of other muscles, fascia and tendons at forearm level

☐ IQ 7 S56.801- Unspecified injury of other muscles, fascia and tendons at forearm level, right arm

☐ IQ 7 S56.802- Unspecified injury of other muscles, fascia and tendons at forearm level, left arm

☐ IQ 7 S56.809- Unspecified injury of other muscles, fascia and tendons at forearm level, unspecified arm

6 S56.81 Strain of other muscles, fascia and tendons at forearm level

☐ SP 7 S56.811- Strain of other muscles, fascia and tendons at forearm level, right arm

☐ SP 7 S56.812- Strain of other muscles, fascia and tendons at forearm level, left arm

☐ IQ 7 S56.819- Strain of other muscles, fascia and tendons at forearm level, unspecified arm

6 S56.82 Laceration of other muscles, fascia and tendons at forearm level

☐ SP 7 S56.821- Laceration of other muscles, fascia and tendons at forearm level, right arm

☐ SP 7 S56.822- Laceration of other muscles, fascia and tendons at forearm level, left arm

☐ IQ 7 S56.829- Laceration of other muscles, fascia and tendons at forearm level, unspecified arm

6 S56.89 Other injury of other muscles, fascia and tendons at forearm level

☐ SP 7 S56.891- Other injury of other muscles, fascia and tendons at forearm level, right arm

☐ SP 7 S56.892- Other injury of other muscles, fascia and tendons at forearm level, left arm

☐ IQ 7 S56.899- Other injury of other muscles, fascia and tendons at forearm level, unspecified arm

5 S56.9 Injury of unspecified muscles, fascia and tendons at forearm level

6 S56.90 Unspecified injury of unspecified muscles, fascia and tendons at forearm level

☐ IQ 7 S56.901- Unspecified injury of unspecified muscles, fascia and tendons at forearm level, right arm

☐ IQ 7 S56.902- Unspecified injury of unspecified muscles, fascia and tendons at forearm level, left arm

☐ IQ 7 S56.909- Unspecified injury of unspecified muscles, fascia and tendons at forearm level, unspecified arm

6 S56.91 Strain of unspecified muscles, fascia and tendons at forearm level

☐ SP 7 S56.911- Strain of unspecified muscles, fascia and tendons at forearm level, right arm

★ New ▲ Revised Px Primary SP PDGM Px SL Low CoM SH High CoM IQ Quest. Encounter H Hospice non-cancer Dx Unspecified M Manifestation

DecisionHealth's FY 2020 Complete Home Health ICD-10-CM Diagnosis Coding Manual
1547

Chapter 19

S00-T88

⊟ SP 7 **S56.912-** Strain of unspecified muscles, fascia and tendons at forearm level, left arm

⊟ SP 7 **S56.919-** Strain of unspecified muscles, fascia and tendons at forearm level, unspecified arm

6 **S56.92** Laceration of unspecified muscles, fascia and tendons at forearm level

⊟ SP 7 **S56.921-** Laceration of unspecified muscles, fascia and tendons at forearm level, right arm

⊟ SP 7 **S56.922-** Laceration of unspecified muscles, fascia and tendons at forearm level, left arm

⊟ SP 7 **S56.929-** Laceration of unspecified muscles, fascia and tendons at forearm level, unspecified arm

6 **S56.99** Other injury of unspecified muscles, fascia and tendons at forearm level

⊟ IQ 7 **S56.991-** Other injury of unspecified muscles, fascia and tendons at forearm level, right arm

⊟ IQ 7 **S56.992-** Other injury of unspecified muscles, fascia and tendons at forearm level, left arm

⊟ IQ 7 **S56.999-** Other injury of unspecified muscles, fascia and tendons at forearm level, unspecified arm

✚ 4 **S57** Crushing injury of elbow and forearm
Use additional code(s) for all associated injuries
EXCLUDES 2 crushing injury of wrist and hand (S67.-)

The appropriate 7th character is to be added to each code from category S57
A   initial encounter
D   subsequent encounter
S   sequela

✚ 5 **S57.0** Crushing injury of elbow

⊟ IQ ✚ 7 **S57.00X-** Crushing injury of unspecified elbow

⊟ SP ✚ 7 **S57.01X-** Crushing injury of right elbow

⊟ SP ✚ 7 **S57.02X-** Crushing injury of left elbow

✚ 5 **S57.8** Crushing injury of forearm

⊟ IQ ✚ 7 **S57.80X-** Crushing injury of unspecified forearm

⊟ SP ✚ 7 **S57.81X-** Crushing injury of right forearm

⊟ SP ✚ 7 **S57.82X-** Crushing injury of left forearm

4 **S58** Traumatic amputation of elbow and forearm
An amputation not identified as partial or complete should be coded to complete
EXCLUDES 1 traumatic amputation of wrist and hand (S68.-)

The appropriate 7th character is to be added to each code from category S58
A   initial encounter
D   subsequent encounter
S   sequela

CODING TIPS ✓ Use these codes only when the amputation was due to trauma. There is no need for adding Z89 with traumatic amputations. See Z47.81 for care of amputations not due to trauma.

5 **S58.0** Traumatic amputation at elbow level

6 **S58.01** Complete traumatic amputation at elbow level

⊟ SP 7 **S58.011-** Complete traumatic amputation at elbow level, right arm

⊟ SP 7 **S58.012-** Complete traumatic amputation at elbow level, left arm

⊟ IQ 7 **S58.019-** Complete traumatic amputation at elbow level, unspecified arm

6 **S58.02** Partial traumatic amputation at elbow level

⊟ SP 7 **S58.021-** Partial traumatic amputation at elbow level, right arm

⊟ SP 7 **S58.022-** Partial traumatic amputation at elbow level, left arm

⊟ IQ 7 **S58.029-** Partial traumatic amputation at elbow level, unspecified arm

5 **S58.1** Traumatic amputation at level between elbow and wrist

6 **S58.11** Complete traumatic amputation at level between elbow and wrist

⊟ SP 7 **S58.111-** Complete traumatic amputation at level between elbow and wrist, right arm

⊟ SP 7 **S58.112-** Complete traumatic amputation at level between elbow and wrist, left arm

⊟ IQ 7 **S58.119-** Complete traumatic amputation at level between elbow and wrist, unspecified arm

6 **S58.12** Partial traumatic amputation at level between elbow and wrist

⊟ SP 7 **S58.121-** Partial traumatic amputation at level between elbow and wrist, right arm

⊟ SP 7 **S58.122-** Partial traumatic amputation at level between elbow and wrist, left arm

⊟ SP IQ 7 **S58.129-** Partial traumatic amputation at level between elbow and wrist, unspecified arm

5 **S58.9** Traumatic amputation of forearm, level unspecified
EXCLUDES 1 traumatic amputation of wrist (S68.-)

6 **S58.91** Complete traumatic amputation of forearm, level unspecified

⊟ SP 7 **S58.911-** Complete traumatic amputation of right forearm, level unspecified

⊟ SP 7 **S58.912-** Complete traumatic amputation of left forearm, level unspecified

⊟ IQ 7 **S58.919-** Complete traumatic amputation of unspecified forearm, level unspecified

6 **S58.92** Partial traumatic amputation of forearm, level unspecified

⊟ SP 7 **S58.921-** Partial traumatic amputation of right forearm, level unspecified

⊟ SP 7 **S58.922-** Partial traumatic amputation of left forearm, level unspecified

4 4th digit required   5 5th digit required   6 6th digit required   7 7th digit required   7 7th digit placeholder   ✚ Additional code   ⊟ Laterality

1548   *DecisionHealth's* FY 2020 Complete Home Health ICD-10-CM Diagnosis Coding Manual

⊟ **IQ** 7 S58.929- **Partial traumatic amputation of unspecified forearm, level unspecified**

4 S59 **Other and unspecified injuries of elbow and forearm**

> **EXCLUDES 2** other and unspecified injuries of wrist and hand (S69.-)

> The appropriate 7th character is to be added to each code from subcategories S59.0, S59.1, and S59.2
>
> A   initial encounter for closed fracture
> D   subsequent encounter for fracture with routine healing
> G   subsequent encounter for fracture with delayed healing
> K   subsequent encounter for fracture with nonunion
> P   subsequent encounter for fracture with malunion
> S   sequela

5 S59.0 **Physeal fracture of lower end of ulna**

6 S59.00 **Unspecified physeal fracture of lower end of ulna**

⊟ **SP** 7 S59.001- **Unspecified physeal fracture of lower end of ulna, right arm**

⊟ **SP** 7 S59.002- **Unspecified physeal fracture of lower end of ulna, left arm**

⊟ **IQ** 7 S59.009- **Unspecified physeal fracture of lower end of ulna, unspecified arm**

6 S59.01 Salter-Harris Type I physeal fracture of lower end of ulna

⊟ **SP** 7 S59.011- Salter-Harris Type I physeal fracture of lower end of ulna, right arm

⊟ **SP** 7 S59.012- Salter-Harris Type I physeal fracture of lower end of ulna, left arm

⊟ **IQ** 7 S59.019- **Salter-Harris Type I physeal fracture of lower end of ulna, unspecified arm**

6 S59.02 Salter-Harris Type II physeal fracture of lower end of ulna

⊟ **SP** 7 S59.021- Salter-Harris Type II physeal fracture of lower end of ulna, right arm

⊟ **SP** 7 S59.022- Salter-Harris Type II physeal fracture of lower end of ulna, left arm

⊟ **IQ** 7 S59.029- **Salter-Harris Type II physeal fracture of lower end of ulna, unspecified arm**

6 S59.03 Salter-Harris Type III physeal fracture of lower end of ulna

⊟ **SP** 7 S59.031- Salter-Harris Type III physeal fracture of lower end of ulna, right arm

⊟ **SP** 7 S59.032- Salter-Harris Type III physeal fracture of lower end of ulna, left arm

⊟ **IQ** 7 S59.039- **Salter-Harris Type III physeal fracture of lower end of ulna, unspecified arm**

6 S59.04 Salter-Harris Type IV physeal fracture of lower end of ulna

⊟ **SP** 7 S59.041- Salter-Harris Type IV physeal fracture of lower end of ulna, right arm

⊟ **SP** 7 S59.042- Salter-Harris Type IV physeal fracture of lower end of ulna, left arm

⊟ **IQ** 7 S59.049- **Salter-Harris Type IV physeal fracture of lower end of ulna, unspecified arm**

6 S59.09 Other physeal fracture of lower end of ulna

⊟ **SP** 7 S59.091- Other physeal fracture of lower end of ulna, right arm

⊟ **SP** 7 S59.092- Other physeal fracture of lower end of ulna, left arm

⊟ **IQ** 7 S59.099- **Other physeal fracture of lower end of ulna, unspecified arm**

5 S59.1 Physeal fracture of upper end of radius

6 S59.10 **Unspecified physeal fracture of upper end of radius**

⊟ **SP** 7 S59.101- **Unspecified physeal fracture of upper end of radius, right arm**

⊟ **SP** 7 S59.102- **Unspecified physeal fracture of upper end of radius, left arm**

⊟ **SP** **IQ** 7 S59.109- **Unspecified physeal fracture of upper end of radius, unspecified arm**

6 S59.11 Salter-Harris Type I physeal fracture of upper end of radius

⊟ **SP** 7 S59.111- Salter-Harris Type I physeal fracture of upper end of radius, right arm

⊟ **SP** 7 S59.112- Salter-Harris Type I physeal fracture of upper end of radius, left arm

⊟ **IQ** 7 S59.119- **Salter-Harris Type I physeal fracture of upper end of radius, unspecified arm**

6 S59.12 Salter-Harris Type II physeal fracture of upper end of radius

⊟ **SP** 7 S59.121- Salter-Harris Type II physeal fracture of upper end of radius, right arm

⊟ **SP** 7 S59.122- Salter-Harris Type II physeal fracture of upper end of radius, left arm

⊟ **IQ** 7 S59.129- **Salter-Harris Type II physeal fracture of upper end of radius, unspecified arm**

6 S59.13 Salter-Harris Type III physeal fracture of upper end of radius

⊟ **SP** 7 S59.131- Salter-Harris Type III physeal fracture of upper end of radius, right arm

⊟ **SP** 7 S59.132- Salter-Harris Type III physeal fracture of upper end of radius, left arm

⊟ **IQ** 7 S59.139- **Salter-Harris Type III physeal fracture of upper end of radius, unspecified arm**

6 S59.14 Salter-Harris Type IV physeal fracture of upper end of radius

⊟ **SP** 7 S59.141- Salter-Harris Type IV physeal fracture of upper end of radius, right arm

Chapter 19

S00-T88

★ New ▲ Revised Px Primary **SP** PDGM Px **SL** Low CoM **SH** High CoM **IQ** Quest. Encounter H Hospice non-cancer Dx | Unspecified | M *Manifestation*

Chapter 19

S00-T88

□ **SP** 7 S59.142- Salter-Harris Type IV physeal fracture of upper end of radius, left arm

□ **!Q** 7 S59.149- Salter-Harris Type IV physeal fracture of upper end of radius, unspecified arm

6 S59.19 Other physeal fracture of upper end of radius

□ **SP** 7 S59.191- Other physeal fracture of upper end of radius, right arm

□ **SP** 7 S59.192- Other physeal fracture of upper end of radius, left arm

□ **!Q** 7 S59.199- Other physeal fracture of upper end of radius, unspecified arm

5 S59.2 Physeal fracture of lower end of radius

6 S59.20 Unspecified physeal fracture of lower end of radius

□ **SP** 7 S59.201- Unspecified physeal fracture of lower end of radius, right arm

□ **SP** 7 S59.202- Unspecified physeal fracture of lower end of radius, left arm

□ **!Q** 7 S59.209- Unspecified physeal fracture of lower end of radius, unspecified arm

6 S59.21 Salter-Harris Type I physeal fracture of lower end of radius

□ **SP** 7 S59.211- Salter-Harris Type I physeal fracture of lower end of radius, right arm

□ **SP** 7 S59.212- Salter-Harris Type I physeal fracture of lower end of radius, left arm

□ **!Q** 7 S59.219- Salter-Harris Type I physeal fracture of lower end of radius, unspecified arm

6 S59.22 Salter-Harris Type II physeal fracture of lower end of radius

□ **SP** 7 S59.221- Salter-Harris Type II physeal fracture of lower end of radius, right arm

□ **SP** 7 S59.222- Salter-Harris Type II physeal fracture of lower end of radius, left arm

□ **!Q** 7 S59.229- Salter-Harris Type II physeal fracture of lower end of radius, unspecified arm

6 S59.23 Salter-Harris Type III physeal fracture of lower end of radius

□ **SP** 7 S59.231- Salter-Harris Type III physeal fracture of lower end of radius, right arm

□ **SP** 7 S59.232- Salter-Harris Type III physeal fracture of lower end of radius, left arm

□ **!Q** 7 S59.239- Salter-Harris Type III physeal fracture of lower end of radius, unspecified arm

6 S59.24 Salter-Harris Type IV physeal fracture of lower end of radius

□ **SP** 7 S59.241- Salter-Harris Type IV physeal fracture of lower end of radius, right arm

□ **SP** 7 S59.242- Salter-Harris Type IV physeal fracture of lower end of radius, left arm

□ **!Q** 7 S59.249- Salter-Harris Type IV physeal fracture of lower end of radius, unspecified arm

6 S59.29 Other physeal fracture of lower end of radius

□ **SP** 7 S59.291- Other physeal fracture of lower end of radius, right arm

□ **SP** 7 S59.292- Other physeal fracture of lower end of radius, left arm

□ **!Q** 7 S59.299- Other physeal fracture of lower end of radius, unspecified arm

5 S59.8 Other specified injuries of elbow and forearm

The appropriate 7th character is to be added to each code in subcategory S59.8
A   initial encounter
D   subsequent encounter
S   sequela

6 S59.80 Other specified injuries of elbow

□ **SP** 7 S59.801- Other specified injuries of right elbow

□ **SP** 7 S59.802- Other specified injuries of left elbow

□ **!Q** 7 S59.809- Other specified injuries of unspecified elbow

6 S59.81 Other specified injuries of forearm

□ **SP** 7 S59.811- Other specified injuries right forearm

□ **SP** 7 S59.812- Other specified injuries left forearm

□ **!Q** 7 S59.819- Other specified injuries unspecified forearm

5 S59.9 Unspecified injury of elbow and forearm

The appropriate 7th character is to be added to each code in subcategory S59.9
A   initial encounter
D   subsequent encounter
S   sequela

6 S59.90 Unspecified injury of elbow

□ **!Q** 7 S59.901- Unspecified injury of right elbow

□ **!Q** 7 S59.902- Unspecified injury of left elbow

□ **!Q** 7 S59.909- Unspecified injury of unspecified elbow

6 S59.91 Unspecified injury of forearm

□ **!Q** 7 S59.911- Unspecified injury of right forearm

□ **!Q** 7 S59.912- Unspecified injury of left forearm

□ **!Q** 7 S59.919- Unspecified injury of unspecified forearm

Injuries to the wrist, hand and fingers (S60-S69)

EXCLUDES 2   burns and corrosions (T20-T32)
                frostbite (T33-T34)
                insect bite or sting, venomous (T63.4)

GUIDELINES   Section I.C.19.c.2)
Multiple fractures are sequenced in accordance with the severity of the fracture.

◨ 4th digit required   ⑤ 5th digit required   ⑥ 6th digit required   ⑦ 7th digit required   ⑦ 7th digit placeholder   ✚ Additional code   □ Laterality

1550   *DecisionHealth's* FY 2020 Complete Home Health ICD-10-CM Diagnosis Coding Manual

Chapter 19

S00-T88

GUIDELINES   Section I.C.19.b.1)-2)

When coding injuries, assign separate codes for each injury unless a combination code is provided, in which case the combination code is assigned ... Traumatic injury codes (S00-T14.9) are not to be used for normal, healing surgical wounds or to identify complications of surgical wounds. The code for the most serious injury, as determined by the provider and the focus of treatment, is sequenced first.

1) Superficial injuries such as abrasions or contusions are not coded when associated with more severe injuries of the same site.

2) When a primary injury results in minor damage to peripheral nerves or blood vessels, the primary injury is sequenced first with additional code(s) for injuries to nerves and spinal cord (such as category S04), and/or injury to blood vessels (such as category S15). When the primary injury is to the blood vessels or nerves, that injury should be sequenced first.

GUIDELINES   Section I.C.19.c

Coding of Traumatic Fractures: The principles of multiple coding of injuries should be followed in coding fractures. Fractures of specified sites are coded individually by site in accordance with both the provisions within categories S02, S12, S22, S32, S42, S49, S52, S59, S62, S72, S79, S82, S89, S92 and the level of detail furnished by medical record content. A fracture not indicated as open or closed should be coded to closed. A fracture not indicated whether displaced or not displaced should be coded to displaced.

CODING TIPS ✓   7th character A is acceptable in home health and hospice when active treatment is provided, such as antibiotics for an infected wound or a wound vac for a dehisced wound. D is used when the complication or injury is now healing. Think of D as aftercare. S is used for sequela of the injury or complication. Sequela is a residual deficit or condition produced as a result of the injury or complication after the original injury or complication has healed.

4 S60   **Superficial injury of wrist, hand and fingers**

> The appropriate 7th character is to be added to each code from category S60
> A   initial encounter
> D   subsequent encounter
> S   sequela

5 S60.0   **Contusion of finger without damage to nail**
> **EXCLUDES 1**   contusion involving nail (matrix) (S60.1)

IQ 7 S60.00X-   Contusion of unspecified finger without damage to nail
> Contusion of finger(s) NOS

6 S60.01   **Contusion of thumb without damage to nail**

IQ 7 S60.011-   Contusion of right thumb without damage to nail

IQ 7 S60.012-   Contusion of left thumb without damage to nail

IQ 7 S60.019-   Contusion of unspecified thumb without damage to nail

6 S60.02   **Contusion of index finger without damage to nail**

IQ 7 S60.021-   Contusion of right index finger without damage to nail

IQ 7 S60.022-   Contusion of left index finger without damage to nail

IQ 7 S60.029-   Contusion of unspecified index finger without damage to nail

6 S60.03   **Contusion of middle finger without damage to nail**

IQ 7 S60.031-   Contusion of right middle finger without damage to nail

IQ 7 S60.032-   Contusion of left middle finger without damage to nail

IQ 7 S60.039-   Contusion of unspecified middle finger without damage to nail

6 S60.04   **Contusion of ring finger without damage to nail**

IQ 7 S60.041-   Contusion of right ring finger without damage to nail

IQ 7 S60.042-   Contusion of left ring finger without damage to nail

IQ 7 S60.049-   Contusion of unspecified ring finger without damage to nail

6 S60.05   **Contusion of little finger without damage to nail**

IQ 7 S60.051-   Contusion of right little finger without damage to nail

IQ 7 S60.052-   Contusion of left little finger without damage to nail

IQ 7 S60.059-   Contusion of unspecified little finger without damage to nail

5 S60.1   **Contusion of finger with damage to nail**

IQ 7 S60.10X-   Contusion of unspecified finger with damage to nail

6 S60.11   **Contusion of thumb with damage to nail**

IQ 7 S60.111-   Contusion of right thumb with damage to nail

IQ 7 S60.112-   Contusion of left thumb with damage to nail

IQ 7 S60.119-   Contusion of unspecified thumb with damage to nail

6 S60.12   **Contusion of index finger with damage to nail**

IQ 7 S60.121-   Contusion of right index finger with damage to nail

IQ 7 S60.122-   Contusion of left index finger with damage to nail

IQ 7 S60.129-   Contusion of unspecified index finger with damage to nail

6 S60.13   **Contusion of middle finger with damage to nail**

IQ 7 S60.131-   Contusion of right middle finger with damage to nail

IQ 7 S60.132-   Contusion of left middle finger with damage to nail

IQ 7 S60.139-   Contusion of unspecified middle finger with damage to nail

6 S60.14   **Contusion of ring finger with damage to nail**

IQ 7 S60.141-   Contusion of right ring finger with damage to nail

IQ 7 S60.142-   Contusion of left ring finger with damage to nail

IQ 7 S60.149-   Contusion of unspecified ring finger with damage to nail

6 S60.15   **Contusion of little finger with damage to nail**

★ New ▲ Revised Px Primary **SP** PDGM Px **SL** Low CoM **SH** High CoM **IQ** Quest. Encounter **H** Hospice non-cancer Dx   Unspecified   **M** *Manifestation*

DecisionHealth's FY 2020 Complete Home Health ICD-10-CM Diagnosis Coding Manual   1551

▣ **IQ** ⑦ **S60.151-** Contusion of right little finger with damage to nail

▣ **IQ** ⑦ **S60.152-** Contusion of left little finger with damage to nail

▣ **IQ** ⑦ **S60.159-** Contusion of unspecified little finger with damage to nail

⑤ **S60.2** Contusion of wrist and hand
EXCLUDES 2 contusion of fingers (S60.0-, S60.1-)

⑥ **S60.21** Contusion of wrist

▣ **IQ** ⑦ **S60.211-** Contusion of right wrist

▣ **IQ** ⑦ **S60.212-** Contusion of left wrist

▣ **IQ** ⑦ **S60.219-** Contusion of unspecified wrist

⑥ **S60.22** Contusion of hand

▣ **IQ** ⑦ **S60.221-** Contusion of right hand

▣ **IQ** ⑦ **S60.222-** Contusion of left hand

▣ **IQ** ⑦ **S60.229-** Contusion of unspecified hand

⑤ **S60.3** Other superficial injuries of thumb

⑥ **S60.31** Abrasion of thumb

▣ **IQ** ⑦ **S60.311-** Abrasion of right thumb

▣ **IQ** ⑦ **S60.312-** Abrasion of left thumb

▣ **IQ** ⑦ **S60.319-** Abrasion of unspecified thumb

⑥ **S60.32** Blister (nonthermal) of thumb

▣ **IQ** ⑦ **S60.321-** Blister (nonthermal) of right thumb

▣ **IQ** ⑦ **S60.322-** Blister (nonthermal) of left thumb

▣ **IQ** ⑦ **S60.329-** Blister (nonthermal) of unspecified thumb

✚ ⑥ **S60.34** External constriction of thumb
Hair tourniquet syndrome of thumb
Use additional cause code to identify the constricting item (W49.0-)

▣ **IQ** ✚ ⑦ **S60.341-** External constriction of right thumb

▣ **IQ** ✚ ⑦ **S60.342-** External constriction of left thumb

▣ **IQ** ✚ ⑦ **S60.349-** External constriction of unspecified thumb

⑥ **S60.35** Superficial foreign body of thumb
Splinter in the thumb

▣ **IQ** ⑦ **S60.351-** Superficial foreign body of right thumb

▣ **IQ** ⑦ **S60.352-** Superficial foreign body of left thumb

▣ **IQ** ⑦ **S60.359-** Superficial foreign body of unspecified thumb

⑥ **S60.36** Insect bite (nonvenomous) of thumb

▣ **IQ** ⑦ **S60.361-** Insect bite (nonvenomous) of right thumb

▣ **IQ** ⑦ **S60.362-** Insect bite (nonvenomous) of left thumb

▣ **IQ** ⑦ **S60.369-** Insect bite (nonvenomous) of unspecified thumb

⑥ **S60.37** Other superficial bite of thumb
EXCLUDES 1 open bite of thumb (S61.05-, S61.15-)

▣ **IQ** ⑦ **S60.371-** Other superficial bite of right thumb

▣ **IQ** ⑦ **S60.372-** Other superficial bite of left thumb

▣ **IQ** ⑦ **S60.379-** Other superficial bite of unspecified thumb

⑥ **S60.39** Other superficial injuries of thumb

▣ **IQ** ⑦ **S60.391-** Other superficial injuries of right thumb

▣ **IQ** ⑦ **S60.392-** Other superficial injuries of left thumb

▣ **IQ** ⑦ **S60.399-** Other superficial injuries of unspecified thumb

⑤ **S60.4** Other superficial injuries of other fingers

⑥ **S60.41** Abrasion of fingers

▣ **IQ** ⑦ **S60.410-** Abrasion of right index finger

▣ **IQ** ⑦ **S60.411-** Abrasion of left index finger

▣ **IQ** ⑦ **S60.412-** Abrasion of right middle finger

▣ **IQ** ⑦ **S60.413-** Abrasion of left middle finger

▣ **IQ** ⑦ **S60.414-** Abrasion of right ring finger

▣ **IQ** ⑦ **S60.415-** Abrasion of left ring finger

▣ **IQ** ⑦ **S60.416-** Abrasion of right little finger

▣ **IQ** ⑦ **S60.417-** Abrasion of left little finger

▣ **IQ** ⑦ **S60.418-** Abrasion of other finger
Abrasion of specified finger with unspecified laterality

▣ **IQ** ⑦ **S60.419-** Abrasion of unspecified finger

⑥ **S60.42** Blister (nonthermal) of fingers

▣ **IQ** ⑦ **S60.420-** Blister (nonthermal) of right index finger

▣ **IQ** ⑦ **S60.421-** Blister (nonthermal) of left index finger

▣ **IQ** ⑦ **S60.422-** Blister (nonthermal) of right middle finger

▣ **IQ** ⑦ **S60.423-** Blister (nonthermal) of left middle finger

▣ **IQ** ⑦ **S60.424-** Blister (nonthermal) of right ring finger

▣ **IQ** ⑦ **S60.425-** Blister (nonthermal) of left ring finger

▣ **IQ** ⑦ **S60.426-** Blister (nonthermal) of right little finger

▣ **IQ** ⑦ **S60.427-** Blister (nonthermal) of left little finger

▣ **IQ** ⑦ **S60.428-** Blister (nonthermal) of other finger
Blister (nonthermal) of specified finger with unspecified laterality

▣ **IQ** ⑦ **S60.429-** Blister (nonthermal) of unspecified finger

✚ ⑥ **S60.44** External constriction of fingers
Hair tourniquet syndrome of finger
Use additional cause code to identify the constricting item (W49.0-)

▣ **IQ** ✚ ⑦ **S60.440-** External constriction of right index finger

▣ **IQ** ✚ ⑦ **S60.441-** External constriction of left index finger

▣ **IQ** ✚ ⑦ **S60.442-** External constriction of right middle finger

▣ **IQ** ✚ ⑦ **S60.443-** External constriction of left middle finger

▣ **IQ** ✚ ⑦ **S60.444-** External constriction of right ring finger

▣ **IQ** ✚ ⑦ **S60.445-** External constriction of left ring finger

▣ **IQ** ✚ ⑦ **S60.446-** External constriction of right little finger

▣ **IQ** ✚ ⑦ **S60.447-** External constriction of left little finger

Chapter 19
S00-T88

④4th digit required   ⑤5th digit required   ⑥6th digit required   ⑦7th digit required   ⑦7th digit placeholder   ✚Additional code   ▣Laterality

1552   *DecisionHealth's* FY 2020 Complete Home Health ICD-10-CM Diagnosis Coding Manual

▣ **IQ** ✚ ⑦ **S60.448-** External constriction of other finger
External constriction of specified finger with unspecified laterality

▣ **IQ** ✚ ⑦ **S60.449-** External constriction of unspecified finger

⑥ **S60.45** Superficial foreign body of fingers
Splinter in the finger(s)

▣ **IQ** ⑦ **S60.450-** Superficial foreign body of right index finger

▣ **IQ** ⑦ **S60.451-** Superficial foreign body of left index finger

▣ **IQ** ⑦ **S60.452-** Superficial foreign body of right middle finger

▣ **IQ** ⑦ **S60.453-** Superficial foreign body of left middle finger

▣ **IQ** ⑦ **S60.454-** Superficial foreign body of right ring finger

▣ **IQ** ⑦ **S60.455-** Superficial foreign body of left ring finger

▣ **IQ** ⑦ **S60.456-** Superficial foreign body of right little finger

▣ **IQ** ⑦ **S60.457-** Superficial foreign body of left little finger

▣ **IQ** ⑦ **S60.458-** Superficial foreign body of other finger
Superficial foreign body of specified finger with unspecified laterality

▣ **IQ** ⑦ **S60.459-** Superficial foreign body of unspecified finger

⑥ **S60.46** Insect bite (nonvenomous) of fingers

▣ **IQ** ⑦ **S60.460-** Insect bite (nonvenomous) of right index finger

▣ **IQ** ⑦ **S60.461-** Insect bite (nonvenomous) of left index finger

▣ **IQ** ⑦ **S60.462-** Insect bite (nonvenomous) of right middle finger

▣ **IQ** ⑦ **S60.463-** Insect bite (nonvenomous) of left middle finger

▣ **IQ** ⑦ **S60.464-** Insect bite (nonvenomous) of right ring finger

▣ **IQ** ⑦ **S60.465-** Insect bite (nonvenomous) of left ring finger

▣ **IQ** ⑦ **S60.466-** Insect bite (nonvenomous) of right little finger

▣ **IQ** ⑦ **S60.467-** Insect bite (nonvenomous) of left little finger

▣ **IQ** ⑦ **S60.468-** Insect bite (nonvenomous) of other finger
Insect bite (nonvenomous) of specified finger with unspecified laterality

▣ **IQ** ⑦ **S60.469-** Insect bite (nonvenomous) of unspecified finger

⑥ **S60.47** Other superficial bite of fingers
EXCLUDES 1 open bite of fingers (S61.25-, S61.35-)

▣ **IQ** ⑦ **S60.470-** Other superficial bite of right index finger

▣ **IQ** ⑦ **S60.471-** Other superficial bite of left index finger

▣ **IQ** ⑦ **S60.472-** Other superficial bite of right middle finger

▣ **IQ** ⑦ **S60.473-** Other superficial bite of left middle finger

▣ **IQ** ⑦ **S60.474-** Other superficial bite of right ring finger

▣ **IQ** ⑦ **S60.475-** Other superficial bite of left ring finger

▣ **IQ** ⑦ **S60.476-** Other superficial bite of right little finger

▣ **IQ** ⑦ **S60.477-** Other superficial bite of left little finger

▣ **IQ** ⑦ **S60.478-** Other superficial bite of other finger
Other superficial bite of specified finger with unspecified laterality

▣ **IQ** ⑦ **S60.479-** Other superficial bite of unspecified finger

⑤ **S60.5** Other superficial injuries of hand
EXCLUDES 2 superficial injuries of fingers (S60.3-, S60.4-)

⑥ **S60.51** Abrasion of hand

▣ **IQ** ⑦ **S60.511-** Abrasion of right hand

▣ **IQ** ⑦ **S60.512-** Abrasion of left hand

▣ **IQ** ⑦ **S60.519-** Abrasion of unspecified hand

⑥ **S60.52** Blister (nonthermal) of hand

▣ **IQ** ⑦ **S60.521-** Blister (nonthermal) of right hand

▣ **IQ** ⑦ **S60.522-** Blister (nonthermal) of left hand

▣ **IQ** ⑦ **S60.529-** Blister (nonthermal) of unspecified hand

⑥ **S60.54** External constriction of hand

▣ **IQ** ⑦ **S60.541-** External constriction of right hand

▣ **IQ** ⑦ **S60.542-** External constriction of left hand

▣ **IQ** ⑦ **S60.549-** External constriction of unspecified hand

⑥ **S60.55** Superficial foreign body of hand
Splinter in the hand

▣ **IQ** ⑦ **S60.551-** Superficial foreign body of right hand

▣ **IQ** ⑦ **S60.552-** Superficial foreign body of left hand

▣ **IQ** ⑦ **S60.559-** Superficial foreign body of unspecified hand

⑥ **S60.56** Insect bite (nonvenomous) of hand

▣ **IQ** ⑦ **S60.561-** Insect bite (nonvenomous) of right hand

▣ **IQ** ⑦ **S60.562-** Insect bite (nonvenomous) of left hand

▣ **IQ** ⑦ **S60.569-** Insect bite (nonvenomous) of unspecified hand

⑥ **S60.57** Other superficial bite of hand
EXCLUDES 1 open bite of hand (S61.45-)

▣ **IQ** ⑦ **S60.571-** Other superficial bite of hand of right hand

▣ **IQ** ⑦ **S60.572-** Other superficial bite of hand of left hand

▣ **IQ** ⑦ **S60.579-** Other superficial bite of hand of unspecified hand

⑤ **S60.8** Other superficial injuries of wrist

⑥ **S60.81** Abrasion of wrist

▣ **IQ** ⑦ **S60.811-** Abrasion of right wrist

▣ **IQ** ⑦ **S60.812-** Abrasion of left wrist

▣ **IQ** ⑦ **S60.819-** Abrasion of unspecified wrist

⑥ **S60.82** Blister (nonthermal) of wrist

⭐ New ▲ Revised **Px** Primary **SP** PDGM Px **SL** Low CoM **SH** High CoM **IQ** Quest. Encounter Ⓗ Hospice non-cancer Dx Unspecified **M** *Manifestation*

DecisionHealth's FY 2020 Complete Home Health ICD-10-CM Diagnosis Coding Manual

1553

☐ !Q 7 **S60.821-** Blister (nonthermal) of right wrist

☐ !Q 7 **S60.822-** Blister (nonthermal) of left wrist

☐ !Q 7 **S60.829-** Blister (nonthermal) of unspecified wrist

6 **S60.84** External constriction of wrist

☐ !Q 7 **S60.841-** External constriction of right wrist

☐ !Q 7 **S60.842-** External constriction of left wrist

☐ !Q 7 **S60.849-** External constriction of unspecified wrist

6 **S60.85** Superficial foreign body of wrist
Splinter in the wrist

☐ !Q 7 **S60.851-** Superficial foreign body of right wrist

☐ !Q 7 **S60.852-** Superficial foreign body of left wrist

☐ !Q 7 **S60.859-** Superficial foreign body of unspecified wrist

6 **S60.86** Insect bite (nonvenomous) of wrist

☐ !Q 7 **S60.861-** Insect bite (nonvenomous) of right wrist

☐ !Q 7 **S60.862-** Insect bite (nonvenomous) of left wrist

☐ !Q 7 **S60.869-** Insect bite (nonvenomous) of unspecified wrist

6 **S60.87** Other superficial bite of wrist
EXCLUDES 1 open bite of wrist (S61.55)

☐ !Q 7 **S60.871-** Other superficial bite of right wrist

☐ !Q 7 **S60.872-** Other superficial bite of left wrist

☐ !Q 7 **S60.879-** Other superficial bite of unspecified wrist

5 **S60.9** Unspecified superficial injury of wrist, hand and fingers

6 **S60.91** Unspecified superficial injury of wrist

☐ !Q 7 **S60.911-** Unspecified superficial injury of right wrist

☐ !Q 7 **S60.912-** Unspecified superficial injury of left wrist

☐ !Q 7 **S60.919-** Unspecified superficial injury of unspecified wrist

6 **S60.92** Unspecified superficial injury of hand

☐ !Q 7 **S60.921-** Unspecified superficial injury of right hand

☐ !Q 7 **S60.922-** Unspecified superficial injury of left hand

☐ !Q 7 **S60.929-** Unspecified superficial injury of unspecified hand

6 **S60.93** Unspecified superficial injury of thumb

☐ !Q 7 **S60.931-** Unspecified superficial injury of right thumb

☐ !Q 7 **S60.932-** Unspecified superficial injury of left thumb

☐ !Q 7 **S60.939-** Unspecified superficial injury of unspecified thumb

6 **S60.94** Unspecified superficial injury of other fingers

☐ !Q 7 **S60.940-** Unspecified superficial injury of right index finger

☐ !Q 7 **S60.941-** Unspecified superficial injury of left index finger

☐ !Q 7 **S60.942-** Unspecified superficial injury of right middle finger

☐ !Q 7 **S60.943-** Unspecified superficial injury of left middle finger

☐ !Q 7 **S60.944-** Unspecified superficial injury of right ring finger

☐ !Q 7 **S60.945-** Unspecified superficial injury of left ring finger

☐ !Q 7 **S60.946-** Unspecified superficial injury of right little finger

☐ !Q 7 **S60.947-** Unspecified superficial injury of left little finger

☐ !Q 7 **S60.948-** Unspecified superficial injury of other finger
Unspecified superficial injury of specified finger with unspecified laterality

☐ !Q 7 **S60.949-** Unspecified superficial injury of unspecified finger

4 **S61** Open wound of wrist, hand and fingers
Code also:
any associated wound infection
EXCLUDES 1 open fracture of wrist, hand and finger
(S62.- with 7th character B)
traumatic amputation of wrist and hand (S68.-)

The appropriate 7th character is to be added to each code from category S61
A   initial encounter
D   subsequent encounter
S   sequela

CODING TIPS ✓ No aftercare code applies, including those indicating dressing changes, drain care, or suture removal. 7th character 'D' is the default for home care and hospice when providing aftercare for a healing or resolving condition; 'A' is used for active treatment such as antibiotics or more than routine wound care; 'S' may be used to indicate a residual condition after the original injury has healed.

CODING TIPS ✓ Open wound codes indicate a wound resulting from a traumatic origin. Do not assign a code for "open wound" unless the etiology of the wound is related to trauma.

5 **S61.0** Open wound of thumb without damage to nail
EXCLUDES 1 open wound of thumb with damage to nail (S61.1-)

6 **S61.00** Unspecified open wound of thumb without damage to nail

☐ SP 7 **S61.001-** Unspecified open wound of right thumb without damage to nail

☐ SP 7 **S61.002-** Unspecified open wound of left thumb without damage to nail

☐ !Q 7 **S61.009-** Unspecified open wound of unspecified thumb without damage to nail

---

4 4th digit required   5 5th digit required   6 6th digit required   7 7th digit required   ⌀ 7th digit placeholder   + Additional code   ☐ Laterality

⑥ **S61.01** **Laceration without foreign body of thumb without damage to nail**

▤ **SP** ⑦ **S61.011-** Laceration without foreign body of right thumb without damage to nail

▤ **SP** ⑦ **S61.012-** Laceration without foreign body of left thumb without damage to nail

▤ **IQ** ⑦ **S61.019-** Laceration without foreign body of unspecified thumb without damage to nail

⑥ **S61.02** **Laceration with foreign body of thumb without damage to nail**

▤ **SP** ⑦ **S61.021-** Laceration with foreign body of right thumb without damage to nail

▤ **SP** ⑦ **S61.022-** Laceration with foreign body of left thumb without damage to nail

▤ **IQ** ⑦ **S61.029-** Laceration with foreign body of unspecified thumb without damage to nail

⑥ **S61.03** **Puncture wound without foreign body of thumb without damage to nail**

▤ **SP** ⑦ **S61.031-** Puncture wound without foreign body of right thumb without damage to nail

▤ **SP** ⑦ **S61.032-** Puncture wound without foreign body of left thumb without damage to nail

▤ **IQ** ⑦ **S61.039-** Puncture wound without foreign body of unspecified thumb without damage to nail

⑥ **S61.04** **Puncture wound with foreign body of thumb without damage to nail**

▤ **SP** ⑦ **S61.041-** Puncture wound with foreign body of right thumb without damage to nail

▤ **SP** ⑦ **S61.042-** Puncture wound with foreign body of left thumb without damage to nail

▤ **IQ** ⑦ **S61.049-** Puncture wound with foreign body of unspecified thumb without damage to nail

⑥ **S61.05** **Open bite of thumb without damage to nail**
Bite of thumb NOS
EXCLUDES 1 superficial bite of thumb (S60.36-, S60.37-)

▤ **SP** ⑦ **S61.051-** Open bite of right thumb without damage to nail

▤ **SP** ⑦ **S61.052-** Open bite of left thumb without damage to nail

▤ **IQ** ⑦ **S61.059-** Open bite of unspecified thumb without damage to nail

⑤ **S61.1** **Open wound of thumb with damage to nail**

⑥ **S61.10** **Unspecified open wound of thumb with damage to nail**

▤ **SP** ⑦ **S61.101-** Unspecified open wound of right thumb with damage to nail

▤ **SP** ⑦ **S61.102-** Unspecified open wound of left thumb with damage to nail

▤ **IQ** ⑦ **S61.109-** Unspecified open wound of unspecified thumb with damage to nail

⑥ **S61.11** **Laceration without foreign body of thumb with damage to nail**

▤ **SP** ⑦ **S61.111-** Laceration without foreign body of right thumb with damage to nail

▤ **SP** ⑦ **S61.112-** Laceration without foreign body of left thumb with damage to nail

▤ **IQ** ⑦ **S61.119-** Laceration without foreign body of unspecified thumb with damage to nail

⑥ **S61.12** **Laceration with foreign body of thumb with damage to nail**

▤ **SP** ⑦ **S61.121-** Laceration with foreign body of right thumb with damage to nail

▤ **SP** ⑦ **S61.122-** Laceration with foreign body of left thumb with damage to nail

▤ **IQ** ⑦ **S61.129-** Laceration with foreign body of unspecified thumb with damage to nail

⑥ **S61.13** **Puncture wound without foreign body of thumb with damage to nail**

▤ **SP** ⑦ **S61.131-** Puncture wound without foreign body of right thumb with damage to nail

▤ **SP** ⑦ **S61.132-** Puncture wound without foreign body of left thumb with damage to nail

▤ **IQ** ⑦ **S61.139-** Puncture wound without foreign body of unspecified thumb with damage to nail

⑥ **S61.14** **Puncture wound with foreign body of thumb with damage to nail**

▤ **SP** ⑦ **S61.141-** Puncture wound with foreign body of right thumb with damage to nail

▤ **SP** ⑦ **S61.142-** Puncture wound with foreign body of left thumb with damage to nail

▤ **IQ** ⑦ **S61.149-** Puncture wound with foreign body of unspecified thumb with damage to nail

⑥ **S61.15** **Open bite of thumb with damage to nail**
Bite of thumb with damage to nail NOS
EXCLUDES 1 superficial bite of thumb (S60.36-, S60.37-)

▤ **SP** ⑦ **S61.151-** Open bite of right thumb with damage to nail

▤ **SP** ⑦ **S61.152-** Open bite of left thumb with damage to nail

▤ **IQ** ⑦ **S61.159-** Open bite of unspecified thumb with damage to nail

⑤ **S61.2** **Open wound of other finger without damage to nail**
EXCLUDES 1 open wound of finger involving nail (matrix) (S61.3-)
EXCLUDES 2 open wound of thumb without damage to nail (S61.0-)

⑥ **S61.20** **Unspecified open wound of other finger without damage to nail**

▤ **SP** ⑦ **S61.200-** Unspecified open wound of right index finger without damage to nail

★ New ▲ Revised **Px** Primary **SP** PDGM Px **SL** Low CoM **SH** High CoM **IQ** Quest. Encounter Ⓗ Hospice non-cancer Dx Unspecified **M** *Manifestation*

DecisionHealth's FY 2020 Complete Home Health ICD-10-CM Diagnosis Coding Manual

1555

Chapter 19

S00-T88

☐ SP 7 S61.201- **Unspecified open wound of left index finger without damage to nail**

☐ SP 7 S61.202- **Unspecified open wound of right middle finger without damage to nail**

☐ SP 7 S61.203- **Unspecified open wound of left middle finger without damage to nail**

☐ SP 7 S61.204- **Unspecified open wound of right ring finger without damage to nail**

☐ SP 7 S61.205- **Unspecified open wound of left ring finger without damage to nail**

☐ SP 7 S61.206- **Unspecified open wound of right little finger without damage to nail**

☐ SP 7 S61.207- **Unspecified open wound of left little finger without damage to nail**

☐ SP 7 S61.208- **Unspecified open wound of other finger without damage to nail**

Unspecified open wound of specified finger with unspecified laterality without damage to nail

☐ IQ 7 S61.209- **Unspecified open wound of unspecified finger without damage to nail**

6 S61.21 **Laceration without foreign body of finger without damage to nail**

☐ SP 7 S61.210- **Laceration without foreign body of right index finger without damage to nail**

☐ SP 7 S61.211- **Laceration without foreign body of left index finger without damage to nail**

☐ SP 7 S61.212- **Laceration without foreign body of right middle finger without damage to nail**

☐ SP 7 S61.213- **Laceration without foreign body of left middle finger without damage to nail**

☐ SP 7 S61.214- **Laceration without foreign body of right ring finger without damage to nail**

☐ SP 7 S61.215- **Laceration without foreign body of left ring finger without damage to nail**

☐ SP 7 S61.216- **Laceration without foreign body of right little finger without damage to nail**

☐ SP 7 S61.217- **Laceration without foreign body of left little finger without damage to nail**

☐ SP 7 S61.218- **Laceration without foreign body of other finger without damage to nail**

Laceration without foreign body of specified finger with unspecified laterality without damage to nail

☐ IQ 7 S61.219- **Laceration without foreign body of unspecified finger without damage to nail**

6 S61.22 **Laceration with foreign body of finger without damage to nail**

☐ SP 7 S61.220- **Laceration with foreign body of right index finger without damage to nail**

☐ SP 7 S61.221- **Laceration with foreign body of left index finger without damage to nail**

☐ SP 7 S61.222- **Laceration with foreign body of right middle finger without damage to nail**

☐ SP 7 S61.223- **Laceration with foreign body of left middle finger without damage to nail**

☐ SP 7 S61.224- **Laceration with foreign body of right ring finger without damage to nail**

☐ SP 7 S61.225- **Laceration with foreign body of left ring finger without damage to nail**

☐ SP 7 S61.226- **Laceration with foreign body of right little finger without damage to nail**

☐ SP 7 S61.227- **Laceration with foreign body of left little finger without damage to nail**

☐ SP 7 S61.228- **Laceration with foreign body of other finger without damage to nail**

Laceration with foreign body of specified finger with unspecified laterality without damage to nail

☐ IQ 7 S61.229- **Laceration with foreign body of unspecified finger without damage to nail**

6 S61.23 **Puncture wound without foreign body of finger without damage to nail**

☐ SP 7 S61.230- **Puncture wound without foreign body of right index finger without damage to nail**

☐ SP 7 S61.231- **Puncture wound without foreign body of left index finger without damage to nail**

☐ SP 7 S61.232- **Puncture wound without foreign body of right middle finger without damage to nail**

☐ SP 7 S61.233- **Puncture wound without foreign body of left middle finger without damage to nail**

☐ SP 7 S61.234- **Puncture wound without foreign body of right ring finger without damage to nail**

☐ SP 7 S61.235- **Puncture wound without foreign body of left ring finger without damage to nail**

☐ SP 7 S61.236- **Puncture wound without foreign body of right little finger without damage to nail**

☐ SP 7 S61.237- **Puncture wound without foreign body of left little finger without damage to nail**

☐ SP 7 S61.238- **Puncture wound without foreign body of other finger without damage to nail**

Puncture wound without foreign body of specified finger with unspecified laterality without damage to nail

4 4th digit required   5 5th digit required   6 6th digit required   7 7th digit required   7 7th digit placeholder   + Additional code   ☐ Laterality

1556   *DecisionHealth's* FY 2020 Complete Home Health ICD-10-CM Diagnosis Coding Manual

Chapter 19

S00-T88

▤ **!Q** 7 **S61.239-** **Puncture wound without foreign body of unspecified finger without damage to nail**

⑥ **S61.24** Puncture wound with foreign body of finger without damage to nail

▤ SP 7 **S61.240-** Puncture wound with foreign body of right index finger without damage to nail

▤ SP 7 **S61.241-** Puncture wound with foreign body of left index finger without damage to nail

▤ SP 7 **S61.242-** Puncture wound with foreign body of right middle finger without damage to nail

▤ SP 7 **S61.243-** Puncture wound with foreign body of left middle finger without damage to nail

▤ SP 7 **S61.244-** Puncture wound with foreign body of right ring finger without damage to nail

▤ SP 7 **S61.245-** Puncture wound with foreign body of left ring finger without damage to nail

▤ SP 7 **S61.246-** Puncture wound with foreign body of right little finger without damage to nail

▤ SP 7 **S61.247-** Puncture wound with foreign body of left little finger without damage to nail

▤ SP 7 **S61.248-** Puncture wound with foreign body of other finger without damage to nail
Puncture wound with foreign body of specified finger with unspecified laterality without damage to nail

▤ **!Q** 7 **S61.249-** **Puncture wound with foreign body of unspecified finger without damage to nail**

⑥ **S61.25** Open bite of finger without damage to nail
Bite of finger without damage to nail NOS
EXCLUDES 1 superficial bite of finger (S60.46-, S60.47-)

▤ SP 7 **S61.250-** Open bite of right index finger without damage to nail

▤ SP 7 **S61.251-** Open bite of left index finger without damage to nail

▤ SP 7 **S61.252-** Open bite of right middle finger without damage to nail

▤ SP 7 **S61.253-** Open bite of left middle finger without damage to nail

▤ SP 7 **S61.254-** Open bite of right ring finger without damage to nail

▤ SP 7 **S61.255-** Open bite of left ring finger without damage to nail

▤ SP 7 **S61.256-** Open bite of right little finger without damage to nail

▤ SP 7 **S61.257-** Open bite of left little finger without damage to nail

▤ SP 7 **S61.258-** Open bite of other finger without damage to nail
Open bite of specified finger with unspecified laterality without damage to nail

▤ **!Q** 7 **S61.259-** **Open bite of unspecified finger without damage to nail**

⑤ **S61.3** Open wound of other finger with damage to nail

⑥ **S61.30** **Unspecified open wound of finger with damage to nail**

▤ SP 7 **S61.300-** **Unspecified open wound of right index finger with damage to nail**

▤ SP 7 **S61.301-** **Unspecified open wound of left index finger with damage to nail**

▤ SP 7 **S61.302-** **Unspecified open wound of right middle finger with damage to nail**

▤ SP 7 **S61.303-** **Unspecified open wound of left middle finger with damage to nail**

▤ SP 7 **S61.304-** **Unspecified open wound of right ring finger with damage to nail**

▤ SP 7 **S61.305-** **Unspecified open wound of left ring finger with damage to nail**

▤ SP 7 **S61.306-** **Unspecified open wound of right little finger with damage to nail**

▤ SP 7 **S61.307-** **Unspecified open wound of left little finger with damage to nail**

▤ SP 7 **S61.308-** **Unspecified open wound of other finger with damage to nail**
Unspecified open wound of specified finger with unspecified laterality with damage to nail

▤ **!Q** 7 **S61.309-** **Unspecified open wound of unspecified finger with damage to nail**

⑥ **S61.31** Laceration without foreign body of finger with damage to nail

▤ SP 7 **S61.310-** Laceration without foreign body of right index finger with damage to nail

▤ SP 7 **S61.311-** Laceration without foreign body of left index finger with damage to nail

▤ SP 7 **S61.312-** Laceration without foreign body of right middle finger with damage to nail

▤ SP 7 **S61.313-** Laceration without foreign body of left middle finger with damage to nail

▤ SP 7 **S61.314-** Laceration without foreign body of right ring finger with damage to nail

▤ SP 7 **S61.315-** Laceration without foreign body of left ring finger with damage to nail

▤ SP 7 **S61.316-** Laceration without foreign body of right little finger with damage to nail

▤ SP 7 **S61.317-** Laceration without foreign body of left little finger with damage to nail

▤ SP 7 **S61.318-** Laceration without foreign body of other finger with damage to nail
Laceration without foreign body of specified finger with unspecified laterality with damage to nail

Chapter 19

S00-T88

★ New ▲ Revised Px Primary SP PDGM Px SL Low CoM SH High CoM !Q Quest. Encounter H Hospice non-cancer Dx ⬚ Unspecified M *Manifestation*

DecisionHealth's FY 2020 Complete Home Health ICD-10-CM Diagnosis Coding Manual

1557

⊟ IQ 7 **S61.319-** **Laceration without foreign body of unspecified finger with damage to nail**

6 **S61.32** Laceration with foreign body of finger with damage to nail

⊟ SP 7 **S61.320-** Laceration with foreign body of right index finger with damage to nail

⊟ SP 7 **S61.321-** Laceration with foreign body of left index finger with damage to nail

⊟ SP 7 **S61.322-** Laceration with foreign body of right middle finger with damage to nail

⊟ SP 7 **S61.323-** Laceration with foreign body of left middle finger with damage to nail

⊟ SP 7 **S61.324-** Laceration with foreign body of right ring finger with damage to nail

⊟ SP 7 **S61.325-** Laceration with foreign body of left ring finger with damage to nail

⊟ SP 7 **S61.326-** Laceration with foreign body of right little finger with damage to nail

⊟ SP 7 **S61.327-** Laceration with foreign body of left little finger with damage to nail

⊟ SP 7 **S61.328-** Laceration with foreign body of other finger with damage to nail
Laceration with foreign body of specified finger with unspecified laterality with damage to nail

⊟ IQ 7 **S61.329-** **Laceration with foreign body of unspecified finger with damage to nail**

6 **S61.33** Puncture wound without foreign body of finger with damage to nail

⊟ SP 7 **S61.330-** Puncture wound without foreign body of right index finger with damage to nail

⊟ SP 7 **S61.331-** Puncture wound without foreign body of left index finger with damage to nail

⊟ SP 7 **S61.332-** Puncture wound without foreign body of right middle finger with damage to nail

⊟ SP 7 **S61.333-** Puncture wound without foreign body of left middle finger with damage to nail

⊟ SP 7 **S61.334-** Puncture wound without foreign body of right ring finger with damage to nail

⊟ SP 7 **S61.335-** Puncture wound without foreign body of left ring finger with damage to nail

⊟ SP 7 **S61.336-** Puncture wound without foreign body of right little finger with damage to nail

⊟ SP 7 **S61.337-** Puncture wound without foreign body of left little finger with damage to nail

⊟ SP 7 **S61.338-** Puncture wound without foreign body of other finger with damage to nail

Puncture wound without foreign body of specified finger with unspecified laterality with damage to nail

⊟ IQ 7 **S61.339-** **Puncture wound without foreign body of unspecified finger with damage to nail**

6 **S61.34** Puncture wound with foreign body of finger with damage to nail

⊟ SP 7 **S61.340-** Puncture wound with foreign body of right index finger with damage to nail

⊟ SP 7 **S61.341-** Puncture wound with foreign body of left index finger with damage to nail

⊟ SP 7 **S61.342-** Puncture wound with foreign body of right middle finger with damage to nail

⊟ SP 7 **S61.343-** Puncture wound with foreign body of left middle finger with damage to nail

⊟ SP 7 **S61.344-** Puncture wound with foreign body of right ring finger with damage to nail

⊟ SP 7 **S61.345-** Puncture wound with foreign body of left ring finger with damage to nail

⊟ SP 7 **S61.346-** Puncture wound with foreign body of right little finger with damage to nail

⊟ SP 7 **S61.347-** Puncture wound with foreign body of left little finger with damage to nail

⊟ SP 7 **S61.348-** Puncture wound with foreign body of other finger with damage to nail
Puncture wound with foreign body of specified finger with unspecified laterality with damage to nail

⊟ IQ 7 **S61.349-** **Puncture wound with foreign body of unspecified finger with damage to nail**

6 **S61.35** Open bite of finger with damage to nail
Bite of finger with damage to nail NOS
EXCLUDES 1 superficial bite of finger (S60.46-, S60.47-)

⊟ SP 7 **S61.350-** Open bite of right index finger with damage to nail

⊟ SP 7 **S61.351-** Open bite of left index finger with damage to nail

⊟ SP 7 **S61.352-** Open bite of right middle finger with damage to nail

⊟ SP 7 **S61.353-** Open bite of left middle finger with damage to nail

⊟ SP 7 **S61.354-** Open bite of right ring finger with damage to nail

⊟ SP 7 **S61.355-** Open bite of left ring finger with damage to nail

⊟ SP 7 **S61.356-** Open bite of right little finger with damage to nail

⊟ SP 7 **S61.357-** Open bite of left little finger with damage to nail

⊟ SP 7 **S61.358-** Open bite of other finger with damage to nail

4 4th digit required   5 5th digit required   6 6th digit required   7 7th digit required   7 7th digit placeholder   + Additional code   ⊟ Laterality

1558   DecisionHealth's FY 2020 Complete Home Health ICD-10-CM Diagnosis Coding Manual

Open bite of specified finger with unspecified laterality with damage to nail

▤ !Q 7 **S61.359-** **Open bite of unspecified finger with damage to nail**

5 **S61.4 Open wound of hand**

6 **S61.40** **Unspecified open wound of hand**

▤ SP 7 **S61.401-** **Unspecified open wound of right hand**

▤ SP 7 **S61.402-** **Unspecified open wound of left hand**

▤ !Q 7 **S61.409-** **Unspecified open wound of unspecified hand**

6 **S61.41** Laceration without foreign body of hand

▤ SP 7 **S61.411-** Laceration without foreign body of right hand

▤ SP 7 **S61.412-** Laceration without foreign body of left hand

▤ !Q 7 **S61.419-** **Laceration without foreign body of unspecified hand**

6 **S61.42** Laceration with foreign body of hand

▤ SP 7 **S61.421-** Laceration with foreign body of right hand

▤ SP 7 **S61.422-** Laceration with foreign body of left hand

▤ !Q 7 **S61.429-** **Laceration with foreign body of unspecified hand**

6 **S61.43** Puncture wound without foreign body of hand

▤ SP 7 **S61.431-** Puncture wound without foreign body of right hand

▤ SP 7 **S61.432-** Puncture wound without foreign body of left hand

▤ !Q 7 **S61.439-** **Puncture wound without foreign body of unspecified hand**

6 **S61.44** Puncture wound with foreign body of hand

▤ SP 7 **S61.441-** Puncture wound with foreign body of right hand

▤ SP 7 **S61.442-** Puncture wound with foreign body of left hand

▤ !Q 7 **S61.449-** **Puncture wound with foreign body of unspecified hand**

6 **S61.45** **Open bite of hand**
Bite of hand NOS
EXCLUDES 1 superficial bite of hand (S60.56-, S60.57-)

▤ SP 7 **S61.451-** Open bite of right hand

▤ SP 7 **S61.452-** Open bite of left hand

▤ !Q 7 **S61.459-** **Open bite of unspecified hand**

5 **S61.5 Open wound of wrist**

6 **S61.50** **Unspecified open wound of wrist**

▤ SP !Q 7 **S61.501-** **Unspecified open wound of right wrist**

▤ SP 7 **S61.502-** **Unspecified open wound of left wrist**

▤ !Q 7 **S61.509-** **Unspecified open wound of unspecified wrist**

6 **S61.51** Laceration without foreign body of wrist

▤ SP 7 **S61.511-** Laceration without foreign body of right wrist

▤ SP 7 **S61.512-** Laceration without foreign body of left wrist

▤ !Q 7 **S61.519-** **Laceration without foreign body of unspecified wrist**

6 **S61.52** Laceration with foreign body of wrist

▤ SP 7 **S61.521-** Laceration with foreign body of right wrist

▤ SP 7 **S61.522-** Laceration with foreign body of left wrist

▤ !Q 7 **S61.529-** **Laceration with foreign body of unspecified wrist**

6 **S61.53** Puncture wound without foreign body of wrist

▤ SP 7 **S61.531-** Puncture wound without foreign body of right wrist

▤ SP 7 **S61.532-** Puncture wound without foreign body of left wrist

▤ !Q 7 **S61.539-** **Puncture wound without foreign body of unspecified wrist**

6 **S61.54** Puncture wound with foreign body of wrist

▤ SP 7 **S61.541-** Puncture wound with foreign body of right wrist

▤ SP 7 **S61.542-** Puncture wound with foreign body of left wrist

▤ !Q 7 **S61.549-** **Puncture wound with foreign body of unspecified wrist**

6 **S61.55** Open bite of wrist
Bite of wrist NOS
EXCLUDES 1 superficial bite of wrist (S60.86-, S60.87-)

▤ SP 7 **S61.551-** Open bite of right wrist

▤ SP 7 **S61.552-** Open bite of left wrist

▤ !Q 7 **S61.559-** **Open bite of unspecified wrist**

4 **S62** **Fracture at wrist and hand level**
Note:
A fracture not indicated as displaced or nondisplaced should be coded to displaced
A fracture not indicated as open or closed should be coded to closed
EXCLUDES 1 traumatic amputation of wrist and hand (S68.-)
EXCLUDES 2 fracture of distal parts of ulna and radius (S52.-)

The appropriate 7th character is to be added to each code from category S62
A   initial encounter for closed fracture
B   initial encounter for open fracture
D   subsequent encounter for fracture with routine healing
G   subsequent encounter for fracture with delayed healing
K   subsequent encounter for fracture with nonunion
P   subsequent encounter for fracture with malunion
S   sequela

★ New ▲ Revised Px Primary SP PDGM Px SL Low CoM SH High CoM !Q Quest. Encounter H Hospice non-cancer Dx   Unspecified   M *Manifestation*

DecisionHealth's FY 2020 Complete Home Health ICD-10-CM Diagnosis Coding Manual   1559

Chapter 19

S00-T88

CODING TIPS ✓ Fractures repaired by joint replacements are NOT coded with Z47.1. Fractures repaired by any other orthopedic surgery are NOT coded with Z47.89. Z codes are not appropriate for fractures of any kind. Code the fracture with 7th character D for fractures undergoing surgical repair.

CODING TIPS ✓ 'D' is the 7th character for home care and hospice unless the physician has documented delayed healing, nonunion or malunion. A sequela is a condition left after the fracture has healed. The Gustilo open fracture classification must be used for open fractures. The default 7th character for open fractures is E.

CODING TIPS ✓ A fracture not indicated as displaced or nondisplaced should be coded to displaced. A fracture not indicated as open or closed should be coded to closed.

⑤ **S62.0** Fracture of navicular [scaphoid] bone of wrist

⑥ **S62.00** Unspecified fracture of navicular [scaphoid] bone of wrist

⊟ SP 7 **S62.001-** Unspecified fracture of navicular [scaphoid] bone of right wrist

⊟ SP 7 **S62.002-** Unspecified fracture of navicular [scaphoid] bone of left wrist

⊟ !Q 7 **S62.009-** Unspecified fracture of navicular [scaphoid] bone of unspecified wrist

⑥ **S62.01** Fracture of distal pole of navicular [scaphoid] bone of wrist
Fracture of volar tuberosity of navicular [scaphoid] bone of wrist

⊟ SP 7 **S62.011-** Displaced fracture of distal pole of navicular [scaphoid] bone of right wrist

⊟ SP 7 **S62.012-** Displaced fracture of distal pole of navicular [scaphoid] bone of left wrist

⊟ !Q 7 **S62.013-** Displaced fracture of distal pole of navicular [scaphoid] bone of unspecified wrist

⊟ SP 7 **S62.014-** Nondisplaced fracture of distal pole of navicular [scaphoid] bone of right wrist

⊟ SP 7 **S62.015-** Nondisplaced fracture of distal pole of navicular [scaphoid] bone of left wrist

⊟ !Q 7 **S62.016-** Nondisplaced fracture of distal pole of navicular [scaphoid] bone of unspecified wrist

⑥ **S62.02** Fracture of middle third of navicular [scaphoid] bone of wrist

⊟ SP 7 **S62.021-** Displaced fracture of middle third of navicular [scaphoid] bone of right wrist

⊟ SP 7 **S62.022-** Displaced fracture of middle third of navicular [scaphoid] bone of left wrist

⊟ !Q 7 **S62.023-** Displaced fracture of middle third of navicular [scaphoid] bone of unspecified wrist

⊟ SP 7 **S62.024-** Nondisplaced fracture of middle third of navicular [scaphoid] bone of right wrist

⊟ SP 7 **S62.025-** Nondisplaced fracture of middle third of navicular [scaphoid] bone of left wrist

⊟ !Q 7 **S62.026-** Nondisplaced fracture of middle third of navicular [scaphoid] bone of unspecified wrist

⑥ **S62.03** Fracture of proximal third of navicular [scaphoid] bone of wrist

⊟ SP 7 **S62.031-** Displaced fracture of proximal third of navicular [scaphoid] bone of right wrist

⊟ SP 7 **S62.032-** Displaced fracture of proximal third of navicular [scaphoid] bone of left wrist

⊟ !Q 7 **S62.033-** Displaced fracture of proximal third of navicular [scaphoid] bone of unspecified wrist

⊟ SP 7 **S62.034-** Nondisplaced fracture of proximal third of navicular [scaphoid] bone of right wrist

⊟ SP 7 **S62.035-** Nondisplaced fracture of proximal third of navicular [scaphoid] bone of left wrist

⊟ !Q 7 **S62.036-** Nondisplaced fracture of proximal third of navicular [scaphoid] bone of unspecified wrist

⑤ **S62.1** Fracture of other and unspecified carpal bone(s)
EXCLUDES 2 fracture of scaphoid of wrist (S62.0-)

⑥ **S62.10** Fracture of unspecified carpal bone
Fracture of wrist NOS

⊟ SP 7 **S62.101-** Fracture of unspecified carpal bone, right wrist

⊟ SP 7 **S62.102-** Fracture of unspecified carpal bone, left wrist

⊟ !Q 7 **S62.109-** Fracture of unspecified carpal bone, unspecified wrist

⑥ **S62.11** Fracture of triquetrum [cuneiform] bone of wrist

⊟ SP 7 **S62.111-** Displaced fracture of triquetrum [cuneiform] bone, right wrist

⊟ SP 7 **S62.112-** Displaced fracture of triquetrum [cuneiform] bone, left wrist

⊟ !Q 7 **S62.113-** Displaced fracture of triquetrum [cuneiform] bone, unspecified wrist

⊟ SP 7 **S62.114-** Nondisplaced fracture of triquetrum [cuneiform] bone, right wrist

⊟ SP 7 **S62.115-** Nondisplaced fracture of triquetrum [cuneiform] bone, left wrist

⊟ !Q 7 **S62.116-** Nondisplaced fracture of triquetrum [cuneiform] bone, unspecified wrist

⑥ **S62.12** Fracture of lunate [semilunar]

⊟ SP 7 **S62.121-** Displaced fracture of lunate [semilunar], right wrist

⊟ SP 7 **S62.122-** Displaced fracture of lunate [semilunar], left wrist

④4th digit required   ⑤5th digit required   ⑥6th digit required   7 7th digit required   ⑦ 7th digit placeholder   ✚Additional code   ⊟Laterality

1560   *DecisionHealth's* FY 2020 Complete Home Health ICD-10-CM Diagnosis Coding Manual

Chapter 19

S00-T88

⊟ !Q 7 **S62.123-** Displaced fracture of lunate [semilunar], unspecified wrist

⊟ SP 7 **S62.124-** Nondisplaced fracture of lunate [semilunar], right wrist

⊟ SP 7 **S62.125-** Nondisplaced fracture of lunate [semilunar], left wrist

⊟ !Q 7 **S62.126-** Nondisplaced fracture of lunate [semilunar], unspecified wrist

6 **S62.13** Fracture of capitate [os magnum] bone

⊟ SP 7 **S62.131-** Displaced fracture of capitate [os magnum] bone, right wrist

⊟ SP 7 **S62.132-** Displaced fracture of capitate [os magnum] bone, left wrist

⊟ !Q 7 **S62.133-** Displaced fracture of capitate [os magnum] bone, unspecified wrist

⊟ SP 7 **S62.134-** Nondisplaced fracture of capitate [os magnum] bone, right wrist

⊟ SP 7 **S62.135-** Nondisplaced fracture of capitate [os magnum] bone, left wrist

⊟ !Q 7 **S62.136-** Nondisplaced fracture of capitate [os magnum] bone, unspecified wrist

6 **S62.14** Fracture of body of hamate [unciform] bone
Fracture of hamate [unciform] bone NOS

⊟ SP 7 **S62.141-** Displaced fracture of body of hamate [unciform] bone, right wrist

⊟ SP 7 **S62.142-** Displaced fracture of body of hamate [unciform] bone, left wrist

⊟ !Q 7 **S62.143-** Displaced fracture of body of hamate [unciform] bone, unspecified wrist

⊟ SP 7 **S62.144-** Nondisplaced fracture of body of hamate [unciform] bone, right wrist

⊟ SP 7 **S62.145-** Nondisplaced fracture of body of hamate [unciform] bone, left wrist

⊟ !Q 7 **S62.146-** Nondisplaced fracture of body of hamate [unciform] bone, unspecified wrist

6 **S62.15** Fracture of hook process of hamate [unciform] bone
Fracture of unciform process of hamate [unciform] bone

⊟ SP 7 **S62.151-** Displaced fracture of hook process of hamate [unciform] bone, right wrist

⊟ SP 7 **S62.152-** Displaced fracture of hook process of hamate [unciform] bone, left wrist

⊟ !Q 7 **S62.153-** Displaced fracture of hook process of hamate [unciform] bone, unspecified wrist

⊟ SP 7 **S62.154-** Nondisplaced fracture of hook process of hamate [unciform] bone, right wrist

⊟ SP 7 **S62.155-** Nondisplaced fracture of hook process of hamate [unciform] bone, left wrist

⊟ !Q 7 **S62.156-** Nondisplaced fracture of hook process of hamate [unciform] bone, unspecified wrist

6 **S62.16** Fracture of pisiform

⊟ SP 7 **S62.161-** Displaced fracture of pisiform, right wrist

⊟ SP 7 **S62.162-** Displaced fracture of pisiform, left wrist

⊟ SP !Q 7 **S62.163-** Displaced fracture of pisiform, unspecified wrist

⊟ SP 7 **S62.164-** Nondisplaced fracture of pisiform, right wrist

⊟ SP 7 **S62.165-** Nondisplaced fracture of pisiform, left wrist

⊟ !Q 7 **S62.166-** Nondisplaced fracture of pisiform, unspecified wrist

6 **S62.17** Fracture of trapezium [larger multangular]

⊟ SP 7 **S62.171-** Displaced fracture of trapezium [larger multangular], right wrist

⊟ SP 7 **S62.172-** Displaced fracture of trapezium [larger multangular], left wrist

⊟ !Q 7 **S62.173-** Displaced fracture of trapezium [larger multangular], unspecified wrist

⊟ SP 7 **S62.174-** Nondisplaced fracture of trapezium [larger multangular], right wrist

⊟ SP 7 **S62.175-** Nondisplaced fracture of trapezium [larger multangular], left wrist

⊟ !Q 7 **S62.176-** Nondisplaced fracture of trapezium [larger multangular], unspecified wrist

6 **S62.18** Fracture of trapezoid [smaller multangular]

⊟ SP 7 **S62.181-** Displaced fracture of trapezoid [smaller multangular], right wrist

⊟ SP 7 **S62.182-** Displaced fracture of trapezoid [smaller multangular], left wrist

⊟ !Q 7 **S62.183-** Displaced fracture of trapezoid [smaller multangular], unspecified wrist

⊟ SP 7 **S62.184-** Nondisplaced fracture of trapezoid [smaller multangular], right wrist

⊟ SP 7 **S62.185-** Nondisplaced fracture of trapezoid [smaller multangular], left wrist

⊟ !Q 7 **S62.186-** Nondisplaced fracture of trapezoid [smaller multangular], unspecified wrist

5 **S62.2** Fracture of first metacarpal bone

6 **S62.20** Unspecified fracture of first metacarpal bone

⊟ SP 7 **S62.201-** Unspecified fracture of first metacarpal bone, right hand

⊟ SP 7 **S62.202-** Unspecified fracture of first metacarpal bone, left hand

⊟ !Q 7 **S62.209-** Unspecified fracture of first metacarpal bone, unspecified hand

6 **S62.21** Bennett's fracture

★ New ▲ Revised Px Primary SP PDGM Px SL Low CoM SH High CoM !Q Quest. Encounter H Hospice non-cancer Dx Unspecified M Manifestation

DecisionHealth's FY 2020 Complete Home Health ICD-10-CM Diagnosis Coding Manual

1561

☐ **SP** 7️⃣ **S62.254-** Nondisplaced fracture of neck of first metacarpal bone, right hand

☐ **SP** 7️⃣ **S62.255-** Nondisplaced fracture of neck of first metacarpal bone, left hand

☐ **!Q** 7️⃣ **S62.256-** Nondisplaced fracture of neck of first metacarpal bone, unspecified hand

DEFINITION An intra-articular fracture dislocation of the base of the first metacarpal bone (thumb) extending into the carpometacarpal joint.

☐ **SP** 7️⃣ **S62.211-** Bennett's fracture, right hand

☐ **SP** 7️⃣ **S62.212-** Bennett's fracture, left hand

☐ **!Q** 7️⃣ **S62.213-** Bennett's fracture, unspecified hand

6️⃣ **S62.22** Rolando's fracture

☐ **SP** 7️⃣ **S62.221-** Displaced Rolando's fracture, right hand

☐ **SP** 7️⃣ **S62.222-** Displaced Rolando's fracture, left hand

☐ **!Q** 7️⃣ **S62.223-** Displaced Rolando's fracture, unspecified hand

☐ **SP** 7️⃣ **S62.224-** Nondisplaced Rolando's fracture, right hand

☐ **SP** 7️⃣ **S62.225-** Nondisplaced Rolando's fracture, left hand

☐ **!Q** 7️⃣ **S62.226-** Nondisplaced Rolando's fracture, unspecified hand

6️⃣ **S62.23** Other fracture of base of first metacarpal bone

☐ **SP** 7️⃣ **S62.231-** Other displaced fracture of base of first metacarpal bone, right hand

☐ **SP** 7️⃣ **S62.232-** Other displaced fracture of base of first metacarpal bone, left hand

☐ **!Q** 7️⃣ **S62.233-** Other displaced fracture of base of first metacarpal bone, unspecified hand

☐ **SP** 7️⃣ **S62.234-** Other nondisplaced fracture of base of first metacarpal bone, right hand

☐ **SP** 7️⃣ **S62.235-** Other nondisplaced fracture of base of first metacarpal bone, left hand

☐ **!Q** 7️⃣ **S62.236-** Other nondisplaced fracture of base of first metacarpal bone, unspecified hand

6️⃣ **S62.24** Fracture of shaft of first metacarpal bone

☐ **SP** 7️⃣ **S62.241-** Displaced fracture of shaft of first metacarpal bone, right hand

☐ **SP** 7️⃣ **S62.242-** Displaced fracture of shaft of first metacarpal bone, left hand

☐ **!Q** 7️⃣ **S62.243-** Displaced fracture of shaft of first metacarpal bone, unspecified hand

☐ **SP** 7️⃣ **S62.244-** Nondisplaced fracture of shaft of first metacarpal bone, right hand

☐ **SP** 7️⃣ **S62.245-** Nondisplaced fracture of shaft of first metacarpal bone, left hand

☐ **!Q** 7️⃣ **S62.246-** Nondisplaced fracture of shaft of first metacarpal bone, unspecified hand

6️⃣ **S62.25** Fracture of neck of first metacarpal bone

☐ **SP** 7️⃣ **S62.251-** Displaced fracture of neck of first metacarpal bone, right hand

☐ **SP** 7️⃣ **S62.252-** Displaced fracture of neck of first metacarpal bone, left hand

☐ **SP** **!Q** 7️⃣ **S62.253-** Displaced fracture of neck of first metacarpal bone, unspecified hand

6️⃣ **S62.29** Other fracture of first metacarpal bone

☐ **SP** 7️⃣ **S62.291-** Other fracture of first metacarpal bone, right hand

☐ **SP** 7️⃣ **S62.292-** Other fracture of first metacarpal bone, left hand

☐ **!Q** 7️⃣ **S62.299-** Other fracture of first metacarpal bone, unspecified hand

5️⃣ **S62.3** Fracture of other and unspecified metacarpal bone

EXCLUDES 2 fracture of first metacarpal bone (S62.2-)

6️⃣ **S62.30** Unspecified fracture of other metacarpal bone

☐ **SP** 7️⃣ **S62.300-** Unspecified fracture of second metacarpal bone, right hand

☐ **SP** 7️⃣ **S62.301-** Unspecified fracture of second metacarpal bone, left hand

☐ **SP** 7️⃣ **S62.302-** Unspecified fracture of third metacarpal bone, right hand

☐ **SP** 7️⃣ **S62.303-** Unspecified fracture of third metacarpal bone, left hand

☐ **SP** 7️⃣ **S62.304-** Unspecified fracture of fourth metacarpal bone, right hand

☐ **SP** 7️⃣ **S62.305-** Unspecified fracture of fourth metacarpal bone, left hand

☐ **SP** 7️⃣ **S62.306-** Unspecified fracture of fifth metacarpal bone, right hand

☐ **SP** 7️⃣ **S62.307-** Unspecified fracture of fifth metacarpal bone, left hand

☐ **!Q** 7️⃣ **S62.308-** Unspecified fracture of other metacarpal bone

Unspecified fracture of specified metacarpal bone with unspecified laterality

☐ **!Q** 7️⃣ **S62.309-** Unspecified fracture of unspecified metacarpal bone

6️⃣ **S62.31** Displaced fracture of base of other metacarpal bone

☐ **SP** 7️⃣ **S62.310-** Displaced fracture of base of second metacarpal bone, right hand

☐ **SP** 7️⃣ **S62.311-** Displaced fracture of base of second metacarpal bone, left hand

☐ **SP** 7️⃣ **S62.312-** Displaced fracture of base of third metacarpal bone, right hand

☐ **SP** 7️⃣ **S62.313-** Displaced fracture of base of third metacarpal bone, left hand

☐ **SP** 7️⃣ **S62.314-** Displaced fracture of base of fourth metacarpal bone, right hand

☐ **SP** 7️⃣ **S62.315-** Displaced fracture of base of fourth metacarpal bone, left hand

☐ **SP** 7️⃣ **S62.316-** Displaced fracture of base of fifth metacarpal bone, right hand

Chapter 19

S00-T88

4️⃣4th digit required   5️⃣5th digit required   6️⃣6th digit required   7️⃣7th digit required   7️⃣7th digit placeholder   ➕Additional code   ☐Laterality

1562   *DecisionHealth's* FY 2020 Complete Home Health ICD-10-CM Diagnosis Coding Manual

▣ SP 7	S62.317-	Displaced fracture of base of fifth metacarpal bone, left hand
▣ SP 7	S62.318-	Displaced fracture of base of other metacarpal bone
		Displaced fracture of base of specified metacarpal bone with unspecified laterality
▣ SP IQ 7	S62.319-	**Displaced fracture of base of unspecified metacarpal bone**

⑥ S62.32 Displaced fracture of shaft of other metacarpal bone

▣ SP 7	S62.320-	Displaced fracture of shaft of second metacarpal bone, right hand
▣ SP 7	S62.321-	Displaced fracture of shaft of second metacarpal bone, left hand
▣ SP 7	S62.322-	Displaced fracture of shaft of third metacarpal bone, right hand
▣ SP 7	S62.323-	Displaced fracture of shaft of third metacarpal bone, left hand
▣ SP 7	S62.324-	Displaced fracture of shaft of fourth metacarpal bone, right hand
▣ SP 7	S62.325-	Displaced fracture of shaft of fourth metacarpal bone, left hand
▣ SP 7	S62.326-	Displaced fracture of shaft of fifth metacarpal bone, right hand
▣ SP 7	S62.327-	Displaced fracture of shaft of fifth metacarpal bone, left hand
▣ SP 7	S62.328-	Displaced fracture of shaft of other metacarpal bone
		Displaced fracture of shaft of specified metacarpal bone with unspecified laterality
▣ IQ 7	S62.329-	**Displaced fracture of shaft of unspecified metacarpal bone**

⑥ S62.33 Displaced fracture of neck of other metacarpal bone

▣ SP 7	S62.330-	Displaced fracture of neck of second metacarpal bone, right hand
▣ SP 7	S62.331-	Displaced fracture of neck of second metacarpal bone, left hand
▣ SP 7	S62.332-	Displaced fracture of neck of third metacarpal bone, right hand
▣ SP 7	S62.333-	Displaced fracture of neck of third metacarpal bone, left hand
▣ SP 7	S62.334-	Displaced fracture of neck of fourth metacarpal bone, right hand
▣ SP 7	S62.335-	Displaced fracture of neck of fourth metacarpal bone, left hand
▣ SP 7	S62.336-	Displaced fracture of neck of fifth metacarpal bone, right hand
▣ SP 7	S62.337-	Displaced fracture of neck of fifth metacarpal bone, left hand
▣ SP 7	S62.338-	Displaced fracture of neck of other metacarpal bone
		Displaced fracture of neck of specified metacarpal bone with unspecified laterality
▣ IQ 7	S62.339-	**Displaced fracture of neck of unspecified metacarpal bone**

⑥ S62.34 Nondisplaced fracture of base of other metacarpal bone

▣ SP 7	S62.340-	Nondisplaced fracture of base of second metacarpal bone, right hand
▣ SP 7	S62.341-	Nondisplaced fracture of base of second metacarpal bone, left hand
▣ SP 7	S62.342-	Nondisplaced fracture of base of third metacarpal bone, right hand
▣ SP 7	S62.343-	Nondisplaced fracture of base of third metacarpal bone, left hand
▣ SP 7	S62.344-	Nondisplaced fracture of base of fourth metacarpal bone, right hand
▣ SP 7	S62.345-	Nondisplaced fracture of base of fourth metacarpal bone, left hand
▣ SP 7	S62.346-	Nondisplaced fracture of base of fifth metacarpal bone, right hand
▣ SP 7	S62.347-	Nondisplaced fracture of base of fifth metacarpal bone, left hand
▣ SP 7	S62.348-	Nondisplaced fracture of base of other metacarpal bone
		Nondisplaced fracture of base of specified metacarpal bone with unspecified laterality
▣ IQ 7	S62.349-	**Nondisplaced fracture of base of unspecified metacarpal bone**

⑥ S62.35 Nondisplaced fracture of shaft of other metacarpal bone

▣ SP 7	S62.350-	Nondisplaced fracture of shaft of second metacarpal bone, right hand
▣ SP 7	S62.351-	Nondisplaced fracture of shaft of second metacarpal bone, left hand
▣ SP 7	S62.352-	Nondisplaced fracture of shaft of third metacarpal bone, right hand
▣ SP 7	S62.353-	Nondisplaced fracture of shaft of third metacarpal bone, left hand
▣ SP 7	S62.354-	Nondisplaced fracture of shaft of fourth metacarpal bone, right hand
▣ SP 7	S62.355-	Nondisplaced fracture of shaft of fourth metacarpal bone, left hand
▣ SP 7	S62.356-	Nondisplaced fracture of shaft of fifth metacarpal bone, right hand
▣ SP 7	S62.357-	Nondisplaced fracture of shaft of fifth metacarpal bone, left hand
▣ SP 7	S62.358-	Nondisplaced fracture of shaft of other metacarpal bone
		Nondisplaced fracture of shaft of specified metacarpal bone with unspecified laterality
▣ IQ 7	S62.359-	**Nondisplaced fracture of shaft of unspecified metacarpal bone**

⑥ S62.36 Nondisplaced fracture of neck of other metacarpal bone

▣ SP 7	S62.360-	Nondisplaced fracture of neck of second metacarpal bone, right hand

★ New ▲ Revised Px Primary SP PDGM Px SL Low CoM SH High CoM IQ Quest. Encounter H Hospice non-cancer Dx Unspecified M *Manifestation*

DecisionHealth's FY 2020 Complete Home Health ICD-10-CM Diagnosis Coding Manual

1563

Chapter 19

S00-T88

⊟ SP 7 **S62.361-** Nondisplaced fracture of neck of second metacarpal bone, left hand

⊟ SP 7 **S62.362-** Nondisplaced fracture of neck of third metacarpal bone, right hand

⊟ SP 7 **S62.363-** Nondisplaced fracture of neck of third metacarpal bone, left hand

⊟ SP 7 **S62.364-** Nondisplaced fracture of neck of fourth metacarpal bone, right hand

⊟ SP 7 **S62.365-** Nondisplaced fracture of neck of fourth metacarpal bone, left hand

⊟ SP 7 **S62.366-** Nondisplaced fracture of neck of fifth metacarpal bone, right hand

⊟ SP 7 **S62.367-** Nondisplaced fracture of neck of fifth metacarpal bone, left hand

⊟ SP 7 **S62.368-** Nondisplaced fracture of neck of other metacarpal bone

Nondisplaced fracture of neck of specified metacarpal bone with unspecified laterality

⊟ !Q 7 **S62.369-** Nondisplaced fracture of neck of unspecified metacarpal bone

6 **S62.39** Other fracture of other metacarpal bone

⊟ SP 7 **S62.390-** Other fracture of second metacarpal bone, right hand

⊟ SP 7 **S62.391-** Other fracture of second metacarpal bone, left hand

⊟ SP 7 **S62.392-** Other fracture of third metacarpal bone, right hand

⊟ SP 7 **S62.393-** Other fracture of third metacarpal bone, left hand

⊟ SP 7 **S62.394-** Other fracture of fourth metacarpal bone, right hand

⊟ SP 7 **S62.395-** Other fracture of fourth metacarpal bone, left hand

⊟ SP 7 **S62.396-** Other fracture of fifth metacarpal bone, right hand

⊟ SP 7 **S62.397-** Other fracture of fifth metacarpal bone, left hand

⊟ SP 7 **S62.398-** Other fracture of other metacarpal bone

Other fracture of specified metacarpal bone with unspecified laterality

⊟ !Q 7 **S62.399-** Other fracture of unspecified metacarpal bone

5 **S62.5** Fracture of thumb

6 **S62.50** Fracture of unspecified phalanx of thumb

⊟ SP 7 **S62.501-** Fracture of unspecified phalanx of right thumb

⊟ SP 7 **S62.502-** Fracture of unspecified phalanx of left thumb

⊟ !Q 7 **S62.509-** Fracture of unspecified phalanx of unspecified thumb

6 **S62.51** Fracture of proximal phalanx of thumb

⊟ SP 7 **S62.511-** Displaced fracture of proximal phalanx of right thumb

⊟ SP 7 **S62.512-** Displaced fracture of proximal phalanx of left thumb

⊟ !Q 7 **S62.513-** Displaced fracture of proximal phalanx of unspecified thumb

⊟ SP 7 **S62.514-** Nondisplaced fracture of proximal phalanx of right thumb

⊟ SP 7 **S62.515-** Nondisplaced fracture of proximal phalanx of left thumb

⊟ !Q 7 **S62.516-** Nondisplaced fracture of proximal phalanx of unspecified thumb

6 **S62.52** Fracture of distal phalanx of thumb

⊟ SP 7 **S62.521-** Displaced fracture of distal phalanx of right thumb

⊟ SP 7 **S62.522-** Displaced fracture of distal phalanx of left thumb

⊟ !Q 7 **S62.523-** Displaced fracture of distal phalanx of unspecified thumb

⊟ SP 7 **S62.524-** Nondisplaced fracture of distal phalanx of right thumb

⊟ SP 7 **S62.525-** Nondisplaced fracture of distal phalanx of left thumb

⊟ !Q 7 **S62.526-** Nondisplaced fracture of distal phalanx of unspecified thumb

5 **S62.6** Fracture of other and unspecified finger(s)

EXCLUDES 2 fracture of thumb (S62.5-)

6 **S62.60** Fracture of unspecified phalanx of finger

⊟ SP 7 **S62.600-** Fracture of unspecified phalanx of right index finger

⊟ SP 7 **S62.601-** Fracture of unspecified phalanx of left index finger

⊟ SP 7 **S62.602-** Fracture of unspecified phalanx of right middle finger

⊟ SP 7 **S62.603-** Fracture of unspecified phalanx of left middle finger

⊟ SP 7 **S62.604-** Fracture of unspecified phalanx of right ring finger

⊟ SP 7 **S62.605-** Fracture of unspecified phalanx of left ring finger

⊟ SP 7 **S62.606-** Fracture of unspecified phalanx of right little finger

⊟ SP 7 **S62.607-** Fracture of unspecified phalanx of left little finger

⊟ SP 7 **S62.608-** Fracture of unspecified phalanx of other finger

Fracture of unspecified phalanx of specified finger with unspecified laterality

⊟ !Q 7 **S62.609-** Fracture of unspecified phalanx of unspecified finger

6 **S62.61** Displaced fracture of proximal phalanx of finger

⊟ SP 7 **S62.610-** Displaced fracture of proximal phalanx of right index finger

⊟ SP 7 **S62.611-** Displaced fracture of proximal phalanx of left index finger

⊟ SP 7 **S62.612-** Displaced fracture of proximal phalanx of right middle finger

⊟ SP 7 **S62.613-** Displaced fracture of proximal phalanx of left middle finger

⊟ SP 7 **S62.614-** Displaced fracture of proximal phalanx of right ring finger

⊟ SP 7 **S62.615-** Displaced fracture of proximal phalanx of left ring finger

⊟ SP 7 **S62.616-** Displaced fracture of proximal phalanx of right little finger

---

4 4th digit required   5 5th digit required   6 6th digit required   7 7th digit required   7 7th digit placeholder   +Additional code   ⊟ Laterality

▤ **SP** 7 **S62.617-** **Displaced fracture of proximal phalanx of left little finger**

▤ **SP** 7 **S62.618-** **Displaced fracture of proximal phalanx of other finger**
Displaced fracture of proximal phalanx of specified finger with unspecified laterality

▤ **IQ** 7 **S62.619-** **Displaced fracture of proximal phalanx of unspecified finger**

6 **S62.62** **Displaced fracture of middle phalanx of finger**

▤ **SP** 7 **S62.620-** **Displaced fracture of middle phalanx of right index finger**

▤ **SP** 7 **S62.621-** **Displaced fracture of middle phalanx of left index finger**

▤ **SP** 7 **S62.622-** **Displaced fracture of middle phalanx of right middle finger**

▤ **SP** 7 **S62.623-** **Displaced fracture of middle phalanx of left middle finger**

▤ **SP** 7 **S62.624-** **Displaced fracture of middle phalanx of right ring finger**

▤ **SP** 7 **S62.625-** **Displaced fracture of middle phalanx of left ring finger**

▤ **SP** 7 **S62.626-** **Displaced fracture of middle phalanx of right little finger**

▤ **SP** 7 **S62.627-** **Displaced fracture of middle phalanx of left little finger**

▤ **SP** 7 **S62.628-** **Displaced fracture of middle phalanx of other finger**
Displaced fracture of middle phalanx of specified finger with unspecified laterality

▤ **IQ** 7 **S62.629-** **Displaced fracture of middle phalanx of unspecified finger**

6 **S62.63** **Displaced fracture of distal phalanx of finger**

▤ **SP** 7 **S62.630-** **Displaced fracture of distal phalanx of right index finger**

▤ **SP** 7 **S62.631-** **Displaced fracture of distal phalanx of left index finger**

▤ **SP** 7 **S62.632-** **Displaced fracture of distal phalanx of right middle finger**

▤ **SP** 7 **S62.633-** **Displaced fracture of distal phalanx of left middle finger**

▤ **SP** 7 **S62.634-** **Displaced fracture of distal phalanx of right ring finger**

▤ **SP** 7 **S62.635-** **Displaced fracture of distal phalanx of left ring finger**

▤ **SP** 7 **S62.636-** **Displaced fracture of distal phalanx of right little finger**

▤ **SP** 7 **S62.637-** **Displaced fracture of distal phalanx of left little finger**

▤ **SP** 7 **S62.638-** **Displaced fracture of distal phalanx of other finger**
Displaced fracture of distal phalanx of specified finger with unspecified laterality

▤ **IQ** 7 **S62.639-** **Displaced fracture of distal phalanx of unspecified finger**

6 **S62.64** **Nondisplaced fracture of proximal phalanx of finger**

▤ **SP** 7 **S62.640-** **Nondisplaced fracture of proximal phalanx of right index finger**

▤ **SP** 7 **S62.641-** **Nondisplaced fracture of proximal phalanx of left index finger**

▤ **SP** 7 **S62.642-** **Nondisplaced fracture of proximal phalanx of right middle finger**

▤ **SP** 7 **S62.643-** **Nondisplaced fracture of proximal phalanx of left middle finger**

▤ **SP** 7 **S62.644-** **Nondisplaced fracture of proximal phalanx of right ring finger**

▤ **SP** 7 **S62.645-** **Nondisplaced fracture of proximal phalanx of left ring finger**

▤ **SP** 7 **S62.646-** **Nondisplaced fracture of proximal phalanx of right little finger**

▤ **SP** 7 **S62.647-** **Nondisplaced fracture of proximal phalanx of left little finger**

▤ **SP** 7 **S62.648-** **Nondisplaced fracture of proximal phalanx of other finger**
Nondisplaced fracture of proximal phalanx of specified finger with unspecified laterality

▤ **IQ** 7 **S62.649-** **Nondisplaced fracture of proximal phalanx of unspecified finger**

6 **S62.65** **Nondisplaced fracture of middle phalanx of finger**

▤ **SP** 7 **S62.650-** **Nondisplaced fracture of middle phalanx of right index finger**

▤ **SP** 7 **S62.651-** **Nondisplaced fracture of middle phalanx of left index finger**

▤ **SP** 7 **S62.652-** **Nondisplaced fracture of middle phalanx of right middle finger**

▤ **SP** 7 **S62.653-** **Nondisplaced fracture of middle phalanx of left middle finger**

▤ **SP** 7 **S62.654-** **Nondisplaced fracture of middle phalanx of right ring finger**

▤ **SP** 7 **S62.655-** **Nondisplaced fracture of middle phalanx of left ring finger**

▤ **SP** 7 **S62.656-** **Nondisplaced fracture of middle phalanx of right little finger**

▤ **SP** 7 **S62.657-** **Nondisplaced fracture of middle phalanx of left little finger**

▤ **SP** 7 **S62.658-** **Nondisplaced fracture of middle phalanx of other finger**
Nondisplaced fracture of middle phalanx of specified finger with unspecified laterality

▤ **IQ** 7 **S62.659-** **Nondisplaced fracture of middle phalanx of unspecified finger**

6 **S62.66** **Nondisplaced fracture of distal phalanx of finger**

▤ **SP** 7 **S62.660-** **Nondisplaced fracture of distal phalanx of right index finger**

▤ **SP** 7 **S62.661-** **Nondisplaced fracture of distal phalanx of left index finger**

▤ **SP** 7 **S62.662-** **Nondisplaced fracture of distal phalanx of right middle finger**

▤ **SP** 7 **S62.663-** **Nondisplaced fracture of distal phalanx of left middle finger**

▤ **SP** 7 **S62.664-** **Nondisplaced fracture of distal phalanx of right ring finger**

▤ **SP** 7 **S62.665-** **Nondisplaced fracture of distal phalanx of left ring finger**

▤ **SP** 7 **S62.666-** **Nondisplaced fracture of distal phalanx of right little finger**

Chapter 19

S00-T88

★ New ▲ Revised Px Primary **SP** PDGM Px **SL** Low CoM **SH** High CoM **IQ** Quest. Encounter ⊞ Hospice non-cancer Dx Unspecified **M** *Manifestation*

DecisionHealth's FY 2020 Complete Home Health ICD-10-CM Diagnosis Coding Manual   1565

⊟ **SP** 7 **S62.667-** **Nondisplaced fracture of distal phalanx of left little finger**

⊟ **SP** 7 **S62.668-** **Nondisplaced fracture of distal phalanx of other finger**
Nondisplaced fracture of distal phalanx of specified finger with unspecified laterality

⊟ **IQ** 7 **S62.669-** **Nondisplaced fracture of distal phalanx of unspecified finger**

5 **S62.9** **Unspecified fracture of wrist and hand**

⊟ **IQ** 7✓ **S62.90X-** **Unspecified fracture of unspecified wrist and hand**

⊟ **SP** 7✓ **S62.91X-** **Unspecified fracture of right wrist and hand**

⊟ **SP** 7✓ **S62.92X-** **Unspecified fracture of left wrist and hand**

4 **S63** **Dislocation and sprain of joints and ligaments at wrist and hand level**

> INCLUDES avulsion of joint or ligament at wrist and hand level
> laceration of cartilage, joint or ligament at wrist and hand level
> sprain of cartilage, joint or ligament at wrist and hand level
> traumatic hemarthrosis of joint or ligament at wrist and hand level
> traumatic rupture of joint or ligament at wrist and hand level
> traumatic subluxation of joint or ligament at wrist and hand level
> traumatic tear of joint or ligament at wrist and hand level

Code also:
any associated open wound

> EXCLUDES 2 strain of muscle, fascia and tendon of wrist and hand (S66.-)

The appropriate 7th character is to be added to each code from category S63
A   initial encounter
D   subsequent encounter
S   sequela

5 **S63.0** **Subluxation and dislocation of wrist and hand joints**

6 **S63.00** **Unspecified subluxation and dislocation of wrist and hand**

Dislocation of carpal bone NOS
Dislocation of distal end of radius NOS
Subluxation of carpal bone NOS
Subluxation of distal end of radius NOS

⊟ **SP** 7 **S63.001-** **Unspecified subluxation of right wrist and hand**

⊟ **SP** 7 **S63.002-** **Unspecified subluxation of left wrist and hand**

⊟ **IQ** 7 **S63.003-** **Unspecified subluxation of unspecified wrist and hand**

⊟ **SP** 7 **S63.004-** **Unspecified dislocation of right wrist and hand**

⊟ **SP** 7 **S63.005-** **Unspecified dislocation of left wrist and hand**

⊟ **IQ** 7 **S63.006-** **Unspecified dislocation of unspecified wrist and hand**

6 **S63.01** **Subluxation and dislocation of distal radioulnar joint**

⊟ **SP** 7 **S63.011-** **Subluxation of distal radioulnar joint of right wrist**

⊟ **SP** 7 **S63.012-** **Subluxation of distal radioulnar joint of left wrist**

⊟ **IQ** 7 **S63.013-** **Subluxation of distal radioulnar joint of unspecified wrist**

⊟ **SP** 7 **S63.014-** **Dislocation of distal radioulnar joint of right wrist**

⊟ **SP** 7 **S63.015-** **Dislocation of distal radioulnar joint of left wrist**

⊟ **IQ** 7 **S63.016-** **Dislocation of distal radioulnar joint of unspecified wrist**

6 **S63.02** **Subluxation and dislocation of radiocarpal joint**

⊟ **SP** 7 **S63.021-** **Subluxation of radiocarpal joint of right wrist**

⊟ **SP** 7 **S63.022-** **Subluxation of radiocarpal joint of left wrist**

⊟ **IQ** 7 **S63.023-** **Subluxation of radiocarpal joint of unspecified wrist**

⊟ **SP** 7 **S63.024-** **Dislocation of radiocarpal joint of right wrist**

⊟ **SP** 7 **S63.025-** **Dislocation of radiocarpal joint of left wrist**

⊟ **IQ** 7 **S63.026-** **Dislocation of radiocarpal joint of unspecified wrist**

6 **S63.03** **Subluxation and dislocation of midcarpal joint**

⊟ **SP** 7 **S63.031-** **Subluxation of midcarpal joint of right wrist**

⊟ **SP** 7 **S63.032-** **Subluxation of midcarpal joint of left wrist**

⊟ **IQ** 7 **S63.033-** **Subluxation of midcarpal joint of unspecified wrist**

⊟ **SP** 7 **S63.034-** **Dislocation of midcarpal joint of right wrist**

⊟ **SP** 7 **S63.035-** **Dislocation of midcarpal joint of left wrist**

⊟ **IQ** 7 **S63.036-** **Dislocation of midcarpal joint of unspecified wrist**

6 **S63.04** **Subluxation and dislocation of carpometacarpal joint of thumb**

> EXCLUDES 2 interphalangeal subluxation and dislocation of thumb (S63.1-)

⊟ **SP** 7 **S63.041-** **Subluxation of carpometacarpal joint of right thumb**

⊟ **SP** 7 **S63.042-** **Subluxation of carpometacarpal joint of left thumb**

⊟ **IQ** 7 **S63.043-** **Subluxation of carpometacarpal joint of unspecified thumb**

⊟ **SP** 7 **S63.044-** **Dislocation of carpometacarpal joint of right thumb**

⊟ **SP** 7 **S63.045-** **Dislocation of carpometacarpal joint of left thumb**

⊟ **IQ** 7 **S63.046-** **Dislocation of carpometacarpal joint of unspecified thumb**

6 **S63.05** **Subluxation and dislocation of other carpometacarpal joint**

---

4 4th digit required   5 5th digit required   6 6th digit required   7 7th digit required   7✓ 7th digit placeholder   ✚ Additional code   ⊟ Laterality

1566   *DecisionHealth's* FY 2020 Complete Home Health ICD-10-CM Diagnosis Coding Manual

EXCLUDES 2 subluxation and dislocation of carpometacarpal joint of thumb (S63.04-)

☐ **SP** 7 S63.051- Subluxation of other carpometacarpal joint of right hand

☐ **SP** 7 S63.052- Subluxation of other carpometacarpal joint of left hand

☐ **IQ** 7 S63.053- Subluxation of other carpometacarpal joint of unspecified hand

☐ **SP** 7 S63.054- Dislocation of other carpometacarpal joint of right hand

☐ **SP** 7 S63.055- Dislocation of other carpometacarpal joint of left hand

☐ **IQ** 7 S63.056- Dislocation of other carpometacarpal joint of unspecified hand

⑥ S63.06 Subluxation and dislocation of metacarpal (bone), proximal end

☐ **SP** 7 S63.061- Subluxation of metacarpal (bone), proximal end of right hand

☐ **SP** 7 S63.062- Subluxation of metacarpal (bone), proximal end of left hand

☐ **IQ** 7 S63.063- Subluxation of metacarpal (bone), proximal end of unspecified hand

☐ **SP** 7 S63.064- Dislocation of metacarpal (bone), proximal end of right hand

☐ **SP** 7 S63.065- Dislocation of metacarpal (bone), proximal end of left hand

☐ **IQ** 7 S63.066- Dislocation of metacarpal (bone), proximal end of unspecified hand

⑥ S63.07 Subluxation and dislocation of distal end of ulna

☐ **SP** 7 S63.071- Subluxation of distal end of right ulna

☐ **SP** 7 S63.072- Subluxation of distal end of left ulna

☐ **IQ** 7 S63.073- Subluxation of distal end of unspecified ulna

☐ **SP** 7 S63.074- Dislocation of distal end of right ulna

☐ **SP** 7 S63.075- Dislocation of distal end of left ulna

☐ **IQ** 7 S63.076- Dislocation of distal end of unspecified ulna

⑥ S63.09 Other subluxation and dislocation of wrist and hand

☐ **SP** 7 S63.091- Other subluxation of right wrist and hand

☐ **SP** 7 S63.092- Other subluxation of left wrist and hand

☐ **IQ** 7 S63.093- Other subluxation of unspecified wrist and hand

☐ **SP** 7 S63.094- Other dislocation of right wrist and hand

☐ **SP** 7 S63.095- Other dislocation of left wrist and hand

☐ **IQ** 7 S63.096- Other dislocation of unspecified wrist and hand

⑤ S63.1 Subluxation and dislocation of thumb

⑥ S63.10 Unspecified subluxation and dislocation of thumb

☐ **SP** 7 S63.101- Unspecified subluxation of right thumb

☐ **SP** 7 S63.102- Unspecified subluxation of left thumb

☐ **IQ** 7 S63.103- Unspecified subluxation of unspecified thumb

☐ **SP** 7 S63.104- Unspecified dislocation of right thumb

☐ **SP** 7 S63.105- Unspecified dislocation of left thumb

☐ **IQ** 7 S63.106- Unspecified dislocation of unspecified thumb

⑥ S63.11 Subluxation and dislocation of metacarpophalangeal joint of thumb

☐ **SP** 7 S63.111- Subluxation of metacarpophalangeal joint of right thumb

☐ **SP** 7 S63.112- Subluxation of metacarpophalangeal joint of left thumb

☐ **IQ** 7 S63.113- Subluxation of metacarpophalangeal joint of unspecified thumb

☐ **SP** 7 S63.114- Dislocation of metacarpophalangeal joint of right thumb

☐ **SP** 7 S63.115- Dislocation of metacarpophalangeal joint of left thumb

☐ **IQ** 7 S63.116- Dislocation of metacarpophalangeal joint of unspecified thumb

⑥ S63.12 Subluxation and dislocation of interphalangeal joint of thumb

☐ **IQ** 7 S63.121- Subluxation of interphalangeal joint of right thumb

☐ **IQ** 7 S63.122- Subluxation of interphalangeal joint of left thumb

☐ **IQ** 7 S63.123- Subluxation of interphalangeal joint of unspecified thumb

☐ **IQ** 7 S63.124- Dislocation of interphalangeal joint of right thumb

☐ **IQ** 7 S63.125- Dislocation of interphalangeal joint of left thumb

☐ **IQ** 7 S63.126- Dislocation of interphalangeal joint of unspecified thumb

⑤ S63.2 Subluxation and dislocation of other finger(s)

EXCLUDES 2 subluxation and dislocation of thumb (S63.1-)

⑥ S63.20 Unspecified subluxation of other finger

☐ **SP** 7 S63.200- Unspecified subluxation of right index finger

☐ **SP** 7 S63.201- Unspecified subluxation of left index finger

☐ **SP** 7 S63.202- Unspecified subluxation of right middle finger

☐ **SP** 7 S63.203- Unspecified subluxation of left middle finger

☐ **SP** 7 S63.204- Unspecified subluxation of right ring finger

Chapter 19

S00-T88

★ New ▲ Revised Px Primary **SP** PDGM Px **SL** Low CoM **SH** High CoM **IQ** Quest. Encounter ⊞ Hospice non-cancer Dx   Unspecified   **M** *Manifestation*

DecisionHealth's FY 2020 Complete Home Health ICD-10-CM Diagnosis Coding Manual   1567

☰ **SP** 7 **S63.205-** **Unspecified subluxation of left ring finger**

☰ **SP** 7 **S63.206-** **Unspecified subluxation of right little finger**

☰ **SP** 7 **S63.207-** **Unspecified subluxation of left little finger**

☰ **SP** 7 **S63.208-** **Unspecified subluxation of other finger**

Unspecified subluxation of specified finger with unspecified laterality

☰ **IQ** 7 **S63.209-** **Unspecified subluxation of unspecified finger**

6 **S63.21** **Subluxation of metacarpophalangeal joint of finger**

☰ **SP** 7 **S63.210-** Subluxation of metacarpophalangeal joint of right index finger

☰ **SP** 7 **S63.211-** Subluxation of metacarpophalangeal joint of left index finger

☰ **SP** 7 **S63.212-** Subluxation of metacarpophalangeal joint of right middle finger

☰ **SP** 7 **S63.213-** Subluxation of metacarpophalangeal joint of left middle finger

☰ **SP** 7 **S63.214-** Subluxation of metacarpophalangeal joint of right ring finger

☰ **SP** 7 **S63.215-** Subluxation of metacarpophalangeal joint of left ring finger

☰ **SP** 7 **S63.216-** Subluxation of metacarpophalangeal joint of right little finger

☰ **SP** 7 **S63.217-** Subluxation of metacarpophalangeal joint of left little finger

☰ **SP** **IQ** 7 **S63.218-** Subluxation of metacarpophalangeal joint of other finger

Subluxation of metacarpophalangeal joint of specified finger with unspecified laterality

☰ **IQ** 7 **S63.219-** **Subluxation of metacarpophalangeal joint of unspecified finger**

6 **S63.22** **Subluxation of unspecified interphalangeal joint of finger**

☰ **IQ** 7 **S63.220-** **Subluxation of unspecified interphalangeal joint of right index finger**

☰ **IQ** 7 **S63.221-** **Subluxation of unspecified interphalangeal joint of left index finger**

☰ **IQ** 7 **S63.222-** **Subluxation of unspecified interphalangeal joint of right middle finger**

☰ **IQ** 7 **S63.223-** **Subluxation of unspecified interphalangeal joint of left middle finger**

☰ **IQ** 7 **S63.224-** **Subluxation of unspecified interphalangeal joint of right ring finger**

☰ **IQ** 7 **S63.225-** **Subluxation of unspecified interphalangeal joint of left ring finger**

☰ **IQ** 7 **S63.226-** **Subluxation of unspecified interphalangeal joint of right little finger**

☰ **IQ** 7 **S63.227-** **Subluxation of unspecified interphalangeal joint of left little finger**

☰ **IQ** 7 **S63.228-** **Subluxation of unspecified interphalangeal joint of other finger**

Subluxation of unspecified interphalangeal joint of specified finger with unspecified laterality

☰ **IQ** 7 **S63.229-** **Subluxation of unspecified interphalangeal joint of unspecified finger**

6 **S63.23** **Subluxation of proximal interphalangeal joint of finger**

☰ **SP** 7 **S63.230-** Subluxation of proximal interphalangeal joint of right index finger

☰ **SP** 7 **S63.231-** Subluxation of proximal interphalangeal joint of left index finger

☰ **SP** 7 **S63.232-** Subluxation of proximal interphalangeal joint of right middle finger

☰ **SP** 7 **S63.233-** Subluxation of proximal interphalangeal joint of left middle finger

☰ **SP** 7 **S63.234-** Subluxation of proximal interphalangeal joint of right ring finger

☰ **SP** 7 **S63.235-** Subluxation of proximal interphalangeal joint of left ring finger

☰ **SP** 7 **S63.236-** Subluxation of proximal interphalangeal joint of right little finger

☰ **SP** 7 **S63.237-** Subluxation of proximal interphalangeal joint of left little finger

☰ **SP** 7 **S63.238-** Subluxation of proximal interphalangeal joint of other finger

Subluxation of proximal interphalangeal joint of specified finger with unspecified laterality

☰ **IQ** 7 **S63.239-** **Subluxation of proximal interphalangeal joint of unspecified finger**

6 **S63.24** **Subluxation of distal interphalangeal joint of finger**

☰ **SP** 7 **S63.240-** Subluxation of distal interphalangeal joint of right index finger

☰ **SP** 7 **S63.241-** Subluxation of distal interphalangeal joint of left index finger

☰ **SP** 7 **S63.242-** Subluxation of distal interphalangeal joint of right middle finger

☰ **SP** 7 **S63.243-** Subluxation of distal interphalangeal joint of left middle finger

4 4th digit required   5 5th digit required   6 6th digit required   7 7th digit required   7 7th digit placeholder   ✚ Additional code   ☰ Laterality

1568   *DecisionHealth's* FY 2020 Complete Home Health ICD-10-CM Diagnosis Coding Manual

⊟ **SP** **7** S63.244- Subluxation of distal interphalangeal joint of right ring finger

⊟ **SP** **7** S63.245- Subluxation of distal interphalangeal joint of left ring finger

⊟ **SP** **7** S63.246- Subluxation of distal interphalangeal joint of right little finger

⊟ **SP** **7** S63.247- Subluxation of distal interphalangeal joint of left little finger

⊟ **SP** **7** S63.248- Subluxation of distal interphalangeal joint of other finger

Subluxation of distal interphalangeal joint of specified finger with unspecified laterality

⊟ **IQ** **7** S63.249- Subluxation of distal interphalangeal joint of unspecified finger

6 S63.25 Unspecified dislocation of other finger

⊟ **SP** **7** S63.250- Unspecified dislocation of right index finger

⊟ **SP** **7** S63.251- Unspecified dislocation of left index finger

⊟ **SP** **7** S63.252- Unspecified dislocation of right middle finger

⊟ **SP** **7** S63.253- Unspecified dislocation of left middle finger

⊟ **SP** **7** S63.254- Unspecified dislocation of right ring finger

⊟ **SP** **7** S63.255- Unspecified dislocation of left ring finger

⊟ **SP** **7** S63.256- Unspecified dislocation of right little finger

⊟ **SP** **7** S63.257- Unspecified dislocation of left little finger

⊟ **SP** **7** S63.258- Unspecified dislocation of other finger

Unspecified dislocation of specified finger with unspecified laterality

⊟ **IQ** **7** S63.259- Unspecified dislocation of unspecified finger

Unspecified dislocation of unspecified finger with unspecified laterality

6 S63.26 Dislocation of metacarpophalangeal joint of finger

⊟ **SP** **7** S63.260- Dislocation of metacarpophalangeal joint of right index finger

⊟ **SP** **7** S63.261- Dislocation of metacarpophalangeal joint of left index finger

⊟ **SP** **7** S63.262- Dislocation of metacarpophalangeal joint of right middle finger

⊟ **SP** **7** S63.263- Dislocation of metacarpophalangeal joint of left middle finger

⊟ **SP** **7** S63.264- Dislocation of metacarpophalangeal joint of right ring finger

⊟ **SP** **7** S63.265- Dislocation of metacarpophalangeal joint of left ring finger

⊟ **SP** **7** S63.266- Dislocation of metacarpophalangeal joint of right little finger

⊟ **SP** **7** S63.267- Dislocation of metacarpophalangeal joint of left little finger

⊟ **SP** **7** S63.268- Dislocation of metacarpophalangeal joint of other finger

Dislocation of metacarpophalangeal joint of specified finger with unspecified laterality

⊟ **IQ** **7** S63.269- Dislocation of metacarpophalangeal joint of unspecified finger

6 S63.27 Dislocation of unspecified interphalangeal joint of finger

⊟ **IQ** **7** S63.270- Dislocation of unspecified interphalangeal joint of right index finger

⊟ **IQ** **7** S63.271- Dislocation of unspecified interphalangeal joint of left index finger

⊟ **IQ** **7** S63.272- Dislocation of unspecified interphalangeal joint of right middle finger

⊟ **IQ** **7** S63.273- Dislocation of unspecified interphalangeal joint of left middle finger

⊟ **IQ** **7** S63.274- Dislocation of unspecified interphalangeal joint of right ring finger

⊟ **IQ** **7** S63.275- Dislocation of unspecified interphalangeal joint of left ring finger

⊟ **IQ** **7** S63.276- Dislocation of unspecified interphalangeal joint of right little finger

⊟ **IQ** **7** S63.277- Dislocation of unspecified interphalangeal joint of left little finger

⊟ **IQ** **7** S63.278- Dislocation of unspecified interphalangeal joint of other finger

Dislocation of unspecified interphalangeal joint of specified finger with unspecified laterality

⊟ **IQ** **7** S63.279- Dislocation of unspecified interphalangeal joint of unspecified finger

Dislocation of unspecified interphalangeal joint of unspecified finger without specified laterality

6 S63.28 Dislocation of proximal interphalangeal joint of finger

⊟ **SP** **7** S63.280- Dislocation of proximal interphalangeal joint of right index finger

⊟ **SP** **7** S63.281- Dislocation of proximal interphalangeal joint of left index finger

---

★ New ▲ Revised Px Primary **SP** PDGM Px **SL** Low CoM **SH** High CoM **IQ** Quest. Encounter **H** Hospice non-cancer Dx Unspecified **M** *Manifestation*

☐ SP 7 **S63.282-** **Dislocation of proximal interphalangeal joint of right middle finger**

☐ SP 7 **S63.283-** **Dislocation of proximal interphalangeal joint of left middle finger**

☐ SP 7 **S63.284-** **Dislocation of proximal interphalangeal joint of right ring finger**

☐ SP 7 **S63.285-** **Dislocation of proximal interphalangeal joint of left ring finger**

☐ SP 7 **S63.286-** **Dislocation of proximal interphalangeal joint of right little finger**

☐ SP 7 **S63.287-** **Dislocation of proximal interphalangeal joint of left little finger**

☐ SP 7 **S63.288-** **Dislocation of proximal interphalangeal joint of other finger**
Dislocation of proximal interphalangeal joint of specified finger with unspecified laterality

☐ !Q 7 **S63.289-** **Dislocation of proximal interphalangeal joint of unspecified finger**

6 **S63.29** **Dislocation of distal interphalangeal joint of finger**

☐ SP 7 **S63.290-** **Dislocation of distal interphalangeal joint of right index finger**

☐ SP 7 **S63.291-** **Dislocation of distal interphalangeal joint of left index finger**

☐ SP 7 **S63.292-** **Dislocation of distal interphalangeal joint of right middle finger**

☐ SP 7 **S63.293-** **Dislocation of distal interphalangeal joint of left middle finger**

☐ SP 7 **S63.294-** **Dislocation of distal interphalangeal joint of right ring finger**

☐ SP 7 **S63.295-** **Dislocation of distal interphalangeal joint of left ring finger**

☐ SP 7 **S63.296-** **Dislocation of distal interphalangeal joint of right little finger**

☐ SP 7 **S63.297-** **Dislocation of distal interphalangeal joint of left little finger**

☐ SP 7 **S63.298-** **Dislocation of distal interphalangeal joint of other finger**
Dislocation of distal interphalangeal joint of specified finger with unspecified laterality

☐ !Q 7 **S63.299-** **Dislocation of distal interphalangeal joint of unspecified finger**

5 **S63.3** **Traumatic rupture of ligament of wrist**

6 **S63.30** **Traumatic rupture of unspecified ligament of wrist**

☐ SP 7 **S63.301-** **Traumatic rupture of unspecified ligament of right wrist**

☐ SP 7 **S63.302-** **Traumatic rupture of unspecified ligament of left wrist**

☐ !Q 7 **S63.309-** **Traumatic rupture of unspecified ligament of unspecified wrist**

6 **S63.31** **Traumatic rupture of collateral ligament of wrist**

☐ SP 7 **S63.311-** **Traumatic rupture of collateral ligament of right wrist**

☐ SP 7 **S63.312-** **Traumatic rupture of collateral ligament of left wrist**

☐ !Q 7 **S63.319-** **Traumatic rupture of collateral ligament of unspecified wrist**

6 **S63.32** **Traumatic rupture of radiocarpal ligament**

☐ SP 7 **S63.321-** **Traumatic rupture of right radiocarpal ligament**

☐ SP 7 **S63.322-** **Traumatic rupture of left radiocarpal ligament**

☐ !Q 7 **S63.329-** **Traumatic rupture of unspecified radiocarpal ligament**

6 **S63.33** **Traumatic rupture of ulnocarpal (palmar) ligament**

☐ SP 7 **S63.331-** **Traumatic rupture of right ulnocarpal (palmar) ligament**

☐ SP 7 **S63.332-** **Traumatic rupture of left ulnocarpal (palmar) ligament**

☐ !Q 7 **S63.339-** **Traumatic rupture of unspecified ulnocarpal (palmar) ligament**

6 **S63.39** **Traumatic rupture of other ligament of wrist**

☐ SP 7 **S63.391-** **Traumatic rupture of other ligament of right wrist**

☐ SP 7 **S63.392-** **Traumatic rupture of other ligament of left wrist**

☐ !Q 7 **S63.399-** **Traumatic rupture of other ligament of unspecified wrist**

5 **S63.4** **Traumatic rupture of ligament of finger at metacarpophalangeal and interphalangeal joint(s)**

6 **S63.40** **Traumatic rupture of unspecified ligament of finger at metacarpophalangeal and interphalangeal joint**

☐ SP 7 **S63.400-** **Traumatic rupture of unspecified ligament of right index finger at metacarpophalangeal and interphalangeal joint**

☐ SP 7 **S63.401-** **Traumatic rupture of unspecified ligament of left index finger at metacarpophalangeal and interphalangeal joint**

☐ SP 7 **S63.402-** **Traumatic rupture of unspecified ligament of right middle finger at metacarpophalangeal and interphalangeal joint**

☐ SP 7 **S63.403-** **Traumatic rupture of unspecified ligament of left middle finger at metacarpophalangeal and interphalangeal joint**

---

4 4th digit required   5 5th digit required   6 6th digit required   7 7th digit required   7 7th digit placeholder   + Additional code   ☐ Laterality

⊟ **SP** 7 **S63.404-** **Traumatic rupture of unspecified ligament of right ring finger at metacarpophalangeal and interphalangeal joint**

⊟ **SP** 7 **S63.405-** **Traumatic rupture of unspecified ligament of left ring finger at metacarpophalangeal and interphalangeal joint**

⊟ **SP** 7 **S63.406-** **Traumatic rupture of unspecified ligament of right little finger at metacarpophalangeal and interphalangeal joint**

⊟ **SP** 7 **S63.407-** **Traumatic rupture of unspecified ligament of left little finger at metacarpophalangeal and interphalangeal joint**

⊟ **SP** 7 **S63.408-** **Traumatic rupture of unspecified ligament of other finger at metacarpophalangeal and interphalangeal joint**

Traumatic rupture of unspecified ligament of specified finger with unspecified laterality at metacarpophalangeal and interphalangeal joint

⊟ **IQ** 7 **S63.409-** **Traumatic rupture of unspecified ligament of unspecified finger at metacarpophalangeal and interphalangeal joint**

6 **S63.41** Traumatic rupture of collateral ligament of finger at metacarpophalangeal and interphalangeal joint

⊟ **SP** 7 **S63.410-** Traumatic rupture of collateral ligament of right index finger at metacarpophalangeal and interphalangeal joint

⊟ **SP** 7 **S63.411-** Traumatic rupture of collateral ligament of left index finger at metacarpophalangeal and interphalangeal joint

⊟ **SP** 7 **S63.412-** Traumatic rupture of collateral ligament of right middle finger at metacarpophalangeal and interphalangeal joint

⊟ **SP** 7 **S63.413-** Traumatic rupture of collateral ligament of left middle finger at metacarpophalangeal and interphalangeal joint

⊟ **SP** 7 **S63.414-** Traumatic rupture of collateral ligament of right ring finger at metacarpophalangeal and interphalangeal joint

⊟ **SP** 7 **S63.415-** Traumatic rupture of collateral ligament of left ring finger at metacarpophalangeal and interphalangeal joint

⊟ **SP** 7 **S63.416-** Traumatic rupture of collateral ligament of right little finger at metacarpophalangeal and interphalangeal joint

⊟ **SP** 7 **S63.417-** Traumatic rupture of collateral ligament of left little finger at metacarpophalangeal and interphalangeal joint

⊟ **SP** 7 **S63.418-** Traumatic rupture of collateral ligament of other finger at metacarpophalangeal and interphalangeal joint

Traumatic rupture of collateral ligament of specified finger with unspecified laterality at metacarpophalangeal and interphalangeal joint

⊟ **IQ** 7 **S63.419-** **Traumatic rupture of collateral ligament of unspecified finger at metacarpophalangeal and interphalangeal joint**

6 **S63.42** Traumatic rupture of palmar ligament of finger at metacarpophalangeal and interphalangeal joint

⊟ **SP** 7 **S63.420-** Traumatic rupture of palmar ligament of right index finger at metacarpophalangeal and interphalangeal joint

⊟ **SP** 7 **S63.421-** Traumatic rupture of palmar ligament of left index finger at metacarpophalangeal and interphalangeal joint

⊟ **SP** 7 **S63.422-** Traumatic rupture of palmar ligament of right middle finger at metacarpophalangeal and interphalangeal joint

⊟ **SP** 7 **S63.423-** Traumatic rupture of palmar ligament of left middle finger at metacarpophalangeal and interphalangeal joint

⊟ **SP** 7 **S63.424-** Traumatic rupture of palmar ligament of right ring finger at metacarpophalangeal and interphalangeal joint

⊟ **SP** 7 **S63.425-** Traumatic rupture of palmar ligament of left ring finger at metacarpophalangeal and interphalangeal joint

⊟ **SP** 7 **S63.426-** Traumatic rupture of palmar ligament of right little finger at metacarpophalangeal and interphalangeal joint

⊟ **SP** 7 **S63.427-** Traumatic rupture of palmar ligament of left little finger at metacarpophalangeal and interphalangeal joint

⊟ **SP** 7 **S63.428-** Traumatic rupture of palmar ligament of other finger at metacarpophalangeal and interphalangeal joint

Traumatic rupture of palmar ligament of specified finger with unspecified laterality at metacarpophalangeal and interphalangeal joint

⊟ **IQ** 7 **S63.429-** **Traumatic rupture of palmar ligament of unspecified finger at metacarpophalangeal and interphalangeal joint**

6 **S63.43** Traumatic rupture of volar plate of finger at metacarpophalangeal and interphalangeal joint

⊟ **SP** 7 **S63.430-** Traumatic rupture of volar plate of right index finger at metacarpophalangeal and interphalangeal joint

---

★ New ▲ Revised **Px** Primary **SP** PDGM Px **SL** Low CoM **SH** High CoM **IQ** Quest. Encounter **H** Hospice non-cancer Dx ⬛ Unspecified **M** *Manifestation*

☐ SP 7 S63.431- Traumatic rupture of volar plate of left index finger at metacarpophalangeal and interphalangeal joint

☐ SP 7 S63.432- Traumatic rupture of volar plate of right middle finger at metacarpophalangeal and interphalangeal joint

☐ SP 7 S63.433- Traumatic rupture of volar plate of left middle finger at metacarpophalangeal and interphalangeal joint

☐ SP 7 S63.434- Traumatic rupture of volar plate of right ring finger at metacarpophalangeal and interphalangeal joint

☐ SP 7 S63.435- Traumatic rupture of volar plate of left ring finger at metacarpophalangeal and interphalangeal joint

☐ SP 7 S63.436- Traumatic rupture of volar plate of right little finger at metacarpophalangeal and interphalangeal joint

☐ SP 7 S63.437- Traumatic rupture of volar plate of left little finger at metacarpophalangeal and interphalangeal joint

☐ SP 7 S63.438- Traumatic rupture of volar plate of other finger at metacarpophalangeal and interphalangeal joint

Traumatic rupture of volar plate of specified finger with unspecified laterality at metacarpophalangeal and interphalangeal joint

☐ IQ 7 S63.439- Traumatic rupture of volar plate of unspecified finger at metacarpophalangeal and interphalangeal joint

6 S63.49 Traumatic rupture of other ligament of finger at metacarpophalangeal and interphalangeal joint

☐ SP 7 S63.490- Traumatic rupture of other ligament of right index finger at metacarpophalangeal and interphalangeal joint

☐ SP 7 S63.491- Traumatic rupture of other ligament of left index finger at metacarpophalangeal and interphalangeal joint

☐ SP 7 S63.492- Traumatic rupture of other ligament of right middle finger at metacarpophalangeal and interphalangeal joint

☐ SP 7 S63.493- Traumatic rupture of other ligament of left middle finger at metacarpophalangeal and interphalangeal joint

☐ SP 7 S63.494- Traumatic rupture of other ligament of right ring finger at metacarpophalangeal and interphalangeal joint

☐ SP 7 S63.495- Traumatic rupture of other ligament of left ring finger at metacarpophalangeal and interphalangeal joint

☐ SP 7 S63.496- Traumatic rupture of other ligament of right little finger at metacarpophalangeal and interphalangeal joint

☐ SP 7 S63.497- Traumatic rupture of other ligament of left little finger at metacarpophalangeal and interphalangeal joint

☐ SP 7 S63.498- Traumatic rupture of other ligament of other finger at metacarpophalangeal and interphalangeal joint

Traumatic rupture of ligament of specified finger with unspecified laterality at metacarpophalangeal and interphalangeal joint

☐ IQ 7 S63.499- Traumatic rupture of other ligament of unspecified finger at metacarpophalangeal and interphalangeal joint

5 S63.5 Other and unspecified sprain of wrist

6 S63.50 Unspecified sprain of wrist

☐ SP 7 S63.501- Unspecified sprain of right wrist

☐ SP 7 S63.502- Unspecified sprain of left wrist

☐ IQ 7 S63.509- Unspecified sprain of unspecified wrist

6 S63.51 Sprain of carpal (joint)

☐ SP 7 S63.511- Sprain of carpal joint of right wrist

☐ SP 7 S63.512- Sprain of carpal joint of left wrist

☐ IQ 7 S63.519- Sprain of carpal joint of unspecified wrist

6 S63.52 Sprain of radiocarpal joint

    EXCLUDES 1 traumatic rupture of radiocarpal ligament (S63.32-)

☐ SP 7 S63.521- Sprain of radiocarpal joint of right wrist

☐ SP 7 S63.522- Sprain of radiocarpal joint of left wrist

☐ IQ 7 S63.529- Sprain of radiocarpal joint of unspecified wrist

6 S63.59 Other specified sprain of wrist

☐ SP 7 S63.591- Other specified sprain of right wrist

☐ SP 7 S63.592- Other specified sprain of left wrist

☐ IQ 7 S63.599- Other specified sprain of unspecified wrist

5 S63.6 Other and unspecified sprain of finger(s)

    EXCLUDES 1 traumatic rupture of ligament of finger at metacarpophalangeal and interphalangeal joint (s) (S63.4-)

6 S63.60 Unspecified sprain of thumb

☐ SP 7 S63.601- Unspecified sprain of right thumb

☐ SP 7 S63.602- Unspecified sprain of left thumb

☐ IQ 7 S63.609- Unspecified sprain of unspecified thumb

6 S63.61 Unspecified sprain of other and unspecified finger(s)

☐ 4th digit required   ⑤ 5th digit required   ⑥ 6th digit required   ⑦ 7th digit required   ☑ 7th digit placeholder   ✚ Additional code   ☐ Laterality

1572   *DecisionHealth's* FY 2020 Complete Home Health ICD-10-CM Diagnosis Coding Manual

▣ **SP** ⑦ S63.610- Unspecified sprain of right index finger

▣ **SP** ⑦ S63.611- Unspecified sprain of left index finger

▣ **SP** ⑦ S63.612- Unspecified sprain of right middle finger

▣ **SP** ⑦ S63.613- Unspecified sprain of left middle finger

▣ **SP** ⑦ S63.614- Unspecified sprain of right ring finger

▣ **SP** ⑦ S63.615- Unspecified sprain of left ring finger

▣ **SP** ⑦ S63.616- Unspecified sprain of right little finger

▣ **SP** ⑦ S63.617- Unspecified sprain of left little finger

▣ **SP** ⑦ S63.618- Unspecified sprain of other finger
　　　　　Unspecified sprain of specified finger with unspecified laterality

▣ **IQ** ⑦ S63.619- Unspecified sprain of unspecified finger

　⑥ S63.62　Sprain of interphalangeal joint of thumb

▣ **SP** ⑦ S63.621- Sprain of interphalangeal joint of right thumb

▣ **SP** ⑦ S63.622- Sprain of interphalangeal joint of left thumb

▣ **IQ** ⑦ S63.629- Sprain of interphalangeal joint of unspecified thumb

　⑥ S63.63　Sprain of interphalangeal joint of other and unspecified finger(s)

▣ **SP** ⑦ S63.630- Sprain of interphalangeal joint of right index finger

▣ **SP** ⑦ S63.631- Sprain of interphalangeal joint of left index finger

▣ **SP** ⑦ S63.632- Sprain of interphalangeal joint of right middle finger

▣ **SP** ⑦ S63.633- Sprain of interphalangeal joint of left middle finger

▣ **SP** ⑦ S63.634- Sprain of interphalangeal joint of right ring finger

▣ **SP** ⑦ S63.635- Sprain of interphalangeal joint of left ring finger

▣ **SP** ⑦ S63.636- Sprain of interphalangeal joint of right little finger

▣ **SP** ⑦ S63.637- Sprain of interphalangeal joint of left little finger

▣ **SP** ⑦ S63.638- Sprain of interphalangeal joint of other finger

▣ **IQ** ⑦ S63.639- Sprain of interphalangeal joint of unspecified finger

　⑥ S63.64　Sprain of metacarpophalangeal joint of thumb

▣ **SP** ⑦ S63.641- Sprain of metacarpophalangeal joint of right thumb

▣ **SP** ⑦ S63.642- Sprain of metacarpophalangeal joint of left thumb

▣ **IQ** ⑦ S63.649- Sprain of metacarpophalangeal joint of unspecified thumb

　⑥ S63.65　Sprain of metacarpophalangeal joint of other and unspecified finger(s)

▣ **SP** ⑦ S63.650- Sprain of metacarpophalangeal joint of right index finger

▣ **SP** ⑦ S63.651- Sprain of metacarpophalangeal joint of left index finger

▣ **SP** ⑦ S63.652- Sprain of metacarpophalangeal joint of right middle finger

▣ **SP** ⑦ S63.653- Sprain of metacarpophalangeal joint of left middle finger

▣ **SP** ⑦ S63.654- Sprain of metacarpophalangeal joint of right ring finger

▣ **SP** ⑦ S63.655- Sprain of metacarpophalangeal joint of left ring finger

▣ **SP** ⑦ S63.656- Sprain of metacarpophalangeal joint of right little finger

▣ **SP** ⑦ S63.657- Sprain of metacarpophalangeal joint of left little finger

▣ **SP** ⑦ S63.658- Sprain of metacarpophalangeal joint of other finger
　　　　　Sprain of metacarpophalangeal joint of specified finger with unspecified laterality

▣ **IQ** ⑦ S63.659- Sprain of metacarpophalangeal joint of unspecified finger

　⑥ S63.68　Other sprain of thumb

▣ **SP** ⑦ S63.681- Other sprain of right thumb

▣ **SP** ⑦ S63.682- Other sprain of left thumb

▣ **IQ** ⑦ S63.689- Other sprain of unspecified thumb

　⑥ S63.69　Other sprain of other and unspecified finger(s)

▣ **SP** ⑦ S63.690- Other sprain of right index finger

▣ **SP** ⑦ S63.691- Other sprain of left index finger

▣ **SP** ⑦ S63.692- Other sprain of right middle finger

▣ **SP** ⑦ S63.693- Other sprain of left middle finger

▣ **SP** ⑦ S63.694- Other sprain of right ring finger

▣ **SP** ⑦ S63.695- Other sprain of left ring finger

▣ **SP** ⑦ S63.696- Other sprain of right little finger

▣ **SP** ⑦ S63.697- Other sprain of left little finger

▣ **SP** ⑦ S63.698- Other sprain of other finger
　　　　　Other sprain of specified finger with unspecified laterality

▣ **IQ** ⑦ S63.699- Other sprain of unspecified finger

　⑤ S63.8　Sprain of other part of wrist and hand

　⑥ S63.8X　Sprain of other part of wrist and hand

▣ **SP** ⑦ S63.8X1- Sprain of other part of right wrist and hand

▣ **SP** ⑦ S63.8X2- Sprain of other part of left wrist and hand

▣ **IQ** ⑦ S63.8X9- Sprain of other part of unspecified wrist and hand

　⑤ S63.9　Sprain of unspecified part of wrist and hand

▣ **IQ** ⑦ S63.90X- Sprain of unspecified part of unspecified wrist and hand

▣ **SP** ⑦ S63.91X- Sprain of unspecified part of right wrist and hand

▣ **SP** ⑦ S63.92X- Sprain of unspecified part of left wrist and hand

　④ S64　Injury of nerves at wrist and hand level
　　　Code also:
　　　　any associated open wound (S61.-)

★ New　▲ Revised　Px Primary　**SP** PDGM Px　**SL** Low CoM　**SH** High CoM　**IQ** Quest. Encounter　**H** Hospice non-cancer Dx　Unspecified　**M** *Manifestation*

DecisionHealth's FY 2020 Complete Home Health ICD-10-CM Diagnosis Coding Manual

Chapter 19

S00-T88

The appropriate 7th character is to be added to each code from category S64

A	initial encounter
D	subsequent encounter
S	sequela

5 S64.0 Injury of ulnar nerve at wrist and hand level

⊟ IQ 7̸ S64.00X- Injury of ulnar nerve at wrist and hand level of unspecified arm

⊟ SP 7̸ S64.01X- Injury of ulnar nerve at wrist and hand level of right arm

⊟ SP 7̸ S64.02X- Injury of ulnar nerve at wrist and hand level of left arm

5 S64.1 Injury of median nerve at wrist and hand level

⊟ IQ 7̸ S64.10X- Injury of median nerve at wrist and hand level of unspecified arm

⊟ SP 7̸ S64.11X- Injury of median nerve at wrist and hand level of right arm

⊟ SP 7̸ S64.12X- Injury of median nerve at wrist and hand level of left arm

5 S64.2 Injury of radial nerve at wrist and hand level

⊟ IQ 7̸ S64.20X- Injury of radial nerve at wrist and hand level of unspecified arm

⊟ SP 7̸ S64.21X- Injury of radial nerve at wrist and hand level of right arm

⊟ SP 7̸ S64.22X- Injury of radial nerve at wrist and hand level of left arm

5 S64.3 Injury of digital nerve of thumb

⊟ IQ 7̸ S64.30X- Injury of digital nerve of unspecified thumb

⊟ SP 7̸ S64.31X- Injury of digital nerve of right thumb

⊟ SP 7̸ S64.32X- Injury of digital nerve of left thumb

5 S64.4 Injury of digital nerve of other and unspecified finger

IQ 7̸ S64.40X- Injury of digital nerve of unspecified finger

6 S64.49 Injury of digital nerve of other finger

⊟ SP 7 S64.490- Injury of digital nerve of right index finger

⊟ SP 7 S64.491- Injury of digital nerve of left index finger

⊟ SP 7 S64.492- Injury of digital nerve of right middle finger

⊟ SP 7 S64.493- Injury of digital nerve of left middle finger

⊟ SP 7 S64.494- Injury of digital nerve of right ring finger

⊟ SP 7 S64.495- Injury of digital nerve of left ring finger

⊟ SP 7 S64.496- Injury of digital nerve of right little finger

⊟ SP 7 S64.497- Injury of digital nerve of left little finger

⊟ SP 7 S64.498- Injury of digital nerve of other finger
Injury of digital nerve of specified finger with unspecified laterality

5 S64.8 Injury of other nerves at wrist and hand level

6 S64.8X Injury of other nerves at wrist and hand level

⊟ SP 7 S64.8X1- Injury of other nerves at wrist and hand level of right arm

⊟ SP 7 S64.8X2- Injury of other nerves at wrist and hand level of left arm

⊟ IQ 7 S64.8X9- Injury of other nerves at wrist and hand level of unspecified arm

5 S64.9 Injury of unspecified nerve at wrist and hand level

⊟ IQ 7̸ S64.90X- Injury of unspecified nerve at wrist and hand level of unspecified arm

⊟ IQ 7̸ S64.91X- Injury of unspecified nerve at wrist and hand level of right arm

⊟ IQ 7̸ S64.92X- Injury of unspecified nerve at wrist and hand level of left arm

4 S65 Injury of blood vessels at wrist and hand level
Code also:
any associated open wound (S61.-)

The appropriate 7th character is to be added to each code from category S65

A	initial encounter
D	subsequent encounter
S	sequela

5 S65.0 Injury of ulnar artery at wrist and hand level

6 S65.00 Unspecified injury of ulnar artery at wrist and hand level

⊟ SP 7 S65.001- Unspecified injury of ulnar artery at wrist and hand level of right arm

⊟ SP 7 S65.002- Unspecified injury of ulnar artery at wrist and hand level of left arm

⊟ IQ 7 S65.009- Unspecified injury of ulnar artery at wrist and hand level of unspecified arm

6 S65.01 Laceration of ulnar artery at wrist and hand level

⊟ SP 7 S65.011- Laceration of ulnar artery at wrist and hand level of right arm

⊟ SP 7 S65.012- Laceration of ulnar artery at wrist and hand level of left arm

⊟ IQ 7 S65.019- Laceration of ulnar artery at wrist and hand level of unspecified arm

6 S65.09 Other specified injury of ulnar artery at wrist and hand level

⊟ SP 7 S65.091- Other specified injury of ulnar artery at wrist and hand level of right arm

⊟ SP 7 S65.092- Other specified injury of ulnar artery at wrist and hand level of left arm

⊟ IQ 7 S65.099- Other specified injury of ulnar artery at wrist and hand level of unspecified arm

5 S65.1 Injury of radial artery at wrist and hand level

6 S65.10 Unspecified injury of radial artery at wrist and hand level

⊟ IQ 7 S65.101- Unspecified injury of radial artery at wrist and hand level of right arm

---

⁴ 4th digit required   ⁵ 5th digit required   ⁶ 6th digit required   ⁷ 7th digit required   7̸ 7th digit placeholder   **+** Additional code   ⊟ Laterality

☐ **IQ** 7 **S65.102-** Unspecified injury of radial artery at wrist and hand level of left arm

☐ **IQ** 7 **S65.109-** Unspecified injury of radial artery at wrist and hand level of unspecified arm

6 **S65.11** Laceration of radial artery at wrist and hand level

☐ **SP** 7 **S65.111-** Laceration of radial artery at wrist and hand level of right arm

☐ **SP** 7 **S65.112-** Laceration of radial artery at wrist and hand level of left arm

☐ **IQ** 7 **S65.119-** Laceration of radial artery at wrist and hand level of unspecified arm

6 **S65.19** Other specified injury of radial artery at wrist and hand level

☐ **SP** 7 **S65.191-** Other specified injury of radial artery at wrist and hand level of right arm

☐ **SP** 7 **S65.192-** Other specified injury of radial artery at wrist and hand level of left arm

☐ **IQ** 7 **S65.199-** Other specified injury of radial artery at wrist and hand level of unspecified arm

5 **S65.2** Injury of superficial palmar arch

6 **S65.20** Unspecified injury of superficial palmar arch

☐ **IQ** 7 **S65.201-** Unspecified injury of superficial palmar arch of right hand

☐ **IQ** 7 **S65.202-** Unspecified injury of superficial palmar arch of left hand

☐ **IQ** 7 **S65.209-** Unspecified injury of superficial palmar arch of unspecified hand

6 **S65.21** Laceration of superficial palmar arch

☐ **SP** 7 **S65.211-** Laceration of superficial palmar arch of right hand

☐ **SP** 7 **S65.212-** Laceration of superficial palmar arch of left hand

☐ **IQ** 7 **S65.219-** Laceration of superficial palmar arch of unspecified hand

6 **S65.29** Other specified injury of superficial palmar arch

☐ **SP** 7 **S65.291-** Other specified injury of superficial palmar arch of right hand

☐ **SP** 7 **S65.292-** Other specified injury of superficial palmar arch of left hand

☐ **IQ** 7 **S65.299-** Other specified injury of superficial palmar arch of unspecified hand

5 **S65.3** Injury of deep palmar arch

6 **S65.30** Unspecified injury of deep palmar arch

☐ **IQ** 7 **S65.301-** Unspecified injury of deep palmar arch of right hand

☐ **IQ** 7 **S65.302-** Unspecified injury of deep palmar arch of left hand

☐ **IQ** 7 **S65.309-** Unspecified injury of deep palmar arch of unspecified hand

6 **S65.31** Laceration of deep palmar arch

☐ **SP** 7 **S65.311-** Laceration of deep palmar arch of right hand

☐ **SP** 7 **S65.312-** Laceration of deep palmar arch of left hand

☐ **IQ** 7 **S65.319-** Laceration of deep palmar arch of unspecified hand

6 **S65.39** Other specified injury of deep palmar arch

☐ **SP** 7 **S65.391-** Other specified injury of deep palmar arch of right hand

☐ **SP** 7 **S65.392-** Other specified injury of deep palmar arch of left hand

☐ **IQ** 7 **S65.399-** Other specified injury of deep palmar arch of unspecified hand

5 **S65.4** Injury of blood vessel of thumb

6 **S65.40** Unspecified injury of blood vessel of thumb

☐ **IQ** 7 **S65.401-** Unspecified injury of blood vessel of right thumb

☐ **IQ** 7 **S65.402-** Unspecified injury of blood vessel of left thumb

☐ **IQ** 7 **S65.409-** Unspecified injury of blood vessel of unspecified thumb

6 **S65.41** Laceration of blood vessel of thumb

☐ **SP** 7 **S65.411-** Laceration of blood vessel of right thumb

☐ **SP** 7 **S65.412-** Laceration of blood vessel of left thumb

☐ **IQ** 7 **S65.419-** Laceration of blood vessel of unspecified thumb

6 **S65.49** Other specified injury of blood vessel of thumb

☐ **SP** 7 **S65.491-** Other specified injury of blood vessel of right thumb

☐ **SP** 7 **S65.492-** Other specified injury of blood vessel of left thumb

☐ **IQ** 7 **S65.499-** Other specified injury of blood vessel of unspecified thumb

5 **S65.5** Injury of blood vessel of other and unspecified finger

6 **S65.50** Unspecified injury of blood vessel of other and unspecified finger

☐ **IQ** 7 **S65.500-** Unspecified injury of blood vessel of right index finger

☐ **IQ** 7 **S65.501-** Unspecified injury of blood vessel of left index finger

☐ **IQ** 7 **S65.502-** Unspecified injury of blood vessel of right middle finger

☐ **IQ** 7 **S65.503-** Unspecified injury of blood vessel of left middle finger

☐ **IQ** 7 **S65.504-** Unspecified injury of blood vessel of right ring finger

☐ **IQ** 7 **S65.505-** Unspecified injury of blood vessel of left ring finger

☐ **IQ** 7 **S65.506-** Unspecified injury of blood vessel of right little finger

☐ **IQ** 7 **S65.507-** Unspecified injury of blood vessel of left little finger

☐ **IQ** 7 **S65.508-** Unspecified injury of blood vessel of other finger

Unspecified injury of blood vessel of specified finger with unspecified laterality

Chapter 19

S00-T88

★ New ▲ Revised Px Primary **SP** PDGM Px **SL** Low CoM **SH** High CoM **IQ** Quest. Encounter **H** Hospice non-cancer Dx ☐ Unspecified **M** *Manifestation*

Chapter 19

S00-T88

☐ **IQ** **7** **S65.509-** Unspecified injury of blood vessel of unspecified finger

6 **S65.51** Laceration of blood vessel of other and unspecified finger

☐ **SP** **7** **S65.510-** Laceration of blood vessel of right index finger

☐ **SP** **7** **S65.511-** Laceration of blood vessel of left index finger

☐ **SP** **7** **S65.512-** Laceration of blood vessel of right middle finger

☐ **SP** **7** **S65.513-** Laceration of blood vessel of left middle finger

☐ **SP** **7** **S65.514-** Laceration of blood vessel of right ring finger

☐ **SP** **7** **S65.515-** Laceration of blood vessel of left ring finger

☐ **SP** **7** **S65.516-** Laceration of blood vessel of right little finger

☐ **SP** **7** **S65.517-** Laceration of blood vessel of left little finger

☐ **SP** **7** **S65.518-** Laceration of blood vessel of other finger
Laceration of blood vessel of specified finger with unspecified laterality

☐ **IQ** **7** **S65.519-** Laceration of blood vessel of unspecified finger

6 **S65.59** Other specified injury of blood vessel of other and unspecified finger

☐ **SP** **7** **S65.590-** Other specified injury of blood vessel of right index finger

☐ **SP** **7** **S65.591-** Other specified injury of blood vessel of left index finger

☐ **SP** **7** **S65.592-** Other specified injury of blood vessel of right middle finger

☐ **SP** **7** **S65.593-** Other specified injury of blood vessel of left middle finger

☐ **SP** **7** **S65.594-** Other specified injury of blood vessel of right ring finger

☐ **SP** **7** **S65.595-** Other specified injury of blood vessel of left ring finger

☐ **SP** **7** **S65.596-** Other specified injury of blood vessel of right little finger

☐ **SP** **7** **S65.597-** Other specified injury of blood vessel of left little finger

☐ **SP** **7** **S65.598-** Other specified injury of blood vessel of other finger
Other specified injury of blood vessel of specified finger with unspecified laterality

☐ **IQ** **7** **S65.599-** Other specified injury of blood vessel of unspecified finger

5 **S65.8** Injury of other blood vessels at wrist and hand level

6 **S65.80** Unspecified injury of other blood vessels at wrist and hand level

☐ **IQ** **7** **S65.801-** Unspecified injury of other blood vessels at wrist and hand level of right arm

☐ **IQ** **7** **S65.802-** Unspecified injury of other blood vessels at wrist and hand level of left arm

☐ **IQ** **7** **S65.809-** Unspecified injury of other blood vessels at wrist and hand level of unspecified arm

6 **S65.81** Laceration of other blood vessels at wrist and hand level

☐ **SP** **7** **S65.811-** Laceration of other blood vessels at wrist and hand level of right arm

☐ **SP** **7** **S65.812-** Laceration of other blood vessels at wrist and hand level of left arm

☐ **IQ** **7** **S65.819-** Laceration of other blood vessels at wrist and hand level of unspecified arm

6 **S65.89** Other specified injury of other blood vessels at wrist and hand level

☐ **SP** **7** **S65.891-** Other specified injury of other blood vessels at wrist and hand level of right arm

☐ **SP** **7** **S65.892-** Other specified injury of other blood vessels at wrist and hand level of left arm

☐ **IQ** **7** **S65.899-** Other specified injury of other blood vessels at wrist and hand level of unspecified arm

5 **S65.9** Injury of unspecified blood vessel at wrist and hand level

6 **S65.90** Unspecified injury of unspecified blood vessel at wrist and hand level

☐ **IQ** **7** **S65.901-** Unspecified injury of unspecified blood vessel at wrist and hand level of right arm

☐ **IQ** **7** **S65.902-** Unspecified injury of unspecified blood vessel at wrist and hand level of left arm

☐ **IQ** **7** **S65.909-** Unspecified injury of unspecified blood vessel at wrist and hand level of unspecified arm

6 **S65.91** Laceration of unspecified blood vessel at wrist and hand level

☐ **SP** **7** **S65.911-** Laceration of unspecified blood vessel at wrist and hand level of right arm

☐ **SP** **7** **S65.912-** Laceration of unspecified blood vessel at wrist and hand level of left arm

☐ **IQ** **7** **S65.919-** Laceration of unspecified blood vessel at wrist and hand level of unspecified arm

6 **S65.99** Other specified injury of unspecified blood vessel at wrist and hand level

☐ **IQ** **7** **S65.991-** Other specified injury of unspecified blood vessel at wrist and hand of right arm

☐ **IQ** **7** **S65.992-** Other specified injury of unspecified blood vessel at wrist and hand of left arm

☐ **IQ** **7** **S65.999-** Other specified injury of unspecified blood vessel at wrist and hand of unspecified arm

4 **S66** Injury of muscle, fascia and tendon at wrist and hand level
Code also:
any associated open wound (S61.-)
EXCLUDES 2 sprain of joints and ligaments of wrist and hand (S63.-)

---

4 4th digit required   **5** 5th digit required   **6** 6th digit required   **7** 7th digit required   **7** 7th digit placeholder   **+** Additional code   ☐ Laterality

1576   *DecisionHealth's* FY 2020 Complete Home Health ICD-10-CM Diagnosis Coding Manual

	The appropriate 7th character is to be added to each code from category S66
	A initial encounter
	D subsequent encounter
	S sequela

⑤ S66.0   Injury of long flexor muscle, fascia and tendon of thumb at wrist and hand level

⑥ S66.00   Unspecified injury of long flexor muscle, fascia and tendon of thumb at wrist and hand level

☰ IQ 7 S66.001-   Unspecified injury of long flexor muscle, fascia and tendon of right thumb at wrist and hand level

☰ IQ 7 S66.002-   Unspecified injury of long flexor muscle, fascia and tendon of left thumb at wrist and hand level

☰ IQ 7 S66.009-   Unspecified injury of long flexor muscle, fascia and tendon of unspecified thumb at wrist and hand level

⑥ S66.01   Strain of long flexor muscle, fascia and tendon of thumb at wrist and hand level

☰ SP 7 S66.011-   Strain of long flexor muscle, fascia and tendon of right thumb at wrist and hand level

☰ SP 7 S66.012-   Strain of long flexor muscle, fascia and tendon of left thumb at wrist and hand level

☰ IQ 7 S66.019-   Strain of long flexor muscle, fascia and tendon of unspecified thumb at wrist and hand level

⑥ S66.02   Laceration of long flexor muscle, fascia and tendon of thumb at wrist and hand level

☰ SP 7 S66.021-   Laceration of long flexor muscle, fascia and tendon of right thumb at wrist and hand level

☰ SP 7 S66.022-   Laceration of long flexor muscle, fascia and tendon of left thumb at wrist and hand level

☰ IQ 7 S66.029-   Laceration of long flexor muscle, fascia and tendon of unspecified thumb at wrist and hand level

⑥ S66.09   Other specified injury of long flexor muscle, fascia and tendon of thumb at wrist and hand level

☰ SP 7 S66.091-   Other specified injury of long flexor muscle, fascia and tendon of right thumb at wrist and hand level

☰ SP 7 S66.092-   Other specified injury of long flexor muscle, fascia and tendon of left thumb at wrist and hand level

☰ IQ 7 S66.099-   Other specified injury of long flexor muscle, fascia and tendon of unspecified thumb at wrist and hand level

⑤ S66.1   Injury of flexor muscle, fascia and tendon of other and unspecified finger at wrist and hand level

EXCLUDES 2   Injury of long flexor muscle, fascia and tendon of thumb at wrist and hand level (S66.0-)

⑥ S66.10   Unspecified injury of flexor muscle, fascia and tendon of other and unspecified finger at wrist and hand level

☰ IQ 7 S66.100-   Unspecified injury of flexor muscle, fascia and tendon of right index finger at wrist and hand level

☰ IQ 7 S66.101-   Unspecified injury of flexor muscle, fascia and tendon of left index finger at wrist and hand level

☰ IQ 7 S66.102-   Unspecified injury of flexor muscle, fascia and tendon of right middle finger at wrist and hand level

☰ IQ 7 S66.103-   Unspecified injury of flexor muscle, fascia and tendon of left middle finger at wrist and hand level

☰ IQ 7 S66.104-   Unspecified injury of flexor muscle, fascia and tendon of right ring finger at wrist and hand level

☰ IQ 7 S66.105-   Unspecified injury of flexor muscle, fascia and tendon of left ring finger at wrist and hand level

☰ IQ 7 S66.106-   Unspecified injury of flexor muscle, fascia and tendon of right little finger at wrist and hand level

☰ IQ 7 S66.107-   Unspecified injury of flexor muscle, fascia and tendon of left little finger at wrist and hand level

☰ IQ 7 S66.108-   Unspecified injury of flexor muscle, fascia and tendon of other finger at wrist and hand level

Unspecified injury of flexor muscle, fascia and tendon of specified finger with unspecified laterality at wrist and hand level

☰ IQ 7 S66.109-   Unspecified injury of flexor muscle, fascia and tendon of unspecified finger at wrist and hand level

⑥ S66.11   Strain of flexor muscle, fascia and tendon of other and unspecified finger at wrist and hand level

☰ SP 7 S66.110-   Strain of flexor muscle, fascia and tendon of right index finger at wrist and hand level

☰ SP 7 S66.111-   Strain of flexor muscle, fascia and tendon of left index finger at wrist and hand level

☰ SP 7 S66.112-   Strain of flexor muscle, fascia and tendon of right middle finger at wrist and hand level

☰ SP 7 S66.113-   Strain of flexor muscle, fascia and tendon of left middle finger at wrist and hand level

★ New ▲ Revised Px Primary SP PDGM Px SL Low CoM SH High CoM IQ Quest. Encounter H Hospice non-cancer Dx Unspecified M *Manifestation*

DecisionHealth's FY 2020 Complete Home Health ICD-10-CM Diagnosis Coding Manual

1577

☐ SP 7 S66.114- Strain of flexor muscle, fascia and tendon of right ring finger at wrist and hand level

☐ SP 7 S66.115- Strain of flexor muscle, fascia and tendon of left ring finger at wrist and hand level

☐ SP 7 S66.116- Strain of flexor muscle, fascia and tendon of right little finger at wrist and hand level

☐ SP 7 S66.117- Strain of flexor muscle, fascia and tendon of left little finger at wrist and hand level

☐ SP 7 S66.118- Strain of flexor muscle, fascia and tendon of other finger at wrist and hand level

Strain of flexor muscle, fascia and tendon of specified finger with unspecified laterality at wrist and hand level

☐ IQ 7 S66.119- **Strain of flexor muscle, fascia and tendon of unspecified finger at wrist and hand level**

6 S66.12 **Laceration of flexor muscle, fascia and tendon of other and unspecified finger at wrist and hand level**

☐ SP 7 S66.120- Laceration of flexor muscle, fascia and tendon of right index finger at wrist and hand level

☐ SP 7 S66.121- Laceration of flexor muscle, fascia and tendon of left index finger at wrist and hand level

☐ SP 7 S66.122- Laceration of flexor muscle, fascia and tendon of right middle finger at wrist and hand level

☐ SP 7 S66.123- Laceration of flexor muscle, fascia and tendon of left middle finger at wrist and hand level

☐ SP 7 S66.124- Laceration of flexor muscle, fascia and tendon of right ring finger at wrist and hand level

☐ SP 7 S66.125- Laceration of flexor muscle, fascia and tendon of left ring finger at wrist and hand level

☐ SP 7 S66.126- Laceration of flexor muscle, fascia and tendon of right little finger at wrist and hand level

☐ SP 7 S66.127- Laceration of flexor muscle, fascia and tendon of left little finger at wrist and hand level

☐ SP 7 S66.128- Laceration of flexor muscle, fascia and tendon of other finger at wrist and hand level

Laceration of flexor muscle, fascia and tendon of specified finger with unspecified laterality at wrist and hand level

☐ IQ 7 S66.129- **Laceration of flexor muscle, fascia and tendon of unspecified finger at wrist and hand level**

6 S66.19 **Other injury of flexor muscle, fascia and tendon of other and unspecified finger at wrist and hand level**

☐ SP 7 S66.190- Other injury of flexor muscle, fascia and tendon of right index finger at wrist and hand level

☐ SP 7 S66.191- Other injury of flexor muscle, fascia and tendon of left index finger at wrist and hand level

☐ SP 7 S66.192- Other injury of flexor muscle, fascia and tendon of right middle finger at wrist and hand level

☐ SP 7 S66.193- Other injury of flexor muscle, fascia and tendon of left middle finger at wrist and hand level

☐ SP 7 S66.194- Other injury of flexor muscle, fascia and tendon of right ring finger at wrist and hand level

☐ SP 7 S66.195- Other injury of flexor muscle, fascia and tendon of left ring finger at wrist and hand level

☐ SP 7 S66.196- Other injury of flexor muscle, fascia and tendon of right little finger at wrist and hand level

☐ SP 7 S66.197- Other injury of flexor muscle, fascia and tendon of left little finger at wrist and hand level

☐ SP 7 S66.198- Other injury of flexor muscle, fascia and tendon of other finger at wrist and hand level

Other injury of flexor muscle, fascia and tendon of specified finger with unspecified laterality at wrist and hand level

☐ IQ 7 S66.199- **Other injury of flexor muscle, fascia and tendon of unspecified finger at wrist and hand level**

5 S66.2 **Injury of extensor muscle, fascia and tendon of thumb at wrist and hand level**

6 S66.20 **Unspecified injury of extensor muscle, fascia and tendon of thumb at wrist and hand level**

☐ IQ 7 S66.201- **Unspecified injury of extensor muscle, fascia and tendon of right thumb at wrist and hand level**

☐ IQ 7 S66.202- **Unspecified injury of extensor muscle, fascia and tendon of left thumb at wrist and hand level**

☐ IQ 7 S66.209- **Unspecified injury of extensor muscle, fascia and tendon of unspecified thumb at wrist and hand level**

6 S66.21 Strain of extensor muscle, fascia and tendon of thumb at wrist and hand level

☐ SP 7 S66.211- Strain of extensor muscle, fascia and tendon of right thumb at wrist and hand level

☐ SP 7 S66.212- Strain of extensor muscle, fascia and tendon of left thumb at wrist and hand level

☐ IQ 7 S66.219- **Strain of extensor muscle, fascia and tendon of unspecified thumb at wrist and hand level**

6 S66.22 Laceration of extensor muscle, fascia and tendon of thumb at wrist and hand level

☐ SP 7 S66.221- Laceration of extensor muscle, fascia and tendon of right thumb at wrist and hand level

☐ SP 7 S66.222- Laceration of extensor muscle, fascia and tendon of left thumb at wrist and hand level

☐ IQ 7 S66.229- **Laceration of extensor muscle, fascia and tendon of unspecified thumb at wrist and hand level**

4 4th digit required   5 5th digit required   6 6th digit required   7 7th digit required   ☑ 7th digit placeholder   + Additional code   ☐ Laterality

1578   *DecisionHealth's* FY 2020 Complete Home Health ICD-10-CM Diagnosis Coding Manual

6 S66.29 Other specified injury of extensor muscle, fascia and tendon of thumb at wrist and hand level

⊟ SP 7 S66.291- Other specified injury of extensor muscle, fascia and tendon of right thumb at wrist and hand level

⊟ SP 7 S66.292- Other specified injury of extensor muscle, fascia and tendon of left thumb at wrist and hand level

⊟ IQ 7 S66.299- Other specified injury of extensor muscle, fascia and tendon of unspecified thumb at wrist and hand level

5 S66.3 Injury of extensor muscle, fascia and tendon of other and unspecified finger at wrist and hand level

> **EXCLUDES 2** Injury of extensor muscle, fascia and tendon of thumb at wrist and hand level (S66.2-)

6 S66.30 Unspecified injury of extensor muscle, fascia and tendon of other and unspecified finger at wrist and hand level

⊟ IQ 7 S66.300- Unspecified injury of extensor muscle, fascia and tendon of right index finger at wrist and hand level

⊟ IQ 7 S66.301- Unspecified injury of extensor muscle, fascia and tendon of left index finger at wrist and hand level

⊟ IQ 7 S66.302- Unspecified injury of extensor muscle, fascia and tendon of right middle finger at wrist and hand level

⊟ IQ 7 S66.303- Unspecified injury of extensor muscle, fascia and tendon of left middle finger at wrist and hand level

⊟ IQ 7 S66.304- Unspecified injury of extensor muscle, fascia and tendon of right ring finger at wrist and hand level

⊟ IQ 7 S66.305- Unspecified injury of extensor muscle, fascia and tendon of left ring finger at wrist and hand level

⊟ IQ 7 S66.306- Unspecified injury of extensor muscle, fascia and tendon of right little finger at wrist and hand level

⊟ IQ 7 S66.307- Unspecified injury of extensor muscle, fascia and tendon of left little finger at wrist and hand level

⊟ IQ 7 S66.308- Unspecified injury of extensor muscle, fascia and tendon of other finger at wrist and hand level
Unspecified injury of extensor muscle, fascia and tendon of specified finger with unspecified laterality at wrist and hand level

⊟ IQ 7 S66.309- Unspecified injury of extensor muscle, fascia and tendon of unspecified finger at wrist and hand level

6 S66.31 Strain of extensor muscle, fascia and tendon of other and unspecified finger at wrist and hand level

⊟ SP 7 S66.310- Strain of extensor muscle, fascia and tendon of right index finger at wrist and hand level

⊟ SP 7 S66.311- Strain of extensor muscle, fascia and tendon of left index finger at wrist and hand level

⊟ SP 7 S66.312- Strain of extensor muscle, fascia and tendon of right middle finger at wrist and hand level

⊟ SP 7 S66.313- Strain of extensor muscle, fascia and tendon of left middle finger at wrist and hand level

⊟ SP 7 S66.314- Strain of extensor muscle, fascia and tendon of right ring finger at wrist and hand level

⊟ SP 7 S66.315- Strain of extensor muscle, fascia and tendon of left ring finger at wrist and hand level

⊟ SP 7 S66.316- Strain of extensor muscle, fascia and tendon of right little finger at wrist and hand level

⊟ SP 7 S66.317- Strain of extensor muscle, fascia and tendon of left little finger at wrist and hand level

⊟ SP 7 S66.318- Strain of extensor muscle, fascia and tendon of other finger at wrist and hand level
Strain of extensor muscle, fascia and tendon of specified finger with unspecified laterality at wrist and hand level

⊟ IQ 7 S66.319- Strain of extensor muscle, fascia and tendon of unspecified finger at wrist and hand level

6 S66.32 Laceration of extensor muscle, fascia and tendon of other and unspecified finger at wrist and hand level

⊟ SP 7 S66.320- Laceration of extensor muscle, fascia and tendon of right index finger at wrist and hand level

⊟ SP 7 S66.321- Laceration of extensor muscle, fascia and tendon of left index finger at wrist and hand level

⊟ SP 7 S66.322- Laceration of extensor muscle, fascia and tendon of right middle finger at wrist and hand level

⊟ SP 7 S66.323- Laceration of extensor muscle, fascia and tendon of left middle finger at wrist and hand level

⊟ SP 7 S66.324- Laceration of extensor muscle, fascia and tendon of right ring finger at wrist and hand level

⊟ SP 7 S66.325- Laceration of extensor muscle, fascia and tendon of left ring finger at wrist and hand level

⊟ SP 7 S66.326- Laceration of extensor muscle, fascia and tendon of right little finger at wrist and hand level

Chapter 19

S00-T88

★ New ▲ Revised Px Primary SP PDGM Px SL Low CoM SH High CoM IQ Quest. Encounter H Hospice non-cancer Dx Unspecified M *Manifestation*

DecisionHealth's FY 2020 Complete Home Health ICD-10-CM Diagnosis Coding Manual 1579

🗏 **SP** **7** **S66.327-** Laceration of extensor muscle, fascia and tendon of left little finger at wrist and hand level

🗏 **SP** **7** **S66.328-** Laceration of extensor muscle, fascia and tendon of other finger at wrist and hand level
Laceration of extensor muscle, fascia and tendon of specified finger with unspecified laterality at wrist and hand level

🗏 **IQ** **7** **S66.329-** Laceration of extensor muscle, fascia and tendon of unspecified finger at wrist and hand level

6 **S66.39** Other injury of extensor muscle, fascia and tendon of other and unspecified finger at wrist and hand level

🗏 **SP** **7** **S66.390-** Other injury of extensor muscle, fascia and tendon of right index finger at wrist and hand level

🗏 **SP** **7** **S66.391-** Other injury of extensor muscle, fascia and tendon of left index finger at wrist and hand level

🗏 **SP** **7** **S66.392-** Other injury of extensor muscle, fascia and tendon of right middle finger at wrist and hand level

🗏 **SP** **7** **S66.393-** Other injury of extensor muscle, fascia and tendon of left middle finger at wrist and hand level

🗏 **SP** **7** **S66.394-** Other injury of extensor muscle, fascia and tendon of right ring finger at wrist and hand level

🗏 **SP** **7** **S66.395-** Other injury of extensor muscle, fascia and tendon of left ring finger at wrist and hand level

🗏 **SP** **7** **S66.396-** Other injury of extensor muscle, fascia and tendon of right little finger at wrist and hand level

🗏 **SP** **7** **S66.397-** Other injury of extensor muscle, fascia and tendon of left little finger at wrist and hand level

🗏 **SP** **7** **S66.398-** Other injury of extensor muscle, fascia and tendon of other finger at wrist and hand level
Other injury of extensor muscle, fascia and tendon of specified finger with unspecified laterality at wrist and hand level

🗏 **IQ** **7** **S66.399-** Other injury of extensor muscle, fascia and tendon of unspecified finger at wrist and hand level

5 **S66.4** Injury of intrinsic muscle, fascia and tendon of thumb at wrist and hand level

6 **S66.40** Unspecified injury of intrinsic muscle, fascia and tendon of thumb at wrist and hand level

🗏 **IQ** **7** **S66.401-** Unspecified injury of intrinsic muscle, fascia and tendon of right thumb at wrist and hand level

🗏 **IQ** **7** **S66.402-** Unspecified injury of intrinsic muscle, fascia and tendon of left thumb at wrist and hand level

🗏 **IQ** **7** **S66.409-** Unspecified injury of intrinsic muscle, fascia and tendon of unspecified thumb at wrist and hand level

6 **S66.41** Strain of intrinsic muscle, fascia and tendon of thumb at wrist and hand level

🗏 **SP** **7** **S66.411-** Strain of intrinsic muscle, fascia and tendon of right thumb at wrist and hand level

🗏 **SP** **7** **S66.412-** Strain of intrinsic muscle, fascia and tendon of left thumb at wrist and hand level

🗏 **IQ** **7** **S66.419-** Strain of intrinsic muscle, fascia and tendon of unspecified thumb at wrist and hand level

6 **S66.42** Laceration of intrinsic muscle, fascia and tendon of thumb at wrist and hand level

🗏 **SP** **7** **S66.421-** Laceration of intrinsic muscle, fascia and tendon of right thumb at wrist and hand level

🗏 **SP** **7** **S66.422-** Laceration of intrinsic muscle, fascia and tendon of left thumb at wrist and hand level

🗏 **IQ** **7** **S66.429-** Laceration of intrinsic muscle, fascia and tendon of unspecified thumb at wrist and hand level

6 **S66.49** Other specified injury of intrinsic muscle, fascia and tendon of thumb at wrist and hand level

🗏 **SP** **7** **S66.491-** Other specified injury of intrinsic muscle, fascia and tendon of right thumb at wrist and hand level

🗏 **SP** **7** **S66.492-** Other specified injury of intrinsic muscle, fascia and tendon of left thumb at wrist and hand level

🗏 **IQ** **7** **S66.499-** Other specified injury of intrinsic muscle, fascia and tendon of unspecified thumb at wrist and hand level

5 **S66.5** Injury of intrinsic muscle, fascia and tendon of other and unspecified finger at wrist and hand level

EXCLUDES 2 injury of intrinsic muscle, fascia and tendon of thumb at wrist and hand level (S66.4-)

6 **S66.50** Unspecified injury of intrinsic muscle, fascia and tendon of other and unspecified finger at wrist and hand level

🗏 **IQ** **7** **S66.500-** Unspecified injury of intrinsic muscle, fascia and tendon of right index finger at wrist and hand level

🗏 **IQ** **7** **S66.501-** Unspecified injury of intrinsic muscle, fascia and tendon of left index finger at wrist and hand level

🗏 **IQ** **7** **S66.502-** Unspecified injury of intrinsic muscle, fascia and tendon of right middle finger at wrist and hand level

🗏 **IQ** **7** **S66.503-** Unspecified injury of intrinsic muscle, fascia and tendon of left middle finger at wrist and hand level

---

4 4th digit required　　**5** 5th digit required　　**6** 6th digit required　　**7** 7th digit required　　**⑦** 7th digit placeholder　　**+** Additional code　　🗏 Laterality

▤ **IQ** **7** **S66.504-** Unspecified injury of intrinsic muscle, fascia and tendon of right ring finger at wrist and hand level

▤ **IQ** **7** **S66.505-** Unspecified injury of intrinsic muscle, fascia and tendon of left ring finger at wrist and hand level

▤ **IQ** **7** **S66.506-** Unspecified injury of intrinsic muscle, fascia and tendon of right little finger at wrist and hand level

▤ **IQ** **7** **S66.507-** Unspecified injury of intrinsic muscle, fascia and tendon of left little finger at wrist and hand level

▤ **IQ** **7** **S66.508-** Unspecified injury of intrinsic muscle, fascia and tendon of other finger at wrist and hand level

Unspecified injury of intrinsic muscle, fascia and tendon of specified finger with unspecified laterality at wrist and hand level

▤ **IQ** **7** **S66.509-** Unspecified injury of intrinsic muscle, fascia and tendon of unspecified finger at wrist and hand level

6 **S66.51** Strain of intrinsic muscle, fascia and tendon of other and unspecified finger at wrist and hand level

▤ **SP** **7** **S66.510-** Strain of intrinsic muscle, fascia and tendon of right index finger at wrist and hand level

▤ **SP** **7** **S66.511-** Strain of intrinsic muscle, fascia and tendon of left index finger at wrist and hand level

▤ **SP** **7** **S66.512-** Strain of intrinsic muscle, fascia and tendon of right middle finger at wrist and hand level

▤ **SP** **7** **S66.513-** Strain of intrinsic muscle, fascia and tendon of left middle finger at wrist and hand level

▤ **SP** **7** **S66.514-** Strain of intrinsic muscle, fascia and tendon of right ring finger at wrist and hand level

▤ **SP** **7** **S66.515-** Strain of intrinsic muscle, fascia and tendon of left ring finger at wrist and hand level

▤ **SP** **7** **S66.516-** Strain of intrinsic muscle, fascia and tendon of right little finger at wrist and hand level

▤ **SP** **7** **S66.517-** Strain of intrinsic muscle, fascia and tendon of left little finger at wrist and hand level

▤ **SP** **7** **S66.518-** Strain of intrinsic muscle, fascia and tendon of other finger at wrist and hand level

Strain of intrinsic muscle, fascia and tendon of specified finger with unspecified laterality at wrist and hand level

▤ **IQ** **7** **S66.519-** Strain of intrinsic muscle, fascia and tendon of unspecified finger at wrist and hand level

6 **S66.52** Laceration of intrinsic muscle, fascia and tendon of other and unspecified finger at wrist and hand level

▤ **SP** **7** **S66.520-** Laceration of intrinsic muscle, fascia and tendon of right index finger at wrist and hand level

▤ **SP** **7** **S66.521-** Laceration of intrinsic muscle, fascia and tendon of left index finger at wrist and hand level

▤ **SP** **7** **S66.522-** Laceration of intrinsic muscle, fascia and tendon of right middle finger at wrist and hand level

▤ **SP** **7** **S66.523-** Laceration of intrinsic muscle, fascia and tendon of left middle finger at wrist and hand level

▤ **SP** **7** **S66.524-** Laceration of intrinsic muscle, fascia and tendon of right ring finger at wrist and hand level

▤ **SP** **7** **S66.525-** Laceration of intrinsic muscle, fascia and tendon of left ring finger at wrist and hand level

▤ **SP** **7** **S66.526-** Laceration of intrinsic muscle, fascia and tendon of right little finger at wrist and hand level

▤ **SP** **7** **S66.527-** Laceration of intrinsic muscle, fascia and tendon of left little finger at wrist and hand level

▤ **SP** **7** **S66.528-** Laceration of intrinsic muscle, fascia and tendon of other finger at wrist and hand level

Laceration of intrinsic muscle, fascia and tendon of specified finger with unspecified laterality at wrist and hand level

▤ **IQ** **7** **S66.529-** Laceration of intrinsic muscle, fascia and tendon of unspecified finger at wrist and hand level

6 **S66.59** Other injury of intrinsic muscle, fascia and tendon of other and unspecified finger at wrist and hand level

▤ **SP** **7** **S66.590-** Other injury of intrinsic muscle, fascia and tendon of right index finger at wrist and hand level

▤ **SP** **7** **S66.591-** Other injury of intrinsic muscle, fascia and tendon of left index finger at wrist and hand level

▤ **SP** **7** **S66.592-** Other injury of intrinsic muscle, fascia and tendon of right middle finger at wrist and hand level

▤ **SP** **7** **S66.593-** Other injury of intrinsic muscle, fascia and tendon of left middle finger at wrist and hand level

▤ **SP** **7** **S66.594-** Other injury of intrinsic muscle, fascia and tendon of right ring finger at wrist and hand level

▤ **SP** **7** **S66.595-** Other injury of intrinsic muscle, fascia and tendon of left ring finger at wrist and hand level

▤ **SP** **7** **S66.596-** Other injury of intrinsic muscle, fascia and tendon of right little finger at wrist and hand level

▤ **SP** **7** **S66.597-** Other injury of intrinsic muscle, fascia and tendon of left little finger at wrist and hand level

★ New ▲ Revised **Px** Primary **SP** PDGM Px **SL** Low CoM **SH** High CoM **IQ** Quest. Encounter **H** Hospice non-cancer Dx   Unspecified   **M** *Manifestation*

DecisionHealth's FY 2020 Complete Home Health ICD-10-CM Diagnosis Coding Manual   1581

Chapter 19

S00-T88

☐ **SP** 7 **S66.598-**   **Other injury of intrinsic muscle, fascia and tendon of other finger at wrist and hand level**
Other injury of intrinsic muscle, fascia and tendon of specified finger with unspecified laterality at wrist and hand level

☐ **IQ** 7 **S66.599-**   **Other injury of intrinsic muscle, fascia and tendon of unspecified finger at wrist and hand level**

5 **S66.8**   **Injury of other specified muscles, fascia and tendons at wrist and hand level**

6 **S66.80**   **Unspecified injury of other specified muscles, fascia and tendons at wrist and hand level**

☐ **IQ** 7 **S66.801-**   **Unspecified injury of other specified muscles, fascia and tendons at wrist and hand level, right hand**

☐ **IQ** 7 **S66.802-**   **Unspecified injury of other specified muscles, fascia and tendons at wrist and hand level, left hand**

☐ **IQ** 7 **S66.809-**   **Unspecified injury of other specified muscles, fascia and tendons at wrist and hand level, unspecified hand**

6 **S66.81**   **Strain of other specified muscles, fascia and tendons at wrist and hand level**

☐ **SP** 7 **S66.811-**   **Strain of other specified muscles, fascia and tendons at wrist and hand level, right hand**

☐ **SP** 7 **S66.812-**   **Strain of other specified muscles, fascia and tendons at wrist and hand level, left hand**

☐ **IQ** 7 **S66.819-**   **Strain of other specified muscles, fascia and tendons at wrist and hand level, unspecified hand**

6 **S66.82**   **Laceration of other specified muscles, fascia and tendons at wrist and hand level**

☐ **SP** 7 **S66.821-**   **Laceration of other specified muscles, fascia and tendons at wrist and hand level, right hand**

☐ **SP** 7 **S66.822-**   **Laceration of other specified muscles, fascia and tendons at wrist and hand level, left hand**

☐ **IQ** 7 **S66.829-**   **Laceration of other specified muscles, fascia and tendons at wrist and hand level, unspecified hand**

6 **S66.89**   **Other injury of other specified muscles, fascia and tendons at wrist and hand level**

☐ **SP** 7 **S66.891-**   **Other injury of other specified muscles, fascia and tendons at wrist and hand level, right hand**

☐ **SP** 7 **S66.892-**   **Other injury of other specified muscles, fascia and tendons at wrist and hand level, left hand**

☐ **IQ** 7 **S66.899-**   **Other injury of other specified muscles, fascia and tendons at wrist and hand level, unspecified hand**

5 **S66.9**   **Injury of unspecified muscle, fascia and tendon at wrist and hand level**

6 **S66.90**   **Unspecified injury of unspecified muscle, fascia and tendon at wrist and hand level**

☐ **IQ** 7 **S66.901-**   **Unspecified injury of unspecified muscle, fascia and tendon at wrist and hand level, right hand**

☐ **IQ** 7 **S66.902-**   **Unspecified injury of unspecified muscle, fascia and tendon at wrist and hand level, left hand**

☐ **IQ** 7 **S66.909-**   **Unspecified injury of unspecified muscle, fascia and tendon at wrist and hand level, unspecified hand**

6 **S66.91**   **Strain of unspecified muscle, fascia and tendon at wrist and hand level**

☐ **SP** 7 **S66.911-**   **Strain of unspecified muscle, fascia and tendon at wrist and hand level, right hand**

☐ **SP** 7 **S66.912-**   **Strain of unspecified muscle, fascia and tendon at wrist and hand level, left hand**

☐ **IQ** 7 **S66.919-**   **Strain of unspecified muscle, fascia and tendon at wrist and hand level, unspecified hand**

6 **S66.92**   **Laceration of unspecified muscle, fascia and tendon at wrist and hand level**

☐ **SP** 7 **S66.921-**   **Laceration of unspecified muscle, fascia and tendon at wrist and hand level, right hand**

☐ **SP** 7 **S66.922-**   **Laceration of unspecified muscle, fascia and tendon at wrist and hand level, left hand**

☐ **IQ** 7 **S66.929-**   **Laceration of unspecified muscle, fascia and tendon at wrist and hand level, unspecified hand**

6 **S66.99**   **Other injury of unspecified muscle, fascia and tendon at wrist and hand level**

☐ **IQ** 7 **S66.991-**   **Other injury of unspecified muscle, fascia and tendon at wrist and hand level, right hand**

☐ **IQ** 7 **S66.992-**   **Other injury of unspecified muscle, fascia and tendon at wrist and hand level, left hand**

☐ **IQ** 7 **S66.999-**   **Other injury of unspecified muscle, fascia and tendon at wrist and hand level, unspecified hand**

✛ 4 **S67**   **Crushing injury of wrist, hand and fingers**
Use additional code for all associated injuries, such as:
fracture of wrist and hand (S62.-)
open wound of wrist and hand (S61.-)

The appropriate 7th character is to be added to each code from category S67
A   initial encounter
D   subsequent encounter
S   sequela

✛ 5 **S67.0**   **Crushing injury of thumb**

---

4 4th digit required   5 5th digit required   6 6th digit required   7 7th digit required   7 7th digit placeholder   ✛ Additional code   ☐ Laterality

1582   *DecisionHealth's* FY 2020 Complete Home Health ICD-10-CM Diagnosis Coding Manual

🔲 🔟 ✚ ☑ **S67.00X-** Crushing injury of unspecified thumb

🔲 **SP** ✚ ☑ **S67.01X-** Crushing injury of right thumb

🔲 **SP** ✚ ☑ **S67.02X-** Crushing injury of left thumb

✚ 🔢 **S67.1** Crushing injury of other and unspecified finger(s)

EXCLUDES 2 crushing injury of thumb (S67.0-)

🔟 ✚ ☑ **S67.10X-** Crushing injury of unspecified finger(s)

✚ 🔢 **S67.19** Crushing injury of other finger(s)

🔲 **SP** ✚ 7 **S67.190-** Crushing injury of right index finger

🔲 **SP** ✚ 7 **S67.191-** Crushing injury of left index finger

🔲 **SP** ✚ 7 **S67.192-** Crushing injury of right middle finger

🔲 **SP** ✚ 7 **S67.193-** Crushing injury of left middle finger

🔲 **SP** ✚ 7 **S67.194-** Crushing injury of right ring finger

🔲 **SP** ✚ 7 **S67.195-** Crushing injury of left ring finger

🔲 **SP** ✚ 7 **S67.196-** Crushing injury of right little finger

🔲 **SP** ✚ 7 **S67.197-** Crushing injury of left little finger

🔲 **SP** ✚ 7 **S67.198-** Crushing injury of other finger
Crushing injury of specified finger with unspecified laterality

✚ 🔢 **S67.2** Crushing injury of hand

EXCLUDES 2 crushing injury of fingers (S67.1-)
crushing injury of thumb (S67.0-)

🔲 🔟 ✚ ☑ **S67.20X-** Crushing injury of unspecified hand

🔲 **SP** ✚ ☑ **S67.21X-** Crushing injury of right hand

🔲 **SP** ✚ ☑ **S67.22X-** Crushing injury of left hand

✚ 🔢 **S67.3** Crushing injury of wrist

🔲 🔟 ✚ ☑ **S67.30X-** Crushing injury of unspecified wrist

🔲 **SP** ✚ ☑ **S67.31X-** Crushing injury of right wrist

🔲 **SP** ✚ ☑ **S67.32X-** Crushing injury of left wrist

✚ 🔢 **S67.4** Crushing injury of wrist and hand

EXCLUDES 1 crushing injury of hand alone (S67.2-)
crushing injury of wrist alone (S67.3-)

EXCLUDES 2 crushing injury of fingers (S67.1-)
crushing injury of thumb (S67.0-)

🔲 🔟 ✚ ☑ **S67.40X-** Crushing injury of unspecified wrist and hand

🔲 **SP** ✚ ☑ **S67.41X-** Crushing injury of right wrist and hand

🔲 **SP** ✚ ☑ **S67.42X-** Crushing injury of left wrist and hand

✚ 🔢 **S67.9** Crushing injury of unspecified part(s) of wrist, hand and fingers

🔲 🔟 ✚ ☑ **S67.90X-** Crushing injury of unspecified part(s) of unspecified wrist, hand and fingers

🔲 **SP** ✚ ☑ **S67.91X-** Crushing injury of unspecified part(s) of right wrist, hand and fingers

🔲 **SP** ✚ ☑ **S67.92X-** Crushing injury of unspecified part(s) of left wrist, hand and fingers

🔢 **S68** Traumatic amputation of wrist, hand and fingers
An amputation not identified as partial or complete should be coded to complete

The appropriate 7th character is to be added to each code from category S68
A initial encounter
D subsequent encounter
S sequela

CODING TIPS ✓ Use these codes only when the amputation was due to trauma. There is no need for adding Z89 with traumatic amputations. See Z47.81 for care of amputations not due to trauma.

🔢 **S68.0** Traumatic metacarpophalangeal amputation of thumb
Traumatic amputation of thumb NOS

🔢 **S68.01** Complete traumatic metacarpophalangeal amputation of thumb

🔲 **SP** 7 **S68.011-** Complete traumatic metacarpophalangeal amputation of right thumb

🔲 **SP** 7 **S68.012-** Complete traumatic metacarpophalangeal amputation of left thumb

🔲 🔟 7 **S68.019-** Complete traumatic metacarpophalangeal amputation of unspecified thumb

🔢 **S68.02** Partial traumatic metacarpophalangeal amputation of thumb

🔲 **SP** 7 **S68.021-** Partial traumatic metacarpophalangeal amputation of right thumb

🔲 **SP** 7 **S68.022-** Partial traumatic metacarpophalangeal amputation of left thumb

🔲 🔟 7 **S68.029-** Partial traumatic metacarpophalangeal amputation of unspecified thumb

🔢 **S68.1** Traumatic metacarpophalangeal amputation of other and unspecified finger
Traumatic amputation of finger NOS

EXCLUDES 2 traumatic metacarpophalangeal amputation of thumb (S68.0-)

🔢 **S68.11** Complete traumatic metacarpophalangeal amputation of other and unspecified finger

🔲 **SP** 7 **S68.110-** Complete traumatic metacarpophalangeal amputation of right index finger

🔲 **SP** 7 **S68.111-** Complete traumatic metacarpophalangeal amputation of left index finger

★ New ▲ Revised Px Primary **SP** PDGM Px **SL** Low CoM **SH** High CoM 🔟 Quest. Encounter 🄷 Hospice non-cancer Dx Unspecified **M** *Manifestation*

DecisionHealth's FY 2020 Complete Home Health ICD-10-CM Diagnosis Coding Manual

1583

⊟ **SP 7** S68.112- **Complete traumatic metacarpophalangeal amputation of right middle finger**

⊟ **SP 7** S68.113- **Complete traumatic metacarpophalangeal amputation of left middle finger**

⊟ **SP 7** S68.114- **Complete traumatic metacarpophalangeal amputation of right ring finger**

⊟ **SP 7** S68.115- **Complete traumatic metacarpophalangeal amputation of left ring finger**

⊟ **SP 7** S68.116- **Complete traumatic metacarpophalangeal amputation of right little finger**

⊟ **SP 7** S68.117- **Complete traumatic metacarpophalangeal amputation of left little finger**

⊟ **SP 7** S68.118- **Complete traumatic metacarpophalangeal amputation of other finger**
Complete traumatic metacarpophalangeal amputation of specified finger with unspecified laterality

⊟ **IQ 7** S68.119- **Complete traumatic metacarpophalangeal amputation of unspecified finger**

6 S68.12 **Partial traumatic metacarpophalangeal amputation of other and unspecified finger**

⊟ **SP 7** S68.120- **Partial traumatic metacarpophalangeal amputation of right index finger**

⊟ **SP 7** S68.121- **Partial traumatic metacarpophalangeal amputation of left index finger**

⊟ **SP 7** S68.122- **Partial traumatic metacarpophalangeal amputation of right middle finger**

⊟ **SP 7** S68.123- **Partial traumatic metacarpophalangeal amputation of left middle finger**

⊟ **SP 7** S68.124- **Partial traumatic metacarpophalangeal amputation of right ring finger**

⊟ **SP 7** S68.125- **Partial traumatic metacarpophalangeal amputation of left ring finger**

⊟ **SP 7** S68.126- **Partial traumatic metacarpophalangeal amputation of right little finger**

⊟ **SP 7** S68.127- **Partial traumatic metacarpophalangeal amputation of left little finger**

⊟ **SP 7** S68.128- **Partial traumatic metacarpophalangeal amputation of other finger**
Partial traumatic metacarpophalangeal amputation of specified finger with unspecified laterality

⊟ **IQ 7** S68.129- **Partial traumatic metacarpophalangeal amputation of unspecified finger**

5 S68.4 **Traumatic amputation of hand at wrist level**
Traumatic amputation of hand NOS
Traumatic amputation of wrist

6 S68.41 **Complete traumatic amputation of hand at wrist level**

⊟ **SP 7** S68.411- **Complete traumatic amputation of right hand at wrist level**

⊟ **SP 7** S68.412- **Complete traumatic amputation of left hand at wrist level**

⊟ **IQ 7** S68.419- **Complete traumatic amputation of unspecified hand at wrist level**

6 S68.42 **Partial traumatic amputation of hand at wrist level**

⊟ **SP 7** S68.421- **Partial traumatic amputation of right hand at wrist level**

⊟ **SP 7** S68.422- **Partial traumatic amputation of left hand at wrist level**

⊟ **IQ 7** S68.429- **Partial traumatic amputation of unspecified hand at wrist level**

5 S68.5 **Traumatic transphalangeal amputation of thumb**
Traumatic interphalangeal joint amputation of thumb

6 S68.51 **Complete traumatic transphalangeal amputation of thumb**

⊟ **SP 7** S68.511- **Complete traumatic transphalangeal amputation of right thumb**

⊟ **SP 7** S68.512- **Complete traumatic transphalangeal amputation of left thumb**

⊟ **IQ 7** S68.519- **Complete traumatic transphalangeal amputation of unspecified thumb**

6 S68.52 **Partial traumatic transphalangeal amputation of thumb**

⊟ **SP 7** S68.521- **Partial traumatic transphalangeal amputation of right thumb**

⊟ **SP 7** S68.522- **Partial traumatic transphalangeal amputation of left thumb**

⊟ **IQ 7** S68.529- **Partial traumatic transphalangeal amputation of unspecified thumb**

5 S68.6 **Traumatic transphalangeal amputation of other and unspecified finger**

6 S68.61 **Complete traumatic transphalangeal amputation of other and unspecified finger(s)**

⊟ **SP 7** S68.610- **Complete traumatic transphalangeal amputation of right index finger**

⊟ **SP 7** S68.611- **Complete traumatic transphalangeal amputation of left index finger**

⊟ **SP 7** S68.612- **Complete traumatic transphalangeal amputation of right middle finger**

4 4th digit required   **5** 5th digit required   **6** 6th digit required   **7** 7th digit required   **7** 7th digit placeholder   **+** Additional code   ⊟ Laterality

1584   *DecisionHealth's* FY 2020 Complete Home Health ICD-10-CM Diagnosis Coding Manual

⊟ SP 7 S68.613- Complete traumatic transphalangeal amputation of left middle finger

⊟ SP 7 S68.614- Complete traumatic transphalangeal amputation of right ring finger

⊟ SP 7 S68.615- Complete traumatic transphalangeal amputation of left ring finger

⊟ SP 7 S68.616- Complete traumatic transphalangeal amputation of right little finger

⊟ SP 7 S68.617- Complete traumatic transphalangeal amputation of left little finger

⊟ SP 7 S68.618- Complete traumatic transphalangeal amputation of other finger
Complete traumatic transphalangeal amputation of specified finger with unspecified laterality

⊟ IQ 7 S68.619- Complete traumatic transphalangeal amputation of unspecified finger

6 S68.62 Partial traumatic transphalangeal amputation of other and unspecified finger

⊟ SP 7 S68.620- Partial traumatic transphalangeal amputation of right index finger

⊟ SP 7 S68.621- Partial traumatic transphalangeal amputation of left index finger

⊟ SP 7 S68.622- Partial traumatic transphalangeal amputation of right middle finger

⊟ SP 7 S68.623- Partial traumatic transphalangeal amputation of left middle finger

⊟ SP 7 S68.624- Partial traumatic transphalangeal amputation of right ring finger

⊟ SP 7 S68.625- Partial traumatic transphalangeal amputation of left ring finger

⊟ SP 7 S68.626- Partial traumatic transphalangeal amputation of right little finger

⊟ SP 7 S68.627- Partial traumatic transphalangeal amputation of left little finger

⊟ SP 7 S68.628- Partial traumatic transphalangeal amputation of other finger
Partial traumatic transphalangeal amputation of specified finger with unspecified laterality

⊟ IQ 7 S68.629- Partial traumatic transphalangeal amputation of unspecified finger

5 S68.7 Traumatic transmetacarpal amputation of hand

6 S68.71 Complete traumatic transmetacarpal amputation of hand

⊟ SP 7 S68.711- Complete traumatic transmetacarpal amputation of right hand

⊟ SP 7 S68.712- Complete traumatic transmetacarpal amputation of left hand

⊟ IQ 7 S68.719- Complete traumatic transmetacarpal amputation of unspecified hand

6 S68.72 Partial traumatic transmetacarpal amputation of hand

⊟ SP 7 S68.721- Partial traumatic transmetacarpal amputation of right hand

⊟ SP 7 S68.722- Partial traumatic transmetacarpal amputation of left hand

⊟ IQ 7 S68.729- Partial traumatic transmetacarpal amputation of unspecified hand

4 S69 Other and unspecified injuries of wrist, hand and finger(s)

The appropriate 7th character is to be added to each code from category S69
A initial encounter
D subsequent encounter
S sequela

5 S69.8 Other specified injuries of wrist, hand and finger(s)

⊟ IQ 7 S69.80X- Other specified injuries of unspecified wrist, hand and finger(s)

⊟ SP 7 S69.81X- Other specified injuries of right wrist, hand and finger(s)

⊟ SP IQ 7 S69.82X- Other specified injuries of left wrist, hand and finger(s)

5 S69.9 Unspecified injury of wrist, hand and finger(s)

⊟ IQ 7 S69.90X- Unspecified injury of unspecified wrist, hand and finger(s)

⊟ IQ 7 S69.91X- Unspecified injury of right wrist, hand and finger(s)

⊟ IQ 7 S69.92X- Unspecified injury of left wrist, hand and finger(s)

Injuries to the hip and thigh (S70-S79)

EXCLUDES 2 burns and corrosions (T20-T32)
frostbite (T33-T34)
snake bite (T63.0-)
venomous insect bite or sting (T63.4-)

GUIDELINES Section I.C.19.c.2)
Multiple fractures are sequenced in accordance with the severity of the fracture.

★ New ▲ Revised Px Primary SP PDGM Px SL Low CoM SH High CoM IQ Quest. Encounter ⊞ Hospice non-cancer Dx Unspecified M Manifestation

DecisionHealth's FY 2020 Complete Home Health ICD-10-CM Diagnosis Coding Manual 1585

GUIDELINES Section I.C.19.b.1)-2)

When coding injuries, assign separate codes for each injury unless a combination code is provided, in which case the combination code is assigned ... Traumatic injury codes (S00-T14.9) are not to be used for normal, healing surgical wounds or to identify complications of surgical wounds. The code for the most serious injury, as determined by the provider and the focus of treatment, is sequenced first.

1) Superficial injuries such as abrasions or contusions are not coded when associated with more severe injuries of the same site.

2) When a primary injury results in minor damage to peripheral nerves or blood vessels, the primary injury is sequenced first with additional code(s) for injuries to nerves and spinal cord (such as category S04), and/or injury to blood vessels (such as category S15). When the primary injury is to the blood vessels or nerves, that injury should be sequenced first.

GUIDELINES Section I.C.19.c

Coding of Traumatic Fractures: The principles of multiple coding of injuries should be followed in coding fractures. Fractures of specified sites are coded individually by site in accordance with both the provisions within categories S02, S12, S22, S32, S42, S49, S52, S59, S62, S72, S79, S82, S89, S92 and the level of detail furnished by medical record content. A fracture not indicated as open or closed should be coded to closed. A fracture not indicated whether displaced or not displaced should be coded to displaced.

CODING TIPS ✓ 7th character A is acceptable in home health and hospice when active treatment is provided, such as antibiotics for an infected wound or a wound vac for a dehisced wound. D is used when the complication or injury is now healing. Think of D as aftercare. S is used for sequela of the injury or complication. Sequela is a residual deficit or condition produced as a result of the injury or complication after the original injury or complication has healed.

4 S70   Superficial injury of hip and thigh

| The appropriate 7th character is to be added to each code from category S70 |
| A   initial encounter |
| D   subsequent encounter |
| S   sequela |

5 S70.0   Contusion of hip

☐ IQ 7x **S70.00X-   Contusion of unspecified hip**

☐ IQ 7x **S70.01X-   Contusion of right hip**

☐ IQ 7x **S70.02X-   Contusion of left hip**

5 S70.1   Contusion of thigh

☐ IQ 7x **S70.10X-   Contusion of unspecified thigh**

☐ IQ 7x **S70.11X-   Contusion of right thigh**

☐ IQ 7x **S70.12X-   Contusion of left thigh**

5 S70.2   Other superficial injuries of hip

6 S70.21   Abrasion of hip

☐ IQ 7 **S70.211-   Abrasion, right hip**

☐ IQ 7 **S70.212-   Abrasion, left hip**

☐ IQ 7 **S70.219-   Abrasion, unspecified hip**

6 S70.22   Blister (nonthermal) of hip

☐ IQ 7 **S70.221-   Blister (nonthermal), right hip**

☐ IQ 7 **S70.222-   Blister (nonthermal), left hip**

☐ IQ 7 **S70.229-   Blister (nonthermal), unspecified hip**

6 S70.24   External constriction of hip

☐ IQ 7 **S70.241-   External constriction, right hip**

☐ IQ 7 **S70.242-   External constriction, left hip**

☐ IQ 7 **S70.249-   External constriction, unspecified hip**

6 S70.25   Superficial foreign body of hip
Splinter in the hip

☐ IQ 7 **S70.251-   Superficial foreign body, right hip**

☐ IQ 7 **S70.252-   Superficial foreign body, left hip**

☐ IQ 7 **S70.259-   Superficial foreign body, unspecified hip**

6 S70.26   Insect bite (nonvenomous) of hip

☐ IQ 7 **S70.261-   Insect bite (nonvenomous), right hip**

☐ IQ 7 **S70.262-   Insect bite (nonvenomous), left hip**

☐ IQ 7 **S70.269-   Insect bite (nonvenomous), unspecified hip**

6 S70.27   Other superficial bite of hip
    EXCLUDES 1   open bite of hip (S71.05-)

☐ IQ 7 **S70.271-   Other superficial bite of hip, right hip**

☐ IQ 7 **S70.272-   Other superficial bite of hip, left hip**

☐ IQ 7 **S70.279-   Other superficial bite of hip, unspecified hip**

5 S70.3   Other superficial injuries of thigh

6 S70.31   Abrasion of thigh

☐ IQ 7 **S70.311-   Abrasion, right thigh**

☐ IQ 7 **S70.312-   Abrasion, left thigh**

☐ IQ 7 **S70.319-   Abrasion, unspecified thigh**

6 S70.32   Blister (nonthermal) of thigh

☐ IQ 7 **S70.321-   Blister (nonthermal), right thigh**

☐ IQ 7 **S70.322-   Blister (nonthermal), left thigh**

☐ IQ 7 **S70.329-   Blister (nonthermal), unspecified thigh**

6 S70.34   External constriction of thigh

☐ IQ 7 **S70.341-   External constriction, right thigh**

☐ IQ 7 **S70.342-   External constriction, left thigh**

☐ IQ 7 **S70.349-   External constriction, unspecified thigh**

6 S70.35   Superficial foreign body of thigh
Splinter in the thigh

☐ IQ 7 **S70.351-   Superficial foreign body, right thigh**

☐ IQ 7 **S70.352-   Superficial foreign body, left thigh**

☐ IQ 7 **S70.359-   Superficial foreign body, unspecified thigh**

6 S70.36   Insect bite (nonvenomous) of thigh

☐ IQ 7 **S70.361-   Insect bite (nonvenomous), right thigh**

☐ IQ 7 **S70.362-   Insect bite (nonvenomous), left thigh**

☐ IQ 7 **S70.369-   Insect bite (nonvenomous), unspecified thigh**

6 S70.37   Other superficial bite of thigh

4 4th digit required   **5** 5th digit required   **6** 6th digit required   **7** 7th digit required   **7x** 7th digit placeholder   **+** Additional code   ☐ Laterality

1586   *DecisionHealth's* FY 2020 Complete Home Health ICD-10-CM Diagnosis Coding Manual

Chapter 19   *S00-T88*

EXCLUDES 1 open bite of thigh (S71.15)

⊟ **IQ** **7** S70.371- Other superficial bite of right thigh

⊟ **IQ** **7** S70.372- Other superficial bite of left thigh

⊟ **IQ** **7** S70.379- Other superficial bite of unspecified thigh

5 S70.9 Unspecified superficial injury of hip and thigh

6 S70.91 Unspecified superficial injury of hip

⊟ **IQ** **7** S70.911- Unspecified superficial injury of right hip

⊟ **IQ** **7** S70.912- Unspecified superficial injury of left hip

⊟ **IQ** **7** S70.919- Unspecified superficial injury of unspecified hip

6 S70.92 Unspecified superficial injury of thigh

⊟ **IQ** **7** S70.921- Unspecified superficial injury of right thigh

⊟ **IQ** **7** S70.922- Unspecified superficial injury of left thigh

⊟ **IQ** **7** S70.929- Unspecified superficial injury of unspecified thigh

4 S71 Open wound of hip and thigh

Code also:
any associated wound infection

EXCLUDES 1 open fracture of hip and thigh (S72.-)
traumatic amputation of hip and thigh (S78.-)

EXCLUDES 2 bite of venomous animal (T63.-)
open wound of ankle, foot and toes (S91.-)
open wound of knee and lower leg (S81.-)

The appropriate 7th character is to be added to each code from category S71
A   initial encounter
D   subsequent encounter
S   sequela

CODING TIPS ✓ Open wound codes indicate a wound resulting from a traumatic origin. Do not assign a code for "open wound" unless the etiology of the wound is related to trauma.

CODING TIPS ✓ No aftercare code applies, including those indicating dressing changes, drain care, or suture removal. 7th character 'D' is the default for home care and hospice when providing aftercare for a healing or resolving condition; 'A' is used for active treatment such as antibiotics or more than routine wound care; 'S' may be used to indicate a residual condition after the original injury has healed.

5 S71.0 Open wound of hip

6 S71.00 Unspecified open wound of hip

⊟ **SP** **7** S71.001- Unspecified open wound, right hip

⊟ **SP** **7** S71.002- Unspecified open wound, left hip

⊟ **IQ** **7** S71.009- Unspecified open wound, unspecified hip

6 S71.01 Laceration without foreign body of hip

⊟ **SP** **7** S71.011- Laceration without foreign body, right hip

⊟ **SP** **7** S71.012- Laceration without foreign body, left hip

⊟ **IQ** **7** S71.019- Laceration without foreign body, unspecified hip

6 S71.02 Laceration with foreign body of hip

⊟ **SP** **7** S71.021- Laceration with foreign body, right hip

⊟ **SP** **7** S71.022- Laceration with foreign body, left hip

⊟ **IQ** **7** S71.029- Laceration with foreign body, unspecified hip

6 S71.03 Puncture wound without foreign body of hip

⊟ **SP** **7** S71.031- Puncture wound without foreign body, right hip

⊟ **SP** **7** S71.032- Puncture wound without foreign body, left hip

⊟ **IQ** **7** S71.039- Puncture wound without foreign body, unspecified hip

6 S71.04 Puncture wound with foreign body of hip

⊟ **SP** **7** S71.041- Puncture wound with foreign body, right hip

⊟ **SP** **7** S71.042- Puncture wound with foreign body, left hip

⊟ **IQ** **7** S71.049- Puncture wound with foreign body, unspecified hip

6 S71.05 Open bite of hip
Bite of hip NOS
EXCLUDES 1 superficial bite of hip (S70.26, S70.27)

⊟ **SP** **7** S71.051- Open bite, right hip

⊟ **SP** **7** S71.052- Open bite, left hip

⊟ **IQ** **7** S71.059- Open bite, unspecified hip

5 S71.1 Open wound of thigh

6 S71.10 Unspecified open wound of thigh

⊟ **SP** **7** S71.101- Unspecified open wound, right thigh

⊟ **SP** **7** S71.102- Unspecified open wound, left thigh

⊟ **IQ** **7** S71.109- Unspecified open wound, unspecified thigh

6 S71.11 Laceration without foreign body of thigh

⊟ **SP** **7** S71.111- Laceration without foreign body, right thigh

⊟ **SP** **7** S71.112- Laceration without foreign body, left thigh

⊟ **IQ** **7** S71.119- Laceration without foreign body, unspecified thigh

6 S71.12 Laceration with foreign body of thigh

⊟ **SP** **7** S71.121- Laceration with foreign body, right thigh

⊟ **SP** **7** S71.122- Laceration with foreign body, left thigh

⊟ **IQ** **7** S71.129- Laceration with foreign body, unspecified thigh

6 S71.13 Puncture wound without foreign body of thigh

★ New ▲ Revised Px Primary **SP** PDGM Px **SL** Low CoM **SH** High CoM **IQ** Quest. Encounter **H** Hospice non-cancer Dx Unspecified **M** *Manifestation*

DecisionHealth's FY 2020 Complete Home Health ICD-10-CM Diagnosis Coding Manual   1587

Chapter 19

S00-T88

☐ SP ⁷ **S71.131-** Puncture wound without foreign body, right thigh

☐ SP ⁷ **S71.132-** Puncture wound without foreign body, left thigh

☐ IQ ⁷ **S71.139-** Puncture wound without foreign body, unspecified thigh

⁶ **S71.14** Puncture wound with foreign body of thigh

☐ SP ⁷ **S71.141-** Puncture wound with foreign body, right thigh

☐ SP ⁷ **S71.142-** Puncture wound with foreign body, left thigh

☐ IQ ⁷ **S71.149-** Puncture wound with foreign body, unspecified thigh

⁶ **S71.15** Open bite of thigh
Bite of thigh NOS
EXCLUDES 1 superficial bite of thigh (S70.37-)

☐ SP ⁷ **S71.151-** Open bite, right thigh

☐ SP ⁷ **S71.152-** Open bite, left thigh

☐ IQ ⁷ **S71.159-** Open bite, unspecified thigh

Gustilo open fracture classification	
Gustilo Grade	**Definition**
I	Open fracture, clean wound, wound <1 cm in length
II	Open fracture, wound > 1 cm but < 10 cm in length without extensive soft-tissue damage, flaps, avulsions
III	Open fracture with extensive soft-tissue laceration (>10 cm), damage, or loss or an open segmental fracture. This type also includes open fractures caused by farm injuries, fractures requiring vascular repair, or fractures that have been open for 8 hr prior to treatment
IIIA	Type III fracture with adequate periosteal coverage of the fracture bone despite the extensive soft-tissue laceration or damage
IIIB	Type III fracture with extensive soft-tissue loss and periosteal stripping and bone damage. Usually associated with massive contamination. Will often need further soft-tissue coverage procedure (i.e. free or rotational flap)
IIIC	Type III fracture associated with an arterial injury requiring repair, irrespective of degree of soft-tissue injury.

http://en.wikipedia.org/wiki/Gustilo_open_fracture_classification

④ **S72** **Fracture of femur**
Note:
A fracture not indicated as displaced or nondisplaced should be coded to displaced
A fracture not indicated as open or closed should be coded to closed
The open fracture designations are based on the Gustilo open fracture classification
EXCLUDES 1 traumatic amputation of hip and thigh (S78.-)
EXCLUDES 2 fracture of lower leg and ankle (S82.-)
fracture of foot (S92.-)
periprosthetic fracture of prosthetic implant of hip (M97.0-)

The appropriate 7th character is to be added to all codes from category S72
A initial encounter for closed fracture
B initial encounter for open fracture type I or II
C initial encounter for open fracture type IIIA, IIIB, or IIIC
D subsequent encounter for closed fracture with routine healing
E subsequent encounter for open fracture type I or II with routine healing
F subsequent encounter for open fracture type IIIA, IIIB, or IIIC with routine healing
G subsequent encounter for closed fracture with delayed healing
H subsequent encounter for open fracture type I or II with delayed healing
J subsequent encounter for open fracture type IIIA, IIIB, or IIIC with delayed healing
K subsequent encounter for closed fracture with nonunion
M subsequent encounter for open fracture type I or II with nonunion
N subsequent encounter for open fracture type IIIA, IIIB, or IIIC with nonunion
P subsequent encounter for closed fracture with malunion
Q subsequent encounter for open fracture type I or II with malunion
R subsequent encounter for open fracture type IIIA, IIIB, or IIIC with malunion
S sequela

CODING TIPS ✓ Fractures repaired by joint replacements are NOT coded with Z47.1. Fractures repaired by any other orthopedic surgery are NOT coded with Z47.89. Z codes are not appropriate for fractures of any kind. Code the fracture with 7th character D for fractures undergoing surgical repair.

CODING TIPS ✓ "D" is the 7th character for home care and hospice unless the physician has documented delayed healing, nonunion or malunion. A sequela is a condition left after the fracture has healed.

CODING TIPS ✓ A fracture not indicated as displaced or nondisplaced should be coded to displaced. A fracture not indicated as open or closed should be coded to closed. The open fracture designations are based on the Gustilo open fracture classification. The 7th characters E, H, M and Q are the default for the Gustilo classification when no information is available. Always query the physician.

④4th digit required ⑤5th digit required ⑥6th digit required ⑦7th digit required ⑦7th digit placeholder ✚Additional code ☐Laterality

1588 *DecisionHealth's* FY 2020 Complete Home Health ICD-10-CM Diagnosis Coding Manual

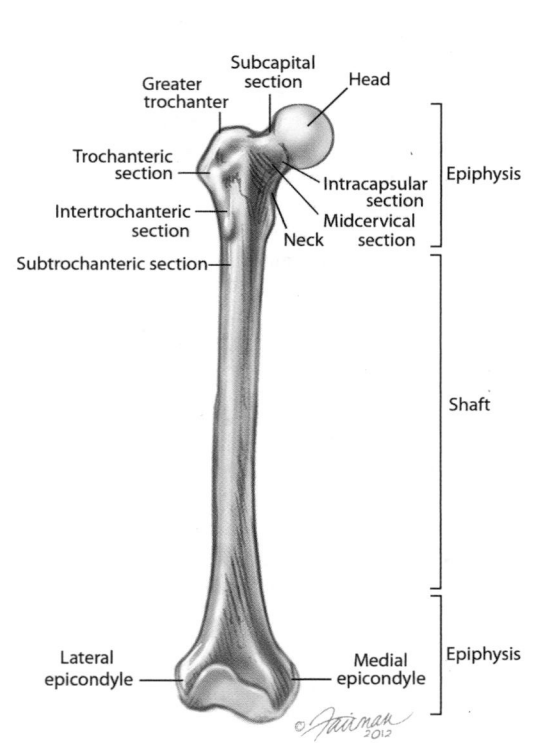

Subcapital section
Greater trochanter
Head
Trochanteric section
Intracapsular section
Intertrochanteric section
Midcervical section
Subtrochanteric section
Neck
Epiphysis
Shaft
Lateral epicondyle
Medial epicondyle
Epiphysis

©Fairman 2012

⑤ S72.0   Fracture of head and neck of femur

> **EXCLUDES 2**   physeal fracture of upper end of femur (S79.0-)

⑥ S72.00   Fracture of unspecified part of neck of femur

Fracture of hip NOS
Fracture of neck of femur NOS

CODING TIPS ✓   A fracture that is only reported as a "hip fracture" should be coded to S72.00- with the appropriate 6th character to indicate laterality, and a 7th character to indicate healing status and episode of care.

⊟ SP 7 **S72.001-   Fracture of unspecified part of neck of right femur**

⊟ SP 7 **S72.002-   Fracture of unspecified part of neck of left femur**

⊟ IQ 7 **S72.009-   Fracture of unspecified part of neck of unspecified femur**

⑥ S72.01   Unspecified intracapsular fracture of femur

Subcapital fracture of femur

⊟ SP 7 **S72.011-   Unspecified intracapsular fracture of right femur**

⊟ SP 7 **S72.012-   Unspecified intracapsular fracture of left femur**

⊟ IQ 7 **S72.019-   Unspecified intracapsular fracture of unspecified femur**

⑥ S72.02   Fracture of epiphysis (separation) (upper) of femur

Transepiphyseal fracture of femur

EXCLUDES 1   capital femoral epiphyseal fracture (pediatric) of femur (S79.01-)
Salter-Harris Type I physeal fracture of upper end of femur (S79.01-)

⊟ SP 7 **S72.021-   Displaced fracture of epiphysis (separation) (upper) of right femur**

⊟ SP 7 **S72.022-   Displaced fracture of epiphysis (separation) (upper) of left femur**

⊟ IQ 7 **S72.023-   Displaced fracture of epiphysis (separation) (upper) of unspecified femur**

⊟ SP 7 **S72.024-   Nondisplaced fracture of epiphysis (separation) (upper) of right femur**

⊟ SP 7 **S72.025-   Nondisplaced fracture of epiphysis (separation) (upper) of left femur**

⊟ IQ 7 **S72.026-   Nondisplaced fracture of epiphysis (separation) (upper) of unspecified femur**

⑥ S72.03   Midcervical fracture of femur

Transcervical fracture of femur NOS

⊟ SP 7 **S72.031-   Displaced midcervical fracture of right femur**

⊟ SP 7 **S72.032-   Displaced midcervical fracture of left femur**

⊟ IQ 7 **S72.033-   Displaced midcervical fracture of unspecified femur**

⊟ SP 7 **S72.034-   Nondisplaced midcervical fracture of right femur**

⊟ SP 7 **S72.035-   Nondisplaced midcervical fracture of left femur**

⊟ IQ 7 **S72.036-   Nondisplaced midcervical fracture of unspecified femur**

⑥ S72.04   Fracture of base of neck of femur

Cervicotrochanteric fracture of femur

⊟ SP 7 **S72.041-   Displaced fracture of base of neck of right femur**

⊟ SP 7 **S72.042-   Displaced fracture of base of neck of left femur**

⊟ IQ 7 **S72.043-   Displaced fracture of base of neck of unspecified femur**

⊟ SP 7 **S72.044-   Nondisplaced fracture of base of neck of right femur**

⊟ SP 7 **S72.045-   Nondisplaced fracture of base of neck of left femur**

⊟ IQ 7 **S72.046-   Nondisplaced fracture of base of neck of unspecified femur**

⑥ S72.05   Unspecified fracture of head of femur

Fracture of head of femur NOS

⊟ SP 7 **S72.051-   Unspecified fracture of head of right femur**

⊟ SP 7 **S72.052-   Unspecified fracture of head of left femur**

⊟ IQ 7 **S72.059-   Unspecified fracture of head of unspecified femur**

⑥ S72.06   Articular fracture of head of femur

⊟ SP 7 **S72.061-   Displaced articular fracture of head of right femur**

★ New ▲ Revised Px Primary SP PDGM Px SL Low CoM SH High CoM IQ Quest. Encounter H Hospice non-cancer Dx   Unspecified   M Manifestation

DecisionHealth's FY 2020 Complete Home Health ICD-10-CM Diagnosis Coding Manual

1589

⊟ SP 7 **S72.062-** Displaced articular fracture of head of left femur

⊟ IQ 7 **S72.063-** Displaced articular fracture of head of unspecified femur

⊟ SP 7 **S72.064-** Nondisplaced articular fracture of head of right femur

⊟ SP 7 **S72.065-** Nondisplaced articular fracture of head of left femur

⊟ SP IQ 7 **S72.066-** Nondisplaced articular fracture of head of unspecified femur

6 **S72.09** Other fracture of head and neck of femur

⊟ SP 7 **S72.091-** Other fracture of head and neck of right femur

⊟ SP 7 **S72.092-** Other fracture of head and neck of left femur

⊟ IQ 7 **S72.099-** Other fracture of head and neck of unspecified femur

5 **S72.1** Pertrochanteric fracture

6 **S72.10** Unspecified trochanteric fracture of femur

Fracture of trochanter NOS

⊟ SP 7 **S72.101-** Unspecified trochanteric fracture of right femur

⊟ SP 7 **S72.102-** Unspecified trochanteric fracture of left femur

⊟ IQ 7 **S72.109-** Unspecified trochanteric fracture of unspecified femur

6 **S72.11** Fracture of greater trochanter of femur

⊟ SP 7 **S72.111-** Displaced fracture of greater trochanter of right femur

⊟ SP 7 **S72.112-** Displaced fracture of greater trochanter of left femur

⊟ IQ 7 **S72.113-** Displaced fracture of greater trochanter of unspecified femur

⊟ SP 7 **S72.114-** Nondisplaced fracture of greater trochanter of right femur

⊟ SP 7 **S72.115-** Nondisplaced fracture of greater trochanter of left femur

⊟ SP IQ 7 **S72.116-** Nondisplaced fracture of greater trochanter of unspecified femur

6 **S72.12** Fracture of lesser trochanter of femur

⊟ SP 7 **S72.121-** Displaced fracture of lesser trochanter of right femur

⊟ SP 7 **S72.122-** Displaced fracture of lesser trochanter of left femur

⊟ IQ 7 **S72.123-** Displaced fracture of lesser trochanter of unspecified femur

⊟ SP 7 **S72.124-** Nondisplaced fracture of lesser trochanter of right femur

⊟ SP 7 **S72.125-** Nondisplaced fracture of lesser trochanter of left femur

⊟ IQ 7 **S72.126-** Nondisplaced fracture of lesser trochanter of unspecified femur

6 **S72.13** Apophyseal fracture of femur

EXCLUDES 1 chronic (nontraumatic) slipped upper femoral epiphysis (M93.0-)

⊟ SP 7 **S72.131-** Displaced apophyseal fracture of right femur

⊟ SP 7 **S72.132-** Displaced apophyseal fracture of left femur

⊟ IQ 7 **S72.133-** Displaced apophyseal fracture of unspecified femur

⊟ SP 7 **S72.134-** Nondisplaced apophyseal fracture of right femur

⊟ SP 7 **S72.135-** Nondisplaced apophyseal fracture of left femur

⊟ IQ 7 **S72.136-** Nondisplaced apophyseal fracture of unspecified femur

6 **S72.14** Intertrochanteric fracture of femur

⊟ SP 7 **S72.141-** Displaced intertrochanteric fracture of right femur

⊟ SP 7 **S72.142-** Displaced intertrochanteric fracture of left femur

⊟ IQ 7 **S72.143-** Displaced intertrochanteric fracture of unspecified femur

⊟ SP 7 **S72.144-** Nondisplaced intertrochanteric fracture of right femur

⊟ SP 7 **S72.145-** Nondisplaced intertrochanteric fracture of left femur

⊟ IQ 7 **S72.146-** Nondisplaced intertrochanteric fracture of unspecified femur

5 **S72.2** Subtrochanteric fracture of femur

⊟ SP 7 **S72.21X-** Displaced subtrochanteric fracture of right femur

⊟ SP 7 **S72.22X-** Displaced subtrochanteric fracture of left femur

⊟ IQ 7 **S72.23X-** Displaced subtrochanteric fracture of unspecified femur

⊟ SP IQ 7 **S72.24X-** Nondisplaced subtrochanteric fracture of right femur

⊟ SP 7 **S72.25X-** Nondisplaced subtrochanteric fracture of left femur

⊟ IQ 7 **S72.26X-** Nondisplaced subtrochanteric fracture of unspecified femur

5 **S72.3** Fracture of shaft of femur

6 **S72.30** Unspecified fracture of shaft of femur

⊟ SP 7 **S72.301-** Unspecified fracture of shaft of right femur

⊟ SP 7 **S72.302-** Unspecified fracture of shaft of left femur

⊟ IQ 7 **S72.309-** Unspecified fracture of shaft of unspecified femur

6 **S72.32** Transverse fracture of shaft of femur

⊟ SP 7 **S72.321-** Displaced transverse fracture of shaft of right femur

⊟ SP 7 **S72.322-** Displaced transverse fracture of shaft of left femur

⊟ IQ 7 **S72.323-** Displaced transverse fracture of shaft of unspecified femur

⊟ SP 7 **S72.324-** Nondisplaced transverse fracture of shaft of right femur

⊟ SP 7 **S72.325-** Nondisplaced transverse fracture of shaft of left femur

⊟ IQ 7 **S72.326-** Nondisplaced transverse fracture of shaft of unspecified femur

6 **S72.33** Oblique fracture of shaft of femur

⊟ SP 7 **S72.331-** Displaced oblique fracture of shaft of right femur

⊟ SP 7 **S72.332-** Displaced oblique fracture of shaft of left femur

⊟ IQ 7 **S72.333-** Displaced oblique fracture of shaft of unspecified femur

4 4th digit required　5 5th digit required　6 6th digit required　7 7th digit required　7 7th digit placeholder　+ Additional code　⊟ Laterality

1590　　　*DecisionHealth's* FY 2020 Complete Home Health ICD-10-CM Diagnosis Coding Manual

☰ **SP** 7 S72.334- Nondisplaced oblique fracture of shaft of right femur

☰ **SP** 7 S72.335- Nondisplaced oblique fracture of shaft of left femur

☰ **!Q** 7 S72.336- Nondisplaced oblique fracture of shaft of unspecified femur

6 S72.34 Spiral fracture of shaft of femur

☰ **SP** 7 S72.341- Displaced spiral fracture of shaft of right femur

☰ **SP** 7 S72.342- Displaced spiral fracture of shaft of left femur

☰ **!Q** 7 S72.343- Displaced spiral fracture of shaft of unspecified femur

☰ **SP** 7 S72.344- Nondisplaced spiral fracture of shaft of right femur

☰ **SP** 7 S72.345- Nondisplaced spiral fracture of shaft of left femur

☰ **!Q** 7 S72.346- Nondisplaced spiral fracture of shaft of unspecified femur

6 S72.35 Comminuted fracture of shaft of femur

☰ **SP** 7 S72.351- Displaced comminuted fracture of shaft of right femur

☰ **SP** 7 S72.352- Displaced comminuted fracture of shaft of left femur

☰ **!Q** 7 S72.353- Displaced comminuted fracture of shaft of unspecified femur

☰ **SP** 7 S72.354- Nondisplaced comminuted fracture of shaft of right femur

☰ **SP** 7 S72.355- Nondisplaced comminuted fracture of shaft of left femur

☰ **SP** **!Q** 7 S72.356- Nondisplaced comminuted fracture of shaft of unspecified femur

6 S72.36 Segmental fracture of shaft of femur

☰ **SP** 7 S72.361- Displaced segmental fracture of shaft of right femur

☰ **SP** 7 S72.362- Displaced segmental fracture of shaft of left femur

☰ **!Q** 7 S72.363- Displaced segmental fracture of shaft of unspecified femur

☰ **SP** 7 S72.364- Nondisplaced segmental fracture of shaft of right femur

☰ **SP** 7 S72.365- Nondisplaced segmental fracture of shaft of left femur

☰ **!Q** 7 S72.366- Nondisplaced segmental fracture of shaft of unspecified femur

6 S72.39 Other fracture of shaft of femur

☰ **SP** 7 S72.391- Other fracture of shaft of right femur

☰ **SP** 7 S72.392- Other fracture of shaft of left femur

☰ **!Q** 7 S72.399- Other fracture of shaft of unspecified femur

5 S72.4 Fracture of lower end of femur
Fracture of distal end of femur
EXCLUDES 2 fracture of shaft of femur (S72.3-)
physeal fracture of lower end of femur (S79.1-)

6 S72.40 Unspecified fracture of lower end of femur

☰ **SP** 7 S72.401- Unspecified fracture of lower end of right femur

☰ **SP** 7 S72.402- Unspecified fracture of lower end of left femur

☰ **!Q** 7 S72.409- Unspecified fracture of lower end of unspecified femur

6 S72.41 Unspecified condyle fracture of lower end of femur
Condyle fracture of femur NOS

☰ **SP** 7 S72.411- Displaced unspecified condyle fracture of lower end of right femur

☰ **SP** 7 S72.412- Displaced unspecified condyle fracture of lower end of left femur

☰ **!Q** 7 S72.413- Displaced unspecified condyle fracture of lower end of unspecified femur

☰ **SP** 7 S72.414- Nondisplaced unspecified condyle fracture of lower end of right femur

☰ **SP** 7 S72.415- Nondisplaced unspecified condyle fracture of lower end of left femur

☰ **!Q** 7 S72.416- Nondisplaced unspecified condyle fracture of lower end of unspecified femur

6 S72.42 Fracture of lateral condyle of femur

☰ **SP** 7 S72.421- Displaced fracture of lateral condyle of right femur

☰ **SP** 7 S72.422- Displaced fracture of lateral condyle of left femur

☰ **!Q** 7 S72.423- Displaced fracture of lateral condyle of unspecified femur

☰ **SP** 7 S72.424- Nondisplaced fracture of lateral condyle of right femur

☰ **SP** 7 S72.425- Nondisplaced fracture of lateral condyle of left femur

☰ **!Q** 7 S72.426- Nondisplaced fracture of lateral condyle of unspecified femur

6 S72.43 Fracture of medial condyle of femur

☰ **SP** 7 S72.431- Displaced fracture of medial condyle of right femur

☰ **SP** 7 S72.432- Displaced fracture of medial condyle of left femur

☰ **!Q** 7 S72.433- Displaced fracture of medial condyle of unspecified femur

☰ **SP** 7 S72.434- Nondisplaced fracture of medial condyle of right femur

☰ **SP** 7 S72.435- Nondisplaced fracture of medial condyle of left femur

☰ **!Q** 7 S72.436- Nondisplaced fracture of medial condyle of unspecified femur

6 S72.44 Fracture of lower epiphysis (separation) of femur
EXCLUDES 1 Salter-Harris Type I physeal fracture of lower end of femur (S79.11-)

☰ **SP** 7 S72.441- Displaced fracture of lower epiphysis (separation) of right femur

☰ **SP** 7 S72.442- Displaced fracture of lower epiphysis (separation) of left femur

★ New ▲ Revised Px Primary **SP** PDGM Px **SL** Low CoM **SH** High CoM **!Q** Quest. Encounter **H** Hospice non-cancer Dx   Unspecified   **M** *Manifestation*

DecisionHealth's FY 2020 Complete Home Health ICD-10-CM Diagnosis Coding Manual   1591

S72.443- Displaced fracture of lower epiphysis (separation) of unspecified femur

S72.444- Nondisplaced fracture of lower epiphysis (separation) of right femur

S72.445- Nondisplaced fracture of lower epiphysis (separation) of left femur

S72.446- Nondisplaced fracture of lower epiphysis (separation) of unspecified femur

S72.45 Supracondylar fracture without intracondylar extension of lower end of femur

Supracondylar fracture of lower end of femur NOS

EXCLUDES 1 supracondylar fracture with intracondylar extension of lower end of femur (S72.46-)

S72.451- Displaced supracondylar fracture without intracondylar extension of lower end of right femur

S72.452- Displaced supracondylar fracture without intracondylar extension of lower end of left femur

S72.453- Displaced supracondylar fracture without intracondylar extension of lower end of unspecified femur

S72.454- Nondisplaced supracondylar fracture without intracondylar extension of lower end of right femur

S72.455- Nondisplaced supracondylar fracture without intracondylar extension of lower end of left femur

S72.456- Nondisplaced supracondylar fracture without intracondylar extension of lower end of unspecified femur

S72.46 Supracondylar fracture with intracondylar extension of lower end of femur

EXCLUDES 1 supracondylar fracture without intracondylar extension of lower end of femur (S72.45-)

S72.461- Displaced supracondylar fracture with intracondylar extension of lower end of right femur

S72.462- Displaced supracondylar fracture with intracondylar extension of lower end of left femur

S72.463- Displaced supracondylar fracture with intracondylar extension of lower end of unspecified femur

S72.464- Nondisplaced supracondylar fracture with intracondylar extension of lower end of right femur

S72.465- Nondisplaced supracondylar fracture with intracondylar extension of lower end of left femur

S72.466- Nondisplaced supracondylar fracture with intracondylar extension of lower end of unspecified femur

S72.47 Torus fracture of lower end of femur

The appropriate 7th character is to be added to all codes in subcategory S72.47

A   initial encounter for closed fracture

D   subsequent encounter for fracture with routine healing

G   subsequent encounter for fracture with delayed healing

K   subsequent encounter for fracture with nonunion

P   subsequent encounter for fracture with malunion

S   sequela

CODING TIPS ✓ Open fractures do not occur with torus fractures and greenstick fractures, therefore the 7th characters for open fractures are not available.

S72.471- Torus fracture of lower end of right femur

S72.472- Torus fracture of lower end of left femur

S72.479- Torus fracture of lower end of unspecified femur

S72.49 Other fracture of lower end of femur

S72.491- Other fracture of lower end of right femur

S72.492- Other fracture of lower end of left femur

S72.499- Other fracture of lower end of unspecified femur

S72.8 Other fracture of femur

S72.8X Other fracture of femur

S72.8X1- Other fracture of right femur

S72.8X2- Other fracture of left femur

S72.8X9- Other fracture of unspecified femur

S72.9 Unspecified fracture of femur

Fracture of thigh NOS
Fracture of upper leg NOS

EXCLUDES 1 fracture of hip NOS (S72.00-, S72.01-)

S72.90X- Unspecified fracture of unspecified femur

S72.91X- Unspecified fracture of right femur

S72.92X- Unspecified fracture of left femur

S73 Dislocation and sprain of joint and ligaments of hip

INCLUDES avulsion of joint or ligament of hip

laceration of cartilage, joint or ligament of hip

---

4 4th digit required   **5** 5th digit required   **6** 6th digit required   **7** 7th digit required   **☑** 7th digit placeholder   **+** Additional code   **⊟** Laterality

sprain of cartilage, joint or
ligament of hip
traumatic hemarthrosis of joint
or ligament of hip
traumatic rupture of joint or
ligament of hip
traumatic subluxation of joint or
ligament of hip
traumatic tear of joint or
ligament of hip

Code also:
any associated open wound
EXCLUDES 2 strain of muscle, fascia and
tendon of hip and thigh
(S76.-)

The appropriate 7th character is to be added to
each code from category S73
A   initial encounter
D   subsequent encounter
S   sequela

⑤ **S73.0   Subluxation and dislocation of hip**
EXCLUDES 2 dislocation and subluxation
of hip prosthesis
(T84.020, T84.021)

⑥ **S73.00   Unspecified subluxation and
dislocation of hip**
Dislocation of hip NOS
Subluxation of hip NOS

⊟ **IQ** 7 S73.001-   **Unspecified subluxation of right
hip**

⊟ **IQ** 7 S73.002-   **Unspecified subluxation of left
hip**

⊟ **IQ** 7 S73.003-   **Unspecified subluxation of
unspecified hip**

⊟ **IQ** 7 S73.004-   **Unspecified dislocation of right
hip**

⊟ **IQ** 7 S73.005-   **Unspecified dislocation of left
hip**

⊟ **IQ** 7 S73.006-   **Unspecified dislocation of
unspecified hip**

⑥ **S73.01   Posterior subluxation and
dislocation of hip**

⊟ **SP** 7 S73.011-   Posterior subluxation of right hip

⊟ **SP** 7 S73.012-   Posterior subluxation of left hip

⊟ **IQ** 7 S73.013-   **Posterior subluxation of
unspecified hip**

⊟ **SP** 7 S73.014-   Posterior dislocation of right hip

⊟ **SP** 7 S73.015-   Posterior dislocation of left hip

⊟ **IQ** 7 S73.016-   **Posterior dislocation of
unspecified hip**

⑥ **S73.02   Obturator subluxation and
dislocation of hip**

⊟ **SP** 7 S73.021-   Obturator subluxation of right
hip

⊟ **SP** 7 S73.022-   Obturator subluxation of left hip

⊟ **IQ** 7 S73.023-   **Obturator subluxation of
unspecified hip**

⊟ **SP** 7 S73.024-   Obturator dislocation of right
hip

⊟ **SP** 7 S73.025-   Obturator dislocation of left hip

⊟ **IQ** 7 S73.026-   **Obturator dislocation of
unspecified hip**

⑥ **S73.03   Other anterior subluxation and
dislocation of hip**

⊟ **SP** 7 S73.031-   Other anterior subluxation of
right hip

⊟ **SP** 7 S73.032-   Other anterior subluxation of left
hip

⊟ **IQ** 7 S73.033-   **Other anterior subluxation of
unspecified hip**

⊟ **SP** 7 S73.034-   Other anterior dislocation of
right hip

⊟ **SP** 7 S73.035-   Other anterior dislocation of left
hip

⊟ **IQ** 7 S73.036-   **Other anterior dislocation of
unspecified hip**

⑥ **S73.04   Central subluxation and dislocation
of hip**

⊟ **SP** 7 S73.041-   Central subluxation of right hip

⊟ **SP** 7 S73.042-   Central subluxation of left hip

⊟ **IQ** 7 S73.043-   **Central subluxation of
unspecified hip**

⊟ **SP** 7 S73.044-   Central dislocation of right hip

⊟ **SP** 7 S73.045-   Central dislocation of left hip

⊟ **IQ** 7 S73.046-   **Central dislocation of
unspecified hip**

⑤ **S73.1   Sprain of hip**

⑥ **S73.10   Unspecified sprain of hip**

⊟ **SP** 7 S73.101-   **Unspecified sprain of right hip**

⊟ **SP** 7 S73.102-   **Unspecified sprain of left hip**

⊟ **IQ** 7 S73.109-   **Unspecified sprain of
unspecified hip**

⑥ **S73.11   Iliofemoral ligament sprain of hip**

⊟ **SP** 7 S73.111-   Iliofemoral ligament sprain of
right hip

⊟ **SP** 7 S73.112-   Iliofemoral ligament sprain of
left hip

⊟ **IQ** 7 S73.119-   **Iliofemoral ligament sprain of
unspecified hip**

⑥ **S73.12   Ischiocapsular (ligament) sprain of
hip**

⊟ **SP** 7 S73.121-   Ischiocapsular ligament sprain of
right hip

⊟ **SP** 7 S73.122-   Ischiocapsular ligament sprain of
left hip

⊟ **IQ** 7 S73.129-   **Ischiocapsular ligament sprain
of unspecified hip**

⑥ **S73.19   Other sprain of hip**

⊟ **SP** 7 S73.191-   Other sprain of right hip

⊟ **SP** 7 S73.192-   Other sprain of left hip

⊟ **IQ** 7 S73.199-   **Other sprain of unspecified hip**

④ **S74   Injury of nerves at hip and thigh level**
Code also:
any associated open wound (S71.-)
EXCLUDES 2 injury of nerves at ankle and
foot level (S94.-)
injury of nerves at lower leg
level (S84.-)

The appropriate 7th character is to be added to
each code from category S74
A   initial encounter
D   subsequent encounter
S   sequela

⑤ **S74.0   Injury of sciatic nerve at hip and thigh
level**

⊟ **IQ** 7 S74.00X-   **Injury of sciatic nerve at hip and
thigh level, unspecified leg**

★ New ▲ Revised Px Primary 🆂🅿 PDGM Px 🆂🅻 Low CoM 🆂🅷 High CoM **IQ** Quest. Encounter Ⓗ Hospice non-cancer Dx   Unspecified   **M** *Manifestation*

DecisionHealth's FY 2020 Complete Home Health ICD-10-CM Diagnosis Coding Manual   1593

🔲 **SP** 🔳 **S74.01X-**   **Injury of sciatic nerve at hip and thigh level, right leg**

🔲 **SP** 🔳 **S74.02X-**   **Injury of sciatic nerve at hip and thigh level, left leg**

🔳 **S74.1**   **Injury of femoral nerve at hip and thigh level**

🔲 **IQ** 🔳 **S74.10X-**   **Injury of femoral nerve at hip and thigh level, unspecified leg**

🔲 **SP** 🔳 **S74.11X-**   **Injury of femoral nerve at hip and thigh level, right leg**

🔲 **SP** 🔳 **S74.12X-**   **Injury of femoral nerve at hip and thigh level, left leg**

🔳 **S74.2**   **Injury of cutaneous sensory nerve at hip and thigh level**

🔲 **IQ** 🔳 **S74.20X-**   **Injury of cutaneous sensory nerve at hip and thigh level, unspecified leg**

🔲 **SP** 🔳 **S74.21X-**   **Injury of cutaneous sensory nerve at hip and high level, right leg**

🔲 **SP** 🔳 **S74.22X-**   **Injury of cutaneous sensory nerve at hip and thigh level, left leg**

🔳 **S74.8**   **Injury of other nerves at hip and thigh level**

🔳 **S74.8X**   **Injury of other nerves at hip and thigh level**

🔲 **SP** 🔳 **S74.8X1-**   **Injury of other nerves at hip and thigh level, right leg**

🔲 **SP** 🔳 **S74.8X2-**   **Injury of other nerves at hip and thigh level, left leg**

🔲 **IQ** 🔳 **S74.8X9-**   **Injury of other nerves at hip and thigh level, unspecified leg**

🔳 **S74.9**   **Injury of unspecified nerve at hip and thigh level**

🔲 **IQ** 🔳 **S74.90X-**   **Injury of unspecified nerve at hip and thigh level, unspecified leg**

🔲 **IQ** 🔳 **S74.91X-**   **Injury of unspecified nerve at hip and thigh level, right leg**

🔲 **IQ** 🔳 **S74.92X-**   **Injury of unspecified nerve at hip and thigh level, left leg**

🔳 **S75**   **Injury of blood vessels at hip and thigh level**
Code also:
any associated open wound (S71.-)
EXCLUDES 2   injury of blood vessels at lower leg level (S85.-)
injury of popliteal artery (S85.0)

The appropriate 7th character is to be added to each code from category S75
A   initial encounter
D   subsequent encounter
S   sequela

🔳 **S75.0**   **Injury of femoral artery**

🔳 **S75.00**   **Unspecified injury of femoral artery**

🔲 **IQ** 🔳 **S75.001-**   **Unspecified injury of femoral artery, right leg**

🔲 **IQ** 🔳 **S75.002-**   **Unspecified injury of femoral artery, left leg**

🔲 **IQ** 🔳 **S75.009-**   **Unspecified injury of femoral artery, unspecified leg**

🔳 **S75.01**   **Minor laceration of femoral artery**
Incomplete transection of femoral artery
Laceration of femoral artery NOS
Superficial laceration of femoral artery

🔲 **SP** 🔳 **S75.011-**   **Minor laceration of femoral artery, right leg**

🔲 **SP** 🔳 **S75.012-**   **Minor laceration of femoral artery, left leg**

🔲 **IQ** 🔳 **S75.019-**   **Minor laceration of femoral artery, unspecified leg**

🔳 **S75.02**   **Major laceration of femoral artery**
Complete transection of femoral artery
Traumatic rupture of femoral artery

🔲 **SP** 🔳 **S75.021-**   **Major laceration of femoral artery, right leg**

🔲 **SP** 🔳 **S75.022-**   **Major laceration of femoral artery, left leg**

🔲 **IQ** 🔳 **S75.029-**   **Major laceration of femoral artery, unspecified leg**

🔳 **S75.09**   **Other specified injury of femoral artery**

🔲 **SP** 🔳 **S75.091-**   **Other specified injury of femoral artery, right leg**

🔲 **SP** 🔳 **S75.092-**   **Other specified injury of femoral artery, left leg**

🔲 **IQ** 🔳 **S75.099-**   **Other specified injury of femoral artery, unspecified leg**

🔳 **S75.1**   **Injury of femoral vein at hip and thigh level**

🔳 **S75.10**   **Unspecified injury of femoral vein at hip and thigh level**

🔲 **IQ** 🔳 **S75.101-**   **Unspecified injury of femoral vein at hip and thigh level, right leg**

🔲 **IQ** 🔳 **S75.102-**   **Unspecified injury of femoral vein at hip and thigh level, left leg**

🔲 **IQ** 🔳 **S75.109-**   **Unspecified injury of femoral vein at hip and thigh level, unspecified leg**

🔳 **S75.11**   **Minor laceration of femoral vein at hip and thigh level**
Incomplete transection of femoral vein at hip and thigh level
Laceration of femoral vein at hip and thigh level NOS
Superficial laceration of femoral vein at hip and thigh level

🔲 **SP** 🔳 **S75.111-**   **Minor laceration of femoral vein at hip and thigh level, right leg**

🔲 **SP** 🔳 **S75.112-**   **Minor laceration of femoral vein at hip and thigh level, left leg**

🔲 **IQ** 🔳 **S75.119-**   **Minor laceration of femoral vein at hip and thigh level, unspecified leg**

🔳 **S75.12**   **Major laceration of femoral vein at hip and thigh level**
Complete transection of femoral vein at hip and thigh level
Traumatic rupture of femoral vein at hip and thigh level

🔲 **SP** 🔳 **S75.121-**   **Major laceration of femoral vein at hip and thigh level, right leg**

🔲 **SP** 🔳 **S75.122-**   **Major laceration of femoral vein at hip and thigh level, left leg**

🔲 **IQ** 🔳 **S75.129-**   **Major laceration of femoral vein at hip and thigh level, unspecified leg**

🔳 **S75.19**   **Other specified injury of femoral vein at hip and thigh level**

---

4 4th digit required   **5** 5th digit required   **6** 6th digit required   **7** 7th digit required   **7** 7th digit placeholder   **+** Additional code   **🔲** Laterality

1594   *DecisionHealth's* FY 2020 Complete Home Health ICD-10-CM Diagnosis Coding Manual

☐ **SP** 7 **S75.191-** Other specified injury of femoral vein at hip and thigh level, right leg

☐ **SP** 7 **S75.192-** Other specified injury of femoral vein at hip and thigh level, left leg

☐ **IQ** 7 **S75.199-** Other specified injury of femoral vein at hip and thigh level, unspecified leg

5 **S75.2** **Injury of greater saphenous vein at hip and thigh level**

> EXCLUDES 1 greater saphenous vein NOS (S85.3)

6 **S75.20** Unspecified injury of greater saphenous vein at hip and thigh level

☐ **IQ** 7 **S75.201-** Unspecified injury of greater saphenous vein at hip and thigh level, right leg

☐ **IQ** 7 **S75.202-** Unspecified injury of greater saphenous vein at hip and thigh level, left leg

☐ **IQ** 7 **S75.209-** Unspecified injury of greater saphenous vein at hip and thigh level, unspecified leg

6 **S75.21** Minor laceration of greater saphenous vein at hip and thigh level
Incomplete transection of greater saphenous vein at hip and thigh level
Laceration of greater saphenous vein at hip and thigh level NOS
Superficial laceration of greater saphenous vein at hip and thigh level

☐ **SP** 7 **S75.211-** Minor laceration of greater saphenous vein at hip and thigh level, right leg

☐ **SP** 7 **S75.212-** Minor laceration of greater saphenous vein at hip and thigh level, left leg

☐ **IQ** 7 **S75.219-** Minor laceration of greater saphenous vein at hip and thigh level, unspecified leg

6 **S75.22** Major laceration of greater saphenous vein at hip and thigh level
Complete transection of greater saphenous vein at hip and thigh level
Traumatic rupture of greater saphenous vein at hip and thigh level

☐ **SP** 7 **S75.221-** Major laceration of greater saphenous vein at hip and thigh level, right leg

☐ **SP** 7 **S75.222-** Major laceration of greater saphenous vein at hip and thigh level, left leg

☐ **IQ** 7 **S75.229-** Major laceration of greater saphenous vein at hip and thigh level, unspecified leg

6 **S75.29** Other specified injury of greater saphenous vein at hip and thigh level

☐ **SP** 7 **S75.291-** Other specified injury of greater saphenous vein at hip and thigh level, right leg

☐ **SP** 7 **S75.292-** Other specified injury of greater saphenous vein at hip and thigh level, left leg

☐ **IQ** 7 **S75.299-** Other specified injury of greater saphenous vein at hip and thigh level, unspecified leg

5 **S75.8** **Injury of other blood vessels at hip and thigh level**

6 **S75.80** Unspecified injury of other blood vessels at hip and thigh level

☐ **IQ** 7 **S75.801-** Unspecified injury of other blood vessels at hip and thigh level, right leg

☐ **IQ** 7 **S75.802-** Unspecified injury of other blood vessels at hip and thigh level, left leg

☐ **IQ** 7 **S75.809-** Unspecified injury of other blood vessels at hip and thigh level, unspecified leg

6 **S75.81** Laceration of other blood vessels at hip and thigh level

☐ **SP** 7 **S75.811-** Laceration of other blood vessels at hip and thigh level, right leg

☐ **SP** 7 **S75.812-** Laceration of other blood vessels at hip and thigh level, left leg

☐ **IQ** 7 **S75.819-** Laceration of other blood vessels at hip and thigh level, unspecified leg

6 **S75.89** Other specified injury of other blood vessels at hip and thigh level

☐ **SP** 7 **S75.891-** Other specified injury of other blood vessels at hip and thigh level, right leg

☐ **SP** 7 **S75.892-** Other specified injury of other blood vessels at hip and thigh level, left leg

☐ **IQ** 7 **S75.899-** Other specified injury of other blood vessels at hip and thigh level, unspecified leg

5 **S75.9** **Injury of unspecified blood vessel at hip and thigh level**

6 **S75.90** Unspecified injury of unspecified blood vessel at hip and thigh level

☐ **IQ** 7 **S75.901-** Unspecified injury of unspecified blood vessel at hip and thigh level, right leg

☐ **IQ** 7 **S75.902-** Unspecified injury of unspecified blood vessel at hip and thigh level, left leg

☐ **IQ** 7 **S75.909-** Unspecified injury of unspecified blood vessel at hip and thigh level, unspecified leg

6 **S75.91** Laceration of unspecified blood vessel at hip and thigh level

☐ **SP** 7 **S75.911-** Laceration of unspecified blood vessel at hip and thigh level, right leg

☐ **SP** 7 **S75.912-** Laceration of unspecified blood vessel at hip and thigh level, left leg

☐ **IQ** 7 **S75.919-** Laceration of unspecified blood vessel at hip and thigh level, unspecified leg

6 **S75.99** Other specified injury of unspecified blood vessel at hip and thigh level

---

★ New ▲ Revised Px Primary **SP** PDGM Px **SL** Low CoM **SH** High CoM **IQ** Quest. Encounter ⊞ Hospice non-cancer Dx Unspecified **M** *Manifestation*

DecisionHealth's FY 2020 Complete Home Health ICD-10-CM Diagnosis Coding Manual

1595

⊟ IQ 7 S75.991- **Other specified injury of unspecified blood vessel at hip and thigh level, right leg**

⊟ IQ 7 S75.992- **Other specified injury of unspecified blood vessel at hip and thigh level, left leg**

⊟ IQ 7 S75.999- **Other specified injury of unspecified blood vessel at hip and thigh level, unspecified leg**

4 S76 **Injury of muscle, fascia and tendon at hip and thigh level**
Code also:
. any associated open wound (S71.-)
EXCLUDES 2 injury of muscle, fascia and tendon at lower leg level (S86)
sprain of joint and ligament of hip (S73.1)

The appropriate 7th character is to be added to each code from category S76
A   initial encounter
D   subsequent encounter
S   sequela

5 S76.0 **Injury of muscle, fascia and tendon of hip**

6 S76.00 **Unspecified injury of muscle, fascia and tendon of hip**

⊟ IQ 7 S76.001- **Unspecified injury of muscle, fascia and tendon of right hip**

⊟ IQ 7 S76.002- **Unspecified injury of muscle, fascia and tendon of left hip**

⊟ IQ 7 S76.009- **Unspecified injury of muscle, fascia and tendon of unspecified hip**

6 S76.01 **Strain of muscle, fascia and tendon of hip**

⊟ SP 7 S76.011- **Strain of muscle, fascia and tendon of right hip**

⊟ SP 7 S76.012- **Strain of muscle, fascia and tendon of left hip**

⊟ IQ 7 S76.019- **Strain of muscle, fascia and tendon of unspecified hip**

6 S76.02 **Laceration of muscle, fascia and tendon of hip**

⊟ SP 7 S76.021- **Laceration of muscle, fascia and tendon of right hip**

⊟ SP 7 S76.022- **Laceration of muscle, fascia and tendon of left hip**

⊟ IQ 7 S76.029- **Laceration of muscle, fascia and tendon of unspecified hip**

6 S76.09 **Other specified injury of muscle, fascia and tendon of hip**

⊟ SP 7 S76.091- **Other specified injury of muscle, fascia and tendon of right hip**

⊟ SP 7 S76.092- **Other specified injury of muscle, fascia and tendon of left hip**

⊟ IQ 7 S76.099- **Other specified injury of muscle, fascia and tendon of unspecified hip**

5 S76.1 **Injury of quadriceps muscle, fascia and tendon**
Injury of patellar ligament (tendon)

6 S76.10 **Unspecified injury of quadriceps muscle, fascia and tendon**

⊟ IQ 7 S76.101- **Unspecified injury of right quadriceps muscle, fascia and tendon**

⊟ IQ 7 S76.102- **Unspecified injury of left quadriceps muscle, fascia and tendon**

⊟ IQ 7 S76.109- **Unspecified injury of unspecified quadriceps muscle, fascia and tendon**

6 S76.11 **Strain of quadriceps muscle, fascia and tendon**

⊟ SP 7 S76.111- **Strain of right quadriceps muscle, fascia and tendon**

⊟ SP 7 S76.112- **Strain of left quadriceps muscle, fascia and tendon**

⊟ IQ 7 S76.119- **Strain of unspecified quadriceps muscle, fascia and tendon**

6 S76.12 **Laceration of quadriceps muscle, fascia and tendon**

⊟ SP 7 S76.121- **Laceration of right quadriceps muscle, fascia and tendon**

⊟ SP 7 S76.122- **Laceration of left quadriceps muscle, fascia and tendon**

⊟ IQ 7 S76.129- **Laceration of unspecified quadriceps muscle, fascia and tendon**

6 S76.19 **Other specified injury of quadriceps muscle, fascia and tendon**

⊟ SP 7 S76.191- **Other specified injury of right quadriceps muscle, fascia and tendon**

⊟ SP 7 S76.192- **Other specified injury of left quadriceps muscle, fascia and tendon**

⊟ IQ 7 S76.199- **Other specified injury of unspecified quadriceps muscle, fascia and tendon**

5 S76.2 **Injury of adductor muscle, fascia and tendon of thigh**

6 S76.20 **Unspecified injury of adductor muscle, fascia and tendon of thigh**

⊟ IQ 7 S76.201- **Unspecified injury of adductor muscle, fascia and tendon of right thigh**

⊟ IQ 7 S76.202- **Unspecified injury of adductor muscle, fascia and tendon of left thigh**

⊟ IQ 7 S76.209- **Unspecified injury of adductor muscle, fascia and tendon of unspecified thigh**

6 S76.21 **Strain of adductor muscle, fascia and tendon of thigh**

⊟ SP 7 S76.211- **Strain of adductor muscle, fascia and tendon of right thigh**

⊟ SP 7 S76.212- **Strain of adductor muscle, fascia and tendon of left thigh**

⊟ IQ 7 S76.219- **Strain of adductor muscle, fascia and tendon of unspecified thigh**

6 S76.22 **Laceration of adductor muscle, fascia and tendon of thigh**

⊟ SP 7 S76.221- **Laceration of adductor muscle, fascia and tendon of right thigh**

⊟ SP 7 S76.222- **Laceration of adductor muscle, fascia and tendon of left thigh**

4 4th digit required   5 5th digit required   6 6th digit required   7 7th digit required   7 7th digit placeholder   + Additional code   ⊟ Laterality

1596   *DecisionHealth's* FY 2020 Complete Home Health ICD-10-CM Diagnosis Coding Manual

Chapter 19

S00-T88

☐ **IQ** 7 **S76.229-** Laceration of adductor muscle, fascia and tendon of unspecified thigh

6 **S76.29** Other injury of adductor muscle, fascia and tendon of thigh

☐ **SP** 7 **S76.291-** Other injury of adductor muscle, fascia and tendon of right thigh

☐ **SP** 7 **S76.292-** Other injury of adductor muscle, fascia and tendon of left thigh

☐ **IQ** 7 **S76.299-** Other injury of adductor muscle, fascia and tendon of unspecified thigh

5 **S76.3** Injury of muscle, fascia and tendon of the posterior muscle group at thigh level

6 **S76.30** Unspecified injury of muscle, fascia and tendon of the posterior muscle group at thigh level

☐ **IQ** 7 **S76.301-** Unspecified injury of muscle, fascia and tendon of the posterior muscle group at thigh level, right thigh

☐ **IQ** 7 **S76.302-** Unspecified injury of muscle, fascia and tendon of the posterior muscle group at thigh level, left thigh

☐ **IQ** 7 **S76.309-** Unspecified injury of muscle, fascia and tendon of the posterior muscle group at thigh level, unspecified thigh

6 **S76.31** Strain of muscle, fascia and tendon of the posterior muscle group at thigh level

☐ **SP** 7 **S76.311-** Strain of muscle, fascia and tendon of the posterior muscle group at thigh level, right thigh

☐ **SP** 7 **S76.312-** Strain of muscle, fascia and tendon of the posterior muscle group at thigh level, left thigh

☐ **IQ** 7 **S76.319-** Strain of muscle, fascia and tendon of the posterior muscle group at thigh level, unspecified thigh

6 **S76.32** Laceration of muscle, fascia and tendon of the posterior muscle group at thigh level

☐ **SP** 7 **S76.321-** Laceration of muscle, fascia and tendon of the posterior muscle group at thigh level, right thigh

☐ **SP** 7 **S76.322-** Laceration of muscle, fascia and tendon of the posterior muscle group at thigh level, left thigh

☐ **IQ** 7 **S76.329-** Laceration of muscle, fascia and tendon of the posterior muscle group at thigh level, unspecified thigh

6 **S76.39** Other specified injury of muscle, fascia and tendon of the posterior muscle group at thigh level

☐ **SP** 7 **S76.391-** Other specified injury of muscle, fascia and tendon of the posterior muscle group at thigh level, right thigh

☐ **SP** 7 **S76.392-** Other specified injury of muscle, fascia and tendon of the posterior muscle group at thigh level, left thigh

☐ **IQ** 7 **S76.399-** Other specified injury of muscle, fascia and tendon of the posterior muscle group at thigh level, unspecified thigh

5 **S76.8** Injury of other specified muscles, fascia and tendons at thigh level

6 **S76.80** Unspecified injury of other specified muscles, fascia and tendons at thigh level

☐ **IQ** 7 **S76.801-** Unspecified injury of other specified muscles, fascia and tendons at thigh level, right thigh

☐ **IQ** 7 **S76.802-** Unspecified injury of other specified muscles, fascia and tendons at thigh level, left thigh

☐ **IQ** 7 **S76.809-** Unspecified injury of other specified muscles, fascia and tendons at thigh level, unspecified thigh

6 **S76.81** Strain of other specified muscles, fascia and tendons at thigh level

☐ **SP** 7 **S76.811-** Strain of other specified muscles, fascia and tendons at thigh level, right thigh

☐ **SP** 7 **S76.812-** Strain of other specified muscles, fascia and tendons at thigh level, left thigh

☐ **IQ** 7 **S76.819-** Strain of other specified muscles, fascia and tendons at thigh level, unspecified thigh

6 **S76.82** Laceration of other specified muscles, fascia and tendons at thigh level

☐ **SP** 7 **S76.821-** Laceration of other specified muscles, fascia and tendons at thigh level, right thigh

☐ **SP** 7 **S76.822-** Laceration of other specified muscles, fascia and tendons at thigh level, left thigh

☐ **IQ** 7 **S76.829-** Laceration of other specified muscles, fascia and tendons at thigh level, unspecified thigh

6 **S76.89** Other injury of other specified muscles, fascia and tendons at thigh level

☐ **SP** 7 **S76.891-** Other injury of other specified muscles, fascia and tendons at thigh level, right thigh

☐ **SP** 7 **S76.892-** Other injury of other specified muscles, fascia and tendons at thigh level, left thigh

☐ **IQ** 7 **S76.899-** Other injury of other specified muscles, fascia and tendons at thigh level, unspecified thigh

5 **S76.9** Injury of unspecified muscles, fascia and tendons at thigh level

6 **S76.90** Unspecified injury of unspecified muscles, fascia and tendons at thigh level

☐ **IQ** 7 **S76.901-** Unspecified injury of unspecified muscles, fascia and tendons at thigh level, right thigh

☐ **IQ** 7 **S76.902-** Unspecified injury of unspecified muscles, fascia and tendons at thigh level, left thigh

---

★ New ▲ Revised **Px** Primary **SP** PDGM Px **SL** Low CoM **SH** High CoM **IQ** Quest. Encounter Ⓗ Hospice non-cancer Dx Unspecified **M** *Manifestation*

☐ !Q 7 S76.909- Unspecified injury of unspecified muscles, fascia and tendons at thigh level, unspecified thigh

6 S76.91 Strain of unspecified muscles, fascia and tendons at thigh level

☐ SP 7 S76.911- Strain of unspecified muscles, fascia and tendons at thigh level, right thigh

☐ SP 7 S76.912- Strain of unspecified muscles, fascia and tendons at thigh level, left thigh

☐ !Q 7 S76.919- Strain of unspecified muscles, fascia and tendons at thigh level, unspecified thigh

6 S76.92 Laceration of unspecified muscles, fascia and tendons at thigh level

☐ SP 7 S76.921- Laceration of unspecified muscles, fascia and tendons at thigh level, right thigh

☐ SP 7 S76.922- Laceration of unspecified muscles, fascia and tendons at thigh level, left thigh

☐ !Q 7 S76.929- Laceration of unspecified muscles, fascia and tendons at thigh level, unspecified thigh

6 S76.99 Other specified injury of unspecified muscles, fascia and tendons at thigh level

☐ !Q 7 S76.991- Other specified injury of unspecified muscles, fascia and tendons at thigh level, right thigh

☐ !Q 7 S76.992- Other specified injury of unspecified muscles, fascia and tendons at thigh level, left thigh

☐ !Q 7 S76.999- Other specified injury of unspecified muscles, fascia and tendons at thigh level, unspecified thigh

+ 4 S77 Crushing injury of hip and thigh
Use additional code(s) for all associated injuries
EXCLUDES 2   crushing injury of ankle and foot (S97.-)
crushing injury of lower leg (S87.-)

The appropriate 7th character is to be added to each code from category S77
A   initial encounter
D   subsequent encounter
S   sequela

+ 5 S77.0 Crushing injury of hip

☐ !Q + 7 S77.00X- Crushing injury of unspecified hip

☐ SP + 7 S77.01X- Crushing injury of right hip

☐ SP + 7 S77.02X- Crushing injury of left hip

+ 5 S77.1 Crushing injury of thigh

☐ !Q + 7 S77.10X- Crushing injury of unspecified thigh

☐ SP + 7 S77.11X- Crushing injury of right thigh

☐ SP + 7 S77.12X- Crushing injury of left thigh

+ 5 S77.2 Crushing injury of hip with thigh

☐ !Q + 7 S77.20X- Crushing injury of unspecified hip with thigh

☐ SP + 7 S77.21X- Crushing injury of right hip with thigh

☐ SP + 7 S77.22X- Crushing injury of left hip with thigh

4 S78 Traumatic amputation of hip and thigh
An amputation not identified as partial or complete should be coded to complete
EXCLUDES 1   traumatic amputation of knee (S88.0-)

The appropriate 7th character is to be added to each code from category S78
A   initial encounter
D   subsequent encounter
S   sequela

CODING TIPS ✓   Use these codes only when the amputation was due to trauma. There is no need for adding Z89 with traumatic amputations. See Z47.81 for care of amputations not due to trauma.

5 S78.0 Traumatic amputation at hip joint

6 S78.01 Complete traumatic amputation at hip joint

☐ SP 7 S78.011- Complete traumatic amputation at right hip joint

☐ SP 7 S78.012- Complete traumatic amputation at left hip joint

☐ !Q 7 S78.019- Complete traumatic amputation at unspecified hip joint

6 S78.02 Partial traumatic amputation at hip joint

☐ SP 7 S78.021- Partial traumatic amputation at right hip joint

☐ SP 7 S78.022- Partial traumatic amputation at left hip joint

☐ !Q 7 S78.029- Partial traumatic amputation at unspecified hip joint

5 S78.1 Traumatic amputation at level between hip and knee
EXCLUDES 1   traumatic amputation of knee (S88.0-)

6 S78.11 Complete traumatic amputation at level between hip and knee

☐ SP 7 S78.111- Complete traumatic amputation at level between right hip and knee

☐ SP 7 S78.112- Complete traumatic amputation at level between left hip and knee

☐ !Q 7 S78.119- Complete traumatic amputation at level between unspecified hip and knee

6 S78.12 Partial traumatic amputation at level between hip and knee

☐ SP 7 S78.121- Partial traumatic amputation at level between right hip and knee

☐ SP 7 S78.122- Partial traumatic amputation at level between left hip and knee

☐ !Q 7 S78.129- Partial traumatic amputation at level between unspecified hip and knee

5 S78.9 Traumatic amputation of hip and thigh, level unspecified

6 S78.91 Complete traumatic amputation of hip and thigh, level unspecified

⁴4th digit required   ⁵5th digit required   ⁶6th digit required   ⁷7th digit required   ⁷7th digit placeholder   +Additional code   ☐Laterality

1598   *DecisionHealth's* FY 2020 Complete Home Health ICD-10-CM Diagnosis Coding Manual

☰ SP 7 S78.911-	**Complete traumatic amputation of right hip and thigh, level unspecified**	
☰ SP 7 S78.912-	**Complete traumatic amputation of left hip and thigh, level unspecified**	
☰ IQ 7 S78.919-	**Complete traumatic amputation of unspecified hip and thigh, level unspecified**	
6 S78.92	**Partial traumatic amputation of hip and thigh, level unspecified**	
☰ SP 7 S78.921-	**Partial traumatic amputation of right hip and thigh, level unspecified**	
☰ SP 7 S78.922-	**Partial traumatic amputation of left hip and thigh, level unspecified**	
☰ IQ 7 S78.929-	**Partial traumatic amputation of unspecified hip and thigh, level unspecified**	

4 S79   Other and unspecified injuries of hip and thigh

Note:
A fracture not indicated as open or closed should be coded to closed

The appropriate 7th character is to be added to each code from subcategories S79.0 and S79.1
A	initial encounter for closed fracture
D	subsequent encounter for fracture with routine healing
G	subsequent encounter for fracture with delayed healing
K	subsequent encounter for fracture with nonunion
P	subsequent encounter for fracture with malunion
S	sequela

5 S79.0   Physeal fracture of upper end of femur
    EXCLUDES 1 apophyseal fracture of upper end of femur (S72.13-)
      nontraumatic slipped upper femoral epiphysis (M93.0-)

6 S79.00	**Unspecified physeal fracture of upper end of femur**
☰ SP 7 S79.001-	**Unspecified physeal fracture of upper end of right femur**
☰ SP 7 S79.002-	**Unspecified physeal fracture of upper end of left femur**
☰ IQ 7 S79.009-	**Unspecified physeal fracture of upper end of unspecified femur**

6 S79.01   Salter-Harris Type I physeal fracture of upper end of femur
Acute on chronic slipped capital femoral epiphysis (traumatic)
Acute slipped capital femoral epiphysis (traumatic)
Capital femoral epiphyseal fracture
    EXCLUDES 1 chronic slipped upper femoral epiphysis (nontraumatic) (M93.02-)

☰ SP 7 S79.011-	**Salter-Harris Type I physeal fracture of upper end of right femur**	
☰ SP 7 S79.012-	**Salter-Harris Type I physeal fracture of upper end of left femur**	
☰ IQ 7 S79.019-	**Salter-Harris Type I physeal fracture of upper end of unspecified femur**	

6 S79.09	**Other physeal fracture of upper end of femur**
☰ SP 7 S79.091-	**Other physeal fracture of upper end of right femur**
☰ SP 7 S79.092-	**Other physeal fracture of upper end of left femur**
☰ IQ 7 S79.099-	**Other physeal fracture of upper end of unspecified femur**

5 S79.1   Physeal fracture of lower end of femur

6 S79.10	**Unspecified physeal fracture of lower end of femur**	
☰ SP 7 S79.101-	**Unspecified physeal fracture of lower end of right femur**	
☰ SP 7 S79.102-	**Unspecified physeal fracture of lower end of left femur**	
☰ IQ 7 S79.109-	**Unspecified physeal fracture of lower end of unspecified femur**	
6 S79.11	**Salter-Harris Type I physeal fracture of lower end of femur**	
☰ SP 7 S79.111-	**Salter-Harris Type I physeal fracture of lower end of right femur**	
☰ SP 7 S79.112-	**Salter-Harris Type I physeal fracture of lower end of left femur**	
☰ IQ 7 S79.119-	**Salter-Harris Type I physeal fracture of lower end of unspecified femur**	
6 S79.12	**Salter-Harris Type II physeal fracture of lower end of femur**	
☰ SP 7 S79.121-	**Salter-Harris Type II physeal fracture of lower end of right femur**	
☰ SP 7 S79.122-	**Salter-Harris Type II physeal fracture of lower end of left femur**	
☰ IQ 7 S79.129-	**Salter-Harris Type II physeal fracture of lower end of unspecified femur**	
6 S79.13	**Salter-Harris Type III physeal fracture of lower end of femur**	
☰ SP 7 S79.131-	**Salter-Harris Type III physeal fracture of lower end of right femur**	
☰ SP 7 S79.132-	**Salter-Harris Type III physeal fracture of lower end of left femur**	
☰ IQ 7 S79.139-	**Salter-Harris Type III physeal fracture of lower end of unspecified femur**	
6 S79.14	**Salter-Harris Type IV physeal fracture of lower end of femur**	
☰ SP 7 S79.141-	**Salter-Harris Type IV physeal fracture of lower end of right femur**	
☰ SP 7 S79.142-	**Salter-Harris Type IV physeal fracture of lower end of left femur**	

Chapter 19

S00-T88

★ New ▲ Revised Px Primary SP PDGM Px SL Low CoM SH High CoM IQ Quest. Encounter H Hospice non-cancer Dx   Unspecified   M *Manifestation*

DecisionHealth's FY 2020 Complete Home Health ICD-10-CM Diagnosis Coding Manual   1599

▤ **IQ** **7** **S79.149-** **Salter-Harris Type IV physeal fracture of lower end of unspecified femur**

6 **S79.19** **Other physeal fracture of lower end of femur**

▤ **SP** **7** **S79.191-** **Other physeal fracture of lower end of right femur**

▤ **SP** **7** **S79.192-** **Other physeal fracture of lower end of left femur**

▤ **IQ** **7** **S79.199-** **Other physeal fracture of lower end of unspecified femur**

5 **S79.8** **Other specified injuries of hip and thigh**

> The appropriate 7th character is to be added to each code in subcategory S79.8
> A   initial encounter
> D   subsequent encounter
> S   sequela

6 **S79.81** **Other specified injuries of hip**

▤ **SP** **7** **S79.811-** **Other specified injuries of right hip**

▤ **SP** **7** **S79.812-** **Other specified injuries of left hip**

▤ **IQ** **7** **S79.819-** **Other specified injuries of unspecified hip**

6 **S79.82** **Other specified injuries of thigh**

▤ **SP** **7** **S79.821-** **Other specified injuries of right thigh**

▤ **SP** **7** **S79.822-** **Other specified injuries of left thigh**

▤ **IQ** **7** **S79.829-** **Other specified injuries of unspecified thigh**

5 **S79.9** **Unspecified injury of hip and thigh**

> The appropriate 7th character is to be added to each code in subcategory S79.9
> A   initial encounter
> D   subsequent encounter
> S   sequela

6 **S79.91** **Unspecified injury of hip**

▤ **IQ** **7** **S79.911-** **Unspecified injury of right hip**

▤ **IQ** **7** **S79.912-** **Unspecified injury of left hip**

▤ **IQ** **7** **S79.919-** **Unspecified injury of unspecified hip**

6 **S79.92** **Unspecified injury of thigh**

▤ **IQ** **7** **S79.921-** **Unspecified injury of right thigh**

▤ **IQ** **7** **S79.922-** **Unspecified injury of left thigh**

▤ **IQ** **7** **S79.929-** **Unspecified injury of unspecified thigh**

Injuries to the knee and lower leg (S80-S89)

EXCLUDES 2   burns and corrosions (T20-T32)
frostbite (T33-T34)
injuries of ankle and foot, except fracture of ankle and malleolus (S90-S99)
insect bite or sting, venomous (T63.4)

GUIDELINES   Section I.C.19.c.2)
Multiple fractures are sequenced in accordance with the severity of the fracture.

GUIDELINES   Section I.C.19.b.1)-2)
When coding injuries, assign separate codes for each injury unless a combination code is provided, in which case the combination code is assigned ... Traumatic injury codes (S00-T14.9) are not to be used for normal, healing surgical wounds or to identify complications of surgical wounds. The code for the most serious injury, as determined by the provider and the focus of treatment, is sequenced first.

1) Superficial injuries such as abrasions or contusions are not coded when associated with more severe injuries of the same site.

2) When a primary injury results in minor damage to peripheral nerves or blood vessels, the primary injury is sequenced first with additional code(s) for injuries to nerves and spinal cord (such as category S04), and/or injury to blood vessels (such as category S15). When the primary injury is to the blood vessels or nerves, that injury should be sequenced first.

GUIDELINES   Section I.C.19.c
Coding of Traumatic Fractures: The principles of multiple coding of injuries should be followed in coding fractures. Fractures of specified sites are coded individually by site in accordance with both the provisions within categories S02, S12, S22, S32, S42, S49, S52, S59, S62, S72, S79, S82, S89, S92 and the level of detail furnished by medical record content. A fracture not indicated as open or closed should be coded to closed. A fracture not indicated whether displaced or not displaced should be coded to displaced.

CODING TIPS ✓   7th character A is acceptable in home health and hospice when active treatment is provided, such as antibiotics for an infected wound or a wound vac for a dehisced wound. D is used when the complication or injury is now healing. Think of D as aftercare. S is used for sequela of the injury or complication. Sequela is a residual deficit or condition produced as a result of the injury or complication after the original injury or complication has healed.

4 **S80** **Superficial injury of knee and lower leg**
     EXCLUDES 2   superficial injury of ankle and foot (S90.-)

> The appropriate 7th character is to be added to each code from category S80
> A   initial encounter
> D   subsequent encounter
> S   sequela

5 **S80.0** **Contusion of knee**

▤ **IQ** **7️** **S80.00X-** **Contusion of unspecified knee**

▤ **IQ** **7️** **S80.01X-** **Contusion of right knee**

▤ **IQ** **7️** **S80.02X-** **Contusion of left knee**

5 **S80.1** **Contusion of lower leg**

▤ **IQ** **7️** **S80.10X-** **Contusion of unspecified lower leg**

▤ **IQ** **7️** **S80.11X-** **Contusion of right lower leg**

▤ **IQ** **7️** **S80.12X-** **Contusion of left lower leg**

5 **S80.2** **Other superficial injuries of knee**

6 **S80.21** **Abrasion of knee**

▤ **IQ** **7** **S80.211-** **Abrasion, right knee**

▤ **IQ** **7** **S80.212-** **Abrasion, left knee**

▤ **IQ** **7** **S80.219-** **Abrasion, unspecified knee**

6 **S80.22** **Blister (nonthermal) of knee**

▤ **IQ** **7** **S80.221-** **Blister (nonthermal), right knee**

---

4 4th digit required   **5** 5th digit required   **6** 6th digit required   **7** 7th digit required   **7️** 7th digit placeholder   **+** Additional code   ▤ Laterality

☐ **!Q** 7 **S80.222-** Blister (nonthermal), left knee

☐ **!Q** 7 **S80.229-** Blister (nonthermal), unspecified knee

6 **S80.24** External constriction of knee

☐ **!Q** 7 **S80.241-** External constriction, right knee

☐ **!Q** 7 **S80.242-** External constriction, left knee

☐ **!Q** 7 **S80.249-** External constriction, unspecified knee

6 **S80.25** Superficial foreign body of knee
Splinter in the knee

☐ **!Q** 7 **S80.251-** Superficial foreign body, right knee

☐ **!Q** 7 **S80.252-** Superficial foreign body, left knee

☐ **!Q** 7 **S80.259-** Superficial foreign body, unspecified knee

6 **S80.26** Insect bite (nonvenomous) of knee

☐ **!Q** 7 **S80.261-** Insect bite (nonvenomous), right knee

☐ **!Q** 7 **S80.262-** Insect bite (nonvenomous), left knee

☐ **!Q** 7 **S80.269-** Insect bite (nonvenomous), unspecified knee

6 **S80.27** Other superficial bite of knee
EXCLUDES 1 open bite of knee (S81.05-)

☐ **!Q** 7 **S80.271-** Other superficial bite of right knee

☐ **!Q** 7 **S80.272-** Other superficial bite of left knee

☐ **!Q** 7 **S80.279-** Other superficial bite of unspecified knee

5 **S80.8** Other superficial injuries of lower leg

6 **S80.81** Abrasion of lower leg

☐ **!Q** 7 **S80.811-** Abrasion, right lower leg

☐ **!Q** 7 **S80.812-** Abrasion, left lower leg

☐ **!Q** 7 **S80.819-** Abrasion, unspecified lower leg

6 **S80.82** Blister (nonthermal) of lower leg

☐ **!Q** 7 **S80.821-** Blister (nonthermal), right lower leg

☐ **!Q** 7 **S80.822-** Blister (nonthermal), left lower leg

☐ **!Q** 7 **S80.829-** Blister (nonthermal), unspecified lower leg

6 **S80.84** External constriction of lower leg

☐ **!Q** 7 **S80.841-** External constriction, right lower leg

☐ **!Q** 7 **S80.842-** External constriction, left lower leg

☐ **!Q** 7 **S80.849-** External constriction, unspecified lower leg

6 **S80.85** Superficial foreign body of lower leg
Splinter in the lower leg

☐ **!Q** 7 **S80.851-** Superficial foreign body, right lower leg

☐ **!Q** 7 **S80.852-** Superficial foreign body, left lower leg

☐ **!Q** 7 **S80.859-** Superficial foreign body, unspecified lower leg

6 **S80.86** Insect bite (nonvenomous) of lower leg

☐ **!Q** 7 **S80.861-** Insect bite (nonvenomous), right lower leg

☐ **!Q** 7 **S80.862-** Insect bite (nonvenomous), left lower leg

☐ **!Q** 7 **S80.869-** Insect bite (nonvenomous), unspecified lower leg

6 **S80.87** Other superficial bite of lower leg
EXCLUDES 1 open bite of lower leg (S81.85-)

☐ **!Q** 7 **S80.871-** Other superficial bite, right lower leg

☐ **!Q** 7 **S80.872-** Other superficial bite, left lower leg

☐ **!Q** 7 **S80.879-** Other superficial bite, unspecified lower leg

5 **S80.9** Unspecified superficial injury of knee and lower leg

6 **S80.91** Unspecified superficial injury of knee

☐ **!Q** 7 **S80.911-** Unspecified superficial injury of right knee

☐ **!Q** 7 **S80.912-** Unspecified superficial injury of left knee

☐ **!Q** 7 **S80.919-** Unspecified superficial injury of unspecified knee

6 **S80.92** Unspecified superficial injury of lower leg

☐ **!Q** 7 **S80.921-** Unspecified superficial injury of right lower leg

☐ **!Q** 7 **S80.922-** Unspecified superficial injury of left lower leg

☐ **!Q** 7 **S80.929-** Unspecified superficial injury of unspecified lower leg

4 **S81** Open wound of knee and lower leg
Code also:
any associated wound infection
EXCLUDES 1 open fracture of knee and lower leg (S82.-)
traumatic amputation of lower leg (S88.-)
EXCLUDES 2 open wound of ankle and foot (S91.-)

The appropriate 7th character is to be added to each code from category S81
A   initial encounter
D   subsequent encounter
S   sequela

CODING TIPS ✓ No aftercare code applies, including those indicating dressing changes, drain care, or suture removal. 7th character 'D' is the default for home care and hospice when providing aftercare for a healing or resolving condition; 'A' is used for active treatment such as antibiotics or more than routine wound care; 'S' may be used to indicate a residual condition after the original injury has healed.

CODING TIPS ✓ Open wound codes indicate a wound resulting from a traumatic origin. Do not assign a code for "open wound" unless the etiology of the wound is related to trauma.

5 **S81.0** Open wound of knee

6 **S81.00** Unspecified open wound of knee

☐ **SP** 7 **S81.001-** Unspecified open wound, right knee

☐ **SP** 7 **S81.002-** Unspecified open wound, left knee

☐ **!Q** 7 **S81.009-** Unspecified open wound, unspecified knee

★ New ▲ Revised Px Primary **SP** PDGM Px **SL** Low CoM **SH** High CoM **!Q** Quest. Encounter H Hospice non-cancer Dx Unspecified **M** Manifestation

DecisionHealth's FY 2020 Complete Home Health ICD-10-CM Diagnosis Coding Manual

1601

⑥ **S81.01** Laceration without foreign body of knee

⊟ SP ⑦ **S81.011-** Laceration without foreign body, right knee

⊟ SP ⑦ **S81.012-** Laceration without foreign body, left knee

⊟ IQ ⑦ **S81.019-** Laceration without foreign body, unspecified knee

⑥ **S81.02** Laceration with foreign body of knee

⊟ SP ⑦ **S81.021-** Laceration with foreign body, right knee

⊟ SP ⑦ **S81.022-** Laceration with foreign body, left knee

⊟ IQ ⑦ **S81.029-** Laceration with foreign body, unspecified knee

⑥ **S81.03** Puncture wound without foreign body of knee

⊟ SP ⑦ **S81.031-** Puncture wound without foreign body, right knee

⊟ SP ⑦ **S81.032-** Puncture wound without foreign body, left knee

⊟ IQ ⑦ **S81.039-** Puncture wound without foreign body, unspecified knee

⑥ **S81.04** Puncture wound with foreign body of knee

⊟ SP ⑦ **S81.041-** Puncture wound with foreign body, right knee

⊟ SP ⑦ **S81.042-** Puncture wound with foreign body, left knee

⊟ IQ ⑦ **S81.049-** Puncture wound with foreign body, unspecified knee

⑥ **S81.05** Open bite of knee
Bite of knee NOS
> **EXCLUDES 1** superficial bite of knee (S80.27-)

⊟ SP ⑦ **S81.051-** Open bite, right knee

⊟ SP ⑦ **S81.052-** Open bite, left knee

⊟ IQ ⑦ **S81.059-** Open bite, unspecified knee

⑤ **S81.8** Open wound of lower leg

⑥ **S81.80** Unspecified open wound of lower leg

⊟ SP ⑦ **S81.801-** Unspecified open wound, right lower leg

⊟ SP ⑦ **S81.802-** Unspecified open wound, left lower leg

⊟ IQ ⑦ **S81.809-** Unspecified open wound, unspecified lower leg

⑥ **S81.81** Laceration without foreign body of lower leg

⊟ SP ⑦ **S81.811-** Laceration without foreign body, right lower leg

⊟ SP ⑦ **S81.812-** Laceration without foreign body, left lower leg

⊟ IQ ⑦ **S81.819-** Laceration without foreign body, unspecified lower leg

⑥ **S81.82** Laceration with foreign body of lower leg

⊟ SP ⑦ **S81.821-** Laceration with foreign body, right lower leg

⊟ SP ⑦ **S81.822-** Laceration with foreign body, left lower leg

⊟ IQ ⑦ **S81.829-** Laceration with foreign body, unspecified lower leg

⑥ **S81.83** Puncture wound without foreign body of lower leg

⊟ SP ⑦ **S81.831-** Puncture wound without foreign body, right lower leg

⊟ SP ⑦ **S81.832-** Puncture wound without foreign body, left lower leg

⊟ IQ ⑦ **S81.839-** Puncture wound without foreign body, unspecified lower leg

⑥ **S81.84** Puncture wound with foreign body of lower leg

⊟ SP ⑦ **S81.841-** Puncture wound with foreign body, right lower leg

⊟ SP ⑦ **S81.842-** Puncture wound with foreign body, left lower leg

⊟ IQ ⑦ **S81.849-** Puncture wound with foreign body, unspecified lower leg

⑥ **S81.85** Open bite of lower leg
Bite of lower leg NOS
> **EXCLUDES 1** superficial bite of lower leg (S80.86-, S80.87-)

⊟ SP ⑦ **S81.851-** Open bite, right lower leg

⊟ SP ⑦ **S81.852-** Open bite, left lower leg

⊟ IQ ⑦ **S81.859-** Open bite, unspecified lower leg

④ **S82** Fracture of lower leg, including ankle
Note:
A fracture not indicated as displaced or nondisplaced should be coded to displaced
A fracture not indicated as open or closed should be coded to closed
The open fracture designations are based on the Gustilo open fracture classification
> **INCLUDES** fracture of malleolus
> **EXCLUDES 1** traumatic amputation of lower leg (S88.-)
> **EXCLUDES 2** fracture of foot, except ankle (S92.-)
> periprosthetic fracture of prosthetic implant of knee (M97.0-)

④4th digit required   ⑤5th digit required   ⑥6th digit required   ⑦7th digit required   ⑦7th digit placeholder   ✚Additional code   ⊟Laterality

1602   *DecisionHealth's* FY 2020 Complete Home Health ICD-10-CM Diagnosis Coding Manual

Chapter 19

S00-T88

The appropriate 7th character is to be added to all codes from category S82

A	initial encounter for closed fracture
B	initial encounter for open fracture type I or II
C	initial encounter for open fracture type IIIA, IIIB, or IIIC
D	subsequent encounter for closed fracture with routine healing
E	subsequent encounter for open fracture type I or II with routine healing
F	subsequent encounter for open fracture type IIIA, IIIB, or IIIC with routine healing
G	subsequent encounter for closed fracture with delayed healing
H	subsequent encounter for open fracture type I or II with delayed healing
J	subsequent encounter for open fracture type IIIA, IIIB, or IIIC with delayed healing
K	subsequent encounter for closed fracture with nonunion
M	subsequent encounter for open fracture type I or II with nonunion
N	subsequent encounter for open fracture type IIIA, IIIB, or IIIC with nonunion
P	subsequent encounter for closed fracture with malunion
Q	subsequent encounter for open fracture type I or II with malunion
R	subsequent encounter for open fracture type IIIA, IIIB, or IIIC with malunion
S	sequela

CODING TIPS ✓ Fractures repaired by joint replacements are NOT coded with Z47.1. Fractures repaired by any other orthopedic surgery are NOT coded with Z47.89. Z codes are not appropriate for fractures of any kind. Code the fracture with 7th character D for fractures undergoing surgical repair.

CODING TIPS ✓ A fracture not indicated as displaced or nondisplaced should be coded to displaced. A fracture not indicated as open or closed should be coded to closed. The open fracture designations are based on the Gustilo open fracture classification. The 7th characters E, H, M and Q are the default for the Gustilo classification when no information is available. Always query the physician.

CODING TIPS ✓ "D" is the 7th character for home care and hospice unless the physician has documented delayed healing, nonunion or malunion. A sequela is a condition left after the fracture has healed.

Patellar tendon

Patella

⑤ **S82.0   Fracture of patella**
Knee cap

⑥ **S82.00   Unspecified fracture of patella**

⊟ **SP** ⑦ **S82.001-   Unspecified fracture of right patella**

⊟ **SP** ⑦ **S82.002-   Unspecified fracture of left patella**

⊟ **IQ** ⑦ **S82.009-   Unspecified fracture of unspecified patella**

⑥ **S82.01   Osteochondral fracture of patella**

⊟ **SP** ⑦ **S82.011-   Displaced osteochondral fracture of right patella**

⊟ **SP** ⑦ **S82.012-   Displaced osteochondral fracture of left patella**

⊟ **IQ** ⑦ **S82.013-   Displaced osteochondral fracture of unspecified patella**

⊟ **SP** ⑦ **S82.014-   Nondisplaced osteochondral fracture of right patella**

⊟ **SP** ⑦ **S82.015-   Nondisplaced osteochondral fracture of left patella**

⊟ **IQ** ⑦ **S82.016-   Nondisplaced osteochondral fracture of unspecified patella**

⑥ **S82.02   Longitudinal fracture of patella**

⊟ **SP** ⑦ **S82.021-   Displaced longitudinal fracture of right patella**

⊟ **SP** ⑦ **S82.022-   Displaced longitudinal fracture of left patella**

⊟ **IQ** ⑦ **S82.023-   Displaced longitudinal fracture of unspecified patella**

★ New ▲ Revised **Px** Primary **SP** PDGM Px **SL** Low CoM **SH** High CoM **IQ** Quest. Encounter 🄷 Hospice non-cancer Dx   Unspecified   **M** *Manifestation*

DecisionHealth's FY 2020 Complete Home Health ICD-10-CM Diagnosis Coding Manual   1603

Chapter 19

S00-T88

Chapter 19

S00-T88

☐ **SP** 7 **S82.024-** Nondisplaced longitudinal fracture of right patella

☐ **SP** 7 **S82.025-** Nondisplaced longitudinal fracture of left patella

☐ **IQ** 7 **S82.026-** Nondisplaced longitudinal fracture of unspecified patella

　　6 **S82.03** Transverse fracture of patella

☐ **SP** 7 **S82.031-** Displaced transverse fracture of right patella

☐ **SP** 7 **S82.032-** Displaced transverse fracture of left patella

☐ **IQ** 7 **S82.033-** Displaced transverse fracture of unspecified patella

☐ **SP** 7 **S82.034-** Nondisplaced transverse fracture of right patella

☐ **SP** 7 **S82.035-** Nondisplaced transverse fracture of left patella

☐ **IQ** 7 **S82.036-** Nondisplaced transverse fracture of unspecified patella

　　6 **S82.04** Comminuted fracture of patella

☐ **SP** 7 **S82.041-** Displaced comminuted fracture of right patella

☐ **SP** 7 **S82.042-** Displaced comminuted fracture of left patella

☐ **IQ** 7 **S82.043-** Displaced comminuted fracture of unspecified patella

☐ **SP** 7 **S82.044-** Nondisplaced comminuted fracture of right patella

☐ **SP** 7 **S82.045-** Nondisplaced comminuted fracture of left patella

☐ **IQ** 7 **S82.046-** Nondisplaced comminuted fracture of unspecified patella

　　6 **S82.09** Other fracture of patella

☐ **SP** 7 **S82.091-** Other fracture of right patella

☐ **SP** 7 **S82.092-** Other fracture of left patella

☐ **IQ** 7 **S82.099-** Other fracture of unspecified patella

　5 **S82.1** Fracture of upper end of tibia
　　　Fracture of proximal end of tibia

　　　EXCLUDES 2 fracture of shaft of tibia (S82.2-)
　　　physeal fracture of upper end of tibia (S89.0-)

　　6 **S82.10** Unspecified fracture of upper end of tibia

☐ **SP** 7 **S82.101-** Unspecified fracture of upper end of right tibia

☐ **SP** 7 **S82.102-** Unspecified fracture of upper end of left tibia

☐ **IQ** 7 **S82.109-** Unspecified fracture of upper end of unspecified tibia

　　6 **S82.11** Fracture of tibial spine

☐ **SP** 7 **S82.111-** Displaced fracture of right tibial spine

☐ **SP** 7 **S82.112-** Displaced fracture of left tibial spine

☐ **IQ** 7 **S82.113-** Displaced fracture of unspecified tibial spine

☐ **SP** 7 **S82.114-** Nondisplaced fracture of right tibial spine

☐ **SP** 7 **S82.115-** Nondisplaced fracture of left tibial spine

☐ **IQ** 7 **S82.116-** Nondisplaced fracture of unspecified tibial spine

　　6 **S82.12** Fracture of lateral condyle of tibia

☐ **SP** 7 **S82.121-** Displaced fracture of lateral condyle of right tibia

☐ **SP** 7 **S82.122-** Displaced fracture of lateral condyle of left tibia

☐ **IQ** 7 **S82.123-** Displaced fracture of lateral condyle of unspecified tibia

☐ **SP** 7 **S82.124-** Nondisplaced fracture of lateral condyle of right tibia

☐ **SP** 7 **S82.125-** Nondisplaced fracture of lateral condyle of left tibia

☐ **IQ** 7 **S82.126-** Nondisplaced fracture of lateral condyle of unspecified tibia

　　6 **S82.13** Fracture of medial condyle of tibia

☐ **SP** 7 **S82.131-** Displaced fracture of medial condyle of right tibia

☐ **SP** 7 **S82.132-** Displaced fracture of medial condyle of left tibia

☐ **IQ** 7 **S82.133-** Displaced fracture of medial condyle of unspecified tibia

☐ **SP** 7 **S82.134-** Nondisplaced fracture of medial condyle of right tibia

☐ **SP** 7 **S82.135-** Nondisplaced fracture of medial condyle of left tibia

☐ **IQ** 7 **S82.136-** Nondisplaced fracture of medial condyle of unspecified tibia

　　6 **S82.14** Bicondylar fracture of tibia
　　　Fracture of tibial plateau NOS

☐ **SP** 7 **S82.141-** Displaced bicondylar fracture of right tibia

☐ **SP** 7 **S82.142-** Displaced bicondylar fracture of left tibia

☐ **IQ** 7 **S82.143-** Displaced bicondylar fracture of unspecified tibia

☐ **SP** 7 **S82.144-** Nondisplaced bicondylar fracture of right tibia

☐ **SP** 7 **S82.145-** Nondisplaced bicondylar fracture of left tibia

☐ **IQ** 7 **S82.146-** Nondisplaced bicondylar fracture of unspecified tibia

　　6 **S82.15** Fracture of tibial tuberosity

☐ **SP** 7 **S82.151-** Displaced fracture of right tibial tuberosity

☐ **SP** 7 **S82.152-** Displaced fracture of left tibial tuberosity

☐ **IQ** 7 **S82.153-** Displaced fracture of unspecified tibial tuberosity

☐ **SP** 7 **S82.154-** Nondisplaced fracture of right tibial tuberosity

☐ **SP** 7 **S82.155-** Nondisplaced fracture of left tibial tuberosity

☐ **IQ** 7 **S82.156-** Nondisplaced fracture of unspecified tibial tuberosity

　　6 **S82.16** Torus fracture of upper end of tibia

---

4 4th digit required　　5 5th digit required　　6 6th digit required　　7 7th digit required　　7 7th digit placeholder　　+ Additional code　　☐ Laterality

1604　　　　*DecisionHealth's* FY 2020 Complete Home Health ICD-10-CM Diagnosis Coding Manual

The appropriate 7th character is to be added to all codes in subcategory S82.16

A   initial encounter for closed fracture

D   subsequent encounter for fracture with routine healing

G   subsequent encounter for fracture with delayed healing

K   subsequent encounter for fracture with nonunion

P   subsequent encounter for fracture with malunion

S   sequela

CODING TIPS ✓ Open fractures do not occur with torus fractures and greenstick fractures, therefore the 7th characters for open fractures are not available.

SP 7 **S82.161-** Torus fracture of upper end of right tibia

SP 7 **S82.162-** Torus fracture of upper end of left tibia

IQ 7 **S82.169-** Torus fracture of upper end of unspecified tibia

6 **S82.19** Other fracture of upper end of tibia

SP 7 **S82.191-** Other fracture of upper end of right tibia

SP 7 **S82.192-** Other fracture of upper end of left tibia

IQ 7 **S82.199-** Other fracture of upper end of unspecified tibia

5 **S82.2** Fracture of shaft of tibia

6 **S82.20** Unspecified fracture of shaft of tibia
Fracture of tibia NOS

SP 7 **S82.201-** Unspecified fracture of shaft of right tibia

SP 7 **S82.202-** Unspecified fracture of shaft of left tibia

IQ 7 **S82.209-** Unspecified fracture of shaft of unspecified tibia

6 **S82.22** Transverse fracture of shaft of tibia

SP 7 **S82.221-** Displaced transverse fracture of shaft of right tibia

SP 7 **S82.222-** Displaced transverse fracture of shaft of left tibia

IQ 7 **S82.223-** Displaced transverse fracture of shaft of unspecified tibia

SP 7 **S82.224-** Nondisplaced transverse fracture of shaft of right tibia

SP 7 **S82.225-** Nondisplaced transverse fracture of shaft of left tibia

IQ 7 **S82.226-** Nondisplaced transverse fracture of shaft of unspecified tibia

6 **S82.23** Oblique fracture of shaft of tibia

SP 7 **S82.231-** Displaced oblique fracture of shaft of right tibia

SP 7 **S82.232-** Displaced oblique fracture of shaft of left tibia

IQ 7 **S82.233-** Displaced oblique fracture of shaft of unspecified tibia

SP 7 **S82.234-** Nondisplaced oblique fracture of shaft of right tibia

SP 7 **S82.235-** Nondisplaced oblique fracture of shaft of left tibia

IQ 7 **S82.236-** Nondisplaced oblique fracture of shaft of unspecified tibia

6 **S82.24** Spiral fracture of shaft of tibia
Toddler fracture

SP 7 **S82.241-** Displaced spiral fracture of shaft of right tibia

SP 7 **S82.242-** Displaced spiral fracture of shaft of left tibia

IQ 7 **S82.243-** Displaced spiral fracture of shaft of unspecified tibia

SP 7 **S82.244-** Nondisplaced spiral fracture of shaft of right tibia

SP 7 **S82.245-** Nondisplaced spiral fracture of shaft of left tibia

IQ 7 **S82.246-** Nondisplaced spiral fracture of shaft of unspecified tibia

6 **S82.25** Comminuted fracture of shaft of tibia

SP 7 **S82.251-** Displaced comminuted fracture of shaft of right tibia

SP 7 **S82.252-** Displaced comminuted fracture of shaft of left tibia

IQ 7 **S82.253-** Displaced comminuted fracture of shaft of unspecified tibia

SP 7 **S82.254-** Nondisplaced comminuted fracture of shaft of right tibia

SP 7 **S82.255-** Nondisplaced comminuted fracture of shaft of left tibia

IQ 7 **S82.256-** Nondisplaced comminuted fracture of shaft of unspecified tibia

6 **S82.26** Segmental fracture of shaft of tibia

SP 7 **S82.261-** Displaced segmental fracture of shaft of right tibia

SP 7 **S82.262-** Displaced segmental fracture of shaft of left tibia

IQ 7 **S82.263-** Displaced segmental fracture of shaft of unspecified tibia

SP 7 **S82.264-** Nondisplaced segmental fracture of shaft of right tibia

SP 7 **S82.265-** Nondisplaced segmental fracture of shaft of left tibia

IQ 7 **S82.266-** Nondisplaced segmental fracture of shaft of unspecified tibia

6 **S82.29** Other fracture of shaft of tibia

SP 7 **S82.291-** Other fracture of shaft of right tibia

SP 7 **S82.292-** Other fracture of shaft of left tibia

IQ 7 **S82.299-** Other fracture of shaft of unspecified tibia

5 **S82.3** Fracture of lower end of tibia

EXCLUDES 1 bimalleolar fracture of lower leg (S82.84-)
fracture of medial malleolus alone (S82.5-)
Maisonneuve's fracture (S82.86-)
pilon fracture of distal tibia (S82.87-)
trimalleolar fractures of lower leg (S82.85-)

★ New ▲ Revised **Px** Primary **SP** PDGM Px **SL** Low CoM **SH** High CoM **IQ** Quest. Encounter **H** Hospice non-cancer Dx   Unspecified   **M** *Manifestation*

DecisionHealth's FY 2020 Complete Home Health ICD-10-CM Diagnosis Coding Manual

1605

Chapter 19

S00-T88

⑥ **S82.30** **Unspecified fracture of lower end of tibia**

⊟ SP ⑦ **S82.301-** **Unspecified fracture of lower end of right tibia**

⊟ SP ⑦ **S82.302-** **Unspecified fracture of lower end of left tibia**

⊟ !Q ⑦ **S82.309-** **Unspecified fracture of lower end of unspecified tibia**

⑥ **S82.31** **Torus fracture of lower end of tibia**

The appropriate 7th character is to be added to all codes in subcategory S82.31

A   initial encounter for closed fracture

D   subsequent encounter for fracture with routine healing

G   subsequent encounter for fracture with delayed healing

K   subsequent encounter for fracture with nonunion

P   subsequent encounter for fracture with malunion

S   sequela

CODING TIPS ✓   Open fractures do not occur with torus fractures and greenstick fractures, therefore the 7th characters for open fractures are not available.

⊟ SP ⑦ **S82.311-** **Torus fracture of lower end of right tibia**

⊟ SP ⑦ **S82.312-** **Torus fracture of lower end of left tibia**

⊟ !Q ⑦ **S82.319-** **Torus fracture of lower end of unspecified tibia**

⑥ **S82.39** **Other fracture of lower end of tibia**

⊟ SP ⑦ **S82.391-** **Other fracture of lower end of right tibia**

⊟ SP ⑦ **S82.392-** **Other fracture of lower end of left tibia**

⊟ !Q ⑦ **S82.399-** **Other fracture of lower end of unspecified tibia**

⑤ **S82.4** **Fracture of shaft of fibula**

EXCLUDES 2   fracture of lateral malleolus alone (S82.6-)

⑥ **S82.40** **Unspecified fracture of shaft of fibula**

⊟ SP ⑦ **S82.401-** **Unspecified fracture of shaft of right fibula**

⊟ SP ⑦ **S82.402-** **Unspecified fracture of shaft of left fibula**

⊟ !Q ⑦ **S82.409-** **Unspecified fracture of shaft of unspecified fibula**

⑥ **S82.42** **Transverse fracture of shaft of fibula**

⊟ SP ⑦ **S82.421-** **Displaced transverse fracture of shaft of right fibula**

⊟ SP ⑦ **S82.422-** **Displaced transverse fracture of shaft of left fibula**

⊟ !Q ⑦ **S82.423-** **Displaced transverse fracture of shaft of unspecified fibula**

⊟ SP ⑦ **S82.424-** **Nondisplaced transverse fracture of shaft of right fibula**

⊟ SP ⑦ **S82.425-** **Nondisplaced transverse fracture of shaft of left fibula**

⊟ !Q ⑦ **S82.426-** **Nondisplaced transverse fracture of shaft of unspecified fibula**

⑥ **S82.43** **Oblique fracture of shaft of fibula**

⊟ SP ⑦ **S82.431-** **Displaced oblique fracture of shaft of right fibula**

⊟ SP ⑦ **S82.432-** **Displaced oblique fracture of shaft of left fibula**

⊟ !Q ⑦ **S82.433-** **Displaced oblique fracture of shaft of unspecified fibula**

⊟ SP ⑦ **S82.434-** **Nondisplaced oblique fracture of shaft of right fibula**

⊟ SP ⑦ **S82.435-** **Nondisplaced oblique fracture of shaft of left fibula**

⊟ !Q ⑦ **S82.436-** **Nondisplaced oblique fracture of shaft of unspecified fibula**

⑥ **S82.44** **Spiral fracture of shaft of fibula**

⊟ SP ⑦ **S82.441-** **Displaced spiral fracture of shaft of right fibula**

⊟ SP !Q ⑦ **S82.442-** **Displaced spiral fracture of shaft of left fibula**

⊟ !Q ⑦ **S82.443-** **Displaced spiral fracture of shaft of unspecified fibula**

⊟ SP ⑦ **S82.444-** **Nondisplaced spiral fracture of shaft of right fibula**

⊟ SP ⑦ **S82.445-** **Nondisplaced spiral fracture of shaft of left fibula**

⊟ SP !Q ⑦ **S82.446-** **Nondisplaced spiral fracture of shaft of unspecified fibula**

⑥ **S82.45** **Comminuted fracture of shaft of fibula**

⊟ SP ⑦ **S82.451-** **Displaced comminuted fracture of shaft of right fibula**

⊟ SP ⑦ **S82.452-** **Displaced comminuted fracture of shaft of left fibula**

⊟ !Q ⑦ **S82.453-** **Displaced comminuted fracture of shaft of unspecified fibula**

⊟ SP ⑦ **S82.454-** **Nondisplaced comminuted fracture of shaft of right fibula**

⊟ SP ⑦ **S82.455-** **Nondisplaced comminuted fracture of shaft of left fibula**

⊟ !Q ⑦ **S82.456-** **Nondisplaced comminuted fracture of shaft of unspecified fibula**

⑥ **S82.46** **Segmental fracture of shaft of fibula**

⊟ SP ⑦ **S82.461-** **Displaced segmental fracture of shaft of right fibula**

⊟ SP ⑦ **S82.462-** **Displaced segmental fracture of shaft of left fibula**

⊟ !Q ⑦ **S82.463-** **Displaced segmental fracture of shaft of unspecified fibula**

⊟ SP ⑦ **S82.464-** **Nondisplaced segmental fracture of shaft of right fibula**

⊟ SP ⑦ **S82.465-** **Nondisplaced segmental fracture of shaft of left fibula**

⊟ !Q ⑦ **S82.466-** **Nondisplaced segmental fracture of shaft of unspecified fibula**

⑥ **S82.49** **Other fracture of shaft of fibula**

⊟ SP ⑦ **S82.491-** **Other fracture of shaft of right fibula**

⊟ SP ⑦ **S82.492-** **Other fracture of shaft of left fibula**

⊟ !Q ⑦ **S82.499-** **Other fracture of shaft of unspecified fibula**

---

④ 4th digit required   ⑤ 5th digit required   ⑥ 6th digit required   ⑦ 7th digit required   ⑦ 7th digit placeholder   ✚ Additional code   ⊟ Laterality

⑤ **S82.5 Fracture of medial malleolus**

> **EXCLUDES 1** pilon fracture of distal tibia
>   (S82.87-)
>   Salter-Harris type III of
>   lower end of tibia
>   (S89.13-)
>   Salter-Harris type IV of
>   lower end of tibia
>   (S89.14-)

▤ **SP** ⑦ **S82.51X-** Displaced fracture of medial malleolus of right tibia

▤ **SP** ⑦ **S82.52X-** Displaced fracture of medial malleolus of left tibia

▤ **IQ** ⑦ **S82.53X-** Displaced fracture of medial malleolus of unspecified tibia

▤ **SP** ⑦ **S82.54X-** Nondisplaced fracture of medial malleolus of right tibia

▤ **SP** ⑦ **S82.55X-** Nondisplaced fracture of medial malleolus of left tibia

▤ **IQ** ⑦ **S82.56X-** Nondisplaced fracture of medial malleolus of unspecified tibia

⑤ **S82.6 Fracture of lateral malleolus**

> **EXCLUDES 1** pilon fracture of distal tibia
>   (S82.87-)

▤ **SP** ⑦ **S82.61X-** Displaced fracture of lateral malleolus of right fibula

▤ **SP** ⑦ **S82.62X-** Displaced fracture of lateral malleolus of left fibula

▤ **IQ** ⑦ **S82.63X-** Displaced fracture of lateral malleolus of unspecified fibula

▤ **SP** ⑦ **S82.64X-** Nondisplaced fracture of lateral malleolus of right fibula

▤ **SP** ⑦ **S82.65X-** Nondisplaced fracture of lateral malleolus of left fibula

▤ **IQ** ⑦ **S82.66X-** Nondisplaced fracture of lateral malleolus of unspecified fibula

⑤ **S82.8 Other fractures of lower leg**

⑥ **S82.81 Torus fracture of upper end of fibula**

> The appropriate 7th character is to be added to all codes in subcategory S82.81
>
> A initial encounter for closed fracture
> D subsequent encounter for fracture with routine healing
> G subsequent encounter for fracture with delayed healing
> K subsequent encounter for fracture with nonunion
> P subsequent encounter for fracture with malunion
> S sequela

CODING TIPS ✓ Open fractures do not occur with torus fractures and greenstick fractures, therefore the 7th characters for open fractures are not available.

▤ **SP** ⑦ **S82.811-** Torus fracture of upper end of right fibula

▤ **SP** ⑦ **S82.812-** Torus fracture of upper end of left fibula

▤ **IQ** ⑦ **S82.819-** Torus fracture of upper end of unspecified fibula

⑥ **S82.82 Torus fracture of lower end of fibula**

> The appropriate 7th character is to be added to all codes in subcategory S82.82
>
> A initial encounter for closed fracture
> D subsequent encounter for fracture with routine healing
> G subsequent encounter for fracture with delayed healing
> K subsequent encounter for fracture with nonunion
> P subsequent encounter for fracture with malunion
> S sequela

CODING TIPS ✓ Open fractures do not occur with torus fractures and greenstick fractures, therefore the 7th characters for open fractures are not available.

▤ **SP** ⑦ **S82.821-** Torus fracture of lower end of right fibula

▤ **SP** ⑦ **S82.822-** Torus fracture of lower end of left fibula

▤ **IQ** ⑦ **S82.829-** Torus fracture of lower end of unspecified fibula

⑥ **S82.83 Other fracture of upper and lower end of fibula**

▤ **SP** ⑦ **S82.831-** Other fracture of upper and lower end of right fibula

▤ **SP** ⑦ **S82.832-** Other fracture of upper and lower end of left fibula

▤ **IQ** ⑦ **S82.839-** Other fracture of upper and lower end of unspecified fibula

⑥ **S82.84 Bimalleolar fracture of lower leg**

▤ **SP** ⑦ **S82.841-** Displaced bimalleolar fracture of right lower leg

▤ **SP** ⑦ **S82.842-** Displaced bimalleolar fracture of left lower leg

▤ **IQ** ⑦ **S82.843-** Displaced bimalleolar fracture of unspecified lower leg

▤ **SP** ⑦ **S82.844-** Nondisplaced bimalleolar fracture of right lower leg

▤ **SP** ⑦ **S82.845-** Nondisplaced bimalleolar fracture of left lower leg

▤ **IQ** ⑦ **S82.846-** Nondisplaced bimalleolar fracture of unspecified lower leg

⑥ **S82.85 Trimalleolar fracture of lower leg**

▤ **SP** ⑦ **S82.851-** Displaced trimalleolar fracture of right lower leg

▤ **SP** ⑦ **S82.852-** Displaced trimalleolar fracture of left lower leg

▤ **IQ** ⑦ **S82.853-** Displaced trimalleolar fracture of unspecified lower leg

▤ **SP** ⑦ **S82.854-** Nondisplaced trimalleolar fracture of right lower leg

▤ **SP** ⑦ **S82.855-** Nondisplaced trimalleolar fracture of left lower leg

▤ **IQ** ⑦ **S82.856-** Nondisplaced trimalleolar fracture of unspecified lower leg

⑥ **S82.86 Maisonneuve's fracture**

▤ **SP** ⑦ **S82.861-** Displaced Maisonneuve's fracture of right leg

▤ **SP** ⑦ **S82.862-** Displaced Maisonneuve's fracture of left leg

Chapter 19

S00-T88

★ New ▲ Revised **Px** Primary **SP** PDGM Px **SL** Low CoM **SH** High CoM **IQ** Quest. Encounter Ⓗ Hospice non-cancer Dx Unspecified **M** *Manifestation*

🔲 **IQ** 7 **S82.863-** **Displaced Maisonneuve's fracture of unspecified leg**

🔲 **SP** 7 **S82.864-** **Nondisplaced Maisonneuve's fracture of right leg**

🔲 **SP** 7 **S82.865-** **Nondisplaced Maisonneuve's fracture of left leg**

🔲 **IQ** 7 **S82.866-** **Nondisplaced Maisonneuve's fracture of unspecified leg**

⑥ **S82.87** **Pilon fracture of tibia**

🔲 **SP** 7 **S82.871-** **Displaced pilon fracture of right tibia**

🔲 **SP** 7 **S82.872-** **Displaced pilon fracture of left tibia**

🔲 **IQ** 7 **S82.873-** **Displaced pilon fracture of unspecified tibia**

🔲 **SP** 7 **S82.874-** **Nondisplaced pilon fracture of right tibia**

🔲 **SP** 7 **S82.875-** **Nondisplaced pilon fracture of left tibia**

🔲 **IQ** 7 **S82.876-** **Nondisplaced pilon fracture of unspecified tibia**

⑥ **S82.89** **Other fractures of lower leg**
Fracture of ankle NOS

🔲 **SP** 7 **S82.891-** **Other fracture of right lower leg**

🔲 **SP** 7 **S82.892-** **Other fracture of left lower leg**

🔲 **IQ** 7 **S82.899-** **Other fracture of unspecified lower leg**

⑤ **S82.9** **Unspecified fracture of lower leg**

🔲 **IQ** ☑ **S82.90X-** **Unspecified fracture of unspecified lower leg**

🔲 **SP** ☑ **S82.91X-** **Unspecified fracture of right lower leg**

🔲 **SP** ☑ **S82.92X-** **Unspecified fracture of left lower leg**

④ **S83** **Dislocation and sprain of joints and ligaments of knee**

> **INCLUDES** avulsion of joint or ligament of knee
> laceration of cartilage, joint or ligament of knee
> sprain of cartilage, joint or ligament of knee
> traumatic hemarthrosis of joint or ligament of knee
> traumatic rupture of joint or ligament of knee
> traumatic subluxation of joint or ligament of knee
> traumatic tear of joint or ligament of knee

Code also:
any associated open wound
> **EXCLUDES 1** derangement of patella (M22.0-M22.3)
> injury of patellar ligament (tendon) (S76.1-)
> internal derangement of knee (M23.-)
> old dislocation of knee (M24.36)
> pathological dislocation of knee (M24.36)
> recurrent dislocation of knee (M22.0)
> **EXCLUDES 2** strain of muscle, fascia and tendon of lower leg (S86.-)

The appropriate 7th character is to be added to each code from category S83
A   initial encounter
D   subsequent encounter
S   sequela

⑤ **S83.0** **Subluxation and dislocation of patella**

⑥ **S83.00** **Unspecified subluxation and dislocation of patella**

🔲 **IQ** 7 **S83.001-** **Unspecified subluxation of right patella**

🔲 **IQ** 7 **S83.002-** **Unspecified subluxation of left patella**

🔲 **IQ** 7 **S83.003-** **Unspecified subluxation of unspecified patella**

🔲 **IQ** 7 **S83.004-** **Unspecified dislocation of right patella**

🔲 **IQ** 7 **S83.005-** **Unspecified dislocation of left patella**

🔲 **IQ** 7 **S83.006-** **Unspecified dislocation of unspecified patella**

⑥ **S83.01** **Lateral subluxation and dislocation of patella**

🔲 **SP** 7 **S83.011-** **Lateral subluxation of right patella**

🔲 **SP** 7 **S83.012-** Lateral subluxation of left patella

🔲 **IQ** 7 **S83.013-** **Lateral subluxation of unspecified patella**

🔲 **SP** 7 **S83.014-** **Lateral dislocation of right patella**

🔲 **SP** 7 **S83.015-** Lateral dislocation of left patella

🔲 **IQ** 7 **S83.016-** **Lateral dislocation of unspecified patella**

⑥ **S83.09** **Other subluxation and dislocation of patella**

🔲 **SP** 7 **S83.091-** **Other subluxation of right patella**

🔲 **SP** 7 **S83.092-** Other subluxation of left patella

🔲 **IQ** 7 **S83.093-** **Other subluxation of unspecified patella**

🔲 **SP** 7 **S83.094-** Other dislocation of right patella

🔲 **SP** 7 **S83.095-** Other dislocation of left patella

🔲 **IQ** 7 **S83.096-** **Other dislocation of unspecified patella**

⑤ **S83.1** **Subluxation and dislocation of knee**
> **EXCLUDES 2** instability of knee prosthesis (T84.022, T84.023)

⑥ **S83.10** **Unspecified subluxation and dislocation of knee**

🔲 **IQ** 7 **S83.101-** **Unspecified subluxation of right knee**

🔲 **IQ** 7 **S83.102-** **Unspecified subluxation of left knee**

🔲 **IQ** 7 **S83.103-** **Unspecified subluxation of unspecified knee**

🔲 **IQ** 7 **S83.104-** **Unspecified dislocation of right knee**

🔲 **IQ** 7 **S83.105-** **Unspecified dislocation of left knee**

🔲 **IQ** 7 **S83.106-** **Unspecified dislocation of unspecified knee**

⑥ **S83.11** **Anterior subluxation and dislocation of proximal end of tibia**

---

④ 4th digit required   ⑤ 5th digit required   ⑥ 6th digit required   ⑦ 7th digit required   ☑ 7th digit placeholder   ✚ Additional code   🔲 Laterality

1608   *DecisionHealth's* FY 2020 Complete Home Health ICD-10-CM Diagnosis Coding Manual

Posterior subluxation and dislocation of distal end of femur

☐ **SP** 7 S83.111- Anterior subluxation of proximal end of tibia, right knee

☐ **SP** 7 S83.112- Anterior subluxation of proximal end of tibia, left knee

☐ **IQ** 7 S83.113- Anterior subluxation of proximal end of tibia, unspecified knee

☐ **SP** 7 S83.114- Anterior dislocation of proximal end of tibia, right knee

☐ **SP** 7 S83.115- Anterior dislocation of proximal end of tibia, left knee

☐ **IQ** 7 S83.116- Anterior dislocation of proximal end of tibia, unspecified knee

6 S83.12 Posterior subluxation and dislocation of proximal end of tibia
Anterior dislocation of distal end of femur

☐ **SP** 7 S83.121- Posterior subluxation of proximal end of tibia, right knee

☐ **SP** 7 S83.122- Posterior subluxation of proximal end of tibia, left knee

☐ **IQ** 7 S83.123- Posterior subluxation of proximal end of tibia, unspecified knee

☐ **SP** 7 S83.124- Posterior dislocation of proximal end of tibia, right knee

☐ **SP** 7 S83.125- Posterior dislocation of proximal end of tibia, left knee

☐ **IQ** 7 S83.126- Posterior dislocation of proximal end of tibia, unspecified knee

6 S83.13 Medial subluxation and dislocation of proximal end of tibia

☐ **SP** 7 S83.131- Medial subluxation of proximal end of tibia, right knee

☐ **SP** 7 S83.132- Medial subluxation of proximal end of tibia, left knee

☐ **IQ** 7 S83.133- Medial subluxation of proximal end of tibia, unspecified knee

☐ **SP** 7 S83.134- Medial dislocation of proximal end of tibia, right knee

☐ **SP** 7 S83.135- Medial dislocation of proximal end of tibia, left knee

☐ **IQ** 7 S83.136- Medial dislocation of proximal end of tibia, unspecified knee

6 S83.14 Lateral subluxation and dislocation of proximal end of tibia

☐ **SP** 7 S83.141- Lateral subluxation of proximal end of tibia, right knee

☐ **SP** 7 S83.142- Lateral subluxation of proximal end of tibia, left knee

☐ **IQ** 7 S83.143- Lateral subluxation of proximal end of tibia, unspecified knee

☐ **SP** 7 S83.144- Lateral dislocation of proximal end of tibia, right knee

☐ **SP** 7 S83.145- Lateral dislocation of proximal end of tibia, left knee

☐ **IQ** 7 S83.146- Lateral dislocation of proximal end of tibia, unspecified knee

6 S83.19 Other subluxation and dislocation of knee

☐ **SP** 7 S83.191- Other subluxation of right knee

☐ **SP** 7 S83.192- Other subluxation of left knee

☐ **IQ** 7 S83.193- Other subluxation of unspecified knee

☐ **SP** 7 S83.194- Other dislocation of right knee

☐ **SP** 7 S83.195- Other dislocation of left knee

☐ **IQ** 7 S83.196- Other dislocation of unspecified knee

5 S83.2 Tear of meniscus, current injury
EXCLUDES 1 old bucket-handle tear (M23.2)

6 S83.20 Tear of unspecified meniscus, current injury
Tear of meniscus of knee NOS

☐ **SP** 7 S83.200- Bucket-handle tear of unspecified meniscus, current injury, right knee

☐ **SP** 7 S83.201- Bucket-handle tear of unspecified meniscus, current injury, left knee

☐ **IQ** 7 S83.202- Bucket-handle tear of unspecified meniscus, current injury, unspecified knee

☐ **SP** 7 S83.203- Other tear of unspecified meniscus, current injury, right knee

☐ **SP** 7 S83.204- Other tear of unspecified meniscus, current injury, left knee

☐ **IQ** 7 S83.205- Other tear of unspecified meniscus, current injury, unspecified knee

☐ **SP** 7 S83.206- Unspecified tear of unspecified meniscus, current injury, right knee

☐ **SP** 7 S83.207- Unspecified tear of unspecified meniscus, current injury, left knee

☐ **IQ** 7 S83.209- Unspecified tear of unspecified meniscus, current injury, unspecified knee

6 S83.21 Bucket-handle tear of medial meniscus, current injury

☐ **SP** 7 S83.211- Bucket-handle tear of medial meniscus, current injury, right knee

☐ **SP** 7 S83.212- Bucket-handle tear of medial meniscus, current injury, left knee

☐ **IQ** 7 S83.219- Bucket-handle tear of medial meniscus, current injury, unspecified knee

6 S83.22 Peripheral tear of medial meniscus, current injury

☐ **SP** 7 S83.221- Peripheral tear of medial meniscus, current injury, right knee

☐ **SP** 7 S83.222- Peripheral tear of medial meniscus, current injury, left knee

☐ **IQ** 7 S83.229- Peripheral tear of medial meniscus, current injury, unspecified knee

6 S83.23 Complex tear of medial meniscus, current injury

☐ **SP** 7 S83.231- Complex tear of medial meniscus, current injury, right knee

★ New ▲ Revised Px Primary **SP** PDGM Px **SL** Low CoM **SH** High CoM **IQ** Quest. Encounter ⊞ Hospice non-cancer Dx Unspecified **M** *Manifestation*

DecisionHealth's FY 2020 Complete Home Health ICD-10-CM Diagnosis Coding Manual

1609

Chapter 19

S00-T88

☐ **SP** ☐7 **S83.232-** **Complex tear of medial meniscus, current injury, left knee**

☐ **IQ** ☐7 **S83.239-** **Complex tear of medial meniscus, current injury, unspecified knee**

☐6 **S83.24** **Other tear of medial meniscus, current injury**

☐ **SP** ☐7 **S83.241-** **Other tear of medial meniscus, current injury, right knee**

☐ **SP** ☐7 **S83.242-** **Other tear of medial meniscus, current injury, left knee**

☐ **IQ** ☐7 **S83.249-** **Other tear of medial meniscus, current injury, unspecified knee**

☐6 **S83.25** **Bucket-handle tear of lateral meniscus, current injury**

☐ **SP** ☐7 **S83.251-** **Bucket-handle tear of lateral meniscus, current injury, right knee**

☐ **SP** ☐7 **S83.252-** **Bucket-handle tear of lateral meniscus, current injury, left knee**

☐ **IQ** ☐7 **S83.259-** **Bucket-handle tear of lateral meniscus, current injury, unspecified knee**

☐6 **S83.26** **Peripheral tear of lateral meniscus, current injury**

☐ **SP** ☐7 **S83.261-** **Peripheral tear of lateral meniscus, current injury, right knee**

☐ **SP** ☐7 **S83.262-** **Peripheral tear of lateral meniscus, current injury, left knee**

☐ **IQ** ☐7 **S83.269-** **Peripheral tear of lateral meniscus, current injury, unspecified knee**

☐6 **S83.27** **Complex tear of lateral meniscus, current injury**

☐ **SP** ☐7 **S83.271-** **Complex tear of lateral meniscus, current injury, right knee**

☐ **SP** ☐7 **S83.272-** **Complex tear of lateral meniscus, current injury, left knee**

☐ **IQ** ☐7 **S83.279-** **Complex tear of lateral meniscus, current injury, unspecified knee**

☐6 **S83.28** **Other tear of lateral meniscus, current injury**

☐ **SP** ☐7 **S83.281-** **Other tear of lateral meniscus, current injury, right knee**

☐ **SP** ☐7 **S83.282-** **Other tear of lateral meniscus, current injury, left knee**

☐ **IQ** ☐7 **S83.289-** **Other tear of lateral meniscus, current injury, unspecified knee**

☐5 **S83.3** **Tear of articular cartilage of knee, current**

☐ **IQ** ☐7 **S83.30X-** **Tear of articular cartilage of unspecified knee, current**

☐ **SP** ☐7 **S83.31X-** **Tear of articular cartilage of right knee, current**

☐ **SP** ☐7 **S83.32X-** **Tear of articular cartilage of left knee, current**

☐5 **S83.4** **Sprain of collateral ligament of knee**

☐6 **S83.40** **Sprain of unspecified collateral ligament of knee**

☐ **SP** ☐7 **S83.401-** **Sprain of unspecified collateral ligament of right knee**

☐ **SP** ☐7 **S83.402-** **Sprain of unspecified collateral ligament of left knee**

☐ **IQ** ☐7 **S83.409-** **Sprain of unspecified collateral ligament of unspecified knee**

☐6 **S83.41** **Sprain of medial collateral ligament of knee**
Sprain of tibial collateral ligament

☐ **SP** ☐7 **S83.411-** **Sprain of medial collateral ligament of right knee**

☐ **SP** ☐7 **S83.412-** **Sprain of medial collateral ligament of left knee**

☐ **IQ** ☐7 **S83.419-** **Sprain of medial collateral ligament of unspecified knee**

☐6 **S83.42** **Sprain of lateral collateral ligament of knee**
Sprain of fibular collateral ligament

☐ **SP** ☐7 **S83.421-** **Sprain of lateral collateral ligament of right knee**

☐ **SP** ☐7 **S83.422-** **Sprain of lateral collateral ligament of left knee**

☐ **IQ** ☐7 **S83.429-** **Sprain of lateral collateral ligament of unspecified knee**

☐5 **S83.5** **Sprain of cruciate ligament of knee**

☐6 **S83.50** **Sprain of unspecified cruciate ligament of knee**

☐ **SP** ☐7 **S83.501-** **Sprain of unspecified cruciate ligament of right knee**

☐ **SP** ☐7 **S83.502-** **Sprain of unspecified cruciate ligament of left knee**

☐ **IQ** ☐7 **S83.509-** **Sprain of unspecified cruciate ligament of unspecified knee**

☐6 **S83.51** **Sprain of anterior cruciate ligament of knee**

☐ **SP** ☐7 **S83.511-** **Sprain of anterior cruciate ligament of right knee**

☐ **SP** ☐7 **S83.512-** **Sprain of anterior cruciate ligament of left knee**

☐ **IQ** ☐7 **S83.519-** **Sprain of anterior cruciate ligament of unspecified knee**

☐6 **S83.52** **Sprain of posterior cruciate ligament of knee**

☐ **SP** ☐7 **S83.521-** **Sprain of posterior cruciate ligament of right knee**

☐ **SP** ☐7 **S83.522-** **Sprain of posterior cruciate ligament of left knee**

☐ **IQ** ☐7 **S83.529-** **Sprain of posterior cruciate ligament of unspecified knee**

☐5 **S83.6** **Sprain of the superior tibiofibular joint and ligament**

☐ **IQ** ☐7 **S83.60X-** **Sprain of the superior tibiofibular joint and ligament, unspecified knee**

☐ **SP** ☐7 **S83.61X-** **Sprain of the superior tibiofibular joint and ligament, right knee**

☐ **SP** ☐7 **S83.62X-** **Sprain of the superior tibiofibular joint and ligament, left knee**

☐5 **S83.8** **Sprain of other specified parts of knee**

☐6 **S83.8X** **Sprain of other specified parts of knee**

☐ **SP** ☐7 **S83.8X1-** **Sprain of other specified parts of right knee**

☐ **SP** ☐7 **S83.8X2-** **Sprain of other specified parts of left knee**

☐4 4th digit required　☐5 5th digit required　☐6 6th digit required　☐7 7th digit required　☐7 7th digit placeholder　✚ Additional code　☐ Laterality

1610　　　*DecisionHealth's* FY 2020 Complete Home Health ICD-10-CM Diagnosis Coding Manual

☰ **IQ** 7 **S83.8X9-** | **Sprain of other specified parts of unspecified knee**

5 **S83.9** **Sprain of unspecified site of knee**

☰ **IQ** 🗗 **S83.90X-** | **Sprain of unspecified site of unspecified knee**

☰ **SP** 🗗 **S83.91X-** | **Sprain of unspecified site of right knee**

☰ **SP** 🗗 **S83.92X-** | **Sprain of unspecified site of left knee**

4 **S84** **Injury of nerves at lower leg level**
Code also:
any associated open wound (S81.-)
EXCLUDES 2 injury of nerves at ankle and foot level (S94.-)

The appropriate 7th character is to be added to each code from category S84
A   initial encounter
D   subsequent encounter
S   sequela

5 **S84.0** **Injury of tibial nerve at lower leg level**

☰ **IQ** 🗗 **S84.00X-** | **Injury of tibial nerve at lower leg level, unspecified leg**

☰ **SP** 🗗 **S84.01X-** Injury of tibial nerve at lower leg level, right leg

☰ **SP** 🗗 **S84.02X-** Injury of tibial nerve at lower leg level, left leg

5 **S84.1** **Injury of peroneal nerve at lower leg level**

☰ **IQ** 🗗 **S84.10X-** | **Injury of peroneal nerve at lower leg level, unspecified leg**

☰ **SP** 🗗 **S84.11X-** Injury of peroneal nerve at lower leg level, right leg

☰ **SP** 🗗 **S84.12X-** Injury of peroneal nerve at lower leg level, left leg

5 **S84.2** **Injury of cutaneous sensory nerve at lower leg level**

☰ **IQ** 🗗 **S84.20X-** | **Injury of cutaneous sensory nerve at lower leg level, unspecified leg**

☰ **SP** 🗗 **S84.21X-** Injury of cutaneous sensory nerve at lower leg level, right leg

☰ **SP** 🗗 **S84.22X-** Injury of cutaneous sensory nerve at lower leg level, left leg

5 **S84.8** **Injury of other nerves at lower leg level**

6 **S84.80** **Injury of other nerves at lower leg level**

☰ **SP** 7 **S84.801-** Injury of other nerves at lower leg level, right leg

☰ **SP** 7 **S84.802-** Injury of other nerves at lower leg level, left leg

☰ **SP** 7 **S84.809-** | **Injury of other nerves at lower leg level, unspecified leg**

5 **S84.9** | **Injury of unspecified nerve at lower leg level**

☰ **IQ** 🗗 **S84.90X-** | **Injury of unspecified nerve at lower leg level, unspecified leg**

☰ **IQ** 🗗 **S84.91X-** | **Injury of unspecified nerve at lower leg level, right leg**

☰ **IQ** 🗗 **S84.92X-** | **Injury of unspecified nerve at lower leg level, left leg**

4 **S85** **Injury of blood vessels at lower leg level**
Code also:
any associated open wound (S81.-)
EXCLUDES 2 injury of blood vessels at ankle and foot level (S95.-)

The appropriate 7th character is to be added to each code from category S85
A   initial encounter
D   subsequent encounter
S   sequela

5 **S85.0** **Injury of popliteal artery**

6 **S85.00** | **Unspecified injury of popliteal artery**

☰ **IQ** 7 **S85.001-** | **Unspecified injury of popliteal artery, right leg**

☰ **IQ** 7 **S85.002-** | **Unspecified injury of popliteal artery, left leg**

☰ **IQ** 7 **S85.009-** | **Unspecified injury of popliteal artery, unspecified leg**

6 **S85.01** **Laceration of popliteal artery**

☰ **SP** 7 **S85.011-** Laceration of popliteal artery, right leg

☰ **SP** 7 **S85.012-** Laceration of popliteal artery, left leg

☰ **IQ** 7 **S85.019-** | **Laceration of popliteal artery, unspecified leg**

6 **S85.09** **Other specified injury of popliteal artery**

☰ **SP** 7 **S85.091-** Other specified injury of popliteal artery, right leg

☰ **SP** 7 **S85.092-** Other specified injury of popliteal artery, left leg

☰ **IQ** 7 **S85.099-** | **Other specified injury of popliteal artery, unspecified leg**

5 **S85.1** **Injury of tibial artery**

6 **S85.10** | **Unspecified injury of unspecified tibial artery**
Injury of tibial artery NOS

☰ **IQ** 7 **S85.101-** | **Unspecified injury of unspecified tibial artery, right leg**

☰ **IQ** 7 **S85.102-** | **Unspecified injury of unspecified tibial artery, left leg**

☰ **IQ** 7 **S85.109-** | **Unspecified injury of unspecified tibial artery, unspecified leg**

6 **S85.11** | **Laceration of unspecified tibial artery**

☰ **SP** 7 **S85.111-** | **Laceration of unspecified tibial artery, right leg**

☰ **SP** 7 **S85.112-** | **Laceration of unspecified tibial artery, left leg**

☰ **IQ** 7 **S85.119-** | **Laceration of unspecified tibial artery, unspecified leg**

6 **S85.12** | **Other specified injury of unspecified tibial artery**

☰ **SP** 7 **S85.121-** | **Other specified injury of unspecified tibial artery, right leg**

☰ **SP** 7 **S85.122-** | **Other specified injury of unspecified tibial artery, left leg**

☰ **IQ** 7 **S85.129-** | **Other specified injury of unspecified tibial artery, unspecified leg**

6 **S85.13** | **Unspecified injury of anterior tibial artery**

☰ **IQ** 7 **S85.131-** | **Unspecified injury of anterior tibial artery, right leg**

Chapter 19

S00-T88

★ New ▲ Revised Px Primary **SP** PDGM Px **SL** Low CoM **SH** High CoM **IQ** Quest. Encounter 🅷 Hospice non-cancer Dx Unspecified M *Manifestation*

DecisionHealth's FY 2020 Complete Home Health ICD-10-CM Diagnosis Coding Manual

1611

Chapter 19

S00-T88

▣ 🔳 7 **S85.132-** Unspecified injury of anterior tibial artery, left leg

▣ 🆂🅿 🔳 7 **S85.139-** Unspecified injury of anterior tibial artery, unspecified leg

6 **S85.14** Laceration of anterior tibial artery

▣ 🆂🅿 7 **S85.141-** Laceration of anterior tibial artery, right leg

▣ 🆂🅿 7 **S85.142-** Laceration of anterior tibial artery, left leg

▣ 🔳 7 **S85.149-** Laceration of anterior tibial artery, unspecified leg

6 **S85.15** Other specified injury of anterior tibial artery

▣ 🆂🅿 7 **S85.151-** Other specified injury of anterior tibial artery, right leg

▣ 🆂🅿 7 **S85.152-** Other specified injury of anterior tibial artery, left leg

▣ 🔳 7 **S85.159-** Other specified injury of anterior tibial artery, unspecified leg

6 **S85.16** Unspecified injury of posterior tibial artery

▣ 🔳 7 **S85.161-** Unspecified injury of posterior tibial artery, right leg

▣ 🔳 7 **S85.162-** Unspecified injury of posterior tibial artery, left leg

▣ 🔳 7 **S85.169-** Unspecified injury of posterior tibial artery, unspecified leg

6 **S85.17** Laceration of posterior tibial artery

▣ 🆂🅿 7 **S85.171-** Laceration of posterior tibial artery, right leg

▣ 🆂🅿 7 **S85.172-** Laceration of posterior tibial artery, left leg

▣ 🔳 7 **S85.179-** Laceration of posterior tibial artery, unspecified leg

6 **S85.18** Other specified injury of posterior tibial artery

▣ 🆂🅿 7 **S85.181-** Other specified injury of posterior tibial artery, right leg

▣ 🆂🅿 7 **S85.182-** Other specified injury of posterior tibial artery, left leg

▣ 🔳 7 **S85.189-** Other specified injury of posterior tibial artery, unspecified leg

5 **S85.2** Injury of peroneal artery

6 **S85.20** Unspecified injury of peroneal artery

▣ 🔳 7 **S85.201-** Unspecified injury of peroneal artery, right leg

▣ 🔳 7 **S85.202-** Unspecified injury of peroneal artery, left leg

▣ 🔳 7 **S85.209-** Unspecified injury of peroneal artery, unspecified leg

6 **S85.21** Laceration of peroneal artery

▣ 🆂🅿 7 **S85.211-** Laceration of peroneal artery, right leg

▣ 🆂🅿 7 **S85.212-** Laceration of peroneal artery, left leg

▣ 🔳 7 **S85.219-** Laceration of peroneal artery, unspecified leg

6 **S85.29** Other specified injury of peroneal artery

▣ 🆂🅿 7 **S85.291-** Other specified injury of peroneal artery, right leg

▣ 🆂🅿 7 **S85.292-** Other specified injury of peroneal artery, left leg

▣ 🔳 7 **S85.299-** Other specified injury of peroneal artery, unspecified leg

5 **S85.3** Injury of greater saphenous vein at lower leg level
Injury of greater saphenous vein NOS
Injury of saphenous vein NOS

6 **S85.30** Unspecified injury of greater saphenous vein at lower leg level

▣ 🔳 7 **S85.301-** Unspecified injury of greater saphenous vein at lower leg level, right leg

▣ 🔳 7 **S85.302-** Unspecified injury of greater saphenous vein at lower leg level, left leg

▣ 🔳 7 **S85.309-** Unspecified injury of greater saphenous vein at lower leg level, unspecified leg

6 **S85.31** Laceration of greater saphenous vein at lower leg level

▣ 🆂🅿 7 **S85.311-** Laceration of greater saphenous vein at lower leg level, right leg

▣ 🆂🅿 7 **S85.312-** Laceration of greater saphenous vein at lower leg level, left leg

▣ 🔳 7 **S85.319-** Laceration of greater saphenous vein at lower leg level, unspecified leg

6 **S85.39** Other specified injury of greater saphenous vein at lower leg level

▣ 🆂🅿 7 **S85.391-** Other specified injury of greater saphenous vein at lower leg level, right leg

▣ 🆂🅿 7 **S85.392-** Other specified injury of greater saphenous vein at lower leg level, left leg

▣ 🔳 7 **S85.399-** Other specified injury of greater saphenous vein at lower leg level, unspecified leg

5 **S85.4** Injury of lesser saphenous vein at lower leg level

6 **S85.40** Unspecified injury of lesser saphenous vein at lower leg level

▣ 🔳 7 **S85.401-** Unspecified injury of lesser saphenous vein at lower leg level, right leg

▣ 🔳 7 **S85.402-** Unspecified injury of lesser saphenous vein at lower leg level, left leg

▣ 🔳 7 **S85.409-** Unspecified injury of lesser saphenous vein at lower leg level, unspecified leg

6 **S85.41** Laceration of lesser saphenous vein at lower leg level

▣ 🆂🅿 7 **S85.411-** Laceration of lesser saphenous vein at lower leg level, right leg

▣ 🆂🅿 7 **S85.412-** Laceration of lesser saphenous vein at lower leg level, left leg

▣ 🔳 7 **S85.419-** Laceration of lesser saphenous vein at lower leg level, unspecified leg

6 **S85.49** Other specified injury of lesser saphenous vein at lower leg level

▣ 🆂🅿 7 **S85.491-** Other specified injury of lesser saphenous vein at lower leg level, right leg

---

4 4th digit required   5 5th digit required   6 6th digit required   7 7th digit required   7 7th digit placeholder   ✛ Additional code   ▣ Laterality

⊟ **SP** **7** **S85.492-** Other specified injury of lesser saphenous vein at lower leg level, left leg

⊟ **IQ** **7** **S85.499-** Other specified injury of lesser saphenous vein at lower leg level, unspecified leg

5 **S85.5** Injury of popliteal vein

  6 **S85.50** Unspecified injury of popliteal vein

⊟ **IQ** **7** **S85.501-** Unspecified injury of popliteal vein, right leg

⊟ **IQ** **7** **S85.502-** Unspecified injury of popliteal vein, left leg

⊟ **IQ** **7** **S85.509-** Unspecified injury of popliteal vein, unspecified leg

  6 **S85.51** Laceration of popliteal vein

⊟ **SP** **7** **S85.511-** Laceration of popliteal vein, right leg

⊟ **SP** **7** **S85.512-** Laceration of popliteal vein, left leg

⊟ **SP** **IQ** **7** **S85.519-** Laceration of popliteal vein, unspecified leg

  6 **S85.59** Other specified injury of popliteal vein

⊟ **SP** **7** **S85.591-** Other specified injury of popliteal vein, right leg

⊟ **SP** **7** **S85.592-** Other specified injury of popliteal vein, left leg

⊟ **IQ** **7** **S85.599-** Other specified injury of popliteal vein, unspecified leg

5 **S85.8** Injury of other blood vessels at lower leg level

  6 **S85.80** Unspecified injury of other blood vessels at lower leg level

⊟ **IQ** **7** **S85.801-** Unspecified injury of other blood vessels at lower leg level, right leg

⊟ **IQ** **7** **S85.802-** Unspecified injury of other blood vessels at lower leg level, left leg

⊟ **IQ** **7** **S85.809-** Unspecified injury of other blood vessels at lower leg level, unspecified leg

  6 **S85.81** Laceration of other blood vessels at lower leg level

⊟ **SP** **7** **S85.811-** Laceration of other blood vessels at lower leg level, right leg

⊟ **SP** **7** **S85.812-** Laceration of other blood vessels at lower leg level, left leg

⊟ **IQ** **7** **S85.819-** Laceration of other blood vessels at lower leg level, unspecified leg

  6 **S85.89** Other specified injury of other blood vessels at lower leg level

⊟ **SP** **7** **S85.891-** Other specified injury of other blood vessels at lower leg level, right leg

⊟ **SP** **7** **S85.892-** Other specified injury of other blood vessels at lower leg level, left leg

⊟ **IQ** **7** **S85.899-** Other specified injury of other blood vessels at lower leg level, unspecified leg

5 **S85.9** Injury of unspecified blood vessel at lower leg level

  6 **S85.90** Unspecified injury of unspecified blood vessel at lower leg level

⊟ **IQ** **7** **S85.901-** Unspecified injury of unspecified blood vessel at lower leg level, right leg

⊟ **IQ** **7** **S85.902-** Unspecified injury of unspecified blood vessel at lower leg level, left leg

⊟ **IQ** **7** **S85.909-** Unspecified injury of unspecified blood vessel at lower leg level, unspecified leg

  6 **S85.91** Laceration of unspecified blood vessel at lower leg level

⊟ **SP** **7** **S85.911-** Laceration of unspecified blood vessel at lower leg level, right leg

⊟ **SP** **7** **S85.912-** Laceration of unspecified blood vessel at lower leg level, left leg

⊟ **IQ** **7** **S85.919-** Laceration of unspecified blood vessel at lower leg level, unspecified leg

  6 **S85.99** Other specified injury of unspecified blood vessel at lower leg level

⊟ **IQ** **7** **S85.991-** Other specified injury of unspecified blood vessel at lower leg level, right leg

⊟ **IQ** **7** **S85.992-** Other specified injury of unspecified blood vessel at lower leg level, left leg

⊟ **IQ** **7** **S85.999-** Other specified injury of unspecified blood vessel at lower leg level, unspecified leg

4 **S86** Injury of muscle, fascia and tendon at lower leg level

Code also:
  any associated open wound (S81.-)

EXCLUDES 2 injury of muscle, fascia and tendon at ankle (S96.-)
  injury of patellar ligament (tendon) (S76.1-)
  sprain of joints and ligaments of knee (S83.-)

The appropriate 7th character is to be added to each code from category S86
A   initial encounter
D   subsequent encounter
S   sequela

5 **S86.0** Injury of Achilles tendon

  6 **S86.00** Unspecified injury of Achilles tendon

⊟ **IQ** **7** **S86.001-** Unspecified injury of right Achilles tendon

⊟ **IQ** **7** **S86.002-** Unspecified injury of left Achilles tendon

⊟ **IQ** **7** **S86.009-** Unspecified injury of unspecified Achilles tendon

  6 **S86.01** Strain of Achilles tendon

⊟ **SP** **7** **S86.011-** Strain of right Achilles tendon

⊟ **SP** **7** **S86.012-** Strain of left Achilles tendon

⊟ **IQ** **7** **S86.019-** Strain of unspecified Achilles tendon

  6 **S86.02** Laceration of Achilles tendon

★ New ▲ Revised Px Primary **SP** PDGM Px **SL** Low CoM **SH** High CoM **IQ** Quest. Encounter **H** Hospice non-cancer Dx Unspecified **M** *Manifestation*

DecisionHealth's FY 2020 Complete Home Health ICD-10-CM Diagnosis Coding Manual

1613

☰ **SP** 7 **S86.021-** Laceration of right Achilles tendon

☰ **SP** 7 **S86.022-** Laceration of left Achilles tendon

☰ **IQ** 7 **S86.029-** Laceration of unspecified Achilles tendon

6 **S86.09** Other specified injury of Achilles tendon

☰ **SP** 7 **S86.091-** Other specified injury of right Achilles tendon

☰ **SP** 7 **S86.092-** Other specified injury of left Achilles tendon

☰ **IQ** 7 **S86.099-** Other specified injury of unspecified Achilles tendon

5 **S86.1** Injury of other muscle(s) and tendon(s) of posterior muscle group at lower leg level

6 **S86.10** Unspecified injury of other muscle(s) and tendon(s) of posterior muscle group at lower leg level

☰ **IQ** 7 **S86.101-** Unspecified injury of other muscle(s) and tendon(s) of posterior muscle group at lower leg level, right leg

☰ **IQ** 7 **S86.102-** Unspecified injury of other muscle(s) and tendon(s) of posterior muscle group at lower leg level, left leg

☰ **IQ** 7 **S86.109-** Unspecified injury of other muscle(s) and tendon(s) of posterior muscle group at lower leg level, unspecified leg

6 **S86.11** Strain of other muscle(s) and tendon(s) of posterior muscle group at lower leg level

☰ **SP** 7 **S86.111-** Strain of other muscle(s) and tendon(s) of posterior muscle group at lower leg level, right leg

☰ **SP** 7 **S86.112-** Strain of other muscle(s) and tendon(s) of posterior muscle group at lower leg level, left leg

☰ **IQ** 7 **S86.119-** Strain of other muscle(s) and tendon(s) of posterior muscle group at lower leg level, unspecified leg

6 **S86.12** Laceration of other muscle(s) and tendon(s) of posterior muscle group at lower leg level

☰ **SP** 7 **S86.121-** Laceration of other muscle(s) and tendon(s) of posterior muscle group at lower leg level, right leg

☰ **SP** 7 **S86.122-** Laceration of other muscle(s) and tendon(s) of posterior muscle group at lower leg level, left leg

☰ **IQ** 7 **S86.129-** Laceration of other muscle(s) and tendon(s) of posterior muscle group at lower leg level, unspecified leg

6 **S86.19** Other injury of other muscle(s) and tendon(s) of posterior muscle group at lower leg level

☰ **SP** 7 **S86.191-** Other injury of other muscle(s) and tendon(s) of posterior muscle group at lower leg level, right leg

☰ **SP** 7 **S86.192-** Other injury of other muscle(s) and tendon(s) of posterior muscle group at lower leg level, left leg

☰ **IQ** 7 **S86.199-** Other injury of other muscle(s) and tendon(s) of posterior muscle group at lower leg level, unspecified leg

5 **S86.2** Injury of muscle(s) and tendon(s) of anterior muscle group at lower leg level

6 **S86.20** Unspecified injury of muscle(s) and tendon(s) of anterior muscle group at lower leg level

☰ **IQ** 7 **S86.201-** Unspecified injury of muscle(s) and tendon(s) of anterior muscle group at lower leg level, right leg

☰ **IQ** 7 **S86.202-** Unspecified injury of muscle(s) and tendon(s) of anterior muscle group at lower leg level, left leg

☰ **IQ** 7 **S86.209-** Unspecified injury of muscle(s) and tendon(s) of anterior muscle group at lower leg level, unspecified leg

6 **S86.21** Strain of muscle(s) and tendon(s) of anterior muscle group at lower leg level

☰ **SP** 7 **S86.211-** Strain of muscle(s) and tendon(s) of anterior muscle group at lower leg level, right leg

☰ **SP** 7 **S86.212-** Strain of muscle(s) and tendon(s) of anterior muscle group at lower leg level, left leg

☰ **IQ** 7 **S86.219-** Strain of muscle(s) and tendon(s) of anterior muscle group at lower leg level, unspecified leg

6 **S86.22** Laceration of muscle(s) and tendon(s) of anterior muscle group at lower leg level

☰ **SP** 7 **S86.221-** Laceration of muscle(s) and tendon(s) of anterior muscle group at lower leg level, right leg

☰ **SP** 7 **S86.222-** Laceration of muscle(s) and tendon(s) of anterior muscle group at lower leg level, left leg

☰ **IQ** 7 **S86.229-** Laceration of muscle(s) and tendon(s) of anterior muscle group at lower leg level, unspecified leg

6 **S86.29** Other injury of muscle(s) and tendon(s) of anterior muscle group at lower leg level

☰ **SP** 7 **S86.291-** Other injury of muscle(s) and tendon(s) of anterior muscle group at lower leg level, right leg

☰ **SP** 7 **S86.292-** Other injury of muscle(s) and tendon(s) of anterior muscle group at lower leg level, left leg

☰ **IQ** 7 **S86.299-** Other injury of muscle(s) and tendon(s) of anterior muscle group at lower leg level, unspecified leg

5 **S86.3** Injury of muscle(s) and tendon(s) of peroneal muscle group at lower leg level

6 **S86.30** Unspecified injury of muscle(s) and tendon(s) of peroneal muscle group at lower leg level

Chapter 19

S00-T88

☐4th digit required   ☐5th digit required   ☐6th digit required   ☐7th digit required   ☑7th digit placeholder   ✚Additional code   ☐Laterality

1614   *DecisionHealth's* FY 2020 Complete Home Health ICD-10-CM Diagnosis Coding Manual

☰ **IQ** ⑦ S86.301- Unspecified injury of muscle(s) and tendon(s) of peroneal muscle group at lower leg level, right leg

☰ **IQ** ⑦ S86.302- Unspecified injury of muscle(s) and tendon(s) of peroneal muscle group at lower leg level, left leg

☰ **IQ** ⑦ S86.309- Unspecified injury of muscle(s) and tendon(s) of peroneal muscle group at lower leg level, unspecified leg

⑥ S86.31 Strain of muscle(s) and tendon(s) of peroneal muscle group at lower leg level

☰ **SP** ⑦ S86.311- Strain of muscle(s) and tendon(s) of peroneal muscle group at lower leg level, right leg

☰ **SP** ⑦ S86.312- Strain of muscle(s) and tendon(s) of peroneal muscle group at lower leg level, left leg

☰ **IQ** ⑦ S86.319- Strain of muscle(s) and tendon(s) of peroneal muscle group at lower leg level, unspecified leg

⑥ S86.32 Laceration of muscle(s) and tendon(s) of peroneal muscle group at lower leg level

☰ **SP** ⑦ S86.321- Laceration of muscle(s) and tendon(s) of peroneal muscle group at lower leg level, right leg

☰ **SP** ⑦ S86.322- Laceration of muscle(s) and tendon(s) of peroneal muscle group at lower leg level, left leg

☰ **IQ** ⑦ S86.329- Laceration of muscle(s) and tendon(s) of peroneal muscle group at lower leg level, unspecified leg

⑥ S86.39 Other injury of muscle(s) and tendon(s) of peroneal muscle group at lower leg level

☰ **SP** ⑦ S86.391- Other injury of muscle(s) and tendon(s) of peroneal muscle group at lower leg level, right leg

☰ **SP** ⑦ S86.392- Other injury of muscle(s) and tendon(s) of peroneal muscle group at lower leg level, left leg

☰ **IQ** ⑦ S86.399- Other injury of muscle(s) and tendon(s) of peroneal muscle group at lower leg level, unspecified leg

⑤ S86.8 Injury of other muscles and tendons at lower leg level

⑥ S86.80 Unspecified injury of other muscles and tendons at lower leg level

☰ **IQ** ⑦ S86.801- Unspecified injury of other muscle(s) and tendon(s) at lower leg level, right leg

☰ **IQ** ⑦ S86.802- Unspecified injury of other muscle(s) and tendon(s) at lower leg level, left leg

☰ **IQ** ⑦ S86.809- Unspecified injury of other muscle(s) and tendon(s) at lower leg level, unspecified leg

⑥ S86.81 Strain of other muscles and tendons at lower leg level

☰ **SP** ⑦ S86.811- Strain of other muscle(s) and tendon(s) at lower leg level, right leg

☰ **SP** ⑦ S86.812- Strain of other muscle(s) and tendon(s) at lower leg level, left leg

☰ **IQ** ⑦ S86.819- Strain of other muscle(s) and tendon(s) at lower leg level, unspecified leg

⑥ S86.82 Laceration of other muscles and tendons at lower leg level

☰ **SP** ⑦ S86.821- Laceration of other muscle(s) and tendon(s) at lower leg level, right leg

☰ **SP** ⑦ S86.822- Laceration of other muscle(s) and tendon(s) at lower leg level, left leg

☰ **IQ** ⑦ S86.829- Laceration of other muscle(s) and tendon(s) at lower leg level, unspecified leg

⑥ S86.89 Other injury of other muscles and tendons at lower leg level

☰ **SP** ⑦ S86.891- Other injury of other muscle(s) and tendon(s) at lower leg level, right leg

☰ **SP** ⑦ S86.892- Other injury of other muscle(s) and tendon(s) at lower leg level, left leg

☰ **IQ** ⑦ S86.899- Other injury of other muscle(s) and tendon(s) at lower leg level, unspecified leg

⑤ S86.9 Injury of unspecified muscle and tendon at lower leg level

⑥ S86.90 Unspecified injury of unspecified muscle and tendon at lower leg level

☰ **IQ** ⑦ S86.901- Unspecified injury of unspecified muscle(s) and tendon(s) at lower leg level, right leg

☰ **IQ** ⑦ S86.902- Unspecified injury of unspecified muscle(s) and tendon(s) at lower leg level, left leg

☰ **IQ** ⑦ S86.909- Unspecified injury of unspecified muscle(s) and tendon(s) at lower leg level, unspecified leg

⑥ S86.91 Strain of unspecified muscle and tendon at lower leg level

☰ **SP** ⑦ S86.911- Strain of unspecified muscle(s) and tendon(s) at lower leg level, right leg

☰ **SP** ⑦ S86.912- Strain of unspecified muscle(s) and tendon(s) at lower leg level, left leg

☰ **IQ** ⑦ S86.919- Strain of unspecified muscle(s) and tendon(s) at lower leg level, unspecified leg

⑥ S86.92 Laceration of unspecified muscle and tendon at lower leg level

☰ **SP** ⑦ S86.921- Laceration of unspecified muscle(s) and tendon(s) at lower leg level, right leg

☰ **SP** ⑦ S86.922- Laceration of unspecified muscle(s) and tendon(s) at lower leg level, left leg

★ New ▲ Revised Px Primary **SP** PDGM Px **SL** Low CoM **SH** High CoM **IQ** Quest. Encounter Ⓗ Hospice non-cancer Dx Unspecified **M** *Manifestation*

DecisionHealth's FY 2020 Complete Home Health ICD-10-CM Diagnosis Coding Manual

1615

Chapter 19

S00-T88

☐ **IQ** ☐ **S86.929-**   **Laceration of unspecified muscle(s) and tendon(s) at lower leg level, unspecified leg**

☐ **S86.99**   **Other injury of unspecified muscle and tendon at lower leg level**

☐ **IQ** ☐ **S86.991-**   **Other injury of unspecified muscle(s) and tendon(s) at lower leg level, right leg**

☐ **IQ** ☐ **S86.992-**   **Other injury of unspecified muscle(s) and tendon(s) at lower leg level, left leg**

☐ **IQ** ☐ **S86.999-**   **Other injury of unspecified muscle(s) and tendon(s) at lower leg level, unspecified leg**

➕ ☐ **S87**   **Crushing injury of lower leg**
Use additional code(s) for all associated injuries
EXCLUDES 2   crushing injury of ankle and foot (S97.-)

The appropriate 7th character is to be added to each code from category S87
A   initial encounter
D   subsequent encounter
S   sequela

➕ ☐ **S87.0**   **Crushing injury of knee**

☐ **IQ** ➕ ☐ **S87.00X-**   **Crushing injury of unspecified knee**

☐ **SP** ➕ ☐ **S87.01X-**   **Crushing injury of right knee**

☐ **SP** ➕ ☐ **S87.02X-**   **Crushing injury of left knee**

➕ ☐ **S87.8**   **Crushing injury of lower leg**

☐ **IQ** ➕ ☐ **S87.80X-**   **Crushing injury of unspecified lower leg**

☐ **SP** ➕ ☐ **S87.81X-**   **Crushing injury of right lower leg**

☐ **SP** ➕ ☐ **S87.82X-**   **Crushing injury of left lower leg**

☐ **S88**   **Traumatic amputation of lower leg**
An amputation not identified as partial or complete should be coded to complete
EXCLUDES 1   traumatic amputation of ankle and foot (S98.-)

The appropriate 7th character is to be added to each code from category S88
A   initial encounter
D   subsequent encounter
S   sequela

CODING TIPS ✓   Use these codes only when the amputation was due to trauma. There is no need for adding Z89 with traumatic amputations. See Z47.81 for care of amputations not due to trauma.

☐ **S88.0**   **Traumatic amputation at knee level**

☐ **S88.01**   **Complete traumatic amputation at knee level**

☐ **SP** ☐ **S88.011-**   **Complete traumatic amputation at knee level, right lower leg**

☐ **SP** ☐ **S88.012-**   **Complete traumatic amputation at knee level, left lower leg**

☐ **IQ** ☐ **S88.019-**   **Complete traumatic amputation at knee level, unspecified lower leg**

☐ **S88.02**   **Partial traumatic amputation at knee level**

☐ **SP** ☐ **S88.021-**   **Partial traumatic amputation at knee level, right lower leg**

☐ **SP** ☐ **S88.022-**   **Partial traumatic amputation at knee level, left lower leg**

☐ **IQ** ☐ **S88.029-**   **Partial traumatic amputation at knee level, unspecified lower leg**

☐ **S88.1**   **Traumatic amputation at level between knee and ankle**

☐ **S88.11**   **Complete traumatic amputation at level between knee and ankle**

☐ **SP** ☐ **S88.111-**   **Complete traumatic amputation at level between knee and ankle, right lower leg**

☐ **SP** ☐ **S88.112-**   **Complete traumatic amputation at level between knee and ankle, left lower leg**

☐ **IQ** ☐ **S88.119-**   **Complete traumatic amputation at level between knee and ankle, unspecified lower leg**

☐ **S88.12**   **Partial traumatic amputation at level between knee and ankle**

☐ **SP** ☐ **S88.121-**   **Partial traumatic amputation at level between knee and ankle, right lower leg**

☐ **SP** ☐ **S88.122-**   **Partial traumatic amputation at level between knee and ankle, left lower leg**

☐ **IQ** ☐ **S88.129-**   **Partial traumatic amputation at level between knee and ankle, unspecified lower leg**

☐ **S88.9**   **Traumatic amputation of lower leg, level unspecified**

☐ **S88.91**   **Complete traumatic amputation of lower leg, level unspecified**

☐ **SP** ☐ **S88.911-**   **Complete traumatic amputation of right lower leg, level unspecified**

☐ **SP** ☐ **S88.912-**   **Complete traumatic amputation of left lower leg, level unspecified**

☐ **IQ** ☐ **S88.919-**   **Complete traumatic amputation of unspecified lower leg, level unspecified**

☐ **S88.92**   **Partial traumatic amputation of lower leg, level unspecified**

☐ **SP** ☐ **S88.921-**   **Partial traumatic amputation of right lower leg, level unspecified**

☐ **SP** ☐ **S88.922-**   **Partial traumatic amputation of left lower leg, level unspecified**

☐ **IQ** ☐ **S88.929-**   **Partial traumatic amputation of unspecified lower leg, level unspecified**

☐ **S89**   **Other and unspecified injuries of lower leg**
Note:
A fracture not indicated as open or closed should be coded to closed
EXCLUDES 2   other and unspecified injuries of ankle and foot (S99.-)

☐ 4th digit required   ☐ 5th digit required   ☐ 6th digit required   ☐ 7th digit required   ☐ 7th digit placeholder   ➕ Additional code   ☐ Laterality

1616   *DecisionHealth's* FY 2020 Complete Home Health ICD-10-CM Diagnosis Coding Manual

The appropriate 7th character is to be added to each code from subcategories S89.0, S89.1, S89.2, and S89.3
A   initial encounter for closed fracture
D   subsequent encounter for fracture with routine healing
G   subsequent encounter for fracture with delayed healing
K   subsequent encounter for fracture with nonunion
P   subsequent encounter for fracture with malunion
S   sequela

CODING TIPS ✓ A fracture not indicated as open or closed should be coded to closed.

⑤ **S89.0 Physeal fracture of upper end of tibia**

⑥ **S89.00 Unspecified physeal fracture of upper end of tibia**

▤ SP 7 **S89.001- Unspecified physeal fracture of upper end of right tibia**

▤ SP 7 **S89.002- Unspecified physeal fracture of upper end of left tibia**

▤ IQ 7 **S89.009- Unspecified physeal fracture of upper end of unspecified tibia**

⑥ **S89.01 Salter-Harris Type I physeal fracture of upper end of tibia**

▤ SP 7 **S89.011- Salter-Harris Type I physeal fracture of upper end of right tibia**

▤ SP 7 **S89.012- Salter-Harris Type I physeal fracture of upper end of left tibia**

▤ IQ 7 **S89.019- Salter-Harris Type I physeal fracture of upper end of unspecified tibia**

⑥ **S89.02 Salter-Harris Type II physeal fracture of upper end of tibia**

▤ SP 7 **S89.021- Salter-Harris Type II physeal fracture of upper end of right tibia**

▤ SP 7 **S89.022- Salter-Harris Type II physeal fracture of upper end of left tibia**

▤ IQ 7 **S89.029- Salter-Harris Type II physeal fracture of upper end of unspecified tibia**

⑥ **S89.03 Salter-Harris Type III physeal fracture of upper end of tibia**

▤ SP 7 **S89.031- Salter-Harris Type III physeal fracture of upper end of right tibia**

▤ SP 7 **S89.032- Salter-Harris Type III physeal fracture of upper end of left tibia**

▤ IQ 7 **S89.039- Salter-Harris Type III physeal fracture of upper end of unspecified tibia**

⑥ **S89.04 Salter-Harris Type IV physeal fracture of upper end of tibia**

▤ SP 7 **S89.041- Salter-Harris Type IV physeal fracture of upper end of right tibia**

▤ SP 7 **S89.042- Salter-Harris Type IV physeal fracture of upper end of left tibia**

▤ IQ 7 **S89.049- Salter-Harris Type IV physeal fracture of upper end of unspecified tibia**

⑥ **S89.09 Other physeal fracture of upper end of tibia**

▤ SP 7 **S89.091- Other physeal fracture of upper end of right tibia**

▤ SP 7 **S89.092- Other physeal fracture of upper end of left tibia**

▤ IQ 7 **S89.099- Other physeal fracture of upper end of unspecified tibia**

⑤ **S89.1 Physeal fracture of lower end of tibia**

⑥ **S89.10 Unspecified physeal fracture of lower end of tibia**

▤ SP 7 **S89.101- Unspecified physeal fracture of lower end of right tibia**

▤ SP 7 **S89.102- Unspecified physeal fracture of lower end of left tibia**

▤ IQ 7 **S89.109- Unspecified physeal fracture of lower end of unspecified tibia**

⑥ **S89.11 Salter-Harris Type I physeal fracture of lower end of tibia**

▤ SP 7 **S89.111- Salter-Harris Type I physeal fracture of lower end of right tibia**

▤ SP 7 **S89.112- Salter-Harris Type I physeal fracture of lower end of left tibia**

▤ IQ 7 **S89.119- Salter-Harris Type I physeal fracture of lower end of unspecified tibia**

⑥ **S89.12 Salter-Harris Type II physeal fracture of lower end of tibia**

▤ SP 7 **S89.121- Salter-Harris Type II physeal fracture of lower end of right tibia**

▤ SP 7 **S89.122- Salter-Harris Type II physeal fracture of lower end of left tibia**

▤ IQ 7 **S89.129- Salter-Harris Type II physeal fracture of lower end of unspecified tibia**

⑥ **S89.13 Salter-Harris Type III physeal fracture of lower end of tibia**
    EXCLUDES 1 fracture of medial malleolus (adult) (S82.5-)

▤ SP 7 **S89.131- Salter-Harris Type III physeal fracture of lower end of right tibia**

▤ SP 7 **S89.132- Salter-Harris Type III physeal fracture of lower end of left tibia**

▤ IQ 7 **S89.139- Salter-Harris Type III physeal fracture of lower end of unspecified tibia**

⑥ **S89.14 Salter-Harris Type IV physeal fracture of lower end of tibia**
    EXCLUDES 1 fracture of medial malleolus (adult) (S82.5-)

▤ SP 7 **S89.141- Salter-Harris Type IV physeal fracture of lower end of right tibia**

▤ SP 7 **S89.142- Salter-Harris Type IV physeal fracture of lower end of left tibia**

▤ IQ 7 **S89.149- Salter-Harris Type IV physeal fracture of lower end of unspecified tibia**

⑥ **S89.19 Other physeal fracture of lower end of tibia**

▤ SP 7 **S89.191- Other physeal fracture of lower end of right tibia**

★ New ▲ Revised Px Primary **SP** PDGM Px **SL** Low CoM **SH** High CoM **IQ** Quest. Encounter ⊞ Hospice non-cancer Dx   Unspecified   **M** *Manifestation*

DecisionHealth's FY 2020 Complete Home Health ICD-10-CM Diagnosis Coding Manual

1617

▤ **SP** ⑦ **S89.192-** Other physeal fracture of lower end of left tibia

▤ **IQ** ⑦ **S89.199-** Other physeal fracture of lower end of unspecified tibia

⑤ **S89.2** Physeal fracture of upper end of fibula

⑥ **S89.20** Unspecified physeal fracture of upper end of fibula

▤ **SP** ⑦ **S89.201-** Unspecified physeal fracture of upper end of right fibula

▤ **SP** ⑦ **S89.202-** Unspecified physeal fracture of upper end of left fibula

▤ **IQ** ⑦ **S89.209-** Unspecified physeal fracture of upper end of unspecified fibula

⑥ **S89.21** Salter-Harris Type I physeal fracture of upper end of fibula

▤ **SP** ⑦ **S89.211-** Salter-Harris Type I physeal fracture of upper end of right fibula

▤ **SP** ⑦ **S89.212-** Salter-Harris Type I physeal fracture of upper end of left fibula

▤ **IQ** ⑦ **S89.219-** Salter-Harris Type I physeal fracture of upper end of unspecified fibula

⑥ **S89.22** Salter-Harris Type II physeal fracture of upper end of fibula

▤ **SP** ⑦ **S89.221-** Salter-Harris Type II physeal fracture of upper end of right fibula

▤ **SP** ⑦ **S89.222-** Salter-Harris Type II physeal fracture of upper end of left fibula

▤ **IQ** ⑦ **S89.229-** Salter-Harris Type II physeal fracture of upper end of unspecified fibula

⑥ **S89.29** Other physeal fracture of upper end of fibula

▤ **SP** ⑦ **S89.291-** Other physeal fracture of upper end of right fibula

▤ **SP** ⑦ **S89.292-** Other physeal fracture of upper end of left fibula

▤ **IQ** ⑦ **S89.299-** Other physeal fracture of upper end of unspecified fibula

⑤ **S89.3** Physeal fracture of lower end of fibula

⑥ **S89.30** Unspecified physeal fracture of lower end of fibula

▤ **SP** ⑦ **S89.301-** Unspecified physeal fracture of lower end of right fibula

▤ **SP** ⑦ **S89.302-** Unspecified physeal fracture of lower end of left fibula

▤ **IQ** ⑦ **S89.309-** Unspecified physeal fracture of lower end of unspecified fibula

⑥ **S89.31** Salter-Harris Type I physeal fracture of lower end of fibula

▤ **SP** ⑦ **S89.311-** Salter-Harris Type I physeal fracture of lower end of right fibula

▤ **SP** ⑦ **S89.312-** Salter-Harris Type I physeal fracture of lower end of left fibula

▤ **IQ** ⑦ **S89.319-** Salter-Harris Type I physeal fracture of lower end of unspecified fibula

⑥ **S89.32** Salter-Harris Type II physeal fracture of lower end of fibula

▤ **SP** ⑦ **S89.321-** Salter-Harris Type II physeal fracture of lower end of right fibula

▤ **SP** ⑦ **S89.322-** Salter-Harris Type II physeal fracture of lower end of left fibula

▤ **IQ** ⑦ **S89.329-** Salter-Harris Type II physeal fracture of lower end of unspecified fibula

⑥ **S89.39** Other physeal fracture of lower end of fibula

▤ **SP** ⑦ **S89.391-** Other physeal fracture of lower end of right fibula

▤ **SP** ⑦ **S89.392-** Other physeal fracture of lower end of left fibula

▤ **IQ** ⑦ **S89.399-** Other physeal fracture of lower end of unspecified fibula

⑤ **S89.8** Other specified injuries of lower leg

The appropriate 7th character is to be added to each code in subcategory S89.8
A   initial encounter
D   subsequent encounter
S   sequela

▤ **IQ** ☑ **S89.80X-** Other specified injuries of unspecified lower leg

▤ **SP** ☑ **S89.81X-** Other specified injuries of right lower leg

▤ **SP** ☑ **S89.82X-** Other specified injuries of left lower leg

⑤ **S89.9** Unspecified injury of lower leg

The appropriate 7th character is to be added to each code in subcategory S89.9
A   initial encounter
D   subsequent encounter
S   sequela

▤ **IQ** ☑ **S89.90X-** Unspecified injury of unspecified lower leg

▤ **IQ** ☑ **S89.91X-** Unspecified injury of right lower leg

▤ **IQ** ☑ **S89.92X-** Unspecified injury of left lower leg

Injuries to the ankle and foot (S90-S99)

EXCLUDES 2 burns and corrosions (T20-T32)
fracture of ankle and malleolus (S82.-)
frostbite (T33-T34)
insect bite or sting, venomous (T63.4)

GUIDELINES Section I.C.19.c.2)
Multiple fractures are sequenced in accordance with the severity of the fracture.

④4th digit required   ⑤5th digit required   ⑥6th digit required   ⑦7th digit required   ☑7th digit placeholder   ➕Additional code   ▤Laterality

1618   *DecisionHealth's* FY 2020 Complete Home Health ICD-10-CM Diagnosis Coding Manual

GUIDELINES Section I.C.19.b.1)-2)

When coding injuries, assign separate codes for each injury unless a combination code is provided, in which case the combination code is assigned ... Traumatic injury codes (S00-T14.9) are not to be used for normal, healing surgical wounds or to identify complications of surgical wounds. The code for the most serious injury, as determined by the provider and the focus of treatment, is sequenced first.

1) Superficial injuries such as abrasions or contusions are not coded when associated with more severe injuries of the same site.

2) When a primary injury results in minor damage to peripheral nerves or blood vessels, the primary injury is sequenced first with additional code(s) for injuries to nerves and spinal cord (such as category S04), and/or injury to blood vessels (such as category S15). When the primary injury is to the blood vessels or nerves, that injury should be sequenced first.

GUIDELINES Section I.C.19.c

Coding of Traumatic Fractures: The principles of multiple coding of injuries should be followed in coding fractures. Fractures of specified sites are coded individually by site in accordance with both the provisions within categories S02, S12, S22, S32, S42, S49, S52, S59, S62, S72, S79, S82, S89, S92 and the level of detail furnished by medical record content. A fracture not indicated as open or closed should be coded to closed. A fracture not indicated whether displaced or not displaced should be coded to displaced.

CODING TIPS ✓ 7th character A is acceptable in home health and hospice when active treatment is provided, such as antibiotics for an infected wound or a wound vac for a dehisced wound. D is used when the complication or injury is now healing. Think of D as aftercare. S is used for sequela of the injury or complication. Sequela is a residual deficit or condition produced as a result of the injury or complication after the original injury or complication has healed.

4 S90 **Superficial injury of ankle, foot and toes**

> The appropriate 7th character is to be added to each code from category S90
> A   initial encounter
> D   subsequent encounter
> S   sequela

5 S90.0 **Contusion of ankle**

S90.00X- Contusion of unspecified ankle

S90.01X- Contusion of right ankle

S90.02X- Contusion of left ankle

5 S90.1 **Contusion of toe without damage to nail**

6 S90.11 Contusion of great toe without damage to nail

S90.111- Contusion of right great toe without damage to nail

S90.112- Contusion of left great toe without damage to nail

S90.119- Contusion of unspecified great toe without damage to nail

6 S90.12 Contusion of lesser toe without damage to nail

S90.121- Contusion of right lesser toe(s) without damage to nail

S90.122- Contusion of left lesser toe(s) without damage to nail

S90.129- Contusion of unspecified lesser toe(s) without damage to nail
Contusion of toe NOS

5 S90.2 **Contusion of toe with damage to nail**

6 S90.21 Contusion of great toe with damage to nail

S90.211- Contusion of right great toe with damage to nail

S90.212- Contusion of left great toe with damage to nail

S90.219- Contusion of unspecified great toe with damage to nail

6 S90.22 Contusion of lesser toe with damage to nail

S90.221- Contusion of right lesser toe(s) with damage to nail

S90.222- Contusion of left lesser toe(s) with damage to nail

S90.229- Contusion of unspecified lesser toe(s) with damage to nail

5 S90.3 **Contusion of foot**
EXCLUDES 2 contusion of toes (S90.1-, S90.2-)

S90.30X- Contusion of unspecified foot
Contusion of foot NOS

S90.31X- Contusion of right foot

S90.32X- Contusion of left foot

5 S90.4 **Other superficial injuries of toe**

6 S90.41 Abrasion of toe

S90.411- Abrasion, right great toe

S90.412- Abrasion, left great toe

S90.413- Abrasion, unspecified great toe

S90.414- Abrasion, right lesser toe(s)

S90.415- Abrasion, left lesser toe(s)

S90.416- Abrasion, unspecified lesser toe(s)

6 S90.42 Blister (nonthermal) of toe

S90.421- Blister (nonthermal), right great toe

S90.422- Blister (nonthermal), left great toe

S90.423- Blister (nonthermal), unspecified great toe

S90.424- Blister (nonthermal), right lesser toe(s)

S90.425- Blister (nonthermal), left lesser toe(s)

S90.426- Blister (nonthermal), unspecified lesser toe(s)

6 S90.44 External constriction of toe
Hair tourniquet syndrome of toe

S90.441- External constriction, right great toe

S90.442- External constriction, left great toe

S90.443- External constriction, unspecified great toe

S90.444- External constriction, right lesser toe(s)

S90.445- External constriction, left lesser toe(s)

S90.446- External constriction, unspecified lesser toe(s)

6 S90.45 Superficial foreign body of toe

★ New ▲ Revised Px Primary SP PDGM Px SL Low CoM SH High CoM IQ Quest. Encounter H Hospice non-cancer Dx   Unspecified   M Manifestation

DecisionHealth's FY 2020 Complete Home Health ICD-10-CM Diagnosis Coding Manual

1619

Splinter in the toe

☰ !Q 7 **S90.451-** Superficial foreign body, right great toe

☰ !Q 7 **S90.452-** Superficial foreign body, left great toe

☰ !Q 7 **S90.453-** Superficial foreign body, unspecified great toe

☰ !Q 7 **S90.454-** Superficial foreign body, right lesser toe(s)

☰ !Q 7 **S90.455-** Superficial foreign body, left lesser toe(s)

☰ !Q 7 **S90.456-** Superficial foreign body, unspecified lesser toe(s)

6 **S90.46** Insect bite (nonvenomous) of toe

☰ !Q 7 **S90.461-** Insect bite (nonvenomous), right great toe

☰ !Q 7 **S90.462-** Insect bite (nonvenomous), left great toe

☰ !Q 7 **S90.463-** Insect bite (nonvenomous), unspecified great toe

☰ !Q 7 **S90.464-** Insect bite (nonvenomous), right lesser toe(s)

☰ !Q 7 **S90.465-** Insect bite (nonvenomous), left lesser toe(s)

☰ !Q 7 **S90.466-** Insect bite (nonvenomous), unspecified lesser toe(s)

6 **S90.47** Other superficial bite of toe
> EXCLUDES 1 open bite of toe (S91.15-, S91.25-)

☰ !Q 7 **S90.471-** Other superficial bite of right great toe

☰ !Q 7 **S90.472-** Other superficial bite of left great toe

☰ !Q 7 **S90.473-** Other superficial bite of unspecified great toe

☰ !Q 7 **S90.474-** Other superficial bite of right lesser toe(s)

☰ !Q 7 **S90.475-** Other superficial bite of left lesser toe(s)

☰ !Q 7 **S90.476-** Other superficial bite of unspecified lesser toe(s)

5 **S90.5** Other superficial injuries of ankle

6 **S90.51** Abrasion of ankle

☰ !Q 7 **S90.511-** Abrasion, right ankle

☰ !Q 7 **S90.512-** Abrasion, left ankle

☰ !Q 7 **S90.519-** Abrasion, unspecified ankle

6 **S90.52** Blister (nonthermal) of ankle

☰ !Q 7 **S90.521-** Blister (nonthermal), right ankle

☰ !Q 7 **S90.522-** Blister (nonthermal), left ankle

☰ !Q 7 **S90.529-** Blister (nonthermal), unspecified ankle

6 **S90.54** External constriction of ankle

☰ !Q 7 **S90.541-** External constriction, right ankle

☰ !Q 7 **S90.542-** External constriction, left ankle

☰ !Q 7 **S90.549-** External constriction, unspecified ankle

6 **S90.55** Superficial foreign body of ankle
Splinter in the ankle

☰ !Q 7 **S90.551-** Superficial foreign body, right ankle

☰ !Q 7 **S90.552-** Superficial foreign body, left ankle

☰ !Q 7 **S90.559-** Superficial foreign body, unspecified ankle

6 **S90.56** Insect bite (nonvenomous) of ankle

☰ !Q 7 **S90.561-** Insect bite (nonvenomous), right ankle

☰ !Q 7 **S90.562-** Insect bite (nonvenomous), left ankle

☰ !Q 7 **S90.569-** Insect bite (nonvenomous), unspecified ankle

6 **S90.57** Other superficial bite of ankle
> EXCLUDES 1 open bite of ankle (S91.05-)

☰ !Q 7 **S90.571-** Other superficial bite of ankle, right ankle

☰ !Q 7 **S90.572-** Other superficial bite of ankle, left ankle

☰ !Q 7 **S90.579-** Other superficial bite of ankle, unspecified ankle

5 **S90.8** Other superficial injuries of foot

6 **S90.81** Abrasion of foot

☰ !Q 7 **S90.811-** Abrasion, right foot

☰ !Q 7 **S90.812-** Abrasion, left foot

☰ !Q 7 **S90.819-** Abrasion, unspecified foot

6 **S90.82** Blister (nonthermal) of foot

☰ !Q 7 **S90.821-** Blister (nonthermal), right foot

☰ !Q 7 **S90.822-** Blister (nonthermal), left foot

☰ !Q 7 **S90.829-** Blister (nonthermal), unspecified foot

6 **S90.84** External constriction of foot

☰ !Q 7 **S90.841-** External constriction, right foot

☰ !Q 7 **S90.842-** External constriction, left foot

☰ !Q 7 **S90.849-** External constriction, unspecified foot

6 **S90.85** Superficial foreign body of foot
Splinter in the foot

☰ !Q 7 **S90.851-** Superficial foreign body, right foot

☰ !Q 7 **S90.852-** Superficial foreign body, left foot

☰ !Q 7 **S90.859-** Superficial foreign body, unspecified foot

6 **S90.86** Insect bite (nonvenomous) of foot

☰ !Q 7 **S90.861-** Insect bite (nonvenomous), right foot

☰ !Q 7 **S90.862-** Insect bite (nonvenomous), left foot

☰ !Q 7 **S90.869-** Insect bite (nonvenomous), unspecified foot

6 **S90.87** Other superficial bite of foot
> EXCLUDES 1 open bite of foot (S91.35-)

☰ !Q 7 **S90.871-** Other superficial bite of right foot

☰ !Q 7 **S90.872-** Other superficial bite of left foot

☰ !Q 7 **S90.879-** Other superficial bite of unspecified foot

5 **S90.9** Unspecified superficial injury of ankle, foot and toe

6 **S90.91** Unspecified superficial injury of ankle

☰ !Q 7 **S90.911-** Unspecified superficial injury of right ankle

☰ !Q 7 **S90.912-** Unspecified superficial injury of left ankle

---

4 4th digit required 5 5th digit required 6 6th digit required 7 7th digit required 7 7th digit placeholder + Additional code ☰ Laterality

☐ 🔢 7 **S90.919-** Unspecified superficial injury of unspecified ankle

6 S90.92 Unspecified superficial injury of foot

☐ 🔢 7 **S90.921-** Unspecified superficial injury of right foot

☐ 🔢 7 **S90.922-** Unspecified superficial injury of left foot

☐ 🔢 7 **S90.929-** Unspecified superficial injury of unspecified foot

6 S90.93 Unspecified superficial injury of toes

☐ 🔢 7 **S90.931-** Unspecified superficial injury of right great toe

☐ 🔢 7 **S90.932-** Unspecified superficial injury of left great toe

☐ 🔢 7 **S90.933-** Unspecified superficial injury of unspecified great toe

☐ 🔢 7 **S90.934-** Unspecified superficial injury of right lesser toe(s)

☐ 🔢 7 **S90.935-** Unspecified superficial injury of left lesser toe(s)

☐ 🔢 7 **S90.936-** Unspecified superficial injury of unspecified lesser toe(s)

4 **S91** Open wound of ankle, foot and toes

Code also:

any associated wound infection

EXCLUDES 1 open fracture of ankle, foot and toes
(S92.-with 7th character B)
traumatic amputation of ankle and foot (S98.-)

The appropriate 7th character is to be added to each code from category S91

A   initial encounter
D   subsequent encounter
S   sequela

CODING TIPS ✓ No aftercare code applies, including those for dressing changes, drain care, or suture removal. 7th character 'D' is the default for home care and hospice when providing aftercare for a healing or resolving condition; 'A' is used for active treatment such as antibiotics or more than routine wound care; 'S' may be used to indicate a residual condition after the original injury has healed.

CODING TIPS ✓ Open wound codes indicate a wound resulting from a traumatic origin. Do not assign a code for "open wound" unless the etiology of the wound is related to trauma.

5 S91.0 Open wound of ankle

6 S91.00 Unspecified open wound of ankle

☐ 💲 7 **S91.001-** Unspecified open wound, right ankle

☐ 💲 7 **S91.002-** Unspecified open wound, left ankle

☐ 💲 🔢 7 **S91.009-** Unspecified open wound, unspecified ankle

6 S91.01 Laceration without foreign body of ankle

☐ 💲 7 **S91.011-** Laceration without foreign body, right ankle

☐ 💲 7 **S91.012-** Laceration without foreign body, left ankle

☐ 🔢 7 **S91.019-** Laceration without foreign body, unspecified ankle

6 S91.02 Laceration with foreign body of ankle

☐ 💲 7 **S91.021-** Laceration with foreign body, right ankle

☐ 💲 7 **S91.022-** Laceration with foreign body, left ankle

☐ 🔢 7 **S91.029-** Laceration with foreign body, unspecified ankle

6 S91.03 Puncture wound without foreign body of ankle

☐ 💲 7 **S91.031-** Puncture wound without foreign body, right ankle

☐ 💲 7 **S91.032-** Puncture wound without foreign body, left ankle

☐ 🔢 7 **S91.039-** Puncture wound without foreign body, unspecified ankle

6 S91.04 Puncture wound with foreign body of ankle

☐ 💲 7 **S91.041-** Puncture wound with foreign body, right ankle

☐ 💲 7 **S91.042-** Puncture wound with foreign body, left ankle

☐ 🔢 7 **S91.049-** Puncture wound with foreign body, unspecified ankle

6 S91.05 Open bite of ankle

EXCLUDES 1 superficial bite of ankle (S90.56-, S90.57-)

☐ 💲 7 **S91.051-** Open bite, right ankle

☐ 💲 7 **S91.052-** Open bite, left ankle

☐ 🔢 7 **S91.059-** Open bite, unspecified ankle

5 S91.1 Open wound of toe without damage to nail

6 S91.10 Unspecified open wound of toe without damage to nail

☐ 💲 7 **S91.101-** Unspecified open wound of right great toe without damage to nail

☐ 💲 7 **S91.102-** Unspecified open wound of left great toe without damage to nail

☐ 🔢 7 **S91.103-** Unspecified open wound of unspecified great toe without damage to nail

☐ 💲 7 **S91.104-** Unspecified open wound of right lesser toe(s) without damage to nail

☐ 💲 7 **S91.105-** Unspecified open wound of left lesser toe(s) without damage to nail

☐ 🔢 7 **S91.106-** Unspecified open wound of unspecified lesser toe(s) without damage to nail

☐ 🔢 7 **S91.109-** Unspecified open wound of unspecified toe(s) without damage to nail

6 S91.11 Laceration without foreign body of toe without damage to nail

☐ 💲 7 **S91.111-** Laceration without foreign body of right great toe without damage to nail

☐ 💲 7 **S91.112-** Laceration without foreign body of left great toe without damage to nail

Chapter 19

S00-T88

★ New ▲ Revised Px Primary 💲 PDGM Px 🟦 Low CoM 🟦 High CoM 🔢 Quest. Encounter ⊞ Hospice non-cancer Dx ▨ Unspecified Ⓜ *Manifestation*

DecisionHealth's FY 2020 Complete Home Health ICD-10-CM Diagnosis Coding Manual

1621

☐ !Q 7 **S91.113-**   Laceration without foreign body of unspecified great toe without damage to nail

☐ SP 7 **S91.114-**   Laceration without foreign body of right lesser toe(s) without damage to nail

☐ SP 7 **S91.115-**   Laceration without foreign body of left lesser toe(s) without damage to nail

☐ !Q 7 **S91.116-**   Laceration without foreign body of unspecified lesser toe(s) without damage to nail

☐ !Q 7 **S91.119-**   Laceration without foreign body of unspecified toe without damage to nail

6 **S91.12**   Laceration with foreign body of toe without damage to nail

☐ SP 7 **S91.121-**   Laceration with foreign body of right great toe without damage to nail

☐ SP 7 **S91.122-**   Laceration with foreign body of left great toe without damage to nail

☐ !Q 7 **S91.123-**   Laceration with foreign body of unspecified great toe without damage to nail

☐ SP 7 **S91.124-**   Laceration with foreign body of right lesser toe(s) without damage to nail

☐ SP 7 **S91.125-**   Laceration with foreign body of left lesser toe(s) without damage to nail

☐ !Q 7 **S91.126-**   Laceration with foreign body of unspecified lesser toe(s) without damage to nail

☐ !Q 7 **S91.129-**   Laceration with foreign body of unspecified toe(s) without damage to nail

6 **S91.13**   Puncture wound without foreign body of toe without damage to nail

☐ SP 7 **S91.131-**   Puncture wound without foreign body of right great toe without damage to nail

☐ SP 7 **S91.132-**   Puncture wound without foreign body of left great toe without damage to nail

☐ !Q 7 **S91.133-**   Puncture wound without foreign body of unspecified great toe without damage to nail

☐ SP 7 **S91.134-**   Puncture wound without foreign body of right lesser toe(s) without damage to nail

☐ SP 7 **S91.135-**   Puncture wound without foreign body of left lesser toe(s) without damage to nail

☐ !Q 7 **S91.136-**   Puncture wound without foreign body of unspecified lesser toe(s) without damage to nail

☐ !Q 7 **S91.139-**   Puncture wound without foreign body of unspecified toe(s) without damage to nail

6 **S91.14**   Puncture wound with foreign body of toe without damage to nail

☐ SP 7 **S91.141-**   Puncture wound with foreign body of right great toe without damage to nail

☐ SP 7 **S91.142-**   Puncture wound with foreign body of left great toe without damage to nail

☐ !Q 7 **S91.143-**   Puncture wound with foreign body of unspecified great toe without damage to nail

☐ SP 7 **S91.144-**   Puncture wound with foreign body of right lesser toe(s) without damage to nail

☐ SP 7 **S91.145-**   Puncture wound with foreign body of left lesser toe(s) without damage to nail

☐ !Q 7 **S91.146-**   Puncture wound with foreign body of unspecified lesser toe(s) without damage to nail

☐ !Q 7 **S91.149-**   Puncture wound with foreign body of unspecified toe(s) without damage to nail

6 **S91.15**   Open bite of toe without damage to nail
Bite of toe NOS
> **EXCLUDES 1**   superficial bite of toe (S90.46-, S90.47-)

☐ SP 7 **S91.151-**   Open bite of right great toe without damage to nail

☐ SP 7 **S91.152-**   Open bite of left great toe without damage to nail

☐ !Q 7 **S91.153-**   Open bite of unspecified great toe without damage to nail

☐ SP 7 **S91.154-**   Open bite of right lesser toe(s) without damage to nail

☐ SP 7 **S91.155-**   Open bite of left lesser toe(s) without damage to nail

☐ !Q 7 **S91.156-**   Open bite of unspecified lesser toe(s) without damage to nail

☐ !Q 7 **S91.159-**   Open bite of unspecified toe(s) without damage to nail

5 **S91.2**   Open wound of toe with damage to nail

6 **S91.20**   Unspecified open wound of toe with damage to nail

☐ SP 7 **S91.201-**   Unspecified open wound of right great toe with damage to nail

☐ SP 7 **S91.202-**   Unspecified open wound of left great toe with damage to nail

☐ !Q 7 **S91.203-**   Unspecified open wound of unspecified great toe with damage to nail

☐ SP 7 **S91.204-**   Unspecified open wound of right lesser toe(s) with damage to nail

☐ SP 7 **S91.205-**   Unspecified open wound of left lesser toe(s) with damage to nail

☐ !Q 7 **S91.206-**   Unspecified open wound of unspecified lesser toe(s) with damage to nail

☐ !Q 7 **S91.209-**   Unspecified open wound of unspecified toe(s) with damage to nail

6 **S91.21**   Laceration without foreign body of toe with damage to nail

☐ SP 7 **S91.211-**   Laceration without foreign body of right great toe with damage to nail

4th digit required   5 5th digit required   6 6th digit required   7 7th digit required   7 7th digit placeholder   +Additional code   ☐ Laterality

1622   *DecisionHealth's* FY 2020 Complete Home Health ICD-10-CM Diagnosis Coding Manual

Chapter 19

S00-T88

☰ SP 7 S91.212- Laceration without foreign body of left great toe with damage to nail

☰ IQ 7 S91.213- Laceration without foreign body of unspecified great toe with damage to nail

☰ SP 7 S91.214- Laceration without foreign body of right lesser toe(s) with damage to nail

☰ SP 7 S91.215- Laceration without foreign body of left lesser toe(s) with damage to nail

☰ IQ 7 S91.216- Laceration without foreign body of unspecified lesser toe(s) with damage to nail

☰ IQ 7 S91.219- Laceration without foreign body of unspecified toe(s) with damage to nail

6 S91.22 Laceration with foreign body of toe with damage to nail

☰ SP 7 S91.221- Laceration with foreign body of right great toe with damage to nail

☰ SP 7 S91.222- Laceration with foreign body of left great toe with damage to nail

☰ IQ 7 S91.223- Laceration with foreign body of unspecified great toe with damage to nail

☰ SP 7 S91.224- Laceration with foreign body of right lesser toe(s) with damage to nail

☰ SP 7 S91.225- Laceration with foreign body of left lesser toe(s) with damage to nail

☰ IQ 7 S91.226- Laceration with foreign body of unspecified lesser toe(s) with damage to nail

☰ IQ 7 S91.229- Laceration with foreign body of unspecified toe(s) with damage to nail

6 S91.23 Puncture wound without foreign body of toe with damage to nail

☰ SP 7 S91.231- Puncture wound without foreign body of right great toe with damage to nail

☰ SP 7 S91.232- Puncture wound without foreign body of left great toe with damage to nail

☰ IQ 7 S91.233- Puncture wound without foreign body of unspecified great toe with damage to nail

☰ SP 7 S91.234- Puncture wound without foreign body of right lesser toe(s) with damage to nail

☰ SP 7 S91.235- Puncture wound without foreign body of left lesser toe(s) with damage to nail

☰ IQ 7 S91.236- Puncture wound without foreign body of unspecified lesser toe(s) with damage to nail

☰ IQ 7 S91.239- Puncture wound without foreign body of unspecified toe(s) with damage to nail

6 S91.24 Puncture wound with foreign body of toe with damage to nail

☰ SP 7 S91.241- Puncture wound with foreign body of right great toe with damage to nail

☰ SP 7 S91.242- Puncture wound with foreign body of left great toe with damage to nail

☰ IQ 7 S91.243- Puncture wound with foreign body of unspecified great toe with damage to nail

☰ SP 7 S91.244- Puncture wound with foreign body of right lesser toe(s) with damage to nail

☰ SP 7 S91.245- Puncture wound with foreign body of left lesser toe(s) with damage to nail

☰ IQ 7 S91.246- Puncture wound with foreign body of unspecified lesser toe(s) with damage to nail

☰ IQ 7 S91.249- Puncture wound with foreign body of unspecified toe(s) with damage to nail

6 S91.25 Open bite of toe with damage to nail
Bite of toe with damage to nail NOS
EXCLUDES 1 superficial bite of toe (S90.46-, S90.47-)

☰ SP 7 S91.251- Open bite of right great toe with damage to nail

☰ SP 7 S91.252- Open bite of left great toe with damage to nail

☰ IQ 7 S91.253- Open bite of unspecified great toe with damage to nail

☰ SP 7 S91.254- Open bite of right lesser toe(s) with damage to nail

☰ SP 7 S91.255- Open bite of left lesser toe(s) with damage to nail

☰ IQ 7 S91.256- Open bite of unspecified lesser toe(s) with damage to nail

☰ IQ 7 S91.259- Open bite of unspecified toe(s) with damage to nail

5 S91.3 Open wound of foot

6 S91.30 Unspecified open wound of foot

☰ SP 7 S91.301- Unspecified open wound, right foot

☰ SP 7 S91.302- Unspecified open wound, left foot

☰ IQ 7 S91.309- Unspecified open wound, unspecified foot

6 S91.31 Laceration without foreign body of foot

☰ SP 7 S91.311- Laceration without foreign body, right foot

☰ SP 7 S91.312- Laceration without foreign body, left foot

☰ IQ 7 S91.319- Laceration without foreign body, unspecified foot

6 S91.32 Laceration with foreign body of foot

☰ SP 7 S91.321- Laceration with foreign body, right foot

☰ SP 7 S91.322- Laceration with foreign body, left foot

☰ IQ 7 S91.329- Laceration with foreign body, unspecified foot

6 S91.33 Puncture wound without foreign body of foot

☰ SP 7 S91.331- Puncture wound without foreign body, right foot

★ New ▲ Revised Px Primary **SP** PDGM Px **SL** Low CoM **SH** High CoM **IQ** Quest. Encounter **H** Hospice non-cancer Dx Unspecified **M** *Manifestation*

DecisionHealth's FY 2020 Complete Home Health ICD-10-CM Diagnosis Coding Manual

1623

⊟ SP 7 **S91.332-** Puncture wound without foreign body, left foot

⊟ !Q 7 **S91.339-** Puncture wound without foreign body, unspecified foot

6 **S91.34** Puncture wound with foreign body of foot

⊟ SP 7 **S91.341-** Puncture wound with foreign body, right foot

⊟ SP 7 **S91.342-** Puncture wound with foreign body, left foot

⊟ !Q 7 **S91.349-** Puncture wound with foreign body, unspecified foot

6 **S91.35** Open bite of foot

EXCLUDES 1   superficial bite of foot (S90.86-, S90.87-)

⊟ SP 7 **S91.351-** Open bite, right foot

⊟ SP 7 **S91.352-** Open bite, left foot

⊟ !Q 7 **S91.359-** Open bite, unspecified foot

Phalange

Metatarsal bone

Cuneiform
  Medial
  Intermediate
  Lateral

Navicular

Talus

Cuboid

Calcaneus

4 **S92** Fracture of foot and toe, except ankle
Note:
A fracture not indicated as displaced or nondisplaced should be coded to displaced
A fracture not indicated as open or closed should be coded to closed

EXCLUDES 1   traumatic amputation of ankle and foot (S98.-)

EXCLUDES 2   fracture of ankle (S82.-)
fracture of malleolus (S82.-)

The appropriate 7th character is to be added to each code from category S92

A   initial encounter for closed fracture
B   initial encounter for open fracture
D   subsequent encounter for fracture with routine healing
G   subsequent encounter for fracture with delayed healing
K   subsequent encounter for fracture with nonunion
P   subsequent encounter for fracture with malunion
S   sequela

CODING TIPS ✓   Fractures are not coded with aftercare. "D" is the 7th character for home care and hospice unless the physician has documented delayed healing, nonunion or malunion. A sequela is a condition left after the fracture has healed. The Gustilo open fracture classification must be used for open fractures.

CODING TIPS ✓   A fracture not indicated as displaced or nondisplaced should be coded to displaced. A fracture not indicated as open or closed should be coded to closed.

5 **S92.0** Fracture of calcaneus
Heel bone
Os calcis

EXCLUDES 2   Physeal fracture of calcaneus (S99.0-)

6 **S92.00** Unspecified fracture of calcaneus

⊟ SP 7 **S92.001-** Unspecified fracture of right calcaneus

⊟ SP 7 **S92.002-** Unspecified fracture of left calcaneus

⊟ !Q 7 **S92.009-** Unspecified fracture of unspecified calcaneus

6 **S92.01** Fracture of body of calcaneus

⊟ SP 7 **S92.011-** Displaced fracture of body of right calcaneus

⊟ SP 7 **S92.012-** Displaced fracture of body of left calcaneus

⊟ !Q 7 **S92.013-** Displaced fracture of body of unspecified calcaneus

⊟ SP 7 **S92.014-** Nondisplaced fracture of body of right calcaneus

⊟ SP 7 **S92.015-** Nondisplaced fracture of body of left calcaneus

⊟ !Q 7 **S92.016-** Nondisplaced fracture of body of unspecified calcaneus

6 **S92.02** Fracture of anterior process of calcaneus

⊟ SP 7 **S92.021-** Displaced fracture of anterior process of right calcaneus

⊟ SP 7 **S92.022-** Displaced fracture of anterior process of left calcaneus

⊟ !Q 7 **S92.023-** Displaced fracture of anterior process of unspecified calcaneus

⊟ SP 7 **S92.024-** Nondisplaced fracture of anterior process of right calcaneus

4 4th digit required   5 5th digit required   6 6th digit required   7 7th digit required   7 7th digit placeholder   ✚ Additional code   ⊟ Laterality

1624   *DecisionHealth's* FY 2020 Complete Home Health ICD-10-CM Diagnosis Coding Manual

☐ SP 7 S92.025- Nondisplaced fracture of anterior process of left calcaneus

☐ IQ 7 S92.026- **Nondisplaced fracture of anterior process of unspecified calcaneus**

6 S92.03 Avulsion fracture of tuberosity of calcaneus

☐ SP 7 S92.031- Displaced avulsion fracture of tuberosity of right calcaneus

☐ SP 7 S92.032- Displaced avulsion fracture of tuberosity of left calcaneus

☐ IQ 7 S92.033- **Displaced avulsion fracture of tuberosity of unspecified calcaneus**

☐ SP 7 S92.034- Nondisplaced avulsion fracture of tuberosity of right calcaneus

☐ SP 7 S92.035- Nondisplaced avulsion fracture of tuberosity of left calcaneus

☐ IQ 7 S92.036- **Nondisplaced avulsion fracture of tuberosity of unspecified calcaneus**

6 S92.04 Other fracture of tuberosity of calcaneus

☐ SP 7 S92.041- Displaced other fracture of tuberosity of right calcaneus

☐ SP 7 S92.042- Displaced other fracture of tuberosity of left calcaneus

☐ IQ 7 S92.043- **Displaced other fracture of tuberosity of unspecified calcaneus**

☐ SP 7 S92.044- Nondisplaced other fracture of tuberosity of right calcaneus

☐ SP 7 S92.045- Nondisplaced other fracture of tuberosity of left calcaneus

☐ IQ 7 S92.046- **Nondisplaced other fracture of tuberosity of unspecified calcaneus**

6 S92.05 Other extraarticular fracture of calcaneus

☐ SP 7 S92.051- Displaced other extraarticular fracture of right calcaneus

☐ SP 7 S92.052- Displaced other extraarticular fracture of left calcaneus

☐ IQ 7 S92.053- **Displaced other extraarticular fracture of unspecified calcaneus**

☐ SP 7 S92.054- Nondisplaced other extraarticular fracture of right calcaneus

☐ SP 7 S92.055- Nondisplaced other extraarticular fracture of left calcaneus

☐ IQ 7 S92.056- **Nondisplaced other extraarticular fracture of unspecified calcaneus**

6 S92.06 Intraarticular fracture of calcaneus

☐ SP 7 S92.061- Displaced intraarticular fracture of right calcaneus

☐ SP 7 S92.062- Displaced intraarticular fracture of left calcaneus

☐ IQ 7 S92.063- **Displaced intraarticular fracture of unspecified calcaneus**

☐ SP 7 S92.064- Nondisplaced intraarticular fracture of right calcaneus

☐ SP 7 S92.065- Nondisplaced intraarticular fracture of left calcaneus

☐ IQ 7 S92.066- **Nondisplaced intraarticular fracture of unspecified calcaneus**

5 S92.1 Fracture of talus
Astragalus

6 S92.10 **Unspecified fracture of talus**

☐ SP 7 S92.101- **Unspecified fracture of right talus**

☐ SP 7 S92.102- **Unspecified fracture of left talus**

☐ IQ 7 S92.109- **Unspecified fracture of unspecified talus**

6 S92.11 Fracture of neck of talus

☐ SP 7 S92.111- Displaced fracture of neck of right talus

☐ SP 7 S92.112- Displaced fracture of neck of left talus

☐ IQ 7 S92.113- **Displaced fracture of neck of unspecified talus**

☐ SP 7 S92.114- Nondisplaced fracture of neck of right talus

☐ SP 7 S92.115- Nondisplaced fracture of neck of left talus

☐ IQ 7 S92.116- **Nondisplaced fracture of neck of unspecified talus**

6 S92.12 Fracture of body of talus

☐ SP 7 S92.121- Displaced fracture of body of right talus

☐ SP 7 S92.122- Displaced fracture of body of left talus

☐ IQ 7 S92.123- **Displaced fracture of body of unspecified talus**

☐ SP 7 S92.124- Nondisplaced fracture of body of right talus

☐ SP 7 S92.125- Nondisplaced fracture of body of left talus

☐ IQ 7 S92.126- **Nondisplaced fracture of body of unspecified talus**

6 S92.13 Fracture of posterior process of talus

☐ SP 7 S92.131- Displaced fracture of posterior process of right talus

☐ SP 7 S92.132- Displaced fracture of posterior process of left talus

☐ IQ 7 S92.133- **Displaced fracture of posterior process of unspecified talus**

☐ SP 7 S92.134- Nondisplaced fracture of posterior process of right talus

☐ SP 7 S92.135- Nondisplaced fracture of posterior process of left talus

☐ IQ 7 S92.136- **Nondisplaced fracture of posterior process of unspecified talus**

6 S92.14 Dome fracture of talus
EXCLUDES 1 osteochondritis dissecans (M93.2)

☐ SP 7 S92.141- Displaced dome fracture of right talus

☐ SP 7 S92.142- Displaced dome fracture of left talus

☐ IQ 7 S92.143- **Displaced dome fracture of unspecified talus**

☐ SP 7 S92.144- Nondisplaced dome fracture of right talus

☐ SP 7 S92.145- Nondisplaced dome fracture of left talus

Chapter 19

S00-T88

★ New ▲ Revised Px Primary SP PDGM Px SL Low CoM SH High CoM IQ Quest. Encounter H Hospice non-cancer Dx   Unspecified   M *Manifestation*

DecisionHealth's FY 2020 Complete Home Health ICD-10-CM Diagnosis Coding Manual

1625

⊟ **IQ** 7 **S92.146-** Nondisplaced dome fracture of unspecified talus

6 **S92.15** Avulsion fracture (chip fracture) of talus

⊟ **SP** 7 **S92.151-** Displaced avulsion fracture (chip fracture) of right talus

⊟ **SP** 7 **S92.152-** Displaced avulsion fracture (chip fracture) of left talus

⊟ **IQ** 7 **S92.153-** Displaced avulsion fracture (chip fracture) of unspecified talus

⊟ **SP** 7 **S92.154-** Nondisplaced avulsion fracture (chip fracture) of right talus

⊟ **SP** 7 **S92.155-** Nondisplaced avulsion fracture (chip fracture) of left talus

⊟ **IQ** 7 **S92.156-** Nondisplaced avulsion fracture (chip fracture) of unspecified talus

6 **S92.19** Other fracture of talus

⊟ **SP** 7 **S92.191-** Other fracture of right talus

⊟ **SP** 7 **S92.192-** Other fracture of left talus

⊟ **IQ** 7 **S92.199-** Other fracture of unspecified talus

5 **S92.2** Fracture of other and unspecified tarsal bone(s)

6 **S92.20** Fracture of unspecified tarsal bone(s)

⊟ **IQ** 7 **S92.201-** Fracture of unspecified tarsal bone(s) of right foot

⊟ **IQ** 7 **S92.202-** Fracture of unspecified tarsal bone(s) of left foot

⊟ **IQ** 7 **S92.209-** Fracture of unspecified tarsal bone(s) of unspecified foot

6 **S92.21** Fracture of cuboid bone

⊟ **SP** 7 **S92.211-** Displaced fracture of cuboid bone of right foot

⊟ **SP** 7 **S92.212-** Displaced fracture of cuboid bone of left foot

⊟ **IQ** 7 **S92.213-** Displaced fracture of cuboid bone of unspecified foot

⊟ **SP** 7 **S92.214-** Nondisplaced fracture of cuboid bone of right foot

⊟ **SP** 7 **S92.215-** Nondisplaced fracture of cuboid bone of left foot

⊟ **IQ** 7 **S92.216-** Nondisplaced fracture of cuboid bone of unspecified foot

6 **S92.22** Fracture of lateral cuneiform

⊟ **SP** 7 **S92.221-** Displaced fracture of lateral cuneiform of right foot

⊟ **SP** 7 **S92.222-** Displaced fracture of lateral cuneiform of left foot

⊟ **IQ** 7 **S92.223-** Displaced fracture of lateral cuneiform of unspecified foot

⊟ **SP** 7 **S92.224-** Nondisplaced fracture of lateral cuneiform of right foot

⊟ **SP** 7 **S92.225-** Nondisplaced fracture of lateral cuneiform of left foot

⊟ **IQ** 7 **S92.226-** Nondisplaced fracture of lateral cuneiform of unspecified foot

6 **S92.23** Fracture of intermediate cuneiform

⊟ **SP** 7 **S92.231-** Displaced fracture of intermediate cuneiform of right foot

⊟ **SP** 7 **S92.232-** Displaced fracture of intermediate cuneiform of left foot

⊟ **IQ** 7 **S92.233-** Displaced fracture of intermediate cuneiform of unspecified foot

⊟ **SP** 7 **S92.234-** Nondisplaced fracture of intermediate cuneiform of right foot

⊟ **SP** 7 **S92.235-** Nondisplaced fracture of intermediate cuneiform of left foot

⊟ **IQ** 7 **S92.236-** Nondisplaced fracture of intermediate cuneiform of unspecified foot

6 **S92.24** Fracture of medial cuneiform

⊟ **SP** 7 **S92.241-** Displaced fracture of medial cuneiform of right foot

⊟ **SP** 7 **S92.242-** Displaced fracture of medial cuneiform of left foot

⊟ **IQ** 7 **S92.243-** Displaced fracture of medial cuneiform of unspecified foot

⊟ **SP** 7 **S92.244-** Nondisplaced fracture of medial cuneiform of right foot

⊟ **SP** 7 **S92.245-** Nondisplaced fracture of medial cuneiform of left foot

⊟ **IQ** 7 **S92.246-** Nondisplaced fracture of medial cuneiform of unspecified foot

6 **S92.25** Fracture of navicular [scaphoid] of foot

⊟ **SP** 7 **S92.251-** Displaced fracture of navicular [scaphoid] of right foot

⊟ **SP** 7 **S92.252-** Displaced fracture of navicular [scaphoid] of left foot

⊟ **IQ** 7 **S92.253-** Displaced fracture of navicular [scaphoid] of unspecified foot

⊟ **SP** 7 **S92.254-** Nondisplaced fracture of navicular [scaphoid] of right foot

⊟ **SP** 7 **S92.255-** Nondisplaced fracture of navicular [scaphoid] of left foot

⊟ **IQ** 7 **S92.256-** Nondisplaced fracture of navicular [scaphoid] of unspecified foot

5 **S92.3** Fracture of metatarsal bone(s)
EXCLUDES 2 Physeal fracture of metatarsal (S99.1-)

6 **S92.30** Fracture of unspecified metatarsal bone(s)

⊟ **SP** **IQ** 7 **S92.301-** Fracture of unspecified metatarsal bone(s), right foot

⊟ **SP** **IQ** 7 **S92.302-** Fracture of unspecified metatarsal bone(s), left foot

⊟ **IQ** 7 **S92.309-** Fracture of unspecified metatarsal bone(s), unspecified foot

6 **S92.31** Fracture of first metatarsal bone

⊟ **SP** 7 **S92.311-** Displaced fracture of first metatarsal bone, right foot

⊟ **SP** 7 **S92.312-** Displaced fracture of first metatarsal bone, left foot

⊟ **IQ** 7 **S92.313-** Displaced fracture of first metatarsal bone, unspecified foot

⊟ **SP** 7 **S92.314-** Nondisplaced fracture of first metatarsal bone, right foot

4 4th digit required   5 5th digit required   6 6th digit required   7 7th digit required   7 7th digit placeholder   ✚ Additional code   ⊟ Laterality

1626   *DecisionHealth's* FY 2020 Complete Home Health ICD-10-CM Diagnosis Coding Manual

☰ **SP** 7 **S92.315-** Nondisplaced fracture of first metatarsal bone, left foot

☰ **IQ** 7 **S92.316-** Nondisplaced fracture of first metatarsal bone, unspecified foot

6 **S92.32** Fracture of second metatarsal bone

☰ **SP** 7 **S92.321-** Displaced fracture of second metatarsal bone, right foot

☰ **SP** 7 **S92.322-** Displaced fracture of second metatarsal bone, left foot

☰ **IQ** 7 **S92.323-** Displaced fracture of second metatarsal bone, unspecified foot

☰ **SP** 7 **S92.324-** Nondisplaced fracture of second metatarsal bone, right foot

☰ **SP** 7 **S92.325-** Nondisplaced fracture of second metatarsal bone, left foot

☰ **IQ** 7 **S92.326-** Nondisplaced fracture of second metatarsal bone, unspecified foot

6 **S92.33** Fracture of third metatarsal bone

☰ **SP** 7 **S92.331-** Displaced fracture of third metatarsal bone, right foot

☰ **SP** 7 **S92.332-** Displaced fracture of third metatarsal bone, left foot

☰ **IQ** 7 **S92.333-** Displaced fracture of third metatarsal bone, unspecified foot

☰ **SP** 7 **S92.334-** Nondisplaced fracture of third metatarsal bone, right foot

☰ **SP** 7 **S92.335-** Nondisplaced fracture of third metatarsal bone, left foot

☰ **IQ** 7 **S92.336-** Nondisplaced fracture of third metatarsal bone, unspecified foot

6 **S92.34** Fracture of fourth metatarsal bone

☰ **SP** 7 **S92.341-** Displaced fracture of fourth metatarsal bone, right foot

☰ **SP** 7 **S92.342-** Displaced fracture of fourth metatarsal bone, left foot

☰ **IQ** 7 **S92.343-** Displaced fracture of fourth metatarsal bone, unspecified foot

☰ **SP** 7 **S92.344-** Nondisplaced fracture of fourth metatarsal bone, right foot

☰ **SP** 7 **S92.345-** Nondisplaced fracture of fourth metatarsal bone, left foot

☰ **IQ** 7 **S92.346-** Nondisplaced fracture of fourth metatarsal bone, unspecified foot

6 **S92.35** Fracture of fifth metatarsal bone

☰ **SP** 7 **S92.351-** Displaced fracture of fifth metatarsal bone, right foot

☰ **SP** 7 **S92.352-** Displaced fracture of fifth metatarsal bone, left foot

☰ **IQ** 7 **S92.353-** Displaced fracture of fifth metatarsal bone, unspecified foot

☰ **SP** 7 **S92.354-** Nondisplaced fracture of fifth metatarsal bone, right foot

☰ **SP** 7 **S92.355-** Nondisplaced fracture of fifth metatarsal bone, left foot

☰ **IQ** 7 **S92.356-** Nondisplaced fracture of fifth metatarsal bone, unspecified foot

5 **S92.4** Fracture of great toe

EXCLUDES 2 Physeal fracture of phalanx of toe (S99.2-)

6 **S92.40** Unspecified fracture of great toe

☰ **SP** 7 **S92.401-** Displaced unspecified fracture of right great toe

☰ **SP** 7 **S92.402-** Displaced unspecified fracture of left great toe

☰ **IQ** 7 **S92.403-** Displaced unspecified fracture of unspecified great toe

☰ **SP** 7 **S92.404-** Nondisplaced unspecified fracture of right great toe

☰ **SP** 7 **S92.405-** Nondisplaced unspecified fracture of left great toe

☰ **IQ** 7 **S92.406-** Nondisplaced unspecified fracture of unspecified great toe

6 **S92.41** Fracture of proximal phalanx of great toe

☰ **SP** 7 **S92.411-** Displaced fracture of proximal phalanx of right great toe

☰ **SP** 7 **S92.412-** Displaced fracture of proximal phalanx of left great toe

☰ **IQ** 7 **S92.413-** Displaced fracture of proximal phalanx of unspecified great toe

☰ **SP** 7 **S92.414-** Nondisplaced fracture of proximal phalanx of right great toe

☰ **SP** 7 **S92.415-** Nondisplaced fracture of proximal phalanx of left great toe

☰ **IQ** 7 **S92.416-** Nondisplaced fracture of proximal phalanx of unspecified great toe

6 **S92.42** Fracture of distal phalanx of great toe

☰ **SP** 7 **S92.421-** Displaced fracture of distal phalanx of right great toe

☰ **SP** 7 **S92.422-** Displaced fracture of distal phalanx of left great toe

☰ **IQ** 7 **S92.423-** Displaced fracture of distal phalanx of unspecified great toe

☰ **SP** 7 **S92.424-** Nondisplaced fracture of distal phalanx of right great toe

☰ **SP** 7 **S92.425-** Nondisplaced fracture of distal phalanx of left great toe

☰ **IQ** 7 **S92.426-** Nondisplaced fracture of distal phalanx of unspecified great toe

6 **S92.49** Other fracture of great toe

☰ **SP** 7 **S92.491-** Other fracture of right great toe

☰ **SP** 7 **S92.492-** Other fracture of left great toe

☰ **IQ** 7 **S92.499-** Other fracture of unspecified great toe

5 **S92.5** Fracture of lesser toe(s)

EXCLUDES 2 Physeal fracture of phalanx of toe (S99.2-)

6 **S92.50** Unspecified fracture of lesser toe(s)

☰ **SP** **IQ** 7 **S92.501-** Displaced unspecified fracture of right lesser toe(s)

☰ **SP** **IQ** 7 **S92.502-** Displaced unspecified fracture of left lesser toe(s)

☰ **IQ** 7 **S92.503-** Displaced unspecified fracture of unspecified lesser toe(s)

☰ **IQ** 7 **S92.504-** Nondisplaced unspecified fracture of right lesser toe(s)

☰ **SP** **IQ** 7 **S92.505-** Nondisplaced unspecified fracture of left lesser toe(s)

★ New ▲ Revised Px Primary **SP** PDGM Px **SL** Low CoM **SH** High CoM **IQ** Quest. Encounter ⊞ Hospice non-cancer Dx Unspecified **M** *Manifestation*

DecisionHealth's FY 2020 Complete Home Health ICD-10-CM Diagnosis Coding Manual

1627

▣ !Q 7 S92.506- Nondisplaced unspecified fracture of unspecified lesser toe(s)

6 S92.51 Fracture of proximal phalanx of lesser toe(s)

▣ SP 7 S92.511- Displaced fracture of proximal phalanx of right lesser toe(s)

▣ SP 7 S92.512- Displaced fracture of proximal phalanx of left lesser toe(s)

▣ !Q 7 S92.513- Displaced fracture of proximal phalanx of unspecified lesser toe(s)

▣ SP 7 S92.514- Nondisplaced fracture of proximal phalanx of right lesser toe(s)

▣ SP 7 S92.515- Nondisplaced fracture of proximal phalanx of left lesser toe(s)

▣ !Q 7 S92.516- Nondisplaced fracture of proximal phalanx of unspecified lesser toe(s)

6 S92.52 Fracture of middle phalanx of lesser toe(s)

▣ SP 7 S92.521- Displaced fracture of middle phalanx of right lesser toe(s)

▣ SP 7 S92.522- Displaced fracture of middle phalanx of left lesser toe(s)

▣ !Q 7 S92.523- Displaced fracture of middle phalanx of unspecified lesser toe(s)

▣ SP 7 S92.524- Nondisplaced fracture of middle phalanx of right lesser toe(s)

▣ SP 7 S92.525- Nondisplaced fracture of middle phalanx of left lesser toe(s)

▣ !Q 7 S92.526- Nondisplaced fracture of middle phalanx of unspecified lesser toe(s)

6 S92.53 Fracture of distal phalanx of lesser toe(s)

▣ SP 7 S92.531- Displaced fracture of distal phalanx of right lesser toe(s)

▣ SP 7 S92.532- Displaced fracture of distal phalanx of left lesser toe(s)

▣ !Q 7 S92.533- Displaced fracture of distal phalanx of unspecified lesser toe(s)

▣ SP 7 S92.534- Nondisplaced fracture of distal phalanx of right lesser toe(s)

▣ SP 7 S92.535- Nondisplaced fracture of distal phalanx of left lesser toe(s)

▣ !Q 7 S92.536- Nondisplaced fracture of distal phalanx of unspecified lesser toe(s)

6 S92.59 Other fracture of lesser toe(s)

▣ SP 7 S92.591- Other fracture of right lesser toe(s)

▣ SP 7 S92.592- Other fracture of left lesser toe(s)

▣ !Q 7 S92.599- Other fracture of unspecified lesser toe(s)

5 S92.8 Other fracture of foot, except ankle

6 S92.81 Other fracture of foot
Sesamoid fracture of foot

CODING TIPS ✓ The sesamoid bones are a pair of small bones located on the bottom surface of the first metatarsal phalangeal joint within the tendons. Sesamoid fractures can be the result of a fall from a height, sports injury or overuse.

▣ SP 7 S92.811- Other fracture of right foot

▣ SP 7 S92.812- Other fracture of left foot

▣ !Q 7 S92.819- Other fracture of unspecified foot

5 S92.9 Unspecified fracture of foot and toe

6 S92.90 Unspecified fracture of foot

▣ SP 7 S92.901- Unspecified fracture of right foot

▣ SP 7 S92.902- Unspecified fracture of left foot

▣ !Q 7 S92.909- Unspecified fracture of unspecified foot

6 S92.91 Unspecified fracture of toe

▣ SP 7 S92.911- Unspecified fracture of right toe(s)

▣ SP 7 S92.912- Unspecified fracture of left toe(s)

▣ !Q 7 S92.919- Unspecified fracture of unspecified toe(s)

4 S93 Dislocation and sprain of joints and ligaments at ankle, foot and toe level

INCLUDES avulsion of joint or ligament of ankle, foot and toe
laceration of cartilage, joint or ligament of ankle, foot and toe
sprain of cartilage, joint or ligament of ankle, foot and toe
traumatic hemarthrosis of joint or ligament of ankle, foot and toe
traumatic rupture of joint or ligament of ankle, foot and toe
traumatic subluxation of joint or ligament of ankle, foot and toe
traumatic tear of joint or ligament of ankle, foot and toe

Code also:
any associated open wound
EXCLUDES 2 strain of muscle and tendon of ankle and foot (S96.-)

The appropriate 7th character is to be added to each code from category S93
A   initial encounter
D   subsequent encounter
S   sequela

5 S93.0 Subluxation and dislocation of ankle joint
Subluxation and dislocation of astragalus
Subluxation and dislocation of fibula, lower end
Subluxation and dislocation of talus
Subluxation and dislocation of tibia, lower end

▣ SP 7 S93.01X- Subluxation of right ankle joint

4 4th digit required   **5** 5th digit required   **6** 6th digit required   **7** 7th digit required   **7** 7th digit placeholder   **+** Additional code   **▣** Laterality

1628   *DecisionHealth's* FY 2020 Complete Home Health ICD-10-CM Diagnosis Coding Manual

Chapter 19

S00-T88

⊟ SP ⑤ S93.02X- Subluxation of left ankle joint

⊟ IQ ⑤ S93.03X- Subluxation of unspecified ankle joint

⊟ SP ⑤ S93.04X- Dislocation of right ankle joint

⊟ SP ⑤ S93.05X- Dislocation of left ankle joint

⊟ IQ ⑤ S93.06X- Dislocation of unspecified ankle joint

⑤ S93.1 Subluxation and dislocation of toe

⑥ S93.10 Unspecified subluxation and dislocation of toe

Dislocation of toe NOS
Subluxation of toe NOS

⊟ IQ ⑦ S93.101- Unspecified subluxation of right toe(s)

⊟ IQ ⑦ S93.102- Unspecified subluxation of left toe(s)

⊟ IQ ⑦ S93.103- Unspecified subluxation of unspecified toe(s)

⊟ IQ ⑦ S93.104- Unspecified dislocation of right toe(s)

⊟ IQ ⑦ S93.105- Unspecified dislocation of left toe(s)

⊟ IQ ⑦ S93.106- Unspecified dislocation of unspecified toe(s)

⑥ S93.11 Dislocation of interphalangeal joint

⊟ SP ⑦ S93.111- Dislocation of interphalangeal joint of right great toe

⊟ SP ⑦ S93.112- Dislocation of interphalangeal joint of left great toe

⊟ IQ ⑦ S93.113- Dislocation of interphalangeal joint of unspecified great toe

⊟ SP ⑦ S93.114- Dislocation of interphalangeal joint of right lesser toe(s)

⊟ SP ⑦ S93.115- Dislocation of interphalangeal joint of left lesser toe(s)

⊟ IQ ⑦ S93.116- Dislocation of interphalangeal joint of unspecified lesser toe(s)

⊟ IQ ⑦ S93.119- Dislocation of interphalangeal joint of unspecified toe(s)

⑥ S93.12 Dislocation of metatarsophalangeal joint

⊟ SP ⑦ S93.121- Dislocation of metatarsophalangeal joint of right great toe

⊟ SP ⑦ S93.122- Dislocation of metatarsophalangeal joint of left great toe

⊟ IQ ⑦ S93.123- Dislocation of metatarsophalangeal joint of unspecified great toe

⊟ SP ⑦ S93.124- Dislocation of metatarsophalangeal joint of right lesser toe(s)

⊟ SP ⑦ S93.125- Dislocation of metatarsophalangeal joint of left lesser toe(s)

⊟ IQ ⑦ S93.126- Dislocation of metatarsophalangeal joint of unspecified lesser toe(s)

⊟ IQ ⑦ S93.129- Dislocation of metatarsophalangeal joint of unspecified toe(s)

⑥ S93.13 Subluxation of interphalangeal joint

⊟ SP ⑦ S93.131- Subluxation of interphalangeal joint of right great toe

⊟ SP ⑦ S93.132- Subluxation of interphalangeal joint of left great toe

⊟ IQ ⑦ S93.133- Subluxation of interphalangeal joint of unspecified great toe

⊟ SP ⑦ S93.134- Subluxation of interphalangeal joint of right lesser toe(s)

⊟ SP ⑦ S93.135- Subluxation of interphalangeal joint of left lesser toe(s)

⊟ IQ ⑦ S93.136- Subluxation of interphalangeal joint of unspecified lesser toe(s)

⊟ IQ ⑦ S93.139- Subluxation of interphalangeal joint of unspecified toe(s)

⑥ S93.14 Subluxation of metatarsophalangeal joint

⊟ SP ⑦ S93.141- Subluxation of metatarsophalangeal joint of right great toe

⊟ SP ⑦ S93.142- Subluxation of metatarsophalangeal joint of left great toe

⊟ IQ ⑦ S93.143- Subluxation of metatarsophalangeal joint of unspecified great toe

⊟ SP ⑦ S93.144- Subluxation of metatarsophalangeal joint of right lesser toe(s)

⊟ SP ⑦ S93.145- Subluxation of metatarsophalangeal joint of left lesser toe(s)

⊟ IQ ⑦ S93.146- Subluxation of metatarsophalangeal joint of unspecified lesser toe(s)

⊟ IQ ⑦ S93.149- Subluxation of metatarsophalangeal joint of unspecified toe(s)

⑤ S93.3 Subluxation and dislocation of foot

EXCLUDES 2 dislocation of toe (S93.1-)

⑥ S93.30 Unspecified subluxation and dislocation of foot

Dislocation of foot NOS
Subluxation of foot NOS

⊟ IQ ⑦ S93.301- Unspecified subluxation of right foot

⊟ IQ ⑦ S93.302- Unspecified subluxation of left foot

⊟ IQ ⑦ S93.303- Unspecified subluxation of unspecified foot

⊟ IQ ⑦ S93.304- Unspecified dislocation of right foot

⊟ IQ ⑦ S93.305- Unspecified dislocation of left foot

⊟ IQ ⑦ S93.306- Unspecified dislocation of unspecified foot

⑥ S93.31 Subluxation and dislocation of tarsal joint

⊟ SP ⑦ S93.311- Subluxation of tarsal joint of right foot

⊟ SP ⑦ S93.312- Subluxation of tarsal joint of left foot

⊟ IQ ⑦ S93.313- Subluxation of tarsal joint of unspecified foot

⊟ SP ⑦ S93.314- Dislocation of tarsal joint of right foot

★ New ▲ Revised Px Primary SP PDGM Px SL Low CoM SH High CoM IQ Quest. Encounter H Hospice non-cancer Dx Unspecified M Manifestation

DecisionHealth's FY 2020 Complete Home Health ICD-10-CM Diagnosis Coding Manual

1629

☰ SP 7 **S93.315-** Dislocation of tarsal joint of left foot

☰ IQ 7 **S93.316-** Dislocation of tarsal joint of unspecified foot

6 **S93.32** Subluxation and dislocation of tarsometatarsal joint

☰ SP 7 **S93.321-** Subluxation of tarsometatarsal joint of right foot

☰ SP 7 **S93.322-** Subluxation of tarsometatarsal joint of left foot

☰ IQ 7 **S93.323-** Subluxation of tarsometatarsal joint of unspecified foot

☰ SP 7 **S93.324-** Dislocation of tarsometatarsal joint of right foot

☰ SP 7 **S93.325-** Dislocation of tarsometatarsal joint of left foot

☰ IQ 7 **S93.326-** Dislocation of tarsometatarsal joint of unspecified foot

6 **S93.33** Other subluxation and dislocation of foot

☰ SP 7 **S93.331-** Other subluxation of right foot

☰ SP 7 **S93.332-** Other subluxation of left foot

☰ IQ 7 **S93.333-** Other subluxation of unspecified foot

☰ SP 7 **S93.334-** Other dislocation of right foot

☰ SP 7 **S93.335-** Other dislocation of left foot

☰ IQ 7 **S93.336-** Other dislocation of unspecified foot

5 **S93.4** Sprain of ankle
> **EXCLUDES 2** injury of Achilles tendon (S86.0-)

6 **S93.40** Sprain of unspecified ligament of ankle

Sprain of ankle NOS
Sprained ankle NOS

☰ SP 7 **S93.401-** Sprain of unspecified ligament of right ankle

☰ SP 7 **S93.402-** Sprain of unspecified ligament of left ankle

☰ IQ 7 **S93.409-** Sprain of unspecified ligament of unspecified ankle

6 **S93.41** Sprain of calcaneofibular ligament

☰ SP 7 **S93.411-** Sprain of calcaneofibular ligament of right ankle

☰ SP 7 **S93.412-** Sprain of calcaneofibular ligament of left ankle

☰ IQ 7 **S93.419-** Sprain of calcaneofibular ligament of unspecified ankle

6 **S93.42** Sprain of deltoid ligament

☰ SP 7 **S93.421-** Sprain of deltoid ligament of right ankle

☰ SP 7 **S93.422-** Sprain of deltoid ligament of left ankle

☰ IQ 7 **S93.429-** Sprain of deltoid ligament of unspecified ankle

6 **S93.43** Sprain of tibiofibular ligament

☰ SP 7 **S93.431-** Sprain of tibiofibular ligament of right ankle

☰ SP 7 **S93.432-** Sprain of tibiofibular ligament of left ankle

☰ IQ 7 **S93.439-** Sprain of tibiofibular ligament of unspecified ankle

6 **S93.49** Sprain of other ligament of ankle
Sprain of internal collateral ligament

Sprain of talofibular ligament

☰ SP 7 **S93.491-** Sprain of other ligament of right ankle

☰ SP 7 **S93.492-** Sprain of other ligament of left ankle

☰ IQ 7 **S93.499-** Sprain of other ligament of unspecified ankle

5 **S93.5** Sprain of toe

6 **S93.50** Unspecified sprain of toe

☰ SP 7 **S93.501-** Unspecified sprain of right great toe

☰ SP 7 **S93.502-** Unspecified sprain of left great toe

☰ IQ 7 **S93.503-** Unspecified sprain of unspecified great toe

☰ SP 7 **S93.504-** Unspecified sprain of right lesser toe(s)

☰ SP 7 **S93.505-** Unspecified sprain of left lesser toe(s)

☰ IQ 7 **S93.506-** Unspecified sprain of unspecified lesser toe(s)

☰ IQ 7 **S93.509-** Unspecified sprain of unspecified toe(s)

6 **S93.51** Sprain of interphalangeal joint of toe

☰ SP 7 **S93.511-** Sprain of interphalangeal joint of right great toe

☰ SP 7 **S93.512-** Sprain of interphalangeal joint of left great toe

☰ IQ 7 **S93.513-** Sprain of interphalangeal joint of unspecified great toe

☰ SP 7 **S93.514-** Sprain of interphalangeal joint of right lesser toe(s)

☰ SP 7 **S93.515-** Sprain of interphalangeal joint of left lesser toe(s)

☰ IQ 7 **S93.516-** Sprain of interphalangeal joint of unspecified lesser toe(s)

☰ IQ 7 **S93.519-** Sprain of interphalangeal joint of unspecified toe(s)

6 **S93.52** Sprain of metatarsophalangeal joint of toe

☰ SP 7 **S93.521-** Sprain of metatarsophalangeal joint of right great toe

☰ SP 7 **S93.522-** Sprain of metatarsophalangeal joint of left great toe

☰ IQ 7 **S93.523-** Sprain of metatarsophalangeal joint of unspecified great toe

☰ SP 7 **S93.524-** Sprain of metatarsophalangeal joint of right lesser toe(s)

☰ SP 7 **S93.525-** Sprain of metatarsophalangeal joint of left lesser toe(s)

☰ IQ 7 **S93.526-** Sprain of metatarsophalangeal joint of unspecified lesser toe(s)

☰ IQ 7 **S93.529-** Sprain of metatarsophalangeal joint of unspecified toe(s)

5 **S93.6** Sprain of foot
> **EXCLUDES 2** sprain of metatarsophalangeal joint of toe (S93.52-)
> sprain of toe (S93.5-)

6 **S93.60** Unspecified sprain of foot

☰ SP 7 **S93.601-** Unspecified sprain of right foot

☰ SP 7 **S93.602-** Unspecified sprain of left foot

☰ IQ 7 **S93.609-** Unspecified sprain of unspecified foot

---

4 4th digit required   5 5th digit required   6 6th digit required   7 7th digit required   7 7th digit placeholder   + Additional code   ☰ Laterality

6 **S93.61** Sprain of tarsal ligament of foot

☰ SP 7 **S93.611-** Sprain of tarsal ligament of right foot

☰ SP 7 **S93.612-** Sprain of tarsal ligament of left foot

☰ IQ 7 **S93.619-** Sprain of tarsal ligament of unspecified foot

6 **S93.62** Sprain of tarsometatarsal ligament of foot

☰ SP 7 **S93.621-** Sprain of tarsometatarsal ligament of right foot

☰ SP 7 **S93.622-** Sprain of tarsometatarsal ligament of left foot

☰ IQ 7 **S93.629-** Sprain of tarsometatarsal ligament of unspecified foot

6 **S93.69** Other sprain of foot

☰ SP 7 **S93.691-** Other sprain of right foot

☰ SP 7 **S93.692-** Other sprain of left foot

☰ IQ 7 **S93.699-** Other sprain of unspecified foot

4 **S94** Injury of nerves at ankle and foot level
Code also:
any associated open wound (S91.-)

The appropriate 7th character is to be added to each code from category S94
A   initial encounter
D   subsequent encounter
S   sequela

5 **S94.0** Injury of lateral plantar nerve

☰ IQ 7 **S94.00X-** Injury of lateral plantar nerve, unspecified leg

☰ SP 7 **S94.01X-** Injury of lateral plantar nerve, right leg

☰ SP 7 **S94.02X-** Injury of lateral plantar nerve, left leg

5 **S94.1** Injury of medial plantar nerve

☰ IQ 7 **S94.10X-** Injury of medial plantar nerve, unspecified leg

☰ SP 7 **S94.11X-** Injury of medial plantar nerve, right leg

☰ SP 7 **S94.12X-** Injury of medial plantar nerve, left leg

5 **S94.2** Injury of deep peroneal nerve at ankle and foot level
Injury of terminal, lateral branch of deep peroneal nerve

☰ IQ 7 **S94.20X-** Injury of deep peroneal nerve at ankle and foot level, unspecified leg

☰ SP 7 **S94.21X-** Injury of deep peroneal nerve at ankle and foot level, right leg

☰ SP 7 **S94.22X-** Injury of deep peroneal nerve at ankle and foot level, left leg

5 **S94.3** Injury of cutaneous sensory nerve at ankle and foot level

☰ IQ 7 **S94.30X-** Injury of cutaneous sensory nerve at ankle and foot level, unspecified leg

☰ SP 7 **S94.31X-** Injury of cutaneous sensory nerve at ankle and foot level, right leg

☰ SP 7 **S94.32X-** Injury of cutaneous sensory nerve at ankle and foot level, left leg

5 **S94.8** Injury of other nerves at ankle and foot level

6 **S94.8X** Injury of other nerves at ankle and foot level

☰ SP 7 **S94.8X1-** Injury of other nerves at ankle and foot level, right leg

☰ SP 7 **S94.8X2-** Injury of other nerves at ankle and foot level, left leg

☰ IQ 7 **S94.8X9-** Injury of other nerves at ankle and foot level, unspecified leg

5 **S94.9** Injury of unspecified nerve at ankle and foot level

☰ IQ 7 **S94.90X-** Injury of unspecified nerve at ankle and foot level, unspecified leg

☰ IQ 7 **S94.91X-** Injury of unspecified nerve at ankle and foot level, right leg

☰ IQ 7 **S94.92X-** Injury of unspecified nerve at ankle and foot level, left leg

4 **S95** Injury of blood vessels at ankle and foot level
Code also:
any associated open wound (S91.-)
EXCLUDES 2 injury of posterior tibial artery and vein (S85.1-, S85.8-)

The appropriate 7th character is to be added to each code from category S95
A   initial encounter
D   subsequent encounter
S   sequela

5 **S95.0** Injury of dorsal artery of foot

6 **S95.00** Unspecified injury of dorsal artery of foot

☰ IQ 7 **S95.001-** Unspecified injury of dorsal artery of right foot

☰ IQ 7 **S95.002-** Unspecified injury of dorsal artery of left foot

☰ IQ 7 **S95.009-** Unspecified injury of dorsal artery of unspecified foot

6 **S95.01** Laceration of dorsal artery of foot

☰ SP 7 **S95.011-** Laceration of dorsal artery of right foot

☰ SP 7 **S95.012-** Laceration of dorsal artery of left foot

☰ IQ 7 **S95.019-** Laceration of dorsal artery of unspecified foot

6 **S95.09** Other specified injury of dorsal artery of foot

☰ SP 7 **S95.091-** Other specified injury of dorsal artery of right foot

☰ SP 7 **S95.092-** Other specified injury of dorsal artery of left foot

☰ IQ 7 **S95.099-** Other specified injury of dorsal artery of unspecified foot

5 **S95.1** Injury of plantar artery of foot

6 **S95.10** Unspecified injury of plantar artery of foot

☰ IQ 7 **S95.101-** Unspecified injury of plantar artery of right foot

☰ IQ 7 **S95.102-** Unspecified injury of plantar artery of left foot

☰ IQ 7 **S95.109-** Unspecified injury of plantar artery of unspecified foot

6 **S95.11** Laceration of plantar artery of foot

☰ SP 7 **S95.111-** Laceration of plantar artery of right foot

☰ SP 7 **S95.112-** Laceration of plantar artery of left foot

★ New   ▲ Revised   Px Primary   SP PDGM Px   SL Low CoM   SH High CoM   IQ Quest. Encounter   H Hospice non-cancer Dx   Unspecified   M *Manifestation*

DecisionHealth's FY 2020 Complete Home Health ICD-10-CM Diagnosis Coding Manual
1631

⊟ IQ 7 **S95.119-** **Laceration of plantar artery of unspecified foot**

6 S95.19   Other specified injury of plantar artery of foot

⊟ SP 7 S95.191-   Other specified injury of plantar artery of right foot

⊟ SP 7 S95.192-   Other specified injury of plantar artery of left foot

⊟ IQ 7 **S95.199-** **Other specified injury of plantar artery of unspecified foot**

5 S95.2   Injury of dorsal vein of foot

6 S95.20   **Unspecified injury of dorsal vein of foot**

⊟ IQ 7 **S95.201-** **Unspecified injury of dorsal vein of right foot**

⊟ IQ 7 **S95.202-** **Unspecified injury of dorsal vein of left foot**

⊟ IQ 7 **S95.209-** **Unspecified injury of dorsal vein of unspecified foot**

6 S95.21   Laceration of dorsal vein of foot

⊟ SP 7 S95.211-   Laceration of dorsal vein of right foot

⊟ SP 7 S95.212-   Laceration of dorsal vein of left foot

⊟ IQ 7 **S95.219-** **Laceration of dorsal vein of unspecified foot**

6 S95.29   Other specified injury of dorsal vein of foot

⊟ SP 7 S95.291-   Other specified injury of dorsal vein of right foot

⊟ SP 7 S95.292-   Other specified injury of dorsal vein of left foot

⊟ IQ 7 **S95.299-** **Other specified injury of dorsal vein of unspecified foot**

5 S95.8   Injury of other blood vessels at ankle and foot level

6 S95.80   **Unspecified injury of other blood vessels at ankle and foot level**

⊟ IQ 7 **S95.801-** **Unspecified injury of other blood vessels at ankle and foot level, right leg**

⊟ IQ 7 **S95.802-** **Unspecified injury of other blood vessels at ankle and foot level, left leg**

⊟ IQ 7 **S95.809-** **Unspecified injury of other blood vessels at ankle and foot level, unspecified leg**

6 S95.81   Laceration of other blood vessels at ankle and foot level

⊟ SP 7 S95.811-   Laceration of other blood vessels at ankle and foot level, right leg

⊟ SP 7 S95.812-   Laceration of other blood vessels at ankle and foot level, left leg

⊟ IQ 7 **S95.819-** **Laceration of other blood vessels at ankle and foot level, unspecified leg**

6 S95.89   Other specified injury of other blood vessels at ankle and foot level

⊟ SP 7 S95.891-   Other specified injury of other blood vessels at ankle and foot level, right leg

⊟ SP 7 S95.892-   Other specified injury of other blood vessels at ankle and foot level, left leg

⊟ IQ 7 **S95.899-** **Other specified injury of other blood vessels at ankle and foot level, unspecified leg**

5 S95.9   **Injury of unspecified blood vessel at ankle and foot level**

6 S95.90   **Unspecified injury of unspecified blood vessel at ankle and foot level**

⊟ IQ 7 **S95.901-** **Unspecified injury of unspecified blood vessel at ankle and foot level, right leg**

⊟ IQ 7 **S95.902-** **Unspecified injury of unspecified blood vessel at ankle and foot level, left leg**

⊟ IQ 7 **S95.909-** **Unspecified injury of unspecified blood vessel at ankle and foot level, unspecified leg**

6 S95.91   **Laceration of unspecified blood vessel at ankle and foot level**

⊟ SP 7 **S95.911-** **Laceration of unspecified blood vessel at ankle and foot level, right leg**

⊟ SP 7 **S95.912-** **Laceration of unspecified blood vessel at ankle and foot level, left leg**

⊟ IQ 7 **S95.919-** **Laceration of unspecified blood vessel at ankle and foot level, unspecified leg**

6 S95.99   **Other specified injury of unspecified blood vessel at ankle and foot level**

⊟ IQ 7 **S95.991-** **Other specified injury of unspecified blood vessel at ankle and foot level, right leg**

⊟ IQ 7 **S95.992-** **Other specified injury of unspecified blood vessel at ankle and foot level, left leg**

⊟ IQ 7 **S95.999-** **Other specified injury of unspecified blood vessel at ankle and foot level, unspecified leg**

4 S96   Injury of muscle and tendon at ankle and foot level
Code also:
   any associated open wound (S91.-)
   EXCLUDES 2   injury of Achilles tendon (S86.0-)
      sprain of joints and ligaments of ankle and foot (S93.-)

The appropriate 7th character is to be added to each code from category S96
A   initial encounter
D   subsequent encounter
S   sequela

5 S96.0   Injury of muscle and tendon of long flexor muscle of toe at ankle and foot level

6 S96.00   **Unspecified injury of muscle and tendon of long flexor muscle of toe at ankle and foot level**

⊟ IQ 7 **S96.001-** **Unspecified injury of muscle and tendon of long flexor muscle of toe at ankle and foot level, right foot**

---

4 4th digit required   5 5th digit required   6 6th digit required   7 7th digit required   ⊘ 7th digit placeholder   + Additional code   ⊟ Laterality

1632   *DecisionHealth's* FY 2020 Complete Home Health ICD-10-CM Diagnosis Coding Manual

Chapter 19

S00-T88

▤ **IQ** **7** S96.002- **Unspecified injury of muscle and tendon of long flexor muscle of toe at ankle and foot level, left foot**

▤ **IQ** **7** S96.009- **Unspecified injury of muscle and tendon of long flexor muscle of toe at ankle and foot level, unspecified foot**

6 S96.01 Strain of muscle and tendon of long flexor muscle of toe at ankle and foot level

▤ **SP** **7** S96.011- Strain of muscle and tendon of long flexor muscle of toe at ankle and foot level, right foot

▤ **SP** **7** S96.012- Strain of muscle and tendon of long flexor muscle of toe at ankle and foot level, left foot

▤ **IQ** **7** S96.019- **Strain of muscle and tendon of long flexor muscle of toe at ankle and foot level, unspecified foot**

6 S96.02 Laceration of muscle and tendon of long flexor muscle of toe at ankle and foot level

▤ **SP** **7** S96.021- Laceration of muscle and tendon of long flexor muscle of toe at ankle and foot level, right foot

▤ **SP** **7** S96.022- Laceration of muscle and tendon of long flexor muscle of toe at ankle and foot level, left foot

▤ **IQ** **7** S96.029- **Laceration of muscle and tendon of long flexor muscle of toe at ankle and foot level, unspecified foot**

6 S96.09 Other injury of muscle and tendon of long flexor muscle of toe at ankle and foot level

▤ **SP** **7** S96.091- Other injury of muscle and tendon of long flexor muscle of toe at ankle and foot level, right foot

▤ **SP** **7** S96.092- Other injury of muscle and tendon of long flexor muscle of toe at ankle and foot level, left foot

▤ **IQ** **7** S96.099- **Other injury of muscle and tendon of long flexor muscle of toe at ankle and foot level, unspecified foot**

5 S96.1 Injury of muscle and tendon of long extensor muscle of toe at ankle and foot level

6 S96.10 **Unspecified injury of muscle and tendon of long extensor muscle of toe at ankle and foot level**

▤ **IQ** **7** S96.101- **Unspecified injury of muscle and tendon of long extensor muscle of toe at ankle and foot level, right foot**

▤ **IQ** **7** S96.102- **Unspecified injury of muscle and tendon of long extensor muscle of toe at ankle and foot level, left foot**

▤ **IQ** **7** S96.109- **Unspecified injury of muscle and tendon of long extensor muscle of toe at ankle and foot level, unspecified foot**

6 S96.11 Strain of muscle and tendon of long extensor muscle of toe at ankle and foot level

▤ **SP** **7** S96.111- Strain of muscle and tendon of long extensor muscle of toe at ankle and foot level, right foot

▤ **SP** **7** S96.112- Strain of muscle and tendon of long extensor muscle of toe at ankle and foot level, left foot

▤ **IQ** **7** S96.119- **Strain of muscle and tendon of long extensor muscle of toe at ankle and foot level, unspecified foot**

6 S96.12 Laceration of muscle and tendon of long extensor muscle of toe at ankle and foot level

▤ **SP** **7** S96.121- Laceration of muscle and tendon of long extensor muscle of toe at ankle and foot level, right foot

▤ **SP** **7** S96.122- Laceration of muscle and tendon of long extensor muscle of toe at ankle and foot level, left foot

▤ **IQ** **7** S96.129- **Laceration of muscle and tendon of long extensor muscle of toe at ankle and foot level, unspecified foot**

6 S96.19 Other specified injury of muscle and tendon of long extensor muscle of toe at ankle and foot level

▤ **SP** **7** S96.191- Other specified injury of muscle and tendon of long extensor muscle of toe at ankle and foot level, right foot

▤ **SP** **7** S96.192- Other specified injury of muscle and tendon of long extensor muscle of toe at ankle and foot level, left foot

▤ **IQ** **7** S96.199- **Other specified injury of muscle and tendon of long extensor muscle of toe at ankle and foot level, unspecified foot**

5 S96.2 Injury of intrinsic muscle and tendon at ankle and foot level

6 S96.20 **Unspecified injury of intrinsic muscle and tendon at ankle and foot level**

▤ **IQ** **7** S96.201- **Unspecified injury of intrinsic muscle and tendon at ankle and foot level, right foot**

▤ **IQ** **7** S96.202- **Unspecified injury of intrinsic muscle and tendon at ankle and foot level, left foot**

▤ **IQ** **7** S96.209- **Unspecified injury of intrinsic muscle and tendon at ankle and foot level, unspecified foot**

6 S96.21 Strain of intrinsic muscle and tendon at ankle and foot level

▤ **SP** **7** S96.211- Strain of intrinsic muscle and tendon at ankle and foot level, right foot

▤ **SP** **7** S96.212- Strain of intrinsic muscle and tendon at ankle and foot level, left foot

▤ **IQ** **7** S96.219- **Strain of intrinsic muscle and tendon at ankle and foot level, unspecified foot**

★ New ▲ Revised Px Primary **SP** PDGM Px **SL** Low CoM **SH** High CoM **IQ** Quest. Encounter Ⓗ Hospice non-cancer Dx   Unspecified   **M** *Manifestation*

DecisionHealth's FY 2020 Complete Home Health ICD-10-CM Diagnosis Coding Manual   1633

6 **S96.22**   Laceration of intrinsic muscle and tendon at ankle and foot level

☲ SP 7 **S96.221-**   Laceration of intrinsic muscle and tendon at ankle and foot level, right foot

☲ SP 7 **S96.222-**   Laceration of intrinsic muscle and tendon at ankle and foot level, left foot

☲ IQ 7 **S96.229-**   Laceration of intrinsic muscle and tendon at ankle and foot level, unspecified foot

6 **S96.29**   Other specified injury of intrinsic muscle and tendon at ankle and foot level

☲ SP 7 **S96.291-**   Other specified injury of intrinsic muscle and tendon at ankle and foot level, right foot

☲ SP 7 **S96.292-**   Other specified injury of intrinsic muscle and tendon at ankle and foot level, left foot

☲ IQ 7 **S96.299-**   Other specified injury of intrinsic muscle and tendon at ankle and foot level, unspecified foot

5 **S96.8**   Injury of other specified muscles and tendons at ankle and foot level

6 **S96.80**   Unspecified injury of other specified muscles and tendons at ankle and foot level

☲ IQ 7 **S96.801-**   Unspecified injury of other specified muscles and tendons at ankle and foot level, right foot

☲ IQ 7 **S96.802-**   Unspecified injury of other specified muscles and tendons at ankle and foot level, left foot

☲ IQ 7 **S96.809-**   Unspecified injury of other specified muscles and tendons at ankle and foot level, unspecified foot

6 **S96.81**   Strain of other specified muscles and tendons at ankle and foot level

☲ SP 7 **S96.811-**   Strain of other specified muscles and tendons at ankle and foot level, right foot

☲ SP 7 **S96.812-**   Strain of other specified muscles and tendons at ankle and foot level, left foot

☲ IQ 7 **S96.819-**   Strain of other specified muscles and tendons at ankle and foot level, unspecified foot

6 **S96.82**   Laceration of other specified muscles and tendons at ankle and foot level

☲ SP 7 **S96.821-**   Laceration of other specified muscles and tendons at ankle and foot level, right foot

☲ SP 7 **S96.822-**   Laceration of other specified muscles and tendons at ankle and foot level, left foot

☲ IQ 7 **S96.829-**   Laceration of other specified muscles and tendons at ankle and foot level, unspecified foot

6 **S96.89**   Other specified injury of other specified muscles and tendons at ankle and foot level

☲ SP 7 **S96.891-**   Other specified injury of other specified muscles and tendons at ankle and foot level, right foot

☲ SP 7 **S96.892-**   Other specified injury of other specified muscles and tendons at ankle and foot level, left foot

☲ IQ 7 **S96.899-**   Other specified injury of other specified muscles and tendons at ankle and foot level, unspecified foot

5 **S96.9**   Injury of unspecified muscle and tendon at ankle and foot level

6 **S96.90**   Unspecified injury of unspecified muscle and tendon at ankle and foot level

☲ IQ 7 **S96.901-**   Unspecified injury of unspecified muscle and tendon at ankle and foot level, right foot

☲ IQ 7 **S96.902-**   Unspecified injury of unspecified muscle and tendon at ankle and foot level, left foot

☲ IQ 7 **S96.909-**   Unspecified injury of unspecified muscle and tendon at ankle and foot level, unspecified foot

6 **S96.91**   Strain of unspecified muscle and tendon at ankle and foot level

☲ SP 7 **S96.911-**   Strain of unspecified muscle and tendon at ankle and foot level, right foot

☲ SP 7 **S96.912-**   Strain of unspecified muscle and tendon at ankle and foot level, left foot

☲ IQ 7 **S96.919-**   Strain of unspecified muscle and tendon at ankle and foot level, unspecified foot

6 **S96.92**   Laceration of unspecified muscle and tendon at ankle and foot level

☲ SP 7 **S96.921-**   Laceration of unspecified muscle and tendon at ankle and foot level, right foot

☲ SP 7 **S96.922-**   Laceration of unspecified muscle and tendon at ankle and foot level, left foot

☲ IQ 7 **S96.929-**   Laceration of unspecified muscle and tendon at ankle and foot level, unspecified foot

6 **S96.99**   Other specified injury of unspecified muscle and tendon at ankle and foot level

☲ IQ 7 **S96.991-**   Other specified injury of unspecified muscle and tendon at ankle and foot level, right foot

☲ IQ 7 **S96.992-**   Other specified injury of unspecified muscle and tendon at ankle and foot level, left foot

☲ IQ 7 **S96.999-**   Other specified injury of unspecified muscle and tendon at ankle and foot level, unspecified foot

➕ 4 **S97**   Crushing injury of ankle and foot
Use additional code(s) for all associated injuries

---

4 4th digit required   5 5th digit required   6 6th digit required   7 7th digit required   7 7th digit placeholder   ➕ Additional code   ☲ Laterality

The appropriate 7th character is to be added to each code from category S97
A   initial encounter
D   subsequent encounter
S   sequela

✚ 5 **S97.0**   **Crushing injury of ankle**

▱ IQ ✚ 7 **S97.00X-**   **Crushing injury of unspecified ankle**

▱ SP ✚ 7 **S97.01X-**   **Crushing injury of right ankle**

▱ SP ✚ 7 **S97.02X-**   **Crushing injury of left ankle**

✚ 5 **S97.1**   **Crushing injury of toe**

✚ 6 **S97.10**   **Crushing injury of unspecified toe(s)**

▱ IQ ✚ 7 **S97.101-**   **Crushing injury of unspecified right toe(s)**

▱ IQ ✚ 7 **S97.102-**   **Crushing injury of unspecified left toe(s)**

▱ IQ ✚ 7 **S97.109-**   **Crushing injury of unspecified toe(s)**
Crushing injury of toe NOS

✚ 6 **S97.11**   **Crushing injury of great toe**

▱ SP ✚ 7 **S97.111-**   **Crushing injury of right great toe**

▱ SP ✚ 7 **S97.112-**   **Crushing injury of left great toe**

▱ IQ ✚ 7 **S97.119-**   **Crushing injury of unspecified great toe**

✚ 6 **S97.12**   **Crushing injury of lesser toe(s)**

▱ SP ✚ 7 **S97.121-**   **Crushing injury of right lesser toe(s)**

▱ SP ✚ 7 **S97.122-**   **Crushing injury of left lesser toe(s)**

▱ IQ ✚ 7 **S97.129-**   **Crushing injury of unspecified lesser toe(s)**

✚ 5 **S97.8**   **Crushing injury of foot**

▱ IQ ✚ 7 **S97.80X-**   **Crushing injury of unspecified foot**
Crushing injury of foot NOS

▱ SP ✚ 7 **S97.81X-**   **Crushing injury of right foot**

▱ SP ✚ 7 **S97.82X-**   **Crushing injury of left foot**

4 **S98**   **Traumatic amputation of ankle and foot**
An amputation not identified as partial or complete should be coded to complete

The appropriate 7th character is to be added to each code from category S98
A   initial encounter
D   subsequent encounter
S   sequela

CODING TIPS ✓   Use these codes only when the amputation was due to trauma. There is no need for adding Z89 with traumatic amputations. See Z47.81 for care of amputations not due to trauma.

5 **S98.0**   **Traumatic amputation of foot at ankle level**

6 **S98.01**   **Complete traumatic amputation of foot at ankle level**

▱ SP 7 **S98.011-**   **Complete traumatic amputation of right foot at ankle level**

▱ SP 7 **S98.012-**   **Complete traumatic amputation of left foot at ankle level**

▱ IQ 7 **S98.019-**   **Complete traumatic amputation of unspecified foot at ankle level**

6 **S98.02**   **Partial traumatic amputation of foot at ankle level**

▱ SP 7 **S98.021-**   **Partial traumatic amputation of right foot at ankle level**

▱ SP 7 **S98.022-**   **Partial traumatic amputation of left foot at ankle level**

▱ IQ 7 **S98.029-**   **Partial traumatic amputation of unspecified foot at ankle level**

5 **S98.1**   **Traumatic amputation of one toe**

6 **S98.11**   **Complete traumatic amputation of great toe**

▱ SP 7 **S98.111-**   **Complete traumatic amputation of right great toe**

▱ SP 7 **S98.112-**   **Complete traumatic amputation of left great toe**

▱ IQ 7 **S98.119-**   **Complete traumatic amputation of unspecified great toe**

6 **S98.12**   **Partial traumatic amputation of great toe**

▱ SP 7 **S98.121-**   **Partial traumatic amputation of right great toe**

▱ SP 7 **S98.122-**   **Partial traumatic amputation of left great toe**

▱ IQ 7 **S98.129-**   **Partial traumatic amputation of unspecified great toe**

6 **S98.13**   **Complete traumatic amputation of one lesser toe**
Traumatic amputation of toe NOS

▱ SP 7 **S98.131-**   **Complete traumatic amputation of one right lesser toe**

▱ SP 7 **S98.132-**   **Complete traumatic amputation of one left lesser toe**

▱ IQ 7 **S98.139-**   **Complete traumatic amputation of one unspecified lesser toe**

6 **S98.14**   **Partial traumatic amputation of one lesser toe**

▱ SP 7 **S98.141-**   **Partial traumatic amputation of one right lesser toe**

▱ SP 7 **S98.142-**   **Partial traumatic amputation of one left lesser toe**

▱ IQ 7 **S98.149-**   **Partial traumatic amputation of one unspecified lesser toe**

5 **S98.2**   **Traumatic amputation of two or more lesser toes**

6 **S98.21**   **Complete traumatic amputation of two or more lesser toes**

▱ SP 7 **S98.211-**   **Complete traumatic amputation of two or more right lesser toes**

▱ SP 7 **S98.212-**   **Complete traumatic amputation of two or more left lesser toes**

▱ IQ 7 **S98.219-**   **Complete traumatic amputation of two or more unspecified lesser toes**

6 **S98.22**   **Partial traumatic amputation of two or more lesser toes**

▱ SP 7 **S98.221-**   **Partial traumatic amputation of two or more right lesser toes**

▱ SP 7 **S98.222-**   **Partial traumatic amputation of two or more left lesser toes**

▱ IQ 7 **S98.229-**   **Partial traumatic amputation of two or more unspecified lesser toes**

5 **S98.3**   **Traumatic amputation of midfoot**

6 **S98.31**   **Complete traumatic amputation of midfoot**

✭ New ▲ Revised   Px Primary   SP PDGM Px   SL Low CoM   SH High CoM   IQ Quest. Encounter   H Hospice non-cancer Dx   Unspecified   M *Manifestation*

⊟ **SP** 7 **S98.311-** Complete traumatic amputation of right midfoot

⊟ **SP** 7 **S98.312-** Complete traumatic amputation of left midfoot

⊟ **IQ** 7 **S98.319-** Complete traumatic amputation of unspecified midfoot

6 **S98.32** Partial traumatic amputation of midfoot

⊟ **SP** 7 **S98.321-** Partial traumatic amputation of right midfoot

⊟ **SP** 7 **S98.322-** Partial traumatic amputation of left midfoot

⊟ **IQ** 7 **S98.329-** Partial traumatic amputation of unspecified midfoot

5 **S98.9** Traumatic amputation of foot, level unspecified

6 **S98.91** Complete traumatic amputation of foot, level unspecified

⊟ **SP** 7 **S98.911-** Complete traumatic amputation of right foot, level unspecified

⊟ **SP** 7 **S98.912-** Complete traumatic amputation of left foot, level unspecified

⊟ **IQ** 7 **S98.919-** Complete traumatic amputation of unspecified foot, level unspecified

6 **S98.92** Partial traumatic amputation of foot, level unspecified

⊟ **SP** 7 **S98.921-** Partial traumatic amputation of right foot, level unspecified

⊟ **SP** 7 **S98.922-** Partial traumatic amputation of left foot, level unspecified

⊟ **IQ** 7 **S98.929-** Partial traumatic amputation of unspecified foot, level unspecified

4 **S99** Other and unspecified injuries of ankle and foot

5 **S99.0** Physeal fracture of calcaneus

The appropriate 7th character is to be added to each code from subcategories S99.0

A	initial encounter for closed fracture
B	initial encounter for open fracture
D	subsequent encounter for fracture with routine healing
G	subsequent encounter for fracture with delayed healing
K	subsequent encounter for fracture with nonunion
P	subsequent encounter for fracture with malunion
S	sequela

6 **S99.00** Unspecified physeal fracture of calcaneus

⊟ **SP** 7 **S99.001-** Unspecified physeal fracture of right calcaneus

⊟ **SP** 7 **S99.002-** Unspecified physeal fracture of left calcaneus

⊟ **IQ** 7 **S99.009-** Unspecified physeal fracture of unspecified calcaneus

6 **S99.01** Salter-Harris Type I physeal fracture of calcaneus

⊟ **SP** 7 **S99.011-** Salter-Harris Type I physeal fracture of right calcaneus

⊟ **SP** 7 **S99.012-** Salter-Harris Type I physeal fracture of left calcaneus

⊟ **IQ** 7 **S99.019-** Salter-Harris Type I physeal fracture of unspecified calcaneus

6 **S99.02** Salter-Harris Type II physeal fracture of calcaneus

⊟ **SP** 7 **S99.021-** Salter-Harris Type II physeal fracture of right calcaneus

⊟ **SP** 7 **S99.022-** Salter-Harris Type II physeal fracture of left calcaneus

⊟ **IQ** 7 **S99.029-** Salter-Harris Type II physeal fracture of unspecified calcaneus

6 **S99.03** Salter-Harris Type III physeal fracture of calcaneus

⊟ **SP** 7 **S99.031-** Salter-Harris Type III physeal fracture of right calcaneus

⊟ **SP** 7 **S99.032-** Salter-Harris Type III physeal fracture of left calcaneus

⊟ **IQ** 7 **S99.039-** Salter-Harris Type III physeal fracture of unspecified calcaneus

6 **S99.04** Salter-Harris Type IV physeal fracture of calcaneus

⊟ **SP** 7 **S99.041-** Salter-Harris Type IV physeal fracture of right calcaneus

⊟ **SP** 7 **S99.042-** Salter-Harris Type IV physeal fracture of left calcaneus

⊟ **IQ** 7 **S99.049-** Salter-Harris Type IV physeal fracture of unspecified calcaneus

6 **S99.09** Other physeal fracture of calcaneus

⊟ **SP** 7 **S99.091-** Other physeal fracture of right calcaneus

⊟ **SP** 7 **S99.092-** Other physeal fracture of left calcaneus

⊟ **IQ** 7 **S99.099-** Other physeal fracture of unspecified calcaneus

5 **S99.1** Physeal fracture of metatarsal

The appropriate 7th character is to be added to each code from subcategories S99.1

A	initial encounter for closed fracture
B	initial encounter for open fracture
D	subsequent encounter for fracture with routine healing
G	subsequent encounter for fracture with delayed healing
K	subsequent encounter for fracture with nonunion
P	subsequent encounter for fracture with malunion
S	sequela

6 **S99.10** Unspecified physeal fracture of metatarsal

⊟ **SP** 7 **S99.101-** Unspecified physeal fracture of right metatarsal

⊟ **SP** 7 **S99.102-** Unspecified physeal fracture of left metatarsal

⊟ **IQ** 7 **S99.109-** Unspecified physeal fracture of unspecified metatarsal

6 **S99.11** Salter-Harris Type I physeal fracture of metatarsal

4 4th digit required   5 5th digit required   6 6th digit required   7 7th digit required   7 7th digit placeholder   ✚ Additional code   ⊟ Laterality

1636   *DecisionHealth's* FY 2020 Complete Home Health ICD-10-CM Diagnosis Coding Manual

⊟ **SP** 7 **S99.111-** Salter-Harris Type I physeal fracture of right metatarsal

⊟ **SP** 7 **S99.112-** Salter-Harris Type I physeal fracture of left metatarsal

⊟ **IQ** 7 **S99.119-** Salter-Harris Type I physeal fracture of unspecified metatarsal

⑥ **S99.12** Salter-Harris Type II physeal fracture of metatarsal

⊟ **SP** 7 **S99.121-** Salter-Harris Type II physeal fracture of right metatarsal

⊟ **SP** 7 **S99.122-** Salter-Harris Type II physeal fracture of left metatarsal

⊟ **IQ** 7 **S99.129-** Salter-Harris Type II physeal fracture of unspecified metatarsal

⑥ **S99.13** Salter-Harris Type III physeal fracture of metatarsal

⊟ **SP** 7 **S99.131-** Salter-Harris Type III physeal fracture of right metatarsal

⊟ **SP** 7 **S99.132-** Salter-Harris Type III physeal fracture of left metatarsal

⊟ **IQ** 7 **S99.139-** Salter-Harris Type III physeal fracture of unspecified metatarsal

⑥ **S99.14** Salter-Harris Type IV physeal fracture of metatarsal

⊟ **SP** 7 **S99.141-** Salter-Harris Type IV physeal fracture of right metatarsal

⊟ **SP** 7 **S99.142-** Salter-Harris Type IV physeal fracture of left metatarsal

⊟ **IQ** 7 **S99.149-** Salter-Harris Type IV physeal fracture of unspecified metatarsal

⑥ **S99.19** Other physeal fracture of metatarsal

⊟ **SP** 7 **S99.191-** Other physeal fracture of right metatarsal

⊟ **SP** 7 **S99.192-** Other physeal fracture of left metatarsal

⊟ **IQ** 7 **S99.199-** Other physeal fracture of unspecified metatarsal

⑤ **S99.2** Physeal fracture of phalanx of toe

The appropriate 7th character is to be added to each code from subcategories S99.2
A   initial encounter for closed fracture
B   initial encounter for open fracture
D   subsequent encounter for fracture with routine healing
G   subsequent encounter for fracture with delayed healing
K   subsequent encounter for fracture with nonunion
P   subsequent encounter for fracture with malunion
S   sequela

⑥ **S99.20** Unspecified physeal fracture of phalanx of toe

⊟ **SP** 7 **S99.201-** Unspecified physeal fracture of phalanx of right toe

⊟ **SP** 7 **S99.202-** Unspecified physeal fracture of phalanx of left toe

⊟ **IQ** 7 **S99.209-** Unspecified physeal fracture of phalanx of unspecified toe

⑥ **S99.21** Salter-Harris Type I physeal fracture of phalanx of toe

⊟ **SP** 7 **S99.211-** Salter-Harris Type I physeal fracture of phalanx of right toe

⊟ **SP** 7 **S99.212-** Salter-Harris Type I physeal fracture of phalanx of left toe

⊟ **IQ** 7 **S99.219-** Salter-Harris Type I physeal fracture of phalanx of unspecified toe

⑥ **S99.22** Salter-Harris Type II physeal fracture of phalanx of toe

⊟ **SP** 7 **S99.221-** Salter-Harris Type II physeal fracture of phalanx of right toe

⊟ **SP** 7 **S99.222-** Salter-Harris Type II physeal fracture of phalanx of left toe

⊟ **IQ** 7 **S99.229-** Salter-Harris Type II physeal fracture of phalanx of unspecified toe

⑥ **S99.23** Salter-Harris Type III physeal fracture of phalanx of toe

⊟ **SP** 7 **S99.231-** Salter-Harris Type III physeal fracture of phalanx of right toe

⊟ **SP** 7 **S99.232-** Salter-Harris Type III physeal fracture of phalanx of left toe

⊟ **IQ** 7 **S99.239-** Salter-Harris Type III physeal fracture of phalanx of unspecified toe

⑥ **S99.24** Salter-Harris Type IV physeal fracture of phalanx of toe

⊟ **SP** 7 **S99.241-** Salter-Harris Type IV physeal fracture of phalanx of right toe

⊟ **SP** 7 **S99.242-** Salter-Harris Type IV physeal fracture of phalanx of left toe

⊟ **IQ** 7 **S99.249-** Salter-Harris Type IV physeal fracture of phalanx of unspecified toe

⑥ **S99.29** Other physeal fracture of phalanx of toe

⊟ **SP** 7 **S99.291-** Other physeal fracture of phalanx of right toe

⊟ **SP** 7 **S99.292-** Other physeal fracture of phalanx of left toe

⊟ **IQ** 7 **S99.299-** Other physeal fracture of phalanx of unspecified toe

⑤ **S99.8** Other specified injuries of ankle and foot

The appropriate 7th character is to be added to each code from subcategory S99.8
A   initial encounter
D   subsequent encounter
S   sequela

⑥ **S99.81** Other specified injuries of ankle

⊟ **SP** 7 **S99.811-** Other specified injuries of right ankle

⊟ **SP** 7 **S99.812-** Other specified injuries of left ankle

⊟ **IQ** 7 **S99.819-** Other specified injuries of unspecified ankle

⑥ **S99.82** Other specified injuries of foot

⊟ **SP** 7 **S99.821-** Other specified injuries of right foot

⊟ **SP** 7 **S99.822-** Other specified injuries of left foot

⊟ **IQ** 7 **S99.829-** Other specified injuries of unspecified foot

Chapter 19

S00-T88

★ New ▲ Revised Px Primary **SP** PDGM Px **SL** Low CoM **SH** High CoM **IQ** Quest. Encounter ⊞ Hospice non-cancer Dx   Unspecified   **M** *Manifestation*

DecisionHealth's FY 2020 Complete Home Health ICD-10-CM Diagnosis Coding Manual   1637

⑤ S99.9   **Unspecified injury of ankle and foot**

The appropriate 7th character is to be added to each code from subcategory S99.9
A   initial encounter
D   subsequent encounter
S   sequela

⑥ S99.91   **Unspecified injury of ankle**

⊟ 🄸🅀 �7 S99.911-   **Unspecified injury of right ankle**

⊟ 🄸🅀 �7 S99.912-   **Unspecified injury of left ankle**

⊟ 🄸🅀 �7 S99.919-   **Unspecified injury of unspecified ankle**

⑥ S99.92   **Unspecified injury of foot**

⊟ 🄸🅀 �7 S99.921-   **Unspecified injury of right foot**

⊟ 🄸🅀 �7 S99.922-   **Unspecified injury of left foot**

⊟ 🄸🅀 �7 S99.929-   **Unspecified injury of unspecified foot**

Injury, poisoning and certain other consequences of external causes (T07-T88)

Injuries involving multiple body regions (T07)

EXCLUDES 1   burns and corrosions (T20-T32)
frostbite (T33-T34)
insect bite or sting, venomous (T63.4)
sunburn (L55.-)

🄸🅀 ✓ T07.XXX-   **Unspecified multiple injuries**

    EXCLUDES 1   injury NOS (T14.90)

The appropriate 7th character is to be added to code T07
A   initial encounter
D   subsequent encounter
S   sequela

Injury of unspecified body region (T14)

❹ T14   **Injury of unspecified body region**

    EXCLUDES 1   multiple unspecified injuries (T07)

The appropriate 7th character is to be added to each code from category T14
A   initial encounter
D   subsequent encounter
S   sequela

🄸🅀 ✓ T14.8XX-   **Other injury of unspecified body region**

Abrasion NOS
Contusion NOS
Crush injury NOS
Fracture NOS
Skin injury NOS
Vascular injury NOS
Wound NOS

⑤ T14.9   **Unspecified injury**

🄸🅀 ✓ T14.90X-   **Injury, unspecified**
Injury NOS

SP ✓ T14.91X-   **Suicide attempt**
Attempted suicide NOS

Effects of foreign body entering through natural orifice (T15-T19)

EXCLUDES 2   foreign body accidentally left in operation wound (T81.5-)
foreign body in penetrating wound - See open wound by body region
residual foreign body in soft tissue (M79.5)
splinter, without open wound - See superficial injury by body region

❹ T15   **Foreign body on external eye**

    EXCLUDES 2   foreign body in penetrating wound of orbit and eye ball (S05.4-, S05.5-)
open wound of eyelid and periocular area (S01.1-)
retained foreign body in eyelid (H02.8-)
retained (old) foreign body in penetrating wound of orbit and eye ball (H05.5-, H44.6-, H44.7-)
superficial foreign body of eyelid and periocular area (S00.25-)

The appropriate 7th character is to be added to each code from category T15
A   initial encounter
D   subsequent encounter
S   sequela

⑤ T15.0   **Foreign body in cornea**

⊟ 🄸🅀 ✓ T15.00X-   **Foreign body in cornea, unspecified eye**

⊟ SP ✓ T15.01X-   **Foreign body in cornea, right eye**

⊟ SP ✓ T15.02X-   **Foreign body in cornea, left eye**

⑤ T15.1   **Foreign body in conjunctival sac**

⊟ 🄸🅀 ✓ T15.10X-   **Foreign body in conjunctival sac, unspecified eye**

⊟ SP ✓ T15.11X-   **Foreign body in conjunctival sac, right eye**

⊟ SP ✓ T15.12X-   **Foreign body in conjunctival sac, left eye**

⑤ T15.8   **Foreign body in other and multiple parts of external eye**
Foreign body in lacrimal punctum

⊟ 🄸🅀 ✓ T15.80X-   **Foreign body in other and multiple parts of external eye, unspecified eye**

⊟ SP ✓ T15.81X-   **Foreign body in other and multiple parts of external eye, right eye**

⊟ SP ✓ T15.82X-   **Foreign body in other and multiple parts of external eye, left eye**

⑤ T15.9   **Foreign body on external eye, part unspecified**

⊟ 🄸🅀 ✓ T15.90X-   **Foreign body on external eye, part unspecified, unspecified eye**

⊟ SP ✓ T15.91X-   **Foreign body on external eye, part unspecified, right eye**

⊟ SP ✓ T15.92X-   **Foreign body on external eye, part unspecified, left eye**

❹ T16   **Foreign body in ear**
    INCLUDES   foreign body in auditory canal

---

❹4th digit required   ⑤5th digit required   ⑥6th digit required   ⑦7th digit required   ✓ 7th digit placeholder   ✚Additional code   ⊟Laterality

The appropriate 7th character is to be added to each code from category T16
A   initial encounter
D   subsequent encounter
S   sequela

⊟ SP 7 T16.1XX-   Foreign body in right ear

⊟ SP 7 T16.2XX-   Foreign body in left ear

⊟ IQ 7 T16.9XX-   Foreign body in ear, unspecified ear

4 T17   Foreign body in respiratory tract

The appropriate 7th character is to be added to each code from category T17
A   initial encounter
D   subsequent encounter
S   sequela

SP 7 T17.0XX-   Foreign body in nasal sinus

SP 7 T17.1XX-   Foreign body in nostril
Foreign body in nose NOS

5 T17.2   Foreign body in pharynx
Foreign body in nasopharynx
Foreign body in throat NOS

   6 T17.20   Unspecified foreign body in pharynx

   SP 7 T17.200-   Unspecified foreign body in pharynx causing asphyxiation

   SP 7 T17.208-   Unspecified foreign body in pharynx causing other injury

   6 T17.21   Gastric contents in pharynx
Aspiration of gastric contents into pharynx
Vomitus in pharynx

   SP 7 T17.210-   Gastric contents in pharynx causing asphyxiation

   SP 7 T17.218-   Gastric contents in pharynx causing other injury

   6 T17.22   Food in pharynx
Bones in pharynx
Seeds in pharynx

   SP 7 T17.220-   Food in pharynx causing asphyxiation

   SP 7 T17.228-   Food in pharynx causing other injury

   6 T17.29   Other foreign object in pharynx

   SP 7 T17.290-   Other foreign object in pharynx causing asphyxiation

   SP 7 T17.298-   Other foreign object in pharynx causing other injury

5 T17.3   Foreign body in larynx

   6 T17.30   Unspecified foreign body in larynx

   SP 7 T17.300-   Unspecified foreign body in larynx causing asphyxiation

   SP 7 T17.308-   Unspecified foreign body in larynx causing other injury

   6 T17.31   Gastric contents in larynx
Aspiration of gastric contents into larynx
Vomitus in larynx

   SP 7 T17.310-   Gastric contents in larynx causing asphyxiation

   SP 7 T17.318-   Gastric contents in larynx causing other injury

   6 T17.32   Food in larynx
Bones in larynx
Seeds in larynx

   SP 7 T17.320-   Food in larynx causing asphyxiation

   SP 7 T17.328-   Food in larynx causing other injury

   6 T17.39   Other foreign object in larynx

   SP 7 T17.390-   Other foreign object in larynx causing asphyxiation

   SP 7 T17.398-   Other foreign object in larynx causing other injury

5 T17.4   Foreign body in trachea

   6 T17.40   Unspecified foreign body in trachea

   SP 7 T17.400-   Unspecified foreign body in trachea causing asphyxiation

   SP 7 T17.408-   Unspecified foreign body in trachea causing other injury

   6 T17.41   Gastric contents in trachea
Aspiration of gastric contents into trachea
Vomitus in trachea

   SP 7 T17.410-   Gastric contents in trachea causing asphyxiation

   SP 7 T17.418-   Gastric contents in trachea causing other injury

   6 T17.42   Food in trachea
Bones in trachea
Seeds in trachea

   SP 7 T17.420-   Food in trachea causing asphyxiation

   SP 7 T17.428-   Food in trachea causing other injury

   6 T17.49   Other foreign object in trachea

   SP 7 T17.490-   Other foreign object in trachea causing asphyxiation

   SP 7 T17.498-   Other foreign object in trachea causing other injury

5 T17.5   Foreign body in bronchus

   6 T17.50   Unspecified foreign body in bronchus

   SP 7 T17.500-   Unspecified foreign body in bronchus causing asphyxiation

   SP 7 T17.508-   Unspecified foreign body in bronchus causing other injury

   6 T17.51   Gastric contents in bronchus
Aspiration of gastric contents into bronchus
Vomitus in bronchus

   SP 7 T17.510-   Gastric contents in bronchus causing asphyxiation

   SP 7 T17.518-   Gastric contents in bronchus causing other injury

   6 T17.52   Food in bronchus
Bones in bronchus
Seeds in bronchus

   SP 7 T17.520-   Food in bronchus causing asphyxiation

   SP 7 T17.528-   Food in bronchus causing other injury

   6 T17.59   Other foreign object in bronchus

   SP 7 T17.590-   Other foreign object in bronchus causing asphyxiation

   SP 7 T17.598-   Other foreign object in bronchus causing other injury

5 T17.8   Foreign body in other parts of respiratory tract
Foreign body in bronchioles
Foreign body in lung

★ New   ▲ Revised   **Px** Primary   **SP** PDGM Px   **SL** Low CoM   **SH** High CoM   **IQ** Quest. Encounter   **H** Hospice non-cancer Dx   Unspecified   **M** *Manifestation*

6 **T17.80** Unspecified foreign body in other parts of respiratory tract

SP 7 **T17.800-** Unspecified foreign body in other parts of respiratory tract causing asphyxiation

SP 7 **T17.808-** Unspecified foreign body in other parts of respiratory tract causing other injury

6 **T17.81** Gastric contents in other parts of respiratory tract
Aspiration of gastric contents into other parts of respiratory tract
Vomitus in other parts of respiratory tract

SP 7 **T17.810-** Gastric contents in other parts of respiratory tract causing asphyxiation

SP 7 **T17.818-** Gastric contents in other parts of respiratory tract causing other injury

6 **T17.82** Food in other parts of respiratory tract
Bones in other parts of respiratory tract
Seeds in other parts of respiratory tract

SP 7 **T17.820-** Food in other parts of respiratory tract causing asphyxiation

SP 7 **T17.828-** Food in other parts of respiratory tract causing other injury

6 **T17.89** Other foreign object in other parts of respiratory tract

SP 7 **T17.890-** Other foreign object in other parts of respiratory tract causing asphyxiation

SP 7 **T17.898-** Other foreign object in other parts of respiratory tract causing other injury

5 **T17.9** Foreign body in respiratory tract, part unspecified

6 **T17.90** Unspecified foreign body in respiratory tract, part unspecified

SP 7 **T17.900-** Unspecified foreign body in respiratory tract, part unspecified causing asphyxiation

SP 7 **T17.908-** Unspecified foreign body in respiratory tract, part unspecified causing other injury

6 **T17.91** Gastric contents in respiratory tract, part unspecified
Aspiration of gastric contents into respiratory tract, part unspecified
Vomitus in trachea respiratory tract, part unspecified

SP 7 **T17.910-** Gastric contents in respiratory tract, part unspecified causing asphyxiation

SP 7 **T17.918-** Gastric contents in respiratory tract, part unspecified causing other injury

6 **T17.92** Food in respiratory tract, part unspecified
Bones in respiratory tract, part unspecified
Seeds in respiratory tract, part unspecified

SP 7 **T17.920-** Food in respiratory tract, part unspecified causing asphyxiation

SP 7 **T17.928-** Food in respiratory tract, part unspecified causing other injury

6 **T17.99** Other foreign object in respiratory tract, part unspecified

SP 7 **T17.990-** Other foreign object in respiratory tract, part unspecified in causing asphyxiation

SP 7 **T17.998-** Other foreign object in respiratory tract, part unspecified causing other injury

4 **T18** Foreign body in alimentary tract
EXCLUDES 2 foreign body in pharynx (T17.2-)

The appropriate 7th character is to be added to each code from category T18
A   initial encounter
D   subsequent encounter
S   sequela

SP 7 **T18.0XX-** Foreign body in mouth

5 **T18.1** Foreign body in esophagus
EXCLUDES 2 foreign body in respiratory tract (T17.-)

6 **T18.10** Unspecified foreign body in esophagus

SP 7 **T18.100-** Unspecified foreign body in esophagus causing compression of trachea
Unspecified foreign body in esophagus causing obstruction of respiration

SP 7 **T18.108-** Unspecified foreign body in esophagus causing other injury

6 **T18.11** Gastric contents in esophagus
Vomitus in esophagus

SP 7 **T18.110-** Gastric contents in esophagus causing compression of trachea
Gastric contents in esophagus causing obstruction of respiration

SP 7 **T18.118-** Gastric contents in esophagus causing other injury

6 **T18.12** Food in esophagus
Bones in esophagus
Seeds in esophagus

SP 7 **T18.120-** Food in esophagus causing compression of trachea
Food in esophagus causing obstruction of respiration

SP 7 **T18.128-** Food in esophagus causing other injury

6 **T18.19** Other foreign object in esophagus

SP 7 **T18.190-** Other foreign object in esophagus causing compression of trachea
Other foreign body in esophagus causing obstruction of respiration

SP 7 **T18.198-** Other foreign object in esophagus causing other injury

SP 7 **T18.2XX-** Foreign body in stomach

SP 7 **T18.3XX-** Foreign body in small intestine

SP 7 **T18.4XX-** Foreign body in colon

SP 7 **T18.5XX-** Foreign body in anus and rectum

Chapter 19

S00-T88

---

4 4th digit required   **5** 5th digit required   **6** 6th digit required   **7** 7th digit required   **7** 7th digit placeholder   **+** Additional code   **⊟** Laterality

Foreign body in rectosigmoid
(junction)

SP ☑ **T18.8XX-** **Foreign body in other parts of alimentary tract**

SP ☑ **T18.9XX-** **Foreign body of alimentary tract, part unspecified**

Foreign body in digestive system NOS

Swallowed foreign body NOS

⁴ T19 **Foreign body in genitourinary tract**

> **EXCLUDES 2** complications due to implanted mesh (T83.7-)
> mechanical complications of contraceptive device (intrauterine) (vaginal) (T83.3-)
> presence of contraceptive device (intrauterine) (vaginal) (Z97.5)

> The appropriate 7th character is to be added to each code from category T19
> A   initial encounter
> D   subsequent encounter
> S   sequela

SP ☑ **T19.0XX-** **Foreign body in urethra**

SP ☑ **T19.1XX-** **Foreign body in bladder**

SP ☑ **T19.2XX-** **Foreign body in vulva and vagina**

SP ☑ **T19.3XX-** **Foreign body in uterus**

SP ☑ **T19.4XX-** **Foreign body in penis**

SP ☑ **T19.8XX-** **Foreign body in other parts of genitourinary tract**

SP ☑ **T19.9XX-** **Foreign body in genitourinary tract, part unspecified**

Burns and corrosions   (T20-T32)

> **INCLUDES** burns (thermal) from electrical heating appliances
> burns (thermal) from electricity
> burns (thermal) from flame
> burns (thermal) from friction
> burns (thermal) from hot air and hot gases
> burns (thermal) from hot objects
> burns (thermal) from lightning
> burns (thermal) from radiation
> chemical burn [corrosion] (external) (internal)
> scalds

> **EXCLUDES 2** erythema [dermatitis] ab igne (L59.0)
> radiation-related disorders of the skin and subcutaneous tissue (L55-L59)
> sunburn (L55.-)

GUIDELINES   Section I.C.19.d.1)-5)

Sequence first the code that reflects the highest degree of burn when more than one burn is present.

a. When the reason for the admission or encounter is for treatment of external multiple burns, sequence first the code that reflects the burn of the highest degree.

b. When a patient has both internal and external burns, the circumstances of admission govern the selection of the principal diagnosis or first-listed diagnosis.

c. When a patient is admitted for burn injuries and other related conditions such as smoke inhalation and/or respiratory failure, the circumstances of admission govern the selection of the principal or first-listed diagnosis.

Classify burns of the same anatomic site and on the same side but of different degrees to the subcategory identifying the highest degree recorded in the diagnosis (e.g., for second and third degree burns of right thigh, assign only code T24.311-).

Non-healing burns are coded as acute burns. Necrosis of burned skin should be coded as a non-healed burn.

For any documented infected burn site, use an additional code for the infection.

When coding burns, assign separate codes for each burn site. Codes for burns of "multiple sites" should only be assigned when the medical record documentation does not specify the individual sites.

GUIDELINES   Section I.C.19.d

The ICD-10-CM makes a distinction between burns and corrosions. The burn codes are for thermal burns, except sunburns, that come from a heat source, such as a fire or hot appliance. The burn codes are also for burns resulting from electricity and radiation. Corrosions are burns due to chemicals. The guidelines are the same for burns and corrosions.

CODING TIPS ✓   When a patient presents with a burn (other than sunburn), an additional code from Chapter 20 (External causes) should be added to indicate the cause (intent) of the burn.

CODING TIPS ✓   A burn that is referred to as "not healing" should be coded as an acute burn using 7th character "A" or "D". Sequelae of a burn, such as contracture or keloid scarring, should be coded by first assigning the code for the residual condition, followed by the appropriate code to identify the burn with the 7th character "S" to indicate sequelae.

Burns and corrosions of external body surface, specified by site   (T20-T25)

> **INCLUDES** burns and corrosions of first degree [erythema]
> burns and corrosions of second degree [blisters][epidermal loss]
> burns and corrosions of third degree [deep necrosis of underlying tissue] [full- thickness skin loss]

Use additional code from category T31 or T32 to identify extent of body surface involved

GUIDELINES   Section I.C.19.d

Current burns (T20-T25) are classified by depth, extent and by agent (X code). Burns are classified by depth as first degree (erythema), second degree (blistering), and third degree (full-thickness involvement). Burns of the eye and internal organs (T26-T28) are classified by site, but not by degree.

⁴ T20 **Burn and corrosion of head, face, and neck**

> **EXCLUDES 2** burn and corrosion of ear drum (T28.41, T28.91)

★ New ▲ Revised Px Primary **SP** PDGM Px **SL** Low CoM **SH** High CoM **IQ** Quest. Encounter **H** Hospice non-cancer Dx   Unspecified   **M** *Manifestation*

DecisionHealth's FY 2020 Complete Home Health ICD-10-CM Diagnosis Coding Manual   1641

Chapter 19

S00-T88

burn and corrosion of eye and
adnexa (T26.-)
burn and corrosion of mouth
and pharynx (T28.0)

The appropriate 7th character is to be added to
each code from category T20
A　　initial encounter
D　　subsequent encounter
S　　sequela

CODING TIPS ✓　Burns are classified according
to degree. When there are multiple burns of
different degrees to the same body part, code
the burn at its highest degree. Remember,
there is a convention requiring the external
cause code at burns. Aftercare codes are not
used for burns, including those for dressing
changes, drain care, suture removal, or skin
grafts. 7th character 'D' is the default for home
care and hospice when providing aftercare for
a healing or resolving condition; 'A' is used for
active treatment such as antibiotics or more
than routine wound care; 'S' is used to identify
residual conditions when the burn has healed.
Different burns heal at differing rates, so a
current burn (with an A or D) can be coded at
the same time as a sequela of a burn. A non-
healing burn is still coded as a burn no matter
how long it has been present.

**+ 5 T20.0　Burn of unspecified degree of head,
face, and neck**

Use additional external cause code to
identify the source, place and intent of
the burn (X00-X19, X75-X77, X96-X98,
Y92)

**!Q + ✓ T20.00X-　Burn of unspecified degree of
head, face, and neck, unspecified
site**

**+ 6 T20.01　Burn of unspecified degree of ear
[any part, except ear drum]**

　　　EXCLUDES 2　burn of ear drum
(T28.41-)

**⊟ !Q + 7 T20.011-　Burn of unspecified degree of
right ear [any part, except ear
drum]**

**⊟ !Q + 7 T20.012-　Burn of unspecified degree of
left ear [any part, except ear
drum]**

**⊟ !Q + 7 T20.019-　Burn of unspecified degree of
unspecified ear [any part,
except ear drum]**

**SP !Q + ✓ T20.02X-　Burn of unspecified degree of
lip(s)**

**!Q + ✓ T20.03X-　Burn of unspecified degree of
chin**

**!Q + ✓ T20.04X-　Burn of unspecified degree of
nose (septum)**

**!Q + ✓ T20.05X-　Burn of unspecified degree of
scalp [any part]**

**!Q + ✓ T20.06X-　Burn of unspecified degree of
forehead and cheek**

**!Q + ✓ T20.07X-　Burn of unspecified degree of
neck**

**!Q + ✓ T20.09X-　Burn of unspecified degree of
multiple sites of head, face, and
neck**

**+ 5 T20.1　Burn of first degree of head, face, and
neck**

Use additional external cause code to
identify the source, place and intent of
the burn (X00-X19, X75-X77, X96-X98,
Y92)

**!Q + ✓ T20.10X-　Burn of first degree of head, face,
and neck, unspecified site**

**+ 6 T20.11　Burn of first degree of ear [any part,
except ear drum]**

　　　EXCLUDES 2　burn of ear drum
(T28.41-)

**⊟ SP + 7 T20.111-　Burn of first degree of right ear
[any part, except ear drum]**

**⊟ SP + 7 T20.112-　Burn of first degree of left ear
[any part, except ear drum]**

**⊟ !Q + 7 T20.119-　Burn of first degree of
unspecified ear [any part,
except ear drum]**

SP + ✓ T20.12X-　Burn of first degree of lip(s)

SP + ✓ T20.13X-　Burn of first degree of chin

**SP + ✓ T20.14X-　Burn of first degree of nose
(septum)**

**SP + ✓ T20.15X-　Burn of first degree of scalp [any
part]**

**SP + ✓ T20.16X-　Burn of first degree of forehead
and cheek**

SP + ✓ T20.17X-　Burn of first degree of neck

**SP + ✓ T20.19X-　Burn of first degree of multiple
sites of head, face, and neck**

**+ 5 T20.2　Burn of second degree of head, face, and
neck**

Use additional external cause code to
identify the source, place and intent of
the burn (X00-X19, X75-X77, X96-X98,
Y92)

**!Q + ✓ T20.20X-　Burn of second degree of head,
face, and neck, unspecified site**

**+ 6 T20.21　Burn of second degree of ear [any
part, except ear drum]**

　　　EXCLUDES 2　burn of ear drum
(T28.41-)

**⊟ SP + 7 T20.211-　Burn of second degree of right
ear [any part, except ear drum]**

**⊟ SP + 7 T20.212-　Burn of second degree of left ear
[any part, except ear drum]**

**⊟ !Q + 7 T20.219-　Burn of second degree of
unspecified ear [any part,
except ear drum]**

SP + ✓ T20.22X-　Burn of second degree of lip(s)

SP + ✓ T20.23X-　Burn of second degree of chin

**SP + ✓ T20.24X-　Burn of second degree of nose
(septum)**

**SP + ✓ T20.25X-　Burn of second degree of scalp
[any part]**

**SP + ✓ T20.26X-　Burn of second degree of forehead
and cheek**

SP + ✓ T20.27X-　Burn of second degree of neck

**SP + ✓ T20.29X-　Burn of second degree of multiple
sites of head, face, and neck**

**+ 5 T20.3　Burn of third degree of head, face, and
neck**

Use additional external cause code to
identify the source, place and intent of
the burn (X00-X19, X75-X77, X96-X98,
Y92)

---

4 4th digit required　　**5** 5th digit required　　**6** 6th digit required　　**7** 7th digit required　　**✓** 7th digit placeholder　　**+** Additional code　　**⊟** Laterality

IQ ✛ ☑ T20.30X- Burn of third degree of head, face, and neck, unspecified site

  ✛ 6 T20.31 Burn of third degree of ear [any part, except ear drum]
      EXCLUDES 2 burn of ear drum (T28.41-)

⊟ SP ✛ 7 T20.311- Burn of third degree of right ear [any part, except ear drum]

⊟ SP ✛ 7 T20.312- Burn of third degree of left ear [any part, except ear drum]

⊟ IQ ✛ 7 T20.319- Burn of third degree of unspecified ear [any part, except ear drum]

SP ✛ ☑ T20.32X- Burn of third degree of lip(s)

SP ✛ ☑ T20.33X- Burn of third degree of chin

SP ✛ ☑ T20.34X- Burn of third degree of nose (septum)

SP ✛ ☑ T20.35X- Burn of third degree of scalp [any part]

SP ✛ ☑ T20.36X- Burn of third degree of forehead and cheek

SP ✛ ☑ T20.37X- Burn of third degree of neck

SP ✛ ☑ T20.39X- Burn of third degree of multiple sites of head, face, and neck

  ✛ 5 T20.4 Corrosion of unspecified degree of head, face, and neck
    Code first:
      (T51-T65) to identify chemical and intent
    Use additional external cause code to identify place (Y92)

IQ ✛ ☑ T20.40X- Corrosion of unspecified degree of head, face, and neck, unspecified site

  ✛ 6 T20.41 Corrosion of unspecified degree of ear [any part, except ear drum]
      EXCLUDES 2 corrosion of ear drum (T28.91-)

⊟ IQ ✛ 7 T20.411- Corrosion of unspecified degree of right ear [any part, except ear drum]

⊟ IQ ✛ 7 T20.412- Corrosion of unspecified degree of left ear [any part, except ear drum]

⊟ IQ ✛ 7 T20.419- Corrosion of unspecified degree of unspecified ear [any part, except ear drum]

IQ ✛ ☑ T20.42X- Corrosion of unspecified degree of lip(s)

IQ ✛ ☑ T20.43X- Corrosion of unspecified degree of chin

IQ ✛ ☑ T20.44X- Corrosion of unspecified degree of nose (septum)

IQ ✛ ☑ T20.45X- Corrosion of unspecified degree of scalp [any part]

IQ ✛ ☑ T20.46X- Corrosion of unspecified degree of forehead and cheek

IQ ✛ ☑ T20.47X- Corrosion of unspecified degree of neck

IQ ✛ ☑ T20.49X- Corrosion of unspecified degree of multiple sites of head, face, and neck

  ✛ 5 T20.5 Corrosion of first degree of head, face, and neck
    Code first:
      (T51-T65) to identify chemical and intent
    Use additional external cause code to identify place (Y92)

IQ ✛ ☑ T20.50X- Corrosion of first degree of head, face, and neck, unspecified site

  ✛ 6 T20.51 Corrosion of first degree of ear [any part, except ear drum]
      EXCLUDES 2 corrosion of ear drum (T28.91-)

⊟ IQ ✛ 7 T20.511- Corrosion of first degree of right ear [any part, except ear drum]

⊟ IQ ✛ 7 T20.512- Corrosion of first degree of left ear [any part, except ear drum]

⊟ IQ ✛ 7 T20.519- Corrosion of first degree of unspecified ear [any part, except ear drum]

IQ ✛ ☑ T20.52X- Corrosion of first degree of lip(s)

IQ ✛ ☑ T20.53X- Corrosion of first degree of chin

IQ ✛ ☑ T20.54X- Corrosion of first degree of nose (septum)

IQ ✛ ☑ T20.55X- Corrosion of first degree of scalp [any part]

IQ ✛ ☑ T20.56X- Corrosion of first degree of forehead and cheek

IQ ✛ ☑ T20.57X- Corrosion of first degree of neck

IQ ✛ ☑ T20.59X- Corrosion of first degree of multiple sites of head, face, and neck

  ✛ 5 T20.6 Corrosion of second degree of head, face, and neck
    Code first:
      (T51-T65) to identify chemical and intent
    Use additional external cause code to identify place (Y92)

IQ ✛ ☑ T20.60X- Corrosion of second degree of head, face, and neck, unspecified site

  ✛ 6 T20.61 Corrosion of second degree of ear [any part, except ear drum]
      EXCLUDES 2 corrosion of ear drum (T28.91-)

⊟ IQ ✛ 7 T20.611- Corrosion of second degree of right ear [any part, except ear drum]

⊟ IQ ✛ 7 T20.612- Corrosion of second degree of left ear [any part, except ear drum]

⊟ IQ ✛ 7 T20.619- Corrosion of second degree of unspecified ear [any part, except ear drum]

IQ ✛ ☑ T20.62X- Corrosion of second degree of lip(s)

IQ ✛ ☑ T20.63X- Corrosion of second degree of chin

IQ ✛ ☑ T20.64X- Corrosion of second degree of nose (septum)

IQ ✛ ☑ T20.65X- Corrosion of second degree of scalp [any part]

IQ ✛ ☑ T20.66X- Corrosion of second degree of forehead and cheek

IQ ✛ ☑ T20.67X- Corrosion of second degree of neck

★ New ▲ Revised Px Primary SP PDGM Px SL Low CoM SH High CoM IQ Quest. Encounter H Hospice non-cancer Dx   Unspecified   M Manifestation

DecisionHealth's FY 2020 Complete Home Health ICD-10-CM Diagnosis Coding Manual   1643

Chapter 19

S00-T88

!Q + ☑ T20.69X- Corrosion of second degree of multiple sites of head, face, and neck

+ ⑤ T20.7 Corrosion of third degree of head, face, and neck
Code first:
(T51-T65) to identify chemical and intent
Use additional external cause code to identify place (Y92)

!Q + ☑ T20.70X- Corrosion of third degree of head, face, and neck, unspecified site

+ ⑥ T20.71 Corrosion of third degree of ear [any part, except ear drum]
EXCLUDES 2 corrosion of ear drum (T28.91-)

⊟ !Q + ⑦ T20.711- Corrosion of third degree of right ear [any part, except ear drum]

⊟ !Q + ⑦ T20.712- Corrosion of third degree of left ear [any part, except ear drum]

⊟ !Q + ⑦ T20.719- Corrosion of third degree of unspecified ear [any part, except ear drum]

!Q + ☑ T20.72X- Corrosion of third degree of lip(s)

!Q + ☑ T20.73X- Corrosion of third degree of chin

!Q + ☑ T20.74X- Corrosion of third degree of nose (septum)

!Q + ☑ T20.75X- Corrosion of third degree of scalp [any part]

!Q + ☑ T20.76X- Corrosion of third degree of forehead and cheek

!Q + ☑ T20.77X- Corrosion of third degree of neck

!Q + ☑ T20.79X- Corrosion of third degree of multiple sites of head, face, and neck

④ T21 Burn and corrosion of trunk
INCLUDES burns and corrosion of hip region
EXCLUDES 2 burns and corrosion of axilla (T22.- with fifth character 4)
burns and corrosion of scapular region (T22.- with fifth character 6)
burns and corrosion of shoulder (T22.- with fifth character 5)

The appropriate 7th character is to be added to each code from category T21
A   initial encounter
D   subsequent encounter
S   sequela

CODING TIPS ✓ Do not use Z codes for skin grafts, dressing changes, drains, etc., for trauma wounds of any type, including burns. Continue to code the burn with the appropriate 7th character.

CODING TIPS ✓ Burns are classified according to degree. When there are multiple burns of different degrees to the same body part, code the burn at its highest degree. Remember, there is a convention requiring the external cause code at burns. Aftercare codes are not used for burns, including those for dressing changes, drain care, suture removal, or skin grafts. 7th character 'D' is the default for home care and hospice when providing aftercare for a healing or resolving condition; 'A' is used for active treatment such as antibiotics or more than routine wound care; 'S' is used to identify residual conditions when the burn has healed. Different burns heal at differing rates, so a current burn (with an A or D) can be coded at the same time as a sequela of a burn. A non-healing burn is still coded as a burn no matter how long it has been present.

+ ⑤ T21.0 Burn of unspecified degree of trunk
Use additional external cause code to identify the source, place and intent of the burn (X00-X19, X75-X77, X96-X98, Y92)

!Q + ☑ T21.00X- Burn of unspecified degree of trunk, unspecified site

!Q + ☑ T21.01X- Burn of unspecified degree of chest wall
Burn of unspecified degree of breast

!Q + ☑ T21.02X- Burn of unspecified degree of abdominal wall
Burn of unspecified degree of flank
Burn of unspecified degree of groin

!Q + ☑ T21.03X- Burn of unspecified degree of upper back
Burn of unspecified degree of interscapular region

!Q + ☑ T21.04X- Burn of unspecified degree of lower back

!Q + ☑ T21.05X- Burn of unspecified degree of buttock
Burn of unspecified degree of anus

!Q + ☑ T21.06X- Burn of unspecified degree of male genital region
Burn of unspecified degree of penis
Burn of unspecified degree of scrotum
Burn of unspecified degree of testis

!Q + ☑ T21.07X- Burn of unspecified degree of female genital region
Burn of unspecified degree of labium (majus) (minus)
Burn of unspecified degree of perineum
Burn of unspecified degree of vulva
EXCLUDES 2 burn of vagina (T28.3)

!Q + ☑ T21.09X- Burn of unspecified degree of other site of trunk

+ ⑤ T21.1 Burn of first degree of trunk
Use additional external cause code to identify the source, place and intent of the burn (X00-X19, X75-X77, X96-X98, Y92)

!Q + ☑ T21.10X- Burn of first degree of trunk, unspecified site

---

④ 4th digit required   ⑤ 5th digit required   ⑥ 6th digit required   ⑦ 7th digit required   ☑ 7th digit placeholder   + Additional code   ⊟ Laterality

1644   *DecisionHealth's* FY 2020 Complete Home Health ICD-10-CM Diagnosis Coding Manual

SP + ☑ T21.11X- **Burn of first degree of chest wall**
Burn of first degree of breast

SP + ☑ T21.12X- **Burn of first degree of abdominal wall**
Burn of first degree of flank
Burn of first degree of groin

SP + ☑ T21.13X- **Burn of first degree of upper back**
Burn of first degree of interscapular region

SP + ☑ T21.14X- **Burn of first degree of lower back**

SP + ☑ T21.15X- **Burn of first degree of buttock**
Burn of first degree of anus

SP + ☑ T21.16X- **Burn of first degree of male genital region**
Burn of first degree of penis
Burn of first degree of scrotum
Burn of first degree of testis

SP + ☑ T21.17X- **Burn of first degree of female genital region**
Burn of first degree of labium (majus) (minus)
Burn of first degree of perineum
Burn of first degree of vulva
EXCLUDES 2 burn of vagina (T28.3)

SP + ☑ T21.19X- **Burn of first degree of other site of trunk**

+ 5 T21.2 **Burn of second degree of trunk**
Use additional external cause code to identify the source, place and intent of the burn (X00-X19, X75-X77, X96-X98, Y92)

!Q + ☑ T21.20X- **Burn of second degree of trunk, unspecified site**

SP + ☑ T21.21X- **Burn of second degree of chest wall**
Burn of second degree of breast

SP + ☑ T21.22X- **Burn of second degree of abdominal wall**
Burn of second degree of flank
Burn of second degree of groin

SP + ☑ T21.23X- **Burn of second degree of upper back**
Burn of second degree of interscapular region

SP + ☑ T21.24X- **Burn of second degree of lower back**

SP + ☑ T21.25X- **Burn of second degree of buttock**
Burn of second degree of anus

SP + ☑ T21.26X- **Burn of second degree of male genital region**
Burn of second degree of penis
Burn of second degree of scrotum
Burn of second degree of testis

SP + ☑ T21.27X- **Burn of second degree of female genital region**
Burn of second degree of labium (majus) (minus)
Burn of second degree of perineum
Burn of second degree of vulva
EXCLUDES 2 burn of vagina (T28.3)

SP + ☑ T21.29X- **Burn of second degree of other site of trunk**

+ 5 T21.3 **Burn of third degree of trunk**

Use additional external cause code to identify the source, place and intent of the burn (X00-X19, X75-X77, X96-X98, Y92)

!Q + ☑ T21.30X- **Burn of third degree of trunk, unspecified site**

SP + ☑ T21.31X- **Burn of third degree of chest wall**
Burn of third degree of breast

SP + ☑ T21.32X- **Burn of third degree of abdominal wall**
Burn of third degree of flank
Burn of third degree of groin

SP + ☑ T21.33X- **Burn of third degree of upper back**
Burn of third degree of interscapular region

SP + ☑ T21.34X- **Burn of third degree of lower back**

SP + ☑ T21.35X- **Burn of third degree of buttock**
Burn of third degree of anus

SP + ☑ T21.36X- **Burn of third degree of male genital region**
Burn of third degree of penis
Burn of third degree of scrotum
Burn of third degree of testis

SP + ☑ T21.37X- **Burn of third degree of female genital region**
Burn of third degree of labium (majus) (minus)
Burn of third degree of perineum
Burn of third degree of vulva
EXCLUDES 2 burn of vagina (T28.3)

SP + ☑ T21.39X- **Burn of third degree of other site of trunk**

+ 5 T21.4 **Corrosion of unspecified degree of trunk**

Code first:
(T51-T65) to identify chemical and intent
Use additional external cause code to identify place (Y92)

!Q + ☑ T21.40X- **Corrosion of unspecified degree of trunk, unspecified site**

!Q + ☑ T21.41X- **Corrosion of unspecified degree of chest wall**
Corrosion of unspecified degree of breast

!Q + ☑ T21.42X- **Corrosion of unspecified degree of abdominal wall**
Corrosion of unspecified degree of flank
Corrosion of unspecified degree of groin

!Q + ☑ T21.43X- **Corrosion of unspecified degree of upper back**
Corrosion of unspecified degree of interscapular region

!Q + ☑ T21.44X- **Corrosion of unspecified degree of lower back**

!Q + ☑ T21.45X- **Corrosion of unspecified degree of buttock**
Corrosion of unspecified degree of anus

!Q + ☑ T21.46X- **Corrosion of unspecified degree of male genital region**
Corrosion of unspecified degree of penis

Chapter 19

S00-T88

☆ New ▲ Revised Px Primary **SP** PDGM Px **SL** Low CoM **SH** High CoM **!Q** Quest. Encounter **H** Hospice non-cancer Dx Unspecified **M** *Manifestation*

Corrosion of unspecified degree of scrotum

Corrosion of unspecified degree of testis

!Q **+** ☑ **T21.47X-** **Corrosion of unspecified degree of female genital region**

Corrosion of unspecified degree of labium (majus) (minus)

Corrosion of unspecified degree of perineum

Corrosion of unspecified degree of vulva

> **EXCLUDES 2** corrosion of vagina (T28.8)

!Q **+** ☑ **T21.49X-** **Corrosion of unspecified degree of other site of trunk**

+ ⑤ **T21.5** **Corrosion of first degree of trunk**

Code first:
(T51-T65) to identify chemical and intent
Use additional external cause code to identify place (Y92)

!Q **+** ☑ **T21.50X-** **Corrosion of first degree of trunk, unspecified site**

!Q **+** ☑ **T21.51X-** **Corrosion of first degree of chest wall**

Corrosion of first degree of breast

!Q **+** ☑ **T21.52X-** **Corrosion of first degree of abdominal wall**

Corrosion of first degree of flank

Corrosion of first degree of groin

!Q **+** ☑ **T21.53X-** **Corrosion of first degree of upper back**

Corrosion of first degree of interscapular region

!Q **+** ☑ **T21.54X-** **Corrosion of first degree of lower back**

!Q **+** ☑ **T21.55X-** **Corrosion of first degree of buttock**

Corrosion of first degree of anus

!Q **+** ☑ **T21.56X-** **Corrosion of first degree of male genital region**

Corrosion of first degree of penis

Corrosion of first degree of scrotum

Corrosion of first degree of testis

!Q **+** ☑ **T21.57X-** **Corrosion of first degree of female genital region**

Corrosion of first degree of labium (majus) (minus)

Corrosion of first degree of perineum

Corrosion of first degree of vulva

> **EXCLUDES 2** corrosion of vagina (T28.8)

!Q **+** ☑ **T21.59X-** **Corrosion of first degree of other site of trunk**

+ ⑤ **T21.6** **Corrosion of second degree of trunk**

Code first:
(T51-T65) to identify chemical and intent
Use additional external cause code to identify place (Y92)

!Q **+** ☑ **T21.60X-** **Corrosion of second degree of trunk, unspecified site**

!Q **+** ☑ **T21.61X-** **Corrosion of second degree of chest wall**

Corrosion of second degree of breast

!Q **+** ☑ **T21.62X-** **Corrosion of second degree of abdominal wall**

Corrosion of second degree of flank

Corrosion of second degree of groin

!Q **+** ☑ **T21.63X-** **Corrosion of second degree of upper back**

Corrosion of second degree of interscapular region

!Q **+** ☑ **T21.64X-** **Corrosion of second degree of lower back**

!Q **+** ☑ **T21.65X-** **Corrosion of second degree of buttock**

Corrosion of second degree of anus

!Q **+** ☑ **T21.66X-** **Corrosion of second degree of male genital region**

Corrosion of second degree of penis

Corrosion of second degree of scrotum

Corrosion of second degree of testis

!Q **+** ☑ **T21.67X-** **Corrosion of second degree of female genital region**

Corrosion of second degree of labium (majus) (minus)

Corrosion of second degree of perineum

Corrosion of second degree of vulva

> **EXCLUDES 2** corrosion of vagina (T28.8)

!Q **+** ☑ **T21.69X-** **Corrosion of second degree of other site of trunk**

+ ⑤ **T21.7** **Corrosion of third degree of trunk**

Code first:
(T51-T65) to identify chemical and intent
Use additional external cause code to identify place (Y92)

!Q **+** ☑ **T21.70X-** **Corrosion of third degree of trunk, unspecified site**

!Q **+** ☑ **T21.71X-** **Corrosion of third degree of chest wall**

Corrosion of third degree of breast

!Q **+** ☑ **T21.72X-** **Corrosion of third degree of abdominal wall**

Corrosion of third degree of flank

Corrosion of third degree of groin

!Q **+** ☑ **T21.73X-** **Corrosion of third degree of upper back**

Corrosion of third degree of interscapular region

!Q **+** ☑ **T21.74X-** **Corrosion of third degree of lower back**

!Q **+** ☑ **T21.75X-** **Corrosion of third degree of buttock**

Corrosion of third degree of anus

!Q **+** ☑ **T21.76X-** **Corrosion of third degree of male genital region**

Corrosion of third degree of penis

Corrosion of third degree of scrotum

Corrosion of third degree of testis

!Q **+** ☑ **T21.77X-** **Corrosion of third degree of female genital region**

Corrosion of third degree of labium (majus) (minus)

Corrosion of third degree of perineum

Corrosion of third degree of vulva

> **EXCLUDES 2** corrosion of vagina (T28.8)

---

④4th digit required   ⑤5th digit required   ⑥6th digit required   ⑦7th digit required   ☑ 7th digit placeholder   **+**Additional code   ⊟Laterality

1646   *DecisionHealth's* FY 2020 Complete Home Health ICD-10-CM Diagnosis Coding Manual

IQ + ☑ T21.79X- Corrosion of third degree of other site of trunk

④ T22 Burn and corrosion of shoulder and upper limb, except wrist and hand

> EXCLUDES 2   burn and corrosion of interscapular region (T21.-)
> burn and corrosion of wrist and hand (T23.-)

> The appropriate 7th character is to be added to each code from category T22
> A   initial encounter
> D   subsequent encounter
> S   sequela

> CODING TIPS ✓   Do not use Z codes for skin grafts, dressing changes, drains, etc., for trauma wounds of any type, including burns. Continue to code the burn with the appropriate 7th character.

> CODING TIPS ✓   Burns are classified according to degree. When there are multiple burns of different degrees to the same body part, code the burn at its highest degree. Remember, there is a convention requiring the external cause code at burns. Aftercare codes are not used for burns, including those for dressing changes, drain care, suture removal, or skin grafts. 7th character 'D' is the default for home care and hospice when providing aftercare for a healing or resolving condition; 'A' is used for active treatment such as antibiotics or more than routine wound care; 'S' is used to identify residual conditions when the burn has healed. Different burns heal at differing rates, so a current burn (with an A or D) can be coded at the same time as a sequela of a burn. A non-healing burn is still coded as a burn no matter how long it has been present.

+ ⑤ T22.0 Burn of unspecified degree of shoulder and upper limb, except wrist and hand

> Use additional external cause code to identify the source, place and intent of the burn (X00-X19, X75-X77, X96-X98, Y92)

IQ + ☑ T22.00X- Burn of unspecified degree of shoulder and upper limb, except wrist and hand, unspecified site

+ ⑥ T22.01 Burn of unspecified degree of forearm

⊟ IQ + ⑦ T22.011- Burn of unspecified degree of right forearm

⊟ IQ + ⑦ T22.012- Burn of unspecified degree of left forearm

⊟ IQ + ⑦ T22.019- Burn of unspecified degree of unspecified forearm

+ ⑥ T22.02 Burn of unspecified degree of elbow

⊟ IQ + ⑦ T22.021- Burn of unspecified degree of right elbow

⊟ IQ + ⑦ T22.022- Burn of unspecified degree of left elbow

⊟ IQ + ⑦ T22.029- Burn of unspecified degree of unspecified elbow

+ ⑥ T22.03 Burn of unspecified degree of upper arm

⊟ IQ + ⑦ T22.031- Burn of unspecified degree of right upper arm

⊟ IQ + ⑦ T22.032- Burn of unspecified degree of left upper arm

⊟ IQ + ⑦ T22.039- Burn of unspecified degree of unspecified upper arm

+ ⑥ T22.04 Burn of unspecified degree of axilla

⊟ IQ + ⑦ T22.041- Burn of unspecified degree of right axilla

⊟ IQ + ⑦ T22.042- Burn of unspecified degree of left axilla

⊟ IQ + ⑦ T22.049- Burn of unspecified degree of unspecified axilla

+ ⑥ T22.05 Burn of unspecified degree of shoulder

⊟ IQ + ⑦ T22.051- Burn of unspecified degree of right shoulder

⊟ IQ + ⑦ T22.052- Burn of unspecified degree of left shoulder

⊟ IQ + ⑦ T22.059- Burn of unspecified degree of unspecified shoulder

+ ⑥ T22.06 Burn of unspecified degree of scapular region

⊟ IQ + ⑦ T22.061- Burn of unspecified degree of right scapular region

⊟ IQ + ⑦ T22.062- Burn of unspecified degree of left scapular region

⊟ IQ + ⑦ T22.069- Burn of unspecified degree of unspecified scapular region

+ ⑥ T22.09 Burn of unspecified degree of multiple sites of shoulder and upper limb, except wrist and hand

⊟ IQ + ⑦ T22.091- Burn of unspecified degree of multiple sites of right shoulder and upper limb, except wrist and hand

⊟ IQ + ⑦ T22.092- Burn of unspecified degree of multiple sites of left shoulder and upper limb, except wrist and hand

⊟ IQ + ⑦ T22.099- Burn of unspecified degree of multiple sites of unspecified shoulder and upper limb, except wrist and hand

+ ⑤ T22.1 Burn of first degree of shoulder and upper limb, except wrist and hand

> Use additional external cause code to identify the source, place and intent of the burn (X00-X19, X75-X77, X96-X98, Y92)

IQ + ☑ T22.10X- Burn of first degree of shoulder and upper limb, except wrist and hand, unspecified site

+ ⑥ T22.11 Burn of first degree of forearm

⊟ SP + ⑦ T22.111- Burn of first degree of right forearm

⊟ SP + ⑦ T22.112- Burn of first degree of left forearm

⊟ IQ + ⑦ T22.119- Burn of first degree of unspecified forearm

+ ⑥ T22.12 Burn of first degree of elbow

⊟ SP + ⑦ T22.121- Burn of first degree of right elbow

⊟ SP + ⑦ T22.122- Burn of first degree of left elbow

⊟ IQ + ⑦ T22.129- Burn of first degree of unspecified elbow

⋆ New ▲ Revised Px Primary SP PDGM Px SL Low CoM SH High CoM IQ Quest. Encounter H Hospice non-cancer Dx Unspecified M Manifestation

DecisionHealth's FY 2020 Complete Home Health ICD-10-CM Diagnosis Coding Manual

1647

Chapter 19

S00-T88

+ ⑥ **T22.13** **Burn of first degree of upper arm**

⊟ SP + ⑦ **T22.131-** **Burn of first degree of right upper arm**

⊟ SP IQ + ⑦ **T22.132-** **Burn of first degree of left upper arm**

⊟ IQ + ⑦ **T22.139-** **Burn of first degree of unspecified upper arm**

+ ⑥ **T22.14** **Burn of first degree of axilla**

⊟ SP + ⑦ **T22.141-** **Burn of first degree of right axilla**

⊟ SP + ⑦ **T22.142-** **Burn of first degree of left axilla**

⊟ IQ + ⑦ **T22.149-** **Burn of first degree of unspecified axilla**

+ ⑥ **T22.15** **Burn of first degree of shoulder**

⊟ SP + ⑦ **T22.151-** **Burn of first degree of right shoulder**

⊟ SP + ⑦ **T22.152-** **Burn of first degree of left shoulder**

⊟ IQ + ⑦ **T22.159-** **Burn of first degree of unspecified shoulder**

+ ⑥ **T22.16** **Burn of first degree of scapular region**

⊟ SP + ⑦ **T22.161-** **Burn of first degree of right scapular region**

⊟ SP + ⑦ **T22.162-** **Burn of first degree of left scapular region**

⊟ IQ + ⑦ **T22.169-** **Burn of first degree of unspecified scapular region**

+ ⑥ **T22.19** **Burn of first degree of multiple sites of shoulder and upper limb, except wrist and hand**

⊟ SP + ⑦ **T22.191-** **Burn of first degree of multiple sites of right shoulder and upper limb, except wrist and hand**

⊟ SP + ⑦ **T22.192-** **Burn of first degree of multiple sites of left shoulder and upper limb, except wrist and hand**

⊟ SP + ⑦ **T22.199-** **Burn of first degree of multiple sites of unspecified shoulder and upper limb, except wrist and hand**

+ ⑤ **T22.2** **Burn of second degree of shoulder and upper limb, except wrist and hand**
Use additional external cause code to identify the source, place and intent of the burn (X00-X19, X75-X77, X96-X98, Y92)

IQ + ⑦ **T22.20X-** **Burn of second degree of shoulder and upper limb, except wrist and hand, unspecified site**

+ ⑥ **T22.21** **Burn of second degree of forearm**

⊟ SP + ⑦ **T22.211-** **Burn of second degree of right forearm**

⊟ SP + ⑦ **T22.212-** **Burn of second degree of left forearm**

⊟ IQ + ⑦ **T22.219-** **Burn of second degree of unspecified forearm**

+ ⑥ **T22.22** **Burn of second degree of elbow**

⊟ SP + ⑦ **T22.221-** **Burn of second degree of right elbow**

⊟ SP + ⑦ **T22.222-** **Burn of second degree of left elbow**

⊟ IQ + ⑦ **T22.229-** **Burn of second degree of unspecified elbow**

+ ⑥ **T22.23** **Burn of second degree of upper arm**

⊟ SP + ⑦ **T22.231-** **Burn of second degree of right upper arm**

⊟ SP + ⑦ **T22.232-** **Burn of second degree of left upper arm**

⊟ IQ + ⑦ **T22.239-** **Burn of second degree of unspecified upper arm**

+ ⑥ **T22.24** **Burn of second degree of axilla**

⊟ SP + ⑦ **T22.241-** **Burn of second degree of right axilla**

⊟ SP + ⑦ **T22.242-** **Burn of second degree of left axilla**

⊟ IQ + ⑦ **T22.249-** **Burn of second degree of unspecified axilla**

+ ⑥ **T22.25** **Burn of second degree of shoulder**

⊟ SP + ⑦ **T22.251-** **Burn of second degree of right shoulder**

⊟ SP + ⑦ **T22.252-** **Burn of second degree of left shoulder**

⊟ IQ + ⑦ **T22.259-** **Burn of second degree of unspecified shoulder**

+ ⑥ **T22.26** **Burn of second degree of scapular region**

⊟ SP + ⑦ **T22.261-** **Burn of second degree of right scapular region**

⊟ SP + ⑦ **T22.262-** **Burn of second degree of left scapular region**

⊟ IQ + ⑦ **T22.269-** **Burn of second degree of unspecified scapular region**

+ ⑥ **T22.29** **Burn of second degree of multiple sites of shoulder and upper limb, except wrist and hand**

⊟ SP + ⑦ **T22.291-** **Burn of second degree of multiple sites of right shoulder and upper limb, except wrist and hand**

⊟ SP + ⑦ **T22.292-** **Burn of second degree of multiple sites of left shoulder and upper limb, except wrist and hand**

⊟ SP + ⑦ **T22.299-** **Burn of second degree of multiple sites of unspecified shoulder and upper limb, except wrist and hand**

+ ⑤ **T22.3** **Burn of third degree of shoulder and upper limb, except wrist and hand**
Use additional external cause code to identify the source, place and intent of the burn (X00-X19, X75-X77, X96-X98, Y92)

IQ + ⑦ **T22.30X-** **Burn of third degree of shoulder and upper limb, except wrist and hand, unspecified site**

+ ⑥ **T22.31** **Burn of third degree of forearm**

⊟ SP + ⑦ **T22.311-** **Burn of third degree of right forearm**

⊟ SP + ⑦ **T22.312-** **Burn of third degree of left forearm**

⊟ IQ + ⑦ **T22.319-** **Burn of third degree of unspecified forearm**

+ ⑥ **T22.32** **Burn of third degree of elbow**

⊟ SP + ⑦ **T22.321-** **Burn of third degree of right elbow**

⊟ SP + ⑦ **T22.322-** **Burn of third degree of left elbow**

⊟ IQ + ⑦ **T22.329-** **Burn of third degree of unspecified elbow**

+ ⑥ **T22.33** **Burn of third degree of upper arm**

---

④4th digit required   ⑤5th digit required   ⑥6th digit required   ⑦7th digit required   ⑦7th digit placeholder   +Additional code   ⊟Laterality

☰ **SP** ✚ **7** T22.331- Burn of third degree of right upper arm

☰ **SP** ✚ **7** T22.332- Burn of third degree of left upper arm

☰ **IQ** ✚ **7** T22.339- Burn of third degree of unspecified upper arm

✚ **6** T22.34 Burn of third degree of axilla

☰ **SP** ✚ **7** T22.341- Burn of third degree of right axilla

☰ **SP** ✚ **7** T22.342- Burn of third degree of left axilla

☰ **IQ** ✚ **7** T22.349- Burn of third degree of unspecified axilla

✚ **6** T22.35 Burn of third degree of shoulder

☰ **SP** ✚ **7** T22.351- Burn of third degree of right shoulder

☰ **SP** ✚ **7** T22.352- Burn of third degree of left shoulder

☰ **IQ** ✚ **7** T22.359- Burn of third degree of unspecified shoulder

✚ **6** T22.36 Burn of third degree of scapular region

☰ **SP** ✚ **7** T22.361- Burn of third degree of right scapular region

☰ **SP** ✚ **7** T22.362- Burn of third degree of left scapular region

☰ **IQ** ✚ **7** T22.369- Burn of third degree of unspecified scapular region

✚ **6** T22.39 Burn of third degree of multiple sites of shoulder and upper limb, except wrist and hand

☰ **SP** ✚ **7** T22.391- Burn of third degree of multiple sites of right shoulder and upper limb, except wrist and hand

☰ **SP** ✚ **7** T22.392- Burn of third degree of multiple sites of left shoulder and upper limb, except wrist and hand

☰ **SP** ✚ **7** T22.399- Burn of third degree of multiple sites of unspecified shoulder and upper limb, except wrist and hand

✚ **5** T22.4 Corrosion of unspecified degree of shoulder and upper limb, except wrist and hand

Code first:
(T51-T65) to identify chemical and intent
Use additional external cause code to identify place (Y92)

IQ ✚ **7** T22.40X- Corrosion of unspecified degree of shoulder and upper limb, except wrist and hand, unspecified site

✚ **6** T22.41 Corrosion of unspecified degree of forearm

☰ **IQ** ✚ **7** T22.411- Corrosion of unspecified degree of right forearm

☰ **IQ** ✚ **7** T22.412- Corrosion of unspecified degree of left forearm

☰ **IQ** ✚ **7** T22.419- Corrosion of unspecified degree of unspecified forearm

✚ **6** T22.42 Corrosion of unspecified degree of elbow

☰ **IQ** ✚ **7** T22.421- Corrosion of unspecified degree of right elbow

☰ **IQ** ✚ **7** T22.422- Corrosion of unspecified degree of left elbow

☰ **IQ** ✚ **7** T22.429- Corrosion of unspecified degree of unspecified elbow

✚ **6** T22.43 Corrosion of unspecified degree of upper arm

☰ **IQ** ✚ **7** T22.431- Corrosion of unspecified degree of right upper arm

☰ **IQ** ✚ **7** T22.432- Corrosion of unspecified degree of left upper arm

☰ **IQ** ✚ **7** T22.439- Corrosion of unspecified degree of unspecified upper arm

✚ **6** T22.44 Corrosion of unspecified degree of axilla

☰ **IQ** ✚ **7** T22.441- Corrosion of unspecified degree of right axilla

☰ **IQ** ✚ **7** T22.442- Corrosion of unspecified degree of left axilla

☰ **IQ** ✚ **7** T22.449- Corrosion of unspecified degree of unspecified axilla

✚ **6** T22.45 Corrosion of unspecified degree of shoulder

☰ **IQ** ✚ **7** T22.451- Corrosion of unspecified degree of right shoulder

☰ **IQ** ✚ **7** T22.452- Corrosion of unspecified degree of left shoulder

☰ **IQ** ✚ **7** T22.459- Corrosion of unspecified degree of unspecified shoulder

✚ **6** T22.46 Corrosion of unspecified degree of scapular region

☰ **IQ** ✚ **7** T22.461- Corrosion of unspecified degree of right scapular region

☰ **IQ** ✚ **7** T22.462- Corrosion of unspecified degree of left scapular region

☰ **IQ** ✚ **7** T22.469- Corrosion of unspecified degree of unspecified scapular region

✚ **6** T22.49 Corrosion of unspecified degree of multiple sites of shoulder and upper limb, except wrist and hand

☰ **IQ** ✚ **7** T22.491- Corrosion of unspecified degree of multiple sites of right shoulder and upper limb, except wrist and hand

☰ **IQ** ✚ **7** T22.492- Corrosion of unspecified degree of multiple sites of left shoulder and upper limb, except wrist and hand

☰ **IQ** ✚ **7** T22.499- Corrosion of unspecified degree of multiple sites of unspecified shoulder and upper limb, except wrist and hand

✚ **5** T22.5 Corrosion of first degree of shoulder and upper limb, except wrist and hand
Code first:
(T51-T65) to identify chemical and intent
Use additional external cause code to identify place (Y92)

IQ ✚ **7** T22.50X- Corrosion of first degree of shoulder and upper limb, except wrist and hand unspecified site

✚ **6** T22.51 Corrosion of first degree of forearm

☰ **IQ** ✚ **7** T22.511- Corrosion of first degree of right forearm

☆ New ▲ Revised Px Primary **SP** PDGM Px **SL** Low CoM **SH** High CoM **IQ** Quest. Encounter **H** Hospice non-cancer Dx Unspecified **M** *Manifestation*

DecisionHealth's FY 2020 Complete Home Health ICD-10-CM Diagnosis Coding Manual

1649

Chapter 19

S00-T88

▤ IQ + 7 T22.512- Corrosion of first degree of left forearm

▤ IQ + 7 T22.519- Corrosion of first degree of unspecified forearm

+ 6 T22.52 Corrosion of first degree of elbow

▤ IQ + 7 T22.521- Corrosion of first degree of right elbow

▤ IQ + 7 T22.522- Corrosion of first degree of left elbow

▤ IQ + 7 T22.529- Corrosion of first degree of unspecified elbow

+ 6 T22.53 Corrosion of first degree of upper arm

▤ IQ + 7 T22.531- Corrosion of first degree of right upper arm

▤ IQ + 7 T22.532- Corrosion of first degree of left upper arm

▤ IQ + 7 T22.539- Corrosion of first degree of unspecified upper arm

+ 6 T22.54 Corrosion of first degree of axilla

▤ IQ + 7 T22.541- Corrosion of first degree of right axilla

▤ IQ + 7 T22.542- Corrosion of first degree of left axilla

▤ IQ + 7 T22.549- Corrosion of first degree of unspecified axilla

+ 6 T22.55 Corrosion of first degree of shoulder

▤ IQ + 7 T22.551- Corrosion of first degree of right shoulder

▤ IQ + 7 T22.552- Corrosion of first degree of left shoulder

▤ IQ + 7 T22.559- Corrosion of first degree of unspecified shoulder

+ 6 T22.56 Corrosion of first degree of scapular region

▤ IQ + 7 T22.561- Corrosion of first degree of right scapular region

▤ IQ + 7 T22.562- Corrosion of first degree of left scapular region

▤ IQ + 7 T22.569- Corrosion of first degree of unspecified scapular region

+ 6 T22.59 Corrosion of first degree of multiple sites of shoulder and upper limb, except wrist and hand

▤ IQ + 7 T22.591- Corrosion of first degree of multiple sites of right shoulder and upper limb, except wrist and hand

▤ IQ + 7 T22.592- Corrosion of first degree of multiple sites of left shoulder and upper limb, except wrist and hand

▤ IQ + 7 T22.599- Corrosion of first degree of multiple sites of unspecified shoulder and upper limb, except wrist and hand

+ 5 T22.6 Corrosion of second degree of shoulder and upper limb, except wrist and hand
Code first:
(T51-T65) to identify chemical and intent
Use additional external cause code to identify place (Y92)

IQ + 7 T22.60X- Corrosion of second degree of shoulder and upper limb, except wrist and hand, unspecified site

+ 6 T22.61 Corrosion of second degree of forearm

▤ IQ + 7 T22.611- Corrosion of second degree of right forearm

▤ IQ + 7 T22.612- Corrosion of second degree of left forearm

▤ IQ + 7 T22.619- Corrosion of second degree of unspecified forearm

+ 6 T22.62 Corrosion of second degree of elbow

▤ IQ + 7 T22.621- Corrosion of second degree of right elbow

▤ IQ + 7 T22.622- Corrosion of second degree of left elbow

▤ IQ + 7 T22.629- Corrosion of second degree of unspecified elbow

+ 6 T22.63 Corrosion of second degree of upper arm

▤ IQ + 7 T22.631- Corrosion of second degree of right upper arm

▤ IQ + 7 T22.632- Corrosion of second degree of left upper arm

▤ IQ + 7 T22.639- Corrosion of second degree of unspecified upper arm

+ 6 T22.64 Corrosion of second degree of axilla

▤ IQ + 7 T22.641- Corrosion of second degree of right axilla

▤ IQ + 7 T22.642- Corrosion of second degree of left axilla

▤ IQ + 7 T22.649- Corrosion of second degree of unspecified axilla

+ 6 T22.65 Corrosion of second degree of shoulder

▤ IQ + 7 T22.651- Corrosion of second degree of right shoulder

▤ IQ + 7 T22.652- Corrosion of second degree of left shoulder

▤ IQ + 7 T22.659- Corrosion of second degree of unspecified shoulder

+ 6 T22.66 Corrosion of second degree of scapular region

▤ IQ + 7 T22.661- Corrosion of second degree of right scapular region

▤ IQ + 7 T22.662- Corrosion of second degree of left scapular region

▤ IQ + 7 T22.669- Corrosion of second degree of unspecified scapular region

+ 6 T22.69 Corrosion of second degree of multiple sites of shoulder and upper limb, except wrist and hand

▤ IQ + 7 T22.691- Corrosion of second degree of multiple sites of right shoulder and upper limb, except wrist and hand

▤ IQ + 7 T22.692- Corrosion of second degree of multiple sites of left shoulder and upper limb, except wrist and hand

▤ IQ + 7 T22.699- Corrosion of second degree of multiple sites of unspecified shoulder and upper limb, except wrist and hand

+ 5 T22.7 Corrosion of third degree of shoulder and upper limb, except wrist and hand
Code first:
(T51-T65) to identify chemical and intent

---

4 4th digit required   5 5th digit required   6 6th digit required   7 7th digit required   ☑ 7th digit placeholder   +Additional code   ▤ Laterality

Use additional external cause code to identify place (Y92)

IQ + ☑ **T22.70X-** Corrosion of third degree of shoulder and upper limb, except wrist and hand, unspecified site

+ ⑥ **T22.71** Corrosion of third degree of forearm

▤ **IQ** + ☑ **T22.711-** Corrosion of third degree of right forearm

▤ **IQ** + ☑ **T22.712-** Corrosion of third degree of left forearm

▤ **IQ** + ☑ **T22.719-** Corrosion of third degree of unspecified forearm

+ ⑥ **T22.72** Corrosion of third degree of elbow

▤ **IQ** + ☑ **T22.721-** Corrosion of third degree of right elbow

▤ **IQ** + ☑ **T22.722-** Corrosion of third degree of left elbow

▤ **IQ** + ☑ **T22.729-** Corrosion of third degree of unspecified elbow

+ ⑥ **T22.73** Corrosion of third degree of upper arm

▤ **IQ** + ☑ **T22.731-** Corrosion of third degree of right upper arm

▤ **IQ** + ☑ **T22.732-** Corrosion of third degree of left upper arm

▤ **IQ** + ☑ **T22.739-** Corrosion of third degree of unspecified upper arm

+ ⑥ **T22.74** Corrosion of third degree of axilla

▤ **IQ** + ☑ **T22.741-** Corrosion of third degree of right axilla

▤ **IQ** + ☑ **T22.742-** Corrosion of third degree of left axilla

▤ **IQ** + ☑ **T22.749-** Corrosion of third degree of unspecified axilla

+ ⑥ **T22.75** Corrosion of third degree of shoulder

▤ **IQ** + ☑ **T22.751-** Corrosion of third degree of right shoulder

▤ **IQ** + ☑ **T22.752-** Corrosion of third degree of left shoulder

▤ **IQ** + ☑ **T22.759-** Corrosion of third degree of unspecified shoulder

+ ⑥ **T22.76** Corrosion of third degree of scapular region

▤ **IQ** + ☑ **T22.761-** Corrosion of third degree of right scapular region

▤ **IQ** + ☑ **T22.762-** Corrosion of third degree of left scapular region

▤ **IQ** + ☑ **T22.769-** Corrosion of third degree of unspecified scapular region

+ ⑥ **T22.79** Corrosion of third degree of multiple sites of shoulder and upper limb, except wrist and hand

▤ **IQ** + ☑ **T22.791-** Corrosion of third degree of multiple sites of right shoulder and upper limb, except wrist and hand

▤ **IQ** + ☑ **T22.792-** Corrosion of third degree of multiple sites of left shoulder and upper limb, except wrist and hand

▤ **IQ** + ☑ **T22.799-** Corrosion of third degree of multiple sites of unspecified shoulder and upper limb, except wrist and hand

④ **T23** Burn and corrosion of wrist and hand

The appropriate 7th character is to be added to each code from category T23
A   initial encounter
D   subsequent encounter
S   sequela

CODING TIPS ✓ Do not use Z codes for skin grafts, dressing changes, drains, etc., for trauma wounds of any type, including burns. Continue to code the burn with the appropriate 7th character.

CODING TIPS ✓ Burns are classified according to degree. When there are multiple burns of different degrees to the same body part, code the burn at its highest degree. Remember, there is a convention requiring the external cause code at burns. Aftercare codes are not used for burns, including those for dressing changes, drain care, suture removal, or skin grafts. 7th character 'D' is the default for home care and hospice when providing aftercare for a healing or resolving condition; 'A' is used for active treatment such as antibiotics or more than routine wound care; 'S' is used to identify residual conditions when the burn has healed. Different burns heal at differing rates, so a current burn (with an A or D) can be coded at the same time as a sequela of a burn. A non-healing burn is still coded as a burn no matter how long it has been present.

+ ⑤ **T23.0** Burn of unspecified degree of wrist and hand

Use additional external cause code to identify the source, place and intent of the burn (X00-X19, X75-X77, X96-X98, Y92)

+ ⑥ **T23.00** Burn of unspecified degree of hand, unspecified site

▤ **IQ** + ☑ **T23.001-** Burn of unspecified degree of right hand, unspecified site

▤ **IQ** + ☑ **T23.002-** Burn of unspecified degree of left hand, unspecified site

▤ **IQ** + ☑ **T23.009-** Burn of unspecified degree of unspecified hand, unspecified site

+ ⑥ **T23.01** Burn of unspecified degree of thumb (nail)

▤ **IQ** + ☑ **T23.011-** Burn of unspecified degree of right thumb (nail)

▤ **IQ** + ☑ **T23.012-** Burn of unspecified degree of left thumb (nail)

▤ **IQ** + ☑ **T23.019-** Burn of unspecified degree of unspecified thumb (nail)

+ ⑥ **T23.02** Burn of unspecified degree of single finger (nail) except thumb

▤ **IQ** + ☑ **T23.021-** Burn of unspecified degree of single right finger (nail) except thumb

▤ **IQ** + ☑ **T23.022-** Burn of unspecified degree of single left finger (nail) except thumb

▤ **IQ** + ☑ **T23.029-** Burn of unspecified degree of unspecified single finger (nail) except thumb

---

★ New ▲ Revised **Px** Primary **SP** PDGM Px **SL** Low CoM **SH** High CoM **IQ** Quest. Encounter **H** Hospice non-cancer Dx | Unspecified | **M** *Manifestation*

Chapter 19

S00-T88

+ ⑥ T23.03 Burn of unspecified degree of multiple fingers (nail), not including thumb

⊟ !Q + ⑦ T23.031- Burn of unspecified degree of multiple right fingers (nail), not including thumb

⊟ !Q + ⑦ T23.032- Burn of unspecified degree of multiple left fingers (nail), not including thumb

⊟ !Q + ⑦ T23.039- Burn of unspecified degree of unspecified multiple fingers (nail), not including thumb

+ ⑥ T23.04 Burn of unspecified degree of multiple fingers (nail), including thumb

⊟ !Q + ⑦ T23.041- Burn of unspecified degree of multiple right fingers (nail), including thumb

⊟ !Q + ⑦ T23.042- Burn of unspecified degree of multiple left fingers (nail), including thumb

⊟ !Q + ⑦ T23.049- Burn of unspecified degree of unspecified multiple fingers (nail), including thumb

+ ⑥ T23.05 Burn of unspecified degree of palm

⊟ !Q + ⑦ T23.051- Burn of unspecified degree of right palm

⊟ !Q + ⑦ T23.052- Burn of unspecified degree of left palm

⊟ !Q + ⑦ T23.059- Burn of unspecified degree of unspecified palm

+ ⑥ T23.06 Burn of unspecified degree of back of hand

⊟ !Q + ⑦ T23.061- Burn of unspecified degree of back of right hand

⊟ !Q + ⑦ T23.062- Burn of unspecified degree of back of left hand

⊟ !Q + ⑦ T23.069- Burn of unspecified degree of back of unspecified hand

+ ⑥ T23.07 Burn of unspecified degree of wrist

⊟ !Q + ⑦ T23.071- Burn of unspecified degree of right wrist

⊟ !Q + ⑦ T23.072- Burn of unspecified degree of left wrist

⊟ !Q + ⑦ T23.079- Burn of unspecified degree of unspecified wrist

+ ⑥ T23.09 Burn of unspecified degree of multiple sites of wrist and hand

⊟ !Q + ⑦ T23.091- Burn of unspecified degree of multiple sites of right wrist and hand

⊟ !Q + ⑦ T23.092- Burn of unspecified degree of multiple sites of left wrist and hand

⊟ !Q + ⑦ T23.099- Burn of unspecified degree of multiple sites of unspecified wrist and hand

+ ⑤ T23.1 Burn of first degree of wrist and hand
Use additional external cause code to identify the source, place and intent of the burn (X00-X19, X75-X77, X96-X98, Y92)

+ ⑥ T23.10 Burn of first degree of hand, unspecified site

⊟ !Q + ⑦ T23.101- Burn of first degree of right hand, unspecified site

⊟ !Q + ⑦ T23.102- Burn of first degree of left hand, unspecified site

⊟ !Q + ⑦ T23.109- Burn of first degree of unspecified hand, unspecified site

+ ⑥ T23.11 Burn of first degree of thumb (nail)

⊟ SP + ⑦ T23.111- Burn of first degree of right thumb (nail)

⊟ SP + ⑦ T23.112- Burn of first degree of left thumb (nail)

⊟ !Q + ⑦ T23.119- Burn of first degree of unspecified thumb (nail)

+ ⑥ T23.12 Burn of first degree of single finger (nail) except thumb

⊟ SP + ⑦ T23.121- Burn of first degree of single right finger (nail) except thumb

⊟ SP + ⑦ T23.122- Burn of first degree of single left finger (nail) except thumb

⊟ !Q + ⑦ T23.129- Burn of first degree of unspecified single finger (nail) except thumb

+ ⑥ T23.13 Burn of first degree of multiple fingers (nail), not including thumb

⊟ SP + ⑦ T23.131- Burn of first degree of multiple right fingers (nail), not including thumb

⊟ SP + ⑦ T23.132- Burn of first degree of multiple left fingers (nail), not including thumb

⊟ !Q + ⑦ T23.139- Burn of first degree of unspecified multiple fingers (nail), not including thumb

+ ⑥ T23.14 Burn of first degree of multiple fingers (nail), including thumb

⊟ SP + ⑦ T23.141- Burn of first degree of multiple right fingers (nail), including thumb

⊟ SP + ⑦ T23.142- Burn of first degree of multiple left fingers (nail), including thumb

⊟ !Q + ⑦ T23.149- Burn of first degree of unspecified multiple fingers (nail), including thumb

+ ⑥ T23.15 Burn of first degree of palm

⊟ SP + ⑦ T23.151- Burn of first degree of right palm

⊟ SP + ⑦ T23.152- Burn of first degree of left palm

⊟ !Q + ⑦ T23.159- Burn of first degree of unspecified palm

+ ⑥ T23.16 Burn of first degree of back of hand

⊟ SP + ⑦ T23.161- Burn of first degree of back of right hand

⊟ SP + ⑦ T23.162- Burn of first degree of back of left hand

⊟ !Q + ⑦ T23.169- Burn of first degree of back of unspecified hand

+ ⑥ T23.17 Burn of first degree of wrist

⊟ SP + ⑦ T23.171- Burn of first degree of right wrist

⊟ SP + ⑦ T23.172- Burn of first degree of left wrist

⊟ !Q + ⑦ T23.179- Burn of first degree of unspecified wrist

+ ⑥ T23.19 Burn of first degree of multiple sites of wrist and hand

---

④4th digit required   ⑤5th digit required   ⑥6th digit required   ⑦7th digit required   ⑦7th digit placeholder   ✚Additional code   ⊟Laterality

☐ **SP** ✚ **7** T23.191- Burn of first degree of multiple sites of right wrist and hand

☐ **SP** ✚ **7** T23.192- Burn of first degree of multiple sites of left wrist and hand

☐ **IQ** ✚ **7** T23.199- Burn of first degree of multiple sites of unspecified wrist and hand

✚ **5** T23.2 Burn of second degree of wrist and hand
Use additional external cause code to identify the source, place and intent of the burn (X00-X19, X75-X77, X96-X98, Y92)

✚ **6** T23.20 Burn of second degree of hand, unspecified site

☐ **IQ** ✚ **7** T23.201- Burn of second degree of right hand, unspecified site

☐ **IQ** ✚ **7** T23.202- Burn of second degree of left hand, unspecified site

☐ **IQ** ✚ **7** T23.209- Burn of second degree of unspecified hand, unspecified site

✚ **6** T23.21 Burn of second degree of thumb (nail)

☐ **SP** ✚ **7** T23.211- Burn of second degree of right thumb (nail)

☐ **SP** ✚ **7** T23.212- Burn of second degree of left thumb (nail)

☐ **IQ** ✚ **7** T23.219- Burn of second degree of unspecified thumb (nail)

✚ **6** T23.22 Burn of second degree of single finger (nail) except thumb

☐ **SP** ✚ **7** T23.221- Burn of second degree of single right finger (nail) except thumb

☐ **SP** ✚ **7** T23.222- Burn of second degree of single left finger (nail) except thumb

☐ **IQ** ✚ **7** T23.229- Burn of second degree of unspecified single finger (nail) except thumb

✚ **6** T23.23 Burn of second degree of multiple fingers (nail), not including thumb

☐ **SP** ✚ **7** T23.231- Burn of second degree of multiple right fingers (nail), not including thumb

☐ **SP** ✚ **7** T23.232- Burn of second degree of multiple left fingers (nail), not including thumb

☐ **IQ** ✚ **7** T23.239- Burn of second degree of unspecified multiple fingers (nail), not including thumb

✚ **6** T23.24 Burn of second degree of multiple fingers (nail), including thumb

☐ **SP** ✚ **7** T23.241- Burn of second degree of multiple right fingers (nail), including thumb

☐ **SP** ✚ **7** T23.242- Burn of second degree of multiple left fingers (nail), including thumb

☐ **IQ** ✚ **7** T23.249- Burn of second degree of unspecified multiple fingers (nail), including thumb

✚ **6** T23.25 Burn of second degree of palm

☐ **SP** ✚ **7** T23.251- Burn of second degree of right palm

☐ **SP** ✚ **7** T23.252- Burn of second degree of left palm

☐ **IQ** ✚ **7** T23.259- Burn of second degree of unspecified palm

✚ **6** T23.26 Burn of second degree of back of hand

☐ **SP** ✚ **7** T23.261- Burn of second degree of back of right hand

☐ **SP** ✚ **7** T23.262- Burn of second degree of back of left hand

☐ **IQ** ✚ **7** T23.269- Burn of second degree of back of unspecified hand

✚ **6** T23.27 Burn of second degree of wrist

☐ **SP** ✚ **7** T23.271- Burn of second degree of right wrist

☐ **SP** ✚ **7** T23.272- Burn of second degree of left wrist

☐ **IQ** ✚ **7** T23.279- Burn of second degree of unspecified wrist

✚ **6** T23.29 Burn of second degree of multiple sites of wrist and hand

☐ **SP** ✚ **7** T23.291- Burn of second degree of multiple sites of right wrist and hand

☐ **SP** ✚ **7** T23.292- Burn of second degree of multiple sites of left wrist and hand

☐ **IQ** ✚ **7** T23.299- Burn of second degree of multiple sites of unspecified wrist and hand

✚ **5** T23.3 Burn of third degree of wrist and hand
Use additional external cause code to identify the source, place and intent of the burn (X00-X19, X75-X77, X96-X98, Y92)

✚ **6** T23.30 Burn of third degree of hand, unspecified site

☐ **IQ** ✚ **7** T23.301- Burn of third degree of right hand, unspecified site

☐ **IQ** ✚ **7** T23.302- Burn of third degree of left hand, unspecified site

☐ **IQ** ✚ **7** T23.309- Burn of third degree of unspecified hand, unspecified site

✚ **6** T23.31 Burn of third degree of thumb (nail)

☐ **SP** ✚ **7** T23.311- Burn of third degree of right thumb (nail)

☐ **SP** ✚ **7** T23.312- Burn of third degree of left thumb (nail)

☐ **IQ** ✚ **7** T23.319- Burn of third degree of unspecified thumb (nail)

✚ **6** T23.32 Burn of third degree of single finger (nail) except thumb

☐ **SP** ✚ **7** T23.321- Burn of third degree of single right finger (nail) except thumb

☐ **SP** ✚ **7** T23.322- Burn of third degree of single left finger (nail) except thumb

☐ **IQ** ✚ **7** T23.329- Burn of third degree of unspecified single finger (nail) except thumb

✚ **6** T23.33 Burn of third degree of multiple fingers (nail), not including thumb

☐ **SP** ✚ **7** T23.331- Burn of third degree of multiple right fingers (nail), not including thumb

☐ **SP** ✚ **7** T23.332- Burn of third degree of multiple left fingers (nail), not including thumb

★ New ▲ Revised Px Primary **SP** PDGM Px **SL** Low CoM **SH** High CoM **IQ** Quest. Encounter ⊞ Hospice non-cancer Dx Unspecified **M** *Manifestation*

DecisionHealth's FY 2020 Complete Home Health ICD-10-CM Diagnosis Coding Manual

1653

☰ **IQ** ✚ **7** **T23.339-** Burn of third degree of unspecified multiple fingers (nail), not including thumb

✚ **6** **T23.34** Burn of third degree of multiple fingers (nail), including thumb

☰ **SP** ✚ **7** **T23.341-** Burn of third degree of multiple right fingers (nail), including thumb

☰ **SP** ✚ **7** **T23.342-** Burn of third degree of multiple left fingers (nail), including thumb

☰ **IQ** ✚ **7** **T23.349-** Burn of third degree of unspecified multiple fingers (nail), including thumb

✚ **6** **T23.35** Burn of third degree of palm

☰ **SP** ✚ **7** **T23.351-** Burn of third degree of right palm

☰ **SP** ✚ **7** **T23.352-** Burn of third degree of left palm

☰ **IQ** ✚ **7** **T23.359-** Burn of third degree of unspecified palm

✚ **6** **T23.36** Burn of third degree of back of hand

☰ **SP** ✚ **7** **T23.361-** Burn of third degree of back of right hand

☰ **SP** ✚ **7** **T23.362-** Burn of third degree of back of left hand

☰ **IQ** ✚ **7** **T23.369-** Burn of third degree of back of unspecified hand

✚ **6** **T23.37** Burn of third degree of wrist

☰ **SP** ✚ **7** **T23.371-** Burn of third degree of right wrist

☰ **SP** ✚ **7** **T23.372-** Burn of third degree of left wrist

☰ **IQ** ✚ **7** **T23.379-** Burn of third degree of unspecified wrist

✚ **6** **T23.39** Burn of third degree of multiple sites of wrist and hand

☰ **SP** ✚ **7** **T23.391-** Burn of third degree of multiple sites of right wrist and hand

☰ **SP** ✚ **7** **T23.392-** Burn of third degree of multiple sites of left wrist and hand

☰ **IQ** ✚ **7** **T23.399-** Burn of third degree of multiple sites of unspecified wrist and hand

✚ **5** **T23.4** Corrosion of unspecified degree of wrist and hand

Code first:
(T51-T65) to identify chemical and intent
Use additional external cause code to identify place (Y92)

✚ **6** **T23.40** Corrosion of unspecified degree of hand, unspecified site

☰ **IQ** ✚ **7** **T23.401-** Corrosion of unspecified degree of right hand, unspecified site

☰ **IQ** ✚ **7** **T23.402-** Corrosion of unspecified degree of left hand, unspecified site

☰ **IQ** ✚ **7** **T23.409-** Corrosion of unspecified degree of unspecified hand, unspecified site

✚ **6** **T23.41** Corrosion of unspecified degree of thumb (nail)

☰ **IQ** ✚ **7** **T23.411-** Corrosion of unspecified degree of right thumb (nail)

☰ **IQ** ✚ **7** **T23.412-** Corrosion of unspecified degree of left thumb (nail)

☰ **IQ** ✚ **7** **T23.419-** Corrosion of unspecified degree of unspecified thumb (nail)

✚ **6** **T23.42** Corrosion of unspecified degree of single finger (nail) except thumb

☰ **IQ** ✚ **7** **T23.421-** Corrosion of unspecified degree of single right finger (nail) except thumb

☰ **IQ** ✚ **7** **T23.422-** Corrosion of unspecified degree of single left finger (nail) except thumb

☰ **IQ** ✚ **7** **T23.429-** Corrosion of unspecified degree of unspecified single finger (nail) except thumb

✚ **6** **T23.43** Corrosion of unspecified degree of multiple fingers (nail), not including thumb

☰ **IQ** ✚ **7** **T23.431-** Corrosion of unspecified degree of multiple right fingers (nail), not including thumb

☰ **IQ** ✚ **7** **T23.432-** Corrosion of unspecified degree of multiple left fingers (nail), not including thumb

☰ **IQ** ✚ **7** **T23.439-** Corrosion of unspecified degree of unspecified multiple fingers (nail), not including thumb

✚ **6** **T23.44** Corrosion of unspecified degree of multiple fingers (nail), including thumb

☰ **IQ** ✚ **7** **T23.441-** Corrosion of unspecified degree of multiple right fingers (nail), including thumb

☰ **IQ** ✚ **7** **T23.442-** Corrosion of unspecified degree of multiple left fingers (nail), including thumb

☰ **IQ** ✚ **7** **T23.449-** Corrosion of unspecified degree of unspecified multiple fingers (nail), including thumb

✚ **6** **T23.45** Corrosion of unspecified degree of palm

☰ **IQ** ✚ **7** **T23.451-** Corrosion of unspecified degree of right palm

☰ **IQ** ✚ **7** **T23.452-** Corrosion of unspecified degree of left palm

☰ **IQ** ✚ **7** **T23.459-** Corrosion of unspecified degree of unspecified palm

✚ **6** **T23.46** Corrosion of unspecified degree of back of hand

☰ **IQ** ✚ **7** **T23.461-** Corrosion of unspecified degree of back of right hand

☰ **IQ** ✚ **7** **T23.462-** Corrosion of unspecified degree of back of left hand

☰ **IQ** ✚ **7** **T23.469-** Corrosion of unspecified degree of back of unspecified hand

✚ **6** **T23.47** Corrosion of unspecified degree of wrist

☰ **IQ** ✚ **7** **T23.471-** Corrosion of unspecified degree of right wrist

☰ **IQ** ✚ **7** **T23.472-** Corrosion of unspecified degree of left wrist

☰ **IQ** ✚ **7** **T23.479-** Corrosion of unspecified degree of unspecified wrist

✚ **6** **T23.49** Corrosion of unspecified degree of multiple sites of wrist and hand

---

4 4th digit required   **5** 5th digit required   **6** 6th digit required   **7** 7th digit required   **☑** 7th digit placeholder   ✚ Additional code   ☰ Laterality

Chapter 19

S00-T88

▤ !Q ✚ 7 **T23.491-** Corrosion of unspecified degree of multiple sites of right wrist and hand

▤ !Q ✚ 7 **T23.492-** Corrosion of unspecified degree of multiple sites of left wrist and hand

▤ !Q ✚ 7 **T23.499-** Corrosion of unspecified degree of multiple sites of unspecified wrist and hand

✚ 5 **T23.5** Corrosion of first degree of wrist and hand
Code first:
(T51-T65) to identify chemical and intent
Use additional external cause code to identify place (Y92)

✚ 6 **T23.50** Corrosion of first degree of hand, unspecified site

▤ !Q ✚ 7 **T23.501-** Corrosion of first degree of right hand, unspecified site

▤ !Q ✚ 7 **T23.502-** Corrosion of first degree of left hand, unspecified site

▤ !Q ✚ 7 **T23.509-** Corrosion of first degree of unspecified hand, unspecified site

✚ 6 **T23.51** Corrosion of first degree of thumb (nail)

▤ !Q ✚ 7 **T23.511-** Corrosion of first degree of right thumb (nail)

▤ !Q ✚ 7 **T23.512-** Corrosion of first degree of left thumb (nail)

▤ !Q ✚ 7 **T23.519-** Corrosion of first degree of unspecified thumb (nail)

✚ 6 **T23.52** Corrosion of first degree of single finger (nail) except thumb

▤ !Q ✚ 7 **T23.521-** Corrosion of first degree of single right finger (nail) except thumb

▤ !Q ✚ 7 **T23.522-** Corrosion of first degree of single left finger (nail) except thumb

▤ !Q ✚ 7 **T23.529-** Corrosion of first degree of unspecified single finger (nail) except thumb

✚ 6 **T23.53** Corrosion of first degree of multiple fingers (nail), not including thumb

▤ !Q ✚ 7 **T23.531-** Corrosion of first degree of multiple right fingers (nail), not including thumb

▤ !Q ✚ 7 **T23.532-** Corrosion of first degree of multiple left fingers (nail), not including thumb

▤ !Q ✚ 7 **T23.539-** Corrosion of first degree of unspecified multiple fingers (nail), not including thumb

✚ 6 **T23.54** Corrosion of first degree of multiple fingers (nail), including thumb

▤ !Q ✚ 7 **T23.541-** Corrosion of first degree of multiple right fingers (nail), including thumb

▤ !Q ✚ 7 **T23.542-** Corrosion of first degree of multiple left fingers (nail), including thumb

▤ !Q ✚ 7 **T23.549-** Corrosion of first degree of unspecified multiple fingers (nail), including thumb

✚ 6 **T23.55** Corrosion of first degree of palm

▤ !Q ✚ 7 **T23.551-** Corrosion of first degree of right palm

▤ !Q ✚ 7 **T23.552-** Corrosion of first degree of left palm

▤ !Q ✚ 7 **T23.559-** Corrosion of first degree of unspecified palm

✚ 6 **T23.56** Corrosion of first degree of back of hand

▤ !Q ✚ 7 **T23.561-** Corrosion of first degree of back of right hand

▤ !Q ✚ 7 **T23.562-** Corrosion of first degree of back of left hand

▤ !Q ✚ 7 **T23.569-** Corrosion of first degree of back of unspecified hand

✚ 6 **T23.57** Corrosion of first degree of wrist

▤ !Q ✚ 7 **T23.571-** Corrosion of first degree of right wrist

▤ !Q ✚ 7 **T23.572-** Corrosion of first degree of left wrist

▤ !Q ✚ 7 **T23.579-** Corrosion of first degree of unspecified wrist

✚ 6 **T23.59** Corrosion of first degree of multiple sites of wrist and hand

▤ !Q ✚ 7 **T23.591-** Corrosion of first degree of multiple sites of right wrist and hand

▤ !Q ✚ 7 **T23.592-** Corrosion of first degree of multiple sites of left wrist and hand

▤ !Q ✚ 7 **T23.599-** Corrosion of first degree of multiple sites of unspecified wrist and hand

✚ 5 **T23.6** Corrosion of second degree of wrist and hand
Code first:
(T51-T65) to identify chemical and intent
Use additional external cause code to identify place (Y92)

✚ 6 **T23.60** Corrosion of second degree of hand, unspecified site

▤ !Q ✚ 7 **T23.601-** Corrosion of second degree of right hand, unspecified site

▤ !Q ✚ 7 **T23.602-** Corrosion of second degree of left hand, unspecified site

▤ !Q ✚ 7 **T23.609-** Corrosion of second degree of unspecified hand, unspecified site

✚ 6 **T23.61** Corrosion of second degree of thumb (nail)

▤ !Q ✚ 7 **T23.611-** Corrosion of second degree of right thumb (nail)

▤ !Q ✚ 7 **T23.612-** Corrosion of second degree of left thumb (nail)

▤ !Q ✚ 7 **T23.619-** Corrosion of second degree of unspecified thumb (nail)

✚ 6 **T23.62** Corrosion of second degree of single finger (nail) except thumb

▤ !Q ✚ 7 **T23.621-** Corrosion of second degree of single right finger (nail) except thumb

▤ !Q ✚ 7 **T23.622-** Corrosion of second degree of single left finger (nail) except thumb

★ New ▲ Revised Px Primary SP PDGM Px SL Low CoM SH High CoM !Q Quest. Encounter ⊞ Hospice non-cancer Dx [Unspecified] M *Manifestation*

DecisionHealth's FY 2020 Complete Home Health ICD-10-CM Diagnosis Coding Manual 1655

☰ **IQ** ✚ **7** **T23.629-** **Corrosion of second degree of unspecified single finger (nail) except thumb**

✚ **6** **T23.63** Corrosion of second degree of multiple fingers (nail), not including thumb

☰ **IQ** ✚ **7** **T23.631-** Corrosion of second degree of multiple right fingers (nail), not including thumb

☰ **IQ** ✚ **7** **T23.632-** Corrosion of second degree of multiple left fingers (nail), not including thumb

☰ **IQ** ✚ **7** **T23.639-** **Corrosion of second degree of unspecified multiple fingers (nail), not including thumb**

✚ **6** **T23.64** Corrosion of second degree of multiple fingers (nail), including thumb

☰ **IQ** ✚ **7** **T23.641-** Corrosion of second degree of multiple right fingers (nail), including thumb

☰ **IQ** ✚ **7** **T23.642-** Corrosion of second degree of multiple left fingers (nail), including thumb

☰ **IQ** ✚ **7** **T23.649-** **Corrosion of second degree of unspecified multiple fingers (nail), including thumb**

✚ **6** **T23.65** Corrosion of second degree of palm

☰ **IQ** ✚ **7** **T23.651-** Corrosion of second degree of right palm

☰ **IQ** ✚ **7** **T23.652-** Corrosion of second degree of left palm

☰ **IQ** ✚ **7** **T23.659-** **Corrosion of second degree of unspecified palm**

✚ **6** **T23.66** Corrosion of second degree of back of hand

☰ **IQ** ✚ **7** **T23.661-** Corrosion of second degree back of right hand

☰ **IQ** ✚ **7** **T23.662-** Corrosion of second degree back of left hand

☰ **IQ** ✚ **7** **T23.669-** **Corrosion of second degree back of unspecified hand**

✚ **6** **T23.67** Corrosion of second degree of wrist

☰ **IQ** ✚ **7** **T23.671-** Corrosion of second degree of right wrist

☰ **IQ** ✚ **7** **T23.672-** Corrosion of second degree of left wrist

☰ **IQ** ✚ **7** **T23.679-** **Corrosion of second degree of unspecified wrist**

✚ **6** **T23.69** Corrosion of second degree of multiple sites of wrist and hand

☰ **IQ** ✚ **7** **T23.691-** Corrosion of second degree of multiple sites of right wrist and hand

☰ **IQ** ✚ **7** **T23.692-** Corrosion of second degree of multiple sites of left wrist and hand

☰ **IQ** ✚ **7** **T23.699-** **Corrosion of second degree of multiple sites of unspecified wrist and hand**

✚ **5** **T23.7** Corrosion of third degree of wrist and hand
Code first:
　(T51-T65) to identify chemical and intent
Use additional external cause code to identify place (Y92)

✚ **6** **T23.70** **Corrosion of third degree of hand, unspecified site**

☰ **IQ** ✚ **7** **T23.701-** **Corrosion of third degree of right hand, unspecified site**

☰ **IQ** ✚ **7** **T23.702-** **Corrosion of third degree of left hand, unspecified site**

☰ **IQ** ✚ **7** **T23.709-** **Corrosion of third degree of unspecified hand, unspecified site**

✚ **6** **T23.71** Corrosion of third degree of thumb (nail)

☰ **IQ** ✚ **7** **T23.711-** Corrosion of third degree of right thumb (nail)

☰ **IQ** ✚ **7** **T23.712-** Corrosion of third degree of left thumb (nail)

☰ **IQ** ✚ **7** **T23.719-** **Corrosion of third degree of unspecified thumb (nail)**

✚ **6** **T23.72** Corrosion of third degree of single finger (nail) except thumb

☰ **IQ** ✚ **7** **T23.721-** Corrosion of third degree of single right finger (nail) except thumb

☰ **IQ** ✚ **7** **T23.722-** Corrosion of third degree of single left finger (nail) except thumb

☰ **IQ** ✚ **7** **T23.729-** **Corrosion of third degree of unspecified single finger (nail) except thumb**

✚ **6** **T23.73** Corrosion of third degree of multiple fingers (nail), not including thumb

☰ **IQ** ✚ **7** **T23.731-** Corrosion of third degree of multiple right fingers (nail), not including thumb

☰ **IQ** ✚ **7** **T23.732-** Corrosion of third degree of multiple left fingers (nail), not including thumb

☰ **IQ** ✚ **7** **T23.739-** **Corrosion of third degree of unspecified multiple fingers (nail), not including thumb**

✚ **6** **T23.74** Corrosion of third degree of multiple fingers (nail), including thumb

☰ **IQ** ✚ **7** **T23.741-** Corrosion of third degree of multiple right fingers (nail), including thumb

☰ **IQ** ✚ **7** **T23.742-** Corrosion of third degree of multiple left fingers (nail), including thumb

☰ **IQ** ✚ **7** **T23.749-** **Corrosion of third degree of unspecified multiple fingers (nail), including thumb**

✚ **6** **T23.75** Corrosion of third degree of palm

☰ **IQ** ✚ **7** **T23.751-** Corrosion of third degree of right palm

☰ **IQ** ✚ **7** **T23.752-** Corrosion of third degree of left palm

☰ **IQ** ✚ **7** **T23.759-** **Corrosion of third degree of unspecified palm**

✚ **6** **T23.76** Corrosion of third degree of back of hand

☰ **IQ** ✚ **7** **T23.761-** Corrosion of third degree of back of right hand

☰ **IQ** ✚ **7** **T23.762-** Corrosion of third degree of back of left hand

☰ **IQ** ✚ **7** **T23.769-** **Corrosion of third degree back of unspecified hand**

✚ **6** **T23.77** Corrosion of third degree of wrist

---

4 4th digit required　**5** 5th digit required　**6** 6th digit required　**7** 7th digit required　**7** 7th digit placeholder　✚ Additional code　☰ Laterality

☐ **IQ** ✚ **7** T23.771- Corrosion of third degree of right wrist

☐ **IQ** ✚ **7** T23.772- Corrosion of third degree of left wrist

☐ **IQ** ✚ **7** T23.779- Corrosion of third degree of unspecified wrist

✚ **6** T23.79 Corrosion of third degree of multiple sites of wrist and hand

☐ **IQ** ✚ **7** T23.791- Corrosion of third degree of multiple sites of right wrist and hand

☐ **IQ** ✚ **7** T23.792- Corrosion of third degree of multiple sites of left wrist and hand

☐ **IQ** ✚ **7** T23.799- Corrosion of third degree of multiple sites of unspecified wrist and hand

4 T24 Burn and corrosion of lower limb, except ankle and foot

> **EXCLUDES 2** burn and corrosion of ankle and foot (T25.-)
> burn and corrosion of hip region (T21.-)

> The appropriate 7th character is to be added to each code from category T24
> A   initial encounter
> D   subsequent encounter
> S   sequela

CODING TIPS ✓ Do not use Z codes for skin grafts, dressing changes, drains, etc., for trauma wounds of any type, including burns. Continue to code the burn with the appropriate 7th character.

CODING TIPS ✓ Burns are classified according to degree. When there are multiple burns of different degrees to the same body part, code the burn at its highest degree. Remember, there is a convention requiring the external cause code at burns. Aftercare codes are not used for burns, including those for dressing changes, drain care, suture removal, or skin grafts. 7th character 'D' is the default for home care and hospice when providing aftercare for a healing or resolving condition; 'A' is used for active treatment such as antibiotics or more than routine wound care; 'S' is used to identify residual conditions when the burn has healed. Different burns heal at differing rates, so a current burn (with an A or D) can be coded at the same time as a sequela of a burn. A non-healing burn is still coded as a burn no matter how long it has been present.

✚ **5** T24.0 Burn of unspecified degree of lower limb, except ankle and foot

> Use additional external cause code to identify the source, place and intent of the burn (X00-X19, X75-X77, X96-X98, Y92)

✚ **6** T24.00 Burn of unspecified degree of unspecified site of lower limb, except ankle and foot

☐ **IQ** ✚ **7** T24.001- Burn of unspecified degree of unspecified site of right lower limb, except ankle and foot

☐ **IQ** ✚ **7** T24.002- Burn of unspecified degree of unspecified site of left lower limb, except ankle and foot

☐ **IQ** ✚ **7** T24.009- Burn of unspecified degree of unspecified site of unspecified lower limb, except ankle and foot

✚ **6** T24.01 Burn of unspecified degree of thigh

☐ **IQ** ✚ **7** T24.011- Burn of unspecified degree of right thigh

☐ **IQ** ✚ **7** T24.012- Burn of unspecified degree of left thigh

☐ **IQ** ✚ **7** T24.019- Burn of unspecified degree of unspecified thigh

✚ **6** T24.02 Burn of unspecified degree of knee

☐ **IQ** ✚ **7** T24.021- Burn of unspecified degree of right knee

☐ **IQ** ✚ **7** T24.022- Burn of unspecified degree of left knee

☐ **IQ** ✚ **7** T24.029- Burn of unspecified degree of unspecified knee

✚ **6** T24.03 Burn of unspecified degree of lower leg

☐ **IQ** ✚ **7** T24.031- Burn of unspecified degree of right lower leg

☐ **IQ** ✚ **7** T24.032- Burn of unspecified degree of left lower leg

☐ **IQ** ✚ **7** T24.039- Burn of unspecified degree of unspecified lower leg

✚ **6** T24.09 Burn of unspecified degree of multiple sites of lower limb, except ankle and foot

☐ **IQ** ✚ **7** T24.091- Burn of unspecified degree of multiple sites of right lower limb, except ankle and foot

☐ **IQ** ✚ **7** T24.092- Burn of unspecified degree of multiple sites of left lower limb, except ankle and foot

☐ **IQ** ✚ **7** T24.099- Burn of unspecified degree of multiple sites of unspecified lower limb, except ankle and foot

✚ **5** T24.1 Burn of first degree of lower limb, except ankle and foot

> Use additional external cause code to identify the source, place and intent of the burn (X00-X19, X75-X77, X96-X98, Y92)

✚ **6** T24.10 Burn of first degree of unspecified site of lower limb, except ankle and foot

☐ **IQ** ✚ **7** T24.101- Burn of first degree of unspecified site of right lower limb, except ankle and foot

☐ **IQ** ✚ **7** T24.102- Burn of first degree of unspecified site of left lower limb, except ankle and foot

☐ **IQ** ✚ **7** T24.109- Burn of first degree of unspecified site of unspecified lower limb, except ankle and foot

✚ **6** T24.11 Burn of first degree of thigh

☐ **SP** ✚ **7** T24.111- Burn of first degree of right thigh

---

☆ New ▲ Revised   **Px** Primary   **SP** PDGM Px   **SL** Low CoM   **SH** High CoM   **IQ** Quest. Encounter   **H** Hospice non-cancer Dx   Unspecified   **M** *Manifestation*

⊟ **SP** ✚ 7 **T24.112-** Burn of first degree of left thigh

⊟ **IQ** ✚ 7 **T24.119-** Burn of first degree of unspecified thigh

✚ 6 **T24.12** Burn of first degree of knee

⊟ **SP** ✚ 7 **T24.121-** Burn of first degree of right knee

⊟ **SP** ✚ 7 **T24.122-** Burn of first degree of left knee

⊟ **IQ** ✚ 7 **T24.129-** Burn of first degree of unspecified knee

✚ 6 **T24.13** Burn of first degree of lower leg

⊟ **SP** ✚ 7 **T24.131-** Burn of first degree of right lower leg

⊟ **SP** ✚ 7 **T24.132-** Burn of first degree of left lower leg

⊟ **IQ** ✚ 7 **T24.139-** Burn of first degree of unspecified lower leg

✚ 6 **T24.19** Burn of first degree of multiple sites of lower limb, except ankle and foot

⊟ **SP** ✚ 7 **T24.191-** Burn of first degree of multiple sites of right lower limb, except ankle and foot

⊟ **SP** ✚ 7 **T24.192-** Burn of first degree of multiple sites of left lower limb, except ankle and foot

⊟ **IQ** ✚ 7 **T24.199-** Burn of first degree of multiple sites of unspecified lower limb, except ankle and foot

✚ 5 **T24.2** Burn of second degree of lower limb, except ankle and foot
> Use additional external cause code to identify the source, place and intent of the burn (X00-X19, X75-X77, X96-X98, Y92)

✚ 6 **T24.20** Burn of second degree of unspecified site of lower limb, except ankle and foot

⊟ **IQ** ✚ 7 **T24.201-** Burn of second degree of unspecified site of right lower limb, except ankle and foot

⊟ **IQ** ✚ 7 **T24.202-** Burn of second degree of unspecified site of left lower limb, except ankle and foot

⊟ **IQ** ✚ 7 **T24.209-** Burn of second degree of unspecified site of unspecified lower limb, except ankle and foot

✚ 6 **T24.21** Burn of second degree of thigh

⊟ **SP** ✚ 7 **T24.211-** Burn of second degree of right thigh

⊟ **SP** ✚ 7 **T24.212-** Burn of second degree of left thigh

⊟ **IQ** ✚ 7 **T24.219-** Burn of second degree of unspecified thigh

✚ 6 **T24.22** Burn of second degree of knee

⊟ **SP** ✚ 7 **T24.221-** Burn of second degree of right knee

⊟ **SP** ✚ 7 **T24.222-** Burn of second degree of left knee

⊟ **IQ** ✚ 7 **T24.229-** Burn of second degree of unspecified knee

✚ 6 **T24.23** Burn of second degree of lower leg

⊟ **SP** ✚ 7 **T24.231-** Burn of second degree of right lower leg

⊟ **SP** ✚ 7 **T24.232-** Burn of second degree of left lower leg

⊟ **IQ** ✚ 7 **T24.239-** Burn of second degree of unspecified lower leg

✚ 6 **T24.29** Burn of second degree of multiple sites of lower limb, except ankle and foot

⊟ **SP** ✚ 7 **T24.291-** Burn of second degree of multiple sites of right lower limb, except ankle and foot

⊟ **SP** ✚ 7 **T24.292-** Burn of second degree of multiple sites of left lower limb, except ankle and foot

⊟ **IQ** ✚ 7 **T24.299-** Burn of second degree of multiple sites of unspecified lower limb, except ankle and foot

✚ 5 **T24.3** Burn of third degree of lower limb, except ankle and foot
> Use additional external cause code to identify the source, place and intent of the burn (X00-X19, X75-X77, X96-X98, Y92)

✚ 6 **T24.30** Burn of third degree of unspecified site of lower limb, except ankle and foot

⊟ **IQ** ✚ 7 **T24.301-** Burn of third degree of unspecified site of right lower limb, except ankle and foot

⊟ **IQ** ✚ 7 **T24.302-** Burn of third degree of unspecified site of left lower limb, except ankle and foot

⊟ **IQ** ✚ 7 **T24.309-** Burn of third degree of unspecified site of unspecified lower limb, except ankle and foot

✚ 6 **T24.31** Burn of third degree of thigh

⊟ **SP** ✚ 7 **T24.311-** Burn of third degree of right thigh

⊟ **SP** ✚ 7 **T24.312-** Burn of third degree of left thigh

⊟ **IQ** ✚ 7 **T24.319-** Burn of third degree of unspecified thigh

✚ 6 **T24.32** Burn of third degree of knee

⊟ **SP** ✚ 7 **T24.321-** Burn of third degree of right knee

⊟ **SP** ✚ 7 **T24.322-** Burn of third degree of left knee

⊟ **IQ** ✚ 7 **T24.329-** Burn of third degree of unspecified knee

✚ 6 **T24.33** Burn of third degree of lower leg

⊟ **SP** ✚ 7 **T24.331-** Burn of third degree of right lower leg

⊟ **SP** ✚ 7 **T24.332-** Burn of third degree of left lower leg

⊟ **IQ** ✚ 7 **T24.339-** Burn of third degree of unspecified lower leg

✚ 6 **T24.39** Burn of third degree of multiple sites of lower limb, except ankle and foot

⊟ **SP** ✚ 7 **T24.391-** Burn of third degree of multiple sites of right lower limb, except ankle and foot

⊟ **SP** ✚ 7 **T24.392-** Burn of third degree of multiple sites of left lower limb, except ankle and foot

⊟ **IQ** ✚ 7 **T24.399-** Burn of third degree of multiple sites of unspecified lower limb, except ankle and foot

Chapter 19

S00-T88

---

4 4th digit required   5 5th digit required   6 6th digit required   7 7th digit required   ✓ 7th digit placeholder   ✚ Additional code   ⊟ Laterality

+ 5 T24.4 **Corrosion of unspecified degree of lower limb, except ankle and foot**
Code first:
(T51-T65) to identify chemical and intent
Use additional external cause code to identify place (Y92)

+ 6 T24.40 **Corrosion of unspecified degree of unspecified site of lower limb, except ankle and foot**

☰ !Q + 7 T24.401- Corrosion of unspecified degree of unspecified site of right lower limb, except ankle and foot

☰ !Q + 7 T24.402- Corrosion of unspecified degree of unspecified site of left lower limb, except ankle and foot

☰ !Q + 7 T24.409- Corrosion of unspecified degree of unspecified site of unspecified lower limb, except ankle and foot

+ 6 T24.41 **Corrosion of unspecified degree of thigh**

☰ !Q + 7 T24.411- Corrosion of unspecified degree of right thigh

☰ !Q + 7 T24.412- Corrosion of unspecified degree of left thigh

☰ !Q + 7 T24.419- Corrosion of unspecified degree of unspecified thigh

+ 6 T24.42 **Corrosion of unspecified degree of knee**

☰ !Q + 7 T24.421- Corrosion of unspecified degree of right knee

☰ !Q + 7 T24.422- Corrosion of unspecified degree of left knee

☰ !Q + 7 T24.429- Corrosion of unspecified degree of unspecified knee

+ 6 T24.43 **Corrosion of unspecified degree of lower leg**

☰ !Q + 7 T24.431- Corrosion of unspecified degree of right lower leg

☰ !Q + 7 T24.432- Corrosion of unspecified degree of left lower leg

☰ !Q + 7 T24.439- Corrosion of unspecified degree of unspecified lower leg

+ 6 T24.49 **Corrosion of unspecified degree of multiple sites of lower limb, except ankle and foot**

☰ !Q + 7 T24.491- Corrosion of unspecified degree of multiple sites of right lower limb, except ankle and foot

☰ !Q + 7 T24.492- Corrosion of unspecified degree of multiple sites of left lower limb, except ankle and foot

☰ !Q + 7 T24.499- Corrosion of unspecified degree of multiple sites of unspecified lower limb, except ankle and foot

+ 5 T24.5 **Corrosion of first degree of lower limb, except ankle and foot**
Code first:
(T51-T65) to identify chemical and intent
Use additional external cause code to identify place (Y92)

+ 6 T24.50 **Corrosion of first degree of unspecified site of lower limb, except ankle and foot**

☰ !Q + 7 T24.501- Corrosion of first degree of unspecified site of right lower limb, except ankle and foot

☰ !Q + 7 T24.502- Corrosion of first degree of unspecified site of left lower limb, except ankle and foot

☰ !Q + 7 T24.509- Corrosion of first degree of unspecified site of unspecified lower limb, except ankle and foot

+ 6 T24.51 Corrosion of first degree of thigh

☰ !Q + 7 T24.511- Corrosion of first degree of right thigh

☰ !Q + 7 T24.512- Corrosion of first degree of left thigh

☰ !Q + 7 T24.519- Corrosion of first degree of unspecified thigh

+ 6 T24.52 Corrosion of first degree of knee

☰ !Q + 7 T24.521- Corrosion of first degree of right knee

☰ !Q + 7 T24.522- Corrosion of first degree of left knee

☰ !Q + 7 T24.529- Corrosion of first degree of unspecified knee

+ 6 T24.53 Corrosion of first degree of lower leg

☰ !Q + 7 T24.531- Corrosion of first degree of right lower leg

☰ !Q + 7 T24.532- Corrosion of first degree of left lower leg

☰ !Q + 7 T24.539- Corrosion of first degree of unspecified lower leg

+ 6 T24.59 Corrosion of first degree of multiple sites of lower limb, except ankle and foot

☰ !Q + 7 T24.591- Corrosion of first degree of multiple sites of right lower limb, except ankle and foot

☰ !Q + 7 T24.592- Corrosion of first degree of multiple sites of left lower limb, except ankle and foot

☰ !Q + 7 T24.599- Corrosion of first degree of multiple sites of unspecified lower limb, except ankle and foot

+ 5 T24.6 **Corrosion of second degree of lower limb, except ankle and foot**
Code first:
(T51-T65) to identify chemical and intent
Use additional external cause code to identify place (Y92)

+ 6 T24.60 **Corrosion of second degree of unspecified site of lower limb, except ankle and foot**

☰ !Q + 7 T24.601- Corrosion of second degree of unspecified site of right lower limb, except ankle and foot

☰ !Q + 7 T24.602- Corrosion of second degree of unspecified site of left lower limb, except ankle and foot

★ New ▲ Revised Px Primary SP PDGM Px SL Low CoM SH High CoM !Q Quest. Encounter H Hospice non-cancer Dx Unspecified M Manifestation

DecisionHealth's FY 2020 Complete Home Health ICD-10-CM Diagnosis Coding Manual

Chapter 19

S00-T88

▤ **!Q** ✚ ⑦ **T24.609-** **Corrosion of second degree of unspecified site of unspecified lower limb, except ankle and foot**

✚ ⑥ **T24.61** Corrosion of second degree of thigh

▤ **!Q** ✚ ⑦ **T24.611-** Corrosion of second degree of right thigh

▤ **!Q** ✚ ⑦ **T24.612-** Corrosion of second degree of left thigh

▤ **!Q** ✚ ⑦ **T24.619-** **Corrosion of second degree of unspecified thigh**

✚ ⑥ **T24.62** Corrosion of second degree of knee

▤ **!Q** ✚ ⑦ **T24.621-** Corrosion of second degree of right knee

▤ **!Q** ✚ ⑦ **T24.622-** Corrosion of second degree of left knee

▤ **!Q** ✚ ⑦ **T24.629-** **Corrosion of second degree of unspecified knee**

✚ ⑥ **T24.63** Corrosion of second degree of lower leg

▤ **!Q** ✚ ⑦ **T24.631-** Corrosion of second degree of right lower leg

▤ **!Q** ✚ ⑦ **T24.632-** Corrosion of second degree of left lower leg

▤ **!Q** ✚ ⑦ **T24.639-** **Corrosion of second degree of unspecified lower leg**

✚ ⑥ **T24.69** Corrosion of second degree of multiple sites of lower limb, except ankle and foot

▤ **!Q** ✚ ⑦ **T24.691-** Corrosion of second degree of multiple sites of right lower limb, except ankle and foot

▤ **!Q** ✚ ⑦ **T24.692-** Corrosion of second degree of multiple sites of left lower limb, except ankle and foot

▤ **!Q** ✚ ⑦ **T24.699-** **Corrosion of second degree of multiple sites of unspecified lower limb, except ankle and foot**

✚ ⑤ **T24.7** Corrosion of third degree of lower limb, except ankle and foot
   Code first:
     (T51-T65) to identify chemical and intent
   Use additional external cause code to identify place (Y92)

✚ ⑥ **T24.70** **Corrosion of third degree of unspecified site of lower limb, except ankle and foot**

▤ **!Q** ✚ ⑦ **T24.701-** **Corrosion of third degree of unspecified site of right lower limb, except ankle and foot**

▤ **!Q** ✚ ⑦ **T24.702-** **Corrosion of third degree of unspecified site of left lower limb, except ankle and foot**

▤ **!Q** ✚ ⑦ **T24.709-** **Corrosion of third degree of unspecified site of unspecified lower limb, except ankle and foot**

✚ ⑥ **T24.71** Corrosion of third degree of thigh

▤ **!Q** ✚ ⑦ **T24.711-** Corrosion of third degree of right thigh

▤ **!Q** ✚ ⑦ **T24.712-** Corrosion of third degree of left thigh

▤ **!Q** ✚ ⑦ **T24.719-** **Corrosion of third degree of unspecified thigh**

✚ ⑥ **T24.72** Corrosion of third degree of knee

▤ **!Q** ✚ ⑦ **T24.721-** Corrosion of third degree of right knee

▤ **!Q** ✚ ⑦ **T24.722-** Corrosion of third degree of left knee

▤ **!Q** ✚ ⑦ **T24.729-** **Corrosion of third degree of unspecified knee**

✚ ⑥ **T24.73** Corrosion of third degree of lower leg

▤ **!Q** ✚ ⑦ **T24.731-** Corrosion of third degree of right lower leg

▤ **!Q** ✚ ⑦ **T24.732-** Corrosion of third degree of left lower leg

▤ **!Q** ✚ ⑦ **T24.739-** **Corrosion of third degree of unspecified lower leg**

✚ ⑥ **T24.79** Corrosion of third degree of multiple sites of lower limb, except ankle and foot

▤ **!Q** ✚ ⑦ **T24.791-** Corrosion of third degree of multiple sites of right lower limb, except ankle and foot

▤ **!Q** ✚ ⑦ **T24.792-** Corrosion of third degree of multiple sites of left lower limb, except ankle and foot

▤ **!Q** ✚ ⑦ **T24.799-** **Corrosion of third degree of multiple sites of unspecified lower limb, except ankle and foot**

④ **T25** **Burn and corrosion of ankle and foot**

The appropriate 7th character is to be added to each code from category T25
A   initial encounter
D   subsequent encounter
S   sequela

CODING TIPS ✓ Do not use Z codes for skin grafts, dressing changes, drains, etc., for trauma wounds of any type, including burns. Continue to code the burn with the appropriate 7th character.

CODING TIPS ✓ Burns are classified according to degree. When there are multiple burns of different degrees to the same body part, code the burn at its highest degree. Remember, there is a convention requiring the external cause code at burns. Aftercare codes are not used for burns, including those for dressing changes, drain care, suture removal, or skin grafts. 7th character 'D' is the default for home care and hospice when providing aftercare for a healing or resolving condition; 'A' is used for active treatment such as antibiotics or more than routine wound care; 'S' is used to identify residual conditions when the burn has healed. Different burns heal at differing rates, so a current burn (with an A or D) can be coded at the same time as a sequela of a burn. A non-healing burn is still coded as a burn no matter how long it has been present.

✚ ⑤ **T25.0** **Burn of unspecified degree of ankle and foot**
   Use additional external cause code to identify the source, place and intent of the burn (X00-X19, X75-X77, X96-X98, Y92)

✚ ⑥ **T25.01** **Burn of unspecified degree of ankle**

---

④ 4th digit required   ⑤ 5th digit required   ⑥ 6th digit required   ⑦ 7th digit required   ⑦ 7th digit placeholder   ✚ Additional code   ▤ Laterality

🔲 **IQ** ✚ 7 T25.011- **Burn of unspecified degree of right ankle**

🔲 **IQ** ✚ 7 T25.012- **Burn of unspecified degree of left ankle**

🔲 **IQ** ✚ 7 T25.019- **Burn of unspecified degree of unspecified ankle**

✚ 6 T25.02 **Burn of unspecified degree of foot**
   EXCLUDES 2 burn of unspecified degree of toe (s) (nail) (T25.03-)

🔲 **IQ** ✚ 7 T25.021- **Burn of unspecified degree of right foot**

🔲 **IQ** ✚ 7 T25.022- **Burn of unspecified degree of left foot**

🔲 **IQ** ✚ 7 T25.029- **Burn of unspecified degree of unspecified foot**

✚ 6 T25.03 **Burn of unspecified degree of toe(s) (nail)**

🔲 **IQ** ✚ 7 T25.031- **Burn of unspecified degree of right toe(s) (nail)**

🔲 **IQ** ✚ 7 T25.032- **Burn of unspecified degree of left toe(s) (nail)**

🔲 **IQ** ✚ 7 T25.039- **Burn of unspecified degree of unspecified toe(s) (nail)**

✚ 6 T25.09 **Burn of unspecified degree of multiple sites of ankle and foot**

🔲 **IQ** ✚ 7 T25.091- **Burn of unspecified degree of multiple sites of right ankle and foot**

🔲 **IQ** ✚ 7 T25.092- **Burn of unspecified degree of multiple sites of left ankle and foot**

🔲 **IQ** ✚ 7 T25.099- **Burn of unspecified degree of multiple sites of unspecified ankle and foot**

✚ 5 T25.1 **Burn of first degree of ankle and foot**
   Use additional external cause code to identify the source, place and intent of the burn (X00-X19, X75-X77, X96-X98, Y92)

✚ 6 T25.11 **Burn of first degree of ankle**

🔲 **SP** ✚ 7 T25.111- **Burn of first degree of right ankle**

🔲 **SP** ✚ 7 T25.112- **Burn of first degree of left ankle**

🔲 **IQ** ✚ 7 T25.119- **Burn of first degree of unspecified ankle**

✚ 6 T25.12 **Burn of first degree of foot**
   EXCLUDES 2 burn of first degree of toe (s) (nail) (T25.13-)

🔲 **SP** ✚ 7 T25.121- **Burn of first degree of right foot**

🔲 **SP** ✚ 7 T25.122- **Burn of first degree of left foot**

🔲 **IQ** ✚ 7 T25.129- **Burn of first degree of unspecified foot**

✚ 6 T25.13 **Burn of first degree of toe(s) (nail)**

🔲 **SP** ✚ 7 T25.131- **Burn of first degree of right toe(s) (nail)**

🔲 **SP** ✚ 7 T25.132- **Burn of first degree of left toe(s) (nail)**

🔲 **IQ** ✚ 7 T25.139- **Burn of first degree of unspecified toe(s) (nail)**

✚ 6 T25.19 **Burn of first degree of multiple sites of ankle and foot**

🔲 **SP** ✚ 7 T25.191- **Burn of first degree of multiple sites of right ankle and foot**

🔲 **SP** ✚ 7 T25.192- **Burn of first degree of multiple sites of left ankle and foot**

🔲 **IQ** ✚ 7 T25.199- **Burn of first degree of multiple sites of unspecified ankle and foot**

✚ 5 T25.2 **Burn of second degree of ankle and foot**
   Use additional external cause code to identify the source, place and intent of the burn (X00-X19, X75-X77, X96-X98, Y92)

✚ 6 T25.21 **Burn of second degree of ankle**

🔲 **SP** ✚ 7 T25.211- **Burn of second degree of right ankle**

🔲 **SP** ✚ 7 T25.212- **Burn of second degree of left ankle**

🔲 **IQ** ✚ 7 T25.219- **Burn of second degree of unspecified ankle**

✚ 6 T25.22 **Burn of second degree of foot**
   EXCLUDES 2 burn of second degree of toe (s) (nail) (T25.23-)

🔲 **SP** ✚ 7 T25.221- **Burn of second degree of right foot**

🔲 **SP** ✚ 7 T25.222- **Burn of second degree of left foot**

🔲 **IQ** ✚ 7 T25.229- **Burn of second degree of unspecified foot**

✚ 6 T25.23 **Burn of second degree of toe(s) (nail)**

🔲 **SP** ✚ 7 T25.231- **Burn of second degree of right toe(s) (nail)**

🔲 **SP** ✚ 7 T25.232- **Burn of second degree of left toe(s) (nail)**

🔲 **IQ** ✚ 7 T25.239- **Burn of second degree of unspecified toe(s) (nail)**

✚ 6 T25.29 **Burn of second degree of multiple sites of ankle and foot**

🔲 **SP** ✚ 7 T25.291- **Burn of second degree of multiple sites of right ankle and foot**

🔲 **SP** ✚ 7 T25.292- **Burn of second degree of multiple sites of left ankle and foot**

🔲 **IQ** ✚ 7 T25.299- **Burn of second degree of multiple sites of unspecified ankle and foot**

✚ 5 T25.3 **Burn of third degree of ankle and foot**
   Use additional external cause code to identify the source, place and intent of the burn (X00-X19, X75-X77, X96-X98, Y92)

✚ 6 T25.31 **Burn of third degree of ankle**

🔲 **SP** ✚ 7 T25.311- **Burn of third degree of right ankle**

🔲 **SP** ✚ 7 T25.312- **Burn of third degree of left ankle**

🔲 **IQ** ✚ 7 T25.319- **Burn of third degree of unspecified ankle**

✚ 6 T25.32 **Burn of third degree of foot**
   EXCLUDES 2 burn of third degree of toe (s) (nail) (T25.33-)

🔲 **SP** ✚ 7 T25.321- **Burn of third degree of right foot**

🔲 **SP** ✚ 7 T25.322- **Burn of third degree of left foot**

🔲 **IQ** ✚ 7 T25.329- **Burn of third degree of unspecified foot**

✚ 6 T25.33 **Burn of third degree of toe(s) (nail)**

🔲 **SP** ✚ 7 T25.331- **Burn of third degree of right toe(s) (nail)**

★ New ▲ Revised Px Primary **SP** PDGM Px **SL** Low CoM **SH** High CoM **IQ** Quest. Encounter 🄷 Hospice non-cancer Dx   Unspecified   **M** *Manifestation*

DecisionHealth's FY 2020 Complete Home Health ICD-10-CM Diagnosis Coding Manual   1661

☐ SP **+** ☑ **T25.332-** Burn of third degree of left toe(s) (nail)

☐ IQ **+** ☑ **T25.339-** **Burn of third degree of unspecified toe(s) (nail)**

+ ☑ **T25.39** Burn of third degree of multiple sites of ankle and foot

☐ SP **+** ☑ **T25.391-** Burn of third degree of multiple sites of right ankle and foot

☐ SP **+** ☑ **T25.392-** Burn of third degree of multiple sites of left ankle and foot

☐ IQ **+** ☑ **T25.399-** **Burn of third degree of multiple sites of unspecified ankle and foot**

+ ☑ **T25.4** **Corrosion of unspecified degree of ankle and foot**

Code first:
  (T51-T65) to identify chemical and intent
Use additional external cause code to identify place (Y92)

+ ☑ **T25.41** **Corrosion of unspecified degree of ankle**

☐ IQ **+** ☑ **T25.411-** **Corrosion of unspecified degree of right ankle**

☐ IQ **+** ☑ **T25.412-** **Corrosion of unspecified degree of left ankle**

☐ IQ **+** ☑ **T25.419-** **Corrosion of unspecified degree of unspecified ankle**

+ ☑ **T25.42** **Corrosion of unspecified degree of foot**

> EXCLUDES 2   corrosion of unspecified degree of toe (s) (nail) (T25.43-)

☐ IQ **+** ☑ **T25.421-** **Corrosion of unspecified degree of right foot**

☐ IQ **+** ☑ **T25.422-** **Corrosion of unspecified degree of left foot**

☐ IQ **+** ☑ **T25.429-** **Corrosion of unspecified degree of unspecified foot**

+ ☑ **T25.43** **Corrosion of unspecified degree of toe(s) (nail)**

☐ IQ **+** ☑ **T25.431-** **Corrosion of unspecified degree of right toe(s) (nail)**

☐ IQ **+** ☑ **T25.432-** **Corrosion of unspecified degree of left toe(s) (nail)**

☐ IQ **+** ☑ **T25.439-** **Corrosion of unspecified degree of unspecified toe(s) (nail)**

+ ☑ **T25.49** **Corrosion of unspecified degree of multiple sites of ankle and foot**

☐ IQ **+** ☑ **T25.491-** **Corrosion of unspecified degree of multiple sites of right ankle and foot**

☐ IQ **+** ☑ **T25.492-** **Corrosion of unspecified degree of multiple sites of left ankle and foot**

☐ IQ **+** ☑ **T25.499-** **Corrosion of unspecified degree of multiple sites of unspecified ankle and foot**

+ ☑ **T25.5** Corrosion of first degree of ankle and foot

Code first:
  (T51-T65) to identify chemical and intent
Use additional external cause code to identify place (Y92)

+ ☑ **T25.51** Corrosion of first degree of ankle

☐ IQ **+** ☑ **T25.511-** Corrosion of first degree of right ankle

☐ IQ **+** ☑ **T25.512-** Corrosion of first degree of left ankle

☐ IQ **+** ☑ **T25.519-** **Corrosion of first degree of unspecified ankle**

+ ☑ **T25.52** Corrosion of first degree of foot

> EXCLUDES 2   corrosion of first degree of toe (s) (nail) (T25.53-)

☐ IQ **+** ☑ **T25.521-** Corrosion of first degree of right foot

☐ IQ **+** ☑ **T25.522-** Corrosion of first degree of left foot

☐ IQ **+** ☑ **T25.529-** **Corrosion of first degree of unspecified foot**

+ ☑ **T25.53** Corrosion of first degree of toe(s) (nail)

☐ IQ **+** ☑ **T25.531-** Corrosion of first degree of right toe(s) (nail)

☐ IQ **+** ☑ **T25.532-** Corrosion of first degree of left toe(s) (nail)

☐ IQ **+** ☑ **T25.539-** **Corrosion of first degree of unspecified toe(s) (nail)**

+ ☑ **T25.59** Corrosion of first degree of multiple sites of ankle and foot

☐ IQ **+** ☑ **T25.591-** Corrosion of first degree of multiple sites of right ankle and foot

☐ IQ **+** ☑ **T25.592-** Corrosion of first degree of multiple sites of left ankle and foot

☐ IQ **+** ☑ **T25.599-** **Corrosion of first degree of multiple sites of unspecified ankle and foot**

+ ☑ **T25.6** Corrosion of second degree of ankle and foot

Code first:
  (T51-T65) to identify chemical and intent
Use additional external cause code to identify place (Y92)

+ ☑ **T25.61** Corrosion of second degree of ankle

☐ IQ **+** ☑ **T25.611-** Corrosion of second degree of right ankle

☐ IQ **+** ☑ **T25.612-** Corrosion of second degree of left ankle

☐ IQ **+** ☑ **T25.619-** **Corrosion of second degree of unspecified ankle**

+ ☑ **T25.62** Corrosion of second degree of foot

> EXCLUDES 2   corrosion of second degree of toe (s) (nail) (T25.63-)

☐ IQ **+** ☑ **T25.621-** Corrosion of second degree of right foot

☐ IQ **+** ☑ **T25.622-** Corrosion of second degree of left foot

☐ IQ **+** ☑ **T25.629-** **Corrosion of second degree of unspecified foot**

+ ☑ **T25.63** Corrosion of second degree of toe(s) (nail)

☐ IQ **+** ☑ **T25.631-** Corrosion of second degree of right toe(s) (nail)

☐ IQ **+** ☑ **T25.632-** Corrosion of second degree of left toe(s) (nail)

☑4th digit required   ☑5th digit required   ☑6th digit required   ☑7th digit required   ☑ 7th digit placeholder   **+**Additional code   ☐Laterality

1662   *DecisionHealth's* FY 2020 Complete Home Health ICD-10-CM Diagnosis Coding Manual

Chapter 19

S00-T88

☐ **IQ** ✚ 7 **T25.639-** Corrosion of second degree of unspecified toe(s) (nail)

✚ 6 **T25.69** Corrosion of second degree of multiple sites of ankle and foot

☐ **IQ** ✚ 7 **T25.691-** Corrosion of second degree of right ankle and foot

☐ **IQ** ✚ 7 **T25.692-** Corrosion of second degree of left ankle and foot

☐ **IQ** ✚ 7 **T25.699-** Corrosion of second degree of unspecified ankle and foot

✚ 5 **T25.7** Corrosion of third degree of ankle and foot

Code first:
(T51-T65) to identify chemical and intent
Use additional external cause code to identify place (Y92)

✚ 6 **T25.71** Corrosion of third degree of ankle

☐ **IQ** ✚ 7 **T25.711-** Corrosion of third degree of right ankle

☐ **IQ** ✚ 7 **T25.712-** Corrosion of third degree of left ankle

☐ **IQ** ✚ 7 **T25.719-** Corrosion of third degree of unspecified ankle

✚ 6 **T25.72** Corrosion of third degree of foot

EXCLUDES 2 corrosion of third degree of toe (s) (nail) (T25.73-)

☐ **IQ** ✚ 7 **T25.721-** Corrosion of third degree of right foot

☐ **IQ** ✚ 7 **T25.722-** Corrosion of third degree of left foot

☐ **IQ** ✚ 7 **T25.729-** Corrosion of third degree of unspecified foot

✚ 6 **T25.73** Corrosion of third degree of toe(s) (nail)

☐ **IQ** ✚ 7 **T25.731-** Corrosion of third degree of right toe(s) (nail)

☐ **IQ** ✚ 7 **T25.732-** Corrosion of third degree of left toe(s) (nail)

☐ **IQ** ✚ 7 **T25.739-** Corrosion of third degree of unspecified toe(s) (nail)

✚ 6 **T25.79** Corrosion of third degree of multiple sites of ankle and foot

☐ **IQ** ✚ 7 **T25.791-** Corrosion of third degree of multiple sites of right ankle and foot

☐ **IQ** ✚ 7 **T25.792-** Corrosion of third degree of multiple sites of left ankle and foot

☐ **IQ** ✚ 7 **T25.799-** Corrosion of third degree of multiple sites of unspecified ankle and foot

---

Burns and corrosions confined to eye and internal organs (T26-T28)

CODING TIPS ✓ Burns to the eyes and internal organs are not coded to degree.

4 **T26** Burn and corrosion confined to eye and adnexa

The appropriate 7th character is to be added to each code from category T26
A   initial encounter
D   subsequent encounter
S   sequela

✚ 5 **T26.0** Burn of eyelid and periocular area

Use additional external cause code to identify the source, place and intent of the burn (X00-X19, X75-X77, X96-X98, Y92)

☐ **IQ** ✚ 7 **T26.00X-** Burn of unspecified eyelid and periocular area

☐ **SP** ✚ 7 **T26.01X-** Burn of right eyelid and periocular area

☐ **SP** ✚ 7 **T26.02X-** Burn of left eyelid and periocular area

✚ 5 **T26.1** Burn of cornea and conjunctival sac

Use additional external cause code to identify the source, place and intent of the burn (X00-X19, X75-X77, X96-X98, Y92)

☐ **IQ** ✚ 7 **T26.10X-** Burn of cornea and conjunctival sac, unspecified eye

☐ **SP** ✚ 7 **T26.11X-** Burn of cornea and conjunctival sac, right eye

☐ **SP** ✚ 7 **T26.12X-** Burn of cornea and conjunctival sac, left eye

✚ 5 **T26.2** Burn with resulting rupture and destruction of eyeball

Use additional external cause code to identify the source, place and intent of the burn (X00-X19, X75-X77, X96-X98, Y92)

☐ **IQ** ✚ 7 **T26.20X-** Burn with resulting rupture and destruction of unspecified eyeball

☐ **SP** ✚ 7 **T26.21X-** Burn with resulting rupture and destruction of right eyeball

☐ **SP** ✚ 7 **T26.22X-** Burn with resulting rupture and destruction of left eyeball

✚ 5 **T26.3** Burns of other specified parts of eye and adnexa

Use additional external cause code to identify the source, place and intent of the burn (X00-X19, X75-X77, X96-X98, Y92)

☐ **IQ** ✚ 7 **T26.30X-** Burns of other specified parts of unspecified eye and adnexa

☐ **SP** ✚ 7 **T26.31X-** Burns of other specified parts of right eye and adnexa

☐ **SP** ✚ 7 **T26.32X-** Burns of other specified parts of left eye and adnexa

✚ 5 **T26.4** Burn of eye and adnexa, part unspecified

Use additional external cause code to identify the source, place and intent of the burn (X00-X19, X75-X77, X96-X98, Y92)

☐ **IQ** ✚ 7 **T26.40X-** Burn of unspecified eye and adnexa, part unspecified

☐ **IQ** ✚ 7 **T26.41X-** Burn of right eye and adnexa, part unspecified

☐ **IQ** ✚ 7 **T26.42X-** Burn of left eye and adnexa, part unspecified

✚ 5 **T26.5** Corrosion of eyelid and periocular area

Code first:
(T51-T65) to identify chemical and intent
Use additional external cause code to identify place (Y92)

☐ **IQ** ✚ 7 **T26.50X-** Corrosion of unspecified eyelid and periocular area

---

★ New ▲ Revised **Px** Primary **SP** PDGM Px **SL** Low CoM **SH** High CoM **IQ** Quest. Encounter 🕀 Hospice non-cancer Dx Unspecified **M** *Manifestation*

☐ !Q + ☑ **T26.51X-** **Corrosion of right eyelid and periocular area**

☐ !Q + ☑ **T26.52X-** **Corrosion of left eyelid and periocular area**

+ ⑤ **T26.6** **Corrosion of cornea and conjunctival sac**
Code first:
(T51-T65) to identify chemical and intent
Use additional external cause code to identify place (Y92)

☐ !Q + ☑ **T26.60X-** **Corrosion of cornea and conjunctival sac, unspecified eye**

☐ !Q + ☑ **T26.61X-** **Corrosion of cornea and conjunctival sac, right eye**

☐ !Q + ☑ **T26.62X-** **Corrosion of cornea and conjunctival sac, left eye**

+ ⑤ **T26.7** **Corrosion with resulting rupture and destruction of eyeball**
Code first:
(T51-T65) to identify chemical and intent
Use additional external cause code to identify place (Y92)

☐ !Q + ☑ **T26.70X-** **Corrosion with resulting rupture and destruction of unspecified eyeball**

☐ !Q + ☑ **T26.71X-** **Corrosion with resulting rupture and destruction of right eyeball**

☐ !Q + ☑ **T26.72X-** **Corrosion with resulting rupture and destruction of left eyeball**

+ ⑤ **T26.8** **Corrosions of other specified parts of eye and adnexa**
Code first:
(T51-T65) to identify chemical and intent
Use additional external cause code to identify place (Y92)

☐ !Q + ☑ **T26.80X-** **Corrosions of other specified parts of unspecified eye and adnexa**

☐ !Q + ☑ **T26.81X-** **Corrosions of other specified parts of right eye and adnexa**

☐ !Q + ☑ **T26.82X-** **Corrosions of other specified parts of left eye and adnexa**

+ ⑤ **T26.9** **Corrosion of eye and adnexa, part unspecified**
Code first:
(T51-T65) to identify chemical and intent
Use additional external cause code to identify place (Y92)

☐ !Q + ☑ **T26.90X-** **Corrosion of unspecified eye and adnexa, part unspecified**

☐ !Q + ☑ **T26.91X-** **Corrosion of right eye and adnexa, part unspecified**

☐ !Q + ☑ **T26.92X-** **Corrosion of left eye and adnexa, part unspecified**

+ ④ **T27** **Burn and corrosion of respiratory tract**
Use additional external cause code to identify the source and intent of the burn (X00-X19, X75-X77, X96-X98)
Use additional external cause code to identify place (Y92)

The appropriate 7th character is to be added to each code from category T27
A   initial encounter
D   subsequent encounter
S   sequela

SP + ☑ **T27.0XX-** **Burn of larynx and trachea**

SP + ☑ **T27.1XX-** **Burn involving larynx and trachea with lung**

SP + ☑ **T27.2XX-** **Burn of other parts of respiratory tract**
Burn of thoracic cavity

!Q + ☑ **T27.3XX-** **Burn of respiratory tract, part unspecified**

SP + ☑ **T27.4XX-** **Corrosion of larynx and trachea**
Code first:
(T51-T65) to identify chemical and intent

▲ SP + ☑ **T27.5XX-** **Corrosion involving larynx and trachea with lung**
Code first:
(T51-T65) to identify chemical and intent

SP + ☑ **T27.6XX-** **Corrosion of other parts of respiratory tract**
Code first:
(T51-T65) to identify chemical and intent

SP !Q + **T27.7XX-** ☑ **Corrosion of respiratory tract, part unspecified**
Code first:
(T51-T65) to identify chemical and intent

+ ④ **T28** **Burn and corrosion of other internal organs**
Use additional external cause code to identify the source and intent of the burn (X00-X19, X75-X77, X96-X98)
Use additional external cause code to identify place (Y92)

The appropriate 7th character is to be added to each code from category T28
A   initial encounter
D   subsequent encounter
S   sequela

SP + ☑ **T28.0XX-** **Burn of mouth and pharynx**

SP + ☑ **T28.1XX-** **Burn of esophagus**

SP + ☑ **T28.2XX-** **Burn of other parts of alimentary tract**

SP + ☑ **T28.3XX-** **Burn of internal genitourinary organs**

▲ + ⑤ **T28.4** **Burns of other and unspecified internal organs**

!Q + ☑ **T28.40X-** **Burn of unspecified internal organ**

+ ⑥ **T28.41** **Burn of ear drum**

☐ SP + ⑦ **T28.411-** **Burn of right ear drum**

☐ SP + ⑦ **T28.412-** **Burn of left ear drum**

☐ !Q + ⑦ **T28.419-** **Burn of unspecified ear drum**

SP + ☑ **T28.49X-** **Burn of other internal organ**

!Q + ☑ **T28.5XX-** **Corrosion of mouth and pharynx**
Code first:
(T51-T65) to identify chemical and intent

④4th digit required   ⑤5th digit required   ⑥6th digit required   ⑦7th digit required   ☑7th digit placeholder   ✚Additional code   ☐Laterality

1664   *DecisionHealth's* FY 2020 Complete Home Health ICD-10-CM Diagnosis Coding Manual

IQ + ☑ T28.6XX- Corrosion of esophagus
Code first:
    (T51-T65) to identify chemical and intent

IQ + ☑ T28.7XX- Corrosion of other parts of alimentary tract
Code first:
    (T51-T65) to identify chemical and intent

IQ + ☑ T28.8XX- Corrosion of internal genitourinary organs
Code first:
    (T51-T65) to identify chemical and intent

+ 5 T28.9 Corrosions of other and unspecified internal organs
Code first:
    (T51-T65) to identify chemical and intent

IQ + ☑ T28.90X- Corrosions of unspecified internal organs

+ 6 T28.91 Corrosions of ear drum
▣ IQ + 7 T28.911- Corrosions of right ear drum
▣ IQ + 7 T28.912- Corrosions of left ear drum
▣ IQ + 7 T28.919- Corrosions of unspecified ear drum

IQ + ☑ T28.99X- Corrosions of other internal organs

Burns and corrosions of multiple and unspecified body regions (T30-T32)

GUIDELINES   Section I.C.19.d.6)-9)
Categories T31 and T32 are based on the classic "rule of nines" in estimating body surface involved: head and neck are assigned nine percent, each arm nine percent, each leg 18 percent, the anterior trunk 18 percent, posterior trunk 18 percent, and genitalia one percent. Providers may change these percentage assignments where necessary to accommodate infants and children who have proportionately larger heads than adults, and patients who have large buttocks, thighs, or abdomen that involve burns.

Encounters for the treatment of the late effects of burns or corrosions (i.e., scars or joint contractures) should be coded with a burn or corrosion code with the 7th character "S" for sequela.

When appropriate, both a code for a current burn or corrosion with 7th character "A" or "D" and a burn or corrosion code with 7th character "S" may be assigned on the same record (when both a current burn and sequelae of an old burn exist). Burns and corrosions do not heal at the same rate and a current healing wound may still exist with sequela of a healed burn or corrosion.

An external cause code should be used with burns and corrosions to identify the source and intent of the burn, as well as the place where it occurred.

▣ T30 Burn and corrosion, body region unspecified

GUIDELINES   Section I.C.19.d.5)
Category T30, Burn and corrosion, body region unspecified is extremely vague and should rarely be used.

CODING TIPS ✓   This code should not be assigned in home health or hospice. The location of the burn should be identifiable by clinical assessment and supported by clinical record documentation. Code the burn to location/site and severity, specifically.

IQ T30.0 Burn of unspecified body region, unspecified degree
This code is not for inpatient use. Code to specified site and degree of burns
Burn NOS
Multiple burns NOS

IQ T30.4 Corrosion of unspecified body region, unspecified degree
This code is not for inpatient use. Code to specified site and degree of corrosion
Corrosion NOS
Multiple corrosion NOS

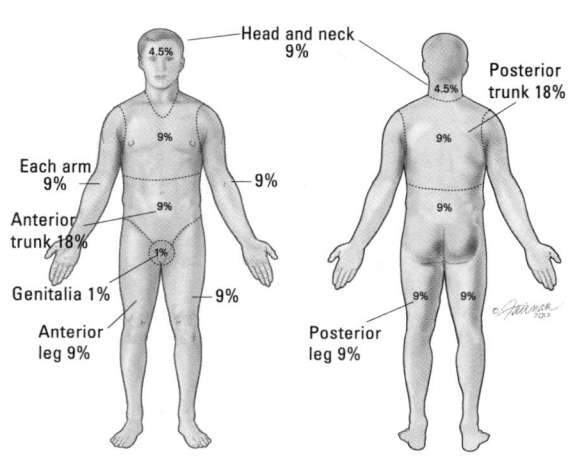

Head and neck 9%
4.5%
Posterior trunk 18%
4.5%
9%
9%
Each arm 9%
9%
Anterior trunk 18%
9%
9%
1%
Genitalia 1%
9%
9% 9%
Anterior leg 9%
Posterior leg 9%

▣ T31 Burns classified according to extent of body surface involved
Note:
This category is to be used as the primary code only when the site of the burn is unspecified. It should be used as a supplementary code with categories T20-T25 when the site is specified.

CODING TIPS ✓   Do not use this code as primary in home care or hospice. T31 is used to identify the extent of a burn estimating body surface affected using the Rule of Nines and is only necessary in home care and hospice for patients who have 3rd degree burns over 20% or more of their bodies.

IQ T31.0 Burns involving less than 10% of body surface
5 T31.1 Burns involving 10-19% of body surface
IQ T31.10 Burns involving 10-19% of body surface with 0% to 9% third degree burns
Burns involving 10-19% of body surface NOS
IQ T31.11 Burns involving 10-19% of body surface with 10-19% third degree burns
5 T31.2 Burns involving 20-29% of body surface

✱ New ▲ Revised   Px Primary   SP PDGM Px   SL Low CoM   SH High CoM   IQ Quest. Encounter   H Hospice non-cancer Dx   Unspecified   M *Manifestation*

DecisionHealth's FY 2020 Complete Home Health ICD-10-CM Diagnosis Coding Manual   1665

IQ T31.20 **Burns involving 20-29% of body surface with 0% to 9% third degree burns**
Burns involving 20-29% of body surface NOS

IQ T31.21 **Burns involving 20-29% of body surface with 10-19% third degree burns**

IQ T31.22 **Burns involving 20-29% of body surface with 20-29% third degree burns**

5 T31.3 **Burns involving 30-39% of body surface**

IQ T31.30 **Burns involving 30-39% of body surface with 0% to 9% third degree burns**
Burns involving 30-39% of body surface NOS

IQ T31.31 **Burns involving 30-39% of body surface with 10-19% third degree burns**

IQ T31.32 **Burns involving 30-39% of body surface with 20-29% third degree burns**

IQ T31.33 **Burns involving 30-39% of body surface with 30-39% third degree burns**

5 T31.4 **Burns involving 40-49% of body surface**

IQ T31.40 **Burns involving 40-49% of body surface with 0% to 9% third degree burns**
Burns involving 40-49% of body surface NOS

IQ T31.41 **Burns involving 40-49% of body surface with 10-19% third degree burns**

IQ T31.42 **Burns involving 40-49% of body surface with 20-29% third degree burns**

IQ T31.43 **Burns involving 40-49% of body surface with 30-39% third degree burns**

IQ T31.44 **Burns involving 40-49% of body surface with 40-49% third degree burns**

5 T31.5 **Burns involving 50-59% of body surface**

IQ T31.50 **Burns involving 50-59% of body surface with 0% to 9% third degree burns**
Burns involving 50-59% of body surface NOS

IQ T31.51 **Burns involving 50-59% of body surface with 10-19% third degree burns**

IQ T31.52 **Burns involving 50-59% of body surface with 20-29% third degree burns**

IQ T31.53 **Burns involving 50-59% of body surface with 30-39% third degree burns**

IQ T31.54 **Burns involving 50-59% of body surface with 40-49% third degree burns**

IQ T31.55 **Burns involving 50-59% of body surface with 50-59% third degree burns**

5 T31.6 **Burns involving 60-69% of body surface**

IQ T31.60 **Burns involving 60-69% of body surface with 0% to 9% third degree burns**
Burns involving 60-69% of body surface NOS

IQ T31.61 **Burns involving 60-69% of body surface with 10-19% third degree burns**

IQ T31.62 **Burns involving 60-69% of body surface with 20-29% third degree burns**

IQ T31.63 **Burns involving 60-69% of body surface with 30-39% third degree burns**

IQ T31.64 **Burns involving 60-69% of body surface with 40-49% third degree burns**

IQ T31.65 **Burns involving 60-69% of body surface with 50-59% third degree burns**

IQ T31.66 **Burns involving 60-69% of body surface with 60-69% third degree burns**

5 T31.7 **Burns involving 70-79% of body surface**

IQ T31.70 **Burns involving 70-79% of body surface with 0% to 9% third degree burns**
Burns involving 70-79% of body surface NOS

IQ T31.71 **Burns involving 70-79% of body surface with 10-19% third degree burns**

IQ T31.72 **Burns involving 70-79% of body surface with 20-29% third degree burns**

IQ T31.73 **Burns involving 70-79% of body surface with 30-39% third degree burns**

IQ T31.74 **Burns involving 70-79% of body surface with 40-49% third degree burns**

IQ T31.75 **Burns involving 70-79% of body surface with 50-59% third degree burns**

IQ T31.76 **Burns involving 70-79% of body surface with 60-69% third degree burns**

IQ T31.77 **Burns involving 70-79% of body surface with 70-79% third degree burns**

5 T31.8 **Burns involving 80-89% of body surface**

IQ T31.80 **Burns involving 80-89% of body surface with 0% to 9% third degree burns**
Burns involving 80-89% of body surface NOS

IQ T31.81 **Burns involving 80-89% of body surface with 10-19% third degree burns**

IQ T31.82 **Burns involving 80-89% of body surface with 20-29% third degree burns**

IQ T31.83 **Burns involving 80-89% of body surface with 30-39% third degree burns**

IQ T31.84 **Burns involving 80-89% of body surface with 40-49% third degree burns**

---

4 4th digit required   5 5th digit required   6 6th digit required   7 7th digit required   7 7th digit placeholder   + Additional code   ⊟ Laterality

!Q **T31.85** **Burns involving 80-89% of body surface with 50-59% third degree burns**

!Q **T31.86** **Burns involving 80-89% of body surface with 60-69% third degree burns**

!Q **T31.87** **Burns involving 80-89% of body surface with 70-79% third degree burns**

!Q **T31.88** **Burns involving 80-89% of body surface with 80-89% third degree burns**

5 **T31.9** **Burns involving 90% or more of body surface**

!Q **T31.90** **Burns involving 90% or more of body surface with 0% to 9% third degree burns**

Burns involving 90% or more of body surface NOS

!Q **T31.91** **Burns involving 90% or more of body surface with 10-19% third degree burns**

!Q **T31.92** **Burns involving 90% or more of body surface with 20-29% third degree burns**

!Q **T31.93** **Burns involving 90% or more of body surface with 30-39% third degree burns**

!Q **T31.94** **Burns involving 90% or more of body surface with 40-49% third degree burns**

!Q **T31.95** **Burns involving 90% or more of body surface with 50-59% third degree burns**

!Q **T31.96** **Burns involving 90% or more of body surface with 60-69% third degree burns**

!Q **T31.97** **Burns involving 90% or more of body surface with 70-79% third degree burns**

!Q **T31.98** **Burns involving 90% or more of body surface with 80-89% third degree burns**

!Q **T31.99** **Burns involving 90% or more of body surface with 90% or more third degree burns**

4 **T32** **Corrosions classified according to extent of body surface involved**

Note:

This category is to be used as the primary code only when the site of the corrosion is unspecified. It may be used as a supplementary code with categories T20-T25 when the site is specified.

!Q **T32.0** **Corrosions involving less than 10% of body surface**

5 **T32.1** **Corrosions involving 10-19% of body surface**

!Q **T32.10** **Corrosions involving 10-19% of body surface with 0% to 9% third degree corrosion**

Corrosions involving 10-19% of body surface NOS

!Q **T32.11** **Corrosions involving 10-19% of body surface with 10-19% third degree corrosion**

5 **T32.2** **Corrosions involving 20-29% of body surface**

!Q **T32.20** **Corrosions involving 20-29% of body surface with 0% to 9% third degree corrosion**

!Q **T32.21** **Corrosions involving 20-29% of body surface with 10-19% third degree corrosion**

!Q **T32.22** **Corrosions involving 20-29% of body surface with 20-29% third degree corrosion**

5 **T32.3** **Corrosions involving 30-39% of body surface**

!Q **T32.30** **Corrosions involving 30-39% of body surface with 0% to 9% third degree corrosion**

!Q **T32.31** **Corrosions involving 30-39% of body surface with 10-19% third degree corrosion**

!Q **T32.32** **Corrosions involving 30-39% of body surface with 20-29% third degree corrosion**

!Q **T32.33** **Corrosions involving 30-39% of body surface with 30-39% third degree corrosion**

5 **T32.4** **Corrosions involving 40-49% of body surface**

!Q **T32.40** **Corrosions involving 40-49% of body surface with 0% to 9% third degree corrosion**

!Q **T32.41** **Corrosions involving 40-49% of body surface with 10-19% third degree corrosion**

!Q **T32.42** **Corrosions involving 40-49% of body surface with 20-29% third degree corrosion**

!Q **T32.43** **Corrosions involving 40-49% of body surface with 30-39% third degree corrosion**

!Q **T32.44** **Corrosions involving 40-49% of body surface with 40-49% third degree corrosion**

5 **T32.5** **Corrosions involving 50-59% of body surface**

!Q **T32.50** **Corrosions involving 50-59% of body surface with 0% to 9% third degree corrosion**

!Q **T32.51** **Corrosions involving 50-59% of body surface with 10-19% third degree corrosion**

!Q **T32.52** **Corrosions involving 50-59% of body surface with 20-29% third degree corrosion**

!Q **T32.53** **Corrosions involving 50-59% of body surface with 30-39% third degree corrosion**

!Q **T32.54** **Corrosions involving 50-59% of body surface with 40-49% third degree corrosion**

!Q **T32.55** **Corrosions involving 50-59% of body surface with 50-59% third degree corrosion**

5 **T32.6** **Corrosions involving 60-69% of body surface**

!Q **T32.60** **Corrosions involving 60-69% of body surface with 0% to 9% third degree corrosion**

!Q **T32.61** **Corrosions involving 60-69% of body surface with 10-19% third degree corrosion**

★ New ▲ Revised Px Primary SP PDGM Px SL Low CoM SH High CoM !Q Quest. Encounter H Hospice non-cancer Dx   Unspecified   M *Manifestation*

DecisionHealth's FY 2020 Complete Home Health ICD-10-CM Diagnosis Coding Manual

1667

Chapter 19

S00-T88

!Q **T32.62** Corrosions involving 60-69% of body surface with 20-29% third degree corrosion

!Q **T32.63** Corrosions involving 60-69% of body surface with 30-39% third degree corrosion

!Q **T32.64** Corrosions involving 60-69% of body surface with 40-49% third degree corrosion

!Q **T32.65** Corrosions involving 60-69% of body surface with 50-59% third degree corrosion

!Q **T32.66** Corrosions involving 60-69% of body surface with 60-69% third degree corrosion

5 **T32.7** Corrosions involving 70-79% of body surface

!Q **T32.70** Corrosions involving 70-79% of body surface with 0% to 9% third degree corrosion

!Q **T32.71** Corrosions involving 70-79% of body surface with 10-19% third degree corrosion

!Q **T32.72** Corrosions involving 70-79% of body surface with 20-29% third degree corrosion

!Q **T32.73** Corrosions involving 70-79% of body surface with 30-39% third degree corrosion

!Q **T32.74** Corrosions involving 70-79% of body surface with 40-49% third degree corrosion

!Q **T32.75** Corrosions involving 70-79% of body surface with 50-59% third degree corrosion

!Q **T32.76** Corrosions involving 70-79% of body surface with 60-69% third degree corrosion

!Q **T32.77** Corrosions involving 70-79% of body surface with 70-79% third degree corrosion

5 **T32.8** Corrosions involving 80-89% of body surface

!Q **T32.80** Corrosions involving 80-89% of body surface with 0% to 9% third degree corrosion

!Q **T32.81** Corrosions involving 80-89% of body surface with 10-19% third degree corrosion

!Q **T32.82** Corrosions involving 80-89% of body surface with 20-29% third degree corrosion

!Q **T32.83** Corrosions involving 80-89% of body surface with 30-39% third degree corrosion

!Q **T32.84** Corrosions involving 80-89% of body surface with 40-49% third degree corrosion

!Q **T32.85** Corrosions involving 80-89% of body surface with 50-59% third degree corrosion

!Q **T32.86** Corrosions involving 80-89% of body surface with 60-69% third degree corrosion

!Q **T32.87** Corrosions involving 80-89% of body surface with 70-79% third degree corrosion

!Q **T32.88** Corrosions involving 80-89% of body surface with 80-89% third degree corrosion

5 **T32.9** Corrosions involving 90% or more of body surface

!Q **T32.90** Corrosions involving 90% or more of body surface with 0% to 9% third degree corrosion

!Q **T32.91** Corrosions involving 90% or more of body surface with 10-19% third degree corrosion

!Q **T32.92** Corrosions involving 90% or more of body surface with 20-29% third degree corrosion

!Q **T32.93** Corrosions involving 90% or more of body surface with 30-39% third degree corrosion

!Q **T32.94** Corrosions involving 90% or more of body surface with 40-49% third degree corrosion

!Q **T32.95** Corrosions involving 90% or more of body surface with 50-59% third degree corrosion

!Q **T32.96** Corrosions involving 90% or more of body surface with 60-69% third degree corrosion

!Q **T32.97** Corrosions involving 90% or more of body surface with 70-79% third degree corrosion

!Q **T32.98** Corrosions involving 90% or more of body surface with 80-89% third degree corrosion

!Q **T32.99** Corrosions involving 90% or more of body surface with 90% or more third degree corrosion

Frostbite　(T33-T34)

EXCLUDES 2　hypothermia and other effects of reduced temperature　(T68, T69.-)

4 **T33** Superficial frostbite

INCLUDES　frostbite with partial thickness skin loss

The appropriate 7th character is to be added to each code from category T33
A　initial encounter
D　subsequent encounter
S　sequela

5 **T33.0** Superficial frostbite of head

6 **T33.01** Superficial frostbite of ear

SP 7 **T33.011-** Superficial frostbite of right ear

SP 7 **T33.012-** Superficial frostbite of left ear

!Q 7 **T33.019-** Superficial frostbite of unspecified ear

SP 7 **T33.02X-** Superficial frostbite of nose

SP 7 **T33.09X-** Superficial frostbite of other part of head

SP 7 **T33.1XX-** Superficial frostbite of neck

SP 7 **T33.2XX-** Superficial frostbite of thorax

SP 7 **T33.3XX-** Superficial frostbite of abdominal wall, lower back and pelvis

5 **T33.4** Superficial frostbite of arm
EXCLUDES 2　superficial frostbite of wrist and hand　(T33.5-)

!Q 7 **T33.40X-** Superficial frostbite of unspecified arm

4 4th digit required　　5 5th digit required　　6 6th digit required　　7 7th digit required　　7 7th digit placeholder　　+ Additional code　　Laterality

1668　　　　　*DecisionHealth's* FY 2020 Complete Home Health ICD-10-CM Diagnosis Coding Manual

☐ **SP** ☑ **T33.41X-** Superficial frostbite of right arm

☐ **SP** ☑ **T33.42X-** Superficial frostbite of left arm

⑤ **T33.5** Superficial frostbite of wrist, hand, and fingers

⑥ **T33.51** Superficial frostbite of wrist

☐ **SP** ⑦ **T33.511-** Superficial frostbite of right wrist

☐ **SP** ⑦ **T33.512-** Superficial frostbite of left wrist

☐ **IQ** ⑦ **T33.519-** Superficial frostbite of unspecified wrist

⑥ **T33.52** Superficial frostbite of hand
EXCLUDES 2 superficial frostbite of fingers (T33.53-)

☐ **SP** ⑦ **T33.521-** Superficial frostbite of right hand

☐ **SP** ⑦ **T33.522-** Superficial frostbite of left hand

☐ **IQ** ⑦ **T33.529-** Superficial frostbite of unspecified hand

⑥ **T33.53** Superficial frostbite of finger(s)

☐ **SP** ⑦ **T33.531-** Superficial frostbite of right finger(s)

☐ **SP** ⑦ **T33.532-** Superficial frostbite of left finger(s)

☐ **IQ** ⑦ **T33.539-** Superficial frostbite of unspecified finger(s)

⑤ **T33.6** Superficial frostbite of hip and thigh

☐ **IQ** ☑ **T33.60X-** Superficial frostbite of unspecified hip and thigh

☐ **SP** ☑ **T33.61X-** Superficial frostbite of right hip and thigh

☐ **SP** ☑ **T33.62X-** Superficial frostbite of left hip and thigh

⑤ **T33.7** Superficial frostbite of knee and lower leg
EXCLUDES 2 superficial frostbite of ankle and foot (T33.8-)

☐ **IQ** ☑ **T33.70X-** Superficial frostbite of unspecified knee and lower leg

☐ **SP** ☑ **T33.71X-** Superficial frostbite of right knee and lower leg

☐ **SP** ☑ **T33.72X-** Superficial frostbite of left knee and lower leg

⑤ **T33.8** Superficial frostbite of ankle, foot, and toe(s)

⑥ **T33.81** Superficial frostbite of ankle

☐ **SP** ⑦ **T33.811-** Superficial frostbite of right ankle

☐ **SP** ⑦ **T33.812-** Superficial frostbite of left ankle

☐ **IQ** ⑦ **T33.819-** Superficial frostbite of unspecified ankle

⑥ **T33.82** Superficial frostbite of foot

☐ **SP** ⑦ **T33.821-** Superficial frostbite of right foot

☐ **SP** ⑦ **T33.822-** Superficial frostbite of left foot

☐ **IQ** ⑦ **T33.829-** Superficial frostbite of unspecified foot

⑥ **T33.83** Superficial frostbite of toe(s)

☐ **SP** ⑦ **T33.831-** Superficial frostbite of right toe(s)

☐ **SP** ⑦ **T33.832-** Superficial frostbite of left toe(s)

☐ **IQ** ⑦ **T33.839-** Superficial frostbite of unspecified toe(s)

⑤ **T33.9** Superficial frostbite of other and unspecified sites

☐ **IQ** ☑ **T33.90X-** Superficial frostbite of unspecified sites
Superficial frostbite NOS

SP ☑ **T33.99X-** Superficial frostbite of other sites
Superficial frostbite of leg NOS
Superficial frostbite of trunk NOS

④ **T34** Frostbite with tissue necrosis

The appropriate 7th character is to be added to each code from category T34
A   initial encounter
D   subsequent encounter
S   sequela

⑤ **T34.0** Frostbite with tissue necrosis of head

⑥ **T34.01** Frostbite with tissue necrosis of ear

☐ **SP** ⑦ **T34.011-** Frostbite with tissue necrosis of right ear

☐ **SP** ⑦ **T34.012-** Frostbite with tissue necrosis of left ear

☐ **IQ** ⑦ **T34.019-** Frostbite with tissue necrosis of unspecified ear

SP ☑ **T34.02X-** Frostbite with tissue necrosis of nose

SP ☑ **T34.09X-** Frostbite with tissue necrosis of other part of head

SP ☑ **T34.1XX-** Frostbite with tissue necrosis of neck

SP ☑ **T34.2XX-** Frostbite with tissue necrosis of thorax

SP ☑ **T34.3XX-** Frostbite with tissue necrosis of abdominal wall, lower back and pelvis

⑤ **T34.4** Frostbite with tissue necrosis of arm
EXCLUDES 2 frostbite with tissue necrosis of wrist and hand (T34.5-)

☐ **IQ** ☑ **T34.40X-** Frostbite with tissue necrosis of unspecified arm

☐ **SP** ☑ **T34.41X-** Frostbite with tissue necrosis of right arm

☐ **SP** ☑ **T34.42X-** Frostbite with tissue necrosis of left arm

⑤ **T34.5** Frostbite with tissue necrosis of wrist, hand, and finger(s)

⑥ **T34.51** Frostbite with tissue necrosis of wrist

☐ **SP** ⑦ **T34.511-** Frostbite with tissue necrosis of right wrist

☐ **SP** ⑦ **T34.512-** Frostbite with tissue necrosis of left wrist

☐ **IQ** ⑦ **T34.519-** Frostbite with tissue necrosis of unspecified wrist

⑥ **T34.52** Frostbite with tissue necrosis of hand
EXCLUDES 2 frostbite with tissue necrosis of finger (s) (T34.53-)

☐ **SP** ⑦ **T34.521-** Frostbite with tissue necrosis of right hand

☐ **SP** ⑦ **T34.522-** Frostbite with tissue necrosis of left hand

☐ **IQ** ⑦ **T34.529-** Frostbite with tissue necrosis of unspecified hand

⑥ **T34.53** Frostbite with tissue necrosis of finger(s)

☐ **SP** ⑦ **T34.531-** Frostbite with tissue necrosis of right finger(s)

☐ **SP** ⑦ **T34.532-** Frostbite with tissue necrosis of left finger(s)

Chapter 19

S00-T88

★ New ▲ Revised Px Primary **SP** PDGM Px **SL** Low CoM **SH** High CoM **IQ** Quest. Encounter ⊞ Hospice non-cancer Dx   Unspecified   **M** Manifestation

DecisionHealth's FY 2020 Complete Home Health ICD-10-CM Diagnosis Coding Manual

1669

⊟ IQ 7 **T34.539-** Frostbite with tissue necrosis of unspecified finger(s)

5 **T34.6** Frostbite with tissue necrosis of hip and thigh

⊟ IQ 7 **T34.60X-** Frostbite with tissue necrosis of unspecified hip and thigh

⊟ SP 7 **T34.61X-** Frostbite with tissue necrosis of right hip and thigh

⊟ SP 7 **T34.62X-** Frostbite with tissue necrosis of left hip and thigh

5 **T34.7** Frostbite with tissue necrosis of knee and lower leg

EXCLUDES 2   frostbite with tissue necrosis of ankle and foot (T34.8-)

⊟ IQ 7 **T34.70X-** Frostbite with tissue necrosis of unspecified knee and lower leg

⊟ SP 7 **T34.71X-** Frostbite with tissue necrosis of right knee and lower leg

⊟ SP 7 **T34.72X-** Frostbite with tissue necrosis of left knee and lower leg

5 **T34.8** Frostbite with tissue necrosis of ankle, foot, and toe(s)

6 **T34.81** Frostbite with tissue necrosis of ankle

⊟ SP 7 **T34.811-** Frostbite with tissue necrosis of right ankle

⊟ SP 7 **T34.812-** Frostbite with tissue necrosis of left ankle

⊟ IQ 7 **T34.819-** Frostbite with tissue necrosis of unspecified ankle

6 **T34.82** Frostbite with tissue necrosis of foot

⊟ SP 7 **T34.821-** Frostbite with tissue necrosis of right foot

⊟ SP 7 **T34.822-** Frostbite with tissue necrosis of left foot

⊟ IQ 7 **T34.829-** Frostbite with tissue necrosis of unspecified foot

6 **T34.83** Frostbite with tissue necrosis of toe(s)

⊟ SP 7 **T34.831-** Frostbite with tissue necrosis of right toe(s)

⊟ SP 7 **T34.832-** Frostbite with tissue necrosis of left toe(s)

⊟ IQ 7 **T34.839-** Frostbite with tissue necrosis of unspecified toe(s)

5 **T34.9** Frostbite with tissue necrosis of other and unspecified sites

IQ 7 **T34.90X-** Frostbite with tissue necrosis of unspecified sites
Frostbite with tissue necrosis NOS

SP 7 **T34.99X-** Frostbite with tissue necrosis of other sites
Frostbite with tissue necrosis of leg NOS
Frostbite with tissue necrosis of trunk NOS

Poisoning by, adverse effects of and underdosing of drugs, medicaments and biological substances (T36-T50)

Note:
The drug giving rise to the adverse effect should be identified by use of codes from categories T36-T50 with fifth or sixth character 5.

INCLUDES   adverse effect of correct substance properly administered
poisoning by overdose of substance
poisoning by wrong substance given or taken in error
underdosing by (inadvertently) (deliberately) taking less substance than prescribed or instructed

Code first, for adverse effects, the nature of the adverse effect, such as:
adverse effect NOS (T88.7)
aspirin gastritis (K29.-)
blood disorders (D56-D76)
contact dermatitis (L23-L25)
dermatitis due to substances taken internally (L27.-)
nephropathy (N14.0-N14.2)

Use additional code(s) to specify:
manifestations of poisoning
underdosing or failure in dosage during medical and surgical care (Y63.6, Y63.8-Y63.9)
underdosing of medication regimen (Z91.12-, Z91.13-)

EXCLUDES 1   toxic reaction to local anesthesia in pregnancy (O29.3-)

EXCLUDES 2   abuse and dependence of psychoactive substances (F10-F19)
abuse of non-dependence-producing substances (F55.-)
drug reaction and poisoning affecting newborn (P00-P96)
pathological drug intoxication (inebriation) (F10-F19)

GUIDELINES   Section I.C.19.e.5)(c)

Underdosing refers to taking less of a medication than is prescribed by a provider or a manufacturer's instruction. Discontinuing the use of a prescribed medication on the patient's own initiative (not directed by the patient's provider) is also classified as an underdosing. For underdosing, assign the code from categories T36-T50 (fifth or sixth character "6").

Codes for underdosing should never be assigned as principal or first-listed codes. If a patient has a relapse or exacerbation of the medical condition for which the drug is prescribed because of the reduction in dose, then the medical condition itself should be coded.

Noncompliance (Z91.12-, Z91.13- and Z91.14-) or complication of care (Y63.6-Y63.9) codes are to be used with an underdosing code to indicate intent, if known.

GUIDELINES   Section I.C.19.e.1)-4)

Codes in categories T36-T65 are combination codes that include the substance that was taken as well as the intent. No additional external cause code is required for poisonings, toxic effects, adverse effects and underdosing codes.

Do not code directly from the Table of Drugs and Chemicals. Always refer back to the Tabular List. Use as many codes as necessary to describe completely all drugs, medicinal or biological substances. If the same code would describe the causative agent for more than one adverse reaction, poisoning, toxic effect or underdosing, assign the code only once. If two or more drugs, medicinal or biological substances are reported, code each individually unless a combination code is listed in the Table of Drugs and Chemicals.

---

4 4th digit required   5 5th digit required   6 6th digit required   7 7th digit required   ✓ 7th digit placeholder   ✚ Additional code   ⊟ Laterality

1670   DecisionHealth's FY 2020 Complete Home Health ICD-10-CM Diagnosis Coding Manual

GUIDELINES Section I.C.19.e.5)(a)

When coding an adverse effect of a drug that has been correctly prescribed and properly administered, assign the appropriate code for the nature of the adverse effect followed by the appropriate code for the adverse effect of the drug (T36-T50). The code for the drug should have a 5th or 6th character "5" (for example T36.0X5-). Examples of the nature of an adverse effect are tachycardia, delirium, gastrointestinal hemorrhaging, vomiting, hypokalemia, hepatitis, renal failure, or respiratory failure.

CODING TIPS ✓ Poisonings are coded as accidental unless there is physician documentation to indicate otherwise. 7th character 'A' means the effect of the drug/chemical requires active treatment. 'D' should be the 7th character if the effect is healing/resolving. 'S' should be used as the 7th character if the condition resulting is still a factor after the medication has long cleared from the body, i.e., glucocorticoids were taken last year resulting in diabetes.

4 T36 Poisoning by, adverse effect of and underdosing of systemic antibiotics

EXCLUDES 1 antineoplastic antibiotics (T45.1-)
locally applied antibiotic NEC (T49.0)
topically used antibiotic for ear, nose and throat (T49.6)
topically used antibiotic for eye (T49.5)

The appropriate 7th character is to be added to each code from category T36
A   initial encounter
D   subsequent encounter
S   sequela

GUIDELINES Section I.C.19.e.5)(b)

When coding a poisoning or reaction to the improper use of a medication (e.g., overdose, wrong substance given or taken in error, wrong route of administration), first assign the appropriate code from categories T36-T50. The poisoning codes have an associated intent as their 5th or 6th character (accidental, intentional self harm, assault and undetermined. If the intent of the poisoning is unknown or unspecified, code the intent as accidental intent. The undetermined intent is only for use if the documentation in the record specifies that the intent cannot be determined.

Use additional code(s) for all manifestations of poisonings. If there is also a diagnosis of abuse or dependence of the substance, the abuse or dependence is assigned as an additional code. *See Section I.C.4. if poisoning is the result of insulin pump malfunctions.*

5 T36.0 Poisoning by, adverse effect of and underdosing of penicillins
6 T36.0X Poisoning by, adverse effect of and underdosing of penicillins
SP IQ 7 T36.0X1- Poisoning by penicillins, accidental (unintentional)
Poisoning by penicillins NOS
SP 7 T36.0X2- Poisoning by penicillins, intentional self-harm
SP 7 T36.0X3- Poisoning by penicillins, assault
SP 7 T36.0X4- Poisoning by penicillins, undetermined

IQ 7 T36.0X5- Adverse effect of penicillins
SP 7 T36.0X6- Underdosing of penicillins
5 T36.1 Poisoning by, adverse effect of and underdosing of cephalosporins and other beta-lactam antibiotics
6 T36.1X Poisoning by, adverse effect of and underdosing of cephalosporins and other beta-lactam antibiotics
SP 7 T36.1X1- Poisoning by cephalosporins and other beta-lactam antibiotics, accidental (unintentional)
Poisoning by cephalosporins and other beta-lactam antibiotics NOS
SP 7 T36.1X2- Poisoning by cephalosporins and other beta-lactam antibiotics, intentional self-harm
SP 7 T36.1X3- Poisoning by cephalosporins and other beta-lactam antibiotics, assault
SP 7 T36.1X4- Poisoning by cephalosporins and other beta-lactam antibiotics, undetermined
IQ 7 T36.1X5- Adverse effect of cephalosporins and other beta-lactam antibiotics
SP 7 T36.1X6- Underdosing of cephalosporins and other beta-lactam antibiotics
5 T36.2 Poisoning by, adverse effect of and underdosing of chloramphenicol group
6 T36.2X Poisoning by, adverse effect of and underdosing of chloramphenicol group
SP 7 T36.2X1- Poisoning by chloramphenicol group, accidental (unintentional)
Poisoning by chloramphenicol group NOS
SP 7 T36.2X2- Poisoning by chloramphenicol group, intentional self-harm
SP 7 T36.2X3- Poisoning by chloramphenicol group, assault
SP 7 T36.2X4- Poisoning by chloramphenicol group, undetermined
IQ 7 T36.2X5- Adverse effect of chloramphenicol group
SP 7 T36.2X6- Underdosing of chloramphenicol group
5 T36.3 Poisoning by, adverse effect of and underdosing of macrolides
6 T36.3X Poisoning by, adverse effect of and underdosing of macrolides
SP 7 T36.3X1- Poisoning by macrolides, accidental (unintentional)
Poisoning by macrolides NOS
SP 7 T36.3X2- Poisoning by macrolides, intentional self-harm
SP 7 T36.3X3- Poisoning by macrolides, assault
SP 7 T36.3X4- Poisoning by macrolides, undetermined
IQ 7 T36.3X5- Adverse effect of macrolides
SP 7 T36.3X6- Underdosing of macrolides
5 T36.4 Poisoning by, adverse effect of and underdosing of tetracyclines
6 T36.4X Poisoning by, adverse effect of and underdosing of tetracyclines
SP 7 T36.4X1- Poisoning by tetracyclines, accidental (unintentional)
Poisoning by tetracyclines NOS

★ New ▲ Revised Px Primary SP PDGM Px SL Low CoM SH High CoM IQ Quest. Encounter H Hospice non-cancer Dx Unspecified M *Manifestation*

DecisionHealth's FY 2020 Complete Home Health ICD-10-CM Diagnosis Coding Manual

1671

SP 7 T36.4X2- Poisoning by tetracyclines, intentional self-harm

SP 7 T36.4X3- Poisoning by tetracyclines, assault

SP 7 T36.4X4- Poisoning by tetracyclines, undetermined

IQ 7 T36.4X5- Adverse effect of tetracyclines

IQ 7 T36.4X6- Underdosing of tetracyclines

5 T36.5 Poisoning by, adverse effect of and underdosing of aminoglycosides
  Poisoning by, adverse effect of and underdosing of streptomycin

6 T36.5X Poisoning by, adverse effect of and underdosing of aminoglycosides

SP 7 T36.5X1- Poisoning by aminoglycosides, accidental (unintentional)
  Poisoning by aminoglycosides NOS

SP 7 T36.5X2- Poisoning by aminoglycosides, intentional self-harm

SP 7 T36.5X3- Poisoning by aminoglycosides, assault

SP 7 T36.5X4- Poisoning by aminoglycosides, undetermined

IQ 7 T36.5X5- Adverse effect of aminoglycosides

SP 7 T36.5X6- Underdosing of aminoglycosides

5 T36.6 Poisoning by, adverse effect of and underdosing of rifampicins

6 T36.6X Poisoning by, adverse effect of and underdosing of rifampicins

SP 7 T36.6X1- Poisoning by rifampicins, accidental (unintentional)
  Poisoning by rifampicins NOS

SP 7 T36.6X2- Poisoning by rifampicins, intentional self-harm

SP 7 T36.6X3- Poisoning by rifampicins, assault

SP 7 T36.6X4- Poisoning by rifampicins, undetermined

IQ 7 T36.6X5- Adverse effect of rifampicins

SP 7 T36.6X6- Underdosing of rifampicins

5 T36.7 Poisoning by, adverse effect of and underdosing of antifungal antibiotics, systemically used

6 T36.7X Poisoning by, adverse effect of and underdosing of antifungal antibiotics, systemically used

SP 7 T36.7X1- Poisoning by antifungal antibiotics, systemically used, accidental (unintentional)
  Poisoning by antifungal antibiotics, systemically used NOS

SP 7 T36.7X2- Poisoning by antifungal antibiotics, systemically used, intentional self-harm

SP 7 T36.7X3- Poisoning by antifungal antibiotics, systemically used, assault

SP 7 T36.7X4- Poisoning by antifungal antibiotics, systemically used, undetermined

IQ 7 T36.7X5- Adverse effect of antifungal antibiotics, systemically used

SP 7 T36.7X6- Underdosing of antifungal antibiotics, systemically used

5 T36.8 Poisoning by, adverse effect of and underdosing of other systemic antibiotics

6 T36.8X Poisoning by, adverse effect of and underdosing of other systemic antibiotics

SP 7 T36.8X1- Poisoning by other systemic antibiotics, accidental (unintentional)
  Poisoning by other systemic antibiotics NOS

SP 7 T36.8X2- Poisoning by other systemic antibiotics, intentional self-harm

SP 7 T36.8X3- Poisoning by other systemic antibiotics, assault

SP 7 T36.8X4- Poisoning by other systemic antibiotics, undetermined

IQ 7 T36.8X5- Adverse effect of other systemic antibiotics

SP 7 T36.8X6- Underdosing of other systemic antibiotics

5 T36.9 Poisoning by, adverse effect of and underdosing of unspecified systemic antibiotic

SP 7 T36.91X- Poisoning by unspecified systemic antibiotic, accidental (unintentional)
  Poisoning by systemic antibiotic NOS

SP 7 T36.92X- Poisoning by unspecified systemic antibiotic, intentional self-harm

SP 7 T36.93X- Poisoning by unspecified systemic antibiotic, assault

SP 7 T36.94X- Poisoning by unspecified systemic antibiotic, undetermined

IQ 7 T36.95X- Adverse effect of unspecified systemic antibiotic

SP 7 T36.96X- Underdosing of unspecified systemic antibiotic

4 T37 Poisoning by, adverse effect of and underdosing of other systemic anti-infectives and antiparasitics

EXCLUDES 1 anti-infectives topically used for ear, nose and throat (T49.6-)
  anti-infectives topically used for eye (T49.5-)
  locally applied anti-infectives NEC (T49.0-)

The appropriate 7th character is to be added to each code from category T37
A   initial encounter
D   subsequent encounter
S   sequela

5 T37.0 Poisoning by, adverse effect of and underdosing of sulfonamides

6 T37.0X Poisoning by, adverse effect of and underdosing of sulfonamides

SP 7 T37.0X1- Poisoning by sulfonamides, accidental (unintentional)
  Poisoning by sulfonamides NOS

SP 7 T37.0X2- Poisoning by sulfonamides, intentional self-harm

SP 7 T37.0X3- Poisoning by sulfonamides, assault

SP 7 T37.0X4- Poisoning by sulfonamides, undetermined

4 4th digit required **5** 5th digit required **6** 6th digit required **7** 7th digit required **7** 7th digit placeholder **+** Additional code **⊟** Laterality

1672   *DecisionHealth's* FY 2020 Complete Home Health ICD-10-CM Diagnosis Coding Manual

Chapter 19

S00-T88

IQ 7 T37.0X5- Adverse effect of sulfonamides

SP 7 T37.0X6- Underdosing of sulfonamides

5 T37.1 Poisoning by, adverse effect of and underdosing of antimycobacterial drugs
> **EXCLUDES 1** rifampicins (T36.6-)
> streptomycin (T36.5-)

6 T37.1X Poisoning by, adverse effect of and underdosing of antimycobacterial drugs

SP 7 T37.1X1- Poisoning by antimycobacterial drugs, accidental (unintentional)
> Poisoning by antimycobacterial drugs NOS

SP 7 T37.1X2- Poisoning by antimycobacterial drugs, intentional self-harm

SP 7 T37.1X3- Poisoning by antimycobacterial drugs, assault

SP 7 T37.1X4- Poisoning by antimycobacterial drugs, undetermined

IQ 7 T37.1X5- Adverse effect of antimycobacterial drugs

SP 7 T37.1X6- Underdosing of antimycobacterial drugs

5 T37.2 Poisoning by, adverse effect of and underdosing of antimalarials and drugs acting on other blood protozoa
> **EXCLUDES 1** hydroxyquinoline derivatives (T37.8-)

6 T37.2X Poisoning by, adverse effect of and underdosing of antimalarials and drugs acting on other blood protozoa

SP 7 T37.2X1- Poisoning by antimalarials and drugs acting on other blood protozoa, accidental (unintentional)
> Poisoning by antimalarials and drugs acting on other blood protozoa NOS

SP 7 T37.2X2- Poisoning by antimalarials and drugs acting on other blood protozoa, intentional self-harm

SP 7 T37.2X3- Poisoning by antimalarials and drugs acting on other blood protozoa, assault

SP 7 T37.2X4- Poisoning by antimalarials and drugs acting on other blood protozoa, undetermined

IQ 7 T37.2X5- Adverse effect of antimalarials and drugs acting on other blood protozoa

SP 7 T37.2X6- Underdosing of antimalarials and drugs acting on other blood protozoa

5 T37.3 Poisoning by, adverse effect of and underdosing of other antiprotozoal drugs

6 T37.3X Poisoning by, adverse effect of and underdosing of other antiprotozoal drugs

SP 7 T37.3X1- Poisoning by other antiprotozoal drugs, accidental (unintentional)
> Poisoning by other antiprotozoal drugs NOS

SP 7 T37.3X2- Poisoning by other antiprotozoal drugs, intentional self-harm

SP 7 T37.3X3- Poisoning by other antiprotozoal drugs, assault

SP 7 T37.3X4- Poisoning by other antiprotozoal drugs, undetermined

IQ 7 T37.3X5- Adverse effect of other antiprotozoal drugs

SP 7 T37.3X6- Underdosing of other antiprotozoal drugs

5 T37.4 Poisoning by, adverse effect of and underdosing of anthelminthics

6 T37.4X Poisoning by, adverse effect of and underdosing of anthelminthics

SP 7 T37.4X1- Poisoning by anthelminthics, accidental (unintentional)
> Poisoning by anthelminthics NOS

SP 7 T37.4X2- Poisoning by anthelminthics, intentional self-harm

SP 7 T37.4X3- Poisoning by anthelminthics, assault

SP 7 T37.4X4- Poisoning by anthelminthics, undetermined

IQ 7 T37.4X5- Adverse effect of anthelminthics

SP 7 T37.4X6- Underdosing of anthelminthics

5 T37.5 Poisoning by, adverse effect of and underdosing of antiviral drugs
> **EXCLUDES 1** amantadine (T42.8-)
> cytarabine (T45.1-)

6 T37.5X Poisoning by, adverse effect of and underdosing of antiviral drugs

SP 7 T37.5X1- Poisoning by antiviral drugs, accidental (unintentional)
> Poisoning by antiviral drugs NOS

SP 7 T37.5X2- Poisoning by antiviral drugs, intentional self-harm

SP 7 T37.5X3- Poisoning by antiviral drugs, assault

SP 7 T37.5X4- Poisoning by antiviral drugs, undetermined

IQ 7 T37.5X5- Adverse effect of antiviral drugs

SP 7 T37.5X6- Underdosing of antiviral drugs

5 T37.8 Poisoning by, adverse effect of and underdosing of other specified systemic anti-infectives and antiparasitics
> Poisoning by, adverse effect of and underdosing of hydroxyquinoline derivatives
> **EXCLUDES 1** antimalarial drugs (T37.2-)

6 T37.8X Poisoning by, adverse effect of and underdosing of other specified systemic anti-infectives and antiparasitics

SP 7 T37.8X1- Poisoning by other specified systemic anti-infectives and antiparasitics, accidental (unintentional)
> Poisoning by other specified systemic anti-infectives and antiparasitics NOS

SP 7 T37.8X2- Poisoning by other specified systemic anti-infectives and antiparasitics, intentional self-harm

SP 7 T37.8X3- Poisoning by other specified systemic anti-infectives and antiparasitics, assault

SP 7 T37.8X4- Poisoning by other specified systemic anti-infectives and antiparasitics, undetermined

Chapter 19

S00-T88

★ New ▲ Revised Px Primary SP PDGM Px SL Low CoM SH High CoM IQ Quest. Encounter H Hospice non-cancer Dx | Unspecified | M Manifestation

DecisionHealth's FY 2020 Complete Home Health ICD-10-CM Diagnosis Coding Manual

1673

!Q 7 T37.8X5- Adverse effect of other specified systemic anti-infectives and antiparasitics

SP 7 T37.8X6- Underdosing of other specified systemic anti-infectives and antiparasitics

5 T37.9 Poisoning by, adverse effect of and underdosing of unspecified systemic anti-infective and antiparasitics

SP ☑ T37.91X- Poisoning by unspecified systemic anti-infective and antiparasitics, accidental (unintentional)

Poisoning by, adverse effect of and underdosing of systemic anti-infective and antiparasitics NOS

SP ☑ T37.92X- Poisoning by unspecified systemic anti-infective and antiparasitics, intentional self-harm

SP ☑ T37.93X- Poisoning by unspecified systemic anti-infective and antiparasitics, assault

SP ☑ T37.94X- Poisoning by unspecified systemic anti-infective and antiparasitics, undetermined

!Q ☑ T37.95X- Adverse effect of unspecified systemic anti-infective and antiparasitic

SP ☑ T37.96X- Underdosing of unspecified systemic anti-infectives and antiparasitics

4 T38 Poisoning by, adverse effect of and underdosing of hormones and their synthetic substitutes and antagonists, not elsewhere classified

> **EXCLUDES 1** mineralocorticoids and their antagonists (T50.0-)
> oxytocic hormones (T48.0-)
> parathyroid hormones and derivatives (T50.9-)

> The appropriate 7th character is to be added to each code from category T38
> A initial encounter
> D subsequent encounter
> S sequela

5 T38.0 Poisoning by, adverse effect of and underdosing of glucocorticoids and synthetic analogues
> **EXCLUDES 1** glucocorticoids, topically used (T49.-)

6 T38.0X Poisoning by, adverse effect of and underdosing of glucocorticoids and synthetic analogues

SP 7 T38.0X1- Poisoning by glucocorticoids and synthetic analogues, accidental (unintentional)
Poisoning by glucocorticoids and synthetic analogues NOS

SP 7 T38.0X2- Poisoning by glucocorticoids and synthetic analogues, intentional self-harm

SP 7 T38.0X3- Poisoning by glucocorticoids and synthetic analogues, assault

SP 7 T38.0X4- Poisoning by glucocorticoids and synthetic analogues, undetermined

!Q 7 T38.0X5- Adverse effect of glucocorticoids and synthetic analogues

SP 7 T38.0X6- Underdosing of glucocorticoids and synthetic analogues

5 T38.1 Poisoning by, adverse effect of and underdosing of thyroid hormones and substitutes

6 T38.1X Poisoning by, adverse effect of and underdosing of thyroid hormones and substitutes

SP 7 T38.1X1- Poisoning by thyroid hormones and substitutes, accidental (unintentional)
Poisoning by thyroid hormones and substitutes NOS

SP 7 T38.1X2- Poisoning by thyroid hormones and substitutes, intentional self-harm

SP 7 T38.1X3- Poisoning by thyroid hormones and substitutes, assault

SP 7 T38.1X4- Poisoning by thyroid hormones and substitutes, undetermined

!Q 7 T38.1X5- Adverse effect of thyroid hormones and substitutes

SP 7 T38.1X6- Underdosing of thyroid hormones and substitutes

5 T38.2 Poisoning by, adverse effect of and underdosing of antithyroid drugs

6 T38.2X Poisoning by, adverse effect of and underdosing of antithyroid drugs

SP 7 T38.2X1- Poisoning by antithyroid drugs, accidental (unintentional)
Poisoning by antithyroid drugs NOS

SP 7 T38.2X2- Poisoning by antithyroid drugs, intentional self-harm

SP 7 T38.2X3- Poisoning by antithyroid drugs, assault

SP 7 T38.2X4- Poisoning by antithyroid drugs, undetermined

!Q 7 T38.2X5- Adverse effect of antithyroid drugs

SP 7 T38.2X6- Underdosing of antithyroid drugs

5 T38.3 Poisoning by, adverse effect of and underdosing of insulin and oral hypoglycemic [antidiabetic] drugs

6 T38.3X Poisoning by, adverse effect of and underdosing of insulin and oral hypoglycemic [antidiabetic] drugs

SP 7 T38.3X1- Poisoning by insulin and oral hypoglycemic [antidiabetic] drugs, accidental (unintentional)
Poisoning by insulin and oral hypoglycemic [antidiabetic] drugs NOS

> **GUIDELINES** Section I.C.4.a.5)(b)
> The principal or first-listed code for an encounter due to an insulin pump malfunction resulting in an overdose of insulin, should also be T85.6-, Mechanical complication of other specified internal and external prosthetic devices, implants and grafts, followed by code T38.3x1-.

SP 7 T38.3X2- Poisoning by insulin and oral hypoglycemic [antidiabetic] drugs, intentional self-harm

---

44th digit required   **5**5th digit required   **6**6th digit required   **7**7th digit required   **☑**7th digit placeholder   **✚**Additional code   **⊟**Laterality

SP **7** **T38.3X3-** Poisoning by insulin and oral hypoglycemic [antidiabetic] drugs, assault

SP **7** **T38.3X4-** Poisoning by insulin and oral hypoglycemic [antidiabetic] drugs, undetermined

IQ **7** **T38.3X5-** Adverse effect of insulin and oral hypoglycemic [antidiabetic] drugs

SP **7** **T38.3X6-** Underdosing of insulin and oral hypoglycemic [antidiabetic] drugs

> **GUIDELINES** Section I.C.4.a.5)(a)
> An underdose of insulin due to an insulin pump failure should be assigned to a code from subcategory T85.6, Mechanical complication of other specified internal and external prosthetic devices, implants and grafts, followed by code T38.3x6-. Additional codes for the type of diabetes mellitus and any associated complications due to the underdosing should also be assigned.

5 **T38.4** Poisoning by, adverse effect of and underdosing of oral contraceptives
Poisoning by, adverse effect of and underdosing of multiple- and single-ingredient oral contraceptive preparations

6 **T38.4X** Poisoning by, adverse effect of and underdosing of oral contraceptives

SP **7** **T38.4X1-** Poisoning by oral contraceptives, accidental (unintentional)
Poisoning by oral contraceptives NOS

SP **7** **T38.4X2-** Poisoning by oral contraceptives, intentional self-harm

SP **7** **T38.4X3-** Poisoning by oral contraceptives, assault

SP **7** **T38.4X4-** Poisoning by oral contraceptives, undetermined

IQ **7** **T38.4X5-** Adverse effect of oral contraceptives

SP **7** **T38.4X6-** Underdosing of oral contraceptives

5 **T38.5** Poisoning by, adverse effect of and underdosing of other estrogens and progestogens
Poisoning by, adverse effect of and underdosing of estrogens and progestogens mixtures and substitutes

6 **T38.5X** Poisoning by, adverse effect of and underdosing of other estrogens and progestogens

SP **7** **T38.5X1-** Poisoning by other estrogens and progestogens, accidental (unintentional)
Poisoning by other estrogens and progestogens NOS

SP **7** **T38.5X2-** Poisoning by other estrogens and progestogens, intentional self-harm

SP **7** **T38.5X3-** Poisoning by other estrogens and progestogens, assault

SP **7** **T38.5X4-** Poisoning by other estrogens and progestogens, undetermined

IQ **7** **T38.5X5-** Adverse effect of other estrogens and progestogens

SP **7** **T38.5X6-** Underdosing of other estrogens and progestogens

5 **T38.6** Poisoning by, adverse effect of and underdosing of antigonadotrophins, antiestrogens, antiandrogens, not elsewhere classified
Poisoning by, adverse effect of and underdosing of tamoxifen

6 **T38.6X** Poisoning by, adverse effect of and underdosing of antigonadotrophins, antiestrogens, antiandrogens, not elsewhere classified

SP **7** **T38.6X1-** Poisoning by antigonadotrophins, antiestrogens, antiandrogens, not elsewhere classified, accidental (unintentional)
Poisoning by antigonadotrophins, antiestrogens, antiandrogens, not elsewhere classified NOS

SP **7** **T38.6X2-** Poisoning by antigonadotrophins, antiestrogens, antiandrogens, not elsewhere classified, intentional self-harm

SP **7** **T38.6X3-** Poisoning by antigonadotrophins, antiestrogens, antiandrogens, not elsewhere classified, assault

SP **7** **T38.6X4-** Poisoning by antigonadotrophins, antiestrogens, antiandrogens, not elsewhere classified, undetermined

IQ **7** **T38.6X5-** Adverse effect of antigonadotrophins, antiestrogens, antiandrogens, not elsewhere classified

SP **7** **T38.6X6-** Underdosing of antigonadotrophins, antiestrogens, antiandrogens, not elsewhere classified

5 **T38.7** Poisoning by, adverse effect of and underdosing of androgens and anabolic congeners

6 **T38.7X** Poisoning by, adverse effect of and underdosing of androgens and anabolic congeners

SP **7** **T38.7X1-** Poisoning by androgens and anabolic congeners, accidental (unintentional)
Poisoning by androgens and anabolic congeners NOS

SP **7** **T38.7X2-** Poisoning by androgens and anabolic congeners, intentional self-harm

SP **7** **T38.7X3-** Poisoning by androgens and anabolic congeners, assault

SP **7** **T38.7X4-** Poisoning by androgens and anabolic congeners, undetermined

IQ **7** **T38.7X5-** Adverse effect of androgens and anabolic congeners

SP **7** **T38.7X6-** Underdosing of androgens and anabolic congeners

Chapter 19

S00-T88

★ New ▲ Revised Px Primary **SP** PDGM Px **SL** Low CoM **SH** High CoM **IQ** Quest. Encounter **H** Hospice non-cancer Dx Unspecified **M** *Manifestation*

Chapter 19

S00-T88

⑤ T38.8 Poisoning by, adverse effect of and underdosing of other and unspecified hormones and synthetic substitutes

⑥ T38.80 Poisoning by, adverse effect of and underdosing of unspecified hormones and synthetic substitutes

SP ⑦ T38.801- Poisoning by unspecified hormones and synthetic substitutes, accidental (unintentional)
Poisoning by unspecified hormones and synthetic substitutes NOS

SP ⑦ T38.802- Poisoning by unspecified hormones and synthetic substitutes, intentional self-harm

SP ⑦ T38.803- Poisoning by unspecified hormones and synthetic substitutes, assault

SP ⑦ T38.804- Poisoning by unspecified hormones and synthetic substitutes, undetermined

!Q ⑦ T38.805- Adverse effect of unspecified hormones and synthetic substitutes

SP ⑦ T38.806- Underdosing of unspecified hormones and synthetic substitutes

⑥ T38.81 Poisoning by, adverse effect of and underdosing of anterior pituitary [adenohypophyseal] hormones

SP ⑦ T38.811- Poisoning by anterior pituitary [adenohypophyseal] hormones, accidental (unintentional)
Poisoning by anterior pituitary [adenohypophyseal] hormones NOS

SP ⑦ T38.812- Poisoning by anterior pituitary [adenohypophyseal] hormones, intentional self-harm

SP ⑦ T38.813- Poisoning by anterior pituitary [adenohypophyseal] hormones, assault

SP ⑦ T38.814- Poisoning by anterior pituitary [adenohypophyseal] hormones, undetermined

!Q ⑦ T38.815- Adverse effect of anterior pituitary [adenohypophyseal] hormones

SP ⑦ T38.816- Underdosing of anterior pituitary [adenohypophyseal] hormones

⑥ T38.89 Poisoning by, adverse effect of and underdosing of other hormones and synthetic substitutes

SP ⑦ T38.891- Poisoning by other hormones and synthetic substitutes, accidental (unintentional)
Poisoning by other hormones and synthetic substitutes NOS

SP ⑦ T38.892- Poisoning by other hormones and synthetic substitutes, intentional self-harm

SP ⑦ T38.893- Poisoning by other hormones and synthetic substitutes, assault

SP ⑦ T38.894- Poisoning by other hormones and synthetic substitutes, undetermined

!Q ⑦ T38.895- Adverse effect of other hormones and synthetic substitutes

SP ⑦ T38.896- Underdosing of other hormones and synthetic substitutes

⑤ T38.9 Poisoning by, adverse effect of and underdosing of other and unspecified hormone antagonists

⑥ T38.90 Poisoning by, adverse effect of and underdosing of unspecified hormone antagonists

SP ⑦ T38.901- Poisoning by unspecified hormone antagonists, accidental (unintentional)
Poisoning by unspecified hormone antagonists NOS

SP ⑦ T38.902- Poisoning by unspecified hormone antagonists, intentional self-harm

SP ⑦ T38.903- Poisoning by unspecified hormone antagonists, assault

SP ⑦ T38.904- Poisoning by unspecified hormone antagonists, undetermined

!Q ⑦ T38.905- Adverse effect of unspecified hormone antagonists

SP ⑦ T38.906- Underdosing of unspecified hormone antagonists

⑥ T38.99 Poisoning by, adverse effect of and underdosing of other hormone antagonists

SP ⑦ T38.991- Poisoning by other hormone antagonists, accidental (unintentional)
Poisoning by other hormone antagonists NOS

SP ⑦ T38.992- Poisoning by other hormone antagonists, intentional self-harm

SP ⑦ T38.993- Poisoning by other hormone antagonists, assault

SP ⑦ T38.994- Poisoning by other hormone antagonists, undetermined

!Q ⑦ T38.995- Adverse effect of other hormone antagonists

SP ⑦ T38.996- Underdosing of other hormone antagonists

④ T39 Poisoning by, adverse effect of and underdosing of nonopioid analgesics, antipyretics and antirheumatics

The appropriate 7th character is to be added to each code from category T39
A   initial encounter
D   subsequent encounter
S   sequela

⑤ T39.0 Poisoning by, adverse effect of and underdosing of salicylates

⑥ T39.01 Poisoning by, adverse effect of and underdosing of aspirin
Poisoning by, adverse effect of and underdosing of acetylsalicylic acid

SP ⑦ T39.011- Poisoning by aspirin, accidental (unintentional)

④4th digit required   ⑤5th digit required   ⑥6th digit required   ⑦7th digit required   ☑7th digit placeholder   ✚Additional code   ⊟Laterality

1676   *DecisionHealth's* FY 2020 Complete Home Health ICD-10-CM Diagnosis Coding Manual

SP **7** T39.012- **Poisoning by aspirin, intentional self-harm**

SP **7** T39.013- **Poisoning by aspirin, assault**

SP **7** T39.014- **Poisoning by aspirin, undetermined**

!Q **7** T39.015- **Adverse effect of aspirin**

SP **7** T39.016- **Underdosing of aspirin**

6 T39.09 **Poisoning by, adverse effect of and underdosing of other salicylates**

SP **7** T39.091- **Poisoning by salicylates, accidental (unintentional)**
Poisoning by salicylates NOS

SP **7** T39.092- **Poisoning by salicylates, intentional self-harm**

SP **7** T39.093- **Poisoning by salicylates, assault**

SP **7** T39.094- **Poisoning by salicylates, undetermined**

!Q **7** T39.095- **Adverse effect of salicylates**

SP **7** T39.096- **Underdosing of salicylates**

5 T39.1 **Poisoning by, adverse effect of and underdosing of 4-Aminophenol derivatives**

6 T39.1X **Poisoning by, adverse effect of and underdosing of 4-Aminophenol derivatives**

SP **7** T39.1X1- **Poisoning by 4-Aminophenol derivatives, accidental (unintentional)**
Poisoning by 4-Aminophenol derivatives NOS

SP **7** T39.1X2- **Poisoning by 4-Aminophenol derivatives, intentional self-harm**

SP **7** T39.1X3- **Poisoning by 4-Aminophenol derivatives, assault**

SP **7** T39.1X4- **Poisoning by 4-Aminophenol derivatives, undetermined**

!Q **7** T39.1X5- **Adverse effect of 4-Aminophenol derivatives**

SP **7** T39.1X6- **Underdosing of 4-Aminophenol derivatives**

5 T39.2 **Poisoning by, adverse effect of and underdosing of pyrazolone derivatives**

6 T39.2X **Poisoning by, adverse effect of and underdosing of pyrazolone derivatives**

SP **7** T39.2X1- **Poisoning by pyrazolone derivatives, accidental (unintentional)**
Poisoning by pyrazolone derivatives NOS

SP **7** T39.2X2- **Poisoning by pyrazolone derivatives, intentional self-harm**

SP **7** T39.2X3- **Poisoning by pyrazolone derivatives, assault**

SP **7** T39.2X4- **Poisoning by pyrazolone derivatives, undetermined**

!Q **7** T39.2X5- **Adverse effect of pyrazolone derivatives**

SP **7** T39.2X6- **Underdosing of pyrazolone derivatives**

5 T39.3 **Poisoning by, adverse effect of and underdosing of other nonsteroidal anti-inflammatory drugs [NSAID]**

6 T39.31 **Poisoning by, adverse effect of and underdosing of propionic acid derivatives**

Poisoning by, adverse effect of and underdosing of fenoprofen
Poisoning by, adverse effect of and underdosing of flurbiprofen
Poisoning by, adverse effect of and underdosing of ibuprofen
Poisoning by, adverse effect of and underdosing of ketoprofen
Poisoning by, adverse effect of and underdosing of naproxen
Poisoning by, adverse effect of and underdosing of oxaprozin

SP **7** T39.311- **Poisoning by propionic acid derivatives, accidental (unintentional)**

SP **7** T39.312- **Poisoning by propionic acid derivatives, intentional self-harm**

SP **7** T39.313- **Poisoning by propionic acid derivatives, assault**

SP **7** T39.314- **Poisoning by propionic acid derivatives, undetermined**

!Q **7** T39.315- **Adverse effect of propionic acid derivatives**

SP **7** T39.316- **Underdosing of propionic acid derivatives**

6 T39.39 **Poisoning by, adverse effect of and underdosing of other nonsteroidal anti-inflammatory drugs [NSAID]**

SP **7** T39.391- **Poisoning by other nonsteroidal anti-inflammatory drugs [NSAID], accidental (unintentional)**
Poisoning by other nonsteroidal anti-inflammatory drugs NOS

SP **7** T39.392- **Poisoning by other nonsteroidal anti-inflammatory drugs [NSAID], intentional self-harm**

SP **7** T39.393- **Poisoning by other nonsteroidal anti-inflammatory drugs [NSAID], assault**

SP **7** T39.394- **Poisoning by other nonsteroidal anti-inflammatory drugs [NSAID], undetermined**

!Q **7** T39.395- **Adverse effect of other nonsteroidal anti-inflammatory drugs [NSAID]**

SP **7** T39.396- **Underdosing of other nonsteroidal anti-inflammatory drugs [NSAID]**

5 T39.4 **Poisoning by, adverse effect of and underdosing of antirheumatics, not elsewhere classified**

EXCLUDES 1 poisoning by, adverse effect of and underdosing of glucocorticoids (T38.0-)
poisoning by, adverse effect of and underdosing of salicylates (T39.0-)

6 T39.4X **Poisoning by, adverse effect of and underdosing of antirheumatics, not elsewhere classified**

SP **7** T39.4X1- **Poisoning by antirheumatics, not elsewhere classified, accidental (unintentional)**
Poisoning by antirheumatics, not elsewhere classified NOS

SP **7** T39.4X2- **Poisoning by antirheumatics, not elsewhere classified, intentional self-harm**

★ New ▲ Revised **Px** Primary **SP** PDGM Px **SL** Low CoM **SH** High CoM **!Q** Quest. Encounter **H** Hospice non-cancer Dx [Unspecified] **M** *Manifestation*

DecisionHealth's FY 2020 Complete Home Health ICD-10-CM Diagnosis Coding Manual

1677

Chapter 19

S00-T88

SP 7 T39.4X3- Poisoning by antirheumatics, not elsewhere classified, assault

SP 7 T39.4X4- Poisoning by antirheumatics, not elsewhere classified, undetermined

IQ 7 T39.4X5- Adverse effect of antirheumatics, not elsewhere classified

SP 7 T39.4X6- Underdosing of antirheumatics, not elsewhere classified

5 T39.8 Poisoning by, adverse effect of and underdosing of other nonopioid analgesics and antipyretics, not elsewhere classified

6 T39.8X Poisoning by, adverse effect of and underdosing of other nonopioid analgesics and antipyretics, not elsewhere classified

SP 7 T39.8X1- Poisoning by other nonopioid analgesics and antipyretics, not elsewhere classified, accidental (unintentional)
Poisoning by other nonopioid analgesics and antipyretics, not elsewhere classified NOS

SP 7 T39.8X2- Poisoning by other nonopioid analgesics and antipyretics, not elsewhere classified, intentional self-harm

SP 7 T39.8X3- Poisoning by other nonopioid analgesics and antipyretics, not elsewhere classified, assault

SP 7 T39.8X4- Poisoning by other nonopioid analgesics and antipyretics, not elsewhere classified, undetermined

IQ 7 T39.8X5- Adverse effect of other nonopioid analgesics and antipyretics, not elsewhere classified

SP 7 T39.8X6- Underdosing of other nonopioid analgesics and antipyretics, not elsewhere classified

5 T39.9 Poisoning by, adverse effect of and underdosing of unspecified nonopioid analgesic, antipyretic and antirheumatic

SP 7 T39.91X- Poisoning by unspecified nonopioid analgesic, antipyretic and antirheumatic, accidental (unintentional)
Poisoning by nonopioid analgesic, antipyretic and antirheumatic NOS

SP 7 T39.92X- Poisoning by unspecified nonopioid analgesic, antipyretic and antirheumatic, intentional self-harm

SP 7 T39.93X- Poisoning by unspecified nonopioid analgesic, antipyretic and antirheumatic, assault

SP 7 T39.94X- Poisoning by unspecified nonopioid analgesic, antipyretic and antirheumatic, undetermined

IQ 7 T39.95X- Adverse effect of unspecified nonopioid analgesic, antipyretic and antirheumatic

SP 7 T39.96X- Underdosing of unspecified nonopioid analgesic, antipyretic and antirheumatic

4 T40 Poisoning by, adverse effect of and underdosing of narcotics and psychodysleptics [hallucinogens]
EXCLUDES 2 drug dependence and related mental and behavioral disorders due to psychoactive substance use (F10.-F19.-)

The appropriate 7th character is to be added to each code from category T40
A   initial encounter
D   subsequent encounter
S   sequela

5 T40.0 Poisoning by, adverse effect of and underdosing of opium

6 T40.0X Poisoning by, adverse effect of and underdosing of opium

SP 7 T40.0X1- Poisoning by opium, accidental (unintentional)
Poisoning by opium NOS

SP 7 T40.0X2- Poisoning by opium, intentional self-harm

SP 7 T40.0X3- Poisoning by opium, assault

SP 7 T40.0X4- Poisoning by opium, undetermined

IQ 7 T40.0X5- Adverse effect of opium

SP 7 T40.0X6- Underdosing of opium

5 T40.1 Poisoning by and adverse effect of heroin

6 T40.1X Poisoning by and adverse effect of heroin

SP 7 T40.1X1- Poisoning by heroin, accidental (unintentional)
Poisoning by heroin NOS

SP 7 T40.1X2- Poisoning by heroin, intentional self-harm

SP 7 T40.1X3- Poisoning by heroin, assault

SP 7 T40.1X4- Poisoning by heroin, undetermined

5 T40.2 Poisoning by, adverse effect of and underdosing of other opioids

6 T40.2X Poisoning by, adverse effect of and underdosing of other opioids

SP 7 T40.2X1- Poisoning by other opioids, accidental (unintentional)
Poisoning by other opioids NOS

SP 7 T40.2X2- Poisoning by other opioids, intentional self-harm

SP 7 T40.2X3- Poisoning by other opioids, assault

SP 7 T40.2X4- Poisoning by other opioids, undetermined

IQ 7 T40.2X5- Adverse effect of other opioids

SP 7 T40.2X6- Underdosing of other opioids

5 T40.3 Poisoning by, adverse effect of and underdosing of methadone

6 T40.3X Poisoning by, adverse effect of and underdosing of methadone

SP 7 T40.3X1- Poisoning by methadone, accidental (unintentional)
Poisoning by methadone NOS

SP 7 T40.3X2- Poisoning by methadone, intentional self-harm

SP 7 T40.3X3- Poisoning by methadone, assault

SP 7 T40.3X4- Poisoning by methadone, undetermined

IQ 7 T40.3X5- Adverse effect of methadone

SP **7** **T40.3X6-** Underdosing of methadone

5 **T40.4** Poisoning by, adverse effect of and underdosing of other synthetic narcotics

6 **T40.4X** Poisoning by, adverse effect of and underdosing of other synthetic narcotics

SP **7** **T40.4X1-** Poisoning by other synthetic narcotics, accidental (unintentional)
Poisoning by other synthetic narcotics NOS

SP **7** **T40.4X2-** Poisoning by other synthetic narcotics, intentional self-harm

SP **7** **T40.4X3-** Poisoning by other synthetic narcotics, assault

SP **7** **T40.4X4-** Poisoning by other synthetic narcotics, undetermined

IQ **7** **T40.4X5-** Adverse effect of other synthetic narcotics

SP **7** **T40.4X6-** Underdosing of other synthetic narcotics

5 **T40.5** Poisoning by, adverse effect of and underdosing of cocaine

6 **T40.5X** Poisoning by, adverse effect of and underdosing of cocaine

SP **7** **T40.5X1-** Poisoning by cocaine, accidental (unintentional)
Poisoning by cocaine NOS

SP **7** **T40.5X2-** Poisoning by cocaine, intentional self-harm

SP **7** **T40.5X3-** Poisoning by cocaine, assault

SP **7** **T40.5X4-** Poisoning by cocaine, undetermined

IQ **7** **T40.5X5-** Adverse effect of cocaine

SP **7** **T40.5X6-** Underdosing of cocaine

5 **T40.6** Poisoning by, adverse effect of and underdosing of other and unspecified narcotics

6 **T40.60** Poisoning by, adverse effect of and underdosing of unspecified narcotics

SP **7** **T40.601-** Poisoning by unspecified narcotics, accidental (unintentional)
Poisoning by narcotics NOS

SP **7** **T40.602-** Poisoning by unspecified narcotics, intentional self-harm

SP **7** **T40.603-** Poisoning by unspecified narcotics, assault

SP **7** **T40.604-** Poisoning by unspecified narcotics, undetermined

IQ **7** **T40.605-** Adverse effect of unspecified narcotics

SP **7** **T40.606-** Underdosing of unspecified narcotics

6 **T40.69** Poisoning by, adverse effect of and underdosing of other narcotics

SP **7** **T40.691-** Poisoning by other narcotics, accidental (unintentional)
Poisoning by other narcotics NOS

SP **7** **T40.692-** Poisoning by other narcotics, intentional self-harm

SP **7** **T40.693-** Poisoning by other narcotics, assault

SP **7** **T40.694-** Poisoning by other narcotics, undetermined

IQ **7** **T40.695-** Adverse effect of other narcotics

SP **7** **T40.696-** Underdosing of other narcotics

5 **T40.7** Poisoning by, adverse effect of and underdosing of cannabis (derivatives)

6 **T40.7X** Poisoning by, adverse effect of and underdosing of cannabis (derivatives)

SP **7** **T40.7X1-** Poisoning by cannabis (derivatives), accidental (unintentional)
Poisoning by cannabis NOS

SP **7** **T40.7X2-** Poisoning by cannabis (derivatives), intentional self-harm

SP **7** **T40.7X3-** Poisoning by cannabis (derivatives), assault

SP **7** **T40.7X4-** Poisoning by cannabis (derivatives), undetermined

IQ **7** **T40.7X5-** Adverse effect of cannabis (derivatives)

SP **7** **T40.7X6-** Underdosing of cannabis (derivatives)

5 **T40.8** Poisoning by and adverse effect of lysergide [LSD]

6 **T40.8X** Poisoning by and adverse effect of lysergide [LSD]

SP **7** **T40.8X1-** Poisoning by lysergide [LSD], accidental (unintentional)
Poisoning by lysergide [LSD] NOS

SP **7** **T40.8X2-** Poisoning by lysergide [LSD], intentional self-harm

SP **7** **T40.8X3-** Poisoning by lysergide [LSD], assault

SP **7** **T40.8X4-** Poisoning by lysergide [LSD], undetermined

5 **T40.9** Poisoning by, adverse effect of and underdosing of other and unspecified psychodysleptics [hallucinogens]

6 **T40.90** Poisoning by, adverse effect of and underdosing of unspecified psychodysleptics [hallucinogens]

SP **7** **T40.901-** Poisoning by unspecified psychodysleptics [hallucinogens], accidental (unintentional)

SP **7** **T40.902-** Poisoning by unspecified psychodysleptics [hallucinogens], intentional self-harm

SP **7** **T40.903-** Poisoning by unspecified psychodysleptics [hallucinogens], assault

SP **7** **T40.904-** Poisoning by unspecified psychodysleptics [hallucinogens], undetermined

IQ **7** **T40.905-** Adverse effect of unspecified psychodysleptics [hallucinogens]

▲ **SP** **7** **T40.906-** Underdosing of unspecified psychodysleptics [hallucinogens]

6 **T40.99** Poisoning by, adverse effect of and underdosing of other psychodysleptics [hallucinogens]

SP **7** **T40.991-** Poisoning by other psychodysleptics [hallucinogens], accidental (unintentional)

★ New ▲ Revised Px Primary **SP** PDGM Px **SL** Low CoM **SH** High CoM **IQ** Quest. Encounter **H** Hospice non-cancer Dx Unspecified **M** *Manifestation*

DecisionHealth's FY 2020 Complete Home Health ICD-10-CM Diagnosis Coding Manual

1679

Poisoning by other
psychodysleptics [hallucinogens]
NOS

SP 7 T40.992- **Poisoning by other
psychodysleptics [hallucinogens],
intentional self-harm**

SP 7 T40.993- **Poisoning by other
psychodysleptics [hallucinogens],
assault**

SP 7 T40.994- **Poisoning by other
psychodysleptics [hallucinogens],
undetermined**

IQ 7 T40.995- **Adverse effect of other
psychodysleptics [hallucinogens]**

▲ **SP 7 T40.996-** **Underdosing of other
psychodysleptics [hallucinogens]**

4 T41 **Poisoning by, adverse effect of and
underdosing of anesthetics and therapeutic
gases**

> **EXCLUDES 1** benzodiazepines (T42.4-)
> cocaine (T40.5-)
> complications of anesthesia
> during pregnancy (O29.-)
> complications of anesthesia
> during labor and delivery
> (O74.-)
> complications of anesthesia
> during the puerperium
> (O89.-)
> opioids (T40.0-T40.2-)

> The appropriate 7th character is to be added to
> each code from category T41
> A   initial encounter
> D   subsequent encounter
> S   sequela

5 T41.0 **Poisoning by, adverse effect of and
underdosing of inhaled anesthetics**
> **EXCLUDES 1** oxygen (T41.5-)

6 T41.0X **Poisoning by, adverse effect of and
underdosing of inhaled anesthetics**

SP 7 T41.0X1- **Poisoning by inhaled anesthetics,
accidental (unintentional)**
Poisoning by inhaled anesthetics
NOS

SP 7 T41.0X2- **Poisoning by inhaled anesthetics,
intentional self-harm**

SP 7 T41.0X3- **Poisoning by inhaled anesthetics,
assault**

SP 7 T41.0X4- **Poisoning by inhaled anesthetics,
undetermined**

IQ 7 T41.0X5- **Adverse effect of inhaled
anesthetics**

SP 7 T41.0X6- **Underdosing of inhaled
anesthetics**

5 T41.1 **Poisoning by, adverse effect of and
underdosing of intravenous anesthetics**
Poisoning by, adverse effect of and
underdosing of thiobarbiturates

6 T41.1X **Poisoning by, adverse effect of and
underdosing of intravenous
anesthetics**

SP 7 T41.1X1- **Poisoning by intravenous
anesthetics, accidental
(unintentional)**
Poisoning by intravenous
anesthetics NOS

SP 7 T41.1X2- **Poisoning by intravenous
anesthetics, intentional self-harm**

SP 7 T41.1X3- **Poisoning by intravenous
anesthetics, assault**

SP 7 T41.1X4- **Poisoning by intravenous
anesthetics, undetermined**

IQ 7 T41.1X5- **Adverse effect of intravenous
anesthetics**

SP 7 T41.1X6- **Underdosing of intravenous
anesthetics**

5 T41.2 **Poisoning by, adverse effect of and
underdosing of other and unspecified
general anesthetics**

6 T41.20 **Poisoning by, adverse effect of and
underdosing of unspecified general
anesthetics**

SP 7 T41.201- **Poisoning by unspecified
general anesthetics, accidental
(unintentional)**
Poisoning by general anesthetics
NOS

SP 7 T41.202- **Poisoning by unspecified
general anesthetics, intentional
self-harm**

SP 7 T41.203- **Poisoning by unspecified
general anesthetics, assault**

SP 7 T41.204- **Poisoning by unspecified
general anesthetics,
undetermined**

IQ 7 T41.205- **Adverse effect of unspecified
general anesthetics**

SP 7 T41.206- **Underdosing of unspecified
general anesthetics**

6 T41.29 **Poisoning by, adverse effect of and
underdosing of other general
anesthetics**

SP 7 T41.291- **Poisoning by other general
anesthetics, accidental
(unintentional)**
Poisoning by other general
anesthetics NOS

SP 7 T41.292- **Poisoning by other general
anesthetics, intentional self-harm**

SP 7 T41.293- **Poisoning by other general
anesthetics, assault**

SP 7 T41.294- **Poisoning by other general
anesthetics, undetermined**

IQ 7 T41.295- **Adverse effect of other general
anesthetics**

SP 7 T41.296- **Underdosing of other general
anesthetics**

5 T41.3 **Poisoning by, adverse effect of and
underdosing of local anesthetics**
Cocaine (topical)
> **EXCLUDES 2** poisoning by cocaine used as
> a central nervous system
> stimulant
> (T40.5X1-T40.5X4)

6 T41.3X **Poisoning by, adverse effect of and
underdosing of local anesthetics**

SP 7 T41.3X1- **Poisoning by local anesthetics,
accidental (unintentional)**
Poisoning by local anesthetics
NOS

SP 7 T41.3X2- **Poisoning by local anesthetics,
intentional self-harm**

4 4th digit required   **5** 5th digit required   **6** 6th digit required   **7** 7th digit required   **7** 7th digit placeholder   **+** Additional code   **⊟** Laterality

1680   *DecisionHealth's* FY 2020 Complete Home Health ICD-10-CM Diagnosis Coding Manual

SP 7 T41.3X3- Poisoning by local anesthetics, assault

SP 7 T41.3X4- Poisoning by local anesthetics, undetermined

IQ 7 T41.3X5- Adverse effect of local anesthetics

SP 7 T41.3X6- Underdosing of local anesthetics

5 T41.4 Poisoning by, adverse effect of and underdosing of unspecified anesthetic

SP ☑ T41.41X- Poisoning by unspecified anesthetic, accidental (unintentional)

Poisoning by anesthetic NOS

SP ☑ T41.42X- Poisoning by unspecified anesthetic, intentional self-harm

SP ☑ T41.43X- Poisoning by unspecified anesthetic, assault

SP ☑ T41.44X- Poisoning by unspecified anesthetic, undetermined

IQ ☑ T41.45X- Adverse effect of unspecified anesthetic

SP ☑ T41.46X- Underdosing of unspecified anesthetics

5 T41.5 Poisoning by, adverse effect of and underdosing of therapeutic gases

6 T41.5X Poisoning by, adverse effect of and underdosing of therapeutic gases

SP 7 T41.5X1- Poisoning by therapeutic gases, accidental (unintentional)

Poisoning by therapeutic gases NOS

SP 7 T41.5X2- Poisoning by therapeutic gases, intentional self-harm

SP 7 T41.5X3- Poisoning by therapeutic gases, assault

SP 7 T41.5X4- Poisoning by therapeutic gases, undetermined

IQ 7 T41.5X5- Adverse effect of therapeutic gases

SP 7 T41.5X6- Underdosing of therapeutic gases

4 T42 Poisoning by, adverse effect of and underdosing of antiepileptic, sedative-hypnotic and antiparkinsonism drugs

> **EXCLUDES 2** drug dependence and related mental and behavioral disorders due to psychoactive substance use (F10.--F19.-)

> The appropriate 7th character is to be added to each code from category T42
> A   initial encounter
> D   subsequent encounter
> S   sequela

5 T42.0 Poisoning by, adverse effect of and underdosing of hydantoin derivatives

6 T42.0X Poisoning by, adverse effect of and underdosing of hydantoin derivatives

SP 7 T42.0X1- Poisoning by hydantoin derivatives, accidental (unintentional)

Poisoning by hydantoin derivatives NOS

SP 7 T42.0X2- Poisoning by hydantoin derivatives, intentional self-harm

SP 7 T42.0X3- Poisoning by hydantoin derivatives, assault

SP 7 T42.0X4- Poisoning by hydantoin derivatives, undetermined

IQ 7 T42.0X5- Adverse effect of hydantoin derivatives

SP 7 T42.0X6- Underdosing of hydantoin derivatives

5 T42.1 Poisoning by, adverse effect of and underdosing of iminostilbenes

Poisoning by, adverse effect of and underdosing of carbamazepine

6 T42.1X Poisoning by, adverse effect of and underdosing of iminostilbenes

SP 7 T42.1X1- Poisoning by iminostilbenes, accidental (unintentional)

Poisoning by iminostilbenes NOS

SP 7 T42.1X2- Poisoning by iminostilbenes, intentional self-harm

SP 7 T42.1X3- Poisoning by iminostilbenes, assault

SP 7 T42.1X4- Poisoning by iminostilbenes, undetermined

IQ 7 T42.1X5- Adverse effect of iminostilbenes

SP 7 T42.1X6- Underdosing of iminostilbenes

5 T42.2 Poisoning by, adverse effect of and underdosing of succinimides and oxazolidinediones

6 T42.2X Poisoning by, adverse effect of and underdosing of succinimides and oxazolidinediones

SP 7 T42.2X1- Poisoning by succinimides and oxazolidinediones, accidental (unintentional)

Poisoning by succinimides and oxazolidinediones NOS

SP 7 T42.2X2- Poisoning by succinimides and oxazolidinediones, intentional self-harm

SP 7 T42.2X3- Poisoning by succinimides and oxazolidinediones, assault

SP 7 T42.2X4- Poisoning by succinimides and oxazolidinediones, undetermined

IQ 7 T42.2X5- Adverse effect of succinimides and oxazolidinediones

SP 7 T42.2X6- Underdosing of succinimides and oxazolidinediones

5 T42.3 Poisoning by, adverse effect of and underdosing of barbiturates

> **EXCLUDES 1** poisoning by, adverse effect of and underdosing of thiobarbiturates (T41.1-)

6 T42.3X Poisoning by, adverse effect of and underdosing of barbiturates

SP 7 T42.3X1- Poisoning by barbiturates, accidental (unintentional)

Poisoning by barbiturates NOS

SP 7 T42.3X2- Poisoning by barbiturates, intentional self-harm

SP 7 T42.3X3- Poisoning by barbiturates, assault

SP 7 T42.3X4- Poisoning by barbiturates, undetermined

IQ 7 T42.3X5- Adverse effect of barbiturates

SP 7 T42.3X6- Underdosing of barbiturates

5 T42.4 Poisoning by, adverse effect of and underdosing of benzodiazepines

6 T42.4X Poisoning by, adverse effect of and underdosing of benzodiazepines

★ New ▲ Revised Px Primary SP PDGM Px SL Low CoM SH High CoM IQ Quest. Encounter H Hospice non-cancer Dx   Unspecified   M Manifestation

DecisionHealth's FY 2020 Complete Home Health ICD-10-CM Diagnosis Coding Manual   1681

SP 7 T42.4X1- **Poisoning by benzodiazepines, accidental (unintentional)**
Poisoning by benzodiazepines NOS

SP 7 T42.4X2- **Poisoning by benzodiazepines, intentional self-harm**

SP 7 T42.4X3- **Poisoning by benzodiazepines, assault**

SP 7 T42.4X4- **Poisoning by benzodiazepines, undetermined**

IQ 7 T42.4X5- **Adverse effect of benzodiazepines**

SP 7 T42.4X6- **Underdosing of benzodiazepines**

5 T42.5 **Poisoning by, adverse effect of and underdosing of mixed antiepileptics**

6 T42.5X **Poisoning by, adverse effect of and underdosing of antiepileptics**

SP 7 T42.5X1- **Poisoning by mixed antiepileptics, accidental (unintentional)**
Poisoning by mixed antiepileptics NOS

SP 7 T42.5X2- **Poisoning by mixed antiepileptics, intentional self-harm**

SP 7 T42.5X3- **Poisoning by mixed antiepileptics, assault**

SP 7 T42.5X4- **Poisoning by mixed antiepileptics, undetermined**

IQ 7 T42.5X5- **Adverse effect of mixed antiepileptics**

SP 7 T42.5X6- **Underdosing of mixed antiepileptics**

5 T42.6 **Poisoning by, adverse effect of and underdosing of other antiepileptic and sedative-hypnotic drugs**
Poisoning by, adverse effect of and underdosing of methaqualone
Poisoning by, adverse effect of and underdosing of valproic acid
EXCLUDES 1 poisoning by, adverse effect of and underdosing of carbamazepine (T42.1-)

6 T42.6X **Poisoning by, adverse effect of and underdosing of other antiepileptic and sedative-hypnotic drugs**

SP 7 T42.6X1- **Poisoning by other antiepileptic and sedative-hypnotic drugs, accidental (unintentional)**
Poisoning by other antiepileptic and sedative-hypnotic drugs NOS

SP 7 T42.6X2- **Poisoning by other antiepileptic and sedative-hypnotic drugs, intentional self-harm**

SP 7 T42.6X3- **Poisoning by other antiepileptic and sedative-hypnotic drugs, assault**

SP 7 T42.6X4- **Poisoning by other antiepileptic and sedative-hypnotic drugs, undetermined**

IQ 7 T42.6X5- **Adverse effect of other antiepileptic and sedative-hypnotic drugs**

SP 7 T42.6X6- **Underdosing of other antiepileptic and sedative-hypnotic drugs**

5 T42.7 **Poisoning by, adverse effect of and underdosing of unspecified antiepileptic and sedative-hypnotic drugs**

SP ✓ T42.71X- **Poisoning by unspecified antiepileptic and sedative-hypnotic drugs, accidental (unintentional)**
Poisoning by antiepileptic and sedative-hypnotic drugs NOS

SP ✓ T42.72X- **Poisoning by unspecified antiepileptic and sedative-hypnotic drugs, intentional self-harm**

SP ✓ T42.73X- **Poisoning by unspecified antiepileptic and sedative-hypnotic drugs, assault**

SP ✓ T42.74X- **Poisoning by unspecified antiepileptic and sedative-hypnotic drugs, undetermined**

IQ ✓ T42.75X- **Adverse effect of unspecified antiepileptic and sedative-hypnotic drugs**

SP ✓ T42.76X- **Underdosing of unspecified antiepileptic and sedative-hypnotic drugs**

5 T42.8 **Poisoning by, adverse effect of and underdosing of antiparkinsonism drugs and other central muscle-tone depressants**
Poisoning by, adverse effect of and underdosing of amantadine

6 T42.8X **Poisoning by, adverse effect of and underdosing of antiparkinsonism drugs and other central muscle-tone depressants**

SP 7 T42.8X1- **Poisoning by antiparkinsonism drugs and other central muscle-tone depressants, accidental (unintentional)**
Poisoning by antiparkinsonism drugs and other central muscle-tone depressants NOS

SP 7 T42.8X2- **Poisoning by antiparkinsonism drugs and other central muscle-tone depressants, intentional self-harm**

SP 7 T42.8X3- **Poisoning by antiparkinsonism drugs and other central muscle-tone depressants, assault**

SP 7 T42.8X4- **Poisoning by antiparkinsonism drugs and other central muscle-tone depressants, undetermined**

IQ 7 T42.8X5- **Adverse effect of antiparkinsonism drugs and other central muscle-tone depressants**

SP 7 T42.8X6- **Underdosing of antiparkinsonism drugs and other central muscle-tone depressants**

4 T43 **Poisoning by, adverse effect of and underdosing of psychotropic drugs, not elsewhere classified**
EXCLUDES 1 appetite depressants (T50.5-)
barbiturates (T42.3-)
benzodiazepines (T42.4-)
methaqualone (T42.6-)

4 4th digit required   **5** 5th digit required   **6** 6th digit required   **7** 7th digit required   **✓** 7th digit placeholder   **+** Additional code   **⊟** Laterality

1682   *DecisionHealth's* FY 2020 Complete Home Health ICD-10-CM Diagnosis Coding Manual

Chapter 19   *S00-T88*

psychodysleptics
[hallucinogens]
(T40.7-T40.9-)

EXCLUDES 2 drug dependence and related
mental and behavioral
disorders due to psychoactive
substance use (F10.- -F19.-)

The appropriate 7th character is to be added to
each code from category T43
A   initial encounter
D   subsequent encounter
S   sequela

⑤ **T43.0 Poisoning by, adverse effect of and
underdosing of tricyclic and tetracyclic
antidepressants**

⑥ **T43.01 Poisoning by, adverse effect of and
underdosing of tricyclic
antidepressants**

SP ⑦ **T43.011- Poisoning by tricyclic
antidepressants, accidental
(unintentional)**
Poisoning by tricyclic
antidepressants NOS

SP ⑦ **T43.012- Poisoning by tricyclic
antidepressants, intentional self-
harm**

SP ⑦ **T43.013- Poisoning by tricyclic
antidepressants, assault**

SP ⑦ **T43.014- Poisoning by tricyclic
antidepressants, undetermined**

IQ ⑦ **T43.015- Adverse effect of tricyclic
antidepressants**

SP ⑦ **T43.016- Underdosing of tricyclic
antidepressants**

⑥ **T43.02 Poisoning by, adverse effect of and
underdosing of tetracyclic
antidepressants**

SP ⑦ **T43.021- Poisoning by tetracyclic
antidepressants, accidental
(unintentional)**
Poisoning by tetracyclic
antidepressants NOS

SP ⑦ **T43.022- Poisoning by tetracyclic
antidepressants, intentional self-
harm**

SP ⑦ **T43.023- Poisoning by tetracyclic
antidepressants, assault**

SP ⑦ **T43.024- Poisoning by tetracyclic
antidepressants, undetermined**

IQ ⑦ **T43.025- Adverse effect of tetracyclic
antidepressants**

SP ⑦ **T43.026- Underdosing of tetracyclic
antidepressants**

⑤ **T43.1 Poisoning by, adverse effect of and
underdosing of monoamine-oxidase-
inhibitor antidepressants**

⑥ **T43.1X Poisoning by, adverse effect of and
underdosing of monoamine-oxidase-
inhibitor antidepressants**

SP ⑦ **T43.1X1- Poisoning by monoamine-
oxidase-inhibitor
antidepressants, accidental
(unintentional)**
Poisoning by monoamine-oxidase-
inhibitor antidepressants NOS

SP ⑦ **T43.1X2- Poisoning by monoamine-
oxidase-inhibitor
antidepressants, intentional self-
harm**

SP ⑦ **T43.1X3- Poisoning by monoamine-
oxidase-inhibitor
antidepressants, assault**

SP ⑦ **T43.1X4- Poisoning by monoamine-
oxidase-inhibitor
antidepressants, undetermined**

IQ ⑦ **T43.1X5- Adverse effect of monoamine-
oxidase-inhibitor antidepressants**

SP ⑦ **T43.1X6- Underdosing of monoamine-
oxidase-inhibitor antidepressants**

⑤ **T43.2 Poisoning by, adverse effect of and
underdosing of other and unspecified
antidepressants**

⑥ **T43.20 Poisoning by, adverse effect of and
underdosing of unspecified
antidepressants**

SP ⑦ **T43.201- Poisoning by unspecified
antidepressants, accidental
(unintentional)**
Poisoning by antidepressants NOS

SP ⑦ **T43.202- Poisoning by unspecified
antidepressants, intentional self-
harm**

SP ⑦ **T43.203- Poisoning by unspecified
antidepressants, assault**

SP ⑦ **T43.204- Poisoning by unspecified
antidepressants, undetermined**

IQ ⑦ **T43.205- Adverse effect of unspecified
antidepressants**
Antidepressant discontinuation
syndrome

SP ⑦ **T43.206- Underdosing of unspecified
antidepressants**

⑥ **T43.21 Poisoning by, adverse effect of and
underdosing of selective serotonin
and norepinephrine reuptake
inhibitors**
Poisoning by, adverse effect of and
underdosing of SSNRI
antidepressants

SP ⑦ **T43.211- Poisoning by selective serotonin
and norepinephrine reuptake
inhibitors, accidental
(unintentional)**

SP ⑦ **T43.212- Poisoning by selective serotonin
and norepinephrine reuptake
inhibitors, intentional self-harm**

SP ⑦ **T43.213- Poisoning by selective serotonin
and norepinephrine reuptake
inhibitors, assault**

SP ⑦ **T43.214- Poisoning by selective serotonin
and norepinephrine reuptake
inhibitors, undetermined**

IQ ⑦ **T43.215- Adverse effect of selective
serotonin and norepinephrine
reuptake inhibitors**

SP ⑦ **T43.216- Underdosing of selective
serotonin and norepinephrine
reuptake inhibitors**

⑥ **T43.22 Poisoning by, adverse effect of and
underdosing of selective serotonin
reuptake inhibitors**

★ New ▲ Revised **Px** Primary **SP** PDGM Px **SL** Low CoM **SH** High CoM **IQ** Quest. Encounter ⊞ Hospice non-cancer Dx | Unspecified | **M** *Manifestation*

DecisionHealth's FY 2020 Complete Home Health ICD-10-CM Diagnosis Coding Manual

1683

Chapter 19

S00-T88

Poisoning by, adverse effect of and underdosing of SSRI antidepressants

SP 7 T43.221- **Poisoning by selective serotonin reuptake inhibitors, accidental (unintentional)**

SP 7 T43.222- **Poisoning by selective serotonin reuptake inhibitors, intentional self-harm**

SP 7 T43.223- **Poisoning by selective serotonin reuptake inhibitors, assault**

SP 7 T43.224- **Poisoning by selective serotonin reuptake inhibitors, undetermined**

IQ 7 T43.225- **Adverse effect of selective serotonin reuptake inhibitors**

SP 7 T43.226- **Underdosing of selective serotonin reuptake inhibitors**

6 T43.29 **Poisoning by, adverse effect of and underdosing of other antidepressants**

SP 7 T43.291- **Poisoning by other antidepressants, accidental (unintentional)**
Poisoning by other antidepressants NOS

SP 7 T43.292- **Poisoning by other antidepressants, intentional self-harm**

SP 7 T43.293- **Poisoning by other antidepressants, assault**

SP 7 T43.294- **Poisoning by other antidepressants, undetermined**

IQ 7 T43.295- **Adverse effect of other antidepressants**

SP 7 T43.296- **Underdosing of other antidepressants**

5 T43.3 **Poisoning by, adverse effect of and underdosing of phenothiazine antipsychotics and neuroleptics**

6 T43.3X **Poisoning by, adverse effect of and underdosing of phenothiazine antipsychotics and neuroleptics**

SP 7 T43.3X1- **Poisoning by phenothiazine antipsychotics and neuroleptics, accidental (unintentional)**
Poisoning by phenothiazine antipsychotics and neuroleptics NOS

SP 7 T43.3X2- **Poisoning by phenothiazine antipsychotics and neuroleptics, intentional self-harm**

SP 7 T43.3X3- **Poisoning by phenothiazine antipsychotics and neuroleptics, assault**

SP 7 T43.3X4- **Poisoning by phenothiazine antipsychotics and neuroleptics, undetermined**

IQ 7 T43.3X5- **Adverse effect of phenothiazine antipsychotics and neuroleptics**

SP 7 T43.3X6- **Underdosing of phenothiazine antipsychotics and neuroleptics**

5 T43.4 **Poisoning by, adverse effect of and underdosing of butyrophenone and thiothixene neuroleptics**

6 T43.4X **Poisoning by, adverse effect of and underdosing of butyrophenone and thiothixene neuroleptics**

SP 7 T43.4X1- **Poisoning by butyrophenone and thiothixene neuroleptics, accidental (unintentional)**

Poisoning by butyrophenone and thiothixene neuroleptics NOS

SP 7 T43.4X2- **Poisoning by butyrophenone and thiothixene neuroleptics, intentional self-harm**

SP 7 T43.4X3- **Poisoning by butyrophenone and thiothixene neuroleptics, assault**

SP 7 T43.4X4- **Poisoning by butyrophenone and thiothixene neuroleptics, undetermined**

IQ 7 T43.4X5- **Adverse effect of butyrophenone and thiothixene neuroleptics**

SP 7 T43.4X6- **Underdosing of butyrophenone and thiothixene neuroleptics**

5 T43.5 **Poisoning by, adverse effect of and underdosing of other and unspecified antipsychotics and neuroleptics**

> **EXCLUDES 1** poisoning by, adverse effect of and underdosing of rauwolfia (T46.5-)

6 T43.50 **Poisoning by, adverse effect of and underdosing of unspecified antipsychotics and neuroleptics**

SP 7 T43.501- **Poisoning by unspecified antipsychotics and neuroleptics, accidental (unintentional)**
Poisoning by antipsychotics and neuroleptics NOS

SP 7 T43.502- **Poisoning by unspecified antipsychotics and neuroleptics, intentional self-harm**

SP 7 T43.503- **Poisoning by unspecified antipsychotics and neuroleptics, assault**

SP 7 T43.504- **Poisoning by unspecified antipsychotics and neuroleptics, undetermined**

IQ 7 T43.505- **Adverse effect of unspecified antipsychotics and neuroleptics**

SP 7 T43.506- **Underdosing of unspecified antipsychotics and neuroleptics**

6 T43.59 **Poisoning by, adverse effect of and underdosing of other antipsychotics and neuroleptics**

SP 7 T43.591- **Poisoning by other antipsychotics and neuroleptics, accidental (unintentional)**
Poisoning by other antipsychotics and neuroleptics NOS

SP 7 T43.592- **Poisoning by other antipsychotics and neuroleptics, intentional self-harm**

SP 7 T43.593- **Poisoning by other antipsychotics and neuroleptics, assault**

SP 7 T43.594- **Poisoning by other antipsychotics and neuroleptics, undetermined**

IQ 7 T43.595- **Adverse effect of other antipsychotics and neuroleptics**

SP 7 T43.596- **Underdosing of other antipsychotics and neuroleptics**

5 T43.6 **Poisoning by, adverse effect of and underdosing of psychostimulants**
> **EXCLUDES 1** poisoning by, adverse effect of and underdosing of cocaine (T40.5-)

---

4 4th digit required   5 5th digit required   6 6th digit required   7 7th digit required   ☑ 7th digit placeholder   ✚ Additional code   ⊟ Laterality

⑥ T43.60   Poisoning by, adverse effect of and underdosing of unspecified psychostimulant

SP 7 T43.601-   Poisoning by unspecified psychostimulants, accidental (unintentional)

Poisoning by psychostimulants NOS

SP 7 T43.602-   Poisoning by unspecified psychostimulants, intentional self-harm

SP 7 T43.603-   Poisoning by unspecified psychostimulants, assault

SP 7 T43.604-   Poisoning by unspecified psychostimulants, undetermined

IQ 7 T43.605-   Adverse effect of unspecified psychostimulants

SP 7 T43.606-   Underdosing of unspecified psychostimulants

⑥ T43.61   Poisoning by, adverse effect of and underdosing of caffeine

SP 7 T43.611-   Poisoning by caffeine, accidental (unintentional)
Poisoning by caffeine NOS

SP 7 T43.612-   Poisoning by caffeine, intentional self-harm

SP 7 T43.613-   Poisoning by caffeine, assault

SP 7 T43.614-   Poisoning by caffeine, undetermined

IQ 7 T43.615-   Adverse effect of caffeine

SP 7 T43.616-   Underdosing of caffeine

⑥ T43.62   Poisoning by, adverse effect of and underdosing of amphetamines
Poisoning by, adverse effect of and underdosing of methamphetamines

SP 7 T43.621-   Poisoning by amphetamines, accidental (unintentional)
Poisoning by amphetamines NOS

SP 7 T43.622-   Poisoning by amphetamines, intentional self-harm

SP 7 T43.623-   Poisoning by amphetamines, assault

SP 7 T43.624-   Poisoning by amphetamines, undetermined

IQ 7 T43.625-   Adverse effect of amphetamines

SP 7 T43.626-   Underdosing of amphetamines

⑥ T43.63   Poisoning by, adverse effect of and underdosing of methylphenidate

SP 7 T43.631-   Poisoning by methylphenidate, accidental (unintentional)
Poisoning by methylphenidate NOS

SP 7 T43.632-   Poisoning by methylphenidate, intentional self-harm

SP 7 T43.633-   Poisoning by methylphenidate, assault

SP 7 T43.634-   Poisoning by methylphenidate, undetermined

IQ 7 T43.635-   Adverse effect of methylphenidate

SP 7 T43.636-   Underdosing of methylphenidate

⑥ T43.64   Poisoning by ecstasy
Poisoning by MDMA
Poisoning by 3,4-methylenedioxymethamphetamine

SP 7 T43.641-   Poisoning by ecstasy, accidental (unintentional)
Poisoning by ecstasy NOS

SP 7 T43.642-   Poisoning by ecstasy, intentional self-harm

SP 7 T43.643-   Poisoning by ecstasy, assault

SP 7 T43.644-   Poisoning by ecstasy, undetermined

⑥ T43.69   Poisoning by, adverse effect of and underdosing of other psychostimulants

SP 7 T43.691-   Poisoning by other psychostimulants, accidental (unintentional)
Poisoning by other psychostimulants NOS

SP 7 T43.692-   Poisoning by other psychostimulants, intentional self-harm

SP 7 T43.693-   Poisoning by other psychostimulants, assault

SP 7 T43.694-   Poisoning by other psychostimulants, undetermined

IQ 7 T43.695-   Adverse effect of other psychostimulants

SP 7 T43.696-   Underdosing of other psychostimulants

⑤ T43.8   Poisoning by, adverse effect of and underdosing of other psychotropic drugs

⑥ T43.8X   Poisoning by, adverse effect of and underdosing of other psychotropic drugs

SP 7 T43.8X1-   Poisoning by other psychotropic drugs, accidental (unintentional)
Poisoning by other psychotropic drugs NOS

SP 7 T43.8X2-   Poisoning by other psychotropic drugs, intentional self-harm

SP 7 T43.8X3-   Poisoning by other psychotropic drugs, assault

SP 7 T43.8X4-   Poisoning by other psychotropic drugs, undetermined

IQ 7 T43.8X5-   Adverse effect of other psychotropic drugs

SP 7 T43.8X6-   Underdosing of other psychotropic drugs

⑤ T43.9   Poisoning by, adverse effect of and underdosing of unspecified psychotropic drug

SP 7 T43.91X-   Poisoning by unspecified psychotropic drug, accidental (unintentional)

Poisoning by psychotropic drug NOS

SP 7 T43.92X-   Poisoning by unspecified psychotropic drug, intentional self-harm

SP 7 T43.93X-   Poisoning by unspecified psychotropic drug, assault

SP 7 T43.94X-   Poisoning by unspecified psychotropic drug, undetermined

IQ 7 T43.95X-   Adverse effect of unspecified psychotropic drug

SP 7 T43.96X-   Underdosing of unspecified psychotropic drug

Chapter 19

S00-T88

★ New ▲ Revised Px Primary SP PDGM Px SL Low CoM SH High CoM IQ Quest. Encounter Ⓗ Hospice non-cancer Dx   Unspecified   M Manifestation

DecisionHealth's FY 2020 Complete Home Health ICD-10-CM Diagnosis Coding Manual   1685

4 T44 **Poisoning by, adverse effect of and underdosing of drugs primarily affecting the autonomic nervous system**

The appropriate 7th character is to be added to each code from category T44
A   initial encounter
D   subsequent encounter
S   sequela

5 T44.0 **Poisoning by, adverse effect of and underdosing of anticholinesterase agents**

6 T44.0X **Poisoning by, adverse effect of and underdosing of anticholinesterase agents**

SP 7 T44.0X1- **Poisoning by anticholinesterase agents, accidental (unintentional)**
Poisoning by anticholinesterase agents NOS

SP 7 T44.0X2- **Poisoning by anticholinesterase agents, intentional self-harm**

SP 7 T44.0X3- **Poisoning by anticholinesterase agents, assault**

SP 7 T44.0X4- **Poisoning by anticholinesterase agents, undetermined**

IQ 7 T44.0X5- **Adverse effect of anticholinesterase agents**

SP 7 T44.0X6- **Underdosing of anticholinesterase agents**

5 T44.1 **Poisoning by, adverse effect of and underdosing of other parasympathomimetics [cholinergics]**

6 T44.1X **Poisoning by, adverse effect of and underdosing of other parasympathomimetics [cholinergics]**

SP 7 T44.1X1- **Poisoning by other parasympathomimetics [cholinergics], accidental (unintentional)**
Poisoning by other parasympathomimetics [cholinergics] NOS

SP 7 T44.1X2- **Poisoning by other parasympathomimetics [cholinergics], intentional self-harm**

SP 7 T44.1X3- **Poisoning by other parasympathomimetics [cholinergics], assault**

SP 7 T44.1X4- **Poisoning by other parasympathomimetics [cholinergics], undetermined**

IQ 7 T44.1X5- **Adverse effect of other parasympathomimetics [cholinergics]**

▲ SP 7 T44.1X6- **Underdosing of other parasympathomimetics [cholinergics]**

5 T44.2 **Poisoning by, adverse effect of and underdosing of ganglionic blocking drugs**

6 T44.2X **Poisoning by, adverse effect of and underdosing of ganglionic blocking drugs**

SP 7 T44.2X1- **Poisoning by ganglionic blocking drugs, accidental (unintentional)**
Poisoning by ganglionic blocking drugs NOS

SP 7 T44.2X2- **Poisoning by ganglionic blocking drugs, intentional self-harm**

SP 7 T44.2X3- **Poisoning by ganglionic blocking drugs, assault**

SP 7 T44.2X4- **Poisoning by ganglionic blocking drugs, undetermined**

IQ 7 T44.2X5- **Adverse effect of ganglionic blocking drugs**

SP 7 T44.2X6- **Underdosing of ganglionic blocking drugs**

5 T44.3 **Poisoning by, adverse effect of and underdosing of other parasympatholytics [anticholinergics and antimuscarinics] and spasmolytics**
Poisoning by, adverse effect of and underdosing of papaverine

6 T44.3X **Poisoning by, adverse effect of and underdosing of other parasympatholytics [anticholinergics and antimuscarinics] and spasmolytics**

SP 7 T44.3X1- **Poisoning by other parasympatholytics [anticholinergics and antimuscarinics] and spasmolytics, accidental (unintentional)**
Poisoning by other parasympatholytics [anticholinergics and antimuscarinics] and spasmolytics NOS

SP 7 T44.3X2- **Poisoning by other parasympatholytics [anticholinergics and antimuscarinics] and spasmolytics, intentional self-harm**

SP 7 T44.3X3- **Poisoning by other parasympatholytics [anticholinergics and antimuscarinics] and spasmolytics, assault**

SP 7 T44.3X4- **Poisoning by other parasympatholytics [anticholinergics and antimuscarinics] and spasmolytics, undetermined**

IQ 7 T44.3X5- **Adverse effect of other parasympatholytics [anticholinergics and antimuscarinics] and spasmolytics**

SP 7 T44.3X6- **Underdosing of other parasympatholytics [anticholinergics and antimuscarinics] and spasmolytics**

5 T44.4 **Poisoning by, adverse effect of and underdosing of predominantly alpha-adrenoreceptor agonists**
Poisoning by, adverse effect of and underdosing of metaraminol

6 T44.4X **Poisoning by, adverse effect of and underdosing of predominantly alpha-adrenoreceptor agonists**

SP 7 T44.4X1- **Poisoning by predominantly alpha-adrenoreceptor agonists, accidental (unintentional)**

4 4th digit required   5 5th digit required   6 6th digit required   7 7th digit required   ☑ 7th digit placeholder   ✚ Additional code   ⊟ Laterality

1686   *DecisionHealth's* FY 2020 Complete Home Health ICD-10-CM Diagnosis Coding Manual

Chapter 19

S00-T88

Poisoning by predominantly alpha-adrenoreceptor agonists NOS

SP 7 **T44.4X2-** **Poisoning by predominantly alpha-adrenoreceptor agonists, intentional self-harm**

SP 7 **T44.4X3-** **Poisoning by predominantly alpha-adrenoreceptor agonists, assault**

SP 7 **T44.4X4-** **Poisoning by predominantly alpha-adrenoreceptor agonists, undetermined**

IQ 7 **T44.4X5-** **Adverse effect of predominantly alpha-adrenoreceptor agonists**

SP 7 **T44.4X6-** **Underdosing of predominantly alpha-adrenoreceptor agonists**

5 **T44.5** **Poisoning by, adverse effect of and underdosing of predominantly beta-adrenoreceptor agonists**

> **EXCLUDES 1**   poisoning by, adverse effect of and underdosing of beta-adrenoreceptor agonists used in asthma therapy (T48.6-)

6 **T44.5X** **Poisoning by, adverse effect of and underdosing of predominantly beta-adrenoreceptor agonists**

SP 7 **T44.5X1-** **Poisoning by predominantly beta-adrenoreceptor agonists, accidental (unintentional)**

Poisoning by predominantly beta-adrenoreceptor agonists NOS

SP 7 **T44.5X2-** **Poisoning by predominantly beta-adrenoreceptor agonists, intentional self-harm**

SP 7 **T44.5X3-** **Poisoning by predominantly beta-adrenoreceptor agonists, assault**

SP 7 **T44.5X4-** **Poisoning by predominantly beta-adrenoreceptor agonists, undetermined**

IQ 7 **T44.5X5-** **Adverse effect of predominantly beta-adrenoreceptor agonists**

SP 7 **T44.5X6-** **Underdosing of predominantly beta-adrenoreceptor agonists**

5 **T44.6** **Poisoning by, adverse effect of and underdosing of alpha-adrenoreceptor antagonists**

> **EXCLUDES 1**   poisoning by, adverse effect of and underdosing of ergot alkaloids (T48.0)

6 **T44.6X** **Poisoning by, adverse effect of and underdosing of alpha-adrenoreceptor antagonists**

SP 7 **T44.6X1-** **Poisoning by alpha-adrenoreceptor antagonists, accidental (unintentional)**

Poisoning by alpha-adrenoreceptor antagonists NOS

SP 7 **T44.6X2-** **Poisoning by alpha-adrenoreceptor antagonists, intentional self-harm**

SP 7 **T44.6X3-** **Poisoning by alpha-adrenoreceptor antagonists, assault**

SP 7 **T44.6X4-** **Poisoning by alpha-adrenoreceptor antagonists, undetermined**

IQ 7 **T44.6X5-** **Adverse effect of alpha-adrenoreceptor antagonists**

SP 7 **T44.6X6-** **Underdosing of alpha-adrenoreceptor antagonists**

5 **T44.7** **Poisoning by, adverse effect of and underdosing of beta-adrenoreceptor antagonists**

6 **T44.7X** **Poisoning by, adverse effect of and underdosing of beta-adrenoreceptor antagonists**

SP 7 **T44.7X1-** **Poisoning by beta-adrenoreceptor antagonists, accidental (unintentional)**

Poisoning by beta-adrenoreceptor antagonists NOS

SP 7 **T44.7X2-** **Poisoning by beta-adrenoreceptor antagonists, intentional self-harm**

SP 7 **T44.7X3-** **Poisoning by beta-adrenoreceptor antagonists, assault**

SP 7 **T44.7X4-** **Poisoning by beta-adrenoreceptor antagonists, undetermined**

IQ 7 **T44.7X5-** **Adverse effect of beta-adrenoreceptor antagonists**

SP 7 **T44.7X6-** **Underdosing of beta-adrenoreceptor antagonists**

5 **T44.8** **Poisoning by, adverse effect of and underdosing of centrally-acting and adrenergic-neuron- blocking agents**

> **EXCLUDES 1**   poisoning by, adverse effect of and underdosing of clonidine (T46.5)
> poisoning by, adverse effect of and underdosing of guanethidine (T46.5)

6 **T44.8X** **Poisoning by, adverse effect of and underdosing of centrally-acting and adrenergic- neuron-blocking agents**

SP 7 **T44.8X1-** **Poisoning by centrally-acting and adrenergic-neuron-blocking agents, accidental (unintentional)**

Poisoning by centrally-acting and adrenergic-neuron-blocking agents NOS

SP 7 **T44.8X2-** **Poisoning by centrally-acting and adrenergic-neuron-blocking agents, intentional self-harm**

SP 7 **T44.8X3-** **Poisoning by centrally-acting and adrenergic-neuron-blocking agents, assault**

SP 7 **T44.8X4-** **Poisoning by centrally-acting and adrenergic-neuron-blocking agents, undetermined**

IQ 7 **T44.8X5-** **Adverse effect of centrally-acting and adrenergic-neuron-blocking agents**

SP 7 **T44.8X6-** **Underdosing of centrally-acting and adrenergic-neuron-blocking agents**

5 **T44.9** **Poisoning by, adverse effect of and underdosing of other and unspecified drugs primarily affecting the autonomic nervous system**

Poisoning by, adverse effect of and underdosing of drug stimulating both alpha and beta-adrenoreceptors

---

★ New ▲ Revised Px Primary **SP** PDGM Px **SL** Low CoM **SH** High CoM **IQ** Quest. Encounter H Hospice non-cancer Dx   Unspecified   **M** *Manifestation*

DecisionHealth's FY 2020 Complete Home Health ICD-10-CM Diagnosis Coding Manual   1687

Chapter 19

S00-T88

6 T44.90 Poisoning by, adverse effect of and underdosing of unspecified drugs primarily affecting the autonomic nervous system

SP 7 T44.901- Poisoning by unspecified drugs primarily affecting the autonomic nervous system, accidental (unintentional)

Poisoning by unspecified drugs primarily affecting the autonomic nervous system NOS

SP 7 T44.902- Poisoning by unspecified drugs primarily affecting the autonomic nervous system, intentional self-harm

SP 7 T44.903- Poisoning by unspecified drugs primarily affecting the autonomic nervous system, assault

SP 7 T44.904- Poisoning by unspecified drugs primarily affecting the autonomic nervous system, undetermined

!Q 7 T44.905- Adverse effect of unspecified drugs primarily affecting the autonomic nervous system

SP 7 T44.906- Underdosing of unspecified drugs primarily affecting the autonomic nervous system

6 T44.99 Poisoning by, adverse effect of and underdosing of other drugs primarily affecting the autonomic nervous system

SP 7 T44.991- Poisoning by other drug primarily affecting the autonomic nervous system, accidental (unintentional)

Poisoning by other drugs primarily affecting the autonomic nervous system NOS

SP 7 T44.992- Poisoning by other drug primarily affecting the autonomic nervous system, intentional self-harm

SP 7 T44.993- Poisoning by other drug primarily affecting the autonomic nervous system, assault

SP 7 T44.994- Poisoning by other drug primarily affecting the autonomic nervous system, undetermined

!Q 7 T44.995- Adverse effect of other drug primarily affecting the autonomic nervous system

SP 7 T44.996- Underdosing of other drug primarily affecting the autonomic nervous system

4 T45 Poisoning by, adverse effect of and underdosing of primarily systemic and hematological agents, not elsewhere classified

The appropriate 7th character is to be added to each code from category T45
A   initial encounter
D   subsequent encounter
S   sequela

5 T45.0 Poisoning by, adverse effect of and underdosing of antiallergic and antiemetic drugs

EXCLUDES 1 poisoning by, adverse effect of and underdosing of phenothiazine-based neuroleptics (T43.3)

6 T45.0X Poisoning by, adverse effect of and underdosing of antiallergic and antiemetic drugs

SP 7 T45.0X1- Poisoning by antiallergic and antiemetic drugs, accidental (unintentional)

Poisoning by antiallergic and antiemetic drugs NOS

SP 7 T45.0X2- Poisoning by antiallergic and antiemetic drugs, intentional self-harm

SP 7 T45.0X3- Poisoning by antiallergic and antiemetic drugs, assault

SP 7 T45.0X4- Poisoning by antiallergic and antiemetic drugs, undetermined

!Q 7 T45.0X5- Adverse effect of antiallergic and antiemetic drugs

SP 7 T45.0X6- Underdosing of antiallergic and antiemetic drugs

5 T45.1 Poisoning by, adverse effect of and underdosing of antineoplastic and immunosuppressive drugs

EXCLUDES 1 poisoning by, adverse effect of and underdosing of tamoxifen (T38.6)

6 T45.1X Poisoning by, adverse effect of and underdosing of antineoplastic and immunosuppressive drugs

SP 7 T45.1X1- Poisoning by antineoplastic and immunosuppressive drugs, accidental (unintentional)

Poisoning by antineoplastic and immunosuppressive drugs NOS

SP 7 T45.1X2- Poisoning by antineoplastic and immunosuppressive drugs, intentional self-harm

SP 7 T45.1X3- Poisoning by antineoplastic and immunosuppressive drugs, assault

SP 7 T45.1X4- Poisoning by antineoplastic and immunosuppressive drugs, undetermined

!Q 7 T45.1X5- Adverse effect of antineoplastic and immunosuppressive drugs

SP 7 T45.1X6- Underdosing of antineoplastic and immunosuppressive drugs

5 T45.2 Poisoning by, adverse effect of and underdosing of vitamins

EXCLUDES 2 poisoning by, adverse effect of and underdosing of nicotinic acid (derivatives) (T46.7)
poisoning by, adverse effect of and underdosing of iron (T45.4)
poisoning by, adverse effect of and underdosing of vitamin K (T45.7)

6 T45.2X Poisoning by, adverse effect of and underdosing of vitamins

SP 7 T45.2X1- Poisoning by vitamins, accidental (unintentional)

---

4 4th digit required   5 5th digit required   6 6th digit required   7 7th digit required   7 7th digit placeholder   ✚ Additional code   ⊟ Laterality

Poisoning by vitamins NOS

SP **7** T45.2X2- **Poisoning by vitamins, intentional self-harm**

SP **7** T45.2X3- **Poisoning by vitamins, assault**

SP **7** T45.2X4- **Poisoning by vitamins, undetermined**

!Q **7** T45.2X5- **Adverse effect of vitamins**

SP **7** T45.2X6- **Underdosing of vitamins**

EXCLUDES 1 vitamin deficiencies (E50-E56)

5 T45.3 **Poisoning by, adverse effect of and underdosing of enzymes**

6 T45.3X **Poisoning by, adverse effect of and underdosing of enzymes**

SP **7** T45.3X1- **Poisoning by enzymes, accidental (unintentional)**

Poisoning by enzymes NOS

SP **7** T45.3X2- **Poisoning by enzymes, intentional self-harm**

SP **7** T45.3X3- **Poisoning by enzymes, assault**

SP **7** T45.3X4- **Poisoning by enzymes, undetermined**

!Q **7** T45.3X5- **Adverse effect of enzymes**

SP **7** T45.3X6- **Underdosing of enzymes**

5 T45.4 **Poisoning by, adverse effect of and underdosing of iron and its compounds**

6 T45.4X **Poisoning by, adverse effect of and underdosing of iron and its compounds**

SP **7** T45.4X1- **Poisoning by iron and its compounds, accidental (unintentional)**

Poisoning by iron and its compounds NOS

SP **7** T45.4X2- **Poisoning by iron and its compounds, intentional self-harm**

SP **7** T45.4X3- **Poisoning by iron and its compounds, assault**

SP **7** T45.4X4- **Poisoning by iron and its compounds, undetermined**

!Q **7** T45.4X5- **Adverse effect of iron and its compounds**

SP **7** T45.4X6- **Underdosing of iron and its compounds**

EXCLUDES 1 iron deficiency (E61.1)

5 T45.5 **Poisoning by, adverse effect of and underdosing of anticoagulants and antithrombotic drugs**

6 T45.51 **Poisoning by, adverse effect of and underdosing of anticoagulants**

SP **7** T45.511- **Poisoning by anticoagulants, accidental (unintentional)**

Poisoning by anticoagulants NOS

SP **7** T45.512- **Poisoning by anticoagulants, intentional self-harm**

SP **7** T45.513- **Poisoning by anticoagulants, assault**

SP **7** T45.514- **Poisoning by anticoagulants, undetermined**

!Q **7** T45.515- **Adverse effect of anticoagulants**

SP **7** T45.516- **Underdosing of anticoagulants**

6 T45.52 **Poisoning by, adverse effect of and underdosing of antithrombotic drugs**

Poisoning by, adverse effect of and underdosing of antiplatelet drugs

EXCLUDES 2 poisoning by, adverse effect of and underdosing of aspirin (T39.01-)
poisoning by, adverse effect of and underdosing of acetylsalicylic acid (T39.01-)

SP **7** T45.521- **Poisoning by antithrombotic drugs, accidental (unintentional)**

Poisoning by antithrombotic drug NOS

SP **7** T45.522- **Poisoning by antithrombotic drugs, intentional self-harm**

SP **7** T45.523- **Poisoning by antithrombotic drugs, assault**

SP **7** T45.524- **Poisoning by antithrombotic drugs, undetermined**

!Q **7** T45.525- **Adverse effect of antithrombotic drugs**

SP **7** T45.526- **Underdosing of antithrombotic drugs**

5 T45.6 **Poisoning by, adverse effect of and underdosing of fibrinolysis-affecting drugs**

6 T45.60 **Poisoning by, adverse effect of and underdosing of unspecified fibrinolysis-affecting drugs**

SP **7** T45.601- **Poisoning by unspecified fibrinolysis-affecting drugs, accidental (unintentional)**

Poisoning by fibrinolysis-affecting drug NOS

SP **7** T45.602- **Poisoning by unspecified fibrinolysis-affecting drugs, intentional self-harm**

SP **7** T45.603- **Poisoning by unspecified fibrinolysis-affecting drugs, assault**

SP **7** T45.604- **Poisoning by unspecified fibrinolysis-affecting drugs, undetermined**

!Q **7** T45.605- **Adverse effect of unspecified fibrinolysis-affecting drugs**

SP **7** T45.606- **Underdosing of unspecified fibrinolysis-affecting drugs**

6 T45.61 **Poisoning by, adverse effect of and underdosing of thrombolytic drugs**

SP **7** T45.611- **Poisoning by thrombolytic drug, accidental (unintentional)**

Poisoning by thrombolytic drug NOS

SP **7** T45.612- **Poisoning by thrombolytic drug, intentional self-harm**

SP **7** T45.613- **Poisoning by thrombolytic drug, assault**

SP **7** T45.614- **Poisoning by thrombolytic drug, undetermined**

!Q **7** T45.615- **Adverse effect of thrombolytic drugs**

SP **7** T45.616- **Underdosing of thrombolytic drugs**

6 T45.62 **Poisoning by, adverse effect of and underdosing of hemostatic drugs**

SP **7** T45.621- **Poisoning by hemostatic drug, accidental (unintentional)**

Chapter 19

S00-T88

✦ New ▲ Revised Px Primary **SP** PDGM Px **SL** Low CoM **SH** High CoM **!Q** Quest. Encounter **H** Hospice non-cancer Dx Unspecified **M** *Manifestation*

DecisionHealth's FY 2020 Complete Home Health ICD-10-CM Diagnosis Coding Manual | 1689

Poisoning by hemostatic drug NOS

SP 7 T45.622- **Poisoning by hemostatic drug, intentional self-harm**

SP 7 T45.623- **Poisoning by hemostatic drug, assault**

SP 7 T45.624- **Poisoning by hemostatic drug, undetermined**

IQ 7 T45.625- **Adverse effect of hemostatic drug**

SP 7 T45.626- **Underdosing of hemostatic drugs**

6 T45.69 **Poisoning by, adverse effect of and underdosing of other fibrinolysis-affecting drugs**

SP 7 T45.691- **Poisoning by other fibrinolysis-affecting drugs, accidental (unintentional)**

Poisoning by other fibrinolysis-affecting drug NOS

SP 7 T45.692- **Poisoning by other fibrinolysis-affecting drugs, intentional self-harm**

SP 7 T45.693- **Poisoning by other fibrinolysis-affecting drugs, assault**

SP 7 T45.694- **Poisoning by other fibrinolysis-affecting drugs, undetermined**

IQ 7 T45.695- **Adverse effect of other fibrinolysis-affecting drugs**

SP 7 T45.696- **Underdosing of other fibrinolysis-affecting drugs**

5 T45.7 **Poisoning by, adverse effect of and underdosing of anticoagulant antagonists, vitamin K and other coagulants**

6 T45.7X **Poisoning by, adverse effect of and underdosing of anticoagulant antagonists, vitamin K and other coagulants**

SP 7 T45.7X1- **Poisoning by anticoagulant antagonists, vitamin K and other coagulants, accidental (unintentional)**

Poisoning by anticoagulant antagonists, vitamin K and other coagulants NOS

SP 7 T45.7X2- **Poisoning by anticoagulant antagonists, vitamin K and other coagulants, intentional self-harm**

SP 7 T45.7X3- **Poisoning by anticoagulant antagonists, vitamin K and other coagulants, assault**

SP 7 T45.7X4- **Poisoning by anticoagulant antagonists, vitamin K and other coagulants, undetermined**

IQ 7 T45.7X5- **Adverse effect of anticoagulant antagonists, vitamin K and other coagulants**

SP 7 T45.7X6- **Underdosing of anticoagulant antagonist, vitamin K and other coagulants**

EXCLUDES 1 vitamin K deficiency (E56.1)

5 T45.8 **Poisoning by, adverse effect of and underdosing of other primarily systemic and hematological agents**

Poisoning by, adverse effect of and underdosing of liver preparations and other antianemic agents

Poisoning by, adverse effect of and underdosing of natural blood and blood products

Poisoning by, adverse effect of and underdosing of plasma substitute

EXCLUDES 2 poisoning by, adverse effect of and underdosing of immunoglobulin (T50.Z1)
poisoning by, adverse effect of and underdosing of iron (T45.4)
transfusion reactions (T80.-)

6 T45.8X **Poisoning by, adverse effect of and underdosing of other primarily systemic and hematological agents**

SP 7 T45.8X1- **Poisoning by other primarily systemic and hematological agents, accidental (unintentional)**

Poisoning by other primarily systemic and hematological agents NOS

SP 7 T45.8X2- **Poisoning by other primarily systemic and hematological agents, intentional self-harm**

SP 7 T45.8X3- **Poisoning by other primarily systemic and hematological agents, assault**

SP 7 T45.8X4- **Poisoning by other primarily systemic and hematological agents, undetermined**

IQ 7 T45.8X5- **Adverse effect of other primarily systemic and hematological agents**

SP 7 T45.8X6- **Underdosing of other primarily systemic and hematological agents**

5 T45.9 **Poisoning by, adverse effect of and underdosing of unspecified primarily systemic and hematological agent**

SP ⊠ T45.91X- **Poisoning by unspecified primarily systemic and hematological agent, accidental (unintentional)**

Poisoning by primarily systemic and hematological agent NOS

SP ⊠ T45.92X- **Poisoning by unspecified primarily systemic and hematological agent, intentional self-harm**

SP ⊠ T45.93X- **Poisoning by unspecified primarily systemic and hematological agent, assault**

SP ⊠ T45.94X- **Poisoning by unspecified primarily systemic and hematological agent, undetermined**

IQ ⊠ T45.95X- **Adverse effect of unspecified primarily systemic and hematological agent**

SP ⊠ T45.96X- **Underdosing of unspecified primarily systemic and hematological agent**

4 T46 **Poisoning by, adverse effect of and underdosing of agents primarily affecting the cardiovascular system**

EXCLUDES 1 poisoning by, adverse effect of and underdosing of metaraminol (T44.4)

---

4 4th digit required   5 5th digit required   6 6th digit required   7 7th digit required   ⊠ 7th digit placeholder   ✛ Additional code   ▣ Laterality

The appropriate 7th character is to be added to each code from category T46
A   initial encounter
D   subsequent encounter
S   sequela

5 **T46.0 Poisoning by, adverse effect of and underdosing of cardiac-stimulant glycosides and drugs of similar action**

  6 **T46.0X Poisoning by, adverse effect of and underdosing of cardiac-stimulant glycosides and drugs of similar action**

SP 7 **T46.0X1- Poisoning by cardiac-stimulant glycosides and drugs of similar action, accidental (unintentional)**
Poisoning by cardiac-stimulant glycosides and drugs of similar action NOS

SP 7 **T46.0X2- Poisoning by cardiac-stimulant glycosides and drugs of similar action, intentional self-harm**

SP 7 **T46.0X3- Poisoning by cardiac-stimulant glycosides and drugs of similar action, assault**

SP 7 **T46.0X4- Poisoning by cardiac-stimulant glycosides and drugs of similar action, undetermined**

IQ 7 **T46.0X5- Adverse effect of cardiac-stimulant glycosides and drugs of similar action**

SP 7 **T46.0X6- Underdosing of cardiac-stimulant glycosides and drugs of similar action**

5 **T46.1 Poisoning by, adverse effect of and underdosing of calcium-channel blockers**

  6 **T46.1X Poisoning by, adverse effect of and underdosing of calcium-channel blockers**

SP 7 **T46.1X1- Poisoning by calcium-channel blockers, accidental (unintentional)**
Poisoning by calcium-channel blockers NOS

SP 7 **T46.1X2- Poisoning by calcium-channel blockers, intentional self-harm**

SP 7 **T46.1X3- Poisoning by calcium-channel blockers, assault**

SP 7 **T46.1X4- Poisoning by calcium-channel blockers, undetermined**

IQ 7 **T46.1X5- Adverse effect of calcium-channel blockers**

SP 7 **T46.1X6- Underdosing of calcium-channel blockers**

5 **T46.2 Poisoning by, adverse effect of and underdosing of other antidysrhythmic drugs, not elsewhere classified**
EXCLUDES 1   poisoning by, adverse effect of and underdosing of beta-adrenoreceptor antagonists (T44.7-)

  6 **T46.2X Poisoning by, adverse effect of and underdosing of other antidysrhythmic drugs**

SP 7 **T46.2X1- Poisoning by other antidysrhythmic drugs, accidental (unintentional)**
Poisoning by other antidysrhythmic drugs NOS

SP 7 **T46.2X2- Poisoning by other antidysrhythmic drugs, intentional self-harm**

SP 7 **T46.2X3- Poisoning by other antidysrhythmic drugs, assault**

SP 7 **T46.2X4- Poisoning by other antidysrhythmic drugs, undetermined**

IQ 7 **T46.2X5- Adverse effect of other antidysrhythmic drugs**

SP 7 **T46.2X6- Underdosing of other antidysrhythmic drugs**

5 **T46.3 Poisoning by, adverse effect of and underdosing of coronary vasodilators**
Poisoning by, adverse effect of and underdosing of dipyridamole
EXCLUDES 1   poisoning by, adverse effect of and underdosing of calcium-channel blockers (T46.1)

  6 **T46.3X Poisoning by, adverse effect of and underdosing of coronary vasodilators**

SP 7 **T46.3X1- Poisoning by coronary vasodilators, accidental (unintentional)**
Poisoning by coronary vasodilators NOS

SP 7 **T46.3X2- Poisoning by coronary vasodilators, intentional self-harm**

SP 7 **T46.3X3- Poisoning by coronary vasodilators, assault**

SP 7 **T46.3X4- Poisoning by coronary vasodilators, undetermined**

IQ 7 **T46.3X5- Adverse effect of coronary vasodilators**

SP 7 **T46.3X6- Underdosing of coronary vasodilators**

5 **T46.4 Poisoning by, adverse effect of and underdosing of angiotensin-converting-enzyme inhibitors**

  6 **T46.4X Poisoning by, adverse effect of and underdosing of angiotensin-converting-enzyme inhibitors**

SP 7 **T46.4X1- Poisoning by angiotensin-converting-enzyme inhibitors, accidental (unintentional)**
Poisoning by angiotensin-converting-enzyme inhibitors NOS

SP 7 **T46.4X2- Poisoning by angiotensin-converting-enzyme inhibitors, intentional self-harm**

SP 7 **T46.4X3- Poisoning by angiotensin-converting-enzyme inhibitors, assault**

SP 7 **T46.4X4- Poisoning by angiotensin-converting-enzyme inhibitors, undetermined**

IQ 7 **T46.4X5- Adverse effect of angiotensin-converting-enzyme inhibitors**

SP 7 **T46.4X6- Underdosing of angiotensin-converting-enzyme inhibitors**

5 **T46.5 Poisoning by, adverse effect of and underdosing of other antihypertensive drugs**

★ New ▲ Revised Px Primary SP PDGM Px SL Low CoM SH High CoM IQ Quest. Encounter H Hospice non-cancer Dx   Unspecified   M *Manifestation*

DecisionHealth's FY 2020 Complete Home Health ICD-10-CM Diagnosis Coding Manual   1691

EXCLUDES 2 poisoning by, adverse effect of and underdosing of beta-adrenoreceptor antagonists (T44.7)
poisoning by, adverse effect of and underdosing of calcium-channel blockers (T46.1)
poisoning by, adverse effect of and underdosing of diuretics (T50.0-T50.2)

6 T46.5X Poisoning by, adverse effect of and underdosing of other antihypertensive drugs

SP 7 T46.5X1- Poisoning by other antihypertensive drugs, accidental (unintentional)
Poisoning by other antihypertensive drugs NOS

SP 7 T46.5X2- Poisoning by other antihypertensive drugs, intentional self-harm

SP 7 T46.5X3- Poisoning by other antihypertensive drugs, assault

SP 7 T46.5X4- Poisoning by other antihypertensive drugs, undetermined

IQ 7 T46.5X5- Adverse effect of other antihypertensive drugs

SP 7 T46.5X6- Underdosing of other antihypertensive drugs

5 T46.6 Poisoning by, adverse effect of and underdosing of antihyperlipidemic and antiarteriosclerotic drugs

6 T46.6X Poisoning by, adverse effect of and underdosing of antihyperlipidemic and antiarteriosclerotic drugs

SP 7 T46.6X1- Poisoning by antihyperlipidemic and antiarteriosclerotic drugs, accidental (unintentional)
Poisoning by antihyperlipidemic and antiarteriosclerotic drugs NOS

SP 7 T46.6X2- Poisoning by antihyperlipidemic and antiarteriosclerotic drugs, intentional self-harm

SP 7 T46.6X3- Poisoning by antihyperlipidemic and antiarteriosclerotic drugs, assault

SP 7 T46.6X4- Poisoning by antihyperlipidemic and antiarteriosclerotic drugs, undetermined

IQ 7 T46.6X5- Adverse effect of antihyperlipidemic and antiarteriosclerotic drugs

SP 7 T46.6X6- Underdosing of antihyperlipidemic and antiarteriosclerotic drugs

5 T46.7 Poisoning by, adverse effect of and underdosing of peripheral vasodilators
Poisoning by, adverse effect of and underdosing of nicotinic acid (derivatives)
EXCLUDES 1 poisoning by, adverse effect of and underdosing of papaverine (T44.3)

6 T46.7X Poisoning by, adverse effect of and underdosing of peripheral vasodilators

SP 7 T46.7X1- Poisoning by peripheral vasodilators, accidental (unintentional)
Poisoning by peripheral vasodilators NOS

SP 7 T46.7X2- Poisoning by peripheral vasodilators, intentional self-harm

SP 7 T46.7X3- Poisoning by peripheral vasodilators, assault

SP 7 T46.7X4- Poisoning by peripheral vasodilators, undetermined

IQ 7 T46.7X5- Adverse effect of peripheral vasodilators

SP 7 T46.7X6- Underdosing of peripheral vasodilators

5 T46.8 Poisoning by, adverse effect of and underdosing of antivaricose drugs, including sclerosing agents

6 T46.8X Poisoning by, adverse effect of and underdosing of antivaricose drugs, including sclerosing agents

SP 7 T46.8X1- Poisoning by antivaricose drugs, including sclerosing agents, accidental (unintentional)
Poisoning by antivaricose drugs, including sclerosing agents NOS

SP 7 T46.8X2- Poisoning by antivaricose drugs, including sclerosing agents, intentional self-harm

SP 7 T46.8X3- Poisoning by antivaricose drugs, including sclerosing agents, assault

SP 7 T46.8X4- Poisoning by antivaricose drugs, including sclerosing agents, undetermined

IQ 7 T46.8X5- Adverse effect of antivaricose drugs, including sclerosing agents

SP 7 T46.8X6- Underdosing of antivaricose drugs, including sclerosing agents

5 T46.9 Poisoning by, adverse effect of and underdosing of other and unspecified agents primarily affecting the cardiovascular system

6 T46.90 Poisoning by, adverse effect of and underdosing of unspecified agents primarily affecting the cardiovascular system

SP 7 T46.901- Poisoning by unspecified agents primarily affecting the cardiovascular system, accidental (unintentional)

SP 7 T46.902- Poisoning by unspecified agents primarily affecting the cardiovascular system, intentional self-harm

SP 7 T46.903- Poisoning by unspecified agents primarily affecting the cardiovascular system, assault

SP 7 T46.904- Poisoning by unspecified agents primarily affecting the cardiovascular system, undetermined

IQ 7 T46.905- Adverse effect of unspecified agents primarily affecting the cardiovascular system

4 4th digit required   **5** 5th digit required   **6** 6th digit required   **7** 7th digit required   ✓ 7th digit placeholder   ✚ Additional code   ⊟ Laterality

1692   DecisionHealth's FY 2020 Complete Home Health ICD-10-CM Diagnosis Coding Manual

SP **7** T46.906- **Underdosing of unspecified agents primarily affecting the cardiovascular system**

6 T46.99 **Poisoning by, adverse effect of and underdosing of other agents primarily affecting the cardiovascular system**

SP **7** T46.991- **Poisoning by other agents primarily affecting the cardiovascular system, accidental (unintentional)**

SP **7** T46.992- **Poisoning by other agents primarily affecting the cardiovascular system, intentional self-harm**

SP **7** T46.993- **Poisoning by other agents primarily affecting the cardiovascular system, assault**

SP **7** T46.994- **Poisoning by other agents primarily affecting the cardiovascular system, undetermined**

IQ **7** T46.995- **Adverse effect of other agents primarily affecting the cardiovascular system**

SP **7** T46.996- **Underdosing of other agents primarily affecting the cardiovascular system**

4 T47 **Poisoning by, adverse effect of and underdosing of agents primarily affecting the gastrointestinal system**

The appropriate 7th character is to be added to each code from category T47
A   initial encounter
D   subsequent encounter
S   sequela

5 T47.0 **Poisoning by, adverse effect of and underdosing of histamine H2-receptor blockers**

6 T47.0X **Poisoning by, adverse effect of and underdosing of histamine H2-receptor blockers**

SP **7** T47.0X1- **Poisoning by histamine H2-receptor blockers, accidental (unintentional)**
Poisoning by histamine H2-receptor blockers NOS

SP **7** T47.0X2- **Poisoning by histamine H2-receptor blockers, intentional self-harm**

SP **7** T47.0X3- **Poisoning by histamine H2-receptor blockers, assault**

SP **7** T47.0X4- **Poisoning by histamine H2-receptor blockers, undetermined**

IQ **7** T47.0X5- **Adverse effect of histamine H2-receptor blockers**

SP **7** T47.0X6- **Underdosing of histamine H2-receptor blockers**

5 T47.1 **Poisoning by, adverse effect of and underdosing of other antacids and anti-gastric-secretion drugs**

6 T47.1X **Poisoning by, adverse effect of and underdosing of other antacids and anti-gastric-secretion drugs**

SP **7** T47.1X1- **Poisoning by other antacids and anti-gastric-secretion drugs, accidental (unintentional)**

Poisoning by other antacids and anti-gastric-secretion drugs NOS

SP **7** T47.1X2- **Poisoning by other antacids and anti-gastric-secretion drugs, intentional self-harm**

SP **7** T47.1X3- **Poisoning by other antacids and anti-gastric-secretion drugs, assault**

SP **7** T47.1X4- **Poisoning by other antacids and anti-gastric-secretion drugs, undetermined**

IQ **7** T47.1X5- **Adverse effect of other antacids and anti-gastric-secretion drugs**

SP **7** T47.1X6- **Underdosing of other antacids and anti-gastric-secretion drugs**

5 T47.2 **Poisoning by, adverse effect of and underdosing of stimulant laxatives**

6 T47.2X **Poisoning by, adverse effect of and underdosing of stimulant laxatives**

SP **7** T47.2X1- **Poisoning by stimulant laxatives, accidental (unintentional)**
Poisoning by stimulant laxatives NOS

SP **7** T47.2X2- **Poisoning by stimulant laxatives, intentional self-harm**

SP **7** T47.2X3- **Poisoning by stimulant laxatives, assault**

SP **7** T47.2X4- **Poisoning by stimulant laxatives, undetermined**

IQ **7** T47.2X5- **Adverse effect of stimulant laxatives**

SP **7** T47.2X6- **Underdosing of stimulant laxatives**

5 T47.3 **Poisoning by, adverse effect of and underdosing of saline and osmotic laxatives**

6 T47.3X **Poisoning by and adverse effect of saline and osmotic laxatives**

SP **7** T47.3X1- **Poisoning by saline and osmotic laxatives, accidental (unintentional)**
Poisoning by saline and osmotic laxatives NOS

SP **7** T47.3X2- **Poisoning by saline and osmotic laxatives, intentional self-harm**

SP **7** T47.3X3- **Poisoning by saline and osmotic laxatives, assault**

SP **7** T47.3X4- **Poisoning by saline and osmotic laxatives, undetermined**

IQ **7** T47.3X5- **Adverse effect of saline and osmotic laxatives**

SP **7** T47.3X6- **Underdosing of saline and osmotic laxatives**

5 T47.4 **Poisoning by, adverse effect of and underdosing of other laxatives**

6 T47.4X **Poisoning by, adverse effect of and underdosing of other laxatives**

SP **7** T47.4X1- **Poisoning by other laxatives, accidental (unintentional)**
Poisoning by other laxatives NOS

SP **7** T47.4X2- **Poisoning by other laxatives, intentional self-harm**

SP **7** T47.4X3- **Poisoning by other laxatives, assault**

SP **7** T47.4X4- **Poisoning by other laxatives, undetermined**

IQ **7** T47.4X5- **Adverse effect of other laxatives**

SP **7** T47.4X6- **Underdosing of other laxatives**

Chapter 19

S00-T88

★ New ▲ Revised **Px** Primary **SP** PDGM Px **SL** Low CoM **SH** High CoM **IQ** Quest. Encounter **H** Hospice non-cancer Dx Unspecified **M** *Manifestation*

⑤ **T47.5 Poisoning by, adverse effect of and underdosing of digestants**

⑥ **T47.5X Poisoning by, adverse effect of and underdosing of digestants**

SP ⑦ **T47.5X1- Poisoning by digestants, accidental (unintentional)**
Poisoning by digestants NOS

SP ⑦ **T47.5X2- Poisoning by digestants, intentional self-harm**

SP ⑦ **T47.5X3- Poisoning by digestants, assault**

SP ⑦ **T47.5X4- Poisoning by digestants, undetermined**

IQ ⑦ **T47.5X5- Adverse effect of digestants**

SP ⑦ **T47.5X6- Underdosing of digestants**

⑤ **T47.6 Poisoning by, adverse effect of and underdosing of antidiarrheal drugs**
EXCLUDES 2 poisoning by, adverse effect of and underdosing of systemic antibiotics and other anti-infectives (T36-T37)

⑥ **T47.6X Poisoning by, adverse effect of and underdosing of antidiarrheal drugs**

SP ⑦ **T47.6X1- Poisoning by antidiarrheal drugs, accidental (unintentional)**
Poisoning by antidiarrheal drugs NOS

SP ⑦ **T47.6X2- Poisoning by antidiarrheal drugs, intentional self-harm**

SP ⑦ **T47.6X3- Poisoning by antidiarrheal drugs, assault**

SP ⑦ **T47.6X4- Poisoning by antidiarrheal drugs, undetermined**

IQ ⑦ **T47.6X5- Adverse effect of antidiarrheal drugs**

SP ⑦ **T47.6X6- Underdosing of antidiarrheal drugs**

⑤ **T47.7 Poisoning by, adverse effect of and underdosing of emetics**

⑥ **T47.7X Poisoning by, adverse effect of and underdosing of emetics**

SP ⑦ **T47.7X1- Poisoning by emetics, accidental (unintentional)**
Poisoning by emetics NOS

SP ⑦ **T47.7X2- Poisoning by emetics, intentional self-harm**

SP ⑦ **T47.7X3- Poisoning by emetics, assault**

SP ⑦ **T47.7X4- Poisoning by emetics, undetermined**

IQ ⑦ **T47.7X5- Adverse effect of emetics**

SP ⑦ **T47.7X6- Underdosing of emetics**

⑤ **T47.8 Poisoning by, adverse effect of and underdosing of other agents primarily affecting gastrointestinal system**

⑥ **T47.8X Poisoning by, adverse effect of and underdosing of other agents primarily affecting gastrointestinal system**

SP ⑦ **T47.8X1- Poisoning by other agents primarily affecting gastrointestinal system, accidental (unintentional)**
Poisoning by other agents primarily affecting gastrointestinal system NOS

SP ⑦ **T47.8X2- Poisoning by other agents primarily affecting gastrointestinal system, intentional self-harm**

SP ⑦ **T47.8X3- Poisoning by other agents primarily affecting gastrointestinal system, assault**

SP ⑦ **T47.8X4- Poisoning by other agents primarily affecting gastrointestinal system, undetermined**

IQ ⑦ **T47.8X5- Adverse effect of other agents primarily affecting gastrointestinal system**

SP ⑦ **T47.8X6- Underdosing of other agents primarily affecting gastrointestinal system**

⑤ **T47.9 Poisoning by, adverse effect of and underdosing of unspecified agents primarily affecting the gastrointestinal system**

SP ☑ **T47.91X- Poisoning by unspecified agents primarily affecting the gastrointestinal system, accidental (unintentional)**
Poisoning by agents primarily affecting the gastrointestinal system NOS

SP ☑ **T47.92X- Poisoning by unspecified agents primarily affecting the gastrointestinal system, intentional self-harm**

SP ☑ **T47.93X- Poisoning by unspecified agents primarily affecting the gastrointestinal system, assault**

SP ☑ **T47.94X- Poisoning by unspecified agents primarily affecting the gastrointestinal system, undetermined**

IQ ☑ **T47.95X- Adverse effect of unspecified agents primarily affecting the gastrointestinal system**

SP ☑ **T47.96X- Underdosing of unspecified agents primarily affecting the gastrointestinal system**

④ **T48 Poisoning by, adverse effect of and underdosing of agents primarily acting on smooth and skeletal muscles and the respiratory system**

The appropriate 7th character is to be added to each code from category T48
A   initial encounter
D   subsequent encounter
S   sequela

⑤ **T48.0 Poisoning by, adverse effect of and underdosing of oxytocic drugs**
EXCLUDES 1 poisoning by, adverse effect of and underdosing of estrogens, progestogens and antagonists (T38.4-T38.6)

⑥ **T48.0X Poisoning by, adverse effect of and underdosing of oxytocic drugs**

SP ⑦ **T48.0X1- Poisoning by oxytocic drugs, accidental (unintentional)**
Poisoning by oxytocic drugs NOS

④4th digit required   ⑤5th digit required   ⑥6th digit required   ⑦7th digit required   ☑7th digit placeholder   ✚Additional code   ⊟Laterality

1694   DecisionHealth's FY 2020 Complete Home Health ICD-10-CM Diagnosis Coding Manual

SP 7 T48.0X2- Poisoning by oxytocic drugs, intentional self-harm

SP 7 T48.0X3- Poisoning by oxytocic drugs, assault

SP 7 T48.0X4- Poisoning by oxytocic drugs, undetermined

IQ 7 T48.0X5- Adverse effect of oxytocic drugs

SP 7 T48.0X6- Underdosing of oxytocic drugs

5 T48.1 Poisoning by, adverse effect of and underdosing of skeletal muscle relaxants [neuromuscular blocking agents]

  6 T48.1X Poisoning by, adverse effect of and underdosing of skeletal muscle relaxants [neuromuscular blocking agents]

SP 7 T48.1X1- Poisoning by skeletal muscle relaxants [neuromuscular blocking agents], accidental (unintentional)
Poisoning by skeletal muscle relaxants [neuromuscular blocking agents] NOS

SP 7 T48.1X2- Poisoning by skeletal muscle relaxants [neuromuscular blocking agents], intentional self-harm

SP 7 T48.1X3- Poisoning by skeletal muscle relaxants [neuromuscular blocking agents], assault

SP 7 T48.1X4- Poisoning by skeletal muscle relaxants [neuromuscular blocking agents], undetermined

IQ 7 T48.1X5- Adverse effect of skeletal muscle relaxants [neuromuscular blocking agents]

SP 7 T48.1X6- Underdosing of skeletal muscle relaxants [neuromuscular blocking agents]

5 T48.2 Poisoning by, adverse effect of and underdosing of other and unspecified drugs acting on muscles

  6 T48.20 Poisoning by, adverse effect of and underdosing of unspecified drugs acting on muscles

SP 7 T48.201- Poisoning by unspecified drugs acting on muscles, accidental (unintentional)
Poisoning by unspecified drugs acting on muscles NOS

SP 7 T48.202- Poisoning by unspecified drugs acting on muscles, intentional self-harm

SP 7 T48.203- Poisoning by unspecified drugs acting on muscles, assault

SP 7 T48.204- Poisoning by unspecified drugs acting on muscles, undetermined

IQ 7 T48.205- Adverse effect of unspecified drugs acting on muscles

SP 7 T48.206- Underdosing of unspecified drugs acting on muscles

  6 T48.29 Poisoning by, adverse effect of and underdosing of other drugs acting on muscles

SP 7 T48.291- Poisoning by other drugs acting on muscles, accidental (unintentional)

Poisoning by other drugs acting on muscles NOS

SP 7 T48.292- Poisoning by other drugs acting on muscles, intentional self-harm

SP 7 T48.293- Poisoning by other drugs acting on muscles, assault

SP 7 T48.294- Poisoning by other drugs acting on muscles, undetermined

IQ 7 T48.295- Adverse effect of other drugs acting on muscles

SP 7 T48.296- Underdosing of other drugs acting on muscles

5 T48.3 Poisoning by, adverse effect of and underdosing of antitussives

  6 T48.3X Poisoning by, adverse effect of and underdosing of antitussives

SP 7 T48.3X1- Poisoning by antitussives, accidental (unintentional)
Poisoning by antitussives NOS

SP 7 T48.3X2- Poisoning by antitussives, intentional self-harm

SP 7 T48.3X3- Poisoning by antitussives, assault

SP 7 T48.3X4- Poisoning by antitussives, undetermined

IQ 7 T48.3X5- Adverse effect of antitussives

SP 7 T48.3X6- Underdosing of antitussives

5 T48.4 Poisoning by, adverse effect of and underdosing of expectorants

  6 T48.4X Poisoning by, adverse effect of and underdosing of expectorants

SP 7 T48.4X1- Poisoning by expectorants, accidental (unintentional)
Poisoning by expectorants NOS

SP 7 T48.4X2- Poisoning by expectorants, intentional self-harm

SP 7 T48.4X3- Poisoning by expectorants, assault

SP 7 T48.4X4- Poisoning by expectorants, undetermined

IQ 7 T48.4X5- Adverse effect of expectorants

SP 7 T48.4X6- Underdosing of expectorants

5 T48.5 Poisoning by, adverse effect of and underdosing of other anti-common-cold drugs
Poisoning by, adverse effect of and underdosing of decongestants
EXCLUDES 2 poisoning by, adverse effect of and underdosing of antipyretics, NEC (T39.9-)
poisoning by, adverse effect of and underdosing of non-steroidal antiinflammatory drugs (T39.3-)
poisoning by, adverse effect of and underdosing of salicylates (T39.0-)

  6 T48.5X Poisoning by, adverse effect of and underdosing of other anti-common-cold drugs

SP 7 T48.5X1- Poisoning by other anti-common-cold drugs, accidental (unintentional)
Poisoning by other anti-common-cold drugs NOS

SP 7 T48.5X2- Poisoning by other anti-common-cold drugs, intentional self-harm

★ New ▲ Revised Px Primary SP PDGM Px SL Low CoM SH High CoM IQ Quest. Encounter H Hospice non-cancer Dx   Unspecified   M *Manifestation*

DecisionHealth's FY 2020 Complete Home Health ICD-10-CM Diagnosis Coding Manual

1695

SP 7 T48.5X3- Poisoning by other anti-common-cold drugs, assault

SP 7 T48.5X4- Poisoning by other anti-common-cold drugs, undetermined

!Q 7 T48.5X5- Adverse effect of other anti-common-cold drugs

SP 7 T48.5X6- Underdosing of other anti-common-cold drugs

5 T48.6 Poisoning by, adverse effect of and underdosing of antiasthmatics, not elsewhere classified

Poisoning by, adverse effect of and underdosing of beta-adrenoreceptor agonists used in asthma therapy

> **EXCLUDES 1** poisoning by, adverse effect of and underdosing of beta-adrenoreceptor agonists not used in asthma therapy (T44.5)
> poisoning by, adverse effect of and underdosing of anterior pituitary [adenohypophyseal] hormones (T38.8)

6 T48.6X Poisoning by, adverse effect of and underdosing of antiasthmatics

SP 7 T48.6X1- Poisoning by antiasthmatics, accidental (unintentional)
Poisoning by antiasthmatics NOS

SP 7 T48.6X2- Poisoning by antiasthmatics, intentional self-harm

SP 7 T48.6X3- Poisoning by antiasthmatics, assault

SP 7 T48.6X4- Poisoning by antiasthmatics, undetermined

!Q 7 T48.6X5- Adverse effect of antiasthmatics

SP 7 T48.6X6- Underdosing of antiasthmatics

5 T48.9 Poisoning by, adverse effect of and underdosing of other and unspecified agents primarily acting on the respiratory system

6 T48.90 Poisoning by, adverse effect of and underdosing of unspecified agents primarily acting on the respiratory system

SP 7 T48.901- Poisoning by unspecified agents primarily acting on the respiratory system, accidental (unintentional)

SP 7 T48.902- Poisoning by unspecified agents primarily acting on the respiratory system, intentional self-harm

SP 7 T48.903- Poisoning by unspecified agents primarily acting on the respiratory system, assault

SP 7 T48.904- Poisoning by unspecified agents primarily acting on the respiratory system, undetermined

!Q 7 T48.905- Adverse effect of unspecified agents primarily acting on the respiratory system

SP 7 T48.906- Underdosing of unspecified agents primarily acting on the respiratory system

6 T48.99 Poisoning by, adverse effect of and underdosing of other agents primarily acting on the respiratory system

SP 7 T48.991- Poisoning by other agents primarily acting on the respiratory system, accidental (unintentional)

SP 7 T48.992- Poisoning by other agents primarily acting on the respiratory system, intentional self-harm

SP 7 T48.993- Poisoning by other agents primarily acting on the respiratory system, assault

SP 7 T48.994- Poisoning by other agents primarily acting on the respiratory system, undetermined

!Q 7 T48.995- Adverse effect of other agents primarily acting on the respiratory system

SP 7 T48.996- Underdosing of other agents primarily acting on the respiratory system

4 T49 Poisoning by, adverse effect of and underdosing of topical agents primarily affecting skin and mucous membrane and by ophthalmological, otorhinorlaryngological and dental drugs

> **INCLUDES** poisoning by, adverse effect of and underdosing of glucocorticoids, topically used

> The appropriate 7th character is to be added to each code from category T49
> A   initial encounter
> D   subsequent encounter
> S   sequela

5 T49.0 Poisoning by, adverse effect of and underdosing of local antifungal, anti-infective and anti-inflammatory drugs

6 T49.0X Poisoning by, adverse effect of and underdosing of local antifungal, anti-infective and anti-inflammatory drugs

SP 7 T49.0X1- Poisoning by local antifungal, anti-infective and anti-inflammatory drugs, accidental (unintentional)
Poisoning by local antifungal, anti-infective and anti-inflammatory drugs NOS

SP 7 T49.0X2- Poisoning by local antifungal, anti-infective and anti-inflammatory drugs, intentional self-harm

SP 7 T49.0X3- Poisoning by local antifungal, anti-infective and anti-inflammatory drugs, assault

SP 7 T49.0X4- Poisoning by local antifungal, anti-infective and anti-inflammatory drugs, undetermined

!Q 7 T49.0X5- Adverse effect of local antifungal, anti-infective and anti-inflammatory drugs

4 4th digit required   **5** 5th digit required   **6** 6th digit required   **7** 7th digit required   **7** 7th digit placeholder   **+** Additional code   **⊟** Laterality

1696   *DecisionHealth's* FY 2020 Complete Home Health ICD-10-CM Diagnosis Coding Manual

SP 7 T49.0X6- Underdosing of local antifungal, anti-infective and anti-inflammatory drugs

5 T49.1 Poisoning by, adverse effect of and underdosing of antipruritics

6 T49.1X Poisoning by, adverse effect of and underdosing of antipruritics

SP 7 T49.1X1- Poisoning by antipruritics, accidental (unintentional)
Poisoning by antipruritics NOS

SP 7 T49.1X2- Poisoning by antipruritics, intentional self-harm

SP 7 T49.1X3- Poisoning by antipruritics, assault

SP 7 T49.1X4- Poisoning by antipruritics, undetermined

IQ 7 T49.1X5- Adverse effect of antipruritics

SP 7 T49.1X6- Underdosing of antipruritics

5 T49.2 Poisoning by, adverse effect of and underdosing of local astringents and local detergents

6 T49.2X Poisoning by, adverse effect of and underdosing of local astringents and local detergents

SP 7 T49.2X1- Poisoning by local astringents and local detergents, accidental (unintentional)
Poisoning by local astringents and local detergents NOS

SP 7 T49.2X2- Poisoning by local astringents and local detergents, intentional self-harm

SP 7 T49.2X3- Poisoning by local astringents and local detergents, assault

SP 7 T49.2X4- Poisoning by local astringents and local detergents, undetermined

IQ 7 T49.2X5- Adverse effect of local astringents and local detergents

SP 7 T49.2X6- Underdosing of local astringents and local detergents

5 T49.3 Poisoning by, adverse effect of and underdosing of emollients, demulcents and protectants

6 T49.3X Poisoning by, adverse effect of and underdosing of emollients, demulcents and protectants

SP 7 T49.3X1- Poisoning by emollients, demulcents and protectants, accidental (unintentional)
Poisoning by emollients, demulcents and protectants NOS

SP 7 T49.3X2- Poisoning by emollients, demulcents and protectants, intentional self-harm

SP 7 T49.3X3- Poisoning by emollients, demulcents and protectants, assault

SP 7 T49.3X4- Poisoning by emollients, demulcents and protectants, undetermined

IQ 7 T49.3X5- Adverse effect of emollients, demulcents and protectants

SP 7 T49.3X6- Underdosing of emollients, demulcents and protectants

5 T49.4 Poisoning by, adverse effect of and underdosing of keratolytics, keratoplastics, and other hair treatment drugs and preparations

6 T49.4X Poisoning by, adverse effect of and underdosing of keratolytics, keratoplastics, and other hair treatment drugs and preparations

SP 7 T49.4X1- Poisoning by keratolytics, keratoplastics, and other hair treatment drugs and preparations, accidental (unintentional)
Poisoning by keratolytics, keratoplastics, and other hair treatment drugs and preparations NOS

SP 7 T49.4X2- Poisoning by keratolytics, keratoplastics, and other hair treatment drugs and preparations, intentional self-harm

SP 7 T49.4X3- Poisoning by keratolytics, keratoplastics, and other hair treatment drugs and preparations, assault

SP 7 T49.4X4- Poisoning by keratolytics, keratoplastics, and other hair treatment drugs and preparations, undetermined

IQ 7 T49.4X5- Adverse effect of keratolytics, keratoplastics, and other hair treatment drugs and preparations

SP 7 T49.4X6- Underdosing of keratolytics, keratoplastics, and other hair treatment drugs and preparations

5 T49.5 Poisoning by, adverse effect of and underdosing of ophthalmological drugs and preparations

6 T49.5X Poisoning by, adverse effect of and underdosing of ophthalmological drugs and preparations

SP 7 T49.5X1- Poisoning by ophthalmological drugs and preparations, accidental (unintentional)
Poisoning by ophthalmological drugs and preparations NOS

SP 7 T49.5X2- Poisoning by ophthalmological drugs and preparations, intentional self-harm

SP 7 T49.5X3- Poisoning by ophthalmological drugs and preparations, assault

SP 7 T49.5X4- Poisoning by ophthalmological drugs and preparations, undetermined

IQ 7 T49.5X5- Adverse effect of ophthalmological drugs and preparations

SP 7 T49.5X6- Underdosing of ophthalmological drugs and preparations

5 T49.6 Poisoning by, adverse effect of and underdosing of otorhinolaryngological drugs and preparations

6 T49.6X Poisoning by, adverse effect of and underdosing of otorhinolaryngological drugs and preparations

★ New ▲ Revised **Px** Primary **SP** PDGM Px **SL** Low CoM **SH** High CoM **IQ** Quest. Encounter **H** Hospice non-cancer Dx ｜ Unspecified ｜ **M** *Manifestation*

DecisionHealth's FY 2020 Complete Home Health ICD-10-CM Diagnosis Coding Manual

1697

Chapter 19

S00-T88

SP 7 T49.6X1- Poisoning by otorhinolaryngological drugs and preparations, accidental (unintentional)
Poisoning by otorhinolaryngological drugs and preparations NOS

SP 7 T49.6X2- Poisoning by otorhinolaryngological drugs and preparations, intentional self-harm

SP 7 T49.6X3- Poisoning by otorhinolaryngological drugs and preparations, assault

SP 7 T49.6X4- Poisoning by otorhinolaryngological drugs and preparations, undetermined

SP IQ 7 T49.6X5- Adverse effect of otorhinolaryngological drugs and preparations

SP IQ 7 T49.6X6- Underdosing of otorhinolaryngological drugs and preparations

5 T49.7 Poisoning by, adverse effect of and underdosing of dental drugs, topically applied

6 T49.7X Poisoning by, adverse effect of and underdosing of dental drugs, topically applied

SP 7 T49.7X1- Poisoning by dental drugs, topically applied, accidental (unintentional)
Poisoning by dental drugs, topically applied NOS

SP 7 T49.7X2- Poisoning by dental drugs, topically applied, intentional self-harm

SP 7 T49.7X3- Poisoning by dental drugs, topically applied, assault

SP 7 T49.7X4- Poisoning by dental drugs, topically applied, undetermined

IQ 7 T49.7X5- Adverse effect of dental drugs, topically applied

SP 7 T49.7X6- Underdosing of dental drugs, topically applied

5 T49.8 Poisoning by, adverse effect of and underdosing of other topical agents
Poisoning by, adverse effect of and underdosing of spermicides

6 T49.8X Poisoning by, adverse effect of and underdosing of other topical agents

SP 7 T49.8X1- Poisoning by other topical agents, accidental (unintentional)
Poisoning by other topical agents NOS

SP 7 T49.8X2- Poisoning by other topical agents, intentional self-harm

SP 7 T49.8X3- Poisoning by other topical agents, assault

SP 7 T49.8X4- Poisoning by other topical agents, undetermined

IQ 7 T49.8X5- Adverse effect of other topical agents

SP 7 T49.8X6- Underdosing of other topical agents

5 T49.9 Poisoning by, adverse effect of and underdosing of unspecified topical agent

SP 7 T49.91X- Poisoning by unspecified topical agent, accidental (unintentional)

SP 7 T49.92X- Poisoning by unspecified topical agent, intentional self-harm

SP 7 T49.93X- Poisoning by unspecified topical agent, assault

SP 7 T49.94X- Poisoning by unspecified topical agent, undetermined

IQ 7 T49.95X- Adverse effect of unspecified topical agent

SP 7 T49.96X- Underdosing of unspecified topical agent

4 T50 Poisoning by, adverse effect of and underdosing of diuretics and other and unspecified drugs, medicaments and biological substances

The appropriate 7th character is to be added to each code from category T50
A   initial encounter
D   subsequent encounter
S   sequela

5 T50.0 Poisoning by, adverse effect of and underdosing of mineralocorticoids and their antagonists

6 T50.0X Poisoning by, adverse effect of and underdosing of mineralocorticoids and their antagonists

SP 7 T50.0X1- Poisoning by mineralocorticoids and their antagonists, accidental (unintentional)
Poisoning by mineralocorticoids and their antagonists NOS

SP 7 T50.0X2- Poisoning by mineralocorticoids and their antagonists, intentional self-harm

SP 7 T50.0X3- Poisoning by mineralocorticoids and their antagonists, assault

SP 7 T50.0X4- Poisoning by mineralocorticoids and their antagonists, undetermined

IQ 7 T50.0X5- Adverse effect of mineralocorticoids and their antagonists

SP 7 T50.0X6- Underdosing of mineralocorticoids and their antagonists

5 T50.1 Poisoning by, adverse effect of and underdosing of loop [high-ceiling] diuretics

6 T50.1X Poisoning by, adverse effect of and underdosing of loop [high-ceiling] diuretics

SP 7 T50.1X1- Poisoning by loop [high-ceiling] diuretics, accidental (unintentional)
Poisoning by loop [high-ceiling] diuretics NOS

SP 7 T50.1X2- Poisoning by loop [high-ceiling] diuretics, intentional self-harm

SP 7 T50.1X3- Poisoning by loop [high-ceiling] diuretics, assault

SP 7 T50.1X4- Poisoning by loop [high-ceiling] diuretics, undetermined

IQ 7 T50.1X5- Adverse effect of loop [high-ceiling] diuretics

---

4 4th digit required   5 5th digit required   6 6th digit required   7 7th digit required   7 7th digit placeholder   ✚ Additional code   ⊟ Laterality

1698   DecisionHealth's FY 2020 Complete Home Health ICD-10-CM Diagnosis Coding Manual

SP **7** **T50.1X6-** Underdosing of loop [high-ceiling] diuretics

5 **T50.2** Poisoning by, adverse effect of and underdosing of carbonic-anhydrase inhibitors, benzothiadiazides and other diuretics
Poisoning by, adverse effect of and underdosing of acetazolamide

6 **T50.2X** Poisoning by, adverse effect of and underdosing of carbonic-anhydrase inhibitors, benzothiadiazides and other diuretics

SP **7** **T50.2X1-** Poisoning by carbonic-anhydrase inhibitors, benzothiadiazides and other diuretics, accidental (unintentional)
Poisoning by carbonic-anhydrase inhibitors, benzothiadiazides and other diuretics NOS

SP **7** **T50.2X2-** Poisoning by carbonic-anhydrase inhibitors, benzothiadiazides and other diuretics, intentional self-harm

SP **7** **T50.2X3-** Poisoning by carbonic-anhydrase inhibitors, benzothiadiazides and other diuretics, assault

SP **7** **T50.2X4-** Poisoning by carbonic-anhydrase inhibitors, benzothiadiazides and other diuretics, undetermined

IQ **7** **T50.2X5-** Adverse effect of carbonic-anhydrase inhibitors, benzothiadiazides and other diuretics

SP **7** **T50.2X6-** Underdosing of carbonic-anhydrase inhibitors, benzothiadiazides and other diuretics

5 **T50.3** Poisoning by, adverse effect of and underdosing of electrolytic, caloric and water-balance agents
Poisoning by, adverse effect of and underdosing of oral rehydration salts

6 **T50.3X** Poisoning by, adverse effect of and underdosing of electrolytic, caloric and water-balance agents

SP **7** **T50.3X1-** Poisoning by electrolytic, caloric and water-balance agents, accidental (unintentional)
Poisoning by electrolytic, caloric and water-balance agents NOS

SP **7** **T50.3X2-** Poisoning by electrolytic, caloric and water-balance agents, intentional self-harm

SP **7** **T50.3X3-** Poisoning by electrolytic, caloric and water-balance agents, assault

SP **7** **T50.3X4-** Poisoning by electrolytic, caloric and water-balance agents, undetermined

IQ **7** **T50.3X5-** Adverse effect of electrolytic, caloric and water-balance agents

SP **7** **T50.3X6-** Underdosing of electrolytic, caloric and water-balance agents

5 **T50.4** Poisoning by, adverse effect of and underdosing of drugs affecting uric acid metabolism

6 **T50.4X** Poisoning by, adverse effect of and underdosing of drugs affecting uric acid metabolism

SP **7** **T50.4X1-** Poisoning by drugs affecting uric acid metabolism, accidental (unintentional)
Poisoning by drugs affecting uric acid metabolism NOS

SP **7** **T50.4X2-** Poisoning by drugs affecting uric acid metabolism, intentional self-harm

SP **7** **T50.4X3-** Poisoning by drugs affecting uric acid metabolism, assault

SP **7** **T50.4X4-** Poisoning by drugs affecting uric acid metabolism, undetermined

IQ **7** **T50.4X5-** Adverse effect of drugs affecting uric acid metabolism

SP **7** **T50.4X6-** Underdosing of drugs affecting uric acid metabolism

5 **T50.5** Poisoning by, adverse effect of and underdosing of appetite depressants

6 **T50.5X** Poisoning by, adverse effect of and underdosing of appetite depressants

SP **7** **T50.5X1-** Poisoning by appetite depressants, accidental (unintentional)
Poisoning by appetite depressants NOS

SP **7** **T50.5X2-** Poisoning by appetite depressants, intentional self-harm

SP **7** **T50.5X3-** Poisoning by appetite depressants, assault

SP **7** **T50.5X4-** Poisoning by appetite depressants, undetermined

IQ **7** **T50.5X5-** Adverse effect of appetite depressants

SP **7** **T50.5X6-** Underdosing of appetite depressants

5 **T50.6** Poisoning by, adverse effect of and underdosing of antidotes and chelating agents
Poisoning by, adverse effect of and underdosing of alcohol deterrents

6 **T50.6X** Poisoning by, adverse effect of and underdosing of antidotes and chelating agents

SP **7** **T50.6X1-** Poisoning by antidotes and chelating agents, accidental (unintentional)
Poisoning by antidotes and chelating agents NOS

SP **7** **T50.6X2-** Poisoning by antidotes and chelating agents, intentional self-harm

SP **7** **T50.6X3-** Poisoning by antidotes and chelating agents, assault

SP **7** **T50.6X4-** Poisoning by antidotes and chelating agents, undetermined

IQ **7** **T50.6X5-** Adverse effect of antidotes and chelating agents

SP **7** **T50.6X6-** Underdosing of antidotes and chelating agents

5 **T50.7** Poisoning by, adverse effect of and underdosing of analeptics and opioid receptor antagonists

6 **T50.7X** Poisoning by, adverse effect of and underdosing of analeptics and opioid receptor antagonists

SP **7** **T50.7X1-** Poisoning by analeptics and opioid receptor antagonists, accidental (unintentional)

Chapter 19

S00-T88

★ New ▲ Revised **Px** Primary **SP** PDGM Px **SL** Low CoM **SH** High CoM **IQ** Quest. Encounter **H** Hospice non-cancer Dx   Unspecified   **M** *Manifestation*

DecisionHealth's FY 2020 Complete Home Health ICD-10-CM Diagnosis Coding Manual

1699

Poisoning by analeptics and opioid receptor antagonists NOS

SP **7** **T50.7X2-** Poisoning by analeptics and opioid receptor antagonists, intentional self-harm

SP **7** **T50.7X3-** Poisoning by analeptics and opioid receptor antagonists, assault

SP **7** **T50.7X4-** Poisoning by analeptics and opioid receptor antagonists, undetermined

IQ **7** **T50.7X5-** Adverse effect of analeptics and opioid receptor antagonists

SP **7** **T50.7X6-** Underdosing of analeptics and opioid receptor antagonists

5 **T50.8** Poisoning by, adverse effect of and underdosing of diagnostic agents

  6 **T50.8X** Poisoning by, adverse effect of and underdosing of diagnostic agents

SP **7** **T50.8X1-** Poisoning by diagnostic agents, accidental (unintentional)

Poisoning by diagnostic agents NOS

SP **7** **T50.8X2-** Poisoning by diagnostic agents, intentional self-harm

SP **7** **T50.8X3-** Poisoning by diagnostic agents, assault

SP **7** **T50.8X4-** Poisoning by diagnostic agents, undetermined

IQ **7** **T50.8X5-** Adverse effect of diagnostic agents

SP **7** **T50.8X6-** Underdosing of diagnostic agents

5 **T50.A** Poisoning by, adverse effect of and underdosing of bacterial vaccines

  6 **T50.A1** Poisoning by, adverse effect of and underdosing of pertussis vaccine, including combinations with a pertussis component

SP **7** **T50.A11-** Poisoning by pertussis vaccine, including combinations with a pertussis component, accidental (unintentional)

SP **7** **T50.A12-** Poisoning by pertussis vaccine, including combinations with a pertussis component, intentional self-harm

SP **7** **T50.A13-** Poisoning by pertussis vaccine, including combinations with a pertussis component, assault

SP **7** **T50.A14-** Poisoning by pertussis vaccine, including combinations with a pertussis component, undetermined

IQ **7** **T50.A15-** Adverse effect of pertussis vaccine, including combinations with a pertussis component

SP **7** **T50.A16-** Underdosing of pertussis vaccine, including combinations with a pertussis component

  6 **T50.A2** Poisoning by, adverse effect of and underdosing of mixed bacterial vaccines without a pertussis component

SP **7** **T50.A21-** Poisoning by mixed bacterial vaccines without a pertussis component, accidental (unintentional)

SP **7** **T50.A22-** Poisoning by mixed bacterial vaccines without a pertussis component, intentional self-harm

SP **7** **T50.A23-** Poisoning by mixed bacterial vaccines without a pertussis component, assault

SP **7** **T50.A24-** Poisoning by mixed bacterial vaccines without a pertussis component, undetermined

IQ **7** **T50.A25-** Adverse effect of mixed bacterial vaccines without a pertussis component

SP **7** **T50.A26-** Underdosing of mixed bacterial vaccines without a pertussis component

  6 **T50.A9** Poisoning by, adverse effect of and underdosing of other bacterial vaccines

SP **7** **T50.A91-** Poisoning by other bacterial vaccines, accidental (unintentional)

SP **7** **T50.A92-** Poisoning by other bacterial vaccines, intentional self-harm

SP **7** **T50.A93-** Poisoning by other bacterial vaccines, assault

SP **7** **T50.A94-** Poisoning by other bacterial vaccines, undetermined

IQ **7** **T50.A95-** Adverse effect of other bacterial vaccines

SP **7** **T50.A96-** Underdosing of other bacterial vaccines

5 **T50.B** Poisoning by, adverse effect of and underdosing of viral vaccines

  6 **T50.B1** Poisoning by, adverse effect of and underdosing of smallpox vaccines

SP **7** **T50.B11-** Poisoning by smallpox vaccines, accidental (unintentional)

SP **7** **T50.B12-** Poisoning by smallpox vaccines, intentional self-harm

SP **7** **T50.B13-** Poisoning by smallpox vaccines, assault

SP **7** **T50.B14-** Poisoning by smallpox vaccines, undetermined

IQ **7** **T50.B15-** Adverse effect of smallpox vaccines

SP **7** **T50.B16-** Underdosing of smallpox vaccines

  6 **T50.B9** Poisoning by, adverse effect of and underdosing of other viral vaccines

SP **7** **T50.B91-** Poisoning by other viral vaccines, accidental (unintentional)

SP **7** **T50.B92-** Poisoning by other viral vaccines, intentional self-harm

SP **7** **T50.B93-** Poisoning by other viral vaccines, assault

SP **7** **T50.B94-** Poisoning by other viral vaccines, undetermined

IQ **7** **T50.B95-** Adverse effect of other viral vaccines

SP **7** **T50.B96-** Underdosing of other viral vaccines

5 **T50.Z** Poisoning by, adverse effect of and underdosing of other vaccines and biological substances

  6 **T50.Z1** Poisoning by, adverse effect of and underdosing of immunoglobulin

---

4 4th digit required   **5** 5th digit required   **6** 6th digit required   **7** 7th digit required   **7** 7th digit placeholder   **+** Additional code   **⊟** Laterality

SP 7 **T50.Z11-** Poisoning by immunoglobulin, accidental (unintentional)

SP 7 **T50.Z12-** Poisoning by immunoglobulin, intentional self-harm

SP 7 **T50.Z13-** Poisoning by immunoglobulin, assault

SP 7 **T50.Z14-** Poisoning by immunoglobulin, undetermined

IQ 7 **T50.Z15-** Adverse effect of immunoglobulin

SP 7 **T50.Z16-** Underdosing of immunoglobulin

6 **T50.Z9** Poisoning by, adverse effect of and underdosing of other vaccines and biological substances

SP 7 **T50.Z91-** Poisoning by other vaccines and biological substances, accidental (unintentional)

SP 7 **T50.Z92-** Poisoning by other vaccines and biological substances, intentional self-harm

SP 7 **T50.Z93-** Poisoning by other vaccines and biological substances, assault

SP 7 **T50.Z94-** Poisoning by other vaccines and biological substances, undetermined

IQ 7 **T50.Z95-** Adverse effect of other vaccines and biological substances

SP 7 **T50.Z96-** Underdosing of other vaccines and biological substances

5 **T50.9** Poisoning by, adverse effect of and underdosing of other and unspecified drugs, medicaments and biological substances

6 **T50.90** Poisoning by, adverse effect of and underdosing of unspecified drugs, medicaments and biological substances

SP 7 **T50.901-** Poisoning by unspecified drugs, medicaments and biological substances, accidental (unintentional)

SP 7 **T50.902-** Poisoning by unspecified drugs, medicaments and biological substances, intentional self-harm

SP 7 **T50.903-** Poisoning by unspecified drugs, medicaments and biological substances, assault

SP 7 **T50.904-** Poisoning by unspecified drugs, medicaments and biological substances, undetermined

IQ 7 **T50.905-** Adverse effect of unspecified drugs, medicaments and biological substances

SP 7 **T50.906-** Underdosing of unspecified drugs, medicaments and biological substances

★ 6 **T50.91** Poisoning by, adverse effect of and underdosing of multiple unspecified drugs, medicaments and biological substances

Multiple drug ingestion NOS
Code also:
  any specific drugs, medicaments and biological substances

★ 7 **T50.911-** Poisoning by multiple unspecified drugs, medicaments and biological substances, accidental (unintentional)

★ 7 **T50.912-** Poisoning by multiple unspecified drugs, medicaments and biological substances, intentional self-harm

★ 7 **T50.913-** Poisoning by multiple unspecified drugs, medicaments and biological substances, assault

★ 7 **T50.914-** Poisoning by multiple unspecified drugs, medicaments and biological substances, undetermined

★ 7 **T50.915-** Adverse effect of multiple unspecified drugs, medicaments and biological substances

★ 7 **T50.916-** Underdosing of multiple unspecified drugs, medicaments and biological substances

6 **T50.99** Poisoning by, adverse effect of and underdosing of other drugs, medicaments and biological substances

SP 7 **T50.991-** Poisoning by other drugs, medicaments and biological substances, accidental (unintentional)

SP 7 **T50.992-** Poisoning by other drugs, medicaments and biological substances, intentional self-harm

SP 7 **T50.993-** Poisoning by other drugs, medicaments and biological substances, assault

SP 7 **T50.994-** Poisoning by other drugs, medicaments and biological substances, undetermined

IQ 7 **T50.995-** Adverse effect of other drugs, medicaments and biological substances

SP 7 **T50.996-** Underdosing of other drugs, medicaments and biological substances

Toxic effects of substances chiefly nonmedicinal as to source   (T51-T65)

Note:
When no intent is indicated code to accidental. Undetermined intent is only for use when there is specific documentation in the record that the intent of the toxic effect cannot be determined.
Use additional code(s):
  for all associated manifestations of toxic effect, such as:
    respiratory conditions due to external agents (J60-J70)
    personal history of foreign body fully removed (Z87.821)
  to identify any retained foreign body, if applicable (Z18.-)
  EXCLUDES 1 contact with and (suspected) exposure to toxic substances (Z77.-)

★ New ▲ Revised Px Primary SP PDGM Px SL Low CoM SH High CoM IQ Quest. Encounter H Hospice non-cancer Dx   Unspecified   M *Manifestation*

DecisionHealth's FY 2020 Complete Home Health ICD-10-CM Diagnosis Coding Manual   1701

Chapter 19

S00-T88

Codes in categories T36-T65 are combination codes that include the substance that was taken as well as the intent. No additional external cause code is required for poisonings, toxic effects, adverse effects and underdosing codes.

Do not code directly from the Table of Drugs and Chemicals. Always refer back to the Tabular List. Use as many codes as necessary to describe completely all drugs, medicinal or biological substances. If the same code would describe the causative agent for more than one adverse reaction, poisoning, toxic effect or underdosing, assign the code only once. If two or more drugs, medicinal or biological substances are reported, code each individually unless a combination code is listed in the Table of Drugs and Chemicals.

GUIDELINES   Section I.C.19.e.5)(d)
When a harmful substance is ingested or comes in contact with a person, this is classified as a toxic effect. The toxic effect codes are in categories T51-T65. Toxic effect codes have an associated intent: accidental, intentional self-harm, assault and undetermined.

CODING TIPS ✓   When coding toxic effects, first assign the code from T51-T65 to identify the substance and intent, followed by an additional code to identify the manifestations of the toxic substance that resulted in the effect(s). If the intent is not documented, accidental intent should be coded. Undetermined intent should only be coded when documentation specifically indicates that the intent cannot be determined.

CODING TIPS ✓   Note there are only codes for poisonings or toxic effects. There are no therapeutic uses for the following substances, therefore there are no codes for adverse effects or underdosing.

4 **T51**   **Toxic effect of alcohol**

> The appropriate 7th character is to be added to each code from category T51
> A   initial encounter
> D   subsequent encounter
> S   sequela

5 **T51.0**   **Toxic effect of ethanol**
Toxic effect of ethyl alcohol
> **EXCLUDES 2**   acute alcohol intoxication or 'hangover' effects (F10.129, F10.229, F10.929)
> drunkenness (F10.129, F10.229, F10.929)
> pathological alcohol intoxication (F10.129, F10.229, F10.929)

6 **T51.0X** **Toxic effect of ethanol**

SP **7** **T51.0X1-** **Toxic effect of ethanol, accidental (unintentional)**
Toxic effect of ethanol NOS
SP **7** **T51.0X2-** **Toxic effect of ethanol, intentional self-harm**
SP **7** **T51.0X3-** **Toxic effect of ethanol, assault**
SP **7** **T51.0X4-** **Toxic effect of ethanol, undetermined**
5 **T51.1** **Toxic effect of methanol**
Toxic effect of methyl alcohol
6 **T51.1X** **Toxic effect of methanol**

SP **7** **T51.1X1-** **Toxic effect of methanol, accidental (unintentional)**
Toxic effect of methanol NOS

SP **7** **T51.1X2-** **Toxic effect of methanol, intentional self-harm**
SP **7** **T51.1X3-** **Toxic effect of methanol, assault**
SP **7** **T51.1X4-** **Toxic effect of methanol, undetermined**
5 **T51.2** **Toxic effect of 2-Propanol**
Toxic effect of isopropyl alcohol
6 **T51.2X** **Toxic effect of 2-Propanol**

SP **7** **T51.2X1-** **Toxic effect of 2-Propanol, accidental (unintentional)**
Toxic effect of 2-Propanol NOS
SP **7** **T51.2X2-** **Toxic effect of 2-Propanol, intentional self-harm**
SP **7** **T51.2X3-** **Toxic effect of 2-Propanol, assault**
SP **7** **T51.2X4-** **Toxic effect of 2-Propanol, undetermined**
5 **T51.3** **Toxic effect of fusel oil**
Toxic effect of amyl alcohol
Toxic effect of butyl [1-butanol] alcohol
Toxic effect of propyl [1-propanol] alcohol
6 **T51.3X** **Toxic effect of fusel oil**

SP **7** **T51.3X1-** **Toxic effect of fusel oil, accidental (unintentional)**
Toxic effect of fusel oil NOS
SP **7** **T51.3X2-** **Toxic effect of fusel oil, intentional self-harm**
SP **7** **T51.3X3-** **Toxic effect of fusel oil, assault**
SP **7** **T51.3X4-** **Toxic effect of fusel oil, undetermined**
5 **T51.8** **Toxic effect of other alcohols**
6 **T51.8X** **Toxic effect of other alcohols**

SP **7** **T51.8X1-** **Toxic effect of other alcohols, accidental (unintentional)**
Toxic effect of other alcohols NOS
SP **7** **T51.8X2-** **Toxic effect of other alcohols, intentional self-harm**
SP **7** **T51.8X3-** **Toxic effect of other alcohols, assault**
SP **7** **T51.8X4-** **Toxic effect of other alcohols, undetermined**
5 **T51.9** **Toxic effect of unspecified alcohol**
SP **7** **T51.91X-** **Toxic effect of unspecified alcohol, accidental (unintentional)**
SP **7** **T51.92X-** **Toxic effect of unspecified alcohol, intentional self-harm**
SP **7** **T51.93X-** **Toxic effect of unspecified alcohol, assault**
SP **7** **T51.94X-** **Toxic effect of unspecified alcohol, undetermined**

4 **T52**   **Toxic effect of organic solvents**
> **EXCLUDES 1**   halogen derivatives of aliphatic and aromatic hydrocarbons (T53.-)

> The appropriate 7th character is to be added to each code from category T52
> A   initial encounter
> D   subsequent encounter
> S   sequela

5 **T52.0** **Toxic effects of petroleum products**
Toxic effects of gasoline [petrol]
Toxic effects of kerosene [paraffin oil]
Toxic effects of paraffin wax
Toxic effects of ether petroleum
Toxic effects of naphtha petroleum

---

4 4th digit required   **5** 5th digit required   **6** 6th digit required   **7** 7th digit required   **7** 7th digit placeholder   **+** Additional code   **⊟** Laterality

Toxic effects of spirit petroleum

⑥ **T52.0X Toxic effects of petroleum products**

[SP] [7] **T52.0X1- Toxic effect of petroleum products, accidental (unintentional)**
Toxic effects of petroleum products NOS

[SP] [7] **T52.0X2- Toxic effect of petroleum products, intentional self-harm**

[SP] [7] **T52.0X3- Toxic effect of petroleum products, assault**

[SP] [7] **T52.0X4- Toxic effect of petroleum products, undetermined**

⑤ **T52.1 Toxic effects of benzene**
EXCLUDES 1 homologues of benzene (T52.2)
nitroderivatives and aminoderivatives of benzene and its homologues (T65.3)

⑥ **T52.1X Toxic effects of benzene**

[SP] [7] **T52.1X1- Toxic effect of benzene, accidental (unintentional)**
Toxic effects of benzene NOS

[SP] [7] **T52.1X2- Toxic effect of benzene, intentional self-harm**

[SP] [7] **T52.1X3- Toxic effect of benzene, assault**

[SP] [7] **T52.1X4- Toxic effect of benzene, undetermined**

⑤ **T52.2 Toxic effects of homologues of benzene**
Toxic effects of toluene [methylbenzene]
Toxic effects of xylene [dimethylbenzene]

⑥ **T52.2X Toxic effects of homologues of benzene**

[SP] [7] **T52.2X1- Toxic effect of homologues of benzene, accidental (unintentional)**
Toxic effects of homologues of benzene NOS

[SP] [7] **T52.2X2- Toxic effect of homologues of benzene, intentional self-harm**

[SP] [7] **T52.2X3- Toxic effect of homologues of benzene, assault**

[SP] [7] **T52.2X4- Toxic effect of homologues of benzene, undetermined**

⑤ **T52.3 Toxic effects of glycols**

⑥ **T52.3X Toxic effects of glycols**

[SP] [7] **T52.3X1- Toxic effect of glycols, accidental (unintentional)**
Toxic effects of glycols NOS

[SP] [7] **T52.3X2- Toxic effect of glycols, intentional self-harm**

[SP] [7] **T52.3X3- Toxic effect of glycols, assault**

[SP] [7] **T52.3X4- Toxic effect of glycols, undetermined**

⑤ **T52.4 Toxic effects of ketones**

⑥ **T52.4X Toxic effects of ketones**

[SP] [7] **T52.4X1- Toxic effect of ketones, accidental (unintentional)**
Toxic effects of ketones NOS

[SP] [7] **T52.4X2- Toxic effect of ketones, intentional self-harm**

[SP] [7] **T52.4X3- Toxic effect of ketones, assault**

[SP] [7] **T52.4X4- Toxic effect of ketones, undetermined**

⑤ **T52.8 Toxic effects of other organic solvents**

⑥ **T52.8X Toxic effects of other organic solvents**

[SP] [7] **T52.8X1- Toxic effect of other organic solvents, accidental (unintentional)**
Toxic effects of other organic solvents NOS

[SP] [7] **T52.8X2- Toxic effect of other organic solvents, intentional self-harm**

[SP] [7] **T52.8X3- Toxic effect of other organic solvents, assault**

[SP] [7] **T52.8X4- Toxic effect of other organic solvents, undetermined**

⑤ **T52.9 Toxic effects of unspecified organic solvent**

[SP] [☑] **T52.91X- Toxic effect of unspecified organic solvent, accidental (unintentional)**

[SP] [☑] **T52.92X- Toxic effect of unspecified organic solvent, intentional self-harm**

[SP] [☑] **T52.93X- Toxic effect of unspecified organic solvent, assault**

[SP] [☑] **T52.94X- Toxic effect of unspecified organic solvent, undetermined**

④ **T53 Toxic effect of halogen derivatives of aliphatic and aromatic hydrocarbons**

The appropriate 7th character is to be added to each code from category T53
A   initial encounter
D   subsequent encounter
S   sequela

⑤ **T53.0 Toxic effects of carbon tetrachloride**
Toxic effects of tetrachloromethane

⑥ **T53.0X Toxic effects of carbon tetrachloride**

[SP] [7] **T53.0X1- Toxic effect of carbon tetrachloride, accidental (unintentional)**
Toxic effects of carbon tetrachloride NOS

[SP] [7] **T53.0X2- Toxic effect of carbon tetrachloride, intentional self-harm**

[SP] [7] **T53.0X3- Toxic effect of carbon tetrachloride, assault**

[SP] [7] **T53.0X4- Toxic effect of carbon tetrachloride, undetermined**

⑤ **T53.1 Toxic effects of chloroform**
Toxic effects of trichloromethane

⑥ **T53.1X Toxic effects of chloroform**

[SP] [7] **T53.1X1- Toxic effect of chloroform, accidental (unintentional)**
Toxic effects of chloroform NOS

[SP] [7] **T53.1X2- Toxic effect of chloroform, intentional self-harm**

[SP] [7] **T53.1X3- Toxic effect of chloroform, assault**

[SP] [7] **T53.1X4- Toxic effect of chloroform, undetermined**

⑤ **T53.2 Toxic effects of trichloroethylene**
Toxic effects of trichloroethene

⑥ **T53.2X Toxic effects of trichloroethylene**

[SP] [7] **T53.2X1- Toxic effect of trichloroethylene, accidental (unintentional)**
Toxic effects of trichloroethylene NOS

[SP] [7] **T53.2X2- Toxic effect of trichloroethylene, intentional self-harm**

★ New ▲ Revised **Px** Primary **SP** PDGM Px **SL** Low CoM **SH** High CoM **IQ** Quest. Encounter **H** Hospice non-cancer Dx   Unspecified   **M** *Manifestation*

DecisionHealth's FY 2020 Complete Home Health ICD-10-CM Diagnosis Coding Manual

1703

SP 7 T53.2X3- Toxic effect of trichloroethylene, assault

SP 7 T53.2X4- Toxic effect of trichloroethylene, undetermined

5 T53.3 Toxic effects of tetrachloroethylene
Toxic effects of perchloroethylene
Toxic effect of tetrachloroethene

  6 T53.3X Toxic effects of tetrachloroethylene

SP 7 T53.3X1- Toxic effect of tetrachloroethylene, accidental (unintentional)
Toxic effects of tetrachloroethylene NOS

SP 7 T53.3X2- Toxic effect of tetrachloroethylene, intentional self-harm

SP 7 T53.3X3- Toxic effect of tetrachloroethylene, assault

SP 7 T53.3X4- Toxic effect of tetrachloroethylene, undetermined

5 T53.4 Toxic effects of dichloromethane
Toxic effects of methylene chloride

  6 T53.4X Toxic effects of dichloromethane

SP 7 T53.4X1- Toxic effect of dichloromethane, accidental (unintentional)
Toxic effects of dichloromethane NOS

SP 7 T53.4X2- Toxic effect of dichloromethane, intentional self-harm

SP 7 T53.4X3- Toxic effect of dichloromethane, assault

SP 7 T53.4X4- Toxic effect of dichloromethane, undetermined

5 T53.5 Toxic effects of chlorofluorocarbons

  6 T53.5X Toxic effects of chlorofluorocarbons

SP 7 T53.5X1- Toxic effect of chlorofluorocarbons, accidental (unintentional)
Toxic effects of chlorofluorocarbons NOS

SP 7 T53.5X2- Toxic effect of chlorofluorocarbons, intentional self-harm

SP 7 T53.5X3- Toxic effect of chlorofluorocarbons, assault

SP 7 T53.5X4- Toxic effect of chlorofluorocarbons, undetermined

5 T53.6 Toxic effects of other halogen derivatives of aliphatic hydrocarbons

  6 T53.6X Toxic effects of other halogen derivatives of aliphatic hydrocarbons

SP 7 T53.6X1- Toxic effect of other halogen derivatives of aliphatic hydrocarbons, accidental (unintentional)
Toxic effects of other halogen derivatives of aliphatic hydrocarbons NOS

SP 7 T53.6X2- Toxic effect of other halogen derivatives of aliphatic hydrocarbons, intentional self-harm

SP 7 T53.6X3- Toxic effect of other halogen derivatives of aliphatic hydrocarbons, assault

SP 7 T53.6X4- Toxic effect of other halogen derivatives of aliphatic hydrocarbons, undetermined

5 T53.7 Toxic effects of other halogen derivatives of aromatic hydrocarbons

  6 T53.7X Toxic effects of other halogen derivatives of aromatic hydrocarbons

SP 7 T53.7X1- Toxic effect of other halogen derivatives of aromatic hydrocarbons, accidental (unintentional)
Toxic effects of other halogen derivatives of aromatic hydrocarbons NOS

SP 7 T53.7X2- Toxic effect of other halogen derivatives of aromatic hydrocarbons, intentional self-harm

SP 7 T53.7X3- Toxic effect of other halogen derivatives of aromatic hydrocarbons, assault

SP 7 T53.7X4- Toxic effect of other halogen derivatives of aromatic hydrocarbons, undetermined

5 T53.9 Toxic effects of unspecified halogen derivatives of aliphatic and aromatic hydrocarbons

SP 7 T53.91X- Toxic effect of unspecified halogen derivatives of aliphatic and aromatic hydrocarbons, accidental (unintentional)

SP 7 T53.92X- Toxic effect of unspecified halogen derivatives of aliphatic and aromatic hydrocarbons, intentional self-harm

SP 7 T53.93X- Toxic effect of unspecified halogen derivatives of aliphatic and aromatic hydrocarbons, assault

SP 7 T53.94X- Toxic effect of unspecified halogen derivatives of aliphatic and aromatic hydrocarbons, undetermined

4 T54 Toxic effect of corrosive substances

> The appropriate 7th character is to be added to each code from category T54
> A   initial encounter
> D   subsequent encounter
> S   sequela

5 T54.0 Toxic effects of phenol and phenol homologues

  6 T54.0X Toxic effects of phenol and phenol homologues

SP 7 T54.0X1- Toxic effect of phenol and phenol homologues, accidental (unintentional)
Toxic effects of phenol and phenol homologues NOS

SP 7 T54.0X2- Toxic effect of phenol and phenol homologues, intentional self-harm

SP 7 T54.0X3- Toxic effect of phenol and phenol homologues, assault

SP 7 T54.0X4- Toxic effect of phenol and phenol homologues, undetermined

4 4th digit required   **5** 5th digit required   **6** 6th digit required   **7** 7th digit required   **7** 7th digit placeholder   **+** Additional code   **=** Laterality

1704   *DecisionHealth's* FY 2020 Complete Home Health ICD-10-CM Diagnosis Coding Manual

⑤ **T54.1** **Toxic effects of other corrosive organic compounds**

⑥ **T54.1X** **Toxic effects of other corrosive organic compounds**

SP ⑦ **T54.1X1-** **Toxic effect of other corrosive organic compounds, accidental (unintentional)**
Toxic effects of other corrosive organic compounds NOS

SP ⑦ **T54.1X2-** **Toxic effect of other corrosive organic compounds, intentional self-harm**

SP ⑦ **T54.1X3-** **Toxic effect of other corrosive organic compounds, assault**

SP ⑦ **T54.1X4-** **Toxic effect of other corrosive organic compounds, undetermined**

⑤ **T54.2** **Toxic effects of corrosive acids and acid-like substances**
Toxic effects of hydrochloric acid
Toxic effects of sulfuric acid

⑥ **T54.2X** **Toxic effects of corrosive acids and acid-like substances**

SP ⑦ **T54.2X1-** **Toxic effect of corrosive acids and acid-like substances, accidental (unintentional)**
Toxic effects of corrosive acids and acid-like substances NOS

SP ⑦ **T54.2X2-** **Toxic effect of corrosive acids and acid-like substances, intentional self-harm**

SP ⑦ **T54.2X3-** **Toxic effect of corrosive acids and acid-like substances, assault**

SP ⑦ **T54.2X4-** **Toxic effect of corrosive acids and acid-like substances, undetermined**

⑤ **T54.3** **Toxic effects of corrosive alkalis and alkali-like substances**
Toxic effects of potassium hydroxide
Toxic effects of sodium hydroxide

⑥ **T54.3X** **Toxic effects of corrosive alkalis and alkali-like substances**

SP ⑦ **T54.3X1-** **Toxic effect of corrosive alkalis and alkali-like substances, accidental (unintentional)**
Toxic effects of corrosive alkalis and alkali-like substances NOS

SP ⑦ **T54.3X2-** **Toxic effect of corrosive alkalis and alkali-like substances, intentional self-harm**

SP ⑦ **T54.3X3-** **Toxic effect of corrosive alkalis and alkali-like substances, assault**

SP ⑦ **T54.3X4-** **Toxic effect of corrosive alkalis and alkali-like substances, undetermined**

⑤ **T54.9** **Toxic effects of unspecified corrosive substance**

SP ⑦ **T54.91X-** **Toxic effect of unspecified corrosive substance, accidental (unintentional)**

SP ⑦ **T54.92X-** **Toxic effect of unspecified corrosive substance, intentional self-harm**

SP ⑦ **T54.93X-** **Toxic effect of unspecified corrosive substance, assault**

SP ⑦ **T54.94X-** **Toxic effect of unspecified corrosive substance, undetermined**

④ **T55** **Toxic effect of soaps and detergents**

The appropriate 7th character is to be added to each code from category T55
A   initial encounter
D   subsequent encounter
S   sequela

⑤ **T55.0** **Toxic effect of soaps**

⑥ **T55.0X** **Toxic effect of soaps**

SP ⑦ **T55.0X1-** **Toxic effect of soaps, accidental (unintentional)**
Toxic effect of soaps NOS

SP ⑦ **T55.0X2-** **Toxic effect of soaps, intentional self-harm**

SP ⑦ **T55.0X3-** **Toxic effect of soaps, assault**

SP ⑦ **T55.0X4-** **Toxic effect of soaps, undetermined**

⑤ **T55.1** **Toxic effect of detergents**

⑥ **T55.1X** **Toxic effect of detergents**

SP ⑦ **T55.1X1-** **Toxic effect of detergents, accidental (unintentional)**
Toxic effect of detergents NOS

SP ⑦ **T55.1X2-** **Toxic effect of detergents, intentional self-harm**

SP ⑦ **T55.1X3-** **Toxic effect of detergents, assault**

SP ⑦ **T55.1X4-** **Toxic effect of detergents, undetermined**

✚ ④ **T56** **Toxic effect of metals**

INCLUDES toxic effects of fumes and vapors of metals
toxic effects of metals from all sources, except medicinal substances

Use additional code to identify any retained metal foreign body, if applicable (Z18.0-, T18.1-)

EXCLUDES 1 arsenic and its compounds (T57.0)
manganese and its compounds (T57.2)

The appropriate 7th character is to be added to each code from category T56
A   initial encounter
D   subsequent encounter
S   sequela

✚ ⑤ **T56.0** **Toxic effects of lead and its compounds**

✚ ⑥ **T56.0X** **Toxic effects of lead and its compounds**

SP ✚ ⑦ **T56.0X1-** **Toxic effect of lead and its compounds, accidental (unintentional)**
Toxic effects of lead and its compounds NOS

SP ✚ ⑦ **T56.0X2-** **Toxic effect of lead and its compounds, intentional self-harm**

SP ✚ ⑦ **T56.0X3-** **Toxic effect of lead and its compounds, assault**

SP ✚ ⑦ **T56.0X4-** **Toxic effect of lead and its compounds, undetermined**

✚ ⑤ **T56.1** **Toxic effects of mercury and its compounds**

Chapter 19

S00-T88

★ New ▲ Revised Px Primary **SP** PDGM Px **SL** Low CoM **SH** High CoM **IQ** Quest. Encounter Ⓗ Hospice non-cancer Dx Unspecified **M** *Manifestation*

DecisionHealth's FY 2020 Complete Home Health ICD-10-CM Diagnosis Coding Manual
1705

☑6 T56.1X Toxic effects of mercury and its compounds

SP+☑7 T56.1X1- Toxic effect of mercury and its compounds, accidental (unintentional)
Toxic effects of mercury and its compounds NOS

SP+☑7 T56.1X2- Toxic effect of mercury and its compounds, intentional self-harm

SP+☑7 T56.1X3- Toxic effect of mercury and its compounds, assault

SP+☑7 T56.1X4- Toxic effect of mercury and its compounds, undetermined

+☑5 T56.2 Toxic effects of chromium and its compounds

+☑6 T56.2X Toxic effects of chromium and its compounds

SP+☑7 T56.2X1- Toxic effect of chromium and its compounds, accidental (unintentional)
Toxic effects of chromium and its compounds NOS

SP+☑7 T56.2X2- Toxic effect of chromium and its compounds, intentional self-harm

SP+☑7 T56.2X3- Toxic effect of chromium and its compounds, assault

SP+☑7 T56.2X4- Toxic effect of chromium and its compounds, undetermined

+☑5 T56.3 Toxic effects of cadmium and its compounds

+☑6 T56.3X Toxic effects of cadmium and its compounds

SP+☑7 T56.3X1- Toxic effect of cadmium and its compounds, accidental (unintentional)
Toxic effects of cadmium and its compounds NOS

SP+☑7 T56.3X2- Toxic effect of cadmium and its compounds, intentional self-harm

SP+☑7 T56.3X3- Toxic effect of cadmium and its compounds, assault

SP+☑7 T56.3X4- Toxic effect of cadmium and its compounds, undetermined

+☑5 T56.4 Toxic effects of copper and its compounds

+☑6 T56.4X Toxic effects of copper and its compounds

SP+☑7 T56.4X1- Toxic effect of copper and its compounds, accidental (unintentional)
Toxic effects of copper and its compounds NOS

SP+☑7 T56.4X2- Toxic effect of copper and its compounds, intentional self-harm

SP+☑7 T56.4X3- Toxic effect of copper and its compounds, assault

SP+☑7 T56.4X4- Toxic effect of copper and its compounds, undetermined

+☑5 T56.5 Toxic effects of zinc and its compounds

+☑6 T56.5X Toxic effects of zinc and its compounds

SP+☑7 T56.5X1- Toxic effect of zinc and its compounds, accidental (unintentional)

Toxic effects of zinc and its compounds NOS

SP+☑7 T56.5X2- Toxic effect of zinc and its compounds, intentional self-harm

SP+☑7 T56.5X3- Toxic effect of zinc and its compounds, assault

SP+☑7 T56.5X4- Toxic effect of zinc and its compounds, undetermined

+☑5 T56.6 Toxic effects of tin and its compounds

+☑6 T56.6X Toxic effects of tin and its compounds

SP+☑7 T56.6X1- Toxic effect of tin and its compounds, accidental (unintentional)
Toxic effects of tin and its compounds NOS

SP+☑7 T56.6X2- Toxic effect of tin and its compounds, intentional self-harm

SP+☑7 T56.6X3- Toxic effect of tin and its compounds, assault

SP+☑7 T56.6X4- Toxic effect of tin and its compounds, undetermined

+☑5 T56.7 Toxic effects of beryllium and its compounds

+☑6 T56.7X Toxic effects of beryllium and its compounds

SP+☑7 T56.7X1- Toxic effect of beryllium and its compounds, accidental (unintentional)
Toxic effects of beryllium and its compounds NOS

SP+☑7 T56.7X2- Toxic effect of beryllium and its compounds, intentional self-harm

SP+☑7 T56.7X3- Toxic effect of beryllium and its compounds, assault

SP+☑7 T56.7X4- Toxic effect of beryllium and its compounds, undetermined

+☑5 T56.8 Toxic effects of other metals

+☑6 T56.81 Toxic effect of thallium

SP+☑7 T56.811- Toxic effect of thallium, accidental (unintentional)
Toxic effect of thallium NOS

SP+☑7 T56.812- Toxic effect of thallium, intentional self-harm

SP+☑7 T56.813- Toxic effect of thallium, assault

SP+☑7 T56.814- Toxic effect of thallium, undetermined

+☑6 T56.89 Toxic effects of other metals

SP+☑7 T56.891- Toxic effect of other metals, accidental (unintentional)
Toxic effects of other metals NOS

SP+☑7 T56.892- Toxic effect of other metals, intentional self-harm

SP+☑7 T56.893- Toxic effect of other metals, assault

SP+☑7 T56.894- Toxic effect of other metals, undetermined

+☑5 T56.9 Toxic effects of unspecified metal

SP+☑ T56.91X- Toxic effect of unspecified metal, accidental (unintentional)

SP+☑ T56.92X- Toxic effect of unspecified metal, intentional self-harm

---

☑4th digit required   ☑5th digit required   ☑6th digit required   ☑7th digit required   ☑7th digit placeholder   +Additional code   ☑Laterality

SP ✛ ☑ T56.93X- Toxic effect of unspecified metal, assault

SP ✛ ☑ T56.94X- Toxic effect of unspecified metal, undetermined

④ T57 Toxic effect of other inorganic substances

> The appropriate 7th character is to be added to each code from category T57
> A   initial encounter
> D   subsequent encounter
> S   sequela

⑤ T57.0 Toxic effect of arsenic and its compounds

⑥ T57.0X Toxic effect of arsenic and its compounds

SP ☑ T57.0X1- Toxic effect of arsenic and its compounds, accidental (unintentional)
Toxic effect of arsenic and its compounds NOS

SP ☑ T57.0X2- Toxic effect of arsenic and its compounds, intentional self-harm

SP ☑ T57.0X3- Toxic effect of arsenic and its compounds, assault

SP ☑ T57.0X4- Toxic effect of arsenic and its compounds, undetermined

⑤ T57.1 Toxic effect of phosphorus and its compounds
EXCLUDES 1   organophosphate insecticides (T60.0)

⑥ T57.1X Toxic effect of phosphorus and its compounds

SP ☑ T57.1X1- Toxic effect of phosphorus and its compounds, accidental (unintentional)
Toxic effect of phosphorus and its compounds NOS

SP ☑ T57.1X2- Toxic effect of phosphorus and its compounds, intentional self-harm

SP ☑ T57.1X3- Toxic effect of phosphorus and its compounds, assault

SP ☑ T57.1X4- Toxic effect of phosphorus and its compounds, undetermined

⑤ T57.2 Toxic effect of manganese and its compounds

⑥ T57.2X Toxic effect of manganese and its compounds

SP ☑ T57.2X1- Toxic effect of manganese and its compounds, accidental (unintentional)
Toxic effect of manganese and its compounds NOS

SP ☑ T57.2X2- Toxic effect of manganese and its compounds, intentional self-harm

SP ☑ T57.2X3- Toxic effect of manganese and its compounds, assault

SP ☑ T57.2X4- Toxic effect of manganese and its compounds, undetermined

⑤ T57.3 Toxic effect of hydrogen cyanide

⑥ T57.3X Toxic effect of hydrogen cyanide

SP ☑ T57.3X1- Toxic effect of hydrogen cyanide, accidental (unintentional)
Toxic effect of hydrogen cyanide NOS

SP ☑ T57.3X2- Toxic effect of hydrogen cyanide, intentional self-harm

SP ☑ T57.3X3- Toxic effect of hydrogen cyanide, assault

SP ☑ T57.3X4- Toxic effect of hydrogen cyanide, undetermined

⑤ T57.8 Toxic effect of other specified inorganic substances

⑥ T57.8X Toxic effect of other specified inorganic substances

SP ☑ T57.8X1- Toxic effect of other specified inorganic substances, accidental (unintentional)
Toxic effect of other specified inorganic substances NOS

SP ☑ T57.8X2- Toxic effect of other specified inorganic substances, intentional self-harm

SP ☑ T57.8X3- Toxic effect of other specified inorganic substances, assault

SP ☑ T57.8X4- Toxic effect of other specified inorganic substances, undetermined

⑤ T57.9 Toxic effect of unspecified inorganic substance

SP ☑ T57.91X- Toxic effect of unspecified inorganic substance, accidental (unintentional)

SP ☑ T57.92X- Toxic effect of unspecified inorganic substance, intentional self-harm

SP ☑ T57.93X- Toxic effect of unspecified inorganic substance, assault

SP ☑ T57.94X- Toxic effect of unspecified inorganic substance, undetermined

④ T58 Toxic effect of carbon monoxide
INCLUDES   asphyxiation from carbon monoxide
toxic effect of carbon monoxide from all sources

> The appropriate 7th character is to be added to each code from category T58
> A   initial encounter
> D   subsequent encounter
> S   sequela

⑤ T58.0 Toxic effect of carbon monoxide from motor vehicle exhaust
Toxic effect of exhaust gas from gas engine
Toxic effect of exhaust gas from motor pump

SP ☑ T58.01X- Toxic effect of carbon monoxide from motor vehicle exhaust, accidental (unintentional)

SP ☑ T58.02X- Toxic effect of carbon monoxide from motor vehicle exhaust, intentional self-harm

SP ☑ T58.03X- Toxic effect of carbon monoxide from motor vehicle exhaust, assault

SP ☑ T58.04X- Toxic effect of carbon monoxide from motor vehicle exhaust, undetermined

⑤ T58.1 Toxic effect of carbon monoxide from utility gas
Toxic effect of acetylene

★ New ▲ Revised Px Primary SP PDGM Px SL Low CoM SH High CoM IQ Quest. Encounter H Hospice non-cancer Dx Unspecified M *Manifestation*

DecisionHealth's FY 2020 Complete Home Health ICD-10-CM Diagnosis Coding Manual   1707

Chapter 19

S00-T88

Toxic effect of gas NOS used for lighting,
    heating, cooking
Toxic effect of water gas

SP ☑ **T58.11X-** Toxic effect of carbon monoxide
from utility gas, accidental
(unintentional)

SP ☑ **T58.12X-** Toxic effect of carbon monoxide
from utility gas, intentional self-
harm

SP ☑ **T58.13X-** Toxic effect of carbon monoxide
from utility gas, assault

SP ☑ **T58.14X-** Toxic effect of carbon monoxide
from utility gas, undetermined

⑤ **T58.2** Toxic effect of carbon monoxide from
incomplete combustion of other
domestic fuels

Toxic effect of carbon monoxide from
incomplete combustion of coal, coke,
kerosene, wood

⑥ **T58.2X** Toxic effect of carbon monoxide
from incomplete combustion of other
domestic fuels

SP ☑ **T58.2X1-** Toxic effect of carbon monoxide
from incomplete combustion of
other domestic fuels, accidental
(unintentional)

SP ☑ **T58.2X2-** Toxic effect of carbon monoxide
from incomplete combustion of
other domestic fuels, intentional
self-harm

SP ☑ **T58.2X3-** Toxic effect of carbon monoxide
from incomplete combustion of
other domestic fuels, assault

SP ☑ **T58.2X4-** Toxic effect of carbon monoxide
from incomplete combustion of
other domestic fuels,
undetermined

⑤ **T58.8** Toxic effect of carbon monoxide from
other source

Toxic effect of carbon monoxide from
blast furnace gas
Toxic effect of carbon monoxide from
fuels in industrial use
Toxic effect of carbon monoxide from kiln
vapor

⑥ **T58.8X** Toxic effect of carbon monoxide
from other source

SP ☑ **T58.8X1-** Toxic effect of carbon monoxide
from other source, accidental
(unintentional)

SP ☑ **T58.8X2-** Toxic effect of carbon monoxide
from other source, intentional
self-harm

SP ☑ **T58.8X3-** Toxic effect of carbon monoxide
from other source, assault

SP ☑ **T58.8X4-** Toxic effect of carbon monoxide
from other source, undetermined

⑤ **T58.9** Toxic effect of carbon monoxide from
unspecified source

SP ☑ **T58.91X-** Toxic effect of carbon monoxide
from unspecified source,
accidental (unintentional)

SP ☑ **T58.92X-** Toxic effect of carbon monoxide
from unspecified source,
intentional self-harm

SP ☑ **T58.93X-** Toxic effect of carbon monoxide
from unspecified source, assault

SP ☑ **T58.94X-** Toxic effect of carbon monoxide
from unspecified source,
undetermined

④ **T59** Toxic effect of other gases, fumes and
vapors

| INCLUDES | aerosol propellants |

| EXCLUDES 1 | chlorofluorocarbons (T53.5) |

The appropriate 7th character is to be added to
each code from category T59
A   initial encounter
D   subsequent encounter
S   sequela

⑤ **T59.0** Toxic effect of nitrogen oxides

⑥ **T59.0X** Toxic effect of nitrogen oxides

SP ☑ **T59.0X1-** Toxic effect of nitrogen oxides,
accidental (unintentional)
Toxic effect of nitrogen oxides
NOS

SP ☑ **T59.0X2-** Toxic effect of nitrogen oxides,
intentional self-harm

SP ☑ **T59.0X3-** Toxic effect of nitrogen oxides,
assault

SP ☑ **T59.0X4-** Toxic effect of nitrogen oxides,
undetermined

⑤ **T59.1** Toxic effect of sulfur dioxide

⑥ **T59.1X** Toxic effect of sulfur dioxide

SP ☑ **T59.1X1-** Toxic effect of sulfur dioxide,
accidental (unintentional)
Toxic effect of sulfur dioxide NOS

SP ☑ **T59.1X2-** Toxic effect of sulfur dioxide,
intentional self-harm

SP ☑ **T59.1X3-** Toxic effect of sulfur dioxide,
assault

SP ☑ **T59.1X4-** Toxic effect of sulfur dioxide,
undetermined

⑤ **T59.2** Toxic effect of formaldehyde

⑥ **T59.2X** Toxic effect of formaldehyde

SP ☑ **T59.2X1-** Toxic effect of formaldehyde,
accidental (unintentional)
Toxic effect of formaldehyde NOS

SP ☑ **T59.2X2-** Toxic effect of formaldehyde,
intentional self-harm

SP ☑ **T59.2X3-** Toxic effect of formaldehyde,
assault

SP ☑ **T59.2X4-** Toxic effect of formaldehyde,
undetermined

⑤ **T59.3** Toxic effect of lacrimogenic gas
Toxic effect of tear gas

⑥ **T59.3X** Toxic effect of lacrimogenic gas

SP ☑ **T59.3X1-** Toxic effect of lacrimogenic gas,
accidental (unintentional)
Toxic effect of lacrimogenic gas
NOS

SP ☑ **T59.3X2-** Toxic effect of lacrimogenic gas,
intentional self-harm

SP ☑ **T59.3X3-** Toxic effect of lacrimogenic gas,
assault

SP ☑ **T59.3X4-** Toxic effect of lacrimogenic gas,
undetermined

⑤ **T59.4** Toxic effect of chlorine gas

⑥ **T59.4X** Toxic effect of chlorine gas

SP ☑ **T59.4X1-** Toxic effect of chlorine gas,
accidental (unintentional)
Toxic effect of chlorine gas NOS

④4th digit required   ⑤5th digit required   ⑥6th digit required   ☑7th digit required   ☑ 7th digit placeholder   ✚Additional code   ▤Laterality

1708   *DecisionHealth's* FY 2020 Complete Home Health ICD-10-CM Diagnosis Coding Manual

SP 7 T59.4X2- Toxic effect of chlorine gas, intentional self-harm

SP 7 T59.4X3- Toxic effect of chlorine gas, assault

SP 7 T59.4X4- Toxic effect of chlorine gas, undetermined

5 T59.5 Toxic effect of fluorine gas and hydrogen fluoride

6 T59.5X Toxic effect of fluorine gas and hydrogen fluoride

SP 7 T59.5X1- Toxic effect of fluorine gas and hydrogen fluoride, accidental (unintentional)
Toxic effect of fluorine gas and hydrogen fluoride NOS

SP 7 T59.5X2- Toxic effect of fluorine gas and hydrogen fluoride, intentional self-harm

SP 7 T59.5X3- Toxic effect of fluorine gas and hydrogen fluoride, assault

SP 7 T59.5X4- Toxic effect of fluorine gas and hydrogen fluoride, undetermined

5 T59.6 Toxic effect of hydrogen sulfide

6 T59.6X Toxic effect of hydrogen sulfide

SP 7 T59.6X1- Toxic effect of hydrogen sulfide, accidental (unintentional)
Toxic effect of hydrogen sulfide NOS

SP 7 T59.6X2- Toxic effect of hydrogen sulfide, intentional self-harm

SP 7 T59.6X3- Toxic effect of hydrogen sulfide, assault

SP 7 T59.6X4- Toxic effect of hydrogen sulfide, undetermined

5 T59.7 Toxic effect of carbon dioxide

6 T59.7X Toxic effect of carbon dioxide

SP 7 T59.7X1- Toxic effect of carbon dioxide, accidental (unintentional)
Toxic effect of carbon dioxide NOS

SP 7 T59.7X2- Toxic effect of carbon dioxide, intentional self-harm

SP 7 T59.7X3- Toxic effect of carbon dioxide, assault

SP 7 T59.7X4- Toxic effect of carbon dioxide, undetermined

5 T59.8 Toxic effect of other specified gases, fumes and vapors

6 T59.81 Toxic effect of smoke
Smoke inhalation
EXCLUDES 2 toxic effect of cigarette (tobacco) smoke (T65.22-)

SP 7 T59.811- Toxic effect of smoke, accidental (unintentional)
Toxic effect of smoke NOS

SP 7 T59.812- Toxic effect of smoke, intentional self-harm

SP 7 T59.813- Toxic effect of smoke, assault

SP 7 T59.814- Toxic effect of smoke, undetermined

6 T59.89 Toxic effect of other specified gases, fumes and vapors

SP 7 T59.891- Toxic effect of other specified gases, fumes and vapors, accidental (unintentional)

SP 7 T59.892- Toxic effect of other specified gases, fumes and vapors, intentional self-harm

SP 7 T59.893- Toxic effect of other specified gases, fumes and vapors, assault

SP 7 T59.894- Toxic effect of other specified gases, fumes and vapors, undetermined

5 T59.9 Toxic effect of unspecified gases, fumes and vapors

SP 7 T59.91X- Toxic effect of unspecified gases, fumes and vapors, accidental (unintentional)

SP 7 T59.92X- Toxic effect of unspecified gases, fumes and vapors, intentional self-harm

SP 7 T59.93X- Toxic effect of unspecified gases, fumes and vapors, assault

SP 7 T59.94X- Toxic effect of unspecified gases, fumes and vapors, undetermined

4 T60 Toxic effect of pesticides
INCLUDES toxic effect of wood preservatives

The appropriate 7th character is to be added to each code from category T60
A   initial encounter
D   subsequent encounter
S   sequela

5 T60.0 Toxic effect of organophosphate and carbamate insecticides

6 T60.0X Toxic effect of organophosphate and carbamate insecticides

SP 7 T60.0X1- Toxic effect of organophosphate and carbamate insecticides, accidental (unintentional)
Toxic effect of organophosphate and carbamate insecticides NOS

SP 7 T60.0X2- Toxic effect of organophosphate and carbamate insecticides, intentional self-harm

SP 7 T60.0X3- Toxic effect of organophosphate and carbamate insecticides, assault

SP 7 T60.0X4- Toxic effect of organophosphate and carbamate insecticides, undetermined

5 T60.1 Toxic effect of halogenated insecticides
EXCLUDES 1 chlorinated hydrocarbon (T53.-)

6 T60.1X Toxic effect of halogenated insecticides

SP 7 T60.1X1- Toxic effect of halogenated insecticides, accidental (unintentional)
Toxic effect of halogenated insecticides NOS

SP 7 T60.1X2- Toxic effect of halogenated insecticides, intentional self-harm

SP 7 T60.1X3- Toxic effect of halogenated insecticides, assault

SP 7 T60.1X4- Toxic effect of halogenated insecticides, undetermined

5 T60.2 Toxic effect of other insecticides

6 T60.2X Toxic effect of other insecticides

★ New ▲ Revised Px Primary SP PDGM Px SL Low CoM SH High CoM IQ Quest. Encounter H Hospice non-cancer Dx Unspecified M *Manifestation*

DecisionHealth's FY 2020 Complete Home Health ICD-10-CM Diagnosis Coding Manual

1709

SP 7 T60.2X1- **Toxic effect of other insecticides, accidental (unintentional)**
Toxic effect of other insecticides NOS

SP 7 T60.2X2- **Toxic effect of other insecticides, intentional self-harm**

SP 7 T60.2X3- **Toxic effect of other insecticides, assault**

SP 7 T60.2X4- **Toxic effect of other insecticides, undetermined**

5 T60.3 Toxic effect of herbicides and fungicides

6 T60.3X Toxic effect of herbicides and fungicides

SP 7 T60.3X1- **Toxic effect of herbicides and fungicides, accidental (unintentional)**
Toxic effect of herbicides and fungicides NOS

SP 7 T60.3X2- **Toxic effect of herbicides and fungicides, intentional self-harm**

SP 7 T60.3X3- **Toxic effect of herbicides and fungicides, assault**

SP 7 T60.3X4- **Toxic effect of herbicides and fungicides, undetermined**

5 T60.4 Toxic effect of rodenticides
EXCLUDES 1 strychnine and its salts (T65.1)
thallium (T56.81-)

6 T60.4X Toxic effect of rodenticides

SP 7 T60.4X1- **Toxic effect of rodenticides, accidental (unintentional)**
Toxic effect of rodenticides NOS

SP 7 T60.4X2- **Toxic effect of rodenticides, intentional self-harm**

SP 7 T60.4X3- **Toxic effect of rodenticides, assault**

SP 7 T60.4X4- **Toxic effect of rodenticides, undetermined**

5 T60.8 Toxic effect of other pesticides

6 T60.8X Toxic effect of other pesticides

SP 7 T60.8X1- **Toxic effect of other pesticides, accidental (unintentional)**
Toxic effect of other pesticides NOS

SP 7 T60.8X2- **Toxic effect of other pesticides, intentional self-harm**

SP 7 T60.8X3- **Toxic effect of other pesticides, assault**

SP 7 T60.8X4- **Toxic effect of other pesticides, undetermined**

5 T60.9 Toxic effect of unspecified pesticide

SP 7 T60.91X- **Toxic effect of unspecified pesticide, accidental (unintentional)**

SP 7 T60.92X- **Toxic effect of unspecified pesticide, intentional self-harm**

SP 7 T60.93X- **Toxic effect of unspecified pesticide, assault**

SP 7 T60.94X- **Toxic effect of unspecified pesticide, undetermined**

4 T61 Toxic effect of noxious substances eaten as seafood
EXCLUDES 1 allergic reaction to food, such as:

anaphylactic reaction or shock due to adverse food reaction (T78.0-)
bacterial foodborne intoxications (A05.-)
dermatitis (L23.6, L25.4, L27.2)
food protein-induced enterocolitis syndrome (K52.21)
food protein-induced enteropathy (K52.22)
gastroenteritis (noninfective) (K52.29)
toxic effect of aflatoxin and other mycotoxins (T64)
toxic effect of cyanides (T65.0-)
toxic effect of harmful algae bloom (T65.82-)
toxic effect of hydrogen cyanide (T57.3-)
toxic effect of mercury (T56.1-)
toxic effect of red tide (T65.82-)

The appropriate 7th character is to be added to each code from category T61
A   initial encounter
D   subsequent encounter
S   sequela

5 T61.0 Ciguatera fish poisoning

SP 7 T61.01X- **Ciguatera fish poisoning, accidental (unintentional)**

SP 7 T61.02X- **Ciguatera fish poisoning, intentional self-harm**

SP 7 T61.03X- **Ciguatera fish poisoning, assault**

SP 7 T61.04X- **Ciguatera fish poisoning, undetermined**

5 T61.1 Scombroid fish poisoning
Histamine-like syndrome

SP 7 T61.11X- **Scombroid fish poisoning, accidental (unintentional)**

SP 7 T61.12X- **Scombroid fish poisoning, intentional self-harm**

SP 7 T61.13X- **Scombroid fish poisoning, assault**

SP 7 T61.14X- **Scombroid fish poisoning, undetermined**

5 T61.7 Other fish and shellfish poisoning

6 T61.77 Other fish poisoning

SP 7 T61.771- **Other fish poisoning, accidental (unintentional)**

SP 7 T61.772- **Other fish poisoning, intentional self-harm**

SP 7 T61.773- **Other fish poisoning, assault**

SP 7 T61.774- **Other fish poisoning, undetermined**

6 T61.78 Other shellfish poisoning

SP 7 T61.781- **Other shellfish poisoning, accidental (unintentional)**

SP 7 T61.782- **Other shellfish poisoning, intentional self-harm**

SP 7 T61.783- **Other shellfish poisoning, assault**

SP 7 T61.784- **Other shellfish poisoning, undetermined**

---

4 4th digit required   5 5th digit required   6 6th digit required   7 7th digit required   ☑ 7th digit placeholder   ✚ Additional code   ▱ Laterality

⑤ **T61.8** Toxic effect of other seafood

⑥ **T61.8X** Toxic effect of other seafood

SP ⑦ **T61.8X1-** Toxic effect of other seafood, accidental (unintentional)

SP ⑦ **T61.8X2-** Toxic effect of other seafood, intentional self-harm

SP ⑦ **T61.8X3-** Toxic effect of other seafood, assault

SP ⑦ **T61.8X4-** Toxic effect of other seafood, undetermined

⑤ **T61.9** Toxic effect of unspecified seafood

SP ⑦ **T61.91X-** Toxic effect of unspecified seafood, accidental (unintentional)

SP ⑦ **T61.92X-** Toxic effect of unspecified seafood, intentional self-harm

SP ⑦ **T61.93X-** Toxic effect of unspecified seafood, assault

SP ⑦ **T61.94X-** Toxic effect of unspecified seafood, undetermined

④ **T62** Toxic effect of other noxious substances eaten as food

> **EXCLUDES 1** allergic reaction to food, such as:
> anaphylactic shock (reaction) due to adverse food reaction (T78.0-)
> bacterial food borne intoxications (A05.-)
> dermatitis (L23.6, L25.4, L27.2)
> food protein-induced enterocolitis syndrome (K52.21)
> food protein-induced enteropathy (K52.22)
> gastroenteritis (noninfective) (K52.29)
> toxic effect of aflatoxin and other mycotoxins (T64)
> toxic effect of cyanides (T65.0-)
> toxic effect of hydrogen cyanide (T57.3-)
> toxic effect of mercury (T56.1-)

> The appropriate 7th character is to be added to each code from category T62
> A   initial encounter
> D   subsequent encounter
> S   sequela

⑤ **T62.0** Toxic effect of ingested mushrooms

⑥ **T62.0X** Toxic effect of ingested mushrooms

SP ⑦ **T62.0X1-** Toxic effect of ingested mushrooms, accidental (unintentional)
Toxic effect of ingested mushrooms NOS

SP ⑦ **T62.0X2-** Toxic effect of ingested mushrooms, intentional self-harm

SP ⑦ **T62.0X3-** Toxic effect of ingested mushrooms, assault

SP ⑦ **T62.0X4-** Toxic effect of ingested mushrooms, undetermined

⑤ **T62.1** Toxic effect of ingested berries

⑥ **T62.1X** Toxic effect of ingested berries

SP ⑦ **T62.1X1-** Toxic effect of ingested berries, accidental (unintentional)
Toxic effect of ingested berries NOS

SP ⑦ **T62.1X2-** Toxic effect of ingested berries, intentional self-harm

SP ⑦ **T62.1X3-** Toxic effect of ingested berries, assault

SP ⑦ **T62.1X4-** Toxic effect of ingested berries, undetermined

⑤ **T62.2** Toxic effect of other ingested (parts of) plant(s)

⑥ **T62.2X** Toxic effect of other ingested (parts of) plant(s)

SP ⑦ **T62.2X1-** Toxic effect of other ingested (parts of) plant(s), accidental (unintentional)
Toxic effect of other ingested (parts of) plant(s) NOS

SP ⑦ **T62.2X2-** Toxic effect of other ingested (parts of) plant(s), intentional self-harm

SP ⑦ **T62.2X3-** Toxic effect of other ingested (parts of) plant(s), assault

SP ⑦ **T62.2X4-** Toxic effect of other ingested (parts of) plant(s), undetermined

⑤ **T62.8** Toxic effect of other specified noxious substances eaten as food

⑥ **T62.8X** Toxic effect of other specified noxious substances eaten as food

SP ⑦ **T62.8X1-** Toxic effect of other specified noxious substances eaten as food, accidental (unintentional)
Toxic effect of other specified noxious substances eaten as food NOS

SP ⑦ **T62.8X2-** Toxic effect of other specified noxious substances eaten as food, intentional self-harm

SP ⑦ **T62.8X3-** Toxic effect of other specified noxious substances eaten as food, assault

SP ⑦ **T62.8X4-** Toxic effect of other specified noxious substances eaten as food, undetermined

⑤ **T62.9** Toxic effect of unspecified noxious substance eaten as food

SP ⑦ **T62.91X-** Toxic effect of unspecified noxious substance eaten as food, accidental (unintentional)
Toxic effect of unspecified noxious substance eaten as food NOS

SP ⑦ **T62.92X-** Toxic effect of unspecified noxious substance eaten as food, intentional self-harm

SP ⑦ **T62.93X-** Toxic effect of unspecified noxious substance eaten as food, assault

SP ⑦ **T62.94X-** Toxic effect of unspecified noxious substance eaten as food, undetermined

④ **T63** Toxic effect of contact with venomous animals and plants

> **INCLUDES** bite or touch of venomous animal
> pricked or stuck by thorn or leaf

★ New ▲ Revised Px Primary **SP** PDGM Px **SL** Low CoM **SH** High CoM **IQ** Quest. Encounter Ⓗ Hospice non-cancer Dx Unspecified **M** *Manifestation*

DecisionHealth's FY 2020 Complete Home Health ICD-10-CM Diagnosis Coding Manual
1711

EXCLUDES 2   ingestion of toxic animal or plant (T61.-, T62.-)

The appropriate 7th character is to be added to each code from category T63
A   initial encounter
D   subsequent encounter
S   sequela

⑤ **T63.0 Toxic effect of snake venom**

⑥ **T63.00 Toxic effect of unspecified snake venom**

SP ⑦ T63.001- **Toxic effect of unspecified snake venom, accidental (unintentional)**
Toxic effect of unspecified snake venom NOS

SP ⑦ T63.002- **Toxic effect of unspecified snake venom, intentional self-harm**

SP ⑦ T63.003- **Toxic effect of unspecified snake venom, assault**

SP ⑦ T63.004- **Toxic effect of unspecified snake venom, undetermined**

⑥ **T63.01 Toxic effect of rattlesnake venom**

SP ⑦ T63.011- **Toxic effect of rattlesnake venom, accidental (unintentional)**
Toxic effect of rattlesnake venom NOS

SP ⑦ T63.012- **Toxic effect of rattlesnake venom, intentional self-harm**

SP ⑦ T63.013- **Toxic effect of rattlesnake venom, assault**

SP ⑦ T63.014- **Toxic effect of rattlesnake venom, undetermined**

⑥ **T63.02 Toxic effect of coral snake venom**

SP ⑦ T63.021- **Toxic effect of coral snake venom, accidental (unintentional)**
Toxic effect of coral snake venom NOS

SP ⑦ T63.022- **Toxic effect of coral snake venom, intentional self-harm**

SP ⑦ T63.023- **Toxic effect of coral snake venom, assault**

SP ⑦ T63.024- **Toxic effect of coral snake venom, undetermined**

⑥ **T63.03 Toxic effect of taipan venom**

SP ⑦ T63.031- **Toxic effect of taipan venom, accidental (unintentional)**
Toxic effect of taipan venom NOS

SP ⑦ T63.032- **Toxic effect of taipan venom, intentional self-harm**

SP ⑦ T63.033- **Toxic effect of taipan venom, assault**

SP ⑦ T63.034- **Toxic effect of taipan venom, undetermined**

⑥ **T63.04 Toxic effect of cobra venom**

SP ⑦ T63.041- **Toxic effect of cobra venom, accidental (unintentional)**
Toxic effect of cobra venom NOS

SP ⑦ T63.042- **Toxic effect of cobra venom, intentional self-harm**

SP ⑦ T63.043- **Toxic effect of cobra venom, assault**

SP ⑦ T63.044- **Toxic effect of cobra venom, undetermined**

⑥ **T63.06 Toxic effect of venom of other North and South American snake**

SP ⑦ T63.061- **Toxic effect of venom of other North and South American snake, accidental (unintentional)**
Toxic effect of venom of other North and South American snake NOS

SP ⑦ T63.062- **Toxic effect of venom of other North and South American snake, intentional self-harm**

SP ⑦ T63.063- **Toxic effect of venom of other North and South American snake, assault**

SP ⑦ T63.064- **Toxic effect of venom of other North and South American snake, undetermined**

⑥ **T63.07 Toxic effect of venom of other Australian snake**

SP ⑦ T63.071- **Toxic effect of venom of other Australian snake, accidental (unintentional)**
Toxic effect of venom of other Australian snake NOS

SP ⑦ T63.072- **Toxic effect of venom of other Australian snake, intentional self-harm**

SP ⑦ T63.073- **Toxic effect of venom of other Australian snake, assault**

SP ⑦ T63.074- **Toxic effect of venom of other Australian snake, undetermined**

⑥ **T63.08 Toxic effect of venom of other African and Asian snake**

SP ⑦ T63.081- **Toxic effect of venom of other African and Asian snake, accidental (unintentional)**
Toxic effect of venom of other African and Asian snake NOS

SP ⑦ T63.082- **Toxic effect of venom of other African and Asian snake, intentional self-harm**

SP ⑦ T63.083- **Toxic effect of venom of other African and Asian snake, assault**

SP ⑦ T63.084- **Toxic effect of venom of other African and Asian snake, undetermined**

⑥ **T63.09 Toxic effect of venom of other snake**

SP ⑦ T63.091- **Toxic effect of venom of other snake, accidental (unintentional)**
Toxic effect of venom of other snake NOS

SP ⑦ T63.092- **Toxic effect of venom of other snake, intentional self-harm**

SP ⑦ T63.093- **Toxic effect of venom of other snake, assault**

SP ⑦ T63.094- **Toxic effect of venom of other snake, undetermined**

⑤ **T63.1 Toxic effect of venom of other reptiles**

⑥ **T63.11 Toxic effect of venom of gila monster**

SP ⑦ T63.111- **Toxic effect of venom of gila monster, accidental (unintentional)**
Toxic effect of venom of gila monster NOS

SP ⑦ T63.112- **Toxic effect of venom of gila monster, intentional self-harm**

SP ⑦ T63.113- **Toxic effect of venom of gila monster, assault**

---

④4th digit required   ⑤5th digit required   ⑥6th digit required   ⑦7th digit required   ⑦7th digit placeholder   ✚Additional code   ▱Laterality

1712   *DecisionHealth's* FY 2020 Complete Home Health ICD-10-CM Diagnosis Coding Manual

SP 7 T63.114- Toxic effect of venom of gila monster, undetermined

6 T63.12 Toxic effect of venom of other venomous lizard

SP 7 T63.121- Toxic effect of venom of other venomous lizard, accidental (unintentional)
Toxic effect of venom of other venomous lizard NOS

SP 7 T63.122- Toxic effect of venom of other venomous lizard, intentional self-harm

SP 7 T63.123- Toxic effect of venom of other venomous lizard, assault

SP 7 T63.124- Toxic effect of venom of other venomous lizard, undetermined

6 T63.19 Toxic effect of venom of other reptiles

SP 7 T63.191- Toxic effect of venom of other reptiles, accidental (unintentional)
Toxic effect of venom of other reptiles NOS

SP 7 T63.192- Toxic effect of venom of other reptiles, intentional self-harm

SP 7 T63.193- Toxic effect of venom of other reptiles, assault

SP 7 T63.194- Toxic effect of venom of other reptiles, undetermined

5 T63.2 Toxic effect of venom of scorpion

6 T63.2X Toxic effect of venom of scorpion

SP 7 T63.2X1- Toxic effect of venom of scorpion, accidental (unintentional)
Toxic effect of venom of scorpion NOS

SP 7 T63.2X2- Toxic effect of venom of scorpion, intentional self-harm

SP 7 T63.2X3- Toxic effect of venom of scorpion, assault

SP 7 T63.2X4- Toxic effect of venom of scorpion, undetermined

5 T63.3 Toxic effect of venom of spider

6 T63.30 Toxic effect of unspecified spider venom

SP 7 T63.301- Toxic effect of unspecified spider venom, accidental (unintentional)

SP 7 T63.302- Toxic effect of unspecified spider venom, intentional self-harm

SP 7 T63.303- Toxic effect of unspecified spider venom, assault

SP 7 T63.304- Toxic effect of unspecified spider venom, undetermined

6 T63.31 Toxic effect of venom of black widow spider

SP 7 T63.311- Toxic effect of venom of black widow spider, accidental (unintentional)

SP 7 T63.312- Toxic effect of venom of black widow spider, intentional self-harm

SP 7 T63.313- Toxic effect of venom of black widow spider, assault

SP 7 T63.314- Toxic effect of venom of black widow spider, undetermined

6 T63.32 Toxic effect of venom of tarantula

SP 7 T63.321- Toxic effect of venom of tarantula, accidental (unintentional)

SP 7 T63.322- Toxic effect of venom of tarantula, intentional self-harm

SP 7 T63.323- Toxic effect of venom of tarantula, assault

SP 7 T63.324- Toxic effect of venom of tarantula, undetermined

6 T63.33 Toxic effect of venom of brown recluse spider

SP 7 T63.331- Toxic effect of venom of brown recluse spider, accidental (unintentional)

SP 7 T63.332- Toxic effect of venom of brown recluse spider, intentional self-harm

SP 7 T63.333- Toxic effect of venom of brown recluse spider, assault

SP 7 T63.334- Toxic effect of venom of brown recluse spider, undetermined

6 T63.39 Toxic effect of venom of other spider

SP 7 T63.391- Toxic effect of venom of other spider, accidental (unintentional)

SP 7 T63.392- Toxic effect of venom of other spider, intentional self-harm

SP 7 T63.393- Toxic effect of venom of other spider, assault

SP 7 T63.394- Toxic effect of venom of other spider, undetermined

5 T63.4 Toxic effect of venom of other arthropods

6 T63.41 Toxic effect of venom of centipedes and venomous millipedes

SP 7 T63.411- Toxic effect of venom of centipedes and venomous millipedes, accidental (unintentional)

SP 7 T63.412- Toxic effect of venom of centipedes and venomous millipedes, intentional self-harm

SP 7 T63.413- Toxic effect of venom of centipedes and venomous millipedes, assault

SP 7 T63.414- Toxic effect of venom of centipedes and venomous millipedes, undetermined

6 T63.42 Toxic effect of venom of ants

SP 7 T63.421- Toxic effect of venom of ants, accidental (unintentional)

SP 7 T63.422- Toxic effect of venom of ants, intentional self-harm

SP 7 T63.423- Toxic effect of venom of ants, assault

SP 7 T63.424- Toxic effect of venom of ants, undetermined

6 T63.43 Toxic effect of venom of caterpillars

SP 7 T63.431- Toxic effect of venom of caterpillars, accidental (unintentional)

SP 7 T63.432- Toxic effect of venom of caterpillars, intentional self-harm

SP 7 T63.433- Toxic effect of venom of caterpillars, assault

★ New ▲ Revised Px Primary SP PDGM Px SL Low CoM SH High CoM IQ Quest. Encounter H Hospice non-cancer Dx Unspecified M Manifestation

DecisionHealth's FY 2020 Complete Home Health ICD-10-CM Diagnosis Coding Manual

1713

SP 7 T63.434- Toxic effect of venom of caterpillars, undetermined

6 T63.44 Toxic effect of venom of bees

SP 7 T63.441- Toxic effect of venom of bees, accidental (unintentional)

SP 7 T63.442- Toxic effect of venom of bees, intentional self-harm

SP 7 T63.443- Toxic effect of venom of bees, assault

SP 7 T63.444- Toxic effect of venom of bees, undetermined

6 T63.45 Toxic effect of venom of hornets

SP 7 T63.451- Toxic effect of venom of hornets, accidental (unintentional)

SP 7 T63.452- Toxic effect of venom of hornets, intentional self-harm

SP 7 T63.453- Toxic effect of venom of hornets, assault

SP 7 T63.454- Toxic effect of venom of hornets, undetermined

6 T63.46 Toxic effect of venom of wasps
Toxic effect of yellow jacket

SP 7 T63.461- Toxic effect of venom of wasps, accidental (unintentional)

SP 7 T63.462- Toxic effect of venom of wasps, intentional self-harm

SP 7 T63.463- Toxic effect of venom of wasps, assault

SP 7 T63.464- Toxic effect of venom of wasps, undetermined

6 T63.48 Toxic effect of venom of other arthropod

SP 7 T63.481- Toxic effect of venom of other arthropod, accidental (unintentional)

SP 7 T63.482- Toxic effect of venom of other arthropod, intentional self-harm

SP 7 T63.483- Toxic effect of venom of other arthropod, assault

SP 7 T63.484- Toxic effect of venom of other arthropod, undetermined

5 T63.5 Toxic effect of contact with venomous fish
EXCLUDES 2   poisoning by ingestion of fish (T61.-)

6 T63.51 Toxic effect of contact with stingray

SP 7 T63.511- Toxic effect of contact with stingray, accidental (unintentional)

SP 7 T63.512- Toxic effect of contact with stingray, intentional self-harm

SP 7 T63.513- Toxic effect of contact with stingray, assault

SP 7 T63.514- Toxic effect of contact with stingray, undetermined

6 T63.59 Toxic effect of contact with other venomous fish

SP 7 T63.591- Toxic effect of contact with other venomous fish, accidental (unintentional)

SP 7 T63.592- Toxic effect of contact with other venomous fish, intentional self-harm

SP 7 T63.593- Toxic effect of contact with other venomous fish, assault

SP 7 T63.594- Toxic effect of contact with other venomous fish, undetermined

5 T63.6 Toxic effect of contact with other venomous marine animals
EXCLUDES 1   sea-snake venom (T63.09)
EXCLUDES 2   poisoning by ingestion of shellfish (T61.78-)

6 T63.61 Toxic effect of contact with Portugese Man-o-war
Toxic effect of contact with bluebottle

SP 7 T63.611- Toxic effect of contact with Portugese Man-o-war, accidental (unintentional)

SP 7 T63.612- Toxic effect of contact with Portugese Man-o-war, intentional self-harm

SP 7 T63.613- Toxic effect of contact with Portugese Man-o-war, assault

SP 7 T63.614- Toxic effect of contact with Portugese Man-o-war, undetermined

6 T63.62 Toxic effect of contact with other jellyfish

SP 7 T63.621- Toxic effect of contact with other jellyfish, accidental (unintentional)

SP 7 T63.622- Toxic effect of contact with other jellyfish, intentional self-harm

SP 7 T63.623- Toxic effect of contact with other jellyfish, assault

SP 7 T63.624- Toxic effect of contact with other jellyfish, undetermined

6 T63.63 Toxic effect of contact with sea anemone

SP 7 T63.631- Toxic effect of contact with sea anemone, accidental (unintentional)

SP 7 T63.632- Toxic effect of contact with sea anemone, intentional self-harm

SP 7 T63.633- Toxic effect of contact with sea anemone, assault

SP 7 T63.634- Toxic effect of contact with sea anemone, undetermined

6 T63.69 Toxic effect of contact with other venomous marine animals

SP 7 T63.691- Toxic effect of contact with other venomous marine animals, accidental (unintentional)

SP 7 T63.692- Toxic effect of contact with other venomous marine animals, intentional self-harm

SP 7 T63.693- Toxic effect of contact with other venomous marine animals, assault

SP 7 T63.694- Toxic effect of contact with other venomous marine animals, undetermined

5 T63.7 Toxic effect of contact with venomous plant

6 T63.71 Toxic effect of contact with venomous marine plant

SP 7 T63.711- Toxic effect of contact with venomous marine plant, accidental (unintentional)

SP 7 T63.712- Toxic effect of contact with venomous marine plant, intentional self-harm

SP 7 T63.713- Toxic effect of contact with venomous marine plant, assault

4 4th digit required   5 5th digit required   6 6th digit required   7 7th digit required   7 7th digit placeholder   + Additional code   Laterality

1714   *DecisionHealth's* FY 2020 Complete Home Health ICD-10-CM Diagnosis Coding Manual

SP 7 T63.714- Toxic effect of contact with venomous marine plant, undetermined

6 T63.79 Toxic effect of contact with other venomous plant

SP 7 T63.791- Toxic effect of contact with other venomous plant, accidental (unintentional)

SP 7 T63.792- Toxic effect of contact with other venomous plant, intentional self-harm

SP 7 T63.793- Toxic effect of contact with other venomous plant, assault

SP 7 T63.794- Toxic effect of contact with other venomous plant, undetermined

5 T63.8 Toxic effect of contact with other venomous animals

6 T63.81 Toxic effect of contact with venomous frog
> **EXCLUDES 1** contact with nonvenomous frog (W62.0)

SP 7 T63.811- Toxic effect of contact with venomous frog, accidental (unintentional)

SP 7 T63.812- Toxic effect of contact with venomous frog, intentional self-harm

SP 7 T63.813- Toxic effect of contact with venomous frog, assault

SP 7 T63.814- Toxic effect of contact with venomous frog, undetermined

6 T63.82 Toxic effect of contact with venomous toad
> **EXCLUDES 1** contact with nonvenomous toad (W62.1)

SP 7 T63.821- Toxic effect of contact with venomous toad, accidental (unintentional)

SP 7 T63.822- Toxic effect of contact with venomous toad, intentional self-harm

SP 7 T63.823- Toxic effect of contact with venomous toad, assault

SP 7 T63.824- Toxic effect of contact with venomous toad, undetermined

6 T63.83 Toxic effect of contact with other venomous amphibian
> **EXCLUDES 1** contact with nonvenomous amphibian (W62.9)

SP 7 T63.831- Toxic effect of contact with other venomous amphibian, accidental (unintentional)

SP 7 T63.832- Toxic effect of contact with other venomous amphibian, intentional self-harm

SP 7 T63.833- Toxic effect of contact with other venomous amphibian, assault

SP 7 T63.834- Toxic effect of contact with other venomous amphibian, undetermined

6 T63.89 Toxic effect of contact with other venomous animals

SP 7 T63.891- Toxic effect of contact with other venomous animals, accidental (unintentional)

SP 7 T63.892- Toxic effect of contact with other venomous animals, intentional self-harm

SP 7 T63.893- Toxic effect of contact with other venomous animals, assault

SP 7 T63.894- Toxic effect of contact with other venomous animals, undetermined

5 T63.9 Toxic effect of contact with unspecified venomous animal

SP ✓ T63.91X- Toxic effect of contact with unspecified venomous animal, accidental (unintentional)

SP ✓ T63.92X- Toxic effect of contact with unspecified venomous animal, intentional self-harm

SP ✓ T63.93X- Toxic effect of contact with unspecified venomous animal, assault

SP ✓ T63.94X- Toxic effect of contact with unspecified venomous animal, undetermined

4 T64 Toxic effect of aflatoxin and other mycotoxin food contaminants

> The appropriate 7th character is to be added to each code from category T64
> A   initial encounter
> D   subsequent encounter
> S   sequela

5 T64.0 Toxic effect of aflatoxin

SP ✓ T64.01X- Toxic effect of aflatoxin, accidental (unintentional)

SP ✓ T64.02X- Toxic effect of aflatoxin, intentional self-harm

SP ✓ T64.03X- Toxic effect of aflatoxin, assault

SP ✓ T64.04X- Toxic effect of aflatoxin, undetermined

5 T64.8 Toxic effect of other mycotoxin food contaminants

SP ✓ T64.81X- Toxic effect of other mycotoxin food contaminants, accidental (unintentional)

SP ✓ T64.82X- Toxic effect of other mycotoxin food contaminants, intentional self-harm

SP ✓ T64.83X- Toxic effect of other mycotoxin food contaminants, assault

SP ✓ T64.84X- Toxic effect of other mycotoxin food contaminants, undetermined

4 T65 Toxic effect of other and unspecified substances

> The appropriate 7th character is to be added to each code from category T65
> A   initial encounter
> D   subsequent encounter
> S   sequela

5 T65.0 Toxic effect of cyanides
> **EXCLUDES 1** hydrogen cyanide (T57.3-)

6 T65.0X Toxic effect of cyanides

SP 7 T65.0X1- Toxic effect of cyanides, accidental (unintentional)
Toxic effect of cyanides NOS

SP 7 T65.0X2- Toxic effect of cyanides, intentional self-harm

★ New ▲ Revised Px Primary **SP** PDGM Px **SL** Low CoM **SH** High CoM **IQ** Quest. Encounter **H** Hospice non-cancer Dx Unspecified **M** *Manifestation*

DecisionHealth's FY 2020 Complete Home Health ICD-10-CM Diagnosis Coding Manual

1715

SP 7 T65.0X3- Toxic effect of cyanides, assault

SP 7 T65.0X4- Toxic effect of cyanides, undetermined

5 T65.1 Toxic effect of strychnine and its salts

  6 T65.1X Toxic effect of strychnine and its salts

SP 7 T65.1X1- Toxic effect of strychnine and its salts, accidental (unintentional)
Toxic effect of strychnine and its salts NOS

SP 7 T65.1X2- Toxic effect of strychnine and its salts, intentional self-harm

SP 7 T65.1X3- Toxic effect of strychnine and its salts, assault

SP 7 T65.1X4- Toxic effect of strychnine and its salts, undetermined

5 T65.2 Toxic effect of tobacco and nicotine
   EXCLUDES 2 nicotine dependence (F17.-)

  6 T65.21 Toxic effect of chewing tobacco

SP 7 T65.211- Toxic effect of chewing tobacco, accidental (unintentional)
Toxic effect of chewing tobacco NOS

SP 7 T65.212- Toxic effect of chewing tobacco, intentional self-harm

SP 7 T65.213- Toxic effect of chewing tobacco, assault

SP 7 T65.214- Toxic effect of chewing tobacco, undetermined

✚ 6 T65.22 Toxic effect of tobacco cigarettes
Toxic effect of tobacco smoke
Use additional code for exposure to second hand tobacco smoke (Z57.31, Z77.22)

SP ✚ 7 T65.221- Toxic effect of tobacco cigarettes, accidental (unintentional)
Toxic effect of tobacco cigarettes NOS

SP ✚ 7 T65.222- Toxic effect of tobacco cigarettes, intentional self-harm

SP ✚ 7 T65.223- Toxic effect of tobacco cigarettes, assault

SP ✚ 7 T65.224- Toxic effect of tobacco cigarettes, undetermined

  6 T65.29 Toxic effect of other tobacco and nicotine

SP 7 T65.291- Toxic effect of other tobacco and nicotine, accidental (unintentional)
Toxic effect of other tobacco and nicotine NOS

SP 7 T65.292- Toxic effect of other tobacco and nicotine, intentional self-harm

SP 7 T65.293- Toxic effect of other tobacco and nicotine, assault

SP 7 T65.294- Toxic effect of other tobacco and nicotine, undetermined

5 T65.3 Toxic effect of nitroderivatives and aminoderivatives of benzene and its homologues
Toxic effect of anilin [benzenamine]
Toxic effect of nitrobenzene
Toxic effect of trinitrotoluene

  6 T65.3X Toxic effect of nitroderivatives and aminoderivatives of benzene and its homologues

SP 7 T65.3X1- Toxic effect of nitroderivatives and aminoderivatives of benzene and its homologues, accidental (unintentional)
Toxic effect of nitroderivatives and aminoderivatives of benzene and its homologues NOS

SP 7 T65.3X2- Toxic effect of nitroderivatives and aminoderivatives of benzene and its homologues, intentional self-harm

SP 7 T65.3X3- Toxic effect of nitroderivatives and aminoderivatives of benzene and its homologues, assault

SP 7 T65.3X4- Toxic effect of nitroderivatives and aminoderivatives of benzene and its homologues, undetermined

5 T65.4 Toxic effect of carbon disulfide

  6 T65.4X Toxic effect of carbon disulfide

SP 7 T65.4X1- Toxic effect of carbon disulfide, accidental (unintentional)
Toxic effect of carbon disulfide NOS

SP 7 T65.4X2- Toxic effect of carbon disulfide, intentional self-harm

SP 7 T65.4X3- Toxic effect of carbon disulfide, assault

SP 7 T65.4X4- Toxic effect of carbon disulfide, undetermined

5 T65.5 Toxic effect of nitroglycerin and other nitric acids and esters
Toxic effect of 1,2,3-Propanetriol trinitrate

  6 T65.5X Toxic effect of nitroglycerin and other nitric acids and esters

SP 7 T65.5X1- Toxic effect of nitroglycerin and other nitric acids and esters, accidental (unintentional)
Toxic effect of nitroglycerin and other nitric acids and esters NOS

SP 7 T65.5X2- Toxic effect of nitroglycerin and other nitric acids and esters, intentional self-harm

SP 7 T65.5X3- Toxic effect of nitroglycerin and other nitric acids and esters, assault

SP 7 T65.5X4- Toxic effect of nitroglycerin and other nitric acids and esters, undetermined

5 T65.6 Toxic effect of paints and dyes, not elsewhere classified

  6 T65.6X Toxic effect of paints and dyes, not elsewhere classified

SP 7 T65.6X1- Toxic effect of paints and dyes, not elsewhere classified, accidental (unintentional)
Toxic effect of paints and dyes NOS

SP 7 T65.6X2- Toxic effect of paints and dyes, not elsewhere classified, intentional self-harm

SP 7 T65.6X3- Toxic effect of paints and dyes, not elsewhere classified, assault

SP 7 T65.6X4- Toxic effect of paints and dyes, not elsewhere classified, undetermined

5 T65.8 Toxic effect of other specified substances

  6 T65.81 Toxic effect of latex

---

4 4th digit required   **5** 5th digit required   **6** 6th digit required   **7** 7th digit required   **7** 7th digit placeholder   **✚** Additional code   **⊟** Laterality

SP 7 T65.811-   **Toxic effect of latex, accidental (unintentional)**
Toxic effect of latex NOS

SP 7 T65.812-   **Toxic effect of latex, intentional self-harm**

SP 7 T65.813-   **Toxic effect of latex, assault**

SP 7 T65.814-   **Toxic effect of latex, undetermined**

6 T65.82   **Toxic effect of harmful algae and algae toxins**
Toxic effect of (harmful) algae bloom NOS
Toxic effect of blue-green algae bloom
Toxic effect of brown tide
Toxic effect of cyanobacteria bloom
Toxic effect of Florida red tide
Toxic effect of pfiesteria piscicida
Toxic effect of red tide

SP 7 T65.821-   **Toxic effect of harmful algae and algae toxins, accidental (unintentional)**
Toxic effect of harmful algae and algae toxins NOS

SP 7 T65.822-   **Toxic effect of harmful algae and algae toxins, intentional self-harm**

SP 7 T65.823-   **Toxic effect of harmful algae and algae toxins, assault**

SP 7 T65.824-   **Toxic effect of harmful algae and algae toxins, undetermined**

6 T65.83   **Toxic effect of fiberglass**

SP 7 T65.831-   **Toxic effect of fiberglass, accidental (unintentional)**
Toxic effect of fiberglass NOS

SP 7 T65.832-   **Toxic effect of fiberglass, intentional self-harm**

SP 7 T65.833-   **Toxic effect of fiberglass, assault**

SP 7 T65.834-   **Toxic effect of fiberglass, undetermined**

6 T65.89   **Toxic effect of other specified substances**

SP 7 T65.891-   **Toxic effect of other specified substances, accidental (unintentional)**
Toxic effect of other specified substances NOS

SP 7 T65.892-   **Toxic effect of other specified substances, intentional self-harm**

SP 7 T65.893-   **Toxic effect of other specified substances, assault**

SP 7 T65.894-   **Toxic effect of other specified substances, undetermined**

5 T65.9   **Toxic effect of unspecified substance**

SP 7 T65.91X-   **Toxic effect of unspecified substance, accidental (unintentional)**
Poisoning NOS

SP 7 T65.92X-   **Toxic effect of unspecified substance, intentional self-harm**

SP 7 T65.93X-   **Toxic effect of unspecified substance, assault**

SP 7 T65.94X-   **Toxic effect of unspecified substance, undetermined**

Other and unspecified effects of external causes (T66-T78)

SP 7 T66.XXX-   **Radiation sickness, unspecified**
EXCLUDES 1   specified adverse effects of radiation, such as:
burns (T20-T31)
leukemia (C91-C95)
radiation gastroenteritis and colitis (K52.0)
radiation pneumonitis (J70.0)
radiation related disorders of the skin and subcutaneous tissue (L55-L59)
sunburn (L55.-)

The appropriate 7th character is to be added to code T66
A   initial encounter
D   subsequent encounter
S   sequela

CODING TIPS ✓   To code a burn or other effect of radiation, other than radiation sickness, code the burn and then the external cause code to indicate the cause, such as Y84.2.

4 T67   **Effects of heat and light**
EXCLUDES 1   erythema [dermatitis] ab igne (L59.0)
malignant hyperpyrexia due to anesthesia (T88.3)
radiation-related disorders of the skin and subcutaneous tissue (L55-L59)
EXCLUDES 2   burns (T20-T31)
sunburn (L55.-)
sweat disorder due to heat (L74-L75)

The appropriate 7th character is to be added to each code from category T67
A   initial encounter
D   subsequent encounter
S   sequela

▲ + 5 T67.0   **Heatstroke and sunstroke**
Use additional code(s) to identify any associated complications of heatstroke, such as:
coma and stupor (R40.-)
rhabdomyolysis (M62.82)
systemic inflammatory response syndrome (R65.1-)

★ + 7 T67.01X-   **Heatstroke and sunstroke**
Heat apoplexy
Heat pyrexia
Siriasis
Thermoplegia

★ + 7 T67.02X-   **Exertional heatstroke**

★ + 7 T67.09X-   **Other heatstroke and sunstroke**

SP 7 T67.1XX-   **Heat syncope**
Heat collapse

SP 7 T67.2XX-   **Heat cramp**

SP 7 T67.3XX-   **Heat exhaustion, anhydrotic**
Heat prostration due to water depletion

★ New   ▲ Revised   Px Primary   **SP** PDGM Px   **SL** Low CoM   **SH** High CoM   **IQ** Quest. Encounter   **H** Hospice non-cancer Dx   Unspecified   **M** *Manifestation*

EXCLUDES 1   heat exhaustion due to salt depletion (T67.4)

SP ☑ T67.4XX- Heat exhaustion due to salt depletion
Heat prostration due to salt (and water) depletion

SP ☑ T67.5XX- Heat exhaustion, unspecified
Heat prostration NOS

SP ☑ T67.6XX- Heat fatigue, transient

SP ☑ T67.7XX- Heat edema

SP ☑ T67.8XX- Other effects of heat and light

SP ☑ T67.9XX- Effect of heat and light, unspecified

SP ✚ ☑ T68.XXX- Hypothermia
Accidental hypothermia
Hypothermia NOS
Use additional code to identify source of exposure:
Exposure to excessive cold of man-made origin (W93)
Exposure to excessive cold of natural origin (X31)

EXCLUDES 1   hypothermia following anesthesia (T88.51)
hypothermia not associated with low environmental temperature (R68.0)
hypothermia of newborn (P80.-)

EXCLUDES 2   frostbite (T33-T34)

The appropriate 7th character is to be added to code T68
A   initial encounter
D   subsequent encounter
S   sequela

✚ ◢ T69 Other effects of reduced temperature
Use additional code to identify source of exposure:
Exposure to excessive cold of man-made origin (W93)
Exposure to excessive cold of natural origin (X31)

EXCLUDES 2   frostbite (T33-T34)

The appropriate 7th character is to be added to each code from category T69
A   initial encounter
D   subsequent encounter
S   sequela

✚ ◢ T69.0 Immersion hand and foot

    ✚ ◢ T69.01 Immersion hand

⊟ SP ✚ ◢ T69.011- Immersion hand, right hand

⊟ SP ✚ ◢ T69.012- Immersion hand, left hand

⊟ SP ✚ ◢ T69.019- Immersion hand, unspecified hand

    ✚ ◢ T69.02 Immersion foot
Trench foot

⊟ SP ✚ ◢ T69.021- Immersion foot, right foot

⊟ SP ✚ ◢ T69.022- Immersion foot, left foot

⊟ SP ✚ ◢ T69.029- Immersion foot, unspecified foot

SP ✚ ☑ T69.1XX- Chilblains

SP ✚ ☑ T69.8XX- Other specified effects of reduced temperature

SP ✚ ☑ T69.9XX- Effect of reduced temperature, unspecified

◢ T70 Effects of air pressure and water pressure

The appropriate 7th character is to be added to each code from category T70
A   initial encounter
D   subsequent encounter
S   sequela

SP ☑ T70.0XX- Otitic barotrauma
Aero-otitis media
Effects of change in ambient atmospheric pressure or water pressure on ears

SP ☑ T70.1XX- Sinus barotrauma
Aerosinusitis
Effects of change in ambient atmospheric pressure on sinuses

◢ T70.2 Other and unspecified effects of high altitude

EXCLUDES 2   polycythemia due to high altitude (D75.1)

SP ☑ T70.20X- Unspecified effects of high altitude

SP ☑ T70.29X- Other effects of high altitude
Alpine sickness
Anoxia due to high altitude
Barotrauma NOS
Hypobaropathy
Mountain sickness

SP ☑ T70.3XX- Caisson disease [decompression sickness]
Compressed-air disease
Diver's palsy or paralysis

SP ☑ T70.4XX- Effects of high-pressure fluids
Hydraulic jet injection (industrial)
Pneumatic jet injection (industrial)
Traumatic jet injection (industrial)

SP ☑ T70.8XX- Other effects of air pressure and water pressure

SP ☑ T70.9XX- Effect of air pressure and water pressure, unspecified

◢ T71 Asphyxiation
Mechanical suffocation
Traumatic suffocation

EXCLUDES 1   acute respiratory distress (syndrome) (J80)
anoxia due to high altitude (T70.2)
asphyxia NOS (R09.01)
asphyxia from carbon monoxide (T58.-)
asphyxia from inhalation of food or foreign body (T17.-)
asphyxia from other gases, fumes and vapors (T59.-)
respiratory distress (syndrome) in newborn (P22.-)

The appropriate 7th character is to be added to each code from category T71
A   initial encounter
D   subsequent encounter
S   sequela

◢ T71.1 Asphyxiation due to mechanical threat to breathing
Suffocation due to mechanical threat to breathing

◢ 4th digit required   ◢ 5th digit required   ◢ 6th digit required   ◢ 7th digit required   ☑ 7th digit placeholder   ✚ Additional code   ⊟ Laterality

1718   *DecisionHealth's* FY 2020 Complete Home Health ICD-10-CM Diagnosis Coding Manual

[6] **T71.11** **Asphyxiation due to smothering under pillow**

[SP] [7] **T71.111-** **Asphyxiation due to smothering under pillow, accidental**
Asphyxiation due to smothering under pillow NOS

[SP] [7] **T71.112-** **Asphyxiation due to smothering under pillow, intentional self-harm**

[SP] [7] **T71.113-** **Asphyxiation due to smothering under pillow, assault**

[SP] [7] **T71.114-** **Asphyxiation due to smothering under pillow, undetermined**

[6] **T71.12** **Asphyxiation due to plastic bag**

[SP] [7] **T71.121-** **Asphyxiation due to plastic bag, accidental**
Asphyxiation due to plastic bag NOS

[SP] [7] **T71.122-** **Asphyxiation due to plastic bag, intentional self-harm**

[SP] [7] **T71.123-** **Asphyxiation due to plastic bag, assault**

[SP] [7] **T71.124-** **Asphyxiation due to plastic bag, undetermined**

[6] **T71.13** **Asphyxiation due to being trapped in bed linens**

[SP] [7] **T71.131-** **Asphyxiation due to being trapped in bed linens, accidental**
Asphyxiation due to being trapped in bed linens NOS

[SP] [7] **T71.132-** **Asphyxiation due to being trapped in bed linens, intentional self-harm**

[SP] [7] **T71.133-** **Asphyxiation due to being trapped in bed linens, assault**

[SP] [7] **T71.134-** **Asphyxiation due to being trapped in bed linens, undetermined**

[6] **T71.14** **Asphyxiation due to smothering under another person's body (in bed)**

[SP] [7] **T71.141-** **Asphyxiation due to smothering under another person's body (in bed), accidental**
Asphyxiation due to smothering under another person's body (in bed) NOS

[SP] [7] **T71.143-** **Asphyxiation due to smothering under another person's body (in bed), assault**

[SP] [7] **T71.144-** **Asphyxiation due to smothering under another person's body (in bed), undetermined**

[6] **T71.15** **Asphyxiation due to smothering in furniture**

[SP] [7] **T71.151-** **Asphyxiation due to smothering in furniture, accidental**
Asphyxiation due to smothering in furniture NOS

[SP] [7] **T71.152-** **Asphyxiation due to smothering in furniture, intentional self-harm**

[SP] [7] **T71.153-** **Asphyxiation due to smothering in furniture, assault**

[SP] [7] **T71.154-** **Asphyxiation due to smothering in furniture, undetermined**

[+] [6] **T71.16** **Asphyxiation due to hanging**
Hanging by window shade cord

Use additional code for any associated injuries, such as:
crushing injury of neck (S17.-)
fracture of cervical vertebrae (S12.0-S12.2-)
open wound of neck (S11.-)

[SP] [+] [7] **T71.161-** **Asphyxiation due to hanging, accidental**
Asphyxiation due to hanging NOS
Hanging NOS

[SP] [+] [7] **T71.162-** **Asphyxiation due to hanging, intentional self-harm**

[SP] [+] [7] **T71.163-** **Asphyxiation due to hanging, assault**

[SP] [+] [7] **T71.164-** **Asphyxiation due to hanging, undetermined**

[6] **T71.19** **Asphyxiation due to mechanical threat to breathing due to other causes**

[SP] [7] **T71.191-** **Asphyxiation due to mechanical threat to breathing due to other causes, accidental**
Asphyxiation due to other causes NOS

[SP] [7] **T71.192-** **Asphyxiation due to mechanical threat to breathing due to other causes, intentional self-harm**

[SP] [7] **T71.193-** **Asphyxiation due to mechanical threat to breathing due to other causes, assault**

[SP] [7] **T71.194-** **Asphyxiation due to mechanical threat to breathing due to other causes, undetermined**

[5] **T71.2** **Asphyxiation due to systemic oxygen deficiency due to low oxygen content in ambient air**
Suffocation due to systemic oxygen deficiency due to low oxygen content in ambient air

[SP] [7] **T71.20X-** **Asphyxiation due to systemic oxygen deficiency due to low oxygen content in ambient air due to unspecified cause**

[SP] [+] [7] **T71.21X-** **Asphyxiation due to cave-in or falling earth**
Use additional code for any associated cataclysm (X34-X38)

[6] **T71.22** **Asphyxiation due to being trapped in a car trunk**

[SP] [7] **T71.221-** **Asphyxiation due to being trapped in a car trunk, accidental**

[SP] [7] **T71.222-** **Asphyxiation due to being trapped in a car trunk, intentional self-harm**

[SP] [7] **T71.223-** **Asphyxiation due to being trapped in a car trunk, assault**

[SP] [7] **T71.224-** **Asphyxiation due to being trapped in a car trunk, undetermined**

[6] **T71.23** **Asphyxiation due to being trapped in a (discarded) refrigerator**

[SP] [7] **T71.231-** **Asphyxiation due to being trapped in a (discarded) refrigerator, accidental**

[SP] [7] **T71.232-** **Asphyxiation due to being trapped in a (discarded) refrigerator, intentional self-harm**

★ New ▲ Revised Px Primary [SP] PDGM Px [SL] Low CoM [SH] High CoM [IQ] Quest. Encounter [H] Hospice non-cancer Dx   Unspecified   [M] *Manifestation*

DecisionHealth's FY 2020 Complete Home Health ICD-10-CM Diagnosis Coding Manual

1719

SP 7 T71.233- Asphyxiation due to being trapped in a (discarded) refrigerator, assault

SP 7 T71.234- Asphyxiation due to being trapped in a (discarded) refrigerator, undetermined

SP 7 T71.29X- Asphyxiation due to being trapped in other low oxygen environment

SP 7 T71.9XX- Asphyxiation due to unspecified cause

Suffocation (by strangulation) due to unspecified cause

Suffocation NOS

Systemic oxygen deficiency due to low oxygen content in ambient air due to unspecified cause

Systemic oxygen deficiency due to mechanical threat to breathing due to unspecified cause

Traumatic asphyxia NOS

4 T73 Effects of other deprivation

The appropriate 7th character is to be added to each code from category T73

A   initial encounter
D   subsequent encounter
S   sequela

SP 7 T73.0XX- Starvation
Deprivation of food

SP 7 T73.1XX- Deprivation of water

SP 7 T73.2XX- Exhaustion due to exposure

SP 7 T73.3XX- Exhaustion due to excessive exertion
Exhaustion due to overexertion

SP 7 T73.8XX- Other effects of deprivation

SP IQ 7 T73.9XX- Effect of deprivation, unspecified

+ 4 T74 Adult and child abuse, neglect and other maltreatment, confirmed
Use additional code, if applicable, to identify any associated current injury
Use additional external cause code to identify perpetrator, if known (Y07.-)

EXCLUDES 1 abuse and maltreatment in pregnancy (O9A.3-, O9A.4-, O9A.5-)
adult and child maltreatment, suspected (T76.-)

The appropriate 7th character is to be added to each code from category T74

A   initial encounter
D   subsequent encounter
S   sequela

GUIDELINES Section I.C.19.f

Sequence first the appropriate code from categories T74.- (Adult and child abuse, neglect and other maltreatment, confirmed) or T76.- (Adult and child abuse, neglect and other maltreatment, suspected) for abuse, neglect and other maltreatment, followed by any accompanying mental health or injury code(s). If the documentation in the medical record states abuse or neglect it is coded as confirmed (T74.-). It is coded as suspected if it is documented as suspected (T76.-).

For cases of confirmed abuse or neglect an external cause code from the assault section (X92-Y09) should be added to identify the cause of any physical injuries. A perpetrator code (Y07) should be added when the perpetrator of the abuse is known. For suspected cases of abuse or neglect, do not report external cause or perpetrator code. If a suspected case of abuse, neglect or mistreatment is ruled out during an encounter code Z04.71, Encounter for examination and observation following alleged physical adult abuse, ruled out, or code Z04.72, Encounter for examination and observation following alleged child physical abuse, ruled out, should be used, not a code from T76.

+ 5 T74.0 Neglect or abandonment, confirmed

SP + 7 T74.01X- Adult neglect or abandonment, confirmed

SP + 7 T74.02X- Child neglect or abandonment, confirmed

+ 5 T74.1 Physical abuse, confirmed
EXCLUDES 2 sexual abuse (T74.2-)

SP + 7 T74.11X- Adult physical abuse, confirmed

SP + 7 T74.12X- Child physical abuse, confirmed
EXCLUDES 2 shaken infant syndrome (T74.4)

+ 5 T74.2 Sexual abuse, confirmed
Rape, confirmed
Sexual assault, confirmed

SP + 7 T74.21X- Adult sexual abuse, confirmed

SP + 7 T74.22X- Child sexual abuse, confirmed

+ 5 T74.3 Psychological abuse, confirmed
Bullying and intimidation, confirmed
Intimidation through social media, confirmed

SP + 7 T74.31X- Adult psychological abuse, confirmed

SP + 7 T74.32X- Child psychological abuse, confirmed

SP + 7 T74.4XX- Shaken infant syndrome

+ 5 T74.5 Forced sexual exploitation, confirmed

SP + 7 T74.51X- Adult forced sexual exploitation, confirmed

SP + 7 T74.52X- Child sexual exploitation, confirmed

+ 5 T74.6 Forced labor exploitation, confirmed

IQ + 7 T74.61X- Adult forced labor exploitation, confirmed

IQ + 7 T74.62X- Child forced labor exploitation, confirmed

+ 5 T74.9 Unspecified maltreatment, confirmed

---

4 4th digit required   5 5th digit required   6 6th digit required   7 7th digit required   7 7th digit placeholder   + Additional code   5 Laterality

1720   *DecisionHealth's* FY 2020 Complete Home Health ICD-10-CM Diagnosis Coding Manual

IQ **+** ☑ **T74.91X-** **Unspecified adult maltreatment, confirmed**

IQ **+** ☑ **T74.92X-** **Unspecified child maltreatment, confirmed**

4 **T75** **Other and unspecified effects of other external causes**

> **EXCLUDES 1** adverse effects NEC (T78.-)
> **EXCLUDES 2** burns (electric) (T20-T31)

The appropriate 7th character is to be added to each code from category T75
A   initial encounter
D   subsequent encounter
S   sequela

5 **T75.0** **Effects of lightning**
Struck by lightning

IQ ☑ **T75.00X-** **Unspecified effects of lightning**
Struck by lightning NOS

SP ☑ **T75.01X-** **Shock due to being struck by lightning**

SP **+** ☑ **T75.09X-** **Other effects of lightning**
Use additional code for other effects of lightning

IQ ☑ **T75.1XX-** **Unspecified effects of drowning and nonfatal submersion**
Immersion
> **EXCLUDES 1** specified effects of drowning- code to effects

5 **T75.2** **Effects of vibration**

IQ ☑ **T75.20X-** **Unspecified effects of vibration**

SP ☑ **T75.21X-** **Pneumatic hammer syndrome**

SP ☑ **T75.22X-** **Traumatic vasospastic syndrome**

SP ☑ **T75.23X-** **Vertigo from infrasound**
> **EXCLUDES 1** vertigo NOS (R42)

SP ☑ **T75.29X-** **Other effects of vibration**

SP **+** ☑ **T75.3XX-** **Motion sickness**
Airsickness
Seasickness
Travel sickness
Use additional external cause code to identify vehicle or type of motion (Y92.81-, Y93.5-)

SP ☑ **T75.4XX-** **Electrocution**
Shock from electric current
Shock from electroshock gun (taser)

5 **T75.8** **Other specified effects of external causes**

SP ☑ **T75.81X-** **Effects of abnormal gravitation [G] forces**

SP ☑ **T75.82X-** **Effects of weightlessness**

SP ☑ **T75.89X-** **Other specified effects of external causes**

+ **4** **T76** **Adult and child abuse, neglect and other maltreatment, suspected**
Use additional code, if applicable, to identify any associated current injury
> **EXCLUDES 1** adult and child maltreatment, confirmed (T74.-)
> suspected abuse and maltreatment in pregnancy (O9A.3-, O9A.4-, O9A.5-)
> suspected adult physical abuse, ruled out (Z04.71)
> suspected adult sexual abuse, ruled out (Z04.41)

suspected child physical abuse, ruled out (Z04.72)
suspected child sexual abuse, ruled out (Z04.42)

The appropriate 7th character is to be added to each code from category T76
A   initial encounter
D   subsequent encounter
S   sequela

> **GUIDELINES** Section I.C.19.f
Sequence first the appropriate code from categories T74.- (Adult and child abuse, neglect and other maltreatment, confirmed) or T76.- (Adult and child abuse, neglect and other maltreatment, suspected) for abuse, neglect and other maltreatment, followed by any accompanying mental health or injury code(s). If the documentation in the medical record states abuse or neglect it is coded as confirmed (T74.-). It is coded as suspected if it is documented as suspected (T76.-).

For cases of confirmed abuse or neglect an external cause code from the assault section (X92-Y09) should be added to identify the cause of any physical injuries. A perpetrator code (Y07) should be added when the perpetrator of the abuse is known. For suspected cases of abuse or neglect, do not report external cause or perpetrator code. If a suspected case of abuse, neglect or mistreatment is ruled out during an encounter code Z04.71, Encounter for examination and observation following alleged physical adult abuse, ruled out, or code Z04.72, Encounter for examination and observation following alleged child physical abuse, ruled out, should be used, not a code from T76.

+ **5** **T76.0** **Neglect or abandonment, suspected**

SP **+** ☑ **T76.01X-** **Adult neglect or abandonment, suspected**

SP **+** ☑ **T76.02X-** **Child neglect or abandonment, suspected**

+ **5** **T76.1** **Physical abuse, suspected**

SP **+** ☑ **T76.11X-** **Adult physical abuse, suspected**

SP **+** ☑ **T76.12X-** **Child physical abuse, suspected**

+ **5** **T76.2** **Sexual abuse, suspected**
Rape, suspected
> **EXCLUDES 1** alleged abuse, ruled out (Z04.7)

SP **+** ☑ **T76.21X-** **Adult sexual abuse, suspected**

SP **+** ☑ **T76.22X-** **Child sexual abuse, suspected**

+ **5** **T76.3** **Psychological abuse, suspected**
Bullying and intimidation, suspected
Intimidation through social media, suspected

SP **+** ☑ **T76.31X-** **Adult psychological abuse, suspected**

SP **+** ☑ **T76.32X-** **Child psychological abuse, suspected**

+ **5** **T76.5** **Forced sexual exploitation, suspected**

SP **+** ☑ **T76.51X-** **Adult forced sexual exploitation, suspected**

SP **+** ☑ **T76.52X-** **Child sexual exploitation, suspected**

★ New ▲ Revised **Px** Primary **SP** PDGM Px **SL** Low CoM **SH** High CoM **IQ** Quest. Encounter **H** Hospice non-cancer Dx   Unspecified   **M** *Manifestation*

DecisionHealth's FY 2020 Complete Home Health ICD-10-CM Diagnosis Coding Manual

1721

+ 5 T76.6   Forced labor exploitation, suspected

IQ + ☑ T76.61X-   Adult forced labor exploitation, suspected

IQ + ☑ T76.62X-   Child forced labor exploitation, suspected

+ 5 T76.9   Unspecified maltreatment, suspected

IQ + ☑ T76.91X-   Unspecified adult maltreatment, suspected

IQ + ☑ T76.92X-   Unspecified child maltreatment, suspected

4 T78   Adverse effects, not elsewhere classified
> EXCLUDES 2   complications of surgical and medical care NEC (T80-T88)

> The appropriate 7th character is to be added to each code from category T78
> A   initial encounter
> D   subsequent encounter
> S   sequela

5 T78.0   Anaphylactic reaction due to food
Anaphylactic reaction due to adverse food reaction
Anaphylactic shock or reaction due to nonpoisonous foods
Anaphylactoid reaction due to food

IQ ☑ T78.00X-   Anaphylactic reaction due to unspecified food

SP ☑ T78.01X-   Anaphylactic reaction due to peanuts

SP ☑ T78.02X-   Anaphylactic reaction due to shellfish (crustaceans)

SP ☑ T78.03X-   Anaphylactic reaction due to other fish

SP ☑ T78.04X-   Anaphylactic reaction due to fruits and vegetables

SP ☑ T78.05X-   Anaphylactic reaction due to tree nuts and seeds
> EXCLUDES 2   anaphylactic reaction due to peanuts (T78.01)

SP ☑ T78.06X-   Anaphylactic reaction due to food additives

SP ☑ T78.07X-   Anaphylactic reaction due to milk and dairy products

SP ☑ T78.08X-   Anaphylactic reaction due to eggs

SP ☑ T78.09X-   Anaphylactic reaction due to other food products

SP + ☑ T78.1XX-   Other adverse food reactions, not elsewhere classified
Use additional code to identify the type of reaction, if applicable
> EXCLUDES 1   anaphylactic reaction or shock due to adverse food reaction (T78.0-)
> anaphylactic reaction due to food (T78.0-)
> bacterial food borne intoxications (A05.-)
> EXCLUDES 2   allergic and dietetic gastroenteritis and colitis (K52.29)
> allergic rhinitis due to food (J30.5)
> dermatitis due to food in contact with skin (L23.6, L24.6, L25.4)

dermatitis due to ingested food (L27.2)
food protein-induced enterocolitis syndrome (K52.21)
food protein-induced enteropathy (K52.22)

SP ☑ T78.2XX-   Anaphylactic shock, unspecified
Allergic shock
Anaphylactic reaction
Anaphylaxis
> EXCLUDES 1   anaphylactic reaction or shock due to adverse effect of correct medicinal substance properly administered (T88.6)
> anaphylactic reaction or shock due to adverse food reaction (T78.0-)
> anaphylactic reaction or shock due to serum (T80.5-)

SP ☑ T78.3XX-   Angioneurotic edema
Allergic angioedema
Giant urticaria
Quincke's edema
> EXCLUDES 1   serum urticaria (T80.6-)
> urticaria (L50.-)

5 T78.4   Other and unspecified allergy
> EXCLUDES 1   specified types of allergic reaction such as:
> allergic diarrhea (K52.29)
> allergic gastroenteritis and colitis (K52.29)
> dermatitis (L23-L25, L27.-)
> food protein-induced enterocolitis syndrome (K52.21)
> food protein-induced enteropathy (K52.22)
> hay fever (J30.1)

SP ☑ T78.40X-   Allergy, unspecified
Allergic reaction NOS
Hypersensitivity NOS

SP ☑ T78.41X-   Arthus phenomenon
Arthus reaction

SP ☑ T78.49X-   Other allergy

SP ☑ T78.8XX-   Other adverse effects, not elsewhere classified

Certain early complications of trauma (T79)

4 T79   Certain early complications of trauma, not elsewhere classified
> EXCLUDES 2   acute respiratory distress syndrome (J80)
> complications occurring during or following medical procedures (T80-T88)
> complications of surgical and medical care NEC (T80-T88)
> newborn respiratory distress syndrome (P22.0)

---

4 4th digit required   5 5th digit required   6 6th digit required   7 7th digit required   ☑ 7th digit placeholder   + Additional code   5 Laterality

The appropriate 7th character is to be added to each code from category T79
A   initial encounter
D   subsequent encounter
S   sequela

SP ☑ T79.0XX- Air embolism (traumatic)
EXCLUDES 1 air embolism complicating abortion or ectopic or molar pregnancy (O00-O07, O08.2)
air embolism complicating pregnancy, childbirth and the puerperium (O88.0)
air embolism following infusion, transfusion, and therapeutic injection (T80.0)
air embolism following procedure NEC (T81.7-)
CODING TIPS ✓ Code T79.0- should not be assigned for an air embolus that is not specified as due to a traumatic cause.

SP ☑ T79.1XX- Fat embolism (traumatic)
EXCLUDES 1 fat embolism complicating:
abortion or ectopic or molar pregnancy (O00-O07, O08.2)
pregnancy, childbirth and the puerperium (O88.8)

SP ☑ T79.2XX- Traumatic secondary and recurrent hemorrhage and seroma

SP ☑ T79.4XX- Traumatic shock
Shock (immediate) (delayed) following injury
EXCLUDES 1 anaphylactic shock due to adverse food reaction (T78.0-)
anaphylactic shock due to correct medicinal substance properly administered (T88.6)
anaphylactic shock due to serum (T80.5-)
anaphylactic shock NOS (T78.2)
anesthetic shock (T88.2)
electric shock (T75.4)
nontraumatic shock NEC (R57.-)
obstetric shock (O75.1)
postprocedural shock (T81.1-)
septic shock (R65.21)
shock complicating abortion or ectopic or molar pregnancy (O00-O07, O08.3)
shock due to lightning (T75.01)
shock NOS (R57.9)

SP ☑ T79.5XX- Traumatic anuria
Crush syndrome
Renal failure following crushing

SP ☑ T79.6XX- Traumatic ischemia of muscle
Traumatic rhabdomyolysis
Volkmann's ischemic contracture
EXCLUDES 2 anterior tibial syndrome (M76.8)
compartment syndrome (traumatic) (T79.A-)
nontraumatic ischemia of muscle (M62.2-)

SP ☑ T79.7XX- Traumatic subcutaneous emphysema
EXCLUDES 1 emphysema NOS (J43)
emphysema (subcutaneous) resulting from a procedure (T81.82)

▲ 5 T79.A Traumatic compartment syndrome
EXCLUDES 1 fibromyalgia (M79.7)
nontraumatic compartment syndrome (M79.A-)
EXCLUDES 2 traumatic ischemic infarction of muscle (T79.6)
CODING TIPS ✓ Do not assign any code from subcategory T79.A- to indicate compartment syndrome that is not specifically stated as due to a traumatic cause. Non-traumatic compartment syndrome is coded to M79.A-.

IQ ☑ T79.A0X- Compartment syndrome, unspecified
Compartment syndrome NOS

6 T79.A1 Traumatic compartment syndrome of upper extremity
Traumatic compartment syndrome of shoulder, arm, forearm, wrist, hand, and fingers

☐ SP 7 T79.A11- Traumatic compartment syndrome of right upper extremity

☐ SP 7 T79.A12- Traumatic compartment syndrome of left upper extremity

☐ IQ 7 T79.A19- Traumatic compartment syndrome of unspecified upper extremity

6 T79.A2 Traumatic compartment syndrome of lower extremity
Traumatic compartment syndrome of hip, buttock, thigh, leg, foot, and toes

☐ SP 7 T79.A21- Traumatic compartment syndrome of right lower extremity

☐ SP 7 T79.A22- Traumatic compartment syndrome of left lower extremity

☐ IQ 7 T79.A29- Traumatic compartment syndrome of unspecified lower extremity

SP ☑ T79.A3X- Traumatic compartment syndrome of abdomen

SP ☑ T79.A9X- Traumatic compartment syndrome of other sites

SP ☑ T79.8XX- Other early complications of trauma

IQ ☑ T79.9XX- Unspecified early complication of trauma

Chapter 19

S00-T88

Complications of surgical and medical care, not elsewhere classified　(T80-T88)

Use additional code for adverse effect, if applicable, to identify drug (T36-T50 with fifth or sixth character 5)

Use additional code(s) to identify the specified condition resulting from the complication

Use additional code to identify devices involved and details of circumstances (Y62-Y82)

EXCLUDES 2 any encounters with medical care for postprocedural conditions in which no complications are present, such as:

artificial opening status (Z93.-)

closure of external stoma (Z43.-)

fitting and adjustment of external prosthetic device (Z44.-)

burns and corrosions from local applications and irradiation (T20-T32)

complications of surgical procedures during pregnancy, childbirth and the puerperium (O00-O9A)

mechanical complication of respirator [ventilator] (J95.850)

poisoning and toxic effects of drugs and chemicals (T36-T65 with fifth or sixth character 1-4 or 6)

postprocedural fever (R50.82)

specified complications classified elsewhere, such as:

cerebrospinal fluid leak from spinal puncture (G97.0)

colostomy malfunction (K94.0-)

disorders of fluid and electrolyte imbalance (E86-E87)

functional disturbances following cardiac surgery (I97.0-I97.1)

intraoperative and postprocedural complications of specified body systems (D78.-, E36.-, E89.-, G97.3-, G97.4, H59.3-, H59.-, H95.2-, H95.3, I97.4-, I97.5, J95.6-, J95.7, K91.6-, L76.-, M96.-, N99.-)

ostomy complications (J95.0-, K94.-, N99.5-)

postgastric surgery syndromes (K91.1)

postlaminectomy syndrome NEC (M96.1)

postmastectomy lymphedema syndrome (I97.2)

postsurgical blind-loop syndrome (K91.2)

ventilator associated pneumonia (J95.851)

GUIDELINES　Section I.B.16

Documentation of Complication of Care: Code assignment is based on the provider's documentation of the relationship between the condition and the care or procedure. The guideline extends to any complications of care, regardless of the chapter the code is located in. It is important to note that not all conditions that occur during or following medical care or surgery are classified as complications. There must be a cause-and-effect relationship between the care provided and the condition, and an indication in the documentation that it is a complication. Query the provider for clarification, if the complication is not clearly documented.

GUIDELINES　Section I.C.19.g.5)

Intraoperative and postprocedural complication codes are found within the body system chapters with codes specific to the organs and structures of that body system. These codes should be sequenced first, followed by a code(s) for the specific complication, if applicable.

CODING TIPS ✓　Conditions classifiable to T80-T88 are classifiable as complications of surgical and medical care. These conditions should only be assigned when diagnostic statements clearly indicate that the condition is a complication. Additional codes may be assigned to fully describe the complication.

◪ T80　Complications following infusion, transfusion and therapeutic injection

INCLUDES　complications following perfusion

EXCLUDES 2　bone marrow transplant rejection (T86.01)

febrile nonhemolytic transfusion reaction (R50.84)

fluid overload due to transfusion (E87.71)

posttransfusion purpura (D69.51)

transfusion associated circulatory overload (TACO) (E87.71)

transfusion (red blood cell) associated hemochromatosis (E83.111)

transfusion related acute lung injury (TRALI) (J95.84)

The appropriate 7th character is to be added to each code from category T80

A　initial encounter

D　subsequent encounter

S　sequela

CODING TIPS ✓　No aftercare code applies, including dressing changes, drain care, and suture removal. 7th character 'D' is the default for home care and hospice when providing aftercare for a healing or resolving condition; 'A' is used for active treatment such as antibiotics or more than routine wound care; 'S' may be used to indicate a residual condition after the original injury has healed. Once complication is repaired in the acute setting, continue to code the complication in home care and hospice with 7th character D if healing/resolving.

SP ☑ T80.0XX-　Air embolism following infusion, transfusion and therapeutic injection

SP ✚ ☑ T80.1XX-　Vascular complications following infusion, transfusion and therapeutic injection

Use additional code to identify the vascular complication

EXCLUDES 2　extravasation of vesicant agent (T80.81-)

infiltration of vesicant agent (T80.81-)

vascular complications specified as due to prosthetic devices, implants and grafts (T82.8-, T83.8-, T84.8-, T85.8-)

postprocedural vascular complications (T81.7-)

✚ ⑤ T80.2　Infections following infusion, transfusion and therapeutic injection

◪ 4th digit required　⑤ 5th digit required　⑥ 6th digit required　☑ 7th digit required　☑ 7th digit placeholder　✚ Additional code　▭ Laterality

1724　　　　　　　*DecisionHealth's* FY 2020 Complete Home Health ICD-10-CM Diagnosis Coding Manual

Use additional code to identify the specific infection, such as:
sepsis (A41.9)

Use additional code (R65.2-) to identify severe sepsis, if applicable

EXCLUDES 2 infections specified as due to prosthetic devices, implants and grafts (T82.6-T82.7, T83.5-T83.6, T84.5-T84.7, T85.7)
postprocedural infections (T81.4-)

CODING TIPS ✓ These codes indicate complications of central lines, including, but not limited to, Hickman catheters, PICC lines, port-a-caths, Swan-Ganz and triple lumen catheters. Do not use Z45.2 for routine care of the venous catheter when it is documented as infected.

✚ 6 T80.21 **Infection due to central venous catheter**
Infection due to pulmonary artery catheter (Swan-Ganz catheter)

SP ✚ 7 T80.211- **Bloodstream infection due to central venous catheter**
Catheter-related bloodstream infection (CRBSI) NOS
Central line-associated bloodstream infection (CLABSI)
Bloodstream infection due to Hickman catheter
Bloodstream infection due to peripherally inserted central catheter (PICC)
Bloodstream infection due to portacath (port-a-cath)
Bloodstream infection due to pulmonary artery catheter
Bloodstream infection due to triple lumen catheter
Bloodstream infection due to umbilical venous catheter

SP ✚ 7 T80.212- **Local infection due to central venous catheter**
Exit or insertion site infection
Local infection due to Hickman catheter
Local infection due to peripherally inserted central catheter (PICC)
Local infection due to portacath (port-a-cath)
Local infection due to pulmonary artery catheter
Local infection due to triple lumen catheter
Local infection due to umbilical venous catheter
Port or reservoir infection
Tunnel infection

SP ✚ 7 T80.218- **Other infection due to central venous catheter**
Other central line-associated infection
Other infection due to Hickman catheter
Other infection due to peripherally inserted central catheter (PICC)

Other infection due to portacath (port-a-cath)
Other infection due to pulmonary artery catheter
Other infection due to triple lumen catheter
Other infection due to umbilical venous catheter

IQ ✚ 7 T80.219- **Unspecified infection due to central venous catheter**
Central line-associated infection NOS
Unspecified infection due to Hickman catheter
Unspecified infection due to peripherally inserted central catheter (PICC)
Unspecified infection due to portacath (port-a-cath)
Unspecified infection due to pulmonary artery catheter
Unspecified infection due to triple lumen catheter
Unspecified infection due to umbilical venous catheter

SP ✚ 7 T80.22X- **Acute infection following transfusion, infusion, or injection of blood and blood products**

SP ✚ 7 T80.29X- **Infection following other infusion, transfusion and therapeutic injection**

5 T80.3 **ABO incompatibility reaction due to transfusion of blood or blood products**
EXCLUDES 1 minor blood group antigens reactions (Duffy) (E) (K) (Kell) (Kidd) (Lewis) (M) (N) (P) (S) (T80.A-)

SP 7 T80.30X- **ABO incompatibility reaction due to transfusion of blood or blood products, unspecified**
ABO incompatibility blood transfusion NOS
Reaction to ABO incompatibility from transfusion NOS

6 T80.31 **ABO incompatibility with hemolytic transfusion reaction**

SP 7 T80.310- **ABO incompatibility with acute hemolytic transfusion reaction**
ABO incompatibility with hemolytic transfusion reaction less than 24 hours after transfusion
Acute hemolytic transfusion reaction (AHTR) due to ABO incompatibility

SP 7 T80.311- **ABO incompatibility with delayed hemolytic transfusion reaction**
ABO incompatibility with hemolytic transfusion reaction 24 hours or more after transfusion
Delayed hemolytic transfusion reaction (DHTR) due to ABO incompatibility

SP 7 T80.319- **ABO incompatibility with hemolytic transfusion reaction, unspecified**

★ New ▲ Revised Px Primary **SP** PDGM Px **SL** Low CoM **SH** High CoM **IQ** Quest. Encounter Ⓗ Hospice non-cancer Dx ⬛ Unspecified **M** *Manifestation*

ABO incompatibility with
hemolytic transfusion reaction at
unspecified time after transfusion

Hemolytic transfusion reaction
(HTR) due to ABO
incompatibility NOS

**SP ☑ T80.39X-   Other ABO incompatibility
reaction due to transfusion of
blood or blood products**
Delayed serologic transfusion
reaction (DSTR) from ABO
incompatibility
Other ABO incompatible blood
transfusion
Other reaction to ABO incompatible
blood transfusion

**⑤ T80.4   Rh incompatibility reaction due to
transfusion of blood or blood products**
Reaction due to incompatibility of Rh
antigens (C) (c) (D) (E) (e)

**SP ☑ T80.40X-   Rh incompatibility reaction due
to transfusion of blood or blood
products, unspecified**
Reaction due to Rh factor in
transfusion NOS
Rh incompatible blood transfusion
NOS

**⑥ T80.41   Rh incompatibility with hemolytic
transfusion reaction**

**SP ☑ T80.410-   Rh incompatibility with acute
hemolytic transfusion reaction**
Acute hemolytic transfusion
reaction (AHTR) due to Rh
incompatibility
Rh incompatibility with hemolytic
transfusion reaction less than 24
hours after transfusion

**SP ☑ T80.411-   Rh incompatibility with delayed
hemolytic transfusion reaction**
Delayed hemolytic transfusion
reaction (DHTR) due to Rh
incompatibility
Rh incompatibility with hemolytic
transfusion reaction 24 hours or
more after transfusion

**SP ☑ T80.419-   Rh incompatibility with
hemolytic transfusion reaction,
unspecified**
Rh incompatibility with hemolytic
transfusion reaction at
unspecified time after transfusion
Hemolytic transfusion reaction
(HTR) due to Rh incompatibility
NOS

**SP ☑ T80.49X-   Other Rh incompatibility reaction
due to transfusion of blood or
blood products**
Delayed serologic transfusion
reaction (DSTR) from Rh
incompatibility
Other reaction to Rh incompatible
blood transfusion

**⑤ T80.A   Non-ABO incompatibility reaction due
to transfusion of blood or blood
products**
Reaction due to incompatibility of minor
antigens (Duffy) (Kell) (Kidd) (Lewis)
(M) (N) (P) (S)

**SP ☑ T80.A0X-   Non-ABO incompatibility
reaction due to transfusion of
blood or blood products,
unspecified**
Non-ABO antigen incompatibility
reaction from transfusion NOS

**⑥ T80.A1   Non-ABO incompatibility with
hemolytic transfusion reaction**

**SP ☑ T80.A10-   Non-ABO incompatibility with
acute hemolytic transfusion
reaction**
Acute hemolytic transfusion
reaction (AHTR) due to non-
ABO incompatibility
Non-ABO incompatibility with
hemolytic transfusion reaction
less than 24 hours after
transfusion

**SP ☑ T80.A11-   Non-ABO incompatibility with
delayed hemolytic transfusion
reaction**
Delayed hemolytic transfusion
reaction (DHTR) due to non-
ABO incompatibility
Non-ABO incompatibility with
hemolytic transfusion reaction 24
or more hours after transfusion

**SP ☑ T80.A19-   Non-ABO incompatibility with
hemolytic transfusion reaction,
unspecified**
Hemolytic transfusion reaction
(HTR) due to non-ABO
incompatibility NOS
Non-ABO incompatibility with
hemolytic transfusion reaction at
unspecified time after transfusion

**SP ☑ T80.A9X-   Other non-ABO incompatibility
reaction due to transfusion of
blood or blood products**
Delayed serologic transfusion
reaction (DSTR) from non-ABO
incompatibility
Other reaction to non-ABO
incompatible blood transfusion

⑤ T80.5   Anaphylactic reaction due to serum
Allergic shock due to serum
Anaphylactic shock due to serum
Anaphylactoid reaction due to serum
Anaphylaxis due to serum
EXCLUDES 1   ABO incompatibility
reaction due to transfusion
of blood or blood products
(T80.3-)
allergic reaction or shock
NOS (T78.2)
anaphylactic reaction or
shock NOS (T78.2)
anaphylactic reaction or
shock due to adverse effect
of correct medicinal
substance properly
administered (T88.6)
other serum reaction
(T80.6-)

**SP ☑ T80.51X-   Anaphylactic reaction due to
administration of blood and blood
products**

**SP ☑ T80.52X-   Anaphylactic reaction due to
vaccination**

☐4th digit required   ☐5th digit required   ☐6th digit required   ☐7th digit required   ☑7th digit placeholder   ✚Additional code   ⊟Laterality

1726   *DecisionHealth's* FY 2020 Complete Home Health ICD-10-CM Diagnosis Coding Manual

SP ⚂ T80.59X- Anaphylactic reaction due to other serum

⑤ T80.6 Other serum reactions

Intoxication by serum
Protein sickness
Serum rash
Serum sickness
Serum urticaria

> **EXCLUDES 2** serum hepatitis (B16-B19)

SP ⚂ T80.61X- Other serum reaction due to administration of blood and blood products

SP ⚂ T80.62X- Other serum reaction due to vaccination

SP ⚂ T80.69X- Other serum reaction due to other serum

Code also:
, if applicable, arthropathy in hypersensitivity reactions classified elsewhere (M36.4)

⑤ T80.8 Other complications following infusion, transfusion and therapeutic injection

⑥ T80.81 Extravasation of vesicant agent

Infiltration of vesicant agent

SP ⑺ T80.810- Extravasation of vesicant antineoplastic chemotherapy

Infiltration of vesicant antineoplastic chemotherapy

SP ⑺ T80.818- Extravasation of other vesicant agent

Infiltration of other vesicant agent

SP ➕ ⚂ T80.89X- Other complications following infusion, transfusion and therapeutic injection

Delayed serologic transfusion reaction (DSTR), unspecified incompatibility

Use additional code to identify graft-versus-host reaction, if applicable, (D89.81-)

⑤ T80.9 Unspecified complication following infusion, transfusion and therapeutic injection

SP ⚂ T80.90X- Unspecified complication following infusion and therapeutic injection

⑥ T80.91 Hemolytic transfusion reaction, unspecified incompatibility

> **EXCLUDES 1** ABO incompatibility with hemolytic transfusion reaction (T80.31-)
> Non-ABO incompatibility with hemolytic transfusion reaction (T80.A1-)
> Rh incompatibility with hemolytic transfusion reaction (T80.41-)

SP ⑺ T80.910- Acute hemolytic transfusion reaction, unspecified incompatibility

SP ⑺ T80.911- Delayed hemolytic transfusion reaction, unspecified incompatibility

SP ⑺ T80.919- Hemolytic transfusion reaction, unspecified incompatibility, unspecified as acute or delayed

Hemolytic transfusion reaction NOS

SP ⑺ T80.92X- Unspecified transfusion reaction

Transfusion reaction NOS

➕ ④ T81 Complications of procedures, not elsewhere classified

Use additional code for adverse effect, if applicable, to identify drug (T36-T50 with fifth or sixth character 5)

> **EXCLUDES 2** complications following immunization (T88.0-T88.1)
> complications following infusion, transfusion and therapeutic injection (T80.-)
> complications of transplanted organs and tissue (T86.-)
> specified complications classified elsewhere, such as:
> complication of prosthetic devices, implants and grafts (T82-T85)
> dermatitis due to drugs and medicaments (L23.3, L24.4, L25.1, L27.0-L27.1)
> endosseous dental implant failure (M27.6-)
> floppy iris syndrome (IFIS) (intraoperative) H21.81
> intraoperative and postprocedural complications of specific body system (D78.-, E36.-, E89.-, G97.3-, G97.4, H59.3-, H59.-, H95.2-, H95.3, I97.4-, I97.5, J95, K91.-, L76.-, M96.-, N99.-)
> ostomy complications (J95.0-, K94.-, N99.5-)
> plateau iris syndrome (post-iridectomy) (postprocedural) H21.82
> poisoning and toxic effects of drugs and chemicals (T36-T65 with fifth or sixth character 1-4 or 6)

The appropriate 7th character is to be added to each code from category T81
A   initial encounter
D   subsequent encounter
S   sequela

CODING TIPS ✓ No aftercare code applies, including dressing changes, drain care, and suture removal. 7th character 'D' is the default for home care and hospice when providing aftercare for a healing or resolving condition; 'A' is used for active treatment such as antibiotics or more than routine wound care; 'S' may be used to indicate a residual condition after the original injury has healed. Once complication is repaired in the acute setting, continue to code the complication in home care and hospice with 7th character D if healing/resolving.

➕ ⑤ T81.1 Postprocedural shock

★ New ▲ Revised Px Primary SP PDGM Px SL Low CoM SH High CoM IQ Quest. Encounter H Hospice non-cancer Dx Unspecified M *Manifestation*

DecisionHealth's FY 2020 Complete Home Health ICD-10-CM Diagnosis Coding Manual

1727

Chapter 19

S00-T88

Shock during or resulting from a procedure, not elsewhere classified

EXCLUDES 1　anaphylactic shock NOS (T78.2)
anaphylactic shock due to correct substance properly administered (T88.6)
anaphylactic shock due to serum (T80.5-)
anesthetic shock (T88.2)
electric shock (T75.4)
obstetric shock (O75.1)
septic shock (R65.21)
shock following abortion or ectopic or molar pregnancy (O00-O07, O08.3)
traumatic shock (T79.4)

SP + ✓ **T81.10X-** **Postprocedural shock unspecified**

Collapse NOS during or resulting from a procedure, not elsewhere classified
Postprocedural failure of peripheral circulation
Postprocedural shock NOS

SP + ✓ **T81.11X-** **Postprocedural cardiogenic shock**

IQ + ✓ **T81.12X-** **Postprocedural septic shock**

Postprocedural endotoxic shock resulting from a procedure, not elsewhere classified
Postprocedural gram-negative shock resulting from a procedure, not elsewhere classified
Code first:
underlying infection
Use additional code, to identify any associated acute organ dysfunction, if applicable

GUIDELINES　Section I.C.1.d.5)(b-c)

For infections following a procedure, a code from T81.40, to T81.43 Infection following a procedure, or a code from O86.00 to O86.03, Infection of obstetric surgical wound, that identifies the site of the infection should be coded first, if known. Assign an additional code for sepsis following a procedure (T81.44) or sepsis following an obstetrical procedure (O86.04). Use an additional code to identify the infectious agent. If the patient has severe sepsis, the appropriate code from subcategory R65.2 should also be assigned with the additional code(s) for any acute organ dysfunction.

If a postprocedural infection has resulted in postprocedural septic shock, assign the codes indicated above for sepsis due to a postprocedural infection, followed by code T81.12-, Postprocedural septic shock. Do not assign code R65.21, Severe sepsis with septic shock. Additional code(s) should be assigned for any acute organ dysfunction.

CODING TIPS ✓　**Documentation:** Only assign T81.12- when the provider diagnostic statements clearly indicate septic shock as a postprocedural complication.

SP + ✓ **T81.19X-** **Other postprocedural shock**
Postprocedural hypovolemic shock

+ 5 **T81.3** **Disruption of wound, not elsewhere classified**

Disruption of any suture materials or other closure methods

EXCLUDES 1　breakdown (mechanical) of permanent sutures (T85.612)
displacement of permanent sutures (T85.622)
disruption of cesarean delivery wound (O90.0)
disruption of perineal obstetric wound (O90.1)
mechanical complication of permanent sutures NEC (T85.692)

CODING TIPS ✓　No aftercare code applies including dressing changes, drain care, and suture removal. The 7th character "D" is the default for home care and hospice when providing aftercare for a healing or resolving condition; "A" is used for active treatment such as antibiotics or more than routine wound care; "S" may be used to indicate a residual condition after the original injury has healed.

SP + ✓ **T81.30X-** **Disruption of wound, unspecified**
Disruption of wound NOS

Chapter 19

S00-T88

---

⁴ 4th digit required　　⁵ 5th digit required　　⁶ 6th digit required　　⁷ 7th digit required　　✓ 7th digit placeholder　　+ Additional code　　⊟ Laterality

1728　　*DecisionHealth's* FY 2020 Complete Home Health ICD-10-CM Diagnosis Coding Manual

CODING TIPS ✓ Code T81.30x- should not be used as it indicates unspecified wound, not unspecified surgical wound.

SP ✚ ☑ T81.31X- Disruption of external operation (surgical) wound, not elsewhere classified

Dehiscence of operation wound NOS

Disruption of operation wound NOS

Disruption or dehiscence of closure of cornea

Disruption or dehiscence of closure of mucosa

Disruption or dehiscence of closure of skin and subcutaneous tissue

Full-thickness skin disruption or dehiscence

Superficial disruption or dehiscence of operation wound

EXCLUDES 1 dehiscence of amputation stump (T87.81)

CODING TIPS ✓ T81.31x- indicates external dehiscence of a surgical wound, as well as dehiscence of a surgical wound unspecified, whether external or internal. Reference the inclusion note for examples of external dehiscence. This code is a NEC code and there may be another more specific code for dehiscence that should be used instead.

SP ✚ ☑ T81.32X- Disruption of internal operation (surgical) wound, not elsewhere classified

Deep disruption or dehiscence of operation wound NOS

Disruption or dehiscence of closure of internal organ or other internal tissue

Disruption or dehiscence of closure of muscle or muscle flap

Disruption or dehiscence of closure of ribs or rib cage

Disruption or dehiscence of closure of skull or craniotomy

Disruption or dehiscence of closure of sternum or sternotomy

Disruption or dehiscence of closure of tendon or ligament

Disruption or dehiscence of closure of superficial or muscular fascia

CODING TIPS ✓ T81.32x- indicates internal dehiscence of a surgical wound. Reference the inclusion note for examples of internal dehiscence.This code is a NEC code and there may be another more specific code for dehiscence that should be used instead. Note the inclusion note at this code.

SP ✚ ☑ T81.33X- Disruption of traumatic injury wound repair

Disruption or dehiscence of closure of traumatic laceration (external) (internal)

CODING TIPS ✓ Assign code T81.33- for a repaired (sutured) traumatic laceration, which has dehisced. Also code the traumatic wound.

✚ S T81.4 Infection following a procedure

Wound abscess following a procedure

Use additional code to identify infection

Use additional code (R65.2-) to identify severe sepsis, if applicable

EXCLUDES 2 bleb associated endophthalmitis (H59.4-)

infection due to infusion, transfusion and therapeutic injection (T80.2-)

infection due to prosthetic devices, implants and grafts (T82.6-T82.7, T83.5-T83.6, T84.5-T84.7, T85.7)

obstetric surgical wound infection (O86.0-)

postprocedural fever NOS (R50.82)

postprocedural retroperitoneal abscess (K68.11)

GUIDELINES Section I.C.1.d.5)(b-c)

For infections following a procedure, a code from T81.40, to T81.43 Infection following a procedure, or a code from O86.00 to O86.03, Infection of obstetric surgical wound, that identifies the site of the infection should be coded first, if known. Assign an additional code for sepsis following a procedure (T81.44) or sepsis following an obstetrical procedure (O86.04). Use an additional code to identify the infectious agent. If the patient has severe sepsis, the appropriate code from subcategory R65.2 should also be assigned with the additional code(s) for any acute organ dysfunction.

If a postprocedural infection has resulted in postprocedural septic shock, assign the codes indicated above for sepsis due to a postprocedural infection, followed by code T81.12-, Postprocedural septic shock. Do not assign code R65.21, Severe sepsis with septic shock. Additional code(s) should be assigned for any acute organ dysfunction.

CODING TIPS ✓ Assign a specific code from the T81.4- category to indicate post-operative infections such as postprocedural sepsis, postoperative wound infections, and intra-abdominal abscess following a procedure. Surgical site infections are commonly classified according to their depth: superficial incisional, deep incisional, and organ/space infection.

Chapter 19

S00-T88

★ New ▲ Revised Px Primary SP PDGM Px SL Low CoM SH High CoM IQ Quest. Encounter H Hospice non-cancer Dx Unspecified M *Manifestation*

DecisionHealth's FY 2020 Complete Home Health ICD-10-CM Diagnosis Coding Manual

1729

CODING TIPS ✓ No aftercare code applies including dressing changes, drain care, and suture removal. The 7th character "D" is the default for home care and hospice when providing aftercare for a healing or resolving condition; "A" is used for active treatment such as antibiotics or more than routine wound care; "S" may be used to indicate a residual condition after the original injury has healed.

SP + ☑ T81.40X- **Infection following a procedure, unspecified**

> **CODING TIPS ✓** Avoid using this code for an infected surgical wound. The default code is T81.49-.

SP + ☑ T81.41X- **Infection following a procedure, superficial incisional surgical site**
Subcutaneous abscess following a procedure
Stitch abscess following a procedure

> **CODING TIPS ✓** A superficial incisional infection involves only the skin and subcutaneous tissue and may be indicated by localized signs such as redness, pain, heat or swelling at the site of the incision or by the drainage of pus.

SP + ☑ T81.42X- **Infection following a procedure, deep incisional surgical site**
Intra-muscular abscess following a procedure

> **CODING TIPS ✓** A deep incisional infection involves deep tissues, such as fascial and muscle layers, and may be indicated by the presence of pus or an abscess, fever with tenderness of the wound, or separation of incision edges exposing deeper tissues.

SP + ☑ T81.43X- **Infection following a procedure, organ and space surgical site**
Intra-abdominal abscess following a procedure
Subphrenic abscess following a procedure

> **CODING TIPS ✓** An organ and space infection involves any part of the anatomy in organs and spaces other than the incision, which was opened or manipulated during operation, such as the joint or the peritoneum, and may be indicated by the drainage of pus or the formation of an abscess detected by histopathological or radiological examination or during re-operation; does not include organ infection.

SP + ☑ T81.44X- **Sepsis following a procedure**
Use additional code to identify the sepsis

> **CODING TIPS ✓** This code is used for postprocedural sepsis. Code the specified infection first, then T81.44-, then the A code for the sepsis.

SP + ☑ T81.49X- **Infection following a procedure, other surgical site**

+ 5 T81.5 **Complications of foreign body accidentally left in body following procedure**

+ 6 T81.50 **Unspecified complication of foreign body accidentally left in body following procedure**

🔲 IQ + 7 T81.500- **Unspecified complication of foreign body accidentally left in body following surgical operation**

🔲 IQ + 7 T81.501- **Unspecified complication of foreign body accidentally left in body following infusion or transfusion**

🔲 IQ + 7 T81.502- **Unspecified complication of foreign body accidentally left in body following kidney dialysis**

🔲 IQ + 7 T81.503- **Unspecified complication of foreign body accidentally left in body following injection or immunization**

🔲 IQ + 7 T81.504- **Unspecified complication of foreign body accidentally left in body following endoscopic examination**

🔲 IQ + 7 T81.505- **Unspecified complication of foreign body accidentally left in body following heart catheterization**

🔲 IQ + 7 T81.506- **Unspecified complication of foreign body accidentally left in body following aspiration, puncture or other catheterization**

🔲 IQ + 7 T81.507- **Unspecified complication of foreign body accidentally left in body following removal of catheter or packing**

🔲 IQ + 7 T81.508- **Unspecified complication of foreign body accidentally left in body following other procedure**

🔲 IQ + 7 T81.509- **Unspecified complication of foreign body accidentally left in body following unspecified procedure**

+ 6 T81.51 **Adhesions due to foreign body accidentally left in body following procedure**

🔲 SP + 7 T81.510- **Adhesions due to foreign body accidentally left in body following surgical operation**

🔲 SP + 7 T81.511- **Adhesions due to foreign body accidentally left in body following infusion or transfusion**

🔲 SP + 7 T81.512- **Adhesions due to foreign body accidentally left in body following kidney dialysis**

🔲 SP + 7 T81.513- **Adhesions due to foreign body accidentally left in body following injection or immunization**

🔲 SP + 7 T81.514- **Adhesions due to foreign body accidentally left in body following endoscopic examination**

---

4 4th digit required   5 5th digit required   6 6th digit required   7 7th digit required   ☑ 7th digit placeholder   + Additional code   🔲 Laterality

1730   *DecisionHealth's* FY 2020 Complete Home Health ICD-10-CM Diagnosis Coding Manual

Chapter 19

S00-T88

☐ SP ✚ ⑦ T81.515- Adhesions due to foreign body accidentally left in body following heart catheterization

☐ SP ✚ ⑦ T81.516- Adhesions due to foreign body accidentally left in body following aspiration, puncture or other catheterization

☐ SP ✚ ⑦ T81.517- Adhesions due to foreign body accidentally left in body following removal of catheter or packing

☐ SP ✚ ⑦ T81.518- Adhesions due to foreign body accidentally left in body following other procedure

☐ IQ ✚ ⑦ T81.519- Adhesions due to foreign body accidentally left in body following unspecified procedure

✚ ⑥ T81.52 Obstruction due to foreign body accidentally left in body following procedure

☐ SP ✚ ⑦ T81.520- Obstruction due to foreign body accidentally left in body following surgical operation

☐ SP ✚ ⑦ T81.521- Obstruction due to foreign body accidentally left in body following infusion or transfusion

☐ SP ✚ ⑦ T81.522- Obstruction due to foreign body accidentally left in body following kidney dialysis

☐ SP ✚ ⑦ T81.523- Obstruction due to foreign body accidentally left in body following injection or immunization

☐ SP ✚ ⑦ T81.524- Obstruction due to foreign body accidentally left in body following endoscopic examination

☐ SP ✚ ⑦ T81.525- Obstruction due to foreign body accidentally left in body following heart catheterization

☐ SP ✚ ⑦ T81.526- Obstruction due to foreign body accidentally left in body following aspiration, puncture or other catheterization

☐ SP ✚ ⑦ T81.527- Obstruction due to foreign body accidentally left in body following removal of catheter or packing

☐ SP ✚ ⑦ T81.528- Obstruction due to foreign body accidentally left in body following other procedure

☐ SP ✚ ⑦ T81.529- Obstruction due to foreign body accidentally left in body following unspecified procedure

✚ ⑥ T81.53 Perforation due to foreign body accidentally left in body following procedure

☐ SP ✚ ⑦ T81.530- Perforation due to foreign body accidentally left in body following surgical operation

☐ SP ✚ ⑦ T81.531- Perforation due to foreign body accidentally left in body following infusion or transfusion

☐ SP ✚ ⑦ T81.532- Perforation due to foreign body accidentally left in body following kidney dialysis

☐ SP ✚ ⑦ T81.533- Perforation due to foreign body accidentally left in body following injection or immunization

☐ SP ✚ ⑦ T81.534- Perforation due to foreign body accidentally left in body following endoscopic examination

☐ SP ✚ ⑦ T81.535- Perforation due to foreign body accidentally left in body following heart catheterization

☐ SP ✚ ⑦ T81.536- Perforation due to foreign body accidentally left in body following aspiration, puncture or other catheterization

☐ SP ✚ ⑦ T81.537- Perforation due to foreign body accidentally left in body following removal of catheter or packing

☐ SP ✚ ⑦ T81.538- Perforation due to foreign body accidentally left in body following other procedure

☐ SP ✚ ⑦ T81.539- Perforation due to foreign body accidentally left in body following unspecified procedure

✚ ⑥ T81.59 Other complications of foreign body accidentally left in body following procedure

EXCLUDES 2 obstruction or perforation due to prosthetic devices and implants intentionally left in body (T82.0-T82.5, T83.0-T83.4, T83.7, T84.0-T84.4, T85.0-T85.6)

☐ SP ✚ ⑦ T81.590- Other complications of foreign body accidentally left in body following surgical operation

☐ SP ✚ ⑦ T81.591- Other complications of foreign body accidentally left in body following infusion or transfusion

☐ SP ✚ ⑦ T81.592- Other complications of foreign body accidentally left in body following kidney dialysis

☐ SP ✚ ⑦ T81.593- Other complications of foreign body accidentally left in body following injection or immunization

☐ SP ✚ ⑦ T81.594- Other complications of foreign body accidentally left in body following endoscopic examination

☐ SP ✚ ⑦ T81.595- Other complications of foreign body accidentally left in body following heart catheterization

☐ SP ✚ ⑦ T81.596- Other complications of foreign body accidentally left in body following aspiration, puncture or other catheterization

☐ SP ✚ ⑦ T81.597- Other complications of foreign body accidentally left in body following removal of catheter or packing

☐ SP ✚ ⑦ T81.598- Other complications of foreign body accidentally left in body following other procedure

Chapter 19

S00-T88

★ New ▲ Revised Px Primary SP PDGM Px SL Low CoM SH High CoM IQ Quest. Encounter H Hospice non-cancer Dx Unspecified M Manifestation

DecisionHealth's FY 2020 Complete Home Health ICD-10-CM Diagnosis Coding Manual

1731

⊟ IQ ✛ 7 T81.599- **Other complications of foreign body accidentally left in body following unspecified procedure**

✛ 5 T81.6 **Acute reaction to foreign substance accidentally left during a procedure**

> EXCLUDES 2   complications of foreign body accidentally left in body cavity or operation wound following procedure (T81.5-)

IQ ✛ 7 T81.60X- **Unspecified acute reaction to foreign substance accidentally left during a procedure**

SP ✛ 7 T81.61X- **Aseptic peritonitis due to foreign substance accidentally left during a procedure**
Chemical peritonitis

SP ✛ 7 T81.69X- **Other acute reaction to foreign substance accidentally left during a procedure**

✛ 5 T81.7 **Vascular complications following a procedure, not elsewhere classified**
Air embolism following procedure NEC
Phlebitis or thrombophlebitis resulting from a procedure

> EXCLUDES 1   embolism complicating abortion or ectopic or molar pregnancy (O00-O07, O08.2)
> embolism complicating pregnancy, childbirth and the puerperium (O88.-)
> traumatic embolism (T79.0)

> EXCLUDES 2   embolism due to prosthetic devices, implants and grafts (T82.8-, T83.81, T84.8-, T85.81-)
> embolism following infusion, transfusion and therapeutic injection (T80.0)

✛ 6 T81.71 **Complication of artery following a procedure, not elsewhere classified**

SP ✛ 7 T81.710- **Complication of mesenteric artery following a procedure, not elsewhere classified**

SP ✛ 7 T81.711- **Complication of renal artery following a procedure, not elsewhere classified**

SP ✛ 7 T81.718- **Complication of other artery following a procedure, not elsewhere classified**

SP ✛ 7 T81.719- **Complication of unspecified artery following a procedure, not elsewhere classified**

SP ✛ 7 T81.72X- **Complication of vein following a procedure, not elsewhere classified**

✛ 5 T81.8 **Other complications of procedures, not elsewhere classified**

> EXCLUDES 2   hypothermia following anesthesia (T88.51)
> malignant hyperpyrexia due to anesthesia (T88.3)

SP ✛ 7 T81.81X- **Complication of inhalation therapy**

SP ✛ 7 T81.82X- **Emphysema (subcutaneous) resulting from a procedure**

SP ✛ 7 T81.83X- **Persistent postprocedural fistula**

SP ✛ 7 T81.89X- **Other complications of procedures, not elsewhere classified**
Use additional code to specify complication, such as:
postprocedural delirium (F05)

> **CODING TIPS ✓** This code is used for non-healing surgical wounds when no other code applies. It is a NEC code so ensure that another complication code is not more appropriate. For example, do not switch from the infected surgical wound or dehisced surgical wound to T81.89x- just because the wound remains open. The 'use additional code' note does not apply when using the code for non-healing surgical wounds.

⊟ IQ ✛ 7 T81.9XX- **Unspecified complication of procedure**

4 T82 **Complications of cardiac and vascular prosthetic devices, implants and grafts**

> EXCLUDES 2   failure and rejection of transplanted organs and tissue (T86.-)

> The appropriate 7th character is to be added to each code from category T82
> A   initial encounter
> D   subsequent encounter
> S   sequela

> **CODING TIPS ✓** No aftercare code applies, including dressing changes, drain care, and suture removal. 7th character 'D' is the default for home care and hospice when providing aftercare for a healing or resolving condition; 'A' is used for active treatment such as antibiotics or more than routine wound care; 'S' may be used to indicate a residual condition after the original injury has healed. Once complication is repaired in the acute setting, continue to code the complication in home care and hospice with 7th character D if healing/resolving.

5 T82.0 **Mechanical complication of heart valve prosthesis**
Mechanical complication of artificial heart valve

> EXCLUDES 1   mechanical complication of biological heart valve graft (T82.22-)

> **CODING TIPS ✓** Do not use Z95.2 when the heart valve is complicated.

SP 7 T82.01X- **Breakdown (mechanical) of heart valve prosthesis**

SP 7 T82.02X- **Displacement of heart valve prosthesis**
Malposition of heart valve prosthesis

SP 7 T82.03X- **Leakage of heart valve prosthesis**

SP 7 T82.09X- **Other mechanical complication of heart valve prosthesis**
Obstruction (mechanical) of heart valve prosthesis
Perforation of heart valve prosthesis
Protrusion of heart valve prosthesis

---

4 4th digit required   5 5th digit required   6 6th digit required   7 7th digit required   7 7th digit placeholder   ✛ Additional code   ⊟ Laterality

1732   DecisionHealth's FY 2020 Complete Home Health ICD-10-CM Diagnosis Coding Manual

Chapter 19

S00-T88

⑤ **T82.1 Mechanical complication of cardiac electronic device**

⑥ **T82.11 Breakdown (mechanical) of cardiac electronic device**

SP ⑦ **T82.110- Breakdown (mechanical) of cardiac electrode**

SP ⑦ **T82.111- Breakdown (mechanical) of cardiac pulse generator (battery)**

SP ⑦ **T82.118- Breakdown (mechanical) of other cardiac electronic device**

!Q ⑦ **T82.119- Breakdown (mechanical) of unspecified cardiac electronic device**

⑥ **T82.12 Displacement of cardiac electronic device**

Malposition of cardiac electronic device

SP ⑦ **T82.120- Displacement of cardiac electrode**

SP ⑦ **T82.121- Displacement of cardiac pulse generator (battery)**

SP ⑦ **T82.128- Displacement of other cardiac electronic device**

!Q ⑦ **T82.129- Displacement of unspecified cardiac electronic device**

⑥ **T82.19 Other mechanical complication of cardiac electronic device**

Leakage of cardiac electronic device
Obstruction of cardiac electronic device
Perforation of cardiac electronic device
Protrusion of cardiac electronic device

SP ⑦ **T82.190- Other mechanical complication of cardiac electrode**

SP ⑦ **T82.191- Other mechanical complication of cardiac pulse generator (battery)**

SP ⑦ **T82.198- Other mechanical complication of other cardiac electronic device**

!Q ⑦ **T82.199- Other mechanical complication of unspecified cardiac device**

⑤ **T82.2 Mechanical complication of coronary artery bypass graft and biological heart valve graft**

EXCLUDES 1 mechanical complication of artificial heart valve prosthesis (T82.0-)

CODING TIPS ✓ Do not use Z95.5 when the bypass graft is complicated.

⑥ **T82.21 Mechanical complication of coronary artery bypass graft**

SP ⑦ **T82.211- Breakdown (mechanical) of coronary artery bypass graft**

SP ⑦ **T82.212- Displacement of coronary artery bypass graft**

Malposition of coronary artery bypass graft

SP ⑦ **T82.213- Leakage of coronary artery bypass graft**

SP ⑦ **T82.218- Other mechanical complication of coronary artery bypass graft**

Obstruction, mechanical of coronary artery bypass graft
Perforation of coronary artery bypass graft
Protrusion of coronary artery bypass graft

⑥ **T82.22 Mechanical complication of biological heart valve graft**

SP ⑦ **T82.221- Breakdown (mechanical) of biological heart valve graft**

SP ⑦ **T82.222- Displacement of biological heart valve graft**

Malposition of biological heart valve graft

SP ⑦ **T82.223- Leakage of biological heart valve graft**

SP ⑦ **T82.228- Other mechanical complication of biological heart valve graft**

Obstruction of biological heart valve graft
Perforation of biological heart valve graft
Protrusion of biological heart valve graft

⑤ **T82.3 Mechanical complication of other vascular grafts**

⑥ **T82.31 Breakdown (mechanical) of other vascular grafts**

SP ⑦ **T82.310- Breakdown (mechanical) of aortic (bifurcation) graft (replacement)**

SP ⑦ **T82.311- Breakdown (mechanical) of carotid arterial graft (bypass)**

SP ⑦ **T82.312- Breakdown (mechanical) of femoral arterial graft (bypass)**

SP ⑦ **T82.318- Breakdown (mechanical) of other vascular grafts**

!Q ⑦ **T82.319- Breakdown (mechanical) of unspecified vascular grafts**

⑥ **T82.32 Displacement of other vascular grafts**

Malposition of other vascular grafts

SP ⑦ **T82.320- Displacement of aortic (bifurcation) graft (replacement)**

SP ⑦ **T82.321- Displacement of carotid arterial graft (bypass)**

SP ⑦ **T82.322- Displacement of femoral arterial graft (bypass)**

SP ⑦ **T82.328- Displacement of other vascular grafts**

!Q ⑦ **T82.329- Displacement of unspecified vascular grafts**

⑥ **T82.33 Leakage of other vascular grafts**

SP ⑦ **T82.330- Leakage of aortic (bifurcation) graft (replacement)**

SP ⑦ **T82.331- Leakage of carotid arterial graft (bypass)**

SP ⑦ **T82.332- Leakage of femoral arterial graft (bypass)**

SP ⑦ **T82.338- Leakage of other vascular grafts**

!Q ⑦ **T82.339- Leakage of unspecified vascular graft**

⑥ **T82.39 Other mechanical complication of other vascular grafts**

Obstruction (mechanical) of other vascular grafts
Perforation of other vascular grafts
Protrusion of other vascular grafts

SP ⑦ **T82.390- Other mechanical complication of aortic (bifurcation) graft (replacement)**

SP ⑦ **T82.391- Other mechanical complication of carotid arterial graft (bypass)**

★ New ▲ Revised Px Primary SP PDGM Px SL Low CoM SH High CoM !Q Quest. Encounter H Hospice non-cancer Dx Unspecified M Manifestation

DecisionHealth's FY 2020 Complete Home Health ICD-10-CM Diagnosis Coding Manual

1733

SP 7 T82.392- Other mechanical complication of femoral arterial graft (bypass)

SP 7 T82.398- Other mechanical complication of other vascular grafts

!Q 7 T82.399- Other mechanical complication of unspecified vascular grafts

5 T82.4 Mechanical complication of vascular dialysis catheter
Mechanical complication of hemodialysis catheter

> **EXCLUDES 1** mechanical complication of intraperitoneal dialysis catheter (T85.62)

> **CODING TIPS ✓** Care for dialysis catheters under the home health benefit is limited to abandoned dialysis catheters. Code the reason that the dialysis catheter cannot be used.

!Q ☑ T82.41X- Breakdown (mechanical) of vascular dialysis catheter

!Q ☑ T82.42X- Displacement of vascular dialysis catheter
Malposition of vascular dialysis catheter

!Q ☑ T82.43X- Leakage of vascular dialysis catheter

!Q ☑ T82.49X- Other complication of vascular dialysis catheter
Obstruction (mechanical) of vascular dialysis catheter
Perforation of vascular dialysis catheter
Protrusion of vascular dialysis catheter

5 T82.5 Mechanical complication of other cardiac and vascular devices and implants

> **EXCLUDES 2** mechanical complication of epidural and subdural infusion catheter (T85.61)

6 T82.51 Breakdown (mechanical) of other cardiac and vascular devices and implants

!Q 7 T82.510- Breakdown (mechanical) of surgically created arteriovenous fistula

!Q 7 T82.511- Breakdown (mechanical) of surgically created arteriovenous shunt

SP 7 T82.512- Breakdown (mechanical) of artificial heart

SP 7 T82.513- Breakdown (mechanical) of balloon (counterpulsation) device

SP 7 T82.514- Breakdown (mechanical) of infusion catheter

SP 7 T82.515- Breakdown (mechanical) of umbrella device

SP 7 T82.518- Breakdown (mechanical) of other cardiac and vascular devices and implants

!Q 7 T82.519- Breakdown (mechanical) of unspecified cardiac and vascular devices and implants

6 T82.52 Displacement of other cardiac and vascular devices and implants
Malposition of other cardiac and vascular devices and implants

!Q 7 T82.520- Displacement of surgically created arteriovenous fistula

!Q 7 T82.521- Displacement of surgically created arteriovenous shunt

SP 7 T82.522- Displacement of artificial heart

SP 7 T82.523- Displacement of balloon (counterpulsation) device

SP 7 T82.524- Displacement of infusion catheter

SP 7 T82.525- Displacement of umbrella device

SP 7 T82.528- Displacement of other cardiac and vascular devices and implants

!Q 7 T82.529- Displacement of unspecified cardiac and vascular devices and implants

6 T82.53 Leakage of other cardiac and vascular devices and implants

!Q 7 T82.530- Leakage of surgically created arteriovenous fistula

!Q 7 T82.531- Leakage of surgically created arteriovenous shunt

SP 7 T82.532- Leakage of artificial heart

SP 7 T82.533- Leakage of balloon (counterpulsation) device

SP 7 T82.534- Leakage of infusion catheter

SP 7 T82.535- Leakage of umbrella device

SP 7 T82.538- Leakage of other cardiac and vascular devices and implants

!Q 7 T82.539- Leakage of unspecified cardiac and vascular devices and implants

6 T82.59 Other mechanical complication of other cardiac and vascular devices and implants
Obstruction (mechanical) of other cardiac and vascular devices and implants
Perforation of other cardiac and vascular devices and implants
Protrusion of other cardiac and vascular devices and implants

!Q 7 T82.590- Other mechanical complication of surgically created arteriovenous fistula

!Q 7 T82.591- Other mechanical complication of surgically created arteriovenous shunt

SP 7 T82.592- Other mechanical complication of artificial heart

SP 7 T82.593- Other mechanical complication of balloon (counterpulsation) device

SP 7 T82.594- Other mechanical complication of infusion catheter

SP 7 T82.595- Other mechanical complication of umbrella device

SP 7 T82.598- Other mechanical complication of other cardiac and vascular devices and implants

!Q 7 T82.599- Other mechanical complication of unspecified cardiac and vascular devices and implants

SP ✚ ☑ T82.6XX- Infection and inflammatory reaction due to cardiac valve prosthesis

---

4 4th digit required   **5** 5th digit required   **6** 6th digit required   **7** 7th digit required   **☑** 7th digit placeholder   **✚** Additional code   **☐** Laterality

1734   *DecisionHealth's* FY 2020 Complete Home Health ICD-10-CM Diagnosis Coding Manual

Chapter 19

S00-T88

Use additional code to identify infection

SP **✛** ☑ **T82.7XX-** **Infection and inflammatory reaction due to other cardiac and vascular devices, implants and grafts**

Use additional code to identify infection

⑤ **T82.8** **Other specified complications of cardiac and vascular prosthetic devices, implants and grafts**

⑥ **T82.81** **Embolism due to cardiac and vascular prosthetic devices, implants and grafts**

SP ⑦ **T82.817-** **Embolism due to cardiac prosthetic devices, implants and grafts**

SP ⑦ **T82.818-** **Embolism due to vascular prosthetic devices, implants and grafts**

⑥ **T82.82** **Fibrosis due to cardiac and vascular prosthetic devices, implants and grafts**

SP ⑦ **T82.827-** **Fibrosis due to cardiac prosthetic devices, implants and grafts**

SP ⑦ **T82.828-** **Fibrosis due to vascular prosthetic devices, implants and grafts**

⑥ **T82.83** **Hemorrhage due to cardiac and vascular prosthetic devices, implants and grafts**

SP ⑦ **T82.837-** **Hemorrhage due to cardiac prosthetic devices, implants and grafts**

SP ⑦ **T82.838-** **Hemorrhage due to vascular prosthetic devices, implants and grafts**

⑥ **T82.84** **Pain due to cardiac and vascular prosthetic devices, implants and grafts**

SP ⑦ **T82.847-** **Pain due to cardiac prosthetic devices, implants and grafts**

SP ⑦ **T82.848-** **Pain due to vascular prosthetic devices, implants and grafts**

⑥ **T82.85** **Stenosis due to cardiac and vascular prosthetic devices, implants and grafts**

CODING TIPS ✓ Approximately 30% of peripheral and bare metal coronary stents will restenose within a year of placement. This condition is variously called restenosis of stent, in-stent stenosis or in-stent restenosis (ISR). The area of in-stent stenosis has a different makeup than is seen in native areas of atherosclerotic plaque and vessel stenosis.

SP ⑦ **T82.855-** **Stenosis of coronary artery stent**
In-stent stenosis (restenosis) of coronary artery stent
Restenosis of coronary artery stent

SP ⑦ **T82.856-** **Stenosis of peripheral vascular stent**
In-stent stenosis (restenosis) of peripheral vascular stent
Restenosis of peripheral vascular stent

SP ⑦ **T82.857-** **Stenosis of other cardiac prosthetic devices, implants and grafts**

SP ⑦ **T82.858-** **Stenosis of other vascular prosthetic devices, implants and grafts**

⑥ **T82.86** **Thrombosis of cardiac and vascular prosthetic devices, implants and grafts**

SP ⑦ **T82.867-** **Thrombosis due to cardiac prosthetic devices, implants and grafts**

SP ⑦ **T82.868-** **Thrombosis due to vascular prosthetic devices, implants and grafts**

⑥ **T82.89** **Other specified complication of cardiac and vascular prosthetic devices, implants and grafts**

SP ⑦ **T82.897-** **Other specified complication of cardiac prosthetic devices, implants and grafts**

SP ⑦ **T82.898-** **Other specified complication of vascular prosthetic devices, implants and grafts**

IQ ☑ **T82.9XX-** **Unspecified complication of cardiac and vascular prosthetic device, implant and graft**

④ **T83** **Complications of genitourinary prosthetic devices, implants and grafts**

EXCLUDES 2 failure and rejection of transplanted organs and tissue (T86.-)

The appropriate 7th character is to be added to each code from category T83
A initial encounter
D subsequent encounter
S sequela

CODING TIPS ✓ No aftercare code applies, including dressing changes, drain care, and suture removal. 7th character 'D' is the default for home care and hospice when providing aftercare for a healing or resolving condition; 'A' is used for active treatment such as antibiotics or more than routine wound care; 'S' may be used to indicate a residual condition after the original injury has healed. Once complication is repaired in the acute setting, continue to code the complication in home care and hospice with 7th character D if healing/resolving.

⑤ **T83.0** **Mechanical complication of urinary catheter**

EXCLUDES 2 complications of stoma of urinary tract (N99.5-)

CODING TIPS ✓ These codes are for mechanical complications of urinary catheters of all kinds. They may be coded with the complication of stoma code, as applicable (N99.5-). Do not use Z46.6 when a complication of the urinary catheter is documented.

⑥ **T83.01** **Breakdown (mechanical) of urinary catheter**

SP ⑦ **T83.010-** **Breakdown (mechanical) of cystostomy catheter**

SP ⑦ **T83.011-** **Breakdown (mechanical) of indwelling urethral catheter**

★ New ▲ Revised **Px** Primary **SP** PDGM Px **SL** Low CoM **SH** High CoM **IQ** Quest. Encounter **H** Hospice non-cancer Dx Unspecified **M** *Manifestation*

DecisionHealth's FY 2020 Complete Home Health ICD-10-CM Diagnosis Coding Manual

1735

SP **7** **T83.012-** **Breakdown (mechanical) of nephrostomy catheter**

SP **7** **T83.018-** **Breakdown (mechanical) of other urinary catheter**
Breakdown (mechanical) of Hopkins catheter
Breakdown (mechanical) of ileostomy catheter
Breakdown (mechanical) urostomy catheter

6 **T83.02** **Displacement of urinary catheter**
Malposition of urinary catheter

SP **7** **T83.020-** **Displacement of cystostomy catheter**

SP **7** **T83.021-** **Displacement of indwelling urethral catheter**

SP **7** **T83.022-** **Displacement of nephrostomy catheter**

SP **7** **T83.028-** **Displacement of other urinary catheter**
Displacement of Hopkins catheter
Displacement of ileostomy catheter
Displacement of urostomy catheter

6 **T83.03** **Leakage of urinary catheter**

SP **7** **T83.030-** **Leakage of cystostomy catheter**

SP **7** **T83.031-** **Leakage of indwelling urethral catheter**

SP **7** **T83.032-** **Leakage of nephrostomy catheter**

SP **7** **T83.038-** **Leakage of other urinary catheter**
Leakage of Hopkins catheter
Leakage of ileostomy catheter
Leakage of urostomy catheter

6 **T83.09** **Other mechanical complication of urinary catheter**
Obstruction (mechanical) of urinary catheter
Perforation of urinary catheter
Protrusion of urinary catheter

SP **7** **T83.090-** **Other mechanical complication of cystostomy catheter**

SP **7** **T83.091-** **Other mechanical complication of indwelling urethral catheter**

SP **7** **T83.092-** **Other mechanical complication of nephrostomy catheter**

SP **7** **T83.098-** **Other mechanical complication of other urinary catheter**
Other mechanical complication of Hopkins catheter
Other mechanical complication of ileostomy catheter
Other mechanical complication of urostomy catheter

5 **T83.1** **Mechanical complication of other urinary devices and implants**

6 **T83.11** **Breakdown (mechanical) of other urinary devices and implants**

SP **7** **T83.110-** **Breakdown (mechanical) of urinary electronic stimulator device**
> **EXCLUDES 2** Breakdown (mechanical) of electrode (lead) for sacral nerve neurostimulator (T85.111)
> Breakdown (mechanical) of implanted electronic sacral neurostimulator, pulse generator or receiver (T85.113)

SP **7** **T83.111-** **Breakdown (mechanical) of implanted urinary sphincter**

SP **7** **T83.112-** **Breakdown (mechanical) of indwelling ureteral stent**

SP **7** **T83.113-** **Breakdown (mechanical) of other urinary stents**
Breakdown (mechanical) of ileal conduit stent
Breakdown (mechanical) of nephroureteral stent

SP **7** **T83.118-** **Breakdown (mechanical) of other urinary devices and implants**

6 **T83.12** **Displacement of other urinary devices and implants**
Malposition of other urinary devices and implants

SP **7** **T83.120-** **Displacement of urinary electronic stimulator device**
> **EXCLUDES 2** Displacement of electrode (lead) for sacral nerve neurostimulator (T85.121)
> Displacement of implanted electronic sacral neurostimulator, pulse generator or receiver (T85.123)

SP **7** **T83.121-** **Displacement of implanted urinary sphincter**

SP **7** **T83.122-** **Displacement of indwelling ureteral stent**

SP **7** **T83.123-** **Displacement of other urinary stents**
Displacement of ileal conduit stent
Displacement of nephroureteral stent

SP **7** **T83.128-** **Displacement of other urinary devices and implants**

6 **T83.19** **Other mechanical complication of other urinary devices and implants**
Leakage of other urinary devices and implants
Obstruction (mechanical) of other urinary devices and implants
Perforation of other urinary devices and implants
Protrusion of other urinary devices and implants

SP **7** **T83.190-** **Other mechanical complication of urinary electronic stimulator device**
> **EXCLUDES 2** Other mechanical complication of electrode (lead) for sacral nerve neurostimulator (T85.191)

44th digit required   **5**5th digit required   **6**6th digit required   **7**7th digit required   **7**7th digit placeholder   **+**Additional code   **☐**Laterality

1736   *DecisionHealth's* FY 2020 Complete Home Health ICD-10-CM Diagnosis Coding Manual

Other mechanical complication of implanted electronic sacral neurostimulator, pulse generator or receiver (T85.193)

SP **7** **T83.191-** **Other mechanical complication of implanted urinary sphincter**

SP **7** **T83.192-** **Other mechanical complication of indwelling ureteral stent**

SP **7** **T83.193-** **Other mechanical complication of other urinary stent**

Other mechanical complication of ileal conduit stent

Other mechanical complication of nephroureteral stent

SP **7** **T83.198-** **Other mechanical complication of other urinary devices and implants**

5 **T83.2** **Mechanical complication of graft of urinary organ**

SP **7** **T83.21X-** **Breakdown (mechanical) of graft of urinary organ**

SP **7** **T83.22X-** **Displacement of graft of urinary organ**

Malposition of graft of urinary organ

SP **7** **T83.23X-** **Leakage of graft of urinary organ**

SP **7** **T83.24X-** **Erosion of graft of urinary organ**

SP **7** **T83.25X-** **Exposure of graft of urinary organ**

SP **7** **T83.29X-** **Other mechanical complication of graft of urinary organ**

Obstruction (mechanical) of graft of urinary organ

Perforation of graft of urinary organ

Protrusion of graft of urinary organ

5 **T83.3** **Mechanical complication of intrauterine contraceptive device**

SP **7** **T83.31X-** **Breakdown (mechanical) of intrauterine contraceptive device**

SP **7** **T83.32X-** **Displacement of intrauterine contraceptive device**

Malposition of intrauterine contraceptive device

Missing string of intrauterine contraceptive device

SP **7** **T83.39X-** **Other mechanical complication of intrauterine contraceptive device**

Leakage of intrauterine contraceptive device

Obstruction (mechanical) of intrauterine contraceptive device

Perforation of intrauterine contraceptive device

Protrusion of intrauterine contraceptive device

5 **T83.4** **Mechanical complication of other prosthetic devices, implants and grafts of genital tract**

6 **T83.41** **Breakdown (mechanical) of other prosthetic devices, implants and grafts of genital tract**

SP **7** **T83.410-** **Breakdown (mechanical) of implanted penile prosthesis**

Breakdown (mechanical) of penile prosthesis cylinder

Breakdown (mechanical) of penile prosthesis pump

Breakdown (mechanical) of penile prosthesis reservoir

SP **7** **T83.411-** **Breakdown (mechanical) of implanted testicular prosthesis**

SP **7** **T83.418-** **Breakdown (mechanical) of other prosthetic devices, implants and grafts of genital tract**

6 **T83.42** **Displacement of other prosthetic devices, implants and grafts of genital tract**

Malposition of other prosthetic devices, implants and grafts of genital tract

SP **7** **T83.420-** **Displacement of implanted penile prosthesis**

Displacement of penile prosthesis cylinder

Displacement of penile prosthesis pump

Displacement of penile prosthesis reservoir

SP **7** **T83.421-** **Displacement of implanted testicular prosthesis**

SP **7** **T83.428-** **Displacement of other prosthetic devices, implants and grafts of genital tract**

6 **T83.49** **Other mechanical complication of other prosthetic devices, implants and grafts of genital tract**

Leakage of other prosthetic devices, implants and grafts of genital tract

Obstruction, mechanical of other prosthetic devices, implants and grafts of genital tract

Perforation of other prosthetic devices, implants and grafts of genital tract

Protrusion of other prosthetic devices, implants and grafts of genital tract

SP **7** **T83.490-** **Other mechanical complication of implanted penile prosthesis**

Other mechanical complication of penile prosthesis cylinder

Other mechanical complication of penile prosthesis pump

Other mechanical complication of penile prosthesis reservoir

SP **7** **T83.491-** **Other mechanical complication of implanted testicular prosthesis**

SP **7** **T83.498-** **Other mechanical complication of other prosthetic devices, implants and grafts of genital tract**

+ **5** **T83.5** **Infection and inflammatory reaction due to prosthetic device, implant and graft in urinary system**

Use additional code to identify infection

CODING TIPS ✓ Do not use Z43 or Z93 codes for routine care when a complication is documented.

+ **6** **T83.51** **Infection and inflammatory reaction due to urinary catheter**

EXCLUDES 2 complications of stoma of urinary tract (N99.5-)

SP **+** **7** **T83.510-** **Infection and inflammatory reaction due to cystostomy catheter**

★ New ▲ Revised Px Primary **SP** PDGM Px **SL** Low CoM **SH** High CoM **IQ** Quest. Encounter **H** Hospice non-cancer Dx   Unspecified   **M** *Manifestation*

SP + 7 T83.511-   **Infection and inflammatory reaction due to indwelling urethral catheter**

SP + 7 T83.512-   **Infection and inflammatory reaction due to nephrostomy catheter**

SP + 7 T83.518-   **Infection and inflammatory reaction due to other urinary catheter**

Infection and inflammatory reaction due to Hopkins catheter

Infection and inflammatory reaction due to ileostomy catheter

Infection and inflammatory reaction due to urostomy catheter

+ 6 T83.59   **Infection and inflammatory reaction due to prosthetic device, implant and graft in urinary system**

SP + 7 T83.590-   **Infection and inflammatory reaction due to implanted urinary neurostimulation device**

> EXCLUDES 2   Infection and inflammatory reaction due to electrode lead of sacral nerve neurostimulator (T85.732)
>
> Infection and inflammatory reaction due to pulse generator or receiver of sacral nerve neurostimulator (T85.734)

SP + 7 T83.591-   **Infection and inflammatory reaction due to implanted urinary sphincter**

SP + 7 T83.592-   **Infection and inflammatory reaction due to indwelling ureteral stent**

SP + 7 T83.593-   **Infection and inflammatory reaction due to other urinary stents**

Infection and inflammatory reaction due to ileal conduit stents

Infection and inflammatory reaction due to nephroureteral stent

SP + 7 T83.598-   **Infection and inflammatory reaction due to other prosthetic device, implant and graft in urinary system**

+ 5 T83.6   **Infection and inflammatory reaction due to prosthetic device, implant and graft in genital tract**

Use additional code to identify infection

SP + ☑ T83.61X-   **Infection and inflammatory reaction due to implanted penile prosthesis**

Infection and inflammatory reaction due to penile prosthesis cylinder

Infection and inflammatory reaction due to penile prosthesis pump

Infection and inflammatory reaction due to penile prosthesis reservoir

SP + ☑ T83.62X-   **Infection and inflammatory reaction due to implanted testicular prosthesis**

SP + ☑ T83.69X-   **Infection and inflammatory reaction due to other prosthetic device, implant and graft in genital tract**

5 T83.7   **Complications due to implanted mesh and other prosthetic materials**

6 T83.71   **Erosion of implanted mesh and other prosthetic materials to surrounding organ or tissue**

SP 7 T83.711-   **Erosion of implanted vaginal mesh to surrounding organ or tissue**

Erosion of implanted vaginal mesh into pelvic floor muscles

SP 7 T83.712-   **Erosion of implanted urethral mesh to surrounding organ or tissue**

Erosion of implanted female urethral sling

Erosion of implanted male urethral sling

Erosion of implanted urethral mesh into pelvic floor muscles

SP 7 T83.713-   **Erosion of implanted urethral bulking agent to surrounding organ or tissue**

SP 7 T83.714-   **Erosion of implanted ureteral bulking agent to surrounding organ or tissue**

SP 7 T83.718-   **Erosion of other implanted mesh to organ or tissue**

SP 7 T83.719-   **Erosion of other prosthetic materials to surrounding organ or tissue**

6 T83.72   **Exposure of implanted mesh and other prosthetic materials into surrounding organ or tissue**

Extrusion of implanted mesh

SP 7 T83.721-   **Exposure of implanted vaginal mesh into vagina**

Exposure of implanted vaginal mesh through vaginal wall

SP 7 T83.722-   **Exposure of implanted urethral mesh into urethra**

Exposure of implanted female urethral sling

Exposure of implanted male urethral sling

Exposure of implanted urethral mesh through urethral wall

SP 7 T83.723-   **Exposure of implanted urethral bulking agent into urethra**

SP 7 T83.724-   **Exposure of implanted ureteral bulking agent into ureter**

SP 7 T83.728-   **Exposure of other implanted mesh into organ or tissue**

SP 7 T83.729-   **Exposure of other prosthetic materials into organ or tissue**

SP ☑ T83.79X-   **Other specified complications due to other genitourinary prosthetic materials**

5 T83.8   **Other specified complications of genitourinary prosthetic devices, implants and grafts**

---

4 4th digit required   **5** 5th digit required   **6** 6th digit required   **7** 7th digit required   ☑ 7th digit placeholder   **+** Additional code   **⊟** Laterality

1738   *DecisionHealth's* FY 2020 Complete Home Health ICD-10-CM Diagnosis Coding Manual

SP ☑ T83.81X- Embolism due to genitourinary prosthetic devices, implants and grafts

SP ☑ T83.82X- Fibrosis due to genitourinary prosthetic devices, implants and grafts

SP ☑ T83.83X- Hemorrhage due to genitourinary prosthetic devices, implants and grafts

SP ☑ T83.84X- Pain due to genitourinary prosthetic devices, implants and grafts

SP ☑ T83.85X- Stenosis due to genitourinary prosthetic devices, implants and grafts

SP ☑ T83.86X- Thrombosis due to genitourinary prosthetic devices, implants and grafts

SP ☑ T83.89X- Other specified complication of genitourinary prosthetic devices, implants and grafts

IQ ☑ T83.9XX- Unspecified complication of genitourinary prosthetic device, implant and graft

4 T84 Complications of internal orthopedic prosthetic devices, implants and grafts

> EXCLUDES 2 failure and rejection of transplanted organs and tissues (T86.-)
> fracture of bone following insertion of orthopedic implant, joint prosthesis or bone plate (M96.6)

The appropriate 7th character is to be added to each code from category T84
A initial encounter
D subsequent encounter
S sequela

CODING TIPS ✓ Code T84 includes all of the complications of orthopedic prostheses, implants and grafts. Most of these codes indicate the joint affected so there is no need to add the Z96.6- code to indicate the prosthesis. Periprosthetic fractures are no longer considered complications and can be found in M97.

CODING TIPS ✓ No aftercare code applies, including dressing changes, drain care, and suture removal. 7th character 'D' is the default for home care and hospice when providing aftercare for a healing or resolving condition; 'A' is used for active treatment such as antibiotics or more than routine wound care; 'S' may be used to indicate a residual condition after the original injury has healed. Once complication is repaired in the acute setting, continue to code the complication in home care and hospice with 7th character D if healing/resolving.

5 T84.0 Mechanical complication of internal joint prosthesis

> CODING TIPS ✓ This subcategory includes complications of internal prosthetic joints. Most include the joint affected, so there is no need to add Z96.6 for the joint unless the complication code does not indicate the joint.

6 T84.01 Broken internal joint prosthesis
Breakage (fracture) of prosthetic joint
Broken prosthetic joint implant
> EXCLUDES 1 periprosthetic joint implant fracture (M97-)

SP 7 T84.010- Broken internal right hip prosthesis

SP 7 T84.011- Broken internal left hip prosthesis

SP 7 T84.012- Broken internal right knee prosthesis

SP 7 T84.013- Broken internal left knee prosthesis

SP + 7 T84.018- Broken internal joint prosthesis, other site
> Use additional code to identify the joint (Z96.6-)

IQ 7 T84.019- Broken internal joint prosthesis, unspecified site

6 T84.02 Dislocation of internal joint prosthesis
Instability of internal joint prosthesis
Subluxation of internal joint prosthesis

SP 7 T84.020- Dislocation of internal right hip prosthesis

SP 7 T84.021- Dislocation of internal left hip prosthesis

SP 7 T84.022- Instability of internal right knee prosthesis

SP 7 T84.023- Instability of internal left knee prosthesis

SP + 7 T84.028- Dislocation of other internal joint prosthesis
> Use additional code to identify the joint (Z96.6-)

IQ 7 T84.029- Dislocation of unspecified internal joint prosthesis

6 T84.03 Mechanical loosening of internal prosthetic joint
Aseptic loosening of prosthetic joint

SP 7 T84.030- Mechanical loosening of internal right hip prosthetic joint

SP 7 T84.031- Mechanical loosening of internal left hip prosthetic joint

SP 7 T84.032- Mechanical loosening of internal right knee prosthetic joint

SP 7 T84.033- Mechanical loosening of internal left knee prosthetic joint

SP + 7 T84.038- Mechanical loosening of other internal prosthetic joint
> Use additional code to identify the joint (Z96.6-)

IQ 7 T84.039- Mechanical loosening of unspecified internal prosthetic joint

+ 6 T84.05 Periprosthetic osteolysis of internal prosthetic joint
> Use additional code to identify major osseous defect, if applicable (M89.7-)

SP + 7 T84.050- Periprosthetic osteolysis of internal prosthetic right hip joint

SP + 7 T84.051- Periprosthetic osteolysis of internal prosthetic left hip joint

SP + 7 T84.052- Periprosthetic osteolysis of internal prosthetic right knee joint

---

★ New ▲ Revised Px Primary SP PDGM Px SL Low CoM SH High CoM IQ Quest. Encounter H Hospice non-cancer Dx Unspecified M *Manifestation*

🔲 **SP** ➕ 7 **T84.053-** **Periprosthetic osteolysis of internal prosthetic left knee joint**

🔲 **SP** ➕ 7 **T84.058-** **Periprosthetic osteolysis of other internal prosthetic joint**
Use additional code to identify the joint (Z96.6-)

🔲 **IQ** ➕ 7 **T84.059-** **Periprosthetic osteolysis of unspecified internal prosthetic joint**

6 **T84.06** **Wear of articular bearing surface of internal prosthetic joint**

🔲 **SP** 7 **T84.060-** **Wear of articular bearing surface of internal prosthetic right hip joint**

🔲 **SP** 7 **T84.061-** **Wear of articular bearing surface of internal prosthetic left hip joint**

🔲 **SP** 7 **T84.062-** **Wear of articular bearing surface of internal prosthetic right knee joint**

🔲 **SP** 7 **T84.063-** **Wear of articular bearing surface of internal prosthetic left knee joint**

🔲 **SP** ➕ 7 **T84.068-** **Wear of articular bearing surface of other internal prosthetic joint**
Use additional code to identify the joint (Z96.6-)

🔲 **IQ** 7 **T84.069-** **Wear of articular bearing surface of unspecified internal prosthetic joint**

6 **T84.09** **Other mechanical complication of internal joint prosthesis**
Prosthetic joint implant failure NOS

🔲 **SP** 7 **T84.090-** **Other mechanical complication of internal right hip prosthesis**

🔲 **SP** 7 **T84.091-** **Other mechanical complication of internal left hip prosthesis**

🔲 **SP** 7 **T84.092-** **Other mechanical complication of internal right knee prosthesis**

🔲 **SP** 7 **T84.093-** **Other mechanical complication of internal left knee prosthesis**

🔲 **SP** ➕ 7 **T84.098-** **Other mechanical complication of other internal joint prosthesis**
Use additional code to identify the joint (Z96.6-)

🔲 **IQ** 7 **T84.099-** **Other mechanical complication of unspecified internal joint prosthesis**

5 **T84.1** **Mechanical complication of internal fixation device of bones of limb**
EXCLUDES 2   mechanical complication of internal fixation device of bones of feet (T84.2-)
mechanical complication of internal fixation device of bones of fingers (T84.2-)
mechanical complication of internal fixation device of bones of hands (T84.2-)
mechanical complication of internal fixation device of bones of toes (T84.2-)

6 **T84.11** **Breakdown (mechanical) of internal fixation device of bones of limb**

🔲 **SP** 7 **T84.110-** **Breakdown (mechanical) of internal fixation device of right humerus**

🔲 **SP** 7 **T84.111-** **Breakdown (mechanical) of internal fixation device of left humerus**

🔲 **SP** 7 **T84.112-** **Breakdown (mechanical) of internal fixation device of bone of right forearm**

🔲 **SP** 7 **T84.113-** **Breakdown (mechanical) of internal fixation device of bone of left forearm**

🔲 **SP** 7 **T84.114-** **Breakdown (mechanical) of internal fixation device of right femur**

🔲 **SP** 7 **T84.115-** **Breakdown (mechanical) of internal fixation device of left femur**

🔲 **SP** 7 **T84.116-** **Breakdown (mechanical) of internal fixation device of bone of right lower leg**

🔲 **SP** 7 **T84.117-** **Breakdown (mechanical) of internal fixation device of bone of left lower leg**

🔲 **IQ** 7 **T84.119-** **Breakdown (mechanical) of internal fixation device of unspecified bone of limb**

6 **T84.12** **Displacement of internal fixation device of bones of limb**
Malposition of internal fixation device of bones of limb

🔲 **SP** 7 **T84.120-** **Displacement of internal fixation device of right humerus**

🔲 **SP** 7 **T84.121-** **Displacement of internal fixation device of left humerus**

🔲 **SP** 7 **T84.122-** **Displacement of internal fixation device of bone of right forearm**

🔲 **SP** 7 **T84.123-** **Displacement of internal fixation device of bone of left forearm**

🔲 **SP** 7 **T84.124-** **Displacement of internal fixation device of right femur**

🔲 **SP** 7 **T84.125-** **Displacement of internal fixation device of left femur**

🔲 **SP** 7 **T84.126-** **Displacement of internal fixation device of bone of right lower leg**

🔲 **SP** 7 **T84.127-** **Displacement of internal fixation device of bone of left lower leg**

🔲 **IQ** 7 **T84.129-** **Displacement of internal fixation device of unspecified bone of limb**

6 **T84.19** **Other mechanical complication of internal fixation device of bones of limb**
Obstruction (mechanical) of internal fixation device of bones of limb
Perforation of internal fixation device of bones of limb
Protrusion of internal fixation device of bones of limb

🔲 **SP** 7 **T84.190-** **Other mechanical complication of internal fixation device of right humerus**

🔲 **SP** 7 **T84.191-** **Other mechanical complication of internal fixation device of left humerus**

🔲 **SP** 7 **T84.192-** **Other mechanical complication of internal fixation device of bone of right forearm**

🔲 **SP** 7 **T84.193-** **Other mechanical complication of internal fixation device of bone of left forearm**

---

4 4th digit required   5 5th digit required   6 6th digit required   7 7th digit required   7 7th digit placeholder   ➕ Additional code   🔲 Laterality

SP 7 T84.194- Other mechanical complication of internal fixation device of right femur

SP 7 T84.195- Other mechanical complication of internal fixation device of left femur

SP 7 T84.196- Other mechanical complication of internal fixation device of bone of right lower leg

SP 7 T84.197- Other mechanical complication of internal fixation device of bone of left lower leg

IQ 7 T84.199- Other mechanical complication of internal fixation device of unspecified bone of limb

5 T84.2 Mechanical complication of internal fixation device of other bones

6 T84.21 Breakdown (mechanical) of internal fixation device of other bones

SP 7 T84.210- Breakdown (mechanical) of internal fixation device of bones of hand and fingers

SP 7 T84.213- Breakdown (mechanical) of internal fixation device of bones of foot and toes

SP 7 T84.216- Breakdown (mechanical) of internal fixation device of vertebrae

SP 7 T84.218- Breakdown (mechanical) of internal fixation device of other bones

6 T84.22 Displacement of internal fixation device of other bones

Malposition of internal fixation device of other bones

SP 7 T84.220- Displacement of internal fixation device of bones of hand and fingers

SP 7 T84.223- Displacement of internal fixation device of bones of foot and toes

SP 7 T84.226- Displacement of internal fixation device of vertebrae

SP 7 T84.228- Displacement of internal fixation device of other bones

6 T84.29 Other mechanical complication of internal fixation device of other bones

Obstruction (mechanical) of internal fixation device of other bones

Perforation of internal fixation device of other bones

Protrusion of internal fixation device of other bones

SP 7 T84.290- Other mechanical complication of internal fixation device of bones of hand and fingers

SP 7 T84.293- Other mechanical complication of internal fixation device of bones of foot and toes

SP 7 T84.296- Other mechanical complication of internal fixation device of vertebrae

SP 7 T84.298- Other mechanical complication of internal fixation device of other bones

5 T84.3 Mechanical complication of other bone devices, implants and grafts

EXCLUDES 2 other complications of bone graft (T86.83-)

6 T84.31 Breakdown (mechanical) of other bone devices, implants and grafts

SP 7 T84.310- Breakdown (mechanical) of electronic bone stimulator

SP 7 T84.318- Breakdown (mechanical) of other bone devices, implants and grafts

6 T84.32 Displacement of other bone devices, implants and grafts

Malposition of other bone devices, implants and grafts

SP 7 T84.320- Displacement of electronic bone stimulator

SP 7 T84.328- Displacement of other bone devices, implants and grafts

6 T84.39 Other mechanical complication of other bone devices, implants and grafts

Obstruction (mechanical) of other bone devices, implants and grafts

Perforation of other bone devices, implants and grafts

Protrusion of other bone devices, implants and grafts

SP 7 T84.390- Other mechanical complication of electronic bone stimulator

SP 7 T84.398- Other mechanical complication of other bone devices, implants and grafts

5 T84.4 Mechanical complication of other internal orthopedic devices, implants and grafts

6 T84.41 Breakdown (mechanical) of other internal orthopedic devices, implants and grafts

SP 7 T84.410- Breakdown (mechanical) of muscle and tendon graft

SP 7 T84.418- Breakdown (mechanical) of other internal orthopedic devices, implants and grafts

6 T84.42 Displacement of other internal orthopedic devices, implants and grafts

Malposition of other internal orthopedic devices, implants and grafts

SP 7 T84.420- Displacement of muscle and tendon graft

SP 7 T84.428- Displacement of other internal orthopedic devices, implants and grafts

6 T84.49 Other mechanical complication of other internal orthopedic devices, implants and grafts

Mechanical complication of other internal orthopedic devices, implants and grafts NOS

Obstruction (mechanical) of other internal orthopedic devices, implants and grafts

Perforation of other internal orthopedic devices, implants and grafts

Protrusion of other internal orthopedic devices, implants and grafts

SP 7 T84.490- Other mechanical complication of muscle and tendon graft

SP 7 T84.498- Other mechanical complication of other internal orthopedic devices, implants and grafts

Chapter 19

S00-T88

★ New ▲ Revised Px Primary SP PDGM Px SL Low CoM SH High CoM IQ Quest. Encounter H Hospice non-cancer Dx Unspecified M Manifestation

DecisionHealth's FY 2020 Complete Home Health ICD-10-CM Diagnosis Coding Manual

1741

+ 5 T84.5   **Infection and inflammatory reaction due to internal joint prosthesis**
Use additional code to identify infection

CODING TIPS ✓   If septic joint or septic arthritis is documented, use an additional code from M00.- to identify the organism.

⊟ !Q + ☑ T84.50X-   Infection and inflammatory reaction due to unspecified internal joint prosthesis

⊟ SP + ☑ T84.51X-   Infection and inflammatory reaction due to internal right hip prosthesis

⊟ SP + ☑ T84.52X-   Infection and inflammatory reaction due to internal left hip prosthesis

⊟ SP + ☑ T84.53X-   Infection and inflammatory reaction due to internal right knee prosthesis

⊟ SP + ☑ T84.54X-   Infection and inflammatory reaction due to internal left knee prosthesis

⊟ SP + ☑ T84.59X-   Infection and inflammatory reaction due to other internal joint prosthesis

+ 5 T84.6   **Infection and inflammatory reaction due to internal fixation device**
Use additional code to identify infection

!Q + ☑ T84.60X-   Infection and inflammatory reaction due to internal fixation device of unspecified site

+ 6 T84.61   Infection and inflammatory reaction due to internal fixation device of arm

⊟ SP + 7 T84.610-   Infection and inflammatory reaction due to internal fixation device of right humerus

⊟ SP + 7 T84.611-   Infection and inflammatory reaction due to internal fixation device of left humerus

⊟ SP + 7 T84.612-   Infection and inflammatory reaction due to internal fixation device of right radius

⊟ SP + 7 T84.613-   Infection and inflammatory reaction due to internal fixation device of left radius

⊟ SP + 7 T84.614-   Infection and inflammatory reaction due to internal fixation device of right ulna

⊟ SP + 7 T84.615-   Infection and inflammatory reaction due to internal fixation device of left ulna

⊟ !Q + 7 T84.619-   Infection and inflammatory reaction due to internal fixation device of unspecified bone of arm

+ 6 T84.62   Infection and inflammatory reaction due to internal fixation device of leg

⊟ SP + 7 T84.620-   Infection and inflammatory reaction due to internal fixation device of right femur

⊟ SP + 7 T84.621-   Infection and inflammatory reaction due to internal fixation device of left femur

⊟ SP + 7 T84.622-   Infection and inflammatory reaction due to internal fixation device of right tibia

⊟ SP + 7 T84.623-   Infection and inflammatory reaction due to internal fixation device of left tibia

⊟ SP + 7 T84.624-   Infection and inflammatory reaction due to internal fixation device of right fibula

⊟ SP !Q + 7 T84.625-   Infection and inflammatory reaction due to internal fixation device of left fibula

⊟ !Q + 7 T84.629-   Infection and inflammatory reaction due to internal fixation device of unspecified bone of leg

SP + ☑ T84.63X-   Infection and inflammatory reaction due to internal fixation device of spine

SP + ☑ T84.69X-   Infection and inflammatory reaction due to internal fixation device of other site

SP + ☑ T84.7XX-   Infection and inflammatory reaction due to other internal orthopedic prosthetic devices, implants and grafts
Use additional code to identify infection

5 T84.8   Other specified complications of internal orthopedic prosthetic devices, implants and grafts

SP ☑ T84.81X-   Embolism due to internal orthopedic prosthetic devices, implants and grafts

SP ☑ T84.82X-   Fibrosis due to internal orthopedic prosthetic devices, implants and grafts

SP ☑ T84.83X-   Hemorrhage due to internal orthopedic prosthetic devices, implants and grafts

SP ☑ T84.84X-   Pain due to internal orthopedic prosthetic devices, implants and grafts

CODING TIPS ✓   A G89.- code may be added to indicate the nature of the pain, e.g. post surgical vs traumatic, and acute vs chronic.

SP ☑ T84.85X-   Stenosis due to internal orthopedic prosthetic devices, implants and grafts

SP ☑ T84.86X-   Thrombosis due to internal orthopedic prosthetic devices, implants and grafts

SP ☑ T84.89X-   Other specified complication of internal orthopedic prosthetic devices, implants and grafts

!Q ☑ T84.9XX-   Unspecified complication of internal orthopedic prosthetic device, implant and graft

4 T85   **Complications of other internal prosthetic devices, implants and grafts**
EXCLUDES 2   failure and rejection of transplanted organs and tissue (T86.-)

The appropriate 7th character is to be added to each code from category T85
A   initial encounter
D   subsequent encounter
S   sequela

---

4 4th digit required   **5** 5th digit required   **6** 6th digit required   **7** 7th digit required   ☑ 7th digit placeholder   **+** Additional code   ⊟ Laterality

CODING TIPS ✓   No aftercare code applies, including dressing changes, drain care, and suture removal. 7th character 'D' is the default for home care and hospice when providing aftercare for a healing or resolving condition; 'A' is used for active treatment such as antibiotics or more than routine wound care; 'S' may be used to indicate a residual condition after the original injury has healed. Once complication is repaired in the acute setting, continue to code the complication in home care and hospice with 7th character D if healing/resolving.

⑤ T85.0   **Mechanical complication of ventricular intracranial (communicating) shunt**

CODING TIPS ✓   Do not use Z98.2 if the ventricular shunt is complicated.

SP ⑦ T85.01X-   **Breakdown (mechanical) of ventricular intracranial (communicating) shunt**

SP ⑦ T85.02X-   **Displacement of ventricular intracranial (communicating) shunt**
Malposition of ventricular intracranial (communicating) shunt

SP ⑦ T85.03X-   **Leakage of ventricular intracranial (communicating) shunt**

SP ⑦ T85.09X-   **Other mechanical complication of ventricular intracranial (communicating) shunt**
Obstruction (mechanical) of ventricular intracranial (communicating) shunt
Perforation of ventricular intracranial (communicating) shunt
Protrusion of ventricular intracranial (communicating) shunt

⑤ T85.1   **Mechanical complication of implanted electronic stimulator of nervous system**

⑥ T85.11   **Breakdown (mechanical) of implanted electronic stimulator of nervous system**

SP ⑦ T85.110-   **Breakdown (mechanical) of implanted electronic neurostimulator of brain electrode (lead)**

SP ⑦ T85.111-   **Breakdown (mechanical) of implanted electronic neurostimulator of peripheral nerve electrode (lead)**
Breakdown of electrode (lead) for cranial nerve neurostimulators
Breakdown of electrode (lead) for gastric neurostimulator
Breakdown of electrode (lead) for sacral nerve neurostimulator
Breakdown of electrode (lead) for vagal nerve neurostimulators

SP ⑦ T85.112-   **Breakdown (mechanical) of implanted electronic neurostimulator of spinal cord electrode (lead)**

SP ⑦ T85.113-   **Breakdown (mechanical) of implanted electronic neurostimulator, generator**

Breakdown (mechanical) of implanted electronic neurostimulator generator, brain, peripheral, gastric, spinal
Breakdown (mechanical) of implanted electronic sacral neurostimulator, pulse generator or receiver

SP ⑦ T85.118-   **Breakdown (mechanical) of other implanted electronic stimulator of nervous system**

⑥ T85.12   **Displacement of implanted electronic stimulator of nervous system**
Malposition of implanted electronic stimulator of nervous system

SP ⑦ T85.120-   **Displacement of implanted electronic neurostimulator of brain electrode (lead)**

SP ⑦ T85.121-   **Displacement of implanted electronic neurostimulator of peripheral nerve electrode (lead)**
Displacement of electrode (lead) for cranial nerve neurostimulators
Displacement of electrode (lead) for gastric neurostimulator
Displacement of electrode (lead) for sacral nerve neurostimulator
Displacement of electrode (lead) for vagal nerve neurostimulators

SP ⑦ T85.122-   **Displacement of implanted electronic neurostimulator of spinal cord electrode (lead)**

SP ⑦ T85.123-   **Displacement of implanted electronic neurostimulator, generator**
Displacement of implanted electronic neurostimulator generator, brain, peripheral, gastric, spinal
Displacement of implanted electronic sacral neurostimulator, pulse generator or receiver

SP ⑦ T85.128-   **Displacement of other implanted electronic stimulator of nervous system**

⑥ T85.19   **Other mechanical complication of implanted electronic stimulator of nervous system**
Leakage of implanted electronic stimulator of nervous system
Obstruction (mechanical) of implanted electronic stimulator of nervous system
Perforation of implanted electronic stimulator of nervous system
Protrusion of implanted electronic stimulator of nervous system

SP ⑦ T85.190-   **Other mechanical complication of implanted electronic neurostimulator of brain electrode (lead)**

SP ⑦ T85.191-   **Other mechanical complication of implanted electronic neurostimulator of peripheral nerve electrode (lead)**
Other mechanical complication of electrode (lead) for cranial nerve neurostimulators

---

★ New   ▲ Revised   Px Primary   **SP** PDGM Px   **SL** Low CoM   **SH** High CoM   **IQ** Quest. Encounter   **H** Hospice non-cancer Dx   Unspecified   **M** *Manifestation*

DecisionHealth's FY 2020 Complete Home Health ICD-10-CM Diagnosis Coding Manual   1743

Other mechanical complication of electrode (lead) for gastric neurostimulator

Other mechanical complication of electrode (lead) for sacral nerve neurostimulator

Other mechanical complication of electrode (lead) for vagal nerve neurostimulators

SP 7 T85.192-   **Other mechanical complication of implanted electronic neurostimulator of spinal cord electrode (lead)**

SP 7 T85.193-   **Other mechanical complication of implanted electronic neurostimulator, generator**

Other mechanical complication of implanted electronic neurostimulator generator, brain, peripheral, gastric, spinal

Other mechanical complication of implanted electronic sacral neurostimulator, pulse generator or receiver

SP 7 T85.199-   **Other mechanical complication of other implanted electronic stimulator of nervous system**

5 T85.2   **Mechanical complication of intraocular lens**

SP ☑ T85.21X-   **Breakdown (mechanical) of intraocular lens**

SP ☑ T85.22X-   **Displacement of intraocular lens**

Malposition of intraocular lens

SP ☑ T85.29X-   **Other mechanical complication of intraocular lens**

Obstruction (mechanical) of intraocular lens

Perforation of intraocular lens

Protrusion of intraocular lens

5 T85.3   **Mechanical complication of other ocular prosthetic devices, implants and grafts**

    EXCLUDES 2   other complications of corneal graft (T86.84-)

6 T85.31   **Breakdown (mechanical) of other ocular prosthetic devices, implants and grafts**

⊟ SP 7 T85.310-   **Breakdown (mechanical) of prosthetic orbit of right eye**

⊟ SP 7 T85.311-   **Breakdown (mechanical) of prosthetic orbit of left eye**

⊟ SP 7 T85.318-   **Breakdown (mechanical) of other ocular prosthetic devices, implants and grafts**

6 T85.32   **Displacement of other ocular prosthetic devices, implants and grafts**

Malposition of other ocular prosthetic devices, implants and grafts

⊟ SP 7 T85.320-   **Displacement of prosthetic orbit of right eye**

⊟ SP 7 T85.321-   **Displacement of prosthetic orbit of left eye**

⊟ SP 7 T85.328-   **Displacement of other ocular prosthetic devices, implants and grafts**

6 T85.39   **Other mechanical complication of other ocular prosthetic devices, implants and grafts**

Obstruction (mechanical) of other ocular prosthetic devices, implants and grafts

Perforation of other ocular prosthetic devices, implants and grafts

Protrusion of other ocular prosthetic devices, implants and grafts

⊟ SP 7 T85.390-   **Other mechanical complication of prosthetic orbit of right eye**

⊟ SP 7 T85.391-   **Other mechanical complication of prosthetic orbit of left eye**

⊟ SP 7 T85.398-   **Other mechanical complication of other ocular prosthetic devices, implants and grafts**

5 T85.4   **Mechanical complication of breast prosthesis and implant**

SP ☑ T85.41X-   **Breakdown (mechanical) of breast prosthesis and implant**

SP ☑ T85.42X-   **Displacement of breast prosthesis and implant**

Malposition of breast prosthesis and implant

SP ☑ T85.43X-   **Leakage of breast prosthesis and implant**

SP ☑ T85.44X-   **Capsular contracture of breast implant**

SP ☑ T85.49X-   **Other mechanical complication of breast prosthesis and implant**

Obstruction (mechanical) of breast prosthesis and implant

Perforation of breast prosthesis and implant

Protrusion of breast prosthesis and implant

5 T85.5   **Mechanical complication of gastrointestinal prosthetic devices, implants and grafts**

6 T85.51   **Breakdown (mechanical) of gastrointestinal prosthetic devices, implants and grafts**

SP 7 T85.510-   **Breakdown (mechanical) of bile duct prosthesis**

SP 7 T85.511-   **Breakdown (mechanical) of esophageal anti-reflux device**

SP 7 T85.518-   **Breakdown (mechanical) of other gastrointestinal prosthetic devices, implants and grafts**

6 T85.52   **Displacement of gastrointestinal prosthetic devices, implants and grafts**

Malposition of gastrointestinal prosthetic devices, implants and grafts

SP 7 T85.520-   **Displacement of bile duct prosthesis**

SP 7 T85.521-   **Displacement of esophageal anti-reflux device**

SP 7 T85.528-   **Displacement of other gastrointestinal prosthetic devices, implants and grafts**

6 T85.59   **Other mechanical complication of gastrointestinal prosthetic devices, implants and**

Obstruction, mechanical of gastrointestinal prosthetic devices, implants and grafts

Perforation of gastrointestinal prosthetic devices, implants and grafts

4 4th digit required   **5** 5th digit required   **6** 6th digit required   **7** 7th digit required   **☑** 7th digit placeholder   **+** Additional code   **⊟** Laterality

1744   *DecisionHealth's* FY 2020 Complete Home Health ICD-10-CM Diagnosis Coding Manual

Protrusion of gastrointestinal prosthetic
devices, implants and grafts

SP 7 T85.590- **Other mechanical complication
of bile duct prosthesis**

SP 7 T85.591- **Other mechanical complication
of esophageal anti-reflux device**

SP 7 T85.598- **Other mechanical complication
of other gastrointestinal
prosthetic devices, implants and
grafts**

5 T85.6 **Mechanical complication of other
specified internal and external
prosthetic devices, implants and grafts**

> **GUIDELINES** Section I.C.4.a.5)(a)-(b)
> An underdose of insulin due to an insulin
> pump failure should be assigned to a code
> from subcategory T85.6 followed by code
> T38.3x6-, Underdosing of insulin and oral
> hypoglycemic [antidiabetic] drugs.
> Additional codes for the type of diabetes
> mellitus and any associated complications
> due to the underdosing should also be
> assigned.
>
> The principal or first-listed code for an
> encounter due to an insulin pump
> malfunction resulting in an overdose of
> insulin, should also be T85.6- followed by
> code T38.3x1-, Poisoning by insulin and
> oral hypoglycemic [antidiabetic] drugs,
> accidental (unintentional).

6 T85.61 **Breakdown (mechanical) of other
specified internal prosthetic devices,
implants and grafts**

SP 7 T85.610- **Breakdown (mechanical) of
cranial or spinal infusion
catheter**
Breakdown (mechanical) of
epidural infusion catheter
Breakdown (mechanical) of
intrathecal infusion catheter
Breakdown (mechanical) of
subarachnoid infusion catheter
Breakdown (mechanical) of
subdural infusion catheter

SP 7 T85.611- **Breakdown (mechanical) of
intraperitoneal dialysis catheter**
> **EXCLUDES 1** mechanical
> complication of
> vascular dialysis
> catheter (T82.4-)

SP 7 T85.612- **Breakdown (mechanical) of
permanent sutures**
> **EXCLUDES 1** mechanical
> complication of
> permanent (wire)
> suture used in bone
> repair (T84.1-
> T84.2)

SP 7 T85.613- **Breakdown (mechanical) of
artificial skin graft and
decellularized allodermis**
Failure of artificial skin graft and
decellularized allodermis
Non-adherence of artificial skin
graft and decellularized
allodermis

Poor incorporation of artificial skin
graft and decellularized
allodermis
Shearing of artificial skin graft and
decellularized allodermis

SP 7 T85.614- **Breakdown (mechanical) of
insulin pump**

SP 7 T85.615- **Breakdown (mechanical) of
other nervous system device,
implant or graft**
Breakdown (mechanical) of
intrathecal infusion pump

SP 7 T85.618- **Breakdown (mechanical) of
other specified internal
prosthetic devices, implants and
grafts**

6 T85.62 **Displacement of other specified
internal prosthetic devices, implants
and grafts**
Malposition of other specified internal
prosthetic devices, implants and
grafts

SP 7 T85.620- **Displacement of cranial or spinal
infusion catheter**
Displacement of epidural infusion
catheter
Displacement of intrathecal
infusion catheter
Displacement of subarachnoid
infusion catheter
Displacement of subdural infusion
catheter

SP 7 T85.621- **Displacement of intraperitoneal
dialysis catheter**
> **EXCLUDES 1** mechanical
> complication of
> vascular dialysis
> catheter (T82.4-)

SP 7 T85.622- **Displacement of permanent
sutures**
> **EXCLUDES 1** mechanical
> complication of
> permanent (wire)
> suture used in bone
> repair (T84.1-
> T84.2)

SP 7 T85.623- **Displacement of artificial skin
graft and decellularized
allodermis**
Dislodgement of artificial skin
graft and decellularized
allodermis

SP 7 T85.624- **Displacement of insulin pump**

SP 7 T85.625- **Displacement of other nervous
system device, implant or graft**
Displacement of intrathecal
infusion pump

SP 7 T85.628- **Displacement of other specified
internal prosthetic devices,
implants and grafts**

6 T85.63 **Leakage of other specified internal
prosthetic devices, implants and
grafts**

SP 7 T85.630- **Leakage of cranial or spinal
infusion catheter**
Leakage of epidural infusion
catheter
Leakage of intrathecal infusion
catheter infusion catheter

★ New ▲ Revised Px Primary **SP** PDGM Px **SL** Low CoM **SH** High CoM **IQ** Quest. Encounter **H** Hospice non-cancer Dx   Unspecified   **M** *Manifestation*

DecisionHealth's FY 2020 Complete Home Health ICD-10-CM Diagnosis Coding Manual

1745

Chapter 19

S00-T88

Leakage of subdural infusion catheter

Leakage of subarachnoid infusion catheter

SP IQ 7 T85.631- **Leakage of intraperitoneal dialysis catheter**

> EXCLUDES 1   mechanical complication of vascular dialysis catheter (T82.4)

SP IQ 7 T85.633- **Leakage of insulin pump**

SP 7 T85.635- **Leakage of other nervous system device, implant or graft**

Leakage of intrathecal infusion pump

SP 7 T85.638- **Leakage of other specified internal prosthetic devices, implants and grafts**

6 T85.69 **Other mechanical complication of other specified internal prosthetic devices, implants and grafts**

Obstruction, mechanical of other specified internal prosthetic devices, implants and grafts

Perforation of other specified internal prosthetic devices, implants and grafts

Protrusion of other specified internal prosthetic devices, implants and grafts

SP 7 T85.690- **Other mechanical complication of cranial or spinal infusion catheter**

Other mechanical complication of epidural infusion catheter

Other mechanical complication of intrathecal infusion catheter

Other mechanical complication of subarachnoid infusion catheter

Other mechanical complication of subdural infusion catheter

SP 7 T85.691- **Other mechanical complication of intraperitoneal dialysis catheter**

> EXCLUDES 1   mechanical complication of vascular dialysis catheter (T82.4)

SP 7 T85.692- **Other mechanical complication of permanent sutures**

> EXCLUDES 1   mechanical complication of permanent (wire) suture used in bone repair (T84.1-T84.2)

SP 7 T85.693- **Other mechanical complication of artificial skin graft and decellularized allodermis**

SP 7 T85.694- **Other mechanical complication of insulin pump**

SP 7 T85.695- **Other mechanical complication of other nervous system device, implant or graft**

Other mechanical complication of intrathecal infusion pump

SP 7 T85.698- **Other mechanical complication of other specified internal prosthetic devices, implants and grafts**

Mechanical complication of nonabsorbable surgical material NOS

+ 5 T85.7 **Infection and inflammatory reaction due to other internal prosthetic devices, implants and grafts**

Use additional code to identify infection

SP + ☑ T85.71X- **Infection and inflammatory reaction due to peritoneal dialysis catheter**

SP + ☑ T85.72X- **Infection and inflammatory reaction due to insulin pump**

+ 6 T85.73 **Infection and inflammatory reaction due to nervous system devices, implants and graft**

SP + 7 T85.730- **Infection and inflammatory reaction due to ventricular intracranial (communicating) shunt**

SP + 7 T85.731- **Infection and inflammatory reaction due to implanted electronic neurostimulator of brain, electrode (lead)**

SP + 7 T85.732- **Infection and inflammatory reaction due to implanted electronic neurostimulator of peripheral nerve, electrode (lead)**

Infection and inflammatory reaction due to electrode (lead) for cranial nerve neurostimulators

Infection and inflammatory reaction due to electrode (lead) for gastric neurostimulator

Infection and inflammatory reaction due to electrode (lead) for sacral nerve neurostimulator

Infection and inflammatory reaction due to electrode (lead) for vagal nerve neurostimulators

SP + 7 T85.733- **Infection and inflammatory reaction due to implanted electronic neurostimulator of spinal cord, electrode (lead)**

SP + 7 T85.734- **Infection and inflammatory reaction due to implanted electronic neurostimulator, generator**

Generator pocket infection

SP + 7 T85.735- **Infection and inflammatory reaction due to cranial or spinal infusion catheter**

Infection and inflammatory reaction due to epidural catheter

Infection and inflammatory reaction due to intrathecal infusion catheter

Infection and inflammatory reaction due to subarachnoid catheter

Infection and inflammatory reaction due to subdural catheter

SP + 7 T85.738- **Infection and inflammatory reaction due to other nervous system device, implant or graft**

---

4 4th digit required   5 5th digit required   6 6th digit required   7 7th digit required   ☑ 7th digit placeholder   + Additional code   ⊟ Laterality

1746   *DecisionHealth's* FY 2020 Complete Home Health ICD-10-CM Diagnosis Coding Manual

Infection and inflammatory reaction due to intrathecal infusion pump

SP **+** ☑ **T85.79X-** **Infection and inflammatory reaction due to other internal prosthetic devices, implants and grafts**

⑤ **T85.8** **Other specified complications of internal prosthetic devices, implants and grafts, not elsewhere classified**

⑥ **T85.81** **Embolism due to internal prosthetic devices, implants and grafts, not elsewhere classified**

SP ⑦ **T85.810-** **Embolism due to nervous system prosthetic devices, implants and grafts**

SP ⑦ **T85.818-** **Embolism due to other internal prosthetic devices, implants and grafts**

⑥ **T85.82** **Fibrosis due to internal prosthetic devices, implants and grafts, not elsewhere classified**

SP ⑦ **T85.820-** **Fibrosis due to nervous system prosthetic devices, implants and grafts**

SP ⑦ **T85.828-** **Fibrosis due to other internal prosthetic devices, implants and grafts**

⑥ **T85.83** **Hemorrhage due to internal prosthetic devices, implants and grafts, not elsewhere classified**

SP ⑦ **T85.830-** **Hemorrhage due to nervous system prosthetic devices, implants and grafts**

SP ⑦ **T85.838-** **Hemorrhage due to other internal prosthetic devices, implants and grafts**

⑥ **T85.84** **Pain due to internal prosthetic devices, implants and grafts, not elsewhere classified**

SP ⑦ **T85.840-** **Pain due to nervous system prosthetic devices, implants and grafts**

SP ⑦ **T85.848-** **Pain due to other internal prosthetic devices, implants and grafts**

⑥ **T85.85** **Stenosis due to internal prosthetic devices, implants and grafts, not elsewhere classified**

SP ⑦ **T85.850-** **Stenosis due to nervous system prosthetic devices, implants and grafts**

SP ⑦ **T85.858-** **Stenosis due to other internal prosthetic devices, implants and grafts**

⑥ **T85.86** **Thrombosis due to internal prosthetic devices, implants and grafts, not elsewhere classified**

SP ⑦ **T85.860-** **Thrombosis due to nervous system prosthetic devices, implants and grafts**

SP ⑦ **T85.868-** **Thrombosis due to other internal prosthetic devices, implants and grafts**

⑥ **T85.89** **Other specified complication of internal prosthetic devices, implants and grafts, not elsewhere classified**

Erosion or breakdown of subcutaneous device pocket

SP ⑦ **T85.890-** **Other specified complication of nervous system prosthetic devices, implants and grafts**

SP ⑦ **T85.898-** **Other specified complication of other internal prosthetic devices, implants and grafts**

IQ ☑ **T85.9XX-** **Unspecified complication of internal prosthetic device, implant and graft**

Complication of internal prosthetic device, implant and graft NOS

+ ④ **T86** **Complications of transplanted organs and tissue**

Use additional code to identify other transplant complications, such as:
graft-versus-host disease (D89.81-)
malignancy associated with organ transplant (C80.2)
post-transplant lymphoproliferative disorders (PTLD) (D47.Z1)

GUIDELINES **Section I.C.19.g.3)(a)**

Codes under category T86, Complications of transplanted organs and tissues, are for use for both complications and rejection of transplanted organs. A transplant complication code is only assigned if the complication affects the function of the transplanted organ. Two codes are required to fully describe a transplant complication: the appropriate code from category T86 and a secondary code that identifies the complication.

Pre-existing conditions or conditions that develop after the transplant are not coded as complications unless they affect the function of the transplanted organs.

GUIDELINES **Section I.C.2.r**

A malignant neoplasm of a transplanted organ should be coded as a transplant complication. Assign first the appropriate code from category T86.-, Complications of transplanted organs and tissue, followed by code C80.2. Use an additional code for the specific malignancy.

CODING TIPS ✓ If the organ must be removed due to failure or rejection, use Z98.85 for removal status.

CODING TIPS ✓ Do not assume dysfunction in a transplanted organ to be a complication of a transplanted organ unless specifically stated by a provider diagnostic statement. The only exception to this is a malignant neoplasm of a transplanted organ. A neoplasm associated with a transplant is coded as an "other complication of transplant" unless specified by the physician as a failure or rejection.

CODING TIPS ✓ This category includes complications for organ transplants, including skin grafts. Note that these complication codes do not require a 7th character.

+ ⑤ **T86.0** **Complications of bone marrow transplant**

IQ **+** **T86.00** **Unspecified complication of bone marrow transplant**

SP **+** **T86.01** **Bone marrow transplant rejection**

SP **+** **T86.02** **Bone marrow transplant failure**

SP **+** **T86.03** **Bone marrow transplant infection**

★ New ▲ Revised Px Primary **SP** PDGM Px **SL** Low CoM **SH** High CoM **IQ** Quest. Encounter ⊞ Hospice non-cancer Dx | Unspecified | **M** *Manifestation*

DecisionHealth's FY 2020 Complete Home Health ICD-10-CM Diagnosis Coding Manual   1747

SP ✚ T86.09   Other complications of bone marrow transplant

✚ 5 T86.1   Complications of kidney transplant

> **GUIDELINES**   Section I.C.19.g.3)(b)
>
> Patients who have undergone kidney transplant may still have some form of chronic kidney disease (CKD) because the kidney transplant may not fully restore kidney function ... Code T86.1- should not be assigned for post kidney transplant patients who have CKD unless a transplant complication such as transplant failure or rejection is documented. If the documentation is unclear as to whether the patient has a complication of the transplant, query the provider.
>
> Conditions that affect the function of the transplanted kidney, other than CKD, should be assigned a code from subcategory T86.1 and a secondary code that identifies the complication. For patients with CKD following a kidney transplant, but who do not have a complication such as failure or rejection, *see section I.C.14. Chronic kidney disease and kidney transplant status.*

!Q ✚ T86.10   Unspecified complication of kidney transplant

SP ✚ T86.11   Kidney transplant rejection

SP ✚ T86.12   Kidney transplant failure

SP ✚ T86.13   Kidney transplant infection
Use additional code to specify infection

SP ✚ T86.19   Other complication of kidney transplant

✚ 5 T86.2   Complications of heart transplant

> **EXCLUDES 1**   complication of:
> artificial heart device (T82.5)
> heart-lung transplant (T86.3)

!Q ✚ T86.20   Unspecified complication of heart transplant

SP ✚ T86.21   Heart transplant rejection

SP ✚ T86.22   Heart transplant failure

SP ✚ T86.23   Heart transplant infection
Use additional code to specify infection

✚ 6 T86.29   Other complications of heart transplant

SP ✚ T86.290   Cardiac allograft vasculopathy

> **EXCLUDES 1**   atherosclerosis of coronary arteries (I25.75-, I25.76-, I25.81-)

SP ✚ T86.298   Other complications of heart transplant

✚ 5 T86.3   Complications of heart-lung transplant

!Q ✚ T86.30   Unspecified complication of heart-lung transplant

SP ✚ T86.31   Heart-lung transplant rejection

SP ✚ T86.32   Heart-lung transplant failure

SP ✚ T86.33   Heart-lung transplant infection
Use additional code to specify infection

SP ✚ T86.39   Other complications of heart-lung transplant

✚ 5 T86.4   Complications of liver transplant

!Q ✚ T86.40   Unspecified complication of liver transplant

SP ✚ T86.41   Liver transplant rejection

SP ✚ T86.42   Liver transplant failure

SP ✚ T86.43   Liver transplant infection
Use additional code to identify infection, such as:
Cytomegalovirus (CMV) infection (B25.-)

SP ✚ T86.49   Other complications of liver transplant

SP ✚ T86.5   Complications of stem cell transplant
Complications from stem cells from peripheral blood
Complications from stem cells from umbilical cord

✚ 5 T86.8   Complications of other transplanted organs and tissues

✚ 6 T86.81   Complications of lung transplant

> **EXCLUDES 1**   complication of heart-lung transplant (T86.3-)

SP ✚ T86.810   Lung transplant rejection

SP ✚ T86.811   Lung transplant failure

SP ✚ T86.812   Lung transplant infection
Use additional code to specify infection

SP ✚ T86.818   Other complications of lung transplant

!Q ✚ T86.819   Unspecified complication of lung transplant

✚ 6 T86.82   Complications of skin graft (allograft) (autograft)

> **EXCLUDES 2**   complication of artificial skin graft (T85.693)

SP ✚ T86.820   Skin graft (allograft) rejection

SP ✚ T86.821   Skin graft (allograft) (autograft) failure

SP ✚ T86.822   Skin graft (allograft) (autograft) infection
Use additional code to specify infection

SP ✚ T86.828   Other complications of skin graft (allograft) (autograft)

!Q ✚ T86.829   Unspecified complication of skin graft (allograft) (autograft)

✚ 6 T86.83   Complications of bone graft

> **EXCLUDES 2**   mechanical complications of bone graft (T84.3-)

SP ✚ T86.830   Bone graft rejection

SP ✚ T86.831   Bone graft failure

SP ✚ T86.832   Bone graft infection
Use additional code to specify infection

SP ✚ T86.838   Other complications of bone graft

!Q ✚ T86.839   Unspecified complication of bone graft

✚ 6 T86.84   Complications of corneal transplant

> **EXCLUDES 2**   mechanical complications of corneal graft (T85.3-)

SP ✚ T86.840   Corneal transplant rejection

SP ✚ T86.841   Corneal transplant failure

SP ✚ T86.842   Corneal transplant infection

4️⃣4th digit required   5️⃣5th digit required   6️⃣6th digit required   7️⃣7th digit required   ☑7th digit placeholder   ✚Additional code   ⬛Laterality

Use additional code to specify
infection

SP ✚ **T86.848** Other complications of corneal
transplant

IQ ✚ **T86.849** Unspecified complication of
corneal transplant

✚ **6** **T86.85** Complication of intestine transplant

SP ✚ **T86.850** Intestine transplant rejection

SP ✚ **T86.851** Intestine transplant failure

SP ✚ **T86.852** Intestine transplant infection
Use additional code to specify
infection

SP ✚ **T86.858** Other complications of intestine
transplant

IQ ✚ **T86.859** Unspecified complication of
intestine transplant

✚ **6** **T86.89** Complications of other transplanted
tissue
Transplant failure or rejection of
pancreas

SP ✚ **T86.890** Other transplanted tissue
rejection

SP ✚ **T86.891** Other transplanted tissue failure

SP ✚ **T86.892** Other transplanted tissue
infection
Use additional code to specify
infection

SP ✚ **T86.898** Other complications of other
transplanted tissue

IQ ✚ **T86.899** Unspecified complication of other
transplanted tissue

✚ **5** **T86.9** Complication of unspecified
transplanted organ and tissue

IQ ✚ **T86.90** Unspecified complication of
unspecified transplanted organ and
tissue

IQ ✚ **T86.91** Unspecified transplanted organ and
tissue rejection

IQ ✚ **T86.92** Unspecified transplanted organ and
tissue failure

IQ ✚ **T86.93** Unspecified transplanted organ and
tissue infection
Use additional code to specify infection

IQ ✚ **T86.99** Other complications of unspecified
transplanted organ and tissue

4 **T87** Complications peculiar to reattachment
and amputation

CODING TIPS ✓   Complications of amputations
include both traumatic amputations with
complications as well as surgical amputations
with complications. Note that most, but not all,
of the complication codes include the extremity
affected. These codes are more specific than
the T81 codes and should be used for any
amputation complications. These
complications do not require 7th characters.

CODING TIPS ✓   A pressure injury on the stump
related to a prosthesis is considered a Medical
Device Related Pressure Injury (MDRPI). This
describes an etiology. Use the L89 codes for
pressure ulcer/injury and the staging system to
stage. A Y79.- code may be added to indicate
the cause as a medical device.

5 **T87.0** Complications of reattached (part of)
upper extremity

6 **T87.0X** Complications of reattached (part of)
upper extremity

☰ **SP** **T87.0X1** Complications of reattached (part
of) right upper extremity

☰ **SP** **T87.0X2** Complications of reattached (part
of) left upper extremity

☰ **IQ** **T87.0X9** Complications of reattached
(part of) unspecified upper
extremity

5 **T87.1** Complications of reattached (part of)
lower extremity

6 **T87.1X** Complications of reattached (part of)
lower extremity

☰ **SP** **T87.1X1** Complications of reattached (part
of) right lower extremity

☰ **SP** **T87.1X2** Complications of reattached (part
of) left lower extremity

☰ **IQ** **T87.1X9** Complications of reattached
(part of) unspecified lower
extremity

SP **T87.2** Complications of other reattached body
part

5 **T87.3** Neuroma of amputation stump

☰ **IQ** **T87.30** Neuroma of amputation stump,
unspecified extremity

☰ **SP** **T87.31** Neuroma of amputation stump, right
upper extremity

☰ **SP** **T87.32** Neuroma of amputation stump, left
upper extremity

☰ **SP** **T87.33** Neuroma of amputation stump, right
lower extremity

☰ **SP** **T87.34** Neuroma of amputation stump, left
lower extremity

5 **T87.4** Infection of amputation stump

CODING TIPS ✓   When a patient presents with
an infected amputation stump wound,
assign the appropriate code from T87.4-.
When both dehiscence and infection are
present, code the dehiscence first (T87.81),
followed by infection. Use an additional
code to specify the infection.

☰ **IQ** **T87.40** Infection of amputation stump,
unspecified extremity

☰ **SP** **T87.41** Infection of amputation stump, right
upper extremity

☰ **SP** **T87.42** Infection of amputation stump, left
upper extremity

☰ **SP** **T87.43** Infection of amputation stump, right
lower extremity

☰ **SP** **T87.44** Infection of amputation stump, left
lower extremity

5 **T87.5** Necrosis of amputation stump

☰ **IQ** **T87.50** Necrosis of amputation stump,
unspecified extremity

☰ **SP** **T87.51** Necrosis of amputation stump, right
upper extremity

☰ **SP** **T87.52** Necrosis of amputation stump, left
upper extremity

☰ **SP** **T87.53** Necrosis of amputation stump, right
lower extremity

☰ **SP** **T87.54** Necrosis of amputation stump, left
lower extremity

5 **T87.8** Other complications of amputation
stump

SP **T87.81** Dehiscence of amputation stump

★ New   ▲ Revised   Px Primary   **SP** PDGM Px   **SL** Low CoM   **SH** High CoM   **IQ** Quest. Encounter   ⊞ Hospice non-cancer Dx   Unspecified   **M** *Manifestation*

DecisionHealth's FY 2020 Complete Home Health ICD-10-CM Diagnosis Coding Manual   1749

CODING TIPS ✓ When a patient presents with a dehiscence of an amputation stump wound, assign code T87.81. When both dehiscence and infection are present, code the dehiscence first (T87.81), followed by infection. Use an additional code to specify the infection.

SP T87.89   Other complications of amputation stump
Amputation stump contracture
Amputation stump contracture of next proximal joint
Amputation stump flexion
Amputation stump edema
Amputation stump hematoma
> **EXCLUDES 2** phantom limb syndrome (G54.6-G54.7)

CODING TIPS ✓ Do not assign a code for complication of an amputation stump for an ulcer (due to pressure, diabetic ulcer, arterial, trauma, stasis, or other) of the amputation stump. Ulcers of the amputation stump are not considered amputation stump complications. A pressure injury on the stump related to a prosthesis is considered a Medical Device Related Pressure Injury (MDRPI). This describes an etiology. Use the L89 codes for pressure ulcer/injury and the staging system to stage. A Y79.- code may be added to indicate the cause as a medical device.

IQ T87.9   Unspecified complications of amputation stump

4 T88   Other complications of surgical and medical care, not elsewhere classified
> **EXCLUDES 2** complication following infusion, transfusion and therapeutic injection (T80.-)
> complication following procedure NEC (T81.-)
> complications of anesthesia in labor and delivery (O74.-)
> complications of anesthesia in pregnancy (O29.-)
> complications of anesthesia in puerperium (O89.-)
> complications of devices, implants and grafts (T82-T85)
> complications of obstetric surgery and procedure (O75.4)
> dermatitis due to drugs and medicaments (L23.3, L24.4, L25.1, L27.0-L27.1)
> poisoning and toxic effects of drugs and chemicals (T36-T65 with fifth or sixth character 1-4 or 6)
> specified complications classified elsewhere

The appropriate 7th character is to be added to each code from category T88
A   initial encounter
D   subsequent encounter
S   sequela

CODING TIPS ✓ No aftercare code applies, including dressing changes, drain care, and suture removal. 7th character 'D' is the default for home care and hospice when providing aftercare for a healing or resolving condition; 'A' is used for active treatment such as antibiotics or more than routine wound care; 'S' may be used to indicate a residual condition after the original injury has healed. Once complication is repaired in the acute setting, continue to code the complication in home care and hospice with 7th character D if healing/resolving.

SP 7 T88.0XX-   Infection following immunization
Sepsis following immunization

SP 7 T88.1XX-   Other complications following immunization, not elsewhere classified
Generalized vaccinia
Rash following immunization
> **EXCLUDES 1** vaccinia not from vaccine (B08.011)
> **EXCLUDES 2** anaphylactic shock due to serum (T80.5-)
> other serum reactions (T80.6-)
> postimmunization arthropathy (M02.2)
> postimmunization encephalitis (G04.02)
> postimmunization fever (R50.83)

SP + 7 T88.2XX-   Shock due to anesthesia
Use additional code for adverse effect, if applicable, to identify drug (T41.- with fifth or sixth character 5)
> **EXCLUDES 1** complications of anesthesia (in):
> labor and delivery (O74.-)
> pregnancy (O29.-)
> puerperium (O89.-)
> postprocedural shock NOS (T81.1-)

SP + 7 T88.3XX-   Malignant hyperthermia due to anesthesia
Use additional code for adverse effect, if applicable, to identify drug (T41.- with fifth or sixth character 5)

SP 7 T88.4XX-   Failed or difficult intubation

+ 5 T88.5   Other complications of anesthesia
Use additional code for adverse effect, if applicable, to identify drug (T41.- with fifth or sixth character 5)

SP + 7 T88.51X-   Hypothermia following anesthesia

SP + 7 T88.52X-   Failed moderate sedation during procedure
Failed conscious sedation during procedure

---

4 4th digit required   5 5th digit required   6 6th digit required   7 7th digit required   7 7th digit placeholder   + Additional code   ⊟ Laterality

1750   DecisionHealth's FY 2020 Complete Home Health ICD-10-CM Diagnosis Coding Manual

Chapter 19

S00-T88

EXCLUDES 2 personal history of
failed moderate
sedation (Z92.83)

SP **+** ☑ **T88.53X-** **Unintended awareness under
general anesthesia during
procedure**

EXCLUDES 2 personal history of
unintended
awareness under
general anesthesia
(Z92.84)

SP **+** ☑ **T88.59X-** **Other complications of anesthesia**

SP **+** ☑ **T88.6XX-** **Anaphylactic reaction due to
adverse effect of correct drug or
medicament properly administered**

Anaphylactic shock due to adverse
effect of correct drug or
medicament properly administered

Anaphylactoid reaction NOS

Use additional code for adverse
effect, if applicable, to identify drug
(T36-T50 with fifth or sixth
character 5)

EXCLUDES 1 anaphylactic reaction
due to serum
(T80.5-)
anaphylactic shock or
reaction due to
adverse food reaction
(T78.0-)

IQ **+** ☑ **T88.7XX-** **Unspecified adverse effect of drug
or medicament**

Drug hypersensitivity NOS

Drug reaction NOS

Use additional code for adverse
effect, if applicable, to identify drug
(T36-T50 with fifth or sixth
character 5)

EXCLUDES 1 specified adverse
effects of drugs and
medicaments
(A00-R94 and T80-
T88.6, T88.8)

SP **+** ☑ **T88.8XX-** **Other specified complications of
surgical and medical care, not
elsewhere classified**

Use additional code to identify the
complication

IQ ☑ **T88.9XX-** **Complication of surgical and
medical care, unspecified**

★ New ▲ Revised Px Primary **SP** PDGM Px **SL** Low CoM **SH** High CoM **IQ** Quest. Encounter ⊞ Hospice non-cancer Dx **Unspecified** **M** *Manifestation*

DecisionHealth's FY 2020 Complete Home Health ICD-10-CM Diagnosis Coding Manual

1751

Chapter 19 Scenarios: Injury, poisoning and certain other consequences of external causes (S00-T88)

Skin graft care, burn

A 62-year-old woman is admitted to home care after having a skin graft onto her right thigh following a third-degree burn that occurred when she accidentally spilled hot oil on herself while cooking. Her doctor has ordered daily dressing changes. The skin donor site has healed and does not require care

Description	Code
Primary: Burn of third degree of right thigh, subsequent encounter	T24.311D
Secondary: Contact with fats and cooking oils, subsequent encounter	X10.2xxD

A burn that is covered with a graft is still considered a burn. Because aftercare codes for injury and trauma do not exist in ICD-10, the acute burn is coded with the appropriate seventh character, "D" to indicate that it is a subsequent encounter. The T24.- category has a "use additional code" note to include the external cause code. That code is included to specify that the burn occurred from contact with hot cooking oil.

Hip fracture

A 72-year-old man was admitted to the hospital following a surgical repair of a left hip fracture. Home physical therapy was initiated for continued aftercare. The referral indicated no other pertinent medical history except for the fall that caused the fracture.

Description	Code
Primary: Fracture of unspecified part of neck of left femur, subsequent encounter for closed fracture with routine healing	S72.002D
Secondary: Unspecified fall, subsequent encounter	W19.xxxD

Even though the fracture was treated surgically, it is still coded with the active fracture code, with a "D" to indicate the subsequent nature of the encounter, per coding guidelines. Code Z91.81 (History of falling) is not included here as there was no indication of any past history or further risks for falls. Without other documentation, a fracture not indicated as open or closed should be coded as closed. A fracture not indicated whether displaced or not displaced should be coded as displaced. Note that it's important to code whether the fracture affects the left or right hip. Unspecified hip fracture is an unacceptable primary diagnosis in PDGM.

Aftercare, amputation

A patient was trimming hedges and dropped the electric trimmer on his right foot, almost severing his foot at the ankle. The patient has a long history of diabetic PVD. The surgeon completed the amputation as a mid-calf (BKA) amputation and home health was ordered for amputation aftercare, including dressing changes.

Description	Code
Primary: Traumatic amputation partial of right foot at ankle level, subsequent encounter	S98.021D
Secondary: Diabetes with peripheral angiopathy without gangrene	E11.51
Secondary: Lower limb amputation status, below the knee	Z89.511
Secondary: Contact with powered garden and outdoor hand tools and machinery, subsequent encounter	W29.3xxD

Aftercare codes for traumatic injuries do not exist in ICD-10. Instead 7th characters are used to indicate the nature of the care provided following an injury. When a 7th character is required and the code has fewer than six characters, a placeholder "x" must be used, according to coding guidelines. The external cause code for how the injury occurred is recommended to further paint the clinical picture. *[I.A.4]*

Wound care and observation, cellulitis

A patient is admitted for wound care and IV antibiotic administration for an abdominal surgical wound infection caused by MSSA. Documentation describes the wound as affecting the organ/space surgical site. The patient had her appendix removed. The wound is also surrounded by cellulitis.

Description	Code
Primary: Infection following a procedure, organ and space surgical site, initial encounter	T81.43xA
Secondary: Cellulitis of abdominal wall	L03.311
Secondary: Methicillin susceptible Staphylococcus aureus infection as the cause of diseases classified elsewhere	B95.61
Secondary: Encounter for adjustment and management of vascular access device	Z45.2
Secondary: Long term (current) use of antibiotics	Z79.2

The surgical wound infection is used first, followed by the cellulitis code and the infecting organism. A Z code for aftercare is not appropriate when the condition is complicated. Because the infection is described as affecting the organ/space surgical site, T81.43- is the correct code. Because the patient is still receiving active treatment for the infection, via IV antibiotics, it requires the seventh character "A." The appendicitis is resolved and thus is not coded. Codes Z45.2 and Z79.2 are assigned to capture the administration and long-term use of antibiotics.

Infected wound

A patient's initial injury was a cat bite on her left hand. When her wound became infected, she was referred to home health for IV antibiotics. The PICC line also became infected. MRSA has grown out of the PICC line. Other diagnoses include diabetes and hypertension.

Description	Code
Primary: Open bite of left hand, initial encounter	S61.452A
Secondary: Other infection due to central venous catheter, initial encounter	T80.218A
Secondary: MRSA	B95.62
Secondary: Diabetes mellitus without mention of complication	E11.9
Secondary: Essential hypertension, unspecified	I10
Secondary: Long term (current) use of antibiotics	Z79.2
Secondary: Encounter for adjustment and management of vascular access device	Z45.2
Secondary: Bitten by cat, initial encounter	W55.01XA

Open wound codes are divided into groups of lacerations, puncture wounds, bites and other wounds. If the skin is unbroken, the bite is coded as a superficial injury. There is no different code to indicate complicated. The MRSA code is included because the open bite code and the catheter infection code both have a "use additional code" note to specify the infection, if known. The seventh character "A" is used for both the injury and infected catheter codes because the patient is still receiving active treatment, via the IV antibiotics. Codes Z45.2 and Z79.2 are additionally assigned to capture the administration of IV antibiotics. An external cause code (W55.01xA) is assigned to capture how the patient sustained the bite and carries the same seventh character as the wound, in accordance with coding guidelines. *[I.C.20.a.2]*

Underdosing

A patient with diagnosis of hypertension continued to experience elevated blood pressure while taking blood pressure meds. Upon patient interview, it was found the patient was taking medication once daily instead of twice daily because of the cost of the drug.

Description	Code
Primary: Essential (primary) hypertension	I10
Secondary: Underdosing of other antihypertensive drugs, subsequent encounter	T46.5x6D
Secondary: Patient's intentional underdosing of medication regimen due to financial hardship	Z91.120

Codes for underdosing should never be assigned as principal or first-listed codes, according to coding guidelines. If a patient has a relapse or exacerbation of the medical condition for which the drug is prescribed because of the reduction in dose, then the medical condition itself should be coded, according to coding guidelines. Report underdosing with codes from T36-T50 with sixth character of "6" to delineate that the adverse effect was due to "underdosing." Finally, report the appropriate Z code for the underdosing reason. *[I.C.19.e.5.c]*

Lasix poisoning

A patient has taken his Lasix 40mg every morning and night for congestive heart failure (CHF). The prescription bottle reads 40mg daily. Patient is dehydrated and hypokalemic.

Description	Code
Primary: Poisoning by diuretics	T50.1x1D
Secondary: Dehydration	E86.0
Secondary: Hypokalemia	E87.6
Secondary: Heart failure, unspecified	I50.9

This is a poisoning because the patient took an incorrect amount of the drug, from what was prescribed. When coding a poisoning or improper use of a medication first assign the appropriate code from categories T36-T50, according to coding guidelines. Use additional code(s) for manifestations of poisonings. The reason for the patient taking the Lasix in the first place, CHF, is also coded, following the manifestations of the poisoning, the dehydration and hypokalemia. *[I.C.19.e.5.b]*

Digoxin adverse effect

A patient has been taking the prescribed amount of Digoxin to treat paroxysmal atrial fibrillation. However, he's began to experience serious side effects, including visual disturbance, a pulse of 42, and bradycardia has been diagnosed. He is toxic according to lab values. Skilled nursing is ordered for observation and assessment, teaching and venipuncture for monitoring levels.

Description	Code
Primary: Other visual disturbances	H53.8
Secondary: Bradycardia	R00.1
Secondary: Adverse effect of cardiac-stimulant glycosides and drugs of similar action, subsequent encounter	T46.0x5D
Secondary: Paroxysmal atrial fibrillation	I48.0
Secondary: Encounter for therapeutic drug level monitoring	Z51.81
Secondary: Other long term (current) drug therapy	Z79.899

When coding an adverse effect of a drug that has been correctly prescribed and properly administered, assign the appropriate code for the nature of the adverse effects (the visual disturbance and bradycardia in this case) followed by the appropriate code for the adverse effect of the drug (T46.0x5D), according to coding guidelines. Do not code bradycardia as the primary diagnosis as it is not an acceptable primary reason for a home health admission. The reason the Digoxin was prescribed in the first place, paroxysmal atrial fibrillation, is also coded following the adverse effect. Codes Z51.81 and Z79.899 capture the venipuncture and drug monitoring. An adverse effect is defined as "hypersensitivity," "reaction," etc. of correct substance properly administered. *[I.C.19.e.5.a]*

Dehisced laceration, diabetic PVD

A 57-year-old woman suffered a deep gash to her right thigh when she accidentally dropped a large kitchen knife. The wound was surgically repaired in the hospital, but later dehisced. She was admitted to home health for wound care, and also has diabetic PVD. She is insulin dependent.

Description	Code
Primary: Disruption of traumatic injury wound repair, initial encounter	T81.33XA
Secondary: Laceration without foreign body, right thigh, initial encounter	S71.111A
Secondary: Type 2 diabetes mellitus with diabetic peripheral angiopathy without gangrene	E11.51
Secondary: Long term (current) use of insulin	Z79.4
Secondary: Contact with knife, initial encounter	W26.0XXA

The patient's dehisced wound is a traumatic wound that was repaired surgically and later reopened. Therefore, it codes to T81.33-. The seventh character "A" is used because there has been dehiscence, which constitutes active treatment according to the Coding Clinic. An additional code for the laceration to her thigh provides the necessary information about the type, location and laterality of the wound. Diabetic PVD is captured with the combination code E11.51. An additional code for insulin use is required because the patient is dependent on insulin but not said to be a Type 1 diabetic. An external cause code is used to help explain how she got the laceration.

Muscle flap failure, wheelchair confinement, obesity

An 80-year-old man underwent surgery to repair a stage 4 pressure ulcer/injury on his left buttocks with a muscle flap, which failed but is still covering the original pressure ulcer/injury. He is now in home health for wound care. He is also obese and confined to his wheelchair and has insulin-dependent diabetes. His BMI is calculated at 42.

Description	Code
Primary: Other transplanted tissue failure	T86.891
Secondary: Pressure ulcer of left buttock, unstageable	L89.320
Secondary: Type 2 diabetes mellitus without complications	E11.9
Secondary: Obesity, unspecified	E66.9
Secondary: Body mass index (BMI) 40.0-44.9, adult	Z68.41
Secondary: Dependence on wheelchair	Z99.3
Secondary: Long term (current) use of insulin	Z79.4

Because the stage 4 pressure ulcer/injury was treated with muscle flap that failed, it should be captured with a complication code that specifies the failure of transplanted tissue. There isn't a specific listing for this type of complication in the index. Thus, the appropriate code choice is found in the "specified tissue NEC" option, which is T86.891 (Other transplanted tissue failure). The pressure ulcer/injury is also coded as unstageable due to the fact that the flap is obscuring the wound bed, according to coding guidelines.

The patient is specified as a diabetic, but with no further information available, the only appropriate code choice is the non-specific E11.9. The patient is diagnosed as obese, and the tabular instruction at E66.9 says to use an additional code for BMI, which can easily be calculated by the assessing clinician. Obesity should always be coded when it's documented, according to Q4 2018 Coding Clinic guidance. Therefore, Z68.41 is coded directly following E66.9. His wheelchair confinement is captured with Z99.3. Insulin dependence in a type 2 diabetic requires the addition of Z79.4 and thus that is coded as well.

Dehiscence following appendectomy, obesity, diabetic kidney disease

A 67-year-old woman is admitted to home health with an abdominal wound resulting from an appendectomy. The wound has dehisced through the skin closures. She is also obese, with a BMI of 37, and has stage 3 chronic kidney disease resulting from her Type 1 diabetes.

Description	Code
Primary: Disruption of external operation (surgical) wound, not elsewhere classified, initial encounter	T81.31XA
Secondary: Type 1 diabetes mellitus with diabetic chronic kidney disease	E10.22
Secondary: Chronic kidney disease, stage 3 (moderate)	N18.3
Secondary: Obesity, unspecified	E66.9
Secondary: Body mass index (BMI) 37.0-37.9, adult	Z68.37

The surgical wound has dehisced, and because it is described as through the skin, it can be coded as an externally dehisced wound, with T81.31XA. The seventh character "A" is used because the wound has dehisced, according to Coding Clinic guidance. Though the diabetic chronic kidney disease can be captured with the combination code E10.22, an additional code, N18.3, is required to specify the stage. As a type 1 diabetic, insulin dependence is assumed and does not have to be stated with a Z code. Obesity should be coded when it's documented, according to Q4 2018 Coding Clinic guidance.

Burn from battery acid

A 59-year-old man was working in his machine shop when he accidentally spilled battery acid on his right thigh, causing a third degree burn over 15 percent of his body area. He was admitted to home health for daily wound care to his thigh.

Description	Code
Primary: Toxic effect of corrosive acids and acid-like substances, accidental (unintentional), subsequent encounter	T54.2x1D
Secondary: Corrosion of third degree of right thigh, subsequent encounter	T24.711D

The burn was caused by a corrosive chemical and should therefore be coded as a corrosion burn. The code identifying the chemical that caused the burn, T54.2x1D, must be coded first, according to tabular instruction. Because the third degree burns have not affected 20 percent or more of the patient's body, a code from the T32.- category isn't necessary.

Puncture wound

A 69-year-old woman slipped and fell while looking in boxes in her basement, suffering a puncture wound when she impaled her left calf on a sharp piece of wood that was sticking out from behind the stairway. She received nine stiches in the emergency room and was discharged to home health for wound care. Skilled nursing will be providing wound care and closely monitoring her recovery as she has diabetic peripheral angiopathy and her doctor is concerned about slow wound healing.

Description	Code
Primary: Puncture wound without foreign body, left lower leg, subsequent encounter	S81.832D
Secondary: Type 2 diabetes mellitus with diabetic peripheral angiopathy without gangrene	E11.51
Secondary: Fall on same level from slipping, tripping and stumbling with subsequent striking against other sharp object, subsequent encounter	W01.118D

The puncture wound is the focus of care and is coded primary. Her diabetes is coded as it will impact her recovery and wound healing. The external cause code is added to help explain the nature of the injury. The external cause code carries the same seventh character as the injury code, in accordance with coding guidelines.

Laceration from hedge trimmer

A 67-year-old man cut his left lower leg while trimming the bushes in front of his home with a powered hedge trimmer, resulting in a deep laceration that required surgery. Following his surgery he was admitted to home health for continue his recovery and for wound care with wet-to-dry dressings. His wound is progressing normally and the care provided is routine. He is also type 1 diabetic with diabetic stage 3 chronic kidney disease.

Description	Code
Primary: Laceration without foreign body, left lower leg, subsequent encounter	S81.812D
Secondary: Type 1 diabetes mellitus with diabetic chronic kidney disease	E10.22
Secondary: Chronic kidney disease, stage 3 (moderate)	N18.3
Secondary: Contact with powered garden and outdoor hand tools and machinery, subsequent encounter	W29.3xxD

Even though the patient underwent surgery to treat the wound, it is still coded as a trauma wound, in accordance with official coding guidelines. His diabetes and diabetic chronic kidney disease have the potential to impact his recovery and ability to fully heal from this trauma wound and therefore they are coded as well. As a type 1 diabetic, insulin dependence is assumed and the code for insulin use is therefore not required. The external cause code to capture how the wound occurred carries the same seventh character as the other codes in the scenario, in accordance with official coding guidelines. *[I.C.21.c.7] [I.C.20.a.2]*

Traumatic periprosthetic fracture

A 74-year-old man was walking down the stairs in his home when he accidentally missed a step and fell the rest of the way down. He was sent to the emergency room and was later admitted to the hospital after undergoing surgery to repair a traumatic periprosthetic fracture of the upper end of his left femur, near his left prosthetic hip joint. The prosthetic hip joint was placed two years ago. Following his hospitalization, he was admitted to home health care for skilled nursing and physical and occupational therapy. He has comorbidities of hypertension and type 2 diabetes. The fracture is the focus of care.

Description	Code
Primary: Fracture of unspecified part of neck of left femur, subsequent encounter for closed fracture with routine healing	S72.002D
Secondary: Periprosthetic fracture around internal prosthetic left hip joint, subsequent encounter	M97.02xD
Secondary: Essential (primary) hypertension	I10
Secondary: Type 2 diabetes mellitus without complications	E11.9
Secondary: Fall (on) (from) unspecified stairs and steps, subsequent encounter	W10.9xxD

As the focus of care, the fracture is coded first, with the code for the traumatic fracture sequenced ahead of the periprosthetic fracture, in accordance with Q4 2016 Coding Clinic guidance. The etiology of the fracture is traumatic and is thus coded as a traumatic fracture with S72.002D. Note that coding the specific location of the fracture (left or right side) is critical as a code for a fracture of an unspecified hip is not an acceptable primary diagnosis code in PDGM. The patient's comorbidities of hypertension and type 2 diabetes have the potential to impact his recovery and thus should be coded. An external cause code, W10.9xxD, is used to describe how the patient suffered the traumatic fracture, in a fall down the stairs.

Shoulder fracture, joint replacement

A 70-year-old man underwent surgery to replace his right shoulder after slipping on an ice-covered walkway and sustaining a fracture of the upper end of his right humerus. He also has comorbid diagnoses of diet-controlled type 2 diabetes and hypertension.

Description	Code
Primary: Unspecified fracture of upper end of right humerus, subsequent encounter for fracture with routine healing	S42.201D
Secondary: Type 2 diabetes mellitus without complications	E11.9
Secondary: Essential (primary) hypertension	I10
Secondary: Presence of right artificial shoulder joint	Z96.611
Secondary: Fall on same level due to ice and snow, subsequent encounter	W00.0xxD

The impetus for the patient's shoulder replacement surgery was a fracture. Because an injury necessitated surgery, a surgical aftercare code is not appropriate. Instead, the fracture itself is coded with the seventh character "D" to denote the subsequent nature of the home health encounter. Diabetes and hypertension are coded as relevant comorbidities that will impact his recovery. A status code to capture the site of the implanted joint is assigned. An external cause code is assigned to help explain how the patient sustained the fracture.

Fibula fracture, infected wound, stitch abscess

A 79-year-old man fractured the shaft of his left fibula and underwent an ORIF procedure to repair it. His fracture is healing normally but the surgical incision site developed a stitch abscess. He arrives in home health with orders for wound care and is still taking oral antibiotics to treat the infection. He will also receive physical and occupational therapy. He also has type 2 diabetes, which is currently stable.

Description	Code
Primary: Infection following a procedure, superficial incisional surgical site, initial encounter	T81.41xA
Secondary: Unspecified fracture of shaft of left fibula, subsequent encounter for closed fracture with routine healing	S82.402D
Secondary: Type 2 diabetes mellitus without complications	E11.9
Secondary: Long term (current) use of antibiotics	Z79.2

The incision site is still requiring active treatment for the infection, which was described as a stitch abscess and thus is coded with T81.41-. The seventh character "A" is assigned because the infection is still being actively treated with antibiotics. The fracture is healing normally and is thus coded with "D." Diabetes is coded as a relevant comorbidity that will require monitoring. The patient continues to take antibiotics and thus Z79.2 is coded to capture this.

HOME HEALTH CODING SCENARIOS

Healing infected surgical wound

A 67-year-old man is being recerted for another episode of home health to continue wound care to a surgical wound. He underwent coronary artery bypass graft (CABG) surgery to treat coronary artery disease and the surgical wound became infected at the superficial incisional surgical site. The infection has now resolved but wound care is still required.

Description	Code
Primary: Infection following a procedure, superficial incisional surgical site, subsequent encounter	T81.41xD
Secondary: Atherosclerotic heart disease of native coronary artery without angina pectoris	I25.10
Secondary: Presence of aortocoronary bypass graft	Z95.1

The infection has resolved and so an infecting organism is not coded. But the wound was previously complicated and thus should still be coded with a complication code, T81.41-. The seventh character "D" signifies that the wound has progressed into the healing phase and is no longer being actively treated. Though the patient had the CABG surgery to treat his coronary artery disease, the operation does not cure the condition; it only treats it. Thus, coronary artery disease is still coded with I25.10. The status of his CABG is captured with Z95.1.

Broken internal hip joint

A 68-year-old woman who has had an internal right hip joint prosthesis for more than three years, was experiencing severe pain in that hip for two days. A trip to the ER revealed a break in her prosthetic hip joint. She recalled falling on some ice on the sidewalk in front of her home several months prior but did not recall any specific injuries from that fall and could not think of any more recent trauma. She was admitted to home health for physical therapy for strengthening until she undergoes surgery to replace the broken prosthetic.

Description	Code
Primary: Broken internal right hip prosthesis, subsequent encounter	T84.010D
Secondary: Fall on same level due to ice and snow, subsequent encounter	W00.0xxD

The internal joint prosthetic itself is broken, necessitating a code from T84.01-. The right hip is affected, making the proper primary diagnosis code T84.010D, with a seventh character "D" for the subsequent nature of the home health encounter. A status code for the replaced joint is not assigned in this scenario as the complication code captures it.

Black widow spider bite

A 67-year-old man sustained a bite on the left forearm from a black widow spider. The focus of care is managing the healing of the bite. He also has diabetes, which is stable and diet-controlled.

Description	Code
Primary: Toxic effect of venom of black widow spider, accidental (unintentional), subsequent encounter	T63.311D
Secondary: Type 2 diabetes mellitus without complications	E11.9

A venous spider bite is coded as a poisoning, with a code from the Table of Drugs and Chemicals, according to the alphabetic index. Diabetes is a relevant comorbidity that could impact his recovery and is thus coded.

Dog bite

A 70-year-old man was mowing his lawn when a dog attacked him and bit his left ankle. The wound is clean without evidence of infection. He also has diagnoses of diabetes and PVD, which could complicate his wound healing. He will receive skilled nursing for wound care.

Description	Code
Primary: Open bite, left ankle, subsequent encounter	S91.052D
Secondary: Type 2 diabetes mellitus with diabetic peripheral angiopathy without gangrene	E11.51
Secondary: Bitten by dog, subsequent encounter	W54.0xxD

The patient has a wound resulting from the dog bite that is the focus of care; thus it is coded as primary. Diabetes and PVD can be assumed to be connected in the absence of another stated etiology. Thus, E11.51 is assigned. While there is no requirement to assign external cause codes, it paints the picture of the patient and his injuries and will help support the care provided.

Revision of right hip prosthesis

A 68-year-old man comes to home health for skilled nursing and physical therapy after undergoing revision surgery to his right prosthetic hip after part of it became dislocated. He has an underlying diagnosis of rheumatoid arthritis.

Description	Code
Primary: Dislocation of internal right hip prosthesis, subsequent encounter	T84.020D
Secondary: Rheumatoid arthritis, unspecified	M06.9

The patient underwent a joint prosthesis revision and thus the complication that necessitated the revision should be coded, not surgical aftercare. In this case, it was a dislocation and thus T84.020D is assigned to capture the dislocation of a right hip prosthesis. His rheumatoid arthritis will impact his recovery and will be a factor in his physical therapy. Therefore it is coded as a relevant comorbidity. No status code is assigned because the complication code identifies the joint.

Mechanical loosening of joint prosthesis

An 82-year-old man comes to home health for surgical aftercare following a revision to his right prosthetic hip joint after a part of it had loosened. He also has severe GERD, which will require monitoring and for which he just started new medications. He will receive skilled nursing and physical therapy.

Description	Code
Primary: Mechanical loosening of internal right hip prosthetic joint, subsequent encounter	T84.030D
Secondary: Gastro-esophageal reflux disease without esophagitis	K21.9

While the patient will be receiving aftercare, the patient underwent a joint prosthetic revision due to a mechanical loosening, which is a complication. Therefore, an aftercare code from Z47.3- (Aftercare following explantation of joint prosthesis) is not appropriate in this scenario. The complication itself is coded instead. The patient's GERD is coded because he is starting new medications and the condition will require monitoring. No status code is required because the complication code identifies the replaced joint.

Traumatic subdural hemorrhage

A 74-year-old patient was diagnosed with Alzheimer's dementia with behavioral problems, dysphagia and hypertension two years ago. Two months ago she suffered a domestic violence assault in which her former husband hit her in the head with a shoe causing her to lose consciousness for about 20 minutes. The patient had a burr hole evacuation procedure to evacuate a hematoma that had increased in size. The surgeon diagnosed a chronic subdural hemorrhage and noted that re-accumulation of blood was likely which would lead to additional hematomas and neurological deficits. Her family opted for no further imaging and has elected the hospice benefit. She requires total care.

Description	Code
Primary: Traumatic subdural hemorrhage with loss of consciousness of 30 minutes or less, subsequent encounter	S06.5x1D
Secondary: Alzheimer's disease, unspecified	G30.9
Secondary: Dementia in other diseases classified elsewhere with behavioral disturbance	F02.81
Secondary: Essential (primary) hypertension	I10
Secondary: Dysphagia, unspecified	R13.10
Secondary: Assault by blunt object, subsequent encounter	Y00.xxxD

The patient's head injury was treated but is not resolved and the patient's family is opting to forgo further investigation. Thus, the head injury is coded in the primary position with the seventh character "D." The Alzheimer's disease with behaviors, dysphagia and hypertension are coded as relevant comorbidities that will impact her care. The external cause code Y00.xxxD is assigned to explain how the patient became injured; in this case, it was an assault.

Infected wound, knee replacement, lupus

A 72-year-old woman recently underwent a right knee replacement to treat osteoarthritis that affects both knees. Her surgical wound incision is documented as infected by the documentation states that the infection is superficial and only affecting the incision itself. The prosthesis is uncomplicated. She was prescribed oral antibiotics for several weeks for the incisional infection. Skilled nursing will provide and teach wound care and dressing changes, medication management, and monitoring PT/INRs. She'll also receive physical and occupational therapy. Other diagnoses include hypertension and systemic lupus erythematosus. She is on an anticoagulant and long-term prednisone due to her lupus.

Description	Code
Primary: Infection following a procedure, superficial incisional surgical site, initial encounter	T81.41xA
Secondary: Unilateral primary osteoarthritis, left knee	M17.12
Secondary: Systemic lupus erythematosus, unspecified	M32.9
Secondary: Essential (primary) hypertension	I10
Secondary: Presence of right artificial knee joint	Z96.651
Secondary: Encounter for therapeutic drug level monitoring	Z51.81
Secondary: Long term (current) use of antibiotics	Z79.2
Secondary: Long term (current) use of anticoagulants	Z79.01
Secondary: Long term (current) use of systemic steroids	Z79.52

Though the surgical wound is infected, it is only affecting the incision and the joint prosthetic is healing normally. Therefore, T81.41- is the appropriate code choice. The seventh character "A" is used because the infection is being actively treated with antibiotics. The patient's comorbidities of lupus and hypertension are coded as secondary diagnoses that will require monitoring. A status code is assigned to denote the replaced knee joint, because the joint prosthetic itself is not complicated. PT/INR monitoring and her use of antibiotics, systemic steroids and anticoagulants are coded as well.

Sepsis due to midline catheter infection

A 66-year-old woman is admitted to home health for treatment, with IV antibiotics, of gram-negative sepsis caused by a midline catheter infection. She is morbidly obese and has insulin-dependent diabetes and hypertension.

Description	Code
Primary: Infection and inflammatory reaction due to other cardiac and vascular devices, implants and grafts, initial encounter	T82.7XXA
Secondary: Gram-negative sepsis, unspecified	A41.50
Secondary: Type 2 diabetes mellitus without complications	E11.9
Secondary: Essential (primary) hypertension	I10
Secondary: Morbid (severe) obesity due to excess calories	E66.01
Secondary: Encounter for adjustment and management of vascular access device	Z45.2
Secondary: Long term (current) use of antibiotics	Z79.2
Secondary: Long term (current) use of insulin	Z79.4

Sepsis due to a midline catheter infection should be coded first with T82.7- followed by the code for the sepsis as the code choice should be driven by the location of the catheter, not its use, according to Q1 2019 Coding Clinic guidance. A seventh character "A" is assigned as the condition is receiving active treatment. Diabetes and hypertension are relevant comorbidities that will impact her care and are thus coded. Morbid obesity is always clinically relevant and should be assigned whether it's the focus of home health treatment, per Q4 2018 Coding Clinic guidance. The administration of IV antibiotics and the dependence on insulin, as a non-type 1 diabetic, are captured with Z45.2, Z79.2 and Z79.4.

HOME HEALTH CODING SCENARIOS

Chapter 20: External Causes of Morbidity (V00-Y99)

Chapter 20 encompasses codes with alpha characters V, W, X and Y, and contains a massive expansion from ICD-9-CM. This chapter permits the classification of environmental events and circumstances as the cause of injury and other adverse effects. Where a code from this section is applicable, it is intended that it shall be used secondary to a code from another ICD-10 chapter indicating the nature of the condition. Most often the condition will be classifiable to Chapter 19, Injury, poisoning and certain other consequences of external causes (S00-T88). Other conditions that may be stated to be due to external causes are classified in Chapters 1 through 18. For these conditions, codes from Chapter 20 may be used to provide additional information as to the cause of the condition.

External cause codes are intended to provide data for injury research and evaluation of injury prevention strategies. However, an external cause code(s) may be used with any code in the range of A00.0-T88.9, Z00-Z99, indicating a health condition due to an external cause such as infections, a disease due to an external source, or another health condition such as a heart attack that occurs during strenuous physical activity.

The codes capture how the injury or health condition happened (cause); the intent (unintentional or accidental; or intentional, such as suicide or assault); the place where the event occurred; the activity of the patient at the time of the event; and the person's status (e.g., civilian, military). The acronym IPAS can be used to remember the sequence of external cause codes – Intent/injury, Place, Activity and Status.

There is no national requirement for mandatory ICD-10-CM external cause code reporting. Unless a provider is subject to a state-based external cause code reporting mandate or these codes are required by a particular payer, reporting of ICD-10-CM codes found in Chapter 20, External Causes of Morbidity, is not required. In the absence of a mandatory reporting requirement, providers are encouraged to voluntarily report external cause codes, as they provide valuable data for injury research and evaluation of injury prevention strategies. (*Source: ICD-10-CM Official Guidelines for Coding and Reporting, 2014*)

Reminder: Within the Official Coding Guidelines, the term provider is used throughout the guidelines to mean physician or any qualified health care practitioner who is legally accountable for establishing the patient's diagnosis.

If an agency chooses to voluntarily report external cause codes, only the code for the intent/cause should be reported. External cause codes for place of encounter, activity and status codes are **used only once at the initial encounter for treatment.** Home health or hospice is never the initial encounter site for treatment (e.g., the patient was seen by a physician in the ER or urgent-care center to diagnose and order treatment first).

External Cause Coding Guidelines

- External cause codes utilize a 7th character to designate the initial encounter, subsequent encounter or sequela for the entire length of treatment for which the injury or condition is being treated.

- The full range of external cause codes is used to completely describe the cause, intent, place of occurrence, and if applicable, the activity of the patient **at the time of the event.**

- No external cause code from Chapter 20 is needed if the external cause and intent are included in the code from another chapter (e.g., T36.0X1, poisoning by penicillins, accidental (unintentional).

Place of Occurrence Guidelines

- Codes from category Y92, Place of occurrence of the external cause, are secondary codes for use after other external cause codes to identify the location of the patient at the time of injury or other condition.

- **A place of occurrence code is used only once, at the initial encounter for treatment.** No 7th characters are used for Y92 and only one Y92 code should be recorded on a medical record. A place of occurrence should be used in conjunction with an activity code, Y93.

- **Do not use** Y92.9, unknown location, if the place of occurrence is not stated or is not applicable.

Activity Code

- Assign a code from category Y93 to describe the activity of the patient at the time the injury or when another health condition occurred, such as a heart attack (I21.3) while shoveling snow (Y93. H1) where the MI resulted from the activity or was contributed to by the activity.

- Activity codes are appropriate for use for both acute injuries, such as those from Chapter 19, and conditions that are due to the long-term, cumulative effects of an activity, such as those from Chapter 13. They are also appropriate for use with external cause and intent codes if identifying the activity provides additional information about the event.

- **An activity code is used only once, at the initial encounter for treatment** and only one code from Y93 should be recorded on a medical record. An activity code should be used in conjunction with codes for external cause status (Y99) and place of occurrence code, Y92.

- The activity codes are not applicable to poisonings, adverse effects, misadventures or sequela.

- **Do not assign** Y93.9, Unspecified activity, if the activity is not stated.

External Cause Status

A code from category Y99, External cause status, should be assigned in all cases when any other external cause code is assigned for an encounter, including an activity code, except for the specific events noted below. Assign a code from category Y99, External cause status, to indicate the work status of the person at the time the event occurred. The status code indicates whether the event occurred during military activity, whether a non-military person was at work, or whether an individual including a student or volunteer was involved in a non-work activity at the time of the causal event.

- A code from Y99, External cause status, should be assigned, when applicable, with other external cause codes, such as transport accidents and falls. The external cause status codes are *not applicable* to poisonings, adverse effects, misadventures or late effects. Do not assign a code from category Y99 if no other external cause codes (cause, activity) are applicable for the encounter.

- *An external cause status code is only used once, at the initial encounter for treatment.* Only one code from Y99 should be reported on a medical record.

- Do not assign code Y99.9, Unspecified external cause status, if the status is not stated.

When applicable, place of occurrence, activity and external cause status codes are sequenced after the main external cause code(s). Regardless of the number of external cause codes assigned, there should be only one place of occurrence code, one activity code, and one external cause status code assigned to an encounter.

Multiple External Cause Coding Guidelines

- If the reporting format permits the capture of additional external cause codes, the cause /intent, including medical misadventures, of the additional events should be reported rather than the codes for place, activity or external status.

- When two or more events cause separate injuries, an external cause code should be assigned for each cause. The assignment of the external cause codes should be sequenced in the following priority:

  - The first-listed external cause code(s) for child and adult abuse takes priority over all other external cause codes.

  - External cause codes for terrorism events take priority over all other external cause codes except child and adult abuse.

  - External cause codes for cataclysmic events take priority over all other external cause codes except child and adult abuse, and terrorism.

  - Activity and external cause status codes are assigned following all causal (intent) external cause codes.

  - The first-listed external cause code should correspond to the cause of the most serious diagnosis due to an assault, accident, or self-harm, following the order of hierarchy listed above.

Adult and child abuse, neglect and maltreatment are classified as assault. Any of the assault codes may be used to indicate the external cause of an injury resulting from confirmed abuse. For confirmed cases of abuse, neglect and maltreatment, when the perpetrator is known, a code from Y07, Perpetrator of maltreatment and neglect, should accompany any other assault codes.

Unknown intent: If the intent (accident, self-harm, assault) of the cause of an injury or other condition is unknown or unspecified, code the intent as accidental intent. All transport accident categories assume accidental intent. External cause codes for events of undetermined intent are only for use if the documentation in the record specifies that the intent cannot be determined.

Sequelae (Late Effects) of External Cause

- Sequelae are reported using the external cause code with the 7th character "S" for sequela. These codes should be used with any report of a late effect or sequela resulting from a previous injury.

- A sequela external cause code should never be used with a related current nature of injury code.

- Use a late effect external cause code for subsequent visits when a late effect of the initial injury is being treated. **Do not use** a late effect external cause code for subsequent visits for follow-up care (e.g., to assess healing, to receive rehabilitative therapy) of the injury when no late effect of the injury has been documented.

Terrorism Guidelines

- When the cause of an injury is **defined by the Federal Government (FBI)** as terrorism, the first-listed external cause code should be a code from category Y38, Terrorism. The definition of terrorism used by the FBI is found at the inclusion note at the beginning of category Y38. An additional code for place of occurrence (Y92.-) also is used. More than one Y38 code may be assigned if the injury is the result of more than one mechanism of terrorism.

- When the cause of the injury is **suspected** to be the result of terrorism, a code from category Y38 should **not** be assigned. Suspected cases should be classified as assault.

- Assign code Y38.9, Terrorism, secondary effects, for conditions occurring subsequent to the terrorist event. This code should not be assigned for conditions that are due to the initial terrorist act.

- It is acceptable to assign code Y38.9 with another code from Y38 if there is an injury due to the initial terrorist event and an injury that is a subsequent result of the terrorist event.

Major Categories in Chapter 20

Transport Accidents (V00-V99) involve a variety of types of injuries that are associated with the various types of transport vehicles, including:

- Pedestrians injured in transport accident (V00-V09)

- Pedal cycle rider injured in transport accidents (V10-V19)

- Motorcycle rider injured in transport accident (V20-V29)

- Occupant of three-wheeled motor vehicle injured in transport accident (V30-V39)

- Car occupant injured in transport accident (V40-V49)

- Occupant of pick-up truck or van injured in transport accident (V50-V59)

- Occupant of heavy transport vehicle injured in transport accident (V60-V69)

- Bus occupant injured in transport accident (V70-V79)

- Other land transport accidents (V80-V89)

- Water transport accidents (V90-V94)

- Air and space transport accidents (V95-V97)

- Other and unspecified transport accidents (V98-V99)

Other external causes of accidental injury (W00-X58)

- Slipping, tripping, stumbling and falls (W00-W19): includes falls from stairs or steps, ladders or scaffolding, out of building or other structures, down manholes or wells, into water, and other tripping, slipping and stumbling.

- Exposure to inanimate mechanical forces (W20-W49)

- Exposure to animate mechanical forces (W50-W64): involves injury by person, rodent, dog, cat, other mammals, nonvenomous marine animal, nonvenomous insect or arthropod, crocodile or alligator, nonvenomous plant thorns, spines or sharp leaves, birds, and nonvenomous amphibians

- Accidental non-transport drowning and submersion (W65-74)

- Exposure to electric current, radiation and extreme ambient temperature and pressure (W85-W99)

- Exposure to smoke, fire and flames (X00-X08)

- Contact with heat and hot substances (X10-X19)

- Exposure to forces of nature (X30-X39)

- Accidental exposure to other specified factors (X52-X58)

- Intentional self-harm (X71-X83)

- Assault (X92-Y09)

- Event of undetermined intent (Y21-Y33)

- Legal intervention, operations of war, military operations, and terrorism (Y35-Y38)

Complications of medical and surgical care (Y62-Y84)

- Misadventures to patients during surgical and medical care (Y62-Y69)

- Medical devices associated with adverse incidents in diagnostic and therapeutic use (Y70-Y82)

- Surgical and other medical procedures as the cause of abnormal reaction of the patient, or later complication, without mention of misadventure at the time of the procedure (Y83-Y84)

- Supplementary factors related to causes of morbidity classified elsewhere (Y90-Y99); physician must determine if this occurred.

CHAPTER 20: EXTERNAL CAUSES OF MORBIDITY (V00-Y99)

Note:

This chapter permits the classification of environmental events and circumstances as the cause of injury, and other adverse effects. Where a code from this section is applicable, it is intended that it shall be used secondary to a code from another chapter of the Classification indicating the nature of the condition. Most often, the condition will be classifiable to Chapter 19, Injury, poisoning and certain other consequences of external causes (S00-T88). Other conditions that may be stated to be due to external causes are classified in Chapters I to XVIII. For these conditions, codes from Chapter 20 should be used to provide additional information as to the cause of the condition.

GUIDELINES ✓ Section I.C.20

The external causes of morbidity codes should never be sequenced as the first-listed or principal diagnosis. External cause codes are intended to provide data for injury research and evaluation of injury prevention strategies. These codes capture how the injury or health condition happened (cause), the intent (unintentional or accidental; or intentional, such as suicide or assault), the place where the event occurred the activity of the patient at the time of the event, and the person's status (e.g., civilian, military).

There is no national requirement for mandatory ICD-10-CM external cause code reporting. Unless a provider is subject to a state-based external cause code reporting mandate or these codes are required by a particular payer, reporting of ICD-10-CM codes in Chapter 20, External Causes of Morbidity, is not required. In the absence of a mandatory reporting requirement, providers are encouraged to voluntarily report external cause codes, as they provide valuable data for injury research and evaluation of injury prevention strategies.

GUIDELINES ✓ Section I.C.20.a.2)

Most categories in chapter 20 have a 7th character requirement for each applicable code. ... While the patient may be seen by a new or different provider over the course of treatment for an injury or condition, assignment of the 7th character for external cause should match the 7th character of the code assigned for the associated injury or condition for the encounter.

CODING TIPS ✓ These codes are used to explain injuries. External cause codes for accidents should not be assigned if there is no injury coded on the claim.

CODING TIPS ✓ These codes can never be placed as primary. Guidelines indicate that they are encouraged, but not required, for home care and hospice. However, if a convention (tabular instruction) indicates to use an additional code, the coder should query for more information and use the code (i.e. for L57 and burns).

CODING TIPS ✓ External cause codes may be coded based on documentation other than the physician's.

This chapter contains the following blocks:

V00-X58	Accidents
V00-V99	Transport accidents
V00-V09	Pedestrian injured in transport accident
V10-V19	Pedal cycle rider injured in transport accident
V20-V29	Motorcycle rider injured in transport accident
V30-V39	Occupant of three-wheeled motor vehicle injured in transport accident
V40-V49	Car occupant injured in transport accident
V50-V59	Occupant of pick-up truck or van injured in transport accident
V60-V69	Occupant of heavy transport vehicle injured in transport accident
V70-V79	Bus occupant injured in transport accident
V80-V89	Other land transport accidents
V90-V94	Water transport accidents
V95-V97	Air and space transport accidents
V98-V99	Other and unspecified transport accidents
W00-X58	Other external causes of accidental injury
W00-W19	Slipping, tripping, stumbling and falls
W20-W49	Exposure to inanimate mechanical forces
W50-W64	Exposure to animate mechanical forces
W65-W74	Accidental non-transport drowning and submersion
W85-W99	Exposure to electric current, radiation and extreme ambient air temperature and pressure
X00-X08	Exposure to smoke, fire and flames
X10-X19	Contact with heat and hot substances
X30-X39	Exposure to forces of nature
X50	Overexertion and strenuous or repetitive movements
X52-X58	Accidental exposure to other specified factors
X71-X83	Intentional self-harm
X92-Y09	Assault
Y21-Y33	Event of undetermined intent
Y35-Y38	Legal intervention, operations of war, military operations, and terrorism
Y62-Y84	Complications of medical and surgical care
Y62-Y69	Misadventures to patients during surgical and medical care
Y70-Y82	Medical devices associated with adverse incidents in diagnostic and therapeutic use
Y83-Y84	Surgical and other medical procedures as the cause of abnormal reaction of the patient, or of later complication, without mention of misadventure at the time of the procedure
Y90-Y99	Supplementary factors related to causes of morbidity classified elsewhere

Accidents   (V00-X58)

Transport accidents   (V00-V99)

Note:

This section is structured in 12 groups. Those relating to land transport accidents (V00-V89) reflect the victim's mode of transport and are subdivided to identify the victim's 'counterpart' or the type of event. The vehicle of which the injured person is an occupant is identified in the first two characters since it is seen as the most important factor to identify for prevention purposes. A transport accident is one in which the vehicle involved must be moving or running or in use for transport purposes at the time of the accident.

Definitions related to transport accidents:

(a) A transport accident (V00-V99) is any accident involving a device designed primarily for, or used at the time primarily for, conveying persons or good from one place to another.

(b) A public highway [trafficway] or street is the entire width between property lines (or other boundary lines) of land open to the public as a matter of right or custom for purposes of moving persons or property from one place to another. A roadway is that part of the public highway designed, improved and customarily used for vehicular traffic.

(c) A traffic accident is any vehicle accident occurring on the public highway [i.e. originating on, terminating on, or involving a vehicle partially on the highway]. A vehicle accident is assumed to have occurred on the public highway unless another place is specified, except in the case of accidents involving only off-road motor vehicles, which are classified as nontraffic accidents unless the contrary is stated.

---

4 4th digit required   **5** 5th digit required   **6** 6th digit required   **7** 7th digit required   **7** 7th digit placeholder   **+** Additional code   **▤** Laterality

(d) A nontraffic accident is any vehicle accident that occurs entirely in any place other than a public highway.

(e) A pedestrian is any person involved in an accident who was not at the time of the accident riding in or on a motor vehicle, railway train, streetcar or animal-drawn or other vehicle, or on a pedal cycle or animal. This includes, a person changing a tire, working on a parked car, or a person on foot. It also includes the user of a pedestrian conveyance such as a baby stroller, ice-skates, skis, sled, roller skates, a skateboard, nonmotorized or motorized wheelchair, motorized mobility scooter, or nonmotorized scooter.

(f) A driver is an occupant of a transport vehicle who is operating or intending to operate it.

(g) A passenger is any occupant of a transport vehicle other than the driver, except a person traveling on the outside of the vehicle.

(h) A person on the outside of a vehicle is any person being transported by a vehicle but not occupying the space normally reserved for the driver or passengers, or the space intended for the transport of property. This includes a person travelling on the bodywork, bumper, fender, roof, running board or step of a vehicle, as well as, hanging on the outside of the vehicle.

(i) A pedal cycle is any land transport vehicle operated solely by nonmotorized pedals including a bicycle or tricycle.

(j) A pedal cyclist is any person riding a pedal cycle or in a sidecar or trailer attached to a pedal cycle.

(k) A motorcycle is a two-wheeled motor vehicle with one or two riding saddles and sometimes with a third wheel for the support of a sidecar. The sidecar is considered part of the motorcycle. This includes a moped, motor scooter, or motorized bicycle.

(l) A motorcycle rider is any person riding a motorcycle or in a sidecar or trailer attached to the motorcycle.

(m) A three-wheeled motor vehicle is a motorized tricycle designed primarily for on-road use. This includes a motor-driven tricycle, a motorized rickshaw, or a three-wheeled motor car.

(n) A car [automobile] is a four-wheeled motor vehicle designed primarily for carrying up to 7 persons. A trailer being towed by the car is considered part of the car. It does not include a van or minivan - see definition (o)

(o) A pick-up truck or van is a four or six-wheeled motor vehicle designed for carrying passengers as well as property or cargo weighing less than the local limit for classification as a heavy goods vehicle, and not requiring a special driver's license. This includes a minivan and a sport-utility vehicle (SUV).

(p) A heavy transport vehicle is a motor vehicle designed primarily for carrying property, meeting local criteria for classification as a heavy goods vehicle in terms of weight and requiring a special driver's license.

(q) A bus (coach) is a motor vehicle designed or adapted primarily for carrying more than 10 passengers, and requiring a special driver's license.

(r) A railway train or railway vehicle is any device, with or without freight or passenger cars couple to it, designed for traffic on a railway track. This includes subterranean (subways) or elevated trains.

(s) A streetcar, is a device designed and used primarily for transporting passengers within a municipality, running on rails, usually subject to normal traffic control signals, and operated principally on a right-of-way that forms part of the roadway. This includes a tram or trolley that runs on rails. A trailer being towed by a streetcar is considered part of the streetcar.

(t) A special vehicle mainly used on industrial premises is a motor vehicle designed primarily for use within the buildings and premises of industrial or commercial establishments. This includes battery-powered airport passenger vehicles or baggage/mail trucks, forklifts, coal-cars in a coal mine, logging cars and trucks used in mines or quarries.

(u) A special vehicle mainly used in agriculture is a motor vehicle designed specifically for use in farming and agriculture (horticulture), to work the land, tend and harvest crops and transport materials on the farm. This includes harvesters, farm machinery and tractor and trailers.

(v) A special construction vehicle is a motor vehicle designed specifically for use on construction and demolition sites. This includes bulldozers, diggers, earth levellers, dump trucks. backhoes, front-end loaders, pavers, and mechanical shovels.

(w) A special all-terrain vehicle is a motor vehicle of special design to enable it to negotiate over rough or soft terrain, snow or sand. Examples of special design are high construction, special wheels and tires, tracks, and support on a cushion of air. This includes snow mobiles, All-terrain vehicles (ATV), and dune buggies. It does not include passenger vehicle designated as Sport Utility Vehicles. (SUV)

(x) A watercraft is any device designed for transporting passengers or goods on water. This includes motor or sail boats, ships, and hovercraft.

(y) An aircraft is any device for transporting passengers or goods in the air. This includes hot-air balloons, gliders, helicopters and airplanes.

(z) A military vehicle is any motorized vehicle operating on a public roadway owned by the military and being operated by a member of the military.

Use additional code to identify:
Airbag injury (W22.1)
Type of street or road (Y92.4-)
Use of cellular telephone and other electronic equipment at the time of the transport accident (Y93.C-)

EXCLUDES 1	agricultural vehicles in stationary use or maintenance (W31.-)
	assault by crashing of motor vehicle (Y03.-)
	automobile or motor cycle in stationary use or maintenance- code to type of accident
	crashing of motor vehicle, undetermined intent (Y32)
	intentional self-harm by crashing of motor vehicle (X82)
EXCLUDES 2	transport accidents due to cataclysm (X34-X38)

Pedestrian injured in transport accident (V00-V09)

INCLUDES	person changing tire on transport vehicle
	person examining engine of vehicle broken down in (on side of) road
EXCLUDES 1	fall due to non-transport collision with other person (W03)
	pedestrian on foot falling (slipping) on ice and snow (W00.-)
	struck or bumped by another person (W51)

+ ⬛4 V00   Pedestrian conveyance accident

Use additional place of occurrence and activity external cause codes, if known (Y92.-, Y93.-)

| **EXCLUDES 1** | collision with another person without fall (W51) |
| | fall due to person on foot colliding with another person on foot (W03) |

★ New ▲ Revised Px Primary **SP** PDGM Px **SL** Low CoM **SH** High CoM **IQ** Quest. Encounter **H** Hospice non-cancer Dx   Unspecified   **M** *Manifestation*

DecisionHealth's FY 2020 Complete Home Health ICD-10-CM Diagnosis Coding Manual

1769

fall from non-moving
wheelchair, nonmotorized
scooter and motorized
mobility scooter without
collision (W05.-)
pedestrian (conveyance)
collision with other land
transport vehicle (V01-V09)
pedestrian on foot falling
(slipping) on ice and snow
(W00.-)

The appropriate 7th character is to be added to
each code from category V00
A   initial encounter
D   subsequent encounter
S   sequela

+ ⑤ V00.0   Pedestrian on foot injured in collision with pedestrian conveyance

!Q + ⑦ V00.01X-   Pedestrian on foot injured in collision with roller-skater

!Q + ⑦ V00.02X-   Pedestrian on foot injured in collision with skateboarder

!Q + ⑦ V00.09X-   Pedestrian on foot injured in collision with other pedestrian conveyance

+ ⑤ V00.1   Rolling-type pedestrian conveyance accident

> EXCLUDES 1   accident with baby stroller
> (V00.82-)
> accident with wheelchair
> (powered) (V00.81-)
> accident with motorized
> mobility scooter
> (V00.83-)

+ ⑥ V00.11   In-line roller-skate accident

!Q + ⑦ V00.111-   Fall from in-line roller-skates

!Q + ⑦ V00.112-   In-line roller-skater colliding with stationary object

!Q + ⑦ V00.118-   Other in-line roller-skate accident

> EXCLUDES 1   roller-skater collision
> with other land
> transport vehicle
> (V01-V09 with 5th
> character 1)

+ ⑥ V00.12   Non-in- line roller-skate accident

!Q + ⑦ V00.121-   Fall from non-in-line roller-skates

!Q + ⑦ V00.122-   Non-in-line roller-skater colliding with stationary object

!Q + ⑦ V00.128-   Other non-in-line roller-skating accident

> EXCLUDES 1   roller-skater collision
> with other land
> transport vehicle
> (V01-V09 with 5th
> character 1)

+ ⑥ V00.13   Skateboard accident

!Q + ⑦ V00.131-   Fall from skateboard

!Q + ⑦ V00.132-   Skateboarder colliding with stationary object

!Q + ⑦ V00.138-   Other skateboard accident

> EXCLUDES 1   skateboarder
> collision with other
> land transport
> vehicle
> (V01-V09 with 5th
> character 2)

+ ⑥ V00.14   Scooter (nonmotorized) accident

> EXCLUDES 1   motor scooter accident
> (V20-V29)

!Q + ⑦ V00.141-   Fall from scooter (nonmotorized)

!Q + ⑦ V00.142-   Scooter (nonmotorized) colliding with stationary object

!Q + ⑦ V00.148-   Other scooter (nonmotorized) accident

> EXCLUDES 1   scooter
> (nonmotorized)
> collision with other
> land transport
> vehicle (V01-V09
> with fifth character
> 9)

+ ⑥ V00.15   Heelies accident
Rolling shoe
Wheeled shoe
Wheelies accident

!Q + ⑦ V00.151-   Fall from heelies

!Q + ⑦ V00.152-   Heelies colliding with stationary object

!Q + ⑦ V00.158-   Other heelies accident

+ ⑥ V00.18   Accident on other rolling-type pedestrian conveyance

!Q + ⑦ V00.181-   Fall from other rolling-type pedestrian conveyance

!Q + ⑦ V00.182-   Pedestrian on other rolling-type pedestrian conveyance colliding with stationary object

!Q + ⑦ V00.188-   Other accident on other rolling-type pedestrian conveyance

+ ⑤ V00.2   Gliding-type pedestrian conveyance accident

+ ⑥ V00.21   Ice-skates accident

!Q + ⑦ V00.211-   Fall from ice-skates

!Q + ⑦ V00.212-   Ice-skater colliding with stationary object

!Q + ⑦ V00.218-   Other ice-skates accident

> EXCLUDES 1   ice-skater collision
> with other land
> transport vehicle
> (V01-V09 with 5th
> character 9)

+ ⑥ V00.22   Sled accident

!Q + ⑦ V00.221-   Fall from sled

!Q + ⑦ V00.222-   Sledder colliding with stationary object

!Q + ⑦ V00.228-   Other sled accident

> EXCLUDES 1   sled collision with
> other land transport
> vehicle
> (V01-V09 with 5th
> character 9)

+ ⑥ V00.28   Other gliding-type pedestrian conveyance accident

!Q + ⑦ V00.281-   Fall from other gliding-type pedestrian conveyance

!Q + ⑦ V00.282-   Pedestrian on other gliding-type pedestrian conveyance colliding with stationary object

④4th digit required   ⑤5th digit required   ⑥6th digit required   ⑦7th digit required   ☑7th digit placeholder   ✚Additional code   ⊟Laterality

1770   *DecisionHealth's* FY 2020 Complete Home Health ICD-10-CM Diagnosis Coding Manual

IQ ✚ 7 V00.288- Other accident on other gliding-type pedestrian conveyance
> EXCLUDES 1 gliding-type pedestrian conveyance collision with other land transport vehicle (V01-V09 with 5th character 9)

✚ 5 V00.3 Flat-bottomed pedestrian conveyance accident

✚ 6 V00.31 Snowboard accident

IQ ✚ 7 V00.311- Fall from snowboard

IQ ✚ 7 V00.312- Snowboarder colliding with stationary object

IQ ✚ 7 V00.318- Other snowboard accident
> EXCLUDES 1 snowboarder collision with other land transport vehicle (V01-V09 with 5th character 9)

✚ 6 V00.32 Snow-ski accident

IQ ✚ 7 V00.321- Fall from snow-skis

IQ ✚ 7 V00.322- Snow-skier colliding with stationary object

IQ ✚ 7 V00.328- Other snow-ski accident
> EXCLUDES 1 snow-skier collision with other land transport vehicle (V01-V09 with 5th character 9)

✚ 6 V00.38 Other flat-bottomed conveyance accident

IQ ✚ 7 V00.381- Fall from other flat-bottomed pedestrian conveyance

IQ ✚ 7 V00.382- Pedestrian on other flat-bottomed pedestrian conveyance colliding with stationary object

IQ ✚ 7 V00.388- Other accident on other flat-bottomed pedestrian conveyance

✚ 5 V00.8 Accident on other pedestrian conveyance

✚ 6 V00.81 Accident with wheelchair (powered)

IQ ✚ 7 V00.811- Fall from moving wheelchair (powered)
> EXCLUDES 1 fall from non-moving wheelchair (W05.0)

IQ ✚ 7 V00.812- Wheelchair (powered) colliding with stationary object

IQ ✚ 7 V00.818- Other accident with wheelchair (powered)

✚ 6 V00.82 Accident with baby stroller

IQ ✚ 7 V00.821- Fall from baby stroller

IQ ✚ 7 V00.822- Baby stroller colliding with stationary object

IQ ✚ 7 V00.828- Other accident with baby stroller

✚ 6 V00.83 Accident with motorized mobility scooter

IQ ✚ 7 V00.831- Fall from motorized mobility scooter
> EXCLUDES 1 fall from non-moving motorized mobility scooter (W05.2)

IQ ✚ 7 V00.832- Motorized mobility scooter colliding with stationary object

IQ ✚ 7 V00.838- Other accident with motorized mobility scooter

✚ 6 V00.89 Accident on other pedestrian conveyance

IQ ✚ 7 V00.891- Fall from other pedestrian conveyance

IQ ✚ 7 V00.892- Pedestrian on other pedestrian conveyance colliding with stationary object

IQ ✚ 7 V00.898- Other accident on other pedestrian conveyance
> EXCLUDES 1 other pedestrian (conveyance) collision with other land transport vehicle (V01-V09 with 5th character 9)

4 V01 Pedestrian injured in collision with pedal cycle

> The appropriate 7th character is to be added to each code from category V01
> A   initial encounter
> D   subsequent encounter
> S   sequela

5 V01.0 Pedestrian injured in collision with pedal cycle in nontraffic accident

IQ 7 V01.00X- Pedestrian on foot injured in collision with pedal cycle in nontraffic accident
> Pedestrian NOS injured in collision with pedal cycle in nontraffic accident

IQ 7 V01.01X- Pedestrian on roller-skates injured in collision with pedal cycle in nontraffic accident

IQ 7 V01.02X- Pedestrian on skateboard injured in collision with pedal cycle in nontraffic accident

IQ 7 V01.09X- Pedestrian with other conveyance injured in collision with pedal cycle in nontraffic accident
> Pedestrian with baby stroller injured in collision with pedal cycle in nontraffic accident
> Pedestrian on ice-skates injured in collision with pedal cycle in nontraffic accident
> Pedestrian on nonmotorized scooter injured in collision with pedal cycle in nontraffic accident
> Pedestrian on sled injured in collision with pedal cycle in nontraffic accident
> Pedestrian on snowboard injured in collision with pedal cycle in nontraffic accident
> Pedestrian on snow-skis injured in collision with pedal cycle in nontraffic accident
> Pedestrian in wheelchair (powered) injured in collision with pedal cycle in nontraffic accident
> Pedestrian in motorized mobility scooter injured in collision with pedal cycle in nontraffic accident

★ New ▲ Revised Px Primary SP PDGM Px SL Low CoM SH High CoM IQ Quest. Encounter H Hospice non-cancer Dx   Unspecified   M Manifestation

DecisionHealth's FY 2020 Complete Home Health ICD-10-CM Diagnosis Coding Manual

1771

⑤ V01.1 Pedestrian injured in collision with pedal cycle in traffic accident

!Q ☑ V01.10X- Pedestrian on foot injured in collision with pedal cycle in traffic accident
Pedestrian NOS injured in collision with pedal cycle in traffic accident

!Q ☑ V01.11X- Pedestrian on roller-skates injured in collision with pedal cycle in traffic accident

!Q ☑ V01.12X- Pedestrian on skateboard injured in collision with pedal cycle in traffic accident

!Q ☑ V01.19X- Pedestrian with other conveyance injured in collision with pedal cycle in traffic accident
Pedestrian with baby stroller injured in collision with pedal cycle in traffic accident
Pedestrian on ice-skates injured in collision with pedal cycle in traffic accident
Pedestrian on nonmotorized scooter injured in collision with pedal cycle in traffic accident
Pedestrian on sled injured in collision with pedal cycle in traffic accident
Pedestrian on snowboard injured in collision with pedal cycle in traffic accident
Pedestrian on snow-skis injured in collision with pedal cycle in traffic accident
Pedestrian in wheelchair (powered) injured in collision with pedal cycle in traffic accident
Pedestrian in motorized mobility scooter injured in collision with pedal cycle in traffic accident

⑤ V01.9 Pedestrian injured in collision with pedal cycle, unspecified whether traffic or nontraffic accident

!Q ☑ V01.90X- Pedestrian on foot injured in collision with pedal cycle, unspecified whether traffic or nontraffic accident
Pedestrian NOS injured in collision with pedal cycle, unspecified whether traffic or nontraffic accident

!Q ☑ V01.91X- Pedestrian on roller-skates injured in collision with pedal cycle, unspecified whether traffic or nontraffic accident

!Q ☑ V01.92X- Pedestrian on skateboard injured in collision with pedal cycle, unspecified whether traffic or nontraffic accident

!Q ☑ V01.99X- Pedestrian with other conveyance injured in collision with pedal cycle, unspecified whether traffic or nontraffic accident
Pedestrian with baby stroller injured in collision with pedal cycle, unspecified whether traffic or nontraffic accident

Pedestrian on ice-skates injured in collision with pedal cycle unspecified, whether traffic or nontraffic accident
Pedestrian on nonmotorized scooter injured in collision with pedal cycle, unspecified whether traffic or nontraffic accident
Pedestrian on sled injured in collision with pedal cycle unspecified, whether traffic or nontraffic accident
Pedestrian on snowboard injured in collision with pedal cycle, unspecified whether traffic or nontraffic accident
Pedestrian on snow-skis injured in collision with pedal cycle, unspecified whether traffic or nontraffic accident
Pedestrian in wheelchair (powered) injured in collision with pedal cycle, unspecified whether traffic or nontraffic accident
Pedestrian in motorized mobility scooter injured in collision with pedal cycle, unspecified whether traffic or nontraffic accident

④ V02 Pedestrian injured in collision with two- or three-wheeled motor vehicle

The appropriate 7th character is to be added to each code from category V02
A   initial encounter
D   subsequent encounter
S   sequela

⑤ V02.0 Pedestrian injured in collision with two- or three-wheeled motor vehicle in nontraffic accident

!Q ☑ V02.00X- Pedestrian on foot injured in collision with two- or three-wheeled motor vehicle in nontraffic accident
Pedestrian NOS injured in collision with two- or three-wheeled motor vehicle in nontraffic accident

!Q ☑ V02.01X- Pedestrian on roller-skates injured in collision with two- or three-wheeled motor vehicle in nontraffic accident

!Q ☑ V02.02X- Pedestrian on skateboard injured in collision with two- or three-wheeled motor vehicle in nontraffic accident

!Q ☑ V02.09X- Pedestrian with other conveyance injured in collision with two- or three-wheeled motor vehicle in nontraffic accident
Pedestrian with baby stroller injured in collision with two- or three-wheeled motor vehicle in nontraffic accident
Pedestrian on ice-skates injured in collision with two- or three-wheeled motor vehicle in nontraffic accident

Chapter 20

V00-Y99

④4th digit required   ⑤5th digit required   ⑥6th digit required   ☑7th digit required   ☑7th digit placeholder   ✚Additional code   ⊟Laterality

1772   *DecisionHealth's* FY 2020 Complete Home Health ICD-10-CM Diagnosis Coding Manual

Pedestrian on nonmotorized scooter injured in collision with two- or three-wheeled motor vehicle in nontraffic accident

Pedestrian on sled injured in collision with two- or three-wheeled motor vehicle in nontraffic accident

Pedestrian on snowboard injured in collision with two- or three-wheeled motor vehicle in nontraffic accident

Pedestrian on snow-skis injured in collision with two- or three-wheeled motor vehicle in nontraffic accident

Pedestrian in wheelchair (powered) injured in collision with two- or three-wheeled motor vehicle in nontraffic accident

Pedestrian in motorized mobility scooter injured in collision with two- or three-wheeled motor vehicle in nontraffic accident

⑤ **V02.1 Pedestrian injured in collision with two- or three-wheeled motor vehicle in traffic accident**

IQ ☑ **V02.10X- Pedestrian on foot injured in collision with two- or three-wheeled motor vehicle in traffic accident**

Pedestrian NOS injured in collision with two- or three-wheeled motor vehicle in traffic accident

IQ ☑ **V02.11X- Pedestrian on roller-skates injured in collision with two- or three-wheeled motor vehicle in traffic accident**

IQ ☑ **V02.12X- Pedestrian on skateboard injured in collision with two- or three-wheeled motor vehicle in traffic accident**

IQ ☑ **V02.19X- Pedestrian with other conveyance injured in collision with two- or three-wheeled motor vehicle in traffic accident**

Pedestrian with baby stroller injured in collision with two- or three-wheeled motor vehicle in traffic accident

Pedestrian on ice-skates injured in collision with two- or three-wheeled motor vehicle in traffic accident

Pedestrian on nonmotorized scooter injured in collision with two- or three-wheeled motor vehicle in traffic accident

Pedestrian on sled injured in collision with two- or three-wheeled motor vehicle in traffic accident

Pedestrian on snowboard injured in collision with two- or three-wheeled motor vehicle in traffic accident

Pedestrian on snow-skis injured in collision with two- or three-wheeled motor vehicle in traffic accident

Pedestrian in wheelchair (powered) injured in collision with two- or three-wheeled motor vehicle in traffic accident

Pedestrian in motorized mobility scooter injured in collision with two- or three-wheeled motor vehicle in traffic accident

⑤ **V02.9 Pedestrian injured in collision with two- or three-wheeled motor vehicle, unspecified whether traffic or nontraffic accident**

IQ ☑ **V02.90X- Pedestrian on foot injured in collision with two- or three-wheeled motor vehicle, unspecified whether traffic or nontraffic accident**

Pedestrian NOS injured in collision with two- or three-wheeled motor vehicle, unspecified whether traffic or nontraffic accident

IQ ☑ **V02.91X- Pedestrian on roller-skates injured in collision with two- or three-wheeled motor vehicle, unspecified whether traffic or nontraffic accident**

IQ ☑ **V02.92X- Pedestrian on skateboard injured in collision with two- or three-wheeled motor vehicle, unspecified whether traffic or nontraffic accident**

IQ ☑ **V02.99X- Pedestrian with other conveyance injured in collision with two- or three-wheeled motor vehicle, unspecified whether traffic or nontraffic accident**

Pedestrian with baby stroller injured in collision with two- or three-wheeled motor vehicle, unspecified whether traffic or nontraffic accident

Pedestrian on ice-skates injured in collision with two- or three-wheeled motor vehicle, unspecified whether traffic or nontraffic accident

Pedestrian on nonmotorized scooter injured in collision with two- or three-wheeled motor vehicle, unspecified whether traffic or nontraffic accident

Pedestrian on sled injured in collision with two- or three-wheeled motor vehicle, unspecified whether traffic or nontraffic accident

Pedestrian on snowboard injured in collision with two- or three-wheeled motor vehicle, unspecified whether traffic or nontraffic accident

Chapter 20

V00-Y99

★ New ▲ Revised Px Primary SP PDGM Px SL Low CoM SH High CoM IQ Quest. Encounter H Hospice non-cancer Dx ⬜ Unspecified M *Manifestation*

DecisionHealth's FY 2020 Complete Home Health ICD-10-CM Diagnosis Coding Manual

1773

Pedestrian on snow-skis injured in collision with two- or three-wheeled motor vehicle, unspecified whether traffic or nontraffic accident

Pedestrian in wheelchair (powered) injured in collision with two- or three-wheeled motor vehicle, unspecified whether traffic or nontraffic accident

Pedestrian in motorized mobility scooter injured in collision with two- or three-wheeled motor vehicle, unspecified whether traffic or nontraffic accident

4 V03   Pedestrian injured in collision with car, pick-up truck or van

The appropriate 7th character is to be added to each code from category V03
A   initial encounter
D   subsequent encounter
S   sequela

5 V03.0   Pedestrian injured in collision with car, pick-up truck or van in nontraffic accident

!Q 7 V03.00X-   Pedestrian on foot injured in collision with car, pick-up truck or van in nontraffic accident

Pedestrian NOS injured in collision with car, pick-up truck or van in nontraffic accident

!Q 7 V03.01X-   Pedestrian on roller-skates injured in collision with car, pick-up truck or van in nontraffic accident

!Q 7 V03.02X-   Pedestrian on skateboard injured in collision with car, pick-up truck or van in nontraffic accident

!Q 7 V03.09X-   Pedestrian with other conveyance injured in collision with car, pick-up truck or van in nontraffic accident

Pedestrian with baby stroller injured in collision with car, pick-up truck or van in nontraffic accident

Pedestrian on ice-skates injured in collision with car, pick-up truck or van in nontraffic accident

Pedestrian on nonmotorized scooter injured in collision with car, pick-up truck or van in nontraffic accident

Pedestrian on sled injured in collision with car, pick-up truck or van in nontraffic accident

Pedestrian on snowboard injured in collision with car, pick-up truck or van in nontraffic accident

Pedestrian on snow-skis injured in collision with car, pick-up truck or van in nontraffic accident

Pedestrian in wheelchair (powered) injured in collision with car, pick-up truck or van in nontraffic accident

Pedestrian in motorized mobility scooter injured in collision with car, pick-up truck or van in nontraffic accident

5 V03.1   Pedestrian injured in collision with car, pick-up truck or van in traffic accident

!Q 7 V03.10X-   Pedestrian on foot injured in collision with car, pick-up truck or van in traffic accident

Pedestrian NOS injured in collision with car, pick-up truck or van in traffic accident

!Q 7 V03.11X-   Pedestrian on roller-skates injured in collision with car, pick-up truck or van in traffic accident

!Q 7 V03.12X-   Pedestrian on skateboard injured in collision with car, pick-up truck or van in traffic accident

!Q 7 V03.19X-   Pedestrian with other conveyance injured in collision with car, pick-up truck or van in traffic accident

Pedestrian with baby stroller injured in collision with car, pick-up truck or van in traffic accident

Pedestrian on ice-skates injured in collision with car, pick-up truck or van in traffic accident

Pedestrian on nonmotorized scooter injured in collision with car, pick-up truck or van in traffic accident

Pedestrian on sled injured in collision with car, pick-up truck or van in traffic accident

Pedestrian on snowboard injured in collision with car, pick-up truck or van in traffic accident

Pedestrian on snow-skis injured in collision with car, pick-up truck or van in traffic accident

Pedestrian in wheelchair (powered) injured in collision with car, pick-up truck or van in traffic accident

Pedestrian in motorized mobility scooter injured in collision with car, pick-up truck or van in traffic accident

5 V03.9   Pedestrian injured in collision with car, pick-up truck or van, unspecified whether traffic or nontraffic accident

!Q 7 V03.90X-   Pedestrian on foot injured in collision with car, pick-up truck or van, unspecified whether traffic or nontraffic accident

Pedestrian NOS injured in collision with car, pick-up truck or van, unspecified whether traffic or nontraffic accident

!Q 7 V03.91X-   Pedestrian on roller-skates injured in collision with car, pick-up truck or van, unspecified whether traffic or nontraffic accident

!Q 7 V03.92X-   Pedestrian on skateboard injured in collision with car, pick-up truck or van, unspecified whether traffic or nontraffic accident

!Q 7 V03.99X-   Pedestrian with other conveyance injured in collision with car, pick-up truck or van, unspecified whether traffic or nontraffic accident

4 4th digit required   5 5th digit required   6 6th digit required   7 7th digit required   7 7th digit placeholder   + Additional code   ⊟ Laterality

1774   *DecisionHealth's* FY 2020 Complete Home Health ICD-10-CM Diagnosis Coding Manual

Chapter 20

V00-Y99

Pedestrian with baby stroller injured in collision with car, pick-up truck or van, unspecified whether traffic or nontraffic accident

Pedestrian on ice-skates injured in collision with car, pick-up truck or van, unspecified whether traffic or nontraffic accident

Pedestrian on nonmotorized scooter injured in collision with car, pick-up truck or van, unspecified whether traffic or nontraffic accident

Pedestrian on sled injured in collision with car, pick-up truck or van in nontraffic accident

Pedestrian on snowboard injured in collision with car, pick-up truck or van, unspecified whether traffic or nontraffic accident

Pedestrian on snow-skis injured in collision with car, pick-up truck or van, unspecified whether traffic or nontraffic accident

Pedestrian in wheelchair (powered) injured in collision with car, pick-up truck or van, unspecified whether traffic or nontraffic accident

Pedestrian in motorized mobility scooter injured in collision with car, pick-up truck or van, unspecified whether traffic or nontraffic accident

4 V04 Pedestrian injured in collision with heavy transport vehicle or bus

> **EXCLUDES 1** pedestrian injured in collision with military vehicle (V09.01, V09.21)

> The appropriate 7th character is to be added to each code from category V04
> A   initial encounter
> D   subsequent encounter
> S   sequela

5 V04.0 Pedestrian injured in collision with heavy transport vehicle or bus in nontraffic accident

IQ ☑ V04.00X- Pedestrian on foot injured in collision with heavy transport vehicle or bus in nontraffic accident
Pedestrian NOS injured in collision with heavy transport vehicle or bus in nontraffic accident

IQ ☑ V04.01X- Pedestrian on roller-skates injured in collision with heavy transport vehicle or bus in nontraffic accident

IQ ☑ V04.02X- Pedestrian on skateboard injured in collision with heavy transport vehicle or bus in nontraffic accident

IQ ☑ V04.09X- Pedestrian with other conveyance injured in collision with heavy transport vehicle or bus in nontraffic accident

Pedestrian with baby stroller injured in collision with heavy transport vehicle or bus in nontraffic accident

Pedestrian on ice-skates injured in collision with heavy transport vehicle or bus in nontraffic accident

Pedestrian on nonmotorized scooter injured in collision with heavy transport vehicle or bus in nontraffic accident

Pedestrian on sled injured in collision with heavy transport vehicle or bus in nontraffic accident

Pedestrian on snowboard injured in collision with heavy transport vehicle or bus in nontraffic accident

Pedestrian on snow-skis injured in collision with heavy transport vehicle or bus in nontraffic accident

Pedestrian in wheelchair (powered) injured in collision with heavy transport vehicle or bus in nontraffic accident

Pedestrian in motorized mobility scooter injured in collision with heavy transport vehicle or bus in nontraffic accident

5 V04.1 Pedestrian injured in collision with heavy transport vehicle or bus in traffic accident

IQ ☑ V04.10X- Pedestrian on foot injured in collision with heavy transport vehicle or bus in traffic accident
Pedestrian NOS injured in collision with heavy transport vehicle or bus in traffic accident

IQ ☑ V04.11X- Pedestrian on roller-skates injured in collision with heavy transport vehicle or bus in traffic accident

IQ ☑ V04.12X- Pedestrian on skateboard injured in collision with heavy transport vehicle or bus in traffic accident

IQ ☑ V04.19X- Pedestrian with other conveyance injured in collision with heavy transport vehicle or bus in traffic accident

Pedestrian with baby stroller injured in collision with heavy transport vehicle or bus in traffic accident

Pedestrian on ice-skates injured in collision with heavy transport vehicle or bus in traffic accident

Pedestrian on nonmotorized scooter injured in collision with heavy transport vehicle or bus in traffic accident

Pedestrian on sled injured in collision with heavy transport vehicle or bus in traffic accident

Pedestrian on snowboard injured in collision with heavy transport vehicle or bus in traffic accident

★ New ▲ Revised Px Primary SP PDGM Px SL Low CoM SH High CoM IQ Quest. Encounter H Hospice non-cancer Dx Unspecified M *Manifestation*

DecisionHealth's FY 2020 Complete Home Health ICD-10-CM Diagnosis Coding Manual

1775

Pedestrian on snow-skis injured in collision with heavy transport vehicle or bus in traffic accident

Pedestrian in wheelchair (powered) injured in collision with heavy transport vehicle or bus in traffic accident

Pedestrian in motorized mobility scooter injured in collision with heavy transport vehicle or bus in traffic accident

⑤ V04.9 **Pedestrian injured in collision with heavy transport vehicle or bus, unspecified whether traffic or nontraffic accident**

IQ ☑ V04.90X- **Pedestrian on foot injured in collision with heavy transport vehicle or bus, unspecified whether traffic or nontraffic accident**

Pedestrian NOS injured in collision with heavy transport vehicle or bus, unspecified whether traffic or nontraffic accident

IQ ☑ V04.91X- **Pedestrian on roller-skates injured in collision with heavy transport vehicle or bus, unspecified whether traffic or nontraffic accident**

IQ ☑ V04.92X- **Pedestrian on skateboard injured in collision with heavy transport vehicle or bus, unspecified whether traffic or nontraffic accident**

IQ ☑ V04.99X- **Pedestrian with other conveyance injured in collision with heavy transport vehicle or bus, unspecified whether traffic or nontraffic accident**

Pedestrian with baby stroller injured in collision with heavy transport vehicle or bus, unspecified whether traffic or nontraffic accident

Pedestrian on ice-skates injured in collision with heavy transport vehicle or bus, unspecified whether traffic or nontraffic accident

Pedestrian on nonmotorized scooter injured in collision with heavy transport vehicle or bus, unspecified whether traffic or nontraffic accident

Pedestrian on sled injured in collision with heavy transport vehicle or bus, unspecified whether traffic or nontraffic accident

Pedestrian on snowboard injured in collision with heavy transport vehicle or bus, unspecified whether traffic or nontraffic accident

Pedestrian on snow-skis injured in collision with heavy transport vehicle or bus, unspecified whether traffic or nontraffic accident

Pedestrian in wheelchair (powered) injured in collision with heavy transport vehicle or bus, unspecified whether traffic or nontraffic accident

Pedestrian in motorized mobility scooter injured in collision with heavy transport vehicle or bus, unspecified whether traffic or nontraffic accident

④ V05 **Pedestrian injured in collision with railway train or railway vehicle**

The appropriate 7th character is to be added to each code from category V05
A   initial encounter
D   subsequent encounter
S   sequela

⑤ V05.0 **Pedestrian injured in collision with railway train or railway vehicle in nontraffic accident**

IQ ☑ V05.00X- **Pedestrian on foot injured in collision with railway train or railway vehicle in nontraffic accident**

Pedestrian NOS injured in collision with railway train or railway vehicle in nontraffic accident

IQ ☑ V05.01X- **Pedestrian on roller-skates injured in collision with railway train or railway vehicle in nontraffic accident**

IQ ☑ V05.02X- **Pedestrian on skateboard injured in collision with railway train or railway vehicle in nontraffic accident**

IQ ☑ V05.09X- **Pedestrian with other conveyance injured in collision with railway train or railway vehicle in nontraffic accident**

Pedestrian with baby stroller injured in collision with railway train or railway vehicle in nontraffic accident

Pedestrian on ice-skates injured in collision with railway train or railway vehicle in nontraffic accident

Pedestrian on nonmotorized scooter injured in collision with railway train or railway vehicle in nontraffic accident

Pedestrian on sled injured in collision with railway train or railway vehicle in nontraffic accident

Pedestrian on snowboard injured in collision with railway train or railway vehicle in nontraffic accident

Pedestrian on snow-skis injured in collision with railway train or railway vehicle in nontraffic accident

④4th digit required   ⑤5th digit required   ⑥6th digit required   ⑦7th digit required   ☑7th digit placeholder   ✚Additional code   ⊟Laterality

1776   *DecisionHealth's* FY 2020 Complete Home Health ICD-10-CM Diagnosis Coding Manual

Pedestrian in wheelchair (powered) injured in collision with railway train or railway vehicle in nontraffic accident

Pedestrian in motorized mobility scooter injured in collision with railway train or railway vehicle in nontraffic accident

⑤ **V05.1** **Pedestrian injured in collision with railway train or railway vehicle in traffic accident**

🔳 ☑ **V05.10X-** **Pedestrian on foot injured in collision with railway train or railway vehicle in traffic accident**
Pedestrian NOS injured in collision with railway train or railway vehicle in traffic accident

🔳 ☑ **V05.11X-** **Pedestrian on roller-skates injured in collision with railway train or railway vehicle in traffic accident**

🔳 ☑ **V05.12X-** **Pedestrian on skateboard injured in collision with railway train or railway vehicle in traffic accident**

🔳 ☑ **V05.19X-** **Pedestrian with other conveyance injured in collision with railway train or railway vehicle in traffic accident**
Pedestrian with baby stroller injured in collision with railway train or railway vehicle in traffic accident
Pedestrian on ice-skates injured in collision with railway train or railway vehicle in traffic accident
Pedestrian on nonmotorized scooter injured in collision with railway train or railway vehicle in traffic accident
Pedestrian on sled injured in collision with railway train or railway vehicle in traffic accident
Pedestrian on snowboard injured in collision with railway train or railway vehicle in traffic accident
Pedestrian on snow-skis injured in collision with railway train or railway vehicle in traffic accident
Pedestrian in wheelchair (powered) injured in collision with railway train or railway vehicle in traffic accident
Pedestrian in motorized mobility scooter injured in collision with railway train or railway vehicle in traffic accident

⑤ **V05.9** **Pedestrian injured in collision with railway train or railway vehicle, unspecified whether traffic or nontraffic accident**

🔳 ☑ **V05.90X-** **Pedestrian on foot injured in collision with railway train or railway vehicle, unspecified whether traffic or nontraffic accident**
Pedestrian NOS injured in collision with railway train or railway vehicle, unspecified whether traffic or nontraffic accident

🔳 ☑ **V05.91X-** **Pedestrian on roller-skates injured in collision with railway train or railway vehicle, unspecified whether traffic or nontraffic accident**

🔳 ☑ **V05.92X-** **Pedestrian on skateboard injured in collision with railway train or railway vehicle, unspecified whether traffic or nontraffic accident**

🔳 ☑ **V05.99X-** **Pedestrian with other conveyance injured in collision with railway train or railway vehicle, unspecified whether traffic or nontraffic accident**
Pedestrian with baby stroller injured in collision with railway train or railway vehicle, unspecified whether traffic or nontraffic
Pedestrian on ice-skates injured in collision with railway train or railway vehicle, unspecified whether traffic or nontraffic
Pedestrian on nonmotorized scooter injured in collision with railway train or railway vehicle, unspecified whether traffic or nontraffic
Pedestrian on sled injured in collision with railway train or railway vehicle, unspecified whether traffic or nontraffic
Pedestrian on snowboard injured in collision with railway train or railway vehicle, unspecified whether traffic or nontraffic
Pedestrian on snow-skis injured in collision with railway train or railway vehicle, unspecified whether traffic or nontraffic
Pedestrian in wheelchair (powered) injured in collision with railway train or railway vehicle, unspecified whether traffic or nontraffic
Pedestrian in motorized mobility scooter injured in collision with railway train or railway vehicle, unspecified whether traffic or nontraffic

④ **V06** **Pedestrian injured in collision with other nonmotor vehicle**
> INCLUDES   collision with animal-drawn vehicle, animal being ridden, nonpowered streetcar
> EXCLUDES 1   pedestrian injured in collision with pedestrian conveyance (V00.0-)

The appropriate 7th character is to be added to each code from category V06
A   initial encounter
D   subsequent encounter
S   sequela

⑤ **V06.0** **Pedestrian injured in collision with other nonmotor vehicle in nontraffic accident**

★ New ▲ Revised Px Primary 🆂🅿 PDGM Px 🆂🅻 Low CoM 🆂🅷 High CoM 🔳 Quest. Encounter Ⓗ Hospice non-cancer Dx Unspecified Ⓜ *Manifestation*

DecisionHealth's FY 2020 Complete Home Health ICD-10-CM Diagnosis Coding Manual

1777

Chapter 20

V00-Y99

[IQ] [✓] V06.00X- **Pedestrian on foot injured in collision with other nonmotor vehicle in nontraffic accident**

Pedestrian NOS injured in collision with other nonmotor vehicle in nontraffic accident

[IQ] [✓] V06.01X- **Pedestrian on roller-skates injured in collision with other nonmotor vehicle in nontraffic accident**

[IQ] [✓] V06.02X- **Pedestrian on skateboard injured in collision with other nonmotor vehicle in nontraffic accident**

[IQ] [✓] V06.09X- **Pedestrian with other conveyance injured in collision with other nonmotor vehicle in nontraffic accident**

Pedestrian with baby stroller injured in collision with other nonmotor vehicle in nontraffic accident

Pedestrian on ice-skates injured in collision with other nonmotor vehicle in nontraffic accident

Pedestrian on nonmotorized scooter injured in collision with other nonmotor vehicle in nontraffic accident

Pedestrian on sled injured in collision with other nonmotor vehicle in nontraffic accident

Pedestrian on snowboard injured in collision with other nonmotor vehicle in nontraffic accident

Pedestrian on snow-skis injured in collision with other nonmotor vehicle in nontraffic accident

Pedestrian in wheelchair (powered) injured in collision with other nonmotor vehicle in nontraffic accident

Pedestrian in motorized mobility scooter injured in collision with other nonmotor vehicle in nontraffic accident

[S] V06.1 **Pedestrian injured in collision with other nonmotor vehicle in traffic accident**

[IQ] [✓] V06.10X- **Pedestrian on foot injured in collision with other nonmotor vehicle in traffic accident**

Pedestrian NOS injured in collision with other nonmotor vehicle in traffic accident

[IQ] [✓] V06.11X- **Pedestrian on roller-skates injured in collision with other nonmotor vehicle in traffic accident**

[IQ] [✓] V06.12X- **Pedestrian on skateboard injured in collision with other nonmotor vehicle in traffic accident**

[IQ] [✓] V06.19X- **Pedestrian with other conveyance injured in collision with other nonmotor vehicle in traffic accident**

Pedestrian with baby stroller injured in collision with other nonmotor vehicle in nontraffic accident

Pedestrian on ice-skates injured in collision with other nonmotor vehicle in traffic accident

Pedestrian on nonmotorized scooter injured in collision with other nonmotor vehicle in traffic accident

Pedestrian on sled injured in collision with other nonmotor vehicle in traffic accident

Pedestrian on snowboard injured in collision with other nonmotor vehicle in traffic accident

Pedestrian on snow-skis injured in collision with other nonmotor vehicle in traffic accident

Pedestrian in wheelchair (powered) injured in collision with other nonmotor vehicle in traffic accident

Pedestrian in motorized mobility scooter injured in collision with other nonmotor vehicle in traffic accident

[S] V06.9 **Pedestrian injured in collision with other nonmotor vehicle, unspecified whether traffic or nontraffic accident**

[IQ] [✓] V06.90X- **Pedestrian on foot injured in collision with other nonmotor vehicle, unspecified whether traffic or nontraffic accident**

Pedestrian NOS injured in collision with other nonmotor vehicle, unspecified whether traffic or nontraffic accident

[IQ] [✓] V06.91X- **Pedestrian on roller-skates injured in collision with other nonmotor vehicle, unspecified whether traffic or nontraffic accident**

[IQ] [✓] V06.92X- **Pedestrian on skateboard injured in collision with other nonmotor vehicle, unspecified whether traffic or nontraffic accident**

[IQ] [✓] V06.99X- **Pedestrian with other conveyance injured in collision with other nonmotor vehicle, unspecified whether traffic or nontraffic accident**

Pedestrian with baby stroller injured in collision with other nonmotor vehicle, unspecified whether traffic or nontraffic accident

Pedestrian on ice-skates injured in collision with other nonmotor vehicle, unspecified whether traffic or nontraffic accident

Pedestrian on nonmotorized scooter injured in collision with other nonmotor vehicle, unspecified whether traffic or nontraffic accident

Pedestrian on sled injured in collision with other nonmotor vehicle, unspecified whether traffic or nontraffic accident

Pedestrian on snowboard injured in collision with other nonmotor vehicle, unspecified whether traffic or nontraffic accident

Chapter 20

V00-Y99

[4] 4th digit required   [S] 5th digit required   [6] 6th digit required   [7] 7th digit required   [✓] 7th digit placeholder   [+] Additional code   [B] Laterality

1778   *DecisionHealth's* FY 2020 Complete Home Health ICD-10-CM Diagnosis Coding Manual

Pedestrian on snow-skis injured in collision with other nonmotor vehicle, unspecified whether traffic or nontraffic accident

Pedestrian in wheelchair (powered) injured in collision with other nonmotor vehicle, unspecified whether traffic or nontraffic accident

Pedestrian in motorized mobility scooter injured in collision with other nonmotor vehicle, unspecified whether traffic or nontraffic accident

4 V09 Pedestrian injured in other and unspecified transport accidents

The appropriate 7th character is to be added to each code from category V09
A   initial encounter
D   subsequent encounter
S   sequela

5 V09.0 Pedestrian injured in nontraffic accident involving other and unspecified motor vehicles

!Q ☑ V09.00X- Pedestrian injured in nontraffic accident involving unspecified motor vehicles

!Q ☑ V09.01X- Pedestrian injured in nontraffic accident involving military vehicle

!Q ☑ V09.09X- Pedestrian injured in nontraffic accident involving other motor vehicles

Pedestrian injured in nontraffic accident by special vehicle

!Q ☑ V09.1XX- Pedestrian injured in unspecified nontraffic accident

5 V09.2 Pedestrian injured in traffic accident involving other and unspecified motor vehicles

!Q ☑ V09.20X- Pedestrian injured in traffic accident involving unspecified motor vehicles

!Q ☑ V09.21X- Pedestrian injured in traffic accident involving military vehicle

!Q ☑ V09.29X- Pedestrian injured in traffic accident involving other motor vehicles

!Q ☑ V09.3XX- Pedestrian injured in unspecified traffic accident

!Q ☑ V09.9XX- Pedestrian injured in unspecified transport accident

Pedal cycle rider injured in transport accident (V10-V19)

INCLUDES   any non-motorized vehicle, excluding an animal-drawn vehicle, or a sidecar or trailer attached to the pedal cycle

EXCLUDES 2   rupture of pedal cycle tire (W37.0)

4 V10 Pedal cycle rider injured in collision with pedestrian or animal

    EXCLUDES 1   pedal cycle rider collision with animal-drawn vehicle or animal being ridden (V16.-)

The appropriate 7th character is to be added to each code from category V10
A   initial encounter
D   subsequent encounter
S   sequela

!Q ☑ V10.0XX- Pedal cycle driver injured in collision with pedestrian or animal in nontraffic accident

!Q ☑ V10.1XX- Pedal cycle passenger injured in collision with pedestrian or animal in nontraffic accident

!Q ☑ V10.2XX- Unspecified pedal cyclist injured in collision with pedestrian or animal in nontraffic accident

!Q ☑ V10.3XX- Person boarding or alighting a pedal cycle injured in collision with pedestrian or animal

!Q ☑ V10.4XX- Pedal cycle driver injured in collision with pedestrian or animal in traffic accident

!Q ☑ V10.5XX- Pedal cycle passenger injured in collision with pedestrian or animal in traffic accident

!Q ☑ V10.9XX- Unspecified pedal cyclist injured in collision with pedestrian or animal in traffic accident

4 V11 Pedal cycle rider injured in collision with other pedal cycle

The appropriate 7th character is to be added to each code from category V11
A   initial encounter
D   subsequent encounter
S   sequela

!Q ☑ V11.0XX- Pedal cycle driver injured in collision with other pedal cycle in nontraffic accident

!Q ☑ V11.1XX- Pedal cycle passenger injured in collision with other pedal cycle in nontraffic accident

!Q ☑ V11.2XX- Unspecified pedal cyclist injured in collision with other pedal cycle in nontraffic accident

!Q ☑ V11.3XX- Person boarding or alighting a pedal cycle injured in collision with other pedal cycle

!Q ☑ V11.4XX- Pedal cycle driver injured in collision with other pedal cycle in traffic accident

!Q ☑ V11.5XX- Pedal cycle passenger injured in collision with other pedal cycle in traffic accident

!Q ☑ V11.9XX- Unspecified pedal cyclist injured in collision with other pedal cycle in traffic accident

4 V12 Pedal cycle rider injured in collision with two- or three-wheeled motor vehicle

The appropriate 7th character is to be added to each code from category V12
A   initial encounter
D   subsequent encounter
S   sequela

!Q ☑ V12.0XX- Pedal cycle driver injured in collision with two- or three-wheeled motor vehicle in nontraffic accident

★ New ▲ Revised Px Primary SP PDGM Px SL Low CoM SH High CoM !Q Quest. Encounter H Hospice non-cancer Dx   Unspecified   M *Manifestation*

DecisionHealth's FY 2020 Complete Home Health ICD-10-CM Diagnosis Coding Manual

1779

!Q ☑ **V12.1XX-** Pedal cycle passenger injured in collision with two- or three-wheeled motor vehicle in nontraffic accident

!Q ☑ **V12.2XX-** Unspecified pedal cyclist injured in collision with two- or three-wheeled motor vehicle in nontraffic accident

!Q ☑ **V12.3XX-** Person boarding or alighting a pedal cycle injured in collision with two- or three-wheeled motor vehicle

!Q ☑ **V12.4XX-** Pedal cycle driver injured in collision with two- or three-wheeled motor vehicle in traffic accident

!Q ☑ **V12.5XX-** Pedal cycle passenger injured in collision with two- or three-wheeled motor vehicle in traffic accident

!Q ☑ **V12.9XX-** Unspecified pedal cyclist injured in collision with two- or three-wheeled motor vehicle in traffic accident

4 **V13** Pedal cycle rider injured in collision with car, pick-up truck or van

> The appropriate 7th character is to be added to each code from category V13
> A   initial encounter
> D   subsequent encounter
> S   sequela

!Q ☑ **V13.0XX-** Pedal cycle driver injured in collision with car, pick-up truck or van in nontraffic accident

!Q ☑ **V13.1XX-** Pedal cycle passenger injured in collision with car, pick-up truck or van in nontraffic accident

!Q ☑ **V13.2XX-** Unspecified pedal cyclist injured in collision with car, pick-up truck or van in nontraffic accident

!Q ☑ **V13.3XX-** Person boarding or alighting a pedal cycle injured in collision with car, pick-up truck or van

!Q ☑ **V13.4XX-** Pedal cycle driver injured in collision with car, pick-up truck or van in traffic accident

!Q ☑ **V13.5XX-** Pedal cycle passenger injured in collision with car, pick-up truck or van in traffic accident

!Q ☑ **V13.9XX-** Unspecified pedal cyclist injured in collision with car, pick-up truck or van in traffic accident

4 **V14** Pedal cycle rider injured in collision with heavy transport vehicle or bus
> **EXCLUDES 1** pedal cycle rider injured in collision with military vehicle (V19.81)

> The appropriate 7th character is to be added to each code from category V14
> A   initial encounter
> D   subsequent encounter
> S   sequela

!Q ☑ **V14.0XX-** Pedal cycle driver injured in collision with heavy transport vehicle or bus in nontraffic accident

!Q ☑ **V14.1XX-** Pedal cycle passenger injured in collision with heavy transport vehicle or bus in nontraffic accident

!Q ☑ **V14.2XX-** Unspecified pedal cyclist injured in collision with heavy transport vehicle or bus in nontraffic accident

!Q ☑ **V14.3XX-** Person boarding or alighting a pedal cycle injured in collision with heavy transport vehicle or bus

!Q ☑ **V14.4XX-** Pedal cycle driver injured in collision with heavy transport vehicle or bus in traffic accident

!Q ☑ **V14.5XX-** Pedal cycle passenger injured in collision with heavy transport vehicle or bus in traffic accident

!Q ☑ **V14.9XX-** Unspecified pedal cyclist injured in collision with heavy transport vehicle or bus in traffic accident

4 **V15** Pedal cycle rider injured in collision with railway train or railway vehicle

> The appropriate 7th character is to be added to each code from category V15
> A   initial encounter
> D   subsequent encounter
> S   sequela

!Q ☑ **V15.0XX-** Pedal cycle driver injured in collision with railway train or railway vehicle in nontraffic accident

!Q ☑ **V15.1XX-** Pedal cycle passenger injured in collision with railway train or railway vehicle in nontraffic accident

!Q ☑ **V15.2XX-** Unspecified pedal cyclist injured in collision with railway train or railway vehicle in nontraffic accident

!Q ☑ **V15.3XX-** Person boarding or alighting a pedal cycle injured in collision with railway train or railway vehicle

!Q ☑ **V15.4XX-** Pedal cycle driver injured in collision with railway train or railway vehicle in traffic accident

!Q ☑ **V15.5XX-** Pedal cycle passenger injured in collision with railway train or railway vehicle in traffic accident

!Q ☑ **V15.9XX-** Unspecified pedal cyclist injured in collision with railway train or railway vehicle in traffic accident

4 **V16** Pedal cycle rider injured in collision with other nonmotor vehicle
> **INCLUDES** collision with animal-drawn vehicle, animal being ridden, streetcar

> The appropriate 7th character is to be added to each code from category V16
> A   initial encounter
> D   subsequent encounter
> S   sequela

!Q ☑ **V16.0XX-** Pedal cycle driver injured in collision with other nonmotor vehicle in nontraffic accident

!Q ☑ **V16.1XX-** Pedal cycle passenger injured in collision with other nonmotor vehicle in nontraffic accident

!Q ☑ **V16.2XX-** Unspecified pedal cyclist injured in collision with other nonmotor vehicle in nontraffic accident

4 4th digit required   5 5th digit required   6 6th digit required   7 7th digit required   ☑ 7th digit placeholder   + Additional code   ⊟ Laterality

1780   *DecisionHealth's* FY 2020 Complete Home Health ICD-10-CM Diagnosis Coding Manual

IQ ☑ V16.3XX- Person boarding or alighting a pedal cycle injured in collision with other nonmotor vehicle in nontraffic accident

IQ ☑ V16.4XX- Pedal cycle driver injured in collision with other nonmotor vehicle in traffic accident

IQ ☑ V16.5XX- Pedal cycle passenger injured in collision with other nonmotor vehicle in traffic accident

IQ ☑ V16.9XX- Unspecified pedal cyclist injured in collision with other nonmotor vehicle in traffic accident

◢ V17 Pedal cycle rider injured in collision with fixed or stationary object

The appropriate 7th character is to be added to each code from category V17
A   initial encounter
D   subsequent encounter
S   sequela

IQ ☑ V17.0XX- Pedal cycle driver injured in collision with fixed or stationary object in nontraffic accident

IQ ☑ V17.1XX- Pedal cycle passenger injured in collision with fixed or stationary object in nontraffic accident

IQ ☑ V17.2XX- Unspecified pedal cyclist injured in collision with fixed or stationary object in nontraffic accident

IQ ☑ V17.3XX- Person boarding or alighting a pedal cycle injured in collision with fixed or stationary object

IQ ☑ V17.4XX- Pedal cycle driver injured in collision with fixed or stationary object in traffic accident

IQ ☑ V17.5XX- Pedal cycle passenger injured in collision with fixed or stationary object in traffic accident

IQ ☑ V17.9XX- Unspecified pedal cyclist injured in collision with fixed or stationary object in traffic accident

◢ V18 Pedal cycle rider injured in noncollision transport accident

| INCLUDES | fall or thrown from pedal cycle (without antecedent collision) overturning pedal cycle NOS overturning pedal cycle without collision |

The appropriate 7th character is to be added to each code from category V18
A   initial encounter
D   subsequent encounter
S   sequela

IQ ☑ V18.0XX- Pedal cycle driver injured in noncollision transport accident in nontraffic accident

IQ ☑ V18.1XX- Pedal cycle passenger injured in noncollision transport accident in nontraffic accident

IQ ☑ V18.2XX- Unspecified pedal cyclist injured in noncollision transport accident in nontraffic accident

IQ ☑ V18.3XX- Person boarding or alighting a pedal cycle injured in noncollision transport accident

IQ ☑ V18.4XX- Pedal cycle driver injured in noncollision transport accident in traffic accident

IQ ☑ V18.5XX- Pedal cycle passenger injured in noncollision transport accident in traffic accident

IQ ☑ V18.9XX- Unspecified pedal cyclist injured in noncollision transport accident in traffic accident

◢ V19 Pedal cycle rider injured in other and unspecified transport accidents

The appropriate 7th character is to be added to each code from category V19
A   initial encounter
D   subsequent encounter
S   sequela

⑤ V19.0 Pedal cycle driver injured in collision with other and unspecified motor vehicles in nontraffic accident

IQ ☑ V19.00X- Pedal cycle driver injured in collision with unspecified motor vehicles in nontraffic accident

IQ ☑ V19.09X- Pedal cycle driver injured in collision with other motor vehicles in nontraffic accident

⑤ V19.1 Pedal cycle passenger injured in collision with other and unspecified motor vehicles in nontraffic accident

IQ ☑ V19.10X- Pedal cycle passenger injured in collision with unspecified motor vehicles in nontraffic accident

IQ ☑ V19.19X- Pedal cycle passenger injured in collision with other motor vehicles in nontraffic accident

⑤ V19.2 Unspecified pedal cyclist injured in collision with other and unspecified motor vehicles in nontraffic accident

IQ ☑ V19.20X- Unspecified pedal cyclist injured in collision with unspecified motor vehicles in nontraffic accident

Pedal cycle collision NOS, nontraffic

IQ ☑ V19.29X- Unspecified pedal cyclist injured in collision with other motor vehicles in nontraffic accident

IQ ☑ V19.3XX- Pedal cyclist (driver) (passenger) injured in unspecified nontraffic accident

Pedal cycle accident NOS, nontraffic
Pedal cyclist injured in nontraffic accident NOS

⑤ V19.4 Pedal cycle driver injured in collision with other and unspecified motor vehicles in traffic accident

IQ ☑ V19.40X- Pedal cycle driver injured in collision with unspecified motor vehicles in traffic accident

IQ ☑ V19.49X- Pedal cycle driver injured in collision with other motor vehicles in traffic accident

⑤ V19.5 Pedal cycle passenger injured in collision with other and unspecified motor vehicles in traffic accident

Chapter 20

V00-Y99

★ New ▲ Revised Px Primary SP PDGM Px SL Low CoM SH High CoM IQ Quest. Encounter H Hospice non-cancer Dx   Unspecified   M *Manifestation*

DecisionHealth's FY 2020 Complete Home Health ICD-10-CM Diagnosis Coding Manual

1781

IQ ☑ V19.50X- Pedal cycle passenger injured in collision with unspecified motor vehicles in traffic accident

IQ ☑ V19.59X- Pedal cycle passenger injured in collision with other motor vehicles in traffic accident

⑤ V19.6 Unspecified pedal cyclist injured in collision with other and unspecified motor vehicles in traffic accident

IQ ☑ V19.60X- Unspecified pedal cyclist injured in collision with unspecified motor vehicles in traffic accident
Pedal cycle collision NOS (traffic)

IQ ☑ V19.69X- Unspecified pedal cyclist injured in collision with other motor vehicles in traffic accident

⑤ V19.8 Pedal cyclist (driver) (passenger) injured in other specified transport accidents

IQ ☑ V19.81X- Pedal cyclist (driver) (passenger) injured in transport accident with military vehicle

IQ ☑ V19.88X- Pedal cyclist (driver) (passenger) injured in other specified transport accidents

IQ ☑ V19.9XX- Pedal cyclist (driver) (passenger) injured in unspecified traffic accident
Pedal cycle accident NOS

Motorcycle rider injured in transport accident (V20-V29)

INCLUDES moped
motorcycle with sidecar
motorized bicycle
motor scooter
EXCLUDES 1 three-wheeled motor vehicle (V30-V39)

④ V20 Motorcycle rider injured in collision with pedestrian or animal
EXCLUDES 1 motorcycle rider collision with animal-drawn vehicle or animal being ridden (V26.-)

The appropriate 7th character is to be added to each code from category V20
A   initial encounter
D   subsequent encounter
S   sequela

IQ ☑ V20.0XX- Motorcycle driver injured in collision with pedestrian or animal in nontraffic accident

IQ ☑ V20.1XX- Motorcycle passenger injured in collision with pedestrian or animal in nontraffic accident

IQ ☑ V20.2XX- Unspecified motorcycle rider injured in collision with pedestrian or animal in nontraffic accident

IQ ☑ V20.3XX- Person boarding or alighting a motorcycle injured in collision with pedestrian or animal

IQ ☑ V20.4XX- Motorcycle driver injured in collision with pedestrian or animal in traffic accident

IQ ☑ V20.5XX- Motorcycle passenger injured in collision with pedestrian or animal in traffic accident

IQ ☑ V20.9XX- Unspecified motorcycle rider injured in collision with pedestrian or animal in traffic accident

④ V21 Motorcycle rider injured in collision with pedal cycle

The appropriate 7th character is to be added to each code from category V21
A   initial encounter
D   subsequent encounter
S   sequela

IQ ☑ V21.0XX- Motorcycle driver injured in collision with pedal cycle in nontraffic accident

IQ ☑ V21.1XX- Motorcycle passenger injured in collision with pedal cycle in nontraffic accident

IQ ☑ V21.2XX- Unspecified motorcycle rider injured in collision with pedal cycle in nontraffic accident

IQ ☑ V21.3XX- Person boarding or alighting a motorcycle injured in collision with pedal cycle

IQ ☑ V21.4XX- Motorcycle driver injured in collision with pedal cycle in traffic accident

IQ ☑ V21.5XX- Motorcycle passenger injured in collision with pedal cycle in traffic accident

IQ ☑ V21.9XX- Unspecified motorcycle rider injured in collision with pedal cycle in traffic accident

④ V22 Motorcycle rider injured in collision with two- or three-wheeled motor vehicle

The appropriate 7th character is to be added to each code from category V22
A   initial encounter
D   subsequent encounter
S   sequela

IQ ☑ V22.0XX- Motorcycle driver injured in collision with two- or three-wheeled motor vehicle in nontraffic accident

IQ ☑ V22.1XX- Motorcycle passenger injured in collision with two- or three-wheeled motor vehicle in nontraffic accident

IQ ☑ V22.2XX- Unspecified motorcycle rider injured in collision with two- or three-wheeled motor vehicle in nontraffic accident

IQ ☑ V22.3XX- Person boarding or alighting a motorcycle injured in collision with two- or three-wheeled motor vehicle

IQ ☑ V22.4XX- Motorcycle driver injured in collision with two- or three-wheeled motor vehicle in traffic accident

IQ ☑ V22.5XX- Motorcycle passenger injured in collision with two- or three-wheeled motor vehicle in traffic accident

IQ ☑ V22.9XX- Unspecified motorcycle rider injured in collision with two- or three-wheeled motor vehicle in traffic accident

④ V23 Motorcycle rider injured in collision with car, pick-up truck or van

Chapter 20

V00-Y99

④ 4th digit required   ⑤ 5th digit required   ⑥ 6th digit required   ⑦ 7th digit required   ☑ 7th digit placeholder   ✚ Additional code   ⊟ Laterality

1782   *DecisionHealth's* FY 2020 Complete Home Health ICD-10-CM Diagnosis Coding Manual

The appropriate 7th character is to be added to each code from category V23
A   initial encounter
D   subsequent encounter
S   sequela

!Q ✓ V23.0XX- Motorcycle driver injured in collision with car, pick-up truck or van in nontraffic accident

!Q ✓ V23.1XX- Motorcycle passenger injured in collision with car, pick-up truck or van in nontraffic accident

!Q ✓ V23.2XX- Unspecified motorcycle rider injured in collision with car, pick-up truck or van in nontraffic accident

!Q ✓ V23.3XX- Person boarding or alighting a motorcycle injured in collision with car, pick-up truck or van

!Q ✓ V23.4XX- Motorcycle driver injured in collision with car, pick-up truck or van in traffic accident

!Q ✓ V23.5XX- Motorcycle passenger injured in collision with car, pick-up truck or van in traffic accident

!Q ✓ V23.9XX- Unspecified motorcycle rider injured in collision with car, pick-up truck or van in traffic accident

4 V24 Motorcycle rider injured in collision with heavy transport vehicle or bus
    EXCLUDES 1 motorcycle rider injured in collision with military vehicle (V29.81)

The appropriate 7th character is to be added to each code from category V24
A   initial encounter
D   subsequent encounter
S   sequela

!Q ✓ V24.0XX- Motorcycle driver injured in collision with heavy transport vehicle or bus in nontraffic accident

!Q ✓ V24.1XX- Motorcycle passenger injured in collision with heavy transport vehicle or bus in nontraffic accident

!Q ✓ V24.2XX- Unspecified motorcycle rider injured in collision with heavy transport vehicle or bus in nontraffic accident

!Q ✓ V24.3XX- Person boarding or alighting a motorcycle injured in collision with heavy transport vehicle or bus

!Q ✓ V24.4XX- Motorcycle driver injured in collision with heavy transport vehicle or bus in traffic accident

!Q ✓ V24.5XX- Motorcycle passenger injured in collision with heavy transport vehicle or bus in traffic accident

!Q ✓ V24.9XX- Unspecified motorcycle rider injured in collision with heavy transport vehicle or bus in traffic accident

4 V25 Motorcycle rider injured in collision with railway train or railway vehicle

The appropriate 7th character is to be added to each code from category V25
A   initial encounter
D   subsequent encounter
S   sequela

!Q ✓ V25.0XX- Motorcycle driver injured in collision with railway train or railway vehicle in nontraffic accident

!Q ✓ V25.1XX- Motorcycle passenger injured in collision with railway train or railway vehicle in nontraffic accident

!Q ✓ V25.2XX- Unspecified motorcycle rider injured in collision with railway train or railway vehicle in nontraffic accident

!Q ✓ V25.3XX- Person boarding or alighting a motorcycle injured in collision with railway train or railway vehicle

!Q ✓ V25.4XX- Motorcycle driver injured in collision with railway train or railway vehicle in traffic accident

!Q ✓ V25.5XX- Motorcycle passenger injured in collision with railway train or railway vehicle in traffic accident

!Q ✓ V25.9XX- Unspecified motorcycle rider injured in collision with railway train or railway vehicle in traffic accident

4 V26 Motorcycle rider injured in collision with other nonmotor vehicle
    INCLUDES collision with animal-drawn vehicle, animal being ridden, streetcar

The appropriate 7th character is to be added to each code from category V26
A   initial encounter
D   subsequent encounter
S   sequela

!Q ✓ V26.0XX- Motorcycle driver injured in collision with other nonmotor vehicle in nontraffic accident

!Q ✓ V26.1XX- Motorcycle passenger injured in collision with other nonmotor vehicle in nontraffic accident

!Q ✓ V26.2XX- Unspecified motorcycle rider injured in collision with other nonmotor vehicle in nontraffic accident

!Q ✓ V26.3XX- Person boarding or alighting a motorcycle injured in collision with other nonmotor vehicle

!Q ✓ V26.4XX- Motorcycle driver injured in collision with other nonmotor vehicle in traffic accident

!Q ✓ V26.5XX- Motorcycle passenger injured in collision with other nonmotor vehicle in traffic accident

!Q ✓ V26.9XX- Unspecified motorcycle rider injured in collision with other nonmotor vehicle in traffic accident

4 V27 Motorcycle rider injured in collision with fixed or stationary object

Chapter 20

V00-Y99

★ New ▲ Revised Px Primary **SP** PDGM Px **SL** Low CoM **SH** High CoM **!Q** Quest. Encounter **H** Hospice non-cancer Dx Unspecified **M** *Manifestation*

DecisionHealth's FY 2020 Complete Home Health ICD-10-CM Diagnosis Coding Manual

1783

The appropriate 7th character is to be added to each code from category V27

A　　initial encounter
D　　subsequent encounter
S　　sequela

!Q ☑ V27.0XX-　**Motorcycle driver injured in collision with fixed or stationary object in nontraffic accident**

!Q ☑ V27.1XX-　**Motorcycle passenger injured in collision with fixed or stationary object in nontraffic accident**

!Q ☑ V27.2XX-　**Unspecified motorcycle rider injured in collision with fixed or stationary object in nontraffic accident**

!Q ☑ V27.3XX-　**Person boarding or alighting a motorcycle injured in collision with fixed or stationary object**

!Q ☑ V27.4XX-　**Motorcycle driver injured in collision with fixed or stationary object in traffic accident**

!Q ☑ V27.5XX-　**Motorcycle passenger injured in collision with fixed or stationary object in traffic accident**

!Q ☑ V27.9XX-　**Unspecified motorcycle rider injured in collision with fixed or stationary object in traffic accident**

4 V28　**Motorcycle rider injured in noncollision transport accident**

> INCLUDES　fall or thrown from motorcycle (without antecedent collision)
> overturning motorcycle NOS
> overturning motorcycle without collision

The appropriate 7th character is to be added to each code from category V28

A　　initial encounter
D　　subsequent encounter
S　　sequela

!Q ☑ V28.0XX-　**Motorcycle driver injured in noncollision transport accident in nontraffic accident**

!Q ☑ V28.1XX-　**Motorcycle passenger injured in noncollision transport accident in nontraffic accident**

!Q ☑ V28.2XX-　**Unspecified motorcycle rider injured in noncollision transport accident in nontraffic accident**

!Q ☑ V28.3XX-　**Person boarding or alighting a motorcycle injured in noncollision transport accident**

!Q ☑ V28.4XX-　**Motorcycle driver injured in noncollision transport accident in traffic accident**

!Q ☑ V28.5XX-　**Motorcycle passenger injured in noncollision transport accident in traffic accident**

!Q ☑ V28.9XX-　**Unspecified motorcycle rider injured in noncollision transport accident in traffic accident**

4 V29　**Motorcycle rider injured in other and unspecified transport accidents**

5 V29.0　**Motorcycle driver injured in collision with other and unspecified motor vehicles in nontraffic accident**

!Q ☑ V29.00X-　**Motorcycle driver injured in collision with unspecified motor vehicles in nontraffic accident**

!Q ☑ V29.09X-　**Motorcycle driver injured in collision with other motor vehicles in nontraffic accident**

5 V29.1　**Motorcycle passenger injured in collision with other and unspecified motor vehicles in nontraffic accident**

!Q ☑ V29.10X-　**Motorcycle passenger injured in collision with unspecified motor vehicles in nontraffic accident**

!Q ☑ V29.19X-　**Motorcycle passenger injured in collision with other motor vehicles in nontraffic accident**

5 V29.2　**Unspecified motorcycle rider injured in collision with other and unspecified motor vehicles in nontraffic accident**

!Q ☑ V29.20X-　**Unspecified motorcycle rider injured in collision with unspecified motor vehicles in nontraffic accident**

Motorcycle collision NOS, nontraffic

!Q ☑ V29.29X-　**Unspecified motorcycle rider injured in collision with other motor vehicles in nontraffic accident**

!Q ☑ V29.3XX-　**Motorcycle rider (driver) (passenger) injured in unspecified nontraffic accident**

Motorcycle accident NOS, nontraffic
Motorcycle rider injured in nontraffic accident NOS

5 V29.4　**Motorcycle driver injured in collision with other and unspecified motor vehicles in traffic accident**

!Q ☑ V29.40X-　**Motorcycle driver injured in collision with unspecified motor vehicles in traffic accident**

!Q ☑ V29.49X-　**Motorcycle driver injured in collision with other motor vehicles in traffic accident**

5 V29.5　**Motorcycle passenger injured in collision with other and unspecified motor vehicles in traffic accident**

!Q ☑ V29.50X-　**Motorcycle passenger injured in collision with unspecified motor vehicles in traffic accident**

!Q ☑ V29.59X-　**Motorcycle passenger injured in collision with other motor vehicles in traffic accident**

5 V29.6　**Unspecified motorcycle rider injured in collision with other and unspecified motor vehicles in traffic accident**

4 4th digit required　　5 5th digit required　　6 6th digit required　　7 7th digit required　　☑ 7th digit placeholder　　+ Additional code　　⊟ Laterality

1784　　　　　　　　　　　　*DecisionHealth's* FY 2020 Complete Home Health ICD-10-CM Diagnosis Coding Manual

IQ ⊘ V29.60X- Unspecified motorcycle rider injured in collision with unspecified motor vehicles in traffic accident

Motorcycle collision NOS (traffic)

IQ ⊘ V29.69X- Unspecified motorcycle rider injured in collision with other motor vehicles in traffic accident

⑤ V29.8 Motorcycle rider (driver) (passenger) injured in other specified transport accidents

IQ ⊘ V29.81X- Motorcycle rider (driver) (passenger) injured in transport accident with military vehicle

IQ ⊘ V29.88X- Motorcycle rider (driver) (passenger) injured in other specified transport accidents

IQ ⊘ V29.9XX- Motorcycle rider (driver) (passenger) injured in unspecified traffic accident

Motorcycle accident NOS

Occupant of three-wheeled motor vehicle injured in transport accident (V30-V39)

INCLUDES motorized tricycle
motorized rickshaw
three-wheeled motor car
EXCLUDES 1 all-terrain vehicles (V86.-)
motorcycle with sidecar (V20-V29)
vehicle designed primarily for off-road use (V86.-)

④ V30 Occupant of three-wheeled motor vehicle injured in collision with pedestrian or animal

EXCLUDES 1 three-wheeled motor vehicle collision with animal-drawn vehicle or animal being ridden (V36.-)

The appropriate 7th character is to be added to each code from category V30
A   initial encounter
D   subsequent encounter
S   sequela

IQ ⊘ V30.0XX- Driver of three-wheeled motor vehicle injured in collision with pedestrian or animal in nontraffic accident

IQ ⊘ V30.1XX- Passenger in three-wheeled motor vehicle injured in collision with pedestrian or animal in nontraffic accident

IQ ⊘ V30.2XX- Person on outside of three-wheeled motor vehicle injured in collision with pedestrian or animal in nontraffic accident

IQ ⊘ V30.3XX- Unspecified occupant of three-wheeled motor vehicle injured in collision with pedestrian or animal in nontraffic accident

IQ ⊘ V30.4XX- Person boarding or alighting a three-wheeled motor vehicle injured in collision with pedestrian or animal

IQ ⊘ V30.5XX- Driver of three-wheeled motor vehicle injured in collision with pedestrian or animal in traffic accident

IQ ⊘ V30.6XX- Passenger in three-wheeled motor vehicle injured in collision with pedestrian or animal in traffic accident

IQ ⊘ V30.7XX- Person on outside of three-wheeled motor vehicle injured in collision with pedestrian or animal in traffic accident

IQ ⊘ V30.9XX- Unspecified occupant of three-wheeled motor vehicle injured in collision with pedestrian or animal in traffic accident

④ V31 Occupant of three-wheeled motor vehicle injured in collision with pedal cycle

The appropriate 7th character is to be added to each code from category V31
A   initial encounter
D   subsequent encounter
S   sequela

IQ ⊘ V31.0XX- Driver of three-wheeled motor vehicle injured in collision with pedal cycle in nontraffic accident

IQ ⊘ V31.1XX- Passenger in three-wheeled motor vehicle injured in collision with pedal cycle in nontraffic accident

IQ ⊘ V31.2XX- Person on outside of three-wheeled motor vehicle injured in collision with pedal cycle in nontraffic accident

IQ ⊘ V31.3XX- Unspecified occupant of three-wheeled motor vehicle injured in collision with pedal cycle in nontraffic accident

IQ ⊘ V31.4XX- Person boarding or alighting a three-wheeled motor vehicle injured in collision with pedal cycle

IQ ⊘ V31.5XX- Driver of three-wheeled motor vehicle injured in collision with pedal cycle in traffic accident

IQ ⊘ V31.6XX- Passenger in three-wheeled motor vehicle injured in collision with pedal cycle in traffic accident

IQ ⊘ V31.7XX- Person on outside of three-wheeled motor vehicle injured in collision with pedal cycle in traffic accident

IQ ⊘ V31.9XX- Unspecified occupant of three-wheeled motor vehicle injured in collision with pedal cycle in traffic accident

④ V32 Occupant of three-wheeled motor vehicle injured in collision with two- or three-wheeled motor vehicle

The appropriate 7th character is to be added to each code from category V32
A   initial encounter
D   subsequent encounter
S   sequela

IQ ⊘ V32.0XX- Driver of three-wheeled motor vehicle injured in collision with two- or three-wheeled motor vehicle in nontraffic accident

Chapter 20

V00-Y99

★ New ▲ Revised Px Primary **SP** PDGM Px **SL** Low CoM **SH** High CoM **IQ** Quest. Encounter **H** Hospice non-cancer Dx **Unspecified** **M** *Manifestation*

DecisionHealth's FY 2020 Complete Home Health ICD-10-CM Diagnosis Coding Manual

1785

!Q ☑ V32.1XX- Passenger in three-wheeled motor vehicle injured in collision with two- or three-wheeled motor vehicle in nontraffic accident

!Q ☑ V32.2XX- Person on outside of three-wheeled motor vehicle injured in collision with two- or three-wheeled motor vehicle in nontraffic accident

!Q ☑ V32.3XX- Unspecified occupant of three-wheeled motor vehicle injured in collision with two- or three-wheeled motor vehicle in nontraffic accident

!Q ☑ V32.4XX- Person boarding or alighting a three-wheeled motor vehicle injured in collision with two- or three-wheeled motor vehicle

!Q ☑ V32.5XX- Driver of three-wheeled motor vehicle injured in collision with two- or three-wheeled motor vehicle in traffic accident

!Q ☑ V32.6XX- Passenger in three-wheeled motor vehicle injured in collision with two- or three-wheeled motor vehicle in traffic accident

!Q ☑ V32.7XX- Person on outside of three-wheeled motor vehicle injured in collision with two- or three-wheeled motor vehicle in traffic accident

!Q ☑ V32.9XX- Unspecified occupant of three-wheeled motor vehicle injured in collision with two- or three-wheeled motor vehicle in traffic accident

4 V33 Occupant of three-wheeled motor vehicle injured in collision with car, pick-up truck or van

The appropriate 7th character is to be added to each code from category V33
A   initial encounter
D   subsequent encounter
S   sequela

!Q ☑ V33.0XX- Driver of three-wheeled motor vehicle injured in collision with car, pick-up truck or van in nontraffic accident

!Q ☑ V33.1XX- Passenger in three-wheeled motor vehicle injured in collision with car, pick-up truck or van in nontraffic accident

!Q ☑ V33.2XX- Person on outside of three-wheeled motor vehicle injured in collision with car, pick-up truck or van in nontraffic accident

!Q ☑ V33.3XX- Unspecified occupant of three-wheeled motor vehicle injured in collision with car, pick-up truck or van in nontraffic accident

!Q ☑ V33.4XX- Person boarding or alighting a three-wheeled motor vehicle injured in collision with car, pick-up truck or van

!Q ☑ V33.5XX- Driver of three-wheeled motor vehicle injured in collision with car, pick-up truck or van in traffic accident

!Q ☑ V33.6XX- Passenger in three-wheeled motor vehicle injured in collision with car, pick-up truck or van in traffic accident

!Q ☑ V33.7XX- Person on outside of three-wheeled motor vehicle injured in collision with car, pick-up truck or van in traffic accident

!Q ☑ V33.9XX- Unspecified occupant of three-wheeled motor vehicle injured in collision with car, pick-up truck or van in traffic accident

4 V34 Occupant of three-wheeled motor vehicle injured in collision with heavy transport vehicle or bus

EXCLUDES 1 occupant of three-wheeled motor vehicle injured in collision with military vehicle (V39.81)

The appropriate 7th character is to be added to each code from category V34
A   initial encounter
D   subsequent encounter
S   sequela

!Q ☑ V34.0XX- Driver of three-wheeled motor vehicle injured in collision with heavy transport vehicle or bus in nontraffic accident

!Q ☑ V34.1XX- Passenger in three-wheeled motor vehicle injured in collision with heavy transport vehicle or bus in nontraffic accident

!Q ☑ V34.2XX- Person on outside of three-wheeled motor vehicle injured in collision with heavy transport vehicle or bus in nontraffic accident

!Q ☑ V34.3XX- Unspecified occupant of three-wheeled motor vehicle injured in collision with heavy transport vehicle or bus in nontraffic accident

!Q ☑ V34.4XX- Person boarding or alighting a three-wheeled motor vehicle injured in collision with heavy transport vehicle or bus

!Q ☑ V34.5XX- Driver of three-wheeled motor vehicle injured in collision with heavy transport vehicle or bus in traffic accident

!Q ☑ V34.6XX- Passenger in three-wheeled motor vehicle injured in collision with heavy transport vehicle or bus in traffic accident

!Q ☑ V34.7XX- Person on outside of three-wheeled motor vehicle injured in collision with heavy transport vehicle or bus in traffic accident

!Q ☑ V34.9XX- Unspecified occupant of three-wheeled motor vehicle injured in collision with heavy transport vehicle or bus in traffic accident

4 V35 Occupant of three-wheeled motor vehicle injured in collision with railway train or railway vehicle

4 4th digit required   **5** 5th digit required   **6** 6th digit required   **7** 7th digit required   **☑** 7th digit placeholder   **+** Additional code   **⊟** Laterality

1786   *DecisionHealth's* FY 2020 Complete Home Health ICD-10-CM Diagnosis Coding Manual

Chapter 20

V00-Y99

The appropriate 7th character is to be added to each code from category V35
A   initial encounter
D   subsequent encounter
S   sequela

IQ ☑ **V35.0XX-** **Driver of three-wheeled motor vehicle injured in collision with railway train or railway vehicle in nontraffic accident**

IQ ☑ **V35.1XX-** **Passenger in three-wheeled motor vehicle injured in collision with railway train or railway vehicle in nontraffic accident**

IQ ☑ **V35.2XX-** **Person on outside of three-wheeled motor vehicle injured in collision with railway train or railway vehicle in nontraffic accident**

IQ ☑ **V35.3XX-** **Unspecified occupant of three-wheeled motor vehicle injured in collision with railway train or railway vehicle in nontraffic accident**

IQ ☑ **V35.4XX-** **Person boarding or alighting a three-wheeled motor vehicle injured in collision with railway train or railway vehicle**

IQ ☑ **V35.5XX-** **Driver of three-wheeled motor vehicle injured in collision with railway train or railway vehicle in traffic accident**

IQ ☑ **V35.6XX-** **Passenger in three-wheeled motor vehicle injured in collision with railway train or railway vehicle in traffic accident**

IQ ☑ **V35.7XX-** **Person on outside of three-wheeled motor vehicle injured in collision with railway train or railway vehicle in traffic accident**

IQ ☑ **V35.9XX-** **Unspecified occupant of three-wheeled motor vehicle injured in collision with railway train or railway vehicle in traffic accident**

④ **V36** **Occupant of three-wheeled motor vehicle injured in collision with other nonmotor vehicle**

    INCLUDES collision with animal-drawn vehicle, animal being ridden, streetcar

The appropriate 7th character is to be added to each code from category V36
A   initial encounter
D   subsequent encounter
S   sequela

IQ ☑ **V36.0XX-** **Driver of three-wheeled motor vehicle injured in collision with other nonmotor vehicle in nontraffic accident**

IQ ☑ **V36.1XX-** **Passenger in three-wheeled motor vehicle injured in collision with other nonmotor vehicle in nontraffic accident**

IQ ☑ **V36.2XX-** **Person on outside of three-wheeled motor vehicle injured in collision with other nonmotor vehicle in nontraffic accident**

IQ ☑ **V36.3XX-** **Unspecified occupant of three-wheeled motor vehicle injured in collision with other nonmotor vehicle in nontraffic accident**

IQ ☑ **V36.4XX-** **Person boarding or alighting a three-wheeled motor vehicle injured in collision with other nonmotor vehicle**

IQ ☑ **V36.5XX-** **Driver of three-wheeled motor vehicle injured in collision with other nonmotor vehicle in traffic accident**

IQ ☑ **V36.6XX-** **Passenger in three-wheeled motor vehicle injured in collision with other nonmotor vehicle in traffic accident**

IQ ☑ **V36.7XX-** **Person on outside of three-wheeled motor vehicle injured in collision with other nonmotor vehicle in traffic accident**

IQ ☑ **V36.9XX-** **Unspecified occupant of three-wheeled motor vehicle injured in collision with other nonmotor vehicle in traffic accident**

④ **V37** **Occupant of three-wheeled motor vehicle injured in collision with fixed or stationary object**

The appropriate 7th character is to be added to each code from category V37
A   initial encounter
D   subsequent encounter
S   sequela

IQ ☑ **V37.0XX-** **Driver of three-wheeled motor vehicle injured in collision with fixed or stationary object in nontraffic accident**

IQ ☑ **V37.1XX-** **Passenger in three-wheeled motor vehicle injured in collision with fixed or stationary object in nontraffic accident**

IQ ☑ **V37.2XX-** **Person on outside of three-wheeled motor vehicle injured in collision with fixed or stationary object in nontraffic accident**

IQ ☑ **V37.3XX-** **Unspecified occupant of three-wheeled motor vehicle injured in collision with fixed or stationary object in nontraffic accident**

IQ ☑ **V37.4XX-** **Person boarding or alighting a three-wheeled motor vehicle injured in collision with fixed or stationary object**

IQ ☑ **V37.5XX-** **Driver of three-wheeled motor vehicle injured in collision with fixed or stationary object in traffic accident**

IQ ☑ **V37.6XX-** **Passenger in three-wheeled motor vehicle injured in collision with fixed or stationary object in traffic accident**

IQ ☑ **V37.7XX-** **Person on outside of three-wheeled motor vehicle injured in collision with fixed or stationary object in traffic accident**

IQ ☑ **V37.9XX-** **Unspecified occupant of three-wheeled motor vehicle injured in collision with fixed or stationary object in traffic accident**

★ New ▲ Revised Px Primary **SP** PDGM Px **SL** Low CoM **SH** High CoM **IQ** Quest. Encounter ℍ Hospice non-cancer Dx Unspecified **M** *Manifestation*

DecisionHealth's FY 2020 Complete Home Health ICD-10-CM Diagnosis Coding Manual

1787

4 V38   Occupant of three-wheeled motor vehicle injured in noncollision transport accident

INCLUDES   fall or thrown from three-wheeled motor vehicle
overturning of three-wheeled motor vehicle NOS
overturning of three-wheeled motor vehicle without collision

The appropriate 7th character is to be added to each code from category V38
A   initial encounter
D   subsequent encounter
S   sequela

!Q ☑ V38.0XX-   Driver of three-wheeled motor vehicle injured in noncollision transport accident in nontraffic accident

!Q ☑ V38.1XX-   Passenger in three-wheeled motor vehicle injured in noncollision transport accident in nontraffic accident

!Q ☑ V38.2XX-   Person on outside of three-wheeled motor vehicle injured in noncollision transport accident in nontraffic accident

!Q ☑ V38.3XX-   Unspecified occupant of three-wheeled motor vehicle injured in noncollision transport accident in nontraffic accident

!Q ☑ V38.4XX-   Person boarding or alighting a three-wheeled motor vehicle injured in noncollision transport accident

!Q ☑ V38.5XX-   Driver of three-wheeled motor vehicle injured in noncollision transport accident in traffic accident

!Q ☑ V38.6XX-   Passenger in three-wheeled motor vehicle injured in noncollision transport accident in traffic accident

!Q ☑ V38.7XX-   Person on outside of three-wheeled motor vehicle injured in noncollision transport accident in traffic accident

!Q ☑ V38.9XX-   Unspecified occupant of three-wheeled motor vehicle injured in noncollision transport accident in traffic accident

4 V39   Occupant of three-wheeled motor vehicle injured in other and unspecified transport accidents

The appropriate 7th character is to be added to each code from category V39
A   initial encounter
D   subsequent encounter
S   sequela

5 V39.0   Driver of three-wheeled motor vehicle injured in collision with other and unspecified motor vehicles in nontraffic accident

!Q ☑ V39.00X-   Driver of three-wheeled motor vehicle injured in collision with unspecified motor vehicles in nontraffic accident

!Q ☑ V39.09X-   Driver of three-wheeled motor vehicle injured in collision with other motor vehicles in nontraffic accident

5 V39.1   Passenger in three-wheeled motor vehicle injured in collision with other and unspecified motor vehicles in nontraffic accident

!Q ☑ V39.10X-   Passenger in three-wheeled motor vehicle injured in collision with unspecified motor vehicles in nontraffic accident

!Q ☑ V39.19X-   Passenger in three-wheeled motor vehicle injured in collision with other motor vehicles in nontraffic accident

5 V39.2   Unspecified occupant of three-wheeled motor vehicle injured in collision with other and unspecified motor vehicles in nontraffic accident

!Q ☑ V39.20X-   Unspecified occupant of three-wheeled motor vehicle injured in collision with unspecified motor vehicles in nontraffic accident

Collision NOS involving three-wheeled motor vehicle, nontraffic

!Q ☑ V39.29X-   Unspecified occupant of three-wheeled motor vehicle injured in collision with other motor vehicles in nontraffic accident

!Q ☑ V39.3XX-   Occupant (driver) (passenger) of three-wheeled motor vehicle injured in unspecified nontraffic accident

Accident NOS involving three-wheeled motor vehicle, nontraffic
Occupant of three-wheeled motor vehicle injured in nontraffic accident NOS

5 V39.4   Driver of three-wheeled motor vehicle injured in collision with other and unspecified motor vehicles in traffic accident

!Q ☑ V39.40X-   Driver of three-wheeled motor vehicle injured in collision with unspecified motor vehicles in traffic accident

!Q ☑ V39.49X-   Driver of three-wheeled motor vehicle injured in collision with other motor vehicles in traffic accident

5 V39.5   Passenger in three-wheeled motor vehicle injured in collision with other and unspecified motor vehicles in traffic accident

!Q ☑ V39.50X-   Passenger in three-wheeled motor vehicle injured in collision with unspecified motor vehicles in traffic accident

!Q ☑ V39.59X-   Passenger in three-wheeled motor vehicle injured in collision with other motor vehicles in traffic accident

5 V39.6   Unspecified occupant of three-wheeled motor vehicle injured in collision with other and unspecified motor vehicles in traffic accident

4 4th digit required   5 5th digit required   6 6th digit required   7 7th digit required   ☑ 7th digit placeholder   ✚ Additional code   ⊟ Laterality

1788   DecisionHealth's FY 2020 Complete Home Health ICD-10-CM Diagnosis Coding Manual

IQ ☑ V39.60X- Unspecified occupant of three-wheeled motor vehicle injured in collision with unspecified motor vehicles in traffic accident

Collision NOS involving three-wheeled motor vehicle (traffic)

IQ ☑ V39.69X- Unspecified occupant of three-wheeled motor vehicle injured in collision with other motor vehicles in traffic accident

⑤ V39.8 Occupant (driver) (passenger) of three-wheeled motor vehicle injured in other specified transport accidents

IQ ☑ V39.81X- Occupant (driver) (passenger) of three-wheeled motor vehicle injured in transport accident with military vehicle

IQ ☑ V39.89X- Occupant (driver) (passenger) of three-wheeled motor vehicle injured in other specified transport accidents

IQ ☑ V39.9XX- Occupant (driver) (passenger) of three-wheeled motor vehicle injured in unspecified traffic accident

Accident NOS involving three-wheeled motor vehicle

Car occupant injured in transport accident (V40-V49)

INCLUDES	a four-wheeled motor vehicle designed primarily for carrying passengers
	automobile (pulling a trailer or camper)
EXCLUDES 1	bus (V50-V59)
	minibus (V50-V59)
	minivan (V50-V59)
	motorcoach (V70-V79)
	pick-up truck (V50-V59)
	sport utility vehicle (SUV) (V50-V59)

④ V40 Car occupant injured in collision with pedestrian or animal

EXCLUDES 1 car collision with animal-drawn vehicle or animal being ridden (V46.-)

The appropriate 7th character is to be added to each code from category V40
A   initial encounter
D   subsequent encounter
S   sequela

IQ ☑ V40.0XX- Car driver injured in collision with pedestrian or animal in nontraffic accident

IQ ☑ V40.1XX- Car passenger injured in collision with pedestrian or animal in nontraffic accident

IQ ☑ V40.2XX- Person on outside of car injured in collision with pedestrian or animal in nontraffic accident

IQ ☑ V40.3XX- Unspecified car occupant injured in collision with pedestrian or animal in nontraffic accident

IQ ☑ V40.4XX- Person boarding or alighting a car injured in collision with pedestrian or animal

IQ ☑ V40.5XX- Car driver injured in collision with pedestrian or animal in traffic accident

IQ ☑ V40.6XX- Car passenger injured in collision with pedestrian or animal in traffic accident

IQ ☑ V40.7XX- Person on outside of car injured in collision with pedestrian or animal in traffic accident

IQ ☑ V40.9XX- Unspecified car occupant injured in collision with pedestrian or animal in traffic accident

④ V41 Car occupant injured in collision with pedal cycle

The appropriate 7th character is to be added to each code from category V41
A   initial encounter
D   subsequent encounter
S   sequela

IQ ☑ V41.0XX- Car driver injured in collision with pedal cycle in nontraffic accident

IQ ☑ V41.1XX- Car passenger injured in collision with pedal cycle in nontraffic accident

IQ ☑ V41.2XX- Person on outside of car injured in collision with pedal cycle in nontraffic accident

IQ ☑ V41.3XX- Unspecified car occupant injured in collision with pedal cycle in nontraffic accident

IQ ☑ V41.4XX- Person boarding or alighting a car injured in collision with pedal cycle

IQ ☑ V41.5XX- Car driver injured in collision with pedal cycle in traffic accident

IQ ☑ V41.6XX- Car passenger injured in collision with pedal cycle in traffic accident

IQ ☑ V41.7XX- Person on outside of car injured in collision with pedal cycle in traffic accident

IQ ☑ V41.9XX- Unspecified car occupant injured in collision with pedal cycle in traffic accident

④ V42 Car occupant injured in collision with two- or three-wheeled motor vehicle

The appropriate 7th character is to be added to each code from category V42
A   initial encounter
D   subsequent encounter
S   sequela

IQ ☑ V42.0XX- Car driver injured in collision with two- or three-wheeled motor vehicle in nontraffic accident

IQ ☑ V42.1XX- Car passenger injured in collision with two- or three-wheeled motor vehicle in nontraffic accident

IQ ☑ V42.2XX- Person on outside of car injured in collision with two- or three-wheeled motor vehicle in nontraffic accident

IQ ☑ V42.3XX- Unspecified car occupant injured in collision with two- or three-wheeled motor vehicle in nontraffic accident

IQ ☑ V42.4XX- Person boarding or alighting a car injured in collision with two- or three-wheeled motor vehicle

★ New ▲ Revised Px Primary 🆂🅿 PDGM Px 🆂🅻 Low CoM 🆂🅷 High CoM IQ Quest. Encounter Ⓗ Hospice non-cancer Dx Unspecified M Manifestation

DecisionHealth's FY 2020 Complete Home Health ICD-10-CM Diagnosis Coding Manual   1789

IQ ☑ V42.5XX- Car driver injured in collision with two- or three-wheeled motor vehicle in traffic accident

IQ ☑ V42.6XX- Car passenger injured in collision with two- or three-wheeled motor vehicle in traffic accident

IQ ☑ V42.7XX- Person on outside of car injured in collision with two- or three-wheeled motor vehicle in traffic accident

IQ ☑ V42.9XX- Unspecified car occupant injured in collision with two- or three-wheeled motor vehicle in traffic accident

4 V43 Car occupant injured in collision with car, pick-up truck or van

The appropriate 7th character is to be added to each code from category V43
A   initial encounter
D   subsequent encounter
S   sequela

5 V43.0 Car driver injured in collision with car, pick-up truck or van in nontraffic accident

IQ ☑ V43.01X- Car driver injured in collision with sport utility vehicle in nontraffic accident

IQ ☑ V43.02X- Car driver injured in collision with other type car in nontraffic accident

IQ ☑ V43.03X- Car driver injured in collision with pick-up truck in nontraffic accident

IQ ☑ V43.04X- Car driver injured in collision with van in nontraffic accident

5 V43.1 Car passenger injured in collision with car, pick-up truck or van in nontraffic accident

IQ ☑ V43.11X- Car passenger injured in collision with sport utility vehicle in nontraffic accident

IQ ☑ V43.12X- Car passenger injured in collision with other type car in nontraffic accident

▲ IQ ☑ V43.13X- Car passenger injured in collision with pick-up truck in nontraffic accident

IQ ☑ V43.14X- Car passenger injured in collision with van in nontraffic accident

5 V43.2 Person on outside of car injured in collision with car, pick-up truck or van in nontraffic accident

IQ ☑ V43.21X- Person on outside of car injured in collision with sport utility vehicle in nontraffic accident

IQ ☑ V43.22X- Person on outside of car injured in collision with other type car in nontraffic accident

IQ ☑ V43.23X- Person on outside of car injured in collision with pick-up truck in nontraffic accident

IQ ☑ V43.24X- Person on outside of car injured in collision with van in nontraffic accident

5 V43.3 Unspecified car occupant injured in collision with car, pick-up truck or van in nontraffic accident

IQ ☑ V43.31X- Unspecified car occupant injured in collision with sport utility vehicle in nontraffic accident

IQ ☑ V43.32X- Unspecified car occupant injured in collision with other type car in nontraffic accident

IQ ☑ V43.33X- Unspecified car occupant injured in collision with pick-up truck in nontraffic accident

IQ ☑ V43.34X- Unspecified car occupant injured in collision with van in nontraffic accident

5 V43.4 Person boarding or alighting a car injured in collision with car, pick-up truck or van

IQ ☑ V43.41X- Person boarding or alighting a car injured in collision with sport utility vehicle

IQ ☑ V43.42X- Person boarding or alighting a car injured in collision with other type car

IQ ☑ V43.43X- Person boarding or alighting a car injured in collision with pick-up truck

IQ ☑ V43.44X- Person boarding or alighting a car injured in collision with van

5 V43.5 Car driver injured in collision with car, pick-up truck or van in traffic accident

IQ ☑ V43.51X- Car driver injured in collision with sport utility vehicle in traffic accident

IQ ☑ V43.52X- Car driver injured in collision with other type car in traffic accident

IQ ☑ V43.53X- Car driver injured in collision with pick-up truck in traffic accident

IQ ☑ V43.54X- Car driver injured in collision with van in traffic accident

5 V43.6 Car passenger injured in collision with car, pick-up truck or van in traffic accident

IQ ☑ V43.61X- Car passenger injured in collision with sport utility vehicle in traffic accident

IQ ☑ V43.62X- Car passenger injured in collision with other type car in traffic accident

IQ ☑ V43.63X- Car passenger injured in collision with pick-up truck in traffic accident

IQ ☑ V43.64X- Car passenger injured in collision with van in traffic accident

5 V43.7 Person on outside of car injured in collision with car, pick-up truck or van in traffic accident

IQ ☑ V43.71X- Person on outside of car injured in collision with sport utility vehicle in traffic accident

IQ ☑ V43.72X- Person on outside of car injured in collision with other type car in traffic accident

IQ ☑ V43.73X- Person on outside of car injured in collision with pick-up truck in traffic accident

IQ ☑ V43.74X- Person on outside of car injured in collision with van in traffic accident

---

4 4th digit required   5 5th digit required   6 6th digit required   7 7th digit required   ☑ 7th digit placeholder   **+** Additional code   ⊟ Laterality

5 V43.9 Unspecified car occupant injured in collision with car, pick-up truck or van in traffic accident

!Q ☑ V43.91X- Unspecified car occupant injured in collision with sport utility vehicle in traffic accident

!Q ☑ V43.92X- Unspecified car occupant injured in collision with other type car in traffic accident

!Q ☑ V43.93X- Unspecified car occupant injured in collision with pick-up truck in traffic accident

!Q ☑ V43.94X- Unspecified car occupant injured in collision with van in traffic accident

4 V44 Car occupant injured in collision with heavy transport vehicle or bus

> EXCLUDES 1   car occupant injured in collision with military vehicle (V49.81)

> The appropriate 7th character is to be added to each code from category V44
> A   initial encounter
> D   subsequent encounter
> S   sequela

!Q ☑ V44.0XX- Car driver injured in collision with heavy transport vehicle or bus in nontraffic accident

!Q ☑ V44.1XX- Car passenger injured in collision with heavy transport vehicle or bus in nontraffic accident

!Q ☑ V44.2XX- Person on outside of car injured in collision with heavy transport vehicle or bus in nontraffic accident

!Q ☑ V44.3XX- Unspecified car occupant injured in collision with heavy transport vehicle or bus in nontraffic accident

!Q ☑ V44.4XX- Person boarding or alighting a car injured in collision with heavy transport vehicle or bus

!Q ☑ V44.5XX- Car driver injured in collision with heavy transport vehicle or bus in traffic accident

!Q ☑ V44.6XX- Car passenger injured in collision with heavy transport vehicle or bus in traffic accident

!Q ☑ V44.7XX- Person on outside of car injured in collision with heavy transport vehicle or bus in traffic accident

!Q ☑ V44.9XX- Unspecified car occupant injured in collision with heavy transport vehicle or bus in traffic accident

4 V45 Car occupant injured in collision with railway train or railway vehicle

> The appropriate 7th character is to be added to each code from category V45
> A   initial encounter
> D   subsequent encounter
> S   sequela

!Q ☑ V45.0XX- Car driver injured in collision with railway train or railway vehicle in nontraffic accident

!Q ☑ V45.1XX- Car passenger injured in collision with railway train or railway vehicle in nontraffic accident

!Q ☑ V45.2XX- Person on outside of car injured in collision with railway train or railway vehicle in nontraffic accident

!Q ☑ V45.3XX- Unspecified car occupant injured in collision with railway train or railway vehicle in nontraffic accident

!Q ☑ V45.4XX- Person boarding or alighting a car injured in collision with railway train or railway vehicle

!Q ☑ V45.5XX- Car driver injured in collision with railway train or railway vehicle in traffic accident

!Q ☑ V45.6XX- Car passenger injured in collision with railway train or railway vehicle in traffic accident

!Q ☑ V45.7XX- Person on outside of car injured in collision with railway train or railway vehicle in traffic accident

!Q ☑ V45.9XX- Unspecified car occupant injured in collision with railway train or railway vehicle in traffic accident

4 V46 Car occupant injured in collision with other nonmotor vehicle

> INCLUDES   collision with animal-drawn vehicle, animal being ridden, streetcar

> The appropriate 7th character is to be added to each code from category V46
> A   initial encounter
> D   subsequent encounter
> S   sequela

!Q ☑ V46.0XX- Car driver injured in collision with other nonmotor vehicle in nontraffic accident

!Q ☑ V46.1XX- Car passenger injured in collision with other nonmotor vehicle in nontraffic accident

!Q ☑ V46.2XX- Person on outside of car injured in collision with other nonmotor vehicle in nontraffic accident

!Q ☑ V46.3XX- Unspecified car occupant injured in collision with other nonmotor vehicle in nontraffic accident

!Q ☑ V46.4XX- Person boarding or alighting a car injured in collision with other nonmotor vehicle

!Q ☑ V46.5XX- Car driver injured in collision with other nonmotor vehicle in traffic accident

!Q ☑ V46.6XX- Car passenger injured in collision with other nonmotor vehicle in traffic accident

!Q ☑ V46.7XX- Person on outside of car injured in collision with other nonmotor vehicle in traffic accident

!Q ☑ V46.9XX- Unspecified car occupant injured in collision with other nonmotor vehicle in traffic accident

4 V47 Car occupant injured in collision with fixed or stationary object

Chapter 20

V00-Y99

★ New ▲ Revised Px Primary SP PDGM Px SL Low CoM SH High CoM !Q Quest. Encounter H Hospice non-cancer Dx   Unspecified   M *Manifestation*

DecisionHealth's FY 2020 Complete Home Health ICD-10-CM Diagnosis Coding Manual

1791

The appropriate 7th character is to be added to each code from category V47
A   initial encounter
D   subsequent encounter
S   sequela

!Q ☑ V47.0XX- Car driver injured in collision with fixed or stationary object in nontraffic accident

!Q ☑ V47.1XX- Car passenger injured in collision with fixed or stationary object in nontraffic accident

!Q ☑ V47.2XX- Person on outside of car injured in collision with fixed or stationary object in nontraffic accident

!Q ☑ V47.3XX- Unspecified car occupant injured in collision with fixed or stationary object in nontraffic accident

!Q ☑ V47.4XX- Person boarding or alighting a car injured in collision with fixed or stationary object

!Q ☑ V47.5XX- Car driver injured in collision with fixed or stationary object in traffic accident

!Q ☑ V47.6XX- Car passenger injured in collision with fixed or stationary object in traffic accident

!Q ☑ V47.7XX- Person on outside of car injured in collision with fixed or stationary object in traffic accident

!Q ☑ V47.9XX- Unspecified car occupant injured in collision with fixed or stationary object in traffic accident

4 V48 Car occupant injured in noncollision transport accident

INCLUDES   overturning car NOS
                overturning car without collision

The appropriate 7th character is to be added to each code from category V48
A   initial encounter
D   subsequent encounter
S   sequela

!Q ☑ V48.0XX- Car driver injured in noncollision transport accident in nontraffic accident

!Q ☑ V48.1XX- Car passenger injured in noncollision transport accident in nontraffic accident

!Q ☑ V48.2XX- Person on outside of car injured in noncollision transport accident in nontraffic accident

!Q ☑ V48.3XX- Unspecified car occupant injured in noncollision transport accident in nontraffic accident

!Q ☑ V48.4XX- Person boarding or alighting a car injured in noncollision transport accident

!Q ☑ V48.5XX- Car driver injured in noncollision transport accident in traffic accident

!Q ☑ V48.6XX- Car passenger injured in noncollision transport accident in traffic accident

!Q ☑ V48.7XX- Person on outside of car injured in noncollision transport accident in traffic accident

!Q ☑ V48.9XX- Unspecified car occupant injured in noncollision transport accident in traffic accident

4 V49 Car occupant injured in other and unspecified transport accidents

The appropriate 7th character is to be added to each code from category V49
A   initial encounter
D   subsequent encounter
S   sequela

5 V49.0 Driver injured in collision with other and unspecified motor vehicles in nontraffic accident

!Q ☑ V49.00X- Driver injured in collision with unspecified motor vehicles in nontraffic accident

!Q ☑ V49.09X- Driver injured in collision with other motor vehicles in nontraffic accident

5 V49.1 Passenger injured in collision with other and unspecified motor vehicles in nontraffic accident

!Q ☑ V49.10X- Passenger injured in collision with unspecified motor vehicles in nontraffic accident

!Q ☑ V49.19X- Passenger injured in collision with other motor vehicles in nontraffic accident

5 V49.2 Unspecified car occupant injured in collision with other and unspecified motor vehicles in nontraffic accident

!Q ☑ V49.20X- Unspecified car occupant injured in collision with unspecified motor vehicles in nontraffic accident

Car collision NOS, nontraffic

!Q ☑ V49.29X- Unspecified car occupant injured in collision with other motor vehicles in nontraffic accident

!Q ☑ V49.3XX- Car occupant (driver) (passenger) injured in unspecified nontraffic accident

Car accident NOS, nontraffic
Car occupant injured in nontraffic accident NOS

5 V49.4 Driver injured in collision with other and unspecified motor vehicles in traffic accident

!Q ☑ V49.40X- Driver injured in collision with unspecified motor vehicles in traffic accident

!Q ☑ V49.49X- Driver injured in collision with other motor vehicles in traffic accident

5 V49.5 Passenger injured in collision with other and unspecified motor vehicles in traffic accident

!Q ☑ V49.50X- Passenger injured in collision with unspecified motor vehicles in traffic accident

!Q ☑ V49.59X- Passenger injured in collision with other motor vehicles in traffic accident

---

4 4th digit required   5 5th digit required   6 6th digit required   7 7th digit required   ☑ 7th digit placeholder   + Additional code   ⊟ Laterality

⑤ **V49.6** **Unspecified car occupant injured in collision with other and unspecified motor vehicles in traffic accident**

IQ ✓ **V49.60X-** **Unspecified car occupant injured in collision with unspecified motor vehicles in traffic accident**

Car collision NOS (traffic)

IQ ✓ **V49.69X-** **Unspecified car occupant injured in collision with other motor vehicles in traffic accident**

⑤ **V49.8** **Car occupant (driver) (passenger) injured in other specified transport accidents**

IQ ✓ **V49.81X-** Car occupant (driver) (passenger) injured in transport accident with military vehicle

IQ ✓ **V49.88X-** Car occupant (driver) (passenger) injured in other specified transport accidents

IQ ✓ **V49.9XX-** **Car occupant (driver) (passenger) injured in unspecified traffic accident**

Car accident NOS

Occupant of pick-up truck or van injured in transport accident   (V50-V59)

INCLUDES a four or six wheel motor vehicle designed primarily for carrying passengers and property but weighing less than the local limit for classification as a heavy goods vehicle
minibus
minivan
sport utility vehicle (SUV)
truck
van

EXCLUDES 1 heavy transport vehicle (V60-V69)

④ **V50** **Occupant of pick-up truck or van injured in collision with pedestrian or animal**

EXCLUDES 1 pick-up truck or van collision with animal-drawn vehicle or animal being ridden (V56.-)

The appropriate 7th character is to be added to each code from category V50
A   initial encounter
D   subsequent encounter
S   sequela

IQ ✓ **V50.0XX-** Driver of pick-up truck or van injured in collision with pedestrian or animal in nontraffic accident

IQ ✓ **V50.1XX-** Passenger in pick-up truck or van injured in collision with pedestrian or animal in nontraffic accident

IQ ✓ **V50.2XX-** Person on outside of pick-up truck or van injured in collision with pedestrian or animal in nontraffic accident

IQ ✓ **V50.3XX-** **Unspecified occupant of pick-up truck or van injured in collision with pedestrian or animal in nontraffic accident**

IQ ✓ **V50.4XX-** Person boarding or alighting a pick-up truck or van injured in collision with pedestrian or animal

IQ ✓ **V50.5XX-** Driver of pick-up truck or van injured in collision with pedestrian or animal in traffic accident

IQ ✓ **V50.6XX-** Passenger in pick-up truck or van injured in collision with pedestrian or animal in traffic accident

IQ ✓ **V50.7XX-** Person on outside of pick-up truck or van injured in collision with pedestrian or animal in traffic accident

IQ ✓ **V50.9XX-** **Unspecified occupant of pick-up truck or van injured in collision with pedestrian or animal in traffic accident**

④ **V51** **Occupant of pick-up truck or van injured in collision with pedal cycle**

The appropriate 7th character is to be added to each code from category V51
A   initial encounter
D   subsequent encounter
S   sequela

IQ ✓ **V51.0XX-** Driver of pick-up truck or van injured in collision with pedal cycle in nontraffic accident

IQ ✓ **V51.1XX-** Passenger in pick-up truck or van injured in collision with pedal cycle in nontraffic accident

IQ ✓ **V51.2XX-** Person on outside of pick-up truck or van injured in collision with pedal cycle in nontraffic accident

IQ ✓ **V51.3XX-** **Unspecified occupant of pick-up truck or van injured in collision with pedal cycle in nontraffic accident**

IQ ✓ **V51.4XX-** Person boarding or alighting a pick-up truck or van injured in collision with pedal cycle

IQ ✓ **V51.5XX-** Driver of pick-up truck or van injured in collision with pedal cycle in traffic accident

IQ ✓ **V51.6XX-** Passenger in pick-up truck or van injured in collision with pedal cycle in traffic accident

IQ ✓ **V51.7XX-** Person on outside of pick-up truck or van injured in collision with pedal cycle in traffic accident

IQ ✓ **V51.9XX-** **Unspecified occupant of pick-up truck or van injured in collision with pedal cycle in traffic accident**

④ **V52** **Occupant of pick-up truck or van injured in collision with two- or three-wheeled motor vehicle**

The appropriate 7th character is to be added to each code from category V52
A   initial encounter
D   subsequent encounter
S   sequela

IQ ✓ **V52.0XX-** Driver of pick-up truck or van injured in collision with two- or three-wheeled motor vehicle in nontraffic accident

IQ ✓ **V52.1XX-** Passenger in pick-up truck or van injured in collision with two- or three-wheeled motor vehicle in nontraffic accident

IQ ✓ **V52.2XX-** Person on outside of pick-up truck or van injured in collision with two- or three-wheeled motor vehicle in nontraffic accident

---

★ New ▲ Revised **Px** Primary **SP** PDGM Px **SL** Low CoM **SH** High CoM **IQ** Quest. Encounter **H** Hospice non-cancer Dx   Unspecified   **M** *Manifestation*

!Q ⊠ V52.3XX- **Unspecified occupant of pick-up truck or van injured in collision with two- or three-wheeled motor vehicle in nontraffic accident**

!Q ⊠ V52.4XX- Person boarding or alighting a pick-up truck or van injured in collision with two- or three-wheeled motor vehicle

!Q ⊠ V52.5XX- Driver of pick-up truck or van injured in collision with two- or three-wheeled motor vehicle in traffic accident

!Q ⊠ V52.6XX- Passenger in pick-up truck or van injured in collision with two- or three-wheeled motor vehicle in traffic accident

!Q ⊠ V52.7XX- Person on outside of pick-up truck or van injured in collision with two- or three-wheeled motor vehicle in traffic accident

!Q ⊠ V52.9XX- **Unspecified occupant of pick-up truck or van injured in collision with two- or three-wheeled motor vehicle in traffic accident**

⊿ V53 **Occupant of pick-up truck or van injured in collision with car, pick-up truck or van**

The appropriate 7th character is to be added to each code from category V53
A   initial encounter
D   subsequent encounter
S   sequela

!Q ⊠ V53.0XX- Driver of pick-up truck or van injured in collision with car, pick-up truck or van in nontraffic accident

!Q ⊠ V53.1XX- Passenger in pick-up truck or van injured in collision with car, pick-up truck or van in nontraffic accident

!Q ⊠ V53.2XX- Person on outside of pick-up truck or van injured in collision with car, pick-up truck or van in nontraffic accident

!Q ⊠ V53.3XX- **Unspecified occupant of pick-up truck or van injured in collision with car, pick-up truck or van in nontraffic accident**

!Q ⊠ V53.4XX- Person boarding or alighting a pick-up truck or van injured in collision with car, pick-up truck or van

!Q ⊠ V53.5XX- Driver of pick-up truck or van injured in collision with car, pick-up truck or van in traffic accident

!Q ⊠ V53.6XX- Passenger in pick-up truck or van injured in collision with car, pick-up truck or van in traffic accident

!Q ⊠ V53.7XX- Person on outside of pick-up truck or van injured in collision with car, pick-up truck or van in traffic accident

!Q ⊠ V53.9XX- **Unspecified occupant of pick-up truck or van injured in collision with car, pick-up truck or van in traffic accident**

⊿ V54 **Occupant of pick-up truck or van injured in collision with heavy transport vehicle or bus**

EXCLUDES 1 occupant of pick-up truck or van injured in collision with military vehicle (V59.81)

The appropriate 7th character is to be added to each code from category V54
A   initial encounter
D   subsequent encounter
S   sequela

!Q ⊠ V54.0XX- Driver of pick-up truck or van injured in collision with heavy transport vehicle or bus in nontraffic accident

!Q ⊠ V54.1XX- Passenger in pick-up truck or van injured in collision with heavy transport vehicle or bus in nontraffic accident

!Q ⊠ V54.2XX- Person on outside of pick-up truck or van injured in collision with heavy transport vehicle or bus in nontraffic accident

!Q ⊠ V54.3XX- **Unspecified occupant of pick-up truck or van injured in collision with heavy transport vehicle or bus in nontraffic accident**

!Q ⊠ V54.4XX- Person boarding or alighting a pick-up truck or van injured in collision with heavy transport vehicle or bus

!Q ⊠ V54.5XX- Driver of pick-up truck or van injured in collision with heavy transport vehicle or bus in traffic accident

!Q ⊠ V54.6XX- Passenger in pick-up truck or van injured in collision with heavy transport vehicle or bus in traffic accident

!Q ⊠ V54.7XX- Person on outside of pick-up truck or van injured in collision with heavy transport vehicle or bus in traffic accident

!Q ⊠ V54.9XX- **Unspecified occupant of pick-up truck or van injured in collision with heavy transport vehicle or bus in traffic accident**

⊿ V55 **Occupant of pick-up truck or van injured in collision with railway train or railway vehicle**

The appropriate 7th character is to be added to each code from category V55
A   initial encounter
D   subsequent encounter
S   sequela

!Q ⊠ V55.0XX- Driver of pick-up truck or van injured in collision with railway train or railway vehicle in nontraffic accident

!Q ⊠ V55.1XX- Passenger in pick-up truck or van injured in collision with railway train or railway vehicle in nontraffic accident

!Q ⊠ V55.2XX- Person on outside of pick-up truck or van injured in collision with railway train or railway vehicle in nontraffic accident

⊿4th digit required ⑤5th digit required ⑥6th digit required ⑦7th digit required ⊠7th digit placeholder ✚Additional code ⊟Laterality

1794 *DecisionHealth's* FY 2020 Complete Home Health ICD-10-CM Diagnosis Coding Manual

Chapter 20 V00-Y99

!Q ✓ V55.3XX- Unspecified occupant of pick-up truck or van injured in collision with railway train or railway vehicle in nontraffic accident

!Q ✓ V55.4XX- Person boarding or alighting a pick-up truck or van injured in collision with railway train or railway vehicle

!Q ✓ V55.5XX- Driver of pick-up truck or van injured in collision with railway train or railway vehicle in traffic accident

!Q ✓ V55.6XX- Passenger in pick-up truck or van injured in collision with railway train or railway vehicle in traffic accident

!Q ✓ V55.7XX- Person on outside of pick-up truck or van injured in collision with railway train or railway vehicle in traffic accident

!Q ✓ V55.9XX- Unspecified occupant of pick-up truck or van injured in collision with railway train or railway vehicle in traffic accident

④ V56 Occupant of pick-up truck or van injured in collision with other nonmotor vehicle

> INCLUDES collision with animal-drawn vehicle, animal being ridden, streetcar

> The appropriate 7th character is to be added to each code from category V56
> A   initial encounter
> D   subsequent encounter
> S   sequela

!Q ✓ V56.0XX- Driver of pick-up truck or van injured in collision with other nonmotor vehicle in nontraffic accident

!Q ✓ V56.1XX- Passenger in pick-up truck or van injured in collision with other nonmotor vehicle in nontraffic accident

!Q ✓ V56.2XX- Person on outside of pick-up truck or van injured in collision with other nonmotor vehicle in nontraffic accident

!Q ✓ V56.3XX- Unspecified occupant of pick-up truck or van injured in collision with other nonmotor vehicle in nontraffic accident

!Q ✓ V56.4XX- Person boarding or alighting a pick-up truck or van injured in collision with other nonmotor vehicle

!Q ✓ V56.5XX- Driver of pick-up truck or van injured in collision with other nonmotor vehicle in traffic accident

!Q ✓ V56.6XX- Passenger in pick-up truck or van injured in collision with other nonmotor vehicle in traffic accident

!Q ✓ V56.7XX- Person on outside of pick-up truck or van injured in collision with other nonmotor vehicle in traffic accident

!Q ✓ V56.9XX- Unspecified occupant of pick-up truck or van injured in collision with other nonmotor vehicle in traffic accident

④ V57 Occupant of pick-up truck or van injured in collision with fixed or stationary object

> The appropriate 7th character is to be added to each code from category V57
> A   initial encounter
> D   subsequent encounter
> S   sequela

!Q ✓ V57.0XX- Driver of pick-up truck or van injured in collision with fixed or stationary object in nontraffic accident

!Q ✓ V57.1XX- Passenger in pick-up truck or van injured in collision with fixed or stationary object in nontraffic accident

!Q ✓ V57.2XX- Person on outside of pick-up truck or van injured in collision with fixed or stationary object in nontraffic accident

!Q ✓ V57.3XX- Unspecified occupant of pick-up truck or van injured in collision with fixed or stationary object in nontraffic accident

!Q ✓ V57.4XX- Person boarding or alighting a pick-up truck or van injured in collision with fixed or stationary object

!Q ✓ V57.5XX- Driver of pick-up truck or van injured in collision with fixed or stationary object in traffic accident

!Q ✓ V57.6XX- Passenger in pick-up truck or van injured in collision with fixed or stationary object in traffic accident

!Q ✓ V57.7XX- Person on outside of pick-up truck or van injured in collision with fixed or stationary object in traffic accident

!Q ✓ V57.9XX- Unspecified occupant of pick-up truck or van injured in collision with fixed or stationary object in traffic accident

④ V58 Occupant of pick-up truck or van injured in noncollision transport accident

> INCLUDES overturning pick-up truck or van NOS
> overturning pick-up truck or van without collision

> The appropriate 7th character is to be added to each code from category V58
> A   initial encounter
> D   subsequent encounter
> S   sequela

!Q ✓ V58.0XX- Driver of pick-up truck or van injured in noncollision transport accident in nontraffic accident

!Q ✓ V58.1XX- Passenger in pick-up truck or van injured in noncollision transport accident in nontraffic accident

!Q ✓ V58.2XX- Person on outside of pick-up truck or van injured in noncollision transport accident in nontraffic accident

!Q ✓ V58.3XX- Unspecified occupant of pick-up truck or van injured in noncollision transport accident in nontraffic accident

★ New ▲ Revised Px Primary **SP** PDGM Px **SL** Low CoM **SH** High CoM **!Q** Quest. Encounter **H** Hospice non-cancer Dx Unspecified **M** *Manifestation*

DecisionHealth's FY 2020 Complete Home Health ICD-10-CM Diagnosis Coding Manual

1795

IQ ☑ V58.4XX- Person boarding or alighting a pick-up truck or van injured in noncollision transport accident

IQ ☑ V58.5XX- Driver of pick-up truck or van injured in noncollision transport accident in traffic accident

IQ ☑ V58.6XX- Passenger in pick-up truck or van injured in noncollision transport accident in traffic accident

IQ ☑ V58.7XX- Person on outside of pick-up truck or van injured in noncollision transport accident in traffic accident

IQ ☑ V58.9XX- Unspecified occupant of pick-up truck or van injured in noncollision transport accident in traffic accident

4 V59 Occupant of pick-up truck or van injured in other and unspecified transport accidents

> The appropriate 7th character is to be added to each code from category V59
> A   initial encounter
> D   subsequent encounter
> S   sequela

5 V59.0 Driver of pick-up truck or van injured in collision with other and unspecified motor vehicles in nontraffic accident

IQ ☑ V59.00X- Driver of pick-up truck or van injured in collision with unspecified motor vehicles in nontraffic accident

IQ ☑ V59.09X- Driver of pick-up truck or van injured in collision with other motor vehicles in nontraffic accident

5 V59.1 Passenger in pick-up truck or van injured in collision with other and unspecified motor vehicles in nontraffic accident

IQ ☑ V59.10X- Passenger in pick-up truck or van injured in collision with unspecified motor vehicles in nontraffic accident

IQ ☑ V59.19X- Passenger in pick-up truck or van injured in collision with other motor vehicles in nontraffic accident

5 V59.2 Unspecified occupant of pick-up truck or van injured in collision with other and unspecified motor vehicles in nontraffic accident

IQ ☑ V59.20X- Unspecified occupant of pick-up truck or van injured in collision with unspecified motor vehicles in nontraffic accident

> Collision NOS involving pick-up truck or van, nontraffic

IQ ☑ V59.29X- Unspecified occupant of pick-up truck or van injured in collision with other motor vehicles in nontraffic accident

IQ ☑ V59.3XX- Occupant (driver) (passenger) of pick-up truck or van injured in unspecified nontraffic accident

> Accident NOS involving pick-up truck or van, nontraffic
> Occupant of pick-up truck or van injured in nontraffic accident NOS

5 V59.4 Driver of pick-up truck or van injured in collision with other and unspecified motor vehicles in traffic accident

IQ ☑ V59.40X- Driver of pick-up truck or van injured in collision with unspecified motor vehicles in traffic accident

IQ ☑ V59.49X- Driver of pick-up truck or van injured in collision with other motor vehicles in traffic accident

5 V59.5 Passenger in pick-up truck or van injured in collision with other and unspecified motor vehicles in traffic accident

IQ ☑ V59.50X- Passenger in pick-up truck or van injured in collision with unspecified motor vehicles in traffic accident

IQ ☑ V59.59X- Passenger in pick-up truck or van injured in collision with other motor vehicles in traffic accident

5 V59.6 Unspecified occupant of pick-up truck or van injured in collision with other and unspecified motor vehicles in traffic accident

IQ ☑ V59.60X- Unspecified occupant of pick-up truck or van injured in collision with unspecified motor vehicles in traffic accident

> Collision NOS involving pick-up truck or van (traffic)

IQ ☑ V59.69X- Unspecified occupant of pick-up truck or van injured in collision with other motor vehicles in traffic accident

5 V59.8 Occupant (driver) (passenger) of pick-up truck or van injured in other specified transport accidents

IQ ☑ V59.81X- Occupant (driver) (passenger) of pick-up truck or van injured in transport accident with military vehicle

IQ ☑ V59.88X- Occupant (driver) (passenger) of pick-up truck or van injured in other specified transport accidents

IQ ☑ V59.9XX- Occupant (driver) (passenger) of pick-up truck or van injured in unspecified traffic accident

> Accident NOS involving pick-up truck or van

Occupant of heavy transport vehicle injured in transport accident   (V60-V69)

INCLUDES	18 wheeler
	armored car
	panel truck
EXCLUDES 1	bus
	motorcoach

4 V60 Occupant of heavy transport vehicle injured in collision with pedestrian or animal

4 4th digit required   **5** 5th digit required   **6** 6th digit required   **7** 7th digit required   ☑ 7th digit placeholder   **+** Additional code   ⊟ Laterality

1796   *DecisionHealth's* FY 2020 Complete Home Health ICD-10-CM Diagnosis Coding Manual

Chapter 20

V00-Y99

EXCLUDES 1 heavy transport vehicle collision with animal-drawn vehicle or animal being ridden (V66.-)

The appropriate 7th character is to be added to each code from category V60
A   initial encounter
D   subsequent encounter
S   sequela

!Q ☑ V60.0XX- Driver of heavy transport vehicle injured in collision with pedestrian or animal in nontraffic accident

!Q ☑ V60.1XX- Passenger in heavy transport vehicle injured in collision with pedestrian or animal in nontraffic accident

!Q ☑ V60.2XX- Person on outside of heavy transport vehicle injured in collision with pedestrian or animal in nontraffic accident

!Q ☑ V60.3XX- Unspecified occupant of heavy transport vehicle injured in collision with pedestrian or animal in nontraffic accident

!Q ☑ V60.4XX- Person boarding or alighting a heavy transport vehicle injured in collision with pedestrian or animal

!Q ☑ V60.5XX- Driver of heavy transport vehicle injured in collision with pedestrian or animal in traffic accident

!Q ☑ V60.6XX- Passenger in heavy transport vehicle injured in collision with pedestrian or animal in traffic accident

!Q ☑ V60.7XX- Person on outside of heavy transport vehicle injured in collision with pedestrian or animal in traffic accident

!Q ☑ V60.9XX- Unspecified occupant of heavy transport vehicle injured in collision with pedestrian or animal in traffic accident

④ V61 Occupant of heavy transport vehicle injured in collision with pedal cycle

The appropriate 7th character is to be added to each code from category V61
A   initial encounter
D   subsequent encounter
S   sequela

!Q ☑ V61.0XX- Driver of heavy transport vehicle injured in collision with pedal cycle in nontraffic accident

!Q ☑ V61.1XX- Passenger in heavy transport vehicle injured in collision with pedal cycle in nontraffic accident

!Q ☑ V61.2XX- Person on outside of heavy transport vehicle injured in collision with pedal cycle in nontraffic accident

!Q ☑ V61.3XX- Unspecified occupant of heavy transport vehicle injured in collision with pedal cycle in nontraffic accident

!Q ☑ V61.4XX- Person boarding or alighting a heavy transport vehicle injured in collision with pedal cycle while boarding or alighting

!Q ☑ V61.5XX- Driver of heavy transport vehicle injured in collision with pedal cycle in traffic accident

!Q ☑ V61.6XX- Passenger in heavy transport vehicle injured in collision with pedal cycle in traffic accident

!Q ☑ V61.7XX- Person on outside of heavy transport vehicle injured in collision with pedal cycle in traffic accident

!Q ☑ V61.9XX- Unspecified occupant of heavy transport vehicle injured in collision with pedal cycle in traffic accident

④ V62 Occupant of heavy transport vehicle injured in collision with two- or three-wheeled motor vehicle

The appropriate 7th character is to be added to each code from category V62
A   initial encounter
D   subsequent encounter
S   sequela

!Q ☑ V62.0XX- Driver of heavy transport vehicle injured in collision with two- or three-wheeled motor vehicle in nontraffic accident

!Q ☑ V62.1XX- Passenger in heavy transport vehicle injured in collision with two- or three-wheeled motor vehicle in nontraffic accident

!Q ☑ V62.2XX- Person on outside of heavy transport vehicle injured in collision with two- or three-wheeled motor vehicle in nontraffic accident

!Q ☑ V62.3XX- Unspecified occupant of heavy transport vehicle injured in collision with two- or three-wheeled motor vehicle in nontraffic accident

!Q ☑ V62.4XX- Person boarding or alighting a heavy transport vehicle injured in collision with two- or three-wheeled motor vehicle

!Q ☑ V62.5XX- Driver of heavy transport vehicle injured in collision with two- or three-wheeled motor vehicle in traffic accident

!Q ☑ V62.6XX- Passenger in heavy transport vehicle injured in collision with two- or three-wheeled motor vehicle in traffic accident

!Q ☑ V62.7XX- Person on outside of heavy transport vehicle injured in collision with two- or three-wheeled motor vehicle in traffic accident

!Q ☑ V62.9XX- Unspecified occupant of heavy transport vehicle injured in collision with two- or three-wheeled motor vehicle in traffic accident

④ V63 Occupant of heavy transport vehicle injured in collision with car, pick-up truck or van

★ New ▲ Revised Px Primary SP PDGM Px SL Low CoM SH High CoM !Q Quest. Encounter 🖽 Hospice non-cancer Dx   Unspecified   M *Manifestation*

DecisionHealth's FY 2020 Complete Home Health ICD-10-CM Diagnosis Coding Manual

1797

The appropriate 7th character is to be added to each code from category V63
A   initial encounter
D   subsequent encounter
S   sequela

!Q ☑ **V63.0XX-** **Driver of heavy transport vehicle injured in collision with car, pick-up truck or van in nontraffic accident**

!Q ☑ **V63.1XX-** **Passenger in heavy transport vehicle injured in collision with car, pick-up truck or van in nontraffic accident**

!Q ☑ **V63.2XX-** **Person on outside of heavy transport vehicle injured in collision with car, pick-up truck or van in nontraffic accident**

!Q ☑ **V63.3XX-** **Unspecified occupant of heavy transport vehicle injured in collision with car, pick-up truck or van in nontraffic accident**

!Q ☑ **V63.4XX-** **Person boarding or alighting a heavy transport vehicle injured in collision with car, pick-up truck or van**

!Q ☑ **V63.5XX-** **Driver of heavy transport vehicle injured in collision with car, pick-up truck or van in traffic accident**

!Q ☑ **V63.6XX-** **Passenger in heavy transport vehicle injured in collision with car, pick-up truck or van in traffic accident**

!Q ☑ **V63.7XX-** **Person on outside of heavy transport vehicle injured in collision with car, pick-up truck or van in traffic accident**

!Q ☑ **V63.9XX-** **Unspecified occupant of heavy transport vehicle injured in collision with car, pick-up truck or van in traffic accident**

4 **V64** **Occupant of heavy transport vehicle injured in collision with heavy transport vehicle or bus**

  EXCLUDES 1 occupant of heavy transport vehicle injured in collision with military vehicle (V69.81)

The appropriate 7th character is to be added to each code from category V64
A   initial encounter
D   subsequent encounter
S   sequela

!Q ☑ **V64.0XX-** **Driver of heavy transport vehicle injured in collision with heavy transport vehicle or bus in nontraffic accident**

!Q ☑ **V64.1XX-** **Passenger in heavy transport vehicle injured in collision with heavy transport vehicle or bus in nontraffic accident**

!Q ☑ **V64.2XX-** **Person on outside of heavy transport vehicle injured in collision with heavy transport vehicle or bus in nontraffic accident**

!Q ☑ **V64.3XX-** **Unspecified occupant of heavy transport vehicle injured in collision with heavy transport vehicle or bus in nontraffic accident**

!Q ☑ **V64.4XX-** **Person boarding or alighting a heavy transport vehicle injured in collision with heavy transport vehicle or bus while boarding or alighting**

!Q ☑ **V64.5XX-** **Driver of heavy transport vehicle injured in collision with heavy transport vehicle or bus in traffic accident**

!Q ☑ **V64.6XX-** **Passenger in heavy transport vehicle injured in collision with heavy transport vehicle or bus in traffic accident**

!Q ☑ **V64.7XX-** **Person on outside of heavy transport vehicle injured in collision with heavy transport vehicle or bus in traffic accident**

!Q ☑ **V64.9XX-** **Unspecified occupant of heavy transport vehicle injured in collision with heavy transport vehicle or bus in traffic accident**

4 **V65** **Occupant of heavy transport vehicle injured in collision with railway train or railway vehicle**

The appropriate 7th character is to be added to each code from category V65
A   initial encounter
D   subsequent encounter
S   sequela

!Q ☑ **V65.0XX-** **Driver of heavy transport vehicle injured in collision with railway train or railway vehicle in nontraffic accident**

!Q ☑ **V65.1XX-** **Passenger in heavy transport vehicle injured in collision with railway train or railway vehicle in nontraffic accident**

!Q ☑ **V65.2XX-** **Person on outside of heavy transport vehicle injured in collision with railway train or railway vehicle in nontraffic accident**

!Q ☑ **V65.3XX-** **Unspecified occupant of heavy transport vehicle injured in collision with railway train or railway vehicle in nontraffic accident**

!Q ☑ **V65.4XX-** **Person boarding or alighting a heavy transport vehicle injured in collision with railway train or railway vehicle**

!Q ☑ **V65.5XX-** **Driver of heavy transport vehicle injured in collision with railway train or railway vehicle in traffic accident**

!Q ☑ **V65.6XX-** **Passenger in heavy transport vehicle injured in collision with railway train or railway vehicle in traffic accident**

!Q ☑ **V65.7XX-** **Person on outside of heavy transport vehicle injured in collision with railway train or railway vehicle in traffic accident**

4 4th digit required   **5** 5th digit required   **6** 6th digit required   **7** 7th digit required   ☑ 7th digit placeholder   **+** Additional code   ⊟ Laterality

1798   *DecisionHealth's* FY 2020 Complete Home Health ICD-10-CM Diagnosis Coding Manual

!Q ✓ V65.9XX- Unspecified occupant of heavy transport vehicle injured in collision with railway train or railway vehicle in traffic accident

◢ V66 Occupant of heavy transport vehicle injured in collision with other nonmotor vehicle

INCLUDES collision with animal-drawn vehicle, animal being ridden, streetcar

The appropriate 7th character is to be added to each code from category V66
A   initial encounter
D   subsequent encounter
S   sequela

!Q ✓ V66.0XX- Driver of heavy transport vehicle injured in collision with other nonmotor vehicle in nontraffic accident

!Q ✓ V66.1XX- Passenger in heavy transport vehicle injured in collision with other nonmotor vehicle in nontraffic accident

!Q ✓ V66.2XX- Person on outside of heavy transport vehicle injured in collision with other nonmotor vehicle in nontraffic accident

!Q ✓ V66.3XX- Unspecified occupant of heavy transport vehicle injured in collision with other nonmotor vehicle in nontraffic accident

!Q ✓ V66.4XX- Person boarding or alighting a heavy transport vehicle injured in collision with other nonmotor vehicle

!Q ✓ V66.5XX- Driver of heavy transport vehicle injured in collision with other nonmotor vehicle in traffic accident

!Q ✓ V66.6XX- Passenger in heavy transport vehicle injured in collision with other nonmotor vehicle in traffic accident

!Q ✓ V66.7XX- Person on outside of heavy transport vehicle injured in collision with other nonmotor vehicle in traffic accident

!Q ✓ V66.9XX- Unspecified occupant of heavy transport vehicle injured in collision with other nonmotor vehicle in traffic accident

◢ V67 Occupant of heavy transport vehicle injured in collision with fixed or stationary object

The appropriate 7th character is to be added to each code from category V67
A   initial encounter
D   subsequent encounter
S   sequela

!Q ✓ V67.0XX- Driver of heavy transport vehicle injured in collision with fixed or stationary object in nontraffic accident

!Q ✓ V67.1XX- Passenger in heavy transport vehicle injured in collision with fixed or stationary object in nontraffic accident

!Q ✓ V67.2XX- Person on outside of heavy transport vehicle injured in collision with fixed or stationary object in nontraffic accident

!Q ✓ V67.3XX- Unspecified occupant of heavy transport vehicle injured in collision with fixed or stationary object in nontraffic accident

!Q ✓ V67.4XX- Person boarding or alighting a heavy transport vehicle injured in collision with fixed or stationary object

!Q ✓ V67.5XX- Driver of heavy transport vehicle injured in collision with fixed or stationary object in traffic accident

!Q ✓ V67.6XX- Passenger in heavy transport vehicle injured in collision with fixed or stationary object in traffic accident

!Q ✓ V67.7XX- Person on outside of heavy transport vehicle injured in collision with fixed or stationary object in traffic accident

!Q ✓ V67.9XX- Unspecified occupant of heavy transport vehicle injured in collision with fixed or stationary object in traffic accident

◢ V68 Occupant of heavy transport vehicle injured in noncollision transport accident

INCLUDES overturning heavy transport vehicle NOS
overturning heavy transport vehicle without collision

The appropriate 7th character is to be added to each code from category V68
A   initial encounter
D   subsequent encounter
S   sequela

!Q ✓ V68.0XX- Driver of heavy transport vehicle injured in noncollision transport accident in nontraffic accident

!Q ✓ V68.1XX- Passenger in heavy transport vehicle injured in noncollision transport accident in nontraffic accident

!Q ✓ V68.2XX- Person on outside of heavy transport vehicle injured in noncollision transport accident in nontraffic accident

!Q ✓ V68.3XX- Unspecified occupant of heavy transport vehicle injured in noncollision transport accident in nontraffic accident

!Q ✓ V68.4XX- Person boarding or alighting a heavy transport vehicle injured in noncollision transport accident

!Q ✓ V68.5XX- Driver of heavy transport vehicle injured in noncollision transport accident in traffic accident

!Q ✓ V68.6XX- Passenger in heavy transport vehicle injured in noncollision transport accident in traffic accident

!Q ✓ V68.7XX- Person on outside of heavy transport vehicle injured in noncollision transport accident in traffic accident

Chapter 20

V00-Y99

★ New ▲ Revised Px Primary SP PDGM Px SL Low CoM SH High CoM !Q Quest. Encounter H Hospice non-cancer Dx   Unspecified   M Manifestation

DecisionHealth's FY 2020 Complete Home Health ICD-10-CM Diagnosis Coding Manual

1799

IQ ✓ V68.9XX- Unspecified occupant of heavy transport vehicle injured in noncollision transport accident in traffic accident

4 V69 Occupant of heavy transport vehicle injured in other and unspecified transport accidents

The appropriate 7th character is to be added to each code from category V69
A   initial encounter
D   subsequent encounter
S   sequela

5 V69.0 Driver of heavy transport vehicle injured in collision with other and unspecified motor vehicles in nontraffic accident

IQ ✓ V69.00X- Driver of heavy transport vehicle injured in collision with unspecified motor vehicles in nontraffic accident

IQ ✓ V69.09X- Driver of heavy transport vehicle injured in collision with other motor vehicles in nontraffic accident

5 V69.1 Passenger in heavy transport vehicle injured in collision with other and unspecified motor vehicles in nontraffic accident

IQ ✓ V69.10X- Passenger in heavy transport vehicle injured in collision with unspecified motor vehicles in nontraffic accident

IQ ✓ V69.19X- Passenger in heavy transport vehicle injured in collision with other motor vehicles in nontraffic accident

5 V69.2 Unspecified occupant of heavy transport vehicle injured in collision with other and unspecified motor vehicles in nontraffic accident

IQ ✓ V69.20X- Unspecified occupant of heavy transport vehicle injured in collision with unspecified motor vehicles in nontraffic accident

Collision NOS involving heavy transport vehicle, nontraffic

IQ ✓ V69.29X- Unspecified occupant of heavy transport vehicle injured in collision with other motor vehicles in nontraffic accident

IQ ✓ V69.3XX- Occupant (driver) (passenger) of heavy transport vehicle injured in unspecified nontraffic accident

Accident NOS involving heavy transport vehicle, nontraffic
Occupant of heavy transport vehicle injured in nontraffic accident NOS

5 V69.4 Driver of heavy transport vehicle injured in collision with other and unspecified motor vehicles in traffic accident

IQ ✓ V69.40X- Driver of heavy transport vehicle injured in collision with unspecified motor vehicles in traffic accident

IQ ✓ V69.49X- Driver of heavy transport vehicle injured in collision with other motor vehicles in traffic accident

5 V69.5 Passenger in heavy transport vehicle injured in collision with other and unspecified motor vehicles in traffic accident

IQ ✓ V69.50X- Passenger in heavy transport vehicle injured in collision with unspecified motor vehicles in traffic accident

IQ ✓ V69.59X- Passenger in heavy transport vehicle injured in collision with other motor vehicles in traffic accident

5 V69.6 Unspecified occupant of heavy transport vehicle injured in collision with other and unspecified motor vehicles in traffic accident

IQ ✓ V69.60X- Unspecified occupant of heavy transport vehicle injured in collision with unspecified motor vehicles in traffic accident

Collision NOS involving heavy transport vehicle (traffic)

IQ ✓ V69.69X- Unspecified occupant of heavy transport vehicle injured in collision with other motor vehicles in traffic accident

5 V69.8 Occupant (driver) (passenger) of heavy transport vehicle injured in other specified transport accidents

IQ ✓ V69.81X- Occupant (driver) (passenger) of heavy transport vehicle injured in transport accidents with military vehicle

IQ ✓ V69.88X- Occupant (driver) (passenger) of heavy transport vehicle injured in other specified transport accidents

IQ ✓ V69.9XX- Occupant (driver) (passenger) of heavy transport vehicle injured in unspecified traffic accident

Accident NOS involving heavy transport vehicle

Bus occupant injured in transport accident (V70-V79)

INCLUDES motorcoach
EXCLUDES 1 minibus (V50-V59)

4 V70 Bus occupant injured in collision with pedestrian or animal
EXCLUDES 1 bus collision with animal-drawn vehicle or animal being ridden (V76.-)

The appropriate 7th character is to be added to each code from category V70
A   initial encounter
D   subsequent encounter
S   sequela

IQ ✓ V70.0XX- Driver of bus injured in collision with pedestrian or animal in nontraffic accident

IQ ✓ V70.1XX- Passenger on bus injured in collision with pedestrian or animal in nontraffic accident

4 4th digit required   5 5th digit required   6 6th digit required   7 7th digit required   ✓ 7th digit placeholder   + Additional code   ⊟ Laterality

!Q ☑ V70.2XX- Person on outside of bus injured in collision with pedestrian or animal in nontraffic accident

!Q ☑ V70.3XX- Unspecified occupant of bus injured in collision with pedestrian or animal in nontraffic accident

!Q ☑ V70.4XX- Person boarding or alighting from bus injured in collision with pedestrian or animal

!Q ☑ V70.5XX- Driver of bus injured in collision with pedestrian or animal in traffic accident

!Q ☑ V70.6XX- Passenger on bus injured in collision with pedestrian or animal in traffic accident

!Q ☑ V70.7XX- Person on outside of bus injured in collision with pedestrian or animal in traffic accident

!Q ☑ V70.9XX- Unspecified occupant of bus injured in collision with pedestrian or animal in traffic accident

4 V71 Bus occupant injured in collision with pedal cycle

The appropriate 7th character is to be added to each code from category V71
A   initial encounter
D   subsequent encounter
S   sequela

!Q ☑ V71.0XX- Driver of bus injured in collision with pedal cycle in nontraffic accident

!Q ☑ V71.1XX- Passenger on bus injured in collision with pedal cycle in nontraffic accident

!Q ☑ V71.2XX- Person on outside of bus injured in collision with pedal cycle in nontraffic accident

!Q ☑ V71.3XX- Unspecified occupant of bus injured in collision with pedal cycle in nontraffic accident

!Q ☑ V71.4XX- Person boarding or alighting from bus injured in collision with pedal cycle

!Q ☑ V71.5XX- Driver of bus injured in collision with pedal cycle in traffic accident

!Q ☑ V71.6XX- Passenger on bus injured in collision with pedal cycle in traffic accident

!Q ☑ V71.7XX- Person on outside of bus injured in collision with pedal cycle in traffic accident

!Q ☑ V71.9XX- Unspecified occupant of bus injured in collision with pedal cycle in traffic accident

4 V72 Bus occupant injured in collision with two- or three-wheeled motor vehicle

The appropriate 7th character is to be added to each code from category V72
A   initial encounter
D   subsequent encounter
S   sequela

!Q ☑ V72.0XX- Driver of bus injured in collision with two- or three-wheeled motor vehicle in nontraffic accident

!Q ☑ V72.1XX- Passenger on bus injured in collision with two- or three-wheeled motor vehicle in nontraffic accident

!Q ☑ V72.2XX- Person on outside of bus injured in collision with two- or three-wheeled motor vehicle in nontraffic accident

!Q ☑ V72.3XX- Unspecified occupant of bus injured in collision with two- or three-wheeled motor vehicle in nontraffic accident

!Q ☑ V72.4XX- Person boarding or alighting from bus injured in collision with two- or three-wheeled motor vehicle

!Q ☑ V72.5XX- Driver of bus injured in collision with two- or three-wheeled motor vehicle in traffic accident

!Q ☑ V72.6XX- Passenger on bus injured in collision with two- or three-wheeled motor vehicle in traffic accident

!Q ☑ V72.7XX- Person on outside of bus injured in collision with two- or three-wheeled motor vehicle in traffic accident

!Q ☑ V72.9XX- Unspecified occupant of bus injured in collision with two- or three-wheeled motor vehicle in traffic accident

4 V73 Bus occupant injured in collision with car, pick-up truck or van

The appropriate 7th character is to be added to each code from category V73
A   initial encounter
D   subsequent encounter
S   sequela

!Q ☑ V73.0XX- Driver of bus injured in collision with car, pick-up truck or van in nontraffic accident

!Q ☑ V73.1XX- Passenger on bus injured in collision with car, pick-up truck or van in nontraffic accident

!Q ☑ V73.2XX- Person on outside of bus injured in collision with car, pick-up truck or van in nontraffic accident

!Q ☑ V73.3XX- Unspecified occupant of bus injured in collision with car, pick-up truck or van in nontraffic accident

!Q ☑ V73.4XX- Person boarding or alighting from bus injured in collision with car, pick-up truck or van

!Q ☑ V73.5XX- Driver of bus injured in collision with car, pick-up truck or van in traffic accident

!Q ☑ V73.6XX- Passenger on bus injured in collision with car, pick-up truck or van in traffic accident

!Q ☑ V73.7XX- Person on outside of bus injured in collision with car, pick-up truck or van in traffic accident

!Q ☑ V73.9XX- Unspecified occupant of bus injured in collision with car, pick-up truck or van in traffic accident

4 V74 Bus occupant injured in collision with heavy transport vehicle or bus
EXCLUDES 1   bus occupant injured in collision with military vehicle (V79.81)

✱ New ▲ Revised Px Primary SP PDGM Px SL Low CoM SH High CoM !Q Quest. Encounter H Hospice non-cancer Dx Unspecified M Manifestation

DecisionHealth's FY 2020 Complete Home Health ICD-10-CM Diagnosis Coding Manual

1801

The appropriate 7th character is to be added to each code from category V74
A   initial encounter
D   subsequent encounter
S   sequela

!Q ☑ V74.0XX-   **Driver of bus injured in collision with heavy transport vehicle or bus in nontraffic accident**

!Q ☑ V74.1XX-   **Passenger on bus injured in collision with heavy transport vehicle or bus in nontraffic accident**

!Q ☑ V74.2XX-   **Person on outside of bus injured in collision with heavy transport vehicle or bus in nontraffic accident**

!Q ☑ V74.3XX-   **Unspecified occupant of bus injured in collision with heavy transport vehicle or bus in nontraffic accident**

!Q ☑ V74.4XX-   **Person boarding or alighting from bus injured in collision with heavy transport vehicle or bus**

!Q ☑ V74.5XX-   **Driver of bus injured in collision with heavy transport vehicle or bus in traffic accident**

!Q ☑ V74.6XX-   **Passenger on bus injured in collision with heavy transport vehicle or bus in traffic accident**

!Q ☑ V74.7XX-   **Person on outside of bus injured in collision with heavy transport vehicle or bus in traffic accident**

!Q ☑ V74.9XX-   **Unspecified occupant of bus injured in collision with heavy transport vehicle or bus in traffic accident**

4 V75   **Bus occupant injured in collision with railway train or railway vehicle**

The appropriate 7th character is to be added to each code from category V75
A   initial encounter
D   subsequent encounter
S   sequela

!Q ☑ V75.0XX-   **Driver of bus injured in collision with railway train or railway vehicle in nontraffic accident**

!Q ☑ V75.1XX-   **Passenger on bus injured in collision with railway train or railway vehicle in nontraffic accident**

!Q ☑ V75.2XX-   **Person on outside of bus injured in collision with railway train or railway vehicle in nontraffic accident**

!Q ☑ V75.3XX-   **Unspecified occupant of bus injured in collision with railway train or railway vehicle in nontraffic accident**

!Q ☑ V75.4XX-   **Person boarding or alighting from bus injured in collision with railway train or railway vehicle**

!Q ☑ V75.5XX-   **Driver of bus injured in collision with railway train or railway vehicle in traffic accident**

!Q ☑ V75.6XX-   **Passenger on bus injured in collision with railway train or railway vehicle in traffic accident**

!Q ☑ V75.7XX-   **Person on outside of bus injured in collision with railway train or railway vehicle in traffic accident**

!Q ☑ V75.9XX-   **Unspecified occupant of bus injured in collision with railway train or railway vehicle in traffic accident**

4 V76   **Bus occupant injured in collision with other nonmotor vehicle**

     INCLUDES   collision with animal-drawn vehicle, animal being ridden, streetcar

The appropriate 7th character is to be added to each code from category V76
A   initial encounter
D   subsequent encounter
S   sequela

!Q ☑ V76.0XX-   **Driver of bus injured in collision with other nonmotor vehicle in nontraffic accident**

!Q ☑ V76.1XX-   **Passenger on bus injured in collision with other nonmotor vehicle in nontraffic accident**

!Q ☑ V76.2XX-   **Person on outside of bus injured in collision with other nonmotor vehicle in nontraffic accident**

!Q ☑ V76.3XX-   **Unspecified occupant of bus injured in collision with other nonmotor vehicle in nontraffic accident**

!Q ☑ V76.4XX-   **Person boarding or alighting from bus injured in collision with other nonmotor vehicle**

!Q ☑ V76.5XX-   **Driver of bus injured in collision with other nonmotor vehicle in traffic accident**

!Q ☑ V76.6XX-   **Passenger on bus injured in collision with other nonmotor vehicle in traffic accident**

!Q ☑ V76.7XX-   **Person on outside of bus injured in collision with other nonmotor vehicle in traffic accident**

!Q ☑ V76.9XX-   **Unspecified occupant of bus injured in collision with other nonmotor vehicle in traffic accident**

4 V77   **Bus occupant injured in collision with fixed or stationary object**

The appropriate 7th character is to be added to each code from category V77
A   initial encounter
D   subsequent encounter
S   sequela

!Q ☑ V77.0XX-   **Driver of bus injured in collision with fixed or stationary object in nontraffic accident**

!Q ☑ V77.1XX-   **Passenger on bus injured in collision with fixed or stationary object in nontraffic accident**

!Q ☑ V77.2XX-   **Person on outside of bus injured in collision with fixed or stationary object in nontraffic accident**

!Q ☑ V77.3XX-   **Unspecified occupant of bus injured in collision with fixed or stationary object in nontraffic accident**

---

4 4th digit required   5 5th digit required   6 6th digit required   7 7th digit required   ☑ 7th digit placeholder   ✚ Additional code   ⊟ Laterality

!Q ✓ V77.4XX- Person boarding or alighting from bus injured in collision with fixed or stationary object

!Q ✓ V77.5XX- Driver of bus injured in collision with fixed or stationary object in traffic accident

!Q ✓ V77.6XX- Passenger on bus injured in collision with fixed or stationary object in traffic accident

!Q ✓ V77.7XX- Person on outside of bus injured in collision with fixed or stationary object in traffic accident

!Q ✓ V77.9XX- Unspecified occupant of bus injured in collision with fixed or stationary object in traffic accident

4 V78 Bus occupant injured in noncollision transport accident

INCLUDES overturning bus NOS
overturning bus without collision

The appropriate 7th character is to be added to each code from category V78
A   initial encounter
D   subsequent encounter
S   sequela

!Q ✓ V78.0XX- Driver of bus injured in noncollision transport accident in nontraffic accident

!Q ✓ V78.1XX- Passenger on bus injured in noncollision transport accident in nontraffic accident

!Q ✓ V78.2XX- Person on outside of bus injured in noncollision transport accident in nontraffic accident

!Q ✓ V78.3XX- Unspecified occupant of bus injured in noncollision transport accident in nontraffic accident

!Q ✓ V78.4XX- Person boarding or alighting from bus injured in noncollision transport accident

!Q ✓ V78.5XX- Driver of bus injured in noncollision transport accident in traffic accident

!Q ✓ V78.6XX- Passenger on bus injured in noncollision transport accident in traffic accident

!Q ✓ V78.7XX- Person on outside of bus injured in noncollision transport accident in traffic accident

!Q ✓ V78.9XX- Unspecified occupant of bus injured in noncollision transport accident in traffic accident

4 V79 Bus occupant injured in other and unspecified transport accidents

The appropriate 7th character is to be added to each code from category V79
A   initial encounter
D   subsequent encounter
S   sequela

5 V79.0 Driver of bus injured in collision with other and unspecified motor vehicles in nontraffic accident

!Q ✓ V79.00X- Driver of bus injured in collision with unspecified motor vehicles in nontraffic accident

!Q ✓ V79.09X- Driver of bus injured in collision with other motor vehicles in nontraffic accident

5 V79.1 Passenger on bus injured in collision with other and unspecified motor vehicles in nontraffic accident

!Q ✓ V79.10X- Passenger on bus injured in collision with unspecified motor vehicles in nontraffic accident

!Q ✓ V79.19X- Passenger on bus injured in collision with other motor vehicles in nontraffic accident

5 V79.2 Unspecified bus occupant injured in collision with other and unspecified motor vehicles in nontraffic accident

!Q ✓ V79.20X- Unspecified bus occupant injured in collision with unspecified motor vehicles in nontraffic accident

Bus collision NOS, nontraffic

!Q ✓ V79.29X- Unspecified bus occupant injured in collision with other motor vehicles in nontraffic accident

!Q ✓ V79.3XX- Bus occupant (driver) (passenger) injured in unspecified nontraffic accident

Bus accident NOS, nontraffic
Bus occupant injured in nontraffic accident NOS

5 V79.4 Driver of bus injured in collision with other and unspecified motor vehicles in traffic accident

!Q ✓ V79.40X- Driver of bus injured in collision with unspecified motor vehicles in traffic accident

!Q ✓ V79.49X- Driver of bus injured in collision with other motor vehicles in traffic accident

5 V79.5 Passenger on bus injured in collision with other and unspecified motor vehicles in traffic accident

!Q ✓ V79.50X- Passenger on bus injured in collision with unspecified motor vehicles in traffic accident

!Q ✓ V79.59X- Passenger on bus injured in collision with other motor vehicles in traffic accident

5 V79.6 Unspecified bus occupant injured in collision with other and unspecified motor vehicles in traffic accident

!Q ✓ V79.60X- Unspecified bus occupant injured in collision with unspecified motor vehicles in traffic accident

Bus collision NOS (traffic)

!Q ✓ V79.69X- Unspecified bus occupant injured in collision with other motor vehicles in traffic accident

5 V79.8 Bus occupant (driver) (passenger) injured in other specified transport accidents

!Q ✓ V79.81X- Bus occupant (driver) (passenger) injured in transport accidents with military vehicle

!Q ✓ V79.88X- Bus occupant (driver) (passenger) injured in other specified transport accidents

---

★ New ▲ Revised Px Primary **SP** PDGM Px **SL** Low CoM **SH** High CoM **!Q** Quest. Encounter **H** Hospice non-cancer Dx   Unspecified   **M** *Manifestation*

IQ ☑ V79.9XX- **Bus occupant (driver) (passenger) injured in unspecified traffic accident**

Bus accident NOS

Other land transport accidents   (V80-V89)

4 V80 **Animal-rider or occupant of animal-drawn vehicle injured in transport accident**

The appropriate 7th character is to be added to each code from category V80
A   initial encounter
D   subsequent encounter
S   sequela

5 V80.0 **Animal-rider or occupant of animal drawn vehicle injured by fall from or being thrown from animal or animal-drawn vehicle in noncollision accident**

6 V80.01 **Animal-rider injured by fall from or being thrown from animal in noncollision accident**

IQ 7 V80.010- **Animal-rider injured by fall from or being thrown from horse in noncollision accident**

IQ 7 V80.018- **Animal-rider injured by fall from or being thrown from other animal in noncollision accident**

IQ ☑ V80.02X- **Occupant of animal-drawn vehicle injured by fall from or being thrown from animal-drawn vehicle in noncollision accident**
Overturning animal-drawn vehicle NOS
Overturning animal-drawn vehicle without collision

5 V80.1 **Animal-rider or occupant of animal-drawn vehicle injured in collision with pedestrian or animal**
EXCLUDES 1   animal-rider or animal-drawn vehicle collision with animal-drawn vehicle or animal being ridden (V80.7)

IQ ☑ V80.11X- **Animal-rider injured in collision with pedestrian or animal**

IQ ☑ V80.12X- **Occupant of animal-drawn vehicle injured in collision with pedestrian or animal**

5 V80.2 **Animal-rider or occupant of animal-drawn vehicle injured in collision with pedal cycle**

IQ ☑ V80.21X- **Animal-rider injured in collision with pedal cycle**

IQ ☑ V80.22X- **Occupant of animal-drawn vehicle injured in collision with pedal cycle**

5 V80.3 **Animal-rider or occupant of animal-drawn vehicle injured in collision with two- or three-wheeled motor vehicle**

IQ ☑ V80.31X- **Animal-rider injured in collision with two- or three-wheeled motor vehicle**

IQ ☑ V80.32X- **Occupant of animal-drawn vehicle injured in collision with two- or three-wheeled motor vehicle**

5 V80.4 **Animal-rider or occupant of animal-drawn vehicle injured in collision with car, pick-up truck, van, heavy transport vehicle or bus**
EXCLUDES 1   animal-rider injured in collision with military vehicle (V80.910)
occupant of animal-drawn vehicle injured in collision with military vehicle (V80.920)

IQ ☑ V80.41X- **Animal-rider injured in collision with car, pick-up truck, van, heavy transport vehicle or bus**

IQ ☑ V80.42X- **Occupant of animal-drawn vehicle injured in collision with car, pick-up truck, van, heavy transport vehicle or bus**

5 V80.5 **Animal-rider or occupant of animal-drawn vehicle injured in collision with other specified motor vehicle**

IQ ☑ V80.51X- **Animal-rider injured in collision with other specified motor vehicle**

IQ ☑ V80.52X- **Occupant of animal-drawn vehicle injured in collision with other specified motor vehicle**

5 V80.6 **Animal-rider or occupant of animal-drawn vehicle injured in collision with railway train or railway vehicle**

IQ ☑ V80.61X- **Animal-rider injured in collision with railway train or railway vehicle**

IQ ☑ V80.62X- **Occupant of animal-drawn vehicle injured in collision with railway train or railway vehicle**

5 V80.7 **Animal-rider or occupant of animal-drawn vehicle injured in collision with other nonmotor vehicles**

6 V80.71 **Animal-rider or occupant of animal-drawn vehicle injured in collision with animal being ridden**

IQ 7 V80.710- **Animal-rider injured in collision with other animal being ridden**

IQ 7 V80.711- **Occupant of animal-drawn vehicle injured in collision with animal being ridden**

6 V80.72 **Animal-rider or occupant of animal-drawn vehicle injured in collision with other animal-drawn vehicle**

IQ 7 V80.720- **Animal-rider injured in collision with animal-drawn vehicle**

IQ 7 V80.721- **Occupant of animal-drawn vehicle injured in collision with other animal-drawn vehicle**

6 V80.73 **Animal-rider or occupant of animal-drawn vehicle injured in collision with streetcar**

IQ 7 V80.730- **Animal-rider injured in collision with streetcar**

IQ 7 V80.731- **Occupant of animal-drawn vehicle injured in collision with streetcar**

6 V80.79 **Animal-rider or occupant of animal-drawn vehicle injured in collision with other nonmotor vehicles**

IQ 7 V80.790- **Animal-rider injured in collision with other nonmotor vehicles**

4 4th digit required   5 5th digit required   6 6th digit required   7 7th digit required   ☑ 7th digit placeholder   + Additional code   ⊟ Laterality

1804   *DecisionHealth's* FY 2020 Complete Home Health ICD-10-CM Diagnosis Coding Manual

IQ 7 V80.791- Occupant of animal-drawn vehicle injured in collision with other nonmotor vehicles

5 V80.8 Animal-rider or occupant of animal-drawn vehicle injured in collision with fixed or stationary object

IQ 7 V80.81X- Animal-rider injured in collision with fixed or stationary object

IQ 7 V80.82X- Occupant of animal-drawn vehicle injured in collision with fixed or stationary object

5 V80.9 Animal-rider or occupant of animal-drawn vehicle injured in other and unspecified transport accidents

6 V80.91 Animal-rider injured in other and unspecified transport accidents

IQ 7 V80.910- Animal-rider injured in transport accident with military vehicle

IQ 7 V80.918- Animal-rider injured in other transport accident

IQ 7 V80.919- Animal-rider injured in unspecified transport accident
Animal rider accident NOS

6 V80.92 Occupant of animal-drawn vehicle injured in other and unspecified transport accidents

IQ 7 V80.920- Occupant of animal-drawn vehicle injured in transport accident with military vehicle

IQ 7 V80.928- Occupant of animal-drawn vehicle injured in other transport accident

IQ 7 V80.929- Occupant of animal-drawn vehicle injured in unspecified transport accident
Animal-drawn vehicle accident NOS

4 V81 Occupant of railway train or railway vehicle injured in transport accident

INCLUDES derailment of railway train or railway vehicle
person on outside of train
EXCLUDES 1 streetcar (V82.-)

The appropriate 7th character is to be added to each code from category V81
A   initial encounter
D   subsequent encounter
S   sequela

IQ 7 V81.0XX- Occupant of railway train or railway vehicle injured in collision with motor vehicle in nontraffic accident
EXCLUDES 1 Occupant of railway train or railway vehicle injured due to collision with military vehicle (V81.83)

IQ 7 V81.1XX- Occupant of railway train or railway vehicle injured in collision with motor vehicle in traffic accident
EXCLUDES 1 Occupant of railway train or railway vehicle injured due to collision with military vehicle (V81.83)

IQ 7 V81.2XX- Occupant of railway train or railway vehicle injured in collision with or hit by rolling stock

IQ 7 V81.3XX- Occupant of railway train or railway vehicle injured in collision with other object
Railway collision NOS

IQ 7 V81.4XX- Person injured while boarding or alighting from railway train or railway vehicle

IQ 7 V81.5XX- Occupant of railway train or railway vehicle injured by fall in railway train or railway vehicle

IQ 7 V81.6XX- Occupant of railway train or railway vehicle injured by fall from railway train or railway vehicle

IQ 7 V81.7XX- Occupant of railway train or railway vehicle injured in derailment without antecedent collision

5 V81.8 Occupant of railway train or railway vehicle injured in other specified railway accidents

IQ 7 V81.81X- Occupant of railway train or railway vehicle injured due to explosion or fire on train

IQ 7 V81.82X- Occupant of railway train or railway vehicle injured due to object falling onto train
Occupant of railway train or railway vehicle injured due to falling earth onto train
Occupant of railway train or railway vehicle injured due to falling rocks onto train
Occupant of railway train or railway vehicle injured due to falling snow onto train
Occupant of railway train or railway vehicle injured due to falling trees onto train

IQ 7 V81.83X- Occupant of railway train or railway vehicle injured due to collision with military vehicle

IQ 7 V81.89X- Occupant of railway train or railway vehicle injured due to other specified railway accident

IQ 7 V81.9XX- Occupant of railway train or railway vehicle injured in unspecified railway accident
Railway accident NOS

4 V82 Occupant of powered streetcar injured in transport accident

INCLUDES interurban electric car
person on outside of streetcar
tram (car)
trolley (car)
EXCLUDES 1 bus (V70-V79)
motorcoach (V70-V79)
nonpowered streetcar (V76.-)
train (V81.-)

The appropriate 7th character is to be added to each code from category V82
A   initial encounter
D   subsequent encounter
S   sequela

★ New ▲ Revised **Px** Primary **SP** PDGM Px **SL** Low CoM **SH** High CoM **IQ** Quest. Encounter **H** Hospice non-cancer Dx Unspecified **M** *Manifestation*

DecisionHealth's FY 2020 Complete Home Health ICD-10-CM Diagnosis Coding Manual

1805

[IQ] [✓] V82.0XX- Occupant of streetcar injured in collision with motor vehicle in nontraffic accident

[IQ] [✓] V82.1XX- Occupant of streetcar injured in collision with motor vehicle in traffic accident

[IQ] [✓] V82.2XX- Occupant of streetcar injured in collision with or hit by rolling stock

[IQ] [✓] V82.3XX- Occupant of streetcar injured in collision with other object

> EXCLUDES 1   collision with animal-drawn vehicle or animal being ridden (V82.8)

[IQ] [✓] V82.4XX- Person injured while boarding or alighting from streetcar

[IQ] [✓] V82.5XX- Occupant of streetcar injured by fall in streetcar

> EXCLUDES 1   fall in streetcar: while boarding or alighting (V82.4) with antecedent collision (V82.0-V82.3)

[IQ] [✓] V82.6XX- Occupant of streetcar injured by fall from streetcar

> EXCLUDES 1   fall from streetcar: while boarding or alighting (V82.4) with antecedent collision (V82.0-V82.3)

[IQ] [✓] V82.7XX- Occupant of streetcar injured in derailment without antecedent collision

> EXCLUDES 1   occupant of streetcar injured in derailment with antecedent collision (V82.0-V82.3)

[IQ] [✓] V82.8XX- Occupant of streetcar injured in other specified transport accidents

Streetcar collision with military vehicle

Streetcar collision with train or nonmotor vehicles

[IQ] [✓] V82.9XX- Occupant of streetcar injured in unspecified traffic accident

Streetcar accident NOS

[4] V83 Occupant of special vehicle mainly used on industrial premises injured in transport accident

> INCLUDES   battery-powered airport passenger vehicle
> battery-powered truck (baggage) (mail)
> coal-car in mine
> forklift (truck)
> logging car
> self-propelled industrial truck
> station baggage truck (powered)
> tram, truck, or tub (powered) in mine or quarry

> EXCLUDES 1   special construction vehicles (V85.-)
> special industrial vehicle in stationary use or maintenance (W31.-)

The appropriate 7th character is to be added to each code from category V83
A   initial encounter
D   subsequent encounter
S   sequela

[IQ] [✓] V83.0XX- Driver of special industrial vehicle injured in traffic accident

[IQ] [✓] V83.1XX- Passenger of special industrial vehicle injured in traffic accident

[IQ] [✓] V83.2XX- Person on outside of special industrial vehicle injured in traffic accident

[IQ] [✓] V83.3XX- Unspecified occupant of special industrial vehicle injured in traffic accident

[IQ] [✓] V83.4XX- Person injured while boarding or alighting from special industrial vehicle

[IQ] [✓] V83.5XX- Driver of special industrial vehicle injured in nontraffic accident

[IQ] [✓] V83.6XX- Passenger of special industrial vehicle injured in nontraffic accident

[IQ] [✓] V83.7XX- Person on outside of special industrial vehicle injured in nontraffic accident

[IQ] [✓] V83.9XX- Unspecified occupant of special industrial vehicle injured in nontraffic accident

Special-industrial-vehicle accident NOS

[4] V84 Occupant of special vehicle mainly used in agriculture injured in transport accident

> INCLUDES   self-propelled farm machinery tractor (and trailer)

> EXCLUDES 1   animal-powered farm machinery accident (W30.8-)
> contact with combine harvester (W30.0)
> special agricultural vehicle in stationary use or maintenance (W30.-)

The appropriate 7th character is to be added to each code from category V84
A   initial encounter
D   subsequent encounter
S   sequela

[IQ] [✓] V84.0XX- Driver of special agricultural vehicle injured in traffic accident

[IQ] [✓] V84.1XX- Passenger of special agricultural vehicle injured in traffic accident

[IQ] [✓] V84.2XX- Person on outside of special agricultural vehicle injured in traffic accident

[IQ] [✓] V84.3XX- Unspecified occupant of special agricultural vehicle injured in traffic accident

[IQ] [✓] V84.4XX- Person injured while boarding or alighting from special agricultural vehicle

[IQ] [✓] V84.5XX- Driver of special agricultural vehicle injured in nontraffic accident

[IQ] [✓] V84.6XX- Passenger of special agricultural vehicle injured in nontraffic accident

[4] 4th digit required   [5] 5th digit required   [6] 6th digit required   [7] 7th digit required   [✓] 7th digit placeholder   [+] Additional code   [≡] Laterality

1806   DecisionHealth's FY 2020 Complete Home Health ICD-10-CM Diagnosis Coding Manual

!Q ☑ V84.7XX- Person on outside of special agricultural vehicle injured in nontraffic accident

!Q ☑ V84.9XX- Unspecified occupant of special agricultural vehicle injured in nontraffic accident

Special-agricultural vehicle accident NOS

④ V85 Occupant of special construction vehicle injured in transport accident

INCLUDES   bulldozer
digger
dump truck
earth-leveller
mechanical shovel
road-roller

EXCLUDES 1   special industrial vehicle (V83.-)
special construction vehicle in stationary use or maintenance (W31.-)

The appropriate 7th character is to be added to each code from category V85
A   initial encounter
D   subsequent encounter
S   sequela

!Q ☑ V85.0XX- Driver of special construction vehicle injured in traffic accident

!Q ☑ V85.1XX- Passenger of special construction vehicle injured in traffic accident

!Q ☑ V85.2XX- Person on outside of special construction vehicle injured in traffic accident

!Q ☑ V85.3XX- Unspecified occupant of special construction vehicle injured in traffic accident

!Q ☑ V85.4XX- Person injured while boarding or alighting from special construction vehicle

!Q ☑ V85.5XX- Driver of special construction vehicle injured in nontraffic accident

!Q ☑ V85.6XX- Passenger of special construction vehicle injured in nontraffic accident

!Q ☑ V85.7XX- Person on outside of special construction vehicle injured in nontraffic accident

!Q ☑ V85.9XX- Unspecified occupant of special construction vehicle injured in nontraffic accident

Special-construction-vehicle accident NOS

④ V86 Occupant of special all-terrain or other off-road motor vehicle, injured in transport accident

EXCLUDES 1   special all-terrain vehicle in stationary use or maintenance (W31.-)
sport-utility vehicle (V50-V59)
three-wheeled motor vehicle designed for on-road use (V30-V39)

The appropriate 7th character is to be added to each code from category V86
A   initial encounter
D   subsequent encounter
S   sequela

⑤ V86.0 Driver of special all-terrain or other off-road motor vehicle injured in traffic accident

!Q ☑ V86.01X- Driver of ambulance or fire engine injured in traffic accident

!Q ☑ V86.02X- Driver of snowmobile injured in traffic accident

!Q ☑ V86.03X- Driver of dune buggy injured in traffic accident

!Q ☑ V86.04X- Driver of military vehicle injured in traffic accident

!Q ☑ V86.05X- Driver of 3- or 4- wheeled all-terrain vehicle (ATV) injured in traffic accident

!Q ☑ V86.06X- Driver of dirt bike or motor/cross bike injured in traffic accident

▲ !Q ☑ V86.09X- Driver of other special all-terrain or other off-road motor vehicle injured in traffic accident

Driver of go cart injured in traffic accident

Driver of golf cart injured in traffic accident

⑤ V86.1 Passenger of special all-terrain or other off-road motor vehicle injured in traffic accident

!Q ☑ V86.11X- Passenger of ambulance or fire engine injured in traffic accident

!Q ☑ V86.12X- Passenger of snowmobile injured in traffic accident

!Q ☑ V86.13X- Passenger of dune buggy injured in traffic accident

!Q ☑ V86.14X- Passenger of military vehicle injured in traffic accident

!Q ☑ V86.15X- Passenger of 3- or 4- wheeled all-terrain vehicle (ATV) injured in traffic accident

!Q ☑ V86.16X- Passenger of dirt bike or motor/cross bike injured in traffic accident

▲ !Q ☑ V86.19X- Passenger of other special all-terrain or other off-road motor vehicle injured in traffic accident

Passenger of go cart injured in traffic accident

Passenger of golf cart injured in traffic accident

⑤ V86.2 Person on outside of special all-terrain or other off-road motor vehicle injured in traffic accident

!Q ☑ V86.21X- Person on outside of ambulance or fire engine injured in traffic accident

!Q ☑ V86.22X- Person on outside of snowmobile injured in traffic accident

!Q ☑ V86.23X- Person on outside of dune buggy injured in traffic accident

!Q ☑ V86.24X- Person on outside of military vehicle injured in traffic accident

!Q ☑ V86.25X- Person on outside of 3- or 4- wheeled all-terrain vehicle (ATV) injured in traffic accident

Chapter 20

V00-Y99

★ New ▲ Revised Px Primary SP PDGM Px SL Low CoM SH High CoM !Q Quest. Encounter Ⓗ Hospice non-cancer Dx   Unspecified   M Manifestation

DecisionHealth's FY 2020 Complete Home Health ICD-10-CM Diagnosis Coding Manual

1807

!Q ☑ V86.26X- Person on outside of dirt bike or motor/cross bike injured in traffic accident

▲ !Q ☑ V86.29X- Person on outside of other special all-terrain or other off-road motor vehicle injured in traffic accident
Person on outside of go cart in traffic accident
Person on outside of golf cart injured in traffic accident

⑤ V86.3 Unspecified occupant of special all-terrain or other off-road motor vehicle injured in traffic accident

!Q ☑ V86.31X- Unspecified occupant of ambulance or fire engine injured in traffic accident

!Q ☑ V86.32X- Unspecified occupant of snowmobile injured in traffic accident

!Q ☑ V86.33X- Unspecified occupant of dune buggy injured in traffic accident

!Q ☑ V86.34X- Unspecified occupant of military vehicle injured in traffic accident

!Q ☑ V86.35X- Unspecified occupant of 3- or 4- wheeled all-terrain vehicle (ATV) injured in traffic accident

!Q ☑ V86.36X- Unspecified occupant of dirt bike or motor/cross bike injured in traffic accident

▲ !Q ☑ V86.39X- Unspecified occupant of other special all-terrain or other off-road motor vehicle injured in traffic accident
Unspecified occupant of go cart injured in traffic accident
Unspecified occupant of golf cart injured in traffic accident

⑤ V86.4 Person injured while boarding or alighting from special all-terrain or other off-road motor vehicle

!Q ☑ V86.41X- Person injured while boarding or alighting from ambulance or fire engine

!Q ☑ V86.42X- Person injured while boarding or alighting from snowmobile

!Q ☑ V86.43X- Person injured while boarding or alighting from dune buggy

!Q ☑ V86.44X- Person injured while boarding or alighting from military vehicle

!Q ☑ V86.45X- Person injured while boarding or alighting from a 3- or 4- wheeled all-terrain vehicle (ATV)

!Q ☑ V86.46X- Person injured while boarding or alighting from a dirt bike or motor/cross bike

▲ !Q ☑ V86.49X- Person injured while boarding or alighting from other special all-terrain or other off-road motor vehicle
Person injured while boarding or alighting from go cart
Person injured while boarding or alighting from golf cart

⑤ V86.5 Driver of special all-terrain or other off-road motor vehicle injured in nontraffic accident

!Q ☑ V86.51X- Driver of ambulance or fire engine injured in nontraffic accident

!Q ☑ V86.52X- Driver of snowmobile injured in nontraffic accident

!Q ☑ V86.53X- Driver of dune buggy injured in nontraffic accident

!Q ☑ V86.54X- Driver of military vehicle injured in nontraffic accident

!Q ☑ V86.55X- Driver of 3- or 4- wheeled all-terrain vehicle (ATV) injured in nontraffic accident

!Q ☑ V86.56X- Driver of dirt bike or motor/cross bike injured in nontraffic accident

▲ !Q ☑ V86.59X- Driver of other special all-terrain or other off-road motor vehicle injured in nontraffic accident
Driver of go cart injured in nontraffic accident
Driver of golf cart injured in nontraffic accident

⑤ V86.6 Passenger of special all-terrain or other off-road motor vehicle injured in nontraffic accident

!Q ☑ V86.61X- Passenger of ambulance or fire engine injured in nontraffic accident

!Q ☑ V86.62X- Passenger of snowmobile injured in nontraffic accident

!Q ☑ V86.63X- Passenger of dune buggy injured in nontraffic accident

!Q ☑ V86.64X- Passenger of military vehicle injured in nontraffic accident

!Q ☑ V86.65X- Passenger of 3- or 4- wheeled all-terrain vehicle (ATV) injured in nontraffic accident

!Q ☑ V86.66X- Passenger of dirt bike or motor/cross bike injured in nontraffic accident

▲ !Q ☑ V86.69X- Passenger of other special all-terrain or other off-road motor vehicle injured in nontraffic accident
Passenger of go cart injured in nontraffic accident
Passenger of golf cart injured in nontraffic accident

⑤ V86.7 Person on outside of special all-terrain or other off-road motor vehicle injured in nontraffic accident

!Q ☑ V86.71X- Person on outside of ambulance or fire engine injured in nontraffic accident

!Q ☑ V86.72X- Person on outside of snowmobile injured in nontraffic accident

!Q ☑ V86.73X- Person on outside of dune buggy injured in nontraffic accident

!Q ☑ V86.74X- Person on outside of military vehicle injured in nontraffic accident

!Q ☑ V86.75X- Person on outside of 3- or 4- wheeled all-terrain vehicle (ATV) injured in nontraffic accident

!Q ☑ V86.76X- Person on outside of dirt bike or motor/cross bike injured in nontraffic accident

▲ !Q ☑ V86.79X- Person on outside of other special all-terrain or other off-road motor vehicles injured in nontraffic accident

④4th digit required ⑤5th digit required ⑥6th digit required ⑦7th digit required ☑7th digit placeholder ✚Additional code ⊟Laterality

1808   DecisionHealth's FY 2020 Complete Home Health ICD-10-CM Diagnosis Coding Manual

Person on outside of go cart injured in nontraffic accident

Person on outside of golf cart injured in nontraffic accident

5 V86.9 **Unspecified occupant of special all-terrain or other off-road motor vehicle injured in nontraffic accident**

IQ ☑ V86.91X- **Unspecified occupant of ambulance or fire engine injured in nontraffic accident**

IQ ☑ V86.92X- **Unspecified occupant of snowmobile injured in nontraffic accident**

IQ ☑ V86.93X- **Unspecified occupant of dune buggy injured in nontraffic accident**

IQ ☑ V86.94X- **Unspecified occupant of military vehicle injured in nontraffic accident**

IQ ☑ V86.95X- **Unspecified occupant of 3- or 4-wheeled all-terrain vehicle (ATV) injured in nontraffic accident**

IQ ☑ V86.96X- **Unspecified occupant of dirt bike or motor/cross bike injured in nontraffic accident**

IQ ☑ V86.99X- **Unspecified occupant of other special all-terrain or other off-road motor vehicle injured in nontraffic accident**

Off-road motor-vehicle accident NOS

Other motor-vehicle accident NOS

Unspecified occupant of go cart injured in nontraffic accident

Unspecified occupant of golf cart injured in nontraffic accident

4 V87 **Traffic accident of specified type but victim's mode of transport unknown**

> **EXCLUDES 1** collision involving:
> pedal cycle (V10-V19)
> pedestrian (V01-V09)

> The appropriate 7th character is to be added to each code from category V87
> A   initial encounter
> D   subsequent encounter
> S   sequela

IQ ☑ V87.0XX- **Person injured in collision between car and two- or three-wheeled powered vehicle (traffic)**

IQ ☑ V87.1XX- **Person injured in collision between other motor vehicle and two- or three-wheeled motor vehicle (traffic)**

IQ ☑ V87.2XX- **Person injured in collision between car and pick-up truck or van (traffic)**

IQ ☑ V87.3XX- **Person injured in collision between car and bus (traffic)**

IQ ☑ V87.4XX- **Person injured in collision between car and heavy transport vehicle (traffic)**

IQ ☑ V87.5XX- **Person injured in collision between heavy transport vehicle and bus (traffic)**

IQ ☑ V87.6XX- **Person injured in collision between railway train or railway vehicle and car (traffic)**

IQ ☑ V87.7XX- **Person injured in collision between other specified motor vehicles (traffic)**

IQ ☑ V87.8XX- **Person injured in other specified noncollision transport accidents involving motor vehicle (traffic)**

IQ ☑ V87.9XX- **Person injured in other specified (collision)(noncollision) transport accidents involving nonmotor vehicle (traffic)**

4 V88 **Nontraffic accident of specified type but victim's mode of transport unknown**

> **EXCLUDES 1** collision involving:
> pedal cycle (V10-V19)
> pedestrian (V01-V09)

> The appropriate 7th character is to be added to each code from category V88
> A   initial encounter
> D   subsequent encounter
> S   sequela

IQ ☑ V88.0XX- **Person injured in collision between car and two- or three-wheeled motor vehicle, nontraffic**

IQ ☑ V88.1XX- **Person injured in collision between other motor vehicle and two- or three-wheeled motor vehicle, nontraffic**

IQ ☑ V88.2XX- **Person injured in collision between car and pick-up truck or van, nontraffic**

IQ ☑ V88.3XX- **Person injured in collision between car and bus, nontraffic**

IQ ☑ V88.4XX- **Person injured in collision between car and heavy transport vehicle, nontraffic**

IQ ☑ V88.5XX- **Person injured in collision between heavy transport vehicle and bus, nontraffic**

IQ ☑ V88.6XX- **Person injured in collision between railway train or railway vehicle and car, nontraffic**

IQ ☑ V88.7XX- **Person injured in collision between other specified motor vehicle, nontraffic**

IQ ☑ V88.8XX- **Person injured in other specified noncollision transport accidents involving motor vehicle, nontraffic**

IQ ☑ V88.9XX- **Person injured in other specified (collision)(noncollision) transport accidents involving nonmotor vehicle, nontraffic**

4 V89 **Motor- or nonmotor-vehicle accident, type of vehicle unspecified**

> The appropriate 7th character is to be added to each code from category V89
> A   initial encounter
> D   subsequent encounter
> S   sequela

IQ ☑ V89.0XX- **Person injured in unspecified motor-vehicle accident, nontraffic**

Motor-vehicle accident NOS, nontraffic

✶ New ▲ Revised Px Primary **SP** PDGM Px **SL** Low CoM **SH** High CoM **IQ** Quest. Encounter 🖽 Hospice non-cancer Dx Unspecified **M** *Manifestation*

DecisionHealth's FY 2020 Complete Home Health ICD-10-CM Diagnosis Coding Manual

1809

!Q ☑ V89.1XX- **Person injured in unspecified nonmotor-vehicle accident, nontraffic**

Nonmotor-vehicle accident NOS (nontraffic)

!Q ☑ V89.2XX- **Person injured in unspecified motor-vehicle accident, traffic**

Motor-vehicle accident [MVA] NOS
Road (traffic) accident [RTA] NOS

!Q ☑ V89.3XX- **Person injured in unspecified nonmotor-vehicle accident, traffic**

Nonmotor-vehicle traffic accident NOS

!Q ☑ V89.9XX- **Person injured in unspecified vehicle accident**

Collision NOS

Water transport accidents   (V90-V94)

4 V90 **Drowning and submersion due to accident to watercraft**

> **EXCLUDES 1** civilian water transport accident involving military watercraft (V94.81-)
> fall into water not from watercraft (W16.-)
> military watercraft accident in military or war operations (Y36.0-, Y37.0-)
> water-transport-related drowning or submersion without accident to watercraft (V92.-)

The appropriate 7th character is to be added to each code from category V90
A   initial encounter
D   subsequent encounter
S   sequela

5 V90.0 **Drowning and submersion due to watercraft overturning**

!Q ☑ V90.00X- **Drowning and submersion due to merchant ship overturning**

!Q ☑ V90.01X- **Drowning and submersion due to passenger ship overturning**

Drowning and submersion due to Ferry-boat overturning
Drowning and submersion due to Liner overturning

!Q ☑ V90.02X- **Drowning and submersion due to fishing boat overturning**

!Q ☑ V90.03X- **Drowning and submersion due to other powered watercraft overturning**

Drowning and submersion due to Hovercraft (on open water) overturning
Drowning and submersion due to Jet ski overturning

!Q ☑ V90.04X- **Drowning and submersion due to sailboat overturning**

!Q ☑ V90.05X- **Drowning and submersion due to canoe or kayak overturning**

!Q ☑ V90.06X- **Drowning and submersion due to (nonpowered) inflatable craft overturning**

!Q ☑ V90.08X- **Drowning and submersion due to other unpowered watercraft overturning**

Drowning and submersion due to windsurfer overturning

!Q ☑ V90.09X- **Drowning and submersion due to unspecified watercraft overturning**

Drowning and submersion due to boat NOS overturning
Drowning and submersion due to ship NOS overturning
Drowning and submersion due to watercraft NOS overturning

5 V90.1 **Drowning and submersion due to watercraft sinking**

!Q ☑ V90.10X- **Drowning and submersion due to merchant ship sinking**

!Q ☑ V90.11X- **Drowning and submersion due to passenger ship sinking**

Drowning and submersion due to Ferry-boat sinking
Drowning and submersion due to Liner sinking

!Q ☑ V90.12X- **Drowning and submersion due to fishing boat sinking**

!Q ☑ V90.13X- **Drowning and submersion due to other powered watercraft sinking**

Drowning and submersion due to Hovercraft (on open water) sinking
Drowning and submersion due to Jet ski sinking

!Q ☑ V90.14X- **Drowning and submersion due to sailboat sinking**

!Q ☑ V90.15X- **Drowning and submersion due to canoe or kayak sinking**

!Q ☑ V90.16X- **Drowning and submersion due to (nonpowered) inflatable craft sinking**

!Q ☑ V90.18X- **Drowning and submersion due to other unpowered watercraft sinking**

!Q ☑ V90.19X- **Drowning and submersion due to unspecified watercraft sinking**

Drowning and submersion due to boat NOS sinking
Drowning and submersion due to ship NOS sinking
Drowning and submersion due to watercraft NOS sinking

5 V90.2 **Drowning and submersion due to falling or jumping from burning watercraft**

!Q ☑ V90.20X- **Drowning and submersion due to falling or jumping from burning merchant ship**

!Q ☑ V90.21X- **Drowning and submersion due to falling or jumping from burning passenger ship**

Drowning and submersion due to falling or jumping from burning Ferry-boat
Drowning and submersion due to falling or jumping from burning Liner

!Q ☑ V90.22X- **Drowning and submersion due to falling or jumping from burning fishing boat**

4 4th digit required   5 5th digit required   6 6th digit required   7 7th digit required   ☑ 7th digit placeholder   ✚ Additional code   ▱ Laterality

1810   DecisionHealth's FY 2020 Complete Home Health ICD-10-CM Diagnosis Coding Manual

IQ ☑ V90.23X- Drowning and submersion due to falling or jumping from other burning powered watercraft

Drowning and submersion due to falling and jumping from burning Hovercraft (on open water)

Drowning and submersion due to falling and jumping from burning Jet ski

IQ ☑ V90.24X- Drowning and submersion due to falling or jumping from burning sailboat

IQ ☑ V90.25X- Drowning and submersion due to falling or jumping from burning canoe or kayak

IQ ☑ V90.26X- Drowning and submersion due to falling or jumping from burning (nonpowered) inflatable craft

IQ ☑ V90.27X- Drowning and submersion due to falling or jumping from burning water-skis

IQ ☑ V90.28X- Drowning and submersion due to falling or jumping from other burning unpowered watercraft

Drowning and submersion due to falling and jumping from burning surf-board

Drowning and submersion due to falling and jumping from burning windsurfer

IQ ☑ V90.29X- Drowning and submersion due to falling or jumping from unspecified burning watercraft

Drowning and submersion due to falling or jumping from burning boat NOS

Drowning and submersion due to falling or jumping from burning ship NOS

Drowning and submersion due to falling or jumping from burning watercraft NOS

⑤ V90.3 Drowning and submersion due to falling or jumping from crushed watercraft

IQ ☑ V90.30X- Drowning and submersion due to falling or jumping from crushed merchant ship

IQ ☑ V90.31X- Drowning and submersion due to falling or jumping from crushed passenger ship

Drowning and submersion due to falling and jumping from crushed Ferry boat

Drowning and submersion due to falling and jumping from crushed Liner

IQ ☑ V90.32X- Drowning and submersion due to falling or jumping from crushed fishing boat

IQ ☑ V90.33X- Drowning and submersion due to falling or jumping from other crushed powered watercraft

Drowning and submersion due to falling and jumping from crushed Hovercraft

Drowning and submersion due to falling and jumping from crushed Jet ski

IQ ☑ V90.34X- Drowning and submersion due to falling or jumping from crushed sailboat

IQ ☑ V90.35X- Drowning and submersion due to falling or jumping from crushed canoe or kayak

IQ ☑ V90.36X- Drowning and submersion due to falling or jumping from crushed (nonpowered) inflatable craft

IQ ☑ V90.37X- Drowning and submersion due to falling or jumping from crushed water-skis

IQ ☑ V90.38X- Drowning and submersion due to falling or jumping from other crushed unpowered watercraft

Drowning and submersion due to falling and jumping from crushed surf-board

Drowning and submersion due to falling and jumping from crushed windsurfer

IQ ☑ V90.39X- Drowning and submersion due to falling or jumping from crushed unspecified watercraft

Drowning and submersion due to falling and jumping from crushed boat NOS

Drowning and submersion due to falling and jumping from crushed ship NOS

Drowning and submersion due to falling and jumping from crushed watercraft NOS

⑤ V90.8 Drowning and submersion due to other accident to watercraft

IQ ☑ V90.80X- Drowning and submersion due to other accident to merchant ship

IQ ☑ V90.81X- Drowning and submersion due to other accident to passenger ship

Drowning and submersion due to other accident to Ferry-boat

Drowning and submersion due to other accident to Liner

IQ ☑ V90.82X- Drowning and submersion due to other accident to fishing boat

IQ ☑ V90.83X- Drowning and submersion due to other accident to other powered watercraft

Drowning and submersion due to other accident to Hovercraft (on open water)

Drowning and submersion due to other accident to Jet ski

IQ ☑ V90.84X- Drowning and submersion due to other accident to sailboat

IQ ☑ V90.85X- Drowning and submersion due to other accident to canoe or kayak

IQ ☑ V90.86X- Drowning and submersion due to other accident to (nonpowered) inflatable craft

IQ ☑ V90.87X- Drowning and submersion due to other accident to water-skis

IQ ☑ V90.88X- Drowning and submersion due to other accident to other unpowered watercraft

Drowning and submersion due to other accident to surf-board

Drowning and submersion due to other accident to windsurfer

★ New ▲ Revised Px Primary SP PDGM Px SL Low CoM SH High CoM IQ Quest. Encounter Ⓗ Hospice non-cancer Dx   Unspecified   M Manifestation

DecisionHealth's FY 2020 Complete Home Health ICD-10-CM Diagnosis Coding Manual

1811

🔲 ☑ V90.89X- **Drowning and submersion due to other accident to unspecified watercraft**

Drowning and submersion due to other accident to boat NOS

Drowning and submersion due to other accident to ship NOS

Drowning and submersion due to other accident to watercraft NOS

4 V91 **Other injury due to accident to watercraft**

| INCLUDES | any injury except drowning and submersion as a result of an accident to watercraft |

| EXCLUDES 1 | civilian water transport accident involving military watercraft (V94.81-) |
| | military watercraft accident in military or war operations (Y36, Y37.-) |

| EXCLUDES 2 | drowning and submersion due to accident to watercraft (V90.-) |

The appropriate 7th character is to be added to each code from category V91

A   initial encounter
D   subsequent encounter
S   sequela

5 V91.0 **Burn due to watercraft on fire**

| EXCLUDES 1 | burn from localized fire or explosion on board ship without accident to watercraft (V93.-) |

🔲 ☑ V91.00X- **Burn due to merchant ship on fire**

🔲 ☑ V91.01X- **Burn due to passenger ship on fire**
Burn due to Ferry-boat on fire
Burn due to Liner on fire

🔲 ☑ V91.02X- **Burn due to fishing boat on fire**

🔲 ☑ V91.03X- **Burn due to other powered watercraft on fire**
Burn due to Hovercraft (on open water) on fire
Burn due to Jet ski on fire

🔲 ☑ V91.04X- **Burn due to sailboat on fire**

🔲 ☑ V91.05X- **Burn due to canoe or kayak on fire**

🔲 ☑ V91.06X- **Burn due to (nonpowered) inflatable craft on fire**

🔲 ☑ V91.07X- **Burn due to water-skis on fire**

🔲 ☑ V91.08X- **Burn due to other unpowered watercraft on fire**

🔲 ☑ V91.09X- **Burn due to unspecified watercraft on fire**
Burn due to boat NOS on fire
Burn due to ship NOS on fire
Burn due to watercraft NOS on fire

5 V91.1 **Crushed between watercraft and other watercraft or other object due to collision**
Crushed by lifeboat after abandoning ship in a collision
Note:
select the specified type of watercraft that the victim was on at the time of the collision

🔲 ☑ V91.10X- **Crushed between merchant ship and other watercraft or other object due to collision**

🔲 ☑ V91.11X- **Crushed between passenger ship and other watercraft or other object due to collision**
Crushed between Ferry-boat and other watercraft or other object due to collision
Crushed between Liner and other watercraft or other object due to collision

🔲 ☑ V91.12X- **Crushed between fishing boat and other watercraft or other object due to collision**

🔲 ☑ V91.13X- **Crushed between other powered watercraft and other watercraft or other object due to collision**
Crushed between Hovercraft (on open water) and other watercraft or other object due to collision
Crushed between Jet ski and other watercraft or other object due to collision

🔲 ☑ V91.14X- **Crushed between sailboat and other watercraft or other object due to collision**

🔲 ☑ V91.15X- **Crushed between canoe or kayak and other watercraft or other object due to collision**

🔲 ☑ V91.16X- **Crushed between (nonpowered) inflatable craft and other watercraft or other object due to collision**

🔲 ☑ V91.18X- **Crushed between other unpowered watercraft and other watercraft or other object due to collision**
Crushed between surfboard and other watercraft or other object due to collision
Crushed between windsurfer and other watercraft or other object due to collision

🔲 ☑ V91.19X- **Crushed between unspecified watercraft and other watercraft or other object due to collision**
Crushed between boat NOS and other watercraft or other object due to collision
Crushed between ship NOS and other watercraft or other object due to collision
Crushed between watercraft NOS and other watercraft or other object due to collision

5 V91.2 **Fall due to collision between watercraft and other watercraft or other object**
Fall while remaining on watercraft after collision
Note:
select the specified type of watercraft that the victim was on at the time of the collision

| EXCLUDES 1 | crushed between watercraft and other watercraft and other object due to collision (V91.1-) |
| | drowning and submersion due to falling from crushed watercraft (V90.3-) |

4 4th digit required   5 5th digit required   6 6th digit required   7 7th digit required   ☑ 7th digit placeholder   ✚ Additional code   ⊟ Laterality

1812   DecisionHealth's FY 2020 Complete Home Health ICD-10-CM Diagnosis Coding Manual

!Q ☑ V91.20X- Fall due to collision between merchant ship and other watercraft or other object

!Q ☑ V91.21X- Fall due to collision between passenger ship and other watercraft or other object

Fall due to collision between Ferry-boat and other watercraft or other object

Fall due to collision between Liner and other watercraft or other object

!Q ☑ V91.22X- Fall due to collision between fishing boat and other watercraft or other object

!Q ☑ V91.23X- Fall due to collision between other powered watercraft and other watercraft or other object

Fall due to collision between Hovercraft (on open water) and other watercraft or other object

Fall due to collision between Jet ski and other watercraft or other object

!Q ☑ V91.24X- Fall due to collision between sailboat and other watercraft or other object

!Q ☑ V91.25X- Fall due to collision between canoe or kayak and other watercraft or other object

!Q ☑ V91.26X- Fall due to collision between (nonpowered) inflatable craft and other watercraft or other object

!Q ☑ V91.29X- Fall due to collision between unspecified watercraft and other watercraft or other object

Fall due to collision between boat NOS and other watercraft or other object

Fall due to collision between ship NOS and other watercraft or other object

Fall due to collision between watercraft NOS and other watercraft or other object

⑤ V91.3 Hit or struck by falling object due to accident to watercraft

Hit or struck by falling object (part of damaged watercraft or other object) after falling or jumping from damaged watercraft

EXCLUDES 2 drowning or submersion due to fall or jumping from damaged watercraft (V90.2-, V90.3-)

!Q ☑ V91.30X- Hit or struck by falling object due to accident to merchant ship

!Q ☑ V91.31X- Hit or struck by falling object due to accident to passenger ship

Hit or struck by falling object due to accident to Ferry-boat

Hit or struck by falling object due to accident to Liner

!Q ☑ V91.32X- Hit or struck by falling object due to accident to fishing boat

!Q ☑ V91.33X- Hit or struck by falling object due to accident to other powered watercraft

Hit or struck by falling object due to accident to Hovercraft (on open water)

Hit or struck by falling object due to accident to Jet ski

!Q ☑ V91.34X- Hit or struck by falling object due to accident to sailboat

!Q ☑ V91.35X- Hit or struck by falling object due to accident to canoe or kayak

!Q ☑ V91.36X- Hit or struck by falling object due to accident to (nonpowered) inflatable craft

!Q ☑ V91.37X- Hit or struck by falling object due to accident to water-skis

Hit by water-skis after jumping off of waterskis

!Q ☑ V91.38X- Hit or struck by falling object due to accident to other unpowered watercraft

Hit or struck by surf-board after falling off damaged surf-board

Hit or struck by object after falling off damaged windsurfer

!Q ☑ V91.39X- Hit or struck by falling object due to accident to unspecified watercraft

Hit or struck by falling object due to accident to boat NOS

Hit or struck by falling object due to accident to ship NOS

Hit or struck by falling object due to accident to watercraft NOS

⑤ V91.8 Other injury due to other accident to watercraft

!Q ☑ V91.80X- Other injury due to other accident to merchant ship

!Q ☑ V91.81X- Other injury due to other accident to passenger ship

Other injury due to other accident to Ferry-boat

Other injury due to other accident to Liner

!Q ☑ V91.82X- Other injury due to other accident to fishing boat

!Q ☑ V91.83X- Other injury due to other accident to other powered watercraft

Other injury due to other accident to Hovercraft (on open water)

Other injury due to other accident to Jet ski

!Q ☑ V91.84X- Other injury due to other accident to sailboat

!Q ☑ V91.85X- Other injury due to other accident to canoe or kayak

!Q ☑ V91.86X- Other injury due to other accident to (nonpowered) inflatable craft

!Q ☑ V91.87X- Other injury due to other accident to water-skis

!Q ☑ V91.88X- Other injury due to other accident to other unpowered watercraft

Other injury due to other accident to surf-board

Other injury due to other accident to windsurfer

!Q ☑ V91.89X- Other injury due to other accident to unspecified watercraft

Other injury due to other accident to boat NOS

Other injury due to other accident to ship NOS

★ New ▲ Revised Px Primary **SP** PDGM Px **SL** Low CoM **SH** High CoM **!Q** Quest. Encounter **H** Hospice non-cancer Dx Unspecified **M** Manifestation

DecisionHealth's FY 2020 Complete Home Health ICD-10-CM Diagnosis Coding Manual

1813

Other injury due to other accident to
watercraft NOS

**4 V92   Drowning and submersion due to accident
on board watercraft, without accident to
watercraft**

> EXCLUDES 1   civilian water transport accident
> involving military watercraft
> (V94.81-)
> drowning or submersion due to
> accident to watercraft
> (V90-V91)
> drowning or submersion of
> diver who voluntarily jumps
> from boat not involved in an
> accident
> (W16.711, W16.721)
> fall into water without
> watercraft (W16.-)
> military watercraft accident in
> military or war operations
> (Y36, Y37)

The appropriate 7th character is to be added to
each code from category V92
A   initial encounter
D   subsequent encounter
S   sequela

**5 V92.0   Drowning and submersion due to fall off
watercraft**
Drowning and submersion due to fall from
gangplank of watercraft
Drowning and submersion due to fall
overboard watercraft

> EXCLUDES 2   hitting head on object or
> bottom of body of water
> due to fall from watercraft
> (V94.0-)

**IQ 7 V92.00X-   Drowning and submersion due to
fall off merchant ship**

**IQ 7 V92.01X-   Drowning and submersion due to
fall off passenger ship**
Drowning and submersion due to fall
off Ferry-boat
Drowning and submersion due to fall
off Liner

**IQ 7 V92.02X-   Drowning and submersion due to
fall off fishing boat**

**IQ 7 V92.03X-   Drowning and submersion due to
fall off other powered watercraft**
Drowning and submersion due to fall
off Hovercraft (on open water)
Drowning and submersion due to fall
off Jet ski

**IQ 7 V92.04X-   Drowning and submersion due to
fall off sailboat**

**IQ 7 V92.05X-   Drowning and submersion due to
fall off canoe or kayak**

**IQ 7 V92.06X-   Drowning and submersion due to
fall off (nonpowered) inflatable
craft**

**IQ 7 V92.07X-   Drowning and submersion due to
fall off water-skis**

> EXCLUDES 1   drowning and
> submersion due to
> falling off burning
> water-skis (V90.27)

drowning and
submersion due to
falling off crushed
water-skis (V90.37)
hit by boat while
water-skiing NOS
(V94.X)

**IQ 7 V92.08X-   Drowning and submersion due to
fall off other unpowered
watercraft**
Drowning and submersion due to fall
off surf-board
Drowning and submersion due to fall
off windsurfer

> EXCLUDES 1   drowning and
> submersion due to
> fall off burning
> unpowered
> watercraft (V90.28)
> drowning and
> submersion due to
> fall off crushed
> unpowered
> watercraft (V90.38)
> drowning and
> submersion due to
> fall off damaged
> unpowered
> watercraft (V90.88)
> drowning and
> submersion due to
> rider of nonpowered
> watercraft being hit
> by other watercraft
> (V94.-)
> other injury due to
> rider of nonpowered
> watercraft being hit
> by other watercraft
> (V94.-)

**IQ 7 V92.09X-   Drowning and submersion due to
fall off unspecified watercraft**
Drowning and submersion due to fall
off boat NOS
Drowning and submersion due to fall
off ship
Drowning and submersion due to fall
off watercraft NOS

**5 V92.1   Drowning and submersion due to being
thrown overboard by motion of
watercraft**

> EXCLUDES 1   drowning and submersion
> due to fall off surf-board
> (V92.08)
> drowning and submersion
> due to fall off water-skis
> (V92.07)
> drowning and submersion
> due to fall off windsurfer
> (V92.08)

**IQ 7 V92.10X-   Drowning and submersion due to
being thrown overboard by motion
of merchant ship**

**IQ 7 V92.11X-   Drowning and submersion due to
being thrown overboard by motion
of passenger ship**
Drowning and submersion due to
being thrown overboard by motion
of Ferry-boat

4 4th digit required   5 5th digit required   6 6th digit required   7 7th digit required   7 7th digit placeholder   + Additional code   ⊟ Laterality

1814   DecisionHealth's FY 2020 Complete Home Health ICD-10-CM Diagnosis Coding Manual

Drowning and submersion due to
being thrown overboard by motion
of Liner

!Q 🗹 V92.12X- **Drowning and submersion due to
being thrown overboard by motion
of fishing boat**

!Q 🗹 V92.13X- **Drowning and submersion due to
being thrown overboard by motion
of other powered watercraft**

Drowning and submersion due to
being thrown overboard by motion
of Hovercraft

!Q 🗹 V92.14X- **Drowning and submersion due to
being thrown overboard by motion
of sailboat**

!Q 🗹 V92.15X- **Drowning and submersion due to
being thrown overboard by motion
of canoe or kayak**

!Q 🗹 V92.16X- **Drowning and submersion due to
being thrown overboard by motion
of (nonpowered) inflatable craft**

!Q 🗹 V92.19X- **Drowning and submersion due to
being thrown overboard by
motion of unspecified watercraft**

Drowning and submersion due to
being thrown overboard by motion
of boat NOS

Drowning and submersion due to
being thrown overboard by motion
of ship NOS

Drowning and submersion due to
being thrown overboard by motion
of watercraft NOS

⑤ V92.2 **Drowning and submersion due to being
washed overboard from watercraft**

Code first:

any associated cataclysm (X37.0-)

!Q 🗹 V92.20X- **Drowning and submersion due to
being washed overboard from
merchant ship**

!Q 🗹 V92.21X- **Drowning and submersion due to
being washed overboard from
passenger ship**

Drowning and submersion due to
being washed overboard from
Ferry-boat

Drowning and submersion due to
being washed overboard from
Liner

!Q 🗹 V92.22X- **Drowning and submersion due to
being washed overboard from
fishing boat**

!Q 🗹 V92.23X- **Drowning and submersion due to
being washed overboard from
other powered watercraft**

Drowning and submersion due to
being washed overboard from
Hovercraft (on open water)

Drowning and submersion due to
being washed overboard from Jet
ski

!Q 🗹 V92.24X- **Drowning and submersion due to
being washed overboard from
sailboat**

!Q 🗹 V92.25X- **Drowning and submersion due to
being washed overboard from
canoe or kayak**

!Q 🗹 V92.26X- **Drowning and submersion due to
being washed overboard from
(nonpowered) inflatable craft**

!Q 🗹 V92.27X- **Drowning and submersion due to
being washed overboard from
water-skis**

EXCLUDES 1 drowning and
submersion due to
fall off water-skis
(V92.07)

!Q 🗹 V92.28X- **Drowning and submersion due to
being washed overboard from
other unpowered watercraft**

Drowning and submersion due to
being washed overboard from surf-
board

Drowning and submersion due to
being washed overboard from
windsurfer

!Q 🗹 V92.29X- **Drowning and submersion due to
being washed overboard from
unspecified watercraft**

Drowning and submersion due to
being washed overboard from boat
NOS

Drowning and submersion due to
being washed overboard from ship
NOS

Drowning and submersion due to
being washed overboard from
watercraft NOS

④ V93 **Other injury due to accident on board
watercraft, without accident to watercraft**

EXCLUDES 1 civilian water transport accident
involving military watercraft
(V94.81-)

other injury due to accident to
watercraft (V91.-)

military watercraft accident in
military or war operations
(Y36, Y37.-)

EXCLUDES 2 drowning and submersion due
to accident on board
watercraft, without accident to
watercraft (V92.-)

The appropriate 7th character is to be added to
each code from category V93
A   initial encounter
D   subsequent encounter
S   sequela

⑤ V93.0 **Burn due to localized fire on board
watercraft**

EXCLUDES 1 burn due to watercraft on fire
(V91.0-)

!Q 🗹 V93.00X- **Burn due to localized fire on board
merchant vessel**

!Q 🗹 V93.01X- **Burn due to localized fire on board
passenger vessel**

Burn due to localized fire on board
Ferry-boat

Burn due to localized fire on board
Liner

!Q 🗹 V93.02X- **Burn due to localized fire on board
fishing boat**

!Q 🗹 V93.03X- **Burn due to localized fire on board
other powered watercraft**

Burn due to localized fire on board
Hovercraft

✱ New ▲ Revised Px Primary SP PDGM Px SL Low CoM SH High CoM !Q Quest. Encounter H Hospice non-cancer Dx   Unspecified   M Manifestation

DecisionHealth's FY 2020 Complete Home Health ICD-10-CM Diagnosis Coding Manual

1815

Burn due to localized fire on board
Jet ski

!Q ☑ V93.04X- **Burn due to localized fire on board sailboat**

!Q ☑ V93.09X- **Burn due to localized fire on board unspecified watercraft**

Burn due to localized fire on board boat NOS

Burn due to localized fire on board ship NOS

Burn due to localized fire on board watercraft NOS

⑤ V93.1 Other burn on board watercraft
Burn due to source other than fire on board watercraft
EXCLUDES 1 burn due to watercraft on fire (V91.0-)

!Q ☑ V93.10X- **Other burn on board merchant vessel**

!Q ☑ V93.11X- **Other burn on board passenger vessel**
Other burn on board Ferry-boat
Other burn on board Liner

!Q ☑ V93.12X- **Other burn on board fishing boat**

!Q ☑ V93.13X- **Other burn on board other powered watercraft**
Other burn on board Hovercraft
Other burn on board Jet ski

!Q ☑ V93.14X- **Other burn on board sailboat**

!Q ☑ V93.19X- **Other burn on board unspecified watercraft**

Other burn on board boat NOS
Other burn on board ship NOS
Other burn on board watercraft NOS

⑤ V93.2 Heat exposure on board watercraft
EXCLUDES 1 exposure to man-made heat not aboard watercraft (W92)
exposure to natural heat while on board watercraft (X30)
exposure to sunlight while on board watercraft (X32)
EXCLUDES 2 burn due to fire on board watercraft (V93.0-)

!Q ☑ V93.20X- **Heat exposure on board merchant ship**

!Q ☑ V93.21X- **Heat exposure on board passenger ship**
Heat exposure on board Ferry-boat
Heat exposure on board Liner

!Q ☑ V93.22X- **Heat exposure on board fishing boat**

!Q ☑ V93.23X- **Heat exposure on board other powered watercraft**
Heat exposure on board hovercraft

!Q ☑ V93.24X- **Heat exposure on board sailboat**

!Q ☑ V93.29X- **Heat exposure on board unspecified watercraft**

Heat exposure on board boat NOS
Heat exposure on board ship NOS
Heat exposure on board watercraft NOS

⑤ V93.3 Fall on board watercraft
EXCLUDES 1 fall due to collision of watercraft (V91.2-)

!Q ☑ V93.30X- **Fall on board merchant ship**

!Q ☑ V93.31X- **Fall on board passenger ship**
Fall on board Ferry-boat
Fall on board Liner

!Q ☑ V93.32X- **Fall on board fishing boat**

!Q ☑ V93.33X- **Fall on board other powered watercraft**
Fall on board Hovercraft (on open water)
Fall on board Jet ski

!Q ☑ V93.34X- **Fall on board sailboat**

!Q ☑ V93.35X- **Fall on board canoe or kayak**

!Q ☑ V93.36X- **Fall on board (nonpowered) inflatable craft**

!Q ☑ V93.38X- **Fall on board other unpowered watercraft**

!Q ☑ V93.39X- **Fall on board unspecified watercraft**

Fall on board boat NOS
Fall on board ship NOS
Fall on board watercraft NOS

⑤ V93.4 Struck by falling object on board watercraft
Hit by falling object on board watercraft
EXCLUDES 1 struck by falling object due to accident to watercraft (V91.3)

!Q ☑ V93.40X- **Struck by falling object on merchant ship**

!Q ☑ V93.41X- **Struck by falling object on passenger ship**
Struck by falling object on Ferry-boat
Struck by falling object on Liner

!Q ☑ V93.42X- **Struck by falling object on fishing boat**

!Q ☑ V93.43X- **Struck by falling object on other powered watercraft**
Struck by falling object on Hovercraft

!Q ☑ V93.44X- **Struck by falling object on sailboat**

!Q ☑ V93.48X- **Struck by falling object on other unpowered watercraft**

!Q ☑ V93.49X- **Struck by falling object on unspecified watercraft**

⑤ V93.5 Explosion on board watercraft
Boiler explosion on steamship
EXCLUDES 2 fire on board watercraft (V93.0-)

!Q ☑ V93.50X- **Explosion on board merchant ship**

!Q ☑ V93.51X- **Explosion on board passenger ship**
Explosion on board Ferry-boat
Explosion on board Liner

!Q ☑ V93.52X- **Explosion on board fishing boat**

!Q ☑ V93.53X- **Explosion on board other powered watercraft**
Explosion on board Hovercraft
Explosion on board Jet ski

!Q ☑ V93.54X- **Explosion on board sailboat**

!Q ☑ V93.59X- **Explosion on board unspecified watercraft**

Explosion on board boat NOS
Explosion on board ship NOS
Explosion on board watercraft NOS

⑤ V93.6 Machinery accident on board watercraft
EXCLUDES 1 machinery explosion on board watercraft (V93.4-)

Chapter 20

V00-Y99

④4th digit required   ⑤5th digit required   ⑥6th digit required   ⑦7th digit required   ☑7th digit placeholder   ✚Additional code   ⊟Laterality

1816   *DecisionHealth's* FY 2020 Complete Home Health ICD-10-CM Diagnosis Coding Manual

machinery fire on board
watercraft (V93.0-)

!Q ☑ V93.60X- **Machinery accident on board merchant ship**

!Q ☑ V93.61X- **Machinery accident on board passenger ship**
Machinery accident on board Ferry-boat
Machinery accident on board Liner

!Q ☑ V93.62X- **Machinery accident on board fishing boat**

!Q ☑ V93.63X- **Machinery accident on board other powered watercraft**
Machinery accident on board Hovercraft

!Q ☑ V93.64X- **Machinery accident on board sailboat**

!Q ☑ V93.69X- **Machinery accident on board unspecified watercraft**
Machinery accident on board boat NOS
Machinery accident on board ship NOS
Machinery accident on board watercraft NOS

⑤ V93.8 **Other injury due to other accident on board watercraft**
Accidental poisoning by gases or fumes on watercraft

!Q ☑ V93.80X- **Other injury due to other accident on board merchant ship**

!Q ☑ V93.81X- **Other injury due to other accident on board passenger ship**
Other injury due to other accident on board Ferry-boat
Other injury due to other accident on board Liner

!Q ☑ V93.82X- **Other injury due to other accident on board fishing boat**

!Q ☑ V93.83X- **Other injury due to other accident on board other powered watercraft**
Other injury due to other accident on board Hovercraft
Other injury due to other accident on board Jet ski

!Q ☑ V93.84X- **Other injury due to other accident on board sailboat**

!Q ☑ V93.85X- **Other injury due to other accident on board canoe or kayak**

!Q ☑ V93.86X- **Other injury due to other accident on board (nonpowered) inflatable craft**

!Q ☑ V93.87X- **Other injury due to other accident on board water-skis**
Hit or struck by object while waterskiing

!Q ☑ V93.88X- **Other injury due to other accident on board other unpowered watercraft**
Hit or struck by object while surfing
Hit or struck by object while on board windsurfer

!Q ☑ V93.89X- **Other injury due to other accident on board unspecified watercraft**
Other injury due to other accident on board boat NOS

Other injury due to other accident on board ship NOS
Other injury due to other accident on board watercraft NOS

④ V94 **Other and unspecified water transport accidents**

> **EXCLUDES 1** military watercraft accidents in military or war operations (Y36, Y37)

The appropriate 7th character is to be added to each code from category V94
A initial encounter
D subsequent encounter
S sequela

!Q ☑ V94.0XX- **Hitting object or bottom of body of water due to fall from watercraft**
> **EXCLUDES 2** drowning and submersion due to fall from watercraft (V92.0-)

⑤ V94.1 **Bather struck by watercraft**
Swimmer hit by watercraft

!Q ☑ V94.11X- **Bather struck by powered watercraft**

!Q ☑ V94.12X- **Bather struck by nonpowered watercraft**

⑤ V94.2 **Rider of nonpowered watercraft struck by other watercraft**

!Q ☑ V94.21X- **Rider of nonpowered watercraft struck by other nonpowered watercraft**
Canoer hit by other nonpowered watercraft
Surfer hit by other nonpowered watercraft
Windsurfer hit by other nonpowered watercraft

!Q ☑ V94.22X- **Rider of nonpowered watercraft struck by powered watercraft**
Canoer hit by motorboat
Surfer hit by motorboat
Windsurfer hit by motorboat

⑤ V94.3 **Injury to rider of (inflatable) watercraft being pulled behind other watercraft**

!Q ☑ V94.31X- **Injury to rider of (inflatable) recreational watercraft being pulled behind other watercraft**
Injury to rider of inner-tube pulled behind motor boat

!Q ☑ V94.32X- **Injury to rider of non-recreational watercraft being pulled behind other watercraft**
Injury to occupant of dingy being pulled behind boat or ship
Injury to occupant of life-raft being pulled behind boat or ship

!Q ☑ V94.4XX- **Injury to barefoot water-skier**
Injury to person being pulled behind boat or ship

⑤ V94.8 **Other water transport accident**

⑥ V94.81 **Water transport accident involving military watercraft**

!Q ☑ V94.810- **Civilian watercraft involved in water transport accident with military watercraft**

★ New ▲ Revised Px Primary SP PDGM Px SL Low CoM SH High CoM !Q Quest. Encounter H Hospice non-cancer Dx Unspecified M *Manifestation*

DecisionHealth's FY 2020 Complete Home Health ICD-10-CM Diagnosis Coding Manual

1817

          Passenger on civilian watercraft injured due to accident with military watercraft

IQ 7 V94.811- Civilian in water injured by military watercraft

IQ 7 V94.818- Other water transport accident involving military watercraft

IQ ☑ V94.89X- Other water transport accident

IQ ☑ V94.9XX- Unspecified water transport accident

          Water transport accident NOS

Air and space transport accidents (V95-V97)

EXCLUDES 1   military aircraft accidents in military or war operations (Y36, Y37)

4 V95   Accident to powered aircraft causing injury to occupant

> The appropriate 7th character is to be added to each code from category V95
> A   initial encounter
> D   subsequent encounter
> S   sequela

5 V95.0   Helicopter accident injuring occupant

IQ ☑ V95.00X- Unspecified helicopter accident injuring occupant

IQ ☑ V95.01X- Helicopter crash injuring occupant

IQ ☑ V95.02X- Forced landing of helicopter injuring occupant

IQ ☑ V95.03X- Helicopter collision injuring occupant

          Helicopter collision with any object, fixed, movable or moving

IQ ☑ V95.04X- Helicopter fire injuring occupant

IQ ☑ V95.05X- Helicopter explosion injuring occupant

IQ ☑ V95.09X- Other helicopter accident injuring occupant

5 V95.1   Ultralight, microlight or powered-glider accident injuring occupant

IQ ☑ V95.10X- Unspecified ultralight, microlight or powered-glider accident injuring occupant

IQ ☑ V95.11X- Ultralight, microlight or powered-glider crash injuring occupant

IQ ☑ V95.12X- Forced landing of ultralight, microlight or powered-glider injuring occupant

IQ ☑ V95.13X- Ultralight, microlight or powered-glider collision injuring occupant

          Ultralight, microlight or powered-glider collision with any object, fixed, movable or moving

IQ ☑ V95.14X- Ultralight, microlight or powered-glider fire injuring occupant

IQ ☑ V95.15X- Ultralight, microlight or powered-glider explosion injuring occupant

IQ ☑ V95.19X- Other ultralight, microlight or powered-glider accident injuring occupant

5 V95.2   Other private fixed-wing aircraft accident injuring occupant

IQ ☑ V95.20X- Unspecified accident to other private fixed-wing aircraft, injuring occupant

IQ ☑ V95.21X- Other private fixed-wing aircraft crash injuring occupant

IQ ☑ V95.22X- Forced landing of other private fixed-wing aircraft injuring occupant

IQ ☑ V95.23X- Other private fixed-wing aircraft collision injuring occupant

          Other private fixed-wing aircraft collision with any object, fixed, movable or moving

IQ ☑ V95.24X- Other private fixed-wing aircraft fire injuring occupant

IQ ☑ V95.25X- Other private fixed-wing aircraft explosion injuring occupant

IQ ☑ V95.29X- Other accident to other private fixed-wing aircraft injuring occupant

5 V95.3   Commercial fixed-wing aircraft accident injuring occupant

IQ ☑ V95.30X- Unspecified accident to commercial fixed-wing aircraft injuring occupant

IQ ☑ V95.31X- Commercial fixed-wing aircraft crash injuring occupant

IQ ☑ V95.32X- Forced landing of commercial fixed-wing aircraft injuring occupant

IQ ☑ V95.33X- Commercial fixed-wing aircraft collision injuring occupant

          Commercial fixed-wing aircraft collision with any object, fixed, movable or moving

IQ ☑ V95.34X- Commercial fixed-wing aircraft fire injuring occupant

IQ ☑ V95.35X- Commercial fixed-wing aircraft explosion injuring occupant

IQ ☑ V95.39X- Other accident to commercial fixed-wing aircraft injuring occupant

5 V95.4   Spacecraft accident injuring occupant

IQ ☑ V95.40X- Unspecified spacecraft accident injuring occupant

IQ ☑ V95.41X- Spacecraft crash injuring occupant

IQ ☑ V95.42X- Forced landing of spacecraft injuring occupant

IQ ☑ V95.43X- Spacecraft collision injuring occupant

          Spacecraft collision with any object, fixed, moveable or moving

IQ ☑ V95.44X- Spacecraft fire injuring occupant

IQ ☑ V95.45X- Spacecraft explosion injuring occupant

IQ ☑ V95.49X- Other spacecraft accident injuring occupant

IQ ☑ V95.8XX- Other powered aircraft accidents injuring occupant

IQ ☑ V95.9XX- Unspecified aircraft accident injuring occupant

          Aircraft accident NOS
          Air transport accident NOS

4 V96   Accident to nonpowered aircraft causing injury to occupant

4th digit required   5 5th digit required   6 6th digit required   7 7th digit required   ☑ 7th digit placeholder   ✚ Additional code   ⊟ Laterality

1818   *DecisionHealth's* FY 2020 Complete Home Health ICD-10-CM Diagnosis Coding Manual

Chapter 20

V00-Y99

The appropriate 7th character is to be added to each code from category V96
A   initial encounter
D   subsequent encounter
S   sequela

⑤ **V96.0 Balloon accident injuring occupant**

🆀 ☑ **V96.00X- Unspecified balloon accident injuring occupant**

🆀 ☑ **V96.01X- Balloon crash injuring occupant**

🆀 ☑ **V96.02X- Forced landing of balloon injuring occupant**

🆀 ☑ **V96.03X- Balloon collision injuring occupant**
Balloon collision with any object, fixed, moveable or moving

🆀 ☑ **V96.04X- Balloon fire injuring occupant**

🆀 ☑ **V96.05X- Balloon explosion injuring occupant**

🆀 ☑ **V96.09X- Other balloon accident injuring occupant**

⑤ **V96.1 Hang-glider accident injuring occupant**

🆀 ☑ **V96.10X- Unspecified hang-glider accident injuring occupant**

🆀 ☑ **V96.11X- Hang-glider crash injuring occupant**

🆀 ☑ **V96.12X- Forced landing of hang-glider injuring occupant**

🆀 ☑ **V96.13X- Hang-glider collision injuring occupant**
Hang-glider collision with any object, fixed, moveable or moving

🆀 ☑ **V96.14X- Hang-glider fire injuring occupant**

🆀 ☑ **V96.15X- Hang-glider explosion injuring occupant**

🆀 ☑ **V96.19X- Other hang-glider accident injuring occupant**

⑤ **V96.2 Glider (nonpowered) accident injuring occupant**

🆀 ☑ **V96.20X- Unspecified glider (nonpowered) accident injuring occupant**

🆀 ☑ **V96.21X- Glider (nonpowered) crash injuring occupant**

🆀 ☑ **V96.22X- Forced landing of glider (nonpowered) injuring occupant**

🆀 ☑ **V96.23X- Glider (nonpowered) collision injuring occupant**
Glider (nonpowered) collision with any object, fixed, moveable or moving

🆀 ☑ **V96.24X- Glider (nonpowered) fire injuring occupant**

🆀 ☑ **V96.25X- Glider (nonpowered) explosion injuring occupant**

🆀 ☑ **V96.29X- Other glider (nonpowered) accident injuring occupant**

🆀 ☑ **V96.8XX- Other nonpowered-aircraft accidents injuring occupant**
Kite carrying a person accident injuring occupant

🆀 ☑ **V96.9XX- Unspecified nonpowered-aircraft accident injuring occupant**
Nonpowered-aircraft accident NOS

④ **V97 Other specified air transport accidents**

The appropriate 7th character is to be added to each code from category V97
A   initial encounter
D   subsequent encounter
S   sequela

🆀 ☑ **V97.0XX- Occupant of aircraft injured in other specified air transport accidents**
Fall in, on or from aircraft in air transport accident
EXCLUDES 1   accident while boarding or alighting aircraft (V97.1)

🆀 ☑ **V97.1XX- Person injured while boarding or alighting from aircraft**

⑤ **V97.2 Parachutist accident**

🆀 ☑ **V97.21X- Parachutist entangled in object**
Parachutist landing in tree

🆀 ☑ **V97.22X- Parachutist injured on landing**

🆀 ☑ **V97.29X- Other parachutist accident**

⑤ **V97.3 Person on ground injured in air transport accident**

🆀 ☑ **V97.31X- Hit by object falling from aircraft**
Hit by crashing aircraft
Injured by aircraft hitting house
Injured by aircraft hitting car

🆀 ☑ **V97.32X- Injured by rotating propeller**

🆀 ☑ **V97.33X- Sucked into jet engine**

🆀 ☑ **V97.39X- Other injury to person on ground due to air transport accident**

⑤ **V97.8 Other air transport accidents, not elsewhere classified**
EXCLUDES 1   aircraft accident NOS (V95.9)
exposure to changes in air pressure during ascent or descent (W94.-)

⑥ **V97.81 Air transport accident involving military aircraft**

🆀 7 **V97.810- Civilian aircraft involved in air transport accident with military aircraft**
Passenger in civilian aircraft injured due to accident with military aircraft

🆀 7 **V97.811- Civilian injured by military aircraft**

🆀 7 **V97.818- Other air transport accident involving military aircraft**

🆀 ☑ **V97.89X- Other air transport accidents, not elsewhere classified**
Injury from machinery on aircraft

Other and unspecified transport accidents (V98-V99)

EXCLUDES 1   vehicle accident, type of vehicle unspecified (V89.-)

④ **V98 Other specified transport accidents**

The appropriate 7th character is to be added to each code from category V98
A   initial encounter
D   subsequent encounter
S   sequela

★ New ▲ Revised Px Primary **SP** PDGM Px **SL** Low CoM **SH** High CoM 🆀 Quest. Encounter Ⓗ Hospice non-cancer Dx   Unspecified   **M** *Manifestation*

DecisionHealth's FY 2020 Complete Home Health ICD-10-CM Diagnosis Coding Manual

1819

!Q ☑ V98.0XX- **Accident to, on or involving cable-car, not on rails**
Caught or dragged by cable-car, not on rails
Fall or jump from cable-car, not on rails
Object thrown from or in cable-car, not on rails

!Q ☑ V98.1XX- **Accident to, on or involving land-yacht**

!Q ☑ V98.2XX- **Accident to, on or involving ice yacht**

!Q ☑ V98.3XX- **Accident to, on or involving ski lift**
Accident to, on or involving ski chair-lift
Accident to, on or involving ski-lift with gondola

!Q ☑ V98.8XX- **Other specified transport accidents**

!Q ☑ V99.XXX- **Unspecified transport accident**

> The appropriate 7th character is to be added to code V99
> A   initial encounter
> D   subsequent encounter
> S   sequela

Other external causes of accidental injury (W00-X58)

CODING TIPS ✓   Do not assign a code for other external causes of accidental injury as an external cause of morbidity when there is no injury coded on the claim.

Slipping, tripping, stumbling and falls (W00-W19)

EXCLUDES 1   assault involving a fall (Y01-Y02)
fall from animal (V80.-)
fall (in) (from) machinery (in operation) (W28-W31)
fall (in) (from) transport vehicle (V01-V99)
intentional self-harm involving a fall (X80-X81)

EXCLUDES 2   at risk for fall (history of fall) Z91.81
fall (in) (from) burning building (X00.-)
fall into fire (X00-X04, X08)

☒ W00   Fall due to ice and snow
> **INCLUDES**   pedestrian on foot falling (slipping) on ice and snow
> **EXCLUDES 1**   fall on (from) ice and snow involving pedestrian conveyance (V00.-)
> fall from stairs and steps not due to ice and snow (W10.-)

> The appropriate 7th character is to be added to each code from category W00
> A   initial encounter
> D   subsequent encounter
> S   sequela

!Q ☑ W00.0XX- **Fall on same level due to ice and snow**

!Q ☑ W00.1XX- **Fall from stairs and steps due to ice and snow**

!Q ☑ W00.2XX- **Other fall from one level to another due to ice and snow**

!Q ☑ W00.9XX- **Unspecified fall due to ice and snow**

☒ W01   Fall on same level from slipping, tripping and stumbling
> **INCLUDES**   fall on moving sidewalk
> **EXCLUDES 1**   fall due to bumping (striking) against object (W18.0-)
> fall in shower or bathtub (W18.2-)
> fall on same level NOS (W18.30)
> fall on same level from slipping, tripping and stumbling due to ice or snow (W00.0)
> fall off or from toilet (W18.1-)
> slipping, tripping and stumbling NOS (W18.40)
> slipping, tripping and stumbling without falling (W18.4-)

> The appropriate 7th character is to be added to each code from category W01
> A   initial encounter
> D   subsequent encounter
> S   sequela

!Q ☑ W01.0XX- **Fall on same level from slipping, tripping and stumbling without subsequent striking against object**
Falling over animal

☐ W01.1 Fall on same level from slipping, tripping and stumbling with subsequent striking against object

!Q ☑ W01.10X- **Fall on same level from slipping, tripping and stumbling with subsequent striking against unspecified object**

☐ W01.11 Fall on same level from slipping, tripping and stumbling with subsequent striking against sharp object

!Q ☑ W01.110- **Fall on same level from slipping, tripping and stumbling with subsequent striking against sharp glass**

!Q ☑ W01.111- **Fall on same level from slipping, tripping and stumbling with subsequent striking against power tool or machine**

!Q ☑ W01.118- **Fall on same level from slipping, tripping and stumbling with subsequent striking against other sharp object**

!Q ☑ W01.119- **Fall on same level from slipping, tripping and stumbling with subsequent striking against unspecified sharp object**

☐ W01.19 Fall on same level from slipping, tripping and stumbling with subsequent striking against other object

!Q ☑ W01.190- **Fall on same level from slipping, tripping and stumbling with subsequent striking against furniture**

!Q ☑ W01.198- **Fall on same level from slipping, tripping and stumbling with subsequent striking against other object**

!Q ☑ W03.XXX- **Other fall on same level due to collision with another person**

☒ 4th digit required   ☐ 5th digit required   ☐ 6th digit required   ☑ 7th digit required   ☑ 7th digit placeholder   ✚ Additional code   ⊟ Laterality

Chapter 20

V00-Y99

1820   DecisionHealth's FY 2020 Complete Home Health ICD-10-CM Diagnosis Coding Manual

Fall due to non-transport collision with other person

> **EXCLUDES 1** collision with another person without fall (W51)
> crushed or pushed by a crowd or human stampede (W52)
> fall involving pedestrian conveyance (V00-V09)
> fall due to ice or snow (W00)
> fall on same level NOS (W18.30)

The appropriate 7th character is to be added to code W03
A   initial encounter
D   subsequent encounter
S   sequela

IQ ☑ W04.XXX- Fall while being carried or supported by other persons
Accidentally dropped while being carried

The appropriate 7th character is to be added to code W04
A   initial encounter
D   subsequent encounter
S   sequela

☑ W05 Fall from non-moving wheelchair, nonmotorized scooter and motorized mobility scooter

> **EXCLUDES 1** fall from moving wheelchair (powered) (V00.811)
> fall from moving motorized mobility scooter (V00.831)
> fall from nonmotorized scooter (V00.141)

The appropriate 7th character is to be added to each code from category W05
A   initial encounter
D   subsequent encounter
S   sequela

IQ ☑ W05.0XX- Fall from non-moving wheelchair

IQ ☑ W05.1XX- Fall from non-moving nonmotorized scooter

IQ ☑ W05.2XX- Fall from non-moving motorized mobility scooter

IQ ☑ W06.XXX- Fall from bed

The appropriate 7th character is to be added to code W06
A   initial encounter
D   subsequent encounter
S   sequela

IQ ☑ W07.XXX- Fall from chair

The appropriate 7th character is to be added to code W07
A   initial encounter
D   subsequent encounter
S   sequela

IQ ☑ W08.XXX- Fall from other furniture

The appropriate 7th character is to be added to code W08
A   initial encounter
D   subsequent encounter
S   sequela

☑ W09 Fall on and from playground equipment

> **EXCLUDES 1** fall involving recreational machinery (W31)

The appropriate 7th character is to be added to each code from category W09
A   initial encounter
D   subsequent encounter
S   sequela

IQ ☑ W09.0XX- Fall on or from playground slide

IQ ☑ W09.1XX- Fall from playground swing

IQ ☑ W09.2XX- Fall on or from jungle gym

IQ ☑ W09.8XX- Fall on or from other playground equipment

☑ W10 Fall on and from stairs and steps

> **EXCLUDES 1** Fall from stairs and steps due to ice and snow (W00.1)

The appropriate 7th character is to be added to each code from category W10
A   initial encounter
D   subsequent encounter
S   sequela

IQ ☑ W10.0XX- Fall (on)(from) escalator

IQ ☑ W10.1XX- Fall (on)(from) sidewalk curb

IQ ☑ W10.2XX- Fall (on)(from) incline
Fall (on) (from) ramp

IQ ☑ W10.8XX- Fall (on) (from) other stairs and steps

IQ ☑ W10.9XX- Fall (on) (from) unspecified stairs and steps

IQ ☑ W11.XXX- Fall on and from ladder

The appropriate 7th character is to be added to code W11
A   initial encounter
D   subsequent encounter
S   sequela

IQ ☑ W12.XXX- Fall on and from scaffolding

The appropriate 7th character is to be added to code W12
A   initial encounter
D   subsequent encounter
S   sequela

☑ W13 Fall from, out of or through building or structure

The appropriate 7th character is to be added to each code from category W13
A   initial encounter
D   subsequent encounter
S   sequela

IQ ☑ W13.0XX- Fall from, out of or through balcony
Fall from, out of or through railing

IQ ☑ W13.1XX- Fall from, out of or through bridge

IQ ☑ W13.2XX- Fall from, out of or through roof

IQ ☑ W13.3XX- Fall through floor

IQ ☑ W13.4XX- Fall from, out of or through window

Chapter 20

V00-Y99

★ New ▲ Revised Px Primary SP PDGM Px SL Low CoM SH High CoM IQ Quest. Encounter H Hospice non-cancer Dx   Unspecified   M Manifestation

DecisionHealth's FY 2020 Complete Home Health ICD-10-CM Diagnosis Coding Manual

1821

EXCLUDES 2 fall with subsequent striking against sharp glass (W01.110)

[IQ] [☑] W13.8XX- Fall from, out of or through other building or structure
Fall from, out of or through viaduct
Fall from, out of or through wall
Fall from, out of or through flag-pole

[IQ] [☑] W13.9XX- Fall from, out of or through building, not otherwise specified
EXCLUDES 1 collapse of a building or structure (W20.-)
fall or jump from burning building or structure (X00.-)

[IQ] [☑] W14.XXX- Fall from tree

The appropriate 7th character is to be added to code W14
A   initial encounter
D   subsequent encounter
S   sequela

[IQ] [☑] W15.XXX- Fall from cliff

The appropriate 7th character is to be added to code W15
A   initial encounter
D   subsequent encounter
S   sequela

[4] W16 Fall, jump or diving into water
EXCLUDES 1 accidental non-watercraft drowning and submersion not involving fall (W65-W74)
effects of air pressure from diving (W94.-)
fall into water from watercraft (V90-V94)
hitting an object or against bottom when falling from watercraft (V94.0)
EXCLUDES 2 striking or hitting diving board (W21.4)

The appropriate 7th character is to be added to each code from category W16
A   initial encounter
D   subsequent encounter
S   sequela

[5] W16.0 Fall into swimming pool
Fall into swimming pool NOS
EXCLUDES 1 fall into empty swimming pool (W17.3)

[6] W16.01 Fall into swimming pool striking water surface

[IQ] [7] W16.011- Fall into swimming pool striking water surface causing drowning and submersion
EXCLUDES 1 drowning and submersion while in swimming pool without fall (W67)

[IQ] [7] W16.012- Fall into swimming pool striking water surface causing other injury

[6] W16.02 Fall into swimming pool striking bottom

[IQ] [7] W16.021- Fall into swimming pool striking bottom causing drowning and submersion

EXCLUDES 1 drowning and submersion while in swimming pool without fall (W67)

[IQ] [7] W16.022- Fall into swimming pool striking bottom causing other injury

[6] W16.03 Fall into swimming pool striking wall

[IQ] [7] W16.031- Fall into swimming pool striking wall causing drowning and submersion
EXCLUDES 1 drowning and submersion while in swimming pool without fall (W67)

[IQ] [7] W16.032- Fall into swimming pool striking wall causing other injury

[5] W16.1 Fall into natural body of water
Fall into lake
Fall into open sea
Fall into river
Fall into stream

[6] W16.11 Fall into natural body of water striking water surface

[IQ] [7] W16.111- Fall into natural body of water striking water surface causing drowning and submersion
EXCLUDES 1 drowning and submersion while in natural body of water without fall (W69)

[IQ] [7] W16.112- Fall into natural body of water striking water surface causing other injury

[6] W16.12 Fall into natural body of water striking bottom

[IQ] [7] W16.121- Fall into natural body of water striking bottom causing drowning and submersion
EXCLUDES 1 drowning and submersion while in natural body of water without fall (W69)

[IQ] [7] W16.122- Fall into natural body of water striking bottom causing other injury

[6] W16.13 Fall into natural body of water striking side

[IQ] [7] W16.131- Fall into natural body of water striking side causing drowning and submersion
EXCLUDES 1 drowning and submersion while in natural body of water without fall (W69)

[IQ] [7] W16.132- Fall into natural body of water striking side causing other injury

[5] W16.2 Fall in (into) filled bathtub or bucket of water

[6] W16.21 Fall in (into) filled bathtub
EXCLUDES 1 fall into empty bathtub (W18.2)

[IQ] [7] W16.211- Fall in (into) filled bathtub causing drowning and submersion

[4] 4th digit required   [5] 5th digit required   [6] 6th digit required   [7] 7th digit required   [☑] 7th digit placeholder   **+** Additional code   [≡] Laterality

1822   *DecisionHealth's* FY 2020 Complete Home Health ICD-10-CM Diagnosis Coding Manual

EXCLUDES 1 drowning and submersion while in filled bathtub without fall (W65)

!Q 7 W16.212- Fall in (into) filled bathtub causing other injury

6 W16.22 Fall in (into) bucket of water

!Q 7 W16.221- Fall in (into) bucket of water causing drowning and submersion

!Q 7 W16.222- Fall in (into) bucket of water causing other injury

5 W16.3 Fall into other water
Fall into fountain
Fall into reservoir

6 W16.31 Fall into other water striking water surface

!Q 7 W16.311- Fall into other water striking water surface causing drowning and submersion

EXCLUDES 1 drowning and submersion while in other water without fall (W73)

!Q 7 W16.312- Fall into other water striking water surface causing other injury

6 W16.32 Fall into other water striking bottom

!Q 7 W16.321- Fall into other water striking bottom causing drowning and submersion

EXCLUDES 1 drowning and submersion while in other water without fall (W73)

!Q 7 W16.322- Fall into other water striking bottom causing other injury

6 W16.33 Fall into other water striking wall

!Q 7 W16.331- Fall into other water striking wall causing drowning and submersion

EXCLUDES 1 drowning and submersion while in other water without fall (W73)

!Q 7 W16.332- Fall into other water striking wall causing other injury

5 W16.4 Fall into unspecified water

!Q 7 W16.41X- Fall into unspecified water causing drowning and submersion

!Q 7 W16.42X- Fall into unspecified water causing other injury

5 W16.5 Jumping or diving into swimming pool

6 W16.51 Jumping or diving into swimming pool striking water surface

!Q 7 W16.511- Jumping or diving into swimming pool striking water surface causing drowning and submersion

EXCLUDES 1 drowning and submersion while in swimming pool without jumping or diving (W67)

!Q 7 W16.512- Jumping or diving into swimming pool striking water surface causing other injury

6 W16.52 Jumping or diving into swimming pool striking bottom

!Q 7 W16.521- Jumping or diving into swimming pool striking bottom causing drowning and submersion

EXCLUDES 1 drowning and submersion while in swimming pool without jumping or diving (W67)

!Q 7 W16.522- Jumping or diving into swimming pool striking bottom causing other injury

6 W16.53 Jumping or diving into swimming pool striking wall

!Q 7 W16.531- Jumping or diving into swimming pool striking wall causing drowning and submersion

EXCLUDES 1 drowning and submersion while in swimming pool without jumping or diving (W67)

!Q 7 W16.532- Jumping or diving into swimming pool striking wall causing other injury

5 W16.6 Jumping or diving into natural body of water
Jumping or diving into lake
Jumping or diving into open sea
Jumping or diving into river
Jumping or diving into stream

6 W16.61 Jumping or diving into natural body of water striking water surface

!Q 7 W16.611- Jumping or diving into natural body of water striking water surface causing drowning and submersion

EXCLUDES 1 drowning and submersion while in natural body of water without jumping or diving (W69)

!Q 7 W16.612- Jumping or diving into natural body of water striking water surface causing other injury

6 W16.62 Jumping or diving into natural body of water striking bottom

!Q 7 W16.621- Jumping or diving into natural body of water striking bottom causing drowning and submersion

EXCLUDES 1 drowning and submersion while in natural body of water without jumping or diving (W69)

!Q 7 W16.622- Jumping or diving into natural body of water striking bottom causing other injury

5 W16.7 Jumping or diving from boat

Chapter 20

V00-Y99

★ New ▲ Revised **Px** Primary **SP** PDGM Px **SL** Low CoM **SH** High CoM **!Q** Quest. Encounter **H** Hospice non-cancer Dx **Unspecified** **M** *Manifestation*

DecisionHealth's FY 2020 Complete Home Health ICD-10-CM Diagnosis Coding Manual

1823

EXCLUDES 1 Fall from boat into water
-see watercraft accident
(V90-V94)

⑥ **W16.71 Jumping or diving from boat striking water surface**

IQ ⑦ **W16.711-** **Jumping or diving from boat striking water surface causing drowning and submersion**

IQ ⑦ **W16.712-** **Jumping or diving from boat striking water surface causing other injury**

⑥ **W16.72 Jumping or diving from boat striking bottom**

IQ ⑦ **W16.721-** **Jumping or diving from boat striking bottom causing drowning and submersion**

IQ ⑦ **W16.722-** **Jumping or diving from boat striking bottom causing other injury**

⑤ **W16.8 Jumping or diving into other water**
Jumping or diving into fountain
Jumping or diving into reservoir

⑥ **W16.81 Jumping or diving into other water striking water surface**

IQ ⑦ **W16.811-** **Jumping or diving into other water striking water surface causing drowning and submersion**
EXCLUDES 1 drowning and submersion while in other water without jumping or diving (W73)

IQ ⑦ **W16.812-** **Jumping or diving into other water striking water surface causing other injury**

⑥ **W16.82 Jumping or diving into other water striking bottom**

IQ ⑦ **W16.821-** **Jumping or diving into other water striking bottom causing drowning and submersion**
EXCLUDES 1 drowning and submersion while in other water without jumping or diving (W73)

IQ ⑦ **W16.822-** **Jumping or diving into other water striking bottom causing other injury**

⑥ **W16.83 Jumping or diving into other water striking wall**

IQ ⑦ **W16.831-** **Jumping or diving into other water striking wall causing drowning and submersion**
EXCLUDES 1 drowning and submersion while in other water without jumping or diving (W73)

IQ ⑦ **W16.832-** **Jumping or diving into other water striking wall causing other injury**

⑤ **W16.9 Jumping or diving into unspecified water**

IQ ⑦ **W16.91X-** **Jumping or diving into unspecified water causing drowning and submersion**

IQ ⑦ **W16.92X-** **Jumping or diving into unspecified water causing other injury**

④ **W17 Other fall from one level to another**

The appropriate 7th character is to be added to each code from category W17
A initial encounter
D subsequent encounter
S sequela

IQ ⑦ **W17.0XX-** **Fall into well**

IQ ⑦ **W17.1XX-** **Fall into storm drain or manhole**

IQ ⑦ **W17.2XX-** **Fall into hole**
Fall into pit

IQ ⑦ **W17.3XX-** **Fall into empty swimming pool**
EXCLUDES 1 fall into filled swimming pool (W16.0-)

IQ ⑦ **W17.4XX-** **Fall from dock**

⑤ **W17.8 Other fall from one level to another**

IQ ⑦ **W17.81X-** **Fall down embankment (hill)**

IQ ⑦ **W17.82X-** **Fall from (out of) grocery cart**
Fall due to grocery cart tipping over

IQ ⑦ **W17.89X-** **Other fall from one level to another**
Fall from cherry picker
Fall from lifting device
Fall from mobile elevated work platform [MEWP]
Fall from sky lift

④ **W18 Other slipping, tripping and stumbling and falls**

The appropriate 7th character is to be added to each code from category W18
A initial encounter
D subsequent encounter
S sequela

⑤ **W18.0 Fall due to bumping against object**
Striking against object with subsequent fall
EXCLUDES 1 fall on same level due to slipping, tripping, or stumbling with subsequent striking against object (W01.1-)

IQ ⑦ **W18.00X-** **Striking against unspecified object with subsequent fall**

IQ ⑦ **W18.01X-** **Striking against sports equipment with subsequent fall**

IQ ⑦ **W18.02X-** **Striking against glass with subsequent fall**

IQ ⑦ **W18.09X-** **Striking against other object with subsequent fall**

⑤ **W18.1 Fall from or off toilet**

IQ ⑦ **W18.11X-** **Fall from or off toilet without subsequent striking against object**
Fall from (off) toilet NOS

IQ ⑦ **W18.12X-** **Fall from or off toilet with subsequent striking against object**

IQ ⑦ **W18.2XX-** **Fall in (into) shower or empty bathtub**
EXCLUDES 1 fall in full bathtub causing drowning or submersion (W16.21-)

⑤ **W18.3 Other and unspecified fall on same level**

---

④4th digit required　⑤5th digit required　⑥6th digit required　⑦7th digit required　⑦ 7th digit placeholder　✚Additional code　⊟Laterality

IQ ☑ W18.30X- Fall on same level, unspecified

IQ ☑ W18.31X- Fall on same level due to stepping on an object

Fall on same level due to stepping on an animal

EXCLUDES 1 slipping, tripping and stumbling without fall due to stepping on animal (W18.41)

IQ ☑ W18.39X- Other fall on same level

⑤ W18.4 Slipping, tripping and stumbling without falling

EXCLUDES 1 collision with another person without fall (W51)

IQ ☑ W18.40X- Slipping, tripping and stumbling without falling, unspecified

IQ ☑ W18.41X- Slipping, tripping and stumbling without falling due to stepping on object

Slipping, tripping and stumbling without falling due to stepping on animal

EXCLUDES 1 slipping, tripping and stumbling with fall due to stepping on animal (W18.31)

IQ ☑ W18.42X- Slipping, tripping and stumbling without falling due to stepping into hole or opening

IQ ☑ W18.43X- Slipping, tripping and stumbling without falling due to stepping from one level to another

IQ ☑ W18.49X- Other slipping, tripping and stumbling without falling

IQ ☑ W19.XXX- Unspecified fall

Accidental fall NOS

The appropriate 7th character is to be added to code W19
A   initial encounter
D   subsequent encounter
S   sequela

Exposure to inanimate mechanical forces (W20-W49)

EXCLUDES 1 assault (X92-Y09)
contact or collision with animals or persons (W50-W64)
exposure to inanimate mechanical forces involving military or war operations (Y36.-, Y37.-)
intentional self-harm (X71-X83)

④ W20 Struck by thrown, projected or falling object

Code first any associated:
cataclysm (X34-X39)
lightning strike (T75.00)

EXCLUDES 1 falling object in machinery accident (W24, W28-W31)
falling object in transport accident (V01-V99)
object set in motion by explosion (W35-W40)
object set in motion by firearm (W32-W34)
struck by thrown sports equipment (W21.-)

The appropriate 7th character is to be added to each code from category W20
A   initial encounter
D   subsequent encounter
S   sequela

IQ ☑ W20.0XX- Struck by falling object in cave-in

EXCLUDES 2 asphyxiation due to cave-in (T71.21)

IQ ☑ W20.1XX- Struck by object due to collapse of building

EXCLUDES 1 struck by object due to collapse of burning building (X00.2, X02.2)

IQ ☑ W20.8XX- Other cause of strike by thrown, projected or falling object

EXCLUDES 1 struck by thrown sports equipment (W21.-)

④ W21 Striking against or struck by sports equipment

EXCLUDES 1 assault with sports equipment (Y08.0-)
striking against or struck by sports equipment with subsequent fall (W18.01)

The appropriate 7th character is to be added to each code from category W21
A   initial encounter
D   subsequent encounter
S   sequela

⑤ W21.0 Struck by hit or thrown ball

IQ ☑ W21.00X- Struck by hit or thrown ball, unspecified type

IQ ☑ W21.01X- Struck by football

IQ ☑ W21.02X- Struck by soccer ball

IQ ☑ W21.03X- Struck by baseball

IQ ☑ W21.04X- Struck by golf ball

IQ ☑ W21.05X- Struck by basketball

IQ ☑ W21.06X- Struck by volleyball

IQ ☑ W21.07X- Struck by softball

IQ ☑ W21.09X- Struck by other hit or thrown ball

⑤ W21.1 Struck by bat, racquet or club

IQ ☑ W21.11X- Struck by baseball bat

IQ ☑ W21.12X- Struck by tennis racquet

IQ ☑ W21.13X- Struck by golf club

IQ ☑ W21.19X- Struck by other bat, racquet or club

⑤ W21.2 Struck by hockey stick or puck

⑥ W21.21 Struck by hockey stick

IQ ☑ W21.210- Struck by ice hockey stick

IQ ☑ W21.211- Struck by field hockey stick

⑥ W21.22 Struck by hockey puck

IQ ☑ W21.220- Struck by ice hockey puck

IQ ☑ W21.221- Struck by field hockey puck

⑤ W21.3 Struck by sports foot wear

IQ ☑ W21.31X- Struck by shoe cleats
Stepped on by shoe cleats

IQ ☑ W21.32X- Struck by skate blades
Skated over by skate blades

IQ ☑ W21.39X- Struck by other sports foot wear

IQ ✚ ☑ W21.4XX- Striking against diving board

★ New ▲ Revised Px Primary SP PDGM Px SL Low CoM SH High CoM IQ Quest. Encounter H Hospice non-cancer Dx   Unspecified   M *Manifestation*

DecisionHealth's FY 2020 Complete Home Health ICD-10-CM Diagnosis Coding Manual

1825

Use additional code for subsequent falling into water, if applicable (W16.-)

⑤ W21.8 Striking against or struck by other sports equipment

!Q ☑ W21.81X- Striking against or struck by football helmet

!Q ☑ W21.89X- Striking against or struck by other sports equipment

!Q ☑ W21.9XX- Striking against or struck by unspecified sports equipment

④ W22 Striking against or struck by other objects
> EXCLUDES 1   striking against or struck by object with subsequent fall (W18.09)

> The appropriate 7th character is to be added to each code from category W22
> A   initial encounter
> D   subsequent encounter
> S   sequela

⑤ W22.0 Striking against stationary object
> EXCLUDES 1   striking against stationary sports equipment (W21.8)

!Q ☑ W22.01X- Walked into wall

!Q ☑ W22.02X- Walked into lamppost

!Q ☑ W22.03X- Walked into furniture

⑥ W22.04 Striking against wall of swimming pool

!Q ⑦ W22.041- Striking against wall of swimming pool causing drowning and submersion
> EXCLUDES 1   drowning and submersion while swimming without striking against wall (W67)

!Q ⑦ W22.042- Striking against wall of swimming pool causing other injury

!Q ☑ W22.09X- Striking against other stationary object

⑤ W22.1 Striking against or struck by automobile airbag

!Q ☑ W22.10X- Striking against or struck by unspecified automobile airbag

!Q ☑ W22.11X- Striking against or struck by driver side automobile airbag

!Q ☑ W22.12X- Striking against or struck by front passenger side automobile airbag

!Q ☑ W22.19X- Striking against or struck by other automobile airbag

!Q ☑ W22.8XX- Striking against or struck by other objects
Striking against or struck by object NOS
> EXCLUDES 1   struck by thrown, projected or falling object (W20.-)

④ W23 Caught, crushed, jammed or pinched in or between objects
> EXCLUDES 1   injury caused by cutting or piercing instruments (W25-W27)
> injury caused by firearms malfunction (W32.1, W33.1-, W34.1-)

injury caused by lifting and transmission devices (W24.-)
injury caused by machinery (W28-W31)
injury caused by nonpowered hand tools (W27.-)
injury caused by transport vehicle being used as a means of transportation (V01-V99)
injury caused by struck by thrown, projected or falling object (W20.-)

> The appropriate 7th character is to be added to each code from category W23
> A   initial encounter
> D   subsequent encounter
> S   sequela

!Q ☑ W23.0XX- Caught, crushed, jammed, or pinched between moving objects

!Q ☑ W23.1XX- Caught, crushed, jammed, or pinched between stationary objects

④ W24 Contact with lifting and transmission devices, not elsewhere classified
> EXCLUDES 1   transport accidents (V01-V99)

> The appropriate 7th character is to be added to each code from category W24
> A   initial encounter
> D   subsequent encounter
> S   sequela

!Q ☑ W24.0XX- Contact with lifting devices, not elsewhere classified
Contact with chain hoist
Contact with drive belt
Contact with pulley (block)

!Q ☑ W24.1XX- Contact with transmission devices, not elsewhere classified
Contact with transmission belt or cable

▲ !Q ☑ W25.XXX- Contact with sharp glass
Code first any associated:
injury due to flying glass from explosion or firearm discharge (W32-W40)
transport accident (V00-V99)
> EXCLUDES 1   fall on same level due to slipping, tripping and stumbling with subsequent striking against sharp glass (W01.110)
> striking against sharp glass with subsequent fall (W18.02)
> EXCLUDES 2   glass embedded in skin (W45)

> The appropriate 7th character is to be added to code W25
> A   initial encounter
> D   subsequent encounter
> S   sequela

④ W26 Contact with other sharp objects
> EXCLUDES 2   sharp object (s) embedded in skin (W45)

---

④ 4th digit required   ⑤ 5th digit required   ⑥ 6th digit required   ⑦ 7th digit required   ☑ 7th digit placeholder   ✚ Additional code   ⊟ Laterality

1826   DecisionHealth's FY 2020 Complete Home Health ICD-10-CM Diagnosis Coding Manual

The appropriate 7th character is to be added to each code from category W26
A   initial encounter
D   subsequent encounter
S   sequela

!Q ☑ W26.0XX- Contact with knife
    EXCLUDES 1   contact with electric knife (W29.1)
!Q ☑ W26.1XX- Contact with sword or dagger
!Q ☑ W26.2XX- Contact with edge of stiff paper
    Paper cut
!Q ☑ W26.8XX- Contact with other sharp object(s), not elsewhere classified
    Contact with tin can lid
!Q ☑ W26.9XX- Contact with unspecified sharp object(s)

④ W27   Contact with nonpowered hand tool

The appropriate 7th character is to be added to each code from category W27
A   initial encounter
D   subsequent encounter
S   sequela

!Q ☑ W27.0XX- Contact with workbench tool
    Contact with auger
    Contact with axe
    Contact with chisel
    Contact with handsaw
    Contact with screwdriver
!Q ☑ W27.1XX- Contact with garden tool
    Contact with hoe
    Contact with nonpowered lawn mower
    Contact with pitchfork
    Contact with rake
!Q ☑ W27.2XX- Contact with scissors
!Q ☑ W27.3XX- Contact with needle (sewing)
    EXCLUDES 1   contact with hypodermic needle (W46.-)
!Q ☑ W27.4XX- Contact with kitchen utensil
    Contact with fork
    Contact with ice-pick
    Contact with can-opener NOS
!Q ☑ W27.5XX- Contact with paper-cutter
!Q ☑ W27.8XX- Contact with other nonpowered hand tool
    Contact with nonpowered sewing machine
    Contact with shovel
!Q ☑ W28.XXX- Contact with powered lawn mower
    Powered lawn mower (commercial) (residential)
    EXCLUDES 1   contact with nonpowered lawn mower (W27.1)
    EXCLUDES 2   exposure to electric current (W86.-)

The appropriate 7th character is to be added to code W28
A   initial encounter
D   subsequent encounter
S   sequela

④ W29   Contact with other powered hand tools and household machinery
    EXCLUDES 1   contact with commercial machinery (W31.82)

contact with hot household appliance (X15)
contact with nonpowered hand tool (W27.-)
exposure to electric current (W86)

The appropriate 7th character is to be added to each code from category W29
A   initial encounter
D   subsequent encounter
S   sequela

!Q ☑ W29.0XX- Contact with powered kitchen appliance
    Contact with blender
    Contact with can-opener
    Contact with garbage disposal
    Contact with mixer
!Q ☑ W29.1XX- Contact with electric knife
!Q ☑ W29.2XX- Contact with other powered household machinery
    Contact with electric fan
    Contact with powered dryer (clothes) (powered) (spin)
    Contact with washing-machine
    Contact with sewing machine
!Q ☑ W29.3XX- Contact with powered garden and outdoor hand tools and machinery
    Contact with chainsaw
    Contact with edger
    Contact with garden cultivator (tiller)
    Contact with hedge trimmer
    Contact with other powered garden tool
    EXCLUDES 1   contact with powered lawn mower (W28)
!Q ☑ W29.4XX- Contact with nail gun
!Q ☑ W29.8XX- Contact with other powered hand tools and household machinery
    Contact with do-it-yourself tool NOS

④ W30   Contact with agricultural machinery
    INCLUDES   animal-powered farm machine
    EXCLUDES 1   agricultural transport vehicle accident (V01-V99)
    explosion of grain store (W40.8)
    exposure to electric current (W86.-)

The appropriate 7th character is to be added to each code from category W30
A   initial encounter
D   subsequent encounter
S   sequela

!Q ☑ W30.0XX- Contact with combine harvester
    Contact with reaper
    Contact with thresher
!Q ☑ W30.1XX- Contact with power take-off devices (PTO)
!Q ☑ W30.2XX- Contact with hay derrick
!Q ☑ W30.3XX- Contact with grain storage elevator
    EXCLUDES 1   explosion of grain store (W40.8)
⑤ W30.8 Contact with other specified agricultural machinery
!Q ☑ W30.81X- Contact with agricultural transport vehicle in stationary use

Chapter 20

V00-Y99

★ New ▲ Revised Px Primary **SP** PDGM Px **SL** Low CoM **SH** High CoM **!Q** Quest. Encounter Ⓗ Hospice non-cancer Dx   Unspecified   **M** *Manifestation*

DecisionHealth's FY 2020 Complete Home Health ICD-10-CM Diagnosis Coding Manual

1827

Contact with agricultural transport vehicle under repair, not on public roadway

> **EXCLUDES 1**   agricultural transport vehicle accident (V01-V99)

IQ ☑ W30.89X- Contact with other specified agricultural machinery

IQ ☑ W30.9XX- Contact with unspecified agricultural machinery

Contact with farm machinery NOS

4 W31 Contact with other and unspecified machinery

> **EXCLUDES 1**   contact with agricultural machinery (W30.-)
> contact with machinery in transport under own power or being towed by a vehicle (V01-V99)
> exposure to electric current (W86)

The appropriate 7th character is to be added to each code from category W31
A   initial encounter
D   subsequent encounter
S   sequela

IQ ☑ W31.0XX- Contact with mining and earth-drilling machinery

Contact with bore or drill (land) (seabed)
Contact with shaft hoist
Contact with shaft lift
Contact with undercutter

IQ ☑ W31.1XX- Contact with metalworking machines

Contact with abrasive wheel
Contact with forging machine
Contact with lathe
Contact with mechanical shears
Contact with metal drilling machine
Contact with milling machine
Contact with power press
Contact with rolling-mill
Contact with metal sawing machine

IQ ☑ W31.2XX- Contact with powered woodworking and forming machines

Contact with band saw
Contact with bench saw
Contact with circular saw
Contact with molding machine
Contact with overhead plane
Contact with powered saw
Contact with radial saw
Contact with sander

> **EXCLUDES 1**   nonpowered woodworking tools (W27.0)

IQ ☑ W31.3XX- Contact with prime movers

Contact with gas turbine
Contact with internal combustion engine
Contact with steam engine
Contact with water driven turbine

5 W31.8 Contact with other specified machinery

IQ ☑ W31.81X- Contact with recreational machinery

Contact with roller coaster

IQ ☑ W31.82X- Contact with other commercial machinery

Contact with commercial electric fan
Contact with commercial kitchen appliances
Contact with commercial powered dryer (clothes) (powered) (spin)
Contact with commercial washing-machine
Contact with commercial sewing machine

> **EXCLUDES 1**   contact with household machinery (W29.-)
> contact with powered lawn mower (W28)

IQ ☑ W31.83X- Contact with special construction vehicle in stationary use

Contact with special construction vehicle under repair, not on public roadway

> **EXCLUDES 1**   special construction vehicle accident (V01-V99)

IQ ☑ W31.89X- Contact with other specified machinery

IQ ☑ W31.9XX- Contact with unspecified machinery

Contact with machinery NOS

4 W32 Accidental handgun discharge and malfunction

> **INCLUDES**   accidental discharge and malfunction of gun for single hand use
> accidental discharge and malfunction of pistol
> accidental discharge and malfunction of revolver
> Handgun discharge and malfunction NOS

> **EXCLUDES 1**   accidental airgun discharge and malfunction (W34.010, W34.110)
> accidental BB gun discharge and malfunction (W34.010, W34.110)
> accidental pellet gun discharge and malfunction (W34.010, W34.110)
> accidental shotgun discharge and malfunction (W33.01, W33.11)
> assault by handgun discharge (X93)
> handgun discharge involving legal intervention (Y35.0-)
> handgun discharge involving military or war operations (Y36.4-)
> intentional self-harm by handgun discharge (X72)
> Very pistol discharge and malfunction (W34.09, W34.19)

4 4th digit required   5 5th digit required   6 6th digit required   7 7th digit required   ☑ 7th digit placeholder   ✚ Additional code   ⊟ Laterality

1828   *DecisionHealth's* FY 2020 Complete Home Health ICD-10-CM Diagnosis Coding Manual

The appropriate 7th character is to be added to each code from category W32
A   initial encounter
D   subsequent encounter
S   sequela

IQ ☑ W32.0XX- **Accidental handgun discharge**

IQ ☑ W32.1XX- **Accidental handgun malfunction**
Injury due to explosion of handgun (parts)
Injury due to malfunction of mechanism or component of handgun
Injury due to recoil of handgun
Powder burn from handgun

④ W33 **Accidental rifle, shotgun and larger firearm discharge and malfunction**

INCLUDES   rifle, shotgun and larger firearm discharge and malfunction NOS

EXCLUDES 1   accidental airgun discharge and malfunction (W34.010, W34.110)
accidental BB gun discharge and malfunction (W34.010, W34.110)
accidental handgun discharge and malfunction (W32.-)
accidental pellet gun discharge and malfunction (W34.010, W34.110)
assault by rifle, shotgun and larger firearm discharge (X94)
firearm discharge involving legal intervention (Y35.0-)
firearm discharge involving military or war operations (Y36.4-)
intentional self-harm by rifle, shotgun and larger firearm discharge (X73)

The appropriate 7th character is to be added to each code from category W33
A   initial encounter
D   subsequent encounter
S   sequela

⑤ W33.0 **Accidental rifle, shotgun and larger firearm discharge**

IQ ☑ W33.00X- **Accidental discharge of unspecified larger firearm**
Discharge of unspecified larger firearm NOS

IQ ☑ W33.01X- **Accidental discharge of shotgun**
Discharge of shotgun NOS

IQ ☑ W33.02X- **Accidental discharge of hunting rifle**
Discharge of hunting rifle NOS

IQ ☑ W33.03X- **Accidental discharge of machine gun**
Discharge of machine gun NOS

IQ ☑ W33.09X- **Accidental discharge of other larger firearm**
Discharge of other larger firearm NOS

⑤ W33.1 **Accidental rifle, shotgun and larger firearm malfunction**

Injury due to explosion of rifle, shotgun and larger firearm (parts)
Injury due to malfunction of mechanism or component of rifle, shotgun and larger firearm
Injury due to piercing, cutting, crushing or pinching due to (by) slide trigger mechanism, scope or other gun part
Injury due to recoil of rifle, shotgun and larger firearm
Powder burn from rifle, shotgun and larger firearm

IQ ☑ W33.10X- **Accidental malfunction of unspecified larger firearm**
Malfunction of unspecified larger firearm NOS

IQ ☑ W33.11X- **Accidental malfunction of shotgun**
Malfunction of shotgun NOS

IQ ☑ W33.12X- **Accidental malfunction of hunting rifle**
Malfunction of hunting rifle NOS

IQ ☑ W33.13X- **Accidental malfunction of machine gun**
Malfunction of machine gun NOS

IQ ☑ W33.19X- **Accidental malfunction of other larger firearm**
Malfunction of other larger firearm NOS

④ W34 **Accidental discharge and malfunction from other and unspecified firearms and guns**

The appropriate 7th character is to be added to each code from category W34
A   initial encounter
D   subsequent encounter
S   sequela

⑤ W34.0 **Accidental discharge from other and unspecified firearms and guns**

IQ ☑ W34.00X- **Accidental discharge from unspecified firearms or gun**
Discharge from firearm NOS
Gunshot wound NOS
Shot NOS

⑥ W34.01 **Accidental discharge of gas, air or spring-operated guns**

IQ ⑦ W34.010- **Accidental discharge of airgun**
Accidental discharge of BB gun
Accidental discharge of pellet gun

IQ ⑦ W34.011- **Accidental discharge of paintball gun**
Accidental injury due to paintball discharge

IQ ⑦ W34.018- **Accidental discharge of other gas, air or spring-operated gun**

IQ ☑ W34.09X- **Accidental discharge from other specified firearms**
Accidental discharge from Very pistol [flare]

⑤ W34.1 **Accidental malfunction from other and unspecified firearms and guns**

IQ ☑ W34.10X- **Accidental malfunction from unspecified firearms or gun**
Firearm malfunction NOS

⑥ W34.11 **Accidental malfunction of gas, air or spring-operated guns**

IQ ⑦ W34.110- **Accidental malfunction of airgun**
Accidental malfunction of BB gun

★ New ▲ Revised Px Primary SP PDGM Px SL Low CoM SH High CoM IQ Quest. Encounter H Hospice non-cancer Dx Unspecified M Manifestation

DecisionHealth's FY 2020 Complete Home Health ICD-10-CM Diagnosis Coding Manual

1829

Accidental malfunction of pellet gun

IQ 7 W34.111- Accidental malfunction of paintball gun
Accidental injury due to paintball gun malfunction

IQ 7 W34.118- Accidental malfunction of other gas, air or spring-operated gun

IQ ✓ W34.19X- Accidental malfunction from other specified firearms
Accidental malfunction from Very pistol [flare]

IQ ✓ W35.XXX- Explosion and rupture of boiler
EXCLUDES 1 explosion and rupture of boiler on watercraft (V93.4)

The appropriate 7th character is to be added to code W35
A   initial encounter
D   subsequent encounter
S   sequela

4 W36 Explosion and rupture of gas cylinder

The appropriate 7th character is to be added to each code from category W36
A   initial encounter
D   subsequent encounter
S   sequela

IQ ✓ W36.1XX- Explosion and rupture of aerosol can

IQ ✓ W36.2XX- Explosion and rupture of air tank

IQ ✓ W36.3XX- Explosion and rupture of pressurized-gas tank

IQ ✓ W36.8XX- Explosion and rupture of other gas cylinder

IQ ✓ W36.9XX- Explosion and rupture of unspecified gas cylinder

4 W37 Explosion and rupture of pressurized tire, pipe or hose

The appropriate 7th character is to be added to each code from category W37
A   initial encounter
D   subsequent encounter
S   sequela

IQ ✓ W37.0XX- Explosion of bicycle tire

IQ ✓ W37.8XX- Explosion and rupture of other pressurized tire, pipe or hose

IQ ✓ W38.XXX- Explosion·and rupture of other specified pressurized devices

The appropriate 7th character is to be added to code W38
A   initial encounter
D   subsequent encounter
S   sequela

IQ ✓ W39.XXX- Discharge of firework

The appropriate 7th character is to be added to code W39
A   initial encounter
D   subsequent encounter
S   sequela

4 W40 Explosion of other materials
EXCLUDES 1 assault by explosive material (X96)

explosion involving legal intervention (Y35.1-)
explosion involving military or war operations (Y36.0-, Y36.2-)
intentional self-harm by explosive material (X75)

The appropriate 7th character is to be added to each code from category W40
A   initial encounter
D   subsequent encounter
S   sequela

IQ ✓ W40.0XX- Explosion of blasting material
Explosion of blasting cap
Explosion of detonator
Explosion of dynamite
Explosion of explosive (any) used in blasting operations

IQ ✓ W40.1XX- Explosion of explosive gases
Explosion of acetylene
Explosion of butane
Explosion of coal gas
Explosion in mine NOS
Explosion of explosive gas
Explosion of fire damp
Explosion of gasoline fumes
Explosion of methane
Explosion of propane

IQ ✓ W40.8XX- Explosion of other specified explosive materials
Explosion in dump NOS
Explosion in factory NOS
Explosion in grain store
Explosion in munitions
EXCLUDES 1 explosion involving legal intervention (Y35.1-)
explosion involving military or war operations (Y36.0-, Y36.2-)

IQ ✓ W40.9XX- Explosion of unspecified explosive materials
Explosion NOS

4 W42 Exposure to noise

The appropriate 7th character is to be added to each code from category W42
A   initial encounter
D   subsequent encounter
S   sequela

IQ ✓ W42.0XX- Exposure to supersonic waves

IQ ✓ W42.9XX- Exposure to other noise
Exposure to sound waves NOS

4 W45 Foreign body or object entering through skin
INCLUDES foreign body or object embedded in skin
nail embedded in skin
EXCLUDES 2 contact with hand tools (nonpowered) (powered) (W27-W29)
contact with other sharp object (s) (W26.-)
contact with sharp glass (W25.-)
struck by objects (W20-W22)

4 4th digit required   **5** 5th digit required   **6** 6th digit required   **7** 7th digit required   **✓** 7th digit placeholder   **+** Additional code   **⊟** Laterality

1830   *DecisionHealth's* FY 2020 Complete Home Health ICD-10-CM Diagnosis Coding Manual

The appropriate 7th character is to be added to each code from category W45
A   initial encounter
D   subsequent encounter
S   sequela

IQ ☑ W45.0XX- **Nail entering through skin**

IQ ☑ W45.8XX- **Other foreign body or object entering through skin**
Splinter in skin NOS

4 W46 **Contact with hypodermic needle**

The appropriate 7th character is to be added to each code from category W46
A   initial encounter
D   subsequent encounter
S   sequela

IQ ☑ W46.0XX- **Contact with hypodermic needle**
Hypodermic needle stick NOS

IQ ☑ W46.1XX- **Contact with contaminated hypodermic needle**

4 W49 **Exposure to other inanimate mechanical forces**
   INCLUDES exposure to abnormal gravitational [G] forces
exposure to inanimate mechanical forces NEC
   EXCLUDES 1 exposure to inanimate mechanical forces involving military or war operations (Y36.-, Y37.-)

The appropriate 7th character is to be added to each code from category W49
A   initial encounter
D   subsequent encounter
S   sequela

5 W49.0 **Item causing external constriction**

IQ ☑ W49.01X- **Hair causing external constriction**

IQ ☑ W49.02X- **String or thread causing external constriction**

IQ ☑ W49.03X- **Rubber band causing external constriction**

IQ ☑ W49.04X- **Ring or other jewelry causing external constriction**

IQ ☑ W49.09X- **Other specified item causing external constriction**

IQ ☑ W49.9XX- **Exposure to other inanimate mechanical forces**

Exposure to animate mechanical forces (W50-W64)

   EXCLUDES 1 Toxic effect of contact with venomous animals and plants (T63.-)

4 W50 **Accidental hit, strike, kick, twist, bite or scratch by another person**
   INCLUDES hit, strike, kick, twist, bite, or scratch by another person NOS
   EXCLUDES 1 assault by bodily force (Y04)
struck by objects (W20-W22)

The appropriate 7th character is to be added to each code from category W50
A   initial encounter
D   subsequent encounter
S   sequela

IQ ☑ W50.0XX- **Accidental hit or strike by another person**
Hit or strike by another person NOS

IQ ☑ W50.1XX- **Accidental kick by another person**
Kick by another person NOS

IQ ☑ W50.2XX- **Accidental twist by another person**
Twist by another person NOS

IQ ☑ W50.3XX- **Accidental bite by another person**
Human bite
Bite by another person NOS

IQ ☑ W50.4XX- **Accidental scratch by another person**
Scratch by another person NOS

IQ ☑ W51.XXX- **Accidental striking against or bumped into by another person**
   EXCLUDES 1 assault by striking against or bumping into by another person (Y04.2)
fall due to collision with another person (W03)

The appropriate 7th character is to be added to code W51
A   initial encounter
D   subsequent encounter
S   sequela

IQ ☑ W52.XXX- **Crushed, pushed or stepped on by crowd or human stampede**
Crushed, pushed or stepped on by crowd or human stampede with or without fall

The appropriate 7th character is to be added to code W52
A   initial encounter
D   subsequent encounter
S   sequela

4 W53 **Contact with rodent**
   INCLUDES contact with saliva, feces or urine of rodent

The appropriate 7th character is to be added to each code from category W53
A   initial encounter
D   subsequent encounter
S   sequela

5 W53.0 **Contact with mouse**

IQ ☑ W53.01X- **Bitten by mouse**

IQ ☑ W53.09X- **Other contact with mouse**

5 W53.1 **Contact with rat**

IQ ☑ W53.11X- **Bitten by rat**

IQ ☑ W53.19X- **Other contact with rat**

5 W53.2 **Contact with squirrel**

IQ ☑ W53.21X- **Bitten by squirrel**

IQ ☑ W53.29X- **Other contact with squirrel**

5 W53.8 **Contact with other rodent**

IQ ☑ W53.81X- **Bitten by other rodent**

IQ ☑ W53.89X- **Other contact with other rodent**

4 W54 **Contact with dog**
   INCLUDES contact with saliva, feces or urine of dog

★ New ▲ Revised **Px** Primary **SP** PDGM Px **SL** Low CoM **SH** High CoM **IQ** Quest. Encounter **H** Hospice non-cancer Dx   Unspecified   **M** *Manifestation*

DecisionHealth's FY 2020 Complete Home Health ICD-10-CM Diagnosis Coding Manual

1831

The appropriate 7th character is to be added to each code from category W54
A   initial encounter
D   subsequent encounter
S   sequela

🔲 ☑ **W54.0XX-** **Bitten by dog**

🔲 ☑ **W54.1XX-** **Struck by dog**
    Knocked over by dog

🔲 ☑ **W54.8XX-** **Other contact with dog**

④ **W55** **Contact with other mammals**

    INCLUDES   contact with saliva, feces or urine of mammal

    EXCLUDES 1   animal being ridden- see transport accidents
        bitten or struck by dog (W54)
        bitten or struck by rodent (W53.-)
        contact with marine mammals (W56.-)

The appropriate 7th character is to be added to each code from category W55
A   initial encounter
D   subsequent encounter
S   sequela

⑤ **W55.0 Contact with cat**

🔲 ☑ **W55.01X-** **Bitten by cat**

🔲 ☑ **W55.03X-** **Scratched by cat**

🔲 ☑ **W55.09X-** **Other contact with cat**

⑤ **W55.1 Contact with horse**

🔲 ☑ **W55.11X-** **Bitten by horse**

🔲 ☑ **W55.12X-** **Struck by horse**

🔲 ☑ **W55.19X-** **Other contact with horse**

⑤ **W55.2 Contact with cow**
    Contact with bull

🔲 ☑ **W55.21X-** **Bitten by cow**

🔲 ☑ **W55.22X-** **Struck by cow**
    Gored by bull

🔲 ☑ **W55.29X-** **Other contact with cow**

⑤ **W55.3 Contact with other hoof stock**
    Contact with goats
    Contact with sheep

🔲 ☑ **W55.31X-** **Bitten by other hoof stock**

🔲 ☑ **W55.32X-** **Struck by other hoof stock**
    Gored by goat
    Gored by ram

🔲 ☑ **W55.39X-** **Other contact with other hoof stock**

⑤ **W55.4 Contact with pig**

🔲 ☑ **W55.41X-** **Bitten by pig**

🔲 ☑ **W55.42X-** **Struck by pig**

🔲 ☑ **W55.49X-** **Other contact with pig**

⑤ **W55.5 Contact with raccoon**

🔲 ☑ **W55.51X-** **Bitten by raccoon**

🔲 ☑ **W55.52X-** **Struck by raccoon**

🔲 ☑ **W55.59X-** **Other contact with raccoon**

⑤ **W55.8 Contact with other mammals**

🔲 ☑ **W55.81X-** **Bitten by other mammals**

🔲 ☑ **W55.82X-** **Struck by other mammals**

🔲 ☑ **W55.89X-** **Other contact with other mammals**

④ **W56** **Contact with nonvenomous marine animal**

    EXCLUDES 1   contact with venomous marine animal (T63.-)

The appropriate 7th character is to be added to each code from category W56
A   initial encounter
D   subsequent encounter
S   sequela

⑤ **W56.0 Contact with dolphin**

🔲 ☑ **W56.01X-** **Bitten by dolphin**

🔲 ☑ **W56.02X-** **Struck by dolphin**

🔲 ☑ **W56.09X-** **Other contact with dolphin**

⑤ **W56.1 Contact with sea lion**

🔲 ☑ **W56.11X-** **Bitten by sea lion**

🔲 ☑ **W56.12X-** **Struck by sea lion**

🔲 ☑ **W56.19X-** **Other contact with sea lion**

⑤ **W56.2 Contact with orca**
    Contact with killer whale

🔲 ☑ **W56.21X-** **Bitten by orca**

🔲 ☑ **W56.22X-** **Struck by orca**

🔲 ☑ **W56.29X-** **Other contact with orca**

⑤ **W56.3 Contact with other marine mammals**

🔲 ☑ **W56.31X-** **Bitten by other marine mammals**

🔲 ☑ **W56.32X-** **Struck by other marine mammals**

🔲 ☑ **W56.39X-** **Other contact with other marine mammals**

⑤ **W56.4 Contact with shark**

🔲 ☑ **W56.41X-** **Bitten by shark**

🔲 ☑ **W56.42X-** **Struck by shark**

🔲 ☑ **W56.49X-** **Other contact with shark**

⑤ **W56.5 Contact with other fish**

🔲 ☑ **W56.51X-** **Bitten by other fish**

🔲 ☑ **W56.52X-** **Struck by other fish**

🔲 ☑ **W56.59X-** **Other contact with other fish**

⑤ **W56.8 Contact with other nonvenomous marine animals**

🔲 ☑ **W56.81X-** **Bitten by other nonvenomous marine animals**

🔲 ☑ **W56.82X-** **Struck by other nonvenomous marine animals**

🔲 ☑ **W56.89X-** **Other contact with other nonvenomous marine animals**

🔲 ☑ **W57.XXX-** **Bitten or stung by nonvenomous insect and other nonvenomous arthropods**

    EXCLUDES 1   contact with venomous insects and arthropods (T63.2-, T63.3-, T63.4-)

The appropriate 7th character is to be added to code W57
A   initial encounter
D   subsequent encounter
S   sequela

④ **W58** **Contact with crocodile or alligator**

The appropriate 7th character is to be added to each code from category W58
A   initial encounter
D   subsequent encounter
S   sequela

⑤ **W58.0 Contact with alligator**

④ 4th digit required   ⑤ 5th digit required   ⑥ 6th digit required   ☑ 7th digit required   ☑ 7th digit placeholder   ✚ Additional code   ⊟ Laterality

1832   *DecisionHealth's* FY 2020 Complete Home Health ICD-10-CM Diagnosis Coding Manual

!Q ☑ **W58.01X-** Bitten by alligator

!Q ☑ **W58.02X-** Struck by alligator

!Q ☑ **W58.03X-** Crushed by alligator

!Q ☑ **W58.09X-** Other contact with alligator

⑤ W58.1 Contact with crocodile

!Q ☑ **W58.11X-** Bitten by crocodile

!Q ☑ **W58.12X-** Struck by crocodile

!Q ☑ **W58.13X-** Crushed by crocodile

!Q ☑ **W58.19X-** Other contact with crocodile

④ W59 Contact with other nonvenomous reptiles

> **EXCLUDES 1** contact with venomous reptile (T63.0-, T63.1-)

> The appropriate 7th character is to be added to each code from category W59
> A   initial encounter
> D   subsequent encounter
> S   sequela

⑤ W59.0 Contact with nonvenomous lizards

!Q ☑ **W59.01X-** Bitten by nonvenomous lizards

!Q ☑ **W59.02X-** Struck by nonvenomous lizards

!Q ☑ **W59.09X-** Other contact with nonvenomous lizards
> Exposure to nonvenomous lizards

⑤ W59.1 Contact with nonvenomous snakes

!Q ☑ **W59.11X-** Bitten by nonvenomous snake

!Q ☑ **W59.12X-** Struck by nonvenomous snake

!Q ☑ **W59.13X-** Crushed by nonvenomous snake

!Q ☑ **W59.19X-** Other contact with nonvenomous snake

⑤ W59.2 Contact with turtles

> **EXCLUDES 1** contact with tortoises (W59.8-)

!Q ☑ **W59.21X-** Bitten by turtle

!Q ☑ **W59.22X-** Struck by turtle

!Q ☑ **W59.29X-** Other contact with turtle
> Exposure to turtles

⑤ W59.8 Contact with other nonvenomous reptiles

!Q ☑ **W59.81X-** Bitten by other nonvenomous reptiles

!Q ☑ **W59.82X-** Struck by other nonvenomous reptiles

!Q ☑ **W59.83X-** Crushed by other nonvenomous reptiles

!Q ☑ **W59.89X-** Other contact with other nonvenomous reptiles

!Q ☑ **W60.XXX-** Contact with nonvenomous plant thorns and spines and sharp leaves

> **EXCLUDES 1** Contact with venomous plants (T63.7-)

> The appropriate 7th character is to be added to code W60
> A   initial encounter
> D   subsequent encounter
> S   sequela

④ W61 Contact with birds (domestic) (wild)

> **INCLUDES** contact with excreta of birds

> The appropriate 7th character is to be added to each code from category W61
> A   initial encounter
> D   subsequent encounter
> S   sequela

⑤ W61.0 Contact with parrot

!Q ☑ **W61.01X-** Bitten by parrot

!Q ☑ **W61.02X-** Struck by parrot

!Q ☑ **W61.09X-** Other contact with parrot
> Exposure to parrots

⑤ W61.1 Contact with macaw

!Q ☑ **W61.11X-** Bitten by macaw

!Q ☑ **W61.12X-** Struck by macaw

!Q ☑ **W61.19X-** Other contact with macaw
> Exposure to macaws

⑤ W61.2 Contact with other psittacines

!Q ☑ **W61.21X-** Bitten by other psittacines

!Q ☑ **W61.22X-** Struck by other psittacines

!Q ☑ **W61.29X-** Other contact with other psittacines
> Exposure to other psittacines

⑤ W61.3 Contact with chicken

!Q ☑ **W61.32X-** Struck by chicken

!Q ☑ **W61.33X-** Pecked by chicken

!Q ☑ **W61.39X-** Other contact with chicken
> Exposure to chickens

⑤ W61.4 Contact with turkey

!Q ☑ **W61.42X-** Struck by turkey

!Q ☑ **W61.43X-** Pecked by turkey

!Q ☑ **W61.49X-** Other contact with turkey

⑤ W61.5 Contact with goose

!Q ☑ **W61.51X-** Bitten by goose

!Q ☑ **W61.52X-** Struck by goose

!Q ☑ **W61.59X-** Other contact with goose

⑤ W61.6 Contact with duck

!Q ☑ **W61.61X-** Bitten by duck

!Q ☑ **W61.62X-** Struck by duck

!Q ☑ **W61.69X-** Other contact with duck

⑤ W61.9 Contact with other birds

!Q ☑ **W61.91X-** Bitten by other birds

!Q ☑ **W61.92X-** Struck by other birds

!Q ☑ **W61.99X-** Other contact with other birds
> Contact with bird NOS

④ W62 Contact with nonvenomous amphibians

> **EXCLUDES 1** contact with venomous amphibians (T63.81-R63.83)

> The appropriate 7th character is to be added to each code from category W62
> A   initial encounter
> D   subsequent encounter
> S   sequela

!Q ☑ **W62.0XX-** Contact with nonvenomous frogs

!Q ☑ **W62.1XX-** Contact with nonvenomous toads

!Q ☑ **W62.9XX-** Contact with other nonvenomous amphibians

!Q ☑ **W64.XXX-** Exposure to other animate mechanical forces

> **INCLUDES** exposure to nonvenomous animal NOS

★ New ▲ Revised Px Primary **SP** PDGM Px **SL** Low CoM **SH** High CoM **!Q** Quest. Encounter **H** Hospice non-cancer Dx Unspecified **M** *Manifestation*

DecisionHealth's FY 2020 Complete Home Health ICD-10-CM Diagnosis Coding Manual

1833

EXCLUDES 1   contact with venomous animal (T63.-)

The appropriate 7th character is to be added to code W64
A   initial encounter
D   subsequent encounter
S   sequela

Accidental non-transport drowning and submersion (W65-W74)

EXCLUDES 1   accidental drowning and submersion due to fall into water (W16.-)
accidental drowning and submersion due to water transport accident (V90.-, V92.-)

EXCLUDES 2   accidental drowning and submersion due to cataclysm (X34-X39)

!Q ☑ W65.XXX-   **Accidental drowning and submersion while in bath-tub**

EXCLUDES 1   accidental drowning and submersion due to fall in (into) bathtub (W16.211)

The appropriate 7th character is to be added to code W65
A   initial encounter
D   subsequent encounter
S   sequela

!Q ☑ W67.XXX-   **Accidental drowning and submersion while in swimming-pool**

EXCLUDES 1   accidental drowning and submersion due to fall into swimming pool (W16.011, W16.021, W16.031)
accidental drowning and submersion due to striking into wall of swimming pool (W22.041)

The appropriate 7th character is to be added to code W67
A   initial encounter
D   subsequent encounter
S   sequela

!Q ☑ W69.XXX-   **Accidental drowning and submersion while in natural water**
Accidental drowning and submersion while in lake
Accidental drowning and submersion while in open sea
Accidental drowning and submersion while in river
Accidental drowning and submersion while in stream

EXCLUDES 1   accidental drowning and submersion due to fall into natural body of water (W16.111, W16.121, W16.131)

The appropriate 7th character is to be added to code W69
A   initial encounter
D   subsequent encounter
S   sequela

!Q ☑ W73.XXX-   **Other specified cause of accidental non-transport drowning and submersion**
Accidental drowning and submersion while in quenching tank
Accidental drowning and submersion while in reservoir

EXCLUDES 1   accidental drowning and submersion due to fall into other water (W16.311, W16.321, W16.331)

The appropriate 7th character is to be added to code W73
A   initial encounter
D   subsequent encounter
S   sequela

!Q ☑ W74.XXX-   **Unspecified cause of accidental drowning and submersion**
Drowning NOS

The appropriate 7th character is to be added to code W74
A   initial encounter
D   subsequent encounter
S   sequela

Exposure to electric current, radiation and extreme ambient air temperature and pressure (W85-W99)

EXCLUDES 1   exposure to:
failure in dosage of radiation or temperature during surgical and medical care (Y63.2-Y63.5)
lightning (T75.0-)
natural cold (X31)
natural heat (X30)
natural radiation NOS (X39)
radiological procedure and radiotherapy (Y84.2)
sunlight (X32)

!Q ☑ W85.XXX-   **Exposure to electric transmission lines**
Broken power line

The appropriate 7th character is to be added to code W85
A   initial encounter
D   subsequent encounter
S   sequela

4 W86   **Exposure to other specified electric current**

The appropriate 7th character is to be added to each code from category W86
A   initial encounter
D   subsequent encounter
S   sequela

!Q ☑ W86.0XX-   **Exposure to domestic wiring and appliances**

!Q ☑ W86.1XX-   **Exposure to industrial wiring, appliances and electrical machinery**
Exposure to conductors

---

4 4th digit required   **5** 5th digit required   **6** 6th digit required   **7** 7th digit required   **☑** 7th digit placeholder   **+** Additional code   **⊟** Laterality

Exposure to control apparatus

Exposure to electrical equipment and machinery

Exposure to transformers

!Q ☑ W86.8XX- Exposure to other electric current

Exposure to wiring and appliances in or on farm (not farmhouse)

Exposure to wiring and appliances outdoors

Exposure to wiring and appliances in or on public building

Exposure to wiring and appliances in or on residential institutions

Exposure to wiring and appliances in or on schools

4 W88 Exposure to ionizing radiation

> EXCLUDES 1 exposure to sunlight (X32)

The appropriate 7th character is to be added to each code from category W88

A   initial encounter
D   subsequent encounter
S   sequela

!Q ☑ W88.0XX- Exposure to X-rays

!Q ☑ W88.1XX- Exposure to radioactive isotopes

!Q ☑ W88.8XX- Exposure to other ionizing radiation

4 W89 Exposure to man-made visible and ultraviolet light

> INCLUDES exposure to welding light (arc)

> EXCLUDES 1 exposure to sunlight (X32)

The appropriate 7th character is to be added to each code from category W89

A   initial encounter
D   subsequent encounter
S   sequela

!Q ☑ W89.0XX- Exposure to welding light (arc)

!Q ☑ W89.1XX- Exposure to tanning bed

!Q ☑ W89.8XX- Exposure to other man-made visible and ultraviolet light

!Q ☑ W89.9XX- Exposure to unspecified man-made visible and ultraviolet light

4 W90 Exposure to other nonionizing radiation

> EXCLUDES 1 exposure to sunlight (X32)

The appropriate 7th character is to be added to each code from category W90

A   initial encounter
D   subsequent encounter
S   sequela

!Q ☑ W90.0XX- Exposure to radiofrequency

!Q ☑ W90.1XX- Exposure to infrared radiation

!Q ☑ W90.2XX- Exposure to laser radiation

!Q ☑ W90.8XX- Exposure to other nonionizing radiation

!Q ☑ W92.XXX- Exposure to excessive heat of man-made origin

The appropriate 7th character is to be added to code W92

A   initial encounter
D   subsequent encounter
S   sequela

4 W93 Exposure to excessive cold of man-made origin

The appropriate 7th character is to be added to each code from category W93

A   initial encounter
D   subsequent encounter
S   sequela

5 W93.0 Contact with or inhalation of dry ice

!Q ☑ W93.01X- Contact with dry ice

!Q ☑ W93.02X- Inhalation of dry ice

5 W93.1 Contact with or inhalation of liquid air

!Q ☑ W93.11X- Contact with liquid air

Contact with liquid hydrogen

Contact with liquid nitrogen

!Q ☑ W93.12X- Inhalation of liquid air

Inhalation of liquid hydrogen

Inhalation of liquid nitrogen

!Q ☑ W93.2XX- Prolonged exposure in deep freeze unit or refrigerator

!Q ☑ W93.8XX- Exposure to other excessive cold of man-made origin

4 W94 Exposure to high and low air pressure and changes in air pressure

The appropriate 7th character is to be added to each code from category W94

A   initial encounter
D   subsequent encounter
S   sequela

!Q ☑ W94.0XX- Exposure to prolonged high air pressure

5 W94.1 Exposure to prolonged low air pressure

!Q ☑ W94.11X- Exposure to residence or prolonged visit at high altitude

!Q ☑ W94.12X- Exposure to other prolonged low air pressure

5 W94.2 Exposure to rapid changes in air pressure during ascent

!Q ☑ W94.21X- Exposure to reduction in atmospheric pressure while surfacing from deep-water diving

!Q ☑ W94.22X- Exposure to reduction in atmospheric pressure while surfacing from underground

!Q ☑ W94.23X- Exposure to sudden change in air pressure in aircraft during ascent

!Q ☑ W94.29X- Exposure to other rapid changes in air pressure during ascent

5 W94.3 Exposure to rapid changes in air pressure during descent

!Q ☑ W94.31X- Exposure to sudden change in air pressure in aircraft during descent

!Q ☑ W94.32X- Exposure to high air pressure from rapid descent in water

!Q ☑ W94.39X- Exposure to other rapid changes in air pressure during descent

!Q ☑ W99.XXX- Exposure to other man-made environmental factors

The appropriate 7th character is to be added to code W99

A   initial encounter
D   subsequent encounter
S   sequela

Chapter 20

V00-Y99

★ New ▲ Revised Px Primary SP PDGM Px SL Low CoM SH High CoM !Q Quest. Encounter H Hospice non-cancer Dx Unspecified M Manifestation

DecisionHealth's FY 2020 Complete Home Health ICD-10-CM Diagnosis Coding Manual

1835

Exposure to smoke, fire and flames (X00-X08)

EXCLUDES 1   arson (X97)
EXCLUDES 2   explosions (W35-W40)
lightning (T75.0-)
transport accident (V01-V99)

4 X00   Exposure to uncontrolled fire in building or structure
> **INCLUDES**   conflagration in building or structure

Code first:
any associated cataclysm
> **EXCLUDES 2**   Exposure to ignition or melting of nightwear (X05)
> Exposure to ignition or melting of other clothing and apparel (X06.-)
> Exposure to other specified smoke, fire and flames (X08.-)

The appropriate 7th character is to be added to each code from category X00
A   initial encounter
D   subsequent encounter
S   sequela

!Q ☑ X00.0XX-   Exposure to flames in uncontrolled fire in building or structure
!Q ☑ X00.1XX-   Exposure to smoke in uncontrolled fire in building or structure
!Q ☑ X00.2XX-   Injury due to collapse of burning building or structure in uncontrolled fire
> **EXCLUDES 1**   injury due to collapse of building not on fire (W20.1)

!Q ☑ X00.3XX-   Fall from burning building or structure in uncontrolled fire
!Q ☑ X00.4XX-   Hit by object from burning building or structure in uncontrolled fire
!Q ☑ X00.5XX-   Jump from burning building or structure in uncontrolled fire
!Q ☑ X00.8XX-   Other exposure to uncontrolled fire in building or structure

4 X01   Exposure to uncontrolled fire, not in building or structure
> **INCLUDES**   exposure to forest fire

The appropriate 7th character is to be added to each code from category X01
A   initial encounter
D   subsequent encounter
S   sequela

!Q ☑ X01.0XX-   Exposure to flames in uncontrolled fire, not in building or structure
!Q ☑ X01.1XX-   Exposure to smoke in uncontrolled fire, not in building or structure
!Q ☑ X01.3XX-   Fall due to uncontrolled fire, not in building or structure
!Q ☑ X01.4XX-   Hit by object due to uncontrolled fire, not in building or structure
!Q ☑ X01.8XX-   Other exposure to uncontrolled fire, not in building or structure

4 X02   Exposure to controlled fire in building or structure
> **INCLUDES**   exposure to fire in fireplace

exposure to fire in stove

The appropriate 7th character is to be added to each code from category X02
A   initial encounter
D   subsequent encounter
S   sequela

!Q ☑ X02.0XX-   Exposure to flames in controlled fire in building or structure
!Q ☑ X02.1XX-   Exposure to smoke in controlled fire in building or structure
!Q ☑ X02.2XX-   Injury due to collapse of burning building or structure in controlled fire
> **EXCLUDES 1**   injury due to collapse of building not on fire (W20.1)

!Q ☑ X02.3XX-   Fall from burning building or structure in controlled fire
!Q ☑ X02.4XX-   Hit by object from burning building or structure in controlled fire
!Q ☑ X02.5XX-   Jump from burning building or structure in controlled fire
!Q ☑ X02.8XX-   Other exposure to controlled fire in building or structure

4 X03   Exposure to controlled fire, not in building or structure
> **INCLUDES**   exposure to bon fire
> exposure to camp-fire
> exposure to trash fire

The appropriate 7th character is to be added to each code from category X03
A   initial encounter
D   subsequent encounter
S   sequela

!Q ☑ X03.0XX-   Exposure to flames in controlled fire, not in building or structure
!Q ☑ X03.1XX-   Exposure to smoke in controlled fire, not in building or structure
!Q ☑ X03.3XX-   Fall due to controlled fire, not in building or structure
!Q ☑ X03.4XX-   Hit by object due to controlled fire, not in building or structure
!Q ☑ X03.8XX-   Other exposure to controlled fire, not in building or structure

!Q ☑ X04.XXX-   Exposure to ignition of highly flammable material
Exposure to ignition of gasoline
Exposure to ignition of kerosene
Exposure to ignition of petrol
> **EXCLUDES 2**   exposure to ignition or melting of nightwear (X05)
> exposure to ignition or melting of other clothing and apparel (X06)

The appropriate 7th character is to be added to code X04
A   initial encounter
D   subsequent encounter
S   sequela

!Q ☑ X05.XXX-   Exposure to ignition or melting of nightwear

---

4 4th digit required   5 5th digit required   6 6th digit required   7 7th digit required   ☑ 7th digit placeholder   + Additional code   ⊟ Laterality

1836   DecisionHealth's FY 2020 Complete Home Health ICD-10-CM Diagnosis Coding Manual

Chapter 20

V00-Y99

EXCLUDES 2 exposure to uncontrolled fire in building or structure (X00.-)
exposure to uncontrolled fire, not in building or structure (X01.-)
exposure to controlled fire in building or structure (X02.-)
exposure to controlled fire, not in building or structure (X03.-)
exposure to ignition of highly flammable materials (X04.-)

The appropriate 7th character is to be added to code X05
A   initial encounter
D   subsequent encounter
S   sequela

☑ **X06** **Exposure to ignition or melting of other clothing and apparel**

EXCLUDES 2 exposure to uncontrolled fire in building or structure (X00.-)
exposure to uncontrolled fire, not in building or structure (X01.-)
exposure to controlled fire in building or structure (X02.-)
exposure to controlled fire, not in building or structure (X03.-)
exposure to ignition of highly flammable materials (X04.-)

The appropriate 7th character is to be added to each code from category X06
A   initial encounter
D   subsequent encounter
S   sequela

!Q ☑ **X06.0XX-** **Exposure to ignition of plastic jewelry**
!Q ☑ **X06.1XX-** **Exposure to melting of plastic jewelry**
!Q ☑ **X06.2XX-** **Exposure to ignition of other clothing and apparel**
!Q ☑ **X06.3XX-** **Exposure to melting of other clothing and apparel**

☑ **X08** **Exposure to other specified smoke, fire and flames**

The appropriate 7th character is to be added to each code from category X08
A   initial encounter
D   subsequent encounter
S   sequela

⑤ X08.0 **Exposure to bed fire**
Exposure to mattress fire

!Q ☑ **X08.00X-** **Exposure to bed fire due to unspecified burning material**
!Q ☑ **X08.01X-** **Exposure to bed fire due to burning cigarette**
!Q ☑ **X08.09X-** **Exposure to bed fire due to other burning material**

⑤ X08.1 **Exposure to sofa fire**

!Q ☑ **X08.10X-** **Exposure to sofa fire due to unspecified burning material**

!Q ☑ **X08.11X-** **Exposure to sofa fire due to burning cigarette**
!Q ☑ **X08.19X-** **Exposure to sofa fire due to other burning material**

⑤ X08.2 **Exposure to other furniture fire**

!Q ☑ **X08.20X-** **Exposure to other furniture fire due to unspecified burning material**

!Q ☑ **X08.21X-** **Exposure to other furniture fire due to burning cigarette**
!Q ☑ **X08.29X-** **Exposure to other furniture fire due to other burning material**
!Q ☑ **X08.8XX-** **Exposure to other specified smoke, fire and flames**

Contact with heat and hot substances (X10-X19)

EXCLUDES 1 exposure to excessive natural heat (X30)
exposure to fire and flames (X00-X08)

☑ **X10** **Contact with hot drinks, food, fats and cooking oils**

The appropriate 7th character is to be added to each code from category X10
A   initial encounter
D   subsequent encounter
S   sequela

!Q ☑ **X10.0XX-** **Contact with hot drinks**
!Q ☑ **X10.1XX-** **Contact with hot food**
!Q ☑ **X10.2XX-** **Contact with fats and cooking oils**

☑ **X11** **Contact with hot tap-water**
INCLUDES contact with boiling tap-water
contact with boiling water NOS
EXCLUDES 1 contact with water heated on stove (X12)

The appropriate 7th character is to be added to each code from category X11
A   initial encounter
D   subsequent encounter
S   sequela

!Q ☑ **X11.0XX-** **Contact with hot water in bath or tub**
EXCLUDES 1 contact with running hot water in bath or tub (X11.1)

!Q ☑ **X11.1XX-** **Contact with running hot water**
Contact with hot water running out of hose
Contact with hot water running out of tap

!Q ☑ **X11.8XX-** **Contact with other hot tap-water**
Contact with hot water in bucket
Contact with hot tap-water NOS

!Q ☑ **X12.XXX-** **Contact with other hot fluids**
Contact with water heated on stove
EXCLUDES 1 hot (liquid) metals (X18)

The appropriate 7th character is to be added to code X12
A   initial encounter
D   subsequent encounter
S   sequela

☑ **X13** **Contact with steam and other hot vapors**

Chapter 20

V00-Y99

⭐ New ▲ Revised Px Primary **SP** PDGM Px **SL** Low CoM **SH** High CoM **!Q** Quest. Encounter Ⓗ Hóspice non-cancer Dx   Unspecified   **M** *Manifestation*

DecisionHealth's FY 2020 Complete Home Health ICD-10-CM Diagnosis Coding Manual

1837

Chapter 20

V00-Y99

The appropriate 7th character is to be added to each code from category X13
A   initial encounter
D   subsequent encounter
S   sequela

IQ ☑ **X13.0XX-**   **Inhalation of steam and other hot vapors**

IQ ☑ **X13.1XX-**   **Other contact with steam and other hot vapors**

⁴ **X14**   **Contact with hot air and other hot gases**

The appropriate 7th character is to be added to each code from category X14
A   initial encounter
D   subsequent encounter
S   sequela

IQ ☑ **X14.0XX-**   **Inhalation of hot air and gases**

IQ ☑ **X14.1XX-**   **Other contact with hot air and other hot gases**

⁴ **X15**   **Contact with hot household appliances**
     EXCLUDES 1   contact with heating appliances (X16)
               contact with powered household appliances (W29.-)
               exposure to controlled fire in building or structure due to household appliance (X02.8)
               exposure to household appliances electrical current (W86.0)

The appropriate 7th character is to be added to each code from category X15
A   initial encounter
D   subsequent encounter
S   sequela

IQ ☑ **X15.0XX-**   **Contact with hot stove (kitchen)**

IQ ☑ **X15.1XX-**   **Contact with hot toaster**

IQ ☑ **X15.2XX-**   **Contact with hotplate**

IQ ☑ **X15.3XX-**   **Contact with hot saucepan or skillet**

IQ ☑ **X15.8XX-**   **Contact with other hot household appliances**
     Contact with cooker
     Contact with kettle
     Contact with light bulbs

IQ ☑ **X16.XXX-**   **Contact with hot heating appliances, radiators and pipes**
     EXCLUDES 1   contact with powered appliances (W29.-)
               exposure to controlled fire in building or structure due to appliance (X02.8)
               exposure to industrial appliances electrical current (W86.1)

The appropriate 7th character is to be added to code X16
A   initial encounter
D   subsequent encounter
S   sequela

IQ ☑ **X17.XXX-**   **Contact with hot engines, machinery and tools**
     EXCLUDES 1   contact with hot heating appliances, radiators and pipes (X16)

contact with hot household appliances (X15)

The appropriate 7th character is to be added to code X17
A   initial encounter
D   subsequent encounter
S   sequela

IQ ☑ **X18.XXX-**   **Contact with other hot metals**
Contact with liquid metal

The appropriate 7th character is to be added to code X18
A   initial encounter
D   subsequent encounter
S   sequela

IQ ☑ **X19.XXX-**   **Contact with other heat and hot substances**
     EXCLUDES 1   objects that are not normally hot, e.g., an object made hot by a house fire (X00-X08)

The appropriate 7th character is to be added to code X19
A   initial encounter
D   subsequent encounter
S   sequela

Exposure to forces of nature (X30-X39)

IQ ☑ **X30.XXX-**   **Exposure to excessive natural heat**
Exposure to excessive heat as the cause of sunstroke
Exposure to heat NOS
     EXCLUDES 1   excessive heat of man-made origin (W92)
               exposure to man-made radiation (W89)
               exposure to sunlight (X32)
               exposure to tanning bed (W89)

The appropriate 7th character is to be added to code X30
A   initial encounter
D   subsequent encounter
S   sequela

IQ ☑ **X31.XXX-**   **Exposure to excessive natural cold**
Excessive cold as the cause of chilblains NOS
Excessive cold as the cause of immersion foot or hand
Exposure to cold NOS
Exposure to weather conditions
     EXCLUDES 1   cold of man-made origin (W93.-)
               contact with or inhalation of dry ice (W93.-)
               contact with or inhalation of liquefied gas (W93.-)

⁴ 4th digit required   ⁵ 5th digit required   ⁶ 6th digit required   ⁷ 7th digit required   ☑ 7th digit placeholder   ✚ Additional code   ⊟ Laterality

1838   *DecisionHealth's* FY 2020 Complete Home Health ICD-10-CM Diagnosis Coding Manual

The appropriate 7th character is to be added to code X31

A   initial encounter
D   subsequent encounter
S   sequela

!Q ☑ X32.XXX-   **Exposure to sunlight**

> EXCLUDES 1   man-made radiation (tanning bed) (W89)
> EXCLUDES 2   radiation-related disorders of the skin and subcutaneous tissue (L55-L59)

The appropriate 7th character is to be added to code X32

A   initial encounter
D   subsequent encounter
S   sequela

!Q ☑ X34.XXX-   **Earthquake**

> EXCLUDES 2   tidal wave (tsunami) due to earthquake (X37.41)

The appropriate 7th character is to be added to code X34

A   initial encounter
D   subsequent encounter
S   sequela

!Q ☑ X35.XXX-   **Volcanic eruption**

> EXCLUDES 2   tidal wave (tsunami) due to volcanic eruption (X37.41)

The appropriate 7th character is to be added to code X35

A   initial encounter
D   subsequent encounter
S   sequela

4 X36   **Avalanche, landslide and other earth movements**

> INCLUDES   victim of mudslide of cataclysmic nature
> EXCLUDES 1   earthquake (X34)
> EXCLUDES 2   transport accident involving collision with avalanche or landslide not in motion (V01-V99)

The appropriate 7th character is to be added to each code from category X36

A   initial encounter
D   subsequent encounter
S   sequela

!Q ☑ X36.0XX-   **Collapse of dam or man-made structure causing earth movement**
!Q ☑ X36.1XX-   **Avalanche, landslide, or mudslide**
4 X37   **Cataclysmic storm**

The appropriate 7th character is to be added to each code from category X37

A   initial encounter
D   subsequent encounter
S   sequela

!Q ☑ X37.0XX-   **Hurricane**
Storm surge
Typhoon
!Q ☑ X37.1XX-   **Tornado**
Cyclone

Twister
!Q ☑ X37.2XX-   **Blizzard (snow)(ice)**
!Q ☑ X37.3XX-   **Dust storm**
5 X37.4   **Tidalwave**
!Q ☑ X37.41X-   **Tidal wave due to earthquake or volcanic eruption**
Tidal wave NOS
Tsunami
!Q ☑ X37.42X-   **Tidal wave due to storm**
!Q ☑ X37.43X-   **Tidal wave due to landslide**
!Q ☑ X37.8XX-   **Other cataclysmic storms**
Cloudburst
Torrential rain

> EXCLUDES 2   flood (X38)

!Q ☑ X37.9XX-   **Unspecified cataclysmic storm**
Storm NOS

> EXCLUDES 1   collapse of dam or man-made structure causing earth movement (X36.0)

!Q ☑ X38.XXX-   **Flood**
Flood arising from remote storm
Flood of cataclysmic nature arising from melting snow
Flood resulting directly from storm

> EXCLUDES 1   collapse of dam or man-made structure causing earth movement (X36.0)
> tidal wave NOS (X37.41)
> tidal wave caused by storm (X37.42)

The appropriate 7th character is to be added to code X38

A   initial encounter
D   subsequent encounter
S   sequela

4 X39   **Exposure to other forces of nature**

The appropriate 7th character is to be added to each code from category X39

A   initial encounter
D   subsequent encounter
S   sequela

5 X39.0   **Exposure to natural radiation**

> EXCLUDES 1   contact with and (suspected) exposure to radon and other naturally occurring radiation (Z77.123)
> exposure to man-made radiation (W88-W90)
> exposure to sunlight (X32)

!Q ☑ X39.01X-   **Exposure to radon**
!Q ☑ X39.08X-   **Exposure to other natural radiation**
!Q ☑ X39.8XX-   **Other exposure to forces of nature**

Overexertion and strenuous or repetitive movements (X50)

4 X50   **Overexertion and strenuous or repetitive movements**

★ New ▲ Revised Px Primary SP PDGM Px SL Low CoM SH High CoM !Q Quest. Encounter H Hospice non-cancer Dx   Unspecified   M Manifestation

DecisionHealth's FY 2020 Complete Home Health ICD-10-CM Diagnosis Coding Manual

1839

The appropriate 7th character is to be added to each code from category X50
A   initial encounter
D   subsequent encounter
S   sequela

!Q ☑ X50.0XX-   Overexertion from strenuous movement or load
Lifting heavy objects
Lifting weights

!Q ☑ X50.1XX-   Overexertion from prolonged static or awkward postures
Prolonged bending
Prolonged kneeling
Prolonged reaching
Prolonged sitting
Prolonged standing
Prolonged twisting
Static bending
Static kneeling
Static reaching
Static sitting
Static standing
Static twisting

!Q ☑ X50.3XX-   Overexertion from repetitive movements
Use of hand as hammer
EXCLUDES 2   Overuse from prolonged static or awkward postures (X50.1)

!Q ☑ X50.9XX-   Other and unspecified overexertion or strenuous movements or postures
Contact pressure
Contact stress

Accidental exposure to other specified factors   (X52-X58)

!Q ☑ X52.XXX-   Prolonged stay in weightless environment
Weightlessness in spacecraft (simulator)

The appropriate 7th character is to be added to code X52
A   initial encounter
D   subsequent encounter
S   sequela

!Q ☑ X58.XXX-   Exposure to other specified factors
Accident NOS
Exposure NOS

The appropriate 7th character is to be added to code X58
A   initial encounter
D   subsequent encounter
S   sequela

Intentional self-harm   (X71-X83)

Purposely self-inflicted injury
Suicide (attempted)
CODING TIPS ✓   Do not assign a code for intentional self harm as an external cause of morbidity when there is no injury coded on the claim.

4 X71   Intentional self-harm by drowning and submersion

The appropriate 7th character is to be added to each code from category X71
A   initial encounter
D   subsequent encounter
S   sequela

!Q ☑ X71.0XX-   Intentional self-harm by drowning and submersion while in bathtub

!Q ☑ X71.1XX-   Intentional self-harm by drowning and submersion while in swimming pool

!Q ☑ X71.2XX-   Intentional self-harm by drowning and submersion after jump into swimming pool

!Q ☑ X71.3XX-   Intentional self-harm by drowning and submersion in natural water

!Q ☑ X71.8XX-   Other intentional self-harm by drowning and submersion

!Q ☑ X71.9XX-   Intentional self-harm by drowning and submersion, unspecified

!Q ☑ X72.XXX-   Intentional self-harm by handgun discharge
Intentional self-harm by gun for single hand use
Intentional self-harm by pistol
Intentional self-harm by revolver
EXCLUDES 1   Very pistol (X74.8)

The appropriate 7th character is to be added to code X72
A   initial encounter
D   subsequent encounter
S   sequela

4 X73   Intentional self-harm by rifle, shotgun and larger firearm discharge
EXCLUDES 1   airgun (X74.01)

The appropriate 7th character is to be added to each code from category X73
A   initial encounter
D   subsequent encounter
S   sequela

!Q ☑ X73.0XX-   Intentional self-harm by shotgun discharge

!Q ☑ X73.1XX-   Intentional self-harm by hunting rifle discharge

!Q ☑ X73.2XX-   Intentional self-harm by machine gun discharge

!Q ☑ X73.8XX-   Intentional self-harm by other larger firearm discharge

!Q ☑ X73.9XX-   Intentional self-harm by unspecified larger firearm discharge

4 X74   Intentional self-harm by other and unspecified firearm and gun discharge

The appropriate 7th character is to be added to each code from category X74
A   initial encounter
D   subsequent encounter
S   sequela

5 X74.0   Intentional self-harm by gas, air or spring-operated guns

!Q ☑ X74.01X-   Intentional self-harm by airgun
Intentional self-harm by BB gun discharge
Intentional self-harm by pellet gun discharge

4 4th digit required   5 5th digit required   6 6th digit required   7 7th digit required   ☑ 7th digit placeholder   ✚ Additional code   ▤ Laterality

1840   *DecisionHealth's* FY 2020 Complete Home Health ICD-10-CM Diagnosis Coding Manual

IQ **☑** **X74.02X-** Intentional self-harm by paintball gun

IQ **☑** **X74.09X-** Intentional self-harm by other gas, air or spring-operated gun

IQ **☑** **X74.8XX-** Intentional self-harm by other firearm discharge

Intentional self-harm by Very pistol [flare] discharge

IQ **☑** **X74.9XX-** Intentional self-harm by unspecified firearm discharge

IQ **☑** **X75.XXX-** Intentional self-harm by explosive material

The appropriate 7th character is to be added to code X75
A   initial encounter
D   subsequent encounter
S   sequela

IQ **☑** **X76.XXX-** Intentional self-harm by smoke, fire and flames

The appropriate 7th character is to be added to code X76
A   initial encounter
D   subsequent encounter
S   sequela

④ X77 Intentional self-harm by steam, hot vapors and hot objects

The appropriate 7th character is to be added to each code from category X77
A   initial encounter
D   subsequent encounter
S   sequela

IQ **☑** **X77.0XX-** Intentional self-harm by steam or hot vapors

IQ **☑** **X77.1XX-** Intentional self-harm by hot tap water

IQ **☑** **X77.2XX-** Intentional self-harm by other hot fluids

IQ **☑** **X77.3XX-** Intentional self-harm by hot household appliances

IQ **☑** **X77.8XX-** Intentional self-harm by other hot objects

IQ **☑** **X77.9XX-** Intentional self-harm by unspecified hot objects

④ X78 Intentional self-harm by sharp object

The appropriate 7th character is to be added to each code from category X78
A   initial encounter
D   subsequent encounter
S   sequela

IQ **☑** **X78.0XX-** Intentional self-harm by sharp glass

IQ **☑** **X78.1XX-** Intentional self-harm by knife

IQ **☑** **X78.2XX-** Intentional self-harm by sword or dagger

IQ **☑** **X78.8XX-** Intentional self-harm by other sharp object

IQ **☑** **X78.9XX-** Intentional self-harm by unspecified sharp object

IQ **☑** **X79.XXX-** Intentional self-harm by blunt object

The appropriate 7th character is to be added to code X79
A   initial encounter
D   subsequent encounter
S   sequela

IQ **☑** **X80.XXX-** Intentional self-harm by jumping from a high place

Intentional fall from one level to another

The appropriate 7th character is to be added to code X80
A   initial encounter
D   subsequent encounter
S   sequela

④ X81 Intentional self-harm by jumping or lying in front of moving object

The appropriate 7th character is to be added to each code from category X81
A   initial encounter
D   subsequent encounter
S   sequela

IQ **☑** **X81.0XX-** Intentional self-harm by jumping or lying in front of motor vehicle

IQ **☑** **X81.1XX-** Intentional self-harm by jumping or lying in front of (subway) train

IQ **☑** **X81.8XX-** Intentional self-harm by jumping or lying in front of other moving object

④ X82 Intentional self-harm by crashing of motor vehicle

The appropriate 7th character is to be added to each code from category X82
A   initial encounter
D   subsequent encounter
S   sequela

IQ **☑** **X82.0XX-** Intentional collision of motor vehicle with other motor vehicle

IQ **☑** **X82.1XX-** Intentional collision of motor vehicle with train

IQ **☑** **X82.2XX-** Intentional collision of motor vehicle with tree

IQ **☑** **X82.8XX-** Other intentional self-harm by crashing of motor vehicle

④ X83 Intentional self-harm by other specified means

EXCLUDES 1 intentional self-harm by poisoning or contact with toxic substance- See Table of Drugs and Chemicals

The appropriate 7th character is to be added to each code from category X83
A   initial encounter
D   subsequent encounter
S   sequela

IQ **☑** **X83.0XX-** Intentional self-harm by crashing of aircraft

IQ **☑** **X83.1XX-** Intentional self-harm by electrocution

IQ **☑** **X83.2XX-** Intentional self-harm by exposure to extremes of cold

IQ **☑** **X83.8XX-** Intentional self-harm by other specified means

Chapter 20

V00-Y99

☆ New ▲ Revised Px Primary **SP** PDGM Px **SL** Low CoM **SH** High CoM **IQ** Quest. Encounter **H** Hospice non-cancer Dx Unspecified **M** *Manifestation*

DecisionHealth's FY 2020 Complete Home Health ICD-10-CM Diagnosis Coding Manual

1841

Assault (X92-Y09)	🔟 **X95.0** Assault by gas, air or spring-operated guns

INCLUDES	homicide
	injuries inflicted by another person with intent to injure or kill, by any means

EXCLUDES 1	injuries due to legal intervention (Y35.-)
	injuries due to operations of war (Y36.-)
	injuries due to terrorism (Y38.-)

CODING TIPS ✓   Do not assign a code for assault as an external cause of morbidity when there is no injury coded on the claim.

4️⃣ **X92**   **Assault by drowning and submersion**

> The appropriate 7th character is to be added to each code from category X92
> A   initial encounter
> D   subsequent encounter
> S   sequela

!Q ☑ **X92.0XX-**   **Assault by drowning and submersion while in bathtub**

!Q ☑ **X92.1XX-**   **Assault by drowning and submersion while in swimming pool**

!Q ☑ **X92.2XX-**   **Assault by drowning and submersion after push into swimming pool**

!Q ☑ **X92.3XX-**   **Assault by drowning and submersion in natural water**

!Q ☑ **X92.8XX-**   **Other assault by drowning and submersion**

!Q ☑ **X92.9XX-**   **Assault by drowning and submersion, unspecified**

!Q ☑ **X93.XXX-**   **Assault by handgun discharge**
Assault by discharge of gun for single hand use
Assault by discharge of pistol
Assault by discharge of revolver

> EXCLUDES 1   Very pistol (X95.8)

> The appropriate 7th character is to be added to code X93
> A   initial encounter
> D   subsequent encounter
> S   sequela

4️⃣ **X94**   **Assault by rifle, shotgun and larger firearm discharge**

> EXCLUDES 1   airgun (X95.01)

> The appropriate 7th character is to be added to each code from category X94
> A   initial encounter
> D   subsequent encounter
> S   sequela

!Q ☑ **X94.0XX-**   **Assault by shotgun**

!Q ☑ **X94.1XX-**   **Assault by hunting rifle**

!Q ☑ **X94.2XX-**   **Assault by machine gun**

!Q ☑ **X94.8XX-**   **Assault by other larger firearm discharge**

!Q ☑ **X94.9XX-**   **Assault by unspecified larger firearm discharge**

4️⃣ **X95**   **Assault by other and unspecified firearm and gun discharge**

> The appropriate 7th character is to be added to each code from category X95
> A   initial encounter
> D   subsequent encounter
> S   sequela

!Q ☑ **X95.01X-**   **Assault by airgun discharge**
Assault by BB gun discharge
Assault by pellet gun discharge

!Q ☑ **X95.02X-**   **Assault by paintball gun discharge**

!Q ☑ **X95.09X-**   **Assault by other gas, air or spring-operated gun**

!Q ☑ **X95.8XX-**   **Assault by other firearm discharge**
Assault by very pistol [flare] discharge

!Q ☑ **X95.9XX-**   **Assault by unspecified firearm discharge**

4️⃣ **X96**   **Assault by explosive material**

> EXCLUDES 1   incendiary device (X97)
> terrorism involving explosive material (Y38.2-)

> The appropriate 7th character is to be added to each code from category X96
> A   initial encounter
> D   subsequent encounter
> S   sequela

!Q ☑ **X96.0XX-**   **Assault by antipersonnel bomb**

> EXCLUDES 1   antipersonnel bomb use in military or war (Y36.2-)

!Q ☑ **X96.1XX-**   **Assault by gasoline bomb**

!Q ☑ **X96.2XX-**   **Assault by letter bomb**

!Q ☑ **X96.3XX-**   **Assault by fertilizer bomb**

!Q ☑ **X96.4XX-**   **Assault by pipe bomb**

!Q ☑ **X96.8XX-**   **Assault by other specified explosive**

!Q ☑ **X96.9XX-**   **Assault by unspecified explosive**

!Q ☑ **X97.XXX-**   **Assault by smoke, fire and flames**
Assault by arson
Assault by cigarettes
Assault by incendiary device

> The appropriate 7th character is to be added to code X97
> A   initial encounter
> D   subsequent encounter
> S   sequela

4️⃣ **X98**   **Assault by steam, hot vapors and hot objects**

> The appropriate 7th character is to be added to each code from category X98
> A   initial encounter
> D   subsequent encounter
> S   sequela

!Q ☑ **X98.0XX-**   **Assault by steam or hot vapors**

!Q ☑ **X98.1XX-**   **Assault by hot tap water**

!Q ☑ **X98.2XX-**   **Assault by hot fluids**

!Q ☑ **X98.3XX-**   **Assault by hot household appliances**

!Q ☑ **X98.8XX-**   **Assault by other hot objects**

!Q ☑ **X98.9XX-**   **Assault by unspecified hot objects**

4️⃣ **X99**   **Assault by sharp object**

> EXCLUDES 1   assault by strike by sports equipment (Y08.0-)

4️⃣4th digit required   5️⃣5th digit required   6️⃣6th digit required   7️⃣7th digit required   ☑7th digit placeholder   ✛Additional code   ⊟Laterality

The appropriate 7th character is to be added to each code from category X99
A   initial encounter
D   subsequent encounter
S   sequela

IQ ☑ X99.0XX-   **Assault by sharp glass**

IQ ☑ X99.1XX-   **Assault by knife**

IQ ☑ X99.2XX-   **Assault by sword or dagger**

IQ ☑ X99.8XX-   **Assault by other sharp object**

IQ ☑ X99.9XX-   **Assault by unspecified sharp object**

Assault by stabbing NOS

IQ ☑ Y00.XXX-   **Assault by blunt object**

> **EXCLUDES 1**   assault by strike by sports equipment (Y08.0-)

The appropriate 7th character is to be added to code Y00
A   initial encounter
D   subsequent encounter
S   sequela

IQ ☑ Y01.XXX-   **Assault by pushing from high place**

The appropriate 7th character is to be added to code Y01
A   initial encounter
D   subsequent encounter
S   sequela

④ Y02   **Assault by pushing or placing victim in front of moving object**

The appropriate 7th character is to be added to each code from category Y02
A   initial encounter
D   subsequent encounter
S   sequela

IQ ☑ Y02.0XX-   **Assault by pushing or placing victim in front of motor vehicle**

IQ ☑ Y02.1XX-   **Assault by pushing or placing victim in front of (subway) train**

IQ ☑ Y02.8XX-   **Assault by pushing or placing victim in front of other moving object**

④ Y03   **Assault by crashing of motor vehicle**

The appropriate 7th character is to be added to each code from category Y03
A   initial encounter
D   subsequent encounter
S   sequela

IQ ☑ Y03.0XX-   **Assault by being hit or run over by motor vehicle**

IQ ☑ Y03.8XX-   **Other assault by crashing of motor vehicle**

④ Y04   **Assault by bodily force**

> **EXCLUDES 1**   assault by:
> submersion (X92.-)
> use of weapon (X93-X95, X99, Y00)

The appropriate 7th character is to be added to each code from category Y04
A   initial encounter
D   subsequent encounter
S   sequela

IQ ☑ Y04.0XX-   **Assault by unarmed brawl or fight**

IQ ☑ Y04.1XX-   **Assault by human bite**

IQ ☑ Y04.2XX-   **Assault by strike against or bumped into by another person**

IQ ☑ Y04.8XX-   **Assault by other bodily force**

Assault by bodily force NOS

④ Y07   **Perpetrator of assault, maltreatment and neglect**

Note:
Codes from this category are for use only in cases of confirmed abuse (T74.-)
Selection of the correct perpetrator code is based on the relationship between the perpetrator and the victim

> **INCLUDES**   perpetrator of abandonment
> perpetrator of emotional neglect
> perpetrator of mental cruelty
> perpetrator of physical abuse
> perpetrator of physical neglect
> perpetrator of sexual abuse
> perpetrator of torture

⑤ Y07.0   **Spouse or partner, perpetrator of maltreatment and neglect**

Spouse or partner, perpetrator of maltreatment and neglect against spouse or partner

IQ Y07.01   **Husband, perpetrator of maltreatment and neglect**

IQ Y07.02   **Wife, perpetrator of maltreatment and neglect**

IQ Y07.03   **Male partner, perpetrator of maltreatment and neglect**

IQ Y07.04   **Female partner, perpetrator of maltreatment and neglect**

⑤ Y07.1   **Parent (adoptive) (biological), perpetrator of maltreatment and neglect**

IQ Y07.11   **Biological father, perpetrator of maltreatment and neglect**

IQ Y07.12   **Biological mother, perpetrator of maltreatment and neglect**

IQ Y07.13   **Adoptive father, perpetrator of maltreatment and neglect**

IQ Y07.14   **Adoptive mother, perpetrator of maltreatment and neglect**

⑤ Y07.4   **Other family member, perpetrator of maltreatment and neglect**

⑥ Y07.41   **Sibling, perpetrator of maltreatment and neglect**

> **EXCLUDES 1**   stepsibling, perpetrator of maltreatment and neglect (Y07.435, Y07.436)

IQ Y07.410   **Brother, perpetrator of maltreatment and neglect**

IQ Y07.411   **Sister, perpetrator of maltreatment and neglect**

⑥ Y07.42   **Foster parent, perpetrator of maltreatment and neglect**

IQ Y07.420   **Foster father, perpetrator of maltreatment and neglect**

IQ Y07.421   **Foster mother, perpetrator of maltreatment and neglect**

⑥ Y07.43   **Stepparent or stepsibling, perpetrator of maltreatment and neglect**

IQ Y07.430   **Stepfather, perpetrator of maltreatment and neglect**

★ New ▲ Revised Px Primary   **SP** PDGM Px   **SL** Low CoM   **SH** High CoM   **IQ** Quest. Encounter   **H** Hospice non-cancer Dx   Unspecified   **M** *Manifestation*

DecisionHealth's FY 2020 Complete Home Health ICD-10-CM Diagnosis Coding Manual

1843

IQ Y07.432 Male friend of parent (co-residing in household), perpetrator of maltreatment and neglect

IQ Y07.433 Stepmother, perpetrator of maltreatment and neglect

IQ Y07.434 Female friend of parent (co-residing in household), perpetrator of maltreatment and neglect

IQ Y07.435 Stepbrother, perpetrator or maltreatment and neglect

IQ Y07.436 Stepsister, perpetrator of maltreatment and neglect

6 Y07.49 Other family member, perpetrator of maltreatment and neglect

IQ Y07.490 Male cousin, perpetrator of maltreatment and neglect

IQ Y07.491 Female cousin, perpetrator of maltreatment and neglect

IQ Y07.499 Other family member, perpetrator of maltreatment and neglect

5 Y07.5 Non-family member, perpetrator of maltreatment and neglect

IQ Y07.50 Unspecified non-family member, perpetrator of maltreatment and neglect

6 Y07.51 Daycare provider, perpetrator of maltreatment and neglect

IQ Y07.510 At-home childcare provider, perpetrator of maltreatment and neglect

IQ Y07.511 Daycare center childcare provider, perpetrator of maltreatment and neglect

IQ Y07.512 At-home adultcare provider, perpetrator of maltreatment and neglect

IQ Y07.513 Adultcare center provider, perpetrator of maltreatment and neglect

IQ Y07.519 Unspecified daycare provider, perpetrator of maltreatment and neglect

6 Y07.52 Healthcare provider, perpetrator of maltreatment and neglect

IQ Y07.521 Mental health provider, perpetrator of maltreatment and neglect

IQ Y07.528 Other therapist or healthcare provider, perpetrator of maltreatment and neglect
  Nurse perpetrator of maltreatment and neglect
  Occupational therapist perpetrator of maltreatment and neglect
  Physical therapist perpetrator of maltreatment and neglect
  Speech therapist perpetrator of maltreatment and neglect

IQ Y07.529 Unspecified healthcare provider, perpetrator of maltreatment and neglect

IQ Y07.53 Teacher or instructor, perpetrator of maltreatment and neglect
  Coach, perpetrator of maltreatment and neglect

IQ Y07.59 Other non-family member, perpetrator of maltreatment and neglect

IQ Y07.6 Multiple perpetrators of maltreatment and neglect

IQ Y07.9 Unspecified perpetrator of maltreatment and neglect

4 Y08 Assault by other specified means

The appropriate 7th character is to be added to each code from category Y08
A   initial encounter
D   subsequent encounter
S   sequela

5 Y08.0 Assault by strike by sport equipment

IQ ✓ Y08.01X- Assault by strike by hockey stick

IQ ✓ Y08.02X- Assault by strike by baseball bat

IQ ✓ Y08.09X- Assault by strike by other specified type of sport equipment

5 Y08.8 Assault by other specified means

IQ ✓ Y08.81X- Assault by crashing of aircraft

IQ ✓ Y08.89X- Assault by other specified means

IQ Y09 Assault by unspecified means
  Assassination (attempted) NOS
  Homicide (attempted) NOS
  Manslaughter (attempted) NOS
  Murder (attempted) NOS

Event of undetermined intent   (Y21-Y33)

Undetermined intent is only for use when there is specific documentation in the record that the intent of the injury cannot be determined. If no such documentation is present, code to accidental (unintentional)

CODING TIPS ✓   Do not assign a code for event of undetermined intent as an external cause of morbidity when there is no injury coded on the claim.

4 Y21 Drowning and submersion, undetermined intent

The appropriate 7th character is to be added to each code from category Y21
A   initial encounter
D   subsequent encounter
S   sequela

IQ ✓ Y21.0XX- Drowning and submersion while in bathtub, undetermined intent

IQ ✓ Y21.1XX- Drowning and submersion after fall into bathtub, undetermined intent

IQ ✓ Y21.2XX- Drowning and submersion while in swimming pool, undetermined intent

IQ ✓ Y21.3XX- Drowning and submersion after fall into swimming pool, undetermined intent

IQ ✓ Y21.4XX- Drowning and submersion in natural water, undetermined intent

IQ ✓ Y21.8XX- Other drowning and submersion, undetermined intent

IQ ✓ Y21.9XX- Unspecified drowning and submersion, undetermined intent

IQ ✓ Y22.XXX- Handgun discharge, undetermined intent
  Discharge of gun for single hand use, undetermined intent
  Discharge of pistol, undetermined intent

---

4 4th digit required   5 5th digit required   6 6th digit required   7 7th digit required   ✓ 7th digit placeholder   ✚ Additional code   ⊟ Laterality

Discharge of revolver, undetermined intent
> **EXCLUDES 2** very pistol (Y24.8)

The appropriate 7th character is to be added to code Y22
A   initial encounter
D   subsequent encounter
S   sequela

4 **Y23   Rifle, shotgun and larger firearm discharge, undetermined intent**
> **EXCLUDES 2** airgun (Y24.0)

The appropriate 7th character is to be added to each code from category Y23
A   initial encounter
D   subsequent encounter
S   sequela

IQ ☑ **Y23.0XX-   Shotgun discharge, undetermined intent**

IQ ☑ **Y23.1XX-   Hunting rifle discharge, undetermined intent**

IQ ☑ **Y23.2XX-   Military firearm discharge, undetermined intent**

IQ ☑ **Y23.3XX-   Machine gun discharge, undetermined intent**

IQ ☑ **Y23.8XX-   Other larger firearm discharge, undetermined intent**

IQ ☑ **Y23.9XX-   Unspecified larger firearm discharge, undetermined intent**

4 **Y24   Other and unspecified firearm discharge, undetermined intent**

The appropriate 7th character is to be added to each code from category Y24
A   initial encounter
D   subsequent encounter
S   sequela

IQ ☑ **Y24.0XX-   Airgun discharge, undetermined intent**
BB gun discharge, undetermined intent
Pellet gun discharge, undetermined intent

IQ ☑ **Y24.8XX-   Other firearm discharge, undetermined intent**
Paintball gun discharge, undetermined intent
Very pistol [flare] discharge, undetermined intent

IQ ☑ **Y24.9XX-   Unspecified firearm discharge, undetermined intent**

IQ ☑ **Y25.XXX-   Contact with explosive material, undetermined intent**

The appropriate 7th character is to be added to code Y25
A   initial encounter
D   subsequent encounter
S   sequela

IQ ☑ **Y26.XXX-   Exposure to smoke, fire and flames, undetermined intent**

The appropriate 7th character is to be added to code Y26
A   initial encounter
D   subsequent encounter
S   sequela

4 **Y27   Contact with steam, hot vapors and hot objects, undetermined intent**

The appropriate 7th character is to be added to each code from category Y27
A   initial encounter
D   subsequent encounter
S   sequela

IQ ☑ **Y27.0XX-   Contact with steam and hot vapors, undetermined intent**

IQ ☑ **Y27.1XX-   Contact with hot tap water, undetermined intent**

IQ ☑ **Y27.2XX-   Contact with hot fluids, undetermined intent**

IQ ☑ **Y27.3XX-   Contact with hot household appliance, undetermined intent**

IQ ☑ **Y27.8XX-   Contact with other hot objects, undetermined intent**

IQ ☑ **Y27.9XX-   Contact with unspecified hot objects, undetermined intent**

4 **Y28   Contact with sharp object, undetermined intent**

The appropriate 7th character is to be added to each code from category Y28
A   initial encounter
D   subsequent encounter
S   sequela

IQ ☑ **Y28.0XX-   Contact with sharp glass, undetermined intent**

IQ ☑ **Y28.1XX-   Contact with knife, undetermined intent**

IQ ☑ **Y28.2XX-   Contact with sword or dagger, undetermined intent**

IQ ☑ **Y28.8XX-   Contact with other sharp object, undetermined intent**

IQ ☑ **Y28.9XX-   Contact with unspecified sharp object, undetermined intent**

IQ ☑ **Y29.XXX-   Contact with blunt object, undetermined intent**

The appropriate 7th character is to be added to code Y29
A   initial encounter
D   subsequent encounter
S   sequela

IQ ☑ **Y30.XXX-   Falling, jumping or pushed from a high place, undetermined intent**
Victim falling from one level to another, undetermined intent

The appropriate 7th character is to be added to code Y30
A   initial encounter
D   subsequent encounter
S   sequela

IQ ☑ **Y31.XXX-   Falling, lying or running before or into moving object, undetermined intent**

The appropriate 7th character is to be added to code Y31
A   initial encounter
D   subsequent encounter
S   sequela

IQ ☑ **Y32.XXX-   Crashing of motor vehicle, undetermined intent**

Chapter 20

V00-Y99

☆ New ▲ Revised Px Primary SP PDGM Px SL Low CoM SH High CoM IQ Quest. Encounter H Hospice non-cancer Dx Unspecified M *Manifestation*

The appropriate 7th character is to be added to code Y32
A   initial encounter
D   subsequent encounter
S   sequela

IQ ☑ Y33.XXX-   Other specified events, undetermined intent

The appropriate 7th character is to be added to code Y33
A   initial encounter
D   subsequent encounter
S   sequela

Legal intervention, operations of war, military operations, and terrorism (Y35-Y38)

4 Y35   Legal intervention

INCLUDES any injury sustained as a result of an encounter with any law enforcement official, serving in any capacity at the time of the encounter, whether on-duty or off-duty. Includes: injury to law enforcement official, suspect and bystander

The appropriate 7th character is to be added to each code from category Y35
A   initial encounter
D   subsequent encounter
S   sequela

5 Y35.0 Legal intervention involving firearm discharge

6 Y35.00   Legal intervention involving unspecified firearm discharge

Legal intervention involving gunshot wound
Legal intervention involving shot NOS

IQ 7 Y35.001-   Legal intervention involving unspecified firearm discharge, law enforcement official injured

IQ 7 Y35.002-   Legal intervention involving unspecified firearm discharge, bystander injured

IQ 7 Y35.003-   Legal intervention involving unspecified firearm discharge, suspect injured

★ 7 Y35.009-   Legal intervention involving unspecified firearm discharge, unspecified person injured

6 Y35.01   Legal intervention involving injury by machine gun

IQ 7 Y35.011-   Legal intervention involving injury by machine gun, law enforcement official injured

IQ 7 Y35.012-   Legal intervention involving injury by machine gun, bystander injured

IQ 7 Y35.013-   Legal intervention involving injury by machine gun, suspect injured

★ 7 Y35.019-   Legal intervention involving injury by machine gun, unspecified person injured

6 Y35.02   Legal intervention involving injury by handgun

IQ 7 Y35.021-   Legal intervention involving injury by handgun, law enforcement official injured

IQ 7 Y35.022-   Legal intervention involving injury by handgun, bystander injured

IQ 7 Y35.023-   Legal intervention involving injury by handgun, suspect injured

★ 7 Y35.029-   Legal intervention involving injury by handgun, unspecified person injured

6 Y35.03   Legal intervention involving injury by rifle pellet

IQ 7 Y35.031-   Legal intervention involving injury by rifle pellet, law enforcement official injured

IQ 7 Y35.032-   Legal intervention involving injury by rifle pellet, bystander injured

IQ 7 Y35.033-   Legal intervention involving injury by rifle pellet, suspect injured

★ 7 Y35.039-   Legal intervention involving injury by rifle pellet, unspecified person injured

6 Y35.04   Legal intervention involving injury by rubber bullet

IQ 7 Y35.041-   Legal intervention involving injury by rubber bullet, law enforcement official injured

IQ 7 Y35.042-   Legal intervention involving injury by rubber bullet, bystander injured

IQ 7 Y35.043-   Legal intervention involving injury by rubber bullet, suspect injured

★ 7 Y35.049-   Legal intervention involving injury by rubber bullet, unspecified person injured

6 Y35.09   Legal intervention involving other firearm discharge

IQ 7 Y35.091-   Legal intervention involving other firearm discharge, law enforcement official injured

IQ 7 Y35.092-   Legal intervention involving other firearm discharge, bystander injured

IQ 7 Y35.093-   Legal intervention involving other firearm discharge, suspect injured

★ 7 Y35.099-   Legal intervention involving other firearm discharge, unspecified person injured

5 Y35.1 Legal intervention involving explosives

6 Y35.10   Legal intervention involving unspecified explosives

IQ 7 Y35.101-   Legal intervention involving unspecified explosives, law enforcement official injured

IQ 7 Y35.102-   Legal intervention involving unspecified explosives, bystander injured

4 4th digit required   5 5th digit required   6 6th digit required   7 7th digit required   ☑ 7th digit placeholder   ➕ Additional code   ⊟ Laterality

1846   *DecisionHealth's* FY 2020 Complete Home Health ICD-10-CM Diagnosis Coding Manual

!Q 7 Y35.103- Legal intervention involving unspecified explosives, suspect injured

★ 7 Y35.109- Legal intervention involving unspecified explosives, unspecified person injured

6 Y35.11 Legal intervention involving injury by dynamite

!Q 7 Y35.111- Legal intervention involving injury by dynamite, law enforcement official injured

!Q 7 Y35.112- Legal intervention involving injury by dynamite, bystander injured

!Q 7 Y35.113- Legal intervention involving injury by dynamite, suspect injured

★ 7 Y35.119- Legal intervention involving injury by dynamite, unspecified person injured

6 Y35.12 Legal intervention involving injury by explosive shell

!Q 7 Y35.121- Legal intervention involving injury by explosive shell, law enforcement official injured

!Q 7 Y35.122- Legal intervention involving injury by explosive shell, bystander injured

!Q 7 Y35.123- Legal intervention involving injury by explosive shell, suspect injured

★ 7 Y35.129- Legal intervention involving injury by explosive shell, unspecified person injured

6 Y35.19 Legal intervention involving other explosives
Legal intervention involving injury by grenade
Legal intervention involving injury by mortar bomb

!Q 7 Y35.191- Legal intervention involving other explosives, law enforcement official injured

!Q 7 Y35.192- Legal intervention involving other explosives, bystander injured

!Q 7 Y35.193- Legal intervention involving other explosives, suspect injured

★ 7 Y35.199- Legal intervention involving other explosives, unspecified person injured

5 Y35.2 Legal intervention involving gas
Legal intervention involving asphyxiation by gas
Legal intervention involving poisoning by gas

6 Y35.20 Legal intervention involving unspecified gas

!Q 7 Y35.201- Legal intervention involving unspecified gas, law enforcement official injured

!Q 7 Y35.202- Legal intervention involving unspecified gas, bystander injured

!Q 7 Y35.203- Legal intervention involving unspecified gas, suspect injured

★ 7 Y35.209- Legal intervention involving unspecified gas, unspecified person injured

6 Y35.21 Legal intervention involving injury by tear gas

!Q 7 Y35.211- Legal intervention involving injury by tear gas, law enforcement official injured

!Q 7 Y35.212- Legal intervention involving injury by tear gas, bystander injured

!Q 7 Y35.213- Legal intervention involving injury by tear gas, suspect injured

★ 7 Y35.219- Legal intervention involving injury by tear gas, unspecified person injured

6 Y35.29 Legal intervention involving other gas

!Q 7 Y35.291- Legal intervention involving other gas, law enforcement official injured

!Q 7 Y35.292- Legal intervention involving other gas, bystander injured

!Q 7 Y35.293- Legal intervention involving other gas, suspect injured

★ 7 Y35.299- Legal intervention involving other gas, unspecified person injured

5 Y35.3 Legal intervention involving blunt objects
Legal intervention involving being hit or struck by blunt object

6 Y35.30 Legal intervention involving unspecified blunt objects

!Q 7 Y35.301- Legal intervention involving unspecified blunt objects, law enforcement official injured

!Q 7 Y35.302- Legal intervention involving unspecified blunt objects, bystander injured

!Q 7 Y35.303- Legal intervention involving unspecified blunt objects, suspect injured

★ 7 Y35.309- Legal intervention involving unspecified blunt objects, unspecified person injured

6 Y35.31 Legal intervention involving baton

!Q 7 Y35.311- Legal intervention involving baton, law enforcement official injured

!Q 7 Y35.312- Legal intervention involving baton, bystander injured

!Q 7 Y35.313- Legal intervention involving baton, suspect injured

★ 7 Y35.319- Legal intervention involving baton, unspecified person injured

6 Y35.39 Legal intervention involving other blunt objects

!Q 7 Y35.391- Legal intervention involving other blunt objects, law enforcement official injured

!Q 7 Y35.392- Legal intervention involving other blunt objects, bystander injured

---

★ New ▲ Revised **Px** Primary **SP** PDGM Px **SL** Low CoM **SH** High CoM **!Q** Quest. Encounter **H** Hospice non-cancer Dx   Unspecified   **M** *Manifestation*

Chapter 20

V00-Y99

!Q 7 Y35.393- Legal intervention involving other blunt objects, suspect injured

★ 7 Y35.399- Legal intervention involving other blunt objects, unspecified person injured

5 Y35.4 Legal intervention involving sharp objects

Legal intervention involving being cut by sharp objects

Legal intervention involving being stabbed by sharp objects

6 Y35.40 Legal intervention involving unspecified sharp objects

!Q 7 Y35.401- Legal intervention involving unspecified sharp objects, law enforcement official injured

!Q 7 Y35.402- Legal intervention involving unspecified sharp objects, bystander injured

!Q 7 Y35.403- Legal intervention involving unspecified sharp objects, suspect injured

★ 7 Y35.409- Legal intervention involving unspecified sharp objects, unspecified person injured

6 Y35.41 Legal intervention involving bayonet

!Q 7 Y35.411- Legal intervention involving bayonet, law enforcement official injured

!Q 7 Y35.412- Legal intervention involving bayonet, bystander injured

!Q 7 Y35.413- Legal intervention involving bayonet, suspect injured

★ 7 Y35.419- Legal intervention involving bayonet, unspecified person injured

6 Y35.49 Legal intervention involving other sharp objects

!Q 7 Y35.491- Legal intervention involving other sharp objects, law enforcement official injured

!Q 7 Y35.492- Legal intervention involving other sharp objects, bystander injured

!Q 7 Y35.493- Legal intervention involving other sharp objects, suspect injured

★ 7 Y35.499- Legal intervention involving other sharp objects, unspecified person injured

5 Y35.8 Legal intervention involving other specified means

6 Y35.81 Legal intervention involving manhandling

!Q 7 Y35.811- Legal intervention involving manhandling, law enforcement official injured

!Q 7 Y35.812- Legal intervention involving manhandling, bystander injured

!Q 7 Y35.813- Legal intervention involving manhandling, suspect injured

★ 7 Y35.819- Legal intervention involving manhandling, unspecified person injured

★ 6 Y35.83 Legal intervention involving a conducted energy device

Electroshock device (taser)

Stun gun

★ 7 Y35.831- Legal intervention involving a conducted energy device, law enforcement official injured

★ 7 Y35.832- Legal intervention involving a conducted energy device, bystander injured

★ 7 Y35.833- Legal intervention involving a conducted energy device, suspect injured

★ 7 Y35.839- Legal intervention involving a conducted energy device, unspecified person injured

6 Y35.89 Legal intervention involving other specified means

!Q 7 Y35.891- Legal intervention involving other specified means, law enforcement official injured

!Q 7 Y35.892- Legal intervention involving other specified means, bystander injured

!Q 7 Y35.893- Legal intervention involving other specified means, suspect injured

5 Y35.9 Legal intervention, means unspecified

!Q 7 Y35.91X- Legal intervention, means unspecified, law enforcement official injured

!Q 7 Y35.92X- Legal intervention, means unspecified, bystander injured

!Q 7 Y35.93X- Legal intervention, means unspecified, suspect injured

★ 7 Y35.99X- Legal intervention, means unspecified, unspecified person injured

4 Y36 Operations of war

INCLUDES injuries to military personnel and civilians caused by war, civil insurrection, and peacekeeping missions

EXCLUDES 1 injury to military personnel occurring during peacetime military operations (Y37.-)

military vehicles involved in transport accidents with non-military vehicle during peacetime (V09.01, V09.21, V19.81, V29.81, V39.81, V49.81, V59.81, V69.81, V79.81)

The appropriate 7th character is to be added to each code from category Y36

A   initial encounter

D   subsequent encounter

S   sequela

5 Y36.0 War operations involving explosion of marine weapons

6 Y36.00 War operations involving explosion of unspecified marine weapon

War operations involving underwater blast NOS

!Q 7 Y36.000- War operations involving explosion of unspecified marine weapon, military personnel

4 4th digit required   5 5th digit required   6 6th digit required   7 7th digit required   7 7th digit placeholder   + Additional code   ⊟ Laterality

1848   *DecisionHealth's* FY 2020 Complete Home Health ICD-10-CM Diagnosis Coding Manual

IQ 7 Y36.001- **War operations involving explosion of unspecified marine weapon, civilian**

6 Y36.01 War operations involving explosion of depth-charge

IQ 7 Y36.010- War operations involving explosion of depth-charge, military personnel

IQ 7 Y36.011- War operations involving explosion of depth-charge, civilian

6 Y36.02 War operations involving explosion of marine mine

War operations involving explosion of marine mine, at sea or in harbor

IQ 7 Y36.020- War operations involving explosion of marine mine, military personnel

IQ 7 Y36.021- War operations involving explosion of marine mine, civilian

6 Y36.03 War operations involving explosion of sea-based artillery shell

IQ 7 Y36.030- War operations involving explosion of sea-based artillery shell, military personnel

IQ 7 Y36.031- War operations involving explosion of sea-based artillery shell, civilian

6 Y36.04 War operations involving explosion of torpedo

IQ 7 Y36.040- War operations involving explosion of torpedo, military personnel

IQ 7 Y36.041- War operations involving explosion of torpedo, civilian

6 Y36.05 War operations involving accidental detonation of onboard marine weapons

IQ 7 Y36.050- War operations involving accidental detonation of onboard marine weapons, military personnel

IQ 7 Y36.051- War operations involving accidental detonation of onboard marine weapons, civilian

6 Y36.09 War operations involving explosion of other marine weapons

IQ 7 Y36.090- War operations involving explosion of other marine weapons, military personnel

IQ 7 Y36.091- War operations involving explosion of other marine weapons, civilian

5 Y36.1 War operations involving destruction of aircraft

6 Y36.10 War operations involving unspecified destruction of aircraft

IQ 7 Y36.100- War operations involving unspecified destruction of aircraft, military personnel

IQ 7 Y36.101- War operations involving unspecified destruction of aircraft, civilian

6 Y36.11 War operations involving destruction of aircraft due to enemy fire or explosives

War operations involving destruction of aircraft due to air to air missile
War operations involving destruction of aircraft due to explosive placed on aircraft
War operations involving destruction of aircraft due to rocket propelled grenade [RPG]
War operations involving destruction of aircraft due to small arms fire
War operations involving destruction of aircraft due to surface to air missile

IQ 7 Y36.110- War operations involving destruction of aircraft due to enemy fire or explosives, military personnel

IQ 7 Y36.111- War operations involving destruction of aircraft due to enemy fire or explosives, civilian

6 Y36.12 War operations involving destruction of aircraft due to collision with other aircraft

IQ 7 Y36.120- War operations involving destruction of aircraft due to collision with other aircraft, military personnel

IQ 7 Y36.121- War operations involving destruction of aircraft due to collision with other aircraft, civilian

6 Y36.13 War operations involving destruction of aircraft due to onboard fire

IQ 7 Y36.130- War operations involving destruction of aircraft due to onboard fire, military personnel

IQ 7 Y36.131- War operations involving destruction of aircraft due to onboard fire, civilian

6 Y36.14 War operations involving destruction of aircraft due to accidental detonation of onboard munitions and explosives

IQ 7 Y36.140- War operations involving destruction of aircraft due to accidental detonation of onboard munitions and explosives, military personnel

IQ 7 Y36.141- War operations involving destruction of aircraft due to accidental detonation of onboard munitions and explosives, civilian

6 Y36.19 War operations involving other destruction of aircraft

IQ 7 Y36.190- War operations involving other destruction of aircraft, military personnel

IQ 7 Y36.191- War operations involving other destruction of aircraft, civilian

5 Y36.2 War operations involving other explosions and fragments

EXCLUDES 1 war operations involving explosion of aircraft (Y36.1-)
war operations involving explosion of marine weapons (Y36.0-)

★ New ▲ Revised **Px** Primary **SP** PDGM Px **SL** Low CoM **SH** High CoM **IQ** Quest. Encounter **H** Hospice non-cancer Dx   Unspecified   **M** *Manifestation*

war operations involving
explosion of nuclear
weapons (Y36.5-)
war operations involving
explosion occurring after
cessation of hostilities
(Y36.8-)

⑥ **Y36.20   War operations involving unspecified explosion and fragments**

War operations involving air blast NOS
War operations involving blast NOS
War operations involving blast
fragments NOS
War operations involving blast wave
NOS
War operations involving blast wind
NOS
War operations involving explosion
NOS
War operations involving explosion of
bomb NOS

!Q ⑦ **Y36.200-   War operations involving unspecified explosion and fragments, military personnel**

!Q ⑦ **Y36.201-   War operations involving unspecified explosion and fragments, civilian**

⑥ **Y36.21   War operations involving explosion of aerial bomb**

!Q ⑦ Y36.210-   War operations involving
explosion of aerial bomb,
military personnel

!Q ⑦ Y36.211-   War operations involving
explosion of aerial bomb, civilian

⑥ **Y36.22   War operations involving explosion of guided missile**

!Q ⑦ Y36.220-   War operations involving
explosion of guided missile,
military personnel

!Q ⑦ Y36.221-   War operations involving
explosion of guided missile,
civilian

⑥ **Y36.23   War operations involving explosion of improvised explosive device [IED]**

War operations involving explosion of
person-borne improvised explosive
device [IED]
War operations involving explosion of
vehicle-borne improvised explosive
device [IED]
War operations involving explosion of
roadside improvised explosive device
[IED]

!Q ⑦ Y36.230-   War operations involving
explosion of improvised explosive
device [IED], military personnel

!Q ⑦ Y36.231-   War operations involving
explosion of improvised explosive
device [IED], civilian

⑥ **Y36.24   War operations involving explosion due to accidental detonation and discharge of own munitions or munitions launch device**

!Q ⑦ Y36.240-   War operations involving
explosion due to accidental
detonation and discharge of own
munitions or munitions launch
device, military personnel

!Q ⑦ Y36.241-   War operations involving
explosion due to accidental
detonation and discharge of own
munitions or munitions launch
device, civilian

⑥ **Y36.25   War operations involving fragments from munitions**

!Q ⑦ Y36.250-   War operations involving
fragments from munitions,
military personnel

!Q ⑦ Y36.251-   War operations involving
fragments from munitions,
civilian

⑥ **Y36.26   War operations involving fragments of improvised explosive device [IED]**

War operations involving fragments of
person-borne improvised explosive
device [IED]
War operations involving fragments of
vehicle-borne improvised explosive
device [IED]
War operations involving fragments of
roadside improvised explosive device
[IED]

!Q ⑦ Y36.260-   War operations involving
fragments of improvised
explosive device [IED], military
personnel

!Q ⑦ Y36.261-   War operations involving
fragments of improvised
explosive device [IED], civilian

⑥ **Y36.27   War operations involving fragments from weapons**

!Q ⑦ Y36.270-   War operations involving
fragments from weapons,
military personnel

!Q ⑦ Y36.271-   War operations involving
fragments from weapons, civilian

⑥ **Y36.29   War operations involving other explosions and fragments**

War operations involving explosion of
grenade
War operations involving explosions of
land mine
War operations involving shrapnel
NOS

!Q ⑦ Y36.290-   War operations involving other
explosions and fragments,
military personnel

!Q ⑦ Y36.291-   War operations involving other
explosions and fragments,
civilian

⑤ **Y36.3   War operations involving fires, conflagrations and hot substances**

War operations involving smoke, fumes,
and heat from fires, conflagrations and
hot substances

EXCLUDES 1   war operations involving
fires and conflagrations
aboard military aircraft
(Y36.1-)

④4th digit required   ⑤5th digit required   ⑥6th digit required   ⑦7th digit required   ⑦7th digit placeholder   ➕Additional code   ⊟Laterality

1850   *DecisionHealth's* FY 2020 Complete Home Health ICD-10-CM Diagnosis Coding Manual

war operations involving
fires and conflagrations
aboard military watercraft
(Y36.0-)
war operations involving
fires and conflagrations
caused indirectly by
conventional weapons
(Y36.2-)
war operations involving
fires and thermal effects of
nuclear weapons
(Y36.53-)

[6] **Y36.30** **War operations involving unspecified fire, conflagration and hot substance**

[!Q] [7] **Y36.300-** **War operations involving unspecified fire, conflagration and hot substance, military personnel**

[!Q] [7] **Y36.301-** **War operations involving unspecified fire, conflagration and hot substance, civilian**

[6] **Y36.31** **War operations involving gasoline bomb**
War operations involving incendiary bomb
War operations involving petrol bomb

[!Q] [7] **Y36.310-** **War operations involving gasoline bomb, military personnel**

[!Q] [7] **Y36.311-** **War operations involving gasoline bomb, civilian**

[6] **Y36.32** **War operations involving incendiary bullet**

[!Q] [7] **Y36.320-** **War operations involving incendiary bullet, military personnel**

[!Q] [7] **Y36.321-** **War operations involving incendiary bullet, civilian**

[6] **Y36.33** **War operations involving flamethrower**

[!Q] [7] **Y36.330-** **War operations involving flamethrower, military personnel**

[!Q] [7] **Y36.331-** **War operations involving flamethrower, civilian**

[6] **Y36.39** **War operations involving other fires, conflagrations and hot substances**

[!Q] [7] **Y36.390-** **War operations involving other fires, conflagrations and hot substances, military personnel**

[!Q] [7] **Y36.391-** **War operations involving other fires, conflagrations and hot substances, civilian**

[5] **Y36.4** **War operations involving firearm discharge and other forms of conventional warfare**

[6] **Y36.41** **War operations involving rubber bullets**

[!Q] [7] **Y36.410-** **War operations involving rubber bullets, military personnel**

[!Q] [7] **Y36.411-** **War operations involving rubber bullets, civilian**

[6] **Y36.42** **War operations involving firearms pellets**

[!Q] [7] **Y36.420-** **War operations involving firearms pellets, military personnel**

[!Q] [7] **Y36.421-** **War operations involving firearms pellets, civilian**

[6] **Y36.43** **War operations involving other firearms discharge**
War operations involving bullets NOS
EXCLUDES 1 war operations involving
munitions fragments
(Y36.25-)
war operations involving
incendiary bullets
(Y36.32-)

[!Q] [7] **Y36.430-** **War operations involving other firearms discharge, military personnel**

[!Q] [7] **Y36.431-** **War operations involving other firearms discharge, civilian**

[6] **Y36.44** **War operations involving unarmed hand to hand combat**
EXCLUDES 1 war operations involving
combat using blunt or
piercing object
(Y36.45-)
war operations involving
intentional restriction
of air and airway
(Y36.46-)
war operations involving
unintentional
restriction of air and
airway (Y36.47-)

[!Q] [7] **Y36.440-** **War operations involving unarmed hand to hand combat, military personnel**

[!Q] [7] **Y36.441-** **War operations involving unarmed hand to hand combat, civilian**

[6] **Y36.45** **War operations involving combat using blunt or piercing object**

[!Q] [7] **Y36.450-** **War operations involving combat using blunt or piercing object, military personnel**

[!Q] [7] **Y36.451-** **War operations involving combat using blunt or piercing object, civilian**

[6] **Y36.46** **War operations involving intentional restriction of air and airway**

[!Q] [7] **Y36.460-** **War operations involving intentional restriction of air and airway, military personnel**

[!Q] [7] **Y36.461-** **War operations involving intentional restriction of air and airway, civilian**

[6] **Y36.47** **War operations involving unintentional restriction of air and airway**

[!Q] [7] **Y36.470-** **War operations involving unintentional restriction of air and airway, military personnel**

[!Q] [7] **Y36.471-** **War operations involving unintentional restriction of air and airway, civilian**

[6] **Y36.49** **War operations involving other forms of conventional warfare**

[!Q] [7] **Y36.490-** **War operations involving other forms of conventional warfare, military personnel**

[!Q] [7] **Y36.491-** **War operations involving other forms of conventional warfare, civilian**

★ New ▲ Revised Px Primary SP PDGM Px SL Low CoM SH High CoM !Q Quest. Encounter H Hospice non-cancer Dx Unspecified M Manifestation

5 Y36.5 War operations involving nuclear weapons
War operations involving dirty bomb NOS

6 Y36.50 War operations involving unspecified effect of nuclear weapon

!Q 7 Y36.500- War operations involving unspecified effect of nuclear weapon, military personnel

!Q 7 Y36.501- War operations involving unspecified effect of nuclear weapon, civilian

6 Y36.51 War operations involving direct blast effect of nuclear weapon
War operations involving blast pressure of nuclear weapon

!Q 7 Y36.510- War operations involving direct blast effect of nuclear weapon, military personnel

!Q 7 Y36.511- War operations involving direct blast effect of nuclear weapon, civilian

6 Y36.52 War operations involving indirect blast effect of nuclear weapon
War operations involving being thrown by blast of nuclear weapon
War operations involving being struck or crushed by blast debris of nuclear weapon

!Q 7 Y36.520- War operations involving indirect blast effect of nuclear weapon, military personnel

!Q 7 Y36.521- War operations involving indirect blast effect of nuclear weapon, civilian

6 Y36.53 War operations involving thermal radiation effect of nuclear weapon
War operations involving direct heat from nuclear weapon
War operation involving fireball effects from nuclear weapon

!Q 7 Y36.530- War operations involving thermal radiation effect of nuclear weapon, military personnel

!Q 7 Y36.531- War operations involving thermal radiation effect of nuclear weapon, civilian

6 Y36.54 War operation involving nuclear radiation effects of nuclear weapon
War operation involving acute radiation exposure from nuclear weapon
War operation involving exposure to immediate ionizing radiation from nuclear weapon
War operation involving fallout exposure from nuclear weapon
War operation involving secondary effects of nuclear weapons

!Q 7 Y36.540- War operation involving nuclear radiation effects of nuclear weapon, military personnel

!Q 7 Y36.541- War operation involving nuclear radiation effects of nuclear weapon, civilian

6 Y36.59 War operation involving other effects of nuclear weapons

!Q 7 Y36.590- War operation involving other effects of nuclear weapons, military personnel

!Q 7 Y36.591- War operation involving other effects of nuclear weapons, civilian

5 Y36.6 War operations involving biological weapons

6 Y36.6X War operations involving biological weapons

!Q 7 Y36.6X0- War operations involving biological weapons, military personnel

!Q 7 Y36.6X1- War operations involving biological weapons, civilian

5 Y36.7 War operations involving chemical weapons and other forms of unconventional warfare
> **EXCLUDES 1** war operations involving incendiary devices (Y36.3-, Y36.5-)

6 Y36.7X War operations involving chemical weapons and other forms of unconventional warfare

!Q 7 Y36.7X0- War operations involving chemical weapons and other forms of unconventional warfare, military personnel

!Q 7 Y36.7X1- War operations involving chemical weapons and other forms of unconventional warfare, civilian

5 Y36.8 War operations occurring after cessation of hostilities
War operations classifiable to categories Y36.0-Y36.8 but occurring after cessation of hostilities

6 Y36.81 Explosion of mine placed during war operations but exploding after cessation of hostilities

!Q 7 Y36.810- Explosion of mine placed during war operations but exploding after cessation of hostilities, military personnel

!Q 7 Y36.811- Explosion of mine placed during war operations but exploding after cessation of hostilities, civilian

6 Y36.82 Explosion of bomb placed during war operations but exploding after cessation of hostilities

!Q 7 Y36.820- Explosion of bomb placed during war operations but exploding after cessation of hostilities, military personnel

!Q 7 Y36.821- Explosion of bomb placed during war operations but exploding after cessation of hostilities, civilian

6 Y36.88 Other war operations occurring after cessation of hostilities

!Q 7 Y36.880- Other war operations occurring after cessation of hostilities, military personnel

!Q 7 Y36.881- Other war operations occurring after cessation of hostilities, civilian

---

4 4th digit required   5 5th digit required   6 6th digit required   7 7th digit required   7 7th digit placeholder   **+**Additional code   ▤ Laterality

⑥ **Y36.89** **Unspecified war operations occurring after cessation of hostilities**

!Q 7 **Y36.890-** **Unspecified war operations occurring after cessation of hostilities, military personnel**

!Q 7 **Y36.891-** **Unspecified war operations occurring after cessation of hostilities, civilian**

⑤ **Y36.9** **Other and unspecified war operations**

!Q ☑ **Y36.90X-** **War operations, unspecified**

!Q ☑ **Y36.91X-** **War operations involving unspecified weapon of mass destruction [WMD]**

!Q ☑ **Y36.92X-** War operations involving friendly fire

④ **Y37** **Military operations**

> INCLUDES   injuries to military personnel and civilians occurring during peacetime on military property and during routine military exercises and operations

> EXCLUDES 1   military aircraft involved in aircraft accident with civilian aircraft (V97.81-)
> military vehicles involved in transport accident with civilian vehicle (V09.01, V09.21, V19.81, V29.81, V39.81, V49.81, V59.81, V69.81, V79.81)
> military watercraft involved in water transport accident with civilian watercraft (V94.81-)
> war operations (Y36.-)

> The appropriate 7th character is to be added to each code from category Y37
> A   initial encounter
> D   subsequent encounter
> S   sequela

⑤ **Y37.0** **Military operations involving explosion of marine weapons**

⑥ **Y37.00** **Military operations involving explosion of unspecified marine weapon**

> Military operations involving underwater blast NOS

!Q 7 **Y37.000-** **Military operations involving explosion of unspecified marine weapon, military personnel**

!Q 7 **Y37.001-** **Military operations involving explosion of unspecified marine weapon, civilian**

⑥ **Y37.01** **Military operations involving explosion of depth-charge**

!Q 7 **Y37.010-** Military operations involving explosion of depth-charge, military personnel

!Q 7 **Y37.011-** Military operations involving explosion of depth-charge, civilian

⑥ **Y37.02** Military operations involving explosion of marine mine

> Military operations involving explosion of marine mine, at sea or in harbor

!Q 7 **Y37.020-** **Military operations involving explosion of marine mine, military personnel**

!Q 7 **Y37.021-** **Military operations involving explosion of marine mine, civilian**

⑥ **Y37.03** **Military operations involving explosion of sea-based artillery shell**

!Q 7 **Y37.030-** **Military operations involving explosion of sea-based artillery shell, military personnel**

!Q 7 **Y37.031-** **Military operations involving explosion of sea-based artillery shell, civilian**

⑥ **Y37.04** **Military operations involving explosion of torpedo**

!Q 7 **Y37.040-** **Military operations involving explosion of torpedo, military personnel**

!Q 7 **Y37.041-** **Military operations involving explosion of torpedo, civilian**

⑥ **Y37.05** **Military operations involving accidental detonation of onboard marine weapons**

!Q 7 **Y37.050-** **Military operations involving accidental detonation of onboard marine weapons, military personnel**

!Q 7 **Y37.051-** **Military operations involving accidental detonation of onboard marine weapons, civilian**

⑥ **Y37.09** **Military operations involving explosion of other marine weapons**

!Q 7 **Y37.090-** **Military operations involving explosion of other marine weapons, military personnel**

!Q 7 **Y37.091-** **Military operations involving explosion of other marine weapons, civilian**

⑤ **Y37.1** **Military operations involving destruction of aircraft**

⑥ **Y37.10** **Military operations involving unspecified destruction of aircraft**

!Q 7 **Y37.100-** **Military operations involving unspecified destruction of aircraft, military personnel**

!Q 7 **Y37.101-** **Military operations involving unspecified destruction of aircraft, civilian**

⑥ **Y37.11** **Military operations involving destruction of aircraft due to enemy fire or explosives**

> Military operations involving destruction of aircraft due to air to air missile
> Military operations involving destruction of aircraft due to explosive placed on aircraft
> Military operations involving destruction of aircraft due to rocket propelled grenade [RPG]
> Military operations involving destruction of aircraft due to small arms fire

Chapter 20

V00-Y99

★ New ▲ Revised Px Primary SP PDGM Px SL Low CoM SH High CoM !Q Quest. Encounter H Hospice non-cancer Dx Unspecified M *Manifestation*

DecisionHealth's FY 2020 Complete Home Health ICD-10-CM Diagnosis Coding Manual

1853

Military operations involving destruction of aircraft due to surface to air missile

!Q 7 Y37.110- **Military operations involving destruction of aircraft due to enemy fire or explosives, military personnel**

!Q 7 Y37.111- **Military operations involving destruction of aircraft due to enemy fire or explosives, civilian**

6 Y37.12 **Military operations involving destruction of aircraft due to collision with other aircraft**

!Q 7 Y37.120- **Military operations involving destruction of aircraft due to collision with other aircraft, military personnel**

!Q 7 Y37.121- **Military operations involving destruction of aircraft due to collision with other aircraft, civilian**

6 Y37.13 **Military operations involving destruction of aircraft due to onboard fire**

!Q 7 Y37.130- **Military operations involving destruction of aircraft due to onboard fire, military personnel**

!Q 7 Y37.131- **Military operations involving destruction of aircraft due to onboard fire, civilian**

6 Y37.14 **Military operations involving destruction of aircraft due to accidental detonation of onboard munitions and explosives**

!Q 7 Y37.140- **Military operations involving destruction of aircraft due to accidental detonation of onboard munitions and explosives, military personnel**

!Q 7 Y37.141- **Military operations involving destruction of aircraft due to accidental detonation of onboard munitions and explosives, civilian**

6 Y37.19 **Military operations involving other destruction of aircraft**

!Q 7 Y37.190- **Military operations involving other destruction of aircraft, military personnel**

!Q 7 Y37.191- **Military operations involving other destruction of aircraft, civilian**

5 Y37.2 **Military operations involving other explosions and fragments**

> **EXCLUDES 1** military operations involving explosion of aircraft (Y37.1-)
> military operations involving explosion of marine weapons (Y37.0-)
> military operations involving explosion of nuclear weapons (Y37.5-)

6 Y37.20 **Military operations involving unspecified explosion and fragments**

Military operations involving air blast NOS

Military operations involving blast NOS

Military operations involving blast fragments NOS

Military operations involving blast wave NOS

Military operations involving blast wind NOS

Military operations involving explosion NOS

Military operations involving explosion of bomb NOS

!Q 7 Y37.200- **Military operations involving unspecified explosion and fragments, military personnel**

!Q 7 Y37.201- **Military operations involving unspecified explosion and fragments, civilian**

6 Y37.21 **Military operations involving explosion of aerial bomb**

!Q 7 Y37.210- **Military operations involving explosion of aerial bomb, military personnel**

!Q 7 Y37.211- **Military operations involving explosion of aerial bomb, civilian**

6 Y37.22 **Military operations involving explosion of guided missile**

!Q 7 Y37.220- **Military operations involving explosion of guided missile, military personnel**

!Q 7 Y37.221- **Military operations involving explosion of guided missile, civilian**

6 Y37.23 **Military operations involving explosion of improvised explosive device [IED]**

Military operations involving explosion of person-borne improvised explosive device [IED]

Military operations involving explosion of vehicle-borne improvised explosive device [IED]

Military operations involving explosion of roadside improvised explosive device [IED]

!Q 7 Y37.230- **Military operations involving explosion of improvised explosive device [IED], military personnel**

!Q 7 Y37.231- **Military operations involving explosion of improvised explosive device [IED], civilian**

6 Y37.24 **Military operations involving explosion due to accidental detonation and discharge of own munitions or munitions launch device**

!Q 7 Y37.240- **Military operations involving explosion due to accidental detonation and discharge of own munitions or munitions launch device, military personnel**

!Q 7 Y37.241- **Military operations involving explosion due to accidental detonation and discharge of own munitions or munitions launch device, civilian**

6 Y37.25 **Military operations involving fragments from munitions**

◪4th digit required   ⑤5th digit required   ⑥6th digit required   ⑦7th digit required   ☑7th digit placeholder   ✚Additional code   ⊟Laterality

1854   *DecisionHealth's* FY 2020 Complete Home Health ICD-10-CM Diagnosis Coding Manual

!Q 7 Y37.250- Military operations involving fragments from munitions, military personnel

!Q 7 Y37.251- Military operations involving fragments from munitions, civilian

6 Y37.26 Military operations involving fragments of improvised explosive device [IED]

Military operations involving fragments of person-borne improvised explosive device [IED]

Military operations involving fragments of vehicle-borne improvised explosive device [IED]

Military operations involving fragments of roadside improvised explosive device [IED]

!Q 7 Y37.260- Military operations involving fragments of improvised explosive device [IED], military personnel

!Q 7 Y37.261- Military operations involving fragments of improvised explosive device [IED], civilian

6 Y37.27 Military operations involving fragments from weapons

!Q 7 Y37.270- Military operations involving fragments from weapons, military personnel

!Q 7 Y37.271- Military operations involving fragments from weapons, civilian

6 Y37.29 Military operations involving other explosions and fragments

Military operations involving explosion of grenade

Military operations involving explosions of land mine

Military operations involving shrapnel NOS

!Q 7 Y37.290- Military operations involving other explosions and fragments, military personnel

!Q 7 Y37.291- Military operations involving other explosions and fragments, civilian

5 Y37.3 Military operations involving fires, conflagrations and hot substances

Military operations involving smoke, fumes, and heat from fires, conflagrations and hot substances

> **EXCLUDES 1** military operations involving fires and conflagrations aboard military aircraft (Y37.1-)
>
> military operations involving fires and conflagrations aboard military watercraft (Y37.0-)
>
> military operations involving fires and conflagrations caused indirectly by conventional weapons (Y37.2-)
>
> military operations involving fires and thermal effects of nuclear weapons (Y36.53-)

6 Y37.30 Military operations involving unspecified fire, conflagration and hot substance

!Q 7 Y37.300- Military operations involving unspecified fire, conflagration and hot substance, military personnel

!Q 7 Y37.301- Military operations involving unspecified fire, conflagration and hot substance, civilian

6 Y37.31 Military operations involving gasoline bomb

Military operations involving incendiary bomb

Military operations involving petrol bomb

!Q 7 Y37.310- Military operations involving gasoline bomb, military personnel

!Q 7 Y37.311- Military operations involving gasoline bomb, civilian

6 Y37.32 Military operations involving incendiary bullet

!Q 7 Y37.320- Military operations involving incendiary bullet, military personnel

!Q 7 Y37.321- Military operations involving incendiary bullet, civilian

6 Y37.33 Military operations involving flamethrower

!Q 7 Y37.330- Military operations involving flamethrower, military personnel

!Q 7 Y37.331- Military operations involving flamethrower, civilian

6 Y37.39 Military operations involving other fires, conflagrations and hot substances

!Q 7 Y37.390- Military operations involving other fires, conflagrations and hot substances, military personnel

!Q 7 Y37.391- Military operations involving other fires, conflagrations and hot substances, civilian

5 Y37.4 Military operations involving firearm discharge and other forms of conventional warfare

6 Y37.41 Military operations involving rubber bullets

!Q 7 Y37.410- Military operations involving rubber bullets, military personnel

!Q 7 Y37.411- Military operations involving rubber bullets, civilian

6 Y37.42 Military operations involving firearms pellets

!Q 7 Y37.420- Military operations involving firearms pellets, military personnel

!Q 7 Y37.421- Military operations involving firearms pellets, civilian

6 Y37.43 Military operations involving other firearms discharge

Military operations involving bullets NOS

> **EXCLUDES 1** military operations involving munitions fragments (Y37.25-)

★ New ▲ Revised **Px** Primary **SP** PDGM Px **SL** Low CoM **SH** High CoM **!Q** Quest. Encounter **H** Hospice non-cancer Dx Unspecified **M** *Manifestation*

military operations
involving incendiary
bullets (Y37.32-)

!Q 7 Y37.430- **Military operations involving
other firearms discharge,
military personnel**

!Q 7 Y37.431- **Military operations involving
other firearms discharge, civilian**

6 Y37.44 **Military operations involving
unarmed hand to hand combat**

> **EXCLUDES 1** military operations
> involving combat using
> blunt or piercing object
> (Y37.45-)
> military operations
> involving intentional
> restriction of air and
> airway (Y37.46-)
> military operations
> involving unintentional
> restriction of air and
> airway (Y37.47-)

!Q 7 Y37.440- **Military operations involving
unarmed hand to hand combat,
military personnel**

!Q 7 Y37.441- **Military operations involving
unarmed hand to hand combat,
civilian**

6 Y37.45 **Military operations involving
combat using blunt or piercing
object**

!Q 7 Y37.450- **Military operations involving
combat using blunt or piercing
object, military personnel**

!Q 7 Y37.451- **Military operations involving
combat using blunt or piercing
object, civilian**

6 Y37.46 **Military operations involving
intentional restriction of air and
airway**

!Q 7 Y37.460- **Military operations involving
intentional restriction of air and
airway, military personnel**

!Q 7 Y37.461- **Military operations involving
intentional restriction of air and
airway, civilian**

6 Y37.47 **Military operations involving
unintentional restriction of air and
airway**

!Q 7 Y37.470- **Military operations involving
unintentional restriction of air
and airway, military personnel**

!Q 7 Y37.471- **Military operations involving
unintentional restriction of air
and airway, civilian**

6 Y37.49 **Military operations involving other
forms of conventional warfare**

!Q 7 Y37.490- **Military operations involving
other forms of conventional
warfare, military personnel**

!Q 7 Y37.491- **Military operations involving
other forms of conventional
warfare, civilian**

5 Y37.5 **Military operations involving nuclear
weapons**

Military operation involving dirty bomb
NOS

6 Y37.50 **Military operations involving
unspecified effect of nuclear weapon**

!Q 7 Y37.500- **Military operations involving
unspecified effect of nuclear
weapon, military personnel**

!Q 7 Y37.501- **Military operations involving
unspecified effect of nuclear
weapon, civilian**

6 Y37.51 **Military operations involving direct
blast effect of nuclear weapon**

Military operations involving blast
pressure of nuclear weapon

!Q 7 Y37.510- **Military operations involving
direct blast effect of nuclear
weapon, military personnel**

!Q 7 Y37.511- **Military operations involving
direct blast effect of nuclear
weapon, civilian**

6 Y37.52 **Military operations involving
indirect blast effect of nuclear
weapon**

Military operations involving being
thrown by blast of nuclear weapon
Military operations involving being
struck or crushed by blast debris of
nuclear weapon

!Q 7 Y37.520- **Military operations involving
indirect blast effect of nuclear
weapon, military personnel**

!Q 7 Y37.521- **Military operations involving
indirect blast effect of nuclear
weapon, civilian**

6 Y37.53 **Military operations involving
thermal radiation effect of nuclear
weapon**

Military operations involving direct
heat from nuclear weapon
Military operation involving fireball
effects from nuclear weapon

!Q 7 Y37.530- **Military operations involving
thermal radiation effect of
nuclear weapon, military
personnel**

!Q 7 Y37.531- **Military operations involving
thermal radiation effect of
nuclear weapon, civilian**

6 Y37.54 **Military operation involving nuclear
radiation effects of nuclear weapon**

Military operation involving acute
radiation exposure from nuclear
weapon
Military operation involving exposure
to immediate ionizing radiation from
nuclear weapon
Military operation involving fallout
exposure from nuclear weapon
Military operation involving secondary
effects of nuclear weapons

!Q 7 Y37.540- **Military operation involving
nuclear radiation effects of
nuclear weapon, military
personnel**

!Q 7 Y37.541- **Military operation involving
nuclear radiation effects of
nuclear weapon, civilian**

6 Y37.59 **Military operation involving other
effects of nuclear weapons**

!Q 7 Y37.590- **Military operation involving
other effects of nuclear weapons,
military personnel**

Chapter 20

V00-Y99

IQ 7 **Y37.591-** Military operation involving other effects of nuclear weapons, civilian

5 **Y37.6** Military operations involving biological weapons

6 **Y37.6X** Military operations involving biological weapons

IQ 7 **Y37.6X0-** Military operations involving biological weapons, military personnel

IQ 7 **Y37.6X1-** Military operations involving biological weapons, civilian

5 **Y37.7** Military operations involving chemical weapons and other forms of unconventional warfare

> **EXCLUDES 1** military operations involving incendiary devices (Y36.3-, Y36.5-)

6 **Y37.7X** Military operations involving chemical weapons and other forms of unconventional warfare

IQ 7 **Y37.7X0-** Military operations involving chemical weapons and other forms of unconventional warfare, military personnel

IQ 7 **Y37.7X1-** Military operations involving chemical weapons and other forms of unconventional warfare, civilian

5 **Y37.9** Other and unspecified military operations

IQ ☑ **Y37.90X-** Military operations, unspecified

IQ ☑ **Y37.91X-** Military operations involving unspecified weapon of mass destruction [WMD]

IQ ☑ **Y37.92X-** Military operations involving friendly fire

✚ 4 **Y38** Terrorism

These codes are for use to identify injuries resulting from the unlawful use of force or violence against persons or property to intimidate or coerce a Government, the civilian population, or any segment thereof, in furtherance of political or social objective

Use additional code for place of occurrence (Y92.-)

> The appropriate 7th character is to be added to each code from category Y38
> A   initial encounter
> D   subsequent encounter
> S   sequela

✚ 5 **Y38.0** Terrorism involving explosion of marine weapons

Terrorism involving depth-charge
Terrorism involving marine mine
Terrorism involving mine NOS, at sea or in harbor
Terrorism involving sea-based artillery shell
Terrorism involving torpedo
Terrorism involving underwater blast

✚ 6 **Y38.0X** Terrorism involving explosion of marine weapons

IQ ✚ 7 **Y38.0X1-** Terrorism involving explosion of marine weapons, public safety official injured

IQ ✚ 7 **Y38.0X2-** Terrorism involving explosion of marine weapons, civilian injured

IQ ✚ 7 **Y38.0X3-** Terrorism involving explosion of marine weapons, terrorist injured

✚ 5 **Y38.1** Terrorism involving destruction of aircraft

Terrorism involving aircraft burned
Terrorism involving aircraft exploded
Terrorism involving aircraft being shot down
Terrorism involving aircraft used as a weapon

✚ 6 **Y38.1X** Terrorism involving destruction of aircraft

IQ ✚ 7 **Y38.1X1-** Terrorism involving destruction of aircraft, public safety official injured

IQ ✚ 7 **Y38.1X2-** Terrorism involving destruction of aircraft, civilian injured

IQ ✚ 7 **Y38.1X3-** Terrorism involving destruction of aircraft, terrorist injured

✚ 5 **Y38.2** Terrorism involving other explosions and fragments

Terrorism involving antipersonnel (fragments) bomb
Terrorism involving blast NOS
Terrorism involving explosion NOS
Terrorism involving explosion of breech block
Terrorism involving explosion of cannon block
Terrorism involving explosion (fragments) of artillery shell
Terrorism involving explosion (fragments) of bomb
Terrorism involving explosion (fragments) of grenade
Terrorism involving explosion (fragments) of guided missile
Terrorism involving explosion (fragments) of land mine
Terrorism involving explosion of mortar bomb
Terrorism involving explosion of munitions
Terrorism involving explosion (fragments) of rocket
Terrorism involving explosion (fragments) of shell
Terrorism involving shrapnel
Terrorism involving mine NOS, on land

> **EXCLUDES 1** terrorism involving explosion of nuclear weapon (Y38.5)
> terrorism involving suicide bomber (Y38.81)

✚ 6 **Y38.2X** Terrorism involving other explosions and fragments

IQ ✚ 7 **Y38.2X1-** Terrorism involving other explosions and fragments, public safety official injured

IQ ✚ 7 **Y38.2X2-** Terrorism involving other explosions and fragments, civilian injured

IQ ✚ 7 **Y38.2X3-** Terrorism involving other explosions and fragments, terrorist injured

★ New ▲ Revised **Px** Primary **SP** PDGM Px **SL** Low CoM **SH** High CoM **IQ** Quest. Encounter ⬚ Hospice non-cancer Dx   Unspecified   **M** *Manifestation*

DecisionHealth's FY 2020 Complete Home Health ICD-10-CM Diagnosis Coding Manual

1857

+ 5 Y38.3 Terrorism involving fires, conflagration and hot substances
Terrorism involving conflagration NOS
Terrorism involving fire NOS
Terrorism involving petrol bomb
> **EXCLUDES 1** terrorism involving fire or heat of nuclear weapon (Y38.5)

+ 6 Y38.3X Terrorism involving fires, conflagration and hot substances

IQ + 7 Y38.3X1- Terrorism involving fires, conflagration and hot substances, public safety official injured

IQ + 7 Y38.3X2- Terrorism involving fires, conflagration and hot substances, civilian injured

IQ + 7 Y38.3X3- Terrorism involving fires, conflagration and hot substances, terrorist injured

+ 5 Y38.4 Terrorism involving firearms
Terrorism involving carbine bullet
Terrorism involving machine gun bullet
Terrorism involving pellets (shotgun)
Terrorism involving pistol bullet
Terrorism involving rifle bullet
Terrorism involving rubber (rifle) bullet

+ 6 Y38.4X Terrorism involving firearms

IQ + 7 Y38.4X1- Terrorism involving firearms, public safety official injured

IQ + 7 Y38.4X2- Terrorism involving firearms, civilian injured

IQ + 7 Y38.4X3- Terrorism involving firearms, terrorist injured

+ 5 Y38.5 Terrorism involving nuclear weapons
Terrorism involving blast effects of nuclear weapon
Terrorism involving exposure to ionizing radiation from nuclear weapon
Terrorism involving fireball effect of nuclear weapon
Terrorism involving heat from nuclear weapon

+ 6 Y38.5X Terrorism involving nuclear weapons

IQ + 7 Y38.5X1- Terrorism involving nuclear weapons, public safety official injured

IQ + 7 Y38.5X2- Terrorism involving nuclear weapons, civilian injured

IQ + 7 Y38.5X3- Terrorism involving nuclear weapons, terrorist injured

+ 5 Y38.6 Terrorism involving biological weapons
Terrorism involving anthrax
Terrorism involving cholera
Terrorism involving smallpox

+ 6 Y38.6X Terrorism involving biological weapons

IQ + 7 Y38.6X1- Terrorism involving biological weapons, public safety official injured

IQ + 7 Y38.6X2- Terrorism involving biological weapons, civilian injured

IQ + 7 Y38.6X3- Terrorism involving biological weapons, terrorist injured

+ 5 Y38.7 Terrorism involving chemical weapons
Terrorism involving gases, fumes, chemicals
Terrorism involving hydrogen cyanide
Terrorism involving phosgene
Terrorism involving sarin

+ 6 Y38.7X Terrorism involving chemical weapons

IQ + 7 Y38.7X1- Terrorism involving chemical weapons, public safety official injured

IQ + 7 Y38.7X2- Terrorism involving chemical weapons, civilian injured

IQ + 7 Y38.7X3- Terrorism involving chemical weapons, terrorist injured

+ 5 Y38.8 Terrorism involving other and unspecified means

IQ + 7 Y38.80X- Terrorism involving unspecified means
Terrorism NOS

+ 6 Y38.81 Terrorism involving suicide bomber

IQ + 7 Y38.811- Terrorism involving suicide bomber, public safety official injured

IQ + 7 Y38.812- Terrorism involving suicide bomber, civilian injured

+ 6 Y38.89 Terrorism involving other means
Terrorism involving drowning and submersion
Terrorism involving lasers
Terrorism involving piercing or stabbing instruments

IQ + 7 Y38.891- Terrorism involving other means, public safety official injured

IQ + 7 Y38.892- Terrorism involving other means, civilian injured

IQ + 7 Y38.893- Terrorism involving other means, terrorist injured

+ 5 Y38.9 Terrorism, secondary effects
Note:
This code is for use to identify conditions occurring subsequent to a terrorist attack not those that are due to the initial terrorist attack

+ 6 Y38.9X Terrorism, secondary effects

IQ + 7 Y38.9X1- Terrorism, secondary effects, public safety official injured

IQ + 7 Y38.9X2- Terrorism, secondary effects, civilian injured

Complications of medical and surgical care (Y62-Y84)

> **INCLUDES** complications of medical devices
> surgical and medical procedures as the cause of abnormal reaction of the patient, or of later complication, without mention of misadventure at the time of the procedure

Misadventures to patients during surgical and medical care   (Y62-Y69)

> **EXCLUDES 1** surgical and medical procedures as the cause of abnormal reaction of the patient, without mention of misadventure at the time of the procedure (Y83-Y84)
> **EXCLUDES 2** breakdown or malfunctioning of medical device (during procedure) (after implantation) (ongoing use) (Y70-Y82)

4 Y62 Failure of sterile precautions during surgical and medical care

---

4 4th digit required   5 5th digit required   6 6th digit required   7 7th digit required   7 7th digit placeholder   + Additional code   5 Laterality

1858   *DecisionHealth's* FY 2020 Complete Home Health ICD-10-CM Diagnosis Coding Manual

IQ Y62.0 **Failure of sterile precautions during surgical operation**

IQ Y62.1 **Failure of sterile precautions during infusion or transfusion**

IQ Y62.2 **Failure of sterile precautions during kidney dialysis and other perfusion**

IQ Y62.3 **Failure of sterile precautions during injection or immunization**

IQ Y62.4 **Failure of sterile precautions during endoscopic examination**

IQ Y62.5 **Failure of sterile precautions during heart catheterization**

IQ Y62.6 **Failure of sterile precautions during aspiration, puncture and other catheterization**

IQ Y62.8 **Failure of sterile precautions during other surgical and medical care**

IQ Y62.9 **Failure of sterile precautions during unspecified surgical and medical care**

4 Y63 **Failure in dosage during surgical and medical care**

> **EXCLUDES 2** accidental overdose of drug or wrong drug given in error (T36-T50)

IQ Y63.0 **Excessive amount of blood or other fluid given during transfusion or infusion**

IQ Y63.1 **Incorrect dilution of fluid used during infusion**

IQ Y63.2 **Overdose of radiation given during therapy**

IQ Y63.3 **Inadvertent exposure of patient to radiation during medical care**

IQ Y63.4 **Failure in dosage in electroshock or insulin-shock therapy**

IQ Y63.5 **Inappropriate temperature in local application and packing**

IQ Y63.6 **Underdosing and nonadministration of necessary drug, medicament or biological substance**

> **GUIDELINES** Section I.C.19.e.5)(c)
> Noncompliance (Z91.12-, Z91.13- and Z91.14-) or complication of care (Y63.6-Y63.9) codes are to be used with an underdosing code to indicate intent, if known.

IQ Y63.8 **Failure in dosage during other surgical and medical care**

> **GUIDELINES** Section I.C.19.e.5)(c)
> Noncompliance (Z91.12-, Z91.13- and Z91.14-) or complication of care (Y63.6-Y63.9) codes are to be used with an underdosing code to indicate intent, if known.

IQ Y63.9 **Failure in dosage during unspecified surgical and medical care**

> **GUIDELINES** Section I.C.19.e.5)(c)
> Noncompliance (Z91.12-, Z91.13- and Z91.14-) or complication of care (Y63.6-Y63.9) codes are to be used with an underdosing code to indicate intent, if known.

4 Y64 **Contaminated medical or biological substances**

IQ Y64.0 **Contaminated medical or biological substance, transfused or infused**

IQ Y64.1 **Contaminated medical or biological substance, injected or used for immunization**

IQ Y64.8 **Contaminated medical or biological substance administered by other means**

IQ Y64.9 **Contaminated medical or biological substance administered by unspecified means**

> Administered contaminated medical or biological substance NOS

4 Y65 **Other misadventures during surgical and medical care**

IQ Y65.0 **Mismatched blood in transfusion**

IQ Y65.1 **Wrong fluid used in infusion**

IQ Y65.2 **Failure in suture or ligature during surgical operation**

IQ Y65.3 **Endotracheal tube wrongly placed during anesthetic procedure**

IQ Y65.4 **Failure to introduce or to remove other tube or instrument**

5 Y65.5 **Performance of wrong procedure (operation)**

IQ Y65.51 **Performance of wrong procedure (operation) on correct patient**

> Wrong device implanted into correct surgical site
> **EXCLUDES 1** performance of correct procedure (operation) on wrong side or body part (Y65.53)

IQ Y65.52 **Performance of procedure (operation) on patient not scheduled for surgery**

> Performance of procedure (operation) intended for another patient
> Performance of procedure (operation) on wrong patient

IQ Y65.53 **Performance of correct procedure (operation) on wrong side or body part**

> Performance of correct procedure (operation) on wrong side
> Performance of correct procedure (operation) on wrong site

IQ Y65.8 **Other specified misadventures during surgical and medical care**

IQ Y66 **Nonadministration of surgical and medical care**

> Premature cessation of surgical and medical care
> **EXCLUDES 1** DNR status (Z66)
> palliative care (Z51.5)

IQ Y69 **Unspecified misadventure during surgical and medical care**

Medical devices associated with adverse incidents in diagnostic and therapeutic use (Y70-Y82)

> **INCLUDES** breakdown or malfunction of medical devices (during use) (after implantation) (ongoing use)
> **EXCLUDES 2** later complications following use of medical devices without breakdown or malfunctioning of device (Y83-Y84)
> misadventure to patients during surgical and medical care, classifiable to (Y62-Y69)

Chapter 20

V00-Y99

★ New ▲ Revised Px Primary SP PDGM Px SL Low CoM SH High CoM IQ Quest. Encounter H Hospice non-cancer Dx Unspecified M Manifestation

DecisionHealth's FY 2020 Complete Home Health ICD-10-CM Diagnosis Coding Manual

1859

surgical and other medical procedures as the cause of abnormal reaction of the patient, or of later complication, without mention of misadventure at the time of the procedure (Y83-Y84)

4️⃣ **Y70** **Anesthesiology devices associated with adverse incidents**

!Q **Y70.0** **Diagnostic and monitoring anesthesiology devices associated with adverse incidents**

!Q **Y70.1** **Therapeutic (nonsurgical) and rehabilitative anesthesiology devices associated with adverse incidents**

!Q **Y70.2** **Prosthetic and other implants, materials and accessory anesthesiology devices associated with adverse incidents**

!Q **Y70.3** **Surgical instruments, materials and anesthesiology devices (including sutures) associated with adverse incidents**

!Q **Y70.8** **Miscellaneous anesthesiology devices associated with adverse incidents, not elsewhere classified**

4️⃣ **Y71** **Cardiovascular devices associated with adverse incidents**

!Q **Y71.0** **Diagnostic and monitoring cardiovascular devices associated with adverse incidents**

!Q **Y71.1** **Therapeutic (nonsurgical) and rehabilitative cardiovascular devices associated with adverse incidents**

!Q **Y71.2** **Prosthetic and other implants, materials and accessory cardiovascular devices associated with adverse incidents**

!Q **Y71.3** **Surgical instruments, materials and cardiovascular devices (including sutures) associated with adverse incidents**

!Q **Y71.8** **Miscellaneous cardiovascular devices associated with adverse incidents, not elsewhere classified**

4️⃣ **Y72** **Otorhinolaryngological devices associated with adverse incidents**

!Q **Y72.0** **Diagnostic and monitoring otorhinolaryngological devices associated with adverse incidents**

!Q **Y72.1** **Therapeutic (nonsurgical) and rehabilitative otorhinolaryngological devices associated with adverse incidents**

!Q **Y72.2** **Prosthetic and other implants, materials and accessory otorhinolaryngological devices associated with adverse incidents**

!Q **Y72.3** **Surgical instruments, materials and otorhinolaryngological devices (including sutures) associated with adverse incidents**

!Q **Y72.8** **Miscellaneous otorhinolaryngological devices associated with adverse incidents, not elsewhere classified**

4️⃣ **Y73** **Gastroenterology and urology devices associated with adverse incidents**

!Q **Y73.0** **Diagnostic and monitoring gastroenterology and urology devices associated with adverse incidents**

!Q **Y73.1** **Therapeutic (nonsurgical) and rehabilitative gastroenterology and urology devices associated with adverse incidents**

!Q **Y73.2** **Prosthetic and other implants, materials and accessory gastroenterology and urology devices associated with adverse incidents**

!Q **Y73.3** **Surgical instruments, materials and gastroenterology and urology devices (including sutures) associated with adverse incidents**

!Q **Y73.8** **Miscellaneous gastroenterology and urology devices associated with adverse incidents, not elsewhere classified**

4️⃣ **Y74** **General hospital and personal-use devices associated with adverse incidents**

!Q **Y74.0** **Diagnostic and monitoring general hospital and personal-use devices associated with adverse incidents**

!Q **Y74.1** **Therapeutic (nonsurgical) and rehabilitative general hospital and personal-use devices associated with adverse incidents**

!Q **Y74.2** **Prosthetic and other implants, materials and accessory general hospital and personal-use devices associated with adverse incidents**

!Q **Y74.3** **Surgical instruments, materials and general hospital and personal-use devices (including sutures) associated with adverse incidents**

!Q **Y74.8** **Miscellaneous general hospital and personal-use devices associated with adverse incidents, not elsewhere classified**

4️⃣ **Y75** **Neurological devices associated with adverse incidents**

!Q **Y75.0** **Diagnostic and monitoring neurological devices associated with adverse incidents**

!Q **Y75.1** **Therapeutic (nonsurgical) and rehabilitative neurological devices associated with adverse incidents**

!Q **Y75.2** **Prosthetic and other implants, materials and neurological devices associated with adverse incidents**

!Q **Y75.3** **Surgical instruments, materials and neurological devices (including sutures) associated with adverse incidents**

!Q **Y75.8** **Miscellaneous neurological devices associated with adverse incidents, not elsewhere classified**

4️⃣ **Y76** **Obstetric and gynecological devices associated with adverse incidents**

!Q **Y76.0** **Diagnostic and monitoring obstetric and gynecological devices associated with adverse incidents**

!Q **Y76.1** **Therapeutic (nonsurgical) and rehabilitative obstetric and gynecological devices associated with adverse incidents**

!Q **Y76.2** **Prosthetic and other implants, materials and accessory obstetric and gynecological devices associated with adverse incidents**

4️⃣4th digit required   5️⃣5th digit required   6️⃣6th digit required   7️⃣7th digit required   7️⃣7th digit placeholder   ➕Additional code   ▱Laterality

1860   *DecisionHealth's* FY 2020 Complete Home Health ICD-10-CM Diagnosis Coding Manual

IQ Y76.3 Surgical instruments, materials and obstetric and gynecological devices (including sutures) associated with adverse incidents

IQ Y76.8 Miscellaneous obstetric and gynecological devices associated with adverse incidents, not elsewhere classified

4 Y77 Ophthalmic devices associated with adverse incidents

IQ Y77.0 Diagnostic and monitoring ophthalmic devices associated with adverse incidents

IQ Y77.1 Therapeutic (nonsurgical) and rehabilitative ophthalmic devices associated with adverse incidents

IQ Y77.2 Prosthetic and other implants, materials and accessory ophthalmic devices associated with adverse incidents

IQ Y77.3 Surgical instruments, materials and ophthalmic devices (including sutures) associated with adverse incidents

IQ Y77.8 Miscellaneous ophthalmic devices associated with adverse incidents, not elsewhere classified

4 Y78 Radiological devices associated with adverse incidents

IQ Y78.0 Diagnostic and monitoring radiological devices associated with adverse incidents

IQ Y78.1 Therapeutic (nonsurgical) and rehabilitative radiological devices associated with adverse incidents

IQ Y78.2 Prosthetic and other implants, materials and accessory radiological devices associated with adverse incidents

IQ Y78.3 Surgical instruments, materials and radiological devices (including sutures) associated with adverse incidents

IQ Y78.8 Miscellaneous radiological devices associated with adverse incidents, not elsewhere classified

4 Y79 Orthopedic devices associated with adverse incidents

IQ Y79.0 Diagnostic and monitoring orthopedic devices associated with adverse incidents

IQ Y79.1 Therapeutic (nonsurgical) and rehabilitative orthopedic devices associated with adverse incidents

> **CODING TIPS ✓** This code may be used to indicate the cause of a pressure injury from a prosthetic limb or other therapeutic orthopedic device.

IQ Y79.2 Prosthetic and other implants, materials and accessory orthopedic devices associated with adverse incidents

IQ Y79.3 Surgical instruments, materials and orthopedic devices (including sutures) associated with adverse incidents

IQ Y79.8 Miscellaneous orthopedic devices associated with adverse incidents, not elsewhere classified

4 Y80 Physical medicine devices associated with adverse incidents

IQ Y80.0 Diagnostic and monitoring physical medicine devices associated with adverse incidents

IQ Y80.1 Therapeutic (nonsurgical) and rehabilitative physical medicine devices associated with adverse incidents

IQ Y80.2 Prosthetic and other implants, materials and accessory physical medicine devices associated with adverse incidents

IQ Y80.3 Surgical instruments, materials and physical medicine devices (including sutures) associated with adverse incidents

IQ Y80.8 Miscellaneous physical medicine devices associated with adverse incidents, not elsewhere classified

4 Y81 General- and plastic-surgery devices associated with adverse incidents

IQ Y81.0 Diagnostic and monitoring general- and plastic-surgery devices associated with adverse incidents

IQ Y81.1 Therapeutic (nonsurgical) and rehabilitative general- and plastic-surgery devices associated with adverse incidents

IQ Y81.2 Prosthetic and other implants, materials and accessory general- and plastic-surgery devices associated with adverse incidents

IQ Y81.3 Surgical instruments, materials and general- and plastic-surgery devices (including sutures) associated with adverse incidents

IQ Y81.8 Miscellaneous general- and plastic-surgery devices associated with adverse incidents, not elsewhere classified

4 Y82 Other and unspecified medical devices associated with adverse incidents

IQ Y82.8 Other medical devices associated with adverse incidents

IQ Y82.9 Unspecified medical devices associated with adverse incidents

---

Surgical and other medical procedures as the cause of abnormal reaction of the patient, or of later complication, without mention of misadventure at the time of the procedure (Y83-Y84)

EXCLUDES 1 misadventures to patients during surgical and medical care, classifiable to (Y62-Y69)

EXCLUDES 2 breakdown or malfunctioning of medical device (after implantation) (during procedure) (ongoing use) (Y70-Y82)

4 Y83 Surgical operation and other surgical procedures as the cause of abnormal reaction of the patient, or of later complication, without mention of misadventure at the time of the procedure

IQ Y83.0 Surgical operation with transplant of whole organ as the cause of abnormal reaction of the patient, or of later complication, without mention of misadventure at the time of the procedure

IQ Y83.1 Surgical operation with implant of artificial internal device as the cause of abnormal reaction of the patient, or of later complication, without mention of misadventure at the time of the procedure

---

★ New ▲ Revised Px Primary SP PDGM Px SL Low CoM SH High CoM IQ Quest. Encounter H Hospice non-cancer Dx Unspecified M Manifestation

DecisionHealth's FY 2020 Complete Home Health ICD-10-CM Diagnosis Coding Manual

1861

!Q Y83.2 Surgical operation with anastomosis, bypass or graft as the cause of abnormal reaction of the patient, or of later complication, without mention of misadventure at the time of the procedure

!Q Y83.3 Surgical operation with formation of external stoma as the cause of abnormal reaction of the patient, or of later complication, without mention of misadventure at the time of the procedure

!Q Y83.4 Other reconstructive surgery as the cause of abnormal reaction of the patient, or of later complication, without mention of misadventure at the time of the procedure

!Q Y83.5 Amputation of limb(s) as the cause of abnormal reaction of the patient, or of later complication, without mention of misadventure at the time of the procedure

!Q Y83.6 Removal of other organ (partial) (total) as the cause of abnormal reaction of the patient, or of later complication, without mention of misadventure at the time of the procedure

!Q Y83.8 Other surgical procedures as the cause of abnormal reaction of the patient, or of later complication, without mention of misadventure at the time of the procedure

!Q Y83.9 Surgical procedure, unspecified as the cause of abnormal reaction of the patient, or of later complication, without mention of misadventure at the time of the procedure

4 Y84 Other medical procedures as the cause of abnormal reaction of the patient, or of later complication, without mention of misadventure at the time of the procedure

!Q Y84.0 Cardiac catheterization as the cause of abnormal reaction of the patient, or of later complication, without mention of misadventure at the time of the procedure

!Q Y84.1 Kidney dialysis as the cause of abnormal reaction of the patient, or of later complication, without mention of misadventure at the time of the procedure

!Q Y84.2 Radiological procedure and radiotherapy as the cause of abnormal reaction of the patient, or of later complication, without mention of misadventure at the time of the procedure

CODING TIPS ✓ This indicates an adverse effect of radiation, such as radiation burns or radiodermatitis from therapeutic use of radiation, e.g. for the treatment of cancer.

!Q Y84.3 Shock therapy as the cause of abnormal reaction of the patient, or of later complication, without mention of misadventure at the time of the procedure

!Q Y84.4 Aspiration of fluid as the cause of abnormal reaction of the patient, or of later complication, without mention of misadventure at the time of the procedure

!Q Y84.5 Insertion of gastric or duodenal sound as the cause of abnormal reaction of the patient, or of later complication, without mention of misadventure at the time of the procedure

!Q Y84.6 Urinary catheterization as the cause of abnormal reaction of the patient, or of later complication, without mention of misadventure at the time of the procedure

!Q Y84.7 Blood-sampling as the cause of abnormal reaction of the patient, or of later complication, without mention of misadventure at the time of the procedure

!Q Y84.8 Other medical procedures as the cause of abnormal reaction of the patient, or of later complication, without mention of misadventure at the time of the procedure

!Q Y84.9 Medical procedure, unspecified as the cause of abnormal reaction of the patient, or of later complication, without mention of misadventure at the time of the procedure

Supplementary factors related to causes of morbidity classified elsewhere   (Y90-Y99)

Note:
These categories may be used to provide supplementary information concerning causes of morbidity. They are not to be used for single-condition coding.

4 Y90 Evidence of alcohol involvement determined by blood alcohol level
Code first:
any associated alcohol related disorders (F10)

!Q Y90.0 Blood alcohol level of less than 20 mg/100 ml

!Q Y90.1 Blood alcohol level of 20-39 mg/100 ml

!Q Y90.2 Blood alcohol level of 40-59 mg/100 ml

!Q Y90.3 Blood alcohol level of 60-79 mg/100 ml

!Q Y90.4 Blood alcohol level of 80-99 mg/100 ml

!Q Y90.5 Blood alcohol level of 100-119 mg/100 ml

!Q Y90.6 Blood alcohol level of 120-199 mg/100 ml

!Q Y90.7 Blood alcohol level of 200-239 mg/100 ml

!Q Y90.8 Blood alcohol level of 240 mg/100 ml or more

!Q Y90.9 Presence of alcohol in blood, level not specified

4 Y92 Place of occurrence of the external cause
The following category is for use, when relevant, to identify the place of occurrence of the external cause. Use in conjunction with an activity code.
Place of occurrence should be recorded only at the initial encounter for treatment

5 Y92.0 Non-institutional (private) residence as the place of occurrence of the external cause

4 4th digit required   5 5th digit required   6 6th digit required   7 7th digit required   7 7th digit placeholder   + Additional code   ⊟ Laterality

1862   DecisionHealth's FY 2020 Complete Home Health ICD-10-CM Diagnosis Coding Manual

Chapter 20

V00-Y99

EXCLUDES 1 abandoned or derelict house
(Y92.89)
home under construction but
not yet occupied (Y92.6-)
institutional place of
residence (Y92.1-)

6 **Y92.00** **Unspecified non-institutional (private) residence as the place of occurrence of the external cause**

!Q **Y92.000** **Kitchen of unspecified non-institutional (private) residence as the place of occurrence of the external cause**

!Q **Y92.001** **Dining room of unspecified non-institutional (private) residence as the place of occurrence of the external cause**

!Q **Y92.002** **Bathroom of unspecified non-institutional (private) residence single-family (private) house as the place of occurrence of the external cause**

!Q **Y92.003** **Bedroom of unspecified non-institutional (private) residence as the place of occurrence of the external cause**

!Q **Y92.007** **Garden or yard of unspecified non-institutional (private) residence as the place of occurrence of the external cause**

!Q **Y92.008** **Other place in unspecified non-institutional (private) residence as the place of occurrence of the external cause**

!Q **Y92.009** **Unspecified place in unspecified non-institutional (private) residence as the place of occurrence of the external cause**
Home (NOS) as the place of
occurrence of the external cause

6 **Y92.01** **Single-family non-institutional (private) house as the place of occurrence of the external cause**
Farmhouse as the place of occurrence
of the external cause
EXCLUDES 1 barn (Y92.71)
chicken coop or hen
house (Y92.72)
farm field (Y92.73)
orchard (Y92.74)
single family mobile
home or trailer
(Y92.02-)
slaughter house
(Y92.86)

!Q **Y92.010** **Kitchen of single-family (private) house as the place of occurrence of the external cause**

!Q **Y92.011** **Dining room of single-family (private) house as the place of occurrence of the external cause**

!Q **Y92.012** **Bathroom of single-family (private) house as the place of occurrence of the external cause**

!Q **Y92.013** **Bedroom of single-family (private) house as the place of occurrence of the external cause**

!Q **Y92.014** **Private driveway to single-family (private) house as the place of occurrence of the external cause**

!Q **Y92.015** **Private garage of single-family (private) house as the place of occurrence of the external cause**

!Q **Y92.016** **Swimming-pool in single-family (private) house or garden as the place of occurrence of the external cause**

!Q **Y92.017** **Garden or yard in single-family (private) house as the place of occurrence of the external cause**

!Q **Y92.018** **Other place in single-family (private) house as the place of occurrence of the external cause**

!Q **Y92.019** **Unspecified place in single-family (private) house as the place of occurrence of the external cause**

6 **Y92.02** **Mobile home as the place of occurrence of the external cause**

!Q **Y92.020** **Kitchen in mobile home as the place of occurrence of the external cause**

!Q **Y92.021** **Dining room in mobile home as the place of occurrence of the external cause**

!Q **Y92.022** **Bathroom in mobile home as the place of occurrence of the external cause**

!Q **Y92.023** **Bedroom in mobile home as the place of occurrence of the external cause**

!Q **Y92.024** **Driveway of mobile home as the place of occurrence of the external cause**

!Q **Y92.025** **Garage of mobile home as the place of occurrence of the external cause**

!Q **Y92.026** **Swimming-pool of mobile home as the place of occurrence of the external cause**

!Q **Y92.027** **Garden or yard of mobile home as the place of occurrence of the external cause**

!Q **Y92.028** **Other place in mobile home as the place of occurrence of the external cause**

!Q **Y92.029** **Unspecified place in mobile home as the place of occurrence of the external cause**

6 **Y92.03** **Apartment as the place of occurrence of the external cause**
Condominium as the place of
occurrence of the external cause
Co-op apartment as the place of
occurrence of the external cause

!Q **Y92.030** **Kitchen in apartment as the place of occurrence of the external cause**

!Q **Y92.031** **Bathroom in apartment as the place of occurrence of the external cause**

!Q **Y92.032** **Bedroom in apartment as the place of occurrence of the external cause**

Chapter 20

V00-Y99

★ New ▲ Revised Px Primary SP PDGM Px SL Low CoM SH High CoM !Q Quest. Encounter H Hospice non-cancer Dx [Unspecified] M *Manifestation*

DecisionHealth's FY 2020 Complete Home Health ICD-10-CM Diagnosis Coding Manual

1863

!Q **Y92.038** Other place in apartment as the place of occurrence of the external cause

!Q **Y92.039** Unspecified place in apartment as the place of occurrence of the external cause

6 **Y92.04** Boarding-house as the place of occurrence of the external cause

!Q **Y92.040** Kitchen in boarding-house as the place of occurrence of the external cause

!Q **Y92.041** Bathroom in boarding-house as the place of occurrence of the external cause

!Q **Y92.042** Bedroom in boarding-house as the place of occurrence of the external cause

!Q **Y92.043** Driveway of boarding-house as the place of occurrence of the external cause

!Q **Y92.044** Garage of boarding-house as the place of occurrence of the external cause

!Q **Y92.045** Swimming-pool of boarding-house as the place of occurrence of the external cause

!Q **Y92.046** Garden or yard of boarding-house as the place of occurrence of the external cause

!Q **Y92.048** Other place in boarding-house as the place of occurrence of the external cause

!Q **Y92.049** Unspecified place in boarding-house as the place of occurrence of the external cause

6 **Y92.09** Other non-institutional residence as the place of occurrence of the external cause

!Q **Y92.090** Kitchen in other non-institutional residence as the place of occurrence of the external cause

!Q **Y92.091** Bathroom in other non-institutional residence as the place of occurrence of the external cause

!Q **Y92.092** Bedroom in other non-institutional residence as the place of occurrence of the external cause

!Q **Y92.093** Driveway of other non-institutional residence as the place of occurrence of the external cause

!Q **Y92.094** Garage of other non-institutional residence as the place of occurrence of the external cause

!Q **Y92.095** Swimming-pool of other non-institutional residence as the place of occurrence of the external cause

!Q **Y92.096** Garden or yard of other non-institutional residence as the place of occurrence of the external cause

!Q **Y92.098** Other place in other non-institutional residence as the place of occurrence of the external cause

CODING TIPS ✓ Assign Y92.098, Other place in other noninstitutional residence, as the place of occurrence of the external cause, for an assisted living facility.

!Q **Y92.099** Unspecified place in other non-institutional residence as the place of occurrence of the external cause

5 **Y92.1** Institutional (nonprivate) residence as the place of occurrence of the external cause

!Q **Y92.10** Unspecified residential institution as the place of occurrence of the external cause

6 **Y92.11** Children's home and orphanage as the place of occurrence of the external cause

!Q **Y92.110** Kitchen in children's home and orphanage as the place of occurrence of the external cause

!Q **Y92.111** Bathroom in children's home and orphanage as the place of occurrence of the external cause

!Q **Y92.112** Bedroom in children's home and orphanage as the place of occurrence of the external cause

!Q **Y92.113** Driveway of children's home and orphanage as the place of occurrence of the external cause

!Q **Y92.114** Garage of children's home and orphanage as the place of occurrence of the external cause

!Q **Y92.115** Swimming-pool of children's home and orphanage as the place of occurrence of the external cause

!Q **Y92.116** Garden or yard of children's home and orphanage as the place of occurrence of the external cause

!Q **Y92.118** Other place in children's home and orphanage as the place of occurrence of the external cause

!Q **Y92.119** Unspecified place in children's home and orphanage as the place of occurrence of the external cause

6 **Y92.12** Nursing home as the place of occurrence of the external cause
Home for the sick as the place of occurrence of the external cause
Hospice as the place of occurrence of the external cause

!Q **Y92.120** Kitchen in nursing home as the place of occurrence of the external cause

!Q **Y92.121** Bathroom in nursing home as the place of occurrence of the external cause

!Q **Y92.122** Bedroom in nursing home as the place of occurrence of the external cause

!Q **Y92.123** Driveway of nursing home as the place of occurrence of the external cause

4 4th digit required   5 5th digit required   6 6th digit required   7 7th digit required   7 7th digit placeholder   + Additional code   Laterality

1864   *DecisionHealth's* FY 2020 Complete Home Health ICD-10-CM Diagnosis Coding Manual

IQ Y92.124 Garage of nursing home as the place of occurrence of the external cause

IQ Y92.125 Swimming-pool of nursing home as the place of occurrence of the external cause

IQ Y92.126 Garden or yard of nursing home as the place of occurrence of the external cause

IQ Y92.128 Other place in nursing home as the place of occurrence of the external cause

IQ Y92.129 Unspecified place in nursing home as the place of occurrence of the external cause

6 Y92.13 Military base as the place of occurrence of the external cause
> **EXCLUDES 1** military training grounds (Y92.83)

IQ Y92.130 Kitchen on military base as the place of occurrence of the external cause

IQ Y92.131 Mess hall on military base as the place of occurrence of the external cause

IQ Y92.133 Barracks on military base as the place of occurrence of the external cause

IQ Y92.135 Garage on military base as the place of occurrence of the external cause

IQ Y92.136 Swimming-pool on military base as the place of occurrence of the external cause

IQ Y92.137 Garden or yard on military base as the place of occurrence of the external cause

IQ Y92.138 Other place on military base as the place of occurrence of the external cause

IQ Y92.139 Unspecified place military base as the place of occurrence of the external cause

6 Y92.14 Prison as the place of occurrence of the external cause

IQ Y92.140 Kitchen in prison as the place of occurrence of the external cause

IQ Y92.141 Dining room in prison as the place of occurrence of the external cause

IQ Y92.142 Bathroom in prison as the place of occurrence of the external cause

IQ Y92.143 Cell of prison as the place of occurrence of the external cause

IQ Y92.146 Swimming-pool of prison as the place of occurrence of the external cause

IQ Y92.147 Courtyard of prison as the place of occurrence of the external cause

IQ Y92.148 Other place in prison as the place of occurrence of the external cause

IQ Y92.149 Unspecified place in prison as the place of occurrence of the external cause

6 Y92.15 Reform school as the place of occurrence of the external cause

IQ Y92.150 Kitchen in reform school as the place of occurrence of the external cause

IQ Y92.151 Dining room in reform school as the place of occurrence of the external cause

IQ Y92.152 Bathroom in reform school as the place of occurrence of the external cause

IQ Y92.153 Bedroom in reform school as the place of occurrence of the external cause

IQ Y92.154 Driveway of reform school as the place of occurrence of the external cause

IQ Y92.155 Garage of reform school as the place of occurrence of the external cause

IQ Y92.156 Swimming-pool of reform school as the place of occurrence of the external cause

IQ Y92.157 Garden or yard of reform school as the place of occurrence of the external cause

IQ Y92.158 Other place in reform school as the place of occurrence of the external cause

IQ Y92.159 Unspecified place in reform school as the place of occurrence of the external cause

6 Y92.16 School dormitory as the place of occurrence of the external cause
> **EXCLUDES 1** reform school as the place of occurrence of the external cause (Y92.15-)
> school buildings and grounds as the place of occurrence of the external cause (Y92.2-)
> school sports and athletic areas as the place of occurrence of the external cause (Y92.3-)

IQ Y92.160 Kitchen in school dormitory as the place of occurrence of the external cause

IQ Y92.161 Dining room in school dormitory as the place of occurrence of the external cause

IQ Y92.162 Bathroom in school dormitory as the place of occurrence of the external cause

IQ Y92.163 Bedroom in school dormitory as the place of occurrence of the external cause

IQ Y92.168 Other place in school dormitory as the place of occurrence of the external cause

IQ Y92.169 Unspecified place in school dormitory as the place of occurrence of the external cause

6 Y92.19 Other specified residential institution as the place of occurrence of the external cause

★ New ▲ Revised Px Primary SP PDGM Px SL Low CoM SH High CoM IQ Quest. Encounter H Hospice non-cancer Dx Unspecified M Manifestation

DecisionHealth's FY 2020 Complete Home Health ICD-10-CM Diagnosis Coding Manual

1865

!Q Y92.190 Kitchen in other specified residential institution as the place of occurrence of the external cause

!Q Y92.191 Dining room in other specified residential institution as the place of occurrence of the external cause

!Q Y92.192 Bathroom in other specified residential institution as the place of occurrence of the external cause

!Q Y92.193 Bedroom in other specified residential institution as the place of occurrence of the external cause

!Q Y92.194 Driveway of other specified residential institution as the place of occurrence of the external cause

!Q Y92.195 Garage of other specified residential institution as the place of occurrence of the external cause

!Q Y92.196 Pool of other specified residential institution as the place of occurrence of the external cause

!Q Y92.197 Garden or yard of other specified residential institution as the place of occurrence of the external cause

!Q Y92.198 Other place in other specified residential institution as the place of occurrence of the external cause

!Q Y92.199 Unspecified place in other specified residential institution as the place of occurrence of the external cause

5 Y92.2 School, other institution and public administrative area as the place of occurrence of the external cause
Building and adjacent grounds used by the general public or by a particular group of the public
> **EXCLUDES 1** building under construction as the place of occurrence of the external cause (Y92.6)
> residential institution as the place of occurrence of the external cause (Y92.1)
> school dormitory as the place of occurrence of the external cause (Y92.16-)
> sports and athletics area of schools as the place of occurrence of the external cause (Y92.3-)

6 Y92.21 School (private) (public) (state) as the place of occurrence of the external cause

!Q Y92.210 Daycare center as the place of occurrence of the external cause

!Q Y92.211 Elementary school as the place of occurrence of the external cause
Kindergarten as the place of occurrence of the external cause

!Q Y92.212 Middle school as the place of occurrence of the external cause

!Q Y92.213 High school as the place of occurrence of the external cause

!Q Y92.214 College as the place of occurrence of the external cause
University as the place of occurrence of the external cause

!Q Y92.215 Trade school as the place of occurrence of the external cause

!Q Y92.218 Other school as the place of occurrence of the external cause

!Q Y92.219 Unspecified school as the place of occurrence of the external cause

!Q Y92.22 Religious institution as the place of occurrence of the external cause
Church as the place of occurrence of the external cause
Mosque as the place of occurrence of the external cause
Synagogue as the place of occurrence of the external cause

6 Y92.23 Hospital as the place of occurrence of the external cause
> **EXCLUDES 1** ambulatory (outpatient) health services establishments (Y92.53-)
> home for the sick as the place of occurrence of the external cause (Y92.12-)
> hospice as the place of occurrence of the external cause (Y92.12-)
> nursing home as the place of occurrence of the external cause (Y92.12-)

!Q Y92.230 Patient room in hospital as the place of occurrence of the external cause

!Q Y92.231 Patient bathroom in hospital as the place of occurrence of the external cause

!Q Y92.232 Corridor of hospital as the place of occurrence of the external cause

!Q Y92.233 Cafeteria of hospital as the place of occurrence of the external cause

!Q Y92.234 Operating room of hospital as the place of occurrence of the external cause

!Q Y92.238 Other place in hospital as the place of occurrence of the external cause

!Q Y92.239 Unspecified place in hospital as the place of occurrence of the external cause

6 Y92.24 Public administrative building as the place of occurrence of the external cause

!Q Y92.240 Courthouse as the place of occurrence of the external cause

!Q Y92.241 Library as the place of occurrence of the external cause

4 4th digit required   5 5th digit required   6 6th digit required   7 7th digit required   7 7th digit placeholder   + Additional code   ⊟ Laterality

1866   *DecisionHealth's* FY 2020 Complete Home Health ICD-10-CM Diagnosis Coding Manual

IQ Y92.242 Post office as the place of occurrence of the external cause

IQ Y92.243 City hall as the place of occurrence of the external cause

IQ Y92.248 Other public administrative building as the place of occurrence of the external cause

6 Y92.25 Cultural building as the place of occurrence of the external cause

IQ Y92.250 Art Gallery as the place of occurrence of the external cause

IQ Y92.251 Museum as the place of occurrence of the external cause

IQ Y92.252 Music hall as the place of occurrence of the external cause

IQ Y92.253 Opera house as the place of occurrence of the external cause

IQ Y92.254 Theater (live) as the place of occurrence of the external cause

IQ Y92.258 Other cultural public building as the place of occurrence of the external cause

IQ Y92.26 Movie house or cinema as the place of occurrence of the external cause

IQ Y92.29 Other specified public building as the place of occurrence of the external cause

Assembly hall as the place of occurrence of the external cause

Clubhouse as the place of occurrence of the external cause

5 Y92.3 Sports and athletics area as the place of occurrence of the external cause

6 Y92.31 Athletic court as the place of occurrence of the external cause

EXCLUDES 1 tennis court in private home or garden (Y92.09)

IQ Y92.310 Basketball court as the place of occurrence of the external cause

IQ Y92.311 Squash court as the place of occurrence of the external cause

IQ Y92.312 Tennis court as the place of occurrence of the external cause

IQ Y92.318 Other athletic court as the place of occurrence of the external cause

6 Y92.32 Athletic field as the place of occurrence of the external cause

IQ Y92.320 Baseball field as the place of occurrence of the external cause

IQ Y92.321 Football field as the place of occurrence of the external cause

IQ Y92.322 Soccer field as the place of occurrence of the external cause

IQ Y92.328 Other athletic field as the place of occurrence of the external cause

Cricket field as the place of occurrence of the external cause

Hockey field as the place of occurrence of the external cause

6 Y92.33 Skating rink as the place of occurrence of the external cause

IQ Y92.330 Ice skating rink (indoor) (outdoor) as the place of occurrence of the external cause

IQ Y92.331 Roller skating rink as the place of occurrence of the external cause

IQ Y92.34 Swimming pool (public) as the place of occurrence of the external cause

EXCLUDES 1 swimming pool in private home or garden (Y92.016)

IQ Y92.39 Other specified sports and athletic area as the place of occurrence of the external cause

Golf-course as the place of occurrence of the external cause

Gymnasium as the place of occurrence of the external cause

Riding-school as the place of occurrence of the external cause

Stadium as the place of occurrence of the external cause

5 Y92.4 Street, highway and other paved roadways as the place of occurrence of the external cause

EXCLUDES 1 private driveway of residence (Y92.014, Y92.024, Y92.043, Y92.093, Y92.113, Y92.123, Y92.154, Y92.194)

6 Y92.41 Street and highway as the place of occurrence of the external cause

IQ Y92.410 Unspecified street and highway as the place of occurrence of the external cause

Road NOS as the place of occurrence of the external cause

IQ Y92.411 Interstate highway as the place of occurrence of the external cause

Freeway as the place of occurrence of the external cause

Motorway as the place of occurrence of the external cause

IQ Y92.412 Parkway as the place of occurrence of the external cause

IQ Y92.413 State road as the place of occurrence of the external cause

IQ Y92.414 Local residential or business street as the place of occurrence of the external cause

IQ Y92.415 Exit ramp or entrance ramp of street or highway as the place of occurrence of the external cause

6 Y92.48 Other paved roadways as the place of occurrence of the external cause

IQ Y92.480 Sidewalk as the place of occurrence of the external cause

IQ Y92.481 Parking lot as the place of occurrence of the external cause

IQ Y92.482 Bike path as the place of occurrence of the external cause

IQ Y92.488 Other paved roadways as the place of occurrence of the external cause

5 Y92.5 Trade and service area as the place of occurrence of the external cause

EXCLUDES 1 garage in private home (Y92.015)
schools and other public administration buildings (Y92.2-)

6 Y92.51 Private commercial establishments as the place of occurrence of the external cause

★ New ▲ Revised Px Primary SP PDGM Px SL Low CoM SH High CoM IQ Quest. Encounter H Hospice non-cancer Dx Unspecified M *Manifestation*

DecisionHealth's FY 2020 Complete Home Health ICD-10-CM Diagnosis Coding Manual

1867

IQ Y92.510 Bank as the place of occurrence of the external cause

IQ Y92.511 Restaurant or café as the place of occurrence of the external cause

IQ Y92.512 Supermarket, store or market as the place of occurrence of the external cause

IQ Y92.513 Shop (commercial) as the place of occurrence of the external cause

6 Y92.52 Service areas as the place of occurrence of the external cause

IQ Y92.520 Airport as the place of occurrence of the external cause

IQ Y92.521 Bus station as the place of occurrence of the external cause

IQ Y92.522 Railway station as the place of occurrence of the external cause

IQ Y92.523 Highway rest stop as the place of occurrence of the external cause

IQ Y92.524 Gas station as the place of occurrence of the external cause

Petroleum station as the place of occurrence of the external cause

Service station as the place of occurrence of the external cause

6 Y92.53 Ambulatory health services establishments as the place of occurrence of the external cause

IQ Y92.530 Ambulatory surgery center as the place of occurrence of the external cause

Outpatient surgery center, including that connected with a hospital as the place of occurrence of the external cause

Same day surgery center, including that connected with a hospital as the place of occurrence of the external cause

IQ Y92.531 Health care provider office as the place of occurrence of the external cause

Physician office as the place of occurrence of the external cause

IQ Y92.532 Urgent care center as the place of occurrence of the external cause

IQ Y92.538 Other ambulatory health services establishments as the place of occurrence of the external cause

IQ Y92.59 Other trade areas as the place of occurrence of the external cause

Office building as the place of occurrence of the external cause

Casino as the place of occurrence of the external cause

Garage (commercial) as the place of occurrence of the external cause

Hotel as the place of occurrence of the external cause

Radio or television station as the place of occurrence of the external cause

Shopping mall as the place of occurrence of the external cause

Warehouse as the place of occurrence of the external cause

5 Y92.6 Industrial and construction area as the place of occurrence of the external cause

IQ Y92.61 Building [any] under construction as the place of occurrence of the external cause

IQ Y92.62 Dock or shipyard as the place of occurrence of the external cause

Dockyard as the place of occurrence of the external cause

Dry dock as the place of occurrence of the external cause

Shipyard as the place of occurrence of the external cause

IQ Y92.63 Factory as the place of occurrence of the external cause

Factory building as the place of occurrence of the external cause

Factory premises as the place of occurrence of the external cause

Industrial yard as the place of occurrence of the external cause

IQ Y92.64 Mine or pit as the place of occurrence of the external cause

Mine as the place of occurrence of the external cause

IQ Y92.65 Oil rig as the place of occurrence of the external cause

Pit (coal) (gravel) (sand) as the place of occurrence of the external cause

IQ Y92.69 Other specified industrial and construction area as the place of occurrence of the external cause

Gasworks as the place of occurrence of the external cause

Power-station (coal) (nuclear) (oil) as the place of occurrence of the external cause

Tunnel under construction as the place of occurrence of the external cause

Workshop as the place of occurrence of the external cause

5 Y92.7 Farm as the place of occurrence of the external cause

Ranch as the place of occurrence of the external cause

EXCLUDES 1 farmhouse and home premises of farm (Y92.01-)

IQ Y92.71 Barn as the place of occurrence of the external cause

IQ Y92.72 Chicken coop as the place of occurrence of the external cause

Hen house as the place of occurrence of the external cause

IQ Y92.73 Farm field as the place of occurrence of the external cause

IQ Y92.74 Orchard as the place of occurrence of the external cause

IQ Y92.79 Other farm location as the place of occurrence of the external cause

5 Y92.8 Other places as the place of occurrence of the external cause

6 Y92.81 Transport vehicle as the place of occurrence of the external cause

EXCLUDES 1 transport accidents (V00-V99)

IQ Y92.810 Car as the place of occurrence of the external cause

IQ Y92.811 Bus as the place of occurrence of the external cause

4 4th digit required   5 5th digit required   6 6th digit required   7 7th digit required   7 7th digit placeholder   + Additional code   ☐ Laterality

1868   *DecisionHealth's* FY 2020 Complete Home Health ICD-10-CM Diagnosis Coding Manual

Chapter 20

V00-Y99

!Q Y92.812 Truck as the place of occurrence of the external cause

!Q Y92.813 Airplane as the place of occurrence of the external cause

!Q Y92.814 Boat as the place of occurrence of the external cause

!Q Y92.815 Train as the place of occurrence of the external cause

!Q Y92.816 Subway car as the place of occurrence of the external cause

!Q Y92.818 Other transport vehicle as the place of occurrence of the external cause

6 Y92.82 Wilderness area

!Q Y92.820 Desert as the place of occurrence of the external cause

!Q Y92.821 Forest as the place of occurrence of the external cause

!Q Y92.828 Other wilderness area as the place of occurrence of the external cause
> Swamp as the place of occurrence of the external cause
> Mountain as the place of occurrence of the external cause
> Marsh as the place of occurrence of the external cause
> Prairie as the place of occurrence of the external cause

6 Y92.83 Recreation area as the place of occurrence of the external cause

!Q Y92.830 Public park as the place of occurrence of the external cause

!Q Y92.831 Amusement park as the place of occurrence of the external cause

!Q Y92.832 Beach as the place of occurrence of the external cause
> Seashore as the place of occurrence of the external cause

!Q Y92.833 Campsite as the place of occurrence of the external cause

!Q Y92.834 Zoological garden (Zoo) as the place of occurrence of the external cause

!Q Y92.838 Other recreation area as the place of occurrence of the external cause

!Q Y92.84 Military training ground as the place of occurrence of the external cause

!Q Y92.85 Railroad track as the place of occurrence of the external cause

!Q Y92.86 Slaughter house as the place of occurrence of the external cause

!Q Y92.89 Other specified places as the place of occurrence of the external cause
> Derelict house as the place of occurrence of the external cause

!Q Y92.9 Unspecified place or not applicable

4 Y93 Activity codes

Note:

Category Y93 is provided for use to indicate the activity of the person seeking healthcare for an injury or health condition, such as a heart attack while shoveling snow, which resulted from, or was contributed to, by the activity. These codes are appropriate for use for both acute injuries, such as those from chapter 19, and conditions that are due to the long-term, cumulative effects of an activity, such as those from chapter 13. They are also appropriate for use with external cause codes for cause and intent if identifying the activity provides additional information on the event. These codes should be used in conjunction with codes for external cause status (Y99) and place of occurrence (Y92).

This section contains the following broad activity categories:

Y93.0 Activities involving walking and running

Y93.1 Activities involving water and water craft

Y93.2 Activities involving ice and snow

Y93.3 Activities involving climbing, rappelling, and jumping off

Y93.4 Activities involving dancing and other rhythmic movement

Y93.5 Activities involving other sports and athletics played individually

Y93.6 Activities involving other sports and athletics played as a team or group

Y93.7 Activities involving other specified sports and athletics

Y93.A Activities involving other cardiorespiratory exercise

Y93.B Activities involving other muscle strengthening exercises

Y93.C Activities involving computer technology and electronic devices

Y93.D Activities involving arts and handcrafts

Y93.E Activities involving personal hygiene and interior property and clothing maintenance

Y93.F Activities involving caregiving

Y93.G Activities involving food preparation, cooking and grilling

Y93.H Activities involving exterior property and land maintenance, building and construction

Y93.I Activities involving roller coasters and other types of external motion

Y93.J Activities involving playing musical instrument

Y93.K Activities involving animal care

Y93.8 Activities, other specified

Y93.9 Activity, unspecified

5 Y93.0 Activities involving walking and running
> **EXCLUDES 1** activity, walking an animal (Y93.K1)
> activity, walking or running on a treadmill (Y93.A1)

!Q Y93.01 Activity, walking, marching and hiking
> Activity, walking, marching and hiking on level or elevated terrain

★ New ▲ Revised Px Primary SP PDGM Px SL Low CoM SH High CoM !Q Quest. Encounter H Hospice non-cancer Dx Unspecified M Manifestation

DecisionHealth's FY 2020 Complete Home Health ICD-10-CM Diagnosis Coding Manual

1869

EXCLUDES 1 activity, mountain climbing (Y93.31)

IQ Y93.02 Activity, running

5 Y93.1 Activities involving water and water craft

EXCLUDES 1 activities involving ice (Y93.2-)

IQ Y93.11 Activity, swimming

IQ Y93.12 Activity, springboard and platform diving

IQ Y93.13 Activity, water polo

IQ Y93.14 Activity, water aerobics and water exercise

IQ Y93.15 Activity, underwater diving and snorkeling
Activity, SCUBA diving

IQ Y93.16 Activity, rowing, canoeing, kayaking, rafting and tubing
Activity, canoeing, kayaking, rafting and tubing in calm and turbulent water

IQ Y93.17 Activity, water skiing and wake boarding

IQ Y93.18 Activity, surfing, windsurfing and boogie boarding
Activity, water sliding

IQ Y93.19 Activity, other involving water and watercraft
Activity involving water NOS
Activity, parasailing
Activity, water survival training and testing

5 Y93.2 Activities involving ice and snow

EXCLUDES 1 activity, shoveling ice and snow (Y93.H1)

IQ Y93.21 Activity, ice skating
Activity, figure skating (singles) (pairs)
Activity, ice dancing

EXCLUDES 1 activity, ice hockey (Y93.22)

IQ Y93.22 Activity, ice hockey

IQ Y93.23 Activity, snow (alpine) (downhill) skiing, snowboarding, sledding, tobogganing and snow tubing

EXCLUDES 1 activity, cross country skiing (Y93.24)

IQ Y93.24 Activity, cross country skiing
Activity, nordic skiing

IQ Y93.29 Activity, other involving ice and snow
Activity involving ice and snow NOS

5 Y93.3 Activities involving climbing, rappelling and jumping off

EXCLUDES 1 activity, hiking on level or elevated terrain (Y93.01)
activity, jumping rope (Y93.56)
activity, trampoline jumping (Y93.44)

IQ Y93.31 Activity, mountain climbing, rock climbing and wall climbing

IQ Y93.32 Activity, rappelling

IQ Y93.33 Activity, BASE jumping
Activity, Building, Antenna, Span, Earth jumping

IQ Y93.34 Activity, bungee jumping

IQ Y93.35 Activity, hang gliding

IQ Y93.39 Activity, other involving climbing, rappelling and jumping off

5 Y93.4 Activities involving dancing and other rhythmic movement

EXCLUDES 1 activity, martial arts (Y93.75)

IQ Y93.41 Activity, dancing

IQ Y93.42 Activity, yoga

IQ Y93.43 Activity, gymnastics
Activity, rhythmic gymnastics

EXCLUDES 1 activity, trampolining (Y93.44)

IQ Y93.44 Activity, trampolining

IQ Y93.45 Activity, cheerleading

IQ Y93.49 Activity, other involving dancing and other rhythmic movements

5 Y93.5 Activities involving other sports and athletics played individually

EXCLUDES 1 activity, dancing (Y93.41)
activity, gymnastic (Y93.43)
activity, trampolining (Y93.44)
activity, yoga (Y93.42)

IQ Y93.51 Activity, roller skating (inline) and skateboarding

IQ Y93.52 Activity, horseback riding

IQ Y93.53 Activity, golf

IQ Y93.54 Activity, bowling

IQ Y93.55 Activity, bike riding

IQ Y93.56 Activity, jumping rope

IQ Y93.57 Activity, non-running track and field events

EXCLUDES 1 activity, running (any form) (Y93.02)

IQ Y93.59 Activity, other involving other sports and athletics played individually

EXCLUDES 1 activities involving climbing, rappelling, and jumping (Y93.3-)
activities involving ice and snow (Y93.2-)
activities involving walking and running (Y93.0-)
activities involving water and watercraft (Y93.1-)

5 Y93.6 Activities involving other sports and athletics played as a team or group

EXCLUDES 1 activity, ice hockey (Y93.22)
activity, water polo (Y93.13)

IQ Y93.61 Activity, american tackle football
Activity, football NOS

IQ Y93.62 Activity, american flag or touch football

IQ Y93.63 Activity, rugby

IQ Y93.64 Activity, baseball
Activity, softball

IQ Y93.65 Activity, lacrosse and field hockey

IQ Y93.66 Activity, soccer

IQ Y93.67 Activity, basketball

IQ Y93.68 Activity, volleyball (beach) (court)

---

4 4th digit required   5 5th digit required   6 6th digit required   7 7th digit required   7 7th digit placeholder   +Additional code   ≣ Laterality

IQ Y93.6A **Activity, physical games generally associated with school recess, summer camp and children**
Activity, capture the flag
Activity, dodge ball
Activity, four square
Activity, kickball

IQ Y93.69 **Activity, other involving other sports and athletics played as a team or group**
Activity, cricket

5 Y93.7 **Activities involving other specified sports and athletics**

IQ Y93.71 **Activity, boxing**

IQ Y93.72 **Activity, wrestling**

IQ Y93.73 **Activity, racquet and hand sports**
Activity, handball
Activity, racquetball
Activity, squash
Activity, tennis

IQ Y93.74 **Activity, frisbee**
Activity, ultimate frisbee

IQ Y93.75 **Activity, martial arts**
Activity, combatives

IQ Y93.79 **Activity, other specified sports and athletics**
> **EXCLUDES 1** sports and athletics activities specified in categories Y93.0-Y93.6

5 Y93.A **Activities involving other cardiorespiratory exercise**
Activities involving physical training

IQ Y93.A1 **Activity, exercise machines primarily for cardiorespiratory conditioning**
Activity, elliptical and stepper machines
Activity, stationary bike
Activity, treadmill

IQ Y93.A2 **Activity, calisthenics**
Activity, jumping jacks
Activity, warm up and cool down

IQ Y93.A3 **Activity, aerobic and step exercise**

IQ Y93.A4 **Activity, circuit training**

IQ Y93.A5 **Activity, obstacle course**
Activity, challenge course
Activity, confidence course

IQ Y93.A6 **Activity, grass drills**
Activity, guerilla drills

IQ Y93.A9 **Activity, other involving cardiorespiratory exercise**
> **EXCLUDES 1** activities involving cardiorespiratory exercise specified in categories Y93.0-Y93.7

5 Y93.B **Activities involving other muscle strengthening exercises**

IQ Y93.B1 **Activity, exercise machines primarily for muscle strengthening**

IQ Y93.B2 **Activity, push-ups, pull-ups, sit-ups**

IQ Y93.B3 **Activity, free weights**
Activity, barbells
Activity, dumbbells

IQ Y93.B4 **Activity, pilates**

IQ Y93.B9 **Activity, other involving muscle strengthening exercises**

> **EXCLUDES 1** activities involving muscle strengthening specified in categories Y93.0-Y93.A

5 Y93.C **Activities involving computer technology and electronic devices**
> **EXCLUDES 1** activity, electronic musical keyboard or instruments (Y93.J-)

IQ Y93.C1 **Activity, computer keyboarding**
Activity, electronic game playing using keyboard or other stationary device

IQ Y93.C2 **Activity, hand held interactive electronic device**
Activity, cellular telephone and communication device
Activity, electronic game playing using interactive device
> **EXCLUDES 1** activity, electronic game playing using keyboard or other stationary device (Y93.C1)

IQ Y93.C9 **Activity, other involving computer technology and electronic devices**

5 Y93.D **Activities involving arts and handcrafts**
> **EXCLUDES 1** activities involving playing musical instrument (Y93.J-)

IQ Y93.D1 **Activity, knitting and crocheting**

IQ Y93.D2 **Activity, sewing**

IQ Y93.D3 **Activity, furniture building and finishing**
Activity, furniture repair

IQ Y93.D9 **Activity, other involving arts and handcrafts**

5 Y93.E **Activities involving personal hygiene and interior property and clothing maintenance**
> **EXCLUDES 1** activities involving cooking and grilling (Y93.G-)
> activities involving exterior property and land maintenance, building and construction (Y93.H-)
> activities involving caregiving (Y93.F-)
> activity, dishwashing (Y93.G1)
> activity, food preparation (Y93.G1)
> activity, gardening (Y93.H2)

IQ Y93.E1 **Activity, personal bathing and showering**

IQ Y93.E2 **Activity, laundry**

IQ Y93.E3 **Activity, vacuuming**

IQ Y93.E4 **Activity, ironing**

IQ Y93.E5 **Activity, floor mopping and cleaning**

IQ Y93.E6 **Activity, residential relocation**
Activity, packing up and unpacking involved in moving to a new residence

IQ Y93.E8 **Activity, other personal hygiene**

IQ Y93.E9 **Activity, other interior property and clothing maintenance**

5 Y93.F **Activities involving caregiving**

Chapter 20

V00-Y99

★ New ▲ Revised Px Primary SP PDGM Px SL Low CoM SH High CoM IQ Quest. Encounter H Hospice non-cancer Dx | Unspecified | M *Manifestation*

DecisionHealth's FY 2020 Complete Home Health ICD-10-CM Diagnosis Coding Manual   1871

Activity involving the provider of caregiving

IQ Y93.F1 Activity, caregiving, bathing

IQ Y93.F2 Activity, caregiving, lifting

IQ Y93.F9 Activity, other caregiving

5 Y93.G Activities involving food preparation, cooking and grilling

IQ Y93.G1 Activity, food preparation and clean up
Activity, dishwashing

IQ Y93.G2 Activity, grilling and smoking food

IQ Y93.G3 Activity, cooking and baking
Activity, use of stove, oven and microwave oven

IQ Y93.G9 Activity, other involving cooking and grilling

5 Y93.H Activities involving exterior property and land maintenance, building and construction

IQ Y93.H1 Activity, digging, shoveling and raking
Activity, dirt digging
Activity, raking leaves
Activity, snow shoveling

IQ Y93.H2 Activity, gardening and landscaping
Activity, pruning, trimming shrubs, weeding

IQ Y93.H3 Activity, building and construction

IQ Y93.H9 Activity, other involving exterior property and land maintenance, building and construction

5 Y93.I Activities involving roller coasters and other types of external motion

IQ Y93.I1 Activity, roller coaster riding

IQ Y93.I9 Activity, other involving external motion

5 Y93.J Activities involving playing musical instrument
Activity involving playing electric musical instrument

IQ Y93.J1 Activity, piano playing
Activity, musical keyboard (electronic) playing

IQ Y93.J2 Activity, drum and other percussion instrument playing

IQ Y93.J3 Activity, string instrument playing

IQ Y93.J4 Activity, winds and brass instrument playing

5 Y93.K Activities involving animal care
EXCLUDES 1   activity, horseback riding (Y93.52)

IQ Y93.K1 Activity, walking an animal

IQ Y93.K2 Activity, milking an animal

IQ Y93.K3 Activity, grooming and shearing an animal

IQ Y93.K9 Activity, other involving animal care

5 Y93.8 Activities, other specified

IQ Y93.81 Activity, refereeing a sports activity

IQ Y93.82 Activity, spectator at an event

IQ Y93.83 Activity, rough housing and horseplay

IQ Y93.84 Activity, sleeping

IQ Y93.85 Activity, choking game
Activity, blackout game
Activity, fainting game

Activity, pass out game

IQ Y93.89 Activity, other specified

IQ Y93.9   Activity, unspecified

IQ Y95 Nosocomial condition

4 Y99 External cause status
Note:
A single code from category Y99 should be used in conjunction with the external cause code(s) assigned to a record to indicate the status of the person at the time the event occurred.

IQ Y99.0 Civilian activity done for income or pay
Civilian activity done for financial or other compensation
EXCLUDES 1   military activity (Y99.1)
volunteer activity (Y99.2)

IQ Y99.1 Military activity
EXCLUDES 1   activity of off duty military personnel (Y99.8)

IQ Y99.2 Volunteer activity
EXCLUDES 1   activity of child or other family member assisting in compensated work of other family member (Y99.8)

IQ Y99.8 Other external cause status
Activity NEC
Activity of child or other family member assisting in compensated work of other family member
Hobby not done for income
Leisure activity
Off-duty activity of military personnel
Recreation or sport not for income or while a student
Student activity
EXCLUDES 1   civilian activity done for income or compensation (Y99.0)
military activity (Y99.1)

IQ Y99.9   Unspecified external cause status

---

4 4th digit required   5 5th digit required   6 6th digit required   7 7th digit required   ✓ 7th digit placeholder   ✚ Additional code   ⊟ Laterality

1872   *DecisionHealth's* FY 2020 Complete Home Health ICD-10-CM Diagnosis Coding Manual

Chapter 20 Scenarios: External causes of morbidity (V00-Y99)

Leukemia due to radiation exposure

A 42-year-old male is admitted to home health for observation and assessment of dehydration, fever and shortness of breath, which are stated to be side effects of experimental chemotherapy taken to treat chronic lymphocytic leukemia. The medical record states that the leukemia resulted from occupational exposure to radiation due to his job as a registered nurse in an emergency room setting.

Description	Code
Primary: Dehydration	E86.0
Secondary: Fever, unspecified	R50.9
Secondary: Shortness of breath	R06.02
Secondary: Adverse effect of antineoplastic and immunosuppressive drugs, subsequent encounter	T45.1X5D
Secondary: Chronic lymphocytic leukemia of B-cell type not having achieved remission	C91.10
Secondary: Exposure to X-rays, sequela	W88.0XXS

Because the dehydration, fever and shortness of breath resulted from the proper use of the experimental drug, they're coded as adverse effects. The dehydration, fever and shortness of breath are coded first, followed by the code for the drug that caused it. The patient's leukemia is still an active condition and so it is included as well. Because it was said to be caused by radiation exposure, an external cause code is assigned to indicate that. The seventh character "S" is assigned to the external cause code to indicate that the leukemia occurred from past radiation exposure.

Burn of palm on hot pan

A 68-year-old man sustained a second degree burn to his left palm after accidently pressing his hand down on a hot skillet on the stove. He was admitted to home health to continue wound care to the site. He is a type 1 diabetic.

Description	Code
Primary: Burn of second degree of left palm, subsequent encounter	T23.252D
Secondary: Type 1 diabetes mellitus without complications	E10.9
Secondary: Contact with hot saucepan or skillet, subsequent encounter	X15.3xxD

The appropriate seventh character "D" is used on the burn code, in accordance with coding conventions, to denote the subsequent nature of the care being given. The external cause code indicating how the wound was sustained carries the same seventh character as the injury code, "D," in accordance with coding guidelines. Two placeholder x's are used here because the external cause code, X15.3-, has only four characters but requires a seventh character. Thus, the two empty places are filled with placeholder x. The patient's type 1 diabetes has the potential to impact his ability to heal from the burn, so it is included as well. An additional code for insulin use is not required because it is assumed in type 1 diabetes.

Gunshot wound, child abuse

A 13-year-old male patient underwent surgery in the hospital for a gunshot wound to the right lower quadrant of his abdomen; the bullet fragment was removed. In a recent domestic violence incident, his father shot and killed his mother with a shotgun, then shot the patient and finally committed suicide. The medical record also documents that prior to the shooting, the patient had suffered severe abuse at the hands of his father which left him underweight with a body mass index (BMI) that is less than the fifth percentile for his age. The patient was admitted to home health for continued wound care and physical therapy to regain strength.

Description	Code
Primary: Child physical abuse, confirmed, subsequent encounter	T74.12xD
Secondary: Puncture wound of abdominal wall with foreign body, right lower quadrant without penetration into peritoneal cavity, subsequent encounter	S31.143D
Secondary: Biological father, perpetrator of maltreatment and neglect	Y07.11
Secondary: Assault by shotgun, subsequent encounter	X94.0xxD
Secondary: Underweight	R63.6
Secondary: Body mass index (BMI) pediatric, less than 5th percentile for age	Z68.51

Because this is a documented case of child abuse, the child abuse code is assigned first, in accordance with coding guidelines. There is a "use additional code" note which gives instructions to code any associated current injury as well as an external cause code to identify the perpetrator. In this case, the injury is a gunshot wound from the shotgun and the perpetrator is the patient's biological father. The patient is coming to home health to continue healing, versus to receive active treatment. Thus, the seventh character "D" is used. The gunshot wound is coded as a puncture wound, according to Q3 2016 Coding Clinic guidance. Since the wound was brought about with a bullet, the code for "with foreign body" is used. The seventh character "D" captures that initial treatment, including removing the bullet fragment, is completed and the patient is now in the healing and recovery phase. An additional code, Y07.11, is assigned the show that the patient's abuse was perpetrated by his father, in accordance with tabular instruction. An external cause code is also assigned to indicate that a shotgun was used to perpetrate the assault/abuse and led to the injuries now needing treatment. The patient was diagnosed as underweight, and thus R63.6 is assigned to capture this. An additional code, Z68.51, is used to show his BMI, which is less than the fifth percentile for his age, in accordance with tabular instruction. Because the patient is between 2-19 years of age, pediatric BMI codes are used.

Radiation burn to chest wall

A 69-year-old woman comes to home health for active treatment to a third degree burn on her chest wall caused by radiation for cancer in the lower inner quadrant of her left breast.

Description	Code
Primary: Burn of third degree of chest wall, initial encounter	T21.31XA
Secondary: Radiological procedure and radiotherapy as the cause of abnormal reaction of the patient, or of later complication, without mention of misadventure at the time of the procedure	Y84.2
Secondary: Malignant neoplasm of lower-inner quadrant of left female breast	C50.312

A radiation burn is treated as a burn, according to the alphabetic index. The seventh character "A" is used because the home health agency will be providing active treatment to the burn. An external cause code, Y84.2, is assigned to indicate that radiation is the source of the burn. Since the cancer is an active diagnosis, it is also coded.

...fluencing Health Status
...th Services (Z00-Z99)

care (Z40-Z53)

...to indicate a
...atients who
...injury, but
...c care, or care
...a residual
...ote for
...ce after
...clude:
...uch as
...and other
...other
...ic

...sions when
...y or external
...are recorded as
...in two main ways:

...y not be sick
...es for some specific
...limited care or service for
...nate an organ or tissue, to
...cination (immunization), or
...which in itself is not a disease or

...mstance or problem is present
...s the person's health status but is
...current illness or injury.

...r use in any healthcare setting and may
...er a first-listed (principal diagnosis code)
...y code, depending on the circumstances of
...er. Certain Z codes may only be used as first-
...rincipal diagnosis.

...er 21 has significant changes from ICD-9-CM,
...ng expansions of some categories, especially the
...ry codes, while eliminating other codes such as
...counter for rehabilitation, aftercare codes for healing
...actures, and aftercare for injury codes. Injuries, including
traumatic and pathological fractures, require assignment of
the acute injury or fracture code with use of the appropriate
7th character extension (for subsequent care).

Don't look for a so-called "rehab code" to capture
a therapy-only case. Instead, capture the therapy a
patient is receiving with ICD-10 codes that describe the
reason for the therapy, such as I50.31 (Acute diastolic
(congestive) heart failure).

As with all coding, it is important to search for codes first
in the Alphabetical Index and confirm the code and read all
of the notes in the Tabular List (code definitions, Excludes 1
and 2 notes, code first and add an additional code).

Z codes are organized by categories. The most important
categories to home health are Status, History and Aftercare.
Here is a look at all of the blocks within chapter 21:

Persons encountering health services for examinations (Z00-Z13)

These codes are primarily used in clinic and physician
offices for examinations and disease and disorder
screenings.

Genetic carrier and genetic susceptibility to disease (Z14-Z15)

These are status codes indicating the person carries a
gene associated with a particular disease, which may be
passed to offspring who may develop that disease. Genetic
carrier codes (Z14.-) indicate the person does not have the
disease and is not at risk of developing the disease. Z15,
Genetic susceptibility to disease, indicates that a person
has a gene that increases the risk of that person developing
the disease. Examples include: Genetic susceptibility to
malignant neoplasm of: breast (Z15.01), ovary, prostate
(Z15.03), endometrium (Z15.04), and other malignant
neoplasm (Z15.09). Codes from Z15 should not be used
as first-listed codes. If the patient has the condition to
which he is susceptible, and that condition is the reason
for the encounter, the code for the current condition
should be sequenced first. If the patient is being seen for
follow-up after completed treatment for the disease, and
the condition no longer exists, a follow-up code should
be sequenced first, followed by the appropriate personal
history and genetic susceptibility codes.

Resistance to antimicrobial drugs (Z16)

This code indicates that a patient has a condition that
is resistant to antimicrobial drug treatment. Z16 includes
a 'code first' note for the infection and a second note that
codes in this category are provided for use as additional
codes to identify the resistance and non-responsiveness
of a condition to antimicrobial drugs. Z16.1- refers to
resistance to beta lactam antibiotics including resistance
to penicillin/amoxicillin/ampicillin (Z16.11). Z16.2- refers
to resistance to other antibiotics such as vancomycin
(Z16.21), resistance to multiple antibiotics (Z16.24), and
other single antibiotics (Z16.29). Z16.3- covers other
antimicrobial drugs such as resistance to antiparasitic,
antifungal, antiviral or antimycobacterial drugs; multiple
and other antimicrobial drugs.

Estrogen receptor status (Z17)

These codes are consolidated to indicate status
codes for **estrogen receptor positive (Z17.0) and
estrogen receptor negative (Z17.1)** with a note to code
first malignant neoplasm of the breast (C50.-).

Retained foreign body fragments (Z18)

A series of 5-character codes describe the nature
of the foreign body fragments as radioactive (Z18.0-),
metal (Z18.1-), plastic (Z18.2), organic such as animal
quills or spines, tooth or wood (Z18.3-), other specified
retained foreign body (Z18.8-), and retained foreign
body fragments of unspecified material (Z18.9).

Hormone sensitivity malignancy status (Z19)

This category was added in FY2017, and contains
codes Z19.1 (Hormone sensitive malignancy status)

and Z19.2 (Hormone resistant malignancy status). This category of codes has a note to code first malignant neoplasm (see Table of Neoplasms).

Persons with potential health hazards related to communicable diseases (Z20-Z29)

These codes indicate contact with, and suspected exposure to, communicable diseases. They are reported for patients who do not show any signs or symptoms of a disease, but are suspected to have been exposed to it by close personal contact with an infected individual or are in an area where the disease is epidemic. These codes may be assigned as principal diagnoses to explain an encounter for testing, or as an additional diagnosis to identify a potential risk.

Codes include contact with and (suspected) exposure to communicable diseases such as intestinal infectious diseases, **contact with/exposure to TB (Z20.1),** sexually transmitted diseases, rabies (Z20.3), rubella (Z20.4), **viral hepatitis (Z20.5), HIV (Z20.6),** pediculosis, acariasis and other infestations (Z20.7), and a number of other bacterial and viral communicable diseases (V20.8-).

Other potential health hazards include HIV status **(Z21) that indicates that a patient has tested positive for HIV, but has not manifested any signs or symptoms of the disease.** Z22.- are carrier status codes indicating that a person harbors the specific organisms of a disease without manifesting symptoms, but is capable of transmitting the infection.

Code Z23 is for encounters for inoculations and vaccinations. It indicates the patient is being seen to receive prophylactic inoculation against a disease. Procedure codes are required to identify the actual administration of the injection and the type(s) of immunizations given.

Codes for immunization not carried out (with reasons) include Z28.0-, Z28.2-, Z28.8-, Z28.9, and **under- immunization status (Z28.3).**

Persons encountering health services in circumstances related to reproduction (Z30-Z39)

This category is used primarily for:

- Counseling on contraceptive management, supervision of normal pregnancy, etc.

- Pregnancy state incidental (Z33.1) is a status code

- Weeks of gestation (Z3A.-) for use only on maternal record to show weeks of gestation of the pregnancy with a note to code first complications of pregnancy, childbirth and the puerperium.

- Outcome of delivery on the mother's record (Z37.-)

- Encounter and care for postpartum care and follow-up (Z39.-).

Encounters for other specific healt[h]

These categories are intended for use reason for care. They may be used for pa already have been treated for a disease o who are receiving aftercare or prophylacti to consolidate the treatment, or to deal wit state. These categories have an Excludes 2 follow-up examination for medical surveillan treatment (Z08-Z09). More specifically, they i

- Z40 Encounter for prophylactic surgery **prophylactic removal of breast (Z40.01)** organs.

- Z41 Encounter for procedures for purposes than remedying health state such as cosme surgery (Z41.1)

- Z42 Encounter for plastic and reconstructive surgery following medical procedure or heale[d] injury such as **breast reconstruction following mastectomy (Z42.1)** or encounter for other plas and reconstructive surgery following medical procedure or healed injury (Z42.8).

- Z43 Encounter for attention to artificial openings includes passage of sounds, reforming the artificial opening, removal of catheter and toileting or cleansing. Examples include: **attention to tracheostomy (Z43.0), colostomy (Z43.3), other artificial opening of urinary tract (Z43.6), other artificial opening (Z43.8).** Note, that once the artificial opening has been closed, codes from category Z43.- are no longer applicable since the patient no longer has the ostomy. If the patient is seen for wound care following closure of the site, assign a code from category Z48.- (Encounter for other postprocedural aftercare).

- Z44 Encounter for fitting and adjustment of external prosthetic device including artificial arm (Z44.0-) or leg (Z44.1-). Fitting and adjustment examples include: Fitting and adjustment complete left artificial arm (Z44.012) or partial artificial right arm (Z44.021), external breast prosthesis (Z44.3-), Fitting and adjustment other external prosthetic device (Z44.8),

- Z45 Encounter for **checking and testing cardiac pacemaker pulse generator (Z45.010), or adjustment and management of automated implantable defibrillator (Z45.02) ; encounter for adjustment and management of vascular access device (Z45.2); encounter for adjustment and management of implanted hearing device (Z45.32); adjustment and management of cerebrospinal fluid drainage device (Z45.41).**

- Z46 Fitting and adjustment of other devices such as **encounter for fitting and adjustment of gastric lap band (Z46.51), fitting and adjustment of urinary device (intermittent or indwelling** catheter) **(Z46.6),** fitting and adjustment of insulin pump, encounter for insulin pump titration **or encounter for insulin pump instruction and training (Z46.81).**

- Z47 Orthopedic aftercare including **aftercare following joint prosthesis (Z47.1); aftercare following explantation of joint prosthesis (Z47.3-); encounter for orthopedic aftercare following surgical amputation (Z47.81) encounter for orthopedic aftercare following scoliosis surgery (Z47.82).** Assign an aftercare code if the condition for which a patient is receiving rehab services is no longer present unless the patient sustained an injury. In these scenarios, assign the injury code with the appropriate 7th character. For example: A hip replacement that was done to treat a right intertrochanteric femur fracture, would be coded with S72.141D (Displaced intertrochanteric fracture of right femur, subsequent encounter for closed fracture with routine healing), not Z47.1 (Aftercare following joint replacement surgery), according to coding guidelines.

- Z48 Encounter for other post-procedural aftercare such as **change/removal nonsurgical wound dressing (Z48.00) or change/removal of surgical wound dressings (Z48.01);** Encounter for aftercare following organ transplant (Z48.2-); **Aftercare following surgery for a neoplasm (Z48.3);** or Aftercare for surgical aftercare following surgery on specific body systems (Z48.81-).

- Z49 Encounter for care involving renal dialysis codes have a note to code also end stage renal disease (N18.6)

- Z51 Encounter for other aftercare and medical care such as: **Z51.11, encounter for antineoplastic chemotherapy or Z51.12, encounter for antineoplastic immunotherapy; and encounter for therapeutic drug level monitoring (Z51.81).**

- Z52 Donors of organs and tissues

- Z53 Persons encountering health services for specific procedures and treatment, not carried out due to specific reasons such as contraindications, patient smoking, reasons of belief and group pressure, and patient's decision.

Persons with potential health hazards related to socioeconomic and psychosocial circumstances (Z55-Z65)

Codes in categories Z55-Z65 (Persons with potential hazards related to socioeconomic and psychosocial circumstances) capture social information, rather than medical diagnoses, and can thus be reported based on information documented by other clinicians, not just the physician, who are involved in the care of the patient, according to Q1 2018 Coding Clinic guidance.

- Z55 includes codes for problems related to education and literacy, while Z56 contains codes related to problems related to employment and unemployment.

- Z57 includes codes for occupational exposure to risk factors such as noise, radiation, dust; tobacco smoke, other air contaminants, toxic agents in agriculture and other industries, extreme temperature, and exposure to other & unspecified risk factors.

- Z59 includes codes for problems related to housing and economic circumstances such as homelessness, inadequate housing, discord with neighbors, lodgers & landlord, problems related to living in residential institution, lack of adequate food & safe drinking water, extreme poverty & low income, and other problems related to housing and economic circumstances.

- Z60 codes describe problems related to social environment such as problems of life style adjustment, living alone, acculturation, social exclusion & rejection and adverse discrimination & persecution.

- Z62, problems relate to upbringing includes inadequate parental supervision & control, parental overprotection, hostility toward & scapegoating of child, personal history of abuse in childhood, and parent-child conflict.

- Z63, Other problems related to primary support group and family circumstances including a variety of stressful life events affecting family and household.

- Z64 and Z65, Problems related to psychosocial circumstances such as unwanted pregnancy, multiparity, conviction without imprisonment, imprisonment & other legal circumstances, etc.

Do not resuscitate status (Z66), Blood Type (Z67) and Body mass Index (Z68)

Code Z66, Do not resuscitate, may only be used when the provider documents that a patient is a "do not resuscitate" at any time during the patient's stay.

Persons encountering health services in other circumstances (Z69-Z76)

- Z69, Encounter for mental health services for victim and perpetrator of abuse

- Z71, Other counseling and medical advice, not elsewhere classified such as counseling and surveillance for dietary, alcohol abuse, drug abuse, tobacco abuse, HIV, and spiritual or religious counseling.

- Z72, Problems related to lifestyle such as tobacco use, lack of physical exercise, inappropriate diet and eating habits, high risk sexual & antisocial behavior, and sleep problems (deprivation, inadequate sleep hygiene).

- Z73, Problems related to life management difficulty such as burn out, Type A behavior pattern, lack of relaxation and leisure, stress NOS, inadequate social skills or social role conflict, limitation of activities due to disability, and other problems relate to life management difficulty.

- Z74, Problems related to care provider dependency such as **bed confinement status (Z74.01)**, need for assistance with personal care, assistance at home and no other household member able to render care, and need for continuous supervision.

- Z75, Problems related to medical facilities and other health care such as person awaiting admission to adequate facility elsewhere, unavailability and inaccessibility of other helping agencies, and holiday relief care.

- Z76, Personal encountering health services in other circumstances such as issue of repeat prescription medications, malingerer, **awaiting organ transplant status (Z76.82).**

Persons with potential health hazards related to family and personal history and certain conditions influencing health status (Z77-Z99)

- Z77, Other contact with and (suspected) exposures hazardous to health such as chiefly nonmedicinal metals & chemicals (e.g., **exposure to lead Z77.011)**, environmental pollution & hazards in the physical environment e.g., **(mold Z77.120)**, and other hazardous substances **(e.g., environmental tobacco smoke, Z77.22).** These codes may be used as first-listed to explain an encounter for testing, or more commonly, as a secondary code to identify a potential risk.

- Z78, Other specified health status, including **physical restraint status (Z78.1).**

- Z79, Long term (current) drug therapy includes **long term use of anticoagulants (Z79.01), antithrombotics/antiplatelets (Z79.02), NSAID (Z79.1), antibiotics Z79.2),** hormonal contraceptives (Z79.3), **insulin (Z79.4),** inhaled steroids (Z79.51), system steroids (Z79.52), aspirin (Z79.82), bisphosphonates (Z79.83); **oral hypoglycemic drugs (Z79.84);** opiate analgesic (Z79.891); use of agents affecting estrogen receptors and estrogen levels – includes both code first and use additional codes notes and six character codes for an expanded list of SERMS, aromatase inhibitors & other agents (Z79.81); and other such as hormone replacement therapy (Z79.890).

Codes from this category indicate a patient's continuous use of a prescription drug (including

aspirin therapy) for the long-term treatment of a condition or for prophylactic use. A code from Z79 is assigned for a patient who is receiving medication for an extended period as a prophylactic measure (such as for the prevention of deep vein thrombosis) or as treatment of a chronic condition (such as arthritis) or a disease requiring a lengthy course of treatment (such as cancer). A code from Z79 is *not assigned for medication being administered for a brief period to treat an acute illness or injury* (such as a course of antibiotics to treat acute bronchitis).

The Z79 codes are *not* for use for patients who have addictions to drugs, or medications for detoxification, or maintenance programs to prevent withdrawal symptoms in patients with drug dependence (e.g., methadone maintenance for opiate dependence). Instead assign the appropriate drug dependence code for those patients.

- Z80, Family history of primary malignant neoplasm by body site. Example: **family history of leukemia (Z80.6)** or **family history of other malignant neoplasms of lymphoid, hematopoietic and related tissue (Z80.7).**

- Z81 – Z84 are all family history codes and are broken into categories as follows: Family history of mental and behavioral disorders (Z81.-), Family history of certain disabilities and chronic diseases (leading to disablement) (Z82.-), Family history of other specific disorders (Z83.-), and Family history of other conditions (Z84.-).

- Z85, Personal history of malignant neoplasm by body system and identification of conditions classifiable to categories in Chapter 2. Be aware of the code first note and use additional codes listed at the top of the category. Examples include: **Z85.110, personal history of malignant carcinoid tumor of bronchus and lung or Z85.820, Personal history of malignant melanoma of skin.**

- Z86, Personal history of certain other diseases includes codes for Personal history of in-situ and benign neoplasm and neoplasms of uncertain behavior (Z86.0-); Personal history of infectious and parasitic diseases (Z86.1-) such as **Personal history of polio (Z86.12) or TB (Z86.11)**; Personal history of endocrine, nutritional and metabolic diseases (Z86.3-) such as **Personal history of diabetic foot ulcer (Z86.31)**; plus Personal history of combat and operational stress reaction (Z86.51) and other mental and behavioral disorder (Z86.59); Personal history of infections of the CNS (Z86.61) or nervous system and sense organs (Z86.69); and Personal history of diseases of the circulatory system (Z86.7-) such as **Personal history of pulmonary embolism (Z86.711) or Personal history of TIA and cerebral infarction without residual deficits (Z86.73).**

- Z87 Personal history of other diseases and conditions may be used in conjunction with follow-up codes. These codes explain a patient's past medical condition that no longer exists and is not receiving any current treatment, but has a potential for recurrence, and therefore may require continued monitoring and may also alter the type of treatment ordered. Examples include: **Personal history of pneumonia (Z87.01), personal history** of other diseases of the respiratory system (Z87.09); **Personal history of peptic ulcer disease (Z87.11)** or Personal history of other diseases of the digestive system (Z87.19); Personal history off diseases of the skin and subcutaneous tissue (Z87.2); Personal history of diseases of the musculoskeletal system and connective tissue (Z87.3-) such **as Personal history of (healed) osteoporosis fracture (Z87.310), or Personal history of other pathological fracture (Z87.311), or Personal history of stress fracture (Z87.312);** Personal history of diseases of genitourinary system (Z87.4-) such as **Personal history of urinary tract infection (Z87.440);** Personal history of other complications of pregnancy, childbirth and the puerperium (Z87.59) or Personal history of pre-term labor (Z87.51); Personal history of other specified conditions (Z87.8-) such as **personal history of (healed) traumatic fracture (Z87.81)** or Personal history of traumatic brain injury (Z87.820) or Personal history of nicotine dependence (Z87.891).

- Z88, Allergy status to drugs, medicaments, and biological substances, such as **Allergy status to penicillin (Z88.0), Allergy status to analgesic agent status (Z88.6) or Allergy status to other anti-infective agents status (Z88.3).**

- Z89, Acquired absence of a limb (amputation status, post-procedural loss of limb, or post-traumatic loss of limb) are status codes that include codes for acquired absence of a thumb, fingers, hand, wrist, upper limb above wrist, upper limb below or above elbow, shoulder, toes, foot, ankle, leg above or below knee, knee, and hip with specific codes for laterality. These codes can *only be used* if there are no complications of the amputation site. For example, **acquired absence of right shoulder (Z89.231) or acquired absence of left great toe (Z89.412) or disarticulation of a right ankle (Z89.441) or acquired absence of left hip joint following explantation of hip joint prosthesis with or without presence of an antibiotic-impregnated spacer (Z89.622).**

- Z90, Acquired absence of organs, not elsewhere classified, are also status codes that can only be used when there are no complications present. Examples include acquired absence of larynx (Z90.02), or **acquired absence of bilateral breasts**

and nipples (Z90.13) or acquired absence of uterus with remaining cervical stump (Z90.711).

- Z91, Personal risk factors, not elsewhere classified, includes status codes for allergy status, other than to drugs and biological substances such as **latex allergy (Z91.040).** Z91.1- codes relate to patient's noncompliance with medical treatment and regimen such as **noncompliance with dietary regimen (Z91.11), or patient's noncompliance with renal dialysis (Z91.15).** Other codes in this category include: **Personal history of falling (Z91.81),** and **Personal history of wandering in diseases classified elsewhere (Z91.83).**

- Z92, Personal history of medical treatment includes the following: **Z92.21, Personal history of antineoplastic chemotherapy; Z92.240, Personal history of inhaled steroid therapy.**

- Z93, Artificial opening status codes *exclude* artificial openings requiring attention or management which are coded to Z43.- and complications of external stoma (J95.0, K94.-, N99.5). These status codes indicate the patient or family caregiver is providing the care for the stoma, not the home health personnel. Some examples of these status codes are: **Z93.3, Colostomy status or Z93.51, Cutaneous-vesicostomy** status.

- Z94, Transplanted organ and tissue status codes indicate an organ or tissue replaced by heterogenous or homogenous transplant. These codes are not to be used in the presence of complications of the transplant organ or tissue. Examples include: **Z94.1, Heart transplant status** that excludes an artificial heart status (Z95.811) or heart-valve replacement status (Z95.2-X95.4); and **Bone marrow transplant status (Z94.81).**

- Z95, Presence of cardiac and vascular implants and grafts includes status codes such as: **Presence of cardiac pacemaker (Z95.0), aortocoronary bypass graft (Z95.1), presence of automatic (implanted) defibrillator (Z95.810).**

- Z96, Presence of orthopedic joint implants are status codes and exclude complications of internal prosthetic devices, implants or grafts, but these codes may be coded in addition to the codes from Z96.6-. Examples include **presence of right artificial hip joint (Z96.641), presence of left artificial knee joint (Z96.652), and presence of right artificial shoulder (Z96.611).** Other functional implants coded at Z96 include: presence of an artificial larynx (Z96.3) or presence of artificial skin (Z96.81).

- Z97, Presence of other devices includes codes for **presence of artificial right arm (complete) or (partial) (Z97.11), presence of bilateral artificial legs, bilateral (complete) (partial) (Z97.16),** and presence of external hearing aid (Z97.4)

- Z98, Other post procedural states has an Excludes 2 note for aftercare (Z43-Z49, Z51), follow-up medical care (Z08-Z09), and post procedural complications. Examples of codes from this category include: **coronary angioplasty status (Z98.61)**, excluding coronary angioplasty status with implant and graft (Z95.5); **breast implant status (Z98.82)**, excluding breast implant removal status (Z98.86); **bariatric surgery status (Z98.84)**; and **transplant organ removal status (Z98.85)** that is used to indicate a transplanted organ has been previously removed due to complication, failure, rejection or infection.

- Z99, Dependence on enabling machines and devices, not elsewhere classified, includes codes such as **Dependence on respirator/ventilator (Z99.1-),** Dependence on renal dialysis (Z99.2), Dependence on wheelchair (Z99.3), and **Dependence on supplemental oxygen** (Z99.81).

Special Instructions related to Z code use

Note: Categories Z89-Z90 and Z93-Z99 can only be used when there are no complications, malfunctions of the organ or tissue replaced, the amputation site or the equipment on which the patient is dependent.

Aftercare codes (Z42-Z49, Z51) are heavily used in home health care for situations when the initial treatment of a disease has been performed and the patient requires continued care during the healing or recovery phase, or for the long-term consequences of the disease. The aftercare Z code should not be used if treatment is directed at a current, acute disease. The diagnosis code is to be used in these cases.

Additional guidance on aftercare codes includes:

- Exceptions to these rules are Z51.0, Encounter for antineoplastic radiation therapy, and Z51.1, Encounter for antineoplastic chemotherapy and immunotherapy. These codes are the first-listed, followed by the diagnosis code when a patient's encounter is solely to receive radiation therapy, chemotherapy or immunotherapy for the treatment of a neoplasm.

- The aftercare Z codes should **not** be used for aftercare for injuries including traumatic fractures. Instead, assign the original (acute) injury code with the appropriate 7th character (for subsequent care).

- The aftercare codes are generally first-listed to explain the specific reason for the encounter. An aftercare code may be used as an additional code when some type of aftercare is provided in addition to the reason for admission and no diagnosis code is applicable. An example of this would be the closure of a colostomy during an encounter for treatment of another condition.

- Aftercare codes should be used in conjunction with other aftercare codes or diagnosis codes to provide better detail on the specifics of an aftercare encounter visit, unless otherwise directed by the classification.

- Certain aftercare Z code categories need a secondary diagnosis code to describe the resolving condition or sequelae. For others, the condition is included in the code title.

- Status Z codes may be used with aftercare Z codes to indicate the nature of the aftercare. For example, Z95.1, Presence of aortocoronary bypass graft, may be used with code Z48.812, Encounter for surgical aftercare following surgery on the circulatory system, to indicate surgery for which the aftercare is being performed. A status code should not be used when the aftercare code indicates the type of status, such as using Z43.0, Encounter for attention to tracheostomy, with Z93.0, Tracheostomy status.

Follow-up codes (Z08-Z09, Z39, follow up-examination after completed treatment for malignant neoplasm, for conditions other than neoplasms and maternal postpartum care) are used to explain continuing surveillance following completed treatment of a disease, condition or injury. They imply that the condition has been fully treated and no longer exists. They should not be confused with aftercare codes, or injury codes with a 7th character for subsequent encounter, that explain ongoing care of a healing condition or its sequelae.

Prophylactic Organ Removal

For encounters specifically for prophylactic removal of an organ, the principal or first-listed code should be a code from category Z40, Encounter for prophylactic surgery.

Note, you would assign code Z48.3 (Aftercare following surgery for neoplasm) if your agency is providing care during the healing and recovery phase, following the initial treatment (surgery) for removal of the breast. You can also assign an additional code from subcategory Z90.1- (Acquired absence of breast and nipple) to provide additional information, according to the Coding Clinic (in a letter dated Aug. 17, 2016).

You would not assign code Z40.01 (Encounter for prophylactic removal of breast) since the home health visit is not the encounter where the breast is actually removed. Also you would not assign an aftercare visit code, such as Z42.1 (Encounter for breast reconstruction following mastectomy) since the breast is not reconstructed during the home health visit, according to Coding Clinic.

CHAPTER 21: FACTORS INFLUENCING HEALTH STATUS AND CONTACT WITH HEALTH SERVICES (Z00-Z99)

Note:

Z codes represent reasons for encounters. A corresponding procedure code must accompany a Z code if a procedure is performed. Categories Z00-Z99 are provided for occasions when circumstances other than a disease, injury or external cause classifiable to categories A00-Y89 are recorded as 'diagnoses' or 'problems'. This can arise in two main ways:

(a) When a person who may or may not be sick encounters the health services for some specific purpose, such as to receive limited care or service for a current condition, to donate an organ or tissue, to receive prophylactic vaccination (immunization), or to discuss a problem which is in itself not a disease or injury.

(b) When some circumstance or problem is present which influences the person's health status but is not in itself a current illness or injury.

ALERT Sometimes payer policy conflicts with official guidelines, rules and conventions, and other official guidance. When a payer refuses to pay based on code(s) used in compliance with that guidance, take the following steps: 1) Determine whether the denial or rejection is truly a coding dispute and not a different coverage or payment issue; 2) Remind the payer that following official guidelines and conventions is required by HIPAA code set standards and provide the official guidance in question. If a payer does have a policy that clearly conflicts with official coding rules or guidelines, every effort should be made to resolve the issue with the payer; 3) If the payer refuses to change its policy, obtain the payer requirements in writing. If the payer refuses to provide their policy in writing, document all discussions, including dates and names of individuals involved; 4) Conform to the payer's policy if the payer continues to deny or reject the claim; 5) Keep a permanent file of the documentation obtained regarding payer coding policies. It may be come in handy in the event of an audit.

GUIDELINES Section I.C.21.a

Z codes are for use in any healthcare setting. Z codes may be used as either a first-listed (principal diagnosis code in the inpatient setting) or secondary code, depending on the circumstances of the encounter. Certain Z codes may only be used as first-listed or principal diagnosis.

CODING TIPS ✓ Aftercare Z codes should not be used for aftercare of injuries. For aftercare of an injury, assign the injury code with the appropriate 7th character, usually "D" if the condition meets the definition of aftercare (patient requires continued care during the healing or recovery phase or long term consequences of the disease/injury). Do not use aftercare Z codes for complications. Continue to code the complication with a D to indicate aftercare.

This chapter contains the following blocks:

Z00-Z13	Persons encountering health services for examinations
Z14-Z15	Genetic carrier and genetic susceptibility to disease
Z16	Resistance to antimicrobial drugs
Z17	Estrogen receptor status
Z18	Retained foreign body fragments
Z19	Hormone sensitivity malignancy status
Z20-Z29	Persons with potential health hazards related to communicable diseases
Z30-Z39	Persons encountering health services in circumstances related to reproduction
Z40-Z53	Encounters for other specific health care
Z55-Z65	Persons with potential health hazards related to socioeconomic and psychosocial circumstances
Z66	Do not resuscitate status
Z67	Blood type
Z68	Body mass index (BMI)
Z69-Z76	Persons encountering health services in other circumstances
Z77-Z99	Persons with potential health hazards related to family and personal history and certain conditions influencing health status

Persons encountering health services for examinations (Z00-Z13)

Note:

Nonspecific abnormal findings disclosed at the time of these examinations are classified to categories R70-R94.

EXCLUDES 1 examinations related to pregnancy and reproduction (Z30-Z36, Z39.-)

4 Z00 Encounter for general examination without complaint, suspected or reported diagnosis

EXCLUDES 1 encounter for examination for administrative purposes (Z02.-)

EXCLUDES 2 encounter for pre-procedural examinations (Z01.81-)

special screening examinations (Z11-Z13)

5 Z00.0 Encounter for general adult medical examination

Encounter for adult periodic examination (annual) (physical) and any associated laboratory and radiologic examinations

EXCLUDES 1 encounter for examination of sign or symptom- code to sign or symptom

general health check-up of infant or child (Z00.12.-)

Px IQ Z00.00 Encounter for general adult medical examination without abnormal findings

Encounter for adult health check-up NOS

Px IQ + Z00.01 Encounter for general adult medical examination with abnormal findings

Use additional code to identify abnormal findings

5 Z00.1 Encounter for newborn, infant and child health examinations

+ 6 Z00.11 Newborn health examination

Health check for child under 29 days old

Use additional code to identify any abnormal findings

EXCLUDES 1 health check for child over 28 days old (Z00.12-)

Px IQ + Z00.110 Health examination for newborn under 8 days old

Health check for newborn under 8 days old

Px IQ + Z00.111 Health examination for newborn 8 to 28 days old

Health check for newborn 8 to 28 days old

Newborn weight check

6 Z00.12 Encounter for routine child health examination

★ New ▲ Revised Px Primary SP PDGM Px SL Low CoM SH High CoM IQ Quest. Encounter H Hospice non-cancer Dx Unspecified M Manifestation

DecisionHealth's FY 2020 Complete Home Health ICD-10-CM Diagnosis Coding Manual

1881

Health check (routine) for child over 28 days old

Immunizations appropriate for age

Routine developmental screening of infant or child

Routine vision and hearing testing

EXCLUDES 1 health check for child under 29 days old (Z00.11-)

health supervision of foundling or other healthy infant or child (Z76.1-Z76.2)

newborn health examination (Z00.11-)

Px IQ ✚ Z00.121 **Encounter for routine child health examination with abnormal findings**

Use additional code to identify abnormal findings

Px IQ Z00.129 **Encounter for routine child health examination without abnormal findings**

Encounter for routine child health examination NOS

Px IQ Z00.2 **Encounter for examination for period of rapid growth in childhood**

Px IQ Z00.3 **Encounter for examination for adolescent development state**

Encounter for puberty development state

Px IQ Z00.5 **Encounter for examination of potential donor of organ and tissue**

IQ Z00.6 **Encounter for examination for normal comparison and control in clinical research program**

Examination of participant or control in clinical research program

S Z00.7 **Encounter for examination for period of delayed growth in childhood**

Px IQ Z00.70 **Encounter for examination for period of delayed growth in childhood without abnormal findings**

Px IQ ✚ Z00.71 **Encounter for examination for period of delayed growth in childhood with abnormal findings**

Use additional code to identify abnormal findings

Px IQ Z00.8 **Encounter for other general examination**

Encounter for health examination in population surveys

4 Z01 **Encounter for other special examination without complaint, suspected or reported diagnosis**

Note:

Codes from category Z01 represent the reason for the encounter. A separate procedure code is required to identify any examinations or procedures performed

INCLUDES routine examination of specific system

EXCLUDES 1 encounter for examination for administrative purposes (Z02.-)

encounter for examination for suspected conditions, proven not to exist (Z03.-)

encounter for laboratory and radiologic examinations as a component of general medical examinations (Z00.0-)

encounter for laboratory, radiologic and imaging examinations for sign (s) and symptom(s) - code to the sign(s) or symptom(s)

EXCLUDES 2 screening examinations (Z11-Z13)

S Z01.0 **Encounter for examination of eyes and vision**

EXCLUDES 1 examination for driving license (Z02.4)

Px IQ Z01.00 **Encounter for examination of eyes and vision without abnormal findings**

Encounter for examination of eyes and vision NOS

Px IQ ✚ Z01.01 **Encounter for examination of eyes and vision with abnormal findings**

Use additional code to identify abnormal findings

★ 6 Z01.02 **Encounter for examination of eyes and vision following failed vision screening**

EXCLUDES 1 examination for examination of eyes and vision with abnormal findings (Z01.01)

examination for examination of eyes and vision without abnormal findings (Z01.00)

★ Z01.020 **Encounter for examination of eyes and vision following failed vision screening without abnormal findings**

★ ✚ Z01.021 **Encounter for examination of eyes and vision following failed vision screening with abnormal findings**

Use additional code to identify abnormal findings

S Z01.1 **Encounter for examination of ears and hearing**

Px IQ Z01.10 **Encounter for examination of ears and hearing without abnormal findings**

Encounter for examination of ears and hearing NOS

6 Z01.11 **Encounter for examination of ears and hearing with abnormal findings**

Px IQ Z01.110 **Encounter for hearing examination following failed hearing screening**

Px IQ ✚ Z01.118 **Encounter for examination of ears and hearing with other abnormal findings**

Use additional code to identify abnormal findings

Px IQ Z01.12 **Encounter for hearing conservation and treatment**

S Z01.2 **Encounter for dental examination and cleaning**

4 4th digit required   **S** 5th digit required   **6** 6th digit required   **7** 7th digit required   **7** 7th digit placeholder   ✚ Additional code   **S** Laterality

1882   *DecisionHealth's* FY 2020 Complete Home Health ICD-10-CM Diagnosis Coding Manual

Px **IQ** **Z01.20** **Encounter for dental examination and cleaning without abnormal findings**
Encounter for dental examination and cleaning NOS

Px **IQ** ✚ **Z01.21** **Encounter for dental examination and cleaning with abnormal findings**
Use additional code to identify abnormal findings

⑤ **Z01.3** **Encounter for examination of blood pressure**

Px **IQ** **Z01.30** **Encounter for examination of blood pressure without abnormal findings**
Encounter for examination of blood pressure NOS

Px **IQ** ✚ **Z01.31** **Encounter for examination of blood pressure with abnormal findings**
Use additional code to identify abnormal findings

⑤ **Z01.4** **Encounter for gynecological examination**
EXCLUDES 2 pregnancy examination or test (Z32.0-)
routine examination for contraceptive maintenance (Z30.4-)

✚ ⑥ **Z01.41** **Encounter for routine gynecological examination**
Encounter for general gynecological examination with or without cervical smear
Encounter for gynecological examination (general) (routine) NOS
Encounter for pelvic examination (annual) (periodic)
Use additional code:
for screening for human papillomavirus, if applicable, (Z11.51)
for screening vaginal pap smear, if applicable (Z12.72)
to identify acquired absence of uterus, if applicable (Z90.71-)
EXCLUDES 1 gynecologic examination status-post hysterectomy for malignant condition (Z08)
screening cervical pap smear not a part of a routine gynecological examination (Z12.4)

Px **IQ** ✚ **Z01.411** **Encounter for gynecological examination (general) (routine) with abnormal findings**
Use additional code to identify abnormal findings

Px **IQ** ✚ **Z01.419** **Encounter for gynecological examination (general) (routine) without abnormal findings**

Px **IQ** **Z01.42** **Encounter for cervical smear to confirm findings of recent normal smear following initial abnormal smear**

⑤ **Z01.8** **Encounter for other specified special examinations**

⑥ **Z01.81** **Encounter for preprocedural examinations**
Encounter for preoperative examinations
Encounter for radiological and imaging examinations as part of preprocedural examination

Px **IQ** **Z01.810** **Encounter for preprocedural cardiovascular examination**

Px **IQ** **Z01.811** **Encounter for preprocedural respiratory examination**

Px **IQ** **Z01.812** **Encounter for preprocedural laboratory examination**
Blood and urine tests prior to treatment or procedure

Px **IQ** **Z01.818** **Encounter for other preprocedural examination**
Encounter for preprocedural examination NOS
Encounter for examinations prior to antineoplastic chemotherapy

Px **IQ** **Z01.82** **Encounter for allergy testing**
EXCLUDES 1 encounter for antibody response examination (Z01.84)

Px **IQ** **Z01.83** **Encounter for blood typing**
Encounter for Rh typing

Px **IQ** **Z01.84** **Encounter for antibody response examination**
Encounter for immunity status testing
EXCLUDES 1 encounter for allergy testing (Z01.82)

Px **IQ** **Z01.89** **Encounter for other specified special examinations**

④ **Z02** **Encounter for administrative examination**

Px **IQ** **Z02.0** **Encounter for examination for admission to educational institution**
Encounter for examination for admission to preschool (education)
Encounter for examination for re-admission to school following illness or medical treatment

Px **IQ** **Z02.1** **Encounter for pre-employment examination**

Px **IQ** **Z02.2** **Encounter for examination for admission to residential institution**
EXCLUDES 1 examination for admission to prison (Z02.89)

Px **IQ** **Z02.3** **Encounter for examination for recruitment to armed forces**

Px **IQ** **Z02.4** **Encounter for examination for driving license**

Px **IQ** **Z02.5** **Encounter for examination for participation in sport**
EXCLUDES 1 blood-alcohol and blood-drug test (Z02.83)

Px **IQ** **Z02.6** **Encounter for examination for insurance purposes**

⑤ **Z02.7** **Encounter for issue of medical certificate**
EXCLUDES 1 encounter for general medical examination (Z00-Z01, Z02.0-Z02.6, Z02.8-Z02.9)

Px **IQ** **Z02.71** **Encounter for disability determination**
Encounter for issue of medical certificate of incapacity
Encounter for issue of medical certificate of invalidity

★ New ▲ Revised Px Primary **SP** PDGM Px **SL** Low CoM **SH** High CoM **IQ** Quest. Encounter **H** Hospice non-cancer Dx Unspecified **M** *Manifestation*

DecisionHealth's FY 2020 Complete Home Health ICD-10-CM Diagnosis Coding Manual

1883

Px **!Q** **Z02.79** **Encounter for issue of other medical certificate**

⑤ **Z02.8** **Encounter for other administrative examinations**

Px **!Q** **Z02.81** **Encounter for paternity testing**

Px **!Q** **Z02.82** **Encounter for adoption services**

Px **!Q** **+** **Z02.83** **Encounter for blood-alcohol and blood-drug test**
Use additional code for findings of alcohol or drugs in blood (R78.-)

Px **!Q** **Z02.89** **Encounter for other administrative examinations**
Encounter for examination for admission to prison
Encounter for examination for admission to summer camp
Encounter for immigration examination
Encounter for naturalization examination
Encounter for premarital examination
EXCLUDES 1 health supervision of foundling or other healthy infant or child (Z76.1-Z76.2)

Px **!Q** **Z02.9** **Encounter for administrative examinations, unspecified**

④ **Z03** **Encounter for medical observation for suspected diseases and conditions ruled out**
This category is to be used when a person without a diagnosis is suspected of having an abnormal condition, without signs or symptoms, which requires study, but after examination and observation, is ruled out. This category is also for use for administrative and legal observation status.
EXCLUDES 1 contact with and (suspected) exposures hazardous to health (Z77.-)
encounter for observation and evaluation of newborn for suspected diseases and conditions ruled out (Z05.-)
person with feared complaint in whom no diagnosis is made (Z71.1)
signs or symptoms under study- code to signs or symptoms

Px **!Q** **Z03.6** **Encounter for observation for suspected toxic effect from ingested substance ruled out**
Encounter for observation for suspected adverse effect from drug
Encounter for observation for suspected poisoning

⑤ **Z03.7** **Encounter for suspected maternal and fetal conditions ruled out**
Encounter for suspected maternal and fetal conditions not found
EXCLUDES 1 known or suspected fetal anomalies affecting management of mother, not ruled out (O26.-, O35.-, O36.-, O40.-, O41.-)

Px **!Q** **Z03.71** **Encounter for suspected problem with amniotic cavity and membrane ruled out**

Encounter for suspected oligohydramnios ruled out
Encounter for suspected polyhydramnios ruled out

Px **!Q** **Z03.72** **Encounter for suspected placental problem ruled out**

Px **!Q** **Z03.73** **Encounter for suspected fetal anomaly ruled out**

Px **!Q** **Z03.74** **Encounter for suspected problem with fetal growth ruled out**

Px **!Q** **Z03.75** **Encounter for suspected cervical shortening ruled out**

Px **!Q** **Z03.79** **Encounter for other suspected maternal and fetal conditions ruled out**

⑤ **Z03.8** **Encounter for observation for other suspected diseases and conditions ruled out**

⑥ **Z03.81** **Encounter for observation for suspected exposure to biological agents ruled out**

Px **!Q** **Z03.810** **Encounter for observation for suspected exposure to anthrax ruled out**

Px **!Q** **Z03.818** **Encounter for observation for suspected exposure to other biological agents ruled out**

Px **!Q** **Z03.89** **Encounter for observation for other suspected diseases and conditions ruled out**

④ **Z04** **Encounter for examination and observation for other reasons**
INCLUDES encounter for examination for medicolegal reasons
This category is to be used when a person without a diagnosis is suspected of having an abnormal condition, without signs or symptoms, which requires study, but after examination and observation, is ruled-out. This category is also for use for administrative and legal observation status.

Px **!Q** **Z04.1** **Encounter for examination and observation following transport accident**
EXCLUDES 1 encounter for examination and observation following work accident (Z04.2)

Px **!Q** **Z04.2** **Encounter for examination and observation following work accident**

Px **!Q** **Z04.3** **Encounter for examination and observation following other accident**

⑤ **Z04.4** **Encounter for examination and observation following alleged rape**
Encounter for examination and observation of victim following alleged rape
Encounter for examination and observation of victim following alleged sexual abuse

Px **!Q** **Z04.41** **Encounter for examination and observation following alleged adult rape**
Suspected adult rape, ruled out
Suspected adult sexual abuse, ruled out

Px **!Q** **Z04.42** **Encounter for examination and observation following alleged child rape**
Suspected child rape, ruled out
Suspected child sexual abuse, ruled out

---

④4th digit required　　⑤5th digit required　　⑥6th digit required　　⑦7th digit required　　⑦7th digit placeholder　　✛Additional code　　⊟Laterality

Px **IQ** Z04.6 **Encounter for general psychiatric examination, requested by authority**

5 Z04.7 **Encounter for examination and observation following alleged physical abuse**

Px **IQ** Z04.71 **Encounter for examination and observation following alleged adult physical abuse**
Suspected adult physical abuse, ruled out
> **EXCLUDES 1** confirmed case of adult physical abuse (T74.-)
> encounter for examination and observation following alleged adult sexual abuse (Z04.41)
> suspected case of adult physical abuse, not ruled out (T76.-)

Px **IQ** Z04.72 **Encounter for examination and observation following alleged child physical abuse**
Suspected child physical abuse, ruled out
> **EXCLUDES 1** confirmed case of child physical abuse (T74.-)
> encounter for examination and observation following alleged child sexual abuse (Z04.42)
> suspected case of child physical abuse, not ruled out (T76.-)

5 Z04.8 **Encounter for examination and observation for other specified reasons**
Encounter for examination and observation for request for expert evidence

Px **IQ** Z04.81 **Encounter for examination and observation of victim following forced sexual exploitation**

Px **IQ** Z04.82 **Encounter for examination and observation of victim following forced labor exploitation**

Px **IQ** Z04.89 **Encounter for examination and observation for other specified reasons**

Px **IQ** Z04.9 **Encounter for examination and observation for unspecified reason**
Encounter for observation NOS

4 Z05 **Encounter for observation and evaluation of newborn for suspected diseases and conditions ruled out**
This category is to be used for newborns, within the neonatal period (the first 28 days of life), who are suspected of having an abnormal condition, but without signs or symptoms, and which, after examination and observation, is ruled out.

IQ Z05.0 **Observation and evaluation of newborn for suspected cardiac condition ruled out**

IQ Z05.1 **Observation and evaluation of newborn for suspected infectious condition ruled out**

IQ Z05.2 **Observation and evaluation of newborn for suspected neurological condition ruled out**

IQ Z05.3 **Observation and evaluation of newborn for suspected respiratory condition ruled out**

5 Z05.4 **Observation and evaluation of newborn for suspected genetic, metabolic or immunologic condition ruled out**

IQ Z05.41 **Observation and evaluation of newborn for suspected genetic condition ruled out**

IQ Z05.42 **Observation and evaluation of newborn for suspected metabolic condition ruled out**

IQ Z05.43 **Observation and evaluation of newborn for suspected immunologic condition ruled out**

IQ Z05.5 **Observation and evaluation of newborn for suspected gastrointestinal condition ruled out**

IQ Z05.6 **Observation and evaluation of newborn for suspected genitourinary condition ruled out**

5 Z05.7 **Observation and evaluation of newborn for suspected skin, subcutaneous, musculoskeletal and connective tissue condition ruled out**

IQ Z05.71 **Observation and evaluation of newborn for suspected skin and subcutaneous tissue condition ruled out**

IQ Z05.72 **Observation and evaluation of newborn for suspected musculoskeletal condition ruled out**

IQ Z05.73 **Observation and evaluation of newborn for suspected connective tissue condition ruled out**

IQ Z05.8 **Observation and evaluation of newborn for other specified suspected condition ruled out**

IQ Z05.9 **Observation and evaluation of newborn for unspecified suspected condition ruled out**

IQ ✚ Z08 **Encounter for follow-up examination after completed treatment for malignant neoplasm**
Medical surveillance following completed treatment
Use additional code to identify any acquired absence of organs (Z90.-)
Use additional code to identify the personal history of malignant neoplasm (Z85.-)
> **EXCLUDES 1** aftercare following medical care (Z43-Z49, Z51)

IQ ✚ Z09 **Encounter for follow-up examination after completed treatment for conditions other than malignant neoplasm**
Medical surveillance following completed treatment
Use additional code to identify any applicable history of disease code (Z86.-. Z87.-)
> **EXCLUDES 1** aftercare following medical care (Z43-Z49, Z51)
> surveillance of contraception (Z30.4-)
> surveillance of prosthetic and other medical devices (Z44-Z46)

4 Z11 **Encounter for screening for infectious and parasitic diseases**

★ New ▲ Revised Px Primary **SP** PDGM Px **SL** Low CoM **SH** High CoM **IQ** Quest. Encounter **H** Hospice non-cancer Dx Unspecified **M** *Manifestation*

DecisionHealth's FY 2020 Complete Home Health ICD-10-CM Diagnosis Coding Manual

1885

Screening is the testing for disease or disease precursors in asymptomatic individuals so that early detection and treatment can be provided for those who test positive for the disease.

> **EXCLUDES 1** encounter for diagnostic examination-code to sign or symptom

!Q Z11.0 Encounter for screening for intestinal infectious diseases

▲ **!Q Z11.1 Encounter for screening for respiratory tuberculosis**
Encounter for screening for active tuberculosis disease

!Q Z11.2 Encounter for screening for other bacterial diseases

!Q Z11.3 Encounter for screening for infections with a predominantly sexual mode of transmission

> **EXCLUDES 2** encounter for screening for human immunodeficiency virus [HIV] (Z11.4)
> encounter for screening for human papillomavirus (Z11.51)

!Q Z11.4 Encounter for screening for human immunodeficiency virus [HIV]

5 Z11.5 Encounter for screening for other viral diseases

> **EXCLUDES 2** encounter for screening for viral intestinal disease (Z11.0)

!Q Z11.51 Encounter for screening for human papillomavirus (HPV)

!Q Z11.59 Encounter for screening for other viral diseases

!Q Z11.6 Encounter for screening for other protozoal diseases and helminthiases

> **EXCLUDES 2** encounter for screening for protozoal intestinal disease (Z11.0)

★ **Z11.7 Encounter for testing for latent tuberculosis infection**

!Q Z11.8 Encounter for screening for other infectious and parasitic diseases
Encounter for screening for chlamydia
Encounter for screening for rickettsial
Encounter for screening for spirochetal
Encounter for screening for mycoses

!Q Z11.9 Encounter for screening for infectious and parasitic diseases, unspecified

+ **4 Z12 Encounter for screening for malignant neoplasms**
Screening is the testing for disease or disease precursors in asymptomatic individuals so that early detection and treatment can be provided for those who test positive for the disease.
Use additional code to identify any family history of malignant neoplasm (Z80.-)

> **EXCLUDES 1** encounter for diagnostic examination-code to sign or symptom

!Q + Z12.0 Encounter for screening for malignant neoplasm of stomach

+ **5 Z12.1 Encounter for screening for malignant neoplasm of intestinal tract**

!Q + Z12.10 Encounter for screening for malignant neoplasm of intestinal tract, unspecified

!Q + Z12.11 Encounter for screening for malignant neoplasm of colon
Encounter for screening colonoscopy NOS

!Q + Z12.12 Encounter for screening for malignant neoplasm of rectum

!Q + Z12.13 Encounter for screening for malignant neoplasm of small intestine

!Q + Z12.2 Encounter for screening for malignant neoplasm of respiratory organs

+ **5 Z12.3 Encounter for screening for malignant neoplasm of breast**

!Q + Z12.31 Encounter for screening mammogram for malignant neoplasm of breast

> **EXCLUDES 1** inconclusive mammogram (R92.2)

!Q + Z12.39 Encounter for other screening for malignant neoplasm of breast

!Q + Z12.4 Encounter for screening for malignant neoplasm of cervix
Encounter for screening pap smear for malignant neoplasm of cervix

> **EXCLUDES 1** when screening is part of general gynecological examination (Z01.4-)
> **EXCLUDES 2** encounter for screening for human papillomavirus (Z11.51)

!Q + Z12.5 Encounter for screening for malignant neoplasm of prostate

!Q + Z12.6 Encounter for screening for malignant neoplasm of bladder

+ **5 Z12.7 Encounter for screening for malignant neoplasm of other genitourinary organs**

!Q + Z12.71 Encounter for screening for malignant neoplasm of testis

!Q + Z12.72 Encounter for screening for malignant neoplasm of vagina
Vaginal pap smear status-post hysterectomy for non-malignant condition
Use additional code to identify acquired absence of uterus (Z90.71-)

> **EXCLUDES 1** vaginal pap smear status-post hysterectomy for malignant conditions (Z08)

!Q + Z12.73 Encounter for screening for malignant neoplasm of ovary

!Q + Z12.79 Encounter for screening for malignant neoplasm of other genitourinary organs

+ **5 Z12.8 Encounter for screening for malignant neoplasm of other sites**

!Q + Z12.81 Encounter for screening for malignant neoplasm of oral cavity

!Q + Z12.82 Encounter for screening for malignant neoplasm of nervous system

!Q + Z12.83 Encounter for screening for malignant neoplasm of skin

!Q + Z12.89 Encounter for screening for malignant neoplasm of other sites

---

4 4th digit required   **5** 5th digit required   **6** 6th digit required   **7** 7th digit required   **7** 7th digit placeholder   **+** Additional code   **8** Laterality

1886   *DecisionHealth's* FY 2020 Complete Home Health ICD-10-CM Diagnosis Coding Manual

!Q **+** **Z12.9** **Encounter for screening for malignant neoplasm, site unspecified**

4 **Z13** **Encounter for screening for other diseases and disorders**

Screening is the testing for disease or disease precursors in asymptomatic individuals so that early detection and treatment can be provided for those who test positive for the disease.

> **EXCLUDES 1** encounter for diagnostic examination-code to sign or symptom

!Q **Z13.0** **Encounter for screening for diseases of the blood and blood-forming organs and certain disorders involving the immune mechanism**

!Q **Z13.1** **Encounter for screening for diabetes mellitus**

5 **Z13.2** **Encounter for screening for nutritional, metabolic and other endocrine disorders**

!Q **Z13.21** **Encounter for screening for nutritional disorder**

6 **Z13.22** **Encounter for screening for metabolic disorder**

!Q **Z13.220** **Encounter for screening for lipoid disorders**

Encounter for screening for cholesterol level

Encounter for screening for hypercholesterolemia

Encounter for screening for hyperlipidemia

!Q **Z13.228** **Encounter for screening for other metabolic disorders**

!Q **Z13.29** **Encounter for screening for other suspected endocrine disorder**

> **EXCLUDES 1** encounter for screening for diabetes mellitus (Z13.1)

5 **Z13.3** **Encounter for screening examination for mental health and behavioral disorders**

!Q **Z13.30** **Encounter for screening examination for mental health and behavioral disorders, unspecified**

!Q **Z13.31** **Encounter for screening for depression**

Encounter for screening for depression, adult

Encounter for screening for depression for child or adolescent

!Q **Z13.32** **Encounter for screening for maternal depression**

Encounter for screening for perinatal depression

!Q **Z13.39** **Encounter for screening examination for other mental health and behavioral disorders**

Encounter for screening for alcoholism

Encounter for screening for intellectual disabilities

5 **Z13.4** **Encounter for screening for certain developmental disorders in childhood**

Encounter for development testing of infant or child

Encounter for screening for developmental handicaps in early childhood

> **EXCLUDES 2** encounter for routine child health examination (Z00.12-)

!Q **Z13.40** **Encounter for screening for unspecified developmental delays**

!Q **Z13.41** **Encounter for autism screening**

!Q **Z13.42** **Encounter for screening for global developmental delays (milestones)**

Encounter for screening for developmental handicaps in early childhood

!Q **Z13.49** **Encounter for screening for other developmental delays**

!Q **Z13.5** **Encounter for screening for eye and ear disorders**

> **EXCLUDES 2** encounter for general hearing examination (Z01.1-)
> encounter for general vision examination (Z01.0-)

!Q **Z13.6** **Encounter for screening for cardiovascular disorders**

5 **Z13.7** **Encounter for screening for genetic and chromosomal anomalies**

> **EXCLUDES 1** genetic testing for procreative management (Z31.4-)

!Q **Z13.71** **Encounter for nonprocreative screening for genetic disease carrier status**

!Q **Z13.79** **Encounter for other screening for genetic and chromosomal anomalies**

5 **Z13.8** **Encounter for screening for other specified diseases and disorders**

> **EXCLUDES 2** screening for malignant neoplasms (Z12.-)

6 **Z13.81** **Encounter for screening for digestive system disorders**

!Q **Z13.810** **Encounter for screening for upper gastrointestinal disorder**

!Q **Z13.811** **Encounter for screening for lower gastrointestinal disorder**

> **EXCLUDES 1** encounter for screening for intestinal infectious disease (Z11.0)

!Q **Z13.818** **Encounter for screening for other digestive system disorders**

6 **Z13.82** **Encounter for screening for musculoskeletal disorder**

!Q **Z13.820** **Encounter for screening for osteoporosis**

!Q **Z13.828** **Encounter for screening for other musculoskeletal disorder**

!Q **Z13.83** **Encounter for screening for respiratory disorder NEC**

> **EXCLUDES 1** encounter for screening for respiratory tuberculosis (Z11.1)

!Q **Z13.84** **Encounter for screening for dental disorders**

6 **Z13.85** **Encounter for screening for nervous system disorders**

!Q **Z13.850** **Encounter for screening for traumatic brain injury**

!Q **Z13.858** **Encounter for screening for other nervous system disorders**

☆ New ▲ Revised **Px** Primary **SP** PDGM Px **SL** Low CoM **SH** High CoM **!Q** Quest. Encounter **H** Hospice non-cancer Dx ▕ Unspecified ▏ **M** *Manifestation*

IQ Z13.88 Encounter for screening for disorder due to exposure to contaminants

> **EXCLUDES 1** those exposed to contaminants without suspected disorders (Z57.-, Z77.-)

IQ Z13.89 Encounter for screening for other disorder

Encounter for screening for genitourinary disorders

IQ Z13.9 Encounter for screening, unspecified

Genetic carrier and genetic susceptibility to disease (Z14-Z15)

4 Z14 Genetic carrier

5 Z14.0 Hemophilia A carrier

IQ Z14.01 Asymptomatic hemophilia A carrier

IQ Z14.02 Symptomatic hemophilia A carrier

IQ Z14.1 Cystic fibrosis carrier

IQ Z14.8 Genetic carrier of other disease

+ 4 Z15 Genetic susceptibility to disease

> **INCLUDES** confirmed abnormal gene

Use additional code, if applicable, for any associated family history of the disease (Z80-Z84)

> **EXCLUDES 1** chromosomal anomalies (Q90-Q99)

> **GUIDELINES** Section I.C.21.c.3)

Codes from category Z15 should not be used as principal or first-listed codes. If the patient has the condition to which he/she is susceptible, and that condition is the reason for the encounter, the code for the current condition should be sequenced first.

+ 5 Z15.0 Genetic susceptibility to malignant neoplasm

Code first:
, if applicable, any current malignant neoplasm (C00-C75, C81-C96)

Use additional code, if applicable, for any personal history of malignant neoplasm (Z85.-)

> **CODING TIPS ✓** These codes should always be used with prophylactic removal of the particular organ, when documented.

IQ + Z15.01 Genetic susceptibility to malignant neoplasm of breast

> **CODING TIPS ✓** Assign Z15.01 for a patient who has prophylactic breast removal due to genetic susceptibility to breast cancer.

IQ + Z15.02 Genetic susceptibility to malignant neoplasm of ovary

IQ + Z15.03 Genetic susceptibility to malignant neoplasm of prostate

IQ + Z15.04 Genetic susceptibility to malignant neoplasm of endometrium

IQ + Z15.09 Genetic susceptibility to other malignant neoplasm

+ 5 Z15.8 Genetic susceptibility to other disease

IQ + Z15.81 Genetic susceptibility to multiple endocrine neoplasia [MEN]

> **EXCLUDES 1** multiple endocrine neoplasia [MEN] syndromes (E31.2-)

IQ + Z15.89 Genetic susceptibility to other disease

Resistance to antimicrobial drugs (Z16)

CODING TIPS ✓ Assign as many codes from Z16 as necessary to identify all antimicrobial resistance documented.

CODING TIPS ✓ When resistance to antibiotics is documented, add the Z16 codes after the codes that indicate the bacteria causing the sepsis (A40-A41), or other bacterial infections (B95-B96), or the combination codes when the bacteria is included in the code (J15.211). Do not use Z16.11 for MRSA because the resistance to penicillins is already included in the MRSA codes. If the MRSA is also documented as resistant to another antibiotic, such as Vancomycin, a Z16 code is added for the other antibiotic.

4 Z16 Resistance to antimicrobial drugs

Note:
The codes in this category are provided for use as additional codes to identify the resistance and non-responsiveness of a condition to antimicrobial drugs.

Code first:
the infection

> **EXCLUDES 1** Methicillin resistant Staphylococcus aureus infection (A49.02)
> Methicillin resistant Staphylococcus aureus pneumonia (J15.212)
> Sepsis due to Methicillin resistant Staphylococcus aureus (A41.02)

> **GUIDELINES** Section I.C.1.c

Many bacterial infections are resistant to current antibiotics. It is necessary to identify all infections documented as antibiotic resistant. Assign a code from category Z16, Resistance to antimicrobial drugs, following the infection code only if the infection code does not identify drug resistance.

5 Z16.1 Resistance to beta lactam antibiotics

IQ Z16.10 Resistance to unspecified beta lactam antibiotics

IQ Z16.11 Resistance to penicillins

Resistance to amoxicillin
Resistance to ampicillin

> **GUIDELINES** Section I.C.e.1)(a)

When a patient is diagnosed with an infection that is due to methicillin resistant Staphylococcus aureus (MRSA), and that infection has a combination code that includes the causal organism (e.g., sepsis, pneumonia) assign the appropriate combination code for the condition.

Do not assign code B95.62, MRSA infection as the cause of diseases classified elsewhere, as an additional code, because the combination code includes the type of infection and the MRSA organism. Do not assign a code from subcategory Z16.11, Resistance to penicillins, as an additional diagnosis.

IQ Z16.12 Extended spectrum beta lactamase (ESBL) resistance

---

4 4th digit required   **5** 5th digit required   **6** 6th digit required   **7** 7th digit required   **⚄** 7th digit placeholder   **+** Additional code   **⊟** Laterality

EXCLUDES 2   Methicillin resistant
              Staphylococcus aureus
              infection in diseases
              classified elsewhere
              (B95.62)

!Q Z16.19   Resistance to other specified beta lactam antibiotics
Resistance to cephalosporins

⑤ Z16.2   Resistance to other antibiotics

!Q Z16.20   Resistance to unspecified antibiotic
Resistance to antibiotics NOS

!Q Z16.21   Resistance to vancomycin

!Q Z16.22   Resistance to vancomycin related antibiotics

!Q Z16.23   Resistance to quinolones and fluoroquinolones

!Q Z16.24   Resistance to multiple antibiotics

!Q Z16.29   Resistance to other single specified antibiotic
Resistance to aminoglycosides
Resistance to macrolides
Resistance to sulfonamides
Resistance to tetracyclines

⑤ Z16.3   Resistance to other antimicrobial drugs
EXCLUDES 1   resistance to antibiotics
              (Z16.1-, Z16.2-)

!Q Z16.30   Resistance to unspecified antimicrobial drugs
Drug resistance NOS

!Q Z16.31   Resistance to antiparasitic drug(s)
Resistance to quinine and related compounds

!Q Z16.32   Resistance to antifungal drug(s)

!Q Z16.33   Resistance to antiviral drug(s)

⑥ Z16.34   Resistance to antimycobacterial drug(s)
Resistance to tuberculostatics

!Q Z16.341   Resistance to single antimycobacterial drug
Resistance to antimycobacterial drug NOS

!Q Z16.342   Resistance to multiple antimycobacterial drugs

!Q Z16.35   Resistance to multiple antimicrobial drugs
EXCLUDES 1   Resistance to multiple
              antibiotics only
              (Z16.24)

!Q Z16.39   Resistance to other specified antimicrobial drug

Estrogen receptor status   (Z17)

CODING TIPS ✓   When a patient has breast cancer and the estrogen receptor status is specified, the appropriate code from category Z17 should be assigned to indicate the ER positive or negative status. Breast cancers that are ER+ may be treated with selective estrogen receptor modulators (SERMs). When SERM therapy is also present in an ER+ breast cancer patient, an additional Z code may be assigned to identify SERM therapy (Z79.81-).

④ Z17   Estrogen receptor status
Code first:
malignant neoplasm of breast (C50.-)

!Q Z17.0   Estrogen receptor positive status [ER+]

!Q Z17.1   Estrogen receptor negative status [ER-]

Retained foreign body fragments   (Z18)

④ Z18   Retained foreign body fragments
INCLUDES   embedded fragment (status)
            embedded splinter (status)
            retained foreign body status
EXCLUDES 1   artificial joint prosthesis status
              (Z96.6-)
              foreign body accidentally left
              during a procedure (T81.5-)
              foreign body entering through
              orifice (T15-T19)
              in situ cardiac device (Z95.-)
              organ or tissue replaced by
              means other than transplant
              (Z96.-, Z97.-)
              organ or tissue replaced by
              transplant (Z94.-)
              personal history of retained
              foreign body fully removed
              Z87.821
              superficial foreign body
              (non-embedded splinter) -
              code to superficial foreign
              body, by site

⑤ Z18.0   Retained radioactive fragments

!Q Z18.01   Retained depleted uranium fragments

!Q Z18.09   Other retained radioactive fragments
Other retained depleted isotope fragments
Retained nontherapeutic radioactive fragments

⑤ Z18.1   Retained metal fragments
EXCLUDES 1   retained radioactive metal
              fragments
              (Z18.01-Z18.09)

!Q Z18.10   Retained metal fragments, unspecified
Retained metal fragment NOS

!Q Z18.11   Retained magnetic metal fragments

!Q Z18.12   Retained nonmagnetic metal fragments

!Q Z18.2   Retained plastic fragments
Acrylics fragments
Diethylhexyl phthalates fragments
Isocyanate fragments

⑤ Z18.3   Retained organic fragments

!Q Z18.31   Retained animal quills or spines

!Q Z18.32   Retained tooth

!Q Z18.33   Retained wood fragments

!Q Z18.39   Other retained organic fragments

⑤ Z18.8   Other specified retained foreign body

!Q Z18.81   Retained glass fragments

!Q Z18.83   Retained stone or crystalline fragments
Retained concrete or cement fragments

!Q Z18.89   Other specified retained foreign body fragments

!Q Z18.9   Retained foreign body fragments, unspecified material

★ New ▲ Revised Px Primary SP PDGM Px SL Low CoM SH High CoM !Q Quest. Encounter H Hospice non-cancer Dx Unspecified M Manifestation

DecisionHealth's FY 2020 Complete Home Health ICD-10-CM Diagnosis Coding Manual   1889

Hormone sensitivity malignancy status (Z19)

4 Z19   Hormone sensitivity malignancy status
Code first:
  malignant neoplasm - see Table of
  Neoplasms, by site, malignant

!Q Z19.1   Hormone sensitive malignancy status
DEFINITION   Identifies cancers that are known to be hormone dependent and for which the use of hormone therapy drugs in treatment is effective.

!Q Z19.2   Hormone resistant malignancy status
Castrate resistant prostate malignancy status

Persons with potential health hazards related to communicable diseases (Z20-Z29)

4 Z20   Contact with and (suspected) exposure to communicable diseases
EXCLUDES 1   carrier of infectious disease (Z22.-)
  diagnosed current infectious or parasitic disease -see Alphabetic Index
EXCLUDES 2   personal history of infectious and parasitic diseases (Z86.1-)
GUIDELINES   Section I.C.21.c.1)
Category Z20 indicates contact with, and suspected exposure to, communicable diseases. These codes are for patients who do not show any sign or symptom of a disease but are suspected to have been exposed to it by close personal contact with an infected individual or are in an area where a disease is epidemic. Category Z77 indicates contact with and suspected exposures hazardous to health.

Contact/exposure codes may be used as a first-listed code to explain an encounter for testing, or, more commonly, as a secondary code to identify a potential risk.

5 Z20.0   Contact with and (suspected) exposure to intestinal infectious diseases
!Q Z20.01   Contact with and (suspected) exposure to intestinal infectious diseases due to Escherichia coli (E. coli)
!Q Z20.09   Contact with and (suspected) exposure to other intestinal infectious diseases
!Q Z20.1   Contact with and (suspected) exposure to tuberculosis
!Q Z20.2   Contact with and (suspected) exposure to infections with a predominantly sexual mode of transmission
!Q Z20.3   Contact with and (suspected) exposure to rabies
!Q Z20.4   Contact with and (suspected) exposure to rubella
!Q Z20.5   Contact with and (suspected) exposure to viral hepatitis

!Q Z20.6   Contact with and (suspected) exposure to human immunodeficiency virus [HIV]
EXCLUDES 1   asymptomatic human immunodeficiency virus [HIV]
  HIV infection status (Z21)
!Q Z20.7   Contact with and (suspected) exposure to pediculosis, acariasis and other infestations
5 Z20.8   Contact with and (suspected) exposure to other communicable diseases
6 Z20.81   Contact with and (suspected) exposure to other bacterial communicable diseases
!Q Z20.810   Contact with and (suspected) exposure to anthrax
!Q Z20.811   Contact with and (suspected) exposure to meningococcus
!Q Z20.818   Contact with and (suspected) exposure to other bacterial communicable diseases
6 Z20.82   Contact with and (suspected) exposure to other viral communicable diseases
!Q Z20.820   Contact with and (suspected) exposure to varicella
!Q Z20.821   Contact with and (suspected) exposure to Zika virus
!Q Z20.828   Contact with and (suspected) exposure to other viral communicable diseases
!Q Z20.89   Contact with and (suspected) exposure to other communicable diseases
!Q Z20.9   Contact with and (suspected) exposure to unspecified communicable disease

!Q Z21   Asymptomatic human immunodeficiency virus [HIV] infection status
HIV positive NOS
Code first:
  Human immunodeficiency virus [HIV] disease complicating pregnancy, childbirth and the puerperium, if applicable (O98.7-)
EXCLUDES 1   acquired immunodeficiency syndrome (B20)
  contact with human immunodeficiency virus [HIV] (Z20.6)
  exposure to human immunodeficiency virus [HIV] (Z20.6)
  human immunodeficiency virus [HIV] disease (B20)
  inconclusive laboratory evidence of human immunodeficiency virus [HIV] (R75)
GUIDELINES   Patients with asymptomatic HIV infection status admitted (or presenting for a health care encounter) during pregnancy, childbirth, or the puerperium should receive codes of O98.7- and Z21.

---

4 4th digit required   5 5th digit required   6 6th digit required   7 7th digit required   7 7th digit placeholder   + Additional code   ⊟ Laterality

GUIDELINES Section I.C.1.a.2)(f)
Patients with any known prior diagnosis of an HIV-related illness should be coded to B20. Once a patient has developed an HIV-related illness, the patient should always be assigned code B20 on every subsequent admission/encounter. Patients previously diagnosed with any HIV illness (B20) should never be assigned to R75 or Z21, Asymptomatic human immunodeficiency virus [HIV] infection status.

GUIDELINES Section I.C.1.a.2)(d)
Z21, Asymptomatic human immunodeficiency virus [HIV] infection status, is to be applied when the patient without any documentation of symptoms is listed as being "HIV positive," "known HIV," "HIV test positive," or similar terminology. Do not use this code if the term "AIDS" is used or if the patient is treated for any HIV-related illness or is described as having any condition(s) resulting from his/her HIV positive status; use B20 in these cases.

4 **Z22** **Carrier of infectious disease**
  INCLUDES colonization status
    suspected carrier
  EXCLUDES 2 carrier of viral hepatitis (B18.-)

IQ **Z22.0** **Carrier of typhoid**

IQ **Z22.1** **Carrier of other intestinal infectious diseases**

IQ **Z22.2** **Carrier of diphtheria**

5 **Z22.3** **Carrier of other specified bacterial diseases**

IQ **Z22.31** **Carrier of bacterial disease due to meningococci**

6 **Z22.32** **Carrier of bacterial disease due to staphylococci**
  GUIDELINES Section I.C.1.e.1)(c)
  Assign code Z22.322 for patients documented as having MRSA colonization. Assign code Z22.321 for patient documented as having MSSA colonization. Colonization is not necessarily indicative of a disease process or as the cause of a specific condition the patient may have unless documented as such by the provider.

IQ **Z22.321** **Carrier or suspected carrier of Methicillin susceptible Staphylococcus aureus**
  MSSA colonization

IQ **Z22.322** **Carrier or suspected carrier of Methicillin resistant Staphylococcus aureus**
  MRSA colonization
  GUIDELINES Section I.C.1.e.1)(d)
  If a patient is documented as having both MRSA colonization and infection during a hospital admission, code Z22.322 and a code for the MRSA infection may both be assigned.

CODING TIPS ✓ This code should be used when "MRSA screen positive" or "nasal swab positive" is documented. Colonization by MRSA makes teaching a patient/caregiver how to do their own wound dressings more difficult and sometimes impractical.

6 **Z22.33** **Carrier of bacterial disease due to streptococci**

IQ **Z22.330** **Carrier of Group B streptococcus**
  EXCLUDES 1 Carrier of streptococcus group B (GBS) complicating pregnancy, childbirth and the puerperium (O99.82-)

IQ **Z22.338** **Carrier of other streptococcus**

IQ **Z22.39** **Carrier of other specified bacterial diseases**

IQ **Z22.4** **Carrier of infections with a predominantly sexual mode of transmission**

IQ **Z22.6** **Carrier of human T-lymphotropic virus type-1 [HTLV-1] infection**

★ **Z22.7** **Latent tuberculosis**
  Latent tuberculosis infection (LTBI)
  EXCLUDES 1 nonspecific reaction to cell mediated immunity measurement of gamma interferon antigen response without active tuberculosis (R76.12)
    nonspecific reaction to tuberculin skin test without active tuberculosis (R76.11)

  DEFINITION Latent tuberculosis infection (LTBI) occurs when a person is infected with the bacteria Mycobacterium tuberculosis, but does not have active tuberculosis (TB) disease. The only sign of a tuberculosis infection is a positive reaction to the tuberculin skin test or tuberculosis blood test. Compared to active tuberculosis, persons with latent tuberculosis infection are not infectious, cannot spread TB and normally do not develop TB disease. But in persons who have a weak immune system, the bacteria can become active, multiply and cause tuberculosis disease.

IQ **Z22.8** **Carrier of other infectious diseases**

IQ **Z22.9** **Carrier of infectious disease, unspecified**

IQ **Z23** **Encounter for immunization**
  Note:
  procedure codes are required to identify the types of immunizations given
  Code first:
  any routine childhood examination

★ New ▲ Revised **Px** Primary **SP** PDGM Px **SL** Low CoM **SH** High CoM **IQ** Quest. Encounter **H** Hospice non-cancer Dx Unspecified **M** *Manifestation*

Chapter 21

Z00-Z99

GUIDELINES   Section I.C.21.c.2)
Code Z23 is for encounters for inoculations and vaccinations. It indicates that a patient is being seen to receive a prophylactic inoculation against a disease. Procedure codes are required to identify the actual administration of the injection and the type(s) of immunizations given. Code Z23 may be used as a secondary code if the inoculation is given as a routine part of preventive health care, such as a well-baby visit.

4 Z28   Immunization not carried out and underimmunization status
INCLUDES   vaccination not carried out

5 Z28.0   Immunization not carried out because of contraindication

IQ Z28.01   Immunization not carried out because of acute illness of patient

IQ Z28.02   Immunization not carried out because of chronic illness or condition of patient

IQ Z28.03   Immunization not carried out because of immune compromised state of patient

IQ Z28.04   Immunization not carried out because of patient allergy to vaccine or component

IQ Z28.09   Immunization not carried out because of other contraindication

IQ Z28.1   Immunization not carried out because of patient decision for reasons of belief or group pressure
Immunization not carried out because of religious belief

5 Z28.2   Immunization not carried out because of patient decision for other and unspecified reason

IQ Z28.20   Immunization not carried out because of patient decision for unspecified reason

IQ Z28.21   Immunization not carried out because of patient refusal

IQ Z28.29   Immunization not carried out because of patient decision for other reason

IQ Z28.3   Underimmunization status
Delinquent immunization status
Lapsed immunization schedule status

5 Z28.8   Immunization not carried out for other reason

IQ Z28.81   Immunization not carried out due to patient having had the disease

IQ Z28.82   Immunization not carried out because of caregiver refusal
Immunization not carried out because of guardian refusal
Immunization not carried out because of parent refusal
EXCLUDES 1   immunization not carried out because of caregiver refusal because of religious belief (Z28.1)

IQ Z28.83   Immunization not carried out due to unavailability of vaccine
Delay in delivery of vaccine
Lack of availability of vaccine
Manufacturer delay of vaccine

IQ Z28.89   Immunization not carried out for other reason

IQ Z28.9   Immunization not carried out for unspecified reason

4 Z29   Encounter for other prophylactic measures
EXCLUDES 1   desensitization to allergens (Z51.6)
prophylactic surgery (Z40.-)

5 Z29.1   Encounter for prophylactic immunotherapy
Encounter for administration of immunoglobulin

IQ Z29.11   Encounter for prophylactic immunotherapy for respiratory syncytial virus (RSV)

IQ Z29.12   Encounter for prophylactic antivenin

IQ Z29.13   Encounter for prophylactic Rho(D) immune globulin

IQ Z29.14   Encounter for prophylactic rabies immune globin

IQ Z29.3   Encounter for prophylactic fluoride administration

IQ Z29.8   Encounter for other specified prophylactic measures

IQ Z29.9   Encounter for prophylactic measures, unspecified

Persons encountering health services in circumstances related to reproduction (Z30-Z39)

4 Z30   Encounter for contraceptive management

5 Z30.0   Encounter for general counseling and advice on contraception

6 Z30.01   Encounter for initial prescription of contraceptives
EXCLUDES 1   encounter for surveillance of contraceptives (Z30.4-)

IQ Z30.011   Encounter for initial prescription of contraceptive pills

IQ Z30.012   Encounter for prescription of emergency contraception
Encounter for postcoital contraception

IQ Z30.013   Encounter for initial prescription of injectable contraceptive

IQ Z30.014   Encounter for initial prescription of intrauterine contraceptive device
EXCLUDES 1   encounter for insertion of intrauterine contraceptive device (Z30.430, Z30.432)

IQ Z30.015   Encounter for initial prescription of vaginal ring hormonal contraceptive

IQ Z30.016   Encounter for initial prescription of transdermal patch hormonal contraceptive device

IQ Z30.017   Encounter for initial prescription of implantable subdermal contraceptive

IQ Z30.018   Encounter for initial prescription of other contraceptives

4 4th digit required   5 5th digit required   6 6th digit required   7 7th digit required   7 7th digit placeholder   + Additional code   Laterality

1892   *DecisionHealth's* FY 2020 Complete Home Health ICD-10-CM Diagnosis Coding Manual

Encounter for initial prescription of
barrier contraception

Encounter for initial prescription of
diaphragm

IQ Z30.019 **Encounter for initial prescription of contraceptives, unspecified**

IQ Z30.02 **Counseling and instruction in natural family planning to avoid pregnancy**

IQ Z30.09 **Encounter for other general counseling and advice on contraception**

Encounter for family planning advice NOS

IQ Z30.2 **Encounter for sterilization**

S Z30.4 **Encounter for surveillance of contraceptives**

IQ Z30.40 **Encounter for surveillance of contraceptives, unspecified**

IQ Z30.41 **Encounter for surveillance of contraceptive pills**

Encounter for repeat prescription for contraceptive pill

IQ Z30.42 **Encounter for surveillance of injectable contraceptive**

6 Z30.43 **Encounter for surveillance of intrauterine contraceptive device**

IQ Z30.430 **Encounter for insertion of intrauterine contraceptive device**

IQ Z30.431 **Encounter for routine checking of intrauterine contraceptive device**

IQ Z30.432 **Encounter for removal of intrauterine contraceptive device**

IQ Z30.433 **Encounter for removal and reinsertion of intrauterine contraceptive device**

Encounter for replacement of intrauterine contraceptive device

IQ Z30.44 **Encounter for surveillance of vaginal ring hormonal contraceptive device**

IQ Z30.45 **Encounter for surveillance of transdermal patch hormonal contraceptive device**

IQ Z30.46 **Encounter for surveillance of implantable subdermal contraceptive**

Encounter for checking, reinsertion or removal of implantable subdermal contraceptive

IQ Z30.49 **Encounter for surveillance of other contraceptives**

Encounter for surveillance of barrier contraception

Encounter for surveillance of diaphragm

IQ Z30.8 **Encounter for other contraceptive management**

Encounter for postvasectomy sperm count

Encounter for routine examination for contraceptive maintenance

EXCLUDES 1 sperm count following sterilization reversal (Z31.42)

sperm count for fertility testing (Z31.41)

IQ Z30.9 **Encounter for contraceptive management, unspecified**

4 Z31 **Encounter for procreative management**

EXCLUDES 1 complications associated with artificial fertilization (N98.-)

female infertility (N97.-)

male infertility (N46.-)

IQ Z31.0 **Encounter for reversal of previous sterilization**

S Z31.4 **Encounter for procreative investigation and testing**

EXCLUDES 1 postvasectomy sperm count (Z30.8)

IQ Z31.41 **Encounter for fertility testing**

Encounter for fallopian tube patency testing

Encounter for sperm count for fertility testing

IQ Z31.42 **Aftercare following sterilization reversal**

Sperm count following sterilization reversal

+ 6 Z31.43 **Encounter for genetic testing of female for procreative management**

Use additional code for recurrent pregnancy loss, if applicable (N96, O26.2-)

EXCLUDES 1 nonprocreative genetic testing (Z13.7-)

IQ + Z31.430 **Encounter of female for testing for genetic disease carrier status for procreative management**

IQ + Z31.438 **Encounter for other genetic testing of female for procreative management**

6 Z31.44 **Encounter for genetic testing of male for procreative management**

EXCLUDES 1 nonprocreative genetic testing (Z13.7-)

IQ Z31.440 **Encounter of male for testing for genetic disease carrier status for procreative management**

IQ Z31.441 **Encounter for testing of male partner of patient with recurrent pregnancy loss**

IQ Z31.448 **Encounter for other genetic testing of male for procreative management**

IQ Z31.49 **Encounter for other procreative investigation and testing**

IQ Z31.5 **Encounter for procreative genetic counseling**

S Z31.6 **Encounter for general counseling and advice on procreation**

IQ Z31.61 **Procreative counseling and advice using natural family planning**

IQ Z31.62 **Encounter for fertility preservation counseling**

Encounter for fertility preservation counseling prior to cancer therapy

Encounter for fertility preservation counseling prior to surgical removal of gonads

IQ Z31.69 **Encounter for other general counseling and advice on procreation**

IQ Z31.7 **Encounter for procreative management and counseling for gestational carrier**

EXCLUDES 1 pregnant state, gestational carrier (Z33.3)

S Z31.8 **Encounter for other procreative management**

★ New ▲ Revised Px Primary SP PDGM Px SL Low CoM SH High CoM IQ Quest. Encounter H Hospice non-cancer Dx Unspecified M Manifestation

DecisionHealth's FY 2020 Complete Home Health ICD-10-CM Diagnosis Coding Manual

1893

Px **IQ** **Z31.81** **Encounter for male factor infertility in female patient**

Px **IQ** **Z31.82** **Encounter for Rh incompatibility status**

Px **IQ** **✚** **Z31.83** **Encounter for assisted reproductive fertility procedure cycle**
Patient undergoing in vitro fertilization cycle
Use additional code to identify the type of infertility
> **EXCLUDES 1**   pre-cycle diagnosis and testing - code to reason for encounter

Px **IQ** **Z31.84** **Encounter for fertility preservation procedure**
Encounter for fertility preservation procedure prior to cancer therapy
Encounter for fertility preservation procedure prior to surgical removal of gonads

IQ **Z31.89** **Encounter for other procreative management**

IQ **Z31.9** **Encounter for procreative management, unspecified**

4 **Z32** **Encounter for pregnancy test and childbirth and childcare instruction**

5 **Z32.0** **Encounter for pregnancy test**

IQ **Z32.00** **Encounter for pregnancy test, result unknown**
Encounter for pregnancy test NOS

IQ **Z32.01** **Encounter for pregnancy test, result positive**

IQ **Z32.02** **Encounter for pregnancy test, result negative**

IQ **Z32.2** **Encounter for childbirth instruction**

IQ **Z32.3** **Encounter for childcare instruction**
Encounter for prenatal or postpartum childcare instruction

4 **Z33** **Pregnant state**

IQ **Z33.1** **Pregnant state, incidental**
Pregnant state NOS
> **EXCLUDES 1**   complications of pregnancy (O00-O9A)
> pregnant state, gestational carrier (Z33.3)

> **GUIDELINES**   Section I.C.15.a.1)
> Should the provider document that the pregnancy is incidental to the encounter, then code Z33.1 should be used in place of any chapter 15 codes. It is the provider's responsibility to state that the condition being treated is not affecting the pregnancy.

Px **IQ** **Z33.2** **Encounter for elective termination of pregnancy**
> **EXCLUDES 1**   early fetal death with retention of dead fetus (O02.1)
> late fetal death (O36.4)
> spontaneous abortion (O03)

IQ **Z33.3** **Pregnant state, gestational carrier**
> **EXCLUDES 1**   encounter for procreative management and counseling for gestational carrier (Z31.7)

4 **Z34** **Encounter for supervision of normal pregnancy**

> **EXCLUDES 1**   any complication of pregnancy (O00-O9A)
> encounter for pregnancy test (Z32.0-)
> encounter for supervision of high risk pregnancy (O09.-)

5 **Z34.0** **Encounter for supervision of normal first pregnancy**

Px **IQ** **Z34.00** **Encounter for supervision of normal first pregnancy, unspecified trimester**

Px **IQ** **Z34.01** **Encounter for supervision of normal first pregnancy, first trimester**

Px **IQ** **Z34.02** **Encounter for supervision of normal first pregnancy, second trimester**

Px **IQ** **Z34.03** **Encounter for supervision of normal first pregnancy, third trimester**

5 **Z34.8** **Encounter for supervision of other normal pregnancy**

Px **IQ** **Z34.80** **Encounter for supervision of other normal pregnancy, unspecified trimester**

Px **IQ** **Z34.81** **Encounter for supervision of other normal pregnancy, first trimester**

Px **IQ** **Z34.82** **Encounter for supervision of other normal pregnancy, second trimester**

Px **IQ** **Z34.83** **Encounter for supervision of other normal pregnancy, third trimester**

5 **Z34.9** **Encounter for supervision of normal pregnancy, unspecified**

Px **IQ** **Z34.90** **Encounter for supervision of normal pregnancy, unspecified, unspecified trimester**

Px **IQ** **Z34.91** **Encounter for supervision of normal pregnancy, unspecified, first trimester**

Px **IQ** **Z34.92** **Encounter for supervision of normal pregnancy, unspecified, second trimester**

Px **IQ** **Z34.93** **Encounter for supervision of normal pregnancy, unspecified, third trimester**

4 **Z36** **Encounter for antenatal screening of mother**
> **INCLUDES**   Encounter for placental sample (taken vaginally)
> Screening is the testing for disease or disease precursors in asymptomatic individuals so that early detection and treatment can be provided for those who test positive for the disease.
> **EXCLUDES 1**   diagnostic examination- code to sign or symptom
> encounter for suspected maternal and fetal conditions ruled out (Z03.7-)
> suspected fetal condition affecting management of pregnancy - code to condition in Chapter 15
> **EXCLUDES 2**   abnormal findings on antenatal screening of mother (O28.-)
> genetic counseling and testing (Z31.43-, Z31.5)
> routine prenatal care (Z34)

---

4 4th digit required   **5** 5th digit required   **6** 6th digit required   **7** 7th digit required   **7** 7th digit placeholder   ✚ Additional code   **⊟** Laterality

1894   *DecisionHealth's* FY 2020 Complete Home Health ICD-10-CM Diagnosis Coding Manual

IQ Z36.0 Encounter for antenatal screening for chromosomal anomalies

IQ Z36.1 Encounter for antenatal screening for raised alphafetoprotein level

Encounter for antenatal screening for elevated maternal serum alphafetoprotein level

IQ Z36.2 Encounter for other antenatal screening follow-up

Non-visualized anatomy on a previous scan

IQ Z36.3 Encounter for antenatal screening for malformations

Screening for a suspected anomaly

IQ Z36.4 Encounter for antenatal screening for fetal growth retardation

Intrauterine growth restriction (IUGR)/small-for-dates

IQ Z36.5 Encounter for antenatal screening for isoimmunization

5 Z36.8 Encounter for other antenatal screening

IQ Z36.81 Encounter for antenatal screening for hydrops fetalis

IQ Z36.82 Encounter for antenatal screening for nuchal translucency

IQ Z36.83 Encounter for fetal screening for congenital cardiac abnormalities

IQ Z36.84 Encounter for antenatal screening for fetal lung maturity

IQ Z36.85 Encounter for antenatal screening for Streptococcus B

IQ Z36.86 Encounter for antenatal screening for cervical length

Screening for risk of pre-term labor

IQ Z36.87 Encounter for antenatal screening for uncertain dates

IQ Z36.88 Encounter for antenatal screening for fetal macrosomia

Screening for large-for-dates

IQ Z36.89 Encounter for other specified antenatal screening

IQ Z36.8A Encounter for antenatal screening for other genetic defects

IQ Z36.9 Encounter for antenatal screening, unspecified

4 Z3A Weeks of gestation

Note:

Codes from category Z3A are for use, only on the maternal record, to indicate the weeks of gestation of the pregnancy, if known.

Code first:

complications of pregnancy, childbirth and the puerperium (O09-O9A)

5 Z3A.0 Weeks of gestation of pregnancy, unspecified or less than 10 weeks

IQ Z3A.00 Weeks of gestation of pregnancy not specified

IQ Z3A.01 Less than 8 weeks gestation of pregnancy

IQ Z3A.08 8 weeks gestation of pregnancy

IQ Z3A.09 9 weeks gestation of pregnancy

5 Z3A.1 Weeks of gestation of pregnancy, weeks 10-19

IQ Z3A.10 10 weeks gestation of pregnancy

IQ Z3A.11 11 weeks gestation of pregnancy

IQ Z3A.12 12 weeks gestation of pregnancy

IQ Z3A.13 13 weeks gestation of pregnancy

IQ Z3A.14 14 weeks gestation of pregnancy

IQ Z3A.15 15 weeks gestation of pregnancy

IQ Z3A.16 16 weeks gestation of pregnancy

IQ Z3A.17 17 weeks gestation of pregnancy

IQ Z3A.18 18 weeks gestation of pregnancy

IQ Z3A.19 19 weeks gestation of pregnancy

5 Z3A.2 Weeks of gestation of pregnancy, weeks 20-29

IQ Z3A.20 20 weeks gestation of pregnancy

IQ Z3A.21 21 weeks gestation of pregnancy

IQ Z3A.22 22 weeks gestation of pregnancy

IQ Z3A.23 23 weeks gestation of pregnancy

IQ Z3A.24 24 weeks gestation of pregnancy

IQ Z3A.25 25 weeks gestation of pregnancy

IQ Z3A.26 26 weeks gestation of pregnancy

IQ Z3A.27 27 weeks gestation of pregnancy

IQ Z3A.28 28 weeks gestation of pregnancy

IQ Z3A.29 29 weeks gestation of pregnancy

5 Z3A.3 Weeks of gestation of pregnancy, weeks 30-39

IQ Z3A.30 30 weeks gestation of pregnancy

IQ Z3A.31 31 weeks gestation of pregnancy

IQ Z3A.32 32 weeks gestation of pregnancy

IQ Z3A.33 33 weeks gestation of pregnancy

IQ Z3A.34 34 weeks gestation of pregnancy

IQ Z3A.35 35 weeks gestation of pregnancy

IQ Z3A.36 36 weeks gestation of pregnancy

IQ Z3A.37 37 weeks gestation of pregnancy

IQ Z3A.38 38 weeks gestation of pregnancy

IQ Z3A.39 39 weeks gestation of pregnancy

5 Z3A.4 Weeks of gestation of pregnancy, weeks 40 or greater

IQ Z3A.40 40 weeks gestation of pregnancy

IQ Z3A.41 41 weeks gestation of pregnancy

IQ Z3A.42 42 weeks gestation of pregnancy

IQ Z3A.49 Greater than 42 weeks gestation of pregnancy

4 Z37 Outcome of delivery

This category is intended for use as an additional code to identify the outcome of delivery on the mother's record. It is not for use on the newborn record.

EXCLUDES 1 stillbirth (P95)

IQ Z37.0 Single live birth

IQ Z37.1 Single stillbirth

IQ Z37.2 Twins, both liveborn

IQ Z37.3 Twins, one liveborn and one stillborn

IQ Z37.4 Twins, both stillborn

5 Z37.5 Other multiple births, all liveborn

IQ Z37.50 Multiple births, unspecified, all liveborn

IQ Z37.51 Triplets, all liveborn

IQ Z37.52 Quadruplets, all liveborn

IQ Z37.53 Quintuplets, all liveborn

IQ Z37.54 Sextuplets, all liveborn

IQ Z37.59 Other multiple births, all liveborn

5 Z37.6 Other multiple births, some liveborn

★ New ▲ Revised **Px** Primary **SP** PDGM Px **SL** Low CoM **SH** High CoM **IQ** Quest. Encounter **H** Hospice non-cancer Dx Unspecified **M** *Manifestation*

DecisionHealth's FY 2020 Complete Home Health ICD-10-CM Diagnosis Coding Manual

1895

IQ Z37.60 **Multiple births, unspecified, some liveborn**

IQ Z37.61 **Triplets, some liveborn**

IQ Z37.62 **Quadruplets, some liveborn**

IQ Z37.63 **Quintuplets, some liveborn**

IQ Z37.64 **Sextuplets, some liveborn**

IQ Z37.69 **Other multiple births, some liveborn**

IQ Z37.7 **Other multiple births, all stillborn**

IQ Z37.9 **Outcome of delivery, unspecified**
Multiple birth NOS
Single birth NOS

4 Z38 **Liveborn infants according to place of birth and type of delivery**
This category is for use as the principal code on the initial record of a newborn baby. It is to be used for the initial birth record only. It is not to be used on the mother's record.

5 Z38.0 **Single liveborn infant, born in hospital**
Single liveborn infant, born in birthing center or other health care facility

Px IQ Z38.00 **Single liveborn infant, delivered vaginally**

Px IQ Z38.01 **Single liveborn infant, delivered by cesarean**

Px IQ Z38.1 **Single liveborn infant, born outside hospital**

Px IQ Z38.2 **Single liveborn infant, unspecified as to place of birth**
Single liveborn infant NOS

5 Z38.3 **Twin liveborn infant, born in hospital**

Px IQ Z38.30 **Twin liveborn infant, delivered vaginally**

Px IQ Z38.31 **Twin liveborn infant, delivered by cesarean**

Px IQ Z38.4 **Twin liveborn infant, born outside hospital**

Px IQ Z38.5 **Twin liveborn infant, unspecified as to place of birth**

5 Z38.6 **Other multiple liveborn infant, born in hospital**

Px IQ Z38.61 **Triplet liveborn infant, delivered vaginally**

Px IQ Z38.62 **Triplet liveborn infant, delivered by cesarean**

Px IQ Z38.63 **Quadruplet liveborn infant, delivered vaginally**

Px IQ Z38.64 **Quadruplet liveborn infant, delivered by cesarean**

Px IQ Z38.65 **Quintuplet liveborn infant, delivered vaginally**

Px IQ Z38.66 **Quintuplet liveborn infant, delivered by cesarean**

Px IQ Z38.68 **Other multiple liveborn infant, delivered vaginally**

Px IQ Z38.69 **Other multiple liveborn infant, delivered by cesarean**

Px IQ Z38.7 **Other multiple liveborn infant, born outside hospital**

Px IQ Z38.8 **Other multiple liveborn infant, unspecified as to place of birth**

4 Z39 **Encounter for maternal postpartum care and examination**

Px IQ Z39.0 **Encounter for care and examination of mother immediately after delivery**
Care and observation in uncomplicated cases when the delivery occurs outside a healthcare facility
EXCLUDES 1 care for postpartum complication- see Alphabetic index

Px IQ Z39.1 **Encounter for care and examination of lactating mother**
Encounter for supervision of lactation
EXCLUDES 1 disorders of lactation (O92.-)

Px IQ Z39.2 **Encounter for routine postpartum follow-up**

Encounters for other specific health care (Z40-Z53)

Categories Z40-Z53 are intended for use to indicate a reason for care. They may be used for patients who have already been treated for a disease or injury, but who are receiving aftercare or prophylactic care, or care to consolidate the treatment, or to deal with a residual state
EXCLUDES 2 follow-up examination for medical surveillance after treatment (Z08-Z09)

4 Z40 **Encounter for prophylactic surgery**
EXCLUDES 1 organ donations (Z52.-) therapeutic organ removal-code to condition

+ 5 Z40.0 **Encounter for prophylactic surgery for risk factors related to malignant neoplasms**
Admission for prophylactic organ removal
Use additional code to identify risk factor

Px IQ + Z40.00 **Encounter for prophylactic removal of unspecified organ**

Px IQ + Z40.01 **Encounter for prophylactic removal of breast**

Px IQ + Z40.02 **Encounter for prophylactic removal of ovary(s)**
Encounter for prophylactic removal of ovary(s) and fallopian tube(s)

IQ + Z40.03 **Encounter for prophylactic removal of fallopian tube(s)**

Px IQ + Z40.09 **Encounter for prophylactic removal of other organ**

Px IQ Z40.8 **Encounter for other prophylactic surgery**

Px IQ Z40.9 **Encounter for prophylactic surgery, unspecified**

4 Z41 **Encounter for procedures for purposes other than remedying health state**

IQ Z41.1 **Encounter for cosmetic surgery**
Encounter for cosmetic breast implant
Encounter for cosmetic procedure
EXCLUDES 1 encounter for plastic and reconstructive surgery following medical procedure or healed injury (Z42.-)
encounter for post-mastectomy breast implantation (Z42.1)

IQ Z41.2 **Encounter for routine and ritual male circumcision**

IQ Z41.3 **Encounter for ear piercing**

IQ Z41.8 **Encounter for other procedures for purposes other than remedying health state**

---

4 4th digit required   **5** 5th digit required   **6** 6th digit required   **7** 7th digit required   **7** 7th digit placeholder   **+** Additional code   **5** Laterality

IQ Z41.9 **Encounter for procedure for purposes other than remedying health state, unspecified**

4 Z42 **Encounter for plastic and reconstructive surgery following medical procedure or healed injury**

> **EXCLUDES 1** encounter for cosmetic plastic surgery (Z41.1)
> encounter for plastic surgery for treatment of current injury - code to relevent injury

Px IQ Z42.1 **Encounter for breast reconstruction following mastectomy**

> **EXCLUDES 1** deformity and disproportion of reconstructed breast (N65.1-)

Px IQ Z42.8 **Encounter for other plastic and reconstructive surgery following medical procedure or healed injury**

4 Z43 **Encounter for attention to artificial openings**

> **INCLUDES** closure of artificial openings
> passage of sounds or bougies through artificial openings
> reforming artificial openings
> removal of catheter from artificial openings
> toilet or cleansing of artificial openings
> **EXCLUDES 1** complications of external stoma (J95.0-, K94.-, N99.5-)
> **EXCLUDES 2** fitting and adjustment of prosthetic and other devices (Z44-Z46)

> **CODING TIPS ✓** Assign codes from category Z43 when the agency is providing active care/intervention to the artificial opening. If the opening has been reversed, codes from category Z43 are no longer applicable since the patient no longer has the ostomy. If the patient is seen for wound care following closure, assign a code from category Z48. If the ostomy is allowed to close on its own, the Z43 codes are appropriate for any care provided.
> Do not use codes in the Z43 category with status ostomy codes (Z93) for the same ostomy or when the ostomy is complicated.

> **CODING TIPS ✓** When assigning a code from Z43 for an encounter for attention to artificial openings, such as a tracheostomy or cystostomy, the plan of care should include interventions for the treatment of the artificial opening.

SP Z43.0 **Encounter for attention to tracheostomy**

SP Z43.1 **Encounter for attention to gastrostomy**

> **EXCLUDES 2** artificial opening status only, without need for care (Z93.-)

SP Z43.2 **Encounter for attention to ileostomy**

SP Z43.3 **Encounter for attention to colostomy**

SP Z43.4 **Encounter for attention to other artificial openings of digestive tract**

SP Z43.5 **Encounter for attention to cystostomy**

SP Z43.6 **Encounter for attention to other artificial openings of urinary tract**
Encounter for attention to nephrostomy
Encounter for attention to ureterostomy
Encounter for attention to urethrostomy

SP Z43.7 **Encounter for attention to artificial vagina**

SP Z43.8 **Encounter for attention to other artificial openings**

IQ Z43.9 **Encounter for attention to unspecified artificial opening**

4 Z44 **Encounter for fitting and adjustment of external prosthetic device**

> **INCLUDES** removal or replacement of external prosthetic device
> **EXCLUDES 1** malfunction or other complications of device - see Alphabetical Index
> presence of prosthetic device (Z97.-)

5 Z44.0 **Encounter for fitting and adjustment of artificial arm**

> **6 Z44.00** **Encounter for fitting and adjustment of unspecified artificial arm**

IQ Z44.001 **Encounter for fitting and adjustment of unspecified right artificial arm**

IQ Z44.002 **Encounter for fitting and adjustment of unspecified left artificial arm**

IQ Z44.009 **Encounter for fitting and adjustment of unspecified artificial arm, unspecified arm**

> **6 Z44.01** **Encounter for fitting and adjustment of complete artificial arm**

IQ Z44.011 **Encounter for fitting and adjustment of complete right artificial arm**

IQ Z44.012 **Encounter for fitting and adjustment of complete left artificial arm**

IQ Z44.019 **Encounter for fitting and adjustment of complete artificial arm, unspecified arm**

> **6 Z44.02** **Encounter for fitting and adjustment of partial artificial arm**

IQ Z44.021 **Encounter for fitting and adjustment of partial artificial right arm**

IQ Z44.022 **Encounter for fitting and adjustment of partial artificial left arm**

IQ Z44.029 **Encounter for fitting and adjustment of partial artificial arm, unspecified arm**

5 Z44.1 **Encounter for fitting and adjustment of artificial leg**

> **6 Z44.10** **Encounter for fitting and adjustment of unspecified artificial leg**

IQ Z44.101 **Encounter for fitting and adjustment of unspecified right artificial leg**

IQ Z44.102 **Encounter for fitting and adjustment of unspecified left artificial leg**

IQ Z44.109 **Encounter for fitting and adjustment of unspecified artificial leg, unspecified leg**

★ New ▲ Revised Px Primary SP PDGM Px SL Low CoM SH High CoM IQ Quest. Encounter H Hospice non-cancer Dx Unspecified M Manifestation

DecisionHealth's FY 2020 Complete Home Health ICD-10-CM Diagnosis Coding Manual

1897

Chapter 21

Z00-Z99

6 **Z44.11 Encounter for fitting and adjustment of complete artificial leg**

⊟ IQ **Z44.111 Encounter for fitting and adjustment of complete right artificial leg**

⊟ IQ **Z44.112 Encounter for fitting and adjustment of complete left artificial leg**

⊟ IQ **Z44.119 Encounter for fitting and adjustment of complete artificial leg, unspecified leg**

6 **Z44.12 Encounter for fitting and adjustment of partial artificial leg**

⊟ IQ **Z44.121 Encounter for fitting and adjustment of partial artificial right leg**

⊟ IQ **Z44.122 Encounter for fitting and adjustment of partial artificial left leg**

⊟ IQ **Z44.129 Encounter for fitting and adjustment of partial artificial leg, unspecified leg**

5 **Z44.2 Encounter for fitting and adjustment of artificial eye**

> **EXCLUDES 1** mechanical complication of ocular prosthesis (T85.3)

⊟ IQ **Z44.20 Encounter for fitting and adjustment of artificial eye, unspecified**

⊟ IQ **Z44.21 Encounter for fitting and adjustment of artificial right eye**

⊟ IQ **Z44.22 Encounter for fitting and adjustment of artificial left eye**

5 **Z44.3 Encounter for fitting and adjustment of external breast prosthesis**

> **EXCLUDES 1** complications of breast implant (T85.4-)
> encounter for adjustment or removal of breast implant (Z45.81-)
> encounter for initial breast implant insertion for cosmetic breast augmentation (Z41.1)
> encounter for breast reconstruction following mastectomy (Z42.1)

⊟ IQ **Z44.30 Encounter for fitting and adjustment of external breast prosthesis, unspecified breast**

⊟ IQ **Z44.31 Encounter for fitting and adjustment of external right breast prosthesis**

⊟ IQ **Z44.32 Encounter for fitting and adjustment of external left breast prosthesis**

IQ **Z44.8 Encounter for fitting and adjustment of other external prosthetic devices**

IQ **Z44.9 Encounter for fitting and adjustment of unspecified external prosthetic device**

4 **Z45 Encounter for adjustment and management of implanted device**

> **INCLUDES** removal or replacement of implanted device
> **EXCLUDES 1** malfunction or other complications of device - see Alphabetical Index
> **EXCLUDES 2** encounter for fitting and adjustment of non-implanted device (Z46.-)

5 **Z45.0 Encounter for adjustment and management of cardiac device**

6 **Z45.01 Encounter for adjustment and management of cardiac pacemaker**
Encounter for adjustment and management of cardiac resynchronization therapy pacemaker (CRT-P)

> **EXCLUDES 1** encounter for adjustment and management of automatic implantable cardiac defibrillator with synchronous cardiac pacemaker (Z45.02)

> **CODING TIPS** ✓ See Z95.0 for presence of cardiac pacemaker.

IQ **Z45.010 Encounter for checking and testing of cardiac pacemaker pulse generator [battery]**
Encounter for replacing cardiac pacemaker pulse generator [battery]

▲ IQ **Z45.018 Encounter for adjustment and management of other part of cardiac pacemaker**

> **EXCLUDES 1** presence of other part of cardiac pacemaker (Z95.0)
> **EXCLUDES 2** presence of prosthetic and other devices (Z95.1-Z95.5, Z95.811-Z97)

IQ **Z45.02 Encounter for adjustment and management of automatic implantable cardiac defibrillator**
Encounter for adjustment and management of automatic implantable cardiac defibrillator with synchronous cardiac pacemaker
Encounter for adjustment and management of cardiac resynchronization therapy defibrillator (CRT-D)

IQ **Z45.09 Encounter for adjustment and management of other cardiac device**

IQ **Z45.1 Encounter for adjustment and management of infusion pump**

> **CODING TIPS** ✓ See also Z46.81, which may be more appropriate to the care being provided.

SP **Z45.2 Encounter for adjustment and management of vascular access device**
Encounter for adjustment and management of vascular catheters

> **EXCLUDES 1** encounter for adjustment and management of renal dialysis catheter (Z49.01)

> **CODING TIPS** ✓ This code is used for routine care of vascular access devices, including peripheral, PICC and central lines. Do not use this code if the line is complicated. See T80 for complications.

5 **Z45.3 Encounter for adjustment and management of implanted devices of the special senses**

---

4 4th digit required   5 5th digit required   6 6th digit required   7 7th digit required   ☑ 7th digit placeholder   ✛ Additional code   ⊟ Laterality

IQ Z45.31   Encounter for adjustment and management of implanted visual substitution device

6 Z45.32   Encounter for adjustment and management of implanted hearing device

> **EXCLUDES 1**   Encounter for fitting and adjustment of hearing aide (Z46.1)

IQ Z45.320   Encounter for adjustment and management of bone conduction device

IQ Z45.321   Encounter for adjustment and management of cochlear device

IQ Z45.328   Encounter for adjustment and management of other implanted hearing device

5 Z45.4   Encounter for adjustment and management of implanted nervous system device

IQ Z45.41   Encounter for adjustment and management of cerebrospinal fluid drainage device

Encounter for adjustment and management of cerebral ventricular (communicating) shunt

▲ IQ Z45.42   Encounter for adjustment and management of neurostimulator

Encounter for adjustment and management of brain neurostimulator

Encounter for adjustment and management of gastric neurostimulator

Encounter for adjustment and management of peripheral nerve neurostimulator

Encounter for adjustment and management of sacral nerve neurostimulator

Encounter for adjustment and management of spinal cord neurostimulator

Encounter for adjustment and management of vagus nerve neurostimulator

IQ Z45.49   Encounter for adjustment and management of other implanted nervous system device

5 Z45.8   Encounter for adjustment and management of other implanted devices

▲ 6 Z45.81   Encounter for adjustment or removal of breast implant

Encounter for elective implant exchange (different material) (different size)

Encounter removal of tissue expander with or without synchronous insertion of permanent implant

> **EXCLUDES 1**   complications of breast implant (T85.4-)
> encounter for initial breast implant insertion for cosmetic breast augmentation (Z41.1)
> encounter for breast reconstruction following mastectomy (Z42.1)

⊟ IQ Z45.811   Encounter for adjustment or removal of right breast implant

⊟ IQ Z45.812   Encounter for adjustment or removal of left breast implant

⊟ IQ Z45.819   Encounter for adjustment or removal of unspecified breast implant

IQ Z45.82   Encounter for adjustment or removal of myringotomy device (stent) (tube)

IQ Z45.89   Encounter for adjustment and management of other implanted devices

IQ Z45.9   Encounter for adjustment and management of unspecified implanted device

4 Z46   Encounter for fitting and adjustment of other devices

> **INCLUDES**   removal or replacement of other device
> **EXCLUDES 1**   malfunction or other complications of device - see Alphabetical Index
> **EXCLUDES 2**   encounter for fitting and management of implanted devices (Z45.-)
> issue of repeat prescription only (Z76.0)
> presence of prosthetic and other devices (Z95-Z97)

IQ Z46.0   Encounter for fitting and adjustment of spectacles and contact lenses

IQ Z46.1   Encounter for fitting and adjustment of hearing aid

> **EXCLUDES 1**   encounter for adjustment and management of implanted hearing device (Z45.32-)

IQ Z46.2   Encounter for fitting and adjustment of other devices related to nervous system and special senses

> **EXCLUDES 2**   encounter for adjustment and management of implanted nervous system device (Z45.4-)
> encounter for adjustment and management of implanted visual substitution device (Z45.31)

IQ Z46.3   Encounter for fitting and adjustment of dental prosthetic device

Encounter for fitting and adjustment of dentures

IQ Z46.4   Encounter for fitting and adjustment of orthodontic device

5 Z46.5   Encounter for fitting and adjustment of other gastrointestinal appliance and device

> **EXCLUDES 1**   encounter for attention to artificial openings of digestive tract (Z43.1-Z43.4)

IQ Z46.51   Encounter for fitting and adjustment of gastric lap band

IQ Z46.59   Encounter for fitting and adjustment of other gastrointestinal appliance and device

SP Z46.6   Encounter for fitting and adjustment of urinary device

---

★ New ▲ Revised Px Primary SP PDGM Px SL Low CoM SH High CoM IQ Quest. Encounter H Hospice non-cancer Dx   Unspecified   M *Manifestation*

DecisionHealth's FY 2020 Complete Home Health ICD-10-CM Diagnosis Coding Manual   1899

EXCLUDES 2 attention to artificial openings of urinary tract (Z43.5, Z43.6)

CODING TIPS ✓ Complications of urinary catheters should be coded to complications, such as T83.0.

CODING TIPS ✓ Code Z46.6 includes removal and intermittent catheterization as well as indwelling catheter care.

⑤ Z46.8 Encounter for fitting and adjustment of other specified devices

IQ Z46.81 Encounter for fitting and adjustment of insulin pump
Encounter for insulin pump instruction and training
Encounter for insulin pump titration

IQ Z46.82 Encounter for fitting and adjustment of non-vascular catheter
CODING TIPS ✓ Non-vascular catheters include subcutaneous infusions, intrathecal infusions, epidural infusions and even NG tubes. Urinary catheters are not included.

IQ Z46.89 Encounter for fitting and adjustment of other specified devices
Encounter for fitting and adjustment of wheelchair

IQ Z46.9 Encounter for fitting and adjustment of unspecified device

④ Z47 Orthopedic aftercare
EXCLUDES 1 aftercare for healing fracture- code to fracture with 7th character D
CODING TIPS ✓ Do not use Z47 codes for surgery for injuries, including fractures. Use the injury code with D as the 7th character.

SP ✛ Z47.1 Aftercare following joint replacement surgery
Use additional code to identify the joint (Z96.6-)
CODING TIPS ✓ Do NOT use Z47.1 for fractures, even if the fracture was treated with a joint replacement. Code the fracture with 7th character D and the appropriate Z96.6- code to indicate the presence of the joint prosthesis.

IQ Z47.2 Encounter for removal of internal fixation device
EXCLUDES 1 encounter for adjustment of internal fixation device for fracture treatment- code to fracture with appropriate 7th character
encounter for removal of external fixation device- code to fracture with 7th character D
infection or inflammatory reaction to internal fixation device (T84.6-)
mechanical complication of internal fixation device (T84.1-)

CODING TIPS ✓ Pay close attention to the Excludes 1 note. Most instances for removal of an internal fixation device are for complications or actual treatment, like an infection. Z47.2 will most often be used for the physician encounter.

⑤ Z47.3 Aftercare following explantation of joint prosthesis
Aftercare following explantation of joint prosthesis, staged procedure
Encounter for joint prosthesis insertion following prior explantation of joint prosthesis
CODING TIPS ✓ Pay close attention to the Excludes 1 note. Most instances for removal of an internal prosthesis are for complications or actual treatment of the fracture. If a mechanical complication has been repaired, continue to code the complication with a D until healed. This code is meant for a staged procedure and is appropriate for a new prosthesis once an infection has resolved.

CODING TIPS ✓ If the joint prosthesis was removed and not replaced, code M96.89 provides additional information regarding instability of the joint, if documented.

SP Z47.31 Aftercare following explantation of shoulder joint prosthesis
EXCLUDES 1 acquired absence of shoulder joint following prior explantation of shoulder joint prosthesis (Z89.23-)
shoulder joint prosthesis explantation status (Z89.23-)

SP Z47.32 Aftercare following explantation of hip joint prosthesis
EXCLUDES 1 acquired absence of hip joint following prior explantation of hip joint prosthesis (Z89.62-)
hip joint prosthesis explantation status (Z89.62-)

SP Z47.33 Aftercare following explantation of knee joint prosthesis
EXCLUDES 1 acquired absence of knee joint following prior explantation of knee prosthesis ()
knee joint prosthesis explantation status (Z89.52-)

⑤ Z47.8 Encounter for other orthopedic aftercare

SP ✛ Z47.81 Encounter for orthopedic aftercare following surgical amputation
Use additional code to identify the limb amputated (Z89.-)
CODING TIPS ✓ If amputation was performed because of a diabetic foot ulcer, use an additional code to indicate the history of diabetic ulcer (Z86.31).

---

④ 4th digit required   ⑤ 5th digit required   ⑥ 6th digit required   ⑦ 7th digit required   ⑦ 7th digit placeholder   ✛ Additional code   ▤ Laterality

CODING TIPS ✓ This code is only used for planned amputations. Do not assign Z47.81 for care following a traumatic amputation or when a surgical amputation is complicated by infection, dehiscence, or other complication.

SP **Z47.82** **Encounter for orthopedic aftercare following scoliosis surgery**

CODING TIPS ✓ If the condition treated by surgery is coded with a M41 code, this aftercare code is correct.

SP **Z47.89** **Encounter for other orthopedic aftercare**

CODING TIPS ✓ Do not use this code for fracture repair. Code the fracture with 7th character D. Do not use this code for trauma to the musculoskeletal system. Use the appropriate trauma code with 7th character D.

CODING TIPS ✓ This code is the best choice for aftercare following musculoskeletal surgery that does not fit into any of the other Z47 codes, such as lumbar fusion or rotator cuff repair resulting from disuse. It is not to be used for aftercare for musculoskeletal injuries. Injuries should continue to be coded with the injury with 7th character D to indicate a healing/resolving injury.

4 **Z48** **Encounter for other postprocedural aftercare**

EXCLUDES 1 encounter for follow-up examination after completed treatment (Z08-Z09)
encounter for aftercare following injury - code to Injury, by site, with appropriate 7th character for subsequent encounter

EXCLUDES 2 encounter for attention to artificial openings (Z43.-)
encounter for fitting and adjustment of prosthetic and other devices (Z44-Z46)

CODING TIPS ✓ Do not use Z48 codes for surgery for injuries. Use the injury code with D as the 7th character.

5 **Z48.0** **Encounter for attention to dressings, sutures and drains**

EXCLUDES 1 encounter for planned postprocedural wound closure (Z48.1)

CODING TIPS ✓ Do not use dressing change codes for complicated wounds. The dressing change should not be primary in home health or hospice. Consider the wound itself or the aftercare following surgery code as the first code.

SP **Z48.00** **Encounter for change or removal of nonsurgical wound dressing**
Encounter for change or removal of wound dressing NOS

SP **Z48.01** **Encounter for change or removal of surgical wound dressing**

SP **Z48.02** **Encounter for removal of sutures**
Encounter for removal of staples

SP **Z48.03** **Encounter for change or removal of drains**

IQ **Z48.1** **Encounter for planned postprocedural wound closure**

EXCLUDES 1 encounter for attention to dressings and sutures (Z48.0-)

5 **Z48.2** **Encounter for aftercare following organ transplant**

CODING TIPS ✓ These aftercare following organ transplant codes do not require a second status code for the organ transplanted. To indicate the status of a transplanted organ, see Z94. If the transplant is documented as complicated (failure, rejection, etc.) then use T86 codes instead.

SP **Z48.21** **Encounter for aftercare following heart transplant**

SP **Z48.22** **Encounter for aftercare following kidney transplant**

SP **Z48.23** **Encounter for aftercare following liver transplant**

SP **Z48.24** **Encounter for aftercare following lung transplant**

6 **Z48.28** **Encounter for aftercare following multiple organ transplant**

SP **Z48.280** **Encounter for aftercare following heart-lung transplant**

SP **Z48.288** **Encounter for aftercare following multiple organ transplant**

6 **Z48.29** **Encounter for aftercare following other organ transplant**

SP **Z48.290** **Encounter for aftercare following bone marrow transplant**

SP **Z48.298** **Encounter for aftercare following other organ transplant**

SP **+** **Z48.3** **Aftercare following surgery for neoplasm**
Use additional code to identify the neoplasm

CODING TIPS ✓ When coding Z48.3, an additional code should be assigned to identify the neoplasm. If it is unclear if the neoplasm has been eradicated or if there are plans to continue treatment for the neoplastic disease, assign the appropriate code from Chapter 2 to indicate the neoplasm. If documentation clearly indicates that the neoplasm has been eradicated, assign the appropriate Z85 or Z86 code to report personal history of neoplasm.

5 **Z48.8** **Encounter for other specified postprocedural aftercare**

6 **Z48.81** **Encounter for surgical aftercare following surgery on specified body systems**
These codes identify the body system requiring aftercare. They are for use in conjunction with other aftercare codes to fully explain the aftercare encounter. The condition treated should also be coded if still present.

EXCLUDES 1 aftercare for injury- code the injury with 7th character D

★ New ▲ Revised **Px** Primary **SP** PDGM Px **SL** Low CoM **SH** High CoM **IQ** Quest. Encounter **H** Hospice non-cancer Dx **Unspecified** **M** *Manifestation*

DecisionHealth's FY 2020 Complete Home Health ICD-10-CM Diagnosis Coding Manual

1901

aftercare following surgery for neoplasm (Z48.3)

EXCLUDES 2 aftercare following organ transplant (Z48.2-) orthopedic aftercare (Z47.-)

CODING TIPS ✓ Use an additional code to indicate the dressing change, if applicable. Status codes may be useful to indicate more fully the post-operative status. Also consider the use of Z90 codes to indicate acquired absence of a body part or organ. Do not use aftercare codes for complications that have been repaired or are resolving. Use the complication code with 7th character D.

SP Z48.810 Encounter for surgical aftercare following surgery on the sense organs

CODING TIPS ✓ Use this aftercare code for pre-operative conditions coded with H codes.

SP Z48.811 Encounter for surgical aftercare following surgery on the nervous system

EXCLUDES 2 encounter for surgical aftercare following surgery on the sense organs (Z48.810)

CODING TIPS ✓ Use this aftercare code for pre-operative conditions coded with G codes.

SP Z48.812 Encounter for surgical aftercare following surgery on the circulatory system

CODING TIPS ✓ Use this aftercare code for pre-operative conditions coded with I codes.

SP Z48.813 Encounter for surgical aftercare following surgery on the respiratory system

CODING TIPS ✓ Use this aftercare code for pre-operative conditions coded with J codes.

IQ Z48.814 Encounter for surgical aftercare following surgery on the teeth or oral cavity

SP Z48.815 Encounter for surgical aftercare following surgery on the digestive system

CODING TIPS ✓ Use this aftercare code for pre-operative conditions coded with K codes.

SP Z48.816 Encounter for surgical aftercare following surgery on the genitourinary system

EXCLUDES 1 encounter for aftercare following sterilization reversal (Z31.42)

CODING TIPS ✓ Use this aftercare code for pre-operative conditions coded with N codes.

SP Z48.817 Encounter for surgical aftercare following surgery on the skin and subcutaneous tissue

CODING TIPS ✓ Use this aftercare code for pre-operative conditions coded with L codes.

IQ Z48.89 Encounter for other specified surgical aftercare

4 Z49 Encounter for care involving renal dialysis

Code also:
associated end stage renal disease (N18.6)

CODING TIPS ✓ These codes are not appropriate for home care or hospice. This care would be considered duplication of services in home health.

5 Z49.0 Preparatory care for renal dialysis

Encounter for dialysis instruction and training

IQ Z49.01 Encounter for fitting and adjustment of extracorporeal dialysis catheter

Removal or replacement of renal dialysis catheter
Toilet or cleansing of renal dialysis catheter

IQ Z49.02 Encounter for fitting and adjustment of peritoneal dialysis catheter

5 Z49.3 Encounter for adequacy testing for dialysis

IQ Z49.31 Encounter for adequacy testing for hemodialysis

IQ Z49.32 Encounter for adequacy testing for peritoneal dialysis

Encounter for peritoneal equilibration test

4 Z51 Encounter for other aftercare and medical care

Code also:
condition requiring care

EXCLUDES 1 follow-up examination after treatment (Z08-Z09)

GUIDELINES Section I.C.2.e.2)

If a patient admission/encounter is solely for the administration of chemotherapy, immunotherapy or external beam radiation therapy, assign code Z51.0, Encounter for antineoplastic radiation therapy, or Z51.11, Encounter for antineoplastic chemotherapy, or Z51.12, Encounter for antineoplastic immunotherapy as the first-listed or principal diagnosis.

The malignancy for which the therapy is being administered should be assigned as a secondary diagnosis.

If a patient admission/encounter is for the insertion or implantation of radioactive elements (e.g., brachytherapy) the appropriate code for the malignancy is sequenced as the principal or first-listed diagnosis. Code Z51.0 should not be assigned.

CODING TIPS ✓ Only the provider administering the radiation, chemotherapy or immunotherapy may assign a code from category Z51 to report encounter for radiation, chemotherapy, or immunotherapy.

Px IQ Z51.0 Encounter for antineoplastic radiation therapy

---

4 4th digit required   5 5th digit required   6 6th digit required   7 7th digit required   ✓ 7th digit placeholder   ✚ Additional code   ▣ Laterality

1902   *DecisionHealth's* FY 2020 Complete Home Health ICD-10-CM Diagnosis Coding Manual

GUIDELINES Section I.C.2.e.3)

When a patient is admitted for the purpose of external beam radiotherapy, immunotherapy or chemotherapy and develops complications such as uncontrolled nausea and vomiting or dehydration, the principal or first-listed diagnosis is Z51.0 or Z51.11 or Z51.12, followed by any codes for the complications.

CODING TIPS ✓ This code is primary only and should only be used if home care or hospice is actually administering the therapy.

S Z51.1 Encounter for antineoplastic chemotherapy and immunotherapy

EXCLUDES 2 encounter for chemotherapy and immunotherapy for nonneoplastic condition - code to condition

Px SP Z51.11 Encounter for antineoplastic chemotherapy

CODING TIPS ✓ This code is primary only and should only be used if home care or hospice is actually administering the therapy.

Px SP Z51.12 Encounter for antineoplastic immunotherapy

CODING TIPS ✓ This code is primary only and should only be used if home care or hospice is actually administering the therapy.

SP Z51.5 Encounter for palliative care

CODING TIPS ✓ This code is appropriate for hospice, end of life care and palliative care as a secondary code.

IQ Z51.6 Encounter for desensitization to allergens

S Z51.8 Encounter for other specified aftercare

EXCLUDES 1 holiday relief care (Z75.5)

IQ Z51.81 Encounter for therapeutic drug level monitoring

Code also:
any long-term (current) drug therapy (Z79.-)

EXCLUDES 1 encounter for blood-drug test for administrative or medicolegal reasons (Z02.83)

CODING TIPS ✓ This code is associated with venipuncture and should only be used if monitoring drug levels. Use a code from Z79 to indicate the drug monitored.

IQ Z51.89 Encounter for other specified aftercare

CODING TIPS ✓ This is not the code for admission for therapy. Assign the appropriate code for the condition for which rehabilitation services are being provided.

4 Z52 Donors of organs and tissues

INCLUDES autologous and other living donors

EXCLUDES 1 cadaveric donor - omit code

examination of potential donor (Z00.5)

5 Z52.0 Blood donor

6 Z52.00 Unspecified blood donor

Px IQ Z52.000 Unspecified donor, whole blood

Px IQ Z52.001 Unspecified donor, stem cells

Px IQ Z52.008 Unspecified donor, other blood

6 Z52.01 Autologous blood donor

Px IQ Z52.010 Autologous donor, whole blood

Px IQ Z52.011 Autologous donor, stem cells

Px IQ Z52.018 Autologous donor, other blood

6 Z52.09 Other blood donor
Volunteer donor

Px IQ Z52.090 Other blood donor, whole blood

Px IQ Z52.091 Other blood donor, stem cells

Px IQ Z52.098 Other blood donor, other blood

5 Z52.1 Skin donor

Px IQ Z52.10 Skin donor, unspecified

Px IQ Z52.11 Skin donor, autologous

Px IQ Z52.19 Skin donor, other

5 Z52.2 Bone donor

Px IQ Z52.20 Bone donor, unspecified

Px IQ Z52.21 Bone donor, autologous

Px IQ Z52.29 Bone donor, other

Px IQ Z52.3 Bone marrow donor

Px IQ Z52.4 Kidney donor

Px IQ Z52.5 Cornea donor

Px IQ Z52.6 Liver donor

5 Z52.8 Donor of other specified organs or tissues

6 Z52.81 Egg (Oocyte) donor

Px IQ Z52.810 Egg (Oocyte) donor under age 35, anonymous recipient
Egg donor under age 35 NOS

Px IQ Z52.811 Egg (Oocyte) donor under age 35, designated recipient

Px IQ Z52.812 Egg (Oocyte) donor age 35 and over, anonymous recipient
Egg donor age 35 and over NOS

Px IQ Z52.813 Egg (Oocyte) donor age 35 and over, designated recipient

Px IQ Z52.819 Egg (Oocyte) donor, unspecified

Px IQ Z52.89 Donor of other specified organs or tissues

IQ Z52.9 Donor of unspecified organ or tissue
Donor NOS

4 Z53 Persons encountering health services for specific procedures and treatment, not carried out

5 Z53.0 Procedure and treatment not carried out because of contraindication

IQ Z53.01 Procedure and treatment not carried out due to patient smoking

IQ Z53.09 Procedure and treatment not carried out because of other contraindication

IQ Z53.1 Procedure and treatment not carried out because of patient's decision for reasons of belief and group pressure

5 Z53.2 Procedure and treatment not carried out because of patient's decision for other and unspecified reasons

---

★ New ▲ Revised Px Primary SP PDGM Px SL Low CoM SH High CoM IQ Quest. Encounter H Hospice non-cancer Dx Unspecified M Manifestation

DecisionHealth's FY 2020 Complete Home Health ICD-10-CM Diagnosis Coding Manual

1903

IQ Z53.20 Procedure and treatment not carried out because of patient's decision for unspecified reasons

IQ Z53.21 Procedure and treatment not carried out due to patient leaving prior to being seen by health care provider

IQ Z53.29 Procedure and treatment not carried out because of patient's decision for other reasons

5 Z53.3 Procedure converted to open procedure

IQ Z53.31 Laparoscopic surgical procedure converted to open procedure

IQ Z53.32 Thoracoscopic surgical procedure converted to open procedure

IQ Z53.33 Arthroscopic surgical procedure converted to open procedure

IQ Z53.39 Other specified procedure converted to open procedure

IQ Z53.8 Procedure and treatment not carried out for other reasons

IQ Z53.9 Procedure and treatment not carried out, unspecified reason

Persons with potential health hazards related to socioeconomic and psychosocial circumstances (Z55-Z65)

4 Z55 Problems related to education and literacy
> EXCLUDES 1 disorders of psychological development (F80-F89)

IQ Z55.0 Illiteracy and low-level literacy

IQ Z55.1 Schooling unavailable and unattainable

IQ Z55.2 Failed school examinations

IQ Z55.3 Underachievement in school

IQ Z55.4 Educational maladjustment and discord with teachers and classmates

IQ Z55.8 Other problems related to education and literacy
> Problems related to inadequate teaching

IQ Z55.9 Problems related to education and literacy, unspecified
> Academic problems NOS

4 Z56 Problems related to employment and unemployment
> EXCLUDES 2 occupational exposure to risk factors (Z57.-)
> problems related to housing and economic circumstances (Z59.-)

IQ Z56.0 Unemployment, unspecified

IQ Z56.1 Change of job

IQ Z56.2 Threat of job loss

IQ Z56.3 Stressful work schedule

IQ Z56.4 Discord with boss and workmates

IQ Z56.5 Uncongenial work environment
> Difficult conditions at work

IQ Z56.6 Other physical and mental strain related to work

5 Z56.8 Other problems related to employment

IQ Z56.81 Sexual harassment on the job

IQ Z56.82 Military deployment status

> Individual (civilian or military) currently deployed in theater or in support of military war, peacekeeping and humanitarian operations

IQ Z56.89 Other problems related to employment

IQ Z56.9 Unspecified problems related to employment
> Occupational problems NOS

4 Z57 Occupational exposure to risk factors

IQ Z57.0 Occupational exposure to noise

IQ Z57.1 Occupational exposure to radiation

IQ Z57.2 Occupational exposure to dust

5 Z57.3 Occupational exposure to other air contaminants

IQ Z57.31 Occupational exposure to environmental tobacco smoke
> EXCLUDES 2 exposure to environmental tobacco smoke (Z77.22)

IQ Z57.39 Occupational exposure to other air contaminants

IQ Z57.4 Occupational exposure to toxic agents in agriculture
> Occupational exposure to solids, liquids, gases or vapors in agriculture

IQ Z57.5 Occupational exposure to toxic agents in other industries
> Occupational exposure to solids, liquids, gases or vapors in other industries

IQ Z57.6 Occupational exposure to extreme temperature

IQ Z57.7 Occupational exposure to vibration

IQ Z57.8 Occupational exposure to other risk factors

IQ Z57.9 Occupational exposure to unspecified risk factor

4 Z59 Problems related to housing and economic circumstances
> EXCLUDES 2 problems related to upbringing (Z62.-)

IQ Z59.0 Homelessness

IQ Z59.1 Inadequate housing
> Lack of heating
> Restriction of space
> Technical defects in home preventing adequate care
> Unsatisfactory surroundings
> EXCLUDES 1 problems related to the natural and physical environment (Z77.1-)

IQ Z59.2 Discord with neighbors, lodgers and landlord

IQ Z59.3 Problems related to living in residential institution
> Boarding-school resident
> EXCLUDES 1 institutional upbringing (Z62.2)

IQ Z59.4 Lack of adequate food and safe drinking water
> Inadequate drinking water supply
> EXCLUDES 1 effects of hunger (T73.0)
> inappropriate diet or eating habits (Z72.4)
> malnutrition (E40-E46)

IQ Z59.5 Extreme poverty

4 4th digit required **5** 5th digit required **6** 6th digit required **7** 7th digit required **7** 7th digit placeholder **+** Additional code **⊟** Laterality

1904

DecisionHealth's FY 2020 Complete Home Health ICD-10-CM Diagnosis Coding Manual

IQ Z59.6 Low income

IQ Z59.7 Insufficient social insurance and welfare support

IQ Z59.8 Other problems related to housing and economic circumstances
Foreclosure on loan
Isolated dwelling
Problems with creditors

IQ Z59.9 Problem related to housing and economic circumstances, unspecified

4 Z60 Problems related to social environment

IQ Z60.0 Problems of adjustment to life-cycle transitions
Empty nest syndrome
Phase of life problem
Problem with adjustment to retirement [pension]

IQ Z60.2 Problems related to living alone

IQ Z60.3 Acculturation difficulty
Problem with migration
Problem with social transplantation

IQ Z60.4 Social exclusion and rejection
Exclusion and rejection on the basis of personal characteristics, such as unusual physical appearance, illness or behavior.
EXCLUDES 1 target of adverse discrimination such as for racial or religious reasons (Z60.5)

IQ Z60.5 Target of (perceived) adverse discrimination and persecution
EXCLUDES 1 social exclusion and rejection (Z60.4)

IQ Z60.8 Other problems related to social environment

IQ Z60.9 Problem related to social environment, unspecified

4 Z62 Problems related to upbringing
INCLUDES current and past negative life events in childhood
current and past problems of a child related to upbringing
EXCLUDES 2 maltreatment syndrome (T74.-)
problems related to housing and economic circumstances (Z59.-)

IQ Z62.0 Inadequate parental supervision and control

IQ Z62.1 Parental overprotection

5 Z62.2 Upbringing away from parents
EXCLUDES 1 problems with boarding school (Z59.3)

IQ Z62.21 Child in welfare custody
Child in care of non-parental family member
Child in foster care
EXCLUDES 2 problem for parent due to child in welfare custody (Z63.5)

IQ Z62.22 Institutional upbringing
Child living in orphanage or group home

IQ Z62.29 Other upbringing away from parents

IQ Z62.3 Hostility towards and scapegoating of child

IQ Z62.6 Inappropriate (excessive) parental pressure

5 Z62.8 Other specified problems related to upbringing

6 Z62.81 Personal history of abuse in childhood

IQ Z62.810 Personal history of physical and sexual abuse in childhood
EXCLUDES 1 current child physical abuse (T74.12, T76.12)
current child sexual abuse (T74.22, T76.22)

IQ Z62.811 Personal history of psychological abuse in childhood
EXCLUDES 1 current child psychological abuse (T74.32, T76.32)

IQ Z62.812 Personal history of neglect in childhood
EXCLUDES 1 current child neglect (T74.02, T76.02)

IQ Z62.813 Personal history of forced labor or sexual exploitation in childhood

IQ Z62.819 Personal history of unspecified abuse in childhood
EXCLUDES 1 current child abuse NOS (T74.92, T76.92)

6 Z62.82 Parent-child conflict

IQ Z62.820 Parent-biological child conflict
Parent-child problem NOS

IQ Z62.821 Parent-adopted child conflict

IQ Z62.822 Parent-foster child conflict

6 Z62.89 Other specified problems related to upbringing

IQ Z62.890 Parent-child estrangement NEC

IQ Z62.891 Sibling rivalry

IQ Z62.898 Other specified problems related to upbringing

IQ Z62.9 Problem related to upbringing, unspecified

4 Z63 Other problems related to primary support group, including family circumstances
EXCLUDES 2 maltreatment syndrome (T74.-, T76)
parent-child problems (Z62.-)
problems related to negative life events in childhood (Z62.-)
problems related to upbringing (Z62.-)

IQ Z63.0 Problems in relationship with spouse or partner
Relationship distress with spouse or intimate partner
EXCLUDES 1 counseling for spousal or partner abuse problems (Z69.1)
counseling related to sexual attitude, behavior, and orientation (Z70.-)

IQ Z63.1 Problems in relationship with in-laws

5 Z63.3 Absence of family member
EXCLUDES 1 absence of family member due to disappearance and death (Z63.4)

⋆ New ▲ Revised Px Primary SP PDGM Px SL Low CoM SH High CoM IQ Quest. Encounter H Hospice non-cancer Dx Unspecified M Manifestation

DecisionHealth's FY 2020 Complete Home Health ICD-10-CM Diagnosis Coding Manual   1905

absence of family member
due to separation and
divorce (Z63.5)

IQ Z63.31 Absence of family member due to military deployment
Individual or family affected by other family member being on military deployment
EXCLUDES 1 family disruption due to return of family member from military deployment (Z63.71)

IQ Z63.32 Other absence of family member

IQ Z63.4 Disappearance and death of family member
Assumed death of family member
Bereavement

IQ Z63.5 Disruption of family by separation and divorce
Marital estrangement

IQ Z63.6 Dependent relative needing care at home

5 Z63.7 Other stressful life events affecting family and household

IQ Z63.71 Stress on family due to return of family member from military deployment
Individual or family affected by family member having returned from military deployment (current or past conflict)

IQ Z63.72 Alcoholism and drug addiction in family

IQ Z63.79 Other stressful life events affecting family and household
Anxiety (normal) about sick person in family
Health problems within family
Ill or disturbed family member
Isolated family

IQ Z63.8 Other specified problems related to primary support group
Family discord NOS
Family estrangement NOS
High expressed emotional level within family
Inadequate family support NOS
Inadequate or distorted communication within family

IQ Z63.9 Problem related to primary support group, unspecified
Relationship disorder NOS

4 Z64 Problems related to certain psychosocial circumstances

IQ Z64.0 Problems related to unwanted pregnancy

IQ Z64.1 Problems related to multiparity

IQ Z64.4 Discord with counselors
Discord with probation officer
Discord with social worker

4 Z65 Problems related to other psychosocial circumstances

IQ Z65.0 Conviction in civil and criminal proceedings without imprisonment

IQ Z65.1 Imprisonment and other incarceration

IQ Z65.2 Problems related to release from prison

IQ Z65.3 Problems related to other legal circumstances

Arrest
Child custody or support proceedings
Litigation
Prosecution

IQ Z65.4 Victim of crime and terrorism
Victim of torture

IQ Z65.5 Exposure to disaster, war and other hostilities
EXCLUDES 1 target of perceived discrimination or persecution (Z60.5)

IQ Z65.8 Other specified problems related to psychosocial circumstances
Religious or spiritual problem

IQ Z65.9 Problem related to unspecified psychosocial circumstances

Do not resuscitate status   (Z66)

IQ Z66 Do not resuscitate
DNR status
CODING TIPS ✓ The use of this code requires a physician's order for Do Not Resuscitate (DNR).

Blood type   (Z67)

4 Z67 Blood type

5 Z67.1 Type A blood

IQ Z67.10 Type A blood, Rh positive

IQ Z67.11 Type A blood, Rh negative

5 Z67.2 Type B blood

IQ Z67.20 Type B blood, Rh positive

IQ Z67.21 Type B blood, Rh negative

5 Z67.3 Type AB blood

IQ Z67.30 Type AB blood, Rh positive

IQ Z67.31 Type AB blood, Rh negative

5 Z67.4 Type O blood

IQ Z67.40 Type O blood, Rh positive

IQ Z67.41 Type O blood, Rh negative

5 Z67.9 Unspecified blood type

IQ Z67.90 Unspecified blood type, Rh positive

IQ Z67.91 Unspecified blood type, Rh negative

Body mass index [BMI]   (Z68)

CODING TIPS ✓ BMI may not be coded without an associated diagnosis from the physician, e.g., overweight, obesity, morbid obesity, or low weight diagnoses. Physician documentation indicating that condition as a diagnosis is required. If suspected, but not present, the coder may query the provider to obtain confirmation of the condition, but may not code obesity without confirmation from the provider. BMI may be calculated and documented based upon nursing documentation(height and weight used to calculate), however the BMI may only be coded if a physician-provided diagnosis, such as overweight, obesity, underweight is coded.

▲ 4 Z68 Body mass index [BMI]
Kilograms per meters squared
Note:
BMI adult codes are for use for persons 20 years of age or older
BMI pediatric codes are for use for persons 2-19 years of age.

4 4th digit required   **5** 5th digit required   **6** 6th digit required   **7** 7th digit required   **7** 7th digit placeholder   **+** Additional code   **⊟** Laterality

1906   *DecisionHealth's* FY 2020 Complete Home Health ICD-10-CM Diagnosis Coding Manual

These percentiles are based on the growth charts published by the Centers for Disease Control and Prevention (CDC)

CODING TIPS ✓ BMI adult codes are for use in persons 20 years of age or older. Pediatric BMI codes (Z68.5-) are for use in persons aged 2-19 years of age. Percentiles are based on growth charts published by the CDC.

IQ Z68.1 Body mass index (BMI) 19.9 or less, adult

S Z68.2 Body mass index (BMI) 20-29, adult

IQ Z68.20 Body mass index (BMI) 20.0-20.9, adult

IQ Z68.21 Body mass index (BMI) 21.0-21.9, adult

IQ Z68.22 Body mass index (BMI) 22.0-22.9, adult

IQ Z68.23 Body mass index (BMI) 23.0-23.9, adult

IQ Z68.24 Body mass index (BMI) 24.0-24.9, adult

IQ Z68.25 Body mass index (BMI) 25.0-25.9, adult

IQ Z68.26 Body mass index (BMI) 26.0-26.9, adult

IQ Z68.27 Body mass index (BMI) 27.0-27.9, adult

IQ Z68.28 Body mass index (BMI) 28.0-28.9, adult

IQ Z68.29 Body mass index (BMI) 29.0-29.9, adult

S Z68.3 Body mass index (BMI) 30-39, adult

IQ Z68.30 Body mass index (BMI) 30.0-30.9, adult

IQ Z68.31 Body mass index (BMI) 31.0-31.9, adult

IQ Z68.32 Body mass index (BMI) 32.0-32.9, adult

IQ Z68.33 Body mass index (BMI) 33.0-33.9, adult

IQ Z68.34 Body mass index (BMI) 34.0-34.9, adult

IQ Z68.35 Body mass index (BMI) 35.0-35.9, adult

IQ Z68.36 Body mass index (BMI) 36.0-36.9, adult

IQ Z68.37 Body mass index (BMI) 37.0-37.9, adult

IQ Z68.38 Body mass index (BMI) 38.0-38.9, adult

IQ Z68.39 Body mass index (BMI) 39.0-39.9, adult

S Z68.4 Body mass index (BMI) 40 or greater, adult

IQ Z68.41 Body mass index (BMI) 40.0-44.9, adult

IQ Z68.42 Body mass index (BMI) 45.0-49.9, adult

▲ IQ Z68.43 Body mass index (BMI) 50.0-59.9, adult

IQ Z68.44 Body mass index (BMI) 60.0-69.9, adult

IQ Z68.45 Body mass index (BMI) 70 or greater, adult

S Z68.5 Body mass index (BMI) pediatric

IQ Z68.51 Body mass index (BMI) pediatric, less than 5th percentile for age

IQ Z68.52 Body mass index (BMI) pediatric, 5th percentile to less than 85th percentile for age

IQ Z68.53 Body mass index (BMI) pediatric, 85th percentile to less than 95th percentile for age

IQ Z68.54 Body mass index (BMI) pediatric, greater than or equal to 95th percentile for age

Persons encountering health services in other circumstances (Z69-Z76)

4 Z69 Encounter for mental health services for victim and perpetrator of abuse
INCLUDES counseling for victims and perpetrators of abuse

S Z69.0 Encounter for mental health services for child abuse problems

6 Z69.01 Encounter for mental health services for parental child abuse

IQ Z69.010 Encounter for mental health services for victim of parental child abuse
Encounter for mental health services for victim of child abuse by parent
Encounter for mental health services for victim of child neglect by parent
Encounter for mental health services for victim of child psychological abuse by parent
Encounter for mental health services for victim of child sexual abuse by parent

IQ Z69.011 Encounter for mental health services for perpetrator of parental child abuse
Encounter for mental health services for perpetrator of parental child neglect
Encounter for mental health services for perpetrator of parental child psychological abuse
Encounter for mental health services for perpetrator of parental child sexual abuse
EXCLUDES 1 encounter for mental health services for non-parental child abuse (Z69.02-)

6 Z69.02 Encounter for mental health services for non-parental child abuse

IQ Z69.020 Encounter for mental health services for victim of non-parental child abuse
Encounter for mental health services for victim of non-parental child neglect
Encounter for mental health services for victim of non-parental child psychological abuse
Encounter for mental health services for victim of non-parental child sexual abuse

IQ Z69.021 Encounter for mental health services for perpetrator of non-parental child abuse

★ New ▲ Revised Px Primary SP PDGM Px SL Low CoM SH High CoM IQ Quest. Encounter H Hospice non-cancer Dx Unspecified M Manifestation

DecisionHealth's FY 2020 Complete Home Health ICD-10-CM Diagnosis Coding Manual

1907

Encounter for mental health services
for perpetrator of non-parental
child neglect
Encounter for mental health services
for perpetrator of non-parental
child psychological abuse
Encounter for mental health services
for perpetrator of non-parental
child sexual abuse

⑤ Z69.1 Encounter for mental health services for spousal or partner abuse problems

🔲 Z69.11 Encounter for mental health services for victim of spousal or partner abuse
Encounter for mental health services
for victim of spouse or partner
neglect
Encounter for mental health services
for victim of spouse or partner
psychological abuse
Encounter for mental health services
for victim of spouse or partner
violence, physical

🔲 Z69.12 Encounter for mental health services for perpetrator of spousal or partner abuse
Encounter for mental health services
for perpetrator of spouse or partner
neglect
Encounter for mental health services
for perpetrator of spouse or partner
psychological abuse
Encounter for mental health services
for perpetrator of spouse or partner
violence, physical
Encounter for mental health services
for perpetrator of spouse or partner
violence, sexual

⑤ Z69.8 Encounter for mental health services for victim or perpetrator of other abuse

▲ 🔲 Z69.81 Encounter for mental health services for victim of other abuse
Encounter for mental health services
for victim of non-spousal adult abuse
Encounter for mental health services
for victim of spouse or partner
violence, sexual
Encounter for rape victim counseling

▲ 🔲 Z69.82 Encounter for mental health services for perpetrator of other abuse
Encounter for mental health services
for perpetrator of non-spousal adult
abuse

④ Z70 Counseling related to sexual attitude, behavior and orientation
> INCLUDES encounter for mental health
> services for sexual attitude,
> behavior and orientation
> EXCLUDES 2 contraceptive or procreative
> counseling (Z30-Z31)

🔲 Z70.0 Counseling related to sexual attitude

🔲 Z70.1 Counseling related to patient's sexual behavior and orientation
Patient concerned regarding impotence
Patient concerned regarding non-
responsiveness
Patient concerned regarding promiscuity
Patient concerned regarding sexual
orientation

🔲 Z70.2 Counseling related to sexual behavior and orientation of third party
Advice sought regarding sexual behavior
and orientation of child
Advice sought regarding sexual behavior
and orientation of partner
Advice sought regarding sexual behavior
and orientation of spouse

🔲 Z70.3 Counseling related to combined concerns regarding sexual attitude, behavior and orientation

🔲 Z70.8 Other sex counseling
Encounter for sex education

🔲 Z70.9 Sex counseling, unspecified

④ Z71 Persons encountering health services for other counseling and medical advice, not elsewhere classified
> EXCLUDES 2 contraceptive or procreation
> counseling (Z30-Z31)
> sex counseling (Z70.-)

🔲 Z71.0 Person encountering health services to consult on behalf of another person
Person encountering health services to
seek advice or treatment for non-
attending third party
> EXCLUDES 2 anxiety (normal) about sick
> person in family (Z63.7)
> expectant (adoptive)
> parent(s) pre-birth
> pediatrician visit (Z76.81)

🔲 Z71.1 Person with feared health complaint in whom no diagnosis is made
Person encountering health services with
feared condition which was not
demonstrated
Person encountering health services in
which problem was normal state
'Worried well'
> EXCLUDES 1 medical observation for
> suspected diseases and
> conditions proven not to
> exist (Z03.-)

🔲 Z71.2 Person consulting for explanation of examination or test findings

🔲 ✚ Z71.3 Dietary counseling and surveillance
Use additional code for any associated
underlying medical condition
Use additional code to identify body mass
index (BMI), if known (Z68.-)

✚ ⑤ Z71.4 Alcohol abuse counseling and surveillance
Use additional code for alcohol abuse or
dependence (F10.-)

🔲 ✚ Z71.41 Alcohol abuse counseling and surveillance of alcoholic

🔲 ✚ Z71.42 Counseling for family member of alcoholic
Counseling for significant other,
partner, or friend of alcoholic

✚ ⑤ Z71.5 Drug abuse counseling and surveillance
Use additional code for drug abuse or
dependence (F11-F16, F18-F19)

🔲 ✚ Z71.51 Drug abuse counseling and surveillance of drug abuser

🔲 ✚ Z71.52 Counseling for family member of drug abuser
Counseling for significant other,
partner, or friend of drug abuser

④4th digit required **⑤**5th digit required **⑥**6th digit required **⑦**7th digit required **☑**7th digit placeholder **✚**Additional code **⑤**Laterality

1908 *DecisionHealth's* FY 2020 Complete Home Health ICD-10-CM Diagnosis Coding Manual

!Q ✚ Z71.6 Tobacco abuse counseling
Use additional code for nicotine
dependence (F17.-)

!Q Z71.7 Human immunodeficiency virus [HIV] counseling

⑤ Z71.8 Other specified counseling
> EXCLUDES 2   counseling for contraception
> (Z30.0-)

!Q Z71.81 Spiritual or religious counseling

!Q Z71.82 Exercise counseling

!Q Z71.83 Encounter for nonprocreative genetic counseling
> EXCLUDES 1   counseling for
> procreative genetics
> (Z31.5)
> counseling for
> procreative
> management (Z31.6)

★ Z71.84 Encounter for health counseling related to travel
Encounter for health risk and safety
counseling for (international) travel
Code also:
, if applicable, encounter for
immunization (Z23)
> EXCLUDES 2   encounter for
> administrative
> examination (Z02.-)
> encounter for other
> special examination
> without complaint,
> suspected or reported
> diagnosis (Z01.-)

!Q Z71.89 Other specified counseling

!Q Z71.9 Counseling, unspecified
Encounter for medical advice NOS

④ Z72 Problems related to lifestyle
> EXCLUDES 2   problems related to life-
> management difficulty
> (Z73.-)
> problems related to
> socioeconomic and
> psychosocial circumstances
> (Z55-Z65)

> CODING TIPS ✓   These codes should be
> assigned only when the documentation
> specifies that the patient has an associated
> problem.

!Q Z72.0 Tobacco use
Tobacco use NOS
> EXCLUDES 1   history of tobacco
> dependence (Z87.891)
> nicotine dependence
> (F17.2-)
> tobacco dependence
> (F17.2-)
> tobacco use during
> pregnancy (O99.33-)

> CODING TIPS ✓   If the physician documents
> "smoker," use code F17.2- instead.

!Q Z72.3 Lack of physical exercise

!Q Z72.4 Inappropriate diet and eating habits
> EXCLUDES 1   behavioral eating disorders
> of infancy or childhood
> (F98.2.-F98.3)
> eating disorders (F50.-)

lack of adequate food
(Z59.4)
malnutrition and other
nutritional deficiencies
(E40-E64)

⑤ Z72.5 High risk sexual behavior
Promiscuity
> EXCLUDES 1   paraphilias (F65)

!Q Z72.51 High risk heterosexual behavior

!Q Z72.52 High risk homosexual behavior

!Q Z72.53 High risk bisexual behavior

!Q Z72.6 Gambling and betting
> EXCLUDES 1   compulsive or pathological
> gambling (F63.0)

⑤ Z72.8 Other problems related to lifestyle

⑥ Z72.81 Antisocial behavior
> EXCLUDES 1   conduct disorders
> (F91.-)

!Q Z72.810 Child and adolescent antisocial behavior
Antisocial behavior (child)
(adolescent) without manifest
psychiatric disorder
Delinquency NOS
Group delinquency
Offenses in the context of gang
membership
Stealing in company with others
Truancy from school

!Q Z72.811 Adult antisocial behavior
Adult antisocial behavior without
manifest psychiatric disorder

⑥ Z72.82 Problems related to sleep

!Q Z72.820 Sleep deprivation
Lack of adequate sleep
> EXCLUDES 1   insomnia (G47.0-)

!Q Z72.821 Inadequate sleep hygiene
Bad sleep habits
Irregular sleep habits
Unhealthy sleep wake schedule
> EXCLUDES 1   insomnia
> (F51.0-, G47.0-)

!Q Z72.89 Other problems related to lifestyle
Self-damaging behavior

!Q Z72.9 Problem related to lifestyle, unspecified

④ Z73 Problems related to life management difficulty
> EXCLUDES 2   problems related to
> socioeconomic and
> psychosocial circumstances
> (Z55-Z65)

!Q Z73.0 Burn-out

!Q Z73.1 Type A behavior pattern

!Q Z73.2 Lack of relaxation and leisure

!Q Z73.3 Stress, not elsewhere classified
Physical and mental strain NOS
> EXCLUDES 1   stress related to employment
> or unemployment (Z56.-)

!Q Z73.4 Inadequate social skills, not elsewhere classified

!Q Z73.5 Social role conflict, not elsewhere classified

!Q Z73.6 Limitation of activities due to disability
> EXCLUDES 1   care-provider dependency
> (Z74.-)

★ New ▲ Revised Px Primary   SP PDGM Px   SL Low CoM   SH High CoM   !Q Quest. Encounter   H Hospice non-cancer Dx   Unspecified   M Manifestation

DecisionHealth's FY 2020 Complete Home Health ICD-10-CM Diagnosis Coding Manual   1909

Chapter 21

Z00-Z99

⑤ **Z73.8** **Other problems related to life management difficulty**

⑥ **Z73.81** **Behavioral insomnia of childhood**

IQ Z73.810 **Behavioral insomnia of childhood, sleep-onset association type**

IQ Z73.811 **Behavioral insomnia of childhood, limit setting type**

IQ Z73.812 **Behavioral insomnia of childhood, combined type**

IQ Z73.819 **Behavioral insomnia of childhood, unspecified type**

IQ Z73.82 **Dual sensory impairment**

IQ Z73.89 **Other problems related to life management difficulty**

IQ Z73.9 **Problem related to life management difficulty, unspecified**

④ **Z74** **Problems related to care provider dependency**

EXCLUDES 2   dependence on enabling machines or devices NEC (Z99.-)

CODING TIPS ✓   These codes are useful to explain the circumstances of the patient and/or the caregiver to assist in explanation of the need for skilled care.

⑤ **Z74.0** **Reduced mobility**

CODING TIPS ✓   These codes are useful to explain reduced mobility for hospice prognosis purposes as well as homebound for home health patients.

IQ Z74.01 **Bed confinement status**
Bedridden

IQ Z74.09 **Other reduced mobility**
Chairridden
Reduced mobility NOS
EXCLUDES 2   wheelchair dependence (Z99.3)

IQ Z74.1 **Need for assistance with personal care**

IQ Z74.2 **Need for assistance at home and no other household member able to render care**

IQ Z74.3 **Need for continuous supervision**

IQ Z74.8 **Other problems related to care provider dependency**

IQ Z74.9 **Problem related to care provider dependency, unspecified**

④ **Z75** **Problems related to medical facilities and other health care**

IQ Z75.0 **Medical services not available in home**
EXCLUDES 1   no other household member able to render care (Z74.2)

IQ Z75.1 **Person awaiting admission to adequate facility elsewhere**

IQ Z75.2 **Other waiting period for investigation and treatment**

IQ Z75.3 **Unavailability and inaccessibility of health-care facilities**
EXCLUDES 1   bed unavailable (Z75.1)

IQ Z75.4 **Unavailability and inaccessibility of other helping agencies**

IQ Z75.5 **Holiday relief care**

IQ Z75.8 **Other problems related to medical facilities and other health care**

IQ Z75.9 **Unspecified problem related to medical facilities and other health care**

④ **Z76** **Persons encountering health services in other circumstances**

IQ Z76.0 **Encounter for issue of repeat prescription**
Encounter for issue of repeat prescription for appliance
Encounter for issue of repeat prescription for medicaments
Encounter for issue of repeat prescription for spectacles
EXCLUDES 2   issue of medical certificate (Z02.7)
repeat prescription for contraceptive (Z30.4-)

Px **IQ Z76.1** **Encounter for health supervision and care of foundling**

Px **IQ Z76.2** **Encounter for health supervision and care of other healthy infant and child**
Encounter for medical or nursing care or supervision of healthy infant under circumstances such as adverse socioeconomic conditions at home
Encounter for medical or nursing care or supervision of healthy infant under circumstances such as awaiting foster or adoptive placement
Encounter for medical or nursing care or supervision of healthy infant under circumstances such as maternal illness
Encounter for medical or nursing care or supervision of healthy infant under circumstances such as number of children at home preventing or interfering with normal care

IQ Z76.3 **Healthy person accompanying sick person**

IQ Z76.4 **Other boarder to healthcare facility**
EXCLUDES 1   homelessness (Z59.0)

IQ Z76.5 **Malingerer [conscious simulation]**
Person feigning illness (with obvious motivation)
EXCLUDES 1   factitious disorder (F68.1-, F68.A)
peregrinating patient (F68.1-)

⑤ **Z76.8** **Persons encountering health services in other specified circumstances**

IQ Z76.81 **Expectant parent(s) prebirth pediatrician visit**
Pre-adoption pediatrician visit for adoptive parent(s)

IQ Z76.82 **Awaiting organ transplant status**
Patient waiting for organ availability

IQ Z76.89 **Persons encountering health services in other specified circumstances**
Persons encountering health services NOS

Persons with potential health hazards related to family and personal history and certain conditions influencing health status (Z77-Z99)

Code also:
any follow-up examination (Z08-Z09)

④ **Z77** **Other contact with and (suspected) exposures hazardous to health**

---

④4th digit required   ⑤5th digit required   ⑥6th digit required   ⑦7th digit required   ⑦7th digit placeholder   ✚Additional code   ▣Laterality

1910   *DecisionHealth's* FY 2020 Complete Home Health ICD-10-CM Diagnosis Coding Manual

INCLUDES contact with and (suspected) exposures to potential hazards to health

EXCLUDES 2 contact with and (suspected) exposure to communicable diseases (Z20.-)

exposure to (parental) (environmental) tobacco smoke in the perinatal period (P96.81)

newborn affected by noxious substances transmitted via placenta or breast milk (P04.-)

occupational exposure to risk factors (Z57.-)

retained foreign body (Z18.-)

retained foreign body fully removed (Z87.821)

toxic effects of substances chiefly nonmedicinal as to source (T51-T65)

GUIDELINES Section I.C.21.c.1)

Category Z20 indicates contact with, and suspected exposure to, communicable diseases. These codes are for patients who do not show any sign or symptom of a disease but are suspected to have been exposed to it by close personal contact with an infected individual or are in an area where a disease is epidemic. Category Z77 indicates contact with and suspected exposures hazardous to health.

Contact/exposure codes may be used as a first-listed code to explain an encounter for testing, or, more commonly, as a secondary code to identify a potential risk.

⑤ Z77.0 **Contact with and (suspected) exposure to hazardous, chiefly nonmedicinal, chemicals**

⑥ Z77.01 **Contact with and (suspected) exposure to hazardous metals**

IQ Z77.010 **Contact with and (suspected) exposure to arsenic**

IQ Z77.011 **Contact with and (suspected) exposure to lead**

IQ Z77.012 **Contact with and (suspected) exposure to uranium**

> **EXCLUDES 1** retained depleted uranium fragments (Z18.01)

IQ Z77.018 **Contact with and (suspected) exposure to other hazardous metals**

Contact with and (suspected) exposure to chromium compounds

Contact with and (suspected) exposure to nickel dust

⑥ Z77.02 **Contact with and (suspected) exposure to hazardous aromatic compounds**

IQ Z77.020 **Contact with and (suspected) exposure to aromatic amines**

IQ Z77.021 **Contact with and (suspected) exposure to benzene**

IQ Z77.028 **Contact with and (suspected) exposure to other hazardous aromatic compounds**

Aromatic dyes NOS
Polycyclic aromatic hydrocarbons

⑥ Z77.09 **Contact with and (suspected) exposure to other hazardous, chiefly nonmedicinal, chemicals**

IQ Z77.090 **Contact with and (suspected) exposure to asbestos**

IQ Z77.098 **Contact with and (suspected) exposure to other hazardous, chiefly nonmedicinal, chemicals**
Dyes NOS

⑤ Z77.1 **Contact with and (suspected) exposure to environmental pollution and hazards in the physical environment**

⑥ Z77.11 **Contact with and (suspected) exposure to environmental pollution**

IQ Z77.110 **Contact with and (suspected) exposure to air pollution**

IQ Z77.111 **Contact with and (suspected) exposure to water pollution**

IQ Z77.112 **Contact with and (suspected) exposure to soil pollution**

IQ Z77.118 **Contact with and (suspected) exposure to other environmental pollution**

⑥ Z77.12 **Contact with and (suspected) exposure to hazards in the physical environment**

IQ Z77.120 **Contact with and (suspected) exposure to mold (toxic)**

IQ Z77.121 **Contact with and (suspected) exposure to harmful algae and algae toxins**

Contact with and (suspected) exposure to (harmful) algae bloom NOS

Contact with and (suspected) exposure to blue-green algae bloom

Contact with and (suspected) exposure to brown tide

Contact with and (suspected) exposure to cyanobacteria bloom

Contact with and (suspected) exposure to Florida red tide

Contact with and (suspected) exposure to pfiesteria piscicida

Contact with and (suspected) exposure to red tide

IQ Z77.122 **Contact with and (suspected) exposure to noise**

IQ Z77.123 **Contact with and (suspected) exposure to radon and other naturally occurring radiation**

> **EXCLUDES 2** radiation exposure as the cause of a confirmed condition (W88-W90, X39.0-)
> radiation sickness NOS (T66)

IQ Z77.128 **Contact with and (suspected) exposure to other hazards in the physical environment**

⑤ Z77.2 **Contact with and (suspected) exposure to other hazardous substances**

IQ Z77.21 **Contact with and (suspected) exposure to potentially hazardous body fluids**

★ New ▲ Revised Px Primary **SP** PDGM Px **SL** Low CoM **SH** High CoM **IQ** Quest. Encounter **H** Hospice non-cancer Dx | Unspecified | **M** *Manifestation*

DecisionHealth's FY 2020 Complete Home Health ICD-10-CM Diagnosis Coding Manual

1911

IQ Z77.22 Contact with and (suspected) exposure to environmental tobacco smoke (acute) (chronic)
Exposure to second hand tobacco smoke (acute) (chronic)
Passive smoking (acute) (chronic)
> EXCLUDES 1   nicotine dependence (F17.-)
> tobacco use (Z72.0)
> EXCLUDES 2   occupational exposure to environmental tobacco smoke (Z57.31)

IQ Z77.29 Contact with and (suspected) exposure to other hazardous substances
> CODING TIPS ✓   This code may be used to indicate passive exposure to e-cigarettes or vaping.

IQ Z77.9 Other contact with and (suspected) exposures hazardous to health

4 Z78 Other specified health status
> EXCLUDES 2   asymptomatic human immunodeficiency virus [HIV] infection status (Z21)
> postprocedural status (Z93-Z99)
> sex reassignment status (Z87.890)

IQ Z78.0 Asymptomatic menopausal state
Menopausal state NOS
Postmenopausal status NOS
> EXCLUDES 2   symptomatic menopausal state (N95.1)

IQ Z78.1 Physical restraint status
> EXCLUDES 1   physical restraint due to a procedure - omit code

IQ Z78.9 Other specified health status

4 Z79 Long term (current) drug therapy
> INCLUDES   long term (current) drug use for prophylactic purposes

Code also:
> any therapeutic drug level monitoring (Z51.81)
> EXCLUDES 2   drug abuse and dependence (F11-F19)
> drug use complicating pregnancy, childbirth, and the puerperium (O99.32-)
> long term (current) use of oral antidiabetic drugs (Z79.84)
> long term (current) use of oral hypoglycemic drugs (Z79.84)

> GUIDELINES   Section I.C.21.c.3)
Codes from this category [Z79] indicate a patient's continuous use of a prescribed drug (including such things as aspirin therapy) for the long-term treatment of a condition or for prophylactic use. It is not for use for patients who have addictions to drugs. This subcategory is not for use of medications for detoxification or maintenance programs to prevent withdrawal symptoms in patients with drug dependence (e.g., methadone maintenance for opiate dependence). Assign the appropriate code for the drug dependence instead.

Assign a code from Z79 if the patient is receiving a medication for an extended period as a prophylactic measure (such as for the prevention of deep vein thrombosis) or as treatment of a chronic condition (such as arthritis) or a disease requiring a lengthy course of treatment (such as cancer). Do not assign a code from category Z79 for medication being administered for a brief period of time to treat an acute illness or injury (such as a course of antibiotics to treat acute bronchitis).

> CODING TIPS ✓   "Long-term use" refers to multiple refills, long term prophylaxis, etc. Use the code if the medication is pertinent to the plan of care.

> CODING TIPS ✓   Codes classifiable to category Z79 should not be assigned as primary diagnoses. When the management of any of these medications is integral to the plan of care, consider the confirmed diagnosis for which the patient is under treatment with the medication. This diagnosis should be coded, with a code from Z79 as an additional diagnosis.

5 Z79.0 Long term (current) use of anticoagulants and antithrombotics/antiplatelets
> EXCLUDES 2   long term (current) use of aspirin (Z79.82)

IQ Z79.01 Long term (current) use of anticoagulants

IQ Z79.02 Long term (current) use of antithrombotics/antiplatelets

IQ Z79.1 Long term (current) use of non-steroidal anti-inflammatories (NSAID)
> EXCLUDES 2   long term (current) use of aspirin (Z79.82)

IQ Z79.2 Long term (current) use of antibiotics
> CODING TIPS ✓   Do not use this code for routine 7-10 days of oral antibiotics.

IQ Z79.3 Long term (current) use of hormonal contraceptives
Long term (current) use of birth control pill or patch

IQ Z79.4 Long term (current) use of insulin

---

4 4th digit required   5 5th digit required   6 6th digit required   7 7th digit required   7 7th digit placeholder   + Additional code   ⊟ Laterality

GUIDELINES Section I.C.4.a.6)(a)
For patients with secondary diabetes mellitus who routinely use insulin or oral hypoglycemic drugs, an additional code from category Z79 should be assigned to identify the long-term (current) use of insulin or oral hypoglycemic drugs. If the patient is treated with both oral medications and insulin, only the code for long-term (current) use of insulin should be assigned. Code Z79.4 should not be assigned if insulin is given temporarily to bring a secondary diabetic patient's blood sugar under control during an encounter.

GUIDELINES Section I.C.4.a.3)
If the documentation in a medical record does not indicate the type of diabetes but does indicate that the patient uses insulin, code E11, Type 2 diabetes mellitus, should be assigned. An additional code should be assigned from category Z79 to identify the long-term (current) use of insulin or oral hypoglycemic drugs. If the patient is treated with both oral medications and insulin, only the code for long-term (current) use of insulin should be assigned if insulin is given temporarily to bring a type 2 patient's blood sugar under control during an encounter.

GUIDELINES Section I.C.15.i
Code Z79.4, Long-term (current) use of insulin or code Z79.84, Long-term (current) use of oral hypoglycemic drugs, should not be assigned with codes from subcategory O24.4.

⑤ Z79.5 **Long term (current) use of steroids**

⚠ Z79.51 **Long term (current) use of inhaled steroids**

⚠ Z79.52 **Long term (current) use of systemic steroids**

⑤ Z79.8 **Other long term (current) drug therapy**

✚ ⑥ Z79.81 **Long term (current) use of agents affecting estrogen receptors and estrogen levels**
　　Code first, if applicable:
　　　malignant neoplasm of breast (C50.-)
　　　malignant neoplasm of prostate (C61)
　　Use additional code, if applicable, to identify:
　　　estrogen receptor positive status (Z17.0)
　　　family history of breast cancer (Z80.3)
　　　genetic susceptibility to malignant neoplasm (cancer) (Z15.0-)
　　　personal history of breast cancer (Z85.3)
　　　personal history of prostate cancer (Z85.46)
　　　postmenopausal status (Z78.0)
　　EXCLUDES 1 hormone replacement therapy (Z79.890)

CODING TIPS ✓ These types of agents are used for both active treatment of malignancies (see the "code first" note) and for prevention of recurring malignancies (see the "use additional code" for history and susceptibility). The clinician/coder should query the physician for further information when the patient is taking one of these drugs to determine whether to code the malignancy, the history of malignant neoplasm or other condition.

⚠ ✚ Z79.810 **Long term (current) use of selective estrogen receptor modulators (SERMs)**
　　Long term (current) use of raloxifene (Evista)
　　Long term (current) use of tamoxifen (Nolvadex)
　　Long term (current) use of toremifene (Fareston)

⚠ ✚ Z79.811 **Long term (current) use of aromatase inhibitors**
　　Long term (current) use of anastrozole (Arimidex)
　　Long term (current) use of exemestane (Aromasin)
　　Long term (current) use of letrozole (Femara)

⚠ ✚ Z79.818 **Long term (current) use of other agents affecting estrogen receptors and estrogen levels**
　　Long term (current) use of estrogen receptor downregulators
　　Long term (current) use of fulvestrant (Faslodex)
　　Long term (current) use of gonadotropin-releasing hormone (GnRH) agonist
　　Long term (current) use of goserelin acetate (Zoladex)
　　Long term (current) use of leuprolide acetate (leuprorelin) (Lupron)
　　Long term (current) use of megestrol acetate (Megace)

⚠ Z79.82 **Long term (current) use of aspirin**

⚠ Z79.83 **Long term (current) use of bisphosphonates**

⚠ Z79.84 **Long term (current) use of oral hypoglycemic drugs**
　　Long term (current) use of oral antidiabetic drugs
　　EXCLUDES 2 long term (current) use of insulin (Z79.4)

⑥ Z79.89 **Other long term (current) drug therapy**

⚠ Z79.890 **Hormone replacement therapy**

⚠ Z79.891 **Long term (current) use of opiate analgesic**
　　Long term (current) use of methadone for pain management
　　EXCLUDES 1 methodone use NOS (F11.9-)
　　　use of methodone for treatment of heroin addiction (F11.2-)

★ New　▲ Revised　**Px** Primary　**SP** PDGM Px　**SL** Low CoM　**SH** High CoM　**⚠** Quest. Encounter　**Ⓗ** Hospice non-cancer Dx　　Unspecified　　**M** *Manifestation*

IQ Z79.899   **Other long term (current) drug therapy**

4 Z80   **Family history of primary malignant neoplasm**

> **GUIDELINES**   Section I.C.21.c.4)
>
> There are two types of history Z codes, personal and family. Personal history codes explain a patient's past medical condition that no longer exists and is not receiving any treatment, but that has the potential for recurrence, and therefore may require continued monitoring.
>
> Family history codes are for use when a patient has a family member(s) who has had a particular disease that causes the patient to be at higher risk of also contracting the disease. Personal history codes may be used in conjunction with follow-up codes and family history codes may be used in conjunction with screening codes to explain the need for a test or procedure. History codes are also acceptable on any medical record regardless of the reason for visit. A history of an illness, even if no longer present, is important information that may alter the type of treatment ordered.

IQ Z80.0   **Family history of malignant neoplasm of digestive organs**
Conditions classifiable to C15-C26

IQ Z80.1   **Family history of malignant neoplasm of trachea, bronchus and lung**
Conditions classifiable to C33-C34

IQ Z80.2   **Family history of malignant neoplasm of other respiratory and intrathoracic organs**
Conditions classifiable to C30-C32, C37-C39

IQ Z80.3   **Family history of malignant neoplasm of breast**
Conditions classifiable to C50.-

5 Z80.4   **Family history of malignant neoplasm of genital organs**
Conditions classifiable to C51-C63

!Q Z80.41   **Family history of malignant neoplasm of ovary**

!Q Z80.42   **Family history of malignant neoplasm of prostate**

!Q Z80.43   **Family history of malignant neoplasm of testis**

!Q Z80.49   **Family history of malignant neoplasm of other genital organs**

5 Z80.5   **Family history of malignant neoplasm of urinary tract**
Conditions classifiable to C64-C68

!Q Z80.51   **Family history of malignant neoplasm of kidney**

!Q Z80.52   **Family history of malignant neoplasm of bladder**

!Q Z80.59   **Family history of malignant neoplasm of other urinary tract organ**

IQ Z80.6   **Family history of leukemia**
Conditions classifiable to C91-C95

IQ Z80.7   **Family history of other malignant neoplasms of lymphoid, hematopoietic and related tissues**
Conditions classifiable to C81-C90, C96.-

IQ Z80.8   **Family history of malignant neoplasm of other organs or systems**
Conditions classifiable to C00-C14, C40-C49, C69-C79

IQ Z80.9   **Family history of malignant neoplasm, unspecified**
Conditions classifiable to C80.1

4 Z81   **Family history of mental and behavioral disorders**

> **GUIDELINES**   Section I.C.21.c.4)
>
> There are two types of history Z codes, personal and family. Personal history codes explain a patient's past medical condition that no longer exists and is not receiving any treatment, but that has the potential for recurrence, and therefore may require continued monitoring.
>
> Family history codes are for use when a patient has a family member(s) who has had a particular disease that causes the patient to be at higher risk of also contracting the disease. Personal history codes may be used in conjunction with follow-up codes and family history codes may be used in conjunction with screening codes to explain the need for a test or procedure. History codes are also acceptable on any medical record regardless of the reason for visit. A history of an illness, even if no longer present, is important information that may alter the type of treatment ordered.

IQ Z81.0   **Family history of intellectual disabilities**
Conditions classifiable to F70-F79

IQ Z81.1   **Family history of alcohol abuse and dependence**
Conditions classifiable to F10.-

IQ Z81.2   **Family history of tobacco abuse and dependence**
Conditions classifiable to F17.-

IQ Z81.3   **Family history of other psychoactive substance abuse and dependence**
Conditions classifiable to F11-F16, F18-F19

IQ Z81.4   **Family history of other substance abuse and dependence**
Conditions classifiable to F55

IQ Z81.8   **Family history of other mental and behavioral disorders**
Conditions classifiable elsewhere in F01-F99

4 Z82   **Family history of certain disabilities and chronic diseases (leading to disablement)**

---

4 4th digit required   5 5th digit required   6 6th digit required   7 7th digit required   7 7th digit placeholder   + Additional code   ⊟ Laterality

GUIDELINES   Section I.C.21.c.4)
There are two types of history Z codes, personal and family. Personal history codes explain a patient's past medical condition that no longer exists and is not receiving any treatment, but that has the potential for recurrence, and therefore may require continued monitoring.

Family history codes are for use when a patient has a family member(s) who has had a particular disease that causes the patient to be at higher risk of also contracting the disease. Personal history codes may be used in conjunction with follow-up codes and family history codes may be used in conjunction with screening codes to explain the need for a test or procedure. History codes are also acceptable on any medical record regardless of the reason for visit. A history of an illness, even if no longer present, is important information that may alter the type of treatment ordered.

IQ Z82.0 **Family history of epilepsy and other diseases of the nervous system**
Conditions classifiable to G00-G99

IQ Z82.1 **Family history of blindness and visual loss**
Conditions classifiable to H54.-

IQ Z82.2 **Family history of deafness and hearing loss**
Conditions classifiable to H90-H91

IQ Z82.3 **Family history of stroke**
Conditions classifiable to I60-I64

5 Z82.4 **Family history of ischemic heart disease and other diseases of the circulatory system**
Conditions classifiable to I00-I52, I65-I99

IQ Z82.41 **Family history of sudden cardiac death**

IQ Z82.49 **Family history of ischemic heart disease and other diseases of the circulatory system**

IQ Z82.5 **Family history of asthma and other chronic lower respiratory diseases**
Conditions classifiable to J40-J47
   EXCLUDES 2   family history of other diseases of the respiratory system (Z83.6)

5 Z82.6 **Family history of arthritis and other diseases of the musculoskeletal system and connective tissue**
Conditions classifiable to M00-M99

IQ Z82.61 **Family history of arthritis**

IQ Z82.62 **Family history of osteoporosis**

IQ Z82.69 **Family history of other diseases of the musculoskeletal system and connective tissue**

5 Z82.7 **Family history of congenital malformations, deformations and chromosomal abnormalities**
Conditions classifiable to Q00-Q99

IQ Z82.71 **Family history of polycystic kidney**

IQ Z82.79 **Family history of other congenital malformations, deformations and chromosomal abnormalities**

IQ Z82.8 **Family history of other disabilities and chronic diseases leading to disablement, not elsewhere classified**

4 Z83 **Family history of other specific disorders**
   EXCLUDES 2   contact with and (suspected) exposure to communicable disease in the family (Z20.-)
   GUIDELINES   Section I.C.21.c.4)
There are two types of history Z codes, personal and family. Personal history codes explain a patient's past medical condition that no longer exists and is not receiving any treatment, but that has the potential for recurrence, and therefore may require continued monitoring.

Family history codes are for use when a patient has a family member(s) who has had a particular disease that causes the patient to be at higher risk of also contracting the disease. Personal history codes may be used in conjunction with follow-up codes and family history codes may be used in conjunction with screening codes to explain the need for a test or procedure. History codes are also acceptable on any medical record regardless of the reason for visit. A history of an illness, even if no longer present, is important information that may alter the type of treatment ordered.

IQ Z83.0 **Family history of human immunodeficiency virus [HIV] disease**
Conditions classifiable to B20

IQ Z83.1 **Family history of other infectious and parasitic diseases**
Conditions classifiable to A00-B19, B25-B94, B99

IQ Z83.2 **Family history of diseases of the blood and blood-forming organs and certain disorders involving the immune mechanism**
Conditions classifiable to D50-D89

IQ Z83.3 **Family history of diabetes mellitus**
Conditions classifiable to E08-E13

5 Z83.4 **Family history of other endocrine, nutritional and metabolic diseases**
Conditions classifiable to E00-E07, E15-E88

IQ Z83.41 **Family history of multiple endocrine neoplasia [MEN] syndrome**

IQ Z83.42 **Family history of familial hypercholesterolemia**

6 Z83.43 **Family history of other disorder of lipoprotein metabolism and other lipidemias**

IQ Z83.430 **Family history of elevated lipoprotein(a)**
Family history of elevated Lp(a)

IQ Z83.438 **Family history of other disorder of lipoprotein metabolism and other lipidemia**
Family history of familial combined hyperlipidemia

IQ Z83.49 **Family history of other endocrine, nutritional and metabolic diseases**

5 Z83.5 **Family history of eye and ear disorders**

6 Z83.51 **Family history of eye disorders**

★ New ▲ Revised Px Primary **SP** PDGM Px **SL** Low CoM **SH** High CoM **IQ** Quest. Encounter **H** Hospice non-cancer Dx   Unspecified   **M** *Manifestation*

DecisionHealth's FY 2020 Complete Home Health ICD-10-CM Diagnosis Coding Manual   1915

Conditions classifiable to H00-H53,
H55-H59

EXCLUDES 2   family history of
blindness and visual
loss (Z82.1)

IQ **Z83.511   Family history of glaucoma**

IQ **Z83.518   Family history of other specified
eye disorder**

IQ **Z83.52   Family history of ear disorders**
Conditions classifiable to H60-H83,
H92-H95

EXCLUDES 2   family history of
deafness and hearing
loss (Z82.2)

IQ **Z83.6   Family history of other diseases of the
respiratory system**
Conditions classifiable to J00-J39, J60-J99

EXCLUDES 2   family history of asthma and
other chronic lower
respiratory diseases
(Z82.5)

5 **Z83.7   Family history of diseases of the
digestive system**
Conditions classifiable to K00-K93

IQ **Z83.71   Family history of colonic polyps**

EXCLUDES 2   family history of
malignant neoplasm of
digestive organs
(Z80.0)

IQ **Z83.79   Family history of other diseases of
the digestive system**

4 **Z84   Family history of other conditions**

GUIDELINES   Section I.C.21.c.4)

There are two types of history Z codes,
personal and family. Personal history codes
explain a patient's past medical condition that
no longer exists and is not receiving any
treatment, but that has the potential for
recurrence, and therefore may require
continued monitoring.

Family history codes are for use when a
patient has a family member(s) who has had a
particular disease that causes the patient to be
at higher risk of also contracting the disease.
Personal history codes may be used in
conjunction with follow-up codes and family
history codes may be used in conjunction with
screening codes to explain the need for a test
or procedure. History codes are also
acceptable on any medical record regardless
of the reason for visit. A history of an illness,
even if no longer present, is important
information that may alter the type of treatment
ordered.

IQ **Z84.0   Family history of diseases of the skin
and subcutaneous tissue**
Conditions classifiable to L00-L99

IQ **Z84.1   Family history of disorders of kidney
and ureter**
Conditions classifiable to N00-N29

IQ **Z84.2   Family history of other diseases of the
genitourinary system**
Conditions classifiable to N30-N99

IQ **Z84.3   Family history of consanguinity**

5 **Z84.8   Family history of other specified
conditions**

IQ **Z84.81   Family history of carrier of genetic
disease**

IQ **Z84.82   Family history of sudden infant
death syndrome**
Family history of SIDS

IQ **Z84.89   Family history of other specified
conditions**

+ 4 **Z85   Personal history of malignant neoplasm**
Code first:
any follow-up examination after treatment
of malignant neoplasm (Z08)
Use additional code to identify:
alcohol use and dependence (F10.-)
exposure to environmental tobacco smoke
(Z77.22)
history of tobacco dependence (Z87.891)
occupational exposure to environmental
tobacco smoke (Z57.31)
tobacco dependence (F17.-)
tobacco use (Z72.0)

EXCLUDES 2   personal history of benign
neoplasm (Z86.01-)
personal history of carcinoma-
in-situ (Z86.00-)

GUIDELINES   Section I.C.2.m

When a primary malignancy has been excised
but further treatment, such as an additional
surgery for the malignancy, radiation therapy or
chemotherapy is directed to that site, the
primary malignancy code should be used until
treatment is completed.

When a primary malignancy has been
previously excised or eradicated from its site,
there is no further treatment (of the
malignancy) directed at that site, and there is
no evidence of any existing primary
malignancy, a code from category Z85 should
be used to indicate the former site of the
malignancy.

Subcategories Z85.0 – Z85.7 should only be
assigned for the former site of a primary
malignancy, not the site of a secondary
malignancy. Codes from subcategory Z85.8-,
may be assigned for the former site(s) of either
a primary or secondary malignancy included in
this subcategory.

4 4th digit required   5 5th digit required   6 6th digit required   7 7th digit required   7 7th digit placeholder   +Additional code   Laterality

1916   *DecisionHealth's* FY 2020 Complete Home Health ICD-10-CM Diagnosis Coding Manual

GUIDELINES Section I.C.21.c.4)
There are two types of history Z codes, personal and family. Personal history codes explain a patient's past medical condition that no longer exists and is not receiving any treatment, but that has the potential for recurrence, and therefore may require continued monitoring.

Family history codes are for use when a patient has a family member(s) who has had a particular disease that causes the patient to be at higher risk of also contracting the disease. Personal history codes may be used in conjunction with follow-up codes and family history codes may be used in conjunction with screening codes to explain the need for a test or procedure. History codes are also acceptable on any medical record regardless of the reason for visit. A history of an illness, even if no longer present, is important information that may alter the type of treatment ordered.

CODING TIPS ✓ The codes in this section are commonly referred to as the "history of cancer" codes. "History" in this case means the cancer has been eradicated from its primary site. It does not necessarily mean the patient no longer has cancer. The cancer may have already metastasized to other sites.

+ ⑤ Z85.0 Personal history of malignant neoplasm of digestive organs

IQ + Z85.00 Personal history of malignant neoplasm of unspecified digestive organ

IQ + Z85.01 Personal history of malignant neoplasm of esophagus
Conditions classifiable to C15

+ ⑥ Z85.02 Personal history of malignant neoplasm of stomach

IQ + Z85.020 Personal history of malignant carcinoid tumor of stomach
Conditions classifiable to C7A.092

IQ + Z85.028 Personal history of other malignant neoplasm of stomach
Conditions classifiable to C16

+ ⑥ Z85.03 Personal history of malignant neoplasm of large intestine

IQ + Z85.030 Personal history of malignant carcinoid tumor of large intestine
Conditions classifiable to C7A.022-C7A.025, C7A.029

IQ + Z85.038 Personal history of other malignant neoplasm of large intestine
Conditions classifiable to C18

+ ⑥ Z85.04 Personal history of malignant neoplasm of rectum, rectosigmoid junction, and anus

IQ + Z85.040 Personal history of malignant carcinoid tumor of rectum
Conditions classifiable to C7A.026

IQ + Z85.048 Personal history of other malignant neoplasm of rectum, rectosigmoid junction, and anus
Conditions classifiable to C19-C21

IQ + Z85.05 Personal history of malignant neoplasm of liver

Conditions classifiable to C22

+ ⑥ Z85.06 Personal history of malignant neoplasm of small intestine

IQ + Z85.060 Personal history of malignant carcinoid tumor of small intestine
Conditions classifiable to C7A.01-

IQ + Z85.068 Personal history of other malignant neoplasm of small intestine
Conditions classifiable to C17

IQ + Z85.07 Personal history of malignant neoplasm of pancreas
Conditions classifiable to C25

IQ + Z85.09 Personal history of malignant neoplasm of other digestive organs

+ ⑤ Z85.1 Personal history of malignant neoplasm of trachea, bronchus and lung

+ ⑥ Z85.11 Personal history of malignant neoplasm of bronchus and lung

IQ + Z85.110 Personal history of malignant carcinoid tumor of bronchus and lung
Conditions classifiable to C7A.090

IQ + Z85.118 Personal history of other malignant neoplasm of bronchus and lung
Conditions classifiable to C34

IQ + Z85.12 Personal history of malignant neoplasm of trachea
Conditions classifiable to C33

+ ⑤ Z85.2 Personal history of malignant neoplasm of other respiratory and intrathoracic organs

IQ + Z85.20 Personal history of malignant neoplasm of unspecified respiratory organ

IQ + Z85.21 Personal history of malignant neoplasm of larynx
Conditions classifiable to C32

IQ + Z85.22 Personal history of malignant neoplasm of nasal cavities, middle ear, and accessory sinuses
Conditions classifiable to C30-C31

+ ⑥ Z85.23 Personal history of malignant neoplasm of thymus

IQ + Z85.230 Personal history of malignant carcinoid tumor of thymus
Conditions classifiable to C7A.091

IQ + Z85.238 Personal history of other malignant neoplasm of thymus
Conditions classifiable to C37

IQ + Z85.29 Personal history of malignant neoplasm of other respiratory and intrathoracic organs

IQ + Z85.3 Personal history of malignant neoplasm of breast
Conditions classifiable to C50.-

+ ⑤ Z85.4 Personal history of malignant neoplasm of genital organs
Conditions classifiable to C51-C63

IQ + Z85.40 Personal history of malignant neoplasm of unspecified female genital organ

IQ + Z85.41 Personal history of malignant neoplasm of cervix uteri

IQ + Z85.42 Personal history of malignant neoplasm of other parts of uterus

---

★ New ▲ Revised **Px** Primary **SP** PDGM Px **SL** Low CoM **SH** High CoM **IQ** Quest. Encounter **H** Hospice non-cancer Dx Unspecified **M** *Manifestation*

IQ + Z85.43 Personal history of malignant neoplasm of ovary

IQ + Z85.44 Personal history of malignant neoplasm of other female genital organs

IQ + Z85.45 Personal history of malignant neoplasm of unspecified male genital organ

IQ + Z85.46 Personal history of malignant neoplasm of prostate

IQ + Z85.47 Personal history of malignant neoplasm of testis

IQ + Z85.48 Personal history of malignant neoplasm of epididymis

IQ + Z85.49 Personal history of malignant neoplasm of other male genital organs

+ 5 Z85.5 Personal history of malignant neoplasm of urinary tract
Conditions classifiable to C64-C68

IQ + Z85.50 Personal history of malignant neoplasm of unspecified urinary tract organ

IQ + Z85.51 Personal history of malignant neoplasm of bladder

+ 6 Z85.52 Personal history of malignant neoplasm of kidney
EXCLUDES 1 personal history of malignant neoplasm of renal pelvis (Z85.53)

IQ + Z85.520 Personal history of malignant carcinoid tumor of kidney
Conditions classifiable to C7A.093

IQ + Z85.528 Personal history of other malignant neoplasm of kidney
Conditions classifiable to C64

IQ + Z85.53 Personal history of malignant neoplasm of renal pelvis

IQ + Z85.54 Personal history of malignant neoplasm of ureter

IQ + Z85.59 Personal history of malignant neoplasm of other urinary tract organ

IQ + Z85.6 Personal history of leukemia
Conditions classifiable to C91-C95
EXCLUDES 1 leukemia in remission C91.0-C95.9 with 5th character 1

+ 5 Z85.7 Personal history of other malignant neoplasms of lymphoid, hematopoietic and related tissues

IQ + Z85.71 Personal history of Hodgkin lymphoma
Conditions classifiable to C81

IQ + Z85.72 Personal history of non-Hodgkin lymphomas
Conditions classifiable to C82-C85

IQ + Z85.79 Personal history of other malignant neoplasms of lymphoid, hematopoietic and related tissues
Conditions classifiable to C88-C90, C96
EXCLUDES 1 multiple myeloma in remission (C90.01)
plasma cell leukemia in remission (C90.11)
plasmacytoma in remission (C90.21)

GUIDELINES Section I.C.2.n
The categories for leukemia, and category C90, Multiple myeloma and malignant plasma cell neoplasms, have codes indicating whether or not the leukemia has achieved remission. There are also codes Z85.6, Personal history of leukemia, and Z85.79, Personal history of other malignant neoplasms of lymphoid, hematopoietic and related tissues. If the documentation is unclear, as to whether the leukemia has achieved remission, the provider should be queried.

+ 5 Z85.8 Personal history of malignant neoplasms of other organs and systems
Conditions classifiable to C00-C14, C40-C49, C69-C75, C7A.098, C76-C79

+ 6 Z85.81 Personal history of malignant neoplasm of lip, oral cavity, and pharynx

IQ + Z85.810 Personal history of malignant neoplasm of tongue

IQ + Z85.818 Personal history of malignant neoplasm of other sites of lip, oral cavity, and pharynx

IQ + Z85.819 Personal history of malignant neoplasm of unspecified site of lip, oral cavity, and pharynx

+ 6 Z85.82 Personal history of malignant neoplasm of skin

IQ + Z85.820 Personal history of malignant melanoma of skin
Conditions classifiable to C43

IQ + Z85.821 Personal history of Merkel cell carcinoma
Conditions classifiable to C4A

IQ + Z85.828 Personal history of other malignant neoplasm of skin
Conditions classifiable to C44

+ 6 Z85.83 Personal history of malignant neoplasm of bone and soft tissue

IQ + Z85.830 Personal history of malignant neoplasm of bone

IQ + Z85.831 Personal history of malignant neoplasm of soft tissue
EXCLUDES 2 personal history of malignant neoplasm of skin (Z85.82-)

+ 6 Z85.84 Personal history of malignant neoplasm of eye and nervous tissue

IQ + Z85.840 Personal history of malignant neoplasm of eye

IQ + Z85.841 Personal history of malignant neoplasm of brain

IQ + Z85.848 Personal history of malignant neoplasm of other parts of nervous tissue

+ 6 Z85.85 Personal history of malignant neoplasm of endocrine glands

IQ + Z85.850 Personal history of malignant neoplasm of thyroid

IQ + Z85.858 Personal history of malignant neoplasm of other endocrine glands

IQ + Z85.89 Personal history of malignant neoplasm of other organs and systems

---

4 4th digit required   5 5th digit required   6 6th digit required   7 7th digit required   7 7th digit placeholder   + Additional code   5 Laterality

IQ + Z85.9   Personal history of malignant neoplasm, unspecified
Conditions classifiable to C7A.00, C80.1

4 Z86   Personal history of certain other diseases
Code first:
any follow-up examination after treatment (Z09)

GUIDELINES   Section I.C.21.c.4)
There are two types of history Z codes, personal and family. Personal history codes explain a patient's past medical condition that no longer exists and is not receiving any treatment, but that has the potential for recurrence, and therefore may require continued monitoring.

Family history codes are for use when a patient has a family member(s) who has had a particular disease that causes the patient to be at higher risk of also contracting the disease. Personal history codes may be used in conjunction with follow-up codes and family history codes may be used in conjunction with screening codes to explain the need for a test or procedure. History codes are also acceptable on any medical record regardless of the reason for visit. A history of an illness, even if no longer present, is important information that may alter the type of treatment ordered.

5 Z86.0   Personal history of in-situ and benign neoplasms and neoplasms of uncertain behavior
EXCLUDES 2   personal history of malignant neoplasms (Z85.-)

6 Z86.00   Personal history of in-situ neoplasm
Conditions classifiable to D00-D09

▲ IQ Z86.000   Personal history of in-situ neoplasm of breast
Conditions classifiable to D05

▲ IQ Z86.001   Personal history of in-situ neoplasm of cervix uteri
Conditions classifiable to D06
Personal history of cervical intraepithelial neoplasia III [CIN III]

☆ Z86.002   Personal history of in-situ neoplasm of other and unspecified genital organs
Conditions classifiable to D07
Personal history of high-grade prostatic intraepithelial neoplasia III [HGPIN III]
Personal history of vaginal intraepithelial neoplasia III [VAIN III]
Personal history of vulvar intraepithelial neoplasia III [VIN III]

☆ Z86.003   Personal history of in-situ neoplasm of oral cavity, esophagus and stomach
Conditions classifiable to D00

☆ Z86.004   Personal history of in-situ neoplasm of other and unspecified digestive organs
Conditions classifiable to D01

Personal history of anal intraepithelial neoplasia (AIN III)

☆ Z86.005   Personal history of in-situ neoplasm of middle ear and respiratory system
Conditions classifiable to D02

☆ Z86.006   Personal history of melanoma in-situ
Conditions classifiable to D03
EXCLUDES 2   sites other than skin - code to personal history of in-situ neoplasm of the site

☆ Z86.007   Personal history of in-situ neoplasm of skin
Conditions classifiable to D04
Personal history of carcinoma in situ of skin

▲ IQ Z86.008   Personal history of in-situ neoplasm of other site
Conditions classifiable to D09

6 Z86.01   Personal history of benign neoplasm

IQ Z86.010   Personal history of colonic polyps

IQ Z86.011   Personal history of benign neoplasm of the brain

IQ Z86.012   Personal history of benign carcinoid tumor

IQ Z86.018   Personal history of other benign neoplasm

IQ Z86.03   Personal history of neoplasm of uncertain behavior

5 Z86.1   Personal history of infectious and parasitic diseases
Conditions classifiable to A00-B89, B99
EXCLUDES 1   personal history of infectious diseases specific to a body system
sequelae of infectious and parasitic diseases (B90-B94)

IQ Z86.11   Personal history of tuberculosis
CODING TIPS ✓   This code is for the patient who has had TB in the past and currently has no residual effects from the TB.

IQ Z86.12   Personal history of poliomyelitis
CODING TIPS ✓   This code is for the patient who has had polio in the past and currently has no residual effects from the polio.

IQ Z86.13   Personal history of malaria

IQ Z86.14   Personal history of Methicillin resistant Staphylococcus aureus infection
Personal history of MRSA infection
CODING TIPS ✓   This code is for the patient who has had a MRSA infection in the past that is resolved and currently is not nasal swab positive. If nasal swab positive, use Z22.322.

☆ Z86.15   Personal history of latent tuberculosis infection

IQ Z86.19   Personal history of other infectious and parasitic diseases

---

☆ New ▲ Revised **Px** Primary **SP** PDGM Px **SL** Low CoM **SH** High CoM **IQ** Quest. Encounter **H** Hospice non-cancer Dx   Unspecified   **M** *Manifestation*

DecisionHealth's FY 2020 Complete Home Health ICD-10-CM Diagnosis Coding Manual   1919

Chapter 21

Z00-Z99

IQ Z86.2 Personal history of diseases of the blood and blood-forming organs and certain disorders involving the immune mechanism
Conditions classifiable to D50-D89

⑤ Z86.3 Personal history of endocrine, nutritional and metabolic diseases
Conditions classifiable to E00-E88

IQ Z86.31 Personal history of diabetic foot ulcer
> **EXCLUDES 2** current diabetic foot ulcer (E08.621, E09.621, E10.621, E11.621, E13.621)

IQ Z86.32 Personal history of gestational diabetes
Personal history of conditions classifiable to O24.4-
> **EXCLUDES 1** gestational diabetes mellitus in current pregnancy (O24.4-)

IQ Z86.39 Personal history of other endocrine, nutritional and metabolic disease
> **CODING TIPS ✓** If the patient no longer has diabetes, either because of loss of weight or pancreatic transplant, use this code to indicate the history.

⑤ Z86.5 Personal history of mental and behavioral disorders
Conditions classifiable to F40-F59

IQ Z86.51 Personal history of combat and operational stress reaction

IQ Z86.59 Personal history of other mental and behavioral disorders

⑤ Z86.6 Personal history of diseases of the nervous system and sense organs
Conditions classifiable to G00-G99, H00-H95

IQ Z86.61 Personal history of infections of the central nervous system
Personal history of encephalitis
Personal history of meningitis

IQ Z86.69 Personal history of other diseases of the nervous system and sense organs

⑤ Z86.7 Personal history of diseases of the circulatory system
Conditions classifiable to I00-I99
> **EXCLUDES 2** old myocardial infarction (I25.2)
> personal history of anaphylactic shock (Z87.892)
> postmyocardial infarction syndrome (I24.1)

⑥ Z86.71 Personal history of venous thrombosis and embolism
> **CODING TIPS ✓** Prior to assigning these codes, ensure that the clot is dissolved. It can take 3-6 months for the clot to dissipate and in the meantime, the acute condition should be coded.

IQ Z86.711 Personal history of pulmonary embolism

IQ Z86.718 Personal history of other venous thrombosis and embolism

IQ Z86.72 Personal history of thrombophlebitis

IQ Z86.73 Personal history of transient ischemic attack (TIA), and cerebral infarction without residual deficits
Personal history of prolonged reversible ischemic neurological deficit (PRIND)
Personal history of stroke NOS without residual deficits
> **EXCLUDES 1** personal history of traumatic brain injury (Z87.820)
> sequelae of cerebrovascular disease (I69.-)

> **GUIDELINES** Section I.C.9.d.3)
Codes from category I69, Sequela of cerebrovascular disease, should not be assigned if the patient does not have neurologic deficits. Assign Z86.73, Personal history of transient ischemic attack (TIA) and cerebral infarction

IQ Z86.74 Personal history of sudden cardiac arrest
Personal history of sudden cardiac death successfully resuscitated

IQ Z86.79 Personal history of other diseases of the circulatory system

④ Z87 Personal history of other diseases and conditions
Code first:
any follow-up examination after treatment (Z09)

> **GUIDELINES** Section I.C.21.c.4)
There are two types of history Z codes, personal and family. Personal history codes explain a patient's past medical condition that no longer exists and is not receiving any treatment, but that has the potential for recurrence, and therefore may require continued monitoring.

Family history codes are for use when a patient has a family member(s) who has had a particular disease that causes the patient to be at higher risk of also contracting the disease. Personal history codes may be used in conjunction with follow-up codes and family history codes may be used in conjunction with screening codes to explain the need for a test or procedure. History codes are also acceptable on any medical record regardless of the reason for visit. A history of an illness, even if no longer present, is important information that may alter the type of treatment ordered.

⑤ Z87.0 Personal history of diseases of the respiratory system
Conditions classifiable to J00-J99

IQ Z87.01 Personal history of pneumonia (recurrent)

IQ Z87.09 Personal history of other diseases of the respiratory system

⑤ Z87.1 Personal history of diseases of the digestive system
Conditions classifiable to K00-K93

IQ Z87.11 Personal history of peptic ulcer disease

④ 4th digit required   ⑤ 5th digit required   ⑥ 6th digit required   ⑦ 7th digit required   ⑦ 7th digit placeholder   ➕ Additional code   ▣ Laterality

1920   *DecisionHealth's* FY 2020 Complete Home Health ICD-10-CM Diagnosis Coding Manual

IQ Z87.19 Personal history of other diseases of the digestive system

IQ Z87.2 Personal history of diseases of the skin and subcutaneous tissue
Conditions classifiable to L00-L99
> **EXCLUDES 2** personal history of diabetic foot ulcer (Z86.31)

S Z87.3 Personal history of diseases of the musculoskeletal system and connective tissue
Conditions classifiable to M00-M99
> **EXCLUDES 2** personal history of (healed) traumatic fracture (Z87.81)

6 Z87.31 Personal history of (healed) nontraumatic fracture
> **CODING TIPS ✓** The patient can have a current fracture and a history of healed fracture at the same time. History of healed osteoporosis fracture qualifies the patient for Calcimar injections. See Z87.81 for history of healed traumatic fracture.

IQ Z87.310 Personal history of (healed) osteoporosis fracture
Personal history of (healed) fragility fracture
Personal history of (healed) collapsed vertebra due to osteoporosis
> **GUIDELINES** Section I.C.13.d.1)
Category M81, Osteoporosis without current pathological fracture, is for use for patients with osteoporosis who do not currently have a pathologic fracture due to the osteoporosis, even if they have had a fracture in the past. For patients with a history of osteoporosis fractures, status code Z87.310, Personal history of (healed) osteoporosis fracture, should follow the code from M81.

IQ Z87.311 Personal history of (healed) other pathological fracture
Personal history of (healed) collapsed vertebra NOS
> **EXCLUDES 2** personal history of osteoporosis fracture (Z87.310)

IQ Z87.312 Personal history of (healed) stress fracture
Personal history of (healed) fatigue fracture

IQ Z87.39 Personal history of other diseases of the musculoskeletal system and connective tissue

S Z87.4 Personal history of diseases of genitourinary system
Conditions classifiable to N00-N99

6 Z87.41 Personal history of dysplasia of the female genital tract
> **EXCLUDES 1** personal history of intraepithelial neoplasia III of female genital tract (Z86.001, Z86.008)

personal history of malignant neoplasm of female genital tract (Z85.40-Z85.44)

IQ Z87.410 Personal history of cervical dysplasia

IQ Z87.411 Personal history of vaginal dysplasia

IQ Z87.412 Personal history of vulvar dysplasia

IQ Z87.42 Personal history of other diseases of the female genital tract

6 Z87.43 Personal history of diseases of male genital organs

IQ Z87.430 Personal history of prostatic dysplasia
> **EXCLUDES 1** personal history of malignant neoplasm of prostate (Z85.46)

IQ Z87.438 Personal history of other diseases of male genital organs

6 Z87.44 Personal history of diseases of urinary system
> **EXCLUDES 1** personal history of malignant neoplasm of cervix uteri (Z85.41)

IQ Z87.440 Personal history of urinary (tract) infections

IQ Z87.441 Personal history of nephrotic syndrome

IQ Z87.442 Personal history of urinary calculi
Personal history of kidney stones

IQ Z87.448 Personal history of other diseases of urinary system

S Z87.5 Personal history of complications of pregnancy, childbirth and the puerperium
Conditions classifiable to O00-O9A
> **EXCLUDES 2** recurrent pregnancy loss (N96)

IQ Z87.51 Personal history of pre-term labor
> **EXCLUDES 1** current pregnancy with history of pre-term labor (O09.21-)

IQ Z87.59 Personal history of other complications of pregnancy, childbirth and the puerperium
Personal history of trophoblastic disease

S Z87.7 Personal history of (corrected) congenital malformations
Conditions classifiable to Q00-Q89 that have been repaired or corrected
> **EXCLUDES 1** congenital malformations that have been partially corrected or repair but which still require medical treatment - code to condition
> **EXCLUDES 2** other postprocedural states (Z98.-)
> personal history of medical treatment (Z92.-)
> presence of cardiac and vascular implants and grafts (Z95.-)
> presence of other devices (Z97.-)

★ New ▲ Revised Px Primary SP PDGM Px SL Low CoM SH High CoM IQ Quest. Encounter H Hospice non-cancer Dx   Unspecified   M *Manifestation*

DecisionHealth's FY 2020 Complete Home Health ICD-10-CM Diagnosis Coding Manual   1921

presence of other functional
implants (Z96.-)
transplanted organ and tissue
status (Z94.-)

⑥ Z87.71 Personal history of (corrected) congenital malformations of genitourinary system

🆀 Z87.710 Personal history of (corrected) hypospadias

🆀 Z87.718 Personal history of other specified (corrected) congenital malformations of genitourinary system

⑥ Z87.72 Personal history of (corrected) congenital malformations of nervous system and sense organs

🆀 Z87.720 Personal history of (corrected) congenital malformations of eye

🆀 Z87.721 Personal history of (corrected) congenital malformations of ear

🆀 Z87.728 Personal history of other specified (corrected) congenital malformations of nervous system and sense organs

⑥ Z87.73 Personal history of (corrected) congenital malformations of digestive system

🆀 Z87.730 Personal history of (corrected) cleft lip and palate

🆀 Z87.738 Personal history of other specified (corrected) congenital malformations of digestive system

🆀 Z87.74 Personal history of (corrected) congenital malformations of heart and circulatory system

🆀 Z87.75 Personal history of (corrected) congenital malformations of respiratory system

🆀 Z87.76 Personal history of (corrected) congenital malformations of integument, limbs and musculoskeletal system

⑥ Z87.79 Personal history of other (corrected) congenital malformations

🆀 Z87.790 Personal history of (corrected) congenital malformations of face and neck

🆀 Z87.798 Personal history of other (corrected) congenital malformations

⑤ Z87.8 Personal history of other specified conditions
> **EXCLUDES 2** personal history of self harm (Z91.5)

🆀 Z87.81 Personal history of (healed) traumatic fracture
> **EXCLUDES 2** personal history of (healed) nontraumatic fracture (Z87.31-)

> **CODING TIPS ✓** The patient can have a current fracture and a history of healed fracture at the same time. See Z87.31 for history of healed pathologic fractures.

⑥ Z87.82 Personal history of other (healed) physical injury and trauma
Conditions classifiable to S00-T88, except traumatic fractures

🆀 Z87.820 Personal history of traumatic brain injury
> **EXCLUDES 1** personal history of transient ischemic attack (TIA), and cerebral infarction without residual deficits (Z86.73)

🆀 Z87.821 Personal history of retained foreign body fully removed

🆀 Z87.828 Personal history of other (healed) physical injury and trauma

⑥ Z87.89 Personal history of other specified conditions

🆀 Z87.890 Personal history of sex reassignment

🆀 Z87.891 Personal history of nicotine dependence
> **EXCLUDES 1** current nicotine dependence (F17.2-)

> **CODING TIPS ✓** Code history of tobacco dependence (Z87.891) for someone who was a smoker but who isn't now. Use this code if the physician uses the term "history." Remission is coded to F17.2 codes.

🆀 Z87.892 Personal history of anaphylaxis
Code also allergy status such as:
allergy status to drugs, medicaments and biological substances (Z88.-)
allergy status, other than to drugs and biological substances (Z91.0-)

🆀 Z87.898 Personal history of other specified conditions

④ Z88 Allergy status to drugs, medicaments and biological substances
> **EXCLUDES 2** Allergy status, other than to drugs and biological substances (Z91.0-)

🆀 Z88.0 Allergy status to penicillin

🆀 Z88.1 Allergy status to other antibiotic agents status

🆀 Z88.2 Allergy status to sulfonamides status

🆀 Z88.3 Allergy status to other anti-infective agents status

🆀 Z88.4 Allergy status to anesthetic agent status

🆀 Z88.5 Allergy status to narcotic agent status

🆀 Z88.6 Allergy status to analgesic agent status

🆀 Z88.7 Allergy status to serum and vaccine status

🆀 Z88.8 Allergy status to other drugs, medicaments and biological substances status

🆀 Z88.9 Allergy status to unspecified drugs, medicaments and biological substances status

④ Z89 Acquired absence of limb
> **INCLUDES** amputation status
postprocedural loss of limb
post-traumatic loss of limb
> **EXCLUDES 1** acquired deformities of limbs (M20-M21)
congenital absence of limbs (Q71-Q73)

---

④4th digit required **⑤**5th digit required **⑥**6th digit required **⑦**7th digit required **⑦**7th digit placeholder **✚**Additional code **⊟**Laterality

CODING TIPS ✓ These codes are used to indicate the absence of the limb after surgical amputation, as well as healed traumatic amputations that no longer require care.

⑤ **Z89.0 Acquired absence of thumb and other finger(s)**

⑥ **Z89.01 Acquired absence of thumb**

▤ **IQ Z89.011 Acquired absence of right thumb**

▤ **IQ Z89.012 Acquired absence of left thumb**

▤ **IQ Z89.019 Acquired absence of unspecified thumb**

⑥ **Z89.02 Acquired absence of other finger(s)**
EXCLUDES 2 acquired absence of thumb (Z89.01-)

▤ **IQ Z89.021 Acquired absence of right finger(s)**

▤ **IQ Z89.022 Acquired absence of left finger(s)**

▤ **IQ Z89.029 Acquired absence of unspecified finger(s)**

⑤ **Z89.1 Acquired absence of hand and wrist**

⑥ **Z89.11 Acquired absence of hand**

▤ **IQ Z89.111 Acquired absence of right hand**

▤ **IQ Z89.112 Acquired absence of left hand**

▤ **IQ Z89.119 Acquired absence of unspecified hand**

⑥ **Z89.12 Acquired absence of wrist**
Disarticulation at wrist

▤ **IQ Z89.121 Acquired absence of right wrist**

▤ **IQ Z89.122 Acquired absence of left wrist**

▤ **IQ Z89.129 Acquired absence of unspecified wrist**

⑤ **Z89.2 Acquired absence of upper limb above wrist**

⑥ **Z89.20 Acquired absence of upper limb, unspecified level**

▤ **IQ Z89.201 Acquired absence of right upper limb, unspecified level**

▤ **IQ Z89.202 Acquired absence of left upper limb, unspecified level**

▤ **IQ Z89.209 Acquired absence of unspecified upper limb, unspecified level**
Acquired absence of arm NOS

⑥ **Z89.21 Acquired absence of upper limb below elbow**

▤ **IQ Z89.211 Acquired absence of right upper limb below elbow**

▤ **IQ Z89.212 Acquired absence of left upper limb below elbow**

▤ **IQ Z89.219 Acquired absence of unspecified upper limb below elbow**

⑥ **Z89.22 Acquired absence of upper limb above elbow**
Disarticulation at elbow

▤ **IQ Z89.221 Acquired absence of right upper limb above elbow**

▤ **IQ Z89.222 Acquired absence of left upper limb above elbow**

▤ **IQ Z89.229 Acquired absence of unspecified upper limb above elbow**

⑥ **Z89.23 Acquired absence of shoulder**
Acquired absence of shoulder joint following explanation of shoulder joint prosthesis, with or without presence of antibiotic-impregnated cement spacer

▤ **IQ Z89.231 Acquired absence of right shoulder**

▤ **IQ Z89.232 Acquired absence of left shoulder**

▤ **IQ Z89.239 Acquired absence of unspecified shoulder**

⑤ **Z89.4 Acquired absence of toe(s), foot, and ankle**

⑥ **Z89.41 Acquired absence of great toe**

▤ **IQ Z89.411 Acquired absence of right great toe**

▤ **IQ Z89.412 Acquired absence of left great toe**

▤ **IQ Z89.419 Acquired absence of unspecified great toe**

⑥ **Z89.42 Acquired absence of other toe(s)**
EXCLUDES 2 acquired absence of great toe (Z89.41-)

▤ **IQ Z89.421 Acquired absence of other right toe(s)**

▤ **IQ Z89.422 Acquired absence of other left toe(s)**

▤ **IQ Z89.429 Acquired absence of other toe(s), unspecified side**

⑥ **Z89.43 Acquired absence of foot**

▤ **IQ Z89.431 Acquired absence of right foot**

▤ **IQ Z89.432 Acquired absence of left foot**

▤ **IQ Z89.439 Acquired absence of unspecified foot**

⑥ **Z89.44 Acquired absence of ankle**
Disarticulation of ankle

▤ **IQ Z89.441 Acquired absence of right ankle**

▤ **IQ Z89.442 Acquired absence of left ankle**

▤ **IQ Z89.449 Acquired absence of unspecified ankle**

⑤ **Z89.5 Acquired absence of leg below knee**

⑥ **Z89.51 Acquired absence of leg below knee**

▤ **IQ Z89.511 Acquired absence of right leg below knee**

▤ **IQ Z89.512 Acquired absence of left leg below knee**

▤ **IQ Z89.519 Acquired absence of unspecified leg below knee**

⑥ **Z89.52 Acquired absence of knee**
Acquired absence of knee joint following explanation of knee joint prosthesis, with or without presence of antibiotic-impregnated cement spacer

▤ **IQ Z89.521 Acquired absence of right knee**

▤ **IQ Z89.522 Acquired absence of left knee**

▤ **IQ Z89.529 Acquired absence of unspecified knee**

⑤ **Z89.6 Acquired absence of leg above knee**

⑥ **Z89.61 Acquired absence of leg above knee**
Acquired absence of leg NOS
Disarticulation at knee

▤ **IQ Z89.611 Acquired absence of right leg above knee**

▤ **IQ Z89.612 Acquired absence of left leg above knee**

★ New ▲ Revised **Px** Primary **SP** PDGM Px **SL** Low CoM **SH** High CoM **IQ** Quest. Encounter ⊞ Hospice non-cancer Dx   Unspecified   **M** *Manifestation*

DecisionHealth's FY 2020 Complete Home Health ICD-10-CM Diagnosis Coding Manual

1923

☐ !Q **Z89.619 Acquired absence of unspecified leg above knee**

6 **Z89.62 Acquired absence of hip**
Acquired absence of hip joint
following explantation of hip joint
prosthesis, with or without presence
of antibiotic-impregnated cement
spacer
Disarticulation at hip

☐ !Q **Z89.621 Acquired absence of right hip joint**

☐ !Q **Z89.622 Acquired absence of left hip joint**

☐ !Q **Z89.629 Acquired absence of unspecified hip joint**

!Q **Z89.9 Acquired absence of limb, unspecified**

4 **Z90 Acquired absence of organs, not elsewhere classified**

> INCLUDES   postprocedural or post-traumatic loss of body part NEC

> EXCLUDES 1   congenital absence - see Alphabetical Index

> EXCLUDES 2   postprocedural absence of endocrine glands (E89.-)

> CODING TIPS ✓   These codes are used to indicate a new or old surgical removal of that particular body part. They are not used for congenital absence.

5 **Z90.0 Acquired absence of part of head and neck**

!Q **Z90.01 Acquired absence of eye**

!Q **Z90.02 Acquired absence of larynx**

!Q **Z90.09 Acquired absence of other part of head and neck**
Acquired absence of nose
> EXCLUDES 2   teeth (K08.1)

5 **Z90.1 Acquired absence of breast and nipple**

☐ !Q **Z90.10 Acquired absence of unspecified breast and nipple**

☐ !Q **Z90.11 Acquired absence of right breast and nipple**

☐ !Q **Z90.12 Acquired absence of left breast and nipple**

☐ !Q **Z90.13 Acquired absence of bilateral breasts and nipples**

!Q **Z90.2 Acquired absence of lung [part of]**

!Q **Z90.3 Acquired absence of stomach [part of]**

5 **Z90.4 Acquired absence of other specified parts of digestive tract**

▲ ✚ 6 **Z90.41 Acquired absence of pancreas**
Code also:
exocrine pancreatic insufficiency
(K86.81)
Use additional code to identify any
associated:
diabetes mellitus,
postpancreatectomy (E13.-)
insulin use (Z79.4)

> GUIDELINES   Section I.C.4.a.6)(b)(i)
For postpancreatectomy diabetes
mellitus (lack of insulin due to the
surgical removal of all or part of the
pancreas), assign code E89.1,
Postprocedural hypoinsulinemia. Assign
a code from category E13 and a code
from subcategory Z90.41-, Acquired
absence of pancreas, as additional
codes.

!Q ✚ **Z90.410 Acquired total absence of pancreas**
Acquired absence of pancreas NOS

!Q ✚ **Z90.411 Acquired partial absence of pancreas**

!Q **Z90.49 Acquired absence of other specified parts of digestive tract**

!Q **Z90.5 Acquired absence of kidney**

!Q **Z90.6 Acquired absence of other parts of urinary tract**
Acquired absence of bladder

5 **Z90.7 Acquired absence of genital organ(s)**
> EXCLUDES 1   personal history of sex reassignment (Z87.890)
> EXCLUDES 2   female genital mutilation status (N90.81-)

6 **Z90.71 Acquired absence of cervix and uterus**

!Q **Z90.710 Acquired absence of both cervix and uterus**
Acquired absence of uterus NOS
Status post total hysterectomy

!Q **Z90.711 Acquired absence of uterus with remaining cervical stump**
Status post partial hysterectomy
with remaining cervical stump

!Q **Z90.712 Acquired absence of cervix with remaining uterus**

6 **Z90.72 Acquired absence of ovaries**

!Q **Z90.721 Acquired absence of ovaries, unilateral**

!Q **Z90.722 Acquired absence of ovaries, bilateral**

!Q **Z90.79 Acquired absence of other genital organ(s)**

5 **Z90.8 Acquired absence of other organs**

!Q **Z90.81 Acquired absence of spleen**

!Q **Z90.89 Acquired absence of other organs**

4 **Z91 Personal risk factors, not elsewhere classified**
> EXCLUDES 2   contact with and (suspected) exposures hazardous to health (Z77.-)
exposure to pollution and other problems related to physical environment (Z77.1-)
female genital mutilation status (N90.81-)
personal history of physical injury and trauma (Z87.81, Z87.82-)
occupational exposure to risk factors (Z57.-)

5 **Z91.0 Allergy status, other than to drugs and biological substances**

4 4th digit required   5 5th digit required   6 6th digit required   7 7th digit required   7 7th digit placeholder   ✚ Additional code   ☐ Laterality

1924   *DecisionHealth's* FY 2020 Complete Home Health ICD-10-CM Diagnosis Coding Manual

EXCLUDES 2 Allergy status to drugs, medicaments, and biological substances (Z88.-)

⑥ **Z91.01 Food allergy status**
EXCLUDES 2 food additives allergy status (Z91.02)

IQ **Z91.010 Allergy to peanuts**

IQ **Z91.011 Allergy to milk products**
EXCLUDES 1 lactose intolerance (E73.-)

IQ **Z91.012 Allergy to eggs**

IQ **Z91.013 Allergy to seafood**
Allergy to shellfish
Allergy to octopus or squid ink

IQ **Z91.018 Allergy to other foods**
Allergy to nuts other than peanuts

IQ **Z91.02 Food additives allergy status**

⑥ **Z91.03 Insect allergy status**

IQ **Z91.030 Bee allergy status**

IQ **Z91.038 Other insect allergy status**

⑥ **Z91.04 Nonmedicinal substance allergy status**

IQ **Z91.040 Latex allergy status**
Latex sensitivity status

IQ **Z91.041 Radiographic dye allergy status**
Allergy status to contrast media used for diagnostic X-ray procedure

IQ **Z91.048 Other nonmedicinal substance allergy status**

IQ **Z91.09 Other allergy status, other than to drugs and biological substances**

⑤ **Z91.1 Patient's noncompliance with medical treatment and regimen**
CODING TIPS ✓ Be careful regarding use of noncompliance codes. Noncompliance may be a reason for initiating care, but continued noncompliance after teaching interventions have been completed usually indicates a lack of medical necessity. The exception is intentional or unintentional underdosing of medications. Underdosing codes are sequenced after the condition not being adequately treated and the T36-T50 code for underdosing, to explain the reason for underdosing.

IQ **Z91.11 Patient's noncompliance with dietary regimen**

⑥ **Z91.12 Patient's intentional underdosing of medication regimen**
Code first:
underdosing of medication (T36-T50) with fifth or sixth character 6
EXCLUDES 1 adverse effect of prescribed drug taken as directed- code to adverse effect poisoning (overdose) -code to poisoning

GUIDELINES Section I.C.19.e.5)(c)
Noncompliance (Z91.12-, Z91.13- and Z91.14-) or complication of care (Y63.6-Y63.9) codes are to be used with an underdosing code to indicate intent, if known.

CODING TIPS ✓ A code from Z91.12- or Z91.13- should be assigned when underdosing has been identified and coded in the plan of care/medical record.

IQ **Z91.120 Patient's intentional underdosing of medication regimen due to financial hardship**

IQ **Z91.128 Patient's intentional underdosing of medication regimen for other reason**

⑥ **Z91.13 Patient's unintentional underdosing of medication regimen**
Code first:
underdosing of medication (T36-T50) with fifth or sixth character 6
EXCLUDES 1 adverse effect of prescribed drug taken as directed- code to adverse effect poisoning (overdose) -code to poisoning

GUIDELINES Section I.C.19.e.5)(c)
Noncompliance (Z91.12-, Z91.13- and Z91.14-) or complication of care (Y63.6-Y63.9) codes are to be used with an underdosing code to indicate intent, if known.

CODING TIPS ✓ A code from Z91.12- or Z91.13- should be assigned when underdosing has been identified and coded in the plan of care/medical record.

IQ **Z91.130 Patient's unintentional underdosing of medication regimen due to age-related debility**

IQ **Z91.138 Patient's unintentional underdosing of medication regimen for other reason**

IQ **Z91.14 Patient's other noncompliance with medication regimen**
Patient's underdosing of medication NOS
GUIDELINES Section I.C.19.e.5)(c)
Noncompliance (Z91.12-, Z91.13- and Z91.14-) or complication of care (Y63.6-Y63.9) codes are to be used with an underdosing code to indicate intent, if known.

IQ **Z91.15 Patient's noncompliance with renal dialysis**

IQ **Z91.19 Patient's noncompliance with other medical treatment and regimen**
Nonadherence to medical treatment

⑤ **Z91.4 Personal history of psychological trauma, not elsewhere classified**

★ New ▲ Revised Px Primary **SP** PDGM Px **SL** Low CoM **SH** High CoM **IQ** Quest. Encounter **H** Hospice non-cancer Dx Unspecified **M** *Manifestation*

DecisionHealth's FY 2020 Complete Home Health ICD-10-CM Diagnosis Coding Manual

1925

GUIDELINES   Section I.C.21.c.4)
There are two types of history Z codes, personal and family. Personal history codes explain a patient's past medical condition that no longer exists and is not receiving any treatment, but that has the potential for recurrence, and therefore may require continued monitoring.

Family history codes are for use when a patient has a family member(s) who has had a particular disease that causes the patient to be at higher risk of also contracting the disease. Personal history codes may be used in conjunction with follow-up codes and family history codes may be used in conjunction with screening codes to explain the need for a test or procedure. History codes are also acceptable on any medical record regardless of the reason for visit. A history of an illness, even if no longer present, is important information that may alter the type of treatment ordered.

6 **Z91.41   Personal history of adult abuse**
> **EXCLUDES 2**   personal history of abuse in childhood (Z62.81-)

IQ **Z91.410   Personal history of adult physical and sexual abuse**
> **EXCLUDES 1**   current adult physical abuse (T74.11, T76.11)
> current adult sexual abuse (T74.21, T76.11)

IQ **Z91.411   Personal history of adult psychological abuse**

IQ **Z91.412   Personal history of adult neglect**
> **EXCLUDES 1**   current adult neglect (T74.01, T76.01)

IQ **Z91.419   Personal history of unspecified adult abuse**

IQ **Z91.42   Personal history of forced labor or sexual exploitation**

IQ **Z91.49   Other personal history of psychological trauma, not elsewhere classified**

IQ **Z91.5   Personal history of self-harm**
> Personal history of parasuicide
> Personal history of self-poisoning
> Personal history of suicide attempt

5 **Z91.8   Other specified personal risk factors, not elsewhere classified**

IQ **Z91.81   History of falling**
> At risk for falling

GUIDELINES   Section I.C.21.c.4)
There are two types of history Z codes, personal and family. Personal history codes explain a patient's past medical condition that no longer exists and is not receiving any treatment, but that has the potential for recurrence, and therefore may require continued monitoring.

Family history codes are for use when a patient has a family member(s) who has had a particular disease that causes the patient to be at higher risk of also contracting the disease. Personal history codes may be used in conjunction with follow-up codes and family history codes may be used in conjunction with screening codes to explain the need for a test or procedure. History codes are also acceptable on any medical record regardless of the reason for visit. A history of an illness, even if no longer present, is important information that may alter the type of treatment ordered.

GUIDELINES   Section I.C.18.d
Code R29.6, Repeated falls, is for use for encounters when a patient has recently fallen and the reason for the fall is being investigated. Code Z91.81, History of falling, is for use when a patient has fallen in the past and is at risk for future falls. When appropriate, both codes R29.6 and Z91.81 may be assigned together.

CODING TIPS ✓   Use this code when a patient has fallen in the past and is at risk for future falls.

IQ **Z91.82   Personal history of military deployment**
> Individual (civilian or military) with past history of military war, peacekeeping and humanitarian deployment (current or past conflict)
> Returned from military deployment

IQ **Z91.83   Wandering in diseases classified elsewhere**
> Code first underlying disorder such as:
> Alzheimer's disease (G30.-)
> autism or pervasive developmental disorder (F84.-)
> intellectual disabilities (F70-F79)
> unspecified dementia with behavioral disturbance (F03.9-)

CODING TIPS ✓   Wandering is considered a behavior when coding dementia.

6 **Z91.84   Oral health risk factors**

IQ **Z91.841   Risk for dental caries, low**

IQ **Z91.842   Risk for dental caries, moderate**

IQ **Z91.843   Risk for dental caries, high**

IQ **Z91.849   Unspecified risk for dental caries**

IQ **Z91.89   Other specified personal risk factors, not elsewhere classified**

4 4th digit required   5 5th digit required   6 6th digit required   7 7th digit required   7 7th digit placeholder   + Additional code   ⊟ Laterality

1926   *DecisionHealth's* FY 2020 Complete Home Health ICD-10-CM Diagnosis Coding Manual

CODING TIPS ✓ Stage A of the ABCD Classification of the American College of Cardiology (ACC)/American Heart Association (AHA) is the presence of heart failure risk factors but no heart disease and no symptoms. This should not be coded to the regular heart failure codes, but rather to code Z91.89, Other specified personal risk factors, not elsewhere classified.

4 **Z92   Personal history of medical treatment**
   EXCLUDES 2   postprocedural states (Z98.-)

IQ **Z92.0   Personal history of contraception**
   EXCLUDES 1   counseling or management of current contraceptive practices (Z30.-)
   long term (current) use of contraception (Z79.3)
   presence of (intrauterine) contraceptive device (Z97.5)

5 **Z92.2   Personal history of drug therapy**
   EXCLUDES 2   long term (current) drug therapy (Z79.-)

IQ **Z92.21   Personal history of antineoplastic chemotherapy**

IQ **Z92.22   Personal history of monoclonal drug therapy**

IQ **Z92.23   Personal history of estrogen therapy**

6 **Z92.24   Personal history of steroid therapy**

IQ **Z92.240   Personal history of inhaled steroid therapy**

IQ **Z92.241   Personal history of systemic steroid therapy**
   Personal history of steroid therapy NOS

IQ **Z92.25   Personal history of immunosupression therapy**
   EXCLUDES 2   personal history of steroid therapy (Z92.24)

IQ **Z92.29   Personal history of other drug therapy**

IQ **Z92.3   Personal history of irradiation**
   Personal history of exposure to therapeutic radiation
   EXCLUDES 1   exposure to radiation in the physical environment (Z77.12)
   occupational exposure to radiation (Z57.1)

5 **Z92.8   Personal history of other medical treatment**

IQ **Z92.81   Personal history of extracorporeal membrane oxygenation (ECMO)**

IQ **Z92.82   Status post administration of tPA (rtPA) in a different facility within the last 24 hours prior to admission to current facility**
   Code first condition requiring tPA administration, such as:
   acute cerebral infarction (I63.-)
   acute myocardial infarction (I21.-, I22.-)

IQ **Z92.83   Personal history of failed moderate sedation**

Personal history of failed conscious sedation
   EXCLUDES 2   failed moderate sedation during procedure (T88.52)

IQ **Z92.84   Personal history of unintended awareness under general anesthesia**
   EXCLUDES 2   unintended awareness under general anesthesia during procedure (T88.53)

IQ **Z92.89   Personal history of other medical treatment**

4 **Z93   Artificial opening status**
   EXCLUDES 1   artificial openings requiring attention or management (Z43.-)
   complications of external stoma (J95.0-, K94.-, N99.5-)

CODING TIPS ✓ Assign codes from category Z93 to indicate artificial openings which are present but do not require intervention or management by the agency. Do not use codes in the Z93 category with attention to artificial opening codes (Z43) codes for the same ostomy or when the ostomy is complicated.

IQ **Z93.0   Tracheostomy status**

IQ **Z93.1   Gastrostomy status**

IQ **Z93.2   Ileostomy status**

IQ **Z93.3   Colostomy status**

IQ **Z93.4   Other artificial openings of gastrointestinal tract status**

5 **Z93.5   Cystostomy status**

IQ **Z93.50   Unspecified cystostomy status**

IQ **Z93.51   Cutaneous-vesicostomy status**

IQ **Z93.52   Appendico-vesicostomy status**

IQ **Z93.59   Other cystostomy status**

IQ **Z93.6   Other artificial openings of urinary tract status**
   Nephrostomy status
   Ureterostomy status
   Urethrostomy status

IQ **Z93.8   Other artificial opening status**

IQ **Z93.9   Artificial opening status, unspecified**

4 **Z94   Transplanted organ and tissue status**
   INCLUDES   organ or tissue replaced by heterogenous or homogenous transplant
   EXCLUDES 1   complications of transplanted organ or tissue - see Alphabetical Index
   EXCLUDES 2   presence of vascular grafts (Z95.-)

CODING TIPS ✓ These are status codes and are used to 1) indicate that a transplant has occurred in the past; and 2) to provide more information as to type of transplant, **if needed**, in the case of aftercare (Z48.2) or transplant complications (T86).

IQ **Z94.0   Kidney transplant status**

IQ **Z94.1   Heart transplant status**
   EXCLUDES 1   artificial heart status (Z95.812)
   heart-valve replacement status (Z95.2-Z95.4)

★ New ▲ Revised Px Primary SP PDGM Px SL Low CoM SH High CoM IQ Quest. Encounter H Hospice non-cancer Dx Unspecified M *Manifestation*

DecisionHealth's FY 2020 Complete Home Health ICD-10-CM Diagnosis Coding Manual

1927

Chapter 21

Z00-Z99

IQ Z94.2   Lung transplant status

IQ Z94.3   Heart and lungs transplant status

IQ Z94.4   Liver transplant status

IQ Z94.5   Skin transplant status
Autogenous skin transplant status

IQ Z94.6   Bone transplant status

IQ Z94.7   Corneal transplant status

5 Z94.8   Other transplanted organ and tissue status

IQ Z94.81   Bone marrow transplant status

IQ Z94.82   Intestine transplant status

IQ Z94.83   Pancreas transplant status

IQ Z94.84   Stem cells transplant status

IQ Z94.89   Other transplanted organ and tissue status

IQ Z94.9   Transplanted organ and tissue status, unspecified

4 Z95   Presence of cardiac and vascular implants and grafts

> **EXCLUDES 2**   complications of cardiac and vascular devices, implants and grafts (T82.-)

> **CODING TIPS ✓**   Assign codes from this category with the aftercare code Z48.812 to provide more information on the aftercare, or alone when aftercare is no longer required. Do not use these codes if there is a complication. If there has been an angioplasty without a stent or implant, see Z98.6.

IQ Z95.0   Presence of cardiac pacemaker
Presence of cardiac resynchronization therapy (CRT-P) pacemaker

> **EXCLUDES 1**   adjustment or management of cardiac device (Z45.0-)
> adjustment or management of cardiac pacemaker (Z45.0)
> presence of automatic (implantable) cardiac defibrillator with synchronous cardiac pacemaker (Z95.810)

IQ Z95.1   Presence of aortocoronary bypass graft
Presence of coronary artery bypass graft

> **CODING TIPS ✓**   Z95.1 and Z95.5 are used to indicate the presence of a coronary bypass grafts and implants without complications. If complications are documented, see T82.2-.

IQ Z95.2   Presence of prosthetic heart valve
Presence of heart valve NOS

> **CODING TIPS ✓**   Code Z95.2 is used to indicate the presence of a heart valve prosthesis without complications. If complications are documented, see T82.0-.

IQ Z95.3   Presence of xenogenic heart valve

IQ Z95.4   Presence of other heart-valve replacement

IQ Z95.5   Presence of coronary angioplasty implant and graft

> **EXCLUDES 1**   coronary angioplasty status without implant and graft (Z98.61)

> **CODING TIPS ✓**   Z95.1 and Z95.5 are used to indicate the presence of a coronary bypass grafts and implants without complications. If complications are documented, see T82.2-.

5 Z95.8   Presence of other cardiac and vascular implants and grafts

6 Z95.81   Presence of other cardiac implants and grafts

> **CODING TIPS ✓**   Do not use these codes if the condition is complicated, unless the status code provides information about the specific type of device. See T82 for complications.

IQ Z95.810   Presence of automatic (implantable) cardiac defibrillator
Presence of automatic (implantable) cardiac defibrillator with synchronous cardiac pacemaker
Presence of cardiac resynchronization therapy defibrillator (CRT-D)
Presence of cardioverter-defibrillator (ICD)

> **CODING TIPS ✓**   This code is generally accepted for the coding of the presence of a "vest."

IQ Z95.811   Presence of heart assist device

> **CODING TIPS ✓**   This code is generally accepted for the coding of the presence of a LVAD.

IQ Z95.812   Presence of fully implantable artificial heart

IQ Z95.818   Presence of other cardiac implants and grafts

> **CODING TIPS ✓**   This code is generally accepted for the coding of the presence of a loop recorder.

6 Z95.82   Presence of other vascular implants and grafts

IQ Z95.820   Peripheral vascular angioplasty status with implants and grafts

> **EXCLUDES 1**   peripheral vascular angioplasty without implant and graft (Z98.62)

IQ Z95.828   Presence of other vascular implants and grafts
Presence of intravascular prosthesis NEC

IQ Z95.9   Presence of cardiac and vascular implant and graft, unspecified

4 Z96   Presence of other functional implants

> **EXCLUDES 2**   complications of internal prosthetic devices, implants and grafts (T82-T85)
> fitting and adjustment of prosthetic and other devices (Z44-Z46)

IQ Z96.0   Presence of urogenital implants

IQ Z96.1   Presence of intraocular lens
Presence of pseudophakia

5 Z96.2   Presence of otological and audiological implants

IQ Z96.20   Presence of otological and audiological implant, unspecified

IQ Z96.21   Cochlear implant status

---

4 4th digit required   **5** 5th digit required   **6** 6th digit required   **7** 7th digit required   **7** 7th digit placeholder   **+** Additional code   **⊟** Laterality

IQ Z96.22 Myringotomy tube(s) status

IQ Z96.29 Presence of other otological and audiological implants
Presence of bone-conduction hearing device
Presence of eustachian tube stent
Stapes replacement

IQ Z96.3 Presence of artificial larynx

5 Z96.4 Presence of endocrine implants

IQ Z96.41 Presence of insulin pump (external) (internal)

CODING TIPS ✓ If the patient uses an insulin pump, use Z96.41 as an secondary code. If there is a complication involving the insulin pump, use a code from T85.6- or T85.7- instead of the Z code.

IQ Z96.49 Presence of other endocrine implants

IQ Z96.5 Presence of tooth-root and mandibular implants

5 Z96.6 Presence of orthopedic joint implants

CODING TIPS ✓ Codes from Z96.6- should be assigned with aftercare code Z47.1. They also may be assigned to indicate the presence of a prosthetic joint even after no care is needed. When a joint replacement is performed to repair a fracture, code the fracture with a 7th character D and use the Z96.6 code to indicate the presence of the joint prosthesis. When a complication is present to a joint prosthesis, assign a complication code from category T84.-, which will identify the joint replaced, as well as the complication. No Z96.6- code is required when a complication is present if the joint is identified in the complication code. If the patient has bilateral joint replacements of the same joint, the coder may assign the bilateral code, or separate codes if the joints were replaced in different encounters.

IQ Z96.60 Presence of unspecified orthopedic joint implant

6 Z96.61 Presence of artificial shoulder joint

IQ Z96.611 Presence of right artificial shoulder joint

IQ Z96.612 Presence of left artificial shoulder joint

IQ Z96.619 Presence of unspecified artificial shoulder joint

6 Z96.62 Presence of artificial elbow joint

IQ Z96.621 Presence of right artificial elbow joint

IQ Z96.622 Presence of left artificial elbow joint

IQ Z96.629 Presence of unspecified artificial elbow joint

6 Z96.63 Presence of artificial wrist joint

IQ Z96.631 Presence of right artificial wrist joint

IQ Z96.632 Presence of left artificial wrist joint

IQ Z96.639 Presence of unspecified artificial wrist joint

6 Z96.64 Presence of artificial hip joint

Hip-joint replacement (partial) (total)

IQ Z96.641 Presence of right artificial hip joint

IQ Z96.642 Presence of left artificial hip joint

IQ Z96.643 Presence of artificial hip joint, bilateral

IQ Z96.649 Presence of unspecified artificial hip joint

6 Z96.65 Presence of artificial knee joint

IQ Z96.651 Presence of right artificial knee joint

IQ Z96.652 Presence of left artificial knee joint

IQ Z96.653 Presence of artificial knee joint, bilateral

IQ Z96.659 Presence of unspecified artificial knee joint

6 Z96.66 Presence of artificial ankle joint

IQ Z96.661 Presence of right artificial ankle joint

IQ Z96.662 Presence of left artificial ankle joint

IQ Z96.669 Presence of unspecified artificial ankle joint

6 Z96.69 Presence of other orthopedic joint implants

IQ Z96.691 Finger-joint replacement of right hand

IQ Z96.692 Finger-joint replacement of left hand

IQ Z96.693 Finger-joint replacement, bilateral

IQ Z96.698 Presence of other orthopedic joint implants

IQ Z96.7 Presence of other bone and tendon implants
Presence of skull plate

5 Z96.8 Presence of other specified functional implants

IQ Z96.81 Presence of artificial skin

★ Z96.82 Presence of neurostimulator
Presence of brain neurostimulator
Presence of gastric neurostimulator
Presence of peripheral nerve neurostimulator
Presence of sacral nerve neurostimulator
Presence of spinal cord neurostimulator
Presence of vagus nerve neurostimulator

IQ Z96.89 Presence of other specified functional implants

IQ Z96.9 Presence of functional implant, unspecified

▲ 4 Z97 Presence of other devices

EXCLUDES 1 complications of internal prosthetic devices, implants and grafts (T82-T85)

EXCLUDES 2 fitting and adjustment of prosthetic and other devices (Z44-Z46)
presence of cerebrospinal fluid drainage device (Z98.2)

IQ Z97.0 Presence of artificial eye

5 Z97.1 Presence of artificial limb (complete) (partial)

★ New ▲ Revised Px Primary **SP** PDGM Px **SL** Low CoM **SH** High CoM **IQ** Quest. Encounter **H** Hospice non-cancer Dx Unspecified **M** *Manifestation*

DecisionHealth's FY 2020 Complete Home Health ICD-10-CM Diagnosis Coding Manual

1929

Chapter 21

Z00-Z99

🔲 **IQ** **Z97.10** **Presence of artificial limb (complete) (partial), unspecified**

🔲 **IQ** **Z97.11** **Presence of artificial right arm (complete) (partial)**

🔲 **IQ** **Z97.12** **Presence of artificial left arm (complete) (partial)**

🔲 **IQ** **Z97.13** **Presence of artificial right leg (complete) (partial)**

🔲 **IQ** **Z97.14** **Presence of artificial left leg (complete) (partial)**

🔲 **IQ** **Z97.15** **Presence of artificial arms, bilateral (complete) (partial)**

🔲 **IQ** **Z97.16** **Presence of artificial legs, bilateral (complete) (partial)**

IQ **Z97.2** **Presence of dental prosthetic device (complete) (partial)**
Presence of dentures (complete) (partial)

IQ **Z97.3** **Presence of spectacles and contact lenses**

IQ **Z97.4** **Presence of external hearing-aid**

IQ **Z97.5** **Presence of (intrauterine) contraceptive device**
> **EXCLUDES 1** checking, reinsertion or removal of implantable subdermal contraceptive (Z30.46)
> checking, reinsertion or removal of intrauterine contraceptive device (Z30.43-)

IQ **Z97.8** **Presence of other specified devices**

4 **Z98** **Other postprocedural states**
> **EXCLUDES 2** aftercare (Z43-Z49, Z51)
> follow-up medical care (Z08-Z09)
> postprocedural complication - see Alphabetical Index

IQ **Z98.0** **Intestinal bypass and anastomosis status**
> **EXCLUDES 2** bariatric surgery status (Z98.84)
> gastric bypass status (Z98.84)
> obesity surgery status (Z98.84)

IQ **Z98.1** **Arthrodesis status**
> **CODING TIPS ✓** Ankylosis of the joint is caused by arthritis, traumatic injury or infection. The joint will assume the least painful position and become permanently fixed. A surgical fusion is coded Z98.1.
> **CODING TIPS ✓** If spinal fusion has taken place, also use a code from M43.2-.

IQ **Z98.2** **Presence of cerebrospinal fluid drainage device**
Presence of CSF shunt
> **CODING TIPS ✓** Do not use this code if the condition is complicated. See T85.0-.

IQ **Z98.3** **Post therapeutic collapse of lung status**
Code first:
> underlying disease

+ **5** **Z98.4** **Cataract extraction status**
Use additional code to identify intraocular lens implant status (Z96.1)
> **EXCLUDES 1** aphakia (H27.0)

🔲 **IQ** **+** **Z98.41** **Cataract extraction status, right eye**

🔲 **IQ** **+** **Z98.42** **Cataract extraction status, left eye**

🔲 **IQ** **+** **Z98.49** **Cataract extraction status, unspecified eye**

5 **Z98.5** **Sterilization status**
> **EXCLUDES 1** female infertility (N97.-)
> male infertility (N46.-)

IQ **Z98.51** **Tubal ligation status**

IQ **Z98.52** **Vasectomy status**

5 **Z98.6** **Angioplasty status**
> **CODING TIPS ✓** Assign codes from this category with the aftercare code Z48.812 to provide more information on the aftercare, or alone when aftercare is no longer required. Do not use these codes if there is a complication.

IQ **Z98.61** **Coronary angioplasty status**
> **EXCLUDES 1** coronary angioplasty status with implant and graft (Z95.5)

IQ **Z98.62** **Peripheral vascular angioplasty status**
> **EXCLUDES 1** peripheral vascular angioplasty status with implant and graft (Z95.820)

5 **Z98.8** **Other specified postprocedural states**

6 **Z98.81** **Dental procedure status**

IQ **Z98.810** **Dental sealant status**

IQ **Z98.811** **Dental restoration status**
Dental crown status
Dental fillings status

IQ **Z98.818** **Other dental procedure status**

IQ **Z98.82** **Breast implant status**
> **EXCLUDES 1** breast implant removal status (Z98.86)

IQ **Z98.83** **Filtering (vitreous) bleb after glaucoma surgery status**
> **EXCLUDES 1** Inflammation (infection) of postprocedural bleb (H59.4-)

IQ **Z98.84** **Bariatric surgery status**
Gastric banding status
Gastric bypass status for obesity
Obesity surgery status
> **EXCLUDES 1** bariatric surgery status complicating pregnancy, childbirth, or the puerperium (O99.84)
> **EXCLUDES 2** intestinal bypass and anastomosis status (Z98.0)
> **CODING TIPS ✓** Code Z98.84 is not appropriate if there is a complication. Use a code from K95 instead.

IQ **Z98.85** **Transplanted organ removal status**
Transplanted organ previously removed due to complication, failure, rejection or infection
> **EXCLUDES 1** encounter for removal of transplanted organ -code to complication of transplanted organ (T86.-)

---

4 4th digit required   **5** 5th digit required   **6** 6th digit required   **7** 7th digit required   **7** 7th digit placeholder   **+** Additional code   🔲 Laterality

1930   *DecisionHealth's* FY 2020 Complete Home Health ICD-10-CM Diagnosis Coding Manual

GUIDELINES Section I.C.21.c.3)

Assign code Z98.85, Transplanted organ removal status, to indicate that a transplanted organ has been previously removed. This code should not be assigned for the encounter in which the transplanted organ is removed. The complication necessitating removal of the transplant organ should be assigned for that encounter.

IQ Z98.86 Personal history of breast implant removal

6 Z98.87 Personal history of in utero procedure

IQ Z98.870 Personal history of in utero procedure during pregnancy
  EXCLUDES 2 complications from in utero procedure for current pregnancy (O35.7)
  supervision of current pregnancy with history of in utero procedure during previous pregnancy (O09.82-)

IQ Z98.871 Personal history of in utero procedure while a fetus

6 Z98.89 Other specified postprocedural states

IQ Z98.890 Other specified postprocedural states
  Personal history of surgery, not elsewhere classified

IQ Z98.891 History of uterine scar from previous surgery
  EXCLUDES 1 Maternal care due to uterine scar from previous surgery (O34.2-)

4 Z99 Dependence on enabling machines and devices, not elsewhere classified
  EXCLUDES 1 cardiac pacemaker status (Z95.0)

SP Z99.0 Dependence on aspirator

5 Z99.1 Dependence on respirator
  Dependence on ventilator

SP Z99.11 Dependence on respirator [ventilator] status

Px IQ Z99.12 Encounter for respirator [ventilator] dependence during power failure
  EXCLUDES 1 mechanical complication of respirator [ventilator] (J95.850)

IQ Z99.2 Dependence on renal dialysis
  Hemodialysis status
  Peritoneal dialysis status
  Presence of arteriovenous shunt for dialysis
  Renal dialysis status NOS
  EXCLUDES 1 encounter for fitting and adjustment of dialysis catheter (Z49.0-)
  EXCLUDES 2 noncompliance with renal dialysis (Z91.15)

IQ Z99.3 Dependence on wheelchair
  Wheelchair confinement status
  Code first cause of dependence, such as:
    muscular dystrophy (G71.0-)
    obesity (E66.-)
  CODING TIPS ✓ Code Z74.09 may be used in conjunction with this code.

5 Z99.8 Dependence on other enabling machines and devices

IQ Z99.81 Dependence on supplemental oxygen
  Dependence on long-term oxygen

IQ Z99.89 Dependence on other enabling machines and devices
  Dependence on machine or device NOS

★ New ▲ Revised Px Primary SP PDGM Px SL Low CoM SH High CoM IQ Quest. Encounter H Hospice non-cancer Dx Unspecified M *Manifestation*

DecisionHealth's FY 2020 Complete Home Health ICD-10-CM Diagnosis Coding Manual

1931

Chapter 21 Scenarios: Factors influencing health status and contact with health services (Z00-Z99)

Joint replacement

A 70-year-old male patient is admitted to home health for physical therapy following a second right knee replacement for bilateral primary osteoarthritis. The patient had previously had a knee replacement but the prosthetic joint became infected and had to be removed. He was treated with antibiotics and the infection completely resolved prior to the placement of the new right knee prosthesis. He still suffers from osteoarthritis in his left knee and will undergo a left knee replacement in the near future.

Description	Code
Primary: Aftercare following explantation of knee joint prosthesis	Z47.33
Secondary: Unilateral primary osteoarthritis, left knee	M17.12
Secondary: Presence of right artificial knee joint	Z96.651

Because the complication (the infection) resolved completely prior to the placement of the second right knee prosthesis and thus the patient's care is routine, Z47.33 is the appropriate primary code choice. The right knee replacement resolved the primary osteoarthritis in his right knee, but it is still in his left knee and will impact his care. Therefore it is coded as a secondary diagnosis. The Z96.651 code is assigned to capture the presence of the right prosthetic knee joint.

Post pulmonary embolectomy

The patient developed chest pain, severe shortness of breath, and was hospitalized. Pulmonary scans and arteriograms revealed that more than half of the major pulmonary arteries were occluded; smaller vessels also were obstructed. Pulmonary embolectomy was performed on major vessels. The patient was sent home on Coumadin. The patient has a history of chronic emphysematous bronchitis and hypertension. Home health orders are for wound care, teaching of the disease process, meds and lab draws for PT/INR.

Description	Code
Primary: Aftercare following surgery of circulatory system	Z48.812
Secondary: Other pulmonary embolism without acute cor pulmonale	I26.99
Secondary: Chronic obstructive pulmonary disease, unspecified	J44.9
Secondary: Essential primary hypertension	I10
Secondary: Therapeutic drug monitoring	Z51.81
Secondary: Long term use of anticoagulants	Z79.01

Although the embolectomy removed occlusions of the major vessels, this patient continues to have occlusions of the small vessels and is undergoing treatment. Thus, I26.99 is still coded. Do not use the history code (Z86.711) in the presence of the acute diagnosis. The chronic emphysematous bronchitis and hypertension are coded as relevant comorbidities. Monitoring of PT/INR and use of anticoagulants are also captured with Z51.81 and Z79.01.

Surgical aftercare, hip replacement

A patient is admitted for surgical aftercare following right hip joint replacement due to primary generalized osteoarthritis.

Description	Code
Primary: Aftercare following joint replacement surgery	Z47.1
Secondary: Primary generalized (osteo)arthritis	M15.0
Secondary: Presence of right artificial hip joint	Z96.641

Code Z47.1 (Aftercare following joint replacement surgery) does not specify the joint replaced. So it does require the use of an additional code to identify the joint (Z96.641). The code title includes laterality. Primary generalized arthritis continues to be assigned even after the joint replacement because it is generalized and therefore occurs in more than just the joint that was just replaced. Thus it is still an active diagnosis.

Surgical aftercare, shoulder replacement

A patient had a right shoulder joint replacement due to localized degenerative joint disease (DJD) in that shoulder. Nursing and therapy are ordered for aftercare.

Description	Code
Primary: Aftercare following joint replacement surgery	Z47.1
Secondary: Presence of right artificial shoulder joint	Z96.611

Aftercare following replacement of a joint (Z47.- category) should be listed as the primary diagnosis. Tabular instructions note this code identifies that a joint has been replaced but a second code needs to be added to identify which joint was replaced. Even though the Z96.611 code is a status code, it is categorized in the Alphabetic Index under the main term "presence." The condition treated also should be coded if still present. In this example, the condition (localized DJD) resolved with the surgery and would not be listed.

Amputation due to PVD

A 70-year-old patient is admitted with a below the knee right leg amputation due to peripheral vascular disease (PVD).

Description	Code
Primary: Encounter for orthopedic aftercare following surgical amputation	Z47.81
Secondary: Peripheral vascular disease, unspecified	I73.9
Secondary: Acquired absence of right leg below knee	Z89.511

The amputation is done because of the PVD but it does not resolve the condition. Therefore, it should still be coded. A code from Z89.- is assigned to identify the amputated limb, according to tabular instruction.

Infected left hip replacement

A 68-year-old female patient was admitted to home care with an infected left hip prosthesis. Home health orders include IV antibiotics, and peak and trough in addition to the wound care.

Description	Code
Primary: Infection and inflammatory reaction due to internal left hip prosthesis, initial encounter	T84.52xA
Secondary: Encounter for adjustment and management of vascular access device	Z45.2
Secondary: Encounter for therapeutic drug level monitoring	Z51.81
Secondary: Long term (current) use of antibiotics	Z79.2

The hip replacement is complicated and therefore an aftercare code is not appropriate. The patient continues to receive active treatment for the complication, necessitating the use of an initial encounter seventh encounter. Codes Z45.2, Z51.81 and Z79.2 are included to capture the IV antibiotics and peak and trough measuring.

New ileostomy, diabetes

A patient is admitted to home health with a newly created ileostomy and is currently unable to independently care for the ostomy. He has a history of prostate cancer, now resolved, and is being treated for diabetes, which is diet-controlled.

Description	Code
Primary: Encounter for attention to ileostomy	Z43.2
Secondary: Type 2 diabetes mellitus without complications	E11.9
Secondary: Personal history of malignant neoplasm of prostate	Z85.46

In this scenario, a code from "encounter for attention to" (Z43.2) is used because the agency will be providing hands-on care and teaching for this patient who needs assistance with his new ileostomy.

Mitral valve replacement

A 72-year-old man complained of increasing shortness of breath during a routine doctor's appointment. A cardiovascular workup revealed severe mitral valve stenosis that a cardiologist determined needed immediate treatment. Shortly thereafter, he underwent surgery to replace the damaged valve with a prosthetic one, which resolved the mitral valve disease. He also has hypertension and is on Coumadin.

Description	Code
Primary: Encounter for surgical aftercare following surgery on the circulatory system	Z48.812
Secondary: Essential (primary) hypertension	I10
Secondary: Presence of prosthetic heart valve	Z95.2
Secondary: Long term (current) use of anticoagulants	Z79.01

The patient underwent heart valve replacement surgery. The condition that necessitated the procedure, mitral valve stenosis, affects the circulatory system. Therefore, the correct surgical aftercare code is Z48.812. As the focus of the home health admission Z48.812 is coded in the primary position. The heart valve replacement surgery resolved the heart valve disease and thus that condition is not coded as an active condition. The status code Z95.2 is assigned to indicate the presence of the patient's prosthetic valve. The fact that the patient is taking Coumadin needs to be captured with Z79.01.

Hip replacement, history of breast cancer, use of Tamoxifen

A 68-year-old woman comes to home health for surgical aftercare following a right hip replacement to treat localized traumatic arthritis. Her medical record states that she has a history of breast cancer in her right breast from five years ago. She underwent a bilateral mastectomy and additional treatment with chemotherapy and radiation. Her treatment was completed four years ago. She continues to take tamoxifen but her history and physical states that it is prescribed prophylactically and she is receiving no active treatment for the cancer.

Description	Code
Primary: Aftercare following joint replacement surgery	Z47.1
Secondary: Presence of right artificial hip joint	Z96.641
Secondary: Personal history of malignant neoplasm of breast	Z85.3
Secondary: Long term (current) use of selective estrogen receptor modulators (SERMs)	Z79.810
Secondary: Acquired absence of bilateral breasts and nipples	Z90.13

As the focus of care the surgical aftercare is coded primary and an additional code to capture the replaced joint is assigned in accordance with tabular instruction. Traumatic arthritis is not coded as it was said to be localized and was thus resolved by the joint replacement procedure. The patient is no longer undergoing treatment for breast cancer and is taking tamoxifen prophylactically, thus making the use of the history code for breast cancer appropriate, versus a code for active cancer. Her long-term use of tamoxifen is captured with Z79.810. Finally, Z90.13 is assigned to capture the absence of her breasts due to bilateral mastectomy.

Out of control diabetes

A 57-year-old man comes to home health with diabetes that is out of control. His history and physician states that the patient admitted to being unable to read and as a result, wasn't able to read his glipizide medication instructions, which led to his dangerously high blood sugar levels because he was taking far less than the prescribed daily dosage. He will receive skilled nursing and medical social work services.

Description	Code
Primary: Type 2 diabetes mellitus with hyperglycemia	E11.65
Secondary: Underdosing of insulin and oral hypoglycemic [antidiabetic] drugs, subsequent encounter	T38.3x6D
Secondary: Patient's unintentional underdosing of medication regimen for other reason	Z91.138
Secondary: Illiteracy and low-level literacy	Z55.0
Secondary: Long term (current) use of oral hypoglycemic drugs	Z79.84

The patient unintentionally underdosed his diabetes medications because he couldn't read the instructions, leading to his diabetes becoming out of control. Out of control diabetes codes to diabetes with hyperglycemia, according to the alphabetic index. The code for underdosing of the drug is coded next, in accordance with coding guidelines. Code Z91.138 helps explain why the patient experienced an underdosing and Z55.0 is assigned to capture that the patient struggles with literacy. Codes in categories Z55 to Z65 can be assigned based on clinician, versus physician, documentation, according to Q1 2018 Coding Clinic guidance. The patient's use of oral hypoglycemic medication is captured with Z79.84.

Old MI with symptoms

An 81-year-old man suffered an ST-elevation MI five weeks ago and is returning home, with home health support, after being in rehab following his hospitalization. He continues to suffer from symptoms related to the MI, including chest pain and dyspnea, which will be the focus of care. His record does not indicate anywhere that he's been diagnosed with coronary artery disease (CAD) or any other form of heart disease. His physician did not return repeated calls for further information on the chest pain and dyspnea symptoms. His panic disorder, newly diagnosed after the heart attack, will be the focus of care.

Description	Code
Primary: Panic disorder [episodic paroxysmal anxiety]	F41.0
Secondary: Chest pain, unspecified	R07.9
Secondary: Dyspnea, unspecified	R06.00
Secondary: Encounter for other specified aftercare	Z51.89

His newly-diagnosed panic disorder is the focus of care and is coded first. He is still receiving care following the MI, though is it no longer considered an acute condition being more than four weeks old, so Z51.89 is coded to indicate that he's still experiencing symptoms related to the MI, in accordance with official coding guidelines and Coding Clinic guidance. Though a diagnosis of CAD is a possibility, it is not coded because the record didn't indicate it and the physician could not be reached to confirm it. Note that symptom codes for chest pain and dyspnea are unacceptable as primary diagnoses under PDGM.

Stage A heart failure

A 77-year-old woman is admitted to home health following hospitalization for exacerbated emphysema and COPD. Her record states she has also been diagnosed with Stage A failure. The emphysema is the focus of care. She is dependent on oxygen and was a smoker for 22 years but quit three years ago.

Description	Code
Primary: Emphysema, unspecified	J43.9
Secondary: Dependence on supplemental oxygen	Z99.81
Secondary: Personal history of nicotine dependence	Z87.891
Secondary: Other specified personal risk factors, not elsewhere classified	Z91.89

A diagnosed specified as "emphysema and COPD" codes to J43.9, according to the alphabetic index. Even though the diagnosis is exacerbated, J43.9 is still the appropriate code, according to Q4 2017 and Q1 2019 Coding Clinic guidance. The fact that the patient used to smoke must be captured with Z87.891, according to tabular instruction. Her use of oxygen is captured with Z99.81. The patient has been diagnosed with Stage A heart failure, which indicates the presence of heart failure risk factors but is not a diagnosis of heart failure. Thus, Z91.89 (Other specified personal risk factors not elsewhere classified) is the correct code for this diagnosis.

Exacerbated heart failure, history of tuberculosis

An 83-year-old man is admitted to home health following hospitalization with acutely exacerbated chronic systolic congestive heart failure. He also has hypertension, chronic obstructive asthma and a history of resolved tuberculosis.

Description	Code
Primary: Hypertensive heart disease with heart failure	I11.0
Secondary: Acute on chronic combined systolic (congestive) and diastolic (congestive) heart failure	I50.43
Secondary: Chronic obstructive pulmonary disease, unspecified	J44.9
Secondary: Personal history of tuberculosis	Z86.11

The ICD-10 classification assumes a relationship between hypertension and heart failure. Thus, the patient's heart failure is coded as hypertensive heart disease, which requires first coding I11.0 followed by I50.43. Chronic obstructive asthma is coded with J44.9, according to the alphabetic index. Finally, Z86.11 is assigned to capture the patient's history of resolved tuberculosis.

HOME HEALTH CODING SCENARIOS

OASIS Guidance

The following is coding guidance from the OASIS Guidance Manual. To view the OASIS Manual and any updates issued, visit: *https://www.cms.gov/Medicare/ Quality-Initiatives-Patient-Assessment-Instruments/ HomeHealthQualityInits/HHQIOASISUserManual.html*

OASIS ITEM

(M1021/1023) Diagnoses and Symptom Control: List each diagnosis for which the patient is receiving home care in Column 1, and enter its ICD-10-CM code at the level of highest specificity in Column 2 (diagnosis codes only – no surgical or procedure codes allowed). Diagnoses are listed in the order that best reflects the seriousness of each condition and supports the disciplines and services provided. Rate the degree of symptom control for each condition in Column 2. ICD-10-CM sequencing requirements must be followed if multiple coding is indicated for any diagnoses.

Code each row according to the following directions for each column.

Column 1: Enter the description of the diagnosis. Sequencing of diagnoses should reflect the seriousness of each condition and support the disciplines and services provided.

Column 2: Enter the ICD-10-CM code for the condition described in Column 1 – no surgical or procedure codes allowed. Codes must be entered at the level of highest specificity and ICD-10-CM coding rules and sequencing requirements must be followed. Note that external cause codes (ICD-10-CM codes beginning with V, W, X, or Y) may not be reported in M1021 (Primary Diagnosis) but may be reported in M1023 (Secondary Diagnoses). Also note that when a Z-code is reported in Column 2, the code for the underlying condition can often be entered in Column 2, as long as it is an active on-going condition impacting home health care.

Rate the degree of symptom control for the condition listed in Column 1. Do not assign a symptom control rating if the diagnosis code is a V, W, X, Y or Z-code. Choose one value that represents the degree of symptom control appropriate for each diagnosis using the following scale:

0– Asymptomatic, no treatment needed at this time

1– Symptoms well controlled with current therapy

2– Symptoms controlled with difficulty, affecting daily functioning; patient needs ongoing monitoring

3– Symptoms poorly controlled; patient needs frequent adjustment in treatment and dose monitoring

4– Symptoms poorly controlled; history of re-hospitalizations

Note that the rating for symptom control in Column 2 should not be used to determine the sequencing of the diagnoses listed in Column 1. These are separate items and sequencing may not coincide.

ITEM INTENT

M1021: the intent of this item is to accurately report and code the patient's primary home health diagnosis and document the degree of symptom control for that diagnosis. The patient's primary home health diagnosis is defined as the chief reason the patient is receiving home care and the diagnosis most related to the current home health Plan of Care.

M1023: the intent of this item is to accurately report and code the patient's secondary home health diagnoses and document the degree of symptom control for each diagnosis. Secondary diagnoses are comorbid conditions that exist at the time of the assessment, that are actively addressed in the patient's Plan of Care, or that have the potential to affect the patient's responsiveness to treatment and rehabilitative prognosis.

TIME POINTS ITEM(S) COMPLETED

Start of care

Resumption of care

Follow-up

RESPONSE-SPECIFIC INSTRUCTIONS

- HHA clinicians and coders must comply with the ICD-10-CM Official Guidelines for Coding and Reporting when assigning primary and secondary diagnoses to the OASIS items M1021 and M1023.

  - The ICD-10-CM is a morbidity classification published by the United States for classifying diagnoses and reason for care in all health care settings. The ICD-10-CM is based on the ICD-10, the international classification of disease published by the World Health Organization (WHO).

- The ICD-10-CM Official Guidelines for Coding and Reporting were developed by the Centers for Medicare & Medicaid Services (CMS) and the National Center for Health Statistics (NCHS). These guidelines are a set of rules that have been developed to accompany and complement the official conventions and instructions provided within the ICD-10-CM itself and should be used as a companion document to the official version of the ICD-10-CM List of Codes and Descriptions.

- Adherence to the ICD-10-CM Official Guidelines for Coding and Reporting when assigning ICD-10-CM diagnosis codes is required under the Health Insurance Portability and Accountability Act (HIPAA). It is expected that each agency will ensure that diagnoses and ICD-10-CM codes reported in the OASIS data set meet these guidelines.

- Identifying the patient's Primary and Secondary Home Health Diagnoses

  - The assessing clinician is expected to complete the patient's comprehensive assessment and understand the patient's overall medical condition and care needs before selecting and assigning diagnoses and may elicit input from other agency staff that have had direct in-person contact with the patient, or have had some other means of gathering information to contribute to the OASIS data collection.

  - The determination of the patient's primary and secondary home health diagnoses must be made by the assessing clinician based on the findings of the assessment, information in the medical record, and input from the physician.

  - As noted in the Item Intent, the patient's primary diagnosis is defined as the chief reason the patient is receiving home care and the diagnosis most related to the current home health Plan of Care. The primary diagnosis may or may not relate to the patient's most recent hospital stay, but must relate to the skilled services (skilled nursing, physical therapy, occupational therapy, and speech language pathology) rendered by the HHA.

  - As noted in the Item Intent, the secondary diagnoses include coexisting conditions actively addressed in the patient's Plan of Care, and any comorbid conditions having the potential to affect the patient's responsiveness to treatment and rehabilitative prognosis. The secondary diagnoses may or may not be related to a patient's recent hospital stay, but must have the potential to impact the skilled services provided by the HHA.

- When determining secondary diagnoses, the assessing clinician should consider diagnoses that are actively addressed in the Plan of Care as well as diagnoses that affect the patient's responsiveness to treatment and rehabilitative prognosis, even if the condition is not the focus of any home health treatment itself.

- Diagnoses may change during the course of the home health stay due to a change in the patient's health status or a change in the focus of home health care. At each required OASIS time point, the clinician must assess the patient's clinical status and determine the primary and secondary diagnoses based on patient status and treatment plan at the time of the assessment.

- Only current medical diagnoses should be reported as primary or secondary diagnoses in M1021 and M1023. Diagnoses should be excluded if they are resolved or do not have the potential to impact the skilled services provided by the HHA. An example of a resolved condition is cholecystitis following a cholecystectomy.

- In addition to following the ICD-10-CM Official Guidelines for Coding and Reporting, selection of home health diagnoses must be performed in compliance with Medicare's rules and regulations for coverage and payment to ensure provider compliance with Section 1862(a)(1)(A) of the Social Security Act. Section 1862(a)(1)(A) excludes provider services from Medicare coverage and payment that "are not reasonable and necessary for diagnosis or treatment of illness or injury or to improve the functioning of a malformed body member."

- Reporting Primary and Secondary Diagnoses in M1021 and M1023

  - At each required OASIS time point, the assessing clinician should enter the patient's current primary and secondary diagnoses in Column 1 of M1021 and M1023. Complete Column 1 from top to bottom, leaving any blank entries at the bottom.

  - The order that secondary diagnoses are entered should be determined by the degree that they impact the patient's health and need for home health care, rather than the degree of symptom control. For example, if a patient is receiving home health care for Type 2 diabetes that is "controlled with difficulty," this diagnosis would be listed above a diagnosis of a fungal infection of a toenail that is receiving treatment, even if the fungal infection is "poorly controlled."

- Reporting ICD-10-CM Codes in Column 2 of M1021 and M1023

  - The assessing clinician can enter the actual numeric ICD-10-CM codes for each diagnosis listed in Column 1 and 2 of M1021 and M1023, once the assessment is completed and the diagnosis is entered in Column 1. Alternatively, a coding specialist in the agency may enter the actual numeric ICD-10-CM codes in Column 2, as long as the assessing clinician has determined the primary and secondary diagnoses in Column 1.

  - The correct process for selecting an ICD-10-CM code using the Alphabetic Index and the Tabular List is described in the ICD-10-CM Official Guidelines for Coding and Reporting. Follow the official conventions and instructions provided within the ICD-10-CM List of Codes and Descriptions and the Official Guidelines to code each row in Column 2.

  - Each ICD-10-CM code must be entered at its highest level of specificity (diagnosis codes only – no surgical or procedure codes allowed).

  - ICD-10-CM does not allow external cause codes (ICD-10-CM codes beginning with V, W, X, or Y) to be reported in M1021 (Primary Diagnosis) but they may be reported in M1023 (Secondary Diagnoses).

  - Also note that when a Z-code is reported in Column 2, the code for the underlying condition may be entered in Column 2, as long as it is a current on-going condition that has a potential to impact the skilled services provided by the HHA. See the ICD-10-CM Official Guidelines for Coding and Reporting for complete instructions on code assignment and sequencing related to the use of Z-codes and use of multiple coding for a single condition (such as manifestation/ etiology pairs).

- Reporting the Symptom Control Rating in Column 2 of M1021 and M1023.

  - At each required time point, the assessing clinician should record the symptom control ratings for each primary and secondary diagnosis in column 2 of M1021 and M1023.

  - Assessing degree of symptom control includes review of presenting signs and symptoms, type and number of medications, frequency of treatment readjustments, and frequency of contact with health care provider. Inquire about the degree to which each condition limits daily activities. Assess the patient to determine if symptoms are controlled by current treatments. Clarify which diagnoses/symptoms have been poorly controlled in the recent past.

  - Choose one value that represents the degree of symptom control appropriate for each diagnosis using the scale provided in the M1021/M1023 instructions.

- Refer to the ICD-10-CM Official Guidelines for Coding and Reporting for instructions on multiple coding for a single condition (such as manifestation/etiology pairs).

DATA SOURCES/RESOURCES

- Patient/caregiver interview
- Physician
- Physician orders
- Referral information
- Current medication list
- The current ICD-10-CM List of Codes and Descriptions and the ICD-10-CM Official Guidelines for Coding and Reporting should be the source for coding (see Chapter 5 for link).
- For degree of symptom control, data sources may include patient/caregiver interview, physician, physical assessment, and review of past health history.

OASIS ITEM

(M1028) Active Diagnoses – Comorbidities and Co-existing Conditions – Check all that apply See OASIS Guidance Manual for a complete list of relevant ICD-10 codes.

> 1 - Peripheral Vascular Disease (PVD) or Peripheral Arterial Disease (PAD)
>
> 2 - Diabetes Mellitus (DM)
>
> 3 - None of the above

Item Intent

This item identifies whether two specific diagnoses are present and active. These diagnoses influence a patient's functional outcomes or increase a patient's risk for development or worsening of pressure ulcer(s).

Time Points Item(s) Completed

Start of care

Resumption of care

Response-Specific Instructions

1. **Identify diagnoses**: The diseases and conditions in this item require a physician (or nurse practitioner, physician assistant, clinical nurse specialist, or other authorized licensed staff if allowable under state licensure laws) documented diagnosis at the time of assessment.

   - Clinical record sources for physician (or nurse practitioner, physician assistant, clinical nurse specialist, or other authorized licensed staff if allowable under state licensure laws) diagnoses include, but are not limited to, transfer documents, physician progress notes, recent history and physical, discharge summary, physician orders, and consults.

     - Available documentation may be limited at admission/start of care. Admission/start of care assessment may indicate symptoms associated with one of this item's listed conditions while a documented diagnosis is not present in available records. The clinician should contact the physician (or other, as listed above) to ask if the patient has the diagnosis. Once a diagnosis has been identified, determine if the diagnosis is active.

     - Although open communication regarding diagnostic information between the physician and other clinical staff is important, it is also essential that diagnoses communicated verbally be documented in the clinical record by the physician (or nurse practitioner, physician assistant, clinical nurse specialist, or other licensed staff if allowable under state licensure laws) to ensure follow-up and coordination of care.

   - Diagnostic information, including past medical and surgical history obtained from family members and close contacts, must also be documented in the clinical record by the physician (or nurse practitioner, physician assistant, clinical nurse specialist, or other authorized licensed staff if allowable under state licensure laws) to ensure validity, follow-up and coordination of care.

   - Only diagnoses confirmed and documented by the physician (or nurse practitioner, physician assistant, clinical nurse specialist, or other authorized licensed staff if allowable under state licensure laws) should be considered when coding this item.

2. **Determine whether diagnoses are active:** Once a diagnosis is identified, determine whether the diagnosis is active.

   - If information regarding active diagnoses is learned after the end of the assessment time frame, the OASIS data set should not be revised to reflect this new information. The OASIS data set should reflect what was known and documented at the time of the assessment.

   - If, however, it comes to light after the data set is submitted that a documented active diagnosis was present but not indicated on the OASIS data set, the Home Health Agency should modify the OASIS data set in accordance with the instructions in the Survey and Certification Memo #15-18-HHA, Outcome and Assessment Information Set (OASIS) transition to the Automated Submission and Processing System (ASAP) and OASIS Correction policy.

     - A copy of this memo is located on CMS.gov under Provider Enrollment and Certification/ Quality Safety & Oversight – General Information/Policy & Memos to States and Regions. For additional details, please reference the OASIS Submission User's Guide and Training site (QTSO site).

ACTIVE DIAGNOSES

Active diagnoses are diagnoses that have a direct relationship to the patient's current functional, cognitive, mood or behavior status; medical treatments; nurse monitoring; or risk of death at the time of assessment. Do not include diseases or conditions that have been resolved or do not affect the patient's current functional, cognitive, or mood or behavior status; medical treatments; nurse monitoring; or risk of death at the time of assessment.

Coding Instructions

Code 1, Peripheral Vascular Disease (PVD) or Peripheral Arterial Disease (PAD), if the patient has an active diagnosis of Peripheral Vascular Disease (PVD) or Peripheral Arterial Disease (PAD), indicated by any of the following diagnosis codes:

Codes that start with the first 4 characters of:

I70.2, Atherosclerosis of native arteries of the extremities

I70.3, Atherosclerosis of unspecified type of bypass graft(s) of the extremities

I70.4, Atherosclerosis of autologous vein bypass graft(s) of the extremities

I70.5, Atherosclerosis of nonautologous biological bypass graft(s) of the extremities

I70.6, Atherosclerosis of nonbiological bypass graft(s) of the extremities

I70.7, Atherosclerosis of other type of bypass graft(s) of the extremities

I70.91, Generalized atherosclerosis

I70.92, Chronic total occlusion of artery of the extremities

Codes that start with the first 3 characters of:

I73, Other peripheral vascular diseases

Code 2, Diabetes Mellitus (DM), if the patient has an active diagnosis of Diabetes Mellitus (DM) indicated by any of the following diagnosis codes:

Codes that start with the first 3 characters of:

E08, Diabetes mellitus due to underlying condition

E09, Drug or chemical induced diabetes mellitus

E10, Type 1 diabetes mellitus

E11, Type 2 diabetes mellitus

E13, Other **specified** diabetes mellitus

Code 3, None of the Above, if the patient does not have any of the active diagnoses listed above.

A dash is a valid response for this item. CMS expects dash use to be a rare occurrence.

Coding Tips

The following tips may assist staff in determining whether a disease or condition should be coded as an active diagnosis.

- The physician (nurse practitioner, physician assistant, clinical nurse specialist, or other authorized licensed staff if allowable under state licensure laws) may specifically indicate that a diagnosis is active.

- If there is documentation in the clinical record that a patient has diabetes mellitus, Select Response 2, Diabetes Mellitus (DM). If there is only documentation in the clinical record of a complication such as nephropathy or neuropathy and there is no documentation that the patient has diabetes, it should not be assumed the complication is associated with diabetes, and Response 2, Diabetes Mellitus, should not be checked.

- The physician (nurse practitioner, physician assistant, clinical nurse specialist or other authorized licensed staff if allowable under state licensure laws) for example, documents at the time of assessment that the patient has inadequately controlled diabetes and requires adjustment of the medication regimen. This would be sufficient documentation of an active diagnosis and would require no additional confirmation because the physician documented the diagnosis and also confirmed that the medication regimen needed to be modified.

Examples

1. Active Diagnosis of Diabetes Mellitus

Mr. A is prescribed insulin for diabetes mellitus. He requires regular blood glucose monitoring to determine whether blood glucose goals are achieved by the current medication regimen. The physician progress note documents diabetes mellitus.

Coding: M1028, Active Diagnoses, would be coded 2, Diabetes Mellitus.

Rationale: This would be considered an active diagnosis because the physician progress note documents the diabetes mellitus diagnosis, and because there is ongoing medication management and glucose monitoring.

2. None of the Above

During the SOC/ROC assessment, Mrs. K told Nurse J, RN that she has had diabetes for 20 years. Nurse J reviewed the transfer documents from the acute care facility and all clinical records on the patient but was unable find a documented diagnosis of Diabetes Mellitus by physician, nurse practitioner, physician assistant or authorized licensed staff member in their state. There is no documented diagnosis of PVD or PAD.

Coding: M1028, Active Diagnoses, would be coded 3, None of the Above.

Rationale: This would be considered a "none of the above" response because the nurse was unable to find the diagnosis of diabetes at the time of assessment, documented by a physician (or nurse practitioner, physician assistant, clinical nurse specialist, or other authorized licensed staff if allowable under state licensure laws). And, there is no documented diagnosis of PVD or PAD.

Data Sources/Resources

- Transfer documents
- Clinical Records
- Referrals

Correcting the OASIS

Recordkeeping Principles, Amendments, Corrections and Delayed Entries

Medicare, other payers and state practice acts require that all relevant documents and entries into the medical record occur at the time the services are rendered. Occasionally, upon review, a provider may discover that certain entries, related to actions that were actually performed at the time of service but not properly documented, need to be amended, corrected or entered after rendering the service. Corrections can include an unintentional omission of documentation of a procedure performed, an error in answering the OASIS that needs to be corrected to ensure compliance with official CMS guidance, and/ or a correction to the coding because it does not comply with the Official Guidelines for Coding and Reporting (official coding guidelines).

Note that this guidance provides direction for corrections to the medical documentation when actions were actually performed. It is always wrong to falsify documentation to indicate some action was taken that was indeed not taken to avoid survey deficiency or to upcode in order to garner more funding when the patient's actual condition does not warrant the option or code chosen. **Important**: Because of the dangers of falsification of documentation, the MACs, CERT, RACs, ZPICs and other government auditors will not accept documentation if it has not been corrected in the manner described below.

The Principles of Document Correction

The following principles apply regardless of whether documentation is on paper or in an electronic health record (EHR):

1. Clearly and permanently identify any amendment, correction or delayed entry as such, and

2. Clearly indicate the date and author of any amendment, correction or delayed entry, and

3. Do not delete, but instead clearly identify all original content

Paper Medical Records: When correcting a paper medical record, these principles are generally accomplished by using a single line strike through so that the original content is still readable. Further, the author of the alteration must sign and date the revision. Similarly, amendments or delayed entries to paper records must be clearly signed and dated upon entry into the record.

Electronic Health Records (EHR): Medical record keeping within an EHR deserves special considerations; however, the principles above remain fundamental and necessary for document submission to MACs, CERT, Recovery Auditors, and ZPICs. Records sourced from electronic systems containing amendments, corrections or delayed entries must:

a. Distinctly identify any amendment, correction or delayed entry, and

b. Provide a reliable means to clearly identify the original content, the modified content, and the date and authorship of each modification of the record.

CMS Manual System, Pub 100-08 Medicare Program Integrity, Transmittal 442, Change Request 8105, December 7, 2012

Diagnoses on the OASIS

CMS expects that the professionals who complete the OASIS be able to choose the primary diagnosis and other diagnoses that should be listed on the POC as part of care planning. However, CMS does not expect that those same professionals be able to actually assign the code. Although home health agencies may expect the clinicians to assign the codes, coding is a specialty and CMS states that a coder may assign the code. If an error is made in coding, there is a professional obligation to correct the error so that coding is in compliance with Official Coding Guidelines and with other professional guidance, i.e., CMS requirements.

So who can make these corrections? CMS states in Category 4 Q37.4 [*Q&A ADDED 01/12; Previously CMS OCCB 07/11 Q&A #2*]:

HHAs should have a policy and procedure for correcting errors that involves the assessing clinician. The policy should follow established clinical record professional practice standards and guidance found in relevant CMS regulations and guidance. Normally, if an error is identified through audit or review, the individual who made the original entry into the patient's record would, whenever possible, make the necessary correction by following agency policy. A correction policy may allow the auditor who found the error to contact the clinician, discuss the discrepancy in the medical record and make the correction following the agency's policy and including information such as who discovered the error, and the date and time of communication with the assessing clinician who agrees that it was an error. Correction of an error will not impact M0090, Date Assessment Completed.

In a case where the original documenter is not available, the clinical supervisor or quality staff may make the correction to the documentation following the correction policy. The supervisor must document why the original assessing clinician is not available to make the correction and how the error was identified and validated as a true error.

When corrections are made to assessments submitted to state, you must determine the impact of the correction on the POC, HHRG, the Plan of Treatment, RAP, and make corrections to those documents and billing, as applicable.

When the comprehensive assessment is corrected, the HHA must maintain the original as well as subsequent corrected assessments in the patient's clinical record per requirements at 42 CFR 484.48. CMS urges HHAs to make corrections and/or submit inactivations as quickly as possible after errors are identified so the state system will be as current and accurate as possible, as the data is used to generate OBQM, OBQI, PBQI, Patient-Related Characteristics Report and HHRG.

So if it's required to ensure the coding is compliant with official guidance, can't a coder correct errors by the clinician? For example, the clinician placed a manifestation code without its required etiology preceding it or the clinician entered a diagnosis that is not supported by documentation.

The determination of the primary and secondary diagnoses must be completed by the assessing clinician, in conjunction with the physician. If the assessing clinician identifies the diagnosis that is the focus of the care and reports it as primary, and coding guidelines required that the selected diagnosis is subject to mandatory multiple coding, the addition of the etiology code and related sequencing is **not** a technical correction because a diagnosis is being added. If any diagnosis is being added, in this case for manifestation coding requirements, the assessing clinician must be contacted and agree to the correction [*Category 4, Q44.1*].

If, based on the review of the comprehensive assessment and plan of care, the auditor questions the accuracy of the primary diagnosis selected by the assessing clinician, this is not considered a "technical" error and the coding specialist may not automatically make the correction without consulting with the assessing clinician [*Category 4, Q44.1*].

If, after discussion of the manifestation coding situation between the assessing clinician and the coding specialist, the assessing clinician agrees with the coding specialist or auditor and that the sequence of the diagnosis codes should be modified to more accurately reflect the diagnosis that is most related to the current POC using current coding guidelines, agency policy will determine how (e.g., by whom) this change is made [*Category 4, Q44.1*].

A diagnosis not supported by documentation may mean that the clinician has decided on a diagnosis not confirmed by the physician or that the clinician has omitted necessary information in the documentation to support why that particular diagnosis is pertinent to the Plan of Care. The assessing clinician should be asked for supporting documentation to substantiate the diagnosis chosen. It may mean that the physician must be queried to confirm the questionable diagnosis and be asked for orders to address the diagnosis when confirmed. Remember, CMS expects that all diagnoses listed have interventions and goals.

What about M0090 (Date assessment completed)?

If the clinician makes a change or agrees to a change in the assessment within the time period for the assessment, e.g., within 5 days after the SOC, then the M0090 date should change. If changes are made after the time period for the assessment, do not necessarily change M0090.

If the original assessing clinician gathers additional information during the SOC five-day assessment time frame that would change a data item response, the M0090 date would be changed to reflect the date the information was gathered and the change was made. If an error is identified at any time, it should be corrected following the agency's correction policy and M0090 would not necessarily be changed [*Category 4, Q19.3*].

Only one clinician can complete the comprehensive assessment, including the OASIS. If the clinician responsible for completing the OASIS assessment gathers new information during the five-day assessment time period, that clinician may change the response to that item and change the M0090 date to reflect the date the latest new information was gathered. This would apply to M2200 [*Category 4, Q19.4*].

If the OASIS is completed by the assessing clinician and then, through an internal review process in the office, it is discovered that the OASIS data contains one or more errors, the identified data item(s) could be corrected by the qualified clinician responsible for performing the review following your agency's correction policy and in such cases of error correction, M0090 would not be changed [*Category 4, Q19.4*].

What if the assessing clinician did not complete the OASIS, e.g., left some items blank, and now is unavailable to finish? Another qualified clinician would have to visit the patient and complete a new comprehensive assessment including OASIS. The other OASIS answers cannot be answered based on a guess or even by another clinician who has seen the patient.

If the comprehensive assessment for a patient requiring OASIS data collection was completed in a non-compliant manner and the OASIS data items were not completed, the agency should send another qualified clinician out during the allowed timeframe for completing the assessment, within five days after the Start of Care (SOC) date, to start and complete an entire comprehensive assessment, not just the OASIS items. It would be required that another qualified clinician complete the entire assessment because only one person can complete an assessment, it is not a collaborative effort between field staff or field staff and supervisors. When a clinician signs the assessment, it is an attestation that everything contained in the assessment is truthful and accurate, based on that clinician's assessment. Information in the medical record cannot be "made up" or "created" in an effort to be compliant with the Comprehensive Assessment of Patient Condition of Participation's (484.55) required timeframes. Careful documentation should be included in the medical record to explain the circumstances that led to the non-compliance [*Category 4, Q37.4*].

Recommendations:

1. Ensure that all qualified clinicians are trained in OASIS data collection to minimize errors.

2. Ensure that all qualified clinicians are able to use care planning skills in order to select the primary and other diagnoses that are appropriate for the Plan of Care of the individual patient.

3. Ensure that coders are qualified and competent to assign the correct codes to the diagnoses selected utilizing official guidance at a minimum and/or be able to review all available information, query the physician when appropriate, request additional documentation from the clinician as needed, and recommend diagnoses and sequencing to the assessing clinician at the optimum.

4. Always request that the assessing clinician approve any changes to the assessment.

   - The best corrections are made by the clinician within the time frame allowed for that assessment. Follow the standards outlined by Medicare for amendments, corrections and delayed entries.

   - The next best method for making changes is to have the clinician approve any changes to that assessment, again within the timeframe for that assessment. Keep in mind that Practice Acts within some states frown on someone who has not assessed the patient making changes to someone else's assessment on the assessment itself. Especially if the documentation is on paper, it is best that the agency has some type of an 'OASIS Correction Worksheet.' Document the original answer, the changed answer and the rationale for making the change (you will not remember why the

change was made next year when that chart is called for medical review). Last, but certainly not least, the assessing clinician must approve the changes before they are entered into the system. If your agency uses an EHR, ensure that the system meets Medicare criteria

5. If the assessing clinician is no longer available (employment has been terminated, vacation, leave, etc.), then have a clear process for how necessary changes are made and by whom they may be made. The error must be a true error and not just a difference in opinion. The supervisor or designated person must document why the original assessing clinician is not available to make the correction and how the error was identified and validated as a true error. Always maintain the original answer, as well as any changes, along with rationale for the change.

6. Implement a data quality audit program to find errors prior to 'locking' and transmitting the OASIS. To be compliant with Medicare Conditions of Participation, the OASIS must be transmitted within 30 days of M0090 (Date Assessment Completed). According to claims processing requirements, the OASIS must be ready for transmission prior to the RAP being submitted. A lot of extra work may be avoided if an agency holds to these principles. If errors are found **after** the OASIS was transmitted or **after** the RAP has been submitted, then there must be a process to determine the impact of the error on the OASIS and the RAP.

   - Any error in OASIS will have impact on outcomes as every item is used in the outcome process, either directly or for risk adjustment.

   - Only errors in case-mix items will impact the RAP. **Any change** to diagnoses will impact claims processing, therefore the RAP will need to be canceled. Remember the diagnoses on the claim must match that on OASIS.

   - The home health agency must cancel a RAP sent in error. RAPs cannot be adjusted. They may be rebilled with appropriate information after cancellation. Type of bill (TOB) 328 is used for a cancel transaction, for both claims and RAPs. [*Home Health Billing Manual, http://www.cms.gov/Regulations-and-Guidance/Guidance/Manuals/Downloads/clm104c10.pdf, 10.1.11 – Payment, Claim Adjustments and Cancellations (Rev. 1, 10-01-03) HH-467.20, A3-3639.20*]

   - OASIS corrections information, once the OASIS has already been submitted can be found on the CMS website. (*See resources below*)

   - Beginning January 1, 2010, home health agencies are required to submit an OASIS as a condition for payment. Contractors may deny the claim as a result of not meeting this regulatory requirement. The assessment must be patient specific, accurate and reflect the current health status of the patient. This status includes certain OASIS elements used for calculation of payment including documentation of clinical needs, functional status, and service utilization.

With promulgation of §484.250 as a condition of payment, entire home health claims are now subject to denial if agencies do not submit start-of-care and recertification assessments for every Medicare.

The HIPPS code on the final claim must match that received on the OASIS validation report, AND OASIS data has to have been submitted prior to the final claim. This requirement is only applicable to those OASIS assessments linked to payment, such as SOC, Recertification and ROC when acting as a Recertification. Please note that *all* OASIS assessments have to be transmitted if the payer is Medicare, Medicare HMO (replacement plans), Medicaid or Medicaid HMO as required by the Conditions of Participation.

A last word from Medicare: Correction of clinical documentation errors is more time consuming because the documentation must be returned to the clinician with an explanation of the error. The clinician must correct the error promptly and return the record to the data entry staff person. The correction is then entered and the record checked again for errors.

In some instances, the correction of one error can cause another error to surface, and the process must be repeated. The agency will benefit from designing a systematic process for correcting clinical documentation errors which functions efficiently despite clinicians' absences or their inability to return to the office. Revising such processes may indicate the need to review and revise the agency policy for correcting clinical records. This process should clearly define each step, identify responsible persons at each step, and estimate the time allowed for each step. If copies of documentation are submitted for data entry, the procedure will need to include steps to ensure the correction is made in the official agency clinical record as well as in the data submitted to the State agency. As with other process changes, once the process is finalized, it must be rigorously enforced. The agency can monitor its own compliance with the 30-day submission requirement by including this component in the tracking system. [*Category 4, Q37.3; Q&A EDITED 01/11; ADDED 09/09; Previously CMS OCCB 01/09 Q&A #2*]

Additional Resources:

- All OASIS official documentation including the Q and A can be found at: *https://www.qtso. com/hhadownload.html*

- Specific information on developing OASIS Data Accuracy programs and correcting OASIS data already submitted may be found in Appendix B to the OASIS manual found at: *www.cms. gov/Medicare/Quality-Initiatives-Patient-Assessment-Instruments/HomeHealthQualityInits/ HHQIOASISUserManual.html* Click on link under Downloads for 2012 OASIS-C Guidance Manual.

Source: Lisa Selman-Holman, JD, BSN, RN, HCS-D, HCS-O, COS-C, AHIMA Approved ICD-10-CM/PCS Trainer, Owner, Selman-Holman & Associates, LLC, and the coding service CoDR – Coding Done Right

Hospice coding primer: Learn to code hospice claims accurately

Code **all** unresolved diagnoses on a hospice patient's claim, not just those that are related to the terminal diagnosis.

Hospices must report all diagnoses of the beneficiary on the hospice claim as a part of the ongoing data collection efforts for possible future hospice payment refinements. Reporting of all diagnoses on the hospice claim aligns with current coding guidelines as well as admission requirements for hospice certifications, CMS stated in its FY2016 Hospice Wage Index rule, and then reiterated in its FY2017 payment hospice rule.

The confusion over how to decide which diagnoses were related or unrelated, and therefore which diagnoses to include on the claim, was resolved in the FY2016 Hospice Wage Index when the rule instructed hospices to include every diagnosis.

The FY2016 rule cited the importance of a comprehensive approach to hospice patients' care, the fact that a large majority of hospice claims still include only one diagnosis and the confusion about "related" versus "unrelated" diagnoses as reasoning for the rule change.

Data reported in the FY2019 proposed hospice payment rule indicates that hospices are acting in compliance with CMS's repeated request that they code every unresolved diagnosis a hospice patient has regardless of its relation to the terminal one.

In fact, analysis of FY2018 hospice claims show that 100% of claims included at least one diagnosis, 90% included at least two diagnoses, and 82% included at least three diagnoses, according to CMS.

Hospices have been spinning from all the changes that have come their way. The recent changes in hospice coding began with the forbidding of assigning debility (R53.81) and adult failure to thrive (R62.7), as well as unspecified dementia (F03.9-) and dementia manifestation codes (F02.8-) as **primary terminal** diagnoses starting Oct. 1, 2014.

Recall that if this directive is not heeded, hospice claims will be returned to provider (RTP'd) for correction.

As a result of this policy, there has been a shift in coding patterns on hospice claims. The top five most commonly reported principal diagnoses in FY2017 were G30.9 (Alzheimer's disease, unspecified), J44.9 (Chronic obstructive pulmonary disease, unspecified), I50.9 (Heart failure, unspecified), G31.1 (Senile degeneration of brain, not elsewhere classified), and C34.90 (Malignant neoplasm of unspecified part of unspecified

bronchus or lung), according to the FY2019 rule. CMS' ongoing analysis of hospice coding trends finds that "neurological and organ-based failure conditions" still are top-reported principal diagnoses, according to the FY2020 proposed hospice rule.

Determine the primary diagnosis

Sometimes the primary hospice diagnosis as well as the documentation necessary to support it, is readily apparent. The patient may have terminal cancer, decompensated COPD, end-stage renal disease or Alzheimer's disease.

But other times it isn't so easy. For some patients, there is no one single diagnosis that is the primary reason for his or her terminal condition.

The patient may have several chronic diagnoses or symptomatic conditions that, when combined, are leading to the patient having a life expectancy of six months or less.

In these cases, it becomes a clinical decision, made by the hospice's interdisciplinary group (IDG), as to which of the diagnoses is the **most contributory** to the terminal prognosis.

Get back to the basics

Adhere to the ICD-10-CM official coding guidelines when coding hospice claims, or risk getting claims denials or additional documentation requests (ADRs).

Although some mistakenly believe that hospice coders don't have to follow these guidelines, they **do** apply to hospice as much as they apply to home health, and closely adhering to them is the best way to steer clear of trouble.

Here are examples of official coding guidelines to which hospice coders must pay particular attention:

- Do **not** report a Z code, such as Z51.5 (Encounter for palliative care) or Z48.812 (Encounter for surgical aftercare following surgery on the circulatory system), as a primary diagnosis, according to Chapter 11 of the Medicare Claims Processing Manual.

- Do **not** report diagnosis codes that cannot be used as the principal diagnosis, such as F02.80 (Dementia in other diseases classified elsewhere without behavioral disturbance). Note that F02.80 is a manifestation code that **can only be sequenced after** its corresponding etiology. *[I.A.13]*

- Follow sequencing instruction provided in the tabular. For example, you must assign E10.22 (Type 1 diabetes mellitus with diabetic chronic kidney disease) ahead of N18.6 (End stage renal disease) when diabetes is the cause of the end-stage renal disease, even if N18.6 is the terminal diagnosis, according to tabular instruction.

- Ensure that the documentation supports the appropriateness for coverage under the hospice benefit.

- Report any mental health disorders or conditions that would affect the patient's plan of care.

Scenario: **Metastatic bone cancer**

The patient is an 88-year-old female with a history of breast cancer that was treated 20 years ago with bilateral mastectomies, chemotherapy and radiation therapy and the cancer was thought to be resolved. She was recently hospitalized for a fracture of the shaft of her right femur that was determined to be the result of metastatic bone cancer consistent with breast cancer primary. She also has COPD, insulin-dependent diabetes and hypertension. She has a history of smoking two packs of cigarettes a day for 30 years, quitting approximately three years ago and has elected to go home with hospice care. Metastatic bone cancer is the primary terminal diagnosis.

Code the scenario:

Primary and Secondary Diagnoses		
Primary	Secondary malignant neoplasm of bone	C79.51
Secondary	Pathological fracture in neoplastic disease, left femur, subsequent encounter for fracture with routine healing	M84.552D
Secondary	Personal history of malignant neoplasm of breast	Z85.3
Secondary	Chronic obstructive pulmonary disease, unspecified	J44.9
Secondary	Essential (primary) hypertension	I10
Secondary	Type 2 diabetes mellitus without complications	E11.9

Additional diagnoses: Z79.4 (Long term (current) use of insulin), Z87.891 (Personal history of nicotine dependence), Z51.5 (Encounter for palliative care)

Rationale:

- ICD-10 guidelines state that when the cancer is the primary focus of care, it is sequenced first followed by the code for the neoplastic fracture.

- Because the primary breast cancer (Z85.3) was stated to be resolved, the code for personal history is assigned.

- Additional codes are assigned to capture all of the patient's current diagnoses, including her insulin-dependent diabetes, hypertension, COPD and smoking history.

- *Tip:* Include a code for a patient's current or past nicotine use when assigning certain respiratory and cardiac codes in ICD-10, including J44.9.

Scenario: **End-stage renal disease**

A male patient is referred to hospice for end stage renal disease. He has refused dialysis and wishes comfort care only. He also has hypertension, type 2 diabetes, PVD, COPD, coronary artery disease and angina. He is tobacco dependent, having smoked one pack of cigarettes per day for 40 years and continues to smoke.

Code the scenario:

Primary and Secondary Diagnoses		
Primary	Hypertensive chronic kidney disease with stage 5 chronic kidney disease or end stage renal disease	I12.0
Secondary	Type 2 diabetes mellitus with diabetic chronic kidney disease	E11.22
Secondary	End stage renal disease	N18.6
Secondary	Type 2 diabetes mellitus with diabetic peripheral angiopathy without gangrene	E11.51
Secondary	Chronic obstructive pulmonary disease, unspecified	J44.9
Secondary	Atherosclerotic heart disease of native coronary artery with unspecified angina pectoris	I25.119
Secondary	Nicotine dependence, cigarettes, uncomplicated	F17.210

Additional diagnoses: Z51.5 (Encounter for palliative care)

Rationale:

- Although the physician states the patient is terminal due to their end stage renal disease, the ICD-10 classification assumes a relationship between the hypertension, diabetes and end-stage renal disease. Hypertension and diabetes must be coded before N18.6, according to coding guidelines.

- The classification also assumes a relationship between diabetes and PVD in the absence of another stated etiology, and thus the diagnosis is coded with E11.51.

- *Tip:* Remember that in ICD-10 there is an assumed relationship between the coronary artery disease and angina and is captured by a combination code, I25.119.

Scenario: End-stage vascular dementia

A female patient comes to hospice care for end stage vascular dementia due to multiple CVAs. She also has oropharyngeal dysphagia and left-side dominant hemiplegia from the CVAs. She also has a history of chronic diastolic heart failure, COPD with chronic hypoxic respiratory failure, is on 4L/min of oxygen via nasal cannula, has a stage three sacral pressure ulcer and an unstageable pressure ulcer on her left heel.

Code the scenario:

Primary and Secondary Diagnoses		
Primary	Other symptoms and signs involving cognitive functions following cerebral infarction	I69.318
Secondary	Vascular dementia without behavioral disturbance	F01.50
Secondary	Hemiplegia and hemiparesis following cerebral infarction affecting left dominant side	I69.352
Secondary	Dysphagia following cerebral infarction	I69.391
Secondary	Dysphagia, oropharyngeal phase	R13.12
Secondary	Chronic obstructive pulmonary disease, unspecified	J44.9

Additional diagnoses: J96.11 (Chronic respiratory failure with hypoxia), L89.153 (Pressure ulcer of sacral region, stage 3), L89.620 (Pressure ulcer of left heel, unstageable), Z99.81 (Dependence on supplemental oxygen), Z51.5 (Encounter for palliative care)

Rationale:

- Coding guidelines require that the cause of the vascular dementia, CVAs in this case, be coded first. Therefore, this patient's terminal condition is coded first with I69.318 and then with F01.50. – *This article was written by guest editor Maurice Frear, HCS-D and is current as of the Manual's publication date.*

Code only confirmed diagnoses on hospice claims, stay in compliance

Hospice coders should not code "probable," "suspected," "likely" or "possible" diagnoses as if they were confirmed diagnoses, according to Q1 2016 Coding Clinic guidance.

This means that hospices may not code lung cancer, for example, in a patient who is suspected of having the disease but either refuses to or cannot undergo further diagnostic testing to confirm it.

Hospice coders are required to following the official coding guidelines. The exception mentioned in Section III, C that allows the coding of unconfirmed diagnosis does not apply to them, according to the Coding Clinic.

That exception is only for inpatient admissions to short-term, acute, long-term care and psychiatric hospitals, the Coding Clinic said.

This guidance aligns with the opinion of CMS's ICD-10 ombudsman Dr. William Rogers, M.D., who previously said that coding unconfirmed diagnoses in hospice is hard to justify and that signs, symptoms and other conditions should be coded in these scenarios to help support the patient's medical necessity for the hospice benefit.

This can be an issue for hospice coders in situations involving patients who elect hospice care due to suspected metastatic cancer, for example. But, the patient is either too frail to undergo further diagnostic testing or refuses it, says Brandi Whitemyer, HCS-D, independent home health & hospice consultant in Canton, Ohio.

Hospice coders have been left wondering how to appropriately capture why the patient is terminally ill, having to choose between an unconfirmed diagnosis and one, such as "lung mass," that is unacceptably vague, Whitemyer says.

Documentation is key to compliance

Ensure that detailed clinical documentation about the patient's health status and his or her appropriateness for hospice care accompanies a hospice record in which a vague diagnosis like "mass" is coded in the primary position due to a lack of diagnostic confirmation.

"Documentation is very critical in the situations when there is no specific diagnosis that can be reported in the principal spot. Therefore, the coder and clinician must be sure any other diagnoses, symptoms, clinical findings, diagnostic studies, etc. that support the patient's eligibility for the hospice benefit are included in the clinical record," says Judy Adams, HCS-D, president of Adams Home Care Consulting in Chapel Hill, N.C.

When hospice coder Maurice Frear comes across records where a patient is either too frail to undergo further diagnostic testing or refuses it, he assigns the diagnosis that is available, such as a "mass" and is sure to include any other diagnoses that are contributing to the patient's decline in six months or less.

These include conditions like malnutrition, anorexia and weight loss. It's also wise to include a code for the patient's BMI (body mass index) along with codes for weight loss, says Frear, HCS-D, coder for Bon Secours Home Health and Hospice in Virginia Beach.

To his knowledge, Frear has never suffered negative consequences, such as claims denials, for taking this approach.

6 more hospice coding tips

Tip: Make sure there's adequate documentation explaining why the patient or the patient's family has refused diagnostic testing or why the patient cannot undergo further testing to determine the etiology of the mass, for example.

Tip: Include a code for a history of cancer, such as Z85.3 (Personal history of malignant neoplasm of breast), if the patient has suspected metastasized cancer resulting from cancer previously thought to be eradicated. This will work together with documentation describing a mass that is suspected but unconfirmed cancer, for example, to further explain the patient's condition.

Tip: Don't assign a code from the F50.0- category (Anorexia nervosa) without a documented diagnosis. These codes refer to a psychiatric disorder, which requires a physician's diagnosis. The loss of appetite experienced by hospice patients, also referred to as anorexia, is a symptom code and is captured with R63.0 (Anorexia/Loss of appetite), according to the alphabetic index.

Tip: Avoid, if possible, coding unspecified diagnoses in the primary position on hospice claims. However, if you cannot get further detail about a diagnosis, make sure the medical record includes supporting information to show why the unspecified diagnosis is the best alternative to use as a principal diagnosis and how the patient qualifies for the hospice benefit.

Tip: Be aware of unspecified diagnoses, such as F03.90 (Unspecified dementia without behavioral disturbance), that CMS has already deemed unacceptable for use as primary hospice diagnoses. For a full list of unallowable terminal diagnosis codes, refer to CMS Transmittal 8877, which you can view at *https://go.cms.gov/1Vh1SBs*.

Tip: Attempt to get an attending physician and/or the medical director of the hospice to make that commitment to the cancer based on what else is going on, e.g. tumor markers, progression of debility.

Scenario: Probable metastatic cancer, anorexia

A 96-year-old woman elected hospice care after her doctor found a large mass on her lung that he believes is metastasized cancer resulting from breast cancer previously treated and believed eradicated 30 years ago. She has refused all further diagnostic testing and wants only comfort care. She has very little appetite, refuses to eat most days and has lost a significant amount of weight. Her BMI is now 16.

Code the scenario:

Primary and Secondary Diagnoses	
Primary diagnosis: Lung mass NOS found on diagnostic imaging of lung	R91.8
Additional diagnosis: Anorexia/Loss of appetite	R63.0
Additional diagnosis: Abnormal weight loss	R63.4
Additional diagnosis: Body mass index (BMI) 19 or less, adult	Z68.1
Additional diagnosis: Personal history of malignant neoplasm of breast	Z85.3

Rationale:

- While the patient's physician suspects metastatic lung cancer, the diagnosis hasn't and won't be confirmed with diagnostic testing, because the patient refused. Therefore, the primary diagnosis is the lung mass.

- Additional diagnoses that are contributing to her terminal status, such as her loss of appetite, weight loss and low BMI, are also coded to further support the admission.

- She has a history of breast cancer that her physician believes is the source of her lung mass. Because it was believed to be eradicated, the history code Z85.3 is assigned.

Do not assign fractures as primary hospice diagnosis, or risk auditor scrutiny

Avoid assigning a fracture code, such as S72.031D (Displaced midcervical fracture of right femur, subsequent encounter for closed fracture with routine healing) as the primary diagnosis on a hospice claim or you could risk a review.

This issue was non-existent in ICD-9 when fractures could only be captured with aftercare V codes (such as with V54.1x, Aftercare for healing traumatic fracture) and V codes weren't eligible to be primary hospice diagnoses.

But now that fracture codes can be assigned, some hospice coders are wondering whether a fracture could ever be appropriate as a primary hospice diagnosis. But it's not a wise choice, experts say.

It's unlikely that a fracture would ever be the main reason for a patient being in hospice care, says Brandi Whitemyer, HCS-D, independent home health & hospice consultant in Canton, Ohio..

Rather, consider what medical issues have resulted from or have been exacerbated by the patient's condition with the fracture and how these may have resulted in a terminal prognosis, says Whitemyer.

For example, a patient with a terminal diagnosis of metastatic bone cancer may have suffered a pathologic hip fracture due to bones that are weakened by the advancing disease, she says.

Scenario: Alzheimer's disease, fracture

A patient with Alzheimer's dementia fractured his hip after falling at home. He is now admitted to hospice as the patient's physician determined that the patient is not appropriate for surgery and the patient is no longer ambulating and his nutritional status has now significantly declined. He is no longer taking in any food by mouth. His terminal diagnosis is reported as Alzheimer's, with related diagnoses of left hip fracture and anorexia/loss of appetite. He is bedfast.

Code the scenario:

Primary and Secondary Diagnoses		
Primary: Alzheimer's disease, unspecified		G30.9
Secondary: Dementia in other diseases classified elsewhere without behavioral disturbance		F02.80
Secondary: Fracture of unspecified part of neck of left femur, subsequent encounter for closed fracture with routine healing		S72.002D
Secondary: Loss of appetite		R63.0
Secondary: Bed confinement status		Z74.01
Secondary: Unspecified fall, subsequent encounter		W19.xxxD

Rationale:

- The primary terminal diagnosis is Alzheimer's diagnosis, which should be reported as G30.9, Alzheimer's disease.

- It should be followed by the manifestation code for dementia in diseases classified elsewhere, F02.80. Note that when coding Alzheimer's, the manifestation code for dementia in diseases classified elsewhere, F02.8-, must always be additionally assigned, according to Coding Clinic.

- The fracture should be listed as well, due to the related nature of the fracture to the terminal condition.

- Also code the anorexia (R63.0) and a Z code for bed confinement status (Z74.01).Do not assign the 7th character "A" when reporting a fracture on a hospice claim.

- An external cause code, W19.xxxD, is also assigned to explain how the patient sustained the fall. It carries the same seventh character as the fracture code, in accordance with coding guidelines.

Use caution when assigning malnutrition as primary hospice diagnosis

Ensure there's adequate documentation explaining how malnutrition is causing a hospice patient's death, or prepare to see those records returned, or even denied.

For example, E46 (Malnutrition NOS) is not specific enough to communicate why a patient's life span is limited to six months or less, which is the requirement for the hospice benefit.

There have been reports of hospices getting denials for using malnutrition codes as a primary hospice diagnoses, says Judy Adams, HCS-D, president of Adams Home Care Consulting in Chapel Hill, N.C., who speculates that it likely began as a reaction from Medicare Administrative Contractors (MACs) to all of the sudden seeing a rash of claims with primary terminal diagnosis codes it hadn't previously seen before.

However, the issue has now become one of inadequate documentation, as the MACs are beginning to deny hospice claims that don't support why malnutrition is causing a patient's death, she says.

Part of the problem is that the hospice industry is not used to documenting at the level that Medicare wants to see to support these diagnoses, Adams says. In the past, their documentation has focused simply on how the patient is doing at each visit.

But what needs to be in the record, if the primary terminal diagnosis is something like severe protein-calorie malnutrition, is measurements of the patient's weight, his or her arm circumference, documentation about how the patient is eating, that his or her muscles are wasting away and skin is hanging, she says.

Additionally, do not assign E41 (Nutritional marasmus) for a patient who is diagnosed with "emaciation" or documented as "emaciated," according to Q3 2017 Coding Clinic guidance. Instead, you should assign R64 (Cachexia).

This is true even though the alphabetic index leads to E41 when searching under "emaciation." The reason for this is that the diagnosis captured by E41 refers to a type of malnutrition that occurs in infants and young children. If that's not applicable to the scenario you're coding, E41 is not the right code, the Coding Clinic said.

Tip: Don't assign a code, even if the alphabetic index leads you there, if it doesn't fit the particulars of the scenario you're working on, according to Coding Clinic guidance.

Hospice FAQ: What you need to know to avoid claim denials

Q: Can I assign "suspected" or "probable" diagnoses on a hospice claim?

A: No. If a hospice has a patient with a suspected or probable diagnosis but no other clinical information to support that diagnosis, the hospice medical director should query the provider who documented the suspected diagnosis for additional clinical information. Hospice coders should not code "probable," "suspected," "likely" or "possible" diagnoses as if they were confirmed diagnoses, according to Q1 2016 Coding Clinic guidance.

If no definitive information can be obtained, the hospice should assign appropriate codes for signs, symptoms and other conditions which lend support for the patient's terminal status and need for hospice care.

Q: Can I code debility or adult failure to thrive as a primary diagnosis on the hospice claim?

A: No, effective Oct. 1, 2014, CMS started to return to provider (RTP) all hospice claims that list in the primary position the vague diagnoses debility (R53.81), adult failure to thrive (R62.7), or an unspecified dementia code (such as F03.90, Unspecified dementia). These diagnoses can still be listed as secondary diagnoses however.

Also claims were returned starting on Oct. 1, 2014, for incorrect assignment of a manifestation code without an appropriate preceding etiology code, such as F02.80 (Dementia in conditions classified elsewhere without behavioral disturbance). CMS added edits to the Medicare Code Editor (MCE) to detect claims that reflect inappropriate assignment of primary and secondary diagnoses and incorrect sequencing of etiology/manifestation pairs.

Keep in mind that coding conventions and guidelines, to which hospices must adhere, require the assignment of an etiology code before its manifestation, such as assigning G30.9 (Alzheimer's disease, unspecified) before F02.80.

Q: What is the etiology-manifestation convention?

A: An etiology is an underlying condition that can cause other diseases, or manifestations. Diabetic chronic kidney disease is an example of an etiology-manifestation pair. Diabetes is the etiology, or underlying cause, of the chronic kidney disease, the manifestation. The etiology-manifestation convention requires you to sequence the code for the etiology (for example, E11.22 for Type 2 diabetes mellitus with diabetic chronic kidney disease) ***immediately before*** you assign the code for the manifestation (such as N18.6 for end-stage renal disease).

Q: What do I do if a hospice patient has multiple diagnoses but none of them is singularly responsible for the patient's life expectancy being six months or less, and the physician says the terminal diagnosis is "debility"?

A: Go back to the hospice interdisciplinary group (IDG), which should include the physician, and explain that CMS will send back the claim if it has a primary diagnosis of debility. Then, have the group list all of the conditions and symptoms that are contributing to the patient's terminal prognosis and decide which of those is the ***most contributory*** toward the patient's terminal state.

For example, a patient may be severely debilitated by end-stage liver disease, congestive heart failure (CHF) and chronic obstructive pulmonary disease (COPD). Though none of the conditions by itself may cause death, together they are leading to her severe debility. In cases like these, if the IDG determines that the CHF is the condition most responsible for exacerbating the other two and therefore causing death, code the CHF in the primary position and include the other diagnoses, including debility if desired, as secondary conditions.

Q: How do I determine whether a condition is "related" to a patient's terminal diagnosis?

A: You don't need to spend time trying to figure this out. In its FY2016 hospice wage index, CMS said to code every unresolved condition a hospice patient has whether it's related or unrelated to the terminal diagnosis. CMS then reiterated this directive in its FY2017 hospice rule. This directive clarifies previous guidance to include comorbid diagnoses that are related to the terminal condition on hospice claims.

Q: Many times hospice patients have a lot of trouble with eating — they either cannot eat or have simply stopped eating. How do I code this? Does R63.0 (Loss of appetite) cover it or is there something else?

A: Search for the most specific diagnosis to capture a hospice patient's eating difficulties. Consider the malnutrition codes available in the code set's nutritional deficiencies section; for example code E43 (Other severe protein calorie malnutrition). Symptom codes, such as R63.0 (Loss of appetite) may be assigned if a definitive diagnosis cannot be reached. You may also want to include codes for weight loss (R63.4) and a low BMI (Z68.-) if these apply.

While the symptom codes mentioned above can be assigned as the primary diagnosis on hospice claims without the risk of being returned to provider, the reason for the loss of appetite, for example, should be determined and coded when known. Be sure to verify all diagnoses with the physician before coding them.

Q: What if the hospice patient's chart indicates that the terminal diagnosis is a fracture; what should I code?

A: Look for another reason, such as a bone cancer, as it's highly unusual that a fracture would be a terminal diagnosis.

Discuss with the physician and the IDG whether there's another condition more appropriate for selection as the terminal diagnosis that may have put the patient at a risk for falls wherein a fracture would be sustained. Investigate what's happened to the patient within the past three to six months that has led to his terminal status.

Q: What if the patient's terminal diagnosis is listed simply as "dementia" with no stated etiology?

A: Seek to change the patient's terminal diagnosis through discussion with the interdisciplinary group.

Look for an underlying condition that may be responsible for the dementia, such as Alzheimer's disease or Parkinson's disease. If there's no known underlying disease, code the dementia as F03.90 or F03.91 depending on whether the patient has behavioral disturbance. Then, look at other conditions the patient may have that are contributing to his or her terminal status, and choose one of those conditions that is most contributory to the terminal status to list as the principal diagnosis making the unspecified dementia a secondary code.

And, remember that patients with unspecified dementia, adult failure to thrive, debility and other vague diagnoses don't have just one condition that is responsible for their terminal status, but rather a combination of conditions and factors that has led to their being terminal. It's the job of the hospice to identify and code every condition and diagnosis that's contributing to the patient's terminal prognosis.

Source: FY2014, 2015, 2016, 2017, 2018, 2019 and 2020 Hospice Wage Index rules; coding experts Brandi Whitemyer, HCS-D, independent home health & hospice consultant, and Judy Adams, HCS-D, president of Adams Home Care Consulting in Asheville, N.C.